ELEVENTH EDITION

# Brenner & Rector's THE KIDNEY

VOLUME ONE

**ALAN S.L. YU, MB, BChir**
Harry Statland and Solon Summerfield Professor of Medicine
Director, Division of Nephrology and Hypertension and the Jared Grantham Kidney Institute
University of Kansas Medical Center
Kansas City, Kansas

**GLENN M. CHERTOW, MD, MPH**
Norman S. Coplon/Satellite Healthcare Professor of Medicine
Department of Medicine
Division of Nephrology
Stanford University School of Medicine
Palo Alto, California

**VALÉRIE A. LUYCKX, MBBCh, MSc**
Affiliate Lecturer
Renal Division
Brigham and Women's Hospital
Harvard Medical School
Boston, Massachusetts;
Institute of Biomedical Ethics and the History of Medicine
University of Zürich
Zürich, Switzerland

**PHILIP A. MARSDEN, MD**
Professor of Medicine
Elisabeth Hofmann Chair in Translational Research
Oreopoulos-Baxter Division Director of Nephrology
University of Toronto
Toronto, Ontario, Canada

**KARL SKORECKI, MD, FRCP(C), FASN**
Dean, Azrieli Faculty of Medicine
Bar-Ilan University
Safed, Israel

**MAARTEN W. TAAL, MBChB, MMed, MD, FCP(SA), FRCP**
Department of Renal Medicine
Royal Derby Hospital
Derby, United Kingdom;
Centre for Kidney Research and Innovation
Division of Medical Sciences and Graduate Entry Medicine
School of Medicine
University of Nottingham
Nottingham, United Kingdom

*Special Assistant to the Editors*
**WALTER G. WASSER, MD**
Attending Physician, Division of Nephrology
Mayanei HaYeshua Medical Center
Bnei Brak, Israel;
Rambam Health Care Campus
Haifa, Israel

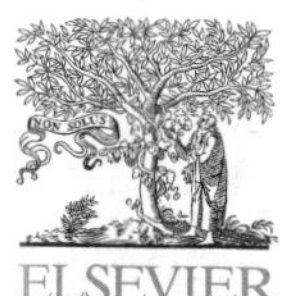

ELSEVIER

Elsevier
1600 John F. Kennedy Blvd.
Ste 1800
Philadelphia, PA 19103-2899

BRENNER & RECTOR'S THE KIDNEY, ELEVENTH EDITION

Set ISBN: 978-0-323-53265-5
Volume 1 ISBN: 978-0-323-75933-5
Volume 2 ISBN: 978-0-323-75934-2



**Notice**

Practitioners and researchers must always rely on their own experience and knowledge in evaluating and using any information, methods, compounds or experiments described herein. Because of rapid advances in the medical sciences, in particular, independent verification of diagnoses and drug dosages should be made. To the fullest extent of the law, no responsibility is assumed by Elsevier, authors, editors or contributors for any injury and/or damage to persons or property as a matter of products liability, negligence or otherwise, or from any use or operation of any methods, products, instructions, or ideas contained in the material herein.

Previous editions copyrighted 2016, 2012, 2008, 2004, 2000, 1996, 1991, 1986, 1981, and 1976.

**Library of Congress Control Number: 2019934877**

*Senior Content Strategist:* Nancy Anastasi Duffy
*Senior Content Development Specialist:* Joanie Milnes
*Publishing Services Manager:* Julie Eddy
*Senior Project Manager:* Rachel E. McMullen
*Design Direction:* Renee Duenow

Printed in India

Last digit is the print number: 9 8 7 6 5 4 3

*Dedicated to*

**Barry M. Brenner, MD**

*our mentor and role model, whose vision continues to challenge and inspire us*

*and to*

**Joan Ryan**

*for her patient stewardship of The Kidney through three wonderful editions*

# Contributors

**Andrew Advani, BSc, MBChB (Hons), PhD, FRCP(UK), FASN**
Associate Professor of Medicine
University of Toronto;
St. Michael's Hospital
Toronto, Ontario, Canada

**Todd Alexander, MD, PhD**
Pediatric Nephrologist and Professor
Department of Paediatrics
University of Alberta
Edmonton, Alberta, Canada

**Michael Allon, MD**
Professor of Medicine
Division of Nephrology
University of Alabama at Birmingham
Birmingham, Alabama

**Gerald B. Appel, MD**
Professor of Clinical Medicine
Department of Medicine
Columbia University Medical Center
New York, New York

**Suheir Assady, MD, PhD**
Director, Department of Nephrology and Hypertension
Rambam Health Care Campus
Haifa, Israel

**Colin Baigent, BMBCh, MA, MSc, FRCP, FFPH**
Professor of Epidemiology
Nuffield Department of Population Health
University of Oxford
Oxford, Great Britain

**George L. Bakris, MD**
Professor and Director
American Heart Association Comprehensive Hypertension Center
Department of Medicine
University of Chicago Medicine
Chicago, Illinois

**Marisa Battistella, PharmD**
Associate Professor
University Health Network/Leslie Dan Faculty of Pharmacy
University of Toronto,
Toronto, Ontario, Canada

**Srinivasan Beddhu, MD**
Professor of Internal Medicine
Department of Internal Medicine
University of Utah School of Medicine
Salt Lake City, Utah

**Aminu K. Bello, MD, PhD**
Assistant Professor/Nephrologist
Department of Medicine
University of Alberta
Edmonton, Alberta, Canada

**Theresa J. Berndt, MD**
Assistant Professor of Medicine
Division of Nephrology and Hypertension
Mayo Clinic College of Medicine
Rochester, Minnesota

**John F. Bertram, BSc, PhD, DSc**
Biomedicine Discovery Institute
Development and Stem Cells Program
Department of Anatomy and Developmental Biology
Monash University
Clayton, Victoria, Australia

**Vivek Bhalla, MD**
Assistant Professor
Medicine/Nephrology
Stanford University School of Medicine
Stanford, California

**Daniel G. Bichet, MD**
Professor
Department of Medicine and Physiology
University of Montreal;
Nephrologist
Department of Medicine
Hôpital du Sacré-Coeur de Montréal
Montréal, Québec, Canada

**Boris Bikbov, MD, PhD**
Researcher
Department of Renal Medicine
Istituto di Ricerche Farmacologiche Mario Negri IRCCS
Ranica, Bergamo, Italy

**Detlef Bockenhauer, MD, PhD**
Professor
Department of Renal Medicine
University College London;
Doctor
Department of Nephrology
Great Ormond Street Hospital for Children
London, Great Britain

**Alain Bonnardeaux, MD, PhD**
Full Professor
Department of Medicine
Université de Montréal
Montréal, Québec, Canada

**Josée Bouchard, MD, FRCPC**
Associate Professor of Medicine
Department of Nephrology
Hôpital du Sacré-Coeur de Montréal
University of Montréal
Montréal, Québec, Canada

**Richard M. Breyer, PhD**
Professor
Division of Nephrology and Hypertension
Vanderbilt University School of Medicine
Nashville, Tennessee

**Stefan Broer, PhD**
Research School of Biology
Australian National University
Canberra, Australian Capital Territory, Australia

**Carlo Brugnara, MD**
Department of Laboratory Medicine
Boston Children's Hospital
Boston, Massachusetts

**Catherine R. Butler, MD**
Fellow
Department of Medicine, Division of Nephrology
University of Washington
Seattle, Washington

**Héloise Cardinal, MD, PhD**
Associate Professor, Division of Nephrology
Department of Medicine
Université de Montréal
Montréal, Québec, Canada

**Juan Jesús Carrero, Pharm, PhD Pharm, PhD Med, MBA**
Professor
Department of Medical Epidemiology and Biostatistics
Karolinska Institutet
Stockholm, Sweden

**Daniel C. Cattran, MD**
Professor of Medicine
Department of Medicine
University Health Network;
Senior Scientist
Toronto General Research Institute
University Health Network
Toronto, Ontario, Canada

**Tak Mao Daniel Chan, MBBS, MD**
Chief of Nephrology
Department of Medicine
University of Hong Kong, Queen Mary Hospital
Hong Kong, Hong Kong

**Tara I. Chang, MD, MS**
Associate Professor of Medicine
Division of Nephrology
Stanford University
Palo Alto, California

**Glenn M. Chertow, MD, MPH**
Norman S. Coplon/Satellite Healthcare Professor of Medicine
Department of Medicine
Division of Nephrology
Stanford University School of Medicine
Palo Alto, California

**Andrew A. Chin, MD**
Division of Nephrology
Department of Internal Medicine
University of California, Davis School of Medicine
Sacramento, California

**Yeoungjee Cho, MBBS(hons), FRACP, PhD**
Consultant Nephrologist
Nephrology
Princess Alexandra Hospital;
Clinical Trialist
Australasian Kidney Trials Network
University of Queensland
Brisbane, Queensland, Australia

**Michel Chonchol, MD**
Professor of Medicine
Division of Renal Diseases and Hypertension
University of Colorado Denver Anschutz Medical Center
Aurora, Colorado

**Marta Christov, MD, PhD**
Assistant Professor of Medicine
Westchester Medical Center and New York Medical College
Valhalla, New York

**William L. Clapp, MD**
Professor of Pathology, Director of Renal Pathology
Department of Pathology, Immunology and Laboratory Medicine
University of Florida College of Medicine
Gainesville, Florida

**Rachel Becker Cohen, MD**
Institute of Pediatric Nephrology
Shaare Zedek Medical Center;
Hadassah-Hebrew University School of Medicine
Jerusalem, Israel

**Kelsey Connelly, MD**
Faculty of Medicine
University of Manitoba
Winnipeg, Manitoba, Canada

**H. Terence Cook, MB BS, FRCPath**
Professor of Renal Pathology
Department of Medicine
Imperial College
London, Great Britain

**Josef Coresh, MD, PhD**
Professor
Epidemiology, Medicine and Biostatistics
Johns Hopkins University;
Director
G.W. Comstock Center for Public Health and Prevention
Johns Hopkins Bloomberg School of Public Health
Baltimore, Maryland

**Ricardo Correa-Rotter, MD**
Head
Department of Nephrology and Mineral Metabolism
Instituto Nacional de Ciencias Médicas y Nutrición Salvador Zubirán
Mexico City, Mexico

**Shawn E. Cowper, MD**
Associate Professor of Dermatology and Pathology
Department of Dermatology
Yale University
New Haven, Connecticut

**Vivette D. D'Agati, MD**
Professor of Pathology
Columbia University College of Physicians and Surgeons;
Director, Renal Pathology Laboratory
Columbia University Medical Center
New York, New York

**Kevin Damman, MD, PhD**
Doctor
Department of Cardiology
University Medical Center Groningen
Groningen, The Netherlands

**Mogamat Razeen Davids, MBChB, FCP(SA), MMed**
Professor
Division of Nephrology, Department of Medicine
Stellenbosch University and Tygerberg Hospital
Cape Town, South Africa

**Sara Davison, BSc, MD, MSc**
Chief of Nephrology
Department of Medicine
University of Alberta
Edmonton, Alberta, Canada

**Aleksander Denic, MD**
Division of Nephrology and Hypertension
Mayo Clinic
Rochester, Minnesota

**Bradley M. Denker, MD**
Associate Professor of Medicine
Department of Medicine
Harvard Medical School;
Clinical Chief
Renal Division
Beth Israel Deaconess Medical Center;
Chief of Nephrology
Harvard Vanguard Medical Associates
Boston, Massachusetts

**Thomas A. Depner, BS, MD**
Division of Nephrology
Department of Internal Medicine
University of California, Davis School of Medicine
Sacramento, California

**Thomas D. DuBose, Jr., MD**
Professor Emeritus of Medicine
Wake Forest School of Medicine
Winston-Salem, North Carolina

**Vinay A. Duddalwar, MD, FRCR**
Professor of Radiology and Urology
Department of Radiology
Keck School of Medicine, University of Southern California
Los Angeles, California

**Kai-Uwe Eckardt, MD**
Professor of Medicine
Director of the Medical Department,
Division of Nephrology and Internal Intensive Care Medicine
Charité–Universitätsmedizin Berlin
Berlin, Germany

**William J. Elliott, MD, PhD**
Professor of Preventive Medicine, Internal Medicine and Pharmacology
Pacific Northwest University of Health Sciences;
Head, Division of Pharmacology
Pacific Northwest University of Health Sciences
Yakima, Washington

**David H. Ellison, MD**
Professor
Department of Internal Medicine
Division of Nephrology and Hypertension
Oregon Health & Science University
Portland, Oregon

**Ronald J. Falk, MD**
Nan and Hugh Cullman Eminent Professor
Chair, Department of Medicine
Director, UNC Kidney Center
Chapel Hill, North Carolina

**Robert Andrew Fenton, BSc, MSc, PhD**
Professor of Molecular Cell Biology
Department of Biomedicine
Aarhus University
Aarhus, Denmark

**Alessia Fornoni, MD, PhD**
Professor of Medicine and Chief
Division of Nephrology and Hypertension
University of Miami Miller School of Medicine;
Director
Katz Family Drug Discovery Center
Miami, Florida

**Benjamin S. Freedman, PhD**
Assistant Professor
Department of Pathology (Adjunct) and Department of Medicine
Division of Nephrology, Kidney Research Institute, and Institute for Stem Cell and Regenerative Medicine
University of Washington School of Medicine
Seattle, Washington

**Yaacov Frishberg, MD**
Institute of Pediatric Nephrology
Shaare Zedek Medical Center;
Hebrew University Hadassah School of Medicine
Jerusalem, Israel

**Jørgen Frøkiaer, MD, DMSci**
Department of Clinical Medicine
Aarhus University
Aarhus, Denmark

**John W. Funder, MD, PhD, FRCP, FRACP**
Distinguished Scholar
Hudson Institute and Monash University
Clayton, Victoria, Australia

**Amit X. Garg, MD**
Professor
Division of Nephrology Department of Medicine
Western University
Institute for Clinical Evaluative Sciences
London, Ontario, Canada

**Marc Ghannoum, MD**
Associate Professor of Medicine
University of Montreal, Verdun Hospital
Montréal, Québec, Canada

**Mohammed Benghanem Gharbi, MD**
Nephrology Department
Faculty of Medicine and Pharmacy of Casablanca
University Hassan II of Casablanca
Casablanca, Morocco

**Richard E. Gilbert, MBBS, PhD, FRACP, FACP, FRCPC**
Professor
Department of Medicine
University of Toronto;
Head
Division of Endocrinology
St. Michael's Hospital
Toronto, Ontario, Canada

**Richard J. Glassock, MD**
Emeritus Professor
Department of Medicine
Geffen School of Medicine at UCLA
Los Angeles, California

**Nimrit Goraya, MD**
Assistant Professor
Division of Nephrology and Hypertension,
Program Director
Nephrology Fellowship Program
Baylor Scott and White Health
Temple, Texas

**Morgan E. Grams, MD, PhD**
Associate Professor
Division of Nephrology
Johns Hopkins University
Baltimore, Maryland

**Per Henrik Groop, MD, DMSc, FRCPE**
Professor
Clinicum
University of Helsinki;
Chief Physician
Abdominal Center Nephrology
Helsinki University Hospital
Helsinki, Finland

**Steven Habbous, MD**
Department of Epidemiology and Biostatistics
Western University
London, Ontario, Canada

**Yoshio N. Hall, MD, MS**
Associate Professor
Department of Medicine/Nephrology
University of Washington;
Investigator
Kidney Research Institute | Medicine
University of Washington
Seattle, Washington

**Mitchell L. Halperin, MD, FRCPC, FRS**
Emeritus Professor of Medicine
Department of Medicine/Nephrology
St. Michaels Hospital
University of Toronto
Toronto, Ontario, Canada

**L. Lee Hamm, MD**
Senior Vice President and Dean
Tulane University School of Medicine
New Orleans, Louisiana

**Peter C. Harris, PhD**
Professor of Medicine and Biochemistry and Molecular Biology
Division of Nephrology and Hypertension
Mayo Clinic
Rochester, Minnesota

**Raymond C. Harris, MD**
Ann and Roscoe R. Robinson Professor of Medicine
Department of Medicine
Vanderbilt University School of Medicine
Nashville, Tennessee

**Richard Haynes, MB, BCh, MRCP(UK)**
Clinical Research Fellow
Nuffield Department of Population Health
University of Oxford;
Honorary Consultant Nephrologist
Oxford Kidney Unit
Oxford University Hospitals NHS Trust
Oxford, Great Britain

**Marie Josée Hébert, MD**
Professor
Vice-Rector of Research
Shire Chair in Nephrology, Transplantation and Renal Regeneration
Department of Medicine
Université de Montréal
Montréal, Québec, Canada

**William G. Herrington, MA, MBBS, MD, MRCP**
Associate Professor and MRC-Kidney Research UK Professor David Kerr Clinician Scientist
MRC Population Health Research Unit
Nuffield Department of Population Health
Oxford, Great Britain

**Ewout J. Hoorn, MD, PhD**
Nephrologist and Associate Professor
Department of Internal Medicine, Division of Nephrology & Transplantation
Erasmus Medical Center
Rotterdam, The Netherlands

**Thomas H. Hostetter, MD**
Professor of Medicine and Vice Chairman for Research
Case Western Reserve University School of Medicine
Cleveland, Ohio

**Susie L. Hu, MD**
Associate Professor of Medicine
Medicine, Division of Kidney Disease and Hypertension
Warren Alpert Medical School of Brown University
Providence, Rhode Island

**Tobias B. Huber, MD**
Professor
Department of Medicine
University Medical Center Hamburg-Eppendorf
Hamburg, Germany

**Hossein Jadvar, MD**
Associate Professor of Radiology
Department of Radiology
Keck School of Medicine, University of Southern California
Los Angeles, California

**Edgar A. Jaimes, MD**
Chief, Renal Service
Department of Medicine
Memorial Sloan Kettering Cancer Center
New York, New York

**Sarbjit Vanita Jassal, MD, MB, MRCP(UK), FRCPC**
Staff Nephrologist and Director, Geriatric Dialysis Program
Division of Nephrology
University Health Network;
Professor of Medicine
University of Toronto
Toronto, Ontario, Canada

**J. Charles Jennette, MD**
Kenneth M. Brinkhous Distinguished Professor and Chair
Department of Pathology and Laboratory Medicine
School of Medicine;
Chief of Pathology and Laboratory Medicine Services, UNC Hospitals;
Executive Director, UNC Nephropathology Division
University of North Carolina at Chapel Hill
Chapel Hill, North Carolina

**David W. Johnson, MBBS (Hons), PhD, DMed(Res), FRACP, FASN**
Director of Nephrology
Department of Nephrology
Princess Alexandra Hospital;
Deputy Chair
Australasian Kidney Trials Network
Brisbane, Queensland, Australia

**Kamel S. Kamel, MD, FRCP(C)**
St. Michael's Hospital
University of Toronto
Toronto, Ontario, Canada

**S. Ananth Karumanchi, MD**
Professor of Medicine
Director, Renovascular Research
Cedars-Sinai Medical Center
Los Angeles, California

**David Kavanagh, MD, PhD**
Professor of Complement Therapeutics
National Renal Complement Therapeutics Centre
Newcastle University
Newcastle upon Tyne, Great Britain

**Frieder Keller, MD, Prof. Dr. Med.**
Internal Medicine
University Hospital
Ulm, Germany

**Christine J. Ko, MD**
Professor of Dermatology and Pathology
Yale University
New Haven, Connecticut

**Harbir Singh Kohli, MD, DM**
Professor
Department of Nephrology
Post Graduate Institute of Medical Education and Research
Chandigarh, Union Territory, India

**Jay L. Koyner, MD**
Associate Professor of Medicine
Department of Medicine
Section of Nephrology
University of Chicago
Chicago, Illinois

**Jordan Kreidberg, MD, PhD**
Division of Nephrology
Boston Children's Hospital
Harvard Medical School
Boston, Massachusetts

**Anoushka Krishnan, MBBS, FRACP**
Department of Nephrology
Sir Charles Gairdner Hospital,
Perth, Western Australia, Australia

**Rajiv Kumar, MD**
Ruth and Vernon Taylor Professor of Medicine, Biochemistry and Molecular Biology,
Distinguished Medical Investigator,
Chair Emeritus
Division of Nephrology and Hypertension
Mayo Clinic College of Medicine
Rochester, Minnesota

**Gabrielle Lafreniere, MD, FRCPC**
Assistant Professor of Medicine
Université Laval;
Geriatrician
Division of Geriatrics
Centre Hospitalier Universitaire de Québec
Québec, Quebec, Canada

**Ngan N. Lam, MD, MSc**
Doctor
Department of Medicine, Nephrology
University of Alberta
Edmonton, Alberta, Canada

**Martin J. Landray, PhD FRCP**
Professor of Medicine and Epidemiology
Clinical Trial Service Unit & Epidemiological Studies Unit
Nuffield Department of Population Health
Oxford, Great Britain

**Harold E. Layton, PhD**
Professor
Department of Mathematics
Duke University
Durham, North Carolina

**Timmy Lee, MD, MSPH**
Associate Professor of Medicine
Department of Medicine
University of Alabama at Birmingham
Birmingham, Alabama

**Colin R. Lenihan, MB BCh BAO, PhD**
Clinical Associate Professor
Department of Nephrology
Stanford University
Palo Alto, California

**Krista L. Lentine, MD, PhD**
Professor of Medicine
Center for Abdominal Transplantation
Saint Louis University
St. Louis, Missouri

**Andrew S. Levey, MD**
Chief Emeritus
William B. Schwartz Division of Nephrology
Tufts Medical Center;
Professor of Medicine
Dr. Gerald J. and Dorothy R. Friedman Professor Emeritus
Tufts University School of Medicine
Boston, Massachusetts

**Adeera Levin, BSc, MD, FRCPC**
Professor
Department of Medicine ( Nephrology)
University of British Columbia;
Director
BC Provincial Renal Agency
Vancouver, British Columbia, Canada

**Christoph Licht, MD**
Pediatric Nephrologist
Department of Paediatrics
Senior Associate Scientist
Program in Cell Biology
Research Institute
The Hospital for Sick Children
Professor
Department of Paediatrics
University of Toronto
Toronto, Ontario, Canada

**Bengt Lindholm, MD, PhD**
Adjunct Professor
Divisions of Baxter Novum and Renal Medicine
Karolinska Institutet
Stockholm, Sweden

**Kathleen Liu, MD, PhD, MAS**
Assistant Professor
Divisions of Nephrology and Critical Care Medicine,
University of California, San Francisco
San Francisco, California

**Valérie A. Luyckx, MBBCh, MSc**
Affiliate Lecturer
Renal Division
Brigham and Women's Hospital
Harvard Medical School
Boston, Massachusetts;
Institute of Biomedical Ethics and the History of Medicine
University of Zürich
Zürich, Switzerland

**David A. Maddox, PhD**
Professor
Department of Internal Medicine
University of South Dakota Sanford School of Medicine;
Senior Research Scientist (WOC)
Research & Development
Sioux Falls VA Health Care System
Sioux Falls, South Dakota

**Yoshiro Maezawa, MD, PhD**
Department of Clinical Cell Biology & Medicine
Chiba University Graduate School of Medicine
Chiba, Japan

**Gary R. Matzke, BS Pharm, PharmD**
Professor Emeritus
Pharmacotherapy and Outcomes Science
School of Pharmacy, Virginia Commonwealth University
Richmond, Virginia

**Ivan D. Maya, MD**
Associate Professor
Department of Medicine
University of Central Florida
Orlando, Florida

**Sharon E. Maynard, MD**
Associate Professor
Department of Medicine
Lehigh Valley Health Network
University of South Florida Morsani College of Medicine
Allentown, Pennsylvania

**James A. McCormick, MD**
Associate Professor
Department of Medicine
Division of Nephrology and Hypertension
Oregon Health and Science University
Portland, Oregon

**Alicia Ann McDonough, PhD**
Professor
Integrative Anatomical Sciences
Department of Cell and Neurobiology
Keck School of Medicine, University of Southern California
Los Angeles, California

**John J.V. McMurray, BSc(Hons), MB ChB(Hons), MD, FESC, FACC, FAHA**
British Heart Foundation Cardiovascular Research Centre
University of Glasgow
Glasgow, Scotland, Great Britain

**Rajnish Mehrotra, MBBS, MD, MS**
Section Head, Nephrology
Harborview Medical Center;
Division of Nephrology
University of Washington
Seattle, Washington

**Timothy W. Meyer, MD**
Professor
Department of Medicine
Stanford University
Stanford, California;
Staff Physician
Department of Medicine
VA Palo Alto HCS
Palo Alto, California

**Catherine Meyer-Schwesinger, MD**
Professor
Institute of Cellular and Integrative Physiology
University Medical Center Hamburg-Eppendorf
Hamburg, Germany

**Orson W. Moe, MD**
Professor
Department of Internal Medicine
Division of Nephrology
UT Southwestern Medical Center;
Director
Charles and Jane Pak Center for Mineral Metabolism and Clinical Research
UT Southwestern Medical Center
Dallas, Texas

**Karen M. Moritz, BSc, MSc, PhD**
Child Health Research Centre and School of Biomedical Sciences
The University of Queensland
St. Lucia, Australia

**Alvin H. Moss, MD**
Director
Center for Health Ethics and Law
West Virginia University;
Professor of Medicine
Department of Medicine
Section of Geriatrics, Palliative Medicine and Hospice
West Virginia University
Morgantown, West Virginia

**David B. Mount, MD**
Clinical Chief
Renal Division
Brigham and Women's Hospital
Boston, Massachusetts

**Karen A. Munger, PhD**
Chief, Research and Development
Sioux Falls VA Health Care System;
Associate Professor of Medicine
Department of Internal Medicine
University of South Dakota
Sioux Falls, South Dakota

**Behzad Najafian, MD**
Associate Professor
Department of Pathology
University of Washington
Seattle, Washington

**Luis Gabriel Navar, PhD**
Professor and Chairman
Department of Physiology
Tulane University
New Orleans, Louisiana

**Robert G. Nelson, MD, PhD**
Senior Investigator
Chief, Chronic Kidney Disease Section
Phoenix Epidemiology and Clinical Research Branch
National Institute of Diabetes and Digestive and Kidney Diseases
Phoenix, Arizona

**Lindsay E. Nicolle, MD**
Professor Emeritus
Department of Internal Medicine
University of Manitoba
Winnipeg, Manitoba, Canada

**Sanjay K. Nigam, MD**
Nancy Kaehr Chair in Research
Pediatrics, Medicine and Cellular Molecular Medicine
University of California, San Diego
La Jolla, California

**Mark Douglas Okusa, MD**
Professor of Medicine, Chief, Division of Nephrology
Department of Medicine
University of Virginia
Charlottesville, Virginia

**Paul M. Palevsky, MD**
Chief, Renal Section
VA Pittsburgh Healthcare System;
Professor of Medicine and Clinical & Translational Science
Renal-Electrolyte Division
Department of Medicine
University of Pittsburgh
Pittsburgh, Pennsylvania

**Suetonia C. Palmer, MB ChB, PhD, FRACP**
Doctor
Department of Medicine
University of Otago Christchurch
Christchurch, New Zealand

**Suzanne L. Palmer, MD**
Professor of Radiology
Department of Radiology
Keck School of Medicine, University of Southern California
Los Angeles, California

**Chirag R. Parikh, MD, PhD**
Director, Division of Nephrology
Ronald Peterson Professor of Medicine
Johns Hopkins School of Medicine
Baltimore, Maryland

**David Pearce, MD**
Professor
Department of Medicine
Division of Nephrology
Department of Cellular and Molecular Pharmacology
University of California San Francisco
San Francisco, California

**Aldo J. Peixoto, MD**
Professor of Medicine
Department of Internal Medicine (Nephrology)
Yale University School of Medicine;
Clinical Chief, Section of Nephrology
Department of Internal Medicine
Yale University School of Medicine
New Haven, Connecticut

**William F. Pendergraft III, MD, PhD**
Assistant Professor of Medicine
Division of Nephrology and Hypertension
Department of Medicine
University of North Carolina School of Medicine
Cambridge, Massachusetts

**Mark A. Perazella, MD, MS**
Professor of Medicine
Section of Nephrology
Yale University School of Medicine;
Director, Acute Dialysis Services
Yale-New Haven Hospital
New Haven, Connecticut

**Norberto Perico, MD**
Istituto di Ricerche Farmacologiche Mario Negri IRCCS
Bergamo, Italy

**Martin R. Pollak, MD**
Division of Nephrology
Beth Israel Deaconess Medical Center
Harvard Medical School
Boston, Massachusetts

**Didier Portilla, MD**
Professor
Department of Medicine
University of Virginia
Charlottesville, Virginia

**Susan E. Quaggin, MD**
Doctor
Feinberg Cardiovascular Research Institute
Northwestern University
Chicago, Illinois

**Jai Radhakrishnan, MD, MS**
Professor of Medicine at Columbia University Medical Center
Division of Nephrology, Department of Medicine
Columbia University Medical Center;
Clinical Chief
Division of Nephrology
New York Presbyterian Hospital
New York, New York

**Rawi Ramadan, MD**
Director, Medical Transplantation Unit
Department of Nephrology and Hypertension
Rambam Health Care Campus
Haifa, Israel

**Heather N. Reich, MD, CM, PhD, FRCPC**
Nephrologist, Clinician Scientist
Department of Nephrology
University Health Network;
Associate Professor
Gabor Zellerman Chair in Nephrology Research
Department of Medicine
University of Toronto
Toronto, Ontario, Canada

**Andrea Remuzzi, MD**
Istituto di Ricerche Farmacologicke Mario Negri IRCCS
Bergamo, Italy

**Giuseppe Remuzzi, MD, FRCP**
Istituto di Ricerche Farmacologicke Mario Negri IRCCS
Bergamo, Italy;
L. Sacco
Department of Biomedical and Clinical Sciences
University of Milan
Milan, Italy

**Leonardo V. Riella, MD, PhD**
Associate Physician
Brigham and Women's Hospital;
Assistant Professor of Medicine
Department of Medicine
Harvard Medical School
Boston, Massachusetts

**Miquel C. Riella, MD, PhD**
Professor of Medicine
Department of Medicine
Catholic University of Parana, Brazil;
Professor of Medicine
Department of Medicine
Evangelic School of Medicine
Curitiba, Brazil

**Choni Rinat III, MD**
Institute of Pediatric Nephrology
Shaare Zedek Medical Center;
Hadassah-Hebrew University School of Medicine
Jerusalem, Israel

**Darren M. Roberts, BPharm, MBBS, PhD, FRACP**
Visiting Medical Officer
NSW Poisons Information Centre
Sydney Children's Hospital Network;
Staff Specialist
Renal Medicine and Clinical Pharmacology and Toxicology
St Vincent's Hospital;
Conjoint Associate Professor
University of New South Wales
Sydney, New South Wales, Australia

**Norman D. Rosenblum, MD**
Paediatric Nephrologist
Department of Paediatrics
The Hospital for Sick Children;
Senior Scientist
Program in Developmental and Stem Cell Biology
The Hospital for Sick Children;
Professor
Department of Paediatrics
University of Toronto
Toronto, Ontario, Canada

**Mitchell H. Rosner, MD**
Professor of Medicine
Chair, Department of Medicine
University of Virginia Health System
Charlottesville, Virginia

**Andrew D. Rule, MD**
Division of Nephrology and Hypertension
Mayo Clinic
Rochester, Minnesota

**Ernesto Sabath, MD**
Department of Natural Sciences
Universidad Autonoma de Queretaro
Queretaro, Mexico

**Manish K. Saha, MD**
Assistant Professor of Medicine
Division of Nephrology and Hypertension
Department of Medicine
UNC Kidney Center
University of North Carolina, Chapel Hill
Chapel Hill, North Carolina

**Khashayar Sakhaee, MD**
Laura Kim Pak Professor in Mineral Metabolism Research
BeautiControl Cosmetics Inc.;
Professor in Mineral Metabolism and Osteoporosis
Chief, Division of Mineral Metabolism
University of Texas, Southwestern Medical Center
Dallas, Texas

**Vinay Sakhuja, MD**
Director of Nephrology and Transplant Medicine
Max Hospital
Mohali, Punjab, India

**Alan D. Salama, MBBS, PhD, FRCP**
UCL Centre for Nephrology
Royal Free Hospital
London, United Kingdom

**Jeff M. Sands, MD**
Juha P. Kokko Professor of Medicine and Physiology
Medicine—Renal Division
Emory University
Atlanta, Georgia

**Anjali Bhatt Saxena, MD**
Director of Peritoneal Dialysis
Department of Internal Medicine
Division of Nephrology
Santa Clara Valley Medical Center
San Jose, California;
Clinical Assistant Professor of Medicine
Department of Internal Medicine
Stanford University
Stanford, California

**Johannes Schlöndorff, MD**
Division of Nephrology
Beth Israel Deaconess Medical Center
Harvard Medical School
Boston, Massachusetts

**Rizaldy Paz Scott, MS, PhD**
Research Assistant Professor
Feinberg School of Medicine
Northwestern University
Chicago, Illinois

**Neil Sheerin, BSc, MBBS, PhD, FRCP**
Professor of Nephrology
Institute of Cellular Medicine
National Renal Complement Therapeutics Centre
Newcastle University
Newcastle upon Tyne, Great Britain

**Prableen Singh, MD**
Associate Professor of Medicine
Division of Nephrology and Hypertension
University of California San Diego & VA San Diego Healthcare System
San Diego, California

**Karl Skorecki, MD, FRCP(C), FASN**
Dean, Azrieli Faculty of Medicine
Bar-Ilan University
Safed, Israel

**Itzchak N. Slotki, MD**
Director
Division of Adult Nephrology
Shaare Zedek Medical Center;
Associate Professor of Medicine
Hadassah Hebrew University of Jerusalem
Jerusalem, Israel

**Miroslaw J. Smogorzewski, MD, PhD**
Associate Professor of Medicine
Division of Nephrology
Department of Medicine
University of Southern California, Keck School of Medicine
Los Angeles, California

**William E. Smoyer, MD**
Vice President and Director
Center for Clinical and Translational Research
Nationwide Children's Hospital;
Professor
Department of Pediatrics
The Ohio State University
Columbus, Ohio

**Stuart M. Sprague, DO**
Chairperson, Division of Nephrology and Hypertension
Department of Medicine
NorthShore University Health System
Evanston, Illinois;
Clinical Professor of Medicine
Department of Medicine
University of Chicago Pritzker School of Medicine
Chicago, Illinois

**Peter Stenvinkel, MD, PhD, FENA**
Professor
Department of Renal Medicine
CLINTEC
Stockholm, Sweden

**Jason R. Stubbs, MD**
Associate Professor of Medicine
Division of Nephrology and Hypertension
The Kidney Institute
University of Kansas Medical Center
Kansas City, Kansas

**Maarten W. Taal, MBChB, MMed, MD, FCP(SA), FRCP**
Department of Renal Medicine
Royal Derby Hospital
Derby, United Kingdom;
Centre for Kidney Research and Innovation
Division of Medical Sciences and Graduate Entry Medicine
School of Medicine
University of Nottingham
Nottingham, United Kingdom

**Manjula Kurella Tamura, MD, MPH**
Professor
Department of Medicine/Nephrology
Stanford University
Palo Alto, California

**Jane C. Tan, MD, PhD**
Department of Medicine
Stanford University
Stanford, California

**Navdeep Tangri, MD, FRCPC, PhD**
University of Manitoba
Department of Medicine
Chronic Disease Innovation Centre, Seven Oaks General Hospital
Winnipeg, Manitoba, Canada

**Stephen C. Textor, MD**
Professor of Medicine
Division of Nephrology and Hypertension
Mayo Clinic
Rochester, Minnesota

**Ravi I. Thadhani, MD, MPH**
Chair, Department of Biomedical Sciences
Cedars-Sinai Medical Center
Los Angeles, California

**Scott Culver Thomson, MD**
Professor
Department of Medicine
University of California;
Chief of Nephrology Section
Department of Medicine
VA San Diego Healthcare System
San Diego, California

**Kathryn Tinckam, MD, MMSc**
Associate Professor
Division of Nephrology
Departments of Medicine and Laboratory Medicine & Pathobiology
University of Toronto
Toronto, Ontario, Canada

**Vicente E. Torres, MD, PhD**
Professor of Medicine
Division of Nephrology and Hypertension
Mayo Clinic
Rochester, Minnesota

**Volker Vallon, MD**
Professor
Division of Nephrology & Hypertension
Departments of Medicine & Pharmacology
University of California San Diego & VA San Diego Healthcare System
San Diego, California

**Joseph G. Verbalis, MD**
Professor
Department of Medicine
Georgetown University
Washington, DC;
Chief
Department of Endocrinology and Metabolism
Georgetown University Hospital
Washington, Maryland

**Jill W. Verlander, DVM**
Scientist
Division of Nephrology, Hypertension, and Renal Transplantation
University of Florida College of Medicine;
Director
College of Medicine Electron Microscopy Core Facility
University of Florida
Gainesville, Florida

**Ron Wald, MDCM, MPH**
Staff Nephrologist
Division of Nephrology
Department of Medicine
Li Ka Shing Knowledge Institute of St. Michael's Hospital and the University of Toronto;
Institute for Clinical Evaluative Sciences
Toronto, Ontario, Canada

**I. David Weiner, MD**
Professor of Medicine and Physiology and Functional Genomics
Division of Nephrology, Hypertension and Transplantation
University of Florida College of Medicine;
Section Chief
Nephrology and Hypertension Section
NF/SGVHS
Gainesville, Florida

**Steven D. Weisbord, MD, MSc**
Staff Physician
Renal Section
VA Pittsburgh Healthcare System;
Associate Professor of Medicine and Clinical and Translational Science
Renal-Electrolyte Division
University of Pittsburgh School of Medicine
Pittsburgh, Pennsylvania

**Robert H. Weiss, MD**
Professor
Department of Nephrology
University of California, Davis
Davis, California

**Donald Everett Wesson, MD, MBA**
President, Baylor Scott and White Health and Wellness Center
Department of Internal Medicine
Baylor Scott and White Health;
Professor of Medicine
Department of Internal Medicine
Texas A&M College of Medicine
Dallas, Texas

**David C. Wheeler, MB ChB, MD**
Professor of Kidney Medicine
Centre for Nephrology, Division of Medicine
University College London
London, Great Britain

**Christopher S. Wilcox, MD, PhD**
Chief
Department of Nephrology and Hypertension
Georgetown University Medical Center
Washington, DC

**Jane Y. Yeun, MD**
Division of Nephrology
Department of Internal Medicine
University of California, Davis School of Medicine
Sacramento, California;
Veterans Affairs Sacramento Health Care System
Mather Field, California

**Brian Young, MD**
Health Sciences Associate Clinical Professor
Division of Nephrology
Department of Internal Medicine, Division of Nephrology
University of California, Davis Medical Center
Sacramento, California

**Alan S.L. Yu, MB, BChir**
Harry Statland and Solon Summerfield Professor of Medicine
Director, Division of Nephrology and Hypertension and the Jared Grantham Kidney Institute
University of Kansas Medical Center
Kansas City, Kansas

**Ming-Zhi Zhang, MD**
Associate Professor
Department of Medicine
Vanderbilt University
Nashville, Tennessee

# Preface

Welcome to the 11th edition of Brenner & Rector's *The Kidney*. Like the summer Olympic games, which it generally precedes by a few months, the emergence of each new edition of *The Kidney* follows a 4-year cycle, which is short enough to keep up with major advances in the field, but just long enough to complete the arduous editorial process. The purpose of this book remains unchanged from what Barry M. Brenner and Floyd C. Rector, Jr. conceived originally in 1973; namely to serve as a compendium of nephrology, from basic science to clinical diagnosis and treatment of kidney disease. The intended audience, now truly international, includes medical students, residents, nephrology fellows and practitioners, adult and pediatric renal scientists, and anyone else fascinated by the mysteries of the kidney. For those of us belonging to a certain generation, the raison d'être for *The Kidney* needs no justification. We grew up with it, considering it the definitive text of nephrology. But the modern era of medicine has been marked by a proliferation of readily accessible online digital tools that promise timely and partially digested answers to highly focused questions, catering to trainees and young physicians accustomed to the rapid pace of the modern digital age, and to established, harried clinicians with limited time for reading. While these tools are invaluable, and I confess that I, too, use them on occasion, there is clearly a place for a more considered exposition of the many complex topics in nephrology, that has both breadth and depth, combining intellectual rigor with the excitement of fresh discoveries.

The 11th edition, as with the previous two, is now edited by an international team of editors, a monumental task that remarkably was once managed singlehandedly by Barry M. Brenner. To introduce fresh perspective, we have added a new editor to the team, Valérie A. Luyckx from University of Zürich and the Brigham and Women's Hospital in Boston, a world-renowned expert in global health and management of kidney disease in underserved populations, and an advisor to the International Society of Nephrology and the World Health Organization on global health-related ethics issues. Almost one third of the chapters in this edition have been rewritten by new authors. In addition, we commissioned four entirely new chapters that address emerging areas in nephrology and are written by authoritative experts in those areas, namely "Cardiorenal Syndromes," "Supportive Care in Advanced Kidney Disease," "Considerations in Live Kidney Donation," and "Global Challenges and Initiatives in Kidney Health." To enhance the reader experience, we have introduced a listing of "Key Points" that appear at the beginning of the chapters, to summarize and highlight the important new information. In addition, some of the chapters that are focused on physiology have "Clinical Relevance" boxes to highlight points in the text that have specific relevance to clinical practice.

While some of us will look forward to the tactile experience of opening the two physical volumes of this new edition when it comes out, many of our readers will inevitably prefer the convenience of perusing our enhanced eBook online. These readers will be rewarded with additional material absent from the print version (a necessity so as to avoid occupational injury while removing from the shelf), including the full list of references for every chapter, board review-style multiple choice questions to encourage active learning and help prepare for certification or recertification, and periodic updates to the content, all of which are fully searchable.

Needless to say, an undertaking of this magnitude requires the combined effort of countless individuals. First and foremost, on behalf of the entire editorial team I would like to express deep gratitude to the 184 authors of the chapters in this edition, all of whom committed time out of their busy schedules as clinicians, scientists, and academic leaders to contribute to this project. I wish to thank my fellow editors, Glenn Chertow, Valérie Luyckx, Phil Marsden, Karl Skorecki, and Maarten Taal for their sterling work, and for entrusting me with the leadership of this edition. I also thank Walter Wasser, who has now come to our rescue twice, at short notice, to assist the editorial team finalize manuscripts, both for this edition and the previous one. All of us, in turn, are grateful to the many staff at Elsevier for shepherding this project along. Joan Ryan, a veteran of many editions of *The Kidney*, was superb as our senior content development specialist, until she had to take a leave of absence and Joanie Milnes graciously stepped in to take over. Nancy Duffy, and before her Maureen Ianuzzi, served expertly as our content strategist, and Rachel McMullen served as our senior project manager.

I would like to thank my family, as well as my trainees, colleagues, and coworkers at the University of Kansas Medical Center, for their patience during the past two years, during which this project consumed far too much of my attention and took me away from spending time with them. Finally, I would like to thank Barry M. Brenner, whose spirit of scientific rigor and exacting intellectual standards continue to guide *The Kidney*. I hope that readers will share our excitement in this new edition and savor all that it has to offer.

*Alan S.L. Yu, MB, BChir*
*Kansas City, Kansas*

# Contents

# NORMAL STRUCTURE AND FUNCTION

SECTION I

# 1 Embryology of the Kidney

Rizaldy Paz Scott | Yoshiro Maezawa | Jordan Kreidberg | Susan E. Quaggin

## CHAPTER OUTLINE



## KEY POINTS

- The development of the kidney relies on reciprocal signaling and inductive interactions between neighboring cells.
- Epithelial cells that comprise the tubular structures of the kidney are derived from two distinct cell lineages: the ureteric epithelia lineage that branches and gives rise to collecting ducts and the nephrogenic mesenchyme lineage that undergoes mesenchyme to epithelial transition to form connecting tubules, distal tubules, the loop of Henle, proximal tubules, parietal epithelial cells, and podocytes.
- Nephrogenesis and nephron endowment requires an epigenetically regulated balance between nephron progenitor self-renewal and epithelial differentiation.
- The timing of incorporation of nephron progenitor cells into nascent nephrons predicts their positional identity within the highly patterned mature nephron.
- Stromal cells and their derivatives coregulate ureteric branching morphogenesis, nephrogenesis, and vascular development.
- Endothelial cells track the development of the ureteric epithelia and establish the renal vasculature through a combination of vasculogenic and angiogenic processes.
- Collecting duct epithelia have an inherent plasticity enabling them to switch between principal and intercalated cell identities.

## MAMMALIAN KIDNEY DEVELOPMENT

### ANATOMIC OVERVIEW OF THE MAMMALIAN KIDNEY

The kidney is a sophisticated, highly vascularized organ that plays a central role in overall body homeostasis. In humans, the kidneys filter as much as 180 liters of blood per day, receiving as much as ~20% of the total cardiac output. Renal filtration of blood removes metabolic waste products (e.g., urea, ammonia, and by-products of bile from the liver) as urine while concomitantly adjusting the levels of water, electrolytes, and pH of tissue fluids. Additionally, the kidneys regulate blood pressure via the renin-angiotensin-aldosterone system, secrete erythropoietin that stimulates erythrocyte production, and contribute to the activation of vitamin D to control calcium and phosphate balance.

The filtration function of the kidneys is accomplished by basic units called nephrons (Fig. 1.1). Humans on average have 1 million nephrons per adult kidney but the range of total nephrons is highly variable across human populations.[4] Each mouse kidney may contain up to 12,000–16,000 nephrons depending on the strain.[5] This wide range in nephron number is influenced by genetic background, fetal nutrition and environment, and maturity at birth.[6,7] Nephron endowment can be clinically important as markedly reduced nephron numbers raises the susceptibility risk to hypertension and chronic kidney disease.[1–3,8,9] At the core of the nephron is the renal corpuscle or glomerulus (see Fig. 1.1). The glomerulus consists of a porous and highly convoluted capillary bed composed of highly fenestrated glomerular endothelial cells. These glomerular capillaries are circumscribed by morphologically elaborate and interdigitating cells called podocytes. These capillaries are further structurally supported by pericytes

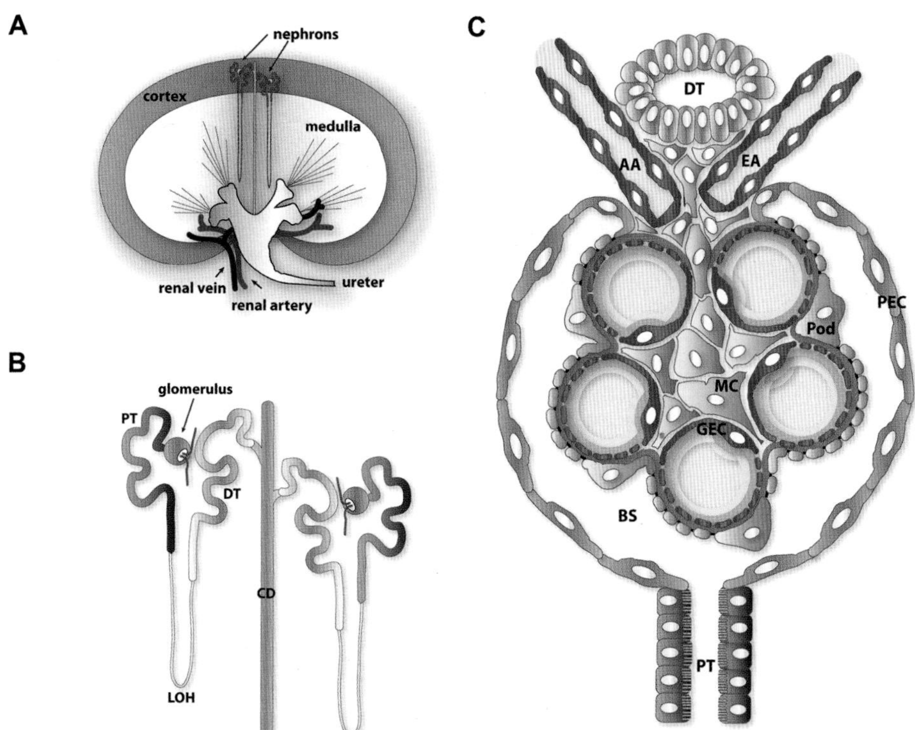


**Fig. 1.1 Anatomic organization of the kidney.** (A) Spatial distribution of nephron within the metanephric kidney. Glomeruli, the filtration compartments of the nephrons, are found in the cortex. (B) Segmental structure of nephrons. The vascularized glomerulus is found at the proximal end and is connected through a series of renal tubules where urinary filtrate composition is refined through resorption and secretion. (C) Cellular organization of the glomeruli. *AA,* Afferent arteriole; *BS,* Bowman space; *CD,* Collecting duct; *DT,* distal tubule; *EA,* efferent arteriole; *GEC,* glomerular endothelial cell; *LOH,* loop of Henle; *MC,* mesangial cell; *PEC,* parietal epithelial cell; *Pod,* podocyte; *PT,* proximal tubule. Reproduced with permission from Scott RP, Quaggin SE. The cell biology of renal filtation. *J Cell Biol.* 2015;209:100–210.

called mesangial cells. Blood filtration occurs through this capillary tuft, generating primary urine that collects within the Bowman capsule, an enclosure formed by parietal epithelial cells. From the Bowman capsule, urine drains through a series of tubules starting with the proximal tubules, the loop of Henle, the distal tubules, and the collecting ducts. These tubules are responsible for dynamic resorption and secretion processes that help recycle filtered small molecules; they also adjust water, electrolyte, and acid–base balance by fine-tuning the composition of the final urine output before it exits the ureter and is excreted via the bladder. Supporting the main functions of the nephrons are interstitial fibroblasts and a heterogenous network of extraglomerular vasculature.

## DEVELOPMENT OF THE UROGENITAL SYSTEM

The vertebrate kidney derives from the intermediate mesoderm of the urogenital ridge, a structure found along the posterior wall of the abdomen in the developing fetus.[10,11] Mammalian kidneys develop in three successive stages, generating three distinct excretory structures known as the pronephros, the mesonephros, and the metanephros (Fig. 1.2). The pronephros and mesonephros are vestigial structures in mammals and degenerate before birth; the metanephros is the definitive mammalian kidney. The early stages of kidney development are required for the development of the adrenal glands and gonads that also form within the urogenital ridge. Furthermore, many of the signaling pathways and genes that play important roles in the metanephric kidney appear to play parallel roles during the development of the pronephros

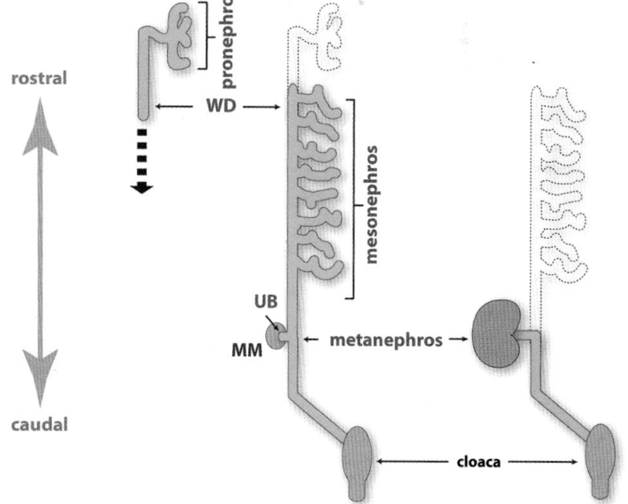


**Fig. 1.2 Three stages of mammalian kidney development.** The pronephros and mesonephros develop in a rostral-to-caudal direction and the tubules are aligned adjacent to the wolffian or nephric duct *(WD)*. The metanephros develops from an outgrowth of the distal end of the wolffian duct known as the ureteric bud epithelium *(UB)* and a cluster of cells known as the metanephric mesenchyme *(MM)*. The pronephros and mesonephros are vestigial structures in mice and humans and are regressed by the time the metanephros is well developed.

and mesonephros. The pronephros consists of pronephric tubules and the pronephric duct (also known as the precursor to the wolffian duct) and develops from the rostral-most region of the urogenital ridge at 22 days of gestation in humans and 8 days post coitum (embryonic stage E8) in mice (Table 1.1). Throughout the rest of this chapter, most timelines of kidney development are with reference to the mouse. The pronephros serves as the principal excretory organ of the larval stages of fishes and amphibians. The mesonephros develops caudal to the pronephric tubules in the midsection of the urogenital ridge. The mesonephros becomes the functional excretory apparatus in lower vertebrates (adult fish and amphibians) and may perform a filtering function during embryonic life in mammals. Prior to its degeneration, endothelial, peritubular myoid, and steroidogenic cells from the mesonephros migrate into the adjacent adrenogonadal primordia, which ultimately form the adrenal gland and gonads.[12] Abnormal mesonephric migration leads to gonadal dysgenesis, a fact that underscores the intricate association between these organ systems during development and explains the common association of gonadal and renal defects in congenital syndromes.[13,14]

## DEVELOPMENT OF THE METANEPHROS

The metanephros is the third and final stage, representing the definitive adult kidney of higher vertebrates. It results from a series of reciprocal inductive interactions that occur between the metanephric mesenchyme (MM) and the epithelial ureteric bud (UB) at the caudal end of the urogenital ridge. The UB is first visible as an outgrowth at the distal end of the wolffian duct approximately between the fourth and fifth week of gestation in humans or E10.5 in mice. The MM becomes histologically distinct from the surrounding mesenchyme and is found adjacent to the UB. Upon invasion of the MM by the UB, signals from the MM cause the UB to branch into a T-tubule (at around E11.5 in mice) and then to undergo iterative dichotomous branching, giving rise to the urinary collecting duct system (Fig. 1.3). Simultaneously, the UB sends reciprocal signals to the MM, which is induced to condense along the surface of the bud. Following condensation, a subset of MM cells aggregates adjacent and inferior to the tips of the branching UB. These collections of cells, known as pretubular aggregates, undergo mesenchymal-to-epithelial conversion to become the renal vesicle (Fig. 1.4).

## URETERIC BRANCHING MORPHOGENESIS

The collecting duct system is composed of hundreds of tubules through which the filtrate produced by the nephrons is conducted out of the kidney, to the ureter, and then to the bladder. Water and salt resorption and excretion, ammonia transport, and $H^+$ ion secretion required for acid–base homeostasis also occur in the collecting ducts, under different regulatory mechanisms, and using different transporters and channels than are active along tubular portions of the nephron. The collecting ducts are all derived from the original

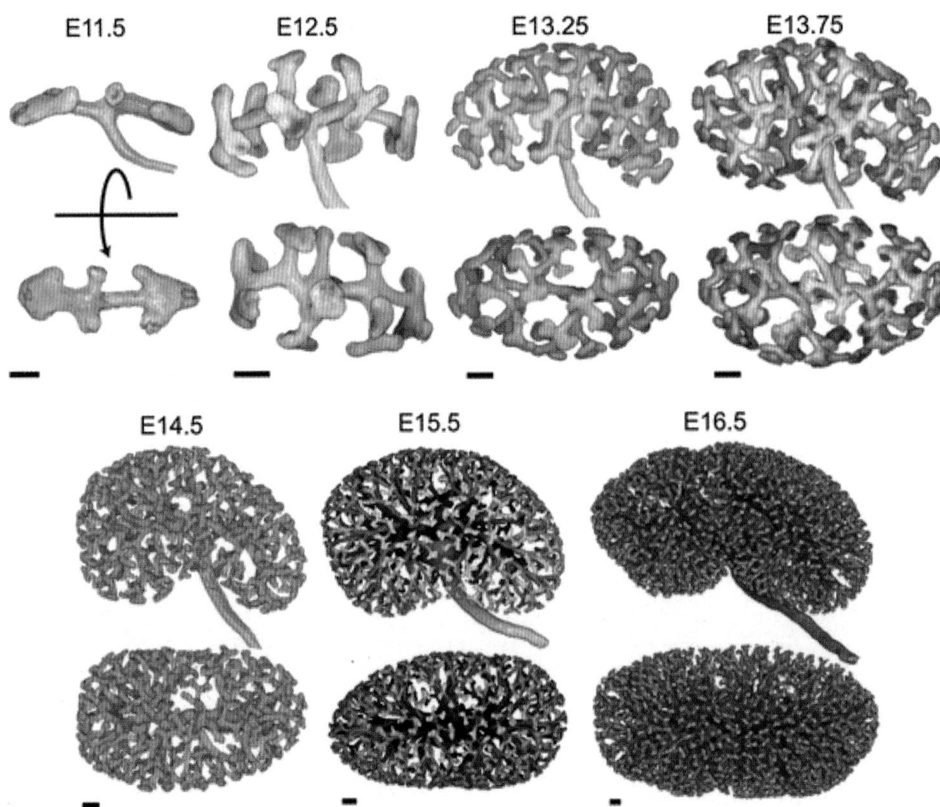


**Fig. 1.3 Ureteric branching morphogenesis.** Rapid reiterative branching of the UB within a 5-day period in mice as imaged with a pan-cytokeratin antibody using optical projection tomography. By E16.5, the renal pelvis, formed by the widening and coalescence of the earliest branches of the ureteric tree, is already apparent. Reproduced with permission from Short KM, Smuth I. Imaging, analyzing and interpreting branching morphogenesis in the developing kidney. *Results Probl Cell Differ.* 2017;60:233–256.

**Table 1.1 Timelines of Human and Mouse Kidney Development**

| Stage/Event | Human[a] | Mouse[b] |
|---|---|---|
| **Pronephros** | | |
| • Emergence | 22nd day | E9 |
| • Disappearance by | 25th day | E10 |
| **Mesonephros** | | |
| • Emergence | 24th day | E10 |
| • Disappearance by | 16th week | E14 |
| **Metanephros** | | |
| • Ureteric bud induction | 28th–32nd day | E10.5 |
| • Nephrogenesis | 44th day | E13 |
| • Glomerulogenesis | 8th–9th week | E14 |
| • Cessation of nephrogenesis | 36th week | P3 |
| **Gestation (Total Length)** | 40 weeks | 19–21 days |

[a]*Human timelines refer to gestational periods.*
[b]*Mouse timelines are indicated as either embryonic days post coitum (E) or postnatal (P).*

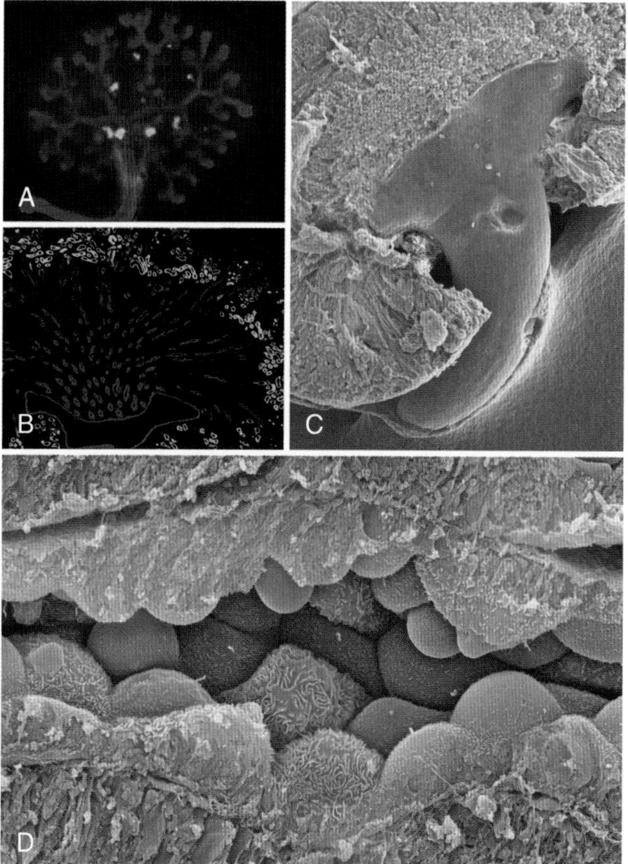


**Fig. 1.4 The collecting duct system.** The branching ureteric epithelia gives rise to the collecting duct system. (A) E12.5 mouse embryonic kidney explant grown for 2 days and (B) neonatal mouse kidney section stained for the ureteric epithelium and collecting ducts (pan-cytokeratin, *red*) and proximal tubules (Lotus lectin, *green*). (C) Scanning electron micrograph of a hemisected adult mouse kidney showing the funnel-shaped renal papilla. (D) Scanning electron micrograph of a collecting duct showing smooth principal cells and reticulated intercalated cells.

UB (Fig. 1.5). Whereas each nephron is an individual unit separately induced and originating from a distinct pretubular aggregate, the collecting ducts are the product of branching morphogenesis from the UB. Considerable remodeling is involved in forming collecting ducts from branches of the UB.[15] The branching is highly patterned, with the first several rounds of branching being somewhat symmetric, followed by additional rounds of asymmetric branching, in which a main trunk of the collecting duct continues to extend toward the nephrogenic zone, while smaller buds branch as they induce new nephrons within the nephrogenic zone. Originally, the UB derivatives are branching within a surrounding mesenchyme. Ultimately, they form a funnel-shaped structure in which cone-shaped groupings of ducts or papillae sit within a funnel or calyx that drains into the ureter. The mouse kidney has a single papilla and calyx, whereas a human kidney has 8 to 10 papillae, each of which drains into a minor calyx, with several minor calyces draining into a smaller number of major calyces.

## DEVELOPMENT OF THE NEPHRON

The renal vesicle undergoes patterned segmentation and proceeds through a series of morphologic changes that include gradual recruitment of mesenchymal progenitors to form the glomerulus and components of the nephrogenic tubules from the proximal convoluted tubule, the loop of Henle, and the distal tubule. The renal vesicles undergo differentiation, passing through morphologically distinct stages starting from the comma-shaped and proceeding to the S-shaped body, capillary loop, and mature stage, each step involving precise proximal-to-distal patterning and structural transformations (see Fig. 1.4). Remarkably, this process is repeated 600,000 to 1 million times in each developing human kidney as new nephrons are sequentially born at the tips of the UB throughout fetal life.

The glomerulus develops from the most proximal end of the renal vesicle that is furthest from the UB tip.[16,17] Distinct cell types of the glomerulus can first be identified in the S-shaped stage, where presumptive podocytes appear as a columnar-shaped epithelial cell layer. A vascular cleft develops and separates the presumptive podocyte layer from more distal cells that will form the proximal tubule. Parietal epithelial cells differentiate and flatten to form the Bowman capsule, a structure that surrounds the urinary space and is continuous with the proximal tubular epithelium. Concurrently, endothelial cells migrate into the vascular cleft. Together with podocytes, the endothelial cells produce the glomerular basement membrane, a major component of the mature filtration barrier. Initially the podocytes are connected by intercellular tightjunctions at their apical surface.[18] As glomerulogenesis proceeds, the podocytes flatten and spread out to cover the increased surface area of the growing glomerular capillary bed. They develop microtubular-based primary processes and actin-based secondary foot processes.[19–21] Foot processes of neighboring podocytes interdigitate and elongate. As podocytes mature, intercellular epithelial tight junctions linking become restricted to the basal aspect of the podocyte, relocate from the cell body to the foot processes, and are eventually replaced by a modified adherens junction-like structure known as the slit diaphragm.[18,22] The slit diaphragms are signaling hubs serving as the final layer of the glomerular filtration barrier.[23] Mesangial cell ingrowth follows

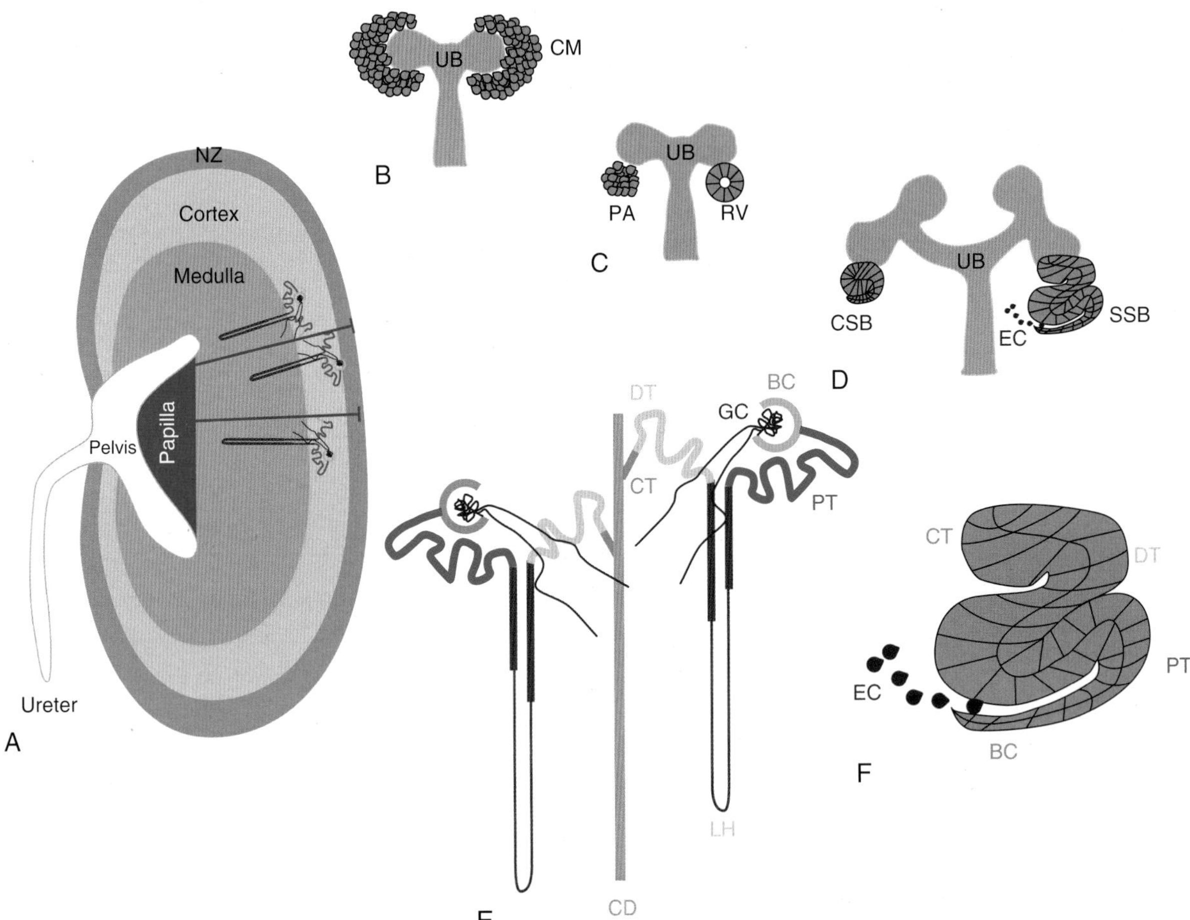


**Fig. 1.5 Overview of nephrogenesis.** (A) Gross kidney histoarchitecture. (B–E) As described in the text, reciprocal interaction between the ureteric bud and metanephric mesenchyme results in a series of well-defined morphologic stages leading to formation of the nephron, including the branching of the UB epithelium and the epithelialization of the metanephric mesenchyme into a highly patterned nephron. (F) Distinctive segmentation of the S-shaped body defines the patterning of the nephron. *BC,* Bowman capsule; *CD,* collecting duct; *CM,* cap mesenchyme; *CSB,* comma-shaped body; *CT,* connecting tubule; *DT,* distal tubule; *EC,* endothelial cells; *LH,* loop of Henle; *NZ,* nephrogenic zone; *PA,* pretubular aggregate; *PT,* proximal tubule; *SSB,* S-shaped body; *UB,* ureteric bud.

the migration of endothelial cells and is required for development and patterning of the capillary loops that are found in normal glomeruli. The endothelial cells also flatten considerably and capillary lumens are formed due to apoptosis of a subset of endothelial cells.[24] At the capillary loop stage, glomerular endothelial cells develop fenestrae, which are semipermeable transcellular pores common in capillary beds exposed to high hemodynamic flux.

In the mature stage glomerulus, the podocytes, fenestrated endothelial cells, and intervening glomerular basement membrane comprise the filtration barrier that separates the urinary from the blood space. Together, these components provide a size- and charge-selective barrier that permits free passage of small solutes and water but prevents the loss of larger molecules such as proteins. The mesangial cells are found between the capillary loops where they are required to provide ongoing structural support to the capillaries and possess smooth-muscle cell-like characteristics that have the capacity to contract, which may account for some of the dynamic properties of the glomerulus. The tubular portion of the nephron becomes segmented in a proximal–distal order, into the proximal convoluted tubule, the descending and ascending loops of Henle, and distal convoluted tubule. The distal tubule is contiguous with the collecting duct, a derivative of the UB. Imaging and fate mapping studies reveal that this interconnection results from the invasion of the UB by cells from the distal segments of nascent nephrons (around the S-shaped body stage).[25]

Although all segments of the nephron are present at birth and filtration occurs prior to birth, maturation of the tubule continues in the postnatal period. Increased expression levels of transporters, switches in transporter isoforms, alterations in paracellular transport mechanisms, and permeability and biophysical properties of tubular membranes have all been observed to occur postnatally.[26] These observations emphasize the importance of considering the developmental stage of the nephron in interpretation of renal transport and may explain the age of onset of symptoms in inherited transport disorders.

## THE NEPHROGENIC ZONE

After the first few rounds of branching of the UB, and the concomitant induction of nephrons from the MM, the kidney subdivides into two major compartments: an outer region called the cortex and an inner region called the medulla. The glomeruli and proximal and distal tubules localize within the cortex, together with the distal part of the nephron that connects directly to the collecting ducts. The loop of Henle and the rest of the collecting duct network comprise the epithelial structures found in the medulla. Kidney growth and nephrogenesis occurs in a radial fashion with new branches of the ureteric tree and newer nephrons added at the outermost periphery of the developing cortex which is called the nephrogenic zone. The nephrogenic zone is morphologically identifiable as a narrow band beneath the renal capsule where the branching UB tips are found together with nascent nephrons (pretubular aggregates, renal vesicles, comma-shaped bodies, and S-shaped bodies) and self-renewing nephron progenitors. Within the developing kidney, the most mature nephrons are found in the innermost layers of the cortex, and the most immature nephrons in the most peripheral regions. The nephrogenic zone, therefore, represents an active site of nephrogenesis. The nephrogenic zone progressively thins out with the gradual depletion of nephrogenic precursors and disappears once the remaining nephron progenitors have completely epithelialized.

## RENAL STROMA AND INTERSTITIAL CELL POPULATIONS

For decades in classic embryologic studies of kidney development, emphasis has been placed on the reciprocal inductive signals between MM and UB. However, in recent years, interest in the stromal cell as a key regulator of nephrogenesis has arisen.[17,27–29] Stromal cells also derive from the MM but are not induced to condense by the UB. Two distinct populations of stromal cells have been described: cortical stromal cells exist as a thin layer beneath the renal capsule while medullary stromal cells populate the interstitial space between the collecting ducts and tubules (Fig. 1.6). Cortical stromal cells also surround the MM condensates and provide signals required for UB branching and patterning of the developing kidney. Disruption or loss of these stromal cells leads to impairment of UB branching, reduction in nephron number, disrupted nephron patterning with failure of cortical–medullary boundary formation, and maldevelopment of the renal vasculature. A reciprocal signaling loop from the UB exists to properly pattern stromal cell populations. Loss of these UB-derived signals leads to a buildup of stromal cells beneath the capsule that are several layers thick. As nephrogenesis proceeds, stromal cells differentiate into peritubular interstitial cells and pericytes that are required for vascular remodeling and the production of extracellular matrix responsible for proper nephric formation.[29] These cells migrate from their position around the condensates to areas between the developing nephrons within the medulla.

## THE RENAL VASCULATURE

The microcirculations of the kidney include the specialized glomerular capillary system responsible for production of the ultrafiltrate, and the vasa recta bundles and peritubular capillaries involved in the countercurrent mechanism for urine osmoregulation (Fig. 1.7). Vasculogenesis and angiogenesis have been described as two distinct processes in blood vessel formation (Fig. 1.8). Vasculogenesis is the de novo differentiation of previously nonvascular endothelial cell precursors into structures that resemble capillary beds, whereas angiogenesis refers to sprouting from these early beds to form mature vessel structures, including arteries, veins, and capillaries. Both processes are involved in development of the renal vasculature. At E11.5 in mice, the UB is tracked by a primitive vessel that elaborates in synchrony with both UB branching and nephrogenesis. A rich capillary network is identifiable by E12.5 while the presence of endothelial cell-containing glomeruli becomes apparent at E14.5.

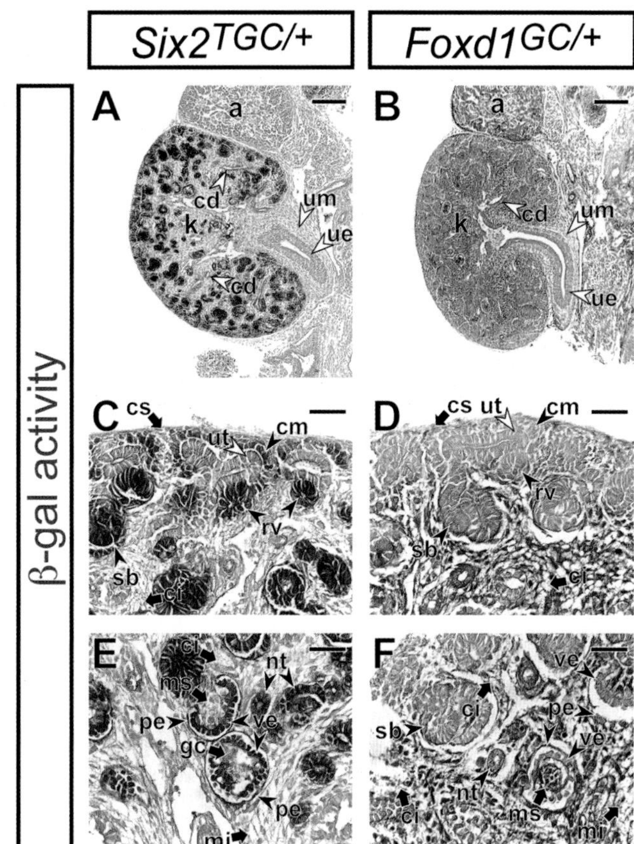


**Fig. 1.6 The nephrogenic and stromal mesenchyme.** Lineage tracing analysis in E14.5 mouse kidneys showing nephrogenic derivatives of *Six2*-expressing condensing mesenchyme (A, C, and E) and the *Foxd1*-expressing stromal mesenchyme (B, D, and F), stained for β-galactosidase activity (*blue*). *a,* Adrenal gland; *cd,* collecting duct; *ci,* renal cortical interstitium; *cm,* cap mesenchyme; *cs,* renal cortical stroma; *gal,* galactosidase; *gc,* glomerular capillary; *k,* kidney; *mi,* renal medullary interstitium; *ms,* mesangium; *nt,* nephrogenic tubule; *pe,* parietal epithelium; *rv,* renal vesicle; *sb,* S-shaped body; *ue,* ureter epithelium; *um,* ureter mesenchyme; *ut,* ureteric tip; *ve,* visceral epithelium (podocyte). Reproduced with permission from Kobayashi A, Mugford JW, Krautzberger Am, et al. Identification of a multipotent self-renewing stromal progenitor population during mammalian kidney organogenesis. *Stem Cell Reports*. 2014;3:650–662.

Transplantation experiments support a model where endogenous endothelial progenitors within the MM give rise to renal vessels in situ through angiogenesis, although the origin of large blood vessels is still not clear.[30–35] At E13, capillaries form networks around the developing nephric tubules and by E14, the hilar artery and first-order interlobar renal artery branches can be identified. These branches will form the corticomedullary arcades and interlobular arteries that branch from these arcades. Further branching produces the glomerular afferent arterioles. From E13.5 onward, endothelial cells migrate into the vascular cleft of developing glomeruli, where they undergo differentiation to form the

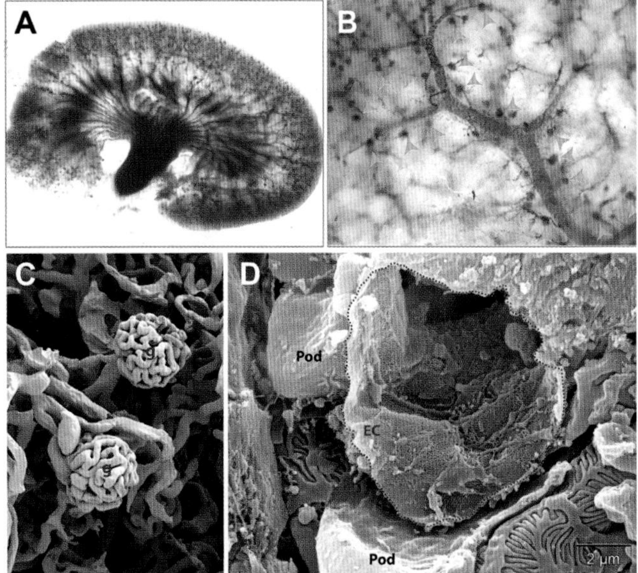


**Fig. 1.7 The renal vasculature.** (A) Visualization of the renal vascular network in a reporter mouse strain expressing prokaryotic β-galactosidase through the promoter of the vascular-specific phosphatase gene *Ptprb*. (B) Higher magnification of the renal cortex in (A) showing endothelial cell distribution in glomeruli (*yellow arrowheads*), arterioles, peritubular capillaries, and arcuate arteries. (C) Corrosion resin cast of the renal vasculature revealing the highly convoluted assembly of the glomerular capillaries *(g)*. (D) Scanning electron micrograph of a glomerulus with an exposed endothelial lumen (*dashed outline*) revealing fenestrations. *EC,* Endothelial cell; *Pod,* podocytes. *Corrosion cast electron micrograph courtesy Fred Hossler, Department of Anatomy and Cell Biology, East Tennessee State University.*

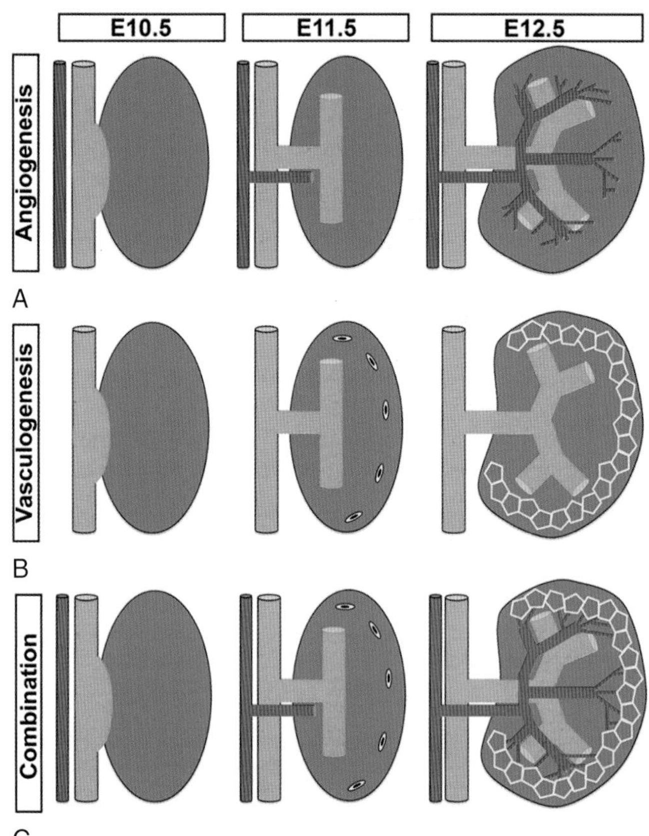


**Fig. 1.8 Angiogenesis and vasculogenesis in renal vascular development.** Schematic overview of early development of the renal vasculature. (A) Angiogenesis generates major blood vessels through sprouting and branching of pioneer vessels (*red*) that follow the branching ureteric bud (*brown*). (B) Scattered endothelial progenitor cells (*yellow*) are distinctly present as early as E11.5 at the periphery of the developing metanephric kidney (*blue*). These sporadic endothelial cells coalesce and organize into a primitive capillary plexus (*yellow*) by E12.5. (C) Major vessels formed via angiogenesis and capillaries that arise by vasculogenesis become interconnected to establish the elaborate renal vascular network. Adapted from Stolz DB, Sims-Lucas S. Unwrapping the origins and roles of the renal endothelium. *Pediatr Nephrol.* 2015;30:865–872.

glomerular capillary loops. The efferent arterioles carry blood away from the glomerulus to a system of fenestrated peritubular capillaries that are in close contact with the adjacent tubules and receive filtered water and solutes reabsorbed from the filtrate.[36] These capillaries have few pericytes. In comparison, the vasa rectae, which surround the medullary tubules and are involved in urinary concentration, are also fenestrated but have more pericytes. They arise from the efferent arterioles of deep glomeruli.[37] The peritubular capillary system surrounding the proximal tubules is well developed in the late fetal period, whereas the vasa rectae mature 1 to 3 weeks postnatally.

## MODEL SYSTEMS TO STUDY KIDNEY DEVELOPMENT

### THE KIDNEY ORGAN CULTURE SYSTEM

From the late 1950s, the method of growing mouse embryonic kidneys as floating cultures on top of filters (Fig. 1.9), a technique pioneered by Clifford Grobstein and improved by Lauri Saxen, accelerated the advancement of the kidney developmental biology field. This classic method, which remains widely in use to this day, has the advantages that the kidney explants are cultivated within an easily manipulated, controlled environment, and there is a possibility of visualizing the pattern of kidney growth by real-time fluorescence microscopy. Although vascularization and functional maturation is largely restricted in embryonic kidney explants, in vitro cultured kidneys display remarkable recapitulation of ureteric branching and epithelialization and segmental patterning of the MM (Fig. 1.10). Historically, kidney explant cultures provided crucial proof for the principle of reciprocal tissue induction in organogenesis. It was used to demonstrate that the UB and the MM exchange inductive cues, driving branching morphogenesis of the UB and epithelialization of the MM.[10,38]

As originally shown by Grobstein, Saxen, and colleagues, the two major components of the metanephric kidney, the MM and the UB, could be separated from each other, and the isolated mesenchyme could be induced to form nephron-like tubules by a selected set of other embryonic tissues, the best example of which is the embryonic neural tube.[10,38] When the neural tube is used to induce the separated mesenchyme, there is terminal differentiation of the mesenchyme into tubules, but not significant tissue expansion. In contrast, intact metanephric rudiments can grow more extensively,

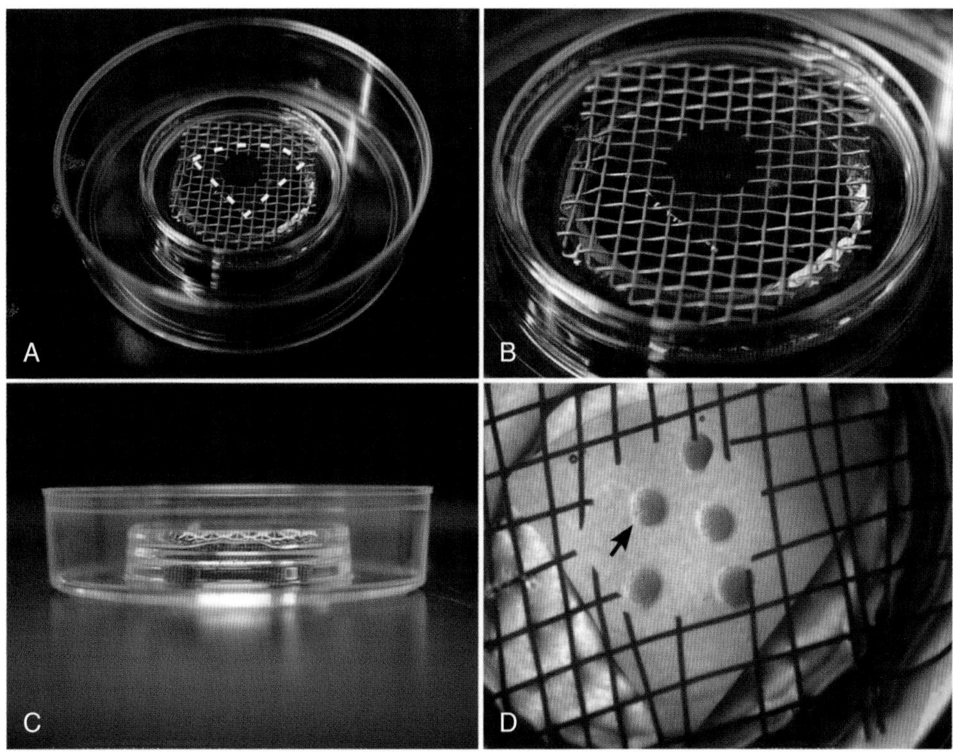


**Fig. 1.9 Metanephric organ explants.** (A, B) Top and (C) lateral view of a kidney organ culture. Embryonic kidney explants are grown at the air–growth medium interface on top of a floating porous polycarbonate filter (*dashed lines* in A) supported on a metal mesh. (D) Kidneys grown after 4 days of culture. *Reproduced with permission from Cold Spring Harbor Protocols.*[741]

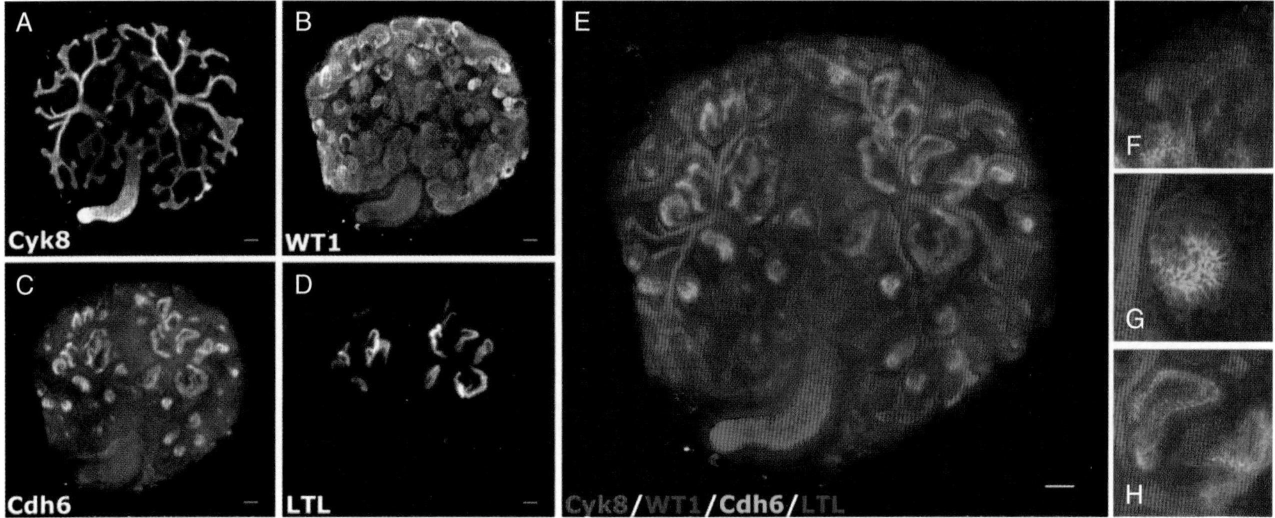


**Fig. 1.10 Recapitulation of branching and nephrogenesis in renal explant cultures.** (A) Ureteric tree stained for cytokeratin 8 *(Cyk8)*. (B) Condensed metanephric mesenchyme stained for WT1. (C) Epithelial derivatives of the metanephric mesenchyme stained for E-cadherin (*Cdh1*). (D) Proximal tubules stained with *Lotus tetraglobulus* lectin *(LTL)*. (E) Merged image of A–D. (F) *WT1*-expressing cells represent the nephron progenitor cells that surround the UB. (G) *Cdh1*-expression marks the mesenchyme-to-epithelial transformation of nephron progenitor cells. (H) Early patterning of nascent nephrons along a proximodistal axis. *Reproduced with permission from Cold Spring Harbor Protocols.*[741]

displaying both sustained UB branching and early induction of nephrons even when cultured for a week. The isolated mesenchyme experiment has proven useful in the analysis of renal agenesis phenotypes, where there is no outgrowth of the UB. In these cases, the mesenchyme can be placed in contact with the neural tube to determine whether it has the intrinsic ability to differentiate. Most often, when renal agenesis is due to the mutation of a transcription factor, tubular induction is not rescued by the neural tube, as could be predicted for transcription factors, which would be expected to act in a cell-autonomous fashion.[39] In the converse situation, in which renal agenesis is caused by loss of a gene function in the UB (e.g., *Emx2*), it is usually possible for the embryonic neural tube to induce tubule formation in isolated mesenchymes.[40] Therefore the organ culture induction assay can be used to test hypotheses concerning whether a particular gene is required in the UB or the MM. Recently, as chemical inhibitors specific for various signal transduction pathways have been synthesized and become available, it has been possible to add these to organ cultures and observe effects that are informative about the roles of specific pathways in development of the kidney. Examples are the use of drugs to block the ERK/MAP kinase, PI3K/Akt, Notch signaling, and Wnt signaling pathways in renal explant cultures.[41–45] Synthetic antisense oligonucleotides and small interfering or silencing RNA (siRNA) have also been successfully used to inhibit gene expression in kidney organ cultures.[45–55]

## GENETIC MOUSE MODELS

Many of the genetic pathways regulating many aspects of development are strongly conserved between mice and humans. Due to the relative ease of manipulating the genome of the mouse, its small size, and shorter gestation period, the mouse has become the primary model organism for the study of mechanism of human development and diseases. Anatomic and functional features of the human kidney are for the most part highly similar in the mouse, albeit at a smaller scale, while a number of genes identified as essential for normal mouse kidney development are also known to be associated with congenital anomalies of the kidney and urinary tract (CAKUT) and other kidney diseases.[56–58]

The wealth of our understanding of metanephric kidney development over the past two decades is owed to the harnessing of homologous gene recombination to introduce targeted mutations and novel alleles into specific genes in cultured mouse embryonic stem cells. This paved the way for the creation of numerous genetically engineered mice that have become highly valuable tools for the study of renal developmental biology and the etiology of certain genetic diseases of the kidneys and the urinary tract (Table e1.2). The technology is applied in many ways. In its simplest is the creation of null mutations within the germline that generate gene knockout mouse models. The limitation of this method is that certain genes are essential for early development and their inactivation in the germline can cause premature lethality, thus precluding the analysis of the function of those genes in organogenesis. A novel improvement to this is the use of a conditional gene-targeting strategy, allowing for the creation of conditional alleles. This involves introducing small recognition sites for recombinase enzymes of which the Cre recombinase is the most routine now (Fig. 1.11). A conditional "floxed" allele of the target gene locus is created by incorporating two *loxP* sites within two separate introns, flanking the exons that can be excised or recombined. In principle, normal transcription from the locus is expected prior to recombination of the floxed allele and should effectively promote a wild type phenotype. The Cre recombinase itself is engineered under the control of a tissue-specific promoter. Breeding between tissue-specific transgenic Cre animals and those harboring a conditional allele for a particular gene ultimately results in a cell- or tissue-type specific inactivation of the gene of interest. This strategy has also been refined in some cases, so that the Cre expression is also temporally regulated by the use of a drug such as doxycycline or tamoxifen. A number of Cre lines are now available to target genes specifically within different subpopulations of renal cells and progenitors. The transgenic Cre lines driven by the *Hoxb7, Six2, Foxd1, and Nphs2* promoters are among the most highly cited gene excision drivers for targeted genetic inactivation in the ureteric, nephrogenic, stromal, and podocyte cell lineages.[59–64] Lately, the introduction of the more precise CRISPR-Cas9 gene editing tool, an ingenious application of the adaptive immune response of prokaryotes against bacteriophages, is facilitating the way researchers create customized mutant cells and animal models to study various aspects of renal development (Fig. 1.12).[65–68]

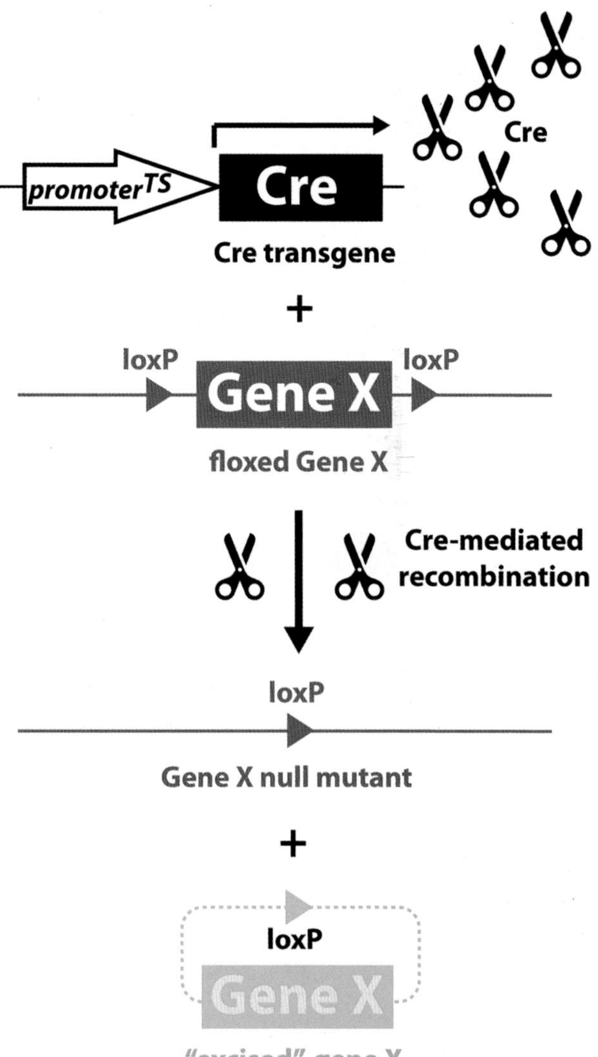


**Fig. 1.11 Cre-lox homologous gene recombination system.** Simplified overview of Cre recombinase–mediated homologous recombination for generation of tissue-specific conditional null mutations of a target gene. Cre recombinase expression is engineered to be driven under the control of tissue specific promoter (promoter$^{TS}$). The target gene (or typically certain exons within the target chromosomal locus) are flanked with loxP sites (recognition sites for Cre recombinase). Cre activity in specific cell types mediates the excision of the loxP-flanked (floxed) target gene, creating a null allele.

The discovery of new kidney-relevant genes or signaling pathways has also been achieved by random chemical mutagenesis in mice. The alkylating agent N-ethyl-N-nitrosourea (ENU) is routinely used to introduce random point mutations in mouse spermatogonia. The introduced mutations can result in loss or gain of function and are either recessive or

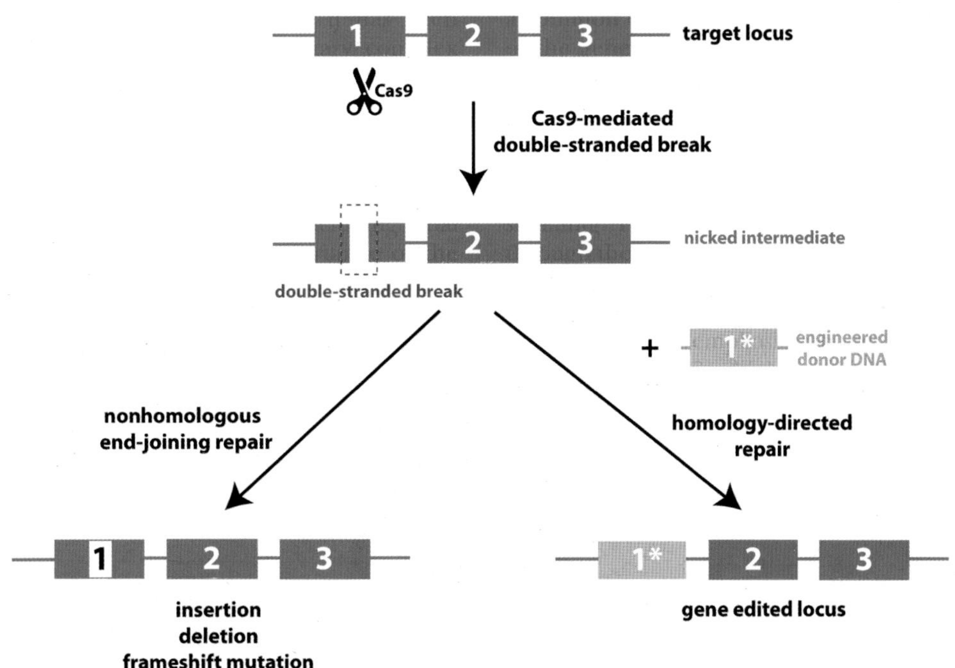


**Fig. 1.12 Gene editing using the CRISPR-Cas9 system.** Simplified overview for targeted introduction of mutations using the CRISPR-Cas9 system. Site-specific cleavage of a target gene locus with the Cas9 endonuclease creates a double-strand DNA break. The nicked target gene can be repaired by an error-prone, nonhomologous repair mechanism resulting in nucleotide insertion, deletion, or frameshift mutations. Introduction of a homologous engineered donor DNA results in a homologous substitution into the target locus which then results in a precisely edited gene.

dominant. Breeding of ENU-injected male mice results in offspring that can then be screened for various renal phenotypes (e.g., dysplasia, cysts, proteinuria) and heritability.[69–71] Some examples of genes whose relevance to kidney development functions was revealed from ENU mutagenesis include *Arhgap23* (ciliogenesis and glomerular cyst defects), *Six1* (renal hypoplasia), *Scl5a2 (SGLT2;* glucosuria), *Pou3f3 (Brn1;* oligonephronia and smaller loop of Henle), and *Aqp11* (proximal tubule vacuolation and cysts).[72–74]

Significant innovations in high-throughput gene sequencing are also facilitating the identification of monogenic mutations associated with heritable kidney diseases.[75,76] Putative disease-causing genes identified from genome-wide association studies can then be validated in corresponding gene-targeted mouse models. Similarly, a gene whose mutation has been identified to cause kidney maldevelopment and dysfunction in mice can be investigated for incidence of mutations across the human genome (e.g., *Arhgdia* in nephrotic syndrome).[77–80] Other genome-wide approaches that have led to the discovery of novel genes in kidney development and disease include gene trap consortia[81,82] and genome-wide transcriptome and proteome projects.[83–85]

## IMAGING AND LINEAGE TRACING STUDIES

Reporter mouse lines are animal models engineered to express transgenes encoding an enzyme (e.g., bacterial β-galactosidase or firefly luciferase) or fluorescent protein tag in a cell lineage–specific manner (Fig. 1.13). In the simplest model, a single transgene comprising the reporter coding region is placed downstream of a cell-specific promoter. Such a model is useful to identify and follow distinct cell lineages where the chosen promoter is active. *Hoxb7-EGFP* is the first fluorescent transgene developed to visualize renal development.[86] Enhanced green fluorescent protein (EGFP), placed under the control of the *Hoxb7* promoter, specifically labels the wolffian duct and the ureteric epithelial lineage. *Hoxb7-EGFP* has therefore proven to be invaluable in studying the rates and pattern of ureteric branching morphogenesis and ureteral development, including disruption of these events in the context of particular mutant backgrounds.[60,87–89] An alternative model uses two separate transgenes, namely a cell-specific Cre driver and an independent reporter transgene (e.g., R26R). With the R26R reporter model, β-galactosidase transgene expression is switched on by a Cre-mediated removal of an upstream stop codon.[90] Inducible reporter systems incorporate genetic regulatory elements that allow for both cell-specific promoter- and drug-dependent activation of the reporter gene. The most commonly used strategies for controlled transgene expression in mice are the Tet-operon/repressor bi-transgenic and the estrogen-receptor ligand binding domain (Cre-ERT2) systems. These inducible reporter systems allow for timed pulse labeling of cell lineages, resulting in permanent tagging of progenitor cells and their direct derivatives. Inducible reporter systems have become valuable tools for the mapping of cell fates. Inducible reporter systems have been used to establish that the *Six2*$^+$ cells are the progenitors of all epithelial structures of the mature nephron.[61] In some cases, the Cre transgene is engineered with an associated fluorophore expression cassette under the control of a shared promoter, thus allowing easy identification of cells with targeted gene mutations. A wide variety of reporter and Cre transgenes (see Table e1.2) are now available to characterize the development and organization of multiple compartments of the kidney.

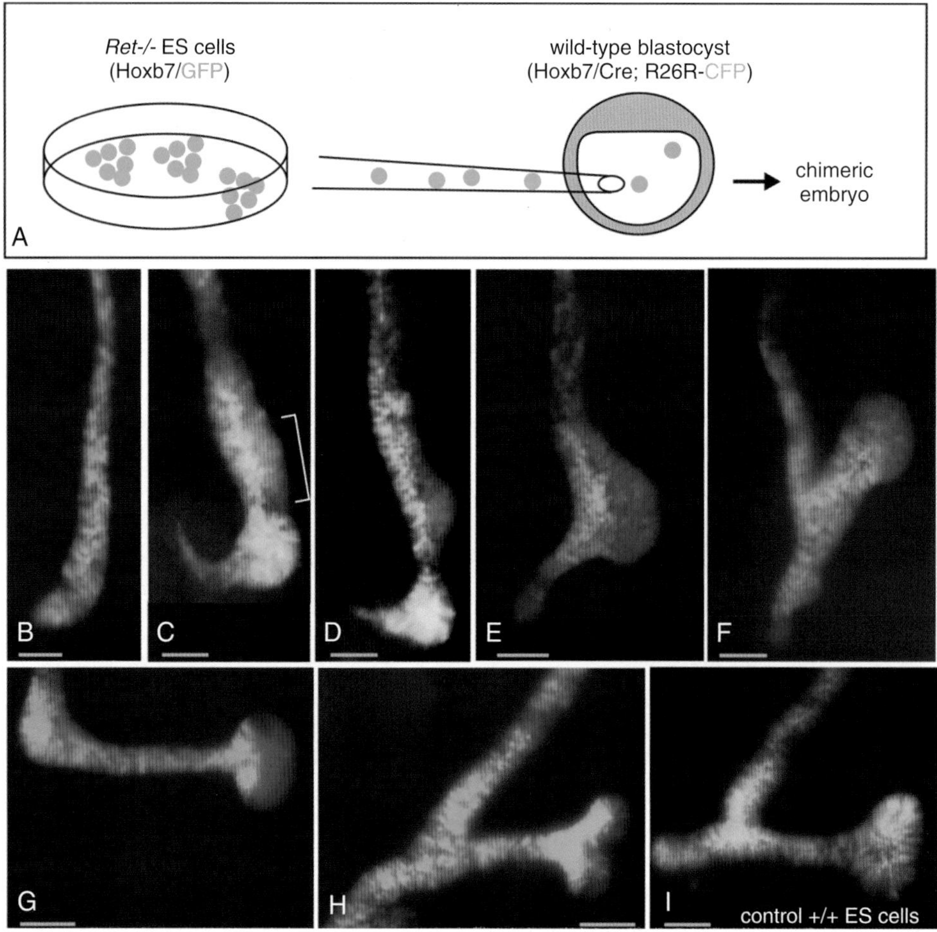


**Fig. 1.13 Cell fate tracing through genetic expression of fluorophores.** Segregation of *Ret*-deficient cells in the outgrowth and branching of the ureteric bud (UB). (A) Ret-null embryonic stem cells *(ES)* expressing *Hoxb7-GFP* were mixed with a wild-type transgenic blastocyst (*Hoxb7-Cre: R26R-CFP*). This generates chimeric animals in which *Ret*-null cells exhibit green fluorescent protein *(GFP)* fluorescence, while wild-type UB cells express cyan fluorescent protein *(CFP)*. (B) At E9.5, *Ret*-null epithelial cells are intermingled with wild-type cells in the wolffian duct *(WD)*. (C) At E10, when the dorsal side of the WD begins to swell, the region where UB will emerge becomes enriched with CFP-expressing but not Ret-null cells. (D, E) At around E10.5 dpc, the UB is exclusively formed by wild-type cells. (F) Upon elongation of the UB at E11, the bulbous distal tip of the UB is formed by wild-type cells but the *Ret*-null cells begin to contribute to the trailing trunk structure. (G, H) During the initial branching of the UB at around E11.5, Ret-null cells are excluded from the distal ampullary UB tips. (I) In contrast, control cells expressing Ret and GFP contribute to the whole branching UB structure. *dpc,* Days post coitum. *Reproduced with permission from Developmental Cell.*[186]

Reporter mice expressing fluorescent tags also come in handy for segregation and isolation of particular cell types on the basis of fluorescence, facilitating global gene expression analysis, elucidation of transcriptional regulatory networks, and epigenetic interactions that orchestrate particular morphogenetic events (Table 1.3). Purified single or bulk populations of fluorescence-tagged cells can be used for high-throughput discovery of transcriptomes, genome-wide DNA-binding protein interactions, histone modifications, and nucleosome complexes through revolutionary next-generation DNA sequencing methods such as RNA-seq (RNA sequencing) and ChIP-seq (chromatin immunoprecipitation sequencing).[91–93]

## NONMAMMALIAN MODEL SYSTEMS FOR KIDNEY DEVELOPMENT

Organisms separated by millions of years of evolution from humans still provide useful models to study the genetic basis and function of mammalian kidney development. This stems from the fact that all of these organisms possess excretory organs designed to remove metabolic wastes from the body, and that genetic pathways involved in other aspects of invertebrate development may serve as templates to dissect pathways in mammalian kidney development. In support of the latter argument, elucidation of the genetic interactions and molecular mechanism of the Kirrel (Neph1) orthologue and nephrin-like molecules SYG1 and SYG2 in synapse formation in the soil nematode *Caenorhabditis elegans* is providing major clues to the function of these genes in glomerular and slit diaphragm formation and function in mammals.[94]

The excretory organs of invertebrates differ greatly in their structure and complexity and range in size from a few cells in *C. elegans,* to several hundred cells in *Drosophila,* to the more recognizable kidneys in amphibians, birds, and mammals. In *C. elegans,* the excretory system consists of a single large H-shaped excretory cell, a pore cell, a duct cell, and a gland cell.[95,96] *C. elegans* provides many benefits as a model system: the availability of powerful genetic tools

**Table 1.3 Mouse Strains for Conditional Gene Targeting and Lineage Marking of Cells**

| Gene Promoter | Cre | rtTA | Cre-ERT2 | Fluorescent Reporter | Renal Expression | Extrarenal Expression | Reference |
|---|---|---|---|---|---|---|---|
| *11Hsd2* | ✓ | | | ✓ | Principal cells of collecting duct, connecting tubules | Amygdala, cerebellum, colon, ovary, uterus, epididymis salivary glands | 696 |
| *Aqp2* | ✓ | | ✓ | | Principal cells of collecting duct | Testis, vas deferens | 697 |
| *Atp6v1b1* | ✓ | | | ✓ | Collecting ducts (intercalated cells), connecting tubule | | 698, 699 |
| *Bmp7* | ✓ | | ✓ | ✓ | Cap mesenchyme | | 700 |
| *Cdh16 (Ksp-Cadherin)* | ✓ | | ✓ | | Renal tubules, collecting ducts, ureteric bud, wolffian duct, mesonephros | Müllerian duct | 701, 702 |
| *Cited1* | | | ✓ | ✓ | Cap mesenchyme | | 703 |
| *Emx1* | ✓ | | ✓ | ✓ | Renal tubules (proximal and distal tubules) | Cerebral cortex, thymus | 704 |
| *Foxd1* | ✓ | | ✓ | ✓ | Stromal cells | | 705 |
| *Gdnf* | | | ✓ | ✓ | Cap mesenchyme | | 706 |
| *Ggt1* | ✓ | | | | Cortical tubules | | 707 |
| *Hoxb6* | ✓ | | ✓ | | Metanephric mesenchyme | Lateral mesoderm, limb buds | 547, 708 |
| *Hoxb7* | ✓ | ✓ | | ✓ | Ureteric bud, wolffian duct, collecting ducts, distal ureter | Spinal cord, dorsal root ganglia | 59 |
| *Kap* | ✓ | | | | Proximal tubules | Brain | 709, 710 |
| *Klf3* | | | ✓ | | Collecting ducts | Gonads | GUDMAP[a] |
| *Nphs1* | ✓ | ✓ | | ✓ | Podocytes | Brain | 711, 712 |
| *Nphs2* | ✓ | ✓ | ✓ | | Podocytes | | 713 |
| *Osr1* | ✓ | | ✓ | ✓ | Metanephric mesenchyme | Intermediate mesoderm | 714, 715 |
| *Osr2* | ✓ | | | | Condensing metanephric mesenchyme; glomeruli | Palatal mesenchyme | 716 |
| *Pax2* | ✓ | | | ✓ | Pronephric duct, wolffian duct, ureteric bud, cap mesenchyme | Inner ear, midbrain, cerebellum, olfactory bulb | 717 |
| *Pax3* | ✓ | | | | Metanephric mesenchyme | Neural tube, neural crest | 713, 718, 719 |
| *Pax8* | ✓ | ✓ | ✓ | ✓ | Renal tubules (proximal and distal tubules) and collecting ducts (Tet-On inducible system) | | 720, 721 |
| *Pck1* | ✓ | | ✓ | ✓ | Proximal tubules | Liver | 630 |
| *Pdgfb* | | | ✓ | | Endothelium | Systemic vascular endothelium | 722 |
| *Pdgfrb* | ✓ | ✓ | ✓ | ✓ | Mesangial cells, vascular smooth muscles | Pericytes, vascular smooth muscles | 396, 510, 723 |
| *Prox1* | ✓ | | ✓ | ✓ | Ascending vasa rectae, lymphatic vessels | Systemic lymphatic vasculature | 724–726 |
| *Rarb* | ✓ | | | ✓ | Metanephric mesenchyme | | 550 |
| *Ren1* | ✓ | | ✓ | ✓ | Juxtaglomerular cells, afferent arterioles, mesangial cells | Adrenal gland, testis, sympathetic ganglia | 420 |
| *Ret* | | | ✓ | | Ureteric bud, collecting ducts | Dorsal root ganglion, neural crest | 727 |
| *Sall1* | | | ✓ | | Metanephric mesenchyme (tamoxifen-inducible system) | Limb buds, central nervous system, heart | 728 |
| *Six2* | ✓ | ✓ | ✓ | ✓ | Cap mesenchyme | | 61 |
| *Slc22a6* | | | ✓ | | Proximal tubules | | 721 |
| *Slc5a2* | ✓ | | | | Proximal tubules | | 729 |
| *Sox18* | | | ✓ | | Cortical and medullary vasculature | Blood vessel and precursor of lymphatic endothelial cells | 730–732 |

*Continued on following page*

**Table 1.3 Mouse Strains for Conditional Gene Targeting and Lineage Marking of Cells (Cont'd)**

| Gene Promoter | Cre | rtTA | Cre-ERT2 | Fluorescent Reporter | Renal Expression | Extrarenal Expression | Reference |
|---|---|---|---|---|---|---|---|
| *Spink3* | ✓ | | | | Medullary tubules (distal or connecting tubules?) | Mesonephric tubules, pancreas, lung, liver, gastrointestinal tract | 718, 719, 733 |
| *T (Brachyury)* | ✓ | | ✓ | | Whole kidney (both ureteric bud and metanephric mesenchyme) | Pan-mesodermal | 286 |
| *Tbx18* | ✓ | | | | Ureteral mesenchyme | Heart, limb buds | 734 |
| *Tcf21* | ✓ | | | | Metanephric mesenchyme, cap mesenchyme, podocytes, stromal cells | Epicardium, lung mesenchyme, gonad, spleen, adrenal gland | 246 |
| *Tek* | ✓ | ✓ | ✓ | ✓ | Endothelium | Systemic vasculature endothelium | 735–737 |
| *Tie1* | ✓ | ✓ | | | Endothelium | Systemic vasculature endothelium | 738 |
| *Umod* | ✓ | | ✓ | | Thick ascending limbs of loops of Henle | Testis, brain | 739 |
| *Wnt4* | ✓ | | ✓ | ✓ | Renal vesicles, nascent nephrons (comma- and S-shaped bodies) | Lungs, developing gonads | 61, 740 |

[a]Genitourinary Development and Molecular Anatomy Project (GUDMAP); http://www.gudmap.org.
Cre (noninducible Cre recombinase transgene); rtTA (reverse tetracycline transactivator, tetracycline inducible expression system); Cre-ERT2 (Cre-estrogen receptor ligand binding domain fusion transgene, tamoxifen-inducible expression system); fluorescent reporter (promoter-driven expression of a fluorescent protein such as green fluorescent protein and its variants.)

including "mutants by mail," a short life and reproductive cycle, a publicly available genome sequence and resource database (http://www.wormbase.org), the ease of performing genetic enhancer-suppressor screens in worms, and the fact that they share many genetic pathways with mammals. Major contributions in our understanding of the function of polycystic and cilia-related genes have been made from studying *C. elegans*. The *Pkd1* and *Pkd2* homologues, *LOV1* and *LOV2* of *C. elegans*, are involved in cilia development and mating behavior.[97,98] Strides in understanding the function of the slit diaphragm have also been made from *C. elegans* as described earlier.

Similar to *C. elegans*, the relative ease of large-scale genetic screens and phenotypic characterization in *Drosophila* makes it another valuable complimentary model for understanding the genetic basis of developmental processes. The excretory system of *Drosophila* consists of two parts, the nephrocytes and the malpighian tubules, which are functionally analogous to podocytes and renal tubules, respectively. A fundamental difference from vertebrate kidneys is that the nephrocytes and malpighian tubules are not physically connected. Nephrocytes either surround the heart (epicardial nephrocytes) or the esophagus (garland cells) and have elaborate membrane invaginations that closely resemble the glomerular filtration barrier. Remarkably, mutations of *Drosophila* homologs of genes known to be essential to form slit diaphragms and maintain podocyte functions also impair nephrocyte morphology and filtration functions.[99–103] Similarly, conserved genes have been identified that regulate normal patterning and function of Malpighian tubules and vertebrate renal tubules.[104–109] Functional readouts such as impaired nephrocyte filtration or uptake of tracers, ultrastructural analysis, and mortality screens can be executed efficiently in *Drosophila*, which can facilitate the characterization of novel gene functions that are vital for renal filtration.[110–112]

The pronephros is the functional kidney of the larva of some fishes (with the exception of jawless fishes which only develop the pronephros) and amphibians, while the mesonephros serve as the kidney in adults of these aquatic animals. The pronephros of the zebrafish (*Danio rerio*) larva consists of two tubules connected to a fused, single, midline glomerulus. The zebrafish pronephric glomerulus expresses many of the same genes found in mammalian glomeruli (e.g., *Vegfa, Nphs1, Nphs2,* and *Wt1*) and contain podocytes and fenestrated endothelial cells.[113] Advantages to the zebrafish as a model system include its short reproductive cycle, transparency of the larvae with easy visualization of defects in pronephric development without sacrificing the organism, the availability of the genome sequence, the ability to rapidly knockdown gene function using morpholino oligonucleotides, and the ability to perform functional studies of filtration using fluorescently tagged labels of varying sizes.[114] These features make zebrafish amenable to both forward and reverse genetic screens. Currently, multiple labs perform knockdown screens of mammalian homologs and genome-wide mutagenesis screens in zebrafish in order to study renal function. The pronephros of the clawed frog *Xenopus laevis* has also been used as a simple model to study early events in nephrogenesis.[115,116] Similar to the fish, the pronephros of the clawed frog consists of a single glomus, paired tubules, and a duct. The fact that *X. laevis* embryos develop rapidly outside the body (all major organ systems are formed by 6 days of age), the ease of injecting DNA, mRNA, and protein, ability to perform grafting, and in vitro culture experiments establish the frog as a valuable model system to dissect early inductive and patterning cues.[117,118] The availability of transgenic zebrafish and *Xenopus* lines that express the fluorescent protein EGFP in pronephric and mesonephric kidneys provide an opportunity to visualize real-time kidney development and function.[119–121]

### STEM CELL DERIVED KIDNEY ORGANOIDS

The discovery that a combination of small molecules and cytokines can effectively induce human pluripotent stem cells (hPSCs) to develop into intermediate mesoderm laid the groundwork for ingenious in vitro methods to generate kidney organoid cultures in which most fundamental processes in early renal development are recapitulated.[65,122–128] These hPSC-derived kidney organoids can form many renal structures, including the glomerulus, proximal tubule, loop of Henle, distal tubule, collecting ducts, interstitium, and a primitive endothelial network. Gene editing of hPSCs through CRISPR-Cas9 technology (see Fig. 1.12) provides a unique opportunity for a time- and cost-effective strategy to interrogate novel gene functions relevant to embryonic kidney development.[66,129–131] One particular example is the study of epithelial cyst pathogenesis in kidney organoids from polycystin-deficient hPSCs.[65] Although their use in renal replacement therapy remains to be realized, kidney organoids have immediate practical application in high-throughput screening of drugs for nephrotoxicity.[132]

## GENETIC ANALYSIS OF MAMMALIAN KIDNEY DEVELOPMENT

### INTERACTION OF THE URETERIC BUD AND THE METANEPHRIC MESENCHYME

The classic studies with the organ culture system that started in the 1950s provided an extensive framework that formed the basis for further studies of organ development.[38,133,134] These elegant studies demonstrated that the epithelialization of the MM requires a UB-derived factor which we now know as Wnt9b.[135] However, the modern era of studies on the early development of the kidney began with the observation of renal agenesis phenotypes in gene-targeted or knockout mice, the earliest among these being the knockout of several transcription factors, including the *Wt1, Pax2, Eya1, Osr1 (Odd1), Six1, Sall1, Lhx1 (Lim1),* and *Emx2*.[39,40,47,136–141] The knockout of genes for several secreted signaling molecules such as GDNF (glial cell line–derived neurotrophic factor), GDF11 (growth differentiation factor 11), gremlin, and the receptors Ret and GFRα1 also resulted in renal agenesis, at least in the majority of embryos.[142–148]

> ***Clinical Relevance***
> Perturbation of cell–cell communication during embryonic kidney development can have wide-ranging detrimental consequences, including renal agenesis, CAKUT, proteinuria, kidney cysts, defective urine osmoregulation, acidosis, and predisposition to hypertension and chronic kidney diseases.

### EARLY LINEAGE DETERMINATION OF THE METANEPHRIC MESENCHYME

In most embryos exhibiting renal agenesis, an appropriately localized putative MM is often uninvaded by a UB outgrowth. Two exceptions are the *Osr1 (Odd1)*- and *Eya1*-mutant embryos, where this distinct patch of MM is absent, suggesting that *Osr1* and *Eya1* represent early determinants of the MM (Fig. 1.14). Together, the phenotypes of these knockout mice have provided an initial molecular hierarchy of early kidney development.[136,149] *Osr1* marks the intermediate mesoderm from which the mesenchymal cells within the mesonephric and metanephric kidney are derived and is subsequently downregulated upon epithelial differentiation. Mice lacking *Osr1* do not form the MM and do not express several other factors required for metanephric kidney formation, including *Eya1, Six2, Pax2, Sall1,* or *Gdnf*.[149]

*Eya1*-mediated specification of the MM cell fate is thought to occur via interaction with another transcription factor, *Six1*. *EYA1* and *SIX1* mutations are found in humans with branchiootorenal (BOR) syndrome.[150] It is now known through in vitro experiments that Eya1 and Six1 form a regulatory complex that appears to be involved in transcriptional regulation.[151,152] Interestingly, Eya1 was shown to have an intrinsic phosphatase activity that regulates the activation of the *Eya1/Six1* complex.[152,153] Moreover, *Eya* and *Six* family genes are coexpressed in several tissues in mammals, *Xenopus* and *Drosophila*, further supporting a functional interaction between these genes.[136,138,139,154,155] Direct transcriptional targets of this complex appear to include the pro-proliferative factor *Myc*.[152] In the *Eya1*-deficient urogenital ridge the putative MM is completely absent.[156] Consistent with this finding, *Six1* is either absent or poorly expressed in the presumptive location of the MM of *Eya1*-null embryos.[152,154–156] *Eya1* is expressed in the *Six1*-null mesenchyme, suggesting that *Eya1* is upstream of *Six1*.[138,139]

The transcription factor *Wt1* is another essential regulator of early MM development. *Wt1* expression is weak in the uninduced MM but increases in the condensed cap mesenchyme surrounding the branching UB tips. *Wt1* expression remains throughout nephrogenesis but eventually becomes restricted to the presumptive podocytes at the proximal end of the S-shaped nephron. Mature podocytes continue to express *Wt1* at high levels. Genetic loss of *Wt1* in mice prevents UB outgrowth and causes apoptosis of the MM, whereas human mutations of *WT1* have been linked to renal tumors.[39,157] Among the numerous identified transcriptional targets of *Wt1* known to be required for kidney development are *Bmp7, Pax2,* and *Sall1*.[48] More recently, it has been shown that *Wt1* regulates antagonistic fibroblast growth factor (FGF) and bone morphogenetic protein (BMP)/SMAD (contraction of homologous Sma and MAD genes of worms and fruitflies) signaling pathways, effectively promoting the proliferation and survival of the MM.[158,159] The absence of *Wt1* significantly downregulates the expression of the genes for several FGF ligands, including *Fgf8, Fgf10, Fgf16,* and *Fgf20,* which support mesenchymal proliferation.[48,159] Furthermore, *Wt1* deficiency in nephron progenitors leads to specific loss of *Gas1*, a gene encoding for an extracellular glycosphingolipid-tethered protein that modulates PI3K-Akt signaling downstream of FGFs.[158] The impairment of FGF signaling upon loss of *Wt1* is exacerbated by the upregulation of BMP/SMAD signaling,

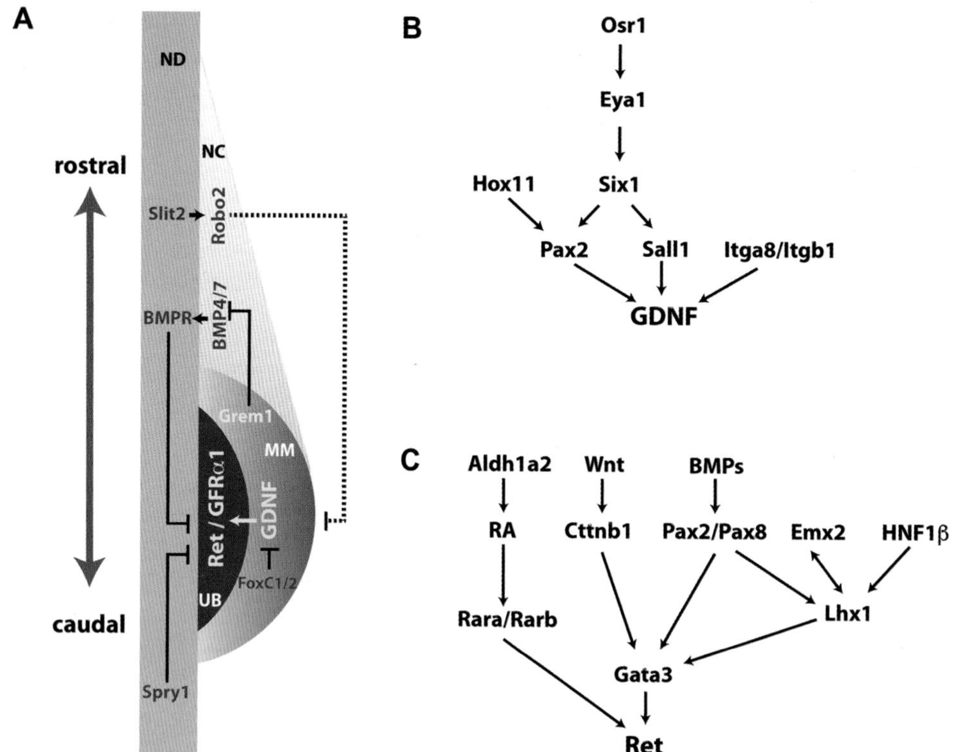


**Fig. 1.14 Genetic interactions during early metanephric kidney development.** (A) Regulatory interactions that control the strategically localized expression of glial cell–derived neurotrophic factor (GDNF) and Ret and the subsequent induction of the ureteric bud. The anterior part of GDNF expression is restricted by Foxc1/2 and Slit2/Robo2 signaling. Spry1 suppresses the postreceptor activity of Ret. BMP4/7-BMPR signaling inhibits the response to GDNF, an effect counteracted by Grem1. Genetic regulatory network that controls the expression of (B) GDNF and (C) Ret. *BMPR,* Bone morphogenetic protein receptor; *MM,* metanephric mesenchyme; *NC,* nephrogenic cord; *ND,* nephric duct; *UB,* ureteric bud.

which promotes apoptosis.[159] This is thought to occur through the loss of *Bmper* expression, a direct target of *Wt1,* which inhibits BMP4 signaling.

## URETERIC BUD INDUCTION

In many cases of renal agenesis, a failure of the GDNF-Ret signaling axis has been identified.[160] GDNF, a member of the TGF-β superfamily and secreted by the MM, activates the Ret-GFRα1 receptor complex that is expressed by cells of the nephric duct and the UB. Activation of the Ret tyrosine kinase is of central importance to UB induction. Most mutant embryos lacking *Gdnf, Ret,* or *Gfra1* exhibit partial or complete renal agenesis due to severe impairment of UB induction while exogenous GDNF is sufficient to induce sprouting of ectopic buds from the nephric duct.[142–144,148,161–164] Consistently, other genes linked to renal agenesis are known to regulate the normal expression of GDNF. These include transcription factors (e.g., *Eya1, Pax2, Six1, Hox11* paralogues, and *Sall1*) and proteins required to stimulate or maintain GDNF expression (e.g., GDF11, Kif26b, nephronectin, α8β1-integrin, and Fras1) (see Fig. 1.14).[136,139,140,145,165–173]

As described earlier, *Eya1* mutants fail to form the MM. *Pax2* is a transcriptional regulator of the paired box family and is expressed widely during the development of both UB and mesenchymal components of the urogenital system.[170] In *Pax2*-null embryos, *Eya1, Six1* and *Sall1* are expressed,[156] suggesting that *Eya1* and *Six1* are likely upstream of *Pax2.* Through a combination of molecular and in vivo studies, it has been demonstrated that *Pax2* appears to act as a transcriptional activator of *Gdnf* and regulates the expression of *Ret.*[171,174] *Pax2* also appears to regulate kidney formation through epigenetic control as it is involved in the assembly of a histone H3–lysine 4 methyltransferase complex through the ubiquitously expressed nuclear factor PTIP, which regulates histone methylation.[175] The *Hox* genes are conserved in all metazoans and specify positional information along the body axis. *Hox11* paralogues include *Hoxa11, Hoxc11,* and *Hoxd11.* Mice carrying mutations in any one of these genes do not have kidney abnormalities; however, triple-mutant mice for these genes demonstrate a complete absence of metanephric kidney induction.[172] Interestingly, in this mutant, the formation of condensing MM and the expression of *Eya1, Pax2,* and *Wt1* remain unperturbed, suggesting that *Hox11* is not upstream of these factors. Although there seems to be some hierarchy, *Eya1, Pax2,* and *Hox11* appear to form a complex to coordinately regulate the expression of *Gdnf.*[176]

*Sall1* indirectly controls the expression of GDNF. *Sall1* is necessary for the expression of the kinesin *Kif26b* by the MM cells.[167] In the absence of either *Sall1* or *Kif26b,* the nephronectin receptor α8β1-integrin expressed by the MM mesenchyme is downregulated. The loss of *Sall1, Kif26b, Itga8* (α8 integrin), *Itgb1* (β1-integrin), and *Npnt* (nephronectin) compromises the adhesion of the MM cells to the UB tips, ultimately causing loss of *Gdnf* expression and failure of UB outgrowth.[168,169,177] The absence of Fras1, an extracellular matrix protein linked to Fraser syndrome, which is expressed selectively in the UB epithelium and nascent epithelialized nephrons but not the MM, causes loss of *Gdnf* expression.[165] Fras1 likely regulates MM induction and GDNF expression via multiple signaling pathways. *Fras1* deficiency results in downregulation of *Gdf11, Hox11, Six2,* and *Itga8,* and an increase in *Bmp4,* which altogether cooperatively controls *Gdnf* expression.[165]

## GENES REQUIRED BY THE URETERIC BUD

Several components of the genetic network supporting the development of the nephric duct and the UB have been identified (see Fig. 1.14). *Pax2* and *Pax8* are required to maintain the expression of *Lhx1*.[178] *Pax2, Pax8,* and *Lhx1* altogether likely coordinate the expression of *Gata3,* which is necessary for elongation of the nephric duct.[179] *Gata3* and *Emx2,* which are required for the expression of *Ret* in the nephric duct, are both regulated by β-catenin (*Ctnnb1*), an effector of the canonical Wnt signaling pathway.[40,180,181] Acting likely in parallel with *Gata3* to maintain *Ret* expression in the UB is *Aldh1a2* (*Raldh2*), a gene in the retinoic acid synthesis pathway.[182] Surprisingly, this genetic regulatory hierarchy cannot fully account for the distinctive phenotypes arising from the mutation of each individual gene, suggesting that additional important components of the nephric duct genetic network have yet to be identified. Nephric duct specification fails in *Pax2/Pax8* mutants but not in the case of *Lhx1* deficiency, where only the caudal portion of the nephric duct degenerates.[178] The absence of *Gata3* or *Aldh1a2* causes misguided elongation of the nephric duct, terminating into either blind-ended ureters or abnormal connections between the bladder and urethra.[179] The curtailed caudal growth of the nephric duct when either *Lhx1* or *Gata3* is lost prevents the formation of the first UB and consequently causes renal agenesis.[179,183,184] The absence of *Aldh1a2* leads to the formation of ectopic ureters and hydronephrotic kidneys.[182] *Emx2* deficiency does not prevent caudal extension of the nephric duct toward the presumptive MM but the evagination of the UB is aborted, thereby resulting in renal agenesis.[40] Without β-catenin, nephric duct cells undergo precocious differentiation into collecting duct epithelia.[185] *Ret* does not affect the nephric duct fate but has importance in later UB development and insertion of the nephric duct to the cloaca.[162,182,186] Identification of additional targets of *Pax2, Pax8, Lhx1, Gata3,* and β-catenin are necessary in order to fully understand these seemingly disparate mutant phenotypes.

UB induction and subsequent branching requires a unique spatial organization of Ret signaling. The bulbous UB tip is a region enriched with proliferative ureteric epithelial cells, in contrast to the emerging stalk regions of the developing ureteric tree.[41,187] It is now well appreciated that receptor tyrosine kinase signaling primarily through Ret is key to the proliferation of UB tip epithelia. Exogenous GDNF supplemented in explanted embryonic kidneys can cause expansion of the UB tip region toward the source of the ligand.[187–189] ERK kinase activation is prominent within the ampullary UB terminals where Ret expression is elevated.[41] Consistently, chimera analysis in mice reveals that Ret-deficient cells do not contribute to the formation of the UB tips.[162] Altogether, these studies underscore the importance of strategic levels of Ret expression and activation of proliferative signaling pathways in the stereotypical sculpting of the nascent collecting duct network.

A ligand-receptor complex formed by GDNF, GFRα1, and Ret is necessary for autophosphorylation of Ret on its intracellular tyrosines (see Fig. 1.12). A number of downstream adaptor molecules and effectors have been identified to interact with active phosphorylated Ret, including Grb2, Grb7, Grb10, ShcA, Frs2, PLCγ1, Shp2, Src, and Dok adaptor family members (Dok4/5/6).[190–201] These downstream Ret effectors altogether are likely contributors to the activation of the Ras/SOS/ERK and PI3K/Akt pathways supporting the proliferation, survival, and migratory behavior of the UB epithelium.[41,43,202] Knock-in mutations of the interaction site for Shc/Frs2/Dok adaptors on the short isoform of Ret lead to the formation of rudimentary kidneys.[203–206] Specific mutation of the PLCγ1 docking site on Ret leads to renal dysplasia and ureter duplications.[203] The loss of *Shp2* and the upstream ERK regulators *Map2k1 (Mek2)* and *Map2k2 (Mek1)* in the UB lineage also cause severe renal hypoplasia phenocopying that is observed in occasional Ret-deficient kidneys.[207,208] UB-specific inactivation of *Pten,* a target of the PI3K/Akt pathway, disrupts UB branching.[209] Taken together, these findings underscore the significance of Ret signaling in normal UB branching.

A number of transcriptional targets of Ret activation in microdissected UB stimulated with GDNF have been elucidated (Fig. 1.15).[210] Among these are *Ret* itself and *Wnt11,* which stimulates *Gdnf* expression in the MM,[211] suggesting that a positive feedback loop exists for the GDNF-Ret signaling pathway. Ret activation also positively regulates the ETS transcription factors *Etv4* and *Etv5,* which are also necessary for normal UB branching morphogenesis. *Etv4*-null homozygous mutants and compound heterozygous mutants for *Etv4* and *Etv5* manifest severe renal hypoplasia or renal agenesis, suggesting that these transcription factors are indispensable targets of Ret for proper UB development.[210] In chimeric animals, *Etv4/Etv5*-deficient cells, like *Ret*-deficient cells, fail to integrate within the UB tip domain.[162,212]

The gene *Sprouty* was identified as a general antagonist of receptor tyrosine kinases and was discovered for inhibiting the FGF and EGF signaling pathways that pattern the *Drosophila* airways, wings, and ovarian follicles.[213–215] Of the four mammalian *Sprouty* homologues, *Spry1, Spry2,* and *Spry4* are expressed in developing kidneys.[216] *Spry1* is expressed strongly at the UB tips, whereas *Spry2* and *Spry4* are found in both the UB and the MM.[217] *Sprouty* molecules are thought to uncouple receptor tyrosine kinases with the activation of ERK pathways either through competitive binding with the Grb2/SOS complex or the kinase Raf, effectively repressing ERK activation. Interestingly, *Spry1* expression is distinctively upregulated upon GDNF activation of Ret.[210] This suggests that Ret activates a negative feedback mechanism via *Spry1* in order to control activated ERK levels and modulate cell proliferation in the UB. Studies on *Spry1* knockout mice reveal some intriguing facets about Ret dependence of UB induction and branching.[87,218–222] *Spry1* deficiency leads to ectopic UB induction and it can rescue renal development in the absence of either GDNF or Ret.[222,223] Germline inactivation of *Spry2* does not overtly affect renal development but can rescue renal hypoplasia in mice engineered to express Ret mutants impaired in activating the Ras/ERK pathway.[217] The transcriptional targets of Ret, such as *Etv4, Etv5,* and *Wnt11,* are retained in *Gdnf/Spry1* or *Ret/Spry1* compound null mutants.[222,223] These findings indicate that Ret signaling is not absolutely required for UB development. In fact,

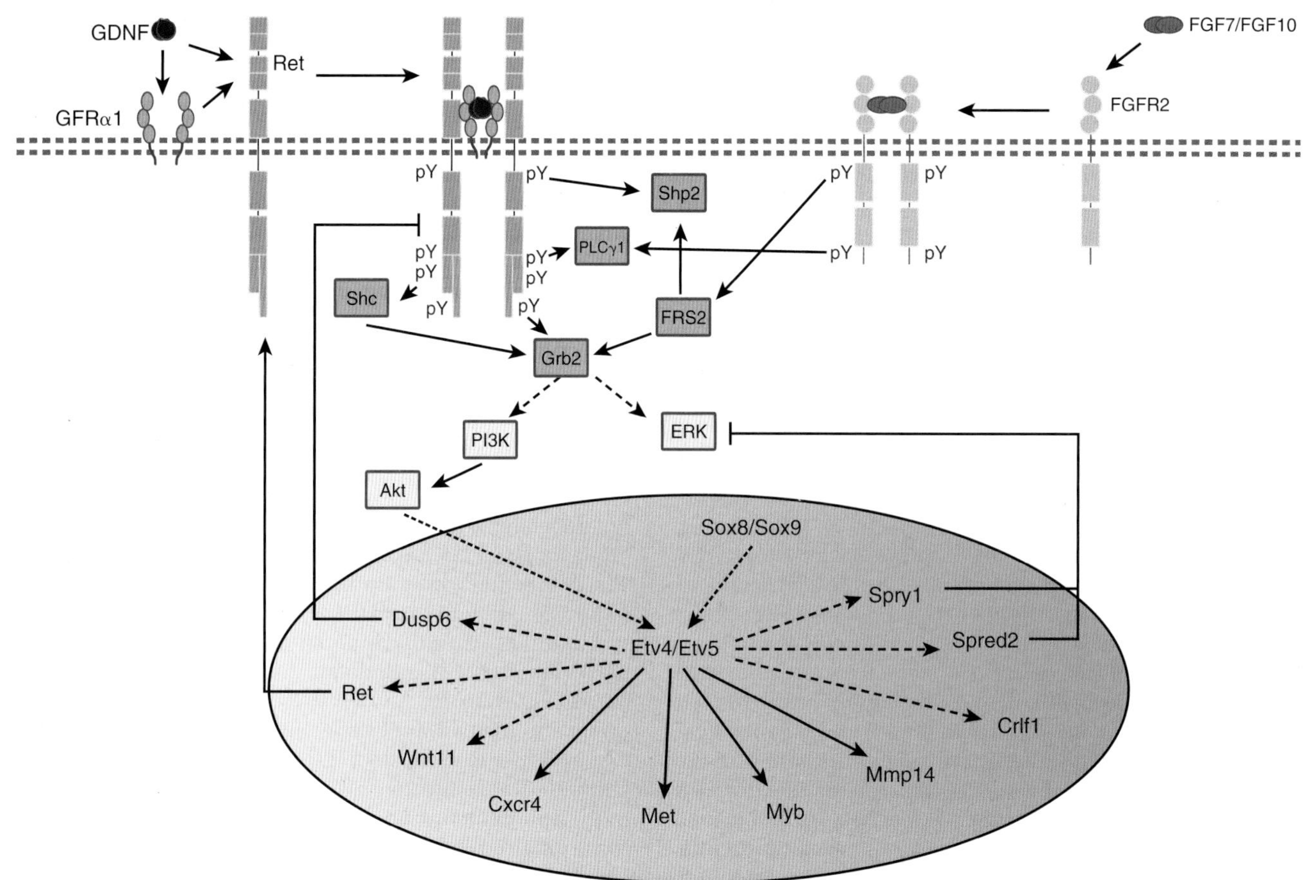


**Fig. 1.15 Ret signaling pathway.** Ret is activated and becomes autophosphorylated on intracellular tyrosine residues upon association with glial cell–derived neurotrophic factor *(GDNF)* and GFRα1. Signaling molecules such as Grb2, Shc, FRS2, PLCγ1, and Shp2 bind directly to the phosphorylated tyrosine residues within the intracellular domain of Ret. Recruitment of Shc, FRS2, and Grb2 leads to activation of ERK and PI3K/Akt pathways. GDNF-Ret signaling leads to the specific activation of a host of genes, some of which are strongly dependent on the upregulation of the transcription factors Etv4 and Etv5 (*solid arrows*). Etv4/Etv5 activation requires activation of the PI3K/Akt but not the ERK pathway. Sox8 and Sox9 are believed to act in parallel to reinforce transcriptional responses to GDNF-Ret engagement. Some of these pathways are shared with the FGF7/10-FGFR2 receptor signaling system. Spry1 and Spred2 negatively regulate ERK signaling, whereas Dusp6 likely mitigates the dephosphorylation of the Ret receptor, thus acting as part of a negative feedback regulatory loop.

signaling via FGF10 and FGFR2 receptors is sufficient for renal development despite the absence of GDNF or Ret, provided *Spry1* is inactivated. Nevertheless, patterns of renal branching are distinctively altered in *Gdnf/Spry1* and *Gdnf//Ret* compound mutants with UB tips often displaying more heterogeneous shapes and orientation. These indicate that there remain some distinctive roles of GDNF-Ret signaling that cannot be fully compensated by FGF10/FGFR2 during UB development.

## ADHESION PROTEINS IN EARLY KIDNEY DEVELOPMENT

A current theme in cell biology is that growth factor signaling often occurs coordinately with signals from the extracellular matrix transduced by adhesion receptors such as members of the integrin family. The α8β1 integrin complex is expressed by cells of the MM interacting with the novel ligand nephronectin (*Npnt*) expressed specifically by UB cells.[169,224] In most *Itga8* (α8 integrin) mutant embryos, UB outgrowth is arrested upon contact with the MM.[169] In a small portion of embryos, this block is overcome, and a single, usually hypoplastic, kidney develops. Knockout mice for *Npnt* exhibit renal agenesis or severe hypoplasia.[168] Thus the interaction of α8β1 integrin with nephronectin must have an important role in the continued growth of the UB toward the MM. Both *Itga8* and *Npnt* knockout phenotypes appear to result from a reduction in *Gdnf* expression.[168] The attraction of the UB to the mesenchyme is also governed by the maintenance of proper cell–cell adhesion within mesenchymal cells. Kif26b, a kinesin specifically expressed in the MM, is important for tight condensation of mesenchymal cells.[167] Genetic inactivation of *Kif26b*-results in renal agenesis resulting from impaired UB induction. In *Kif26b*-mutant mice, the compact aggregation of mesenchymal cells is compromised, resulting in distinctive loss of polarized expression of integrin α8 and severe downregulation of *Gdnf* expression. Hence, dysregulation of mesenchymal cell adhesion causes the failure to attract and induce the ureteric epithelia. Genetic evidence further shows that nephronectin localization at the basement membrane of the UB is critical for *Gdnf* expression by the MM. Genetic inactivation of basement membrane proteins associated with Fraser syndrome (*Fras1*, *Frem1/Qbrick*, and *Frem2*) lead to renal agenesis characterized by severe downregulation of *Gdnf* expression.[165,166,225–228] On the basis of interaction of nephronectin with *Fras1*, *Frem1*, and *Frem2*, it has been proposed that the Fras1/Frem1/Frem2 ternary complex anchor nephronectin to the UB basement membrane, thus stabilizing engagement with α8β1 integrin expressed by the MM (Fig. 1.16).[225] Grip1, a PDZ-domain protein known to interact with Fras1, is required to localize the Fras1/Frem1/Frem2 complex on the basal aspect of the UB epithelium.[229] *Grip1* mutations phenocopy Fraser syndrome, including renal agenesis, thus further highlighting the importance of the strategic localization of nephronectin on the UB surface towards the opposing MM.[229–231]

The establishment of epithelial basement membranes during metanephric kidney development involves the stage-specific assembly of different laminin α and β subunits with a common laminin γ1 subunit. The UB-specific inactivation of the gene *Lamc1*, which encodes for laminin γ1, leads to impaired UB induction and branching, ultimately causing either renal agenesis or hypomorphic kidneys with water transport deficits.[232] *Lamc1* deficiency prevents the formation of basement membranes, causing downregulation of both growth factor (GDNF, Wnt11, and FGF2) and integrin-based signaling. This highlights another example of how signaling through the extracellular matrix intersects with growth factor signaling to influence morphogenesis. The importance of basement membrane assembly in the development of other renal structures is emphasized by genetic studies on the genes *Lama5* and *Lamb2*, which encode for laminins α5 and β2, respectively. Loss of *Lama5* causes either renal agenesis or

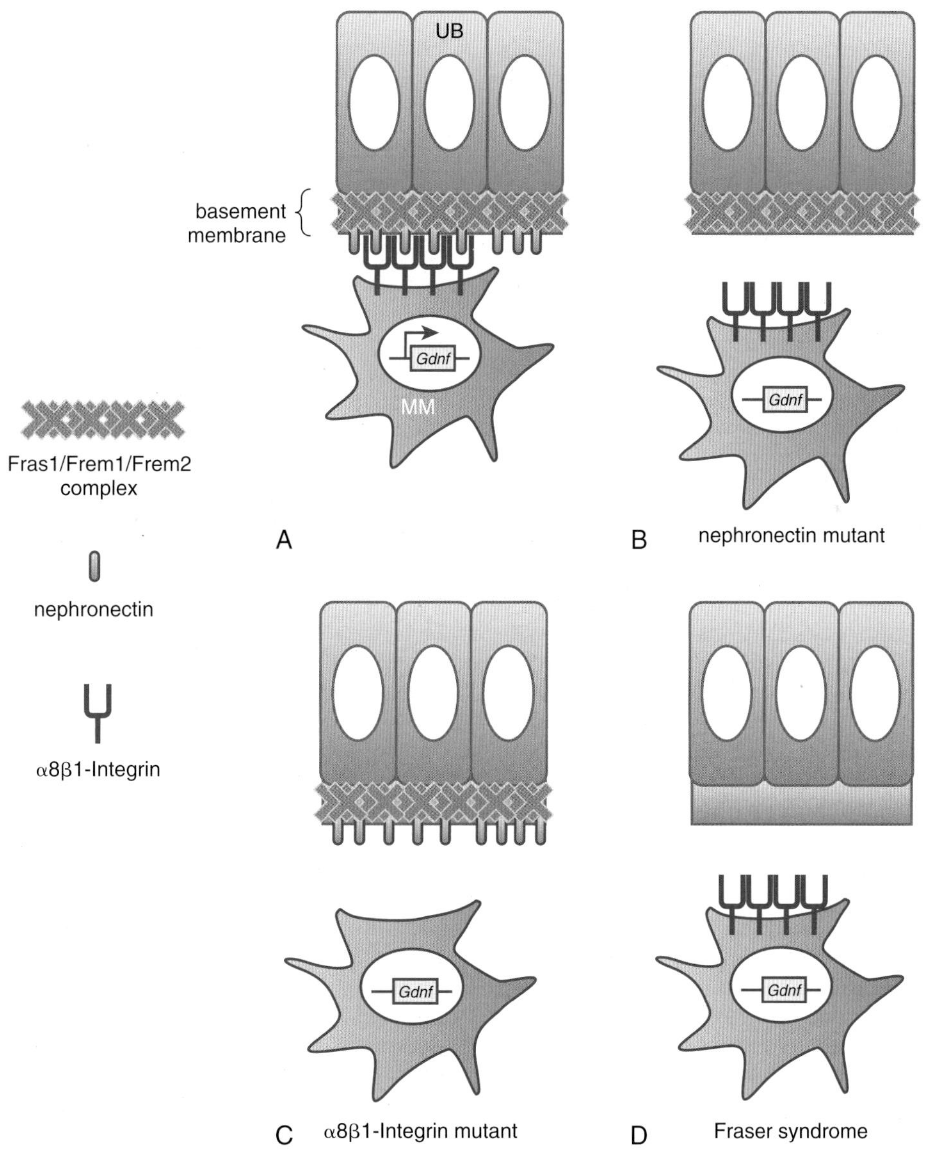


**Fig. 1.16 Molecular model of renal defect in Fraser syndrome.** (A) Adhesion to the ureteric bud (UB) epithelium positively regulates the expression of glial cell–derived neurotrophic factor *(GDNF)* by the metanephric mesenchyme *(MM)*. Adhesion and GDNF expression are impaired in the absence of (B) nephronectin (expressed by the UB), (C) α8β1 integrin (expressed by the MM), (D) or the Fras1/Frem1/Frem2 complex. Fras1, Frem1, and Frem2 are implicated in Fraser syndrome, and are believed to coordinately anchor nephronectin to the UB basement membrane and stabilize the conjugation with α8β1 integrin. Modified from Kiyosumi, Takeichi M, Nakano I, et al.: Basement membrane assembly of the integrin α8β1 ligand nephronectin requires Fraser syndrome-associated proteins. *J Cell Biol.* 2012;197:677–689.

disruption of glomerulogenesis, whereas deficiency for *Lamb2* leads to a defective glomerular filtration barrier.[233,234]

The UB branching program is stereotypically organized such that the proliferative UB epithelial cells are largely confined to the bulbous UB tips, whereas cell division is dampened within the elongated nonbranching UB stalks of the growing ureteric tree. TROP2/Tacstd2, an adhesion molecule related to EpCAM, is expressed prominently in the UB stalks where it colocalizes with collagen-1.[235] TROP2, unlike EpCAM, which is expressed throughout the UB tree, is not expressed at the UB ampullary tips. Consistently, dissociated and sorted UB cells expressing high levels of TROP2 are nonproliferative and express low levels of *Ret*, *Gfra1*, and *Wnt11*, which are notable UB tip markers. Elevated expression of TROP2 is also associated with poor attachment of epithelial cells to collagen matrix and suppression of cell spreading and motility, thus emphasizing the importance of this adhesion molecule in negative regulation of UB branching and the sculpting of the nascent collecting duct network. The formation of patent lumens within epithelial tubules of the kidney is also dependent on coordinated cell adhesion. β1 Integrin is tethered to the actin cytoskeleton via a ternary complex formed between integrin-like kinase (ILK) and parvin. ILK has been shown to be important in mediating cell cycle arrest and cell contact inhibition in the collecting duct epithelia.[236] The targeted ablation of the *Ilk* gene in the UB did not cause remarkable defects in UB branching but eventually caused postnatal lethality due to obstruction of collecting ducts arising from dysregulated intraluminal cell proliferation. Thus cell adhesion molecules may suppress cell division to regulate distinctive aspects of renal branching and tubulogenesis.

## POSITIONING OF THE URETERIC BUD

A crucial aspect of kidney development that is of great relevance to renal and urological congenital defects in humans relates to the positioning of the UB (see Fig. 1.14). Incorrect positioning of the bud, or duplication of the bud, results in abnormally shaped kidneys and incorrect insertion of the ureter into the bladder, with a resultant ureteral reflux that can predispose to infection and scarring of the kidneys and urological tract.

*Foxc1* is a transcription factor of the Forkhead family, expressed in the intermediate mesoderm and the MM adjacent to the wolffian duct. In the absence of *Foxc1*, the expression of GDNF adjacent to the wolffian duct is less restricted than in wild type embryos. *Foxc1* deficiency results in ectopic UBs, hypoplastic kidneys, and duplicated ureters.[237] Additional molecules that regulate the location of UB outgrowth are Slit2 and Robo2, signaling molecules best known for their role in axon guidance in the developing nervous system. Slit2 is a secreted factor, and Robo2 is its cognate receptor. Slit2 is mainly expressed in the Wolffian duct, whereas Robo2 is expressed in the mesenchyme.[238] UBs form ectopically in embryos deficient in either *Slit2* or *Robo2*, similar to the *Foxc1* mutant. However, in contrast to the *Foxc1* phenotype, none of the ureters in *Slit2/Robo2* mutants failed to undergo the normal remodeling that results in insertion in the bladder.[238] Instead, the ureters remained connected to the nephric duct in *Slit2* or *Robo2* mutants. The domain of *Gdnf* expression is expanded anteriorly in the absence of either *Slit2* or *Robo2*. Indeed, mutations in *Robo2* have been identified in patients with vesicoureteral junction defects and vesicoureteral reflux.[239] The expression of *Pax2*, *Eya1*, *Foxc1*, and *Six2*, all thought to regulate *Gdnf* expression, was not dramatically different in the absence of *Slit2* or *Robo2*, suggesting that Slit2-Robo2 signaling was not upstream of these genes. Instead, recent findings strongly suggest that Slit2-Robo2 signaling, as in other systems, acts as a repulsive guidance cue.[240] Consistent with this are findings that *Slit2* is most strongly expressed at an increasing gradient, at regions more anterior from the normal site of UB induction. Thus the absence of *Robo2* most likely compromises normal separation of the wolffian duct from the nephrogenic mesenchyme, ultimately broadening the nephrogenic zone and provoking ectopic UB induction.

*Spry1*, as described earlier in this chapter, negatively regulates the Ras/Erk signaling pathway and is expressed strongly in the posterior wolffian duct and the UB tips.[241] Embryos lacking *Spry1* develop supernumerary UBs, but unlike mutants of *Foxc1*, *Slit2*, or *Robo2* they do not display changes in *Gdnf* expression.[218] The phenotype of *Spry1* mutants can be rescued by reducing the *Gdnf* expression dosage.[218] *Spry1* deletion also rescues the renal agenesis defect in mice lacking either *Ret* or *Gdnf*.[222] Consistently, renal agenesis and severe renal hypoplasia in mice expressing Ret specifically mutated on a tyrosine phosphorylation site known to couple with the Ras/ERK pathway can be reversed in the absence of *Spry1*.[223] Thus *Spry1* appears to regulate UB induction sites by dampening receptor tyrosine kinase–dependent proliferative signaling.

Another negative regulator of branching is BMP4, which is expressed in the mesenchyme surrounding the wolffian duct. *Bmp4* heterozygous mutants have duplicated ureters, and, in organ culture, BMP4 blocks the induction of ectopic UBs by GDNF-soaked beads.[242] Furthermore, knockout of *Grem1*, which encodes for the secreted BMP inhibitor Gremlin, causes renal agenesis, supporting a role for BMP in the suppression of UB formation.[243]

## FORMATION OF THE COLLECTING DUCT SYSTEM

The overall shape, structure, and size of the kidneys are largely guided by the stereotypical branching of the UB and the subsequent patterning of the collecting duct system. During late gestation, past embryonic stage E15.5 in the mouse, the trunks of the UB tree undergo extensive elongation to establish the array of collecting ducts found in the renal medulla and papilla. The radial arrangement of elongated collecting ducts together with the loops of Henle (derived from the nephrogenic mesenchyme) establishes the corticomedullary axis by which nephron distributions are patterned. After birth, further elongation of the newly formed collecting duct network is partly responsible for the postnatal growth of the kidney.

Elongation of the collecting duct involves oriented cell division characterized by the parallel alignment of the mitotic spindle of proliferating ductal epithelia with the longitudinal axis of the duct.[244] Oriented cytokinesis, therefore, guarantees that the daughter cells contribute to lengthening of the duct with minimal effect on tubular lumen diameter. The renal medulla and pelvis are nonexistent in mice lacking *Wnt7b*.[245] Notably, the collecting ducts and loops of Henle are stubbier due to reorientation of cell division toward a radial instead of a longitudinal axis. *Wnt7b* expression is restricted within the nonbranching stalk of the ureteric tree and is absent in the ampullary UB tips. Failed development of the renal medullary and papillary regions is also recapitulated in mice where *Cttnb1* is ablated in the renal stroma, suggesting that Wnt7b activates the canonical β-catenin–dependent Wnt signaling pathway involving the ureteric epithelia and the surrounding stroma.[245–247] However, the relevant reverse signal from the interstitial stroma to the collecting duct that drives oriented cell division in the duct epithelia remains unknown.

The normal development of the collecting ducts is also dependent on cell survival cues provided by diverse ligands, such as Wnt7b, EGF, HGF, and interactions with the extracellular matrix.[245,248,249] Papillary collecting ducts display higher incidences of apoptosis in mice lacking Wnt7b or EGFR.[245,248] Conversely, loss of Dkk1 (Dickkopf1), a secreted antagonist of Wnt7b, results in overgrowth of the renal papilla.[250] Conditional inactivation of *Dkk1* using the *Pax8-Cre* transgene (expressed in renal tubules and the collecting ducts) causes increased proliferation of papillary epithelial cells. The HGF-receptor Met, α3β1 integrin (*Itga3/Itgb1*), and laminin α5 (*Lama5*) are all required to maintain the expression of Wnt7b, and thus likely support the viability of collecting duct cells.[177,249,251]

Poor development of the renal medulla and papilla are also observed in mutant mice lacking *Fgf7, Fgf10, Fgfr2, Bmpr1a* (*Alk3*), the components of the renin-angiotensin system, *Shh* (Sonic hedgehog), or the orphan nuclear steroid hormone receptor gene *Esrrg*. FGF7 and FG10 are the cognate ligands of FGFR2. Renal hypoplasia is observed when *Fgfr2* is conditionally removed from the ureteric lineage and is more severe than in mutants lacking *Fgf7* or *Fgf10,* suggesting that these related ligands may have some functional redundancy in the development of the UB and collecting ducts.[60,252,253] Kidneys lacking *Bmp1ra* show an attenuated phosphorylation of SMAD1, an effector of the BMP and TGFβ ligands, and a concomitant increase in Myc and β-catenin levels.[254] Although the significance of these results is not clear, the elevated expression of β-catenin indicates a novel crosstalk between BMP and Wnt signaling pathways in collecting ducts. Signaling through angiotensin is relevant to both early UB branching and the morphogenesis of medullary collecting ducts.[255] Genetic inactivation of angiotensinogen, its processing enzyme ACE, and its target angiotensin-II AT1R receptors (Agtr1a and Agtr1b) results in similar phenotypes characterized by hypoplastic kidneys with modestly sized renal papillae.[256–261] Furthermore, the postnatal growth and survival of renal papilla grown ex vivo are dependent on the presence of AT1R.[262] Interestingly, in cultures of renal papilla explants, angiotensin appears to regulate the Wnt7b, FGF7, and α3β1 integrin signaling pathways such that the loss of endogenous angiotensin or pharmacologic inhibition of AT1R causes significant dampening of the expression of *Wnt7b, Fgf7, Cttnb1, Itga3,* and *Itgb1.*[262] *Shh* is expressed in the more distal derivatives of the UB, the medullary collecting ducts, and the ureter.[59] The germline deletion of *Shh* results in either bilateral renal agenesis or a single ectopic dysplastic kidney.[263,264] It has been shown that *Shh* controls the expression of early inductive and patterning genes (*Pax2* and *Sall1*), cell cycle regulators (*Mycn* and *Ccnd1*), and signaling effectors of the Hedgehog pathway (*Gli1* and *Gli2*). Interestingly, genetic removal of *Gli3* in an *Shh*-null background restores the expression of *Pax2, Sall1, Cdnd1, Mycn, Gli1,* and *Gli2,* providing physiologic proof for the role of *Gli3* as a repressor of the Shh pathway in renal development.[264] Frameshift mutations resulting in truncation of the expressed Gli3 protein are linked to Pallister-Hall syndrome and the presence of hydronephrosis and hydroureter in both humans and mice.[265,266] *Esrrg* has a strong and localized expression within collecting duct epithelia later in gestation and its inactivation in mice causes complete aplasia of the renal medulla and papillae. However, the ligand of *Esrrg* remains to be identified and little is known regarding its downstream targets.

The mature collecting duct epithelia consist of two major cell subtypes: the abundant principal cells which strongly express the aquaporins, ion channels, and pumps mediating $Na^+$ and $K^+$ transport; and the fewer intercalated cells which are responsible for secretion of protons and bicarbonate ions (see Fig. 1.14). A third collecting duct cell subtype, now called the transition cell, has been recently identified and coexpresses principal and intercalated cell-specific genes.[267] Fate mapping analyses in an *Aqp2-Cre* and *Atp6v1b1-Cre* fluorescent reporter mouse line estimate that principal cells constitute ~60% of collecting duct epithelia, while intercalated cells and transition cells constitute ~30% and ~10%, respectively. Genetic studies suggest a cell type plasticity among collect duct epithelia with gene mutations identified as leading to disproportionate increase in one cell at the expense of the other with detrimental consequences in the maintenance of fluid, electrolyte, and acid balance.[267–272] Lineage tracing analyses indicate that both principal and intercalated cells can dynamically switch fates, transforming into an intermediate cell type, the transition cell.[267] Gene expression analyses implicate the Notch signaling pathway as an important regulator of collecting duct cell composition and patterning. Intercalated cells strongly express the Notch ligand Jag1, whereas principal cells express the Notch2 receptor.[267,273] Genetic induction of Notch signaling within collecting ducts in adult mice notably increased the amount of *Aqp2*$^+$ principal cells while the number of *Atp6v1b1*$^+$ intercalated cells decreased in parallel, without altering the number of transition cells.[267] Similarly, loss of the transcription factors Tfcp2l1, Foxi1, or the p53-related Trp63 results in the paucity of intercalated cells.[268,269] Tfcp2l1 induces the expression of intercalated cell-specific genes including *Jag1* and *Atp6v1b1.*[273] It has been proposed that Notch activation in the UB suppresses *Foxi1,* while the identification of putative Trp63 binding sites in the promoters of several Notch ligands suggests that Trp63 may repress Notch signaling.[270,271] Conversely, inhibition of Notch signaling in ureteric epithelia leads to a disproportionate predominance of intercalated cells at the expense of principal cells, and the onset of polyuria, urinary concentration defects, and hydronephrosis.[271,272,274] A specific target of Notch signaling in principal cells is the transcription factor Elf5, which positively regulates expression of principal cell-specific genes *Aqp2* and *Avpr2.*[274] One other identified epigenetic regulator of principal cell fate is the histone methyltransferase encoded by *Dot1l,* which normally represses the aquaporin gene *Aqp5* and the intercalated cell-specific gene *Atp6v1b1.*[275–277] *Dot1l* deficiency elevates the expression of both *Aqp5,* whose product interferes with cell surface localization of the principal cell-specific aquaporin Aqp2 while concomitantly promoting the acquisition of intercalated cell traits with the upregulation of *Atp6v1b1.*

## MOLECULAR GENETICS OF NEPHROGENESIS

### EPITHELIALIZATION OF THE METANEPHRIC MESENCHYME

The generation of a sufficient number of nephrons requires a highly regulated balance between the expansion of progenitor compartments and the commitment toward epithelial fate to become renal vesicles. This has important clinical implications as the impaired renewal of nephron precursors or their perturbed differentiation can ultimately cause a wide range of renal pathologies due to significant paucity of functional nephrons. Signaling through Wnt, FGF, the BMP family of ligands, and Fat4 have been identified as important regulators of the delicate balance between progenitor self-renewal and differentiation.

All nephrogenic structures (podocytes, parietal epithelial cells, proximal tubules, loop of Henle, distal tubules, and the connecting tubule directly conjoined with the collecting duct) descend from a common progenitor pool that expresses the transcription factor *Six2*.[61] *Six2* expression is notably elevated in the cap mesenchyme that condenses adjacent to the UB and is downregulated once this cap mesenchyme organizes into pretubular aggregates. It is now recognized that *Six2* activity is required to keep these nephron progenitor cells in a naïve, proliferative precursor state.[61,278] Six2 has been demonstrated to function as both a transcriptional activator that promotes cell cycling and proliferation, and as part of a repressor complex silencing differentiation-related genes.[279,280] Six2 can synergize with Sall1, to promote transcription of genes relevant to progenitor status (e.g., *Wt1, Eya1,* and *Gdnf*). Six2 and Sall1 also co-occupy promoters of their own genes, thus acting as positive feedback regulators of progenitor fate. Six2 also interacts with Osr1, Tcf (Lef), and Aes (Groucho/TLE) to form a repressor complex that antagonizes expression of genes related to epithelialization (e.g., *Fgf8* and *Wnt4*).[281,282] Complete loss of *Six2* causes premature ectopic formation of renal vesicles at E12.5 and the untimely depletion of nephron precursors.[61,278] In contrast, overexpression of *Six2* prevented epithelialization of the cap mesenchyme.[278]

*Six2*$^+$ nephron progenitors respond to stimulation with the UB-secreted factor Wnt9b and transition into epithelial renal vesicles.[283] During the transition from cap mesenchyme to renal vesicles, expressions of a second Wnt family member Wnt4 and an FGF family member Fgf8 are activated. Canonical Wnt signaling involving β-catenin–dependent gene transcription is necessary and sufficient for the early inductive actions of Wnt9b and Wnt4, although it is also known that Wnt4 can activate a noncanonical alternative pathway during the final phase of nephrogenic epithelialization.[284–289] The interaction between Six2- and Wnt-signaling pathways appears to be intricately dosage- and context-dependent.[280,282,283] When *Six2* expression remains high, Wnt signaling promotes progenitor renewal.[290] In this situation, the stabilization of β-catenin promotes the association of *Six2* downstream target Myc with β-catenin, favoring precursor proliferation.[283,291] However, with a sustained canonical Wnt-signaling pathway, β-catenin accumulates and displaces Aes converting the Tcf complex into a differentiation driver.[280] The stabilization of β-catenin eventually interferes with *Six2* expression, thus attenuating *Six2* expression. Notch signaling is required to prime nephron progenitors for differentiation and contributes to the silencing of *Six2* expression.[292] All nephron segments fail to form when Notch signaling is lost within the *Six2*$^+$ precursor lineage.[293]

The growth factor BMP7 is also required for the formation of the nephrogenic compartment.[294–296] Activation of the Jnk pathway mediates the proliferative effect of BMP7 in uncommitted nephron precursors.[297,298] BMP7, through activation of the p38-MAPK, causes upregulation of the transcriptional repressor *Trps1*.[299] Loss of *Trps1* severely impairs the formation of renal vesicles. It has been speculated that *Trps1* may indirectly relieve repression of *Cdh1* expression. Additionally, BMP7-dependent phosphorylation and nuclear translocation of SMAD1/5/8 is required for Wnt9b-induced epithelialization.[300] Thus BMP7 has dual essential roles in promoting both progenitor replenishment and priming for epithelialization. How these pathways integrate with *Six2*-dependent signaling complexes remains poorly understood. BMP signaling could either positively or negatively modulate β-catenin signaling. In other systems, SMAD proteins can associate and synergize with β-catenin and Tcf.[301] BMP signaling can also activate the PTEN pathway, which indirectly suppresses β-catenin activity.[302,303]

The FGFs FGF2, FGF8, FGF9, and FGF20, and their cognate receptors FGFR1 and FGFR2, are essential to form nephrons. Compound loss of FGFR1 and FGFR2 in the MM leads to renal agenesis.[304] FGF9 and FGF20 are required to maintain the multipotency and proliferative state of nephron precursors.[305] FGF2 is required for the condensation of the cap mesenchyme.[306] FGF8 is not needed for the formation of renal vesicles but is required for the survival of the newly formed nephrogenic epithelia. Renal vesicles lacking *Fgf8* fail to express *Wnt4* and *Lhx1*, and do not progress into S-shaped intermediate nephrons.[286,287] Potential downstream targets of FGFR1/FGFR2 relevant to nephrogenesis are the closely related MAGUK family proteins encoded by the genes *Cask* and *Dlg1*.[307] The absence of *Cask* and *Dlg1* causes impaired proliferation and cell death in nephron precursors, with a distinctive dampening of the Ras/ERK signaling pathway.[308] *Fgf8* expression is severely attenuated when both *Cask* and *Dlg1* are absent. Moreover, *Cask/Dlg1* deficiency causes the formation of a loose cluster of cap mesenchyme around the UB. As *Dlg1* has been implicated in the directed migration of Schwann cells,[309,310] it is tempting to speculate that *Cask* and *Dlg1* may play a supportive role in the UB-directed condensation of the cap mesenchyme.

### NEPHRON SEGMENTATION AND TUBULOGENESIS

The mature nephron is a highly compartmentalized structure with individual segments having distinguishable molecular, cellular, and anatomic attributes. Nephron segments are organized along a proximal-distal axis, from the most proximal renal corpuscle or glomerulus, followed by the proximal tubule, the loop of Henle, the distal tubule, and the most distal connecting tubule that links directly to the UB-derived collecting duct. The segmental patterning of nephrons involves a complex series of events instructed by inductive cues between neighboring cells and controlled by epigenetic signaling mechanisms. A variety of human diseases result from the mispatterning of nephrons.[311]

Elegant imaging studies combined with high-throughput single-cell gene expression analysis demonstrate that nephron patterning is determined as early as the recruitment of mesenchymal nephron progenitors from the cap mesenchyme.[312] Recent evidence indicates that renal vesicle arises not from a single event in time. Instead, nephron progenitors progressively incorporate into the nascent nephrons, with the timing of their recruitment predicting their acquisition of proximal–distal fates (i.e., initial recruits commit to distal fates while the last recruits contribute to the formation of more proximal fates) (Fig. 1.17).

By the renal vesicle stage, gene expression asymmetry highlights an early establishment of proximal and distal domains. Genes such as *Fgf8, Lhx1, Dll1, Dkk1, Hnf1b, Sox9,* and *Pou3f3* are markedly elevated in the distal portion of the renal vesicles, whereas *Wt1, Foxc2,* and *Mafb* are largely restricted in the proximal end.[57,313] Some genes are expressed in both regions, such as *Wnt4, Jag1, Cdh6,* and *Ccnd1,* albeit nonuniformly and more elevated in the distal domain.[313] By the S-shaped body stage, nephron segmentation has become more evident, with several more marker genes having distinctively regionalized expression patterns.

As the earliest nephron precursors that interact with the UB become destined to acquire distal fates, it can be speculated that localized Wnt9b signaling orients the proximal–distal axis. Interestingly, in chick mesonephros, overexpression of Wnt3 in the coelomic lining redirects the glomerular development farthest away from the coelomic lining while the distal nephron occasionally become fused with the coelomic lining.[314] During nephrogenesis, a gradient of β-catenin activity is established along the nephron's longitudinal axis with the highest β-catenin activity found in the distal end, progressively decreasing towards the proximal end.[45] Although β-catenin is absolutely required to initiate nephron induction, its activity must be attenuated in order to complete an epithelial differentiation program.[289] Indeed, a β-catenin gradient is already established within renal vesicles and a persistent constitutive activation of β-catenin prevents epithelialization.[45,289] In organ cultures, pharmacologic manipulation of β-catenin activity can alter proximal and distal fate acquisition. Attenuation of β-catenin activity accelerates glomerular development. Conversely, augmentation of β-catenin activity favors the expression of *Lgr5,* a marker of distal fate, while repressing proximal identity. Additionally, it has been identified that modulation of β-catenin activity involves an integration of Wnt, Notch, and BMP signaling pathways.

Although many genes are now known as marking nephron segments, only a few other genes and pathways have been characterized that strongly influence proximal versus distal fate determination. Loss of *Hnf1b* in the nephrogenic precursors causes marked loss of proximal and median domain markers at the S-shaped body stage, causing the formation of immature and cystic glomeruli connected to the collecting duct by a severely truncated renal tubule.[315–317] A mutation in *Sall1* that prevents Sall1-NuRD interaction downregulates the distal marker *Lgr5,* and specifically impairs the development of the loop of Henle and distal tubules.[318] Other genes

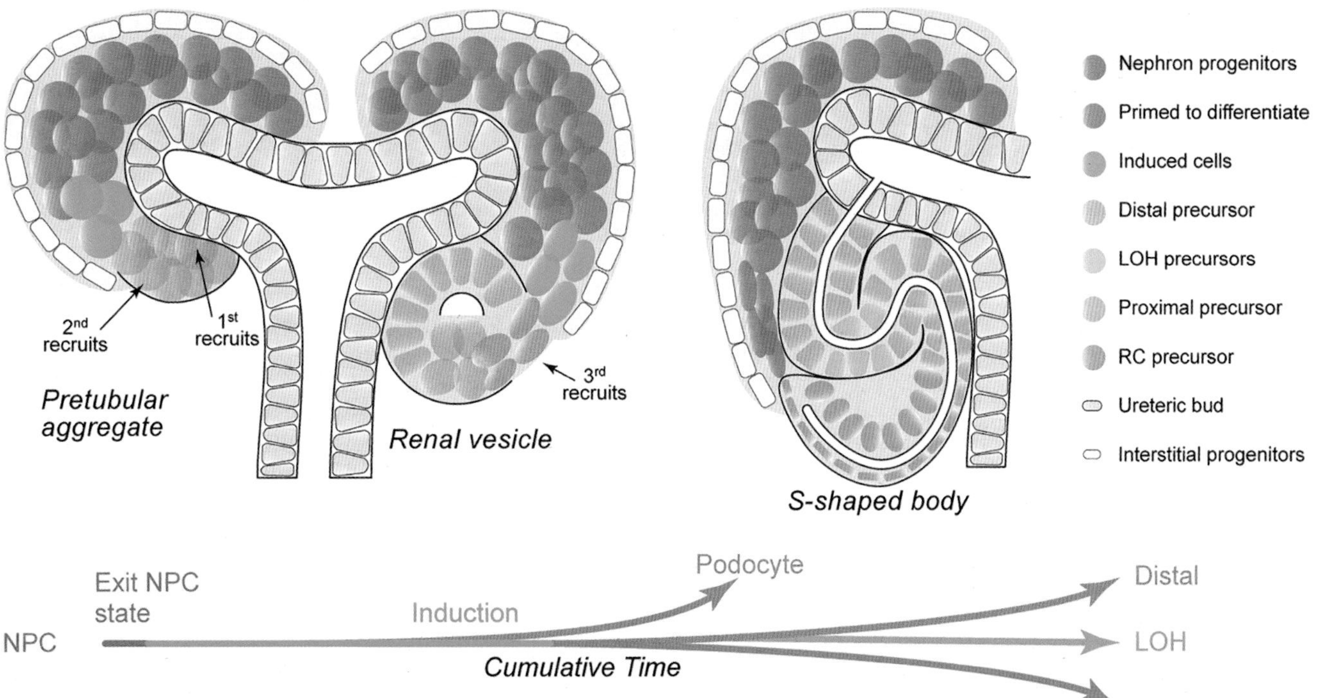


**Fig. 1.17** Gradual recruitment of progenitor cells during nephrogenesis. Early recruited nephron progenitors clustering around the ureteric bud give rise to pretubular aggregates. New progenitors continue to be recruited and incorporate to the proximal end of the renal vesicle. Distal, medial, and proximal domains are established by the S-shaped body stage. *NPC,* Nephron progenitor cell; *LOH,* loop of Henle; *RC,* renal corpuscle. Adapted from Lindström NO, De Sena Brandine G, Tran T, et al. Progressive recruitment of mesenchymal progenitors reveals a time-dependent process of cell fate acquisition in mouse and human nephrogenesis. *Dev Cell* 2018;45:651–660.

required to generate distal tubules and the loop of Henle are *Pou3f3* and *Adamts1*.[319–321]

In addition to cell differentiation, the spatial orientation of cells is essential for tubule elongation and morphogenesis. In epithelia, cells are uniformly organized along an apical–basal plane of polarity. However, in addition, cells in most tissues require positional information in the plane perpendicular to the apical–basal axis. This type of polarization is referred to as planar cell polarity and is critical for the morphogenesis of metazoans.[322,323] Using cell lineage analysis and close examination of the mitotic axis of dividing cells, it has been shown that the lengthening of renal tubules is associated with mitotic orientation of cells along the tubule axis, demonstrating intrinsic planar cell polarity.[244] Dysregulation of oriented cell division can give rise to cysts due to abnormal widening of tubule diameters.[324] To date, molecules implicated in planar cell polarity and nephrogenic tubule elongation include *Wnt9b, Hnf1b, Pkhd1, Fat4, Celsr1, and Vangl2.*[244,246,325–332]

## CESSATION OF NEPHROGENESIS

Nephrogenesis is a time-limited event that is not reactivated postinjury to the kidneys of humans and mice at adulthood. The last wave of nephrogenesis is observed around the 36th wave of gestation in humans and shortly after birth in mice.[333,334] Cessation of nephron generation is characterized by the exhaustion of nephron progenitor cells and the completion of epithelial differentiation of the remaining nephrogenic precursor. Although various morphologic and molecular changes occurring at this time have been characterized in mouse kidneys, the exact trigger is not fully understood.[333,335,336]

In mice, the nephrogenic zone progressively shrivels after birth and is replaced by mature tubules by P6. The precursor markers *Six2* and *Cited1* are significantly downregulated at P2 and are undetectable by P3, concomitant with the disappearance of the cap mesenchyme. Multiple newly induced nephrons are found associated with each UB tip at P3 that are no longer found at P7. Ureteric branching also ends between birth and P3 accompanied by a significant reduction of *Ret* and *Wnt11* and loss of the UB ampullary shape.[333,335] In contrast, *Wnt9b* expression in the UB remains high even at P4, consistent with findings that the UB tips isolated from P3 kidneys remain competent in promoting survival and inducing epithelialization of recombined mesenchyme taken from embryonic kidneys.[333] This strongly argues against the possibility that weakened trophic support from the UB contributes to the progressive decline of the nephrogenic precursor population and is supported by the rarity of apoptosis within the postnatal nephrogenic zone. *Foxd1* expression is also downregulated by P3, but given the expansion of the cap mesenchyme in *Foxd1*- or stroma-deficient kidneys, it is unlikely that postnatal loss of the *Foxd1*$^+$ stromal compartment provokes the abrupt halting of nephrogenesis.[333] There is also no evidence that nephrogenic progenitors have switched to stromal fates. Instead, what is now apparent is that the remaining cap mesenchyme becomes globally committed to epithelialize. Interestingly, when nephron progenitor proliferation is enhanced and kidney size is increased as seen in *Six2* haploinsufficient mice, the timing of nephrogenesis cessation is unaltered.[337]

Two opposing factors appear more likely to contribute to the termination of nephrogenesis: (1) a rapid decline in the proliferation rate of the *Six2*$^+$ cell compartment, which was observed between E15.5 and P0; and (2) an acceleration of nephrogenic differentiation postnatally.[333,335] One model proposed posits that the novel spatial relationship between cell types in the kidney around birth (as compared to early embryonic stages) dramatically alters the molecular context of the nephrogenic niche, thus shifting the balance between progenitor self-renewal and commitment to differentiation.[335,336,338] Another proposed model argues that increased oxygen tension after birth, which turns on the expression of glycolysis-related genes, could act as an active trigger that ends nephrogenesis.[336] However, this latter model, although applicable in mice, may not be a shared mechanism in humans where nephrogenesis ceases before parturition. A thorough understanding of the mechanism of nephrogenesis cessation is necessary to better assess the potential of regenerative therapies for the kidney.

## MOLECULAR GENETICS OF THE STROMAL CELL LINEAGE

The maintenance of reiterative ureteric branching and nephron induction largely accounts for the growth and enlargement of embryonic kidneys. Genetic studies reveal that interstitial stroma provide additional inductive cues that regulate UB branching and nephrogenesis (Fig. 1.18). These studies also underscore the pivotal role played by the stroma in establishing the stereotypical radial patterning of the kidney. In embryonic kidneys, the stroma is organized into two distinct zones: an outer stromal region within the nephrogenic zone expressing the winged helix transcription factor *Foxd1*, and a deeper region expressing the basic-helix–loop–helix (bHLH) transcription factor *Tcf21* (*Pod1*).[28,29,339,340] Without either *Foxd1* or *Tcf21*, UB branching and nephrogenesis are notably impaired, resulting in a distinctive perturbation of the corticomedullary renal histoarchitecture.[28,29,339]

The most prominent features of the genetic loss of *Foxd1* include the thickening of the renal capsule and the formation of large metanephric mesenchymal condensates.[28,341] The morphologically altered renal capsule in *Foxd1*-mutant kidneys has notably lost expression of *Aldh1a2 (Raldh2)* and *Sfrp1* (a regulator of Wnt signaling), and is abnormally interspersed with endothelial cells and *Bmp4*-positive cells.[341] The identity of these *Bmp4*-expressing cells populating the renal capsule in *Foxd1*-deficient kidneys is unknown, although they are clearly distinct from the presumptive medullary stroma based on lineage tracing for *Foxd1*-promoter expression. As BMP4 is a known chemotactic agent for endothelial cells,[342] it is very likely that the ectopic *Bmp4*-positive cells account for the presence of endothelial cells within the broadened renal capsule of *Foxd1*-mutant kidneys. The accumulation of the cap mesenchyme is also likely contributed in part by ectopic *Bmp4* signaling in the absence of *Foxd1* because *Bmp4* has been shown to antagonize epithelialization of the cap mesenchyme.[342] Transcriptome analysis reveals that the gene *Dcn*, which encodes for the collagen-binding proteoglycan decorin, is a specific target that is repressed by *Foxd1* in the cortical interstitium.[343] *Dcn* expression is normally localized within the medullary stroma but is normally absent in the cortical stroma of wild type kidneys. In the absence of *Foxd1*, *Dcn*

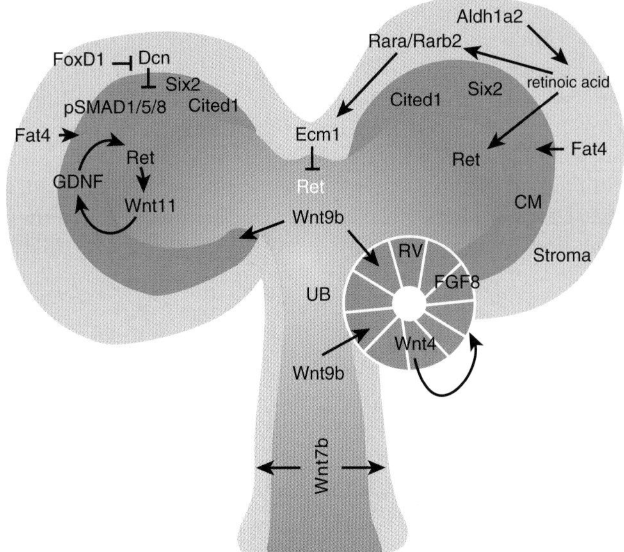


**Fig. 1.18** Tripartite inductive interactions regulating ureteric branching and nephrogenesis. Six2 and Cited1 are expressed in the self-renewing nephron progenitors within the cap mesenchyme *(CM)* surrounding the ureteric bud *(UB)*. The UB tip domains express high levels of Ret, which is activated by glial cell–derived neurotrophic factor *(GDNF)* from the surrounding CM. Wnt11 is upregulated in response to Ret activation and stimulates GDNF synthesis in the CM. Wnt9b expressed by the UB, and Fat4 by the Foxd1-positive stroma are required to initiate nephrogenesis from a subset of the CM. This results in the formation of a transient renal vesicle *(RV)* expressing FGF8 and Wnt4, factors that sustain epithelialization. The stroma expresses *Aldh1a2*, a gene required for retinoic acid synthesis, and genes for the retinoic acid receptors (*Rara* and *Rarb*). Retinoic acid signaling stimulates elevated expression of Ret in the UB tip domain while at the same time suppressing Ret expression via Rara/Rarb2 and Ecm1 in the stroma to initiate bifurcation of the UB tip to generate new branches. Foxd1 in the cortical stroma also represses Dcn, thus relieving the Dcn-mediated suppression of BMP7-dependent signaling, which results in phosphorylation of SMAD1/5/8 (pSMAD1/5/8) and epithelialization of the cap mesenchyme.

becomes abundantly expressed in the presumptive cortical stromal region. Functional cell-culture–based assays and epithelialization assays of mesenchymal aggregates reveals that Dcn inhibits Bmp7 signaling and mesenchyme-to-epithelial transformation. The antagonistic effect of *Dcn* on epithelial differentiation is further enhanced in vitro when the mesenchymal aggregates are grown in collagen IV, thus recapitulating the persistence of the cap mesenchyme as seen in *Foxd1*-mutant kidneys where both *Dcn* and collagen IV are upregulated in the cortical interstitium. These findings are corroborated by the partial rescue of the *Foxd1*-null phenotype through genetic inactivation of *Dcn*. Fate mapping studies also reveal that the *Foxd1*$^+$ stromal mesenchyme are the precursors of renal mural cells (renin cells, smooth muscle cells, pericytes, perivascular fibroblasts, and glomerular mesangial cells) and endothelial cells comprising peritubular capillaries.[32,33,344,345]

*Tcf21* is expressed in the medullary stroma as well as in the condensing MM.[339,340] *Tcf21* is also expressed in a number of differentiated renal cell types that derive from these mesenchymal cells and include developing and mature podocytes of the renal glomerulus, cortical and medullary peritubular interstitial cells, pericytes surrounding small renal vessels, and adventitial cells surrounding larger blood vessels (see Fig. 1.6).[246] The defect in nephrogenesis observed in *Tcf21*-null mice is similar to the defect seen in *Foxd1* knockout mice, with a disruption of branching morphogenesis with an associated arrest and delay in nephrogenesis.[339,341,346] Interestingly, as with *Foxd1*, *Tcf21* also represses *Dcn*, although the significance of *Dcn* upregulation in *Tcf21*-null mutant mice has not been formally addressed.[347] The analysis of chimeric mice that are derived from *Tcf21*-mutant embryonic stem cells and GFP-expressing embryos demonstrated both cell autonomous and noncell-autonomous roles for *Tcf21* in nephrogenesis.[346] Most strikingly, the glomerulogenesis defect is rescued by the presence of wild type stromal cells (i.e., mutant cells will epithelialize and form nephrons normally as long as they are surrounded by wild-type stromal cells). In addition, there is a cell-autonomous requirement for *Tcf21* in stromal mesenchymal cells to allow differentiation into interstitial and pericyte cell lineages of the cortex and medulla as *Tcf21*-null cells were unable to contribute to these populations.

Although many of the defects in the *Tcf21*-mutant kidneys phenocopy those seen in the *Foxd1*-mutant kidneys, there are important differences. Kidneys from *Tcf21*-null mice have vascular anomalies and defective pericyte differentiation that were not reported in *Foxd1*-mutant mice.[339,346] These differences might result from the broader domain of *Tcf21* expression, which also includes the condensing mesenchyme, podocytes, and medullary stromal cells, in addition to the stromal cells that surround the condensates. In contrast to *Foxd1*, *Tcf21* is not highly expressed in the thin rim of stromal cells found immediately beneath the capsule, suggesting that *Foxd1* and *Tcf21* might mark early and late stromal cell lineages, respectively, with overlap in the stroma that surrounds the condensates.[29] However, definitive co-labeling studies to address this issue have not been performed. As both *Tcf21* and *Foxd1* are transcription factors, it is interesting to speculate that they might interact or regulate the expression of a common stromal "inducing factor."

Retinoids secreted by the renal stroma are also recognized as important for the maintenance of a high level of *Ret* receptor expression in the UB tip, promoting the proliferation of UB epithelial cells and the growth of the ureteric tree.[17,348–350] The defective UB branching seen in *Foxd1*-null mutants is most likely a direct consequence of the loss of cortical expression of *Aldh1a2*, a gene involved in retinol synthesis.[341] More recently, it has been shown that renal stroma immediately around the UB tips is also important in regulating the bifurcation of the tips and the creation of new UB branches.[351] Autocrine retinoid signaling in the stromal cells juxtaposed to the UB tips stimulates the expression of extracellular matrix 1 (*Ecm1*). *Ecm1* is specifically expressed at the UB cleft, where it suppresses and restricts *Ret* expression domains within the UB tips. In the absence of *Ecm1*, *Ret* expression in the UB tips broadens, effectively attenuating UB branching due to impaired formation of UB bifurcation clefts. Thus stromal retinoids promote and confine *Ret* expression domains and more likely cell proliferation patterns within the UB tips.

Recent studies provide valuable insight on how stroma-based signaling intersects with UB-derived inductive cues to promote proper differentiation of the nephrogenic mesenchyme.[352–356] When the stromal lineage is selectively annihilated by

*Foxd1-Cre*–driven expression of diphtheria toxin, the zone of condensing mesenchymal cells capping the UBs is abnormally broadened while the development of pretubular aggregates is strongly hindered. This reiterates findings from the *Foxd1*-null mice suggesting that regulation of nephrogenesis involves a crosstalk between stroma and UB-derived inductive signals. In particular, it was shown that Fat4-dependent Hippo signaling initiated by the stroma integrates with canonical Wnt signaling derived from the ureteric lineage in order to balance the nephron precursor propagation and differentiation. The absence of Fat4 in the stromal compartment or its ligands Dchs1 and Dchs2 from the cap mesenchyme phenocopies the expansion of the nephrogenic precursor domain and failed epithelial differentiation of nephron progenitors seen in stroma-deficient kidneys.[353,356] It was postulated that Fat4, acting through the Hippo pathway, promotes the differentiation of the epithelial transition of nephrogenic precursors.[353–356] This was further reiterated by the rescue of the depletion of nephrogenic precursors by *Fat4* deficiency in *Wnt9b* knockouts.[352] Interestingly, the loss of Vangl2, a signaling partner of Fat4 known to regulate renal tubular diameter, fails to rescue the loss of nephron progenitors in *Wnt9b* knockouts, suggesting that Fat4-mediated signaling during early differentiation of nephrogenic precursors is likely independent of the planar cell polarity pathway.[330,352] Transcriptional regulation of stroma-dependent restriction of nephron progenitor expansion involves the transcription factors *Sall1, Foxd1,* and *Pbx1.*[28,341,357] More importantly, *Sall1* is likely a major upstream regulator of many of the stroma functions as Sall1 binds directly to several stroma-related gene loci, including *Fat4, Dcn, Pbx1, Tcf21, Meis1,* and *Hoxd10.*[358] Loss of *Sall1* in the stroma downregulates *Fat4* expression and results in an excess of *Six2*$^+$ nephron precursors.

The T-box transcription factor *Tbx18* is strongly expressed during early urogenital tract development in the ureteral mesenchyme and a subset of kidney stromal mesenchyme originating from *Foxd1* positive precursor cells.[359,360] Later in renal development, *Tbx18* expression is also found in the renal capsule, vascular smooth muscle cells, pericytes, mesangial cells, and the mesenchyme surrounding the renal papillae and calyces.[360] The most overt phenotype of *Tbx18*-inactivation is the onset of hydronephrosis and hydroureter as a result of impaired development of the ureteral smooth muscle cells.[359,361] This underscores the importance of *Tbx18* in the normal differentiation of the ureteral mesenchyme. A more recent detailed phenotypic characterization of *Tbx18*-null mutant kidneys reveals an additional significance of this transcription factor in the overall development of the renal vasculature.[360] The branching and overall density of the renal vasculature are notably reduced in the absence of *Tbx18. Tbx18* is also specifically required in the normal development of the glomerular microvasculature. Loss of *Tbx18* causes significant oligonephronia and dilation of glomerular capillaries. These vascular phenotypes likely result from the degeneration of the stromal mesenchyme adjacent to the developing vasculature and the failure to sustain the proliferation of mesangial precursors.

Mice carrying a hypomorphic allele of *Notch2* that is missing two epidermal growth factor (EGF) motifs are born with a reduced number of glomeruli that lack both endothelial and mesangial cells, as discussed in the section on nephron segmentation.[362,363] The downstream Notch signaling target, *Rbpj*, has also been described as crucial for the proper development of the renal vasculature and the glomerular mesangium. Conditional inactivation of *Rbpj* in the *Foxd1*-expressing stromal lineage leads to profound renal maldevelopment and early postnatal death.[364] *Rbpj* deficiency in the renal stroma results in poor branching and simplification of the renal vascular network. *Rbpj* conditional mutant kidneys have a greater proportion of larger vessels and a concomitant reduction in microvascular density. Glomeruli are dilated and lack mesangial cells in *Rbpj* conditional knockouts. Furthermore, loss of *Rbpj* results in loss of renin cells, abnormal thickening of blood vessels, and renal fibrosis. Altogether, these studies highlight the distinctive significance of Notch signaling within the stromal mesenchyme in the establishment and organization of the renal vasculature.

## MOLECULAR GENETICS OF VASCULAR FORMATION

Although we now have a comprehensive if not complete understanding of the mechanisms underlying ureteric branching and nephrogenesis, we still know little how the complex vascularization of the kidney is coordinated with epithelial and stromal development. During kidney development, the formation and elaborate patterning of an arterial, venous, and capillary blood vascular network involves a combination of both vasculogenesis and angiogenesis (see Fig. 1.8). In addition, lymphangiogenesis underlies the development of the lymphatic vasculature from veins. The major renal vessels align close to the branching UB and likely elaborate through angiogenesis into large-caliber afferent and efferent distributaries.[33] Vasculogenesis in the kidney likely arises from sporadic endothelial cells within the MM that organize to form a primitive vascular network and then give rise to most of the peritubular capillaries.[32,365,33] Additionally, vasculogenesis within the S-shaped nephron intermediates establishes the glomerular capillaries.[34,35,366,367]

Grafting studies demonstrate that transplanted embryonic kidneys can become vascularized from the invasion of host-derived extrinsic blood vessels.[368,369] However, more recent fate mapping studies provide compelling evidence for the existence of endogenous endothelial precursors within the kidney.[31–35] Cultured mouse embryonic kidneys contain a heterogenous intrinsic pool of endothelial cells that express the endothelial-specific markers Kdr, Cd31, and Cd146.[33] As early as E11.5 embryonic stage in the mouse, *Kdr*$^+$ cells are readily identifiable as either single-cell clusters or primitive capillaries. The primitive capillaries consist of *Cd31*$^+$/*Cd146*$^+$ cells, whereas the single cells predominantly express *Cd146*$^+$ but not *Cd31.* At E12.5, *Cd31*$^+$ cells have formed an elaborate chain-like network, including being found adjacent to *Pax2*$^+$ cap mesenchyme while singular *Cd146*$^+$ cells have become scarce. Lineage tracing analysis demonstrates that a subset of endogenous renal endothelial cells that give rise to peritubular capillaries but not glomerular endothelial cells are derived from *Foxd1*$^+$ stromal cells.[32,33]

Isolated E11.5, E12.5, and E13.5 kidneys, and also cultured E11.5 kidneys, produce VEGF-A, a potent factor known to promote vascularization.[33] Indeed, the pharmacologic inhibition of VEGFR signaling completely abolishes the establishment of endothelial cell networks in cultured embryonic kidney explants, suggesting that VEGF-A signaling is essential for renal vascular development. More recent imaging studies reveal that kidney vascularization is initiated at E11 in the mouse, when systemic vessels from embryonic circulation circumscribe around the UB.[370,371] From E13.5, the endothelial network surrounds the cap mesenchyme and UB in a cyclical manner by which endothelia form across and in close contact with the bifurcating UB, which begs the question as to whether endothelial development coregulate ureteric branching. It is, however, easily conceivable that given the importance of oxygen levels in nephrogenesis,[372–374] the intimate integration of the renal vascular plexus, which carries oxygen-delivering erythrocytes, is essential for nephron maturation.

Conditional gene targeting experiments and cell-selective deletion of *Vegfa* from podocytes demonstrates that VEGF-A signaling is required for formation and maintenance of the glomerular filtration barrier.[375,376] Glomerular endothelial cells express VEGFR2 as they migrate into the vascular cleft. Although a few endothelia migrate into the developing glomeruli of *Vegfa* podocyte conditional knockout mutants (likely due to a small amount of VEGF-A produced by presumptive podocytes at the S-shaped stage of glomerular development prior to Cre-mediated genetic deletion), the endothelia fail to develop fenestrations and rapidly disappear, leaving capillary "ghosts" (Fig. 1.19). Deletion of a single *Vegfa* allele from podocytes leads to glomerular endothelial defects known as endotheliosis, a phenomenon involving hypertrophy of glomerular endothelial cells and loss of fenestrations (endotheliosis), progressing to capillary occlusion and thrombosis (thrombotic microangiopathy).[375] Inactivation of *Vegfr2* phenocopies endotheliosis and thrombotic microangiopathy, indicating that VEGFA primarily signals through VEGFR2 in supporting the development and maintenance of the glomerular endothelium.[377] As the dose of *Vegfa* decreased, the associated endothelial phenotypes became more severe. Upregulation of the major 164 angiogenic VEGF-A isoform in developing podocytes of transgenic mice led to massive proteinuria and collapse of the glomerular tuft by 5 days of age. Taken together, these results show a requirement for VEGF-A for development and maintenance of the specialized glomerular endothelia and demonstrate a major paracrine signaling function for VEGF-A in the glomerulus. Furthermore, tight regulation of the dose of VEGF-A is essential for proper formation of the glomerular capillary system. The molecular basis and mechanism of dosage sensitivity is unclear at present and is particularly intriguing given the documented inducible regulation of VEGF-A by hypoxia-inducible factors (HIFs) at a transcriptional level. Despite this, it is clear that in vivo, a single *Vegfa* allele is unable to compensate for loss of the other. Similarly, VEGF-A signaling is essential for the development of the

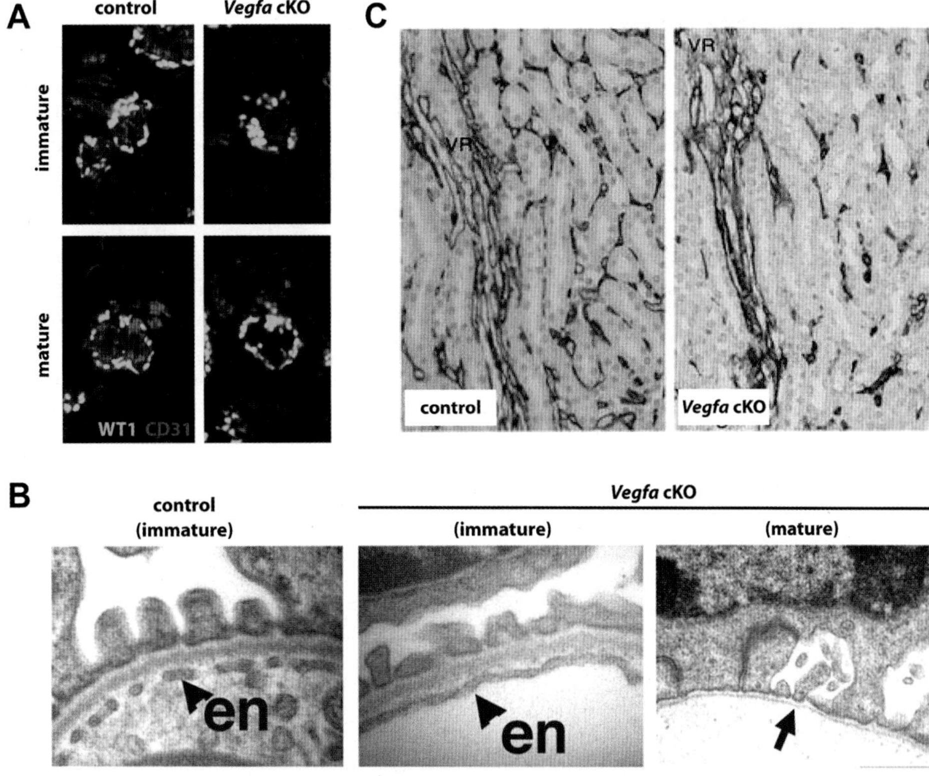


**Fig. 1.19 VEGF-A is essential for the development of the glomerular and peritubular capillaries.** (A) *Vegfa* inactivation in podocytes leads to recruitment of fewer endothelial cells in the glomerulus which are subsequently lost. Podocytes and endothelial cells are stained with WT1 (*green*) and CD31 (*red*), respectively. (B) Transmission electron micrograph showing that in podocyte-specific *Vegfa* knockouts, the glomerular endothelium *(en)* lack fenestrae (*arrowheads*) and eventually detach leaving the glomerular basement membrane bare (*arrow*). (C) *Vegfa* ablation in renal tubules leads to a significant reduction in peritubular capillaries (stained *brown* for CD34). *VR,* Vasa recta. Panels (A) and (B) were adapted from Eremina V, et al. Glomerular-specific alterations of VEGF-A expression lead to distinct congenital and acquired renal diseases. *J Clin Invest.* 2003;111:707–716. Panel (C) adapted from Dimke H. Tubulovascular cross-talk by vascular endothelial growth factor A maintains peritubular microvasculature in kidney. *J Am Soc Nephrol.* 2014;26:1027–1038.

peritubular capillaries. Ablation of *Vegfa* in renal tubules did not cause gross histologic disturbance in the kidney but lead to a dramatic reduction of peritubular capillaries and an abnormal elevation in renal erythropoietin production (see Fig. 1.19).[378] This uncovered an important tubulo vascular crosstalk involved in the promotion of erythrocyte development by the kidney.

A second major receptor tyrosine kinase (RTK) signaling pathway required for maturation of developing blood vessels is the angiopoietin–Tie signaling system. Angiopoietin 1 (*Angpt1*) stabilizes newly formed blood vessels and is associated with loss of vessel plasticity and concurrent recruitment of pericytes or vascular support cells to the vascular wall.[379] The molecular switch or pathway leading to vessel maturation through the activation of Tie2 (encoded by the gene *Tek*, the major receptor for Angpt1) is not known and appears to be independent of the platelet-derived growth factor (PDGF) signaling system that is required for pericyte recruitment. The importance of Angpt1 in promoting the development of the renal microvasculature was first suggested based on observations that exogenous Angpt1 enhances the growth of interstitial capillaries in mouse metanephric organ cultures.[380] Because *Angpt1*-null mice perish embryonically at around E12.5, the in vivo role of *Angpt1* during renal development was gleaned using an inducible knockout strategy.[381,382] Ablation of *Angpt1* deletion at around E10.5 results in general dilation of renal blood vessels, including the glomerular capillaries sometimes observed as simplified single enlarged loops.[382] A marked reduction of mesangial cells was also observed in *Angpt1*-deficient mutants. Without *Angpt1*, a few endothelial cells are seen detached from the glomerular basement membrane. In contrast, it is proposed that angiopoietin 2 (*Angpt2*) functions as a context-dependent antagonist of the Tie2 receptor.[383,384] Consistent with this hypothesis is the fact that overexpression of *Angpt2* in transgenic mice results in a phenotype similar to the *Angpt1* or *Tek* knockout mice. Angpt1, Angpt2, Tie2, and the orphan receptor Tie1 are all expressed in the developing kidney.[385–389] Whereas, *Angpt1* is quite broadly expressed in condensing mesenchyme, podocytes, and tubular epithelial cells, *Angpt2* is more restricted to pericytes and smooth muscle cells surrounding cortical and large vessels as well as in the mesangium. *Angpt2*-null mice are viable but exhibit defects in peritubular cortical capillary development.[390] Podocyte-specific overexpression of *Angpt2* causes proteinuria and increased apoptosis in glomerular capillaries.[391] Both angiopoietin ligands function in concert with VEGF-A, although the precise degree of crosstalk between these pathways is still under investigation. VEGF-A and Angpt2, for example, have been shown to cooperate in promoting endothelial sprouting. Chimeric studies showed that Tie1 is required for the development of the glomerular capillary system because *Tie1*-null cells fail to incorporate in the glomerular endothelium.[392]

Renal vascular development also relies on a third tyrosine kinase–dependent signaling mediated by ephrins and Eph family receptors, which are better known for their involvement in axon guidance and specification of arterial and venous cell fates.[393,394] Ephrins and their cognate receptors are expressed widely during renal development. Overexpression of *Ephb4* leads to defects in glomerular arteriolar formation, whereas conditional deletion of *Efnb2* (*EphrinB2*) from perivascular smooth muscle cells and mesangial cells leads to glomerular vascular abnormalities.[395,396] How this occurs is not entirely clear as *Efnb2* has a dynamic pattern of expression in the developing glomerulus, beginning in podocyte precursors and rapidly switching to glomerular endothelial cells and mesangial cells.[397]

Dysregulation of BMP within the podocyte compartment also results in glomerular vascular defects. Overexpression of BMP4 leads to defects in endothelial and mesangial recruitment, wheras overexpression of noggin, a natural BMP2 antagonist, leads to collapse of the glomerular tuft.[398,399] *Bmp4* haploinsufficiency, on the other hand, leads to dysplastic kidneys and glomerular cysts with collapsed capillary tufts.[399] Additional studies are required to fully understand the role of this family of growth factors in glomeruli.

An additional pathway that is likely to play a role in glomerular endothelial development and perhaps of the entire renal vasculature is the SDF1-CXCR4 axis. CXCR4, a G-protein–coupled chemokine receptor, is strongly expressed in endothelial cells. SDF1 (encoded by the gene *Cxcl12*), the only known ligand for CXCR4, is expressed in a dynamic segmental pattern in podocytes and later in the mesangial cells of the glomerulus.[400] Embryonic deletion of either *Cxcl12* or *Cxcr4* does not preclude nephrogenesis but results in the defective formation of blood vessels, notably an abnormal patterning of the renal vasculature and the development of a simplified and dilated glomerular capillary tuft.[401] Genetic loss of CXCR7, which is thought to act as a decoy receptor for SDF1, interestingly phenocopies defective development seen in SDF1 and CXCR4-mutant mice. Unlike CXCR4, CXCR7 is specifically expressed by podocytes and not endothelial cells.[402] It has been proposed that CXCR7, acting as a scavenger receptor, establishes an SDF1 morphogen gradient preventing feedback inhibition of CXCR4 receptor expression in target cells such as the endothelium. Consistent with this, inactivation of *Cxcr7* distinctively causes downregulation of *Cxcr4* expression in the renal cap mesenchyme and the glomerular tuft. Thus the spatial regulation of SDF1-CXCR4 signaling appears to be important for the normal development of the glomerular vasculature.

Two transcription factors belonging to the large Sry-related HMG box (Sox) gene family, named *Sox17* and *Sox18*, have distinctive and overlapping expression in vascular endothelial cells.[403] Complete loss of *Sox17* is embryonic lethal in mice due to endodermal dysmorphogenesis.[404] In mice, *Sox18* ablation results in a mild coat defect but does not cause cardiovascular abnormalities.[405] Nevertheless, a point mutation in *SOX18* in humans has been implicated in HLT (hypotrichosis-lymphedema-telangiectasia) syndrome, which affects hair, lymph, and blood vessel vasculature.[406] The more severe consequence of the human *SOX18* mutation compared to the null mutation in mice was suggested to be due to a dominant-negative effect. *Sox17*, however, shows haploinsufficiency in a homozygous *Sox18* background, affecting neovascularization in kidneys, liver, and the reproductive system and causing early postnatal lethality.[403] Kidneys from *Sox17/Sox18* double-null mutant mice have hypoplastic and atrophying medullary regions. In these compound *Sox17/Sox18* mutants, the radiating outer medullary vascular bundles of the vasa recta are missing without apparent abnormalities in the inner medullary or cortical regions. These defects within the outer medullary region result in variable degrees of hydronephrosis. Interestingly, midgestational loss of both Angpt1 and Angpt2 ligands or their cognate receptor Tie2 leads to rarefaction of the medullary capillary plexus and the absence of outer medullary vascular bundles, particularly the fenestrated ascending vasa recta, leading to urinary concentration defects and interstitial fluid retention that culminates in the formation of interstitium-derived medullary cysts (Fig. 1.20).[407] This raises an intriguing possibility that Sox17 and Sox18 pathways either converge or intersect with Angpt1/Angpt2-Tie2 signaling in coordinating late-stage angiogenesis in kidneys.

A least understood component of the renal vasculature are the lymphatic vessels. Similar to other organs, the renal lymphatics play important roles in interstitial fluid homeostasis and the regulation of the immune response. Lymphatic vessels have been identified surrounding the renal artery in the hilum, in the arcuate and interlobular arteries in the cortex, and are also found in the renal capsule.[408–410] These lymphatic vessels are known to express the hyaluronan receptor Lyve1.[407,411] The medulla was previously thought to lack lymphatic vessels. However, more recently a study of angiopoietin-Tie2 signaling in the kidney reveals that the ascending vasa rectae represent hybrid vessels that express markers of both blood (*Cd34, Emcn, Pecam1,* and *Plvap*) and lymphatic endothelial cells (*Prox1* and *Vegfr3*) (see Fig. 1.19).[407] This underscores a novel lymphatic circuit for the drainage of medullary interstitial fluid as part of the osmoregulation of urine. VEGF-C signaling via the receptor VEGFR3 is essential for lymphangiogenesis.[412–415] *Vegfr3* deficiency in adult mice causes the extravasation of fibrinogen into the renal interstitium.[416] How the renal lymphatic vasculature is particularly remodeled upon inactivation of VEGF-C/VEGFR3 signaling remains unknown.

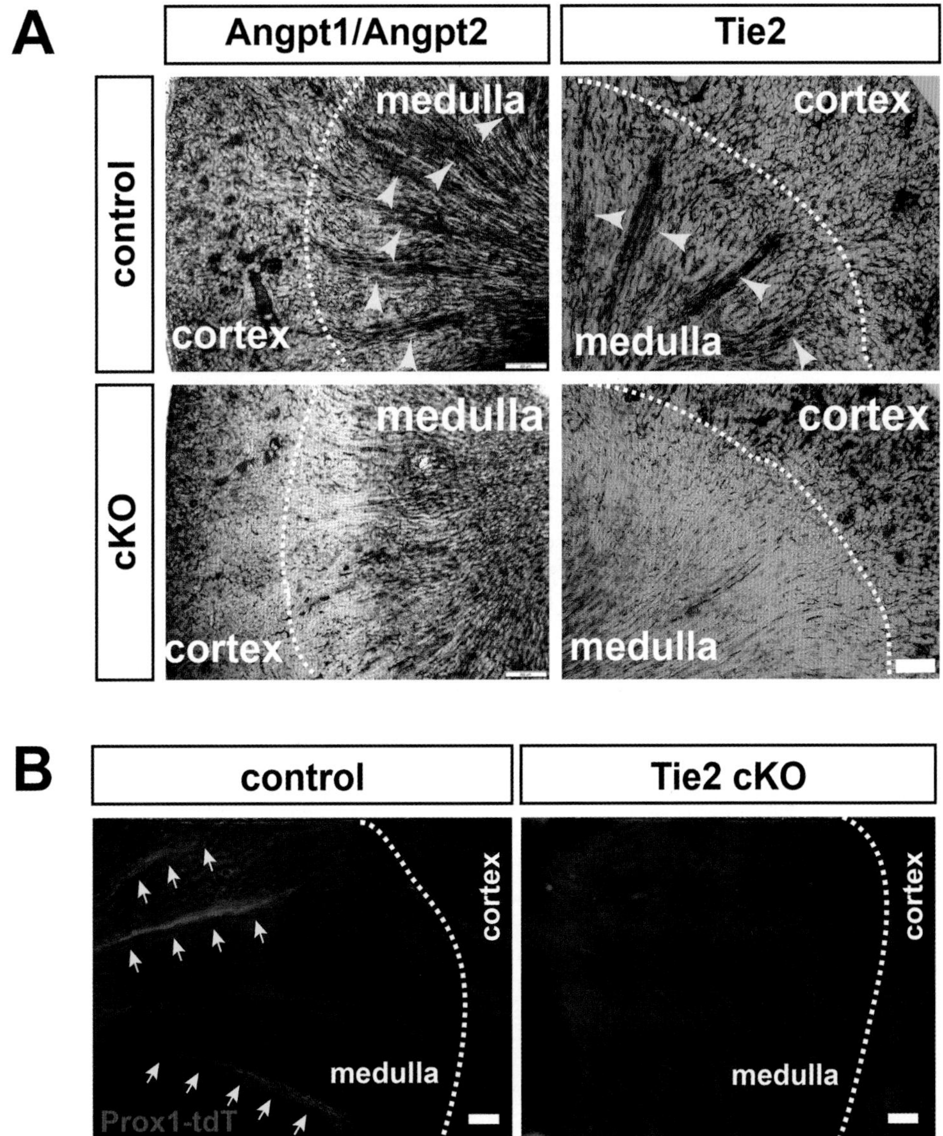


**Fig. 1.20 Ascending vasa recta development depends on angiopoietin-Tie2 signaling.** (A) Midgestational (E16.5) loss of both Angpt1 and Angpt2 or their cognate receptor Tie2 (Tek) leads to loss of vasa recta bundles (*yellow arrowheads*) in the outer renal medulla, particularly the ascending vasa rectae. (B) Ascending vasa rectae are novel lymphatic-like vessels expressing the lymphatic-specific Prox1 transcription factor as seen in transgenic reporter mice expressing the fluorophore tdTomato under the control of the *Prox1* promoter. *Prox1-tdT*$^+$ vascular bundles representing the ascending vasa rectae are absent in kidneys of Tie2-deficient mouse mutants. *cKO,* Conditional knockout; *Prox1-tdT,* Prox1-tdTomato transgene. Adapted with permission from Kenig-Kozlovsky, Scott RP, Onay T, et al. Ascending vasa recta are angiopoietin/Tie2-dependent lymphatic-like vessels. *J Am Soc Nephrol.* 2018;29:1097–1107.

## RENIN CELLS AND THE JUXTAGLOMERULAR APPARATUS

The juxtaglomerular apparatus consists of cells that line the afferent arteriole, the macula densa cells of the distal tubule, and the extraglomerular mesangial cells that are in contact with intraglomerular mesangium.[417] Renin-expressing cells may be seen in arterioles in early mesonephric kidneys in 5-week human fetuses and in metanephric kidneys by week 8, at a stage prior to hemodynamic flow changes within the kidney, and are derived from *Foxd1*-expressing stromal mesenchyme.[418] Renin-expressing cells reside within the MM and give rise not only to juxtaglomerular cells but also to mesangial cells.[419,420]

The only known substrate for renin, angiotensinogen, is converted to angiotensin I and angiotensin II by angiotensin-converting enzyme (ACE).[421] The renin–angiotensin–aldosterone axis is required for normal renal development. In humans, the use of ACE inhibitors during pregnancy has been associated with congenital defects including renal anomalies.[422,423] Two subtypes of angiotensin receptors exist: AT1 receptors are responsible for most of the classically recognized functions of the renin–angiotensin system (RAS), including pressor effects and aldosterone release mediated through angiotensin; functions of the type 2 receptors have been more difficult to characterize, but generally seem to oppose the actions of the AT1 receptors.[424] Genetic deletion of angiotensinogen or ACE results in hypotension and defects in formation of the renal papilla and pelvis.[256–259] Humans have one *AT1* gene whereas mice have two: *Agtr1a* and *Agtr1b*. Mice carrying a knockout for either AT1 receptor alone exhibit no major defects,[425,426] whereas combined deficiency phenocopies the angiotensinogen and ACE phenotypes.[260,261] Although AT2 receptor (*Agtr2*) expression is markedly upregulated in the embryonic kidney, genetic deletion of the AT2 receptor does not cause major impairment of renal development.[427,428] However, an association between *Agtr2*-deficiency and malformations of the collecting duct system, including vesicoureteral reflux and ureteropelvic junction obstruction, has been reported.[429]

MicroRNAs (miRNAs) are regulatory RNAs that act as antisense posttranscriptional repressors by binding the 3′ untranslated region of target mRNAs. Eukaryotes express hundreds of miRNAs that can regulate thousands of mRNAs, and they have been shown to play an important role in development and disease, including in differentiation, signaling pathways, proliferation, apoptosis, and tumorigenicity. Dicer1 is an endoribonuclease that processes precursor miRNAs. Deletion of *Dicer1* from renin-expressing cells results in severely reduced number of juxtaglomerular cells, reduced renin production, and lower blood pressure. The kidney develops severe vascular abnormalities and striped fibrosis along the affected blood vessels, suggesting that miRNAs are required for normal morphogenesis and function of the kidney.[430]

Gene promoter analysis indicates that renin expression is dependent on the Notch signaling pathway. The intracellular domain of Notch (NIC) and the transcription factor Rbpj bind and cooperatively stimulate reporter gene expression from the renin promoter.[431] Genetic studies, however, indicate that Notch signaling has a broader role in the juxtaglomerular apparatus.[432] The conditional ablation of *Rbpj* in renin cells results in severe paucity of juxtaglomerular cells with consequential decrease in overall renin expression and the development of lower blood pressure. Lack of increase in apoptosis in *Rbpj* conditional mutant kidneys suggests that *Rbpj* may have altered the cell fate specification of renin cell precursors.

## PODOCYTE DEVELOPMENT

Presumptive podocytes are located at the proximal end of the S-shaped body, lining the emerging vascular cleft (Fig. 1.21). Immature podocytes are simple columnar epithelia expressing E-cadherin (Fig. 1.22). Postmitotic mature podocytes, on the other hand, normally lose E-cadherin expression and atypically express vimentin, an intermediate filament protein more common among mesenchymal cells but absent in most epithelial cells. The most distinctive morphologic feature of a fully differentiated podocyte is its arborized and stellate appearance (Fig. 1.22). Podocytes ensheathe the glomerular capillaries with their foot processes, effectively forming the final layer of the glomerular filtration barrier. Foot processes emanating from adjacent podocytes interdigitate in *trans* and form a unique and porous intercellular junction called the slit diaphragm through which primary urinary filtrate passes. Three-dimensional reconstruction of podocyte ultrastructure obtained by block-face scanning electron microscopy reveals the morphologic transformation of podocytes during development and the formation of interdigitating foot processes.[22,433] Columnar-shaped immature podocytes are linked by tight and adherens junctions that progressively migrate from the apical to the basal side. Once the junctional complex has descended close to the basement membrane, podocytes begin to flatten, spread, and interdigitate with short primitive foot processes underneath the junctions. As the primitive processes grow, the tight and adherens junctions relocate from the cell body to between the processes forming the immature foot processes. Finally, the junctional complexes are gradually replaced with slit diaphragms, resulting in mature foot processes.

The transcription factors *Wt1*, *Tcf21*, *Mafb*, *Foxc2*, and *Lmx1b* are highly expressed by developing podocytes and are important for the elaboration of podocyte foot processes and the establishment of slit diaphragms.* Complete loss of *Wt1* leads to renal agenesis.[39] However, specific loss of a *Wt1* splice isoform results in poor development of podocyte foot processes.[436] The *Wt1*-null phenotype in mice can also be rescued using a yeast artificial chromosome containing the human *WT1* gene and, depending on the level of expression of WT1, the mice developed a range of glomerular pathologies ranging from crescentic glomerulonephritis to mesangial sclerosis, clinical features observed in Denys-Drash syndrome arising from a mutant *WT1* allele in humans.[437] Transgenic mice expressing a Denys-Drash–mutant *Wt1* allele under the regulation of a podocyte-specific promoter also developed glomerular disease with abnormalities observed in the adjacent endothelium.[438] Genome-wide analysis of the *Wt1* targets in podocytes reveals that *Wt1* autoregulates its own transcription and acts as master regulator of a complex transcriptional network that regulates podocyte development, structure, and function, including transcription factors (*Lmx1b, Tcf21, Mafb,*

*References 39, 83, 339, 340, 434, and 435.

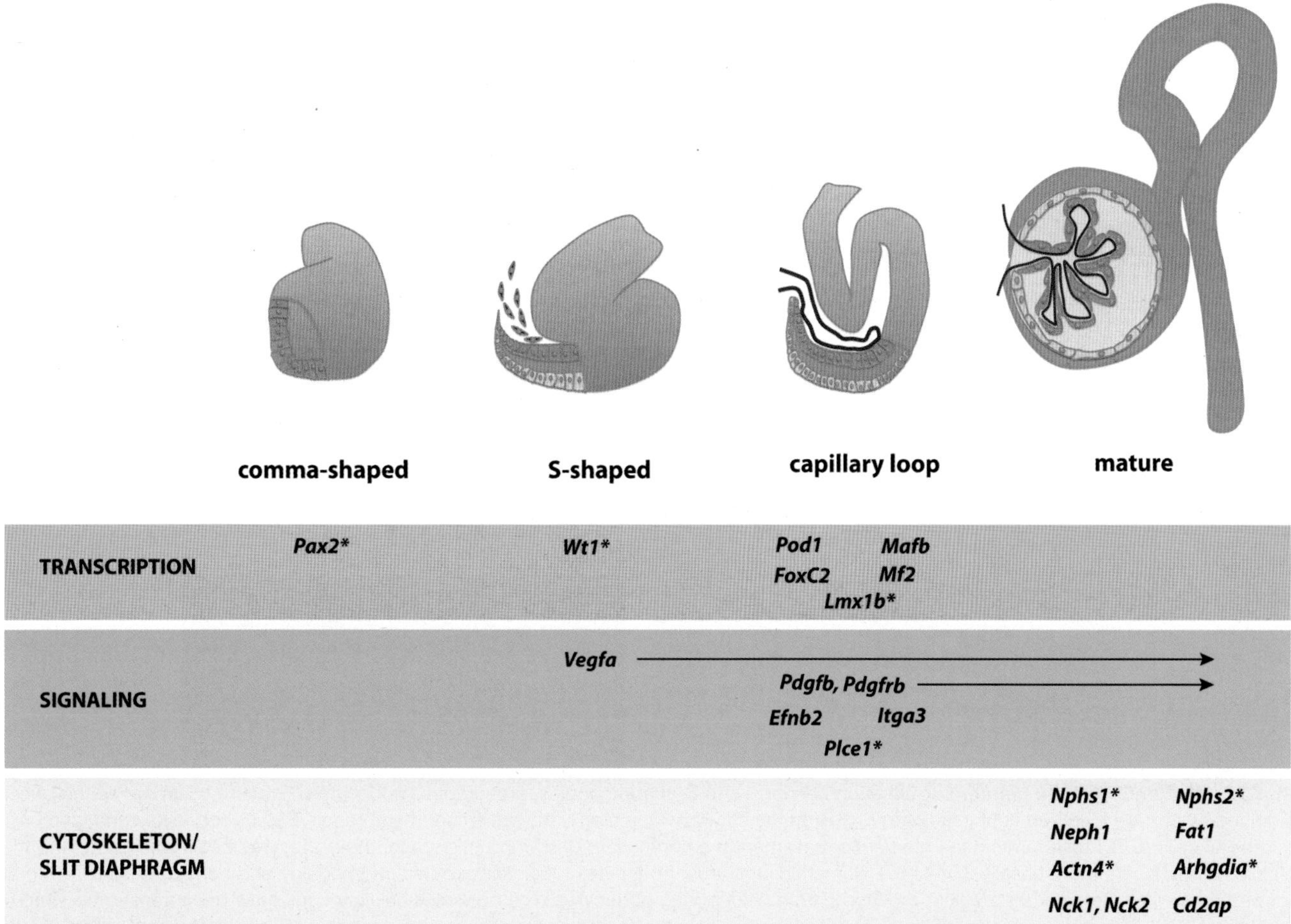


**Fig. 1.21 Molecular basis of glomerular development.** Key factors are shown along with the time point where major effects were observed in knockout or transgenic mouse studies. Many factors play roles at more than one time point. Genes identified as mutated in patients with glomerular disease are marked by asterisks.

*Tead1, Foxc1,* and *Foxc2*) and genes strongly linked to podocyte dysfunction and nephrotic diseases (*Actn4, Arhgap24, Cd2ap, Col4a3, Col4a4, Lamb2, Nphs1, Nphs2,* and *Plce1*).[439] Inactivation of *Lmx1b, Tcf21, Mafb,* and *Foxc2* causes podocytes to remain as cuboidal epithelia and failure to spread on the glomerular capillary bed.[83,339,434,440] *Tcf21* likely acts upstream of *Mafb* as the latter is downregulated in *Tcf21*-null mice.[434] Loss of *Mafb* and *Lmx1b* reduces the expression of *Nphs1* (nephrin) and *Nphs2* (podocin), whereas the absence of *Foxc2* causes the specific downregulation of *Nphs2* and $\alpha3\alpha4\alpha5$ (IV) collagen.[83,434,441] *Lmx1b* mutations are linked to nail-patella syndrome in humans, with a subset of affected individuals manifesting nephrotic disease.[435,442] *Wt1, Tcf21, Mafb, Foxc2* and *Lmx1b* are expressed from the S-shape stage onward and remain constitutively expressed in adult glomeruli. Proteinuria develops from loss of these genes, thus underscoring the importance of normal podocyte maturation in the establishment of the glomerular filtration barrier.

Genetic studies have also led to the identification of structural proteins crucial for normal podocyte function and the integrity of the glomerular filtration barrier. The seminal discoveries of the causal link between nephrotic diseases and mutations in podocyte-specific genes *Nphs1* and *Nphs2* set the stage for vigorous investigations that led to the appreciation of the key importance of podocytes in renal filtration.[443,444]

Mutations in *Nphs1,* the gene that encodes for the protein nephrin, are associated with congenital nephropathy of the Finnish variety (CNF), a serious condition that requires early renal replacement therapy.[444] Glomeruli obtained from infants affected by CNF are devoid of slit diaphragms. Nephrin, a huge transmembrane adhesion molecule with multiple immunoglobulin-like motifs, was shown to be a structural component of the slit diaphragm. *Nphs2,* whose product is the intracellular membrane-bound protein podocin, and is the first gene identified as being linked to steroid-resistant nephrotic syndrome (SRNS).[443] Podocin, which interacts with nephrin in cholesterol-rich membrane microdomains (also called lipid rafts), is also a vital and indispensable component of the slit diaphragm.[445–449] A number of other genes specifically expressed by podocytes have been associated with proteinuric diseases, including *Cd2ap, Kirrel (Neph1), Fat1, Actn4, Trpc6, Myo1e, Arhgap24, Arhgdia, Rhpn1, Inf2, Coq2, Coq6, Plce1,* and *APOL1.*[77,78,80,82,450–464] The products of these genes are either integral parts of the slit diaphragm complex or direct interacting partners of the complex, while the remainder are important in regulating the development, viability, cytoskeleton, and distinctive morphology of podocytes (Fig. 1.23).

The topologic organization of slit diaphragm components remains unknown, but it is likely that the larger adhesion molecules nephrin and Fat1 could be bridging juxtaposed

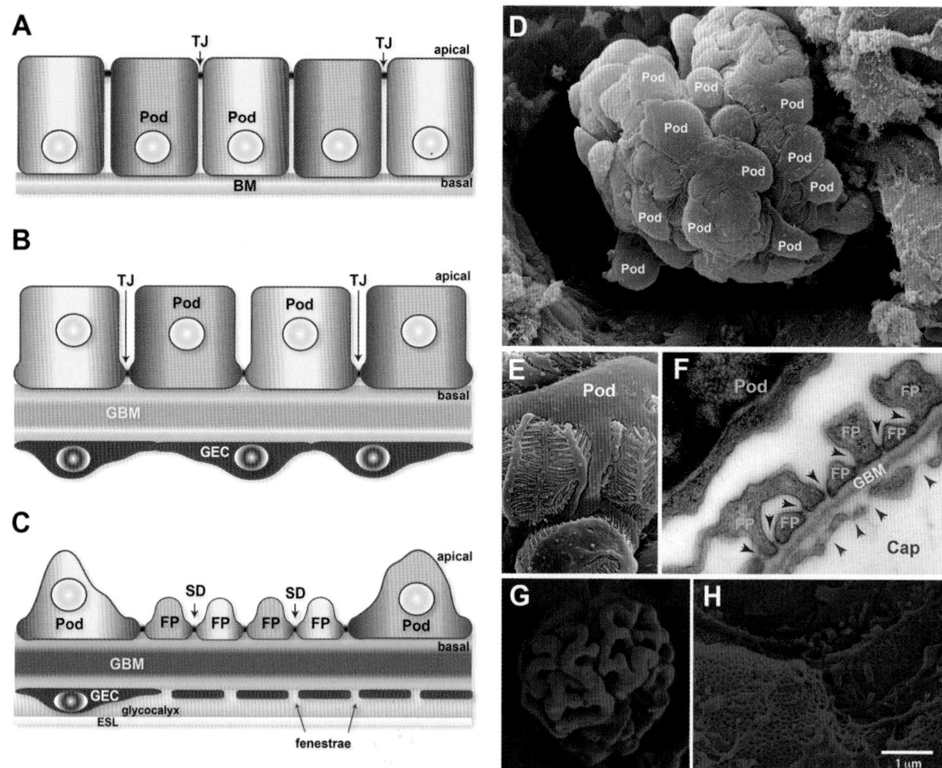


**Fig. 1.22 Maturation of the glomerular filtration barrier.** (A) In S-shaped bodies, presumptive podocytes *(Pod)* are columnar epithelial cells conjoined by apically localized tight junctions *(TJ)*. (B) At the capillary loop stage, the basement membranes *(BM)* of podocytes and glomerular endothelial cells *(GEC)* fuse forming the glomerular basement membrane *(GBM)*. During this stage, the podocytes begin to spread, and their cell junctions relocate more basally. (C) As the glomerulus matures, podocytes lose their cuboidal morphology and have developed elaborate foot processes *(FP)* that interdigitate with processes from neighboring podocytes. The podocyte cell junctions have been transformed into slit diaphragms *(SD)* that link juxtaposed FPs. GECs also flatten, develop fenestrae, and become covered by a glycocalyx that, together with absorbed plasma components, form the endothelial cell surface layer *(ESL)*. The GBM is now a unified BM between podocytes and the GECs. (D) Scanning electron micrograph (SEM) of a cracked glomerulus exposing the capillary tuft covered by podocytes (gold). (E) Higher magnification view of a podocyte in situ revealing the elaborate FPs interdigitated with FPs from other podocytes. (F) Transmission electron micrograph of a glomerulus showing the SD (*blue arrows*) between interdigitating FPs and the endothelial fenestrae (*red arrows*) on the opposite side of the GBM (Cap, glomerular capillary lumen). (G) SEM of a resin cast of the renal vasculature demonstrating the highly convoluted glomerular capillary tuft. (*Courtesy of Fred E. Hossler, East Tennessee State University*). (H) A view inside an exposed glomerular endothelial lumen showing its highly fenestrated surface. Adapted from Scott RP, Quaggin SE. Formation and maintenance of a functional glomerulus. In Little, M. H. (ed.). *Kidney Development, Disease, Repair and Regeneration.* San Diego: Academic Press; 2016.

foot processes (see Fig. 1.22).[459,465–467] Smaller adhesion molecules within the slit diaphragms such as Neph1, Neph3, and P-cadherin may more likely associate in *cis* (within the same foot process surface).[468–470] Nephrin and the related protein Neph1 are known to interact with the polarity complex proteins Par3, Par6, and aPKCλ/ι, indicating a coregulation between the polarized cell structure of podocytes and the compartmentalized assembly of the slit diaphragm complex along the foot processes.[471] Conditional inactivation in podocytes of aPKCλ/ι or the small GTPase Cdc42, which positively regulates the Par3/Par6/ aPKCλ/ι complex, causes proteinuria characterized by abnormal pseudo-slit diaphragms formed between effaced foot processes (Fig. 1.24).[472–474] It has also been shown that inactivation of aPKCλ/ι can specifically inhibit the localization of nephrin to the cell surface.[475]

Terminal foot processes of podocytes are longitudinally supported by parallel bundles of actin, setting them apart from the larger primary processes that have a microtubule-based backbone.[21] The stereotypical response of podocytes to injury either through chemical insults or a detrimental gene mutation is effacement of foot processes. In effaced foot processes, the actin cytoskeleton has been remodeled into a mesh-like network of randomly oriented filaments.[476] Genetic and biochemical studies provide evidence that the slit diaphragm is functionally coupled to the actin cytoskeleton, and that perturbation of this relationship results in compromised renal filtration and proteinuric disease. Nck adaptor molecules (Nck1 and Nck2) are known to link tyrosine kinase receptors to signaling molecules that regulate the actin cytoskeleton. Podocytes lacking *Nck1* and *Nck2* are effaced and form abnormal slit diaphragms.[64] Cell culture studies reveal that clustered nephrin is phosphorylated at its cytoplasmic tail by the kinase Fyn, creating distinctive phosphotyrosine sites where Nck1 and Nck2 adaptors can bind directly. The association between nephrin and Nck adaptors consequently recruits N-WASP and the Arp2/3 protein complex to mediate localized polymerization of actin.[64,477] Loss of Fyn causes congenital nephrosis, whereas podocyte-specific inactivation of *Wasl*, the gene encoding for N-WASP, leads to proteinuric disease.[478,479] It is also very likely that Nck adaptors can mediate the adhesion of podocytes to the glomerular basement membrane by virtue of their ability to interact with the PINCH–ILK–integrin complex.[480–482] Cdc42, in addition to its role in podocyte polarization, has also been shown to be

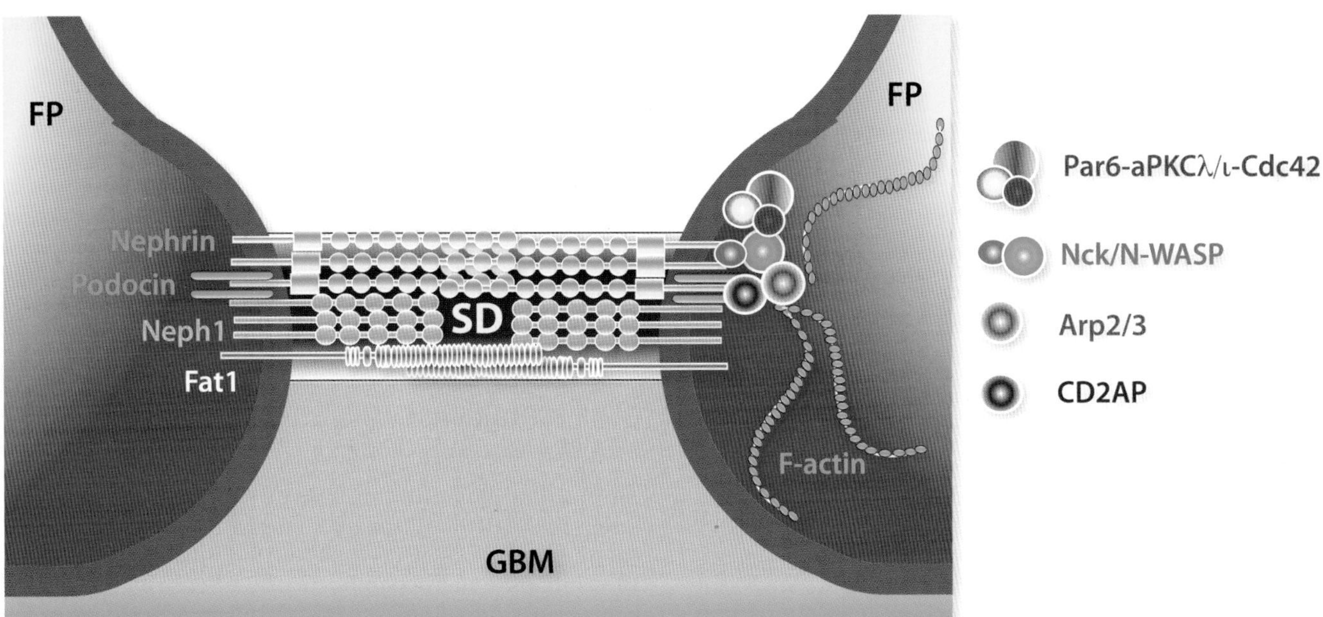


**Fig. 1.23 Structural overview of the slit diaphragm.** An oversimplified diagram depicting the major adhesion receptors comprising the SD and how they are possibly integrated with the actin cytoskeleton of podocyte foot processes. *FP,* Podocyte foot process; *SD,* slit diaphragm; *GBM,* glomerular basement membrane. Adapted from Scott RP, Quaggin SE. Formation and maintenance of a functional glomerulus. In Little, M. H. (ed.). *Kidney Development, Disease, Repair and Regeneration.* San Diego: Academic Press; 2016.

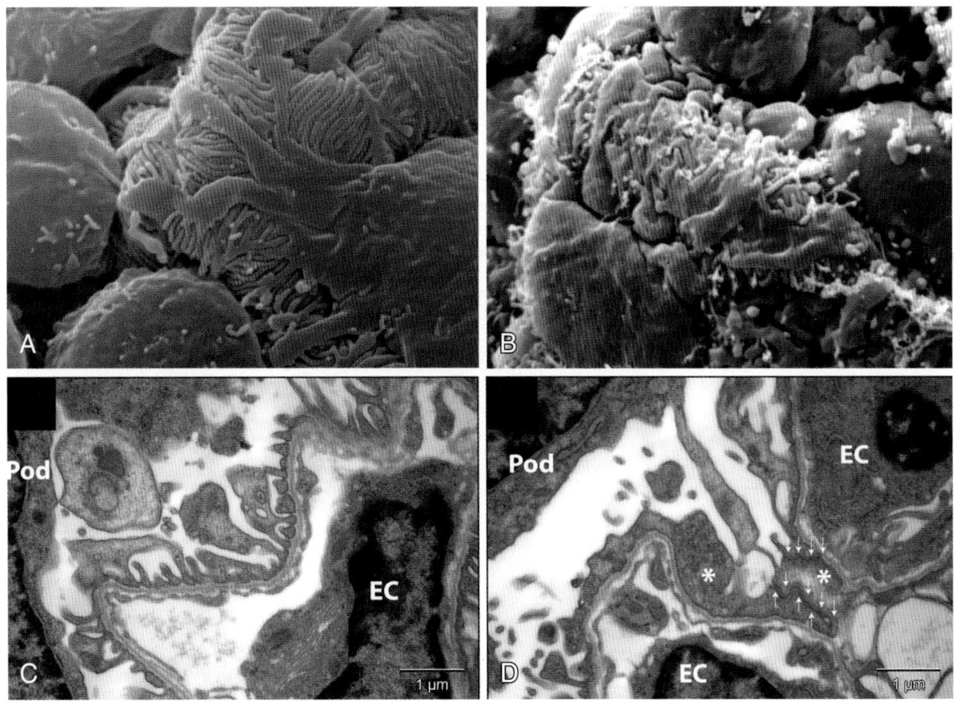


**Fig. 1.24 Cdc42 is required for normal podocyte development.** (A, B) False-colored scanning electron micrographs of glomeruli from neonatal kidneys: (A) wild-type control podocytes showing normal interdigitated podocytes; and (B) Cdc42-deficient mutant podocytes showing total effacement of foot processes. (C, D) Transmission electron micrographs of sectioned glomeruli: (C) wild-type control showing regularly interdigitating podocyte foot processes and basolateral slit diaphragms; and (D) podocyte-specific Cdc42-deficient mutant showing mislocalized cell junctions (*arrows*) between effaced foot processes (*asterisk*). *EC,* Endothelial cell; *Pod,* podocyte. Adapted from Scott RP, Hawley SP, Ruston J, et al. Podocyte-specific loss of Cdc42 leads to congenital nephropathy. *J Am Soc Nephrol.* 2012;23:1149–1154.

required for the coupling of actin polymerization to nephrin. CD2AP, a molecule known to stabilize actin microfilaments, is also indispensable in podocytes.[483–485] Mutations in *Actn4, Arhgdia, Arhgap24, Inf2,* and *Myo1e,* whose protein products are established regulators of the actin cytoskeleton, are also implicated in pathologic transformation of podocytes and proteinuric diseases.[77,78,80,451–453,455–458]

It has been proposed that the slit diaphragm likely functions in mechanotransduction in podocytes, allowing them to modulate renal filtration in response to hemodynamic changes within the glomerular microenvironment.[486,487] *MEC-2*, the *C. elegans* homologue of podocin, is a component of the touch receptor complex coupled to the ion channel MEC-4/MEC-10.[488] Loss of *MEC-2* in worms leads to insensitivity to touch.[488] In podocytes, the ion channel *Trpc6* forms an integral component of the slit diaphragm directly interacting with podocin.[487] In diverse cell types such as myocytes, cochlear hair cells, and sensory neurons, the Trpc6 channel opening is gated by mechanical stimuli. Human mutations in *TRPC6* have been strongly linked to proteinuria.[460,489,490]

A novel lipid-dependent signaling pathway involving the VEGF receptor Flt1 (VEGFR1) has been described recently as crucial for the regulation of podocyte actin cytoskeleton and the maintenance of slit diaphragms. Genetic removal of *Flt1* from podocytes leads to foot process effacement and proteinuria.[491] Intriguingly, a kinase-inactive mutant of Flt1 is able to support normal podocyte development and function. In vivo, Flt1 is cleaved, releasing a soluble ectodomain (sFlt1). The secreted sFlt1 has been shown to act as an autocrine factor in podocytes, associating with glycosphingolipids, and mediating podocyte cell adhesion, nephrin phosphorylation, and actin polymerization. It has been proposed that sFlt1 may function physiologically to stabilize the slit diaphragms and the attachment of podocytes to the glomerular basement membrane.

Three groups generated mice carrying a podocyte-specific deletion of *Dicer1*, thereby interfering with the production of functional miRNAs.[492–494] Podocyte-specific *Dicer1* knockout mice develop albuminuria by 3 weeks of age and rapidly progress to end-stage renal failure by approximately 6 weeks. A number of potential miRNA targets were identified, but their functional significance in the podocyte in vivo is yet unknown.

From all of these studies, it follows that intrinsic proteins and functions of podocytes play a key role in the development and maintenance of the permselective properties of the glomerular filtration barrier. Podocytes also function as vasculature support cells producing VEGF-A and other angiogenic growth factors. It is likely that endothelial cells also produce hitherto unknown trophic factors that promote terminal differentiation and survival of podocytes.

## GLOMERULAR BASEMENT MEMBRANE DEVELOPMENT

The mature glomerular basement membrane (GBM) is a fusion of the extracellular matrices (ECM) of podocytes and glomerular endothelial cells. The GBM is a highly organized and compositionally complex matrix whose abundant components include collagens (types I, IV, VI, and XVIII), laminins (α5, β2, and γ1), nidogen-1, heparan sulfate proteoglycans (agrin and perlecan), and tubulointerstitial nephritis antigen-like protein (Fig. 1.25).[495–497] The GBM is an essential part of the glomerular filtration barrier, functioning as an intermediary sieving matrix and a sink for secreted trophic and signaling factors, as well as mediating cellular communication between the glomerular endothelium and podocytes. Furthermore, adhesive cell–ECM interactions among the

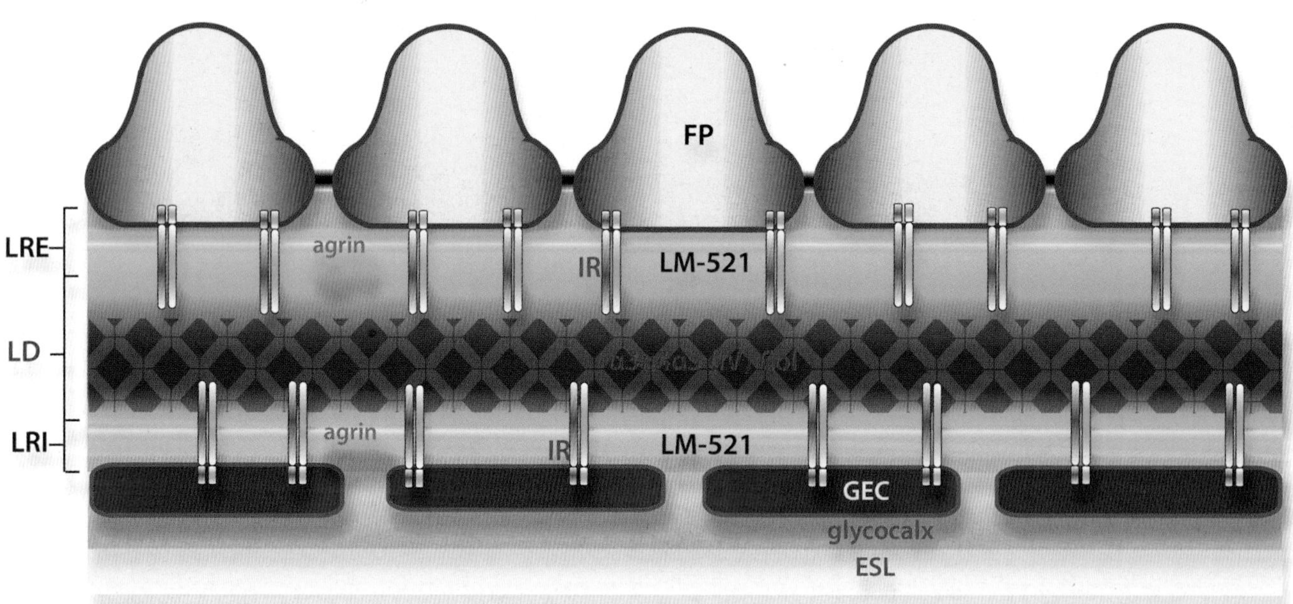


**Fig. 1.25 Stratified organization of the glomerular basement membrane.** A model of the organization of a mature GBM. The laminin complex LM-521 (*pale cyan*) and agrin (*yellow*) form two distinct layers underneath the basal aspects of podocytes and GECs. α3α4α5-Type IV collagens (*hatched brown area*) are more centrally distributed but are thought to be closer to the GEC. The laminin and type IV collagen complexes have significant overlap. Epitope mapping of integrin-β1 suggests that integrin receptors *(IR)* on podocytes are normally separate and less likely to interact with the type IV collagens in the mature human GBM. The morphologically distinct layers of the GBM in transmission electron micrographs are roughly demarcated. *ESL,* Endothelial surface layer; *FP,* podocyte foot process; *GBM,* glomerular basement membrane; *GEC,* glomerular endothelial cell; *LD,* lamina densa; *LM,* laminin; *LRE,* lamina rare externa; *LRI,* lamina rara interna. Based on STORM imaging by Suleiman HL, Zhang L, Roth R, et al. Nanoscale protein architecture of the kidney glomerular basement membrane. Elife 2013;2:e01149. Adapted from Scott RP, Quaggin SE. Formation and maintenance of a functional glomerulus. In Little MH (ed.). *Kidney Development, Disease, Repair and Regeneration.* San Diego: Academic Press; 2016.

GBM, the podocytes, and the glomerular endothelial cells maintain the structural integrity of the glomerular filtration barrier.

Among the major components of the GBM, type IV collagens and laminins have been shown to be the most indispensable, highlighted by proteinuric kidney diseases such as Alport syndrome, Goodpasture disease, and Pierson syndrome. Alport syndrome is linked to a growing list of mutations in the genes *COL4A3, COL4A4,* and *COL4A5* encoding for type IV collagen subunits α3, α4, and α5, respectively.[498,499] Maturation of the GBM requires the replacement of juvenile α1α1α2 with α3α4α5 type IV collagen trimers, a developmental switch improving the structural resilience of the GBM.[500] In Alport syndrome, the assembly of heterotrimeric α3α4α5 type IV collagen complex is compromised while the α1α1α2 type IV collagen complexes persists. Because α3α4α5 type IV collagen trimers constitute about half the total proteins in the mature GBM, it is not surprising that Alport syndrome GBM is severely distorted.[501] The importance of type IV collagens in the GBM is further underscored in Goodpasture disease, an autoimmune disorder targeting α3 type IV collagen subunit.[502] In Pierson syndrome, mutations in *LAMB2* encoding the laminin β2 subunit impair the assembly of the laminin complex LM-521 (a trimer formed among laminin-α5, -β2, and -γ1 subunits).[503,504] Deformation of the GBM and proteinuria results from loss of *Lamb2* and *Lama5* (laminin-α5) in mice.[234,505–507]

## DEVELOPMENT OF THE MESANGIUM

Mesangial cells grow into the developing glomerulus and come to sit between the capillary loops. Gene deletion studies have demonstrated a critical role for PDGF-B/PDGFR-β signaling in this process (Fig. 1.26). Deletion of the *Pdgfb* gene, which is expressed by glomerular endothelia, or the PDGFR-β receptor gene (*Pdgfrb*), which is expressed by mesangial cells, results in glomeruli with a single balloon-like capillary loop, instead of the intricately convoluted glomerular capillaries of wild-type kidneys. Furthermore, the glomeruli contain no mesangial cells.[508] Endothelial-cell–specific deletion of *Pdgfb* results in the same glomerular phenotype and shows that production of PDGF-B by the endothelium is required for mesangial migration.[509] PDGF-B–dependent recruitment of mesangial cells into nascent glomeruli also requires the coreceptor neuropilin-1 (Nrp1).[510] *Nrp1*-deficiency within the *Pdgfrb*$^+$-cell lineage in mice phenocopies glomerular aneurysm seen upon loss of either *Pdgfb* or *Pdgfrb* (Fig. 1.27). In vitro, mesangial cell chemotaxis, but not cell proliferation and survival in response to PDGF-B, strongly requires the mesangial expression of *Nrp1*. Furthermore, loss of the mesangium resulting from *Nrp1* ablation results in the delamination of the glomerular endothelium and inward buckling of the GBM. These findings altogether underscore the key supportive role of the mesangium for the development and maintenance of a highly convoluted glomerular capillary tuft. Indeed, targeted injury to the mesangium, either with snake venom or with antibodies against *Thy1*, results in secondary damage to the glomerular endothelium and glomerular aneurysms.[511–515] Mesangial cells and the matrix they produce are required to pattern the glomerular capillary system. Loss of podocyte-derived factors such as VEGF-A also leads to failure of mesangial cell ingrowth, likely through the primary loss of endothelial cells and failure of PDGF-B signaling.[376]

A

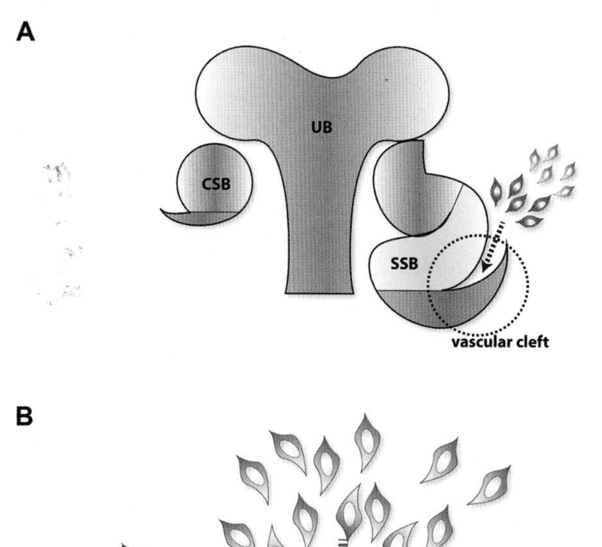


B

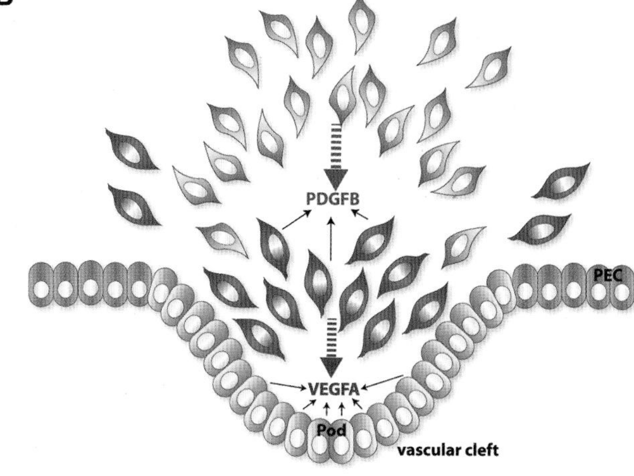


**Fig. 1.26 Sequential recruitment of endothelial and mesangial cells into the developing glomerulus.** (A) The glomerulus forms around the vascular cleft at the proximal end of S-shaped intermediate nephrons. (B) Within the vascular cleft, presumptive podocytes *(Pod)* secrete VEGFA that attracts VEGFR2-expressing angioblasts (*red*), which are the precursors of GECs. The angioblasts are followed by mesangial cell precursors expressing PDGFR-β (*green*), which are attracted by PDGFB secreted by the endothelial cells. *UB,* Ureteric bud; *CSB,* comma-shaped body; *PEC,* parietal epithelial cell; *SSB,* S-shaped body. Adapted from Scott RP, Quaggin SE. Formation and maintenance of a functional glomerulus. In Little MH (ed.). *Kidney Development, Disease, Repair and Regeneration.* San Diego: Academic Press; 2016.

A number of other knockouts demonstrate defects in both vascular development and mesangial cell ingrowth. Loss of the transcription factors *Tcf21* and *Foxc2* causes defective migration of mesangial cells.[83,339] Mesangial abnormalities in *Tcf21*- and *Foxc2*-deficient mice are poorly understood in terms of mesangium-specific transcriptional targets of *Tcf21* and *Foxc2.* Nevertheless, these mutant phenotypes highlight the importance of crosstalk between cell compartments within the glomerulus.

## DEVELOPMENT OF THE BOWMAN CAPSULE

The outermost cells of the proximal end of the S-shaped nascent nephron are the presumptive parietal epithelial cells that eventually form the Bowman capsule that enclose the glomerular tuft and where primary urinary filtrate collects. Similar to podocytes, parietal precursors are originally cuboidal epithelial cells that progressively flatten and become

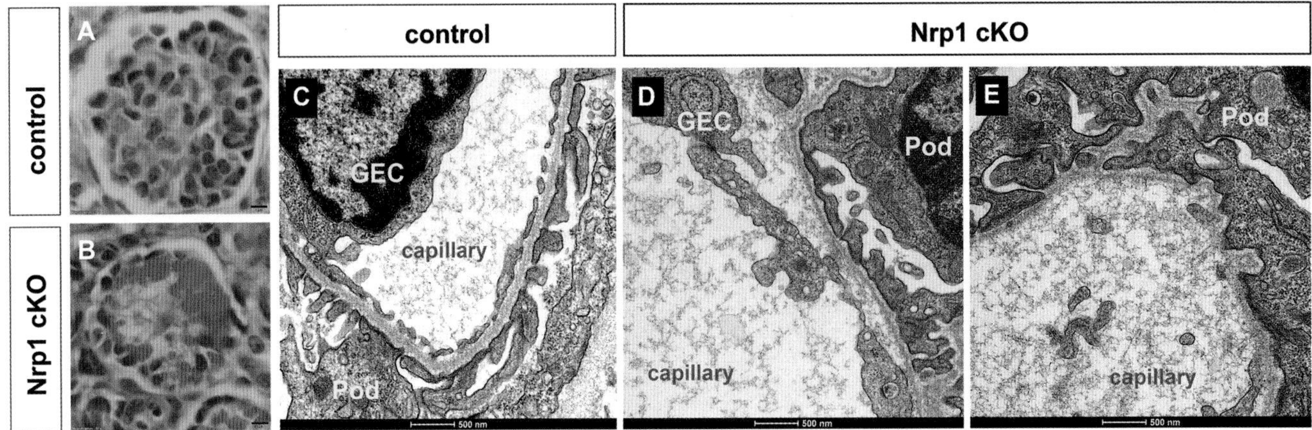


**Fig. 1.27 Nrp1 is required for mesangial cell recruitment in the glomerulus.** (A, B) Hypocellularity and glomerular aneurysm due to the absence of the mesangium in Nrp1-deficient mice. Representative histological sections of normal control (A) and *Nrp1* conditional knockout *(cKO)*-mutant kidneys. (C–E) Transmission electron micrographs of glomeruli showing the delamination (D) or complete detachment (E) of the glomerular endothelium from the glomerular basement membrane in *Nrp1*-cKO kidneys. In the absence of *Nrp1* in the *Pdgfrb*$^+$ lineage, the glomerular endothelium has impaired development of fenestrae. *GEC,* Glomerular endothelial cell; *Pod,* podocyte. Adapted from Bartlett CS, Scott RP, Carota IA, et al. Glomerular mesangial recruitment and function require the co-receptor neuropilin-1. *Am J Physiol Renal Physiol.* 2017;313:F1232-F1242.

squamous. Parietal epithelia express the proteins claudin-1 (*Cldn1*) and claudin-2 (*Cldn2*) that form part of tight junctions, which help contain urinary filtrate.[516,517] Parietal epithelial cells like podocytes express *Wt1,* although at a reduced level. Whether this differential level of *Wt1* expression affects cell fate commitment to either the podocyte or parietal cell lineage warrants further investigation. WT1 is known to attenuate canonical Wnt signaling through an epigenetic mechanism that suppresses *Cttnb1* expression.[518] Specific loss of *Cttnb1* in nephrogenic epithelia from the S-shaped stage causes the formation of glomerular cysts where the Bowman capsule lacks parietal epithelia and are instead formed by podocytes containing notably containing foot processes and slit diaphragms.[519] Parietal cell specification is therefore strongly dependent on canonical Wnt-β–catenin signaling, which sets it apart from podocytes where *Cttnb1* expression is dispensable.[520] In the absence of parietal epithelial cells, glomerular capillaries develop poorly while the mislocalized *Vegfa*-expressing podocytes cause formation of ectopic capillaries next to the abnormal Bowman capsule.[519] It can therefore be inferred that parietal epithelial cells may function in compartmentalizing the podocyte–glomerular endothelial cell crosstalk, ensuring that glomerular endothelial cells form a well elaborated capillary tuft covered by an adequate number of podocytes.

## NEURAL DEVELOPMENT

Renal vascular tone and urinary functions are regulated by a dense neural network in the kidney that relays bidirectional signals to the brain.[521] Glomerular filtration rate, renal blood flow, tubular resorption of fluid, electrolytes, and urinary solutes, as well as the secretion of renin, are regulated by sympathetic innervations of the glomeruli, renal tubules and blood vessels.[522] Over the past decade, the renal sympathetic innervation has attracted considerable attention after it has been recognized that persistently elevated renal sympathetic nerve activity contributes to the pathogenesis of renal hypertension.[523,524] In particular, it has been shown that surgical excision of sympathetic input to the kidneys can alleviate refractory hypertension.[525,526] The distribution of afferent and efferent nerves to the kidney has been partially mapped but the developmental program involved in establishing them is largely unknown.[527–529] Fate mapping and molecular studies specifically addressing the origin and development of renal nerves have yet to be reported, although many lessons have been learned about guidance pathways in play in both neural and vascular development in other systems. Neurons, like early blood vessels, appear to closely track the branching UB in cultured embryonic kidneys.[33,370,530] It can be speculated that the sympathetic innervation and vascularization of the kidney are coordinately synchronized with better known inductive events between the UB and the MM.

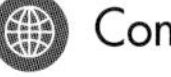 Complete reference list available at ExpertConsult.com.

## KEY REFERENCES

5. Short KM, Combes AN, Lefevre J, et al. Global quantification of tissue dynamics in the developing mouse kidney. *Dev Cell.* 2014;29:188–202.
10. Saxen L. *Organogenesis of the Kidney.* Cambridge: Cambridge University Press; 1987.
41. Grobstein C. Trans-filter induction of tubules in mouse metanephrogenic mesenchyme. *Exp Cell Res.* 1956;10:424–440.
48. Lindstrom NO, Lawrence ML, Burn SF, et al. Integrated beta-catenin, BMP, PTEN, and Notch signaling patterns the nephron. *Elife.* 2015;3:e04000.
59. Lindstrom NO, McMahon JA, Guo J, et al. Conserved and divergent features of human and mouse kidney organogenesis. *J Am Soc Nephrol.* 2018;29:785–805.
64. Kobayashi A, Valerius MT, Mugford JW, et al. Six2 defines and regulates a multipotent self-renewing nephron progenitor population throughout mammalian kidney development. *Cell Stem Cell.* 2008;3:169–181.
65. Kobayashi A, Mugford JW, Krautzberger AM, et al. Identification of a multipotent self-renewing stromal progenitor population during mammalian kidney organogenesis. *Stem Cell Reports.* 2014;3:650–662.
136. Carroll TJ, Park JS, Hayashi S, et al. Wnt9b plays a central role in the regulation of mesenchymal to epithelial transitions underlying organogenesis of the mammalian urogenital system. *Dev Cell.* 2005;9:283–292.

143. Moore MW, Klein RD, Farinas I, et al. Renal and neuronal abnormalities in mice lacking GDNF. *Nature.* 1996;382:76–79.
144. Pichel JG, Shen L, Sheng HZ, et al. Defects in enteric innervation and kidney development in mice lacking GDNF. *Nature.* 1996;382:73–76.
145. Sanchez MP, Silos-Santiago I, Frisen J, et al. Renal agenesis and the absence of enteric neurons in mice lacking GDNF. *Nature.* 1996;382:70–73.
162. Schuchardt A, D'Agati V, Larsson-Blomberg L, et al. Defects in the kidney and enteric nervous system of mice lacking the tyrosine kinase receptor Ret. *Nature.* 1994;367:380–383.
165. Vega QC, Worby CA, Lechner MS, et al. Glial cell line-derived neurotrophic factor activates the receptor tyrosine kinase RET and promotes kidney morphogenesis. *Proc Natl Acad Sci U S A.* 1996;93:10657–10661.
187. Chi X, Michos O, Shakya R, et al. Ret-dependent cell rearrangements in the Wolffian duct epithelium initiate ureteric bud morphogenesis. *Dev Cell.* 2009;17:199–209.
212. Majumdar A, Vainio S, Kispert A, et al. Wnt11 and Ret/Gdnf pathways cooperate in regulating ureteric branching during metanephric kidney development. *Development.* 2003;130:3175–3185.
219. Basson MA, Akbulut S, Watson-Johnson J, et al. Sprouty1 is a critical regulator of GDNF/RET-mediated kidney induction. *Dev Cell.* 2005;8:229–239.
223. Michos O, Cebrian C, Hyink D, et al. Kidney development in the absence of Gdnf and Spry1 requires Fgf10. *PLoS Genet.* 2010;6: e1000809.
225. Brandenberger R, Schmidt A, Linton J, et al. Identification and characterization of a novel extracellular matrix protein nephronectin that is associated with integrin alpha8beta1 in the embryonic kidney. *J Cell Biol.* 2001;154:447–458.
239. Grieshammer U, Le M, Plump AS, et al. SLIT2-mediated ROBO2 signaling restricts kidney induction to a single site. *Dev Cell.* 2004;6: 709–717.
246. Yu J, Carroll TJ, Rajagopal J, et al. A Wnt7b-dependent pathway regulates the orientation of epithelial cell division and establishes the cortico-medullary axis of the mammalian kidney. *Development.* 2009;136:161–171.
258. Niimura F, Labosky PA, Kakuchi J, et al. Gene targeting in mice reveals a requirement for angiotensin in the development and maintenance of kidney morphology and growth factor regulation. *J Clin Invest.* 1995;96:2947–2954.
268. Park J, Shrestha R, Qiu C, et al. Single-cell transcriptomics of the mouse kidney reveals potential cellular targets of kidney disease. *Science.* 2018;360:758–763.
274. Werth M, Schmidt-Ott KM, Leete T, et al. Transcription factor TFCP2L1 patterns 2604 cells in the mouse kidney collecting ducts. *Elife.* 2017;6.
279. Self M, Lagutin OV, Bowling B, et al. Six2 is required for suppression of nephrogenesis and progenitor renewal in the developing kidney. *EMBO J.* 2006;25:5214–5228.
281. Park JS, Ma W, O'Brien LL, et al. Six2 and Wnt regulate self-renewal and commitment of nephron progenitors through shared gene regulatory networks. *Dev Cell.* 2012;23:637–651.
283. Xu J, Liu H, Park JS, et al. Osr1 acts downstream of and interacts synergistically with Six2 to maintain nephron progenitor cells during kidney organogenesis. *Development.* 2014;141:1442–1452.
284. Karner CM, Das A, Ma Z, et al. Canonical Wnt9b signaling balances progenitor cell expansion and differentiation during kidney development. *Development.* 2011;138:1247–1257.
285. Tanigawa S, Wang H, Yang Y, et al. Wnt4 induces nephronic tubules in metanephric mesenchyme by a non-canonical mechanism. *Dev Biol.* 2011;352:58–69.
286. Stark K, Vainio S, Vassileva G, et al. Epithelial transformation of metanephric mesenchyme in the developing kidney regulated by Wnt-4. *Nature.* 1994;372:679–683.
290. Park JS, Valerius MT, McMahon AP. Wnt/beta-catenin signaling regulates nephron induction during mouse kidney development. *Development.* 2007;134:2533–2539.
293. Chung E, Deacon P, Marable S, et al. Notch signaling promotes nephrogenesis by downregulating Six2. *Development.* 2016;143: 3907–3913.
294. Chung E, Deacon P, Park JS. Notch is required for the formation of all nephron segments and primes nephron progenitors for differentiation. *Development.* 2017;144:4530–4539.
313. Lindstrom NO, De Sena Brandine G, Tran T, et al. Progressive recruitment of mesenchymal progenitors reveals a time-dependent process of cell fate acquisition in mouse and human nephrogenesis. *Dev Cell.* 2018;45:651–660, e654.
326. Karner CM, Chirumamilla R, Aoki S, et al. Wnt9b signaling regulates planar cell polarity and kidney tubule morphogenesis. *Nat Genet.* 2009;41:793–799.
331. Saburi S, Hester I, Fischer E, et al. Loss of Fat4 disrupts PCP signaling and oriented cell division and leads to cystic kidney disease. *Nat Genet.* 2008;40:1010–1015.
334. Hartman HA, Lai HL, Patterson LT. Cessation of renal morphogenesis in mice. *Dev Biol.* 2007;310:379–387.
336. Rumballe BA, Georgas KM, Combes AN, et al. Nephron formation adopts a novel spatial topology at cessation of nephrogenesis. *Dev Biol.* 2011;360:110–122.
353. Das A, Tanigawa S, Karner CM, et al. Stromal-epithelial crosstalk regulates kidney progenitor cell differentiation. *Nat Cell Biol.* 2013;15:1035–1044.
354. Bagherie-Lachidan M, Reginensi A, Pan Q, et al. Stromal Fat4 acts non-autonomously with Dchs1/2 to restrict the nephron progenitor pool. *Development.* 2015;142:2564–2573.
357. Mao Y, Francis-West P, Irvine KD. Fat4/Dchs1 signaling between stromal and cap mesenchyme cells influences nephrogenesis and ureteric bud branching. *Development.* 2015;142:2574–2585.
371. Munro DAD, Hohenstein P, Davies JA. Cycles of vascular plexus formation within the nephrogenic zone of the developing mouse kidney. *Sci Rep.* 2017;7:3273.
372. Daniel E, Azizoglu DB, Ryan AR, et al. Spatiotemporal heterogeneity and patterning of developing renal blood vessels. *Angiogenesis.* 2018.
376. Eremina V, Sood M, Haigh J, et al. Glomerular-specific alterations of VEGF-A expression 2819 lead to distinct congenital and acquired renal diseases. *J Clin Invest.* 2003;111:707–716.
379. Dimke H, Sparks MA, Thomson BR, et al. Tubulovascular crosstalk by vascular endothelial growth factor a maintains peritubular microvasculature in kidney. *J Am Soc Nephrol.* 2014.
433. Ichimura K, Kakuta S, Kawasaki Y, et al. Morphological process of podocyte development revealed by block-face scanning electron microscopy. *J Cell Sci.* 2017;130:132–142.
443. Boute N, Gribouval O, Roselli S, et al. NPHS2, encoding the glomerular protein podocin, is mutated in autosomal recessive steroid-resistant nephrotic syndrome. *Nat Genet.* 2000;24:349–354.
444. Kestila M, Lenkkeri U, Mannikko M, et al. Positionally cloned gene for a novel glomerular protein—nephrin—is mutated in congenital nephrotic syndrome. *Mol Cell.* 1998;1:575–582.
497. Suleiman H, Zhang L, Roth R, et al. Nanoscale protein architecture of the kidney glomerular basement membrane. *Elife.* 2013;2:e01149.
508. Lindahl P, Hellstrom M, Kalen M, et al. Paracrine PDGF-B/PDGF-Rbeta signaling controls mesangial cell development in kidney glomeruli. *Development.* 1998;125:3313–3322.
509. Bjarnegard M, Enge M, Norlin J, et al. Endothelium-specific ablation of PDGFB leads to pericyte loss and glomerular, cardiac and placental abnormalities. *Development.* 2004;131:1847–1857.

# 2 Anatomy of the Kidney

Jill W. Verlander | William L. Clapp

CHAPTER OUTLINE



The structure of the kidney, including the ultrastructure of individual cell types, their axial distribution, and arrangement within the kidney, is essential to normal renal function. In this chapter, we describe normal mammalian renal structure, including gross anatomy, histology, and ultrastructure.

## GROSS FEATURES

Normal mammalian kidneys are paired and retroperitoneal. In the human, the kidneys are located approximately between the twelfth thoracic and third lumbar vertebrae on opposite sides of the vertebral column. The right kidney is usually slightly more caudal in position than the left. Each kidney normally weighs between 125 to 170 g in adult males and 115 to 155 g in adult females, and measures approximately 11 to 12 cm long, 5.0 to 7.5 cm wide, and 2.5 to 3.0 cm thick. By magnetic resonance imaging, the mean kidney lengths are 12.4 +/− 0.9 cm for men and 11.6 +/− 1.1 cm for women, and the mean kidney volumes are 202 +/− 36 mL for men and 154 +/− 33 mL for women.[1] Located on the medial or concave surface of each kidney is the hilum, an indentation where the renal pelvis, the renal artery and vein, the lymphatics, and a nerve plexus pass into the sinus of the kidney. A thin tough fibrous capsule covers the surface of the kidney.

In humans and most mammals, each kidney is normally supplied by a single renal artery, although one or more accessory renal arteries may be present. The renal artery enters the hilum and usually divides into an anterior and a posterior branch. Three segmental or lobar arteries arise from the anterior branch and supply the upper, middle, and lower thirds of the anterior surface of the kidney (Fig. 2.1). The posterior branch supplies more than half of the posterior surface and occasionally gives rise to a small apical segmental branch. However, the apical segmental or lobar branch arises most commonly from the anterior division. No collateral circulation exists between individual segmental or lobar arteries or their subdivisions. The kidneys often receive aberrant arteries from the superior mesenteric, suprarenal, testicular, or ovarian arteries. True accessory arteries that arise from the abdominal aorta usually supply the lower pole of the kidney. The arterial and venous circulations in the kidney are described in detail in Chapter 3.

On the cut surface of a bisected human kidney, two main regions are visible, a granular outer region, the cortex, and a striated inner region, the medulla (Fig. 2.2). In humans, the medulla is composed of renal pyramids, conical tissue masses with the base of each pyramid at the corticomedullary boundary, and the apex extending toward the renal pelvis, forming a papilla. On the tip of each papilla is the area cribrosa (Fig. 2.3), where the distal ends of collecting ducts (ducts of Bellini) open into the renal pelvis. A single renal pyramid and its surrounding cortex comprise a renal lobe. In contrast to the human kidney, the kidney of the rat and many other laboratory animals has a single renal pyramid with its overlying cortex and is therefore termed “unipapillate.” Otherwise, these kidneys resemble the human kidney in their gross appearance. In humans, the renal cortex is about 1 cm in thickness, forms a cap over the base of each renal pyramid, and extends downward between the individual pyramids to form the columns of Bertin (see Figs. 2.2 and 2.4). From the base of the renal pyramid, at the corticomedullary junction, the “medullary rays” extend into the cortex. The medullary rays are formed by the cortical collecting ducts, the straight segments of the proximal tubules, and the cortical thick ascending limbs (TALs) of loop of Henle, aligned together. These straight segments are interposed among the convoluted tubules and appear to radiate from the medulla into the cortex, hence the name.

The renal pelvis represents the expanded portion of the upper urinary tract. In humans, transitional epithelium or urothelium, composed of multiple cell layers, lines the pelvis and ureter. In rodents, cuboidal epithelium lines the renal pelvis and also covers the urinary surface of the papilla. Two and sometimes three extensions of the renal pelvis, the major calyces, reach outward from the upper dilated part of the pelvis, which further divides into several minor calyces. These receive the urine discharged at the area cribrosa of each renal pyramid. In unipapillate kidneys, the papilla is directly surrounded by the renal pelvis. The ureters originate from the distal renal pelvis at the ureteropelvic junction and discharge into the fundus of the urinary bladder. In adult humans, the ureters are approximately 28 to 34 cm long and have a mean diameter of 1.8 mm, with a maximum of 3 mm considered normal.[2] The walls of the calyces, pelvis, and ureters contain smooth muscle-related cells and interstitial cells, which serve a pacemaker function to propel the urine to the bladder.

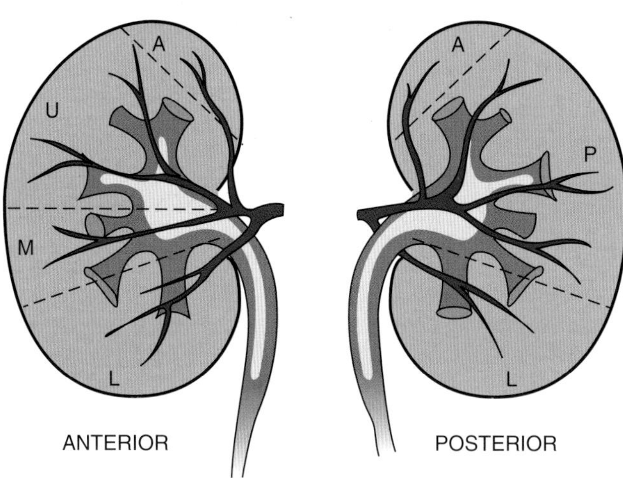


**Fig. 2.1** Diagram of the vascular supply of the human kidney. The anterior half of the kidney can be divided into upper *(U)*, middle *(M)*, and lower *(L)* segments, each supplied by a segmental branch of the anterior division of the renal artery. A small apical segment *(A)* is usually supplied by a division from the anterior segmental branch. The posterior half of the kidney is divided into apical *(A)*, posterior *(P)*, and lower *(L)* segments, each supplied by branches of the posterior division of the renal artery. (Modified from Graves FT. The anatomy of the intrarenal arteries and its application to segmental resection of the kidney. *Br J Surg.* 1954;42:132–139.)

## THE NEPHRON

The nephron is the functional unit of the kidney, composed of the renal corpuscle (the term renal or Malpighian corpuscle comprises the glomerulus and Bowman's capsule) and the associated renal tubules from the proximal tubule through the connecting segment (CNT) (Fig. 2.5). Although the average nephron number in adult humans is approximately 900,000 to 1 million per kidney, numbers for individual human kidneys range from approximately 200,000 to more than 2.5 million,[3–6] contrasting with the approximately 30,000 nephrons in each adult rat kidney.[7–9] The origin of the nephron is the metanephric blastema. Although there has not been universal agreement on the origin of the connecting tubule, it is now generally believed also to derive from the metanephric

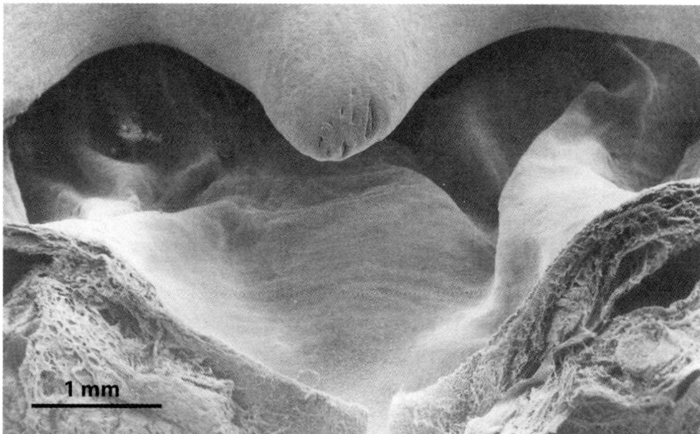


**Fig. 2.3** Scanning electron micrograph of papilla from a rat kidney *(upper center),* illustrating the area cribrosa formed by slit-like openings where the ducts of Bellini terminate. The renal pelvis *(below)* surrounds the papilla.

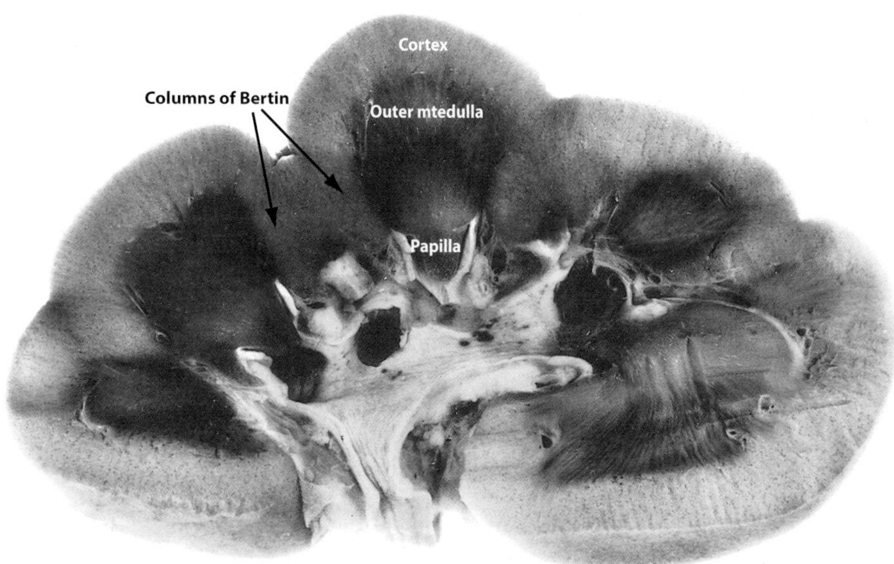


**Fig. 2.2** Bisected kidney from a 4-year-old child demonstrating the difference in appearance between the light-staining cortex and the dark-staining outer medulla. The inner medulla and papillae are less dense than the outer medulla. The columns of Bertin can be seen extending downward to separate the papillae.

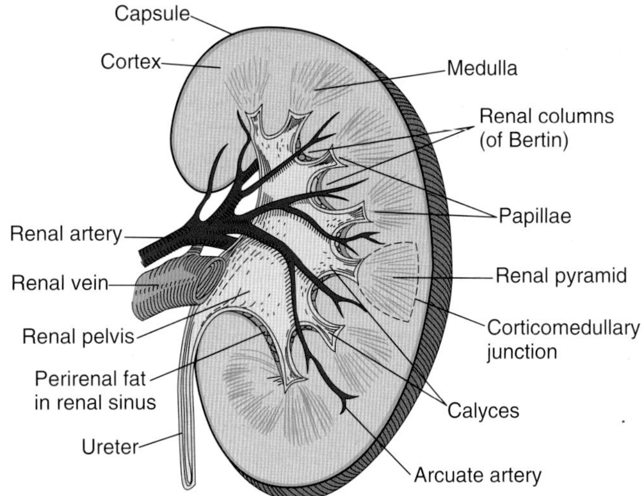


**Fig. 2.4** Diagram of the cut surface of a bisected kidney, depicting important anatomic structures.

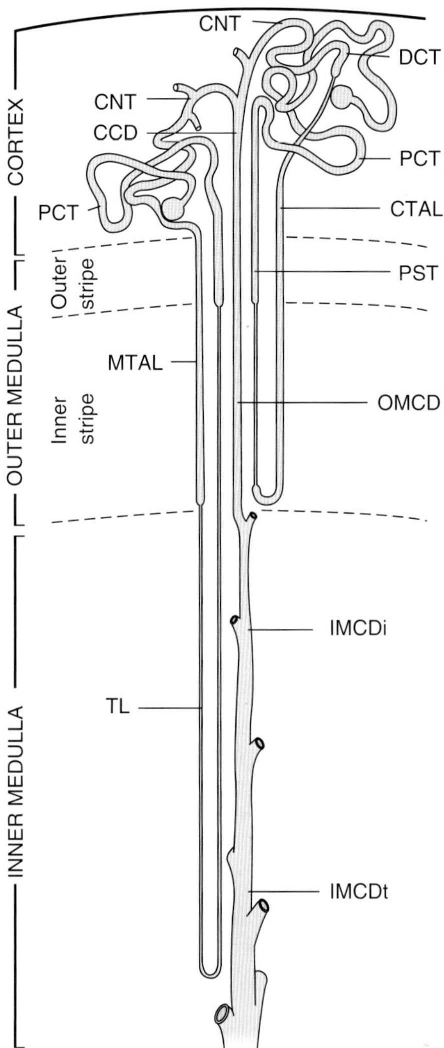


**Fig. 2.5** Diagram illustrating superficial and juxtamedullary nephron. *CCD*, Cortical collecting duct; *CNT*, connecting tubule; *CTAL*, cortical thick ascending limb; *DCT*, distal convoluted tubule; *IMCDi*, initial inner medullary collecting duct; *IMCDt*, terminal inner medullary collecting duct; *MTAL*, medullary thick ascending limb; *OMCD*, outer medullary collecting duct; *PCT*, proximal convoluted tubule; *PST*, proximal straight tubule; *TL*, thin limb of loop of Henle. (Modified from Madsen KM, Tisher CC. Structural-functional relationship along the distal nephron. *Am J Physiol.* 1986;250:F1–F15.)

blastema.[10] The collecting duct system, which includes the initial collecting tubule (ICT), the cortical collecting duct (CCD), the outer medullary collecting duct (OMCD), and the inner medullary collecting duct (IMCD), is not considered part of the nephron because it has a different embryonic origin, the ureteric bud, multiple nephrons merge into the system, and the collecting duct was formerly considered simply a conduit for the tubule fluid. Thus, the collecting duct classically has not been included as a component of an individual functional unit. Nonetheless, the collecting ducts make critical contributions to renal function and the components of the nephron and the collecting duct system are functionally interrelated.

The various tubule segments are composed of structurally distinct epithelial cells along a basement membrane that faces the interstitium on the blood side of the cell. A tubule lumen is formed at the apical side of the cell, which contains the glomerular filtrate that is modified by transport processes to ultimately produce urine. With the exception of intercalated cells and the IMCD cell in the terminal portion of the IMCD, all epithelial cells in the renal tubules and glomeruli contain a single cilium that extends into the tubule lumen or Bowman's space. Many epithelial cells of the renal tubules exhibit significant structural alterations in response to physiologic stimuli, such as changes in cell size, the complexity of the plasma membrane compartments, the abundance of cytoplasmic vesicles, and the abundance and appearance of lysosomes and multivesicular bodies. As such, the specific descriptions of epithelial cell ultrastructure that follow are based on observations of the cells under basal conditions, with added examples of structural alterations induced by changes in diet or physiologic stimuli.

Individual nephrons are classified as superficial, midcortical, and juxtamedullary, based on the position of the glomerulus in the cortex. These typically have differences in the length of loop of Henle and are subject to variations in blood supply under different physiologic states. The loop of Henle contains the straight portion of the proximal tubule (pars recta), descending and ascending thin limb segments, and the straight portion of the distal tubule (TAL, or pars recta) (see Fig. 2.5). The length of the loop of Henle is generally related to the position of its parent glomerulus in the cortex. Most nephrons originating from superficial and midcortical locations have shorter loops of Henle that bend within the inner stripe of the outer medulla close to the inner medulla; these nephrons have no, or very short, ascending thin limbs, as the hairpin turn connects descending thin limb to TAL. A few species, including humans, also possess cortical nephrons with extremely short loops that never enter the medulla but turn back within the cortex.[11] Juxtamedullary nephrons have long loops of Henle with long descending and ascending thin limb segments that extend into the inner medulla. Many variations exist, however, between the two basic types of nephrons, depending on their relative positions in the cortex. The ratio of long- and short-loop nephrons varies among species. Humans and rodents have more short-looped than long-looped nephrons.[12–16] Renal tubules that are located on the surface of the renal cortex, where they are accessible for micropuncture experiments, belong almost exclusively to superficial, hence short-looped, nephrons.

The medulla is divided into inner and outer regions; the outer medulla is subdivided into inner and outer stripes (Figs. 2.5 and 2.6). These distinctions are based on the populations of specific renal tubule segments. The inner medulla is easily distinguished from the outer medulla by the absence of TALs. There is a distinct border between the two regions, visible in histologic sections, where the thin ascending limbs make an abrupt transition to TALs (Fig. 2.6). The inner medulla contains both descending and ascending thin limbs and collecting ducts, but no TALs. In the outer medulla, the inner and outer stripes are easily distinguished by the presence of proximal tubules in the outer stripe and their absence in the inner stripe; the border is marked by the abrupt transition from proximal straight tubules (PSTs) to descending thin limbs (Fig. 2.6). Thus, the inner stripe contains TALs, descending thin limbs, and collecting ducts, but no proximal tubules. The outer stripe contains the terminal portion of PSTs, TALs, and collecting ducts. By contrast, the renal cortex contains the glomeruli, both convoluted and PSTs, TALs, distal convoluted tubules (DCTs), CNTs, and collecting ducts, but not thin limbs of loop of Henle.

## GLOMERULUS

The nephron begins with the glomerulus, which is composed of a capillary network lined by a thin layer of endothelial cells, a central region of mesangial cells with surrounding matrix material, and the visceral epithelial cells (podocytes) overlying the capillaries (Figs. 2.7–2.10). The parietal layer of Bowman's capsule with its basement membrane encases the glomerulus. Bowman's space, or the urinary space, is the cavity between the visceral and parietal epithelia. Although "renal corpuscle" is strictly the correct terminology to refer to the glomerulus and Bowman's capsule, glomerulus is used throughout this chapter because of its common use. At the vascular pole, where the afferent and efferent arterioles enter and exit the glomerulus, the visceral epithelium is continuous with the parietal epithelium. The parietal epithelium transitions to proximal tubule epithelium at or near the urinary pole. The average diameter of a glomerulus is approximately 200 μm in the human kidney and 120 μm in the rat kidney. However, the size and number of glomeruli vary significantly with age, gender, birth weight, and renal health. The average glomerular volume is 0.6 to 1 million $\mu m^3$ in rats[7,8] and 3 to 7 million $\mu m^3$ in humans,[3,4,6] although individual glomerular volume within single human kidneys can vary as much as eightfold.[5] Rat juxtamedullary glomeruli are larger than superficial glomeruli; this is not the case in the human kidney.[17]

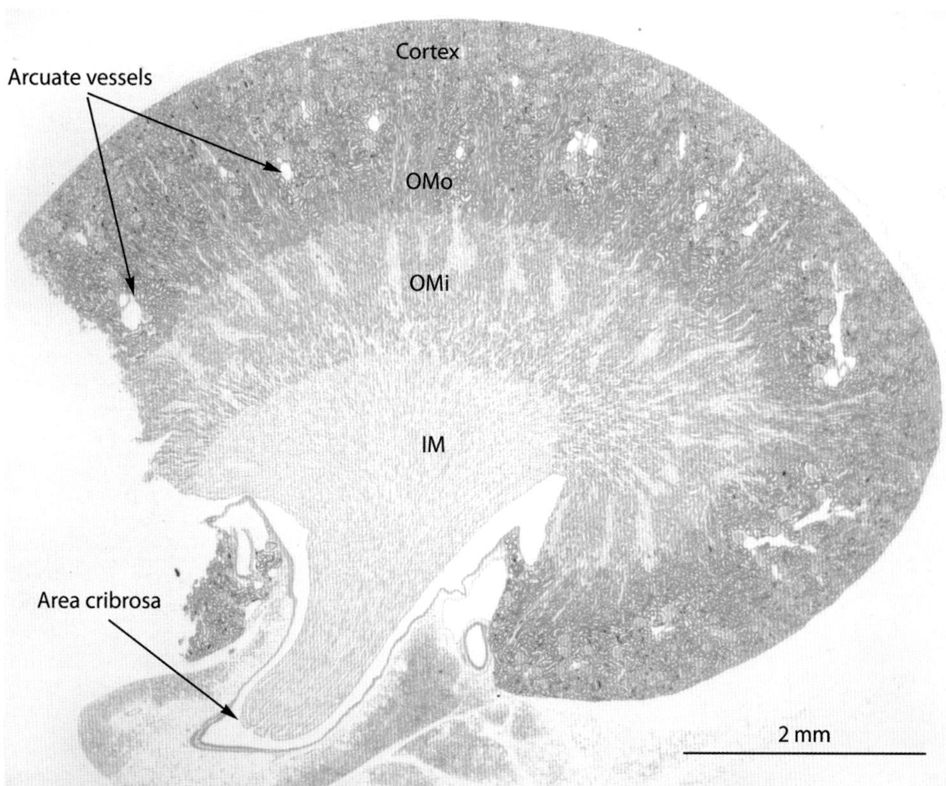


**Fig. 2.6** Light micrograph of a sagittal section of normal mouse kidney. The renal cortex is the region between the arcuate vessels and the renal capsule. The borders between the outer stripe of the outer medulla *(OMo)*, inner stripe or the outer medulla *(OMi)*, and inner medulla *(IM)* are easily distinguished by the changes in the staining intensity. The OMo, which contains proximal tubules, has a similar staining intensity as the cortex. OMi by comparison, has paler staining due to the absence of proximal tubules. IM stains even more weakly due to the absence of thick ascending limbs in this region. The tip of the papilla, identified by the area cribrosa, extends into the proximal ureter in mouse kidneys. Hematoxylin and eosin stain.

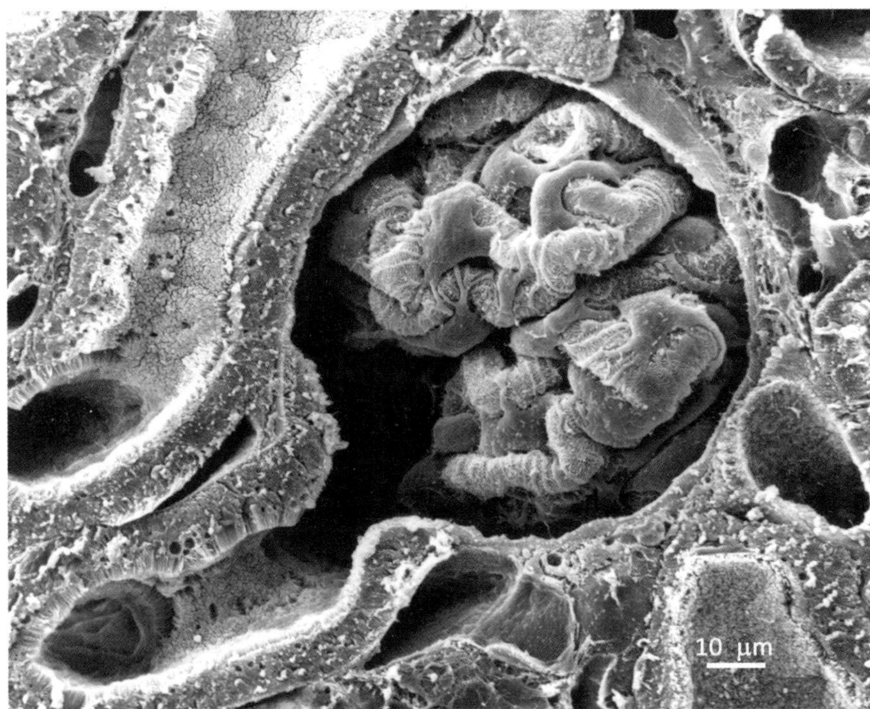


**Fig. 2.7** Scanning electron micrograph of a rat glomerulus. The glomerular tuft is encased by Bowman's capsule. Podocytes, with their interdigitating foot processes, cover the capillaries. The glomerular filtrate drains into the proximal tubule at the urinary pole. (From Sands JM, Verlander JW. Functional anatomy of the kidney. In: McQueen C, ed. *Comprehensive Toxicology,* 3rd ed. St. Louis: Elsevier; 2017.)

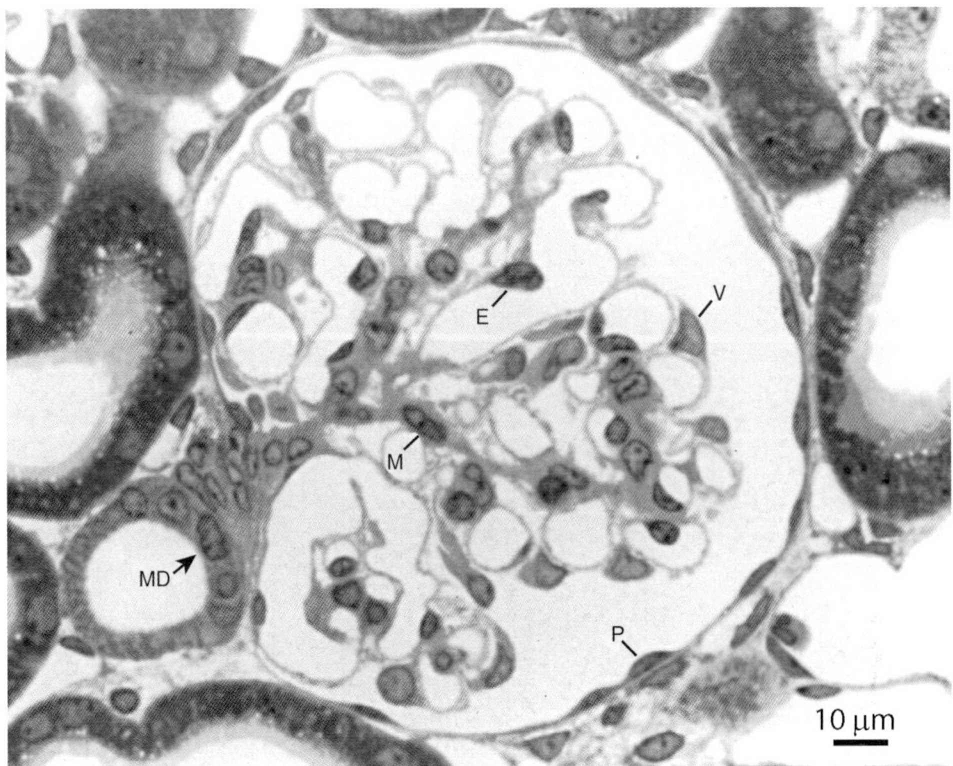


**Fig. 2.8** Light micrograph of a normal glomerulus from a rat, demonstrating the four major cellular components: endothelial cell *(E)*, mesangial cell *(M)*, parietal epithelial cell *(P)*, and visceral epithelial cell or podocyte *(V)*. The macula densa *(MD)* is located in the thick ascending limb at the vascular pole.

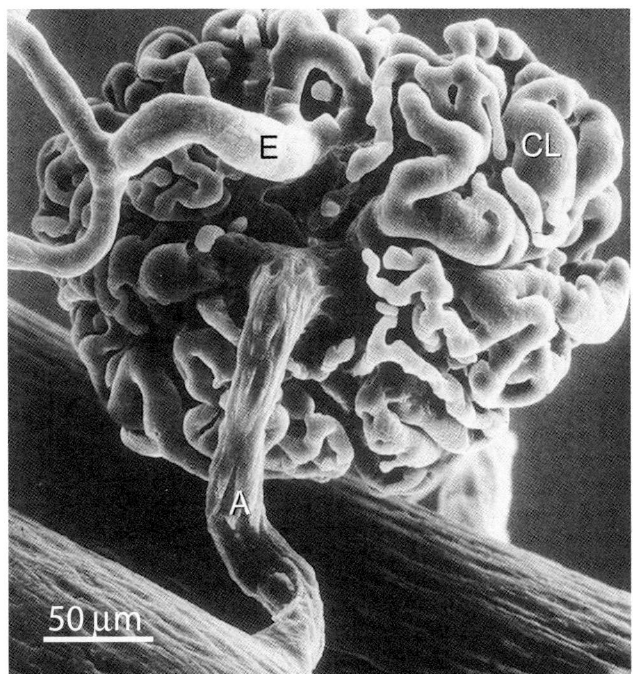


**Fig. 2.9** Scanning electron micrograph of a cast of a glomerulus with its many capillary loops *(CL)* and adjacent renal vessels. The afferent arteriole *(A)* takes its origin from an interlobular artery at lower left. The efferent arteriole *(E)* branches to form the peritubular capillary plexus *(upper left)*. (Courtesy Waykin Nopanitaya, PhD.)

The main function of the glomerulus is filtration of the plasma. The layers of the glomerular capillary wall, the fenestrated capillary endothelium, the glomerular basement membrane (GBM), and the filtration slit diaphragm between the foot processes of the visceral epithelial cells form the filtration barrier between the blood and the urinary space (Fig. 2.11). To cross the capillary wall, a molecule must pass sequentially through the fenestrated endothelium, the GBM, and the filtration slit diaphragm. Although the glomerular capillary wall allows passage of small molecules, the prevailing view is that it normally restricts the passage of cells and larger molecules, such as albumin, due to its size- and charge-selective properties.[18]

## ENDOTHELIAL CELLS

The glomerular capillaries are lined by a thin fenestrated endothelium (Figs. 2.11 and 2.12). These endothelial cells form the initial barrier to the passage of blood constituents from the capillary lumen to Bowman's space. Under normal conditions, the formed elements of the blood, including erythrocytes, leukocytes, and platelets, do not gain access to the subendothelial space.

The endothelial cell nucleus lies adjacent to the mesangium, with the remainder of the cell irregularly attenuated around the capillary lumen (see Fig. 2.10). The endothelium contains pores or fenestrae that range from 70 to 100 nm in diameter in human (see Figs. 2.11 and 2.12).[19] Nonfenestrated,

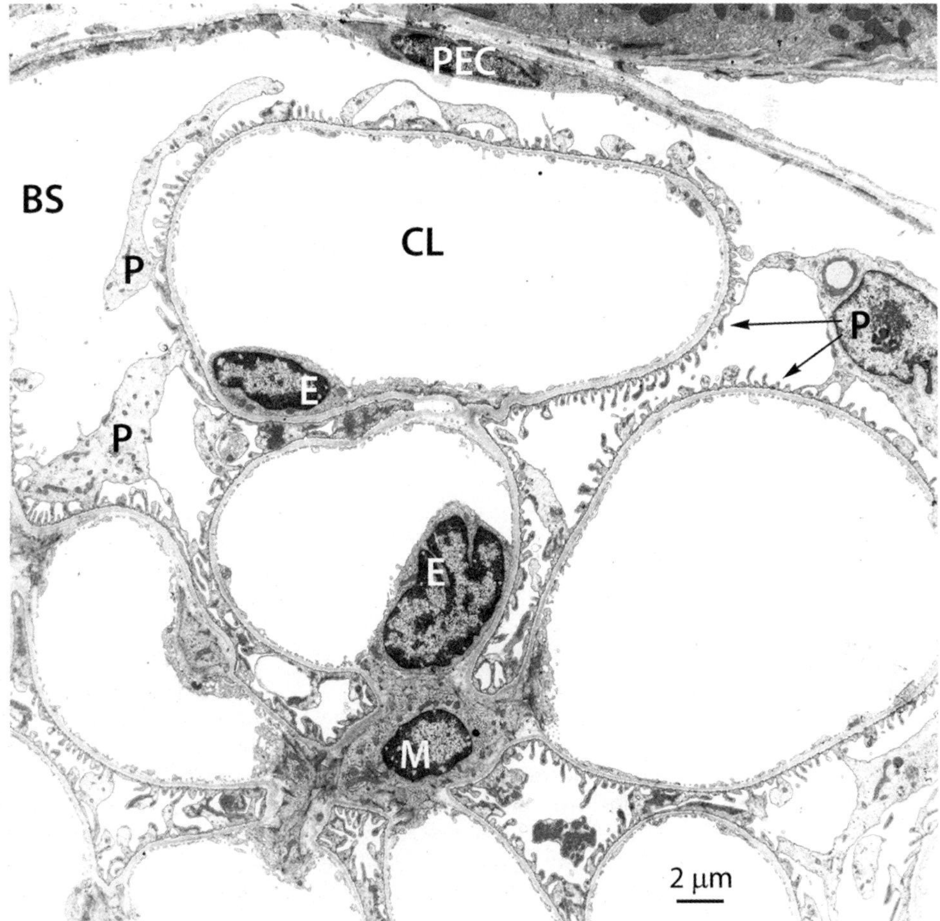


**Fig. 2.10** Transmission electron micrograph of a normal rat glomerulus. The capillary loops are lined by fenestrated endothelial cells *(E)*, facing the capillary lumen *(CL)*. Mesangial cells *(M)* lie beneath the endothelial cells, among the capillary loops. Podocytes *(P)* and their extensive, interdigitating primary and secondary foot processes *(arrows)*, cover the surface of the capillaries, facing the glomerular filtrate in Bowman's space *(BS)*. Parietal epithelial cells *(PEC)* line Bowman's capsule facing Bowman's space.

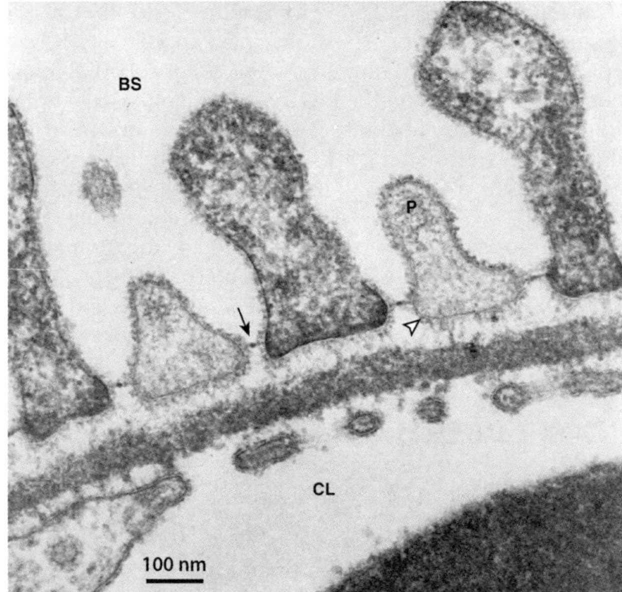


**Fig. 2.11** Transmission electron micrograph of normal rat glomerular capillary wall fixed in a 1% glutaraldehyde solution containing tannic acid. Note the relationship among the three layers of the glomerular basement membrane and the presence of the pedicels *(P)* embedded in the lamina rara externa *(arrowhead)*. The filtration slit diaphragm with the central dense spot *(thin arrow)* is especially evident between the individual pedicels. The fenestrated endothelial lining of the capillary loop is shown below the basement membrane. A portion of an erythrocyte is located in the extreme lower right corner. *BS*, Bowman's space; *CL*, capillary lumen.

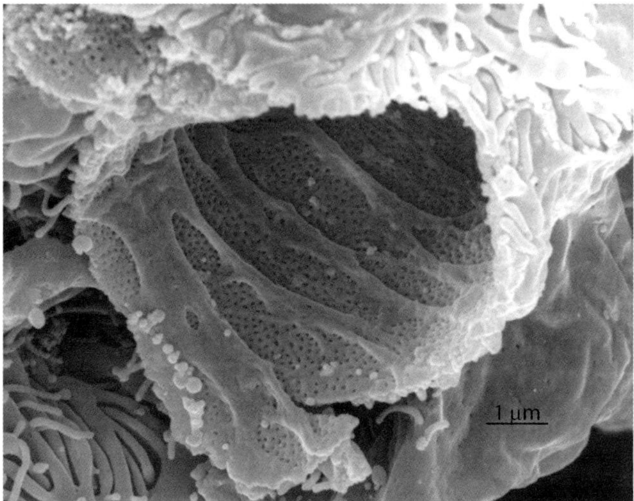


**Fig. 2.12** Scanning electron micrograph of a glomerular capillary from the kidney of a normal rat. Numerous endothelial pores, or fenestrae, are present in the endothelial cells lining the capillary lumen. The ridgelike structures are localized thickenings of the endothelial cells. Interdigitating foot processes of the podocytes cover the urinary side of the capillaries.

ridgelike structures termed "cytofolds" are found near the cell borders. An extensive network of intermediate filaments and microtubules is present in the endothelial cells, and microfilaments surround the fenestrations.[20] Most studies indicate adult glomerular endothelial cells lack diaphragms across the fenestrae, whereas diaphragmed fenestrae are present in the embryo, where they may compensate for the functional immaturity of the embryonic glomerular filtration barrier.[21] The glomerular endothelium is covered by a glycocalyx layer, the visualization of which requires special methods such as electron microscopy with cationic dyes or lipid particles.[22–24] The glycocalyx also fills the endothelial fenestrae forming "sieve plugs," the exact function of which is unknown.[25] The glycocalyx consists of membrane-bound proteoglycans (syndecan and glypican) with attached glycosaminoglycans (GAGs), secreted glycoproteins (perlecan and versican), and secreted GAGs (hyaluronan), which provide a negative charge.[26]

Classic ultrastructural studies demonstrated that endogenous albumin is largely confined to the glomerular capillary lumen and does not pass through the endothelium.[27] In recent years, more studies have addressed the potential role of the glomerular endothelium, and particularly its glycocalyx, in filtration. Studies in rats showed that eluting molecular components of the glomerular endothelial glycocalyx with hypertonic sodium chloride induced a 12-fold increase in proteinuria.[28] Injection of hyaluronidase, a hyaluronan-degrading enzyme, in mice led to disruption of the glomerular endothelial glycocalyx and leakage of albumin across the endothelium.[29] Using isolated human and rodent glomeruli, enzymatic disruption of the glomerular endothelial glycocalyx resulted in increased glomerular albumin permeability.[30] Thus, experimental evidence supports that the glomerular endothelial glycocalyx is an important component of the filtration barrier.

Signaling between glomerular cells is critical for the development and maintenance of the filtration barrier.[31] The surfaces of glomerular endothelial cells express receptors for the vascular endothelial growth factor (VEGF) family.[32] VEGF is synthesized by podocytes (glomerular visceral epithelial cells) and is an important regulator of microvascular permeability.[32,33] VEGF increases endothelial cell permeability and induces the formation of endothelial fenestrations.[34,35] VEGF-A is the best characterized podocyte growth factor, and its principal receptor is VEGFR2, expressed on endothelial cells. Podocyte-specific alterations of VEGF-A have demonstrated that it is required for normal differentiation of glomerular endothelial cells.[36,37] Moreover, drug inhibition of VEGF-A in patients or podocyte-specific deletion of VEGF-A in adult mice results in severe glomerular endothelial injury and thrombotic microangiopathy.[38] Thus, VEGF produced by podocytes plays a critical role in the differentiation and maintenance of glomerular endothelial cells and is an important regulator of endothelial cell permeability.

Several other cell–cell communication pathways exist between glomerular cells. For example, angiopoietin–TIE signaling regulates endothelial homeostasis in an intricate manner.[31] Angiopoietin-1 (ANGPT1) produced in podocytes binds to endothelial-expressed tyrosine kinase receptor TIE2, the phosphorylation of which promotes endothelial survival. In contrast, angiopoietin-2 secreted by endothelial cells is an antagonist of ANGPT1-mediated TIE2 activation in endothelial cells.

## GLOMERULAR BASEMENT MEMBRANE

By transmission electron microscopy, the GBM is composed of a central dense layer, the lamina densa, and two thinner, more electron-lucent layers, the lamina rara externa and the lamina rara interna (see Fig. 2.11). The latter two layers measure approximately 20 to 40 nm in thickness.[19] Although in the rat the width of the GBM has been found to be 132 nm,[39] the width of the human GBM has consistently been reported to be more than 300 nm[40,41] with a slightly thicker basement membrane in men (373 nm) than in women (326 nm).[42] Compared with other basement membranes, the GBM is thicker, likely at least in part from fusion of endothelial and epithelial basement membranes during development.[43] Mass spectrometry–based proteomic analysis has revealed at least 212 proteins in the normal human glomerular extracellular matrix; however, like other basement membranes in the body, the GBM is composed primarily of type IV collagen, laminin, nidogen (entactin), and heparan sulfate proteoglycans (HSPGs).[44–49]

Type IV collagen consists of six chains, α1(IV) through α6(IV). Three α(IV) chains self-associate intracellularly to form triple helical molecules called protomers. Three types of promoters are formed: α1α2α1, α3α4α5, and α5α6α5. Upon secretion into the extracellular space, the protomers self-associate via their amino- and carboxy-terminal domains to form polymerized networks. Three sets of collagen IV networks form: α1α2α1(IV)-α1α2α1(IV), α3α4α5(IV)-α3α4α5(IV), and α1α2α1(IV)-α5α6α5(IV). The networks undergo specific extracellular modifications to form an elaborate scaffold that tethers other molecules, serve as a cell-signaling interface, and provide support for adjacent cells.[50] Halogens facilitate the assembly of the collagen IV scaffold. For example, extracellular chloride ions activate a molecular switch that enables individual promoter carboxy domains to oligomerize,[51] and ionic bromide is essential for enzymatic cross-linking to stabilize the protomer–protomer connections.[52] The α3α4α5(IV)-α3α4α5(IV) network predominates in the GBM, whereas the α1α2α1(IV)-α5α6α5(IV) network is in Bowman's capsule. Whereas α1α2α1(IV) protomers are synthesized from both endothelial cells and podocytes, α3α4α5(IV) protomers are secreted only by podocytes.[53] Mutations in the genes encoding α3, α4, and α5(IV) chains cause Alport syndrome, and autoantibodies against the carboxy terminal a3(IV) chain are responsible for anti-GBM disease.[54]

Laminins (LMs) are large heterotrimeric glycoproteins composed of three chains; α, β, and γ. The major laminin in the adult GBM is LM-521 (containing the α5, β2, and γ1 chains). Both glomerular endothelial cells and podocytes synthesize laminin α5 and β2.[55] Mutations of laminin β2 result in a congenital nephrotic syndrome called Pierson syndrome in humans.[56]

Nidogens, also known as entactins, are glycoproteins. Nidogen-1 binds to both collagen IV and laminin but does not appear essential for GBM formation.[57] HSPGs consist of a core protein linked to sulfated GAG side chains. Agrin, perlecan, and type XVIII collagen are HSPGs found in the GBM.[58] Agrin is the major HSPG in the GBM, whereas perlecan and type XVIII collagen are found mainly in the mesangium.

Subdiffraction resolution stochastic optical reconstruction microscopy has provided a precise view of the nanoscale organization of these molecular networks within the GBM.[59] The α3α4α5(IV) network localizes to the center of the GBM, whereas the α1α2α1(IV) network maps near the endothelial side of the GBM. Laminin-521 is situated in two layers near the endothelial and podocyte sides of the GBM and also in the central portion of the GBM. Agrin localizes in two layers along the endothelial and podocyte surfaces of the GBM, with more detected near the podocytes.

The contribution of the GBM to the glomerular filtration barrier has been studied for decades.[60,61] Ultrastructural tracer studies provided evidence to suggest that the GBM constitutes both a size-selective and a charge-selective barrier.[62–64] Additional studies revealed a lattice of anionic sites with a spacing between them of approximately 60 nm (Fig. 2.13) throughout the lamina rara interna and lamina rara externa.[65,66] The anionic sites in the GBM consist of heparan sulfate GAG side chains of the proteoglycans rich in heparan sulfate.[67,68] Removal of the heparan sulfate side chains by enzymatic digestion resulted in an increase in the in vitro permeability of the GBM to ferritin[69] and to bovine serum albumin,[70] suggesting that HSPGs play a role in establishing the permeability properties of the GBM to plasma proteins (see Fig. 2.13). However, in vivo studies have addressed the role of proteoglycans and charge selectivity in the GBM. Overexpression of heparanase in transgenic mice led to a fivefold reduction in GAG-associated sites in the GBM but no proteinuria.[71] Moreover, podocyte-specific deletion of agrin alone or in combination with deletion of perlecan heparan sulfate side chains in mice resulted in a dramatic reduction in GBM anionic sites but did not alter the filtration barrier to albumin or a negatively charged tracer.[72,73] Thus, more recent data suggest the role of GBM anionic charge, at least that contributed by proteoglycans, is minimal in the function of the glomerular filtration barrier.

Nevertheless, a variety of genetic findings in humans and studies in mice indicate that an intact GBM serves a barrier function to protein permeability. The absence of an intact α3α4α5(IV) network in the GBM of Alport syndrome eventually results in proteinuria. In humans and animal models of Alport syndrome, there is a compensatory increase in the α1α2α1(IV) network, laminin α5 chain, and ectopic laminin isoforms (α1, α2, and β1 chains) in the defective GBM.[74,75] These secondary changes alter cell matrix signaling, are accompanied by characteristic splitting and "basket-weave" lamellation of the GBM, and produce proteinuria.

Strong evidence for a specific role of the GBM in the filtration barrier is the presence of laminin β2 mutations in humans or mice resulting in massive proteinuria.[76,77] Laminin-β2–deficient (*Lamb2*$^{-/-}$) mice develop severe proteinuria and ectopic laminin chains (α1,α2,α3, β3, and γ2) that accumulate in the GBM, but this ectopic deposition fails to compensate for the absence of laminin β2.[78] Importantly, the albuminuria in the mice precedes podocyte foot process effacement and filtration slit diaphragm abnormalities, indicating the GBM has an essential role in the filtration barrier. Remarkably, injection of recombinant human LM-521 accumulates in the correct orientation in the GBM and delays the onset of proteinuria in *Lamb2*$^{-/-}$ mice, which lack LM-521.[79]

## PODOCYTES

Podocytes (visceral epithelial cells) are the largest cells in the glomerulus and are positioned on the outside of the glomerular capillary wall (see Figs. 2.7, 2.10–2.12, and 2.14). Mature podocytes are terminally differentiated and generally

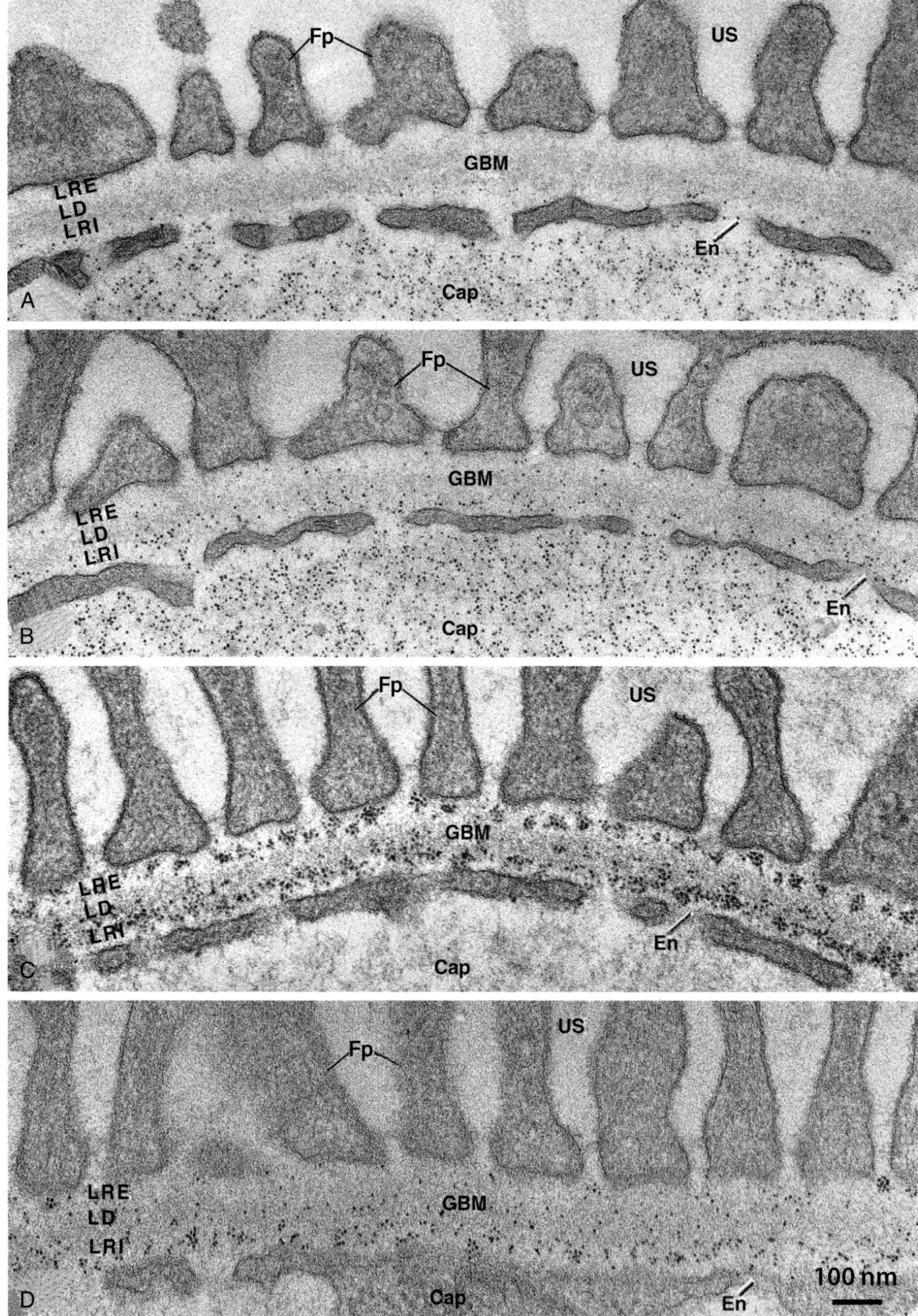


**Fig. 2.13** Transmission electron micrographs of the glomerular filtration barrier in normal rats perfused with native anionic ferritin (A) or cationic ferritin (C) and in rats treated with heparitinase before perfusion with anionic (B) or cationic ferritin (D). In normal animals, anionic ferritin is present in the capillary *(Cap)* but does not enter the glomerular basement membrane *(GBM)*, as shown in (A). In contrast, cationic ferritin binds to the negatively charged sites in the lamina rara interna *(LRI)* and lamina rara externa *(LRE)* of the GBM (see C). After treatment with heparitinase, both anionic (B) and cationic (D) ferritin penetrate into the GBM, but there is no labeling of negatively charged sites by cationic ferritin. *En*, Endothelial fenestrae; *Fp*, foot processes; *LD*, lamina densa; *US*, urinary space. (Modified from Kanwar YS. Biophysiology of glomerular filtration and proteinuria. *Lab Invest.* 1984;51:7–21.)

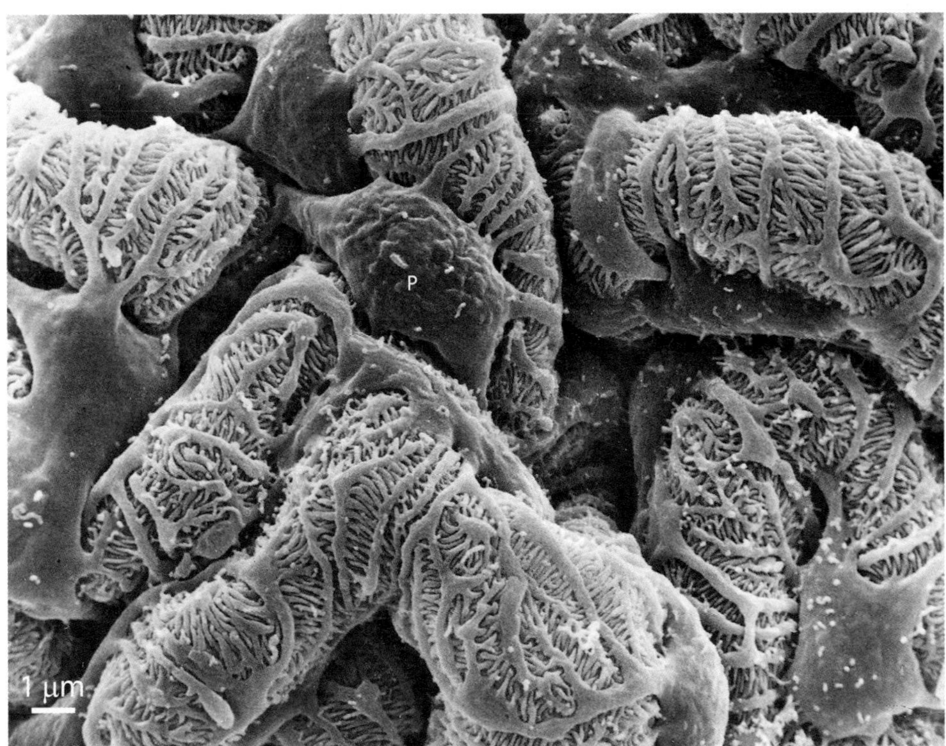


**Fig. 2.14** Scanning electron micrograph of a glomerulus from the kidney of a normal rat. The visceral epithelial cells, or podocytes *(P)*, extend multiple processes outward from the main cell body to wrap around individual capillary loops. Immediately adjacent pedicels, or foot processes, arise from different podocytes.

do not replicate. They have a prominent cell body containing nuclei, endoplasmic reticulum, Golgi apparatus, and an endocytic–lysosomal system. The cell bodies give rise to long cytoplasmic primary processes that branch into secondary and tertiary processes, surround the capillaries, and finally divide into foot processes. The foot processes come into direct contact with the lamina rara externa of the GBM (see Figs. 2.11 and 2.13). By scanning electron microscopy (SEM), it is apparent that adjacent foot processes are derived from different podocytes (Fig. 2.14). The gap between adjacent foot processes is bridged by a thin structure called the "filtration slit diaphragm." Advanced techniques, including serial block-face SEM (SBF-SEM) and focused ion beam SEM (FIB-SEM), show that foot processes emerge directly from the podocyte cell body as well as the elongated cytoplasmic processes.[80,81] These studies reveal tortuous ridgelike prominences along the basal surface of the cell body and the cytoplasmic processes, from which the proximal portions of the foot processes emerge.

A series of studies using three-dimensional (3D) electron microscopic reconstruction and SBF-SEM have supported the existence of a subpodocyte space (SPS) under the podocyte cell body and a narrow interpodocyte space, which interconnects the SPS with the peripheral Bowman's space.[82,83] Whether these spaces act as a resistance pathway across the filtration barrier remains to be determined.

Podocytes have an elaborate cytoskeleton that underlies their shape, stability, adhesion, and response to stress.[84] Large numbers of microtubules and intermediate filaments (vimentin) are present in the cell body and primary processes,[85] whereas actin filaments are especially abundant in the foot processes.[86] Ultrastructural studies have demonstrated two distinct actin filament networks in foot processes of rat podocytes.[87,88] "Actin bundles," containing α-actinin and synaptopodin, extend along the longitudinal axis of the foot processes above the level of the slit diaphragm. The cortical actin network, containing cortactin, lies between the actin bundle and the plasma membrane. In glomerular diseases associated with proteinuria, the podocyte cytoskeleton is disrupted, slit diaphragms are lost, and the interdigitating foot processes are replaced by broad regions of podocyte processes covering the GBM.[89] This "foot process effacement" is often accompanied by aggregated filaments appearing as a cytoplasmic mat juxtaposed to the GBM.

Actin fibers are composed of bundles of actin filaments. Both contractile and noncontractile actin fibers are present in most cells, and the former (actin stress fibers) are characterized by periodic alternating bands of α-actinin and myosin.[90] Studies using superresolution microscopic methods have revealed a detailed model of the podocyte actin cytoskeleton in both mice and humans.[91] Actin fibers in the center of the foot process contain α-actinin and synaptopodin but lack myosin IIA, whereas actin fibers in the podocyte cell body and primary processes contain myosin IIA but lack synaptopodin. These findings suggest the actin fibers in the foot process are noncontractile, whereas the actin fibers in the cell body and primary processes are contractile. In podocyte injury models with foot process effacement and proteinuria, myosin IIA translocates to cytoplasm adjacent to the GBM, forming sarcomere-like structures with alternating synaptopodin and α-actinin staining. Thus, podocytes contain distinct actin filament networks that appear to provide tensional integrity (tensegrity) and can redistribute in response to injury.[92]

Foot processes contain two structures, focal adhesions (FAs) and filtration slit diaphragms (SDs), that interact with and control the actin cytoskeleton.[93] FAs anchor the base of the foot processes to the GBM. They consist of transmembrane protein complexes through which the actin cytoskeleton is regulated by extracellular signaling.[94] Cell adhesions rich in integrins and their interacting proteins are known as the "integrin adhesome."[95] FAs are a form of integrin adhesome and, at the foot process–GBM interface, consist of α3β1 integrin and various adaptor proteins, kinases, and phosphatases and guanosine triphosphatases (GTPases). The α3β1 integrin interconnects laminin in the GBM with the talin, paxillin, and vinculin adaptor cytoplasmic complex, which link to the actin cytoskeleton. Mutations of the integrin α3 subunit in humans are associated with massive proteinuria.[96] Podocyte adhesion to the GBM is supported by the interaction of integrin α3β1 with the tetraspanin protein CD151, the absence of which leads to severe proteinuria.[97] FA kinase and integrin-linked kinase localize to FAs and mediate signaling with the actin cytoskeleton.

The Rho family of small GTPases, including RhoA, Rac1, and Cdc42, regulate actin cytoskeleton dynamics.[98] Activation of podocyte RhoA and Rac1 in transgenic mice leads to proteinuria and podocyte foot process effacement.[99–102] In contrast, podocyte deletion of C4dc42 results in proteinuria and foot process effacement.[103,104] Rho GTPases cycle between an active GTP-bound form and an inactive guanosine diphosphate (GDP)-bound form.[105] Rho GTPases are inactivated by GTPase-activating proteins (GAPs), which increase GTP hydrolysis or by guanine nucleotide dissociation inhibitors (GDIs), which sequester their inactive GDP-bound form in the cytoplasm. Mutations in the genes that encode Arhgap24, a GAP, and Arhgdia, a GDI, result in Rac1 activation and proteinuria in humans.[106,107] Moreover, mutations in Kank2 (kidney ankyrin repeat-containing protein), an *Arhgdia*-interacting protein that localizes to FAs, leads to RhoA activation and proteinuria.[108] Dynamin is a large GTPase that has a role in clathrin-mediated endocytosis but also directly binds actin filaments and promotes actin polymerization.[109] Dynamin regulates FA maturation in podocytes in vitro, and its conditional deletion in mouse podocytes results in foot process effacement and severe proteinuria.[110,111] These studies suggest dynamin serves as a molecular link between endocytosis and actin remodeling in podocytes. Thus, an intricate physiologic balance of the various GTPases is required for normal podocyte homeostasis.

The filtration SD is the second structure that controls the actin cytoskeleton. It appears as a thin line on electron microscopy (see Fig. 2.11) and bridges the 30–40 nm space (called the filtration slit) between adjacent foot processes. A central dot within the SD may occasionally be seen on ultrastructural cross-sections, and it appears as a continuous central filament on sections parallel to the plane of the GBM (see Fig. 2.15). Based on these observations, Rodewald and Karnovsky proposed a porous zipper-like model for the SD.[112] In this model, there are regularly spaced cross-bridges that extend from the membranes of two adjacent foot processes to a linear central filament that runs equidistant and parallel to the cell membranes. The cross-bridge structures measuring 7 × 14 nm are separated by pores measuring 4 × 40 nm. Advanced microscopy techniques have provided alternative models and insights into the SD structure. Based on a freeze-etching replica ultrastructural method, it was proposed the SD has a sheetlike rather than a zipper-like substructure.[113] Electron microscope tomography showed the SD to consist of a network of winding cross strands, 30–35 nm in length, which merge centrally into a longitudinal density.[114] Although this study generally concurred with the zipper-like model, the pores surrounding the strands appeared more irregular than originally proposed. In contrast, an investigation using enhanced SEM revealed variable-shape pores in the center of the SD and no central filament.[115] This finding is more consistent with the SD as a heteroporous structure rather than the zipper-like model. High-resolution helium-ion SEM studies demonstrate the SD with cross-bridging filaments and surrounding pores forming a ladderlike structure in the middle of the filtration slit, also without a distinct central midline, thus generally supporting the heteroporous model.[116,117] The complexity of the SD is further illustrated by cryo-EM tomographic studies showing distinct cross-bridging strands are composed of different molecules.[118] Bridging shorter strands in the lower part of the SD closest to the GBM consist of the nephrin-related protein, Neph1, whereas longer strands in the top part of the SD toward the apical side contain nephrin. This study supports

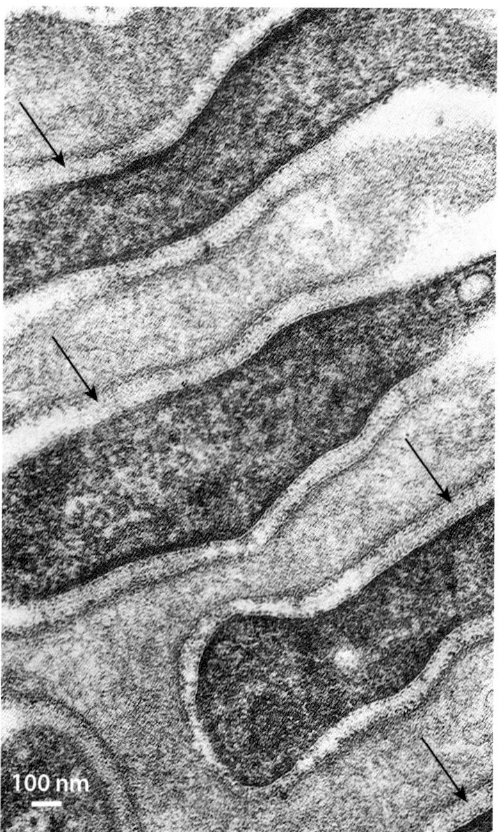


**Fig. 2.15** Electron micrograph showing the epithelial foot processes of normal rat glomerulus preserved in a 1% glutaraldehyde solution containing tannic acid. In several areas, the slit diaphragm has been sectioned parallel to the plane of the basement membrane, revealing a highly organized substructure. The thin central filament corresponding to the central dot observed on cross-section (see Fig. 2.11) is indicated by the arrows.

the existence of a layered bipartite molecular assembly within the SD.

Our understanding of the podocyte role and its SD in the filtration barrier was accelerated with identification of the protein nephrin, encoded by *NPHS1*, the gene mutated in congenital nephrotic syndrome of the Finnish type.[119] Nephrin normally localizes to the SD, and its absence in the human congenital syndrome or in transgenic mice leads to loss of the SD, foot process effacement, and massive proteinuria. The SD area or domain of the podocyte includes the SD itself and the adjacent foot process membrane and cytoplasm. An expanding number of proteins localize to the SD domain, where they interact with nephrin and other partners, forming a multiprotein complex. Mutations in over 30 genes, many of which localize to the SD domain and the podocyte actin cytoskeleton, cause human nephrotic syndrome.[120] For example, mutations or deficiencies of genes encoding SD domain proteins, such as podocin, CD2-associated protein, phospholipase Cε1, and transient receptor potential cation channel type 6, result in SD loss, foot process effacement, and proteinuria. Thus, there is convincing genetic evidence for the essential role of the SD, likely as a size-selective element, in the filtration barrier.

In addition to functioning as a critical structural barrier in filtration, the SD also functions as a signaling hub to regulate actin dynamics.[121] Although the signaling pathways are incompletely understood, nephrin plays a central role. For example, phosphorylation of tyrosine residues within the intracellular domain of nephrin by Fyn kinase results in the recruitment of actin adaptor proteins such as Nck proteins (Nck1 and Nck2), which, in turn, induce actin polymerization.[122,123] Moreover, Nck protein binding to Fyn promotes increased phosphorylation of nephrin.[124] Downstream of its interaction with nephrin, Nck directly binds to and activates the neuronal Wiskott-Aldrich syndrome protein (N-WASP), an actin nucleation protein. N-WASP binds and activates the ubiquitously expressed Arp2/3 multiprotein complex, which induces actin polymerization.[125,126] The importance of this signaling pathway is highlighted by studies showing that intact nephrin phosphorylation and the presence of podocyte Nck and N-WASP proteins are required for an intact filtration barrier of foot processes and stabilization of foot processes.[127–129] There is also increasing evidence that the phosphorylation state of nephrin plays a role in its endocytic trafficking within the podocyte and is important for turnover and maintenance of the SD.[130]

## MESANGIAL CELLS

The mesangial cells and their surrounding matrix constitute the mesangium, which provides a scaffold for the surrounding glomerular capillaries.[19,131,132] The mesangium is separated from the capillary lumens by the endothelium and is surrounded by the GBM between capillary loops (see Figs. 2.8 and 2.10). Thus, the mesangium directly abuts both the endothelium and the GBM. The points where the GBM no longer encircles the capillary and starts to surround the mesangium are called the "mesangial angles." Three-dimensional reconstruction studies reveal continuity of the entire mesangium as a continuous arborizing structure within the glomerulus.[133] Mesangial cells are located within the central axial region of the mesangium and are irregular in shape with a dense nucleus. They have elongated cytoplasmic processes that extend toward the endothelium and the adjacent GBM (paramesangial GBM). At the endothelial interface, the fingerlike mesangial cell processes may extend a short distance into the space between the endothelium and GBM. In certain forms of glomerular injury, the mesangial processes may insinuate between the endothelium and GBM for a noticeable distance along the peripheral capillary wall (mesangial interposition). In addition to the usual complement of organelles, mesangial cells possess an extensive array of microfilaments containing actin, myosin, and α-actinin.[134] The mesangial processes, containing bundles of microfilaments, appear to bridge the gap in the GBM encircling the capillary, adhere to endothelial cells, and interconnect opposing mesangial angles of the GBM. This cell–matrix interconnection is believed to prevent capillary wall distention secondary to elevation of the intracapillary hydraulic pressure.[134–136]

Several studies have elucidated molecules that mediate the interactions between mesangial cells and other glomerular cells and also the GBM.[137] Afadin, an F-actin binding protein, localizes to cell contacts between mesangial and endothelial cells, also colocalizes with β-catenin, and may play a role in mesangial cell migration.[138] Integrin α3β1 and Lu/BCAM are mesangial receptors that mediate adhesion of mesangial cells to the laminin α5 chain in the GBM.[139] An actin cross-linking protein, EPLIN, is highly expressed in mesangial cell processes at the mesangial angles, where they attach to the GBM.[140] Nephronectin, a protein within the GBM, binds to its receptor a8b1 integrin, produced by mesangial cells to form a GBM–mesangial adhesion at the lateral base (near the mesangial angles) of the capillary loops.[141]

The mesangium is continuous with the extraglomerular mesangium, a component of the juxtaglomerular apparatus (JGA). The intraglomerular and extraglomerular cells are similar, and gap junctions exist between them.[142] Cells of renin lineage within the extraglomerular mesangium have been shown to migrate and repopulate the mesangium after glomerular injury.[143]

As proposed by Schlondorff,[144] the mesangial cell may have some specialized features of pericytes and possesses many of the functional properties of smooth muscle cells. In addition to providing structural support for the glomerular capillary loops, the mesangial cell has contractile properties and is thought to play a role in the regulation of glomerular filtration.[144] The local generation of autacoids, such as prostaglandin $E_2$, by the mesangial cell may provide a counterregulatory mechanism to oppose the effect of vasoconstrictors.

Mesangial cells exhibit phagocytic properties and participate in the clearance of macromolecules from the mesangium,[144,145] as evidenced by the uptake of tracers such as ferritin,[131] colloidal carbon,[146] and aggregated proteins.[147] Mesangial cells are also involved in the generation and metabolism of the extracellular mesangial matrix.[144,148] Because of both their distinct anatomic localization and their production of various vasoactive substances (e.g., nitric oxide), growth factors (e.g., VEGF, platelet-derived growth factor [PDGF], transforming growth factor [TGF]), and cytokines and chemokines (interleukins, chemokine [C-X-C motif] ligand 1, chemokine [C-C motif] ligand [CCLs]), mesangial cells are also perfectly suited to mediate an extensive crosstalk to both endothelial cells and podocytes to control and maintain glomerular function.[149] The PDGF-B isoform, the main ligand for the receptor PDGFR-β, is a potent mitogen for mesangial cell proliferation, and genetic deletion of PDGF-B and PDGFR-β results in an absence of mesangial cells and mesangium.[150] As such, the mesangial cells also importantly contribute to a number of glomerular diseases, including IgA nephropathy and diabetic nephropathy.

The mesangial cell is surrounded by a matrix that is similar to but not identical with the GBM; the mesangial matrix is more coarsely fibrillar and slightly less electron dense. The presence of abundant thin microfibrils, best observed with tannic acid staining, likely explains the fibrillary character of the mesangial matrix.[151] Fibrillin-1 is the major protein of the microfibrils, but other associated proteins include microfibril-associated glycoproteins 1 and 2 and latent TGF-binding protein-1.[152,153] Fibrillin-1 and α8 integrin colocalize in the mesangium and appear to interact to regulate mesangial adhesion.[154]

The mesangial matrix also contains fibronectin, type IV collagen α1 and α2 chains (not type IV α3, α4, or α5 chains, which are present in the GBM), type V collagen, various laminin isoforms (not laminin-521, which is present in the GBM), and the proteoglycan perlecan (not the proteoglycan agrin, which is present in the GBM). For example, laminin α1 is present in the mesangial matrix (not the GBM), and studies suggest it regulates mesangial cell homeostasis and matrix deposition by inhibiting TGF-β/Smad pathway signaling.[155] Several cell surface receptors of the β-integrin family have been identified on the mesangial cells, including α1β1, α3β1, and the fibronectin receptor, α5β1.[156–158] These integrins mediate attachment of the mesangial cells to specific molecules in the extracellular mesangial matrix and link the matrix to the cytoskeleton. The attachment to the mesangial matrix is important for cell anchorage, contraction, and migration; ligand–integrin binding also serves as a signal transduction mechanism that regulates the production of extracellular matrix as well as the synthesis of various vasoactive mediators, growth factors, and cytokines.[148,159]

## PARIETAL EPITHELIAL CELLS

The parietal epithelium, which lines the inner aspect of Bowman's capsule, consists of flat squamous-like cells known as PECs (parietal epithelial cells) (Fig. 2.10).[19] At the urinary pole, there is an abrupt transition from the PECs to the taller cuboidal cells of the proximal tubule, which has a well-developed brush border (Fig. 2.16). The PECs are 0.1 to 0.3 μm in height, except at the nucleus, where they increase to 2.0 to 3.5 μm. Each cell has a long cilium, and organelles are generally sparse but include small mitochondria, numerous vesicles of 40 to 90 nm in diameter, and the Golgi apparatus. Large vacuoles and multivesicular bodies are rare. PECs express Pax-2 and claudin-1. The thickness of the basement membrane of Bowman's capsule varies from 1200 to 1500 nm.[19] The basement membrane often has a lamellated appearance and increases in thickness with disease processes. At both the vascular pole and the urinary pole, the thickness of Bowman's capsule decreases markedly. In contrast to the GBM, the basement membrane of the capsule contains the α6 chain of type IV collagen, which is part of the α1α2α1(IV)-α5α6α5(IV) protomer network.

PECs function as a permeability barrier for the urinary filtrate. In experimental glomerulonephritis, this barrier is

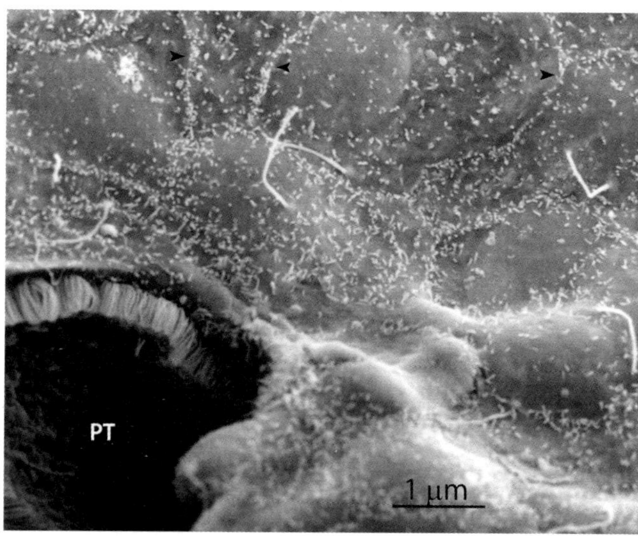


**Fig. 2.16** Scanning electron micrograph showing the surface of the parietal epithelial cells adjacent to the early proximal tubule *(PT)* at the urinary pole. Parietal epithelial cells have single cilia, and their lateral cell margins are accentuated by short microvilli *(arrowheads)*.

compromised, and macromolecules can leak into the space between the PECs and the basement membrane of Bowman's capsule and subsequently into the periglomerular space.[160] Several investigations suggest different populations of PECs exist.[161] Cells located at the glomerular vascular pole interposed between the PECs and podocytes have been called "peripolar cells."[162] By electron microscopy, these cells have prominent cytoplasmic granules, and display an immunophenotype between PECs and podocytes and are currently called "transitional cells."[163,164] Their function is unknown. Other cells lining Bowman's capsule near the vascular pole expressing podocyte markers and forming interdigitating foot processes are called "parietal podocytes" (or "ectopic podocytes").[163,165] In glomerular disease, PECs may transform into cuboidal cells with enlarged nuclei and express CD44.[166] These "activated PECs" demonstrate proliferation, migration, and matrix deposition and play a role in diseases such as focal segmental glomerulosclerosis.

Several studies have addressed the role of PECs as possible progenitor cells to renew podocytes.[167] These various investigations using different experimental mouse models of podocyte depletion and genetic labeling methods have shown that PECs may serve as podocyte progenitor cells, transdifferentiating into podocytes, which repopulate the glomerular tuft.[164,168–170] In some studies of experimental glomerular injury, a subpopulation of podocytes actually migrates to Bowman's capsule and expresses PEC markers.[171–173] An understanding of these bidirectional differentiation pathways involving PECs and podocytes awaits further investigations.

## JUXTAGLOMERULAR APPARATUS

The JGA is located at the vascular pole of the glomerulus, where the TAL of loop of Henle comes into contact with its parent glomerulus. It represents a major structural component of the renin–angiotensin system and contributes to the regulation of glomerular arteriolar resistance and glomerular filtration.[174]

The JGA has vascular and tubular components. The vascular components are the terminal portion of the afferent arteriole, the initial portion of the efferent arteriole, and the extraglomerular mesangium. The tubular component is the macula densa, located in the terminal portion of the TAL that lies between the afferent and efferent arterioles, in contact with the extraglomerular mesagium.[175–177] The extraglomerular mesangium, also called the polar cushion (polkissen) or the lacis, is bounded by the macula densa, the specialized regions of the afferent and efferent glomerular arterioles at their junction with the glomerular tuft, and the mesangial cells of the glomerular tuft (the intraglomerular mesangial cells). Specialized cell types of the JGA include the juxtaglomerular granular cells, the agranular extraglomerular mesangial cells, and the epithelial cells that make up the macula densa.

## JUXTAGLOMERULAR GRANULAR CELLS

The juxtaglomerular granular cells are located primarily in the walls of the afferent and, less commonly, the efferent arterioles.[176–179] They exhibit features of both smooth muscle cells and secretory epithelial cells and therefore have been called epithelioid or myoepithelial cells.[176] They contain myofilaments in the cytoplasm, a well-developed endoplasmic reticulum, and small "protogranules" with a crystalline substructure in the Golgi complex.[176,180] The signature feature of juxtaglomerular cells is the numerous electron-dense, membrane-bound granules of variable size and shape (Fig. 2.17),[179] which contain the aspartyl protease renin.[179,181] In addition to renin granules, lipofuscin-like granules are common in juxtaglomerular cells in the human kidney, as well as in extraglomerular mesangial cells.[178,180]

In addition to renin, the juxtaglomerular granular cells express angiotensin II, which localizes in the same granules as renin [179] and has highest activity in the afferent arteriole.[182] Like lysosomes, renin-containing granules have an acid pH and contain lysosomal enzymes, including acid phosphatases and cathepsin B, and have the capacity to take up and degrade internalized material.[142,179,183] During kidney development, renin expression is present in the intrarenal arteries, but by adulthood in normal conditions, renin granules are largely found only in juxtaglomerular granular cells in the distal afferent arteriole.[184] Nonetheless, in adults, renin expression may again extend into more proximal arterial portions in some conditions, such as extravascular volume depletion, hypotension, and hemorrhage.[185–187]

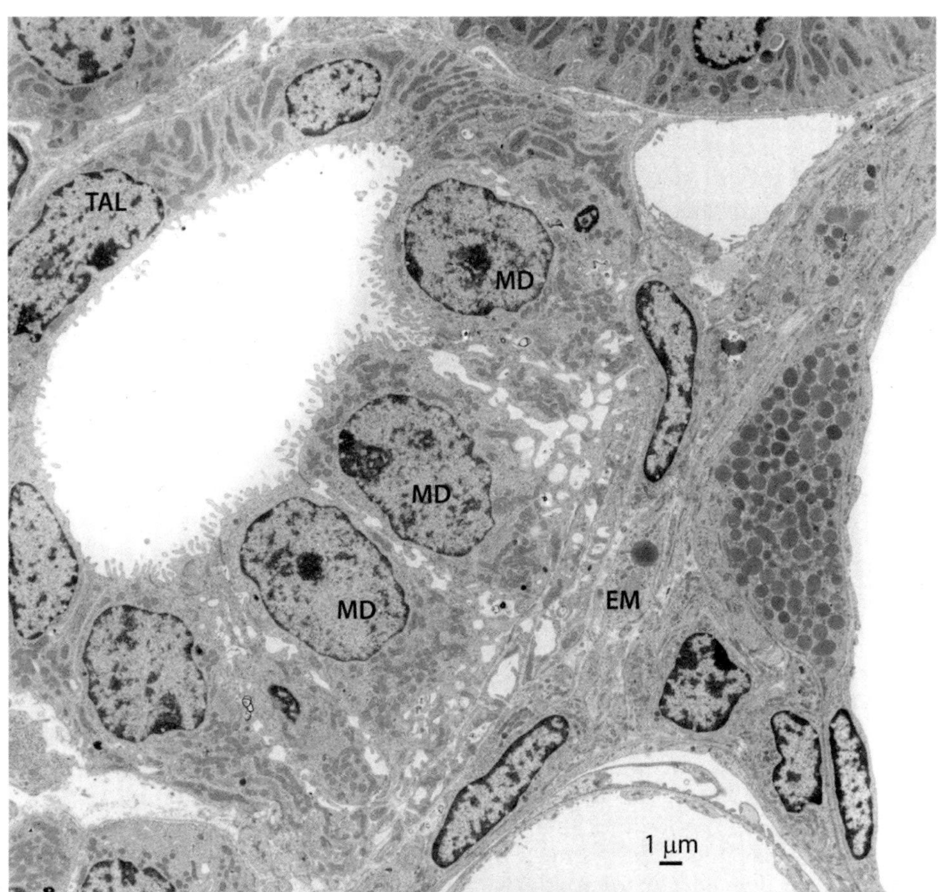


**Fig. 2.17** Transmission electron micrograph of juxtaglomerular apparatus from a rabbit kidney, illustrating macula densa *(MD)*, extraglomerular mesangium *(EM)*, and a portion of an arteriole *(on the right)*, containing numerous electron-dense granules. Macula densa cells are significantly taller and narrower than the adjacent thick ascending limb *(TAL)* cells.

## EXTRAGLOMERULAR MESANGIUM

Located between the afferent and efferent arterioles in close contact with the macula densa (see Fig. 2.17), the extraglomerular mesangium is continuous with the intraglomerular mesangium and is composed of cells that are similar in ultrastructure to the mesangial cells.[176,177] The extraglomerular mesangial cells possess long, thin cytoplasmic processes separated by basement membrane material. Although not typical, extraglomerular mesangial cells occasionally contain renin granules. The extraglomerular mesangial cells are in contact with the afferent and efferent arterioles and the macula densa, and gap junctions are commonly observed between the various cells of the vascular portion of the JGA.[142,188] Gap junctions, formed at least in part from connexin 40,[189] exist between extraglomerular and intraglomerular mesangial cells, enabling signaling to be conveyed from the macula densa through the extraglomerular mesangium to the glomerulus.[142,190] Moreover, there is evidence that altered gap junction structure and function may eliminate the tubuloglomerular feedback response.[190,191]

## MACULA DENSA

The macula densa is a specialized region in the TAL adjacent to the hilum of the parent glomerulus (see Figs. 2.8 and 2.17). Macula densa cells are morphologically distinct from the surrounding cells of the TAL. They are columnar cells with large, apically placed nuclei, although there are considerable species differences in the height of macula densa cells. Compared with TAL cells, macula densa cells have relatively little cytoplasm, few basolateral plasma membrane infoldings, and lower mitochondrial density; mitochondria are small and either scattered (rat) or basal to the nucleus (human), and rarely enclosed within basolateral plasma membrane infoldings. The Golgi apparatus is lateral to and beneath the cell nucleus and other cell organelles, including lysosomes, autophagic vacuoles, ribosomes, and smooth and rough endoplasmic reticulum, and also is located principally beneath the cell nucleus. Basal cytoplasmic extensions contact the vascular elements, and at these points, the macula densa basement membrane is fused with basement membrane of the vascular elements.[175,176] Macula densa cells lack the lateral cell processes and interdigitations that are characteristic of the TAL, and the width of the lateral intercellular spaces varies with the physiologic state of the animal.[192]

# PROXIMAL TUBULE

The proximal tubule consists of the proximal convoluted tubule (PCT, pars convoluta), which originates at the glomerular urinary pole and is located in the cortical labyrinth, and the PST, pars recta, which is distal to the PCT and located in the medullary ray in the cortex and extending through the outer stripe of the outer medulla (see Fig. 2.5). The proximal tubule length varies among species, measured at ~10 mm in rabbits,[193] ~8 mm in rats, 4 to 5 mm in mice,[15] and ~14 mm in humans.[194] The volume density of proximal tubules in the cortex is greater in males than females in rats and mice[195,196]; in mice, proximal tubules account for ~60% of the cortical volume in males and only ~40% in females.[195] These structural differences correlate with sexual dimorphism in proximal tubule transporter expression.[197]

In the rat[198] and the rhesus monkey,[199] three morphologically distinct segments—S1, S2, and S3—have been identified based on their ultrastructural characteristics[198,200,201] (Figs. 2.18–2.20). The S1 segment is the initial portion of the proximal tubule; it begins at the glomerulus (see Figs. 2.7 and 2.16) and constitutes approximately two-thirds of the PCT in rat. The S2 segment contains the distal third of the PCT and the initial portion of the PST. The S3 segment is the remainder of the PST, located in the deep inner cortex and the outer stripe of the outer medulla.

Ultrastructurally, S1 cells have a tall brush border, a well-developed vacuolar–lysosomal system, and extensive lateral plasma membrane invaginations and lateral cell processes, which extend from the apical to the basal surface and interdigitate with processes from adjacent cells. Elongated mitochondria are located in the lateral cell processes near the plasma membrane. The ultrastructure of S2 cells is similar, except the brush border is shorter, the basolateral invaginations are less prominent, and the mitochondria are smaller. Numerous small processes, termed "micropedici" (little feet), are located close to the base of the cell. The endocytic compartment is less prominent than in the S1 segment, with the number and size of the lysosomes varying among species and between males and females, being more abundant and larger in males.[193,198]

In rat kidney, where the S1, S2, and S3 designations were first described, S3 cells are characterized by a long brush border; few lateral cell processes and invaginations; small, randomly distributed mitochondria; and small and sparse endocytic vacuoles and lysosomes.[198] Peroxisomes are present throughout the proximal tubule, although they are more abundant in the straight portion of S2 and in S3 compared with S1.[198]

The S1, S2, and S3 designations were originally defined based on ultrastructural characteristics in the rat kidney, and due to variations in the ultrastructure among species, these terms are only properly applied to particular species. For example, the late PST has a relatively short brush border in humans[194] and large endocytic vacuoles and numerous small lysosomes in rabbits.[193] In rabbits, the S2 segment represents a transition between the S1 and S3 segments.[202,203] A morphometric study in mice found no structural segmentation in the cortical segments of the proximal tubule[15]; however, variations in the length of the brush border are evident among mouse proximal tubule profiles in the cortex, and the PST in the outer stripe of the outer medulla typically has a longer brush border compared with most cortical segments. Furthermore, the mouse proximal tubule exhibits clear axial heterogeneity in expression of certain proteins, such as the electrogenic sodium bicarbonate cotransporter splice variant 1-A (NBCe1-A), which is abundant in the basolateral plasma membrane in the PCT and early PST in the cortex, but undetectable in the PST in the outer medulla[204] and the basolateral glutamine transporter, SN1 (SNAT3), which is confined to the PST in the outer medulla and medullary ray under basal conditions, but not detectable in PCT.[205,206] In the nondiseased human kidney, only the PCT and the PST have been positively identified and described.[194] Thus, the terms PCT and PST will be used hereafter unless the S1–S3 terminology is specifically intended.

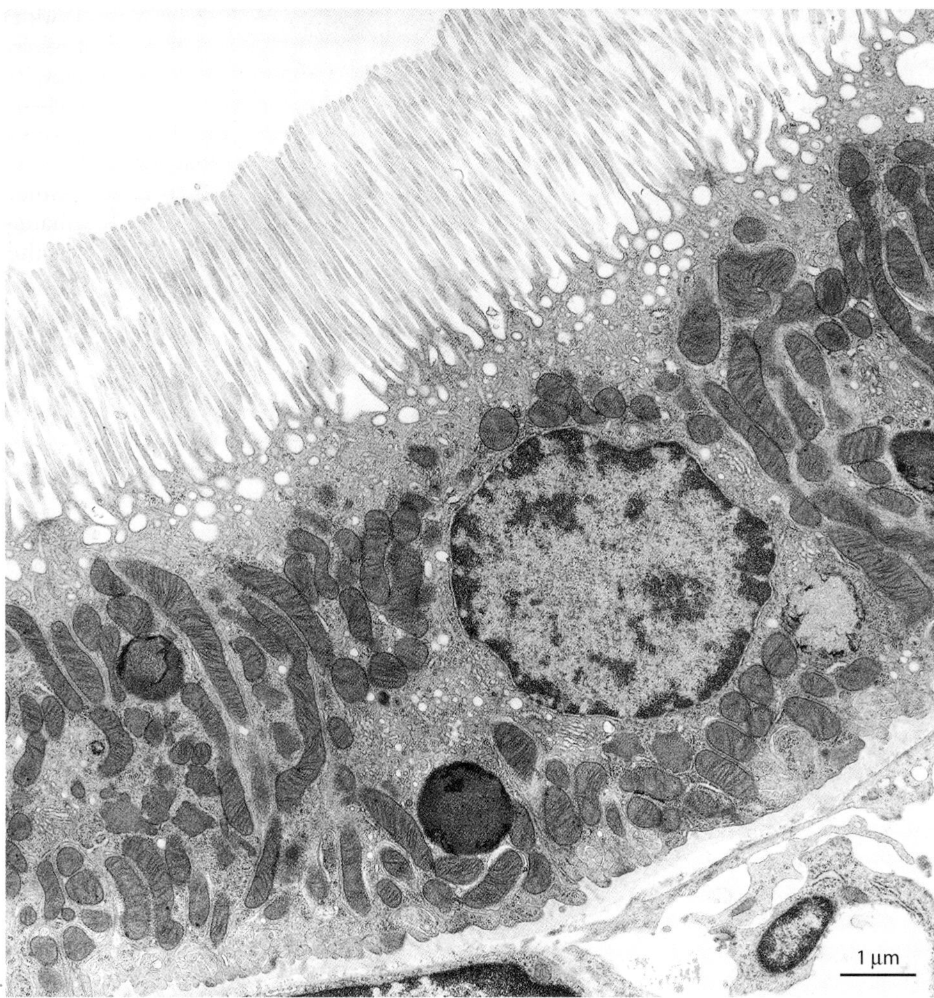


**Fig. 2.18** Transmission electron micrograph of the S1 segment of a rat proximal tubule. The cells are characterized by a tall brush border, a prominent endocytic–lysosomal apparatus, and extensive invaginations of the basolateral plasma membrane with numerous long mitochondria aligned among the basolateral plasma membrane infoldings.

## PROXIMAL CONVOLUTED TUBULE

Cells of the PCT are structurally complex.[202,207,208] Large primary ridges extend laterally from the apical to the basal surfaces of the cells. Large lateral processes, often containing mitochondria, extend outward from the primary ridges and interdigitate with similar processes in adjacent cells (Fig. 2.21). Near the luminal surfaces of the cells, smaller lateral processes extend from the primary ridges to interdigitate with those of adjacent cells. Small basal villi that do not contain mitochondria are found along the basal cell surfaces (Figs. 2.18, 2.19, 2.21, and 2.22). These extensive interdigitations result in a complex extracellular compartment, the basolateral intercellular space (Figs. 2.21–2.23), which is separated from the tubule lumen (apical cell surface) by the tight junctions (zonula occludens).[209] Proximal tubule tight junctions express specific claudin proteins, which confer specific ion permeabilities and likely contribute to the high rates of paracellular sodium and water transport.[210–212] Below the tight junction lies the belt-like intermediate junction, the zonula adherens,[209] followed by several desmosomes distributed randomly at variable distances beneath the intermediate junction. In mammalian and invertebrate renal proximal tubules, gap junctions are present in small numbers[213] and can provide a pathway for the movement of ions between cells and for cell–cell communication via a family of proteins known as connexins.[214] The lateral intercellular space of each PCT cell is open at the basement membrane, which separates the cell from the peritubular interstitium and capillaries. The thickness of the basement membrane gradually decreases along the proximal tubule. For example, in the rhesus monkey, the basement membrane thickness is approximately 250 nm, 145 nm, and 70 nm in the S1, S2, and S3 segments, respectively.[199]

The lateral cell processes of PCT cells combined with extensive invaginations of the plasma membrane increase both the intercellular space and surface area of the basolateral plasma membrane. In rabbits, the area of the lateral surface equals that of the luminal surface and amounts to 2.9 $mm^2$ per mm of tubule.[215] Elongated mitochondria are located in the lateral cell processes near the plasma membrane (see Figs. 2.18 and 2.23), where sodium–potassium adenosine triphosphatase ($Na^+$-$K^+$-ATPase) resides.[216,217] Although mitochondria often appear rod-shaped in two-dimensional images, many mitochondria are branched and connected with one another.[218] A system of smooth membranes, the

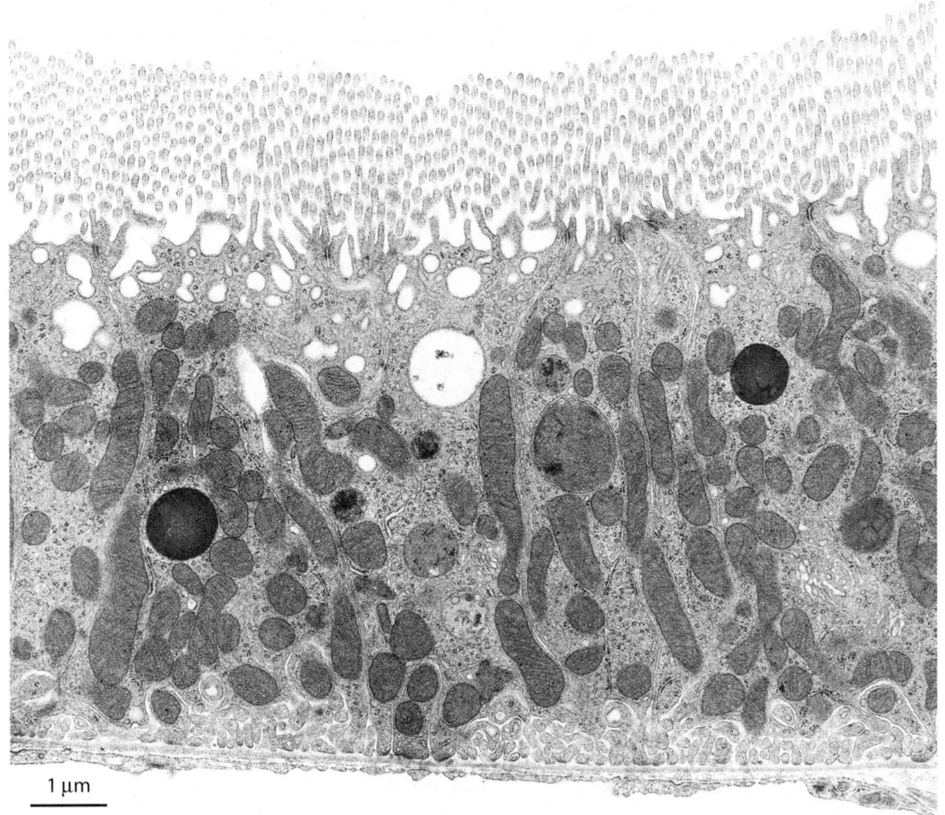


**Fig. 2.19** Transmission electron micrograph of the S2 segment of a rat proximal tubule. The brush border is shorter than in the S1 segment. Mitochondria are numerous and generally aligned with the basolateral plasma membrane infoldings. There are numerous small lateral processes at the base of the cell.

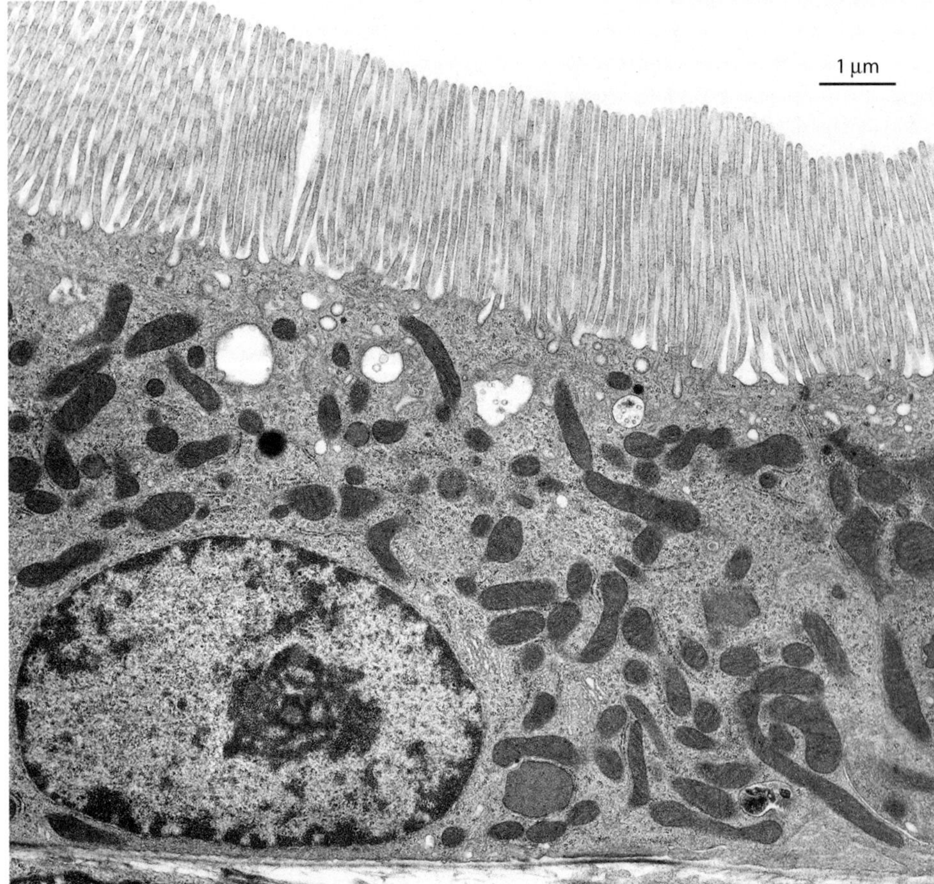


**Fig. 2.20** Transmission electron micrograph of the S3 segment of a rat proximal tubule. The brush border is tall, but the endocytic–lysosomal apparatus is less prominent than in the S1 and S2 segments. Basolateral invaginations are sparse, and mitochondria are scattered randomly throughout the cytoplasm.

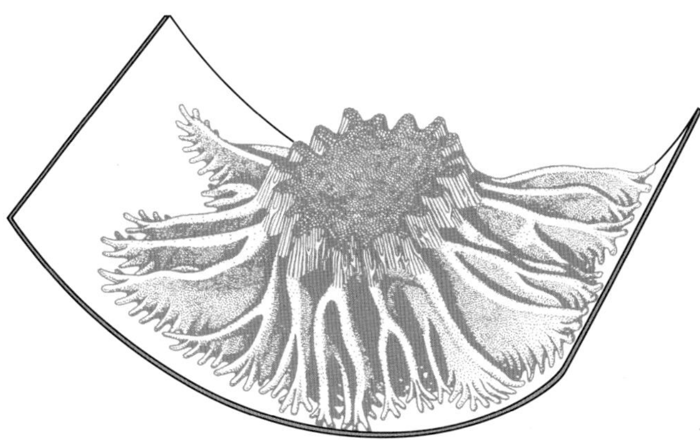

**Fig. 2.21** Schematic drawing illustrating the three-dimensional configuration of the proximal convoluted tubule cell. (From Welling LW, Welling DJ. Shape of epithelial cells and intercellular channels in the rabbit proximal nephron. *Kidney Int.* 1976;9:385–394.)

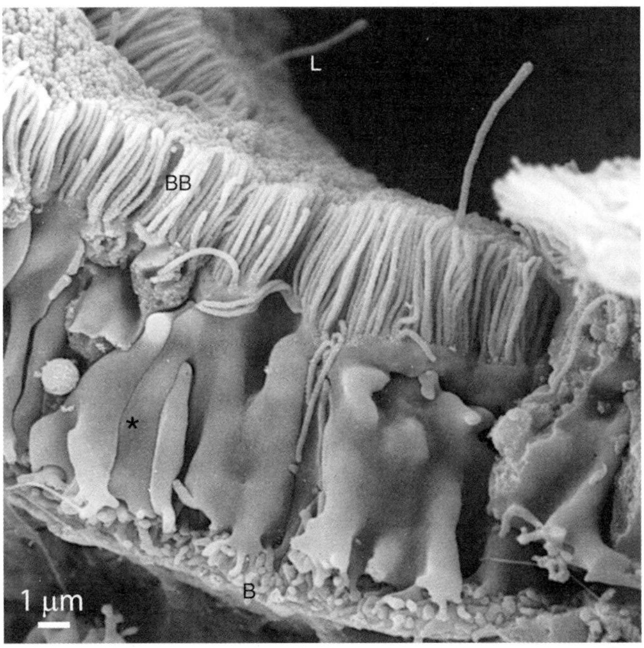


**Fig. 2.22** Scanning electron micrograph of rat proximal convoluted tubule, illustrating the lush brush border *(BB)*, primary cilia extending into the lumen, prominent lateral cell processes, and multiple small basal processes *(B)*, called micropedici. (Modified from Verlander JW. Solute reabsorption. In *Cunningham's Veterinary Physiology,* 6th ed. St Louis: Elsevier; In press.)

paramembranous cisternal system, which may be in continuity with the smooth endoplasmic reticulum, is often observed between the plasma membrane and mitochondria. PCT cells contain large quantities of smooth and rough endoplasmic reticulum, and free ribosomes are abundant. A well-developed Golgi apparatus, composed of smooth-surfaced sacs or cisternae, coated vesicles, uncoated vesicles, and larger vacuoles, is located above and lateral to the nucleus. In addition, an extensive system of microtubules is located throughout the cytoplasm of proximal tubule cells.

PCT cells have lush luminal brush borders formed by densely packed, fingerlike projections of the apical plasma membranes, the microvilli. The brush border greatly increases the apical cell surface,[215] increasing the absorptive surface facing the luminal fluid. Each microvillus contains 6 to 10 actin filaments of approximately 6 nm in diameter that extend variable distances into the cell body. A network of filaments containing myosin and spectrin,[219] the terminal web, is located in the apical cytoplasm just beneath and perpendicular to the microvilli.[220] Each PCT cell has a well-developed endocytic–lysosomal apparatus that is involved in the reabsorption of macromolecules from the ultrafiltrate and their degradation.[221,222] The endocytic compartment includes an extensive system of coated pits, small coated vesicles, apical dense tubules, and larger endocytic vacuoles without a cytoplasmic coat (Fig. 2.24). The coated pits are invaginations of the apical plasma membrane at the base of the microvilli and contain clathrin,[219] megalin,[223–225] and cubilin,[225] proteins that are involved in receptor-mediated endocytosis. The cytoplasmic coat of the small vesicles is similar in ultrastructure to the coat that is present on the cytoplasmic side of the coated pits.

PCT cells contain numerous lysosomes of variable size, shape, and ultrastructural appearance (Fig. 2.25).[221,226] Lysosomes are membrane-bound, heterogeneous organelles that contain proteases, lipases, glycosidases, and acid hydrolases, including acid phosphatases. Lysosomes degrade material absorbed by endocytosis (heterophagocytosis) and often contain electron-dense deposits that are believed to represent reabsorbed substances such as proteins (see Figs. 2.19 and 2.25). Lysosomes also participate in the normal turnover of intracellular constituents by autophagocytosis, and autophagic vacuoles containing fragments of cell organelles are often seen in PCT cells.[226] Lysosomes containing nondigestible substances are called residual bodies; these can empty their contents into the tubule lumen by exocytosis. Multivesicular bodies (MVBs), which are part of the vacuolar–lysosomal system, are often observed in the cytoplasm of PCT cells. MVBs were originally thought to be involved in membrane retrieval and/or membrane disposal, but later studies suggest that MVBs may provide an exit route for plasma membrane vesicles formed by endocytosis and could function as a signaling mechanism to downstream nephron segments.[227,228] The extensive vacuolar–lysosomal system of proximal tubule cells plays an important role in the reabsorption and degradation of albumin and low-molecular-weight plasma proteins from the glomerular filtrate.[221,229,230] Under normal conditions, the vacuolar–lysosomal system is most prominent in the PCT, but in proteinuric states, large vacuoles and extensive lysosomes can be observed in the PST as well.[193,198]

## PROXIMAL STRAIGHT TUBULE

In the rat, the proximal straight tubule (PST, pars recta) includes the terminal portion of the S2 segment, located in the medullary ray, and the entire S3 segment. PST morphology varies considerably among species. For example, the rat S3 brush border measures up to 4 µm long, whereas in the rabbit and human PST, the brush border is relatively short. The S3 epithelium is simpler than both the S1 and S2 segments.[198,202] Basolateral plasma membrane invaginations are virtually absent, mitochondria are small and randomly scattered throughout the cytoplasm, and intercellular spaces

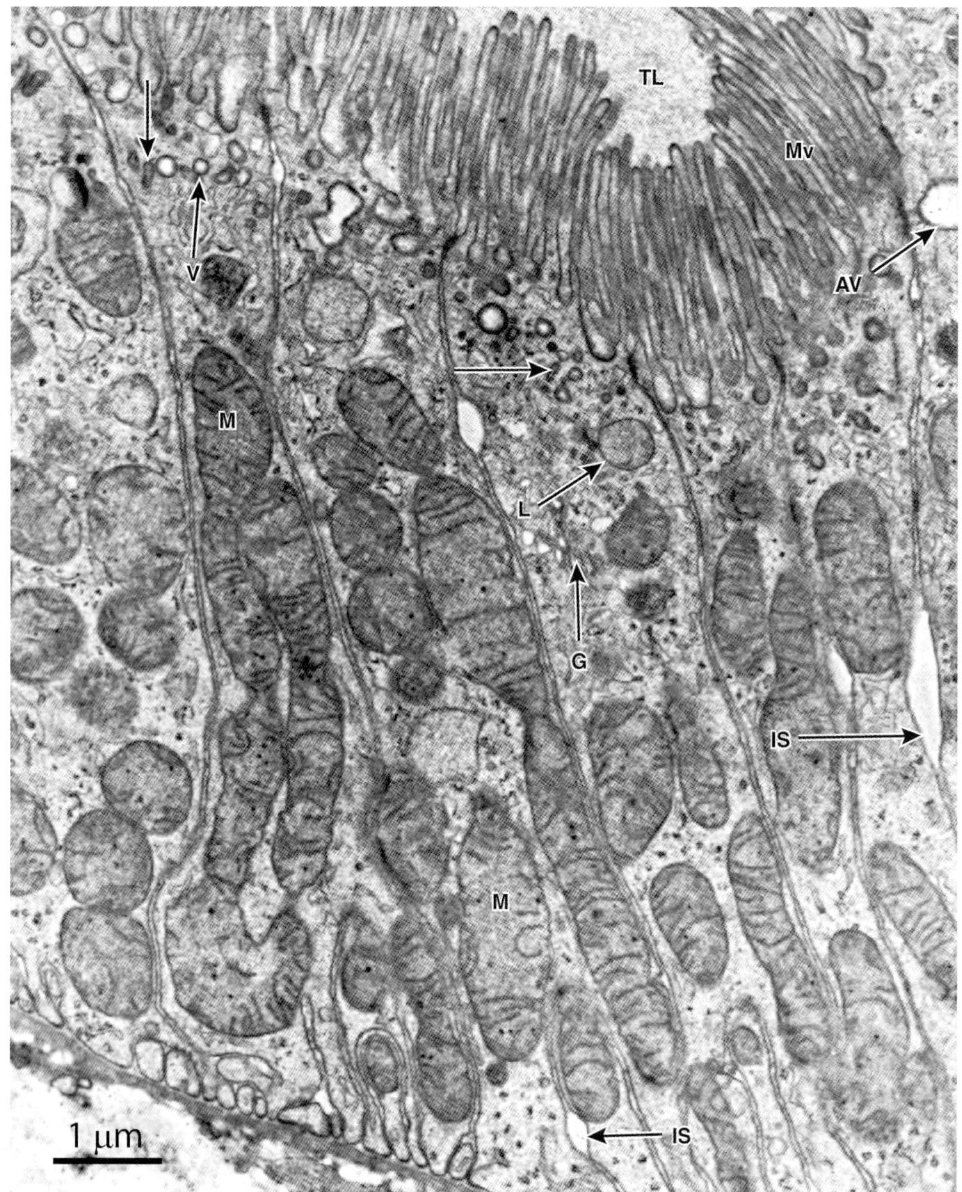


**Fig. 2.23** Transmission electron micrograph of the proximal convoluted tubule from a normal human kidney. The mitochondria *(M)* are elongated and tortuous, occasionally doubling back on themselves. The endocytic apparatus, composed of apical vacuoles *(AV)*, apical vesicles *(V)*, and apical dense tubules *(arrows)*, is well developed. *G*, Golgi apparatus; *IS*, intercellular space; *L*, lysosome; *Mv*, microvilli forming the brush border; *TL*, tubule lumen.

are smaller and less complex (Figs. 2.20 and 2.26). These morphologic characteristics are in agreement with studies demonstrating that $Na^+$-$K^+$-ATPase activity is significantly less in the PST compared to PCT.[231] In contrast to PCT cells, the vacuolar–lysosomal system is less prominent in rat S3 cells, although in both rabbits and humans, many small lysosomes containing electron-dense membranelike material are present in the late PST.[193,194,232] Peroxisomes are common in the PST (Fig. 2.27). In contrast to lysosomes, peroxisomes are irregular in shape, are surrounded by a 6.5-nm-thick membrane, and do not contain acid hydrolases.[226] Peroxisomes within the PST vary considerably in appearance among species. In the rat, small, circular profiles are visible by transmission electron microscopy just inside the limiting membrane, and rod-shaped structures often project outward from the organelle. In addition, a small nucleoid is often present in peroxisomes in the PST. Peroxisomes contain abundant catalase, which is involved in the degradation of hydrogen peroxide, and various oxidative enzymes, including l-α-hydroxy-acid oxidase and D-amino acid oxidase.[233,234]

The proximal tubule plays a major role in the reabsorption of $Na^+$, $HCO_3^-$, $Cl^-$, $K^+$, $Ca^{2+}$, $PO_4^{3-}$, water, and organic solutes such as vitamins, glucose, and amino acids; secretion of protons, ammonia, and organic anions; and uptake of filtered peptides and proteins. The ultrastructural features of proximal tubule cells aid in these transport processes, most notably the high surface density of both the apical and basolateral plasma membrane compartments, the high mitochondrial

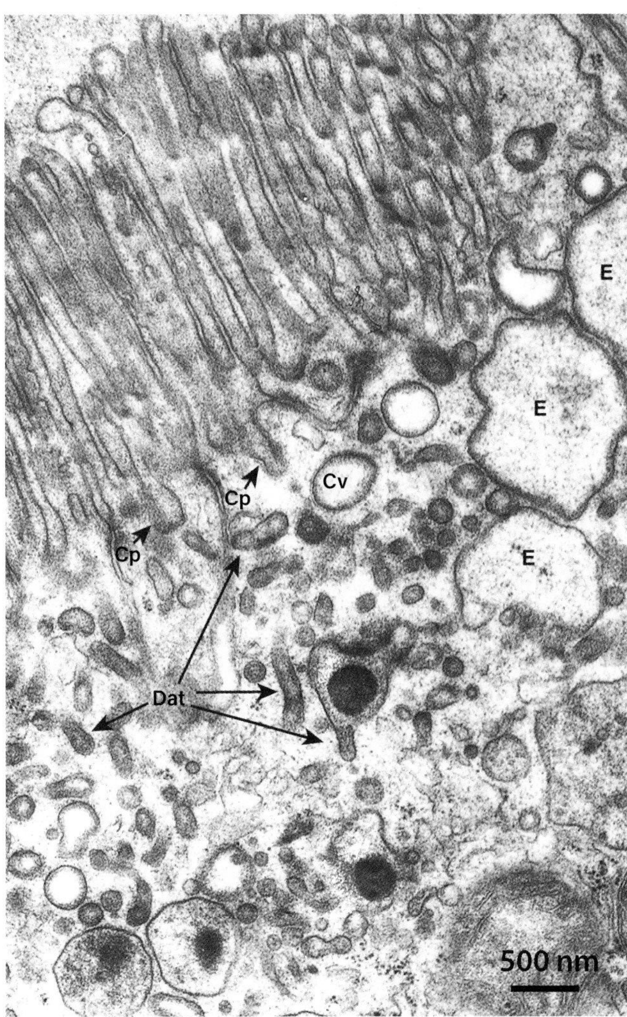


**Fig. 2.24** Transmission electron micrograph of the apical region of a human proximal tubule, illustrating the endocytic apparatus, including coated pits *(Cp)*, coated vesicles *(Cv)*, apical dense tubules *(Dat)*, and endosomes *(E)*.

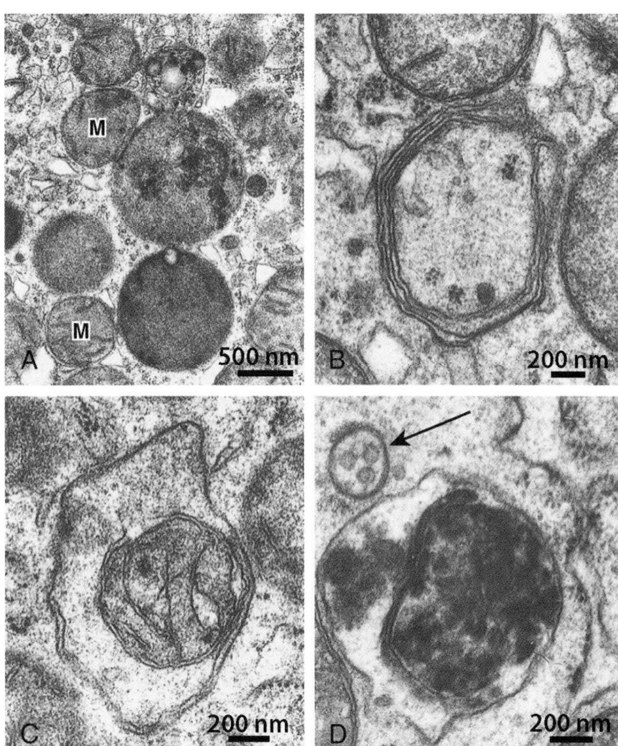


**Fig. 2.25** Transmission electron micrographs illustrating the appearance of different types of lysosomes from human proximal tubules. (A) Lysosomes. Several mitochondria *(M)* are also shown. (B) Early stage of formation of an autophagic vacuole. (C) Fully formed autolysosome containing a mitochondrion undergoing digestion. (D) Autolysosome containing a microbody undergoing digestion. A multivesicular body *(arrow)* is also shown. (From Tisher CC, Bulger RE, Trump BF. Human renal ultrastructure. I: Proximal tubule of healthy individuals. *Lab Invest.* 1966;15:1357–1394.)

density in early proximal tubule segments, and the abundant endocytic vesicles and lysosomal system. Proximal tubule cells alter transport capacity in some instances by redistribution of specific transporters located in the brush border. For example, the apical sodium–hydrogen exchanger, NHE3, is rapidly redistributed between the brush border microvilli and the base of the microvilli in models that alter proximal tubule sodium uptake,[235,236] whereas parathyroid hormone stimulates redistribution of the sodium phosphate transporter, NaPi-2, from the microvilli to endosomes.[236] Changes in the hydraulic and oncotic pressures across the tubule and capillary wall cause significant ultrastructural changes in the proximal tubule, especially in the configuration of the lateral intercellular spaces.[237,238]

## THIN LIMBS OF THE LOOP OF HENLE

The thin limbs of the loop of Henle connect the proximal and distal tubules of the nephron. The thin limbs arise abruptly from the distal end of the PST, descend a variable distance, make a hairpin turn, and ascend to the abrupt transition to the TAL. The transition from the proximal tubule to the descending thin limb (Figs. 2.5, 2.6, 2.28, and 2.29) defines the boundary between the outer and inner stripes of the outer medulla, and the transition from the thin ascending limb to the thick ascending limb defines the boundary between the outer and inner medulla (see Figs. 2.5 and 2.6). Short-looped nephrons, which originate from superficial and midcortical glomeruli, have a short descending thin limb that transitions to the TAL at the hairpin turn near the border of the outer and inner medulla. Long-looped nephrons, which originate from juxtamedullary glomeruli, have long descending and ascending thin limbs connected by a hairpin turn located at variable depths in the inner medulla. Nephrons arising in the extreme outer cortex have only short cortical loops that do not extend into the medulla. Although these features are generally consistent among mammalian species, detailed studies of the organization of the renal medulla in several laboratory animals, including 3D reconstruction studies, have described variations among species in the length and ultrastructure of the thin-limb segments.[13,239]

There are four types of thin-limb epithelia, types I through IV, based on ultrastructural characteristics[240–244] (Fig. 2.30).

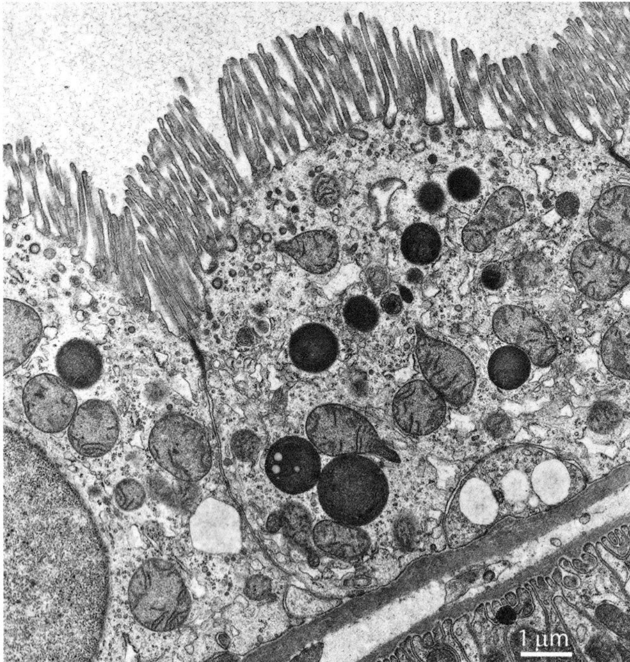


**Fig. 2.26** Low-magnification transmission electron micrograph of a segment of the proximal straight tubule from a human kidney. The microvilli on the convex apical cell surface are not as long as those in the rat proximal straight tubule. The lysosomes are extremely electron dense. The clear, single membrane–limited structures at the base of the cell to the right represent lipid droplets. (Courtesy R.E. Bulger, PhD.)

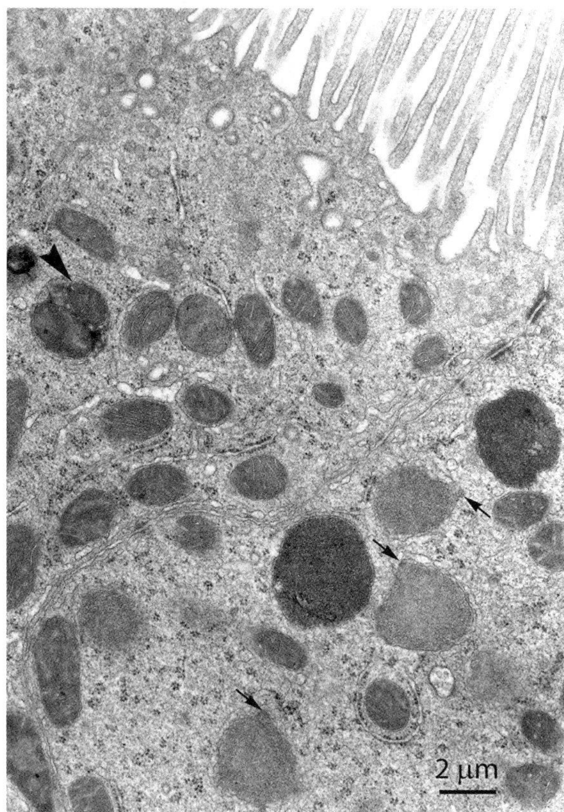


**Fig. 2.27** Transmission electron micrograph of the rat proximal straight tubule, S3 segment. Endocytic vesicles, lysosomes, and autophagic vacuoles *(arrowhead)* are less abundant than in S1 and S2 segments. However, peroxisomes are abundant and identified by their irregular, angular shape and small, circular protuberances along the edges *(arrows)*.

Type I epithelium is found exclusively in the descending thin limb of short-looped nephrons. It is extremely thin, and both the apical and basolateral plasma membranes are relatively smooth, with few apical microprojections and few basolateral infoldings. Lateral interdigitations and cellular organelles are sparse. Tight junctions are intermediate in depth with several junctional strands, characteristics of a tight epithelium.[245–247]

The descending thin limb of long-looped nephrons contains type II epithelium in the outer medulla and type III epithelium in the inner medulla. Type II epithelium is taller than type I epithelium and exhibits considerable species differences. In the rat,[248] mouse,[240] *Psammomys obesus,*[244] and hamster,[242] the type II epithelium has extensive lateral and basal interdigitations (Fig. 2.31). The tight junctions are extremely shallow and contain a single junctional strand, characteristics of a "leaky" epithelium. Short, blunt microvilli cover the luminal surface. Cell organelles, including mitochondria, are more prominent than in other segments of the thin limb. In the rabbit the type II epithelium is less complex,[202] lateral interdigitations are less prominent, and tight junctions are deeper.[247]

Compared with type II epithelium, type III epithelium is thinner and simpler in structure. The cells do not interdigitate, the tight junctions are intermediate in depth, and there are fewer luminal surface microprojections (Figs. 2.30 and 2.32). Type IV epithelium forms the bends of the long loops and the entire ascending thin limb. Type IV epithelium (Figs. 2.30 and 2.32) is generally low and flat and has relatively few organelles. It has few surface microprojections but abundant lateral cell processes and interdigitations. The tight junctions are shallow, characteristic of a leaky epithelium.

Thin limb segments exhibit specific expression patterns for several transport proteins, including $Na^+$-$K^+$-ATPase, the water channel, aquaporin-1 (AQP1), and the urea transporter, UT-A2. Correlating to its more complex structural features, the rat type II epithelium has significantly greater $Na^+$-$K^+$-ATPase protein expression[249] and activity[250] compared with other descending thin limb segments. In rabbit, the type II thin limb does not have complex basolateral plasma membrane infoldings and, like all segments of the rabbit thin limb, has very low $Na^+$-$K^+$-ATPase activity.[251] AQP1[239,252,253] and the urea transporter, UT-A2,[254–256] are expressed in specific segmental patterns, exclusively in the descending thin limbs. However, in the Munich-Wistar rat, segments with structural features and immunoreactivity for AQP1 and UT-A2 typical of descending thin limbs are intermingled with segments typical of ascending limbs.[257]

The 3D arrangement of the inner medulla has been characterized in detailed structural studies, documenting the spatial organization of specific thin limb segments relative to vasa recta and collecting ducts in the medulla, which, along with the specific transport properties of the thin limb segments, is believed to be a necessary element of the urine concentrating mechanism.[13,258–267]

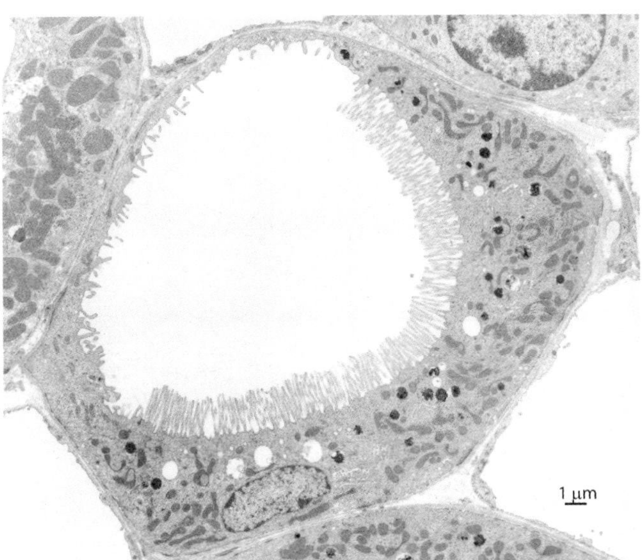


**Fig. 2.28** Transmission electron micrograph from rabbit kidney illustrating the abrupt transition from the proximal straight tubule to the descending thin limb of the loop of Henle. (Modified from Madsen KM, Park CH. Lysosome distribution and cathepsin B and L activity along the rabbit proximal tubule. *Am J Physiol.* 1987;253:F1290–F1301.)

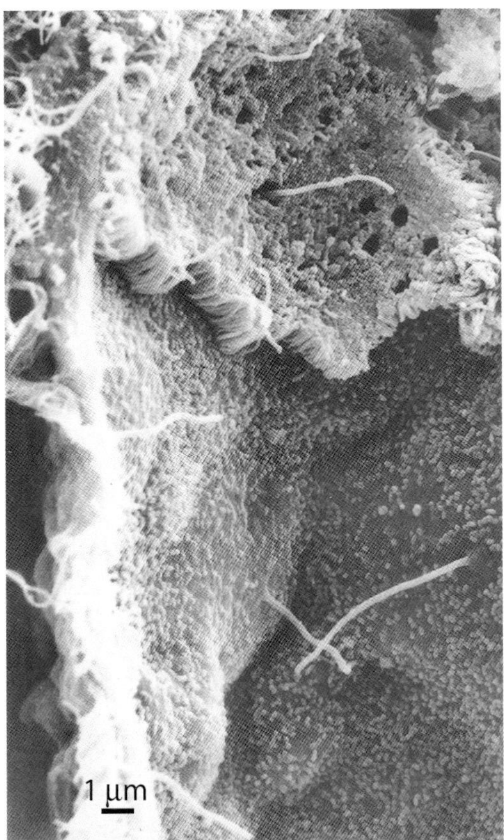


**Fig. 2.29** Scanning electron micrograph depicting the abrupt transition from the terminal S3 segment of the rat proximal tubule *(top)* to the descending thin limb *(bottom)*. Elongated cilia project into the lumen from cells of the proximal tubule and the thin limb.

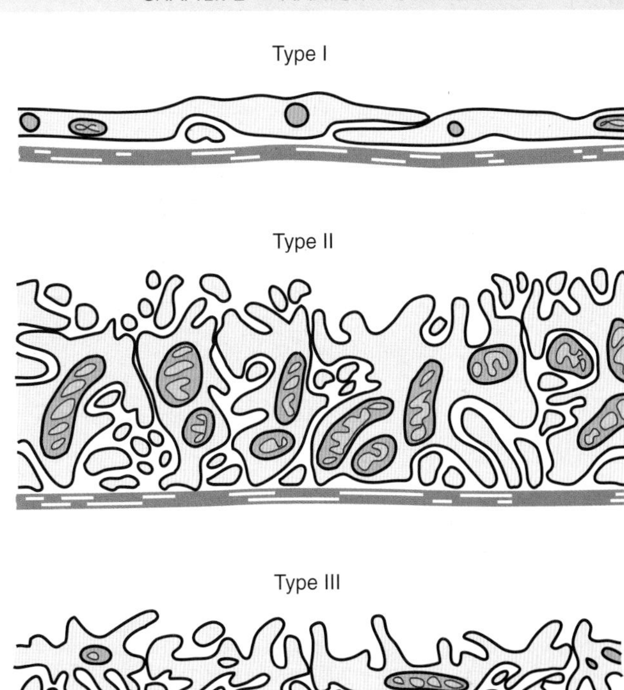


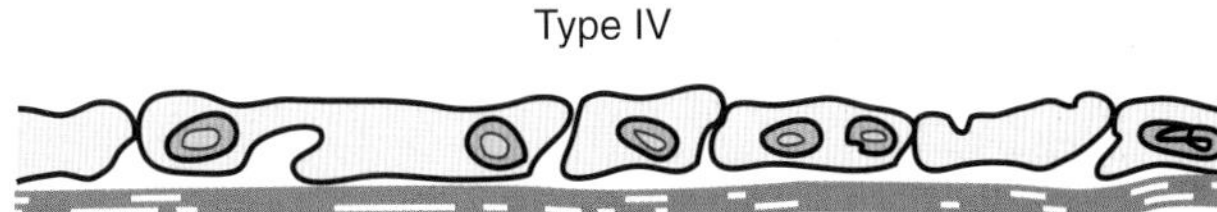


**Fig. 2.30** Diagram depicting the appearance of the four types of thin limb segments in a rat kidney. (See text for explanation.)

## DISTAL TUBULE

The term "distal tubule" has been used in different ways to encompass different segments of the distal nephron. According to the standard nomenclature of renal anatomists, the "distal tubule" includes the TAL of loop of Henle (pars recta or distal straight tubule), which contains the macula densa and the distal convoluted tubule (pars convoluta).[268] However, in micropuncture studies and more common usage, the distal tubule includes the segments from just distal to the macula densa to the first confluence of two tubules. By this definition, the distal tubule may include up to four different epithelial segments, a short portion of TAL, DCT, connecting tubule (CNT), and ICT.[202,269,270] The lengths of the segments that make up the distal tubule vary among species and rat strains. The length of the tubule from the macula densa to the first tubule junction in the rat is reported to be 2.4–2.5 mm.[269] In Sprague-Dawley and Brattleboro rats, DCT accounts for ~75%–77% of distal tubule accessible by micropuncture, whereas in Wistar rats, DCT constitutes only ~48% of the distal tubule, with the remainder being CNT and ICT.[269] In studies of microdissected rabbit distal tubule, segments designated as DCTb, DCTg, and DCTl, likely correlating to DCT, CNT, and ICT, measured 0.49 mm, 0.42 mm, and 0.41 mm, respectively.[271] However, the rabbit DCT was measured at ~1 mm long in structural studies.[202]

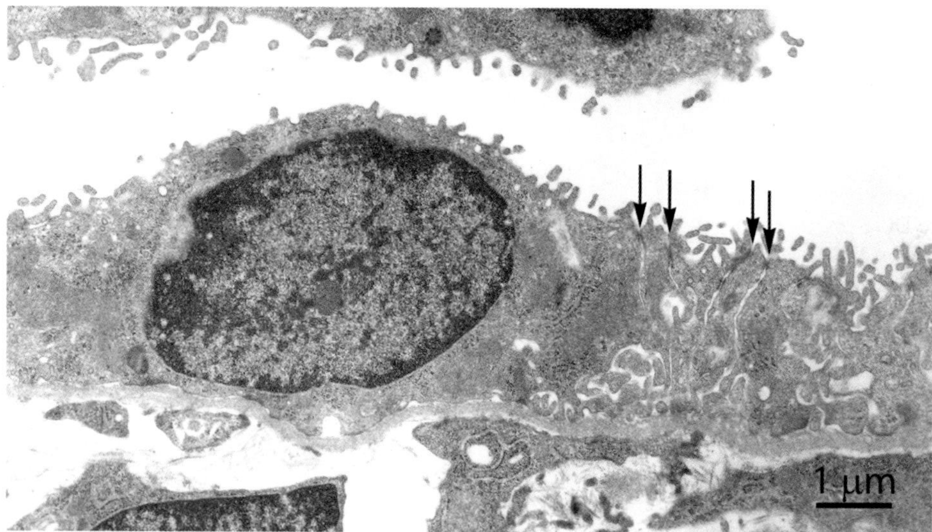


**Fig. 2.31** Transmission electron micrograph of type II epithelium of the thin limb of loop of Henle in the inner stripe of the outer medulla of a rat kidney. Compared with other thin limb types, type II epithelium is taller and has more organelles, prominent apical plasma membrane microprojections, and complex basolateral plasma membrane infoldings. The cells have extensive lateral interdigitations attached near the apical surface by short tight junctions *(arrows)*. (Modified from Verlander JW. Normal ultrastructure of the kidney and lower urinary tract. *Toxicol Pathol.* 1998;Jan-Feb;26(1):1–17.)

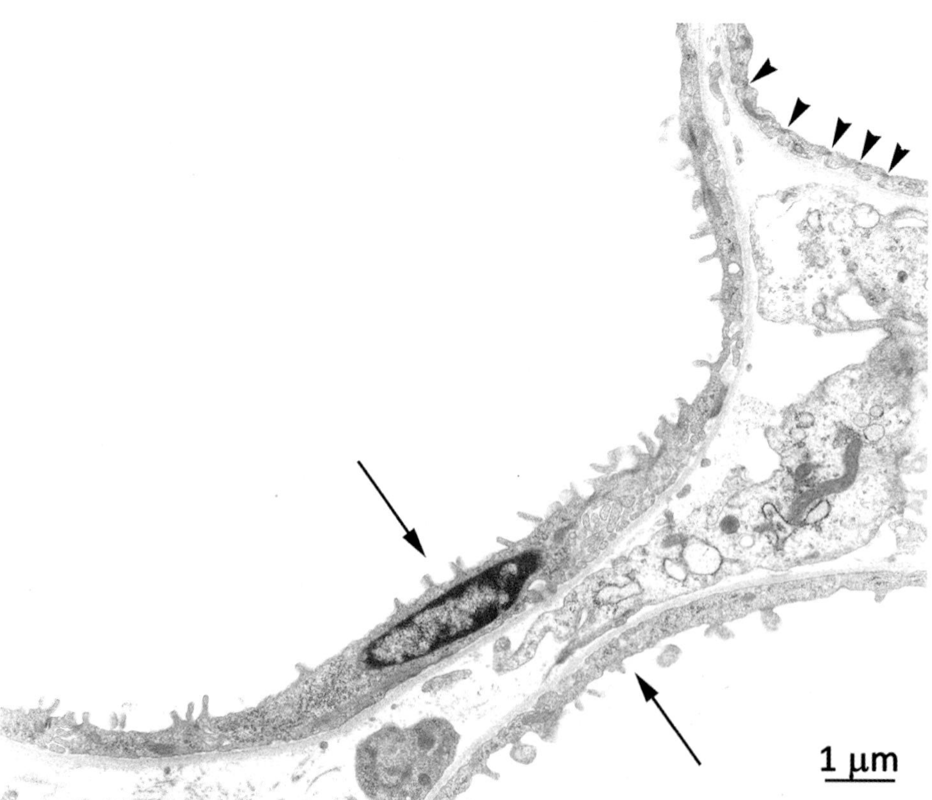


**Fig. 2.32** Transmission electron micrograph of thin limbs of the loop of Henle in the initial inner medulla of rat kidney. Type III epithelium *(arrows)* has prominent apical plasma membrane microprojections. It is a very low, flat epithelium with relatively few basolateral plasma membrane infoldings compared with type II epithelium. A small portion of type IV thin limb epithelium is also visible, which also is very flat but has numerous tight junctions *(arrowheads)* due to the abundant lateral interdigitations. (From Sands JM, Verlander JW. Functional anatomy of the kidney. In: McQueen C, ed. *Comprehensive toxicology,* 3rd ed. St Louis: Elsevier; 2017.)

## THICK ASCENDING LIMB

The TAL arises abruptly from the thin limbs of loop of Henle, spans the inner and outer stripes of the outer medulla, extends through the cortex in the medullary rays, contacts the glomerulus of its own nephron at the macula densa, and extends a short distance beyond the macula densa before the transition to the DCT[202,270] (see Fig. 2.5). In short-looped nephrons, the transition to the TAL can occur shortly before the hairpin turn, but this is not the case in all species.[15] In the outer medulla, TAL cells are taller in the inner stripe, beginning at ~11 μm and declining to between 7 and 8 μm in height.[202,270,272] As the tubule ascends toward the cortex, cell height gradually decreases further to ~5 μm in the cortical TAL (cTAL) of the rat.[272] In rabbits also, the cTAL is lower than the medullary TAL (mTAL) in height, averaging 4.5 μm but declining to ~2 μm in the terminal part.[202,273]

TAL cells have extensive infoldings of the basolateral plasma membrane and interdigitations between adjacent cells (Figs. 2.33 and 2.34). The basolateral infoldings often extend from the base to two-thirds or more of the cell height, particularly in the mTAL in the inner stripe. The cell nucleus is centrally located, with little cytoplasm or organelles between the nucleus and either the apical or basal surface. Abundant elongated mitochondria are located in lateral cell processes, generally oriented perpendicularly to the basement membrane, similar to the S1 segment of the proximal tubule, and they contain prominent granules in the matrix. The TAL also has a well-developed Golgi complex; small, subapical cytoplasmic vesicles and tubulovesicles; multivesicular bodies and lysosomes; and abundant smooth and rough endoplasmic reticulum. The tight junctions are 0.1 to 0.2 μm in depth in the rat[209]; in rabbit, the length of the tight junctions increases from the mTAL to the cTAL.[202] Intermediate junctions are also present, but desmosomes appear to be lacking.

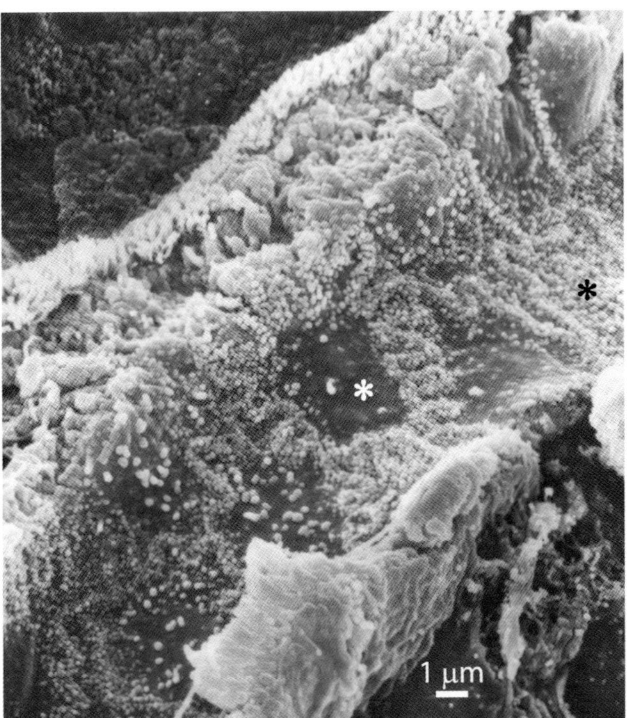


**Fig. 2.33** Scanning electron micrograph illustrating the luminal surface of rat medullary thick ascending limb. The *white asterisk* denotes smooth-surfaced cells; the *black asterisk* identifies rough-surfaced cells. (Modified from Madsen KM, Verlander, Tisher CC. Relationship between structure and function in distal tubule and collecting duct. *J Electron Micros Tech.* 1988;9:187–208.)

By SEM, the TAL of the rat kidney has two morphologically distinct cells, designated "smooth" and "rough," distinguished by the appearance of the luminal plasma membrane and lateral cell borders.[270] Rough TAL cells have numerous small apical microprojections, whereas the apical surface of smooth TAL cells has few microprojections except along the cell borders (Fig. 2.33); both types have a single, central primary cilium. In the inner stripe of the outer medulla, rough TAL cells generally have prominent lateral processes that interdigitate with neighboring cells, producing an undulating cell border, whereas smooth TAL cells typically have only shallow lateral processes and hence a relatively simple cell border; these differences are not present in the cTAL.[270] However, compared with rough TAL cells, smooth TAL cells have a more prominent subapical cytoplasmic vesicle and tubulovesicle compartment. The smooth surface pattern predominates in the mTAL, but as the thick limb ascends, the number of rough TAL cells increases, and luminal microprojections and apical lateral invaginations become more prominent. Consequently, the surface area of the luminal plasma membrane is significantly greater in the cTAL than in the mTAL.[272]

The structural characteristics of the TAL, notably the high density of mitochondria interposed between extensive basolateral plasma membrane infoldings, contribute to its important role in active reabsorption of NaCl via the $Na^+$, $K^+$,$2Cl^-$ cotransporter located in the apical plasma membrane[274] driven by abundant basolateral $Na^+$-$K^+$-ATPase. Within the TAL, axial heterogeneity in the ultrastructural features correlates with $Na^+$-$K^+$-ATPase activity, with the mTAL in the inner stripe having the greatest basolateral plasma membrane area, mitochondrial density, and $Na^+$-$K^+$-ATPase activity.[249,272,275,276] However, functional correlations with the observed axial and cellular structural heterogeneity are limited.[277] Some physiologic studies using the isolated perfused tubule technique found that NaCl transport is greater in the medullary segment than in the cortical segment of the TAL,[278] consistent with the structural differences, but others did not observe this.[279,280] Similarly, functional differences between the smooth and rough forms of TAL cells have not been defined. Although cellular heterogeneity in the expression of various transport proteins, including ROMK, $H^+$ATPase, and NKCC2, has been observed in the TAL, these variations in protein expression have not yet been correlated with the apical surface patterns described using electron microscopy.[277]

## DISTAL CONVOLUTED TUBULE

The abrupt transition from the TAL to the DCT occurs a short distance distal to the macula densa and is located in the cortical labyrinth (Figs. 2.5 and 2.35). Like TAL cells, DCT cells contain extensive basolateral plasma membrane infoldings and a dense array of long mitochondria aligned with the plasma membrane infoldings perpendicular to the basement membrane (Fig. 2.36). However, DCT cells are significantly taller than TAL cells, and the cell nuclei are

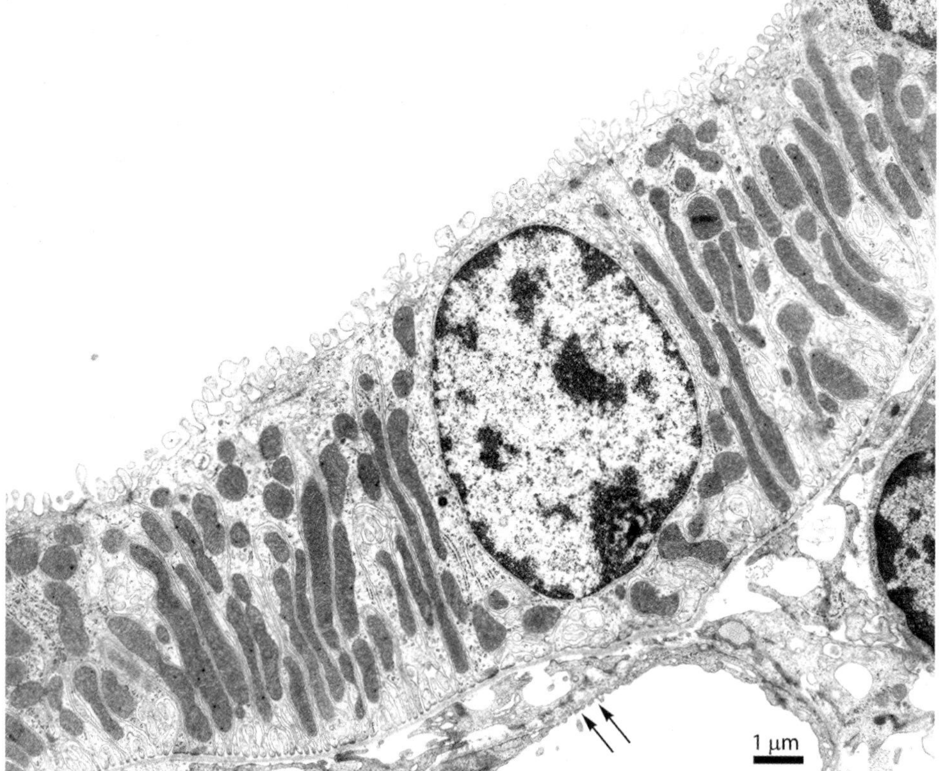


**Fig. 2.34** Transmission electron micrograph of cortical thick ascending limb (TAL) in rat kidney. The apical surface has numerous short apical microprojections, typical of the rough TAL cells common in the cortical TAL, and deep, complex invaginations of the basal plasma membrane extend into the apical region of the cell and enclose elongated mitochondrial profiles. There are few organelles and little cytoplasm between the nucleus and the apical and basal aspects of the cell compared with the distal convoluted tubule (see Fig. 2.36). A peritubular capillary with fenestrated endothelium *(arrows)* is adjacent to the basal side of the TAL cell.

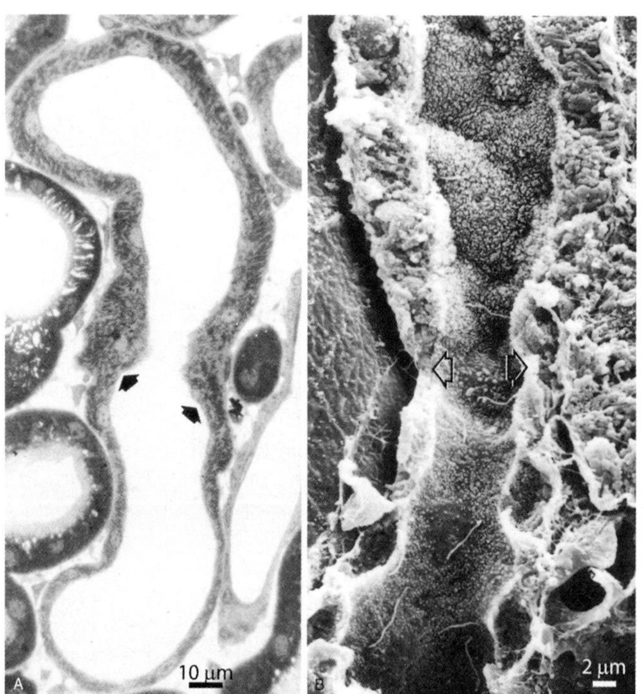


**Fig. 2.35** Micrographs depicting the abrupt transition *(arrows)* from the thick ascending limb of Henle *(below)* to the distal convoluted tubule *(above)*. (A) Light micrograph of normal rat kidney. (B) Scanning electron micrograph of normal rabbit kidney. (B, Courtesy Ann LeFurgey, PhD.)

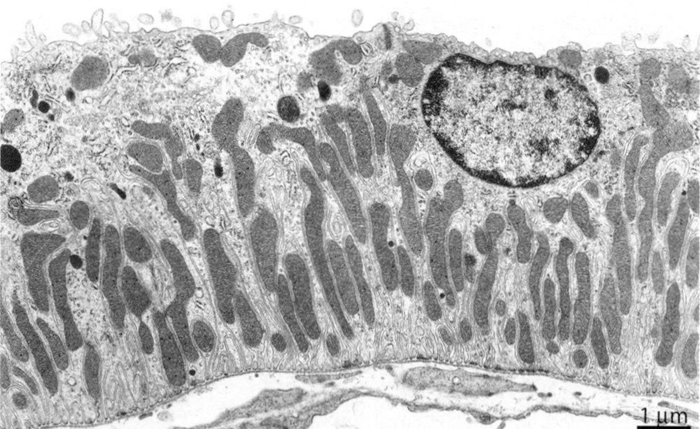


**Fig. 2.36** Transmission electron micrograph of rat distal convoluted tubule (DCT). Although the structure of DCT cells is similar to thick ascending limb (TAL) cells in many ways, DCT cells are considerably taller, with numerous basal plasma membrane infoldings and mitochondria interposed between the nucleus and the basement membrane. Compare with the TAL cell in Fig. 2.34.

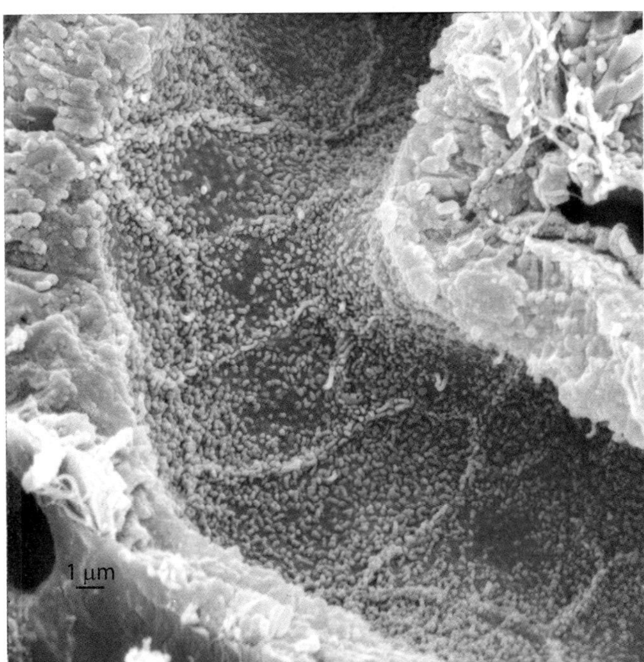


**Fig. 2.37** Scanning electron micrograph showing the luminal surface of a distal convoluted tubule from a rat kidney. Short microvilli are prominent, cell borders are accentuated by longer and more abundant microvilli, and the cell borders in the apical region are simple, lacking the interdigitations seen in the thick ascending limb (TAL). (Compare with Fig. 2.33.)

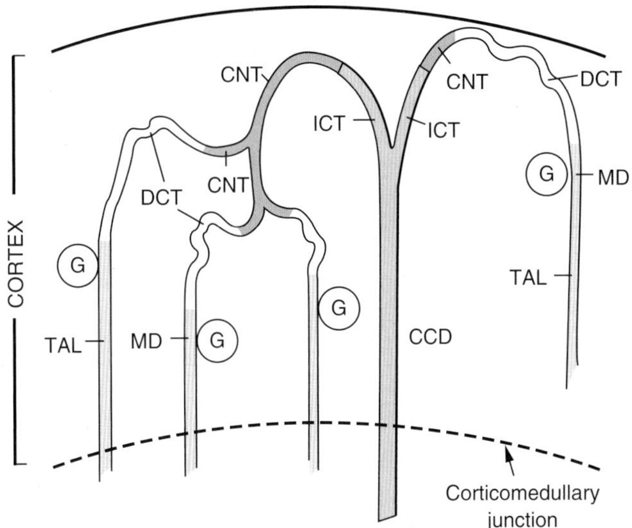


**Fig. 2.38** Diagram of the various anatomic arrangements of the distal tubule and cortical collecting duct in superficial and juxtamedullary nephrons. (See text for detailed explanation.) *CCD*, Cortical collecting duct; *CNT*, connecting segment; *DCT*, distal convoluted tubule; *G*, glomerulus; *ICT*, initial collecting tubule; *MD*, macula densa; *TAL*, ascending thick limb (of Henle).

close to the apical plasma membrane with basolateral plasma membrane infoldings and mitochondria interposed between the nucleus and basement membrane. On the luminal surface, DCT cells have a single central cilium and numerous small microprojections, which are more prominent at the lateral cell borders; the lateral borders are simple compared with TAL cells (Fig. 2.37). The junctional complex is composed of a tight junction, which is approximately 0.3 µm in depth, and an intermediate junction.[209] The Golgi complex is well-developed, and lysosomes and multivesicular bodies are present but less common than in the proximal tubule. The cells contain numerous small subapical vesicles, microtubules, free ribosomes, and rough and smooth endoplasmic reticulum.

As mentioned previously, in micropuncture studies, the "distal tubule" includes tubule segments from immediately distal to the macula densa to the first junction with another renal tubule, which includes as many as four different types of epithelia (Fig. 2.38). In general, the "early" or "bright" distal tubule corresponds largely to the DCT plus a short segment of TAL, whereas the "late" or "granular" distal tubule corresponds to the connecting tubule and the initial portion of the collecting duct in the cortical labyrinth, the ICT.[269,281] In several species, the DCT exhibits axial heterogeneity with respect to cell morphology and transporter expression.[282] In rabbits, the transition from DCT to CNT is morphologically distinct, but in rats, mice, and humans, the late portion of the DCT shares features of the CNT, including the presence of intercalated cells and several proteins expressed in CNT cells. In fact, two DCT segments, DCT1 and DCT2, have been defined in the rat based on protein expression characteristics. Expression of the apical thiazide-sensitive NaCl cotransporter, NCC, is definitive for DCT cells and is present throughout the entire DCT. The initial DCT segment, DCT1, is distinguished from the late segment, DCT2, by the presence in DCT2 of the $Na^+$–$Ca^{2+}$ exchanger (NCX1) and vitamin D–dependent calcium-binding protein, calbindin-D28K,[283] proteins that are also expressed in CNT cells.[284] In mice[285,286] and humans,[287] NCX and calbindin-D28K are expressed throughout most of the DCT; thus, DCT1 and DCT2 are not distinguishable, at least not as originally defined. Nonetheless, in rat, mouse, and human, the early DCT is distinct from the late DCT in that the latter portion expresses the epithelial sodium channel (ENaC),[286] which is also expressed in CNT cells, and in mice and rats, the late DCT expresses the apical calcium channel TRPV5, which is absent from the early DCT.[288,289] Furthermore, in rat and mouse, the late portion of the DCT also contains intercalated cells, predominantly the so-called non-A, non-B subtype, which is described in detail in the section on the collecting duct.

The DCT has the highest $Na^+$-$K^+$-ATPase activity of all nephron segments,[231,251] which drives ion transport and correlates with the high mitochondrial density and elaborate basolateral plasma membrane infoldings in this segment. The NCC is present in the apical plasma membrane and subapical vesicles.[290–292] A number of studies have demonstrated structural changes in the DCT in response to physiologic stimuli that alter the transport activity in this segment.[293–297] For example, treatment with furosemide, an inhibitor of the TAL transporter NKCC2, causes a marked increase in DCT cell size, basolateral plasma membrane area, and cell proliferation, along with increased NCC expression and sodium uptake, suggesting structural adaptations correlating with functional adaptations to conserve sodium when NKCC2 is inhibited and NaCl delivery to the DCT is increased.[293,298] In animals fed a low-salt diet, NCC is largely expressed in the apical plasma membrane where it mediates apical NaCl uptake, whereas feeding a high-salt diet or acute induction of hypertension causes redistribution of NCC to the subapical cytoplasmic vesicles.[299,300] Conversely, angiotensin II administration acutely causes a significant increase in the apical plasma membrane expression of NCC and a reduction in NCC expression in apical cytoplasmic membrane vesicles, whereas treatment with captopril, an angiotensin-converting enzyme inhibitor, has the opposite effect on NCC distribution,[301] although under these conditions, phosphorylated NCC is found exclusively in the apical plasma membrane and not in cytoplasmic vesicles.[302] Similarly, estradiol administration in ovariectomized rats, which increases NCC phosphorylation and activity,[303] causes an increase in apical plasma membrane complexity and apical plasma membrane NCC expression along with depletion of apical cytoplasmic vesicles.[304] Thus, structural changes occur in the DCT in response to stimuli that alter NCC transporter expression and functional activity.

## CONNECTING SEGMENT

The CNT constitutes the main portion of the "late" or "granular" distal tubule as defined in the micropuncture literature. The CNTs of superficial nephrons continue directly into ICTs, whereas CNTs from midcortical and juxtamedullary nephrons join to form arcades that ascend in the cortex and continue into ICTs (see Fig. 2.38).[202,271] CNTs are present throughout the cortical labyrinth but are present in higher density surrounding interlobular vessels; the CNT makes contact with the afferent arteriole of its own glomerulus, upstream of the JGA.[305,306] These contacts enable crosstalk between the CNT and renal vasculature, which regulates renal perfusion in addition to the classic tubuloglomerular feedback mechanism mediated through the JGA.[307–310]

In the rabbit, the CNT is a well-defined segment composed of two cell types: the CNT cell and the intercalated cell.[202,297] However in other species, including rats,[269,281] mice,[297] and humans,[178,311] the transition from DCT to CNT is not structurally distinct. More distally, the rat and mouse CNT clearly differs from the late DCT in the increased frequency of intercalated cells and the structural characteristics of the majority cell type, the CNT cell (Fig. 2.39). The CNT transitions to the ICT, which is located in the cortical labyrinth and connects the CNT to the CCD, which is located in the medullary ray. The ICT is a lower epithelium than the CNT, and like the CCD, is made up of principal cells and intercalated cells (Fig. 2.40). In rabbit kidney, the CNT to ICT transition is distinct. In rat kidney, although there is some intermingling of CNT cells and principal cells in the late portion of the CNT, the CNT and ICT are largely distinguishable by the morphologic characteristics of CNT cells versus principal cells. In mouse, the transition from CNT to ICT is more gradual, and only the early CNT and late ICT are clearly identifiable as such based on cellular morphology.

The CNT contains primarily two cell types: the majority cell type, the CNT cell, which occurs only in this segment, and intercalated cells, which account for approximately 40% of the cells. The CNT cell is tall with an apically located nucleus like the DCT cell, but has a rounder nucleus, more cytoplasm and organelles between the apical plasma membrane and the nucleus, shallower and less uniform basolateral plasma membrane infoldings, and fewer, more randomly arranged mitochondria.[312]

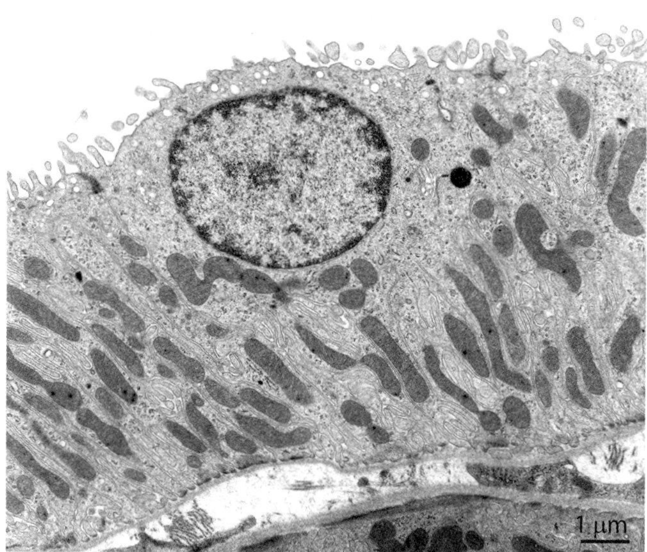


**Fig. 2.39** Transmission electron micrograph of rat connecting segment (CNT) cell. The CNT cell has deep basolateral plasma membrane infoldings with numerous mitochondria, but a lower mitochondrial density than distal convoluted tubule (DCT) cells, and the nucleus is typically rounder than DCT cell nuclei. (Compare with Fig. 2.36.)

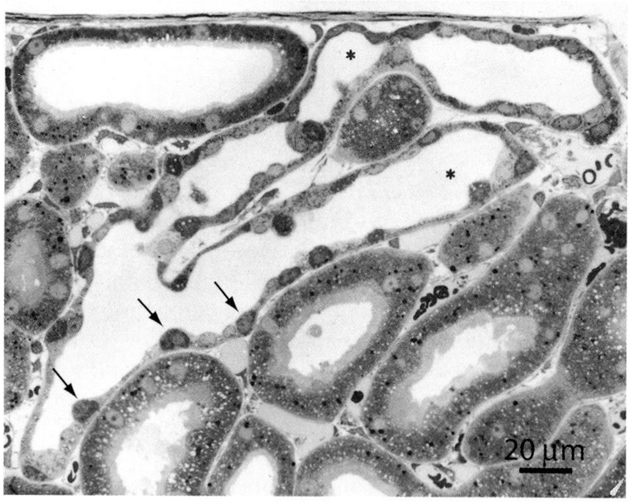


**Fig. 2.40** Light micrograph of initial collecting tubules *(asterisks)* in toluidine blue–stained rat kidney. One tubule lies just beneath the renal capsule *(top of picture)*, where it would be easily accessible to micropuncture. Dark staining cells *(arrows)* are intercalated cells. This segment of the collecting duct corresponds to the so-called late distal tubule as defined in micropuncture studies.

Three distinct intercalated cell subtypes are present in the CNT, based on not only morphologic characteristics but also distinct patterns of transporter expression: type A, type B, and non A, non B.[313–316] In rat and mouse CNT, the so-called non A, non B intercalated cell is the most prevalent subtype, followed by type A cells and type B cells.[313] The morphologic characteristics and localization of specific ion transporters distinguishing these three intercalated cell subtypes and their axial distribution are detailed in the following section.

The CNT contributes to regulated reabsorption of sodium, calcium, and water via specific proteins expressed in CNT cells. In addition to basolateral $Na^+$-$K^+$-ATPase, CNT cells and principal cells in the ICT express the ENaC[282,286,287] and the apical potassium channel, ROMK.[317] Proteins mediating calcium transport expressed by CNT cells include the basolateral $Na^+$-$Ca^{2+}$ exchanger, NCX1, $Ca^{2+}$-ATPase, apical TRPV5, and calbindin-D28K.[292,318–323] In rats, mice, and humans, the CNT, like the collecting duct, expresses the vasopressin-sensitive AQP2,[287,324,325] although AQP2 appears to be absent from the rabbit CNT.[326]

In rat kidney, a small population of cells in the late DCT at the transition to the CNT expresses both the NCC and the $Na^+$-$Ca^{2+}$ exchanger, which have been considered specific for DCT cells and CNT cells, respectively.[284,318] In rabbit kidney, the CNT is distinct from the DCT in both structure and function, and cells coexpressing NCC and the $Na^+$-$Ca^{2+}$ exchanger are not evident in either segment.[291] The CNT makes a transition to the ICT, a segment composed of principal cells and intercalated cells located in the cortical labyrinth before joining with the CCD in the medullary ray. Expression of the $Na^+$-$Ca^{2+}$ exchanger is abundant in the basolateral plasma membrane of CNT cells but undetectable in CCD principal cells.[282]

Potassium loading in rats stimulates potassium secretion in the CNT and increases the basolateral plasma membrane surface area of CNT cells and principal cells of both the CNT and the ICT[327] where $Na^+$-$K^+$-ATPase resides, as well as the apical expression of the potassium channel, ROMK.[317] In rabbits, feeding a low-sodium, high-potassium diet induces a similar increase in CNT basolateral plasma membrane.[297] These structural changes are consistent with increased basolateral $Na^+$-$K^+$-ATPase expression and activity driving apical potassium secretion.

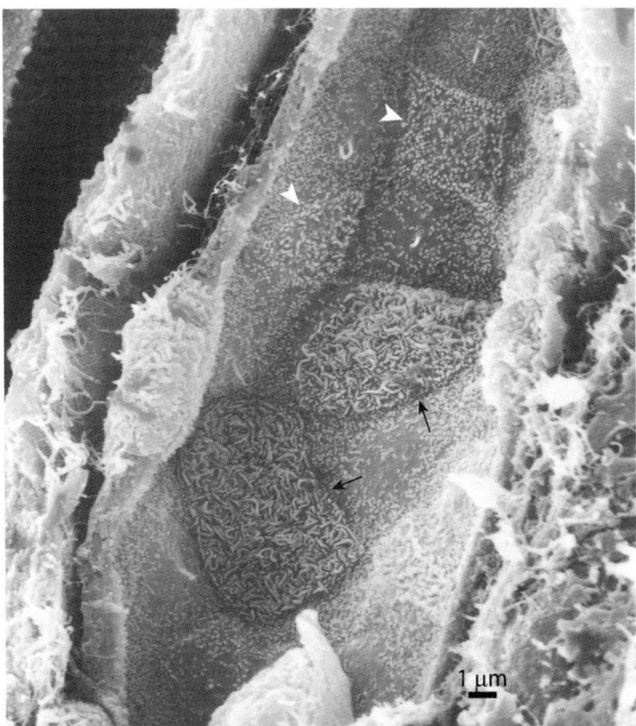


**Fig. 2.41** Scanning electron micrograph showing the luminal surface of a rat cortical collecting duct. Principal cells have small, stubby apical microprojections, and a single cilium. Two configurations of intercalated cells are present: type A *(arrows)*, with a large luminal surface covered mostly with microplicae, and type B *(arrowhead)*, with a more angular outline and a surface covered mostly with small microvilli. (Modified from Madsen KM, Verlander JW, Tisher CC. Relationship between structure and function in distal tubule and collecting duct. *J Electron Microsc Tech.* 1988;9:187–208.)

## COLLECTING DUCT

The collecting duct extends from the initial connecting tubule in the cortex to the tip of the papilla. Subsegments of the collecting duct are defined by their location in the kidney: ICT, CCD, OMCD, and IMCD. The CCD is the portion of the collecting duct located in the medullary ray in the cortex and runs parallel with the cortical PST and TAL. The CCD begins at the fusion of the ICT, located in the cortical labyrinth, with the collecting duct in the medullary ray. The OMCD includes a portion in the outer stripe of the outer medulla, OMCDo, and in the inner stripe, OMCDi. IMCD subsegments in the rat kidney are designated as $IMCD_1$, $IMCD_2$, and $IMCD_3$, corresponding to the proximal, middle, and distal thirds of the IMCD,[328,329] or initial IMCD (IMCDi) and terminal IMCD (IMCDt). In rats, IMCDi corresponds to $IMCD_1$, which is the portion in the base of the inner medulla, whereas IMCDt corresponds to $IMCD_2$ and $IMCD_3$, the papillary portion of the IMCD. The IMCDs terminate as the ducts of Bellini, which open at the tip of the papilla to form the area cribrosa (see Figs. 2.3 and 2.6).

In the ICT, CCD, OMCD, and IMCDi, there are two major cell types: principal cells and intercalated cells (Fig. 2.41). Principal cells are the majority cell type, normally accounting for ~60%–65% of cells in the rat and mouse CCD and OMCD[313,314,330] and ~90% of cells in the rat $IMCD_1$.[328,329] Intercalated cells account for the remainder, with axial heterogeneity in the incidence of the different intercalated cell subtypes. However, the number of intercalated cells is not fixed, even in adult wild-type animals, as several studies have documented increased numbers and percentage of intercalated cells during chronic carbonic anhydrase inhibition,[331] chronic potassium depletion,[332,333] and chronic lithium administration,[334–337] the latter producing even an atypical distribution of intercalated cell subtypes in mice.[334] The terminal portion of the IMCD is made up of a distinct epithelial cell type, the IMCD cell.

### CORTICAL COLLECTING DUCT

The collecting duct in the cortex includes ICT in the cortical labyrinth and the CCD in the medullary ray (see Fig. 2.5). The cells of the ICT are taller than those of the CCD and generally have more complex plasma membrane microprojections and infoldings (Fig. 2.42) and more intense plasma membrane transporter expression, but otherwise these two subsegments are morphologically similar. Nonetheless, because of these subtle differences in ultrastructure, it is important to distinguish between ICT and CCD when quantifying morphologic components or subcellular immunolabeling.

Principal cells account for approximately 60%–65% of cells in the CCD of rabbit,[338] as in rat and mouse.[313,314,330] The nucleus in principal cells is located close to the apical surface, a feature that helps distinguish principal cells from intercalated cells, which have a central or basal nucleus. By transmission electron microscopy, principal cells have relatively few small cytoplasmic vesicles between the nucleus and the apical plasma membrane, a light-staining cytoplasm, and few apical plasma membrane microprojections. By SEM, these apical microprojections appear as short, stubby microvilli that are less numerous near the single central cilium than at the periphery of the cell (see Fig. 2.41). Principal cells have numerous basal plasma membrane infoldings, without interposition of mitochondria or other organelles (see Fig. 2.42). Lateral cell processes and interdigitations are virtually absent.[339] Cell organelles are relatively sparse: mitochondria are small and scattered randomly in the cytoplasm; there are few lysosomes, autophagic vacuoles, and multivesicular bodies; and the Golgi body, rough and smooth endoplasmic reticulum, and free ribosomes are present but not prominent.

Intercalated cells in the CCD are distinguishable from principal cells by several morphologic features. As mentioned earlier, intercalated cells lack cilia and have a more centrally or basally located nucleus versus the apical nucleus of principal cells. Under basal conditions, intercalated cells have more abundant apical plasma membrane microprojections, higher mitochondrial density, abundant cytoplasmic vesicles, numerous polyribosomes, and a prominent Golgi apparatus. In the CNT through CCD, intercalated cells in plastic sections stain more intensely with toluidine blue than principal cells, partly due to cytoplasmic staining and partly due to the high mitochondrial density. This characteristic earned them the designation "dark cells," in early morphologic studies (see Fig. 2.40). By transmission electron microscopy, the electron density of intercalated cell cytoplasm varies with the subtype but generally is somewhat darker than surrounding principal and CNT cells.

In the rat, mouse, and human kidney, three distinct intercalated cell subtypes are present in the CNT, ICT, and CCD. These subtypes are recognizable by ultrastructural features and cell-specific expression and subcellular distribution of various membrane and cytoplasmic proteins. Ultrastructural studies characterized two distinct populations of intercalated cells in the rat CCD, types A and type B, with ~60% of intercalated cells identified as type A and ~40% as type B (Fig. 2.43).[340] The existence of a third distinct intercalated cell subtype was recognized later, the so-called non-A, non-B intercalated cell, which occurs almost exclusively in the CNT and ICT (Fig. 2.44).[313,315,341–344]

By transmission electron microscopy under basal conditions, type A intercalated cells are characterized by moderate apical plasma membrane microprojections, a prominent apical cytoplasmic vesicle compartment, numerous mitochondria, a centrally located nucleus, and moderate basolateral plasma membrane infoldings (see Fig. 2.43). Profiles of the subapical vesicles appear as spherical vesicles and elongated tubulovesicles, which occasionally can be seen in contact with, or invaginating from, the apical plasma membrane (Fig. 2.45). Both the apical plasma membrane and the apical cytoplasmic vesicles are relatively electron-dense, in part due to coating of the cytoplasmic surfaces with characteristic club-shaped particles or "studs," which are also present in the structurally similar OMCD intercalated cells[340,343–346] and which are associated with the vacuolar proton pump, $H^+$-ATPase.[347] By SEM, the apical plasma membrane microprojections are mostly in the form of small folds, "microplicae," rather than microvilli, again similar to OMCD intercalated cells.[330,340,348]

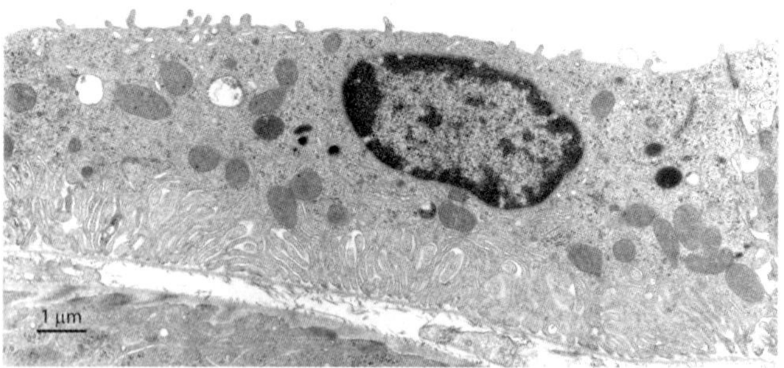


**Fig. 2.42** Transmission electron micrograph of a principal cell from the initial collecting tubule (ICT) from normal rat kidney. Principal cells in the ICT are similar to those in the cortical collecting duct, but typically are slightly taller and have more extensive infoldings of the basal plasma membrane.

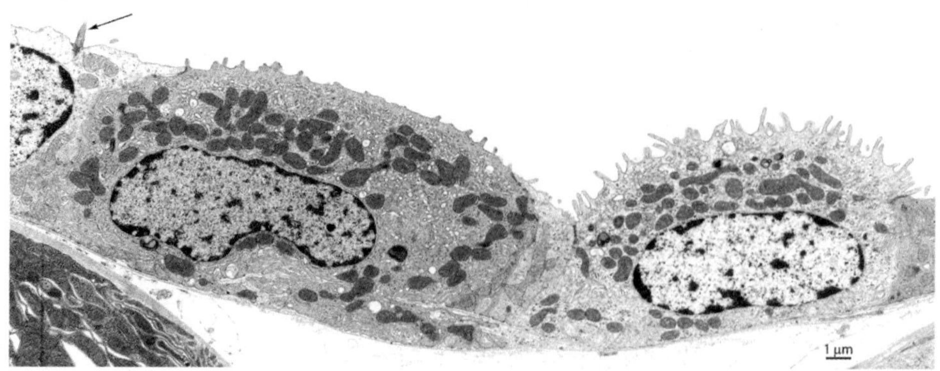


**Fig. 2.43** Transmission electron micrograph from rat cortical collecting duct illustrating type A *(right)* and type B *(left)* intercalated cells under basal conditions. Note differences in the density of the cytoplasm the location of the nuclei, the distribution of the mitochondria and cytoplasmic vesicles, and the number of apical projections between the two cell types. (Modified from Madsen KM, Verlander JW, Tisher CC. Relationship between structure and function in distal tubule and collecting duct. *J Electron Microsc Tech.* 1988;9:187–208.)

By SEM under basal conditions, type B intercalated cells typically have a smaller, more angular luminal cell outline than type A cells and only sparse microprojections, mostly in the form of short microvilli (see Fig. 2.41).[340] By transmission electron microscopy, the type B intercalated cell has a denser cytoplasm and more abundant, frequently clustered mitochondria, and the cell nucleus is typically eccentric, rather than centered (see Fig. 2.43). Numerous vesicles are present throughout the cytoplasm, but the cytoplasmic vesicle membranes are more delicate in appearance and less electron-dense compared with those in type A cells, and few membrane "studs" are evident. The apical plasma membrane is relatively smooth, with small, short microprojections, and a band of dense cytoplasm without organelles or vesicles typically is present just beneath the apical plasma membrane. The basolateral plasma membrane infoldings are more elaborate than in type A cells, except in regions of cytoplasmic extensions filled with vesicles that frequently contact the basement membrane. In the rat under basal conditions, the surface density of the basolateral plasma membrane in type B intercalated cells is significantly greater, and that of the apical plasma membrane is significantly less than in type A cells.[340]

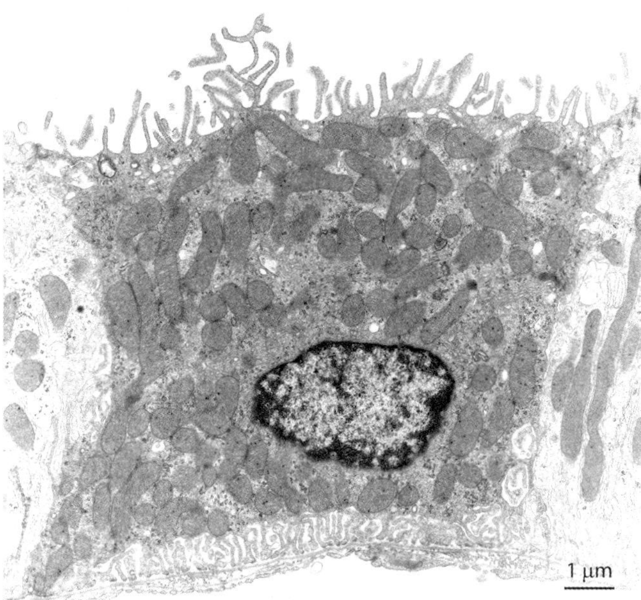


**Fig. 2.44** Transmission electron micrograph of a non-A, non-B intercalated cell in rat kidney. This intercalated cell subtype has a very high mitochondrial density compared with type A and type B intercalated cells, complex basolateral plasma membrane infoldings, and abundant long apical microprojections under basal conditions.

The so-called non-A, non-B intercalated cell represents approximately half of the intercalated cells in the mouse CNT and ICT but is less common in the rat.[313] This cell was initially dubbed "non-A, non-B" because it exhibited protein expression patterns different from the recognized A and B cell types, but it was unclear whether it was a distinct cell type. It now appears clear that this cell is indeed a distinct cell type that can be characterized and differentiated from A and B cells by specific protein expression patterns, in addition to its structural features (Figs. 2.44 and 2.46).

In rabbit kidney, intercalated cells are generally similar to those of rat and mouse. Early studies described "light" and "dark" forms of intercalated cells, with the dark form predominantly in the cortex and the light form predominantly in the outer medulla, suggesting that "light" and "dark" forms may correspond to type A and type B cells, respectively.[202] Four different surface configurations by SEM were described in rabbit collecting duct, based on the presence of microplicae, long and short microvilli, and combinations of these. The precise correlation of the surface configurations to type A and B intercalated cells is not known. However, cells with microplicae were most prevalent in the outer medulla and inner portion of the CCD[338]; this distribution and similarity to the morphology of type A intercalated cells of rat suggest they are type A cells in rabbit as well.

It is well established that intercalated cells contribute to acid–base homeostasis by transport of protons, bicarbonate,

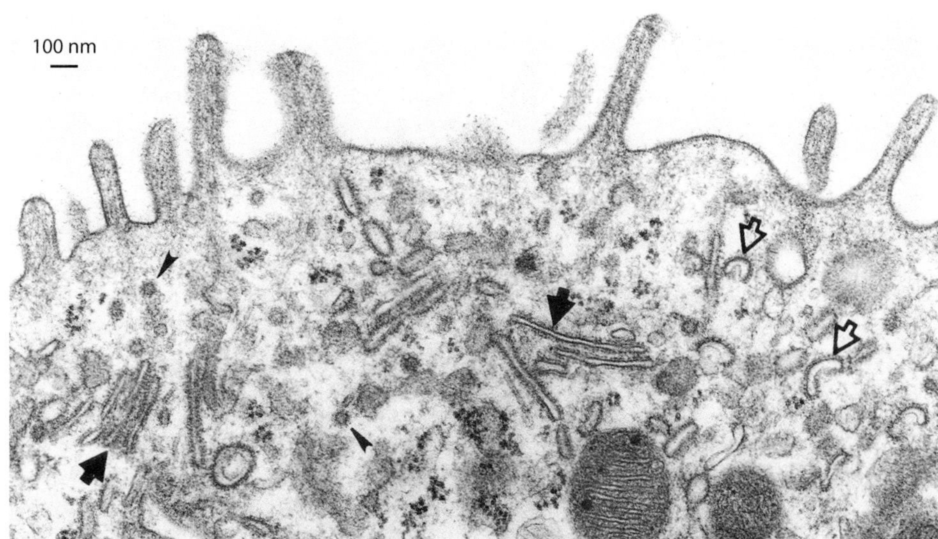


**Fig. 2.45** Transmission electron micrograph illustrating the apical region of a type A intercalated cell from a rat kidney. Note the large number of tubulovesicles *(solid arrows)*, invaginated vesicles *(open arrows)*, and small coated vesicles with the appearance of clathrin vesicles *(arrowheads)*.

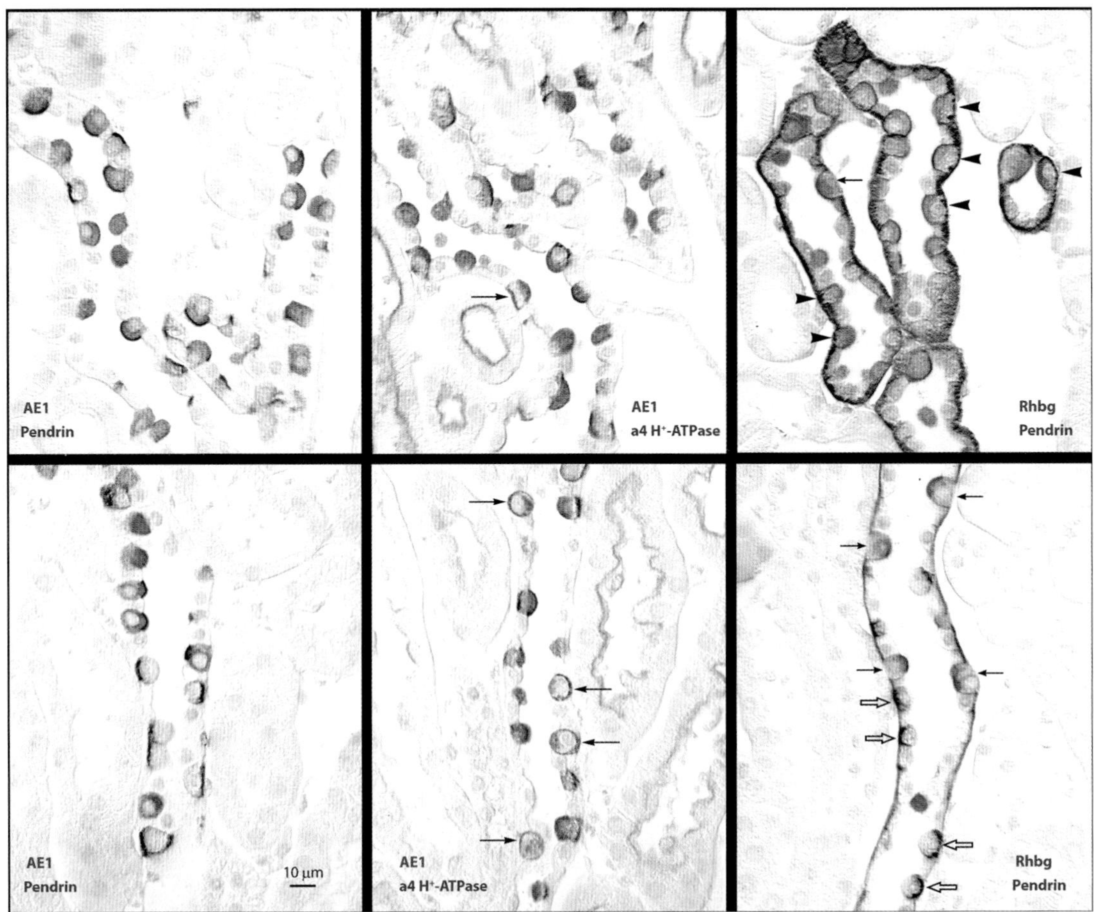


**Fig. 2.46** Characteristic immunolabeling of three distinct intercalated cell subtypes in the connecting segment (CNT, *top panels*) and cortical collecting duct (CCD, *bottom panels*) by differential interference contrast microscopy (DIC). Type A intercalated cells express the basolateral anion exchanger, AE1, apical $H^+$-ATPase, and the basolateral ammonia transporter, Rhbg. Type B intercalated cells express the apical anion exchanger, pendrin, and basolateral $H^+$-ATPase, but no AE1 or Rhbg. The third type, the so-called non-A, non-B intercalated cell (or type C intercalated cell), expresses apical pendrin and basolateral Rhbg, but no AE1. Left column: Double labeling for AE1 *(brown)*, which is definitive for type A intercalated cells, and apical pendrin *(blue)*, which is present in type B and non-A, non-B intercalated cells. Pendrin labeling is exclusively in AE1-negative cells. Middle column: Double labeling for AE1 *(brown)* and the a4 subunit of $H^+$-ATPase *(blue)*. Type A intercalated cells (AE1-positive) have apical $H^+$-ATPase label. Type B intercalated cells have basolateral $H^+$-ATPase label *(arrows)*, as well as diffuse apical label, which correlates with cytoplasmic vesicle labeling shown by immunogold electron microscopy. Type B intercalated cells are uncommon in the connecting segment (CNT), but represent virtually all of the non-A intercalated cells in the cortical collecting duct (CCD). In the CNT, the majority of non-A intercalated cells have apical $H^+$-ATPase label but no basolateral label. These are non-A, non-B (type C) intercalated cells. Right column: Double labeling for pendrin *(blue)* and Rhbg *(brown)*. Type B intercalated cells and non-A, non-B intercalated cells, both pendrin-positive, can be discriminated by basolateral Rhbg expression. Non-A, non-B intercalated cells, which express basolateral Rhbg *(arrowheads)*, are the predominant pendrin-positive cell type in the CNT. Type B intercalated cells do not express detectable Rhbg *(arrows)* and comprise virtually all of the pendrin-positive cells in the CCD. Rhbg immunolabel is also present in type A intercalated cells *(open arrows)*, CNT cells, and CCD principal cells.

and ammonia. All intercalated cell subtypes express carbonic anhydrase type II (CA II) throughout the cytoplasm, although the different subtypes exhibit varied patterns of expression.[341,349,350] Type A intercalated cells have the most intense immunolabeling for CA II, with more intense labeling near the apical and basolateral plasma membrane domains. CA II expression in type B intercalated cells is diffuse and relatively weak, whereas the level in non-A, non-B cells is intermediate.[341]

The electrogenic proton pump, $H^+$-ATPase, is also strongly expressed in all intercalated cells, but the subcellular distribution determined by immunogold electron microscopy varies among the subtypes.[314,351–353] In type A intercalated cells, $H^+$-ATPase is present in the apical plasma membrane and apical cytoplasmic vesicle membranes. In type B intercalated cells, $H^+$-ATPase is present in the basolateral plasma membrane but not in the apical plasma membrane, and in cytoplasmic vesicles throughout the cell, including subapical vesicles, which likely accounts for cells with "bipolar" $H^+$-ATPase immunolabeling, have been observed by light (Fig. 2.46).[313] Like A cells, non-A, non-B intercalated cells have $H^+$-ATPase in the apical plasma membrane and subapical cytoplasmic vesicles. These distinctions in $H^+$-ATPase distribution may not be discernible by light microscopy techniques, depending on the resolution of the method and the characteristics of the anti-$H^+$-ATPase antibody used (Fig. 2.46). In rabbits, cells with the subcellular distribution of $H^+$-ATPase typical of type A and type B intercalated cells are present in the CNT, ICT, and CCD, but in CCD under basal conditions, the most prevalent distribution pattern is exclusively in intracytoplasmic vesicles in small intercalated cells with relatively uncomplicated plasma membrane compartments, suggestive of an inactive cell.[353] Intercalated cells in the rabbit CNT and ICT have the typical polarized distribution of $H^+$-ATPase seen in rat and mouse intercalated cells.[353]

Expression of the $Cl^-/HCO_3^-$ anion exchanger, AE1, is definitive for type A intercalated cells, as it is the only renal epithelial cell that expresses this protein. In rat and mouse kidney, AE1 is almost entirely expressed in the basolateral plasma membrane,[314,342,354,355] whereas in rabbit kidney under basal conditions, a large portion of AE1 is intracellular in multivesicular bodies and cytoplasmic vesicles, in addition to the basolateral plasma membrane.[356,357]

In addition to being devoid of AE1, type B and non-A, non-B intercalated cells are distinguished from type A cells by the expression of the apical $Cl^-/HCO_3^-$ exchanger, pendrin (Slc26a4).[313,315,358–360] In both type B and non-A, non-B intercalated cells, pendrin is present in the apical plasma membrane and subapical cytoplasmic vesicles, although in basal conditions, the subcellular distribution is significantly different; pendrin is predominantly in the apical plasma membrane of non-A, non-B cells but predominantly in subapical vesicles in type B cells, with little apical plasma membrane expression.[315]

The three recognized intercalated cell subtypes also have cell-specific expression of other transporters and enzymes, particularly those involved in ammonia metabolism. Type A and non-A, non-B intercalated cells express the ammonia transporters, Rhbg and Rhcg, and cytoplasmic glutamine synthetase.[361,362] In both cell types, Rhbg is exclusively in the basolateral plasma membrane, whereas Rhcg is expressed in both the apical and basolateral plasma membranes in type A cells, in the apical plasma membrane in non-A, non-B cells, and in apical cytoplasmic vesicles in both cell types.[316,353,363–365] In contrast, type B intercalated cells do not express detectable Rhcg, Rhbg, or glutamine synthetase.[361,362,366]

The pattern of transporter and enzyme expression in intercalated cell subtypes combined with physiologic studies and morphologic studies documenting cell-specific alterations in ultrastructural features and transporter distribution in response to physiologic maneuvers together have established that type A intercalated cells secrete acid, whereas type B intercalated cells secrete bicarbonate, indicating that the existence of these functionally distinct intercalated cells subtypes is responsible for the ability of the CCD to accomplish both net acid secretion and net bicarbonate secretion.[367,368] Many structural studies have documented intercalated cell subtype-specific changes in ultrastructure and subcellular distribution of ion and ammonia transporters in response to physiologic disturbances.[340,352,357,369–372] Such studies have demonstrated an increase in apical plasma membrane surface area and diminished apical cytoplasmic vesicles and redistribution of $H^+$-ATPase and Rhcg to the apical plasma membrane in type A intercalated cells in models of acidosis[340,357,369] and increased basolateral plasma membrane surface area along with redistribution of AE1 from intracellular compartments to the basolateral plasma membrane in type A cells of acid-loaded rabbits,[357] consistent with activation of acid and ammonia secretion by type A cells during acidosis. In contrast, chloride-depletion metabolic alkalosis decreases apical plasma membrane complexity and increases the abundance of apical cytoplasmic vesicles concomitant with internalization of $H^+$-ATPase in type A cells, suggesting inactivation of acid secretion.[352] In type B intercalated cells, various models in mice that enhance bicarbonate secretion and chloride uptake increase apical plasma membrane surface area, decrease apical cytoplasmic vesicles, and cause redistribution of pendrin from the cytoplasmic vesicles to the apical plasma membrane.[370–372] In rats, chloride-depletion metabolic alkalosis increases type B intercalated cell size, basolateral plasma membrane complexity, and basolateral plasma membrane $H^+$-ATPase expression.[352]

Non-A, non-B intercalated cells have the ability to secrete bicarbonate via apical pendrin and to secrete protons via apical $H^+$-ATPase, but the net effect of these processes is poorly understood because the anatomy of the CNT, where most non-A, non-B cells reside, makes in vitro studies of these specific cells extremely difficult if not impossible. Type B and non-A, non-B intercalated cells appear to have an important role in transcellular chloride reabsorption via coordination of apical pendrin-mediated $Cl^-/HCO_3^-$ exchange and basolateral chloride exit via ClC-K2 channels.[373,374] In mouse models that increase pendrin activity in type B intercalated cells, described above, non-A, non-B cells typically exhibit increased apical plasma membrane area and pendrin expression as well, although the relative distribution of pendrin between cytoplasmic vesicles and the apical plasma membrane frequently does not change.[370–372,375]

The functions of type A, **a**cid-secreting, and type B, **b**icarbonate-secreting, intercalated cells correspond well to their names. Although changes in nomenclature can create confusion initially, because the "non-A, non-B" cell is primarily found in the **C**NT and is believed to have an important role in **c**hloride transport, designating it as a "type C" intercalated cell would be logical.

In contrast to intercalated cells, principal cells express abundant $Na^+K^+$-ATPase in the basolateral plasma membrane, the ENaC, and the potassium channel, ROMK, in the apical plasma membrane. AQP2 is present in the apical plasma membrane and cytoplasmic vesicles, as well as in the basolateral plasma membrane.[324,376,377] The ammonia transporters Rhbg and Rhcg are less abundant than in intercalated cells in the basal state but otherwise are expressed in a pattern similar to type A intercalated cells. These transporters enable principal cells to reabsorb sodium and secrete potassium, to reabsorb water when vasopressin is present, and to contribute to ammonia secretion.

Structural correlates in principal cells in cortical segments to changes in the physiologic state are typically not as dramatic as those seen in intercalated cells. In rats and rabbits, feeding a high-potassium diet[297,327] or treating with aldosterone or the mineralocorticoid analog deoxycorticosterone[378–380] significantly increases the basolateral plasma membrane surface area of principal cells. Furthermore, models that enhance sodium reabsorption in the CCD cause redistribution and increased apical plasma membrane expression of ENaC subunits.[381–384] These structural and immunolocalization studies correlate with the roles of principal cells in regulated sodium reabsorption and potassium secretion.

## OUTER MEDULLARY COLLECTING DUCT

Like the CCD, the OMCD epithelium is made up of principal cells and intercalated cells. In rat and mouse kidney, intercalated cells represent 35%–40% of the cells in both the OMCDo and the OMCDi.[314,330] In rabbit kidney, the percentage of intercalated cells in the OMCD is less, approximately 18%, with the percentage declining axially from the OMCDo to the deep OMCDi.[338] However, some investigators did not observe distinct epithelial cell heterogeneity in the rabbit OMCDi based on morphologic criteria, although the cells varied in mitochondrial content, subapical vesicle abundance, and density of rod-shaped particles in the apical plasma membrane.[385]

Principal cells of the OMCD are structurally similar to those in the CCD, although they become slightly taller, and the number of organelles and basal infoldings decreases as the collecting duct descends through the outer medulla. Like principal cells in the CCD, those in the OMCDo express apical plasma membrane ENaC and AQP2 and basolateral plasma membrane $Na^+K^+$-ATPase, consistent with their function in sodium and water reabsorption.[217,377,381,386] The ammonia transporters, Rhbg and Rhcg, are also expressed in a similar pattern as in CCD principal cells, with basolateral Rhbg and apical and basolateral Rhcg, consistent with a role in ammonia secretion.[361,365]

The majority of intercalated cells of the OMCD are structurally similar to type A intercalated cells of the CCD (Fig. 2.47), although with more prominent apical plasma membrane microprojections and fewer apical cytoplasmic vesicles under basal conditions. They also have similar transporter expression patterns, including $H^+$ATPase and Rhcg in the apical plasma membrane and apical cytoplasmic vesicles and AE1, Rhbg, and Rhcg in the basolateral plasma membrane.[351–354,361] In the OMCDi, the intercalated cells are taller, there are generally fewer apical cytoplasmic tubulovesicles, and the cytoplasm is less electron-dense such that it is similar to that of principal cells. Type B intercalated cells, identified by pendrin expression, are generally absent, but when present are typically sparse and limited to the OMCDo near the corticomedullary junction. The presence of only the acid-secreting intercalated cell subtype in the OMCD is consistent with this segment's ability to secrete acid and inability to secrete bicarbonate.[367]

Under basal conditions, intercalated cells in the outer medulla exhibit moderate apical plasma membrane surface microplicae and cytoplasmic tubulovesicles; the cytoplasmic face of the tubulovesicles is coated with electron-dense stud-like particles[343,344] associated with the vacuolar $H^+$-ATPase (see Fig. 2.45).[347] After induction of acute respiratory acidosis, metabolic acidosis, or hypokalemia, the apical cytoplasmic tubulovesicles are depleted, and apical plasma membrane microplicae proliferate and protrude into the lumen, producing a marked increase in apical plasma membrane surface area[330,343,344,387] and an increase in apical plasma membrane exhibiting studs on the cytoplasmic face, visible by transmission electron microscopy.[343,344] These ultrastructural changes coincide with increased apical plasma membrane expression of $H^+$ATPase and Rhcg and decreased expression of these transporters in the apical cytoplasmic vesicle compartment, consistent with enhanced proton and ammonia secretion during these conditions.[369,388,389] Conversely, during chloride-depletion metabolic acidosis, apical plasma membrane surface area and $H^+$ATPase expression decrease, whereas apical cytoplasmic vesicles and $H^+$ATPase expression increase, consistent with reduced acid secretion in response to alkalosis.[352] Similar responses have been documented in type A intercalated cells in the CCD.[340,352,357]

In rabbit kidney, additional structural changes are associated with acid-loading involving the redistribution of expression of AE1, the basolateral $Cl^-/HCO_3^-$ exchanger. Under basal conditions, rabbit OMCD intercalated cells contain prominent intracytoplasmic multivesicular bodies that express AE1.[356] After acid loading, these multivesicular bodies are reduced in number, and basolateral plasma membrane boundary

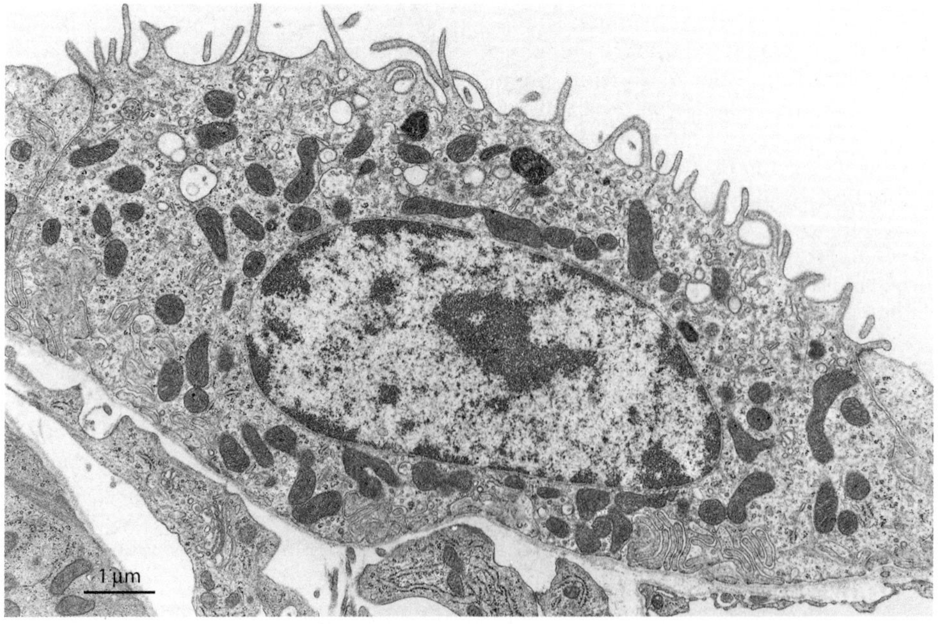


**Fig. 2.47** Transmission electron micrograph of an intercalated cell in the outer medullary collecting duct of a normal rat kidney. The cell has a prominent tubulovesicular membrane compartment and many microprojections on the apical surface. (Modified from Madsen KM, Tisher CC. Response of intercalated cells of rat outer medullary collecting duct to chronic metabolic acidosis. *Lab Invest.* 1984;51:268–276.)

length and AE1 expression increase, along with the development of prominent basolateral extensions that give the cells a stellate appearance by light microscopy.[357] These findings suggest that in rabbits, acidosis stimulates not only redistribution of proton pumps from the cytoplasmic pool to the apical plasma membrane but also redistribution of intracellular AE1 to the basolateral plasma membrane, thus enabling enhanced proton secretion and bicarbonate reabsorption.

## INNER MEDULLARY COLLECTING DUCT

The IMCD extends from the boundary between the outer and inner medulla, defined by the transitions from thin to thick ascending limbs, to the papillary tip. In rat and rabbit, the transition from thin to thick ascending limbs, and thus the beginning of the IMCD, occurs within the renal parenchyma proximal to the papilla, forming the base of the inner medulla. However, in some mice, the TALs arise in the proximal portion of the papilla, in which case the IMCD is entirely contained within the papilla.

The IMCDs fuse successively as they descend in the inner medulla, such that few tubules remain at the papillary tip (Fig. 2.48). Cell height and tubule diameter increase distally, and the most distal portion, the ducts of Bellini, are composed of relatively tall, columnar epithelium. The IMCDt opens on the tip of the papilla at the area cribrosa (see Figs. 2.3 and 2.6). The length of the papilla, the number of collecting duct fusions, and cell height vary among species.[241,390] In the rabbit, the cell height gradually increases from ~10 μm initially to ~50 μm near the papillary tip, whereas in the rat, the height increases from ~6 μm to ~15 μm at the papillary tip.[241,391] In the rabbit and rat, the papillary tip is located in the renal pelvis at or near the renal hilum, whereas in the mouse, the papilla extends beyond the hilum, turning and extending a short distance into the ureter.

For ultrastructural characterization in the rat, the inner medulla was subdivided arbitrarily into thirds, and the IMCD in each region designated accordingly.[328,329,391] The outer third, $IMCD_1$, is the portion in the base of the inner medulla. The middle and terminal thirds, $IMCD_2$ and $IMCD_3$, are the portions in the proximal and terminal halves of the papilla, respectively. $IMCD_1$ is similar in ultrastructure to the OMCDi (Fig. 2.49), although the percentage of intercalated cells is only ~10% in rat $IMCD_1$.[328,329] In rabbit, the IMCDi is essentially composed of only one cell type, similar in ultrastructure to the principal cell in the OMCDi, with intercalated cells typically representing only 1% or less of cells.[202,338] Rat $IMCD_2$ contains a mixture of ciliated cells similar to the principal cells in $IMCD_1$, a population of nonciliated cells, termed IMCD cells, and only rare intercalated cells (Fig. 2.50).[328,329] Ciliated cells disappear in the distal $IMCD_2$, and $IMCD_3$ is composed entirely of IMCD cells, similar to those in $IMCD_2$ but taller (Fig. 2.51). In physiologic studies, the rat IMCD segments are often divided into an initial portion, the IMCDi, corresponding to $IMCD_1$, and a terminal or papillary portion, the IMCDt, which includes $IMCD_2$ and $IMCD_3$. Such studies in the rat have demonstrated that the structurally defined IMCD segments are also functionally distinct in comparisons of IMCDi ($IMCD_1$) to IMCDt ($IMCD_2$ and $IMCD_3$).[392–394]

The IMCD cell of $IMCD_2$ and $IMCD_3$ is structurally distinct from principal cells (compare Figs. 2.52 and 2.49).[328,391] It is one of the two epithelial cell types in the kidney (the other being intercalated cells) that has no central cilium. The luminal surface is covered with abundant, small, stubby plasma membrane microprojections that are covered with a prominent glycocalyx. Basal plasma membrane infoldings are relatively sparse, whereas lateral plasma membrane infoldings are prominent. Although both the apical and basal plasma membrane surface densities decrease progressively from $IMCD_1$ to $IMCD_3$, the absolute area of these membrane compartments does not change. In contrast, the lateral plasma membrane surface density and absolute area progressively increase. IMCD cells typically have a light-staining cytoplasm, few cell organelles, numerous free ribosomes, and many

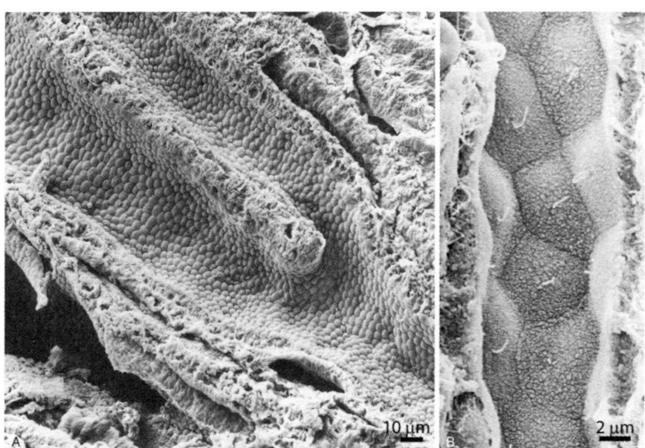


**Fig. 2.48** Scanning electron micrographs of the normal papillary collecting duct of a rabbit. (A) The junction between two subdivisions at low magnification. (B) Higher-magnification view illustrating the luminal surfaces of individual cells with prominent microvilli and single cilia. (A, Courtesy Ann LeFurgey, PhD; B, modified from LeFurgey A, Tisher CC. Morphology of rabbit collecting duct. *Am J Anat.* 1979;155: 111–124.)

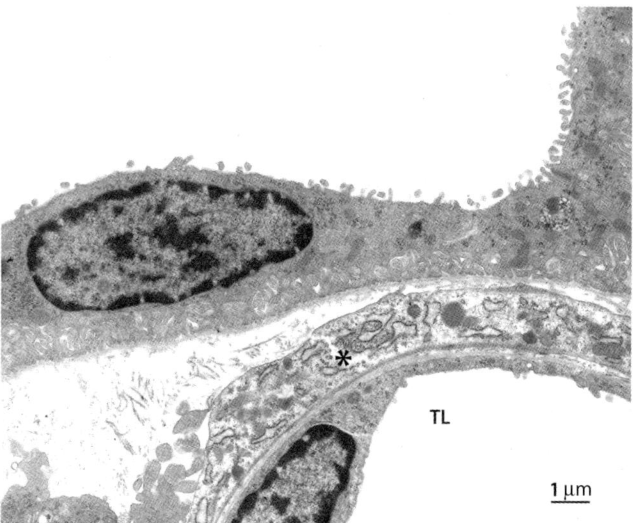


**Fig. 2.49** Transmission electron micrograph of a principal cell from the initial portion of the rat inner medullary collecting duct. There are few organelles in the cytoplasm, and apical microprojections are sparse. An interstitial fibroblast *(asterisk)* with dilated rough endoplasmic reticulum and a thin limb *(TL)* of loop of Henle are also illustrated.

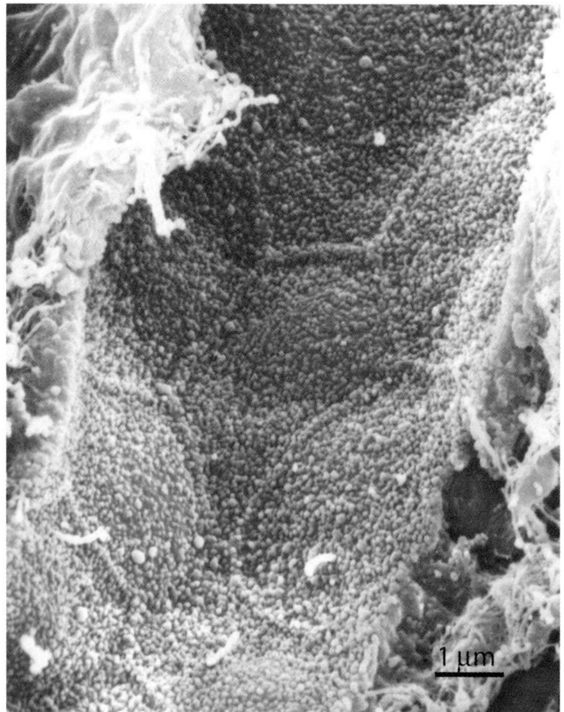


**Fig. 2.50** Scanning electron micrograph from the middle portion of the rat inner medullary collecting duct. The luminal surface is covered with small microvilli, and some cells have single cilia, whereas others do not. (Modified from Madsen KM, Clapp WL, Verlander JW. Structure and function of the inner medullary collecting duct. *Kidney Int.* 1988;34: 441–454.)

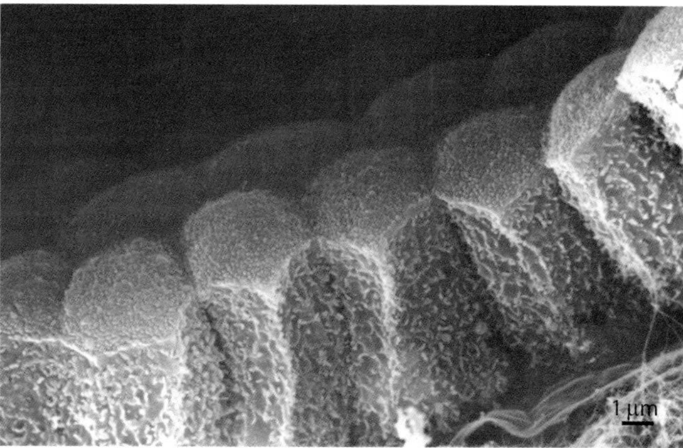


**Fig. 2.51** Scanning electron micrograph of the terminal portion of rabbit inner medullary collecting duct. The cells are tall and covered with small microvilli on their luminal surfaces, but lack cilia. Small lateral cell processes project into the lateral intercellular spaces. (Modified from Madsen KM, Clapp WL, Verlander JW. Structure and function of the inner medullary collecting duct. *Kidney Int.* 1988;34:441.)

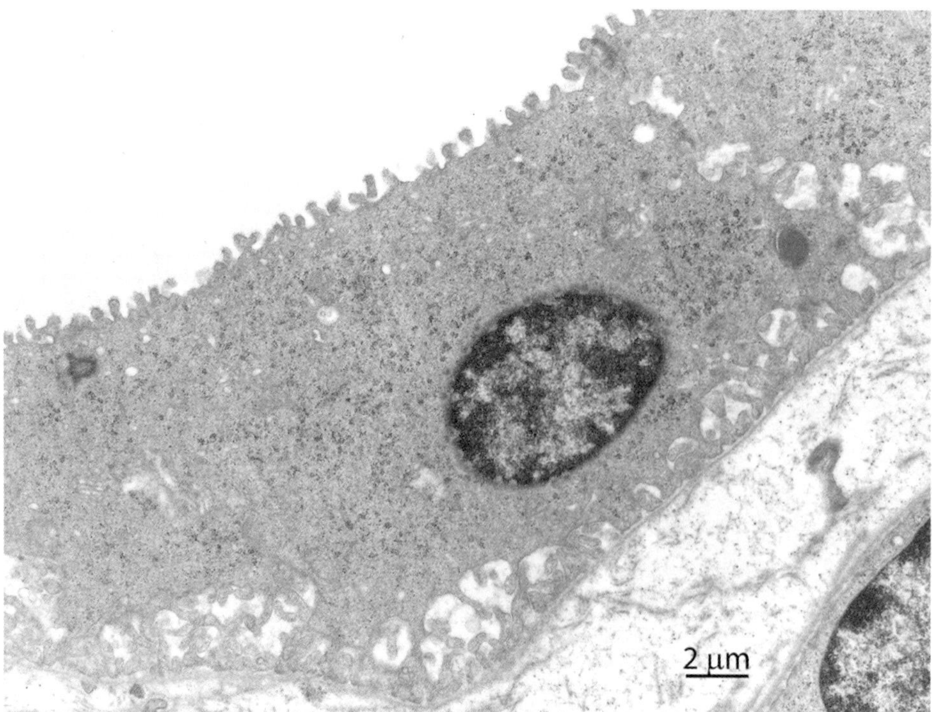


**Fig. 2.52** Transmission electron micrograph of rat inner medullary collecting duct (IMCD) cell. IMCD cells are tall, possess few organelles, and have small microprojections on their apical surfaces. Ribosomes are abundant, and small vesicles are scattered throughout the cytoplasm.

small, coated vesicles resembling clathrin-coated vesicles (Fig. 2.52). IMCD cells, particularly those in $IMCD_3$, contain electron-dense, intracytoplasmic bodies representing lysosomes or lipid inclusions, often located beneath the nucleus.[328]

$IMCD_1$ and OMCDi principal and intercalated cells have similar transporter expression patterns and are believed to be functionally similar. However, $IMCD_2$ and $IMCD_3$ (IMCDt) not only have distinct structural features but also are distinct with respect to transporter expression. Notably, IMCD cells, present only in $IMCD_2$ and $IMCD_3$, express the urea transporters UT-A1 and UT-A3, whereas principal cells in $IMCD_1$ do not.[395] Although few studies have correlated structural and functional responses in the IMCD, the rat $IMCD_1$ principal cell responds to chronic low-protein diet with a marked increase in basolateral plasma membrane area and enhanced urea transport, whereas IMCD cells in $IMCD_2$ show no change in ultrastructure or urea transport.[392] Later studies identified a sodium-dependent, active urea transport process present in $IMCD_1$ but absent in $IMCD_2$ and $IMCD_3$.[393] IMCD cells also express AQP2 and regulation of its subcellular distribution occurs in response to vasopressin and water restriction, which stimulate redistribution of AQP2 from intracytoplasmic vesicles to the apical plasma membrane, thus enabling enhanced water uptake.[377,378,396–398]

## PAPILLARY SURFACE EPITHELIUM

The papilla is covered by a simple cuboidal epithelium, aptly named the papillary surface epithelium (PSE). PSE cells typically have a relatively smooth apical surface, numerous cytoplasmic vesicles, few mitochondria, and moderate basolateral infoldings. Multiple immunolocalization studies have detected expression of various transporters and other proteins, including the urea transporter, UT-B1, $Na^+$-$K^+$-ATPase, $H^+$-$K^+$-ATPase $\alpha_{2c}$, NKCC1, and osteopontin.[399–402] PSE cellular expression of $H^+$-$K^+$-ATPase $\alpha_{2c}$ is heterogeneous, suggesting heterogeneity in the epithelial cell types.[401] Limited physiologic studies have demonstrated transport activity consistent with the reported protein expression,[403–405] and the presence of osteopontin supports the concept that PSE has a role in inhibiting urinary crystal deposition.[399]

## INTERSTITIUM

The renal interstitium is composed of the structures interposed between the basement membranes of the renal tubules, glomeruli, and the vascular elements.[406,407] Included in this space are several types of interstitial cells, extracellular matrix, interstitial fluid, lymphatics, and nerves.[406–408] The interstitial volume in the rat and rabbit kidney constitutes approximately 13% and 18% of the total kidney volume, respectively.[409] There is a considerable difference in the abundance of interstitium in the cortex compared with the medulla. In the rat kidney cortex, the peritubular interstitium constitutes 4% to 9% of the tissue volume.[45,410,411] Interstitial volume increases from 10% to 20% in the outer medulla to approximately 30% to 40% at the papillary tip in both the rat and the rabbit.[390,412]

The interstitium may be subdivided into different compartments, primarily the peritubular interstitium and the periarterial connective tissue.[407] Although the glomerular and extraglomerular mesangium may be considered part of the interstitium, based on their location, the makeup of the cells, and their communication with the peritubular interstitium,[407] they are a specialized component of the glomerulus and JGA, discussed in a previous section, and are not included here.

The peritubular interstitium includes the interstitial cells, extracellular matrix, and interstitial fluid interposed between the basement membranes of the renal tubules and peritubular capillaries; it is continuous with the connective tissue of the renal capsule.[411] The periarterial interstitium is a layer of connective tissue and interstitial cells surrounding the arteries in the renal cortex and may account for half of the cortical interstitial volume.[407,411] It is most abundant around the interlobular and arcuate arteries and communicates with the peritubular interstitium[407] and with the connective tissue underlying the epithelium of the renal pelvis.[411] The periarterial interstitium is composed of a network of fibroblasts, similar to those in the peritubular interstitium, amid loose connective tissue; embedded in this are lymphatics and nerve fibers. The periarterial interstitium diminishes along the smaller arterioles and ends at the vascular pole of the glomerulus.

Interstitial cells can be classified most simply into two types: fibroblasts and cells of the immune system[411,413]; these cell types correspond to the earlier designations, type 1 and type 2 interstitial cells.[408,413–415] Fibroblasts, also known as "stellate" or "sustentacular cells," are resident cells and are the most abundant cell type in the peritubular interstitium.[407,411,413,416] In healthy kidney, interstitial fibroblasts are interconnected by intermediate junctions and form a network throughout the renal parenchyma, spanning between the capillaries and renal tubules. Interstitial fibroblasts form a scaffold, maintaining the architecture of the kidney, in part through attachments of their cellular extensions, "attachment plaques" filled with actin fibers, to the basement membranes of the capillaries and tubules and also by synthesis of collagen fibers of the extracellular matrix and microfilaments. The morphology of "quiescent" fibroblasts in the cortical interstitium of healthy kidney is typical of fibroblasts in other tissues, characterized by an elongated cell shape, angular nucleus, long cytoplasmic extensions, and abundant intracellular actin filaments (Fig. 2.53). The larger cytoplasmic extensions are flattened, perforated "leaflike" extensions or longer filiform processes. The cytoplasm contains numerous mitochondria and free ribosomes and prominent rough endoplasmic reticulum with dilated cisterns containing flocculent material. In inflammatory disease, interstitial fibroblasts increase in number, and the morphology of these "activated" fibroblasts differs from the fibroblasts of healthy kidney interstitium. These are termed "myofibroblasts" due to characteristics in common with smooth muscle cells, particularly formation of bundles of myofilaments and increased expression of α-smooth muscle actin. In the deep inner stripe of the outer medulla and the inner medulla, the fibroblast morphology differs from those in the cortex, containing numerous lipid inclusions, such that they have been called "lipid-laden" cells. These cells have relatively few mitochondria, rough endoplasmic reticulum with widely dilated cisterns and frequent contacts with the plasma membrane, and a more prominent cytoskeleton near the plasma membrane and extending into the cytoplasmic extensions, containing α-smooth muscle actin and vimentin filaments.[411,417]

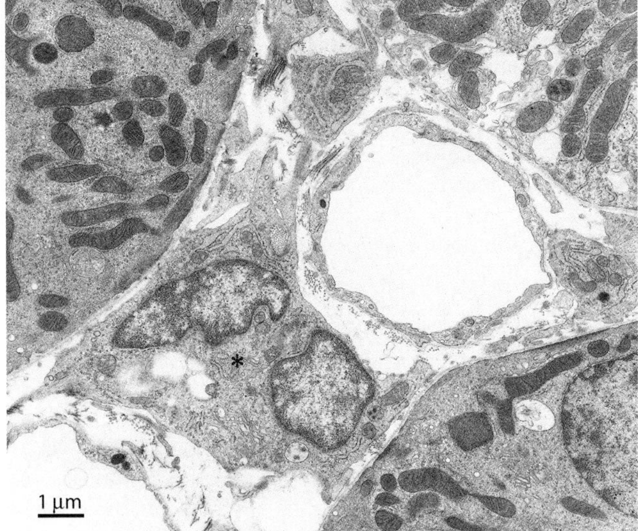


**Fig. 2.53** Transmission electron micrograph of cortical interstitial fibroblast *(asterisk)* from a rat. A peritubular capillary is located at right center.

Pericytes are contractile cells intimately associated with the capillaries in both the renal cortex and medulla and may be considered a component of the renal interstitium.[407,417–419] These cells correspond to cells previously identified in the medullary interstitium and designated "type 3 interstitial cells." They are most abundant in the inner stripe of the outer medulla in association with descending vasa recta, but are also present in the renal cortex. Pericytes are attached to or embedded in the basement membrane of capillaries and wrap long cytoplasmic extensions around the vessel. In the renal medulla, they frequently contain lipid inclusions, which are less abundant than in medullary fibroblasts. Multiphoton imaging of pericytes using cell-specific markers recently demonstrated that pericyte density is greatest at branch points of the microvasculature where shear stress is greatest, with the cell bodies downstream of the branch point and cellular extensions reaching upstream, wrapping around the capillaries at the branch point.[420] Pericytes proliferate during inflammation and appear to be the progenitors of the interstitial myofibroblasts, leading to increased matrix deposition and fibrosis.[421]

The other major category of cells in the interstitium includes various cells of the immune system.[411] Of these, the most common are dendritic cells. Dendritic cells in the kidney have a typical stellate shape, long cytoplasmic extensions, few lysosomes, and abundant mitochondria and rough endoplasmic reticulum. Dendritic cells are distinguished from fibroblasts by the lack of actin filament bundles under the plasma membrane and within cytoplasmic extensions; furthermore, the organelles in dendritic cells are clustered around the nucleus and absent from the cytoplasmic extensions.[411,413,416] Less commonly found in the interstitium are transitory cells of the immune system, mainly macrophages and lymphocytes. In the healthy kidney, macrophages are mostly located in the periarterial interstitium, but they are not abundant. Lymphocytes are uncommon, and granulocytes are rare.[411]

The extracellular matrix of the interstitium consists of collagen fibrils within a ground substance of sulfated and nonsulfated GAGs and interstitial fluid.[407,408] Collagen fibrils of types I, III, V, VI, VII, and XV have been identified in the extracellular matrix[407,418,422,423] as well as fibronectin and laminin.[407,422]

## CORTICAL INTERSTITIUM

In the renal cortex, the peritubular interstitium is compartmentalized into a wide interstitial space, between two or more adjacent renal tubules, and a narrow or slit-like interstitial space between the basement membrane of a single tubule and the adjacent peritubular capillary.[415,424] Approximately two-thirds of the total peritubular capillary wall faces the narrow compartment, and this portion of the vessel wall is fenestrated.[410]

Fibroblasts and dendritic cells constitute the majority of interstitial cells in the peritubular interstitium, are distributed homogeneously, and are in close proximity to each other.[411] The cell types can be discriminated by light microscopy by immunolabeling, as the cortical fibroblasts express the enzyme, ecto-5′-nucleotidase (5′NT), whereas dendritic cells express MHC class II.[411] Under basal conditions, 5′NT expression in cortical fibroblasts is strongest in the cortical labyrinth in the deep inner cortex.[411,425] As 5′NT mediates production of extracellular adenosine, a signaling molecule implicated in control of renal vascular resistance, cortical interstitial fibroblasts may contribute to regulation of renal hemodynamics.[406,416] Peritubular interstitial fibroblasts and/or pericytes in the deep inner cortex are also the renal source of erythropoietin,[417,426] and perivascular interstitial cells associated with the afferent arteriole can be recruited to produce renin during salt and volume depletion, renal hypoperfusion, or inhibition of the renin–angiotensin–aldosterone system.[417]

## MEDULLARY INTERSTITIUM

As in the cortex, fibroblasts and dendritic cells constitute the vast majority of interstitial cells in the healthy renal medulla.[411,413,427] As described earlier, the fibroblasts of the medullary interstitium differ most notably from the cortical fibroblasts in the abundance of intracytoplasmic lipid inclusions, with an average diameter of 0.4 to 0.5 µm; the lipid droplets are homogeneous in density and have no limiting membrane (Figs. 2.54 and 2.55).[415,424,427,428] Only occasional cortical fibroblasts contain lipid droplets; the incidence of these "lipid-laden" fibroblasts increases in the inner stripe of the outer medulla and they are present throughout the inner medulla.[411] Unlike the fibroblasts of the cortex, medullary interstitial fibroblasts do not express erythropoietin messenger RNA or 5′NT.[425,426]

Medullary interstitial fibroblasts form a ladderlike structure between the loops of Henle and vasa recta, arranged in columns along the corticomedullary axis and oriented perpendicular to the adjacent tubules and vessels (see Fig. 2.54). The elongated cell processes are in close contact with the thin limbs of Henle and the vasa recta, but direct contact with collecting ducts is rarely observed. Often, a single cell is in contact with several vessels and thin limbs.[424] The long cytoplasmic processes from different cells are often connected by specialized cell junctions that vary in both size and shape

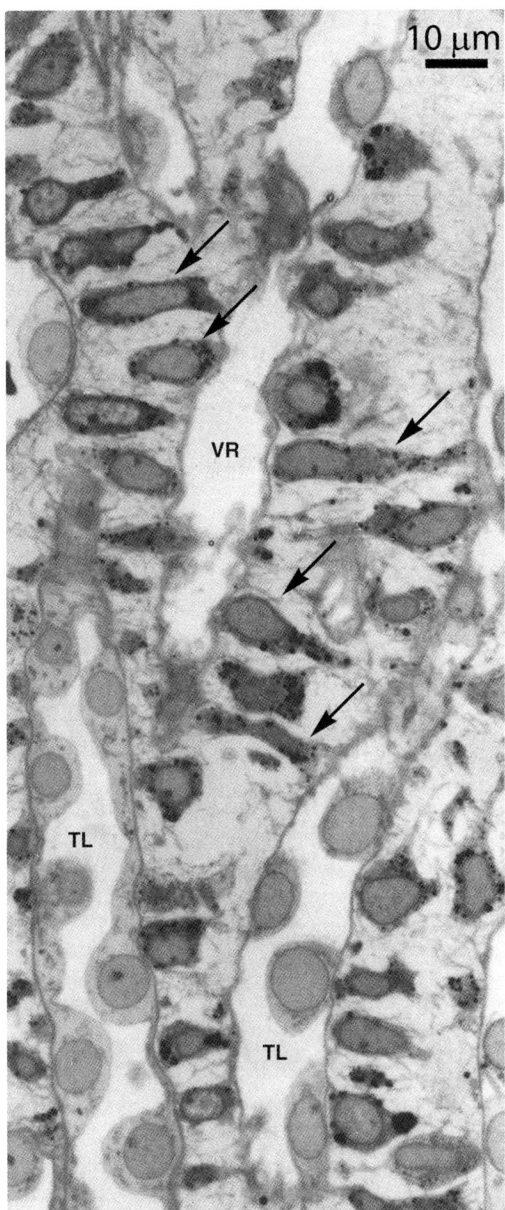


**Fig. 2.54** Light micrograph of the renal medullary interstitium from a normal rat. The lipid-laden interstitial fibroblasts bridge the interstitial space between adjacent thin limbs of Henle *(TL)* and vasa recta *(VR)*.

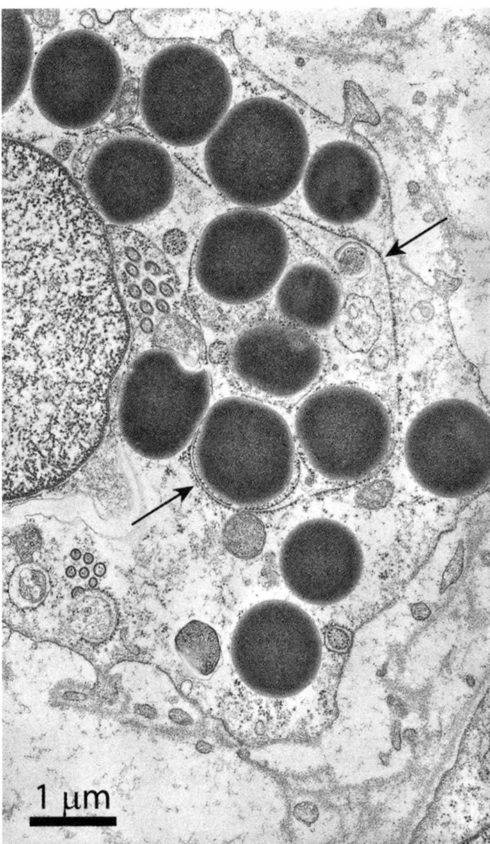


**Fig. 2.55** Higher-magnification electron micrograph illustrating the relationship between the electron-dense lipid droplets, which almost fill the medullary interstitial fibroblasts, and the granular endoplasmic reticulum *(arrows)*. Wisps of basement membrane–like material adjacent to the surfaces of the cells are contiguous with the basement membranes of the adjacent tubules *(lower right)*.

and contain elements of tight junctions, intermediate junctions, and gap junctions.[429,430] The cells likely provide structural support in the medulla because of their special arrangement perpendicular to the tubules and vessels. The close relationship between medullary interstitial fibroblasts and the thin limbs and capillaries also suggests a possible interaction with these structures. Three-dimensional reconstructions of the inner medulla have demonstrated arrangements of ascending thin limbs, ascending vasa recta, and collecting ducts to form interstitial nodal spaces or microdomains, which are abundant in rodent kidney but relatively infrequent in human inner medulla.[12,265,431] The interstitial nodal spaces align in stacks along the corticomedullary axis and are believed to be divided by the interstitial fibroblasts.[12,431,432] Peritubular interstitial fibroblasts in the medulla express cyclooxygenase-2 and are a major site of prostaglandin synthesis, with the major product being $PGE_2$.[417,433]

Dendritic cells are also present in the medullary interstitium and can be identified at the light microscopic level by immunoreactivity for MHC II. However, their prevalence varies among the regions of the medulla. They are most abundant in the inner stripe of the outer medulla, frequently aligned with collecting ducts. They are less abundant in the upper third of the inner medulla, and disappear in the distal portions of the inner medulla in the healthy kidney.[411]

## LYMPHATICS

The renal lymphatic circulation includes capsular, subcapsular, and intrarenal components.[434,435] The subcapsular component consists of a network of lymphatics in the space between the renal capsule and the renal parenchyma. The intrarenal component includes lymphatic capillaries and channels that coalesce and drain via bundles of lymphatic vessels at the hilum of the kidney. Subcapsular lymphatics may drain directly to the lymphatics at the hilum or may communicate with intrarenal lymphatic vessels. Intrarenal

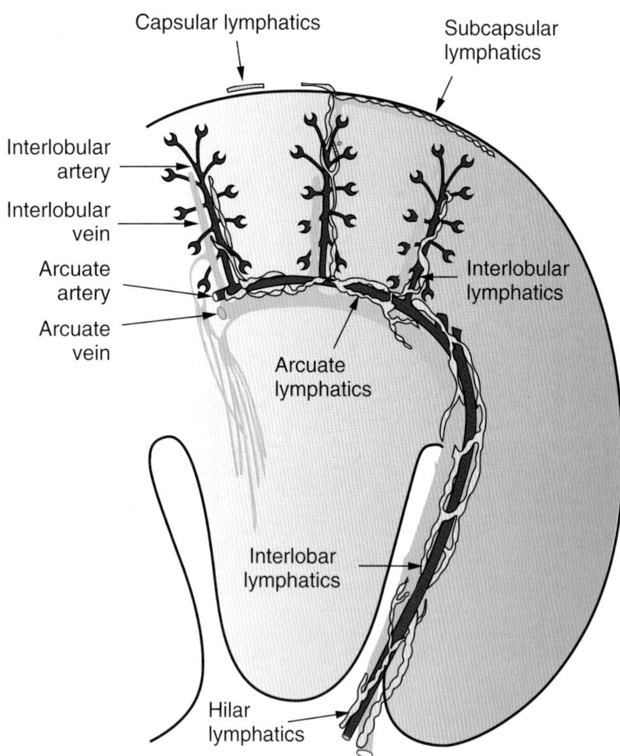


**Fig. 2.56** Diagram of the lymphatic circulation in the mammalian kidney. (Modified from Kriz W, Dieterich HJ. The lymphatic system of the kidney in some mammals. Light and electron microscopic investigations. *Z Anat Entwicklungsgesch.* 1970;131:111–147.)

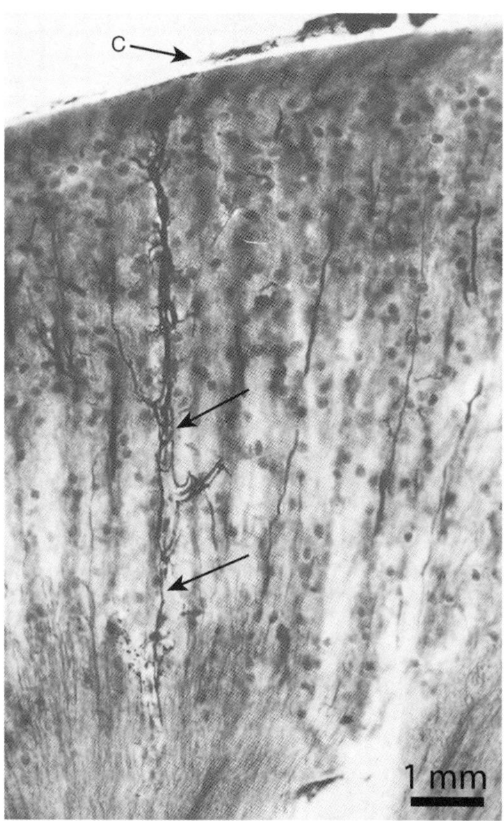


**Fig. 2.57** Light micrograph of a sagittal section through the cortex and outer medulla of a dog kidney. A capsular lymphatic *(C)* was injected with India ink. Intrarenal lymphatics *(arrows)* follow the distribution of the interlobular arteries in the cortex. (Modified from Bell RD, Keyl MJ, Shrader FR, et al. Renal lymphatics: the internal distribution. *Nephron.* 1968;5:454–463.)

lymphatics neighboring the interlobular blood vessels drain into the arcuate lymphatic vessels near the corticomedullary junction, which drain through interlobar lymphatics to hilar lymphatic vessels (Fig. 2.56).[436]

Communications between the capsular lymphatics and intrarenal lymphatics have been described in some animals, such that the lymphatic vessels of the renal capsule drain into subcapsular lymphatic channels, providing continuous lymphatic drainage from the renal capsule, through the cortex, and into the hilar region (Fig. 2.57). In dog kidney, "communicating" and "perforating" lymphatic channels that transverse the renal capsule have been described.[437] In these studies, a small number of communicating lymphatic channels were found, usually associated with an interlobular artery and vein; these lymphatics penetrated the capsule and appeared to represent a connection between the hilar and capsular systems. The perforating lymphatic channel penetrated the capsule alone or in association with a small vein; these channels appeared to represent a primary pathway for lymph drainage from the superficial cortex.

The intrarenal lymphatics represent a small fraction of the renal tissue, with the lymphatic volume density in the cortex ranging from 0.02%–0.37%, depending on the species.[438,439] In normal human, rat, mouse, and pig kidney, the majority of lymphatic capillaries in the renal parenchyma cluster in the adventitia around the interlobular and arcuate arteries (Fig. 2.58),[434,436,440] and in the mouse, they also extend along the afferent arteriole.[440] In most animal species, lymphatic capillaries are rarely found among renal tubules and glomeruli, but in the horse and dog, lymphatics are abundant around glomeruli,[434] and in dog kidney, small lymphatics are found in proximity to proximal and distal tubules.[438,441] Studies of normal human kidney using immunolabeling to detect lymphatics found lymphatic capillaries most commonly in the adventitia surrounding interlobular and arcuate vessels, as in other species[442,443]; lymphatic capillaries among renal tubules were rare in one study[443] and in another were described as interspersed among renal tubules in the cortex, though they were less common than vascular capillaries and were sporadic near glomeruli.[442] Lymphatics are rarely found in the medulla of healthy kidneys, a finding that is consistent among species.[440,442,444,445]

Lymphatic capillaries, including the interlobular lymphatics, are composed of a layer of lymphatic endothelial cells, but unlike capillaries of the vascular system, they lack a basement membrane and fenestrations.[436,445] Lymphatic capillary endothelial cells are anchored by filaments attached to basal cytoplasmic projections.[435,445] The interlobar and hilar lymphatic channels are *collecting* lymphatic vessels and contain numerous valves,[434,436] semilunar projections in the lumen of the lymphatic vessels that limit backflow of lymph. Collecting lymphatics also are distinguished from lymphatic capillaries by the presence of a continuous basement membrane and pericytes around the interstitial face of the lymphatic.[445]

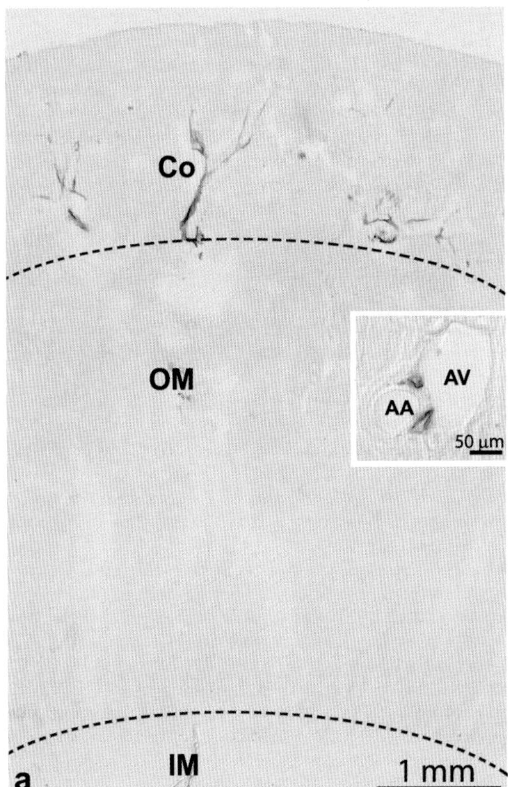


**Fig. 2.58** Light micrograph of 50-µm-thick section of adult mouse kidney labeled for lymphatic endothelium-specific hyaluronan receptor LYVE-1, which marks lymphatic endothelial cells almost exclusively. The lymphatics are largely clustered around the arcuate and interlobular vessels. *Co*, Cortex; *OM*, outer medulla; *IM*, inner medulla; *AA*, arcuate artery; *AV*, arcuate vein (Modified from Lee HW, Qin YX, Kim YM, et al. Expression of lymphatic endothelium-specific hyaluronan receptor LYVE-1 in the developing mouse kidney. *Cell Tissue Res.* 2011;343:429–444.)

The majority of efferent renal hilar lymphatics drain to regional lymph nodes. The right kidney lymphatics drain into the paracaval, precaval, interaortocaval, and retrocaval nodes, and the left kidney lymphatics drain into the preaortic, paraaortic, and retroaortic nodes. In addition, posterior efferent renal lymphatic vessels may communicate directly with the thoracic duct.[446–448] Finally, in some rat and primate species, lymphovenous drainage has been detected, with direct connections between the lymphatic system and the renal veins or the vena cava near the renal veins. These multiple and variable drainage patterns may have important clinical implications in the pathogenesis, staging, and diagnosis of renal cell carcinoma metastases.[449,450]

Until relatively recently, identification of the intrarenal lymphatics relied on structural studies using lymphatic injections, microradiography, and electron microscopy. These laborious techniques limited the examination of the effects of physiologic and pathologic processes on the lymphatic system. However, the discovery of specific proteins expressed by lymphatic endothelial cells has enabled immunodetection of these cells (Fig. 2.58). The various markers used to detect intrarenal lymphatic endothelial cells include the hyaluronate receptor, LYVE-a; the lymphatic transcription factor, Prox-1; vascular endothelial growth factor receptor 3; the integral membrane glycoprotein, podoplanin; and the sialoglycoprotein, D2-40.[435,440,451] Lymphatic endothelial cells also express AQP1.[253,452] Using immunolabeling for lymphatic endothelial cell markers, several studies have reported proliferation of intrarenal lymphatics in the renal parenchyma in forms of hypertension,[453] tubulointerstitial nephritis,[443] transplant rejection,[454,455] ureteral obstruction,[456] and diabetic nephropathy[457] and in the tissue surrounding renal cell carcinomas.[442] The role of lymphangiogenesis in these nephropathies is not well understood. It has been implicated in the pathogenesis of renal inflammation,[435] but some studies suggest it may be beneficial and limit renal injury, at least in some conditions.[453,456]

## INNERVATION

The sympathetic innervation of the kidney arises from the intermediolateral column of the spinal cord between T6 and L2,[458] although some report a narrower range, between T9 and T13.[459] Neurons from the brain project to this region of the spinal cord primarily from the raphe nucleus and rostral ventrolateral medulla in the vasomotor center of the brain, the pontine A5 noradrenergic cell group, and the paraventricular nucleus in the hypothalamus;[460,461] these areas in the brain determine the sympathetic signaling to the kidney.[459] The sympathetic preganglionic fibers exit the spinal cord between T11 and L3 or L4 and connect with postganglionic fibers in both paravertebral and prevertebral ganglia, the latter including the aorticorenal, splanchnic, celiac, and mesenteric ganglia, and in the renal plexus[459,462–464] and postganglionic fibers arising from different ganglia appear to innervate different regions of the kidney.[464] There is considerable variation among species and among individuals in the spinal cord segment that supplies the preganglionic fibers and in the ganglia where the postganglionic fibers to the kidney originate.[459,460]

The postganglionic fibers form the extrinsic nerves to the kidney, which contain both unmyelinated and myelinated fibers. The vast majority of renal nerve fibers in rat and mouse are unmyelinated, 96%–98% in the rat,[465,466] and 99.5% unmyelinated fibers in the mouse.[467] The diameter of the renal nerves differs considerably between these species, measuring ~98 µm in diameter in the rat[466] and ~35 µm in diameter in the mouse,[467] due to a greater number of fibers in the rat extrinsic renal nerves rather than a significant difference in the diameter of unmyelinated nerve fibers between species.[466,467] Nerve fibers in the rabbit renal cortex fall into two groups based on fiber diameters,[468,469] but morphometric studies of rat and mouse extrinsic renal nerves have not consistently found this pattern.[459] Although a bimodal distribution of unmyelinated nerve fiber diameter was found in the renal nerve of Sprague-Dawley rats,[465] in Wistar rats[466] and C57BL/6J mice,[467] the average diameter of unmyelinated fibers ranged between 0.5 and 0.7 µm in a unimodal size distribution.

The renal nerves enter the kidney at the hilum and run with the renal arteries into the kidney, where they continue along the arterial circulation as it subdivides, lying within the perivascular interstitium and penetrating the vessel walls to innervate vascular smooth muscle cells in interlobar, arcuate, and interlobular arteries and in afferent and efferent arterioles, including juxtaglomerular cells.[176,458,459,470–473]

Nerve endings are in contact with approximately one-third of the cells of the efferent arteriole and somewhat less of the afferent arteriole,[474] and synapses between autonomic nerve endings and granular and agranular cells of the JGA are visible by transmission electron microscopy.[475] Consistent with these observations, renin secretion is modulated by renal sympathetic nerve activity.[462,476] Neuroeffector junctions at the macula densa are infrequent in comparison to the afferent and efferent arterioles.[474]

Single nerve fibers penetrate the cortical and juxtamedullary renal parenchyma and parts of the medulla.[213,459,477–479] Unmyelinated nerve fibers accompanying the efferent arterioles of juxtamedullary glomeruli extend with the vasculature to the level of the inner stripe of the outer medulla.[480] Sympathetic nerve terminals make contact with the basement membranes of the tubule epithelial cells at nerve varicosities containing dense-cored vesicles, which contain norepinephrine[213,470,479] and tyrosine hydroxylase, the rate-limiting enzyme in norepinephrine production.[462] Although neuroeffector junctions are present on all renal tubule types, the density of nerve varicosities varies among the renal tubules; the TAL has the highest density, followed by the DCT, the proximal tubule, and the collecting duct.[213]

The majority of the renal innervation is efferent. However, afferent nerves are also present, principally innervating the renal pelvis, but also the interlobar, arcuate, and interlobular arteries, and afferent arterioles.[458,470,481–483] Approximately 75%–80% of afferent renal nerves are unmyelinated.[458,484,485] Unlike efferent nerve fibers, which express tyrosine hydroxylase, afferent nerve fibers express calcitonin gene-related peptide, and thus, efferent and afferent fibers can be discriminated using immunolocalization for these enzymes.[470,483,486]

## ACKNOWLEDGMENTS

Portions of this chapter are adapted from the chapters written previously by Kirsten M. Madsen, Soren Nielsen, and C. Craig Tisher (8th edition), Søren Nielsen, Tae-Hwan Kwon, Robert A. Fenton, and Jeppe Praetorius (9th edition), and Robert A. Fenton and Jeppe Praetorius (10th edition).

The authors are grateful for the support and encouragement of our families, for our mentors in our early careers, particularly Dr. C. Craig Tisher and Dr. Kirsten Madsen, and for our collaborators and colleagues. The work of our laboratories over the years was only possible due to the dedication of many talented microscopists, particularly Dr. Sharon W. Matthews, Chao Chen, Wendy Wilber, and Fred Kopp, and the support of the National Institutes of Health, American Heart Association, and Gatorade Research Fund.

 Complete reference list available at ExpertConsult.com.

## KEY REFERENCES

5. Bertram JF, Douglas-Denton RN, Diouf B, et al. Human nephron number: implications for health and disease. *Pediatr Nephrol.* 2011;26(9):1529–1533. doi:10.1007/s00467-011-1843-8. [doi].

11. Christensen EI, Wagner CA, Kaissling B. Uriniferous tubule: structural and functional organization. *Compr Physiol.* 2012;2(2):805–861. doi:10.1002/cphy.c100073. [doi].

22. Dane MJ, van den Berg BM, Lee DH, et al. A microscopic view on the renal endothelial glycocalyx. *Am J Physiol Renal Physiol.* 2015;308(9):F956–F966. doi:10.1152/ajprenal.00532.2014. [doi].

31. Bartlett CS, Jeansson M, Quaggin SE. Vascular growth factors and glomerular disease. *Annu Rev Physiol.* 2016;78:437–461. doi:10.1146/annurev-physiol-021115-105412. [doi].

49. Miner JH. The glomerular basement membrane. *Exp Cell Res.* 2012;318(9):973–978. doi:10.1016/j.yexcr.2012.02.031. [doi].

53. Abrahamson DR, Hudson BG, Stroganova L, et al. Cellular origins of type IV collagen networks in developing glomeruli. *J Am Soc Nephrol.* 2009;20(7):1471–1479. doi:10.1681/ASN.2008101086. [doi].

59. Suleiman H, Zhang L, Roth R, et al. Nanoscale protein architecture of the kidney glomerular basement membrane. *Elife.* 2013;2:e01149. doi:10.7554/eLife.01149. [doi].

78. Jarad G, Cunningham J, Shaw AS, et al. Proteinuria precedes podocyte abnormalities in Lamb2-/- mice, implicating the glomerular basement membrane as an albumin barrier. *J Clin Invest.* 2006;116(8):2272–2279. doi:10.1172/JCI28414. [doi].

80. Ichimura K, Miyazaki N, Sadayama S, et al. Three-dimensional architecture of podocytes revealed by block-face scanning electron microscopy. *Sci Rep.* 2015;5:8993. doi:10.1038/srep08993. [doi].

81. Burghardt T, Hochapfel F, Salecker B, et al. Advanced electron microscopic techniques provide a deeper insight into the peculiar features of podocytes. *Am J Physiol Renal Physiol.* 2015;309(12):F1082–F1089. doi:10.1152/ajprenal.00338.2015. [doi].

84. Schell C, Huber TB. The evolving complexity of the podocyte cytoskeleton. *J Am Soc Nephrol.* 2017;28(11):3166–3174. doi:10.1681/ASN.2017020143. [doi].

91. Suleiman HY, Roth R, Jain S, et al. Injury-induced actin cytoskeleton reorganization in podocytes revealed by super-resolution microscopy. *JCI Insight.* 2017;2(16):doi:10.1172/jci.insight.94137. [doi].

116. Rice WL, Van Hoek AN, Paunescu TG, et al. High resolution helium ion scanning microscopy of the rat kidney. *PLoS ONE.* 2013;8(3):e57051. doi:10.1371/journal.pone.0057051. [doi].

117. Tsuji K, Paunescu TG, Suleiman H, et al. Re-characterization of the glomerulopathy in CD2AP deficient mice by high-resolution helium ion scanning microscopy. *Sci Rep.* 2017;7(1):8321-017-08304-3. doi:10.1038/s41598-017-08304-3. [doi].

118. Grahammer F, Wigge C, Schell C, et al. A flexible, multilayered protein scaffold maintains the slit in between glomerular podocytes. *JCI Insight.* 2016;1(9). doi: 10.1172/jci.insight.86177 [pii].

121. New LA, Martin CE, Jones N. Advances in slit diaphragm signaling. *Curr Opin Nephrol Hypertens.* 2014;23(4):420–430. doi:10.1097/01.mnh.0000447018.28852.b6. [doi].

149. Schlondorff D, Banas B. The mesangial cell revisited: no cell is an island. *J Am Soc Nephrol.* 2009;20(6):1179–1187. doi:10.1681/ASN.2008050549. [doi].

161. Shankland SJ, Smeets B, Pippin JW, et al. The emergence of the glomerular parietal epithelial cell. *Nat Rev Nephrol.* 2014;10(3):158–173. doi:10.1038/nrneph.2014.1. [doi].

167. Shankland SJ, Freedman BS, Pippin JW. Can podocytes be regenerated in adults? *Curr Opin Nephrol Hypertens.* 2017;26(3):154–164. doi:10.1097/MNH.0000000000000311. [doi].

179. Hackenthal E, Paul M, Ganten D, et al. Morphology, physiology, and molecular biology of renin secretion. *Physiol Rev.* 1990;70(4):1067–1116. doi:10.1152/physrev.1990.70.4.1067. [doi].

198. Maunsbach AB. Observations on the segmentation of the proximal tubule in the rat kidney. comparison of results from phase contrast, fluorescence and electron microscopy. *J Ultrastruct Res.* 1966;16(3):239–258.

202. Kaissling B, Kriz W. Structural analysis of the rabbit kidney. *Adv Anat Embryol Cell Biol.* 1979;56:1–123.

236. Yang LE, Maunsbach AB, Leong PK, et al. Differential traffic of proximal tubule Na+ transporters during hypertension or PTH: NHE3 to base of microvilli vs. NaPi2 to endosomes. *Am J Physiol Renal Physiol.* 2004;287(5):F896–F906. doi:10.1152/ajprenal.00160.2004. [doi].

259. Christensen EI, Grann B, Kristoffersen IB, et al. Three-dimensional reconstruction of the rat nephron. *Am J Physiol Renal Physiol.* 2014;306(6):F664–F671. doi:10.1152/ajprenal.00522.2013. [doi].

265. Wei G, Rosen S, Dantzler WH, et al. Architecture of the human renal inner medulla and functional implications. *Am J Physiol Renal Physiol.* 2015;309(7):F627–F637. doi:10.1152/ajprenal.00236.2015. [doi].

266. Pannabecker TL. Structure and function of the thin limbs of the loop of henle. *Compr Physiol.* 2012;2(3):2063–2086. doi:10.1002/cphy.c110019. [doi].

268. Kriz W, Bankir L. A standard nomenclature for structure of the kidney. the renal commission of the international union of physiological sciences(IUPS). *Anat Embryol (Berl).* 1988;178(2):N1–N8.

269. Woodhall PB, Tisher CC. Response of the distal tubule and cortical collecting duct to vasopressin in the rat. *J Clin Invest.* 1973; 52(12):3095–3108. doi:10.1172/JCI107509. [doi].
285. Campean V, Kricke J, Ellison D, et al. Localization of thiazide-sensitive Na(+)-Cl(-) cotransport and associated gene products in mouse DCT. *Am J Physiol Renal Physiol.* 2001;281(6):F1028–F1035. doi:10.1152/ajprenal.0148.2001. [doi].
305. Dorup J, Morsing P, Rasch R. Tubule-tubule and tubule-arteriole contacts in rat kidney distal nephrons. A morphologic study based on computer-assisted three-dimensional reconstructions. *Lab Invest.* 1992;67(6):761–769.
306. Ren Y, Garvin JL, Liu R, et al. Crosstalk between the connecting tubule and the afferent arteriole regulates renal microcirculation. *Kidney Int.* 2007;71(11):1116–1121. doi: S0085-2538(15)52273-4 [pii].
314. Teng-umnuay P, Verlander JW, Yuan W, et al. Identification of distinct subpopulations of intercalated cells in the mouse collecting duct. *J Am Soc Nephrol.* 1996;7(2):260–274.
328. Clapp WL, Madsen KM, Verlander JW, et al. Morphologic heterogeneity along the rat inner medullary collecting duct. *Lab Invest.* 1989;60(2):219–230.
340. Verlander JW, Madsen KM, Tisher CC. Effect of acute respiratory acidosis on two populations of intercalated cells in rat cortical collecting duct. *Am J Physiol.* 1987;253(6 Pt 2):F1142–F1156.
344. Madsen KM, Tisher CC. Response of intercalated cells of rat outer medullary collecting duct to chronic metabolic acidosis. *Lab Invest.* 1984;51(3):268–276.
357. Verlander JW, Madsen KM, Cannon JK, et al. Activation of acid-secreting intercalated cells in rabbit collecting duct with ammonium chloride loading. *Am J Physiol.* 1994;266(4 Pt 2):F633–F645.
369. Seshadri RM, Klein JD, Smith T, et al. Changes in subcellular distribution of the ammonia transporter, Rhcg, in response to chronic metabolic acidosis. *Am J Physiol Renal Physiol.* 2006;290(6):F1443–F1452. doi: 00459.2005 [pii].
371. Verlander JW, Kim YH, Shin W, et al. Dietary Cl(-) restriction upregulates pendrin expression within the apical plasma membrane of type B intercalated cells. *Am J Physiol Renal Physiol.* 2006;291(4):F833–F839. doi: 00474.2005 [pii].
380. Kaissling B, Le Hir M. Distal tubular segments of the rabbit kidney after adaptation to altered Na- and K-intake. I. structural changes. *Cell Tissue Res.* 1982;224(3):469–492.
387. Elger M, Bankir L, Kriz W. Morphometric analysis of kidney hypertrophy in rats after chronic potassium depletion. *Am J Physiol.* 1992;262(4 Pt 2):F656–F667. doi:10.1152/ajprenal.1992.262.4.F656. [doi].
389. Brown D, Paunescu TG, Breton S, et al. Regulation of the V-ATPase in kidney epithelial cells: dual role in acid-base homeostasis and vesicle trafficking. *J Exp Biol.* 2009;212(Pt 11):1762–1772. doi:10.1242/jeb.028803. [doi].
407. Lemley KV, Kriz W. Anatomy of the renal interstitium. *Kidney Int.* 1991;39(3):370–381. doi: S0085-2538(15)57139-1 [pii].
411. Kaissling B, Hegyi I, Loffing J, et al. Morphology of interstitial cells in the healthy kidney. *Anat Embryol (Berl).* 1996;193(4):303–318.
419. Takahashi-Iwanaga H. The three-dimensional cytoarchitecture of the interstitial tissue in the rat kidney. *Cell Tissue Res.* 1991;264(2):269–281.
426. Bachmann S, Le Hir M, Eckardt KU. Co-localization of erythropoietin mRNA and ecto-5′-nucleotidase immunoreactivity in peritubular cells of rat renal cortex indicates that fibroblasts produce erythropoietin. *J Histochem Cytochem.* 1993;41(3):335–341. doi:10.1177/41.3.8429197. [doi].
432. Gilbert RL, Pannabecker TL. Architecture of interstitial nodal spaces in the rodent renal inner medulla. *Am J Physiol Renal Physiol.* 2013;305(5):F745–F752. doi:10.1152/ajprenal.00239.2013. [doi].
435. Yazdani S, Navis G, Hillebrands JL, et al. Lymphangiogenesis in renal diseases: passive bystander or active participant? *Expert Rev Mol Med.* 2014;16:e15. doi:10.1017/erm.2014.18. [doi].
442. Ishikawa Y, Akasaka Y, Kiguchi H, et al. The human renal lymphatics under normal and pathological conditions. *Histopathology.* 2006;49(3):265–273. doi: HIS2478 [pii].
467. Fazan VP, Ma X, Chapleau MW, et al. Qualitative and quantitative morphology of renal nerves in C57BL/6j mice. *Anat Rec.* 2002;268(4):399–404. doi:10.1002/ar.10174. [doi].
470. Barajas L, Liu L, Powers K. Anatomy of the renal innervation: intrarenal aspects and ganglia of origin. *Can J Physiol Pharmacol.* 1992;70(5):735–749.

3

# The Renal Circulations and Glomerular Filtration

Luis Gabriel Navar | David A. Maddox | Karen A. Munger

## CHAPTER OUTLINE



## KEY POINTS

- Renal blood flow and GFR increase with protein intake in men and women and, at any given level of protein intake, GFR is greater in younger (20–50 years of age) than in older subjects (55–88 years of age) and greater in men than in women, even when factored for body surface area.
- The decline in hydraulic pressure between the renal artery and glomerular capillaries is greatest along the afferent arteriole, whereas 70% of the decline in postglomerular hydraulic pressure occurs at the efferent arteriole. The last 50 to 150 μm of the afferent arteriole and the first early part of the efferent arteriole (first 50–150 μm) provide most of the preglomerular and postglomerular resistances.
- Glomerular capillary blood pressure, $P_{GC}$, declines only slightly within the capillary network, thus maintaining the transcapillary hydraulic pressure gradient ($\Delta P = P_{GC}$ minus Bowman's space pressure, $P_{BS}$) at a relatively constant rate. However, glomerular capillary protein oncotic pressure ($\pi_{GC}$) rises along the length of the glomerular capillaries as protein-free fluid is filtered into Bowman's space, thus reducing the net filtration pressure, with $\pi g$ reaching and becoming equal to $\Delta P$ in some cases such as hydropenia.
- The barrier to the filtration of fluid and macromolecules includes the glycocalyx lining the endothelial cells, the fenestrations of the endothelial layer of the glomerular capillaries, the layers of the glomerular basement membrane, the filtration slits between the podocytes surrounding the capillaries, and the filtration slit diaphragm extending along the filtration slits to connect adjacent foot processes. Breakdown or injury in any of the restrictive barriers may lead to increased passage of albumin and other proteins.
- The high resistance of the afferent and efferent arterioles leads to a large drop in vascular hydraulic pressure prior to the peritubular capillaries so that peritubular capillary pressure is much lower than glomerular capillary pressure (15–20 mm Hg). The oncotic pressure of fluid entering the peritubular capillaries is elevated because of the filtration of protein-free fluid out of the glomerular capillaries. The net balance between the transcapillary oncotic and hydraulic pressure gradients thus favors entry of the fluid reabsorbed by the tubules into the peritubular capillaries.
- The finding that both renal blood flow and GFR are autoregulated indicates that the principal resistance change due to autoregulatory adjustments is primarily localized to the preglomerular vasculature. The autoregulation mechanisms provide a powerful mechanism to maintain the intrarenal hemodynamic environment in balance with the metabolically determined tubular transport function.

**KEY POINTS**—cont'd

- The myogenic and tubuloglomerular feedback mechanisms are primarily responsible for the autoregulatory responses. The myogenic mechanism refers to the ability of arterial smooth muscle to contract and relax in response to increases and decreases in vascular wall tension. The tubuloglomerular feedback mechanism provides signals from the macula densa to the afferent arteriole. Paracrine mediators include ATP, adenosine, nitric oxide and arachidonic acid metabolites.
- Overall renal hemodynamic function is regulated by complex interactions between extrinsic and intrinsic mechanisms, including the sympathetic nervous system, circulating vasoactive factors, endothelial nitric oxide, intrarenal angiotensin II, arachidonic acid metabolites, purinergic factors and other paracrine systems, which exert direct effects and modulate the sensitivity of the tubuloglomerular feedback mechanism.

## INTRODUCTION

The kidneys are unique in having three distinct microvascular networks identified as the glomerular capillary microcirculation, the cortical peritubular capillary microcirculation, and the unique medullary microcirculation, which nourishes the medullary tissues and maintains the interstitial environment. Each of these circulations has specialized functions that allow filtration of a large volume of fluid at the glomerular capillaries, the consequent reabsorption of most of the filtrate back into the circulation, and the establishment of a medullary environment having a high interstitial osmolality. These renal circulations not only provide the renal cells and tissues with oxygen and nutrients, but also maintain and regulate the hemodynamic environment to achieve their designated functions. Under resting conditions, blood flow to the kidneys represents approximately 20% of cardiac output in humans, even though these organs constitute less than 1% of body mass. This renal blood flow (RBF), approximately 400 mL/100 g of tissue per minute, is significantly greater than that observed in other vascular beds considered to be well perfused, such as the heart, liver, and brain.[1,2] From this enormous blood flow (1.0–1.2 L/min), approximately 20% of the plasma flow is filtered and becomes the glomerular filtrate, but only a small volume of urine, about 1%, is formed from that filtrate. Although the metabolic energy requirements of tubular transport processes are relatively high, the renal arteriovenous $O_2$ difference reveals that blood flow far exceeds that needed for metabolic demands. In fact, the high blood flow is essential to provide the appropriate hemodynamic environments necessary for the filtration at the glomeruli and the reabsorption into the postglomerular capillaries.[3,4]

In Chapter 2, the gross anatomy of the kidney and arrangement of tubular segments are described in detail. In this chapter, we consider the intrarenal organization of the discrete microcirculatory networks, as shown in Fig. 3.1. We will also consider the differences in regional blood flows and how the structure of the microcirculation contributes to the regulation of the intrarenal hemodynamic environment, thus maintaining appropriate levels of RBF and glomerular filtration rate (GFR).

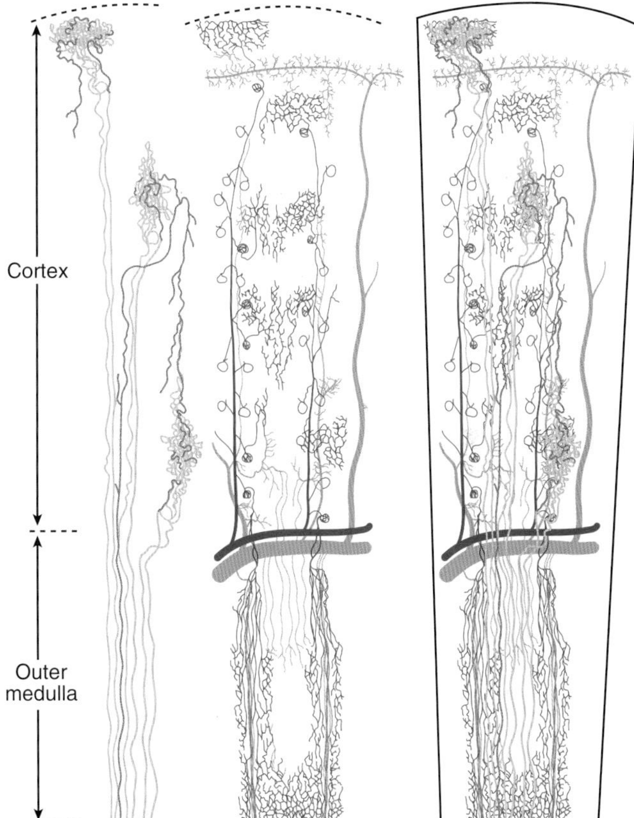


**Fig. 3.1** Renal vasculature and tubule organization. *Left,* Three nephrons are shown without accompanying vascular structures. Vascular structures are shown in the *central portion* of the figure. *Right,* Vascular and tubular structures are superimposed. Configurations of tubular segments were generalized from patterns found by silicone rubber injections. For clarity, more distal parts of the nephron are shown in deeper colors. Arterial components of the vascular system are shown in *red*, venous components in *blue*. Only representative venous connections are shown. (From Beeuwkes R III, Bonventre JV. Tubular organization and vascular tubular relations in the dog kidney. *Am J Physiol.* 1975;229:695–713.)

## RENAL BLOOD FLOW AND GLOMERULAR FILTRATION RATE

Historically, GFR and renal plasma flow (RPF) have been estimated using the clearance of inulin for the determination of GFR and of *p*-aminohippuric acid (PAH) for the determinations of RPF, from which RBF can be calculated using RPF and hematocrit.[5] Whereas inulin is only filtered across the glomerular capillaries, PAH is both filtered at the glomerulus and actively secreted by the tubules. This results in the renal extraction of 80% to 90% of PAH from the blood. PAH is not completely extracted from the blood because of flow through regions of the kidney, in particular the medulla, that do not perfuse proximal tubule segments, where secretion occurs, and limitations of the secretory process of PAH in cortical regions, along with the presence of a few periglomerular shunts (Fig. 3.2). Thus, PAH clearance is an approximation often termed "effective" or "estimated" renal plasma flow (ERPF) and provides an estimate of RPF without the need for a renal venous blood sample.[5] However, this estimate of RPF is much less accurate in renal disease because extraction is further reduced by damage to proximal tubule segments or rarefaction of the peritubular capillaries involved in PAH secretion.[6] Values taken from a composite of studies in normal human subjects[5] are shown in Table 3.1. As indicated in the data presented, RBF and GFR are lower in women than in men, even when corrected for body surface area. Values for normal subjects vary considerably in different studies, as reflected in Fig. 3.3, which shows more recently obtained data on ERPF and GFR in adult humans from various studies that were not corrected for body surface area. The data also reveal marked differences in GFR and ERPF between obese and lean subjects. These differences are likely the result of increased food intake and, hence, increased protein consumption.[7] Indeed, as shown in Fig. 3.4, GFR increases with protein intake in men and women and, at any given level of protein intake, GFR is higher in young people (20–50 years of age; mean, 31 years) than in older subjects (55–88 years of age; mean, 70 years). Improved methods of RBF

**Table 3.1 Renal Blood Flow, Renal Plasma Flow, Glomerular Filtration Rates and Filtration Fractions in Healthy Men and Women[a]**

| Subject(s) | RBF, mL/min | RPF, mL/min | GFR, mL/min | Filtration Fraction |
|---|---|---|---|---|
| Men | 1166 | 655 | 127 | 0.193 |
| Women | 940 | 600 | 118 | 0.197 |
| Combined | 1165 | 634 | 123 | .197 |

[a]Data for RPF based on clearances of Diodrast as well as *p*-aminohippuric acid (PAH) and for GFR based on clearance of inulin. Clearances are corrected to 1.73 $m^2$ and suggest lower normalized RBF, RPF, and GFR values in women

*GFR*, glomerular filtration rate; *RBF*, renal blood flow; *RPF*, renal plasma flow.

Data from Smith HW. *The kidney: Structure and function in health and disease.* New York: Oxford University Press; 1951:544–545.

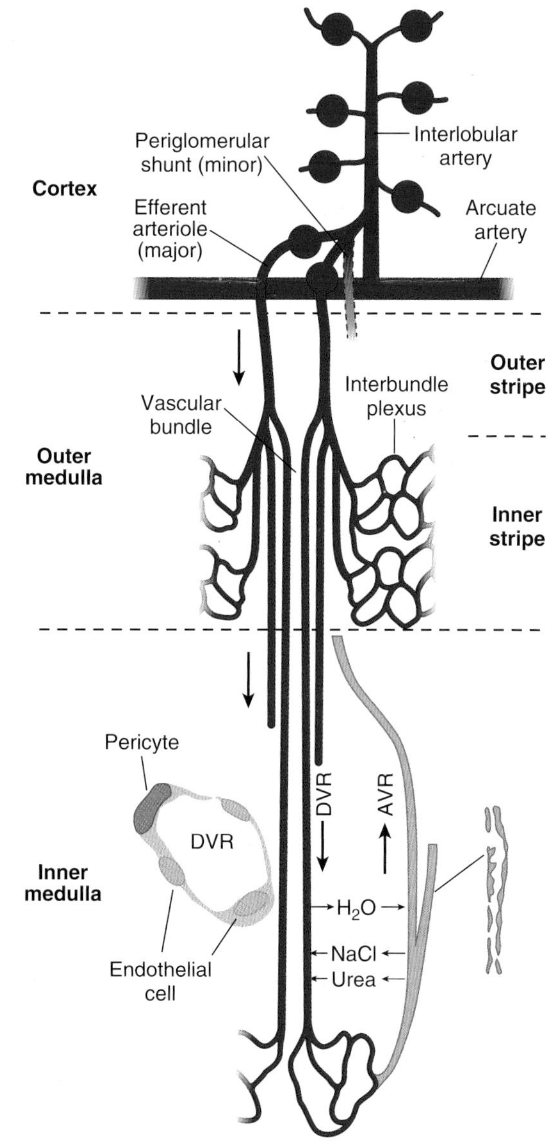


**Fig. 3.2** The medullary microcirculation. In the cortex, interlobular arteries arise from the arcuate artery and ascend toward the cortical surface. Cortical and juxtamedullary afferent arterioles leading to glomeruli branch from the interlobular artery. Most of the blood flow reaches the medulla through juxtamedullary efferent arterioles; however, a small fraction may also arise from periglomerular shunt pathways. In the outer medulla, juxtamedullary efferent arterioles in the outer stripe give rise to descending vasa recta *(DVR),* which coalesce to form vascular bundles in the inner stripe. DVR on the periphery of vascular bundles give rise to the interbundle capillary plexus that surrounds nephron segments—thick ascending limb, collecting duct, long looped thin descending limbs (not shown). DVR in the center continue across the inner-outer medullary junction to perfuse the inner medulla. Vascular bundles disappear in the inner medulla, and vasa recta become dispersed with nephron segments. Ascending vasa recta *(AVR)* that arise from the sparse capillary plexus of the inner medulla return to the cortex by passing through outer medullary vascular bundles. *Inset,* DVR have a continuous endothelium. (From Pallone TL, Zhang Z, Rhinehart K. Physiology of the renal medullary microcirculation. *Am J Physiol.* 2003;284:F253–F266, 2003.)

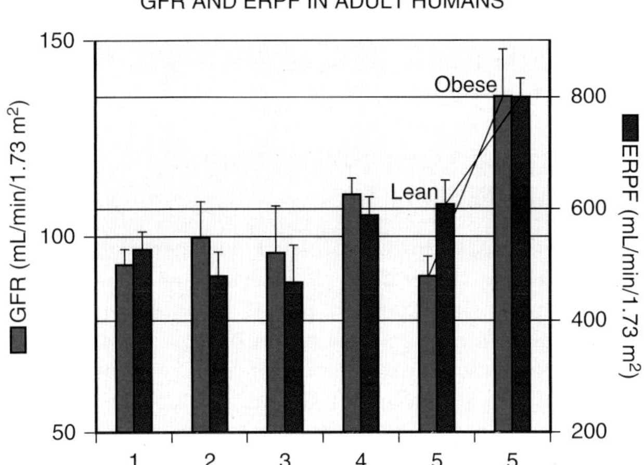


**Fig. 3.3** Typical values for glomerular filtration rate *(GFR)* and estimated renal plasma flow *(ERPF)* from five studies in adults. Values from men and women were pooled. Numbers under each set of bars refer to the following studies: 1, Giordano and DeFronzo[517]; 2, Winetz et al[518]; 3, Hostetter[519]; 4, Deen et al[520]; 5, Chagnac et al.[521] For studies 1 through 3 and 5, values were obtained after approximately 12 hours of fasting; subjects in study 4 were allowed food ad lib. For study 5, values from lean subjects (average body mass index [BMI] = 22) were compared with those from obese nondiabetic individuals (BMI >38) after a 10-hour fast but are not corrected for body surface area.

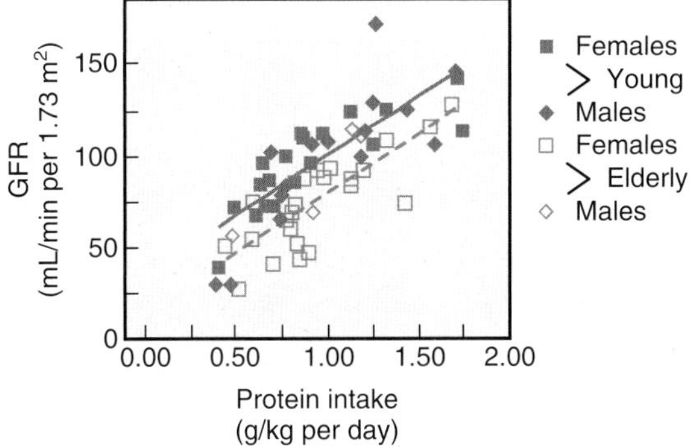


**Fig. 3.4** Relationship between protein intake and glomerular filtration rate *(GFR)*. Data from younger (mean age, 31 years; range, 20–50 years) and older (mean age, 70 years; range, 55–88 years) healthy humans. *Closed symbols,* younger subjects; *open symbols,* older subjects; *squares,* women; *diamonds,* men. (From Lew SQ, Bosch P. Effect of diet on creatinine clearance in young and elderly healthy subjects and in patients with renal disease. *J Am Soc Nephrol.* 1991;2:856–865.)

measurement include laser Doppler flowmetry, video microscopy, and imaging techniques such as positron emission tomography (PET), high-speed computed tomography (CT), and magnetic resonance imaging (MRI).[6,8–12] These methods have been especially useful in determining changes in regional blood flow.

## MAJOR ARTERIES AND VEINS

Blood supply to each kidney is provided by a renal artery that branches directly from the abdominal aorta. The renal artery typically branches into multiple segmental vessels at a point just before entry into the renal parenchyma and continues to branch in a nonanastomotic manner to supply the glomeruli prior to entering the postglomerular microcirculation (see Fig. 3.1).[3] Therefore, complete obstruction of an arterial segmental vessel results in ischemia and infarction of the tissue in its area of distribution. Ligation of individual segmental arteries has frequently been performed in experimental studies to reduce renal mass and produce the remnant kidney model of chronic renal failure.[13,14] Morphologic studies in this model have revealed the presence of ischemic zones adjacent to the totally infarcted areas. These regions contain viable glomeruli that appear shrunken and crowded together, demonstrating that some portions of the renal cortex may have partial dual perfusion.[15] The anatomic distribution just described is most common; however, other patterns may occur.[16,17] Secondary renal arteries found in 20% to 30% of normal individuals may result from division of the renal artery at the aorta. These vessels, which most often supply the lower pole,[18] may be the sole arterial supply of some part of the kidney.[19]

Within the renal sinus of the human kidney, division of the segmental arteries gives rise to the interlobar arteries. These vessels, in turn, give rise to the arcuate arteries, whose several divisions lie at the border between the cortex and medulla. The interlobular arteries branch from the arcuate arteries more or less sharply, usually as a common trunk that divides two to five times as it extends toward the kidney surface[20,21] (see Fig. 3.1). Afferent arterioles leading to glomeruli arise from the interlobular arteries (see Figs. 3.1 and 3.2). Glomeruli are classified according to their position within the cortex as superficial (i.e., near the kidney surface), midcortical, or juxtamedullary, near the corticomedullary border (see Fig. 3.1). The capillary network of each glomerulus originates from the afferent arteriole as it enters into a manifold-like chamber. The glomerular capillaries coalesce into an efferent chamber leading to an efferent arteriole that delivers blood to the postglomerular capillary circulation, forming both the cortical peritubular capillaries and complex medullary capillaries. The arrangement of the medullary microcirculation plays an important role in the process of concentration of urine.

Venous drainage of the peritubular capillaries from the superficial cortex is via superficial cortical veins.[20,22] In the middle and inner cortices, venous drainage is achieved mainly by the interlobular veins. The dense peritubular capillary network surrounding the interlobular vessels drains directly into the interlobular veins through multiple connections, whereas the less dense, long-meshed network of the medullary rays appears to anastomose with the interlobular network and thus drains laterally (see Fig. 3.1). The medullary circulation also shows two different types of drainage. The outer medullary networks typically extend into the medullary rays before joining interlobular veins, whereas the long vascular bundles of the inner medulla (vasa recta) converge abruptly and join the arcuate veins.

## OXYGEN CONSUMPTION

Because of the unique juxtaposition of the arteriolar and venular network, much of the abundant oxygen supply to the kidneys diffuses from the arterioles to the venules.[23] The shunting of oxygen, coupled with the very high rate of oxygen consumption (~4 μmol/min/g), leaves the oxygen tension ($pO_2$) in the cortex much lower than what would be predicted from the $pO_2$ in renal venous blood. Tissue $pO_2$ values in the cortex border on hypoxia, varying from 40 to 45 mm Hg in the outer and mid cortices and even lower (30 mm Hg) in the deep cortex.[13,24,25] As shown in Fig. 3.5, the countercurrent arrangement between the descending and ascending vasa recta permits further shunting of oxygen, leaving $pO_2$ values in the medullary tissues of 20 mm Hg or lower toward the papillary tip.[23,25–27]

About 75% of the oxygen consumption by the kidneys provides the energy required by the $Na^+$-$K^+$-ATPase, which is the major active transport system of the tubules. Changes in oxygen consumption rate vary proportionally with the changes in net Na transport by the tubules. Reduced tissue oxygen levels occur in hypertension, which can compromise renal function.[24,28] The shunting of oxygen from arterioles to venules suggests that diffusible gas molecules that are formed in the kidney, including $CO_2$, NO, and hydrogen sulfide ($H_2S$), may also undergo shunting, but from venules to arterioles, thus making it more difficult to wash out unwanted substances such as $CO_2$ but also accentuating intrarenal retention of protective molecules such as nitric oxide (NO; see Fig. 3.5).[29]

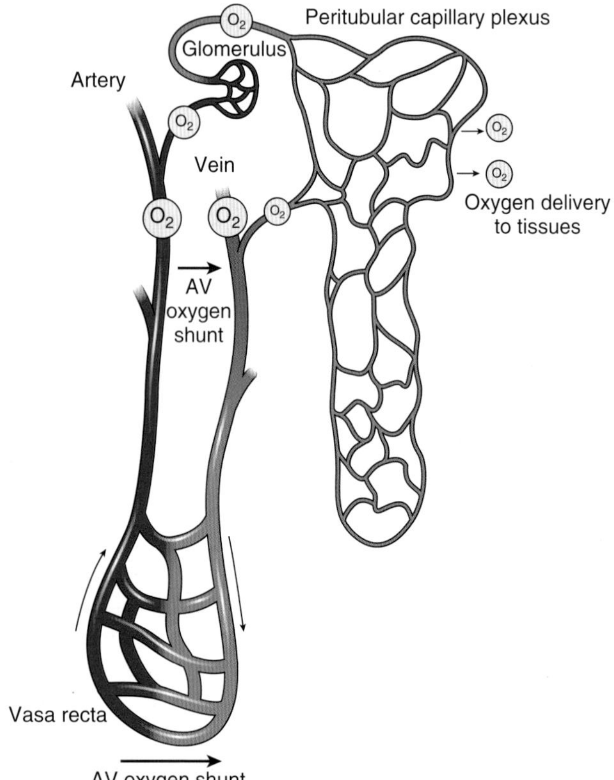


**Fig. 3.5** The arterial to venous *(AV)* oxygen shunt. Oxygen is delivered by red blood cells in the artery. Red blood cells release oxygen in the capillaries, which diffuses into the interstitium to reach target cells. Blood with low oxygen tension passes into the vein. The juxtaposition of the arteries and veins present in the kidney facilitates oxygen diffusion from the artery to the vein. Oxygen tensions in the capillaries are relatively low when red blood cells reach the peritubular capillary plexus, which indicate that the kidney is inefficient in extracting oxygen. The relative oxygen tensions are represented by the size of the circles surrounding $O_2$. (From Mimura I, Nangaku M. The suffocating kidney: tubulointerstitial hypoxia in end-stage renal disease. *Nat Rev Nephrol.* 2010;6:667–678.)

## HYDRAULIC PRESSURE PROFILE AND VASCULAR RESISTANCES

The decline in hydraulic pressure between the systemic vasculature and the end of the interlobular artery in both the superficial and juxtamedullary microvasculatures can be as much as 25 mm Hg at normal perfusion pressures, with most of that pressure drop occurring along the interlobular arteries (Fig. 3.6). Based on studies of the vasculature of juxtamedullary nephrons, most of the preglomerular pressure drop between the arcuate artery and the glomerulus occurs along the afferent arteriole.[30,31] Approximately 70% of the postglomerular hydraulic pressure drop occurs along the efferent arterioles. The very late portion of the afferent arteriole (last 50–150 μm) and the early portion of the efferent arteriole (first 50–150 μm) provide the major fraction of the total preglomerular and postglomerular resistance (see Fig. 3.6).[30,31] Multiphoton imaging studies have indicated the presence of an intraglomerular precapillary sphincter at the terminal end of afferent arterioles (Fig. 3.7).[32,33] Collectively, the total resistance ($R_T$) consists of two major sites, the afferent (Ra) and efferent (Re) arterioles and a minor contribution

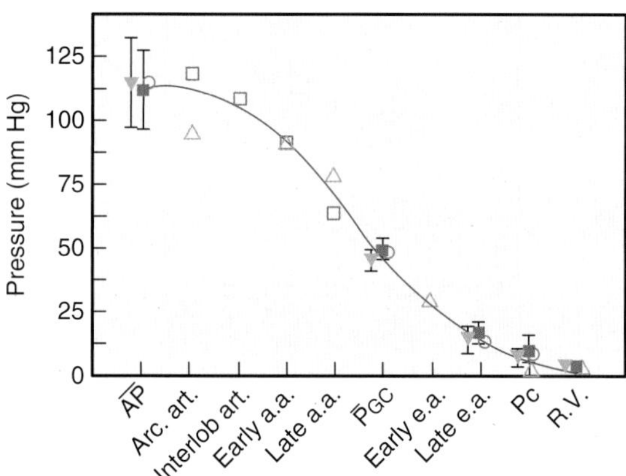


**Fig. 3.6** Hydraulic pressure profile in the kidney. Filled squares and triangles denote values (mean ± 2 standard deviation) obtained from euvolemic and hydropenic Munich-Wistar rats. Values from studies in the squirrel monkey[78] are shown as *open diamonds*. *Open inverted triangles* and *open squares* are from studies in the Sprague Dawley rat in juxtamedullary nephrons perfused with whole blood. These nephrons are located inside the cortical surface opposed to the pelvic lining and arcuate veins, in which entire pressure profiles can be obtained from the interlobular artery *(Interlob Art)*, the proximal *(Early a.a.)* and distal *(Late a.a.)* portions of the afferent arteriole, the glomerular capillaries *($P_{GC}$)*, the proximal *(Early e.a.)* and late *(Late e.a.)* segments of the efferent arteriole, the peritubular capillaries *($P_c$)*, and the renal vein *(R.V.)*. *AP,* Arterial pressure; *Arc. art.,* arcuate artery; *$P_{GC}$,* glomerular capillary pressure. (Modified from Maddox DA, Brenner BM. Glomerular ultrafiltration. In *Brenner and Rector's The Kidney*, 7th Edition. Philadelphia: W.B. Saunders Company; 2004, pp 353–412; Casellas D, Navar LG. In vitro perfusion of juxtamedullary nephrons in rats. *Am J Physiol.* 1984;246:F349–F358; Imig JD, Roman RJ. Nitric oxide modulates vascular tone in preglomerular arterioles. *Hypertension.* 1992;19(6 Pt 2):770–774.)

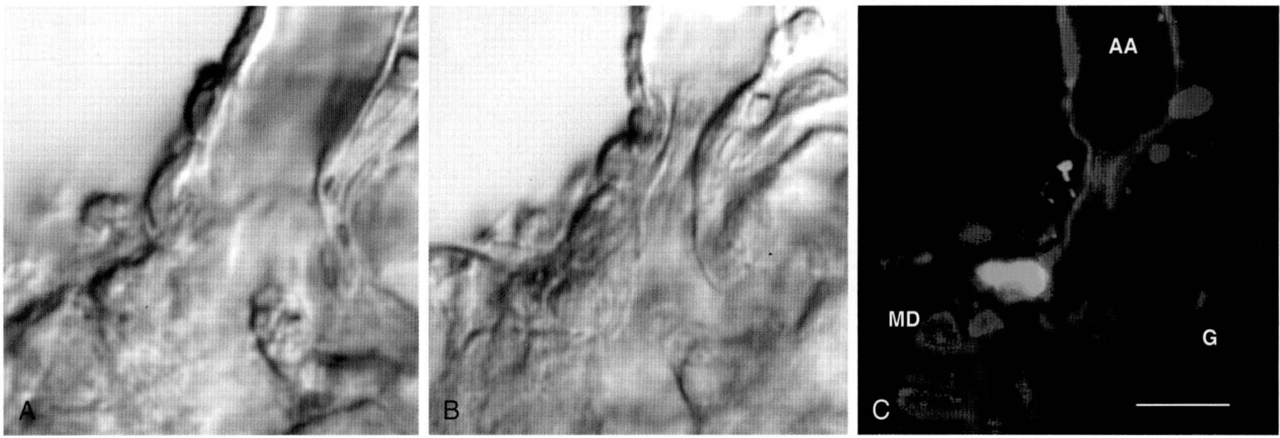


**Fig. 3.7** Constriction of the terminal afferent arteriole *(AA)* via an intraglomerular precapillary sphincter in response to elevations in distal tubular NaCl content. (A, B) Transmitted light differential interference contrast (DIC) images. (A) Control, with NaCl concentration at the macula densa at 10 mM. (B) NaCl concentration is increased to 60 mM, resulting in an almost complete closure of the AA. (C) Fluorescence image of the same preparation as shown in B. Vascular endothelium and tubular epithelium are labeled with R18 *(red),* renin granules with quinacrine *(green),* and cell nuclei with Hoechst 33342 *(blue).* Note that renin-positive granular cells constitute the sphincter, demonstrating contractile responses in glomerular cells. *G;*Glomerulus; *MD,* macula densa. Scale bar = 10 μm. (From Peti-Peterdi J. Multiphoton imaging of renal tissues in vitro. *Am J Physiol Renal Physiol.* 2005;288:F1079–F1083.)

from the outflowing venules and veins (Rv). Accordingly, the following relationships describe the intrarenal cortical vascular resistances:

$$R_T = Ra + Re + Rv \quad (1)$$

$$Ra = (AP - P_{GC})/RBF \quad (2)$$

$$Re = (P_{GC} - P_C)/EABF \quad (3)$$

where EABF = RBF − GFR

$$Rv = (P_C - P_V)/RBF \quad (4)$$

where AP = arterial pressure; $P_{GC}$ = glomerular capillary pressure; $P_C$ = peritubular capillary pressure; $P_V$ = renal vein pressure; and EABF = efferent arteriolar blood flow.

## INTRARENAL BLOOD FLOW DISTRIBUTION

The cortex accounts for filtration at the glomeruli and most of the reabsorption from proximal and distal nephron cortical tubules, whereas the medulla reabsorbs less than 20% of the total reabsorbate, in keeping with its primary function to maintain a hypertonic interstitial gradient when needed to excrete a concentrated urine. Blood flow to these regions is differentially regulated in response to the differing functions and demands of these two kidney regions.[34] Approximately 80% of the RBF perfuses the cortex and is under the control of numerous intrinsic paracrine vasoactive factors, as well as extrinsic humoral and neural influences. Vasoconstrictors, including angiotensin II (Ang II), endothelin, purinergic agents, and norepinephrine, as well as vasodilators, including bradykinin and nitric oxide, interact to regulate cortical blood flow and medullary blood flow.[34,35] There can be extensive redistribution of blood flow in the kidney under various conditions that may be important in physiologic and pathophysiologic conditions.[36]

Structural differences in vascular components of the cortex and the medulla may account for differences in RBF—namely, the organization of the afferent and efferent arterioles of the cortical and juxtamedullary glomeruli. The cortical afferent arterioles have larger internal diameters than the efferent arterioles, whereas juxtamedullary afferent and efferent arterioles are larger than the outer cortical arterioles, and efferent arterioles of juxtamedullary nephrons are more muscular compared with the cortical arterioles.[34,37] In addition, the cortical peritubular capillaries, derived from efferent arterioles of cortical glomeruli, are about half the diameter of the medullary vasa recta derived from efferent arterioles of the juxtamedullary glomeruli (Fig. 3.8).[34] These features may partially explain the differential control of medullary and cortical blood flows.

### VASCULAR-TUBULE RELATIONS

Cortical vascular-tubule relations have been described extensively (see Figs. 3.1 and 3.2).[20,38,39] The efferent peritubular capillary network and the tubules arising from each glomerulus in the outermost region of the cortex are tightly associated, but this relationship becomes dissociated in deeper regions of the cortex. This close association does not mean that each vessel adjacent to a given tubule necessarily arises from the same glomerulus. Although superficial nephron segments and peritubular capillaries arising from the same glomerulus are closely associated, each postglomerular efferent arteriole may serve segments of more than one nephron.[40] However, the loops of Henle of all nephrons, as they descend into the medullary ray, are supplied by postglomerular blood vessels emerging from midcortical and deep nephrons, with some of the branches from deep nephrons descending into the medullary ray, termed the *vasa recta* (see Figs. 3.1 and 3.2). The dissociation between individual tubules and the corresponding postglomerular capillary network is most apparent in the inner cortex. The convoluted tubule segments of these nephrons lie above the glomeruli surrounded by the dense network close to the interlobular vessels or by capillary networks arising from other inner cortical glomeruli. With regard to efferent vessel patterns and vascular-tubule relationships,[39,41] there is a close association between the initial portions of peritubular capillaries and early and late proximal tubule segments of the same glomerulus.[42–44]

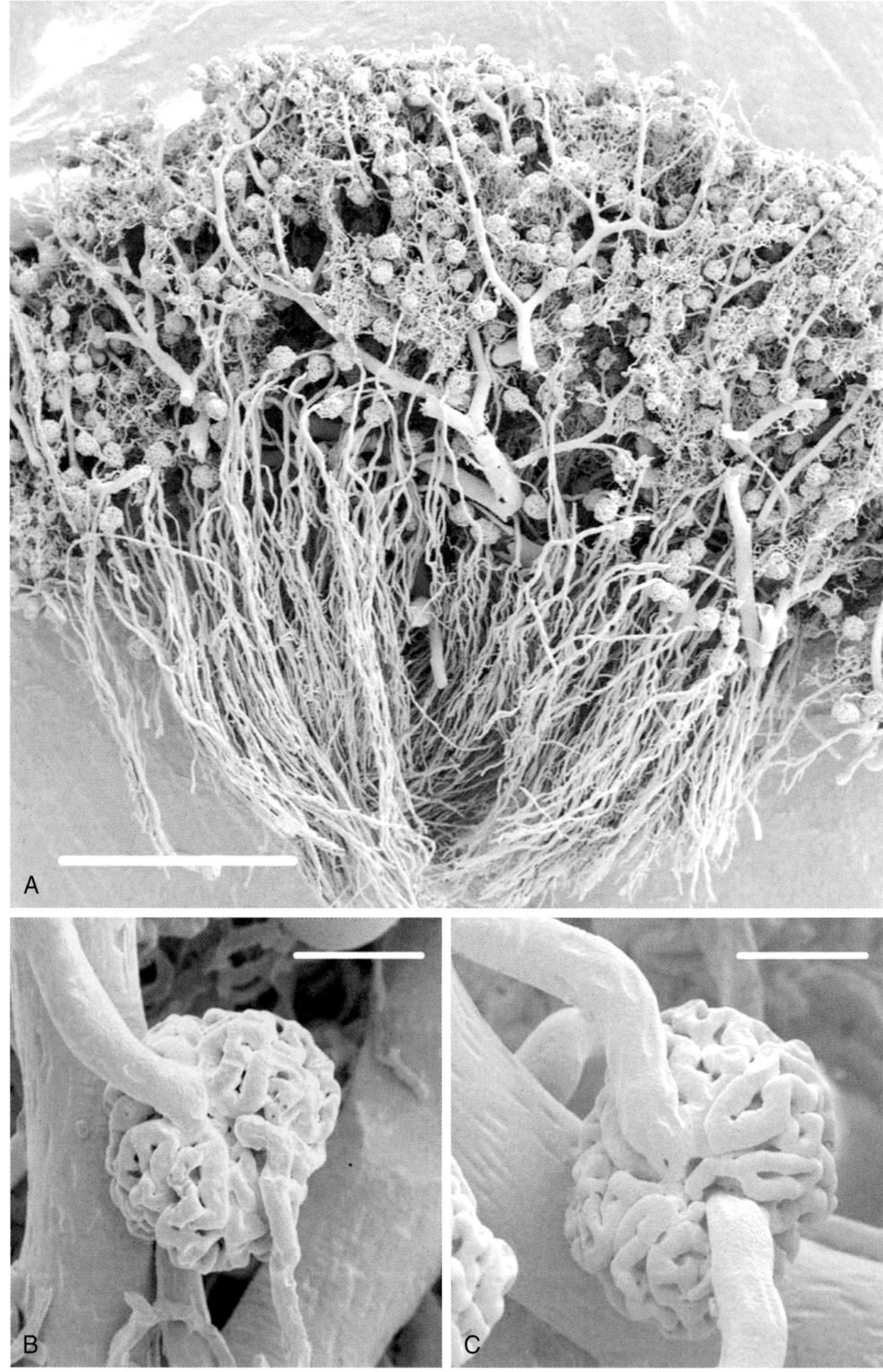


**Fig. 3.8** A, Resin casts of renal glomeruli of a rabbit, depicting both cortical and medullary glomeruli. For Panel A, the scale bar represents 1 mm. B, Cortical glomerulus showing afferent (upper vessel) and efferent arterioles and the capillary tuft (scale bar = 60 μm). C, A juxtamedullary glomerulus showing afferent (upper vessel) and efferent arterioles and the capillary tuft (scale bar 60 = μm). Note that the juxtamedullary arterioles are larger in diameter than the cortical glomerular arterioles, particularly the efferent arterioles. (From Evans RG, Eppel GA, Anderson WP, Denton KM: Mechanisms underlying the differential control of blood flow in the renal medulla and cortex. *J Hypertens.* 2004;22:1439–1451.)

## STRUCTURAL AND FUNCTIONAL ASPECTS OF THE GLOMERULAR MICROCIRCULATION

Some of the structural relationships of the glomerular microcirculation are seen in Fig. 3.8, which shows a scanning electron micrograph of a resin-filled cast of a kidney. The afferent arteriole branching from the interlobular artery, the many loops of the glomerular capillaries, and the efferent arteriole as it emerges from the glomerular tuft can be seen in B and C. An ultrastructural analysis of the vascular pole of the renal glomerulus has revealed differences in the structure and branching patterns of the afferent and efferent arterioles as these vessels enter and exit the tuft.[45] Afferent arterioles lose their internal elastic layer and smooth muscle cell layer prior to entering the glomerular tuft. Smooth muscle cells are replaced by renin-positive, myosin-negative granular cells that are in close contact with the extraglomerular mesangium (Fig. 3.9).[32,46] On entering Bowman's space, afferent arterioles undergo a transition into a vascular chamber that has a manifold-like structure distributing primary branches along the surface of the glomerular tuft, which branch further into the individual glomerular capillaries.[45,47]

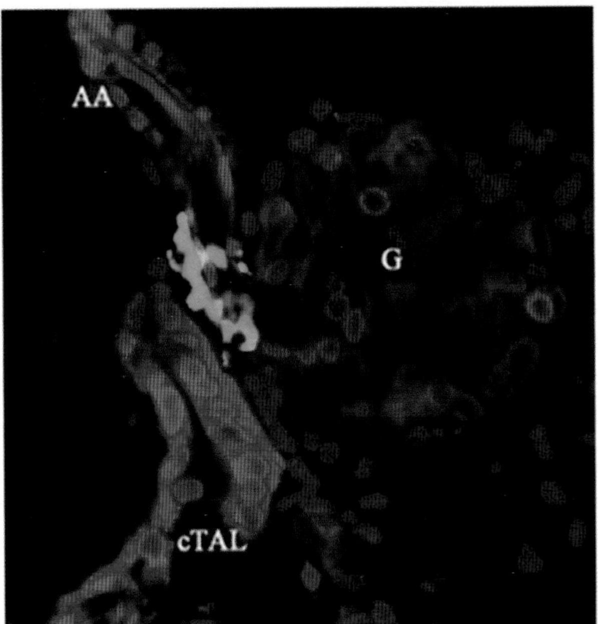


**Fig. 3.9** Multicolor labeling of the in vitro microperfused juxtaglomerular apparatus with attached glomerulus. Cell membranes of tubular epithelium (cortical thick ascending limb, *[cTAL]* containing the macula densa), vascular endothelium of the afferent arteriole *(AA),* and glomerulus *(G)* are labeled with R18 *(red),* renin granules with quinacrine *(green),* and cell nuclei with Hoechst 33342 *(blue).* (From Peti-Peterdi J. Multiphoton imaging of renal tissues in vitro. *Am J Physiol Renal Physiol.* 2005;288:F1079–F1083.)

The primary branches have wide lumens and immediately acquire features of glomerular capillaries, including a fenestrated endothelium, characteristic glomerular basement membrane, and epithelial foot processes. In human glomeruli, however, these primary branches serve as conduit vessels that branch into the filtering capillaries (Fig. 3.10).[47] In contrast, the efferent arteriole originates deep within the tuft, from the convergence of capillaries into multiple lobules that exit into an efferent vascular chamber, which narrows into an efferent arteriole. Additional tributaries join the efferent arteriole as it travels toward the vascular pole. The structure of the capillary wall begins to change, even before the vessels coalesce to form the efferent arteriole, losing fenestrae progressively until a smooth epithelial lining is formed. At the arteriole's terminal portion within the tuft, endothelial cells may bulge into the lumen, reducing its internal diameter.[45] Efferent arterioles acquire a smooth muscle cell layer, which is observed distal to the entry point of the final glomerular capillary. The efferent arteriole is also in close contact with the glomerular mesangium as it forms inside the tuft and with the extraglomerular mesangium as it exits the tuft. This precise and close anatomic relationship between the afferent and efferent arterioles and mesangium with the macula densa cells of the ascending loop of Henle provides the structural basis for the presence of an intraglomerular signaling system, known as the "tubuloglomerular feedback mechanism," which participates in the regulation of blood flow and GFR.[32,45,48]

The appearance of the vascular pathways within the glomerulus may change under different physiologic conditions. The glomerular mesangium (Fig. 3.11) has been shown to contain contractile elements[45,49] and to exhibit contractile activity when exposed to Ang II.[50] Mesangial cells, which possess AT1 receptors for Ang II, undergo contraction when exposed to this peptide in vitro.[51] Three-dimensional

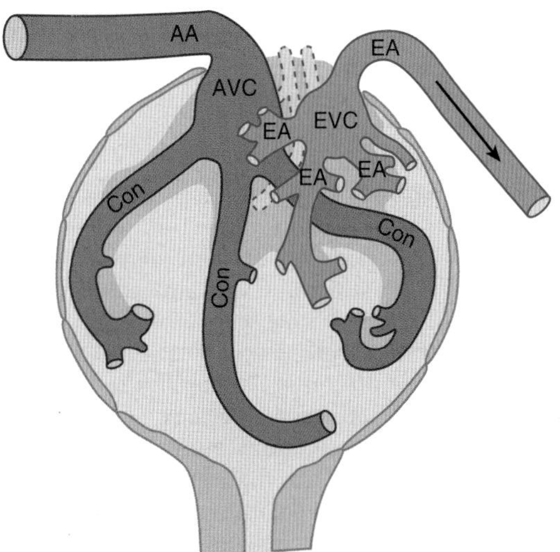


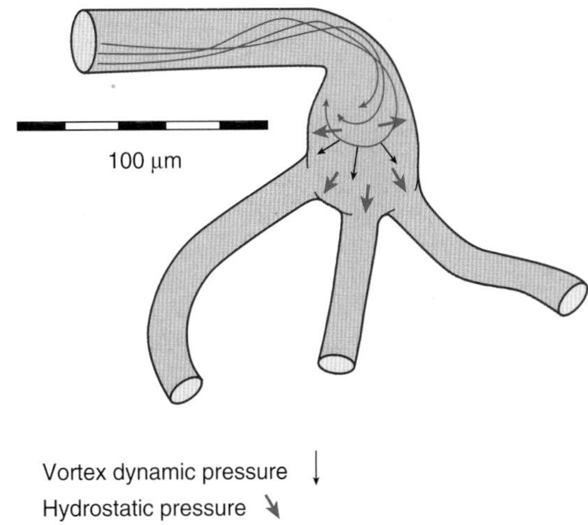


**Fig. 3.10** Structure of the human glomerulus. Note the sharp turn made by the afferent arteriole *(AA)* as it enters the afferent vascular chamber *(AVC),* which flows into the conduit afferent capillaries *(Con).* Efferent first-order vessels (E1) and the efferent vascular chamber *(EVC)* transition into the efferent arteriole *(EA). Right,* Distribution of hydraulic forces in the AVC. (From Neal CR, Arkill K, Bell JS, et al. Novel hemodynamic structures in the human glomerulus. *Am J Physiol Renal Physiol.* 2018;315(5):F1370–F1384; color figures courtesy Dr. Christopher Neal.)

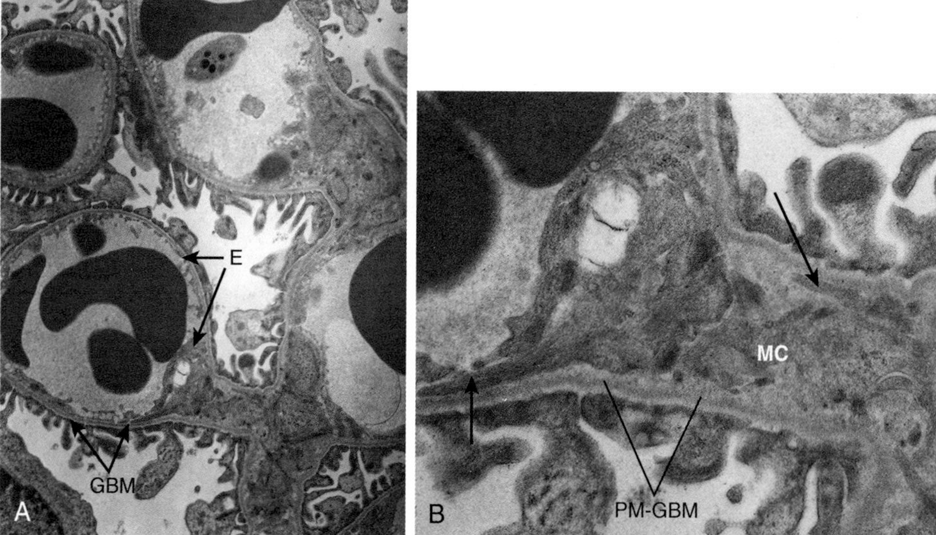


**Fig. 3.11** Electron micrographs of glomerular capillaries of a Munich-Wistar rat. (A) Overview of several capillaries (≈×14,500). Most of the glomerular capillary endothelium *(E)* is in contact with the glomerular basement membrane *(GBM)*, with only a small portion in contact with the mesangium (M). At its outer aspect, the GBM is covered by podocyte foot processes. There is no basement membrane separating the endothelium from the mesangium at their interface. (B) Mesangial cell *(MC)* extends outward to meet the glomerular capillary (≈×42,000). Kriz and co-workers have suggested that such cylinder-like stalks appear to be contractile filament bundles (*short arrow*) that attach to the perimesangial glomerular basement membranes *(PM-GBM)* and extend to the GBM at the mesangial angles (*long arrow*). For this preparation the nephron was perfusion-fixed by micropuncture with 1.25% glutaraldehyde through Bowman's space, thereby yielding the fixation of glomerular structures, as well as the red cells in the capillaries. (Modified from Kriz W, Elger M, Mundel P, Lemley KV. Structure-stabilizing forces in the glomerular tuft. *J Am Soc Nephrol.* 1995;5(10):1731–1739; Kriz W, Kaissling B. *Structural organization of the mammalian kidney.* Third Edition ed: Lippincott, Williams & Wilkins; 2000; Drenckhahn D, Schnittler H, Nobiling R, Kriz W. Ultrastructural organization of contractile proteins in rat glomerular mesangial cells. *Am J Pathol.* 1990;137(6):1343–1351.)

reconstruction of the entire mesangium in the rat has suggested that approximately 15% of capillary loops may be entirely enclosed within armlike extensions of mesangial cells that are anchored to the extracellular matrix.[52] Contraction of these cells might alter local blood flow and filtration rate, as well as the intraglomerular distribution of blood flow and total filtration surface area. Many hormones and other vasoactive substances capable of altering glomerular filtration may bring about this adjustment, in part by altering the state of contraction of mesangial cells.

## DETERMINANTS OF GLOMERULAR FILTRATION

A critical function of the mechanisms regulating renal hemodynamics is to maintain the blood flow and pressure profile within the glomerular tufts at levels such that the filtration rate allows optimum function of reabsorptive and secretory processes by the tubular network. The exquisite differential regulation of the preglomerular (afferent) and postglomerular (efferent) resistances exert fine control of the intraglomerular hemodynamic environment and thus the GFR. This nesting of the glomerular capillary system between the afferent and efferent arterioles allows for precise regulation of the intraglomerular forces governing filtration. These forces, coupled with the unique restrictive molecular permeability of the glomerular capillary structure, lead to the formation of a nearly protein-free filtrate, from the glomerular capillaries into Bowman's space, as the first step in the process of urine formation.

### PERMEABILITY OF THE GLOMERULAR FILTRATION BARRIER

In addition to the unique role of the glomerular capillary wall and surrounding glomerular epithelial cells in regulating fluid movement from the glomerular capillary into Bowman's space, these structures also regulate the movement of macromolecules. Molecules the size of inulin or smaller are normally able to cross the glomerular capillary wall without restriction. However, the transglomerular permeation of molecules of increasing size becomes limited, so that molecules the size of albumin or larger are almost completely prevented from crossing into Bowman's space.

As shown in Fig. 3.12, the composite filtration barrier includes the glycocalyx lining the endothelial cells, the fenestrations of the endothelial layer of the glomerular capillaries, the three layers of the glomerular basement membrane, the filtration slits between adjacent foot processes of the visceral epithelial cells (podocytes) that surround the capillaries, and the filtration slit diaphragm that extends along the filtration slits and connects adjacent foot processes to form the ultimate barrier to filtration[53] (see Fig. 3.12). This complex barrier has a high permeability to small molecules such as water, electrolytes, amino acids, glucose, and other endogenous or exogenous compounds with molecular radii smaller than 20 Å. This allows these compounds to be freely filtered from the blood into Bowman's space while virtually excluding molecules larger than around 50 Å.[54–61] In studies using fractional clearances of neutral

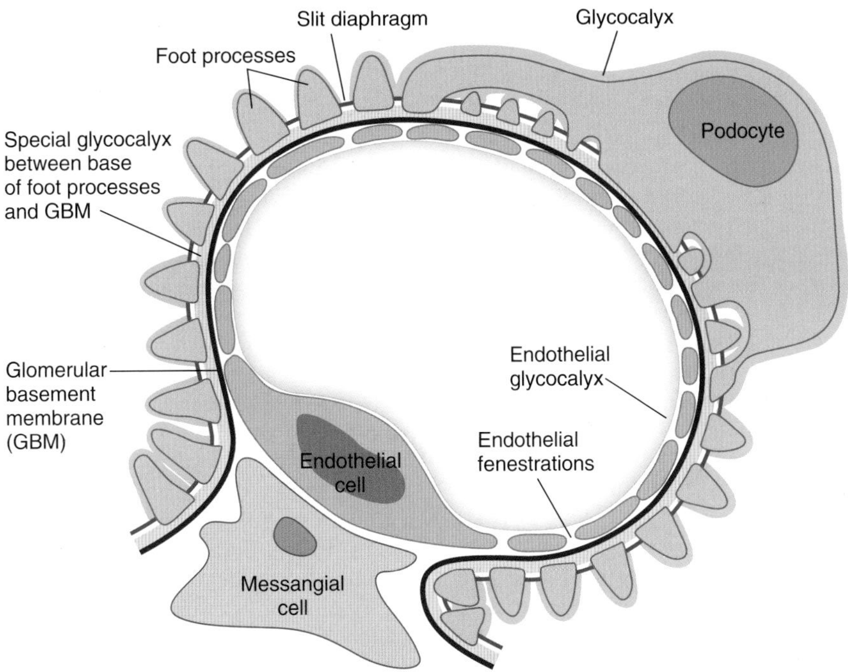


**Fig. 3.12** Schematic drawing of a glomerular capillary. The elements considered as part of the glomerular filtration barrier include the following: endothelial glycocalyx, fenestrated endothelium, basement membrane, specialized glycocalyx between the foot processes and basement membrane, and podocyte and slit diaphragm. (From Schlöndorff D, Wyatt CM, Campbell KN. Revisiting the determinants of glomerular filtration barrier: what goes round must come round, *Kidney Int.* 2017;92:533–536.)

dextran, comparable size selectivity[62] was observed in rats,[63] dogs,[64] and humans.[65] As recently emphasized,[53] there has been considerable controversy regarding the component primarily responsible for the exclusion of macromolecules from the filtrate. The size selectivity of the glomerular filtration barrier is determined largely by a combination of the slit diaphragms between podocyte foot processes and the glomerular basement membrane (GBM). Although there is some controversy regarding glomerular charge selectivity, there is good evidence for a role of charge in restricting the transmural movement of negatively charged macromolecules such as albumin at the level of the GBM, which contains negatively charged heparan sulfate proteoglycans, as well as laminin, type IV collagen, and nidogen.[66,67]

Other studies have now demonstrated the presence of a fine meshwork of glycosaminoglycans covering the luminal endothelial layer and bridging the endothelial fenestrations so that the endothelial layer is now considered the initial coarse barrier for macromolecular exclusion.[68] Further studies using negatively charged gold nanoparticles have confirmed that the lamina densa of the basement membrane serves as an exclusion barrier for molecules the size of immunoglobulin G (IgG) and albumin. Small particles permeated into the lamina densa and accumulated upstream, covering the base of the foot processes.[60]

## HYDRAULIC AND ONCOTIC FORCES IN THE GLOMERULAR CAPILLARIES AND BOWMAN'S SPACE

The process of filtration of fluid at any given point of the glomerular capillary is governed by the net balance among the transcapillary hydraulic pressure gradient ($\Delta P$), the transcapillary colloid osmotic pressure gradient ($\Delta\pi$), and the hydraulic conductivity of the filtration barrier per surface area unit (Lp), coupled with the surface area (Sf). The product of Lp and Sf is called the "filtration coefficient" ($K_f$). Fluid flow ($J_v$) at any given point in the capillary is determined by the Starling equation:

$$J_v = Lp\,[(P_{GC} - P_{BS}) - (\pi_{GC} - \pi_{BS})] \tag{5}$$

where $P_{GC}$ and $P_{BS}$ are the hydraulic pressures in the glomerular capillaries and Bowman's space, respectively, and $\pi_{GC}$ and $\pi_{BS}$ are the corresponding colloid osmotic pressures at any given point. Because the protein concentration of the fluid in Bowman's space is very low, $\pi_{BS}$ approaches zero and can be disregarded. The total GFR of fluid for a single nephron (SNGFR) is equal to the product of the surface area for filtration ($S_f$) and the hydraulic conductivity (Lp), defined as the filtration coefficient ($K_f$) and the values of the right-hand terms in Eq.5 averaged along the length of the glomerular capillaries yielding the expression:

$$SNGFR = LpS_f\,[(P_{GC} - P_{BS}) - (\pi_{GC})] \text{ or } SNGFR = K_f\,(\Delta P - \pi_{GC}) \tag{6}$$

Thus,

$$SNGFR = K_f \times P_{UF} \tag{7}$$

where $P_{UF}$ = the mean filtration pressure, the difference between the mean transcapillary hydraulic and colloid osmotic pressure gradients, $\Delta P$ and $\pi_{GC}$, respectively.

It is important to emphasize the difference between Lp, the hydraulic conductivity, and the macromolecular permeability. These are regulated differently and are not closely coupled. Based on known ultrastructural detail and the hydrodynamic properties of the individual components of the filtration barrier, mathematical modeling suggests that only around 2% of the total hydraulic resistance is accounted for by the fenestrated capillary endothelium, whereas the basement membrane accounts for nearly 50%.[66,69,70] The remaining hydraulic resistance resides in the diaphragm of the filtration slits, which are complex structures containing numerous proteins, including nephrin and podocin.[66,70–72] Disruption of these slit diaphragm proteins leads to substantial proteinuria.[72] A reduction in the frequency of intact filtration slits is an important factor in the deterioration of filtration in some disease states.[66,73] In the case of macromolecule permeability, mathematical modeling efforts contend that the sieving efficiency of the layers of the glomerular filtration barrier are interdependent. Moreover, whereas hydraulic resistances are additive, macromolecule sieving coefficients are multiplicative; thus, a small change in the macromolecule permeability of one layer can significantly change the overall permeability of the filtration barrier.[62,66]

Because surface glomeruli are not present in most experimental animals, indirect approaches to measure glomerular pressure have been used in many experimental studies to evaluate the responses of glomerular pressure. The stop-flow technique has been used by many investigators to estimate $P_{GC}$.[2,35,74,75] When fluid movement in the early proximal tubule is blocked, intratubular pressure upstream from the block increases until net filtration at the glomerulus ceases.[76] At that point, the sum of this hydrostatic pressure in the early proximal tubule plus the systemic colloid oncotic pressure is equal to the pressure in the glomerular capillaries ($P_{GCSF}$). The stop-flow technique has been used in different strains of rats, as well as in dogs and mice, with the $P_{GCSF}$ averaging 55 to 60 mm Hg in the dog and about 50 mm Hg in the rat.[4,55] Glomerular capillary pressures calculated using this stop-flow have been compared with values obtained by direct micropuncture of glomerular capillaries in a number of studies; these indicate that $P_{GCSF}$, measured at normal APs, provides a close estimate of $P_{GC}$ measured directly.[35,55,74,75]

Direct measurements of glomerular capillary hydraulic pressure in vertebrates ($P_{GC}$) became possible when it was discovered that a mutant strain of the Munich-Wistar rat had surface glomeruli that allowed direct puncture of glomerular capillaries.[77] Subsequent studies have confirmed the original observations, demonstrating that values for $P_{GC}$ in surface glomeruli average 43 to 49 mm Hg in this strain of rats (Fig. 3.13), and similar values were found in the squirrel monkey, which also has some superficial glomeruli.[78] Because the glomerular capillaries are nested between the afferent and efferent arterioles, $P_{GC}$ is nearly constant along the length

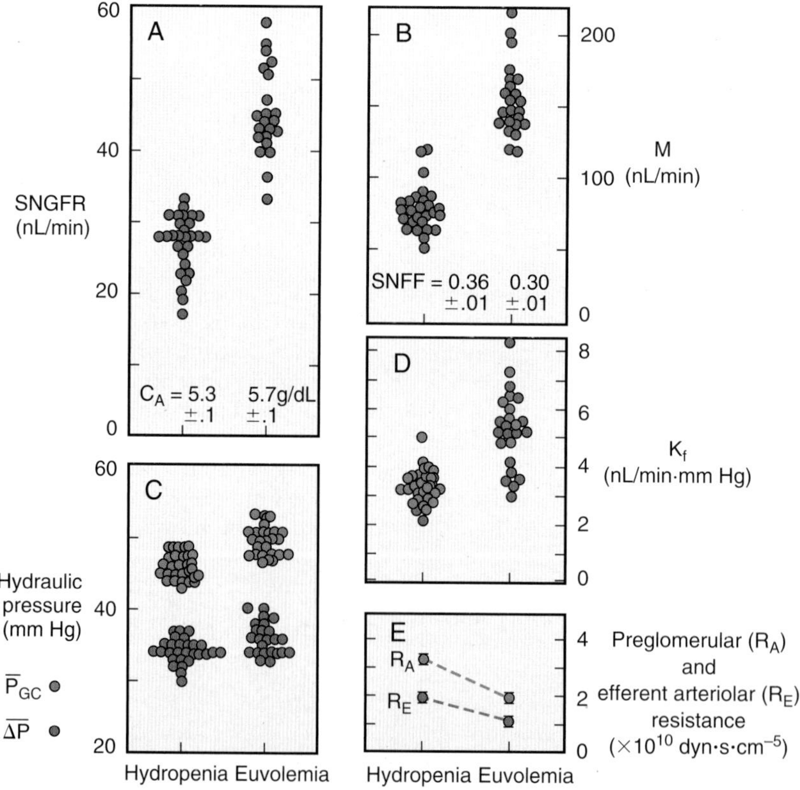


**Fig. 3.13** Glomerular filtration in the Munich-Wistar rat. (A–E) Each point represents the mean value reported for studies in hydropenic and euvolemic rats provided food and water ad lib until the time of study. Data from euvolemic rats are thought to be representative of nonanesthesia conditions. Only data from studies using male or a mix of male and female rats are shown. Values of the ultrafiltration coefficient, $K_f$ (*red circles* in D), denote minimum values because the animals were in filtration pressure equilibrium. *Blue circles* represent unique values of $K_f$ calculated under conditions of filtration pressure disequilibrium ($\pi_E/\Delta P \leq 0.95$). $C_A$, Concentration in the afferent arteriole; $\Delta P$, pressure gradient; $P_{GC}$, pressure in the glomerular capillaries; $Q_A$, glomerular plasma flow rate; *SNFF*, single-nephron filtration fraction; *SNGFR*, single-nephron glomerular filtration. (From Maddox DA, Brenner BM. Glomerular ultrafiltration. In: Brenner BM, ed. *The kidney*. 7th ed. Philadelphia: Saunders; 2004:353–412; Maddox DA, Deen WM, Brenner BM. *Handbook of physiology: Section 8; Renal physiology* Vol 1. New York: Oxford University Press; 1992, pp. 545–638.)

GLOMERULAR PRESSURES IN THE MUNICH-WISTAR RAT

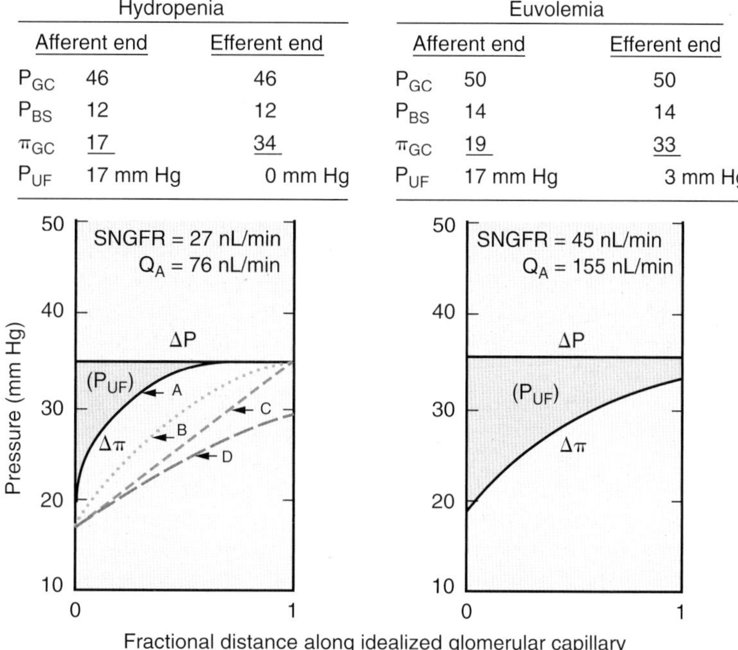

| | Hydropenia | | Euvolemia | |
|---|---|---|---|---|
| | Afferent end | Efferent end | Afferent end | Efferent end |
| $P_{GC}$ | 46 | 46 | 50 | 50 |
| $P_{BS}$ | 12 | 12 | 14 | 14 |
| $\pi_{GC}$ | 17 | 34 | 19 | 33 |
| $P_{UF}$ | 17 mm Hg | 0 mm Hg | 17 mm Hg | 3 mm Hg |



**Fig. 3.14** Hydraulic and colloid osmotic pressure profiles along idealized glomerular capillaries in hydropenic and euvolemic rats. Values shown are mean values derived from the studies shown in Fig. 3.13. The transcapillary hydraulic pressure gradient, $\Delta P$, is equal to $P_{GC}$ – PT, and the transcapillary colloid osmotic pressure gradient, $\Delta\pi$, is equal to $\pi_{GC} - \pi_{BS}$, where $P_{GC}$ and $P_{BS}$ are the hydraulic pressures in the glomerular capillary and Bowman's space, respectively, and $\pi_{GC}$ and $\pi_{BS}$ are the corresponding colloid osmotic pressures. Because the value of $\pi_{BS}$ is negligible, $\Delta\pi$ essentially equals $\pi_{GC}$. $P_{UF}$ is the ultrafiltration pressure at any point. The area between the $\Delta P$ and $\Delta\pi$ curves represents the net ultrafiltration pressure, $P_{UF}$. *Left,* Lines A and B represent two of the many possible profiles under conditions of filtration pressure equilibrium; line D represents disequilibrium and line C represents the hypothetic linear $\Delta\pi$ profile. *Right,* Pressure profile after correction for surgical induced loss of plasma volume depicts a small positive $\Delta P$ at the efferent level indicative of disequilibrium conditions. *$Q_A$,* Glomerular plasma flow; *SNGFR,* single-nephron glomerular filtration rate.

of the capillary bed, resulting in a transcapillary hydraulic pressure gradient that averages 34 mm Hg in hydropenic Munich-Wistar rats (see Fig. 3.13). Coupling these hydraulic pressure measurements with determinations of systemic plasma protein concentration and efferent arteriolar protein concentrations of superficial nephrons has permitted an opportunity to determine the hydraulic and oncotic pressures that govern glomerular filtration at the beginning and end of the capillary network.

The early direct measurements of $P_{GC}$ made in hydropenic rats were under conditions of surgically induced reductions in plasma volume and GFR. Subsequent studies, in which plasma volume was restored to a euvolemic state, equal to that of the awake animal,[79] by infusion of iso-oncotic plasma, yielded SNGFR values substantially higher than in hydropenic rats. This is primarily as a consequence of increases in glomerular plasma flow ($Q_A$) associated with a fall in preglomerular ($R_A$) and efferent arteriolar ($R_E$) resistance values (see Fig. 3.13), indicating that the early studies in hydropenic rats were performed under conditions of elevated activity of the sympathetic nervous system. Collectively, the experimental studies in Munich-Wistar rats (see Fig. 3.13) and several other strains of rats studied under euvolemic conditions have indicated that glomerular pressure in rats is in the range of 50 mm Hg, leading to higher transglomerular capillary pressures.

Glomerular capillary hydraulic and oncotic pressure profiles for rats under hydropenic and euvolemic conditions are shown in Fig. 3.14, using the mean values determined from the studies shown in Fig. 3.13. In hydropenic animals, by the time the blood reaches the efferent end of the glomerular capillaries, plasma oncotic pressure ($\pi_E$) rises to a value that, on average, equals ΔP. As a consequence, the net local filtration pressure, $P_{UF}$ ($P_{GC} - [P_T + \pi_{GC}]$), is reduced from approximately 17 mm Hg at the afferent end of the glomerular capillary network to essentially zero by the efferent end (referred to as "filtration pressure equilibrium"). The value of ΔP is nearly constant along the glomerular capillaries, and the decline in $P_{UF}$ along the capillary network is due to a rise in $\pi_{GC}$ (see Fig. 3.14). An exact profile of the $\Delta\pi$ curve cannot be ascertained under conditions of filtration pressure equilibrium, and hence only maximum estimates of $P_{UF}$ and minimum estimates of $K_f$ can be obtained by assuming a linear rise in the $\Delta\pi$ curve. To obtain accurate measurements of the $\Delta\pi$ curve, Deen and colleagues plasma-expanded rats to increase plasma flow to obtain filtration pressure disequilibrium (Fig. 3.14, curve D), permitting an exact determination of $P_{UF}$ and hence $K_f$.[80] Filtration pressure disequilibrium is present in about 60% of the studies in the euvolemic Munich-Wistar rat (see Fig. 3.13) and in most of the studies in Sprague-Dawley rats and in dogs,[4,74,75,81] permitting exact determinations of $P_{UF}$ along the entire length of the glomerular capillaries and hence an accurate $K_f$ reflecting the total surface area.

### DETERMINATION OF THE FILTRATION COEFFICIENT

As shown in Eq. 7, SNGFR equals the filtration coefficient ($K_f$) times the net driving force for filtration averaged over the length of the glomerular capillaries ($P_{UF}$). The values of $K_f$ from many studies in euvolemic Munich-Wistar rats studied under conditions of filtration pressure disequilibrium (see Fig. 3.13) averaged 5.0 ± 0.3 nL/(min·mm Hg). These are values similar to those found in other rat strains and in dogs (3–5 nL/[min·mm Hg]).[4,55,74,75] Because this value remains essentially unchanged over a twofold range of changes in $Q_A$, the data suggest that changes in $Q_A$ per se do not affect $K_f$.[80]

In the rat, total capillary basement membrane surface area per glomerulus ($A_s$) has been determined to be around 0.003 $cm^2$ in superficial nephrons and 0.004 $cm^2$ in deep nephrons.[82] A large portion of the capillary surface area faces the mesangium and, as a consequence, only the peripheral area of the capillaries surrounded by podocytes participates in filtration. This peripheral area available for filtration ($A_p$) is only about half that of $A_s$ (~0.0016–0.0018; 0.0019–0.0022 $cm^2$ in the superficial and deep glomeruli, respectively).[82] Using a value of $K_f$ of around 5 nL/min mm Hg, as determined by micropuncture techniques, with these estimates of $A_{p,}$, yields a hydraulic conductivity (Lp) of 45 to 48 nL/(sec·mm Hg·$cm^2$). These estimates of k for the rat glomerulus are all one or two orders in magnitude higher than those reported for capillary networks in mesentery, skeletal muscle, omentum or peritubular capillaries of the kidney,[55,83] thus supporting the premise of very high glomerular hydraulic permeability of the glomerular capillaries.

### DETERMINANTS OF GLOMERULAR FILTRATION COEFFICIENT IN HUMAN SUBJECTS

Hydraulic pressure in the glomerular capillaries of human kidneys cannot be measured using micropuncture of glomerular capillaries or measurements of stop-flow pressures in proximal tubules or free-flow pressures in Bowman's space. From determinations of plásma protein concentrations, and thus the afferent arteriolar oncotic pressure together with the whole-kidney filtration fraction, efferent arteriolar oncotic pressure can be calculated, generally yielding values around 37 mm Hg. In addition, peritubular capillary pressure has been estimated from intrarenal venous pressure measurements, yielding estimates of proximal tubule hydraulic pressure of 20 to 25 mm Hg.[84,85] Coupled with an efferent oncotic pressure of 37 mm Hg, this indicates that the minimal value for glomerular capillary pressure in humans is in the range of 57 to 62 mm Hg. Glomerular volumes and diameters of human kidneys are larger than in the experimental species, suggesting that the single-nephron $K_f$ is greater than in the experimental animals. It is thought that in humans, filtration pressure disequilibrium is normally present, and GFR exhibits less plasma flow dependency than in rats.[2] The molecular sieving approach has been used as an alternative noninvasive means for the evaluation of the hydraulic conductivity characteristics and filtration coefficient in studies of glomerular dynamics in humans. By using uncharged macromolecules with varying molecular radii, which are partially restricted, the sieving coefficients for molecules of different sizes can be obtained.[63,86,87] Combining the sieving data with mathematical models, estimated data for $K_f$ values can be derived. Values for single-nephron $K_f$ in normal human subjects have varied from 3.6 to 9.4 nL/min mm Hg, with an average value of about 6 to 7 nL/min mm Hg.[2,4,75,88,89]

### SELECTIVE ALTERATIONS IN THE PRIMARY DETERMINANTS OF GLOMERULAR FILTRATION

The four primary determinants of filtration are $Q_A$, ΔP, $K_f$, and $\pi_A$, and alterations in each of these will affect the GFR. The degree to which such alterations will modify SNGFR has been examined by mathematical modeling[80] and compared with values obtained experimentally (see Arendshorst and Navar,[2] Navar et al.,[4] and Lowenstein et al.[84]).

#### Glomerular Plasma Flow ($Q_A$)

Because protein is normally excluded from the glomerular filtrate, the total amount of protein entering the glomerular capillary network from the afferent arteriole is maintained, leading to progressively increasing protein concentration as the plasma traverses the glomerular capillaries to the efferent arteriole. Thus, there is a substantial increase in the plasma colloid osmotic pressure (πg) in the glomerular capillaries as the plasma traverses from the inlet to the outlet. This increase in πg counteracts the net hydraulic filtration pressure and may completely offset the ΔP, so that πg = ΔP if equilibrium is reached before the plasma reaches the efferent arteriole, preventing further net filtration of fluid into Bowman's space. Under this condition of filtration pressure equilibrium, where ΔP = $\pi_E$, SNGFR will vary directly with changes in $Q_A$ as a greater filtering surface area is recruited. Once $Q_A$ increases enough to produce disequilibrium, $\pi_E$ becomes less than ΔP, and the SNGFR will no longer vary linearly with $Q_A$.[90] However, there is still an effect of increases in plasma flow to increase GFR, although to a lesser extent, because the filtration fraction will decrease and there will be a lesser overall increase in πg. As shown in Fig. 3.15, increases in plasma flow are associated with increases in GFR in a number of studies in rats, dogs, nonhuman primates, and humans.

#### Transcapillary Hydraulic Pressure Difference (ΔP)

Mathematical modeling indicates that isolated changes in the glomerular transcapillary hydraulic pressure gradient exert strong effects on SNGFR.[2,4,80] In particular, when ΔP exceeds the colloid osmotic pressure at the efferent end of the glomerular capillary, filtration occurs throughout the glomerular capillary network, and SNGFR increases as ΔP increases. The relationship between SNGFR and ΔP is nonlinear, however, because the rise in SNGFR at any given fixed value of $Q_A$ results in a concurrent increase in Δπ. Because net effective filtration pressure is a small fraction of $P_{GC}$, small isolated changes in $P_{GC}$ can cause large percentile changes in net filtration pressure.

#### Glomerular Capillary Filtration Coefficient ($K_f$)

Glomerular damage from a variety of kidney diseases and various hormonal and pharmacologic influences can result in alterations in the glomerular filtration coefficient ($K_f$) due to reductions in surface area available for filtration and/or to reductions in the hydraulic conductivity because of thickening of the basement membrane or other derangements.

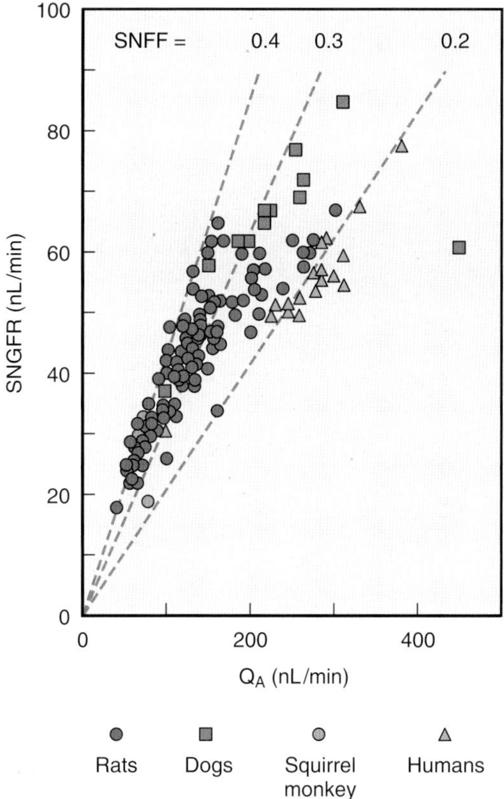


**Fig. 3.15** Association between single-nephron glomerular filtration rate *(SNGFR)* and glomerular plasma flow ($Q_A$); data are from rats, dogs, squirrel monkeys, and humans. The values for SNGFR and $Q_A$ for humans were calculated by dividing the whole-kidney GFR and renal plasma flow by the estimated total number of nephrons/kidney (1 million). Each point represents the mean value for a given study. *SNFF,* Single-nephron filtration fraction. (Data from Maddox DA, Brenner BM. Glomerular ultrafiltration. In: Brenner BM, ed. *The kidney*. 7th ed. Philadelphia: Saunders; 2004:353–412; Maddox DA, Deen WM, Brenner BM. *Handbook of physiology: Section 8; Renal physiology* Vol 1. New York: Oxford University Press; 1992.)

Hydraulic conductivity of the glomerular basement membrane demonstrates an inverse relationship to ΔP, indicating that $K_f$ may be directly influenced by ΔP.[91] $K_f$ is also affected by the plasma protein concentration.[81,92] Under conditions of filtration pressure equilibrium, reductions in $K_f$ do not affect SNGFR until $K_f$ is reduced enough to produce filtration pressure disequilibrium. However, increases in $K_f$ above normal will increase SNGFR until equilibrium conditions occur.[80,83] When plasma flow is high, and disequilibrium exists, there is a more direct relationship between $K_f$ and SNGFR.[80,83]

#### Colloid Osmotic Pressure ($\pi_A$)

SNGFR and the single-nephron filtration fraction (SNFF) are each theoretically predicted to vary reciprocally as a function of $\pi_A$.[80] If $Q_A$, ΔP, and $K_f$ are held constant, reductions in $\pi_A$ are predicted to increase $P_{UF}$, leading to an increase in SNGFR. An increase in $\pi_A$ should produce a decrease in SNGFR until $\pi_A$ equals ΔP (normally, ~35 mm Hg), at which point filtration stops. In contrast to theoretic predictions, experimentally induced reductions in $\pi_A$ do not lead to a rise in SNGFR because there are changes in $P_{BS}$ and $K_f$ so that a reduction in $\pi_A$ results in a reduction in $K_f$, thereby offsetting variations in $P_{UF}$ that occur with changes in $\pi_A$.[83] Studies in isolated glomeruli have indicated that extremely low concentrations of albumin produce an increase in $K_f$, whereas extremely high concentrations of albumin result in a decrease in $K_f$.[83] However, in vivo studies have shown that increases in plasma π will increase $K_f$ in both rats[92] and dogs.[81] These divergent results of the effects of protein concentration or $\pi_A$ on $K_f$ can be partially explained by the results from studies of isolated glomerular basement membranes, which have shown a biphasic relationship between albumin concentration and hydraulic permeability.[91] There were lower values of hydraulic permeability at an albumin concentration of 4 g/dL than at either 0 or 8 g/dL.

## POSTGLOMERULAR CIRCULATION

### PERITUBULAR CAPILLARY DYNAMICS

The same Starling forces that control fluid movement across all capillary beds govern the rate of fluid movement across the peritubular capillary walls of the renal cortex. Owing to the high resistance of the afferent and efferent arterioles, a large drop in hydraulic pressure occurs prior to the peritubular capillaries so that peritubular capillary pressure is 15 to 20 mm Hg. In addition, because protein-free fluid is filtered out of the glomerular capillaries and into Bowman's space, the plasma proteins become concentrated, yielding an elevated oncotic pressure of blood flowing into the peritubular capillaries. As a consequence, the balance between the transcapillary oncotic and hydraulic pressure gradients favors movement of the tubular reabsorbate into the capillaries. However, variations in these forces have significant effects on net proximal reabsorption.[35,54,93] The absolute amount of movement resulting from this driving force also depends on the peritubular capillary surface area available for fluid uptake and the hydraulic conductivity of the peritubular capillary wall. Values for the hydraulic conductivity of the peritubular capillaries are not as great as those for the glomerular capillaries, but this difference is offset by the much greater total surface area of the peritubular capillary network.

The peritubular capillary surface contains fenestrations that are bridged by a thin diaphragm and glycocalyx that is negatively charged.[3,94] Beneath the fenestrae of the endothelial cells lies a thin basement membrane that surrounds the capillary. The peritubular capillaries are closely opposed to cortical tubules (Fig. 3.16), so that the extracellular space between the tubules and capillaries constitutes only about 5% of the cortical volume.[95] The tubular epithelial cells are surrounded by the tubular basement membrane, which is distinct from and wider than the capillary basement membrane (see Fig. 3.16). Numerous microfibrils connect the tubular and capillary basement membranes, a feature that may help limit expansion of the interstitium and maintain close contact between tubular epithelial cells and the peritubular capillaries during periods of high fluid flux.[96] Thus, the pathway for fluid reabsorption from the tubular lumen to the peritubular capillary is composed, in series, from the epithelial cell, lateral spaces, tubular basement membrane, a narrow interstitial region containing microfibrils, the capillary basement membrane, and the thin membrane bridging the endothelial fenestrae.[96]

Like the endothelial cells, the basement membrane of the peritubular capillaries possesses anionic sites.[94,97] The

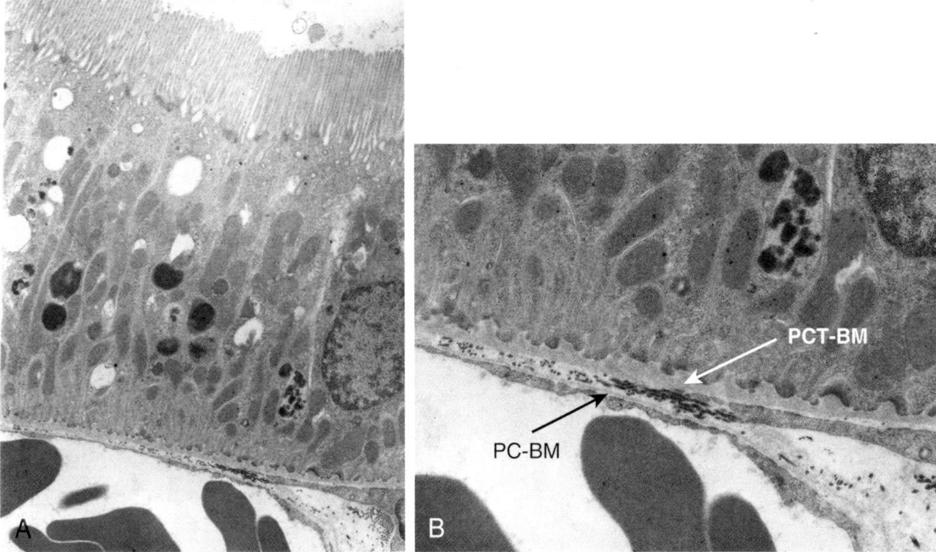


**Fig. 3.16** Apposition of peritubular capillaries with basolateral tubular membranes. Shown are electron micrographs of a proximal tubule of a Munich-Wistar rat. The tubule was perfusion-fixed with 1.25% glutaraldehyde, thereby also fixing red cells in adjacent capillaries. (A) The apposition of the basolateral surface of the tubular cells with the adjacent peritubular capillaries is close, leaving little interstitial space where the two come in contact (magnification ≈×13,000). (B) The proximal tubule basement membrane *(PCT-BM)* is relatively thick in comparison with the peritubular capillary endothelial basement membrane (*PC-BM*; magnification ≈×25,000). (Courtesy D. Maddox.)

electronegative charge density of the peritubular capillary basement membrane is significantly greater than that observed in the unfenestrated capillaries of skeletal muscle and similar to that observed in the glomerular capillary bed. These anionic sites in the peritubular capillaries compensate for the greater permeability of fenestrated capillaries, allowing free exchange of water and small molecules while restricting anionic plasma proteins to the circulation. The renal peritubular capillaries are reported to be more permeable to both small and large molecules than are other beds,[98] but this may be an artifact of the experimental conditions used. Indeed, other studies have indicated that the permeability of the peritubular vessels to dextrans and albumin is extremely low.[97,99]

## MEDULLARY MICROCIRCULATION

Similar to cortical peritubular vessels, the functional role of the medullary peritubular vasculature is to supply the metabolic needs of nearby tissues, but this unique vasculature is also responsible for the uptake and removal of water extracted from collecting ducts during the process of urine concentration. Because the urinary concentration process requires the development and maintenance of a hypertonic interstitium, the countercurrent arrangement of vasa recta plays a vital role in maintaining the medullary solute gradient through passive countercurrent exchange.

Medullary blood flow constitutes only about 10% to 15% of total RBF[3,6,100,101] and is derived entirely from efferent arterioles of the juxtamedullary nephrons (see Figs. 3.1 and 3.2).[22,37,102–105] Depending on the species and the method of evaluation, from 7% to 18% of glomeruli give rise to efferent arterioles that supply the medulla.[22,106] Efferent arterioles of juxtamedullary nephrons are larger in diameter, possess thicker endothelium, and have more prominent smooth muscle layers than efferent arterioles originating from superficial glomeruli.[34,107]

Despite the fact that medullary flow is less than 20% of the cortical flow, it is still relatively high compared with other tissues per gram of tissue; outer medullary flow exceeds that of liver, and inner medullary flow is comparable to that of resting muscle or brain.[108] The high efficiency of countercurrent mechanisms in this area permits the existence and maintenance of the inner medullary solute concentration gradients in the presence of such large flows. The descending vasa recta have a continuous endothelium, in which water moves across water channels, and urea moves through endothelial carriers.[109,110] The ascending vasa recta are fenestrated, with a high hydraulic conductivity, and water movement is governed by transcapillary hydraulic and oncotic pressure gradients.[110] Medullary blood flow is highest under conditions of water diuresis and declines during antidiuresis.[100] A direct vasoconstrictive effect of vasopressin on the medullary microcirculation contributes to this decrease during antidiuresis.[111] Vasodilatory factors act to preserve medullary blood flow and prevent ischemia. Acetylcholine,[112] vasodilator prostaglandins,[113] kinins,[114] adenosine,[115] atrial peptides,[116] bradykinin,[9] and nitric oxide[117] increase medullary RBF. In contrast to their vasoconstrictor effects in the renal cortex, Ang II[118–121] and endothelin[118] increase medullary blood flow, effects mediated in part by vasodilatory prostaglandins,[119,120] whereas vasopressin decreases medullary blood flow.[111,122] Alterations in medullary blood flow may be a key determinant of medullary fluid tonicity and, thereby, of solute transport in the loops of Henle and the control of sodium excretion and blood pressure.[123] During hemorrhage, there is primarily cortical ischemia, with maintained blood flow through the medulla.[124]

The precise location of the boundary between the renal cortex and medulla is difficult to discern because the medullary rays of the cortex merge imperceptibly with the medulla. In general, the arcuate arteries or sites at which the interlobular arteries branch into arcuate arteries mark this boundary. When considering the medullary circulation, most studies have focused on its relation to the countercurrent mechanism, as facilitated by the parallel array of descending and ascending vasa recta. This configuration is characteristic of the inner medulla, but the medulla also contains an outer zone consisting of two morphologically distinct regions, the outer and inner stripes of the outer medulla (see Fig. 3.2). The boundary between the outer medulla and inner medulla is defined by the beginning of the thick ascending limbs of Henle (see Fig. 3.1). In addition to the thick ascending limbs, the outer medulla contains descending straight segments of proximal tubules (pars recta), descending thin limbs, and collecting ducts. The nephron segments of the inner stripe of the outer medulla include thick ascending limbs, thin descending limbs, and collecting ducts. Each of these morphologically distinct medullary regions is supplied and drained by a specific vascular system.

Both the outer and inner stripes contain two distinct circulatory regions—the vascular bundles, formed by the coalescence of the descending and ascending vasa recta, and the interbundle capillary plexus. Vascular bundles of the descending and ascending vasa recta arise from the efferent arterioles of juxtamedullary glomeruli and descend through the outer stripe of the outer medulla to supply the inner stripe of the outer medulla and inner medulla (see Fig. 3.2). Within the outer stripe, nutrient flow is provided by the ascending vasa recta rising from the inner stripe. This notion is supported by the large area of contact between the ascending vasa recta and descending proximal straight tubules within this zone.[103,106,125]

The outer medulla includes the metabolically active thick ascending limbs. Nutrients and $O_2$ to this energy-demanding tissue in the inner stripe are delivered by a dense capillary plexus arising from a few descending vasa recta at the periphery of the bundles. Of the 10% to 15% of total RBF directed to the medulla, the largest portion perfuses this inner stripe capillary plexus. The descending vasa recta possess a contractile layer composed of smooth muscle cells in the early segments that evolve into pericytes by the more distal portions of the vessels. These pericytes contain smooth muscle $\alpha$-actin, suggesting that they serve as contractile elements and participate in the regulation of medullary blood flow,[126] as well as in vascular-tubular crosstalk.[127] Each of these vessels also displays a continuous endothelium that persists until the hairpin turn is reached, and the vessels divide to form the medullary capillaries. In contrast, ascending vasa recta, like true capillaries, lack a contractile layer and are characterized by a highly fenestrated endothelium.[128,129] The smooth muscle cells of the descending vasa recta are replaced by pericytes surrounding the endothelium, with subsequent loss of the pericytes and transformation into medullary capillaries accompanied by endothelial fenestrations.[102,125]

The rich capillary network of the inner stripe drains into numerous veins, which, for the most part, do not join the vascular bundles but ascend directly to the outer stripe. These veins subsequently rise to the cortical-medullary junction and join with cortical veins at the level of the inner cortex.[130] A few veins may extend within the medullary rays to regions near the kidney surface.[20,104,130] Thus, the capillary network of the inner stripe makes no contact with the vessels draining the inner medulla.

The inner medulla contains the thin descending and thin ascending limbs of Henle, together with collecting ducts (see Fig. 3.2). Within this region, the straight, unbranching vasa recta descend in bundles, with individual vessels leaving at every level to divide into a simple capillary network characterized by elongated links (see Figs. 3.1 and 3.2).[102,106,130] These capillaries converge to form the venous vasa recta. Within the inner medulla, the descending and ascending vascular pathways remain in close apposition, although distinct vascular regions can no longer be clearly discerned. The venous vasa recta rise toward the outer medulla in parallel with the supply vessels to join the vascular bundles. Within the outer stripe of the outer medulla, the vascular bundles spread out and traverse the outer stripe as wide tortuous channels that lie in close apposition to the tubules, eventually emptying into arcuate or deep interlobular veins.[106] The venous pathways in the bundles are both larger and more numerous than the arterial vessels, suggesting lower flow velocities in the ascending (venous) than in the descending (arterial) vessels.[131] The close apposition of the arterial and venous pathways in the vascular bundles is important for maintaining the hypertonicity of the inner medulla.

The mechanism of urine concentration requires coordinated function of the vascular and tubular components of the medulla. In species capable of marked concentrating ability, medullary vascular-tubular relationships show a high degree of organization favoring particular exchange processes by the juxtaposition of specific tubular segments and blood vessels.[130,132] In addition to anatomic proximity, the absolute magnitude of these exchanges is greatly influenced by the permeability characteristics of the structures involved, which may vary significantly among species.[133]

## PARACRINE AND ENDOCRINE FACTORS REGULATING RENAL HEMODYNAMICS AND GLOMERULAR FILTRATION RATE

### EXTRINSIC AND INTRINSIC REGULATION OF THE RENAL MICROCIRCULATIONS

A variety of hormonal, neural, and paracrine factors exert regulating influences on RBF and GFR.[35,55,83] Renal blood vessels from the arcuate arteries and interlobular arteries to the afferent and efferent arterioles are influenced to a greater or lesser extent by these intrinsic and extrinsic influences. As a result, the vascular tones of preglomerular and postglomerular resistance vessels are regulated to control RBF, glomerular hydraulic pressure, and the transcapillary hydraulic pressure gradient. The glomerular mesangium is the site of action and production of many such substances. Vasoactive compounds may elicit acute alterations in $K_f$ by changing the effective surface area for filtration through contraction of mesangial cells, causing shunting of blood to fewer capillary loops.[35,134,135] In addition, contraction of glomerular epithelial cells (podocytes), which contain filamentous actin molecules, may decrease the size of the filtration slit pores, thereby altering hydraulic conductivity of the filtration pathway and reducing $K_f$.[136] Various growth factors influence chronic changes in renal hemodynamics by promoting mesangial cell proliferation and expansion of the extracellular matrix, leading to obliteration of capillary loops and a reduction in the filtration coefficient.

Our understanding of afferent and efferent arteriolar vascular responses to neural, paracrine hormonal, and vasoactive substances have, to a large extent, come from micropuncture studies of glomerular hemodynamics. Various other methods have been used to examine the effects of vasoactive substances on the preglomerular and postglomerular vasculature.[35,55,83,137–144] The results using these different techniques have provided important insights into the vasoactive properties of the preglomerular and postglomerular vasculature that control renal hemodynamics and glomerular filtration rate.

The renal vasculature and glomerular mesangium respond to numerous endogenous hormones and vasoactive peptides, such as Ang II, by vasoconstriction, reductions in RBF and GFR, and reductions in the glomerular capillary filtration coefficient. Among the vasoconstrictors are Ang II, norepinephrine, leukotrienes C4 and D4, platelet-activating factor (PAF), adenosine 5'-triphosphate (ATP), endothelin, vasopressin, serotonin, and epidermal growth factor.[35,55,83] Similarly, vasodilatory substances, such as NO and prostaglandin E2 (PGE2), and PGI2, histamine, bradykinin, acetylcholine, insulin, insulin-like growth factor, calcitonin gene-related peptide, cyclic adenosine monophosphate, and relaxin can increase RBF and GFR.[35,55,83] However, in addition to having their own direct effects on RBF and GFR, a number of these complex vasoactive systems, such as the renin-angiotensin-aldosterone system (RAAS) and arachidonic acid metabolites, produce both vasoconstriction and vasodilator effects and can also stimulate production and release of other factors thus, masking their primary effect. Furthermore, vasoconstrictor agents such as Ang II may result in a feedback stimulation of vasodilatory compensatory factors yielding a complex interactive balance regulating renal hemodynamics.

## INTRINSIC MECHANISMS: RENAL AUTOREGULATION

Renal autoregulation refers to the intrinsic ability of the kidney to respond to a perturbation that elicits a vasoactive response, which alters renal vascular resistance in the direction that maintains RBF and GFR. Changes in perfusion pressure are the manipulation most commonly used to demonstrate autoregulatory efficiency. Although the efficiency with which blood flow is maintained differs from organ to organ (being most efficient in brain and kidney), all organs and tissues exhibit autoregulation. As shown in Fig. 3.17, the kidney autoregulates renal blood flow over a wide range of renal perfusion pressures. Autoregulation of blood flow in response to changes in perfusion pressure requires parallel changes in resistance.

The finding that both RBF and GFR are autoregulated with a high efficiency indicates that the principal resistance change due to autoregulatory adjustments is localized to the preglomerular vasculature. Studies of single-nephron function of superficial nephrons have demonstrated that SNGFR also exhibits efficient autoregulation, as long as the tubular fluid collections do not block flow to the macula densa. Furthermore, direct measurements of glomerular pressures in the Munich-Wistar rat, which has glomeruli on the renal cortical surface that is accessible to micropuncture, have demonstrated autoregulation of glomerular pressure in response to variations in renal arterial perfusion pressure. Fig. 3.18 summarizes the effects of graded reductions in renal perfusion pressure

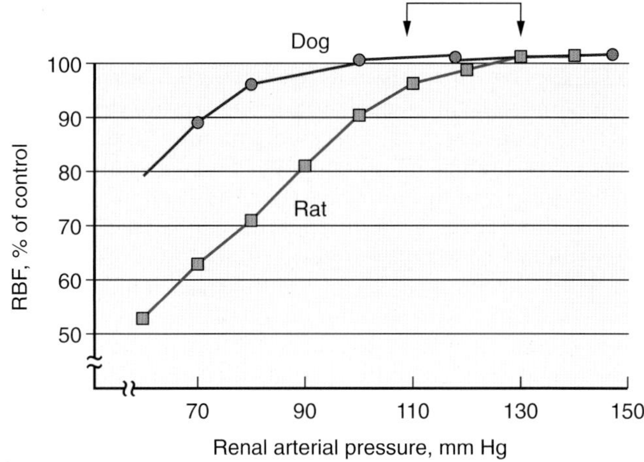


**Fig. 3.17** Autoregulatory response of total renal blood flow *(RBF)* to changes in renal perfusion pressure in the dog and rat. In general, the normal anesthetized dog exhibits greater autoregulatory capability to maintain RBF and glomerular filtration rate to lower arterial pressures than the rat. (From Navar LG, Bell PD, Burke TJ: Role of a macula densa feedback mechanism as a mediator of renal autoregulation. *Kidney Int.* 1982;22:S157–S164.)

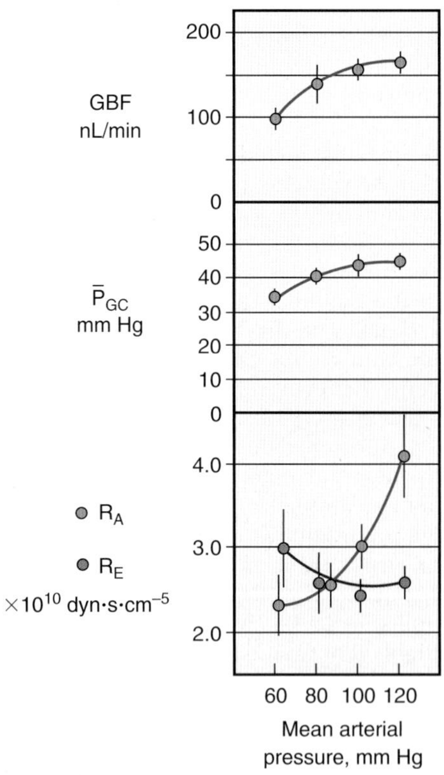


**Fig. 3.18** Glomerular dynamics in response to reductions of renal arterial pressure in the normal hydropenic rat. As can be seen, glomerular blood flow *(GBF)* and glomerular capillary hydraulic pressure ($P_{GC}$) remained relatively constant as blood pressure was lowered from ≈120 to ≈80 mm Hg over the range of perfusion pressure examined, primarily as a result of reductions in afferent arteriolar resistance *($R_A$)*. Efferent arteriolar resistance *($R_E$)* was relatively constant but increased slightly at lower pressures. (Modified from Robertson CR, Deen WM, Troy JL, Brenner BM: Dynamics of glomerular ultrafiltration in the rat. III: hemodynamics and autoregulation. *Am J Physiol.* 1972;223:1191, 1972.)

on $P_{GC}$ and preglomerular ($R_A$) and efferent arteriolar ($R_E$) resistance.[145] Graded reductions in renal perfusion pressure from 120 to 80 mm Hg result in only a modest decline in glomerular capillary blood flow, whereas a further reduction in perfusion pressure to 60 mm Hg leads to a more pronounced decline (see Fig. 3.18).

Autoregulation of glomerular capillary blood flow and $P_{GC}$ as perfusion pressure decreased from 120 to 80 mm Hg is the result primarily of a pronounced decrease in $R_A$, with little or no change in $R_E$. Over the range of renal perfusion pressures from 120 to 60 mm Hg, $R_E$ tended to increase slightly at the lower perfusion pressure. Under conditions of modest plasma volume expansion, $R_A$ declines while $R_E$ increases slightly as renal perfusion pressure is lowered so that $P_{GC}$ and $\Delta P$ are virtually unchanged over the entire range of renal perfusion pressures.[145] The mean glomerular transcapillary hydraulic pressure difference ($\Delta P$) exhibits almost perfect autoregulation over the entire range of perfusion pressures.[145] These results indicate that autoregulation of GFR is the consequence of the autoregulation of glomerular blood flow and glomerular capillary pressure. Similar results have been obtained in other rat strains and in dogs, where proximal and distal tubular pressures and peritubular capillary pressure also demonstrated autoregulation.[146]

Although more controversial, autoregulation also occurs in the medullary circulation,[147–149] an effect that may be influenced by the volume status of the animal.[148] In the split hydronephrotic rat kidney preparation,[150] reductions in perfusion pressure from 120 to 95 mm Hg elicited dilation of all preglomerular vessels, including the arcuate and interlobular arteries. The large preglomerular arterioles, including the interlobular arteries, contribute to the constancy of outer cortical blood flow in the upper autoregulatory range.[151] These responses notwithstanding, most evidence has indicated that the major preglomerular resistance components are the afferent arterioles.[33,152–154] Direct observations of perfused juxtamedullary nephrons have revealed parallel reductions in the luminal diameters of arcuate, interlobular, and afferent arterioles in response to elevations in perfusion pressure. However, because quantitatively similar reductions in vessel diameter produce much greater elevations in resistance in smaller than in larger vessels, the predominant effect of these changes is an increase in afferent arteriolar resistance.[30,152]

Under conditions of substantial plasma volume expansion, medullary blood flow autoregulation efficiency is diminished, whereas cortical blood flow autoregulatory responses are maintained. This loss of medullary blood flow autoregulation is thought to contribute to the exaggerated pressure natriuresis during plasma volume expansion.[36,155]

### Cellular Mechanisms Involved in Renal Autoregulation

Autoregulation of the afferent arteriole and interlobular artery is blocked by administration of L-type calcium channel blockers, inhibition of mechanosensitive cation channels, and a calcium-free perfusate.[156–159] Thus, the autoregulatory response involves gating of mechanosensitive channels, which produces membrane depolarization and activation of voltage-dependent calcium channels and leads to an increase in intracellular calcium concentration and vasoconstriction.[156,160,161] Indeed, calcium channel blockade almost completely blocks the autoregulation of RBF.[162,163] Intrinsic metabolites of the cytochrome P450 epoxygenase pathway attenuate the autoregulatory capacity of the afferent arteriole, whereas metabolites of the cytochrome P450 hydroxylase pathway enhance autoregulatory responsiveness.[164]

Inhibition of nitric oxide (NO) does not prevent autoregulation of GFR and RBF, but values for RBF are reduced at any given renal perfusion pressure as compared with control values.[165–168] In the isolated, perfused, juxtamedullary afferent arteriole, the initial vasodilatation observed when pressure was increased was of shorter duration when endogenous NO formation was blocked, but the autoregulatory response was unaffected.[161] Cortical and juxtamedullary preglomerular vessels in the split hydronephrotic kidney also autoregulate in the presence of NO inhibition.[169] Thus, the evidence indicates that NO is not essential for the manifestation of renal autoregulation, although it does greatly influence the plateau of the autoregulatory response. Furthermore, NO plays a role in tubuloglomerular feedback, as will be discussed.[35,170]

### Myogenic and Tubuloglomerular Feedback Mechanisms

There is general consensus that both myogenic and tubuloglomerular feedback mechanisms contribute to autoregulatory responses. The myogenic mechanism refers to the ability of arterial smooth muscle to contract and relax in response to increases and decreases in vascular wall tension.[153,156,171,172] Thus, an increase in perfusion pressure, which initially distends the vascular wall, is followed by contraction of a resistance vessel, resulting in a recovery of blood flow from an initial elevation to a value comparable to the control level. Evidence that the renal vasculature is intrinsically responsive to changes in the transmural hydraulic pressure difference and exhibits myogenic responses has been obtained in isolated afferent arterioles. Myogenic control of renal vascular resistance has been estimated to contribute up to 50% of the total autoregulatory response.[153,173]

Autoregulation of renal blood flow is observed, even when tubuloglomerular feedback is inhibited by furosemide, suggesting an important role for a myogenic mechanism.[174] This myogenic mechanism of autoregulation occurs very rapidly, reaching a full response in 3 to 10 seconds.[174,175] Autoregulation occurs in all the preglomerular resistance vessels of the in vitro, blood-perfused, juxtamedullary nephron preparation.[152,153,164,175–177] Of note, the afferent arterioles in this preparation constricted in response to rapid increases in perfusion pressure, even when flow to the macula densa was prevented by resection of the papilla, indicating a myogenic response.[175] Isolated perfused rabbit afferent arterioles respond to step increases of intraluminal pressure with a decrease in luminal diameter.[143] In contrast, efferent arteriolar segments showed vasodilation when submitted to the same procedure, probably reflecting simple passive physical properties.

Autoregulation is also observed in the afferent arteriole and arcuate and interlobular arteries of the nonfiltering hydronephrotic kidney preparation but, again, the efferent arteriole does not autoregulate in this model.[156,158,159,169,178] However, it should be noted that efferent arteriolar resistance in vivo may increase in response to prolonged reductions in AP.[145,179] This may result from increased activity of the intrarenal renin-angiotensin system (RAS). These data may also explain why autoregulation of GFR is more efficient than autoregulation of RBF.

The autoregulatory threshold can be reset in response to a variety of perturbations. Autoregulation in the afferent arteriole is attenuated in diabetic kidneys and may contribute to the hyperfiltration seen early in this disease.[178] Autoregulation is partially restored by insulin treatment and/or by inhibition of endogenous prostaglandin production.[178] Autoregulation in the remnant kidney is markedly attenuated 24 hours after the reduction in renal mass but is restored by cyclooxygenase inhibition, suggesting that release of vasodilatory prostaglandins may be involved in the initial response to increased SNGFR in the remaining nephrons after an acute partial nephrectomy.[180] Much higher pressures than normal are required to evoke a vasoconstrictor response in the afferent arteriole during the development of spontaneous hypertension.[181] Both the afferent arterioles and the interlobular arteries of Dahl salt-sensitive hypertensive rats exhibit reduced myogenic responsiveness to increases in perfusion pressure when fed a high-salt diet.[182] Thus, alterations in autoregulatory responses of the renal vasculature occur in a variety of disease states and may influence the kidney's ability to alter excretory responses to increased plasma volume expansion.

During development of the nephron, the tubule develops a segment that descends from the cortex into the medulla, but the connection with the originating glomerulus remains throughout the developmental process and provides the structural basis for the regulatory mechanism known as "tubuloglomerular feedback" (TGF; Fig. 3.19). A specialized nephron segment macula densa, at the end of the thick ascending limb of the loop of Henle, has distinct morphologic characteristics, including the presence of a primary cilium.[183] Macula densa cells are adjacent to the cells of the glomerulus and connect with the extraglomerular mesangium and afferent and efferent arterioles of the glomerulus (see Fig. 3.19). This anatomic arrangement of macula densa cells, extraglomerular mesangial cells, arteriolar smooth muscle cells, and renin-secreting cells of the afferent arteriole is known as the "juxtaglomerular apparatus" (JGA).[184]

The JGA is ideally suited to serve as a feedback system whereby a physicochemical stimulus in the tubular fluid activates the macula densa cells, which in turn transmit signals to the arterioles to alter the degree of contraction, thus regulating afferent arteriolar resistance. Changes in the volume flow and composition of the fluid flowing past the macula densa elicit rapid alterations in afferent arteriolar resistance and glomerular filtration, with increases in delivery of fluid resulting in decreases in SNGFR and $P_{GC}$ of the same nephron.[35,185,186] The TGF system senses delivery of fluid to the macula densa and "feeds back" signals to control filtration rate, thus providing a powerful feedback mechanism to regulate the pressures and flows that govern GFR in response to acute perturbations in delivery of fluid to the macula densa. The TGF mechanism is thus another important mechanism that helps explain the very high efficiency of autoregulation of RBF and GFR. Increased RBF or glomerular capillary pressure leads to increased GFR and, therefore, greater delivery of volume and solute to the distal tubule. Increased distal delivery is sensed by the macula densa, which activates effector mechanisms that increase preglomerular resistance, reducing RBF, glomerular pressure, and GFR.[48]

Increased perfusion of the late proximal tubule into the distal tubule causes a reduction in glomerular blood flow, glomerular pressure, and GFR.[187] Furthermore, experimental maneuvers that decrease distal tubule fluid flow induce afferent arteriolar vasodilation and interfere with the normal autoregulatory response.[35,170,188] In addition, perfusion with furosemide-containing solutions into the macula densa segment abrogate the normal constrictor response of afferent arterioles to increased perfusion pressure,[189] presumably by blocking the $Na^+$-$K^+$-$2Cl^-$ transporter on the luminal membrane of the macula densa cells.[153,190] These studies have suggested that the autoregulatory response in juxtamedullary nephrons is also highly dependent on the TGF mechanism. Moreover, deletion of the $A_1$ adenosine receptor gene in mice to block TGF results in less efficient autoregulation, again indicating the role for TGF in the autoregulatory response.[191]

To examine the role of TGF in autoregulation, investigators have studied spontaneous oscillations in proximal tubule pressure and RBF and the response of the renal circulation to high-frequency oscillations in tubule flow or renal perfusion pressure.[192] Oscillations in tubule pressure have been observed in anesthetized rats at a rate of about three cycles/min that are sensitive to small changes in delivery of fluid to the macula densa.[193] These spontaneous oscillations are eliminated by loop diuretics.[194] To examine this hypothesis,[192] sinusoidal oscillations were induced in distal tubule flow in rats at a frequency similar to that of the spontaneous fluctuations in tubule pressure. Varying distal delivery at this rate caused parallel fluctuations in stop-flow pressure (an index of glomerular capillary pressure), probably mediated by alterations in afferent resistance, again consistent with dynamic regulation of glomerular blood flow by the TGF system. To investigate the role of this system in autoregulation,[195] the effects of sinusoidal variations in AP at varying frequencies on renal blood flow were examined. Two separate components of autoregulation were identified, one operating at about the same frequency as the spontaneous fluctuations in tubule pressure, the TGF component, and one operating at a much higher frequency consistent with spontaneous fluctuations in vascular smooth muscle tone by the myogenic component.[196] These data have suggested that slow pressure changes elicit a predominant TGF response, whereas the rapid response reflects the myogenic mechanism.

The TGF mechanism stabilizes delivery of volume and solute to the distal nephron. Under normal conditions, flow-related changes in the tubular fluid composition at the macula densa are sensed, and signals are transmitted to the afferent arterioles to regulate the filtered load. Early distal tubular fluid is hypotonic (~120 mOsm/kg $H_2O$), and its composition is closely coupled to fluid flow along the ascending loop of Henle, so that increases in flow cause increases in tubular fluid osmolality and NaCl concentration at the macula densa, which lead to vasoconstriction of the afferent arteriole. At the cellular level, increases in tubular fluid osmolality elicit increases in cytosolic $[Ca^{2+}]$ in macula densa cells, which result in release of a vasoconstrictive factor from these cells.[197] As depicted in Fig. 3.20, suggested mediators of TGF include purinergic compounds, such as adenosine and ATP, and one or more of the eicosanoids, such as prostaglandin E2 (PGE2) or 20-hydroxyeicosatetraenoic acid (20-HETE). The factor mediating TGF responses vasoconstricts

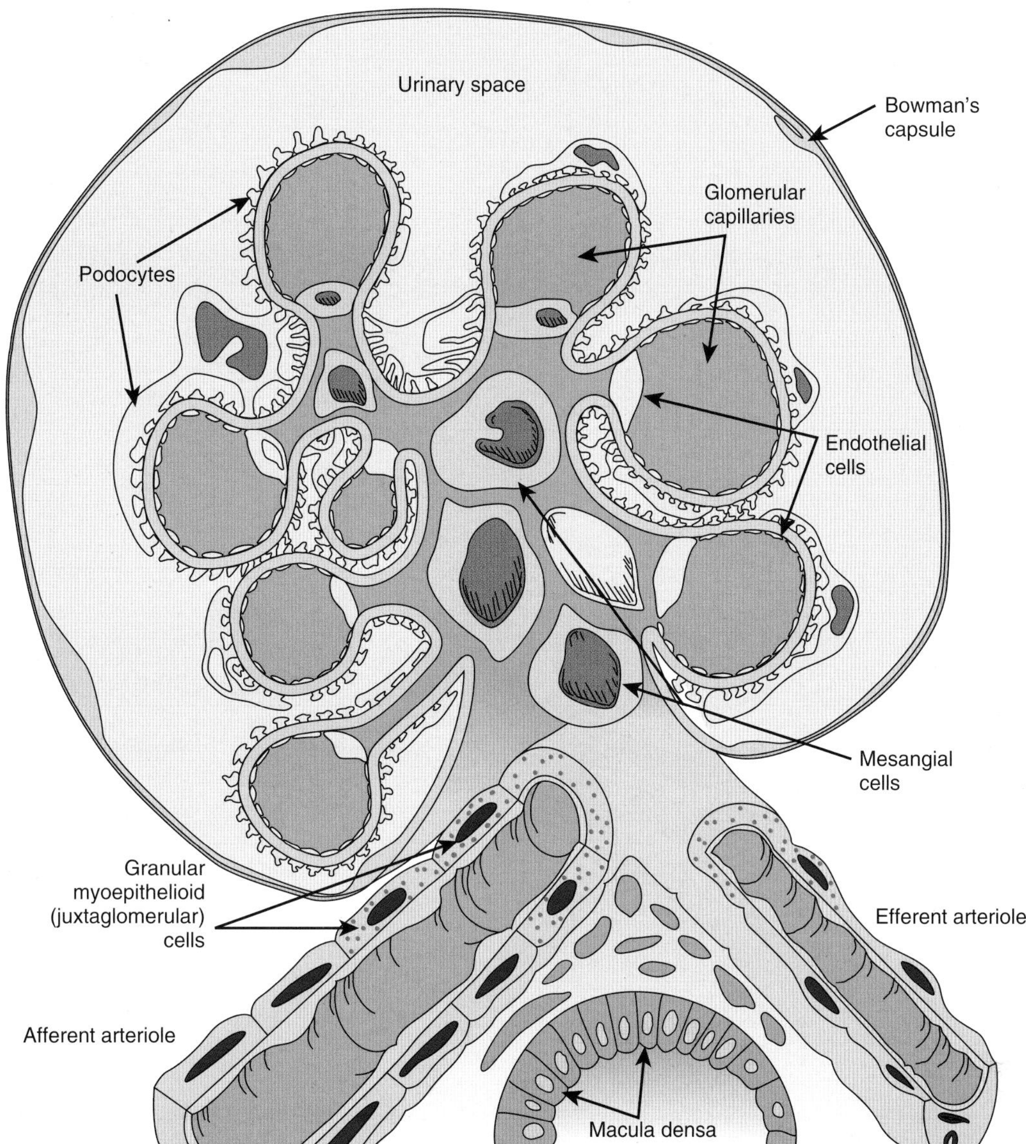


**Fig. 3.19.** Schematic drawing of a cross-section of a glomerulus, vascular pole, and macula densa cells forming the juxtaglomerular apparatus. As the afferent arteriole enters the glomerular tuft (large vessel, *lower left*), it breaks into a capillary network, and blood leaves the glomerular tuft via the efferent arteriole (large vessel, *lower right*). The glomerular capillaries have a fenestrated endothelium. The capillary network and mesangium located between the capillaries are bound together by a common basement membrane (*blue line* between the podocytes and capillaries). The basement membrane is absent between the capillary lumen and mesangial cells. The outer side of the basement membrane is surrounded by interdigitating visceral epithelial cells known as podocytes. Kriz and coworkers[184] have pointed out that the glomerular mesangium is continuous with the extraglomerular mesangium (consisting of extraglomerular mesangial cells and matrix) at the vascular pole. The extraglomerular mesangium, along with the macula densa cells of the distal tubule and the afferent arteriole, form the juxtaglomerular apparatus. (Courtesy D.A. Maddox.)

afferent arteriolar vessels through the opening of voltage-gated $Ca^{2+}$ channels in vascular smooth muscle cells.[35]

The sensitivity of the TGF mechanism can be modulated by many agents and circumstances. TGF sensitivity is diminished during volume expansion, thus allowing a greater delivery of fluid and electrolytes to the distal nephron for any given level of GFR. Reductions in TGF sensitivity allow correction of volume expansion. In contrast, contraction of extracellular fluid and blood volume is associated with an enhanced sensitivity of the TGF mechanism, which together with an augmented proximal reabsorption helps conserve fluid and electrolytes. A major regulator of TGF sensitivity is Ang II. In states of low Ang II activity (e.g., extracellular volume expansion, salt loading), the TGF mechanism is less responsive, whereas feedback sensitivity is enhanced during conditions of high Ang II activity, such as occurs during dehydration, hypotension, or hypovolemia.

The interactions between the myogenic mechanism and the TGF are complex and not simply additive. Contributions from other systems add additional complexity. For example, glomerulotubular balance, whereby proximal tubule reabsorption increases as GFR rises, blunts the effects of alterations in GFR on distal delivery. In addition, the persistence of some autoregulatory behavior in nonfiltering kidneys[198] and

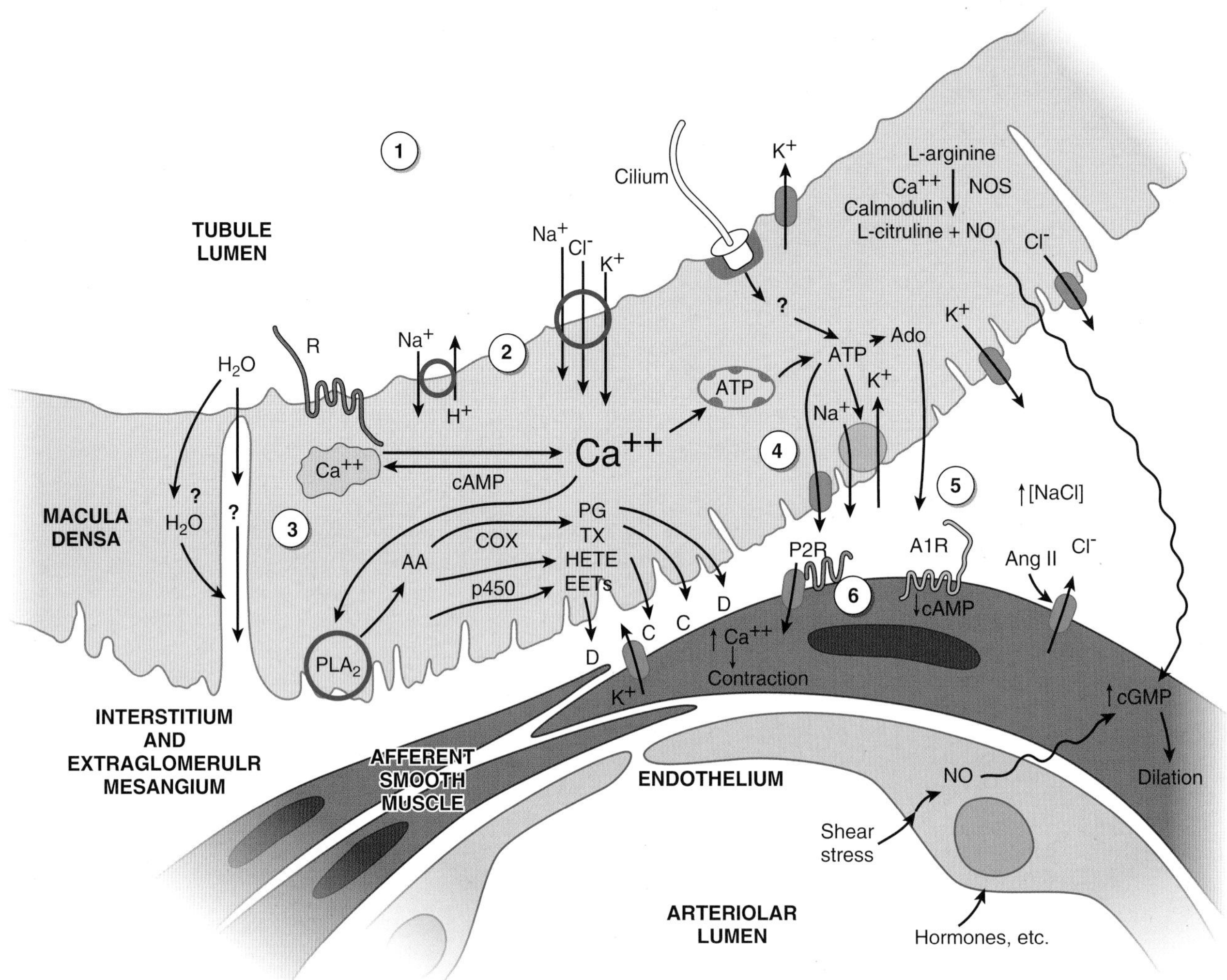


**Fig. 3.20** Proposed macula densa tubuloglomerular feedback (TGF) signaling mechanisms. Numbers in circles refer to the following sequence of events: 1, Flow-dependent changes in tubular fluid composition, including $Na^+$, $Cl^-$, osmolality, signals from intratubular paracrine agents, and cilia disturbance; 2, membrane activation step, including membrane depolarization, enhanced $Na^+$, $Cl^-$, $K^+$ uptake, or other sensing mechanism; 3, transmission from membrane to intracellular signal mobilization; 4, formation and release of TGF mediators, including ATP and adenosine *(Ado),* arachidonic acid *(AA)* metabolites, and nitric oxide *(NO)*; 5, receptor activation by released agents, membrane depolarization, and activation of $Ca^{2+}$ channels in vascular smooth muscle cells; 6, afferent arteriolar vasoconstriction partially countered by NO-stimulated increases in cGMP and other released mediators—local angiotensin II (Ang II) and neuronal nitric oxide synthase (nNOS) activity modulate the response. *ATP,* Adenosine triphosphate; *A1R,* adenosine A1 receptor; *C,* constriction; *cGMP*, cyclic guanosine monophosphate; *COX,* cyclooxygenase; *D,* dilation; *EET,* epoxyeicosatrienoic acid; *HETE,* hydroxyeicosatetraenoic acid; *P2R,* P2 purinergic receptors; *p450,* cytochrome P 450; *PG,* prostaglandins; *PLA2,* phospholipase A2; *TX,* thromboxanes. (Modified from Navar LG, Bell PD, Burke TJ: Role of a macula densa feedback mechanism as a mediator of renal autoregulation. *Kidney Int.* 1982;22:S157–S164.)

in isolated blood vessels has suggested that the delivery of filtrate to the distal tubule is not absolutely required for constancy of blood flow. Nevertheless, the myogenic and TGF mechanisms are not mutually exclusive, and various models of renal autoregulation incorporate both systems.[172,199] Because the myogenic and TGF responses share the same effector site, the afferent arteriole, interactions between these two systems are unavoidable, and each response is capable of modulating the other. The prevailing view is that these two mechanisms act in concert to accomplish the same end, a stabilization of renal function when blood pressure is altered.[35,173,200] Furthermore, the time constraints are different; the myogenic component of autoregulation requires less than 10 seconds for completion and normally follows first-order kinetics without rate-sensitive components.[173] The response time for the tubuloglomerular feedback may occur as rapidly as 5 seconds,[154] although others have suggested that it takes 30 to 60 seconds and shows spontaneous oscillations at 0.025 to 0.033 Hz.[173] The myogenic and tubuloglomerular feedback mechanisms account for most of the autoregulatory responses, but additional systems have been suggested.[173] Furthermore, the nature of their interaction may be complex, with the TGF primarily influencing the sensitivity of the myogenic mechanism.[35]

### Mechanisms of Tubuloglomerular Feedback Control of Renal Blood Flow and Glomerular Filtration Rate

There appear to be several factors that have been identified as tubular signals for TGF.[201] Changes in delivery of $Na^+$, $Cl^-$, and $K^+$ are thought to be sensed by the macula densa through the $Na^+$-$K^+$-$2Cl^-$ cotransporter on the luminal cell membrane of the macula densa cells.[202] Alterations in $Na^+$, $K^+$, and $Cl^-$ reabsorption result in inverse changes in SNGFR and renal vascular resistance, primarily due to changes in preglomerular resistance. For example, when salt concentration increases at the macula densa, the feedback mechanism increases afferent arteriolar resistance, thus decreasing glomerular pressure and SNGFR. Agents such as furosemide that interfere with the $Na^+$-$K^+$-$2Cl^-$ cotransporter in the macula densa cells[190] inhibit the feedback response.[203]

Additional studies have been performed in which macula densa segments were perfused with solutions that contained minimal concentrations of essential ions needed to maintain the integrity of the $Na^+$-$K^+$-$2Cl^-$ cotransporter, with the remaining solute being deficient in $Na^+$ (choline chloride) or deficient in $Cl^-$ (Na isocyanate). These solutions clearly elicited normal TGF responses.[204] Furthermore, orthograde perfusion with nonelectrolyte solutes also elicited TGF responses.[35,205] Collectively, these results indicate that the integrity of the $Na^+$-$K^+$-$2Cl^-$ cotransporter must be maintained for the sensing mechanism to function normally. However, the actual sensing mechanism may be activated by changes in total solute concentration. Furthermore, studies evaluating the possible role of the primary cilium in macula densa cells have suggested that flow-dependent signals may stimulate the cilium and alter the magnitude of the TGF response.[183,206]

Another area of uncertainty involves the intracellular signaling cascade to generate a vasoactive agent that is secreted. Some studies have suggested that the luminal signal activates release of $Ca^{2+}$ from the intracellular stores that then lead to the formation of ATP, which is secreted and plays a central role in mediating the signal from the luminal cell membrane of the macula densa. This is illustrated in Fig. 3.20, which is derived from based on several sources.[35,186] According to this scheme, increased delivery of solute to the macula densa results in concentration-dependent increases in solute uptake by the $Na^+$-$K^+$-$2Cl^-$ cotransporter and may separately generate a signal to initiate the cascade. This, in turn, stimulates mitochondrial activity in the macula densa cells, leading to the formation of ATP. Macula densa cells respond to an increase in luminal [NaCl] or total solute concentration by releasing ATP at the basolateral cell membrane through ATP-permeable, large-conductance anion channels, possibly providing a communication link between macula densa cells and adjacent mesangial cells via purinoceptors receptors on the latter.[207] The ATP can exert direct actions on the vascular smooth muscle cells and is also metabolized further, with ultimate degradation to the metabolites, adenosine diphosphate (ADP) and adenosine monophosphate (AMP). Activity of cytosolic 5'-nucleotidase or endo-5'-nucleotidase bound to the cell membrane results in the formation of adenosine.[186] In addition to the ATP metabolites, the macula densa cells also produce arachidonic acid metabolites, including PGE2 and PGI2, and nitric oxide and reactive oxygen species. Thus, there are several vasoactive substances that are secreted and may alter afferent arteriolar vascular tone. Although ATP and adenosine are formed in macula densa cells or in the adjacent interstitium, ATP interacts with purinergic (P2) receptors on the extraglomerular mesangial and vascular cells, resulting in an increase in $[Ca^{2+}]_i$.[208] The increase in $[Ca^{2+}]_i$ may occur, in part, via basolateral membrane depolarization through receptor operated channels, followed by a further increase in $Ca^{2+}$ entry into the cells via voltage-gated $Ca^{2+}$ channels.[209] As indicated in Fig. 3.20, gap junctions then transmit the calcium transient to the adjacent afferent arteriole, or ATP can exert similar effects directly on vascular smooth muscle cells, thus leading to vasoconstriction. Some of the ATP elicited by macula densa cells is metabolized to adenosine, which also can directly constrict the afferent arteriole through activation of purinergic P1 receptors.[210]

Although there is general consensus that ATP is secreted by macula densa cells, some investigators have suggested that the ATP metabolite, adenosine, is primarily responsible for mediating tubuloglomerular feedback. Intraluminal administration of an adenosine A1 receptor agonist enhances the TGF response.[211] In addition, TGF is attenuated in adenosine A1 receptor-deficient mice.[212,213] Blocking adenosine A1 receptors, or inhibition of adenosine synthesis via inhibition of 5'-nucleotidase, reduces TGF efficiency.[214] Addition of adenosine to the afferent arteriole causes vasoconstriction via activation of the adenosine A1 receptor, and addition of an A1 receptor antagonist blocks both the effects of adenosine and of high macula densa [NaCl].[215] These results are consistent with the hypothesis that adenosine is also a mediator of TGF responses invoking an effect of $Na^+/K^+$-ATPase activity and leading to increased adenosine synthesis.[215] However, adenosine also activates adenosine A2 receptors, which cause afferent arteriolar dilation and apparently abrogate the actions of A1 receptors.[216,217]

Efferent arterioles also respond to adenosine but they vasodilate in response to an increase in NaCl concentration at the macula densa or to direct application due to actions of the adenosine A2 receptors, which antagonize the effects of A1 receptors.[217,218] The changes in efferent arteriolar resistance tend to be in an opposite direction to that of the afferent arterioles, which vasoconstrict in response to increased NaCl at the macula densa.[215,219] The net result, however, is decreased glomerular blood flow, decreased glomerular hydraulic pressure, and a reduction in SNGFR.

There are many additional paracrine agents produced and secreted by macula densa cells, as shown in Fig. 3.20. These include metabolites of the arachidonic acid cascade, including prostaglandins PGE2 and PGI2, and other products of the cyclooxygenase pathway, products of the cytochrome P450 pathway, including epoxygenases and the cytochrome P450 4A HETEs.[35,164,220] Another very important regulating paracrine regulator is NO, which exerts vasodilatory responses when released by the macula densa cells. Under normal circumstances, when the NaCl concentration of tubular fluid is increased, there are increases in ATP release coupled with reductions in PGE2 formation until the ATP release reaches a plateau, and the $PGE_2$ release is markedly reduced. With further increases in [NaCl], NO release is augmented to counteract the effects of increased ATP.[35]

In addition to the paracrine factors released by macula densa cells, there are also many modulatory agents that influence the sensitivity of TGF responses. Ang II is one of the more important factors. TGF is blunted by Ang II antagonists and Ang II synthesis inhibitors, and TGF is markedly reduced in knockout mice lacking the AT1A Ang II receptors or angiotensin-converting enzyme (ACE).[221,222] Furthermore, systemic infusion of Ang II in ACE knockout mice restores TGF.[221,223–228] Ang II also enhances TGF via activation of AT1 receptors on the luminal membrane of the macula densa.[229] Acute inhibition of the AT1 receptor in normal mice reduces TGF responses and reduces autoregulatory efficiency.[224] Several studies have shown the interactions between adenosine and Ang in the TGF mechanism. In these studies, adenosine $A_1$ receptor antagonist administration results in decreased afferent arteriolar resistance and increased transcapillary hydraulic pressure differences ($\Delta P$), whereas pretreatment with an angiotensin AT1 receptor antagonist prevented these changes.[230] Although it is known that Ang II is not the primary regulator of TGF, these results indicate that Ang II plays a prominent role in modulating tubuloglomerular feedback sensitivity, and that this response is mediated through the AT1 receptor.

Neuronal NO synthase (nNOS or NOS I) is present in macula densa cells.[231] NO derived from nNOS in the macula densa provides a vasodilatory influence on tubuloglomerular feedback, decreasing the amount of vasoconstriction of the afferent arteriole that otherwise would occur.[231,232] Increased distal sodium chloride delivery to the macula densa stimulates nNOS activity and also increases activity of the inducible form of cyclooxygenase (COX-2), which forms PGE2 and counteracts TGF-mediated constriction of the afferent arteriole.[231,232] Macula densa cell pH increases in response to increased luminal sodium concentration and may be related to the stimulation of nNOS.[233] Inhibition of macula densa guanylate cyclase increases the TGF response to high luminal [NaCl], further indicating the importance of NO in modulating TGF.[219] In an isolated perfused JGA preparation, microperfusion of the macula densa with an inhibitor of NO production led to constriction of the adjacent afferent arteriole.[234] When the macula densa was perfused with a solution low in Na concentration, however, the response was blocked, indicating that Na reabsorption is required.[234] Microperfusion of the macula densa with the precursor of NO, L-arginine, blunts TGF responses, especially in salt-depleted animals.[235–237] These results indicate that NO released from macula densa cells or endothelial cells causes afferent arteriolar vasodilation acutely or may blunt TGF responses. An increase in NO production may also inhibit renin release by increasing cyclic guanosine monophosphate (cGMP) in the granular cells of the afferent arteriole,[238] thereby accentuating its vasodilatory effects. When NO production was chronically blocked in knockout mice lacking nNOS, TGF in response to acute perturbations in distal sodium delivery was normal.[225] However, the presence of intact nNOS in the JGA is required for sodium chloride–dependent renin secretion.[225] The TGF system, which elicits vasoconstriction and a reduction in SNGFR in response to acute increases in sodium and solute delivery to the macula densa, appears to activate a vasodilatory response secondarily via NO release.[239] Stimulation of NO production in response to increased distal salt delivery under conditions of volume expansion would be advantageous by resetting TGF and limiting TGF-mediated vasoconstrictor responses.

The dynamics of the TGF mechanism can be temporally divided into two or more responses with different time constants. The initial rapid response occurs within a few seconds and elicits a rapid vasoconstriction and decrease in GFR and $P_{GC}$ when sodium delivery to the macula densa cells is acutely increased. A second vasoconstrictor response occurs in seconds to minutes and changes the slope of the response to a slower time constant. This may be due to modulation of the initial response by some of the modulating agents mentioned. The rapid TGF system prevents large changes in GFR under conditions such as spontaneous fluctuations in blood pressure, thereby maintaining tight control of distal sodium delivery in the short term. Over the long term, renin secretion, controlled by the JGA in accordance with the requirements for sodium balance and the TGF system, resets to a new sodium delivery rate.[225] In the uninephrectomized rat with sustained elevations of the GFR, the TGF system appears to be reset.[240]

### Connecting Tubule Glomerular Feedback Mechanism

There is also growing interest in a second feedback loop that links the connecting tubule, which has been shown to be in apposition to its own glomerulus and in close contact with the afferent arteriole.[241] In vitro perfusion of the connecting tubule has shown that increases in luminal NaCl elicit vasodilation of preconstricted afferent arterioles.[242] This action is opposite to the effect of macula densa TGF signaling, in which increases in NaCl cause vasoconstriction, raising the question of how these two opposing systems interact. Additional studies demonstrating that the addition of amiloride to the perfusion solution prevents the action of increased luminal $Na^+$, have suggested that the epithelial sodium channel mediates the connecting TGF (CTGF).[242] The afferent vasodilator effect of increased $E_{Na}C$ activity appears to be mediated by PGE2 acting on an EP4 receptor on the afferent arteriole.[243] An additional role of epoxyeicosatrienoic acid (EET) has also been suggested.[244] Furthermore, the presence of Ang II in the luminal fluid enhances the afferent arteriolar vasodilator effect caused by increases in luminal $Na^+$ concentration.[245] This CTGF mechanism is thought to mediate resetting of the macula densa TGF mechanism by partially reducing its sensitivity.[246] A modulating role of CTGF has been observed in experimental hypertension,[247] during high salt intake,[248] and in the renal vasodilatory response that occurs in the remaining kidney after unilateral nephrectomy.[249]

## ENDOTHELIAL FACTORS AND GASEOUS TRANSMITTERS CONTROLLING RENAL HEMODYNAMICS AND GLOMERULAR FILTRATION RATE

A particularly intriguing and growing area of research involves the paracrine interactions between endothelial cells and the underlying smooth muscle cells. As shown in Fig. 3.21, endothelial cells respond to various physical and chemical stimuli, including pressure, flow, shear stress, and circumferential strain, as well as vasoactive factors normally present in the blood. Under normal conditions, an increase in shear stress may activate endothelial cells to produce NO and the prostanoids PGE2 and PGI2, which help adjust vascular tone to accommodate the increased load. However, during conditions of tissue injury or inflammation, the endothelial cells may also be stimulated to produce endothelin, thromboxane,

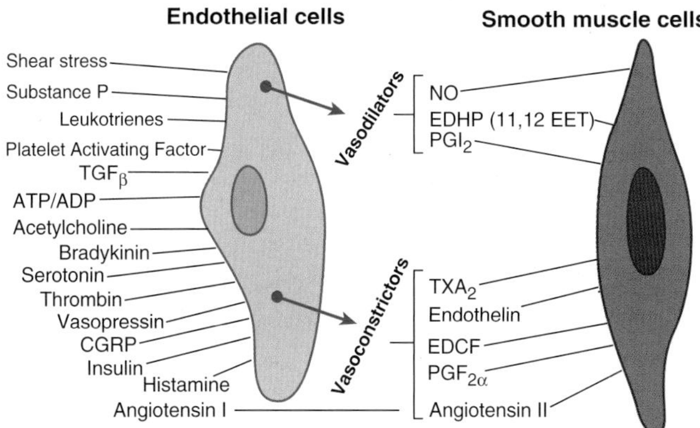


**Fig. 3.21** Interaction of endothelial cells with smooth muscle or mesangial cells. As indicated in the text, several agents interact with endothelial cells to produce the vasodilator nitric oxide *(NO)*. Others yield vasoconstriction (see text and other sources). Angiotensin-converting enzyme converts angiotensin I to the potent vasoconstrictor angiotensin II. *ATP–ADP*, Adenosine trisphosphate–adenosine diphosphate; *CGRP,* calcitonin gene-related peptide; *EDCF,* endothelial-derived constricting factor; *EDHP,* endothelial-derived hyperpolarizing factor; *EET,* epoxyeicosatrienoic acid; *PGF*$_{2\alpha}$, prostaglandin $F_{2\alpha}$; *PGI*$_2$, prostaglandin I2; *TGF*$_\beta$, transforming growth factor beta; *TXA*$_2$, thromboxane A2. (Modified from Arendshorst W, Navar LG. Renal circulation and glomerular hemodyanamics. In: Schrier RW, Coffman TM, Falk RJ, Molitoris BA, Neilson EG, eds. *Schrier's diseases of the kidney*. Philadelphia: Lippincott Williams & Wilkins; 2013:74–131; Navar LG, Arendshorst WJ, Pallone TL, Inscho EW, Imig JD, Bell PD. The renal microcirculation. In: Tuma RF, Duran WN, Ley K, eds. *Handbook of physiology: Microcirculation.* Vol 2: Academic Press; 2008:550–683; Maddox, DA, Deen WL, and Brenner BM. Glomerular Filtration; *Handbook of Physiology: Section 8 Renal Physiology*. American Physiological Society, New York: Oxford University Press; 1992, 545–638; Maddox DA, Brenner BM. Glomerular ultrafiltration. In: Brenner BM, ed. *The kidney*. 7th ed. Philadelphia: Saunders; 2004:353–412.)

certain growth and profibrotic factors that elicit vasoconstriction, and/or additional paracrine factors associated with tissue injury and fibrosis. Several of these factors associated with regulation of the renal microcirculation are gaseous physiologic transmitters, called "gasotransmitters," which have been identified over the last 2 decades. NO is the first such gasotransmitter discovered, but carbon monoxide (CO) and hydrogen sulfide ($H_2S$) have also been shown to influence the renal microcirculation.

### Nitric Oxide and Nitric Oxide Synthases

In 1980, Furchgott and Zawadzki[250] demonstrated that the vasodilatory action of acetylcholine requires the presence of an intact endothelium. Acetylcholine binds to receptors on endothelial cells, leading to the formation and release of an "endothelial-derived relaxing factor," now known to be NO.[251,252] Many cell types, including the endothelium, produce NO from the amino acid L-arginine[35,83,253] by a family of nitric oxide synthases (NOSs) that are present in many cell types, including vascular endothelial cells, macrophages, neurons, glomerular mesangial cells, macula densa, and renal tubular cells.[35,254–256] Three main NOS isoforms have been isolated. Neuronal NOS, also termed "NOS I" or "nNOS," and endothelial NOS, also called "NOS III" or "eNOS," are constitutively present in the kidney. A third NOS, iNOS or NOS II, is inducible, is expressed after transcriptional induction, and remains active for prolonged periods.[35,83] All three isoforms of NOS are found in the kidney. The arcuate and interlobular arteries, as well as the afferent and efferent arterioles, all produce NO, which regulates basal vascular tone, as indicated by the constriction that occurs in response to inhibition of endogenous NO production.[35,83]

Once released by the endothelium, NO diffuses into adjacent and downstream vascular smooth muscle cells,[257] where it stimulates the activity of soluble guanylate cyclase and increases cGMP formation.[83,258–263] cGMP reduces calcium influx, intracellular calcium release, and intracellular calcium concentration. This occurs, in part, through a cGMP-dependent protein kinase (PKG)-mediated phosphorylation of targets, which include inositol trisphosphate (IP3) receptors, calcium channels, and phospholipase A2,[264] thereby reducing the amount of free calcium available for contraction, hence promoting relaxation.[265]

In addition to stimulation by acetylcholine, NO formation in the vascular endothelium increases in response to bradykinin,[262,266–269] thrombin,[270] platelet-activating factor,[271] endothelin,[272] and calcitonin gene-related peptide.[267,273–276] Elevation of blood flow through vessels with intact endothelium or across cultured endothelial cells results in increased shear stress and increased NO release. Both the pulse frequency and pulse pressure modulate flow-induced NO release.[259,266,268,277–281] Elevated perfusion pressure and shear stress also increase NO release from afferent arterioles.[282]

NO plays a major role in modulation of renal hemodynamics, regulation of medullary perfusion, modulation of the sensitivity of the TGF mechanism, inhibition of tubular sodium reabsorption, modulation of renal sympathetic neural activity, and mediation of pressure natriuresis.[35,283–287] NO dominates integrated renal hyperemic responses to acetylcholine and bradykinin, and renal endothelium-dependent vasodilation is diminished in diabetes due to impaired NO function.[288] Pressure natriuresis in experimental models using stepwise increases of both renal perfusion pressure and medullary blood flow involve increased NO release, which can exert direct tubular effects to promote sodium and water excretion.[289,290] Tubular epithelial cells are capable of releasing NO but, during increased medullary flow, the vasa recta may be a primary source of the NO, as suggested by the fact that flow-dependent increases of NO also occur, even during microperfusion of isolated outer medullary vasa recta.[291]

There are important interactions among NO, Ang II, and renal nerves in the control of renal function and blood pressure.[292] Nonselective NOS inhibition using competitive inhibitors of NO results in decreases in RPF, increases in mean arterial blood pressure (AP), and generally a reduction in GFR.[165,293,294] These effects are largely prevented by the simultaneous administration of excess L-arginine, the NOS substrate.[293] Selective inhibition of neuronal NOS (nNOS or type I NOS), which is found in the thick ascending limb of the loop of Henle, the macula densa, and efferent arterioles,[256,285] decreases GFR without affecting blood pressure or RBF.[295] Because eNOS is found in the endothelium of renal blood vessels, including both the afferent and efferent arterioles and glomerular capillary endothelial cells,[256] differences in the effects of generalized NOS inhibition versus specific inhibition of nNOS on NO formation and RBF appear to be related to the distinct distribution of eNOS versus nNOS in the kidney. Both acute and chronic inhibition of

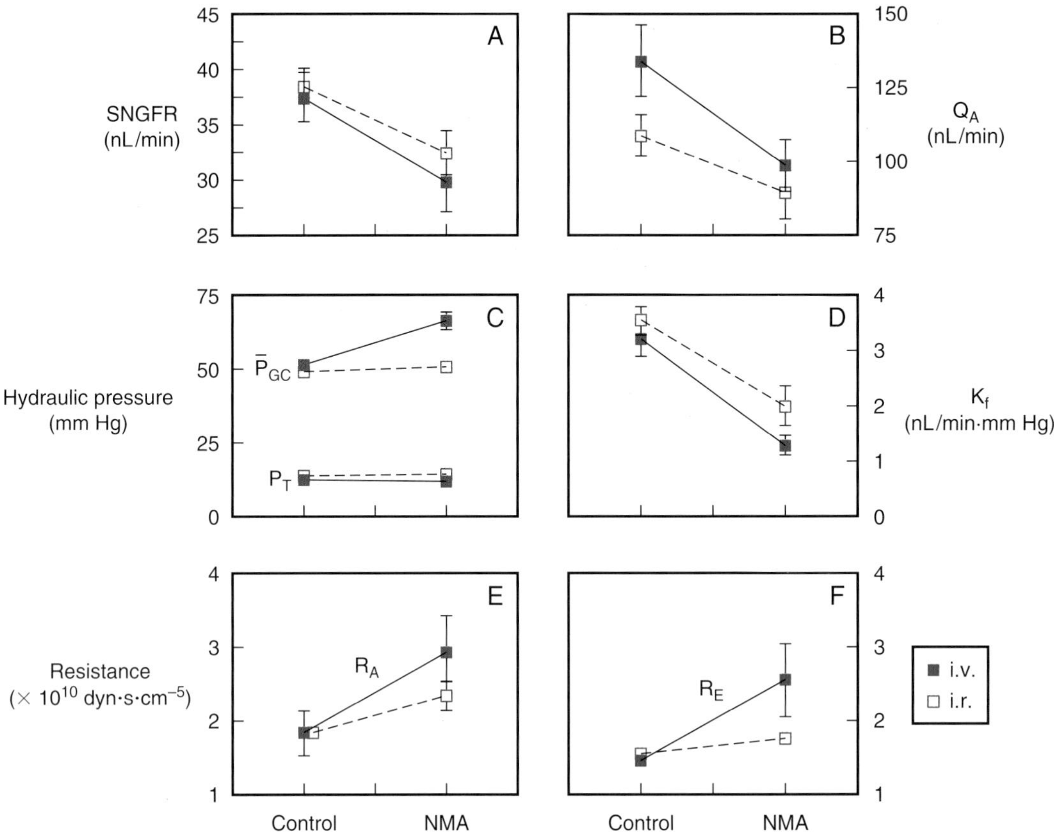


**Fig. 3.22** (A–F) Role of nitric oxide in the control of glomerular filtration dynamics. Studies were performed in euvolemic Munich-Wistar rats receiving intravenous pressor doses of the nonselective nitric oxide synthase (NOS) blocker, *N*-monomethyl-L-arginine (*NMA;* i.v., *filled squares*) or nonpressor doses of NMA at the origin of the renal artery (i.r., *open squares*). $K_f$, Filtration coefficient; $P_{GC}$, pressure in the glomerular capillaries; $P_T$, pressure in the tubules; $Q_A$, glomerular plasma flow rate; $R_A$, preglomerular arteriolar resistance; $R_E$, efferent arteriolar resistance; *SNGFR,* single-nephron glomerular filtration rate. (Data [mean ± SE] obtained from Deng A, Baylis C: Locally produced NO controls preglomerular resistance and filtration coefficient. *Am J Physiol.* 1993;264:F212–F215.)

NO production result in systemic and glomerular capillary hypertension, an increase in preglomerular ($R_A$) and efferent arteriolar ($R_E$) resistance, a decrease in $K_f$, and decreases in both single-nephron plasma flow and GFR.[296–300]

As shown in Fig. 3.22, acute administration of pressor doses of a blocker of NO production results in a decline in SNGFR, $Q_A$, and $K_f$ and increases in both preglomerular and efferent arteriolar resistances. Administration of nonpressor doses of the inhibitor of NO formation through the renal artery yielded an increase in preglomerular resistance and a decrease in SNGFR and $K_f$ but no effect on efferent resistance[297] These studies suggest that the cortical afferent, but not efferent, arterioles are under tonic control by NO. However, others have found that the renal artery, arcuate and interlobular arteries, and afferent and efferent arterioles all produce NO and constrict in response to inhibition of endogenous NO production.[144,169,234,257,301–304] In agreement with this finding, investigators[31,302] have reported that NO dilates both efferent and afferent arterioles in perfused juxtamedullary nephrons. Interestingly, the modulatory influence of nNOS on afferent arteriolar tone is dependent on the maintenance of distal tubular fluid, indicative of a critical interaction with the TGF mechanism.[304]

Controversy exists regarding the role of the RAS in the genesis of the increase in vascular resistance that follows blockade of NOS. Studies of in vitro perfused nephrons[302] and of anesthetized rats in vivo[305] suggest that the increase in renal vascular resistance that follows NOS blockade is blunted when Ang II formation or receptor binding is blocked. NO inhibits renin release, whereas acute Ang II infusion increases cortical NOS activity and protein expression, and chronic Ang II infusion increases mRNA levels for eNOS and nNOS.[305,306] Ang II increases NO production in isolated perfused afferent arterioles via activation of the AT1 Ang II receptors.[307] In contrast, nonselective NOS inhibition increases renal oxygen consumption, independently of Ang II.[308] Additionally, inhibition of NOS in conscious rats had similar effects on renal hemodynamics in the intact and Ang II–blocked state.[309] This suggests that the vasoconstrictor response to NOS blockade is not mediated by Ang II. Further studies[310] have shown that when the Ang II levels are acutely raised by the infusion of Ang II, acute NO blockade amplifies the renal vasoconstrictor actions of Ang II. An observation in agreement with this finding is that intrarenal inhibition of NO enhances Ang II–induced afferent, but not efferent, arteriolar vasoconstriction.[144,311] In the juxtaglomerular nephron, however, blockade of nNOS enhanced efferent but not afferent arteriolar responsiveness to Ang II.[304] These data suggest that NO modulates the vasoconstrictor effects of Ang II on glomerular arterioles in vivo, perhaps blunting

Ang II's vasoconstrictor response in the afferent arteriole, with some results showing similar responses on the efferent arteriole.

### Effects of Heme Oxygenase and Carbon Monoxide on Renal Function

Heme is degraded by heme oxygenase (HO) enzymes (HO-1 and HO-2) producing carbon monoxide (CO), biliverdin, and bilirubin and by the release of free iron.[2,35,312–315] Induction of HO-1 with hemin in anesthetized rats resulted in significant increases in RBF and GFR, a lower renal vascular resistance, and an increase in sodium excretion in untreated control rats without affecting blood pressure. Furthermore, autoregulatory responses to acute Ang II infusion were blunted, and these studies suggested a vasodilatory influence of HO-1 induction and hence CO production.[313] When a heme oxygenase inhibitor was administered either alone or to rats receiving an NOS inhibitor—N(ω)-nitro-L-arginine methyl ester (L-NAME)—for 4 days, blockade of HO in control rats decreased CO, HO-1 levels, urine volume, and sodium excretion, but did not affect AP, RBF, or GFR. In rats undergoing NOS inhibition with L-NAME, blockade of HO decreased endogenous CO and renal HO-1 levels, urine volume, and sodium excretion, but again had no effect on AP, RBF, or GFR. An increase in plasma renin activity was observed in untreated rats but not in L-NAME–treated rats, indicating that the effects on urine volume and sodium excretion are associated, even when NO was inhibited. This suggests that inhibition of HO promotes water and sodium excretion by a direct tubular action. independently of renal hemodynamics or the NO system.[314]

Inhibition of renal medullary HO activity and CO production decreases medullary blood flow and sodium excretion; the abundance of both the HO-1 and HO-2 isoforms of HO are higher in the inner medulla and lower in the cortex.[316] Inhibition of HO significantly reduces renal medullary cGMP concentrations when infused into the renal medullary interstitial space. These results suggest that both HO-1 and HO-2 are highly expressed in the renal medulla that HO, and its products play a key role in maintaining the constancy of blood flow to the renal medulla; cGMP may mediate the vasodilator effect of HO and CO in the renal medullary circulation.[316] In anesthetized rats, increases in renal perfusion pressure were found to increase CO concentrations in the renal medulla. An HO inhibitor reduced HO activity and pressure-dependent increases in CO in the medulla and blunted pressure natriuresis.[317] In conscious rats fed a normal-sodium diet, chronic infusion of an HO inhibitor into the renal medulla increased mean AP. When rats were placed on a high-salt diet, inhibition of HO activity caused a further increase in AP. Thus, renal medullary HO activity plays a key role in the control of arterial blood pressure and the control of pressure natriuresis.[317]

Using a CO-releasing molecule (CORM-A1), Ryan and coworkers demonstrated that increases in CO in the mouse increase RBF, with comparable results obtained from infusion of the vasodilator acetylcholine.[318] Pretreatment with an inhibitor of guanylate cyclase to block acetylcholine reduced the increase in RBF by CORM-A1. In isolated vasoconstricted renal interlobular arteries, CORM-A1–induced vasodilation was attenuated with the guanylate cyclase inhibitor, as observed in vivo. Inhibition of calcium-activated potassium channels ($K_{Ca}$) with iberiotoxin completely blocked CORM-A1 vasodilation. Thus, CO released from CORM-AI increases RBF and decreases vascular resistance by activating guanylate cyclase and opening $K_{Ca}$ channels.[318]

The vascular effects of HO may be related to CO synthesis and are affected by NO release linked to the HO-CO system. Administration of a CO donor into the renal artery of rats increased RBF, GFR urinary cGMP excretion, and blood carboxyhemoglobin levels.[319] Inhibition of HO induced acute renal failure, with decreases in RBF, GFR, and cGMP excretion. These effects were nearly eliminated by the addition of a CO donor, which also decreased renal cortical NO concentration, urinary excretion of nitrates and nitrites, and urinary cGMP excretion and increased blood carboxyhemoglobin levels. Inhibition of renal HO resulted in acute renal failure, characterized by a large drop (–77%) in RBF and GFR (–93%). Supplementing HO inhibition with CO donor administration reversed the effects of HO inhibition on RBF and GFR, suggesting that the deleterious effects of HO on RBF and GFR were caused by the inhibition of CO. HO inhibition also decreased cortical NO concentration and increased urinary nitrate and/or nitrite excretion of the HO-CO system, whereas a CO donor increased renal NO levels and decreased nitrate and nitrite excretion. These results have suggested that changes in NO release contribute to the renal effects of the HO-CO system.[319]

Administration of heme decreases vascular resistance and increases RBF and sodium excretion, excretion of 6-keto-PGF1α, and the concentration of CO in renal cortical microdialysate. Pretreatment with an inhibitor of HO blunted heme-induced renal vasodilation and increased RBF. Pretreatment with sodium meclofenamate blunted the renal vasodilatory effect of heme, suggesting that heme-induced renal vasodilation is cyclooxygenase-dependent, yielding increased synthesis of PGI2.

### Hydrogen Sulfide

A growing body of evidence has shown that $H_2S$, an endogenous bioactive gas synthesized in nearly all organs, plays an important role in the regulation of kidney function. $H_2S$ generation by kidney cells is reduced in acute and chronic disease states, and $H_2S$ donors ameliorate injury[320] but, under some conditions, $H_2S$ may lead to kidney injury.[321] $H_2S$ is produced by cystathionine beta-synthase (CBS) and cystathionine gamma-lyase (CGL) by the transsulfuration of homocysteine.[322,323] Incubation of renal tissue homogenates with L-cysteine as a substrate yields $H_2S$. This response was prevented by inhibitors of both CBS and CGL in combination, whereas either inhibitor alone induced only a small decrease in $H_2S$.[322]

$H_2S$ plays a role in renal hemodynamics, as shown by the effects of intrarenal infusion of a donor of $H_2S$ (NaHS), which increased renal blood flow and GFR, as well as urinary sodium and potassium excretion. Infusion of L-cysteine also increases endogenous $H_2S$ production.[322] Simultaneous infusion of both an inhibitor of CBS and CGL to decrease $H_2S$ production decreased GFR and sodium and potassium excretion, but either inhibitor alone did not affect these renal functions.[322] $H_2S$ causes endothelium-dependent/cytochrome P450– dependent vasodilation and vascular smooth muscle hyperpolarization of small arterial vessels, increasing ryanodine-mediated $Ca^{2+}$ release through the activation of large conductance calcium activated potassium channels, causing membrane hyperpolarization and vasodilation.[324] The involvement of cGMP-dependent protein kinase-I in $H_2S$-induced vasorelaxation was shown in preconstricted aortic rings, with or without intact endothelium.[325] Treatment of the aortic rings with NaHS (an $H_2S$ donor) indicated that a cGMP-dependent protein kinase (PKG) is activated by $H_2S$. Incubation with a PKG-1 inhibitor blocked NaHS-stimulated vasodilation.[325] NaHS-induced vasorelaxation was reduced by removal of the endothelium and by inhibitors of either NO or cGMP production.[326] $H_2S$ also relaxes smooth muscle by activating ATP-sensitive potassium channels.[327]

Increases in TGF-β1 are associated with the development of tubulointerstitial fibrosis and glomerular sclerosis in other renal diseases and are mediated, at least in part, by Ang II. Ang II- and transforming growth factor beta 1 (TGF-β1)–induced renal tubular epithelial-mesenchymal transition (EMT) plays a pivotal role leading to renal sclerosis. One study has demonstrated that Ang II stimulates EMT in renal tubular epithelial cells by increasing the level of α-smooth actin and decreasing E-cadherin.[328] This effect was blocked by a TGF-β receptor kinase inhibitor. Ang II stimulated TGF-β activation and exogenous TGF-β1–induced EMT. The $H_2S$ donor NaHS blocked the promotion of EMT by Ang II and TGF-β1 and reduced TGF-β activity. $H_2S$ cleaves the disulfide bond in dimeric active TGF-β1, promoting the formation of inactive TGF- β1 monomer.[328] These results have suggested the potential to treat sclerosis in the kidney (both glomerular sclerosis and tubulointerstitial fibrosis), as well as other diseases associated with fibrosis and TGF-β1 (e.g., pulmonary fibrosis) by stimulating $H_2S$ or using another means to form the inactive TGF-β1 monomer.

## REACTIVE OXYGEN SPECIES

Reactive oxygen species (ROS) are products of a one-electron reduction of dioxygen (oxygen gas, $O_2$) to form the anionic form of $O_2$, superoxide, $O_2^-$ . Superoxide is generated by the catalytic actions of oxidative enzymes, such as nicotinamide adenine dinucleotide (NADH)/reduced NADPH oxidase (NOX) and cytochrome oxidase.[2,35] Superoxide is toxic and organisms creating $O_2^-$ have developed isoforms of superoxide dismutase (SOD), which catalyzes the conversion of superoxide to hydrogen peroxide ($H_2O_2$). Other enzymes degrade $H_2O_2$, protecting against the deleterious actions of this ROS.[2,35] ROS are produced in the kidney by endothelial cells, epithelial cells, vascular smooth muscle cells, mesangial cells, podocytes, and other cell types and have effects on the kidney vasculature.[329]

Normally, oxidative and antioxidative enzymes in the kidney yield a balanced production of NO and the superoxide anion. ROS are formed in the arteries, arterioles, glomeruli, and juxtaglomerular apparatus and other nephron segments, and the oxidases NOX 1, 2, and 4, NOS, and COX are also found in the kidney.[2,35] In the renal vasculature, NOX 1 and NOX 2 produce $O_2^-$, whereas NOX 4 in epithelial cells produces $H_2O_2$. Superoxide dismutase converts superoxide to $H_2O_2$; catalase and glutathione peroxidase degrade $H_2O_2$.

Stimulants of $O_2^-$ production include Ang II,[330–332] endothelin,[333] norepinephrine,[2] TGF-β1,[334] and stretch of vascular walls by increased intravascular pressure.[335,336] Ang II activates NADPH oxidases in afferent arterioles to form $O_2^-$, leading to calcium release from intracellular stores by activation of the inositol trisphosphate receptor (IP3R).[330] Superoxide also enhances calcium entry pathways into afferent arterioles through L-type channels by membrane depolarization.[337] NOX2 NADPH oxidase is activated by Ang II, promoting the generation of ROS, which scavenge NO and cause subsequent NO-deficiency.[331] $O_2^-$ and $H_2O_2$ activate different signaling pathways in vascular smooth muscle cells linked to discrete membrane channels, with opposite effects on membrane potential and voltage-operated $Ca^{2+}$ channels, and therefore have opposite effects on myogenic contractions.[335]

Increased perfusion pressure and Ang II increase $O_2^-$ production and increase myogenic responses in arterioles of superoxide gene-deleted mice compared with controls.[338] In the macula densa of blood-perfused juxtamedullary nephrons, $O_2^-$ was undetectable in control normotensive mice, but was markedly elevated in Ang II-induced hypertensive animals. NO was found in the macula densa of control mice but was undetectable in the macula densa of hypertensive animals.[339] These data suggest that under normal conditions, NO generated in the macula densa reduces tubuloglomerular feedback sensitivity, but in Ang II-induced hypertension, the TGF response is augmented by $O_2^-$ generated by the macula densa.[339] Increased perfusion pressure causes vascular $O_2^-$ production from NADPH oxidase, enhancing myogenic contractions independently of NO, whereas $H_2O_2$ impairs pressure-induced contractions but is not involved in the normal myogenic response.[340]

In the remnant kidney model, COX-2 is induced, leading to activation of thromboxane prostanoid receptors (TP-Rs), which enhance ET-1, ROS generation, and contractions.[333] Compared with controls, diabetic mouse afferent arterioles also have increased production of $O_2^-$ and $H_2O_2$ and enhanced responses to ET-1. These responses are accompanied by reduced protein expression and activities for catalase and superoxide dismutase-2. ET-1 further increases $O_2^-$, whereas $H_2O_2$ is unchanged by ET-1. Increased ROS in diabetes (notably $H_2O_2$) contributes to the enhanced arteriolar responses to ET-1.[341] TGF-β1, a growth factor involved in glomerular and tubular injury in diabetes, blocks autoregulation of afferent arterioles, an effect prevented with an ROS scavenger or an NADPH oxidase inhibitor. In smooth muscle cells, TGF-β1 stimulated ROS formation that was inhibited by NADPH oxidase inhibitors.[334]

In afferent arterioles from rats with spontaneous hypertension, pressure-induced increases in ROS were four times greater in SHR than in WKY rats. Both a scavenger of $O_2^-$ and an NOX2-based (NADPH oxidase) inhibitor attenuated pressure-induced constriction in SHR vessels but not in WKY. Thus, NOX2-derived $O_2^-$ may contribute to an enhanced myogenic response in SHR afferent arterioles.[342] Of note, arterioles from rats with ischemia-reperfusion injury had a 38% increase in $H_2O_2$, which could act to buffer the effect of Ang II and be a protective mechanism.[343]

### Endothelin

Endothelin is a potent vasoconstrictor agent derived primarily from vascular endothelial cells.[344] There are three distinct genes for endothelin, each encoding distinct 21–amino acid isopeptides, ET-1, ET-2, and ET-3.[344–346] Proteolytic cleavage of a 212–amino acid preproendothelin by furin yields a 38- to 40-amino acid proendothelin, which in turn is cleaved by endothelin-converting enzyme to yield endothelin peptides.[347,348] ET-1, the primary endothelin produced in the kidney, is formed in arcuate arteries and veins, interlobular arteries, afferent and efferent arterioles, glomerular capillary endothelial cells, glomerular epithelial cells, and glomerular mesangial cells.[349–360] ET-1 acts in an autocrine or paracrine fashion, or both,[361] to alter a variety of biologic processes in these cells. Endothelins are potent vasoconstrictors, and the renal vasculature is highly sensitive to these agents.[362] Once released from endothelial cells, endothelins bind to specific receptors on vascular smooth muscle, the $ET_A$ receptors that bind both ET-1 and ET-2.[361,363–366] $ET_B$ receptors are expressed in the glomerulus on mesangial cells and podocytes and have equal affinity for ET-1, ET-2, and ET-3.[365,366] There are two subtypes of $ET_B$ receptors, the $ET_{B1}$ linked to vasodilation and the $ET_{B2}$ linked to vasoconstriction.[367] An endothelin-specific protease modulates endothelin levels in the kidney.[368–370]

Endothelin production is stimulated by physical factors, including shear stress and vascular stretch.[371,372] A variety of hormones, growth factors, and vasoactive peptides increase endothelin production, including TGF-β, platelet-derived growth factor, tumor necrosis factor-α, Ang II, arginine vasopressin, insulin, bradykinin, thromboxane A2, and thrombin.[349,353,355,359,373–376] Endothelin production is inhibited by atrial and brain natriuretic peptides acting through a cGMP-dependent process[368,377] and by factors that increase intracellular cAMP and protein kinase A activation, such as β-adrenergic agonists.[355] ATP-binding renal purinergic (P2) receptors may regulate ET-1 production.[378]

Intravenous infusion of ET-1 induces a marked, prolonged pressor response[344,379] accompanied by increases in preglomerular and efferent arteriolar resistances and a decrease in RBF and GFR, without changes in fractional Na excretion.[379] As shown in Fig. 3.23, infusion of subpressor doses of ET-1 decreases SNGFR, $Q_A$, and whole-kidney RBF and GFR,[380–384] accompanied by increases in preglomerular and postglomerular resistances and filtration fraction.[380,382,385] Vasoconstriction of afferent and efferent arterioles by endothelin has been confirmed in the split hydronephrotic rat kidney preparation[386,387] and in isolated perfused arterioles.[301,388,389] Endothelin also causes mesangial cell contraction.[346,390] The vasoconstrictor effects of the endothelins can be modulated by several factors,[364,391] including NO,[301,392] bradykinin,[393] prostaglandin E2,[394] and prostacyclin.[394,395] The endothelin pathways demonstrate significant sexual dimorphisms that may affect the progression of renal disease and treatment choices.[396]

The $ET_A$ and $ET_B$ receptors have been cloned and characterized.[366,397,398] $ET_A$ receptors are abundant on vascular smooth muscle, have a high affinity for ET-1, and play a prominent role in the pressor response to endothelin.[399] $ET_B$ receptors are present on endothelial cells, where they may mediate NO release and relaxation.[398] Both $ET_A$ and $ET_B$ receptors are expressed in the media of interlobular arteries and afferent and efferent arterioles. Only $ET_A$ receptors are present on vascular smooth muscle cells of interlobar and arcuate arteries.[400] There is strong labeling of $ET_B$ receptors on peritubular and glomerular capillaries, as well as the vasa

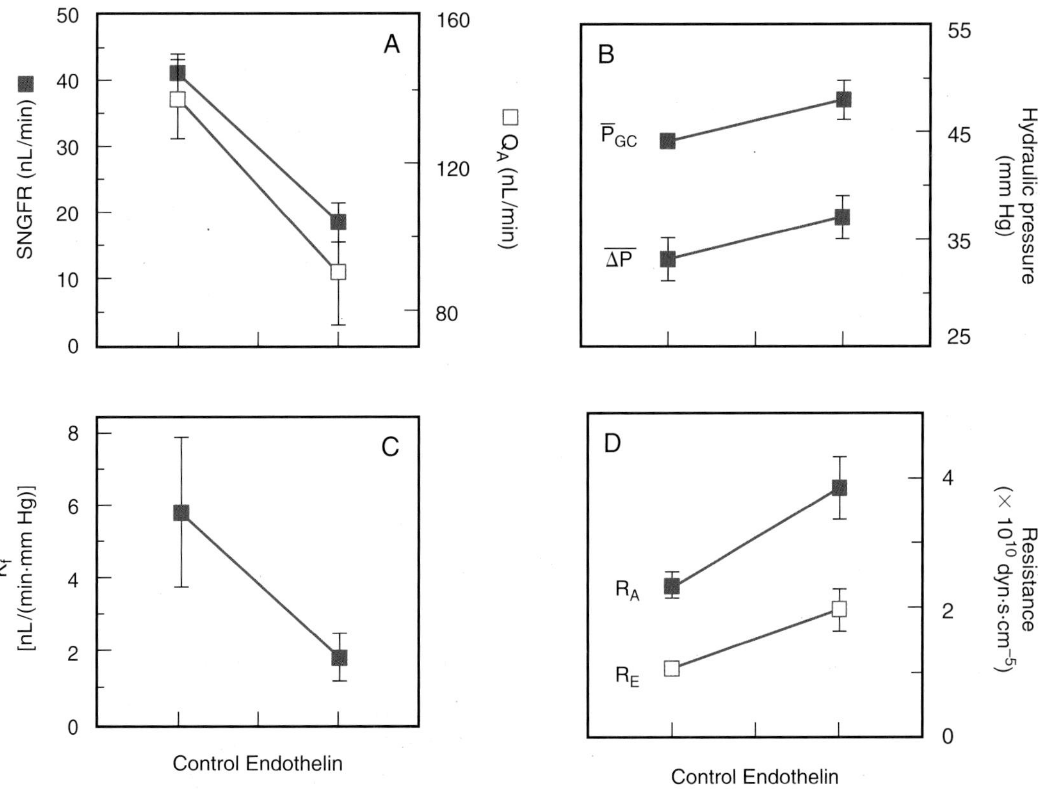


**Fig. 3.23** (A–D) Effects of intravenous administration of endothelin (subpressor dose) on glomerular dynamics. $K_f$, Filtration coefficient; $\Delta P$, mean transcapillary pressure gradient; $P_{GC}$, mean glomerular capillary pressure; $Q_A$, single-nephron glomerular plasma flow; $R_A$, afferent arteriolar resistance; $R_E$, efferent arteriolar resistance; *SNGFR,* single-nephron glomerular filtration rate. (Data [mean ± SE] obtained in Munich-Wistar rats from Badr KF, et al. Mesangial cell, glomerular and renal vascular responses to endothelin in the rat kidney. Elucidation of signal transduction pathways. *J Clin Invest.* 1989;83(1):336–342.)

recta endothelium.[400] $ET_A$ receptors are evident on glomerular mesangial cells and pericytes of descending vasa recta bundles.[400] Endogenous endothelin may actually dilate the afferent arteriole and lower $K_f$ via $ET_B$ receptors.[401]

$ET_A$ receptor antagonists may be useful for patients with diabetic nephropathy.[402] These $ET_A$ receptor antagonists have been shown to reduce albuminuria in diabetic nephropathy, although the albuminuria returns on cessation of the drug. It has been used alone and in conjunction with renin-angiotensin blockade.[403,404] However, $ET_A$ receptor antagonists have been associated with edema and heart failure, so patients already manifesting these conditions should be excluded from this type of medication.[405]

Endothelin stimulates the production of vasodilatory prostaglandins,[383,392,395,406,407] yielding a feedback loop to dampen the vasoconstrictor effects of endothelin. ET-1, ET-2, and ET-3 also stimulate NO production in the arterioles and glomerular mesangium via activation of the $ET_B$ receptor.[270,272,301,392,408] Resistance in the renal and systemic vasculature is markedly increased during inhibition of NO production. There is a dynamic interrelationship between NO and endothelin effects, so that $ET_A$ blockade or inhibition of endothelin-converting enzyme leads to increased renal resistance caused by NO inhibition.[409,410] The vasoconstrictive effects of Ang II may be mediated, in part, by stimulation of ET-1 production, which acts on $ET_A$ receptors to produce vasoconstriction.[373,376] Chronic administration of Ang II reduces renal blood flow, an effect reduced by a mixed $ET_A$-$ET_B$ receptor antagonist, suggesting that endothelin contributes to the renal vasoconstrictive effects of Ang II.[373]

Blood flow through the renal medulla is influenced by ET-1 as well as by Ang II, norepinephrine, nitric oxide, and vasodilatory prostaglandins. Medullary vasodilation measured by laser Doppler techniques was seen to occur at low doses of endothelin when cortical blood flow was decreased.[411] An $ET_A$ receptor antagonist blocked cortical vasoconstriction by ET-1 but failed to prevent medullary dilation. The endothelin-induced medullary vasodilation was blocked by an $ET_{A/B}$ receptor antagonist and was mimicked by an $ET_B$ receptor agonist. Inhibition of NO completely blocked the endothelin-induced vasodilation of medullary blood flow, and inhibition of prostaglandins attenuated the response. These results have indicated that endothelin causes cortical vasoconstriction mediated by $ET_A$ receptors, whereas activation of $ET_B$ receptors causes medullary vasodilation mediated by the release of NO.[411]

Medullary blood flow occurs through vasa recta capillaries, and most regions of the vasa recta are covered by pericytes capable of vasoconstriction. The role of these pericytes in controlling blood flow through the vasa recta has been examined with confocal microscopy and pericyte-mediated vasoconstriction and vasodilation were visualized. Ang II, endothelin, and norepinephrine all caused vasoconstriction at pericyte locations.[412] These effects were attenuated by an NO donor and enhanced with inhibitors of NO production or inhibition of prostaglandin release by nonselective cyclo-oxygenase inhibition with indomethacin. Because of the narrow diameter of the vasa recta (normally, ~10 μm), constriction of pericytes can cause impairment of the movement of red cells and hence blood flow through the medulla. These results suggest an important role for pericytes in the control of the medullary circulation.[412]

## ROLE OF THE RENIN-ANGIOTENSIN-ALDOSTERONE SYSTEM IN THE CONTROL OF RENAL BLOOD FLOW AND GLOMERULAR FILTRATION RATE

The RAS exerts major autocrine, paracrine, and endocrine functions regulating RBF and GFR. As presented in detail in several recent reviews,[2,35,55,83] renin is a proteolytic enzyme synthesized, stored, and released from the kidney, and also synthesized in the liver. In the kidney, it is synthesized and secreted primarily by the granulated epithelioid cells of the JGA adjacent to the terminal portion of the afferent arteriole; renin is also formed in the proximal tubules and in the principal cells of the connecting tubule and collecting duct.[2,35,413–415] Renin release from the kidneys is stimulated by a decrease in sodium intake, a reduction in extracellular fluid volume and blood volume, a decrease in arterial blood pressure, and increased sympathetic nerve activity.[416] Renin cleaves a decapeptide, angiotensin I (Ang I) from angiotensinogen, a glycoprotein formed in the proximal tubules of the kidney[415] and the liver. Circulating angiotensinogen is present in the $\alpha_2$-globulin fraction of plasma. Subsequent conversion of Ang I by angiotensin-converting enzyme (ACE), identical to kininase II, yields the octapeptide Ang II. ACE is present in many tissues, including lung. In the kidney, it is bound to the luminal sides of endothelial cells of blood vessels and tubular cells, including the brush border of the proximal tubule. All components needed for the production and degradation (the latter by angiotensinase A) of Ang II are present in the immediate region of the juxtaglomerular region of the nephron, allowing direct local regulation of glomerular blood flow and filtration rate.[35,55]

Ang II is a potent vasoconstrictor, and numerous studies have demonstrated that preglomerular vessels, including the arcuate arteries, interlobular arteries, and afferent arterioles, as well as the postglomerular efferent arterioles, constrict in response to exogenous and endogenous Ang II.[144,174,303,389,417,418]

Some studies have indicated that efferent arterioles have a greater sensitivity to Ang II, whereas others have shown similar effects on both afferent and efferent arterioles.[35,144,303,389,418] Fig. 3.24 shows the effects of Ang II on diameters in these vessels. As shown in Fig. 3.24, both L-type and T-type $Ca^{++}$ channels are involved in the afferent arteriolar responses to Ang II while the T-type $Ca^{++}$ channels are predominate at the efferent arterioles.[522,523] In addition to constricting vascular smooth muscle cells, Ang II increases myocardial contractility, stimulates aldosterone release, increases salt appetite and thirst, and helps regulate sodium transport by the kidney tubules and intestine.[419] The overall effect of Ang II is to minimize renal fluid and sodium losses and maintain extracellular fluid volume (ECFV) and arterial blood pressure.[416]

There are two major classes of Ang II receptors, AT1 and AT2, but the hypertensinogenic and vasoconstrictive actions of Ang II are primarily due to the AT1 receptor, which is widely distributed throughout all segments of the renal microvasculature in the cortical and medullary circulatory beds and are also present in the glomeruli, including mesangial cells, glomerular capillary endothelial cells, and podocytes.[35,83,420] In rodents, afferent arterioles have both AT1a and AT1b receptors, whereas efferent arterioles have only AT1a receptors.[420,421] AT1 receptors are also present in the proximal and distal tubules, loop of Henle and macula densa

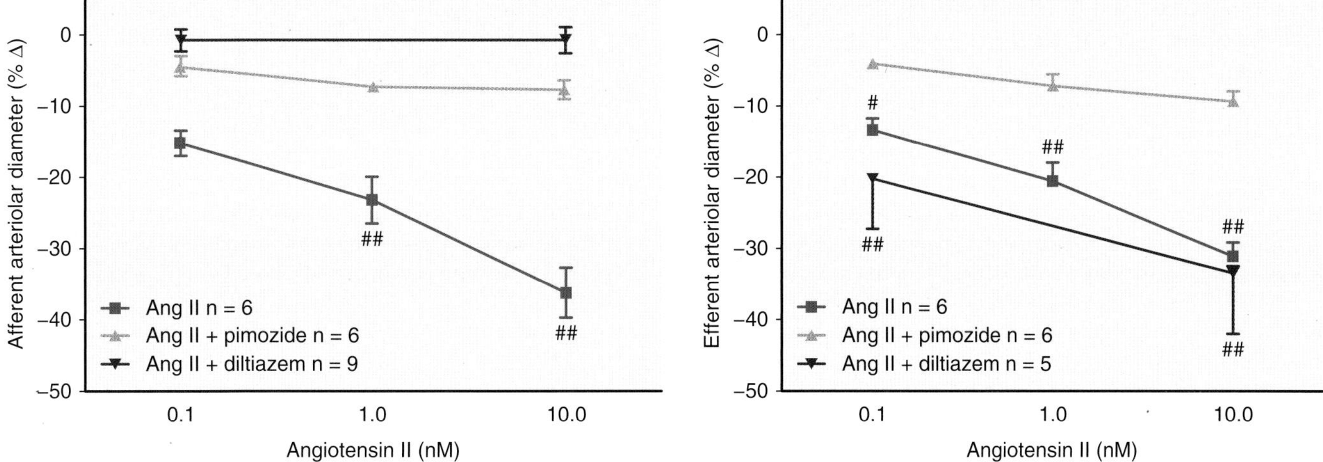


**Fig. 3.24** Role of L- and T-type $Ca^{2+}$ channels in angiotensin II (Ang II)–mediated afferent and efferent arteriolar vasoconstriction. Ang II constricts both afferent and efferent arterioles. The vasoconstrictor effects of Ang II on afferent arterioles are blocked by both L-type and T-type $Ca^{2+}$ channel blockers. In contrast, the efferent vasoconstrictor effects of Ang II are not blocked by L-type $Ca^{2+}$ channel blockers, but are blocked by T-type $Ca^{2+}$ channel blockers.[35,522,523] (From Carmines PK, Navar LG. Disparate effects of Ca channel blockade on afferent and efferent arteriolar responses to Ang II. *Am J Physiol Renal Physiol.* 1989;256(6 Pt 2):F1015–F1020; Feng MG, Navar LG. Angiotensin II-mediated constriction of afferent and efferent arterioles involves T-type $Ca^{2+}$ channel activation. *Am J Nephrol.* 2004;24(6):641–648.)

cells, cortical and medullary collecting ducts, glomerular podocytes, and mesangial cells.[419]

The vasoconstrictor effects of Ang II are blunted by the endogenous production of vasodilators including NO, cyclooxygenase, and cytochrome P450 epoxygenase metabolites in the afferent but not the efferent arterioles.[140,144,303,311,422–425] Ang II-simulated release of NO in the afferent arterioles occurs through activation of the AT1 receptors.[307,426] Ang II increases the production of prostaglandins (both PGE2 and PGI2) in afferent arteriolar smooth muscle cells, and PGE2, PGI2, and cAMP all blunt Ang II-induced calcium entry into these cells,[423] potentially explaining, at least in part, the different effects of Ang II on vasoconstriction of the afferent and efferent arterioles.[422,423] In contrast to effects on the afferent arteriole, PGE2 had no effect on Ang II-induced vasoconstriction of the efferent arteriole.[140] The effects of PGE2 on Ang II-induced vasoconstriction of the afferent arteriole are concentration-dependent, with low concentrations acting as a vasodilator via interaction with prostaglandin EP4 receptors and high concentrations of PGE2 acting on prostaglandin EP3 receptors to restore the Ang II effects in that segment.[140] Ang II infusion alone produces decreases in renal blood flow, with lesser effects on GFR resulting in an increase in filtration fraction.[35] However, when combined with cyclooxygenase inhibition, Ang II causes marked reductions in SNGFR and $Q_A$, suggesting an important role for endogenous vasodilatory prostaglandins in ameliorating the vasoconstrictor effects of Ang II.[427] Because Ang II increases renal production of vasodilatory prostaglandins, this serves as a feedback loop to modulate the vasoconstrictor effects on Ang II under chronic conditions when the RAAS is stimulated.[83]

Ang II decreases $K_f$[427] and contracts mesangial cells.[428] One possible cause for the changes in $K_f$ is that contraction of the mesangial cells reduces effective filtration area by blocking flow through some glomerular capillaries, but no direct evidence has been obtained to support this hypothesis. Alternatively, Ang II might decrease hydraulic conductivity, rather than or as well as reducing the surface area available for filtration, thereby reducing $K_f$.[429] Glomerular epithelial cells possess both AT1 and AT2 receptors and respond to Ang II by increasing cAMP production, suggesting a possible role for these cells in reducing $K_f$.[430] Alterations in epithelial structure or the size of the filtration slits, however, have not been detected following infusion of Ang II at a dose sufficient to decrease GFR and $K_f$.[431]

The vasoconstrictive effect of Ang II on glomerular mesangial cells is markedly reduced by NO. Release of NO from endothelial cells stimulated by bradykinin increases cGMP production in co-incubated mesangial cells. Comparable results were obtained when mesangial cells were incubated with NO alone.[262] Ang II alone caused constriction of the mesangial cells, but this effect was largely eliminated when the cells were co-incubated with both Ang II and NO. These studies suggest that local NO production from endothelial cells can modify the effects of Ang II on glomerular mesangial cells.[262] Glomerular epithelial cells contain Ang II receptors and, together with mesangial cells, may play an important role in Ang II-mediated control of the glomerular filtration barrier.[430]

Blockade of the AT1 receptors caused a dose-dependent dilation when Ang II was added to the lumen or bath of isolated afferent arterioles preconstricted by norepinephrine. This effect was blocked by pretreatment with an AT2 receptor antagonist, suggesting that activation of the AT2 causes vasodilation of afferent arterioles. Disruption of the endothelium or simultaneous inhibition of the cytochrome P450 pathway also abolished the vasodilation by Ang II. Thus, activation of AT2 receptors may cause endothelium-dependent vasodilation via a cytochrome P450 pathway, counteracting the vasoconstrictor effects of Ang II at AT1 receptors.[432,433]

As indicated, Ang II produces prohypertensive and renal vasoconstrictor effects via the activation of AT1 receptors, whereas activation of AT2 receptors results in modest vasodilation.[35,433] Several metabolic fragments of the octapeptide

Ang II, once believed to be inactive, have now been shown to have physiologic effects on the kidney, often opposing the actions of Ang II. The related peptide, Ang 1-7, has been shown to induce vasodilation of preconstricted renal arterioles.[434] These effects of Ang 1-7 occur independently of binding to AT1 or AT2 receptors and appear to involve activation of the G protein–coupled Mas receptor,[435] which has been shown to be expressed on the afferent arteriole.[436] In addition, an isoform of ACE, known as "ACE2,"[437,438] is involved in the formation of Ang 1-7.[439] Ang 1-7, ACE2, and the Mas receptor have all been detected in the kidney. The balance between opposing actions of the vasoconstrictor peptide, Ang II, and the vasodilator peptide, Ang 1-7, may be influenced by the ratio of ACE to ACE2 and AT1 to Mas receptor content in specific vascular regions (and tubular segments) of the kidney. Cardiovascular and renal diseases may involve an imbalance of these peptides, enzymes, or receptors.[436]

Additional mechanisms involved in Ang II-induced hypertension have been proposed. The principal cells of the connecting tubule and collecting duct express prorenin receptors and produce renin, which, coupled with delivery of angiotensinogen from the proximal tubule,[414] allows for the local formation of Ang I.[2,413,433] Luminal ACE in the collecting duct is then available to produce Ang II, which in turn can increase sodium reabsorption by enhancing activity of $E_{Na}C$ and other transporters in the collecting duct, an effect that may be important in the progression of diabetes and Ang II-induced hypertension.[413,414,433,440]

## ROLE OF ANGIOTENSIN II IN GLOMERULAR AND TISSUE INJURY

Chronic renal failure is characterized by a progressive decline in renal function, with glomerular and tubular injury and systemic hypertension. An important demonstration of an elevation of glomerular hydraulic pressure in kidney disease was in a model of nephrotoxic serum nephritis (NSN),[441] where Ang II is thought to have a key role in the renal complications that develop. Intravenous infusion of Ang II increases $P_{GC}$ and $\Delta P$ in rats with reduced renal mass.[442] In the remnant kidney model of renal failure, inhibition of Ang II production by an ACE inhibitor lowered $P_{GC}$ and $\Delta P$ toward normal and prevented proteinuria and glomerular injury.[443] Over the last 30 years, the efficacy of blockade of the RAAS with ACE inhibitors and/or Ang II type 1 receptor antagonists (angiotensin receptor blockers [ARBs]) in limiting or slowing the progression of some types of kidney disease has been established.[444] ACE inhibitors and ARBs also are effective in the treatment of spontaneous glomerulosclerosis associated with aging.[445,446] Both ACE inhibitors and ARBs prevented hypertension, limited proteinuria, and ameliorated sclerosis in several experimental models of glomerulonephritis.[447] In one study, ACE inhibition was suggested to promote regeneration of new renal tissue.[448] Similarly, in the remnant kidney model of renal disease, there is evidence that chronic treatment with an ACE inhibitor causes reversal of renal injury.[449]

Accumulation of extracellular matrix proteins, including collagen and fibronectin, leads to glomerular and tubular injury.[450] Enhanced production of TGF-β1 in the remnant kidney increases matrix formation by stimulating the production of TGF-β1. Administration of a neutralizing antibody or an Ang II receptor antagonist reduces plasma TGF-β1 levels and blood pressure toward normal.[451] ACE inhibition in the obese Zucker rat has significantly reduced proteinuria compared with untreated obese animals, downregulated expression of nephrin, and decreased expression of TGB-β1, collagen IV, and fibronectin.[452] Similarly, in an animal model of myocardial infarction (MI), rats with MI had significant renal injury, and treatment by ACE inhibition exerted beneficial effects.[453]

Ang II induces upregulation and activation of a transcription factor called "sterol-responsive element-binding protein" (SREBP-1), leading to upregulation of TGF-β1 and increased production of matrix collagen and fibronectin.[450] An ARB prevented the increase in TGF-β1 formation and the induction of SREBP-1. Inhibition of SREBP-1 prevented Ang II-induced glomerular upregulation of TGF-β1 and matrix synthesis, demonstrating a significant role of the transcription factor in glomerular injury and indicating that TGF-β1 plays a role in the stimulation of matrix production.[450] SREBP-1 upregulation is observed in diabetic kidneys; SREBP-1 is activated by high glucose levels and mediates profibrogenic responses in primary rat mesangial cells.[454] In these cells, high glucose levels activated SREBP-1, which binds to the TGF-β1 promoter, resulting in TGF-β1 upregulation.[454]

Treatment with an ARB in rats with NSN protected against interstitial inflammation, tubular degeneration, and segmental glomerulosclerosis.[455] NSN rats were treated with pirfenidone (an antifibrotic, antiinflammatory compound first used to treat pulmonary fibrosis) or with pirfenidone plus an ARB. Pirfenidone alone yielded a decrease in proteinuria and the ARB a slightly greater decrease; the two together had additive effects on proteinuria, interstitial inflammation, tubular degeneration, and segmental glomerulosclerosis.[455] Transgenic mice overexpressing active renin from the liver develop progressive pulmonary fibrosis, much like that seen in humans with pulmonary fibrosis. There was increased extracellular matrix deposition of fibronectin and collagens and increased production of TGF-β1 and connective tissue growth factor (CTGF).[456] Two weeks of treatment with a renin inhibitor or an ARB reduced production of TGF-β1 and CTGF and decreased deposition of matrix proteins.

## ARACHIDONIC ACID METABOLITES REGULATING RENAL BLOOD FLOW AND GLOMERULAR FILTRATION RATE

The processing of the essential polyunsaturated fatty acid, linoleic acid, in the liver yields the polyunsaturated fatty acid arachidonic acid, which is stored in membrane phospholipids. Biologically active eicosanoids, C20 metabolites of arachidonic acid, are produced by three primary enzymatic pathways, including the following: cyclooxygenase-generating prostaglandins (PGs) and thromboxanes (TBXs); lipoxygenase (OX) yielding leukotrienes (LTs) and HETEs; and cytochrome P450 pathways synthesizing HETEs and EETs. Arachidonic acid (AA) is released from cell membranes, predominantly by phospholipase A2 (PLA2).[457–461] These eicosanoids regulate the renal microcirculation, in part by activating G protein–coupled receptors in the endothelium and vascular smooth muscles.[458,462]

### Prostaglandins

Following the interaction of various hormones and vasoactive substances with their membrane receptors, PLA2 is activated, resulting in the release of AA from the cell membranes. This allows the enzymatic action of cyclooxygenase to process AA into prostaglandins—PGG2 and subsequently PGH2. PGH2 is then converted into a number of biologically active prostaglandins, including PGE2, prostacyclin (PGI2), PGF2α, PGE1, PGD2, and thromboxane (TxA2). Prostaglandins play important roles in healthy and diseased kidneys.[93,463–466] PGE2 receptors are the most abundant prostaglandin receptors in the kidney. The effects of PGE2 on the kidneys depend on the location of the receptor subtype and interaction with other active compounds. PGE2 activates at least four receptors, EP1 to EP4. Prostaglandin EP1 receptor activation results in contractile effects in smooth muscle through the Gq alpha protein linkage, whereas EP2 and EP4 are relaxant via the Gs alpha subunit. EP3 is an inhibitory receptor (Gi alpha), decreasing cAMP, which causes vasoconstriction.[35,463,464]

In the kidneys, PGE1, PGI2, and PGE2 are vasodilator prostaglandins that generally increase renal plasma flow yet produce little or no increase in GFR and SNGFR, in part due to a decline in $K_f$.[93,464–466] TxA2 generally results in contraction of the glomerular mesangial cells via the Gq alpha subunit. During blockade of endogenous prostaglandin production, infusion of PGE2 or PGI2 decreases SNGFR and $Q_A$, accompanied by an increase in renal vascular resistance (particularly $R_E$), increases in $P_{GC}$ and ΔP, and a decline in $K_f$.[467] Additional blockade of Ang II receptors during cyclooxygenase inhibition results in vasodilation in response to PGE2 or PGI2, resulting in a return of SNGFR and $Q_A$ equal to or more than control values, a fall in $P_{GC}$ below control values, and a return of $K_f$ to normal.[467] Thus, the renal vasoconstriction induced by exogenous PGE2 or PGI2 appears to be mediated by induction of renin and Ang II production.

Vasodilation at the whole-kidney level resulting from PGI2 infusion during cyclooxygenase and Ang II inhibition has not always been observed.[468] Topical application (but not luminal) of PGE2 to the afferent arteriole increased the vasoconstrictive effect of Ang II and norepinephrine, whereas PGI2 only attenuated norepinephrine-induced vasoconstriction.[469] PGE2 also constricted interlobular arteries but neither prostaglandin produced vasodilation of vessels preconstricted by Ang II.[469] Indomethacin alone induced vasoconstriction of preglomerular and postglomerular resistance vessels of superficial and juxtamedullary nephrons, indicating that vasodilatory prostaglandins normally modulate endogenous vasoconstrictors.[470] However, there appears to be gender-dependent differences in mechanisms, because indomethacin treatment results in net renal vasodilation in female rats.[471] The combination of cyclooxygenase inhibition with an ACE inhibitor caused vasodilation of preglomerular but not postglomerular vessels of the cortical nephrons due to the effects of continued NO production in the preglomerular vessels.[470] Additionally, the PGE2 EP3 receptor regulates COX-2 through a negative feedback loop in the thick ascending limb of the loop of Henle.[472] These data, taken together, indicate that differences in the response to vasoactive prostaglandins between superficial and deep nephrons may be due to prostaglandin receptor subtypes and cyclooxygenase activity.

### Leukotrienes and Lipoxins

Leukotrienes are a class of lipid products formed from AA via the lipoxygenase pathway. Leukotrienes that affect glomerular filtration and renal blood flow are leukotriene C4 (LTC4), leukotriene D4 (LTD4), and leukotriene B4 (LTB4). LTC4 and LTD4 are potent vasoconstrictors,[473] whereas LTB4 produces moderate renal vasodilation and an increase in RBF, with no change in GFR in the normal rat.[474] Intravenous infusion of LTC4 increases renal vascular resistance, leading to a decrease in RBF and GFR, as well as a decrease in plasma volume and cardiac output.[475,476] The decline in RBF is diminished by saralasin, an Ang II receptor antagonist, and indomethacin, an inhibitor of cyclooxygenase, indicating the involvement of Ang II and cyclooxygenase products in the response to LTC4, as well as a direct effect of LTC4 on the renal resistance vessels.[475] Similarly, LTD4 decreased $K_f$, but increased renal vascular resistance, particularly, $R_E$, a fall in $Q_A$ and SNGFR, and a rise in $P_{GC}$ and ΔP during blockade of Ang II and control of renal perfusion pressure, demonstrating a direct effect of this leukotriene on renal hemodynamics.[477] Leukotrienes often mediate drug-associated nephrotoxicity in some models of kidney disease.[478]

Inflammatory injury also activates the 5-, 12-, and 15-lipoxygenase pathways in neutrophils and platelets to form acyclic eicosanoids called lipoxins (LXs), of which there are two main types, LXA4 and LXB4.[479] LXB4 and 7-*cis*-11-*trans*-LXA4 produce renal vasoconstriction.[478,480] By contrast, intrarenal infusion of LXA4 induces a reduction in preglomerular resistance ($R_A$) without affecting $R_E$, thereby resulting in an increase in $P_{GC}$ and ΔP.[477] The specific vasodilation of the preglomerular vessels by LXA4 was blocked by cyclooxygenase inhibition, indicating that vasodilatory prostaglandins are responsible for this effect.[477,480] Unique to this compound, LXA4 produced vasodilation while simultaneously causing a reduction in $K_f$.[480] Because $P_{GC}$, ΔP, and $Q_A$ were increased, SNGFR also increased.[477] Furthermore, transfection of rat kidney with the 15-lipoxygenase gene suppressed inflammation and preserved function in experimental glomerulonephritis.[481] The lipoxins have also been used to treat acute renal failure in mice.[482,483]

### Cytochrome P450

A rapidly growing field of study is that of eicosanoids formed through the cytochrome P 450 (CYP450) monooxygenase pathway. AA is metabolized via the CYP450 enzymes to other active metabolites, including EETs, dihydrooxyeicosatetraenoic acids (DiHETEs), and HETEs, which act locally in a paracrine manner.[35] Early researchers demonstrated the role of one metabolite, 20-HETE, involved in regulating renal hemodynamics through direct actions, as well as exerting modulatory actions on the TGF mechanism.[460] In addition to its vascular effects, 20-HETE inhibits sodium transport in the proximal tubule and the thick ascending loop of Henle. 20-HETE elicits an enhancement of myogenic tone and vasoconstricts afferent arterioles, which may be partially mediated through the augmentation of the TGF mechanism.[484] Blockade of 20-HETE formation attenuated vascular responses to Ang II, endothelin, norepinephrine, NO, and CO.[222,484] NO inhibits the production of 20-HETE, which contributes to the vasodilatory effect of NO.[222,460,463,485–487]

In contrast to the contractile responses of 20-HETE, some of the EETs mentioned also formed via the CYP450 pathway are potent vasodilators.[35,488] EETs are formed locally and serve as both autocrine and paracrine factors. EETs are endothelium-derived hyperpolarizing factors that elicit potent vasodilation of the afferent arteriole.[488] These actions are mediated in part by activating large conductance potassium channels.

## NEURAL REGULATION OF RENAL CIRCULATION

The renal vasculature, including the afferent and efferent arterioles, macula densa cells of the distal tubule, and glomerular mesangium are richly innervated.[83,489] Innervation primarily includes renal efferent sympathetic adrenergic nerves[489,490] and renal afferent sensory fibers containing peptides, including calcitonin gene-related peptide (CGRP) and substance P.[83,489] Sympathetic efferent nerves are found in all segments of the vascular tree, from the main renal artery to the afferent arteriole (including the renin-containing juxtaglomerular cells) and efferent arteriole.[489,490] They play an important role in the regulation of renal hemodynamics, sodium transport, and renin secretion.[491] Afferent nerves containing CGRP and substance P are localized primarily in the main renal artery and interlobar arteries, with some innervation also observed in the arcuate artery, interlobular artery, afferent arteriole, and juxtaglomerular apparatus.[489,490] Peptidergic nerve fibers immunoreactive for neuropeptide Y (NPY), neurotensin, vasoactive intestinal polypeptide, and somatostatin are also found in the kidney.[55] Neuronal NOS-immunoreactive neurons have been identified in the kidney.[489] The NOS-containing neuronal stomata are seen in the wall of the renal pelvis, at the renal hilus close to the renal artery, along the interlobar arteries, the arcuate arteries, and extending to the afferent arteriole, supporting their role in the control of RBF.[489] They are also present in nerve bundles that have vasomotor and sensory fibers, suggesting that they modulate renal neural function.[489]

In micropuncture studies of the effects of renal nerve stimulation (RNS), RNS alone increased $R_A$ and $R_E$, resulting in a decrease in plasma flow and SNGFR, without any effect on $K_f$.[492] When prostaglandin production was inhibited by indomethacin, however, the same level of RNS produced even greater increases in $R_A$ and $R_E$, accompanied by very large declines in plasma flow and SNGFR and decreases in $K_f$, $P_{GC}$, and $\Delta P$.[492] When saralasin was administered as a competitive inhibitor of endogenous Ang II in conjunction with indomethacin, RNS had no effect on $K_f$, but both $R_A$ and $R_E$ were still increased, and $\Delta P$ was slightly reduced.[492] The release of norepinephrine by RNS enhances Ang II production and results in arteriolar vasoconstriction and reductions in $K_f$. The increase in Ang II production may then enhance vasodilator prostaglandin production,[492,493] which partially ameliorates the constriction.

Continued vasoconstriction by RNS during the blockade of endogenous prostaglandins and Ang II has indicated that norepinephrine has vasoconstrictive properties by itself. The findings that norepinephrine causes constriction of preglomerular vessels support the direct effects of norepinephrine on renal microvessels.[422] Inhibition of NOS results in a decline in SNGFR in normal rats but not in rats with surgical renal denervation, suggesting that NO normally modulates the effects of renal adrenergic activity.[494] However, this modulation does not appear to be related to the sympathetic modulation of renin secretion.[495] Under conditions of renal injury and inflammation, the effects of increased renal nerve activity are exacerbated.[496] The actions of increased sympathetic activity to decrease renal cortical perfusion are attenuated by temporally mediated reductions in ROS.[497]

Renal denervation in animals undergoing acute water deprivation (48-hour duration) or with congestive heart failure produces increases in SNGFR, plasma flow, and $K_f$.[498] This indicates that the natural activity of the renal nerves in these settings plays an important role in the constriction of the arterioles and reductions in $K_f$ that were observed with water deprivation and in congestive heart failure.[498] The vasoconstrictive effects of the renal nerves in both settings were mediated in part by a stimulatory effect on Ang II release, together with direct vasoconstrictive effects on the preglomerular and postglomerular blood vessels.[498] These studies have demonstrated the important role of the renal nerves in pathophysiologic settings.

Clinical trials have focused on whether catheter-based renal artery denervation reduces blood pressure in patients with resistant hypertension. Some studies have demonstrated sustained reduction in blood pressure in patients who underwent renal denervation; however, the blood pressure response did not differ from the sham-treated patients at 6 months after treatment.[499] More recent clinical trials using improved catheters have provided more promising long-term effects.[500]

## GLOMERULAR HEMODYNAMICS IN THE AGING KIDNEY

Aging is commonly associated with the progressive development of chronic renal disease characterized by global glomerulosclerosis, tubular atrophy, interstitial fibrosis, and arteriosclerosis. Over 75 years ago, Davies and Shock demonstrated that beyond 40 to 50 years of age, inulin clearance in humans declined approximately 8 mL/min/1.73 $m^2$ in each subsequent decade of age.[501] In healthy adult living kidney donors, the prevalence of glomerulosclerosis, followed by local tubular atrophy and interstitial fibrosis, was found to increase progressively from 2.7% for patients aged 18 to 29 years to 73% for patients aged 70 to 77 years.[502] Despite these changes, the age-related decline in GFR was not fully explained by these age-related histologic changes.[502,503] Fig. 3.25 shows the declines in GFR beyond the ages of 40 to 50 years[83,504–506] Kidney disease associated with aging is generally accompanied by declines in GFR, RPF, and RBF associated with an increase in filtration fraction. In one study, the calculated filtration coefficient, $K_f$, was lower in older than in younger subjects (4.9 ± 1.7 nL/[min·mm Hg] in older subjects vs 7.0 ± 2.9 nL/[min·mm Hg] in younger subjects).[507] However, age-related declines in GFR and RBF do not necessarily occur in everyone.[502,506,508] As shown in Fig. 3.25, associated with the decline in GFR and RBF is the fact that systolic blood pressure increases with age,[507,509] which may contribute to a further decline in renal function. Nevertheless, in disease-free older individuals, GFR is generally adequate to sustain quality of life (see Fig. 3.25).

Factors likely involved in the decline in renal function associated with aging include eating high-protein meals, which may lead to episodes of hyperfiltration and glomerular capillary hypertension, development of diabetes, with associated

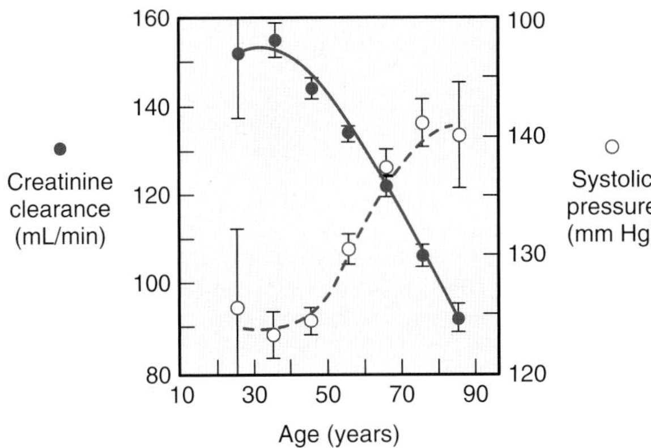


**Fig. 3.25** Correlation of aging with systolic blood pressure and creatinine clearance ($C_{Cr}$) in normal adults. (From Lindeman R, Tobin J, Shock N. Association between blood pressure and the rate of decline in renal function with age. *Kidney Int.* 1984;26: 861–868.)

advanced glycosylated end products, obesity, oxidative stress due to chronic exposure to oxygen free radicals, dyslipidemia, excessive exposure to some drugs that reduce renal function, infections, atherosclerotic disease, male gender, genetic and racial differences, and environmental factors.[506,510–512] Sclerotic glomeruli seen with aging are smaller than functional glomeruli, leading to a decline in average glomerular size. With the progressive loss of filtering glomeruli, unaffected glomeruli undergo compensatory hypertrophy, which helps preserve GFR.[502] As has been shown in studies of the rat, following removal of 50% to 80% of total renal mass, the remaining nephrons undergo compensatory hypertrophy and increases in SNGFR and glomerular capillary hydraulic pressures.[14,513,514] In the aging human, progressive loss of functioning nephrons and hypertrophy of remaining filtering units would also result in glomerular capillary hypertension and damage to these remaining nephrons. Because these alterations use renal reserve capacity, there is a reduced capability of the renal vasculature in older individuals to respond to amino acid infusion, so that there is only an increase in GFR and filtration fraction and RPF remains unchanged.[508,515] In contrast, the vasoconstrictive response to Ang II is identical in younger and older people.[516] These data suggest that there is a blunted renal vasodilatory response but a vasoconstrictive response is maintained in older subjects, indicating that the aged kidney has used reserve capacity and is in a state of compensatory renal vasodilation to compensate for the chronic glomerular injury and loss of functional glomeruli.[515]

 Complete reference list available at ExpertConsult.com.

## KEY REFERENCES


2. Arendshorst W, Navar LG. Renal circulation and glomerular hemodyanamics. In: Schrier RW, Coffman TM, Falk RJ, et al, eds. *Schrier's Diseases of the Kidney*. Philadelphia: Lippincott Williams & Wilkins; 2013:74–131.
4. Navar LG, Bell PD, Evan AP. The regulation of glomerular filtration rate in mammalian kidneys. In: Andreoli TE, Hoffman J, Fanestil D, et al, eds. *Physiology of Membrane Disorders*. New York: Plenum Medical Book Co.; 1986:637–667.
5. Smith HW. *The Kidney: Structure and Function in Health and Disease*. Vol 4. New York: Oxford University Press; 1951.
25. Evans RG, Harrop GK, Ngo JP, et al. Basal renal O2 consumption and the efficiency of O2 utilization for Na+ reabsorption. *Am J Physiol Renal Physiol.* 2014;306(5):F551–F560.
26. Mimura I, Nangaku M. The suffocating kidney: tubulointerstitial hypoxia in end-stage renal disease. *Nat Rev Nephrol.* 2010;6(11): 667–678.
35. Navar LG, Arendshorst WJ, Pallone TL, et al. The renal microcirculation. In: Tuma RF, Duran WN, Ley K, eds. *Handbook of Physiology: Microcirculation*. Vol 2. Academic Press; 2008:550–683.
41. Beeuwkes R 3rd. The vascular organization of the kidney. *Annu Rev Physiol.* 1980;42:531–542.
47. Neal CR, Arkill K, Bell JS, et al. Novel haemodynamic structures in the human glomerulus. *Am J Physiol Renal Physiol.* 2018;315:F1370–F1384.
60. Lawrence MG, Altenburg MK, Sanford R, et al. Permeation of macromolecules into the renal glomerular basement membrane and capture by the tubules. *Proc Natl Acad Sci USA.* 2017;114(11): 2958–2963.
62. Haraldsson B, Nystrom J, Deen WM. Properties of the glomerular barrier and mechanisms of proteinuria. *Physiol Rev.* 2008;88(2): 451–487.
67. Suh JH, Miner JH. The glomerular basement membrane as a barrier to albumin. *Nat Rev Nephrol.* 2013;9(8):470–477.
74. Arendshorst WJ, Gottschalk CW. Glomerular ultrafiltration dynamics: historical perspective. *Am J Physiol Renal Physiol.* 1985;248(2 Pt 2): F163–F174.
75. Oken DE. An analysis of glomerular dynamics in rat, dog, and man. *Kidney Int.* 1982;22(2):136–145.
89. Lenihan CR, Busque S, Derby G, et al. Longitudinal study of living kidney donor glomerular dynamics after nephrectomy. *J Clin Invest.* 2015;125(3):1311–1318.
102. Pallone TL, Zhang Z, Rhinehart K. Physiology of the renal medullary microcirculation. *Am J Physiol Renal Physiol.* 2003;284(2):F253–F266.
127. Peppiatt-Wildman CM. The evolving role of renal pericytes. *Curr Opin Nephrol Hypertens.* 2013;22(1):10–16.
132. Pannabecker TL, Dantzler WH. Three-dimensional architecture of inner medullary vasa recta. *Am J Physiol Renal Physiol.* 2006; 290(6):F1355–F1366.
154. Peti-Peterdi J, Morishima S, Bell PD, et al. Two-photon excitation fluorescence imaging of the living juxtaglomerular apparatus. *Am J Physiol Renal Physiol.* 2002;283(1):F197–F201.
163. Griffin KA, Hacioglu R, Abu-Amarah I, et al. Effects of calcium channel blockers on "dynamic" and "steady-state step" renal autoregulation. *Am J Physiol Renal Physiol.* 2004;286(6):F1136–F1143.
191. Hashimoto S, Huang Y, Briggs J, et al. Reduced autoregulatory effectiveness in adenosine 1 receptor-deficient mice. *Am J Physiol Renal Physiol.* 2006;290(4):F888–F891.
200. Loutzenhiser R, Griffin K, Williamson G, et al. Renal autoregulation: new perspectives regarding the protective and regulatory roles of the underlying mechanisms. *Am J Physiol Regul Integr Comp Physiol.* 2006;290(5):R1153–R1167.
202. Schnermann J, Briggs JP. Tubuloglomerular feedback: mechanistic insights from gene-manipulated mice. *Kidney Int.* 2008;74(4):418–426.
217. Feng MG, Navar LG. Afferent arteriolar vasodilator effect of adenosine predominantly involves adenosine A2B receptor activation. *Am J Physiol Renal Physiol.* 2010;299:F310–F315.
220. Fan F, Roman RJ. Effect of cytochrome P450 metabolites of arachidonic acid in nephrology. *J Am Soc Nephrol.* 2017;28(10): 2845–2855.
222. Schnermann J. Concurrent activation of multiple vasoactive signaling pathways in vasoconstriction caused by tubuloglomerular feedback: a quantitative assessment. *Annu Rev Physiol.* 2015;77:301–322.
239. Kovacs G, Komlosi P, Fuson A, et al. Neuronal nitric oxide synthase: its role and regulation in macula densa cells. *J Am Soc Nephrol.* 2003;14(10):2475–2483.
313. Botros FT, Dobrowolski L, Navar LG. Renal heme oxygenase-1 induction with hemin augments renal hemodynamics, renal autoregulation, and excretory function. *Int J Hypertens.* 2012;2012:189512.
320. Kasinath BS, Feliers D, Lee HJ. Hydrogen sulfide as a regulatory factor in kidney health and disease. *Biochem Pharmacol.* 2018;149:29–41.
330. Fellner SK, Arendshorst WJ. Angiotensin II, reactive oxygen species, and Ca2+ signaling in afferent arterioles. *Am J Physiol Renal Physiol.* 2005;289(5):F1012–F1019.
336. Li L, Lai EY, Luo Z, et al. Superoxide and hydrogen peroxide counterregulate myogenic contractions in renal afferent arterioles from a mouse model of chronic kidney disease. *Kidney Int.* 2017;92(3):625–633.

337. Vogel PA, Yang X, Moss NG, et al. Superoxide enhances Ca2+ entry through L-type channels in the renal afferent arteriole. *Hypertension.* 2015;66(2):374–381.
339. Song J, Lu Y, Lai EY, et al. Oxidative status in the macula densa modulates tubuloglomerular feedback responsiveness in angiotensin II-induced hypertension. *Acta Physiol (Oxf).* 2015;213(1):249–258.
341. Zhang S, Huang Q, Wang Q, et al. Enhanced renal afferent arteriolar reactive oxygen species and contractility to endothelin-1 are associated with canonical wnt signaling in diabetic mice. *Kidney Blood Press Res.* 2018;43(3):860–871.
370. De Miguel C, Speed JS, Kasztan M, et al. Endothelin-1 and the kidney: new perspectives and recent findings. *Curr Opin Nephrol Hypertens.* 2016;25(1):35–41.
378. Gohar EY, Kasztan M, Pollock DM. Interplay between renal endothelin and purinergic signaling systems. *Am J Physiol Renal Physiol.* 2017;313(3):F666–F668.
413. Prieto MC, Gonzalez AA, Navar LG. Evolving concepts on regulation and function of renin in distal nephron. *Pflugers Arch.* 2013;465(1):121–132.
414. Ramkumar N, Kohan DE. Role of collecting duct renin in blood pressure regulation. *Am J Physiol Regul Integr Comp Physiol.* 2013;305(2):R92–R94.
420. Navar LG. Intrarenal renin-angiotensin system in regulation of glomerular function. *Curr Opin Nephrol Hypertens.* 2014;23(1):38–45.
440. Gonzalez AA, Lara LS, Prieto MC. Role of Collecting Duct Renin in the Pathogenesis of Hypertension. *Curr Hypertens Rep.* 2017;19(8):62.
450. Wang TN, Chen X, Li R, et al. SREBP-1 mediates angiotensin II-induced TGF-beta1 upregulation and glomerular fibrosis. *J Am Soc Nephrol.* 2015;26(8):1839–1854.
457. Navar LG, Inscho EW, Majid SA, et al. Paracrine regulation of the renal microcirculation. *Physiol Rev.* 1996;76(2):425–536.
464. Carlstrom M, Wilcox CS, Arendshorst WJ. Renal autoregulation in health and disease. *Physiol Rev.* 2015;95(2):405–511.
472. Vio CP, Quiroz-Munoz M, Cuevas CA, et al. Prostaglandin E2 EP3 receptor regulates cyclooxygenase-2 expression in the kidney. *Am J Physiol Renal Physiol.* 2012;303(3):F449–F457.
478. Rubinstein M, Dvash E. Leukotrienes and kidney diseases. *Curr Opin Nephrol Hypertens.* 2018;27(1):42–48.
483. Chandrasekharan JA, Sharma-Walia N. Lipoxins: nature's way to resolve inflammation. *J Inflamm Res.* 2015;8:181–192.
484. Roman RJ, Fan F. 20-HETE: hypertension and beyond. *Hypertension.* 2018;72(1):12–18.
488. Imig JD. Epoxyeicosatrienoic acids, hypertension, and kidney injury. *Hypertension.* 2015;65(3):476–482.
499. Bhatt DL, Kandzari DE, O'Neill WW, et al. A controlled trial of renal denervation for resistant hypertension. *N Engl J Med.* 2014;370(15):1393–1401.
502. Glassock RJ, Rule AD. The implications of anatomical and functional changes of the aging kidney: with an emphasis on the glomeruli. *Kidney Int.* 2012;82(3):270–277.
505. Maddox DA, Alavi FK, Zawada ET Jr. The kidney and aging. In: Massry SG, Glassock RJ, eds. *Textbook of Nephrology.* Baltimore: Lippincott Williams & Wilkins; 2001:1094–1105.

# 4 Glomerular Cell Biology and Podocytopathies

Catherine Meyer-Schwesinger | Tobias B. Huber

**CHAPTER OUTLINE**



**KEY POINTS**

- The glomerulus represents a functional and integrated syncytium of four types of glomerular cells, which together ascertain glomerular filtration.
- Together, podocytes and glomerular endothelial cells allow for a size- and charge-selective glomerular filtration due to their specialized three-dimensional structure, extensive glycocalyx coating, and the coordinated synthesis of the unique glomerular basement membrane.
- Mesangial cells provide structural support of the glomerular capillaries, regulate glomerular filtration, and maintain glomerular endothelial health.
- Parietal epithelial cells build the Bowman's capsule to prevent leakage of the primary urine filtrate to the tubulointerstitium, contribute to glomerular scarring, and are thought to constitute a potential reservoir for podocytes in development, maturation, and eventually in adulthood.
- The hallmarks of diseases related to primary podocyte injury of genetic or autoimmune origin are proteinuria (often nephrotic range), foot process effacement, podocyte hypertrophy, and depletion.
- Crosstalk between glomerular cell types attenuates and/or perpetuates glomerular injury.
- Most forms of glomerular injury result from humoral and cellular immunologic mechanisms to which the glomerulus reacts by basic responses such as cellular proliferation, changes in glomerular cell phenotypes, and increased deposition of extracellular matrix.

## GLOMERULAR CELL ANATOMY AND INJURY RESPONSE PATTERNS

Loss of protein into the urine (proteinuria), especially albumin (albuminuria), is the hallmark of glomerular disease and an important prognostic marker for a wide variety of kidney diseases, including the numerically and economically increasing challenge of diabetic nephropathy.[1] Albuminuria is also an independent risk factor for cardiovascular mortality.[2] Therefore, understanding the pathophysiology of albuminuria and therapeutic approaches to its modification has major clinical and health economic significance.

The kidney of a healthy 70-kg adult filters approximately 180 L of plasma per day. Filtration and urine production takes place in the smallest functional unit of the kidney, called the nephron. The ultimate site of filtration is located at the beginning of the nephron in the renal corpuscule. The renal corpuscule (Fig. 4.1) is composed of the glomerulus, a network (tuft) of capillaries, which is surrounded by parietal epithelial cells (PECs) of Bowman's capsule (BC), and is thereby separated from the tubular system. As described and depicted in detail in Chapter 3, blood enters the glomerulus at the vascular pole through an afferent arteriole of the renal circulation and is drained into an efferent arteriole. The unique resistance of these arterioles generates a high pressure within the capillary convolute of the glomerulus, ultimately driving the ultrafiltration of a primary urinary filtrate through the glomerular filtration barrier into Bowman's space with an effective filtration pressure of approximately 50 mm Hg.[3]

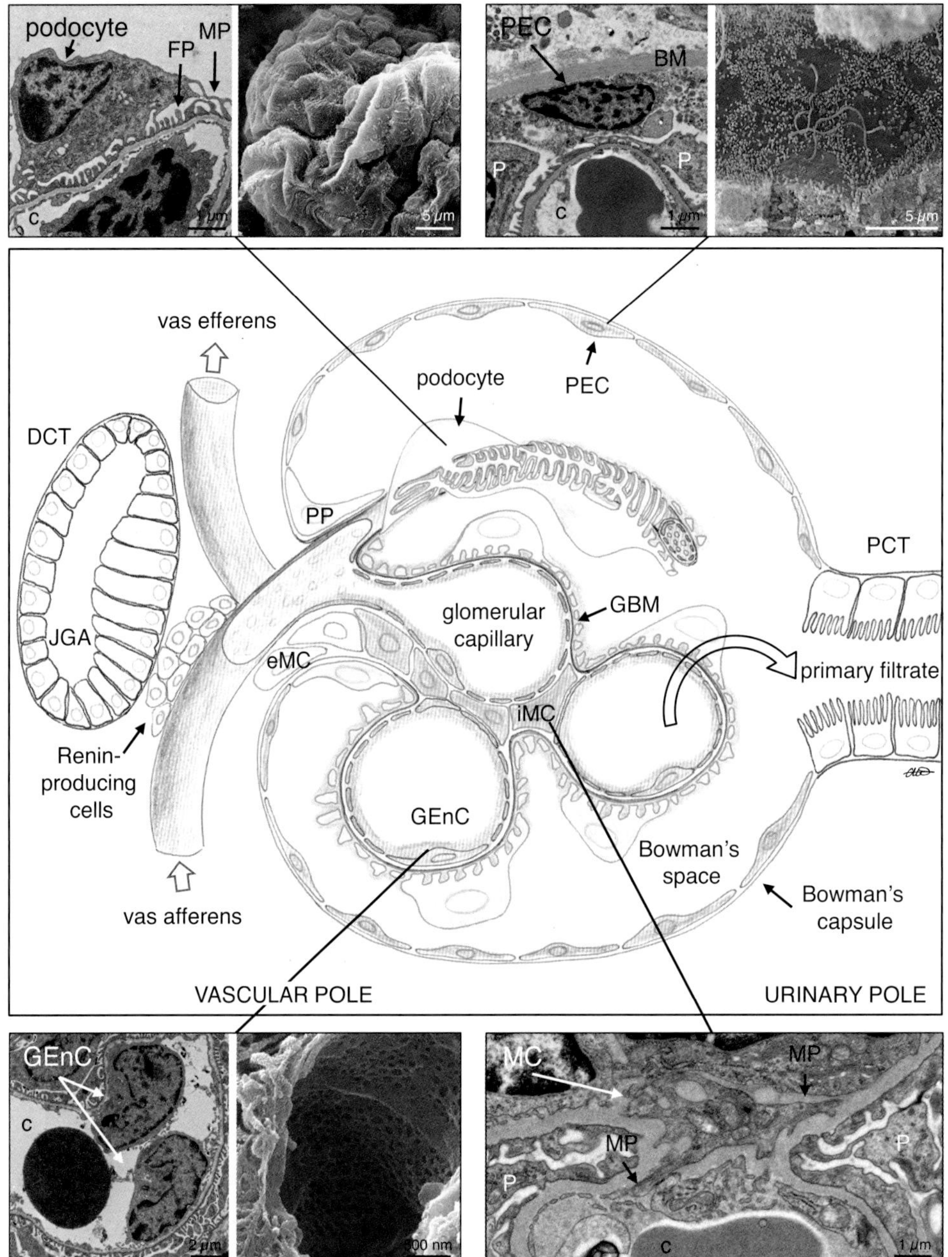


**Fig. 4.1 Scheme of the glomerulus depicting the localization of the four resident glomerular cell types.** The four types are podocytes, parietal epithelial cells (PEC), glomerular endothelial cells (GEnC), and mesangial cells (MC). Transmission and scanning electron micrographs show the typical ultrastructure of the glomerular cells. *BM,* Bowman's membrane; *c*, capillary lumen; *DCT*, distal convoluted tubule; *eMC*, extraglomerular mesangial cell; *FP*, foot process; *GBM*, glomerular basement membrane; *JGA*, juxtaglomerular apparatus; *iMC*, intraglomerular mesangial cell; *MP*, major process; *P*, podocyte; *PCT*, proximal convoluted tubule; *PP*, parietal podocyte. (All transmission electron microscopy and scanning electron microscope are from Oliver Kretz, Hamburg, Germany.)

Tracer studies point to a charge selectivity favoring the filtration of positively charged solutes.[4,5] Furthermore, an electrokinetic model of filtration has been proposed. In this model, filtration pressure establishes a streaming potential across the glomerular filtration barrier with Bowman's space being more negatively charged than the endothelial lumen. This might establish a retrograde electrophoretic field that acts opposite to diffusive and convective fluxes and tends to exclude negatively charged macromolecules away from the glomerular filtration barrier in the course of active filtration.[6] The primary urine exits the renal corpuscule at the urinary pole to be further processed to final urine in the downstream tubular system. While water and small molecules such as glucose, salt, and amino acids freely pass across the glomerular filtration barrier, a partial impermeability to large molecules, such as albumin, into the primary urine is maintained. The degree of fractional albumin filtration has been a matter of debate, but more recent two-photon in vivo imaging studies indicate values for a glomerular sieving coefficient of 0.02–0.04 for albumin filtration into the primary urine, which for the most part is reabsorbed by the proximal tubule.[7] This partial impermeability to large molecules is achieved by a highly complex interplay of two types of glomerular cells: the visceral epithelial cells (podocytes) and the glomerular endothelial cells, which ultimately compose the three-layered glomerular filtration barrier (podocyte—the 250–400 nm thick glomerular basement membrane [GBM]—endothelial cell). The GBM is composed of several types of extracellular matrix (ECM) macromolecules (laminin, type IV collagen, the heparan sulfate proteoglycan agrin, and nidogen), which produce an interwoven meshwork thought to impart both size-selective and charge-selective properties.[8] Finally, intraglomerular mesangial cells (MCs) occupy the space between the glomerular filtration barrier to provide structural support. As specialized pericytes, MCs indirectly participate in filtration by reducing the glomerular surface area by contraction and are also thought to participate in matrix turnover and innate immune function.[9] Although all glomerular cells form a functional and integrated syncytium, in this chapter each component is described in brief.

*Clinical Relevance*

The glomerulus is a functional syncytium of four cell types, which interact in physiologic and also pathologic situations, thereby perpetuating and extending the site of glomerular injury.

## PODOCYTES

### STRUCTURE

Podocytes are highly differentiated, mesenchymal-derived cells.[10] An apicobasal polarity axis allows for podocyte orientation between the urinary space and the GBM.[11] Podocytes reside in the urinary space and embrace the glomerular capillaries with their flat cell body, from which they extend long-branching major processes. Major processes give rise to secondary processes (often called foot processes), which interdigitate in a zipper-like fashion with secondary processes of neighboring podocytes[12] (Fig. 4.2). Foot processes attach podocytes to the underlying ECM of the GBM by specific proteins, such as adhesion receptors, including integrins, syndecans, vinculin, talin, and dystroglycan.[13] Foot processes are interconnected by slit diaphragms, which represent highly sophisticated cell–cell contacts that form an adjustable, nonclogging barrier through which glomerular filtration occurs. Although the term "diaphragm" implicates a thin-layered sieve, recent studies revealed that the slit diaphragm is composed of multiple layers of flexible transmembrane molecules to limit the passage of macromolecules.[14] Structurally, the slit diaphragm combines components of several types of cell–cell junctions, including tight, adhesion, neuronal, and gap junctions. Proteins from tight (ZO-1, JAM4, occludin, and cingulin) and adherens junctions (P-cadherin, FAT1, and the catenin family of proteins) are associated with the immunoglobulin superfamily members nephrin and neph1.[15] Nephrin and neph1 form the core component of the slit diaphragm by a bipartite assembly with neph1 molecules spanning the lower part of the slit close to the GBM and nephrin molecules positioned in the apical side.[14] The stomatin protein family member podocin (NPHS2) helps anchor nephrin to the plasma membrane and generates a signaling hub in lipid rich membrane compartments, e.g., for the $Ca^{2+}$-permeable transient receptor potential channel (TRPC) 6[16]—that might translate mechanical tension to ion channel action and cytoskeletal regulation.[17] On their intracellular C-terminal parts, nephrin and neph1 are associated with several signaling adaptor molecules and scaffold proteins linking the slit diaphragm to the actin cytoskeleton.[14,18] In general, the podocyte cytoskeleton is highly elaborate. The podocyte cell body and major and secondary processes contain vimentin-rich intermediate filaments that assist in maintaining cell shape and rigidity. Large microtubules form organized structures along major processes. Foot processes contain long actin fiber bundles that run cortically and contiguously to link adjacent podocytes. Actin, α-actinin-4, and myosin form a contractile system in foot processes, which is regulated by the interplay of the actin binding proteins synaptopodin[19] and α-actinin-4 with rho GTPases. This well-orchestrated actin and microtubule cytoskeleton ensures the high plasticity of the podocyte process network.[20,21] The apical surfaces of podocytes are covered by the surface sialomucin podocalyxin,[22] whose highly negative charge functions to keep adjacent foot processes separated, thereby keeping the urinary filtration barrier open.[23]

### FUNCTION

The main podocyte function is to build, maintain, and regulate the three-layered glomerular filtration barrier.

1. **The synthesis of the mature GBM** requires the crosstalk of podocytes with endothelial cells.[24] Podocytes and endothelial cells both secrete laminin 111 and type IV collagen α1α2α1 in GBM development and the final laminin 521 isoforms after maturation. However, only podocytes secrete type IV collagen α3α4α5 of the fully mature GBM.[25]
2. **Podocytes maintain the glomerular filtration barrier** by secreting survival factors such as angiopoietin-1 (Angpt1, which binds to Tie2 on glomerular endothelial cells [GEnC] and MCs),[26] normosialylated angiopoietin-like-4 (which binds to integrin αVβ5 on GEnC),[27] vascular endothelial growth factor A (binds to vascular endothelial growth factor receptor 2 [VEGFR2] on GEnC),[28] and stromal derived factor 1 (which binds to CXCR4 on GEnC)[29]; these factors exert paracrine effects across the filtration barrier on glomerular endothelial and MCs supporting their respective migration, differentiation, and survival.[30]
3. **Podocytes stabilize the glomerular filtration barrier** by expressing cell–matrix adhesion receptors such as integrin α3β1, which connects laminin 521 in the GBM through various adaptor proteins to the intracellular actin cytoskeleton or integrins α2β1 and αVβ3, α-dystroglycan, syndecan-4, and type XVII collagen.[31]
4. **Podocytes regulate glomerular filtration**[32] by presumably compressing the GBM through their adhesion to the GBM and the tensile forces of their cytoskeleton, which in turn reduces the permeability to macromolecules.[33] Furthermore, they regulate glomerular filtration through the formation of the slit diaphragm and by sensing the glomerular filtration pressure by a mechanoreceptor complex situated at the slit diaphragm.[34]

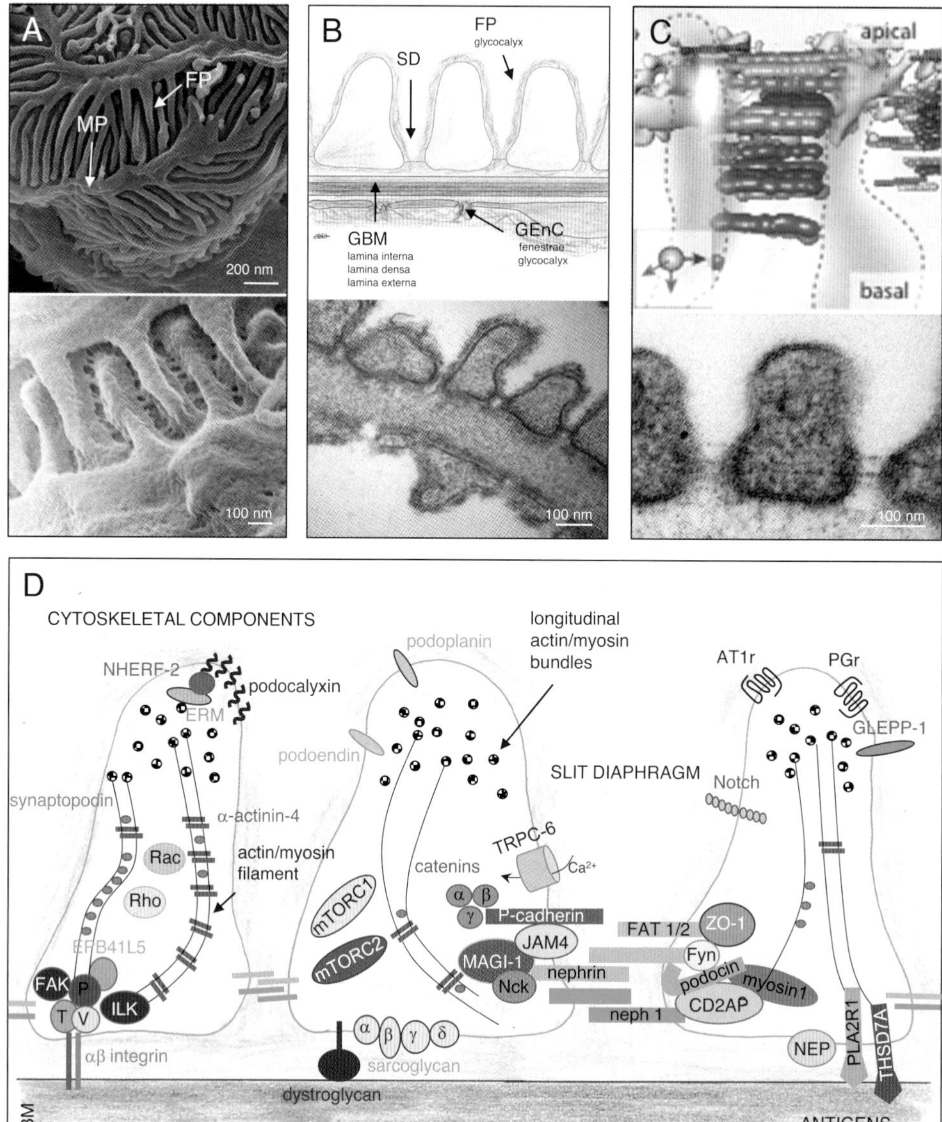


**Fig. 4.2 Anatomy of the glomerular filter.** (A) Scanning electron microscopy (SEM) of podocyte major processes (*MP*) and secondary interdigitating foot processes (*FP*). (B) Scheme and transmission electron microscopy (TEM) of three-layered glomerular filtration barrier consisting of (1) podocyte FPs covered by a glycocalyx, the specialized cell–cell contact called slit diaphragm (*SD*) connecting the interdigitating foot processes; (2) the three-layered glomerular basement membrane (*GBM*) consisting of podocyte-derived lamina interna, the podocyte/endothelial cell–derived lamina densa, and the endothelial-derived lamina externa; and (3) the glomerular endothelial cells (*GEnC*) with the large fenestrae and thick glycocalyx. (C) Scheme of the typical sagittal view of two FPs, showing three layers of ~25 nm long strands that are attributed to neph1 (*blue*, and 5 IG repeats) and one layer of ~40 nm long strands that represent nephrin (*red*, and 9 IG repeats). (D) Scheme of podocyte FP proteins constituting the (1) FP cytoskeleton (actin/myosin filaments, the actin binding proteins synaptopodin, α-actinin-4); (2) the podocyte adhesion complex (α3/β1 integrin connecting the GBM to focal adhesions constituted of focal adhesion kinase [*FAK*], integrin linked kinase [*ILK*], talin [*T*], vinculin [*V*], paxillin [*P*], FERM domain protein EPB41L5); (3) matrix interacting proteins dystroglycan, sarcoglycan; (4) the slit diaphragm (with the transmembrane proteins nephrin, neph1, FAT1/2, P-cadherin, and the scaffolding protein *ZO-1* [zonula occludens 1], the intracellular signaling hub constituted of podocin, *TRPC6* [transient receptor potential cation channel, subfamily C, member 6, and the connection to the actin cytoskeleton through *CD2AP*, CD2-associated protein, the cytoskeletal adaptor protein Nck, the multidomain scaffolding protein MAGI-1 and the junctional cell adhesion protein JAM4); (5) the negatively-charged sialoprotein podocalyxin (which is connected to the plasma membrane by NHERF-1 = Na+/H+ exchanger regulatory factor 1 and ERM [ezrin/moesin/radixin proteins]) localizes to the surface of the plasma membrane, as do GLEPP-1 (glomerular epithelial cell membrane protein-tyrosine phosphatase 1), podoplanin, and podoendin; (6) the G-coupled receptors angiotensin receptor 1 (*AT1r*) and prostaglandin receptor (*PGr*); (7) the podocyte antigens neutral endopeptidase (*NEP*); phospholipase A2 receptor 1 (*PLA$_2$R1*), and thrombospondin type 1 domain containing 7A (THSD7A) identified in antenatal and adult membranous nephropathy; and (8) intracellular signaling molecules *Rho, Rac, mTORC1/2* (mammalian target of rapamycin complex 1 and 2), *Notch,* and *Fyn*. ([A, C] All TEM and SEM from mouse glomeruli are from Oliver Kretz, Hamburg, Germany. [B] TEM from mouse glomerulus exhibiting glycocalyx from K. Betteridge, K. Onions, and R. Foster, Bristol, UK. [C] Scheme from Grahammer F, Wigge C, Schell C, et al: A flexible, multilayered protein scaffold maintains the slit in between glomerular podocytes. *JCI Insight* 1, 2016.[14] [D] Drawn by C. Meyer-Schwesinger.)

## PODOCYTE PATHOPHYSIOLOGY

Due to their molecular setup and localization, podocytes are permanently targeted by, and required to respond to, various physiologic and pathophysiologic stressors. If exposure is too excessive in time and dosage, this leads to complex adaptive and maladaptive intracellular changes, which then lead to the typical histopathologic sequence of foot process effacement, podocyte hypertrophy, and podocyte detachment from the GBM with loss into the urine (Fig. 4.3). Podocyte dysfunction results in clinical proteinuria and in a variety of glomerular responses, such as disruption of podocyte-endothelial crosstalk and activation of podocyte–parietal cell interactions culminating in glomerulosclerosis.

Over 80 pathways have been described that result in podocyte distress, including circulating factors, cell-surface signaling, metabolism, fibrosis, inflammation, and the actin cytoskeleton.[35] As a general theme, podocyte injury appears to involve reactivation of developmental programs such as those engaged by Notch,[36] Wnt,[37–40] and mTOR pathways.[41] Overactivation, imbalance, and impairment of these central intracellular signaling pathways disrupt normal podocyte energy metabolism[42] and protein homeostasis,[43] thus initiating a mostly irreversible dedifferentiation process.

### Podocyte Foot Process Effacement

Podocyte function largely depends on its complex three-dimensional cytoskeletal structure. The identification of over 50 monogenic causes of podocyte disease[44] has immensely increased our understanding of podocyte function and dysfunction. Regardless of the underlying disease, a characteristic and almost predictable response to podocyte injury is a change in shape, called effacement.[45] Numerous studies have shown that effacement is an active process, due to

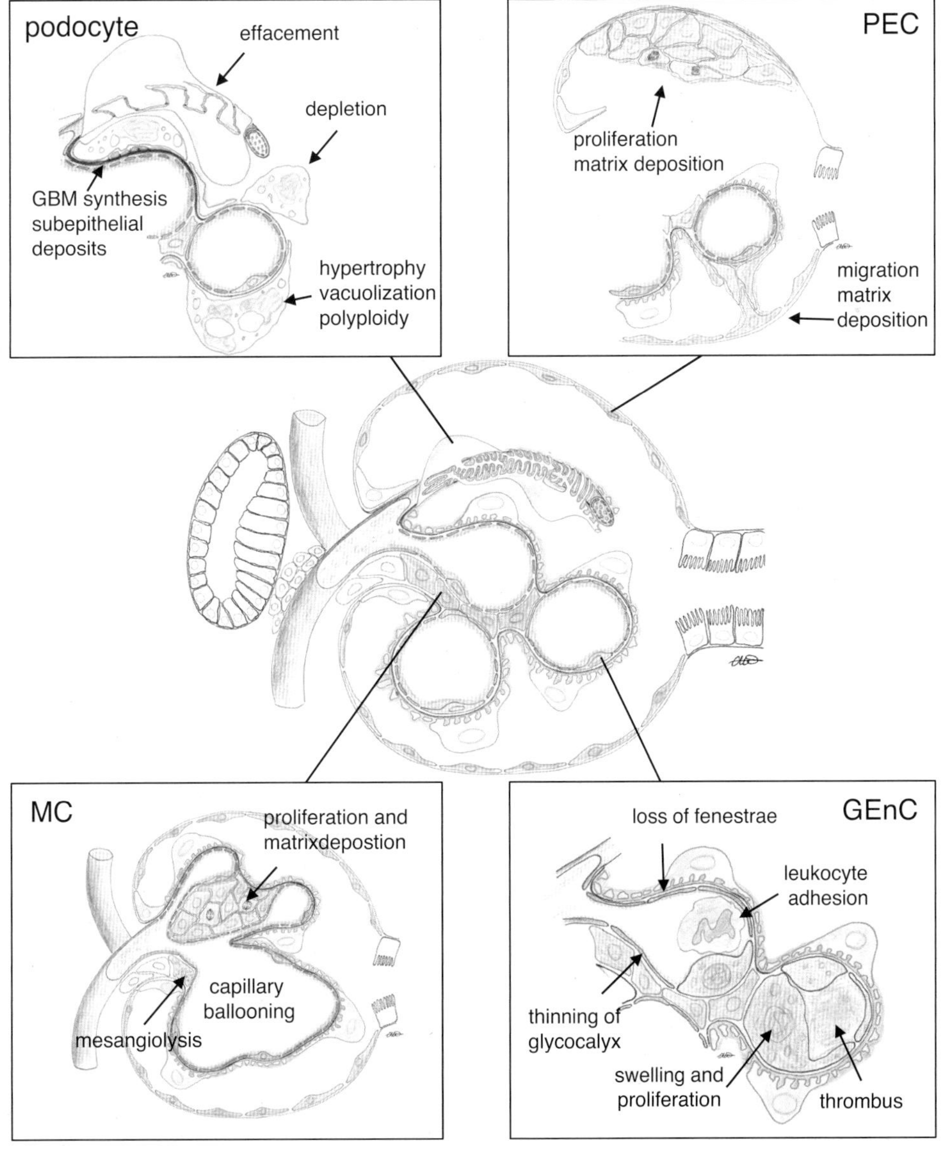


**Fig. 4.3 Pathophysiological reaction patterns of glomerular cells.** *GEnC,* Glomerular endothelial cell; *MC,* mesangial cell; *PEC,* parietal epithelial cell.

changes in the actin cytoskeleton of the podocyte, which forms the "backbone" of these highly specialized cells.[46] Further evidence that effacement is an active process is that in some instances it can be reversed, such as in treatment-responsive patients with minimal change disease (MCD). There has been debate as to whether effacement per se causes proteinuria, because proteinuria due to podocyte damage can occur independent of this change in shape. The relationship between podocyte foot process effacement and proteinuria has been questioned,[47] and it is clear that there is still much to learn about this long-recognized but still poorly understood ultrastructural phenomenon. Confusingly, effacement has also been reported (in the absence of proteinuria) in the protein-malnutrition state kwashiorkor,[48] suggesting that it may be a feature of hypoalbuminemia rather than of proteinuria per se. However, it is generally accepted that effacement is a manifestation of serious podocyte injury, and that this histologic finding implies changes in either slit diaphragm proteins (i.e., nephrin[49] and podocin[50]), actin binding and regulating proteins (i.e., α-actinin-4[51] and CD2AP[52]), podocyte attachment to the GBM (i.e., laminin β2[53] and integrin β4[54]), nuclear proteins (WT1[55] and LMX1B[56]), mitochondrial[57] and lysosomal[58] components, and/or other events, as genetic studies in humans suggest. Therefore teasing out precisely the biologic role of effacement in the development and maintenance of proteinuria may not be important.

### Podocyte Hypertrophy

Podocytes are terminally differentiated epithelial cells and unable to adequately proliferate to cover denuded areas of the GBM in situations of glomerular (GBM) distention (i.e., in case of renal hyperfiltration) or podocyte loss. Despite the virtual absence of podocyte mitosis and regeneration, current knowledge suggests that differentiated podocytes do have at least some capacity to adjust to an altered glomerular architecture by hypertrophy. Therefore hypertrophy can be adaptive in the setting of glomerular development, growth, and numerical minimal podocyte depletion (up to 20%), or can reflect a multifactorial maladaptive response of podocytes due to persistent injury promoting stimuli such as high glucose in diabetic nephropathy or subepithelial deposits in membranous nephropathy.[59] Recent findings highlight mammalian target of rapamycin (mTOR) and its downstream target, the translational repressor protein 4E-BP1,[60] as a key regulator of both adaptive and maladaptive podocyte hypertrophy, whereby the timing, extent, and duration of mTOR activation decide whether hypertrophy is adaptive or maladaptive.[41] Inhibition of mTOR by rapamycin in the setting of adaptive hypertrophy results in proteinuria and glomerulosclerosis, whereas inhibition of mTOR in the setting of maladaptive hypertrophy could be therapeutically beneficial.[61] Besides an imbalance of mTOR signaling pathways,[62,63] podocyte hypertrophy in response to hyperglycemia and stretch have been shown to be also mediated by the cyclin-dependent kinase inhibitor p27Kip1.[64,65] Hypertrophy in membranous nephropathy seems to originate in part from altered protein degradation and subsequent cytoplasmic accumulation of proteins.[66]

### Podocyte Depletion

Many podocyte diseases such as focal segmental glomerulosclerosis (FSGS), membranous nephropathy (MN), and diabetic kidney disease are accompanied by a progressive decline in overall kidney function, measured clinically by a decrease in glomerular filtration rate. This is largely due to glomerulosclerosis, with or without tubulointerstitial fibrosis. Patterns of glomerulosclerosis histologically include a segmental form (a portion of an individual glomerulus is scarred) and the more extensive global form (the majority of an individual glomerulus scars). Podocyte depletion is a major contributor to the development of age-related glomerulosclerosis in humans and rodents.[67–70] A decrease in podocyte number is one of the best predictors for a poor outcome in clinical diabetic kidney disease. A loss of 20% of podocytes is tolerated by rats[71] and mice[72] and is accompanied by MC proliferation and expansion. Segmental glomerulosclerosis ensues when 40% of podocytes are depleted, and global glomerulosclerosis occurs when the podocyte number is below 60% of normal.[71] There has been a long-standing debate on the underlying mechanisms for podocyte depletion, ranging from necrosis, apoptosis, and necroptosis to the detachment of viable cells from the GBM.[73] Interestingly, viable podocytes can be isolated from the urine of proteinuric patients, emphasizing the importance of podocyte detachment as a mechanism of podocyte depletion in glomerular diseases.

Studies have suggested that despite a lack of proliferation, podocyte number can be restored following certain therapies such as angiotensin-converting enzyme inhibition.[74] Despite compelling data, however, it remains unclear whether podocyte regeneration exists in renal aging or in pathophysiologic situations and, if podocyte regeneration exists, from what source of resident progenitor cells the novel podocytes originate.[75] Possible sources discussed might be progenitor cells derived from glomerular parietal epithelial cells[76] and/or cells of renin lineage,[77] although further studies are needed to fully validate these findings.

### Podocyte-Related Mechanisms of Proteinuria

Proteinuria is the clinical hallmark of podocyte injury, ensuing from a disruption of their most important biologic function, which is namely to limit the passage of plasma proteins into the urinary space. In general, any kind of injury affecting podocyte function results in proteinuria, either selective as albuminuria (mostly loss of the 60-kDa protein albumin) or nonselective as global proteinuria (loss of a multitude of proteins over 60 kDa of size, including immunoglobulins of 150 kDa) in case of major breakdown of the glomerular filtration barrier. Genetic studies and animal studies have demonstrated that podocyte-dependent proteinuria originates from at least six distinct mechanisms.

**Mechanism 1:** Alteration of the slit membrane as the size- and charge-selective barrier to proteins through hereditary or acquired defects of one or more structural slit diaphragm proteins, such as nephrin or podocin, leads to increased passage of proteins across this barrier. Either an absolute decrease in slit diaphragm protein levels or a change in their subcellular location is associated with proteinuria. Moreover, given the complex interplay between proteins comprising the slit diaphragm, a change in one slit diaphragm protein often leads to a cascading dysfunction of one or more of the other proteins.[78]

**Mechanism 2:** Alteration of the podocyte cytoskeletal network either through mutations of structural proteins and adaptor proteins or through an imbalance of signaling through actin-regulating enzymes and of converging signaling pathways culminate in enhanced or decreased actin polymerization, ultimately leading to proteinuria through a loss of the complex three-dimensional structure and flexibility of the podocyte cytoskeleton.

**Mechanism 3:** Although no known hereditary mutations of podocalyxin have been described, loss of podocalyxin results in reduced negative surface charge of podocyte processes and proteinuria.[23]

**Mechanism 4:** Podocyte depletion (i.e., through loss of adhesion)[79] results in denuded GBM areas through which proteins escape.

**Mechanism 5:** Alteration in GBM composition by podocytes through increased secretion of ECM proteins is typically observed in membranous and diabetic nephropathy. These ECM proteins are laid down along the GBM and eventually lead to the characteristic thickening of the GBM in these diseases.[80] The altered ECM composition leads to secondary changes (loss) in negative charge to the GBM, thereby enabling increased passage of proteins. In addition, increased production and secretion of reactive oxygen species and metalloproteinases from podocytes leads to degradation of the GBM and proteinuria.

**Mechanism 6:** Effect on the glomerular endothelial cell whose survival is dependent in part on the VEGFA produced and secreted from podocytes.[81] A decrease in production by podocytes, such as when podocyte number decreases, leads to secondary apoptosis of glomerular endothelial cells, which in turn is accompanied by a decrease in resistance of this layer of the glomerular filtration barrier.

## MESANGIAL CELLS

### STRUCTURE

MCs are divided into intraglomerular and extraglomerular MCs. MCs are mainly derived from the metanephric mesenchyme[82] and migrate into the cleft of the comma and S-shaped bodies as well as the maturing glomerulus under the chemotactic control of platelet-derived growth factor B[83] and the survival factor VEGF, both secreted from the progenitors of podocytes and GEnC.[84] In the mature glomerulus, MCs constitute the central stalk and are in continuity with the extraglomerular mesangium and the juxtaglomerular apparatus. Extraglomerular MCs are in close connection to afferent and efferent arteriolar cells by gap junctions, allowing for intercellular communication.[85] MCs are highly branched with processes extending in all directions. First, MCs have major processes that contain abundant bundles of microfilaments, microtubules, and intermediate filaments.[86] These major processes contain actin, myosin and α-actinin, and connect MCs with anchoring filaments to the GBM opposite podocyte foot processes and at paramesangial angles, giving them contractile properties.[87] Second, MCs have abundant microvillus-like projections arising from the cell body or from the major processes. Within the cell body microfilament bundles are less frequent and the perinuclear region is free of microfilaments.[86] MCs are in direct contact with GEnC without an intervening basement membrane on the capillary lumen side, where the cell membranes of both cell types interdigitate.[88] MCs do not express highly cell-specific markers; however, they express genes that classify MCs as a special form of microvascular pericytes.[89] MCs are positive for vimentin and desmin.

### FUNCTION

MCs, together with their matrix, form a functional unit with GEnC and podocytes.[9]

1. MCs are required for the development and for the mechanical (structural) support of glomerular capillary loops.[90,91] Mechanical support is in part mediated by attachment of MCs to the carboxy-terminus globular domain of laminin α5 in the GBM.[92]
2. MCs regulate the glomerular capillary flow and ultrafiltration surface and hence the fine-tuning of glomerular filtration by cell contraction at the single nephron level.[93] Contraction of MCs is regulated by vasoactive substances[94] and is dependent on the calcium signaling response and membrane permeability.[94,95] Relaxation of MCs, on the other hand, is mediated by paracrine factors, hormones, and cyclic adenosine monophosphate (cAMP), with a role for growth factor priming.[94]
3. MCs are responsible for the homeostasis of the mesangial matrix through synthesis and degradation of their own matrix components (type IV collagen α1α2, type V collagen, laminin fibronectin, proteoglycans [heparan and chondroitin sulfate, decorin, and biglycan], entactin, and nidogen).[83,96–98] The mesangial matrix provides structural support to the glomerulus[9] and regulates the behavior of MCs, such as growth and proliferation,[99] partly by binding and sequestering growth factors and thereby influencing their activation and release.[9] Furthermore, the mesangial matrix signals to MCs in response to mechanical stretch.[100]
4. MCs are sources and targets of growth factors, cytokines, and vasoactive agents.[9] For example, MCs produce transforming growth factor (TGF)-1, VEGF, and CTGF[9] in response to capillary stretching resulting from glomerular hypertension. MC proliferation, along with eicosanoid and matrix production, is influenced by PDGF-B,[101] PDGF-C,[102] fibroblast growth factor (FGF),[96] hepatocyte growth factor (HGF),[97] connective growth factor (CTGF),[103] epidermal growth factor (EFG),[104] and TGF-β.[98]
5. MCs keep the mesangial space free from accumulating macromolecules, which trespass from the capillary lumen through the fenestrated endothelium. For this purpose, MCs phagocytose glomerular basal lamina or immune complexes formed at or delivered to the glomerular capillaries,[105,106] and aid neutrophils to phagocytose apoptotic cells.[107] Macromolecules are removed by both receptor-dependent and independent mechanisms, depending on the size, charge, concentration, and affinity for MC receptors.[9,108]
6. MCs are involved in the tubuloglomerular feedback by communicating with vascular smooth muscle cells over gap junctions.[109]
7. MCs maintain endothelial health and function by cross communication via the mediators and pathways described above.

### PATHOPHYSIOLOGY

As of yet, no discrete primary disease of MCs has been described. However, MCs react to changes of the intravascular milieu (soluble factors), immunoglobulin deposition, and to changes affecting GEnC and podocytes. Glomerular MC injury is commonly associated with mesangial immune deposit formation in IgA nephropathy, lupus nephritis, and Henoch-Schönlein purpura (also designated as IgA vasculitis).[110] Even though IgA nephropathy primarily affects the mesangium (mesangioproliferative disease), it produces marked hematuria and proteinuria, indicating changes in the permeability of endothelial cells, GBM, and podocytes. The myriad biologic responses of MCs to injury range from mesangiolysis to mesangial hypercellularity, mesangial expansion, and the promotion of glomerular inflammation (see Fig. 4.3). Overall, these biologic responses of MCs to injury are elicited (1) by structural abnormalities of the basement membrane that are either acquired (as in diabetes mellitus) or genetic (as in Alport syndrome); (2) by factors either released from neighboring MCs in an autocrine manner; or (3) from circulating factors affecting MCs in an endocrine manner.

**Mesangiolysis** is defined as a dissolution or attenuation of mesangial matrix and degeneration of MCs either by apoptosis or lysis without obvious damage to the capillary basement membranes. The matrix swells, loosens, and eventually dissolves; the MCs may show swelling and vacuolization. Mesangiolysis results in a dilation of the glomerular capillary lumina, as the mechanic support of capillaries provided by the anchoring points of MCs to the GBM is lost.[111] Loss of intraglomerular MCs can be replenished by ingrowth of extraglomerular MCs.[112]

**Mesangial hypercellularity** is characterized by an increase of intraglomerular MC number by hypertrophy, proliferation, and migration[82] as in IgA nephropathy. In cases where the proliferative insult is limited, mesangial hypercellularity is limited by apoptosis and phagocytosis of these apoptotic cells by adjacent MCs or by infiltrating inflammatory cells.[113]

**Mesangial expansion** is a term characterizing the widening of the intraglomerular mesangium. Mesangial expansion occurs in diabetic nephropathy by excess mesangial matrix production such as fibronectin by MCs[114] or by decreased degradation of the mesangial matrix by metalloproteinases.[115] Mesangial expansion also occurs through the deposition of immune complexes, light chains, amyloid, fibrils, complement, and worn-out GBM material.[116]

**Promotion of glomerular inflammation:** Injured MCs generate reactive oxygen species, proinflammatory activators such as platelet activating factor,[117] cytokines (TNF-α, CSF-1 and IL-6), and chemokines,[9] thus sustaining and perpetuating glomerular inflammation.

## GLOMERULAR ENDOTHELIAL CELLS

### STRUCTURE

The glomerular microcirculation is unique as unlike other capillary circulations, glomerular capillaries are highly permeable to water and small solutes while maintaining relative impermeability to macromolecules potentially even as small as albumin.[118] GEnCs are highly specialized cells that form the continuous inner layer of glomerular capillaries. GEnCs have a particular embryonic origin, with the majority of GEnCs arising by vasculogenesis from mesenchymal precursors in combination with a minority of GEnCs arising from introgression of existing vessels.[119,120] In the mature glomerulus, the nucleus of GEnCs bulges into the capillary lumen. The cytoplasm of GEnCs is 200 nm thin at its slimmest areas and punctuated by numerous fenestrae. The fenestrae of GEnCs are the largest in comparison to the fenestrae of endothelial cells of other organs and represent circular pores of 60 to 80 nm in diameter, which cover 20% of the glomerular endothelial surface.[121] Under special fixation conditions, a diaphragm is visible that spans the fenestrae.[122] GEnCs are covered by a 200- to 400-nm–thick glycocalyx, which represents a negatively charged gel-like surface structure of proteoglycans with their covalently bound polysaccharide chains named glycosaminoglycans (GAGs), glycoproteins, and glycolipids. The main carbohydrate constituents are heparan sulfate (HS), chondroitin sulfate (CS), and hyaluronan (HA), bound to the HA binding surface proteins such as CD44. The glycocalyx is attached to the GEnC by charge–charge interactions,[123] rendering GEnC very sensitive to hemodynamic factors[118] such as shear stress.[124] The glycocalyx covers the fenestrae and the interfenestral domains of GEnC equally[125]; however, the thickness of the glycocalyx differs between fenestrated and nonfenestrated GEnCs.[126] The GEnC fenestrae are plugged by a high content of HA[126] and are considered to be a key component of the glomerular permeability barrier. Like other endothelial cells, GEnCs express the specific markers platelet endothelial cell adhesion molecule 1 (PECAM1, CD31), intercellular adhesion molecule 2 (ICAM2), VEGFR2, growth factor receptor Tie2, von Willebrand factor, and vascular endothelial (VE)-cadherin (CD144).[127]

### FUNCTION

1. GEnCs are involved in the GBM production together with podocytes but to a lesser extent than podocytes as seen in mice with podocyte-specific type IV collagen α5 chain deletion (Alport model), which exhibit marked thinning and alteration of the GBM.[128,129]
2. GEnCs contribute to the hydraulic conductivity of the glomerular filtration barrier through GEnC fenestrations,[130] which are formed in response to VEGF.[127,131]
3. GEnCs contribute to the size and charge selectivity of the glomerular filtration barrier by the endothelial surface lining composed of the membrane-bound glycocalyx and the loosely bound endothelial cell coat.[126,132] The glycocalyx adds to size and charge selectivity, most likely by forming a mesh-like structure of negatively charged HSs and the less charged HA,[133] as infusion of enzymes that degrade the glycocalyx increases albumin passage through the GEnC.[134]
4. The glycocalyx of GEnC protects against protein leakage, inflammation, and coagulation.[134] With properties like a hydrogel, the glycocalyx acts as a size barrier to protein. With the high negative charge of polyanions, the glycocalyx electrically repels proteins.[135–137] GAG-degrading enzymes such as chondroitinase and heparanase alter glomerular permeability.[138,139] The gel-like, antiadhesive properties of the glycocalyx preclude the interaction of leukocytes with adhesion molecules.

### PATHOPHYSIOLOGY

GEnCs are primarily targeted in several forms of vasculitis, in hemolytic uremic syndrome, and in preeclampsia.[140] Even though GEnCs are primarily affected, these conditions are associated with mesangiolysis and proteinuria, indicating endothelium-dependent changes in MCs and podocytes. Injury of the GEnC induces the release of vasoactive substances and changes the composition of the endothelial glycocalyx and endothelial adhesion molecules, resulting in a net prothrombotic state (see Fig. 4.3).[141,142] Furthermore, GEnCs hypertrophy, proliferate, go into apoptosis, and detach, further accelerating the thrombosis of glomerular capillaries.[141] Experimental models indicate that recovery from glomerular injury is dependent on GEnC angiogenesis.[143–145] Visualization of GEnC injury remains challenging. Morphologic signs of GEnC injury are swelling of the cell body, thinning of the glycocalyx,[146,147] loss of fenestrations, and enhanced expression of adhesion markers such as CD34[148] and E-selectin (CD62E), an adhesion receptor for leukocytes. GEnC injury has been demonstrated to arise from an altered crosstalk with podocytes.

> ***Clinical Relevance***
> Proteinuria is a hallmark of glomerular injury and should usually initiate a workup by a nephrologist to identify eventual underlying genetic, inflammatory, toxic, tumor, and infectious causes.

**Endotheliosis:** Glomerular capillary endotheliosis describes the swelling of GEnC with the deposition of fibrous material in and beneath GEnC, a condition typically seen in preeclamptic glomerular injury. The net result of GEnC swelling and deposition of fibrous material is capillary occlusion.

**Changes of glycocalyx and their sequelae** because the glycocalyx functions as a molecular scaffold and binds (1) circulating proteins such as growth factors and chemokines; (2) proteins involved in cell attachment, migration, and differentiation; and (3) proteins involved in blood coagulation and inflammation, alterations of the glycocalyx are central to the pathology of GEnC and glomerular injury. GEnC injury induces changes both in the thickness and in the molecular composition of the endothelial glycocalyx. Changes in glycocalyx thickness are mainly due to upregulation of glycocalyx-degrading enzymes such as hyaluronidase, heparanase, and proteinases, thereby shedding glycocalyx fragments into the glomerular circulation. Alteration of glycocalyx composition such as decreased levels of HA or changes in HS sulfation patterns change the antiadhesive and anticoagulative properties of the glycocalyx. In total, loss of glycocalyx thickness and glycocalyx modification result in enhanced permeability of the filtration barrier to proteins, inflammation, and coagulation.[134]

**Mediation of the inflammatory reaction:** Injured GEnCs release vasoactive substances (nitric oxide and endothelin), which regulate glomerular filtration. Furthermore, GEnCs promote glomerular inflammation by attracting leukocytes by means of shed glycocalyx fragments and by expressing leukocyte adhesion molecules. Upon perturbation of the glycocalyx, these adhesion molecules become unmasked and allow leukocyte interactions with the endothelial surface. HS of the glycocalyx acts as a direct ligand for L-selectin.[149] Upon stimulation with inflammatory stimuli, GEnCs increase the expression of HS domains,[150] which facilitates leukocyte extravasation.[151] The endothelium binds chemokines, which regulate the extravasation of leukocytes upon a chemo attractant gradient.[152] Alterations of glycocalyx composition ensue in enhanced binding of chemokines by way of positive charge interactions.[153]

## PARIETAL EPITHELIAL CELLS

PECs are derived from the metanephric mesenchyme and line Bowman's capsule of the renal glomerulus. During the vesicle and comma stages in glomerular development, PECs share a common phenotype with the other epithelial cells of the later glomerulus—namely, podocytes and proximal tubular cells. With the formation of the Bowman's space in the S-shaped body, the phenotypes of PECs, podocytes, and proximal tubular cells diverge. In the mature kidney, PECs are a heterogeneous population of cells as PECs at the urinary pole maintain features of proximal tubular cells and PECs at the vascular pole maintain features of podocytes and are therefore termed parietal podocytes.[154]

### STRUCTURE

PECs resemble squamous epithelial cells with their small thin cell body ranging in thickness from 0.1 to 0.3 μm and increasing to 2.0 to 3.5 μm at the nucleus. The surface of some PECs is lined by microvilli and cilia in a range from zero to two cilia per cell.[155] They are interconnected by "labyrinth-like" delicate tight junctions located at the apical surface, which consist of claudin-1, -2, -3, K-cadherin (Cdh6), kidney specific cadherin (Cdh16), occludin, and zonula-occludens 1 (ZO-1).[156] PECs have a simple cytoskeleton with filaments at the basal membrane region.[157] They express the intermediate filament protein cytokeratin 8.[158] PECs have the transcriptional prerequisite to express podocyte markers.[159] The expression of podocyte proteins is negatively regulated through protein degradation[159] and by microRNA-193a,[160] which represses Wilms tumor protein 1 (WT1) mRNA levels.[161] PECs express the transcription factor Pax2 from the paired box family, which is involved in regulating genes governing proliferation, cell growth, and survival. Furthermore, PECs can be differentiated from podocytes through the expression of EPH receptor A7 belonging to the ephrin receptor subfamily, ladinin (a proposed anchoring filament that is a component of basement membranes), and scinderin (a calcium-dependent protein that regulates cortical actin networks).[162]

### FUNCTION

1. PECs at the vascular pole constitute a potential reservoir for podocytes in glomerular development, maturation,[72,163] and eventually even adulthood.[164]
2. PECs presumably form the basement membrane of Bowman's capsule, which consists of laminin-111, laminin-511,[165,166] type IV collagen α1 α2, and type IV collagen α5 α6[167,168]; however, this is not definitely proven.
3. PECs prevent the leakage of urine from the urinary space into the periglomerular compartment.[169]

### PATHOPHYSIOLOGY

To date there is no evidence for glomerular injuries related to primary PEC injury. However, PECs have taken the center stage of attention for their contribution to glomerular diseases such as rapid progressive glomerulonephritis (RPGN) and

FSGS. Activated PECs exhibit a larger cytoplasm and larger rounder nuclei. Further signs of PEC activation are a de novo expression of CD44[170] and the phosphorylation of signaling molecules.[171,172] The predominant reactions of PECs to glomerular injury are proliferation, migration, and synthesis of a matrix that results in the development of crescents or glomerular tuft scars (see Fig. 4.3). There is an ongoing debate whether PECs serve as an intrinsic fixed progenitor population to replenish podocytes or proximal tubular progenitor cells in glomerular regeneration.[173] PECs respond to injury with the expression of podocyte markers such as synaptopodin and WT1.[174,175]

**Proliferation and migration:** Activation of PECs as in rapid progressive glomerulonephritis (RPGN) results in their proliferation and the formation of extracapillary proliferations, also called cellular glomerular crescents, of which PECs are the major constituents.[176] Crescent formation is not only the result of PEC proliferation but also in part the result of the transdifferentiation of PECs to myofibroblasts,[170,177] the deposition of matrix, and the infiltration with inflammatory cells. Crescents can occlude the tubular outlet of the glomerulus, resulting in entire nephron degeneration,[178] and are generally associated with a poor prognosis. PEC proliferation is usually associated with glomerular endothelial cell, GBM, or podocyte injury, as leakage of plasma components such as fibrin from the blood circulation is a strong inducer of PEC proliferation.[179,180] Additionally, PEC depletion initiates PEC proliferation and crescent formation.[181] Migration of PECs from Bowman's capsule onto the glomerular tuft is the predominant reaction of PECs in focal segmental glomerulosclerosis (FSGS).[176] In this scenario, PECs are activated and invade the glomerulus at focal areas via adhesions connecting sclerotic capillary areas with Bowman's capsule.[182] PECs are then present in the sclerotic regions[183,184] and can be visualized by staining for CD44.[185]

**Matrix deposition:** Thickening of Bowman's capsule due to matrix production can be observed in aging glomeruli[186] and glomerular injury. Matrix deposition by PECs is observed in glomerular crescents and in the sclerotic glomerular tuft regions in FSGS. PECs that migrate to the glomerular tuft produce and deposit ECM proteins. The composition of this ECM is related to that of Bowman's capsule[183] and contains specific heparan sulfate moieties of heparan sulfate proteoglycans.[187]

## GLOMERULAR CELL CROSSTALK

Podocytes, glomerular endothelial cells, MCs, and PECs with their respective matrix must be considered as a functional unit, in which every cell plays its part in ensuring proper glomerular filtration. As a consequence, 30 years of isolated cell-type–based research is now being replaced by systems biology approaches to integrate the role and contribution of each individual glomerular cell type for the proper glomerular biology and function. Recent advances have demonstrated that glomerular cell crosstalk is the prerequisite for normal glomerular development and health. Furthermore, primary injury of one glomerular cell type affects the other glomerular cell types by crosstalk. Clinical and experimental observations suggest that crosstalk exists between podocytes and GEnC, between GEnC and MCs, between MCs and podocytes, and finally between podocytes and PECs (Fig. 4.4).

### PODOCYTES AND GLOMERULAR ENDOTHELIAL CELLS

Podocytes are essential for GEnC development and maintenance, and the first glomerular cell crosstalk to be identified was the cross communication from podocytes to GEnC. Podocytes secrete vascular growth factors, such as VEGFA, which bind to its cognate receptor VEGFR2 on GEnC, a crosstalk crucial for GEnC health[81] and which, if disrupted, results in glomerular injury. A tight control of VEGFA levels is essential for correct glomerular barrier function, and even though other podocyte-specific proteins such as the transcription factor Pod1/Tcf21[188] or the TGF-β activated kinase 1 (Tak1)[189] have been shown to be essential for GEnC development and health, it remains to be established whether this is a direct effect or a consequence of altered VEGFA levels. Podocyte progenitors also express ephrin B2, another vascular growth factor, and by this might contribute to EphB4 receptor expressing GEnC development and health.[190] Angptl is expressed by both podocytes and MCs and binds to the tyrosine-protein kinase receptor (Tie2/Tek) expressed on GEnC. This crosstalk is thought to stabilize the glomerular capillaries, as mice with induced deletion of Angptl at embryonic day 10.5 exhibit dilated capillary loops and disrupted subendothelial GBM structures and reduced MCs, whereas podocytes appear intact.[191] Podocytes also secrete the chemokine CXCL12 (SDF1), which binds to its receptor CXCR4 on GEnC, a crosstalk important for the formation of glomerular capillaries.[29]

Despite their importance in glomerular development and maintenance, some podocyte-derived signals have been shown to perpetuate or attenuate GEnC injury in pathologic settings. Therefore, enhanced circulation of endothelin-1 or enhanced podocyte expression of endothelin-1, which binds in a paracrine way to the endothelin receptor A on GEnC, mediates mitochondrial oxidative stress and dysfunction in adjacent GEnC.[192,193] Furthermore, endothelin 1 induces podocytes to release the GEnC glycocalyx-degrading enzyme heparanase, contributing to GEnC injury in diabetic nephropathy.[194] Another example for disease-perpetuating crosstalk is the podocyte-specific expression of angiopoietin-2, which results in GEnC apoptosis without affecting podocytes.[195] The CXCL12/CXCR4 crosstalk enhances GEnC injury in diabetic nephropathy[171] and in Shiga toxin–associated hemolytic uremic syndrome.[172] A GEnC-protective crosstalk with podocytes was suggested for podocyte-derived angiopoeitin-like-4 (Angptl4), which is structurally similar to angiopoietins but does not signal over Tie2. Angptl4 was suggested to protect GEnC from oxidative injury in nephrotic syndrome by binding to αVβ5 integrins.[27] A protective reverse signaling from GEnCs to podocytes has been demonstrated for vasohibin secreted from GEnC, which is thought to counteract VEGFA signaling in situations of pathologic elevated VEGFA levels such as in diabetic nephropathy.[196]

### GLOMERULAR ENDOTHELIAL CELLS AND MESANGIAL CELLS

The fate of MCs and GEnCs is tightly linked. Both communicate directly at the paramesangial areas of glomerular capillaries, where their plasma membranes are in direct contact. Even though MCs secrete a multitude of factors in vitro, which could affect GEnC, only a few MCs secreted factors have been identified that partake in GEnC crosstalk in

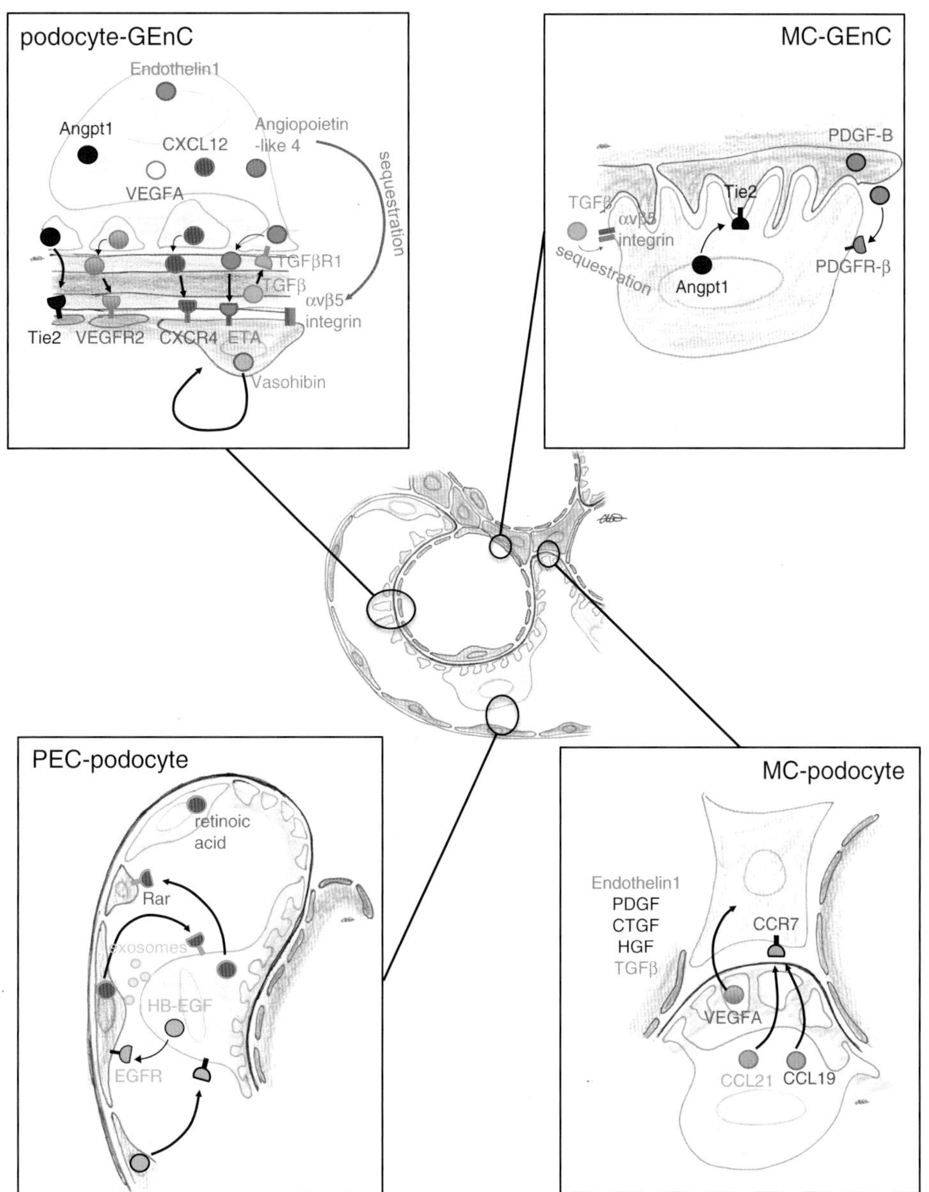


**Fig. 4.4 Examples of intra glomerular crosstalk.** *Angpt1,* angiopoietin 1; *CTGF,* connective tissue growth factor; *CXCL12,* C-X-C chemokine ligand 12, *CXCR4,* chemokine receptor 4; *EGFR,* epidermal growth factor receptor; *Eta,* endothelin-1 receptor A; *HB-EGF,* heparin-binding epidermal growth factor–like growth factor; *HGF,* hepatocyte growth factor; *PDGF,* platelet-derived growth factor; *PDGF-B,* platelet-derived growth factor B; *PDGFRβ,* platelet-derived growth factor receptor β; *Rar,* retinoic acid receptor; *Tie2,* tyrosine-protein kinase receptor 2; *TGFβ,* transforming growth factor β; *TGF-βR1,* transforming growth factor-β receptor 1; *VEGFA*, vascular endothelial growth factor A; *VEGFR2*, vascular endothelial growth factor receptor 2.

vivo. This is in part a consequence of the lack of glomerular endothelial cell and also of MC-specific gene targeting strategies in vivo, which is a prerequisite for such investigations. Endothelial derived PDGF-B and its receptor PDGFR-β, localized on MCs, have been demonstrated to be of crucial importance for the development and maintenance of glomerular capillaries.[9] Consequently, injury and loss of GEnCs—for example, due to toxin- or antibody-related GEnC injury—results in decreased PDGF-B levels and MC death (mesangiolysis). MCs maintain endothelial health and function through integrin α5β8-dependent sequestering of TGF-β, thereby reducing the amount of active TGF-β.[197] Furthermore, like podocytes, MCs synthesize angiopoietin-1, which binds to its receptor Tie2 on GEnC[191] to stabilize the vasculature.

## PODOCYTES AND MESANGIAL CELLS

It is not clear to date at which sites podocytes communicate with MCs and the in vivo evidence of podocyte–MC crosstalk is scarce. Nonetheless, experimental data and clinical observations in several hereditary forms of nephrotic syndrome due to mutations in podocyte-specific genes[198] suggest that such a communication exists. For example, in glomerular development, mutations in podocyte genes such as the transcription factor Pod1/tcf21,[199] phospholipase Cε[200] laminin α5,[92] and Wilms tumor antigen[55] result in a failure of MCs to migrated into glomeruli. The podocyte-specific deletion of collagen type IV α3 (Alport mouse) results in enhanced expression of integrin α1 by MCs,[201] possibly affecting MCs cell adhesion and cell signaling at the GBM. The chemokines CCL19 and CCL21, generated by podocytes, bind to CCR7 on MCs and are thought to regulate local MC migration and adherence to the GBM.[202] Also, a decrease of VEGFA secretion from podocytes results in mesangiolysis,[30] supporting the idea of a podocyte-MC crosstalk, which is of relevance in glomerular development. In glomerular injury, experimental data support a communication of podocytes with MCs, although it cannot be excluded that the observed effects on MCs in podocyte injury are not the result from altered PDGF-B levels related to podocyte-dependent GEnC injury. Several signaling pathways might be involved in podocyte-MC crosstalk in the setting of injury, such as endothelin 1, PDGF, CTGF, HGF, and TGF-β.[28]

### PODOCYTES AND PARIETAL EPITHELIAL CELLS

Under physiologic conditions podocytes and PECs are in close proximity at the vascular pole, where transitional cells called parietal podocytes carry both the characteristics of PECs and podocytes.[154] Another theoretical site of cross communication is across Bowman's space, where the apical membranes of podocytes and PECs can overcome the physical separation given by the primary filtrate and touch. Controlled depletion of PECs results in transient proteinuria with focal podocyte foot process effacement,[181] and podocytopenia is associated with PEC hyperplasia,[203] suggesting interdependence of both cells. Communication between PECs and podocytes could also ensue from the uptake of podocyte-derived proteins from the primary urine by PECs.[204] Furthermore, podocytes release exosomes to the urine[205,206] that in turn could affect PECs.

In glomerular injury, podocytes are in close contact to PECs by bridges formed between the capillary tuft and Bowman's capsule[207] and in intraglomerular crescents, of which they are both constituents.[176,208] In glomerulonephritis, mathematical multiscale modeling studies[209] and experimental data suggest that podocyte and PEC cross communication might regulate proliferation of both cells and regulate regeneration of podocytes from PECs. Proliferation of both cell types and thereby crescent formation was shown to be dependent of the heparin-binding EGF-like growth factor (HB-EGF), which is de novo expressed by podocytes and PECs in RPGN and the EGF receptor, which is found on both cells.[210] Lineage tracing experiments suggest that podocyte regeneration in glomerulonephritis occurs from renal progenitor cells located in Bowman's capsule[76] and that this process can be enhanced by retinoic acid.[211] Therefore, retinoic acid synthesized in glomeruli promotes renal progenitor cells to differentiate toward a podocyte phenotype.[212]

## COMMON MECHANISMS OF GLOMERULAR DISEASES

There appear to be several basic responses of the glomerulus to injury such as cellular proliferation, changes in glomerular cell phenotypes, and increased deposition of extracellular matrix. Any cause of severe glomerulonephritis (GN) can cause a crescent formation (typical for rapid progressive GN), which is composed of parietal cells,[181,213] podocytes,[208] and inflammatory cells.[214,215] Most forms of glomerular injury result from immunologic mechanisms,[216–220] which include both humoral and cellular components. Only little is known about the origin of the etiologic agents that induce the immunologic mechanisms, with the exception of infection-related forms of disease such as beta-hemolytic streptococci in poststreptococcal GN, or hepatitis C and hepatitis B virus in cryoglobulinemic membranoproliferative GN. However, it is likely that drugs, toxins, and other infectious agents induce similar immune responses that result in GN via shared common pathways.

The humoral response is often a T helper cell 2 (Th2) mediated response resulting in B-cell activation, antibody generation and deposition, and complement activation. Immunoglobulin and complement component deposition is found in most human glomerular diseases, suggesting that the humoral response is crucial in the development of glomerular injury, which has been the rationale for the use of therapeutic B-cell depletion in various glomerular diseases. There are three patterns of immunoglobulin deposition in the glomerulus: (1) immune deposits at the GBM and in the subepithelial space (underneath podocytes) are typical for membranous nephropathy and usually do not initiate a strong inflammatory reaction, as the deposits are separated from the circulation by the GBM; (2) immune deposits in the subendothelial space (lupus nephritis and membranoproliferative GN); or (3) in the mesangium (IgA nephropathy and lupus nephritis), on the other hand, initiate multiple inflammatory processes. The final pattern of immunoglobulin deposition is determined by the biologic properties of the immunoglobulins (IgG subtype) deposited, the absolute amount of immunoglobulins deposited, and lastly the mechanisms whereby the deposits are formed. Deposition of the complement-fixing IgG1 or IgG3 subtypes ensues in stronger glomerular injury than deposition of IgA or IgG4, which both poorly activate complement.[221] Principally, antibody–antigen binding that takes place within the glomerulus to glomerular self or nonself antigens (termed in situ binding) induces stronger complement activation than when preformed immune complexes are deposited in glomeruli. Typical glomerular self-antigens are the phospholipase A2 receptor ($PLA_2R1$)[222] and thrombospondin type-1 domain-containing 7A (THSD7A)[223] in membranous nephropathy, or the noncollagenous domain of the α3 chain of type IV collagen known as the Goodpasture antigen.[224,225] Nonself antigens localize to glomerular capillaries by mechanisms such as charge affinity for glomerular structures or pure passive trapping in the glomerular sieve in the form of the antigen alone (termed as planted antigens) or as antigen-antibody complexes formed outside the kidney. In situ antibody binding to planted nonself antigens is typical in lupus nephritis to DNA nucleosome complexes[226,227] or in IgA nephropathy to abnormally glycosylated IgA.[228] Glomerular deposition of preformed immune complexes to nonself antigens has been demonstrated in early childhood MN, where immune complexes containing cationic bovine serum albumin are deposited,[229] or in hepatitis C virus–associated membranoproliferative GN where hepatitis C virus–containing cryoglobulins are deposited.[230] There is little experimental evidence that immunoglobulin binding alone induces significant tissue injury, except for when the antibodies bind to podocyte antigens such as nephrin[231,232] of the slit membrane or to THSD7A.[233] Of note, severe inflammation can occur with only little antibody deposited, as in antineutrophil cytoplasmic antibody (ANCA)-associated GN.

The cellular response is a largely T helper cell 1 (Th1)-mediated response characterized by the infiltration of circulating mononuclear cells such as lymphocytes and macrophages into glomeruli and the formation of crescents. Neutrophils are the earliest cells to be found in inflamed glomeruli in human biopsies and are strong inducers of glomerular injury.[234] Animal studies demonstrate that their strongest attractants to inflamed glomeruli are interleukin (IL) 8 and complement factor C5a,[235] bound to the glomerular endothelium via HS proteoglycans.[150,236] Neutrophils are activated by phagocytosis of immune complex aggregates, which induces them to undergo a respiratory burst with generation of reactive oxygen species such as hydrogen peroxide. Hydrogen peroxide interacts with the neutrophil cationic enzyme myeloperoxidase (MPO) to halogenate the glomerular capillary wall.[237] Furthermore, neutrophils store other cationic enzymes such as proteinase 3 (PR3), elastase, and cathepsin G, which upon release further degrade the glomerular capillary wall. Lastly, neutrophils release extracellular traps, web-like DNA structures expulsed from nuclei with adherent histones, proteases, peptides, and enzymes, which show a modest contribution to glomerular injury in anti-GBM glomerulonephritis,[238] but could be more injurious in ANCA-associated GN and lupus nephritis.[239]

Macrophages are typically found in glomerular lesions with crescents and serve as effector cells of both humoral and cell-mediated forms of immune glomerular injury, because their localization to inflamed glomeruli is induced by interactions with immunoglobulins through their Fc receptors and through chemokines, such as CCLS, and CCL2. Similar to neutrophils, macrophages generate direct tissue injury by the release of oxidants and proteases. Additionally, they release tissue factor to induce glomerular fibrin deposition and crescent formation and TGF-β to induce the synthesis of the extracellular matrix, culminating in glomerular sclerosis.[240]

T cells are rarely found in injured glomeruli except for GNs primarily mediated by macrophages such as crescentic GN. T-cell–mediated glomerular injury is mostly the result from released chemokines and the recruitment of macrophages.[241] However, ovalbumin-specific CD4+ and CD8+ T cells together can induce glomerular injury in transgenic mice that express the antigen ovalbumin in podocytes.[204] Among the known T-cell subtypes, there is strong experimental evidence for the importance of T helper cell 17 (Th17) in crescentic GN.[242,243] Th17 cells produce and secrete IL-17 A, IL-17F, IL-21, IL-22, which promotes inflammation by directly causing tissue injury and enhancing secretion of proinflammatory cytokines and chemokines by resident cells. This results in augmented infiltration of leukocytes, in particular neutrophils, recruited by CXCL5[244] to the affected kidney where they induce further inflammation and injury.[245] The kidney-infiltrating Th17 cells are partly recruited from the gut.[246]

Platelets are present in glomerular lesions in which intracapillary thrombosis is involved, typically observed in thrombotic microangiopathies and antiphospholipid syndrome. Platelets are important players in the formation of thrombi and in the recruitment of leukocytes to the inflamed glomerulus.[247] In addition, they release factors that enhance glomerular permeability to proteins, enhance immune complex deposition,[248–250] and induce MC proliferation (PDGF)[251] and MC sclerosis (TGF-β).[252]

Dendritic cells (DCs) are restricted to the tubulointerstitium and are absent from glomeruli.[253] However, proteins that pass the glomerular filter are captured by renal DCs or reach the renal lymph nodes by lymphatic drainage[254] to induce immune tolerance[255] to innocuous proteins, such as food antigens or hormones, or to stimulate infiltrating T cells to produce proinflammatory cytokines.[204]

The site of glomerular injury, especially when glomerular cell is involved, determines whether the patient has an inflammatory or a noninflammatory injury (Fig. 4.5). Because glomerular endothelial and MCs are in contact with circulating factors such as complement and inflammatory cells, they are prone to react to injury via a principally more dramatic inflammatory response. In contrast, PECs and podocytes are separated by the GBM from the circulation; thus podocyte injury is rarely associated with activation of circulating inflammatory cells. Clinically the distinction between inflammatory and noninflammatory injury is crucial for the adequate diagnosis and management of patients. The clinical characteristics of inflammatory injury are hematuria with dysmorphic erythrocytes with or without red blood cell casts and occasional leukocyturia. Inflammatory injury is accompanied by varying degrees of proteinuria, which ranges from mild to nephrotic range proteinuria and a normal

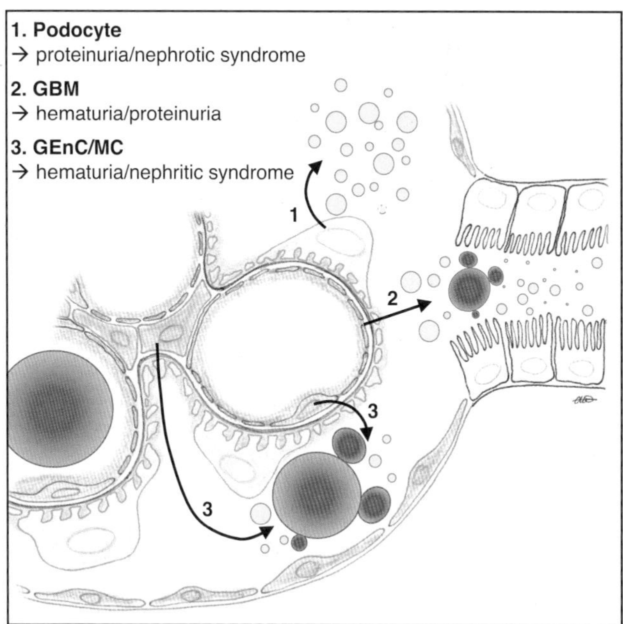


**Fig. 4.5 The clinical presentation reflects the localization of glomerular injury.** Injury of podocytes results in proteinuria (*yellow droplets*) eventually leading to the clinical manifestation of nephrotic syndrome. Injury of the glomerular basement membrane (*GBM*) commonly results in proteinuria and hematuria with dysmorphic erythrocytes. Injury of glomerular endothelial cells (*GEnC*) and mesangial cells (*MC*) usually leads to hematuria with dysmorphic erythrocytes and only little proteinuria.

or reduced glomerular filtration rate, depending on the severity of disease. Morphologically, inflammatory injury is characterized by glomerular hypercellularity that results from proliferating resident glomerular (mostly MCs and PECs) and from infiltrating hematopoietic cells (mostly neutrophils and macrophages), phenotype change, and visible structural injury. Glomerular injury arises from the release of inflammatory substances from infiltrating hematopoietic cells and from glomerular cells or from the impairment of protective mediators such as complement factor H[256] or complement factor H–related protein 5[257] as negative regulators of the complement pathway. The release of inflammatory substances, such as cytokines, growth factors, proteases, products resulting from complement activation (C5a, C5b-9), vasoactive agents, and oxidants,[217,258,259] initiates thrombosis, necrosis, and crescent formation which, if extensive, leads to the serious clinical condition of rapid progressive glomerulonephritis. Noninflammatory lesions usually involve podocytes and are termed podocytopathies. They are characterized by proteinuria and (if proteinuria is extensive) nephrotic syndrome (a triad consisting of proteinuria over 3.5 g/day, edema, and hypertriglyceridemia) without hematuria.

> ***Clinical Relevance***
> The site of glomerular injury determines the clinical picture. Whereas involvement of podocytes presents as glomerular injury with proteinuria or nephrotic syndrome, involvement of glomerular endothelial cells, the GBM, and/or MCs typically presents with microhematuria or nephritic syndrome.

## MECHANISMS OF INJURY IN COMMON PODOCYTOPATHIES

The most common causes of noninflammatory immune-mediated glomerular injury are minimal change disease (MCD), primary focal segmental glomerulosclerosis (FSGS), and membranous nephropathy (MN). All three entities exhibit a dramatic increase in glomerular permeability with little to significant structural abnormalities by light microscopy in common. These diseases are classified as podocytopathies, as podocytes are thought to be the primary glomerular cell affected in the pathogenesis. In contrast, "nontraditional" podocyte diseases include diabetic kidney disease, human immunodeficiency virus nephropathy, amyloidosis, Fabry disease, membranoproliferative glomerulonephritis, and postinfectious glomerulonephritis. Diabetic nephropathy (covered in detail in Chapter 39) is the numerically and economically most important form of progressive kidney disease worldwide, involving the podocyte, endothelial, and MCs with a perturbation of glomerular cell crosstalk. The inciting causes of each podocyte disease differ, and therefore each disease affects podocytes in different ways; in turn, the response to injury in each disease differs, leading to different histologic and clinical manifestations. Yet, regardless of the inciting causes and their mediators, several common clinical and pathologic responses occur in podocyte injury, as highlighted earlier—namely, hypertrophy, foot process effacement, loss, and proteinuria.

### MINIMAL CHANGE DISEASE AND FOCAL SEGMENTAL GLOMERULOSCHLEROSIS

Characteristics of MCD: In MCD the glomerulus is per definition mostly normal by light microscopy with absence of complement or immunoglobulin deposition. In light of the histologic "minimal changes," pathologic diagnosis is primarily based on electron microscopic evaluations of podocytes, which exhibit foot process effacement, microvillous transformation, and vacuolization. The absence of glomerular sclerosis differentiates MCD from FSGS. MCD typically presents as a steroid-sensitive nephrotic syndrome (SSNS), contrasting with FSGS, which often presents with steroid-resistant nephrotic syndrome (SRNS). Whether steroid-resistant MCD exists as its own disease entity, or whether steroid resistance in histologic MCD represents an early form of FSGS is a matter of debate, considering the high rate of sampling error on renal biopsies, possibly missing present (but rare) glomeruli with sclerosis. It is likely that patients with MCD can progress to FSGS due to a consistent pathologic agent.[260]

Characteristics of FSGS: FSGS is a generic term for a histologic injury pattern defined by segmental glomerular consolidation into a scar that affects some but not all glomeruli with a wide range of etiologic interpretations. FSGS describes both a disease characterized by a primary podocyte injury (primary FSGS), and a lesion that occurs secondarily in any type of chronic kidney disease (secondary FSGS).[261] There is abundant evidence that classical FSGS is the consequence of podocyte loss in experimental models,[262] which is accompanied by proliferation and migration of PECs to the glomerular tuft (both discussed earlier in the chapter). The underlying causes or mechanisms of FSGS are broadly considered as hereditary/congenital and sporadic/acquired in nature. Primary FSGS presents either with SSNS if triggered by causative circulating agents that increase the permeability of the glomerular filtration barrier (as discussed later) or with SRNS in case of an underlying genetic cause. Secondary FSGS, on the other hand, is associated with nephron loss, drug toxicity, or viral infections and rarely presents with nephrotic syndrome, but is steroid resistant.

#### PATHOPHYSIOLOGIC CONCEPTS OF MCD AND PRIMARY FSGS

MCD and primary FSGS might represent different histologic patterns of the same disease entity. At least there is a significant overlap in the factors causing these podocytopathies, which are the following:

1. **Soluble serum factors:** Based on experimental data, soluble serum factors are thought to be causative in MCD and FSGS, as nephrotic plasma has direct cellular effects on cultured podocytes[263] or in single perfused kidneys.[264] Many efforts have been undertaken to unravel "the increasing or missing circulating permeability factor" in SSNS and SRNS.[265] Roles have been indicated for TNFα,[266,267] circulating cardiotrophin-like cytokine factor 1 (member of the IL-6 family), circulating hemopexin,[268,269] and the soluble urokinase-type plasminogen activator receptor (suPAR)[270] in the development of nephrotic syndrome.[271] These factors, however, need further verification in the context of human disease activity,[272,273] disease specificity,[274–276] and therapeutic effects.[277]

2. **Immune dysfunction:** Considerable clinical and experimental evidence point toward an immune dysfunction on the T- and B-cell side in MCD. Clinically, MCD is not only very responsive to steroids but also to rituximab,[278,279] a monoclonal antibody against plasma cell CD20, and a significant association of HLA-DQA1 (a major histocompability complex class II) missense coding variants exists.[280] Additionally, MCD is associated with Hodgkin disease and with allergies.[281] On the experimental side, mice develop proteinuria if they receive CD34+ peripheral stem cells from MCD patients[282] or following the injection of the supernatant derived from T cells or from peripheral blood mononuclear cells.[283] T- and B-cell dysfunction is further suggested by a different DNA methylation pattern of Th0 cells in MCD patients,[284] an altered Th17/regulatory T-cell balance,[285] and an upregulation of T-cell–derived IL-13 in patients[160] that can cause proteinuria and foot process effacement in rats.[286,287] Further pointing toward an immune dysfunction as the origin of nephrotic syndrome is the finding that abatacept, an antibody challenging the CD80 (B7-1)–CTLA-4-axis has been shown to reduce proteinuria in FSGS,[288] an effect requiring still further confirmation.[289–291] Recent experimental findings have given rise to the idea of a disease-specific expression of CD80[288,292] or of the expression of a hyposialylated form of angiopoietin-like-4 by podocytes, which might contribute to glomerular disease.[293–295]
3. **Genetic inheritance:** Familial cases are rare in MCD, making genetic causes for MCD unlikely. Nonetheless, whole-exome sequencing in SSNS patients revealed mutations in epithelial membrane protein 2 (EMP2), which is involved in regulating endocytosis and transcytosis,[296] shedding new light into possible causes for podocyte disruption in SSNS. There are changes in expression patterns of podocyte-specific transcripts[297] and proteins[298] in MCD, but it is difficult to determine whether these are cause or effect. There is strong evidence for genetic causes leading to FSGS. Inheritance of genetic causes of primary FSGS may be autosomal dominant or recessive, with a subset of autosomal recessive SRNS presenting as congenital nephrotic syndrome. The biologic functions altered in podocytes by the gene mutations involved in FSGS are broad, ranging from cytoskeletal regulation, slit membrane function, lysosomal function, mitochondrial function, and attachment to the GBM.[44] In the late 1990s positional cloning of the gene responsible for congenital nephrotic syndrome of the Finnish type led to the identification of the archetypal podocyte-specific protein, nephrin.[49] This was rapidly followed by the identification of other proteinuric diseases linked to podocyte-specific single-gene disorders, including those affecting podocin,[50] Wilms tumor 1,[299] CD2AP,[300] α-actinin-4,[51] TRPC6,[301] phospholipase Cε1 (PLCE1),[200] WW and PDZ domain-containing 2 (MAGI2),[302] kidney ankyrin repeat-containing protein (KANK), and others.[303,304] In each of these conditions it is generally accepted that proteinuria results directly from the disruption of these constitutively expressed genes in the podocyte, leading to FSGS.

   It is becoming increasingly clear that monogenic inheritance of abnormalities in podocyte-specific genes is only one aspect of FSGS. Even though the amount of over 50 known mutations of podocyte genes involved in SRNS is steadily increasing, these mutations are rare and explain less than 30% of patients with hereditary cases and only 20% of patients with sporadic cases of FSGS.[44] Studies of the increased susceptibility of African Americans to FSGS have implicated variants of another gene expressed in podocytes, apolipoprotein L1 (APOL1).[305,306] Experimental expression of the APOL1 risk alleles in a podocyte specific manner demonstrated that these were causal for podocyte foot process effacement, proteinuria, and glomerulosclerosis.[307] Mechanistically, the risk-variant APOL1 alleles interfere with endosomal trafficking and block autophagic flux, ultimately leading to inflammatory-mediated podocyte death and glomerular scarring.[307] A key question for practicing nephrologists is whether podocyte-specific gene mutations or polymorphisms play a role as predisposing factors for the much more common "sporadic" forms of proteinuric disease. In human disease an opportunity to study the very earliest features of FSGS is afforded by studies of FSGS recurrence in transplanted kidneys; changes in podocytes can be seen in reperfusion biopsies and are predictive of full-blown FSGS recurrence.[308] Chapter 43 includes an in-depth discussion of inherited glomerular diseases.
4. **Altered posttranslational regulation of podocyte proteins:** Besides abnormalities in podocyte genes, altered posttranslational regulation of podocyte mRNA by small noncoding RNA molecules, termed microRNAs, have been shown to result in FSGS, such as the transcription factor Wilms tumor protein 1 (WT1) by microRNA-193a[161] or of Notch1 and p53 by microRNA-30.[309]

## MEMBRANOUS NEPHROPATHY

Membranous nephropathy is an autoimmune disease with the morphologic hallmarks of GBM thickening, granular staining for human IgG and complement components along the glomerular filtration barrier, and subepithelial (subpodocyte) electron-dense deposits by electron microscopy. Although this histologic pattern can arise from the deposition of preformed immune complexes as in lupus nephritis type 5 or from subepithelial antigen trapping in hepatitis B virus and hepatitis C virus–associated secondary forms of MN, primary MN is thought to be the consequence of in situ binding of autoantibodies to podocyte-expressed antigens. The concept that primary MN is an antibody-mediated disease has been supported by the discoveries of autoantibodies to podocyte membrane antigens such as neutral endopeptidase (NEP),[310] the phospholipase $A_2$ receptor ($PLA_2R1$),[222] and thrombospondin type 1 domain-containing 7A (THSD7A).[223] $PLA_2R1$ and THSD7A are targets for a malfunctioning immune system in 70% and 5% of adult cases, respectively, and NEP is important in a small number of neonates with MN caused by alloimmunization due to vertical transfer of antibodies from a genetically NEP-deficient mother.[221] $PLA_2R1$ polymorphisms influence the susceptibility to MN, and the association between certain HLA-DQA1 alleles and MN suggests that these HLA class II molecules could facilitate autoimmunity against $PLA_2R1$.[311] In contrast to $PLA_2R1$-associated MN, THSD7A-associated MN has a high coincidence of malignancy.[312,313] The direct pathogenicity of autoantibodies is suggested by the observations that $PLA_2R1$ or THSD7A autoantibodies are present in patients with a rapid recurrence of MN in renal transplants,[223,314,315] the finding that anti-$PLA_2R1$ antibody levels are associated with disease remission[316,317] and progression,[317–319] and the finding that MN can be induced in mice that normally express THSD7A on podocytes[320,321] by injection of human autoantibodies[233] or rabbit antibodies to THSD7A.[322] So far there is no proof that $PLA_2R1$-specific autoantibodies are pathogenic, related to the fact that rodents necessary for such studies normally do not express $PLA_2R1$ on podocytes. The role of complement in the pathogenesis of human MN remains unclear. First, the deposited IgG in idiopathic MN is typically of the noncomplement fixing IgG4 subtype. Second, in rodent models of MN, clinical and morphologic MN can be induced in the absence of detectable complement deposition,[233,322] as well as in rodents with genetic deficiency in complement components.[323,324] On the other hand, C3 and the membrane attack complex C5b9 are usually constituents of the deposits[325]; C5b9 inserts into the podocyte membrane and is transported across the cell[326] and excreted into the urine, where high levels of C5b9 can be measured in humans.[327] Experimental studies allow for an injurious as well as a protective function of C5b9. Sublytic C5b9 has been shown to induce podocyte injury by multiple pathways such as the activation of kinases, the induction of endoplasmic reticulum stress, and the production of extracellular matrix.[328] On the other hand, C5b9 enhances the ubiquitin proteasome system,[329] which supports a protective removal of damaged proteins.

## EFFECTS OF EXISTING THERAPIES ON PODOCYTES

The basis for therapy of primary nephrotic syndrome (reviewed in Chapter 33) is mostly of a supportive nature, including antihypertensive and antiproteinuric therapy and dietary recommendations.[330] Regrettably, no therapeutic approaches are currently available that specifically target podocytes in disease. However, several therapies have, in addition to their systemic effects, direct biologic actions on podocytes (i.e., pleiotropic actions), and these will be considered in the following sections.

### RENIN ANGIOTENSIN SYSTEM BLOCKADE

Blockade of the renin angiotensin system belongs to the standard supportive therapy regimen for primary podocytopathies with proteinuria and remains unchallenged. Systemic and glomerular overactivation of the renin angiotensin system (RAS) through its main effector angiotensin II is central to the pathogenesis of proteinuric glomerular diseases; levels of tissue angiotensin II and the angiotensin subtype 1 receptor are increased in glomeruli[331] and podocytes[332] in primary podocytopathies. Activation of RAS is detrimental to glomerular cells including podocytes as it promotes multiple trophic effects, such as apoptosis, ECM protein accumulation, reactive oxygen species production, oxidative stress, alteration in slit diaphragm proteins partly by epigenetic modulation of nephrin promoter methylation,[333] increased calcium influx through TRPC6 channels,[334,335] cell cycle inhibition, detachment, and inflammatory cytokine production.[332,336] Blocking the RAS with angiotensin-converting enzyme inhibitors, angiotensin 1 receptor (AT1R) antagonists, and mineralocorticoid receptor blockers reduces proteinuria resulting in renoprotection, an effect that is attributed to a reduction in glomerular hydrostatic pressure and an abolishment of the detrimental trophic glomerular effects mentioned earlier.[32] For these reasons, inhibition of the renin angiotensin aldosterone system is currently the standard of care for lowering proteinuria.

### GLUCOCORTICOIDS

Steroids are immunomodulatory drugs widely used in the treatment of proteinuric diseases, but their modes of action, especially in the noninflammatory forms of nephrotic syndrome such as MCD and primary FSGS, remain completely unknown. Glucocorticoid receptor (GR) expression is ubiquitous; therefore, these drugs could affect any glomerular cell type. It has been shown that GR-induced signaling pathways are functional in murine podocytes, having transcriptional and posttranscriptional effects on podocyte genes.[337] Initial reports in murine[338] and human[339] podocytes showed that dexamethasone had potent biologic effects directly on podocyte structure and function. These include limiting podocyte apoptosis,[340] induction of podocyte differentiation by restoring the actin cytoskeleton,[338] increasing levels of the transcription factors Kruppel-like factor 15 (KLF15),[341] and by preventing the downregulation of protective microRNA-30.[309] Specifically, the slit membrane protein nephrin is affected by steroids, as steroids enhance the transport of nephrin from the ER[342] and induce the phosphorylation of nephrin,[343] which is reduced in MCD[344] and important for the function of nephrin and therefore of the slit membrane.

### EVIDENCE FOR DIRECT ACTIONS OF IMMUNOSUPPRESSANTS ON PODOCYTES

The calcineurin inhibitors cyclosporine and tacrolimus are widely used in nephrotic syndrome, either alone or in combination with other therapies. Calcineurin is a $Ca^{2+}$-dependent phosphatase, which dephosphorylates nuclear factor of activated T cells (NFAT), a transcription factor. Dephosphorylation of NFAT initiates its cytoplasmic to nuclear translocation, resulting in an increased transcription of genes such as TRCP6,[345] whose gain of function mutations in podocytes induce FSGS.[301] In accordance, podocyte-expressed NFAT is a strong inducer of glomerulosclerosis in mice.[346] Besides their known immunomodulatory effects in T cells, calcineurin inhibitors affect the podocyte cytoskeleton by transcriptional downregulation of the earlier mentioned calcium channel TRPC6,[347] and by preventing the degradation of the actin-organizing protein synaptopodin[348] in an NFAT-independent manner. Together, these mechanisms appear to result in a stabilization of the podocyte actin cytoskeleton and direct reduction of proteinuria.

The specific anti–B-cell monoclonal antibody rituximab, increasingly thought to be effective in proteinuric diseases even when they are not all obviously immune mediated,[349] has been shown to have direct effects on podocytes, including stabilizing their actin cytoskeleton.[350] Although monoclonal antibodies are assumed to have very specific binding targets, they can also have "off-target" effects. In this case it seems that rituximab, as well as binding to the CD20 molecule that is its accepted molecular target, also binds to a podocyte protein called sphingomyelin phosphodiesterase acid-like-3b (SMPDL-3b) and this protein stabilizes the actin cytoskeleton.[350]

## IDENTIFICATION OF CANDIDATE THERAPEUTIC APPROACHES FOR THE FUTURE

End-stage renal disease constitutes an enormous burden of morbidity, both to patients who suffer a lifelong chronic disease and to health services that are challenged by high costs arising from dialysis and transplantation. Despite major advances over the past 15 years in unraveling genetic and biologic causes of podocyte dysfunction as the origin of most forms of nephrotic syndrome, glomerular target cell-directed therapies are still in their infancy. Especially in comparison to other specialties in medicine, only a few new drugs have been approved for renal failure in comparison to many new drugs for cancer therapy or for heart diseases. Nonetheless, the separation of monogenic causes of podocyte dysfunction from other causes is now used to stratify those patients in whom immunosuppression can be minimized due to low potential of success. Furthermore, the discovery of the genes involved in hereditary proteinuric disease unraveled critical (and in the future potentially drug able) pathways required for podocyte maintenance, for stabilization of the podocyte actin cytoskeleton and slit diaphragm, and for restoration of metabolic and mitochondrial function.[351] Several experimental approaches of recent years have aimed at finding podocyte-specific interventions, which stabilize the actin cytoskeletal backbone of podocyte foot processes and by this also of the slit diaphragm.[352–355] Targeting the metabolic and mitochondrial function in podocytes seems to be another therapeutic option for many forms of podocyte injury. Even though mTOR inhibition is known to induce proteinuria as a typical side effect,[356,357] inhibition of an overactivated mTOR pathway in the setting of metabolic super fluency, as in diabetic nephropathy, is beneficial for podocyte function and proteinuria.[61] Other examples with therapeutic potential targeting metabolic pathways include lipid lowering (e.g., statins),[358,359] antidiabetic agents such as thiazolidinediones (TZDs), or glitazones that activate the peroxisome proliferator-activated receptor $\gamma$(PPAR$\gamma$),[360–363] and manipulation of VEGF levels[364] or autophagy.[365]

## SUMMARY

Kidney diseases with glomerular involvement account for the vast majority of end-stage renal diseases. In the past two decades much has been learned about the glomerulus, a functional and integrated syncytium of four types of glomerular cells, which together ascertain glomerular filtration. Podocytes and GEnC comprise the glomerular filtration barrier. Together, both cells allow for a size- and charge-selective glomerular filtration due to their specialized three-dimensional structure, extensive glycocalyx coating, and synthesis of the unique GBM. MCs regulate glomerular filtration by means of contraction and release of vasoactive substances and maintain the health of glomerular endothelial cells. PECs, built Bowman's capsule to prevent leakage of the primary urine to the tubulointerstitium, can contribute to glomerular scarring, and are thought to constitute a potential reservoir for podocytes in development, maturation, and eventually in adulthood. A cell type–specific view of glomerular physiology and pathophysiology has enhanced our understanding of glomerular cell biology immensely in the past decades. However, the intricate interactions of glomerular cell types are getting more and more center stage attention as clinical and experimental observations demonstrate that the normal functioning of glomerular filtration requires a coordinated interaction of all four cell types and that injury of one glomerular cell type usually affects the others. Several clinical and experimental challenges and opportunities lie ahead. Identification, designing, and delivering glomerular cell specific therapeutic agents is actively being pursued, both to enhance efficacy and to reduce systemic side effects. Noninvasive diagnostic testing is being keenly studied, such as measuring glomerular cell products in the urine, and markers in the serum and urine, which will hopefully translate into clinical practice. The past two decades have witnessed phenomenal advances in understanding glomerular cell biology in health and disease, which hopefully soon translates into better therapeutic options for progressive glomerular and renal kidney disease.

## ACKNOWLEDGMENTS

The authors would like to thank Dr. Stuart Shankland and Dr. Peter Mathieson, who contributed to earlier versions of this topic review, and Dr. Pierre Ronco and Dr. William Couser for inspiring our chapter on "common mechanisms of glomerular injury."

 Complete reference list available at ExpertConsult.com.

## KEY REFERENCES

5. Farquhar MG, Wissig SL, Palade GE. Glomerular permeability. I. ferritin transfer across the normal glomerular capillary wall. *J Exp Med.* 1961;113:47–66.
10. Abrahamson DR. Structure and development of the glomerular capillary wall and basement membrane. *Am J Physiol.* 1987;253: F783–F794.
14. Grahammer F, Wigge C, Schell C, et al. A flexible, multilayered protein scaffold maintains the slit in between glomerular podocytes. *JCI Insight.* 2016;1.
16. Huber TB, Schermer B, Muller RU, et al. Podocin and MEC-2 bind cholesterol to regulate the activity of associated ion channels. *Proc Natl Acad Sci USA.* 2006;103:17079–17086.
19. Asanuma K, Yanagida-Asanuma E, Faul C, et al. Synaptopodin orchestrates actin organization and cell motility via regulation of RhoA signalling. *Nat Cell Biol.* 2006;8:485–491.
22. Kerjaschki D, Sharkey DJ, Farquhar MG. Identification and characterization of podocalyxin—the major sialoprotein of the renal glomerular epithelial cell. *J Cell Biol.* 1984;98:1591–1596.
25. Abrahamson DR, Hudson BG, Stroganova L, et al. Cellular origins of type IV collagen networks in developing glomeruli. *J Am Soc Nephrol.* 2009;20:1471–1479.
30. Eremina V, Cui S, Gerber H, et al. Vascular endothelial growth factor a signaling in the podocyte-endothelial compartment is required for mesangial cell migration and survival. *J Am Soc Nephrol.* 2006;17:724–735.
49. Kestila M, Lenkkeri U, Mannikko M, et al. Positionally cloned gene for a novel glomerular protein—nephrin—is mutated in congenital nephrotic syndrome. *Mol Cell.* 1998;1:575–582.
50. Boute N, Gribouval O, Roselli S, et al. NPHS2, encoding the glomerular protein podocin, is mutated in autosomal recessive steroid-resistant nephrotic syndrome. *Nat Genet.* 2000;24:349–354.
51. Kaplan JM, Kim SH, North KN, et al. Mutations in ACTN4, encoding alpha-actinin-4, cause familial focal segmental glomerulosclerosis. *Nat Genet.* 2000;24:251–256.
52. Kim JM, Wu H, Green G, et al. CD2-associated protein haploinsufficiency is linked to glomerular disease susceptibility. *Science.* 2003;300:1298–1300.

55. Pelletier J, Bruening W, Kashtan CE, et al. Germline mutations in the Wilms' tumor suppressor gene are associated with abnormal urogenital development in Denys-Drash syndrome. *Cell.* 1991;67:437–447.
57. Diomedi-Camassei F, Di Giandomenico S, Santorelli FM, et al. COQ2 nephropathy: a newly described inherited mitochondriopathy with primary renal involvement. *J Am Soc Nephrol.* 2007;18:2773–2780.
69. Wiggins JE, Goyal M, Sanden SK, et al. Podocyte hypertrophy, "adaptation," and "decompensation" associated with glomerular enlargement and glomerulosclerosis in the aging rat: prevention by calorie restriction. *J Am Soc Nephrol.* 2005;16:2953–2966.
72. Wanner N, Hartleben B, Herbach N, et al. Unraveling the role of podocyte turnover in glomerular aging and injury. *J Am Soc Nephrol.* 2014;25:707–716.
81. Eremina V, Sood M, Haigh J, et al. Glomerular-specific alterations of VEGF-a expression lead to distinct congenital and acquired renal diseases. *J Clin Invest.* 2003;111:707–716.
86. Drenckhahn D, Schnittler H, Nobiling R, et al. Ultrastructural organization of contractile proteins in rat glomerular mesangial cells. *Am J Pathol.* 1990;137:1343–1351.
87. Kriz W, Elger M, Lemley K, et al. Structure of the glomerular mesangium: a biomechanical interpretation. *Kidney Int Suppl.* 1990;30:S2–S9.
90. Leveen P, Pekny M, Gebre-Medhin S, et al. Mice deficient for PDGF B show renal, cardiovascular, and hematological abnormalities. *Genes Dev.* 1994;8:1875–1887.
92. Kikkawa Y, Virtanen I, Miner JH. Mesangial cells organize the glomerular capillaries by adhering to the G domain of laminin alpha5 in the glomerular basement membrane. *J Cell Biol.* 2003;161:187–196.
93. Blantz RC, Gabbai FB, Tucker BJ, et al. Role of mesangial cell in glomerular response to volume and angiotensin II. *Am J Physiol.* 1993;264:F158–F165.
101. Ostendorf T, Kunter U, Grone HJ, et al. Specific antagonism of PDGF prevents renal scarring in experimental glomerulonephritis. *J Am Soc Nephrol.* 2001;12:909–918.
130. Deen WM. What determines glomerular capillary permeability? *J Clin Invest.* 2004;114:1412–1414.
135. Chang RL, Deen WM, Robertson CR, et al. Permselectivity of the glomerular capillary wall: III. Restricted transport of polyanions. *Kidney Int.* 1975;8:212–218.
139. Jeansson M, Haraldsson B. Morphological and functional evidence for an important role of the endothelial cell glycocalyx in the glomerular barrier. *Am J Physiol Renal Physiol.* 2006;290:F111–F116.
160. Kietzmann L, Guhr SS, Meyer TN, et al. MicroRNA-193a regulates the transdifferentiation of human parietal epithelial cells toward a podocyte phenotype. *J Am Soc Nephrol.* 2015;26:1389–1401.
161. Gebeshuber CA, Kornauth C, Dong L, et al. Focal segmental glomerulosclerosis is induced by microRNA-193a and its downregulation of WT1. *Nat Med.* 2013;19:481–487.
163. Appel D, Kershaw DB, Smeets B, et al. Recruitment of podocytes from glomerular parietal epithelial cells. *J Am Soc Nephrol.* 2009;20:333–343.
165. Miner JH, Patton BL, Lentz SI, et al. The laminin alpha chains: expression, developmental transitions, and chromosomal locations of alpha1-5, identification of heterotrimeric laminins 8-11, and cloning of a novel alpha3 isoform. *J Cell Biol.* 1997;137:685–701.
185. Smeets B, Stucker F, Wetzels J, et al. Detection of activated parietal epithelial cells on the glomerular tuft distinguishes early focal segmental glomerulosclerosis from minimal change disease. *Am J Pathol.* 2014;184:3239–3248.
204. Heymann F, Meyer-Schwesinger C, Hamilton-Williams EE, et al. Kidney dendritic cell activation is required for progression of renal disease in a mouse model of glomerular injury. *J Clin Invest.* 2009;119:1286–1297.
207. Le Hir M, Keller C, Eschmann V, et al. Podocyte bridges between the tuft and Bowman's capsule: an early event in experimental crescentic glomerulonephritis. *J Am Soc Nephrol.* 2001;12:2060–2071.
212. Lasagni L, Angelotti ML, Ronconi E, et al. Podocyte regeneration driven by renal progenitors determines glomerular disease remission and can be pharmacologically enhanced. *Stem Cell Reports.* 2015;5:248–263.
217. Nangaku M, Couser WG. Mechanisms of immune-deposit formation and the mediation of immune renal injury. *Clin Exp Nephrol.* 2005;9:183–191.
222. Beck LH Jr, Bonegio RG, Lambeau G, et al. M-type phospholipase A2 receptor as target antigen in idiopathic membranous nephropathy. *N Engl J Med.* 2009;361:11–21.
223. Tomas NM, Beck LH Jr, Meyer-Schwesinger C, et al. Thrombospondin type-1 domain-containing 7A in idiopathic membranous nephropathy. *N Engl J Med.* 2014;371:2277–2287.
225. Hudson BG, Tryggvason K, Sundaramoorthy M, et al. Alport's syndrome, Goodpasture's syndrome, and type IV collagen. *N Engl J Med.* 2003;348:2543–2556.
233. Tomas NM, Hoxha E, Reinicke AT, et al. Autoantibodies against thrombospondin type 1 domain-containing 7A induce membranous nephropathy. *J Clin Invest.* 2016;126:2519–2532.
242. Paust HJ, Turner JE, Steinmetz OM, et al. The IL-23/th17 axis contributes to renal injury in experimental glomerulonephritis. *J Am Soc Nephrol.* 2009;20:969–979.
246. Krebs CF, Paust HJ, Krohn S, et al. Autoimmune renal disease is exacerbated by S1P-receptor-1-dependent intestinal th17 cell migration to the kidney. *Immunity.* 2016;45:1078–1092.
270. Wei C, El Hindi S, Li J, et al. Circulating urokinase receptor as a cause of focal segmental glomerulosclerosis. *Nat Med.* 2011;17:952–960.
301. Winn MP, Conlon PJ, Lynn KL, et al. A mutation in the TRPC6 cation channel causes familial focal segmental glomerulosclerosis. *Science.* 2005;308:1801–1804.
310. Debiec H, Guigonis V, Mougenot B, et al. Antenatal membranous glomerulonephritis due to anti-neutral endopeptidase antibodies. *N Engl J Med.* 2002;346:2053–2060.
313. Hoxha E, Wiech T, Stahl PR, et al. A mechanism for Cancer-associated membranous nephropathy. *N Engl J Med.* 2016;374:1995–1996.
317. Hoxha E, Thiele I, Zahner G, et al. Phospholipase A2 receptor autoantibodies and clinical outcome in patients with primary membranous nephropathy. *J Am Soc Nephrol.* 2014;25:1357–1366.
326. Kerjaschki D, Schulze M, Binder S, et al. Transcellular transport and membrane insertion of the C5b-9 membrane attack complex of complement by glomerular epithelial cells in experimental membranous nephropathy. *J Immunol.* 1989;143:546–552.
348. Faul C, Donnelly M, Merscher-Gomez S, et al. The actin cytoskeleton of kidney podocytes is a direct target of the antiproteinuric effect of cyclosporine A. *Nat Med.* 2008;14:931–938.
350. Fornoni A, Sageshima J, Wei C, et al. Rituximab targets podocytes in recurrent focal segmental glomerulosclerosis. *Sci Transl Med.* 2011;3:85ra46.
355. Schiffer M, Teng B, Gu C, et al. Pharmacological targeting of actin-dependent dynamin oligomerization ameliorates chronic kidney disease in diverse animal models. *Nat Med.* 2015;21:601–609.

# 5 Metabolic Basis of Solute Transport

Prabhleen Singh | Scott Culver Thomson | Alicia Ann McDonough

CHAPTER OUTLINE



Metabolism refers to the entire set of interconnected chemical reactions within living organisms that form and maintain tissue and govern the storage and release of energy in order to sustain life. This chapter is dedicated to one aspect of kidney metabolism—namely, the storage, release, and utilization of energy by the nephron as it transforms the glomerular filtrate into urine.

How much energy is required to make the urine? Of the major body organs, the kidney consumes the second highest amount of oxygen per gram of tissue (2.7 mmol/kg/min vs. 4.3 mmol/kg/min for the heart).[1] Most of the potential energy provided by renal oxidative metabolism is committed to epithelial transport, which determines the volume and composition of the urine. It has been asserted that, because the kidney reabsorbs 99% of the glomerular filtrate, it must use a lot of energy. But this logic is incorrect. The minimum net energy required for reabsorption does not depend on the amount of fluid that is reabsorbed. Forming a volume of urine with a solute composition equal to that of the body fluid from which it is formed is the thermodynamic equivalent of partitioning a bucket into two compartments by the use of a divider, which requires no net energy. On the other hand, energy is required to form a urine that differs in solute composition from that of the body fluids (i.e., plasma). To appreciate this, consider that the hypothetical remixing of urine with plasma would cause the formation of entropy, known as mixing entropy. Thus, energy is required to form urine from plasma and attain a state of reduced entropy. The minimum amount of energy required for this is equal to the temperature multiplied by the decrease in mixing entropy associated with the differential solute composition of urine versus plasma.

This chapter provides an overview of the interdependence of renal solute transport and renal metabolism, including (1) the role of the sodium pump, $Na^+$-$K^+$-adenosine triphosphatase (ATPase), in epithelial transport; (2) the metabolic substrates fueling active transport along the nephron and regional metabolic considerations; (3) the role of renal blood flow, the glomerular filtration rate (GFR), and tubuloglomerular feedback in controlling fluid and electrolyte filtration and tissue oxygenation; (4) the amount of oxygen consumed per sodium reabsorbed ($Qo_2/T_{Na}$); and (5) the metabolic efficiency of transport during normal perturbations and disease.

## THERMODYNAMIC APPROACH TO METABOLISM AND TRANSPORT

### THERMODYNAMIC ANALYSIS OF KIDNEY FUNCTION

Interest in kidney metabolism antedates most knowledge of the kidney's inner workings or of biochemistry. The theoretical minimum amount of energy required to make urine was determined from the laws of equilibrium thermodynamics nearly a century ago. For a human in balance on a typical diet, the cost of converting the glomerular filtrate into urine by an idealized process that is 100% efficient, infinitely slow, completely reversible, involves no back-leak, and generates no entropy and heat is about 0.5 cal/min/1.73 $m^2$.[2] In reality, the kidney consumes more than 50-fold this amount of energy. On this basis alone, one might argue that the kidney is horribly inefficient, even after one subtracts the cost of the kidney maintaining itself. On the other hand, added costs are imposed by the requirement to make urine in a finite amount of time, the need for flexibility to rapidly alter the volume and composition of the urine, the stoichiometric constraints of biochemistry, the known limits on the thermodynamic efficiency of oxidative phosphorylation, and the intrinsic permeabilities of tissues to electrolytes, gases, and urea.

The thermodynamic requirement may be a small fraction of the actual expenditure, but before one concludes that the body is unconcerned with thermodynamics, it may be noted that the thermodynamic energy required of the kidney to maintain salt and nitrogen balance with consumption of a typical diet is minimized with the usual water intake of 1 to 2 L/day. This suggests that the human body evolved to minimize the thermodynamic energy requirements of the kidney.

Moreover, the thermodynamic cost of excreting urea declines as blood urea nitrogen (BUN) concentration increases. Thus, as BUN rises in kidney disease, less energy is required to maintain the nitrogen balance. In kidney disease, the urine composition is also restricted to a narrower range. Using a classical thermodynamic approach, Newburgh suggested that the composition of the urine and the body fluids in kidney disease is determined by the available free energy; he noted that the declining flexibility of the diseased kidney to vary the urine composition could be predicted from the reduced free energy available for transport.[3]

### APPLICATION OF THE LAWS OF THERMODYNAMICS TO KIDNEY FUNCTION

The macroscopic laws of equilibrium thermodynamics apply to kidney metabolism; any theory of metabolism is necessarily incorrect if it violates these laws. The laws of thermodynamics essentially describe transitions of a system from one state to another. The first law of thermodynamics states that total energy is conserved during any process that occurs in a closed system. When a system is open to its environment, the combined energy of the system + environment remains constant. When the total internal energy, temperature, pressure, and volume of a system remain constant, any process that yields a change in free energy also yields reciprocal changes in entropy. Doing work on the system is equivalent to adding free energy to the system, which determines the upper limit of how much useful work the system can do against its environment.

The first law stipulates that total energy is conserved throughout any process but provides no other indication of whether a given process will occur spontaneously. The glomerular filtrate contains a mixture of salt and urea. The tubule partitions this into urine and reabsorbate. The urine has a different ratio of urea to salt than the reabsorbate, so the entropy has decreased. But the total internal energy of the combined urine and reabsorbate is the same as the original filtrate. Hence, the first law would be satisfied if the urine were to form spontaneously from the filtrate. The fact that NaCl and urea never sort themselves spontaneously into regions of higher and lower concentration is a consequence of the second law of thermodynamics, which states that all spontaneous processes generate entropy. Conversely, all spontaneous processes dissipate free energy and will cease when the supply of free energy is exhausted. It is possible to reduce entropy or elevate free energy in a system, but only if the system imports energy from its surroundings, in which case, there will be an increase in entropy of the surroundings that exceeds the decrease in entropy of the system. Some processes in the kidney, such as conversion of chemical to mechanical energy by the $Na^+$-$K^+$-ATPase, are highly efficient and generate almost no entropy. Other processes, such as the countercurrent multiplier, are inefficient and generate a lot of entropy. As a rule, those processes that generate the least entropy work over short distances and short times.

The laws of equilibrium thermodynamics determine the direction of any spontaneous process, but they do not address the rate of change. Hence the laws of equilibrium thermodynamics are not adequate for a full description of a living system that is displaced from equilibrium and characterized by flow of matter and energy within the system itself, as well as between the system and its environment. Thermodynamic principles are extended to incorporate time as a variable by the theory of nonequilibrium thermodynamics. Nonequilibrium thermodynamics entails certain assumptions and approximations that make it more of a tool and less of an edifice than classical equilibrium thermodynamics, but the theory performs well in many areas of physiology, including transport physiology. Basically, the theory asserts that the flow of any extensive property (e.g., mass, volume, charge) is the product of a driving force and a proportionality constant, which has units of conductance. It applies to both macro- and microprocesses involved in forming the urine. Examples include all mechanisms for secondary active transport and the conversion of chemical to translational free energy by ATPases.

## ENERGY AND THE SODIUM PUMP

$Na^+$-$K^+$-ATPase, also referred to as the sodium pump, is a ubiquitous plasma membrane protein that transports intracellular sodium out of the cell and extracellular potassium into the cell, thereby generating opposite concentration gradients for sodium and potassium ions across the cell membrane. This process of separating sodium from potassium across the cell membrane is fueled by the hydrolysis of adenosine triphosphate (ATP).[4,5] Each cycle of the pump consumes 1 ATP molecule while transporting 3 $Na^+$ and 2 $K^+$ ions across the cell membrane. The hydrolysis of ATP and the associated transport of ions are mutually dependent[4,5] and constitute an example of primary active transport. In this process there is nearly full conversion from chemical to mechanical energy, with minimal dissipation. The translational energy that develops after ATP hydrolysis results from electrostatic repulsion between the product ions, ADP and Pi, in accordance with Coulomb's law. Although this energy could be dissipated through subsequent collisions, such events are unlikely over very short time scales and short distances. For a relative kinetic energy of the phosphate of 0.6 eV, for example, the phosphate ion moves about 0.1 nm in 0.3 ps. If no other collisions occur in that short time interval, the phosphate can then transfer its entire kinetic energy to the sodium pump in the form of a molecular strain. Given the intrinsic free energy of ATP hydrolysis, the pump can generate gradients that store up to approximately 0.6 eV of electrochemical potential per 3 $Na^+$ plus 2 $K^+$ ions. For a typical cell in a typical environment, about 0.4 eV is required to cycle the pump against the existing Na and K gradients, which means that cells tend to operate with some reserve to further reduce their sodium or increase their potassium concentrations.

### STRUCTURE OF THE SODIUM PUMP

The sodium pump is composed of an α catalytic subunit, which hydrolyzes ATP and transports $Na^+$ and $K^+$ across the

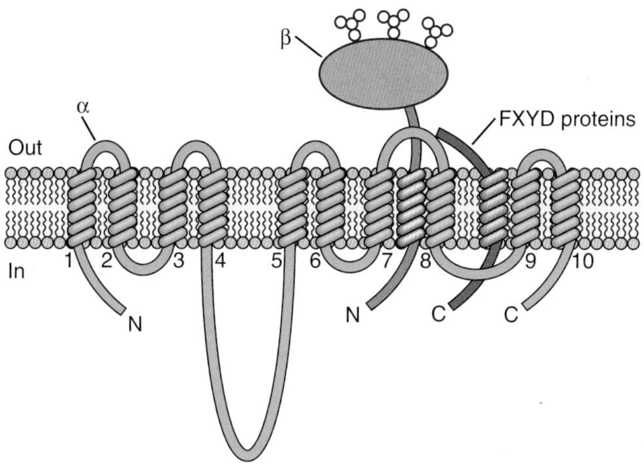


**Fig. 5.1** Na$^+$-K$^+$-ATPase is composed of a catalytic α-subunit (*teal*), an obligatory β-subunit (*pink*), and tissue-specific FXYD proteins (*blue*). The α-submit has 10 transmembrane segments. It hydrolyzes ATP, is phosphorylated in the large cytoplasmic loop, and transports sodium and potassium. The β-subunit is a type II glycoprotein that is located close to M7/M10 and interacts with the extracellular loop between transmembrane segments M7 and M8 and with intracellular regions of the α-subunit.[3] FXYD proteins are type I membrane proteins that interact with M9 with the β-subunit,[4] and in the case of FXYD1 with the intracellular lipid surface and the cytoplasmic domain of the α-subunit [5•]. (From Geering K. Functional roles of Na,K-ATPase subunits. *Curr Opin Nephrol Hypertens.* 2008;17[5]:526–532.)

membrane, a β-subunit that is critical for functional maturation and delivery of Na$^+$-K$^+$-ATPase to the plasma membrane, and an FXYD protein that can modulate the kinetics of Na$^+$-K$^+$-ATPase in a tissue-specific manner[6] (Fig. 5.1). There are multiple isoforms of each subunit. The α1β1 heterodimer is likely the exclusive Na$^+$-K$^+$-ATPase in renal epithelia,[7] whereas several FXYD protein subunits are expressed differentially along the nephron.[6–9] Biophysical models describing the turnover of the sodium pump through its functional cycle are described in a review by Horisberger.[4]

## OTHER ADENOSINE TRIPHOSPHATASES

Besides Na$^+$-K$^+$-ATPase, additional ion-translocating ATPases are expressed in renal epithelia along the nephron,[10] including H$^+$-K$^+$-ATPase,[11,12] Ca$^{2+}$-ATPases,[13] and H$^+$-ATPases.[14,15] These transport ATPases play important roles in maintaining urinary acidification and calcium homeostasis as discussed in Chapters 6, 7, and 9. These ATPases do not contribute significantly to the reabsorption of the bulk of the filtrate.

## PUMP LEAK PROCESS AND THE SODIUM POTENTIAL

For a cell in a steady state, the pumping of ions by the Na$^+$-K$^+$-ATPase must be offset by an equal and opposite diffusion of those ions back across the cell membrane. The back-leak of ions is an example of electrodiffusion. This diffusion of ions generates an electric field to retard diffusion of the most mobile charged species, thereby transferring free energy from the chemical potential of the mobile species to an electrical potential acting on the less mobile species. If the electric field is constant within the cell membrane, then the electrical potential difference across the membrane is given by the Goldman voltage equation, which is shown here for a membrane that is permeable to Na, K, and Cl:

$$\psi = \frac{RT}{F}\ln\left(\frac{P_K[K]_o + P_{Na}[Na]_o - P_{Cl}[Cl]_o}{P_K[K]_i + P_{Na}[Na]_i - P_{Cl}[Cl]_i}\right)$$

where $P_X$ is the permeability to $X$, $[X]o$ is the concentration of $X$ outside the cell, and $[X]i$ is the concentration inside the cell. If the permeability to one ion dominates the others, then the membrane voltage approaches the Nernst potential for that ion and the free energy is transferred to electrochemical potential of the other ions. If chloride is not actively transported, then the second law of thermodynamics dictates that no free energy exists in the chloride gradient. Thus, for a membrane that actively transports Na and K and is primarily permeable to K, the membrane voltage approaches the Nernst potential for K and the free energy provided by active transport is all transferred to the transmembrane Na difference.

To summarize, because cell membranes are generally more permeable to potassium than to sodium, potassium diffusion contributes more to the cell voltage than sodium diffusion, even though three sodium ions leak into the cell for every two potassium ions that leak out. Thus, diffusion of potassium out of the cell dominates the cell voltage, making it negative. The negative cell voltage, in turn, neutralizes the net driving force for further potassium egress and augments the net driving force for sodium entry. Because cell membranes are poor capacitors, an imperceptible charge imbalance suffices to form the entire membrane voltage. This allows the transmembrane concentration differences for sodium and potassium to remain nearly equal and opposite despite the much greater permeability to potassium. The net outcome of this pump-leak process is that electrochemical potential, which originates with ATP hydrolysis, becomes concentrated in the transmembrane sodium gradient, whereas potassium resides near electrochemical equilibrium.

## HARNESSING THE SODIUM POTENTIAL FOR WORK

The difference in electrochemical potential for sodium across the cell membrane is available to drive the unfavorable passage of other solutes across the membrane by a variety of exchangers and cotransporters. Examples include the proximal tubule Na$^+$/H$^+$ exchanger, sodium-glucose cotransporters (SGLTs), the basolateral Na/α-ketoglutarate (α-KG) cotransporter, the furosemide-sensitive Na-K-2Cl cotransporter, (NKCC2), and the thiazide-sensitive Na-Cl cotransporter (NCC). Generically, transport that directly uses free energy from the sodium gradient to drive uphill flux of another solute is referred to as secondary active transport[16] (α-KG cotransport in Fig. 5.2). Tertiary active transport refers to the net flux of a solute against its electrochemical potential gradient coupled indirectly to the Na$^+$ gradient (three transport processes working in parallel). An example of tertiary active transport is the uptake of various organic anions from the peritubular blood into the proximal tubular cell by the so-called organic anion transporters (OATs). Energy from the sodium gradient is converted into a gradient for α-KG to diffuse out of the cell

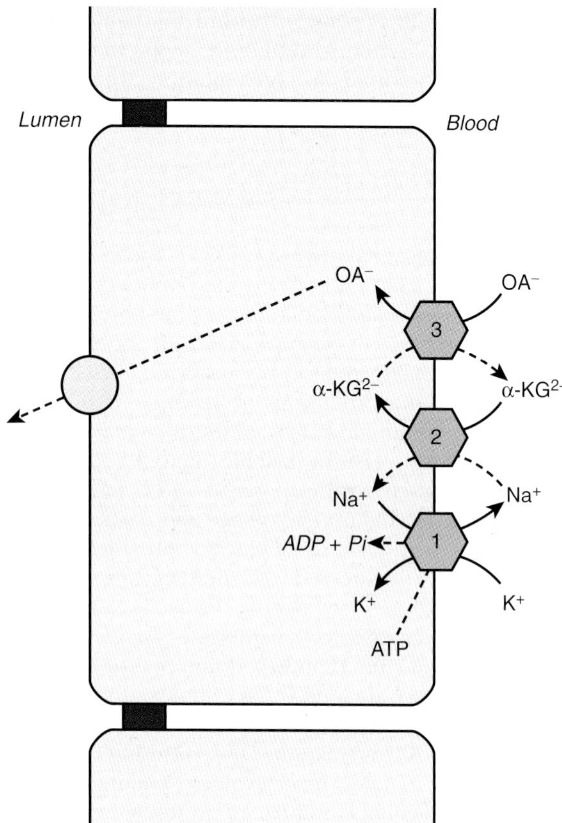


**Fig. 5.2** Different modes of active uphill transport as exemplified by organic acid (*OA*) secretion in proximal tubule epithelial cells. Transport across the basolateral membrane involves three steps functioning in parallel. Primary active transport (1) of Na and K by $Na^+$-$K^+$-ATPase coupled to the hydrolysis of ATP establishes the inwardly directed Na gradient. Secondary active transport (2) of α-ketoglutarate (*α-KG*) with Na on an Na/α-KG cotransporter uses the inwardly directed Na gradient to drive α-KG into the cell. Tertiary active transport (3) of OA with α-KG on an OA/α-KG antiporter uses the outward downhill transport of α-KG to drive the inward uphill transport of OA. The α-KG is recycled through the Na/α-KG cotransporter, which thus links the uphill transport of OA to the generation of the Na gradient by the $Na^+$-$K^+$-ATPase. Ultimately OAs are secreted down the OA concentration gradient into the tubular lumen. (From Dantzler WH, Wright SH. The molecular and cellular physiology of basolateral organic anion transport in mammalian renal tubules. *Biochim Biophys Acta.* 2003;1618[2]:185–193.)

by Na/α-KG cotransport. OATs use this potential difference to exchange α-KG for another organic anion[17] (see Fig. 5.2).

For tubular cells that actively reabsorb chloride, free energy is transferred from the Na potential to drive apical chloride entry and raise cell chloride above equilibrium. In the proximal tubule, the energy for apical chloride entry is derived circuitously via sodium-hydrogen exchange that is coupled to oxalate, formate, or hydroxyl ion transport (see Chapter 5). In the thick ascending loop of Henle (TALH) and distal convoluted tubule (DCT), the energy transfer occurs by direct cotransport with Na via NKCC2 or NCC. In each case, raising cell chloride above equilibrium provides a driving force for chloride to diffuse out of the cell across the basolateral membrane, which is permeable to chloride. Raising cell chloride also makes the basolateral membrane voltage less negative, as is apparent from the Goldman equation. Because luminal voltage is the sum of voltage steps across the basolateral and apical membranes, raising cell chloride in a cell with basolateral chloride conductance will raise the lumen voltage (make it more positive), thus providing free energy that can either be dissipated by the intercellular back-leak of chloride, which would increase entropy, or be applied to do the useful work of cation reabsorption, which would decrease entropy. The kidney uses the latter mechanism of energy transfer to augment Na reabsorption in the proximal tubule as well as calcium and magnesium reabsorption in the TALH.

For cells that express ENaC, opening these channels will depolarize the apical membrane, as can be seen from the Goldman equation. K ions, which enter the cell via the basolateral Na pump, can leave the cell by K conductances in either basolateral or apical membranes. Depolarizing the apical membrane will increase the fraction of K ions leaving by way of the apical membrane conductance. This represents the transfer of free energy from the $Na^+$-$K^+$-ATPase and the apical Na potential to the useful work of K secretion.

## CELL POLARITY AND VECTORIAL TRANSPORT

The polar arrangement of transporters in renal cells is essential for vectorial transport. Wherever it is expressed along the nephron, the sodium pump, which removes sodium from the cell, is restricted to the basolateral membrane. Meanwhile, the variety of exchangers, cotransporters, and sodium channels through which sodium enters the tubular cell are restricted to the apical membrane. These include the principal $Na^+/H^+$ exchanger (NHE3) and SGLTs in the proximal tubule, the NKCC2 in the thick ascending limb (TAL) of the loop of Henle, the NCC in the distal convoluted tubule, and epithelial sodium channels in the connecting tubule and collecting duct (see Chapter 5). These apical sodium transporters effect secondary active transport coupled to the primary active transporter, $Na^+$-$K^+$-ATPase.

Close coordination of sodium uptake across the apical membrane with sodium extrusion across the basolateral membrane is required to avoid osmotic swelling and shrinking of the cell. Assuming ATP is not limiting for basolateral exit, the magnitude of transepithelial transport is a function of (1) the number of transporters in the plasma membrane, which can be varied by changes in synthesis or degradation rates and/or trafficking between intracellular and plasma membranes, and (2) the activity per transporter, which can be varied by covalent modification (e.g., phosphorylation or proteolysis) or protein–protein interaction (e.g., $Na^+$-$K^+$-ATPase kinetics are influenced by FXYD subunit association).[6] The rate of apical sodium entry is also subject to influence by the availability of substrates for cotransport. For example, the amount of sodium–glucose cotransport depends on the availability of glucose in proximal tubular fluid, and the sodium entry at a given point along the TAL is subject to variations in the local chloride concentration, because NKCC2 has a relatively low affinity for chloride.

Many factors and hormones known to regulate renal sodium reabsorption (including angiotensin II, aldosterone, dopamine, parathyroid hormone, and blood pressure) act in parallel to affect the activity, distribution, or abundance of apical transporters and basolateral sodium pumps.[7,18] The molecular basis of this apical–basolateral crosstalk is not clearly understood, especially in the light of close cell volume control; however, there is evidence for a role of elevated cellular calcium level in response to depressed sodium transport.[19] There is also recent evidence for a salt-inducible kinase that responds to slight elevations in cell Na and Ca,[20] as well as evidence for coupling of $Na^+$-$K^+$-ATPase to apical channel activity.[21]

## METABOLIC SUBSTRATES FUELING ACTIVE TRANSPORT ALONG THE NEPHRON

Mitchell has noted that:

*"Biochemists generally accept the idea that metabolism is the cause of membrane transport."*

The underlying idea of the hypothesis put forward here is that if the processes that we call metabolism and transport represent events in a sequence, not only can metabolism be the cause of transport, but also transport can be the cause of metabolism. Thus, we might be inclined to recognize that transport and metabolism, as usually understood by biochemists, may be conceived advantageously as different aspects of one and the same process of vectorial metabolism.[22]

### METABOLISM BASICS

Detailed accounts of cellular metabolism are provided in many excellent texts[23]; nonetheless, an abbreviated overview relevant to renal metabolism is warranted. Substrates enter the kidney by renal blood flow (RBF) and GFR and enter renal epithelial cells by substrate transporters, often facilitated by the inward-directed $Na^+$ gradient created by the sodium pump (see Fig. 5.2), as discussed thoroughly in Chapter 8. Oxygen is likewise delivered by RBF to the epithelial cells. Once in the cell, substrates face one of three fates: (1) transport across the epithelium back into the blood (reabsorption); (2) conversion into another substrate (e.g., lactate to pyruvate); or (3) oxidization to $CO_2$ in the process of cellular ATP production.[24] This section traces the roadmap that connects substrates to production of ATP in the mitochondrion and to ATP utilization by the sodium pump, and the feedback connections between production and utilization.

Renal epithelia, except in the descending and thin ascending limbs of the loop of Henle, are packed with mitochondria (see Chapter 2). All the pathways of fuel oxidation take place in the mitochondrial matrix, except for glycolysis, which occurs in the cytosol. Substrates in the cytosol can freely cross the outer mitochondrial membrane through integral membrane porins. These substrates, as well as adenosine diphosphate (ADP) and phosphate (the building blocks of ATP), cross the inner mitochondrial membrane into the mitochondrial matrix via specific substrate transporters driven by their respective concentration gradients or by the $H^+$ gradient created by the electron transport chain (ETC; Fig. 5.3).

As illustrated in Fig. 5.4, amino acids, fatty acids, and pyruvate are metabolized to acetyl–coenzyme A and enter the citric acid cycle. With each turn of the cycle, three molecules of reduced nicotinamide adenine dinucleotide

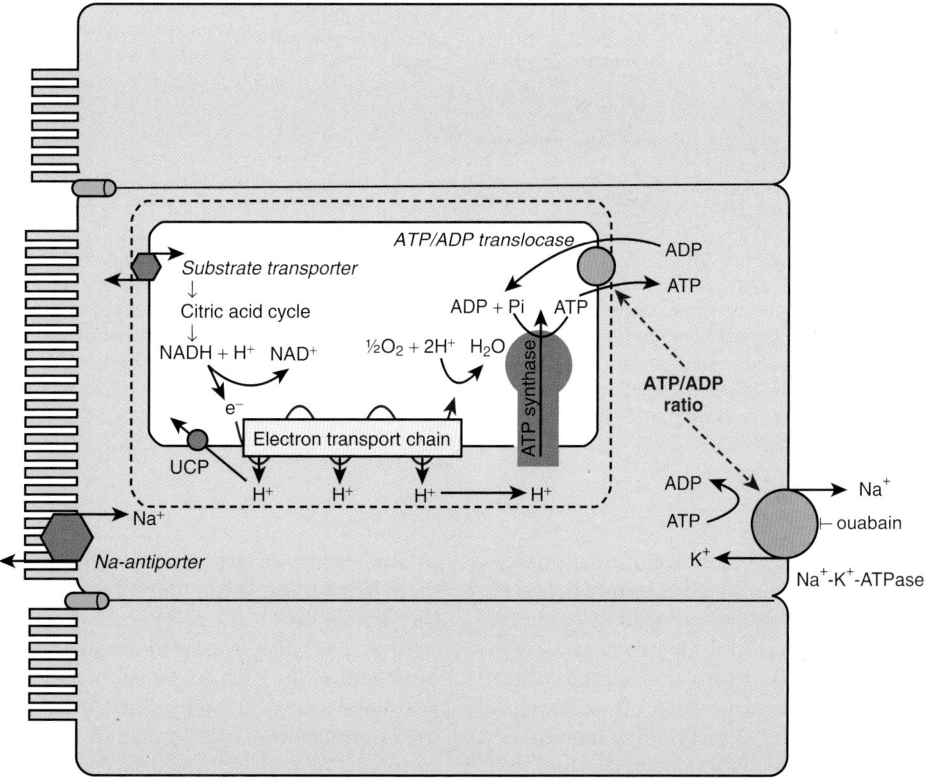


**Fig. 5.3** Whittam model. Coupling of ATP utilization by $Na^+$-$K^+$-ATPase to ATP production by mitochondrial oxygen consumption ($Qo_2$). Hydrolysis of ATP produces ADP plus inorganic phosphate (*Pi*), which lowers the ATP/ADP ratio, a signal to increase ADP uptake into the mitochondria and increase ATP synthesis.

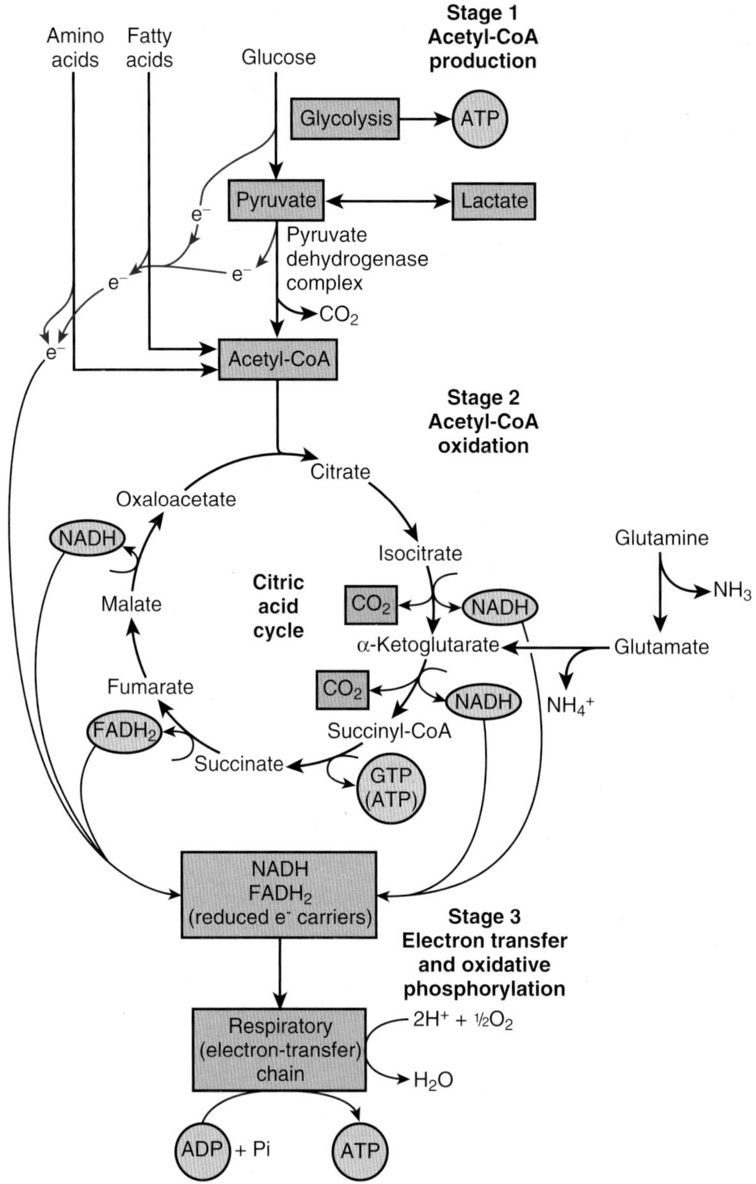


**Fig. 5.4** Catabolism of proteins, fats, and carbohydrates in three stages of cellular respiration. Stage 1: oxidation of fatty acids, glucose, and some amino acids yields acetyl–coenzyme A (*CoA*). Stage 2: oxidation of acetyl groups in the citric acid cycle includes four steps in which electrons are abstracted. Stage 3: electrons carried by reduced nicotinamide adenine dinucleotide (*NADH*) and reduced flavin adenine dinucleotide (*$FADH_2$*) are funneled into a chain of mitochondrial (or, in bacteria, plasma membrane–bound) electron carriers (the respiratory chain) that ultimately reduces $O_2$ to $H_2O$. This electron flow drives the production of ATP. Also indicated are two proximal tubule pathways: (1) oxidation of lactate through pyruvate and acetyl-CoA, and (2) glutamine conversion to glutamate and α-ketoglutarate in the mitochondria with the production of two molecules of $NH_3$, which is the main source of $NH_3$ secreted during acidosis. (Modified from Nelson DL, Cox MM. *Lehninger principles of biochemistry,* 5th ed. New York: WH Freeman; 2008.)

(NADH), one molecule of reduced flavin adenine dinucleotide ($FADH_2$), one molecule of guanosine triphosphate (GTP) or ATP, and two molecules of $CO_2$ are released in oxidative decarboxylation reactions (Table 5.1). Electrons carried by NADH and $FADH_2$ are transferred into the mitochondrial electron transport chain, a series of integral membrane complexes located within the inner mitochondrial membrane, where the electrons are sequentially transferred, ultimately to oxygen, which is reduced to $H_2O$. NADH and $FADH_2$ oxidization provoke the transport of $H^+$ from the matrix to the inner mitochondrial space.

The release of the potential energy stored in the $H^+$ gradient across the inner mitochondrial membrane provides the driving force for ATP synthesis from ADP by the ATP synthase: $H^+$ is transported into the matrix coupled to the production of ATP from ADP and inorganic phosphate (Pi) (see Fig. 5.3). These are the fundamental pieces of the chemiosmotic mechanism of oxidative phosphorylation proposed by Peter Mitchell in 1961.[22] The newly synthesized ATP is extruded from the matrix into the intermembrane space via the ADP–ATP countertransporter known as adenine nucleotide translocase and then exits the mitochondria

**Table 5.1 Adenosine Triphosphate (ATP) Yield From Metabolism of One Glucose Molecule**

| Process | Direct Product | Final ATP |
|---|---|---|
| **ATP Yield from Complete Oxidation of Glucose** | | |
| Glycolysis | 2 NADH (cytosol) | 5[a] |
| | 2 ATP | 2 |
| Pyruvate oxidation (two per glucose) | 2 NADH (mitochondrial matrix) | 5 |
| Acetyl–coenzyme A oxidation in citric acid cycle (two per glucose) | 6 NADH (mitochondrial matrix) | 18 |
| | 2 FADH2 | 4 |
| Total yield per glucose | | 30 |
| **ATP Yield from Glycolysis of Glucose** | | |
| Glycolysis | 2 ATP, 2 NADH | 2 |

[a]Via malate–aspartate shuttle.

across the permeable outer membrane. In the cytosol, ATP is available to bind to ATPases such as plasma membrane $Na^+$-$K^+$-ATPase.

In summary, the flow of electrons through the ETC generates a proton gradient across the inner mitochondrial membrane that provides the energy to drive ATP synthesis from ADP + Pi by ATP synthase and is also sufficient to extrude the ATP across the mitochondrial membrane.[23] Thus, the oxidation of substrates is coupled to ATP synthesis by an electrochemical proton gradient. This coupling can be influenced by uncoupling protein isoforms (UCPs) located in the mitochondrial inner membrane and expressed in a tissue-specific manner. Simply stated, UCPs create a proton leak that dissipates the proton gradient available to drive oxidative phosphorylation (see Fig. 5.3). It has been reported that UCP-2 is expressed in the renal proximal tubule and TAL (not in glomerulus or the distal nephron) and that its expression is elevated in kidneys of diabetic rats.[25] However, the physiologic consequences of the expression and regulation of UCP in kidneys has not been explored much experimentally.

## WHITTAM MODEL

In the early 1960s, the coupling between active transport, respiration, and $Na^+$-$K^+$-ATPase activity was recognized by Whittam and Blond,[69,70] who tested the idea that inhibition of active ion transport at the plasma membrane would cause a fall in oxygen consumption ($Qo_2$) in the mitochondria. Using brain or kidney samples studied in vitro, they demonstrated that inhibition of $Na^+$-$K^+$-ATPase activity by removal of sodium or addition of the sodium pump–specific inhibitor ouabain (neither of which directly inhibits mitochondrial respiration) markedly reduced $Qo_2$, which led the investigators to conclude that an extramitochondrial ATPase, sensitive to $Na^+$ and ouabain, as well as to $K^+$ and $Ca^{++}$, is one of the pacemakers of respiration of the kidney cortex.[26,27]

A careful study by Balaban and colleagues two decades later[28] used a suspension of renal cortical tubules to reexamine this Whittam model (see Fig. 5.3) in more detail by measuring the redox state of mitochondrial nicotinamide adenine dinucleotide (NAD), cellular ATP and ADP concentrations, ATP/ADP ratio, and $Qo_2$ in the same samples. If transport and respiration are assumed to be coupled, inhibition of transport is predicted to provoke a mitochondrial transition to a resting state[29] accompanied by an increase in NADH/$NAD^+$ (reduced to oxidized NAD), increase in [ATP], decrease in [ADP] and [Pi], increase in ATP/ADP ratio, and decrease in $Qo_2$. Stimulation of active transport would provoke the opposite pattern: decreased NADH, ATP, and ATP/ADP ratio, and increased $Qo_2$. Predictably, incubating the renal cortical tubule suspension with the $Na^+$-$K^+$-ATPase inhibitor ouabain caused a 50% decline in $Qo_2$, reduction of NAD to NADH, and a 30% increase in the ATP/ADP ratio, all evidence for coupling of mitochondrial ATP production to ATP consumption via $Na^+$-$K^+$-ATPase. Similarly, in tubules deprived of $K^+$ (which is required for $Na^+$-$K^+$-ATPase turnover), adding 5 mmol/L $K^+$ increased $Qo_2$ by more than 50%, oxidized NADH to $NAD^+$, and decreased the cellular ATP/ADP ratio by 50%. These results provide evidence for the coupling of both $Na^+$-$K^+$-ATPase and ATP production via ATP synthase to the cellular ATP/ADP ratio (see Fig. 5.3).

## ENERGY REQUIREMENTS AND SUBSTRATE USE ALONG THE NEPHRON

In all renal epithelial cells from the proximal convoluted tubule to the inner medullary collecting duct (IMCD), the basolateral sodium pump uses the hydrolysis of ATP to drive primary active transport of $Na^+$ out of and $K^+$ into the cell, and the gradients created are used to drive coupled transport of ions and substrates across both the apical and basolateral membranes.

Despite consistent distribution and function, the relative abundance of Na,K-ATPase as a function of tubular location along the nephron is highly variable. Na,K-ATPase activity, ouabain binding, and Na,K-ATPase subunit abundance have been studied in dissected tubules and with imaging techniques. Na,K-ATPase expression patterns and ouabain binding patterns along the nephron are very similar.[10,30] The pronounced differences in activity can largely be accounted for by differences in sodium pump number measured either by ouabain binding or by immunoblot of subunits in dissected nephron segments (Fig. 5.5).[31]

The patterns of $Na^+$-$K^+$-ATPase protein expression and activity as a function of tubule length are what is to be expected from what is understood of the physiology of the nephron segments: moderate levels are expressed in the proximal tubule where two-thirds of the sodium is reabsorbed across a leaky epithelium, and lower levels are expressed in the straight than in the convoluted segments, reflecting the amount of sodium transported in these two regions. Very low levels are detected in the thin limbs of the loop of Henle, whereas high levels are expressed in the medullary and cortical TAL ("diluting segments") that must reabsorb a significant fraction of NaCl without water against an increasingly steep transepithelial gradient. The $Na^+$-$K^+$-ATPase activity and expression in the DCT, which is responsible for reabsorbing another 5% to 7% of the filtered load against a very steep transepithelial gradient, is very high. In the collecting duct, which reabsorbs a smaller fraction of $Na^+$ via channels electrically coupled to the secretion of $K^+$ or $H^+$ and has variable

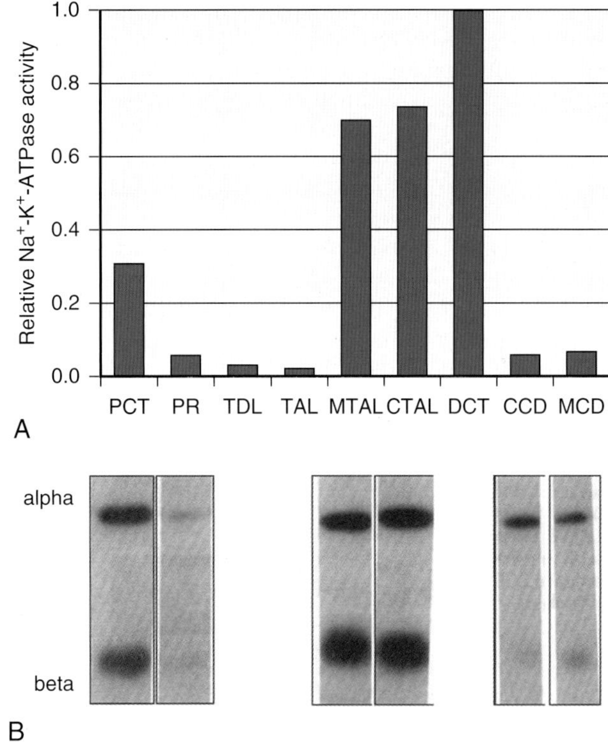


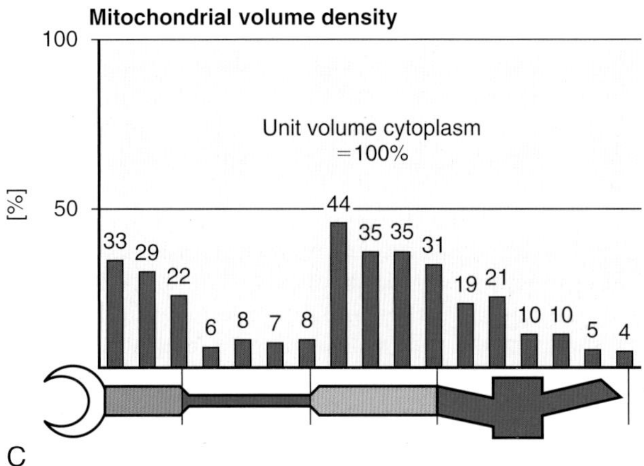


**Fig. 5.5** (A) Relative levels of Na⁺-K⁺ATPase activity measured in individual segments of the rat nephron. (Data are normalized to that of the distal convoluted tubule and expressed per unit length of tubule segment.) (B) Detection of $Na^+$-$K^+$-ATPase $\alpha_1$- and $\beta_1$-subunits along the nephron. Tubule segments 40 mm long were resolved by sodium dodecyl sulfate–polyacrylamide gel electrophoresis and subjected to immunoblotting with subunit-specific antisera. Blots placed below corresponding tubule label indicated in (A). (C) Morphologic analysis of mitochondrial density relative to a unit of cytoplasm. *CCD,* Cortical collecting duct; *CTAL,* cortical thick ascending limb of the loop of Henle; *DCT,* distal convoluted tubule; *MCD,* outer medullary collecting duct; *MTAL,* medullary thick ascending limb of the loop of Henle; *PCT,* proximal convoluted tubule; *PR,* pars recta (proximal straight tubule); *TAL,* thin ascending limb of the loop of Henle; *TDL,* thin descending limb of the loop of Henle. ([A] redrawn from Katz AI, Doucet A, Morel F. Na⁺-K⁺-ATPase activity along the rabbit, rat, and mouse nephron. *Am J Physiol.* 1979;237:F114–F120; [B] based on data from McDonough AA, Magyar CE, Komatsu Y. Expression of Na[+]-K[+]-ATPase alpha- and beta-subunits along rat nephron: isoform specificity and response to hypokalemia. *Am J Physiol.* 1994;267:C901–C908; [C] based on data from Pfaller W, Rittinger M. Quantitative morphology of the rat kidney. *Int J Biochem.* 1980;12[1-2]:17–22.)

$H_2O$ permeability, the $Na^+$-$K^+$-ATPase is quite low, albeit sufficient to drive sodium reabsorption in this region. The distribution of the ATP-producing mitochondria along the nephron, reported as percent of cytoplasmic volume,[32] parallels the distribution of the ATP-consuming sodium pumps but is somewhat less variable, ranging from 10% or less of the cell volume in the thin loop of Henle and medullary collecting duct to 20% in the cortical collecting duct (CCD) and proximal straight tubule to 30% to 40% of cell volume in the proximal tubule and TAL[32] (Fig. 5.5*C*).

Determining which substrates support ATP production and $Na^+$-$K^+$-ATPase activity along the nephron has been the subject of many studies and reviews.[24,33,34] To obtain nephron-specific information, investigators have dissected nephron segments and assayed for either metabolic pathway enzyme distribution or examined how specific substrates affected ATP levels. Although these in vitro approaches lack the in vivo realities of blood flow, tubular flow, and autocrine–paracrine, hormonal, and nervous system inputs that are evident in the whole kidney, the studies do provide information about the metabolic potential of each segment under defined conditions.

Isolated nephron segments had been reported to have low levels of cellular ATP, so Uchida and Endou[35] reasoned that if the segments were incubated with fuels that could be used by the segment, their ATP levels should increase toward physiologic levels. They examined a range of substrates for their ability to maintain cellular ATP levels in microdissected glomeruli and nephron segments (excluding thin sections of loop of Henle and papillary duct). The substrates studied (all at 2 mmol/L) included L-glutamine, D-glucose, β-hydroxybutyrate (HBA), and DL-lactate. Because the preincubation did not fully deplete the TAL and distal nephron segments of ATP, the ionophore monensin was included in the incubation with the substrate to dissipate the $Na^+$ gradient and promote ATP consumption.

The change in ATP per millimeter of tubule (or glomerulus) as a function of substrate addition, shown in Fig. 5.6, illustrates that each segment had a distinct ability to use these substrates. Lactate was very effective at maintaining ATP levels in all nephron segments tested, notably in the proximal tubule. The S1, S2, and S3 segments of the proximal tubule all used glutamine effectively as a fuel, which is consistent with the role of the proximal tubule in ammoniagenesis. Glutamine is the main amino acid oxidized by the proximal tubule, where it is deaminated and converted to α-KG, yielding 2 $NH_3$ molecules that are secreted during acidosis, as illustrated in Fig. 5.4 and discussed in Chapter 9. Glutamine is not a preferred fuel in the more distal nephron segments. Glucose is completely reabsorbed along the proximal tubule yet, glucose is not an effective metabolic fuel for the S1 or S2 regions of the proximal tubule. In contrast, all of the more distal segments tested readily used glucose to maintain cellular ATP. The ketone HBA was used effectively in all nephron segments tested; however, in S1 and S2 of the proximal tubule the capacity of HBA to support ATP production was far less than that provided by glutamine or lactate.

The distribution along the nephron of numerous enzymes involved in metabolic pathways, collated from many studies, has been summarized by Guder and Ross.[33] Their description of glycolytic (Fig. 5.7A) and gluconeogenic (Fig. 5.7B) enzymes along the rat nephron[36–38] demonstrates very low

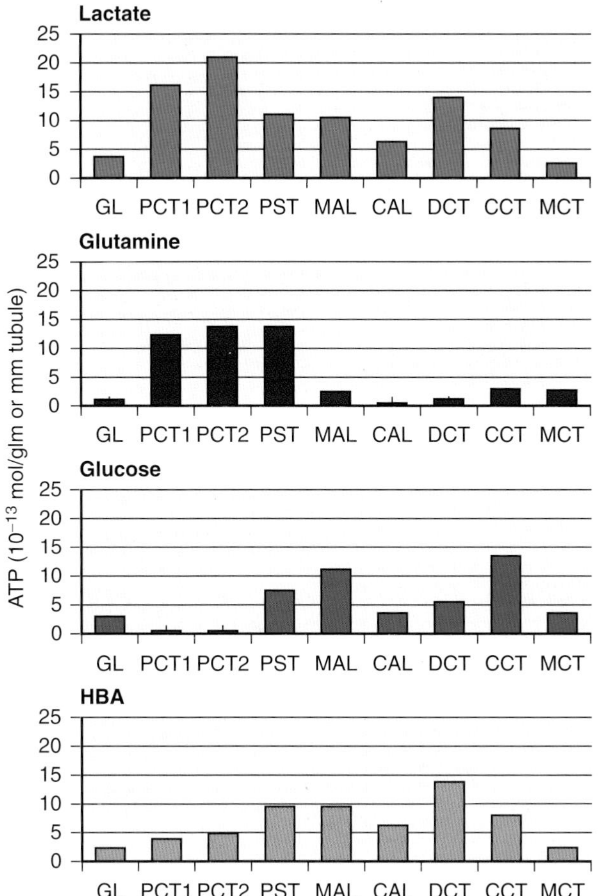


**Fig. 5.6** ATP production in glomeruli and dissected nephron segments as a function of substrates. In glomeruli and PCT1, PCT2, and PST segments, the values equal the differences in ATP content between samples incubated with and without each substrate for 30 minutes. In MAL, CAL, DCT, CCT, and MCT, the values equal the differences in ATP content between samples incubated with and without each substrate in the presence of monensin (10 pg/mL) for 15 minutes. *CAL,* Cortical ascending limb; *CCT,* cortical collecting tubule; *DCT,* distal convoluted tubule; *GL,* glomerulus; *MAL,* medullary thick ascending limb; *MCT,* medullary collecting tubule; *PCT1,* early proximal convoluted tubule; *PCT2,* late proximal convoluted tubule; *PST,* proximal straight tubule. (Data from Uchida S, Endou H. Substrate specificity to maintain cellular ATP along the mouse nephron. *Am J Physiol.* 1988;255: F977–F983.)

glycolytic potential in the proximal tubule and high glycolytic potential from medullary ascending limb to medullary collecting tubule. In contrast, gluconeogenic enzymes are found almost exclusively in the proximal tubule.

In summary, the proximal tubule reabsorbs glucose and can synthesize glucose biosynthetically but does not metabolize glucose. There are both practical and theoretical explanations for the lack of glucose metabolism in this segment. The proximal tubule is specialized to reabsorb the filtered load of glucose from the tubular fluid back into the blood. Because of the enormous load of glucose moving through these cells, a proximal tubule hexokinase would need to have exceedingly low affinity for glucose, which would be difficult to regulate. In contrast, more distal regions of the nephron such as the loop of Henle and distal nephron normally have little or no glucose in their tubular fluid, have no Na–glucose cotransporters in their apical membranes, and cannot synthesize glucose, but these regions use glucose delivered via RBF as a metabolic fuel (which could be provided by gluconeogenesis in the proximal tubule during fasting). A summary of substrate preferences along the nephron is provided in Fig. 5.8.[34]

## RENAL GLUCONEOGENESIS AND LACTATE HANDLING

In a review of renal gluconeogenesis, Gerich and colleagues[39] comment that the kidney can be considered two separate organs, because the proximal tubule makes and releases glucose from noncarbohydrate precursors, whereas glucose utilization occurs primarily in the medulla. Because the kidney is both a consumer and a producer of glucose, net arteriovenous glucose differences across the kidney can be uninformative, because glucose consumption in the medulla can mask glucose release by the cortex.

Gerich and colleagues[39] also make the case that the kidney is a significant gluconeogenic organ in normal humans based on the following: (1) in humans fasted overnight, proximal tubule gluconeogenesis can be as much as 40% of whole-body gluconeogenesis[39]; (2) during liver transplantation, endogenous glucose release falls to only 50% of control levels by 1 hour after liver removal[40]; and (3) pathologically in type 2 diabetes, renal glucose release is increased by about the same fraction as hepatic glucose release.[41] Zucker diabetic fatty rats also exhibit marked stimulation of gluconeogenesis compared with their lean litter mate controls.[42]

Lactate can reach the nephron by filtration or blood flow and can also be produced along the nephron. Within the kidney, lactate can be (1) oxidized to produce energy with generation of $CO_2$, a process that consumes oxygen but generates ATP; or (2) converted to glucose via gluconeogenesis in the proximal tubule, a process that consumes oxygen and ATP. This is shown in Fig. 5.9. Studies by Cohen[43] in an isolated whole kidney perfused with just lactate as substrate demonstrated a change in $^{14}$C–lactate utilization as a function of its concentration in the perfusate: at low concentrations, all the lactate was oxidized (detected as $CO_2$) in order to fuel transport and basal metabolism; when lactate in perfusate was raised above 2 mmol/L some of the lactate was used for synthesis of glucose (gluconeogenesis); and at high lactate in perfusate the metabolic and synthetic rates approach maximum, and some lactate is conserved (reabsorbed). However, it is not the normal circumstance that lactate is the sole substrate, and it is now appreciated that the metabolism of lactate is affected by the presence of other substrates—for example, lactate uptake and oxidation are inhibited in the presence of fatty acids.[24,44]

The kidney's ability to convert lactate to glucose provides evidence that it can participate in cell–cell lactate shuttle, also known as the Cori cycle.[45] This cycle is important when oxidative phosphorylation is inhibited in vigorously exercising muscle, which becomes hypoxic. In the muscle, pyruvate is reduced to lactate to regenerate $NAD^+$ from NADH, which is necessary for ATP production by glycolysis to continue. Lactate is released into the blood and can be taken up by tissues capable of gluconeogenesis, such as the liver and kidney. In the proximal tubule, the lactate that is not oxidized can be converted to glucose, and because this substrate is

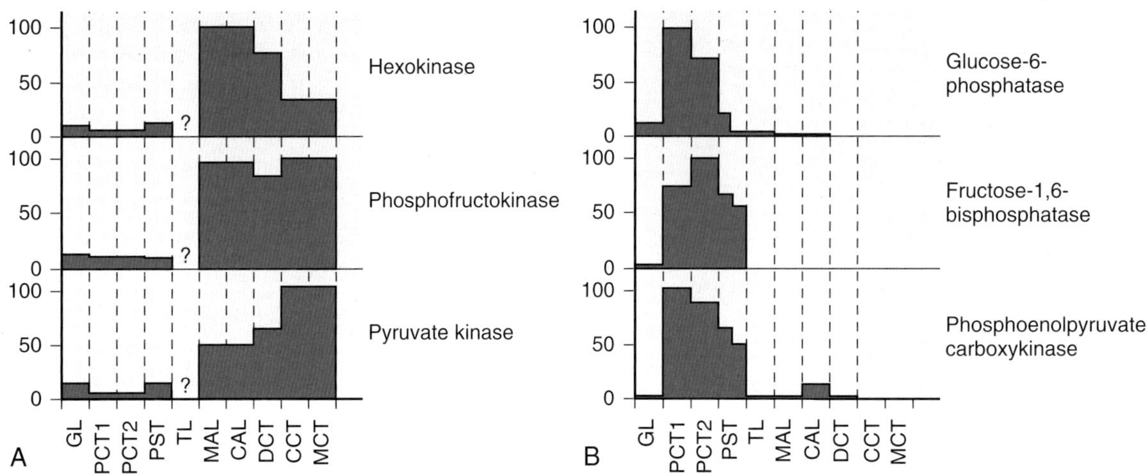


**Fig. 5.7** Distribution of glycolytic and gluconeogenic enzymes along the rat nephron. Nephron segments were dissected from fed (A) and starved (B) rats, respectively. The activity of hexokinase, phosphofructokinase, pyruvate kinase, glucose-6-phosphatase, fructose 1,6-bisphosphatase, and phosphoenolpyruvate carboxykinase was determined in individual segments. Enzyme activities are expressed as a percentage of the maximal value observed, based on the original activity per gram of dry weight. *CAL,* Cortical ascending limb; *CCT,* cortical collecting tubule; *DCT,* distal convoluted tubule; *GL,* glomerulus; *MAL,* medullary thick ascending limb; *MCT,* medullary collecting tubule; *PCT1,* early proximal convoluted tubule; *PCT2,* late proximal convoluted tubule; *PST,* proximal straight tubule; *TL,* loop of Henle, thin limbs. (Modified from Guder WG, Ross BD. Enzyme distribution along the nephron. *Kidney Int.* 1984;26[2]:101–111.)

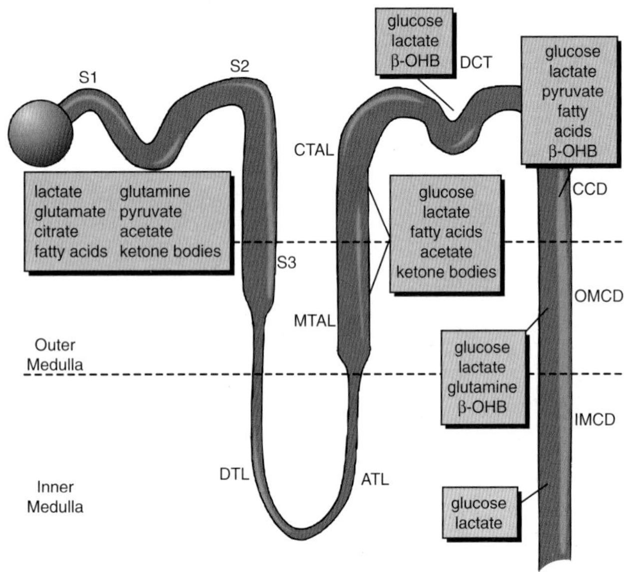


**Fig. 5.8** Substrate preferences along the nephron. Summary of preferred substrates to fuel active transport in nephron segments as gleaned primarily from studies using oxygen consumption ($Qo_2$), ion fluxes, radioactive carbon ($^{14}C$)-labeled carbon dioxide generation from $^{14}C$-labeled substrates, ATP contents, and reduced nicotinamide adenine dinucleotide fluorescence. *ATL,* Ascending thin limb; *β-OHB,* β-Hydroxybutyrate; *CCD,* cortical collecting duct; *CTAL,* cortical thick ascending limb of the loop of Henle; *DCT,* distal convoluted tubule; *DTL,* descending thin limb; *IMCD,* inner medullary collecting duct; *MTAL,* medullary thick ascending limb of the loop of Henle; *OMCD,* outer medullary collecting duct; *S1, S2, S3,* successive segments of proximal tubule. (From Kone BC. Metabolic basis of solute transport. In *Brenner and Rector's the kidney,* 5th ed. St Louis: Saunders; 2008.)

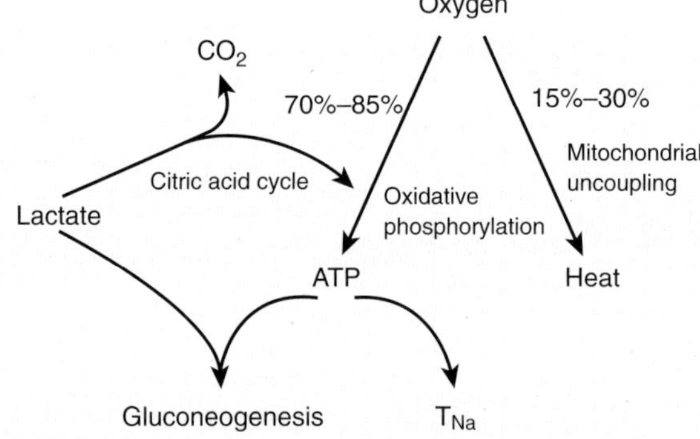


**Fig. 5.9** Fate of lactate and oxygen in renal metabolism. Oxygen can be used to generate ATP via oxidative phosphorylation or heat if mitochondrial uncoupling occurs. Lactate can act as a substrate for gluconeogenesis, which consumes energy, or can enter into the citric acid cycle to generate energy. ATP is either used for Na transport ($T_{Na}$) or consumed in the process of gluconeogenesis.

not used by the proximal tubule, glucose will be reabsorbed back into the blood, where it will be available for metabolism by the exercising muscle. Overall, this cycle is metabolically costly: glycolysis produces 2 ATP molecules at a cost of 6 ATP molecules consumed in the gluconeogenesis. Thus, the Cori cycle is an energy-requiring process that shifts the metabolic burden away from the exercising muscle during hypoxia. This cell–cell lactate shuttle could also operate within the kidney between nephron segments that produce lactate anaerobically and the proximal tubule.

Renal medullary lactate concentration was explored in a 1965 study in rats by Scaglione and colleagues[46] to test the idea that the medulla used glycolysis in the low-oxygen environment. Medullary lactate concentration is a function of delivery via the blood flow, production in the medulla, and removal by the blood flow, because there is no gluconeogenesis in this region to consume lactate. Because of the countercurrent arrangement of the vasa recta, lactate would be expected to concentrate in the medulla somewhat. The study results indicated that lactate concentration was twice as high in the inner medulla as in the cortex and

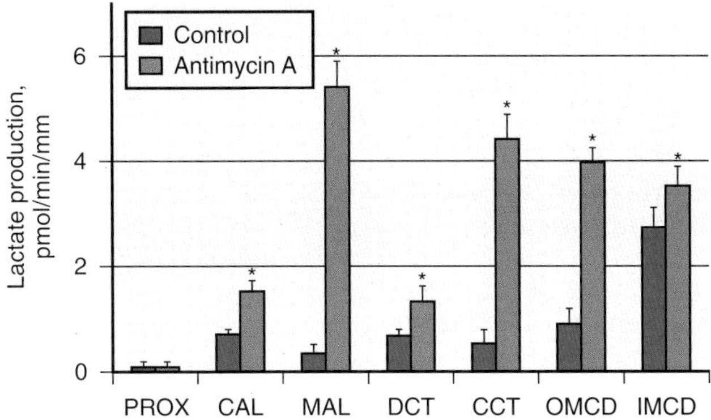


**Fig. 5.10** Lactate production by rat nephron segments under control conditions and in the presence of antimycin A. *CAL,* Cortical ascending limb; *CCT,* cortical collecting tubule; *DCT,* distal convoluted tubule; *IMCD,* inner medullary collecting duct; *MAL,* medullary thick ascending limb; *OMCD,* outer medullary collecting duct; *PROX,* proximal tubule. (From Bagnasco S, Good D, Balaban R, et al. Lactate production in isolated segments of the rat nephron. *Am J Physiol.* 1985;248:F522–F526.)

that during osmotic diuresis the medullary lactate doubled, whereas cortical lactate remained unchanged. The authors postulated that increased medullary lactate was evidence for increased glycolysis during osmotic diuresis because the diuresis and increased flow through the vasa recta would be expected to decrease medullary lactate if synthesis rates were unchanged. Sodium delivery to the distal nephron would also increase during osmotic diuresis and the accompanying increased $Na^+$ reabsorption could drive the increased glycolysis.

Twenty years later, Bagnasco and colleagues[47] studied lactate production along the nephron in dissected rat nephron segments incubated in vitro with glucose with or without an inhibitor of oxidative metabolism, antimycin A. The only pathway for lactate production in the kidney is from pyruvate via lactate dehydrogenase. Proximal tubules produced no lactate with or without antimycin A. The distal segments all produced lactate, and the production was significantly increased (approximately 10-fold in TAL) during antimycin A incubation (Fig. 5.10), which led the authors to conclude that significant amounts of lactate can be produced by anaerobic glycolysis during anoxia in the distal segments. The IMCD, a region with low oxygen tension under control conditions, had high levels of lactate production even without antimycin A, which indicates that it is primed for anaerobic glycolysis.

# NEPHRON-REGION–SPECIFIC METABOLIC CONSIDERATIONS

## PROXIMAL TUBULE

Studies carried out in a number of laboratories provide evidence that sodium transport and gluconeogenesis compete for ATP in the proximal convoluted tubule.[48–50] Friedrichs and Schoner[49] studied both processes in rat renal tubules and slices and found that ouabain inhibition of $Na^+$-$K^+$-ATPase increased renal gluconeogenesis by 10% to 40% depending on the substrate, and that stimulating $Na^+$-$K^+$-ATPase activity with high extracellular $K^+$ inhibited gluconeogenesis. The authors concluded that inhibition of the sodium pump induced a higher energy state of the cell, which would favor energy-requiring synthetic processes.

Nagami and Lee[50] used an isolated perfused mouse proximal tubule preparation to address this issue. When tubules were perfused at higher rates, delivering more sodium to the proximal tubule, the glucose production rate was decreased by 50%, whereas when tubules were incubated with ouabain in the bath or perfused with amiloride (to inhibit apical transport), the glucose production rate increased above that seen in nonperfused tubules. These authors also verified that the reduction in glucose production seen at elevated perfusion rates does not result from increased glucose utilization and is not dependent on the presence of specific substrates. Related to the topic of proximal tubule gluconeogenesis, two studies suggest that the blood glucose–lowering effects of sodium glucose cotransporter isoform 2 (SGLT2) inhibitors are due, in part, to reduced proximal gluconeogenesis: inhibiting SGLT2-mediated glucose uptake in diabetic mice reduced gluconeogenic gene expression, including PEPCK, a principal regulator of gluconeogenesis.[51,52]

Recent studies and mathematical models have evaluated the effects of inhibiting proximal tubule transport routes on metabolism and transport efficiency (sodium transport/oxygen consumption, $T_{Na}/Qo_2$, discussed further under the section regarding metabolic cost of sodium reabsorption). Proximal tubule transport, $T_{Na}$, is the sum of transcellular reabsorption (e.g., via $Na^+/H^+$ exchanger isoform 3 [NHE3]) and sodium glucose cotransporter isoform 2 (SGLT2), and paracellular reabsorption (e.g., via claudin 2 [cldn2]). Mathematical models predict that $T_{Na}/Qo_2$ is 80% higher in the S3 segment of the proximal tubule due to the larger paracellular contribution to $T_{Na}$, which is highly energy efficient. In these models, inhibiting NHE3 (the main sodium transporter in the proximal tubule), or Na,K-ATPase reduced $T_{Na}$, $Qo_2$, and transport efficiency.[53] Inhibiting SGLT2 also lowered $T_{Na}$ but increased $Qo_2$ in part by activating NHE3 and SGLT1 and in part by blunting the driving force for paracellular transport of $T_{Na}$ due to tubular glucose buildup.[51,53] Regarding paracellular reabsorption, $Qo_2$ is markedly increased in proximal tubule claudin-2 null mice as $T_{Na}$ is shifted from the energy efficient paracellular route to the Na,K-ATPase driven transcellular routes. Consequently, cldn2 mice exhibit medullary hypoxia and increased susceptibility to tubular injury.[54,55] How (or if) the increase in the metabolic cost of transport affects metabolic pathways and substrate utilization in the proximal tubule remains to be determined.

## THICK ASCENDING LIMB

The TAL has a very high rate of $Na^+$ transport against a steep concentration gradient, very high levels of $Na^+$-$K^+$-ATPase activity and expression, and, perhaps not unexpectedly, 40% of its cytosolic volume occupied by mitochondria (see Fig. 5.5). Although the TALs have a far greater capacity for anaerobic metabolism than the proximal tubules, this region still requires oxidative metabolism to maintain cellular ATP levels and active $Na^+$ reabsorption.[35,56]

## CORTICAL COLLECTING DUST

CCD metabolism is particularly interesting because it is made up of distinctly different cell types: principal cells that reabsorb sodium and intercalated cells that can secrete bicarbonate ($HCO_3^-$). Hering-Smith and Hamm microperfused rabbit CCD and measured $Na^+$ reabsorption (with $22Na^+$) from lumen to bath, and $HCO_3^-$ transport by microcalorimetry in the presence of substrates and with or without inhibitors. Both $Na^+$ reabsorption and $HCO_3^-$ secretion were inhibited by antimycin A, which provides evidence for dependence on oxidative phosphorylation. However, neither was dependent on either glycolysis or the hexose–monophosphate shunt pathways. A small component of $Na^+$ transport was supported by endogenous substrates. $Na^+$ reabsorption was supported best by a mixture of basolateral glucose and acetate, whereas $HCO_3^-$ secretion was fully supported by either glucose or acetate. $HCO_3^-$ secretion (but not $Na^+$ transport) was supported to some extent by luminal glucose. In sum, this study indicates that principal cells and intercalated cells have distinct metabolic phenotypes.

## MEDULLARY COLLECTING DUCT

Medullary collecting ducts contribute to final urinary acidification. Comparing the outer medullary collecting duct (OMCD) with the CCD, Hering-Smith and Hamm[57] found that bicarbonate secretion in the OMCD could be fully supported by endogenous substrates. This region has far less sodium transport and few mitochondria (see Fig. 5.5). Stokes and colleagues[58] isolated IMCDs and examined their metabolic characteristics. In the absence of exogenous substrate, IMCD can maintain cellular ATP and respire normally, which is evidence for the presence of significant endogenous substrate. In the presence of rotenone, an inhibitor of oxidative phosphorylation, glycolysis increased 56%, which provides evidence for anaerobic metabolism, as supported by enzymatic profiles. Inhibition of sodium pump activity reduced $Q_{O_2}$ by 25% to 35%, which provides evidence for a requirement for a linkage between sodium pump activity and oxidative metabolism.

In studies that examined the metabolic determinants of $K^+$ transport in isolated IMCD,[12] glucose increased both oxygen consumption and cell $K^+$ content by more than 10%, whereas an inhibitor of glycolysis promoted a release of cell $K^+$. Nor could cell $K^+$ content be maintained during inhibition of mitochondrial oxidative phosphorylation. Thus, in the IMCD, both glycolysis and oxidative phosphorylation are required to maintain optimal $Na^+$-$K^+$-ATPase activity to preserve cellular $K^+$ gradients. Given the low $P_{O_2}$ and low density of mitochondria in this region, the collecting ducts have a higher reliance on anaerobic metabolism, but still take advantage of oxidative metabolism to fully support transport.

## SEXUAL DIMORPHIC PATTERN OF TRANSPORTERS ALONG THE NEPHRON AND METABOLIC CONSIDERATIONS

For 30 years, sex differences in renal hemodynamics, including lower GFR and higher RVR in females, and similar blood pressures between sexes, have been recognized in experimental rodents.[59] Immunoblots coupled to physiologic assays in rats indicate that females, versus males, exhibit a distinct transporter profile of lower proximal transporters' abundance and $HCO_3^-$ reabsorption coupled to higher distal NCC and ENaC activation[60] (Fig. 5.11). This shift in $T_{Na}$ from the energetically efficient PT to the costlier distal nephron is predicted to decrease sodium transport energy efficiency ($T_{Na}/Q_{O_2}$) in females. A rationale for this downstream shift in $T_{Na}$ can be found in female biology. Pregnancy, and even more so lactation, represent major challenges to fluid homeostasis in females. The proximal tubule, which is shorter at baseline in females versus males,[61] lengthens during lactation, driving a proportional increase in $T_{Na}$ in a region where transport efficiency is very high due to paracellular $T_{Na}$.[61,62] These significant sex- and reproduction-dependent differences in renal transport function likely necessitate differences in nephron region–specific metabolism that warrant serious future consideration.

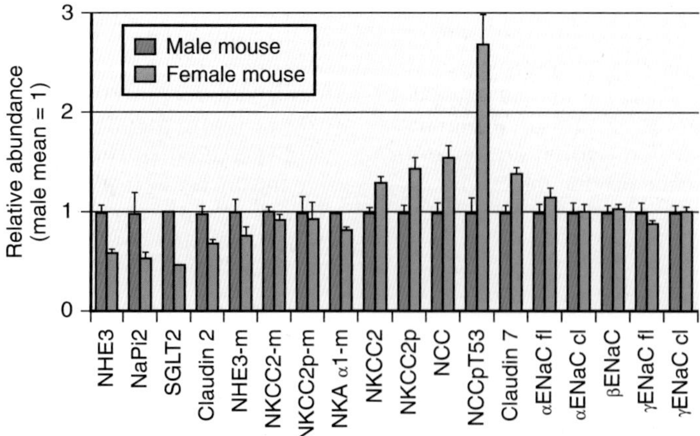


**Fig. 5.11** Profile of renal sodium transporter protein abundance in female C57BL/6 mice expressed relative to abundance in male mice (defined as 1.0). Cortical and medullary (*-m*) samples were detected by immunoblot: $Na^+/H^+$ exchanger isoform 3 (*NHE3*), $Na^+$-phosphate cotransporter isoform 2 (NaPi2), $Na^+$-glucose cotransporter (*SGLT2*), claudin 2, $Na^+$-$K^+$-$2Cl^-$ cotransporter isoform 2 (*NKCC2* and activated phosphorylated form *NKCC2p*), Na,K-ATPase α catalytic isoform, $Na^+$- $Cl^-$ cotransporter (*NCC* and activated phosphorylated form NCCp), claudin 7, epithelial $Na^+$ channel α,β,γ subunits full length (*fl*), and activated cleaved (*cl*) forms. (Adapted from Veiras et al.[60] and Pastor-Soler and Hallows KR[192]).

## CONTROL OF RENAL OXYGENATION

The kidneys are faced with the challenge of maintaining intrarenal oxygen levels so as to avoid both hypoxia, which leads to energy failure, and hyperoxia, which promotes oxidant damage.[63] Determinants of renal oxygenation and tissue oxygen tension ($Po_2$) include (1) RBF and oxygen content of arterial blood; (2) the oxygen consumed by the cells; and (3) arterial-to-venous (AV) oxygen shunting, which entails the diffusion of oxygen from preglomerular arteries to postglomerular veins without being available to the cell for consumption.

### RENAL BLOOD FLOW, OXYGEN CONSUMPTION, AND AV OXYGEN SHUNTING

The kidney enjoys a high blood flow, nearly 25% of the cardiac output, which is needed to sustain GFR. Compared with other major body organs, renal $Qo_2$ (product of RBF and renal oxygen extraction) per gram of tissue is high, second only to the heart (2.7 mmol/kg/min vs. 4.3 mmol/kg/min for the heart).[1] Renal $Qo_2$ is largely driven by the high RBF because renal oxygen extraction itself is low. Although RBF is high and renal oxygen extraction is low, the renal cortex is vulnerable to hypoxia.[64] It has been hypothesized that renal AV oxygen shunting is an adaptation to prevent hyperoxia in the setting of the high renal perfusion needed to sustain GFR. However, such shunting can be detrimental in conditions of oxygen demand-supply mismatch.[63]

The phenomenon of $O_2$ shunting from descending to ascending vasa recta in the medulla has been accepted,[65] yet little else is known regarding the location of shunting in the cortex or its impact on oxygenation. Evidence for AV $O_2$ shunting in the kidney cortex was provided when it was shown, using oxygen-sensing microelectrodes, that the oxygen tension is substantially higher in the renal vein (50 mm Hg) than in efferent arterioles (45 mm Hg) or tubules (40 mm Hg).[67,68] The fraction of oxygen subject to preglomerular AV $O_2$ shunting and impact on delivery of $O_2$ to the renal cortex was recently examined by independent groups using computer model simulations. A 2015 study concluded that preglomerular $O_2$ shunting was negligible and unlikely to impact renal oxygenation.[69] The issue was raised that the model may not have sufficiently considered the impact of wrapped artery–vein pairs (with short diffusion and no $O_2$ sink) that would facilitate AV $O_2$ shunting.[70] A 2017 study examining the preglomerular AV $O_2$ shunting concluded that although the AV shunting would have only a small impact under baseline conditions, it would exacerbate hypoxia during renal ischemia.[71]

Noting the similarity of tissue $Po_2$ in the kidney and in other organs, some have argued that the renal AV $O_2$ shunt is an adaptive mechanism for preventing the exposure of cortical tubules to toxic levels of oxygen while permitting a high RBF, which is needed for clearance.[72] As mentioned earlier, there is substantial shunting of oxygen from descending to ascending vasa recta in the renal medulla due to countercurrent flow in these vessels. Countercurrent flow in "hairpin loops" formed by the vasa recta facilitates the recycling of solutes to the inner medulla, where a high osmolarity is essential to the formation of concentrated urine (see Chapter 10). As an inherent consequence of this countercurrent mechanism for maintaining a medullary osmotic gradient, there arises a negative oxygen gradient from cortex to inner medulla, where $Po_2$ falls to 10 mm Hg.[73] This results from the combination of slow blood flow through the vasa recta, $O_2$ consumption by active transport in the outer medullary TAL, and diffusion of $O_2$ from descending to ascending vasa recta.[73] This leaves the medullary tissue at the brink of hypoxia, especially the stripe of outer medulla where the S3 segment of the proximal tubule and medullary TAL lie, making these segments most vulnerable to ischemic injury as they reabsorb significant fractions of filtered $Na^+$.

Consideration of $O_2$ transport was incorporated into a mathematical model of the rat outer medulla by Chen and colleagues.[74,75] The model takes into account fine details of the medullary anatomy, which includes positioning of the long descending vasa recta in the center of vascular bundles and the positioning of the TAL and collecting ducts at some distance from those vascular bundles. The model predicts steeply declining $O_2$ gradients from vascular bundles to the corresponding TALs and a compromise between the TAL and inner medulla with respect to the provision of oxygen.[76]

In most organs, tissue oxygen can be stabilized by metabolic regulation of blood flow. In such an arrangement, vasoactive end products of metabolism due to increased metabolic activity and oxygen utilization produce a signal that results in more blood flow to that organ. A unique feature of renal oxygenation is that the kidney cannot rely on this simple mode of metabolic autoregulation because, unlike other organs that receive blood solely to supply the metabolic needs of the organ, the kidney also receives blood to perform the functions of glomerular filtration and tubule transport.

RBF creates its own demand because it determines GFR, which in turn determines the rate of sodium reabsorption, which is the main determinant of $Qo_2$.[77,78] If the kidneys were to modulate RBF as a means of stabilizing renal $O_2$ content, this would create a vicious cycle of positive feedback in which increased $O_2$ delivery would increase $O_2$ consumption, which would call for more $O_2$ delivery. Positive feedback is inherently destabilizing, so this arrangement alone could not work to stabilize either RBF or renal $O_2$ content. Hence, the kidney is compelled to invoke mechanisms that are more complex. There are two generic routes for the kidney to stabilize its $O_2$ content. One is to dissociate RBF from GFR. The other is to alter the metabolic efficiency of $Na^+$ transport (Table 5.2). Further details are discussed shortly.

Ultimately, the rate at which the kidney consumes oxygen must be linked to GFR. This is true because the main use

**Table 5.2 Mechanisms for Changing the Amount of Oxygen Consumed per Work Performed**

| |
|---|
| Dissociate glomerular filtration rate from renal blood flow. |
| Alter the amount of $O_2$ consumed per $Na^+$ reabsorbed. |
| Shift transport between tubular segments that make more or less use of passive reabsorption. |
| Alter back-leak permeability of the tubule. |
| Change the coupling ratio of adenosine triphosphate generated to $O_2$ consumed by mitochondria. |

of oxygen is to support the reabsorption of the filtered sodium, which is linked to GFR by glomerulotubular balance (GTB). GTB describes the direct effect of the filtered load on tubular reabsorption, and it operates in all nephron segments, although the mechanism differs between segments. In the proximal tubule, shear strain tied to increased tubular flow exerts torque on the apical microvilli, which leads to upregulation of apical sodium transporters.[79,80] In cases in which filtration fraction increases, the parallel increase in peritubular capillary oncotic pressure will increase the Starling force driving fluid reabsorption. In the TAL, flux through NKCC2 is limited by chloride concentration, which declines more slowly along the TAL at high flow rates. But although GTB applies to net reabsorption, increased flow rate in the tubule also shortens the time that a given sodium ion is exposed to the reabsorptive machinery. This leads to the prediction that GTB can do no better than maintain constant fractional reabsorption.[78]

## TUBULOGLOMERULAR FEEDBACK

Significant fluctuations in RBF, GFR, and filtered $Na^+$ load would overwhelm the kidney's ability to accurately match $Na^+$ and volume output to input and compromise homeostasis of extracellular fluid volume. This does not normally occur because RBF and GFR are tightly controlled by the tubuloglomerular feedback (TGF) mechanism (described in detail in Chapter 3). In short, if RBF and/or GFR increases and GTB maintains a constant fractional reabsorption along the proximal tubule, an increasing amount of salt will be delivered to the macula densa, which sets off the TGF response. Specifically, increases in apical NaCl delivery or flow to this region provoke the cells of the macula densa to release ATP into the interstitium surrounding the afferent arterioles. This response is dependent on the basolateral $Na^+$-$K^+$-ATPase to maintain the inward-directed $Na^+$ gradient.[81] ATP release is via maxi-anion channels.[82] Some fraction of the released ATP is converted to adenosine by local ecto-nucleoside triphosphate diphosphohydrolase 1 (ecto-NTPDase1) and ecto-5′-nucleotidase.[83] This adenosine activates $A_1$ adenosine receptors on the afferent arteriole, causing vasoconstriction. The arteriolar constriction reduces RBF and GFR in concert until $Na^+$ delivery to the macula densa is realigned. Thus, an inverse relationship is established between tubular NaCl load and the GFR of the same nephron.[77]

Due to the time it takes for information to pass through the TGF system, the system is prone to oscillate with a period of around 30 seconds. Rhythmic oscillations of kidney $Po_2$ occur at the same frequency as TGF-mediated oscillations in tubular flow. This illustrates the simultaneous influence of TGF over minute-to-minute tubular flow rate and oxygen levels in the kidney.[84]

Adenosine mediates TGF as a vasoconstrictor. Adenosine-mediated vasoconstriction is unique to the afferent arteriole. In all other beds where adenosine is vasoactive, it exerts a vasodilatory effect mediated by $A_2$ receptors. In addition to adenosine receptors, the afferent arteriole expresses $P_{2X}$ purinergic receptors that also mediate a vasoconstrictor response, in this case to interstitial ATP. These $P_{2X}$ receptors are essential to pressure-mediated RBF autoregulation,[85] but adenosine $A_1$ receptors are sufficient to explain the TGF response.[83]

Adenosine also plays an important role in stabilizing medullary energy balance through local adjustments in blood flow and transport along with other autocrine and paracrine factors, including vasodilatory prostaglandins and nitric oxide, which increase medullary blood flow while inhibiting sodium transport in the TAL.[48,86,87] Adenosine, in particular, is a case study in local metabolic regulation by negative feedback in the medulla. When ATP levels decline, adenosine is released from TAL cells into the renal interstitium, where it binds to adenosine $A_1$ receptors and inhibits $Na^+$ reabsorption in the TAL and IMCD. This has the effect of increasing $Po_2$ by reducing $Qo_2$. The same pool of adenosine also activates vascular adenosine $A_2$ receptors in the deep cortex and medullary vasa recta to increase blood flow.[88,89]

By these mechanisms, the TAL looks after its own interest. But because TAL sodium reabsorption normally exceeds the urinary sodium excretion by 40-fold, any significant decline in TAL reabsorption must be compensated for by increasing active transport somewhere else or by reducing GFR through TGF. Activation of $A_1$ receptors in the glomerulus, proximal tubule, or TAL contributes to lessening the amount of work imposed on the hypoxic outer medulla, whereas activating $A_2$ receptors in the vasa recta supports $O_2$ delivery to the medulla (summarized in Fig. 5.12).

## METABOLIC COST OF SODIUM REABSORPTION

The cost of renal sodium transport can be estimated from the sodium pump stoichiometry and the amount of oxygen required to produce ATP. Sodium pump stoichiometry dictates that hydrolysis of one ATP molecule is coupled to the transport of 3 $Na^+$ ions out of the cell and 2 $K^+$ ions into the cell,[4] and oxidative metabolism generates approximately 6 ATP molecules per $O_2$ molecule consumed (see Table 5.1 and Fig. 5.4). In the 1960s, several investigators undertook measuring the metabolic cost of tubular reabsorption in various species of mammals. There is fair consensus among four oft-cited studies published between 1961 and 1966 that the relationship between $Qo_2$ and $T_{Na}$ is linear and that the kidney reabsorbs 25 to 29 $Na^+$ ions per molecule of $O_2$ consumed in the process.[90–93] A representative figure from one of these studies is shown in Fig. 5.13.

If one assumes that kidney mitochondria make 6 molecules of ATP per molecule of $O_2$, the kidney must then reabsorb 4 to 5 $Na^+$ per ATP molecule. This exceeds the 3:1 stoichiometry of the $Na^+$-$K^+$-ATPase, which was known at the time (reviewed in Burg and Good).[94] Because there are thermodynamic difficulties with the idea of an undiscovered basolateral sodium pump capable of forcing 5 $Na^+$ from a tubular cell with energy from a single ATP molecule, it was surmised that a considerable fraction of overall sodium reabsorption must be passive and paracellular, as is now accepted.

It was later suggested, by Cohen[43] and others, that these calculated ratios of $Qo_2/T_{Na}$ actually underestimate the true efficiency of sodium reabsorption because a fraction of the oxygen consumed during $Na^+$ transport is also spent metabolizing organic substrates that enter the cell by Na cotransport. The most important example of this is lactate, which is converted to glucose in the proximal tubule via the Cori cycle. The capacity for renal gluconeogenesis from lactate is large, and it has been estimated that the kidney can consume

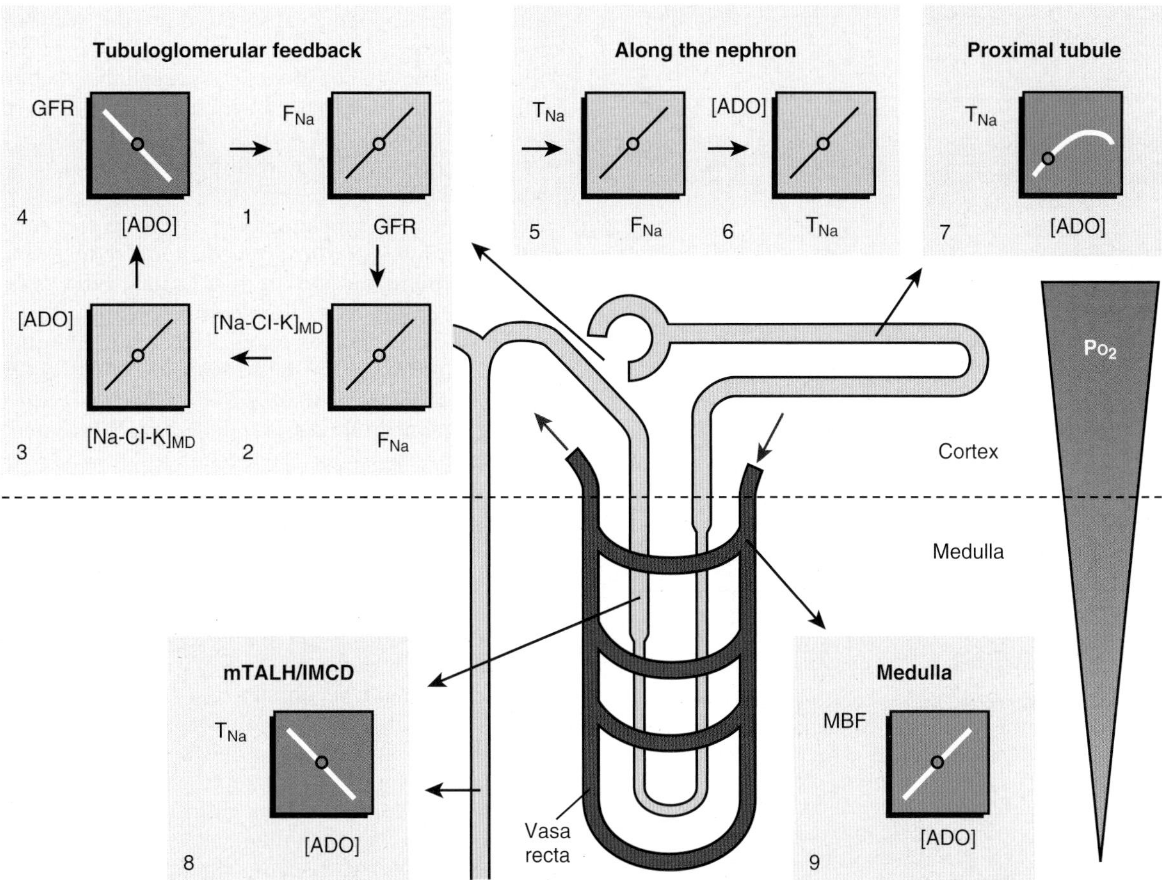


**Fig. 5.12** Role of extracellular adenosine (*ADO*) in protecting the renal medulla from hypoxia. The line plots illustrate the relationships between the given parameters. *Small circles* on these lines indicate ambient physiologic conditions. (1) A rise in glomerular filtration rate (*GFR*) increases the $Na^+$ load ($F_{Na}$) to the tubular system in cortex and medulla. (2) This rise in $F_{Na}$ increases the salt concentration sensed by the macula densa (*[Na-Cl-K]$_{MD}$*). (3) The increase in [Na-Cl-K]$_{MD}$, in turn, enhances local ADO. (4) ADO lowers GFR and thus $F_{Na}$, which closes a negative feedback loop and thus provides a basis for an oscillating system. (5) $F_{Na}$ determines $Na^+$ transport work ($T_{Na}$) and $O_2$ consumption in every nephron segment, and thus oscillations in $F_{Na}$ may help protect the medulla. (6) A rise in $T_{Na}$ increases ADO along the nephron. (7) In the cortical proximal tubule, ADO stimulates $T_{Na}$ and thus lowers the $Na^+$ load to segments residing in the medulla. (8) In contrast, ADO inhibits transport work in the medulla, including medullary thick ascending limb (*mTAL*) and inner medullary collecting duct (*IMCD*). (9) In addition, ADO enhances medullary blood flow (*MBF*), which increases $O_2$ delivery and further limits $O_2$-consuming transport in the medulla. (Modified from Vallon V, et al. Adenosine and kidney function. *Physiol Rev.* 2006;86:901–940.)

up to 25% as much energy converting lactate to glucose as it spends reabsorbing sodium.[43]

The metabolic cost of active sodium transport is expected to vary along the nephron. As reviewed earlier, the overall stoichiometry of $Na^+$ reabsorbed to $O_2$ consumed is estimated at 25 to 30 (microequivalents $Na^+$/micromoles $O_2$).[90,92] This ratio translates to 5 $Na^+$ reabsorbed for every ATP molecule consumed, which is much higher than the ratio of 3 $Na^+$ to every ATP molecule predicted by sodium pump stoichiometry. In fact, one might expect a ratio lower than 3 because of the basal metabolic functions of the kidney that are independent of sodium transport (i.e., insensitive to the $Na^+$-$K^+$-ATPase inhibitor ouabain) (Fig. 5.14) and because of tubular back-leak.

One reason for this higher than expected efficiency of sodium reabsorption is that the kidney can leverage excess free energy in the gradients created by primary and secondary active transport to drive passive paracellular reabsorption of sodium chloride. The paracellular route in the proximal tubule responsible for sodium reabsorption is the tight junction protein channel claudin-2.[95] Free energy for paracellular reabsorption is available in the mid-proximal tubule and early TAL.[94] In the proximal tubule, the driving force for the passive transport develops as a result of the preferential absorption of bicarbonate over chloride earlier in the tubule.[96,97]

The decline in tubular bicarbonate concentration is paralleled by a rise in chloride concentration as water follows $Na^+$, $HCO_3^-$, and organic osmoles across the leaky proximal tubule (see Chapter 5). This favorable lumen-to-blood $Cl^-$ gradient drives passive paracellular chloride reabsorption. The transepithelial voltage that arises from electrodiffusion of chloride, in turn, drives passive sodium reabsorption. Because the NaCl reflection coefficient is less than that for $NaHCO_3$ in this region,[96] coupled sodium chloride reabsorption also occurs secondary to solvent drag.[98] Although estimates vary, this passive reabsorption may increase the number of $Na^+$ ions reabsorbed to $O_2$ molecules consumed in the proximal tubule from 18 to 48.[99] As discussed in a previous section,

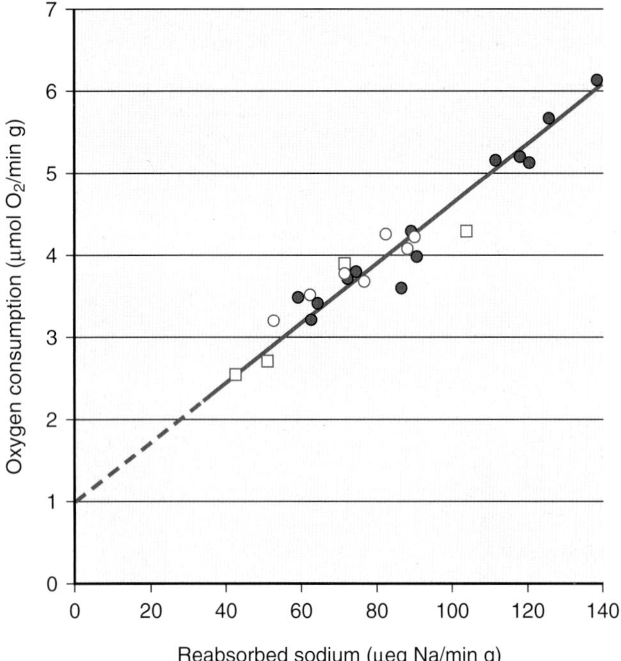


**Fig. 5.13** Oxygen consumption as a function of net sodium reabsorption in whole dog kidney. *Filled circles*, control; *open circles*, hypoxia; *squares*, hydrochlorothiazide. The slope of the line fitted to the data points represents $Q_{O_2}/T_{Na}$ and is approximately 1/28. (Modified from Thurau K. Renal Na-reabsorption and $O_2$-uptake in dogs during hypoxia and hydrochlorothiazide infusion. *Proc Soc Exp Biol Med.* 1961;106:714–717; and Mandel LJ, Balaban RS. Stoichiometry and coupling of active transport to oxidative metabolism in epithelial tissues. *Am J Physiol.* 1981;240[5]:F357–F371.)

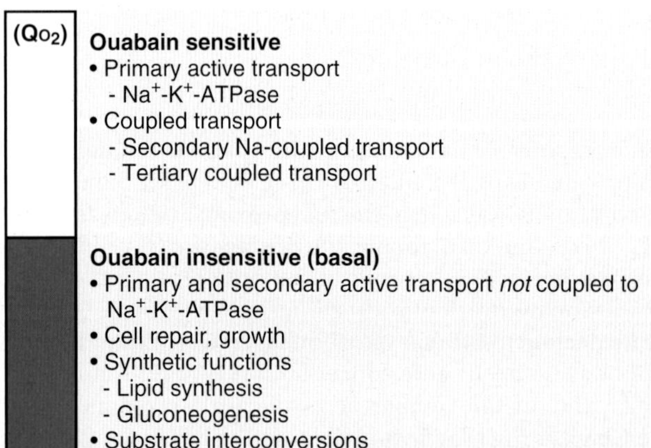


**Fig. 5.14** A large fraction of renal epithelial oxygen consumption ($Q_{O_2}$) in renal cells is sensitive to the $Na^+$-$K^+$-ATPase–specific inhibitor ouabain, and this $Q_{O_2}$ drives primary active transport and transport coupled to sodium pump activity. The fraction of renal oxygen consumption that does not change in the presence of ouabain is, by definition, independent of $Na^+$-$K^+$-ATPase activity in the cell and is roughly equivalent to the basal $Q_{O_2}$, which fuels transport not coupled to sodium gradients, cell repair and growth, biosynthesis, and substrate interconversions.

blunting paracellular reabsorption in the claudin-2–null mouse increases the oxygen consumption cost of $T_{Na}$ by shifting it from paracellular to transcellular reabsorption, supporting the idea that paracellular transport is required for energy efficiency of oxygen utilization in the service of the large fraction of $Na^+$ reabsorption that occurs in the proximal tubule.[55]

Simultaneously blocking both cytosolic and membrane carbonic anhydrase with acetazolamide reduces bicarbonate reabsorption and $Q_{O_2}$ in a 16:1 molar ratio as expected for simple coupling to the sodium pump.[100] But inhibiting bicarbonate reabsorption with a membrane-specific carbonic anhydrase inhibitor, which acidifies the tubular lumen, paradoxically increases $Q_{O_2}$ both in vivo and in isolated proximal tubules, an effect that is prevented by also blocking the apical $Na^+/H^+$ exchanger NHE3.[101] A simple explanation is lacking for why increasing the cell-to-lumen proton gradient should increase $Q_{O_2}$ in the proximal tubule, but these results establish the phenomenon in vitro and in vivo.

The early portion of the TAL is also capable of paracellular $Na^+$ reabsorption. In this region, $Na^+$ can be transported transcellularly by the apical Na-K-2Cl cotransporter or apical $Na^+/H^+$ exchanger, secondary to a high density of $Na^+$-$K^+$-ATPase extruding $Na^+$ across the basolateral membranes. In addition, $Na^+$ can be reabsorbed paracellularly as long as there is a lumen-positive transepithelial voltage sufficient to overcome the force for back diffusion associated with an unfavorable concentration difference. A lumen-positive voltage develops in the TAL because the apical membrane has a high concentration of $K^+$ channels, whereas the basolateral membrane has both $K^+$ and $Cl^-$ channels. As predicted by the Goldman-Hodgkin-Katz voltage equation, the chloride conductance causes the basolateral membrane potential to be less negative than the apical membrane potential, which results in a positive transepithelial gradient.[102,103]

Further along the nephron in the distal tubule and collecting duct, the tubular fluid sodium concentration is too low to allow paracellular reabsorption of sodium. In those segments, a lower limit on the cost of $Na^+$ reabsorption is set by the 3 $Na^+$/1 ATP ratio of the sodium pump. Although active transport of sodium is a pacemaker for renal respiration, there are ways to reset the relationship of $Q_{O_2}$ to sodium pump activity. Examples of this were provided by Silva and Epstein, who measured both $O_2$ consumption and $Na^+$-$K^+$-ATPase activity in rat kidney slices in which an increase in the latter had been induced by prior treatment of the animals with triiodothyronine ($T_3$), methylprednisolone, potassium loading, or subtotal nephrectomy. Although each of these maneuvers increased ex vivo sodium pump activity, only $T_3$ and methylprednisolone increased $Q_{O_2}$.[104]

It has also been shown that the thermogenic effect of catecholamines, normally associated with brown fat and striated muscle, also occurs in the kidney, which responds to dopamine infusion with a near doubling of overall metabolic rate, but minimal change in sodium reabsorption.[105] Dopamine inhibits $Na^+$ reabsorption in the proximal tubule,[106,107] thereby shifting the reabsorptive burden to less efficient downstream segments. However, heat accumulates in both cortex and medulla during dopamine infusion, which suggests that the mechanism may be a direct effect of catecholamines on renal metabolism. In addition, an increase in RBF by dopamine could be responsible for the increased renal oxygen consumption, which is the product of RBF and renal oxygen extraction.

Weinstein and Szyjewicz[108,109] also examined $Qo_2/T_{Na}$ using 10% body weight short-term saline expansion as another way to inhibit proximal $Na^+$ reabsorption in rats. This maneuver reduced fractional $Na^+$ reabsorption by 30% in the proximal tubule, leading to a GTB-mediated increase in net reabsorption downstream of the proximal tubule. Yet overall $Qo_2$ did not increase but actually fell. It was conjectured that energy for this increase in downstream reabsorption was derived anaerobically, but the full details of this remain to be clarified. It appears that the energy cost of transport in the proximal versus distal nephron during inhibition of proximal tubule transport depends on the nature of the stimulus provoking the change in transport as well as the metabolic environment.

Energetic efficiency of $Na^+$ reabsorption is highly variable along the nephron, in large part due to the presence of paracellular pathways for reabsorption in "leaky" epithelia such as the proximal tubule that can take advantage of favorable concentration and electrochemical gradients to reabsorb $Na^+$ without requiring ATP hydrolysis. Thus, if proximal reabsorption is lower (as in females) or reduced, the shift of $T_{Na}$ to more distal sites should provoke an increase in $Qo_2$ driven by higher active uphill transcellular $Na^+$ reabsorption. The example of the cldn-2 null mouse is provided earlier as an example.[55] Layton et al. now provide computational models that assess how shifting $T_{Na}$ from one region to another or inhibiting $T_{Na}$ in a region-specific manner alters overall $Qo_2$.[110,111] In this model, increasing single-nephron GFR did not alter the efficiency of reabsorbing $Na^+$ in the proximal tubule ($T_{Na}/Qo_2$) while it increased $T_{Na}/Qo_2$ downstream secondary to higher paracellular $T_{Na}$ due to higher luminal [$Na^+$]. This finding suggests that the proximal S3 segment and medullary thick ascending limb (which are vulnerable to hypoxia) are buffered from higher $Qo_2$ in response to increased flow and substrate delivery.[110] When the model was applied to an examination of the effects of inhibiting individual transporters, the impact of inhibiting the proximal tubule NHE3 was most pronounced, not unexpected given the fact that the NHE3 reabsorbs 36% of filtered $Na^+$ at baseline. Overall, inhibiting NHE3 by 80% reduced GFR by 30% (mediated by TGF) and reduced whole kidney $T_{Na}/Qo_2$ by 20%, explained by far less proximal paracellular $T_{Na}$ and the shift of $T_{Na}$ to less efficient distal regions. Interestingly, the model predicts that NHE3 and NKCC2 inhibition increase CNT and CD ENaC-mediated $T_{Na}/Qo_2$ secondary to increased luminal $Na^+$. Inhibition of NKCC2, NCC, or ENaC, although changing urine volume, $Na^+$ and $K^+$ excretion as predicted, did not change whole kidney $T_{Na}/Qo_2$.[111]

## RENAL OXYGENATION AND METABOLISM DURING NORMAL PERTURBATIONS AND DISEASE

The kidneys have developed multiple mechanisms to minimize changes in oxygen delivery and to cope with a reduction in $Po_2$. Some of these are specific to the kidney, whereas others are generic to many tissues as discussed next.

### PHYSIOLOGIC REGULATION: FILTRATION FRACTION AND $Qo_2/T_{NA}$

As reviewed earlier, there are two generic routes for the kidney to achieve a stable content of $O_2$: dissociation of RBF from GFR, and alteration of $Qo_2/T_{Na}$ (see Table 5.2). Both routes are subject to regulation. Dissociating RBF from GFR equates to changing the glomerular filtration fraction. This can work to stabilize kidney $O_2$ because lowering the filtration fraction increases the ratio of supply to demand for $O_2$. For nephrons in filtration equilibrium, this requires independent control of the afferent and efferent arterioles, which can be achieved by modulating relative activities of purinergic, angiotensin, nitric oxide, and other signaling systems in the glomerulus. A full discussion of glomerular hemodynamics is available in Chapter 3, but a few features are noted here.

To begin, filtration fraction can be lowered by constricting the afferent arteriole (which reduces net $O_2$ delivery) or dilating the efferent arteriole (which increases net $O_2$ delivery). Constricting the afferent arteriole confers initial energy savings by reducing GFR faster than RBF, but there is diminishing return as $O_2$ delivery declines toward the basal requirement. Dilating the efferent arteriole reduces GFR only when glomerular capillary pressure is low to begin with, such as during hypotension or with high afferent resistance.[112] When angiotensin II acts on the afferent and efferent arterioles to stabilize GFR in the face of low blood pressure or high upstream resistance by preferentially constricting efferent arterioles, the kidney is accepting a decrease in the ratio of $O_2$ supply to $O_2$ demand. Conversely, adenosine signaling in the glomerulus decreases filtration fraction and so manages to stabilize nephron function without compromising the $O_2$ supply–demand balance. Adenosine in the nanomolar range constricts the afferent arteriole via high-affinity $A_1$ adenosine receptors. Higher adenosine concentration dilates the efferent arteriole via low-affinity $A_2$ adenosine receptors. Interstitial adenosine concentration rises as more NaCl is delivered into the nephron. The prototype for this is the TGF signaling through the macula densa, although other sources are not precluded (see Fig. 5.12). When the kidney is operating in the domain of modest distal delivery, increasing the TGF signal constricts the afferent arteriole. When the kidney is operating in the domain of high distal delivery, further increase causes the efferent arteriole to dilate,[113] which can be viewed as a shift in priority toward maintaining the $O_2$ supply as the supply diminishes.

The second generic means for stabilizing kidney $O_2$ is to alter $Qo_2/T_{Na}$. As mentioned earlier, studies in the 1960s established the linear relationship between $Qo_2$ and $T_{Na}$. Each adopted a similar standard, which was to express suprabasal renal $Qo_2$ as a function of $T_{Na}$. Suprabasal $O_2$ consumption was obtained by subtracting from total $O_2$ consumption the amount required for basal metabolism. The latter was determined by various methods. One method was to plot $Qo_2$ against $T_{Na}$ and then extrapolate to the *y*-intercept to obtain basal $Qo_2$. Another approach was to reduce renal perfusion pressure to the point that glomerular filtration ceased, then ascribe the residual measured $Qo_2$ to basal metabolism. These approaches for obtaining basal $O_2$ consumption have their unique limitations, and both require the dubious assumption that basal metabolism is static under most conditions and is unaffected by $T_{Na}$ per se. Nonetheless, these studies attempted to measure and incorporate the contribution of basal $Qo_2$ to the total $Qo_2$. In the recent literature, the ratio of total $Qo_2$ to $T_{Na}$ has been represented as an index of metabolic efficiency of transport, ignoring the contribution of basal $Qo_2$ to the total $Qo_2$. This can lead to inaccuracies as estimates of basal metabolism have varied widely in the published literature, indicating its susceptibility to different experimental conditions.[114] For example, the proximal tubule can devote considerable energy to gluconeogenesis, especially in the postabsorptive or fasting states, and in diabetes.[41,115,116] In light of the fact that oxygen can be diverted to do other work, an increase in $Qo_2/T_{Na}$ is not necessarily due to "decreased transport efficiency."

The specific factors contributing to this $Qo_2/T_{Na}$ stoichiometry as well as to the basal metabolic rate in the kidney have been the subject of numerous reviews.[117,118] It is theoretically possible to alter $Qo_2/T_{Na}$ in a number of ways (see Table 5.2):

1. Transport could be shifted from the proximal tubule, where efficient use of energy from the $Na^+$-$K^+$-ATPase drives passive transport, to other segments where all $Na^+$ reabsorbed passes through the $Na^+$-$K^+$-ATPase.
2. Tubular back-leak permeability could change, which would affect the number of times that a given $Na^+$ ion must be reabsorbed to escape excretion into the urine.
3. The ratio of ATP produced per $O_2$ consumed could be altered by the regulated activity of UCPs (see Fig. 5.3).[25]
4. ATP could be diverted to gluconeogenesis, such as during fasting.

The same neurohumoral factors that exert well-known effects on glomerular hemodynamics and $O_2$ supply, including nitric oxide, angiotensin II, adenosine, and catecholamines, also appear to participate in the regulation of kidney metabolism and $Qo_2$ by the tubule. It has been shown[119,120] that the administration of nonselective nitric oxide synthase (NOS) inhibitors increases $Qo_2/T_{Na}$. Other experiments suggested that NOS-1 is the specific isoform that regulates this action in vivo.[119] The changes in $Qo_2$ with NOS inhibition may occur due to (1) a shift in the site of sodium reabsorption to a less efficient nephron segment; (2) decreased efficiency of transport in the proximal tubule (i.e., decrease in the passive component of reabsorption); or (3) less efficient use of $O_2$ by mitochondria. For example, nitric oxide given directly to a proximal tubular cell is both a proximal diuretic[121] and a competitive inhibitor of $O_2$ flux through the ETC in mitochondria.[122]

Most effects of nitric oxide are mediated by cyclic guanosine monophosphate, but the mitochondrial effect is presumed to occur through the competitive inhibition of cytochrome *c* oxidase.[122–124] Studies in normal rats,[125] in rats with experimental diabetes,[126] and in rats with untreated hypertension[127,128] have found an antagonistic relationship between nitric oxide and angiotensin II in terms of both glomerular hemodynamics and tubular reabsorption. Specifically, systemic NOS blockade causes renal vasoconstriction and activation of TGF, which can be prevented by angiotensin II blockers.

A similar antagonistic relationship appears to exist in control of kidney metabolism as well. Angiotensin II was recently shown to be capable of increasing $Qo_2$ despite lowering $T_{Na}$.[129] Rats and mice with angiotensin-induced hypertension exhibit stimulation of sodium transporters from the cortical TAL to the CD, in regions with higher $Qo_2/T_{Na}$, and inhibition or no stimulation of sodium transporters in the proximal nephron, where $Qo_2/T_{Na}$ is lower.[130,131] Studies in spontaneous hypertensive rats have suggested opposing effects of angiotensin II and nitric oxide on the $Qo_2/T_{Na}$ ratio in the kidney.[132] Rats with angiotensin-induced hypertension demonstrated an increased $Qo_2/T_{Na}$ that was reversed by a mimetic of superoxide dismutase, which is consistent with the theory that many angiotensin II effects are mediated by upregulating the activity of reduced nicotinamide adenine dinucleotide phosphate (NADPH) oxidase.[129] In addition, there is evidence that angiotensin II contributes to mitochondrial dysfunction and oxygen consumption in aging rats.[133]

There is also evidence for a self-contained, intrarenal renin-angiotensin system that operates independently of the systemic renin–angiotensin system (RAS).[134–137] It is possible to dissociate tubular and whole-kidney angiotensin II in the regulation of proximal reabsorption and salt homeostasis.[137] For example, a low-salt diet activates the systemic RAS and increases renal sodium reabsorption without any measurable increase in intrarenal synthesis of angiotensin II,[138] whereas a high-salt diet has a predictable inhibitory effect on plasma and whole-kidney angiotensin II but, surprisingly, leads to increased angiotensin II content of proximal tubular fluid. This finding explains why the tonic influence of endogenous angiotensin II over proximal reabsorption fails to decline with consumption of a high-salt diet. Thus, whereas the systemic RAS is oriented toward salt homeostasis, it appears that the tubular angiotensin II system is oriented toward a stable salt delivery beyond the proximal tubule.[137]

The role of angiotensin II in kidney metabolism is implicated in the ablation/infarction remnant kidney model of chronic kidney disease (CKD). Oxygen consumption factored for nephron number or $T_{Na}$ has been shown to be elevated in this model[139–141] and lowered by various treatments including angiotensin blockade.[139] A connection has also been established recently between local accumulation of the Krebs cycle intermediate succinate and activation of the RAS.[142] Succinate can accumulate extracellularly when oxygen supply does not match demand. In the extracellular fluid, it can bind to its G protein–coupled receptor, GPR91. $Po_2$ in the juxtaglomerular region is reduced in the hyperglycemia of diabetes, and succinate levels are very high in urine and renal tissue of diabetic animals. Inhibition of the Krebs cycle's succinate dehydrogenase complex causes robust renin release. This effect is amplified in high-glucose conditions or with added succinate. In summary, GPR91-mediated signaling in the juxtaglomerular apparatus could modulate glomerular filtration rate and RAS activity in response to changes in metabolism (especially after a meal when glucose level is elevated). Pathologically, GPR91-mediated signaling could link metabolic diseases (such as diabetes) with RAS activation, systemic hypertension, and organ injury.

## HYPOXIA AND ISCHEMIA

Intrarenal hypoxia has been proposed as a final common pathway to progression of CKD.[143] In late stages of CKD, rarefaction of capillaries and other structural changes have been implicated in the decrease in oxygen supply leading to hypoxia. However, intrarenal hypoxia has been demonstrated in the early stages before any structural changes.[144] High

$Qo_2/T_{Na}$ has been postulated to be the etiology of tubular hypoxia in the early stages of CKD.[139] In early experimental diabetes, decreased tissue oxygen tension ($Po_2$) has also been demonstrated prior to any structural changes associated with diabetic nephropathy.[145] Various forms of kidney injury, acute and chronic, have demonstrated tissue hypoxia in early and late stages as discussed later in the chapter.

Blood oxygen level–dependent magnetic resonance imaging (BOLD MRI) has been used to measure blood flow, oxygen tension, and regional tissue oxygenation in kidney cortex and medulla in humans with hypertension. The following were compared: kidneys with atherosclerotic renal artery stenosis, the kidneys contralateral with the stenotic kidneys, and kidneys in individuals with essential hypertension with no accompanying stenosis.[146,147] In the stenotic kidneys, as expected, tissue volume was decreased and blood flow was compromised; however, there was no significant decrease in $Po_2$ in the cortex or deep medulla compared with the contralateral kidney in the same person or compared with kidneys in individuals with essential hypertension. This led the authors to postulate that there was reduced oxygen consumption in the stenotic kidneys. Consistent with this interpretation, furosemide-suppressible $Qo_2$ in the medulla was significantly less in the stenotic kidney than in the contralateral kidney or kidneys in individuals with essential hypertension.[147] The association between tissue hypoxia and renal damage has also been assessed in patients with renal artery stenosis.[148]

In diabetic and nondiabetic CKD patients, intrarenal hypoxia correlates with renal pathology.[149,150] Alterations in renal oxygenation in acute transplant rejection have also been described.[151] Recently, the effect of sodium intake on renal tissue oxygenation was investigated.[152] In brief, 1 week of low-$Na^+$ intake increased renal medullary oxygenation in both normotensive and hypertensive subjects, whereas a high-$Na^+$ diet reduced medullary oxygenation. Another recent study in patients with CKD and hypertension compared with healthy controls revealed tight regulation of renal oxygenation at rest but altered response to furosemide in both CKD and hypertension groups, suggesting early metabolic changes in hypertension.[153,154] In many of these studies, furosemide was administered to inhibit tubular reabsorption, which improved medullary oxygenation, demonstrating the significant role of Na reabsorption-driven $Qo_2$, even in established disease with structural alterations, which impact oxygen delivery.

Assessment of tissue hypoxia in acute kidney injury has largely been described in animal studies. Studies in an ischemia–reperfusion model in rats and pigs demonstrated reduced oxygenation and persistent tissue hypoxia in the early stages after reperfusion,[155,156] which was more prominent in the outer medullary regions. These studies were limited to early stages after reperfusion (3–4 hours post ischemia). Assessment of tissue oxygenation in later stages could provide important information regarding the role of hypoxia in repair or recovery from AKI and/or transition to CKD. In animal studies of sepsis associated AKI, variability in tissue oxygenation has been reported depending on the animal model, species, or time point after injury.[157–161] However, increased renal oxygen extraction despite reduction in GFR and filtered load has been described,[160,161] indicating inefficiency of oxygen utilization and/or changes in basal metabolism of tubular cells. Clinical studies assessing renal oxygenation in AKI are limited. However, in a set of elegant studies in postcardiac surgery patients with or without AKI, increased renal $O_2$ extraction and $Qo_2/T_{Na}$ was demonstrated in the AKI group.[162] Improvement in renal oxygenation with loop diuretics due to reduction in tubular transport related $Qo_2$ was also demonstrated.[163]

## HYPOXIA-INDUCIBLE FACTOR

One of the major transcription factors mediating the cellular adaptation to hypoxia is the oxygen-sensitive, hypoxia-inducible factor (HIF).[164] A great body of work by Semenza have described the role of HIF as a primary oxygen sensor and regulator of cellular oxygen homeostasis.[164–167] It accumulates in hypoxic cells, where it acts to regulate gene expression. HIF consists of a labile α subunit (HIF1α, HIF2α, HIF3α) and a constitutive β subunit. These subunits heterodimerize to form a transcriptional complex that translocates to the nucleus and binds to hypoxia response elements of various hypoxia responsive genes.[168,169] HIF1α and HIF2α have been well studied, have similar structures, and have significant overlap in their actions on target genes; however, some target genes appear to be exclusively under the regulation of one or the other. Their renal tissue expression patterns also differ, with predominant expression of HIF1α in the tubular epithelial cells and HIF2α in the interstitial fibroblasts and peritubular endothelial cells in the hypoxic kidney.[170,171] There is limited information regarding the function and actions of HIF-3α.

During adaptation to hypoxia, HIF1α and 2α regulate the expression of many genes that regulate oxygen delivery and consumption. Changes that culminate in a rise in erythropoiesis, vasodilation, and tissue vascularization all increase oxygen delivery.[172,173] Another set of responses conserve energy by decreasing substrate movement into the tricarboxylic acid cycle, increasing cellular glucose uptake and glycolytic enzymes to increase anaerobic ATP production and shifting the cell towards glycolytic metabolism.[167] HIF-1α also has significant effects on mitochondrial metabolism; specifically, it diminishes NADH supply to the ETC, induces a subunit switch in complex IV of ETC to optimize its efficiency in hypoxia, and represses mitochondrial biogenesis and respiration.[174,175] Finally, HIF-1α also induces mitochondrial autophagy as an adaptive metabolic response to prevent increased levels of reactive oxygen species (ROS) generation and cell death in hypoxia.[176]

Recently, HIF-1 α has also been recognized as a regulator of salt transport. High-salt intake increased HIF-1 α expression in the renal medulla.[177] Inhibition of HIF-1α in the renal medulla decreased medullary blood flow, and blunted urine flow and urinary Na excretion. In the presence of HIF-1α inhibitor, rats on a high-salt intake developed positive cumulative salt balance and higher blood pressure. Thus, medullary HIF-1α inhibition on a high-salt intake leads to resetting of pressure natriuresis, Na retention, and salt-sensitive hypertension.[178] HIF-1α expression has been reported in the medulla in a normal rat,[179] where selective inhibition of medullary HIF-1 induced significant tubulointerstitial damage. Interestingly, HIF-1 expression appeared to correlate with salt transport—an increase noted after an increase in medullary workload and a decrease in expression noted after inhibiting Na transport in the TAL by furosemide administration, which also increased medullary $Po_2$.[179]

HIF activity is regulated by proteasomal degradation during normoxia by von Hippel-Lindau-E3 ubiquitin ligase complex after being hydroxylated by prolyl 4 hydroxylase domains (PHD). Of the three main identified PHDs (1, 2, and 3), PHD2 is the main enzyme that targets HIF for degradation under normoxia.[170] All three PHDs are expressed in the kidney and are found predominantly in the distal convoluted tubule, collecting duct, and podocytes, and levels are depressed during ischemia and reperfusion.[169,170] HIF activity is also regulated by factor inhibiting HIF (FIH), which inhibits its transcriptional activity by hydroxylating an asparagine residue within the transactivation domain and prevents the binding of coactivators to the HIF transcriptional complex.[166]

A tremendous amount of progress has been made in understanding how HIF helps to maintain $O_2$ homeostasis, and the study of this factor in the kidney under normal physiologic and pathophysiologic conditions. Particularly, the role of HIF stabilization and activation in the kidney to stimulate erythropoietin production has been targeted therapeutically. Structural analogs of 2-oxyglutarate, which are the substrates used by PHDs for HIF hydroxylation, have been developed to reversibly inhibit PHD activity. These analogs are in phase 2 and 3 clinical trials for treatment of anemia by endogenous erythropoietin production in CKD.[180] Recently, the efficacy of Vadadustat, an oral PHD inhibitor, was evaluated in a 20-week, double-blind, randomized, placebo-controlled, phase IIb study in patients with stage 3–5 CKD.[181] Hemoglobin levels were increased and maintained in the treatment arm without major adverse effects. Moreover, increased iron mobilization was also reported in patients treated with Vadadustat. Another oral PHD inhibitor, Roxadustat, was evaluated in an open-label, phase IIb study in patients with CKD using different starting doses and frequencies of administration for 16 or 24 weeks.[182] The various dosing regimens were well tolerated and effective in achieving target hemoglobin levels, without the need for additional iron supplementation. The same agent has also shown effectiveness in patients on incident hemodialysis or peritoneal dialysis.[183] A third agent, GSK1278863, was evaluated in both CKD patients not on dialysis and ESRD patients on dialysis in a 4-week, phase IIa study.[184] It was safe and well tolerated in both populations and produced dose-dependent increases in hemoglobin concentrations in the CKD patients, whereas only the higher dose was effective in maintaining hemoglobin concentrations in the ESRD patients on dialysis. The ease of administration, lower peak plasma erythropoietin levels, and beneficial effects on iron homeostasis make these oral HIF stabilizers attractive alternatives for anemia management in CKD. However, longer-duration trials to study efficacy and safety of these agents in CKD and ESRD patients are needed.

## ADENOSINE MONOPHOSPHATE–ACTIVATED PROTEIN KINASE

The energy status of the cell can be detected by the ultrasensitive 5′-adenosine monophosphate (AMP)–activated protein kinase (AMPK), which is a ubiquitously expressed, highly conserved, key energy sensor and regulator of cellular metabolic activity.[185] AMPK consists of a heterotrimer of a catalytic subunit (α1 or α2), together with a beta (β1 or β2) and a gamma (γ1, γ2, or γ3) regulatory subunit.[185] Cellular energy stress, which can be due to a variety of conditions, such as nutrient or glucose deprivation, exercise, hypoxia, or ischemia, is detected as a rising concentration of AMP and an increase in the AMP/ATP ratio. AMPK is activated by phosphorylation of the α catalytic subunit on threonine-172 (Thr172) by upstream kinases.[186] The binding of AMP to the γ-regulatory subunit of AMPK increases its activity in three ways: (1) conformational change in AMPK, which allows enhanced phosphorylation of the α catalytic subunit on Thr172 by upstream kinases, thus, activating AMPK; (2) inhibition of dephosphorylation of the catalytic subunit; and (3) direct allosteric activation. These three effects, working in concert, render the system exquisitely sensitive to changes in AMP, and all are antagonized by ATP; thus the importance of the AMP/ATP ratio. AMPK acts as a metabolic checkpoint to facilitate metabolic adaptation to cellular energetic stress by triggering ATP producing pathways such as fatty acid oxidation, glucose uptake, and glycolysis, while inhibiting ATP consuming pathways such as fatty acid synthesis, protein synthesis, and potentially active transport[187] (see Fig. 5.15). AMPK also promotes cellular autophagy, an energy conserving survival mechanism in low energy states by inhibiting mTOR.[188,189]

There is abundant AMPK expression in the kidney, but the understanding of its impact on energy metabolism and transport in the kidney is just emerging. The role of AMPK

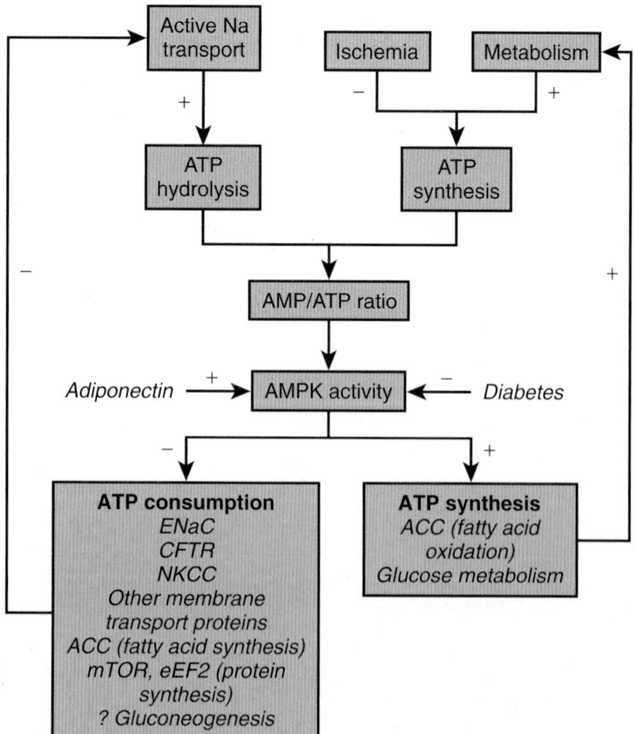


**Fig. 5.15** Proposed role of adenosine monophosphate–activated protein kinase (*AMPK*) in the kidney in coupling catabolic pathways requiring ATP hydrolysis (primarily sodium transport) with metabolic pathways leading to ATP synthesis (primarily fatty acid and glucose oxidation). +, Activating pathway; –, inhibitory pathway. *ACC*, acetyl-CoA carboxylase. (From Hallows KR, et al. Role of the energy sensor AMP-activated kinase in renal physiology and disease. *Am J Physiol Renal Physiol.* 2010;298:F1067–F1077.)

in ion transport in the kidney has been recently reviewed.[190,191] Overall, AMPK becomes activated when ATP is limiting, that is, when the AMP/ATP ratio increases, and once activated it decreases ATP consumption and increases ATP synthesis. In the kidney, sodium transport is the major energy-consuming process and there is increasing evidence regarding the role of AMPK in sodium transport in the kidney and other epithelial cells. AMPK has been shown to inhibit the activity of various transport proteins in the lung, gut, and kidney, including epithelial Na channel (ENaC) in the kidney collecting duct, Na-K-2Cl cotransporter (NKCC2) in the thick ascending limb, and $Na^+$-$K^+$-ATPase in the alveolar epithelial cells, particularly during hypoxia (as reviewed[191,192]). Hallows and colleagues have determined that AMPK activation depresses transport mediated by the cystic fibrosis transmembrane conductance regulator, the epithelial sodium channel, the vacuolar $H^+$-ATPase, and NKCC (see Fig. 5.15). A key question is whether renal AMPK activation suppresses $Na^+$-$K^+$-ATPase activity along the nephron. AMPK activation has been reported to inhibit lung cell $Na^+$-$K^+$-ATPase transport activity mediated by endocytosis,[193] but AMPK activation had no apparent effect on skeletal muscle $Na^+$-$K^+$-ATPase activity or distribution,[194] which leaves the question open for the kidney, where one report demonstrates that inhibition of AMPK induces the endocytosis of $Na^+$-$K^+$-ATPase in Madin-Darby canine kidney cells.[195]

AMPK expression in the kidney is seen mainly in the cortical thick ascending limb and macula densa cells, and in some distal convoluted tubules and collecting ducts.[196] Recently, AMPK expression in the proximal tubule has also been reported.[197] Differing results in pAMPK expression in response to high salt intake has been observed with increased pAMPK in one study[196] and reduced expression in another.[198] In vivo, pharmacologic activation of AMPK in rats fed a high salt diet was shown to enhance TGF response and reduce sodium reabsorption in the proximal and distal tubule but had no effects on these parameters in rats fed a normal salt diet.[198] Whether these effects are driven by a change in cellular metabolism that results in an increase in AMP/ATP levels is not clear. Consumption of a high salt diet does decrease the fraction of the filtered load of $Na^+$ that is absorbed. Given the effect of AMPK activation in inhibiting transporters, the findings suggest that AMPK participates in salt and water homeostasis. The AMPK pathway may provide another important layer of regulation between ATP production by mitochondria and ATP consumption by transporters. In the Whittam model illustrated in Fig. 5.3, increased active transport provokes a decrease in the ATP/ADP ratio, which drives increased ATP production by the mitochondria. When ATP production by the mitochondria becomes limiting, however, AMPK is likely to be activated, which would drive a reduction in ATP consumption by active membrane transporters. Thus, AMPK may regulate the coupling of ion transport and energy metabolism in the kidney.

Regulation of glucose and lipid metabolism by AMPK in pathophysiologic conditions such as diabetic nephropathy and CKD has been elucidated in recent publications. In animal models of CKD, diabetes, and obesity, reduced AMPK activity has been described.[199–202] Endogenous AMPK activation by targeting adiponectin (adipose tissue–derived cytokine) as well as pharmacologic AMPK activation (metformin, AICAR) has been shown to improve glucose and lipid homeostasis in diabetes and obesity-associated kidney disease. In a recent paper, significant changes in renal metabolism with the deletion of a major upstream AMPK activator, liver kinase B1 (LKB1), in kidney distal tubules were observed.[203] Expression of AMPK and other key regulators of metabolism were significantly diminished and accompanied by tubular epithelial injury and interstitial fibrosis. In cultured epithelial cells, loss of LKB1 was associated with diminished fatty acid oxidation and glycolysis, leading to energy depletion and apoptotic cell death. In human kidney samples, lower levels of phosphorylated LKB1 and AMPK $\alpha 2$ subunit were seen in CKD patients. Thus, the important role of AMPK in regulating kidney metabolism is being increasingly recognized.

Acute renal ischemia provokes a rapid and powerful activation of AMPK, but its functional role in the response to ischemia remains unclear. There is conflicting evidence in the literature regarding the effects of AMPK activation in renal ischemia–reperfusion injury.[204–207] Similarly, while several studies show a beneficial effect of AMPK activation in myocardial ischemia–reperfusion, there are some conflicting studies demonstrating deleterious effects of AMPK activation in ischemic injury in the heart and brain (as reviewed[185]). Hence, the effects of AMPK activation are likely to be time, tissue, and cell-dependent. Whether AMPK abundance or its phosphorylation is higher in the hypoxia-prone medulla than in the cortex has not yet been investigated, nor have studies been conducted examining the effect of AMPK activation on renal gluconeogenesis or glycolysis.[193–195]

## TUBULAR METABOLISM

Until recently there were limited studies exploring cellular metabolism in pathophysiologic conditions. Several recent publications have highlighted metabolic alterations in various forms of CKD. Moreover, alterations in glucose and fatty acid metabolism as early events in the course of diabetic and other forms of CKD place metabolic reprogramming central to the pathophysiology of CKD.

In mouse models of autosomal dominant polycystic kidney disease (ADPKD) and in kidney tissue from patients with ADPKD, defective glucose metabolism—specifically, increased aerobic glycolysis—was observed.[208] Moreover, treatment with 2-deoxyglucose, an inhibitor of glycolysis, lowered kidney weight, volume, cystic index, and proliferation rates in mouse models of ADPKD.[209] This phenotypic feature of enhanced aerobic glycolysis, also known as Warburg effect, is typically seen in proliferating cancer cells. In these mice models of PKD1 gene inactivation, there was inhibition of liver kinase B1(LKB1)-AMPK axis along with activation of mTOR complex I pathway, leading to increased glycolysis.[208]

Besides altered glucose metabolism, changes in fatty acid metabolism in the kidney have been described in CKD. In a recent paper, Kang et al. described reduced levels of enzymes and regulators involved in fatty acid oxidation in mouse models of fibrosis.[210] In transcriptional analyses of microdissected human kidney samples from patients with diabetic or hypertensive CKD changes in fatty acid metabolism, β-oxidation, amino acid catabolism, and carbohydrate metabolism were observed. Genes related to fatty acid metabolism and their key transcriptional regulator complex, PPARA–PPARGC1A, were markedly lower in CKD samples compared with samples obtained from people with normal kidney function. This was associated with higher lipid accumulation in renal tubular epithelial cells. Key regulators of glucose utilization were also lower in CKD samples. Using elegant experiments with genetic and pharmacologic approaches, the reduction in fatty acid oxidation was shown to be directly implicated in the pathogenesis of renal fibrosis in CKD. Although lipid accumulation in tubular cells in CKD patients has been reported before, these findings showed convincingly that it is the reduction in fatty acid oxidation rather than just the accumulation of lipid in tubular cells that plays a role in the development of renal fibrosis.

Metabolic reprogramming has also been recently reported in diabetic CKD.[211] As discussed earlier, proximal tubules are largely dependent on mitochondrial oxidative metabolism for energy with limited glycolytic capacity. Under physiologic conditions, proximal tubules mainly use fatty acids, lactate, and glutamine as substrates for energy generation. In diabetes, there are increases in plasma concentration of glucose and fatty acids. These changes are also found intracellularly in various tissues including the kidneys, particularly proximal tubules. In an elegant study, Sas et al. provided a comprehensive assessment of substrate metabolism in diabetes using a systems-based approach that included transcriptomics, metabolomics, and metabolic flux analyses to determine alterations in glucose and fatty acid metabolism.[211] In the kidney cortex in a type 2 diabetic mouse model (db/db mice), transcriptomic and metabolomic profiling demonstrated an increase in glycolysis, fatty acid β-oxidation, and tricarboxylic acid (TCA) cycle flux. Increased renal metabolism was associated with increased protein acetylation, which is a nutrient sensing posttranslational modification. There was also evidence for mitochondrial dysfunction as discussed later. Remarkably, transcriptomic analysis of kidney biopsy samples in patients with type 2 diabetes identified significant enrichment of many pathways involved in fatty acid, glucose, and amino acid metabolism and network analysis showed results similar to those obtained in db/db mice. In another cohort of type 1 diabetic patients enrolled in the Finnish Diabetic Nephropathy (FinnDiane) Study, increased glycolytic (hexose-6-phosphates, 2,3-phosphoglycerate) and TCA cycle metabolites (succinate, fumarate, malate) were detected in the urine compared with healthy control subjects. Urine samples from a subset of patients from the Family Investigation of Nephropathy and Diabetes (FIND) study, showed increased glycolytic intermediates at baseline in diabetic subjects compared with control subjects. TCA cycle intermediates in the urine were also elevated in diabetic subjects and predicted diabetic kidney disease progression, demonstrating their potential as prognostic biomarkers of diabetic kidney disease progression. These and previously discussed studies highlight the adaptive and maladaptive metabolic reprogramming and its role in the pathophysiology of diabetic and nondiabetic CKD.

## MITOCHONDRIAL DISORDERS

Given the central role of mitochondria in producing ATP via oxidative phosphorylation, it is not surprising that genetic mutations affecting mitochondrial function have renal manifestations. Moreover, several lines of investigation support the significant role of early mitochondrial dysfunction in the pathophysiology of acute and chronic kidney diseases. The mitochondrial genome is distinct from the nuclear genome, and it encodes 13 of the 88 protein subunits of ETC complexes I through V as well as 22 mitochondrial-specific transfer RNAs (tRNAs) and two RNA components of the translational apparatus. The nuclear genome encodes the remaining respiratory chain subunits as well as most of the mitochondrial DNA replication and expression components.

Disorders affecting mitochondrial oxidative phosphorylation can arise from mutations in either mitochondrial genes or nuclear genes encoding respiratory chain components or ancillary factors involved in maintenance of ETC function or the overall number of mitochondria.[212] The incidence of genetic mitochondrial disorders is estimated at about 1 in 5000 births, with the most common affecting the sequence of a mitochondrial tRNA for leucine. Such mutations affect mitochondrial function in all tissues. Symptoms are evident before 2 months of age, and the number of organ systems affected increases with age.

Impairment of mitochondrial oxidative phosphorylation results in increased levels of reducing equivalents (NADH, FADH), which, in the mitochondria, transform acetoacetate to 3-hydroxybutyrate and, in the cytosol, transform pyruvate to lactate. Thus, elevated levels of lactic acid, ketone bodies, and impaired redox status are suggestive of a mitochondrial defect disorder.[213] If the genetic cause of the impairment can be pinpointed, then an appropriate therapy, if available, can be implemented to treat these life-threatening disorders; for example, coenzyme $Q_{10}$ enzyme defects can be treated with coenzyme $Q_{10}$ supplementation.[212]

Myopathies and cardiomyopathies are the most common manifestations of mitochondrial disease, and central nervous system symptoms, including encephalopathies, are very common. Renal system impairment can be present but is not seen without other system deficiencies and is usually reported in children. Although glomerular disease and tubulointerstitial nephropathy have both been reported, the most frequently observed is impairment of proximal tubule reabsorption, known as de Toni–Debré–Fanconi syndrome, in which there are urinary losses of bicarbonate, amino acids, glucose, phosphate, uric acid, potassium, and water. All of these symptoms can be explained by a lack of ATP to fuel $Na^+$-$K^+$-ATPase sufficiently to drive transepithelial transport. The symptoms can range from mild to more severe and present in the neonatal period in most patients. Biopsy specimens show tubular dilations, casts, dedifferentiation, and cellular vacuolization. At the cellular level there are enlarged mitochondria. Supplements of sodium bicarbonate, potassium, vitamin D, phosphorus, and water are called for if these symptoms are evident.[212,213]

Significant changes in mitochondrial function in diabetic kidneys have been described and recently reviewed in detail.[214,215] Early changes in mitochondrial energetics, increased mitochondrial fragmentation, and reduced levels of PGC1a have been described in diabetic kidneys. In diabetic nephropathy, increased metabolism has been shown to be associated with mitochondrial dysfunction.[211] Assessment of oxidative phosphorylation in mitochondria isolated from renal cortexes of 24-week-old control and diabetic mice showed increased proton leak and diminished mitochondrial ATP production. Additionally, total mitochondrial capacity was decreased in diabetic mitochondria, and the expression of mitochondrial uncoupling protein 2 was increased fourfold.

In renal cortexes from diabetic mice, expression of proteins in complexes I, II, III, and complex IV subunit cytochrome *c* oxidase subunit 4 (COX4) were significantly decreased at 24 weeks. The results of these studies suggested that dysfunction of ETC proteins in mitochondria from diabetic kidneys lead to less efficient ATP production and compensatory increases in glucose and fatty acid metabolic flux. This may be the primary metabolic abnormality in the diabetic kidney cortex as it precedes other markers of renal injury. Another study compared urine metabolites in patients with diabetes, but with or without CKD and in healthy controls.[216] Bioinformatic analyses revealed that 12 of the 13 differentially expressed metabolites were linked to mitochondrial metabolism. Kidney sections in patients with diabetes and CKD showed lower expression of mitochondrial proteins and lower gene expression of PGC1a, which is a major regulator of mitochondrial biogenesis. Urine exosomes in these patients also showed less mitochondrial DNA. Evidence of mitochondrial dysfunction in nondiabetic CKD is also emerging. Early changes in mitochondrial function and structure in animal models of CKD has been reported.[217] In patients with CKD, mRNA levels of several mitochondrial enzymes and transcription factors were found to be lower, although no differences in mitochondrial copy number was seen.[210] In another clinical study, mitochondrial DNA copy number was evaluated in peripheral blood in a population cohort.[218] Participants with higher mitochondrial DNA copy numbers had a lower rate of prevalent diabetes and lower risk of incident CKD, even after adjusting for various risk factors for CKD.

The role of mitochondrial dysfunction in AKI has received significant attention. Several publications have elucidated the underlying mechanisms of mitochondrial dysfunction in various etiologies of AKI (reviewed in details[215]). In ischemic and nephrotoxic AKI, decreased mitochondrial mass, disruption of cristae, and significant mitochondrial swelling has been observed.[219] In ischemic AKI, increase in mitochondrial NADH and dissipation of mitochondrial membrane potential in proximal tubules has been demonstrated.[220] In ischemic and myoglobulinuric AKI, reduction in various ETC proteins in the proximal tubule was shown.[221] Other studies have uncovered the crucial role of mitochondrial biogenesis using stimulators of PGC1α, master regulator of mitochondrial biogenesis in recovery from ischemic AKI[222] and sepsis-associated AKI.[158] The role of mitochondrial dynamics has also been elucidated in some forms of AKI. In an elegant study, Brooks et al. described the disruption of mitochondrial dynamics and its pathogenic role in ischemic and nephrotoxic AKI.[219] Mitochondrial fragmentation was shown to precede tubular cell injury and death and pharmacologic inhibition of Drp1 prevented fragmentation and ameliorated AKI. Further highlighting the role of mitochondrial dysfunction, several pharmacologic targets to improve mitochondrial function in AKI and CKD have been investigated and found to be effective.[223]

## SUMMARY

Most of the energy consumed by the kidney is traceable to the energy requirements for sodium reabsorption. Although all sodium reabsorption is linked to $Na^+$-$K^+$-ATPase, efficiency is achieved by leveraging $Na^+$-$K^+$-ATPase into transepithelial chloride or voltage gradients that allow some sodium to be reabsorbed without passing through the $Na^+$-$K^+$-ATPase itself. ATP production in the proximal tubule is solely by aerobic metabolism, whereas the medullary segments have additional capacity to produce energy by glycolysis. Transport activity regulates metabolism, metabolism may be rate limiting for transport, and the efficiency of transport can be made to vary at multiple levels from back-leak permeability to the efficiency of mitochondrial respiration. With regard to metabolic autoregulation, the kidney faces a particular challenge because the usual mechanism for delivering more oxygen to the kidney also increases the demand for that oxygen. Several intermediaries have been identified as parts of the complex network of interactions between transport and metabolism that allow the kidney to meet this challenge while balancing the risk of hypoxia against the risk of oxygen toxicity. A partial list of these includes adenosine, nitric oxide, prostaglandins, angiotensin II, dopamine, succinate, uncoupling proteins, HIF, and AMPK. A multiscale systems model that incorporates these elements along with renal anatomy to recapitulate renal metabolism is expected in the future.

 Complete reference list available at ExpertConsult.com.

## KEY REFERENCES

24. Mandel LJ. Metabolic substrates, cellular energy production, and the regulation of proximal tubular transport. *Annu Rev Physiol.* 1985;47:85–101.
48. Epstein FH. Oxygen and renal metabolism. *Kidney Int.* 1997;51:381–385.
60. Veiras LC, Girardi ACC, Curry J, et al. Sexual dimorphic pattern of renal transporters and electrolyte homeostasis. *J Am Soc Nephrol.* 2017;28:3504–3517.
78. Thomson SC, Blantz RC. Glomerulotubular balance, tubuloglomerular feedback, and salt homeostasis. *J Am Soc Nephrol.* 2008;19:2272–2275.
95. Yu ASL. Paracellular transport and energy utilization in the renal tubule. *Curr Opin Nephrol Hypertens.* 2017;26:398–404.
165. Semenza GL. Hypoxia-inducible factors in physiology and medicine. *Cell.* 2012;148:399–408.
180. Sugahara M, Tanaka T, Nangaku M. Prolyl hydroxylase domain inhibitors as a novel therapeutic approach against anemia in chronic kidney disease. *Kidney Int.* 2017;92:306–312.
185. Steinberg GR, Kemp BE. AMPK in health and disease. *Physiol Rev.* 2009;89:1025–1078.
210. Kang HM, Ahn SH, Choi P, et al. Defective fatty acid oxidation in renal tubular epithelial cells has a key role in kidney fibrosis development. *Nat Med.* 2015;21:37–46.
211. Sas KM, Kayampilly P, Byun J, et al. Tissue-specific metabolic reprogramming drives nutrient flux in diabetic complications. *JCI Insight.* 2016;1:e86976.

# 6 Transport of Sodium, Chloride, and Potassium

James A. McCormick | David B. Mount | David H. Ellison

CHAPTER OUTLINE



## INTRODUCTION TO NA, CL, AND K TRANSPORT

### SODIUM AND CHLORIDE TRANSPORT

Daily sodium ($Na^+$) intake for adults in the United States is approximately 180 mmol (4.2 g) for men and 150 mmol (3.5 g) for women (https://www.cdc.gov/nchs/nhanes/wweia.htm). As $Na^+$ is the principal osmole in extracellular fluid, the total body content of $Na^+$ and chloride ($Cl^-$), its primary anion, determine the extracellular fluid volume. Renal excretion or retention of salt ($Na^+$-$Cl^-$) is thus the major determinant of the extracellular fluid volume, such that genetic loss- or gain-of-function in renal $Na^+$-$Cl^-$ transport can be associated with relative hypotension or hypertension, respectively. On a quantitative level, at a glomerular filtration rate (GFR) of 180 L/day and serum $Na^+$ of about 140 mmol/L, the kidney filters some 25,000 mmol/day of $Na^+$; this is equivalent to about 1.5 kg of salt, which would occupy roughly 10 times the extracellular space.[1] Minute changes in renal $Na^+$-$Cl^-$ excretion can thus have massive effects on the extracellular fluid volume. In addition, 99.6% of filtered $Na^+$-$Cl^-$ must be reabsorbed to excrete 140 mmol/L per day. Energetically, this renal absorption of $Na^+$ consumes 1 molecule of adenosine triphosphate (ATP) per five molecules of $Na^+$.[1] This is gratifyingly economical, given that the absorption of $Na^+$-$Cl^-$ is primarily, but not exclusively, driven by basolateral $Na^+$-$K^+$-ATPase, which has a stoichiometry of three molecules of transported $Na^+$ per molecule of ATP.[2] This estimate reflects a net expenditure, however, because the cost of transepithelial $Na^+$-$Cl^-$ transport varies considerably along the nephron, from a predominance of passive transport by thin ascending limbs to the purely active transport mediated by the "aldosterone-sensitive distal nephron" (distal convoluted tubule [DCT], connecting tubule [CNT], and collecting duct).

As much as 60% to 70% of filtered $Na^+$-$Cl^-$ is reabsorbed along the proximal tubule (PT), and approximately 25% along the thick ascending limb (TAL; Fig. 6.1). Whereas the PT can theoretically absorb as much as nine $Na^+$ molecules for each hydrolyzed ATP, paracellular $Na^+$ transport by the TAL doubles the efficiency of transepithelial $Na^+$-$Cl^-$ transport (six $Na^+$ molecules per ATP).[1,3] By the time filtered fluid reaches the macula densa, more than 90% of filtered $Na^+$ has been reabsorbed,[4] a percentage that varies only slightly, when dietary NaCl intake ranges from very low to very high.[5] Thus the terminal segments of the nephron, while reabsorbing only 5% to 10% of filtered $Na^+$, are a primary site of transport regulation. Here, renal $Na^+$-$Cl^-$ absorption occurs at full cost (3 $Na^+$ per ATP) in the aldosterone-sensitive distal nephron while affording the generation of considerable transepithelial gradients.[1]

The nephron thus constitutes a serial arrangement of tubule segments with considerable heterogeneity in the physiologic consequences, mechanisms, and regulation of transepithelial $Na^+$-$Cl^-$ transport. These issues will be reviewed in this section in anatomic order.

### PROXIMAL TUBULE

A primary function of the renal PT is the near-isosmotic reabsorption of two-thirds to three-quarters of the glomerular ultrafiltrate. This encompasses the reabsorption of at least 60% of filtered $Na^+$ with accompanying anions (Fig. 6.1), such that this nephron segment plays a critical role in the maintenance of extracellular fluid volume. Although all segments of the PT share the ability to transport a variety of inorganic and organic solutes, there are considerable differences in the transport characteristics and capacity of early, mid, and late segments of the PT. There is thus a gradual reduction in the volume of transported fluid and solutes as one proceeds along the proximal nephron. This corresponds to distinct ultrastructural characteristics in the tubular epithelium, moving from the S1 segment (early proximal convoluted tubule [PCT]) to the S2 segment (late PCT and beginning of the proximal straight tubule) and the S3 segment (remainder of the proximal straight tubule). Cells of the S1 segment are thus characterized by a tall brush

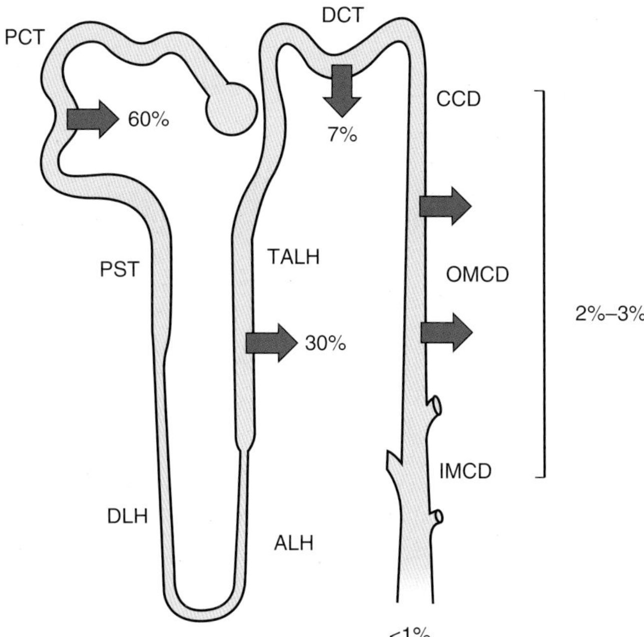


**Fig. 6.1** Percentage reabsorption of filtered $Na^+$-$Cl^-$ along the euvolemic nephron. *ALH,* Thin ascending limb of the loop of Henle; *CCD,* cortical collecting duct; *DCT,* distal convoluted tubule; *DLH,* descending thin limb of the loop of Henle; *IMCD,* inner medullary collecting duct; *OMCD,* outer medullary collecting duct; *PCT,* proximal convoluted tubule; *PST,* proximal straight tubule; *TALH,* thick ascending limb of the loop of Henle. (From Moe OW, Baum M, Berry CA, Rector Jr FC. Renal transport of glucose, amino acids, sodium, chloride, and water. In: Brenner BM, ed. *Brenner and Rector's the Kidney.* Philadelphia: WB Saunders; 2004:413–452.)

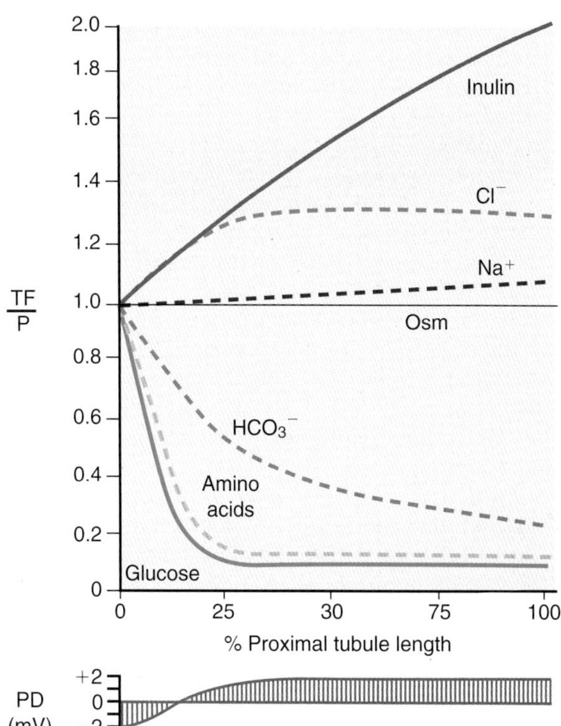


**Fig. 6.2** Reabsorption of solutes along the proximal tubule in relation to the transepithelial potential difference *(PD). Osm,* Osmolality; *TF/P,* ratio of tubule fluid to plasma concentration. (From Rector Jr FC. Sodium, bicarbonate, and chloride absorption by the proximal tubule. *Am J Physiol.* 1983;244:F461–F471.)

border, with extensive lateral invaginations of the basolateral membrane.[6] Numerous elongated mitochondria are located in lateral cell processes, with a proximity to the plasma membrane that is characteristic of epithelial cells involved in active transport. Ultrastructure of the S2 segment is similar, albeit with a shorter brush border, fewer lateral invaginations, and less prominent mitochondria. In epithelial cells of the S3 segment, lateral cell processes and invaginations are essentially absent, with small mitochondria that are randomly distributed within the cell.[6] The extensive brush border of proximal tubular cells serves to amplify the apical cell surface that is available for reabsorption; again, this amplification is axially distributed, increasing the apical area 36-fold in S1 and 15-fold in S3.[7] At the functional level, bicarbonate reabsorption rates decline by at least 80% between the first and last portions of the PT, whereas $Cl^-$ reabsorption declines by approximately 50%.[8]

There is also considerable axial heterogeneity in the quantitative capacity of the proximal nephron for organic solutes such as glucose and amino acids, with predominant reabsorption of these substrates in S1 segments.[9] The $Na^+$-dependent reabsorption of glucose, amino acids, and other solutes in S1 segments results in a transepithelial potential difference (PD) that is initially lumen negative due to electrogenic removal of $Na^+$ from the lumen (Fig. 6.2).[10] This is classically considered the first phase of volume reabsorption by the PT.[11] The lumen-negative PD serves to drive both paracellular $Cl^-$ absorption and a backleak of $Na^+$ from the peritubular space to the lumen. Paracellular $Cl^-$ absorption in this setting accomplishes the net transepithelial absorption of a solute such as glucose, along with equal amounts of $Na^+$ and $Cl^-$; by contrast, backleak of $Na^+$ leads only to reabsorption of the organic solute, with no net transepithelial transport of $Na^+$ or $Cl^-$. The amount of $Cl^-$ reabsorption that is driven by this lumen-negative PD thus depends on the relative permeability of the paracellular pathway to $Na^+$ and $Cl^-$. There appears to be considerable heterogeneity in the relative paracellular permeability to $Na^+$ and $Cl^-$; for example, whereas superficial PCTs and proximal straight tubules in the rabbit are $Cl^-$ selective, juxtamedullary PTs in this species are reportedly $Na^+$ selective.[12,13] Regardless, the component of paracellular $Cl^-$ transport that is driven by this lumen-negative PD is restricted to the very early PT.

The second phase of volume reabsorption by the PT is dominated by $Na^+$-$Cl^-$ reabsorption via paracellular and transcellular pathways.[11] In addition to the $Na^+$-dependent reabsorption of organic solutes, the early PT has a much higher capacity for $HCO_3^-$ absorption via the coupling of apical $Na^+$-$H^+$ exchange, carbonic anhydrase, and basolateral $Na^+$-$HCO_3^-$ cotransport.[9] As the luminal concentrations of $HCO_3^-$ and other solutes begin to drop, the concentration of $Na^+$-$Cl^-$ rises to a value greater than that of the peritubular space.[14] This is accompanied by a reversal of the lumen-negative PD to a lumen-positive value generated by passive $Cl^-$ diffusion (Fig. 6.2).[15] This lumen-positive PD serves to drive paracellular $Na^+$ transport, whereas the chemical gradient between the lumen and peritubular space provides the driving force for paracellular reabsorption of $Cl^-$. This passive paracellular pathway is thought to mediate about 40% of transepithelial $Na^+$-$Cl^-$ reabsorption by the mid to late PT.[12] Of note, however, there may be heterogeneity in the relative importance of this paracellular pathway, with evidence that active (i.e., transcellular) reabsorption predominates in PCTs from juxtamedullary versus superficial nephrons.[16] Regardless, the combination of passive and active transport of $Na^+$-$Cl^-$ explains how the PT is able to reabsorb about 60% of filtered $Na^+$-$Cl^-$, despite $Na^+$-$K^+$-ATPase activity that is considerably lower than that of distal segments of the nephron (Fig. 6.3).[17]

The transcellular component of $Na^+$-$Cl^-$ reabsorption initially emerged from studies of the effect of cyanide, ouabain, luminal anion transport inhibitors, cooling, and luminal-peritubular $K^+$ removal.[11] For example, the luminal addition of SITS (4-acetamido-4′-isothiocyanostilbene-2,2′-disulfonic acid), an inhibitor of anion transporters, reduces volume reabsorption of PCTs perfused with a high $Cl^-$, low $HCO_3^-$ solution that mimics the luminal composition of the late PT; this occurs in the absence of an effect on carbonic anhydrase.[14] This transcellular component of $Na^+$-$Cl^-$ reabsorption is clearly electroneutral. For example, in the absence of anion gradients across the perfused PT, there is no change in transepithelial PD after the inhibition of active transport by ouabain, despite a marked reduction in volume reabsorption.[18] Transcellular $Na^+$-$Cl^-$ reabsorption is accomplished by the coupling of luminal $Na^+$-$H^+$ exchange or $Na^+$-$SO_4^{2-}$ cotransport with a heterogeneous population of anion exchangers, as reviewed later.

## PARACELLULAR NA⁺-CL⁻ TRANSPORT

A number of factors serve to optimize the conditions for paracellular $Na^+$-$Cl^-$ transport by the mid to late PT. First, the PT is a low-resistance, so-called leaky epithelium, with tight junctions that are highly permeable to both $Na^+$ and $Cl^-$.[12,13] Second, these tight junctions are preferentially permeable to $Cl^-$ over $HCO_3^-$, a feature that helps generate the lumen-positive PD in the mid to late PT.[14] Third, the increase in luminal $Na^+$-$Cl^-$ concentrations in the mid to late PT generates a chemical driving force for paracellular reabsorption of $Cl^-$.[15] This increase in luminal $Na^+$-$Cl^-$ is the direct result of the robust reabsorption of $HCO_3^-$ and other solutes by the early S1 segment, combined with the isosmotic reabsorption of filtered water.[9,19]

A highly permeable paracellular pathway is a consistent feature of epithelia that function in the near-isosmolar reabsorption of $Na^+$-$Cl^-$, including the small intestine, PT, and gallbladder. Morphologically, the apical tight junction of proximal tubular cells and other leaky epithelia is considerably less complex than that of tight epithelia. Freeze-fracture microscopy thus reveals that the tight junction of proximal tubular cells is comparatively shallow, with as few as one junctional strand (Fig. 6.4); by contrast, high-resistance

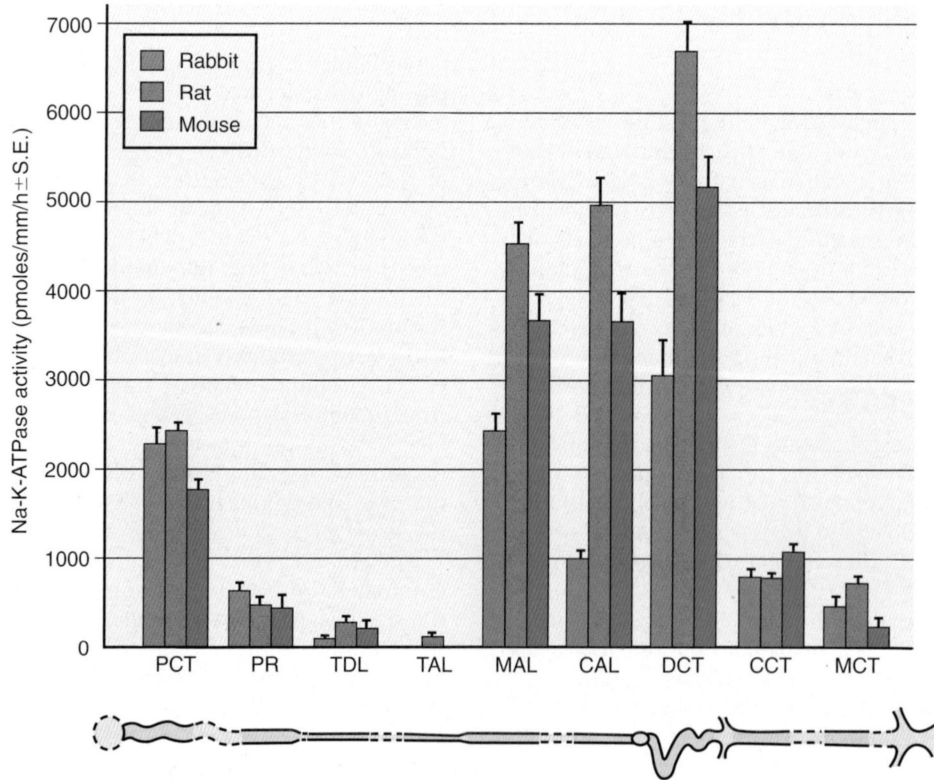


**Fig. 6.3** Distribution of $Na^+$-$K^+$-ATPase activity along the nephron. *CCD,* Cortical collecting duct; *cTAL,* cortical thick ascending limb; *DCT,* distal convoluted tubule; *MCD,* medullary collecting duct; *mTAL,* medullary thick ascending limb; *PCT,* proximal convoluted tubule; *PST,* proximal straight tubule; *tAL,* thin ascending limb of the loop of Henle; *tDL,* descending thin limb of the loop of Henle. (From Katz AI, Doucet A, Morel F. Na-K-ATPase activity along the rabbit, rat, and mouse nephron. *Am J Physiol.* 1979;237:F114–F120.)

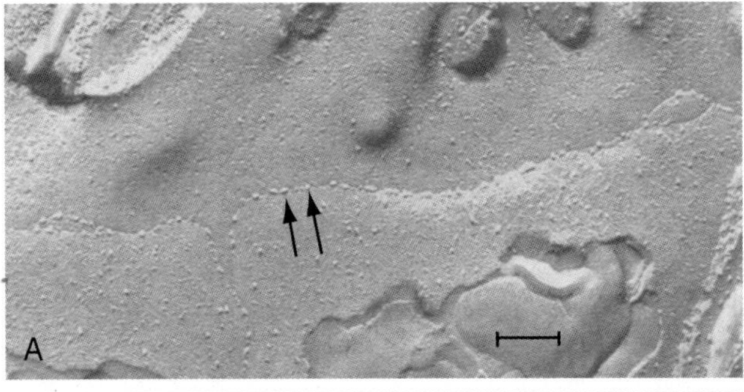


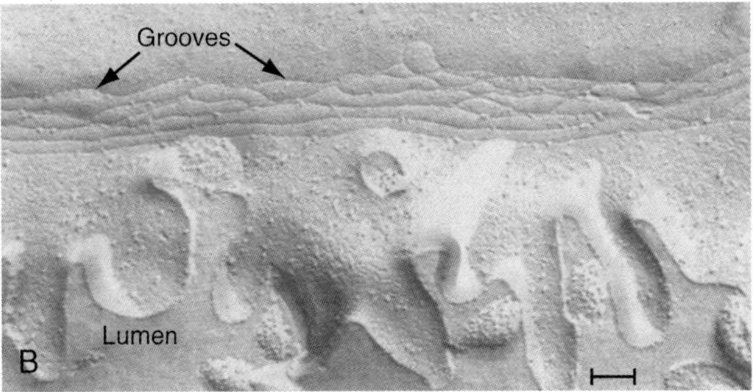


**Fig. 6.4** Freeze-fracture electron microscopy images of tight junctions in mouse proximal and distal nephron. (A) Proximal convoluted tubule, a "leaky" epithelium; the tight junction contains only one junctional strand, seen as a groove in the fracture face *(arrows).* (B) Distal convoluted tubule, a "tight" epithelium. The tight junction is deeper and contains several anastamosing strands, seen as grooves in the fracture face. (From Claude P, Goodenough DA. Fracture faces of zonulae occludentes from "tight" and "leaky" epithelia. *J Cell Biol.* 1973;58: 390–400.)

epithelia have deeper tight junctions, with a complex and extensive network of junctional strands.[20] At the functional level, tight junctions of epithelia function as charge- and size-selective paracellular tight junction channels, physiologic characteristics that are thought to be conferred by integral membrane proteins that cluster together at the tight junction. Changes in the expression of these proteins can have marked effects on permeability without affecting the number of junctional strands.[14,21,22] In particular, the charge and size selectivity of tight junctions appears to be conferred in large part by the claudins, a large (>20) gene family of tetraspan transmembrane proteins,[23–25] one of which was recently crystallized.[26] The repertoire of claudins expressed by proximal tubular epithelial cells may thus determine the high paracellular permeability of this nephron segment. At a minimum, proximal tubular cells coexpress claudin-2, claudin-10, and claudin-17.[14,27,28]

The robust expression of claudin-2 in the PT is of particular interest because this claudin can dramatically decrease the resistance of transfected epithelial cells.[22] Overexpression of claudin-2, but not claudin-10, also increases $Na^+$-dependent water flux in epithelial cell lines, suggesting that claudin-2 directly modulates paracellular water permeability.[29] Consistent with this cellular phenotype, targeted deletion of claudin-2 in mice generates a tight epithelium in the PT, with a reduction in $Na^+$, $Cl^-$, and fluid absorption.[30] Loss of claudin-2 expression does not affect the ultrastructure of tight junctions, but leads to a reduction in paracellular cation permeability and secondary reduction in transepithelial $Cl^-$ transport.[30] This action enhances the energy efficiency of proximal solute reabsorption. Although reabsorption is lower in claudin-2 knockout mice, overall sodium handling is normal because solute transport is increased along more distal segments. This requirement for more transcellular solute transport along the loop of Henle contributes to lower medullary oxygen tension, and increased susceptibility to renal ischemia.[31] Terminal differentiation of proximal tubular claudin-2 expression requires the integrin $\beta_1$-subunit, such that deletion of this protein in mice converts the PT to a tight epithelium expressing low levels of claudin-2.[32]

The molecular identification of anion-selective claudins in the PT has lagged, but claudin-17 has been shown to generate a predominantly anion-selective paracellular conductance in Madin-Darby canine kidney (MDCK) C7 cells, whereas knockdown of the protein was able to reverse a predominantly cation-selective LLC-PK(1) epithelial cell line to an anion-selective cell line.[28] Claudin-17 is expressed along the PT, suggesting a significant role in paracellular chloride absorption by this nephron segment. Recently, it has been suggested that a form of claudin-10, claudin-10a, is another anion-selective paracellular pathway along the PT.[33]

The reabsorption of $HCO_3^-$ and other solutes from the glomerular ultrafiltrate would be expected to generate an osmotic gradient across the epithelium, resulting in a hypotonic lumen. This appears to be the case, although the absolute difference in osmolality between the lumen and peritubular space has been a source of considerable controversy.[19] Another controversial issue has been the relative importance of paracellular versus transcellular water transport from this hypotonic lumen. These issues have been elegantly addressed through characterization of knockout mice with a targeted deletion of aquaporin-1, a water channel protein expressed at the apical and basolateral membranes of the PT. Mice deficient in aquaporin-1 have an 80% reduction in water permeability in perfused S2 segments, with a 50% reduction in transepithelial fluid transport.[34] Aquaporin-1 deficiency also results in a marked increase in luminal hypotonicity, providing definitive proof that near-isosmotic reabsorption by the PT requires transepithelial water transport via aquaporin-1.[19] The residual water transport in the PTs of aquaporin-1 knockout mice is mediated in part by aquaporin-7 and/or by claudin-2–dependent paracellular water transport.[30,35] Combined knockout of aquaporin-1 and claudin-2 in mice demonstrates sustained PT water reabsorption (25% of wild type), suggestive of compensation from other pathways.[36] Alternative pathways for water reabsorption may include cotransport of $H_2O$ via the multiple $Na^+$-dependent solute transporters in the early PT; this novel hypothesis is, however, a source of considerable controversy.[37,38] A related issue is the relative importance of diffusional versus convective (solvent drag) transport of $Na^+$-$Cl^-$ across the paracellular tight junction; convective transport of $Na^+$-$Cl^-$ with water would seem to play a lesser role than diffusion, given the evidence that the transcellular pathway is the dominant transepithelial pathway for water in the PT.[12,19,34,35]

## TRANSCELLULAR $Na^+$-$Cl^-$ TRANSPORT

### Apical Mechanisms

Apical $Na^+$-$H^+$ exchange plays a critical role in the transcellular and paracellular reabsorption of $Na^+$-$Cl^-$ by the PT. In addition to providing an entry site in the transcellular transport of $Na^+$, $Na^+$-$H^+$ exchange plays a dominant role in the functional "absorption" of $HCO_3^-$ by the early PT ($HCO_3^-$ does not actually move across the apical membrane, but rather is generated within cells together with $H^+$); as the movement of $Na^+$ and $HCO_3^-$ drives osmotic water movement, it also acts to increase the luminal concentration of $Cl^-$, which in turn increases the driving forces for the passive paracellular transport of $Cl^-$.[39] Increases in luminal $Cl^-$ also help drive the apical uptake of $Cl^-$ during transcellular transport. Not surprisingly, there is a considerable reduction in fluid transport of perfused PTs exposed to concentrations of amiloride that are sufficient to inhibit proximal tubular $Na^+$-$H^+$ exchange.[14]

$Na^+$-$H^+$ exchange is predominantly mediated by the NHE proteins, encoded by the nine members of the *SLC9* gene family; NHE3 in particular plays an important role in proximal tubular physiology.[40] The NHE3 protein is expressed at the apical membrane of S1, S2, and S3 segments.[41] The apical membrane of the PT also expresses alternative $Na^+$-dependent $H^+$ transporters, including NHE8.[40,42] NHE8 predominates over NHE3 in the neonatal PT, with subsequent induction of NHE3 and downregulation of NHE8 in mature, adult nephrons.[40] The primacy of NHE3 in mature PTs is illustrated by the renal phenotype of NHE3 knockout mice, which have a 62% reduction in proximal fluid absorption and a 54% reduction in baseline chloride absorption.[43,44] A recent study in which *Nhe3* was disrupted specifically in the kidney showed that it plays a role in maintaining blood pressure at baseline, and plasma $Na^+$ in response to increased or reduced dietary $Na^+$-$Cl^-$, with compensatory upregulation of $Na^+$-$Cl^-$ cotransporter (NCC) and epithelial $Na^+$ channel (ENaC) occurring.[45] The severe salt-wasting phenotype seen in global *Nhe3* knockout mice occurs due to its deletion in intestine.

Much as amiloride and other inhibitors of $Na^+$-$H^+$ exchange have revealed an important role for this transporter in transepithelial salt transport by the PT, evidence for the involvement of an apical anion exchanger first came from the use of anion transport inhibitors; DIDS (4,4′-diisothiocyanostilbene-2,2′-disulfonic acid), furosemide, and SITS all reduce fluid absorption from the lumen of PT segments perfused with solutions containing $Na^+$-$Cl^-$.[14] In the simplest arrangement for the coupling of $Na^+$-$H^+$ exchange to $Cl^-$ exchange, $Cl^-$ would be exchanged with the $OH^-$ ion during $Na^+$-$Cl^-$ transport (Fig. 6.5). Evidence for such a $Cl^-$-$OH^-$ exchanger was reported by a number of groups in the early 1980s that used membrane vesicles isolated from

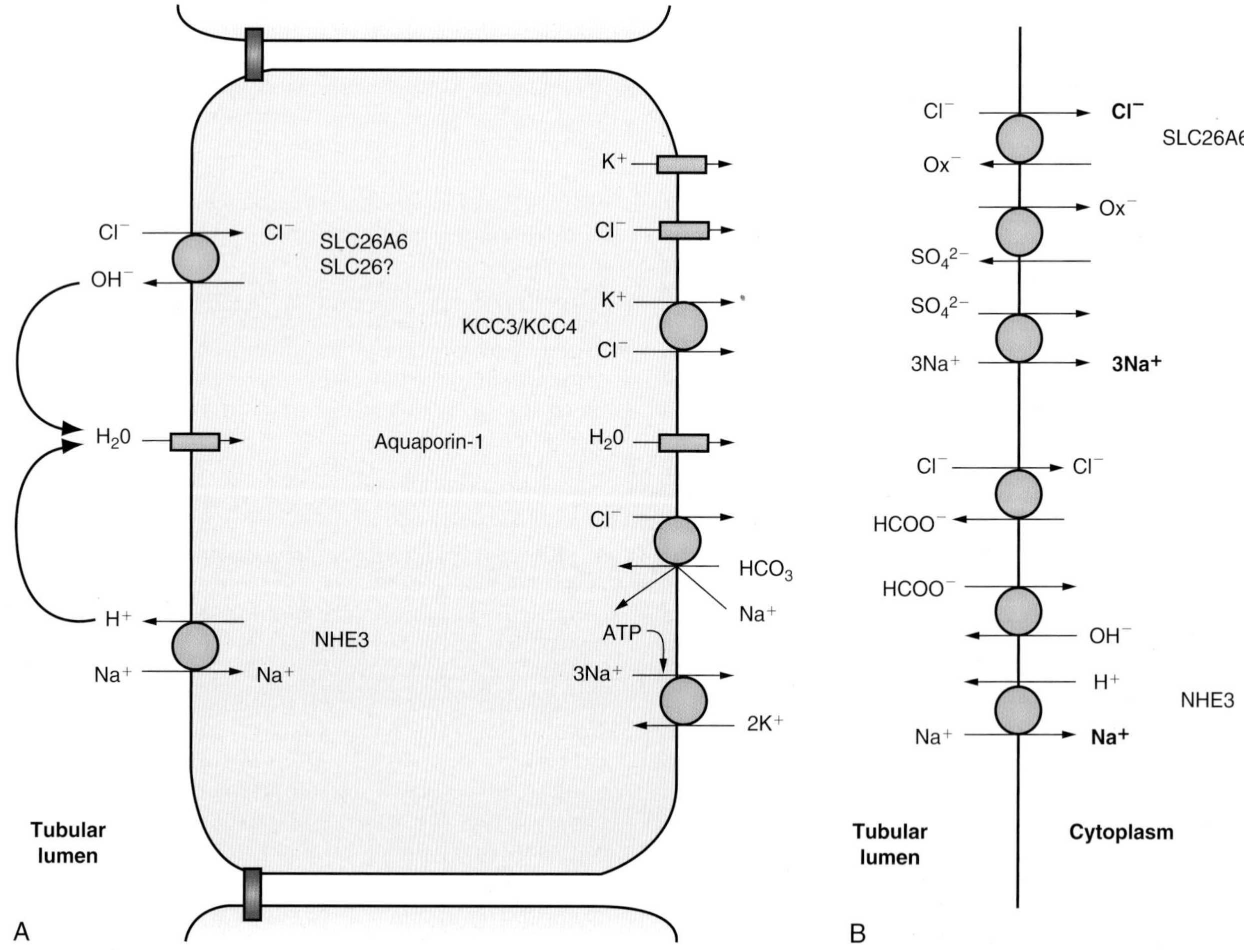


**Fig. 6.5** Transepithelial $Na^+$-$Cl^-$ transport in the proximal tubule. (A) In the simplest scheme, $Cl^-$ enters the apical membrane via a $Cl^-$-$OH^-$ exchanger, coupled to $Na^+$ entry via NHE3. (B) Alternative apical anion exchange activities that couple to $Na^+$-$H^+$ exchange and $Na^+$-$SO_4^{2-}$ cotransport. See text for details.

the PT.[46] These findings could not, however, be replicated in similar studies from other groups.[46,47] Moreover, experimental evidence was provided for the existence of a dominant $Cl^-$-formate exchange activity in brush border vesicles in the absence of significant $Cl^-$-$OH^-$ exchange.[47] It was postulated that recycling of formate by the back diffusion of formic acid would sustain the net transport of $Na^+$-$Cl^-$ across the apical membrane. Vesicle formate transport stimulated by a pH gradient ($H^+$-formate cotransport or formate-$OH^-$ exchange) is saturable, consistent with a carrier-mediated process rather than diffusion of formic acid across the apical membrane of the PT.[48] Transport studies using brush border vesicles have also detected the presence of $Cl^-$-oxalate exchange mechanisms in the apical membrane of the PT, in addition to $SO_4^{2-}$-oxalate exchange.[39,49] Based on differences in the affinities and inhibitor sensitivity of the $Cl^-$-oxalate and $Cl^-$-formate exchange activities, it was suggested that there are two separate apical exchangers in the proximal nephron, a $Cl^-$-formate exchanger and a $Cl^-$-formate-oxalate exchanger capable of transporting both formate and oxalate (Fig. 6.5).

The physiological relevance of apical $Cl^-$-formate and $Cl^-$-oxalate exchange has been addressed by perfusing individual PT segments with solutions containing $Na^+$-$Cl^-$ and formate or oxalate. Both formate and oxalate significantly increased fluid transport under these conditions in rabbit, rat, and mouse PTs.[44] This increase in fluid transport was inhibited by DIDS, suggesting involvement of the DIDS-sensitive anion exchanger(s) detected in brush border vesicle studies. A similar mechanism for $Na^+$-$Cl^-$ transport in the DCT has also been detected, independent of thiazide-sensitive $Na^+$-$Cl^-$ cotransport.[50] Further experiments have indicated that the oxalate- and formate-dependent anion transporters in the PT are coupled to distinct $Na^+$ entry pathways, to $Na^+$-$SO_4^{2-}$ cotransport and $Na^+$-$H^+$ exchange, respectively.[51] The coupling of $Cl^-$-oxalate transport to $Na^+$-$SO_4^{2-}$ cotransport requires the additional presence of $SO_4^{2-}$-oxalate exchange, which has been demonstrated in brush border membrane vesicle studies.[52] The obligatory role for NHE3 in formate-stimulated $Cl^-$ transport was illustrated using *Nhe3* null mice, in which the formate effect is abolished; as expected, oxalate stimulation of $Cl^-$ transport is preserved in the *Nhe3* null mice.[44] Finally, tubular perfusion data from superficial and juxtamedullary PCTs have suggested that there is heterogeneity in the dominant mode of anion exchange along the PT, such that $Cl^-$-formate exchange is absent in juxtamedullary PCT, in which $Cl^-$-$OH^-$ exchange may instead be dominant.[14]

The molecular identity of the apical anion exchanger(s) involved in transepithelial $Na^+$-$Cl^-$ reabsorption by the PT has been the object of almost 3 decades of investigation. A key breakthrough was the observation that the SLC26A4 anion exchanger, also known as pendrin, is capable of $Cl^-$-formate exchange when expressed in *Xenopus laevis* oocytes.[53] However, expression of SLC26A4 in the PT is minimal or absent in several species, and formate-stimulated $Na^+$-$Cl^-$ transport in this nephron segment is unimpaired in *Slc26a4* null mice.[14] There is, however, robust expression of SLC26A4 in distal type B intercalated cells; the role of this exchanger in $Cl^-$ transport by the distal nephron is reviewed elsewhere in this chapter (see the "Connecting Tubules and the Cortical Collecting Duct: $Cl^-$ Transport" section).[54] Regardless, these data for SLC26A4 led to the identification and characterization of SLC26A6, a widely expressed member of the SLC26 family that is expressed at the apical membrane of proximal tubular cells. Murine SLC26A6, when expressed in *Xenopus* oocytes, mediates the multiple modes of anion exchange that have been implicated in transepithelial $Na^+$-$Cl^-$ by the PT, including $Cl^-$-formate, $Cl^-$-$OH^-$, $Cl^-$-$SO_4^{2-}$, and $SO_4^{2-}$-oxalate exchange.[55] However, tubule perfusion experiments in mice deficient in SLC26A6 did not reveal a reduction in baseline $Cl^-$ or fluid transport, indicative of considerable heterogeneity in apical $Cl^-$ transport by the PT.[56] Candidates for the residual $Cl^-$ transport in SLC26A6-deficient mice include SLC26A7 and SLC26A9, which are expressed at the apical membrane of PTs; however, these members of the SLC26 family appear to function as $Cl^-$ channels rather than as exchangers.[57–59] SLC26A2 may also contribute to apical anion exchange in the PT.[60] It does, however, appear that SLC26A6 is the dominant $Cl^-$-oxalate exchanger of the proximal brush border; the usual increase in tubular fluid transport induced by oxalate is abolished in *Slc26a6* knockout mice, with an attendant loss of $Cl^-$-oxalate exchange in brush border membrane vesicles.[56,61]

Somewhat surprisingly, SLC26A6 mediates electrogenic $Cl^-$-$OH^-$ and $Cl^-$-$HCO_3^-$ exchange, and most if not all the members of this family are electrogenic in at least one mode of anion transport.[14,55,58,62,63] This begs the question of how the electroneutrality of transcellular $Na^+$-$Cl^-$ transport is preserved. Notably, however, the stoichiometry and electrophysiology of $Cl^-$-base exchange differ for individual members of the family; for example, SLC26A6 exchanges one $Cl^-$ for two $HCO_3^-$ anions, whereas SLC26A3 exchanges two $Cl^-$ anions for one $HCO_3^-$ anion.[14,63] Coexpression of two or more electrogenic SLC26 exchangers in the same membrane may thus yield a net electroneutrality of apical $Cl^-$ exchange. Alternatively, apical $K^+$ channels in the PT may function to stabilize membrane potential during $Na^+$-$Cl^-$ absorption.[64]

Another puzzle is why $Cl^-$-formate exchange preferentially couples to $Na^+$-$H^+$ exchange mediated by NHE3 (Fig. 6.5), without evident coupling of $Cl^-$-oxalate exchange to $Na^+$-$H^+$ exchange or $Cl^-$-formate exchange to $Na^+$-$SO_4^{2-}$ cotransport; it is evident that SLC26A6 is capable of mediating $SO_4^{2-}$-formate exchange, which would be necessary to support coupling between $Na^+$-$SO_4^{2-}$ cotransport and formate.[44,55] Scaffolding proteins may serve to cluster these different transporters together in separate microdomains, leading to preferential coupling. Notably, whereas both SLC26A6 and NHE have been reported to bind to the scaffolding protein PDZK1, distribution of SLC26A6 is selectively impaired in *Pdzk1* knockout mice.[65] Petrovic and colleagues have also reported a novel activation of proximal $Na^+$-$H^+$ exchange by luminal formate, suggesting a direct effect of formate per se on NHE3; this may in part explain the preferential coupling of $Cl^-$-formate exchange to NHE3.[66] Despite these intriguing observations, the relative importance of transcellular versus passive paracellular $Cl^-$ reabsorption in the PT remains to be established with certainty.

### Basolateral Mechanisms

As in other absorptive epithelia, basolateral $Na^+$-$K^+$-ATPase activity establishes the $Na^+$ gradient for transcellular $Na^+$-$Cl^-$ transport by the PT and provides a major exit pathway for $Na^+$. To preserve the electroneutrality of transcellular $Na^+$-$Cl^-$ transport, this exit of $Na^+$ across the basolateral membrane must be balanced by an equal exit of $Cl^-$.[18] Several exit pathways for $Cl^-$ have been identified in proximal tubular cells, including $K^+$-$Cl^-$ cotransport, $Cl^-$ channels, and various modalities of $Cl^-$-$HCO_3^-$ exchange (Fig. 6.5).

Several lines of evidence support the existence of a swelling-activated basolateral $K^+$-$Cl^-$ cotransporter (KCC) in the PT.[67] The KCC proteins are encoded by four members of the cation-chloride cotransporter gene family; *Kcc1, Kcc3,* and *Kcc4* are all expressed in the kidney. In particular, there is very heavy coexpression of KCC3 and KCC4 at the basolateral membrane of the PT, from S1 to S3.[68] At the functional level, basolateral membrane vesicles from the renal cortex reportedly contain $K^+$-$Cl^-$ cotransport activity.[67] The use of ion-sensitive microelectrodes, combined with luminal charge injection and manipulation of bath $K^+$ and $Cl^-$, suggest the presence of an electroneutral KCC at the basolateral membrane of proximal straight tubules. Increases or decreases in basolateral $K^+$ increase or decrease intracellular $Cl^-$ activity, respectively, with reciprocal effects of basolateral $Cl^-$ on $K^+$ activity; these data are consistent with coupled $K^+$-$Cl^-$ transport.[69,70] Notably, a 1-mmol/L concentration of furosemide, sufficient to inhibit all four of the KCCs, does not inhibit this $K^+$-$Cl^-$ cotransport under baseline conditions.[69] However, only 10% of baseline $K^+$ efflux in the PT is mediated by furosemide-sensitive $K^+$-$Cl^-$ cotransport, which is likely quiescent in the absence of cell swelling. Thus the activation of apical $Na^+$-glucose transport in proximal tubular cells strongly activates a barium-resistant ($Ba^{2+}$) $K^+$ efflux pathway that is 75% inhibited by 1-mmol/L furosemide.[71] In addition, a volume regulatory decrease (VRD) in $Ba^{2+}$-blocked PTs swollen by hypotonic conditions is blocked by 1-mmol/L furosemide.[67] Cell swelling in response to apical $Na^+$ absorption is postulated to activate a volume-sensitive basolateral KCC, which participates in transepithelial absorption of $Na^+$-$Cl^-$.[14] Notably, targeted deletion of *Kcc3* and *Kcc4* in the respective knockout mice reduces VRD in the PT.[72] Furthermore, perfused PTs from KCC3-deficient mice have a considerable reduction in transepithelial fluid transport, suggesting an important role for basolateral $K^+$-$Cl^-$ cotransport in transcellular $Na^+$-$Cl^-$ reabsorption.[73]

The basolateral chloride conductance of mammalian proximal tubular cells is relatively low, suggesting a lesser role for $Cl^-$ channels in transepithelial $Na^+$-$Cl^-$ transport. Basolateral anion substitutions have minimal effect on the membrane potential, despite considerable effects on intracellular $Cl^-$ activity, nor for that matter do changes in basolateral membrane potential affect intracellular $Cl^-$.[69,70,74] However, as with basolateral $K^+$-$Cl^-$ cotransport, basolateral $Cl^-$ channels in the PT may be relatively inactive in the absence of cell swelling. Cell swelling thus activates both $K^+$ and $Cl^-$ channels at the basolateral membranes of proximal tubular cells.[14,75,76] Seki and associates have reported the presence of a basolateral $Cl^-$ channel in S3 segments of the rabbit nephron, wherein they did not see an effect of the KCC inhibitor H74 on intracellular $Cl^-$ activity.[77] The molecular identity of these and other basolateral $Cl^-$ channels in the proximal nephron is not known with certainty, although S3 segments have been shown to express messenger RNA (mRNA) exclusively for the swelling-activated CLC-2 $Cl^-$ channel; the role of this channel in transcellular $Na^+$-$Cl^-$ reabsorption is not as yet clear.[78]

Finally, there is functional evidence for $Na^+$-dependent and $Na^+$-independent $Cl^-$-$HCO_3^-$ exchange at the basolateral membrane of proximal tubular cells.[13,74,79] The impact of $Na^+$-independent $Cl^-$-$HCO_3^-$ exchange on basolateral exit is thought to be minimal.[74] First, this exchanger is expected to mediate $Cl^-$ entry under physiologic conditions.[79] Second, there is only a modest difference between the rate of decrease in intracellular $Cl^-$ activity and the combined removal of $Na^+$ and $Cl^-$ versus $Cl^-$ and $HCO_3^-$, suggesting that pure $Cl^-$-$HCO_3^-$ exchange does not contribute significantly to $Cl^-$ exit. By contrast, there is a 75% reduction in the rate of decrease in intracellular $Cl^-$ activity after the removal of basolateral $Na^+$.[74] The $Na^+$-dependent $Cl^-$-$HCO_3^-$ exchanger may thus play a considerable role in basolateral $Cl^-$ exit, with recycled exit of $Na^+$ and $HCO_3^-$ via the basolateral $Na^+$-$HCO_3^-$ cotransporter NBC1 (Fig. 6.5). The molecular identity of this proximal tubular $Na^+$-dependent $Cl^-$-$HCO_3^-$ exchanger is not as yet known.

## REGULATION OF PROXIMAL TUBULAR $NA^+$-$CL^-$ TRANSPORT

### Glomerulotubular Balance

A fundamental property of the kidney is the phenomenon of glomerulotubular balance, wherein changes in the GFR are offset by changes in tubular reabsorption, thus maintaining a constant fractional reabsorption of fluid and $Na^+$-$Cl^-$ (Fig. 6.6). Although the distal nephron is capable of adjusting reabsorption in response to changes in tubular flow, the impact of GFR on $Na^+$-$Cl^-$ reabsorption by the PT is particularly pronounced (Fig. 6.7).[80] Glomerulotubular balance is independent of direct neuronal and systemic hormonal control, and is thought to be mediated by the additive effects of luminal and peritubular factors.[81]

Until recently, there was some controversy regarding the role of luminal factors in glomerulotubular balance because experiments performed using isolated rabbit PTs failed to demonstrate a significant effect of tubular flow on fluid absorption.[82] This issue has largely been resolved, however,

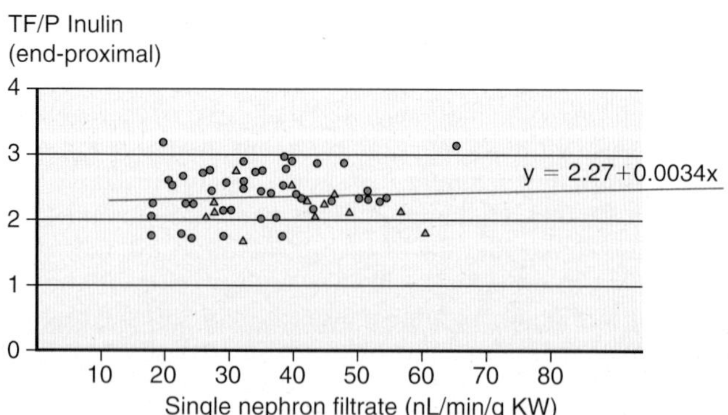


**Fig. 6.6** Glomerulotubular balance. The tubular fluid-to-plasma ratio of the nonreabsorbable marker, inulin (TF/P inulin), at the end of the proximal tubule, which is used as a measure of fractional water absorption by the proximal tubule, does not change as a function of single-nephron glomerular filtration rate. Measurements were done during antidiuresis *(triangles)* and water diuresis *(circles)*. (From Schnermann J, Wahl M, Liebau G, Fischbach H. Balance between tubular flow rate and net fluid reabsorption in the proximal convolution of the rat kidney. I. Dependency of reabsorptive net fluid flux upon proximal tubular surface area at spontaneous variations of filtration rate. *Pflugers Arch.* 1968;304:90–103.)

with clear evidence that fluid shear stress (FSS) increases solute and water absorption.[83] Du and coworkers reported linear flow dependence of fluid and $HCO_3^-$ transport in isolated perfused murine PTs (Fig. 6.8),[81,84] mediated by NHE3 and the $H^+$-ATPase, as discussed later. These data were analyzed using a mathematical model that estimated microvillus torque as a function of tubular flow; accounting for increases in tubular diameter, which reduce torque, there is a linear relationship between calculated torque and fluid and $HCO_3^-$ absorption.[81,84] Consistent with an effect of torque rather than flow per se, increasing viscosity of the perfusate by the addition of dextran increases the effect on fluid transport; the extra viscosity increases the hydrodynamic effect of flow and thus increases torque. The mathematical analysis of Du and associates provides an excellent explanation of the discrepancy between their results and those of Burg and Orloff.[82] Whereas Burg and Orloff performed their experiments in rabbits, the more recent report used mice; other studies that had found an effect of flow used perfusion of rat PTs, presumably more similar to mouse than rabbit.[80–82,84] Increased flow has a considerably greater effect on tubular diameter in the rabbit PT, thus reducing the increase in torque. Mathematical analysis of the rabbit data thus predicts a 43% increase in torque due to a 41% increase in tubule diameter at a threefold increase in flow; this corresponds to the statistically insignificant 36% increase in volume reabsorption reported by Burg and Orloff.[82]

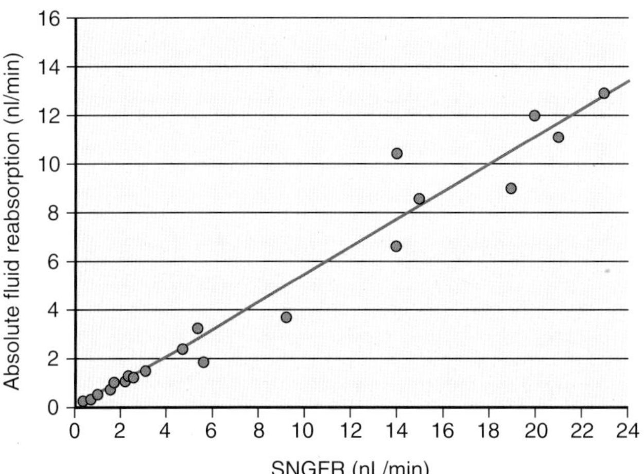


**Fig. 6.7** Glomerulotubular balance. Shown is the linear increase in absolute fluid reabsorption by the late proximal tubule as a function of single-nephron glomerular filtration rate *(SNGFR)*. (From Spitzer A, Brandis M. Functional and morphologic maturation of the superficial nephrons. Relationship to total kidney function. *J Clin Invest.* 1974;53: 279–287.)

Pharmacologic inhibition reveals that tubular flow activates proximal $HCO_3^-$ reabsorption mediated by NHE3 and apical $H^+$-ATPase.[81] The flow-dependent increase in proximal fluid and $HCO_3^-$ reabsorption is also attenuated in NHE3-deficient knockout mice.[81,84] Inhibition of the actin cytoskeleton with cytochalasin D reduces the effect of flow on fluid and $HCO_3^-$ transport. This maneuver blocked the effects of flow on NHE3 and $Na^+/K^+$-ATPase, but not on $H^+$-ATPase. It also blocks the effects of FSS on movement of these transporters to the plasma membranes, suggesting that flow-dependent movement of microvilli activates these transport proteins via their linkage to the cytoskeleton (see Fig. 6.12 for NHE3).[85] FSS induces densely distributed peripheral actin bands and increases the formation of tight junctions and adherens junctions in cultured tubule cells; this junctional buttressing is hypothesized to maximize flow-activated transcellular salt and water absorption.[86]

The roles of dopamine, angiotensin II (Ang II), and calcium on FSS-induced sodium and bicarbonate transport have been examined. Luminal dopamine completely inhibited the flow-induced increase in $Na^+$ transport,[83] with the major effects being mediated through the $D_{1A}$ receptor. Deletion of $AT_{1A}$ receptors in mice also abrogated flow-induced increments in $Na^+$ transport,[87] but these effects may be related to the profound basal reductions in NHE3 activity. When $AT_1$ receptor blockers are employed, flow-induced $Na^+$ transport remained.[87,88] Intracellular activation of IP3 through a local calcium signal may mediate the effects of flow on NHE3 activity, although increased calcium influx does not appear to play a role.[89] Flow and torque were not found to have any effects on chloride absorption, suggesting no convective flow of chloride through the paracellular pathway.

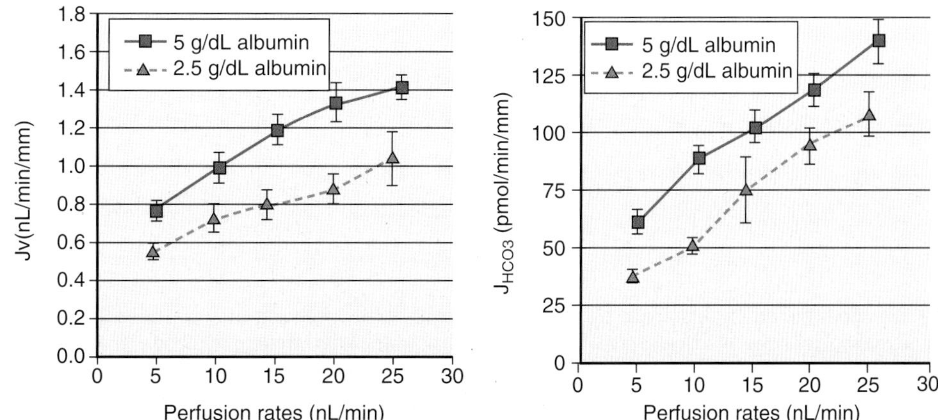


**Fig. 6.8** Glomerulotubular balance; flow-dependent increases in fluid *($J_v$)* and $HCO_3^-$ *($J_{HCO3}$)* absorption by perfused mouse proximal tubules. Absorption also increases when bath albumin concentration increases from 2.5 to 5 g/dL. (From Du Z, Yan Q, Duan Y, et al. Axial flow modulates proximal tubule NHE3 and H-ATPase activities by changing microvillus bending moments. *Am J Physiol Renal Physiol.* 2006;290:F289–F296.)

Another mechanism for glomerulotubular balance operating from the luminal side involves limiting solute concentration. Solutes, such as bicarbonate, amino acids, and glucose, that are reabsorbed coupled to sodium will be depleted earlier along the PT when flow is low, thereby limiting reabsorption rates along the segment as a whole.[90]

Peritubular factors also play an important additive role in glomerulotubular balance, perhaps accounting for the difficulties in documenting flow-induced alterations using isolated rabbit PTs. Specifically, increases in GFR result in an increase in filtration fraction and an attendant increase in postglomerular protein and peritubular oncotic pressure. It has long been appreciated that changes in peritubular protein concentration have important effects on proximal tubular $Na^+$-$Cl^-$ reabsorption; these effects are also seen in combined capillary and tubular perfusion experiments.[81,91] Peritubular protein also has an effect in isolated perfused PT segments, where the effect of hydrostatic pressure is abolished.[81] Increases in peritubular protein concentration have an additive effect on the flow-dependent activation of proximal fluid and $HCO_3^-$ absorption (Fig. 6.8). The effect of peritubular protein on $HCO_3^-$ absorption, which is a predominantly transcellular phenomenon, suggests that changes in peritubular oncotic pressure do not affect transport via the paracellular pathway.[14] However, the mechanism of the stimulatory effect of peritubular protein on transcellular transport is still not completely clear.[81] There are also changes in absorption that correlate with changes in peritubular hydrostatic pressure, as occurs during expansion or contraction of the extracellular fluid volume.[91]

### Neurohumoral Influences

Fluid and $Na^+$-$Cl^-$ reabsorption by the PT are affected by a number of hormones and neurotransmitters. The major hormonal influences on renal $Na^+$-$Cl^-$ transport are shown in Fig. 6.9. Renal sympathetic tone exerts a particularly important stimulatory influence, as does Ang II; dopamine is a major inhibitor of proximal tubular $Na^+$-$Cl^-$ reabsorption.

Unilateral denervation of the rat kidney causes a marked natriuresis and a 40% reduction in proximal $Na^+$-$Cl^-$ reabsorption, without effects on single-nephron GFR or on the contralateral innervated kidney.[92] By contrast, low-frequency electrical stimulation of renal sympathetic nerves increases proximal tubular fluid absorption, with a 32% drop in natriuresis and no change in GFR.[93] Basolateral epinephrine and/or norepinephrine stimulate proximal $Na^+$-$Cl^-$ reabsorption via both α- and β-adrenergic receptors. Several lines of evidence suggest that $\alpha_1$-adrenergic receptors exert a

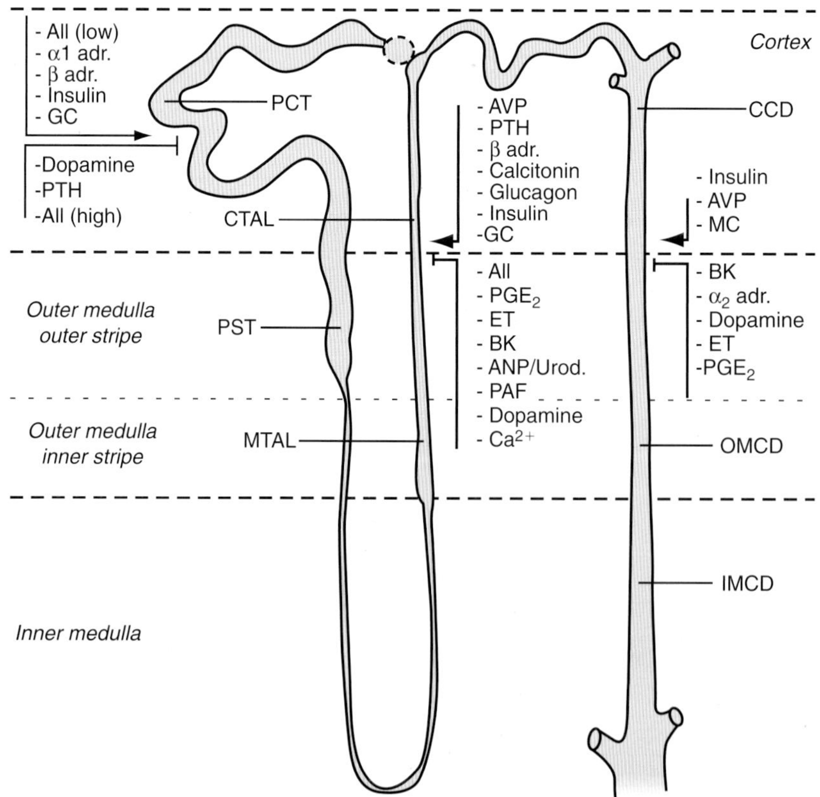


**Fig. 6.9** Neurohumoral influences on $Na^+$-$Cl^-$ absorption by the proximal tubule, thick ascending limb, and collecting duct. Factors that stimulate (→) and inhibit (|–) sodium reabsorption are as follows: *ANG II,* Angiotensin II (low and high referring to picomolar and micromolar concentrations, respectively); *ANP/Urod,* atrial natriuretic peptide and urodilatin; *AVP,* arginine vasopressin; *BK,* bradykinin; *CCD,* cortical collecting duct; *cTAL,* cortical thick ascending limb; *ET,* endothelin; *GC,* glucocorticoids; *IMCD,* inner medullary collecting duct; *MC,* mineralocorticoids; *mTAL,* medullary thick ascending limb of the loop of Henle; *OMCD,* outer medullary collecting duct; *PAF,* platelet-activating factor; *PCT,* proximal convoluted tubule; *$PGE_2$,* prostaglandin $E_2$; *PST,* proximal straight tubule; *PTH,* parathyroid hormone; *α1 adr,* $\alpha_1$-adrenergic agonist; *β adr,* β-adrenergic agonist. (From Feraille E, Doucet A. Sodium-potassium-adenosine triphosphatase-dependent sodium transport in the kidney: hormonal control. *Physiol Rev.* 2001;81:345–418.)

stimulatory effect on proximal $Na^+$-$Cl^-$ transport via activation of basolateral $Na^+$-$K^+$-ATPase and apical $Na^+$-$H^+$ exchange; the role of $\alpha_2$-adrenergic receptors is more controversial.[94] Ligand-dependent recruitment of the scaffolding protein NHE regulatory factor-1 (NHERF-1) by $\beta_2$-adrenergic receptors results in direct activation of apical NHE3, bypassing the otherwise negative effect of downstream cyclic adenosine monophosphate (cAMP; see later).[95,96] Ang II has potent effects on proximal $Na^+$-$Cl^-$ reabsorption and therefore on blood pressure. Genetic deletion of $AT_{1A}$ receptors from PT cells reduced proximal fluid reabsorption, lowered basal blood pressure, shifted the pressure natriuresis, and attenuated the hypertensive response to Ang II infused chronically.[96] Although basal abundances of NHE3 and NaPi2 were similar in PTs from control and knockout mice, the abundance of NHE3 and NaPi2 was lower following Ang II infusion in mice lacking $AT_{1A}$, suggesting that these effects are mediated, at least in part, through these two prominent $Na^+$ transport pathways.

Despite this clear stimulatory effect, it has also been appreciated for 3 decades that Ang II has a bimodal (sometimes called "biphasic") effect on the PT $Na^+$ transport in rats, rabbits, and mice; stimulation of $Na^+$-$Cl^-$ reabsorption occurs at $10^{-12}$ to $10^{-10}$ M, whereas inhibition of $Na^+$-$Cl^-$ reabsorption occurs at concentrations greater than $10^{-7}$ M (Fig. 6.10).[97] Note, however, that plasma Ang II concentrations typically do not exceed $10^{-9}$ M, even during pathological states, such as 2 kidney/1 clip Goldblatt hypertension.[98] Furthermore, this biphasic role of Ang II may not hold true for all species, and in human PT samples, obtained during nephrectomy, concentrations up to $10^{-6}$ M Ang II stimulate $Na^+$-$Cl^-$ reabsorption, primarily owing to a stimulatory effect of the nitric oxide (NO)–cyclic guanosine monophosphate

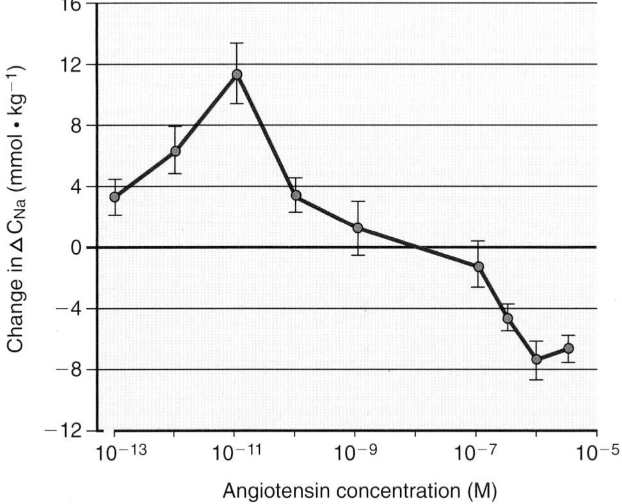


**Fig. 6.10** Biphasic effect of angiotensin II (Ang II) on $Na^+$ reabsorption in microperfused proximal tubules. The steady-state transepithelial $Na^+$ concentration gradient (peritubular-luminal), $\Delta C_{Na}$, that developed in a stationary split droplet is used as an indication of the rate of active $Na^+$ reabsorption. This is plotted as a function of peritubular Ang II concentration; low concentrations activate $Na^+$ absorption by the proximal tubule, whereas higher concentrations inhibit it. (From Harris PJ, Navar LG. Tubular transport responses to angiotensin. *Am J Physiol.* 1985;248:F621–F630)

(cGMP) pathway on extracellular signal–regulated kinase (ERK) phosphorylation.[99] Although the plasma Ang II concentration is typically below the inhibitory concentration, it should be noted, as discussed further later, that the concentration of Ang II in the lumen of the PT frequently exceeds that in plasma, and thus plasma concentrations may not be the sole determining factor. Given the substantial effects of proximal $AT_{1A}$ receptor deletion to reduce blood pressure and shift the pressure natriuresis,[96] it seems likely that the predominant effect of Ang II is stimulatory along the PT under most physiological conditions.

Further complexity of Ang II signaling arises from the presence of $AT_1$ receptors at both the luminal and basolateral membranes in the PT.[100] Ang II application to the luminal or peritubular side of perfused tubules has a similar bimodal effect on fluid transport, albeit with more potent effects at the luminal side.[101] Traditionally, experiments using receptor antagonists and knockout mice have indicated that the stimulatory and inhibitory effects of Ang II are both mediated via $AT_1$ receptors due to signaling at the luminal and basolateral membranes.[102] However, other work has identified that $AT_2$ receptors working through NO-cGMP pathway are able to downregulate NHE3 and $Na^+$-$K^+$-ATPase, leading to natriuresis and reduced blood pressure.[103] Finally, Ang II is also synthesized and secreted by the PT, exerting a potent autocrine effect on proximal tubular $Na^+$-$Cl^-$ reabsorption.[104] Proximal tubular cells thus express mRNA for angiotensinogen, renin, and angiotensin-converting enzyme (ACE),[94] allowing for the autocrine generation of Ang II. Indeed, luminal concentrations of Ang II can be 100- to 1000-fold higher than circulating levels of the hormone.[94] Proximal tubular and systemic synthesis of Ang II may be subject to different control. In fact, intrarenal Ang II appears to stimulate proximal $Na^+$-$Cl^-$ and fluid reabsorption even when dietary salt intake is high, thereby helping to prevent rises in glomerular filtration from increasing late proximal flow.[105] It should be recalled, however, that in this, as in many salt loading studies in rodents, animals received 1% saline as drinking solution. Thus the high salt load was accompanied by free water deprivation, a circumstance shown recently to lead to stress and inflammation.[106]

The PT is also a target for natriuretic hormones; in particular, dopamine synthesized in the PT has negative autocrine effects on proximal $Na^+$-$Cl^-$ reabsorption.[94] Proximal tubular cells have the requisite enzymatic machinery for the synthesis of dopamine, using L-dopa reabsorbed from the glomerular ultrafiltrate. Dopamine synthesis by proximal tubular cells and release into the tubular lumen are increased after volume expansion or a high-salt diet, resulting in a considerable natriuresis.[107,108] Luminal dopamine antagonizes the stimulatory effect of epinephrine on volume absorption in perfused PCTs, consistent with an autocrine effect of dopamine released into the tubular lumen.[107,109] Dopamine primarily exerts its natriuretic effect via $D_1$-like dopamine receptors ($D_1$ and $D_5$ in humans); as is the case for the $AT_1$ receptors for Ang II, $D_1$ receptors are expressed at the apical and luminal membranes of PTs.[100,110] Targeted deletion of the $D_{1A}$ and $D_5$ receptors in mice leads to hypertension by mechanisms that include reduced proximal tubular natriuresis.[111,112] The proximal tubular-specific deletion of aromatic amino acid decarboxylase, which produces dopamine, generates mice that are a vivid demonstration of the role of intrarenal dopamine. This intrarenal dopamine deficiency leads to upregulation of sodium transporters along the nephron, upregulation of the intrarenal renin–angiotensin axis, decreased natriuresis in response to L-dopa, and reduced medullary cyclooxygenase-2 (COX-2) expression, with reduced urinary prostaglandin levels. These mice also exhibit salt-sensitive hypertension and ultimately a significantly shorter life span compared with wild type mice.[113]

The natriuretic effect of dopamine in the PT is modulated by atrial natriuretic peptide (ANP), which inhibits apical $Na^+$-$H^+$ exchange via a dopamine-dependent mechanism.[14] ANP appears to induce recruitment of the $D_1$ dopamine receptor to the plasma membrane of proximal tubular cells, thus sensitizing the tubule to the effect of dopamine.[114] The inhibitory effect of ANP on basolateral $Na^+$-$K^+$-ATPase occurs via a $D_1$-dependent mechanism, with a synergistic inhibition of $Na^+$-$K^+$-ATPase by the two hormones.[114] Furthermore, dopamine and $D_1$ receptors appear to play critical permissive roles in the in vivo natriuretic effect of ANP.[14]

Finally, there is considerable crosstalk between the major antinatriuretic and natriuretic influences on the PT. For example, ANP inhibits Ang II–dependent stimulation of proximal tubular fluid absorption, presumably via the dopamine-dependent mechanisms discussed earlier.[14,115] Dopamine also decreases the expression of $AT_1$ receptors for Ang II in cultured proximal tubular cells.[116] Furthermore, the provision of L-dopa in the drinking water of rats decreases $AT_1$ receptor expression in the PT, suggesting that dopamine synthesis in the PT resets the sensitivity to Ang II.[116] Ang II signaling through $AT_1$ receptors decreases expression of the $D_5$ dopamine receptor, whereas renal cortical expression of $AT_1$ receptors is in turn increased in knockout mice deficient in the $D_5$ receptor.[117] Similar interactions have been found between proximal tubular $AT_1$ receptors and the $D_2$-like $D_3$ receptor.[118]

### Regulation of Proximal Tubular Transporters

The apical $Na^+$-$H^+$ exchanger NHE3 and the basolateral $Na^+$-$K^+$-ATPase are primary targets for signaling pathways elicited by the various antinatriuretic and natriuretic stimuli discussed earlier; NHE3 mediates the rate-limiting step in transepithelial $Na^+$-$Cl^-$ absorption and, as such, is the dominant target for regulatory pathways.[84] NHE3 is regulated by the combined effects of direct phosphorylation and dynamic, carboxyl-terminal interaction with scaffolding proteins and signal transduction proteins, which primarily regulate transport via changes in trafficking of the exchanger protein to and from the brush border membrane (Fig. 6.11).[40,119] Basal activity of the exchanger is also dependent on carboxyl-terminal binding of casein kinase 2 (CK2); phosphorylation of serine 719 by CK2 contributes significantly to the transport activity of NHE3 by modulating membrane trafficking of the transport protein.[120]

Increases in cAMP have a profound inhibitory effect on apical $Na^+$-$H^+$ exchange in the PT. Intracellular cAMP is increased in response to dopamine signaling via $D_1$-like receptors and/or parathyroid hormone (PTH)–dependent signaling via the PTH receptor, whereas Ang II–dependent activation of NHE3 is associated with a reduction in cAMP.[121] PTH is a potent inhibitor of NHE3, presumably so as to promote the distal delivery of $Na^+$-$HCO_3^-$ and an attendant stimulation of distal calcium reabsorption.[122] The activation of protein kinase A (PKA) by increased cAMP results in direct phosphorylation of NHE3; although several sites in NHE3 are phosphorylated by PKA, the phosphorylation of serine 552 (S552) and 605 (S605) has been specifically implicated in the inhibitory effect of cAMP on $Na^+$-$H^+$ exchange.[123] So-called phospho-specific antibodies, which specifically recognize the phosphorylated forms of S552 and S605, have demonstrated dopamine-dependent increases in the phosphorylation of both these serines.[124] Moreover,

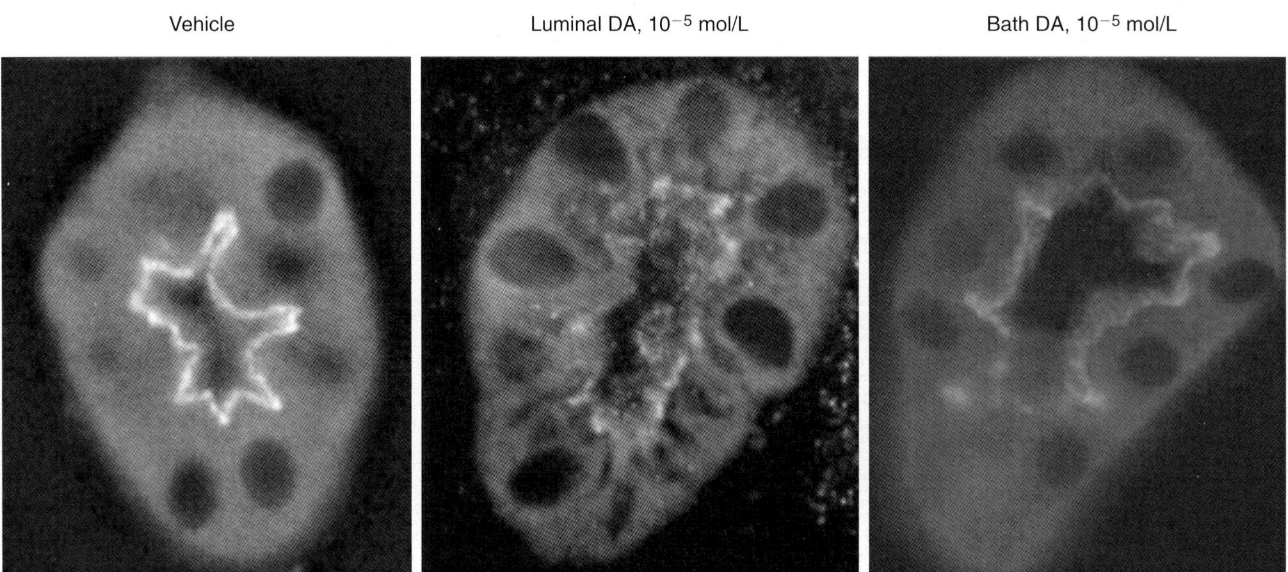


**Fig. 6.11** Effect of dopamine on trafficking of the $Na^+$-$H^+$ exchanger NHE3 in the proximal tubule. Microdissected proximal convoluted tubules were perfused for 30 minutes with $10^{-5}$ mol/L dopamine *(DA)*, in the lumen or the bath, inducing a retraction of immunoreactive NHE3 protein from the apical membrane. (From Bacic D, Kaissling B, McLeroy P, et al. Dopamine acutely decreases apical membrane Na/H exchanger NHE3 protein in mouse renal proximal tubule. *Kidney Int.* 2003;64:2133–2141.)

immunostaining of rat kidney has revealed that S552-phosphorylated NHE3 localizes at the coated pit region of the brush border membrane, where the oligomerized inactive form of NHE3 predominates.[124,125] The cAMP-stimulated phosphorylation of NHE3 by PKA thus results in a redistribution of the transporter from the microvillar membrane to an inactive submicrovillar population (Fig. 6.11). Notably, however, phosphorylation of these residues appears to be necessary but not sufficient for regulation of NHE3.[40] A number of regulators of NHE3, including gastrin and uroguanylin, have been found to exert a functional effect through phosphorylation of S552 and/or S605.[126,127]

The regulation of NHE3 by cAMP also requires the participation of a family of homologous scaffolding proteins that contain protein–protein interaction motifs known as PDZ domains (named for the PSD95, *Drosophila* disc large, and ZO-1 proteins in which these domains were first discovered; Fig. 6.12). The first of these proteins, NHERF-1, was purified as a cellular factor required for the inhibition of NHE3 by PKA.[128] NHERF-2 was in turn cloned by yeast two-hybrid screens as a protein that interacts with the carboxyl-terminus of NHE3; NHERF-1 and NHERF-2 have very similar effects on the regulation of NHE3 in cultured cells. The related protein PDZK1 interacts with NHE3 and a number of other epithelial transporters and is required for expression of the anion exchanger SLC26A6 at brush border membranes of the PT.[65]

NHERF-1 and NHERF-2 are both expressed in human and mouse PT cells; NHERF-1 colocalizes with NHE3 in microvilli of the brush border, whereas NHERF-2 is predominantly expressed at the base of microvilli in the vesicle-rich domain.[128] The NHERFs assemble a multiprotein, dynamically regulated signaling complex that includes NHE3 and several other transport proteins. In addition to NHE3, they bind to the actin-associated protein, ezrin, thus linking NHE3 to the cytoskeleton; this linkage to the cytoskeleton may be particularly important for the mechanical activation of NHE3 by microvillar bending, as has been implicated in glomerulotubular balance (see earlier discussion).[81,84,128] Ezrin also interacts directly with NHE3, binding to a separate binding site within the carboxyl-terminus of the transport protein.[119] Ezrin functions as an anchoring protein for PKA, bringing PKA into close proximity with NHE3 and facilitating its phosphorylation (Fig. 6.12).[128] Analysis of knockout mice for *Nherf-1* has revealed that it is not required for baseline activity of NHE3; as expected, however, it is required for cAMP-dependent regulation of the exchanger by PTH.[128] One long-standing paradox has been that β-adrenergic receptors, which increase cAMP in the PT, cause an activation of apical $Na^+$-$H^+$ exchange.[94] This was resolved by the observation that the first PDZ domain of NHERF-1 interacts with the $\beta_2$-adrenergic receptor in an agonist-dependent fashion; this interaction serves to disrupt the interaction between the second PDZ domain and NHE3, resulting in a stimulation of the exchanger, despite the catecholamine-dependent increase in cAMP.[128]

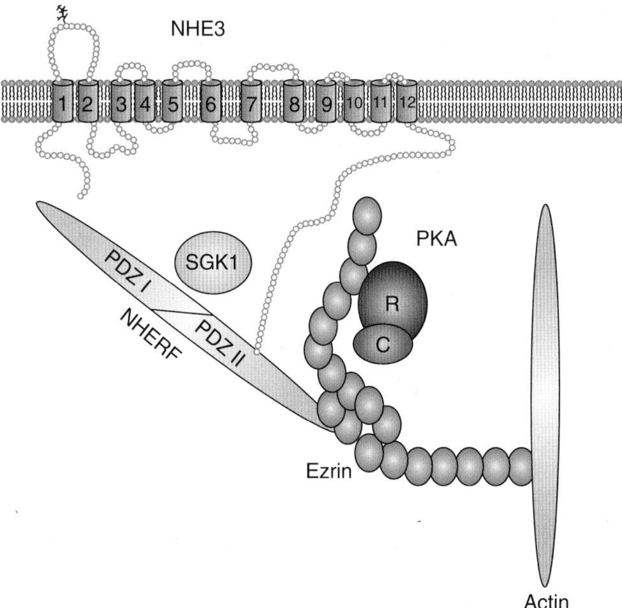


**Fig. 6.12** Scaffolding protein NHERF ($Na^+$-$H^+$ exchanger regulatory factor) links the $Na^+$-$H^+$ exchanger NHE3 to the cytoskeleton and signaling proteins. NHERF binds to ezrin, which in turn links to protein kinase A *(PKA)* and the actin cytoskeleton. NHERF also binds to SGK1 (serum- and glucocorticoid-regulated kinase 1), which activates NHE3. *C,* Catalytic; *PDZ,* domain named for the PSD95, *Drosophila* disc large (*Drosophila*), and ZO-1 proteins; *R,* regulatory.

As discussed earlier, at concentrations higher than $10^{-7}$ M (Fig. 6.10), Ang II has an inhibitory effect on proximal tubular $Na^+$-$Cl^-$ absorption.[97] This inhibition is dependent on the activation of brush border phospholipase $A_2$ ($PLA_2$), which results in the liberation of arachidonic acid.[101] Metabolism of arachidonic acid by cytochrome P450 monooxygenases, in turn, generates 20-hydroxyeicosatetraenoic acid (20-HETE) and epoxyeicosatrienoic acids (EETs), compounds that inhibit NHE3 and the basolateral $Na^+$-$K^+$-ATPase.[94,129] EETs and 20-HETE have also been implicated in the reduction in proximal $Na^+$-$Cl^-$ absorption that occurs during pressure natriuresis, inhibiting $Na^+$-$K^+$-ATPase and retracting NHE3 from the brush border membrane.[130]

Antinatriuretic stimuli such as Ang II acutely increase the expression of NHE3 at the apical membrane, at least in part by inhibiting the generation of cAMP.[121] Low-dose Ang II 0.1 nmol/L ($10^{-10}$ M) also increases exocytic insertion of NHE3 into the plasma membrane via a mechanism that is dependent on phosphatidylinositol-3-kinase (PI3K).[131] Treatment of rats with captopril thus results in a retraction of NHE3 and associated proteins from the brush border of PT cells.[132] Glucocorticoids also increase NHE3 activity due to transcriptional induction of the *Nhe3* gene and an acute stimulation of exocytosis of the exchanger to the plasma membrane.[40] Glucocorticoid-dependent exocytosis of NHE3 appears to require NHERF-2, which acts in this context as a scaffolding protein for the glucocorticoid-induced serine-threonine kinase SGK1 (see the "Regulation of $Na^+$-$Cl^-$ Transport in the Connecting Tubule and Cortical Collecting Duct: Aldosterone" section).[133] The acute effect of dexamethasone has thus been shown to require direct phosphorylation of serine 663 in the NHE3 protein by SGK1.[134]

Finally, many of the natriuretic and antinatriuretic pathways that influence NHE3 have parallel effects on the basolateral $Na^+$-$K^+$-ATPase (see Feraille and Doucet[94] for a detailed review). The molecular mechanisms underlying inhibition of $Na^+$-$K^+$-ATPase by dopamine have been particularly well characterized.

Inhibition by dopamine is associated with removal of active $Na^+$-$K^+$-ATPase units from the basolateral membrane, somewhat analogous to the effect on NHE3 expression at the apical membrane.[135] This inhibitory effect is primarily mediated by protein kinase C (PKC), which directly phosphorylates the $\alpha_1$-subunit of $Na^+$-$K^+$-ATPase, the predominant $\alpha$-subunit in the kidney.[94] The effect of dopamine requires phosphorylation of serine 18 of the $\alpha_1$-subunit by PKC; this phosphorylation does not affect enzymatic activity of the $Na^+$-$K^+$-ATPase, but rather induces a conformational change that enhances the binding of PI3K to an adjacent, proline-rich domain. The PI3K recruited by this phosphorylated $\alpha_1$-subunit then stimulates the dynamin-dependent endocytosis of the $Na^+$-$K^+$-ATPase complex via clathrin-coated pits.[135]

## LOOP OF HENLE

The loop of Henle encompasses the thin descending limb, thin ascending limb, and TAL. The descending and ascending thin limbs function in passive absorption of water and $Na^+$-$Cl^-$, respectively, whereas the TAL reabsorbs about 30% of filtered $Na^+$-$Cl^-$ via active transport.[136,137] There is considerable cellular and functional heterogeneity along the entire length of the loop of Henle, with consequences for the transport of water, $Na^+$-$Cl^-$, and other solutes. The thin descending limb begins in the outer medulla after an abrupt transition from S3 segments of the PT, marking the boundary between the outer and inner stripes of the outer medulla. Thin descending limbs end at a hairpin turn at the end of the loop of Henle. Short-looped nephrons that originate from superficial and midcortical nephrons have a short descending limb within the inner stripe of the outer medulla; these tubules merge abruptly into the TAL close to the hairpin turn of the loop (see also discussion later). Long-looped nephrons originating from juxtamedullary glomeruli have a long ascending thin limb that then merges with the TAL. The TALs of long-looped nephrons begin at the boundary between the inner and outer medulla, whereas the TALs of short-looped nephrons may be entirely cortical. The ratio of medullary to cortical TAL for a given nephron is a function of the depth of its origin, such that superficial nephrons are primarily composed of cortical TALs, whereas juxtamedullary nephrons primarily possess medullary TALs.

The TAL begins abruptly after the thin ascending limb of long-looped nephrons and after the aquaporin-negative segment of short-limbed nephrons.[138] The TAL extends into the renal cortex, where it meets its parent glomerulus at the vascular pole; the plaque of cells at this junction form the macula densa, which function as the tubular sensor for tubuloglomerular feedback (TGF) and tubular regulation of renin release by the juxtaglomerular apparatus. Cells in the medullary TAL are 7 to 8 μm in height, with extensive invaginations of the basolateral plasma membrane and interdigitations between adjacent cells.[6] As in the PT, these lateral cell processes contain numerous elongated mitochondria, perpendicular to the basement membrane. Cells in the cortical TAL are considerably shorter, 2 μm in height at the end of the cortical TAL in rabbits, with fewer mitochondria and a simpler basolateral membrane.[6] Macula densa cells also lack the lateral cell processes and interdigitations characteristic of medullary TAL cells.[6] However, scanning electron microscopy has revealed that the TAL of rat and hamster contains two morphologic subtypes, a rough-surfaced cell type (R cells) with prominent apical microvilli and a smooth-surfaced cell type (S cells) with an abundance of subapical vesicles.[6,139–141] In the hamster TAL, cells can also be separated into those with high apical and low basolateral $K^+$ conductance and weak basolateral $Cl^-$ conductance (LBC cells) versus a second population with low apical and high basolateral $K^+$ conductance combined with high basolateral $Cl^-$ conductance (HBC).[140,142] The relative frequency of the morphologic and functional subtypes in the cortical and medullary TAL suggests that HBC cells correspond to S cells and LBC cells to R cells.[140]

### TRANSPORT CHARACTERISTICS OF THE DESCENDING THIN LIMB

It has long been appreciated that the osmolality of tubular fluid increases progressively between the corticomedullary junction and papillary tip due to active secretion of solutes or passive absorption of water along the descending thin limb.[143] Subsequent reports have revealed a very high water permeability of perfused outer medullary thin descending limbs in the absence of significant permeability to $Na^+$-$Cl^-$.[144] Notably, however, the permeability properties of descending thin limbs vary as a function of depth in the inner medulla and inclusion in short- versus long-looped nephrons.[145,146] Descending thin limbs from short-looped nephrons contain type I cells, very flat, endothelial-like cells, with intermediate-depth tight junctions suggesting a relative tight epithelium.[145,146] The epithelium of descending limbs from long-looped nephrons is initially more complex, with taller type II cells possessing more elaborate apical microvilli and more prominent mitochondria. In the lower medullary portion of long-looped nephrons, these cells change into a type III morphology, endothelial-like cells similar to the type I cells from short-looped nephrons.[145] The permeability properties appear to change as a function of cell type, with a progressive axial drop in water permeability of long-looped descending limbs; the water permeability of descending thin limbs in the middle part of the inner medulla is thus about 42% that of outer medullary thin descending limbs.[147] Furthermore, the distal 20% of descending thin limbs have a very low water permeability.[147] These changes in water permeability along the descending thin limb are accompanied by a progressive increase in $Na^+$-$Cl^-$ permeability, although the ionic permeability remains considerably less than that of the ascending thin limb.[146]

Consistent with a primary role in passive water and solute absorption, $Na^+$-$K^+$-ATPase activity in the descending thin limb is almost undetectable,[17] suggesting that these cells do not actively transport $Na^+$-$Cl^-$; those ion transport pathways that have been identified in descending thin limb cells are thought to contribute primarily to cellular volume regulation.[148] In contrast to the relative lack of $Na^+$-$Cl^-$ transport, transcellular water reabsorption by the thin descending limb is a critical component of the renal countercurrent concentrating mechanism (see Chapter 10).[136,144]

### $NA^+$-$CL^-$ TRANSPORT BY THE THIN ASCENDING LIMB

Fluid entering the thin ascending limb has a very high concentration of $Na^+$-$Cl^-$ due to osmotic equilibration by the water-permeable descending limbs. The passive reabsorption of this delivered $Na^+$-$Cl^-$ by the thin ascending limb is a critical component of the passive equilibration model of the renal countercurrent multiplication system (see Chapter 10). Consistent with this role, the permeability properties of the thin ascending limb are dramatically different from those of the descending thin limb, with a much higher permeability to $Na^+$-$Cl^-$ and vanishingly low water permeability.[146,149] Passive $Na^+$-$Cl^-$ reabsorption by thin ascending limbs occurs via a combination of paracellular $Na^+$ transport and transcellular $Cl^-$ transport.[137,142,150–153] The inhibition of paracellular conductance by protamine thus selectively inhibits $Na^+$ transport across perfused thin ascending limbs, consistent with paracellular transport of $Na^+$.[150] As in the descending limb, thin ascending limbs have a modest $Na^+$-$K^+$-ATPase activity (Fig. 6.3); however, the active transport of $Na^+$ across thin ascending limbs accounts for only an estimated 2% of $Na^+$ reabsorption by this nephron segment.[154] Chloride channel blockers reduce $Cl^-$ permeability of the thin ascending limb, consistent with passive transcellular $Cl^-$ transport.[153] Direct measurement of the membrane potential of impaled hamster thin ascending limbs has also yielded evidence for apical and basolateral $Cl^-$ channel activity.[142] This transepithelial transport of $Cl^-$, but not $Na^+$, is activated by vasopressin, with a pharmacologic profile that is consistent with direct activation of thin ascending limb $Cl^-$ channels.[155]

Both apical and basolateral $Cl^-$ transport in the thin ascending limb appear to be mediated by the CLC-K1 $Cl^-$ channel in cooperation with the Barttin subunit (see also the "$Na^+$-$Cl^-$ Transport by the Thick Ascending Limb: Basolateral Mechanisms" section). Immunofluorescence and in situ hybridization indicate a selective expression of CLC-K1 (homologous to the human chloride channel Kb, CLC-NKB) in thin ascending limbs, although single-tubule, reverse transcriptase-polymerase chain reaction (RT-PCR) studies have suggested additional expression in the TAL, DCT, and cortical collecting duct (CCD).[156–158] Notably, immunofluorescence and immunogold labeling indicate that CLC-K1 is expressed exclusively at both the apical and basolateral membranes of thin ascending limbs, such that both the luminal and basolateral $Cl^-$ channels of this nephron segment are encoded by the same gene.[142,156] Homozygous knockout mice with a targeted deletion of *Clc-k1* have a vasopressin-resistant nephrogenic diabetes insipidus, reminiscent of the phenotype of aquaporin-1 knockout mice.[136,159] Given that CLC-K1 is potentially expressed in the TAL, dysfunction of this nephron segment might also contribute to the renal phenotype of *Clc-k1* knockout mice; however, the closely homologous channel CLC-K2 (CLC-NKB) is clearly expressed in the TAL, where it can likely substitute for CLC-K1.[158] Furthermore, loss-of-function mutations in *CLC-NKB* cause Bartter syndrome, which is phenocopied in *Clc-k2* knockout mice, indicating that CLC-K2, rather than CLC-K1, is critical for transport function of the TAL.[160–162]

Detailed characterization of *Clc-k1* knockout mice has revealed a selective impairment in $Cl^-$ transport by the thin ascending limb.[137] Whereas $Cl^-$ absorption is profoundly reduced, $Na^+$ absorption by thin ascending limbs is not significantly impaired (Fig. 6.13). The diffusion voltage induced by a transepithelial $Na^+$-$Cl^-$ gradient is reversed by the absence of CLC-K1, from +15.5 mV in homozygous wild type controls (+/+) to −7.6 mV in homozygous knockout mice (−/−). This change in diffusion voltage is due to the dominance of paracellular $Na^+$ transport in the CLC-K1-deficient −/− mice, leading to a lumen-negative potential; this corresponds to a marked reduction in the relative permeability of $Cl^-$ to that of $Na^+$ ($P_{Cl}/P_{Na}$), from 4.02 to 0.63 (Fig. 6.13). Protamine, an inhibitor of paracellular $Na^+$ transport, has a comparable effect on

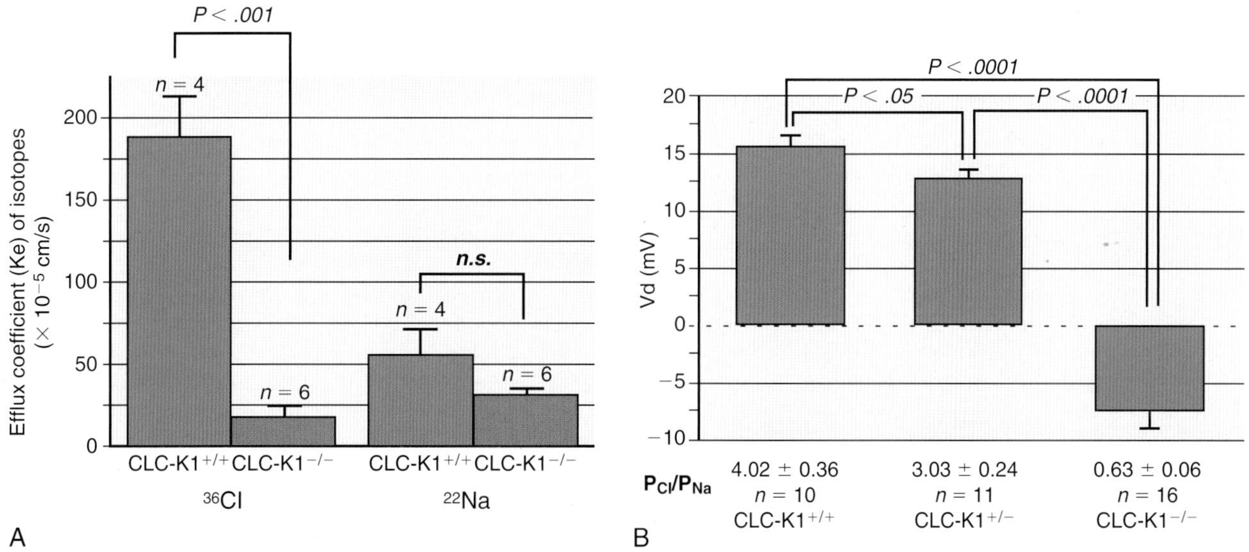


**Fig. 6.13** Role of the CLC-K1 chloride channel in $Na^+$ and $Cl^-$ transport by the thin ascending limbs. Homozygous knockout mice (CLC-K1$^{-/-}$) are compared with their littermate controls (CLC-K1$^{+/+}$). (A) Efflux coefficients for $^{36}Cl^-$ and $^{22}Na^+$ in the thin ascending limbs. $Cl^-$ absorption is essentially abolished in the knockout mice, whereas there is no significant effect of CLC-K1 deficiency on $Na^+$ transport. (B) The diffusion voltage (VD), induced by a transepithelial $Na^+$-$Cl^-$ gradient, is reversed by the absence of CLC-K1, from +15.5 mV in controls to −7.6 mV in homozygous knockout mice. This change in diffusion voltage is due to the dominance of paracellular $Na^+$ transport in the CLC-K1–deficient −/− mice, leading to a lumen-negative potential; this corresponds to a marked reduction in the relative permeability of $Cl^-$ to that of $Na^+$ ($P_{Cl}/P_{Na}$), from 4.02 to 0.63. (From Liu W, Morimoto T, Kondo Y, et al. Analysis of NaCl transport in thin ascending limb of the loop of Henle in CLC-K1 null mice. *Am J Physiol Renal Physiol.* 2002;282:F451–F457.)

the diffusion voltage in −/− mice versus +/− and +/+ mice that have been treated with 5-nitro-2-(3-phenylpropylamino)-benzoate (NPPB) to inhibit CLC-K1; the respective diffusion voltages are 7.9 mV (−/− plus protamine), 8.6 mV (+/− plus protamine and NPPB), and 9.8 (+/+ plus protamine and NPPB). Therefore the paracellular $Na^+$ conductance is unimpaired and essentially the same in *Clc-k1* knockout mice when compared with littermate controls. This study thus provided elegant proof for the relative independence of paracellular and transcellular conductances for $Na^+$ and $Cl^-$, respectively, in thin ascending limbs.[137]

CLC-K1 associates with Barttin, an accessory subunit identified via positional cloning of the gene for Bartter syndrome with sensorineural deafness (see the "$Na^+$-$Cl^-$ Transport by the Thick Ascending Limb: Basolateral Mechanisms" section).[163] Barttin is expressed with CLC-K1 in thin ascending limbs, in addition to the TAL, DCT, and α-intercalated cells.[158,163] Rat CLC-K1 is unique among the CLC-K orthologs and paralogs (CLC-K1/2 in rodents, CLC-NKB/NKA in humans) in that it can generate $Cl^-$ channel activity in the absence of coexpression with Barttin; however, its human ortholog CLC-NKA is nonfunctional in the absence of Barttin.[156,158,164] Regardless, Barttin coimmunoprecipitates with CLC-K1 and increases expression of the channel protein at the cell membrane.[158,164] This so-called chaperone function seems to involve the transmembrane core of Barttin, whereas domains within the cytoplasmic carboxy terminus modulate channel properties (open probability and unitary conductance).[164]

With respect to regulation in this nephron segment, vasopressin has stimulatory effects on $Cl^-$ transport by the thin ascending limb, acting as in principal cells and TAL through V2 receptors and cAMP.[155] Water deprivation induces a fourfold increase in CLC-K1 mRNA, indicating transcriptional effects of vasopressin or medullary tonicity.[165] Basolateral calcium in turn inhibits $Cl^-$ and $Na^+$ transport in the thin ascending limb via activation of the calcium-sensing receptor (CaSR).[166]

## NA+-CL− TRANSPORT BY THE THICK ASCENDING LIMB

### Apical Na+-Cl− Transport

The TAL reabsorbs about 30% of filtered $Na^+$-$Cl^-$ (Fig. 6.1). In addition to an important role in the defense of the extracellular fluid volume, $Na^+$-$Cl^-$ reabsorption by the water-impermeable TAL is a critical component of the renal countercurrent multiplication system. The separation of $Na^+$-$Cl^-$ and water by the TAL is thus responsible for the capability of the kidney to dilute or concentrate the urine. In concert with the countercurrent mechanism, $Na^+$-$Cl^-$ reabsorption by the thin ascending limb and TAL increases medullary tonicity, facilitating water absorption by the collecting duct.

Notwithstanding the morphological heterogeneity described earlier, the cells of the medullary TAL, cortical TAL, and macula densa share the same basic transport mechanisms (Fig. 6.14). $Na^+$-$Cl^-$ reabsorption by the TAL is thus a secondarily active process, driven by the favorable electrochemical gradient for $Na^+$ established by the basolateral $Na^+$-$K^+$-ATPase.[14,167] $Na^+$, $K^+$, and $Cl^-$ are cotransported across the apical membrane by an electroneutral $Na^+$-$K^+$-$2Cl^-$ cotransporter, which generally requires the simultaneous presence of all three ions.[14] Of note, under certain circumstances,

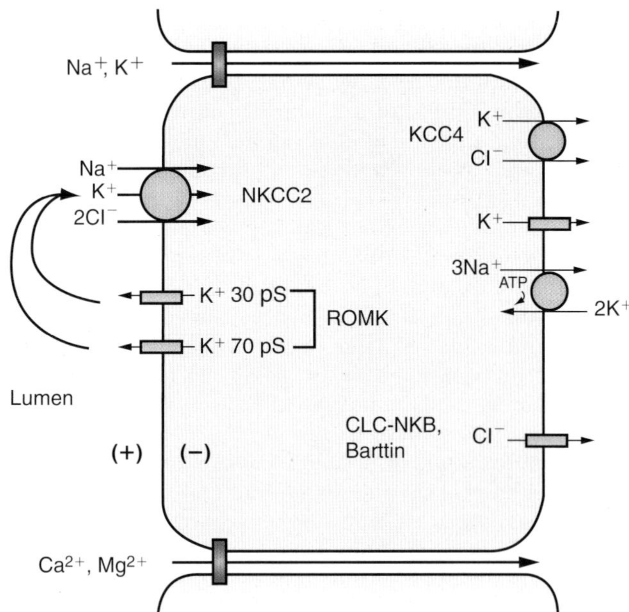


**Fig. 6.14** Transepithelial $Na^+$-$Cl^-$ transport pathways in the thick ascending limb. *CLC-K2,* $Cl^-$ channel, Barttin; *KCC4,* $K^+$-$Cl^-$ cotransporter-4; *NKCC2,* $Na^+$-$K^+$-$2Cl^-$ cotransporter-2; *ROMK,* renal outer medullary $K^+$ channel.

apical $Na^+$-$Cl^-$ transport in the TAL appears to be $K^+$ independent; this issue is reviewed later (see the "Regulation of $Na^+$-$Cl^-$ Transport by the Thick Ascending Limb" section). Apical $Na^+$-$K^+$-$2Cl^-$ cotransport is mediated by the cation-chloride cotransporter NKCC2, encoded by *SLC12A1*.[168] This is a member of the cation chloride cotransporter family of proteins that includes the thiazide-sensitive transporter NCC, and the potassium chloride cotransporters. Functional expression of NKCC2 in *Xenopus* oocytes yields $Cl^-$- and $Na^+$-dependent uptake of $Rb^+$ (a radioactive substitute for $K^+$) and $Cl^-$- and $K^+$-dependent uptake of $^{22}Na^+$.[97,168–170] As expected, NKCC2 is sensitive to micromolar concentrations of furosemide, bumetanide, and other loop diuretics.[168]

Immunofluorescence indicates expression of NKCC2 protein along the entire length of the TAL.[168] In particular, immunoelectron microscopy reveals expression in both rough (R) and smooth (S) cells of the TAL (see earlier discussion).[141] NKCC2 expression in subapical vesicles is particularly prominent in smooth cells, suggesting a role for vesicular trafficking in the regulation of NKCC2 (see the "Regulation of $Na^+$-$Cl^-$ Transport by the Thick Ascending Limb" section).[141] NKCC2 is also expressed in macula densa cells, which have been shown to possess apical $Na^+$-$K^+$-$2Cl^-$ cotransport activity.[141,171] This latter observation is of considerable significance, given the role of the macula densa in TGF and renal renin secretion; luminal loop diuretics block TGF and the suppression of renin release by luminal $Cl^-$.[14]

Alternative splicing of exon 4 of the *SLC12A1* gene yields NKCC2 proteins that differ within transmembrane domain 2 and the adjacent intracellular loop; the functional significance of these variants appears primarily related to differences in binding to chloride.[172] There are thus three different variants of exon 4, denoted "A," "B," and "F"; the variable inclusion of these cassette exons yields NKCC2-A, NKCC2-B, and NKCC2-F proteins.[168,170] Kinetic characterization reveals that these isoforms differ dramatically in ion affinities.[168,170] In particular, NKCC2-F has a very low affinity for $Cl^-$ ($K_m$ = 113 mmol/L) and NKCC2-B has a very high affinity ($K_m$ = 8.9 mmol/L); NKCC2-A has an intermediate affinity for $Cl^-$ ($K_m$ = 44.7 mmol/L).[170] These isoforms differ in axial distribution along the tubule, with the F cassette expressed in the inner stripe of the outer medulla, the A cassette in the outer stripe, and the B cassette in cortical TAL.[14] There is thus an axial distribution of the anion affinity of NKCC2 along the TAL, from a low-affinity, high-capacity transporter (NKCC2-F) to a high-affinity, low-capacity transporter (NKCC2-B). Although technically compromised by the considerable homology between the 3′ end of these 96-base pair exons, in situ hybridization has suggested that rabbit macula densa exclusively expresses the NKCC2-B isoform.[14] Notably, however, selective knockout of the B cassette exon 4 does not eliminate NKCC2 expression in the murine macula densa, which also seems to express NKCC2-A by in situ hybridization.[173] The comparative phenotypes of NKCC2-A and NKCC2-B knockout mice are consistent with the relative $Cl^-$ affinity of each isoform, with NKCC2-B functioning as a high-affinity, low-capacity isoform and NKCC2-A functioning as a low-affinity, high-capacity isoform. Thus targeted deletion of NKCC2-A selectively reduces TGF responses at the higher range of tubular flow rates (a low-affinity, high-capacity situation), whereas NKCC2-B deletion reduces responses at low flow rates.[174] Loss of NKCC2-A almost abolishes the suppression of plasma renin activity by isotonic saline infusion, which is, if anything, more robust in NKCC2-B knockout mice than wild type littermates.[174]

It should be mentioned in this context that the $Na^+$-$H^+$ exchanger NHE3 functions as an alternative mechanism for apical $Na^+$ absorption by the TAL. There is also evidence in mouse cortical TAL for $Na^+$-$Cl^-$ transport via parallel $Na^+$-$H^+$ and $Cl^-$-$HCO_3^-$ exchange, although the role of this mechanism in transepithelial $Na^+$-$Cl^-$ transport seems less prominent than in the PT.[14] Indeed, apical $Na^+$-$H^+$ exchange mediated by NHE3 appears to function primarily in $HCO_3^-$ absorption by the TAL.[175] There is thus a considerable upregulation of both apical $Na^+$-$H^+$ exchange and NHE3 protein in the TAL of acidotic animals, paired with an induction of AE2, a basolateral $Cl^-$-$HCO_3^-$ exchanger.[176,177] NHE3 in the TAL is also upregulated by increased flow. However, this is not via shear stress, as demonstrated in the PT, but by the production of endogenous $O_2^-$ and activation of PKC, a potential pathway for flow-stimulated bicarbonate reabsorption.[178]

### Apical $K^+$ Channels

Microperfused TALs develop a lumen-positive PD during perfusion with $Na^+$-$Cl^-$.[179,180] This lumen-positive PD plays a critical role in the physiology of the TAL, driving the paracellular transport of $Na^+$, $Ca^{2+}$, and $Mg^{2+}$ (Fig. 6.14). Originally attributed to electrogenic $Cl^-$ transport, the lumen-positive transepithelial PD in the TAL is generated by the combination of apical $K^+$ channels and basolateral $Cl^-$ channels.[14,167,180] The conductivity of the apical membrane of TAL cells is predominantly, if not exclusively, $K^+$ selective. Luminal recycling of $K^+$ via $Na^+$-$K^+$-$2Cl^-$ cotransport and apical $K^+$ channels, along with basolateral depolarization due to $Cl^-$ exit through $Cl^-$ channels, results in the lumen-positive transepithelial PD.[14,167]

Several lines of evidence have indicated that apical $K^+$ channels are required for transepithelial $Na^+$-$Cl^-$ transport by the TAL.[14,167] First, the removal of $K^+$ from luminal perfusate results in a marked decrease in $Na^+$-$Cl^-$ reabsorption by the TAL, as measured electrophysiologically; the residual $Na^+$-$Cl^-$ transport in the absence of luminal $K^+$ is sustained by $K^+$ movement into the luminal fluid apical $K^+$ channels, because the combination of $K^+$ removal and a luminal $K^+$ channel inhibitor (barium) almost abolishes the equivalent short circuit current.[14] Apical $K^+$ channels are thus required for continued functioning of NKCC2, the apical $Na^+$-$K^+$-$2Cl^-$ cotransporter; the low luminal concentration of $K^+$ in this nephron segment would otherwise become limiting for transepithelial $Na^+$-$Cl^-$ transport.

Second, the net transport of $K^+$ across perfused TAL is less than 10% that of $Na^+$ and $Cl^-$; about 90% of the $K^+$ transported by NKCC2 is recycled across the apical membrane via $K^+$ channels, resulting in minimal net $K^+$ absorption by the TAL.[14,181]

Third, the intracellular $K^+$ activity of perfused TAL cells is about 15 to 20 mV above equilibrium due to furosemide-sensitive entry of $K^+$ via NKCC2.[182] Given an estimated apical $K^+$ conductivity of about 12 $mS/cm^2$, this intracellular $K^+$ activity yields a calculated $K^+$ current of about 200 $\mu A/cm^2$, which corresponds quantitatively to the uptake of $K^+$ by the apical $Na^+$-$K^+$-$2Cl^-$ cotransporter.[167]

Fourth, the observation that Bartter syndrome can be caused by mutations in renal outer medullary potassium (ROMK, encoded by *KCNJ1*) provides genetic proof for the importance of $K^+$ channels in $Na^+$-$Cl^-$ absorption by the TAL (see later).[183] Finally, a novel ROMK inhibitor functions as a potent diuretic in vivo, primarily due to inhibition of TAL $Na^+$-$Cl^-$ transport.[184]

Three types of apical $K^+$ channels have been identified in the TAL, a channel with a conductance of 30 picosiemen (30 pS), a channel with a conductance of 70 pS, and a high-conductance, calcium-activated maxi-$K^+$ channel (Fig. 6.14).[185–187] The higher $P_o$ and greater density of the 30-pS and 70-pS channels versus the maxi-$K^+$ channel suggest that these are the primary routes for $K^+$ recycling across the apical membrane; the 70-pS channel in turn appears to mediate about 80% of the apical $K^+$ conductance of TAL cells.[188] The low-conductance, 30-pS channel shares several electrophysiologic and regulatory characteristics with ROMK, the cardinal inward-rectifying $K^+$ channel that was initially cloned from renal outer medulla.[14] In humans, three isoforms of ROMK (ROMK1, 2, and 3) are generated by alternative splicing of the *KCNJ1* gene; ROMK3 has not been detected in rat or mouse.[189] ROMK2 has the shortest amino terminus, ROMK1 has an additional 16 residues, and ROMK3 an additional 22 residues (compared with ROMK2). ROMK1 mRNA is expressed in the mid and late distal tubule and the CCD, and in the outer medullary collecting duct (OMCD), but not along the TAL (see later). ROMK2 mRNA is expressed from the medullary TAL through the CCD, but is absent from the OMCD.[189] ROMK3 is expressed from the medullary TAL through the DCT. ROMK protein has been identified at the apical membrane of medullary TAL, cortical TAL, and macula densa.[190] Furthermore, the 30-pS channel is also absent from the apical membrane of mice with homozygous deletion of the gene encoding ROMK.[191] Notably, not all cells in the TAL are labeled with ROMK antibody, suggesting that ROMK might be absent in the so-called HBC cells with HBC and low apical $K^+$ conductance (also see earlier discussion).[140,142] HBC cells are thought to correspond to the smooth-surfaced morphologic subtype of TAL cells (S cells)[140]; however, distribution of ROMK protein by immunoelectron microscopy has not as yet been reported.

ROMK clearly plays a critical role in $Na^+$-$Cl^-$ absorption by the TAL, given that loss-of-function mutations in this gene are associated with Bartter syndrome.[183] The role of ROMK in Bartter syndrome was initially discordant with the data, suggesting that the 70-pS $K^+$ channel is the dominant conductance at the apical membrane of TAL cells; heterologous expression of the ROMK protein in *Xenopus* oocytes had yielded a channel with a conductance of about 30 pS, suggesting that the 70-pS channel was distinct from ROMK.[14,188] This paradox has been resolved by the observation that the 70-pS channel is absent from the TAL of ROMK knockout mice, indicating that ROMK proteins form a subunit of the 70-pS channel.[192] A recent study specifically examined the effects of ROMK1 disruption in mice, and consistent with its absence along the TAL, discussed earlier, these mice did not display a Bartter syndrome phenotype.[193]

ROMK activity in the TAL is clearly modulated by association with other proteins, such that coassociation with other subunits to generate the 70-pS channel is perfectly compatible with the known physiology of this protein. ROMK thus associates with scaffolding proteins NHERF-1 and NHERF-2 (see the "Regulation of Proximal Tubular $Na^+$-$Cl^-$ Transport: Neurohumoral Influences" section) via the carboxyl-terminal PDZ-binding motif of ROMK; NHERF-2 is coexpressed with ROMK in the TAL.[194] The association of ROMK with NHERFs serves to bring ROMK into closer proximity to the cystic fibrosis transmembrane regulator protein (CFTR).[194] This ROMK–CFTR interaction is, in turn, required for the native ATP and glibenclamide sensitivity of apical $K^+$ channels in the TAL.[195]

### Paracellular Transport

TALs perfused with $Na^+$-$Cl^-$ develop a lumen-positive, transepithelial PD generated by the combination of apical $K^+$ secretion and basolateral $Cl^-$ efflux.[14,167,179,180,182] This lumen-positive PD plays a critical role in the paracellular reabsorption of $Na^+$, $Ca^{2+}$, and $Mg^{2+}$ by the TAL (Fig. 6.14). In the transepithelial transport of $Na^+$, the stoichiometry of NKCC2 ($1Na^+$:$1K^+$:$2Cl^-$) is such that other mechanisms are necessary to balance the exit of $Cl^-$ at the basolateral membrane; consistent with this requirement, data from mouse TAL have indicated that about 50% of transepithelial $Na^+$ transport occurs via the paracellular pathway.[3,196] For example, the ratio of net $Cl^-$ transepithelial absorption to net $Na^+$ absorption through the paracellular pathway is $2.4 \pm 0.3$ in microperfused mouse medullary TAL segments, and the expected ratio of 50% of $Na^+$ transport occurs via the paracellular pathway. In the absence of vasopressin, apical $Na^+$-$Cl^-$ cotransport is not $K^+$ dependent (see the "Regulation of $Na^+$-$Cl^-$ Transport by the Thick Ascending Limb" section), reducing the lumen-positive PD; switching to $K^+$-dependent $Na^+$-$K^+$-$2Cl^-$ cotransport in the presence of vasopressin results in a doubling of $Na^+$-$Cl^-$ reabsorption, without an effect on oxygen consumption.[3,196] Therefore, the combination of a cation-permeable paracellular pathway and an "active transport," lumen-positive PD,[167] generated indirectly by the basolateral $Na^+$-$K^+$-ATPase, results in a doubling of active $Na^+$-$Cl^-$ transport for a given level of oxygen consumption.[3,197]

Unlike in the PT, the voltage-positive PD in the TAL is generated almost entirely by transcellular transport, rather than by diffusion across the lateral tight junction.[15] Mouse TAL segments primarily express claudin-14, -16, -19, and -10.[14,198–200] In vasopressin-stimulated mouse TAL segments, with a lumen-positive PD of 10 mV, the maximal increase in $Na^+$-$Cl^-$ in the lateral interspace is about 10 mmol/L.[196] Tight junctions in the TAL are cation selective, with $P_{Na}/P_{Cl}$ ratios of 2 to 5.[167,196] Notably, however, $P_{Na}/P_{Cl}$ ratios can be highly variable in individual tubules, ranging from 2 to 5 in a single study of perfused mouse TAL.[196] Recently, it has been suggested that the claudin profile of cells along the TAL represents a mosaic, with some cell interfaces expressing the $Na^+$-selective claudin-10, whereas others express claudin-3, -16, or -19. It was suggested that this mosaic pattern reveals the existence of spatially separated paracellular routes for $Na^+$ and $Ca^{2+}/Mg^{2+}$.[201] Regardless, assuming a net $P_{Na}/P_{Cl}$ ratio of about 3, the maximal dilution potential in the mouse TAL is between 0.7 and 1.1 mV, consistent with a dominant effect of transcellular processes on the lumen-positive PD.[196]

The reported transepithelial resistance in the TAL is between 10 and 50 $\Omega \cdot cm^2$; although this resistance is higher than that of the PT, the TAL is not considered a tight epithelium.[14,167] Notably, however, water permeability of the TAL is extremely low, less than 1% that of the PT.[167] These hybrid characteristics—relatively low resistance and very low water permeability—allow the TAL to generate and sustain $Na^+$-$Cl^-$ gradients of up to 120 mmol/L.[14,167] Not unexpectedly, given its lack of water permeability, the TAL does not express aquaporin water channels; as in the PT, the particular repertoire of claudins expressed in the TAL determines the resistance and ion selectivity of this nephron segment.

Mutations in human claudin-16 (previously called paracellin-1) and claudin-19 are associated with hereditary hypomagnesemia, suggesting that these claudins are particularly critical for the cation selectivity of TAL tight junctions.[14,199] Heterologous expression of claudin-16 (paracellin-1) in the anion-selective LLC-PK1 cell line markedly increases $Na^+$ permeability without affecting $Cl^-$ permeability; this generates a significant increase in the $P_{Na}/P_{Cl}$ ratio (Fig. 6.15).[202] LLC-PK1 cells expressing claudin-16 also have increased permeability to other monovalent cations. There is, however, only a modest increase in $Mg^{2+}$ permeability, suggesting that claudin-16 does not form an $Mg^{2+}$-specific pathway in the tight junction; rather, it may serve to increase the overall cation selectivity of the tight junction. Claudin-19 appears in turn to reduce $P_{Cl}$ in LLC-PK1 cells, without having much effect on $Mg^{2+}$ or $Na^+$ permeability.[203] The claudin-16 and claudin-19 proteins interact in multiple systems, and coexpression of claudin-16 and claudin-19 synergistically increases the $P_{Na}/P_{Cl}$ ratio in LLC-PK1 cells.[203,204] Knockdown of claudin-16 in transgenic mice increases $Na^+$ absorption in the downstream collecting duct, with the development of hypovolemic hyponatremia after treatment with amiloride; claudin-19 knockdown mice exhibit an increase in fractional excretion of $Na^+$ and a doubling in serum aldosterone levels.[204,205] In summary, therefore, claudin-16 and claudin-19 interact to confer the cation selectivity of tight junctions in the TAL, contributing significantly to the transepithelial absorption of $Na^+$ in this nephron segment.

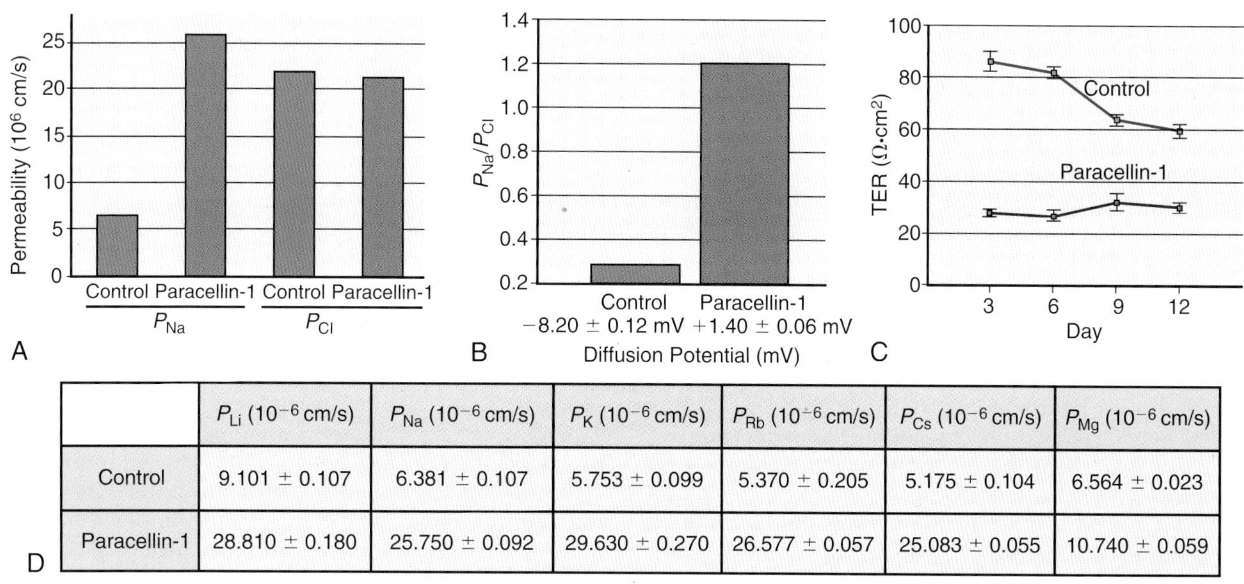


| | $P_{Li}$ ($10^{-6}$ cm/s) | $P_{Na}$ ($10^{-6}$ cm/s) | $P_K$ ($10^{-6}$ cm/s) | $P_{Rb}$ ($10^{-6}$ cm/s) | $P_{Cs}$ ($10^{-6}$ cm/s) | $P_{Mg}$ ($10^{-6}$ cm/s) |
|---|---|---|---|---|---|---|
| Control | 9.101 ± 0.107 | 6.381 ± 0.107 | 5.753 ± 0.099 | 5.370 ± 0.205 | 5.175 ± 0.104 | 6.564 ± 0.023 |
| Paracellin-1 | 28.810 ± 0.180 | 25.750 ± 0.092 | 29.630 ± 0.270 | 26.577 ± 0.057 | 25.083 ± 0.055 | 10.740 ± 0.059 |

**Fig. 6.15** Effect of claudin-16 (formerly called paracellin-1) overexpression in LLC-PK1 cells. (A) Effects of claudin-16 on the permeability of $Na^+$ and $Cl^-$ in LLC-PK1 cells. (B) Ratio of $P_{Na}$ to $P_{Cl}$ and diffusion potential *(bottom)* across an LLC-PK1 cell monolayer. (C) Transepithelial resistance across an LLC-PK1 cell monolayer over a period of 12 days in cells expressing claudin-16 and control cells. (D) Summary of the effects of claudin-16 on permeability of various cations in LLC-PK1 cells. (From Hou J, Paul DL, Goodenough DA. Paracellin-1 and the modulation of ion selectivity of tight junctions. *J Cell Sci.* 2005;118:5109–5118.)

Other claudins expressed in the TAL modulate the function of claudin-16–claudin-19 heterodimers or have independent effects. Claudin-14 interacts with claudin-16, disrupting cation selectivity of the paracellular barrier in cells that also coexpress claudin-19.[206] Claudin-14 expression in the TAL is calcium dependent via the CaSR, providing a novel axis for calcium-dependent regulation of paracellular calcium transport (see later).[206–208] Claudin-10 appears to modulate paracellular $Na^+$ permeability specifically, with impaired paracellular $Na^+$ transport in claudin-10 knockout mice and a salt-wasting nephropathy in humans bearing compound heterozygous claudin-10 mutations.[33,209]

### Basolateral Mechanisms

The basolateral $Na^+$-$K^+$-ATPase is the primary exit pathway for $Na^+$ at the basolateral membrane of TAL cells. The $Na^+$ gradient generated by $Na^+$-$K^+$-ATPase activity is also thought to drive the apical entry of $Na^+$, $K^+$, and $Cl^-$ via NKCC2, the furosemide-sensitive $Na^+$-$K^+$-$2Cl^-$ cotransporter.[14] Inhibition of $Na^+$-$K^+$-ATPase with ouabain thus collapses the lumen-positive PD and abolishes transepithelial $Na^+$-$Cl^-$ transport in the TAL.[179,180,197] Basolateral exit of $Cl^-$ from TAL cells is primarily but not exclusively electrogenic, mediated by an approximately 10-pS $Cl^-$ channel.[14,167,210] Reductions in basolateral $Cl^-$ depolarize the basolateral membrane, whereas decreases in intracellular $Cl^-$ induced by luminal furosemide have a hyperpolarizing effect.[14] Intracellular $Cl^-$ activity during transepithelial $Na^+$-$Cl^-$ transport is above its electrochemical equilibrium,[14] with an intracellular negative voltage of −40 to −70 mV that drives basolateral $Cl^-$ exit.[14,167]

At least two CLC chloride channels, CLC-K1 and CLC-K2 (CLC-NKA and CLC-NKB in humans), are coexpressed in this nephron segment.[158,163] However, an increasing body of evidence has indicated that the dominant $Cl^-$ channel in the TAL is encoded by CLC-K2. First, CLC-K1 is heavily expressed at the apical and basolateral membranes of the thin ascending limb, and the phenotype of the corresponding knockout mouse is consistent with primary dysfunction of thin ascending limbs, rather than the TAL (see $Na^+$-$Cl^-$ transport by the thin ascending limb).[3,137,156,159] Second, loss-of-function mutations in CLC-NKB are associated with Bartter syndrome, providing genetic evidence for a dominant role of this channel in $Na^+$-$Cl^-$ transport in the TAL.[160] More recently, a very common T481S polymorphism in human CLC-NKB was shown to increase channel activity by a factor of 20; preliminary data have indicated an association with hypertension, suggesting that this gain-of-function in CLC-NKB increases $Na^+$-$Cl^-$ transport by the TAL and/or other segments of the distal nephron.[211–213] Finally, CLC-K2 protein is heavily expressed at the basolateral membrane of the mouse TAL, with additional expression in the DCT, CNT, and α-intercalated cells.[214] Recently, *Clc-k2* was deleted from mice, leading to salt wasting, resembling Bartter syndrome, and to a loss of the around 10-pS chloride channel in TAL cells.[162] Deletion of this gene also abrogated the response to furosemide, indicating the central role that this channel plays in transepithelial NaCl transport. This approach also permitted conclusions to be drawn regarding the location of ClC-K1 and ClC-K2 in the kidney, even though antibodies cross-react against the two related chloride channels. In the *Clc-k2* knockout mice, the reaction product could be seen to extend beyond the thin ascending limb into the medullary TAL, suggesting that ClC-K1 plays a role there.

A key advance was the characterization of the Barttin subunit of CLC-K channels, which is coexpressed with CLC-K1 and CLC-K2 in several nephron segments, including TAL.[158,163] Unlike rat CLC-K1, the rat CLC-K2, human CLC-NKA, and human CLC-NKB paralogs are not functional in the absence of Barttin coexpression.[163,164] CLC-NKB coexpressed with Barttin is highly selective for $Cl^-$, with a permeability series of $Cl^- \gg Br^- = NO_3^- > I^-$.[14,158,163] CLC-NKB/Barttin channels are activated by increases in extracellular $Ca^{2+}$ and are pH sensitive, with activation at an alkaline extracellular pH and marked inhibition at an acidic pH.[163] CLC-NKA/Barttin channels have similar pH and calcium sensitivities, but exhibit higher permeability to $Br^-$.[163] Strikingly, despite the considerable homology between the CLC-NKA/NKB proteins, these channels also differ considerably in pharmacologic sensitivity to various $Cl^-$ channel blockers, potential lead compounds for the development of paralog-specific inhibitors.[215]

Correlation between functional characteristics of CLC-K proteins with native $Cl^-$ channels in TAL has been problematic, but the recent knockout work discussed earlier has begun to provide clarity. Wide variation in single-channel conductance has been reported for basolateral $Cl^-$channels in the TAL.[216] This is perhaps due to the use of collagenase and other conditions for the preparation of tubule fragments and/or basolateral vesicles, manipulations that potentially affect channel characteristics.[216] Notably, single-channel conductance has not been reported for CLC-NKB/Barttin channels because of the difficulty in expressing the channel in heterologous systems; this complicates the comparison of CLC-NKB/Barttin with native $Cl^-$ channels. Single-channel conductance has, however, been reported for the V166E mutant of rat CLC-K1, which alters gating of the channel without expected effects on single-channel amplitude – coexpression with Barttin increases the single-channel conductance of V166E CLC-K1 from about 7 to 20 pS.[164] Therefore, part of the reported variability in native single-channel conductance may reflect heterogeneity in the interaction between CLC-NKB and/or CLC-NKA with Barttin. Regardless, a study using whole-cell recording techniques has suggested that CLC-K2 (CLC-NKB in humans) is the dominant $Cl^-$ channel in TAL and other segments of the distal nephron.[216] Like CLC-NKB/Barttin, this native channel is highly $Cl^-$ selective, with considerably weaker conductance for $Br^-$ and $I^-$; CLC-NKA/Barttin channels exhibit higher permeability to $Br^-$.[14,158,163,216] TAL cells from wild type mice exhibited a dominant basolateral chloride conductance of 8 pS, which was entirely absent in *Clc-k2* knockout mice. Coupled with the strong Bartter syndrome phenotype, these results support the key role of this chloride channel in driving transepithelial NaCl transport along the TAL.

Electroneutral $K^+$-$Cl^-$ cotransport has also been implicated in transepithelial $Na^+$-$Cl^-$ transport in the TAL (Fig. 6.14), functioning in $K^+$-dependent $Cl^-$ exit at the basolateral membrane.[14] The KCC KCC4 is thus expressed at the basolateral membrane of medullary and cortical TAL, in addition to the macula densa.[217,218] There is also functional evidence for $K^+$-$Cl^-$ cotransport at the basolateral membrane of this section of the nephron. First, TAL cells contain a $Cl^-$-dependent $NH_4^+$ transport mechanism that is sensitive to 1.5-mmol/L furosemide and 10-mmol/L barium ($Ba^{2+}$).[219] $NH_4^+$ ions have the same ionic radius as $K^+$ and are transported by KCC4 and other KCCs; KCC4 is also sensitive to $Ba^{2+}$ and millimolar furosemide, consistent with the pharmacology of $NH_4^+$-$Cl^-$ cotransport in the TAL.[219–221] Second, to account for the effects on the transmembrane PD of basolateral $Ba^{2+}$ and/or increased $K^+$, it has been suggested that the basolateral membrane of TAL contains a $Ba^{2+}$-sensitive $K^+$-$Cl^-$ transporter; this is also consistent with the known expression of $Ba^{2+}$-sensitive KCC4 at the basolateral membrane.[14,217,218,221] Third, increases in basolateral $K^+$ cause $Cl^-$-dependent cell swelling in *Amphiuma* early distal tubule, an analog of the mammalian TAL; in *Amphiuma* LBC cells with low basolateral conductance, analogous to mammalian LBC cells (see the "$Na^+$-$Cl^-$ Transport by the Thick Ascending Limb: Apical $Na^+$-$Cl^-$ Transport" section), this cell swelling was not accompanied by changes in basolateral membrane voltage or resistance, consistent with $K^+$-$Cl^-$ transport.[140,142,222]

There is thus considerable evidence for basolateral $K^+$-$Cl^-$ cotransport in the TAL, mediated by KCC4.[217,218] However, direct confirmation of a role for basolateral $K^+$-$Cl^-$ cotransport in transepithelial $Na^+$-$Cl^-$ transport is lacking. Indeed, KCC4-deficient mice do not have a prominent defect in function of the TAL, but exhibit instead a renal tubular acidosis.[217] The renal tubular acidosis in these mice has been attributed to defects in acid extrusion by $H^+$-ATPase in α-intercalated cells; however, this phenotype is conceivably the result of a reduction in medullary $NH_4^+$ reabsorption by the TAL due to the loss of basolateral $NH_4^+$ exit mediated by KCC4.[217,220,223]

Finally, there is also evidence for the existence of $Ba^{2+}$-sensitive $K^+$ channel activity at the basolateral membrane of the TAL, providing an alternative exit pathway for $K^+$ to that mediated by KCC4.[224–226] Such channel activity may help stabilize the basolateral membrane potential above the equilibrium potential for $Cl^-$, thus maintaining a continuous driving force for $Cl^-$ exit via CLC-NKB/Barttin $Cl^-$ channels.[226] Patch-clamp experiments have identified two types of $K^+$ channels in the basolateral membrane of the TAL: a 40-pS inwardly rectifying $K^+$ channel and an $Na^+$- and $Cl^-$-activated, 80- to 150-pS K channel (Kca4.1 or slo2.2).[225,227] The 40-pS $K^+$ channel was absent in the TAL of *Kcnj10* knockout mice, suggesting that the 40-pS $K^+$ channel is a KIR4.1 and KIR4.5 heterotetramer.[227] Although KIR4.1 is also detected in human TAL, loss-of-function *KCNJ10* mutations do not show the phenotype of Bartter syndrome, suggesting that the disruption of KIR4.1 has no significant effect on transport function in the TAL.[228] This may reflect secondary activation of alternative $K^+$ channels along TAL, as *Kcnj10* knockout mice demonstrate vasopressin-induced stimulation of the 80- to 150-pS K channel. Basolateral $K^+$ channels may also attenuate the increases in intracellular $K^+$ that are generated by the basolateral $Na^+$-$K^+$-ATPase, thus maintaining transepithelial $Na^+$-$Cl^-$ transport.[224–226]

## REGULATION OF $NA^+$-$CL^-$ TRANSPORT BY THE THICK ASCENDING LIMB

### Activating Influences

Transepithelial $Na^+$-$Cl^-$ transport by the TAL is regulated by a complex blend of competing neurohumoral influences, which are required to maintain the urinary concentrating capacity, and modulate salt balance. In particular, increases in intracellular cAMP tonically stimulate ion transport in the TAL; the stimulatory hormones and mediators that increase cAMP in this nephron segment include vasopressin, PTH, glucagon, calcitonin, and β-adrenergic activation (Fig. 6.9). These overlapping cAMP-dependent stimuli are thought to result in maximal baseline stimulation of transepithelial $Na^+$-$Cl^-$ transport.[94] For example, characterization of the in vivo effect of these hormones requires the prior simultaneous suppression or absence of circulating vasopressin, PTH, calcitonin, and glucagon.[94] This baseline activation is, in turn, modulated by a number of negative influences, most prominently prostaglandin $E_2$ ($PGE_2$) and extracellular $Ca^{2+}$ (Fig. 6.9). Other hormones and autocoids working through cGMP-dependent signaling, including NO, have potent negative effects on $Na^+$-$Cl^-$ transport within the TAL.[230] By contrast, Ang II has a stimulatory effect on $Na^+$-$Cl^-$ transport within the TAL.[231]

Vasopressin is perhaps the most extensively studied positive modulator of transepithelial $Na^+$-$Cl^-$ transport in the TAL. The TAL, with the exception of macula densa cells,[232] expresses type 2 vasopressin receptors ($V_2Rs$) at both the mRNA and protein levels, and microdissected TALs respond to the hormone with an increase in intracellular cAMP.[233] Vasopressin activates apical $Na^+$-$K^+$-$2Cl^-$ cotransport within minutes in perfused mouse TAL segments and also exerts a longer-term influence on NKCC2 expression and function. The acute activation of apical $Na^+$-$K^+$-$2Cl^-$ cotransport is achieved at least in part by the stimulated exocytosis of NKCC2 proteins, from subapical vesicles to the plasma membrane.[234] This trafficking-dependent activation is abrogated by treatment of perfused tubules with tetanus toxin, which cleaves the vesicle-associated membrane proteins VAMP-2 and VAMP-3.[234] As $V_2Rs$ are prominently expressed along the collecting duct, as well as along the TAL and DCT, it has been difficult to separate the roles of vasopressin signaling in the two sites. This limitation was recently overcome by introducing a dominant-negative $V_2R$ mutant into TAL cells of rat. The rats demonstrated polyuria and defective urinary concentration, as well as hypercalciuria, reminiscent of mild Bartter syndrome.[232] The absence of $V_2R$ expression by macula densa cells was suggested to maintain TGF independent of vasopressin signaling.

Activation of NKCC2 by vasopressin is also associated with the phosphorylation of a cluster of amino-terminal threonines in the transporter protein; treatment of rats with the $V_2$ agonist desmopressin (DDAVP) induces phosphorylation of these residues in vivo, as measured with a phosphospecific antibody.[234] These threonine residues are substrates for SPAK (STE20/SPS1-related proline/alanine-rich kinase) and OSR1 (oxidative stress–responsive kinase 1), first identified by Gagnon and colleagues as key regulatory kinases for NKCC1 and other cation-chloride cotransporters.[235] SPAK and OSR1 are in turn activated by upstream WNK (*with no lysine [K]* kinases), such that SPAK or OSR1 requires coexpression with WNK4 to activate NKCC1 fully, at least in in vitro systems.[235] By contrast, two reports of *Wnk4* knockout mice suggested that WNK4 does not regulate NKCC2 in vivo.[236,237] Regardless, expression of WNK3 in *Xenopus* oocytes results in activatory phosphorylation of the amino-terminal threonines in NKCC2 that are phosphorylated in TAL cells after treatment with DDAVP.[234,238]

The amino-terminal phosphorylation of NKCC2 by SPAK and/or OSR1 kinases appears to be important for activity of the transporter in the native TAL. The amino-terminus of NKCC2 contains a predicted binding site for SPAK,[239] proximal to the sites of regulatory phosphorylation; the analogous binding site is required for activation of the NKCC1 cotransporter.[240] SPAK also requires the sorting receptor SORLA (sorting protein-related receptor with A-type repeats) for proper trafficking within TAL cells, such that targeted deletion of *Sorla* results in a marked reduction in amino-terminal NKCC2 phosphorylation.[241] The role of the upstream WNK kinases is illustrated by the phenotype of a "knock-in" mouse strain, in which the knocked-in mutant SPAK cannot be activated by upstream WNK kinases; these mice have a marked reduction in amino-terminal phosphorylation of both NKCC2 and the thiazide-sensitive NCC, with associated salt-sensitive hypotension.[242] The upstream WNK kinases appear to regulate SPAK and NKCC2 in a chloride-dependent fashion, phosphorylating and activating SPAK and the transporter in response to a reduction in intracellular chloride concentration (see the "Integrated $Na^+$-$Cl^-$ and $K^+$ Transport in the Distal Nephron" section).[243]

Of the two kinases, SPAK and OSR1, OSR1 is perhaps more critical for NKCC2 function in the TAL, because pan-renal epithelial-specific deletion of *Osr1* leads to decreased amino-terminal phosphorylation of NKCC2, and a Bartter syndrome-like phenotype.[244] Several groups reported an increase in NKCC2 amino-terminal phosphorylation and an increased response to furosemide in *Spak* knockout mice, suggesting overcompensation by OSR1.[245–247] By contrast, it was reported that baseline $Na^+$ absorption by isolated perfused TAL segments is profoundly impaired in SPAK-deficient mice, though this may reflect an absence of activating factors present in vivo.[248] Truncated species of SPAK protein have also been detected in kidney due to generation of alternative mRNA species that lack the amino-terminal kinase domain and to proteolytic degradation; both forms of SPAK function as dominant-negative inhibitors of the full-length kinase, abrogating the usual stimulatory effect on coexpressed NKCC2 or NKCC1.[247,249] A lack of these species in SPAK knockout mice may also contribute to the increased amino-terminal NKCC2 phosphorylation observed, due to the removal of a dominant-negative effect on OSR1. Further complexity arises from the influence of the adaptor protein calcium-binding protein 39 (CAB39, also called mouse protein-25, MO25[250]), which can both increase SPAK/OSR1-driven phosphorylation of NKCC2 and also activate SPAK/OSR1 directly, without the need for upstream phosphorylation by WNK kinases, by promoting dimerization of the kinases.[250,251] WNK4 is also capable of direct interaction with CAB39, promoting activation of NKCC2 in the absence of SPAK or OSR1 expression.[252] In support of SPAK/OSR1-independent activation of NKCC2, in mice in which both SPAK and OSR1 were disrupted in the kidney, significant amino-terminal phosphorylation of NKCC2 was still detected. However, although this could reflect a direct effect of WNK4 on NKCC2, it could also result from phosphorylation by an as-yet unidentified kinase. Therefore, there appear to be at least three potential pathways for NKCC2 activation—a WNK4-dependent SPAK/OSR1 pathway, a WNK4-independent SPAK/OSR1 pathway, and a SPAK/OSR1-independent WNK4 pathway.[252] It should be noted, however, that amino-terminal phosphorylation has a smaller effect on NKCC2 activity than it does on NKCC1 and NCC.[238] Thus changes in NKCC2 phosphorylation may not always reflect changes in NKCC2 activity.[253]

Vasopressin has also been shown to alter the stoichiometry of furosemide-sensitive apical $Cl^-$ transport in the TAL, from a $K^+$-independent $Na^+$-$Cl^-$ mode to the classic $Na^+$-$K^+$-$2Cl^-$ cotransport stoichiometry.[3] In the absence of vasopressin, $^{22}Na^+$ uptake by mouse medullary TAL cells is not dependent on the presence of extracellular $K^+$, whereas the addition of the hormone induces a switch to $K^+$-dependent $^{22}Na^+$ uptake. Underscoring the metabolic advantages of paracellular $Na^+$ transport, which is critically dependent on the apical entry of $K^+$ via $Na^+$-$K^+$-$2Cl^-$ cotransport (see previously), vasopressin accomplishes a doubling of transepithelial $Na^+$-$Cl^-$ transport without affecting $^{22}Na^+$ uptake (an indicator of transcellular $Na^+$-$Cl^-$ transport); this doubling in transepithelial absorption occurs without an increase in $O_2$ consumption, highlighting the energy efficiency of ion transport by the TAL.[3] The mechanism of this shift in the apparent stoichiometry of NKCC2 is not completely clear. However, splice variants of mouse NKCC2 with a novel, shorter carboxyl-terminus have been found to confer sensitivity to cAMP when coexpressed with full-length NKCC2.[254] Notably, these shorter splice variants appear to encode furosemide-sensitive, $K^+$-independent NCCs when expressed alone in *Xenopus* oocytes.[255] The in vivo relevance of these phenomena is not clear, however, nor is it known whether similar splice variants exist in species other than mouse.

In addition to its acute effects on NKCC2, the apical $Na^+$-$K^+$-$2Cl^-$ cotransporter, vasopressin increases transepithelial $Na^+$-$Cl^-$ transport by activating apical $K^+$ channels and basolateral $Cl^-$ channels in the TAL.[94,233] Details have yet to emerge of the regulation of the basolateral CLC-K2/Barttin $Cl^-$ channel complex by vasopressin, cAMP, and related pathways. However, the apical $K^+$ channel ROMK is directly phosphorylated by PKA on three serine residues (S25, S200, and S294 in the ROMK2 isoform). Phosphorylation of at least two of these three serines is required for detectable $K^+$ channel activity in *Xenopus* oocytes; mutation of all three serines to alanine abolishes phosphorylation and transport activity, and all three serines are required for full channel activity.[256] These three phospho acceptor sites have distinct effects on ROMK activity and expression.[257] Phosphorylation of the amino-terminal S25 residue appears to regulate trafficking of the channel to the cell membrane, without effects on channel gating; this serine is also a substrate for the SGK1 kinase, which activates the channel via an increase in expression at the membrane.[257] By contrast, phosphorylation of the two carboxyl-terminal serines modulates open channel probability via effects on pH-dependent gating and on activation by the binding of phosphatidylinositol 4,5-bisphosphate (PIP2) to the carboxyl-terminal domain of the channel.[258,259]

Vasopressin also has considerable long-term effects on transepithelial $Na^+$-$Cl^-$ transport by the TAL. Sustained increases in circulating vasopressin result in marked hypertrophy of medullary TAL cells, accompanied by a doubling in baseline active $Na^+$-$Cl^-$ transport.[233] Water restriction or treatment with DDAVP also results in an increase in abundance of the NKCC2 protein in rat TAL cells. Consistent with a direct effect of vasopressin-dependent signaling, expression of NKCC2 is reduced in mice with a heterozygous deletion of the $G_s$ stimulatory G protein, through which the $V_2R$ activates cAMP generation.[233] Increases in cAMP are thought to induce transcription of the *Slc12a1* gene that encodes NKCC2 directly, given the presence of a cAMP-response element in the 5′ promoter.[233,234] Abrogation of the tonic negative effect of $PGE_2$ on cAMP generation with indomethacin also results in a considerable increase in abundance of the NKCC2 protein.[233] Finally, in addition to these effects on NKCC2 expression, water restriction or DDAVP treatment increases abundance of the ROMK protein at the apical membrane of TAL cells.[260]

Recently, a role for β3-adrenergic receptors in activation of NKCC2 was proposed, with administration of the selective agonist BRL37344 increasing NKCC2 phosphorylation ex vivo in wild type but not β3-adrenergic receptor knockout mice, which also displayed a mild $Na^+$- and $K^+$-wasting phenotype.[261]

### Inhibitory Influences

The stimulation of transepithelial $Na^+$-$Cl^-$ transport by cAMP-generating hormones (e.g., vasopressin, PTH) is modulated by a number of negative neurohumoral influences (Fig. 6.9).[94] In particular, extracellular $Ca^{2+}$ and $PGE_2$ exert dramatic inhibitory effects on ion transport by this and other segments of the distal nephron through a plethora of synergistic mechanisms. Extracellular $Ca^{2+}$ and $PGE_2$ both activate the $G_i$ inhibitory G protein in TAL cells, opposing the stimulatory, $G_s$-dependent effects of vasopressin on intracellular levels of cAMP.[262,263] Extracellular $Ca^{2+}$ exerts its effect through the CaSR, which is heavily expressed at the basolateral membrane of TAL cells; $PGE_2$ primarily signals through $EP_3$ prostaglandin receptors.[94,263,264] The increases in intracellular $Ca^{2+}$ due to the activation of the CaSR and other receptors directly inhibit cAMP generation by a $Ca^{2+}$-inhibitable adenylate cyclase that is expressed in the TAL, accompanied by an increase in phosphodiesterase-dependent degradation of cAMP (Fig. 6.16).[263,265] These negative stimuli likely inhibit baseline transport in the TAL; abrogation of the negative effect of $PGE_2$ with indomethacin results in a considerable increase in abundance of the NKCC2 protein, whereas targeted deletion of the CaSR in mouse TAL activates NKCC2 via increased amino-terminal phosphorylation.[189,209]

Activation of the CaSR and other receptors in the TAL also results in the downstream generation of arachidonic acid metabolites, with potent negative effects on $Na^+$-$Cl^-$ transport (Fig. 6.16). Extracellular $Ca^{2+}$ thus activates $PLA_2$ in TAL cells, leading to the liberation of arachidonic acid. This arachidonic acid is in turn metabolized by cytochrome P450 ω-hydroxylase to 20-HETE or by COX-2 to $PGE_2$; cytochrome P450 ω-hydroxylation generally predominates in response to activation of the CaSR in TAL.[263] 20-HETE has very potent negative effects on apical $Na^+$-$K^+$-$2Cl^-$ cotransport, apical $K^+$ channels, and the basolateral $Na^+$-$K^+$-ATPase.[94,263] $PLA_2$-dependent generation of 20-HETE also underlies in part the negative effect of bradykinin and Ang II on $Na^+$-$Cl^-$ transport.[94,263] Activation of the CaSR also induces tumor necrosis factor-α expression in the TAL, which activates COX-2 and thus generation of $PGE_2$ (Fig. 6.16); this $PGE_2$ in turn results in additional inhibition of $Na^+$-$Cl^-$ transport.[263]

The relative importance of the CaSR in the regulation of $Na^+$-$Cl^-$ transport by the TAL is dramatically illustrated by the phenotype of a handful of patients with gain-of-function mutations in this receptor. In addition to suppressed PTH and hypocalcemia, the usual phenotype caused by gain-of-function mutations in the CaSR (autosomal dominant hypoparathyroidism), these patients manifest a hypokalemic alkalosis, polyuria, and increases in circulating renin and aldosterone.[266,267] Therefore, the persistent inhibition of $Na^+$-$Cl^-$ transport in the TAL by these overactive mutants of the CaSR causes a rare subtype of Bartter syndrome, type V, in the genetic classification of this disease.[263]

Activation of the CaSR also affects claudin expression in TAL cells via downregulation of microRNAs, leading to PTH-independent hypercalciuria (see Chapter 7).[206–208,268]

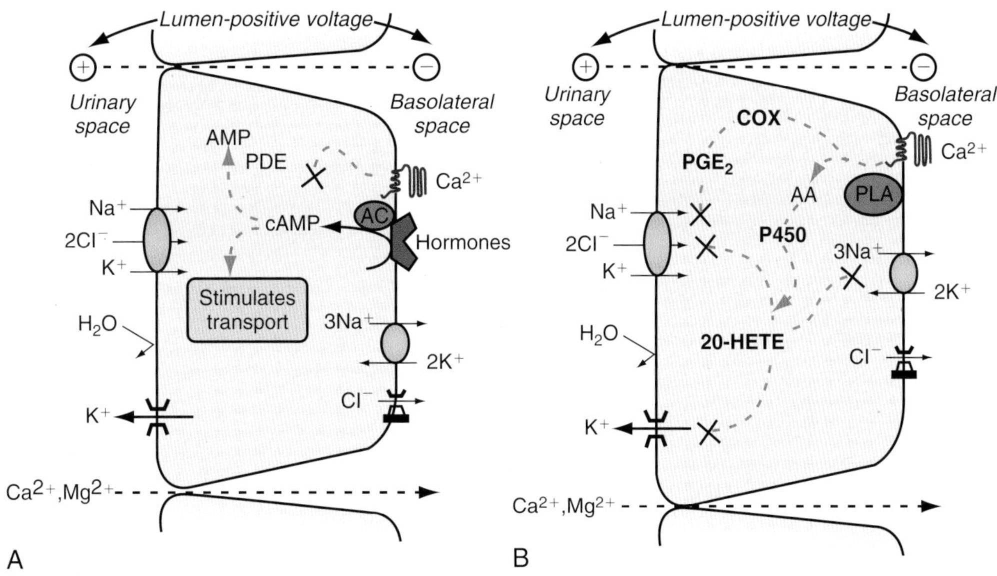


**Fig. 6.16** Inhibitory effects of the calcium-sensing receptor (CaSR) on transepithelial $Na^+$-$Cl^-$ transport in the thick ascending limb. (A) Activation of the basolateral CaSR inhibits the generation of cAMP in response to vasopressin and other hormones (see text for details). (B) Stimulation of phospholipase $A_2$ by the CaSR leads to liberation of arachidonic acid, which is in turn metabolized by cytochrome P450 ω-hydroxylase to 20-HETE (20-hydroxyeicosatetraenoic acid), or by cyclooxygenase-2 (COX-2) to prostaglandin $E_2$ ($PGE_2$). 20-HETE is a potent natriuretic factor, inhibiting apical $Na^+$-$K^+$-$2Cl^-$ cotransport, apical $K^+$ channels, and the basolateral $Na^+$-$K^+$-ATPase. Activation of the CaSR also induces tumor necrosis factor-α (TNF-α) expression in the TAL, which activates COX-2 and thus generation of $PGE_2$, leading to additional inhibition of $Na^+$-$Cl^-$ transport. (From Hebert SC. Calcium and salinity sensing by the thick ascending limb: a journey from mammals to fish and back again. *Kidney Int Suppl.* 2004;91:S28–S33.)

### Uromodulin

TAL cells are unique in expressing the membrane-bound, glycosylphosphatidylinositol (GPI)–anchored protein, uromodulin (Tamm-Horsfall glycoprotein), which is not expressed by macula densa cells or the downstream DCT. Uromodulin is released by proteolytic cleavage at the apical membrane and is secreted as the most abundant protein in normal human urine (20 to 100 mg/day).[269] Uromodulin has a host of emerging roles in the physiology and biology of the TAL. A high-salt diet increases uromodulin expression, suggesting a role in ion transport.[269] In this regard, uromodulin facilitates membrane trafficking and function of the NKCC2 protein, with similar effects on apical ROMK protein.[270,271]

Autosomal dominant mutations in the *UMOD* gene encoding uromodulin are associated with medullary cystic disease type 2 and familial juvenile hyperuricemic nephropathy. Now referred to as uromodulin-associated kidney disease, this syndrome includes progressive tubulointerstitial damage and chronic kidney disease (CKD), variably penetrant hyperuricemia and gout, and variably penetrant renal cysts that are typically confined to the corticomedullary junction.[269] The causative mutations tend to affect conserved cysteine residues within the amino-terminal half of the protein, leading to protein misfolding and retention within the endoplasmic reticulum.[269,272] More common genetic variants in the *UMOD* promoter have recently been linked in genomewide association studies with a risk of CKD and hypertension.[269] These susceptibility variants have a high frequency (≈0.8) and confer an approximately 20% higher risk for CKD and a 15% risk for hypertension.[273] These polymorphisms are associated with more abundant renal uromodulin transcript and higher urinary uromodulin excretion due to activating effects on the *UMOD* promoter.[273,274] Overexpression of uromodulin in transgenic mice leads to distal tubular injury, with segmental dilation and an increased tubular cast area relative to wild type mice; similar lesions are increased in frequency in older adults homozygous for susceptibility variants in *UMOD* when compared with those homozygous for protective variants.[273]

Uromodulin-transgenic mice also manifest salt-sensitive hypertension due to activation of the SPAK kinase and activating amino-terminal phosphorylation of NKCC2. Human hypertensive individuals homozygous for susceptibility variants in *UMOD* appear to have an analogous phenotype, with exaggerated natriuresis in response to furosemide compared with those who are homozygous for protective variants.[273] These findings are compatible with the stimulatory effects of uromodulin on NKCC2 and ROMK—that is, a net gain of function in TAL transport.[270,271] Uromodulin excretion also appears to parallel transport activity of the TAL, with common polymorphisms in the *KCNJ1* gene encoding ROMK and two genes involved in regulating SPAK and OSR1 kinase activity (*SORL1* and *CAB39*).[274]

## ANATOMY OF THE DISTAL NEPHRON

The distal nephron that extends beyond the TAL is the final arbiter of urinary $Na^+$-$Cl^-$ excretion and a critical target for natriuretic and antinatriuretic stimuli. The understanding of the cellular organization and molecular phenotype of the distal nephron continues to evolve and merits a brief review in this context. The DCT begins at a variable distance after the macula densa, with an abrupt transition between NKCC2-positive cortical TAL cells and DCT cells that express the thiazide-sensitive NCC. Considerable progress has been made in the phenotypic classification of cell types in the DCT and adjacent nephron segments, based on the expression of an expanding list of transport proteins and other markers.[275] This analysis has revealed considerable differences in the organization of the DCT, CNT, and CCD in rodent, rabbit, and human kidneys. In general, rabbit kidneys are unique in the axial demarcation of DCT, CNT, and CCD segments, at both a molecular and morphologic level; the organization of the DCT to CCD is considerably more complex in other species, with boundaries that are much less absolute.[275] Notably, however, the overall repertoire of transport proteins expressed does not vary among these species; what differs is the specific cellular and molecular organization of this segment of the nephron.

The early DCT (DCT1) of mouse kidney expresses NCC and a specific marker, parvalbumin, which also distinguishes the DCT1 from the adjacent cortical TAL (Fig. 6.17).[276] Targeted deletion of parvalbumin in mice reveals that this intracellular $Ca^{2+}$-binding protein is required for full activity of NCC in the DCT.[277] Cells of the late DCT (DCT2) in mice coexpress NCC with proteins involved in transcellular $Ca^{2+}$ transport, including the apical calcium channel, TRPV5 (previously ECaC1), the cytosolic calcium-binding protein calbindin $D_{28K}$, and the basolateral $Na^+$-$Ca^{2+}$ exchanger NCX1.[276] NCC is coexpressed with ENaC in the late DCT2 of mouse, where the two proteins physically and may functionally interact,[278] with robust expression of ENaC continuing in the downstream CNT and CCD.[276] By contrast, rabbit kidney does not have a DCT1 or DCT2 and exhibits abrupt transitions between NCC- and ENaC-positive DCT and CNT segments, respectively.[275] Human kidneys that have been studied thus far exhibit expression of calbindin $D_{28K}$ all along the DCT and CNT, extending into the CCD; however, the intensity of expression varies at these sites. Approximately 30% of cells in the distal convolution of human kidney express NCC, with 70% expressing ENaC (CNT cells); ENaC and NCC overlap in expression at the end of the human DCT segment. Finally, cells of the early CNT of human kidneys express ENaC in the absence of aquaporin-2, the apical vasopressin-sensitive water channel.[275]

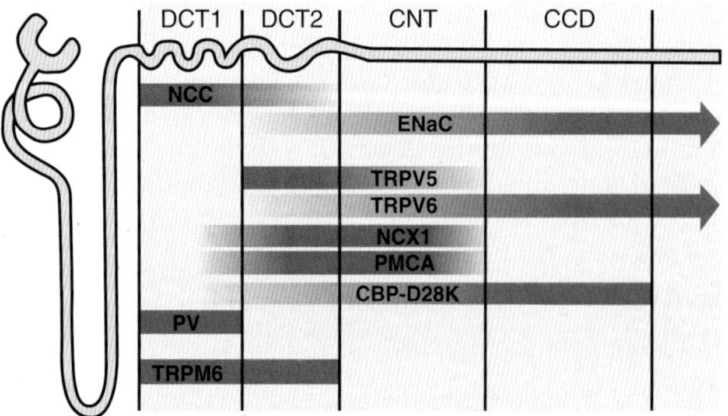


**Fig. 6.17** Schematic representation of the segmentation of the mouse distal nephron and distribution and abundance of $Na^+$-, $Ca^{2+}$-, and $Mg^{2+}$-transporting proteins. *CBP-D28K,* calbindin-D28K; *CCD,* cortical collecting duct; *CNT,* connecting tubule; *DCT1* and *DCT 2,* distal convoluted tubules 1 and 2, respectively; *ENaC,* epithelial $Na^+$ channel; *NCC,* thiazide-sensitive $Na^+$-$Cl^-$ cotransporter; *NCX1,* $Na^+$-$Ca^{2+}$ exchanger; *PMCA,* plasma membrane $Ca^{2+}$-ATPase; *PV,* parvalbumin; *TRPM6,* apical $Mg^{2+}$ entry channel; *TRPV5* and *TRPV6,* apical $Ca^{2+}$ entry channels.[276,614,615]

Although primarily contiguous with the DCT, CNT cells share several traits with principal cells of the CCD, including apical expression of ENaC and ROMK, the $K^+$ secretory channel; the capacity for $Na^+$-$Cl^-$ reabsorption and $K^+$ secretion in this nephron segment is as much as 10 times higher than that of the CCD.[279] Intercalated cells are the minority cell type in the distal nephron, emerging within the DCT and CNT and extending into the early inner medullary collecting duct (IMCD).[280] Three subtypes of intercalated cells have been defined, based on differences in the subcellular distribution of the $H^+$-ATPase and the presence or absence of the basolateral AE1 $Cl^-$-$HCO_3^-$ exchanger. Type A intercalated cells extrude protons via an apical $H^+$-ATPase in series with basolateral AE1; type B intercalated cells secrete $HCO_3^-$ and $OH^-$ via an apical anion exchanger (SLC26A4 or pendrin) in series with basolateral $H^+$-ATPase.[280] In rodents, the most prevalent subtype of intercalated cells in the CNT is the non-A, non-B intercalated cell, which possesses an apical $Cl^-$-$HCO_3^-$ exchanger (SLC26A4 or pendrin) along with apical $H^+$-ATPase.[280] Although intercalated cells play a dominant role in acid–base homeostasis, $Cl^-$ transport by type B intercalated cells performs an increasingly appreciated role in distal nephron $Na^+$-$Cl^-$ transport (see the "Connecting Tubules and the Cortical Collecting Duct: $Cl^-$ Transport" section).

The OMCD encompasses two separate subsegments corresponding to the outer and inner stripes of the outer medulla, OMCDo and OMCDi, respectively. OMCDo and OMCDi contain principal cells with apical amiloride-sensitive $Na^+$ channels (ENaCs); however, the primary role of this nephron segment is renal acidification, with a particular dominance of type A intercalated cells in OMCDi.[6,281] The OMCD may also play a role in $K^+$ reabsorption via the activity of apical $H^+$-$K^+$-ATPase pumps,[282–284] although deletion of this transport protein does not alter the ability to conserve $K^+$ substantially.[285]

Finally, the IMCD begins at the boundary between the outer and inner medulla and extends to the tip of the papilla. The IMCD is arbitrarily separated into three equal zones, denoted IMCD1, IMCD2, and IMCD3; at the functional level, an early IMCD (IMCDi) and a terminal portion (IMCDt) can be appreciated.[6] The IMCD plays a particularly prominent role in vasopressin-sensitive water and urea transport.[6] The early IMCD contains principal cells and intercalated cells; all three subsegments (IMCD1–3) express apical ENaC protein, albeit considerably weaker expression than in the CNT and CCD.[286] The roles of the IMCD and OMCD in $Na^+$-$Cl^-$ homeostasis have been more elusive than those of the CNT and CCD; however, to the extent that ENaC is expressed in the IMCD and OMCD, homologous mechanisms are expected to function in $Na^+$-$Cl^-$ reabsorption by the CNT, CCD, OMCD, and IMCD segments.

## DISTAL CONVOLUTED TUBULE

### Mechanisms of $Na^+$-$Cl^-$ Transport in the Distal Convoluted Tubule

Earlier micropuncture studies that did not distinguish between early and late DCT indicated that this nephron segment reabsorbs about 10% of filtered $Na^+$-$Cl^-$.[5,287] The apical absorption of $Na^+$ and $Cl^-$ by the DCT is mutually dependent; ion substitution does not affect transepithelial voltage, suggesting electroneutral transport.[288] The absorption of $Na^+$ by perfused

DCT segments is also inhibited by chlorothiazide, localized proof that this nephron segment is the target for thiazide diuretics.[289] Similar thiazide-sensitive $Na^+$-$Cl^-$ cotransport exists in the urinary bladder of winter flounder, the species in which the thiazide-sensitive NCC was first identified by expression cloning.[290] Functional characterization of rat NCC indicates very high affinities for both $Na^+$ and $Cl^-$ (Michaelis–Menten constants of 7.6 ± 1.6 and 6.3 ± 1.1 mmol/L, respectively); equally high affinities had previously been obtained by Velázquez and associates in perfused rat DCT.[288,291] The measured Hill coefficients of rat NCC are about 1 for each ion, consistent with electroneutral cotransport.[291]

NCC expression is the defining characteristic of the DCT (Fig. 6.18).[275] There is also evidence for expression of this transporter in osteoblasts, peripheral blood mononuclear cells, and intestinal epithelium; however, the functional significance of expression reported for these sites remains unclear.[168,292] The human SLC12A3 gene encodes three isoforms (NCC1, NCC2, and NCC3), but only NCC3 has been studied extensively, because NCC1 and NCC2 are not expressed in rats or mice.[293] These isoforms may undergo differential regulation. For example, NCC1 and NCC2 contain a region in their carboxyl-termini that is absent from NCC3 and contain a serine (S811), which undergoes phosphorylation and contributes to cotransporter activity.[294] Loss-of-function mutations in the *SLC12A3* gene encoding human NCC cause Gitelman syndrome, familial hypokalemic alkalosis with hypomagnesemia, and hypocalciuria (see Chapter 44). Mice with homozygous deletion of the *Slc12a3* gene encoding NCC exhibit marked morphologic defects in the early DCT, with a reduction in the absolute number of DCT cells and changes in ultrastructural appearance.[295,296] Similarly, thiazide treatment promotes marked apoptosis of the proximal part of DCT, suggesting that thiazide-sensitive $Na^+$-$Cl^-$ cotransport plays an important role in modulating growth and regression of this nephron segment.[297]

Coexpression of NCC and ENaC occurs in the "late DCT" (DCT2) and CNT segments of many species, either in the same cells or in adjacent cells in the same tubule.[275] Notably, ENaC is the primary $Na^+$ transport pathway of CNT and CCD cells, rather than DCT. There is, however, evidence for other $Na^+$ and $Cl^-$ entry pathways in DCT cells. In particular, the $Na^+$-$H^+$ exchanger NHE2 (SLC9A2) is coexpressed with NCC at the apical membrane of rat DCT cells.[298] As in the PT, perfusion of the DCT with formate and oxalate stimulates DIDS-sensitive $Na^+$-$Cl^-$ transport that is distinct from the thiazide-sensitive transport mediated by NCC.[50] Therefore a parallel arrangement of $Na^+$-$H^+$ exchange and $Cl^-$ anion exchangers may play an important role in electroneutral $Na^+$-$Cl^-$ absorption by the DCT (Fig. 6.18). The $Na^+$-$H^+$ antiporter NHA2 (SLC9B2) has been localized to the DCT, and the anion exchanger SLC26A6 may be expressed in DCT cells; NHE2, NHA2, and SLC26A6 are thus candidate mechanisms for this alternative pathway of DCT $Na^+$-$Cl^-$ absorption.[298–300]

At the basolateral membrane, as in other nephron segments, $Na^+$ exits via $Na^+$-$K^+$-ATPase; bearing in mind the considerable caveats in morphologic identification of the DCT, this nephron segment appears to have the highest $Na^+$-$K^+$-ATPase activity of the entire nephron (Fig. 6.3).[17,275] Basolateral membranes of DCT cells in both rabbit and mouse express the KCC KCC4, a potential exit pathway for

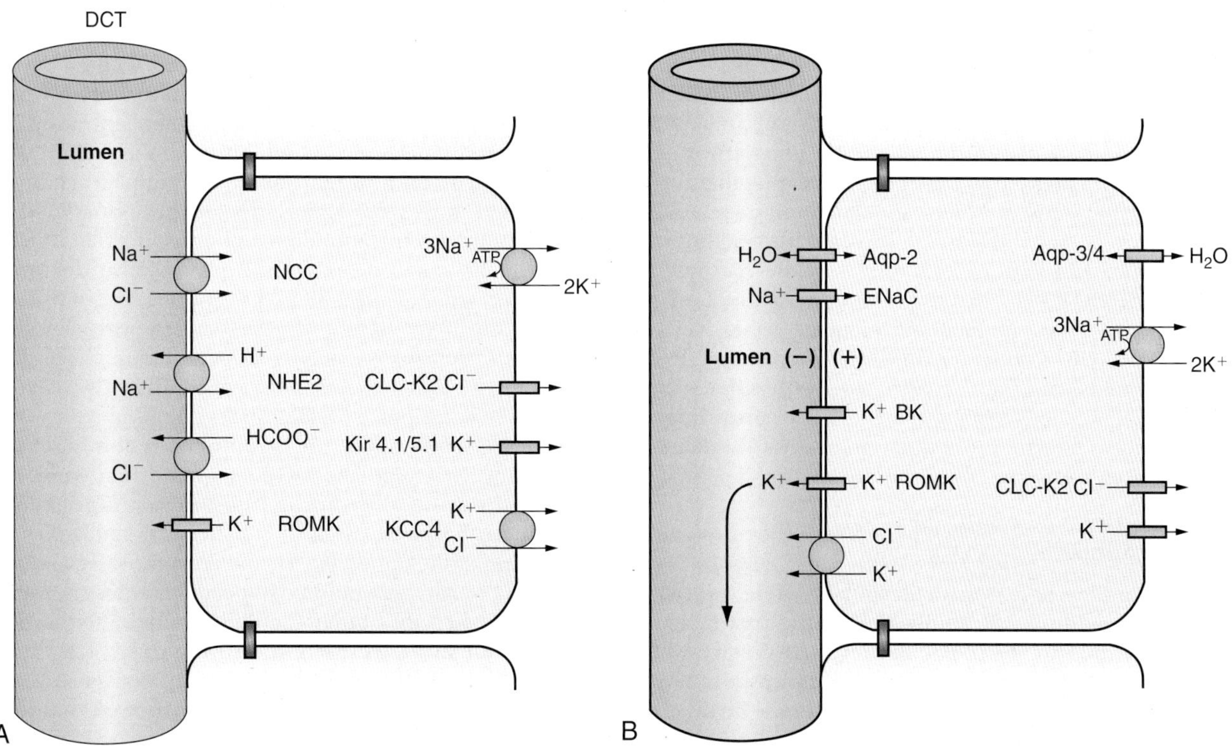


**Fig. 6.18** Transport pathways for $Na^+$-$Cl^-$ and $K^+$ in distal convoluted tubule *(DCT)* cells (A) and principal cells of the connecting tubule (CNT) and cortical collecting duct (CCD) (B). *Aqp-2, 3/4,* Aquaporin-2, aquaporin-3/4; *ENaC,* epithelial $Na^+$ channel; *KCC4,* $K^+$-$Cl^-$ cotransporter-4; *NCC,* thiazide-sensitive $Na^+$-$Cl^-$ cotransporter; *NHE-2,* $Na^+$-$H^+$ exchanger-2; *ROMK,* renal outer medullary $K^+$ channel.

$Cl^-$.[218,301] However, several lines of evidence have indicated that $Cl^-$ primarily exits DCT cells via basolateral $Cl^-$ channels. First, the basolateral membrane of rabbit DCT contains $Cl^-$ channel activity, with functional characteristics similar to those of CLC-K2.[216,302] Second, CLC-K2 protein is expressed at the basolateral membrane of DCT and CNT cells. Although mRNA for CLC-K1 can also be detected by RT-PCR of microdissected DCT segments,[158,214] recent data show that deletion of CLC-K2 from mice leads to a loss of response to furosemide, and a markedly blunted one to thiazide, implicating this channel in chloride reabsorption along both the TAL and the DCT.[162] Finally, loss-of-function mutations in CLC-NKB, the human ortholog of CLC-K2, cause classic Bartter syndrome; this Bartter subtype has a phenotype that is typically intermediate between Bartter syndrome type I, and Gitelman syndrome, consistent with loss of function of DCT segments.[160,162,303]

$K^+$ channels at the basolateral membrane of DCT cells play a critical role in the function of this nephron segment. Cell-attached patches in basolateral membranes of microdissected DCTs detect an inward rectifying $K^+$ channel, with characteristics similar to those of heteromeric KIR4.1/KIR5.1 and KIR4.2/KIR5.1 channels.[228,304–306] Basolateral membranes of the DCT express immunoreactive KIR4.1 and KIR5.1 protein, and DCT cells express KIR4.2 mRNA.[228,304–306] Patients with loss-of-function mutations in the *KCNJ10* gene that encodes KIR4.1 develop a syndrome encompassing epilepsy, ataxia, sensorineural deafness, and tubulopathy (EAST or SeSAME syndrome).[228,307] The associated tubulopathy includes hypokalemia, metabolic alkalosis, hypocalciuria, and hypomagnesemia.[228,307] Mice in which *Kcnj10* has been deleted following development demonstrate hypokalemic alkalosis with hypocalciuria, and suppression of NCC abundance,[308] indicating a key role of this channel in supporting transepithelial NaCl transport.[228,308,309] While KIR4.1 activity is detected in the TAL, KIR4.1 disruption in mice has no significant effect on TAL membrane potential or NKCC2 expression, so the physiological relevance of this is unclear.[310] By contrast, *Kcnj10* disruption markedly depolarizes the basolateral cell membrane of DCT cells, indicating that these $K^+$ channels play a key role in setting the membrane potential in the DCT.[308,311] In addition to sensing the membrane potential, the KIR4.1/KIR5.1 channels at the basolateral membrane of DCT cells are hypothesized to function in basolateral $K^+$ recycling, maintaining adequate $Na^+$-$K^+$-ATPase activity for $Na^+$-$Cl^-$ absorption and other aspects of DCT function. Notably, the CaSR coassociates with KIR4.1 and KIR4.2 proteins and inhibits their activity, providing a mechanism for the dynamic modulation of $Na^+$-$Cl^-$, calcium, and magnesium transport by the DCT.[305]

### Regulation of $Na^+$-$Cl^-$ Transport in the Distal Convoluted Tubule

Our understanding of factors that regulate solute transport by the DCT has advanced rapidly, during the past 5 years. Studies performed in the 1990s showed that dietary NaCl deprivation activates thiazide-sensitive NaCl transport along the DCT.[5] When distal salt delivery was increased further, by administering loop diuretics continuously and administering saline, as drinking solution, additional increases in transport capacity were observed, together with considerable hypertrophy of DCT cells. One contributor to this phenotype is Ang II. DCT cells express $AT_1$ receptors, and Ang II activates NCC, through a mechanism that requires the kinase WNK4 (see discussion later).[237,312–316]

Aldosterone has also been suggested as a factor that modulates NCC, which would make the DCT part of the aldosterone-sensitive distal nephron. Aldosterone, given to adrenalectomized rats, activated NCC.[317] Dietary salt restriction and exogenous mineralocorticoids were also shown to increase the abundance of NCC, and phosphorylated NCC.[318] DCT cells, at least in rats, were shown to express 11 beta hydroxysteroid dehydrogenase type 2 (11β-HSD2),[319] at least at low levels, and its deletion from mice resulted in a phenotype that includes hypertrophy of DCT cells, and increases in the abundance of phosphorylated NCC.[320] Aldosterone has been reported to enhance NCC activity acutely in cultured DCT cells.[321] Roy and colleagues identified two alternatively spliced exons in WNK1 that contain PY motifs, which bind the E3 ubiquitin ligase NEDD4-2. These motifs were suggested to mediate NCC activation by aldosterone.[322]

It was only the recognition that dietary potassium intake is a powerful NCC and DCT regulatory factor that has modified the view of aldosterone's role. Vallon and colleagues documented that dietary potassium deprivation increased the abundance of phosphorylated NCC in mice.[323] Two groups subsequently showed that low potassium intake can increase NCC abundance and activity even in the setting of high salt intake, and another showed that high potassium intake can suppress NCC, even when dietary salt intake is low.[324] Thus it appears that the effects of potassium predominate over those of sodium. These effects of high potassium intake raised the possibility that aldosterone may not be playing a dominant role in NCC regulation, as high potassium diets are associated with high aldosterone secretion and low NCC activity.[324] Increasingly, it has become apparent that DCT cells, and NCC, are exquisitely sensitive to plasma $[K^+]$. These effects occur very rapidly, as a short-term gavage with high potassium solution leads to rapid dephosphorylation of the NCC.[325] Similarly, raising the plasma potassium concentration, either by potassium infusion,[326] by administering the sodium channel blocking drug amiloride,[327] or by deleting $Na^+$ channels,[328] strikingly reduces the abundance of phosphorylated NCC. These effects on the abundance of phosphorylated NCC are functionally relevant, as several groups have documented that directional changes in pNCC abundance, in the setting of potassium challenge, are associated with concordant changes in thiazide-sensitive NaCl excretion.[329] The mechanisms involved in the potassium effect will be discussed later, with the discussion of WNK kinases.

The recognition that potassium plays a dominant role in regulating NCC and the DCT suggested that some effects observed during aldosterone infusion might be secondary to induced potassium imbalance. Mice with nephron-specific disruption of the mineralocorticoid receptor (MR) did exhibit low NCC activity, as would be expected if aldosterone stimulates NCC directly, but NCC could be stimulated to normal levels by dietary $K^+$ restriction, proving that it was effects of MR deletion on potassium balance that were responsible for changes in NCC.[329,330] A second group showed that in mice with deletion of MR in approximately 20% of renal tubule cells, which allowed side-by-side comparison of cells in the same segment, no differences in NCC abundance and phosphorylation were observed between DCT cells that did and did not express mineralocorticoid receptors; dietary $Na^+$ restriction upregulated NCC to similar extent in both types of cell.[331] By contrast, along the collecting duct ENaC expression and apical membrane localization were not detected on control diet nor in response to dietary $Na^+$ restriction in knockout cells. Finally, studies in adult mice with inducible disruption of the MR target α-ENaC showed that a high $Na^+$/low $K^+$ diet, which normalized plasma [$K^+$], also normalized the reduced abundances of total and phosphorylated NCC seen on a normal diet.[328] In summary, the preponderance of evidence suggests that the effects of plasma [$K^+$] are dominant, and that aldosterone plays only a modifying role in regulating NCC; the effects of potassium on NCC and aldosterone on ENaC appear to comprise a potassium switch in the kidney (see later).

A central role in the regulation of DCT $Na^+$ and $Cl^-$ transport is played by WNK1 and WNK4, key regulatory kinases in the distal nephron that were initially identified as two of the causative genes for familial hyperkalemic hypertension (FHHt; also known as pseudohypoaldosteronism type II or Gordon syndrome). FHHt is in every respect the mirror image of Gitelman syndrome, encompassing hypertension, hyperkalemia, hyperchloremic metabolic acidosis, suppressed plasma renin activity and aldosterone, and hypercalciuria.[332] Furthermore, FHHt behaves like a gain-of-function in NCC and/or the DCT in that treatment with thiazides typically results in resolution of the entire syndrome[332]; however, simple transgenic overexpression of NCC in DCT cells does not replicate the phenotype in mice, indicating specific effects of the mutant WNK1 and WNK4 alleles.[332,333]

WNK kinases have pleiotropic effects, and initial experiments involving WNK expression in heterologous systems have often produced results that now seem contradictory. Yet, a consensus view of the predominant effects of WNK kinases in regulating NCC has begun to emerge. According to a highly simplified scheme (Fig. 6.19), WNK kinases activate the downstream kinases SPAK and/or OSR1 by binding to them along their conserved carboxyl-terminal domains, and directly phosphorylating them. When so activated, and enhanced by interactions with MO25 (Cab39),[250] these secondary kinases bind to and activate NCC by enhancing phosphorylation of key residues in the NCC amino terminal cytoplasmic domain.[334]

Mutations in both WNK1 and WNK4 can cause FHHt. Intronic mutations in WNK1 enhance the expression of a full-length kinase-active form of WNK1 along the DCT, where it is normally expressed only at low levels[335]; WNK4-point mutations cluster around an acid-rich conserved region of

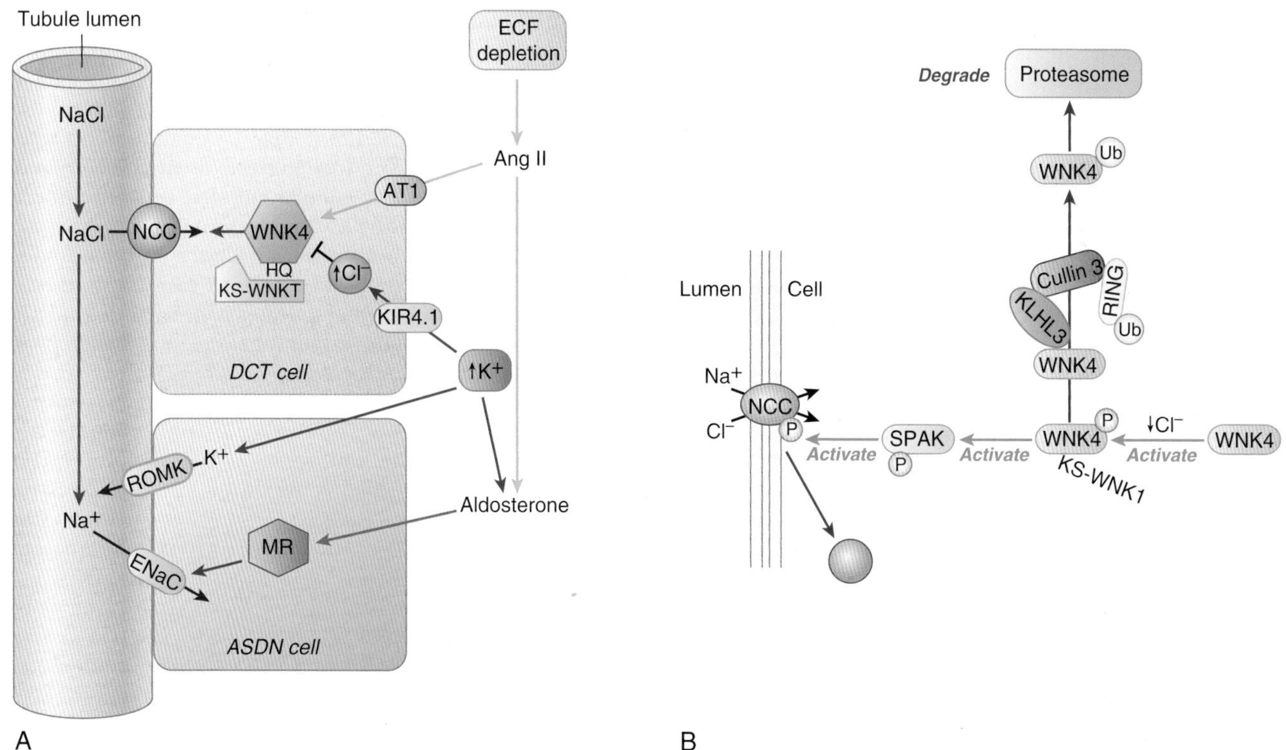


**Fig. 6.19** Regulation of distal transport by WNK kinases. (A) Comparison of effects of extracellular fluid *(ECF)* volume depletion and hyperkalemia (↑[$K^+$]) on transport along the distal nephron. In the lumen, $Na^+$ delivery to the aldosterone-sensitive distal nephron *(ASDN)* is determined by entry into the distal convoluted tubule *(DCT)* and reabsorption by the thiazide-sensitive NaCl cotransporter *(NCC)*. WNK4, likely together with WNK1-S [also known as kidney-specific (KS)-WNK1], activates NCC.[616] This process is stimulated by angiotensin II *(Ang II)*, which also enhances aldosterone secretion by the adrenal gland to stimulate the epithelial $Na^+$ channel *(ENaC)*, via the mineralocorticoid receptor *(MR)*. Sodium reabsorption along both the DCT and ASDN corrects ECF volume depletion. During hyperkalemia, NCC is turned off via increased intracellular chloride (modulated by $K^+$ flux through KIR4.1 channels), and $Na^+$ is reabsorbed primarily by ENaC, favoring $K^+$ secretion. (B) Detailed scheme of WNK kinase regulation. NCC is phosphorylated and activated by STE20/SPS1-related proline/alanine-rich kinase *(SPAK)*, which is phosphorylated and activated by WNK4, which is activated by low intracellular chloride concentration. WNKs can interact with a cullin-ring ligase, via the adaptor Kelch-Like 3 *(KLHL3)*, leading to WNK ubiquitination and subsequent degradation by the proteasome. When dephosphorylated, NCC can be removed from the apical plasma membrane.

the protein, or near the carboxyl-terminal domain.[336] These mutations disrupt WNK binding to adaptor proteins that are essential for WNK degradation (see later).[337–339] Thus both WNK mutant forms of FHHt result in increased abundance of WNKs along the DCT.

The WNK1 and WNK4 proteins are coexpressed within the distal nephron in DCT and CCD cells, where they both localize to the cytoplasm (diffusely, and also in punctate structures) and apical membrane.[340,341] Although both WNK4 and WNK1 can stimulate NCC activity in expression systems, only deletion of WNK4 has been shown to reduce NCC activity in mice.[236,237] In mice in which an FHHt-like phenotype has been generated by mutation of the protein KLHL3 (see later), increased WNK1 abundance does not compensate for deletion of WNK4, suggesting a key role for WNK4.[33] Generation of mice with WNK1 deletion specifically in the kidney may shed more light on its contribution to NCC regulation in vivo.

WNKs, especially WNK4, appear to be sensitive to inhibition by chloride,[342,343] so that when intracellular chloride concentration is low, the stimulatory effect is maximal; when intracellular chloride concentration is higher, there is less stimulation.[344] For WNK1, chloride binds to the catalytic site of the kinase and inhibits autophosphorylation and activation of the kinase.[342] This chloride binding has a major role in the potassium-sensing function of DCT cells. Reduction in potassium intake and/or hypokalemia lead to reduced basolateral $K^+$ concentration in the DCT; the subsequent hyperpolarization is dependent on basolateral KIR4.1-containing $K^+$ channels.[308,311,327] Hyperpolarization has been proposed to lead to chloride exit via basolateral CLC-K2 chloride channels and a reduction in intracellular chloride; the reduction in intracellular chloride activates the SPAK and OSR1-WNK cascade, resulting in phosphorylation of NCC and activation of the transporter.[327] This model helps explain the activating effect of potassium depletion on NCC and the inhibitory effect of potassium loading on NCC, and they go a long way to explain the critical role of the DCT and NCC in potassium homeostasis.[327]

To develop in vivo models relevant to FHHt, two groups developed mice expressing WNK4 carrying a mutation that causes the disease. Lalioti and coworkers generated BAC-transgenic mice that is an FHHt mutant of WNK4 (TgWnk-$4^{PHAII}$, bearing a Q562E mutation associated with the disease),[345] and Yang and colleagues developed a knock-in mouse expressing D568. Both models were hypertensive,[345a] with biochemical phenotypes similar to that of FHHt (i.e., hyperkalemia, acidosis, and hypercalciuria). $TgWnk4^{PHAII}$ mice also exhibit marked hyperplasia of the DCT. Of particular significance, the DCT hyperplasia of $TgWnk4^{PHAII}$ mice was completely suppressed on an NCC-deficient background, generated by mating $TgWnk4^{PHAII}$ mice with NCC knockout mice.[295,296] Therefore the DCT is the primary target for FHHt-associated mutations in WNK4. In addition, as suggested by prior studies, changes in $Na^+$-$Cl^-$ entry via NCC can evidently modulate hyperplasia or regression of the DCT.[275,295,296,345] Vidal-Petiot and colleagues have also generated mice that lack the orthologous intron of WNK1 involved in patients with FHHt, recapitulating the phenotype.[335] Treatment with the calcineurin inhibitor tacrolimus has a similar effect as in FHHt.[348]

WNK proteins are regulated by Cullin 3 (CUL3) and Kelch-like 3 (KLHL3), components of an E3 ubiquitin ligase complex that targets the WNKs for degradation.[339,349,350] Mutations in the *CUL3* and *KLHL3* genes also cause FHHt and account for the majority of cases. Disease-associated mutations in KLHL3 abrogate binding to WNK4 and vice versa.[339] In turn, disease-associated mutations in CUL3 may deplete levels of KLHL3, preventing WNK degradation.[351] Physiologically, phosphorylation of KLHL3 by PKC, downstream of Ang II, also abrogates the interaction between KLHL3 and WNK4, leading to NCC activation.[352] More information about the mechanisms of FHHt, and the roles of regulatory proteins can be found in Chapters 17 and 44.

The various mechanistic models for the regulation of NCC by upstream WNK1, WNK4, and the SPAK-OSR1 kinases have recently been reviewed; interactions between WNK4 and both WNK3 and SGK1 also contribute to the complexity, as do CUL3 and KLH3.[339,349–356] Competing divergent mechanisms can be reconciled by the likelihood that the physiologic context determines whether WNK4 will have an activating or inhibitory effect on NCC. For example, the activation of NCC by the Ang II receptor type 1 appears to require the downstream activation of SPAK by WNK4.[315,357] Changes in circulating and local levels of Ang II, aldosterone, vasopressin, and $K^+$ are thus expected to have different and often opposing effects on the activity of NCC in the DCT (see also Fig. 6.19 and the "Integrated $Na^+$-$Cl^-$ and $K^+$ Transport in the Distal Nephron" section).[315,353,357–361]

WNK kinases exhibit effects in expression systems that may seem anomalous, but which likely reflect their pleiotropic properties. In *Xenopus* oocytes, for example, WNK4 can inhibit NCC, through its carboxyl-terminal domain, which binds to protein phosphatase 1.[362] It now appears that this effect results from WNK4 inhibiting endogenously expressed WNK kinases in the setting of high intracellular chloride concentrations.[363] WNK4 coexpression with NCC reduces transporter expression at the membrane of both *Xenopus* oocytes and mammalian cells, suggesting a prominent effect on membrane trafficking.[353,357] The WNK4 kinase activates lysosomal degradation of the transporter protein, rather than inducing dynamin- and clathrin-dependent endocytosis.[364,365] This occurs through effects of WNK4 on the interaction of NCC with the lysosomal targeting receptor sortilin and AP-3 adaptor complex.[364,365] Dynamin-dependent endocytosis of NCC is induced by ERK1/2 phosphorylation via activation of H-Ras, Raf, and MEK1/2, resulting in ubiquitination of NCC and endocytosis of the transporter, suggesting a significant role in the downregulation of NCC by PTH.[366–368] Ubiquitination of NCC is catalyzed by the ubiquitin-ligase NEDD4-2, causing downregulation of NCC.[321] NCC is highly ubiquitinated at multiple specific sites, but it is unclear whether ubiquitination at all of these sites involves NEDD4-2.[369] Ubiquitination at these different sites has different effects on NCC, either modulating its endocytosis or degradation. The full implications of these effects observed in cell culture systems regarding in vivo behavior awaits additional study.

## CONNECTING TUBULES AND THE CORTICAL COLLECTING DUCT

### Apical $Na^+$ Transport

The apical membrane of CNT cells and principal cells contain prominent $Na^+$ and $K^+$ conductances, without a measurable apical conductance for $Cl^-$.[216,279,370,371] The entry

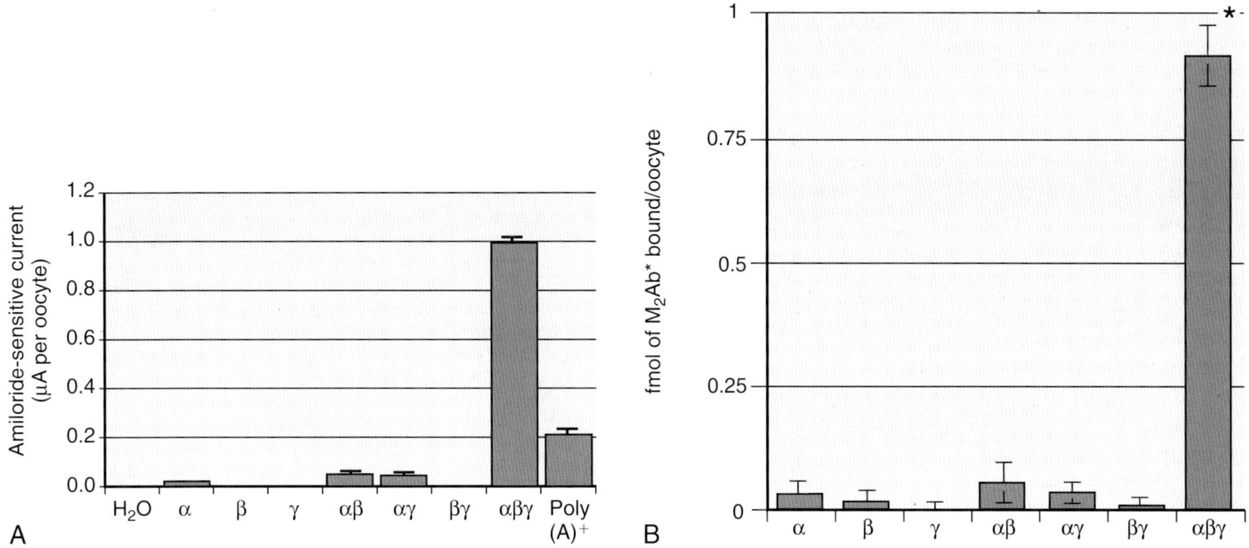


**Fig. 6.20** Maximal expression of the amiloride-sensitive epithelial $Na^+$ channel (ENaC) at the plasma membrane requires the coexpression of all three subunits (α-, β-, and γ-ENaC). (A) Amiloride-sensitive current in *Xenopus* oocytes expressing the individual subunits and various combinations thereof. (B) Surface expression is markedly enhanced in *Xenopus* oocytes that coexpress all three subunits. The individual complementary DNAs (cDNAs) were engineered with an external epitope tag; expression of the channel proteins at the cell surface is measured by binding of a monoclonal antibody ($M_2Ab^*$) to the tag. *Poly $A^+$,* Polyadenylated messenger RNA (mRNA). (A from Canessa CM, Schild L, Buell G, et al. Amiloride-sensitive epithelial $Na^+$ channel is made of three homologous subunits. *Nature.* 1994;367:463–467; B from Firsov, D, Schild L, Gautschi I, et al. Cell surface expression of the epithelial Na channel and a mutant causing Liddle syndrome: a quantitative approach. *Proc Natl Acad Sci U S A.* 1996;93:15370–15375.)

of $Na^+$ occurs via the highly selective epithelial $Na^+$ channel (ENaC), which is sensitive to micromolar concentrations of amiloride (Fig. 6.20).[372] This selective absorption of positive charge generates a lumen-negative PD, the magnitude of which varies considerably as a function of mineralocorticoid status and other factors. This lumen-negative PD serves to drive the following critical processes: (1) $K^+$ secretion via apical $K^+$ channels; (2) paracellular $Cl^-$ transport through the adjacent tight junctions; and/or (3) electrogenic $H^+$ secretion via adjacent type A intercalated cells.[373]

ENaC is a heteromeric channel complex formed by the assembly of separate, homologous subunits, denoted α-, β-, and γ-ENaC.[14] These channel subunits share a common structure, with intracellular amino- and carboxyl-terminal domains, two transmembrane segments, and a large glycosylated extracellular loop.[14] *Xenopus* oocytes expressing α-ENaC alone have detectable $Na^+$ channel activity (Fig. 6.20), which facilitated the initial identification of this subunit by expression cloning; functional complementation of this modest activity was then used to clone the other two subunits by expression cloning.[14] Full channel activity requires the coexpression of all three subunits, which causes a dramatic increase in expression of the channel complex at the plasma membrane (Fig. 6.20).[374] The subunit stoichiometry has been a source of considerable controversy, with some reports favoring a tetramer with ratios of two α-ENaC proteins to one each of β- and γ-ENaC (2α:1β:1γ) and others favoring a higher-order assembly with a stoichiometry of 3α:3β:3γ.[375] Regardless, the single-channel characteristics of heterologously expressed ENaC are essentially identical to those of the amiloride-sensitive channel detectable at the apical membrane of CCD cells.[14,372]

ENaC plays a critical role in renal $Na^+$-$Cl^-$ reabsorption and maintenance of the extracellular fluid volume. In particular, recessive loss-of-function mutations in the three subunits of ENaC are a cause of pseudohypoaldosteronism type I.[14,376] Patients with this syndrome typically present with severe neonatal salt wasting, hypotension, acidosis, and hyperkalemia; this dramatic phenotype underscores the critical roles of ENaC activity in renal $Na^+$-$Cl^-$ reabsorption, $K^+$ secretion, and $H^+$ secretion. Gain-of-function mutations in all three ENaC subunits have been reported to cause Liddle syndrome, an autosomal dominant hypertensive syndrome accompanied by suppressed aldosterone and variable hypokalemia.[377] The majority of ENaC mutations associated with Liddle syndrome disrupt interactions between a PPxY motif in the carboxyl-terminus of channel subunits with the NEDD4-2 ubiquitin-ligase leading to increased surface expression of the channel. Mutations in the extracellular loops of α-ENaC and γ-ENaC have also been identified,[378,379] with the α-ENaC mutation increasing intrinsic activity of the channel.[379]

The ENaC protein is detectable at the apical membrane of CNT cells and principal cells in the CCD, OMCD, and IMCD.[281,286] Notably, however, several lines of evidence have supported the hypothesis that the CNT makes the dominant contribution to amiloride-sensitive $Na^+$ reabsorption by the distal nephron:

1. Amiloride-sensitive $Na^+$ currents in the CNT are twofold to fourfold higher than in the CCD; the maximal capacity of the CNT for $Na^+$ reabsorption is estimated to be about 10 times higher than that of the CCD.[279]
2. Targeted deletion of α-ENaC in the collecting duct abolishes amiloride-sensitive currents in CCD principal

cells, but does not affect $Na^+$ or $K^+$ homeostasis; the residual ENaC expression in the late DCT and CNT of these knockout mice easily compensates for the loss of the channel in CCD cells.[380]

3. $Na^+$-$K^+$-ATPase activity in the CCD is considerably less than that of the DCT (see also Fig. 6.4); this speaks to a greater capability for transepithelial $Na^+$-$Cl^-$ absorption by the DCT and CNT.[17]
4. The apical recruitment of ENaC subunits in response to dietary $Na^+$ restriction begins in the CNT, with progressive recruitment of subunits in the downstream CCD at lower levels of dietary $Na^+$; although the CNT plays a dominant role in ENaC-mediated sodium transport, it does so primarily in an aldosterone-independent mechanism, with aldosterone-mediated sodium transport in the CCD involved in the finely tuned regulation of sodium transport.[381,382]
5. Patch-clamp analysis of knock-in mice homozygous for a Liddle syndrome ENaC mutant showed that the primary site of increased $Na^+$ reabsorption is the DCT2/CNT rather than the CNT/CCD.[383]

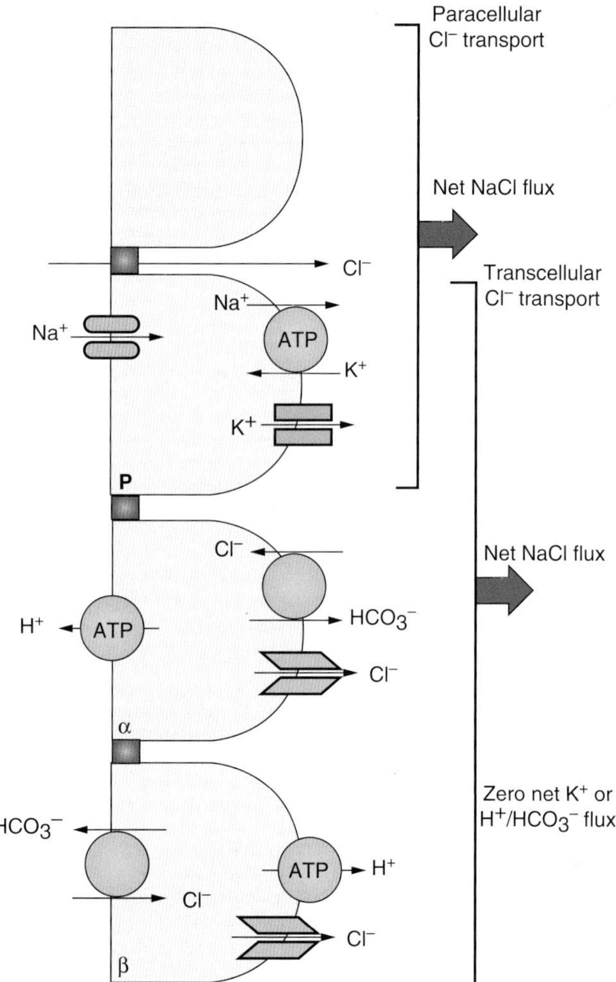


**Fig. 6.21** Transepithelial $Cl^-$ transport by principal and intercalated cells. The lumen-negative potential difference (PD) generated by principal cells drives paracellular $Cl^-$ absorption. Alternatively, transepithelial transport occurs in type B intercalated cells via apical $Cl^-$-$HCO_3^-$ exchange (SLC26A4/pendrin) and basolateral $Cl^-$ exit via CLC-K2. (Modified from Moe OW, Baum M, Berry CA, Rector Jr FC. Renal transport of glucose, amino acids, sodium, chloride, and water. In: Brenner BM, ed. *Brenner and Rector's the Kidney.* Philadelphia: WB Saunders; 2004:413–452.)

## $Cl^-$ Transport

There are two major pathways for $Cl^-$ absorption in the CNT and CCD – paracellular transport across the tight junction and transcellular transport across type B intercalated cells (Fig. 6.21).[280,384] The CNT and CCD are "tight" epithelia, with comparatively low paracellular permeability that is not selective for $Cl^-$ over $Na^+$; however, voltage-driven, paracellular $Cl^-$ transport in the CCD may play a considerable role in transepithelial $Na^+$-$Cl^-$ absorption.[385] The CNT, DCT, and collecting duct coexpress claudin-3, -4, and -8; claudin-8 in particular may function as a paracellular cation barrier that prevents backleak of $Na^+$, $K^+$, and $H^+$ in this segment of the nephron.[14,386] Several lines of evidence have indicated that claudin-4 and claudin-8 interact to form a paracellular pathway for $Cl^-$ in the collecting duct, thus mediating transcellular $Cl^-$ absorption via the paracellular pathway.[387] CCD-specific knockout of claudin-4 in mice leads to NaCl wasting and hypotension,[388] while CCD-specific disruption of claudin-8 causes hypotension, hypokalemia, and metabolic alkalosis, which resembles Gitelman syndrome.[389] Regulated changes in paracellular permeability may also contribute to $Cl^-$ absorption by the CNT and CCD. In particular, wild type WNK4 appears to increase paracellular $Cl^-$ permeability in transfected MDCK II cell lines; a WNK4 FHHt mutant has a much larger effect, with no effect seen in cells expressing kinase-dead WNK4 constructs.[390] Yamauchi and colleagues have also reported that FHHt-associated WNK4 increases paracellular permeability, due perhaps to an associated hyperphosphorylation of claudin proteins.[391] The claudin-4-mediated chloride conductance is also negatively regulated by cleavage in its second extracellular loop by channel-activating protease 1 (cap1).[388] Similar to WNK4-mediated degradation by CUL 3/KLHL3 (see the "Regulation of $Na^+$-$Cl^-$ Transport in the Distal Convoluted Tubule" section), claudin-8 was shown to be a target of KLHL3-mediated degradation, with FHHt-associated KLHL3 displaying impaired interaction.[389]

Transcellular $Cl^-$ absorption across intercalated cells is thought to play a quantitatively greater role in the CNT and CCD than that of paracellular transport.[384] In the simplest scheme, this process requires the concerted function of type A and type B intercalated cells, achieving net electrogenic $Cl^-$ absorption without affecting $HCO_3^-$ or $H^+$ excretion (see also Fig. 6.21).[384] Chloride thus enters type B intercalated cells via apical $Cl^-$-$HCO_3^-$ exchange, followed by exit from the cell via basolateral $Cl^-$ channels. Recycling of $Cl^-$ at the basolateral membrane of adjacent type A intercalated cells also results in $HCO_3^-$ absorption and extrusion of $H^+$ at the apical membrane. The net effect of apical $Cl^-$-$HCO_3^-$ exchange in type B intercalated cells, leading to apical secretion of $HCO_3^-$, and recycling of $Cl^-$ at the basolateral membrane type A intercalated cells, leading to apical secretion of $H^+$, is electrogenic $Cl^-$ absorption across type B intercalated cells (Fig. 6.21).

At the basolateral membrane, intercalated cells have a very robust $Cl^-$ conductance, with transport characteristics similar to those of CLC-K2/Barttin.[216,392] CLC-K2 protein is also detected at the basolateral membrane of type A intercalated cells, and CLC-K2 activity has been observed in type B cells.[214,393] The basolateral $Na^+$-$K^+$-$2Cl^-$ cotransporter NKCC1 in adjacent type A intercalated cells also plays an evident role in transepithelial $Cl^-$ absorption by the CCD.[394] At the apical membrane, the SLC26A4 exchanger (also known as pendrin) has been conclusively identified as the elusive $Cl^-$-$HCO_3^-$ exchanger of type B and non-A, non-B intercalated cells; this exchanger functions as the apical entry site during transepithelial $Cl^-$ transport by the distal nephron.[280] Human *SLC26A4* is mutated in Pendred syndrome, which encompasses sensorineural hearing loss and goiter; these patients do not have an appreciable renal phenotype.[280] However, *Slc26a4* knockout mice are sensitive to restriction of dietary $Na^+$-$Cl^-$, developing hypotension during severe restriction.[395] *Slc26a4* knockout mice are also resistant to mineralocorticoid-induced hypertension.[396] Pendrin has indirect effects on ENaC abundance and activity, apparently by modulating luminal ATP and $HCO_3^-$ concentrations; pendrin and ENaC are also both coactivated by Ang II[397–400] and pendrin expression is also induced by aldosterone.[401] The overexpression of pendrin in intercalated cells thus causes hypertension in transgenic mice, with an increase in ENaC activity and activity of electroneutral $Na^+$-$Cl^-$ absorption (see later).[402] Conversely, disruption of pendrin in mice decreased ENaC-mediated $Na^+$ absorption by reducing channel open probability and channel density at the apical membrane.[403] Finally, dietary $Cl^-$ restriction with provision of $Na^+$-$HCO_3^-$ results in $Cl^-$ wasting in *Slc26a4* knockout mice and increased apical expression of SLC26A4 protein in the type B intercalated cells of normal littermate controls.[404] Several groups have reported that SLC26A4 expression is exquisitely responsive to changes in distal chloride delivery.[405] Therefore SLC26A4 plays a critical role in distal nephron $Cl^-$ absorption, underlining the particular importance of transcellular $Cl^-$ transport in this process. Of broader relevance, these studies have served to underline the important role for $Cl^-$ homeostasis in the maintenance of extracellular volume and pathogenesis of hypertension.[405]

### Electroneutral $Na^+$-$Cl^-$ Cotransport

Thiazide-sensitive $Na^+$-$Cl^-$ cotransport is considered the exclusive provenance of the DCT, which expresses the canonical thiazide-sensitive transporter NCC (see the "Mechanisms of $Na^+$-$Cl^-$ Transport in the Distal Convoluted Tubule" section). However, Tomita and coworkers demonstrated many years ago that approximately 50% of $Na^+$-$Cl^-$ transport in rat CCD is electroneutral, amiloride resistant, and thiazide sensitive.[406,407] Thiazide-sensitive electroneutral $Na^+$-$Cl^-$ transport has also been demonstrated in mouse CCD.[408] This transport activity is preserved in CCDs from mice with genetic disruption of NCC and ENaC, indicating independence from the dominant apical $Na^+$ transport pathways in the distal nephron. This thiazide-sensitive, electroneutral $Na^+$-$Cl^-$ transport appears to be mediated by the parallel activity of the $Na^+$-driven SLC4A8 $Cl^-$-$HCO_3^-$ exchanger and SLC26A4 $Cl^-$-$HCO_3^-$ exchanger (pendrin; see earlier discussion).[408] *Slc4a8* knockout mice display only a mild perturbation of $Na^+$-$Cl^-$ and water balance due to compensation by NCC; combined SLC4A8 and NCC disruption caused intravascular volume contraction and hypokalemia.[409] Notably, however, heterologously expressed recombinant SLC4A8 and SLC26A4 are resistant and partially sensitive to thiazide, respectively, such that the in vivo pharmacology of this electroneutral $Na^+$-$Cl^-$ absorption is not completely explained. Immunolocalization of Slc4a8 within the CCD has been problematic; hence, it is unknown whether SLC4A8 and SLC26A4 are coexpressed in type B intercalated cells. Regardless, the combined activity of SLC4A8 and SLC26A4 appears to play a major role in $Na^+$-$Cl^-$ transport within the CCD, with significant implications for $Na^+$-$Cl^-$ and $K^+$ homeostasis (see also the "Integrated $Na^+$-$Cl^-$ and $K^+$ Transport in the Distal Nephron" section).

The apical entry of $Na^+$ via SLC4A8 requires a basolateral exit of $Na^+$ in type B intercalated cells, evidently mediated by the basolateral $Na^+$-$HCO_3^-$ transporter SLC4A9.[2] Another puzzle was the energetics of transcellular $Na^+$-$Cl^-$ transport in intercalated cells, which possess minimal, if any, detectable $Na^+$-$K^+$-ATPase activity. A series of elegant experiments have revealed that electroneutral $Na^+$-$Cl^-$ transport in type B intercalated cells is energized by and thus dependent on the activity of the basolateral $H^+$-ATPase.[2] Type B intercalated cells are therefore unique among mammalian renal epithelial cells in that transcellular ion transport is driven by $H^+$-ATPase rather than $Na^+$-$K^+$-ATPase activity.

## REGULATION OF $NA^+$-$CL^-$ TRANSPORT IN THE CONNECTING TUBULE AND CORTICAL COLLECTING DUCT

### Aldosterone

The DCT, CNT, and collecting ducts collectively constitute the aldosterone-sensitive distal nephron, expressing the mineralocorticoid receptor and 11β-HSD2 enzyme that protects against illicit activation by glucocorticoids.[275] Aldosterone plays a dominant positive role in the regulation of distal nephron $Na^+$-$Cl^-$ transport, with a plethora of mechanisms and transcriptional targets.[410] For example, aldosterone increases the expression of the $Na^+$-$K^+$-ATPase $\alpha_1$- and $\beta_1$-subunits in the CCD, in addition to inducing SLC26A4, the apical $Cl^-$-$HCO_3^-$ exchanger of intercalated cells.[396,411] Aldosterone may also affect paracellular permeability of the distal nephron via posttranscriptional modification of claudins and other components of the tight junction.[412] However, particularly impressive progress has been made in the understanding of the downstream effects of aldosterone on synthesis, trafficking, and membrane-associated activity of ENaC subunits. A detailed discussion of aldosterone's actions may be found in Chapter 12; here we summarize the major findings of relevance to $Na^+$-$Cl^-$ transport.

Aldosterone increases abundance of α-ENaC via a glucocorticoid response element in the promoter of the *SCNN1A* gene that encodes this subunit.[413] Aldosterone also relieves a tonic inhibition of the *SCNN1A* gene by a complex that includes the Dot1a (disruptor of telomere silencing splicing variant *a*) and AF9 and AF17 transcription factors.[414] An aldosterone-dependent reduction in promoter methylation is also involved.[415] This transcriptional activation results in an increased abundance of α-ENaC protein in response to exogenous aldosterone or dietary $Na^+$-$Cl^-$ restriction (Fig. 6.22); the response to $Na^+$-$Cl^-$ restriction is blunted by spironolactone, indicating involvement of the mineralocorticoid receptor.[416–418] At baseline, α-ENaC transcripts in the kidney are less abundant than those encoding β- and γ-ENaC[419] (Fig. 6.22). All three subunits are required for efficient processing

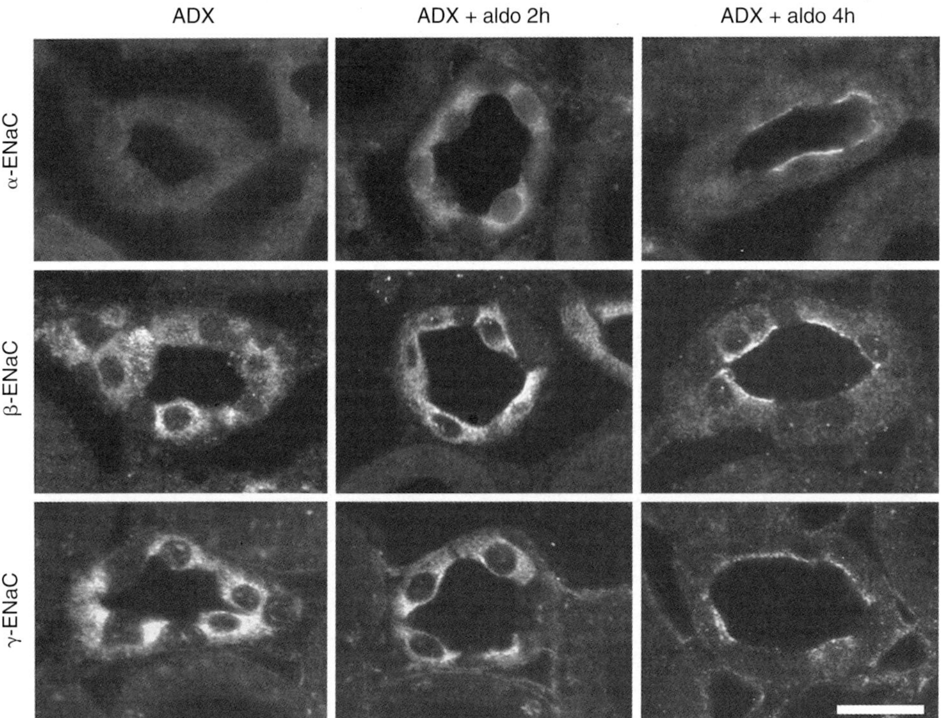


**Fig. 6.22** Immunofluorescence images of connecting tubule profiles in kidneys from adrenalectomized rats *(ADX)* and from ADX rats 2 and 4 hours after aldosterone (aldo) injection. Antibodies against the α, β, and γ subunits of epithelial $Na^+$ channel *(ENaC)* reveal absent expression of the former in ADX rats, with progressive induction by aldosterone. All three subunits traffic to the apical membrane in response to aldosterone. This coincides with rapid aldosterone induction of the SGK kinase in the same cells; SGK is known to increase the expression of ENaC at the plasma membrane (see text for details). Bar ≅ 15 μm. (From Loffing J, Zecevic M, Féraille E, et al. Aldosterone induces rapid apical translocation of ENaC in early portion of renal collecting system: possible role of SGK. *Am J Physiol Renal Physiol.* 2001;280:F675–F682.)

of heteromeric channels in the endoplasmic reticulum and trafficking to the plasma membrane (Fig. 6.20), such that the induction of α-ENaC is thought to relieve a major bottleneck in the processing and trafficking of active ENaC complexes.[419]

Aldosterone also plays an indirect role in the regulated trafficking of ENaC subunits to the plasma membrane via the regulation of accessory proteins that interact with preexisting ENaC subunits. Aldosterone rapidly induces expression of a serine-threonine kinase denoted SGK1 (serum and glucocorticoid-induced kinase-1); coexpression of SGK1 with ENaC subunits in *Xenopus* oocytes results in a dramatic activation of the channel due to increased expression at the plasma membrane.[418,420,421] Notably, an analogous redistribution of ENaC subunits occurs in the CNT and early CCD, from a largely cytoplasmic location during dietary $Na^+$-$Cl^-$ excess to a purely apical distribution after aldosterone or $Na^+$-$Cl^-$ restriction (Fig. 6.22).[381,416,418] Furthermore, there is a temporal correlation between the appearance of induced SGK1 protein in the CNT and the redistribution of ENaC protein to the plasma membrane.[418]

SGK1 modulates membrane expression of ENaC by interfering with regulated endocytosis of its channel subunits. Specifically, the kinase interferes with interactions between ENaC subunits and the ubiquitin ligase NEDD4-2.[419] PPxY domains in the C termini of all three ENaC subunits bind to WW domains of NEDD4-2[422]; these PPxY domains are deleted, truncated, or mutated in patients with Liddle syndrome, leading to a gain of function in channel activity.[374,377] Coexpression of NEDD4-2 with the wild type ENaC channel results in a marked inhibition of channel activity due to retrieval from the cell membrane, whereas channels bearing Liddle syndrome mutations are resistant; NEDD4-2 is thought to ubiquitinate ENaC subunits, resulting in the removal of channel subunits from the cell membrane and degradation in lysosomes and the proteosome.[419] A PPxY domain in SGK1 also binds to NEDD4-2, which is a phosphorylation substrate for the kinase; phosphorylation of NEDD4-2 by SGK1 abrogates its inhibitory effect on ENaC subunits.[423,424] Aldosterone also stimulates NEDD4-2 phosphorylation in vivo.[425] NEDD4-2 phosphorylation in turn results in ubiquitin-mediated degradation of SGK1, suggesting that there is considerable feedback regulation in this system.[426] Aldosterone also reduces NEDD4-2 protein expression in cultured CCD cells, and acetylation of ENaC antagonizes ENaC ubiquitination, suggesting additional levels of in vivo regulation.[427,428]

The induction of SGK1 by aldosterone thus appears to stimulate the redistribution of ENaC subunits from the cytoplasm to the apical membrane of CNT and CCD cells. This phenomenon involves SGK1-dependent phosphorylation of the NEDD4-2 ubiquitin ligase, which is coexpressed with ENaC and SGK1 in the distal nephron.[427] Of note, there is considerable axial heterogeneity in the recruitment and redistribution of ENaC to the plasma membrane, which begins in the CNT and only extends into the CCD and OMCD in $Na^+$-$Cl^-$–restricted or aldosterone-treated animals.[275,418] The underlying causes of this progressive axial recruitment are not as yet clear.[275] However, NEDD4-2 expression is inversely related to the apical distribution of ENaC, with low expression in the CNT and increased expression levels in the CCD. In all likelihood, the relative balance among SGK1, ENaC, and NEDD4-2 figures prominently in the recruitment of the channel subunits to the apical membrane.[427]

NEDD4-2 and ENaC are part of a larger regulatory complex that includes the signaling protein Raf-1, stimulatory aldosterone-induced chaperone GILZ1 (glucocorticoid-induced leucine zipper-1), and scaffolding protein CNK3.[429,430] The mTORC2 (mammalian target of rapamycin complex 2) kinase complex is another component, catalyzing upstream activation of SGK1 and thus inducing activation of ENaC.[431,432]

Although many studies have supported a central role for SGK1 in mediating the effects of aldosterone on ENaC, a recent study found that despite altered apical trafficking of ENaC in SGK1 knockout mice, ENaC activity is normal even after aldosterone administration. This suggests that other aldosterone-induced proteins play a role in ENaC activation via mineralocorticoid receptors.[433,434] For example, another aldosterone-induced protein, Ankyrin G, a cytoskeletal protein involved in vesicular trafficking, increases ENaC activity in cultured CCD cells by promoting its plasma membrane insertion from recycling endosomes.[435]

Finally, aldosterone indirectly activates ENaC channels through the induction of channel-activating proteases, which increase open channel probability by cleavage of the extracellular domains of α- and γ-ENaC. Western blotting of renal tissue from rats subjected to $Na^+$-$Cl^-$ restriction or treatment with aldosterone has revealed α- and γ-ENaC subunits of lower molecular mass than those detected in control animals, indicating that aldosterone induces proteolytic cleavage.[417,436] Proteases that have been implicated in the processing of ENaC include furin, elastase, and three membrane-associated proteases denoted CAP1–3 (channel activating proteases-1, -2, and -3).[437–439] Filtered proteases such as plasmin may also contribute to ENaC activation in nephrotic syndrome.[439] CAP1 was initially identified from *Xenopus* A6 cells as an ENaC-activating protease; the mammalian ortholog is an aldosterone-induced protein in principal cells.[440,441] Urinary excretion of CAP1, also known as prostasin, is increased in hyperaldosteronism, with a reduction after adrenalectomy.[441] CAP1 is tethered to the plasma membrane by a GPI linkage, whereas CAP2 and CAP3 are transmembrane proteases.[438,440] All three of these proteases activate ENaC by increasing the $P_o$ of the channel, without increasing expression at the cell surface.[438] However, analysis of CAP2 knockout mice indicates that it does not play a role in ENaC regulation and sodium balance in vivo.[442] Proteolytic cleavage of ENaC appears to activate the channel by removing the self-inhibitory effect of external $Na^+$; in the case of furin-mediated proteolysis of α-ENaC, this appears to involve the removal of an inhibitory domain from within the extracellular loop.[438,443] Extracellular $Na^+$ appears to interact with a specific acidic cleft in the extracellular loop of α-ENaC, causing inhibition of the channel.[444] The structures of the extracellular domains of ENaC and related channels resemble an outstretched hand holding a ball, with defined subdomains termed the "wrist," "finger," "thumb," "palm," "β-ball," and "knuckle"; functionally relevant proteolytic events target the finger domains of ENaC subunits.[439] Unprocessed channels at the plasma membrane are thought to function as a reserve pool, capable of rapid activation by membrane-associated luminal proteases.[437]

### Vasopressin and Other Factors

Although not typically considered an antinatriuretic hormone, vasopressin has well-characterized stimulatory effects on $Na^+$-$Cl^-$ transport by the CCD.[94,445] Vasopressin directly activates ENaC in murine CCD, increasing the open probability ($P_o$) of the channel.[446] In perfused rat CCD segments, vasopressin and aldosterone can have synergistic effects on $Na^+$ transport, with a combined effect that exceeds that of the individual hormones.[445] In addition, water and $Na^+$ restriction synergistically increase the $P_o$ of ENaC in murine CCDs.[446] Prostaglandins inhibit this effect of vasopressin, particularly in the rabbit CCD; this inhibition occurs at least in part through reductions in vasopressin-generated cAMP.[94,445] There are, however, considerable species-dependent differences in the interactions between vasopressin and negative modulators of $Na^+$-$Cl^-$ transport in the CCD, which include prostaglandins, bradykinin, endothelin, and $\alpha_2$-adrenergic tone.[94,445] Regardless, cAMP causes a rapid increase in the $Na^+$ conductance of apical membranes in the CCD; this effect appears to be due to increases in the surface expression of ENaC subunits at the plasma membrane[447] in addition to effects on open channel probability.[446,448] Notably, cAMP inhibits retrieval of ENaC subunits from the plasma membrane via PKA-dependent phosphorylation of the phosphoacceptor sites in NEDD4-2 that are targeted by SGK1; therefore both aldosterone and vasopressin converge on NEDD4-2 in the regulation of ENaC activity in the distal nephron.[449] Analogous to the effect on trafficking of aquaporin-2 in principal cells, cAMP also seems to stimulate exocytosis of ENaC subunits to the plasma membrane.[448] Finally, similar to the long-term effects of vasopressin on aquaporin-2 expression and NKCC2 expression, chronic treatment with DDAVP results in an increase in abundance of the β- and γ-ENaC subunits.[233,450]

The activation of ENaC by vasopressin appears to have additional direct effects on water homeostasis. Hypernatremic mice treated with the ENaC inhibitor benzamil thus exhibit further increases in tonicity due to a reduction in urinary osmolality.[451] In adrenalectomized mice, which lack circulating aldosterone, vasopressin maintains ENaC activity in the distal nephron.[452] This vasopressin-dependent activation of ENaC may, by extension, play a role in generating hyponatremia in the setting of primary adrenal failure. Systemic generation of circulating Ang II induces aldosterone release by the adrenal gland, with downstream activation of ENaC. However, Ang II also directly activates amiloride-sensitive $Na^+$ transport in perfused CCDs; blockade by losartan or candesartan suggests that this activation is mediated by Ang II receptors type 1.[453] Of particular significance, the effect of luminal Ang II ($10^{-9}$ M) was greater than that of bath Ang II, suggesting that intratubular Ang II may regulate ENaC in the distal nephron. Ang II also activates chloride absorption across intercalated cells via a pendrin (SLC26A4) and an $H^+$-ATPase-dependent mechanism.[454] Stimulation of ENaC is seen when tubules are perfused with Ang I; this effect is blocked by ACE inhibition with captopril, suggesting that intraluminal conversion of Ang I to Ang II can occur in the CCD.[455] Notably, CNT cells express considerable amounts of immunoreactive renin versus the vanishingly low expression of renin mRNA in the PT.[456] Angiotensinogen secreted into the tubule by PT cells may thus be converted to Ang II in the CNT via locally generated renin and ACE and/or related proteases.[456]

Luminal perfusion with ATP or uridine triphosphate (UTP) inhibits amiloride-sensitive $Na^+$ transport and reduces ENaC $P_o$ in the CCD via activation of luminal $P2Y_2$ purinergic receptors.[457,458] Targeted deletion of the murine $P2Y_2$ receptor results in salt-resistant hypertension due in part to an upregulation of NKCC2 activity in the TAL; resting ENaC activity is also increased, but suppressed aldosterone and downregulation of the α-subunit of ENaC blunts the role of amiloride-sensitive transport.[458,459] Clamping mineralocorticoid activity at higher levels, via the administration of exogenous mineralocorticoid, reveals that $P2Y_2$ receptor activation may be a major mechanism for the modulation of ENaC $P_o$ in response to changes in dietary $Na^+$-$Cl^-$.[323] Increased dietary $Na^+$-$Cl^-$ thus leads to increased urinary ATP and UTP excretion in mice[458]; endogenous ATP from principal cells inhibits ENaC, and ENaC activity is not responsive to increased dietary $Na^+$-$Cl^-$ in $P2Y_2$ receptor knockout mice.[323,458] In addition, the activation of apical ionotropic purinergic receptors, likely $P2X_4$ and/or $P2X_4/P2X_6$, can inhibit or activate ENaC, depending on luminal $Na^+$ concentration; these receptors may also participate in fine-tuning ENaC activity in response to dietary $Na^+$-$Cl^-$.[460]

As in other segments of the nephron, $Na^+$-$Cl^-$ transport by the CNT and CCD is modulated by metabolites of arachidonic acid generated by cytochrome P450 monooxygenases. In particular, arachidonic acid inhibits ENaC channel activity in the rat CCD via generation of the epoxygenase product 11,12-EET by the CYP2C23 enzyme expressed in principal cells.[461] Targeted deletion of the murine *Cyp4a10* gene, encoding, another P450 monooxygenase, results in salt-sensitive hypertension; urinary excretion of 11,12-EET is reduced in these knockout mice, with a blunted effect of arachidonic acid on ENaC channel activity in the CCD.[462] These mice also became normotensive after treatment with amiloride, indicative of in vivo activation of ENaC. It appears that deletion of *Cyp4a10* reduces activity of the murine ortholog of rat CYPC23 (*Cyp2c44* in mouse) and/or related epoxygenases via reduced generation of a ligand for PPARα (peroxisome proliferator–activated receptor α) that induces epoxygenase activity.[462] The mechanism(s) whereby 11,12-EET inhibits ENaC are unknown as yet. However, renal 11,12-EET production is known to be salt-sensitive, suggesting that generation of this mediator may serve to reduce ENaC activity during high dietary $Na^+$-$Cl^-$ intake.[461]

Finally, activation of PPARγ by thiazolidinediones (TZDs) results in amiloride-sensitive hypertension, suggesting in vivo activation of ENaC.[463,464] TZDs (e.g., rosiglitazone, pioglitazone, troglitazone) are insulin-sensitizing drugs used for the treatment of type II diabetes. Treatment with these agents is frequently associated with fluid retention, suggesting an effect on renal $Na^+$-$Cl^-$ transport. Given robust expression of PPARγ in the collecting duct, activation of ENaC was an attractive hypothesis for this TZD-associated edema syndrome.[463,464] This appears to be the case, in that selective deletion of the murine PPARγ gene in principal cells abrogates the increase in amiloride-sensitive transport seen in response to TZDs.[463,464] Conversely, mice with disruption of α-ENaC specifically along CNT/CCD display blunted increases in total body water and extracellular fluid volume in response to rosiglitazone administration, providing direct evidence that the effects of PPARγ are mediated through ENaC.[465] TZDs appear to induce transcription of the *Sccn1g* gene encoding γ-ENaC in addition to inducing SGK1; targeted deletion of SGK1 in knockout mice attenuates but does not abolish TZD-associated edema.[463,466,467] Notably, however, other studies have failed to detect an effect of TZDs on ENaC activity, which may instead activate a nonspecific cation channel within the IMCD.[468,469] Regardless, the beneficial effect of spironolactone in type II diabetics with TZD-associated volume expansion is consistent with in vivo activation of $Na^+$-$Cl^-$ absorption in the aldosterone-responsive distal nephron.[470] In addition, the risk of peripheral edema is increased considerably in patients treated with both TZDs and insulin therapy. Notably, insulin appears to activate ENaC via SGK1-dependent mechanisms; PPARγ is required for the full activating effect of insulin on ENaC, such that this clinical observation may reflect synergistic activation of ENaC by insulin and TZDs.[468,471,472]

## POTASSIUM TRANSPORT

Maintenance of $K^+$ balance is important for a multitude of physiologic processes. Changes in intracellular $K^+$ affect cell volume regulation, regulation of intracellular pH, enzymatic function, protein synthesis, DNA synthesis, and apoptosis.[14] Changes in the ratio of intracellular to extracellular $K^+$ affect the resting membrane potential, leading to depolarization in hyperkalemia and hyperpolarization in hypokalemia. Thus, disorders of extracellular $K^+$ have a dominant effect on excitable tissues, chiefly heart and muscle. In addition, a growing body of evidence has implicated hypokalemia and/or reduced dietary $K^+$ in the pathobiology of hypertension, heart failure, and stroke; these and other clinical consequences of $K^+$ disorders are reviewed in Chapter 17.

Potassium is predominantly an intracellular cation, with only 2% of total body $K^+$ residing in the extracellular fluid. Extracellular $K^+$ is maintained within a very narrow range by three primary mechanisms. First, the distribution of $K^+$ between the intracellular and extracellular space is determined by the activity of a number of transport pathways—namely, $Na^+$-$K^+$-ATPase, the $Na^+$-$K^+$-$2Cl^-$ cotransporter NKCC1, the four KCCs, and a plethora of $K^+$ channels. In particular, skeletal muscle contains as much as 75% of total body potassium and exerts considerable influence on extracellular $K^+$. Short-term and long-term regulation of muscle $Na^+$-$K^+$-ATPase play a dominant role in determining the distribution of $K^+$ between the intracellular and extracellular spaces; the various hormones and physiologic conditions that affect the uptake of $K^+$ by skeletal muscle are reviewed in Chapter 17. Second, the colon has the ability to absorb and secrete $K^+$, with considerable mechanistic and regulatory similarities to renal $K^+$ secretion. $K^+$ secretion in the distal colon is increased after dietary loading and in end-stage renal disease.[14,473,474] However, the colon has a relatively limited capacity for $K^+$ excretion, such that changes in renal $K^+$ excretion play the dominant role in responding to changes in $K^+$ intake. In particular, regulated $K^+$ secretion by the CNT and CCD plays a critical role in the response to hyperkalemia and $K^+$ loading; increases in the reabsorption of $K^+$ by intercalated cells of the CCD and OMCD function in the response to hypokalemia or $K^+$ deprivation.

This section reviews the mechanisms and regulation of transepithelial $K^+$ transport along the nephron. As in other sections of this chapter, the emphasis is on particularly recent developments in the molecular physiology of renal $K^+$ transport. Of note, transport pathways for $K^+$ play important roles in renal $Na^+$-$Cl^-$ transport, particularly within the TAL. Furthermore, $Na^+$ absorption via ENaC in the aldosterone-sensitive distal nephron generates a lumen-negative PD that drives distal $K^+$ excretion. These pathways are primarily discussed in the section on renal $Na^+$-$Cl^-$ transport; related issues relevant to $K^+$ homeostasis per se will be specifically addressed in this section.

## PROXIMAL TUBULE

The PT reabsorbs some 50% to 70% of filtered $K^+$ (Fig. 6.23). PTs generate minimal transepithelial $K^+$ gradients, and fractional reabsorption of $K^+$ is similar to that of $Na^+$.[282] $K^+$ absorption follows that of fluid, $Na^+$, and other solutes, such that this nephron segment does not play a direct role in regulated renal excretion.[475,476] Notably, however, changes in $Na^+$-$Cl^-$ reabsorption by the PT have considerable effects on distal tubular flow and distal tubular $Na^+$ delivery, with attendant effects on the excretory capacity for $K^+$ (see the section "Distal Nephron, $K^+$ secretion" below).

The mechanisms involved in transepithelial $K^+$ transport by the PT are not completely clear, although active transport does not appear to play a major role.[476,477] Luminal barium has modest effects on transepithelial $K^+$ transport by the PT, suggesting a component of transcellular transport via barium-sensitive $K^+$ channels.[478] However, the bulk of $K^+$ transport is thought to occur via the paracellular pathway, driven by the lumen-positive PD in the mid to late PT (Fig. 6.2).[478,479] The total $K^+$ permeability of the PT is thus rather high, apparently due to features of the paracellular pathway.[478,479] The combination of luminal $K^+$ concentrations that are about 10% higher than that of plasma, a lumen-positive PD of about 2 mV (Fig. 6.2), and high paracellular permeability leads to considerable paracellular absorption in the PT. This absorption is thought to primarily proceed via convective transport—solvent drag due to frictional interactions between water and $K^+$—rather than diffusional transport.[480] Notably, however, the primary pathway for water movement in the PT is conclusively transcellular via aquaporin-1 and aquaporin-7 water channels in the apical and basolateral membrane.[19,34,35] Therefore the apparent convective transport of $K^+$ would have to constitute so-called pseudosolvent drag, with hypothetical uncharacterized interactions between water traversing the transcellular route and diffusion of $K^+$ along the paracellular pathway.[480]

## LOOP OF HENLE

Transport by the loop of Henle plays a critical role in medullary $K^+$ recycling (Fig. 6.24). Several lines of evidence have indicated that a considerable fraction of $K^+$ secreted by the CCD is reabsorbed by the medullary collecting ducts and then secreted into the late PT and/or descending thin

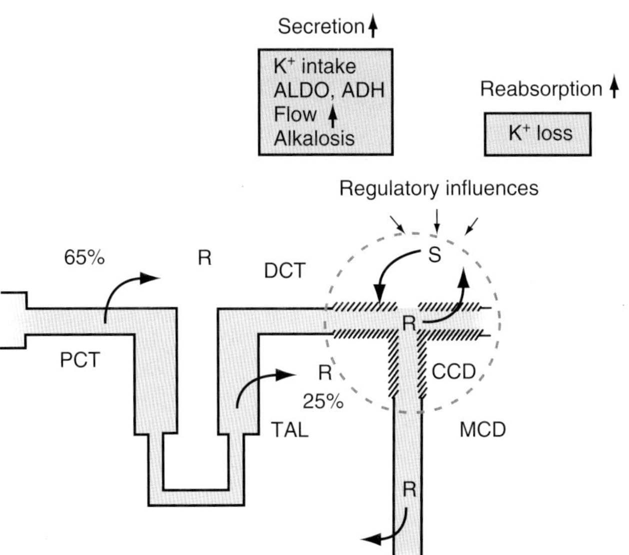


**Fig. 6.23** $K^+$ transport along the nephron. Approximately 90% of filtered $K^+$ is reabsorbed by the proximal tubule and the loop of Henle. $K^+$ is secreted along the initial and cortical collecting duct. Net reabsorption occurs in response to $K^+$ depletion, primarily within the medullary collecting duct. *ADH,* Antidiuretic hormone; *ALDO,* aldosterone; *CCD,* cortical collecting duct; *DCT,* distal convoluted tubule; *MCD,* medullary collecting duct; *PCT,* proximal convoluted tubule; *R,* reabsorption; *S,* secretion; *TAL,* thick ascending limb.

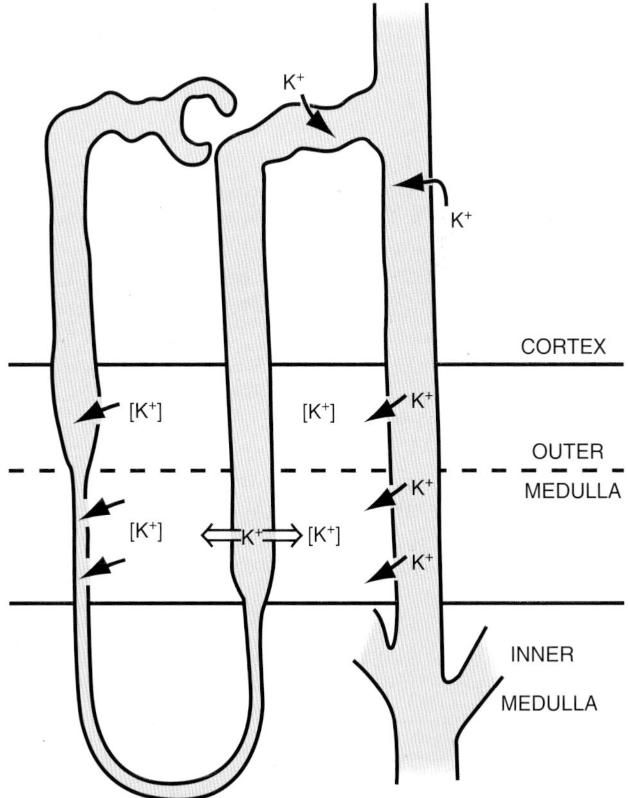


**Fig. 6.24** Schematic representation of medullary $K^+$ recycling. Medullary interstitial $K^+$ increases considerably after dietary $K^+$ loading due to the combined effects of secretion in the cortical collecting duct, absorption in the outer medullary collecting duct, thick ascending limb, and inner medullary collecting duct, and secretion in the descending thin limb. See text for details. (From Stokes JB. Consequences of potassium recycling in the renal medulla. Effects of ion transport by the medullary thick ascending limb of the loop of Henle. *J Clin Invest.* 1982;70:219–229.)

limbs of long-looped nephrons.[481] In potassium-loaded rats, there is thus a doubling of luminal $K^+$ in the terminal thin descending limbs, with a sharp drop after inhibition of CCD $K^+$ secretion by amiloride.[482] Enhancement of CCD $K^+$ secretion by treatment with DDAVP also results in an increase in luminal $K^+$ in the descending thin limbs.[483] This recycling pathway (secretion in CCD, absorption in OMCD and IMCD, secretion in descending thin limb) is associated with a marked increase in medullary interstitial $K^+$. Passive transepithelial $K^+$ absorption by the thin ascending limb and active absorption by the TAL also contribute to this increase in interstitial $K^+$ (Fig. 6.24).[181] Specifically, the absorption of $K^+$ by the ascending thin limb, TAL, and OMCD exceeds the secretion by the descending thin limbs, thus trapping $K^+$ in the interstitium.

The physiologic significance of medullary $K^+$ recycling is not completely clear. However, an increase in interstitial $K^+$ concentration from 5 to 25 mmol/L dramatically inhibits $Cl^-$ (and to a lesser extent, $Na^+$) transport by perfused TALs.[181] By inhibiting $Na^+$-$Cl^-$ absorption by the TAL, increases in interstitial $K^+$ contribute to the well-documented diuretic effects of a high-$K^+$ diet,[484] and would increase $Na^+$ delivery to the CNT and CCD, thus enhancing the lumen-negative PD in these tubules and increasing $K^+$ secretion.[181] Alternatively, the marked increase in medullary interstitial $K^+$ after dietary $K^+$ loading serves to limit the difference between luminal and peritubular $K^+$ in the CCD, thus minimizing passive $K^+$ loss from the collecting duct.

$K^+$ is secreted into the descending thin limbs by passive diffusion, driven by the high medullary interstitial $K^+$ concentration. Descending thin limbs thus have a very high-$K^+$ permeability, without evidence for active transepithelial $K^+$ transport.[485] Transepithelial $K^+$ transport by ascending thin limbs has not to our knowledge been measured; however, as is the case for $Na^+$-$Cl^-$ transport (see the "$Na^+$-$Cl^-$ Transport by the Thin Ascending Limb" section), the absorption of $K^+$ by the thin ascending limbs is presumably passive. Active transepithelial $K^+$ transport across the TAL includes a transcellular component, via apical $Na^+$-$K^+$-$2Cl^-$ cotransport mediated by NKCC2, and a paracellular pathway (Fig. 6.14). Luminal $K^+$ channels play a critical role in generating the lumen-positive PD in the TAL, as summarized earlier (see the "$Na^+$-$Cl^-$ Transport by the Thick Ascending Limb: Apical $K^+$ Channels" section). Secretion of $K^+$ through these may also play a role in the response to high dietary $K^+$. Patch-clamp analysis of split-open TALs revealed that 70-pS ROMK exhibited a higher open probability (Po) in mice placed on a low-$Na^+$/high-$K^+$ diet.[486] This may be dependent on NKCC2 activity, because micropuncture showed that furosemide increased $K^+$ secretion in the early distal tubule in mice on a normal diet, but decreased it in mice on the low-$Na^+$/high-$K^+$ diet.

## DISTAL NEPHRON

### $K^+$ SECRETION

Approximately 90% of filtered $K^+$ is reabsorbed by the PT and loop of Henle (Fig. 6.23); the fine-tuning of renal $K^+$ excretion occurs in the remaining distal nephron. The bulk of regulated secretion occurs in principal cells within the CNT and CCD, whereas $K^+$ reabsorption primarily occurs in the OMCD (see later). A low rate of $K^+$ secretion is initially detectable in the early DCT, in which NCC-positive cells express ROMK, the apical $K^+$ secretory channel.[190,487] Generally, the CCD is considered the primary site for distal $K^+$ secretion, partially due to the greater ease with which this segment is perfused and studied. However, as is the case for $Na^+$-$Cl^-$ absorption (see the "Connecting Tubules and the Cortical Collecting Duct: Apical $Na^+$ Transport" section), the bulk of distal $K^+$ secretion appears to occur prior to the CCD, within the CNT.[282,371]

In principal cells, apical $Na^+$ entry via ENaC generates a lumen-negative PD, which drives passive $K^+$ exit through apical $K^+$ channels. Distal $K^+$ secretion is therefore dependent on delivery of adequate luminal $Na^+$ to the CNT and CCD, essentially ceasing when luminal $Na^+$ drops below 8 mmol/L.[488–490] Dietary $Na^+$ intake also influences $K^+$ excretion, such that excretion is enhanced by excess $Na^+$ intake and reduced by $Na^+$ restriction.[488,489] Secreted $K^+$ enters principal cells via the basolateral $Na^+$-$K^+$-ATPase, which also generates the gradient that drives apical $Na^+$ entry via ENaC (Fig. 6.23).

Two major subtypes of apical $K^+$ channels function in secretion by the CNT and CCD, with or without the DCT; a small-conductance (SK), 30-pS channel and a large-conductance, $Ca^{2+}$-activated, 150-pS (maxi-K or BK) channel.[191,371,491] The density and high $P_o$ of the SK channel indicates that this pathway alone is sufficient to mediate the bulk of $K^+$ secretion in the CCD under baseline conditions—hence, its designation as the secretory $K^+$ channel.[492] Notably, SK channel density is considerably higher in the CNT than in the CCD, consistent with the greater capacity for $Na^+$ absorption and $K^+$ secretion in the CNT.[36] The characteristics of the SK channel are similar to those of the ROMK $K^+$ channel, and ROMK protein has been localized at the apical membrane of principal cells.[188,493] SK channel activity is absent from apical membranes of the CCD in homozygous knockout mice with a targeted deletion of the *Kcnj1* gene that encodes ROMK, definitive proof that ROMK is the SK channel.[191] The observation that these knockout mice are normokalemic, with an increased excretion of $K^+$, illustrates the considerable redundancy in distal $K^+$ secretory pathways; distal $K^+$ secretion in these mice is mediated by apical BK channels (see later).[191,494] However, dietary $K^+$ loading induced hyperkalemia in ROMK1 knockout mice, consistent with a role in $K^+$ secretion along the CCD.[193] Of interest, loss-of-function mutations in human *KCNJ1* genes are associated with Bartter syndrome; ROMK expression is critical for the 30- and 70-pS channels that generate the lumen-positive PD in the TAL (Fig. 6.14).[191,192] These patients typically have slightly higher serum $K^+$ levels than those with other genetic forms of Bartter syndrome, and affected patients with severe neonatal hyperkalemia have also been described; this neonatal hyperkalemia is presumably the result of a transient developmental deficit in apical BK channel activity.[14,183] Note that Bartter syndrome due to *KCNJ1* disruption may specifically reflect a defect in ROMK2 and/or ROMK3 function since mice with disruption of ROMK1, consistent with its absence along the TAL, do not display a Bartter syndrome phenotype.[193]

The apical $Ca^{2+}$-activated BK channel plays a critical role in flow-dependent $K^+$ secretion by the CNT and CCD.[491] BK channels have a heteromeric structure, with α-subunits that form the ion channel pore and modulatory β-subunits that affect the biophysical, regulatory, and pharmacologic characteristics of the channel complex.[491] BK α-subunit transcripts are expressed in multiple nephron segments, and channel protein is detectable at the apical membrane of principal and intercalated cells in the CCD and CNT.[491] The β-subunits are differentially expressed within the distal nephron. Thus $\beta_1$-subunits are restricted to the CNT, with no expression in intercalated cells, whereas $\beta_4$-subunits are detectable at the apical membranes of the TAL, DCT, and intercalated cells.[491,495] Increased distal flow has a well-established stimulatory effect on $K^+$ secretion, due in part to enhanced delivery and absorption of $Na^+$ and to increased removal of secreted $K^+$.[488,489] The pharmacology of flow-dependent $K^+$ secretion in the CCD is consistent with dominant involvement of BK channels, and flow-dependent $K^+$ secretion is reduced in mice with targeted deletion of the $\alpha_1$- and $\beta_1$-subunits.[491,496–498] Both mice strains develop hyperaldosteronism that is exacerbated by a high-$K^+$ diet, leading to hypertension in the $\alpha_1$-subunit knockout.[498] Disruption of the β2 subunit also leads to hyperaldosteronism, but flow-induced $K^+$ secretion is normal, suggesting compensation by other isoforms.[499] $Ca^{2+}$-dependence of BK activation involves TRPV4.[500–502] A high-$K^+$ diet increases TRPV4 expression, and leads to its redistribution to the apical membrane in CCD. The importance of this process in BK activation was demonstrated in TRPV4 knockout mice, which display decreased BK activity in CCD, and hyperkalemia after dietary $K^+$ loading.

One enigma has been the greater density of BK channels in intercalated cells in both the CCD and CNT.[503,504] This has suggested a major role for intercalated cells in $K^+$ secretion; however, the much lower density of $Na^+$-$K^+$-ATPase activity in intercalated cells has been considered inadequate to support $K^+$ secretion across the apical membrane.[505] More recent evidence has revealed a major role for the basolateral $Na^+$-$K^+$-$2Cl^-$ cotransporter NKCC1 in $K^+$ secretion mediated by apical BK channels. NKCC1 is expressed almost exclusively at the basolateral membrane of intercalated cells, providing an alternative entry pathway for basolateral $K^+$ secreted at the apical membrane.[506,507] This still begs the question of how basolateral $Na^+$ recycles across the basolateral membrane in the absence of significant $Na^+$-$K^+$-ATPase activity; one possibility is an alternative basolateral $Na^+$ pump, the ouabain-insensitive furosemide-sensitive $Na^+$-ATPase, a transport activity that has been detected in cell culture models of intercalated cells.[506] At the apical membrane, BK-mediated $K^+$ secretion is only partially dependent on luminal $Na^+$; $K^+$ secretion would eventually hyperpolarize the membrane in the absence of apical $Na^+$ entry, which is mediated by ENaC in principal cells.[508] An intriguing possibility is that apical $Cl^-$ channels allow for the parallel secretion of $K^+$ and $Cl^-$ in intercalated cells.[509]

BK channels also play a critical role in cell volume regulation by intercalated cells, with indirect, flow-mediated influences on distal $K^+$ secretion. MDCK-C11 cells have an intercalated cell phenotype and express BK α- and $\beta_4$-subunits, as do intercalated cells; shear stress activates BK channels in these cells, leading to loss of $K^+$ and cell shrinkage.[495,510] Mice with a targeted deletion of the $\beta_4$-subunit exhibit normal $K^+$ excretion on a normal diet.[505] However, when fed a high-$K^+$ diet, which increases urinary and tubular flow rates and tubular shear stress, the $\beta_4$-knockout mice develop hyperkalemia with a blunted increase in $K^+$ excretion and urinary flow rates. Intercalated cells from $\beta_4$-knockouts fail to significantly decrease cell volume in response to high-$K^+$ diet. Intercalated cells thus function as so-called speed bumps that protrude into the lumen of distal tubules; flow-activated BK channels reduce the cell volume of intercalated cells after $K^+$ loading, reducing tubular resistance, increasing tubular flow rates, and increasing distal $K^+$ secretion.[505]

The physiologic rationale for the presence of two apical secretory $K^+$ channels, ROMK/SK and BK channels, is not completely clear. However, the high density and higher $P_o$ of ROMK/SK channels are perhaps better suited for a role in basal $K^+$ secretion, with additional recruitment of the higher capacity, flow-activated BK channels when additional $K^+$ secretion is required.[491] Evolving evidence has also indicated that BK channels function in partially $Na^+$-independent $K^+$ secretion by intercalated cells, with ROMK functioning in ENaC- and $Na^+$-dependent $K^+$ excretion by DCT, CNT, and CCD cells. Regardless, at the whole-organ level, the two $K^+$ channels can substitute for one another, with BK-dependent $K^+$ secretion in ROMK knockout mice and an upregulation of ROMK in the distal nephron of $\alpha_1$-subunit BK knockouts.[494,497]

Other $K^+$ channels reportedly expressed at the luminal membranes of the CNT and CCD include voltage-sensitive channels such as Kv1.3, the calcium-activated, small-conductance SK3 channel, and double-pore $K^+$ channels, such as TWIK-1 and KCNQ1.[511–514] KCNQ1 mediates $K^+$ secretion in the inner ear and is expressed at the apical membrane of principal cells in the CCD, whereas TWIK-1 is expressed at the apical membrane of intercalated cells.[514,515] The roles of these channels in renal $K^+$ secretion or absorption are not fully characterized. However, Kv1.3 may play a role in distal $K^+$ secretion in that luminal margatoxin, a specific blocker of this channel, reduces $K^+$ secretion in CCDs of rat kidneys from animals on a high-$K^+$ diet.[516] Other apical $K^+$ channels in the distal nephron may subserve other physiologic functions. For example, the apical Kv1.1 channel is critically involved in $Mg^{2+}$ transport by the DCT, likely by hyperpolarizing the apical membrane and increasing the driving force for $Mg^{2+}$ influx via TRPM6 (transient receptor potential cation channel 6); missense mutations in *KV1.1* are a cause of genetic hypomagnesemia.[517]

$K^+$ channels present at the basolateral membrane of principal cells appear to set the resting potential of the basolateral membrane and function in $K^+$ secretion and $Na^+$ absorption at the apical membrane, the latter via $K^+$ recycling at the basolateral membrane to maintain activity of the $Na^+$-$K^+$-ATPase. A variety of different $K^+$ channels have been described in the electrophysiologic characterization of the basolateral membrane of principal cells, which has a number of technical barriers to overcome.[518] However, a single predominant activity has been identified in principal cells from the rat CCD using whole-cell recording techniques under conditions in which ROMK is inhibited (low intracellular pH or presence of the ROMK inhibitor tertiapin-Q).[518] This basolateral current is tetraethylammonium-insensitive, barium-sensitive, and acid-sensitive ($pK_a \cong 6.5$), with a conductance of about 17 pS and weak inward rectification. These properties do not correspond exactly to specific characterized $K^+$ channels or combinations thereof. However, candidate inward-rectifying $K^+$ channel subunits that have been localized at the basolateral membrane of the CCD include KIR4.1, KIR5.1, KIR7.1, and KIR2.3.[518] KIR4.1 and KIR5.1 channels generate a predominant 40-pS basolateral $K^+$ channel in murine principal cells,[519] with both KIR4.1 and KIR5.1 participating in generating the membrane potential that permits $Na^+$ entry through ENaC.[227,520] Notably, basolateral $K^+$ channel activity increases on a high-$K^+$ diet, suggesting a role in transepithelial $K^+$ secretion.[518] Disruption of KIR5.1 in rats reveals it plays a critical role in mediating collecting duct function, particularly with respect to maintenance of $K^+$ homeostasis.[520] Activation of KIR4.1/5.1 by insulin and insulin-like growth factor-1 (IGF-1) may also facilitate $Na^+$ reabsorption along the CCD by hyperpolarizing the basolateral membrane.[521]

In addition to apical $K^+$ channels, considerable evidence has implicated apical $K^+$-$Cl^-$ cotransport (or functionally equivalent pathways) in distal $K^+$ secretion.[67,488,522,523] Thus, in rat distal tubules, a reduction in luminal $Cl^-$ markedly increases $K^+$ secretion; the replacement of luminal $Cl^-$ with $SO_4^-$ or gluconate has an equivalent stimulatory effect on $K^+$ secretion.[524] This anion-dependent component of $K^+$ secretion is not influenced by luminal $Ba^{2+}$, suggesting that it does not involve apical $K^+$ channel activity.[524] Perfused surface distal tubules are a mixture of the DCT, connecting segment, and initial collecting duct; however, $Cl^-$-coupled $K^+$ secretion is detectable in the DCT and in early CNT.[525] In addition, similar pathways are detectable in rabbit CCD, where a decrease in luminal $Cl^-$ concentration from 112 to 5 mmol/L increases $K^+$ secretion by 48%.[526] A reduction in basolateral $Cl^-$ also decreases $K^+$ secretion without an effect on transepithelial voltage or $Na^+$ transport, and the direction of $K^+$ flux can be reversed by a lumen to bath $Cl^-$ gradient, resulting in $K^+$ absorption.[526] In perfused CCDs from rats treated with mineralocorticoid, vasopressin increases $K^+$ secretion; because this increase in $K^+$ secretion is resistant to luminal $Ba^{2+}$ (2 mmol/L), vasopressin may stimulate $Cl^-$-dependent $K^+$ secretion.[14,527] Pharmacologic study results of perfused tubules are consistent with $K^+$-$Cl^-$ cotransport mediated by the KCCs; however, of the three renal KCCs, only KCC1 is apically expressed along the nephron.[67,523] Other functional possibilities for $Cl^-$-dependent $K^+$ secretion include parallel operation of apical $H^+$-$K^+$-exchange and $Cl^-$-$HCO_3^-$ exchange in type B intercalated cells.[522]

A provocative study by Frindt and Palmer serves to underline the importance of ENaC-independent $K^+$ excretion, whether it is mediated by apical $K^+$-$Cl^-$ cotransport and/or by other mechanisms (see also the "Integrated $Na^+$-$Cl^-$ and $K^+$ Transport in the Distal Nephron" section).[528] Rats were infused with amiloride via osmotic minipumps, generating urinary concentrations considered sufficient to inhibit more than 98% of ENaC activity. Whereas amiloride almost abolished $K^+$ excretion in rats on a normal $K^+$ intake, acute and long-term high-$K^+$ diets led to an increasing fraction of $K^+$ excretion that was independent of ENaC activity (≈50% after 7–9 days on a high-$K^+$ diet).

## $K^+$ REABSORPTION BY THE COLLECTING DUCT

In addition to $K^+$ secretion, the distal nephron is capable of considerable reabsorption, primarily during restriction of dietary $K^+$.[282–284] This reabsorption is accomplished largely by intercalated cells in the OMCD via the activity of apical $H^+/K^+$-ATPase pumps. Under $K^+$-replete conditions, apical $H^+/K^+$-ATPase activity recycles $K^+$ with an apical $K^+$ channel, without an effect on transepithelial $K^+$ absorption. Under $K^+$-restricted basolateral conditions, $K^+$ absorbed via apical $H^+/K^+$-ATPase appears to exit intercalated cells via a $K^+$ channel, thus achieving the transepithelial transport of $K^+$.[529]

$H^+$-$K^+$-ATPase holoenzymes are members of the P-type family of ion transport ATPases, which also includes subunits of the basolateral $Na^+$-$K^+$-ATPase.[530] $HK\alpha_1$ and $HK\alpha_2$ are also referred to as the gastric and colonic subunits, respectively; humans also have an $HK\alpha_4$-subunit.[530,531] A specific $HK\beta$ subunit interacts with the $HK\alpha$ subunits to ensure delivery to the cell surface and complete expression of $H^+$-$K^+$-ATPase activity; $HK\alpha_2$ and $HK\alpha_4$ subunits are also capable of interaction with $Na^+$-$K^+$-ATPase β-subunits.[14,532] The pharmacology of $H^+$-$K^+$-ATPase holoenzymes differs considerably, such that the gastric $HK\alpha_1$ subunit is typically sensitive to the $H^+$-$K^+$-ATPase inhibitors SCH-28080 and omeprazole and resistant to ouabain; the colonic $HK\alpha_2$ subunit is usually sensitive to ouabain and resistant to SCH-28080.[532] Within the kidney, the $HK\alpha_1$ subunit is expressed at the apical membrane of at least a subset of type A intercalated cells in the distal nephron.[531] $HK\alpha_2$-subunit distribution in the distal nephron is more diffuse, with robust expression at the apical membrane of types A and B intercalated cells and connecting segment cells and lesser expression in principal cells.[533–535] The human $HK\alpha_4$ subunit is reportedly expressed in intercalated cells.[531]

$HK\alpha_1$ and $HK\alpha_2$ subunits are both constitutively expressed in the distal nephron. However, tubule perfusion of $K^+$-replete animals suggests a functional dominance of omeprazole/SCH-28080-sensitive, ouabain-resistant $H^+$-$K^+$-ATPase activity, consistent with holoenzymes containing the $HK\alpha_1$ subunit.[536] $K^+$ deprivation increases the overall activity of $H^+$-$K^+$-ATPase in the collecting duct, with the emergence of ouabain-sensitive $H^+$-$K^+$-ATPase activity; this is consistent with a relative dominance of the $HK\alpha_2$ subunit during $K^+$-restricted conditions.[14] $K^+$ restriction also induces a dramatic upregulation of the $HK\alpha_2$-subunit transcript and protein in the outer and inner medulla during $K^+$ depletion; $HK\alpha_1$-subunit expression is unaffected.[14] Mice with targeted deletion of the $HK\alpha_2$ subunit exhibit lower plasma and muscle $K^+$ than wild type littermates when maintained on a $K^+$-deficient diet. However, this appears to be due to marked loss of $K^+$ in the colon rather than in the kidney, because renal $K^+$ excretion is appropriately reduced in the $K^+$-depleted knockout mice.[285] Presumably the lack of an obvious renal phenotype in $HK\alpha_1$- or $HK\alpha_2$-subunit knockout mice reflects the marked redundancy in the expression of $HK\alpha$ subunits in the distal nephron.[285,537] Indeed, collecting ducts from the $HK\alpha_1$-subunit knockout mice have significant residual ouabain-resistant and SCH-28080-sensitive $H^+$-$K^+$-ATPase activities, consistent with the expression of other $HK\alpha$-subunits that confer characteristics similar to the "gastric" $H^+$-$K^+$-ATPase.[538] However, data from $HK\alpha_1$- and $HK\alpha_2$-subunit knockout mice have suggested that compensatory mechanisms in these mice are not accounted for by ATPase-type mechanisms.[539]

The importance of $K^+$ reabsorption mediated by the collecting duct is dramatically illustrated by the phenotype of transgenic mice with generalized overexpression of a gain-of-function mutation in $H^+$-$K^+$-ATPase, effectively bypassing the redundancy and complexity of this reabsorptive pathway. This transgene expresses a mutant form of the $HK\beta$-subunit, in which a tyrosine-to-alanine mutation within the carboxyl-terminal tail abrogates regulated endocytosis from the plasma membrane; these mice have higher plasma $K^+$ than their wild type littermates, with approximately half the fractional excretion of $K^+$.[540]

The $H^+$,$K^+$-ATPase may also serve to recycle $K^+$, facilitating downregulation of ENaC by the purinergic signaling system during high dietary $Na^+$ intake. ENaC activity in $HK\alpha_1$ knockout mice is uncoupled from dietary $Na^+$ intake, and urinary [ATP] is not increased by a high-$Na^+$ diet, as in wild type mice.[541]

## REGULATION OF DISTAL $K^+$ TRANSPORT

### MODULATION OF RENAL OUTER MEDULLARY POTASSIUM CHANNEL ACTIVITY

ROMK and other Kir channels are inward-rectifying—that is, $K^+$ flows inward more readily than outward (Kir, inward rectifying renal $K^+$ channel). Even though outward conductance is usually less than inward conductance, $K^+$ efflux through the ROMK predominates in the CNT and CCD because the membrane potential is more positive than the equilibrium potential for $K^+$. Intracellular magnesium ($Mg^{2+}$) and polyamines play key roles in inward rectification, binding, and blocking the pore of the channel from the cytoplasmic side.[542–544] A single transmembrane residue, asparagine-171 in ROMK1, controls the affinity and blocking effect of $Mg^{2+}$ and polyamines.[542,543] Intracellular $Mg^{2+}$ in the TAL, DCT, CNT, and principal cells is thought to have a significant effect on ROMK activity because it inhibits outward ROMK-dependent currents in principal cells.[545] The blocking affinity of $Mg^{2+}$ is enhanced at lower extracellular $K^+$ concentrations, which should aid in reducing $K^+$ secretion during hypokalemia and $K^+$ deficiency.[545] A reduction of this intracellular $Mg^{2+}$ block may also explain the hypokalemia associated with hypomagnesemia, wherein distal $K^+$ secretion is enhanced.[544,545]

In addition to inward rectification, the endogenous ROMK channels in the TAL and principal cells exhibit a very high channel $P_o$. The high $P_o$ of ROMK is maintained by the combined effects of binding of PIP2 to the channel protein, direct channel phosphorylation by PKA, ATP binding to the ROMK–CFTR complex, and cytoplasmic pH. PIP2 binding to ROMK is thus required to maintain the channel in an open state, whereas cytoplasmic acidification inhibits the channel.[546] PKA phosphorylates ROMK protein at one amino-terminal serines and two carboxyl-terminal serines—S25, S200, and S294 in the ROMK2 isoform.[256] Phosphorylation of all three sites is required for full channel function. Phosphorylation of the amino-terminal site overrides the effect of a carboxy-terminal endoplasmic reticulum retention signal, thus increasing expression of the channel protein at the cell membrane.[547] Phosphorylation of S200 and S294 maintains the channel in a high $P_o$ state, in part by modulating the effects of PIP2, ATP, and pH.[195,258,259]

Because ROMK channels exhibit such a high $P_o$, physiologic regulation of the channel is primarily achieved by regulated changes in the number of active channels on the plasma membrane. The associated mechanisms are discussed in the context of the adaptation to $K^+$ loading and hyperkalemia and $K^+$ deprivation and hypokalemia.

### ALDOSTERONE AND $K^+$ LOADING

Aldosterone has a potent kaliuretic effect, with important interrelationships between circulating $K^+$ and aldosterone.[548] Aldosterone release by the adrenal is thus induced by hyperkalemia and/or a high-$K^+$ diet, suggesting an important feedback effect of aldosterone on $K^+$ homeostasis.[549] Aldosterone also has clinically relevant effects on $K^+$ homeostasis, with a clear relationship at all levels of serum $K^+$ between circulating levels of the hormone and the ability to excrete $K^+$.

Aldosterone has no effect on the density of apical ROMK channels in the CCD; it does, however, induce a marked increase in the density of apical $Na^+$ channels in the CNT and CCD.[550] This hormone activates ENaC via interrelated effects on the synthesis, trafficking, and membrane-associated activity of the subunits encoding the channel (see the "Regulation of $Na^+$-$Cl^-$ Transport in the Connecting Tubule and Cortical Collecting Duct" section). Aldosterone is thus induced by a high-$K^+$ diet and strongly stimulates apical ENaC activity, which provides the lumen-negative PD that stimulates $K^+$ secretion by principal cells.

The important relationships between $K^+$ and aldosterone notwithstanding, it is increasingly clear that much of the adaptation to a high-$K^+$ intake is aldosterone independent. For example, a high-$K^+$ diet in adrenalectomized animals increases apical $Na^+$ reabsorption and $K^+$ secretion in the CCD.[551] At the tubular level, when basolateral $K^+$ is increased, there is significant activation of $Na^+$-$K^+$-ATPase, accompanied by a secondary activation of apical $Na^+$ and $K^+$ channels.[552] Increased dietary $K^+$ also markedly increases the density of ROMK channels in the CCD, along with a modest increase in $Na^+$ channel (ENaC) density; this is associated with changes in the subcellular distribution of the ROMK protein, with an increase in apical expression.[550,553] Notably, this increase in ENaC and ROMK density in the CCD occurs within hours of consuming a high-$K^+$ diet, with a minimal associated increase in circulating aldosterone (Table 6.1).[554] By contrast, a week of low $Na^+$-$Cl^-$ intake, with almost a 1000-fold increase in aldosterone, has no effect on ROMK channel density, nor for that matter does 2 days of aldosterone infusion, despite the development of hypokalemia (Table 6.1).[554] Unlike the marked increase seen in the CCD, the density of ROMK channels in the CNT is not increased by high dietary $K^+$,[371,550,554] but this may reflect difficulties in estimating channel densities in small membrane patches. Measurement of whole cell currents using the ROMK inhibitor tertiapin-Q indicates an upregulation of ROMK activity in the CNT by a high-$K^+$ diet.[555]

BK channels in the CNT and CCD play an important role in the flow-activated component of distal $K^+$ excretion; these channels are also activated by dietary $K^+$ loading.[491] Flow-stimulated $K^+$ secretion by the CCD of mice and rats is thus enhanced on a high-$K^+$ diet, with an absence of flow-dependent $K^+$ secretion in rats on a low-$K^+$ diet.[494,556] This is accompanied by the appropriate changes in transcript levels for $\alpha$ and $\beta_{2-4}$ subunits of the BK channel proteins in microdissected CCDs ($\beta_1$ subunits are restricted to the CNT).[491] Trafficking of BK subunits is also affected by dietary $K^+$, with a largely intracellular distribution of $\alpha$ subunits in $K^+$-restricted rodents and prominent apical expression in $K^+$-loaded rodents.[500,556] Aldosterone does not contribute to the regulation of BK channel activity or expression in response to a high-$K^+$ diet.[557]

The changes in trafficking and/or activity of the ROMK channel that are induced by dietary $K^+$ appear in large part to involve tyrosine phosphorylation and dephosphorylation of the ROMK protein (see later). However, a series of reports have linked changes in expression of WNK1 kinase subunits

**Table 6.1 Effect of High-K⁺ Diet, Aldosterone, and/or Na⁺-Cl⁻ Restriction on SK Channel Density in the Rat Cortical Collecting Duct**

| Parameter | K⁺ Channel Density (μm²) | Plasma Aldosterone (ng/dL) | Plasma K (mmol/L) |
|---|---|---|---|
| Control | 0.41 | 15 | 3.68 |
| High-K⁺ diet, 6 hours | 1.51 | 36 | NM |
| High-K⁺ diet, 48 hours | 2.13 | 98 | 4.37 |
| Low-Na⁺ diet, 7 days | 0.48 | 1260 | NM |
| Aldosterone infusion, 48 hours | 0.44 | 550 | 2.44 |
| Aldosterone + high-K⁺ diet | 0.32 | 521 | 3.80 |

*NM,* Not measured.

Modified from Palmer LG, Frindt G. Regulation of apical K channels in rat cortical collecting tubule during changes in dietary K intake. *Am J Physiol.* 1999;277:F805–F812.

in the response to a high-$K^+$ diet. WNK1 and WNK4 were initially identified as causative genes for FHHt (see also the "Regulation of $Na^+$-$Cl^-$ Transport in the Distal Convoluted Tubule" section). ROMK expression at the membrane of *Xenopus* oocytes is dramatically reduced by coexpression of WNK4; FHHt-associated mutations dramatically increase this effect, suggesting a direct inhibition of SK channels in FHHt.[558] This is further supported by a recent patch-clamp study that showed DCT2/CNT isolated from transgenic mice expressing FHHt-causing mutant WNK4 has lower ENaC and ROMK activity, suggesting direct, NCC-independent effects of the mutant.[559] The aldosterone-induced SGK1 is activated by the upstream kinase mTORC2. Disruption of mTORC2 in renal epithelia in mice causes profound hyperkalemia when they are placed on a high-$K^+$ diet. Patch-clamp analysis showed that in CNT/CCD, while ENaC activity was unaltered, $Ba^{2+}$-sensitive $K^+$ currents were almost absent. SGK1 phosphorylation was ablated, suggesting that hyperkalemia may result from unchecked WNK4-mediated ROMK endocytosis.[560]

The study of WNK1 is further complicated by the transcriptional complexity of its gene, which has at least three separate promoters and a number of alternative splice forms. In particular, the predominant intrarenal WNK1 isoform is generated by a distal nephron transcriptional site that bypasses the amino-terminal exons that encode the kinase domain, yielding a kinase-deficient short form of the protein (WNK1-S, also known as kidney-specific [KS]-WNK1).[561] Full-length WNK1 (WNK1-L) inhibits ROMK activity by inducing endocytosis of the channel protein; kinase activity and/or the amino-terminal kinase domain of WNK1 appear to be required for this effect, although Cope and colleagues have reported that a kinase-dead mutant of WNK1 is unimpaired.[562–564] WNK1 and WNK4 induce endocytosis of ROMK via interaction with intersectin, a multimodular endocytic scaffold protein.[565] Additional binding of ROMK to the clathrin adaptor protein termed "autosomal recessive hypercholesterolemia" (ARH) is required for basal and WNK1-stimulated endocytosis of the channel protein.[566] Ubiquitination of ROMK protein is also involved in clathrin-dependent endocytosis, requiring interaction between the channel and the U3 ubiquitin ligase POSH (***p****lenty* ***o****f* ***SH*** domains).[567]

The shorter WNK1-S isoform, which lacks the kinase domain, appears to inhibit the effect of WNK1-L.[563,564] The ratio of WNK1-S to WNK1-L transcripts is reduced by $K^+$ restriction (greater endocytosis of ROMK) and increased by $K^+$ loading (reduced endocytosis of ROMK), suggesting that this ratio between WNK1-S and WNK1-L functions as a type of switch to regulate distal $K^+$ secretion.[563,564,568] The inhibitory effect of WNK1-S tracks to the first 253 amino acids of the protein, encompassing the initial 30 amino acids unique to this isoform and an adjacent autoinhibitory domain.[569] Transgenic mice that overexpress this inhibitory domain of WNK1-S have lower serum $K^+$ concentrations, higher fractional excretion of $K^+$, and increased expression of ROMK protein at the apical membrane of CNT and CCD cells—all consistent with an important inhibitory effect of WNK1-S.[569]

The BK channel is also regulated by the WNK kinases. WNK4 thus inhibits BK channel activity and protein expression, whereas FHHt-associated mutations in WNK4 also enhance the inhibitory effect via ubiquitination.[570–572] A high-$K^+$ diet increases WNK1-L expression selectively in intercalated cells,[573] and activates BK by reducing ERK1/2 signaling–mediated lysosomal degradation of the channel protein.[229]

## $K^+$ DEPRIVATION

A reduction in dietary $K^+$ leads within 24 hours to a dramatic drop in urinary $K^+$ excretion.[568,574] This drop in excretion is due to both an induction of reabsorption by intercalated cells in the OMCD and to a reduction in SK channel activity in principal cells.[14,283,284] The mechanisms involved in $K^+$ reabsorption by intercalated cells are discussed earlier; notably, $H^+/K^+$-ATPase activity in the collecting duct does not appear to be regulated by aldosterone.[575]

Considerable progress has been made in defining the signaling pathways that regulate the activity of the SK channel (ROMK) in response to changes in dietary $K^+$. Dietary $K^+$ intake modulates trafficking of the ROMK channel protein to the plasma membrane of principal cells, with a marked increase in the relative proportion of intracellular channel protein in $K^+$-depleted animals and clearly defined expression at the plasma membrane of CCD cells from animals on a high-$K^+$ diet.[553,576] The membrane insertion and activity of ROMK are modulated by tyrosine phosphorylation of the channel protein, such that phosphorylation of tyrosine residue 337 stimulates endocytosis and dephosphorylation induces exocytosis; this tyrosine phosphorylation appears to play a key role in the regulation of ROMK by dietary $K^+$.[577–579] Whereas the levels of protein tyrosine phosphatase-1D do not vary with $K^+$ intake, intrarenal activity of the cytoplasmic tyrosine kinases c-src and c-yes are inversely related to dietary $K^+$ intake, with a decrease under high-$K^+$ conditions and a marked increase after several days of $K^+$ restriction.[14,580] Localization studies have indicated coexpression of c-src with ROMK in the TAL and principal cells of the CCD.[553] Moreover, inhibition of protein tyrosine phosphatase activity, leading to a dominance of tyrosine phosphorylation, dramatically increases the proportion of intracellular ROMK in the CCD of animals on a high-$K^+$ diet.[553]

The neurohumoral factors that induce the $K^+$-dependent trafficking and expression of apical ROMK and BK channels have only come into focus rather recently.[553,556,576] Several studies have implicated the intrarenal generation of superoxide anions in the activation of cytoplasmic tyrosine kinases.[581–583] Potential candidates for the upstream kaliuretic factor include Ang II and growth factors such as IGF-1.[581] Ang II inhibits ROMK activity in $K^+$-restricted rats, but not rats on a normal $K^+$ diet.[584] This inhibition involves downstream activation of superoxide production and c-src activity, such that the well-known induction of Ang II by a low-$K^+$ diet appears to play a major role in reducing distal tubular $K^+$ secretion.[585]

Reports of transient postprandial kaliuresis in sheep, independent of changes in plasma $K^+$ or aldosterone, have suggested that an enteric or hepatoportal $K^+$ sensor controls kaliuresis via a sympathetic reflex; tissue kallikrein (TK) has recently emerged as a candidate mediator for this postprandial kaliuresis (see later).[586] Regardless of the signaling involved, changes in dietary $K^+$ absorption have a direct anticipatory effect on $K^+$ homeostasis in the absence of changes in plasma $K^+$. Such a feed-forward control has the theoretical advantage of greater stability because it operates prior to changes in plasma $K^+$.[587] Notably, changes in ROMK phosphorylation status and insulin-sensitive muscle uptake can be seen in $K^+$-deficient animals in the absence of a change in plasma $K^+$, suggesting that upstream activation of the major mechanisms that serve to reduce $K^+$ excretion (reduced $K^+$ secretion in the CNT and CCD, decreased peripheral uptake, and increased $K^+$ reabsorption in the OMCD) does not require changes in plasma $K^+$.[588] Consistent with this hypothesis, moderate $K^+$ restriction, without an associated drop in plasma $K^+$, is sufficient to induce Ang II–dependent superoxide generation and c-src activation, leading to inhibition of ROMK channel activity.[585]

### VASOPRESSIN

Vasopressin has a well-characterized stimulatory effect on $K^+$ secretion by the distal nephron.[483,589] From an evolutionary viewpoint, this vasopressin-dependent activation serves to preserve $K^+$ secretion during dehydration and extracellular volume depletion, when circulating levels of vasopressin are high and tubular delivery of $Na^+$ and fluid is reduced. The stimulation of basolateral $V_2Rs$ results in an activation of ENaC, which increases the driving force for $K^+$ secretion by principal cells; the relevant mechanisms have been discussed earlier in this chapter (see the "Regulation of $Na^+$-$Cl^-$ Transport in the Connecting Tubule and Cortical Collecting Duct: Vasopressin and Other Factors" section). In addition, vasopressin activates SK channels directly in the CCD, as does cAMP.[492,590] The ROMK is directly phosphorylated by PKA on three serine residues (S25, S200, and S294 in the ROMK2 isoform), with phosphorylation of all three sites required for full activity in *Xenopus* oocytes (see the "Regulation of $Na^+$-$Cl^-$ Transport by the Thick Ascending Limb: Activating Influences" section). Finally, the stimulation of luminal $V_1$ receptors also stimulates $K^+$ secretion in the CCD, apparently via activation of BK channels.[591]

### TISSUE KALLIKREIN

The serine protease TK is involved in the generation of kinins, ultimately stimulating the formation of bradykinin.[592] Within the kidney, TK is synthesized in CNT cells and released into the tubular lumen and peritubular interstitium. Although TK-induced bradykinin has a number of effects on distal tubular physiology, more recent data have revealed a provocative role in postprandial kaliuresis.[592] Thus oral $K^+$-$Cl^-$ loading leads to a spike in urinary $K^+$ and TK excretion in rats, mice, and humans.[592] The increase in urinary TK after $K^+$ loading is not accompanied by changes in urinary aldosterone and can be detected in aldosterone synthase knockout mice.[593] Mice deficient in TK demonstrate postprandial hyperkalemia, indicating a role for the protease in postprandial kaliuresis. This transient hyperkalemia is accompanied by a marked increase in $K^+$ reabsorption by perfused CCDs due to an upregulation of $H^+/K^+$-ATPase activity and an increase in $HK\alpha_2$-subunit transcript. The addition of luminal but not basolateral TK inhibits the activated CCD $H^+/K^+$-ATPase activity in the TK knockout mice, consistent with direct proteolytic activation. There is also a marked increase in $Na^+$ reabsorption by perfused CCDs from TK knockout mice, without development of a lumen-negative PD; this is consistent with an increased activity of the electroneutral $Na^+$-$Cl^-$ cotransport mediated by the $Na^+$-driven SLC4A8 $Cl^-$-$HCO_3^-$ exchanger and the SLC26A4 $Cl^-$-$HCO_3^-$ exchanger (see later discussion as well).[408] This electroneutral transport pathway had previously been shown to be inhibited by bradykinin; hence the activation by TK deletion presumably reflected loss of tonic inhibition by TK-generated bradykinin.[406] Previous data had indicated that TK mediates proteolytic cleavage of the $\gamma$ subunit of ENaC, with reduced ENaC activity in TK-deficient mice; net $Na^+$ balance is thus neutral in these mice.[594]

In summary, TK secretion from CNT cells is induced by oral $K^+$-$Cl^-$ loading, causing proteolytic activation of ENaC and thus an increase in ENaC-driven $K^+$ secretion, bradykinin-dependent inhibition of electroneutral $Na^+$-$Cl^-$ cotransport in the CCD.[406,408,594] There is consequently a further augmentation of electrogenic $Na^+$ transport (favoring $K^+$ secretion), and direct luminal inhibition of $H^+/K^+$-ATPase activity and thus a decrease or tonic inhibition of $K^+$ reabsorption. TK may very well be the postprandial factor that functions in feed-forward control of plasma $K^+$.[586,587]

## INTEGRATED $NA^+$-$CL^-$ AND $K^+$ TRANSPORT IN THE DISTAL NEPHRON

Segmentation of the renal epithelia into distinct sections does not mean that different segments function independently. Increasing evidence from in vivo studies in mice with multiple genes disrupted, or from studies in which knockout mice are subjected to drug treatment or dietary manipulation, shows that effects in one segment exert compensatory effects to maintain homeostasis. For example, *Slc26a4* knockout mice with combined genetic ablation of NCC[595] or administration of hydrochlorothiazide[596] display salt wasting and volume contraction. Similarly, ENaC blockade with amiloride leads to enhanced natriuresis in NCC knockout mice.[597] In mice with disruption of MR specifically in renal epithelia, while activities of both ENaC and NCC are diminished, the effect on NCC is secondary to the hyperkalemia induced by lower ENaC activity.[329,330] These mice are hypotensive, but normalization of plasma [$K^+$] by dietary $K^+$ restriction stimulates NCC activity resulting in normalization of blood pressure. Grimm and colleagues performed microarray studies on SPAK knockout mice, which display lower NCC activity, and proposed that α-ketoglutarate may serve as a downstream signaling molecule that mediates compensatory responses.[598] These interactions between segments are likely to be similar to those seen with diuretic treatment and may contribute to diuretic resistance (see Chapter 50). In the following sections, other examples of this intersegment crosstalk are described in more depth.

In the classic model of renal $K^+$ secretion, the lumen-negative PD generated by $Na^+$ entry via ENaC induces the exit of $K^+$ via apical $K^+$-selective channels. This general scheme explains much of the known physiology and pathophysiology of renal $K^+$ secretion, yet has several key consequences that bear emphasis. First, enhanced $Na^+$-$Cl^-$ reabsorption upstream of the CNT and CCD will reduce the delivery of luminal $Na^+$ to the CNT and CCD, decrease the lumen-negative PD, and thus decrease $K^+$ secretion; $K^+$ secretion by the CCD essentially stops when luminal $Na^+$ drops below 8 mmol/L.[488–490] In this respect, the increasingly refined phenotypic understanding of FHHt, caused by kinase-induced gain of function of the DCT, has served to underscore that variation in NCC-dependent $Na^+$-$Cl^-$ absorption, just upstream of the CNT, has truly profound effects on the ability to excrete dietary $K^+$ (Fig. 6.19).[345] Second, aldosterone is a kaliuretic hormone, induced by hyperkalemia. However, under certain circumstances associated with marked induction of aldosterone, such as dietary sodium restriction, sodium balance is maintained without effects on $K^+$ homeostasis. This so-called aldosterone paradox—how the kidney independently regulates $Na^+$-$Cl^-$ and $K^+$ handling by the aldosterone-sensitive distal nephron—is only recently beginning to yield to investigative efforts. The major factors in the integrated control of $Na^+$-$Cl^-$ and $K^+$ transport appear to include electroneutral thiazide-sensitive $Na^+$-$Cl^-$ transport within the CCD, ENaC-independent $K^+$ excretion within the distal nephron, and the differential regulation of various signaling pathways by aldosterone, Ang II, and dietary $K^+$.[406–408,528,599,600]

Thiazide-sensitive electroneutral $Na^+$-$Cl^-$ transport within the CCD is evidently mediated by the parallel activity of the $Na^+$-driven SLC4A8 $Cl^-$-$HCO_3^-$ exchanger and the SLC26A4 $Cl^-$-$HCO_3^-$ exchanger.[408] The molecular identity of this transport mechanism has only emerged rather recently, so regulatory influences are not fully characterized.[408] However, electroneutral $Na^+$-$Cl^-$ transport within the CCD is evidently induced by volume depletion and mineralocorticoid treatment.[406–408] This mechanism appears to mediate about 50% of $Na^+$ reabsorption in the CCD under these conditions, all without affecting the luminal PD and thus without direct effect on $K^+$ excretion. Therefore electroneutral, thiazide-sensitive $Na^+$-$Cl^-$ transport affords the ability to increase the reabsorption of $Na^+$ within the CCD without affecting $K^+$ excretion. The converse occurs after several days of accommodation to a high-$K^+$ diet, which increases the fraction of ENaC-independent, amiloride-resistant $K^+$ excretion to about 50%. Again, this presumptively electroneutral, aldosterone-independent pathway for $K^+$ excretion serves to uncouple distal tubular $Na^+$ and $K^+$ excretion.[528]

WNK-dependent signaling constitutes a major pathway for integrating $Na^+$-$Cl^-$ and $K^+$ transport within the distal nephron, and is regulated by the differential influence of $K^+$ intake on circulating Ang II, ROMK activity (i.e., $K^+$ secretory capacity), ratio of WNK1 isoforms, and activity of NCC in the DCT. Thus Ang II activates NCC via the WNK4-SPAK pathway, reducing delivery of $Na^+$ to the CNT and limiting $K^+$ secretion.[312,315,601] By contrast, Ang II inhibits ROMK activity via several mechanisms, including downstream activation of c-src tyrosine kinases.[583–585] Whereas $K^+$ restriction induces renin and circulating Ang II, increases in dietary $K^+$ are suppressive.[585,602] A decrease in circulating and local Ang II partially explains why NCC phosphorylation and activity are downregulated by a high-$K^+$ diet; teleologically, this serves to increase delivery of $Na^+$ to the CNT, thus increasing $K^+$ secretion.[361]

The DCT also clearly functions as a potassium sensor, directly responding to changes in circulating potassium (Fig. 6.19). Evidence that a key role of the DCT is to act as a plasma [$K^+$] sensor, rather than to maintain plasma [$Na^+$], is demonstrated by the observation that acute $K^+$ loading dephosphorylates NCC even in $Na^+$-restricted mice.[603] Reduction in potassium intake and/or hypokalemia thus lead to reduced basolateral [$K^+$] in the DCT; the subsequent hyperpolarization of DCT cells is dependent on basolateral KIR4.1-containing $K^+$ channels.[308,327] Hyperpolarization leads to chloride exit via basolateral CLC-K2 chloride channels; the resulting decrease in intracellular chloride disinhibits WNK kinases, resulting in phosphorylation of NCC and activation of the transporter by SPAK/OSR1.[327] Ex vivo studies (microperfusion and kidney slices) have provided evidence that increased phosphorylation of NCC resulting in response to lower extracellular [$K^+$] is dependent on increased intracellular chloride.[604] Along the DCT, WNK4 appears to be the major WNK activating NCC,[236] and WNK4 is also more sensitive to changes in intracellular chloride than WNK1 or WNK3.[343] The essential role of this pathway in mediating responses to dietary $K^+$ restriction is clearly demonstrated by the development of severe hypokalemia in mice lacking KIR4.1,[311] WNK4,[605] SPAK/OSR1,[606] and NCC (D.H. Ellison, unpublished observations; see Fig. 6.19 for summary of model). An alternative mechanism has been proposed in which KLHL3, part of the ubiquitin ligase complex that degrades WNK4, is phosphorylated in response to $K^+$ depletion. This prevents WNK4 binding to the complex, decreasing WNK4 degradation, which promotes NCC activation.[607]

NCC undergoes rapid dephosphorylation in response to $K^+$ loading,[604,608] a process that appears to be largely independent of increased intracellular chloride, which would inhibit WNKs.[604] This suggests a role for protein phosphatases; one study suggested that PP3 (calcineurin) is responsible for NCC dephosphorylation,[608] while another found no role for PP1, PP2A, or PP3.[604] Glucocorticoid-induced leucine zipper protein (GILZ) may also play a role in the response to high dietary $K^+$ by inhibiting SPAK activity and hence NCC. Compared with wild type mice, *Gilz* knockout mice are more sensitive to NCC inhibition by thiazides and have greater abundance of phosphorylated NCC. *Gilz* knockout mice display elevated plasma [$K^+$] at baseline, with dietary $Na^+$ restriction increasing it further. When plasma [$K^+$] increases, GILZ-mediated inhibition of NCC may serve to maintain distal $Na^+$ delivery to ENaC to drive kaliuresis.[609] Most studies have used diets completely almost deficient in $K^+$, or with very high levels, for example, 5% KCl, to examine NCC activation status. Relatively small changes in plasma [$K^+$] also alter the degree of NCC phosphorylation in vivo, suggesting that the role of NCC to maintain plasma [$K^+$] is homeostatically important under dietary $K^+$ levels that do not show extreme deviation from normal.[343]

A mouse model in which NCC activity was increased specifically along DCT1, by expressing a constitutively active SPAK mutant only in this segment, suggests that altering NCC activity may affect distal $K^+$ secretion by inducing remodeling of the CNT, and not just by altering $Na^+$ delivery to ENaC.[610] These mice displayed hyperkalemia, which was associated with lower volume of the CNT and lower ROMK abundance, which may limit $K^+$ secretion. Chronic blockade of NCC led to increased CNT volume and ROMK abundance, and normalized plasma $K^+$, suggesting that altered $Na^+$ delivery to the CNT may induce remodeling.

Finally, within principal cells, increases in aldosterone induce the SGK1 kinase, which phosphorylates WNK4 and attenuates the effect of WNK4 on ROMK, while activating ENaC via NEDD4-2-dependent effects.[611] However, when dietary $K^+$ intake is reduced, c-src tyrosine kinase activity increases under the influence of increased Ang II, causing direction inhibition of ROMK activity via tyrosine phosphorylation of the channel.[577,579,612] The increase in c-src tyrosine kinase activity also abrogates the effect of SGK1 on WNK4.[600,613] While NEDD4-2 can regulate NCC during $K^+$ restriction,[321] ENaC regulation may be more important. In NEDD4-2 knockout mice, chronic $K^+$ restriction led to hypokalemia and urinary $K^+$ wasting that was reversed with the ENaC blocker benzamil.[340] Higher phosphorylation of NCC and lower ROMK abundance were observed, but not sufficient to compensate for the effect on ENaC activation. While both insulin and IGF-1 activate ENaC, insulin promotes kaliuresis whereas IGF-1 exerts an antikaliuretic response. Patch-clamp analysis of isolated mouse CCD cells showed that this differential effect on $K^+$ secretion may be due to differential effects on CLC-K2 (which is expressed in intercalated cells).[392] IGF-1 stimulates ClC-K2, which may promote net $Na^+$-$Cl^-$ reabsorption, thus reducing the driving force for $K^+$ secretion by the CCD. By contrast, insulin inhibits ClC-K2, which would enhance the generation of the electrogenic drive for $K^+$ secretion.

 Complete reference list available at ExpertConsult.com.

## KEY REFERENCES


2. Chambrey R, Kurth I, Peti-Peterdi J, et al. Renal intercalated cells are rather energized by a proton than a sodium pump. *Proc Natl Acad Sci USA.* 2013;110:7928–7933.
3. Sun A, Grossman EB, Lombardi M, et al. Vasopressin alters the mechanism of apical Cl- entry from Na+:Cl- to Na+:K+:2Cl- cotransport in mouse medullary thick ascending limb. *J Membr Biol.* 1991;120:83–94.
10. Kokko JP. Proximal tubule potential difference. Dependence on glucose, $HCO_3$, and amino acids. *J Clin Invest.* 1973;52:1362–1367.
11. Alpern RJ, Howlin KJ, Preisig PA. Active and passive components of chloride transport in the rat proximal convoluted tubule. *J Clin Invest.* 1985;76:1360–1366.
15. Barratt LJ, Rector FC Jr, Kokko JP, et al. Factors governing the transepithelial potential difference across the proximal tubule of the rat kidney. *J Clin Invest.* 1974;53:454–464.
17. Katz AI, Doucet A, Morel F. Na-K-ATPase activity along the rabbit, rat, and mouse nephron. *Am J Physiol.* 1979;237:F114–FF120.
30. Muto S, Hata M, Taniguchi J, et al. Claudin-2-deficient mice are defective in the leaky and cation-selective paracellular permeability properties of renal proximal tubules. *Proc Natl Acad Sci USA.* 2010;107:8011–8016.
34. Schnermann J, Chou CL, Ma T, et al. Defective proximal tubular fluid reabsorption in transgenic aquaporin-1 null mice. *Proc Natl Acad Sci USA.* 1998;95:9660–9664.
36. Schnermann J, Huang Y, Mizel D. Fluid reabsorption in proximal convoluted tubules of mice with gene deletions of claudin-2 and/or aquaporin1. *Am J Physiol Renal Physiol.* 2013;305:F1352–F1364.
41. Bacic D, Kaissling B, McLeroy P, et al. Dopamine acutely decreases apical membrane Na/H exchanger NHE3 protein in mouse renal proximal tubule. *Kidney Int.* 2003;64:2133–2141.
43. Schultheis PJ, Clarke LL, Meneton P, et al. Renal and intestinal absorptive defects in mice lacking the NHE3 Na+/H+ exchanger. *Nat Genet.* 1998;19:282–285.
50. Wang T, Agulian SK, Giebisch G, et al. Effects of formate and oxalate on chloride absorption in rat distal tubule. *Am J Physiol.* 1993;264:F730–F736.
80. Wang T. Flow-activated transport events along the nephron. *Curr Opin Nephrol Hypertens.* 2006;15:530–536.
105. Thomson SC, Deng A, Wead L, et al. An unexpected role for angiotensin II in the link between dietary salt and proximal reabsorption. *J Clin Invest.* 2006;116:1110–1116.
113. Zhang MZ, Yao B, Wang S, et al. Intrarenal dopamine deficiency leads to hypertension and decreased longevity in mice. *J Clin Invest.* 2011;121:2845–2854.
158. Waldegger S, Jeck N, Barth P, et al. Barttin increases surface expression and changes current properties of ClC-K channels. *Pflugers Arch.* 2002;444:411–418.
160. Simon DB, Bindra RS, Mansfield TA, et al. Mutations in the chloride channel gene, CLCNKB, cause Bartter syndrome type III. *Nat Genet.* 1997;17:171–178.
163. Estevez R, Boettger T, Stein V, et al. Barttin is a Cl- channel beta-subunit crucial for renal Cl- reabsorption and inner ear K+ secretion. *Nature.* 2001;414:558–561.
180. Rocha AS, Kokko JP. Sodium chloride and water transport in the medullary thick ascending limb of Henle. Evidence for active chloride transport. *J Clin Invest.* 1973;52:612–623.
181. Stokes JB. Consequences of potassium recycling in the renal medulla. Effects of ion transport by the medullary thick ascending limb of Henle's loop. *J Clin Invest.* 1982;70:219–229.
190. Xu JZ, Hall AE, Peterson LN, et al. Localization of the ROMK protein on apical membranes of rat kidney nephron segments. *Am J Physiol.* 1997;F739–F748.
192. Lu M, Wang T, Yan Q, et al. ROMK is required for expression of the 70-pS K channel in the thick ascending limb. *Am J Physiol Renal Physiol.* 2004;286:F490–F495.
235. Gagnon KB, England R, Delpire E. Volume sensitivity of cation-Cl- cotransporters is modulated by the interaction of two kinases: Ste20-related proline-alanine-rich kinase and WNK4. *Am J Physiol Cell Physiol.* 2006;290:C134–C142.
264. Riccardi D, Hall AE, Chattopadhyay N, et al. Localization of the extracellular Ca2+/polyvalent cation-sensing protein in rat kidney. *Am J Physiol.* 1998;274:F611–F622.
273. Trudu M, Janas S, Lanzani C, et al; Swiss Kidney Project on Genes in Hypertension (SKIPOGH) team. Common noncoding UMOD gene variants induce salt-sensitive hypertension and kidney damage by increasing uromodulin expression. *Nat Med.* 2013;19:1655–1660.
275. Loffing J, Kaissling B. Sodium and calcium transport pathways along the mammalian distal nephron: from rabbit to human. *Am J Physiol Renal Physiol.* 2003;284:F628–F643.
309. Zhang C, Wang L, Zhang J, et al. KCNJ10 determines the expression of the apical Na-Cl cotransporter (NCC) in the early distal convoluted tubule (DCT1). *Proc Natl Acad Sci USA.* 2014;111:11864–11869.
327. Terker AS, Zhang C, McCormick JA, et al. Potassium modulates electrolyte balance and blood pressure through effects on distal cell voltage and chloride. *Cell Metab.* 2015;21:39–50.
335. Vidal-Petiot E, Elvira-Matelot E, Mutig K, et al. WNK1-related familial hyperkalemic hypertension results from an increased expression

of L-WNK1 specifically in the distal nephron. *Proc Natl Acad Sci USA*. 2013;110:14366–14371.
345. Lalioti MD, Zhang J, Volkman HM, et al. Wnk4 controls blood pressure and potassium homeostasis via regulation of mass and activity of the distal convoluted tubule. *Nat Genet*. 2006;38: 1124–1132.
349. Boyden LM, Choi M, Choate KA, et al. Mutations in Kelch-like 3 and cullin 3 cause hypertension and electrolyte abnormalities. *Nature*. 2012;482:98–102.
404. Verlander JW, Kim YH, Shin W, et al. Dietary Cl(−) restriction upregulates pendrin expression within the apical plasma membrane of type B intercalated cells. *Am J Physiol Renal Physiol*. 2006;291: F833–F839.
423. Snyder PM, Olson DR, Thomas BC. Serum and glucocorticoid-regulated kinase modulates Nedd4-2-mediated inhibition of the epithelial Na+ channel. *J Biol Chem*. 2002;277:5–8.
430. Soundararajan R, Ziera T, Koo E, et al. Scaffold protein connector enhancer of kinase suppressor of Ras isoform 3 (CNK3) coordinates assembly of a multiprotein epithelial sodium channel (ENaC)-regulatory complex. *J Biol Chem*. 2012;287:33014–33025.
439. Kleyman TR, Carattino MD, Hughey RP. ENaC at the cutting edge: regulation of epithelial sodium channels by proteases. *J Biol Chem*. 2009;284:20447–20451.
444. Kashlan OB, Blobner BM, Zuzek Z, et al. Na+ inhibits the epithelial Na+ channel by binding to a site in an extracellular acidic cleft. *J Biol Chem*. 2015;290:568–576.
446. Bugaj V, Pochynyuk O, Stockand JD. Activation of the epithelial Na+ channel in the collecting duct by vasopressin contributes to water reabsorption. *Am J Physiol Renal Physiol*. 2009;297:F1411–F1418.
451. Mironova E, Chen Y, Pao AC, et al. Activation of ENaC by AVP contributes to the urinary concentrating mechanism and dilution of plasma. *Am J Physiol Renal Physiol*. 2015;308:F237–F243.
462. Nakagawa K, Holla VR, Wei Y, et al. Salt-sensitive hypertension is associated with dysfunctional Cyp4a10 gene and kidney epithelial sodium channel. *J Clin Invest*. 2006;116:1696–1702.
463. Guan Y, Hao C, Cha DR, et al. Thiazolidinediones expand body fluid volume through PPARgamma stimulation of ENaC-mediated renal salt absorption. *Nat Med*. 2005;11:861–866.
504. Palmer LG, Frindt G. High-conductance K channels in intercalated cells of the rat distal nephron. *Am J Physiol Renal Physiol*. 2007;292:F966–F973.
505. Holtzclaw JD, Grimm PR, Sansom SC. Intercalated cell BK-alpha/beta4 channels modulate sodium and potassium handling during potassium adaptation. *J Am Soc Nephrol*. 2010;21:634–645.
523. Amorim JB, Bailey MA, Musa-Aziz R, et al. Role of luminal anion and pH in distal tubule potassium secretion. *Am J Physiol Renal Physiol*. 2003;284:F381–F388.
545. Yang L, Frindt G, Palmer LG. Magnesium modulates ROMK channel-mediated potassium secretion. *J Am Soc Nephrol*. 2010;21:2109–2116.
549. Palmer LG, Frindt G. Aldosterone and potassium secretion by the cortical collecting duct. *Kidney Int*. 2000;57:1324–1328.
550. Palmer LG, Antonian L, Frindt G. Regulation of apical K and Na channels and Na/K pumps in rat cortical collecting tubule by dietary K. *J Gen Physiol*. 1994;104:693–710.
554. Palmer LG, Frindt G. Regulation of apical K channels in rat cortical collecting tubule during changes in dietary K intake. *Am J Physiol*. 1999;277:F805–F812.
600. Yue P, Lin DH, Pan CY, et al. Src family protein tyrosine kinase (PTK) modulates the effect of SGK1 and WNK4 on ROMK channels. *Proc Natl Acad Sci USA*. 2009;106:15061–15066.
604. Penton D, Czogalla J, Wengi A, et al. Extracellular K+ rapidly controls NaCl cotransporter phosphorylation in the native distal convoluted tubule by Cl- -dependent and independent mechanisms. *J Physiol*. 2016;594(21):6319–6331.

7

# The Regulation of Calcium, Magnesium, and Phosphate Excretion by the Kidney

Theresa J. Berndt | Rajiv Kumar

## CHAPTER OUTLINE



## KEY POINTS

- $1\alpha,25(OH)_2D_3$, parathyroid hormone (PTH), and the phosphatonin, FGF-23, regulate renal tubule function to maintain homeostasis of serum calcium and phosphate concentrations, whereas magnesium handling is regulated largely by dietary magnesium load.
- The hypocalciuric effect of PTH is mediated by increased paracellular $Ca_2^+$ reabsorption in the thick ascending limb of Henle, via inhibition of claudin-14 and by changes in the expression of apical channels in the distal tubule.
- Sclerostin is an osteocyte-derived glycoprotein that has calciuric effects and appears to serve as a counterbalance to PTH and $1\alpha,25(OH)_2$ in calcium homeostasis.
- Claudin-10b is a tight junction protein that mediates paracellular $Na^+$ reabsorption in the medullary thick ascending limb, thereby limiting $Ca_2^+$ reabsorption further downstream in the cortical thick ascending limb.
- Mutations in claudin-10b cause hypermagnesemia and hypokalemic alkalosis, together with various extrarenal manifestations.
- PTH and FGF-23 converge on a common signaling pathway in the proximal tubule, involving phosphorylation of NHERF-1 and dissociation and internalization of the NaPi-IIa cotransporter, to cause phosphaturia.
- $1\alpha,25(OH)_2D$ stimulates the synthesis of FGF-23, which in turn inhibits 25-hydroxyvitamin D $1\alpha$-hydroxylase, serving as a negative feedback loop to limit vitamin D effects on phosphate turnover.

## CALCIUM TRANSPORT IN THE KIDNEY

### THE ROLE OF CALCIUM IN CELLULAR PROCESSES

Calcium is an abundant cation in the body (Table 7.1). Several biochemical and physiologic processes, including nerve conduction and function, coagulation, enzyme activity, exocytosis, and bone mineralization, are critically dependent on normal calcium concentrations in extracellular fluid.[1–3] Not unexpectedly, significant decreases or increases in serum calcium concentrations are associated with marked symptoms and signs. Intricate mechanisms exist to maintain extracellular fluid calcium concentrations within a narrow range and to maintain calcium balance. Decreases in serum calcium concentrations are associated with numbness and tingling of the extremities and peri-oral region, cramping, Chvostek and Trousseau signs, tetany, and when profound, generalized seizures.[4–6] A negative calcium balance that is present when calcium absorption in the intestine is reduced is associated with secondary hyperparathyroidism, hypophosphatemia, and rickets or osteomalacia.[5,6] Hypercalcemia, especially when severe, is associated with lethargy, confusion, irritability, depression, hallucinations, and in extreme cases, stupor and coma, anorexia, nausea, vomiting and constipation, cardiac ectopy,

**Table 7.1 Composition of the Whole Body as Determined by Chemical Analysis (Values per Kilogram Fat-Free Tissue Unless Otherwise Indicated)**

| Body Weight (kg) | Water[a] (g) | Fat[a] (g) | Water (g) | N (g) | Na (mEq) | K (mEq) | Cl (mEq) | Mg (g) | Ca (g) | P (g) | Fe (mg) | Cu (mg) | Zn (mg) | B (mg) | Co (mg) |
|---|---|---|---|---|---|---|---|---|---|---|---|---|---|---|---|
| 70 | 605 | 160 | 720 | 34 | 80 | 69 | 50 | 0.47 | 22.4 | 12.0 | 74 | 1.7 | 28 | 0.37 | 0.02 |

[a]Per kilogram whole body weight.

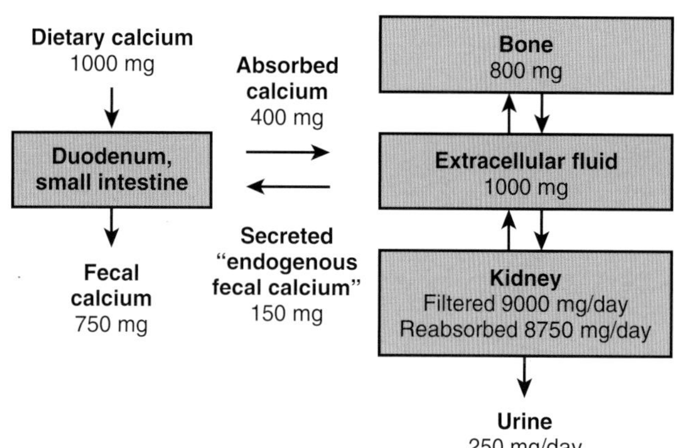


**Fig. 7.1** Calcium homeostasis in normal humans showing the amounts of calcium absorbed in the intestine and reabsorbed by the kidney.

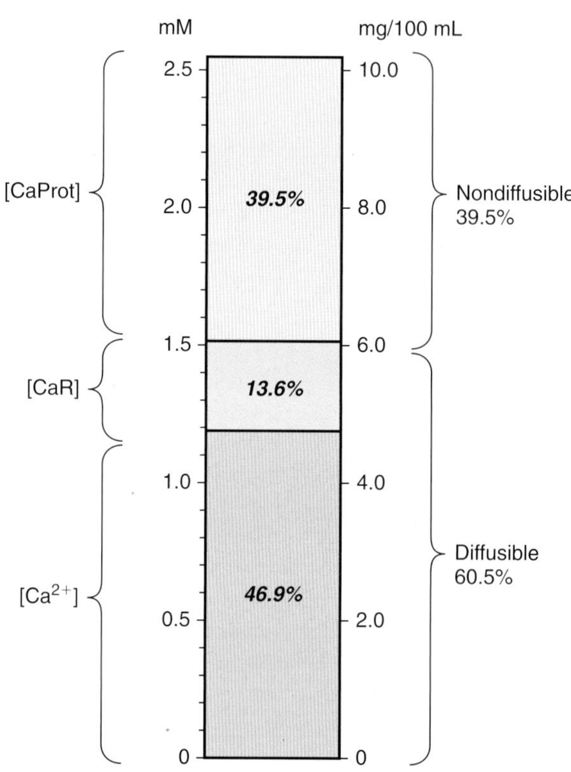


**Fig. 7.2 Components of serum total calcium assessed by ultrafiltration data in normal human patients.** *CaR,* Diffuse of both calcium complexes; *$Ca^{2+}$,* ionized calcium, *CaProt,* protein-bound calcium. Redrawn from Moore, EW. Ionized calcium in normal serum, ultrafiltrates, and whole blood determined by ion-exchange electrodes. *J Clin Invest.* 1970;49:318–334, with permission of the publisher.

and polyuria and renal colic from the passage of renal stones.[7] The attendant hypercalciuria is associated with a reduced capacity to concentrate urine,[8–11] volume depletion, and nephrocalcinosis and renal stones.[12,13] Hypercalcemia occurs as a result of parathyroid hormone (PTH)-dependent or PTH-independent processes, and changes in laboratory values depend on the etiology of hypercalcemia.[7] Thus, in PTH-dependent hypercalcemia, elevated serum PTH concentrations are present and are the cause of hypercalcemia, whereas in PTH-independent hypercalcemia, PTH concentrations are suppressed, sometimes in association with increases in various vitamin D metabolites.[7] As shown in Fig. 7.1, the intestine and kidney are important in the absorption and the reabsorption and excretion of calcium. Following the absorption in the intestine, calcium in the extracellular fluid space is deposited in bone (the major repository of calcium in the body) and is filtered in the kidney. The concentration of calcium in serum varies with age and gender, with higher values present in children and adolescent subjects than in adults.

## CALCIUM IS PRESENT IN SERUM IN BOUND AND FREE FORMS

Calcium is present in plasma in filterable (60% of total calcium) and bound (40% of total calcium) forms. Filterable calcium is composed of calcium complexed to anions, such as citrate, sulfate, and phosphate (~10% of total calcium) and ionized calcium (~50% of total calcium) (Fig. 7.2).[14] The percentage of calcium bound to proteins (predominantly albumin, and to a lesser extent, globulins), and the amount of filterable calcium, is dependent on plasma pH.[14] Alkalemia is associated with a reduction in free calcium, whereas acidemia is associated with an increase in free calcium. A 1-g/dL change in serum albumin is associated with a 0.8-mg/dL change in total serum calcium, and a 1-g/dL change in globulins is associated with a 0.16-mg/dL change in total serum calcium. An equation defining the amount of calcium (mmol/L) bound to albumin and globulins (g/L) as a function of pH is as follows[14]:

$$[\mathrm{CaProt}] = 0.019[\mathrm{Alb}] - [(0.42)([\mathrm{Alb}]/47.3)(7.42 - \mathrm{pH})] + 0.004[\mathrm{Glob}] - [(0.42)([\mathrm{Glob}]/25.0)(7.42 - \mathrm{pH})]$$

If one assumes that all calcium is bound to albumin, the following equation applies:

$$[\mathrm{CaProt}] = 0.0211[\mathrm{Alb}] - [(0.42)([\mathrm{Alb}]/47.3)(7.42 - \mathrm{pH})],$$

where Alb is albumin, CaProt is protein-bound calcium, and Glob is globulins.

A nomogram describing this relationship is shown in Fig. 7.3.

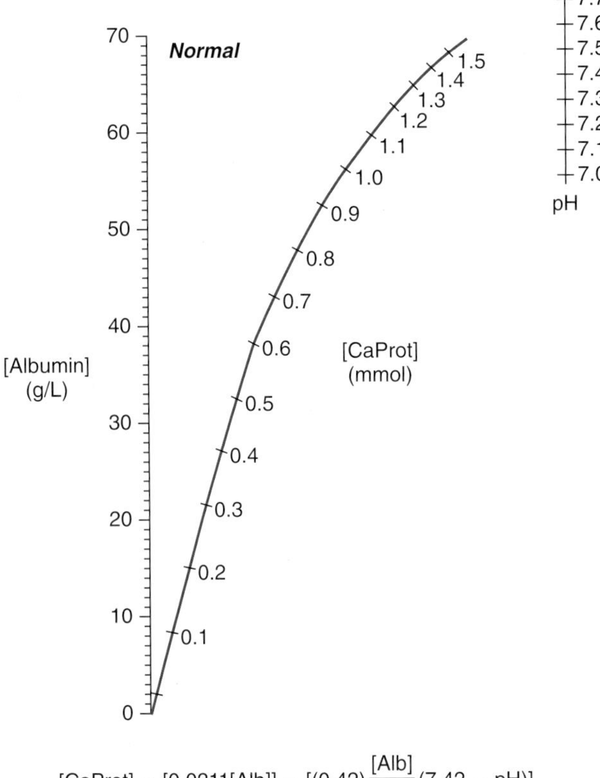


$$[CaProt] = [0.0211[Alb]] - [(0.42)\frac{[Alb]}{47.3}(7.42 - pH)]$$

**Fig. 7.3 A nomogram for estimating protein-bound calcium levels [CaProt] in normal humans.** [CaProt] is obtained by connecting observed albumin and pH values with a straight line and reading the point at which it intersects the curve. The equation describing the relationship between [CaProt] (protein-bound calcium), serum albumin concentrations, and pH is shown at the bottom of the graph. Redrawn from Moore EW. Ionized calcium in normal serum, ultrafiltrates, and whole blood determined by ion-exchange electrodes. *J Clin Invest.* 1970;49:318–334, with permission of the publisher.

## REGULATION OF CALCIUM HOMEOSTASIS BY THE PARATHYROID HORMONE–VITAMIN D ENDOCRINE SYSTEM

In states of neutral calcium balance, the amount of calcium absorbed by the intestine is equivalent to the amount excreted by the kidney. The central role of the vitamin D–PTH endocrine system in the regulation of calcium homeostasis is well recognized.[15–17] The major physiologic role of vitamin D through the activity of its active metabolite 1α,25-dihydroxyvitamin $D_3$ (1α,25$(OH)_2D_3$) is the maintenance of normal calcium and phosphorus balance.[18–21] In Fig. 7.4 the metabolism of vitamin D and the adaptations that occur in response to changes in serum calcium are illustrated. Fig. 7.4A summarizes the salient biochemical transformations that occur endogenously during the formation and metabolism of vitamin $D_3$. Vitamin $D_3$ (cholecalciferol) is formed in the skin by the ultraviolet light–mediated photolysis of the B-ring of the sterol precursor, 7-dehydrocholesterol, which gives rise to pre-vitamin $D_3$ that rapidly undergoes thermal equilibration to vitamin $D_3$.[22–30] Vitamin $D_2$, or ergocalciferol, derived by photolysis of the plant sterol, ergosterol, is ingested orally, after which it is metabolized in a similar manner to vitamin $D_3$.[31] Although vitamin $D_2$ is less active in birds than mammals, when compared with vitamin $D_3$, the metabolic transformations of vitamin $D_2$ and vitamin $D_3$ are similar.[32] Vitamin $D_3$, bound to vitamin D–binding protein, to which it preferentially binds relative to its precursor, pre-vitamin $D_3$,[29] exits the skin, enters the circulation, and is metabolized in the liver microsomes and mitochondria to 25-hydroxyvitamin $D_3$ (25(OH)$D_3$) by the vitamin $D_3$-25-hydroxylase.[16,33–43] The CYP2R1 is the cytochrome P450 of the microsomal vitamin $D_3$-25 hydroxylase.[41] Other vitamin $D_3$-25-hydroxylases play a role in the transformation of vitamin $D_3$ to 25(OH)$D_3$ because deletion of the *Cyp2r1* gene in mice results in reduced (>50% reduction) but detectable serum 25(OH)$D_3$ concentrations.[43]

The subsequent metabolism of 25(OH)$D_3$ is dependent on the calcium and phosphorus requirements of the individual. In states of calcium demand, 25(OH)$D_3$ is metabolized by the 25-hydroxyvitamin $D_3$-1α-hydroxylase to the biologically active vitamin D metabolite, 1α,25-dihydroxyvitamin $D_3$ (1α,25$(OH)_2D_3$), in mitochondria of kidney proximal and distal tubule cells by PTH-dependent processes (see Fig. 7.4B).[18,26,44–56] In response to reductions in calcium intake and subsequent decreases in serum calcium, PTH release from the parathyroid glands is increased. The change in serum calcium concentrations is detected by the parathyroid gland calcium-sensing receptor, a G-protein–coupled receptor, which alters PTH release from the parathyroid cell.[57–60] PTH enhances calcium transport in the distal tubule of the kidney directly,[61–63] and indirectly through changes in sclerostin expression,[55,56,64,65] and increases the activity of the renal 25-hydroxyvitamin D 1α-hydroxylase, and attendant increases in the synthesis of 1α,25$(OH)_2D_3$.[52] 1α,25$(OH)_2D_3$ increases calcium transport in the intestine[49,50,66] and kidney.[67–71] At the same time, both PTH[72–74] and 1α,25$(OH)_2$D[75,76] increase bone calcium mobilization and help to maintain serum calcium concentrations. The converse series of events occurs in hypercalcemic circumstances. In states of calcium sufficiency, the synthesis of 1α,25$(OH)_2D_3$ is reduced, and the synthesis of 24*R*,25-dihydroxyvitamin $D_3$ (24*R*,25$(OH)_2D_3$), a vitamin D metabolite with reduced bioactivity, is increased.[77–79] The synthesis of 24*R*,25$(OH)_2D_3$ is mediated by a 1α,25$(OH)_2D_3$-inducible enzyme, the 25(OH) $D_3$-24-hydroxylase, that is present in several target tissues of 1α,25$(OH)_2D_3$ including the intestine and the kidney.[77,80–84]

1α,25$(OH)_2D_3$, PTH, and the phosphatonin, fibroblast growth factor-23 (FGF-23), regulate and maintain normal phosphorus concentrations.[85–87] Serum phosphate concentrations also regulate the synthesis of 1α,25$(OH)_2D_3$ by PTH independent mechanisms.[88] In states of phosphorus demand, 25(OH)$D_3$ is metabolized to 1α,25$(OH)_2D_3$ and the synthesis of 24*R*,25$(OH)_2D_3$ is reduced.[16,46,89–92] The enhanced synthesis of 1α,25$(OH)_2D_3$ in hypophosphatemic states is induced directly by reductions in serum phosphate,[88,93–95] an increase in the expression of IGF-1,[96,97] and by inhibition of FGF-23.[98] The converse occurs in hyperphosphatemic states. A decrease in serum phosphate concentrations is associated with an increase in ionized calcium, a decrease in PTH secretion, and a subsequent decrease in renal phosphate excretion. An increase in renal 25-hydroxyvitamin D-1α-hydroxylase activity, increased 1α,25$(OH)_2D_3$ synthesis, and increased phosphorus absorption in the intestine and reabsorption in the kidney occur.[88,92,94,99–105] In the intestine and kidney, 1α,25$(OH)_2D_3$ increases the expression of the sodium–phosphate cotransporters IIb, and IIa and IIc, respectively, thereby regulating

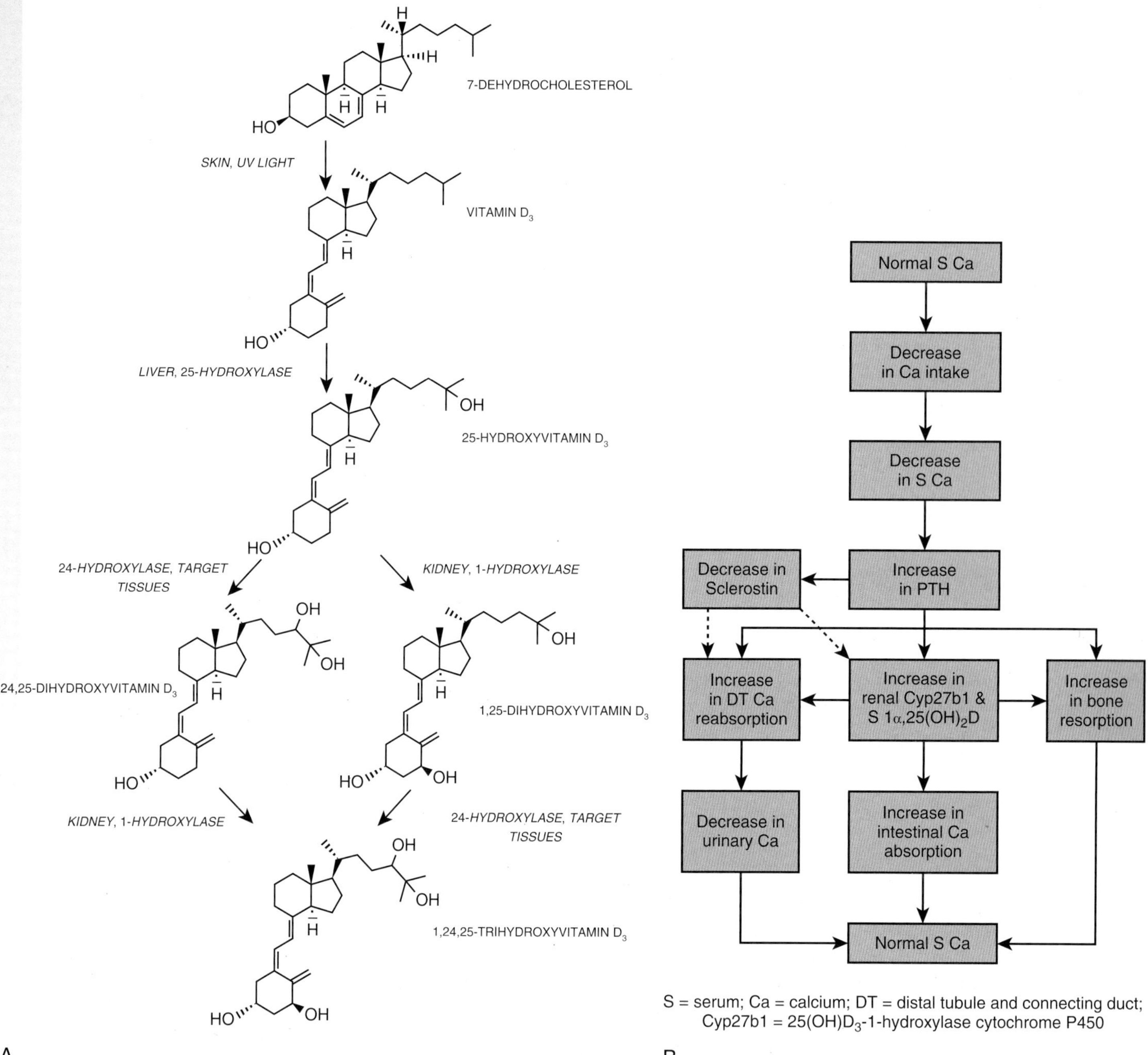


**Fig. 7.4 A. The formation and metabolism of vitamin D3. B.** Physiologic changes in response to decreases in serum calcium concentrations. *Ca,* Calcium; *Cyp27b1,* 25(OH)$D_3$-1-hydroxylase cytochrome P450; *DT,* distal tubule and connection duct; *PTH,* parathyroid hormone; *S,* serum; *UV,* ultraviolet. From Tebben PJ, Singh RJ, Kumar R. Vitamin D-mediated hypercalcemia: mechanisms, diagnosis, and treatment. *Endocr Rev.* 2016;37:521–547.

the efficiency of Pi absorption in enterocytes and proximal tubule (PT) cells.[87,106–108] In hyperphosphatemic states, renal 25-hydroxyvitamin D-1α-hydroxylase activity and 1α,25(OH)$_2$D$_3$ synthesis are diminished, and 25-hydroxyvitamin D-24-hydroxylase activity is increased in association with elevations in FGF-23.[7,98] Numerous other factors other than calcium and phosphorus alter the activity of the 25(OH)D-1α-hydroxylase and the reader is referred to reviews on this matter.[47,109–113]

The bioactivity of vitamin $D_3$ depends on the formation of 1α,25(OH)$_2$D$_3$ as pharmacologic amounts of vitamin $D_3$ or 25(OH)$D_3$ are required to elicit a biological response in anephric animals and patients,[53,75,114] whereas 1α,25(OH)$_2$D$_3$ readily increases intestinal calcium transport[49,50] and mobilizes calcium from bone[75] when given in physiologic amounts. The actions of 1α,25(OH)$_2$D$_3$ require the presence of the vitamin D receptor (VDR), a steroid hormone receptor, that binds 1α,25(OH)$_2$D$_3$ with high affinity.[115–118] Following binding of 1α,25(OH)$_2$D$_3$ to the ligand binding domain of the VDR, a conformational change in the receptor occurs and is associated with the recruitment of RXRα and coactivator (or corepressor) proteins to DNA binding elements within the transcription start site or other areas of genes regulated by

1α,25(OH)$_2$D$_3$.[20,119–139] The efficiency of calcium absorption increases or decreases inversely with the amount of dietary calcium, and adaptations to changes in calcium intake are dependent on 1α,25(OH)$_2$D$_3$.[140,141] Calcium is absorbed by the intestine by passive paracellular and active transcellular mechanisms.[141–143] Active calcium absorption initially involves the movement of calcium across the apical border of the intestinal cell into the cell down a concentration and electrical gradient and does not require the expenditure of energy.[17,144] The extrusion of calcium out of the intestinal cell at the basolateral membrane is against an electrical and concentration gradient and requires the energy expenditure.[17,144] Essential to the process of active calcium transport are several vitamin D–dependent proteins, including the TRPV 5/6 (transient receptor potential vanilloid 5/6) epithelial calcium channels, calbindin $D_{9K}$ and $D_{28K}$, and the plasma membrane calcium pump.[87] In the duodenal enterocyte, apically situated TRPV 5/6 cation channels mediate the increase in Ca uptake from the lumen into the cell[145]; intracellular Ca binding proteins such as calbindin $D_{9K}$ and $D_{28K}$ facilitate the movement of Ca across the cell[17,143]; and the basolateral plasma membrane Ca pump (PMCA)[2,146,147] and the Na-Ca exchanger (NCX)[148] assist in the extrusion of Ca from within the cell into the extracellular fluid (ECF). The Na gradient for the activity of the NCX is maintained by the Na-K-ATPase. Intestinal transcellular Ca transport is regulated by 1α,25(OH)$_2$D$_3$, which increases the expression of TRPV 6 channels,[149] the intracellular concentrations of calbindin $D_{9K}$ and $D_{28K}$,[17,150–152] and the expression of the plasma membrane pump, isoform 1.[153,154] The requirement of various intestinal Ca transporter proteins in transcellular Ca transport in vivo has been examined in knockout mice. Deletions of *TrpV6* and *calbindin $D_{9K}$* genes are not associated with alterations in intestinal Ca transport in vivo in the basal state and following the administration of 1α,25(OH)$_2$D$_3$,[155,156] although one report suggests that basal Ca transport on an adequate Ca diet is normal in *TrpV6* knockout mice but adaptations to a low-Ca diet are impaired.[157] We recently showed that deletion of the *Pmca1* in the intestine is associated with reduced growth and bone mineralization and a failure to upregulate calcium absorption in response to 1α,25(OH)$_2$D$_3$, thereby establishing the essential role of the pump in transcellular intestinal Ca transport.[158]

## REABSORPTION OF CALCIUM ALONG THE TUBULE

The kidney reabsorbs filtered calcium in amounts that are subject to regulation by calciotropic hormones, PTH and 1α,25(OH)$_2$D.[16,145,159–164] Between 9000 and 10,000 mg of complexed and ionized calcium are filtered by the glomerulus in a 24-hour period. The amount of calcium appearing in the urine is approximately 250 mg/day, and it is therefore evident that a large percentage of filtered calcium is reabsorbed. As a result of reabsorption processes that occur in both the proximal and distal tubule, only 1%–2% of calcium filtered at the glomerulus appears in the urine.[145,161,164] Fig. 7.5 shows the percentages of calcium reabsorbed along different segments of the nephron.

### $CA^{2+}$ REABSORPTION IN THE PROXIMAL TUBULE

As noted earlier, about 60%–70% of total plasma calcium is free (not protein bound) and is filtered at the glomerulus.[165,166]

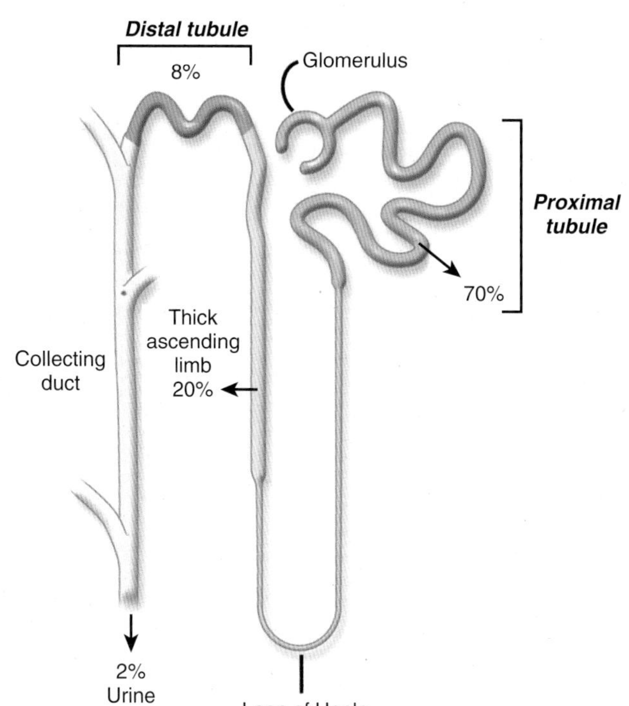


**Fig. 7.5** Percentages of filtered calcium reabsorbed along the tubule.

A large percentage (~70%) of filtered calcium ($Ca^{2+}$) is reabsorbed in the PT mainly by paracellular processes that are linked with sodium ($Na^+$) reabsorption.[165,167–170] In this nephron segment, the reabsorption of $Na^+$ and $Ca^{2+}$ is proportional under a variety of conditions[169,171] and is not dissociated following the administration of several factors that are known to alter renal $Ca^{2+}$ reabsorption, such as PTH, cyclic AMP, chlorothiazide, furosemide, acetazolamide, or changes in the hydrogen ion content.[168,169,172,173] The precise cellular and molecular machinery responsible for the movement of $Ca^{2+}$ from the lumen of the PT into the interstitial space is not clearly defined. A majority of $Ca^{2+}$ is believed to move in between cells (paracellular movement) with a smaller, but significant, transcellular component (Fig. 7.6). The components of the paracellular pathway likely include the tight junction protein, claudin-2, which functions as a paracellular cation channel. $Ca^{2+}$ permeates through claudin-2[174] and simultaneously competitively inhibits $Na^+$ conductance.[175] A transcellular component of $Ca^{2+}$ reabsorption may also be present in the PT. Undefined $Ca^{2+}$ channels and intracellular $Ca^{2+}$-binding proteins influence the movement of $Ca^{2+}$ into and across the cell. The Na-K-ATPase has been implicated in transcellular $Ca^{2+}$ transport in the PT,[176] and both the $Na^+$-$Ca^{2+}$ exchanger[177] and isoforms 1 and 4 of the plasma membrane $Ca^{2+}$ pump[178,179] are expressed in the PT, and could be important in the movement of $Ca^{2+}$ out of the PT cell. Although the PT reabsorbs large amounts of $Ca^{2+}$, primarily by paracellular processes, the rate of $Ca^{2+}$ reabsorption is not influenced by factors or hormones that regulate calcium balance.[168,169,172] Extracellular volume status is the major factor that influences $Ca^{2+}$ reabsorption in the PT, via its effects on $Na^+$ reabsorption (see later).

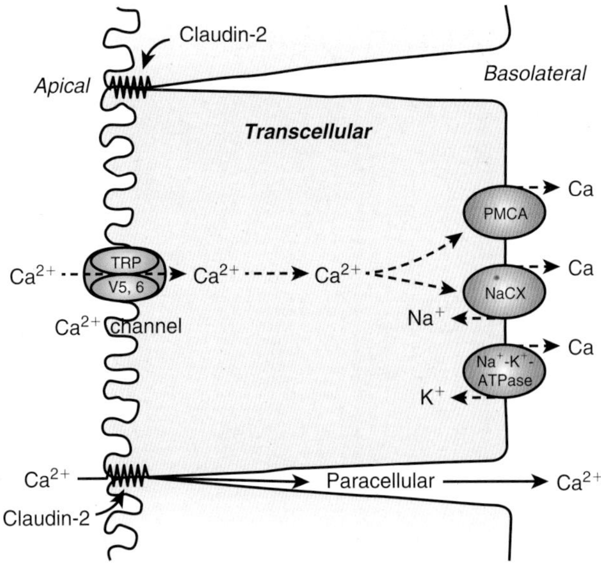


**Fig. 7.6 Mechanisms by which calcium is transported in the proximal tubule.** The majority of calcium is reabsorbed by paracellular mechanisms. A smaller percentage is reabsorbed by transcellular mechanisms.

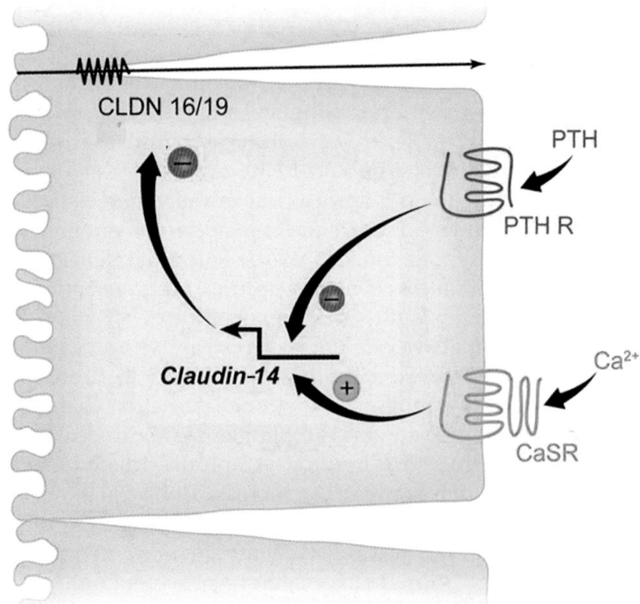


**Fig. 7.7 Mechanisms and regulation of calcium transport in the thick ascending limb of Henle *(TALH)*.** In the TALH, calcium is reabsorbed via paracellular mechanisms through a pore composed in part by claudin-16 and claudin-19. The activity of the latter proteins is suppressed by claudin-14, whose expression is controlled by parathyroid hormone *(PTH)* and $Ca^{2+}$. PTH binds to its receptor and inhibits the expression of claudin-14, whereas extracellular fluid $Ca^{2+}$ activates the calcium-sensing receptor (CaSR) and increases claudin-14 expression. The reabsorption of $Ca^{2+}$ in the TALH is the result of opposing activities of PTH and $Ca^{2+}$ through their receptors. *CLDN 16/19*, Claudin-16 and -19; *PTH,* parathyroid hormone; *PTH R,* parathyroid receptor.

## CA²⁺ REABSORPTION IN THE LOOP OF HENLE

The thin descending and thin ascending limbs of the loop of Henle do not transport significant amounts of $Ca^{2+}$.[197,198] Between 20%–25% of filtered $Ca^{2+}$ is reabsorbed in the thick ascending loop of Henle, primarily by the paracellular route involving claudin-16 and -19.[165,180–191] Thick ascending limb cells express the furosemide-sensitive Na-K-Cl cotransporter, NKCC2,[192–195] which mediates the reabsorption of $Na^+$ and thereby contributes to the driving force for paracellular $Ca^{2+}$ transport. A lumen-positive transepithelial potential is generated in the thick ascending limb of the loop of Henle (TALH) through the activity of the NKCC2 (Na-K-2Cl cotransporter)[196] by two mechanisms: secondary apical recycling of $K^+$ via ROMK, and a NaCl diffusion potential generated by reabsorbed NaCl establishing a concentration gradient across the Na-selective paracellular pathway. This transepithelial voltage provides the driving force for passive $Ca^{2+}$ reabsorption through the paracellular pathway.

Claudins, located in the tight junction between cells of the TALH play a role in the paracellular movement of $Ca^{2+}$ (and $Mg^{2+}$ reabsorption, as discussed in the next section)[197,198] (Fig. 7.7). Claudin-16 (also known as paracellin), together with claudin-19, forms a paracellular pore. A heteromeric claudin-16 and claudin-19 interaction is required to assemble and traffic to the tight junction and to generate cation-selective paracellular channels.[199,200] It has been postulated that these channels are themselves responsible for permeating divalent cations, $Ca^{2+}$ and $Mg^{2+}$, via the paracellular route.[197,198] An alternative hypothesis is that claudin-16 and -19 form $Na^+$ channels and act primarily to establish the transepithelial NaCl diffusion potential, thus contributing to the driving force for divalent cation reabsorption.[199–202] Regardless of the mechanism, loss-of-function mutations in the genes encoding claudin-16 and -19 result in familial hypomagnesemia with hypercalciuria and nephrocalcinosis (FHHNC), which is characterized by renal $Ca^{2+}$ and $Mg^{2+}$ wasting due to defective thick ascending limb divalent cation reabsorption. Hou et al. generated claudin-16 and claudin-19 knockdown mouse models using transgenic siRNAs and demonstrated that these mice have significantly reduced plasma $Mg^{2+}$ concentrations and excessive urinary excretion of $Mg^{2+}$ and $Ca^{2+}$.[380] Calcium deposits were observed in the basement membranes of the medullary tubules and the interstitium in the kidney of claudin-16 knockdown mice. Thus, the phenotypes of *Cldn16* and *Cldn19* knockdown mice recapitulate the phenotype of human FHHNC patients. Similarly, mutations of NKCC2 are associated with the common form of Bartter syndrome and can be associated with hypercalciuria[203] (see also Chapters 18 and 44).

Calcium-regulating hormones can regulate reabsorption of $Ca^{2+}$ by the thick ascending limb, but there is considerable species heterogeneity. In the mouse, PTH and calcitonin (CT) stimulate $Ca^{2+}$ transport in the cortical thick ascending limb,[184,186,204,205] whereas in the rabbit CT stimulates calcium reabsorption in the medullary thick ascending limb but not in the cortical thick ascending limb.[189] Extracellular fluid calcium also regulates calcium reabsorption in this segment through the $Ca^{2+}$-sensing receptor (see later).

## CA²⁺ REABSORPTION IN THE DISTAL TUBULE

In the distal convoluted tubule (primarily DCT2) and connecting tubule (together abbreviated as DT), 5%–10% of filtered $Ca^{2+}$ is reabsorbed[206–208] by active transport processes against both an electrical and concentration gradient. $Ca^{2+}$ reabsorption in the DT occurs via a transcellular pathway. The apically situated, transient receptor potential cation channels, subfamily V, type 5 and 6 channels (TRPV5, TRPV6) mediate the increase in $Ca^{2+}$ uptake from the lumen into the cell.[164,209–214] Micropuncture studies in knockout mice indicate that TRPV5 is the gatekeeper of $Ca^{2+}$ reabsorption in the accessible DT in mice (Fig. 7.8A).[211] The intracellular $Ca^{2+}$-binding proteins, calbindin $D_{9K}$ and $D_{28K}$, facilitate the movement of $Ca^{2+}$ across the cell.[160,215] The basolateral plasma membrane calcium ATPase (PMCA) pump,[159,160,162] $Na^+$-$Ca^{2+}$ exchanger (NaCX),[216–219] and the $Na^+$-$Ca^{2+}$-$K^+$ exchanger (NaCKX)[220] mediate the active extrusion of $Ca^{2+}$ across the basolateral membrane (see Fig. 7.8B and 7.8C). The $Na^+$ gradient for the activity of the NaCX and the NaCKX is provided by the Na-K ATPase situated at the basolateral cell membrane (not shown). $Ca^{2+}$ reabsorption in the DT is increased by PTH,[61–63] CT,[204,205] and $1\alpha,25(OH)_2D_3$.[67–71]

## REGULATION OF $CA^{2+}$ TRANSPORT IN THE KIDNEY

### CALCIUM-REGULATING HORMONES

The calcium-regulating hormones, PTH and $1\alpha,25(OH)_2D_3$, regulate the expression or activity of calcium channels, calcium-binding proteins, calcium pumps, and exchangers in the kidney to increase tubule retention of filtered calcium via the transcellular pathway. PTH increases the activity of TRPV5 channels in the DT by activating cAMP-PKA signaling, and phosphorylating a threonine residue within the channel, resulting in an increase in the open probability of the channel.[220] PTH also activates the PKC pathway, thereby increasing the numbers of TRPV5 channels on the surface of tubular cells by inhibiting endocytosis of caveolae in which the channels are located.[221] $1\alpha,25(OH)_2D_3$ enhances the expression of TRPV5 and TRPV6 channels present in the distal and connecting tubule and cortical collecting duct by increasing respective mRNA concentrations through increased binding of the VDR to response elements in the gene promoters.[70,213] $1\alpha,25(OH)_2D_3$ increases the expression of calbindin $D_{9K}$ and $D_{28K}$ and the PMCA pump in the kidney and cultured renal cells.[70,179,222–231] The effect of PTH and $1\alpha,25(OH)_2D_3$ is to increase the expression of $Ca^{2+}$ channels, binding proteins, pumps and exchangers, thereby increasing the retention of calcium by the kidney.

PTH has also been well described to increase renal tubule $Ca^{2+}$ reabsorption by increasing its passive permeability in the TALH, predominantly in the cortical segment.[232,233] The mechanism has now been elucidated. PTH, acting through the PTH/PTHrP receptor, has been shown to inhibit the transcription and subcellular trafficking of claudin 14, thereby increasing paracellular $Ca^{2+}$ reabsorption in the TALH[234] (see Fig. 7.7). Claudin-14 binds to claudin-16 and functions to inhibit the paracellular pore comprised of claudins 16 and 19. Tissue-specific knockout of the renal tubule PTH/PTHrP receptor in mice caused hypercalciuria and hypocalcemia, which was completely rescued by claudin-14 deletion, suggesting that the effect of PTH on paracellular $Ca^{2+}$ transport in the TALH may be more important than previously appreciated.

### EXTRACELLULAR CALCIUM AND DIET

The level of extracellular calcium regulates renal $Ca^{2+}$ reabsorption by signaling though the Ca-sensing receptor (CaSR). In the kidney, the CaSR is primarily expressed on the basolateral membrane of the TALH. Activation of CaSR reduces renal tubular $Ca^{2+}$ reabsorption and induces calciuresis

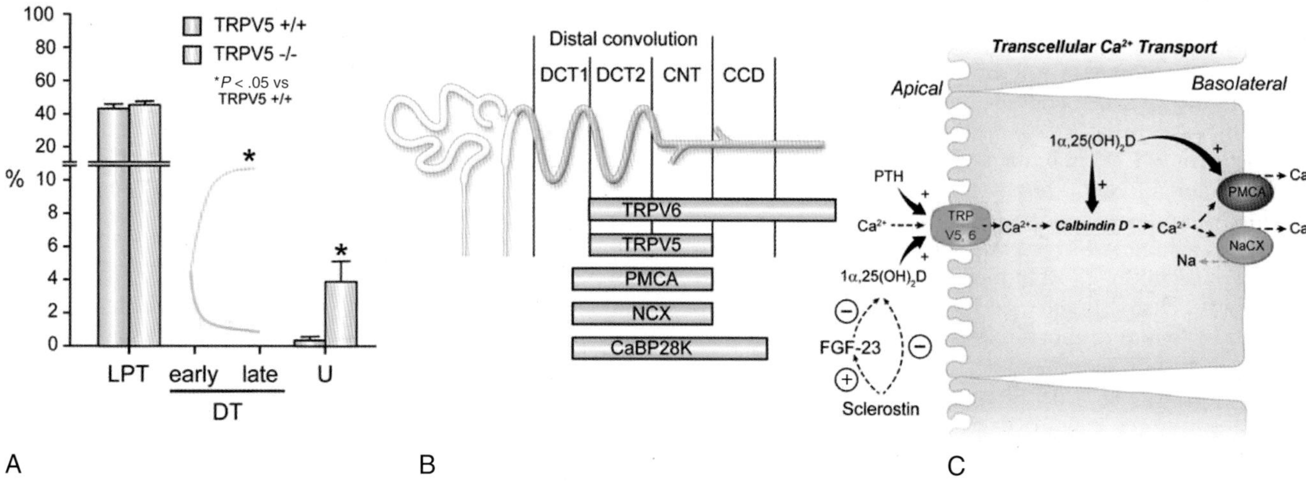


**Fig. 7.8 Mechanisms of calcium transport in the distal convoluted tubule. A.** Role of TRPV5 investigated by micropuncture of kidneys from TRPV5 knockout mice. The figure shows fractional $Ca^{2+}$ delivery to micropuncture sites in the late proximal tubule *(LPT)* to sites located along the distal convolution *(DC)* from early to late DC (as localized using tubule $K^+$ concentrations) and to the urine. Deletion of TRPV5 in mice prevents $Ca^{2+}$ reabsorption along the DT and there is even evidence for $Ca^{2+}$ leaking back into the lumen, possibly by paracellular routes; TRPV6 may partially compensate in the collecting duct. **B.** Distribution of $1\alpha,25(OH)_2D$ or parathyroid hormone–sensitive channels and transporters along the distal convoluted tubule (*DCT1* and *DCT2*), connecting tubule *(CNT)*, and cortical and medullary collecting ducts (*CCD* and *MCD*). **C.** Ca transport in the DT occurs by transcellular mechanisms. Transcellular Ca transport is mediated by several channels, pumps, and exchangers located at the apical and basolateral portions of the cell. Modified from Kumar R, Vallon V. Reduced renal calcium excretion in the absence of sclerostin expression: evidence for a novel calcium-regulating bone kidney axis. *J Am Soc Nephrol.* 2014;25:2159–2168, with permission of the publisher.

in response to a Ca load.[235,236] One mechanism is by inhibition of NKCC2 expression[236] or activity. More recently, it has been suggested that CaSR acts primarily by regulating paracellular permeability. Loupy et al. showed that a CaSR antagonist increased $Ca^{2+}$ permeability in isolated perfused TALH with no change in transepithelial voltage or Na flux.[237] This appears to be mediated by regulation of the expression of claudin-14. Activation of the CaSR causes robust upregulation of claudin-14,[238,239] which through physical interaction, inhibits paracellular cation channels formed by claudin-16 and claudin-19[238] (see Fig. 7.7). The signaling mechanism seems to involve CaSR inhibiting calcineurin, a phosphatase that normally activates NFAT to increase transcription of two micro-RNAs miR-9 and miR-374, thereby downregulating claudin-14 expression.[240,241] The central role of claudin-14 is further supported by the finding that claudin-14 knockout mice are unable to increase their fractional excretion of calcium in response to a high $Ca^{2+}$ diet,[238] and exhibit complete loss of regulation of urinary $Ca^{2+}$ excretion in response to either a CaSR agonist or antagonist.[240,242] Of note, claudin-14 expression is also decreased in kidney of mice fed a low-calcium diet compared with those fed a high-calcium diet,[234] providing a mechanism by which calcium excretion is matched to dietary intake.

### DIURETICS

Loop diuretics such as furosemide increase urinary calcium losses. The mechanism by which furosemide causes hypercalciuria is linked to its ability to bind to and inhibit the furosemide-sensitive Na-K-Cl cotransporter, NKCC2,[192–195] present in the TALH. NaCl absorption is diminished, as is potassium recycling, resulting in a reduction in lumen positivity that drives $Ca^{2+}$ reabsorption. Subjects with the common form of Bartter syndrome have inactivating mutations of the NKCC2 and associated with calciuria.[203] Compensatory increases occur in the expression of distal tubule transport channels and proteins such as the TRPV5 and TRPV6 channels and calbindin $D_{28K}$ following the administration of furosemide, but fail to compensate for the increase in excretion that occurs in the TALH.[242] Thiazide diuretics, on the other hand, cause hypocalciuria[213,243–245] and the effect appears to be independent of PTH in humans and rodents. Thiazides bind to and inhibit the Na-Cl cotransporter in the distal tubule.[192,246] Chronic thiazide use is associated with a reduction in extracellular fluid volume, which secondarily enhances $Na^+$ and $Ca^{2+}$ reabsorption in the PT of in the kidney.[173] Distal tubule $Ca^{2+}$ transport is clearly unaffected by "chronic" thiazide use,[173] in contrast to older reports that thiazide "acutely" increases $Ca^{2+}$ reabsorption in isolated perfused DCT.[247] The development of hypocalciuria parallels a compensatory increase in $Na^+$ reabsorption secondary to an initial natriuresis following thiazide administration. These observations are supported by the upregulation of the $Na^+/H^+$ exchanger, responsible for the majority of $Na^+$ and associated $Ca^{2+}$ reabsorption in the PT, whereas the expression of proteins involved in active $Ca^{2+}$ transport in the distal tubule was unaltered. Indeed, thiazide administration was associated with hypocalciuria in *Trpv5*-knockout mice. Humans with Gitelman syndrome and inactivating mutations of the thiazide-sensitive Na-Cl transporter have hypocalciuria, hypomagnesemia, and volume depletion,[208,248–250] findings that are recapitulated in the Na-Cl cotransporter knockout mouse.[251]

*Clinical Relevance*

**Hypomagnesemia With Epidermal Growth Factor (EGF) Receptor Inhibitors**

Because EGF activates TRPM6 in the distal convoluted tubules, EGF receptor inhibitors, which are widely used as chemotherapeutic agents, cause hypomagnesemia. Monoclonal antibodies targeting the EGF receptor, such as cetuximab and panitumumab, are frequently associated with this complication, whereas the incidence with small-molecule tyrosine kinase inhibitors such as erlotinib seems to be less.

**Diuretics in Calcium Disorders**

Because of their hypercalciuric effect, loop diuretics are used for the acute treatment of hyperkalemia. Conversely, in patients with idiopathic hypercalciuria, thiazide diuretics are effective at lowering urine calcium concentration and thereby reducing the risk of kidney stone formation.

### ESTROGENS

Estrogens influence calcium transport in the kidney as postmenopausal women have higher urinary $Ca^{2+}$ excretion than premenopausal women.[252] In the early postmenopausal period the administration of estrogen is associated with a decrease in urine $Ca^{2+}$ excretion and an increase in serum PTH and $1\alpha,25(OH)_2D$.[253,254] Estradiol increases the expression of the TRPV5 channel in the kidney in a manner independent of $1\alpha,25(OH)_2D_3$.[255] These observations are supported by reduced duodenal TRPV5 channel expression in mice lacking the estrogen receptor $\alpha$.[256]

### EXTRACELLULAR FLUID VOLUME

In conditions such as volume depletion, where PT $Na^+$ reabsorption is increased, one also observes enhanced $Ca^{2+}$ reabsorption that can contribute to the hypercalcemia that is sometimes seen in such situations. Conversely, the salutary effects of isotonic saline administration in hypercalcemic patients are attributable to a reduction in $Ca^{2+}$ reabsorption as a result of reduced $Na^+$ reabsorption.

### METABOLIC ACIDOSIS AND ALKALOSIS

Metabolic acidosis is associated with hypercalciuria, and when prolonged, often results in bone loss and osteoporosis.[257] Metabolic acidosis and metabolic alkalosis decrease or increase the reabsorption of $Ca^{2+}$ in the distal tubule,[172,258–261] the expression TrpV5 in the distal tubule,[262] and the activity of TrpV5 channels.[263–265]

## REGULATION OF RENAL CALCIUM TRANSPORT BY NOVEL PROTEINS

### KLOTHO

Klotho is a coreceptor for the phosphaturic peptide, FGF 23, with $\beta$-glucuronidase activity.[266–269] It is a kidney- and parathyroid gland–specific protein, which influences epithelial $Ca^{2+}$ transport by deglycosylating TRPV5, thereby trapping the channel in the plasma membrane and sustaining the activity of the channel.[270] Further evaluation of serum Klotho concentrations and their association with changes in renal calcium excretion is required to establish a role of this factor in regulation of renal calcium transport.

### SCLEROSTIN

Sclerostin is an osteocyte-derived glycoprotein that influences bone mass.[271] Patients with sclerosteosis and its milder variant, van Buchem disease,[272–274] have exceptionally dense bones and skeletal overgrowth that often constricts cranial nerve foramina and the foramen magnum, resulting in premature death. Sclerosteosis is due to inactivating mutations of the sclerostin (*SOST*) gene, and the milder van Buchem disease is due to a 52-kb deletion of a downstream enhancer element of the sclerostin gene.[275] Mouse models of sclerosteosis have increases in skeletal mass similar to those found in patients with the disease.[55,276–278] By using a *Sost* gene knockout model generated in our laboratory[55] we have demonstrated that sclerostin, either directly or indirectly, through an alteration in the synthesis of 1α,25-dihydroxyvitamin D (1α,25$(OH)_2$D), influences renal calcium reabsorption in the kidney. Urinary calcium excretion and renal fractional excretion of calcium are decreased in *Sost*$^{-/-}$ mice.[55] Serum 1α,25$(OH)_2$D concentrations are increased without attendant hypercalcemia; renal 25(OH)D-1α hydroxylase (*Cyp27b1*) mRNA and protein expression are also increased in *Sost*$^{-/-}$ mice, strongly suggesting that the increase in serum 1α,25$(OH)_2$D concentrations was due to increased 1α,25$(OH)_2$D synthesis. When recombinant sclerostin is added to cultures of proximal tubular cells the expression of the messenger RNA for *Cyp27b1,* the 1α-hydroxylase cytochrome P450, is diminished. Serum 24, 25$(OH)_2$D concentrations were diminished in *Sost*$^{-/-}$ mice, and PTH concentrations were similar in knockout and wild-type mice. The lack of change in PTH is consistent with previous studies in humans.[279] The data suggest that in addition to the hormones traditionally thought to alter calcium reabsorption in the kidney (PTH and 1α,25$(OH)_2$D), sclerostin plays a significant role in altering renal calcium excretion. Wheras PTH and 1α,25$(OH)_2$D decrease fractional excretion of calcium by increasing the efficiency of calcium reabsorption in the DT, sclerostin increases fractional excretion of calcium (the absence of sclerostin expression being associated with a reduced fractional excretion of calcium).[55] Thus, the adaptation to a reduction in calcium intake and resultant downstream alterations in hormones may need to be amended to include changes in sclerostin expression (see Fig. 7.4B and Fig.7.8C).

## MAGNESIUM TRANSPORT IN THE KIDNEY

### THE ROLE OF MAGNESIUM IN CELLULAR PROCESSES

Magnesium is an abundant cation in the human body (Table 7.1).[280–285] Magnesium is required for a variety of biochemical functions.[286] The activities of magnesium-dependent enzymes are modulated by the metal as a result of binding to the substrate or as a result of direct binding to the enzyme.[286–289] Enzymes of the glycolytic and citric acid pathways, exonuclease, topoisomerase, RNA and DNA polymerases, and adenylate cyclase are among the many enzymes regulated by magnesium.[286–290] Additionally, magnesium regulates channel activity.[286]

**Table 7.2 Distribution and Concentrations of Magnesium in a Healthy Adult**

| Site | % total-body Mg | Concentration/content |
|---|---|---|
| Bone | 53 | 0.5% of bone ash |
| Muscle | 27 | 9 mmol/kg wet weight |
| Soft tissue | 19 | 9 mmol/kg wet weight |
| Adipose tissue | 0.012 | 0.8 mmol/kg wet weight |
| Erythrocytes | 0.5 | 1.65–2.73 mmol/L |
| Serum | 0.3 | 0.69–0.94 mmol/L |

Given its role in such diverse biological processes, it is not surprising that a deficiency or increase in serum magnesium concentrations is associated with important clinical symptoms.[291] For example, low magnesium concentrations are associated with muscular weakness, fasciculations, Chvostek and Trousseau signs, and sometimes frank tetany.[291] The tetany of hypomagnesemia is independent of changes in serum calcium. On occasion, personality changes, anxiety, delirium and psychoses may manifest. Hypocalcemia,[292–298] reduced PTH secretion,[299–304] and hypokalemia[305–308] are sometimes present in hypomagnesemic subjects. Cardiac arrhythmias and prolongation of the corrected QT interval[309,310] are sometimes observed. Conversely, hypermagnesemia seen in association with the administration of excessive amounts of magnesium in diseases such as eclampsia and in patients with renal failure is manifest as weakness of the voluntary muscles.

### MAGNESIUM IS PRESENT IN SERUM IN BOUND AND FREE FORMS

Most magnesium within the body is present in bone or within the cells (Table 7.2).[286] Approximately 60% of magnesium is stored in bone. Serum magnesium concentrations vary slightly with age and in adults are 1.6–2.3 mg/dL (0.66–0.94 mmol/L). Within plasma, about 70% of Mg is ultrafiltrable, 55% is free, and about 14% of Mg is in the form of soluble complexes with citrate and phosphate.[311] Because Mg is present largely within cells and bone, there is some interest as to whether serum Mg concentrations reflect tissue stores, especially when Mg is depleted or deficient. When rats[312–314] and humans[291,315] are fed Mg-deficient diets, serum Mg decreases within 1 day in rats and in 5–6 days in humans. Bone Mg and blood mononuclear cell Mg concentrations correlate well with total body Mg and serum Mg.[315–318] The correlations between total body Mg stores and muscle or cardiac Mg, however, are not precise.[315]

### REGULATION OF MG HOMEOSTASIS

The intestine and the kidney regulate magnesium balance (Fig. 7.9).[286] A diet adequate in magnesium normally contains 200–300 mg of magnesium.[319] Between 75 and 150 mg of ingested dietary magnesium is absorbed in the jejunum and ileum, primarily by paracellular passive processes.[320–325] The TRPM6 protein (a mutant form of this protein is present in patients with familial hypomagnesemia) is localized to

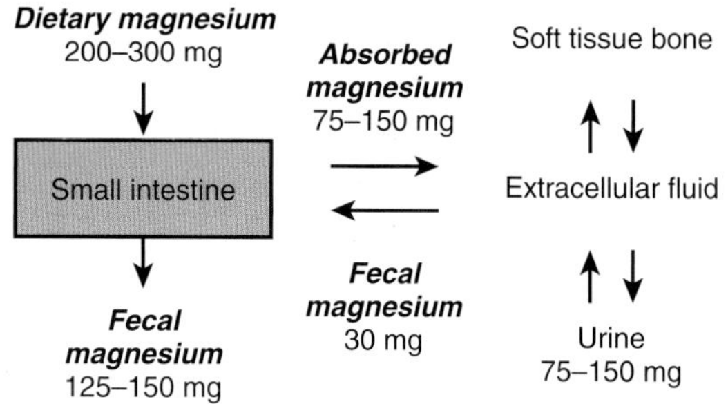


**Fig. 7.9** Magnesium homeostasis in normal humans showing the amounts of magnesium absorbed in the intestine and reabsorbed by the kidney.

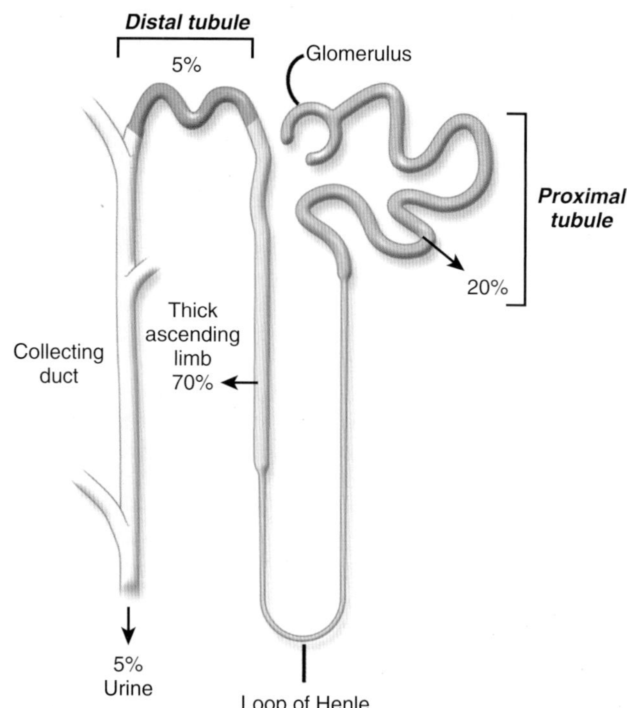


**Fig. 7.10** Percentages of filtered magnesium reabsorbed along the tubule.

the apical membrane of intestinal and renal epithelial cells and mediates transcellular magnesium absorption.[145,326] A homolog of TRPM6, TRPM7 is ubiquitously expressed and plays a role in whole-body magnesium homeostasis and many cellular functions, ranging from control of cell proliferation and cellular magnesium homeostasis to cell adhesion and cell migration.[327–335] It forms a heteromeric complex with TRPM6 and is necessary for TRPM6 activity and epithelial magnesium absorption.[336,337] About 30 mg of magnesium is secreted into the intestine via pancreatic and intestinal secretions, giving a net magnesium absorption of approximately 130 mg/24 h. Magnesium that is not absorbed in the intestine and is secreted into the intestinal lumen eventually appears in the feces (125–150 mg). Absorbed magnesium enters the extracellular fluid pool and moves in and out of bone and soft tissues. Approximately 130 mg of magnesium (equivalent to the net and amount absorbed in the intestine) is excreted in the urine.

In experimental animals and humans, feeding a diet low in magnesium results in a rapid decrease in urinary and fecal magnesium and the occurrence of a negative magnesium balance.[338–347] Conversely, the administration of magnesium is associated with an increase in the renal excretion of magnesium.[348–350] Unlike the cases of calcium and phosphorus, however, no hormones or molecules have been identified that alter magnesium transport in the intestine or that alter the renal excretion of magnesium in response to changes in magnesium balance.[286,351,352]

## REABSORPTION OF MAGNESIUM ALONG THE TUBULE

Approximately 10% of total body magnesium is filtered daily by the glomeruli (approximately 3000 mg/24 hr). About 75% of total plasma magnesium is filterable. Because urinary magnesium excretion is about 150 mg/24 hr, a substantial fraction of filtered magnesium is reabsorbed along the tubule (approximately 95%).

### MG$^{2+}$ REABSORPTION IN THE PROXIMAL TUBULE

Between 15% and 20% of filtered magnesium is reabsorbed in the PT (Fig. 7.10). The cellular and molecular mechanisms by which magnesium is reabsorbed in the proximal nephron are unknown. However, it is speculated that reabsorption of magnesium in the proximal nephron occurs by paracellular mechanisms, likely driven by the concentration gradient resulting from reabsorption of $Na^+$ and water. However, magnesium permeability in this segment is likely to be quite low, as the tubular fluid-to-ultrafiltrate magnesium ratio can rise to 1.65 in the late PT.[353]

### MG$^{2+}$ REABSORPTION IN THE THICK ASCENDING LIMB

The bulk of the filtered magnesium is reabsorbed in the TALH, again by a paracellular mechanism of which claudin-16 is a critical component.[199,201,354–361] As discussed earlier for $Ca^{2+}$ transport, claudin-16 and claudin-19 form cation-selective paracellular channels[199,200] that either directly mediate paracellular $Mg^{2+}$ reabsorption or facilitate the generation of an NaCl diffusion potential that provides the driving force for paracellular $Mg^{2+}$ reabsorption. Mutations of the *CLDN16* and *CLDN19* genes, and the *SLC12A1, KCNJ1,* and *CLCNKB* genes that encode proteins required for normal thick ascending limb function, result in excessive magnesium losses in the urine and hypomagnesemia. Claudin-10 is also highly expressed in the TALH. The predominant isoform, claudin-10b, acts as a paracellular $Na^+$ channel and is spatially distinct from claudin-16/19, being expressed mainly in the medullary TALH.[362] Deletion of the *Cldn10* gene in mice is associated with decreased paracellular sodium reabsorption, hypermagnesemia, and nephrocalcinosis.[363] In isolated perfused TAL tubules of claudin-10–deficient mice, paracellular permeability of sodium is decreased and the relative permeability of calcium and magnesium is increased. This suggests that claudin-10b uses the lumen-positive voltage in the early TALH to drive paracellular $Na^+$ reabsorption and thereby reduces the electrical potential available for divalent cation reabsorption later on in the cortical TALH. Mutations in claudin-10, or specifically in claudin-10b, have recently been described in several families with variable degrees of hypermagnesemia, hypocalciuria, and hypokalemic metabolic alkalosis, together with several unusual extrarenal manifestations, including anhidrosis, alacrima, xerostomia, and ichthyosis.[364–366] Fig. 7.11 shows the mechanism by which magnesium is transported in the TALH.

Magnesium reabsorption in the TALH is inhibited by hypermagnesemia, presumably because it reduces the concentration gradient for paracellular diffusion.[367] Conversely, hypomagnesemia and magnesium depletion stimulate magnesium reabsorption in the TALH.[368] These are also the main physiological regulators of renal magnesium excretion.

## $MG^{2+}$ REABSORPTION IN THE DISTAL TUBULE

Between 5% and 10% of filtered magnesium is reabsorbed transcellularly in the distal convoluted tubule. The rate-limiting step is thought to be apical entry of $Mg^{2+}$ through an $Mg^{2+}$ channel that is formed by a complex of TRPM6 and TRPM7.[326,336,337] Epidermal growth factor (EGF) promotes TRPM6 trafficking to the plasma membrane.[369] The driving force for apical $Mg^{2+}$ entry is the lumen-negative electrical membrane potential, the set point of which is likely determined by the conductance of an apical voltage-gated potassium channel, Kv1.1.[370] These explain why mutations in TRPM6, pro-EGF, and Kv1.1 are all genetic causes of hypomagnesemia (see Chapter 44 for a detailed discussion of inherited hypomagnesemia).

It is unclear as to the mode of basolateral exit of magnesium from the cell into the interstitial space. CNNM2 is suspected to play a role because it encodes a transmembrane protein localized at the basolateral membrane that is regulated by $Mg^{2+}$ deficiency and when mutated causes renal $Mg^{2+}$ wasting.[371] It has been proposed to function as an $Mg^{2+}$ channel or $Mg^{2+}$-sensitive $Na^+$ channel,[372,373] but others have not found evidence that it transports $Mg^{2+}$.[374]

Another intriguing possibility is SLC41A1, a homolog of bacterial MgtE $Mg^{2+}$ transporters[375] that functions as an $Na^+$-$Mg^{2+}$ exchanger when expressed in mammalian cells.[376] Interestingly, mutations in SLC41A1 have recently been found to cause a form of nephronopthisis.[377] Because basolateral extrusion of $Mg^{2+}$ in the DT must involve energetically active transport, it is likely that the Na-K-ATPase plays a role, albeit indirectly. FXYD2 likely participates in this because it is the gamma subunit of the Na-K-ATPase and, when mutated, causes dominant isolated hypomagnesemia. Likewise, the transcription cofactors, hepatocyte nuclear factor 1B (HNF1B) and pterin-4 alpha-carbinolamine dehydratase (PCBD1) costimulate the promoter of FXYD2, and so mutations in either of them are associated with hypomagnesemia.[378,379] Finally, mutations in the basolateral potassium channel in the DT, Kir4.1, cause a syndrome called SeSAME or EAST that is associated with hypomagnesemia.[380,381] Kir4.1 is thought to facilitate $Mg^{2+}$ reabsorption in the DT by recycling $K^+$ across the basolateral membrane, thus enabling the Na-K-ATPase to transport $Na^+$. Fig. 7.12 shows the cellular localization of these proteins in the distal convoluted tubule into the cell.

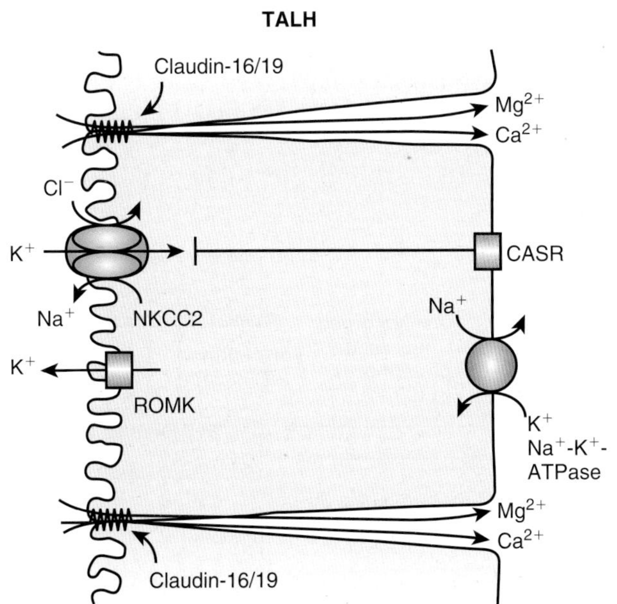


**Fig. 7.11 Mechanism by which magnesium is transported in cells of the thick ascending limb of the loop of Henle *(TALH)*.** The majority of magnesium is reabsorbed by paracellular mechanisms. Claudin-16 and claudin-19 are depicted as directly transporting $Ca^{2+}$ and $Mg^{2+}$, but it has also been hypothesized that their primary role is to allow backleak of reabsorbed $Na^+$ and thus establish an NaCl diffusion potential, thereby indirectly facilitating divalent cation reabsorption. *CaSR,* Calcium-sensing receptor; *NKCC2,* Na-K-Cl cotransporter; *ROMK,* renal outer medullary potassium channel.

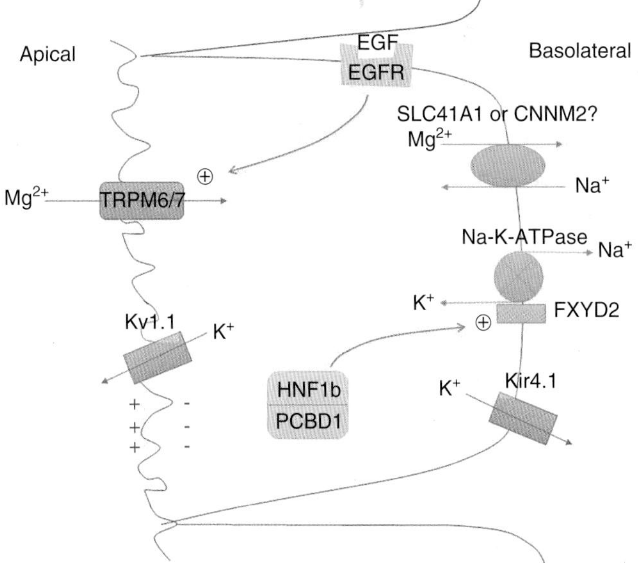


**Fig. 7.12 Mechanism by which magnesium is transported in distal tubule cells.** The majority of magnesium is reabsorbed by transcellular mechanisms. $Mg^{2+}$ enters apically via the TRPM6/7 heteromeric channel, driven by the membrane voltage set by the $K^+$ channel, Kv1.1. Its exit pathway is unknown but may be via CNNM2 or SLC41A1, perhaps acting as a basolateral Na–Mg exchanger. Active extrusion is likely driven by the $Na^+$ gradient generated by the Na-K-ATPase alpha subunit and accessory subunit, FXYD2. The basolateral $K^+$ channel Kir 4.1 recycles $K^+$ that enters via the Na-K-ATPase. See text for role of other regulators. *EGF,* Epidermal growth factor; *EGFR, epidermal growth factor receptor.*

## REGULATION OF MAGNESIUM TRANSPORT IN THE KIDNEY

A variety of factors alter magnesium reabsorption in the kidney (Table 7.3)*. With the exception of magnesium excess and depletion, it is unclear whether any of these are physiologically important regulators. Thus, although effects on magnesium excretion in the urine are noted following the infusion of various substances or following blockade of their activity, it is not clear that such changes occur with physiologic changes in concentrations of these factors in vivo. Furthermore, the concentrations of the effector substances do not change in the physiologically appropriate manner following changes in serum concentrations of magnesium. Thus, hormonal homeostasis, in which concentrations of a hormone (PTH, glucagon, arginine vasopressin, and so on) change following changes in the concentration of magnesium, and in turn, alter the retention or concentrations of magnesium, is difficult to demonstrate.

# PHOSPHORUS TRANSPORT IN THE KIDNEY

## THE ROLE OF PHOSPHORUS IN CELLULAR PROCESSES

Phosphorus is a key component of hydroxyapatite, the major component of bone mineral, nucleic acids, bioactive signaling proteins, phosphorylated enzymes, and cellular membranes.[411–414] Prolonged deficiency of phosphorus and inorganic phosphate results in serious biological problems, including impaired bone mineralization, resulting in osteomalacia or rickets, abnormal erythrocyte, leukocyte and platelet function, impaired cell membrane integrity that can result in rhabdomyolysis, and impaired cardiac function.[415–417] Phosphate balance is maintained through a series of complex hormonally and locally regulated metabolic adjustments. In states of neutral phosphate balance, net intake equals net output. The major organs involved in the absorption, excretion, and reabsorption of phosphate are the intestine and the kidney (Fig. 7.13). A normal diet adequate in phosphorus normally contains ~1500 mg of phosphorus. Approximately 1100 mg of ingested dietary phosphate is absorbed in the proximal intestine predominantly in the jejunum. About 200 mg of phosphorus is secreted into the intestine via pancreatic and intestinal secretions, giving a net phosphorus absorption of approximately 900 mg/24 hr. Phosphorus that is not absorbed in the intestine or is secreted into the intestinal lumen eventually appears in the feces. Absorbed phosphorus enters the extracellular fluid pool and moves in and out of bone (and to a smaller extent in and out of soft tissues) as needed (~200 mg). Approximately 900 mg of phosphorus (equivalent to the amount absorbed in the intestine) is excreted in the urine.

**Table 7.3 Factors Altering the Reabsorption of Magnesium in the Kidney**

| Substance | Effect |
|---|---|
| **Peptide hormones** | |
| Parathyroid hormone[205,383–387] | Increase |
| Calcitonin[387–395] | Increase |
| Glucagon[396,397] | Increase |
| Arginine vasopressin[398] | Increase |
| Insulin[399] | Increase |
| **β-Adrenergic agonists** | |
| Isoproterenol[382] | Increase |
| **Prostaglandins PGE$_2$**[400] | Decrease |
| **Mineralocorticoids** | |
| Aldosterone | Increase |
| **1, 25-dihydroxyvitamin D$_3$**[401] | Decrease |
| **Magnesium** | |
| Restriction[338–341,343] | Increase |
| Increase[348–350] | Decrease |
| **Metabolic alkalosis**[261,402,403] | Increase |
| **Metabolic acidosis**[261,402,403] | Decrease |
| **Hypercalcemia**[404] | Decrease |
| **Phosphate depletion**[405,406] | Decrease |
| **Diuretics** | |
| Furosemide | Decrease |
| Amiloride[408,409] | Increase |
| Chlorothiazide[407,410] | Increase |

*PGE$_2$*, Prostaglandin E$_2$.
From Dai LJ, Ritchie G, Kerstan D, et al. Magnesium transport in the renal distal convoluted tubule. *Physiol Rev.* 2001;81:51–84.

*References 205, 261, 338–341, 343, 348–350, and 382–410.

## PHOSPHORUS IS PRESENT IN BLOOD IN MULTIPLE FORMS

About 85% of phosphorus in the body is present in bones, 14% exists in cells from soft tissues, and 1% is present in extracellular fluids. In mammals, bone contains a substantial amount of phosphorus (approximately 10 g/100 g dry fat free tissue); in comparison, muscle contains 0.2 g/100 g fat free tissue, and the brain 0.33 g/100 g fresh tissue.[418] Phosphorus is present in virtually every bodily fluid. In human plasma

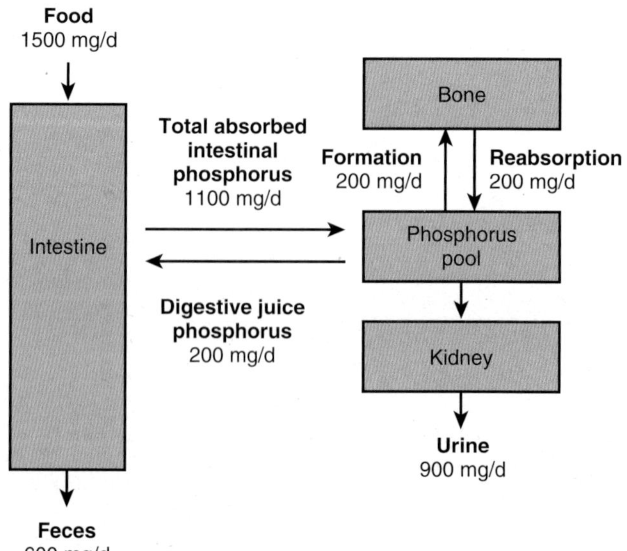


**Fig. 7.13 Phosphorus homeostasis in humans.** The major organs involved in the absorption, excretion, and reabsorption of phosphate are the intestine and the kidney.

**Table 7.4 Distribution of and Concentrations of Phosphorus (mmol/L) in Adult Human Blood**

| Phosphorus Compounds | Erythrocytes | Plasma |
|---|---|---|
| Phosphate ester | 12.3–19.0 | 0.86–1.45 |
| Phospholipids | 4.13–4.81 | 2.23–3.13 |
| Inorganic phosphate | 0.03–0.13 | 0.71–1.36 |

or serum, phosphorus exists in the form of inorganic phosphorus or phosphate (Pi), lipid phosphorus, and phosphoric ester phosphorus. Total serum phosphorus concentrations range between 8.9 and 14.9 mg/dL (2.87–4.81 mmol/L), inorganic phosphorus (phosphate, Pi) concentrations between 2.56 and 4.16 mg/dL (0.83–1.34 mmol/L) (this is what is usually measured clinically and referred to as the serum phosphorus, and the normal range changes with age),[419] phosphoric ester phosphorus concentrations between 2.5 and 4.5 mg/dL (0.81–1.45 mmol/L), and lipid phosphorus concentration between 6.9 and 9.7 mg/dL (2.23–3.13 mmol/L) (Table 7.4).[418]

## REGULATION OF PHOSPHATE HOMEOSTASIS—AN INTEGRATED VIEW

Intestinal feed-forward and hormonal feedback systems (PTH–vitamin D endocrine system and the phosphatonins) are likely to be responsible for the control of phosphorus homeostasis (Fig. 7.14). The short-term responses that occur within minutes to hours of feeding of a high-Pi meal are important in regulating phosphorus homeostasis via feed-forward mechanisms, whereas the longer-term changes occur as a result of alterations in circulating concentrations of PTH, $1\alpha,25(OH)_2D_3$, and the phosphatonins such as fibroblast growth factor 23.[86,420–423] Intestinal signals have been shown in rodents to rapidly alter renal Pi excretion in response to changes in duodenal Pi concentrations.[421]

PTH, $1\alpha,25(OH)_2D_3$, and the phosphatonin FGF-23 control phosphorus homeostasis on longer-term basis (hours to days).[85,86] Concentrations of these hormones and factors are regulated by phosphorus in a manner that is conducive to the maintenance of normal phosphorus concentrations. Fig. 7.15 shows the physiologic changes known to occur with low or high dietary intakes of phosphate. A decrease in serum phosphate concentrations, as would occur with a reduced intake of phosphorus, results in increased ionized calcium concentrations, decreased PTH secretion, and a subsequent decrease in renal phosphate excretion. At the same time, by PTH-independent mechanisms, there is an increase in renal 25-hydroxyvitamin D 1α-hydroxylase activity, increased $1\alpha,25(OH)_2D_3$ synthesis, and increased phosphorus absorption in the intestine and reabsorption in the kidney.[88,92,94,99–105] Conversely, with elevated phosphate intake, there are decreased calcium concentrations and increased PTH release from the parathyroid gland. PTH actually has two opposing effects: it increases urinary phosphate excretion but also increases the synthesis of $1\alpha,25(OH)_2D_3$ by stimulating the activity of the renal 25-hydroxyvitamin D 1α-hydroxylase; the net effect is to increase renal phosphate excretion. Increased serum phosphate concentrations simultaneously inhibit renal 25-hydroxyvitamin D 1α-hydroxylase and decrease $1\alpha,25(OH)_2D_3$ synthesis. Reduced $1\alpha,25(OH)_2D_3$ concentrations decrease intestinal phosphorus absorption as well as renal

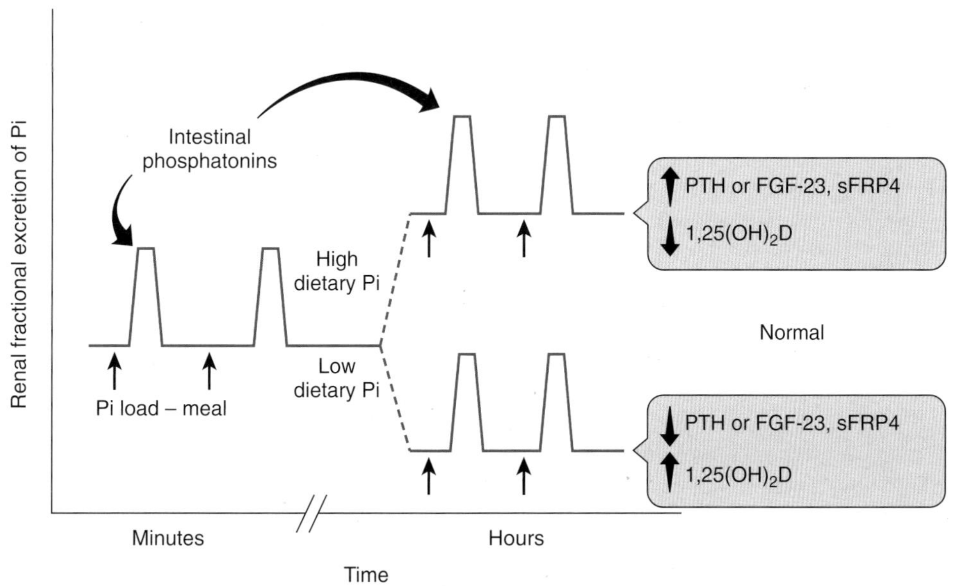


**Fig. 7.14 Intestinal feed-forward and hormonal feedback systems are responsible for the control of phosphorus homeostasis.** Changes in intestinal luminal phosphate concentrations *(Pi load – meal)* result in the elaboration of chemical signals *(Intestinal phosphatonins)* that alter the fractional excretion of phosphate in the kidney over a time frame of minutes. Long-term changes in the amount of phosphate in the diet result in changes in the concentrations of PTH, 1α,25-dihydroxyvitamin D, and phosphatonins, which influence the fractional excretion of phosphate in the kidney over a time frame of hours, as shown. Short-term changes mediated by feed-forward intestinal signals are proposed to be superimposed on this chronic baseline. *PTH,* Parathyroid hormone.

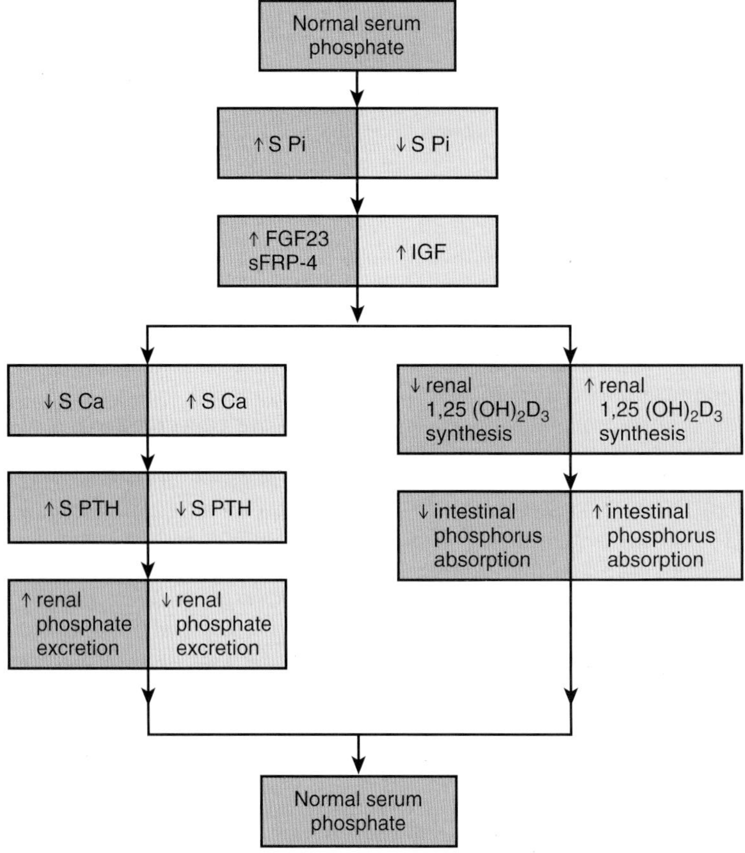


**Fig. 7.15** Changes in growth factors (fibroblast growth factor 23 *[FGF 23]*, *sFRP-4* (secreted frizzled related protein 4) insulin-like growth factor *(IGF)*, parathyroid hormone *(PTH)*, and 1α,25-dihydroxyvitamin D, and the subsequent physiologic changes in intestinal phosphate absorption or renal phosphate reabsorption following perturbations in serum phosphate.

phosphate reabsorption. All of these factors tend to bring serum phosphate concentrations back into the normal range.

The phosphatonins FGF-23 and sFRP-4 inhibit renal phosphate reabsorption.[98,424–432] They also decrease,[424,430,433–438] and IGF-1 increases[96] the activity of the 25-hydroxyvitamin D 1α-hydroxylase ("growth factors" in Fig. 7.15). FGF-23 induces renal phosphate wasting in patients with tumor-induced osteomalacia (TIO),[427,439–441] autosomal dominant hypophosphatemic rickets (ADHR), X-linked hypophosphatemic rickets (XLH), and autosomal recessive hypophosphatemic rickets (ARHR).[425,430,432,442] From a physiologic perspective, it would be appropriate for FGF-23 and sFRP-4 concentrations to be regulated by the intake of dietary phosphorus and by serum phosphate concentrations. In humans, in the short-term the feeding of meals containing increased amounts of phosphate does not increase serum FGF-23 concentrations despite the induction of a robust and dose-dependent phosphaturia.[422,443] Other human studies conducted over a period of days or weeks, however, have shown changes in serum FGF-23 concentrations following alterations in the content of phosphate in the diet.[444,445] In mice, Perwad et al. have shown that a high-phosphate diet increased and a low-phosphate diet decreased serum FGF-23 levels in these animals within 5 days of a changing dietary phosphate intake.[446] The changes in serum FGF-23 correlated with changes in serum phosphate concentrations. Studies from our laboratory performed in rats fed a low-, normal, or high-phosphate diet demonstrate that serum FGF-23 levels significantly decrease in animals fed a low-phosphate diet, and increase in animals fed a high-phosphate diet within 24 hours of altering dietary phosphate intake but do not correlate with serum phosphate in the animals fed a high-phosphate diet.[98]

## REABSORPTION OF PHOSPHATE ALONG THE NEPHRON

Virtually all serum phosphate is filtered at the glomerulus.[447] Under conditions of normal dietary phosphate intake, and in the presence of intact parathyroid glands, approximately 20% of the filtered phosphate load is excreted. The other 80% of the filtered load of phosphate is reabsorbed by the renal tubules. The PTs are the major sites of phosphate reabsorption along the nephron (Fig. 7.16).[447] Little phosphate reabsorption occurs between the late PT and the early distal tubule in animals with intact parathyroid glands.[448–456] In the absence of PTH, however, phosphate is avidly reabsorbed between the late PT and early distal tubule, reflecting phosphate reabsorption by the proximal straight tubule.[451] Phosphate transport rates are approximately three times higher in the proximal convoluted than in the proximal straight tubules.[457] Renal phosphate handling is characterized by intranephronal heterogeneity, reflecting segmental differences in phosphate handling within an individual nephron as well as internephronal heterogeneity.[448,452,457,458]

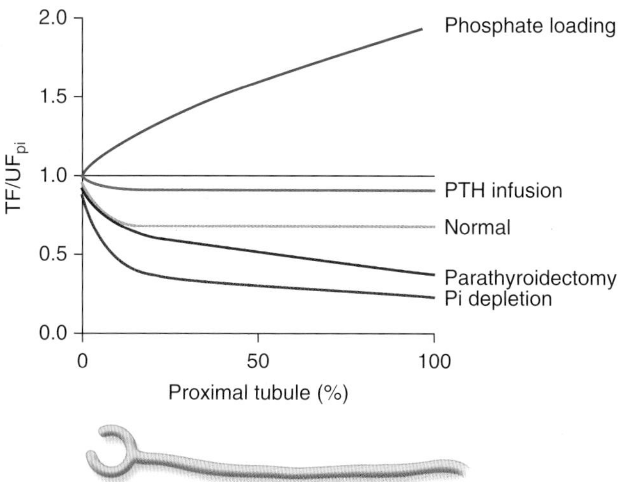


**Fig. 7.16 The proximal tubule is the major site of phosphate reabsorption along the nephron.** The effects of dietary phosphate loading or deprivation, parathyroid hormone *(PTH)* infusion, or parathyroidectomy on phosphate absorption along the proximal tubule are shown. *Proximal tubule %,* Distance along the proximal tubule as a percentage of total length; *PTH,* parathyroid hormone; *TF/UFPi,* ratio of tubular fluid-to-ultrafiltrate phosphate concentration.

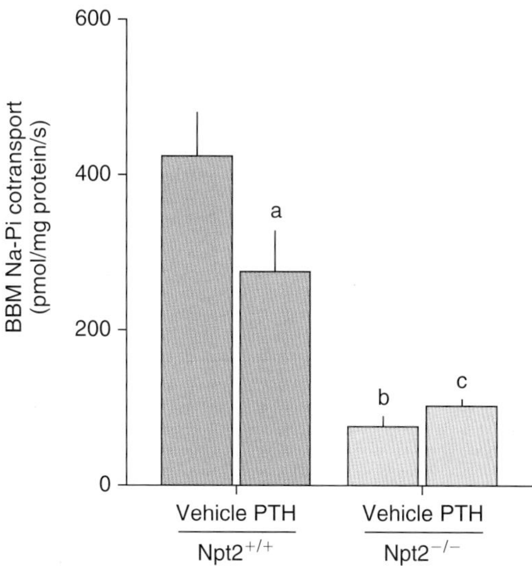


**Fig. 7.17 Mice with ablation of the *NaPi-IIa* gene exhibit renal phosphate wasting and fail to respond to parathyroid hormone (PTH).** The effect of PTH or vehicle on brush border membrane (BBM) Na-Pi cotransport in *Npt2*$^{+/+}$ and *Npt2*$^{-/-}$ mice is shown. [a]Effect of PTH in *Npt2*$^{+/+}$ mice, $P < .0015$. [b]Effect of genotype in vehicle-treated mice, $P < .0001$; [c]Effect of genotype in PTH-treated mice, $P < .0041$. Reproduced from Zhao N, Tenenhouse HS. Npt2 gene disruption confers resistance to the inhibitory action of parathyroid hormone on renal sodium-phosphate cotransport. *Endocrinology* 2000;141:2159–2165.

The uptake of phosphate is mediated by Na–phosphate cotransporters located at the apical border of PT cells (NaPi-IIa/Slc34A1 and NaPi IIc/Slc34a3).[459–482] The structure and physiology of these phosphate transport molecules have been extensively reviewed, and the reader is directed to other publications in this regard.[459–482] The Na–phosphate cotransporters are highly homologous and are predicted to have similar structures. Mice with ablation of the *NaPi-IIa/Slc34a1* gene exhibit renal phosphate wasting and reduced PT brush border membrane vesicle phosphate uptake (Fig. 7.17).[483] In humans, *SLC34A1* mutations are associated with hypophosphatemia and urinary phosphate losses with urolithiasis or bone demineralization.[484] It is estimated that the NaPi-IIa transporter is responsible for approximately 85% of proximal tubular phosphate transport and contributes to the adaptive increases in tubular phosphate transport in animals fed a low-phosphate diet.[483,485] Mice with constitutive or renal-specific deletions of the *NaPi-IIc/Slc34a3* gene do not display abnormalities in phosphate excretion or phosphate serum concentrations.[486,487] This is in contrast to humans, in whom *SLC34A3* mutations are associated with hypophosphatemic rickets with hypercalciuria.[488,489] The extrusion of phosphate at the basolateral membrane of the proximal tubular cell may be mediated by the xenotropic and polytropic retroviral receptor (Xpr1).[490] Mice with conditional deletions of *Xpr1* exhibited tubular dysfunction with glycosuria, amino-aciduria, hypercalciuria, and phosphaturia and developed hypophosphatemic rickets. In primary cultures of proximal tubular cells, Xpr1 deficiency significantly reduced phosphate uptake and decreased the expression of NaPi-IIa and NaPi-IIc cotransporters.

Interactions between the NaPi-IIa/Slc34A1 and the intracellular protein, the sodium-hydrogen exchanger regulatory factor-1 (NHERF-1), modulate the amount of NaPi-IIa/Slc34A1 and NaPi IIc/Slc34a3 present on the surface of the proximal tubular cell.[491–510] By binding to the NaPi-IIa/Slc34A1 protein, NHERF-1 functions to retain the NaPi-IIa/Slc34A1 protein on the surface of the proximal tubular cell; phosphate uptake diminishes as a consequence of endocytosis of the NaPi-IIa/Slc34A1 when it dissociates from NHERF-1, a process that is activated by the hormonal induction of protein kinase C and the phosphorylation of specific serine and threonine residues on the PDZ domain of NHERF-1.[495,500,506,511–514] Ezrin, a protein that facilitates the association of NHERF-1 to the actin cytoskeleton, also plays a role in the regulation of proximal tubular phosphate transport and the expression of NaPi-IIa/Slc34A1 in proximal tubular cells.[515,516] Ezrin knockdown mice exhibit hypophosphatemia and osteomalacia and a reduction in NaPi-IIa/Slc34A1 and NHERF-1 expression at the apical membrane of PTs. Cellular events associated with uptake of Pi into the cell and extrusion of Pi out of the cell are shown in Fig. 7.18.

## REGULATION OF PHOSPHATE TRANSPORT IN THE KIDNEY

### DIETARY PHOSPHATE

The influence of dietary phosphate intake on the urinary excretion of phosphate has been known for many years.[448,517–532] The reabsorption of phosphate is decreased in animals fed a high-phosphate diet, whereas animals with a low intake of phosphate reabsorb almost 100% of the filtered load of phosphate.* These changes in phosphate reabsorption are associated with parallel changes in the abundance of NaPi-IIa and IIc.[535,536] In infants and children, phosphate reabsorption is high so as to maintain a positive phosphate balance required for growth.[537,538] Conversely, decreased phosphate reabsorption has been demonstrated in the elderly.[539]

*References 182, 219–228, 234, 240, 241, 354, 533, and 534.

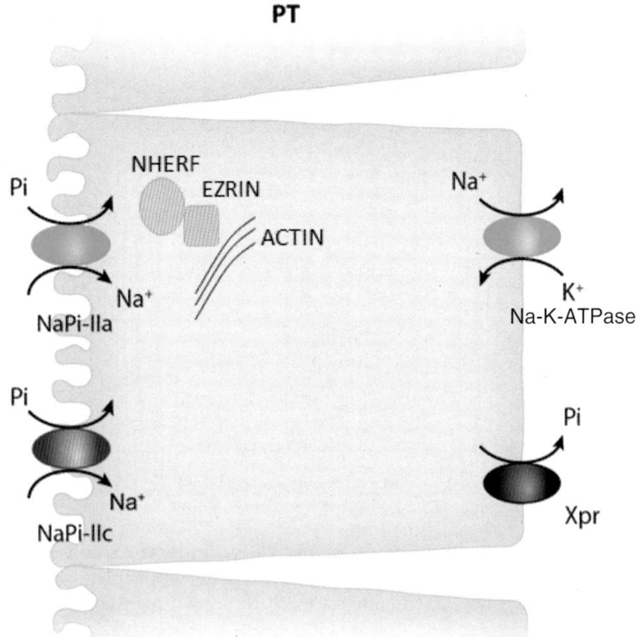


**Fig. 7.18 Mechanisms by which phosphate is transported across the proximal tubular cell.** Apical uptake is mediated by the sodium-phosphate cotransporters IIa and IIc. The Na-K ATPase located at the basolateral aspect of the cell provides a sodium gradient within the cell that permits these sodium-phosphate cotransporters to take up sodium and phosphate. By binding to the NaPi-IIa protein, NHERF-1 retains the NaPi-IIa protein on the surface of the proximal tubular cell thereby enhancing phosphate uptake; phosphate uptake diminishes as a consequence of endocytosis of the NaPi-IIa when it dissociates from NHERF-1, a process that is activated by the hormonal induction of protein kinase C and the phosphorylation of specific serine and threonine residues on the PDZ domain of NHERF-1. Ezrin, a protein that facilitates the association of NHERF-1 to the actin cytoskeleton also regulates proximal tubular phosphate transport. Ezrin knock down mice exhibit hypophosphatemia and osteomalacia and a reduction in NaPi-IIa/Slc34A1 and NHERF-1 expression at the apical membrane of proximal tubules. The xenotropic and polytropic retroviral receptor (Xpr1) plays a role in the extrusion of phosphate at the basolateral cell surface. *PT,* Proximal tubule.

Although dietary phosphate deprivation and excess results in marked changes in the plasma concentrations of several hormones (see Fig. 7.15) that contribute to the increase or decrease in renal phosphate reabsorption, acute changes in tubular reabsorption can also be demonstrated independent of changes in these hormones.[421,540–543] When a bolus of phosphate is instilled into the duodenum of intact rats, renal phosphate excretion increases within 10 minutes without changes in serum Pi concentrations.[421] The change in Pi reabsorption in response to a high-Pi meal is independent of plasma Pi concentrations and filtered Pi load. Such changes are not elicited upon the administration of NaCl into the duodenum. The increase in renal phosphate excretion is independent of PTH as thyro-parathyroidectomy does not alter the process. Serum concentrations of PTH do not change, and serum concentrations of other phosphaturic peptides, such as FGF-23 and sFRP-4, are unchanged following the infusion of intraduodenal phosphate. Aqueous duodenal extracts contain a phosphaturic substance that is likely to be a protein. The processes or pathways by which changes in luminal phosphate concentrations within the bowel are detected have not been defined, although the presence of a "phosphate sensor" has been postulated.[544] A recent study, though, suggests that such an intestinal phosphate-sensing mechanism may be absent in humans.[545]

Studies using cultured renal proximal tubular cells provide evidence of an intrinsic ability of these cultured cells to increase phosphate transport when exposed to a low phosphate concentration in the medium.[540–543] The mechanism of upregulation of Na/Pi cotransport in OK cells by low-Pi media involves two regulatory mechanisms: an immediate (early) increase (after 2 hours) in the expression of Na/Pi cotransporter, independent of mRNA synthesis or stability, and a delayed (late) effect (after 4–6 hours), resulting in an increase in NaPi-4 mRNA abundance.[542,546] The enhanced Pi reabsorption of short-term Pi deprivation has been linked to decreased intrarenal synthesis of dopamine and/or stimulation of beta adrenoreceptors, because infusion of dopamine or propranolol restores the phosphaturic response to PTH in short-term (less than 3 days) Pi deprivation.[547–549] Conversely, dopamine may also mediate the acute phosphaturic effect of a high-Pi diet.[499] The NaPi-IIa transporter is expressed in the brain and is regulated by dietary Pi, suggesting that dietary Pi could regulate neural outputs and regulate renal Pi excretion.[550] Increasing cerebrospinal fluid Pi concentrations in the presence of low plasma Pi concentrations reversed the adaptations to feeding a low-Pi diet, suggesting that the Pi concentration in the brain regulates not only central but also renal expression of NaPi-IIa transporters. It should be remembered that alterations in serum Pi concentrations also alter $1\alpha,25(OH)_2D_3$ synthesis and serum concentrations.[88,92,94,99–105] Infusions of $1\alpha,25(OH)_2D_3$ increase the renal reabsorption Pi, predominantly in the proximal nephron.[68,551–557]

## PARATHYROID HORMONE

Parathyroidectomy decreases renal Pi excretion and, conversely, injection of PTH increases urinary Pi excretion[558–562] by altering Pi reabsorption along the PT (see Fig. 7.16).[450–454,563] The proximal straight tubule is an important site of PTH action with respect to Pi transport and may be critical in the final regulation of Pi excretion.[449,455,458,564] PTH maintains Pi homeostasis by regulating NaPi cotransporters in the kidney. This is mediated by PTH/PTHrP receptors on the apical membrane that signal through protein kinase C (PKC), and on the basolateral membrane that signal through both cAMP/PKA and PKC. This leads to endocytosis of NaPi-IIa and -IIc cotransporters, which are degraded within the lysosomes.[469,474,565,566] The transporters are reduced in number along the apical borders of proximal tubular cells following the administration of PTH 1-34 but not by the administration of PTH 3-34.[479,480] Disruption of the *NaPi-IIa* (*Slc34a1*) gene in mice resulted in increased Pi excretion compared with wild-type mice and a resistance to the phosphaturic effect of PTH (see Fig. 7.17), although the cyclic adenosine monophosphate (cAMP) response is normal.[567] It has been proposed that the primary mechanism for PTH action is PKC-mediated phosphorylation of a PDZ domain on NHERF-1. This leads to dissociation of NaPi-IIa/NHERF-1 complexes, freeing NaPi-IIa from the apical surface for internalization.[500,506]

Under certain conditions, the phosphaturic effect of PTH is blunted or absent. These include short-term Pi deprivation or acute respiratory alkalosis. In these situations, the inhibitory effect of PTH on Pi reabsorption by the proximal convoluted tubule remains intact. However, the increased delivery of Pi leads to enhanced downstream reabsorption by the proximal straight tubule.[455,458,564] These studies suggest that the regulation of Pi reabsorption by PTH in the proximal convoluted and proximal straight tubules may be mediated by different mechanisms. It should be noted that PTH has two opposing effects: PTH increases urinary Pi excretion but also increases the synthesis of 1α,25(OH)$_2$D$_3$ by stimulating the activity of the 25(OH)D$_3$ 1α-hydroxylase enzyme in the kidney.[88,92,94,99–105]

## VITAMIN D AND VITAMIN D METABOLITES

Dietary Pi deprivation or hypophosphatemia induces 25-hydroxyvitamin D$_3$ 1α-hydroxylase.[88,92,94,99–105] Mice or rats, but not pigs, fed a low-Pi diet show a decrease in the activity of the 25-hydroxyvitamin D$_3$ 24-hydroxylase (a renal enzyme involved in the catabolism of 1,25(OH)$_2$D$_3$) compared with rats fed a normal Pi diet within 24 hours of Pi restriction.[83,568,569] 1,25(OH)$_2$D$_3$ decreases renal Pi excretion,[62,68,551–554] but the mechanism remains unknown. VDR-mutant mice exhibit decreased serum Pi; however, Pi transport or by renal cortical brush border membranes, Pi excretion, or NaPi-IIa or NaPi IIc mRNA levels were not different between VDR-null or wild-type mice, whereas NaPi-IIa protein expression and NaPi-IIa cotransporter immunoreactive signals were slightly but significantly decreased in the VDR mice compared with the wild-type mice.[536] When VDR knockout mice were fed a low-Pi diet, serum Pi concentrations were more markedly decreased in the VDR knockout mice than in the wild-type mice. Other studies performed in VDR and 25(OH)D 1α-hydroxylase–null mutant mice show that both these knockout mice adapt to Pi deprivation with increased NaPi-IIa protein in a manner similar to that found in wild-type mice.[570] However, when these mice were fed a high-Pi diet, Pi excretion was less in the VDR and 25-hydroxyvitamin D 1α-hydroxylase–null mutant mice compared with the wild-type mice. In vitamin D–deprived rats, NaPi-IIa transporter protein and mRNA were reported to be decreased in juxtamedullary but not superficial renal cortical tubules compared with normal rats.[571]

## INSULIN, GROWTH HORMONE, AND INSULIN-LIKE GROWTH FACTOR

Insulin decreases plasma Pi and Pi excretion in human and animal models.[572–575] This enhanced renal Pi reabsorption can be demonstrated in the absence of changes in blood glucose, PTH, and Pi levels or urinary Na excretion. Micropuncture studies[573] demonstrate enhanced Pi reabsorption in hyperinsulinemic dogs and somatostatin infusion, which decreases plasma insulin levels and increases Pi excretion.[576] Growth hormone decreases Pi excretion and has been postulated to contribute to increased Pi reabsorption and positive Pi balance demonstrated in growing animals.[577,578] Administration of a growth hormone antagonist for 4 days to immature rats is associated with increased Pi excretion and a decreased transport capacity for Pi reabsorption.[579,580] In juvenile rats suppression of growth hormone is associated with an increase in Pi excretion as a result of decreased NaPi-IIa expression.[581] Growth hormone administration increases Pi uptake by brush border membrane vesicles.[582] Because growth hormone increases renal insulin-like growth factor-1 (IGF-1 synthesis),[583] the effects of growth hormone on Pi reabsorption may also be due to IGF-1.[577,583–588]

## RENAL NERVES, CATECHOLAMINES, DOPAMINE, AND SEROTONIN

Numerous studies have demonstrated that acute renal denervation or the administration of catecholamines alters Pi reabsorption regardless of PTH.[547,589–601] The increase in urinary Pi excretion after acute renal denervation could be due to both increased production of dopamine and decreased α- or β-adrenoreceptor activity, because acute renal denervation has been shown to initially increase renal dopamine excretion and almost completely abolish renal norepinephrine and epinephrine levels.[602,603] Epinephrine decreases plasma Pi, presumably by shifting Pi from the extracellular into the intracellular space. The hypophosphatemic response to isoproterenol infusion is blocked by propranolol, suggesting involvement of the beta adrenoreceptors. Infusion of isoproterenol markedly enhances renal Pi reabsorption in normal rats and in hypophosphatemic mice.[600,604] The enhanced Pi reabsorption and attenuated phosphaturic response to PTH observed in acute respiratory alkalosis and Pi deprivation is blocked by infusion of propranolol, suggesting a possible role for stimulation of β-adrenoreceptors in these conditions. Stimulation of α-adrenoreceptors by the addition of epinephrine to OK cells blunts the PTH-induced increase in cAMP levels and the inhibition of Pi transport.[605] Stimulation of α2-adrenoreceptors in vivo has also been demonstrated to attenuate the phosphaturic response to PTH.[548] Dopamine infusion and the infusion of L-dopa or gludopa, or dopamine precursors, increase Pi excretion in the absence of PTH.[606–608] Dopamine administration decreases Pi transport in OK cells and rabbit proximal straight tubules.[599,609–614] Increasing dietary Pi intake increases urinary dopamine excretion and Pi excretion.[615] Inhibition of endogenous dopamine synthesis by the administration of carbidopa to rats results in decreased dopamine and Pi excretion, suggesting a role for endogenous dopamine in Pi regulation.[595,603] A paracrine role for dopamine in Pi regulation is strengthened by studies in OK cells showing that the addition of dopamine or L-dopa selectively decreases Pi uptake. Furthermore, Pi-replete OK cells produce more dopamine from L-dopa than Pi-deprived cells.[611] Dopamine inhibits Pi transport by multiple mechanisms, including activation of DA1 and DA2 receptors.[610,613,614] Dopamine induces the internalization of NaPi-IIa cotransporter molecules by activation of luminal DA1 receptors.[609] Renal PTs also synthesize serotonin from 5-hydroxytryptophan using the same enzyme that converts L-dopa to dopamine. Incubation of OK cells with either serotonin or 5-hydroxytryptophan enhances Pi transport and raises the possibility that serotonin may also be involved in the physiologic regulation of renal Pi transport.[606,612,616,617]

## PHOSPHATOMINS (FGF-23, sFRP-4)

The term "phosphatonin" was introduced to describe a factor or factors responsible for the inhibition of renal phosphate reabsorption and altered 25(OH)D 1α- hydroxylase regulation observed in patients with tumor-induced osteomalacia.[440] Cai et al.[439] described a patient with TIO in whom the biochemical characteristics of hypophosphatemia, renal phosphate wasting, and reduced serum 1α,25(OH)$_2$D disappeared following removal of the tumor. Several factors have been identified that are associated with phosphate wasting, including FGF-23 sFRP-4, fibroblast growth factor 7 (FGF-7), and matrix extracellular phosphoglycoprotein (MEPE).

The most extensively studied phosphatonin is FGF-23, a 251–amino acid–secreted protein.[419,425,431,618] Recombinant FGF-23 administered intraperitoneally to mice or rats induces phosphaturia and inhibits 25-hydroxyvitamin D 1α-hydroxylase activity.[419,425,431,618] The minimal sequence needed for phosphaturic activity resides between amino acids 176 and 210.[431] Transgenic animals overexpressing FGF-23 are hypophosphatemic, phosphaturic, and show the presence of rickets and reduced serum 1α,25(OH)$_2$D concentrations or 25-hydroxyvitamin D 1α-hydroxylase activity.[433,434,619] Conversely, mice in which the *FGF-23* gene has been ablated demonstrate hyperphosphatemia, reduced phosphate excretion, markedly elevated serum 1α,25(OH)$_2$D concentrations and renal 25-hydroxyvitamin D 1α-hydroxylase mRNA expression, vascular calcification, and early mortality.[434,620] The ablation of the VDR in FGF-23–null mice has been reported to rescue this phenotype, supporting an important role for vitamin D in the pathogenesis of the abnormal phenotype seen in FGF-23–null mice.[621]

FGF-23 binds and signals through FGF receptors 1c, 3c, and FGFR4[269]; the role of Fgfr3 and Fgfr4 has not been established in mice in vivo.[622] Han et al. recently demonstrated that mice with deletion of *Fgfr1* in the PT had an increase in sodium-dependent phosphate cotransporter expression, hyperphosphatemia and refractoriness to the phosphaturic action of FGF-23, suggesting that FGFR1c plays a key role in its effects in the PT.[623] Deletion of the *Fgfr1* in the distal tubule resulted in hypercalciuria and secondary hyperparathyroidism. A coreceptor, klotho, is necessary for FGF-23 to exhibit bioactivity.[269,624] The role of klotho in FGF-23 signaling is supported by the observation that klotho knockout mice have a phenotype identical to that of FGF-23 knockout mice,[625] whereas a human mutation that increases klotho levels phenocopies TIO and X-linked hypophosphatemic rickets.[626]

The mechanism for FGF-23 action is thought to involve downstream signaling through ERK1/2 and serum and glucocorticoid kinase-1 (SGK1).[627] SGK1 in turn phosphorylates NHERF1, leading to the dissociation of NaPi-IIa transporters that become internalized and degraded, analogous to its regulation by PTH.[628] This model is supported by the observation that FGF-23 is no longer phosphaturic when given to NHERF1-null mice.[629] Recent evidence suggests that Jak3 may also be involved because Jak3-null mice have renal phosphate wasting and elevated FGF-23 levels.[630]

FGF-23 synthesis is regulated by 1α,25(OH)$_2$D. Increasing doses of 1α,25(OH)$_2$D increase FGF-23 concentrations in the serum within 24 hours, but statistically significant changes are observed 4 hours after 1α,25(OH)$_2$D treatment.[631,632] In the physiologic sense, it is possible that FGF-23 is a negative feedback regulator of the 25-hydroxyvitamin D 1α-hydroxylase enzyme.

The Wnt antagonist, sFRP-4, is highly expressed in tumors associated with renal phosphate wasting and osteomalacia.[429] Recombinant sFRP-4 is phosphaturic in rats and prevents the upregulation of the 25-hydroxyvitamin D 1α-hydroxylase enzyme seen in the presence of hypophosphatemia.[424] sFRP-4 decreases Na$^+$-Pi cotransporter abundance in the brush border membrane of the PT, and reduces the surface expression of the Na$^+$-Pi-IIa cotransporter in PTs of the kidney, as well as on the surface of OK cells.[438] sFRP-4 expression is increased in bone samples and serum from X-linked hypophosphatemic mice in mice with a global knockout of the *phex* gene but not in mice in which the *phex* gene has been knocked out in bone alone.[633] sFRP-4 protein concentrations are increased in the kidneys of rats fed a high-phosphate diet for 2 weeks but not in animals fed a low-phosphate diet, suggesting a possible role for sFRP-4 during increases in phosphate intake.[634] This suggests in turn that sFRP-4 concentrations are altered in the kidney of animals fed a high-phosphate diet and could play a role in the long-term adaptations to high-phosphate intake.

MEPE is abundantly overexpressed in tumors associated with renal phosphate wasting and osteomalacia.[635] Recombinant MEPE is phosphaturic and reduces serum phosphate concentrations when administered to mice in vivo.[636] The protein has been shown to inhibit phosphate reabsorption in the proximal convoluted tubule,[637] to inhibit Na-dependent phosphate uptake in opossum kidney cells, and to reduce PT expression of NaPi-IIa protein.[638] The protein has also been demonstrated to reduce intestinal Pi absorption directly.[638] MEPE also inhibits bone mineralization in vitro, and MEPE-null mice have increased bone mineralization.[639] Thus, it is possible that MEPE is important in the pathogenesis of hypophosphatemia in renal phosphate wasting observed in patients with TIO. However, MEPE infusion does not recapitulate the defect in vitamin D metabolism seen in patients with TIO.[636] Infusion of MEPE reduces serum phosphate concentrations, and serum 1α,25(OH)$_2$D concentrations increase following MEPE as would be expected in the face of hypophosphatemia. Thus, in patients with TIO, it is likely that MEPE contributes to the hypophosphatemia, but other products such as FGF-23 and sFRP-4 inhibit 1α,25(OH)$_2$D concentrations by inhibiting the activity of the 25-hydroxyvitamin D 1α-hydroxylase. MEPE may play a role in the pathogenesis of X-linked hypophosphatemic rickets, in which there is phosphate wasting, and evidence for a mineralization defect that is independent of low phosphate concentrations in the extracellular fluid.[633] MEPE expression is increased in mice with the *Hyp* mutation, and mice with a global knockout of the *phex* gene but not in mice with a bone specific knockout of the *phex* gene. It is not known whether MEPE is regulated by phosphate concentrations although Jain et al. have demonstrated that it is correlated with serum Pi concentration in normal humans.[640] Another growth factor, FGF-7, also known as keratinocyte growth factor, is overexpressed in tumors associated with phosphate wasting and osteomalacia.[488] FGF-7 inhibits Na-dependent phosphate transport in OK cells, and we have demonstrated that FGF-7 inhibits renal phosphate reabsorption in vivo. FGF-7 is present in normal plasma and is significantly increased in patients with renal failure (personal observations). Whether or not FGF-7 is regulated by phosphate concentrations is unknown.

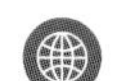 Complete reference list available at ExpertConsult.com.

## KEY REFERENCES


2. Brini M, Carafoli E. Calcium pumps in health and disease. *Physiol Rev.* 2009;89:1341–1378.
10. Marx SJ, Attie MF, Stock JL, et al. Maximal urine-concentrating ability: familial hypocalciuric hypercalcemia versus typical primary hyperparathyroidism. *J Clin Endocrinol Metab.* 1981;52:736–740.
14. Moore EW. Ionized calcium in normal serum, ultrafiltrates, and whole blood determined by ion-exchange electrodes. *J Clin Invest.* 1970;49:318–334.
15. DeLuca HF, Schnoes HK. Metabolism and mechanism of action of vitamin D. *Annu Rev Biochem.* 1976;45:631–666.
17. Wasserman RH, Smith CA, Brindak ME, et al. Vitamin D and mineral deficiencies increase the plasma membrane calcium pump of chicken intestine. *Gastroenterology.* 1992;102:886–894.
55. Ryan ZC, Ketha H, McNulty MS, et al. Sclerostin alters serum vitamin D metabolite and fibroblast growth factor 23 concentrations and the urinary excretion of calcium. *Proc Natl Acad Sci U S A.* 2013;110:6199–6204.
60. Brown EM, Pollak M, Hebert SC. The extracellular calcium-sensing receptor: its role in health and disease. *Annu Rev Med.* 1998;49: 15–29.
145. Dimke H, Hoenderop JG, Bindels RJ. Molecular basis of epithelial Ca2+ and Mg2+ transport: insights from the TRP channel family. *J Physiol.* 2011;589:1535–1542.
159. Borke JL, Minami J, Verma A, et al. Monoclonal antibodies to human erythrocyte membrane Ca++-Mg++ adenosine triphosphatase pump recognize an epitope in the basolateral membrane of human kidney distal tubule cells. *J Clin Invest.* 1987;80:1225–1231.
165. Lassiter WE, Gottschalk CW, Mylle M. Micropuncture study of renal tubular reabsorption of calcium in normal rodents. *Am J Physiol.* 1963;204:771–775.
168. Agus ZS, Gardner LB, Beck LH, et al. Effects of parathyroid hormone on renal tubular reabsorption of calcium, sodium, and phosphate. *Am J Physiol.* 1973;224:1143–1148.
175. Yu AS, Cheng MH, Coalson RD. Calcium inhibits paracellular sodium conductance through claudin-2 by competitive binding. *J Biol Chem.* 2010;285:37060–37069.
192. Gamba G, Miyanoshita A, Lombardi M, et al. Molecular cloning, primary structure, and characterization of two members of the mammalian electroneutral sodium-(potassium)-chloride cotransporter family expressed in kidney. *J Biol Chem.* 1994;269:17713–17722.
199. Konrad M, Schaller A, Seelow D, et al. Mutations in the tight-junction gene claudin 19 (CLDN19) are associated with renal magnesium wasting, renal failure, and severe ocular involvement. *Am J Hum Genet.* 2006;79:949–957.
203. Hebert SC. Bartter syndrome. *Curr Opin Nephrol Hypertens.* 2003;12: 527–532.
206. Costanzo LS, Windhager EE. Calcium and sodium transport by the distal convoluted tubule of the rat. *Am J Physiol.* 1978;235: F492–F506.
208. Dimke H, Hoenderop JG, Bindels RJ. Hereditary tubular transport disorders: implications for renal handling of Ca2+ and Mg2+. *Clin Sci.* 2010;118:1–18.
210. Hoenderop JG, Nilius B, Bindels RJ. Calcium absorption across epithelia. *Physiol Rev.* 2005;85:373–422.
211. Hoenderop JG, van Leeuwen JP, van der Eerden BC, et al. Renal Ca2+ wasting, hyperabsorption, and reduced bone thickness in mice lacking TRPV5. *J Clin Invest.* 2003;112:1906–1914.
216. Magyar CE, White KE, Rojas R, et al. Plasma membrane Ca2+-ATPase and NCX1 Na+/Ca2+ exchanger expression in distal convoluted tubule cells. *Am J Physiol Renal Physiol.* 2002;283:F29–F40.
219. Yu AS, Hebert SC, Lee SL, et al. Identification and localization of renal Na(+)-Ca2+ exchanger by polymerase chain reaction. *Am J Physiol.* 1992;263:F680–F685.
246. Gamba G, Saltzberg SN, Lombardi M, et al. Primary structure and functional expression of a cDNA encoding the thiazide-sensitive, electroneutral sodium-chloride cotransporter. *Proc Natl Acad Sci U S A.* 1993;90:2749–2753.
270. Chang Q, Hoefs S, van der Kemp AW, et al. The beta-glucuronidase klotho hydrolyzes and activates the TRPV5 channel. *Science.* 2005; 310:490–493.
298. Wiegmann T, Kaye M. Hypomagnesemic hypocalcemia. Early serum calcium and late parathyroid hormone increase with magnesium therapy. *Arch Intern Med.* 1977;137:953–955.
300. Sherwood LM, Herrman I, Bassett CA. Parathyroid hormone secretion in vitro: regulation by calcium and magnesium ions. *Nature.* 1970;225:1056–1058.
301. Chase LR, Slatopolsky E. Secretion and metabolic efficacy of parthyroid hormone in patients with severe hypomagnesemia. *J Clin Endocrinol Metab.* 1974;38:363–371.
308. Whang R, Chrysant S, Dillard B, et al. Hypomagnesemia and hypokalemia in 1,000 treated ambulatory hypertensive patients. *J Am Coll Nutr.* 1982;1:317–322.
326. Voets T, Nilius B, Hoefs S, et al. TRPM6 forms the Mg2+ influx channel involved in intestinal and renal Mg2+ absorption. *J Biol Chem.* 2004;279:19–25.
359. Simon DB, Lu Y, Choate KA, et al. Paracellin-1, a renal tight junction protein required for paracellular Mg2+ resorption. *Science.* 1999;285:103–106.
378. Ferre S, de Baaij JH, Ferreira P, et al. Mutations in PCBD1 cause hypomagnesemia and renal magnesium wasting. *J Am Soc Nephrol.* 2014;25:574–586.
416. Knochel JP. The pathophysiology and clinical characteristics of severe hypophosphatemia. *Arch Intern Med.* 1977;137:203–220.
419. Berndt T, Kumar R. Phosphatonins and the regulation of phosphate homeostasis. *Annu Rev Physiol.* 2007;69:341–359.
421. Berndt T, Thomas LF, Craig TA, et al. Evidence for a signaling axis by which intestinal phosphate rapidly modulates renal phosphate reabsorption. *Proc Natl Acad Sci U S A.* 2007;104:11085–11090.
427. Bowe AE, Finnegan R, Jan de Beur SM, et al. FGF-23 inhibits renal tubular phosphate transport and is a PHEX substrate. *Biochem Biophys Res Commun.* 2001;284:977–981.
428. De Beur SM, Finnegan RB, Vassiliadis J, et al. Tumors associated with oncogenic osteomalacia express genes important in bone and mineral metabolism. *J Bone Miner Res.* 2002;17:1102–1110.
430. Schiavi SC, Kumar R. The phosphatonin pathway: new insights in phosphate homeostasis. *Kidney Int.* 2004;65:1–14.
431. Berndt TJ, Craig TA, McCormick DJ, et al. Biological activity of FGF-23 fragments. *Pflugers Arch.* 2007;454:615–623.
439. Cai Q, Hodgson SF, Kao PC, et al. Brief report: inhibition of renal phosphate transport by a tumor product in a patient with oncogenic osteomalacia. *N Engl J Med.* 1994;330:1645–1649.
441. Shimada T, Mizutani S, Muto T, et al. Cloning and characterization of FGF23 as a causative factor of tumor-induced osteomalacia. *Proc Natl Acad Sci U S A.* 2001;98:6500–6505.
451. Greger R, Lang F, Marchand G, et al. Site of renal phosphate reabsorption. Micropuncture and microinfusion study. *Pflugers Arch.* 1977;369:111–118.
452. Haramati A, Haas JA, Knox FG. Nephron heterogeneity of phosphate reabsorption: effect of parathyroid hormone. *Am J Physiol.* 1984;246:F155–F158.
474. Murer H, Hernando N, Forster I, et al. Proximal tubular phosphate reabsorption: molecular mechanisms. *Physiol Rev.* 2000;80:1373–1409.
482. Werner A, Moore ML, Mantei N, et al. Cloning and expression of cDNA for a Na/Pi cotransport system of kidney cortex. *Proc Natl Acad Sci U S A.* 1991;88:9608–9612.
483. Beck L, Karaplis AC, Amizuka N, et al. Targeted inactivation of Npt2 in mice leads to severe renal phosphate wasting, hypercalciuria, and skeletal abnormalities. *Proc Natl Acad Sci U S A.* 1998;95:5372–5377.
618. ADHR Consortium. Autosomal dominant hypophosphataemic rickets is associated with mutations in FGF23. *Nat Genet.* 2000;26:345–348.
633. Yuan B, Takaiwa M, Clemens TL, et al. Aberrant Phex function in osteoblasts and osteocytes alone underlies murine X-linked hypophosphatemia. *J Clin Invest.* 2008.
635. Rowe PS, de Zoysa PA, Dong R, et al. MEPE, a new gene expressed in bone marrow and tumors causing osteomalacia. *Genomics.* 2000; 67:54–68.

# 8 Renal Handling of Organic Solutes

Volker Vallon | Stefan Broer | Sanjay K. Nigam

CHAPTER OUTLINE



KEY POINTS

- In a normoglycemic adult, the kidneys filter 160–180 g/day of glucose (~30% of daily energy expenditure), which is reabsorbed by the sodium glucose cotransporter SGLT2 (~97%) and SGLT1 (~3%) in the early and late proximal tubule, respectively.
- The basal overall glucose tubular reabsorption capacities for SGLT2 versus SGLT1 is in the range of 3:1 to 5:1. The transport capacity of tubular SGLT1 is unmasked (up to ~80 g/day) when more glucose is delivered to the late proximal tubule (e.g., in diabetes or with SGLT2 inhibition).
- The good correlation between the level of basolateral GLUT1 expression and the glycolytic activity of the different nephron segments indicates that the more distal tubule segments in particular are taking up glucose for energy supply via basolateral GLUT1.
- One of the major roles of organic anionic transporters, long considered mainly drug and toxin transporters, now appears to be to regulate many aspects of endogenous physiology.
- OAT1 and OAT3 appear to be the major renal basolateral transporters involved in the elimination of numerous uremic toxins originating in the gut microbiome, although OCT2 is likely the main route of TMAO elimination.
- The Remote Sensing and Signaling Hypothesis is a systems biology theory about the role of SLC and ABC transporters in the interorgan and interorganismal (e.g., host gut microbiome) "remote" communication via transporter-mediated movement of metabolites, signaling molecules, gut microbiome products, nutrients, uric acid, and uremic toxins into different body tissues and fluid compartments. It provides a framework for understanding uremia and hyperuricemia.
- Amino acid transporters often form heterodimers with ancillary subunits that are essential for trafficking of the transporters to the cell surface. Genetic complexity is observed in renal aminoacidurias due to heterodimer formation and transporter redundancy.
- Rare inherited aminoacidurias define four major routes of amino acid reabsorption. Amino acid antiporters play an important role in the apical and basolateral transport of cationic and neutral amino acids.

## GLUCOSE

The kidneys are a major site of glucose handling. This includes the continuous glomerular filtration of large amounts of glucose, almost all of which is subsequently reabsorbed by the proximal tubule, such that the formed urine in a healthy individual is nearly glucose free. The glucose reabsorbed by the proximal tubule is primarily taken up into the peritubular capillaries and provided as an energy source to further distal tubular segments or returned to the systemic circulation. Moreover and in addition to the liver, the kidneys contribute to the endogenous production of glucose or gluconeogenesis. Thus, the kidneys use glucose as fuel but also contribute to maintaining blood glucose levels and overall metabolic balance by reabsorbing filtered glucose and generating new glucose.

This is relevant in healthy individuals, in particular in the fasting state, and becomes pathophysiologically important in diabetes and hyperglycemic conditions. As a consequence, new antihyperglycemic drugs have been developed that target renal glucose reabsorption, induce urinary glucose loss, and have clinical efficacy with regard to lowering blood glucose, and even more importantly, they have protective effects on the kidney and cardiovascular system.

## PHYSIOLOGY OF RENAL GLUCOSE TRANSPORT

In many organisms including human, the cellular uptake and metabolism of D-glucose serves as an important energy source.[1,2] The brain primarily runs on glucose and depends on its continuous uptake, which alone requires ~125 g of glucose every day. As a consequence, glucose homeostasis is finely regulated, and blood glucose levels are maintained in a range of 4–9 mmol/L by various hormones, including insulin and glucagon, that regulate glucose uptake into target cells as well as glucose storage and endogenous glucose production.[1,2]

Glucose is a small molecule that is freely filtered by the glomeruli of the kidneys. Under conditions of normal blood glucose levels (~5.5 mmol/L or 100 mg/dL) and normal glomerular filtration rate (GFR, ~180 L/day), the kidneys filter 160–180 g of glucose each day. This is equal to ~30% of the daily energy expenditure, which would be lost into the urine if not regained by the renal tubules. Instead, more than 99% of the filtered glucose is reabsorbed by the tubules, primarily in the proximal tubule (Fig. 8.1). As described in more detail below, glucose reabsorption in the proximal tubule involves the two $Na^+$-glucose cotransporters SGLT2 and SGLT1, which are expressed in the brush border membrane of the early and later proximal tubule, respectively. $Na^+$–glucose cotransport is a saturable process and has a maximum transport capacity (Tmax). The Tmax of the kidneys for glucose can vary among individuals and averages ~430 g and ~500 g/day (300 and 350 mg/min) in female and male healthy human subjects, respectively.[3,4] This equals ~threefold the normal tubular glucose load of 160–180 g/day so that the renal glucose reabsorption capacity is not saturated under conditions of normal blood glucose levels and GFR. Theoretically, at a normal GFR, the Tmax should be reached, and glucose should begin to be excreted in the urine at a plasma glucose threshold of ~15.5 mmol/L (280 mg/dL). The Tmax for glucose of individual nephrons is variable, however, and thus, low-level urinary glucose spilling begins in a normal, glucose-tolerant individual at modestly elevated plasma glucose levels of ~10–11 mmol/L (180–200 mg/dL; see "Splay," Fig. 8.2). A robust and linear increase in urinary glucose excretion occurs when blood glucose levels rise above 15–16 mmol/L. GFR is a determinant of the filtered glucose load, and as a consequence, glucosuria can occur at lower plasma glucose concentrations when GFR is elevated (e.g., in pregnancy or in diabetes), or at higher blood glucose levels when GFR is reduced (e.g., in chronic kidney disease; CKD). In addition, changes in the transport activity and expression level of SGLT2 and SGLT1 (see later) are expected to further modify this relationship.

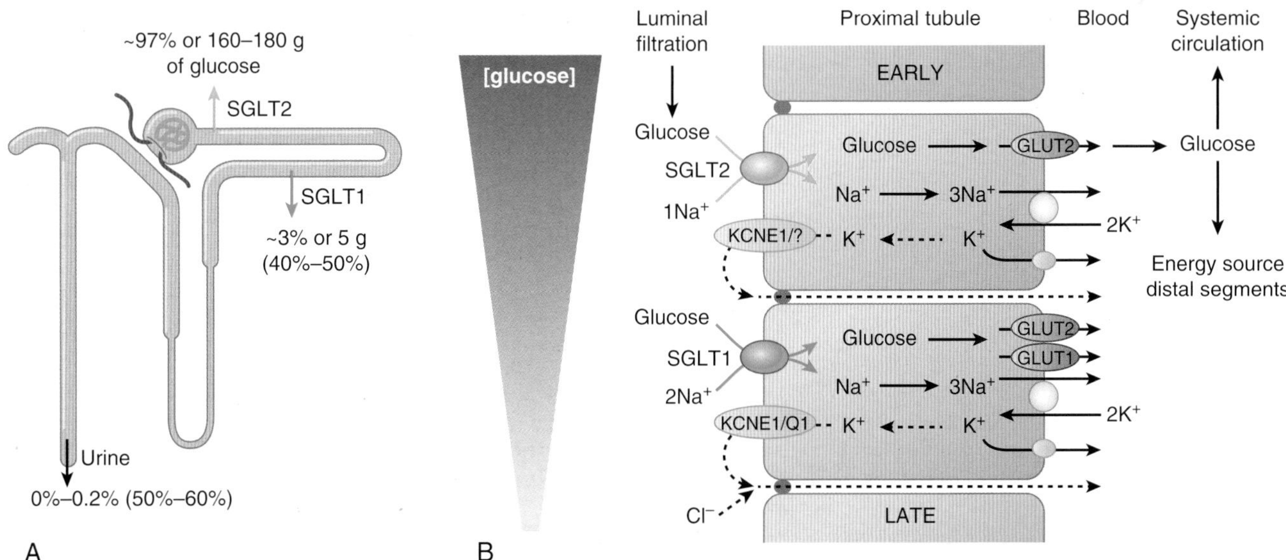


**Fig. 8.1 Glucose transport in the kidney.** (A) Under normoglycemia, ~97% of filtered glucose is reabsorbed via SGLT2 in the early segments of the proximal tubule. The remaining ~3% of glucose is reabsorbed by SGLT1 in the late proximal tubule such that the urine is nearly free of glucose. SGLT2 inhibition shifts glucose reabsorption downstream and unmasks the capacity of SGLT1 to reabsorb glucose (~40% of filtered glucose, depending on glucose load; see numbers in parentheses). (B) Cell model of glucose transport: The basolateral $Na^+$-$K^+$-ATPase lowers cytosolic $Na^+$ concentrations and generates a negative interior voltage, thereby providing the driving force for $Na^+$-coupled glucose uptake through SGLT2 and SGLT1 across the apical membrane. The facilitative glucose transporters GLUT2 and GLUT1 mediate glucose transport across the basolateral membrane down its chemical gradient. $Na^+$–glucose cotransport is electrogenic and accompanied by paracellular $Cl^-$ reabsorption or transcellular $K^+$ secretion to stabilize membrane potential; $K^+$ channels KCNE1/unknown $\alpha$ subunit and KCNE1/KCNQ1 in early and late proximal tubule, respectively. (This figure was modified with permission from Vallon V. Molecular determinants of renal glucose transport. *Am J Physiol Cell Physiol.* 2011;300:C6–C8.)

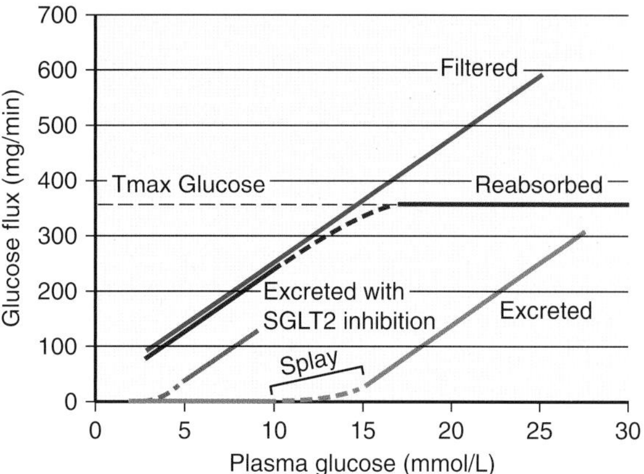


**Fig. 8.2 Tubular reabsorption and urinary excretion of glucose as a function of filtered glucose.** Tubular reabsorption of glucose increases linearly with the filtered glucose load until reabsorption reaches the tubular reabsorption capacity *(Tmax Glucose)* and glucose starts appearing in the urine. Theoretically, a Tmax of ~350 mg/min and normal glomerular filtration rate would result in a plasma glucose threshold of ~15.5 mmol/L. However, due to variability of Tmax in individual nephrons, the plasma glucose concentration that results in glucosuria in a normal individual is ~10–11.1 mmol/L (see "*Splay*"). SGLT2 inhibition reduces the renal glucose reabsorption to the transport capacity of SGLT1 and shifts the function to the left—that is, it reduces the renal glucose threshold (~3 mM) and Tmax (~150 mg/min).

## A PRIMARY ROLE FOR SGLT2 IN RENAL GLUCOSE REABSORPTION

Experiments performed on isolated nephron segments of rabbit kidneys in the early 1980s identified differences in the rate of uptake and affinity for glucose between the early and late proximal tubule segments, respectively.[5] Subsequent studies confirmed that the heterogeneity in glucose transport across the proximal tubule was attributed to the presence of two different glucose transporters in the brush border membrane.[6] These studies and transport studies in membrane vesicles and analyses of mRNA expression in isolated nephron segments of rat and rabbit kidneys as well as the cloning of the responsible genes, performed largely between 1981 and 1995, identified the $Na^+$–glucose cotransporters SGLT2 (SLC5A2) and SGLT1 (SLC5A1) as the primary genes and pathways for renal glucose reabsorption.[5–14] These studies established the concept that the "bulk" of tubular glucose uptake across the apical membrane occurs in the "early" proximal tubule (S1/2 segment) and is mediated by the low-affinity and high-capacity SGLT2. In comparison, the higher-affinity and lower-capacity SGLT1 is thought to "clean up" most of the remaining luminal glucose in "later" parts of the proximal tubule (S2/S3 segment) (see Fig. 8.1). In accordance, SGLT2 and SGLT1 have been localized with the use of well-validated antibodies in both rodents and humans to the brush border membrane primarily of the early and late proximal tubule, respectively.[15–18] In the mouse kidney, the levels of SGLT1 protein expression in the brush border were highest in S2 segments and somewhat lower in S3 segments in medullary rays and in the outer stripe.[19] In the human kidney, the strongest expression of SGLT1 was found in the S3 segment.[18] In accordance and demonstrating the functional role of SGLT2, free-flow renal micropuncture showed that glucose reabsorption in the early proximal tubule is completely absent in mice lacking SGLT2[15] (Fig. 8.3). In comparison, fractional glucose reabsorption along the proximal convoluted tubule (PCT) was only slightly reduced from 97% to 94% in mice lacking SGLT1.[20]

The phenotype of humans carrying mutations in the genes for SGLT1 (*SLC5A1*) and SGLT2 (*SLC5A2*) demonstrated their distinct quantitative contribution to renal glucose reabsorption. Mutations in SGLT1 cause "Intestinal Glucose Galactose Malabsorption" [Online Mendelian Inheritance in Man (OMIM) 182380] because the active intestinal reabsorption of glucose is mediated by SGLT1.[21,22] Newborns with mutations in SGLT1 as well as mice lacking SGLT1[20] can present with life-threatening diarrhea when exposed to dietary galactose or glucose; however, they show little or no glucosuria. In contrast, individuals with mutations in SGLT2 present persistent "Familial Renal Glucosuria" (OMIM 233100) ranging from 1 to >100 g per day, but they have no intestinal phenotype.[23] Although mutations in SGLT2 are rare and therefore the consequences are not well studied or fully understood, it is remarkable that no other complications (e.g., urinary infections or impaired kidney function) have been consistently observed in these subjects.[21,23] This information added to the rationale of developing SGLT2 inhibitors as potentially safe antihyperglycemic drugs (see later). Consistent with the described phenotypes in humans, genetic and pharmacologic studies in mice showed that under normoglycemic conditions, SGLT2 reabsorbs ~97% of the filtered glucose, whereas SGLT1 mediates the reabsorption of the remaining ~2%–3%[15,20,24] (see Figs. 8.1 and 8.3).

## UNMASKING A SIGNIFICANT GLUCOSE TRANSPORT CAPACITY OF SGLT1 IN THE LATE PROXIMAL TUBULE

In healthy human subjects, similar to the phenotype in rodents, SGLT2 is thought to reabsorb >90% of filtered glucose, yet they maintain a fractional glucose reabsorption of 40%–50% following application of a selective SGLT2 inhibitor[25–27] (see Fig. 8.1). This observation is mimicking the phenotype of normoglycemic mice lacking *Sglt2* (*Sglt2–/–*), in which fractional renal glucose reabsorption varied between 10% and 60%, inversely with the amount of filtered glucose, with a mean value of ~40%[15] (see Fig. 8.3). Follow-up studies demonstrated that the persisting glucose reabsorption is mediated in the downstream late proximal tubule by SGLT1, whose transport capacity is unmasked by SGLT2 inhibition (Figs. 8.1 and 8.3). First and indirect evidence came from micropuncture studies in *Sglt2–/– mice*: these mice have no net glucose reabsorption in the early proximal tubule; however, their glucose reabsorption in the later parts of the PCT accessible to micropuncture, where SGLT1 is expressed in S2 segments, is increased compared with wild-type (WT) mice[15] (Fig. 8.3). Metabolic cage studies further showed that the dose–response curve for glucosuria of a selective SGLT2 inhibitor was shifted leftward in *Sglt1–/–* mice; that is, glucosuria initiated at lower doses, and the maximum glucosuric response doubled compared with WT mice[24] (Fig. 8.3). Renal clearance studies found that concentrations of the SGLT2 inhibitor in early proximal tubule fluid close to the reported half maximal inhibitory concentration ($IC_{50}$) for mouse SGLT2 were associated with fractional renal glucose reabsorption

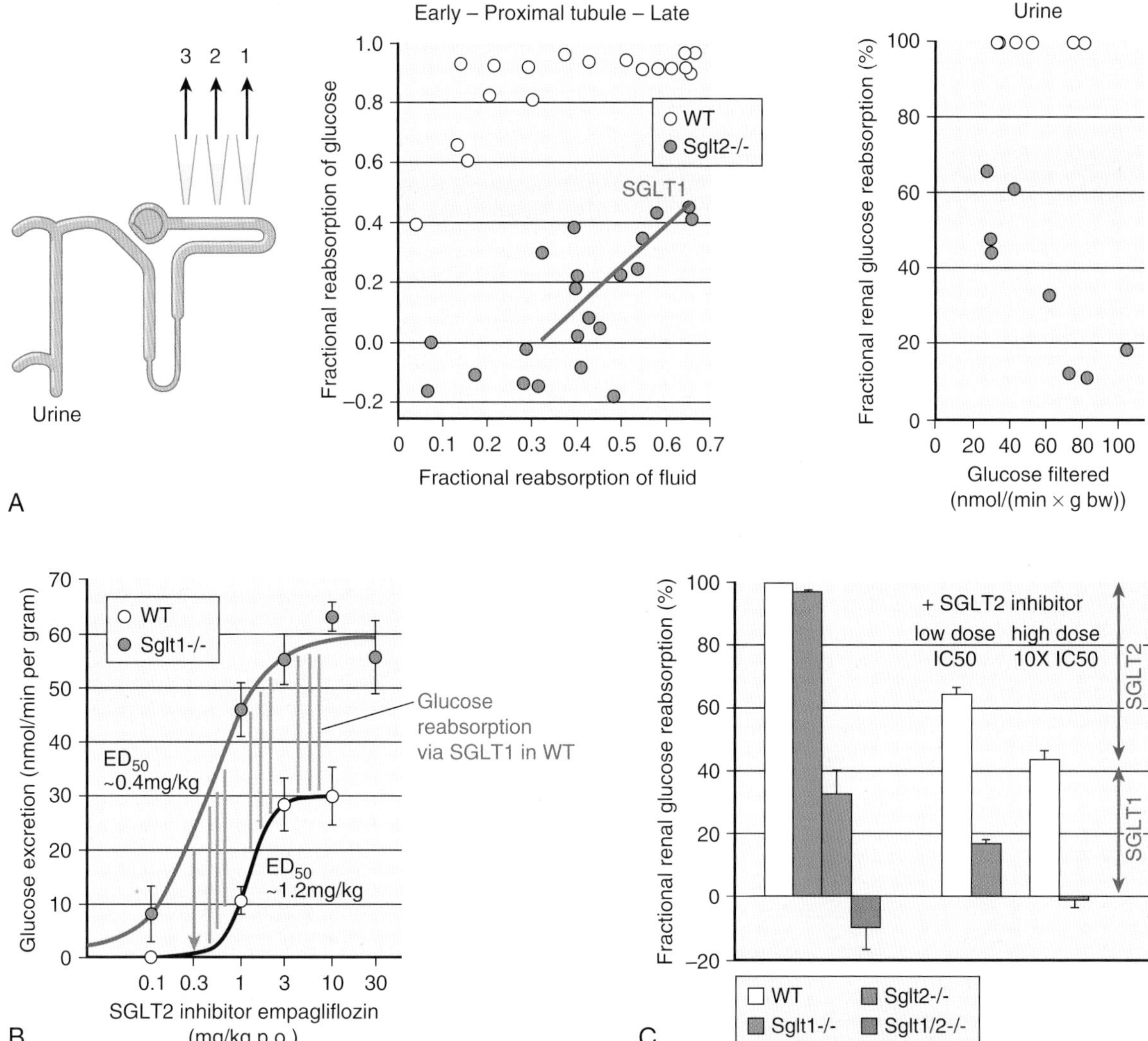


**Fig. 8.3 Contribution of SGLT2 and SGLT1 to renal glucose reabsorption.** (A) *Left panels:* Free-flow collections of tubular fluid performed by micropuncture to establish a profile for fractional reabsorption of glucose versus fluid along accessible proximal tubules at the kidney surface. Glucose reabsorption is absent in the early proximal tubule of *Sglt2–/–* mice but enhanced in the later proximal tubule, potentially reflecting compensation by SGLT1-mediated transport. Right panel: Renal inulin clearance studies revealed that the reduction in fractional renal glucose reabsorption in *Sglt2–/–* mice was inversely related to the amount of filtered glucose. (B) In metabolic cage studies, the SGLT2 inhibitor empagliflozin dose dependently increased glucose excretion in wild-type *(WT)* mice. The response curve was shifted leftward, and the maximum response doubled in *Sglt1–/–* mice. The difference between dose–response curves, which reflects glucose reabsorption via SGLT1 in WT mice, was maintained for higher doses (all vertical lines have same length), consistent with selectivity of the inhibitor for SGLT2 versus SGLT1 in this dose range. Glucosuria is initiated in WT mice when SGLT1-mediated glucose uptake is saturate *(red arrow)*. (C) Renal inulin clearance studies in mice lacking *Sglt1, Sglt2, or both Sglt1 and Sglt2* indicated that the glucose reabsorption preserved in *Sglt2–/–* (~40%) is mediated by SGLT1. Application of the SGLT2 inhibitor empagliflozin at low and high doses to establish free plasma concentrations (corresponding to early tubular concentrations) close to $IC_{50}$ for mouse SGLT2 (~1–2 nM) or 10-fold this concentration confirmed the role of SGLT1 during pharmacologic SGLT2 inhibition. (Data from Vallon V, Platt KA, Cunard R, et al. SGLT2 mediates glucose reabsorption in the early proximal tubule. *J Am Soc Nephrol.* 2011;22:104–112; and Rieg T, Masuda T, Gerasimova M, et al. Increase in SGLT1-mediated transport explains renal glucose reabsorption during genetic and pharmacological SGLT2 inhibition in euglycemia. *Am J Physiol Renal Physiol.* 2014;306:F188–F193.)

of 64% in WT and 17% in *Sglt1–/–* mice. Dosing the SGLT2 inhibitor to fully inhibit SGLT2 reduced fractional renal glucose reabsorption to 44% in WT and eliminated net renal glucose reabsorption in *Sglt1–/–* mice (Fig. 8.3). Finally, the absence of net renal glucose reabsorption was confirmed in male and female mice lacking both *Sglt1 and Sglt2*[24] (Fig. 8.3). These studies demonstrated that SGLT1 provides a significant glucose transport capacity in the late proximal tubule, which, in the normal kidney, remains mostly unused due to upstream glucose reabsorption by SGLT2. Inhibition of the latter, however, delivers more glucose downstream and unmasks the transport capacity of SGLT1 (Fig. 8.1). This is also consistent with a high maximal glucose transport rate proposed for human SGLT1 based on in vitro studies.[28] As a consequence, combined inhibition of renal SGLT2 and SGLT1 is more glucosuric than inhibition of SGLT2 alone. This has been observed in nondiabetic and diabetic mice[24,29] and in studies using a potent dual SGLT2/SGLT1 inhibitor.[30]

The studies further indicated that SGLT2 and SGLT1 can account for all net glucose reabsorption in the kidney under normoglycemic conditions[24] (Fig. 8.3). Moreover, the data allowed estimating that the basal overall glucose reabsorption capacities for SGLT2 versus SGLT1 in a nondiabetic mouse kidney is in the range of 3:1 to 5:1.[31]

*Clinical Relevance*

**Inhibition of Renal Glucose Reabsorption as a New Antihyperglycemic Therapy**

SGLT2 inhibitors are a new class of antihyperglycemic drugs that have been approved in T2DM, work independently of insulin, improve glycemic control in all stages of diabetes mellitus in the absence of clinically relevant hypoglycemia, and can be combined with other antidiabetic agents. SGLT2 inhibition lowers glomerular hyperfiltration by a blood glucose–independent mechanism. By acting as a diuretic and lowering blood pressure and diabetic glomerular hyperfiltration, SGLT2 inhibitors have the potential to induce protective effects on the kidney and cardiovascular system beyond blood glucose control.

## MOLECULAR CHARACTERIZATION OF PROXIMAL TUBULAR GLUCOSE TRANSPORT

### APICAL GLUCOSE TRANSPORTERS

Crane first proposed in 1960 that active glucose transport in the intestinal epithelium (which expresses SGLT1) was energized by the $Na^+$ gradient across cell membranes, the so-called $Na^+$–glucose cotransport hypothesis (for review, see Wright et al.[21]). The $Na^+/K^+$-ATPase located on the basolateral membrane is the primary active and ATP-consuming transport step, which lowers cytosolic $Na^+$ concentrations and establishes the concentration gradient that drives $Na^+$ uptake, and, secondary, the uptake of other molecules from the luminal surface into proximal tubule cells (Figs. 8.1 and 8.4). This concept was rapidly refined and extended to active transport processes of a diverse range of molecules and ions including $Na^+$–glucose cotransport in the kidney.[21]

SGLT1 and SGLT2 have been the most intensively studied members of the human SLC5 solute carrier (SLC) family, which now includes 12 members. Six of these are named as SGLTs, varying in their preferences for binding of glucose, galactose, mannose, fructose, myoinositol, choline, short-chain fatty acids, and other anions.[21] All SGLTs have 15 exons, spanning from 8 to 72 kb, which code for 60- to 80-kDa proteins composed of 580–718 amino acids.[21] The molecular nature of SGLTs has been largely pioneered by studies in

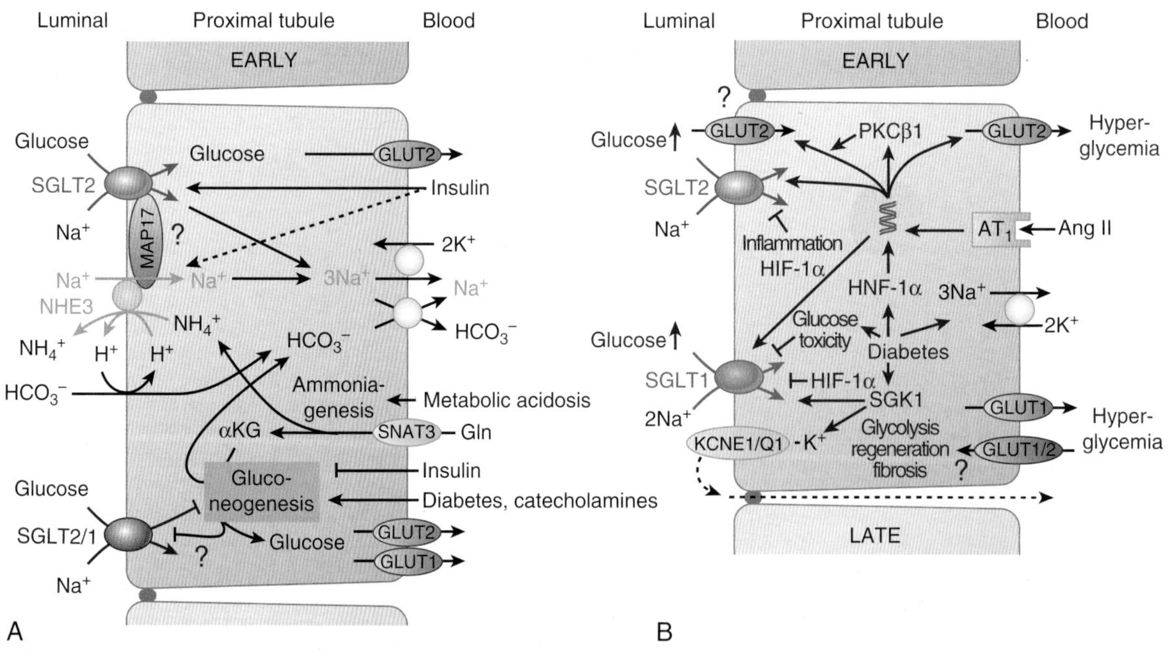


**Fig. 8.4 Regulation of glucose transport in the proximal tubule.** (A) Insulin is a physiologic stimulator of SGLT2, which may serve to maximize renal glucose reabsorption capacity in situations of increased blood glucose levels (e.g., after a meal). At the same time, enhanced $Na^+$–glucose uptake and insulin suppress renal gluconeogenesis. The latter, in contrast, is stimulated by fasting, which may involve increased catecholamine levels. In metabolic acidosis, the increase in gluconeogenesis from glutamine *(Gln)* is linked to the formation of (1) ammonium *($NH_4^+$)*, a renally excreted acid equivalent, and (2) new bicarbonate, which is taken up into the circulation. The $Na^+$-$H^+$ exchanger NHE3 contributes to apical $H^+/NH_4^+$ secretion and $Na^+$/bicarbonate reabsorption. SGLT2 and NHE3 are both stimulated by insulin to enhance $Na^+$ and glucose reabsorption, and their functions may be positively linked through the scaffolding protein MAP17. (B) Diabetes increases luminal glucose delivery to both SGLT2- and SGLT1-expressing segments. Glucose transporters GLUT2 and GLUT1 mediate glucose transport across the basolateral membrane, but GLUT2 may also translocate to the apical membrane in diabetes. Angiotensin II *(Ang I)*, serum, glucocorticoid-inducible kinase SGK1, hepatocyte nuclear factor HNF-1α, and protein kinase C PKCβ1 promote glucose reabsorption in the diabetic kidney, whereas hypoxia-induced HIF-1α, inflammation, and excessive intracellular glucose levels may be inhibitory. Basolateral glucose uptake via GLUT1/2 may be involved in glycolysis and tubule regeneration after injury as well as hyperglycemia-induced TGF-β.

the laboratory of Wright and colleagues (see Wright et al.[21] for review). This involved identifying and cloning SGLT1, identifying that defects in SGLT1 were associated with intestinal malabsorption of glucose–galactose and cloning of SGLT2. Wright's group also defined the crystal structure of a sodium galactose bacterial isoform in *Vibrio parahaemolyticus* (vSGLT), which allowed better characterization of how $Na^+$ and sugar transport is coupled: $Na^+$ binds first to the outside of the transport protein to open the outside gate, thereby permitting outside sugar to bind and be trapped; this is followed by a conformational change and the subsequent opening of the inward gate releases the $Na^+$ and sugar into the cell cytoplasm. The transport cycle is completed by the change in conformation from an inward-facing ligand-free state to an outward-facing ligand-free state.[21,32]

The sugar selectivity and transport kinetics of cloned SGLTs were determined using electrophysiologic techniques in various expression systems. The affinity of SGLT1 is similar for glucose and galactose, whereas SGLT2 does not transport galactose, and neither transports fructose.[21] More recent studies in transfected human embryonic kidney (HEK) 293T cells indicated that the apparent affinities ($K_m$) for D-glucose are rather similar for human SGLT1 and human SGLT2, with values of 2 mM and 5 mM, respectively.[28] Sugar binding occurs in a $Na^+$-dependent manner, and the $K_m$ values for $Na^+$ transport by human SGLT1 and human SGLT2 are 70 mM and 25 mM, respectively.[28] Thus, under euglycemic conditions, the glucose concentration in the tubular fluid of the very early proximal tubule (reflecting blood glucose levels) is similar to the $K_m$ of SGLT2, whereas the luminal $Na^+$ concentration of ~140 mM is higher than the $K_m$ of SGLT2 and not rate limiting.

SGLT1 and SGLT2 transport $Na^+$ and glucose with an $Na^+$–glucose coupling ratio of 2:1 and 1:1, respectively.[28] The greater $Na^+$–glucose coupling ratio of SGLT1 enhances its glucose concentration power and thereby the ability of the late proximal tubule to effectively reabsorb glucose despite falling luminal glucose concentrations (see Fig. 8.1). $Na^+$–glucose transport is electrogenic, and the membrane potential and driving force are maintained by paracellular $Cl^-$ reabsorption or transcellular $K^+$ secretion, the latter involving KCNE1/KCNQ1 channels in the luminal membrane of the proximal tubule[33,34] (Fig. 8.1).

The mRNA expression of three other members of the SLC5 family that can transport glucose based on in vitro substrate studies has been detected in the kidney.[35] SGLT3 (*SLC5A4*) is not a glucose transporter, but glucose can depolarize the plasma membrane in its presence in a saturable, $Na^+$-dependent manner, and this effect is inhibited by phlorizin. As such, it has been proposed to be a glucose sensor; however, its expression and function in the kidney remain unclear.[36] SGLT4 (*SLC5A9*) is expressed in the kidney, and transports glucose in COS-7 cells but with a lower apparent affinity than mannose (Ki 8 vs. 0.15 mM).[37] Thus, SGLT4 may primarily be involved in mannose homeostasis. SGLT5 (*SLC5A10*) is an $Na^+$-dependent sugar transporter that has a relatively high affinity and capacity for mannose and fructose relative to glucose and galactose.[38,39] SGLT5 mRNA is highly kidney abundant and expressed in kidney cortex,[38,40] and recent studies in knockout mice indicated that SGLT5 is the major luminal transporter for fructose reabsorption in the kidney.[41]

## BASOLATERAL GLUCOSE TRANSPORTERS

In the healthy kidney, the glucose that is being reabsorbed by proximal tubule cells is not linked to appreciable glucose metabolism in these cells. This is due to the fact that most glucose is reabsorbed in the early PCT (S1 segment), but these cells lack significant capacity for aerobic and anaerobic glycolysis.[42–44] Thus, glucose that is taken up across the luminal membrane or formed within proximal tubule cells (see later) exits across the basolateral membrane into the interstitium by concentration–driven facilitative glucose transporters, GLUT2 and GLUT1 (see Fig. 8.1) and subsequently enters the peritubular capillaries by convection through fenestrated endothelial cells. GLUT2, the low-affinity (Km; 15–20 mM) "liver" transporter is primarily expressed in the PCT (S1/S2 segments), but GLUT2 mRNA has also been detected in the proximal straight tubule (PST) (S3 segment).[45] GLUT2 is thought to be the dominant transporter involved in basolateral exit of glucose derived from apical glucose uptake or gluconeogenesis in the PCT.[46–48] In comparison, GLUT1, the high-affinity (1–2 mM) "erythroid/brain" transporter is expressed along the entire proximal tubule and has been implicated in transcellular glucose transport, particularly in the S3 segments.[46–48] Notably, GLUT1 is also expressed in the basolateral membrane of further distal tubule segments and at higher levels than in S3 segments. This includes expression in the medullary thin and thick ascending limbs (TAL) of the rat kidney and at the highest levels in connecting segments and collecting ducts. In the latter, GLUT1 was expressed at the highest level in intercalated cells and to a lesser extent in principal cells.[48] These findings indicated a good correlation between the level of GLUT1 expression and the glycolytic activity of the different nephron segments, indicating that, in particular, the more distal tubule segments are taking up glucose for energy supply via basolateral GLUT1. Recent studies used positron emission tomography and α-methyl-4-[F-18]-fluoro-4-deoxy-d-glucopyranoside to monitor glucose transport in mouse kidneys lacking either SGLT1, SGLT2, or GLUT2. The studies confirmed prominent contributions of SGLT2 and SGLT1 to renal glucose uptake. Moreover, renal glucose reabsorption appeared absent in mice lacking GLUT2, consistent with a more prominent role of GLUT2 versus GLUT1 with regard to basolateral glucose exit of glucose in the proximal tubule[49] (Fig. 8.1). This is in line with the renal phenotype of patients with mutations in GLUT2 and GLUT1. Loss of function mutations in GLUT2 are the basis of the Fanconi–Bickel syndrome, which includes a renal Fanconi syndrome, a proximal tubulopathy consisting of glycosuria, phosphaturia, aminoaciduria, proteinuria, and hyperuricemia.[50–52] The observed proximal tubulopathy may be due to intracellular glucose accumulation and glucotoxicity that occurs when basolateral glucose exit is blocked. In comparison, patients with GLUT1 mutations have primarily neurologic symptoms, and no renal phenotype has been documented.[50,53]

In addition to GLUT1 and GLUT2, some of the other 12 members of the SLC2 gene family have been found in the kidney and may contribute to glucose transport, but little is known about their quantitative contribution.[54] For example, GLUT4 mRNA and immunoreactivity were focally localized in the TALH of the loop of Henle, coexpressed with IGF-I and increased by vasopressin treatment, indicating a potential role in local fuel control.[45] GLUT5 is strongly expressed in the apical membrane of the S3 segment in the rat kidney but proposed to transport primarily fructose.[45,55] GLUT12 can transport glucose, and an apical localization has been reported in distal tubules and collecting ducts, but its quantitative role remains to be determined.[56]

### RENAL FORMATION OF GLUCOSE

The kidneys not only reabsorb the filtered glucose and use glucose as an energy source, but they also generate new glucose. Gluconeogenesis involves the formation of glucose-6-phosphate from precursors such as lactate, glutamine, alanine, and glycerol with its subsequent hydrolysis by glucose-6-phosphatase to generate free glucose that can exit the cell. The healthy human kidneys produce ~15–55 g glucose per day by gluconeogenesis. In fact, the human liver and kidneys provide about equal amounts of glucose via gluconeogenesis in the postabsorptive state (i.e., 12–16 hours after the last meal).[57] Renal gluconeogenesis occurs along the entire proximal tubule, but its activity is usually higher in the earlier segments.[43,58]

Renal gluconeogenesis is stimulated by epinephrine and inhibited by insulin[57] (see Fig. 8.4). Insulin-induced suppression of gluconeogenic gene expression in the proximal tubule was accompanied by phosphorylation and inactivation of forkhead box transcription factor 1 (FoxO1).[59] In contrast to the liver, renal gluconeogenesis is probably insensitive to glucagon.[57] Studies in humans indicated that in the postabsorptive state, renal gluconeogenesis uses primarily lactate as substrate, followed by glutamine, glycerol, and alanine.[60]

In contrast to the uniform stimulation of gluconeogenesis along the entire proximal tubule by starvation, metabolic acidosis enhances gluconeogenesis primarily in S1 and S2 segments.[43,58,61] Furthermore, gluconeogenesis in response to metabolic acidosis primarily uses glutamine as substrate. During the process of renal gluconeogenesis from glutamine, the conversion of glutamine to glutamate and α-ketoglutarate produces ammonium ($NH_4^+$), which is excreted into the urine as an acid equivalent. The subsequent pathway from α-ketoglutarate to glucose forms new bicarbonate, which is returned as buffer to the systemic circulation (see Fig. 8.4). The described link between proximal tubular ammonium, bicarbonate, and glucose formation explains why acidosis is a prominent stimulus for renal gluconeogenesis.[57,60]

Apical glucose uptake via SGLT1 or SGLT2 can have an inhibitory influence on the expression of renal gluconeogenic genes (see Fig. 8.4). This effect may serve to prevent glucose overload in the cells of the proximal tubule, and has been proposed to involve glucose-induced and sirtuin 1–mediated deacetylation of peroxisome proliferator–activated receptor gamma coactivator 1-α, a coactivator of FoxO1.[59]

In general, it is expected that cytosolic glucose in proximal tubule S3 segments is used for metabolism or leaves the cell via basolateral GLUT1. It has also been hypothesized that glucose generated from lactate in the medullary S3 segment forms part of an intrarenal Cori cycle[62]; glucose enters the lumen by reversed transport through SGLT1 and is taken up by downstream tubular segments, where it is used as energy substrate for glycolysis (e.g., in medullary TAL), and the formed lactate is being returned to the neighboring S3 segment as a substrate for gluconeogenesis. Studies in human proximal tubule segments indicated that in contrast to S1 segments, lactate appears to be a better gluconeogenic precursor than glutamine in S2 and S3 segments.[63] Moreover, studies in mice indicated that the luminal membrane of the thick ascending limb in the outer stripe of the outer medulla and in the cortex (including the macula densa) express SGLT1.[19] The rat appears to express SGLT1 also in the cortical TAL and macula densa.[17] Further studies are needed to clarify whether the TAL (and macula densa) in human also express SGLT1, and determine the potential role of SGLT1 in these structures, including a proposed Cori cycle.

Taken together and under normal conditions, the PCT is the site of greatest renal glucose reabsorption and generation. The ability of early proximal tubular segments for gluconeogenesis but inability to metabolize glucose prevents a futile cycle. The reabsorption of filtered glucose and renal gluconeogenesis provide an energy source to distal tubular segments, primarily in the renal medulla, and returning the glucose to the systemic circulation helps to maintain blood glucose levels, particularly in the postabsorptive state. In addition, renal gluconeogenesis is closely linked to the renal response to metabolic acidosis. See Chapter 5 for additional discussion of the role of gluconeogenesis in renal metabolism.

## RENAL GLUCOSE TRANSPORT IN DISEASE STATES

### GLUCOSE TRANSPORT IS INCREASED IN THE DIABETIC KIDNEY

Lowering hyperglycemia is vital in diabetic patients to attenuate the progression of the underlying metabolic dysfunction[64] and to reduce the risk of diabetic complications including nephropathy and cardiovascular disease.[65] Current therapies for type 2 diabetes mellitus (T2DM) include drugs that target the liver, small intestine, adipose tissue, skeletal muscle, and/or pancreas. Many of these therapies, including insulin, have difficulties to establish adequate glycemic control without the potential for relevant unwanted side effects, including hypoglycemia and weight gain, and may not reduce cardiovascular complications.[66] The following sections outline how glucose transport changes in the diabetic kidney, its implications for diabetic kidney function, and how targeting renal glucose transport can serve as a new antihyperglycemic therapy.

Diabetes mellitus is associated with increased blood glucose levels. This enhances the amounts of glucose filtered by the kidneys, as long as GFR is preserved. In fact, the early phase of diabetes is often associated with an increase in GFR or glomerular hyperfiltration (see later), which further increases the tubular glucose load. At the same time, the tubular capacity to reabsorb glucose increases by ~20%–30% to ~500–600 g/day in patients with T2DM[67,68] and type 1 diabetes (T1DM).[3] Thus, diabetes often increases the glomerular filtration and tubular reabsorption of glucose. Moreover and despite increased blood glucose levels, diabetes also enhances renal gluconeogenesis.[57] The latter can be the consequence of diabetes-associated metabolic acidosis, and the induced gluconeogenesis involves metabolism of glutamine to glucose associated with the generation of ammonia and bicarbonate[57] (see Fig. 8.4). Other potential triggers for gluconeogenesis in diabetes include the activation of the sympathetic nervous system, the reduced insulin levels observed in T1DM, enhanced circulating fatty acids, or the kidneys receive another signal from insulin-dependent cells that cannot take up glucose due to low insulin levels (T1DM) or insulin resistance (T2DM) and are glucose "starved."

Increasing renal glucose reabsorption in response to a rise in filtered glucose makes sense with regard to energy substrate conservation. Moreover, the further distal segments may need/use more glucose as an energy substrate to reabsorb the load of salt and other compounds, which is increased due to glomerular hyperfiltration. Renal glucose retention and enhanced glucose formation become maladaptive in diabetes, however, when they sustain hyperglycemia (see Fig. 8.4). In this regard, the kidney provides a safety valve that can prevent extreme hyperglycemia. When blood glucose levels increase to the point that the filtered load exceeds the Tm or tubular transport capacity for glucose, then the surplus is excreted in the urine. The safety valve, however, only opens at rather high blood glucose levels (>15 mmol/L) (see Fig. 8.2) and only works as long as glomerular filtration is maintained, and its threshold depends on the level of expression and activity of the involved glucose transporter, and its functionality may thus vary from patient to patient.

## GLUCOSE TRANSPORTERS IN THE DIABETIC KIDNEY

The levels of protein expression and activity of SGLT2, SGLT1, GLUT2, and potentially GLUT1 determine the capacity of renal glucose reabsorption, and their upregulation may explain the increased glucose transport maximum that can be observed in diabetes. The available preclinical and human studies reported increased, unchanged, or reduced renal glucose transporter expression and/or activity in diabetes or under high-glucose conditions.[69] The observed different responses may reflect different diabetes models, metabolic states, levels of kidney injury, other factors that regulate the expression of these transporters, the use of nonselective antibodies, or dissociations between mRNA and protein expression.

## SGLT2 AND GLUT2

Using knockout mice as gold standard negative antibody controls, the renal protein expression of SGLT2 was found to be increased by 40%–80% in the early hyperglycemic stages of genetic mouse models of T2DM (db/db) and T1DM (Akita).[70,71] The proximal tubule, like many nephron segments, expresses insulin receptors and binds insulin.[72] Application of insulin to HEK-293T cells phosphorylated SGLT2 at Ser624, which increased $Na^+$–glucose transport.[73] Thus, the insulin release following a meal may act on the PCT to enhance SGLT2 activity and conserve filtered glucose (see Fig. 8.4). Moreover, hyperinsulinemia associated with insulin resistance in obesity and T2DM may enhance renal SGLT2 activity[72] (Fig. 8.4). This may be coordinated with a stimulatory effect of insulin on other $Na^+$-coupled transporters in the proximal tubule, including the $Na^+$–proton exchanger NHE3.[72,74] Recent studies indicated that SGLT2 may be functionally linked to NHE3[75–77] such that SGLT2 inhibition may, to some extent, inhibit NHE3 in the proximal tubule (Fig. 8.4). A similar interaction has been proposed for the coregulation of SGLT1 and NHE3 in the small intestine.

Consistent with a potential concerted regulation of luminal and basolateral glucose transport, upregulation of GLUT2 expression has been reported in renal proximal tubules in diabetic rats.[78–81] Notably, studies in streptozotocin (STZ)-induced T1DM in rats proposed targeting of GLUT2 (but not GLUT1) also to the brush border membrane of proximal tubules.[82,83] The latter may be linked to protein kinase C PKCβ1 activation[83–85] and may implicate facilitative glucose transport, together with SGLT2 and SGLT1 in the increased glucose reabsorption across the apical membrane of proximal tubules in the diabetic kidney (Fig. 8.4).

The available data on changes in glucose transporters in diabetic patients are sparse and also variable. Primary cultures of human exfoliated proximal tubular epithelial cells harvested from fresh urine of patients with T2DM showed an increased glucose uptake associated with increased protein expression of SGLT2 and GLUT2.[86] An increase in SGLT2 protein expression has also been reported in fresh kidney biopsies of patients with T2DM and advanced nephropathy.[87] On the other hand, the mRNA expression of SGLT2 and GLUT2 was slightly lower in 19 patients with T2DM and preserved kidney function as compared with 20 nondiabetic patients matched for age and estimated GFR (eGFR), all being subjected to nephrectomy.[88] Similar results were reported for SGLT2 and GLUT2 mRNA in another set of patients with T2DM, but the results did not reach statistical significance.[89]

If an increase in SGLT2 expression occurs in the diabetic kidney, then it may simply reflect overall growth and hypertrophy of the diabetic proximal tubule and the associated increase in transport machinery,[90,91] and this may be exaggerated with advanced nephropathy when nephrons are lost and the remaining nephrons aim to compensate. Moreover, upregulation of SGLT2 expression in diabetic rats has been linked to activation of Ang II AT1 receptors[92] and the transcription factor, hepatocyte nuclear factor HNF-1α.[93] The latter as well as HNF-3β have also been implicated in renal GLUT2 upregulation[79] (see Fig. 8.4). Notably, pharmacologic inhibition of SGLT2 in normoglycemic mice also increased renal membrane SGLT2 protein expression,[71] possibly reflecting a negative feedback regulation of SGLT2 expression by intracellular glucose levels. Along this line, if renal SGLT2 expression is reduced in the diabetic kidney, this may be due to enhanced diabetes-induced proximal tubular gluconeogenesis (Fig. 8.4) or reflect more severe tubular hypoxia or inflammation.[94–96]

## SGLT1 AND GLUT1

The renal expression of SGLT1 protein appears to vary among genetic mouse models of diabetes: renal SGLT1 protein expression was found to be increased in leptin-deficient ob/ob mice,[97] a model of T2DM, and reduced in Akita mice, a model of T1DM[70]; the latter study used knockout mice as negative antibody control. In contrast to SGLT2 (see earlier), insulin stimulation slightly decreased SGLT1-mediated $Na^+$–glucose transport in HEK-293T cells,[73] indicating differences in the regulation of these two transporters. In contrast to the strong increase in SGLT2 (see earlier), SGLT1 protein was not significantly changed in fresh kidney biopsies of patients with T2DM and nephropathy in comparison with nondiabetic controls.[87] The interpretation of renal SGLT1 mRNA expression data may be complicated by the observation that mRNA and protein expression can dissociate, at least in mouse kidney.[98]

GLUT1 protein expression was downregulated in proximal tubules isolated from rat cortices at 2 and 4 weeks after STZ,[81] but increased in kidneys of rats at 30 weeks after STZ.[56] A study in patients with T2DM and preserved kidney function reported that in whole renal tissue, GLUT1 mRNA expression were slightly lower as compared with nondiabetic patients.[88]

Why should diabetes reduce renal SGLT1 expression? Although this would make the renal glucose valve to open earlier (and make SGLT2 inhibitors more efficacious, see later), this may not be the kidneys' intention. A reduced renal SGLT1 protein expression was also observed in response to genetic or pharmacologic SGLT2 inhibition in nondiabetic mice.[15,71] These conditions and diabetes share an enhanced glucose load to the late proximal tubule. In vitro studies in proximal tubule cells indicated that high glucose can reduce SGLT expression and $Na^+$–glucose cotransport activity via enhanced oxidative stress.[99] Studies in a model of pig epithelial tubular cells (LLC-PK1) showed that hypoxia can diminish SGLT1 (and SGLT2) protein expression by activation of hypoxia-inducible factor-1α (HIF-1α).[95] Thus, an increased glucose load to the outer medullary S3 segment enhances $Na^+$–glucose reabsorption and thereby hypoxia, which may downregulate SGLT1 to limit oxygen-consuming transport work and glucotoxicity in this segment, which has a high sensitivity to acute injury[94] (see Fig. 8.4).

In comparison, an increase in SGLT1 expression in the diabetic kidney would further increase the renal glucose reabsorption capacity but may put the S3 segment at risk of hypoxia and enhanced glucotoxicity. Studies in Akita diabetic mice indicated that the serum and glucocorticoid-inducible kinase SGK1 may stimulate SGLT1 activity and glucose reabsorption in PSTs.[100] SGK1 could also promote proximal tubular glucose reabsorption by enhancing the activity of luminal $K^+$ channels (KCNE1/KCNQ1), which maintain the electrical driving force during electrogenic $Na^+$–glucose cotransport[33,34,101] (see Fig. 8.4). SGK1 was upregulated in proximal tubules in patients with diabetic nephropathy.[102]

Transport functions in proximal tubules require high turnover of ATP, which, under normal conditions, is derived primarily through mitochondrial oxidative phosphorylation.[43,103] This may change in pathophysiologic situations with impaired mitochondrial function, when glycolysis may be enhanced and contribute to maintaining ATP. For example, a shift to glycolysis has been proposed in proximal tubules regenerating from acute kidney injury (AKI) as well as proximal tubules undergoing atrophy.[104] This metabolic switch to glycolysis occurred early during proximal tubule regeneration and was reversed during successful tubular recovery, but persisted and became progressively more severe in tubule cells that failed to redifferentiate. Tubular upregulation of HIF-1α in mice enhanced renal GLUT1 mRNA expression; this was associated with less oxygen consumption and increased glycolysis.[105] Thus, hypoxia may increase basolateral GLUT1-mediated facilitative uptake of glucose, which is then used for glycolysis and recovery. Hypoxia-induced GLUT1 likely applies to distal tubule segments but may also be relevant for medullary S3 segments.[104] In this regard, studies in the proximal tubular cell line LLC-PK1, which was cultured and polarized on porous tissue culture inserts, showed that basolateral exposure to 25 mmol/L D-glucose enhanced glucose uptake via GLUT1 and the subsequent intracellular metabolism of glucose enhanced TGF-β 1 synthesis and secretion; this was not observed in response to apical glucose exposure.[106] These in vitro studies suggest that it may be the hyperglycemia-induced persistent uptake of glucose via basolateral GLUT1 (or GLUT2), rather than the filtered glucose, that affects the tubular synthesis of TGF-β 1 and thereby the development of tubulointerstitial fibrosis and tubular growth (Fig. 8.4).

## INHIBITION OF RENAL GLUCOSE REABSORPTION AS A NEW ANTIHYPERGLYCEMIC THERAPY

When blood glucose levels increase to the point that the filtered load exceeds the transport capacity of the tubular system, then the surplus is excreted in the urine. This renal safety valve can prevent extreme hyperglycemia. As outlined earlier, most capacity for renal glucose reabsorption is provided by SGLT2 in the early proximal tubule. When SGLT2 is inhibited, the reabsorptive capacity for glucose declines to the residual capacity of SGLT1, which equals ~80 g/day. In other words, SGLT2 inhibition causes the renal safety valve to open at a lower threshold (see Fig. 8.2) and makes it also relevant to glucose homeostasis in the euglycemic and moderately hyperglycemic range. Several SGLT2 inhibitors have now been approved as glucose-lowering agents for subjects with T2DM and preserved kidney function. Previously, the presence of glucosuria in a diabetic patient indicated inappropriate blood glucose control, as it showed that blood glucose was so high that the filtered glucose overwhelmed the glucose reabsorption capacity. In contrast and with the use of SGLT2 inhibitors, glucosuria is purposely induced to improve blood glucose control. The following sections discuss the role of SGLT2 in the pathophysiology of renal glucose reabsorption and outline the unexpected logic of inhibiting SGLT2 in the diabetic kidney.[90] This includes the counterproductive enhancement of renal glucose reabsorption via SGLT2 in diabetes as well as a brief discussion of the basic mechanisms that link a primary inhibition of $Na^+$–glucose cotransport in the kidney to secondary beneficial consequences on the metabolism, the kidneys, and the cardiovascular system.

Long-term access to excessive exogenous energy resources is not part of human evolution. As a consequence, it may not come as a surprise that the body's responses to excess exogenous energy resources can be maladaptive. In contrast, the body's responses to environments with scarce energy resources have been intensively tested and refined during evolution for the survival of the organism. Therefore, targeting metabolism in the "periphery" by inhibiting renal glucose reabsorption and spilling glucose as an energy resource into the urine and then using the central metabolic counterregulatory mechanisms to readjust the metabolism, may provide unique benefits as an antihyperglycemic approach.[90] This is supported by clinical outcome studies using an SGLT2 inhibitor on top of standard of care in patients with high cardiovascular risk that demonstrated protective effects with regard to clinically relevant renal and cardiovascular outcomes.[107–109]

Phlorizin is a flavonoid contained in the bark of various fruit trees and was discovered to cause glucosuria more than 100 years ago.[110] Phlorizin competitively inhibits SGLT2 and SGLT1, the former with a 10-fold higher affinity.[21,28] SGLT1 is expressed in many other organs and is the primary pathway for glucose reabsorption in the intestine.[111] As a consequence, oral administration of phlorizin is burdened by extrarenal side effects, most prominently diarrhea. In comparison and in healthy subjects, SGLT2 appears to be expressed only in kidney proximal tubule,[18,98] with a proposed expression and function in α cells of the pancreas[112] needing confirmation. Inhibition of renal glucose transport became practical when phlorizin derivates were developed that are specific for SGLT2, have good oral bioavailability, and are suitable for once-daily dosing.[113] Three members in this class, dapagliflozin (Forxiga or Farxiga in the United States), canagliflozin (Invokana), and empagliflozin (Jardiance) are approved in the United States and Europe for use in T2DM with preserved kidney function. Others, including ipragliflozin (Suglat), luseogliflozin (Lusefi), and tofogliflozin (0) are approved in Japan. SGLT2 inhibitors are under clinical investigation as add-on therapies to insulin in T1DM.

SGLT2 inhibitors act on their target from the extracellular surface of the cell membrane[114] and reach their target by glomerular filtration and, as indicated for empagliflozin, also by tubular secretion.[115] SGLT2 inhibitors induce a sustained urinary glucose loss of 40–80 g/day.[113,116,117] In patients with T2DM, this is associated with a decrease in Hb A1C levels by 0.5%–0.7% at 12 weeks of treatment, and this effect persisted for up to 52 weeks.[118] The higher the blood glucose level and GFR, the more glucose is filtered and reabsorbed and, as a consequence, can be excreted in response to SGLT2 blockade. Thus, SGLT2 blockers naturally have a greater efficacy when it is desirable for them to be more efficacious.[15,119,120] By lowering blood glucose levels and body weight, SGLT2 inhibitors improve β-cell function and sensitivity to insulin in patients and rodent models with T2DM.[119,121–124] Because the renal mechanism of action of SGLT2 inhibitors is independent of insulin, their efficacy is not declining with progressive β-cell dysfunction and/or insulin resistance, and SGLT2 inhibitors act synergistically with other blood glucose–lowering agents.[113]

Two SGLT2 inhibitors have now been evaluated in major clinical trials in patients with T2DM: empagliflozin in the 7,020-patient EMPA-REG OUTCOME trial[107,109] and, more recently, canagliflozin in 10,142 patients in the CANVAS program.[108] In addition to cardiovascular endpoints, both trials also included measurement of albuminuria and eGFR. The outcomes of the EMPA-REG OUTCOME and the CANVAS program are similar in most regards. Both went beyond the requisite safety parameters to show ~35% reductions in the incidence of heart failure. Both trials also reported beneficial effects on the kidney, including 40%–50% reductions in the hazard ratios for albuminuria or decline in eGFR. The relative risk of cardiovascular death was significantly reduced by SGLT2 inhibition in the EMPA-REG OUTCOME trial but not in the CANVAS program. This difference might be due to the higher prevalence of cardiovascular disease in the EMPA-REG OUTCOME cohort at baseline. The main cardiovascular effect of SGLT2 inhibition was on heart failure, rather than ischemic events, and both trials showed tangible benefits on heart failure outcomes. These benefits occurred when added to standard care, which included ~80% of patients being treated with an angiotensin-converting enzyme inhibitor or angiotensin AT1 receptor antagonist. The main side effect of SGLT2 inhibitors is an increased risk of genitourinary infections due to the glucosuric effect.[125]

**How can inhibition of renal glucose transport protect the kidney and cardiovascular system?** By reducing hyperglycemia, SGLT2 inhibitors have the potential to reduce glucotoxicity in the kidney and extrarenal organs.[126,127] In accordance, studies in diabetic rodents have shown that SGLT2 inhibition can reduce growth, lipid accumulation, inflammation, and injury of the diabetic kidney secondary to a strong blood glucose–lowering effect[70,71,87,97,128–131] (Fig. 8.5). The observed small effect of SGLT2 inhibitors on blood glucose control in the EMPA-REG OUTCOME trial and the CANVAS program alone, however, appears insufficient to fully explain the rapid beneficial effect on heart failure detectable within a few months. Although other mechanisms are likely to contribute (see later), it is also possible that, in contrast to SGLT2 inhibitors, these other agents have simultaneous countervailing effects that offset the benefits of better glycemic control, including increased obesity or an increased hypoglycemia risk.

**SGLT2 inhibition lowers body weight and has a low hypoglycemia risk.** In patients with T2DM, including those in the EMPA-REG OUTCOME trial and the CANVAS program, the glucosuric effect of SGLT2 inhibition was associated with a 2- to 3-kg lower body weight. Although the diuretic effect and fluid loss may contribute to the initial weight loss, the majority of the steady-state weight loss with SGLT2 inhibitor treatment is due to fat loss, including lesser visceral and subcutaneous fat[132–134] (see Fig. 8.5), due to a shift in substrate utilization from carbohydrates to lipids.[119,135,136] The released free fatty acids are used by the liver to form ketone bodies and thus increase ketogenesis.[137] SGLT2 inhibitors may improve cardiac outcomes in part by increasing plasma levels of ketone bodies like β-hydroxybutyrate, which are used as energy substrate to improve the performance of cardiac myocytes (or the kidney) in diabetes mellitus[138,139] (Fig. 8.5). SGLT2 inhibitors can increase the risk of diabetic ketoacidosis,[137] particularly when the drugs are used off-label in patients with T1DM.[137]

SGLT2 inhibitors do not increase the incidence of hypoglycemia.[107–109,118] This is because they become ineffective at lowering blood glucose any further once the filtered glucose load falls to ~80 g/day, which can be handled by renal SGLT1 (see Fig. 8.1). In addition, SGLT2 inhibitors leave the metabolic counterregulation intact and increase plasma glucagon concentrations and subsequently endogenous hepatic glucose production (gluconeogenesis) in patients with T2DM.[119,122] This is potentially relevant for cardiovascular outcome, because episodes of hypoglycemia can impair the cardioprotective effects of antihyperglycemic therapy.[140]

**SGLT2 inhibition lowers blood pressure and improves hyperuricemia.** A meta-analysis of patients with T2DM treated with SGLT2 inhibitors found a consistent decrease in systolic blood pressure of 3–6 mm Hg,[118] similar to preclinical data and the EMPA-REG OUTCOME trial and the CANVAS program. The magnitude of this blood pressure effect is expected to have cardiovascular protective consequences, particularly in high-risk patients.[141] The blood pressure–lowering effect of SGLT2 inhibition relates to the reduction in body weight and a modest glucose-based osmotic diuresis (100–470 mL/day) and a small natriuretic effect.[126,142–145] The lower blood pressure and an associated modest reduction in plasma volume[146] may quickly reduce cardiac pre- and afterload and thereby contribute to the rapid beneficial effects in heart failure patients[107] (see Fig. 8.5).

Beneficial renal and cardiovascular effects of SGLT2 inhibition may also be due to a plasma uric acid–lowering effect.[147] The uricosuric effect of SGLT2 inhibitors is positively

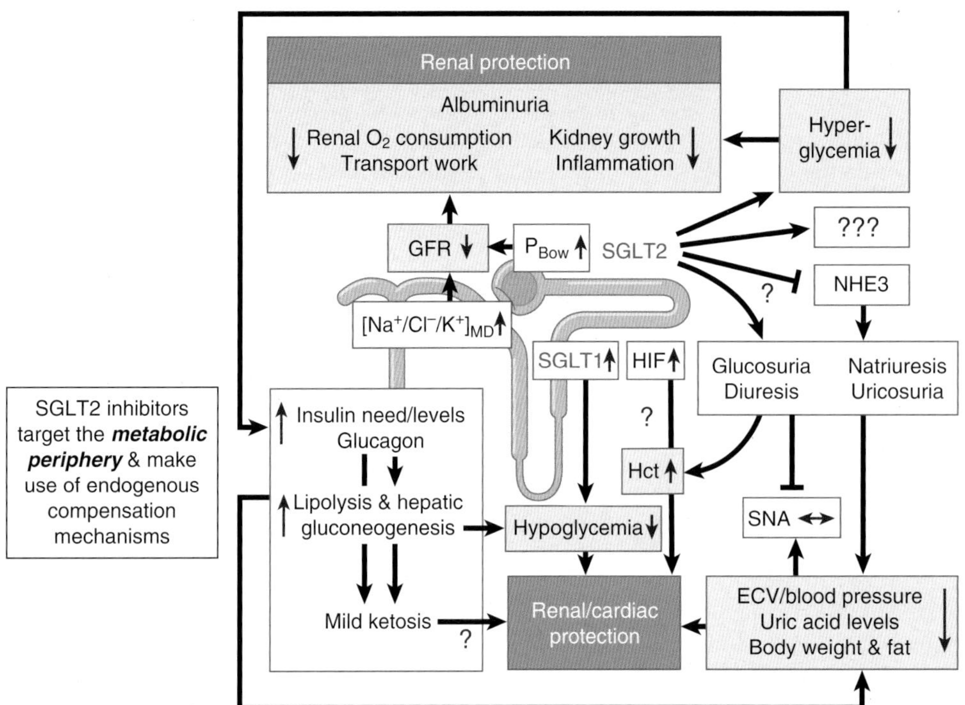


**Fig. 8.5 Proposed mechanisms of kidney and heart protection by SGLT2 inhibition in type 1 and type 2 diabetes.** SGLT2 inhibition attenuates the primary proximal tubular hyperreabsorption in the diabetic kidney, which increases/restores (1) the signal of the tubuloglomerular feedback at the macula densa (*$[Na^+/Cl^-/K^+]_{MD}$*) and (2) the hydrostatic pressure in the Bowman space (*$P_{Bow}$*). This lowers glomerular hyperfiltration with beneficial effects on tubular transport work and thus oxygen consumption and the filtration of albumin. By lowering blood glucose, SGLT2 inhibitors can reduce kidney growth and inflammation and albuminuria. SGLT2 inhibitors have a modest osmotic diuretic, natriuretic, and uricosuric effect, which can reduce extracellular volume *(ECV)*, blood pressure, serum uric acid levels, and body weight. SGLT2 inhibition blunts an expected reactive increase in sympathetic nerve activity *(SNA)*. SGLT2 may be functionally linked to the $Na^+$-$H^+$-exchanger 3 *(NHE3)* such that SGLT2 inhibition may also inhibit NHE3 in the proximal tubule. SGLT2 inhibition lowers insulin levels (therapeutic need and/or endogenous) and increases glucagon levels, which increases lipolysis and hepatic gluconeogenesis. These metabolic adaptations reduce fat tissue/body weight and the hypoglycemia risk and induce a mild ketosis, which all may be beneficial for the kidney and cardiovascular system. The hypoglycemia risk is further reduced by SGLT1-mediated glucose reabsorption. SGLT2 enhances active glucose and $Na^+$ reabsorption in the outer medulla; this may enhance hypoxia-inducible factor *(HIF)*–induced genes and have kidney and cardiac protective effects through enhancing erythropoietin, hematocrit, and oxygen transport. *Black arrows* indicate consequences of SGLT2 inhibition, and *red arrows* demonstrate direction of changes in the associated variables. "?" indicates hypotheses that need further confirmation. (This figure was modified with permission from Vallon V, Thomson SC. Targeting renal glucose reabsorption to treat hyperglycaemia: the pleiotropic effects of SGLT2 inhibition. *Diabetologia* 2017;60:215–225.)

related to the increase in tubular and urinary glucose delivery, as observed in healthy subjects and patients with T2DM[148,149] (see Fig. 8.5) and may involve an interaction with the luminal urate transporter URAT1.[149]

**SGLT2 inhibition lowers diabetic glomerular hyperfiltration.** Glomerular hyperfiltration, which is observed in a subset of patients at the onset of T1DM and T2DM, can increase the risk for developing diabetic nephropathy later on.[150] Less than 1% of filtered $Na^+$ is excreted in the urine in normal human subjects to match urinary excretion to dietary $Na^+$ intake (i.e., almost all the filtered $Na^+$ is reabsorbed). As a consequence, GFR, as the primary determinant of filtered $Na^+$, also becomes the primary determinant of renal $Na^+$ reabsorption. The latter, however, determines transport work and, thereby, renal oxygen consumption and requirement. Therefore, glomerular hyperfiltration increases transport work and oxygen consumption in the diabetic kidney, and lowering GFR has opposite effects.[142]

According to the "tubular hypothesis," glomerular hyperfiltration in diabetes is explained by primary tubular hyperreabsorption (for review, see Vallon and Thomson[69]). Moderate levels of hyperglycemia increase proximal tubular reabsorption by providing more substrate for $Na^+$–glucose cotransport via SGLT2 and SGLT1 and by causing the tubule to grow, which enhances the transport machinery and capacity. The increased reabsorption reduces the NaCl and fluid delivery to the downstream macula densa, which senses this reduction and causes GFR to increase through the normal physiologic action of tubuloglomerular feedback (TGF) (Fig. 8.6). The primary effect of the TGF is to adjust the tone of the afferent arteriole and thereby GFR of the same nephron to stabilize the NaCl and fluid delivery downstream of the macula densa. This facilitates the fine regulation of NaCl and fluid balance in the distal nephron by neurohumoral control. A secondary consequence of this TGF physiology is that the mechanism contributes to the autoregulation of GFR and renal blood flow. Moreover, it makes GFR responsive to primary changes in tubular transport upstream of the macula densa, like in the diabetic kidney. A primary increase in proximal reabsorption also reduces distal tubular flow rate, which increases GFR by lowering tubular back pressure—i.e., the hydrostatic pressure in Bowman space—and thereby increasing the effective glomerular filtration pressure (Fig. 8.6). Mathematical modeling indicates that TGF and the

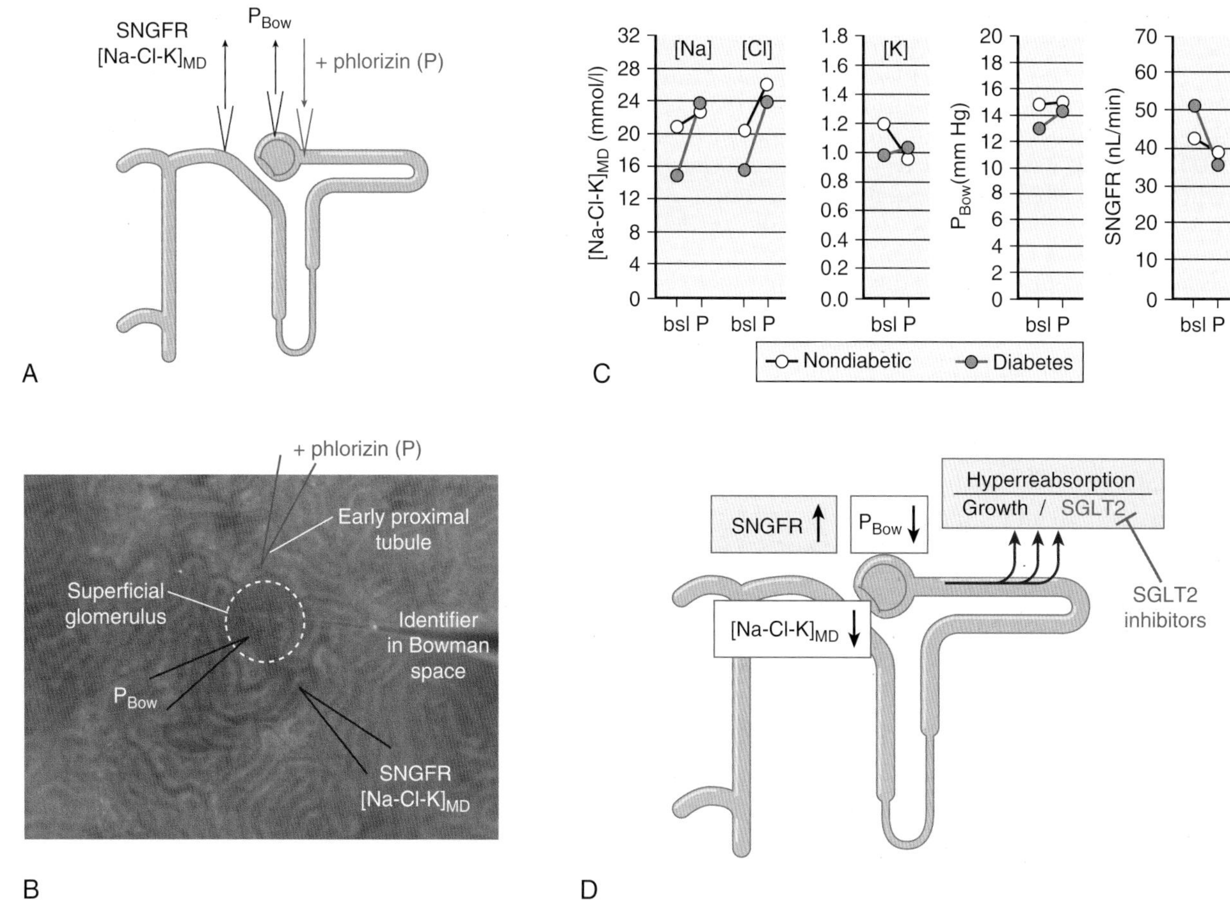


**Fig. 8.6 The tubular hypothesis of diabetic glomerular hyperfiltration: effect of SGLT2 inhibition.** (A, B) In vivo micropuncture studies in rats with superficial glomeruli were performed in nondiabetic and streptozotocin diabetic rats.[152] Small amounts of blue dye were injected into the Bowman space to determine nephron configuration, including the first proximal tubular loop and the early distal tubule close to the macula densa. Tubular fluid was collected close to the macula densa to determine (1) the tubuloglomerular feedback signal *($[Na\text{-}Cl\text{-}K]_{MD}$)*, and (2) single-nephron glomerular filtration rate *(SNGFR)* by inulin clearance. The Bowman space was punctured to determine the hydrostatic pressure *($P_{Bow}$)*. Measurements were performed under control conditions and following application of the SGLT2/SGLT1 inhibitor phlorizin into the early proximal tubule (i.e., without changing systemic blood glucose levels). (C) Basal measurements *(bsl)* revealed that glomerular hyperfiltration in diabetes was associated with reductions in $[Na\text{-}Cl\text{-}K]_{MD}$ and $P_{Bow}$. Adding phlorizin *(P)* had a small effect in nondiabetic rats but normalized $[Na\text{-}Cl\text{-}K]_{MD}$, $P_{Bow}$, and SNGFR in diabetes. (D) Diabetes induces a primary hyperreabsorption in the proximal tubule due to tubular growth and enhanced $Na^+$–glucose cotransport, which, through tubuloglomerular feedback ($[Na\text{-}Cl\text{-}K]_{MD}$) and reducing tubular back pressure ($P_{Bow}$), causes glomerular hyperfiltration. SGLT2 contributes to the tubular hyperreabsorption, and as a consequence, SGLT2 inhibition mitigates these changes and lowers glomerular hyperfiltration. (This figure was modified with permission from Vallon V, Thomson SC. Targeting renal glucose reabsorption to treat hyperglycaemia: the pleiotropic effects of SGLT2 inhibition. *Diabetologia* 2017;60:215–225.)

changes in tubular back pressure contribute equally to the increase in GFR in diabetes.[151]

Vice versa, SGLT2 inhibition attenuates proximal tubule hyperreabsorption in the diabetic kidney and thereby lowers diabetic glomerular hyperfiltration (see Figs. 8.5 and 8.6). This has been shown in micropuncture studies in rats using direct application of phlorizin into the Bowman space[152] and by acute or chronic systemic application of selective SGLT2 inhibitors.[153] In accordance, pharmacologic or genetic inhibition of SGLT2 suppressed hyperfiltration on the whole-kidney level in diabetic mice.[70,71] Consistent with the proposed local mechanism, the suppression of diabetic hyperfiltration in response to SGLT2 inhibition was associated with an increase in the NaCl concentration at the macula densa[152,153] and in the hydrostatic pressure in the Bowman space,[152] and was independent of effects on blood glucose[70,152,153] (Fig. 8.5). The GFR-lowering effect has more recently been confirmed in humans. The SGLT2 inhibitor empagliflozin decreased GFR by 19% in T1DM patients with baseline hyperfiltration independently of lowering blood glucose levels.[120] The SGLT2 inhibitor canagliflozin initially lowered eGFR in patients with T2DM and basal eGFR of ≥55 mL/min/1.73 $m^2$. Following this initial dip, eGFR increased over the following weeks and months in the canagliflozin-treated group such that eGFR was better preserved after 2 years of follow-up and associated with reduced urinary albumin-to-creatinine ratios than in the control group, which had been treated with glimepiride to achieve similar blood glucose control.[154]

Surviving nephrons in advanced stages of CKD are assumed to hyperfilter as a way of compensation for the reduced nephron number and thus maintain a high glucose load on the level of the single nephron. This should preserve the acute GFR-lowering effect of SGLT2 inhibition, even if the effect on overall glucose homeostasis was attenuated. In accordance, the SGLT2 inhibitor canagliflozin modestly reduced eGFR together with proteinuria within 3 weeks in patients with T2DM and basal eGFR values between 30 and 50 mL/min/1.73 $m^2$ (CKD3).[155] Empagliflozin also induced a small decline in eGFR in patients with T2DM and CKD2 and CKD3; this effect was maintained at 52 weeks, associated with reduced urine albumin-to-creatinine ratios and, most importantly, full reversibility after a 3-week washout period, indicating a functional GFR reduction.[156]

Lowering single-nephron glomerular hyperfiltration in CKD and thereby the oxygen-consuming transport work may help to preserve the integrity of the remaining nephrons and overall kidney function in the long term (see Fig. 8.5). This has been proposed for blockers of angiotensin II[157] and may also apply to SGLT2 inhibitors. Because ~80% of patients were also treated with a form of angiotensin II blockade, the EMPA-REG OUTCOME trial and CANVAS program provided evidence that the two strategies are additive and apply to patients with initial GFRs of at least 30 mL/min/1.73 $m^2$ of body surface area.[108,109] The additive effect is consistent with the concept that angiotensin II blockade is primarily dilating the efferent arteriole, whereas SGLT2 inhibition primarily constricts the afferent arteriole.

**SGLT2 inhibition has distinct effects on renal cortical and medullary $O_2$ requirements.** Mathematical modeling predicted that inhibition of SGLT2 in the diabetic kidney reduces oxygen consumption in the PCT and renal cortex, in part by lowering GFR[142,143] (Fig. 8.5). The predicted increase in cortical $O_2$ pressure and availability has been observed in a diabetic rat model using phlorizin, a dual SGLT1/SGLT2 inhibitor.[158] Interestingly, preserving renal cortical oxygenation may be important to preserve kidney function in patients with CKD.[159]

SGLT2 inhibition also shifts glucose uptake downstream to the S3 segments (see earlier) and enhances transcellular $Na^+$ reabsorption in distal segments, including the S3 segment and medullary TAL. This may further reduce the already physiologically low $O_2$ availability in the renal outer medulla. The latter has been proposed for SGLT2 inhibition using mathematical modeling[142,143] and was shown in vivo in rats in response to acute dual SGLT2/SGLT1 inhibition by phlorizin in nondiabetic and diabetic rats.[158] The effect on medullary transport and oxygenation would be attenuated by the reduction in blood glucose and GFR in response to SGLT2 inhibition.[142,143] Moreover, the proposed SGLT2 inhibitor–induced reduction in oxygen pressure in the deep cortex and outer medulla may stimulate hypoxia-inducible factors HIF-1 and HIF-2 (see Fig. 8.5). Gene knockout of SGLT2 increased the renal mRNA expression of hemoxygenase,[1,7] a tissue-protective gene that is induced by HIF-1α. On the other hand, activation of HIF-2 may explain an enhanced erythropoietin release from renal interstitial cells in response to SGLT2 inhibition.[160] Together with the diuretic effect, the latter may contribute to the observed modest increase in hematocrit and hemoglobin in response to SGLT2 inhibition. This may improve the oxygenation of the kidney outer medulla and cortex but also facilitate oxygen delivery to the heart and other organs (Fig. 8.5). Notably, changes in hematocrit and hemoglobin from baseline explained 51.8% and 48.9%, respectively, of the effect of the SGLT2 inhibitor empagliflozin versus placebo on the risk of cardiovascular death.[161] In other words and in addition to its volume effect, SGLT2 inhibition may simulate systemic hypoxia to the oxygen sensor in the deep cortex and outer medulla of the kidney, and the induced response then helps the failing heart and also the kidney. In accordance with an overall nephroprotective effect, SGLT2 inhibitor use reduced the risk of AKI in an analysis of >3000 patients with T2DM by ~50%.[162] Nevertheless, caution is warranted, as excessive volume depletion and the transport shift to the outer medulla may increase the AKI risk in individual sensitive patients.

**Preservation of blood pressure–lowering and heart failure–protective effects of SGLT2 inhibitors in CKD despite attenuated antihyperglycemic effects.** The amount of filtered glucose determines the glucosuric and blood glucose–lowering effect of SGLT2 inhibition. As a consequence, the antihyperglycemic effects of SGLT2 inhibitors are attenuated in patients with reduced GFR. In contrast, the blood pressure–lowering and heart failure–protective effects are preserved in patients with CKD and reduced GFR (eGFR ≥30 mL/min 1.73 $m^2$).[163,164] Modeling studies of CKD and nephron loss predicted that the increase in single-nephron GFR in remaining nephrons and the reduction of glucose reabsorption by SGLT2 inhibition increase paracellular $Na^+$ secretion in the proximal tubule.[165] Thus, the model predicted that the chronic natriuretic and diuretic effects of SGLT2 inhibition persist in CKD. The modeling approach also predicted that the SGLT2 inhibition–induced changes in the oxygen signal at the renal sensor are preserved in CKD.[165]

Ongoing trials with different SGLT2 inhibitors, also including studies in nondiabetic patients with heart failure and/or CKD, will provide further data for comparison between SGLT2 inhibitors and are expected to further refine our understanding of the therapeutic potential and safety of SGLT2 inhibition.

## ORGANIC CATIONS AND ANIONS

### ORGANIC ANION TRANSPORTERS AND ORGANIC CATION TRANSPORTERS

Historically, the renal organic anion transport system has been one of the best studied in physiology.[166–173] Essentially, it has been operationally characterized as the probenecid-sensitive para-aminohippurate (PAH) transport system. Classically, it is described as a proximal tubule transport system of small organic anions (e.g., PAH) bound with low affinity to plasma proteins (mainly albumin). Because, with an intact glomerular filtration barrier, albumin-bound molecules would not be filtered, they move into the peritubular capillaries. Molecules like PAH are efficiently extracted on a "first pass" by a high-capacity transport system with selectivity for organic anions. This explains why PAH clearance can be used as a measure of renal plasma flow. Operationally, the system can be blocked by the organic anion drug probenecid, which has seen considerable clinical use in the setting of hyperuricemia and to increase blood levels of other organic anion drugs like penicillins and cidofovir.[174–176]

The main gene responsible for this probenecid-inhibited PAH transport is a SLC transporter known as OAT1 (SLC22A6) and was originally called NKT (novel kidney transporter).[177,178] Like most other members of the mammalian SLC family, it has 12 membrane-spanning segments (Fig. 8.7A). At the time of its discovery, NKT was proposed to function as either

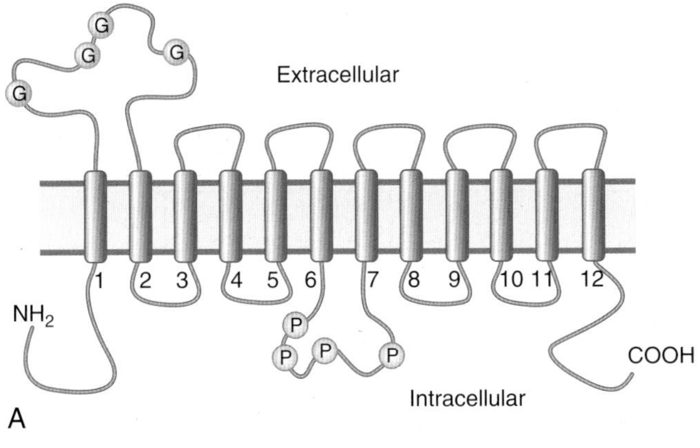


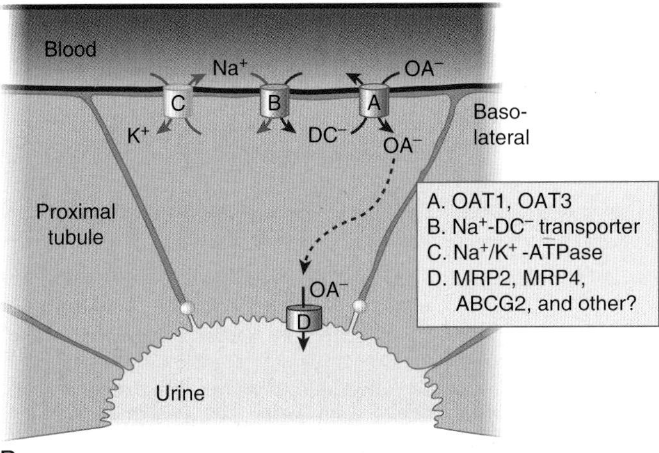


**Fig. 8.7 Topology of OAT1 and schematic of OAT1-mediated organic anion influx uptake as a "tertiary" transport process.** (A) An intracellular loop links two six-transmembrane domains yielding 12 membrane-spanning regions similar to many other SLC transporters (*G*, glycosylation sites; *P*, PKC, phosphorylation sites). (B) Schematic depicting a proximal tubule cell showing OAT-mediated influx of organic anions *(OA⁻)* from the plasma to the lumen. OAT1 (A), OA- influx by OAT1 at the basolateral membrane via antiport of dicarboxylates *(DC⁻)* down a gradient. OAT-mediated influx is connected to the transmembrane gradient of dicarboxylates created as a result $Na^+$/dicarboxylate cotransporter and mitochondrial TCA cycle (B). This "tertiary" process depends upon the ATP hydrolyzed by the $Na^+$-$K^+$-ATPase to create an extracellular-to-intracellular sodium gradient (C). Transport of OA-into urinary space (D) probably occurs through a number of apical membrane transporters, including the MRPs. (Modified from Nigam SK, Bush KT, Martovetsky G, et al. The organic anion transporter (OAT) family: a systems biology perspective. *Physiol Rev.* 2015;95:83–123; and Eraly SA, Bush KT, Sampogna RV, et al. The molecular pharmacology of organic anion transporters: from DNA to FDA? *Mol. Pharmacol.* 2004;65:479–487.)

an organic anion or organic cation transporter; numerous studies have since confirmed that, although OAT1 and other members of the OAT subfamily are predominantly organic anion transporters, they can also transport organic cations and zwitterions.[179,180]

The current view of how a prototypical organic anion—PAH in this case—is taken up across the basolateral membrane (blood side) of the proximal tubule cell involves three different transporters: OAT1, the sodium–dicarboxylate cotransporter (NaDC3, SLC13A3), and the sodium–potassium ATPase (Fig. 8.7B). This "tertiary" transport system is believed to operate through the following mechanisms: (1) exchange (antiport) of PAH in the plasma with α-ketoglutarate by OAT1; (2) cotransport (symport) of sodium and α-ketoglutarate into the cell by NaDC3; and (3) extrusion of sodium into the plasma, creating a sodium gradient, through the ATP-dependent action of the sodium–potassium ATPase (Na-K-ATPase). Thus, organic anion transport is ATP dependent only in an indirect way and depends on two other gradients: (1) a sodium gradient generated by the Na-K-ATPase, among other factors, that enables cotransport of sodium with α-ketoglutarate into the cell by NaDC3; and (2) a high intracellular α-ketoglutarate level that is partly due to the aforementioned NaDC3 cotransport and partly contributed by aerobic mitochondrial metabolism resulting in the generation of tricarboxylic acid (TCA) cycle intermediates such as α-ketoglutarate. Blocking any of these processes, for example, ouabain inhibition of the Na-K-ATPase, lithium inhibition of NaDC3, or probenecid inhibition of OAT1, markedly diminishes or even completely abolishes PAH transport via OAT1. In general, OAT3 appears to function via an analogous tertiary transport system, although it is not entirely clear that the linkage to α-ketoglutarate exchange is as tight.

When OAT1 was originally discovered (as NKT), two other homologous transporters, NLT (now OAT2, SLC22A7)[181] and OCT1, organic cation transporter 1 (SLC22A1)[182] were also found in the sequence database, and it was proposed that this was a new family of SLC transporters, which is now known as SLC22.[178] Since then, the SLC22 family has grown to roughly 30 transporters in humans and mice.[183,184]

A new evolutionary-based classification of SLC22 has been proposed, which divides the family into a major OAT clade and a major OCT clade, which further divide into six subclades (Fig. 8.8). The assumption is that the various SLC22 subclades defined by phylogenetic relationships will lead to a better functional classification and help deorphanize SLC22 transporters of unclear function. Accordingly, subclades within the OAT clade include the OAT subclade, the OAT-like subclade, and the OAT-related subclade; within the OCT clade is the OCT subclade, OCT-like (OCTN) subclade, and the OCT-related subclade.[183,185] The specific details of many of these transporters are beyond the scope of this chapter, and, indeed, many remain "orphans" with respect to endogenous substrate preference. Nevertheless, it is important to point out that, with the exception of certain subclades, the predominant expression for most of the other SLC22 transporters tends to be in the kidney proximal tubule, choroid plexus, or the liver. Even so, SLC22 transporters are expressed throughout the body, and there are even members with highly selective localization to the olfactory epithelium and brain substructures (OAT6, SLC22A20).[186] SLC22 is thus a very interesting SLC family involved in the transport of anionic, cationic, and zwitterionic drugs; toxins; metabolites; signaling molecules; antioxidants; dietary components; vitamins; gut microbiome products; and uremic toxins.[183]

Here we focus on OAT1 (SLC22A6) and OAT3 (SLC22A8), which are the major renal metabolite, drug, and toxin (including uremic toxin) organic anion transporters (Table 8.1); OCT2 (SLC22A2), the major transporter of cationic drugs and metabolites; and URAT1 (SLC22A12), the latter being the most extensively studied of several urate transporters in the OAT subclade. Along with a number of other SLC and ABC transporters, these SLC22 transporters are the most

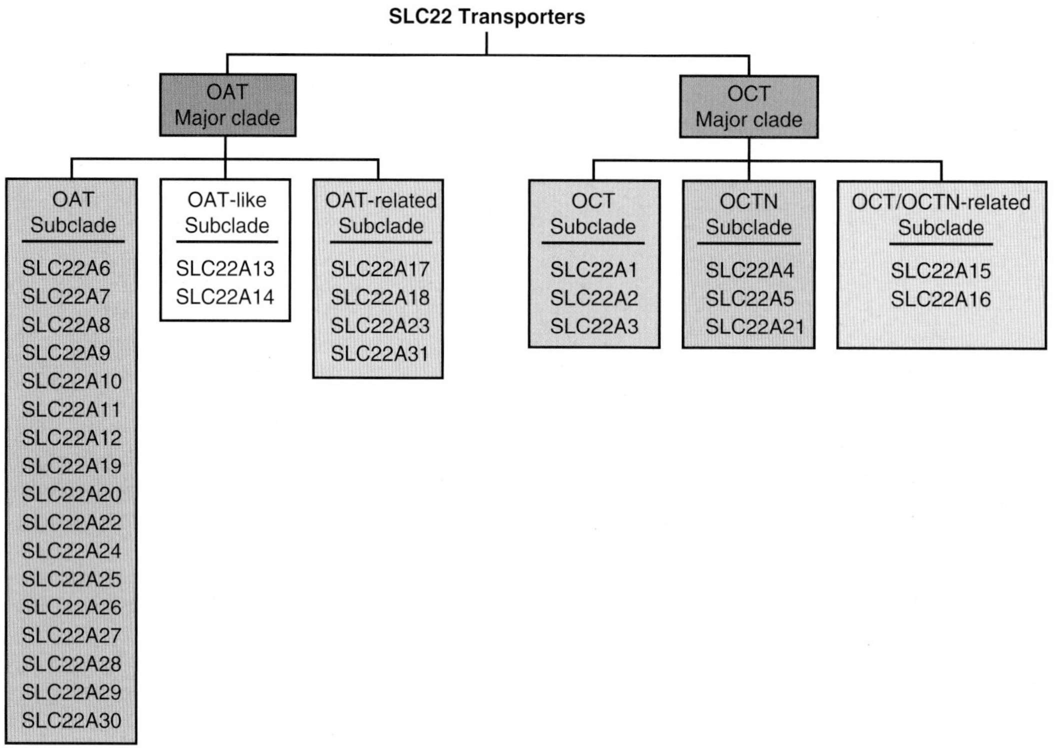


**Fig. 8.8 The six subfamilies of SLC22 transporters.** Evolutionary analysis indicates that SLC22 transporters are highly conserved and found in fly, worm, sea urchin, and other organisms. The SLC22 family is composed of two major clades, which are the organic anion transporter (*OAT*) major clade and organic cation transporter (*OCT*) major clade. Each of these clades is divided into three subclades, designated as *OAT*, *OAT-like*, *OAT-related*, *OCT*, *OCTN* (organic cation/carnitine transporter), and *OCT/OCTN*-related. (Modified from Nigam SK. The SLC22 transporter family: a paradigm for the impact of drug transporters on metabolic pathways, signaling, and disease. *Ann Rev Pharmacol Toxicol.* 2018;58:32.31–32.25; and Zhu C, Nigam KB, Date RC, et al. Evolutionary analysis and classification of OATS, OCTS, OCTNS, and other SLC22 transporters: structure-function implications and analysis of sequence motifs. *PLoS ONE.* 2015;10:e0140569.)

clinically relevant and quantitatively important organic anion and organic cation transporters in the proximal tubule of the kidney.[184,187]

## OAT1 (SLC22A6) AND OAT3 (SLC22A8)

Both OAT1 and OAT3 were among the original seven drug transporters that regulatory agencies identified as important for analysis of the possibility of transport of new drug entities.[188] This regulatory attention has perpetuated the notion that these transporters primarily transport drugs. Although it is true that the OATs transport drugs (e.g., antibiotics, antivirals, nonsteroidal antiinflammatory drugs, diuretics) and toxins (e.g., organic mercurials, aristolochic acid), it is now clear that they, as well as the other five SLC and ABC transporters highlighted by regulatory agencies, transport many endogenous metabolites, signaling molecules, vitamins, gut microbiome, and dietary products.[184]

Indeed, there is a growing appreciation that the primary function of these multispecific transporters may not be the handling of drugs and toxins but rather the modulation of local and systemic metabolism and signaling.[189,190] Much of this change in our understanding of "what drug transporters really do" is the result of "omics" analyses of knockout mice, human genome-wide association studies (GWAS), and the identification of heritable mutations that cause or modulate well-known metabolic diseases.[184]

According to this new systems biology view (explained in more detail later), the multispecificity of these transporters for endogenous substrates enables a range of drugs and toxins to coopt these transporters expressed in the gut, liver, kidney, and many other tissues. But the pharmaceutical and commercial relevance of these transporters can create the misconception that these widely expressed and evolutionarily conserved genes primarily exist to handle synthetic drugs. Although this is apparently their key role from the perspective of clinical pharmacology and pharmacokinetics, it is becoming clear that this lens is extremely limited even from the clinical point of view, because it is now evident that OAT1, OAT3, and other "drug" transporters are central to endogenous physiology and are important for understanding the pathophysiology of uremia, hyperuricemia, and a number of genetic conditions.

## OAT1 KNOCKOUT AND OAT3 KNOCKOUT MICE

Our understanding of in vivo OAT function has changed with the application of omics (e.g., metabolomics, transcriptomics) analyses to *Oat* knockout mice. The *Oat1* and *Oat3* knockout mice were first analyzed over a decade ago and have continued to yield considerable insight into the in vivo function of these two major organic anion transporters, particularly their endogenous function.[191–196]

As expected, the *Oat1* knockout mouse tissue has defective uptake of the classic organic anion transporter probe PAH, whereas the *Oat3* knockout mouse tissue has defective uptake of estrone sulfate.[191,197] Consistent with in vitro data, the *Oat1* and/or *Oat3* knockout mice have altered in vivo or ex vivo (e.g., embryonic kidney organ cultures) handling of diuretics

**Table 8.1 Some SLC22 Transporter Substrates**

| Substrate | SLC22 Transporter | | | |
|---|---|---|---|---|
| | SLC22A6 OAT1 | SLC22A8 OAT3 | SLC22A1 OCT1 | SLC22A2 OCT2 |
| Nonsteroidal antiinflammatory drugs | ✓ | ✓ | | |
| Ibuprofen | | | | |
| Naproxen | | | | |
| Antivirals | ✓ | ✓ | | |
| Tenofovir | | | | |
| Adefovir | | | | |
| Cidofovir | | | | |
| β-lactam antibiotics | ✓ | ✓ | | |
| Ampicillin | | | | |
| Benzylpenicillin | | | | |
| Diuretics | ✓ | ✓ | | |
| Bumetanide | | | | |
| Furosemide | | | | |
| TCA cycle intermediates | ✓ | ✓ | | |
| Short-chain fatty acids | ✓ | ✓ | | |
| Bile acids | | ✓ | | |
| Flavonoids | ✓ | ✓ | | |
| Gut microbiome products | ✓ | ✓ | ✓ | ✓ |
| Organic mercurials | ✓ | ✓ | | |
| Cisplatin | | | ✓ | ✓ |
| Metformin | | | ✓ | ✓ |
| Cimetidine | | ✓ | ✓ | ✓ |
| Thiamine | | | ✓ | ✓ |

*TCA*, Tricarboxylic acid.

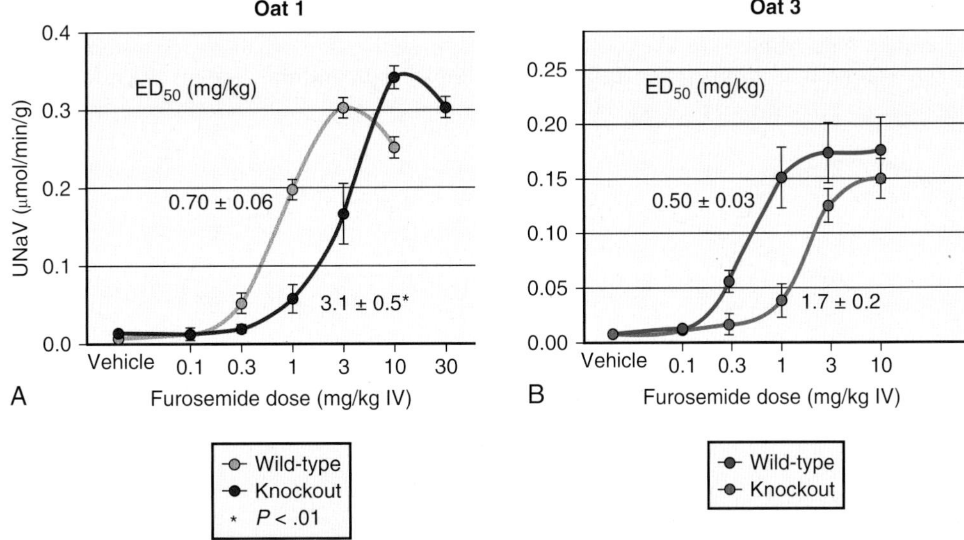


**Fig. 8.9** Marked attenuation of thiazide and loop diuretic effects in *Oat1* and *Oat3* knockout mice. In *Oat1* or *Oat3* knockout, which transport diuretics (Table 8.1), luminal sodium elimination is markedly attenuated. *ED50*, Half-maximal effective dose; *IV*, intravenous; *UNa*V, urinary sodium excretion. (Modified from Eraly SA, Vallon V, Vaughn DA, et al. Decreased renal organic anion secretion and plasma accumulation of endogenous organic anions in OAT1 knock-out mice. *J Biol Chem* 2006;281:5072–5083; and Vallon V, Rieg T, Ahn SY, et al. Overlapping in vitro and in vivo specificities of the organic anion transporters OAT1 and OAT3 for loop and thiazide diuretics. *Am J Physiol Renal Physiol.* 2008;294:F867–F873.)

(e.g., loop, thiazides), antibiotics (e.g., penicillin, ciprofloxacin), a wide range of antiviral agents, and methotrexate.[198–204]

Knockout mice responses to loop and thiazide diuretics provide a useful illustration (Fig. 8.9). These albumin-bound drugs in the peritubular capillaries must be transported by basolateral uptake transporters OAT1 and OAT3 in the proximal tubule, transit the cell, and exit through apical transporters (including members of the ABCC or MRP families)—all before flowing down the luminal (urinary) space to be excreted or, for the loop and thiazide diuretics, to inhibit salt reabsorption in later nephron segments. Three to five times more diuretic is required to achieve the same degree of natriuresis after deletion of either *Oat1* or *Oat3* in mice.[191,198]

OATs are implicated in renal organic mercurial toxicity because mercury binds to glutathione and other thiol-containing compounds, many of which are "effectively" seen as organic anions by the transporter.[205] When the *Oat1* knockout mouse was treated with high-dose mercury, the kidneys were surprisingly well protected from injury (histologically and by renal indices), consistent with the inability of the organic mercurial to be taken up by the proximal tubule due to the absence of Oat1.[206]

Perhaps most interesting, and somewhat unexpected, have been the results from performing metabolomics analyses on the plasma of the *Oat* knockout animals[191,193–195,207] (Fig. 8.10). These have revealed a somewhat surprising range of endogenous OAT substrates.

Generally speaking, both OAT1 and OAT3 appear to play a key role in regulating the flow of organic anions through the so-called gut–liver–kidney axis.[194] This includes the renal handling of many compounds derived from the gut microbiome—either products of the gut microbiome or due to the action of the gut microbiome on dietary components such as phytochemicals. For example, in the *Oat3* knockout, among the greatest changes are in flavonoids that have been acted upon by phase 2 liver enzymes (e.g., glucuronidation). This highlights the important connection between OATs (especially OAT3) with liver metabolism (via so-called drug-metabolizing enzymes) of endogenous compounds as well as drugs and toxins.

Other groups of metabolites elevated in the *Oat3* knockout include primary and secondary bile acids.[194] In *Oat1* and *Oat3* knockouts, fatty acids, TCA cycle intermediates, and vitamins are also elevated. Nevertheless, unlike the case of FDA-approved drugs—where it is difficult to distinguish molecular properties of drug substrates that predispose to interaction with OAT1 or OAT3[208]—the sets of metabolites appear fairly distinct, although there is still much overlap.[194]

These chemical properties of drugs and metabolites interacting with OAT1 versus OAT3 deserve further mention. With respect to drugs, OAT1 and OAT3 strongly favor anionic drug substrates, but both transporters (especially OAT3) can bind a limited number of cationic/zwitterionic drugs.[180] Cimetidine is an example.[179] Importantly, chemical properties of metabolites interacting with the OATs appear substantially different from the drug data. This could partly be due to a selection factor related to which drugs make it to market. However, it remains that, more than for drugs, the molecular and chemical properties of metabolites appear to distinguish, in a general way, between OAT1 and OAT3 substrates—with OAT3 substrates being larger, less polar, more chemically complex, and containing more ring structures.[194] Nevertheless, it is worth mentioning again that there is overlap between OAT1 and OAT3 metabolite substrates.

In addition, metabolic reconstructions based on changes in gene expression in the knockouts have been performed.[207–209] These metabolic reconstructions are generally consistent with metabolomics data; the reconstructions indicate that OATs regulate many systemic biochemical pathways as well as those in the proximal tubule (Table 8.2). For example, among the top biochemical pathways revealed in reconstructions are purine metabolism, TCA cycle, fatty acid metabolism, eicosanoid metabolism, amino acid metabolism (tryptophan, tyrosine, arginine), and a variety of vitamin-dependent pathways. Together, the reconstructions and the metabolomics data support the view that OATs are not simply "drug" transporters but impact many aspects of systemic and proximal tubule physiology.

Together, the metabolic reconstructions based on knockout omics data and the analysis of endogenous substrates (e.g.,

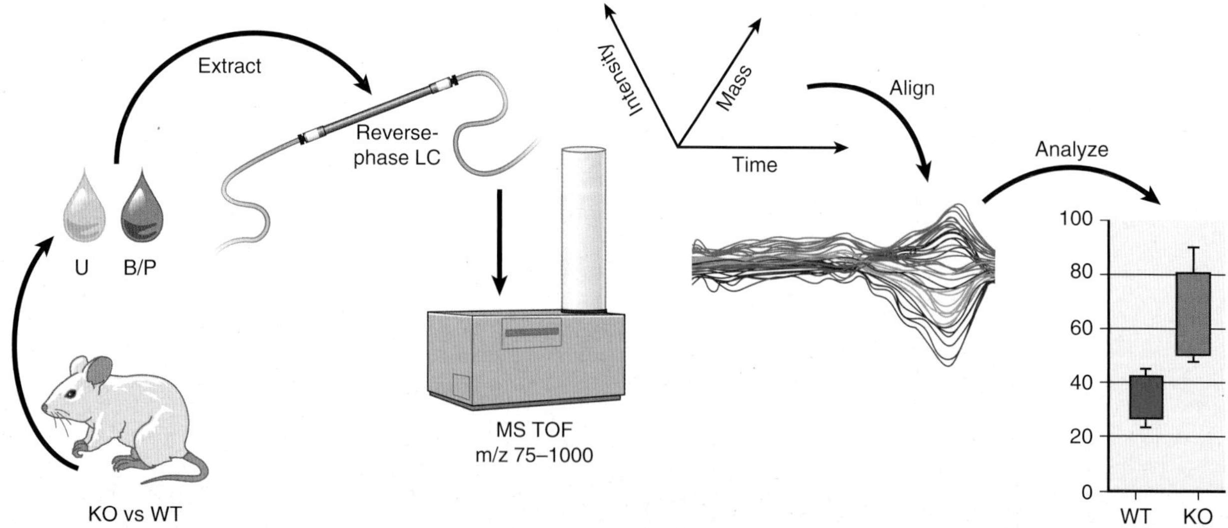


**Fig. 8.10 Schematic of approach to metabolomic analysis of *Oat1* knockout mice.** Schematic of strategy for untargeted metabolomic analysis of metabolites, gut microbiome (enterobiome) products, vitamins, and signaling molecules, many of which have been shown to directly interact with Oat1 as determined by in vitro assays. Wild-type and *Oat1–/–* mice plasma and urine were profiled using liquid chromatography with tandem mass spectrometry (LC/MS/MS). Importantly, untargeted metabolomics identifies gut microbiome and uremic toxins 1 (Oat1). Subsequently, *Oat3* knockouts were also profiled; gut microbiome products and uremic toxins were also identified, as well as a number of bile acids and flavonoid metabolites. *KO,* Knockout; *WT,* wild-type. (Modified from Wikoff WR, Nagle MA, Kouznetsova VL, et al. Untargeted metabolomics identifies enterobiome metabolites and putative uremic toxins as substrates of organic anion transporter 1 (Oat1). *J Proteome Res.* 2011;10:2842–2851.)

**Table 8.2 Top Pathways Affected by Oat1 Loss in Knockout Mice**

| |
|---|
| TCA cycle |
| Tyrosine metabolism |
| Alanine, aspartate, and glutamate metabolism |
| Butanoate metabolism |
| Arginine and proline metabolism |
| Tryptophan metabolism |
| Nicotinate and nicotinamide metabolism |
| Valine, leucine, and isoleucine degradation |
| Nitrogen metabolism |
| Glyoxylate and dicarboxylate metabolism |
| Propanoate metabolism |
| Glycine, serine, and threonine metabolism |
| Purine metabolism |
| Pyrimidine metabolism |

*TCA,* Tricarboxylic acid.
Adapted from Liu HC, Jamshidi N, Chen Y, et al. An organic anion transporter 1 (OAT1)-centered metabolic network. *J Biol Chem*. 2016;291:19474-19486.

metabolites, signaling molecules) from the perspective of chemical properties calls into question the oft-discussed "redundancy" of OAT1 and OAT3 in the proximal tubule. From a practical pharmacokinetic perspective, this view may still be a useful first approximation for many drugs that can interact with both OAT1 and OAT3. But considering the endogenous metabolite preferences alone (without considering drugs), a more appropriate view might be that the two transporters have distinct roles in many metabolic processes, although they work together to handle certain substrates like uric acid. Based on current data, OAT1 appears more linked to local and systemic aerobic metabolism, whereas OAT3 appears more linked to flow of metabolites that originate in the gut or liver (e.g., primary and secondary bile acids). There is also some evidence to suggest that OAT3 could modify phenotypes, for instance, in diabetic disease,[210] blood pressure,[192] and in the setting of treatment with SGLT2 inhibitors.[115]

## OAT1 AND OAT3 SINGLE-NUCLEOTIDE POLYMORPHISMS

Nonsynonymous coding region single-nucleotide polymorphisms (SNPs) in the OATs are uncommon compared with noncoding region SNPs.[211] Although SNPs in OATs have received less attention than OCT SNPs—because OCTs appear to be more polymorphic in humans—associations have, in recent years, been reported that affect diuretic responsiveness, mercury toxicity, antibiotic levels, and hyperuricemia.[212–216] A noncoding SNP in the OAT1 gene appears to be associated with the progression of renal disease; whether or not this is related to altered handling of one or more uremic or other toxins is not clear.[217] Based on animal and human data, it would not be surprising if OAT3 SNPs are found to be associated with glucose homeostasis or diabetic renal disease. Because there is considerable overlap in drugs transported by OAT1 and OAT3, it may be that SNPs in both OATs (or in an OAT and the "corresponding" apical transporter such as MRP2 or MRP4) are required for pronounced drug, toxin, and metabolite phenotypes.[218] This question needs to be examined in more detail.

## OCT2 (SLC22A2)

Unlike the OAT subclade (of the SLC22 OAT major clade), which is large, the OCT subclade (one of three subclades of the SLC22 OCT major clade) consists of three highly homologous (both protein sequence and function) transporters: OCT1, OCT2, and OCT3.[183] OCTs are generally held to be electrogenic uniporters.[219] Organic cation transporter 2 (OCT2) is the main renal uptake transporter on the basolateral membrane (blood side) of the proximal tubule cell that is involved in the elimination of organic cationic drugs such as metformin and *cis*-platinum.[220,221] On the luminal (apical, urine side) of the cell, it appears that MATE (SLC47) transporter family members efflux organic cations into the urinary space.[222] Recently, the primary liver OCT, OCT1—one of the drug transporters that, along with OAT1 and OAT3, has been highlighted by regulatory agencies as important for new drug testing to identify transport mechanisms—has been shown to be a thiamine transporter.[223]

Thus, as with the OATs, OCTs may function primarily in regulating metabolite flow into and out of tissues, and as with OATs, the best in vivo functional information regarding endogenous function comes from analysis of metabolites altered in the knockout mice. On the whole, the known drug and metabolite substrates for the OCTs appear less diverse than for the OATs, and it appears that, based on molecular property analysis of drug substrates, OCT1 and OCT2 have largely overlapping specificities, at least for drugs.[180]

## OCT2 SINGLE NUCLEOTIDE POLYMORPHISMS

The OCTs appear more polymorphic than the OATs; SNPs in OCT2 have received considerable clinical attention because, consistent with in vitro studies, they can affect levels of the antidiabetic agent metformin and the chemotherapeutic agent *cis*-platinum.[224–227] These associations are much better established than the SNP associations mentioned above for the OATs.[228] Because metformin and *cis*-platinum have been so widely used, and because of the potential for toxicity, it is important for the clinician to be aware of the possibility that SNPs in OCT2 can affect drug levels.

***Clinical Relevance***

**The Remote Sensing and Signaling Hypothesis: A Framework for Understanding Hyperuricemia and Uremia**

The OATs and OCTs have recently garnered a great deal of attention because of regulatory concerns due to transporter-mediated drug–drug interactions. Much more is likely on the way regarding drug-metabolite interactions (DMI) with the advent of better techniques to analyze metabolites in tissues and body fluids. With new approaches to uremia and hyperuricemia (especially in CKD) being considered, one expects more clinical studies and trials aimed at decreasing the burden of uremic toxins and uric acid—and prolonging time to severe CKD and dialysis. In this regard, the Remote Sensing and Signaling Hypothesis should be useful for considering approaches to ameliorate perturbed inter-organ and interorganismal communication via metabolites and signaling molecules, including those derived from the gut microbiome.

## APICAL MEMBRANE PROXIMAL TUBULE TRANSPORTERS INVOLVED IN THE HANDLING OF ORGANIC ANIONS, ORGANIC CATIONS, AND ORGANIC ZWITTERIONS

In the proximal tubule, the OAT1, OAT3, and OCT2 function in basolateral side uptake (influx) of organic anions and cations from the blood. Although what happens to these charged organic molecules inside the cell remains poorly defined, their exit, usually in unchanged form, has become better understood in recent years. Many of the organic anions taken up by OAT1 and OAT3, for example, are effluxed across the apical membrane by members of the ABCC family, MRP2 (ABCC2) and MRP4 (ABCC4).[168] These are not the only apical transporters of organic anions in the proximal tubule; for example, OAT4 and the well-known ABC transporters, P-glycoprotein and ABCG2, appear to play a role for certain substrates.[168] Although in simplified representations, there is a tendency to match basolateral OAT1 and OAT3 with apical MRP2 and MRP4, it is likely that, depending on the anionic substrate taken up by OAT1 and OAT3, one or several apical transporters are involved in apical efflux into the proximal tubule lumen.

With respect to the apical efflux of organic cations, in recent years, MATEs, particularly MATE-2K, have received attention.[168,222] MATEs are members of the SLC47 family, and it is well established that they transport many cationic drugs taken up by OCT2. Other apical transporters might also transport some OCT2 substrates, but their contribution is not well defined. It is also important to mention the organic cation/zwitterion transporters OCTN1 (SLC22A4) and OCTN2 (SLC22A5). Although they are sometimes listed along with drug transporters, their endogenous substrates—ergothioneine and carnitine, respectively—are well established.[229,230] Indeed, mutations in OCTN2 cause systemic carnitine deficiency, which can lead to severe cardiac and skeletal myopathy. Ergothioneine, on the other hand, is considered an important antioxidant. Nevertheless, OCTNs have some ability to interact with cation drugs.

## RENAL TRANSPORT OF SPECIFIC ORGANIC SUBSTRATES IN DISEASE

### UREMIC TOXIN TRANSPORT

The importance of OATs in renal handling of gut microbiome–derived metabolites merits further discussion. Many of the metabolites accumulating in the *Oat* knockouts, such as indoxyl sulfate, kynurenine, p-cresol sulfate, and hippurate, are among the sets of gut microbiome–derived small molecules (organic anions); they are also frequently implicated as "uremic toxins"[193,195] (Table 8.3).

The list of small molecules implicated in uremic toxicity is long and much debated.[231,232] These uremic toxins are thought to play a role in many tissue and organ toxicities and dysfunctions that occur in the uremic syndrome associated with severe CKD. It is unlikely that any single uremic toxin on the list is the key to all the manifestations of the uremic syndrome, although there is growing evidence that certain uremic toxins play a role in particular tissue toxicities. These include TMAO (trimethylamine-N-oxide), which has been implicated in cardiovascular toxicity,[233,234] and indoxyl sulfate, which has been implicated in multiple aspects of the uremic syndrome.[235]

**Table 8.3 Uremic Toxins Accumulating in *Oat1* and/or *Oat3* Knockout Mice**

| | |
|---|---|
| Indoxyl sulfate | Indolelactate |
| p-Cresol sulfate | Kynurenate |
| Hippurate | Putrescine |
| CMPF | Uric acid |
| Phenyl sulfate | Creatinine |
| Xanthurenate | |

*CMPF,* 3-Carboxy-4-methyl-5-propyl-2-furanpropanoate.
Adapted from Wikoff WR, Nagle MA, Kouznetsova VL, et al. Untargeted metabolomics identifies enterobiome metabolites and putative uremic toxins as substrates of organic anion transporter 1 (Oat1). *J Proteome Res.* 2011;10:2842-2851; and Wu W, Bush KT, Nigam SK. Key role for the organic anion transporters, OAT1 and OAT3, in the in vivo handling of uremic toxins and solutes. *Sci Rep.* 2017;7:4939.

Some of these uremic toxins (e.g., indoxyl sulfate) may play a role in the actual progression of renal disease, presumably via OAT-mediated uptake into proximal tubule cells.[195,236] The pathophysiology of uremia is beyond the scope of this chapter, and readers are referred instead to Chapter 52. But it is important to emphasize the growing appreciation of the role of OAT1 and OAT3 in regulating levels of many molecules considered uremic toxins. Thus, it will be interesting to determine whether SNPs, or other factors that affect the expression or function of OAT1 and OAT3, alter the time at which the uremic syndrome develops or the progression of renal disease.

OCT2 also appears to be a transporter of certain cationic uremic toxins, notably TMAO, a molecule accumulating in CKD that is associated with cardiovascular disease.[237] The apical transporters of organic anions, the MATEs, appear to be involved in the efflux of TMAO. Of note, the deletion in mice of OAT3, which can transport a few organic cations despite being an organic anion transporter, results in elevated levels of TMAO, although it is not clear whether TMAO is actually transported by OAT3.[195]

### URIC ACID TRANSPORT

Uric acid is an antioxidant that also has deleterious effects.[238] It is also on the list of "uremic toxins." Apart from gout and kidney stones, hyperuricemia has been associated with cardiovascular disease, metabolic syndrome, hypertension, and progression of renal disease.[239] Metabolism of purines by enzymes primarily in the liver (e.g., xanthine oxidase) results in uric acid formation. On the other hand, uric acid elimination and retention in the body is largely determined by the kidney and, to a lesser extent (in the absence of kidney disease), by the intestine.

One of the unexpected results of GWAS and knockout mouse studies from the perspective of uric acid homeostasis was the number of SLC and ABC "drug" transporters that were implicated in regulating serum uric acid levels and then shown to transport urate.[238,240] These transporters include ABCG2 (also known as BCRP), URAT1 (a close relative of OAT1 and OAT3), OAT1 and OAT3, as well as other OATs. In murine knockouts of OAT1, OAT3, and URAT1 (SLC22A12, originally discovered as Rst in mice[241]), there are alterations in renal urate handling, although they are not as great as might have been expected if these genes were, as was thought by many at the time, the major contributors to renal urate handling.[196] Subsequently, another SLC transporter, related to the glucose transporters, known as GLUT9 (SLC2A9), was found to be very important for renal urate handling.[242] Other transporters implicated in uric acid transport are MRP2 (ABCC2), MRP4 (ABCC4), NPT1 (SLC17A1), NPT4 (SLC17A3), OAT4 (SLC22A11), and OAT10 (SLC22A13).[243] The list of associated genes, which includes nontransporters as well, continues to grow as more analyses are done in different ethnic groups. Indeed, based on GWAS and other studies, it appears that different subsets of the aforementioned genes may be more or less important in urate handling, depending on ethnicity and gender.

Together, these transporters are responsible for the complex handling of uric acid by the kidney, but it is important to emphasize that ABCG2 is increasingly perceived as the main intestinal uric acid efflux transporter.[244] Intestinal extrusion of urate becomes particularly important in the setting of severe renal insufficiency, and in this regard, it has been found that SNPs in ABCG2 become more highly associated with uric acid levels in CKD patients[215] (Fig. 8.11). This seems to be an example of remote organ communication (i.e., between injured kidney to intestine; see also later) with the apparent "objective" of optimizing uric acid levels as transport in another organ (intestinal efflux) takes over from the declining kidney, thereby reducing the plasma uric acid levels. From studies in animal models, it is believed that the high uric acid level itself in CKD leads to increased expression and/or function of intestinal ABCG2, and if so, this may be a case of substrate induction of the transporter.[245]

## CREATININE TRANSPORT

Although new measures may soon become routinely used in hospitals, serum creatinine continues to be considered an index of renal function both in primary care and hospital settings. A number of members of the SLC22 family (containing OATs and OCTs) transport creatinine. These include OCT2, OAT2, OAT3, and possibly OAT1.[246–248] All of these are considered key transporters of organic cation drugs, organic anion drugs, and zwitterionic drugs. Their relative importance in renal creatinine handling is debated, but it is likely that all play some role in the renal handling of creatinine, with OCT2 and OAT2 being particularly important, at least based on more recent

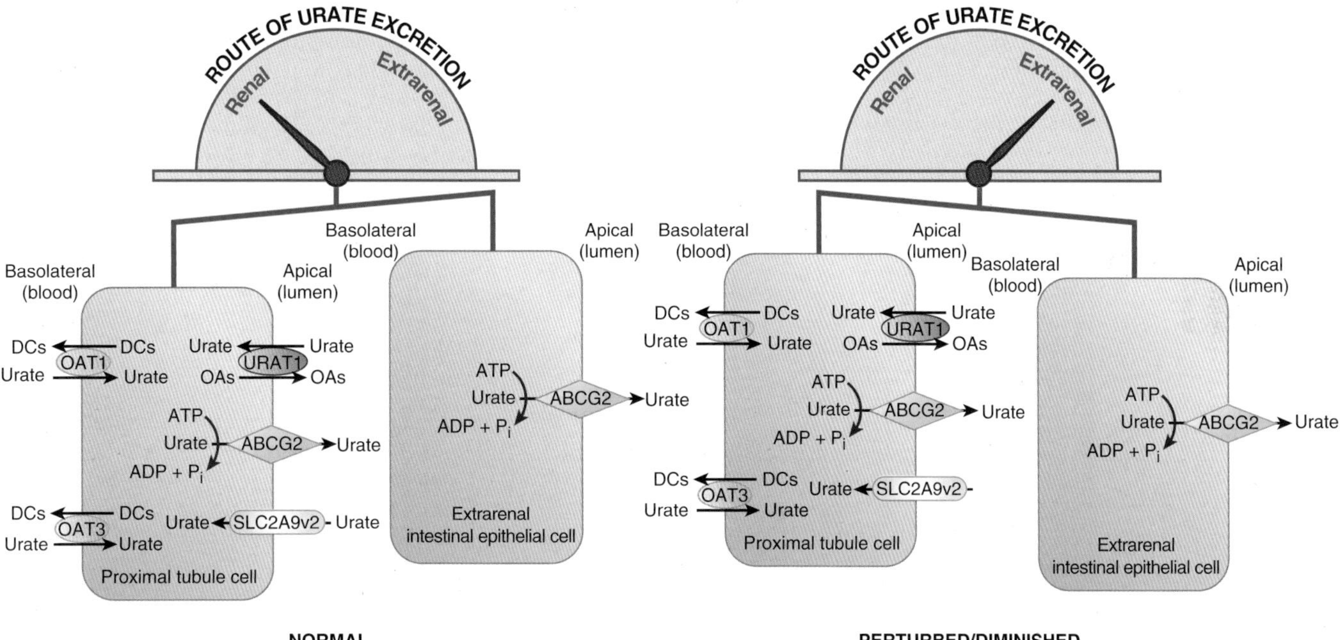


**Fig. 8.11 In chronic kidney disease, the intestinal role of uric acid transporters (mainly ABCG2) becomes much more important.** Schematic of urate excretion in the setting of normal renal function versus that in which there is diminished renal function. In the normal situation, the majority of urate excretion (~70%) is performed mainly in the proximal tubule of the kidney and is mediated by a number of transporters found on the apical and basolateral membranes of the proximal tubule cell. The illustration depicts only some of the transporters involved and includes members of the SLC and ABC families of membrane transporters. On the basolateral surface, the uptake of uric acid from the blood is mediated mainly by OAT1 (SLC22A6) and OAT3 (SLC22A8). These solute carrier transporters exchange dicarboxylates *(DCs)* for urate resulting in the net movement of this organic anion into the proximal tubular cell. At the apical surface, a number of transporters, including ABCG2 (depicted here), NPT1 (SLC17A1), and NPT4 (SLC17A3), as well as ABCC family members, work to secrete urate into the tubular lumen for excretion via the urine. The relative importance of the aforementioned apical transporters in urate secretion remains unclear. Transport of urate via ABCG2 is driven through ATP hydrolysis. Several other apical membrane transporters are well established in the reabsorption of urate, including URAT1 and SLC2A9v2. URAT1, or SLC22A12, exchanges intercellular organic anions for urate, resulting in the movement of uric acid back into the proximal tubule cell. Meanwhile, under normal physiologic conditions, up to 30% of uric acid is excreted via extrarenal transporters, believed to largely be driven by ABCG2 expressed in intestinal epithelial cells. The results of the analysis of human data—as well as physiologic data from rodent models with renal dysfunction—support the view that urate transport by ABCG2, most likely in intestine, compensates for poor renal urate handling in the setting of diminished kidney function. (Modified from Bhatnagar V, Richard EL, Wu W, et al. Analysis of ABCG2 and other urate transporters in uric acid homeostasis in chronic kidney disease: potential role of remote sensing and signaling. *Clin Kidney J.* 2016;9:444–453.)

studies. The issue is clinically relevant, because a number of drugs (e.g., trimethoprim) are thought to "artificially" create the impression of renal dysfunction when creatinine is the primary measure used because of drug–metabolite interactions at the level of the transporter.[168]

## THE REMOTE SENSING AND SIGNALING HYPOTHESIS: A FRAMEWORK FOR UNDERSTANDING HYPERURICEMIA AND UREMIA

It is evident from in vitro transport studies, metabolomics analyses of knockout animals, GWAS studies, and metabolic diseases due to transporter mutations that multispecific "drug" transporters of both the SLC and ABC transporter family are critical in the local and systemic regulation of levels of a huge array of metabolites.[183,184,189,190,249]

The Remote Sensing and Signaling Hypothesis—which began to be formulated in 2004–2007[186]—argues that the physiologic role of multispecific "drug" transporters and their close (often mono- or oligo-specific) relatives is the regulation of "remote" interorgan and interorganismal communication via metabolites and signaling molecules by these SLC and ABC transporters (Fig. 8.12).

The system is hypothesized to be actively regulated through transcriptional mechanisms (e.g., nuclear receptors) and posttranslational mechanisms (e.g., kinases regulating transporter internalization or PDZ domain association). It is envisioned to work in parallel with the neuroendocrine, growth factor cytokine, and autonomic systems. The argument is that this type of SLC and ABC transporter-mediated remote interorgan and remote interorganismal communication via small molecules of "high informational content" (e.g., rate-limiting metabolites, signaling molecules, antioxidants, vitamins) is as critical as these other homeostatic systems and, as such, deserves comparable consideration for understanding health and disease states.

The hypothesis seems to be particularly relevant to renal disease. Consider, for instance, the previously discussed example of apparent interorgan remote communication—in order to reestablish uric acid homeostasis.[243] An injured organ—the malfunctioning kidney in CKD—is involved in a kind of "organ cross-talk" with the intestine, whereby intestinal ABCG2 transporters, and possibly others, appear to "take over" from many renal SLC uric acid transporters as tubular function declines. As discussed earlier, high urate, certain uremic toxins, or both—accumulating as a consequence of renal disease—are thought to induce expression of intestinal transporters.

More generally, considering the uremic syndrome as partly due to "pathologic" transporter-mediated remote interorgan and interorganismal communication of uremic toxins—which includes signaling molecules that bind G-protein–coupled

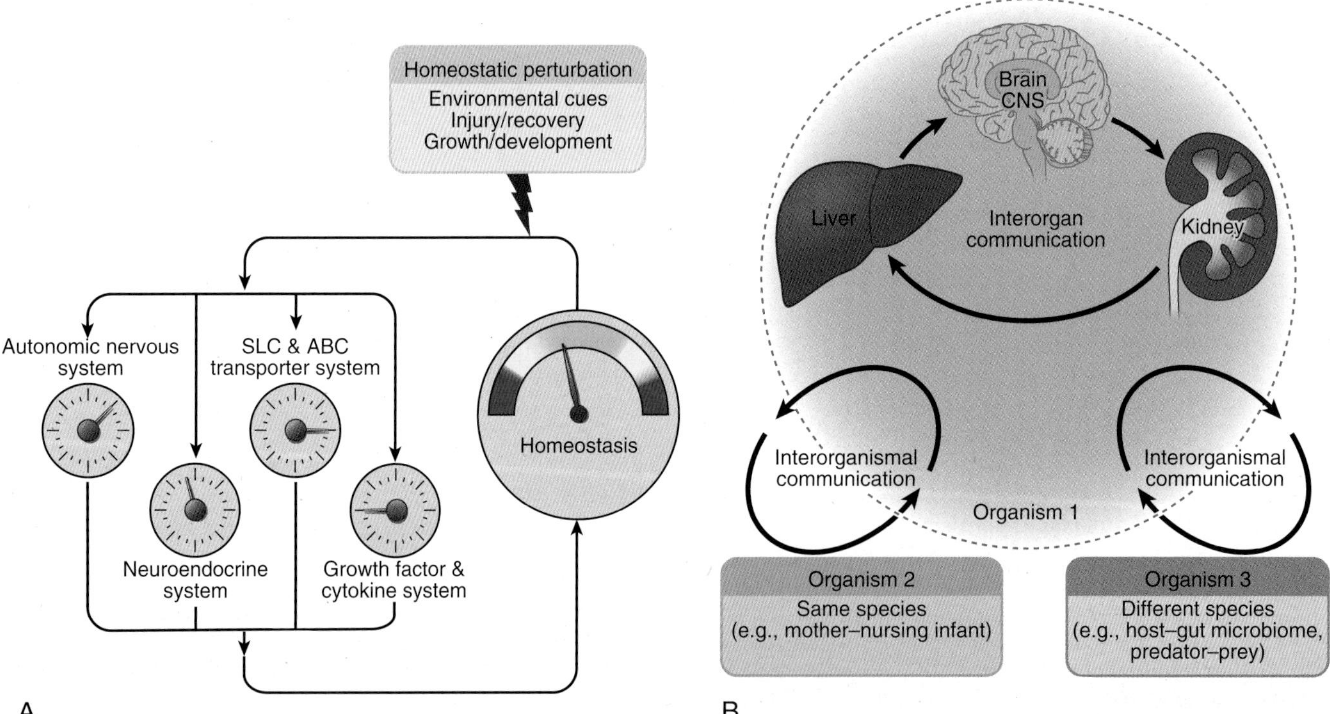


**Fig. 8.12 The Remote Sensing and Signaling Hypothesis as it relates to multispecific and more selective SLC and ABC transporters as well as drug-metabolizing enzymes (*DMEs*) in different tissues communicating "remotely" (interorgan and interorganismal) in part due to differentially expressed transporters via the gut–liver–kidney axis in health and disease.** The Remote Sensing and Signaling Hypothesis emphasizes the role of multispecific ("drug" transporters like OAT1, OAT3, ABCG2, and MRPs) and more selective SLC22 transporters as well other SLC and ABC drug and DMEs in a remote interorgan and interorganism communication network involving transporters and DMEs in epithelial and nonepithelial tissues as well as various body fluid spaces, such cerebrospinal fluid, breast milk, and urine. This remote sensing and signaling system works in concert with more classic systems involved in homeostasis and resetting homeostasis in the setting of diseases like hyperuricemia and uremia. These other systems include the neuroendocrine, growth factor cytokine, autonomic nervous systems, and increasing evidence indicates that it is intertwined with these classic homeostatic systems. *CNS*, Central nervous system. (Adapted from Nigam SK. What do drug transporters really do? *Nat Rev Drug Discov.* 2015;14:29–44.)

receptors (e.g., kynurenine) and nuclear receptors (e.g., indoxyl sulfate)—provides a different lens on the numerous biochemical and cellular aberrations found in the uremic syndrome, which affect many tissues and body compartments. Moreover, the source of many uremic toxins in the body is the gut microbiome—the result of interorganismal communication—and these toxins affect signaling and metabolism in multiple organs before, in many cases, being eliminated by proximal tubule multispecific "drug" transporters, such as the OAT1, OAT3, OCT2, and the MATEs.

The Remote Sensing and Signaling Hypothesis provides a systems pathophysiology framework for thinking about the many metabolic and signaling aberrations of the uremic syndrome in the context of remote interorgan and interorganismal small molecule communication. Such a systems-level view may lead to the consideration of new therapeutic approaches aimed at altering remote sensing and signaling mechanisms as they become better understood—with the hope of ameliorating some of the many harmful manifestations of the uremic syndrome.

### DRUG–METABOLITE INTERACTIONS

As more is learned about the endogenous substrates of OATs, OCTs, and other drug transporters, and as more is learned through metabolomics and metabolic reconstructions (such as those described above) regarding the regulation of tissue-specific metabolism by these transporters, it will become possible to consider new ways to modulate complex metabolic diseases like uremia and to understand the implications of drug–metabolite interactions (DMI) beyond simple competition at the level of the transporter itself.[168,208] For example, currently the thinking on DMI is largely limited to looking at the transporter-level competition between the drug trimethoprim, which binds OCT2 and thereby raises the plasma concentration of a single OCT2-transported metabolite such as creatinine. But in the case of OAT1, it is now well established from knockout studies that loss of OAT1 function affects many metabolic pathways.[208,209] The implication is that a drug that competes for OAT1 binding with endogenous metabolites normally transported by OAT1 (e.g., probenecid) will have broad effects on metabolism, affecting metabolites and signaling molecules that may themselves not be direct OAT1 substrates. This type of DMI may help partly explain the broad metabolic syndrome–like effects seen in the setting of chronic use of certain OAT-transported drugs, such as diuretics and HIV antivirals.[250,251] Much work needs to be done in this area of DMI where competition for transport by the drug may affect a wide range of metabolic pathways; this would seem particularly relevant in the setting of moderate CKD where the affected metabolites would likely include certain uremic toxins.[168]

## AMINO ACIDS

### PHYSIOLOGY OF RENAL AMINO ACID TRANSPORT

Rare inherited defects of renal amino acid transport have been instrumental for our understanding of renal metabolite reabsorption.[252,253] Four disorders associated with apical amino acid transporters define four major renal transport pathways, namely, a transporter for neutral amino acids (mutated in Hartnup disorder), a transporter for cationic amino acids and cystine (mutated in cystinuria), a transporter for anionic amino acids (mutated in dicarboxylic aminoaciduria), and a transporter for glycine and proline (mutated in iminoglycinuria)[254] (see Chapter 44 for a detailed discussion of these inherited disorders). With the exception of iminoglycinuria, aminoacidurias also affect intestinal transport. Genetic complexity is observed in cystinuria and iminoglycinuria, demonstrating the involvement of more than one gene in the transport process. Apart from intestinal transport, aminoacidurias affecting apical transport have little effect on other organs, indicating that expression of these transporters is largely specific to the apical membrane in the kidney and intestine, although some renal amino acid transporters are also found in the brain. The four major amino acid transport activities were verified further by in vitro studies using a variety of methods such as microperfusion studies, brush border membrane vesicles, cortical slices, and cell lines.[254,255] In vitro studies, in addition, identified a fifth transport activity, namely for β-amino acids, for which no corresponding disorder exists. Transport across the basolateral membrane has been more challenging to delineate, and it is unclear whether the five apical pathways are matched by five basolateral exit routes. A clear pathway for the release of cationic amino acids has been genetically identified through the rare amino aciduria lysinuric protein intolerance (LPI) and through functional studies.[256,257] A release pathway for neutral amino acids was defined functionally using vesicles derived from the basolateral membrane.[258] Release of anionic amino acids is difficult to measure, due to significant metabolism of glutamate by epithelial cells[259] (see also Fig. 8.4). Glycine is likely to join other neutral amino acids for efflux, but the efflux pathways for proline and β-amino acids remain unclear. More than 98% of all filtered amino acids are reabsorbed in the proximal tubule; other parts of the tubule thus do not significantly contribute to amino acid reabsorption and are not discussed here.[260] Some differences in transporter expression are observed between the PCT and the PST; these are illustrated in Fig. 8.13. Species differences may occur in the kidney and are mentioned where relevant.

### MOLECULAR BIOLOGY OF RENAL AMINO ACID TRANSPORTERS

Molecular cloning, human genetics, and mouse models have helped to identify almost all amino acid transporters in the apical and basolateral membrane.[254,261] Renal epithelial amino acid transporters are found in a variety of SLC families (Table 8.4). The SLC nomenclature is generally used for the genes, whereas acronyms are typically used for the proteins that describe some of the properties of the transporter. Expression cloning using *Xenopus laevis* oocytes or mammalian cell lines has been instrumental in the identification of renal amino acid transporters.[262] Additional transporters were identified by sequence similarity. As a result of these efforts, the amino acid transporter endowment of renal epithelial cells is now well understood, and an overview is depicted in Fig. 8.13. In the following, transporters for each group of amino acids are described in detail.

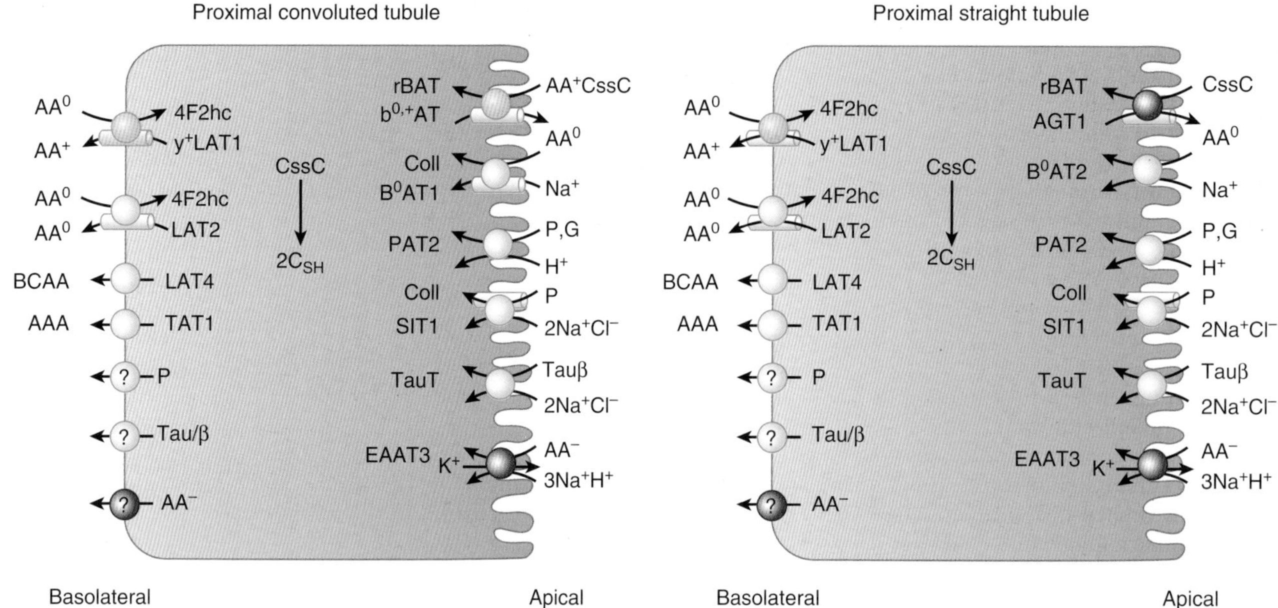


**Fig. 8.13 Amino acid transporters in the proximal tubule.** The common name of amino acid transporters in the proximal convoluted tubule and proximal straight tubule are shown next to each transporter. Transporter requirement for ancillary subunits are indicated by a tubelike structure. Transporters for anionic amino acids are shown in *red*; transporters for cationic amino acid are shown in *yellow*. *AA⁰*, neutral amino acids; *AA⁺*, cationic amino acids; *AA⁻*, anionic amino acids; *AAA*, aromatic amino acids; *BCAA*, branched-chain amino acids; $C_{SH}$, cystine; *CssC*, cystine; *G*, glycine; *P*, proline; *Tau/β*, taurine and β-amino acids.

**Table 8.4 Human Tubular Amino Acid Transporters Properties and Distribution of Human Renal Tubular Transporters**

| Amino Acid Transporter | SLC | PCT/PST | Substrates | Affinities | Disease | Structure class |
|---|---|---|---|---|---|---|
| **Apical** | | | | | | |
| $B^0AT1$ | SLC6A19 | PCT | All neutral | 800–15,000 μM | Hartnup disorder (OMIM 234500) | LeuT |
| $B^0AT2$ | SLC6A15 | PCT | BCAA, Met, Pro | 50–200 μM | n.r. | LeuT |
| Collectrin | TMEM27 | PCT | N/A | Ancillary | n.r. | 1TM |
| rBAT | SLC3A1 | PCT < PST | N/A | Ancillary | Cystinuria (OMIM 220100) | 1TM |
| $b^{0,+}AT$ | SLC7A9 | PCT > PST | Arg, Lys, Orn, CssC, Met, Leu, Ala | 100 μM | Cystinuria (OMIM 220100), isolated cystinuria (OMIM 238200) | LeuT |
| EAAT3 | SLC1A1 | PCT < PST | Glu, Asp, CssC | 20–80 μM | Dicarboxylic amino aciduria (OMIM 222730) | Glt |
| AGT1 | SLC7A13 | PCT = PST | Glu, Asp, CssC | 20–60 μM | n.r. | LeuT |
| PAT2 | SLC36A2 | PCT | | | Iminoglycinuria (OMIM 242600), Hyperglycinuria (OMIM138500) | LeuT |
| SIT | SLC36A2 | PCT < PST | | | Iminoglycinuria (modifier) (OMIM 242600) | LeuT |
| TauT | SLC6A6 | PCT, PST | | | n.r. | LeuT |
| **Basolateral** | | | | | | |
| LAT2 | SLC7A8 | PCT | | | n.r. | LeuT |
| 4F2hc | SLC3A2 | PCT = PST | | Ancillary | Lethal | 1TM |
| $y^+LAT1$ | SLC7A7 | PCT = PST | | | Lysinuric protein intolerance (OMIM 222700) | LeuT |
| TAT1 | SLC16A10 | PCT | | | n.r. | MFS |
| LAT4 | SLC43A2 | PCT = PST | BCAA, Met, Phe | 5000 μM | n.r. | MFS |

*BCAA*, Branched-chain amino acids; *CssC*, cystine; *1TM*, single transmembrane-helix protein; *MFS*, multifacilitator superfamily; *n.r.*, not reported; *OMIM*, Online Mendelian Inheritance in Man; *PCT*, proximal convoluted tubule; *PST*, proximal straight tubule.
Links to Diseases Refer to the OMIM Database.

## TRANSPORTERS FOR NEUTRAL AMINO ACIDS

### APICAL TRANSPORTERS

The presence of a dominant transporter for neutral amino acids can be inferred from the aminoaciduria observed in Hartnup disorder, which is restricted to neutral amino acids, but affecting every member of this group.[263] This transporter was identified as the amino acid transporter $B^0AT1$ (*B*road neutral (0) *A*mino acid *T*ransporter 1, SLC6A19).[264,265] Although Hartnup disorder shows simple recessive inheritance and therefore is monogenic, the transporter protein requires association with ancillary proteins to traffic to the apical membrane and to be fully functional.[266] In the kidney, this is facilitated by collectrin (TMEM27),[267] whereas in the intestine, this role is served by angiotensin-converting enzyme 2 (ACE2).[268] Both proteins are type I transmembrane (TM) proteins with a single TM domain. Although ACE2 is expressed in the kidney, its expression levels in the proximal tubule are too small to make a significant contribution to $B^0AT1$ surface expression. $B^0AT1$ and TMEM27 are both expressed in the PCT.[267] Consistent with the monogenic inheritance, mutations in TMEM27 have not been observed in Hartnup disorder and would be expected to show an amino acid transporter defect in the kidney but not intestine. Thus far, more than 20 different causative mutations have been identified in the *SLC6A19* gene.[269] Interestingly, rare variants in *SLC6A19* have been associated with low serum creatinine levels and may have a kidney protective effect or affect creatinine synthesis.[270] $B^0AT1$ transports all neutral amino acids in symport with $1Na^+$; in contrast to many other members of the SLC6 family, chloride ions are not cotransported.[271] Substrate affinities range from 1–12 mM, with a preference for branched-chain amino acids (BCAA) and methionine, followed by large hydrophilic and aromatic amino acids.[272] In in vitro systems proline and tryptophan are very poor substrates of $B^0AT1$, but in vivo data suggest a significant contribution to the transport of both amino acids.[273] Mice lacking $B^0AT1$ replicate the human aminoaciduria of Hartnup disorder but do not show any additional pathology (Table 8.5). In addition to the low-affinity $B^0AT1$ transporter in the PCT, functional studies suggest the presence of a high-affinity transporter for neutral amino acids in the PST. A candidate could be $B^0AT2$ (SLC6A15), which is expressed at low levels in the proximal tubule.[274] $B^0AT2$ has a narrower substrate specificity than $B^0AT1$, showing a strong preference for BCAA and methionine with substrate affinities $<100\ \mu M$. Like $B^0AT1$, the transporter is $Na^+$ dependent and chloride independent.[275]

#### Specific Apical Transporters for Proline and Glycine

Proline and glycine have unusual physicochemical properties, which cause these amino acids to be inefficiently transported by more broadly specific amino acid transporters. Glycine is lacking a side chain, reducing its affinity to side-chain binding pockets, whereas proline has a secondary amino group and restricted flexibility. As a result, proline is a poor substrate for $B^0AT1$ and is not recognized by the basolateral neutral amino acid transporter LAT2 (see later). A common transporter for glycine, proline, and hydroxyproline in humans is supported by two lines of evidence. First, in the rare disorder iminoglycinuria, all three amino acids are found in the urine.[273] Second, prolinemia, when passing the renal threshold, causes prolinuria, hydroxyprolinuria, and glycinuria.[276] Although iminoglycinuria is an autosomal recessive disorder, it shows clear signs of genetic complexity.[277] For instance, some cases of iminoglycinuria show malabsorption of proline in the intestine. Moreover, in some cases, heterozygotes are normal, whereas in other pedigrees, hyperglycinuria is observed. These cases can all be explained by the combined action of proton–amino acid transporter 2 (PAT2, SLC36A2), the system IMINO

**Table 8.5 Physiologic Characteristics of Knockout Mice of Renal Amino Acid Transporters**

| Transporter | Plasma AA | Urine AA | Renal Pathology | Other Features |
|---|---|---|---|---|
| rBAT | Normal | +++: Lys, Arg, Orn, CssC | Nephritis, kidney stones | None |
| $b^{0,+}AT$ | +: His, Ser, Glu/n | +++: Lys, Arg, Orn, CssC, + Glu/n | Glomerular fibrosis, nephritis, kidney stones | None |
| $B^0AT1$ | Normal | +++ Neutral AA | None<br>Reduced serum creatinine | Propensity for colitis, improved glycemic control |
| $B^0AT3$ | Normal | +++: Gly<br>++: Ala, Val, Leu, Ile, Met, Ser, Thr, Gln, Phe, Tyr | None | Stress-induced increase of blood pressure |
| TAT1 | +: Phe, Tyr, Trp<br>-: Gly, Ala, Met, Ser, Thr, Asn, Gln<br>HPD +: Phe, Tyr, Trp | +: Phe, Tyr, Trp<br>HPD +: Val, Ile, Leu, Thr, Gln, His, Phe, Tyr, Trp | None | None |
| LAT4 | -: Ala, Pro, His, Ser | Not available | None reported | Liver inflammation, malnutrition |
| LAT2 | +: Gly, Ala, Ser, Thr, Gln, Val, Lys | +: Gly, Ser, Thr, Gln, Leu, Val | None | None |
| $y^+LAT1$ | Not available | +++: Lys, Arg, Orn | None | Failure to thrive, intrauterine growth restriction |
| TauT | –: Taurine<br>-: Glu | +++: Taurine | Enlarged kidney, glomerulosclerosis, nephropathy | Muscle weakness, cardiomyopathy, retinal degeneration, hearing loss, chronic liver disease |

*CssC*, Cystine; *Glu/n*, glutamate or glutamine; *HPD*, high-protein diet; +, elevated, ++ significantly elevated, +++ highly elevated; -, reduced, –, significantly reduced.

transporter SIT1 (SLC6A20), and the general neutral amino acid transporter $B^0AT1$ (SLC6A19).[273] Homozygous mutations in PAT2 account for iminoglycinuria, whereas heterozygous mutations cause selective hyperglycinuria. SIT1 mutations contribute to the iminoglycinuria phenotype and also explain a sporadically observed reduced proline absorption in the intestine. $B^0AT1$ provides the baseload for proline and glycine reabsorption, explaining why the extent of aminoaciduria is well below the filtered amounts.[273] The related glycine and alanine transporter $B^0AT3$ (SLC6A18) is only functional in mouse[278,279] (Table 8.5) but not in higher mammalian species, where its function has been replaced by PAT2.

PAT2 (SLC36A2) has been identified as the specific transporter for small neutral amino acids, specifically alanine, glycine, and proline. Single N-methylation of amino acids is tolerated such as in sarcosine or proline. PAT2 is mutated in all cases of iminoglycinuria and is expressed in the proximal tubule of the kidney.[273] The $K_M$ values for its substrates range from 0.1–0.6 mM.[280]

SIT1 (SLC6A20) accepts only amino acids with secondary, tertiary, or quaternary amines, such as proline, sarcosine, betaine, and methylaminoisobutyric acid.[281,282] SIT1 is an $Na^+$ and $Cl^-$ dependent transporter, transporting 1 substrate, $2Na^+$ and $1Cl^-$ ion. This generates a net positive transporter current, which can be observed when expressed heterologously. Expression of the transporter at the cell surface requires collectrin (TMEM27).[283]

$B^0AT3$ (SLC6A18) preferentially transports alanine and glycine.[279] SLC6A18 knockout mice have hyperglycinuria and slightly elevated urine levels of other neutral amino acids,[278] but humans with homozygous mutations in SLC6A18 are normal because even the normal allele is nonfunctional.[273,284] The mouse transporter requires collectrin coexpression for trafficking and also for its catalytic function.[284]

#### Specific Apical Transporters for B-Amino Acids

This group of amino acids consists of taurine, β-alanine, and its homolog gamma-aminobutyric acid (GABA). Plasma concentration of GABA is very low (about 0.1 μM), while taurine levels are significantly higher (about 50 μM). Both amino acids are often accepted by the same transporters, but in the kidney, specific GABA transporters are observed as well. Reabsorption of these amino acids is mainly mediated by the taurine transporter TauT (SLC6A6).[285] PAT2 shows weak affinity for these substrates but is probably physiologically irrelevant. TauT translocates taurine with a $K_M$ of 20 μM in a process that involves the cotransport of $2Na^+$ and $1Cl^-$. Urinary taurine excretion in TauT-deficient mice reaches the filtered amounts.[286]

### BASOLATERAL TRANSPORTERS

Functional studies identified an $Na^+$-independent transporter broadly specific for neutral amino acids also in the basolateral membrane. The heteromeric amino acid transporter 4F2hc-LAT2 (SLC3A2-SLC7A8) matches with regard to the substrate specificity but mechanistically is an antiporter.[287–289] A uniporter has been identified for aromatic amino acids (TAT1, SLC16A10),[290] but this transporter cannot explain the net flux of amino acids across the renal epithelium as illustrated by *Tat1* knockout mice.[291] These mice show elevated levels of aromatic amino acids in the urine but normal levels of other amino acids. Only on a high-protein diet, a more general aminoaciduria was observed, suggesting cooperation between LAT2 and TAT1. LAT4 (SLC43A2) allows efflux of BCAA, methionine, and phenylalanine, thus covering large neutral amino acids.[292] A specific efflux pathway for small neutral amino acids has not been identified and thus is likely to occur through cooperation between LAT2, TAT1, and LAT4: efflux of small neutral AA in exchange for large neutral AA or aromatic AA, which is supported by the appearance of small neutral amino acids in the urine of *Lat2* knockout mice.[293]

LAT2 (SLC3A2-SLC7A8) shows a distinct asymmetry with regard to affinity on the two faces of the membrane. The $K_M$ values on the outside range from 40–200 μM, while on the inside, $K_M$ values range from 3–30 mM.[294] The transporter accepts all neutral amino acids except proline. TAT1 (SLC16A10) shows very low affinity for its substrates, ranging from 3–7 mM.[295] Although the transporter is related to monocarboxylate transporters, it does not cotransport protons.[290] Apart from aromatic amino acids, TAT1 also transports the N-methylated derivatives of these amino acids and L-dopa.

LAT4 (SLC43A2) belongs to a separate transporter family than 4F2hc-LAT2. It does not require additional subunits and transports its substrates with low affinity ($K_M$ for phenylalanine is 5 mM) on both sides of the membrane.[296]

The kidney contributes to gluconeogenesis and pH regulation. The glutamine, asparagine, and histidine transporter SNAT3 (SLC38A3) is located in the basolateral membrane but is typically expressed at low levels. During chronic acidosis, it is upregulated and glutamine imported for deamination by phosphate-activated glutaminase.[297] The resulting glutamate is further deaminated to 2-oxoglutarate, which serves as a substrate for gluconeogenesis[298] (see also Fig. 8.4). Ammonia is released into the urine, thereby disposing of protons. Upregulation of SNAT3 mRNA during chronic metabolic acidosis involves promoter regulation and mRNA stability.[299] The related transporter SNAT (SLC38A5) is also expressed in the kidney and may contribute to glutamine uptake.[300] Its subcellular localization is unknown.

There is no clear pathway for the basolateral exit of proline. Although glycine is inefficiently transported by many neutral amino acid transporters, including 4F2hc-LAT2, the latter does not accept proline. Release of taurine also remains unclear. The GABA/betaine transporter BGT1 (SLC6A12) has been identified in the basolateral membrane of renal epithelial cells but accumulates its substrates in the cytosol and therefore is not a feasible efflux pathway.

## TRANSPORTERS FOR CATIONIC AMINO ACIDS AND CYSTINE

### APICAL TRANSPORTERS

The presence of a transporter for cationic amino acids that is shared with cystine can be deduced from the aminoaciduria observed in cystinuria, which includes both groups of amino acids.[301] Renal cystine clearance is close to GFR in cystinuria, whereas cationic amino acids remain partially reabsorbed. Cationic amino acids and cystine are transported in the proximal tubule by the heteromeric transporter rBAT/$b^{0,+}AT$ (broad neutral and cationic amino acid transporter).[302] Cystinuria is an autosomal recessive disorder. Homozygous (or compound heterozygous) mutations in the rBAT encoding gene SLC3A1 are classified as type A cystinuria, whereas homozygous (or compound heterozygous) mutations in the $b^{0,+}AT$ encoding gene SLC7A9 are classified as type B.[303] This genetic heterogeneity can be detected in the heterozygous state, where rBAT heterozygotes do not show residual aminoaciduria, while $b^{0,+}$AT heterozygotes show some release of cystine and lysine into the urine. Cystinuria causes formation of kidney stones due to the low solubility of cystine.[301] The distribution of rBAT along the proximal tubule shows increasing expression toward the PST, whereas $b^{0,+}$AT shows the opposite trend. This suggested that rBAT may have a different partner in the PST, which was shown to be the aspartate/glutamate transporter AGT1.[304] Initially AGT1 was thought to have a basolateral localization; however, follow-up studies using more specific antibodies demonstrated an apical localization. Functionally, AGT1 operates as a cystine transporter, exchanging cystine for glutamate. Interestingly, this suggests that cystine is transported as a neutral amino acid in the PCT and as an anionic amino acid in the PST. In $b^{0,+}$AT knockout mice fractional excretion of arginine reaches 80%, while only 11% of the tubular cystine load is excreted.[305] This is consistent with the presence of additional cystine transporters, such as AGT1 and EAAT3 (see anionic amino acid transporters later). The rBAT protein is a highly glycosylated type II membrane protein that is connected by a disulfide bridge to the transporter subunit $b^{0,+}$AT just outside the membrane.[306] Heterodimer formation is essential for the exit of the complex from the endoplasmic reticulum.[307] Transport properties of rbat/$b^{0,+}$AT have been largely elucidated using the oocyte endogenous transporter that associates with rbat when its cRNA is expressed in this system.[308] These experiments show that rbat/$b^{0,+}$AT is an obligatory antiporter that preferentially takes up cationic amino acids from the lumen in exchange for neutral amino acids. This directionality is imposed by the inside-negative cell membrane potential, and it is also confirmed by the lack of neutral amino acids in cystinuria.[309] Affinities for cationic amino acids and cystine are approximately 100 μM; neutral amino acids have slightly higher apparent $K_M$ values.[310] The acidic amino acid–cystine exchanger AGT1 transports cystine with a $K_M$ of 68 μM.[304] In mice, the gene is only expressed in males and thus is unlikely to be essential for renal cystine reabsorption. In humans, isolated cystinuria, a rare disorder in which only cystine is elevated in urine, is caused by selected mutations in $b^{0,+}$AT that affect the substrate selectivity of the transport subunit.[311] Mutations in AGT1 have not been identified thus far.

> ***Clinical Relevance***
>
> **Transporters for Cationic Amino Acids and Cystine Apical Transporters**
>
> Urolithiasis occurs in most cases of cystinuria. The generation of kidney stones is managed through the combination of several treatments. Tiopronin (α-mercaptopropionylglycine) is administered to form adducts with cysteine, which have a higher solubility than cystine. Potassium citrate is used to increase the pH of urine >7.5. Reduction of animal protein intake and nocturnal fluid intakes are recommended. All treatments are aimed to reduce cysteine formation and precipitation.

### BASOLATERAL TRANSPORTERS

A basolateral exit pathway for cationic amino acids is defined by the disease LPI.[256,312] LPI is caused by mutations in the SLC7A7 light chain of the heteromeric transporter 4F2hc-SLC7A7.[313,314] The disease is very rare, with less than 200 cases reported, mainly from the Finnish population, where a founder mutation exists. In contrast to apical transport disorders, which are often benign, LPI can be a very severe disease, although clinical symptoms vary widely.[256] It also has a number of extrarenal pathologies, such as alveolar proteinosis and immune defects, which are not well understood. Plasma levels of cationic amino acids are reduced, which affects urea cycle function, causing the adverse reaction to protein ingestion. Urine levels of cationic amino acids are very high, particularly that of lysine. Intestinal absorption of cationic amino acids is also affected. Although a functionally redundant transporter exists (4F2hc-SLC7A6), its expression is low and cannot replace malfunction of SLC7A7.[315] Functionally, SLC7A6 and SLC7A7 are characterized as system $y^{+}$L, indicating a transporter that exchanges neutral and cationic amino acids, which was initially discovered in placenta and erythrocytes.[316] The $y^{+}$LAT1 (SLC7A7) transporter accepts neutral and cationic amino acids with high affinity ($K_m$ values about 20 μM), but the affinity for neutral amino acids is two orders of magnitude lower in the absence of $Na^{+}$.[317] As a result, the preferential mode of operation is an efflux of cationic amino acids in exchange for extracellular neutral amino acids. The $y^{+}$LAT1 transporter is widely expressed in the basolateral membrane of the proximal tubulus.

The prevalence of exchangers for the transport of cationic and neutral amino acids sets these mechanisms apart from the paradigm set by glucose reabsorption. One possible reason could be the maintenance of cytosolic amino acid pools that are significantly higher than those observed in blood plasma and which are required for protein biosynthesis and amino acid homeostasis.[318] In the presence of basolateral facilitators, cytosolic amino acid pools would be close to those observed in the blood.

## TRANSPORTERS FOR ANIONIC AMINO ACIDS

The main apical transporter for anionic amino acids in the proximal tubule is EAAT3 (named EAAC1 in rodents, SLC1A3).[319] EAAT3 transports both glutamate ($K_M$ = 14 μM) and aspartate and shows a preference of D-aspartate over L-aspartate.[320] As pointed out earlier, EAAT3 also contributes to cystine transport,[321] but cystine is only marginally elevated in individuals with dicarboxylic aminoaciduria.[322] The latter is a rare condition caused by mutations in EAAT3.[322] It is readily detected by highly elevated urine levels of aspartate and glutamate; excretion can reach or even exceed the filtered amounts. In addition to the kidney, EAAT3 is expressed in neurons and the intestine and allows high cytosolic accumulation due to the cotransport of $3Na^{+}$ and $1H^{+}$ and the antiport of $1K^{+}$.[323] Despite expression of EAAT3 in neurons, dicarboxylic aminoaciduria is considered a benign disorder.[324] However, an association of EAAT3 mutations with obsessive-compulsive disorder has been reported.[325] Expression of EAAT3 is relatively low in the PCT, increases toward the PST, and is also observed in the distal parts of the tubule.[319] Nevertheless, 90% of the filtered anionic amino acid load is reabsorbed in the PCT. The transporter is regulated by osmolarity and amino acid deprivation.[326] A dedicated efflux pathway for glutamate in renal epithelial cells has not been identified. In fact, there is evidence for an accumulative glutamate transporter in the basolateral membrane, which would prevent efflux.[259] In accordance, glutamate is intensively metabolized in epithelial cells, and efflux may be limited. Moreover, members of the SLC22 family are nonspecific anion transporters, and those located in the basolateral membrane may serve as efflux pathways for glutamate.[327]

## STRUCTURAL INFORMATION OF AMINO ACID TRANSPORTERS

Plasma membrane amino acid transporters thus far fall into three different protein folds, namely the LeuT-fold, the Glt-fold, and the multifacilitator superfamily (MFS)-fold[328] (see Table 8.4). Functionally, it has long been established that transporters must be able to adopt an inward-facing and an outward-facing conformation.[329,330] All transporters analyzed thus far operate in an alternating access mode in which the substrate and cosubstrates (if applicable) bind on one side of the membrane (e.g., outside). Subsequently, weak interactions between substrate and the transporter cause the transporter to enclose the substrate, resulting in the occluded conformation. The transporter transitions further into an inside–open conformation to release the substrate.[328] In the case of antiporters, the energy barrier for a substrate-less translocation is too high; thus, the return to the initial conformation is only possible in a substrate-bound state. In the case of symporters and uniporters, the empty transporter can transition back through a substrate-free occluded state, back to the outside–open conformation, thereby closing the catalytic cycle. However, at least in the case of the LeuT protein fold, a pseudosubstrate in the form of a leucine side chain residing close to the substrate binding site occupies the empty binding site, thereby facilitating the transition back to the outside conformation.[331]

For the LeuT-fold, high-resolution structures have been identified for all but one stage of the transport cycle (Fig.

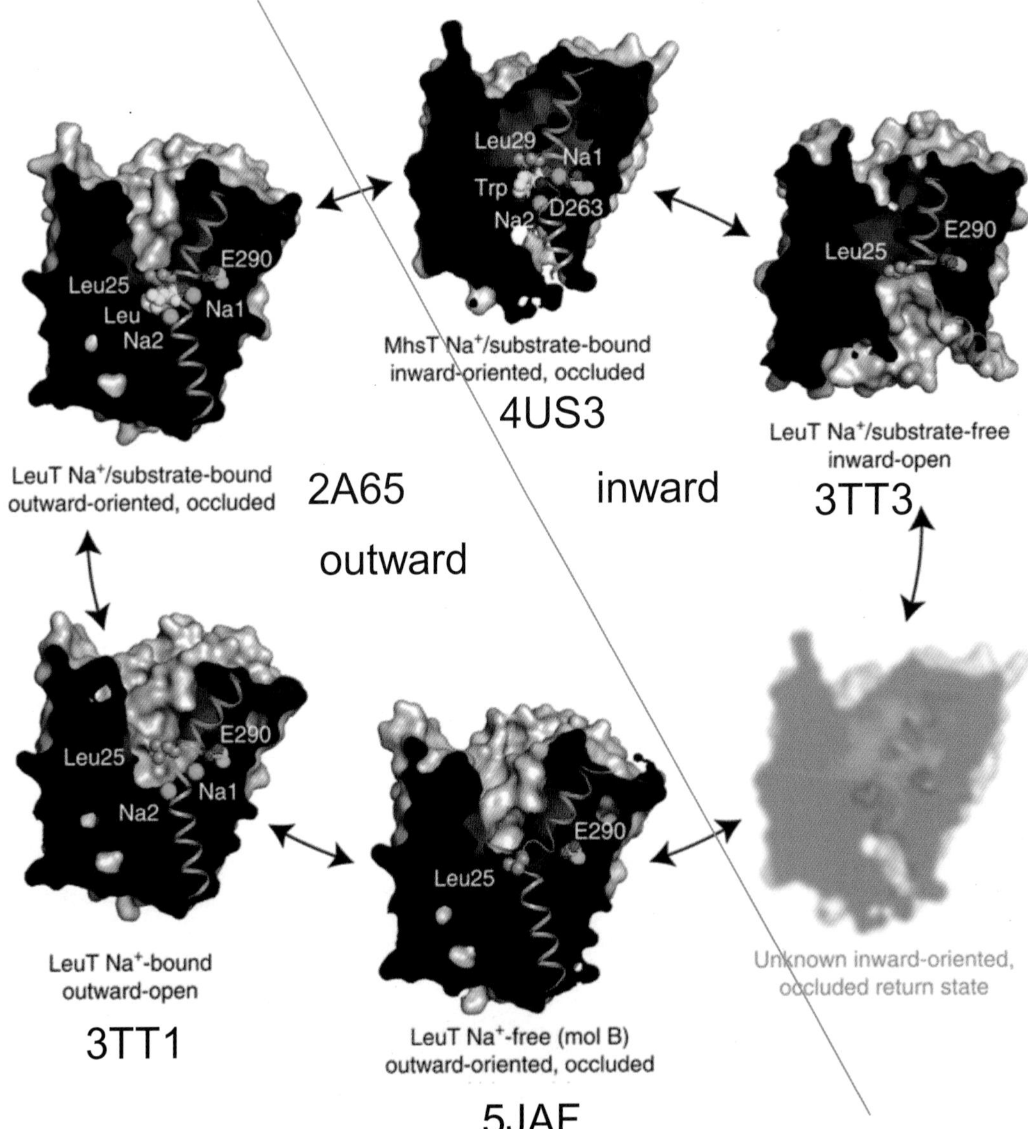


**Fig. 8.14** Transport cycle of LeuT-fold proteins. TM1 helix and pseudosubstrate Leu25 (Leu29$^{MhsT}$) are shown in *pink*, the $Na^+$ ions are shown as *green spheres*, and Glu290 (or Asp263$^{MhsT}$) as *cyan*, and substrate at the binding site as *yellow spheres*. (Reused from Malinauskaite L, Said S, Sahin C, et al. A conserved leucine occupies the empty substrate site of LeuT in the Na(+)-free return state. *Nat Commun.* 2016;7:11673, under creative common license.)

8.14). The first structure of LeuT revealed an internal symmetry, whereby helix 1-5 can be superimposed onto helix 1-6 in a twofold rotation.[332] This internal symmetry provides the structural basis for the adoption of an inward- and outward-facing conformation.[333] Further investigation of this protein fold revealed that part of the protein remains rather immobile—an arrangement of helices 3,5 and 7,8 named the hash (#)—whereas others move significantly—the bundle—composed of helices 1,2 and 6,7.[333] The hydrogen bond network is interrupted in the center of helices 1 and 6, allowing the helix to bend and to use these hydrogen bonds to interact with substrates and cotransported ions. A key feature in most transporters with a LeuT-fold is a motion of the bundle relative to the hash or vice versa, thereby alternatively closing and opening alternating sites of the transporter.[328] Another common feature is the presence of one or more aromatic amino acids adjacent to the substrate binding site, which insulate the substrate during the transition to the occluded state. These residues are referred to as "thin" gates in contrast to subsequent enclosure of the substrate by more substantial parts of the protein (thick gates).

The transport process in $Na^+$-driven glutamate transporters is quite different, as it involves an elevator-like movement of the transport domain relative to a rigid scaffold domain.[334] $Glt_{Ph}$ is composed of eight TM segments and two helical hairpins (HP1 and HP2).[335] The six N-terminal helices form a large bracket that holds TM7, TM8, HP1, and HP2. Two large loops, one connecting TM2 and TM3 and the other TM5 and TM6, serve as the hinge to allow elevator-like movement of the substrate binding domain.[336] Reminiscent of similar features in LeuT, the structure and ions are bound by unwound regions of TM7, TM8, HP1, and HP2. Alternating access is mediated by opening of helical HPs on the respective side of the membrane. Glutamate transporters form trimers, which are likely to be important to stabilize the scaffold against the movement of the elevator domain.

In the MFS fold, the protein has a symmetry axis perpendicular to the membrane between helices 1–6 and 7–12.[337,338] During the transport cycle, the two halves of the protein move against each other. This rocker-switch mode needs to be modified to accommodate initial occlusion of the substrate by the bending of the outer ends of helices 1 and 7 on the outside or 4 and 10 on the inside. Binding of amino acids remains unclear due to the lack of high-resolution structures of amino acid–translocating members.

As pointed out earlier, several renal amino acid transporters form heterodimers with ancillary proteins—for instance, SLC7 transporters with 4F2hc and rBAT and SLC6 transporter $B^0AT1$ with collectrin. The main role of ancillary subunits is to facilitate the exit of the complex from the endoplasmic reticulum.[307] Collectrin, in addition, is also essential for the catalytic activity of the transporter.[284] The structure of the ectodomains of transporter ancillary proteins is known for 4F2hc,[339] but the precise heteromeric arrangement is only partially understood.[340] The structure of the 4F2hc ectodomain, which is related to bacterial α-amylases, is composed of two subdomains, namely domain A, a triosphosphate isomerase barrel domain $(\alpha\beta)_8$, and domain C, made up of eight antiparallel β-strands.[339] However, neither 4F2hc nor rBAT has glycosidase activity and they both lack conservation of critical catalytic residues. The glycosylation of the ancillary proteins could be important to help with quality control in the endoplasmic reticulum. In addition to its role in amino acid transport, collectrin is thought be involved in kidney development and vesicle exocytosis, but these functions are mechanistically less well understood.[341] The 4F2 heavy chain has additional functions in integrin signaling, which are well understood in cancer cells but not in epithelial cells.[266,306,342]

 Complete reference list available at ExpertConsult.com.

## KEY REFERENCES


5. Barfuss DW, Schafer JA. Differences in active and passive glucose transport along the proximal nephron. *Am J Physiol.* 1981;241:F322–F332.
6. Turner RJ, Moran A. Heterogeneity of sodium-dependent D-glucose transport sites along the proximal tubule: evidence from vesicle studies. *Am J Physiol.* 1982;242:F406–F414.
7. Wells RG, Pajor AM, Kanai Y, et al. Cloning of a human kidney cDNA with similarity to the sodium-glucose cotransporter. *Am J Physiol.* 1992;263:F459–F465.
8. Hediger MA, Coady MJ, Ikeda TS, et al. Expression cloning and cDNA sequencing of the Na+/glucose co-transporter. *Nature.* 1987;330:379–381.
15. Vallon V, Platt KA, Cunard R, et al. SGLT2 mediates glucose reabsorption in the early proximal tubule. *J Am Soc Nephrol.* 2011;22:104–112.
20. Gorboulev V, Schurmann A, Vallon V, et al. Na(+)-D-glucose cotransporter SGLT1 is pivotal for intestinal glucose absorption and glucose-dependent incretin secretion. *Diabetes.* 2012;61:187–196.
21. Wright EM, Loo DD, Hirayama BA. Biology of human sodium glucose transporters. *Physiol Rev.* 2011;91:733–794.
22. Martin MG, Turk E, Lostao MP, et al. Defects in Na+/glucose cotransporter (SGLT1) trafficking and function cause glucose-galactose malabsorption. *Nat Genet.* 1996;12:216–220.
24. Rieg T, Masuda T, Gerasimova M, et al. Increase in SGLT1-mediated transport explains renal glucose reabsorption during genetic and pharmacological SGLT2 inhibition in euglycemia. *Am J Physiol Renal Physiol.* 2014;306:F188–F193.
28. Hummel CS, Lu C, Loo DD, et al. Glucose transport by human renal Na+/D-glucose cotransporters SGLT1 and SGLT2. *Am J Physiol Cell Physiol.* 2011;300:C14–C21.
32. Faham S, Watanabe A, Besserer GM, et al. The crystal structure of a sodium galactose transporter reveals mechanistic insights into Na+/sugar symport. *Science.* 2008;321:810–814.
41. Fukuzawa T, Fukazawa M, Ueda O, et al. SGLT5 reabsorbs fructose in the kidney but its deficiency paradoxically exacerbates hepatic steatosis induced by fructose. *PLoS ONE.* 2013;8:e56681.
57. Gerich JE. Role of the kidney in normal glucose homeostasis and in the hyperglycaemia of diabetes mellitus: therapeutic implications. *Diabet Med.* 2010;27:136–142.
90. Vallon V, Thomson SC. Targeting renal glucose reabsorption to treat hyperglycaemia: the pleiotropic effects of SGLT2 inhibition. *Diabetologia.* 2017;60:215–225.
109. Wanner C, Inzucchi SE, Lachin JM, et al. Empagliflozin and progression of kidney disease in type 2 diabetes. *N Engl J Med.* 2016;375:323–334.
120. Cherney DZ, Perkins BA, Soleymanlou N, et al. Renal hemodynamic effect of sodium-glucose cotransporter 2 inhibition in patients with type 1 diabetes mellitus. *Circulation.* 2014;129:587–597.
152. Vallon V, Richter K, Blantz RC, et al. Glomerular hyperfiltration in experimental diabetes mellitus: potential role of tubular reabsorption. *J Am Soc Nephrol.* 1999;10:2569–2576.
161. Inzucchi SE, Zinman B, Fitchett D, et al. How does empagliflozin reduce cardiovascular mortality? Insights from a mediation analysis of the EMPA-REG OUTCOME trial. *Diabetes Care.* 2018;41:356–363.
167. You G. Structure, function, and regulation of renal organic anion transporters. *Med Res Rev.* 2002;22:602–616.
169. Emami RA, Nies AT, Schaeffeler E, et al. Organic anion transporters and their implications in pharmacotherapy. *Pharmacol Rev.* 2012;64:421–449.
172. Saito H. Pathophysiological regulation of renal SLC22A organic ion transporters in acute kidney injury: pharmacological and toxicological implications. *Pharmacol Ther.* 2010;125:79–91.
178. Lopez-Nieto CE, You G, Bush KT, et al. Molecular cloning and characterization of NKT, a gene product related to the organic cation transporter family that is almost exclusively expressed in the kidney. *J Biol Chem.* 1997;272:6471–6478.

182. Grundemann D, Gorboulev V, Gambaryan S, et al. Drug excretion mediated by a new prototype of polyspecific transporter. *Nature.* 1994;372:549–552.
183. Nigam SK. The SLC22 transporter family: a paradigm for the impact of drug transporters on metabolic pathways, signaling, and disease. *Annu Rev Pharmacol Toxicol.* 2018;58:663–687.
184. Nigam SK. What do drug transporters really do? *Nat Rev Drug Discov.* 2015;14:29–44.
187. U.S. Food and Drug Administration. *Guidance for Industry: Drug Interaction Studies—Study Design, Data Analysis, Implications for Dosing, and Labeling Recommendations.* Silver Spring, MD: US Department of Health and Human Services, Food Drug Administration Center for Drug Evaluation and Research CDER; 2012. http://www.fda.gov/downloads/Drugs/GuidanceComplianceRegulatoryInformation/Guidances/UCM292362.pdf.
193. Wikoff WR, Nagle MA, Kouznetsova VL, et al. Untargeted metabolomics identifies enterobiome metabolites and putative uremic toxins as substrates of organic anion transporter 1 (Oat1). *J Proteome Res.* 2011;10:2842–2851.
194. Bush KT, Wu W, Lun C, et al. The drug transporter OAT3 (SLC22A8) and endogenous metabolite communication via the gut-liver-kidney axis. *J Biol Chem.* 2017;292:15789–15803.
195. Wu W, Bush KT, Nigam SK. Key role for the organic anion transporters, OAT1 and OAT3, in the in vivo handling of uremic toxins and solutes. *Sci Rep.* 2017;7:4939.
198. Vallon V, Rieg T, Ahn SY, et al. Overlapping in vitro and in vivo specificities of the organic anion transporters OAT1 and OAT3 for loop and thiazide diuretics. *Am J Physiol Renal Physiol.* 2008;294:F867–F873.
199. Vanwert AL, Bailey RM, Sweet DH. Organic anion transporter 3 (Oat3/Slc22a8) knockout mice exhibit altered clearance and distribution of penicillin G. *Am J Physiol Renal Physiol.* 2007;293:F1332–F1341.
203. Miyajima M, Kusuhara H, Fujishima M, et al. Organic anion transporter 3 mediates the efflux transport of an amphipathic organic anion, dehydroepiandrosterone sulfate, across the blood-brain barrier in mice. *Drug Metab Dispos.* 2011;39:814–819.
206. Torres AM, Dnyanmote AV, Bush KT, et al. Deletion of multispecific organic anion transporter Oat1/Slc22a6 protects against mercury-induced kidney injury. *J Biol Chem.* 2011;286:26391–26395.
208. Liu HC, Jamshidi N, Chen Y, et al. An organic anion transporter 1 (OAT1)-centered metabolic network. *J Biol Chem.* 2016;291:19474–19486.
215. Bhatnagar V, Richard EL, Wu W, et al. Analysis of ABCG2 and other urate transporters in uric acid homeostasis in chronic kidney disease: potential role of remote sensing and signaling. *Clin Kidney J.* 2016;9:444–453.
222. Nies AT, Koepsell H, Damme K, et al. Organic cation transporters (OCTs, MATEs), in vitro and in vivo evidence for the importance in drug therapy. *Handb Exp Pharmacol.* 2011;105–167.
223. Chen L, Shu Y, Liang X, et al. OCT1 is a high-capacity thiamine transporter that regulates hepatic steatosis and is a target of metformin. *Proc Natl Acad Sci U. S. A.* 2014;111:9983–9988.
238. Mandal AK, Mount DB. The molecular physiology of uric acid homeostasis. *Annu Rev Physiol.* 2015;77:323–345.
257. Rajantie J, Simell O, Perheentupa J. Lysinuric protein intolerance. Basolateral transport defect in renal tubuli. *J Clin Invest.* 1981;67:1078–1082.
264. Seow HF, Broer S, Broer A, et al. Hartnup disorder is caused by mutations in the gene encoding the neutral amino acid transporter SLC6A19. *Nat Genet.* 2004;36:1003–1007.
265. Kleta R, Romeo E, Ristic Z, et al. Mutations in SLC6A19, encoding B0AT1, cause Hartnup disorder. *Nat Genet.* 2004;36:999–1002.
267. Danilczyk U, Sarao R, Remy C, et al. Essential role for collectrin in renal amino acid transport. *Nature.* 2006;444:1088–1091.
273. Broer S, Bailey CG, Kowalczuk S, et al. Iminoglycinuria and hyperglycinuria are discrete human phenotypes resulting from complex mutations in proline and glycine transporters. *J Clin Invest.* 2008;118:3881–3892.
301. Chillaron J, Font-Llitjos M, Fort J, et al. Pathophysiology and treatment of cystinuria. *Nat Rev Nephrol.* 2010;6:424–434.
304. Nagamori S, Wiriyasermkul P, Guarch ME, et al. Novel cystine transporter in renal proximal tubule identified as a missing partner of cystinuria-related plasma membrane protein rBAT/SLC3A1. *Proc Natl Acad Sci U. S. A.* 2016;113:775–780.
313. Torrents D, Mykkanen J, Pineda M, et al. Identification of SLC7A7, encoding y+LAT-1, as the lysinuric protein intolerance gene. *Nat Genet.* 1999;21:293–296.
314. Borsani G, Bassi MT, Sperandeo MP, et al. SLC7A7, encoding a putative permease-related protein, is mutated in patients with lysinuric protein intolerance. *Nat Genet.* 1999;21:297–301.
322. Bailey CG, Ryan RM, Thoeng AD, et al. Loss-of-function mutations in the glutamate transporter SLC1A1 cause human dicarboxylic aminoaciduria. *J Clin Invest.* 2011;121:446–453.

# 9 Renal Acidification Mechanisms

I. David Weiner | Jill W. Verlander

## CHAPTER OUTLINE



## KEY POINTS

- Proximal tubule filtered bicarbonate reabsorption involves apical $H^+$ secretion by NHE3 and $H^+$-ATPase, and in the neonatal kidney NHE8 substitutes for NHE3.
- Proximal tubule bicarbonate reabsorption is regulated by peritubular $HCO_3^-$ and $CO_2$, but not directly by peritubular pH.
- Proximal tubule basolateral NBCe1 is necessary for bicarbonate reabsorption and regulates both ammonia metabolism and citrate reabsorption.
- Aquaporins transport $CO_2$ and $NH_3$ in addition to $H_2O$.
- Renal ammonia transport involves selective transport of $NH_3$ and $NH_4^+$ by specific membrane proteins that exhibit significant axial and apical versus basolateral plasma membrane heterogeneity along the nephron and collecting duct.
- Ammonia metabolism involves both ammonia generation (ammoniagenesis) and ammonia recycling; the latter occurs through the protein glutamine synthetase.
- Renal interstitial sulfatides, probably by reversibly binding interstitial $NH_4^+$, are necessary for normal ammonia metabolism.
- The bicarbonate secreting anion exchanger, pendrin, which is necessary for recovery from metabolic alkalosis, has a critical role in volume homeostasis and blood pressure regulation through roles both as a $Cl^-$ reabsorbing protein and through indirect interactions with the $Na^+$-reabsorbing protein, ENaC.

Maintaining normal acid–base homeostasis is critical for normal health. Acid–base disorders can lead to a number of clinical problems, such as growth retardation, nausea, and vomiting; increased susceptibility to cardiac arrhythmias; decreased cardiovascular catecholamine sensitivity; bone disorders, including osteoporosis and osteomalacia; recurrent nephrolithiasis, skeletal muscle atrophy; paresthesia; and coma.[266] In people with chronic kidney disease (CKD), metabolic acidosis leads to more rapid progression of worsened renal function and increased risk of requiring renal replacement therapy.[97,216] Finally, the presence of either metabolic acidosis or metabolic alkalosis correlates with increased mortality in patients both with and without CKD.[214,289,327]

Acid–base homeostasis involves two separate but related processes, bicarbonate reabsorption and new bicarbonate generation. The first relates to the reabsorption of bicarbonate filtered by the glomerulus. The second relates to the need to generate "new bicarbonate" to replenish bicarbonate that neutralizes endogenous and exogenous fixed acid loads. Finally, a number of pathophysiologic conditions generate acid or alkali loads to which the kidneys must respond to in order to maintain acid–base homeostasis.

## BICARBONATE REABSORPTION

Bicarbonate reabsorption involves coordinated transport events in multiple nephron segments (Fig. 9.1). The proximal tubule reabsorbs the majority of filtered bicarbonate. Little-to-no bicarbonate reabsorption occurs in the thin descending limb of the loop of Henle, moderate reabsorption occurs in the thick ascending limb (TAL) of Henle loop, and the

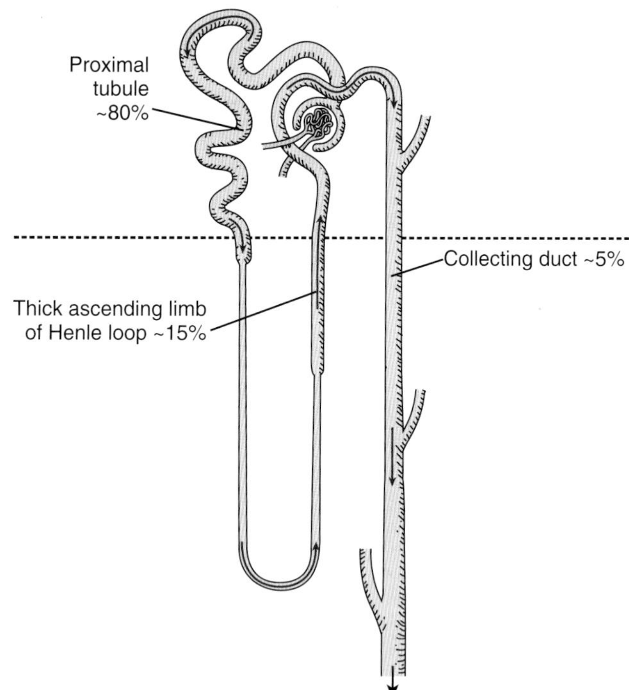


**Fig. 9.1** Summary of sites of bicarbonate reabsorption. The proximal tubule is the primary site quantitatively for filtered bicarbonate reabsorption. Minimal reabsorption occurs in the thin limb of the loop of Henle. The thick ascending limb of the loop of Henle reabsorbs the majority of the bicarbonate not reabsorbed in the proximal tubule. The collecting duct is the primary site for reabsorption of the remaining filtered bicarbonate.

remaining filtered bicarbonate is reabsorbed in the distal convoluted tubule (DCT), connecting segment (CNT), initial collecting tubule (ICT), and the collecting duct.

## PROXIMAL TUBULE

### GENERAL TRANSPORT MECHANISMS

Proximal tubule bicarbonate reabsorption involves several distinct, but interconnected, processes (Fig. 9.2). First, protons ($H^+$) are secreted into the luminal fluid. Multiple proteins mediate $H^+$ secretion; the apical $Na^+/H^+$ exchanger, NHE3, and an apical $H^+$-ATPase are the primary mechanisms of proton secretion in the adult kidney. In the neonatal kidney, the $Na^+/H^+$ exchanger, NHE8, appears to substitute for NHE3 as the primary $Na^+/H^+$ exchanger (NHE) isoform.[30] In the adult kidney, NHE3 is responsible for 60%–70% of $H^+$ secretion and $H^+$-ATPase accounts for the majority of the remainder.

Secreted $H^+$ combines with luminal $HCO_3^-$ to form carbonic acid ($H_2CO_3$). Luminal carbonic acid dissociates to water ($H_2O$) and carbon dioxide ($CO_2$). Although this can occur spontaneously, the spontaneous dehydration rate is inadequate to support normal rates of proximal tubule bicarbonate reabsorption. The dehydration reaction is catalyzed by carbonic anhydrase IV (CA IV), a membrane-bound carbonic anhydrase isoform present in the proximal tubule brush border.

Luminal $CO_2$ then moves across the apical plasma membrane into the cell. Although this process has traditionally been thought to occur through lipid-phase diffusion, the integral membrane protein, aquaporin 1 (AQP1), may mediate ~50% of $CO_2$ transport across the apical plasma membrane.[46] Cytosolic $CO_2$ is then hydrated, forming carbonic acid, through a process accelerated by the cytosolic carbonic anhydrase, carbonic anhydrase II (CA II). Cytosolic carbonic acid spontaneously dissociates to $H^+$ and $HCO_3^-$. This "replenishes" the $H^+$ secreted across the apical plasma membrane by apical NHE3 and $H^+$-ATPase.

Cytosolic $HCO_3^-$ is transported across the basolateral plasma membrane. In the S1 and S2 segments of the proximal tubule the primary $HCO_3^-$ transport mechanism is a sodium-coupled, electrogenic bicarbonate cotransporter, NBCe1-A.[1,256] Because NBCe1-A is electrogenic, generation and regulation of the transmembrane voltage between cytoplasm and interstitium is important, and appears to be related to extracellular pH-dependent activation of the basolateral TWIK-related acid-sensitive $K^+$ channel, TASK2.[445] In the S3 segment, an $Na^+$-dependent, $Cl^-/HCO_3^-$ exchanger appears to be the primary mechanism of basolateral $HCO_3^-$ transport,[217] although NBCe1 may also contribute.[284]

In addition to active $H^+$ secretion–mediated luminal bicarbonate reabsorption, the proximal tubule also exhibits passive $H^+$ and bicarbonate transport. Because bicarbonate reabsorption decreases the luminal bicarbonate concentration and increases the luminal $H^+$ concentration relative to the peritubular space, passive bicarbonate transport results in bicarbonate secretion, which limits net bicarbonate reabsorption. The molecular mechanisms of bicarbonate backleak are unclear, but several functional aspects are known. It is quantitatively less in the newborn than in the adult kidney,[323] is decreased by angiotensin II (AngII),[242] involves both paracellular and transcellular components, and involves membrane proteins, but not NHE3.[158,315] Quantitatively, the bicarbonate backleak rate is less than that of bicarbonate reabsorption in the initial portions of the proximal tubule. However, in more distal portions, particularly when luminal bicarbonate concentrations have decreased as a result of more proximal bicarbonate reabsorption, bicarbonate backleak rates are greater as a result of the greater transepithelial bicarbonate gradient. Simultaneously, the lower luminal pH limits NHE3-mediated proton secretion and bicarbonate reabsorption. This can result in the bicarbonate backleak rate becoming equivalent to the bicarbonate reabsorption rate. When this occurs, there is no further net bicarbonate reabsorption. Under typical circumstances, this occurs when luminal bicarbonate concentrations have decreased to approximately 6 mmol/L, corresponding to a luminal pH of 6.8.

#### Proteins Involved in Proximal Tubule Bicarbonate Reabsorption

**$Na^+/H^+$ Exchangers.** $Na^+/H^+$ exchangers are expressed widely in the kidney, where they function in intracellular pH regulation, transepithelial bicarbonate reabsorption, and vacuolar acidification. All use the extracellular-to-intracellular $Na^+$ gradient to enable secondary active, electroneutral $H^+$ secretion. Although the preferred ions are $Na^+$ and $H^+$, $Li^+$ can substitute for $Na^+$ and $NH_4^+$ can substitute for $H^+$.[204] The latter process, which enables $Na^+/NH_4^+$ exchange, appears to be important for proximal tubule $NH_4^+$ secretion.[274]

NHE3 (SLC9A3) is the primary apical $Na^+/H^+$ exchanger in the proximal tubule and mediates the majority of

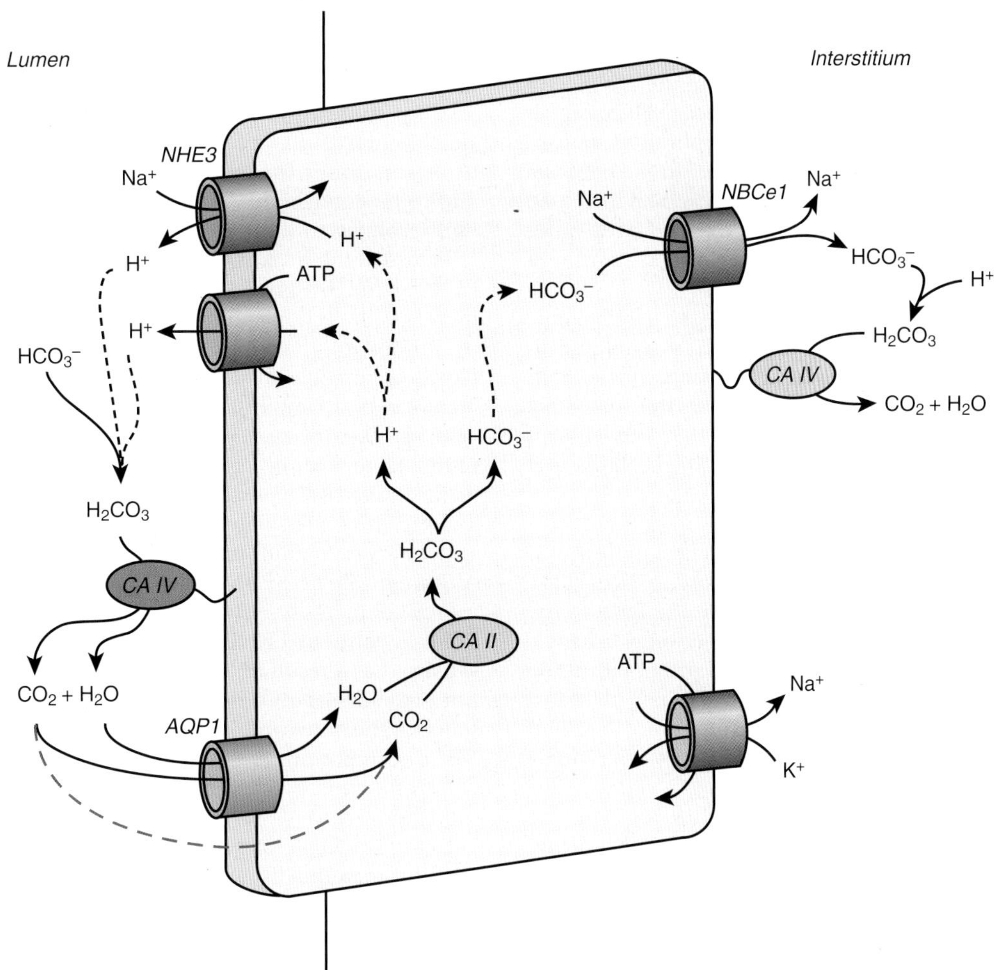


**Fig. 9.2** Bicarbonate reabsorption in the proximal tubule. Proximal tubule $HCO_3^-$ reabsorption involves integrated function of multiple proteins. Protons are secreted by the $Na^+/H^+$ exchanger, *NHE3*, and by $H^+$-ATPase, and titrate luminal $HCO_3^-$ to $H_2CO_3$. Luminal $H_2CO_3$ dehydration to $H_2O$ and $CO_2$ is accelerated by luminal carbonic anhydrase activity mediated by CA IV. $CO_2$ enters the cell via aquaporin I *(AQP1)* and most likely also via passive lipid-phase diffusion, where its hydration to $H_2CO_3$ is accelerated by cytoplasmic CA II. $H_2CO_3$ rapidly dissociates to $H^+$ and $HCO_3^-$, thereby "replenishing" the secreted cytosolic $H^+$. Cytosolic $HCO_3^-$ exits across the basolateral plasma membrane primarily by the electrogenic sodium-bicarbonate cotransporter, *NBCe1-A*. In the PST, a basolateral $Cl^-/HCO_3^-$ exchange activity (not shown) is the primary basolateral $HCO_3^-$ exit mechanism. *ATP,* Adenosine triphosphate; *CA IV*, carbonic anhydrase 4; *PST*, proximal straight tubule.

luminal bicarbonate reabsorption. Multiple mechanisms regulate NHE3; the best studied are parathyroid hormone (PTH), dopamine, and AngII. Both PTH and dopamine inhibit NHE3 activity, whereas AngII has a biphasic effect, stimulatory at low concentrations and inhibitory at high concentrations. Both PTH and dopamine increase intracellular cyclic adenosine monophosphate (cAMP) levels, leading to decreased NHE3 activity,[87] and dopamine also has protein kinase C- (PKC)-dependent effects.[137] AngII decreases cAMP levels and activates PKC, tyrosine kinase, and phosphatidylinositol-3-kinase.[178]

NHE3 phosphorylation is an important regulatory mechanism. Serine-552 (in the rat sequence) is a consensus protein kinase A (PKA) phosphorylation site, and phosphorylation of this site causes localization to the coated pit region of the brush-border membrane, where NHE3 cannot contribute to bicarbonate reabsorption.[211] Similarly, phosphorylation of serine-719 regulates insertion into the plasma membrane.[345] This phosphorylation affects interactions of multiple signaling proteins with NHE3, alters the size of the NHE3 protein binding complex, and alters NHE3 lipid raft distribution, which cause changes in specific aspects of basal as well as acutely regulated NHE exchange activity.[346] Dephosphorylation, mediated by the serine/threonine phosphatase PP1, but not PP2, at serines 552 and 605, and at other novel phosphorylation sites, stimulates NHE3 activity.[105] Ang II counteracts the effects of cAMP/PKA by dephosphorylating NHE3 at serine 552, which may be a key event in the regulation of renal proximal tubule sodium handling.[89]

Movement of NHE3 between different subcellular locations, including microvilli, intermicrovillar clefts, endosomes, and the cytoplasm, is an important regulatory mechanism. Only NHE3 in microvilli contributes to bicarbonate reabsorption. Redistribution within these domains is regulated by a variety of factors, including renal sympathetic nerve activity, glucocorticoids, insulin, AngII, dopamine, and PTH.[22,39,87,260,334] This process involves a number of cellular proteins, including dynamin, NHERF-1, clathrin-coated vesicles, calcineurin homologous protein-1, ezrin phosphorylation, G-protein alpha subunits, and G-protein beta-gamma dimers.[8,100,179]

NHE8 (SLC9A8) is a second $Na^+/H^+$ exchanger found in the proximal tubule.[149] Under normal conditions in the adult kidney, NHE8 is mostly intracellular,[38] but in the absence of NHE3 and during acid-loading in normal mice, NHE8 protein expression increases in brush border membrane fractions and contributes to bicarbonate reabsorption.[30] In the neonatal kidney, brush border membrane NHE8 expression is increased and NHE3 expression is decreased compared with adult kidneys, suggesting that NHE8 is the primary mechanism of apical NHE activity in the neonatal kidney.[30,31,309,406]

NHE1 (SLC9A1) is a third member of the NHE family that is present in the proximal tubule. NHE1 is a ubiquitous sodium hydrogen exchanger present in essentially all cells in mammalian organs and is located in the proximal tubule in the basolateral plasma membrane.[34] Its role in the proximal tubule appears to be acute intracellular pH regulation.[60]

**$H^+$-ATPase.** A second mechanism of proximal tubule apical $H^+$ secretion involves the vacuolar $H^+$-ATPase.[443] $H^+$-ATPase is expressed in the brush border microvilli, the base of the brush border, and apical invaginations between clathrin-coated domains.[52] $H^+$-ATPase also acidifies proximal tubule endosomes and lysosomes, senses endosomal pH, and is involved in recruiting trafficking proteins to acidified vesicles, thereby ensuring appropriate progression from early endosomes to lysosomes.[54] Proximal tubule $H^+$-ATPase activity is increased by AngII, increased axial flow, and chronic metabolic acidosis.[74,103,427] $H^+$-ATPase has a direct binding interaction with aldolase, which may underlie the development of proximal RTA in individuals with hereditary fructose intolerance.[247] In addition, PKA stimulates and the adenosine monophosphate–activated protein kinase (AMPK) inhibits apical plasma membrane $H^+$-ATPase insertion and activity.[7]

**NBCe1 (SLC4A4).** Basolateral bicarbonate exit largely is mediated by the electroneutral sodium-bicarbonate cotransporter, NBCe1. In humans, three splice variants of the NBCe1 gene are known; NBCe1-A, also known as kNBC1, is the primary splice variant expressed in the kidney, where it is found exclusively in the basolateral plasma membrane in the proximal convoluted tubule.[61,256] In mice, there are a total of five known splice variants.[219] NBCe1-A has large cytoplasmic amino- and carboxy-termini tails, 14 transmembrane domains, and two glycosylation sites.[45,244,335,490]

NBCe1-A in the proximal tubule mediates the coupled net movement of $Na^+$ and $HCO_3^-$. The majority of evidence suggests this involves a 1:3 ratio of $Na^+$ and $HCO_3^-$ equivalents.[151,336] Because the cytoplasm is negatively charged relative to the peritubular compartment, this electrical gradient provides the driving gradient to enable the coupled movement of $Na^+$ and $HCO_3^-$ out of the cell, against their concentration gradient. The coupling ratio of $Na^+$ and $HCO_3^-$ is likely to be critically important: a 1:3 coupling mediates net $HCO_3^-$ efflux, whereas with a 1:2 ratio, depending on the assumptions of intracellular $Na^+$ and $HCO_3^-$ concentration and of basolateral membrane voltage, the net electrochemical gradient may favor $HCO_{3q}$ influx. Indeed, some proximal renal tubular acidosis (RTA) cases may result from NBCe1 mutations that alter the coupling ratio.[491] However, the specific molecular mechanisms of this 1:3 coupling ratio are only partially understood. In nonrenal cells, NBCe1-A appears to have a 1:2 coupling ratio.[151,173,232] Moreover, it appears that when NBCe1-A is expressed in a proximal tubule cell line, Ser-982 phosphorylation shifts the stoichiometry from 1:3 to 1:2.[152] Two aspartate residues near Ser-982 are necessary for this stoichiometry shift.[153] Thus, the coupling ratio of 1:3 appears to be important for NBCe1-A to facilitate bicarbonate exit and to be determined, at least in part, by phosphorylation–dephosphorylation of specific amino acid residues.

Proximal tubule NBCe1-A–mediated bicarbonate transport is regulated by physiologic conditions. Transport activity increases in response to metabolic acidosis and to a variety of stimuli that increase bicarbonate reabsorption.[130,314,373] However, changes in steady-state protein expression do not appear to be an important regulatory mechanism, as metabolic acidosis does not appear to alter NBCe1-A expression.[220] Other factors known to regulate NBCe1-A activity include intracellular ATP, possibly through an as yet unidentified kinase,[173] and a regulated recycling pathway involving PKC[305] and calcium/calmodulin-dependent protein kinase II.[306] Although Ste20/SPS1-related proline-alanine-rich kinase (SPAK)-dependent Ser65 phosphorylation and IRBIT- and SPAK-dependent Thr49 phosphorylation regulate NBCe1-B activity,[176] as a result of alternative splicing these residues are not present in NBCe1-A. Moreover, because of differential splicing, the auto-inhibitory domain present in NBCe1-B and NBCe1-C is not present in NBCe1-A, which results in approximately fourfold greater basal activity of NBCe1-A compared with the –B and –C variants.[259]

Defects in NBCe1 are the most common cause of autosomal recessive proximal RTA (pRTA).[186,219,491] In addition to causing severe pRTA, NBCe1 defects can cause growth and mental retardation, basal ganglia calcification, cataracts, corneal opacities (band keratopathy), glaucoma, elevated serum amylase and lipase, and defects in the enamel suggestive of amelogenesis imperfecta.[186,219] In mice, homozygous NBCe1 deletion causes a very severe phenotype, with severe metabolic acidosis, marked volume depletion, and death within a few weeks after birth. Heterozygous deletion causes a milder phenotype but still causes development of pRTA.[129,167]

NBCe1, in addition to its role in proximal tubule bicarbonate reabsorption, also has a critical role regulating other proximal tubule acid–base functions. NBCe1 gene deletion causes abnormal renal ammonia and organic anion metabolism, and these effects appear to be mediated through alterations in proximal tubule proteins involved in the metabolism and/or transport of these acid–base components.[167,293] This critical role of NBCe1 appears to be due, at least in part, to the A splice variant, NBCe1-A. Recent studies show that mice with NBCe1-A-specific deletion live to adulthood, have spontaneous metabolic acidosis without increased ammonia excretion, an abnormal physiologic response, and have greatly impaired ammonia metabolism and excretion response to acid loading.[228] The abnormal ammonia excretion correlates with abnormal expression of critical proteins involved in ammoniagenesis, including PDG, PEPCK, and GS.[228]

**Carbonic Anhydrase.** Carbonic anhydrases are a family of zinc metalloenzymes that catalyze the reversible hydration of $CO_2$ to form carbonic acid ($H_2CO_3$), reaction A in the equation:

$$CO_2 + H_2O \overset{A}{\Leftrightarrow} H_2CO_3 \overset{B}{\Leftrightarrow} H^+ + HCO_3^-.$$

In the absence of carbonic anhydrase, the hydration/dehydration reaction (reaction A) is rate limiting, whereas reaction B occurs essentially instantaneously.

*CA II.* CA II is the predominant carbonic anhydrase in the kidney and in the proximal tubule. It is located in the cytoplasm of the proximal tubule, in addition to multiple other sites in the kidney, including thin descending limb, thick ascending limb of the loop of Henle (TAL), and intercalated cells. In the mouse kidney, CA II is also expressed in collecting duct principal cells.

*CA IV.* CA IV is found in the proximal tubule and in intercalated cells in the collecting duct.[352] CA IV is linked to the plasma membrane via a glycosylphosphatidylinositol (GPI) anchor and extends into the extracellular compartment; the active site is thus extracellular, not intracellular.[492] In the proximal tubule, CA IV is expressed in both apical and basolateral plasma membranes where, by facilitating $HCO_3^-$ interconversion with $CO_2$, it contributes to transepithelial bicarbonate reabsorption.[53]

## REGULATION OF PROXIMAL TUBULE BICARBONATE REABSORPTION

### Systemic Acid–Base

Changes in extracellular acid–base status profoundly alter proximal tubule bicarbonate reabsorption. Both metabolic and respiratory acidosis increase bicarbonate reabsorption, and alkalosis decreases it. This occurs with both acute and chronic pH changes, although the effects are substantially greater with chronic changes. It is important to note that these effects are mediated through changes in interstitial (i.e., peritubular) $HCO_3^-$, and $pCO_2$. Changes in luminal $HCO_3^-$ have the opposite effect on proximal tubule bicarbonate transport, a manifestation of glomerular–tubular balance.

Recent studies have begun to elucidate the mechanisms through which extracellular bicarbonate and $CO_2$ regulate proximal tubule bicarbonate reabsorption. Changes in either peritubular $CO_2$ or $HCO_3^-$ concentration, but not pH when the other two components are constant, alter bicarbonate reabsorption.[489] These effects are specific to bicarbonate reabsorption, as fluid reabsorption rates do not change. The basolateral plasma membrane protein, protein–tyrosine phosphatase, receptor-type, gamma (PTPRG), is necessary for this molecular sensing.[488] PTPRG may couple to the ErbB tyrosine kinases, ErbB1 and ErbB2, as inhibitors of these proteins block these responses, and phosphorylation of ErbB1 and ErbB2 is regulated by both bicarbonate and $CO_2$ concentration.[370] An additional mechanism may involve the intrarenal angiotensin system, as peritubular $CO_2$ stimulates intracellular AngII production and luminal secretion, which acts through an apical $AT_1$ receptor to stimulate bicarbonate reabsorption.[485,487]

Chronic metabolic acidosis increases proximal tubule bicarbonate reabsorption more than acute metabolic acidosis. This adaptive increase involves increased NHE3 expression and activity and increased $H^+$-ATPase activity,[16,74,314] but not detectable changes in NBCe1 or NBCe1-A expression.[220,228] Glucocorticoid levels rise with chronic metabolic acidosis,[464] and glucocorticoid receptor activation enhances acidosis-induced increases in NHE3 expression and apical trafficking.[14]

**Luminal Flow Rate.** Renal bicarbonate reabsorption changes in parallel with glomerular filtration rate and luminal flow.[310] Increased luminal flow enhances apical plasma membrane NHE3 activity.[312] In addition, increased flow minimizes changes in the luminal bicarbonate concentration, thereby maintaining a higher mean luminal bicarbonate concentration, which facilitates bicarbonate reabsorption.[13] Proximal tubule brush border microvilli may function as flow sensors, with drag force transmitted through the actin filament, altering cytoskeletal elements and regulating transport.[103]

**AngII.** AngII is an important regulator of proximal tubule ion transport, including bicarbonate reabsorption. Low AngII concentrations increase but high concentrations inhibit bicarbonate reabsorption.[78,442] Both luminal and peritubular low-dose AngII stimulate bicarbonate reabsorption, mediated predominantly through apical and basolateral $AT_1$ receptors. Acidosis increases $AT_1$ receptor expression, which may contribute to adaptive changes in bicarbonate reabsorption.[279]

**Potassium.** Chronic hypokalemia stimulates and hyperkalemia inhibits proximal tubule bicarbonate reabsorption.[328] This is associated with parallel changes in apical $Na^+/H^+$ exchange and basolateral sodium–bicarbonate cotransport activity,[372] and involves increased apical and basolateral plasma membrane $AT_1$ receptor expression.[126] Acute changes in extracellular potassium concentration, however, do not alter proximal tubule bicarbonate transport.[77]

**Endothelin.** Endothelin has important and direct effects on ion transport in a variety of renal epithelial cells, including the proximal tubule. Endothelin can be produced in the proximal tubule and exhibits an autocrine effect to stimulate NHE3.[240] In particular, metabolic acidosis–induced increases in NHE3 expression may require endothelin B (ET-B) receptor activation.[222]

**PTH.** PTH acutely inhibits proximal tubule bicarbonate reabsorption through activation of adenylyl cyclase and increased intracellular cAMP production.[263] Systemic PTH administration leads acutely to metabolic acidosis, but chronically leads to metabolic alkalosis.[183] The acute effect is due primarily to increased urinary bicarbonate excretion, likely due to changes in proximal tubule bicarbonate reabsorption; the chronic effect is due to increased titratable acid excretion, which is likely due to increased excretion of dihydrogen and hydrogen phosphate.[183]

**Calcium Sensing Receptor.** The calcium sensing receptor (CaSR) is present in the apical membrane in the proximal tubule. CaSR activation, either by increased luminal calcium or through calcimimetic agents, increases bicarbonate reabsorption through a mechanism likely involving the activation of apical NHE3.[66] CaSR activation may modulate the effects of PTH in proximal tubule bicarbonate reabsorption; hypercalcemia resulting from excess PTH has the opposite effect of PTH alone on bicarbonate transport.

## LOOP OF HENLE

The TAL of the loop of Henle reabsorbs ~15% of the filtered bicarbonate load. The overall schema is fundamentally similar to that in the proximal tubule. Apical $Na^+/H^+$ exchange and vacuolar $H^+$-ATPase secrete $H^+$. Quantitatively, apical $Na^+/H^+$ exchange activity is the major $H^+$ secretory mechanism;

vacuolar $H^+$-ATPase activity is present, but has at most a minor role in bicarbonate reabsorption.[67,148] Two $Na^+/H^+$ exchanger isoforms are present in the TAL, NHE2, and NHE3, and NHE3 appears to be the predominant isoform.[409,444] Secreted $H^+$ reacts with luminal $HCO_3^-$, forming $H_2CO_3$, which dissociates to $CO_2$ and $H_2O$. Whether luminal CA IV is present is unclear, with conflicting reports in the literature.[53,402] Luminal $CO_2$ moves down its concentration gradient across the apical plasma membrane into the cell cytoplasm. Cytoplasmic CA II catalyzes $CO_2$ hydration to form $H_2CO_3$, which dissociates to $H^+$ and $HCO_3^-$, thereby regenerating the $H^+$ secreted across the apical plasma membrane. Several basolateral bicarbonate exit mechanisms are present. These include basolateral $Cl^-/HCO_3^-$ exchange, possibly AE2,[11] and a coupled $K^+$-$HCO_3^-$ cotransport activity that may be mediated by KCC4.[270] Although an electroneutral sodium–bicarbonate cotransporter (NBCn1) is present,[424] electrochemical gradients for its transport favor bicarbonate uptake, not extrusion, suggesting that it is unlikely to contribute significantly to basolateral bicarbonate exit.

Several plasma membrane proteins either directly or indirectly alter bicarbonate reabsorption. Inhibiting the apical $Na^+$-$K^+$-$2Cl^-$ cotransporter, NKCC2, increases bicarbonate reabsorption.[67] This may occur because inhibiting NKCC2 decreases $Na^+$ entry, which decreases intracellular $Na^+$, increasing the $Na^+$ uptake gradient for apical $Na^+/H^+$ exchange and thereby increasing bicarbonate reabsorption. Inhibiting basolateral $Na^+/H^+$ exchange activity decreases bicarbonate reabsorption through cytoskeletal alterations that decrease apical NHE3 expression.[145,447]

#### Regulation of TAL Bicarbonate Reabsorption

A variety of stimuli regulate TAL bicarbonate reabsorption. Metabolic acidosis increases TAL bicarbonate reabsorption,[69,138] but whether the effects are specific to metabolic acidosis or due to other mechanisms is not clear. One study reported that metabolic acidosis induced with $NH_4Cl$ and that chloride loading with NaCl had similar effects on bicarbonate transport, raising the possibility that chloride loads, not acid loads, regulate TAL bicarbonate transport.[138] Data in favor of acidosis regulating TAL bicarbonate transport are that $NH_4Cl$-induced metabolic acidosis, but not equivalent chloride loading with NaCl, increases TAL NHE3 expression.[198] Further supporting a role of the TAL in acid–base regulation is that experimental models of metabolic alkalosis decrease bicarbonate reabsorption.[141]

Several hormones regulate bicarbonate reabsorption. AngII stimulates TAL bicarbonate reabsorption, likely through activation of $AT_1$ receptors.[68,272] Glucocorticoid receptors are present in the TAL and glucocorticoids are necessary for normal bicarbonate reabsorption.[408] Mineralocorticoids, at high concentrations, stimulate bicarbonate reabsorption,[141] but their absence does not alter basal transport.[408] Arginine vasopressin (AVP) inhibits bicarbonate reabsorption through prostaglandin E2-mediated inhibition of apical $Na^+/H^+$ exchange activity.[44,139] PTH inhibits bicarbonate reabsorption, but the effect is less than the effect of AVP.[139]

Cytokines also regulate bicarbonate transport. Lipopolysaccharide (LPS) inhibits transport; this effect involves the cytokine receptor, TLR4, and separate pathways activated by luminal and peritubular LPS. Luminal LPS involves the mTOR pathway, whereas peritubular LPS functions through the mitogen-activated protein kinase kinase (MAP) extracellular signal-related kinase (ERK) pathway.[146,448] High-mobility group box 1 (HMGB1) is a nuclear protein released extracellularly in response to infection or injury, where it interacts with toll-like receptor 4 (TLR4) and other receptors to mediate inflammation. It inhibits TAL bicarbonate reabsorption through a receptor for advanced glycation end products (RAGE)-dependent mechanism that involves signaling through Rho and Rho-associated kinase (ROCK).[147,446]

Another important regulatory factor is medullary osmolality. Increased tonicity inhibits and decreased tonicity stimulates bicarbonate reabsorption; this occurs through phosphatidylinositol 3-kinase–mediated changes in apical $Na^+/H^+$ exchange activity.[140,144] In addition, AVP, which contributes to the development of the medullary osmotic gradient, discussed elsewhere in this textbook, inhibits bicarbonate reabsorption.[139]

### ACID–BASE TRANSPORTERS IN THE TAL

Many of the major $H^+$ and $HCO_3^-$ transporters were discussed earlier in relation to the proximal tubule and are not repeated here.

#### NBCn1 (SLC4A7)

NBCn1 facilitates the electroneutral, coupled transport of $Na^+$ and $HCO_3^-$ in a 1 : 1 ratio. In the kidney, NBCn1 is found in the basolateral plasma membrane in the TAL, outer medullary collecting duct (OMCD) intercalated cells, and terminal inner medullary collecting duct (IMCD).[220,311] Because the concentrations of $Na^+$ and $HCO_3^-$ are generally lower in the cytoplasm than in the interstitium, basolateral NBCn1 likely mediates peritubular $HCO_3^-$ uptake. Moreover, both metabolic acidosis and hypokalemia increase TAL NBCn1 expression.[189,220] Thus, NBCn1 is unlikely to mediate a critical role in bicarbonate reabsorption. Instead, it is likely to contribute to ammonia reabsorption, which will be discussed later.

### DISTAL CONVOLUTED TUBULE

The DCT consists of two cell types, DCT cells and intercalated cells, and the mechanisms involved in bicarbonate reabsorption appear to differ between DCT and intercalated cells. DCT cells express apical NHE2[75] and NHE2 inhibitors decrease bicarbonate reabsorption.[444] Basolateral $HCO_3^-$ exit likely involves AE2.[11] A basolateral $Cl^-$ channel that has limited $HCO_3^-$ permeability may also contribute.[463] Cytosolic CA II is present, but not apical CA IV.[53] In the late DCT intercalated cells are present.[251] Quantitatively, intercalated cells constitute only a very small proportion of all cells in the DCT, ~4% and 7% in the mouse and rat kidneys, respectively.[201] The majority of intercalated cells in the DCT are type A and non-A, non-B intercalated cells.[201]

### COLLECTING DUCT

The renal collecting duct is the final site of bicarbonate reabsorption and both reabsorbs and secretes luminal bicarbonate.[261] Specific proteins in specific epithelial cell types, which vary in type and frequency in different collecting duct segments, mediate these processes.

#### Collecting Duct Segments

Technically, the collecting duct begins with the ICT, immediately distal to the CNT, and extends through the IMCD. The

CNT arises from a different embryonic origin than the ICT and the remainder of the collecting duct. However, the CNT is included in the discussion of the role of the collecting duct in acid–base regulation because it has cell types and acid–base transport mechanisms similar to the collecting duct. Different portions of the collecting duct are identified by where they reside: ICT, cortical collecting duct (CCD), outer medullary collecting duct in the outer stripe (OMCDo), outer medullary collecting duct in the inner stripe (OMCDi), and the IMCD.

### Cell Composition

Collecting duct segments contain several distinct epithelial cell types, and the cellular composition differs in the various collecting duct segments. Two distinct cell types, intercalated cells and principal cells, are present. Principal cells account for ~60%–65% of cells and intercalated cells account for the remainder in the ICT, CCD, and OMCD. In the IMCD, the proportion of intercalated cells is less, about 10% of cells in the initial portion of the rat IMCD, and it decreases progressively from the outer medullary–inner medullary junction distally, completing disappearing by the middle of the papilla. In the terminal IMCD, the epithelium is composed of IMCD cells, a cell distinct from both intercalated cells and principal cells. The CNT contains both intercalated cells and a cell type specific to the CNT, termed the CNT cell; in some species, principal cells are also present.

At least three distinct intercalated cell subtypes exist: the type A (or α) intercalated cell, the type B (or β) intercalated cell, and the non-A, non-B intercalated cell (Fig. 9.3). In the CNT, both type A and non-A, non-B intercalated cells are present, and type B intercalated cells are infrequent. In the CCD, both type A and type B intercalated cells are present, and the non-A, non-B cell is infrequent. In the OMCD and IMCD, only the type A intercalated cell is present under normal conditions.

### Type A Intercalated Cell

The type A intercalated cell is involved in $H^+$ secretion, $HCO_3^-$ reabsorption, and ammonia secretion. The proteins involved in these processes are, in general, different from those in the proximal tubule and TAL (Fig. 9.4).

Both vacuolar $H^+$-ATPase and P-type $H^+$-$K^+$-ATPases are involved in apical $H^+$ secretion. $H^+$-ATPase is abundant in the apical plasma membrane and in apical cytoplasmic tubulovesicles in type A intercalated cells. $H^+$-ATPase undergoes trafficking between the cytoplasmic compartment and the apical plasma membrane; this mechanism, rather than changes in total protein expression, appears to be the major adaptive response to acid–base disturbances.[27] In addition to having a major role in $H^+$ secretion, $H^+$-ATPase also has an essential role in cell volume regulation and maintenance of intracellular electronegativity, replacing the $Na^+$-$K^+$-ATPase that provides these functions in most other cell types.[73]

A second means of $H^+$ secretion involves electroneutral, $K^+$-dependent $H^+$-$K^+$-ATPase activity that is mediated by P-type $H^+$-$K^+$-ATPase proteins.[155] At least two $H^+$-$K^+$-ATPase α-isoforms are present. One, $HK\alpha_1$, is similar to the α-isoform involved in gastric acid secretion. The other, $HK\alpha_2$, is similar to the α-isoform in the colon. $K^+$ reabsorbed via apical $H^+$-$K^+$-ATPase can either recycle across the apical plasma membrane or exit the cell across the basolateral plasma membrane, and relative movement across the apical versus basolateral plasma membranes is regulated by dietary $K^+$ intake.[484]

A truncated isoform of the erythrocyte anion exchanger, termed kAE1, is present in the basolateral plasma membrane and mediates basolateral bicarbonate exit.[9] $Cl^-$ that enters the cell via basolateral $Cl^-/HCO_3^-$ exchange exits via the KCl cotransporter, KCC4[41,264]; a basolateral $Cl^-$ channel, presumably ClC-Kb in humans and ClC-K2 in rodents, also contributes to $Cl^-$ recycling.[210]

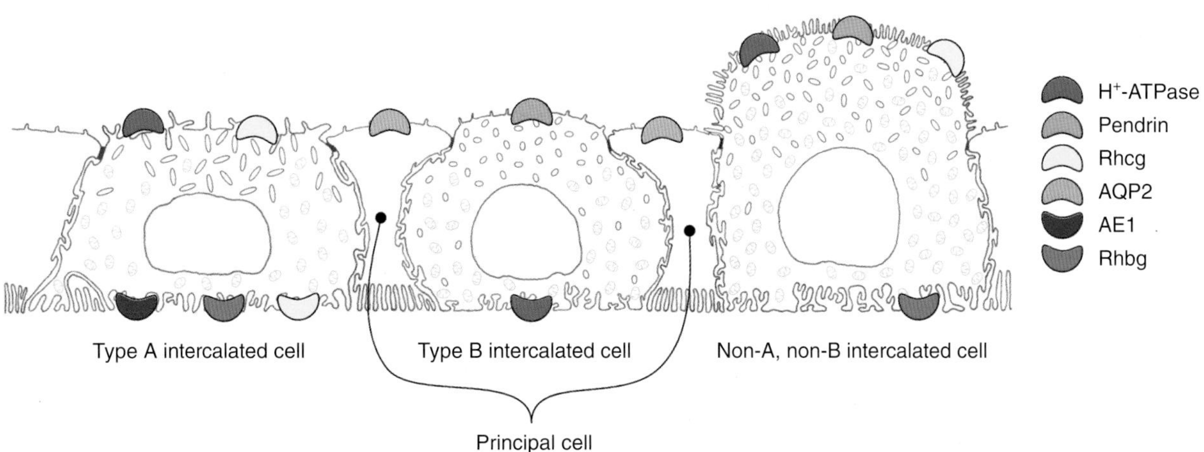


**Fig. 9.3** Intercalated cell subtypes in the distal nephron and collecting duct. The late DCT, connecting segment, initial collecting tubule, CCD, OMCD, and IMCD have multiple distinct cell types. Three intercalated cell types can be distinguished based on ultrastructural features and differential expression in plasma membrane domains of several proteins involved in renal acid–base transport, including $H^+$-ATPase, AE1, pendrin, Rhbg, and Rhcg. $H^+$-ATPase is present in the apical portion of the type B intercalated cell, where it is found in cytoplasmic vesicles; ultrastructural analysis shows it is not in the apical plasma membrane. These specific intercalated cell subtypes occur at different frequencies specific to the various tubule segments. *CCD*, Collecting duct system; *DCT*, distal convoluted tubule; *IMCD*, inner medullary collecting duct; *OMCD*, outer medullary collecting duct.

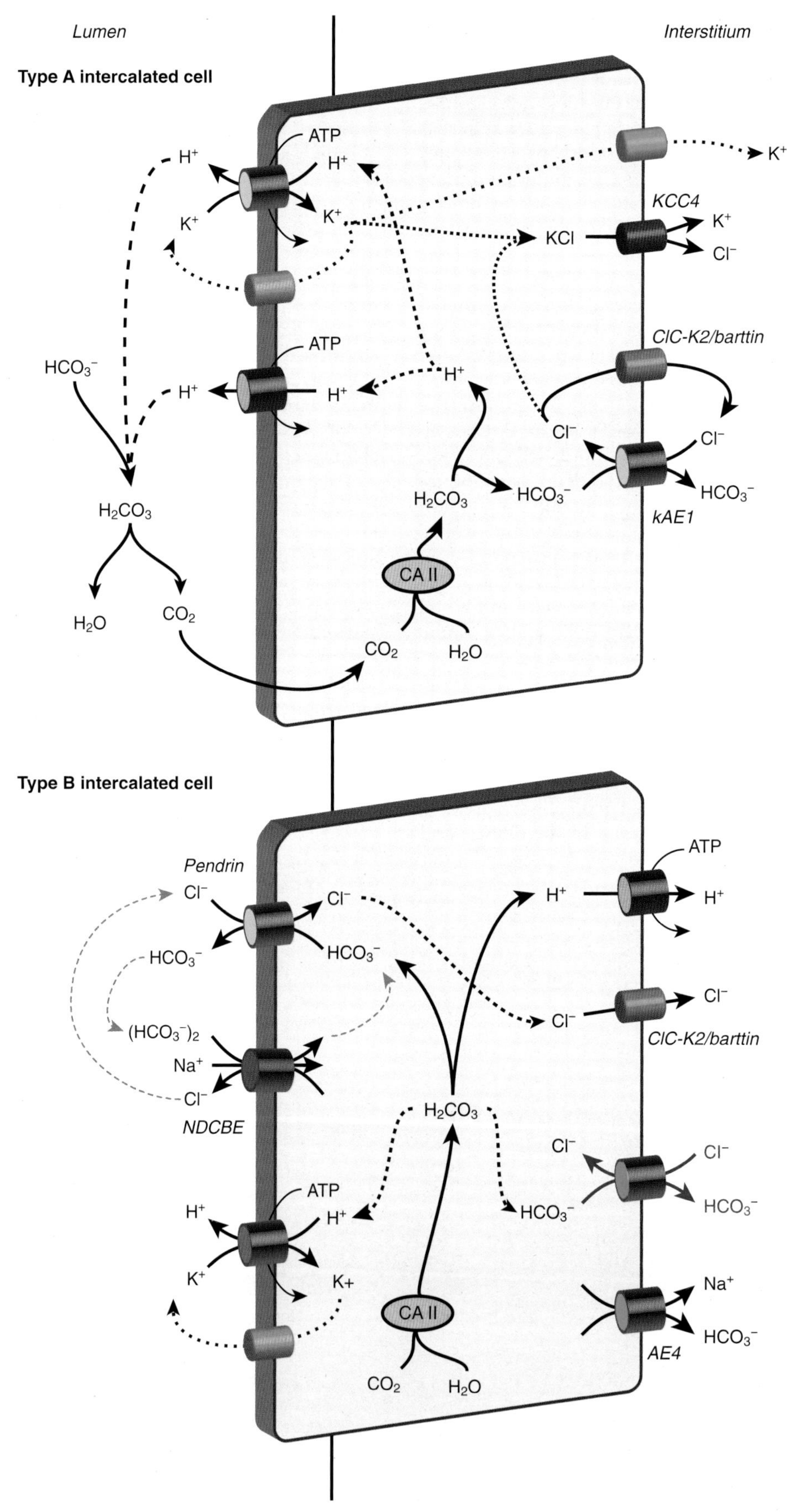

Lumen
Interstitium
Type A intercalated cell
ATP
H+
K+
K+
KCl
KCC4
Cl−
ClC-K2/barttin
HCO3−
ATP
H+
H+
H+
Cl−
Cl−
H2CO3
HCO3−
HCO3−
kAE1
H2CO3
CA II
H2O
CO2
CO2
H2O
Type B intercalated cell
Pendrin
Cl−
Cl−
HCO3−
HCO3−
ATP
H+
H+
(HCO3−)2
Na+
Cl−
NDCBE
Cl−
Cl−
ClC-K2/barttin
H2CO3
Cl−
Cl−
ATP
H+
H+
HCO3−
HCO3−
K+
K+
Na+
CA II
HCO3−
AE4
CO2
H2O

Cytoplasmic CA II is abundant in type A intercalated cells and enables intracellular generation of $H^+$ for apical secretion and $HCO_3^-$ for basolateral transport. In addition, membrane-associated carbonic anhydrases are present in the apical region (CA IV) and, at least in mouse and rabbit, in the basolateral region (CA XII) of intercalated cells.[316]

### Type B Intercalated Cell

The type B intercalated cell mediates a major role in $HCO_3^-$ secretion and luminal $Cl^-$ reabsorption. It contains basolateral $H^+$-ATPase and an apical $Cl^-/HCO_3^-$ exchanger, pendrin.[10] $H^+$-ATPase is also present in vesicles throughout the cell, but it is not present in the apical plasma membrane. Similar to the type A intercalated cell, $H^+$-ATPase, rather than $Na^+$-$K^+$-ATPase, maintains intracellular electronegativity and prevents cell swelling.[73] Type B intercalated cells also express $H^+$-$K^+$-ATPase.[421,473] In the rabbit and mouse an apical $H^+$-$K^+$-ATPase activity is present,[250,456] whereas in the rat a basolateral $H^+$-$K^+$-ATPase activity may be present.[133] The type B cell also has cytoplasmic CA II, which facilitates intracellular $H^+$ and $HCO_3^-$ production. Fig. 9.4 summarizes the proteins involved in type B intercalated cell acid–base transport.

There is functional evidence that pendrin-mediated apical $Cl^-/HCO_3^-$ exchange works in concert with an apical $Na^+$-dependent $Cl^-/HCO_3^-$ exchanger, NDCBE (*Slc4a8*), to mediate net NaCl absorption,[237] and NDCBE protein and mRNA have been reported in renal cortical homogenates.[237,468] However, in recent studies using single-cell RNA-seq NDCBE transcripts were virtually undetectable in type B intercalated cells.[80] Basolateral $Na^+$ and $Cl^-$ exits are mediated by the basolateral $NaHCO_3$ cotransporter, AE4,[73] and a $Cl^-$ channel, ClC-K2/Barttin, or ClC-Kb.[170]

The type B intercalated cell also has the ability to secrete $H^+$ and reabsorb luminal $HCO_3^-$. As noted earlier, most studies indicate the type B intercalated cell has an apical $H^+$-$K^+$-ATPase activity that may mediate proton secretion, and functional studies have shown that CCD intercalated cells with apical $Cl^-/HCO_3^-$ exchange activity (i.e., all type B intercalated cells) also have basolateral $Cl^-/HCO_3^-$ exchange activity that is functionally distinct from the kAE1 activity that present in type A intercalated cells.[459]

The type B intercalated cell has several roles in acid–base and ion transport homeostasis. Genetic deletion of the apical $Cl^-/HCO_3^-$ exchanger, pendrin, impairs $HCO_3^-$ secretion, luminal $Cl^-$ reabsorption, and, through a mechanism involving coordinated function with principal cell luminal $Na^+$ reabsorption.[203,339,413] The type B intercalated cell may also contribute to $H^+$ secretion and luminal $HCO_3^-$ reabsorption. Ammonia, which is increased in metabolic acidosis and hypokalemia, increases type B intercalated cell apical $H^+$-$K^+$-ATPase and basolateral $Cl^-/HCO_3^-$ exchange activity, which would result in increased net $HCO_3^-$ reabsorption.[121]

### Non-A, Non-B, or Type C Intercalated Cell

A third intercalated cell subtype, generally termed the non-A, non-B cell, is present in the CNT and ICT.[201,391] This cell has several features that distinguish it from both the type A intercalated cell and the type B intercalated cell. These differences include the expression of both pendrin and $H^+$-ATPase in the apical plasma membrane and in apical cytoplasmic vesicles, the absence of basolateral plasma membrane $H^+$-ATPase and AE1, the presence of apical, but not basolateral Rhcg, and the absence of basolateral Rhbg (see Fig. 9.3). Thus, it differs significantly from both type A and type B intercalated cells. Studies of the developing kidney show that non-A, non-B cells and type B intercalated cells arise simultaneously, but from different foci.[164,374] This cell type was termed "non-A, non-B cell" in early studies. However, its unique transporter expression, distribution, and developmental origin suggest this is a third distinct intercalated cell subtype.

### Principal Cells

Principal cells have indirect and direct roles in acid secretion. Indirectly, principal cell–mediated $Na^+$ reabsorption leads to luminal electronegativity; this facilitates $H^+$ secretion by the electrogenic, and thus voltage-sensitive, $H^+$-ATPase. In addition, principal cells have direct roles. Functional studies show that principal cells have apical $H^+$ secretory and basolateral $Cl^-/HCO_3^-$ exchange activities,[452,460] and they express $H^+$-ATPase[102,425] and both the $HK\alpha_1$ and $HK\alpha_2$ isoforms of $H^+$-$K^+$-ATPase.[155] In the mouse and rat kidney, principal cells in the OMCDi and initial IMCD express both carbonic anhydrase activity and CA II protein.[101,205] Finally, the ammonia transporters, Rhcg and Rhbg, are both present in principal cells in the rat and mouse CCD and OMCD.[199]

### IMCD Cell

The IMCD cell is a distinct cell type and is the predominant cell present in the terminal IMCD. It exhibits carbonic anhydrase activity,[205] both $H^+$-ATPase and $H^+$-$K^+$-ATPase activity,[155,435] and basolateral $Cl^-/HCO_3^-$ exchange.[449] In vitro microperfusion studies have demonstrated directly that the IMCD secretes $H^+$ and reabsorbs luminal $HCO_3^-$.[437]

**Fig. 9.4** Bicarbonate transport by the type A and the type B intercalated cell. *Top panel* shows a model of acid–base transport by the type A intercalated cell. Two families of $H^+$ transporters, $H^+$-ATPase and $H^+$-$K^+$-ATPase, are present in the apical plasma membrane. Secreted $H^+$ titrates luminal $HCO_3^-$ to form $H_2CO_3$, which dehydrates to water *($H_2O$)* and carbon dioxide *($CO_2$)*. Luminal carbonic anhydrase activity, most likely mediated by CA IV, is variably present in the collecting duct (see text for details). Cytosolic $H^+$ and $HCO_3^-$ are formed from CA II-accelerated hydration of $CO_2$ and rapid dissociation of $H_2CO_3$. Cytosolic $HCO_3^-$ exits across the basolateral plasma membrane via the anion exchanger, kAE1. $Cl^-$ that enters via kAE1 recycles via a basolateral $Cl^-$ channel. $K^+$ that enters via apical $H^+$-$K^+$-ATPase can either recycle via an apical, $Ba^+$-sensitive $K^+$ channel or be reabsorbed via a basolateral $Ba^+$-sensitive $K^+$ channel. A basolateral $Na^+/H^+$ exchanger is present but does not contribute to bicarbonate reabsorption and is not shown. *Bottom panel* shows a model of acid–base transport by the type B intercalated cell. Apical pendrin is the primary mechanism of bicarbonate secretion. Chloride enters the cell via pendrin and exits across a basolateral chloride channel, ClC-K2/barttin. Basolateral $H^+$-ATPase extrudes protons into the peritubular compartment. Cytoplasmic bicarbonate and protons are produced from $CO_2$ and water in a CA II–catalyzed reaction. In addition, an apical $H^+$-$K^+$-ATPase in series with a basolateral $Cl^-/HCO_3^-$ exchange activity is present and may contribute to bicarbonate reabsorption by the type B intercalated cell. Apical NDCBE is present and mediates $Na^+$-$(HCO_3^-)_2$ exchange for $Cl^-$. When coupled with pendrin this can enable coupled $Na^+$-$Cl^-$ reabsorption. *CA II*, Carbonic anhydrase II.

## FUNCTIONAL ROLE OF DIFFERENT COLLECTING DUCT SEGMENTS

### CNT-ICT

Relatively little information is available on the functional role of the CNT and ICT in acid–base homeostasis. Morphologic and immunolocalization studies suggest that the CNT and ICT contain type A and type B intercalated cell types and non-A, non-B cells.[201,391,419] Under basal conditions, the CNT, at least in the rabbit, secretes bicarbonate through a $Cl^-$-, carbonic anhydrase–, and $H^+$-ATPase–dependent mechanism[404]; this likely involves apical pendrin, cytosolic CA II, and basolateral $H^+$-ATPase.

### CCD

Unlike the OMCD and IMCD, which can secrete only acid (i.e., reabsorb bicarbonate), the CCD both reabsorbs and secretes bicarbonate. The basal direction of bicarbonate transport varies among species, but both bicarbonate absorption and secretion can be induced in response to systemic acid or alkali loading.[18,245,261] The ability to secrete bicarbonate, which is not found in the OMCD or IMCD, correlates with the presence of type B intercalated cells in the CCD, but not in the OMCD or IMCD. Mineralocorticoids stimulate CCD bicarbonate secretion, likely related to generation of metabolic alkalosis and to stimulation of pendrin expression[128,413]; however, mineralocorticoid receptors are present in type B intercalated cells,[288,363] and thus direct stimulation of type B cell ion transport by mineralocorticoids is possible.

### OMCD

The OMCD is responsible for approximately 40%–50% of the net acid secretion that occurs in the collecting duct. Both intercalated cells and principal cells contribute to acid secretion, although intercalated cells are believed to be the primary cell responsible for OMCD acid secretion.[452,460]

### IMCD

The IMCD secretes $H^+$ and reabsorbs luminal bicarbonate.[433] However, the number of type A intercalated cells is substantially less than in other collecting duct segments. In the rat they account for only 10% of cells in IMCD1[86] and in all species examined the prevalence diminishes distally such that almost no intercalated cells exist in the distal portion of IMCD (IMCD3). Nonetheless, bicarbonate reabsorption occurs in the terminal IMCD and basolateral $Cl^-/HCO_3^-$ exchange is present in cultured IMCD cells.[449] $H^+$ secretion is partly mediated by $H^+$-$K^+$-ATPase.[439] In rats fed a potassium-deficient diet, $H^+$-$K^+$-ATPase activities were upregulated,[435] but $H^+$-$K^+$-ATPase accounted for only ~50% of bicarbonate reabsorption in the IMCD, indicating that other mechanisms of luminal acidification also contribute, likely including $H^+$-ATPase. The IMCD expresses CA IV and luminal, cytoplasmic, and lateral membrane–associated carbonic anhydrase activity has been reported.[205,432]

## PROTEINS INVOLVED IN COLLECTING DUCT $H^+$/BICARBONATE TRANSPORT

Collecting duct $H^+$ and $HCO_3^-$ transport involves the coordinated activity of multiple transporters in conjunction with specific carbonic anhydrase isoforms. Later in this chapter we review the specific proteins involved.

### $H^+$-ATPase

Electrogenic apical $H^+$ secretion in acid-secreting intercalated cells and basolateral proton transport by bicarbonate-secreting intercalated cells is mediated by the vacuolar $H^+$-ATPase. Intercalated cells in the OMCD and initial IMCD, type A intercalated cells in the CCD, and non-A, non-B intercalated cells in the CNT and CCD, contain $H^+$-ATPase in the apical plasma membrane and in an apical cytoplasmic vesicle pool, and redistribution between the cytoplasmic vesicle pool and the apical plasma membrane is a major mechanism regulating $H^+$ secretion. $H^+$-ATPase is also present in the apical region of principal cells and CNT cells, but expression is much less than in intercalated cells. In Type B intercalated cells, H-ATPase is present in the basolateral plasma membrane and in sub-apical vesicles, but not in the apical plasma membrane. The role of apical $H^+$-ATPase in nonintercalated cells has not been clearly defined; it may be involved in endosomal trafficking and fusion,[184] and in the OMCDi it can also mediate apical $H^+$ secretion.[452]

Vacuolar $H^+$-ATPase is an assembly of multiple subunits that form two main domains, the $V_1$ domain, which is extramembranous and hydrolyzes ATP, and the $V_0$ domain, which is a transmembranous portion and transports protons. The $V_0$ domain is composed of six subunits; the $V_1$ domain is composed of eight subunits and is linked to the $V_0$ domain via a stalk region composed of subunits from both $V_0$ and $V_1$. Distinct isoforms and splice variants have been identified for many of these $H^+$-ATPase subunits and their cell-specific distribution may contribute to cell-specific regulation of proton and bicarbonate transport.

Genetic defects in several $H^+$-ATPase subunits have been shown to cause distal RTA (dRTA), also known as Type I RTA, in humans. Defects in the B1 subunit of the hydrolytic $V_1$ domain resulting from ATP6V1B1 gene mutations can produce early-onset hearing loss in combination with autosomal recessive, severe dRTA.[194,195,382] Mice with B1 subunit deletion have incomplete distal RTA.[116] In these mice, the B2 subunit appears to substitute partially for the B1 subunit, enabling partial compensation.[301] Mutations in the a4 subunit (ATP6V0A4) in the $H^+$-translocating $V_0$ domain also produce recessive, severe early onset of dRTA, with variable onset of hearing loss.[371,382,411]

Normal $H^+$-ATPase function appears to involve coexpression of the Atp6ap2/(pro)renin receptor. This is a type 1 transmembrane protein and an accessory subunit of $H^+$-ATPase and may also function in the renin-angiotensin system. Its deletion results in decreased $H^+$-ATPase activity and impaired renal acid–base homeostasis.[399] Although Atp6ap2 is a cell surface protein capable of binding and nonproteolytically activating prorenin, prorenin does not acutely regulate $H^+$-ATPase activity.[96] Atp6ap2 also appears to regulate NKCC2 and AQP2 expression, and this may occur through the autophagosomal substrate p62.[399]

### $H^+$-$K^+$-ATPase

The second mechanism of collecting duct $H^+$ secretion involves electroneutral $H^+$-$K^+$ exchange.[155] The active protein is a heterodimer composed of α- and β-subunits. The α-subunit is an integral membrane protein with multiple membrane spanning domains and contains the catalytic portion of the enzyme. Two α-subunit isoforms have been identified. $HK\alpha_1$, also termed the gastric isoform, was identified originally in the stomach. $HK\alpha_1$ forms heterodimers with its specific β-subunit, HKβ. The β-subunit has only a single membrane-spanning region and is necessary for targeting of the α-subunit to the plasma membrane and for transport function.[155] $HK\alpha_2$ was identified originally in the colon and is sometimes referred to as the colonic isoform. Three splice variants of $HK\alpha_2$ have been identified in the kidney. $HK\alpha_2$ forms heterodimers with the $\beta_1$-subunit of $Na^+$-$K^+$-ATPase.

$HK\alpha_1$, $HK\alpha_2$, and HKβ are expressed throughout the collecting duct, with greater expression in intercalated cells than in principal cells.[4,6,64] Functional studies suggest that both $HK\alpha_1$ and $HK\alpha_2$ are present in type A as well as type B intercalated cells.[250,265,456] However, immunohistochemistry studies have yielded variable results with respect to the precise cellular distribution of the $HK\alpha_1$ and $HK\alpha_2$ isoforms. $HK\alpha_1$ immunoreactivity was found in both AE1-positive (type A) and AE1-negative intercalated cells in both rat and rabbit collecting ducts,[473] but in human kidneys, diffuse $HK\alpha_1$ immunoreactivity was present in both intercalated and principal cells.[215] $HK\alpha_2$ immunoreactivity was consistently apical, but in different cell types in different studies. It was found exclusively in the CNT cell in rabbits in one study[114] and exclusively in the OMCD principal cell in rats in another.[343] A third study found the splice variant, $HK\alpha_{2c}$, in intercalated cells, principal cells, and CNT cells from the CNT through the initial IMCD in rabbit kidney.[421] In situ hybridization studies have shown both intercalated cell and principal cell expression of HKα1, HKα2, and HKβ mRNA in the rat kidney, although principal cell signal was less intense than intercalated cell signal.[5,64]

Multiple physiologic conditions alter $H^+$-$K^+$-ATPase expression and activity. Metabolic acidosis increases $H^+$-$K^+$-ATPase activity in the CCD and $HK\alpha_1$ and $HK\alpha_2$ mRNA expression in the OMCD, suggesting that $H^+$-$K^+$-ATPase contributes to $H^+$ secretion.[155] Specific studies have identified apical, but not basolateral, $H^+$-$K^+$-ATPase activity in both types A and B intercalated cells in mouse and rabbit kidneys.[265,456,483] Extracellular ammonia, which increases with both metabolic acidosis and hypokalemia, enhances apical $H^+$-$K^+$-ATPase–mediated $H^+$ secretion in both type A and type B intercalated cells in the CCD.[121,123]

## Pendrin (SLC26A4)

Pendrin is an electroneutral $Cl^-/HCO_3^-$ exchanger present in the kidney exclusively in type B and non-A, non-B intercalated cells. It is found in the apical plasma membrane and in apical cytoplasmic vesicles in type B and non-A, non-B intercalated cells in the CNT, ICT, and CCD. Under basal conditions, pendrin is predominantly expressed in the apical plasma membrane in non-A, non-B intercalated cells and in subapical cytoplasmic vesicles in type B intercalated cells, and redistribution between these two subcellular sites is an important regulatory mechanism.[441] Pendrin is regulated by AngII, nitric oxide, and cAMP.[393,414] In addition to bicarbonate secretion, pendrin also mediates an important role in extracellular fluid volume and blood pressure regulation. This appears to involve roles in both transcellular $Cl^-$ reabsorption and, through luminal alkalinization due to $HCO_3^-$ secretion, activation of the principal cell epithelial $Na^+$ transporter, ENaC[108,436] and involving the $Na^+$-dependent, chloride–bicarbonate exchanger (NDCBE, SLC4A8).[237]

## Carbonic Anhydrase

Three carbonic anhydrase isoforms, CA II, CA IV, and CA XII, are present in the collecting duct. CA II is cytosolic in proximal tubule cells, discussed earlier, in intercalated cells, and in principal cells in the collecting ducts of mice.[420] CA II is present in all intercalated cell types, but expression is generally greater in the type A than in type B intercalated cells.

CA IV is an extracellular, membrane-associated carbonic anhydrase tethered to the membrane through a glycosylphosphatidylinositol lipid (GPI) anchoring protein. It is expressed apically in the majority of cells in rabbit OMCD and IMCD and in type A intercalated cells in the CCD.[356] In the OMCDi, luminal carbonic anhydrase inhibition decreases bicarbonate absorption, suggesting an important role for CA IV in acid–base homeostasis.[403]

Carbonic anhydrase XII (CA XII) is another extracellular, membrane-associated carbonic anhydrase found in the collecting duct.[316] In contrast to CA IV, CA XII is an integral membrane protein with a single transmembrane spanning region.[316] Basolateral CA XII immunoreactivity has been reported in principal cells in the human kidney, and in the mouse, basolateral CA XII immunoreactivity is found in type A intercalated cells in the CCD and OMCD.[316,319]

## kAE1

The major basolateral anion exchanger in type A intercalated cells is kAE1, a truncated form of the erythrocyte anion exchanger AE1. In the human, rat, and mouse kidneys, kAE1 is expressed almost entirely in the basolateral plasma membrane. In the rabbit kidney under basal conditions, kAE1 is present in intracytoplasmic multivesicular bodies, as well as in the basolateral plasma membrane; metabolic acidosis decreases intracellular kAE1 and increases basolateral kAE1, suggesting regulated trafficking contributes to bicarbonate reabsorption.[416]

Several mutations in AE1 cause human autosomal dominant and autosomal recessive dRTA. Autosomal dominant dRTA can be caused by a trafficking defect leading either to mistargeting to the apical plasma membrane or failure of plasma membrane insertion.[324,362] Autosomal recessive dRTA due to defective AE1 is commonly due to mutations that lead to intracellular protein retention.[388]

## KCC4

KCC4 is a member of the SLC12 family of solute transporters and mediates electroneutral, coupled transport of $K^+$ and $Cl^-$. Basolateral KCC4 expression has been shown in the proximal convoluted tubule (PCT), TAL, DCT, CNT, and type A intercalated cells.[41,412] In the type A intercalated cell, KCC4 likely contributes to basolateral $Cl^-$ recycling. Metabolic acidosis increases KCC4 expression in type A intercalated cells in the OMCD, suggesting a role in the response to metabolic acidosis[264] by facilitating basolateral $Cl^-/HCO_3^-$ exchange, and KCC4 deletion causes development of distal RTA,[41] suggesting KCC4 is necessary for both basal and acidosis-stimulated acid–base homeostasis.

## $Cl^-$ Channel

$Cl^-$ entry via basolateral kAE1 recycles across the basolateral plasma membrane. In addition to KCC4, the $Cl^-$ channel, ClC-K2, is present in the basolateral plasma membrane of type A intercalated cells and likely contributes to this recycling.[296]

### Other Anion Exchangers

Several other anion transporters, including anion exchangers and sodium bicarbonate cotransporters (NBCs), are present in the collecting duct, but their roles in acid–base homeostasis are less completely understood. AE2 is expressed in collecting ducts, particularly in the basolateral plasma membrane of IMCD cells.[125] Another $Cl^-/HCO_3^-$ exchanger, Slc26a7, is found in the basolateral plasma membrane of OMCD intercalated cells.[307] Slc26a7 mRNA and protein expression increases with acid loading, suggesting it may contribute to regulated bicarbonate reabsorption.[384] AE4 (Slc4a9) is present in the collecting duct, but both its location and function are in question. Although originally thought to be an anion exchanger, other evidence suggests AE4 functions in type B intercalated cells as a $NaHCO_3$ cotransporter.[73] Studies of the rabbit kidney have variously reported that AE4 immunoreactivity is exclusively apical in type B intercalated cells,[401] apical and lateral in type A intercalated cells,[209] and exclusively lateral in type B intercalated cells.[318] In both rat and mouse kidneys, only basolateral AE4 protein expression has been detected in both type A[80,209] and type B intercalated cells.[73,80,209] In the mouse, both mRNA and basolateral protein expression are significantly stronger in type B than in type A intercalated cells.[80]

### Sodium Bicarbonate Cotransporters

Several NBCs are expressed in the collecting duct. NBC3 (Slc4a7) is found in the apical region of OMCD intercalated cells and type A intercalated cells in the CCD and in the basolateral region of type B intercalated cells.[221,320] It appears to contribute to intracellular pH regulation, but not to transepithelial bicarbonate transport.[482] NBCn1, another SLC4A7 gene product, is an electroneutral NBC, and basolateral expression is found in the terminal IMCD and in OMCD intercalated cells.[311] Finally, recent evidence indicates AE4 (SLC4A9), discussed earlier, functions as a $Na^+$-$HCO_3^-$ cotransporter.[73]

### NBCe2 (SLC4A5)

The electrogenic, $Na^+$-$HCO_3^-$ cotransporter, isoform 2 (NBCe2, SLC4A5) appears to contribute to acid–base homeostasis, but its specific cellular expression remains unclear. An initial study suggested there was only apical expression in collecting duct intercalated cells in the CCD and OMCD,[95] whereas a different study identified NBCe2 in microdissected mouse CNT segments.[466] Genetic deletion in one study induced metabolic acidosis,[150] whereas in a second study, NBCe2 deletion did not alter basal acid–base homeostasis, but did impair the ability to respond to exogenous acid loading.[466] The mechanism through which NBCe2 contributes to acid–base homeostasis, given the evidence for its apical localization, is unclear. There is evidence that NBCe2 deletion leads to increased pendrin expression, which could, by increasing $HCO_3^-$ secretion, contribute to the acid–base phenotype observed.[95] NBCe2 deletion is also associated with increased expression of the $\beta_1$-subunit of $H^+$-ATPase, which may serve as an adaptive response that minimizes the extent of the acid–base disturbance.[466] However, the possibility of additional mechanisms through which NBCe2 contributes to acid–base homeostasis cannot be excluded at present.

Other studies suggest NBCe2 is present in the proximal tubule, not the distal nephron. In a study examining the human kidney under basal conditions, NBCe2 mRNA was found in the proximal tubule by in situ hybridization, and protein expression was observed in subcellular fractionation enriched for apical brush-border proteins.[135]

## REGULATION OF COLLECTING DUCT ACID–BASE TRANSPORT

The collecting duct is the final site controlling renal acid–base regulation. It responds quickly to physiologic conditions to increase acid or bicarbonate excretion as needed to maintain systemic acid–base homeostasis.

## ACIDOSIS

The collecting duct response to metabolic acidosis includes adaptations in all segments of the collecting duct and the CNT. Increased acid secretion in the collecting duct during acidosis is mediated primarily by $H^+$-ATPase. Both metabolic and respiratory acidosis increase apical plasma membrane $H^+$-ATPase expression and activity in acid-secreting collecting duct intercalated cells. Redistribution of $H^+$-ATPase from a subapical vesicle pool to the apical plasma membrane is the primary means of activation of proton secretion, and involves vesicular trafficking that requires soluble NSF-attachment protein receptor (SNARE) proteins and Rab GTPases.[102,425] In most models of metabolic acidosis, total renal $H^+$-ATPase mRNA and protein expression do not change,[379,425] but a study examining OMCD segments from acid-loaded mice found increased mRNA expression of several $H^+$-ATPase subunits, including the B1 and a4 subunits.[82]

During chronic metabolic acidosis, AE1 mRNA and AE1 protein expression in the basolateral plasma membrane in OMCD and CCD type A intercalated cells is increased.[181,341] In rats and mice, AE1 is present in the basolateral plasma membrane under basal conditions, and the subcellular distribution does not change with metabolic acidosis.[181,341] In rabbits fed a normal diet, AE1 is in both intracellular multivesicular bodies and the basolateral plasma membrane in type A intercalated cells. Metabolic acidosis increases the basolateral plasma membrane boundary length and the amount of AE1 immunoreactivity in the basolateral plasma membrane and reduces intracellular AE1.[416]

During metabolic acidosis, both net $HCO_3^-$ secretion and type B intercalated cell-mediated unidirectional $HCO_3^-$ secretion decrease. This is associated with decreased pendrin expression in type B and non-A, non-B cells as well as decreased apical $Cl^-/HCO_3^-$ exchange activity in type B intercalated cells in the CCD.[124,426,475] Reduced bicarbonate secretion by B cells during acid loading thus contributes to increased net bicarbonate reabsorption.

Carbonic anhydrase activity and the expression of CA II and CA IV in the collecting duct are increased by metabolic acidosis.[316] CA IV expression is upregulated in the OMCD, whereas CA II expression is upregulated in the CNT, CCD, and OMCD.

The collecting duct response to respiratory acidosis appears to be similar to that of metabolic acidosis. Respiratory acidosis stimulates structural changes in OMCD and CCD type A intercalated cells consistent with translocation of $H^+$-ATPase-bearing membrane from the apical vesicle pool to the apical plasma membrane.[418] Respiratory acidosis also stimulates N-ethylmaleimide-sensitive ATPase activity, a measure of H-ATPase activity[106,425] and bicarbonate reabsorption in isolated

CCDs,[262] consistent with activation of $H^+$-ATPase mediated proton secretion. In addition, chronic respiratory acidosis increases kAE1 mRNA.[94] Pendrin expression decreases during respiratory acidosis,[98] which likely mediates decreased bicarbonate secretion.

## ALKALOSIS

Metabolic alkalosis induces coordinated changes in acid–base transport throughout the collecting duct. In the OMCD of bicarbonate-loaded animals, bicarbonate reabsorption is decreased compared with control animals[245] and in the IMCD, bicarbonate loading abolishes acid secretion.[32] In the CCD, bicarbonate loading in animals produces net bicarbonate secretion.[261] However, no studies have shown the development of $HCO_3^-$ secretion by the OMCD or the IMCD in response to metabolic alkalosis, and this correlates with the lack of pendrin-expressing type B and non-A, non-B intercalated cells in these segments.

The cellular response to alkalosis in OMCD and CCD type A cells entails essentially the reverse of processes that occur to stimulate acid secretion. $H^+$-ATPase is redistributed from the apical plasma membrane into the apical vesicle pool, and basolateral AE1 immunoreactivity decreases.[26,341,417] Depending on the animal model, alkalosis increases pendrin expression and its apical distribution in type B and non-A, non-B intercalated cells and increases pendrin-mediated CCD bicarbonate secretion.[124,426] However, pendrin expression, subcellular location, and functional activity are regulated by other factors independent of acid–base status, including pregnancy, aldosterone, AngII, activation of AT1a and AT1b receptors, nitric oxide, and cAMP,* in addition to chloride balance and luminal chloride delivery.[321,415]

## HORMONAL REGULATION OF COLLECTING DUCT ACID–BASE TRANSPORT

In addition to extracellular pH, multiple other factors regulate collecting duct acid–base transport. Importantly, in vivo acid–base changes cause greater adaptations than equivalent in vitro changes, suggesting that in vivo regulatory mechanisms mediate a critical role in the response to acid–base disturbances.[134] Several hormones and receptors regulate bicarbonate transport in the collecting duct, particularly aldosterone and its analogs, and AngII.

Aldosterone is an important regulator of collecting duct bicarbonate transport.[381] Both in vivo and in vitro mineralocorticoids increase OMCD bicarbonate reabsorption.[381] This involves, at least when studied in vitro, increased $H^+$-ATPase activity and apical translocation in OMCD intercalated cells, stimulated through a non-genomic pathway not inhibited by mineralocorticoid receptor blockade.[474] Mineralocorticoids also increase CCD bicarbonate secretion; this is dependent on luminal chloride, mediated by pendrin, and involves increased pendrin mRNA and protein expression and pendrin redistribution from cytoplasmic vesicles to the apical plasma membrane in type B intercalated cells.[339,413] Likely because of parallel stimulation of both acid and bicarbonate secretion, mineralocorticoid therapy usually has modest effects on systemic acid–base homeostasis.

AngII exerts effects on the proximal tubule, TAL, DCT and collecting ducts. The collecting duct expresses apical AT1 (AT1a) receptors in both principal cells and intercalated cells.[338] In mouse OMCD and CCD, AngII in vitro increases $H^+$-ATPase activity in acid-secreting intercalated cells by trafficking $H^+$-ATPase to the apical plasma membrane.[304,338] In mouse OMCD, AngII stimulates $H^+$-ATPase activity through a G-protein–coupled phosphokinase C pathway.[338] However, in other studies, in vivo and in vitro AngII decreased bicarbonate reabsorption in rat OMCD and in vitro AngII decreased $H^+$-ATPase activity via AT1 receptors[394,440]; this apparent discrepancy has not been resolved. AngII also increases pendrin-dependent $Cl^-$ absorption,[302] apical $Cl^-/HCO_3^-$ exchange in type B intercalated cells,[457] and pendrin protein expression in the apical plasma membrane in non-A, non-B intercalated cells in the CNT, an effect mediated through activation of the angiotensin type 1a receptor (Agtr1a).[414]

Endothelin has important effects on collecting duct acid–base transport that are mediated partly by nitric oxide. Dietary protein intake stimulates urinary acidification through a process involving $H^+$-ATPase activation, mediated by endothelin and nitric oxide.[467] Endothelin-1 (ET-1) is synthesized by the collecting duct,[364,383] and endothelin receptors A and B (ET-A and ET-B) are present in the collecting duct.[212] ET-B activation regulates both type A and type B intercalated cell responses to metabolic acidosis.[405]

The CaSR is apical in IMCD cells and in type A intercalated cells[331] and mediates luminal $Ca^{+2}$-stimulation of $H^+$-ATPase.[330] Luminal acidification stimulated by this pathway may inhibit calcium precipitation and minimize development of nephrolithiasis.[330]

Activation of the vasopressin type 1A (V1a) receptor is an additional regulatory mechanism. The V1a receptor is expressed in the medullary TAL (mTAL) and throughout the collecting duct,[70,481] with expression in both intercalated cells and principal cells in the CCD and only in intercalated cells in the OMCD.[70] Metabolic acidosis increases V1a receptor expression in the mTAL and the OMCD in the inner stripe.[70,389] Genetic deficiency of the V1a receptor causes development of type IV RTA and diminishes mineralocorticoid stimulation of $H^+$-$K^+$-ATPase and Rhcg.[187]

Several other hormones and drugs also alter collecting duct acid–base transport. Kallikrein inhibits bicarbonate secretion.[253] Calcitonin stimulates $H^+$-ATPase–dependent bicarbonate reabsorption in the rabbit CCD.[365] Isoproterenol stimulates bicarbonate secretion by type B intercalated cells.[351]

## PARACRINE REGULATION

Several compounds produced and/or transported in the proximal tubule and TAL have downstream effects that regulate collecting duct acid–base transport. Presumably, this enables these segments, which exist in an area with very high blood flow and thus rapid exposure to changes in systemic acid–base and potassium, to regulate transport in collecting duct segments in the outer medulla and inner medulla, sites of low blood flow and thus reduced exposure to changes in systemic acid–base and potassium homeostasis. The paracrine molecules most extensively studied are ammonia and alpha-ketoglutarate.

Ammonia, discussed in detail later regarding its role in net acid excretion, also appears to function as an intrarenal, paracrine signaling molecule that regulates collecting duct transport.[451] It is produced primarily in the proximal tubule and undergoes regulated transport in both the proximal

*References 302, 303, 393, 413, 414, 468.

tubule and the TAL in response to both acid loading and hypokalemia. In addition to its roles in bicarbonate generation, ammonia stimulates CCD bicarbonate reabsorption in a concentration-dependent fashion.[123] Ammonia stimulates type A intercalated cell acid secretion and inhibits type B intercalated cell bicarbonate secretion.[121,123] Its stimulation of proton secretion involves stimulation of $H^+$-$K^+$-ATPase, not $H^+$-ATPase, activity.[122,123]

The Krebs cycle intermediate, 2-oxoglutarate (alpha-ketoglutarate), may have an important role in acid–base homeostasis. Changes in acid–base loading change the net direction of transport in the proximal tubule and the loop of Henle from reabsorption, seen with acid loading, to net secretion, seen with alkali loading.[79,115,395] In the CNT and CCD, luminal 2-oxoglutarate enhances net bicarbonate and sodium chloride reabsorption, acting through its receptor, Oxgr1, in type B and non-A, non-B intercalated cells.[395] Thus, 2-oxoglutarate can function as a paracrine mediator enabling functional coordination of the proximal tubule and the TAL with the collecting duct.

### CELLULAR ADAPTATIONS TO ACID–BASE PERTURBATIONS

In addition to changes in the abundance and subcellular distribution of membrane transporters, adaptive responses to some physiologic disturbances may involve changes in the numbers of intercalated cells. Several studies have shown that chronic metabolic acidosis and chronic hypokalemia increase intercalated cell numbers in medullary collecting ducts,* whereas others find no change in intercalated cell number in these conditions.[168,181,419] Chronic administration of lithium and acetazolamide also increases intercalated cell numbers in the OMCD.[23,85,398]

Increases in intercalated cell numbers could result from intercalated cell proliferation or from principal cell proliferation followed by conversion into intercalated cells. Studies using proliferation markers show that metabolic acidosis, hypokalemia, and lithium administration are each associated with increased proliferation of collecting duct cells,[84,297,465] some showing increased proliferation in type A intercalated cells,[410,465] and others showing the proliferating cells are principal cells.[84,202,297,398] The latter studies suggested that principal cells and OMCD intercalated cells may interconvert based on observations of rare cells with immunohistochemical and ultrastructural characteristics of both cell types[84,297,398] and through genetic studies that irreversibly identify principal cells as cells that express genes under the control of the AQP2 promoter.[202] The histone H3 K79 methyltransferase, Dot1L, may be involved in preventing transformation of principal cells into intercalated cells; Dot1L deletion decreases the number of principal cells and increases the number of collecting duct intercalated cells.[479] Other studies show that principal cells respond to acid by producing the cytokine SDF1, also known as CXCL12, which then acts on adjacent intercalated cells via its receptor, CXCR4.[355] SDF1is transcriptionally regulated and is a target of the hypoxia-sensing transcription factor HIF1α in principal cells.[355]

With respect to the CCD, some studies suggested there may be interconversion of type A and type B intercalated cells. An early paper examining the rabbit isolated perfused CCD equated apical endocytosis with alpha (type A) intercalated cells and used apical peanut lectin binding as a marker of beta (type B) intercalated cells. Chronic $NH_4Cl$ loading in vivo increased the number of intercalated cells exhibiting apical endocytosis in microperfused CCDs and decreased the number of cells that bound peanut lectin; the interpretation was that intercalated cell subtypes in the CCD could interconvert, with the type B intercalated cells reversing polarity to meet the physiologic demand for increased acid secretion.[353] Subsequently, some studies reported that acidosis, lithium administration, and carbonic anhydrase inhibition each alter the relative numbers of intercalated cells identifiable as type A or type B, although none have shown cells in native tissue with either apical AE1, basolateral pendrin, or coexpression of these two transporters.[23,85,124,317,465] Other studies of acid–base disturbances find regulation of the abundance and distribution of transport proteins specific to the A and B intercalated cell types and changes in cell morphology, but no change in the relative or absolute numbers of specific intercalated cell subtypes.[27,341,418,419] The explanation for these different findings could include differences in the experimental models, species examined, sensitivity and specificity of intercalated cell identification, and cell quantitation methods.

In vitro studies have implicated the extracellular matrix protein, hensin, and the prolyl isomerase activity of cyclophilin in the process of intercalated cell remodeling.[354,387] In mice with intercalated cell-specific hensin deletion there is development of a distal RTA, lack of type A intercalated cells, and an increased number of type B intercalated cells.[127] Hensin's effects on type A intercalated cell development appears to require the activation of beta-1 integrin.[127]

*References 23, 85, 297, 398, 410, and 465.

## BICARBONATE GENERATION

Acid–base homeostasis requires not only reabsorption of filtered bicarbonate, but also the generation of new bicarbonate to replace the bicarbonate used for buffering of endogenous and exogenous fixed acids. There are two major components of bicarbonate generation, titratable acid excretion and ammonia excretion. In addition, organic anion excretion is biologically important. Organic anions can be metabolized to form $HCO_3^-$; accordingly, their excretion is physiologically equivalent to bicarbonate excretion.

### TITRATABLE ACID EXCRETION

Titratable acids are urinary solutes that buffer secreted protons, enabling $H^+$ excretion without substantial changes in urine pH. Titratable acid excretion constitutes ~40% of net acid excretion under basal conditions. Metabolic acidosis increases titratable acid excretion by as much as 50% above baseline[159,347] (Fig. 9.5).

Multiple buffers contribute to titratable acid excretion. An ideal urinary buffer has a $pK_a$ lower than systemic pH, so that the majority of the filtered component is in the base form, and a $pK_a$ higher than urine pH, so that the majority of the urinary form is in the acid form. Phosphate is the predominant titratable acid and typically accounts for more than 50% of total titratable acid.[159,478] Citrate and creatinine also contribute to titratable acid excretion, but to a lesser

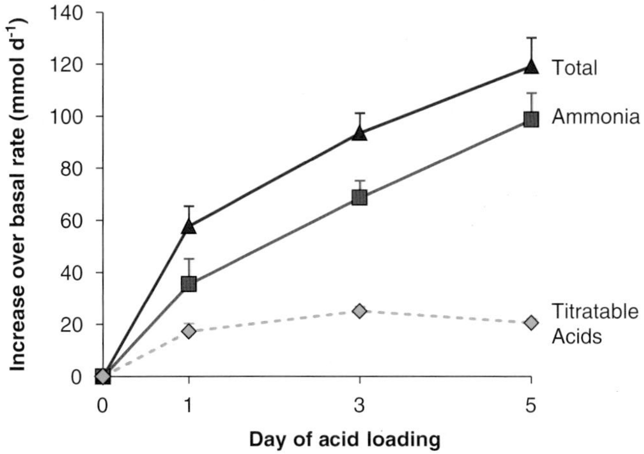


**Fig. 9.5** Relative contribution of titratable acid and ammonia excretion in the response to metabolic acidosis. Normal human volunteers were acid-loaded with ~2 mmol/kg of ammonium chloride and changes in urinary ammonia and titratable acid excretion were quantified. Data recalculated from Elkinton et al.[109]

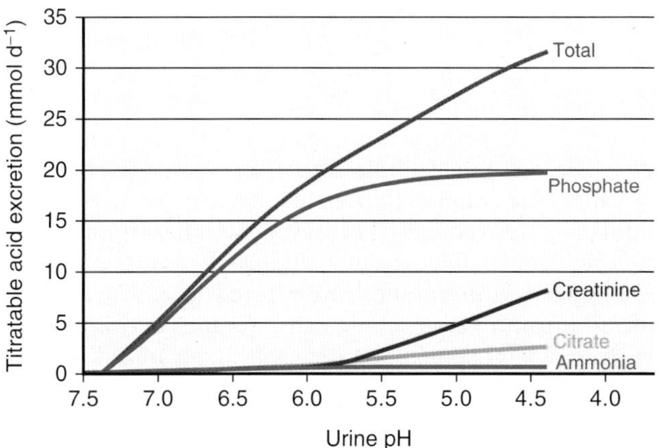


**Fig. 9.6** Relative contribution of various urinary buffers to titratable acid excretion. Ability of various urinary buffers to contribute to titratable acid excretion depends on the amount excreted in the urine, their $pK_a$, and final urine pH. Figure shows titratable acid excretion accounted for by each of the four major urinary buffers, phosphate, creatinine, citrate, and ammonia, at differing urine pH. Rates were calculated with daily excretion rate and $pK_a$, respectively, for phosphate, 25 mmol/d and 6.8; creatinine, 11 mmol/d and 4.9; citrate, 3 mmol/d and 5.6; and ammonia, 40 mmol/d and 9.15.

extent. Although ammonia is frequently termed a urinary buffer, because of its high $pK_a$ it does not contribute substantially to titratable acid excretion. The role of ammonia in new bicarbonate generation is considered separately later in the chapter. Fig. 9.6 shows the relative contributions of major urinary buffers to titratable acid excretion and shows the effect of changes in urine pH after taking into account the amount excreted under normal conditions and the $pK_a$ of each buffer.

## PHOSPHATE AS A TITRATABLE ACID

Titratable acid excretion in the form of phosphate is the amount of $HPO_4^{-2}$ that is filtered, not reabsorbed, and that buffers secreted $H^+$, forming $H_2PO_4^-$. Phosphate exists, under physiologically relevant conditions, in equilibrium between two forms: $H_2PO_4^-$ and $HPO_4^{-2}$. The relative amount of these two forms is given by

$$10^{pH-6.8} = \frac{[HPO_4^{-2}]}{[H_2PO_4^-]}.$$

The amount of $H_2PO_4^-$ in the urine ($H_2PO_4^-{}_{Urine}$) at any given pH can be calculated as

$$H_2PO_{4\,Urine}^- = \frac{U_{Phos}V}{10^{(pH_U-6.8)}+1},$$

where $U_{Phos}$ is the urinary concentration of total phosphate. Filtered phosphate, at the typical serum pH of 7.4, is ~80% in the form of $HPO_4^{-2}$ and 20% in the form of $H_2PO_4^-$. Thus, at any urine pH ($pH_U$), titratable acid excretion in the form of phosphate ($TA_{Phos}$) is given by the formula

$$TA_{Phos} = U_{Phos}V * \left(\frac{1}{10^{(pH_U-6.8)}+1} - 0.2\right).$$

These considerations indicate that titratable acid excretion as phosphoric acid is determined by phosphate excretion and by the ability to lower urine pH. Phosphate excretion is determined by the difference between the filtered load of phosphate and tubular phosphate reabsorption. Regulation of renal tubular phosphate transport is a complex process and is discussed in detail elsewhere in this text. Here, we review only the factors that regulate this process in response to acid–base disorders.

The proximal tubule is the primary site of phosphate reabsorption and is where metabolic acidosis and other acid–base disorders regulate phosphate transport. Acid loading decreases proximal tubule phosphate reabsorption, leading to increased excretion. However, absolute changes in urinary phosphate excretion are usually rather modest, less than a twofold increase. The decrease involves decreased NaPi-IIa protein and mRNA expression and changes in its subcellular distribution.[15,15,156] Acid loading alters NaPi-IIa expression even if the acid load is completely compensated and there are no changes in systemic pH, suggesting that factors that precede changes in systemic pH regulate this response.[423] Metabolic acidosis also lowers luminal pH in the proximal tubule, which directly inhibits phosphate uptake.[174,4C7] Finally, metabolic acidosis increases PTH release, which also inhibits phosphate reabsorption.

Other phosphate transporters besides NaPi-IIa, such as NaPi-IIc and Pit-2, are present in the proximal tubule apical plasma membrane. Whether NaPi-IIc changes with metabolic acidosis is unclear as some studies find decreased expression[423] and others do not.[292] Pit-2 expression, although regulated by dietary phosphate availability, is not altered in metabolic acidosis in phosphate replete conditions, but does increase in response to metabolic acidosis in conditions of phosphate depletion.[423]

Acidosis-induced changes in phosphate excretion depend on systemic phosphate availability. In the presence of dietary phosphate restriction, basal phosphate excretion is reduced, and the increase in urinary phosphate excretion in response to metabolic acidosis is blunted.[423] Similarly, changes in NaPi-IIa abundance are blunted.[15] In contrast to NaPi-IIa, and to their response to metabolic acidosis in phosphate-replete animals, NaPi-IIc and Pit-2 expression actually increase in phosphate-restricted animals exposed to metabolic acidosis.[423]

Increased renal phosphate excretion with metabolic acidosis is balanced by parallel increases in extrarenal phosphate transport. Metabolic acidosis increases small intestinal $Na^+$-dependent phosphate transport, and this is associated with increased expression of NaPi-IIb.[378] There is also increased phosphate release from bone in response to both acute and chronic metabolic acidosis.[234] These extrarenal effects minimize the changes in systemic phosphate levels that could otherwise develop from the increased phosphate excretion.

### OTHER URINARY BUFFERS

Creatinine, which is used typically to assess glomerular filtration, has a $pK_a$ of ~4.9 and is excreted in sufficient amounts, ~11 mmol $d^{-1}$, that it can contribute to titratable acid excretion. This is particularly true in conditions when urinary pH is 5.5 or less.[159] Uric acid, although it can function as a buffer, is typically excreted in such small amounts, ~4 mmol $d^{-1}$, as to limit is role as a titratable acid. In ketoacidosis, β-hydroxybutyric acid and acetoacetic acid excretion increases, which increases titratable acid excretion. However, because ketoacids can be metabolized to bicarbonate, their loss in the urine has no net effect on acid–base homeostasis.

## ORGANIC ANION EXCRETION

Multiple organic anions in the urine can contribute to acid–base homeostasis. At least 95 different urinary organic anions have been identified, and many, including hippuric, erythronic, threonic, tartaric, and uric acids, are excreted in substantial quantities.[72] In general, their role in acid–base homeostasis is not as a titratable acid. Instead, because their metabolism produces bicarbonate, their excretion enables alkali excretion without altering urine pH.

### CITRATE EXCRETION

Citrate plays an important role in both acid–base homeostasis and preventing calcium nephrolithiasis. The latter function relates to citrate's ability to form reversible, noncovalent complexes with urinary and luminal calcium, thereby decreasing ionized calcium and decreasing the rate of calcium deposition into renal stones. Citrate may also inhibit calcium oxalate nucleation by colloidal stabilization of early-stage calcium oxalate complexes.[340] A complete description of citrate's role in nephrolithiasis can be found elsewhere in this text. In this chapter we discuss citrate's role in acid–base homeostasis.

Citrate has two roles in acid–base homeostasis: (1) as a urinary buffer contributing to titratable acid excretion, and (2) as a substrate in the tricarboxylic acid cycle. The two primary molecular forms of citrate, $citrate^{-3}$ and $citrate^{-2}$, exist in equilibrium with each other:

$$Citrate^{-3} + H^+ \leftrightarrow Citrate^{-2}$$

The $pK_a$ of this buffer reaction is ~6.4. Other molecular forms, $citrate^{-1}$ and $citrate^0$, because of the $pK_a$ of the appropriate buffer reactions, are at such sufficiently low concentrations that they appear to not be transported to a significant extent. Thus, at a normal physiologic pH of 7.4, ~91% of total citrate is in the form of $citrate^{-3}$ and only ~9% is $citrate^{-2}$. Because glomerular filtrate has a pH essentially identical to systemic arterial pH, essentially all filtered citrate is in the form of $citrate^{-3}$. In contrast, only 29% of urinary citrate at a typical urine pH of ~6.0 is in the form of $citrate^{-3}$, meaning that ~71% has been protonated and converted to $citrate^{-2}$. This difference in $citrate^{-2}$ between filtrate and final urine enables citrate to serve as a titratable acid (see Fig. 9.6).

The second mechanism through which citrate contributes to acid–base homeostasis relates to its function as a metabolic substrate for the tricarboxylic acid cycle. Its complete metabolism, as occurs in the proximal tubule, results in $HCO_3^-$ generation. Thus, citrate excretion, which is the difference between its filtration and its reabsorption, with subsequent metabolism that forms $HCO_3^-$, is functionally equivalent to $HCO_3^-$ excretion. Citrate excretion thereby enables base excretion without altering urine pH, which may be beneficial for minimization of pH-dependent calcium nucleation and calcium-containing stone growth.

Multiple factors regulate renal citrate excretion. Metabolic acidosis decreases and alkalosis increases citrate excretion.[25] Hypokalemia reduces citrate excretion.[2,120] This effect is likely independent of systemic pH. The carbonic anhydrase inhibitor, acetazolamide, and a high dietary intake of either NaCl or protein decrease citrate excretion.[157,213] Lithium chloride administered at therapeutic doses in animal models increases citrate excretion,[42] but studies in humans have not confirmed this finding.[43]

Renal tubular citrate transport is the primary determinant of citrate excretion. In humans, plasma citrate levels average ~0.1 mM, and changes in plasma levels are not an important regulatory mechanism. The proximal tubule reabsorbs a variable proportion, typically 65%–90%, of filtered citrate, and reabsorption parallels the filtered load. Citrate transported into proximal tubule cells, whether across apical or basolateral plasma membranes, is fully metabolized, enabling citrate to serve as a significant component of renal oxidative metabolism.[157] There does not appear to be significant transepithelial citrate transport, and there does not appear to be significant citrate transport in other renal sites.

Apical citrate transport is mediated primarily by the sodium–dicarboxylate cotransporter, NaDC1, an integral membrane protein highly expressed in the apical plasma membrane in the proximal tubule.[223,294,357] This conclusion is based on the finding that NaDC1 expression parallels citrate reabsorption in metabolic acidosis,[17] by the similarity of NaDC1 transport activity to the transport activity identified in brush border membrane vesicles,[294,357] and by results of NaDC1 gene deletion studies. Specifically, NaDC1 deletion increases citrate excretion, along with excretion of several other Krebs cycle intermediates known to be transported by NaDC1.[171]

However, NaDC1 may not be the only protein involved in filtered citrate reabsorption. Preliminary studies report the presence of a residual citrate reabsorption process in NaDC1-knockout mice.[392] This additional citrate transport activity may be the calcium-regulated transport activity that has been identified in cultured proximal tubule cells.[171,172] At present, the gene and gene product responsible for this citrate transport activity have not been identified.

Multiple mechanisms regulate proximal tubule citrate transport. First, the transported citrate form is $citrate^{-2}$, not $citrate^{-3}$. Because the $pK_a$ of the citrate buffer reaction is 6.4, luminal acidification, resulting from increased apical $H^+$

secretion, directly increases luminal citrate$^{-2}$ concentration, which increases citrate reabsorption. Because many conditions stimulate luminal acidification, this provides a mechanism to increase filtered citrate reabsorption without altering the number or activity of citrate transporters. Second, metabolic acidosis increases apical citrate transport capacity,[190] most likely by increasing NaDC-1 expression.[17] Both hypokalemia and starvation decrease citrate excretion, likely through stimulation of proximal tubule citrate transport.[236,472] Several cellular signaling proteins regulate NaDC1. One is the calcineurin inhibitor target protein, cyclophilin,[33] which likely mediates the effects of calcineurin inhibitors to increase citrate reabsorption.[375] Others include protein kinase C, sodium–hydrogen exchanger regulating factor 2, serum and glucocorticoid-inducible kinase, and protein kinase B.[40,295] Finally, recent studies have implicated the proximal tubule basolateral bicarbonate transporter, NBCe1, as a critical determinant of NaDC1 expression.[293]

Basolateral citrate transport in the proximal tubule has different characteristics than apical transport. Uptake is pH-independent, $Na^+$-dependent, and electroneutral, appears to involve 3 $Na^+$ and 1 citrate$^-$,[157,191] and appears to be mediated by NaDC3.[59] Approximately 20% of proximal tubule citrate uptake appears to be mediated by basolateral uptake. However, because the proximal tubule does not secrete citrate, basolateral citrate uptake does not regulate renal citrate excretion.

### OTHER ORGANIC ANIONS

Humans excrete 26–52 mEq $d^{-1}$ of organic anions other than citrate. Because organic anions can be metabolized to bicarbonate, organic anion excretion is functionally equivalent to alkali excretion and thereby can contribute to acid–base regulation. The extent of change in these organic anions with acid–base disturbances is not clear. Some studies show acid or alkali loading does not alter urinary organic anion excretion,[235] whereas other studies show alkali loading increases and acid loading decreases organic anion excretion[177]

Quantitatively, there are important species-dependent differences in the magnitude of organic anion excretion. In humans, basal organic anion excretion averages 0.3–0.7 mEq $kg^{-1}$ $d^{-1}$,[235] whereas in the rat organic anion excretion is 2–8 mEq $kg^{-1}$ $d^{-1}$.[56,333] Studies in the dog report 1–2 mEq $kg^{-1}$ $d^{-1}$ [290] and in the rabbit average 4 mEq $kg^{-1}$ $d^{-1}$.[333] This species-dependent variation may in part reflect differences in intestinal organic anion absorption[333] or in the intestinal biome.

## AMMONIA METABOLISM

Renal ammonia metabolism and transport is a predominant mechanism of the renal response to most acid–base disorders (see Fig. 9.5). Ammonia metabolism involves integrated function of multiple portions of the kidney. Only a minimal amount of urinary ammonia derives from glomerular filtration, making urinary ammonia excretion unique among the major compounds present in the urine. Instead, the kidney produces ammonia, which is then selectively transported either into the urine or the renal vein, where it is transported to the systemic circulation. Importantly, renal vein ammonia content exceeds arterial content, indicating the kidney is a net producer of ammonia, even when there is significant urinary ammonia excretion. Selective ammonia transport involves integrated transport in the proximal tubule, TAL of the loop of Henle, and the collecting duct (Fig. 9.7).

### AMMONIA CHEMISTRY

Ammonia exists in two molecular forms, $NH_3$ and $NH_4^+$. The relative amounts of each are governed by the buffer reaction: $NH_3 + H^+ \leftrightarrow NH_4^+$. This reaction occurs essentially instantaneously and has a $pK_a$ under biologically relevant conditions of ~9.15. Accordingly, the majority of ammonia is present as $NH_4^+$; at pH 7.4 only ~1.7% is present as $NH_3$. Because most biological fluids exist at a pH substantially below this pKa', small changes in pH cause exponential changes in $NH_3$ concentration, but almost no change in $NH_4^+$ concentration (Fig. 9.8).

$NH_3$, although uncharged, has an asymmetric arrangement of positively charged hydrogen nuclei around a central nitrogen; this results in significant polarity (Fig. 9.9). As a consequence, $NH_3$ has limited lipid permeability. Consequently, diffusion across plasma membranes is limited, and $NH_3$ transporters both accelerate $NH_3$ transport and provide important regulatory control.

$NH_4^+$ also has limited permeability across lipid bilayers in the absence of specific transport proteins. However, in aqueous solutions $NH_4^+$ and $K^+$ have nearly identical biophysical characteristics, which enables $NH_4^+$ to be transported at the $K^+$-transport site of essentially all $K^+$ transporters.[453] Several $Na^+/H^+$ exchanger (NHE) family members also appear to transport $NH_4^+$ at the $H^+$ binding site, resulting in $Na^+/NH_4^+$ exchange activity.

### AMMONIA PRODUCTION

Almost all renal epithelial cells can produce ammonia, but the proximal tubule is the primary site for physiologically relevant ammoniagenesis.[143] The renal isoform of glutaminase (KGA), also known as phosphate-dependent glutaminase (PDG), is involved in this process.[91] The proximal tubule accounts for 60%–70% of total renal ammonia production under basal conditions and at least 70%–80% in response to metabolic acidosis[143] (Fig. 9.10).

Although multiple pathways for ammoniagenesis are present in the proximal tubule (Fig. 9.11), the predominant pathway involves PDG.[92,461] PDG is an inner mitochondrial membrane-bound enzyme that metabolizes glutamine to glutamate, producing $NH_4^+$. Glutamate then undergoes further metabolism through multiple pathways. The major pathways involve glutamate dehydrogenase (GDH) with production of α-ketoglutarate (α-KG, also known as 2-oxoglutarate) and release of $NH_4^+$. GDH-mediated metabolism is regulated in parallel with changes in total renal ammoniagenesis. Because glutamate is a negative regulator of PDG activity, changes in GDH activity, by changing mitochondrial glutamate levels, indirectly regulates PDG functional activity.

Glutamate can be converted back to glutamine via the enzyme glutamine synthetase. This reaction uses $NH_4^+$ as a cosubstrate, decreasing net $NH_4^+$ formation. Glutamine synthetase is expressed in the proximal tubule and in intercalated cells, and its expression decreases in response to metabolic acidosis[88,226] and, in the proximal tubule, with hypokalemia.[422] Dietary protein restriction, which decreases ammonia excretion, increases glutamine synthetase expression, likely resulting in increased ammonia recycling and thereby

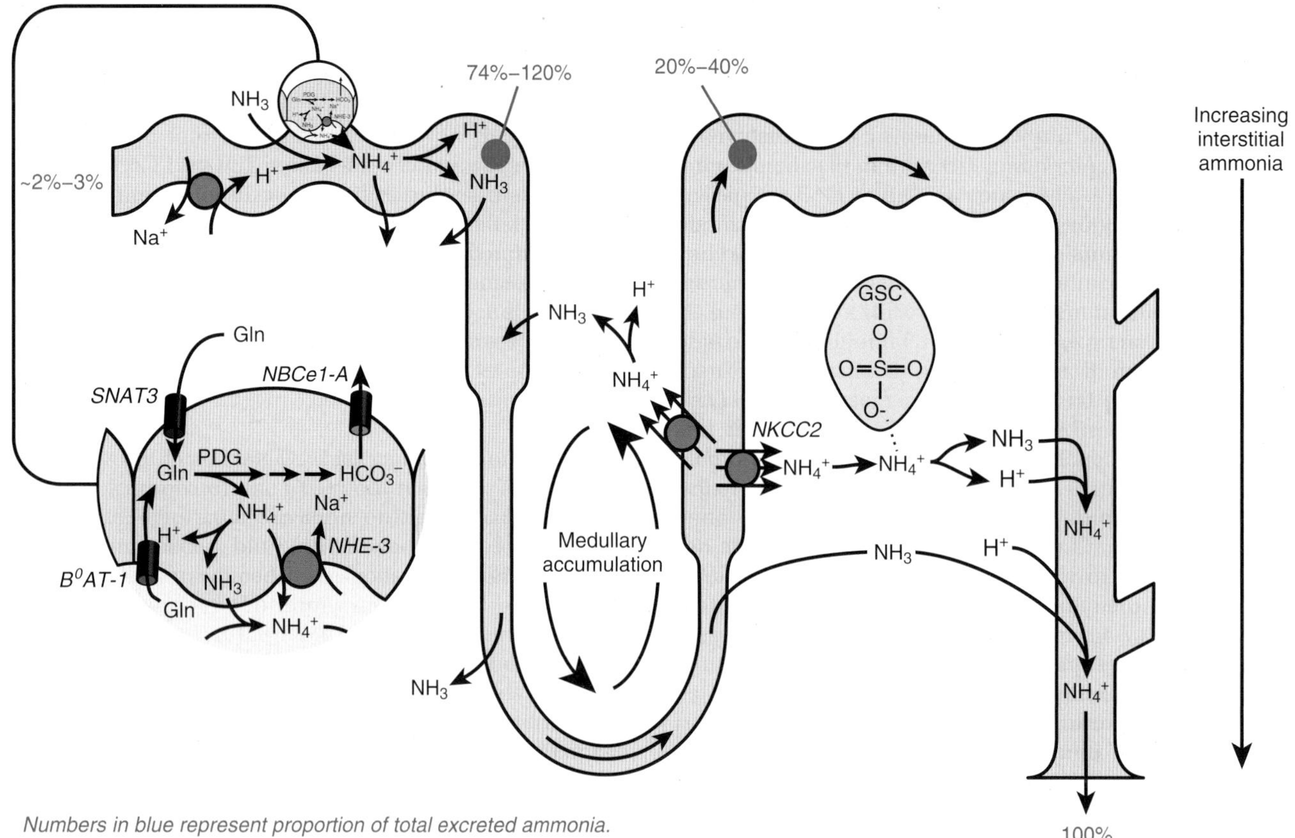


**Fig. 9.7** Integrated overview of renal ammonia metabolism. Renal ammoniagenesis occurs primarily in the proximal tubule, involving glutamine uptake by SNAT3 (SN1) and $B^0AT$-1, glutamine metabolism forming ammonium and bicarbonate, and apical $NH_4^+$ secretion involving NHE3 and parallel $H^+$ and $NH_3$ transport. Ammonia reabsorption in the thick ascending limb, involving apical NKCC2-mediated uptake, results in medullary ammonia accumulation. Medullary sulfatides (*highlighted in green*) reversibly bind $NH_4^+$, contributing to medullary accumulation. Ammonia is secreted in the collecting duct via parallel $H^+$ and $NH_3$ secretion. Numbers in blue represent the proportion of total excreted ammonia at each location. *GSC*, Galactosylceramide backbone.

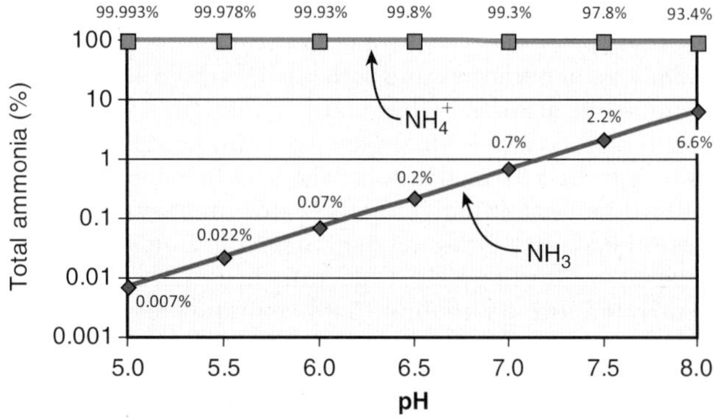


**Fig. 9.8** Relative changes in $NH_3$ and $NH_4^+$ concentration as pH changes. $NH_3$ and $NH_4^+$ contributions to total ammonia were determined from the buffer reaction, $NH_3 + H^+ \leftrightarrow NH_4^+$. A $pK_a$ of 9.15 was used for calculations. Amounts shown are proportion of total ammonia present as $NH_3$ and $NH_4^+$. Note that the *y*-axis log transformed. Reprinted from Weiner ID, JW Verlander. Renal ammonia metabolism and transport. *Compr. Physiol.* 2013;3:201–220 with permission.

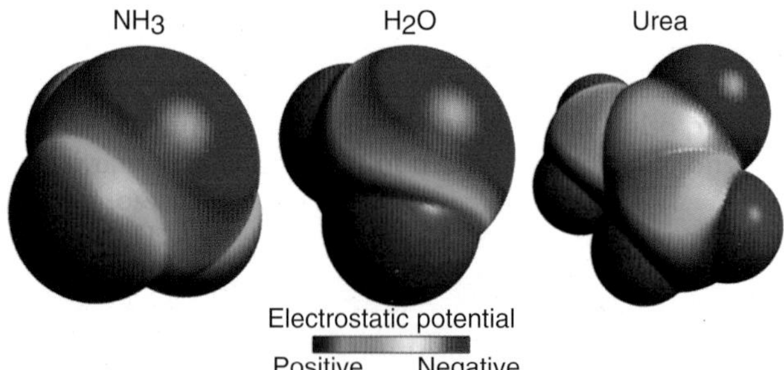


**Fig. 9.9** Electrostatic charge distribution in $NH_3$, $H_2O$, and urea molecules. Models of $NH_3$, $H_2O$, and urea showing space-filling representation and surface pseudocolored to show surface charge. Each molecule, although an uncharged molecule, is polar. This polarity results in limited permeability across plasma membranes. Models generated using Avogadro software (Avogadro Chemistry, Inc.) v1.0.3.

diminishing net ammoniagenesis. Proximal tubule-specific glutamine synthetase deletion blunts the decrease in ammonia excretion in response to dietary protein restriction.[227] Thus, glutamine synthetase–mediated ammonia recycling, which exhibits regulation counter to that of PDG in conditions that alter ammonia excretion, is an important component of renal ammonia metabolism.

α-KG can be metabolized through α-KG dehydrogenase and succinate dehydrogenase to form oxaloacetic acid (OAA). OAA can serve as a substrate for phosphoenolpyruvate carboxykinase (PEPCK) to form phosphoenolpyruvate (PEP), which can be used as a substrate for gluconeogenesis.

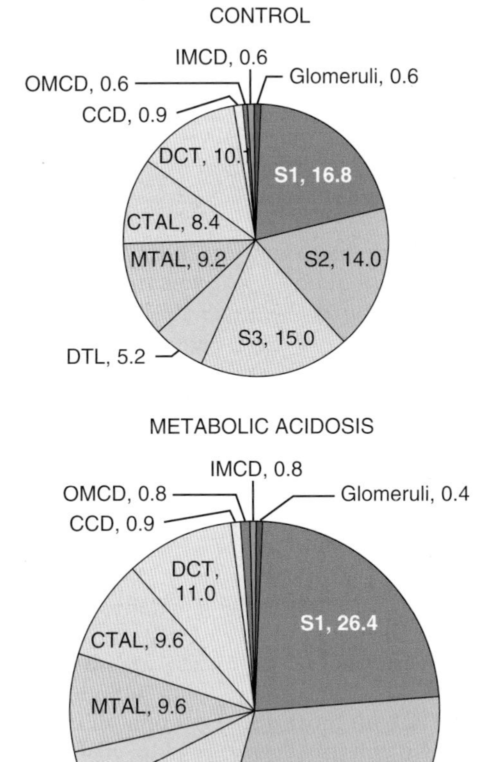


**Fig. 9.10** Ammonia production in various renal segments. Ammonia production rates in different renal components measured in microdissected components from rats on control diets and after inducing metabolic acidosis. All segments tested produced ammonia. Metabolic acidosis increases total renal ammoniagenesis, but only through increased production in proximal tubule segments (S1, S2, and S3). Rates (pmol/mm) were calculated from measured ammonia production rates and mean length per segment as described in Good and Burg.[143] The size of the pie graph is proportional to total renal ammoniagenesis rates. *CCD,* Cortical collecting duct; *CTAL*, cortical thick ascending limb of Henle loop; *DCT*, distal convoluted tubule; *DTL*, descending thin limb of Henle loop; *IMCD*, inner medullary collecting duct; *MTAL,* medullary thick ascending limb of Henle loop; *OMCD,* outer medullary collecting duct.

Conditions that increase ammonia increase flux through this pathway and stimulate renal gluconeogenesis. Alternatively, PEP can be converted to pyruvate in an ATP-dependent reaction by pyruvate kinase. Pyruvate can then enter the TCA cycle, where its metabolism leads to ATP generation. The net result is that complete glutamine metabolism results in production of 2 $NH_4^+$ and 2 $HCO_3^-$ molecules per glutamine molecule in association with a variable extent of glucose production. Conversion of PEP to pyruvate with subsequent entry into the TCA cycle results in more ATP production than utilization of PEP for gluconeogenesis.[458]

## GLUTAMINE TRANSPORT IN AMMONIAGENESIS

Glutamine is the primary substrate for renal ammoniagenesis. Under normal acid–base balance conditions, the kidneys extract less than 3% of the glutamine present in arterial blood flow to the kidneys. Acute metabolic acidosis induces a rapid, ~twofold increase in plasma glutamine levels; this results primarily from increased skeletal muscle and hepatic glutamine release.[390] In parallel, renal glutamine uptake increases to as much as 20% of delivered glutamine.[182,390] With chronic metabolic acidosis, renal extraction can increase to as much as 50% of delivered glutamine.[182] Because glutamine uptake can exceed filtered glutamine, the presence of and ability to increase basolateral glutamine uptake is an important component of the regulation of ammoniagenesis.

Filtered glutamine is almost completely reabsorbed in the PCT.[366] Multiple glutamine transporters are expressed in the apical membrane in the proximal tubule, including the $Na^+$-dependent neutral amino acid transporters $B^0AT1$ (SLC6A19) and $B^0AT3$ (SLC6A18). Under basal conditions, luminal glutamine reabsorbed in the proximal tubule not used for ammoniagenesis can be transported across the basolateral plasma membrane. This appears to involve LAT2-4F2hc (SLC7A8-SLC3A2) and $Y^+LAT1$-4F2hc (SLC7A7-SLC3A2).[29,308,337] LAT2-4F2hc and $Y^+LAT1$-4F2hc are obligatory amino acid exchangers, and the amino acid transported into the cell likely exits via basolateral TAT1 (Slc16a10), a facilitated aromatic amino acid transporter.[29,325,326]

Basolateral glutamine uptake into proximal tubule cells appears to occur through the $Na^+$-coupled, neutral amino acid transporter, SN1 (SLC38A3, also known as SNAT3).[196] Under basal conditions, basolateral SN1 is detectable only in the S3 proximal tubule segments, conditions that increase ammoniagenesis, such as metabolic acidosis and hypokalemia, increase S3 segment expression and induce expression in the S2 proximal tubule segment.[62,269]

Because the initial enzyme involved in ammonia, PDG, is a mitochondrial enzyme, glutamine movement across the mitochondrial membrane is necessary. This process involves a specific transporter-mediated mechanism, is trans-stimulated and cis-inhibited by alanine, and is stimulated by metabolic acidosis.[348] The gene and the gene product that mediate this activity are unknown at present.

## AMMONIA TRANSPORT

Ammonia produced in the proximal tubule is secreted preferentially into the tubule lumen. Preferential apical secretion is due to multiple factors, including NHE3-mediated $Na^+/NH_4^+$ exchange and luminal acidification, which facilitates “trapping” of secreted $NH_3$ as $NH_4^+$.[275,368] However, a recent study examining the effect of proximal tubule NHE3 deletion on acid–base homeostasis found no alteration in renal ammonia excretion.[238]

The proximal tubule also can reabsorb luminal ammonia; this appears to occur primarily in the late proximal tubule.[160] These portions of the proximal tubule express glutamine synthetase, which catalyzes the reaction of $NH_4^+$ with glutamate to form glutamine.[57] Metabolic acidosis converts late proximal tubule ammonia transport from net reabsorption to net secretion[160]; the molecular mechanisms that underlie this conversion involve decreased glutamine synthetase–mediated $NH_4^+$ metabolism.[88,329]

The TAL reabsorbs luminal ammonia. The apical $Na^+$-$K^+$-$2Cl^-$ cotransporter, NKCC2, mediates the majority of ammonia reabsorption.[19] Metabolic acidosis increases both TAL ammonia reabsorption and NKCC2 expression.[20] Intracellular

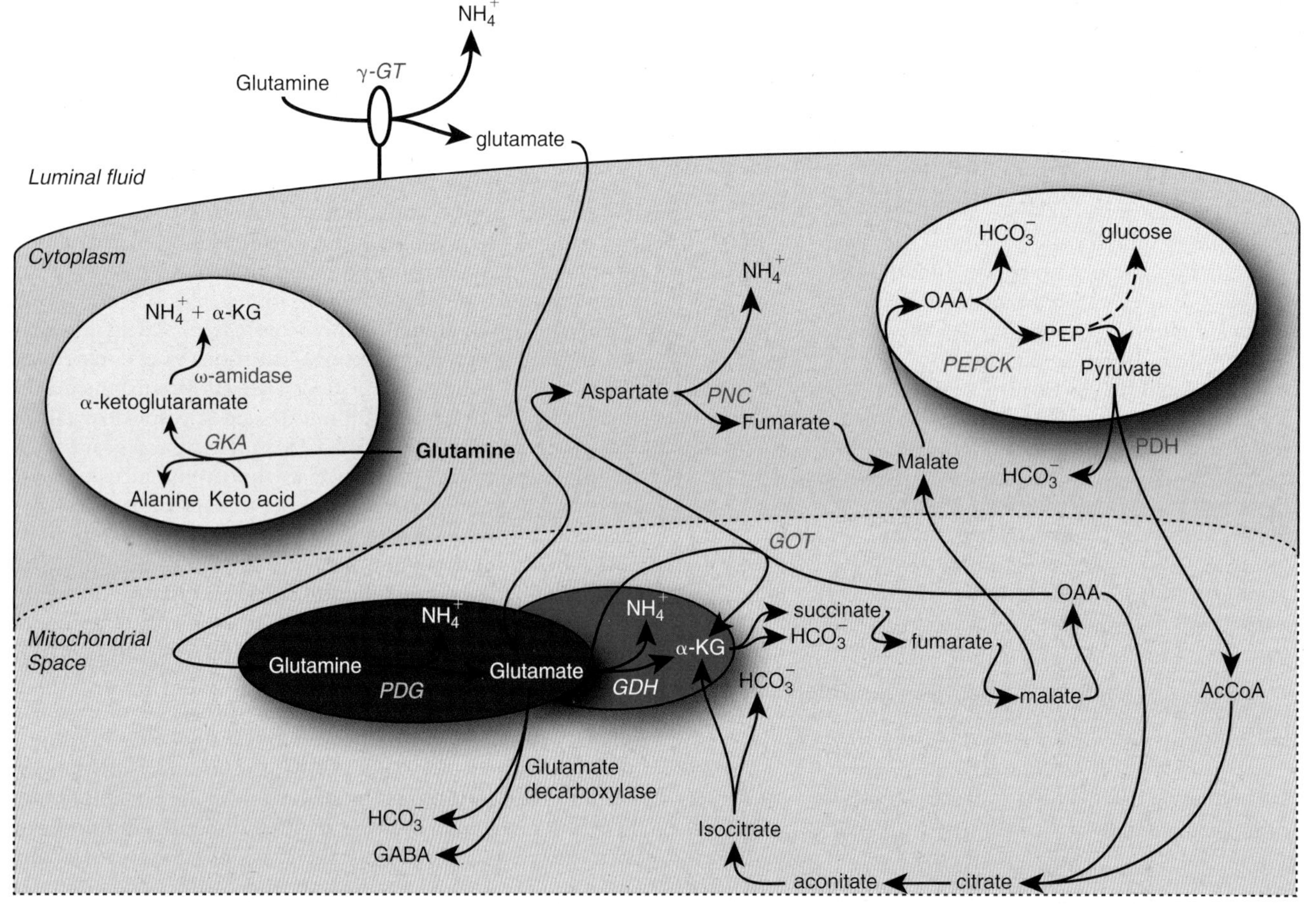


**Fig. 9.11** Mechanisms of ammoniagenesis. Multiple pathways for enzymatic ammonia production originating from glutamine metabolism are present in the proximal tubule. Glutamine metabolism through PDG and GDH and involving PEPCK is the quantitatively most significant component of renal ammoniagenesis and is the primary pathway stimulated in response to metabolic acidosis. *GDH*, Glutamate dehydrogenase; *PDG*, phosphate-dependent glutaminase; *PEPCK*, phosphoenolpyruvate carboxykinase. Reprinted from Weiner ID, JW Verlander. Renal ammonia metabolism and transport. *Compr. Physiol.* 2013:201–2013 with permission.

$NH_4^+$ can dissociate into $NH_3$ and $H^+$, resulting in intracellular acidification. One major mechanism of ammonia exit across the basolateral plasma membrane involves basolateral $NH_4^+$ transport involves NHE4-mediated $Na^+/NH_4^+$ exchange activity.[50,461] In addition, $NH_4^+$ transported into the cell by NKCC2 can dissociate into $NH_3$ and $H^+$. $NH_3$ appears to exit across the basolateral plasma membrane via an unidentified mechanism. Basolateral $HCO_3^-$ entry via the electroneutral sodium–bicarbonate cotransporter, isoform 1 (NBCn1, SLC4A7), enables buffering of the released $H^+$, preventing development of progressive intracellular acidosis, and facilitating continued ammonia transport.[189,233]

Some of the ammonia absorbed by the medullary TAL undergoes recycling into the thin descending limb of the loop of Henle. This results in counter current amplification of medullary interstitial ammonia concentration. Ammonia recycling predominantly involves $NH_3$ transport, with a smaller component of $NH_4^+$ transport.[118]

The net effect of ammonia absorption by the TAL of the loop of Henle and passive ammonia secretion into the thin descending limb of the loop of Henle is development of an axial ammonia concentration gradient that parallels the hypertonicity gradient. Moreover, ammonia absorption by the medullary TAL results in ammonia delivery to the distal tubule accounting for only ~20%–40% of final urinary ammonia content.[104,159] Thus, tubule segments farther downstream secrete the majority of ammonia excreted by the kidneys.

There is likely to be a small component of ammonia secretion in the regions of the distal tubule prior to the CCD (i.e., the DCT, CNT, and ICT). Studies in the rat show ammonia secretion in the micropuncturable distal tubule could account for ~10%–15% of ammonia excretion.[367,471]

Collecting duct ammonia secretion involves the integrated function of several proteins (Fig. 9.12). Several studies of the CCD, OMCD, and the IMCD have shown that collecting duct ammonia secretion involves parallel $NH_3$ and $H^+$ transport, with little-to-no transepithelial $NH_4^+$ permeability.[104,206] $H^+$ secretion likely involves both $H^+$-ATPase and $H^+$-$K^+$-ATPase. Carbonic anhydrase is necessary for ammonia secretion, probably through a role in supplying cytosolic $H^+$ for secretion.[430] Transepithelial ammonia secretion involves both basolateral uptake and apical secretion, and specific proteins are involved in each process.

The primary basolateral ammonia transporters involved in ammonia secretion appear to differ depending on the

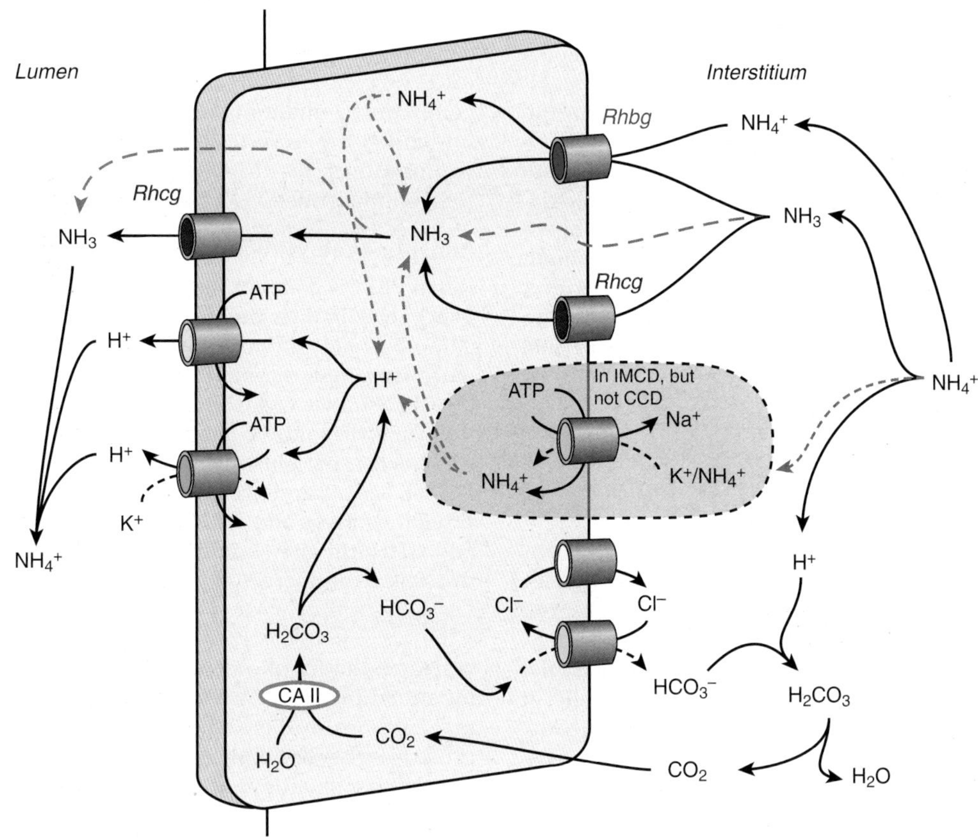


**Fig. 9.12** Mechanisms of collecting duct ammonia secretion. Rhbg and Rhcg likely both contribute to basolateral ammonia uptake. As described in the text, whether Rhbg transports ammonia in the molecular form of $NH_4^+$ or $NH_3$, or even both, remains controversial, but the likely electrochemical gradients result in uptake of both ammonia molecular species across the basolateral membrane. Rhcg mediates electroneutral $NH_3$ uptake across the basolateral plasma membrane. $NH_3$ is then secreted across the apical plasma membrane down its electrochemical gradient through processes involving both apical Rhcg transport and through a separate, undefined mechanism that may reflect lipid-phase diffusion. $H^+$ ions are secreted across the apical plasma membrane by both $H^+$-ATPase and $H^+$-$K^+$-ATPase. Cytoplasmic $H^+$ is supplied either by dissociation of $NH_4^+$ or via a carbonic anhydrase II *(CA II)*-dependent bicarbonate shuttle mechanism involving basolateral chloride–bicarbonate exchange and basolateral chloride channel—mediated bicarbonate shuttling. Also shown is $NH_4^+$ uptake by basolateral $Na^+$-$K^+$-ATPase, which contributes to ammonia secretion in the IMCD where the majority of cells do not express Rh glycoproteins. *IMCD*, Inner medullary collecting duct.

collecting duct location. In the CCD and OMCD, the Rhesus glycoproteins, Rhbg (SLC42A2) and Rhcg (SLC42A3), appear to be the primary transport mechanisms. A hyperpolarization-activated cyclic nucleotide-gated HCN2 channel may also enable basolateral $NH_4^+$ uptake.[71] In the IMCD basolateral $Na^+$-$K^+$-ATPase contributes to basolateral $NH_4^+$ uptake.[428,429,438] In contrast, in the CCD inhibiting $Na^+$-$K^+$-ATPase does not alter ammonia secretion, suggesting either that it is uninvolved in ammonia secretion in this region of the collecting duct or that other transport mechanisms compensate when it is inhibited.[207] Another possible $NH_4^+$ transport mechanism involves NKCC1. Basolateral NKCC1, which can transport $NH_4^+$ at the $K^+$ binding site, is present in both OMCD intercalated cells and IMCD cells.[136,193] However, inhibiting NKCC1 does not alter OMCD ammonia secretion, suggesting either NKCC1 does not contribute to transepithelial ammonia secretion or that alternative transport mechanisms compensate in its absence.[430] There may also be a component of $NH_3$-gradient driven, diffusive $NH_3$ uptake, at least as has been identified in cultured IMCD cells.[165]

Apical ammonia secretion appears to occur only by $NH_3$ movement. The primary protein involved is Rhcg. In studies of CCD and OMCD from acid-loaded mice examined with in vitro microperfusion, Rhcg deletion decreased apical $NH_3$ transport by ~65%.[37] A significant component of the remaining $NH_3$ permeability may involve diffusive $NH_3$ transport.[166] Additionally, some studies have raised the possibility that, at least in response to dietary $K^+$ restriction, the colonic isoform of $H^+$-$K^+$-ATPase, HKα2, secretes $NH_4^+$.[282]

A substantial component of collecting duct ammonia secretion appears to involve cytosolic $HCO_3^-$ production by CA II. Studies using microperfused collecting duct segments show that inhibiting CA-II essentially abolishes ammonia secretion.[430] Presumably, CA II–mediated acceleration of the reaction

$$CO_2 + H_2O \xleftrightarrow{CA-II} H_2CO_3 \leftrightarrow H^+ + HCO_3^-$$

provides the $H^+$ needed for the apical $H^+$ secretion. The $HCO_3^-$ is transported across the basolateral plasma membrane, in most cases likely by a basolateral $Cl^-/HCO_3^-$ exchanger. This results either in the generation of "new" $HCO_3^-$ or, if cytosolic $NH_3$ resulted from basolateral $NH_3$ uptake, buffering of the $H^+$ released from $NH_4^+$ as a result of the decrease in peritubular $NH_3$ concentration.

The absence or presence of carbonic anhydrase activity at the apical membrane also impacts collecting duct ammonia secretion. In the absence of luminal carbonic anhydrase, $H^+$ secretion increases the luminal [$H^+$] above equilibrium because of relatively slow spontaneous dehydration of $H_2CO_3$ to $CO_2$ and $H_2O$. This is termed a luminal "disequilibrium pH." This increased luminal acidification shifts the $H^+ + NH_3 \leftrightarrow NH_4^+$ reaction toward $NH_4^+$, thereby decreasing luminal [$NH_3$]. The decreased luminal [$NH_3$] increases the gradient for $NH_3$ secretion and increases net ammonia secretion. A luminal disequilibrium pH has been found and shown to accelerate ammonia secretion in the rat OMCD and terminal IMCD[119,432] and in the rabbit CCD and OMCDo,[207,376,377] but not in the rabbit OMCDi.[376]

## SPECIFIC PROTEINS INVOLVED IN RENAL AMMONIA METABOLISM

### Phosphate-Dependent Glutaminase

PDG is the initial enzymatic step in renal ammoniagenesis. It is located in mitochondria and catalyzes the reaction, L-glutamine + $H_2O \rightarrow$ L-glutamate + $NH_4^+$. In the kidney, PDG activity is found primarily in the proximal tubule, although a lesser degree of activity is found in essentially all renal epithelial cells.[91,197,477] The physiologic role of this activity outside of the proximal tubule is unclear. Some studies have found that metabolic acidosis increases PDG activity in the DTL, mTAL in the outer stripe, and DCT,[197] whereas others have found no change in activity in sites other than the proximal tubule.[477] Quantitative analyses suggest that the proximal tubule is the primary site of ammonia production, and accounts for the majority of the increase in ammoniagenesis with metabolic acidosis.[92,461]

Multiple PDG isoforms exist. In humans, the gene for the kidney-type isoform gives rise to at least two transcripts, human kidney-type glutaminase (KGA) and the glutaminase C splice variant (GAC).[255] A separate gene gives rise to a liver-type glutaminase isoform (LGA). The KGA protein is expressed ubiquitously in the kidney, including the renal proximal tubule, and is the source of the majority of renal PDG.

Metabolic acidosis increases proximal tubule PDG activity; these increases derive from multiple mechanisms. There is increased protein expression, and this appears to be transcriptionally mediated.[396,397] The increase in PDG mRNA results from mRNA stabilization, not increased transcription rates.[185] A second regulatory mechanism likely involves changes in intra-mitochondrial glutamate. Glutamate is a competitive inhibitor of PDG,[360] and decreases in intra-mitochondrial glutamate concentration, which occur during metabolic acidosis as a consequence of increased glutamate dehydrogenase activity, increase PDG activity.[3]

### Glutamate Dehydrogenase (GDH)

GDH is a mitochondrial enzyme that catalyzes the reaction, L-glutamate + $H_2O$ + $NAD^+$ (or $NADP^+$) $\rightarrow \alpha\text{-KG}^{-2} + NH_4^+ +$ NADH (or NADPH) + $H^+$. Two GDH isoforms exist and are products of two different genes; GLUD1 is widely expressed, including in the kidney, whereas GLUD2 appears to be a neural and testicular-specific isoform.[257,361]

Metabolic acidosis stimulates renal GDH activity,[476] both by altering its affinity for glutamate and by increasing protein and mRNA (GLUD1) expression.[3,90,93] Acidosis also decreases intramitochondrial α-ketoglutarate (α-KG) concentration, which contributes to increased GDH activity.[360] Decreased α-KG accelerates GDH activity by relieving α-KG–mediated competitive inhibition of the enzymatic reaction and by inhibiting the reverse reaction.[349,350] Changes in mRNA expression occur through changes in mRNA stability, not transcription rate.[192]

### Phosphoenolpyruvate Carboxykinase (PEPCK)

Renal PEPCK is a cytosolic enzyme that is the product of the PCK1 gene. In the kidney, as in extrarenal sites, including liver, adipose tissue, and small intestine, PEPCK is a key enzyme in gluconeogenesis through its role in conversion of oxaloacetate into PEP and $CO_2$. It also mediates an important role in the renal response to metabolic acidosis,[58] coincident with increased renal gluconeogenesis. The adaptive increase in PEPCK activity and protein expression result from increased protein synthesis and mRNA expression.[90] In contrast to PDG and GDH, the increased PEPCK mRNA expression appears to result from increased gene transcription.[169]

### γ-GT

γ-GT accounts for phosphate-independent glutaminase activity identified in many early enzymatic studies of renal ammoniagenesis. However, γ-GT is expressed primarily in the proximal straight tubule (PST),[91] and micropuncture studies suggest that glutamine is completely reabsorbed in the PCT, making PST ammoniagenesis via γ-GT unlikely to contribute significantly to renal ammoniagenesis.

### NHE3

Multiple lines of evidence suggest that the apical $Na^+/H^+$ exchanger, NHE3, secretes $NH_4^+$ through binding of $NH_4^+$ at the $H^+$ binding site. These data include evidence that proximal tubule brush border membrane vesicles exhibit $NH_4^+/Na^+$ exchange activity;[204] that combining a low luminal $Na^+$ concentration with $Na^+/H^+$ exchange inhibitor, amiloride, decreases ammonia secretion;[274] and that the $Na^+/H^+$ exchange inhibitor, EIPA, blunts ammonia secretion when alternative secretory pathways are blocked.[368] Against a role of NHE3 in ammonia secretion, however, is that proximal tubule–specific NHE3 deletion does not alter either basal or acidosis-stimulated ammonia excretion.[238]

Changes in NHE3 expression and activity during metabolic acidosis may be an important component of ammonia regulation and may be regulated by AngII and ET-1. Specific studies show that NHE3 expression and activity parallel changes in ammonia secretion in response to chronic metabolic acidosis, changes in extracellular potassium and exposure to AngII.[16,110,276,280] In S2 and S3 segments, chronic metabolic acidosis increases AT1 receptor–mediated stimulation of NHE3.[277,278,281] ET-1 expression increases during metabolic acidosis and subsequent activation of the ET-B receptor increases NHE3 expression and renal ammonia excretion.[222]

NHE3 is also present in the apical plasma membrane of the TAL. However, because NHE3 secretes $NH_4$,$^+$ and the TAL reabsorbs $NH_4$,$^+$ NHE3 appears unlikely to mediate an important role in loop of Henle ammonia transport.

## POTASSIUM CHANNELS

At a molecular level, $K^+$ and $NH_4^+$ have nearly identical biophysical characteristics. This enables essentially all $K^+$

transporters to also transport $NH_4^+$, albeit at transport rates that are often 10%–20% of that observed for $K^+$.[453] The primary evidence that apical $K^+$ channels contribute to proximal tubule ammonia transport comes from in vitro microperfusion studies showing that barium, a nonspecific $K^+$ channel inhibitor, inhibits proximal tubule ammonia transport.[368] Multiple $K^+$ channels are present in the apical plasma membrane of the proximal tubule, including KCNA10, TWIK-1, and KCNQ1; it is not known currently which of these mediates ammonia transport. In the TAL, $K^+$ channels can contribute to luminal $NH_4^+$ uptake when apical $Na^+$-$K^+$-$2Cl^-$ cotransport is inhibited.[19] However, NKCC2 inhibitors completely inhibit TAL ammonia transport, suggesting that apical $K^+$ channels are unlikely to mediate a quantitatively important role in TAL ammonia transport.[142]

### $Na^+$-$K^+$-$2Cl^-$ Cotransport

NKCC1 (SLC12A2), also known as $Na^+$-$K^+$-$2Cl^-$ cotransporter, isoform 1, is present in the basolateral plasma membrane of intercalated cells in the OMCD and IMCD and in IMCD cells.[83,136,193] However pharmacologic inhibitors do not alter either OMCD ammonia secretion or IMCD basolateral ammonia uptake.[429,430] Thus, NKCC1 appears unlikely to mediate a substantial role in ammonia secretion.

NKCC2 (SLC12A1), also known as $Na^+$-$K^+$-$2Cl^-$ cotransporter, isoform 2, is a kidney-specific isoform expressed in the apical plasma membrane of the TAL and is the major mechanism for ammonia reabsorption in the TAL of the loop of Henle.[142] Luminal $NH_4^+$ competes for binding with $K^+$ to the $K^+$-transport site, enabling alterations in luminal $K^+$ in hypokalemia and in hyperkalemia to alter net $NH_4^+$ transport and leading to alterations in medullary interstitial ammonia concentration in conditions of altered potassium homeostasis. Metabolic acidosis increases NKCC2 expression, which likely contributes to the increased ammonia reabsorption observed.[20,138] Acidosis-induced increases in glucocorticoid levels appear to mediate increased NKCC2 expression and activity.[21]

### $Na^+$-$K^+$-ATPase

$Na^+$-$K^+$-ATPase is present in the basolateral plasma membrane of essentially all renal epithelial cells. $NH_4^+$ binds to and is transported at the $K^+$-binding site, enabling $Na^+$ for $NH_4^+$ exchange.[218,434] In the IMCD, $Na^+$-$K^+$-ATPase-mediated basolateral $NH_4^+$ uptake is critical for IMCD ammonia and acid secretion.[218,434] Decreases in interstitial $K^+$ levels during hypokalemia facilitate increased basolateral $NH_4^+$ uptake by $Na^+$-$K^+$-ATPase, and contribute to increased $NH_4^+$ secretion rates.[431] In the CCD, in contrast, basolateral $Na^+$-$K^+$-ATPase does not appear to contribute to CCD ammonia secretion.[207]

### $H^+$-$K^+$-ATPase

$H^+$-$K^+$-ATPase proteins are members of the P-type ATPase family and transport $NH_4^+$. The majority of evidence suggests $NH_4^+$ is transported at the $K^+$ binding site, such that these proteins mediate $H^+/NH_4^+$ exchange. Thus, $H^+$-$K^+$-ATPase is unlikely to contribute to collecting duct ammonia secretion. However, potassium deficiency increases expression of the colonic $H^+$-$K^+$-ATPase and it has been postulated that this mediates increased $NH_4^+$ secretion via transport at the $H^+$ binding site.[282]

### Aquaporins

$H_2O$ and $NH_3$ have a similar molecular size and charge distribution. This has led to several studies examining whether aquaporin water channels transport $NH_3$. These studies have demonstrated that some, but not all, aquaporin-family members can transport ammonia. Table 9.1 summarizes the results of these studies. With the exception of AQP8, discussed later, experimental evidence regarding the role of these proteins in renal ammonia metabolism is not available.

Substantial evidence, but not without a degree of controversy, indicates that AQP8 contributes to renal ammonia metabolism. It is found in intracellular sites in the proximal tubule, CCD, and OMCD in the kidney, but not the plasma membrane.[111] The majority of ammonia generation occurs inside mitochondria in the proximal tubule. Thus, ammonia must be transported from mitochondria to cytoplasm. Several studies using heterologous expression show AQP8 can transport ammonia[132,175,243,344] and it is able to complement ammonia transport defects in yeast lacking endogenous ammonia transporters.[188] In cultured proximal tubule cells, AQP8 is located in the inner mitochondrial membrane and AQP8 knockdown decreases ammonia secretion.[268] In vivo, metabolic acidosis increases AQP8 expression.[268] All of these findings suggest AQP8 has an important role in proximal tubule mitochondrial ammonia transport. However, studies examining mice with AQP8 gene deletion found normal ammonia excretion, under basal conditions and following acute or chronic acid loading.[480]

## CARBONIC ANHYDRASE

Carbonic anhydrase, in addition to its role in bicarbonate reabsorption, also contributes to ammonia secretion. Direct studies have shown that carbonic anhydrase inhibition, presumably through effects on CA II, blocks OMCD ammonia secretion.[430] Fig. 9.12 shows the putative role of cytoplasmic CA II in facilitating transepithelial ammonia secretion.

CA IV, although functioning to increase bicarbonate reabsorption, likely decreases collecting duct ammonia secretion because it prevents a luminal disequilibrium pH. Apical CA IV expression has been demonstrated in the

**Table 9.1 Ammonia Transport by Aquaporins**

| Aquaporin | Finding | Citation |
|---|---|---|
| AQP1 | $NH_3$ transport | 132, 285 |
| | No transport | 175 |
| AQP2 | No transport | 132 |
| AQP3 | $NH_3$ transport | 132 |
| | Both $NH_3$ and $NH_4^+$ transport | 175 |
| AQP4 | No transport | 132, 273 |
| AQP5 | No transport | 132, 273 |
| AQP6 | $NH_3$ transport | 132 |
| AQP7 | $NH_3$ transport | 132 |
| AQP8 | $NH_3$ transport | 132, 344 |
| | Both $NH_3$ and $NH_4^+$ transport | 175 |
| | Transport present, $NH_3$ vs. $NH_4^+$ not differentiated | 243 |
| AQP9 | $NH_3$ transport | 132 |
| | $NH_3$ and $NH_4^+$ transport | 175 |
| AQP0 | No transport | 132 |

rabbit CCD type A intercalated cell, in the rabbit OMCD and IMCD,[356] in the human CCD and OMCD,[246] but not in the rat collecting duct.[53] This pattern is inconsistent with evidence of luminal disequilibrium pH in the rat CCD and OMCD,[119,208] but is consistent with the evidence of luminal disequilibrium pH in the rabbit CCD and OMCD outer stripe segments.[376,377]

## Rh GLYCOPROTEINS

Rh glycoproteins are mammalian orthologs of Mep/AMT proteins, ammonia transporter family proteins present in yeast, plants, bacteria, and many other organisms. Three mammalian Rh glycoproteins are known: Rh A glycoprotein (RhAG/Rhag), Rh B glycoprotein (RhBG/Rhbg), and Rh C glycoprotein (RhCG/Rhcg).

### Rhag/RhAG (SLC42A1)

Rhag is an essential component of the erythrocyte "Rhesus complex," which consists of Rhag in association with RhD and RhCE subunits in what appears to be a 1:1:1 stoichiometric ratio.[154] Rhag transports ammonia in the form of $NH_3$, whereas RhD and RhCE do not.[254,470] In humans, RhAG deficiency leads to $Rh_{null}$ disease, which is characterized by hemolytic anemia, spherocytosis, and lack of erythrocyte expression of RhAG, RhD, and RhCE.[180,469] Rhag protein is present in erythrocytes and in erythrocyte precursor cells present in the bone marrow and in rodent spleen, but does not appear to be expressed in nonerythroid tissues. In particular, Rhag is not found in the kidney, except in residual erythrocytes.[450,455]

### Rhbg/RhBG (SLC42A2)

Rhbg in the kidney is found exclusively in distal epithelial cell populations, with low-level basolateral expression in the DCT, and higher-level basolateral expression in the CNT, CCD, OMCD, and IMCD.[162,322,420] The CNT and the collecting duct have heterogeneous epithelial cell populations; type A and non-A, non-B intercalated cells, principal cells, and CNT cells express Rhbg, but expression is greater in intercalated cells. Type B intercalated cells do not express detectable Rhbg immunolabel. Although an initial study detected Rhbg mRNA but not Rhbg protein in the human kidney,[51] subsequent studies identified Rhbg protein expression in a pattern nearly identical to that observed in the studies of the rat and mouse kidney.[162]

The majority of evidence indicates that Rhbg contributes significantly to renal ammonia excretion during basal conditions and conditions that increase ammonia excretion. Intercalated cell-specific Rhbg deletion, while not altering ammonia excretion, induces adaptive changes in other enzymes involved in ammonia metabolism that appear to compensate for its absence, indicating a role for Rhbg under basal conditions.[36] Both metabolic acidosis and hypokalemia, common conditions associated with increased ammonia excretion, increase Rhbg protein expression, and genetic deletion of Rhbg from intercalated cells impairs changes in ammonia excretion in response to these stimuli.[35,36] However, a study that used a different method of acid loading, which produced less stimulation of ammonia excretion, found no effect of Rhbg deletion.[76] This suggests that other mechanisms can compensate for the lack of Rhbg, such as those identified by Bishop et al,[36] if only modest increases in ammonia

**Table 9.2 $NH_3$ and $NH_4^+$ Transport Characteristics of Rhbg and Rhcg**

| | Electroneutral | | Electrogenic | | |
|---|---|---|---|---|---|
| | $NH_3$ Transport | $CH_3NH_2$ transport | $NH_4^+$ Transport | $CH_3NH_3^+$ Transport | Citation |
| Rhbg | Absent | | Present | | 287 |
| | | Present | | Absent | 248 |
| | Present | | Absent | | 493 |
| | | Present | | Absent | 252 |
| | | Present | Present | Present | 283 |
| | Absent | Present | Present | Present | 286 |
| | Present | | | | 131 |
| | Present | | Present | | 65 |
| Rhcg | Present | | Present | | 24 |
| | | Present | | Absent | 493 |
| | | Present | | Absent | 252 |
| | | Present | | Absent | 258 |
| | | Present | | Absent | 37 |
| | | Present | | Absent | 271 |
| | Present | | Absent | | 154 |
| | Present | | Absent | | 48 |
| | Present | | | | 131 |
| | Absent | | Present | | 65 |

excretion are needed, whereas greater degrees of adaptation require Rhbg expression.

A number of studies have addressed the issue as to whether Rhbg transports $NH_3$, $NH_4^+$, or both, and have resulted in conflicting results. Table 9.2 summarizes these studies. The more recent studies suggest that Rhbg can transport both $NH_3$ and $NH_4^+$. The molecular mechanism through which $NH_4^+$ is transported has not been identified, but is likely to be a form of $NH_3$-$H^+$ cotransport rather than direct transport of the molecular species $NH_4^+$. Importantly, the electrochemical gradient across the basolateral plasma membrane is such that both electroneutral $NH_3$ transport and electrogenic $NH_4^+$ transport modes will result in ammonia transport from the interstitium into the cell cytoplasm.[462]

### Rhcg/RhCG

Rhcg is expressed in the kidney exclusively in epithelial cells of distal segments.[107,161,358,359,420] Rhcg expression is prominent in the CNT, ICT, CCD, OMCD, and IMCD, weakly expressed in late DCT cells, and exhibits both apical and basolateral expression.[161,199,358,359] Rhcg expression differs among renal epithelial cell types. In general, type A intercalated cells express higher levels of Rhcg than do principal cells. Rhcg is not detectable by immunohistochemistry in type B intercalated cells. In the CNT, non-A, non-B intercalated cells express apical Rhcg but have very little or no basolateral Rhcg immunolabel. IMCD cells do not express detectable Rhcg.

Rhcg has an important role in renal ammonia excretion in a wide variety of conditions, including basal acid–base homeostasis, metabolic acidosis, hypokalemia, and several other conditions. Gene deletion studies show that the absence of Rhcg impairs basal ammonia excretion.[37,224] Metabolic acidosis, hypokalemia, and high dietary protein intake increase Rhcg expression, and Rhcg expression is necessary for the normal increase in ammonia excretion.* In contrast to high dietary protein intake, during dietary protein restriction Rhcg expression is not needed for the decreased ammonia excretion that occurs.[225] With reduced renal mass there is increased single-nephron ammonia excretion, and this increase involves increased polarization of Rhcg to the apical and basolateral plasma membrane.[200] Cyclosporine A can induce renal tubular acidosis, and this involves altered Rhcg expression.[241] Aldosterone and chronic lithium administration increase renal ammonia excretion, and both are associated with increased Rhcg expression.[187,454] Finally, the critical role of Rhcg in collecting duct ammonia secretion has been shown in studies using in vitro microperfusion that show that Rhcg deletion, at least in CCD and OMCD from mice with chronic metabolic acidosis, impairs transepithelial ammonia secretion and impairs both apical and basolateral plasma membrane $NH_3$ transport.[37,48]

Rhcg expression appears to be regulated through a variety of mechanisms. There are changes in total protein expression in a variety of conditions, as detailed earlier. In metabolic acidosis, this increase is not associated with changes in steady-state mRNA expression, indicating at least a component of posttranscriptional regulation.[358] During a high protein diet there is a transient increase in Rhcg mRNA expression, indicating that there can also be a component of transcriptional regulation.[47] In addition, Rhcg is found in both the apical and basolateral plasma membrane and in subapical cytoplasmic vesicles, and changes in subcellular distribution and expression are a prominent component of the response to metabolic acidosis, hypokalemia, and reduced renal mass.[35,163,200,359]

Rhcg may regulate collecting duct ammonia secretion in part through effects on $H^+$-ATPase expression. Recent studies show that Rhcg and $H^+$-ATPase are located within the same cellular protein complex and that Rhcg may modulate $H^+$-ATPase activity and expression.[49] However, $H^+$-ATPase does not appear to affect Rhcg function. This mechanism may help to coordinate ammonia and proton secretion beyond physicochemical driving forces.

Multiple studies have addressed the molecular form of ammonia that Rhcg transports. Table 9.2 summarizes the results of these studies. Essentially all studies have found that Rhcg transports ammonia in the form of $NH_3$. This selective transport of $NH_3$ is critical for Rhcg to facilitate ammonia secretion across the apical plasma membrane in the collecting duct. Under normal conditions, the high luminal $NH_4^+$ concentrations present throughout the collecting duct in combination with intracellular electronegativity relative to the luminal fluid result in a substantial electrochemical gradient for electrogenic $NH_4^+$ transport from the lumen to the cytoplasm. Thus, if Rhcg were an electrogenic $NH_4^+$ transporter, it would facilitate collecting duct $NH_4^+$ reabsorption, and would be highly unlikely to contribute to collecting duct ammonia secretion.

#### $CO_2$ Transport by Rh Glycoproteins

Rhesus glycoproteins can transport molecules other than ammonia, specifically $CO_2$. Quantitative studies using human erythrocytes deficient in RhAG show that the absence of RhAG decreases $CO_2$ transport.[112,113] Studies using heterologous expression in *Xenopus* oocytes show all Rh glycoproteins can transport $CO_2$.[131,273] However, the physiologic role of Rhbg- or Rhcg-mediated $CO_2$ transport in the kidney is not clear. Intercalated cells use cytoplasmic $CO_2$ to generate, through a CA II-catalyzed process, the intracellular $H^+$ used for urinary acidification. Several studies using Rhbg and/or Rhcg deletion show that Rhbg and Rhcg expression are not necessary for urine acidification.† However, these studies cannot exclude the possibility of either altered intrarenal $CO_2$ concentrations, which enable diffusive $CO_2$ movement in the absence of Rhbg and Rhcg, or adaptive changes in other $CO_2$ transport mechanisms.

### SULFATIDES

Sulfatides, highly charged anionic glycosphingolipids, appear to have an important role in renal ammonia metabolism. Sulfatides can reversibly bind $NH_4^+$. They are expressed throughout the kidney, but levels are highest in the outer and inner medulla and metabolic acidosis increases medullary interstitial sulfatide content.[380] Sulfatides appear to have an important role in maintaining the high inner medullary ammonia and increase in urinary acid elimination that develop during metabolic acidosis. Disruption of renal sulfatide synthesis, by a genetic approach along the entire renal tubule, led to lower urinary pH accompanied by lower ammonium excretion.[380] After acid loading, mice deficient in renal sulfatide synthesis showed impaired ammonia excretion, decreased ammonia accumulation in the papilla, and chronic hyperchloremic metabolic acidosis.[380] Thus, sulfatides, likely through their ability to reversibly bind interstitial $NH_4^+$, have an important role in renal ammonia, handling, urinary acidification, and acid–base homeostasis.

## ACID–BASE SENSORS

Several studies have begun to elucidate the molecular mechanisms through which the kidney recognizes altered systemic pH. Candidate molecular sensors have included acid-/alkali-sensing receptors, tyrosine kinases, and bicarbonate-stimulated adenylyl cyclase.

### ACID-/ALKALI-SENSING RECEPTORS

#### GPR4

Several G-protein–coupled receptors are sensitive to extracellular pH, which results in pH-dependent intracellular cAMP or IP3 production.[249] Of these, GPR4 has been studied most extensively. It is expressed in the kidney, and GPR4 deletion results in mild metabolic acidosis, less acidic urine, and decreased ability to excrete an acid load.[386] In acid-loaded mice, GPR4 deletion blunted the ability to increase expression of the intercalated cell basolateral protein AE1, and it blunted the acidosis-induced increase in type A and decrease in type B cells that were detectable in the CCD.[385] Which renal cells express GPR4 has not been determined, but a preliminary report suggests that GPR4 is expressed in renal interstitial cells, not tubule epithelial cells.[267]

*References 37, 47, 224, 230, 358, and 359.

†References 36, 37, 76, 224, 229, 231.

### INSULIN RECEPTOR–RELATED RECEPTOR (InsR-RR)

InsR-RR is a member of the insulin receptor family and may have a role regulating collecting duct acid–base transport. It is found in the kidney in the basolateral plasma membrane of type B cell and non-A, non-B intercalated cells,[28] and is activated by alkaline pH.[99] InsR-RR–deficient mice express lower levels of pendrin and have decreased ability to excrete an alkali load.[99]

## KINASES

### Pyk2/ETB RECEPTOR PATHWAY

The nonreceptor tyrosine kinase, Pyk2, may function as a pH sensor in renal epithelial cells.[239] In cultured proximal tubule cells, Pyk2 is activated by extracellular acidosis, and through activation of c-Src, leads to NHE3 activation.[239,400] A parallel pathway for proximal tubule NHE3 activation exists, involving ERK1/2 and c-fos activation, but does not involve Pyk2.[55] These two pathways both increase expression of the endothelin gene, ET-1, which in turn activates the ETB receptor and increases apical plasma membrane NHE3 expression.[313] In cultured OMCD cells, Pyk2 is required for acidosis-induced activation of $H^+$-ATPase through a signaling mechanism that involves the MAPK signaling pathway ERK1/2.[117]

### RECEPTOR TYROSINE KINASE

The proximal tubule responds to changes in peritubular $HCO_3^-$ and $CO_2$ with altered rates of luminal $HCO_3^-$ reabsorption. This activation involves a receptor tyrosine kinase, possibly a member of the ErbB family,[486] and may involve ErbB1/2 heterodimerization and activation of receptor tyrosine phosphatase-γ.[55] Acute acidosis increases tyrosine phosphorylation of ErbB1 and ErbB2, consistent with a role in a signaling cascade regulating $HCO_3^-$ reabsorption.[370]

## BICARBONATE-STIMULATED ADENYLYL CYCLASE

Another mechanism regulating renal acid–base homeostasis involves the soluble adenylyl cyclase (sAC). Its production of cAMP is directly stimulated by increases in cytoplasmic $HCO_3^-$,[81] and cAMP stimulates collecting duct $H^+$ secretion.[300] sAC is widely expressed in the kidney, including the TAL, DCT, and collecting duct.[298,299] In collecting duct intercalated cells, sAC colocalizes with $H^+$-ATPase in both the type A and type B intercalated cell and it coimmunoprecipitates with $H^+$-ATPase, implicating it in regulation of $H^+$ secretion.[299] In clear cells of the epididymis, used as a model system of collecting duct intercalated cells, sAC regulates apical $H^+$-ATPase expression through changes in cAMP production.[298] Changes in cAMP levels also alter the expression of pendrin protein in type B and non-A, non-B intercalated cells in cultured CCD and CNT.[393] Increased cAMP increases pendrin expression in these cells, whereas nitric oxide reduces pendrin expression through hydrolysis of intracellular cAMP.

# DIURNAL VARIATION IN ACID EXCRETION

There is a diurnal variation in renal acid excretion, which involves ammonia and titratable acid excretion and urine pH.[369] Circadian changes in NHE3 expression have been identified, particularly in the TAL in the outer medulla,[291] and are likely mediated by Clock and BMAL1 genes.[342] There are also circadian changes in ENaC expression,[332] which by altering luminal electronegativity may alter voltage-sensitive $H^+$ secretion and urine acidification. Diurnal variation in net acid excretion is altered in uric acid stone formers and may contribute to the pathogenesis of nephrolithiasis in this condition.[63]

## ACKNOWLEDGMENTS

The authors thank the many talented investigators with whom we have been fortunate to work; the superb mentors who have supported, encouraged, and enabled our scientific endeavors; and our wonderful spouses and families who have supported all aspects of our lives. The preparation of this chapter was supported by funds from NIH R01-DK-045788 and R01-DK107798.

 Complete reference list available at ExpertConsult.com.

## KEY REFERENCES

30. Baum M, Twombley K, Gattineni J, et al. Proximal tubule Na+/H+ exchanger activity in adult NHE8-/-, NHE3-/-, and NHE3-/-/NHE8-/- mice. *Am J Physiol Renal Physiol*. 2012;303:F1495–F1502.
36. Bishop JM, Verlander JW, Lee HW, et al. Role of the rhesus glycoprotein, Rh B glycoprotein, in renal ammonia excretion. *Am J Physiol Renal Physiol*. 2010;299:F1065–F1077.
37. Biver S, Belge H, Bourgeois S, et al. A role for Rhesus factor rhcg in renal ammonium excretion and male fertility. *Nature*. 2008;456:339–343.
38. Bobulescu IA, Moe OW. Luminal Na+/H+ exchange in the proximal tubule. *Pflugers Arch*. 2009;458:5–21.
41. Boettger T, Hubner CA, Maier H, et al. Deafness and renal tubular acidosis in mice lacking the K-CL co-transporter Kcc4. *Nature*. 2002;416:874–878.
50. Bourgeois S, Meer LV, Wootla B, et al. NHE4 is critical for the renal handling of ammonia in rodents. *J Clin Invest*. 2010;120:1895–1904.
52. Brown D, Hirsch S, Gluck SL. Localization of a proton-pumping ATPase in rat kidney. *J Clin Invest*. 1988;82:2114–2126.
54. Brown D, Paunescu TG, Breton S, et al. Regulation of the v-ATPase in kidney epithelial cells: dual role in acid-base homeostasis and vesicle trafficking. *J Exp Biol*. 2009;212:1762–1772.
62. Busque SM, Wagner CA. Potassium restriction, high protein intake, and metabolic acidosis increase expression of the glutamine transporter SNAT3 (Slc38a3) in mouse kidney. *Am J Physiol Renal Physiol*. 2009;297:F440–F450.
73. Chambrey R, Kurth I, Peti-Peterdi J, et al. Renal intercalated cells are rather energized by a proton than a sodium pump. *Proc Natl Acad Sci U S A*. 2013;110:7928–7933.
80. Chen L, Lee JW, Chou CL, et al. Transcriptomes of major renal collecting duct cell types in mouse identified by single-cell RNA-seq. *Proc Natl Acad Sci U S A*. 2017;114:E9989–E9998.
81. Chen Y, Cann MJ, Litvin TN, et al. Soluble adenylyl cyclase as an evolutionarily conserved bicarbonate sensor. *Science*. 2000;289:625–628.
84. Christensen BM, Kim YH, Kwon TH, et al. Lithium treatment induces a marked proliferation of primarily principal cells in rat kidney inner medullary collecting duct. *Am J Physiol Renal Physiol*. 2006;291:F39–F48.
92. Curthoys NP, Moe OW. Proximal tubule function and response to acidosis. *Clin J Am Soc Nephrol*. 2014;9:1627–1638.
97. de Brito-Ashurst I, Varagunam M, Raftery MJ, et al. Bicarbonate supplementation slows progression of CKD and improves nutritional status. *J Am Soc Nephrol*. 2009;20:2075–2084.
116. Finberg KE, Wagner CA, Bailey MA, et al. The B1-subunit of the H+ ATPase is required for maximal urinary acidification. *Proc Natl Acad Sci U S A*. 2005;102:13616–13621.
132. Geyer RR, Musa-Aziz R, Qin X, et al. Relative CO2/NH3 selectivities of mammalian aquaporins 0-9. *Am J Physiol Cell Physiol*. 2013;304:C985–C994.

154. Gruswitz F, Chaudhary S, Ho JD, et al. Function of human Rh based on structure of RhCG at 2.1 A. *Proc Natl Acad Sci U S A.* 2010;107:9638–9643.
155. Gumz ML, Lynch IJ, Greenlee MM, et al. The renal H+-K+-ATPases: physiology, regulation, and structure. *Am J Physiol Renal Physiol.* 2010;298:F12–F21.
167. Handlogten ME, Osis G, Lee HW, et al. NBCe1 expression is required for normal renal ammonia metabolism. *Am J Physiol Renal Physiol.* 2015;309:F658–F666.
186. Igarashi T, Inatomi J, Sekine T, et al. Mutations in SLC4a4 cause permanent isolated proximal renal tubular acidosis with ocular abnormalities. *Nat Genet.* 1999;23:264–266.
189. Jakobsen JK, Odgaard E, Wang W, et al. Functional up-regulation of basolateral Na+-dependent HCO3-transporter NBCn1 in medullary thick ascending limb of K+-depleted rats. *Pflugers Arch.* 2004;448:571–578.
195. Karet FE, Finberg KE, Nelson RD, et al. Mutations in the gene encoding B1 subunit of H+-ATPase cause renal tubular acidosis with sensorineural deafness. *Nat Genet.* 1999;21:84–90.
202. Kim WY, Nam S, Choi A, et al. Aquaporin 2-labeled cells differentiate to intercalated cells in response to potassium depletion. *Histochem Cell Biol.* 2016;145:17–24.
216. Kraut JA, Madias NE. Metabolic acidosis of CKD: an update. *Am J Kidney Dis.* 2016;67:307–317.
219. Kurtz I, Zhu Q. Structure, function, and regulation of the SLC4 NBCe1 transporter and its role in causing proximal renal tubular acidosis. *Curr Opin Nephrol Hypertens.* 2013;22:572–583.
226. Lee HW, Osis G, Handlogten ME, et al. Proximal tubule-specific glutamine synthetase deletion alters basal and acidosis-stimulated ammonia metabolism. *Am J Physiol Renal Physiol.* 2016;310:F1229–F1242.
228. Lee HW, Osis G, Harris AN, et al. NBCe1-A regulates proximal tubule ammonia metabolism under basal conditions and in response to metabolic acidosis. *J Am Soc Nephrol.* 2018;29:1182–1187.
273. Musa-Aziz R, Chen LM, Pelletier MF, et al. Relative $CO_2/NH_3$ selectivities of AQP1, AQP4, AQP5, AmtB, and RhAG. *Proc Natl Acad Sci U S A.* 2009;106:5406–5411.
293. Osis G, Handlogten ME, Lee H-W, et al. Effect of NBCe1 deletion on renal citrate and 2-oxoglutarate handling. *Physiol Rep.* 2016;4:e12778,.
302. Pech V, Kim YH, Weinstein AM, et al. Angiotensin II increases chloride absorption in the cortical collecting duct in mice through a pendrin-dependent mechanism. *Am J Physiol Renal Physiol.* 2007;292:F914–F920.
303. Pech V, Thumova M, Dikalov SI, et al. Nitric oxide reduces Cl-absorption in the mouse cortical collecting duct through an ENaC-dependent mechanism. *Am J Physiol Renal Physiol.* 2013;304:F1390–F1397.
339. Royaux IE, Wall SM, Karniski LP, et al. Pendrin, encoded by the pendred syndrome gene, resides in the apical region of renal intercalated cells and mediates bicarbonate secretion. *Proc Natl Acad Sci U S A.* 2001;98:4221–4226.
342. Saifur RM, Emoto N, Nonaka H, et al. Circadian clock genes directly regulate expression of the Na(+)/H(+) exchanger NHE3 in the kidney. *Kidney Int.* 2005;67:1410–1419.
355. Schwartz GJ, Gao X, Tsuruoka S, et al. SDF1 induction by acidosis from principal cells regulates intercalated cell subtype distribution. *J Clin Invest.* 2015;125:4365–4374.
380. Stettner P, Bourgeois S, Marsching C, et al. Sulfatides are required for renal adaptation to chronic metabolic acidosis. *Proc Natl Acad Sci U S A.* 2013;110:9998–10003.
386. Sun X, Yang LV, Tiegs BC, et al. Deletion of the pH sensor GPR4 decreases renal acid excretion. *J Am Soc Nephrol.* 2010;21:1745–1755.
395. Tokonami N, Morla L, Centeno G, et al. α-ketoglutarate regulates acid-base balance through an intrarenal paracrine mechanism. *J Clin Invest.* 2013;123:3166–3171.
413. Verlander JW, Hassell KA, Royaux IE, et al. Deoxycorticosterone upregulates PDS (Slc26a4) in mouse kidney: role of pendrin in mineralocorticoid-induced hypertension. *Hypertension.* 2003;42:356–362.
418. Verlander JW, Madsen KM, Tisher CC. Effect of acute respiratory acidosis on two populations of intercalated cells in rat cortical collecting duct. *Am J Physiol.* 1987;253:F1142–F1156.
420. Verlander JW, Miller RT, Frank AE, et al. Localization of the ammonium transporter proteins, Rh B glycoprotein and rh C glycoprotein, in the mouse kidney. *Am J Physiol Renal Physiol.* 2003;284:F323–F337.
436. Wall SM, Pech V. The interaction of pendrin and the epithelial sodium channel in blood pressure regulation. *Curr Opin Nephrol Hypertens.* 2008;17:18–24.
447. Watts BA III, George T, Good DW. The basolateral NHE1 Na+/H+ exchanger regulates transepithelial HCO3- absorption through actin cytoskeleton remodeling in renal thick ascending limb. *J Biol Chem.* 2005;280:11439–11447.
458. Weiner ID, Verlander JW. Ammonia transporters and their role in acid-base balance. *Physiol Rev.* 2017;97:465–494.
466. Wen D, Yuan Y, Cornelius RJ, et al. Deficient acid handling with distal RTA in the NBCe2 knockout mouse. *Am J Physiol Renal Physiol.* 2015;309:F523–F530.
467. Wesson DE. Regulation of kidney acid excretion by endothelins. *Kidney Int.* 2006;70:2066–2073.
470. Westhoff CM, Ferreri-Jacobia M, Mak DO, et al. Identification of the erythrocyte Rh-blood group glycoprotein as a mammalian ammonium transporter. *J Biol Chem.* 2002;277:12499–12502.
479. Wu H, Chen L, Zhou Q, et al. Aqp2-expressing cells give rise to renal intercalated cells. *J Am Soc Nephrol.* 2013;24:243–252.
481. Yasuoka Y, Kobayashi M, Sato Y, et al. The intercalated cells of the mouse kidney OMCD are the target of the vasopressin V1a receptor axis for urinary acidification. *Clin Exp Nephrol.* 2013;17:783–792.
489. Zhou Y, Zhao J, Bouyer P, et al. Evidence from renal proximal tubules that $HCO_3^-$ and solute reabsorption are acutely regulated not by pH but by basolateral $HCO_3^-$ and $CO_2$. *Proc Natl Acad Sci U S A.* 2005;102:3875–3880.

# 10 Urine Concentration and Dilution

Jeff M. Sands | Harold E. Layton | Robert Andrew Fenton

## CHAPTER OUTLINE



## KEY POINTS

- Nephron segments and vasculature in the renal medulla are arranged in complex but specific anatomic relationships, both in terms of which segment leads to the next segment and in terms of which segments are adjacent to one another, that play an important role in the concentrating and diluting process. The recently discovered interstitial nodal spaces in the inner medulla may participate in this three-dimensional architecture.
- The urinary concentrating mechanism is dependent on two independent processes: (1) generation of a hypertonic medullary interstitium by concentration of NaCl and urea via countercurrent multiplication processes; and (2) osmotic equilibration of the tubule fluid within the medullary collecting ducts with the hypertonic medullary interstitium under the control of vasopressin.
- Vasopressin and the type 2 vasopressin receptor ($V_2R$) play a central role in the urinary concentrating mechanism. $V_2R$ activation stimulates NaCl reabsorption by the thick ascending limbs of Henle, urea transport in terminal portions of the inner medullary collecting duct (IMCD), and accumulation of the water channel, AQP2, on the apical plasma membrane of collecting duct principal cells.
- Vasopressin binding to $V_2R$ stimulates adenylyl cyclase, predominantly isoform 6, to increase cytosolic cyclic adenosine monophosphate (cAMP) levels as well as intracellular calcium. This stimulates AQP2 accumulation at the apical plasma membrane by inducing depolymerization of the actin cytoskeleton, and by protein phosphorylation, with S256 being an essential site.
- Vasopressin stimulates phosphorylation of the urea transporters (UTs), UT-A1 (at serines 486 and 499), and UT-A3, and their apical plasma membrane accumulation in the inner medullary collecting duct (IMCD) through two cAMP-dependent pathways: protein kinase A (PKA) and Epac (exchange protein activated by cAMP). This leads to increased urea permeability in the IMCD, which facilitates urea reabsorption, increasing medullary interstitial osmolality and the osmotic gradient promoting water reabsorption through AQP2.
- Urea is lost from the inner medullary interstitium, largely via the vasa recta, but urea recycling pathways play a major role in limiting this loss.
- Metformin, an AMP-activated kinase (AMPK) activator, increases UT-A1 and AQP2 phosphorylation and urine-concentrating ability in rodents. Thus, drugs that activate AMPK may be a future therapy for nephrogenic diabetes insipidus.
- Controversy persists as to the nature of the mechanism that generates the inner medullary osmolality, particularly the NaCl gradient, because there is no active NaCl transport in the thin ascending limb. Several recent and ingenious hypotheses have been advanced that depend on the peristalsis of the renal pelvis and the compressibility of the hyaluronan matrix that constitutes the medullary interstitial matrix as integral components of the concentrating mechanism.

## INDEPENDENT REGULATION OF WATER AND SALT EXCRETION

The kidney is responsible for numerous homeostatic functions. For example, body fluid tonicity is tightly controlled by the regulation of water excretion, extracellular fluid volume is controlled by regulation of NaCl excretion, systemic acid–base balance is controlled by regulation of net acid excretion, systemic $K^+$ balance is controlled by regulation of $K^+$ excretion, and body nitrogen balance[1] is maintained through regulation of urea excretion.

The independent regulation of water and solute excretion is essential for the homeostatic functions of the kidney to be performed simultaneously. This means that in the absence of changes in solute intake or in the metabolic production of waste solutes, the kidney is able to excrete different volumes of water upon changes in water intake. This ability to excrete the appropriate amount of water without marked perturbations in solute excretion (without disturbing the other homeostatic functions of the kidney) is dependent on renal concentrating and diluting mechanisms and forms the basis of this chapter.

Renal water excretion is tightly regulated by the peptide hormone arginine vasopressin (AVP; also named antidiuretic hormone, ADH). Under normal circumstances, the circulating vasopressin level is determined by osmoreceptors in the hypothalamus that trigger increases in vasopressin secretion (by the posterior pituitary gland) when the osmolality of the blood rises above a threshold value, about 292 mOsm/kg $H_2O$ (reviewed by Sands et al.[2]). This mechanism can be modulated when other inputs to the hypothalamus (e.g., arterial underfilling, severe fatigue, or physical stress) override the osmotic mechanism. Upon an increase in plasma osmolality, vasopressin is secreted from the posterior pituitary gland into the peripheral plasma. The kidney responds to the variable vasopressin levels by varying urine flow (i.e., water excretion). For example, during extreme antidiuresis (high vasopressin), water excretion is greater than 100-fold lower than during major water diuresis (low vasopressin). These major changes in water excretion are obtained without substantial changes in steady-state solute excretion (Fig. 10.1). This phenomenon is dependent on the kidney's ability to concentrate and dilute the urine. During low circulating vasopressin levels, urine osmolality is less than that of plasma (290 mOsm/kg $H_2O$): the diluting function of the kidney. In contrast, when the circulating vasopressin level is high, urine osmolality is much higher than that of plasma: the concentrating function of the kidney.

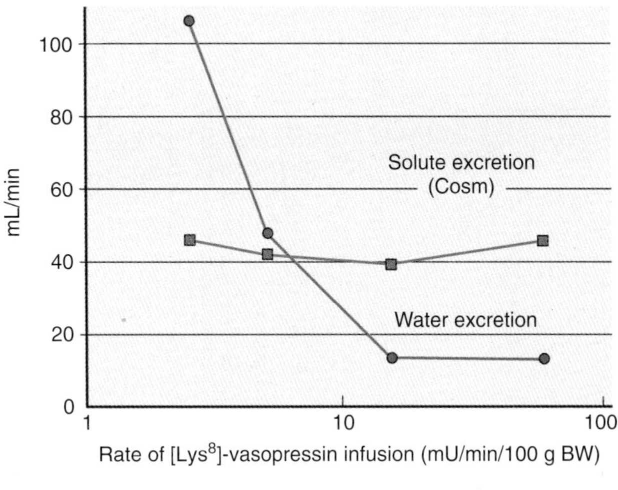


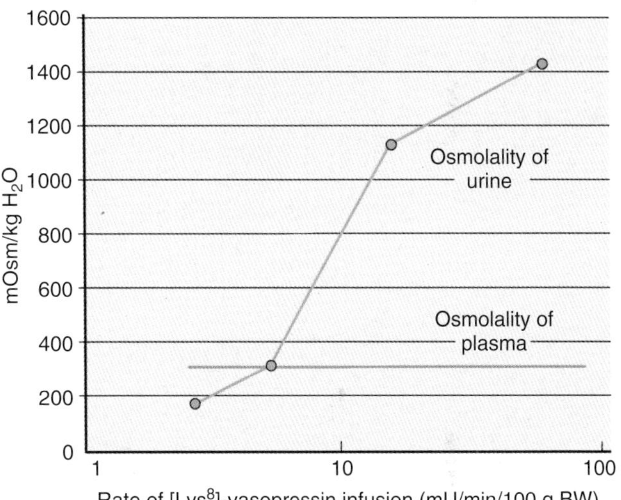


**Fig. 10.1** Steady-state renal response to varying rates of vasopressin infusion in conscious rats. A water load (4% of body weight) was maintained throughout the experiments to suppress endogenous vasopressin secretion. Although the urine flow rate was markedly reduced at higher vasopressin infusion rates, the osmolar clearance (solute excretion) changed little. Concordantly, at higher vasopressin infusion rates, the osmolality of the urine increases significantly, whereas plasma osmolality remains constant. *BW,* Body weight. Data from Atherton JC, Hai MA, Thomas S. The time course of changes in renal tissue composition during water diuresis in the rat. *J Physiol.* 1068; 197:429–443.

## ORGANIZATION OF STRUCTURES IN THE KIDNEY RELEVANT TO URINARY CONCENTRATING AND DILUTING PROCESS

The kidney's ability to vary water excretion over a wide physiologic range, without altering steady-state solute excretion, cannot be simply explained as a consequence of the sequential transport processes along the nephron.[3] The independent regulation of water and sodium excretion occurs in the renal medulla, where the nephron segments and vasculature (vasa recta) are arranged in complex but specific anatomic relationships, both in terms of which segments connect to which segments and their three-dimensional configuration. Thus, it is necessary to consider the parallel interactions between nephron segments that occur as a result of its looped or hairpin structure. Fig. 10.2 illustrates the regional architecture of the renal medulla and medullary rays.[4]

Fig. 10.3 shows a schematic representation of the mammalian nephron with the localization of major water channels (aquaporins; AQPs), urea transporters (UTs), and ion transporters important to the urinary concentrating process. Fig. 10.4 shows which of these transporters and channels are molecular targets for regulated vasopressin action, either in abundance or activity, and thus likely to play a role in urine

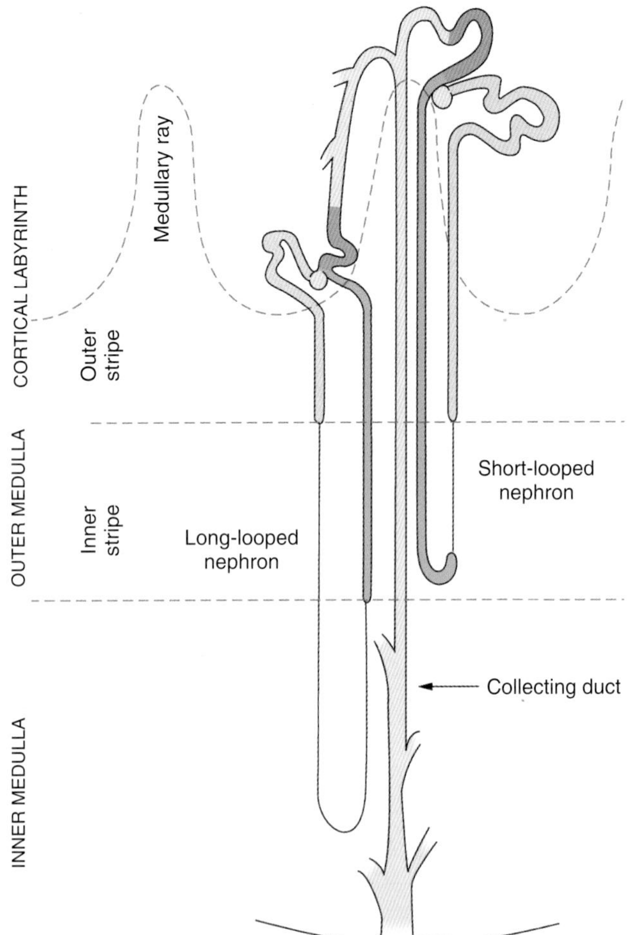


**Fig. 10.2** Mammalian renal structure. Major regions of the kidney are shown on the left. Configurations of a long-looped and a short-looped nephron are depicted. The major portions of the nephron are proximal tubules *(medium blue)*, thin limbs of loops of Henle *(single line)*, thick ascending limbs of loops of Henle *(green)*, distal convoluted tubules *(lavender)*, and the collecting duct system *(yellow)*. Modified from Knepper MA, Stephenson JL. Urinary concentrating and diluting processes. In: Andreoli TE, Fanestil DD, Hoffman JF, Schultz SG, eds. *Physiology of Membrane Disorders.* New York: Plenum; 1986:713–726.

concentration. The functions of several of the transporters and channels shown in Fig. 10.3 have been evaluated in mice using gene deletion techniques (reviewed by Fenton et al.[5]). The phenotypes of these mice have been informative with regard to the role of these proteins and their nephron segments in the urinary concentrating and diluting mechanisms.

## RENAL TUBULE

### LOOPS OF HENLE

The kidney generally contains two populations of nephrons, long-looped and short-looped, which merge to form a common collecting duct system (see Fig. 10.2). Both types of nephrons have loops of Henle that are arranged in a folded or hairpin configuration. Short-looped nephrons generally have glomeruli that are located more superficially in the cortex and have loops that bend in the outer medulla. Long-looped nephrons generally have glomeruli that are located more deeply within the cortex and have loops that bend at various levels of the inner medulla. Long-looped nephrons also contain a thin ascending limb, a segment that is not present in short-looped nephrons. Thin ascending limbs are found only in the inner medulla. The inner-outer medullary border is defined by the transition from thin to thick ascending limbs. Thus, the outer medulla contains only thick ascending limbs, regardless of the type of loop. The long-looped nephrons bend at various levels of the inner medulla from the inner-outer medullary border to the papillary tip. Thus, progressively fewer loops of Henle extend to deeper levels of the inner medulla. Some mammalian kidneys, such as human kidneys, also contain cortical nephrons, which are nephrons whose loops of Henle do not reach into the medulla.

The loops of Henle receive tubular fluid from the proximal convoluted tubules. Tubular fluid exits the thick ascending limbs of both long- and short-looped nephrons, and from cortical nephrons in species that have them, and flows into distal convoluted tubules. Thus, the descending and ascending limbs of the loops of Henle have a countercurrent flow configuration and are composed of several different nephron segments (see Fig. 10.2). The descending portion of the loop of Henle consists of the S2 proximal straight tubule in the medullary ray, the S3 proximal straight tubule (or pars recta) in the outer stripe of the outer medulla, and the thin descending limb in the inner stripe of the outer medulla and the inner medulla. The descending thin limb of short-looped nephrons differs structurally and functionally from the descending thin limb of long-looped nephrons.[6,7]

The location of the descending thin limb of short-looped nephrons within the outer medulla is illustrated in Fig. 10.5 (labeled in green).[8] The descending thin limbs of short-looped nephrons surround the vascular bundles in the outer medulla and tend to be organized in a ring-like pattern (see Fig. 10.5, inset). Thin descending limbs of long-looped nephrons in the outer medulla differ morphologically and functionally from thin descending limbs of long-looped nephrons in the inner medulla.[9–12] The histologic transition from the outer medullary to the inner medullary type of thin descending limbs of long-looped nephrons is gradual and often occurs at some distance into the inner medulla, rather than strictly at the inner-outer medullary border as is the case for the transition between thin and thick ascending limbs.

Pannabecker and coworkers used immunohistochemical labeling and computer-assisted reconstruction to provide new detail about the functional architecture of the rat inner medulla.[13–15] Fig. 10.6 shows a computerized reconstruction of the inner medullary portion of several long-looped nephrons from rats that are labeled using antibodies to the water channel aquaporin-1 (AQP1, shown in red) and the chloride channel ClC-K1 (shown in green) (reviewed by Pannabecker et al.[13–16]). AQP1 is a marker of thin descending limbs of long-looped nephrons in the outer medulla, and it is detected in thin descending limbs of long-looped nephrons in the inner medulla for a variable distance. However, AQP1 was not found in the thin descending limbs of the loops of Henle that turn within the upper millimeter of the inner medulla. Correspondingly, Zhai and colleagues determined that AQP1 was not detectable along the entire length of thin descending limbs of short-looped rat nephrons.[17] In contrast, the upper 40% of thin descending limbs that turn below the first millimeter express AQP1, whereas the lower 60% do

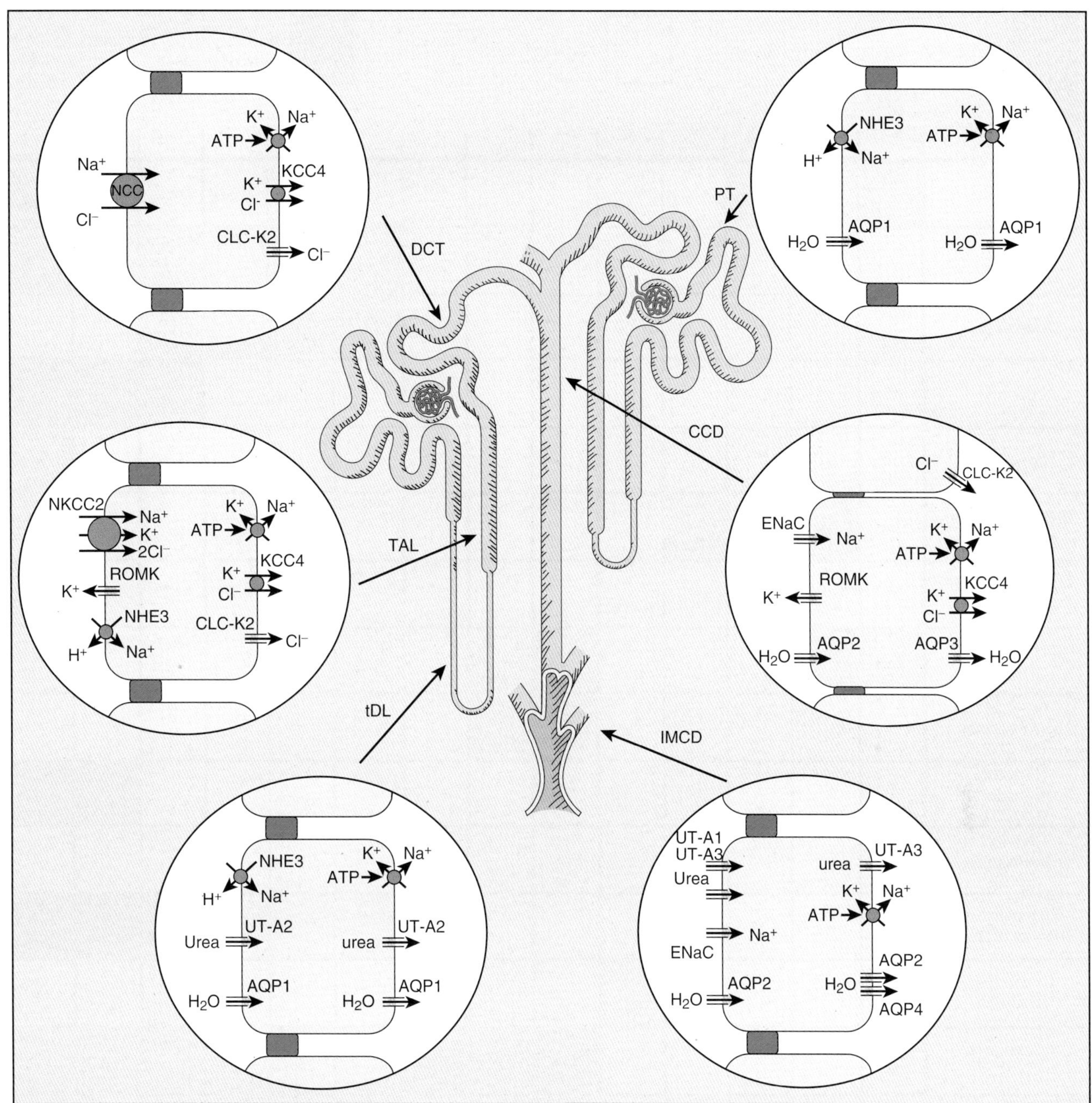


**Fig. 10.3** Major aquaporins, urea transporters, and ion transporters/channels that are important to the urinary concentrating and diluting process. Figure depicts a schematic overview of a mammalian kidney tubule, showing the solute and water transport pathways in the proximal tubule *(PT)*, thin descending limb of Henle loop *(tDL)*, thick ascending limb *(TAL)*, distal convoluted tubule *(DCT)*, cortical collecting duct *(CCD)*, and inner medullary collecting duct *(IMCD)*. Tubule lumen side is always on the left-hand side of the cell, whereas the interstitium is on the right-hand side. Arrows represent direction of movement. Adapted from Fenton RA, Knepper MA. Mouse models and the urinary concentrating mechanism in the new millennium. *Physiol Rev.* 2007;87:1083–1112.

not. ClC-K1 is a marker of the thin ascending limb-type epithelium. It is first detected just before the bend of the loops of Henle, consistent with several morphologic studies demonstrating that the descending limb to ascending limb transition occurs before the loop bend. A substantial portion of the inner medullary thin descending limb of long-looped nephrons did not express either AQP1 or ClC-K1, as indicated in gray in Fig. 10.6.

The deepest portions of descending thin limbs have low water permeability and reduced AQP1.[18] It has been proposed, but not demonstrated experimentally, that urine concentration would be improved by the presence of a urea-$Na^+$ or urea-$Cl^-$ cotransporter in the AQP1-null portion of the thin descending limb.[19] These deep AQP1-null, prebend segments and thin ascending limbs lie equally near the collecting ducts.[18] However, the distal 30% of thin ascending limbs of the longest loops of Henle lie distant from collecting ducts.[18] Urea permeability is lower in the upper portion of thin descending limbs than in the lower portion or in thin ascending limbs in Munich-Wistar rats.[20] Because phloretin does not inhibit urea

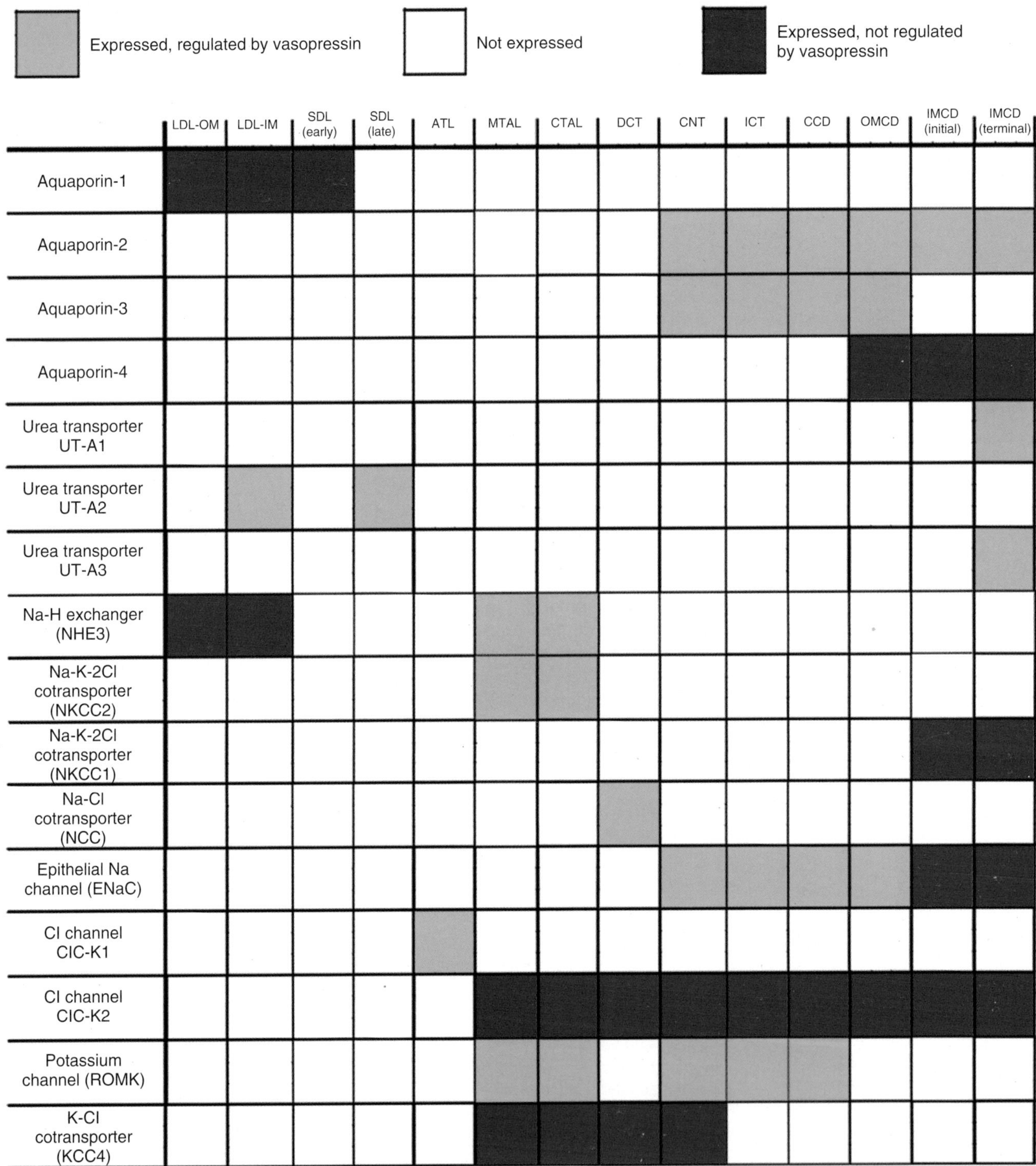


**Fig. 10.4** Grid showing sites of expression of water channels, urea transporters, and ion transporters important to the urinary concentrating process. (See text for details).

permeability, urea transport is not mediated by the UT-A2 urea transporter in these segments.[20] Two novel variants of UT-A2, UT-A2c, and UT-A2d, and a variant of the sodium-glucose cotransporter 1, SGLT1a, are expressed in the lower portion of thin descending and thin ascending limb segments, and may mediate urea transport.[21]

Pannabecker and Dantzler[22] identified three population groups of loops of Henle in Munich-Wistar rats that can be distinguished by the position of the thin ascending limb at the base of the inner medulla and by differing loop length (Fig. 10.7). Group 1 loops have thin ascending limbs that are interposed between collecting ducts; group 2 loops have thin ascending limbs that are adjacent to just one collecting duct; and group 3 loops have thin ascending limbs that lie more than 0.5 tubule diameters from a collecting duct. As the collecting ducts coalesce and the shorter loops of Henle

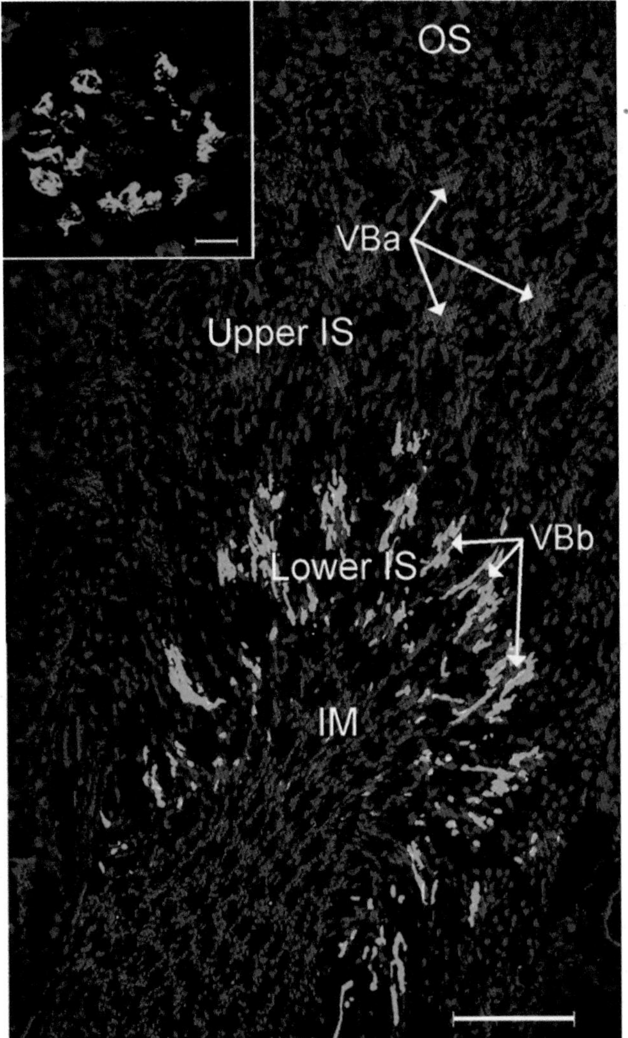


**Fig. 10.5** Triple immunolabeling of rat renal medulla showing localization of UT-A2 *(green)*, marking late thin descending limbs from short-looped nephrons, von Willebrand factor *(blue)* marking endothelial cells of vasa recta, and aquaporin-1 *(red)* marking thin descending limbs from outer medullary long-looped nephrons and early short-looped nephrons. Inset shows a cross-section of a vascular bundle demonstrating that UT-A2–positive thin descending limbs from short-looped nephrons surround the vascular bundles in the deep part of the outer medulla. *IM*, Inner medulla; *IS*, inner stripe of outer medulla; *OS*, outer stripe of outer medulla: *VBa*, vascular bundles in outer part of inner stripe; *VBb*, vascular bundles in inner part of inner stripe. Reproduced with permission from Wade JB, Lee AJ, Liu J, et al. UT-A2. A 55 kDa urea transporter protein in thin descending limb of Henle loop whose abundance is regulated by vasopressin. *Am J Physiol Renal Physiol.* 2002;278:F52–F62.

disappear, the originating portions of the longer thin ascending limbs run alongside the collecting ducts for a substantial distance.[22]

Detailed studies of inner medullary structure, both by Kriz and colleagues[23–26] and more recently by Pannabecker and colleagues,[16,19,22,27–30] found that the inner medullary collecting ducts in the inner medullary base (initial inner medullary collecting ducts) form clusters that coalesce along the cortico-medullary axis. The thin descending limbs are predominantly present at the periphery of these clusters and appear to form an asymmetric ring around each collecting duct cluster, whereas the thin ascending limbs are distributed relatively uniformly among the collecting ducts and thin descending limbs.[27,31]

In the rat, each collecting duct is surrounded by approximately four ascending vasa recta.[32] One or two thin ascending limbs lie between each ascending vasa recta, and opposite to the collecting duct.[32] Pannabecker and colleagues hypothesized that descending and ascending thin limbs enter and exit collecting duct clusters in a manner that is important for the generation and maintenance of the osmolality gradient within the inner medulla.[18] These structures form an interstitial nodal space that runs axially through the inner medulla and that may carry water, urea, and NaCl.[32] These anatomic relationships may facilitate the preferential mixing of solutes and fluid within the interstitial nodal space.[33] In humans, interstitial nodal spaces are relatively infrequent.[30]

### Kidney-Specific Chloride Channel 1 (ClC-K1)

ClC-K1 localizes to both the apical and basolateral plasma membranes of thin ascending limbs.[34] Additionally, ClC-K1 mRNA has been detected in both the thick ascending limb and distal convoluted tubule.[35] In isolated perfused tubules, the chloride conductance of thin ascending limbs is increased by vasopressin exposure: either as a result of increased unit conductance or altered cellular localization of ClC-K1 chloride channels.[36] Microperfusion studies of ClC-K1– null mice (*Clcnk1–/–*) determined that there was drastically reduced transepithelial chloride transport in the thin ascending limbs of knockout mice.[37] *Clcnk1–/–* mice had significantly greater urine volume and lower urine osmolality compared with controls, and even after water deprivation or vasopressin administration, knockout mice were unable to concentrate their urine. This observed polyuria was due to water diuresis and not osmotic diuresis. Inner medullary concentrations of $Na^+$ and $Cl^-$ from *Clcnk1–/–* mice were approximately half those of controls, resulting in a significantly reduced osmolality of the papilla. These studies demonstrate that ClC-K1 is necessary for maintenance of maximal osmolality in the inner medullary tissue. The findings in the *Clcnk1–/–* mice emphasize the importance of rapid chloride exit (and presumably sodium exit) from thin ascending limbs in the inner medullary concentrating process and provide support for the "passive mechanism" (see later).

### Na-K-2Cl Cotransporter Type 2 (NKCC2) and $Na^+$-$H^+$-Exchanger Isoform Type 3 (NHE3)

NKCC2 and NHE3 are the major apical transporters mediating $Na^+$ entry in the thick ascending limb.[38–41] However, knockout of NKCC2 or NHE3 results in drastically different effects on the urinary concentrating mechanism.[42,43] Total NHE3 knockout mice have a marked reduction in proximal tubule fluid absorption, with a compensatory decrease in glomerular filtration rate owing to an intact tubuloglomerular feedback mechanism.[44] On *ad libitum* water intake, total NHE3 knockout mice manifest a moderate increase in water intake associated with lower urinary osmolality.[45] In addition, renal tubule-selective NHE3 knockout mice have only small increases in fluid intake and urinary flow under basal conditons and a minor urinary concentrating defect.[46] In contrast, NKCC2 knockout mice die before weaning due to renal fluid wasting

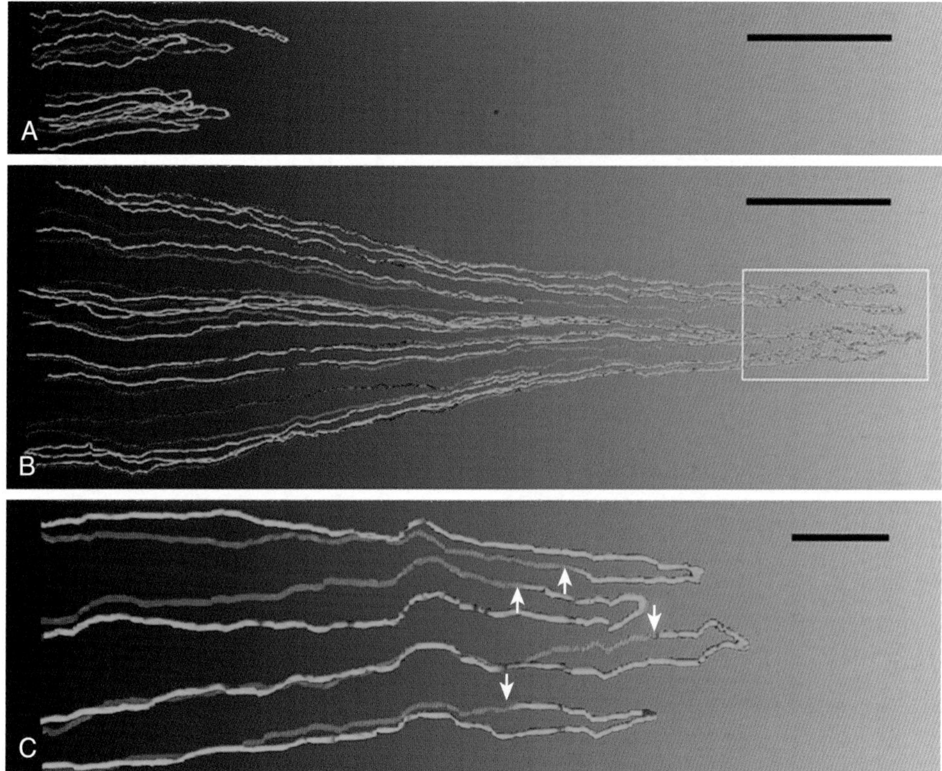


**Fig. 10.6** Computer-assisted reconstruction of loops of Henle from rat inner medulla showing expression of aquaporin-1 (AQP1; *red*) and ClC-K1 *(green)*; *gray regions* (B-crystallin) express undetectable levels of AQP1 and ClC-K1. Loops are oriented along the corticopapillary axis, with the *left* edge of each image nearer the base of the inner medulla. (A) Thin limbs that have their bends within the first millimeter beyond the outer-inner medullary boundary. Descending segments lack detectable AQP1. ClC-K1 is expressed continuously along the prebend segment and the thin ascending limb. (B) Loops that have their bends beyond the first millimeter of the inner medulla. AQP1 is expressed along the initial 40% of each thin descending limb and is absent from the remainder of each loop. ClC-K1 is expressed continuously along the prebend segment and the thin ascending limb. Boxed area is enlarged in (C). (C) Enlargement of near-bend regions of four thin limbs from box in (B). ClC-K1 expression, corresponding to thin descending limb prebend segment, begins, on average, 165 μm before the loop bend *(arrows)*. Scale bars, 500 μm (A) and (B) and 100 μm (C). Reproduced with permission from: Pannabecker TL, Dantzler WH, Layton HE, et al. Role of three-dimensional architecture in the urine concentrating mechanism of the rat renal inner medulla. *Am J Physiol Renal Physiol.* 2008;295:F1271–F1285.

and dehydration,[43] highlighting the essential role of NKCC2 in the urinary concentrating mechanism.

Why does the deletion of NKCC2 result in such a severe phenotype, when the deletion of NHE3, a transporter responsible for reabsorption of far more $Na^+$, results in a viable mouse capable of maintaining extracellular fluid volume? The answer appears to be in the special role that NKCC2 plays in the macula densa in the mediation of tubuloglomerular feedback. Tubuloglomerular feedback allows NHE3 knockout mice to maintain a relatively normal distal delivery through a decrease in glomerular filtration rate, whereas NKCC2 mice cannot compensate in this manner because the transporter is necessary for tubuloglomerular feedback to occur.[47,48]

#### Renal Outer Medullary Potassium Channel (ROMK, Kir 1.1)

ROMK is an ATP-sensitive inwardly rectifier potassium channel that localizes to the thick ascending limb, distal convoluted tubule, connecting tubule, and collecting duct system, where it is predominantly associated with the apical plasma membrane.[49–53] Chronic vasopressin treatment increases ROMK abundance in thick ascending limbs, thus contributing to vasopressin's long-term effect to increase NaCl transport in this segment.[54,55] The majority of ROMK knockout mice die before weaning due to hydronephrosis and severe dehydration.[56] Although 5% of these mice survive the perinatal period, adult mice manifest polydipsia, polyuria, impaired urinary concentrating ability, hypernatremia, and reduced blood pressure, consistent with the known role of ROMK in active NaCl absorption in the thick ascending limb. From these animals, a line of mice has been derived that has a greater survival rate and no hydronephrosis in adult animals; yet the urine concentrating defect persists.

### DISTAL TUBULE SEGMENTS IN THE CORTICAL LABYRINTH

After tubular fluid exits the loop of Henle through the cortical thick ascending limb, it enters the distal convoluted tubule, which is located in the cortical labyrinth. In most mammalian species, several distal tubules merge to form a connecting tubule arcade.[57] The connecting tubule cells express both the vasopressin-regulated water channel, aquaporin-2 (AQP2), and the type 2 vasopressin receptor ($V_2R$),[58] suggesting that

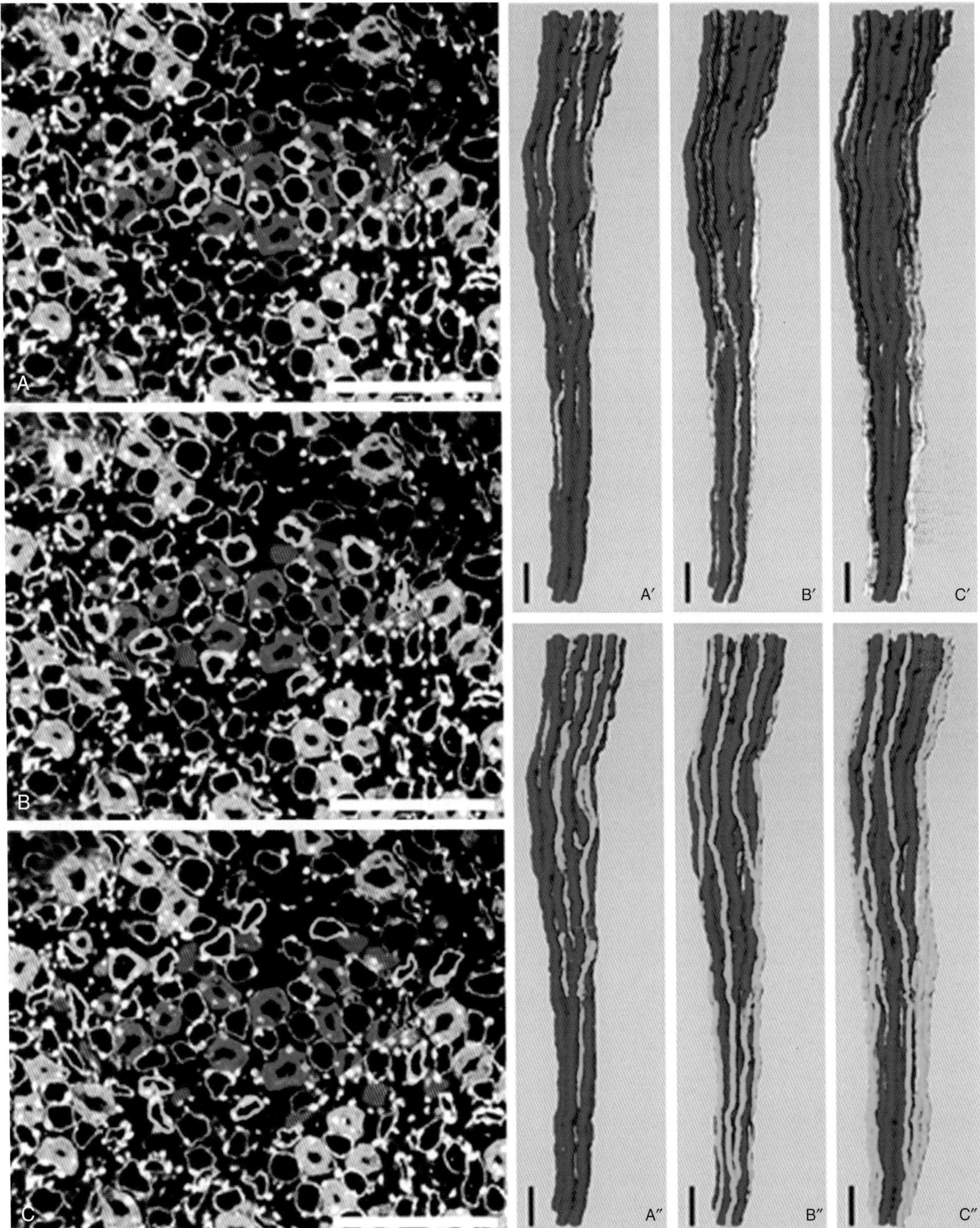


**Fig. 10.7** Spatial relationships between thin descending limbs *(red tubules)*, thin ascending limbs *(green tubules)*, and collecting ducts *(dark blue tubules)*. Thin ascending limbs were categorized into three groups related to their lateral proximity to collecting ducts. Members of each group are shown in a transverse section located at the base of the inner medulla: (A) group 1; (B) group 2; and (C) group 3. In (A), (B), and (C), *open red figures* represent aquaporin-1 (AQP1)-null thin descending limbs, *solid red figures* represent AQP1-expressing thin descending limbs, *white outlined figures* represent thin ascending limbs not associated with the collecting duct cluster, and *light blue figures* represent collecting ducts not associated with the collecting duct cluster. Two prebend segments from group 1 are included in (A). One thin ascending limb from each of groups 2 and 3 (B) and (C) extends below the region of reconstruction, and their thin descending limbs were therefore not reconstructed. (A′), (B′), and (C′) show thin descending limbs and collecting ducts; (A″), (B″), and (C″) show thin ascending limbs and collecting ducts. Gray tubules in (A′), (B′), and (C′) represent AQP1-null thin descending limbs. Scale bars, 100 μm. Reproduced with permission from Pannabecker TL, Dantzler WH. Three-dimensional lateral and vertical relationships of inner medullary loops of Henle and collecting ducts. *Am J Physiol Renal Physiol.* 2004;287:F767–F774.

the arcades are sites of vasopressin-regulated water reabsorption, similar to collecting ducts (see later). Tubular fluid exits the connecting tubules within the arcades and enters the initial collecting tubules, located in the superficial cortex, and then into the cortical collecting ducts. In most rodent species that have been studied, several nephrons merge to form a single cortical collecting duct.[6,59]

### COLLECTING DUCT SYSTEM

The collecting duct system spans all regions of the kidney, starting in the cortex and running to the tip of the inner medulla (see Fig. 10.2). The collecting ducts are the major site of vasopressin-regulated water and urea transport. The transport of water and urea is crucial to the urine-concentrating mechanism, and these are discussed in detail later in this chapter. The collecting ducts are arranged in parallel to the loops of Henle in the medullary rays, outer medulla, and inner medulla. Like the loops of Henle, several morphologically and functionally discrete segments are contained within the collecting duct system. In general, the collecting ducts descend straight through the medullary rays and outer medulla without joining with other collecting ducts. However, several collecting ducts merge as they descend within the inner medulla, resulting in a progressive reduction in the number of inner medullary collecting ducts from the inner-outer medullary border to the papillary tip.[59] The tapered structure of the renal papilla results from the reduction in collecting duct number, accompanied by a progressive reduction in the number of loops of Henle, reaching the deepest levels of the inner medulla.

The epithelial sodium channel (ENaC) is localized to the late distal convoluted tubule, connecting tubule, initial collecting tubule, and throughout the collecting duct.[60,61] Vasopressin treatment increases the protein abundance of the beta- and gamma-subunits of ENaC.[62–64] Acute vasopressin exposure also increases $Na^+$ reabsorption in the cortical collecting duct by increasing apical $Na^+$ entry via ENaC,[65–67] due to adenylyl cyclase (AC) 6–dependent stimulation of ENaC open probability and apical membrane channel number.[68] Deletion of any of the ENaC subunits results in a severe phenotype with neonatal death.[69–72] Alpha ENaC deletion from the collecting ducts alone, leaving intact ENaC expression in the connecting tubule and nonrenal tissues, results in viable mice that have little or no difficulty in maintaining salt and fluid homeostasis.[73] In contrast, alpha ENaC deletion from the connecting tubule and collecting duct together results in a mouse model with increased urine volume and decreased urine osmolality,[74] indicating that alpha ENaC expression within the connecting tubule and collecting duct is crucial for sodium and water homeostasis.

## VASCULATURE

For detailed description of the renal vasculature, see Chapter 2 (Anatomy of the Kidney). The major blood vessels that carry blood into and out of the renal medulla are named the vasa recta. Blood enters the descending vasa recta from the efferent arterioles of juxtamedullary nephrons and supplies it to the capillary plexuses at each level of the medulla. The outer medullary capillary plexus is denser and better perfused than the plexus in the inner medulla.[75] Blood from the inner medullary capillary plexus feeds into the ascending vasa recta (ascending vasa recta are never formed directly from descending vasa recta in a loop-like structure). Inner medullary ascending vasa recta traverse the inner stripe of the outer medulla in close physical association with the descending vasa recta in vascular bundles.[23] In many animal species, thin descending limbs of short-looped nephrons surround the vascular bundles, as shown in Fig. 10.5. Here the thin descending limb segments are labeled with an antibody to the UT-A2 urea transporter,[8] suggesting a route for urea recycling from the vasa recta to the thin descending limbs of short-looped nephrons. The outer medullary capillary plexus is drained by vasa recta that ascend through the outer stripe of the outer medulla, separate from the descending vasa recta.[26] Recent computer-assisted digital tracing of the mouse kidney combined with AQP1 immunohistochemistry shows that the arrangement of tubules and vessels in the vascular bundles is important for providing a pathway for lateral osmolality heterogeneity for urine concentration.[76]

The counterflow arrangement of the vasa recta in the medulla promotes countercurrent exchange of solutes and water, which is facilitated by the presence of AQP1[77,78] and UT-B UTs[79–81] in the endothelial cells of the descending portion of the vasa recta. In rats, UT-B is expressed in both the outer medullary and inner medullary descending vasa recta.[81,82] In humans, UT-B is also expressed in the descending vasa recta, but its expression decreases with depth in the inner medulla.[30]

Countercurrent exchange provides a means of reducing the effective blood flow to the medulla while maintaining a high absolute perfusion rate.[83] The low effective blood flow that results from countercurrent exchange is thought to be important for the preservation of solute concentration gradients in the medullary tissue (see later).

In contrast to the medulla, the cortical labyrinth has a high effective blood flow. The rapid vascular perfusion to this region promotes the rapid return of solutes and water reabsorbed from the nephron to the general circulation. The rapid perfusion is thought to maintain the interstitial concentrations of most solutes at levels close to those in the peripheral plasma. The medullary rays of the cortex have a capillary plexus that is considerably sparser than that of the cortical labyrinth. Consequently, the effective blood flow to the medullary rays has been postulated to be lower than that of the cortical labyrinth.[3]

## MEDULLARY INTERSTITIUM

The renal medullary interstitium connects the tubules and vasculature.[84] It is a complex space that includes the medullary interstitial cells, microfibrils, extracellular matrix, and fluid.[31,84–86] The interstitium is relatively small in volume in the outer medulla and the outer portion of the inner medulla, which may be important in limiting the diffusion of solutes upward along the medullary axis.[3,27,84] In contrast, the interstitial space is much larger in the inner half of the inner medulla.[3,27,84] Within this region, it consists of a gelatinous matrix containing large amounts of highly polymerized hyaluronic acid, consisting of alternating N-acetyl-D-glucosamine and D-glucuronate moieties.[87] Theories have been proposed in which the hyaluronic acid interstitial matrix plays a direct role in the generation of an inner medullary osmotic gradient through its ability to store and transduce energy from the smooth muscle contractions of the renal pelvis (see later).[87]

## RENAL PELVIS

Urine exits the collecting duct system through the ducts of Bellini at the papillary tip and enters the renal pelvis (Fig. 10.8). The renal pelvis (or calyx in multipapillate kidneys) is a complex intrarenal urinary space that surrounds the papilla. The renal pelvis has portions that extend into the outer medulla, which are called fornices and secondary pouches. Although a transitional epithelium lines most of the pelvic space, the renal parenchyma is separated from the pelvic space by a simple cuboidal epithelium.[88] In humans, the UT-B urea transporter is expressed within this papillary surface epithelium.[30] It has been proposed that water and solute transport could occur across this epithelium, thereby modifying the composition of the renal medullary interstitial fluid.[89] There are two smooth muscle layers within the renal pelvic (calyceal) wall.[90] Contractions of these smooth muscle layers generate powerful peristaltic waves that appear to displace the renal papilla downward with a "milking" action.[91] These peristaltic waves may intermittently propel urine along the collecting ducts. The contractions compress all structures within the renal inner medulla, including the interstitium, loops of Henle, vasa recta, and collecting ducts.[92] Theories have been proposed whereby these contractions furnish part of the energy for concentrating solutes, and hence concentrating urine, within the inner medulla (see later).[87]

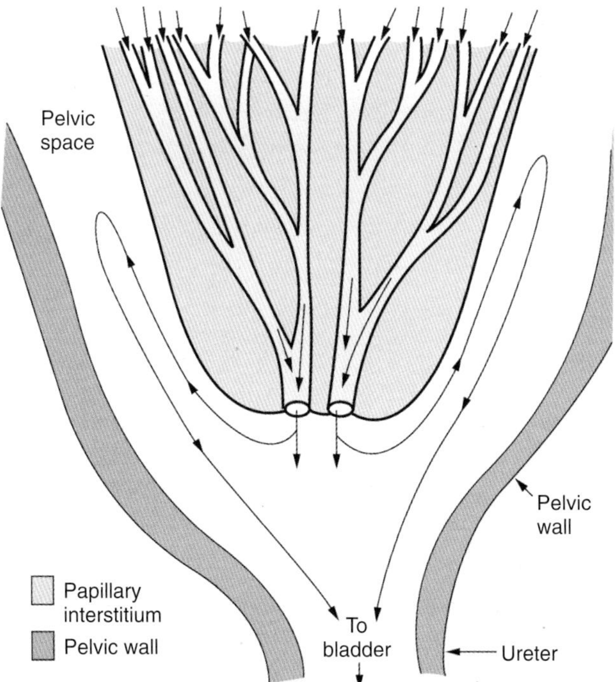


**Fig. 10.8** Pattern of urine flow in papillary collecting ducts and renal pelvis. Urine exits the papillary collecting ducts (ducts of Bellini) at the tip of the renal papilla and is carried to the urinary bladder by the ureter. Under some circumstances, a fraction of the urine may reflux backward in the pelvic space and contact the outer surface of the renal papilla. Solute and water exchange across the papillary surface epithelium has been postulated (see text).

# VASOPRESSIN AND THE TYPE 2 VASOPRESSIN RECEPTOR

The small peptide hormone vasopressin and the $V_2R$ play a central role in the urinary concentrating mechanism. $V_2R$ activation stimulates NaCl reabsorption by the thick ascending limbs of Henle, urea transport in terminal portions of the inner medullary collecting duct, and accumulation of a water channel, AQP2, on the plasma membrane of collecting duct principal cells. These events permit the collecting duct luminal fluid to equilibrate osmotically with the surrounding interstitium in the kidney, resulting in water reabsorption and urine concentration. Dysfunction of this reabsorption mechanism in the collecting duct results in the production of large amounts of dilute urine, up to 18 L/d, a disease known as diabetes insipidus. In the following we address how the $V_2R$ and AQP2 interact via intracellular signaling pathways to regulate collecting duct water reabsorption and urine concentration.

> *Clinical Relevance*
>
> **Nephrogenic Diabetes Insipidus**
>
> Nephrogenic diabetes insipidus (NDI) results from the inability of the kidney to respond to vasopressin and produce a concentrated urine. Congenital NDI results from mutations in the $V_2R$ in 90% of families (in which the mutation is known) and in AQP2 in most of the other 10% (reviewed in Sands and Bichet[469]). Acquired forms of NDI occur much more frequently and arise as a consequence of drug treatments, electrolyte disturbances, and urinary tract obstruction. In most manifestations of acquired NDI, dysregulation of AQP2, either in terms of protein abundance or in AQP2 membrane targeting, plays a fundamental role in the development of polyuria.[470,471] Downregulation of AQP2 observed in acquired NDI is most likely the primary cause of the NDI, rather than being a secondary event (e.g., as a consequence of the increased urine production or reduction in interstitial osmolality). For example, in models of hypokalemic and lithium-induced NDI, the changes in AQP2 expression in the kidney cortex are identical to those seen in the inner medulla,[472–474] which indicates that interstitial tonicity is not a major factor. Moreover, washout of the medullary osmotic gradient for 1 or 5 days using the loop diuretic furosemide has no effect on AQP2 expression,[474,475] which indicates that high urine flow in itself is not responsible for the reduced AQP2 expression in experimental NDI. Studies investigating the molecular physiology and signaling pathways regulating water and urea transport have identified several novel therapeutic possibilities for treating NDI (reviewed in Sands and Klein[403]).

## VASOPRESSIN

The ADH of most mammals is a nine–amino acid peptide, vasopressin. Secretion of vasopressin from the posterior pituitary is stimulated by an increase in plasma osmolality, but also by a reduction in plasma volume (reviewed in Sands et al.[2]). Vasopressin activates regulatory systems necessary to retain water and restore osmolality to normal.[93] The effects of vasopressin occur through the stimulation of receptors that are located on different cell types.[94,95] Here we focus on the $V_2R$ activation of a cyclic adenosine monophosphate (cAMP) pathway in renal epithelial cells for modulation of collecting duct water transport.

## TYPE 2 VASOPRESSIN RECEPTOR

The $V_2R$ is a seven transmembrane–spanning domain receptor that couples to heterotrimeric G proteins (GPCRs).[96,97] In the kidney it is expressed from the thick ascending limb of the loop of Henle through to the collecting duct principal cells.[98–102] When vasopressin binds to the $V_2R$, AC activity is stimulated and cytosolic cAMP levels increase.[103] This ultimately leads to an accumulation of AQP2 in the apical plasma membrane of collecting duct principal cells, thus increasing transepithelial water permeability and facilitating osmotically driven water reabsorption (Fig. 10.9). Intracellular calcium is also increased by vasopressin via a mechanism involving calmodulin[104]; this is also involved in the regulated trafficking of AQP2.[105,106] A critical role of the $V_2R$ for urinary concentration has been demonstrated in two mouse models of X-linked nephrogenic diabetes insipidus (XNDI). Upon constitutive deletion,[107] male mutant mice ($V_2R^{-/y}$) die within 7 days after birth, with 3-day-old mice displaying severe hypernatremia,

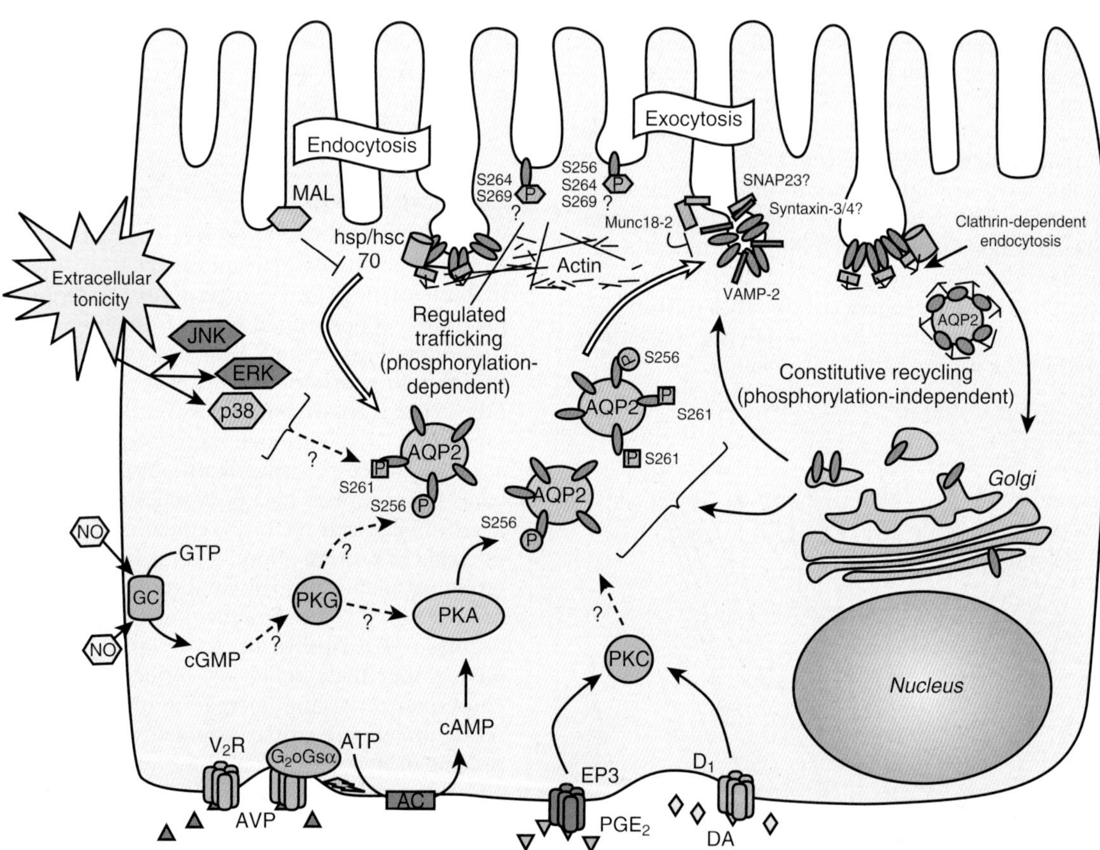


**Fig. 10.9** Key events that contribute to the regulation of aquaporin-2 (AQP2) trafficking. The canonical pathway involves interaction of vasopressin with the type 2 receptor *($V_2R$)* on the basolateral surface of the principal cell. This increases cyclic adenosine monophosphate *(cAMP)* formation after $G_{\alpha s}$ stimulation of adenylyl cyclase *(AC)*. Phosphorylation of AQP2 occurs initially on residue S256, via protein kinase A *(PKA)* activation. After vasopressin stimulation, residue S261 on AQP2 is dephosphorylated, and residue S264 and S269 phosphorylation is increased. During exocytosis AQP2 interacts with soluble *N*-ethylmaleimide–sensitive factor attachment protein receptor *(SNARE)* proteins and their regulatory proteins such as Munc18-2, and these interactions may be regulated by phosphorylation. At the cell surface, phosphorylated AQP2 is present in endocytosis-resistant domains, and its interaction with heat shock protein/heat shock cognate 70 (hsp/hsc70), which is required for clathrin-mediated endocytosis, is inhibited. The myeloid and lymphocyte protein (MAL) also is involved in AQP2 endocytosis by an as-yet-unknown mechanism. Endocytosis of AQP2 is also facilitated by protein kinase C *(PKC)* activation (but possibly not by direct phosphorylation of AQP2), as well as by activation of dopamine *(DA, $D_1$)*, prostaglandin $E_2$ *($PGE_2$)*, and $PGE_2$ receptor type 3 *(EP3)*. However, constitutive exocytosis of AQP2 occurs without vasopressin stimulation and does not require AQP2 phosphorylation on residue S256. Accumulation of AQP2 at the plasma membrane is increased by inhibiting clathrin-mediated endocytosis. AQP2 phosphorylation can also be increased by stimulating the cyclic guanosine monophosphate/protein kinase G *(cGMP/PKG)* pathways using, for example, nitric oxide *(NO)*. Extracellular hypertonicity activates the mitogen-activated protein (MAP) kinase pathway, and c-Jun N-terminal kinase *(JNK)*, extracellular signal–regulated kinase *(ERK)*, and p38 MAP kinase activities are all required for AQP2 surface accumulation after acute hypertonic shock. Finally, AQP2 trafficking involves the actin cytoskeleton, and actin depolymerization results in cell surface accumulation of AQP2 without the need for vasopressin stimulation. *ATP*, Adenosine triphosphate; *GC*, guanylyl cyclase; *GTP*, guanosine triphosphate; *SNAP23*, synaptosomal-associated protein 23; *VAMP-2,* vesicle-associated membrane protein 2.

drastically increased serum $Na^+$ and $Cl^-$ levels, and significantly lower urine osmolality. In mice with conditional deletion of the $V_2R$,[108,109] adult mice display all of the characteristic symptoms of XNDI,[110,111] including polyuria, polydipsia, and resistance to the antidiuretic actions of vasopressin.

The function of the $V_2R$ depends on interaction with GPCRs and β-arrestin. Upon vasopressin binding, the $V_2R$ assumes an active configuration and the bound heterotrimeric G protein, Gs, dissociates into Gsα and Gsβγ subunits.[103] This G protein is localized on the basolateral plasma membrane of the thick ascending limb of Henle, distal convoluted tubule, and collecting duct principal cells.[112,113] AC is stimulated by activated Gsα, and cAMP levels are increased. The predominant AC isoform in the kidney is AC-6,[114] and knockout mice lacking the AC-6 isoform have significant nephrogenic diabetes insipidus (NDI).[115,116] After vasopressin binding,[117] the $V_2R$ is internalized, delivered to, and degraded in lysosomes, thus terminating the response. Many accessory proteins are involved in $V_2R$ downregulation, including inhibitory $G_i$ proteins,[103,118,119] proteins involved in clathrin-mediated endocytosis,[120,121] and proteins of the so-called retromer complex.[122,123] Destruction of cAMP by cytosolic phosphodiesterases is also associated with limiting $V_2R$ responses,[124] but cAMP levels in vasopressin target cells remain elevated for a considerable time after stimulation, and the $V_2R$ continues to signal from endosomes after internalization.[122]

A critical step in $V_2R$ internalization is the binding of β-arrestin to the $V_2R$,[125] which is triggered by phosphorylation of the $V_2R$ by kinases, including G-protein–coupled receptor kinases (GRKs).[126] Following β-arrestin–dependent ubiquitination of the $V_2R$.[127] arrestin-receptor complexes recruit the clathrin adaptor protein AP-2,[119] and the complex is then internalized via clathrin-mediated endocytosis.[120,128,129] Arrestins also uncouple GPCRs from GPCRs, producing a desensitized receptor.[130] Restoration of prestimulation levels of $V_2R$ at the cell surface requires several hours.[131–133] The majority of the $V_2R$ that is internalized with vasopressin enters a lysosomal degradation compartment.[127,134,135] Delivery of both the ligand and receptor to lysosomes may be required to terminate the physiologic response to vasopressin.[136] Restoration of prestimulation levels of the $V_2R$ at the cell surface partly requires new protein synthesis.[134]

## VASOPRESSIN-REGULATED WATER TRANSPORT

### COLLECTING DUCT WATER ABSORPTION AND OSMOTIC EQUILIBRATION

The urinary concentrating mechanism is dependent on two independent processes: (1) generation of a hypertonic medullary interstitium by concentration of NaCl and urea via countercurrent processes, and (2) osmotic equilibration of the tubule fluid within the medullary collecting ducts with the hypertonic medullary interstitium. As discussed, vasopressin is essential for determining the degree of water excretion because it increases NaCl reabsorption via the thick ascending limb and thus the hypertonicity of the medullary interstitium and it regulates collecting duct water permeability. When circulating vasopressin levels are low the water permeability of the collecting ducts is also extremely low; relatively little water is reabsorbed from the tubule fluid and large volumes of hypotonic urine are produced. In contrast, high circulating levels of vasopressin increase the permeability of the apical membrane of the thick ascending limb to NaCl, leading to an increase in the osmolality of the peritubular interstitium (due to countercurrent multiplication) and increasing the water permeability of the collecting ducts to very high levels. Combined, this results in water being rapidly reabsorbed from the cortical and outer medullary portions of the collecting duct system via AQP water channels,[137–139] resulting in the production of a small volume of hypertonic urine, with osmolality approaching that of the inner medullary interstitium.

The late distal tubule (the late distal convoluted tubule, the connecting tubule, and the initial collecting tubule) is the earliest site along the renal tubule where water absorption increases during antidiuresis (Fig. 10.10).[140] Although the

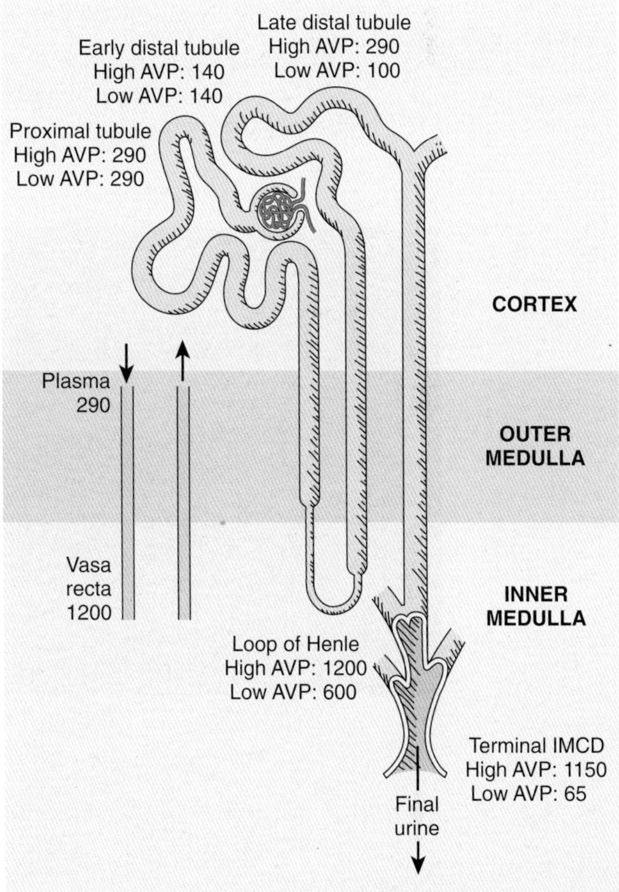


**Fig. 10.10** Typical osmolalities (in mOsm/kg $H_2O$) found in various vascular *(left)* and renal tubule *(right)* sites in rat kidneys. Fluid in the proximal tubule is always isosmotic with plasma (290 mOsm/kg $H_2O$). Fluid emerging from the loop of Henle (entering the early distal tubule) is always hypotonic. Osmolality in the late distal tubule increases to plasma level only during antidiuresis. Final urine is hypertonic when the circulating vasopressin level is high, and hypotonic when the vasopressin level is low. A high osmolality is always maintained in the loop of Henle and vasa recta. During antidiuresis, osmolalities in all inner medullary structures are nearly equal. Osmolalities are somewhat attenuated in the loop and vasa recta during water diuresis (not shown). Based on micropuncture studies; see text. *AVP,* Vasopressin; *IMCD,* inner medullary collecting duct.

distal convoluted tubule does not express any water channels, it does express the $V_2R$ and vasopressin regulates NaCl transport in this segment via increasing activity of the Na-Cl cotransport protein, NCC.[141,142] In contrast, the connecting tubule and the cortical collecting duct express the $V_2R$ and the vasopressin-regulated water channel AQP2.[143] Thus, it is likely that the connecting tubule and the cortical collecting duct segments are the earliest sites of distal tubular osmotic equilibration.

The volume of water absorption in the connecting segment and initial collecting tubule required to raise tubule fluid to isotonicity is considerably greater than the additional amount required to concentrate the urine above the osmolality of plasma in the medullary portion of the collecting duct system.[3] Consequently, during antidiuresis, most of the water reabsorbed from the collecting duct system enters the cortical labyrinth, where the effective blood flow is high enough to return the reabsorbed water to the general circulation without diluting the interstitium. In contrast, if such a large volume of water was reabsorbed along the medullary collecting ducts, it would have a significant dilution effect on the medullary interstitium and thus impair concentrating ability).[144,145]

During water diuresis, a modest corticomedullary osmolality gradient persists,[146,147] and the water permeability of the collecting ducts is low but not zero.[148,149] Consequently, some water is reabsorbed by the collecting ducts during water diuresis, driven by the small transepithelial osmolality gradient. The majority of this water reabsorption occurs in the terminal inner medullary collecting ducts, where the transepithelial osmolality gradient is highest. In fact, more water is absorbed from the terminal inner medullary collecting ducts during water diuresis than during antidiuresis, owing to a much greater transepithelial osmolality gradient.[144,145,150]

## AQUAPORIN-2: THE VASOPRESSIN-SENSITIVE COLLECTING DUCT WATER CHANNEL

The first water channel, AQP1 was identified in 1991 by Peter Agre and his associates.[151–154] AQP1 is expressed in proximal tubules and thin descending limbs of long-loop nephrons[10,155,156] but not short-loop nephrons.[17] AQP2, cloned in 1993, is the vasopressin-regulated water channel in kidney collecting duct principal cells.[157] Vasopressin stimulation of the collecting duct results in the accumulation of AQP2 on the plasma membrane of principal cells (Fig. 10.11). This involves the recycling of AQP2 between intracellular vesicles and the cell surface.[137,158–164] However, aquaporin-3 (AQP3) and aquaporin-4 (AQP4), both of which are found in the

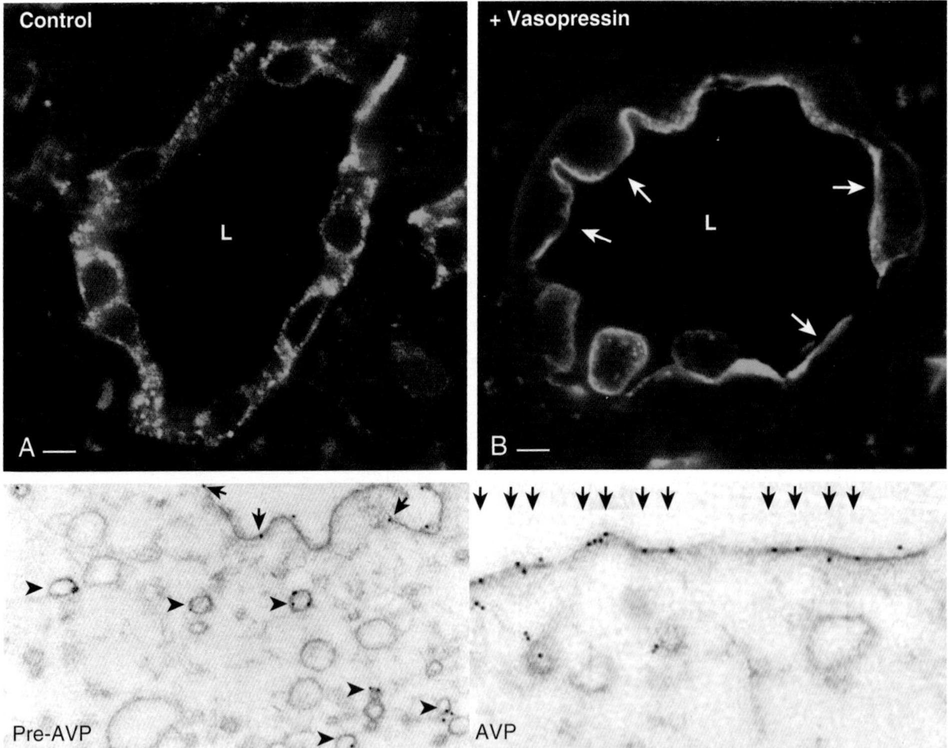


**Fig. 10.11** Increased plasma membrane expression of AQP2 in principal cells of AVP-deficient Brattleboro rat kidney inner medullary collecting duct injected with vasopressin for 15 minutes. Kidneys were then fixed, sectioned and immunostained using anti-AQP2 antibodies. Under control conditions (A), AQP2 has a cytosolic distribution in principal cells. After perfusion with AVP (B), AQP2 shows an increased apical localization in principal cells *(arrows)*. A weaker basolateral localization of AQP2 in principal cells is also visible in this section. The lower two panels show the effect of AVP on AQP2 distribution by immunogold electron microscopy. Tubules were perfused with 4 nM DDAVP for 60 minutes. The *left panel* (pre-AVP) shows the apical region of a principal cell, with gold particles (detecting AQP2) distributed on cytoplasmic vesicles, as well as a few on the apical plasma membrane *(arrows)*. After AVP treatment, the number of gold particles on the apical plasma membrane is greatly increased *(arrows)*, and the number of labeled cytoplasmic vesicles *(arrowheads)* is decreased. *L*, Tubule lumen. Scale bar, 5 µm. (Lower panels adapted from Nielsen S, Chou CL, Marples D, et al. Vasopressin increases water permeability of kidney collecting duct by inducing translocation of aquaporin-CD water channels to plasma membrane. *Proc Natl Acad Sci U S A.* 1995;92:1013–1017.)

basolateral membrane of principal cells,[165,166] are also regulated at the expression, and possibly functional level, by vasopressin and/or dehydration.[166–169]

## OVERVIEW OF VASOPRESSIN-REGULATED AQP2 TRAFFICKING IN COLLECTING DUCT PRINCIPAL CELLS

The vasopressin-induced change from a low-to-high permeability state of collecting duct principal cells, and vice versa, involves the reversible redistribution of AQP2 from cytoplasmic vesicles to the apical plasma membrane. Early freeze-fracture electron microscopy studies using amphibian urinary bladder and skin suggested that clusters of water channels are located on intracellular vesicles that fuse with the apical plasma membrane upon vasopressin stimulation. The water channels are internalized back into the cell by endocytosis after vasopressin washout.[170–174] Antibodies against AQP2 demonstrated that it is located in the apical plasma membrane of collecting duct principal cells, as well as in intracellular vesicles.[157,175,176] In vitro and in vivo studies correlated the vasopressin-stimulated increase in collecting duct water permeability and urinary concentration with relocalization of AQP2 from intracellular vesicles to the plasma membrane of principal cells (see Fig. 10.11).[176–179] This relocation was reversible upon vasopressin washout and in animals either infused with a $V_2R$ antagonist or subjected to water loading to reduce circulating vasopressin levels.[180–182] One unexpected observation from initial studies was that significant amounts of AQP2 were present on principal cell basolateral membranes in some kidney regions, and that this staining tended to increase after vasopressin treatment. Recent studies have suggested that basolateral AQP2 is not only a potential pathway for water transport across the basolateral membrane, but may also have a role in cell migration and tubulogenesis due to interaction with β1 integrin.[183,184]

Some of the internalized AQP2 that accumulates in endosomes after vasopressin withdrawal follows a complex intracellular pathway before reinsertion into the plasma membrane.[164,185–187] Unlike the $V_2R$,[134] de novo protein synthesis is not required for sequential responses to vasopressin stimulation.[188] A significant amount of AQP2 also accumulates in multivesicular bodies (MVBs).[180,189] This pool of AQP2 can then be directed to lysosomes for degradation, be transferred to a recycling compartment, or be directly transported to the cell surface via transport vesicles that derive from the MVBs. The fate of internalized AQP2 seems to be at least in part regulated by ubiquitylation.[190,193] Under certain conditions AQP2 can also be degraded in autophagosomes.[194,195]

Some of the MVBs can fuse with the apical membrane of principal cells and release small nanovesicles known as exosomes into the tubule lumen. These exosomes contain a variety of different proteins,[196] including AQP2 on their limiting membranes,[197,198] in addition to AQP2 mRNA and many other mRNAs and microRNAs within their lumen.[199,200] AQP2 protein can be detected in urine, and the amount increases in conditions of antidiuresis, when more AQP2 is present in the apical membrane of principal cells. The physiologic relevance of this urinary excretion of AQP2 remains unknown, but the amount of exosomal AQP2 can be increased by vasopressin and urinary alkalinization,[201] and a role in cell-cell communication has been proposed.[200]

## BASOLATERAL AQUAPORINS IN PRINCIPAL CELLS

The presence of AQP3 and/or AQP4 renders the basolateral plasma membranes of collecting duct principal cells constitutively permeable to water.[202,203] AQP3 expression is predominant in the cortex and decreases toward the inner medulla, with the reverse pattern for AQP4 (see Fig. 10.12), which is most abundant in the inner medulla.[166,203] The abundances of AQP3 and AQP4 can be increased by the long-term action of vasopressin.[202–204] AQP2 is also localized in the basolateral plasma membrane of these cells in some regions of the collecting duct.[175,177,205–208] Basolateral expression of AQP2 is greatly increased by vasopressin[209,210] or long-term (6 days) aldosterone.[207,211,212] A proportion of basolateral AQP2 likely represents a transient step in an indirect apical targeting pathway for the AQP2 protein.[213,214]

## AQUAPORIN KNOCKOUT MICE

The physiological roles of various AQPs in the urinary concentrating mechanism have been uncovered by the use of various genetically modified mouse models.

### AQUAPORIN-1 KNOCKOUT MICE

AQP1 knockout mice have increased urine volume and reduced urinary osmolality that does not increase in response to water deprivation.[215] Proximal tubule fluid absorption is markedly impaired in AQP1 knockout mice, but distal delivery of water and NaCl is not impaired due to a reduction in glomerular filtration rate via the tubular–glomerular feedback mechanism.[216] The osmotic water permeability of isolated perfused thin descending limbs from AQP1 knockout mice was markedly reduced compared with control animals.[217] As rapid water absorption from long-loop thin descending limbs is essential for countercurrent multiplication processes in the outer medulla, the reduced water reabsorption is one factor responsible for the concentrating defect in AQP1 knockout mice. Descending vasa recta, a second renal medullary site of AQP1 expression, also displayed a marked reduction in osmotic water permeability in AQP1 knockout mice,[77,78] and thus countercurrent exchange processes are also likely to be impaired in AQP1 knockout mice. The results from studies in these mice show that AQP1 in the renal medulla is essential for the urine-concentrating mechanism.

### AQUAPORIN-2 KNOCKOUT MICE

A number of different genetic models have been generated to assess the role of AQP2 in the urinary concentrating mechanism, including inducible and nephron-specific models of AQP2 deletion, models where essential phosphorylation sites in AQP2 are modified, and models of autosomal dominant NDI.[192,218–226] The major phenotype in these models is severe polyuria; however, with free-access to water, plasma concentrations of electrolytes, urea, and creatinine are not different in knockout mice compared to controls. In contrast, a mouse model with connecting tubule-specific AQP2 deletion[227] has indicated a role of the connecting tubule in regulating body water balance under basal conditions, but not for maximal concentration of the urine during antidiuresis. Taken together, these mouse models confirm that AQP2 is responsible for the

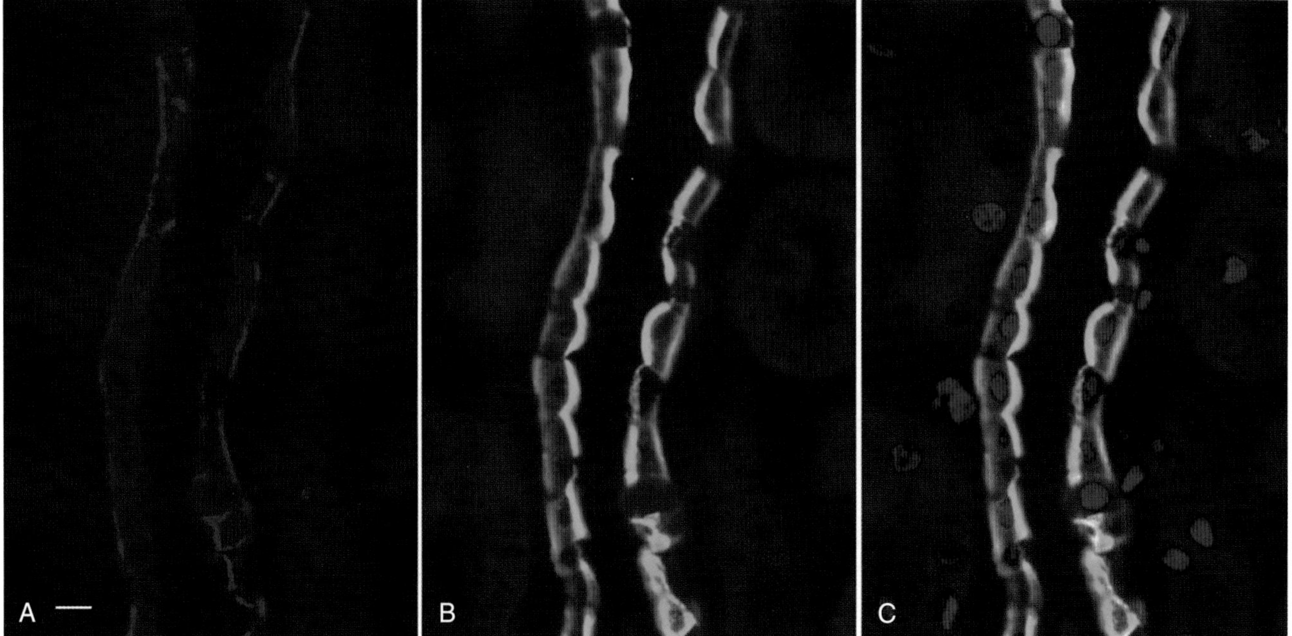


**Fig. 10.12** Localization of aquaporins in the outer medullary collecting duct (outer stripe) of rat kidney. Images show sections immunostained in (A) for aquaporin-4 (AQP4) *(red)* and (B) for aquaporin-2 (AQP2) *(green)*. The merged image in (C) shows that AQP2 is largely apical in this region, but both AQP2 and AQP4 are present on basolateral membranes. Intercalated cells are not stained with either antibody and appear as darker gaps among the other cells. In (C), nuclei are stained with 4′,6-diamidino-2-phenylindole (DAPI). Scale bar, 10 μm.

majority of transcellular water reabsorption in the connecting tubule and collecting duct system.

### AQUAPORIN-3 AND AQUAPORIN-4 KNOCKOUT MICE

The osmotic water permeability of the basolateral membrane of cortical collecting duct cells from AQP3 knockout mice is reduced by greater than threefold compared with wild type control mice.[228] Consequently, AQP3 knockout mice are markedly polyuric (10-fold greater daily urine volume than controls), but they can slightly increase their urine osmolality after either water deprivation or vasopressin treatment.[3] AQP4 knockout mice have a fourfold decrease in inner medullary collecting duct osmotic water permeability, indicating that AQP4 is responsible for the majority of water movement across the basolateral membrane in this segment.[229,230] Despite this reduced inner medullary collecting duct water permeability, AQP4 knockout mice have no difference in urine osmolality. However, after 36 hours of water deprivation, AQP4 knockout mice have a significantly reduced maximal urine osmolality that cannot be further increased by AVP administration. This modest decrease in urinary concentrating ability in AQP4 knockout mice, compared with the profound concentrating defect in AQP3 knockout mice, is likely due to the normal distribution of water transport along the collecting duct,[3] with much greater osmotic reabsorption of water in the cortical portion of the collecting duct system (where AQP3 is predominant), than in the medullary collecting ducts (where AQP4 is the predominant basolateral water channel).

## MECHANISMS OF AQUAPORIN-2 TRAFFICKING

A wealth of information regarding the regulated trafficking, function, structure, and water transport capacity of AQP2 has been generated by the use of various in vitro or ex vivo experimental systems.[154,178,188,231–250] In the following sections, we discuss the various mechanisms of AQP2 trafficking that are continually evolving in parallel with new discoveries related to the targeting and trafficking of membrane proteins in general.

### AQUAPORIN-2 RECYCLING

Clathrin-coated pits are critical for the internalization of both AQP2 and the $V_2R$,[119,120,128,251,252] with inhibition of clathrin-mediated endocytosis causing AQP2 plasma membrane accumulation (Fig. 10.13).[159,185,186,251,253–256] Although caveolae have been proposed as an alternative endocytotic pathway for AQP2 in cultured cells,[257] caveolae and caveolin are not present on the apical pole of principal cells in vivo.[258,259] After internalization, AQP2 enters a subapical recycling compartment distinct from organelles such as the Golgi, the trans-Golgi network (TGN), and lysosomes,[188,260,261] but it likely recycles via the classic endosomal recycling compartments[186,262,263] with the vacuolar protein sorting–associated protein 35 (Vps35) playing an important role.[264]

### ROLE OF THE CYTOSKELETON IN AQUAPORIN-2 TRAFFICKING

The cytoskeleton and soluble *N*-ethylmaleimide-sensitive factor attachment protein receptor (SNARE) complex play important roles in multiple aspects of vesicle trafficking, including exocytosis, endocytosis, and vesicle docking and fusion.[265–273] Thus, it is no surprise that they are important for AQP2 trafficking.

Actin associates directly with AQP2[274–276] or AQP2-containing vesicles[277] and upon vasopressin-mediated depolymerization, AQP2 accumulates in the plasma membrane.[278–281] Apical fluid shear stress also depolymerizes the apical actin cytoskeleton and causes AQP2 membrane accumulation.[282,283] A

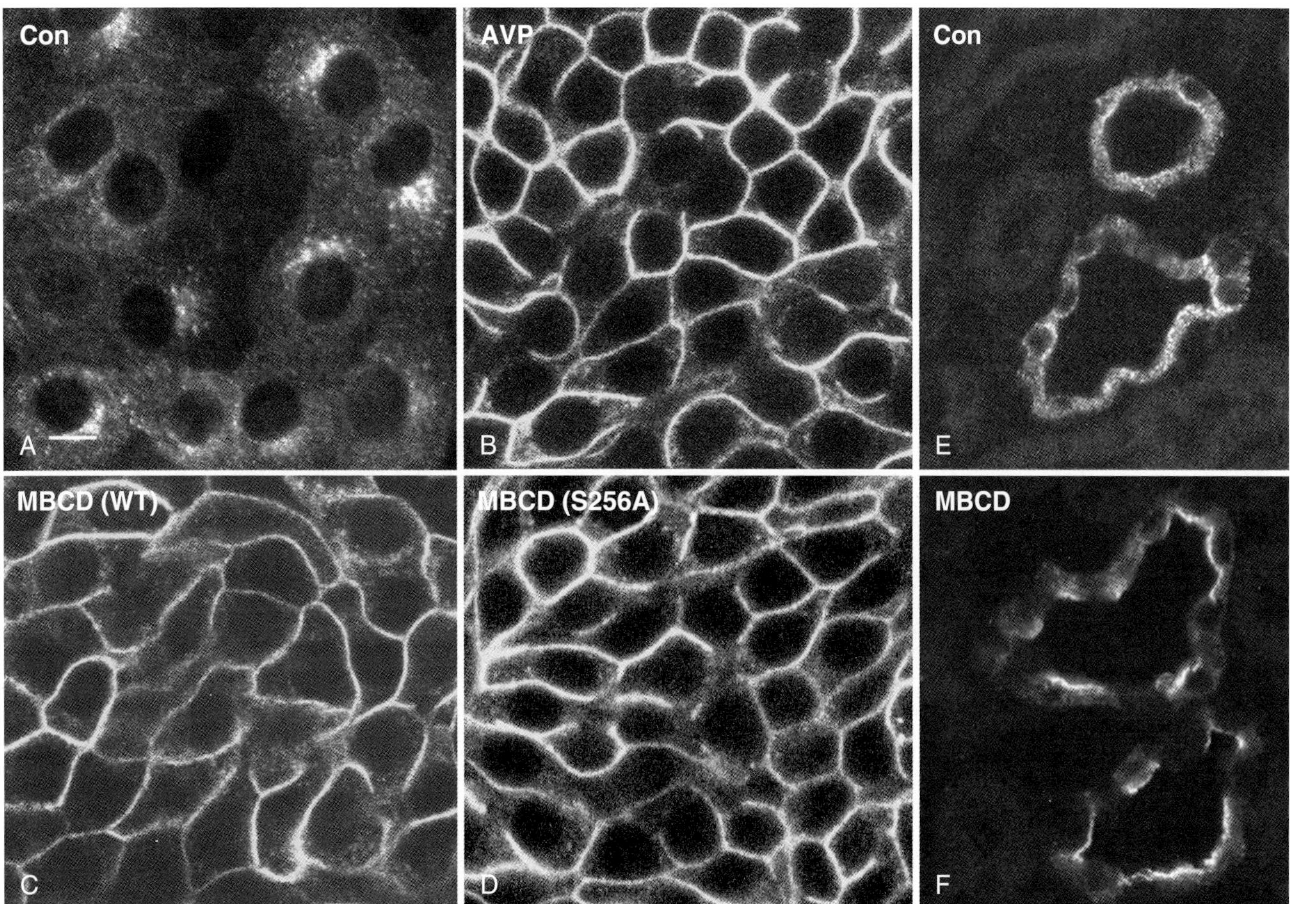


**Fig. 10.13** Methyl-β-cyclodextrin *(MBCD)* stimulates aquaporin-2 (AQP2) membrane accumulation in LLC-PK$_1$ cells (A) to (D) and collecting duct principal cells in situ (E) and (F). Immunofluorescence staining for AQP2 in LLC-PK$_1$ cells expressing wild type AQP2 (A) to (C) or a mutant in which the S256 residue has been replaced by alanine (S256A) (D). Under baseline conditions, wild type AQP2 is located mainly on intracellular vesicles, often concentrated in the perinuclear region of the cell (A). After vasopressin (AVP) treatment, wild type AQP2 relocates to the plasma membrane (B). When endocytosis is inhibited by application of the cholesterol-depleting drug MBCD, both wild type and S256A AQP2 accumulate at the cell surface in the absence of AVP (C) and (D). This result shows that both wild type AQP2 and S256A AQP2 are constitutively recycling between intracellular vesicles and the plasma membrane, and that inhibiting endocytosis with MBCD is sufficient to cause membrane accumulation, even in the absence of S256 phosphorylation of AQP2. In collecting duct principal cells (inner stripe of outer medulla) in situ, AQP2 is located on vesicles scattered throughout the cytoplasm after perfusion of intact kidneys in vitro (E). However, after perfusion of kidneys for 60 minutes with 5 mmol/L MBCD, increased apical plasma membrane expression of AQP2 is seen (F). This finding indicates that AQP2 is constitutively recycling through the apical plasma membrane in principal cells in situ, and that membrane accumulation can be induced by blocking endocytosis (with MBCD) even in the absence of vasopressin. *Con*, Control; *WT,* wild type.

role for A-kinase anchoring protein 220 (AKAP220) and Rho GTPases in modulating the actin effects on AQP2 have been proposed.[280,284–288] AQP2 also complexes with various other actin-associated proteins including myosins,[277,281,289–291] Rab proteins,[262,292] members of the ERM (ezrin-radixin-moesin) family,[293,294] and the signal-induced proliferation–associated gene 1 (SPA-1).[288] Although the mechanisms behind actin depolymerization and AQP2 trafficking are not clear (see Fig. 10.14), only vasopressin induces significant actin depolymerization in cells expressing AQP2,[283] suggesting a novel mechanism of protein trafficking in which the channel protein itself critically regulates local actin reorganization to initiate its movement.[275] The integrin-linked kinase (ILK) is also important in orchestrating cytoskeletal organization during AQP2 recycling and entry into the exocytotic pathway.[295,296]

Dynein and dynactin, a protein complex linking microtubules and vesicles, are associated with AQP2-bearing vesicles[297] and depolymerization of microtubules partially inhibits vasopressin-induced water permeability in target epithelia[298–300] and apical localization of AQP2.[176,249,301,302] A role of microtubules in the basolateral to apical transcytosis of AQP2 has also been suggested.[214] Together, the data on microtubules indicate that they are predominantly responsible for long-range trafficking of AQP2 vesicles toward the plasma membrane and localization of AQP2 inside the cell after internalization, but that the final steps of vesicle approach and fusion are microtubule independent.[303]

A variety of SNARE proteins are associated with AQP2-containing vesicles or colocalize with AQP2 in collecting duct cells, including VAMP-2 (vesicle-associated membrane protein 2, synaptobrevin-2), VAMP-3 (cellubrevin), VAMP-8, SNAP23 (synaptosomal-associated protein 23), the ATPase Hrs-2, syntaxin 3, syntaxin 4, syntaxin 7, syntaxin 12, and syntaxin 13.[277,304–310] Of these, VAMP-2, VAMP-3, syntaxin 3,

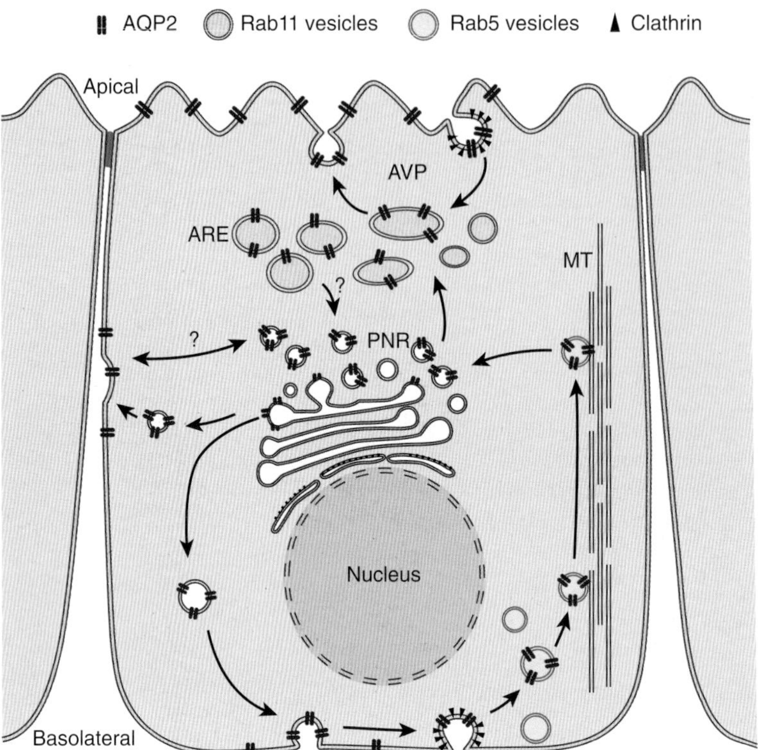


**Fig. 10.14** Aquaporin-2 (AQP2) follows a transcytotic pathway before apical membrane delivery. From vesicles in the perinuclear region *(PNR)*, probably originating from the trans-Golgi network, AQP2 can be delivered to the basolateral plasma membrane before reaching the apical surface of epithelial cells. From there, it is retrieved by clathrin-mediated endocytosis into Rab5-positive endosomes *(green)*, which move in a microtubule *(MT)*-dependent manner to the PNR and ultimately to Rab11-positive apical recycling endosomes *(AREs; purple)*. These Rab11-positive vesicles are involved in recycling AQP2 constitutively to and from the apical plasma membrane. The endocytotic branch of this recycling pathway is inhibited by the methyl-β-cyclodextrin treatment shown in Fig. 10.13, resulting in cell surface accumulation of AQP2. The physiologic stimulus, vasopressin *(AVP)*, increases apical AQP2 expression in two ways. It increases exocytosis from the Rab11 compartment and also inhibits clathrin-mediated endocytosis of AQP2 from the apical plasma membrane. The delivery of AQP2 to the basolateral membrane of collecting duct principal cells may be important for collecting duct tubulogenesis,[183] whereas apical AQP2 is necessary for urine concentration. From Yui N, Lu HA, Chen Y, et al. Basolateral targeting and microtubule-dependent transcytosis of the aquaporin-2 water channel. *Am J Physiol Cell Physiol.* 2013;304:C38–C48.

and SNAP23 are the ones that have been functionally shown to be important for AQP2 trafficking.[306,309,311] Interaction of AQP2 and the SNARE complex may be mediated by the protein snapin[312] and/or by the angiotensin-converting enzyme 2 homolog collectrin, which has been implicated in salt-sensitive hypertension.[313]

## ESSENTIAL ROLE OF AQUAPORIN-2 PHOSPHORYLATION

The rise in intracellular cAMP following $V_2R$ stimulation is important for modulating the abundance of AQP2 by modulation of AQP2 gene transcription.[242,314] cAMP also plays a role in AQP2 trafficking by affecting the phosphorylation status of AQP2,[262,315–317] with phosphatase inhibitors increasing cell surface accumulation of AQP2.[318,319] However, $V_2R$-mediated increases in cAMP are not absolutely necessary for receptor-mediated AQP2 membrane targeting and alternative pathways to increase AQP2 membrane targeting exist.[320–323]

AQP2 contains several phosphorylation sites for protein kinases,[138,324–326] several of which are important for AQP2 trafficking alongside AQP2 ubiquitylation.[190–193] Whether any of the phosphorylation sites are important for modulation of AQP2 unit water permeability is controversial.[327–329] Early work focused on the involvement of S256 phosphorylation in AQP2 trafficking, with the current consensus being that S256 phosphorylation is necessary for vasopressin-induced cell-surface accumulation of AQP2[222,330–334] (Fig. 10.15). The importance of this site is highlighted by a mutation (S254L), which destroys the PKA phosphorylation site at S256 resulting in NDI in humans.[334,335] The roles of S261, S264, and S269 (threonine in humans) are slowly being uncovered.[328] All three phosphorylated forms are localized to some degree in the plasma membrane in vivo.[169,189,336,337] Vasopressin decreases the abundance of pS261, whereas AMP-activated kinase (AMPK) activation increases the levels.[338] However, this site alone is not required for AQP2 trafficking.[339,340] Interestingly, activation of AMPK with metformin increases AQP2 phosphorylation in general,[341] whereas levels of phosphorylation are significantly attenuated under acidic conditions.[342] The pS269 form of AQP2 is exclusively detected in the apical plasma membrane, and a regulatory role of this phosphorylation site directly in the plasma membrane for inhibiting AQP2 endocytosis has been shown.[*]

[*]References 169, 189, 191, 336, 337, and 343.

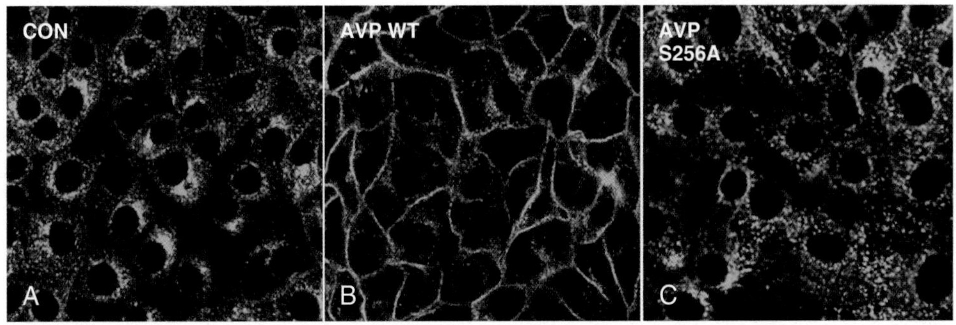


**Fig. 10.15** Immunofluorescence staining showing aquaporin-2 *(AQP2)* expressed in LLC-$PK_1$ cells. Under control *(CON)* conditions (A), AQP2 is located on perinuclear and more diffusely distributed intracellular vesicles, with very little plasma membrane staining. After vasopressin *(AVP)* treatment for 10 minutes, AQP2 accumulates on the plasma membrane of cells expressing wild type *(WT)* AQP2 (B) but remains mainly on intracellular vesicles after vasopressin treatment of cells expressing AQP2-S256A, a mutation that prevents protein kinase A–mediated phosphorylation of this critical amino acid (C).

### ROLE OF PHOSPHORYLATION IN EXOCYTOSIS AND ENDOCYTOSIS OF AQUAPORIN-2

Although S256 phosphorylation is necessary for vasopressin-induced cell-surface accumulation of AQP2, the role that phosphorylation plays in AQP2 exocytosis is complex. An AQP2 S256A mutant accumulates on the plasma membrane upon inhibition of endocytosis (see Fig. 10.13),[253] suggesting that the exocytotic pathway is intact under these conditions. Vasopressin also increases exocytosis of vesicles in AQP2-expressing cells whether or not AQP2 is phosphorylated at S256.[344] Thus, although vasopressin-induced accumulation of AQP2 at the cell surface requires S256 phosphorylation, and AQP2 is present in "endocytosis-resistant" membrane domains after vasopressin treatment,[253,345,346] exocytotic insertion of AQP2 into the plasma membrane is probably independent of this phosphorylation event. Furthermore, the regulated endocytosis of AQP2 may not be dependent on its phosphorylation state.[347] For example, prostaglandin $E_2$ ($PGE_2$)[348] can induce AQP2 internalization independent of S256 phosphorylation, but other studies indicate that the effects of $PGE_2$ on AQP2 and urine concentration depend on which $PGE_2$ receptor it acts upon.[109,250,344,349–351]

Accumulating evidence suggests that phosphorylation-mediated interaction of AQP2 with other regulatory proteins is important for modulating cell-surface accumulation of AQP2. For example, AQP2 phosphorylation modifies its interaction with key proteins of the vesicle docking/fusion apparatus or endocytotic machinery, including heat shock cognate/heat shock protein 70 (hsc/hsp70)[345,352] dynamin and clathrin,[340,352] annexin 2,[169] the myelin and lymphocyte protein (MAL),[353] or 14-3-3ζ.[354]

## VASOPRESSIN-REGULATED UREA TRANSPORT IN THE INNER MEDULLA

### UREA TRANSPORTER PROTEINS

Urea plays a central role in the urinary concentrating mechanism. Urea importance has been appreciated since 1934, when Gamble and colleagues initially described "an economy of water in renal function referable to urea,"[355] findings which were recently confirmed and advanced in UT-A1/A3 knockout mice[356] (discussed later). Many studies show that maximal urine-concentrating ability is decreased in protein-deprived or malnourished humans (and other mammals), and that urea infusion restores urine-concentrating ability (reviewed in Sands and Layton[357]). Urine-concentrating defects have been demonstrated in UT-A1/A3,[358] UT-A2,[359] UT-B,[360–362] and UT-A2/UT-B knockout mice.[363] Thus, an effect due to urea or UTs must be part of the mechanism by which the inner medulla concentrates urine.

Two urea transporter genes have been cloned in mammals: the UT-A (*Slc14A2*) gene encodes 6 protein and 9 cDNA isoforms (reviewed in Sands and Layton[357]), and the UT-B (*Slc14A1*) gene encodes 2 protein isoforms.[364] The UT-A gene, which has been cloned from rodents and humans, has two promoter elements: one upstream of exon 1 and a second that is located within intron 12 and drives the transcription of UT-A2 and UT-A2b (see references 365–368; also reviewed in Sands and Layton[357]). UT-B, which is also the Kidd blood group antigen in humans, has been cloned from humans and rodents[369] (also reviewed by Sands and Layton[357]).

UT-A promoter I contains a tonicity enhancer (TonE) element and hyperosmolality increases its activity.[366,370] UT-A1 is expressed in the terminal inner medullary collecting duct and is detected in the apical plasma membrane.[367,371,372] UT-A3 is also expressed in the terminal inner medullary collecting duct; it is primarily detected in the basolateral plasma membrane but has been detected in the apical plasma membrane.[373–375] UT-A2 is expressed in thin descending limbs.[8,371,372,376] UT-B is expressed in descending vasa recta and red blood cells (reviewed by Sands and Layton[357]) (Fig. 10.16).

Vasopressin increases the phosphorylation and the apical plasma membrane accumulation of UT-A1 and of UT-A3 in rat inner medullary collecting ducts.[375,377] UT-A1 is phosphorylated by vasopressin at serines 486 and 499.[325,378] Both phospho-S486-UT-A1 and phospho-S499-UT-A1 are expressed predominantly in the apical plasma membrane in vasopressin-treated rat inner medullary collecting ducts.[379,380] The site in UT-A3 that is phosphorylated by vasopressin has not been determined, except that neither of the two PKA consensus sites is involved.[381] Vasopressin stimulates urea transport, UT-A1 phosphorylation, and apical plasma membrane accumulation through two cAMP-dependent pathways: PKA and Epac (exchange protein activated by cAMP).[382] Epac increases UT-A1 phosphorylation but not at either serine 486 or 499.[380]

UT-A1 is dephosphorylated by multiple phosphatases, including calyculin and calcineurin.[383] 14-3-3 proteins bind

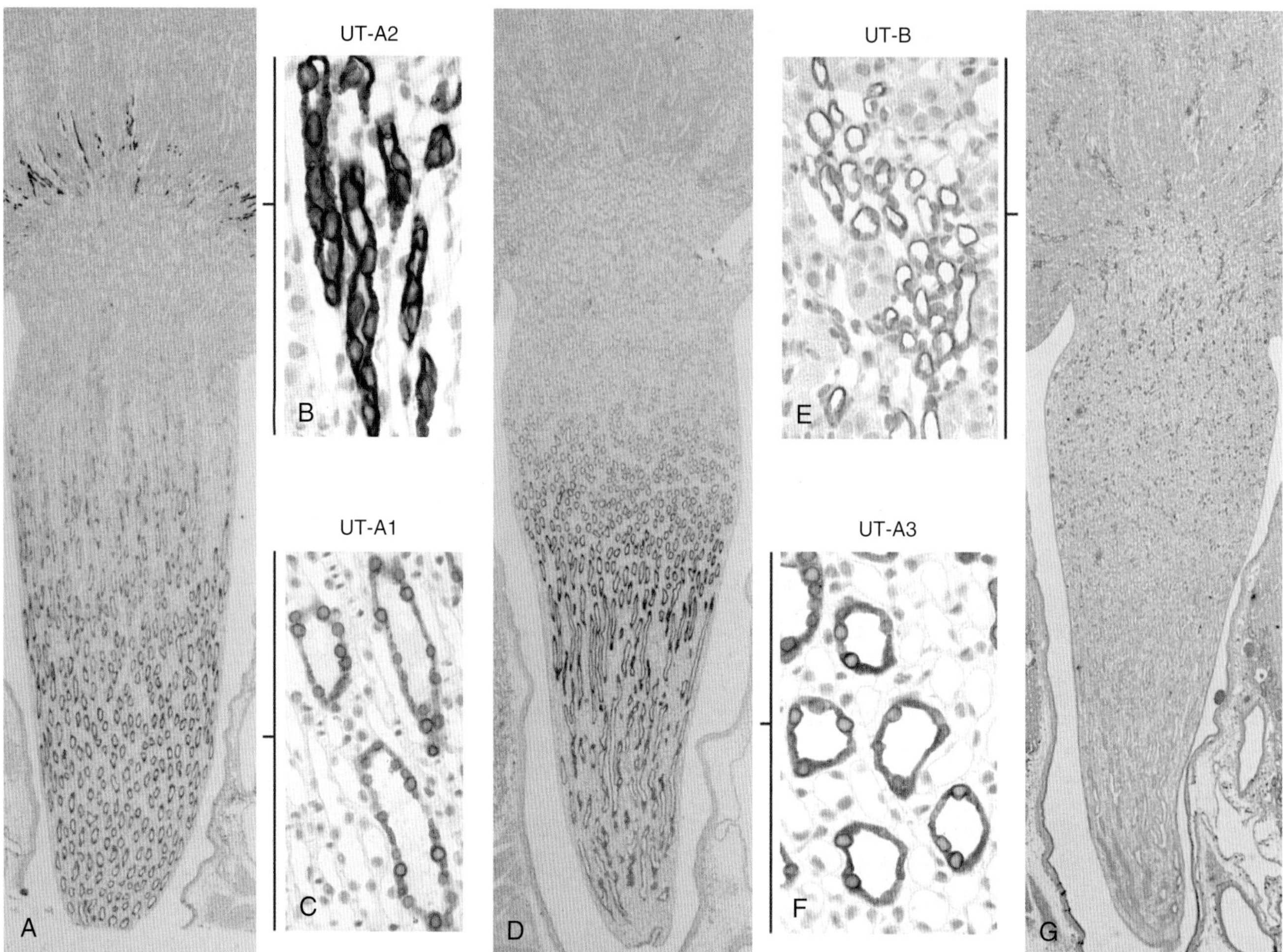


**Fig. 10.16** Localization of urea transporters. UT-A1 is localized to the terminal portion of the inner medullary collecting duct, whereas UT-A2 is localized to the thin descending limbs of Henle loop in the inner stripe of outer medulla (A). Higher magnification shows that both UT-A2 (B) and UT-A1 (C) are predominantly intracellular. UT-A3 is localized to the terminal portion of the inner medullary collecting duct (D) and is both intracellular and in the basolateral membrane domains (F). UT-B is expressed in the descending vasa recta (G), where it is localized to the basolateral and apical regions (E). Adapted from Fenton RA, Knepper MA. Urea and renal function in the 21st century: insights from knockout mice. *J Am Soc Nephrol.* 2007;18: 679–688.

to phosphorylated serine or threonine residues and regulate protein function. UT-A1 and 14-3-3γ bind, and PKA activation enhances this binding.[384] 14-3-3γ increases UT-A1 ubiquitination and degradation by interacting with the E3 ubiquitin ligase, MDM2, and decreases urea transport.[384] Thus, UT-A1 phosphorylation is increased by PKA, and UT-A1 degradation is enhanced by subsequent binding to 14-3-3γ, potentially providing a negative feedback mechanism to return UT-A1 function to its basal state following vasopressin stimulation.[384] Although data showing these opposite effects of vasopressin/PKA are established, the physiologic significance remains to be determined.

Hyperosmolality increases urea permeability in rat terminal inner medullary collecting ducts, even in the absence of vasopressin,[385–387] suggesting that it is an independent activator of urea transport. Hyperosmolality stimulates urea permeability via activation of PKCα and intracellular calcium,[388–391] whereas vasopressin stimulates urea permeability via increases in cAMP.[392] Hyperosmolality increases the phosphorylation and the plasma membrane accumulation of both UT-A1 and UT-A3,[375,377,393,394] similar to the effect of vasopressin. UT-A1 is phosphorylated by PKCα at serine 494.[390,395–397]

Genetic knockout of PKCα in mice results in a urine-concentrating defect.[395,398,399] PKCα knockout mice have reduced levels of UT-A1 protein abundance[395] and UT-A1 sialylation.[400] PKCα activation increases UT-A1 sialylation and UT-A1 accumulation in the apical plasma membrane, an effect mediated by Src kinase.[400] PKCα also enhances UT-A3 sialylation, an effect mediated by ST6GalI.[401]

Metformin, an AMPK activator, increases UT-A1 and AQP2 phosphorylation in inner medullary collecting duct suspensions, urea and water transport in perfused terminal inner medullary collecting ducts, and urine-concentrating ability in two rodent models of congenital NDI: tolvaptan-treated rats and V2R knockout mice.[341,402] Thus, drugs that activate AMPK may be a future therapy for NDI.[341,402,403]

## UREA TRANSPORTER KNOCKOUT MICE

### UT-A1/A3 KNOCKOUT MICE

A mouse model where the two inner medullary collecting duct UTs, UT-A1 and UT-A3, are deleted (*UT-A1/A3*$^{-/-}$ mice) have a complete absence of phloretin-sensitive and vasopressin-regulated urea transport in the inner medullary collecting duct.[358,404–406] These *UT-A1/A3*$^{-/-}$ mice fed a normal or high protein diet have a significantly greater fluid intake and urine flow, resulting in a decreased urine osmolality, compared with wild type mice.[358,407] Under these dietary conditions, after an 18-hour water restriction, *UT-A1/A3*$^{-/-}$ mice are unable to reduce their urine flow to levels below those observed under basal conditions, resulting in volume depletion and loss of body weight. In contrast, on a low-protein diet (4%), *UT-A1/A3*$^{-/-}$ mice do not show a substantial degree of polyuria and can reduce their urine volume to a similar level as control mice after water restriction. On a low-protein diet, hepatic urea production is low and urea delivery to the inner medullary collecting duct is predicted to be low, thus rendering collecting duct urea transport largely immaterial to water balance. Thus, the concentrating defect in *UT-A1/A3*$^{-/-}$ mice is due to a urea-dependent osmotic diuresis, results that are compatible with a model of urea handling proposed in the 1950s by Berliner and colleagues.[83]

*UT-A1/A3*$^{-/-}$ mice have also been exploited to study the "passive mechanism for urine concentration models" proposed in 1972 by Kokko and Rector and by Stephenson for concentration of $Na^+$ and $Cl^-$ in the inner medulla in the absence of active transport[408,409] (see later). In these models, the passive electrochemical gradient that drives $Na^+$ and $Cl^-$ to exit from the thin ascending limb is indirectly dependent on rapid reabsorption of urea from the inner medullary collecting duct. However, despite a profound decrease in inner medulla urea accumulation in *UT-A1/A3*$^{-/-}$ mice, three independent studies failed to demonstrate the predicted decline in $Na^+$ and $Cl^-$ concentrations in the inner medulla.[355,358,405,406] Based on these results alone, the passive concentrating model in the form originally proposed does not appear to be the only mechanism by which NaCl is concentrated in the inner medulla. However, mathematical modeling analysis of these same data concluded that the results found in the *UT-A1/A3*$^{-/-}$ mice are consistent with what one would predict for the passive mechanism.[410] Thus, the issue remains unresolved at present.

Another hypothesis regarding urea and the urinary concentrating mechanism was described over 80 years ago as "an economy of water in renal function referable to urea" and affectionately known as the Gamble phenomenon.[355] Gamble described that (1) the water requirement for excretion of urea is less than for excretion of an osmotically equivalent amount of NaCl, and (2) less water is required for the excretion of urea and NaCl together than the water needed to excrete an osmotically equivalent amount of either urea or NaCl alone. In *UT-A1/A3*$^{-/-}$ mice, both elements of the Gamble phenomenon were absent, indicating that inner medullary collecting duct UTs play an essential role.[356] When wild type mice were given progressively increasing amounts of urea or NaCl in the diet, both substances induced osmotic diuresis, but at different excretion levels (6000 μosmol/day for urea; 3500 μosmol/day for NaCl). Mice were unable to increase urinary NaCl concentrations above 420 mM. Thus, the second component of the Gamble phenomenon derives from the fact that both urea and NaCl excretion are saturable, presumably resulting from an ability to exceed the respective reabsorptive capacity for urea and NaCl, rather than a specific interaction of urea transport and NaCl transport at an epithelial level.

A mouse lacking UT-A3 but expressing UT-A1 was created by transgenic restoration of UT-A1 into the *UT-A1/A3*$^{-/-}$ knockout mouse in order to determine the effect of UT-A1 alone.[411] Basal urea permeability in the inner medullary collecting duct of the UT-A1-only mouse was normal, but unlike wild type mice, vasopressin did not stimulate urea permeability above basal levels.[411] Surprisingly, urine-concentrating ability was restored to wild type levels in the UT-A1 only mice.[411]

## UT-B AND UT-A2 KNOCKOUT MICE

UT-B knockout mice have a reduced urine-concentrating ability that is similar to humans lacking UT-B (reviewed by Fenton and Knepper[406] and Klein et al.[412]). In humans, UT-B is the Kidd blood group antigen, and people lacking the Kidd antigen are unable to concentrate their urine above 800 mOsm/kg $H_2O$, even following overnight water deprivation and exogenous vasopressin administration.[413]

Mice lacking UT-A2 also have reduction in urine-concentrating ability (reviewed in Fenton and Knepper[406] and Klein et al.[412]). The urine-concentrating defect is thought to result from impairment of urea recycling (reviewed in Fenton and Knepper[406] and Klein et al.[412]). Because UT-B knockout may also interfere with urea recycling, a mouse lacking both UT-B and UT-A2 was generated.[363] Unexpectedly, UT-A2 deletion appeared to partially correct the concentrating defect in mice lacking only UT-B.[363] These results suggest that rather than playing a role in maintaining urea concentration during the normal steady state, UT-A2 may function to move urea during the acute transition from diuresis to antidiuresis.[363]

## MICE LACKING ALL UREA TRANSPORTERS

Mice lacking all UTs have a 3.5-fold increase in urine output, produce dilute urine, and have reduced blood pressure.[414] The all-UT knockout mice do not increase urine osmolality or urea following water restriction, acute urea loading, or a high protein intake.[414] The all-UT knockout mice do not exhibit physiological abnormalities in extrarenal tissues.[414]

***Clinical Relevance***

**Urearetics**

In recent years, urea transporter inhibitors have been developed as potential novel diuretics (reviewed in references 476 through 478). Dimethylthiourea (DMTU), a urea analog, inhibits UT-A1 and UT-B, results in a sustained and reversible reduction in urine osmolality, an increase in urine volume, and mild hypokalemia in rats.[479,480] Other thiourea analogs are being investigated for selective inhibition of UT-A1 or UT-B.[479] Another class of inhibitors, an indole thiazole or γ-sultambenzosulfonamide, is selective for UT-A and results in diuresis with more urea than salt excretion in rats, even when the rats were given dDAVP.[481] Another potential class of inhibitors are 2,7-distributed fluorenones, the most potent of which inhibited UT-A1 and UT-B with an IC50 of 1 μM.[482] A fourth class are thienoquinolins that inhibit both UT-A and UT-B, PU-14, results in a diuresis in rats.[483,484] The thienoquinolin PU-48 results in a diuresis in both wild type and UT-B knockout mice, indicating that its effect was to inhibit UT-A, and inhibits urea permeability in perfused rat inner medullary collecting ducts.[485] Because the diuresis induced by PU-48 did not change serum sodium, chloride, or potassium levels, it supports the hypothesis that an agent that targets UT-A1, which is expressed in the last portion of the inner medullary collecting duct, may have less risk for side effects, such as hypokalemia, than conventional diuretics that act in more proximal portions of the nephron.[485]

## ACCUMULATION OF UREA IN RENAL INNER MEDULLA

Urea accumulation within the inner medulla is partly dependent on variable urea permeabilities along the collecting duct system (Fig. 10.17). Within the collecting duct system, only the terminal inner medullary collecting duct possesses high urea permeability,[415] which can be further increased by vasopressin.[148,416,417] UT-A1 and UT-A3 UTs are localized to the apical and basolateral plasma membranes of the inner medullary collecting duct cells and are responsible for the high urea permeability of the terminal portion of the inner medullary collecting duct. The mechanisms of urea accumulation in the renal medulla are depicted in Fig. 10.18. Accumulation of urea is predominantly a result of passive urea reabsorption from the inner medullary collecting duct. Tubular fluid entering the collecting duct system in the renal cortex has a relatively low urea concentration. However, during antidiuresis, water is osmotically reabsorbed from the urea-impermeable parts of the collecting duct system in the cortex and outer medulla, causing a progressive increase in the luminal urea concentration along the connecting tubules, cortical collecting ducts, and outer medullary collecting ducts. Thus, when the tubule fluid reaches the highly urea permeable terminal inner medullary collecting duct (due to the presence of UTs), urea rapidly exits from the lumen to the inner medullary interstitium, where it is "trapped" by countercurrent urea exchange between descending and ascending flows in both the vasa recta and loops of Henle. Under steady-state conditions, and in the continued presence of vasopressin, urea nearly equilibrates across the inner medullary collecting duct epithelium and thus osmotically balances the urea in the collecting duct lumen, preventing possible instances of osmotic diuresis (Fig. 10.19).

The descending and ascending vasa recta are in close association with each other in the inner medulla, facilitating countercurrent exchange of urea between the two structures.[83] In the ascending vasa recta, aided by the extremely high ($>40 \times 10^{-5}$ cm/sec) permeability to urea, the concentration of urea exiting the inner medulla is similar to the concentration of urea in the descending vasa recta.[79,416] This minimizes the washout of urea from the inner medulla. However, countercurrent exchange cannot completely eliminate loss of urea from the inner medullary interstitium, because the volume flow rate of blood in the ascending vasa recta exceeds that in the descending vasa recta.[418] During antidiuresis, water is added to the vasa recta from both inner medullary collecting ducts and descending limbs, resulting in a higher volume flow rate and an increased mass flow rate of urea. This ensures that the inner medullary vasculature continually removes urea from the inner medulla. Quantitatively, the most important loss of urea from the inner medullary interstitium is thought to occur via the vasa recta,[419] but urea recycling pathways play a major role in limiting the loss of urea from the inner medulla. Three major urea recycling pathways are described later in this section, and an overview of these is shown in Fig. 10.20).

### 1. Recycling of Urea Through the Ascending Limbs, Distal Tubules, and Collecting Ducts

Urea that escapes the inner medulla in the ascending limbs of the long loops of Henle is carried back through the thick ascending limbs, distal convoluted tubules, and early portions of the collecting duct system by the flow of tubule fluid.[420] When it reaches the urea-permeable part of the inner medullary collecting ducts, it passively exits into the inner medullary interstitium and starts the cycle again.

### 2. Recycling of Urea Through the Vasa Recta, Short Loops of Henle, and Collecting Ducts

The delivery of urea to the superficial distal tubule exceeds the delivery out of the superficial proximal tubule.[420–422] This

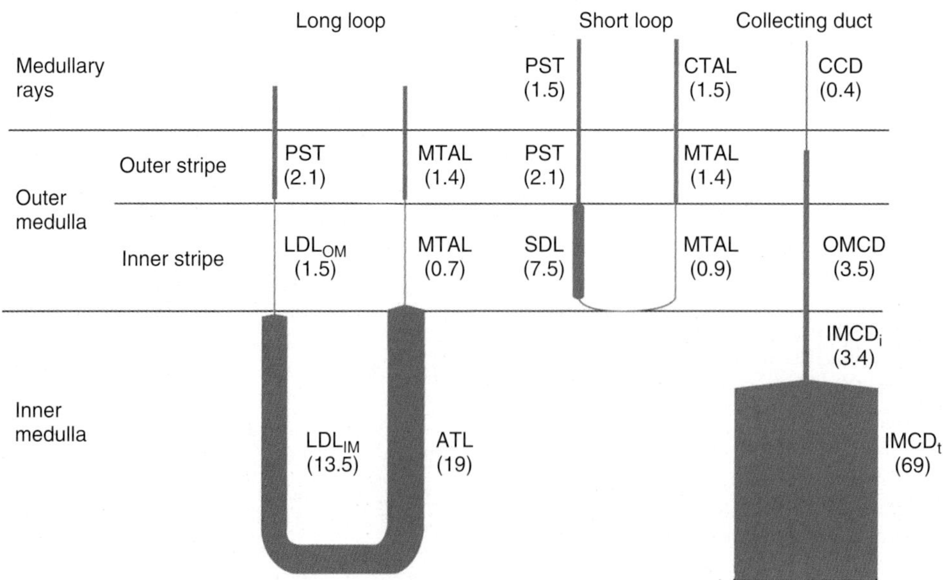


**Fig. 10.17** Urea permeabilities of mammalian renal tubule segments. The width of each segment in the diagram is distorted to be proportional to the urea permeability of that segment. Numbers in parentheses are measured values for the permeability coefficient ($\times 10^{-5}$ cm/sec). Values are from isolated perfused tubule studies. *ATL,* Ascending thin limb; *CTAL,* cortical thick ascending limb; *IMCD$_i$,* initial inner medullary collecting duct; *IMCD$_t$,* terminal inner medullary collecting duct; *LDL,* thin descending limb of long-looped nephron; *MTAL,* medullary thick ascending limb; *OMCD,* outer medullary collecting duct; *PST,* proximal straight tubule; *SDL,* thin descending limb of short-looped nephron.

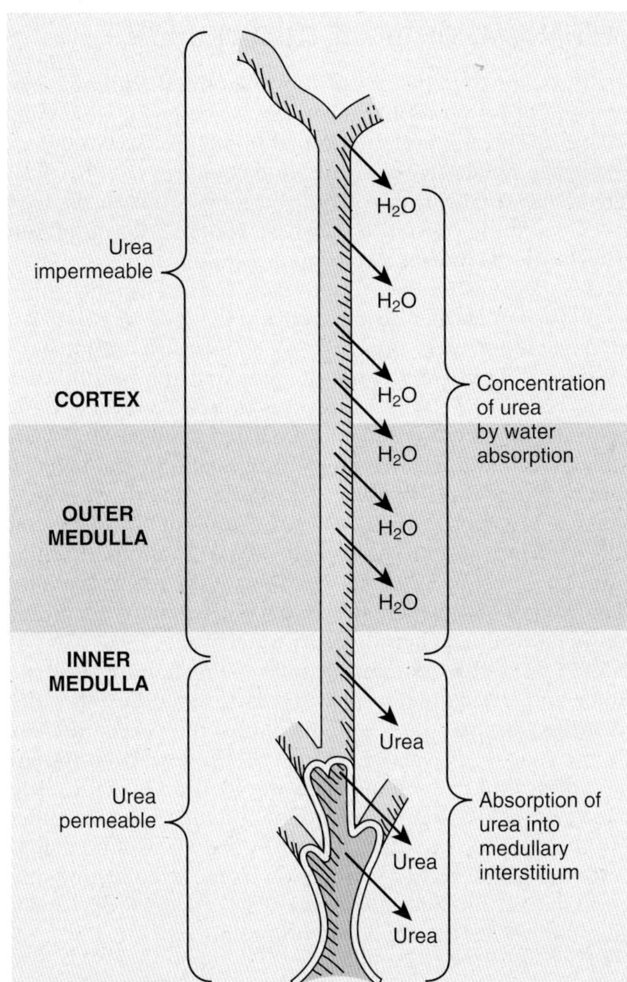


**Fig. 10.18** Schematic representation of the mammalian collecting duct system showing principal sites of water absorption and urea absorption. Water is absorbed in the early part of the collecting duct system, driven by an osmotic gradient. Because urea permeabilities of cortical collecting duct, outer medullary collecting duct, and initial inner medullary collecting duct are very low, the water absorption concentrates urea in the lumen of these segments. When the tubule fluid reaches the terminal inner medullary collecting duct, which is highly permeable to urea, urea rapidly exits from the lumen. This urea is trapped in the inner medulla as a result of countercurrent exchange.

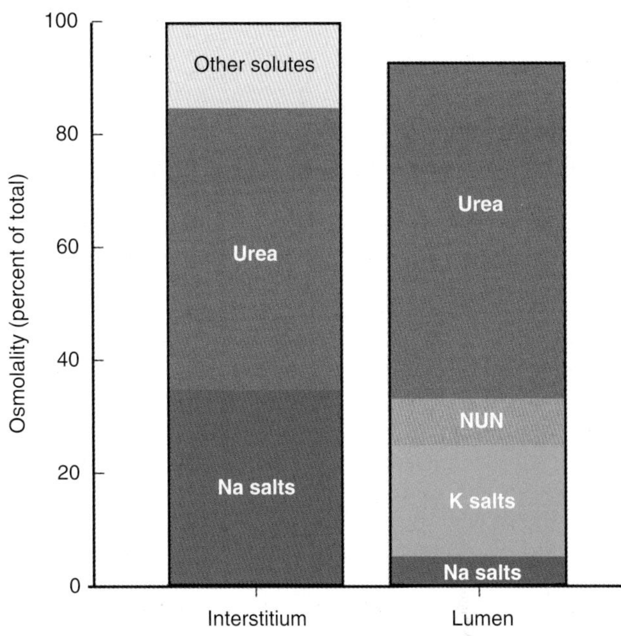


**Fig. 10.19** Solutes that account for osmolality of medullary interstitium and tubule fluid in the inner medullary collecting duct during antidiuresis in rats. Urea nearly equilibrates across the inner medullary collecting duct epithelium as a result of rapid facilitated urea transport. Although the osmolalities of the fluid in the two spaces are nearly equal, the nonurea solutes can differ considerably between the two compartments. Typical values in untreated rats are presented. Values can differ considerably in other species and in the same species with different diets. *NUN*, Nonurea nitrogen.

implies that net urea addition occurs somewhere along the short loops of Henle. One possible mechanism is that the urea leaving the inner medulla in the vasa recta is transferred to the descending limbs of the short loops of Henle[421] and is subsequently carried through the superficial distal tubules back to the urea-permeable part of the inner medullary collecting ducts, where it passively exits, completing the recycling pathway. The close physical association between the vasa recta and the descending limbs of the short loops in the vascular bundles of the inner stripe of the outer medulla would facilitate this transfer of urea from the vasa recta to the short loops of Henle.[26,423] Furthermore, the existence of a facilitative UT, UT-A2, in the thin descending limb of short loops of Henle[8,371] provides further support for this mechanism. However, as discussed earlier, recent studies on UT-A2

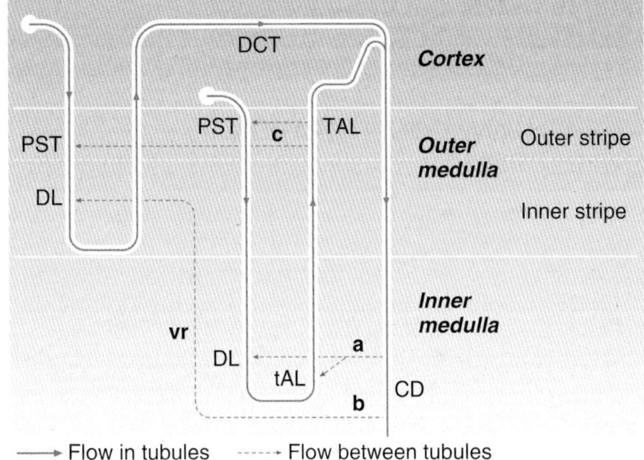


**Fig. 10.20** Pathways of urea recycling in renal medulla. *Solid blue lines* represent a short-looped nephron *(left)* and a long-looped nephron *(right)*. Transfer of urea between nephron segments is indicated by *dashed red arrows* labeled a, b, and c corresponding to recycling pathways described in the text. *CD*, Collecting duct; *DCT*, distal convoluted tubule; *DL*, descending limb; *PST*, proximal straight tubule; *tAL*, thin ascending limb; *TAL*, thick ascending limb; *vr*, vasa recta. Reproduced with permission from Knepper MA, Roch-Ramel F. Pathways of urea transport in the mammalian kidney. *Kidney Int.* 1987;31: 629–633.

knockout mice and UT-A2/UT-B knockout mice have raised doubts about the importance of this pathway.[5,359]

#### 3. Urea Recycling Between Ascending and Descending Limbs of the Loops of Henle

The urea permeability of thick ascending limbs from the inner stripe of the outer medulla is low.[424,425] However, the urea permeability of thick ascending limbs from the outer stripe of the outer medulla and the medullary rays is relatively high.[424,426] Based on this, a urea recycling pathway has been proposed in which urea is reabsorbed from thick ascending limbs and is secreted into neighboring proximal straight tubules, forming a recycling pathway between the ascending limb and descending limbs of the loop of Henle.[3,419] Urea recycling from the thick ascending limbs and the proximal straight tubules is facilitated by the parallel relationship of these two structures in the outer stripe of the outer medulla and in the medullary rays. This transfer of urea is also likely to depend on a relatively attenuated effective blood flow in these regions. Urea secretion into the proximal straight tubules can occur by passive diffusion,[426] active transport,[427] or a combination of both. Urea presumably enters the proximal straight tubules of both short- and long-looped nephrons. The urea that enters the short-looped nephrons will be carried back to the inner medulla by the flow of tubule fluid through the superficial distal tubules and cortical collecting ducts, reentering the inner medullary interstitium by reabsorption from the terminal inner medullary collecting duct. The urea that enters proximal straight tubules of long-looped nephrons returns to the inner medulla directly through the descending limbs of the loops of Henle.[419]

## URINE CONCENTRATION AND DILUTION PROCESSES ALONG THE MAMMALIAN NEPHRON

### SITES OF URINE CONCENTRATION AND DILUTION

Micropuncture studies of the mammalian nephron have determined the major sites of tubule fluid concentration and dilution (see Fig. 10.10). Regardless of whether the kidney is diluting or concentrating the urine, proximal tubule fluid is always isosmotic with plasma.[428] Whereas early distal convoluted tubule fluid is always hypotonic, the earliest nephron segment where significant differences in tubule fluid osmolality can be detected is the late distal tubule. During water diuresis, the fluid in the distal tubule fluid remains hypotonic. During antidiuresis, the fluid in the distal tubule becomes isosmotic with plasma, and the osmolality between the end of the late distal tubule and the inner medullary collecting ducts rises to a level greater than that of plasma. Thus, the conclusion from micropuncture studies is that the loop of Henle is the major site of dilution of tubule fluid, and that dilution processes in the loop occur regardless of whether the final urine is dilute or concentrated. Further dilution of the tubule fluid can occur in the collecting ducts during water diuresis.[429] In contrast, the chief site of urine concentration is beyond the distal tubule (i.e., in the collecting duct system). The mechanisms of urinary dilution and of urinary concentration are discussed in the subsequent sections.

### MECHANISMS OF TUBULE FLUID DILUTION

Micropuncture studies in rats show that the fluid in the early distal tubule is hypotonic, due mainly to a reduction in luminal NaCl concentration relative to that in the proximal tubule.[430] The low luminal NaCl concentration could result either from active NaCl reabsorption from the loop of Henle or from water secretion into the loop of Henle. Micropuncture measurements in rats, performed using inulin as a volume marker, demonstrate net water reabsorption from the superficial loops of Henle during antidiuresis, thereby ruling out water secretion as a potential mechanism of tubule fluid dilution.[420] Thus, one can conclude that luminal dilution occurs because of NaCl reabsorption from the loops of Henle, in excess of water reabsorption. Classic studies of isolated perfused rabbit thick ascending limbs established the mechanism of tubule fluid dilution.[431,432] NaCl is rapidly reabsorbed by active transport, which lowers the luminal osmolality and NaCl concentration to levels below those in the peritubular fluid. The osmotic water permeability of the thick ascending limb is very low, which prevents dissipation of the transepithelial osmolality gradient by water flux.

The tubule fluid remains hypotonic throughout the distal tubule and collecting duct system during water diuresis, aided by the low osmotic water permeability of the collecting ducts when circulating levels of vasopressin are low. Even though the tubule fluid remains hypotonic in the collecting duct system, the solute composition of the tubule fluid is modified within the collecting duct, mainly by $Na^+$ absorption and $K^+$ secretion. Active NaCl reabsorption from the collecting duct results in a further dilution of the collecting duct fluid, beyond that achieved in the thick ascending limbs.[429]

### MECHANISM OF TUBULE FLUID CONCENTRATION

When circulating vasopressin levels are high, net water absorption occurs between the late distal tubule and the collecting ducts.[420] Because water is absorbed in excess of solutes, with a resulting rise in osmolality along the collecting ducts toward the papillary tip,[433] it can be concluded that collecting duct fluid is concentrated chiefly by water absorption, rather than by solute addition.

An axial osmolality gradient in the renal medullary tissue, with the highest degree of hypertonicity at the papillary tip, provides the osmotic driving force for water absorption along the collecting ducts. This osmolality gradient was initially reported by Wirz and colleagues.[434] In a classic study, they demonstrated, in antidiuretic rats, the existence of a continuously increasing osmolality gradient along the outer and inner medulla, with the highest osmolality in the deepest part of the inner medulla, the papillary tip. In addition, within the medulla the osmolality of the collecting ducts was as high as in the loops of Henle and the osmolality of vasa recta blood, sampled from near the papillary tip, was virtually equal to that of the final urine.[434] Taken together these results demonstrate that the high tissue osmolality was not simply a manifestation of a high osmolality in a single structure, namely, the collecting duct. Micropuncture studies by Gottschalk and Mylle[428] based on the superficial and thus accessible tubules and vessels confirmed that the osmolality of the fluid in the loops of Henle, the vasa recta, and the collecting ducts is approximately the same (see Fig. 10.10); thus, these studies support the hypothesis that the collecting duct fluid is concentrated by osmotic equilibration with a hypertonic medullary interstitium. Furthermore, in vitro studies demonstrated that collecting ducts have a high water permeability in the presence of vasopressin,[99,416] as is required for osmotic equilibration. The mechanism by which the corticomedullary osmolality gradient is generated is considered later.

Although the final axial osmolality gradient within the renal medulla is due to the combined gradients of several individual solutes, as initially demonstrated using tissue slice analysis by Ullrich and Jarausch,[435] the principal solutes responsible for the osmolality gradient are NaCl and urea (Fig. 10.21). The increase in the NaCl concentration gradient along the corticomedullary axis occurs predominantly in the outer medulla, with only a small increase in the inner medulla. In contrast, the increase in urea concentration occurs predominantly in the inner medulla, with little or no increase in the initial outer medulla. The mechanisms for generating the NaCl gradient in the outer medulla and urea accumulation in the inner medulla are discussed later.

## GENERATION OF THE AXIAL NaCl GRADIENT IN THE RENAL OUTER MEDULLA

In both diuresis and antidiuresis, an osmolality gradient is maintained along the corticomedullary axis of the outer medulla (see Fig. 10.21).[436] That gradient arises mostly from an accumulation of NaCl and is generated by the concentrating mechanism of the outer medulla. Because the axial osmolality gradient is present in both diuresis and antidiuresis (in which the outer medullary collecting duct is water-permeable to varying degrees), the accumulation of NaCl in the outer medulla cannot depend on a sustained osmolality difference across the collecting duct epithelium. Thus, the concentrating mechanism must depend on the loops of Henle, on the vasculature, and on their interactions within the outer medulla. Moreover, a mass balance of water and NaCl must be maintained. Thus, for example, concentrated fluid that flows into the inner medulla must be balanced by dilute fluid that, in the presence of vasopressin, is absorbed from the cortical collecting duct, dilutes the cortical interstitial fluid, enters the cortical vasculature, and thus participates in maintaining an appropriate systemic level of blood plasma osmolality.

It has long been believed that the osmolality gradient of the outer medulla is generated by means of countercurrent multiplication of a single effect ("Vervielf\;a:ltigung des Einzeleffektes"). In this paradigm, proposed by Kuhn and Ryffle in 1942,[437] osmotic pressure is raised along parallel but opposing flows in nearby tubes that are made contiguous by a hairpin turn (Fig. 10.22); a transfer of solute from one tubule to another (i.e., a single effect) would augment (multiply), or reinforce, the osmotic pressure in the parallel flows. Thus, by means of the countercurrent configuration, a small transverse osmotic difference would be multiplied into a relatively large difference along the axes of flow. In support of this paradigm, Kuhn and Ryffle provided both a mathematical model and an apparatus that exemplified countercurrent multiplication.

As anatomic and physiologic understanding of the renal medulla increased, the countercurrent multiplication paradigm was reinterpreted and modified. In 1951, Hargitay and Kuhn[438] put the paradigm in the context of specific renal tubules. The loop of Henle was identified with the parallel

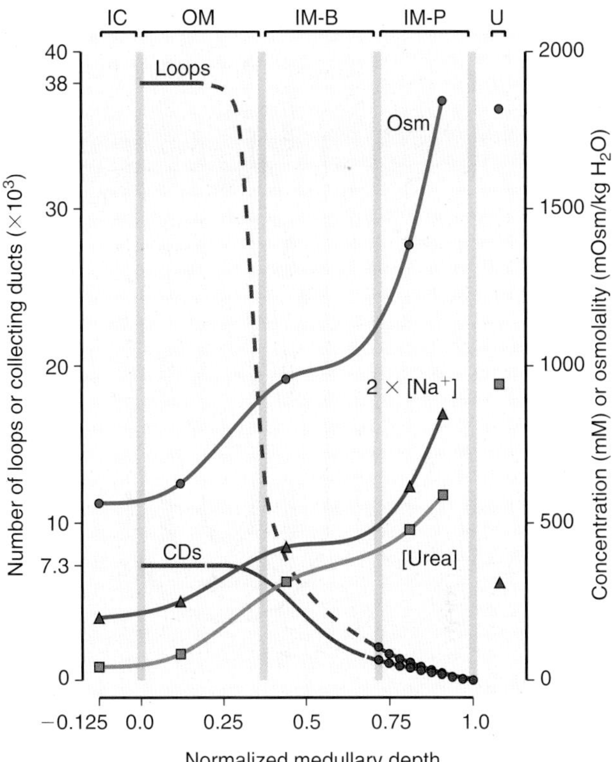


**Fig. 10.21** Data from rat kidney in an antidiuretic state. Osmolality, urea concentration, and sodium concentration plus its anion are shown *(scale at right)*, in addition to the loop of Henle and collecting duct populations *(scale at left)*. Loop of Henle and collecting duct populations decrease in inner medulla because collecting ducts merge and loops turn back. The osmolality gradient is larger in the outer medulla and papilla than in the outer part of the inner medulla. The gradient is largest in the papilla, where the osmolality and concentration profiles appear to increase exponentially. The shape of the sodium profile has been corroborated by electron microprobe measurements.[486] *IC*, Inner cortex; *IM*, outer part (base) of inner medulla; *OM*, outer medulla; *P*, papilla or inner part (tip) of inner medulla; *U*, urine. Figure based on published data. Curves connecting data points are natural cubic splines, computed by standard algorithms.[487] Dashed curve segments are interpolations without supporting measurements. Tubule populations in papilla are from Hans et al.[488] tubule populations in outer medulla are based on estimates in Knepper et al.[59] Concentrations and osmolalities are from tissue slices and urine samples collected 4.5 hours after onset of vasopressin infusion at 15 μU/min per 100 g body weight. Data are from Fig. 5 in Atherton et al.[489] and Figs. 1, 3, 9 in Hai and Thomas[436]; slice locations were given in Wade et al.[8] The osmolality reported in the inner cortex seems high relative to the reported plasma concentration of 314 mOsm/kg $H_2O$. The osmolality and concentration profiles, as drawn in the study by Hai and Thomas,[436] apparently do not take into account relative distances between tissue sample sites. (From Sands JM, Layton HE. The urine-concentrating mechanism and urea transporters. In: Alpern RJ, Caplan MJ, Moe OW, eds. *The Kidney: Physiology and Pathophysiology,* ed 5. San Diego: Academic Press; 2013:1463–1510.)

tubes joined by a hairpin turn as proposed by Kuhn and Ryffle. Thus, the loops of Henle were proposed as the source of the outer medullary gradient, and that gradient was hypothesized to draw water out of water-permeable collecting ducts. In 1959, Kuhn and Ramel[439] used a mathematical model to show that active transport of NaCl from thick ascending

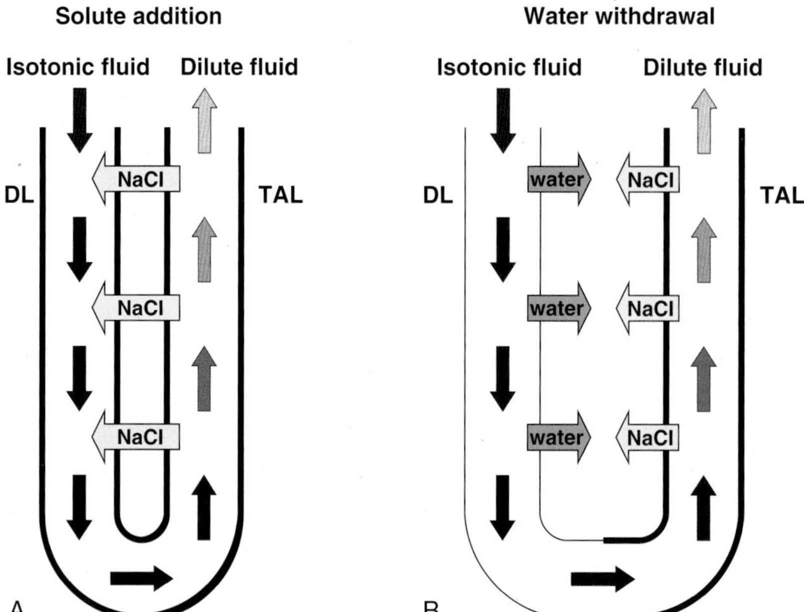


**Fig. 10.22** (A) Countercurrent multiplication by means of NaCl transfer from an ascending flow to a descending flow. (B) Countercurrent multiplication by means of water withdrawal from a descending flow. NaCl transport from the ascending flow into the interstitium raises interstitial osmolality; this results in passive water transport from the descending flow, which has lower osmolality than the interstitium. In both panels, tubular fluid flow direction is indicated by *blue arrows*; increasing osmolality is indicated by *darkening shades of blue*. Ascending flow may be considered to be in the thick ascending limb of Henle *(TAL)*; descending flow in the descending limb of Henle *(DL)*. *Thick black lines* indicate that a tubule is impermeable to water; *thin lines* indicate high permeability to water. (From Layton AT, Layton HE. Countercurrent multiplication may not explain the axial osmolality gradient in the outer medulla of the rat kidney. *Am J Physiol Renal Physiol.* 2011; 301:F1047-F1056.)

limbs could serve as the single effect. Subsequent physiologic experiments confirmed the active NaCl transport and the osmotic absorption of water from collecting ducts.[420,431–433] Experiments indicating high water permeability in hamster descending limbs of short loops[440] and in descending limbs of long loops[9,10,12] suggested that the accumulation of NaCl from thick limbs concentrated descending limb tubular fluid by osmotic water withdrawal, rather than by NaCl addition (see Fig. 10.22).

In more recent years, as anatomic details of the medulla emerged, it has become necessary to refine the paradigm of countercurrent multiplication to provide an accurate representation of the means by which the gradient is generated in the mammalian outer medulla. In particular, the descending limbs of short loops have been shown to be anatomically separated from ascending limbs, with inner stripe portions of short loops near (or within) the vascular bundles and thick limbs near the collecting ducts.[23,441] This configuration is not consistent with direct interactions between counterflowing limbs. Furthermore, in short-looped rat nephrons, Wade et al.[8] found that AQP1 is not expressed in portions of descending limb segments in the distal inner stripe. Zhai et al.[17] found that AQP1 is not expressed in descending limbs of short loops in the inner stripes of mice, rats, and humans. The absence of AQP1 suggests that the assumption of high water permeability in descending limbs of short loops merits further experimental study.

From these considerations, it seems reasonable to hypothesize that the outer medullary osmolality gradient arises principally from vigorous active transport of NaCl, without accompanying water, from the thick ascending limbs of short- and long-looped nephrons. The tubular fluid of the thick limbs that enters the cortex is diluted well below plasma osmolality, and thus the requirement of mass balance is met. In rats and mice, the thick limbs are localized near the collecting ducts[442]; mathematical models suggest that at a given level of the outer medulla, the interstitial osmolality will be higher near the collecting ducts than near the vascular bundles.[443,444] This higher osmolality will facilitate water withdrawal from the descending limbs of long loops and from collecting ducts. Descending vasa recta are thought to be found only in the vascular bundles. Thus, the ascending vasa recta will act as the collectors of any NaCl that is absorbed from the loops of Henle and water that is absorbed from the descending limbs of long loops and from collecting ducts.

The countercurrent configuration of the ascending vasa recta, relative to the descending limbs and collecting ducts, is likely to participate in sustaining the axial gradient: as ascending vasa recta fluid ascends toward the cortex, its osmolality will exceed that in the descending limbs of long loops and in the collecting ducts. Thus, ascending vasa recta fluid will be progressively diluted as that fluid contributes to the concentrating of fluid in descending limbs of long loops and in collecting ducts, by giving up NaCl to, and absorbing water from, the interstitium (Fig. 10.23).

The previous summary appears to account for the elevation of osmolality in the outer medulla without invoking a role for countercurrent multiplication. However, a question remains: why does the osmolality gradient increase along the outer

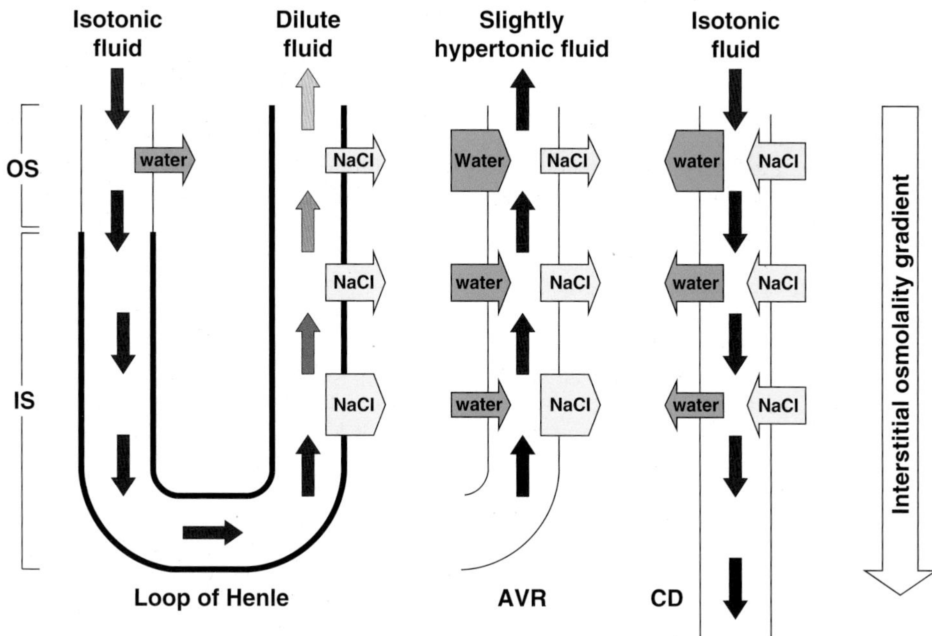


**Fig. 10.23** Outer medullary concentrating mechanism based on NaCl addition to the interstitium but without water absorption from descending limbs of short loops. Arrows indicate water *(cyan)* and NaCl *(yellow)* transepithelial transport; arrow widths suggest relative transport magnitudes. Isotonic fluid is considered to have the same osmolality as blood plasma. Flow entering the AVR is assumed to arise from a descending vas rectum that is in, or near, a vascular bundle. Outflow from the collecting duct enters the inner medullary collecting duct. Tubular fluid flow direction is indicated by *blue arrows;* increasing osmolality is indicated by *darkening shades of blue*. *Thick black lines* indicate that a tubule is impermeable to water; *thin lines* indicate high permeability to water. *AVR*, Ascending vas rectum; *CD*, collecting duct; *IS*, inner stripe; *OS*, outer stripe. (From Layton AT, Layton HE. Countercurrent multiplication may not explain the axial osmolality gradient in the outer medulla of the rat kidney. *Am J Physiol Renal Physiol.* 2011; 301:F1047-F1056.)

medulla as a function of increasing medullary depth? The answer likely lies in the local balance of NaCl absorption from thick limbs and water absorption from descending limbs of long loops and from collecting ducts. At deeper medullary levels, the rate of NaCl absorption from thick limbs may be higher than at shallow levels, owing to a higher Na-K-ATPase activity at deeper levels[445] and to a saturation of transport proteins by the higher NaCl concentration in thick limb tubular fluid before dilution. Moreover, because of the water already absorbed in the upper outer medulla, the load of water presented to the thick limbs deep in the outer medulla by descending limbs of long loops and by the collecting ducts is much reduced.

A caveat is in order: our understanding of the outer medulla is mostly based on information obtained from heavily studied laboratory animals, especially rats and mice. Outer medullary function and structure are likely to vary substantially in other species. For example, the human kidney has limited concentrating capability (relative to many other mammals) and only about one seventh of the loops of Henle are long[446]; the mountain beaver (*Aplodontia rufa*) has mostly cortical loops of Henle and essentially no inner medulla.[447] It seems likely that the outer medullary structure in these species differ substantially from that in rats and mice. Finally, it should be acknowledged that the paradigm formulated above is similar to that proposed by Berliner et al. in 1958.[83]

## DETERMINANTS OF CONCENTRATING ABILITY

The overall concentrating ability of the kidney arises from interactions among several differing components. In addition to the active transport of NaCl from the thick ascending limbs and the water permeability of the collecting ducts, two other factors play a significant role in determining the osmolality of the final urine. One important determinant is the delivery rate of NaCl and water to the loop of Henle, which sets an upper limit on the amount of NaCl actively reabsorbed by the thick ascending limb to drive the outer medullary concentrating mechanism. Another important determinant is the volume of tubular fluid delivered to the medullary collecting duct, which has an underappreciated effect on the concentrating process. Too much fluid delivery saturates water reabsorption processes along the medullary collecting ducts, leading to interstitial dilution due to rapid osmotic water transport. In contrast, too little fluid delivery to the medullary collecting ducts, even in the absence of vasopressin, results in sustained osmotic equilibration across the collecting duct epithelium owing to the nonzero osmotic water permeability of the inner medullary collecting duct.[144,148,149]

## AN UNRESOLVED QUESTION: CONCENTRATION OF NaCl IN THE RENAL INNER MEDULLA

Tissue slice studies demonstrate that the corticomedullary osmolality gradient is made up largely of a NaCl gradient in the outer medulla and a urea gradient in the inner medulla (see Fig. 10.21). Accordingly, in the previous sections we have emphasized the processes that concentrate NaCl in the outer medulla and the processes responsible for urea accumulation in the inner medulla (passive urea absorption from the inner medullary collecting duct plus countercurrent exchange of urea via diffusion). The concentrating mechanism described previously functions only in the renal outer medulla and medullary rays of the cortex. The ascending limbs of loops of Henle that reach into the inner medulla are thin-walled and do not actively transport NaCl[416,448,449]; nonetheless, in antidiuresis a substantial axial osmolality gradient is generated in the inner medulla of many mammals. For nearly 50 years, controversy has persisted regarding the nature of the mechanism that generates the inner medullary osmolality gradient. Moreover, the energy source for the concentrating of nonurea solutes in the inner medullary interstitium is not known. General analysis of inner medullary concentrating processes indicates that, to satisfy mass balance requirements, either an ascending stream (thin ascending limbs or ascending vasa recta) must be diluted relative to the inner medullary interstitium, or a descending stream (descending thin limbs, descending vasa recta, or collecting ducts) must be concentrated locally relative to the inner medulla.[87,450]

Three major hypotheses have been proposed for the concentrating mechanism of the inner medulla.

#### 1. The "Passive Mechanism"

Kokko and Rector[408] and Stephenson[409] independently proposed a model by which the osmolality in the thin ascending limb could be lowered below that of the interstitium entirely by passive transport processes in the inner medulla. This mechanism is generally referred to as the "passive model" or the "passive countercurrent multiplier mechanism." The passive mechanism depends on the separation of urea and NaCl that is accomplished by NaCl absorption from the thick ascending limbs; indeed, this absorption is the hypothesized energy source for the passive mechanism. In this model, rapid urea reabsorption from the inner medullary collecting duct generates and maintains a high urea concentration in the inner medullary interstitium, causing the osmotic withdrawal of water from the thin descending limb. This concentrates NaCl in the descending limb lumen and results in a transepithelial gradient favoring the passive reabsorption of NaCl from the thin ascending limb of Henle loop. Additionally, if the ascending limbs have extremely low urea permeability, then any NaCl that has been reabsorbed from the thin ascending limb will not be replaced by urea. Thus, the ascending limb fluid will be dilute relative to the fluid in other nephron segments, generating a "single effect" analogous to active NaCl absorption from thick ascending limbs. This single effect can then be multiplied by the counterflow between the ascending and descending limbs of Henle loops. This model requires that the thin descending limbs are highly permeable to water but not NaCl or urea, whereas the thin ascending limb would have to be permeable to NaCl but not water or urea. However, several objections to the passive mechanism have since been made. Contrary to the permeability requirements of the passive model, high urea permeabilities have been measured in the thin descending limb and thin ascending limb (summarized in Gamba and Knepper[451]), whereas little or no osmotic water permeability has been measured in the lower portions of thin descending limbs in the inner medulla.[20] In addition, studies in UT-A1/A3 urea transporter knockout mice found that urea accumulation in the inner medulla was largely eliminated, but inner medullary NaCl accumulation was not affected[143,358,407] (see "UT-A1/A3 knockout mice" in earlier section).

Layton and colleagues reevaluated the passive mechanism by incorporating measured loop NaCl, urea, and water permeabilities into a mathematical model.[19,452,453] These studies suggest that water absorption from descending limbs is not a requirement for the passive mechanism to generate an osmolality gradient, and that the urea-permeable loops of Henle can serve as a highly effective countercurrent urea exchanger. However, the model was able to fully account for the high urine osmolalities attained by some animals.

#### 2. Concentrating Mechanism Driven by External Solute

Jen and Stevenson[454] proposed that the concentrating mechanism of the inner medulla depends on a solute other than NaCl and urea. By means of a mathematical model, they demonstrated, in principle, that the continuous addition of small amounts of an unspecified, but osmotically active, solute to the inner medullary interstitium could produce a substantial axial osmolality gradient. Such a solute would have to be generated in the inner medulla by a chemical reaction that produces more osmotically active particles than it consumes. The mechanism of concentration is similar to that driven by urea in the "passive" models proposed by Kokko and Rector and by Stephenson[408,409]: the thin descending limbs in the inner medulla are assumed impermeable to the solute (thus it is an "external" solute), and as a result, water is withdrawn from the descending limbs and the concentration of NaCl is raised in descending limb tubular fluid. Beginning at the loop bend, elevated NaCl concentration within the loop will result in a substantial NaCl efflux that will dilute the ascending flow and that is sufficient to generate the axial gradient.

The feasibility of this mechanism was subsequently confirmed by Thomas and Wexler[455] in the context of a more detailed mathematical model. In further modeling studies, Thomas,[456] and Hervy and Thomas[457] proposed that lactate, generated by anaerobic glycolysis (the predominant means of ATP generation in the inner medulla), could serve as the solute. Two lactate ions are generated per glucose consumed:

$$\text{glucose} \rightarrow 2\ \text{lactate-} + 2\ \text{H}^{+}$$

However, as pointed out by Knepper et al.,[87] the net generation of osmotically active particles depends on which buffering anions are titrated by the protons. If the protons titrate bicarbonate, there may be a net removal of osmotically active particles; if instead the protons titrate other buffers (e.g., phosphate or $NH_3$), there will be a net generation of osmotically active particles. Mathematical models developed by Zhang and Edwards[458] and by Chen et al.[459] predicted that vascular countercurrent exchange would tend to restrict significant glucose availability into the outer medulla and the upper inner medulla, thus limiting the rate of lactate generation in the deep inner medulla where the highest osmolalities are found.

#### 3. Hyaluronan as a Mechano-osmotic Transducer

In the mechano-osmotic induction hypothesis,[87,460] in which energy from the peristaltic contractions of the renal pelvic wall is used to concentrate solutes in the descending limbs and collecting ducts by water withdrawal, or, alternatively, the peristaltic contractions reduce sodium activity in the hyaluronan matrix of the interstitium, resulting in the reabsorption of hypotonic fluid from that matrix into ascending vasa recta. Hyaluronan (or "hyaluronic acid") is a glycosaminoglycan[461,462] that is abundant in the interstitium of the renal inner medulla.[463,464] The hyaluronan in the inner medulla is produced by a specialized interstitial cell (the type 1 interstitial cell), which forms characteristic "bridges" between the thin limbs of Henle and the vasa recta.[465] These bridges may delimit, above and below, the nodal compartments identified by Pannabecker and Dantzler,[28] which were discussed previously. Thus, the inner medullary interstitium may be considered to be composed of a compressible, viscoelastic, hyaluronan matrix.

Several hypotheses have been advanced that depend on the peristalsis of the papilla as an integral component of the concentrating mechanism of the inner medulla.[87,357,466] In one hypothesis, which was suggested in part by Schmidt-Nielsen,[467] compression of the hyaluronan matrix stores some of the mechanical energy from the smooth muscle contraction that gives rise to the peristaltic wave. In the postwave decompression, the matrix exerts an elastic force that promotes water absorption from thin descending limbs and collecting ducts, and thereby increases tubular fluid osmolality. Water absorption from the descending limbs would raise tubular fluid NaCl concentration and thus promote a vigorous NaCl absorption from the loop bends and early ascending limbs. However, if, as is apparently the case in rat, the lower 60% of inner medullary descending limbs are water impermeable,[20] water is unlikely to be absorbed from descending limbs in the deep portion of the inner medulla where the highest osmolalities are achieved.

Another hypothesis involves special properties of hyaluronan.[468] Hyaluronan is a large polyanion (1000 to 10,000 kDa). Its charge is due to the carboxylate (COO) groups of the glucuronic subunits. Hyaluronan is hydrophilic and assumes a highly expanded, random coil confirmation that occupies a large volume of space relative to its mass. This extended state arises partly from electrostatic repulsion between carboxylate groups (which maximize the distances between neighboring negative charges), and partly from the extended conformations of the glycosidic bonds.

Knepper et al. proposed that the periodic compression of the papilla, and the effects of that compression on the hyaluronan matrix, could explain the osmolality gradient along the inner medulla.[87] When hyaluronan is compressed, the repulsive forces of neighboring carboxylate groups are overcome, in part, by a condensation of cations (mainly $Na^+$), and a localized crystalloid structure is formed. Thus, compression of the hyaluronan gel results in a decrease of the local sodium ion activity in the gel.[87] In aqueous solutions that are in equilibrium with the gel, the NaCl concentration will decrease as a consequence of the compression-induced reduction in $Na^+$ activity within the gel. Therefore, the free fluid that is expressed from the hyaluronan matrix during the contraction phase will have a lower total solute concentration than that of the gel as a whole. The slightly hypotonic fluid expressed from the matrix is likely to escape the inner medulla via the ascending vasa recta, the only structure that remains open during the compressive phase of the contraction cycle.[467] As a consequence, the ascending fluid within the ascending vasa recta would have a lower osmolality than the local interstitium, and as a result, fluid in collecting ducts and descending vasa recta would be concentrated.

This mechanism is consistent with the nodal compartments found by Pannabecker and Dantzler[28]: these compartments, which are likely rich in hyaluronan, are in contact with collecting ducts, thin ascending limbs, and ascending vasa recta. Thus, they are well-configured to be sites of transduction (i.e., sites where the mechanical energy of peristalsis is harnessed to generate an ascending flow that is dilute relative to average local osmolality). However, no quantitative analyses or mathematical models have examined the mass balance consistency or the thermodynamic adequacy of hypotheses that depend on the peristaltic contractions.

## ACKNOWLEDGMENTS

This work was supported by National Institutes of Health grant R01-DK41707 to JMS. RAF is supported by the Danish Medical Research Council, the Novo Nordisk Foundation, the Carlsberg Foundation (Carlsbergfondet) and the Lundbeck Foundation.

Drs. Dennis Brown and Robert A. Fenton were coauthors of a chapter on the cell biology of vasopressin action in the 10th edition and some of the material in that chapter is incorporated into this chapter in the present edition.

 Complete reference list available at ExpertConsult.com.

## KEY REFERENCES

5. Fenton RA, Knepper MA. Mouse models and the urinary concentrating mechanism in the new millennium. *Physiol Rev.* 2007;87:1083–1112.
15. Pannabecker TL. Comparative physiology and architecture associated with the mammalian urine concentrating mechanism: role of inner medullary water and urea transport pathways in the rodent medulla. *Am J Physiol Regul Integr Comp Physiol.* 2013;304(7):R488–R503.
18. Westrick KY, Serack B, Dantzler WH, et al. Axial compartmentation of descending and ascending thin limbs of Henle's loops. *Am J Physiol Renal Physiol.* 2013;304(3):F308–F316.
87. Knepper MA, Saidel GM, Hascall VC, et al. Concentration of solutes in the renal inner medulla: interstitial hyaluronan as a mechano-osmotic transducer. *Am J Physiol Renal Physiol.* 2003;284(3):F433–F446.
97. Lolait SJ, O'Carroll A-M, McBride OW, et al. Cloning and characterization of a vasopressin V2 receptor and possible link to nephrogenic diabetes insipidus. *Nature.* 1992;357:336–339.
116. Roos KP, Strait KA, Raphael KL, et al. Collecting duct-specific knockout of adenylyl cyclase type VI causes a urinary concentration defect in mice. *Am J Physiol Renal Physiol.* 2012;302(1):F78–F84.
126. Ren XR, Reiter E, Ahn S, et al. Different G protein-coupled receptor kinases govern G protein and beta-arrestin-mediated signaling of V2 vasopressin receptor. *Proc Natl Acad Sci U S A.* 2005;102(5):1448–1453.
138. Fenton RA, Pedersen CN, Moeller HB. New insights into regulated aquaporin-2 function. *Curr Opin Nephrol Hypertens.* 2013;22(5):551–558.
148. Sands JM, Nonoguchi H, Knepper MA. Vasopressin effects on urea and $H_2O$ transport in inner medullary collecting duct subsegments. *Am J Physiol.* 1987;253:F823–F832.
154. Preston GM, Carroll TP, Guggino WB, et al. Appearance of water channels in *Xenopus* oocytes expressing red cell CHIP28 protein. *Science.* 1992;256:385–387.
167. Poulsen SB, Kim YH, Frokiaer J, et al. Long-term vasopressin-v2-receptor stimulation induces regulation of aquaporin 4 protein in renal inner medulla and cortex of Brattleboro rats. *Nephrol Dial Transplant.* 2013;28(8):2058–2065.
169. Zwang NA, Hoffert JD, Pisitkun T, et al. Identification of phosphorylation-dependent binding partners of aquaporin-2 using protein mass spectrometry. *J Proteome Res.* 2009;8(3):1540–1554.
178. Nielsen S, Chou C-L, Marples D, et al. Vasopressin increases water permeability of kidney collecting duct by inducing translocation of aquaporin-CD water channels to plasma membrane. *Proc Natl Acad Sci U S A.* 1995;92:1013–1017.

185. Bouley R, Hasler U, Lu HA, et al. Bypassing vasopressin receptor signaling pathways in nephrogenic diabetes insipidus. *Semin Nephrol.* 2008;28(3):266–278.
191. Moeller HB, Aroankins TS, Slengerik-Hansen J, et al. Phosphorylation and ubiquitylation are opposing processes that regulate endocytosis of the water channel aquaporin-2. *J Cell Sci.* 2014;127(Pt 14):3174–3183.
195. Khositseth S, Charngkaew K, Boonkrai C, et al. Hypercalcemia induces targeted autophagic degradation of aquaporin-2 at the onset of nephrogenic diabetes insipidus. *Kidney Int.* 2017;91(5):1070–1087.
227. Kortenoeven ML, Pedersen NB, Miller RL, et al. Genetic ablation of aquaporin-2 in the mouse connecting tubules results in defective renal water handling. *J Physiol.* 2013;591(Pt 8):2205–2219.
243. Boone M, Kortenoeven ML, Robben JH, et al. Counteracting vasopressin-mediated water reabsorption by ATP, dopamine, and phorbol esters: mechanisms of action. *Am J Physiol Renal Physiol.* 2011;300(3):F761–F771.
248. Bouley R, Soler NP, Cohen O, et al. Stimulation of AQP2 membrane insertion in renal epithelial cells in vitro and in vivo by the cGMP phosphodiesterase inhibitor sildenafil citrate (Viagra). *Am J Physiol Renal Physiol.* 2005;288(6):F1103–F1112.
264. Lee MS, Choi HJ, Park EJ, et al. Depletion of vacuolar protein sorting-associated protein 35 is associated with increased lysosomal degradation of aquaporin-2. *Am J Physiol Renal Physiol.* 2016;311(6): F1294–F1307.
285. Li W, Zhang Y, Bouley R, et al. Simvastatin enhances aquaporin-2 surface expression and urinary concentration in vasopressin-deficient Brattleboro rats through modulation of Rho GTPase. *Am J Physiol Renal Physiol.* 2011;301(2):F309–F318.
320. Olesen ET, Moeller HB, Assentoft M, et al. The vasopressin type 2 receptor and prostaglandin receptors EP2 and EP4 can increase aquaporin-2 plasma membrane targeting through a cAMP-independent pathway. *Am J Physiol Renal Physiol.* 2016;311(5): F935–F944.
322. Cheung PW, Nomura N, Nair AV, et al. EGF receptor inhibition by erlotinib increases aquaporin 2-mediated renal water reabsorption. *J Am Soc Nephrol.* 2016;27(10):3105–3116.
326. Hoffert JD, Pisitkun T, Saeed F, et al. Dynamics of the G protein-coupled vasopressin V2 receptor signaling network revealed by quantitative phosphoproteomics. *Mol Cell Proteomics.* 2012;11(2): doi:10.1074/mcp.M111.014613.
328. Moeller HB, MacAulay N, Knepper MA, et al. Role of multiple phosphorylation sites in the COOH-terminal tail of aquaporin-2 for water transport: evidence against channel gating. *Am J Physiol Renal Physiol.* 2009;296(3):F649–F657.
340. Moeller HB, Praetorius J, Rutzler MR, et al. Phosphorylation of aquaporin-2 regulates its endocytosis and protein-protein interactions. *Proc Natl Acad Sci U S A.* 2010;107(1):424–429.
341. Klein JD, Wang Y, Blount MA, et al. Metformin, an AMPK activator, stimulates the phosphorylation of aquaporin 2 and urea transporter A1 in inner medullary collecting ducts. *Am J Physiol Renal Physiol.* 2016;310(10):F1008–F1012.
349. Olesen ET, Fenton RA. Is there a role for PGE2 in urinary concentration? *J Am Soc Nephrol.* 2013;24(2):169–178.
355. Gamble JL, McKhann CF, Butler AM, et al. An economy of water in renal function referable to urea. *Am J Physiol.* 1934;109:139–154.
358. Fenton RA, Chou C-L, Stewart GS, et al. Urinary concentrating defect in mice with selective deletion of phloretin-sensitive urea transporters in the renal collecting duct. *Proc Natl Acad Sci U S A.* 2004;101(19):7469–7474.
367. Bagnasco SM, Peng T, Janech MG, et al. Cloning and characterization of the human urea transporter UT-a1 and mapping of the human *Slc14a2* gene. *Am J Physiol Renal Physiol.* 2001;281:F400–F406.
371. Nielsen S, Terris J, Smith CP, et al. Cellular and subcellular localization of the vasopressin-regulated urea transporter in rat kidney. *Proc Natl Acad Sci U S A.* 1996;93:5495–5500.
376. You G, Smith CP, Kanai Y, et al. Cloning and characterization of the vasopressin-regulated urea transporter. *Nature.* 1993;365: 844–847.
378. Blount MA, Mistry AC, Fröhlich O, et al. Phosphorylation of UT-a1 urea transporter at serines 486 and 499 is important for vasopressin-regulated activity and membrane accumulation. *Am J Physiol Renal Physiol.* 2008;295(1):F295–F299.
391. Wang Y, Klein JD, Fröhlich O, et al. Role of protein kinase C-α in hypertonicity-stimulated urea permeability in mouse inner medullary collecting ducts. *Am J Physiol Renal Physiol.* 2013;304:F233–F238.
402. Efe O, Klein JD, LaRocque LM, et al. Metformin improves urine concentration in rodents with nephrogenic diabetes insipidus. *JCI Insight.* 2016;1(11).
403. Sands JM, Klein JD. Physiological insights into novel therapies for nephrogenic diabetes insipidus. *Am J Physiol Renal Physiol.* 2016;doi:10.1152/ajprenal.00418.2016.
408. Kokko JP, Rector FC. Countercurrent multiplication system without active transport in inner medulla. *Kidney Int.* 1972;2:214–223.
409. Stephenson JL. Concentration of urine in a central core model of the renal counterflow system. *Kidney Int.* 1972;2:85–94.
410. Pannabecker TL, Dantzler WH, Layton HE, et al. Role of three-dimensional architecture in the urine concentrating mechanism of the rat renal inner medulla. *Am J Physiol Renal Physiol.* 2008;295(5):F1271–F1285.
428. Gottschalk CW, Mylle M. Micropuncture study of the mammalian urinary concentrating mechanism: evidence for the countercurrent hypothesis. *Am J Physiol.* 1959;196:927–936.
431. Burg MB, Green N. Function of the thick ascending limb of Henle's loop. *Am J Physiol.* 1973;224:659–668.
432. Rocha AS, Kokko JP. Sodium chloride and water transport in the medullary thick ascending limb of Henle. Evidence for active chloride transport. *J Clin Invest.* 1973;52:612–623.
434. Wirz H, Hargitay B, Kuhn W. Lokalisation des konzentrierungsprozesses in der niere durch direkte kryoskopie. *Helv Physiol Pharmacol Acta.* 1951;9:196–207.
437. Kuhn W, Ryffel K. Herstellung konzentrierter lösungen aus verdünnten durch blosse membranwirkung: ein modellversuch zur funktion der niere. *Hoppe Seylers Z Physiol Chem.* 1942;276: 145–178.
453. Layton AT. A mathematical model of the urine concentrating mechanism in the rat renal medulla. I. Formulation and base-case results. *Am J Physiol Renal Physiol.* 2011;300(2):F356–F371.
454. Jen JF, Stephenson JL. Externally driven countercurrent multiplication in a mathematical model of the urinary concentrating mechanism of the renal inner medulla. *Bull Math Biol.* 1994;56(3): 491–514.
457. Hervy S, Thomas SR. Inner medullary lactate production and urine-concentrating mechanism: a flat medullary model. *Am J Physiol Renal Physiol.* 2003;284(1):F65–F81.
467. Schmidt-Nielsen B. The renal concentrating mechanism in insects and mammals: a new hypothesis involving hydrostatic pressures. *Am J Physiol.* 1995;268:R1087–R1100.
478. Klein JD, Sands JM. Urea transport and clinical potential of urearetics. *Curr Opin Nephrol Hypertens.* 2016;25(5):444–451.

# 11 Vasoactive Molecules and the Kidney

Richard E. Gilbert | Andrew Advani

## CHAPTER OUTLINE



## KEY POINTS

- Beyond the classical endocrine renin–angiotensin system (RAS) that pivots around the actions of systemically circulating angiotensin II, an additional, quasi-independent local RAS operates within the kidney in paracrine, autocrine, and possibly even intracrine modes.
- Although much of our understanding of the RAS relates to the actions of angiotensin II, a range of other angiotensin-related proteins, enzymes, and receptors also have important biological actions in both kidney physiology and disease.
- Therapies that block the RAS have been employed to slow renal decline in chronic kidney disease for decades and agents that either prevent (e.g., endothelin receptor antagonists) or augment (e.g., neprilysin inhibitors in combination with angiotensin receptor blockade) the actions of other vasoactive molecules are under investigation.
- Endothelin type A receptor blockade is undergoing phase III evaluation for the treatment of diabetic nephropathy, although earlier clinical trials were hampered by dose-dependent fluid retention.
- Inhibition of neprilysin prevents the degradation of the natriuretic peptides atrial natriuretic peptide and brain natriuretic peptide, but its effects are limited by an unopposed RAS. Concurrent angiotensin receptor blockade and neprilysin inhibition improves outcomes in patients with heart failure, although its effects on hard renal outcomes are currently unknown.
- Concurrent angiotensin-converting enzyme inhibition and neprilysin inhibition are associated with an increased risk of angioedema.
- The development of therapies that affect other vasoactive molecules (e.g., the kallikrein–kinin system, urotensin II, guanylin, uroguanylin, and adrenomedullin) has been limited.

Vasoactive peptides, arising from both the systemic circulation and from local tissue-based generation, play important roles in kidney physiology, not only in the regulation of renal blood flow (RBF) but also in electrolyte exchange, acid–base balance, and diuresis. More recent interest has focused on the role of these peptide systems in kidney development and in the pathogenesis of organ injury.

## RENIN–ANGIOTENSIN–ALDOSTERONE SYSTEM

In their now seminal 1898 report, *Niere und Kreislauf*, Robert Tigerstedt and Per Bergman, while working at the Karolinska Institute in Sweden, described the prolonged vasopressor effects of crude kidney extracts.[1] Although recognizing the impurity of the extract, Tigerstedt named the unidentified active substance, "renin," based on its organ of origin. More than 110 years later, our understanding of the renin–angiotensin system (RAS) continues to evolve with recent insights into its pivotal role in pathophysiological as well as physiological processes. Underlying this effort to fully understand the RAS is not only a desire for knowledge but also a profound appreciation of the therapeutic importance of its blockade that emanates from the renoprotective effects of angiotensin-converting enzyme inhibition first described by Anderson, Meyer, Rennke, and Brenner in 1985 in a rodent model of progressive kidney disease.[2]

*Clinical Relevance*

The renin–angiotensin system (RAS) plays a fundamental role in blood pressure, plasma volume, electrolyte, and acid–base homeostasis. Beyond its function in kidney physiology, however, angiotensin II, the primary effector molecule of the RAS, raises intraglomerular pressure, induces proteinuria, and stimulates the production of extracellular matrix that leads to glomerulosclerosis and interstitial fibrosis. Accordingly, blockade of angiotensin II synthesis by angiotensin-converting enzyme inhibition or antagonizing its action at the angiotensin I receptor with an angiotensin receptor blocker is at the cornerstone of strategies that attenuate progressive kidney function decline in most forms of chronic kidney disease.

## CLASSICAL RENIN–ANGIOTENSIN–ALDOSTERONE SYSTEM

The classical view of the RAS focuses on the endocrine aspects of this peptidergic system. Angiotensinogen synthesized by the liver enters the circulation where it is cleaved to form angiotensin I by renin, a peptidase that is secreted from the juxtaglomerular apparatus (JGA) of the kidney. The terminal two amino acids of angiotensin I are then removed to form angiotensin II, as it traverses through the circulation, exposed to angiotensin-converting enzyme (ACE), a peptidase robustly expressed on endothelial cells of the pulmonary vasculature. Angiotensin II, the principal effector molecule of the RAS, then binds to its type 1 receptor ($AT_1R$), resulting in vasoconstriction, sodium retention, thirst, and aldosterone secretion. This traditional view of the RAS is still valid but has been considerably augmented in recent years, not only by the discovery of new enzymes, peptides, and receptors, but also by an appreciation that the RAS has an independently functioning local tissue–based component that acts through paracrine, autocrine, and possibly intracrine mechanisms (Fig. 11.1).

### ANGIOTENSINOGEN

Angiotensinogen is primarily, although by no means exclusively, synthesized in the liver, particularly the pericentral zone of the hepatic lobules.[3] In humans, it is coded by a single gene, composed of five exons and four introns, that spans about 13 kb of genomic sequence on chromosome 1 (1q42-q43). It is translated to a 453 amino acid globular glycoprotein with a molecular weight between 45 and 65 kDa, depending on the extent of its glycosylation, that then undergoes posttranslational cleavage of a 24– or 33–amino acid signal peptide,[4] giving rise to the mature circulating form of angiotensinogen.[5]

Structurally, angiotensinogen bears substantial homology to the serpin superfamily of protease inhibitors and like many members of its family behaves as an acute phase reactant in the inflammatory setting,[6] reflecting the presence of an acute-phase response element that binds the transcription factor, NF-κB (nuclear factor kappa-light-chain-enhancer of activated B cells).[7]

### RENIN

Like angiotensinogen, the gene encoding renin is also located on the long arm of chromosome 1 (1q32) and contains 10 exons and 9 introns, similar to other aspartyl proteases.[8] Unlike humans and rats that have only a single renin gene, the mouse has two genes, *Ren1* and *Ren2*, expressed primarily in the submandibular gland and kidney, respectively.

Following its synthesis as a 406–amino acid preprohormone, the 23–amino acid leader sequence of preprorenin is cleaved in the rough endoplasmic reticulum, giving rise to prorenin (also called inactive renin and "big" renin), which may be then rapidly secreted directly from the Golgi apparatus or from protogranules.[4] Alternatively, and virtually exclusively in the JGA, prorenin may be packaged into mature, dense granules that instead of being immediately secreted, undergo further processing to the active enzyme, renin (active renin). Contrasting with the more constitutive secretion of prorenin, the release of renin-containing granules is tightly regulated.[8]

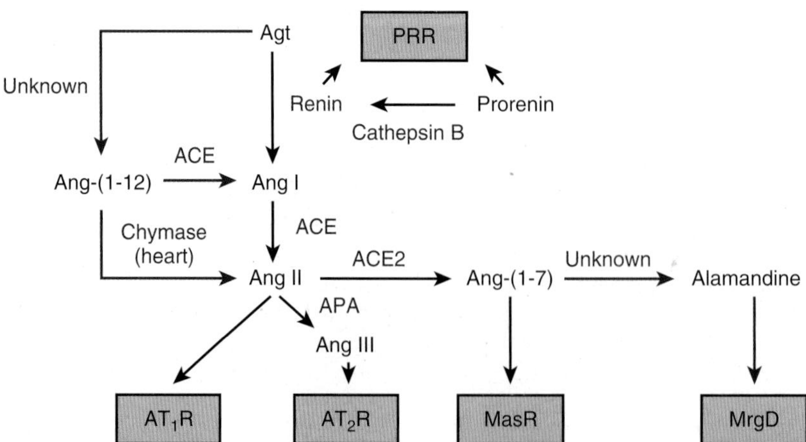


**Fig. 11.1** Schematic depiction of the renin–angiotensin system components and selected actions. The enzymes of the system are shown in *red*. Newly described enzymatic pathways are shown as *red arrows*. Receptors are shown in the *boxes*. *ACE*, Angiotensin-converting enzyme; *Agt*, angiotensinogen; *Ang*, angiotensin; *APA*, aminopeptidase A; *$AT_1R$*, angiotensin type-1 receptor; *$AT_2R$*, angiotensin type-2 receptor; *MasR*, *Mas* receptor; *MrgD*, *Mas*-related G-protein–coupled receptor; *PRR*, (pro)renin receptor. (Modified from Carey RM. Newly discovered components and actions of the renin-angiotensin system. *Hypertension.* 2013;62: 818–822.)

Mature, active renin is a variably glycosylated 340–amino acid 37–40-kDa aspartyl protease that is active at neutral pH, and in contrast to the more promiscuous activities of most other proteases in this class, has only a single known substrate, cleaving the decapeptide angiotensin I from the amino terminal of angiotensinogen. Although the kidney produces both renin and prorenin, a range of extrarenal tissues including the adrenals, gonads, and placenta produce prorenin and contribute to its presence in plasma. However, as evidenced by the near total absence of active renin in anephric patients, the kidney, and the JGA in particular, appears to be the only source of circulating renin in humans.

Factors that chronically stimulate renin secretion, such as a low sodium diet and ACE inhibition, lead to an increase in the number of renin secreting cells rather than an increase in cell size or the number of granules that each JGA cell contains. This expansion of the renin secreting mass occurs proximally by metaplastic transformation of smooth muscle cells within the walls of the afferent arteriole. Although sometimes mentioned, ectopic renin expression within the extraglomerular mesangium appears to be an uncommon event.[9]

## PRORENIN ACTIVATION

Prorenin is maintained as an inactive zymogen through the occupation of its catalytic cleft by its prosegment. Removing this prosegment by either proteolytic or nonproteolytic means yields active renin, a term that denotes its enzymatic activity rather than its amino acid sequence (Fig. 11.2).

Within the dense core secretory granules of the JGA, acidification by vacuolar adenosine triphosphatases (ATPases) provides the optimal pH for the prosegment cleaving enzymes (proconvertase 1 and cathepsin B), and may also assist the pH-dependent, nonenzymatic activation of prorenin as well.[9–11] Although various peptidases such as trypsin, plasmin, and kallikrein can also cleave the prosegment of prorenin in vitro, these do not appear to contribute to the generation of renin in the in vivo setting. Although traditionally viewed as occurring only in the JGA, recent cell culture–based studies suggest that proteolytic activation of renin can also occur in cardiac and vascular smooth muscle cells by as yet unidentified serine proteases.[12–14] The significance of these findings in the intact organism, however, remains to be established.

In addition to proteolytic cleavage of its prosegment, prorenin can also be reversibly activated nonenzymatically by a conformational change such that the prosegment no longer occupies the enzymatic cleft. Under usual circumstances, less than 2% of prorenin is in this open active conformation. This process can, however, be induced by acid (pH 4.0)[15,16] and to a lesser extent by cold.[17] More recently, the putative (pro)renin receptor (PRR; discussed later) has also been shown to nonproteolytically activate prorenin.[18]

## REGULATION OF RENIN SECRETION

Mechanical, neurological, and chemical factors regulate the activity of the RAS by modulating renin secretion.

### Renal Baroreceptor

The existence of a renal baroreceptor mechanism was first conceptualized by Skinner and colleagues to explain how renin secretion increases when afferent arteriolar perfusion pressure falls.[19] Studies in conscious dogs show that changes in renal perfusion pressure have only a small effect on renin secretion until a threshold of about 90 mm Hg is reached, below which renin secretion abruptly increases, doubling with every 2 to 3 mm Hg fall in pressure.[20] Accordingly, reduction in pressure below this level profoundly stimulates renin secretion, thereby acutely activating the RAS and resulting in a range of angiotensin II–dependent phenomena that collectively serve to restore systemic pressure. Despite the importance of the baroreceptor function, several decades of research have not identified precisely how the pressure signal is transduced into renin release, though postulated mediators include stretch-activated calcium channels, endothelins (ETs), and prostaglandins.

### Neural Control

The JGA is endowed with a rich network of noradrenergic nerve endings and their β1 receptors. Stimulation of the

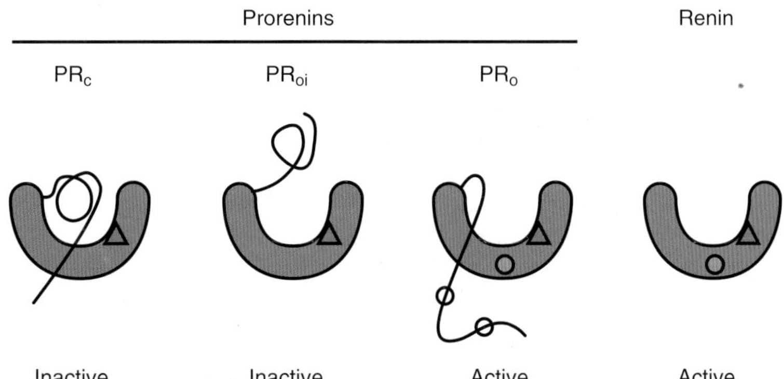


**Fig. 11.2** The conformational changes and the expression of immunoreactive epitopes associated with the activation of prorenin are depicted. The main body of the molecule *(blue)*, the substrate-binding cleft, and the prosegment *(black line)* are shown. The closed triangle represents the epitope of the main body expressed by $PR_c$ (prorenin in the inactive closed conformation), $PR_{oi}$ (prorenin in the inactive intermediary open conformation), $PR_o$ (prorenin in the active open conformation), and renin. The closed circle *(yellow)* represents the epitope of the main body, expressed by $PR_o$ and renin, but not by $PR_c$ and $PR_{oi}$. The *open circles* represent epitopes of the prosegment expressed by $PR_o$ but not by $PR_c$ and $PR_{oi}$. (Modified from Schalekamp MA, Derkx FH, Deinum J, et al. Newly developed renin and prorenin assays and the clinical evaluation of renin inhibitors. *J Hypertension.* 2008;26:928–937.)

renal sympathetic nerve activity leads to renin secretion that is independent of changes in RBF, glomerular filtration rate (GFR), or $Na^+$ reabsorption. Moreover, this effect can be blocked surgically (denervation) and pharmacologically, by the administration of β-adrenoreceptor blockers.[20] The role of cholinergic, dopaminergic, and adrenergic activation is controversial, though these agents have also been shown to modulate renin release under certain circumstances.

### Tubule Control

Chronic diminution in luminal NaCl delivery to the macula densa is a potent stimulus for renin secretion, reflecting a coordinate interaction between a range of mediators including adenosine, nitric oxide (NO), and prostaglandins that not only affect renin release but also its transcription.[21] This mechanism is thought to account for the chronically high plasma renin activity (PRA) in subjects ingesting a low-salt diet.[22]

### Metabolic Control

The tricarboxylic acid (TCA) cycle provides a final common pathway by which carbohydrates, fatty acids, and amino acids converge in the process of adenosine triphosphate (ATP) generation by aerobic electron transfer. Although the TCA cycle operates within mitochondria, its intermediates can be detected within the extracellular space, increasing in abundance when local energy supply and demand are mismatched or when cells are exposed to hypoxia, toxins, or injury.[23] Succinate, for instance, has been shown to stimulate renin release and its intravenous administration leads to hypertension, though the mechanisms underlying this effect have only recently been unraveled. In 2004, He and colleagues reported that alpha keto-glutarate and succinate are ligands for the previously orphaned G protein–coupled receptors (GPCRs), GPR99 and GPR91, respectively, and that succinate-induced hypertension is abolished in GPR91-deficient mice.[24] Indeed, in follow-up studies from this group, GPR91 was localized to the apical plasma membrane of macula densa cells where succinate stimulation was shown to activate p38 and Erk 1/2 mitogen-activated protein (MAP) kinases (MAPKs), inducing cyclooxygenase-2 (COX-2)-dependent synthesis of prostaglandin E2, a well-established paracrine mediator of renin release.[25] Moreover, the ability of tubule succinate to induce JG renin secretion suggests that this phenomenon is likely an important determinant of JGA function in both physiological and pathophysiological settings. In diabetic rats, for instance, elevated succinate has been detected in both plasma and urine.[25]

### Vitamin D Receptor

The vitamin D receptor (VDR) is a negative regulator of the RAS such that VDR-null mice display a marked increase in renin expression and angiotensin II production in conjunction with hypertension and cardiac hypertrophy.[26] Importantly, these effects occurred independently of calcium and parathyroid hormone, both of which have been reported to also modulate renin expression. The molecular basis for the interaction between vitamin D and renin expression has also been, at least partly, unraveled in a series of studies by Yuan et al.[27] Under usual circumstances, activation of the cyclic adenosine monophosphate (cAMP)–protein kinase A pathway by the sympathetic nervous system or macula densa leads to phosphorylation of a cAMP response element (CRE) binding protein (CREB) and recruitment of CREB-binding protein/p300 to the CRE in the promoter region of the renin gene. VDR-bound 1,25 $(OH)_2D_3$, however, blocks binding of CREB to the CRE DNA *cis*-element, leading to a reduction in renin gene transcription (Fig. 11.3).

From a clinical perspective, this interaction between vitamin D and renin may explain the well-documented inverse relationship between plasma vitamin $D_3$, blood pressure, and PRA. While several studies examining the effects of vitamin D supplementation as a renoprotective or antihypertensive measure have been undertaken, their findings have been mixed and long-term, randomized controlled trials with clinically meaningful endpoints are awaited.

### Other Local Factors

In addition to the factors discussed earlier, a large range of locally produced biologically active molecules have also been shown to alter renin secretion. These include peptides [ANP, kinins, vasoactive intestinal polypeptide, ET, calcitonin gene–related peptide (CGRP)], amines (dopamine and histamine), and arachidonic acid derivatives.[20]

## PLASMA PRORENIN AND RENIN

Under usual circumstances, the plasma concentration of prorenin is approximately 10 times greater than renin. In some patients with diabetes, however, plasma prorenin is disproportionately increased, where it predicts the development of diabetic nephropathy (including microalbuminuria) and retinopathy.[28,29]

In addition to its role in the research setting, measurement of plasma renin is an important clinical assay, providing important information, for example, when evaluating patients with possible hyperaldosteronism, assessing volume status, and in predicting the response to, or monitoring drug

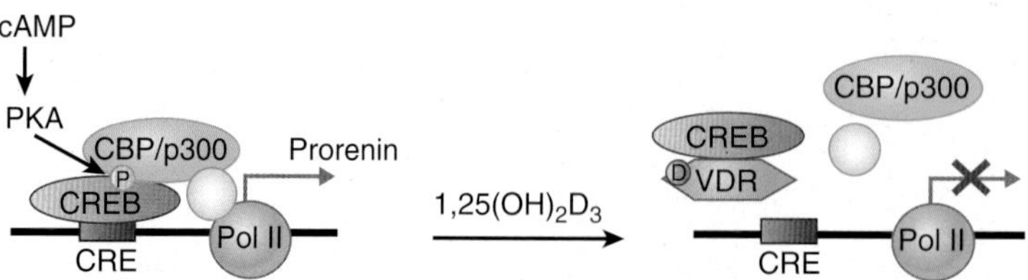


**Fig. 11.3** Model of $1,25(OH)_2D_3$-induced transrepression of renin gene expression. The cAMP–PKA pathway activates CREB by phosphorylation, leading to recruitment of CBP/p300. In the presence of $1,25(OH)_2D_3$, liganded VDR interacts with CREB and blocks its binding to CRE, leading to reduction of renin gene transcription. *cAMP,* Cyclic AMP; *CBP,* CREB-binding protein; *CRE,* cAMP response element; *CREB,* CRE-binding protein; *D,* $1,25(OH)_2D_3$; *P,* phosphorylation; *PKA,* protein kinase A; *Pol II,* RNA polymerase II; *VDR,* vitamin D receptor. (Modified from Yuan W, Pan W, Kong J, et al. 1,25-Dihydroxyvitamin $D_3$ suppresses renin gene transcription by blocking the activity of the cyclic AMP response element in the renin gene promoter. *J Biol Chem.* 2007;282:29821–29830.)

adherence to, an ACE inhibitor or angiotensin receptor blocker (ARB). In broad terms, plasma renin is determined by either activity or immunological assay methods.[30] The most commonly used method involves the measurement of PRA. With this method, the rate at which angiotensin I is produced from plasma angiotensinogen is assayed. To prevent angiotensin I's degradation or its conversion to angiotensin II, inhibitors of angiotensinase and ACE are added to the assay. Accordingly, PRA is not only dependent on renin and endogenous angiotensinogen concentrations but will also overestimate the extent of inhibition by renin inhibitors due to the displacement of protein-bound drug by the peptidase inhibitors. The latter scenario may be diminished by using an antibody capture method in which antiangiotensin I antibody, instead of peptidase inhibitors, is used to protect angiotensin I from further catabolism.[31]

The nomenclature of renin assays can be quite confusing in that plasma renin concentration (PRC) may be measured by both activity and immunological assays. With the activity method (PRCa), exogenous angiotensinogen is added to the assay, thereby avoiding the influence that endogenous levels of the substrate might have. However, PRCa may also be affected by the presence of renin inhibitors, though like PRA may take advantage of antibody capture methodology.[30] In the immunological assay for renin (PRCi), the concentrations of renin and prorenin in its active, open conformation are assessed, so that like PRA and PRCa, the PRCi assay is also time and temperature dependent because lower temperatures will increase the proportion of prorenin in its active conformation. Moreover, renin inhibitors, by binding to the active site of prorenin in its open conformation, prevent the refolding of the prosegment and may therefore lead to an overestimation of PRCi.[30,31]

## ANGIOTENSIN-CONVERTING ENZYME

ACE is a zinc-containing dipeptidyl carboxypeptidase that cleaves the terminal histidyl-leucine from angiotensin I to form the octapeptide angiotensin II. In contrast to the single-substrate specificity of renin, ACE is not specific, cleaving the two terminal acids from peptides with the C′-terminal sequence $R_1$-$R_2$-$R_3$-OH, where $R_1$ is the protected (noncleaved) amino acid, $R_2$ is any nonproline L-amino acid, and $R_3$ is any nondicarboxylic (cysteine, ornithine, lysine, arginine) L-amino acid with a free carboxyl terminal.[4] Importantly, therefore, ACE also catalyzes the inactivation of bradykinin. Although encoded by a single ACE gene, two distinct tissue-specific messenger RNAs (mRNAs) are transcribed, each with different initiation and alternative splice sites.[32] The somatic form, present in almost all tissues, is a 1306–amino acid, 140–160-kDa glycoprotein with two active sites, whereas the 90- to 100- kDa testicular or germinal form is found exclusively in postmeiotic male germ cells, and contains a single active site and appears to be involved in spermatogenesis.[4,33,34] The somatic form of ACE is widely distributed with activity present not only in tissues but also in most biological fluids. In the human kidney, ACE is present to the greatest extent within proximal and distal tubules, however, both its magnitude of expression and its site-specific distribution may be altered by disease.[35]

## ANGIOTENSIN TYPE 1 RECEPTOR

The $AT_1R$ mediates most of the known physiological effects of angiotensin II. The gene for this widely distributed 359–amino acid, 40-kDa, seven-transmembrane GPCR is located on chromosome 3 in humans.[36]

Within the kidney, $AT_1Rs$ are widely expressed. In the glomerulus, they are found in both afferent and efferent arterioles as well as in the mesangium, endothelium, and on podocytes.[37] Consistent with angiotensin II's role in $Na^+$ reabsorption, $AT_1Rs$ are highly abundant on the brush borders of proximal tubule epithelial cells.[38] Prominent expression has also been found in renal medullary interstitial cells, located between the renal tubules and vasa recta, where angiotensin II is purported to have a potential role in the regulation of medullary blood flow.[39]

Angiotensin II binding to $AT_1R$ initiates cell signaling by several different pathways that have been mostly studied in vascular smooth muscle cells.[40] These include G protein–mediated pathways, and the activation of tyrosine kinases, NADH/NADPH oxidases, and serine/threonine kinases.[36]

### G Protein–Mediated Signaling

In the classical G protein–mediated pathway, $AT_1R$ ligand binding leads to activation of phospholipases C, D, and $A_2$. Phospholipase C rapidly hydrolyses phosphatidylinositol bisphosphate to inositol trisphosphate and diacylglycerol (DAG), initiating calcium release from intracellular stores and protein kinase C (PKC) activation, respectively. Phospholipase D similarly generates DAG and activates PKC, whereas phospholipase A2 ($PLA_2$) leads to the formation of various vasoactive and proinflammatory arachidonic acid derivatives.

### Reactive Oxygen Species

Although previously regarded as toxic waste products, emerging evidence indicates that reactive oxygen species may also act as second messengers, not only activating other cell signaling cascades such as p38 MAPK but also a number of transcription pathways implicated in the pathogeneses of inflammatory and degenerative disease.[36] Although the mechanisms by which the $AT_1R$ stimulates NADH/NADPH are not well understood, angiotensin II binding to this receptor results in the generation of both superoxide and hydrogen peroxide.

### Tyrosine Kinases

Angiotensin II binding to the $AT_1R$ "transactivates" a number of nonreceptor tyrosine kinases [Src, Pyk2, Focal adhesion kinase (FAK), and Janus kinase (JAK)] as well as the growth factor receptor tyrosine kinases for epidermal growth factor (EGF)[41,42] and platelet-derived growth factor (PDGF).[43,44] By binding to the $AT_1R$, angiotensin II initiates the translocation of tumor necrosis factor-alpha (TNF-$\alpha$)–converting enzyme (TACE, ADAM17) to the cell surface. TACE then cleaves TNF-$\alpha$ from its membrane-associated precursor (pro-TNF-$\alpha$), allowing it to bind to the EGF receptor (EGFR) on the cell surface. This ligand–receptor interaction then induces EGFR autophosphorylation and activates its downstream signaling pathways that include Akt, Erk-1/2, and mammalian target of rapamycin (Fig. 11.4). The in vivo relevance of this transactivation pathway has been recently confirmed. Using mice that express a dominant negative form of EGFR, Lautrette and colleagues showed that despite similar blood pressures, mutant mice infused with angiotensin II had less proteinuria and renal fibrosis than did their wild-type

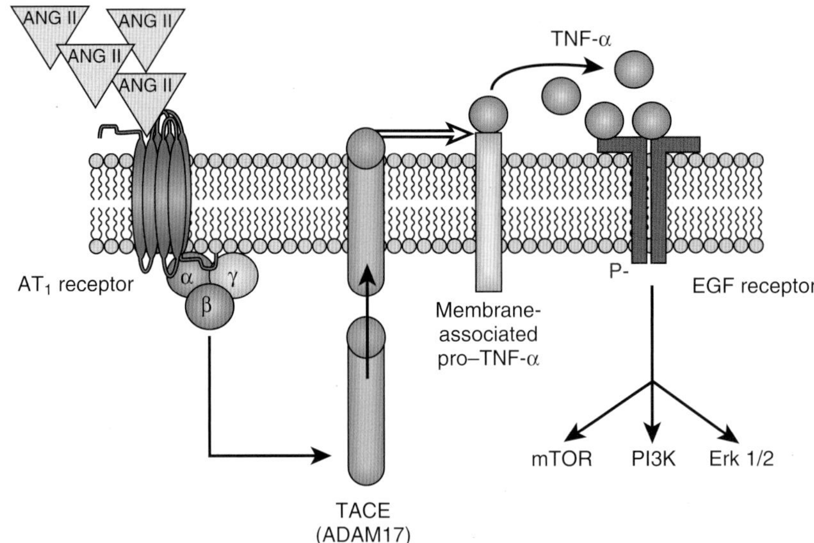


**Fig. 11.4** Angiotensin II *(ANG II)* binds to its angiotensin II type 1 *(AT$_1$)* receptor, a G protein–coupled receptor lacking intrinsic tyrosine kinase activity. Through as-yet-undescribed mechanisms, this interaction leads to the translocation of the metalloprotease tumor necrosis factor-α *(TNF-α)*–converting enzyme *(TACE)* from the cytosol to the cell surface, where it cleaves TNF-α from its membrane-associated promolecule, allowing it to bind and activate the epidermal growth factor (EGF) receptor. *Erk 1/2,* Extracellular signal–regulated kinases 1 and 2; *mTOR,* mammalian target of rapamycin; *P13K,* phosphatidylinositol-3-kinase. (Modified from Wolf G. "As time goes by": angiotensin II–mediated transactivation of the EGF receptor comes of age. *Nephrol Dial Transplant.* 2005;20:2050–2053.)

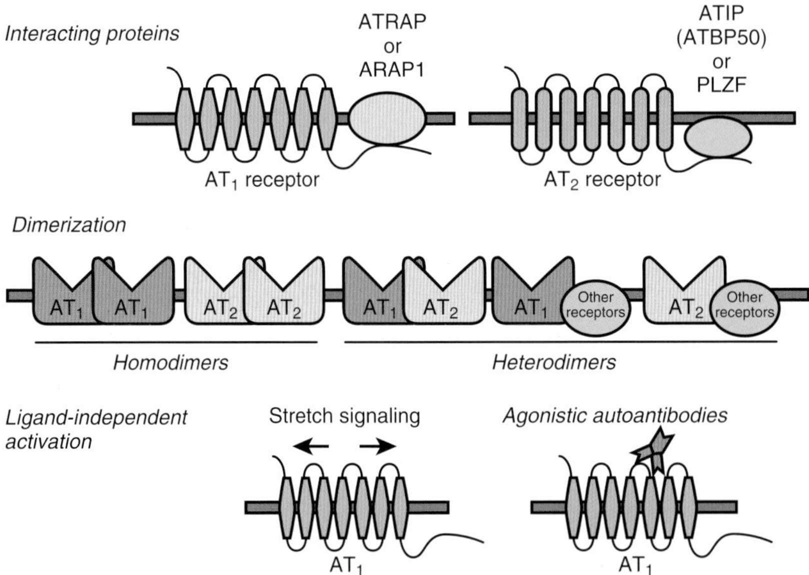


**Fig. 11.5** Regulation of angiotensin receptors. *ARAP1,* AT$_1$ receptor–associated protein 1; *ATBP50,* AT$_2$ receptor–binding protein of 50 kDa; *ATIP,* angiotensin type 2 receptor–interacting protein; *AT$_1$ receptor,* angiotensin type 1 receptor; *AT$_2$ receptor,* angiotensin type 2 receptor; *ATRAP,* AT$_1$ receptor–associated protein; *PLZF,* promyelocytic leukemia zinc finger. (Modified from Mogi M, Iwai M, Horiuchi M. New insights into the regulation of angiotensin receptors. *Curr Opin Nephrol Hypertens.* 2009;18:138–143.)

counterparts.[45] Consistent with these findings and the pivotal role of the RAS in diabetic nephropathy, studies using a specific EGFR tyrosine kinase inhibitor (i.e., PKI 166) have also shown a reduction in early structural injury in a rat model of diabetic nephropathy.[46]

Like EGFR, the transactivation of the PDGF receptor (PDGFR) by AT$_1$R is also complex, involving the adaptor protein Shc.[43,44] In addition to studies that have explored the angiotensin–PDGFR interaction in cell culture or organ baths,[47] a more recent report has shown that despite continued hypertension, inhibition of the PDGFR kinase in vivo can also dramatically attenuate angiotensin II–induced vascular remodeling.[48]

### Angiotensin Type 1 Receptor Internalization

In addition to the conventional ligand–receptor mediated pathways, a range of other signaling mechanisms that involve the AT$_1$R have also been described. These include the discovery of receptor interacting proteins, heterologous receptor dimerization, and ligand-independent activation (Fig. 11.5).[49]

These new insights, although adding greater complexity to our understanding of the RAS, also provide the potential for new therapeutic targets in disease prevention and management.

Following ligand binding and the initiation of signal transduction, $AT_1Rs$ are rapidly internalized, followed by either lysosomal degradation or recycling back to the plasma membrane. Several mechanisms account for $AT_1R$ internalization, including interaction with caveolae, phosphorylation of its carboxyl terminal by G-protein receptor kinases,[36] and association with the newly described $AT_1R$ interacting proteins.[49] To date, two such interacting proteins, *$AT_1$ receptor–associated protein* (ATRAP)[50] and *$AT_1$ receptor–associated protein-1* (ARAP1),[51] have been described. ATRAP interacts with the C terminal of $AT_1R$, downregulating cell surface $AT_1R$ expression and attenuating angiotensin II–mediated effects.[49] ARAP1, though somewhat similar to ATRAP, promotes $AT_1R$ recycling to the plasma membrane such that its kidney-specific overexpression induces hypertension and renal hypertrophy.[51]

### Angiotensin Type 1 Receptor Dimerization

In addition to their ability to induce cell signaling in their monomeric state, GPCRs like $AT_1R$ may also associate to form both homodimers and heterodimers.[52] Beyond its constitutive homodimerization,[53] $AT_1R$ may dimerize with angiotensin type 2 receptor ($AT_2R$) and also form hetero-oligomers with receptors for bradykinin (B2), epinephrine (β2), dopamine (D1,3,5), ET (B), Mas, and EGF that modulate their function.[54–57]

### Ligand-Independent Angiotensin Type 1 Receptor Activation

Without involvement of angiotensin II, cell stretch induces a conformational switch that initiates $AT_1R$'s intracellular signaling pathways.[58,59] As might be expected from an understanding of this mechanism, an $AT_1R$ blocker, acting as an inverse agonist, will abrogate these effects, as described in both cardiac[59] and mesangial cells.[60] A similar means of ligand-independent activation has also been shown to result from the binding of agonist antibodies to $AT_1R$ in some women with preeclampsia[61] and in certain cases of renal allograft rejection.[62]

## PHYSIOLOGIC EFFECTS OF ANGIOTENSIN II IN THE KIDNEY

The traditional actions of angiotensin II relate primarily to its effects on vascular tone and fluid balance that are mediated by its actions on the vasculature, heart, kidney, brain, and adrenal glands by the $AT_1R$. In vascular smooth muscle, stimulation of $AT_1Rs$ by angiotensin II induces cell contraction and consequent vasoconstriction. In the adrenal cortex, this ligand– receptor interaction stimulates aldosterone release, thereby promoting sodium reabsorption in the distal nephron. Moreover, angiotensin II will directly enhance sodium retention by the proximal tubule and in the brain it will stimulate thirst and salt craving. Additional effects include sympathoadrenal stimulation and the augmentation of cardiac contractility. Together, these effects serve to maintain extracellular fluid volume and systemic blood pressure. Given the central role that the kidney has in the regulation of these key aspects of mammalian homeostasis, it is not surprising that angiotensin II should have profound effects on renal physiology.

## HEMODYNAMIC ACTIONS

The effects of exogenously administered angiotensin II are dose dependent. At low doses, angiotensin II infusion increases renal vascular resistance (RVR) and lowers RBF without affecting GFR so that the filtration fraction is increased. At higher doses of angiotensin II, RVR is further increased, leading to an augmented reduction in RBF and fall in GFR.[63] However, because GFR is reduced to a lesser extent than renal plasma flow, the filtration fraction remains elevated. Such studies are consistent with the view that limited stimulation of the RAS would mostly serve to enhance tubule sodium, as is seen, for instance, in societies unaccustomed to contemporary diets.[22] Greater activation of the RAS, by contrast, as might be found in the setting of severe volume depletion, would result in angiotensin II–dependent reduction in RBF that would aid in sustaining systemic blood pressure while further stimulating sodium reabsorption.

Kidney micropuncture has been used extensively to explore the intrarenal sites of angiotensin II's effects on vascular resistance. These studies demonstrate that although angiotensin II increases both afferent and efferent arteriolar resistance, intraglomerular capillary pressure ($P_{GC}$) is consistently elevated[64] and the ultrafiltration coefficient ($K_f$) is reduced.[63] Moreover, as predicted by mathematical modeling, the glomerular hypertension induced by angiotensin II does not lead to acute proteinuria, because the structural barriers to macromolecular passage remain intact.[63] Chronic angiotensin II infusion with sustained intraglomerular hypertension, by contrast, leads to glomerular capillary damage and substantial proteinuria.

## TUBULE TRANSPORT

### Sodium

Consistent with its importance in the regulation of volume status, angiotensin II has profound effects on renal $Na^+$ handling. The proximal tubule is responsible for the reabsorption of approximately two-thirds of the sodium from the glomerular filtrate and binding sites for angiotensin II are particularly abundant in the proximal tubule with immunohistochemical localization of the $AT_1R$ to both apical and basolateral surfaces.[65] At picomolar concentrations, angiotensin II stimulates the luminal $Na^+/H^+$ exchanger, the basolateral $Na^+/HCO3^-$ cotransporter, and the $Na^+$–$K^+$ ATPase. However, at concentrations greater than $10^{-9}$ M, angiotensin II inhibits the very same transporters. The mechanisms underlying this dose-dependent effect of angiotensin II on $Na^+$ transport, that seem to also occur in the loop of Henle,[65] are incompletely understood. In the distal tubule, the effects of angiotensin II on $Na^+$ transport are site dependent. In the early distal tubule, for instance, angiotensin II stimulates apical $Na^+/H^+$ exchange while in the late distal tubule it stimulates the amiloride-sensitive sodium channel.[65]

### Acid–Base Regulation

The kidney has a key role in the maintenance of physiological pH by regulating the secretion/reabsorption of acids and bases. As for $Na^+$, angiotensin II also has substantial effects on acid–base transport in the proximal tubule, distal tubule, and collecting duct. Recent interest has focused, in particular, on its actions in the collecting duct. In the collecting duct, angiotensin II not only stimulates $Na^+/H^+$ exchangers and $Na^+/HCO3^-$ cotransporters but has also been shown to stimulate the vacuolar $H^+$-ATPase in intercalated A-cells via its $AT_1R$ receptor.[66] Moreover, elegant and detailed electron microscopic studies have helped to unravel the mechanisms by which angiotensin II exerts its effects at this site, revealing translocation of the $H^+$-ATPase from the cytoplasm to the apical surface in response to ligand stimulation.[67]

## EXPANDED RENIN–ANGIOTENSIN–ALDOSTERONE SYSTEM: ENZYMES, ANGIOTENSIN PEPTIDES, AND RECEPTORS

### ANGIOTENSIN TYPE 2 RECEPTOR

In humans, the $AT_2R$ is a 363–amino acid protein that maps to the X chromosome and is highly homologous to its rat and mouse counterparts.[68] Like $AT_1R$, $AT_2R$ is also a seven-transmembrane GPCR, though it shares only 34% homology.

Despite substantial research, the actions of $AT_2R$ are still not well understood and remain somewhat controversial.[69] In general, however, the actions of $AT_2R$ stimulation oppose those of $AT_1R$. For instance, whereas $AT_1R$ vasoconstricts and promotes $Na^+$ retention, $AT_2R$ stimulation leads to vasodilation[70] and natriuresis,[71] consistent with its abundance on the epithelium of the proximal tubule.[72] The vasodilatory effects of $AT_2R$ stimulation are mediated by increasing NO synthesis and cyclic guanosine monophosphate (cGMP) by bradykinin-dependent and -independent mechanisms.[73] Its natriuretic effects, however, seem to be dependent on angiotensin II's conversion to angiotensin III by aminopeptidase N.[74]

Like the $AT_1R$, the activity of $AT_2R$ may also be modulated by oligomerization, in association with various interacting proteins and ligand-independent effects.[73]

### (PRO)RENIN RECEPTOR

In 2002 an apparently novel, 350-amino acid, single-transmembrane protein that binds both renin and prorenin with high affinity was identified.[18] Ligand binding to this protein was shown to induce a fourfold increase in the catalytic cleavage of angiotensinogen as well as stimulating intracellular signaling with activation of MAPKs extracellular signal–regulated kinases 1 and 2 (ERK1/2),[18] leading to it being named the (pro)renin receptor [(P)RR]. The designation (pro)renin refers to its ability to interact with both renin and prorenin.

Given its localization to the mesangium in initial studies, its actions in augmenting local angiotensin II production, and its ability to increase mesangial transforming growth factor-β (TGF-β) production,[75] the (P)RR was understandably implicated in the pathogenesis of kidney disease.[76] However, despite the appeal, it has been difficult to reconcile this view of the (P)RR with a number of other experimental findings, regarding not only its potentially pathogenetic role, but also its pattern of distribution within the kidney and its homology to other proteins. For instance, given the purported pathogenetic role of the (P)RR, the increased abundance of renin that follows the use of ACE inhibitors and ARBs would be expected to be adverse, yet these classes of drugs have been repeatedly shown to be renoprotective. Second, although the (P)RR was initially localized to the glomerular mesangium, more recent detailed studies have shown that (P)RR is primarily expressed in the collecting duct.[77] Third, although initially reported as having no homology with any known membrane protein,[18] database interrogation shows that the (P)RR is identical to two other proteins: CAPER (endoplasmic reticulum–localized type 1 transmembrane adaptor precursor) and ATP6ap2 (ATPase, $H^+$ transporting, lysosomal accessory protein 2),[78–82] a protein that associates with the vacuolar $H^+$-ATPase.[83] Indeed, the predominant expression of the (P)RR at the apex of acid secreting cells in the collecting duct, in conjunction with its colocalization and homology with an accessory subunit of the vacuolar $H^+$-ATPase, suggests that the (P)RR may function primarily in urinary acidification.[77] However, the vacuolar $H^+$-ATPase is not restricted to the kidney but is widely distributed in the plasma membrane and the membranes of organelles in several tissues where it functions, not only in urinary acidification but also in endocytosis, conversion of proinsulin to insulin, and osteoclast bone resorption.[84] Whereas the prevailing data indicate that (P)RR is an accessory subunit of the vacuolar $H^+$-ATPase that also binds renin and prorenin, the precise functions of the prorenin- and renin-binding subunit remain to be unraveled in the kidney and elsewhere.

### ANGIOTENSIN-CONVERTING ENZYME 2

In 2000, two groups independently reported the existence of the first ACE homolog, ACE2, an apparently novel zinc metalloprotease but with considerable homology (40% identity and 61% similarity) to ACE.[85,86] The gene-encoding ACE2, located on the X chromosome (Xp22), contains 18 exons, several of which bear considerable similarity to the first 17 exons of human *ACE*. Its transcript is 3.4 kb, generating an 805–amino acid peptide that is most highly expressed in kidney, heart, and testis but is also present in plasma and urine.[87,88] In contrast to ACE, ACE2 functions as a carboxypeptidase, removing the terminal phenylalanine from angiotensin II to yield the vasodilatory heptapeptide, angiotensin 1-7 [Ang (1-7)]. ACE2 may also indirectly lead to the formation of Ang (1-7) by cleaving the C-terminal leucine from angiotensin I, thereby generating angiotensin 1-9 [Ang (1-9)] which may then give rise to Ang (1-7) under the influence of ACE or neutral endopeptidase (NEP).[88] Thus ACE2 contributes to both angiotensin II degradation and Ang (1-7) synthesis. Accordingly, ACE and ACE2 were initially viewed as having opposing actions with regard to vascular tone and tissue injury. However, emerging data suggest that the situation is far from clear. For instance, while lentivirus-induced overexpression of ACE2 in the heart exerted a protective influence following experimental myocardial infarction,[89] ACE2 overexpression led to cardiac dysfunction and fibrosis, despite lowering systemic blood pressure.[90]

In the kidney, ACE2 colocalizes with ACE and angiotensin receptors in the proximal tubule while in the glomerulus it is predominantly expressed within podocytes and to a lesser extent in mesangial cells, contrasting the endothelial predilection of ACE at that site.[91] Numerous studies have explored changes in ACE2 expression in human kidney disease as well as in a range of animal models, reporting both increased and decreased levels.[92] As such, it is uncertain whether increased ACE2 might be detrimental or a beneficial response to injury. With this in mind, the findings of intervention studies are of particular importance.

In experimental diabetic nephropathy, for instance, pharmacological ACE2 inhibition with MLN-4760 led to worsening albuminuria and glomerular injury[91]; similar findings were reported in ACE2 knockout mice that were crossed with the Akita model of type 1 diabetes.[93] As might be expected from these findings, augmenting ACE2 activity by the infusion of human recombinant protein (hrACE2) was shown to attenuate diabetic kidney injury in the Akita mouse. In this study, hrACE2 not only improved kidney structure and function but also showed that the protective effects were likely due to reduction in angiotensin II and an increase in Ang (1-7) signaling.[94] In addition to its role in the RAS, ACE2 has been shown to be the receptor for the severe adult respiratory syndrome (SARS) coronavirus.[95] The relevance of some of these findings to the human setting will hopefully be clarified when results of the recently initiated clinical trials of a recombinant human ACE2 peptide (GSK2586881) become available.

## ANGIOTENSIN PEPTIDES

### Angiotensin III, or Angiotensin-(2-8)

Formed by the actions of aminopeptidase A, the heptapeptide angiotensin III (angiotensin 2-8), like angiotensin II (angiotensin 1-8), exerts its effects by binding to the $AT_1R$ and $AT_2R$.[96] Initially, angiotensin III was thought to have a predominant role in regulating vasopressin release.[97] However, more recent studies indicate that while angiotensin III is equipotent to angiotensin II with regard to its effects on blood pressure, aldosterone secretion, and renal function, its metabolic clearance rate is approximately five times as rapid.[98]

### Angiotensin IV, or Angiotensin-(3–8)

Angiotensin IV is generated from angiotensin III by the actions of aminopeptidase M. Although some of its actions are mediated by the $AT_1R$, the majority of angiotensin IV's biological effects are thought to result from its binding to insulin-regulated aminopeptidase.[99] Previously viewed as inactive, there has been considerable recent interest in angiotensin IV with regard to its actions in the central nervous system (CNS), where it not only enhances learning and memory but also possesses anticonvulsant properties and protects the brain from ischemic injury.[99]

In addition to its CNS effects, angiotensin IV has also been implicated in atherogenesis, principally related to its ability to activate NF-κB and upregulate several proinflammatory factors that include monocyte chemoattractant protein-1 (MCP-1), intercellular adhesion molecule-1, interleukin-6 (IL-6), and TNF-α, as well as enhancing the synthesis of the prothrombotic factor plasminogen activator inhibitor-1.[100,101] In the kidney, angiotensin IV is reported to have variable effects on blood flow and natriuresis.[99]

### Angiotensin-(1-7)

The ostensibly vasodilatory and antitrophic angiotensin 1-7 may be formed by the actions of several endopeptidases that include removal of the terminal tripeptide of angiotensin I by NEP, cleavage of the C-terminal phenylalanine of angiotensin II by ACE2, and the excision of the dipeptidyl group from the C terminal of angiotensin 1-9 by ACE. Evolving evidence indicates that the actions of this heptapeptide are mediated by its binding to the orphan GPCR *masR*.[102] Angiotensin 1-7 induces vasodilation by a number of mechanisms that include the amplification of bradykinin's effects, stimulating cGMP synthesis, and inhibiting the release of norepinephrine.[103] Additionally, angiotensin 1-7 inhibits vascular smooth muscle proliferation and prevents neo-intima formation following balloon injury of the carotid arteries.[104] Contrasting these findings, however, is a recent report that exogenous angiotensin-(1-7), rather than ameliorating diabetic nephropathy, as might have been predicted based on the prevailing paradigm, actually accelerated the progression of the disease.[93]

### Angiotensin-(2-10)

In addition to angiotensin II and the other C-terminal cleavage products discussed earlier, angiotensin I (1-10) may also give rise to a number of other potentially biologically active peptides that result from removal of amino acids from its N terminus. Of these, angiotensin 2-10, produced by the actions of aminopeptidase A has been found to modulate the pressor activity of angiotensin II in rodents.[105]

### Angiotensin-(1-12)

Angiotensin-(1-12) is a dodecapeptide, first isolated in rat intestine but also found to be present in the kidney and heart, that is cleaved from angiotensinogen by a heretofore unidentified nonrenin enzyme.[106] Notably, in the kidney, angiotensin-(1-12), akin to other components of the intrarenal RAS, is primarily localized to the proximal tubule epithelium.[107] Although its biological activity is incompletely understood, its main mode of action is thought to be mediated by its ability to serve as a precursor to angiotensin II by the site- and possibly species-specific actions of ACE and chymase.[108] Other pathways may, however, also contribute to the overall effects of angiotensin-(1-12), which in the rat kidney may also include the formation of angiotensin-(1-7) and angiotensin-(1-4) by neprilysin.[107]

### Angiotensin A and Alamandine

Identified by mass spectroscopy, angiotensin A and alamandine are characterized by the decarboxylation of N-terminal aspartic acid to alanine in angiotensin II and angiotensin-(1-7), respectively.[109] While the extremely low concentrations of angiotensin A suggest that it is unlikely to play a physiological role, this may not be the case for alamandine, which circulates in human plasma and at increased concentrations in patients with end-stage renal disease (ESRD).[109] With its ability to lower blood pressure and reduce fibrosis, the actions of alamandine resemble those of angiotensin-(1-7). However, rather than exerting its effects via the *Mas* receptor, alamandine's actions occur through a related receptor, the *Mas*-related GPCR (*Mrg*D).[110]

## INTRARENAL RENIN–ANGIOTENSIN–ALDOSTERONE SYSTEM

In the traditional view of the RAS, angiotensin II functions as a hormone that, in classical endocrine fashion, circulates systemically to act at sites distant from those where it was formed. However, since the cloning of its components, it has become increasingly clear that there is an additional local, tissue-based RAS that functions quasi-independently from its systemic counterpart, acting in paracrine, autocrine, and possibly even intracrine modes.[1] This is most clearly seen in the kidney where pioneering work of Navar and others[111–113] has shown that the kidney possesses all the necessary molecular machinery to synthesize angiotensin II and other bioactive angiotensin peptides. Moreover, their concentrations in glomerular filtrate, tubule fluid, and interstitium are between 10- and 1000-fold higher than in plasma.[38,114]

Within the kidney, renin-expressing cells have traditionally been considered to be terminally differentiated and confined to the JGA. However, in a series of elegant studies using a fate-mapping cre-loxP system, Sequeira López and coworkers showed that renin-expressing cells are precursors to a range of other cell types in the kidney, including those of the arteriolar media, mesangium, Bowman's capsule, and proximal tubule.[115] While normally quiescent, these cells may undergo metaplastic transformation to synthesize renin when homeostasis is challenged.[115] Such threats include not only those related to volume depletion but also tissue injury. For instance, in the setting of single nephron hyperfiltration and consequent progressive dysfunction that follows renal mass reduction, Gilbert and colleagues noted the de novo expression of renin mRNA and angiotensin II peptide in tubule epithelial cells.[116]

In addition to resident kidney cells, infiltrating mast cells may also contribute to activation of the local RAS in disease. Traditionally associated with allergic reactions and host responses to parasite infestation, mast cells have been increasingly recognized for their role in inflammation, immunomodulation, and chronic disease. In the kidney, interstitial mast cell infiltration accompanies most forms of CKD where their abundance correlates with the extent of tubulointerstitial fibrosis and declining GFR, though not proteinuria.[117] Notably, mast cells have been shown to synthesize renin,[118] such that their degranulation will release large quantities of both renin and chymase, accelerating angiotensin II formation in the local environment.

### Intracrine Renin–Angiotensin–Aldosterone System

Peptide hormones traditionally bind to their cognate receptors on the plasma membrane and produce their effects through the generation of secondary intermediates. However, emerging evidence suggests that certain peptides may also act directly within the cell's interior, having arrived there by either internalization or intracellular synthesis. For instance, angiotensin II has not only been localized within the cytoplasm and nucleus but its introduction into the cytoplasm was shown more than a decade ago to have major effects on intracellular calcium currents.[119] Uptake of angiotensin II from the extracellular space likely contributes to its intracellular activity; however, recent studies have focused predominantly on its endogenous synthesis. Consistent with the potential role for intracellular angiotensin II, transgenic mice that express an enhanced cyan fluorescent protein–angiotensin II fusion protein that lacks a secretory signal so that it is retained intracellularly develop hypertension with microthrombi in glomerular capillaries and small vessels.[120] To date, numerous canonical and noncanonical pathways in the cytoplasm, nucleus, and mitochondria have been implicated in the intracrine RAS,[121,122] providing a new forefront for the role of the RAS in physiology, pathophysiology, and therapeutics.

## RENIN–ANGIOTENSIN–ALDOSTERONE SYSTEM IN KIDNEY PATHOPHYSIOLOGY

In a critical series of experiments in the 1980s, Brenner, Hostetter, and colleagues studied the hemodynamic effects of renal mass ablation in 5/6 nephrectomized rats, a now well-established model of progressive kidney disease.[123] In the setting of nephron loss, those glomeruli that remain undergo compensatory enlargement with increased single nephron GFR (SNGFR) and elevations in intraglomerular pressure ($P_{GC}$), argued to initiate glomerulosclerosis and loss of function. That this phenomenon might be related to angiotensin II was suggested by previous work in which angiotensin II infusion was demonstrated to also result in elevated $P_{GC}$.[124] Together, these studies suggested that intraglomerular hypertension, as a consequence of angiotensin II's action, was a pivotal factor underlying the inexorable progression of kidney disease and that strategies to reduce $P_{GC}$ would lead to its amelioration. Indeed, in proof-of-concept studies, blockade of angiotensin II formation with the ACE inhibitor, enalapril, was shown to dilate the glomerular efferent arteriole, reduce $P_{GC}$, and disease progression in 5/6 nephrectomized rats.[125] By contrast, combination therapy with hydralazine, reserpine, and hydrochlorothiazide, though equally effective in lowering systemic blood pressure, failed to ameliorate intraglomerular hypertension and disease progression.[125] These studies were soon followed by similar ones in other disease models, particularly diabetes, which like the 5/6 nephrectomized rat is also characterized by increased SNGFR and elevated $P_{GC}$.[126]

### FIBROSIS

During the past 20 years considerable research has focused on many of the nonhemodynamic effects of angiotensin II. For instance, in addition to their effects on $P_{GC}$, ACE inhibitors and ARBs are also highly effective in reducing interstitial fibrosis and tubule atrophy, each close correlates of progressive kidney dysfunction. Underlying these effects is the ability of angiotensin II to potently induce expression of the profibrotic and proapoptotic growth factor and TGF-β in a range of kidney cell types.[127,128] Consistent with these in vitro studies, TGF-β overexpression is seen in both the glomerular and tubulointerstitial compartments in 5/6 nephrectomized rats and diabetic rats, where studies also showed that both ACE inhibitors and ARBs were effective at reducing TGF-β and disease progression.[129,130] Similarly, in human diabetic nephropathy, the ACE inhibitor perindopril was found to reduce TGF-β mRNA in a sequential renal biopsy study[131] and losartan was shown to lower urinary TGF-β excretion.[132]

### PROTEINURIA

The development of proteinuria is both a cardinal manifestation of glomerular injury and a pathogenetic factor in the progression of renal dysfunction. While $P_{GC}$ remains an important factor in determining the transglomerular passage of albumin, more recent work has focused on the potential contribution of the podocyte. Indeed, podocyte injury is a cardinal manifestation of proteinuric renal disease where foot process effacement has been shown to be prevented by both ACE inhibition and angiotensin receptor blockade.[133] In consideration of its crucial role in the development and function of the glomerular filtration barrier, other studies have focused on the podocyte slit pore membrane protein nephrin. Of note, podocytes express the $AT_1R$ and respond to the addition of angiotensin II to the cell culture medium by dramatically decreasing their expression of nephrin.[134] Consistent with these findings, the reduction in nephrin expression in patients with diabetic nephropathy was shown to be ameliorated by ACE inhibitor treatment for 2 years.[135]

### INFLAMMATION, IMMUNITY, AND THE RENIN–ANGIOTENSIN–ALDOSTERONE SYSTEM

Inflammatory cell infiltration is a long-recognized feature of CKD that is attenuated in rodent models by agents that block the RAS.[136] In the in vitro setting, angiotensin II activates NF-κB by both $AT_1R$- and $AT_2R$-dependent pathways, stimulating the expression of a number of potent chemokines such as MCP-1 and regulated on activation, normal T cell expressed and secreted (RANTES) as well as cytokines, like IL-6.[137] In addition to angiotensin II, angiotensin-(1-7), acting via the Mas receptor, activates NF-κB, inducing proinflammatory effects in the kidney under both basal and disease settings.[138]

In addition to macrophages, mast cells, and other components of the innate immune system, the adaptive immune system also appears to be involved in the pathogenesis of angiotensin II–mediated organ injury. Of note, suppression of the adaptive immune system prevents the development of angiotensin II–dependent hypertension in experimental models[139] and adoptive transfer of $CD4^+CD25^+$ regulatory T cells is able to ameliorate angiotensin II–dependent injury.[140]

### DIABETES PARADOX

Despite the fact that patients with long-standing diabetes characteristically have low plasma renin,[141–143] suggesting that the RAS is not activated by the disease, agents that block the RAS are the mainstay of therapy in diabetic nephropathy. Compounding this apparent paradox, although PRA is normal or low in diabetes, plasma prorenin is characteristically elevated. This dichotomy suggests differences in cell-specific responses to diabetes since the JGA is the primary source of renin secretion while prorenin is secreted by a much wider range of cell types. In a recent commentary, Peti-Peterdi et al. have ventured to explain the (pro)renin paradox of diabetes.[144] Although early diabetes would lead to augmented succinate and enhanced JGA renin release, elevated angiotensin II levels would thereafter suppress JGA renin secretion. Contrasting this negative feedback at the JGA, angiotensin II has been shown to have the opposite effect in the tubule, with diabetes causing a 3.5-fold increase in collecting duct renin that could be reduced by $AT_1R$ blockade.[145]

## ENDOTHELIN

*Clinical Relevance*

The actions of the endothelins (ETs) are mediated by two receptors: ET types A (ET-A) and B (ET-B). ET receptor antagonists (particularly ET-A receptor antagonists) are being investigated for their efficacy in slowing renal decline in chronic kidney diseases, especially diabetic kidney disease. However, whereas ET receptor antagonists lower proteinuria, their development has been hampered by fluid retention and a narrow therapeutic window.

ETs are potent vasoconstrictors that, although expressed primarily in the vascular endothelium, are also notably present within the renal medulla. The biologic effects of the ET system are mediated by two receptors: ET types A (ET-A) and B (ET-B). In the kidneys, these receptors contribute to the regulation of RBF, salt and water balance, and acid–base homeostasis, as well as potentially mediating tissue inflammation and fibrosis. An important therapeutic role has emerged for ET receptor antagonism in the treatment of pulmonary hypertension;[146–149] ET receptor antagonists have been granted regulatory authority approval for this indication in the United States and in Europe.[150] ET receptor blockade as a therapeutic strategy has been investigated in a range of renal diseases. Recent clinical trials have demonstrated the antiproteinuric and antihypertensive properties of ET receptor antagonists, which have a relatively narrow therapeutic window for the treatment of CKD.

## STRUCTURE, SYNTHESIS, AND SECRETION OF THE ENDOTHELINS

ETs consist of three 21–amino acid isoforms that are structurally and pharmacologically distinct: ET-1, ET-2, and ET-3. The dominant isoform in the cardiovascular system is ET-1. Differences in the amino acid sequence among the isopeptides are minor. All three isoforms share a common structure with a typical hairpin-loop configuration that results from two disulfide bonds at the amino terminus and a hydrophobic carboxy terminus that contains an aromatic indol side chain at $Trp_{21}$ (Fig. 11.6). Both the carboxy terminus and the two disulfide bonds are responsible for the biologic activity of the peptide. ETs are synthesized from preprohormones by posttranslational proteolytic cleavage mediated by furin and other enzymes. Dibasic pair–specific processing endopeptidases, which recognize Arg-Arg or Lys-Arg paired amino acids, cleave preproETs, reducing their size from approximately 203 to 39 amino acids. Subsequent proteolytic cleavage of the largely biologically inactive big ETs is mediated by endothelin-converting enzymes (ECEs), the key enzymes in the ET biosynthetic pathway. ECE1 and ECE2 are type II membrane-bound metalloproteases whose amino acid sequence is significantly homologous to that of neprilysin (NEP 24.11).

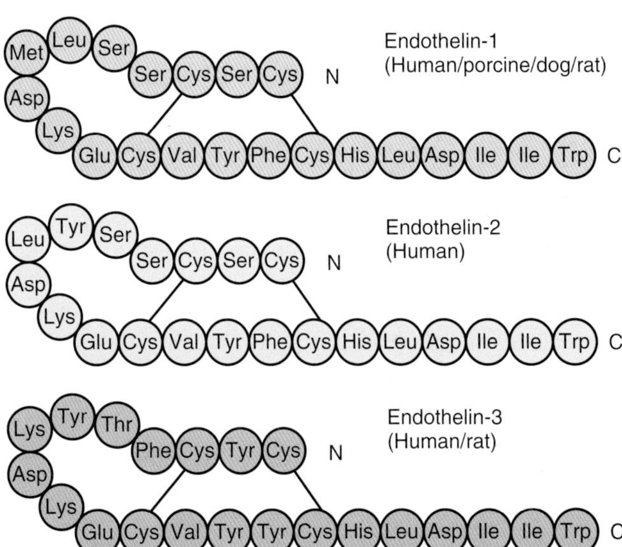


**Fig. 11.6** Molecular structure of the three endothelin isoforms. (Modified from Schiffrin EL. Vascular endothelin in hypertension. *Vascul Pharmacol.* 2005;43:19–29.)

**Table 11.1 Endothelin Gene and Protein Expression**

| Stimulation | |
|---|---|
| **Vasoactive Peptides** | **Growth Factors** |
| Angiotensin II | Epidermal growth factor |
| Bradykinin | Insulin-like growth factor |
| Vasopressin | Transforming growth factor-β |
| Endothelin-1 | **Coagulation** |
| Epinephrine | Thromboxane $A_2$ |
| Insulin | Tissue plasminogen activator |
| Glucocorticoids | **Other** |
| Prolactin | Calcium |
| **Inflammatory Mediators** | Hypoxia |
| Endotoxin | Shear stress |
| Interleukin-1 | Phorbol esters |
| Tumor necrosis factor-α | Oxidized low-density lipoproteins |
| Interferon-β | |
| **Inhibition** | |
| Atrial natriuretic peptide | Prostacyclin |
| Brain natriuretic peptide | Protein kinase A activators |
| Bradykinin | Nitric oxide |
| Heparin | Angiotensin-converting enzyme inhibitors |

Secretion of ET-1 is dependent on de novo protein synthesis, which is constitutive. However, a range of stimuli may also increase ET synthesis through both transcriptional and posttranscriptional regulation (Table 11.1). Once it is synthesized, ET-1 is secreted by endothelial cells into the basolateral compartment, toward the adjacent smooth muscle cells. Because of its abluminal secretion, plasma levels of ET-1 do not necessarily reflect its production.[151]

Within the kidneys, ET-1 expression is most abundant in the inner medulla. In fact, this region possesses the highest concentration of ET-1 of any tissue bed.[152] In addition to their presence in the inner medullary collecting ducts (IMCDs), ETs have also been described in glomerular endothelial cells,[153] glomerular epithelial cells,[154] mesangial cells,[155] vasa recta,[156] and tubule epithelial cells.[157] The kidneys also synthesize ET-2 and ET-3, although at much lower levels than they do ET-1.[158] As with ET-1, ECE1 mRNA is also more abundant in the renal medulla than in the cortex under normal conditions. However, in disease states such as chronic heart failure, ECE1 mRNA is upregulated primarily within the cortex.[159] In human kidneys, ECE1 has been localized to endothelial cells and tubule epithelial cells in the cortex and medulla.[160]

## ENDOTHELIN RECEPTORS

ETs bind to two seven-transmembrane domain GPCRs, ET-A and ET-B. Within the vasculature, ET-A receptors are found on smooth muscle cells, where they mediate vasoconstriction. Although ET-B receptors localized on vascular smooth muscle cells can also mediate vasoconstriction, they are also expressed on endothelial cells, where their activation results in vasodilation through the production of NO and prostacyclin.[161] In addition to their role in mediating vascular tone, ET-B receptors also act as clearance receptors for ET-1,[162] particularly in the lung, where ET-B receptor binding accounts for approximately 80% of clearance.[163] Because of its natriuretic and vasodilatory actions, the ET-B receptor is generally considered to confer predominantly renoprotective effects.

In the kidneys, expression of both ET-A and ET-B receptors is most prominent within the IMCDs, although binding of ET-1 also occurs in smooth muscle cells, endothelial cells, renomedullary interstitial cells, thin descending limbs, and medullary thick ascending limbs.[156] ET-A receptors are localized to several renovascular structures, including vascular smooth muscle cells, arcuate arteries, and pericytes of descending vasa recta, as well as glomeruli. ET-B receptors, although prominently represented within the medullary collecting system, have also been demonstrated in proximal convoluted tubules, collecting ducts of the inner cortex, medullary thick ascending limbs, and podocytes.[164]

## PHYSIOLOGIC ACTIONS OF ENDOTHELIN IN THE KIDNEY

The ETs have several effects on normal renal function, including regulation of RBF, sodium and water balance, and acid–base homeostasis. Although ET-1 has hemodynamic effects in almost all vessels, the sensitivity of different vascular beds varies. The renal vasculature, along with the mesenteric vessels, is the most sensitive: vasoconstriction occurs at picomolar concentrations of ET-1,[165,166] increasing RVR and decreasing RBF. However, long-lasting vasoconstriction that is mediated by the ET-A receptor may be preceded by a transient ET-B receptor–mediated vasodilation.[167] Because of the site-specific distribution of ET receptors, ET-1 may exert different vasoconstrictive and vasodilatory effects in different regions of the kidneys. For example, by inducing NO release from adjacent tubule epithelial cells, ET-1 may actually increase blood flow in the renal medulla, where ET-B receptors predominate.[168]

In addition to effects on RBF, the ET system also plays a direct role in renal sodium and water handling.[169] In the renal medulla, ET is regulated by sodium intake and exerts its natriuretic and diuretic effects through the ET-B receptor.[170–172] In addition to natriuretic and diuretic effects, the ET-B receptor may also contribute to acid–base homeostasis by stimulating proximal tubule sodium/proton exchanger isoform 3 (NHE3).[173] Although the role of ET-B receptor activation in urinary sodium excretion has been appreciated for some time, more recent evidence suggests that renal medullary ET-A receptors may also mediate natriuresis.[174] This may partly explain the edema that can occur as a side effect of ET-A or dual ET receptor antagonism.

### ROLE OF ENDOTHELIN IN ESSENTIAL HYPERTENSION

In view of its potent vasoconstrictive properties, it is not surprising that ET-1 has been implicated in the pathogenesis of hypertension. In preclinical models of hypertension, ET antagonism may ameliorate heart failure, vascular injury, and renal failure, as well as reduce the incidence of stroke.[175,176] ET-A receptor antagonism has also been shown to normalize blood pressure in rats exposed to eucapnic intermittent hypoxia, which is analogous to sleep apnea in humans.[177]

PreproET-1 mRNA is increased in the endothelium of subcutaneous resistance arteries in patients with moderate to severe hypertension[178] and according to a recent meta-analysis, plasma ET-1 concentrations are increased in individuals with hypertension.[179] However, plasma ET-1 levels are not universally elevated[175]; an increase is found more commonly in the presence of end-organ damage or in salt-depleted, salt-sensitive patients with a blunted renin response.[180] A major component of this increase in disease is often decreased clearance by the kidneys. These findings suggest that certain patient subgroups may be more responsive than others to ET receptor blockade. Females appear to be relatively protected from the pressor effects of ET-1 by virtue of both increased ET-B expression and a blunted hemodynamic response to ET-A receptor activation.[181]

Clinical trials of the antihypertensive effects of ET receptor antagonism have been hampered by difficulties with selectivity for the ET-A receptor, study design, dosing regimens, and adverse events.[182] Because the ET-B receptor exerts diuretic and natriuretic effects, induces vasodilation, and clears ET-1, selective ET-A receptor antagonists may be expected to demonstrate a more favorable antihypertensive profile.[182] Mixed ET-A/B and specific ET-A receptor antagonists are distinguished by their in vitro binding affinities with mixed ET-A/B receptor antagonists demonstrating a selectivity for ET-A of <100-fold, and ET-A selective antagonists having an affinity for the ET-A receptor of 100-fold or higher. However, it has been suggested that a 1000-fold or higher affinity may be required in order to induce ET-A receptor-specific effects in vivo.[183,184] In an early study, treatment of patients with essential hypertension with the nonselective ET receptor antagonist bosentan decreased blood pressure as effectively as enalapril, without reflex neurohumoral activation, over a 4-week period.[185] Similarly, in 115 patients with resistant hypertension who were taking three or more agents, the selective ET-A receptor antagonist darusentan significantly reduced blood pressure at 10 weeks.[186] In a subsequent study of 379 individuals with resistant hypertension, darusentan treatment for 14 weeks reduced blood pressure by approximately 18/10 mm Hg with no evidence of dose dependence across a range of 50 to 100 mg/day.[187] However, in a second study of similar design a large placebo effect meant that darusentan treatment failed to achieve its primary endpoint of change in office blood pressure and the development of the drug for this indication was halted.[188] Interestingly, in both of these studies ambulatory blood pressure monitoring revealed a reduction in systolic blood pressure with active treatment.[183,189] However, also in both studies, peripheral edema or fluid retention was more common in patients treated with darusentan than those receiving placebo.[187,188]

## ROLE OF ENDOTHELIN IN RENAL INJURY

Beyond its effects on the regulation of vascular tone, the ET system also likely plays a direct role in the pathogenesis of fibrotic injury in CKD.[190] In patients with CKD, plasma ET-1 concentrations are elevated, as a result of both increased production and decreased renal clearance.[191] Urinary levels of ET-1 are also increased, which is indicative of increased renal ET-1 expression.[192] One mechanism for increased renal ET-1 in CKD is a direct effect of urinary protein on ET-1 expression in tubule epithelial cells.[193,194] Beyond direct effects of urine protein, a number of proinflammatory factors induce ET-1 expression in the kidneys, including hypoxia, angiotensin II, thrombin, thromboxane $A_2$, TGF-β, and shear stress (Table 11.1).

Several distinct mechanisms may account for the injurious effects of ET-1 on the kidneys. Locally derived ET-1 has direct hemodynamic effects, increasing $P_{GC}$ at high doses and causing vasoconstriction of the vasa recta and peritubular capillaries, with a resultant reduction in tissue oxygen tension. ET-1 acts as a chemoattractant for inflammatory cells, which may express the peptide themselves, stimulating interstitial fibroblast and mesangial cell proliferation and mediating the production of a number of factors associated with collagenous matrix deposition, including TGF-β, matrix metalloproteinase-1, and tissue inhibitors of metalloproteinases-1 and -2. In mesangial cells, ET-1 can induce cytoskeletal remodeling and cell contraction[195] and, in these cells, ET-A receptor activation appears to be important to the development of Alport glomerular disease.[196]

A particularly important role of ET-1 in mediating injury of glomerular podocytes is also beginning to emerge. For instance, increased passage of protein across the filtration barrier causes podocyte cytoskeletal rearrangements and coincident upregulation of ET-1, which may act in an autocrine manner to further propagate ultrastructural injury in the same cells.[197–199] ET-1 promotes podocyte dedifferentiation and migration by activating ET-A and increasing β-arrestin-1 expression which ultimately results in EGFR transactivation, phosphorylation of β-catenin, and increased expression of the transcription factor Snail, an inducer of epithelial–mesenchymal transition.[200] ET-1 induces calcium signaling in podocytes through both the ET-A and ET-B receptors, and mice with deletion of both the ET-A receptor and ET-B receptor from podocytes are protected from the glomerular injury associated with streptozotocin-induced diabetes.[201] Using these mice, investigators have subsequently gone on to demonstrate that ET-1 causes podocytes to release heparanase that damages the endothelial glycocalyx facilitating albumin passage across the filtration barrier.[202]

## THE ENDOTHELIN SYSTEM IN CHRONIC KIDNEY DISEASE AND DIABETIC NEPHROPATHY

### PRECLINICAL STUDIES OF ET RECEPTOR ANTAGONISTS IN DIABETIC KIDNEY DISEASE

ET receptor antagonists have been employed to study the role of ETs in renal pathophysiology in a range of experimental models, including the rat remnant kidney, lupus nephritis, and diabetes. In the remnant kidney model of progressive renal disease, although beneficial effects have been reported with nonselective ET receptor antagonists,[203] selective ET-A receptor inhibition appears to yield superior outcomes with concomitant inhibition of ET-B receptors, potentially abrogating any beneficial effects.[204]

Data with regard to an effect of high glucose concentrations on ET synthesis and secretion are conflicting. Mesangial cell p38 MAPK activation in response to ET-1, angiotensin II, and PDGF is enhanced in the presence of high glucose levels.[205] By contrast, mesangial contraction in response to ET-1 is diminished under high-glucose conditions.[206,207] Circulating ET-1 concentrations are elevated in animal models of both type 1 and type 2 diabetes. Increased expression of

ET-1 and its receptors has been found in glomeruli and in tubule epithelial cells,[194,208] although increased expression of ET receptors has not been a universal finding.[209] Diabetes also causes an increase in renal ECE1 expression, the effect being synergistic with that of radiocontrast media.[210]

A number of researchers have investigated the effect of both nonselective and selective ET-A receptor antagonists in experimental diabetic nephropathy. In streptozotocin-diabetic rats, the nonselective ET receptor antagonist bosentan has yielded conflicting results,[211,212] whereas another nonselective ET receptor antagonist, PD142893, improved renal function when administered to streptozotocin-diabetic rats that were already proteinuric.[194] More recently, acute ET-A receptor antagonism was shown to improve oxygen availability in the kidneys of streptozotocin-diabetic rats.[213] In Otsuka Long Evans Tokushima Fatty (OLETF) rats with type 2 diabetes, selective ET-A receptor blockade attenuated albuminuria, without affecting blood pressure, whereas ET-B receptor blockade had no effect.[214] In a study of streptozotocin-diabetic apolipoprotein E knockout mice, the renoprotective effects of the predominant ET-A receptor antagonist avosentan were comparable or superior to the ACE inhibitor quinapril.[215] Supporting a protective role for the ET-B receptor, diabetic ET-B receptor–deficient rats developed severe hypertension and progressive renal failure.[216]

Accumulation of reactive oxygen species plays a major role in the pathogenesis of diabetic complications, particularly diabetic nephropathy,[217,218] and several observations suggest that the ET system may contribute to oxidative stress. In low-renin hypertension, ET-1 increases superoxide in carotid arteries,[219] and ET-A receptor blockade decreases vascular superoxide generation.[220,221] Similarly, ET-1 infusion increased urinary excretion of 8-isoprostane prostaglandin $F_2\alpha$ in rats, which is indicative of increased generation of reactive oxygen species.[222] By contrast, however, other preclinical studies have suggested a predominantly proinflammatory role for ET-1 in diabetic nephropathy. For instance, the selective ET-A receptor antagonist ABT-627 prevented the development of albuminuria in streptozotocin-diabetic rats without an improvement in markers of oxidative stress but with a reduction in macrophage infiltration and urinary excretion of TGF-$\beta$ and prostaglandin $E_2$ metabolites.[223]

## CLINICAL STUDIES OF ET RECEPTOR ANTAGONISTS IN CKD AND DIABETIC NEPHROPATHY

Both plasma and urinary ET-1 levels are increased in patients with CKD[191,224,225] with plasma ET-1 levels inversely correlating with estimated GFR. In a study of hypertensive patients with CKD, both selective ET-A receptor blockade and nonselective ET receptor blockade lowered blood pressure.[226] However, ET-A receptor blockade increased both RBF and effective filtration fraction and decreased RVR, whereas dual blockade had no effect.[226]

In a study of 22 nondiabetic individuals with CKD, intravenous infusion of the ET-A receptor antagonist BQ-123 reduced pulse wave velocity and proteinuria to a greater extent than the calcium channel antagonist nifedipine which comparably lowered blood pressure.[227] These findings suggest a potentially blood pressure–independent mechanism of action for the antiproteinuric effect observed. In a subsequent study by the same investigators, 27 subjects with proteinuric CKD were treated with the ET-A receptor antagonist sitaxsentan for 6 weeks in a three-way crossover study design. Sitaxsentan treatment was associated with a reduction in blood pressure, proteinuria, and pulse-wave velocity, whereas nifedipine reduced pulse-wave velocity and blood pressure but had no effect on urine protein excretion.[228] Subsequently, sitaxsentan was also shown to restore the nocturnal dip in blood pressure in people with CKD.[229] A fall in GFR with sitaxsentan therapy observed in this study is analogous to that seen with RAS blockade.[228] Although no clinically significant adverse effects were seen, sitaxsentan development has subsequently been halted due to hepatotoxicity.

The effect of the ET-A receptor antagonist avosentan was examined, in addition to standard treatment with an ACE inhibitor or ARB, in a placebo-controlled trial of 286 patients with diabetic nephropathy and macroalbuminuria.[230] At 12 weeks, avosentan was found to decrease urine albumin excretion rate without affecting blood pressure. These results led to the initiation of the ASCEND trial (a randomised, double blind, placebo controlled, parallel group study to assess the effect of the endothelin receptor antagonist avosentan on time to doubling of serum creatinine, end-stage renal disease or death in patients with type 2 diabetes mellitus and diabetic nephropathy).[231] ASCEND set out to examine the effects of avosentan, on top of RAS blockade, in 1392 individuals with type 2 diabetes and nephropathy but was terminated after a median duration of 4 months due to adverse events.[231] In that study, despite a more than 40% reduction in urine albumin-to-creatinine ratio with avosentan, adverse events, predominantly fluid overload and congestive heart failure, occurred more frequently in those receiving active therapy than placebo.[231]

Since the publication of ASCEND, it has become increasingly apparent that the outcome of that study was hampered by the relatively high dose of avosentan that was selected and that ET-A receptor antagonists likely have a relatively narrow therapeutic window. However, if this therapeutic window is appropriately targeted and patients carefully selected, then ET-A receptor antagonists may still find a clinical niche for the treatment of diabetic nephropathy. The Reducing Residual Albuminuria in Subjects with Diabetes and Nephropathy with Atrasentan trial and an identical study conducted in Japan (RADAR/JAPAN) explored the effects of two different doses of the ET-A receptor antagonist atrasentan (0.75 and 1.25 mg/day, respectively) in 211 patients with type 2 diabetes and albuminuria (estimated GFR [eGFR] 30–75 mL/min/1.73 m$^2$).[232] In comparison with placebo, 0.75 and 1.25 mg/day atrasentan, on top of maximum tolerated doses of ACE inhibitor or ARB, reduced urine albumin-to-creatinine ratio by an average of 35% and 38%, respectively, without major side effects.[232] Atrasentan treatment was also associated with decreases in 24-hour blood pressure, low-density lipoprotein cholesterol, and triglycerides.[232] Importantly, despite a comparable lowering of albuminuria to the 0.75 mg/day dose of atrasentan, the 1.25 mg/day atrasentan dose was accompanied by more fluid retention.[232] In a post hoc analysis, fluid retention was more likely in participants with lower eGFR and a higher dose of atrasentan, whereas the degree of urinary albumin lowering was not linked to the degree of fluid retention.[233] Thus it is likely that the antiproteinuric and fluid retaining effects of ET receptor antagonists are mediated by different mechanisms; plausibly the former by vascular or glomerular actions, and the latter by direct effects of ET receptor blockade on sodium transport in the renal tubule.[233] Regardless, based on the promising results of RADAR/JAPAN, the 0.75 mg/day dose of atrasentan is currently being investigated in the phase 3 Study of Diabetic Nephropathy with Atrasentan (SONAR) trial, which has a primary outcome of hard renal endpoints (time to doubling of serum creatinine or ESRD, including renal death; NCT01858532). This study aims to recruit over 4000 participants and is estimated to complete at the end of 2018.

### COMBINED ECE AND NEPRILYSIN INHIBITION

Distinct from ET receptor antagonism, blockade of ET-1-induced signaling has been explored in the clinical setting with the use of the combined ECE and neprilysin inhibitor daglutril.[234] In an 8-week, crossover design study of participants with type 2 diabetes, blood pressure <140/90 mm Hg, and urinary albumin excretion 20–999 μg/min, daglutril (300 mg/day) did not significantly reduce albuminuria compared with placebo, although blood pressure was reduced.[234] The failure to reach the primary endpoint of albuminuria reduction may relate to concurrent neprilysin inhibition, which may diminish ET-1 degradation.[235] Alternatively, it may reflect an overall diminution of ET-1 with consequent decreased activation of ET-B as well as ET-A.[236]

## THE ENDOTHELIN SYSTEM AND OTHER KIDNEY DISEASES

In addition to diabetic and nondiabetic CKD, the role of the ET system has also been investigated in a number of other kidney diseases. Overall, these studies have suggested some degree of renoprotection with either selective ET-A or nonselective ET receptor inhibitors.

### SICKLE CELL DISEASE-ASSOCIATED NEPHROPATHY

Administration of the selective ET-A receptor antagonist ambrisentan preserved GFR and prevented the development of albuminuria in a humanized mouse model of sickle cell disease (SCD).[237] However, the renoprotective effects of ambrisentan were only partially recapitulated by treatment with the combined ET-A/ET-B receptor antagonist A-182086, highlighting the importance of selectively targeting the ET-A receptor in SCD.[237]

### RENOVASCULAR DISEASE

A series of recent studies in pigs provide support for ET-A receptor blockade in the treatment of renovascular disease. In an initial study, investigators treated pigs with unilateral renal artery stenosis with an ET-A receptor antagonist beginning at the onset of renovascular disease and continuing for 6 weeks.[238] In these experiments, researchers observed that ET-A receptor blockade preserved renal hemodynamics, renal function, and microvascular architecture in the stenotic kidney.[238] Similarly, ET-A receptor blockade (but not ET-B receptor blockade) reversed microvascular rarefaction and diminished renal inflammation and fibrosis when it was initiated 6 weeks after the induction of renal artery stenosis.[239] Finally, ET-A receptor blockade also led to an improvement in microvascular density and renal function recovery compared with placebo when it was administered following percutaneous transluminal renal angioplasty/stenting.[240]

### ACUTE KIDNEY INJURY

ET-1 may play a role in sepsis-mediated acute renal failure,[241] although experimental findings have been conflicting, dependent to some extent on the ET receptor antagonist employed. For example, in a rat model of early normotensive endotoxemia, neither an ET-A receptor antagonist nor a combined ET-A/ET-B receptor blockade improved GFR,[242] whereas ET-B receptor blockade alone resulted in a marked reduction in RBF.[242] By contrast, in a porcine model of endotoxemic shock, the dual ET receptor antagonist tezosentan attenuated the decrease in RBF and increase in plasma creatinine.[243] Pointing to a role of ET-1/ET-A signaling in the progression from acute kidney injury to CKD, transient unilateral renal ischemia induced upregulation of ET-1 and ET-A receptor in mice and ET-A receptor antagonism (but not ET-B receptor antagonism) prevented progressive kidney injury.[244]

### SYSTEMIC LUPUS ERYTHEMATOSUS

Urinary ET-1 excretion is correlated with disease activity in patients with systemic lupus erythematosus (SLE),[245] and serum from such patients has been shown to stimulate ET-1 release from endothelial cells in culture.[246] In accordance with a pathogenetic role for the ET system in SLE, the ET-A receptor antagonist FR139317 attenuated renal injury in a murine model of lupus nephritis.[247]

### PRIMARY FOCAL AND SEGMENTAL GLOMERULOSCLEROSIS

Sparsentan is a dual ET-A receptor/ARB antagonist being developed for the treatment of primary focal and segmental glomerulosclerosis (FSGS) by Retrophin Inc. In late 2016, the company reported results from the phase 2 DUET study that examined the effect of three different doses of sparsentan (200, 400, and 800 mg/day) when compared with the ARB irbesartan (300 mg/day) in 96 participants over an 8-week period. The mean reduction in proteinuria in sparsentan-treated patients was 45% in comparison to a 19% reduction in those receiving irbesartan.[248]

### SCLERODERMA

The Zibotentan Better Renal Scleroderma Outcome Study (ZEBRA) is a 3-part phase 2 study (ZEBRA 1, ZEBRA 2A, and ZEBRA 2B) exploring the safety and therapeutic potential of the ET-A receptor antagonist zibotentan in acute and chronic renal complications of scleroderma (NCT02047708). The primary outcome measure is the plasma level of soluble vascular cell adhesion molecule-1 as a biomarker of scleroderma renal involvement.

### HEPATORENAL SYNDROME

Plasma ET-1 concentrations are increased in individuals with cirrhosis and ascites and in patients with type 2 hepatorenal syndrome (diuretic-resistant or refractory ascites with slowly progressive renal decline) in whom systemic vasodilation accompanies paradoxical renal vasoconstriction.[249] To investigate the therapeutic potential of ET receptor antagonism in this setting, the combined ET-A/ET-B receptor blocker tezosentan was administered to six patients in an early phase clinical trial.[250] In this study, treatment was discontinued early in five patients, in one case because of systemic hypotension and in four because of concerns about worsening renal function.[250] These adverse effects are consistent with a dose-dependent decline in renal function in patients with acute heart failure treated with tezosentan, and they highlight the need for caution with the use of ET receptor antagonists in certain patient populations.

### PREECLAMPSIA

A role for ET-1 in the development of preeclampsia is suggested by the observations that infusion of fms-like tyrosine kinase-1 and TNF-α into pregnant rats induced ET-A-dependent hypertension,[251–253] whereas ET-A receptor antagonism attenuated placental ischemia-induced hypertension in a rat model.[254] Despite the mechanistic role of ET-1 in the pathogenesis of preeclampsia, however, ET receptor antagonists are very unlikely to be used in this condition given their known teratogenicity.[251]

## SAFETY PROFILE OF ENDOTHELIN RECEPTOR ANTAGONISTS

The therapeutic development of ET receptor antagonists has been slowed by the adverse side effect profile of available agents, particularly the dose dependency of certain adverse effects. Most notable has been the development of fluid retention, peripheral edema, and congestive heart failure despite the use of predominant ET-A receptor antagonists. The mechanisms that underlie the fluid retention associated with ET-A receptor antagonism have not been fully resolved. It has been suggested that the use of comparatively high doses of ET-A receptor antagonists may have resulted in concurrent ET-B receptor blockade. However, inhibition of nephron ET-A receptors may also be implicated.[167,255] For instance, mice with nephron or collecting duct ET-A receptor deletion were protected from the fluid retention associated with ET-A receptor blockade.[256] Hepatotoxicity may be a class effect or may be restricted to particular subclasses of ET receptor antagonist. A rise in hepatic transaminases has been observed with both bosentan and sitaxsentan, which are both sulfonamide-based agents, but not with ambrisentan or darusentan, which are propionic acid based.[183,186,187,257,258] As discussed earlier, teratogenicity would preclude the use of this class of agents in pregnancy, whereas the potential for testicular toxicity has also been described, although testicular damage has not been reported in patients taking ET receptor antagonists for the treatment of pulmonary hypertension.[236]

# NATRIURETIC PEPTIDES

***Clinical Relevance***

Neprilysin inhibitors prevent the enzymatic degradation of the natriuretic peptides. When used alone they do not produce sustained antihypertensive effects, likely a consequence of compensatory upregulation of the renin–angiotensin system. The combination of neprilysin inhibition and angiotensin-converting enzyme inhibition is associated with an increased risk of angioedema. The combination of angiotensin receptor blockade and an inhibitor of neprilysin has a more favorable side-effect profile and has demonstrated efficacy in the treatment of heart failure. The effect of combination angiotensin receptor blockade/neprilysin inhibition on hard renal outcomes is currently unknown.

The NPs are a family of vasoactive hormones that play a role in salt and water homeostasis. The family consists of at least five structurally related peptides: ANP, BNP, CNP, *Dendroaspis* natriuretic peptide (DNP), and urodilatin. ANP was originally isolated from human and rat atrial tissues in 1984.[259] Since then, the NP family has been found to include several other members, all of which share a common 17–amino acid ring structure that is stabilized by a cysteine bridge and that contains several invariant amino acids.[260] Both BNP[261] and CNP[262] were originally identified in porcine brain tissue, and DNP was first isolated from the venom of the green mamba snake *Dendroaspis angusticeps*.[263] Urodilatin is an NH2-terminally extended form of ANP that was initially described in human urine.[264] NP inactivation occurs through at least two distinct pathways: binding to a clearance receptor (natriuretic peptide receptor [NPR]-C) and enzymatic degradation. Other peptides that may be involved in salt and water balance include guanylin, uroguanylin, and adrenomedullin.

ANP and BNP act as endogenous antagonists of the RAS-mediating natriuresis, diuresis, vasodilation, and suppression of sympathetic activity, as well as inhibiting cell growth and decreasing secretion of aldosterone and renin.[265] The role of NPs in cardiovascular and renal disease, particularly BNP, has led to their adoption into clinical practice as indicators of disease states and, to some extent, as therapeutic agents.

## STRUCTURE AND SYNTHESIS OF THE NATRIURETIC PEPTIDES

### ATRIAL NATRIURETIC PEPTIDE

ANP is a 28–amino acid peptide comprising a 17–amino acid ring linked by a disulfide bond between two cysteine residues and a COOH-terminal extension that confers its biologic activity (Fig. 11.7). The gene for ANP, *NPPA*, is found on chromosome 1p36 and encodes the precursor preproANP, which is between 149 and 153 amino acids in length according to the species of origin. Human preproANP consists of 151 amino acids and is rapidly processed to the 126–amino acid proANP. ANP is identical in mammalian species except for a single amino acid substitution at residue 110, which is isoleucine in rat, rabbit, and mouse and methionine in human, pig, dog, sheep, and cow.

ANP synthesis occurs primarily within atrial cardiomyocytes, in which it is stored as proANP, the main constituent of the atrial secretory granules. The major stimulus to ANP release is mechanical stretch of the atria that is secondary to increased wall tension. In addition to atrial stretch, ANP synthesis and release may be stimulated by neurohumoral factors such as glucocorticoids, ET, vasopressin, and angiotensin II, partly through changes in atrial pressure and partly through direct cellular effects. Although ANP mRNA levels are approximately 30- to 50-fold higher in the cardiac atria than in the ventricles, ventricular expression is dramatically increased in the developing heart and in conditions of hemodynamic overload such as heart failure and hypertension. Beyond the heart, ANP has also been demonstrated in the kidneys, brain, lungs, adrenal glands, and liver. In the kidneys, alternate processing of proANP adds four amino acids to the $NH_2$ terminus of the ANP peptide to generate a 32–amino acid peptide: proANP 95-126, or urodilatin.

ANP is stored, primarily as proANP, in the secretory granules of the atrial cardiomyocytes and is released by fusion of the granules with the cell surface. During this process, proANP is cleaved to an $NH_2$-terminal 98–amino acid peptide (ANP

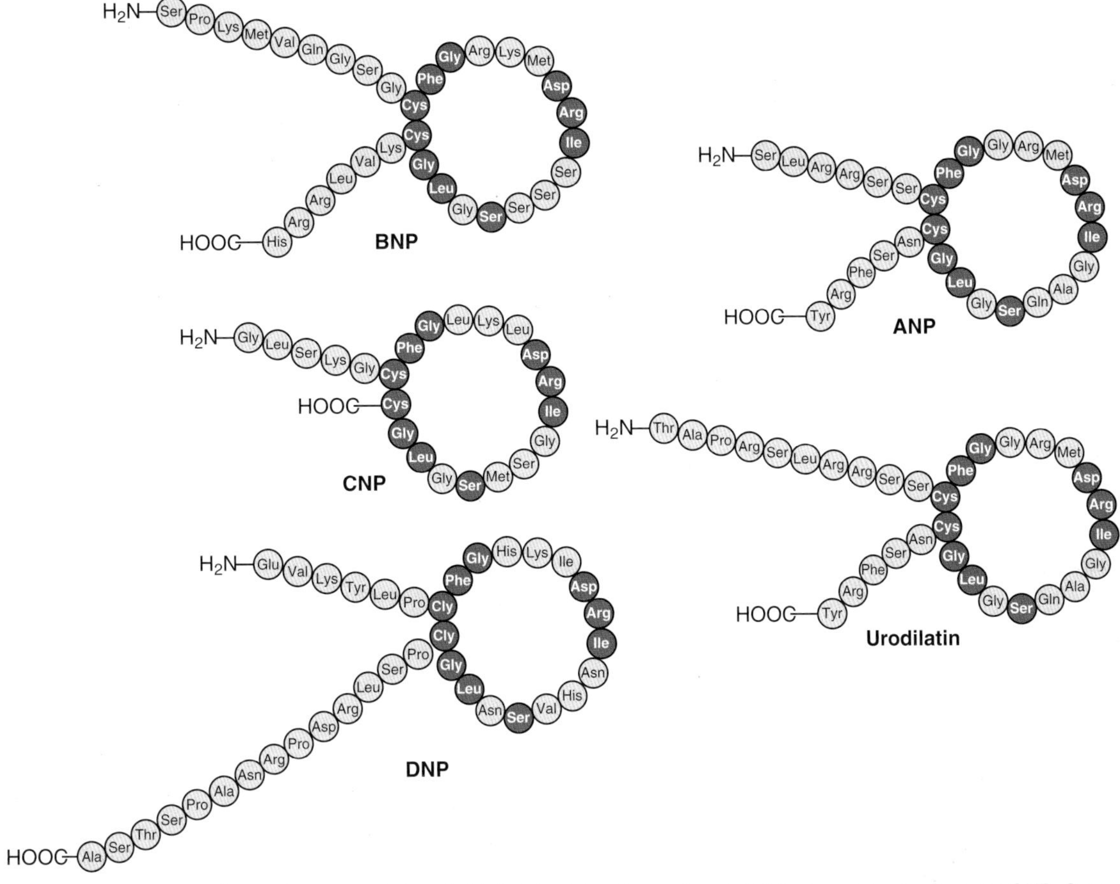


**Fig. 11.7** Molecular structure of the natriuretic peptides. *ANP,* Atrial natriuretic peptide; *BNP,* brain natriuretic peptide; *CNP,* C-type natriuretic peptide; *DNP, Dendroaspis* natriuretic peptide. (Modified from Cea LB. Natriuretic peptide family: new aspects. *Curr Med Chem Cardiovasc Hematol Agents.* 2005;3:87–98.)

1-98) and the COOH-terminal 28–amino acid biologically active fragment (ANP 99-126). Both fragments circulate in the plasma; further processing of the $NH_2$-terminal fragment leads to the generation of peptides ANP 1-30 (long-acting NP), ANP 31-67 (vessel dilator), and ANP 79-98 (kaliuretic peptide), all of whose biologic actions may be similar to those of ANP.[266]

## BRAIN NATRIURETIC PEPTIDE

The BNP gene, NPPB, is located only about 8 kb upstream of the ANP gene on the short arm of chromosome 1 in humans, which suggests that the two genes may share both evolutionary origin and transcriptional regulation. By contrast, NPPC, the gene encoding CNP, is found separately, on chromosome 2. CNP is highly conserved across species; thus it may represent the evolutionary ancestor of ANP and BNP. BNP, like ANP, is synthesized as a preprohormone, between 121 and 134 amino acids in length, according to species of origin. Human preproBNP (134 amino acids) is cleaved to produce the 108–amino acid precursor proBNP. Further processing leads to the production of the 32–amino acid, biologically active BNP (which corresponds to the C terminal of the precursor), as well as a 76–amino acid N-terminal fragment (NT-proBNP).[267] Active BNP, NT-proBNP, and pro-BNP all circulate in the plasma. Circulating BNP contains the characteristic 17–amino acid ring structure closed by a disulfide bond between two cysteine residues, along with a nine–amino acid N-terminal tail and a six–amino acid C-terminal tail (Fig. 11.7).[268]

The term *brain natriuretic peptide* is somewhat misleading, given that the primary sites of synthesis of BNP are the cardiac ventricles, and expression also occurs, to a lesser extent, in atrial cardiomyocytes. Like ANP, expression of BNP is regulated by changes in intracardiac pressure and stretch. However, unlike ANP, which is stored and released from secretory granules, BNP is regulated at the gene expression level and is synthesized and secreted in bursts. BNP expression is increased in heart failure, hypertension, and renal failure. Its plasma half-life is approximately 22 minutes; by contrast, the half-life of circulating ANP is 3 to 5 minutes, and the half-life of the biologically inactive NT-proBNP is 120 minutes. This difference is relevant to the utility of NP measurement as a biologic marker of cardiorenal disease. Changes in pulmonary capillary wedge pressure may be reflected by plasma BNP concentrations every 2 hours and by NT-proBNP levels every 12 hours.[269,270] The physiologic actions of BNP are similar to those of ANP, including effects on the kidneys (natriuresis and diuresis), vasculature (hypotension), endocrine system (inhibition of plasma renin and aldosterone secretion), and the brain (central vasodepressor activity).

## C-TYPE NATRIURETIC PEPTIDE

As is the case for ANP and BNP, CNP is derived from a prepropeptide that undergoes posttranslational proteolytic cleavage. The initial translation product preproCNP is 126 amino acids in length and is cleaved to produce the 103–amino acid prohormone. Cleavage of proCNP yields two mature peptides made up of 22 and 53 amino acids: CNP and $NH_2$-terminally extended form of CNP, respectively. Of the 17 amino acids within the CNP ring structure, 11 are identical to those in the other NPs, although, uniquely, CNP lacks an amino tail at the carboxy terminus (Fig. 11.7). Whereas ANP and BNP are ligands for a guanylyl cyclase–coupled receptor, the NPR-A receptor, CNP is a specific ligand for the NPR-B receptor. CNP primarily functions in an autocrine/paracrine manner with effects on vascular tone and muscle cell growth.[271] Expression of the CNP gene by the endothelial cells, the presence of CNP receptors on vascular smooth muscle cell, and the antiproliferative effect of CNP on vascular smooth muscle cells suggest that CNP is produced by the endothelium and acts on adjacent cells, serving as an autocrine/paracrine endothelium-derived locally active vasoregulatory system. Accordingly, plasma concentrations of CNP are very low, although they are increased in the conditions of heart failure and renal failure. CNP is present in the heart, kidneys, and endothelium, and its receptor is also expressed in abundance in the hypothalamus and pituitary gland, which suggests that the peptide may also play a role as a neuromodulator or neurotransmitter. Regulation of CNP expression is distinct from that of ANP and BNP and is controlled by a number of vasoactive mediators, including insulin, vascular endothelial growth factor, TGF-β, TNF-α, and IL-1β.[271]

The principle enzymes responsible for the conversion of proANP, proBNP, and proCNP to their active forms are the serine proteases, corin and furin.[272] Corin converts proANP to ANP,[273] furin converts proCNP to CNP[274] and both corin and furin cleave proBNP.[275] Corin is highly expressed in the heart and to a lesser extent in the kidney[272] and it is the rate-limiting enzyme in ANP activation.[276] In response to pressure overload, corin-deficient mice develop hypertension together with cardiac hypertrophy and dysfunction.[277,278] In the kidneys, corin colocalizes with ANP[279] and decreased urinary corin excretion has been observed in patients with CKD.[280] Interestingly, studies combining observations made in organ-specific corin-deficient mice together with human correlative experiments have identified a role for impaired uterine corin/ANP function in the pathogenesis of preeclampsia.[281]

### *DENDROASPIS* NATRIURETIC PEPTIDE

The physiologic role of DNP has been controversial since its original identification in the venom of the Green Mamba snake, *D. angusticeps,* in 1992.[263,282] DNP is a 38–amino acid peptide that shares the 17–amino acid ring structure common to all NPs, except that it has unique N- and C-terminal regions (Fig. 11.7).[270] Immunoreactivity for DNP has been reported in human plasma and atrial myocardium, and DNP has also been described in rat[283] and rabbit[284] kidneys, rat colon,[285] rat aortic vascular smooth muscle cells,[286] and pig ovarian granulosa cells.[287] DNP binds to NPR-A[288] and the clearance receptor NPR-C,[289] which may be of particular relevance in view of the peptide's apparent resistance to enzymatic degradation.[290] In dogs, either under normal conditions or in a pacing-induced heart failure model, administration of synthetic DNP decreased cardiac filling pressures; increased GFR, natriuresis, and diuresis; and lowered blood pressure, suppressing renin release and increasing plasma and urine cGMP levels.[291,292] Despite these propitious findings, several aspects of the biologic role of DNP remain contentious. In particular, the gene for the peptide has not been identified in mammals and the fractionation of DNP from human samples has not been reported.[282] These uncertainties have led some authors to question whether DNP is, in fact, expressed at all in humans.[282]

### URODILATIN

Urodilatin is a structural homolog of ANP that shares the same 17–amino acid ring structure and COOH-terminal tail. It is synthesized in renal distal tubule cells and differentially processed to a 32–amino acid $NH_2$-terminally extended form of ANP.[293] Urodilatin is not found in plasma; instead, it acts in a paracrine manner within the kidneys on receptors in the glomeruli and IMCDs to promote natriuresis and diuresis. Urodilatin is upregulated in diabetic animals[294] and in the remnant kidney[295] and is relatively resistant to enzymatic degradation, which may explain its more potent renal effects.

## NATRIURETIC PEPTIDE RECEPTORS

NPs mediate their biologic effects by binding to three distinct guanylyl cyclase NPRs. The terminology can be somewhat confusing: NPR-A binds ANP and BNP, and NPR-B binds CNP, whereas NPR-C acts as a clearance receptor for all three peptides.

NPR-A and NPR-B are structurally similar but share only 44% homology in the extracellular ligand-binding segment; this difference is probably responsible for the differences in ligand specificity. Both NPR-A and NPR-B have a molecular weight of approximately 120 kDa and consist of a ligand-binding extracellular domain, a single transmembrane segment, an intracellular kinase domain, and an enzymatically active guanylyl cyclase domain.[260] The kinase homology domain of NPR-A and NPR-B shares 30% homology with protein kinases but has no kinase activity. Ligand binding of NPR-A and NPR-B prevents the normal inhibitory action exerted by the kinase homology domain on the guanylyl cyclase domain, allowing the generation of cGMP, which acts as a second messenger responsible for most of the biologic effects of the NPs. NPR-C, in contrast to NPR-A and -B, lacks both the kinase homology domain and the catalytic guanylyl cyclase domain and therefore does not signal through a second-messenger system. Instead, the receptor contains the extracellular ligand-binding segment, a transmembrane domain, and a 37–amino acid cytoplasmic domain containing a G protein–activating sequence.[296] In NPR-C–knockout mice, blood pressure is reduced and the plasma half-life of ANP is increased; this finding supports the role of NPR-C as a clearance receptor.[297]

NPR-C binds all members of the NP family with high affinity. It is the most abundantly expressed of the NPRs—present in the kidneys, vascular endothelium, smooth muscle cells, and heart—and represents approximately 95% of the total receptor population. Preferential binding of NPR-C to ANP over BNP may explain the relatively increased plasma half-life of BNP.[270] NPR-C clears NPs from the circulation through a process of receptor-mediated endocytosis and lysosomal degradation before rapid recycling of the internalized receptor to the cell surface. Although the primary function of NPR-C is as a clearance receptor, ligand binding may exert biologic effects on the cell through G protein–mediated inhibition of cAMP.[298] The biologic effects of NPs are largely dependent on the distribution of their receptors. NPR-A mRNA is present mainly in the kidneys, especially in the IMCD cells, although the receptor is also notably present within the glomeruli, renal vasculature, and proximal tubules. The distribution of NPR-B overlaps with that of NPR-A; the receptor is found in the kidneys, vasculature, and brain. However, in accordance with the paracrine effects of CNP on vascular tone, mitogenesis, and cell migration, NPR-B is expressed in greater abundance than is NPR-A within the vascular endothelium and smooth muscle, whereas expression levels are relatively lower within the kidneys.

## NEPRILYSIN

Receptor-mediated endocytosis probably accounts for about 50% of clearance of the NPs from the circulation; catalytic degradation by the enzyme neprilysin (NEP 24.11) is responsible for the majority of the rest, and direct renal excretion accounts for only a minor contribution.[270] Receptor clearance probably plays an even smaller role in conditions associated with chronically elevated NP levels, because of increased receptor occupancy and downregulation of NPR-C expression.

Neprilysin is a membrane-bound zinc metalloproteinase, originally termed *enkephalinase* because of its ability to degrade opioid receptors in the brain. The enzyme has structural and catalytic similarity to other metallopeptidases, including aminopeptidase; ACE; ECE; and carboxypeptidases A, B, and E and, in addition to the NPs, numerous other substrates have been described for neprilysin (Table 11.2). The primary mechanism of action of neprilysin is to hydrolyze peptide bonds on the $NH_2$ side of hydrophobic amino acid residues. In the case of ANP, neprilysin cleaves the $Cys^{105}$-$Phe^{106}$ bond to disrupt the ring structure and inactivate the peptide. The Cys-Phe bond of BNP is relatively insensitive to enzymatic cleavage. Neprilysin has a nearly ubiquitous tissue distribution; expression has been demonstrated in the kidneys, liver, heart, brain, lungs, gut, and adrenal glands. The metallopeptidase is present not only on the surface of endothelial cells but also on smooth muscle cells, fibroblasts, and cardiac myocytes[299]; it is most abundant in the brush border of the proximal tubules of the kidneys, where it rapidly degrades filtered ANP, preventing the peptide from reaching more distal luminal receptors.

## ACTIONS OF THE NATRIURETIC PEPTIDES

### RENAL EFFECTS OF THE NATRIURETIC PEPTIDES

The natriuretic and diuretic actions of the NPs are consequences of both vasomotor effects and direct effects on the renal tubule. Both ANP and BNP cause an increase in glomerular capillary hydrostatic pressure and a rise in GFR by inducing afferent arteriolar vasodilation and efferent arteriolar vasoconstriction. These contrasting effects of the NPs on the afferent and efferent arterioles differ from the actions of classical vasodilators such as bradykinin. In addition to direct effects on vascular tone, ANP can increase GFR through cGMP-mediated mesangial cell relaxation and consequent changes in the ultrafiltration coefficient. Plasma levels of ANP that do not increase GFR can induce natriuresis, indicating the potential for direct tubule effects, which may involve either locally produced NPs acting in a paracrine manner, such as urodilatin, or circulating NPs. A number of mechanisms may be responsible for the natriuresis, including direct effects on sodium transport in tubule epithelial cells and indirect effects through inhibition of renin secretion after increased sodium delivery to the macula densa.

NPs also antagonize vasopressin in the cortical collecting ducts. Similar mechanisms probably underlie the response to ANP, BNP, and urodilatin. By contrast, CNP has little natriuretic or diuretic effect, which may indicate a requirement for the presence of the C-terminal extension of the peptide for renal effects. The NPs may have antifibrotic effects within the kidneys, as evidenced by an increase in renal fibrosis in NPR-A–knockout mice after unilateral ureteric obstruction.[300] In cultured proximal tubule cells, ANP attenuates high glucose–induced activation of TGF-$\beta_1$, Smad, and collagen synthesis, which illustrates the potentially antifibrotic properties of the peptide in the context of diabetic nephropathy.[301]

**Table 11.2 Peptides That Have Been Described as Substrates for Neprilysin**[393,547]

| | | |
|---|---|---|
| Atrial natriuretic peptide | Cholecystokinin | Interleukin-1β |
| Brain natriuretic peptide | Corticotropin-releasing hormone | β-Lipotropin |
| C-type natriuretic peptide | Dynorphins | Luliberin |
| Endothelin-1 | Endorphins | Luteinizing hormone-releasing hormone |
| Bradykinin and kallidin | Endothelin-2 | α-Melanocyte-stimulating hormone |
| Substance P | Endothelin-3 | Neurokinin A |
| Angiotensin I | Enkephalins | Neuropeptide Y |
| Angiotensin II | N-Formylmethionine-leucyl-phenylalanine | Neurotensin |
| Angiotensin 1-7 | Fibroblast growth factor-2 | Oxytocin |
| Adrenocorticotrophic hormone | Gastric-inhibitory peptide | Peptide YY |
| Adrenomedullin | Gastrin-releasing peptide | Secretin |
| Amyloid-β peptide | Glucagon | Somatostatin |
| Big endothelin-1 | Gonadotropin-releasing hormone | Thymopentin |
| Bombesin-like peptides | Incretins | Vasoactive intestinal peptide |
| Calcitonin gene–related peptide | Insulin B chain | Vasopressin |

### CARDIOVASCULAR EFFECTS OF THE NATRIURETIC PEPTIDES

All NPs have vasodilatory and hypotensive properties. Heterozygous mutant mice with a disrupted proANP gene display evidence of salt-sensitive hypertension,[302] whereas hypotension is a feature of transgenic mice overexpressing ANP.[303] In a human patient population, a variant in the ANP promoter was associated with both lower levels of plasma ANP and increased susceptibility to early development of hypertension.[304] However, infusion of high concentrations of ANP can actually induce a rise in blood pressure, which suggests that counterregulatory baroreceptors may be activated.[305]

ANP lowers blood pressure through two major direct mechanisms. First, it increases vascular permeability with a shift of fluid from the intravascular to extravascular compartments by capillary hydraulic pressure. Second, ANP increases venous capacitance and lowers preload.[306] In addition, ANP and BNP antagonize the vasoconstrictive effects of the RAS, ET, and the sympathetic nervous system[265] by decreasing sympathetic peripheral vascular tone, thereby suppressing the release of catecholamines and reducing central sympathetic outflow.[267] By lowering the activation threshold of vagal afferents, ANP prevents the vasoconstriction and tachycardia that normally follow a reduction in preload and thereby produces a sustained drop in blood pressure. CNP is a more potent vasodilator than either ANP or BNP. In fact, CNP relaxes human subcutaneous resistance arteries, whereas ANP and BNP have no effect.[307]

NPs have a number of other effects on the cardiovascular system distinct from their action on vasomotor tone. For example, NPs play a major role in cardiac remodeling. Mice with genetic deficiencies of ANP exhibit an increase in cardiac mass,[302] whereas heart size is diminished in mice transgenically overexpressing ANP.[303] The antimitogenic and antitrophic effects of NPs, which appear to be mediated by cGMP, have also been demonstrated in a range of cultured cell types, including cultured vascular cells, fibroblasts, and myocytes, and in vivo in response to balloon angioplasty. Further evidence for the role of ANP in mediating cardiac hypertrophy was obtained from population studies, in which variants in either the *NPPA* promoter (associated with reduced circulating ANP) or the NPR-A gene, NPR1, have been associated with left ventricular hypertrophy.[308,309] BNP has been shown to have antifibrotic properties within the heart. In vitro, BNP antagonizes TGF-β–induced fibrosis in cardiac fibroblasts,[310] and in vivo, targeted genetic disruption of BNP in mice is associated with an increase in cardiac fibrosis, in the absence of either hypertension or ventricular hypertrophy.[311]

Cardiac CNP is increased in heart failure where it may play a role in ventricular remodeling.[312] Comparison of plasma CNP levels in samples taken from the aorta and renal vein, at the time of diagnostic heart catheterization, has demonstrated that CNP is indeed synthesized and secreted by the kidney.[313] Moreover, this effect was found to be blunted in patients with heart failure, potentially contributing to renal sodium retention.[313] In rats subjected to unilateral ureteric obstruction, recombinant CNP decreased blood urea nitrogen and creatinine levels and attenuated renal fibrosis.[314]

### OTHER EFFECTS OF THE NATRIURETIC PEPTIDES

Even though they do not cross the blood–brain barrier, NPs exert important CNS effects that may augment their peripheral actions. ANP, BNP, and particularly CNP are all expressed within the brain. Circulating NPs may also exert central effects through actions at sites that are outside the blood–brain barrier. The NPR-B receptor is expressed throughout the CNS, which reflects the wide distribution of CNP, whereas the NPR-A receptor is expressed in areas adjacent to the third ventricle, which is indicative of a role of peripherally circulating ANP and BNP, as well as centrally expressed peptides. Complementing their natriuretic and diuretic effects, NPs inhibit both salt appetite and water drinking. ANP also prevents release of vasopressin and possibly adrenocorticotropic hormone from the pituitary gland, whereas sympathetic tone is increased by the actions of the NPs on the brain stem.

Clinical and experimental evidence suggests that NPs play a role in mediating metabolism. Circulating levels of NPs are decreased in obese individuals[315] and among patients with the metabolic syndrome,[316,317] correlating inversely with both plasma glucose and fasting insulin levels.[318] In accordance with these epidemiologic observations, infusion of ANP activates hormone-sensitive lipase from fat cells, which is indicative of lipolysis.[319] In vitro, ANP inhibits preadipocyte proliferation,[320] the lipolytic properties of the peptide being mediated by cGMP phosphorylation.[321,322]

Knockout mouse studies have revealed that CNP plays a predominant role in the regulation of skeletal growth, specifically cartilage homeostasis and endochondral bone formation.[323] Mice with genetic deficiencies of either CNP or its receptor NPR-B lack growth of longitudinal bones and vertebrae and have a shortened life span as a consequence of respiratory insufficiency secondary to abnormal ossification of the skull and vertebrae.[324,325] Transgenic mice that overexpress CNP are relatively protected from glucocorticoid-induced growth retardation.[326] Mutations in the NPR-B gene have also been reported in patients with the autosomal recessive skeletal dysplasia and acromesomelic dysplasia–type Maroteaux, and obligate carriers of the mutations have heights that are below predicted levels.[325] Accordingly, CNP analog therapy is being investigated as a possible treatment for achondroplasia.[327]

## NATRIURETIC PEPTIDES AS BIOMARKERS OF DISEASE

Both ANP and BNP have been studied as clinical biomarkers of heart failure and renal failure. The short half-life of ANP (2–5 minutes) restricts its applicability.[328] However, the biologically inactive $NH_2$-terminal 98–amino acid peptide ANP 1-98 does not bind to NPR-A or NPR-C and so remains in the circulation longer than ANP does. In heart failure, ANP 1-98 levels closely reflect the degree of renal function.[329] Plasma concentrations of the midregional epitopes of the stable prohormones of both ANP and adrenomedullin are predictive of the progression of renal decline in patients with nondiabetic CKD.[330] The prognostic performance of midregional proANP is not superior to that of NT-proBNP or BNP in hemodialysis patients[331] and measurement of ANP or one of its prohormone derivatives is currently not part of routine clinical care. Signal peptides from both ANP and BNP are present in venous blood and rise rapidly following myocardial infarction, suggesting that their detection may aid in the diagnosis of cardiac ischemia.[332,333] Commercial assays are widely available for measurement of either BNP or the biologically inactive peptide fragment NT-proBNP. Correspondingly, since 2000, measurement of circulating BNP and NT-proBNP levels has been incorporated into several clinical practice guidelines for the management of heart failure. Important differences distinguish BNP and NT-proBNP from each other as clinical biomarkers. NT-proBNP is not removed from the circulation by binding to the clearance receptor NPR-C, and hence its circulating half-life of approximately 2 hours is significantly longer than that of BNP (approximately 20 minutes). In addition, both BNP and NT-proBNP are affected by renal impairment,[334] but the magnitude of the effect is greater for NT-proBNP.[335]

## BRAIN NATRIURETIC PEPTIDE AND N-TERMINAL PROBRAIN NATRIURETIC PEPTIDE AS BIOMARKERS OF HEART FAILURE

Measurement of circulating levels of either BNP or NT-proBNP has effectively helped guide clinical practice in several aspects of the management of heart failure, including diagnosis, screening, prognosis, and monitoring of therapy.[260] The primary role of BNP measurement in the assessment of dyspnea is as a "ruling out" test: A plasma BNP level lower than 100 pg/mL has a negative predictive value for heart failure of 90%.[336] In the ProBNP Investigation of Dyspnea in the Emergency Department (PRIDE) study, an NT-proBNP level lower than 300 pg/mL was optimal in ruling out heart failure, with a negative predictive value of 99%.[337] Screening for BNP[338] and NT-BNP[339] levels has also proven useful in identifying individuals at risk for heart failure for whom aggressive medical therapy should be targeted. The utility of serial BNP or NT-BNP measurements in guiding the treatment of patients with heart failure was the subject of a 2016 Cochrane Review.[340] This review concluded that low-quality evidence shows that NP-guided treatment is associated with a reduction in hospital admissions for heart failure and that low-quality evidence shows uncertainty with respect to the effect of NP-guided treatment on mortality or all-cause hospital admissions.[340] In the interpretation of plasma levels of BNP and NT-proBNP, a number of other biologic variables should be taken into account. NP levels rise with age and are higher in women, the latter effect possibly secondary to estrogen regulation, inasmuch as hormone replacement therapy increases BNP levels.[341] Conversely, NP levels fall with increasing obesity. Although BNP levels of heart failure patients are higher in Asian or African American patients than in Caucasian or Hispanic patients, they provide prognostic value regardless of race or ethnicity.[342]

## ROLE OF BRAIN NATRIURETIC PEPTIDE AND N-TERMINAL PROBRAIN NATRIURETIC PEPTIDE AS BIOMARKERS IN RENAL DISEASE

The interpretation of NP concentrations in patients with renal disease merits special consideration. NP levels are increased in individuals with impaired renal function. This increase is probably multifactorial in origin and not solely the consequence of increased intravascular volume. Other factors that contribute to increased NP levels include decreased NP responsiveness, subclinical ventricular dysfunction, hypertension, left ventricular hypertrophy, subclinical ischemia, myocardial fibrosis, and RAS activation,[343] as well as decreased filtration and reduced clearance by NPR-C and NEP.[344] Although, on the basis of observational studies, it has been widely considered that renal clearance plays a greater role in the removal of NT-proBNP from the circulation than removal of BNP, one study has challenged this view. By measuring both NT-proBNP and BNP in the renal arteries and veins of 165 subjects undergoing renal arteriography, investigators found that both NT-proBNP and BNP are equally dependent on renal clearance.[345] However, the NT-proBNP-to-BNP ratio did increase with declining GFR, which suggests that the two peptides may be differentially cleared at GFRs lower than 30 mL/min/1.73 $m^2$.[345]

Even though both BNP and NT-proBNP are affected by renal impairment, their clinical utility for the prediction of heart failure persists in CKD patients in the context of appropriately adjusted reference ranges. For example in the Breathing Not Properly study, BNP cut point values were approximately threefold higher to diagnose heart failure in patients with an estimated GFR lower than 60 mL/min relative to the conventional cut point value of 100 pg/mL.[346] In a cohort of 831 patients with dyspnea and a GFR less than 60 mL/min, both BNP and NT-proBNP were effective predictors of heart failure, although NT-proBNP was superior in predicting mortality.[347] In asymptomatic patients with CKD, both BNP and NT-proBNP were equivalent and effective in indicating the presence of left ventricular hypertrophy or coronary artery disease.[348] In patients with CKD, BNP and NT-proBNP may be predictive of the progression of renal decline[349,350] and cardiovascular disease and mortality. In a nondialysis CKD population, NT-proBNP, but not BNP, was an independent predictor of death[351]; in 994 black patients with hypertensive renal disease (GFR = 20 to 65 mL/min/1.73 $m^2$), NT-proBNP was predictive of cardiovascular disease and mortality, particularly among individuals with proteinuria.[352] In pediatric CKD patients, both BNP and pro-BNP (but not troponins I and T) were indicative of left ventricular hypertrophy or dysfunction.[353]

BNP and NT-proBNP have been studied extensively in dialysis recipients both as prognostic indicators and as markers of volume status. The molecular weights of BNP (3.5 kDa) and NT-proBNP (8.35 kDa) are low enough that both peptides may be cleared by high-flux dialysis.[354,355] Nevertheless, in contrast to ANP, which falls sharply after either hemodialysis or peritoneal dialysis, levels of BNP and NT-proBNP are less affected.[354,356] The role of NP levels as indicators of volume status in either hemodialysis or peritoneal dialysis recipients is confounded by the common coexistence of left ventricular abnormalities.[334,346,357–360] Both BNP and NT-proBNP levels are predictive of mortality, heart failure, and coronary artery disease in the population undergoing dialysis.[361–366] However, no definite cut point values for diagnosing heart failure in dialysis patients have been defined.[346]

## CIRCULATING C-TYPE NATRIURETIC PEPTIDE LEVELS AS A BIOMARKER FOR RISK OF MYOCARDIAL INFARCTION

Although CNP usually functions in a paracrine manner, its presence in the plasma may provide utility as a biomarker of cardiovascular risk. In a study of 1841 individuals from the general population, individuals with plasma CNP levels in the highest quartile were at increased risk of myocardial infarction and, unlike BNP levels, plasma CNP levels were unaffected by sex and only weakly associated with age.[367]

## THERAPEUTIC USES OF NATRIURETIC PEPTIDES

Even though NP levels are increased in heart failure, their biologic effects are blunted. Intravenous administration of recombinant NPs increases their circulating levels several-fold, overcoming this resistance. As such, two recombinant NPs are currently available as therapeutic agents for the treatment of heart failure: recombinant ANP (carperitide), which is available in Japan for the treatment of pulmonary edema, and recombinant BNP (nesiritide), which is licensed in several countries, including the United States, for the treatment of acute decompensated heart failure.

### RECOMBINANT ATRIAL NATRIURETIC PEPTIDE

ANP has a short half-life and a high total body clearance. Its intravenous administration causes a reduction in blood pressure, diuresis, and natriuresis in healthy individuals; this response is reduced in the setting of acute heart failure. In a 6-year open-label study of 3777 patients with acute heart failure treated with carperitide, clinical improvement was reported in 82%.[368] Whereas early experimental studies were suggestive of a potential benefit of exogenous ANP in acute renal failure, results in patients have generally been disappointing. Nevertheless, the peptide may have a limited role in selected patient populations. For example, low-dose carperitide preserved renal function in patients undergoing repair of abdominal aortic aneurysm[369] and reduced the incidence of contrast-induced nephropathy in patients after coronary angiography.[370] However, a meta-analysis suggested that recombinant ANP has no effect on mortality in patients with acute renal injury, although a trend toward a reduction in the need for renal replacement therapy was shown.[371] In a separate meta-analysis of studies conducted in cardiovascular surgery patients, ANP infusion decreased peak serum creatinine, incidence of arrhythmia, and need for renal replacement therapy, whereas both ANP and BNP decreased the length of intensive care unit and hospital stay.[372] Among 367 high-risk individuals undergoing coronary artery bypass grafting (CABG), recombinant ANP decreased the incidence of major adverse cardiovascular and cerebrovascular events and the need for dialysis, immediately and up to 2 years postoperatively, although survival was unaffected.[373] Similarly, among CKD patients undergoing CABG, those receiving recombinant ANP experienced a smaller rise in serum creatinine, fewer cardiac events, and lower requirement for dialysis, although mortality did not differ from those that did not receive ANP.[374] However, when employed in an effort to treat rather than prevent acute kidney injury following cardiac surgery, recombinant ANP had no significant effect on renal function, the need for renal replacement, length of stay, or medical costs.[375]

### RECOMBINANT BRAIN NATRIURETIC PEPTIDE

Nesiritide is recombinant human BNP, manufactured from *Escherichia coli* and identical in structure to native human BNP, with a mean terminal half-life of 18 minutes in patients with heart failure.[376] Intravenous administration of nesiritide lowers pulmonary and systemic vascular resistance, decreases right atrial pressure, and increases cardiac output (presumably through effects on ventricular afterload) in a concentration-dependent fashion.[377] In the kidneys, nesiritide increases RBF and GFR through both direct vasodilatory effects and indirect effects on cardiac output and norepinephrine inhibition.[378] Diuresis and natriuresis may also occur, although these effects are modest and may not be seen at the approved doses. Additional effects of nesiritide may also include inhibition of renin secretion in the kidneys and aldosterone production in the heart and adrenal glands.

In response to meta-analysis data suggesting that nesiritide treatment may be associated with a worsening of renal function and an increase in the rate of early death,[379,380] the Acute Study of Clinical Effectiveness of Nesiritide in Decompensated Heart Failure (ASCEND-HF) trial was initiated.[381] In this study of 7141 patients hospitalized with acute heart failure, nesiritide neither increased nor decreased the rate of death or rehospitalization, rates of worsening renal function were unaffected, and there was a small but nonsignificant improvement in self-reported rates of dyspnea.[381] Based on these results, the investigators concluded that nesiritide cannot be recommended for routine use in the broad population of patients with acute heart failure.[381]

### THERAPEUTIC USES OF OTHER NATRIURETIC PEPTIDES

The effects of urodilatin (ularitide) have been assessed in both heart failure and acute renal failure. However, the diuretic effect of urodilatin appears to be attenuated in heart failure patients, which reflects a blunted response, as observed for ANP and BNP.[382,383] Similarly, as with ANP and BNP, hypotension appears to be a dose-limiting side effect of ularitide therapy.[383,384] In the Safety and Efficacy of an Intravenous Placebo-Controlled Randomized Infusion of Ularitide in a Prospective Double-blind Study in Patients with Symptomatic, Decompensated Chronic Heart Failure (SIRIUS II) study, a phase II trial of 221 patients hospitalized for decompensated heart failure, a single 24-hour infusion of ularitide preserved short-term renal function.[385] The NP vessel dilator may offer theoretical advantages for the treatment of acute decompensated heart failure in comparison with current NP-based therapies.[386,387] In particular, vessel dilator may produce a greater and more sustained natriuresis than does ANP or BNP, without a blunted response in patients with heart failure, and may also improve renal function in the setting of experimental acute renal injury.[388] An alternative therapeutic approach is the development of novel chimeric peptides. For example, researchers have synthesized a peptide (cenderitide) that represents fusion of the 22–amino acid peptide CNP together with the 15–amino acid linear C terminus of DNP.[389] In vitro, this peptide activates cGMP and attenuates cardiac fibroblast proliferation. In vivo, cenderitide is both natriuretic and diuretic and increases GFR with less hypotension than does BNP.[389,390] Cenderitide is more resistant to degradation by neprilysin than the naturally occurring NPs and is eightfold more potent in inducing glomerular cGMP production than CNP.[391]

### COMBINATION ANGIOTENSIN RECEPTOR BLOCKADE AND NEPRILYSIN INHIBITION

Notwithstanding concerns regarding the efficacy and cost effectiveness of recombinant NP therapy, a major limitation is the requirement for systemic administration, which is unsuitable for chronic treatment. Alternative methods to increase the biologic activity of NPs may offer a more feasible approach for chronic therapy. In particular, inhibition of the enzymatic degradation of NPs by neprilysin has been the focus of drug discovery efforts for a number of years. Neprilysin is a zinc metallopeptidase with catalytic similarity to ACE and with a wide tissue distribution, although abundant at the proximal tubule brush border. Several pharmacologic neprilysin inhibitors have been investigated (e.g., candoxatril, thiorphan, and phosphoramidon). Although these agents, in general, lead to an increase in plasma levels of the NPs and, under some experimental conditions, induce natriuresis and diuresis with peripheral vasodilation, results of clinical trials in hypertension and heart failure have generally been disappointing. Specifically, sustained antihypertensive effects have not been demonstrated, and some researchers have reported a paradoxical rise in blood pressure. This may be a consequence of the induction of both neprilysin and ACE expression with neprilysin inhibition[392] and a consequent increase in angiotensin II levels.[393] The biologic actions of the NPs are, however, restored in the presence of an inhibited RAS and this has led to the development of two classes of agent: (1) vasopeptidase inhibitors that inhibit both neprilysin and ACE and (2) combined angiotensin receptor blockade/neprilysin inhibition, the latter having gained regulatory authority approval for the treatment of heart failure.

The rational design of vasopeptidase inhibitors—such as mixanpril (S21402), CGS30440, aladotril, MDL 100173, sampatrilat, and omapatrilat—was made possible because of the similar structural characteristics of the catalytic sites of both neprilysin and ACE.[299] Despite the theoretical advantages of vasopeptidase inhibitors, phase III clinical studies have not been able to demonstrate superiority of vasopeptidase inhibition over ACE inhibition, and an increase in the incidence of angioedema has raised safety concerns. For instance, in the Omapatrilat Cardiovascular Treatment vs. Enalapril (OCTAVE) trial of 25,302 hypertensive patients, angioedema occurred in 2.17% of omapatrilat-treated patients, in comparison with 0.68% of patients treated with the ACE inhibitor enalapril.[394] In the Omapatrilat Versus Enalapril Randomized Trial of Utility in Reducing Events (OVERTURE) study, the incidence of angioedema was, again, increased among subjects receiving omapatrilat in comparison with those receiving enalapril (0.8% vs. 0.5%).[395] The increased angioedema with vasopeptidase inhibition is likely a consequence of decreased degradation of bradykinin and substance P with combined inhibition of the two metallopeptidases.[396]

The rationale that concurrent RAS blockade may potentiate the therapeutic effects of neprilysin inhibition yet concurrent ACE inhibition increases the risk of angioedema encouraged the development of a new class of drug that combines an ARB and neprilysin inhibitor. This class has been termed ARNi (i.e., angiotensin receptor-neprilysin inhibitor), although ARBs do not inhibit enzymatic activity. In July 2015, the first in the class, valsartan/sacubitril gained approval from the U.S. Food and Drug Administration for the treatment of heart failure with reduced ejection fraction. Valsartan/sacubitril is a single molecule composed of molecular moieties of the ARB, valsartan, and the neprilysin inhibitor prodrug sacubitril (formerly AHU-377) in a 1:1 ratio.[397] During development, the combination drug of valsartan/sacubitril was referred to as LCZ696. After ingestion, valsartan/sacubitril dissociates into valsartan and sacubitril, and sacubitril is subsequently converted to its active form sacubitrilat (LBQ657) by esterases.[396] In a study of 1328 patients, valsartan/sacubitril conferred greater blood pressure lowering than valsartan alone with no cases of angioedema reported.[398] In the Prospective comparison of ARNi with ARB on Management Of heart failUre with preserved ejectioN fracTion (PARAMOUNT) study of 301 individuals with heart failure with preserved ejection fraction, valsartan/sacubitril lowered NT-proBNP levels to a greater extent than valsartan after 12 weeks of treatment and was well tolerated.[399] Although the reduction in NT-proBNP was sustained at 36 weeks, the difference in NT-proBNP levels between participants randomized to valsartan/sacubitril and valsartan was no longer significant.[399] However, left atrial remodeling and heart failure symptoms were improved.[399]

The case for regulatory authority approval for valsartan/sacubitril was based on the findings of the phase III prospective comparison of ARNi with ACEi (Determine Impact on Global Mortality and Morbidity in Heart Failure [PARADIGM-HF] trial).[400] PARADIGM-HF compared the effects of valsartan/sacubitril (200 mg twice daily) and enalapril (10 mg twice daily) in 8442 patients with heart failure (New York Heart Association class II–IV) and a reduced ejection fraction (≤40%).[400] The primary outcome, a composite of cardiovascular death and hospitalization for heart failure, occurred in 21.8% of participants treated with valsartan/sacubitril and 26.5% of participants treated with enalapril (hazard ratio 0.80, confidence interval 0.73–0.87, $P < .001$). Hypotension was more common in participants receiving valsartan/sacubitril, whereas cough, hyperkalemia, and renal impairment were more common in those receiving enalapril.[400] Importantly, there was no significant difference in the number of cases of angioedema between participants receiving valsartan/sacubitril than those receiving enalapril, although the number of cases of angioedema was numerically higher in the valsartan/sacubitril group (19 vs. 10, $P = .13$). The effect of valsartan/sacubitril in patients with heart failure and preserved ejection fraction is currently being evaluated in the Prospective Comparison of ARNI with ARB Global Outcomes in Heart Failure with preserved Ejection Fraction (PARAGON-HF) trial (NCT01920711), and other molecules combining ARB and NEP inhibition are also currently under development.[401,402]

Despite the promising findings of PARADIGM-HF, there are some difficulties with the design of the study and there are some theoretical considerations around the use of neprilysin inhibitors in a broad population. In terms of the active comparator in PARADIGM-HF, it is noteworthy that valsartan/sacubitril was not compared with valsartan alone and that the dose of enalapril (10 mg twice daily) may have been insufficient. For instance, in the Cooperative North Scandinavian Enalapril Survival Study (CONSENSUS) of patients with heart failure, the target dose of enalapril was up to 20 mg twice daily.[403] Separately, whether the apparently low risk of angioedema observed in PARADIGM-HF translates to the real-world setting remains to be determined. Only 5% of participants in PARADIGM-HF were black, a group at increased risk of angioedema associated with ACE inhibition or neprilysin inhibition.[396] Furthermore, 78% of participants in PARADIGM-HF had been previously treated with an ACE inhibitor and inclusion of a run-in period where all participants were exposed to enalapril may have resulted in an underrepresentation in the number of cases of angioedema.[400]

Other theoretical risk concerns surrounding chronic neprilysin inhibition largely relate to the other substrates that are normally degraded by neprilysin (Table 11.2). Based on the breadth of activity of these substrates, the possibility has been raised that long-term neprilysin inhibition could have deleterious effects on bronchial reactivity, pain, inflammation, tumorigenesis, and neuronal function.[393] Of particular note has been the recognition that neprilysin is important in the metabolism of amyloid-β peptides and that its inhibition could predispose to the development of Alzheimer's disease, age-related macular degeneration, and cerebral amyloid angiopathy which may take many years to manifest.[393] A trial comparing the efficacy and safety of valsartan/sacubitril with valsartan on cognitive function in patients with heart failure and preserved ejection fraction is ongoing (NCT02884206).

### RENAL EFFECTS OF VALSARTAN/SACUBITRIL IN PATIENTS WITH HEART FAILURE AND PRESERVED EJECTION FRACTION

The renal effects of valsartan/sacubitril were assessed in a post hoc analysis of participants in the PARAMOUNT trial of individuals with heart failure and preserved ejection fraction.[404] Participants received treatment with valsartan/sacubitril titrated to 200 mg twice daily or valsartan titrated to 160 mg twice daily, which each give similar levels of systemic exposure to valsartan.[397,398] In the PARAMOUNT trial, eGFR declined less with valsartan/sacubitril treatment than it did with valsartan treatment over a 36-week period (−1.5 vs. −5.2 mL/min/1.73 m$^2$, $P$ = .002), whereas the geometric mean of the urinary albumin-to-creatinine ratio increased from baseline in the valsartan/sacubitril group (2.4–2.9 mg/mmol) and was unchanged in the valsartan group (2.1–2.0 mg/mmol; $P$ value for difference between groups = .016).[404] The finding of a relative preservation in eGFR with valsartan/sacubitril is consistent with the observation from the PARADIGM-HF trial that valsartan/sacubitril-treated patients experienced less renal impairment that necessitated cessation of therapy than enalapril-treated patients.[400] Both the effect on eGFR and albuminuria are reminiscent of the effect of systemic ANP administration, raising the possibility that they are a consequence of increased levels of biologically active ANP with neprilysin inhibition.[404] Participants in the PARAMOUNT trial were required to have an eGFR of at least 30 mL/min/1.73 m$^2$ at enrollment[399] and thus the effects of combination ARB and neprilysin inhibition in more advanced renal disease are currently unknown, as are the effects on hard renal endpoints in at-risk populations.

## OTHER NATRIURETIC PEPTIDES

### GUANYLIN AND UROGUANYLIN

The existence of intestinal NPs has been suggested by initial observations that sodium excretion is greater after an oral salt load than after an intravenous salt load.[405,406] These intestinal peptides include guanylin and uroguanylin. However, a study of 15 healthy volunteers found that sodium excretion was similar in response to either oral or intravenous sodium load during either a low- or high-sodium–containing diet.[407] Moreover, serum concentrations of either prouroguanylin or proguanylin were unchanged following either oral or intravenous sodium load and showed no correlation with sodium excretion.[407] Collectively, these observations challenge the notion of a gastrointestinal–renal natriuretic axis mediated by the guanylin peptide family.[407,408] It thus appears likely that the natriuretic, kaliuretic, and diuretic effects of guanylin and uroguanylin, which occur without change in GFR or RBF, are mediated by local production of the peptides within the kidney.[408]

### ADRENOMEDULLIN

Adrenomedullin is a 52–amino acid peptide originally isolated from human pheochromocytoma cells,[409] although it is synthesized mainly by vascular smooth muscle cells, endothelial cells, and macrophages[410] and is present in the plasma, vasculature, lungs, heart, and adipose tissue. The peptide is upregulated in patients with cardiovascular disease and has positive inotropic and vasodilatory properties. Systemic administration of adrenomedullin induces an NO-dependent natriuresis and an increase in GFR both under normal conditions and in patients with congestive heart failure; it also decreases plasma aldosterone levels without affecting renin activity. Individuals with type 2 diabetes and plasma levels of midregional proadrenomedullin (MR-proADM) peptide in the highest tertile are at an increased risk of severe nephropathy (doubling of plasma creatinine and/or ESRD), which may reflect a reactive rise in MR-proADM.[411]

# KALLIKREIN–KININ SYSTEM

The KKS is a complex network of peptide hormones, receptors, and peptidases that is evolutionarily conserved with homologs in nonmammalian species.[412] Discovery of the KKS is attributed to Abelous and Bardier, who reported in 1909 that experimental injection of urine resulted in an acute fall in systemic blood pressure.[412a] Since that time, investigators have recognized that the physiologic actions of the KKS also include regulation of tissue blood flow, transepithelial water and electrolyte transport, cellular growth, capillary permeability, and inflammatory responses. The main components of the KKS are the enzyme kallikrein, its substrate kininogen, effector hormones known as *kinins* (especially bradykinin and kallidin [also termed *lys-bradykinin*]) and their inactivating enzymes, which include kininases I and II (ACE) and neprilysin.

Kinins exert their biologic effects through binding to two receptors: the bradykinin B1 receptor (B1R) and bradykinin B2 receptor (B2R). The B2R is widely expressed and mediates all the physiologic actions of the kinins under normal conditions. The B1R is activated predominantly by des-Arg-bradykinin, a natural degradation product of bradykinin, generated by cleavage of the peptide by kininase I. The KKS may be subdivided into a circulatory (plasma) KKS and a tissue (including renal) KKS, which may be distinguished by their principal effector molecules, bradykinin and kallidin, respectively. In the kidneys, the kinins play a significant role in the modulation of renal hemodynamics and salt and water homeostasis.

## COMPONENTS OF THE KALLIKREIN–KININ SYSTEM

### KININOGEN

Humans possess a single kininogen gene, *KNG1*, which is localized to chromosome 3q26 and encodes both high–molecular weight (HMW) kininogens (626 amino acids, 88 to 120 kDa) and low–molecular weight (LMW) kininogens (409 amino acids, 50–68 kDa) through alternate splicing from 11 exons spread over a 27-kb genomic region. A second kininogen gene has been identified in mice.[413] In humans, kininogen deficiency may be relatively asymptomatic[414]; the kininogen-deficient Brown Norway Katholiek rat strain, however, shows increased sensitivity to the pressor effects of salt, angiotensin II, and mineralocorticoid.[415,416]

## KALLIKREIN

HMW and LMW kininogen are cleaved by the serine protease kallikrein. The name "kallikrein" is derived from the Greek term *kallikreas,* meaning "pancreas," after the work of Frey and others, in the 1930s, who extracted a kinin-producing enzyme from the pancreas of dogs.[416a] Since then, 15 tissue kallikreins have been identified, although, in humans, only one (KLK1) is involved in local kinin production. The human kallikrein genes are clustered on chromosome 19 at loci q13.3-13.4. Plasma kallikrein is found in the circulation and is involved largely with the coagulation cascade and activation of neutrophils. The tissue kallikreins are acid glycoproteins that are variably and extensively glycosylated. Human renal kallikrein is synthesized as a zymogen (prekallikrein) with a 17–amino acid signal peptide and a 7–amino acid activation sequence, which must be cleaved in order to activate the enzyme. In most mammals, including humans, tissue kallikrein cleaves kallidin (lys-bradykinin) from kininogens, whereas plasma kallikrein releases bradykinin.

Although the physiologic effects of kallikrein have been attributed to increased kinin generation, the enzyme may also have direct effects on the B2R, as well as actions independent of the kinin receptors.[417,418] For example, in kininogen-deficient Brown Norway Katholiek rats, local injection of kallikrein into the myocardium after coronary artery ligation had a cardioprotective effect that was abolished by the NO synthase inhibitor Nω-nitro-L-arginine methyl ester and the selective B2R inhibitor icatibant (Hoe 140).[417] As a serine protease, kallikrein may also elicit kinin receptor–independent effects on endothelial cell migration and survival through cleavage of growth factors and matrix metalloproteinases.[419] Transgenic mice overexpressing human kallikrein exhibit a sustained reduction in systemic blood pressure throughout their life span, which is indicative of the lack of sufficient compensatory mechanisms to reverse the hypotensive effect of kallikrein.[420] In humans, polymorphisms of the kallikrein gene *KLK1* or its promoter can impair enzymatic activity, potentially influencing both kinin-dependent and kinin-independent effects. Among normotensive men with a common loss-of-function *KLK1* polymorphism (R53H), an increase in wall shear stress and a paradoxical reduction in artery diameter and lumen were noted, although flow-mediated and endothelium-independent vasodilation were unaffected.[421]

### KININS

The kinins are bradykinin and kallidin in humans and bradykinin and kallidin-like peptide in rodents.[422] Plasma aminopeptidase can convert kallidin (10 amino acids: Lys-Arg-Pro-Pro-Gly-Phe-Ser-Pro-Phe-Arg) to bradykinin (9 amino acids: Arg-Pro-Pro-Gly-Phe-Ser-Pro-Phe-Arg) by cleavage of the first N-terminal lysine residue. Cleavage of the carboxy-terminal arginine residue by kininase I (carboxypeptidase-N) and carboxypeptidase-M generates their des-Arg derivatives, which are agonists of the B1R.[422] Removal of two C-terminal amino acids (Phe and Arg) by ACE (kininase II), neprilysin, or ECE is responsible for inactivation of the peptides.[422]

### BRADYKININ RECEPTORS

B1R and B2R share 36% homology, and both are GPCRs with seven transmembrane domains. The genes for the two receptors are in tandem on a compact locus (14q23) separated by only 12 kb.[423] The B2R is the principal receptor mediating the actions of both kinins, is expressed in abundance by vascular endothelial cells, and is present in most tissues, including those of the kidneys, heart, skeletal muscle, CNS, vas deferens, trachea, intestines, uterus, and bladder. In general, the distribution and action of B1Rs are similar to those of the B2Rs. The B1R, by contrast, is expressed at low levels under normal conditions but is upregulated in response to inflammatory stimuli (e.g., lipopolysaccharide, endotoxins, and cytokines such as IL-1β and TNF-α)[424] and in the setting of diabetes[425] and ischemia-reperfusion injury.[426] B2R binds both bradykinin and kallidin, whereas bradykinin has almost no effect at the B1R. The carboxypeptidase required to generate the des-Arg B1R-active kinin fragments is closely associated with the B1R on the cell surface.[427] This association would enable B2R agonists to rapidly activate B1Rs, particularly in response to inflammation.[427]

Ligand binding of both receptor subtypes induces activation of phospholipase C, which results in intracellular calcium mobilization through production of inositol 1,4,5-triphosphate and DAG via activation of G proteins, including $G\alpha_q$ and $G\alpha_i$. The physiologic effects of bradykinin receptor activation are mediated through generation of both endothelial NO synthase–derived NO and prostaglandins. B2R activation leads to a rise in intracellular calcium concentrations in vascular endothelial cells.[422] However, bradykinin-induced vasodilation is not abolished by coadministration of NO synthase and COX inhibitors, which indicates that additional effectors are also likely to be involved, possibly an endothelium-derived hyperpolarizing factor. In addition, through binding to both B1R[428] and B2R,[429] bradykinin also increases the expression of inducible NO synthase (iNOS), at least in rodents. It is very difficult to induce the iNOS gene in human tissues, especially the vascular endothelium. Mice that have genetic deficiencies of B2R,[430] B1R,[431] or both receptors[432] have been generated; the reported phenotypes of the different knockout strains have been varied, which may be a result of different genetic backgrounds, or, in the case of the single knockouts, differing compensatory effects of the remaining receptor. For example, some studies of B2R-deficient mice revealed an increase in resting systemic blood pressure, an exaggerated pressor response to angiotensin II[433] and salt sensitivity,[434] whereas others revealed no difference in resting blood pressure between B2R- or B1R-deficient mice and wild-type animals.[431,435] Double B2R-/B1R-knockout mice were also reported to have resting blood pressure identical to that in wild-type mice and were resistant to lipopolysaccharide-induced hypotension.[432,436] By contrast, transgenic mice expressing the human B2R had a lower resting blood pressure than did wild-type controls.[437] Transgenic mice expressing the rat B1R (as well as their native murine B2R) were normotensive but showed an exaggerated hypotensive response to lipopolysaccharide and, unexpectedly, a hypertensive response to des-Arg bradykinin.[438]

### KALLISTATIN

Kallistatin is an endogenous serpin inhibitor of kallikrein that acts by forming a heat-stable complex with the enzyme. Surprisingly, administration of human kallistatin to rodents induced vasodilation and a decline in systemic blood pressure, which was unaltered by either an NO synthase inhibitor or the B2R antagonist icatibant; this suggests that the vasodilatory properties of kallistatin may be mediated through a smooth muscle mechanism independent of bradykinin receptor activation.[439]

### KININASES

With the exception of the metabolites des-Arg-bradykinin and des-Arg-kallidin, kinin-cleavage products are biologically inactive. Kinins are cleaved by a number of enzymes, including carboxypeptidases, ACE, and neprilysin. ACE also truncates its own reaction product, bradykinin-(1–7), further to form bradykinin-(1–5). Neprilysin, like ACE, cleaves bradykinin at the 7 to 8 position and has a broad substrate specificity (Table 11.2). The amino-terminal of bradykinin possesses two proline residues and is susceptible to cleavage by the proline-specific exopeptidase aminopeptidase P. The resultant peptide, bradykinin-(2–9), may be further cleaved by proteases that include the endothelial enzyme dipeptidyl peptidase-4, which reduces this metabolite to bradykinin-(4–9).

## PLASMA AND TISSUE KALLIKREIN–KININ SYSTEM

The two independent KKSs in humans (plasma and tissue) can be distinguished by the specific subtypes of kallikreins, kininogens, and kinins involved. The circulating plasma KKS includes HMW kininogen and plasma prekallikrein, both of which are synthesized in the liver and secreted in the plasma, in which kallikrein is generated by the cell matrix–associated prekallikrein activator prolylcarboxypeptidase.[440] Of importance is that bradykinin is the main effector molecule of the plasma KKS. The tissue-specific KKS consists of locally synthesized or liver-derived kininogen (HMW and LMW), tissue kallikrein, and the effector molecules kallidin in humans and kallidin-like peptide in rodents. The half-life of kinins is 10 to 30 seconds, but in tissues with high kallikrein content, including the kidneys, local and plasma-derived LMW kininogen can be continuously cleaved to produce kallidin. Fig. 11.8 illustrates the enzymatic cascades of the plasma and tissue KKSs.

## RENAL KALLIKREIN–KININ SYSTEM

The tissue KKS contributes to the physiologic functions of the kidneys with effects on RVR, natriuresis, diuresis, and other vasoactive mediators, such as renin and angiotensin, eicosanoids, catecholamines, NO, vasopressin, and ET. In the kidneys, large quantities of kininogen and kallikrein are synthesized by the tubule epithelium and are excreted in the urine. Locally formed kinin is also detectable in the urine,

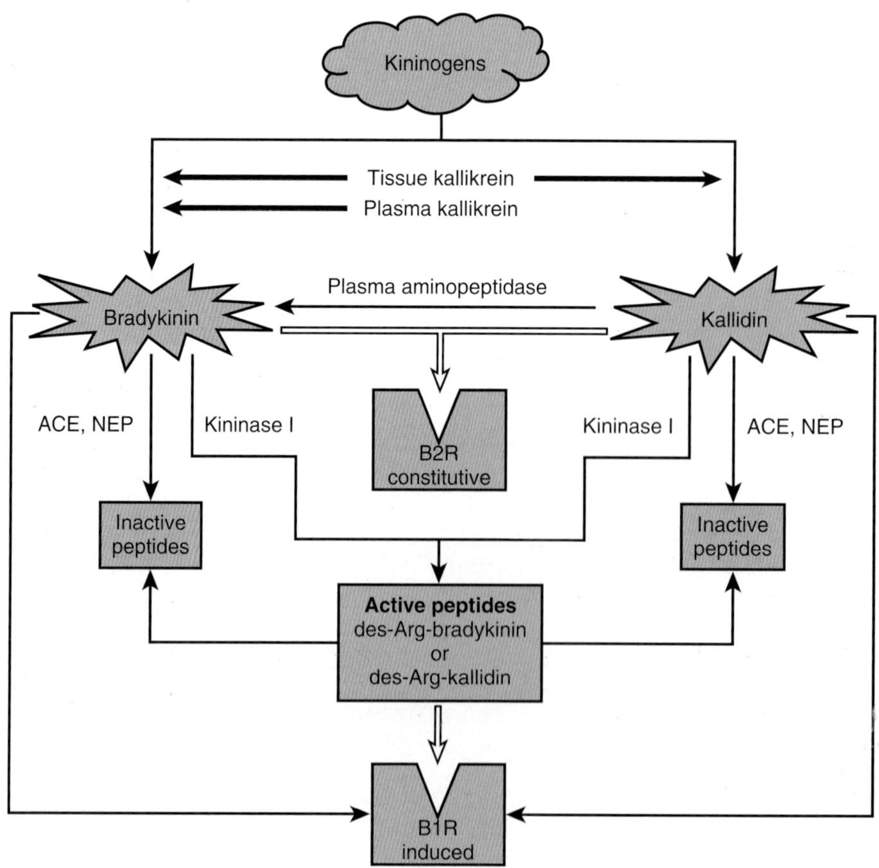


**Fig. 11.8** Enzymatic cascade of the kallikrein–kinin system. *ACE,* Angiotensin-converting enzyme; *B1R,* bradykinin B1 receptor; *B2R,* bradykinin B2 receptor; *NEP,* neutral endopeptidase.

renal interstitial fluid, and renal venous blood. In the human kidneys, kallikrein is localized to the connecting tubules with close anatomic association between the kallikrein-expressing tubules and the afferent arterioles of the JGA. Results of some studies suggest that renal kallikrein mRNA is also detectable by in situ hybridization at the glomerular vascular pole. This anatomic association highlights the physiologic relationship between the KKS and the RAS and is consistent with a paracrine function for the KKS in the regulation of RBF, GFR, and renin release. In this regard, it has been suggested that, through effects on prostaglandin production, kinins may lower tubuloglomerular feedback sensitivity.

Expression of kallikrein within the kidneys is altered during development and is regulated by estrogen and progesterone, salt intake, thyroid hormone, and glucocorticoid.[441–444] The enzyme is not normally filtered at the glomerulus in the absence of glomerular injury. Kininogens are localized mostly to connecting tubule principal cells near kallikrein, which can be found in the connecting tubules of the same nephron. Once activated, renal kallikrein cleaves both HMW and LMW kininogens to release kallidin. The majority of the physiologic effects of kinins are mediated through activation of constitutively expressed B2Rs, with little or no B1R mRNA detectable in normal kidneys. In rats, administration of lipopolysaccharide, however, induces expression of B1R throughout the nephron (except the outer medullary collecting ducts), with strong expression in the efferent arteriole, medullary limb, and distal tubule.[445]

The KKS is involved in the regulation of both renal hemodynamics and tubule function. Diuretic and natriuretic effects play a pivotal role in the contribution of the renal KKS to fluid and electrolyte balance. Kinins have been reported to increase RBF and papillary blood flow and to mediate the hyperfiltration induced by a high-protein diet. Kinins also inhibit conductive sodium entry in the IMCDs,[446] and B2R-deficient mice demonstrate increased urinary concentration in response to vasopressin, which indicates that, through the B2R, endogenous kinins oppose the antidiuretic effect of vasopressin.[447] Kinins may therefore affect sodium reabsorption through direct effects on sodium transport along the nephron, through vasodilatory effects, and through changes in the osmotic gradient of the renal medulla. In addition to the effects on renal vascular tone, salt homeostasis, and water homeostasis, experiments with the B2R antagonist icatibant have yielded evidence that kinins may also have antihypertrophic and antiproliferative properties in mesangial cells, fibroblasts, and renomedullary interstitial cells. The antiproliferative effect of bradykinin in mesangial cells may be mediated through interaction of the B2R with the protein-tyrosine phosphatase SH2 domain–containing phosphatase-2.[448]

### REGULATION OF TUBULE TRANSPORT BY TISSUE KALLIKREIN

Independent of its ability to generate kinin, tissue kallikrein also exerts separate effects on tubule solute transport by regulating the activity of the epithelial $Na^+$ channel (ENaC), the colonic $H^+$, $K^+$ ATPase, and the epithelial calcium channel TRPV5 (transient receptor potential channel vanilloid subtype 5).[449] The connecting tubules secrete a large amount of tissue kallikrein which, through its enzymatic activity, can alter the function of ion transporters expressed on the luminal surface of cells downstream of its site of secretion.[449] For instance, tissue kallikrein may participate in the proteolytic processing of ENaC increasing its activity, whereas tissue kallikrein–deficient mice have decreased ENaC activity.[450] Despite decreased ENaC activity, however, coincident upregulation of ENaC-independent electroneutral NaCl absorption ensures that tissue kallikrein is not essential for sodium homeostasis.[449,451] The cortical collecting ducts from tissue kallikrein–deficient mice also demonstrate enhanced activity of the colonic $H^+$, $K^+$ ATPase in intercalated cells, resulting in net $K^+$ absorption.[449,452] Finally, tissue kallikrein functions to stabilize the TRPV5 channel at the plasma membrane, promoting $Ca^{2+}$ reabsorption, whereas tissue kallikrein knockout mice exhibit robust hypercalciuria.[453] Distal tubule defects in potassium[454] and calcium[455] handling have also been reported in humans with the loss-of-function R53H polymorphism in the tissue kallikrein gene.

## THE KALLIKREIN–KININ SYSTEM IN RENAL DISEASE

### HYPERTENSION

Although it has been known for many years that kinin infusion results in an acute drop in systemic blood pressure by reducing peripheral resistance, the role of the KKS in mediating primary or secondary hypertension has yet to be fully established. Decreased activity of kallikrein has been reported in the urine of hypertensive patients and hypertensive rats. An inverse relationship between urinary kallikrein excretion and blood pressure in humans may be suggestive of a role for the renal KKS in protecting against hypertension.[456] However, an alternative interpretation may be that preexisting or hypertension-induced renal disease may itself lead to a reduction in renal kallikrein excretion. In the Dahl salt-sensitive rat model of hypertension, ACE inhibitors attenuate the progression of proteinuria and hypertensive nephrosclerosis better than do ARBs.[457] That this difference may be mediated by enhanced kinin activity with ACE inhibition is supported by the observations that infusion of either kallikrein[458] or bradykinin[459] in this model attenuated glomerulosclerosis without affecting blood pressure. Studies in two-kidney, one-clip hypertension have yielded conflicting results. The incidence of two-kidney, one-clip hypertension was increased in B2R-deficient mice, in comparison with wild-type animals.[460] By contrast, with regard to the response between tissue kallikrein–deficient mice and wild-type animals, there was no difference with respect to kidney size, renin release, systemic blood pressure increase, and cardiac remodeling.[461]

Despite the uncertainty about the role of the KKS in mediating the pathogenesis of hypertension, a variety of genetic mutations of the KKS have been associated with hypertension in animal models and in humans.[462] Inactivating mutations in the kallikrein gene have been identified in spontaneously hypertensive rats,[463] and an association between mutations in the regulatory region of the kallikrein gene *KLK1* and hypertension has also been described in African Americans[464] and Chinese Han people.[465] The loss-of-function *KLK1* R53H mutation is found in 5% to 7% of the Caucasian population,[466] but this one single-nucleotide polymorphism (SNP) has not in itself been found to markedly alter blood pressure.[467] ACE polymorphisms, responsible for different plasma levels of the enzyme and, accordingly, altered kinin levels, have been identified as independent risk factors for progression of various diseases, including diabetic nephropathy, but they do not affect blood pressure. Finally, a number of SNPs in both the B2R and B1R genes have been associated with hypertension[468,469] and coronary risk in hypertensive individuals.[470]

## DIABETIC NEPHROPATHY

Observations in both experimental animal models and in humans indicate a role for altered KKS activity in the pathogenesis of diabetic nephropathy, although results in experimental studies have been conflicting. The KKS is markedly altered in rats with streptozotocin-induced diabetes and changes are correlated with those in renal plasma flow and GFR.[471] Renal and urinary levels of active kallikrein are increased in rats with moderate hyperglycemia in association with reduced RVR, increased GFR, and increased renal plasma flow and treatment of diabetic rats with the kallikrein inhibitor aprotinin or with a B2R antagonist reduced RBF and GFR.[471] By contrast, in non–insulin-treated streptozotocin-treated rats with severe hyperglycemia and hypofiltration, kallikrein excretion and expression were reduced.[471,472] In addition to its hemodynamic effects, the KKS may also play a renoprotective role in diabetic nephropathy through its antiinflammatory and antiproliferative properties.[424]

Results of receptor antagonist studies initially suggested that the KKS had a limited role in preserving renal structure and function in diabetic nephropathy: Treatment of diabetic rats with icatibant had no effect on glomerular structure or on albuminuria, nor did it alter the attenuating effect of ACE inhibition on either of these parameters.[473] In contrast to this finding, however, the results of more contemporary work suggest that the beneficial effects of ACE inhibitors in experimental diabetic nephropathy may be attenuated by coadministration of a B2R antagonist.[474–476] In Akita diabetic mice lacking the B2R, there was a marked increase in mesangial sclerosis and a worsening of albuminuria,[477] in association with an increase in oxidative stress and mitochondrial damage[478]; however, another study reported contrary results in that B2R-knockout mice were relatively protected from the renal injury caused by streptozotocin-induced diabetes.[479] Upregulation of B1R occurs in response to B2R knockout and could plausibly contribute to renal pathology or alternatively confer a renoprotective benefit. In support of the latter thesis, Akita-diabetic mice deficient in both B2R and B1R exhibited augmented renal injury in comparison to those lacking B2R alone.[480]

In further support of a renoprotective effect of the KKS in diabetic nephropathy, one study showed that induction of diabetes by streptozotocin in mice caused a twofold increase in mRNA for kininogen, tissue kallikrein, kinins, and kinin receptors, with a doubling in albumin excretion in kallikrein-knockout mice in comparison with wild-type animals.[481] In another study, gene delivery of human tissue kallikrein with an adeno-associated virus vector attenuated renal injury in diabetes and decreased urinary albumin excretion.[482] When exogenous pancreatic kallikrein was administered to diabetic mice, it caused a reduction in albuminuria, renal fibrosis, inflammation, and oxidative stress.[483] Conversely, however, kallistatin, which decreases kallikrein activity, also attenuated renal injury in diabetic mice when it was overexpressed using ultrasound microbubble-mediated gene transfer.[484]

Urinary kallikrein excretion in patients with type 1 diabetes demonstrates a similar association with GFR as observed in rats with streptozotocin-induced diabetes.[485] Active kallikrein excretion is increased in hyperfiltering individuals in comparison with both patients with type 1 diabetes who have a normal GFR and normal controls, and it is correlated with both GFR and distal tubule sodium reabsorption.[485] Results of genetic association studies in patients with diabetes have, however, been conflicting: One study demonstrated an association between B2R polymorphisms and albuminuria in 49 patients with type 1 diabetes and 112 patients with type 2 diabetes,[486] whereas another revealed no association between either B1R or B2R polymorphisms and incipient or overt nephropathy in 285 patients with type 2 diabetes.[487] Plasma levels of HMW kininogen fragments were observed to be elevated among individuals with type 1 diabetes and progressive renal decline.[488]

## ISCHEMIC RENAL INJURY

In models of ischemia-reperfusion injury, ACE inhibitors appear to be superior to ARBs in protecting against tubule necrosis, loss of endothelial function, and excretory dysfunction.[489] This superiority may be attributed to enhanced kinin activity with ACE inhibition, inasmuch as the effect is negated by B2R antagonists and inhibitors of NO synthase.[490,491] Bradykinin suppresses the opening of mitochondrial pores,[492] and NO suppresses oxidative metabolism; both observations indicate that the KKS may exert its protective effects in ischemia-reperfusion injury through attenuation of oxidative damage. In mice with genetic deficiencies in either the B2R alone or both B1R and B2R, ischemic damage was enhanced in comparison with wild-type mice; injury was most severe in mice that lacked both receptors.[436] By contrast, tissue kallikrein infusion aggravated renal ischemia-reperfusion injury in rats,[493] whereas expression of the human kallistatin gene with an adenoviral vector protected mice from renal ischemia-reperfusion injury.[494] Thus although physiologic kinin levels may be protective in this setting, higher levels may be detrimental, possibly through pathologic reperfusion.[422]

## CHRONIC KIDNEY DISEASE

In the remnant kidney model of progressive renal disease, adenovirus-mediated or adeno-associated virus–mediated gene delivery of kallikrein attenuated the decline in renal function.[495] In the model of unilateral ureteric obstruction, both genetic ablation of the B2R and pharmacologic blockade of the B2R increased tubulointerstitial fibrosis.[496] By contrast, expression of the B1R is increased after unilateral ureteric obstruction,[497] and treatment with a nonpeptide B1R antagonist reduced macrophage infiltration and fibrosis.[497] In the same model, B1R-deficient mice similarly showed less upregulation of inflammatory cytokines, reduced albumin excretion, and diminished fibrosis in comparison with wild-type mice.[498] In an Adriamycin-induced mouse model of FSGS, B1R antagonist therapy attenuated and B1R agonist therapy aggravated renal dysfunction.[499] Together, these observations suggest that although the B2R is renoprotective, under some circumstances (and in contrast to the observations made in Akita-diabetic B1R/B2R knockout mice) compensatory B1R upregulation may contribute to the pathogenesis of renal fibrosis. In humans, polymorphisms in both the B1R gene[500,501] and the B2R gene[500,502] have been associated with the development of ESRD.

### LUPUS NEPHRITIS/ANTI–GLOMERULAR BASEMENT MEMBRANE DISEASE

Evidence has linked the KKS to the pathogenesis of the immune-mediated nephritides, SLE, Goodpasture syndrome (antiglomerular basement membrane [GBM] disease), and spontaneous lupus nephritis. Mice strains differ in their susceptibility to anti-GBM antibody–induced nephritis. Comparison of disease-sensitive and control strains, by microarray analysis of renal cortical tissue, revealed that 360 gene transcripts were differentially expressed.[503] Of the underexpressed genes, one-fifth belonged to the kallikrein gene family.[503] Furthermore, in disease-sensitive mice, B2R antagonism augmented proteinuria after anti-GBM challenge, whereas bradykinin administration attenuated disease.[503] In the same study, SNPs in the *KLK1* and *KLK3* promoters were also described in patients with SLE and lupus nephritis.[503] Extending their work further, the same investigators showed that adenoviral delivery of the *KLK1* gene attenuated renal injury in congenic mice possessing a lupus-susceptibility interval on chromosome 7.[504]

### ANTINEUTROPHIL CYTOPLASMIC ANTIBODY–ASSOCIATED VASCULITIS

Granulomatosis with polyangiitis (GPA) may be associated with a necrotizing glomerulonephritis. The major antigenic target in GPA is neutrophil-derived proteinase 3 (PR3). Incubation of PR3 with HMW kininogen resulted in the generation of a novel tridecapeptide kinin, termed "PR3-kinin."[505] PR3-kinin binds to B1R directly and can also activate B2R after further processing to form bradykinin.[505] These observations suggest that, in GPA, PR3 may activate the kinin pathway in a kallikrein-independent manner. B1R upregulation has been observed in biopsies from patients with Henoch–Schönlein purpura nephropathy or with antineutrophil cytoplasmic antibody–associated vasculitis.[506] Similarly, B1R upregulation was also observed in a murine serum–induced glomerulonephritis model, whereas treatment with a B1R antagonist attenuated renal decline.[506]

## UROTENSIN II

Urotensin II (U-II) is a potent vasoactive cyclic undecapeptide originally isolated from the caudal neurosecretory organ of teleost fish. The system is now known to be present in humans. The two principal regulatory peptides derived from this organ are urotensin I (U-I), which is homologous to mammalian corticotropin-releasing factor, and U-II, which bears sequence similarity to somatostatin[507] and has notable hemodynamic, gastrointestinal, reproductive, osmoregulatory, and metabolic functions in fish. Homologs of U-II have been identified in many species, including humans.

## SYNTHESIS, STRUCTURE, AND SECRETION OF UROTENSIN II

Human U-II is derived from two prepropeptide alternate splice variants of 124 and 139 amino acids, differing only in the N-terminal sequence.[508,509] The C terminus is cleaved by prohormone convertases to yield the mature 11–amino acid U-II peptide. U-II contains a cyclic Cys-Phe-Trp-Lys-Tyr-Cys hexapeptide sequence that is conserved across species and is essential for its biologic activity[510] (Fig. 11.9). The N-terminal region of the precursor is highly variable across species. Prepro–U-II mRNA has been described in a range of cell types, including vascular smooth muscle cells, endothelial cells, neuronal cells, and cardiac fibroblasts. Multiple monobasic and polybasic amino acid sequences have been identified as posttranslational cleavage sites of the prohormone. However, a specific U-II–converting enzyme has not yet been described. With respect to its tissue distribution, immunohistochemical staining has identified U-II protein in the blood vessels of various organs and also within the tubule epithelial

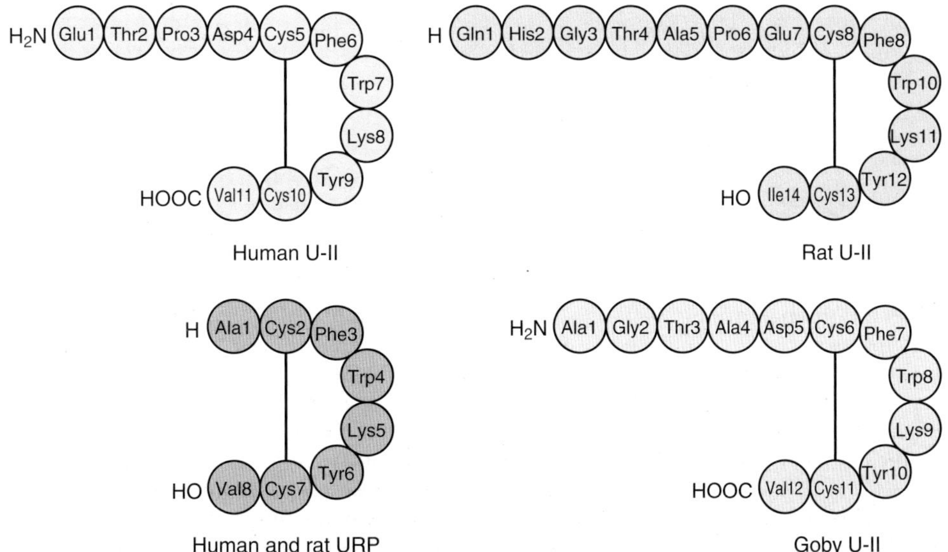


**Fig. 11.9** Molecular structure of human, rat, and goby urotensin II (U-II). *URP,* Urotensin-related peptide. (Modified from Ashton N. Renal and vascular actions of urotensin II. *Kidney Int.* 2006;70:624–629.)

cells of the kidneys.[507,511,512] A significant arteriovenous gradient exists across the heart, liver, and kidneys, which indicates that these organs are important sites of U-II production.[513]

In 1999, Ames and colleagues[509] identified U-II as the ligand for the previously orphan rat receptor GPR14/SENR. The U-II receptor (commonly referred to as the UT receptor) is a seven-transmembrane, GPCR, encoded on chromosome 17q25.3 in humans,[514] that bears structural similarity to both somatostatin receptor subtype 4 and the opioid receptors. Ligand binding of the receptor results in G protein–mediated activation of PKC, calmodulin, and phospholipase C; evidence also links MAPKs ERK1/2, the Rho kinase pathway, and peroxisome proliferator-activated receptor α in the intracellular signaling cascade.[515–518]

The relationship between U-II and the UT receptor is not exclusive; the receptor also binds alternative U-II fragments such as U-II(4-11) and U-II(5-11), as well as urotensin-related peptide (URP).[519,520] URP was originally isolated from rat brain and binds with high affinity to the UT receptor.[520] Although this 8–amino acid peptide retains the cyclic hexapeptide sequence, it is derived from a different precursor to U-II and may have different physiologic properties.[521]

## PHYSIOLOGIC ROLE OF UROTENSIN II

U-II is the most potent vasoconstrictor known, being 16 times more potent than ET-1 in the isolated rat thoracic aorta.[509] However, its vasoconstrictive properties are not universal, varying between species and between vascular beds. For example, U-II has little or no effect on venous tone, and it does not cause constriction of rat abdominal aorta, femoral arteries, or renal arteries.[522] It also lacks systemic pressor activity when administered intravenously to anesthetized rats.[509,523] In cynomolgus monkeys, bolus intravenous injection of U-II induced myocardial depression, circulatory collapse, and death.[509] In contrast to the vasoconstrictive properties of vascular smooth muscle UT receptor, endothelial UT receptor may mediate vasodilation in pulmonary and mesenteric vessels.[524] The response to U-II may be dependent on the caliber of the artery; a small-vessel response is more endothelium mediated, and a large-vessel response is more dependent on vascular smooth muscle.[507] These disparities are among many examples of how the role of U-II may be influenced by a number of factors, including animal model, vascular bed, method of exogenous U-II administration, and the presence of comorbid conditions.

## UROTENSIN II IN THE KIDNEY

The kidneys are major sites of U-II production; this is indicated by both the arteriovenous gradient of plasma U-II across the kidneys and the observation that urinary U-II clearance exceeds urinary creatinine clearance.[507,513] In fact, in humans, urinary concentrations of U-II are approximately three orders of magnitude higher than plasma concentrations.[525] U-II is present in a number of kidney cell types, including the smooth muscle cells and endothelium of arteries, proximal convoluted tubules, and particularly the distal tubules and collecting ducts.[512] UT receptor mRNA is also present in the kidneys, especially within the renal medulla,[525–527] which suggests that the peptide may have autocrine or paracrine functions at this site. In addition, URP mRNA has been described in both rat and human kidneys.[520,526,527] Studies of the role of U-II in normal renal physiology have yielded conflicting findings. In one report, continuous infusion of U-II into the renal artery of anesthetized rats caused NO-dependent increases in GFR, urinary water excretion, and urinary sodium excretion.[528] By contrast, another study showed that bolus injection of picomolar concentrations of U-II produced a dose-dependent decrease in GFR and a reduction in urine flow and urinary sodium excretion.[527] Furthermore, a third group of researchers reported that intravenous bolus injection of U-II in nanomolar amounts induced only a minor reduction in GFR and had no effect on sodium excretion.[529] These researchers also investigated the effect of U-II administration in the context of experimental congestive heart failure, in which the peptide induced an almost 30% increase in GFR.[529]

## OBSERVATIONAL STUDIES OF UROTENSIN II IN RENAL DISEASE

Variations in the concentration of U-II in the plasma and urine have been found in a number of diseases with, again, sometimes conflicting results. U-II levels in plasma may be increased in hypertensive individuals in comparison with normotensive controls and are correlated with systolic blood pressure.[530] In one study, U-II concentrations in plasma were increased twofold in patients with renal disease not on hemodialysis and threefold in patients on hemodialysis.[531] In a separate study, the same investigators observed U-II levels in both plasma and urine to be higher in patients with type 2 diabetes and renal disease than in such patients with normal renal function.[532] Higher U-II levels in urine have been described in patients with essential hypertension, in patients with glomerular disease and hypertension, and in patients with renal tubule disorders, but not in normotensive patients with glomerular disease.[525] Increased expression of both U-II and the UT receptor have also been demonstrated in biopsy samples of patients with diabetic nephropathy[533]; increased U-II levels have also been described in glomerulonephritis[534] and in minimal change disease.[535] By contrast, a more recent study described a reduction in U-II levels with CKD. Here, investigators reported that plasma U-II concentrations were highest in healthy individuals, lower in individuals with ESRD, and lowest in subjects with non-ESRD CKD, while hypothesizing that the discordance with earlier work may reflect the different populations studied or the assays used.[536]

## INTERVENTIONAL STUDIES OF UROTENSIN II IN THE KIDNEY

Both peptide and nonpeptide UT receptor antagonists have been studied. Urantide is a derivative of human U-II.[537] Continuous infusion of urantide into rats induces an increase in GFR and natriuresis,[527] although it is not clear whether the natriuresis is a consequence of altered renal vascular tone or a direct effect of U-II on the tubule epithelium. Whereas urantide is a potent antagonist of the rat UT receptor,[537] it has been found to have agonist properties in cells expressing the human UT receptor.[538] An alternative U-II peptide antagonist, UFP-803, also has partial agonist properties in human UT receptor–expressing cells,[539] which complicates the interpretation of a peptide-based approach to U-II inhibition. Two compounds in the nonpeptide group of U-II antagonists have been studied: palosuran (ACT-058362) and SB-611812. Intravenous administration of palosuran protected against renal ischemia in a rat model.[540] The same compound was also studied in rats with streptozotocin-induced diabetes, in which it was found to significantly reduce the severity of albuminuria.[541] In a study of 19 individuals with type 2 diabetes and macroalbuminuria, palosuran attenuated urine albumin excretion after 2 weeks.[542] However, in a subsequent 4-week study of 54 individuals with type 2 diabetes, hypertension, and nephropathy, palosuran had no effect on albuminuria, blood pressure, GFR, or renal plasma flow,[543] effectively halting the development of this drug for this indication. SB-611812 decreased the carotid intima-to-media ratio in a rat model of balloon angioplasty–induced stenosis.[544] The same compound attenuated myocardial remodeling and was associated with a reduced rate of mortality in a rat model of ischemic cardiomyopathy.[545,546] At present, there are no reports of the effect of SB-611812 in renal disease.

 Complete reference list available at ExpertConsult.com.

## KEY REFERENCES


1. Paul M, Poyan Mehr A, Kreutz R. Physiology of local renin-angiotensin systems. *Physiol Rev.* 2006;86:747–803.
2. Anderson S, Meyer TW, Rennke HG, et al. Control of glomerular hypertension limits glomerular injury in rats with reduced renal mass. *J Clin Invest.* 1985;76:612–619.
4. Griendling KK, Murphy TJ, Alexander RW. Molecular biology of the renin-angiotensin system. *Circulation.* 1993;87:1816–1828.
18. Nguyen G, Delarue F, Burckle C, et al. Pivotal role of the renin/prorenin receptor in angiotensin II production and cellular responses to renin. *J Clin Invest.* 2002;109:1417–1427.
25. Vargas SL, Toma I, Kang JJ, et al. Activation of the succinate receptor GPR91 in macula densa cells causes renin release. *J Am Soc Nephrol.* 2009;20:1002–1011.
30. Campbell DJ, Nussberger J, Stowasser M, et al. Activity assays and immunoassays for plasma Renin and prorenin: information provided and precautions necessary for accurate measurement. *Clin Chem.* 2009;55:867–877.
37. Gloy J, Henger A, Fischer KG, et al. Angiotensin II modulates cellular functions of podocytes. *Kidney Int Suppl.* 1998;67:S168–S170.
38. Velez JC. The importance of the intrarenal renin-angiotensin system. *Nat Clin Pract Nephrol.* 2009;5:89–100.
45. Lautrette A, Li S, Alili R, et al. Angiotensin II and EGF receptor cross-talk in chronic kidney diseases: a new therapeutic approach. *Nat Med.* 2005;11:867–874.
48. Kelly DJ, Cox AJ, Gow RM, et al. Platelet-derived growth factor receptor transactivation mediates the trophic effects of angiotensin II in vivo. *Hypertension.* 2004;44:195–202.
65. Kennedy CR, Burns KD. Angiotensin II as a mediator of renal tubular transport. *Contrib Nephrol.* 2001;47–62.
77. Advani A, Kelly DJ, Cox AJ, et al. The (Pro)renin receptor: site-specific and functional linkage to the vacuolar H+-ATPase in the kidney. *Hypertension.* 2009;54:261–269.
86. Donoghue M, Hsieh F, Baronas E, et al. A novel angiotensin-converting enzyme-related carboxypeptidase (ACE2) converts angiotensin I to angiotensin 1-9. *Circ Res.* 2000;87:E1–E9.
91. Soler MJ, Wysocki J, Batlle D. Angiotensin-converting enzyme 2 and the kidney. *Exp Physiol.* 2008;93:549–556.
100. Esteban V, Ruperez M, Sanchez-Lopez E, et al. Angiotensin IV activates the nuclear transcription factor-kappaB and related proinflammatory genes in vascular smooth muscle cells. *Circ Res.* 2005;96:965–973.
103. Ferrario CM. Angiotensin-converting enzyme 2 and angiotensin-(1-7): an evolving story in cardiovascular regulation. *Hypertension.* 2006; 47:515–521.
108. Dell'Italia LJ, Ferrario CM. The never-ending story of angiotensin peptides: beyond angiotensin I and II. *Circ Res.* 2013;112:1086–1087.
109. Carey RM. Newly discovered components and actions of the renin-angiotensin system. *Hypertension.* 2013;62:818–822.
112. Braam B, Mitchell KD, Fox J, et al. Proximal tubular secretion of angiotensin II in rats. *Am J Physiol.* 1993;264:F891–F898.
123. Taal MW, Brenner BM. Renoprotective benefits of RAS inhibition: from ACEI to angiotensin II antagonists. *Kidney Int.* 2000;57: 1803–1817.
125. Anderson S, Rennke HG, Brenner BM. Therapeutic advantage of converting enzyme inhibitors in arresting progressive renal disease associated with systemic hypertension in the rat. *J Clin Invest.* 1986;77:1993–2000.
127. Kagami S, Border WA, Miller DE, et al. Angiotensin II stimulates extracellular matrix protein synthesis through induction of transforming growth factor-beta expression in rat glomerular mesangial cells. *J Clin Invest.* 1994;93:2431–2437.
130. Gilbert RE, Cox A, Wu LL, et al. Expression of transforming growth factor-beta1 and type IV collagen in the renal tubulointerstitium in experimental diabetes: effects of ACE inhibition. *Diabetes.* 1998;47:414–422.
131. Langham RG, Kelly DJ, Gow RM, et al. Transforming growth factor-beta in human diabetic nephropathy: effects of ACE inhibition. *Diabetes Care.* 2006;29:2670–2675.
132. Houlihan CA, Akdeniz A, Tsalamandris C, et al. Urinary transforming growth factor-beta excretion in patients with hypertension, type 2 diabetes, and elevated albumin excretion rate: effects of angiotensin receptor blockade and sodium restriction. *Diabetes Care.* 2002;25:1072–1077.
133. Mifsud SA, Allen TJ, Bertram JF, et al. Podocyte foot process broadening in experimental diabetic nephropathy: amelioration with renin-angiotensin blockade. *Diabetologia.* 2001;44:878–882.
135. Langham RG, Kelly DJ, Cox AJ, et al. Proteinuria and the expression of the podocyte slit diaphragm protein, nephrin, in diabetic nephropathy: effects of angiotensin converting enzyme inhibition. *Diabetologia.* 2002;45:1572–1576.
185. Krum H, Viskoper RJ, Lacourciere Y, et al. The effect of an endothelin-receptor antagonist, bosentan, on blood pressure in patients with essential hypertension. Bosentan Hypertension Investigators. *N Engl J Med.* 1998;338:784–790.
187. Weber MA, Black H, Bakris G, et al. A selective endothelin-receptor antagonist to reduce blood pressure in patients with treatment-resistant hypertension: a randomised, double-blind, placebo-controlled trial. *Lancet.* 2009;374:1423–1431.
227. Dhaun N, Macintyre IM, Melville V, et al. Blood pressure-independent reduction in proteinuria and arterial stiffness after acute endothelin-a receptor antagonism in chronic kidney disease. *Hypertension.* 2009;54:113–119.
228. Dhaun N, MacIntyre IM, Kerr D, et al. Selective endothelin-A receptor antagonism reduces proteinuria, blood pressure, and arterial stiffness in chronic proteinuric kidney disease. *Hypertension.* 2011;57:772–779.
230. Wenzel RR, Littke T, Kuranoff S, et al. Avosentan reduces albumin excretion in diabetics with macroalbuminuria. *J Am Soc Nephrol.* 2009;20:655–664.
231. Mann JF, Green D, Jamerson K, et al. Avosentan for overt diabetic nephropathy. *J Am Soc Nephrol.* 2010;21:527–535.
232. de Zeeuw D, Coll B, Andress D, et al. The endothelin antagonist atrasentan lowers residual albuminuria in patients with type 2 diabetic nephropathy. *J Am Soc Nephrol.* 2014;25:1083–1093.
233. Kohan DE, Lambers Heerspink HJ, Coll B, et al. Predictors of atrasentan-associated fluid retention and change in albuminuria in patients with diabetic nephropathy. *Clin J Am Soc Nephrol.* 2015; 10:1568–1574.
337. Januzzi JL Jr, Camargo CA, Anwaruddin S, et al. The N-terminal Pro-BNP investigation of dyspnea in the emergency department (PRIDE) study. *Am J Cardiol.* 2005;95:948–954.
338. Ledwidge M, Gallagher J, Conlon C, et al. Natriuretic peptide-based screening and collaborative care for heart failure: the STOP-HF randomized trial. *JAMA.* 2013;310:66–74.
339. Huelsmann M, Neuhold S, Resl M, et al. PONTIAC (NT-proBNP selected prevention of cardiac events in a population of diabetic patients without a history of cardiac disease): a prospective randomized controlled trial. *J Am Coll Cardiol.* 2013;62:1365–1372.
380. Sackner-Bernstein JD, Skopicki HA, Aaronson KD. Risk of worsening renal function with nesiritide in patients with acutely decompensated heart failure. *Circulation.* 2005;111:1487–1491.
381. O'Connor CM, Starling RC, Hernandez AF, et al. Effect of nesiritide in patients with acute decompensated heart failure. *N Engl J Med.* 2011;365:32–43.

393. Campbell DJ. Long-term neprilysin inhibition - implications for ARNIs. *Nat Rev Cardiol.* 2017;14:171–186.
394. Kostis JB, Packer M, Black HR, et al. Omapatrilat and enalapril in patients with hypertension: the Omapatrilat Cardiovascular Treatment vs. Enalapril (OCTAVE) trial. *Am J Hypertens.* 2004;17:103–111.
395. Packer M, Califf RM, Konstam MA, et al. Comparison of omapatrilat and enalapril in patients with chronic heart failure: the Omapatrilat Versus Enalapril Randomized Trial of Utility in Reducing Events (OVERTURE). *Circulation.* 2002;106:920–926.
396. Hubers SA, Brown NJ. Combined angiotensin receptor antagonism and neprilysin inhibition. *Circulation.* 2016;133:1115–1124.
398. Ruilope LM, Dukat A, Bohm M, et al. Blood-pressure reduction with LCZ696, a novel dual-acting inhibitor of the angiotensin II receptor and neprilysin: a randomised, double-blind, placebo-controlled, active comparator study. *Lancet.* 2010;375:1255–1266.
399. Solomon SD, Zile M, Pieske B, et al. The angiotensin receptor neprilysin inhibitor LCZ696 in heart failure with preserved ejection fraction: a phase 2 double-blind randomised controlled trial. *Lancet.* 2012;380:1387–1395.
400. McMurray JJ, Packer M, Desai AS, et al. Angiotensin-neprilysin inhibition versus enalapril in heart failure. *N Engl J Med.* 2014;371:993–1004.
404. Voors AA, Gori M, Liu LC, et al. Renal effects of the angiotensin receptor neprilysin inhibitor LCZ696 in patients with heart failure and preserved ejection fraction. *Eur J Heart Fail.* 2015;17:510–517.
436. Kakoki M, McGarrah RW, Kim HS, et al. Bradykinin B1 and B2 receptors both have protective roles in renal ischemia/reperfusion injury. *Proc Natl Acad Sci USA.* 2007;104:7576–7581.
488. Merchant ML, Niewczas MA, Ficociello LH, et al. Plasma kininogen and kininogen fragments are biomarkers of progressive renal decline in type 1 diabetes. *Kidney Int.* 2013;83:1177–1184.

12

# Aldosterone and Mineralocorticoid Receptors: Renal and Extrarenal Roles

David Pearce | Vivek Bhalla | John W. Funder

## CHAPTER OUTLINE



## KEY POINTS

- Inappropriate aldosterone hypersecretion relative to sodium status is much more common in hypertensives (5%–15%) than is generally appreciated and is even found in a significant percentage of normotensives.
- Most unilateral aldosterone-producing adenomas harbor disease-causing gene mutations, the most common of which is in the $K^+$ channel gene, *KCNJ5*. Germline mutations in *KCNJ5* cause familial bilateral adrenal hyperplasia. Most recently, the chloride channel gene, *CLCN2,* has been implicated in early-onset primary aldosteronism, with clinical findings most consistent with bilateral hyperplasia.
- Recent evidence supports the idea that the actions of aldosterone on the distal convoluted tubule are indirect and mediated by changes in $K^+$. Aldosterone stimulates ENaC in connecting tubule and cortical collecting ducts, and the ensuing hypokalemia acts directly in DCT cells to stimulate the Na-Cl cotransporter, NCC.
- SGK1 gene transcription is regulated by aldosterone, and it in turn stimulates ENaC, thereby enhancing $Na^+$ reabsorption and $K^+$ secretion. SGK1 also responds to and integrates a variety of other hormonal and nonhormonal signals, including insulin and IL-17, which stimulate SGK1 activity and contribute to salt-sensitive hypertension.
- Studies in mice demonstrate a role for T cells in the pathogenesis of hypertension through a mechanism involving IL-17A and SGK1. Mice lacking T cell SGK1 are protected from angiotensin II induced hypertension and renal inflammation.
- The classic thinking that $Na^+$ is dissolved, fully exchangeable, and osmotically active in both intracellular and extracellular compartments has been proving inadequate. Recent studies have identified a nonexchangeable pool of $Na^+$ in extracellular compartments, most notably in subcutaneous tissues in an osmotically inactive form, perhaps sequestered within negatively charged glycosaminoglycans.

In mammals, the control of extracellular fluid volume and blood pressure is intimately intertwined with the regulation of epithelial ion transport. Aldosterone, which is essential for survival, is the central hormone regulating the relevant epithelial transport processes, particularly of ions such as $Na^+$, $K^+$, and $Cl^-$. All circulating aldosterone is generated in the adrenal glomerulosa, where its synthesis and secretion are under the control of angiotensin II and potassium, and its major epithelial actions occur in the distal nephron and colon. The former extends from the late distal convoluted tubule (DCT) through the connecting segment and the entire cortical and medullary collecting ducts. These segments, rich in mineralocorticoid receptor (MR), are often referred to as the "aldosterone-sensitive distal nephron" (ASDN).[1] Most, if not all, effects of aldosterone are mediated by MR, a hormone-regulated transcription factor related closely to the glucocorticoid receptor and more distantly to other members of the nuclear receptor superfamily. The physiologic effects of aldosterone on epithelia entail direct gene-regulatory actions of MR. Thus, a sound foundation for understanding aldosterone's physiologic effects on the extracellular fluid, blood pressure, and electrolyte concentrations can be understood through familiarity with the MR-dependent effects on the transcription of various genes, which, in turn, alter epithelial ion transport. Aldosterone actions in certain disease states involve both genomic and nongenomic effects in epithelial and nonepithelial tissues. Furthermore, physiologic and pathophysiologic effects of cortisol are also mediated in part by MR, which binds cortisol with high affinity. This chapter addresses the cellular and molecular mechanisms underlying aldosterone—and, to some extent, cortisol—action, focusing primarily on effects on ion transport in epithelia but also highlighting key aspects of nonepithelial actions, which are of substantial importance to its pathophysiologic effects.

## GENERAL INTRODUCTION TO ALDOSTERONE AND MINERALOCORTICOID RECEPTORS

Steroid hormones are derived from cholesterol and produced in systemically relevant amounts in a relatively narrow range of tissues (e.g., adrenal glands, gonads, placenta, skin). In mammalian physiology, six classes of steroid hormones are commonly recognized— mineralocorticoid, glucocorticoid, androgen, estrogen, progestin, and the secosteroid vitamin $D_3$. This classification was based on observed effects of these hormones and has proven robust, despite current appreciation of a much more diverse physiology of steroid hormones over and above their classic roles. In further support of this original classification is the characterization of six intracellular receptors—MR; glucocorticoid, GR; androgen, AR; estrogen, ER; progestin, PR; and vitamin $D_3$, VDR. As further addressed later, it is now appreciated that a one-to-one relationship between receptor and hormone does not hold, and this is particularly the case for MR.

Aldosterone was isolated and characterized in 1953. Crucial for its isolation was the application of radioisotopic techniques to measure [$Na^+$] and [$K^+$] flux across epithelia in the laboratory of Sylvia Simpson, a biologist, and Jim Tait, a physicist.[2,3] Because of this, the active principle was initially called "electrocortin"; the name was soon changed to aldosterone when its unique aldehyde (rather than methyl) group at carbon 18 was discovered in collaborative studies between investigators in London and Basel.[4] Aldosterone is commonly depicted so as to highlight this aldehyde group (Fig. 12.1, *right*). In vivo, the very reactive aldehyde group cyclizes with the β-hydroxyl group at carbon 11 to form the 11,18- hemiacetal and, in addition, may exist in an 11,18-hemiketal form. This cyclization of the 11β-hydroxyl group protects aldosterone from dehydrogenation by the enzyme 11β-hydroxysteroid dehydrogenase in epithelial tissue and by some neuronal and smooth muscle cells, which enables it to activate epithelial MR and thus regulate ion transport at very low (subnanomolar) circulating levels.[5,6]

There is broad evidence that aldosterone is not the only cognate ligand for MR, its essential effects via MR on epithelial ion transport notwithstanding. MR is found in high abundance in the hippocampus and cardiomyocytes and, in these nonepithelial tissues—which lack 11β-hydroxysteroid dehydrogenase type 2 (11β-HSD2; see later, "11β-Hydroxysteroid Dehydrogenase Type 2")—they are essentially constitutively occupied by glucocorticoids (cortisol in humans, corticosterone in rodents). This is due to the comparable affinity and markedly higher plasma free levels (≥100-fold) of endogenous

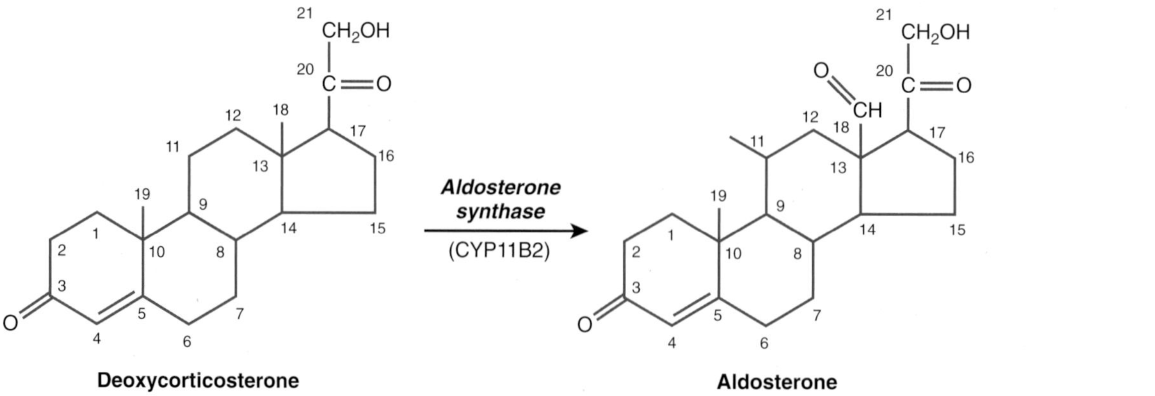

**Fig. 12.1 Final step in aldosterone synthesis.** Note that the aldehyde form of aldosterone is shown. Most aldosterone (>99%) exists as the hemiacetal form, which is cyclized and does not allow access of 11β-hydroxysteroid dehydrogenase type 2 (11β-HSD2) to the 11-hydroxyl. See text for details.

glucocorticoids compared with those of aldosterone. In terms of evolution, MR appeared well before aldosterone synthase (e.g., in fish).[7] It was commonly assumed that MR and GR share a common immediate evolutionary precursor,[8] although this has been challenged on sequence grounds,[9] which implicate MR as the first of the MR-GR-AR-PR subfamily to branch off an ancestral receptor. A final reason not to equate MR and aldosterone action derives from a comparison of the MR knockout and aldosterone synthase knockout ($AS^{-/-}$) phenotypes. MR knockout mice (which lack all functional MR) cannot survive sodium restriction; $AS^{-/-}$ mice (which have no detectable aldosterone) survive even stringent sodium restriction but die when their fluid intake is restricted to that of wild-type animals.[10] The survival of $AS^{-/-}$ mice on a low-$Na^+$ intake may reflect, in part, $Na^+$ retention via renal tubular intercalated cells, in which MRs (not 11β-HSD2–protected) are activated by glucocorticoids in the context of high ambient angiotensin concentrations.[11,12] Their inability to survive fluid restriction suggests an as yet poorly defined dependence on aldosterone for vasopressin action.[13] Potassium homeostasis is also surprisingly intact in $AS^{-/-}$ mice, although they do not tolerate extremes of $K^+$ loading.[13a]

## ALDOSTERONE SYNTHESIS

Aldosterone is synthesized in the adrenal cortex, which has three functional zones. The outermost layer of cells represents the zona glomerulosa, which is the unique site of aldosterone biosynthesis in normal physiology (see later; aldosterone is produced in excessive amounts in patients with glucocorticoid-remediable aldosteronism). Cortisol is synthesized in the middle zone, the zona fasciculata, and the innermost zona reticularis secretes adrenal androgens in many species, including humans, but not in rats or mice. Normally, the glomerulosa secretes aldosterone at the rate of 50 to 200 μg/day to give plasma levels of 4 to 21 μg/dL; in contrast, secretion of cortisol is at levels 200- to 500-fold higher. Underlying the separate synthesis of cortisol and aldosterone is expression of the enzyme 17α-hydroxylase uniquely in the zona fasciculata and that of aldosterone synthase uniquely in the glomerulosa.

In most species, aldosterone synthase, or cytochrome P450 (CYP) enzyme 11B2, is responsible for the conversion of deoxycorticosterone to aldosterone in a three-step process of sequential 11β-hydroxylation, 18-hydroxylation, and 18-methyl oxidation, to produce the characteristic C18-aldehyde from which aldosterone derives its name (see Fig. 12.1, *left*). Although CYP11B2 is distinct from CYP11B1 (11β-hydroxylase) in most species,[14,15] in some species (e.g., bovine), only a single CYP11B is expressed. How this enzyme is responsible for the three-step process of aldosterone synthesis in the glomerulosa but not the fasciculata has yet to be determined.

Fig. 12.2 also illustrates key steps in the biosynthesis of cortisol to illustrate the overlap and similarities with those of aldosterone. The genes encoding CYP11B1 and CYP11B2 lie close to one another on human chromosome band 8q24.3, so that an unequal crossing over at meiosis has been shown to be responsible for the syndrome of glucocorticoid-remediable aldosteronism (now known as "familial hyperaldosteronism type I"), in which the 5′ end of the CYP11B1 is fused to the 3′ end of CYP11B2. The chimeric gene product[16] is expressed in the fasciculata and responds to adrenocorticotropic hormone (ACTH) with aldosterone synthesis, producing a syndrome of juvenile-onset hyperaldosteronism and hypertension.

Normal glomerulosa secretion of aldosterone is primarily regulated by angiotensin II in response to posture and acute

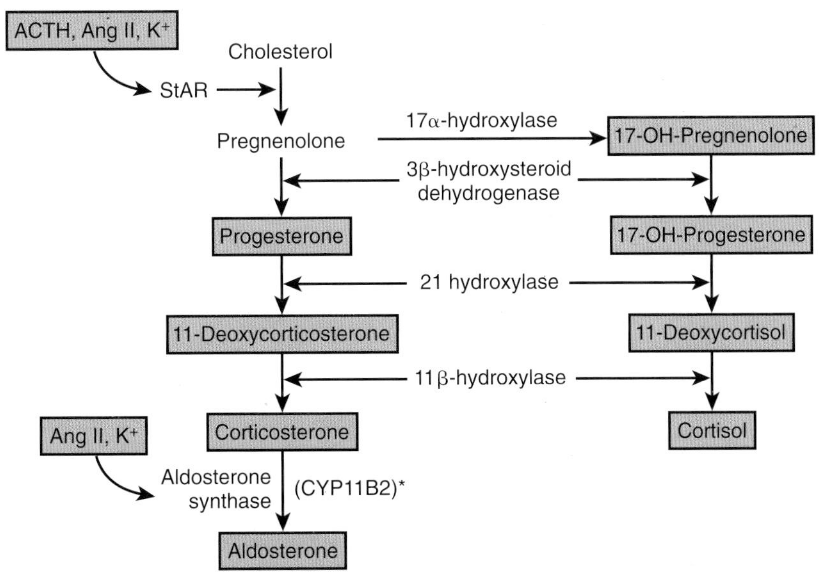


**Fig. 12.2 Overview of aldosterone synthetic pathway showing key regulatory nodes.** Note that adrenocorticotropic hormone *(ACTH)*, angiotensin II *(Ang II)*, and $K^+$ regulate steroidogenic acute regulatory protein *(StAR)*, which stimulates cholesterol uptake by mitochondria and thus substrate availability for synthesis of all of the steroid hormones. Aldosterone synthase (gene name, *CYP11B2*), which is selectively expressed in the adrenal glomerulosa, mediates the final step in aldosterone synthesis. It is also regulated by Ang II and $K^+$. Aldosterone synthesis is shown on the left. Cortisol synthesis is also shown *(right)* to emphasize the interconnections and similarities between these pathways.

lowering of circulating volume, to plasma [$K^+$] in response to elevated potassium levels, particularly in settings of $Na^+$ deficiency,[17] and to ACTH to the extent of entrainment of the circadian fluctuation in plasma aldosterone levels with those of cortisol. Aldosterone secretion is lowered by high levels of atrial natriuretic peptide and by the administration of heparin, somatostatin, and dopamine. As yet, incompletely characterized molecules of adipocyte origin have been shown to stimulate aldosterone secretion in vitro, and roles in the metabolic syndrome have been proposed on this basis.[18]

Angiotensin and plasma [$K^+$] stimulate aldosterone secretion primarily by increasing the expression and activity of key steroidogenic enzymes, as well as the steroidogenic acute regulatory protein (StAR).[19] StAR is required for cholesterol transport into mitochondria and hence for its availability for steroid synthesis.[20] Regulated steroidogenic enzymes include side chain cleavage enzyme 3β-hydroxysteroid dehydrogenase and, most notably, aldosterone synthase. Common to the mechanism of stimulation by angiotensin II and [$K^+$] is elevation of intracellular [$Ca^{2+}$]. Angiotensin II activates the G-protein–coupled angiotensin type I receptor (AT1R) in the glomerulosa cell membrane, which in turn activates phospholipase C, which catalyzes the hydrolysis of phosphatidylinositol 4,5-bisphosphate (PIP2) to inositol trisphosphate (IP3) and diacylglycerol (DAG). DAG stimulates protein kinase C, whereas IP3 stimulates $Ca^{2+}$ release from intracellular stores, both of which affect the aldosterone biosynthetic pathway. AT1R also separately stimulates $Ca^{2+}$ influx, which is important for sustained stimulation of aldosterone secretion.[21] Elevated [$K^+$] increases intracellular [$Ca^{2+}$] by depolarizing the cell membrane and activating voltage-sensitive $Ca^{2+}$ channels.[22,23] Patients taking angiotensin-converting enzyme inhibitors or angiotensin receptor blockers usually show a degree of suppression of aldosterone secretion, reflected in a modest (0.2–0.3 mEq/L) elevation in plasma [$K^+$] levels. This is often sufficient to establish a new steady state, with plasma aldosterone levels rising into the normal range, a process best termed "breakthrough" rather than "escape," given the time-honored usage of the latter to refer to the escape from progression of the salt and water effect of mineralocorticoid excess in the medium and long term.[24]

Studies have shed new light on the regulation of aldosterone production by the adrenal glomerulosa in health and disease. Choi and associates have found recurrent somatic mutations in the $K^+$ channel Kir3.4 (encoded by the gene *KCNJ5*), which were present in more than one-third of spontaneous human aldosterone-producing adenomas studied.[25] These mutations increased $Na^+$ conductance through Kir3.4 and resulted in increased $Ca^{2+}$ entry and enhanced aldosterone production and glomerulosa cell proliferation. Interestingly, an inherited mutation in *KCNJ5* is associated with hypertension associated with marked bilateral adrenal hyperplasia (now known as "familial hyperaldosteronism type III" [FH-III]).[26] These findings suggest that *KCNJ5* may provide tonic inhibition of aldosterone production and glomerulosa cell proliferation. In glomerulosa cells harboring the mutant channel, both proliferation rate and aldosterone synthesis are increased. These initial studies were continued and extended by a much wider survey by Boulkroun and colleagues[27]; subsequently, less common but similarly somatic mutations in the adrenal cortex *(ATP1A1, ATP2A3, CACNA1D,* and *CTNNB1)* have been associated with hyperaldosteronism caused by adrenal adenomas.[28,29]

## MECHANISMS OF MINERALOCORTICOID RECEPTOR FUNCTION AND GENE REGULATION

Mammals cannot survive without MR, except with substantial NaCl supplementation. This member of the nuclear receptor superfamily appears to have both genomic and nongenomic actions; however, the latter do not appear to play a significant role in the control of epithelial ion transport. This section thus focuses exclusively on the function of MR as a hormone-regulated transcription factor.

### MINERALOCORTICOID RECEPTOR FUNCTION AS A HORMONE-REGULATED TRANSCRIPTION FACTOR: GENERAL FEATURES AND SUBCELLULAR LOCALIZATION

In the presence of agonists, MR binds to specific genomic sites and alters the transcription rate of a subset of genes. Fig. 12.3 shows the fundamental paradigm of MR function. All nuclear receptors shuttle in and out of the nucleus; however, in the absence of hormone, some, such as the estrogen and vitamin D receptors, are predominantly nuclear, whereas others, like GR, are almost exclusively cytoplasmic. In the absence of hormone, MR is distributed relatively evenly between nuclear and cytoplasmic compartments but, in the presence of hormone, it is highly concentrated in the nucleus (Fig. 12.4).[30,31] It is also notable that in addition to this marked

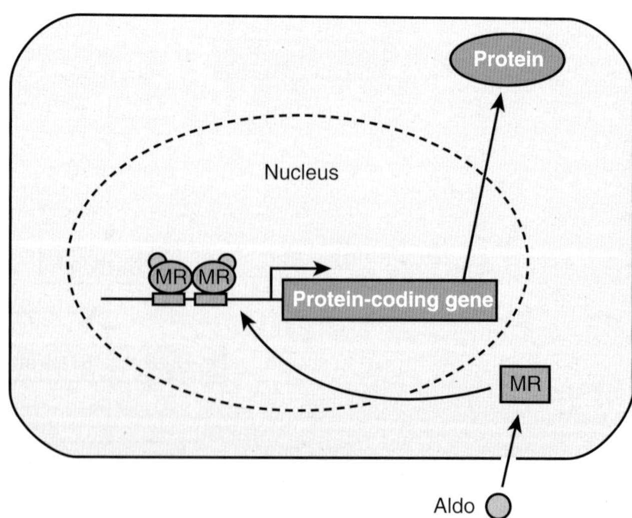


**Fig. 12.3 General mechanism of aldosterone action through the mineralocorticoid receptor *(MR)*.** This simple schematic shows the general features of MR regulation of a "simple" hormone response element (HRE), common to a large subset (but not all) of aldosterone-stimulated genes. Note that in the absence of hormone, MR is found in both nucleus and cytoplasm (see Fig. 12.4). Aldosterone *(Aldo)* triggers nuclear translocation of cytoplasmic MR, binding as a dimer to HREs, and stimulation of transcription initiation complex formation (*arrow,* upstream of the so-called protein-coding gene, defines the site of transcription initiation). See text for further details.

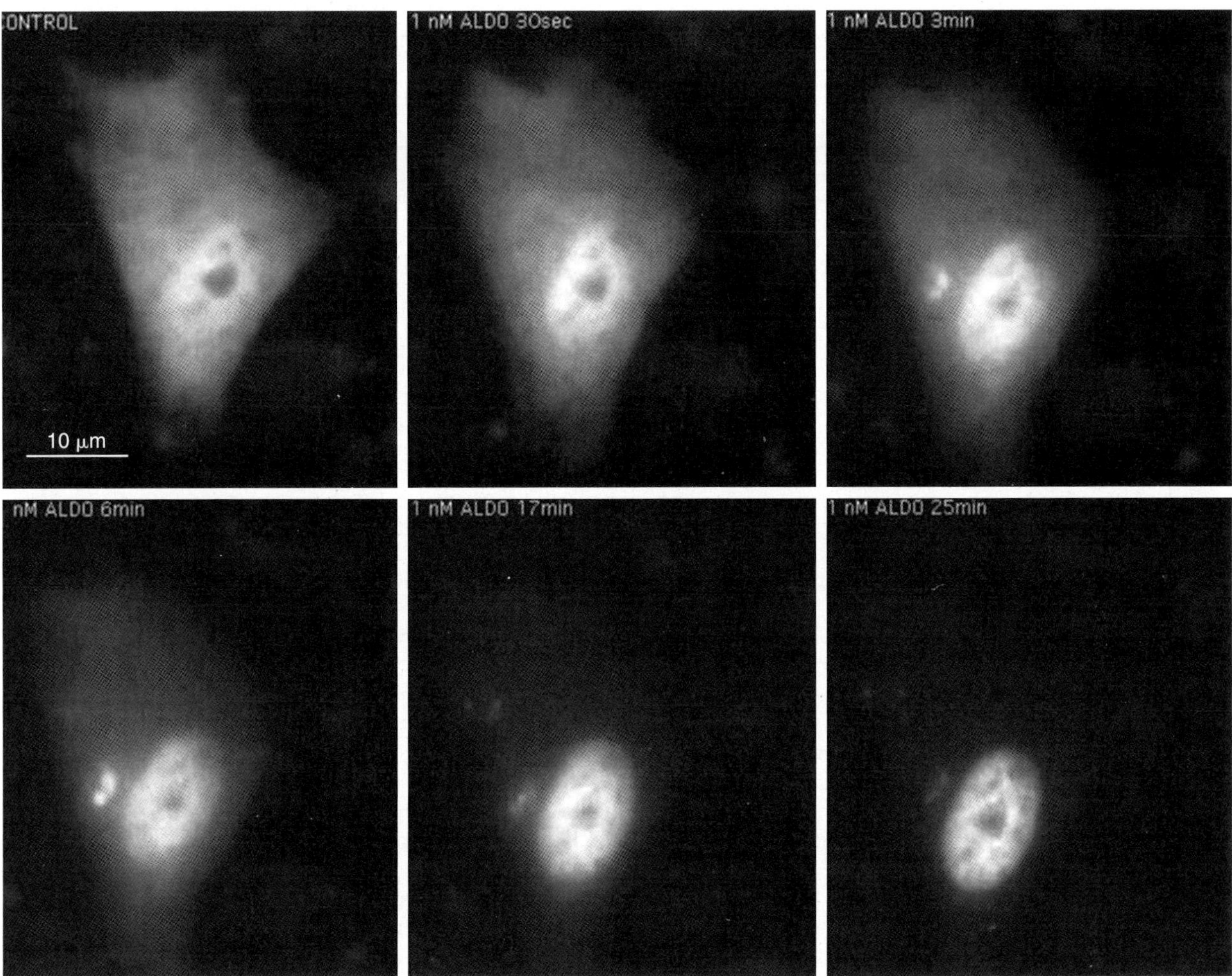


**Fig. 12.4 Time-dependent nuclear translocation of the mineralocorticoid receptor (MR) in the presence of aldosterone.** Cultured cells expressing green fluorescent protein–MR fusion protein (GFP-MR) were grown in a steroid-free medium and treated with 1 nmol/L aldosterone. Translocation of GFP-MR was followed in real time, and images were captured at indicated times. It is notable that the nuclear accumulation of GFP-MR started within 30 seconds, was half-maximal at 7.5 minutes, and was complete by 10 minutes. Control: MR distribution before addition of aldosterone. (From Fejes-Toth G, Pearce D, Naray-Fejes-Toth A. Subcellular localization of mineralocorticoid receptors in living cells: effects of receptor agonists and antagonists. *Proc Natl Acad Sci U. S. A.* 1998; 95[6]:2973–2978.)

change in MR cellular distribution, its subnuclear organization and protein-protein interactions are also changed.[31] Like its close cousin the GR, the unliganded MR (in the absence of hormone) is complexed with a set of chaperone proteins, which include the heat shock proteins hsp90, hsp70, and hsp56 and immunophilins.[32,33] This chaperone complex is essential for several aspects of MR function, notably high-affinity hormone binding and trafficking to the nucleus.[33] It was thought for many years that after binding hormone, the hsp90-containing chaperone complex is jettisoned. However, it has become clear that this complex remains associated with the receptor and plays an important role in nuclear trafficking.[32] Several members of the immunophilin family, including FKBP52, FKBP51, and CyP40, are present in the chaperone complex and provide a bridge between hsp90 and the cytoplasmic motor protein dynein, which moves the receptor-hsp90 complex retrogradely along microtubules to the nuclear envelope.[33] Here, the receptor is handed off to the nuclear pore protein, importin-α, and translocated into the nucleus, where it functions as a transcription factor, stimulating the transcription of certain genes and repressing the transcriptional activity of others. In the regulation of ion transport, stimulation of key target genes is paramount. Transcriptional repression may be essential for effects in nonepithelial cells, including neurons, cardiomyocytes, smooth muscle cells, and macrophages.[34]

## DOMAIN STRUCTURE OF MINERALOCORTICOID RECEPTORS

The MRs of all vertebrates are highly conserved. There are only minor differences between MRs in rodents and MRs in humans.[34] In general, the steroid and nuclear receptors have been divided into three major domains (Fig. 12.5):

1. An N-terminal transcriptional regulatory domain
2. A central DNA-binding domain (DBD)
3. A C-terminal ligand/hormone-binding domain (LBD)

Each of these broadly defined domains has more than one function, and not all the functions can be neatly assigned to separate distinct domains; however, much of the action

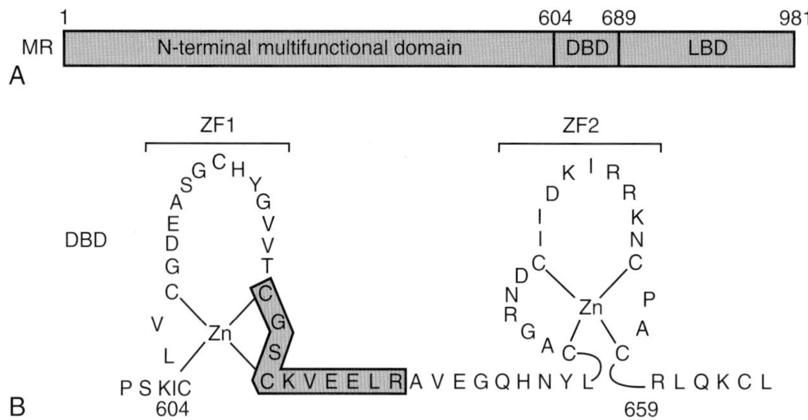


**Fig. 12.5 Domain structure of the mineralocorticoid receptor *(MR)*.** Three major domains have been defined, which are common to all steroid and nuclear receptors. Further refinements have led some to use a six-letter system, which is shown; however, this adds little to the understanding of receptor structure or function, and we prefer the three–global domain system. These large receptor sections should not be confused with the many small functional domains that have been identified, as discussed in the text. The size and amino acid designations used here are for rat MR (981 amino acids total); they apply with minor variations to human MR (984 amino acids total). (A) Strip diagram of MR. The N-terminus is to the *left,* C-terminus to the *right.* (B) Schematic of MR DNA-binding domain *(DBD)*, showing the two zinc fingers and the positions of the coordinating Zn ions. *Boxed region* is the alpha helix, which intercalates into the major groove of the DNA and provides the major protein–DNA interaction contacts. The dimerization interface comprises amino acids within the second zinc finger, which form van der Waals and salt bridge interactions. *LBD,* Ligand/hormone–binding domain.

of MRs can be understood from this point of view. In the following sections, the domains are described roughly in the historical order in which they were characterized, which also parallels the clarity of functional and structural knowledge about them.

## DNA-BINDING DOMAIN

The essential quality of MR function as a transcription factor is its ability to bind specifically to DNA. This protein-DNA interaction is mediated by the receptor's compact modular DBD (amino acids 603–688 of human MR; Fig. 12.5 shows a strip diagram and two-dimensional structure), which forms a variety of contacts with a specific 15-nucleotide DNA sequence termed a "hormone response element" (HRE). Receptor binding to the HRE in the vicinity of regulated genes promotes the recruitment of coactivators and components of the general transcription machinery, such as the TATA-binding protein, which binds to the thymidine- and adenosine-rich DNA sequence found upstream of many genes and is required for correct transcription initiation. These types of HREs have been identified near or in many of the key MR-regulated genes, such as serum- and glucocorticoid-regulated kinase 1 *(SGK1),* glucocorticoid-induced leucine zipper *(GILZ),* and amiloride-sensitive sodium channel subunit α *(α-ENaC).* Although, in many cases, differential binding to HREs is a key determinant of the specificity of many transcription factors, it should be noted that some steroid receptors (notably MR and GR) have only minor (<10%) differences within this domain and have identical DNA-binding properties.[35] Specificity in these cases is determined through other mechanisms.[34,36]

The canonical MR HRE is a 15-nucleotide sequence that forms a partial palindrome (inverted repeat), which binds a receptor homodimer. A dimer interface embedded within the DBD is essential for MR to form these requisite homodimers, as well as to form heterodimers with GR.[37,38] Mutations that disrupt this interface have complex effects on receptor activity in animals[39] and cultured cells,[40] and similar mutations in other receptors (AR in particular) result in disease states.[41] Also, in at least one kindred of the autosomal dominant form of pseudohypoaldosteronism type I, an MR DBD mutation appears to be causative, although the mechanistic basis has not been elucidated.[42]

In addition to supporting DNA binding and dimerization, the DBD also harbors a nuclear localization signal,[43,44] as well as surfaces that contact distant parts of the receptor and that mediate interactions with other proteins, as has been shown for GR and, in some cases, MR.[45–47]

## LIGAND/HORMONE-BINDING DOMAIN

The MR LBD comprises amino acids 689 to 981 (see Fig. 12.5A). Like the DBD, the LBD has multiple functions; in addition to binding with high affinity to various MR agonists and antagonists, it also harbors interaction surfaces for coactivators, dimerization, and N-C interactions.[48–50] MR is distinct from GR in that it binds with equally high affinity to cortisol, corticosterone (the physiologic glucocorticoid in rats and mice), and aldosterone. Indeed, as discussed later, MR appears to function as a high-affinity glucocorticoid receptor in some tissues, including the brain and heart.

High-resolution representations of the crystal structures of wild-type and mutant MR have identified the structural features of the LBD and specific amino acid contacts involved in binding to the mineralocorticoid desoxycorticosterone (Fig. 12.6).[51,52] Key features include the following:

1. The LBD of MR, like that of other nuclear receptors, is arranged into 11 α-helices and four small β-strands.
2. The C-terminal alpha helix (α-helix), H12, contains the activation function AF2.
3. Ligand is deeply embedded into a pocket comprising α-helices H3, H4, H5, H7, and H10 and two beta strands (β-strands); numerous contacts are made between amino acids of the pocket and hormone.

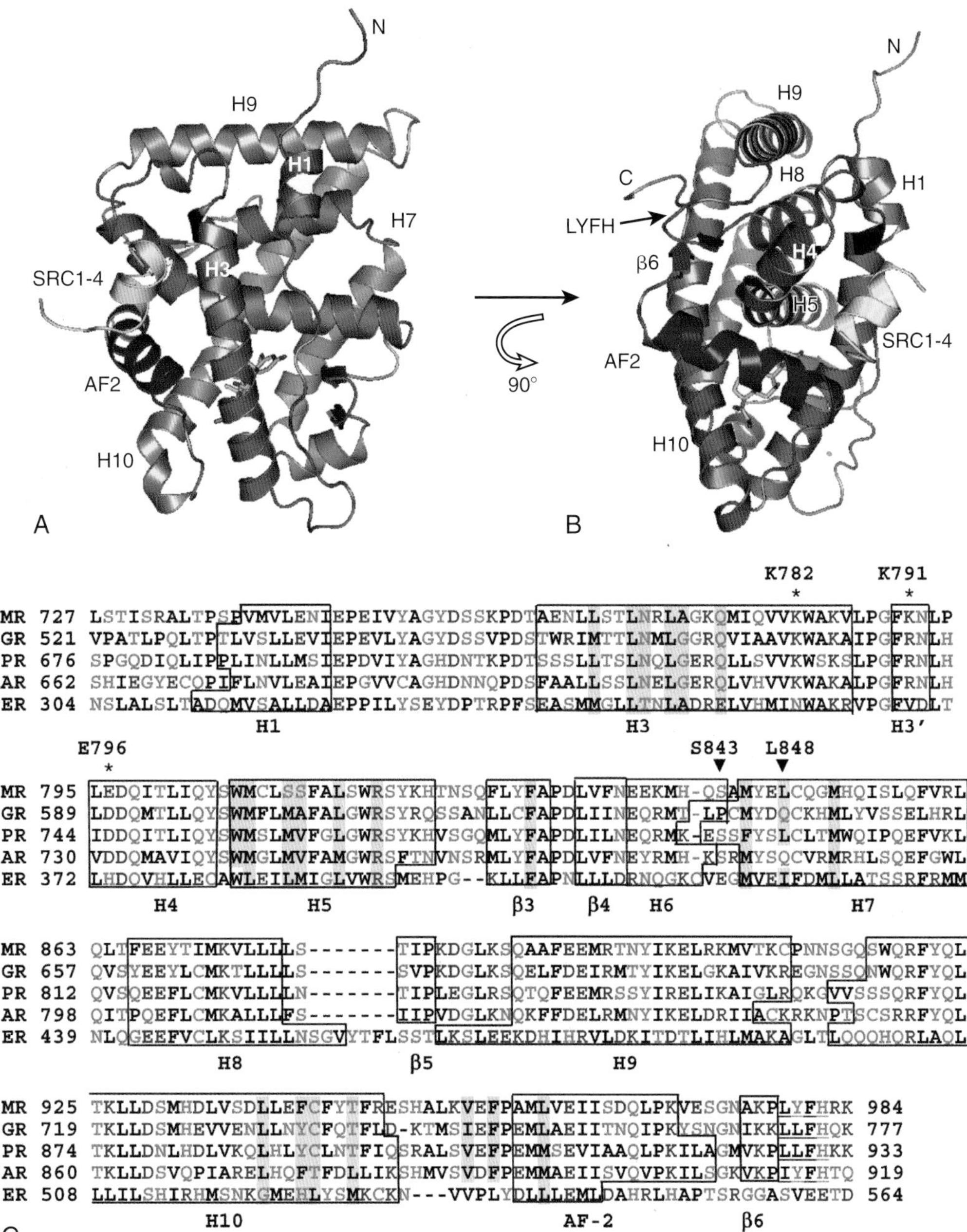


**Fig. 12.6** Mineralocorticoid receptor *(MR)* ligand/hormone–binding domain (LBD) crystal structure. Structure of the MR LBD bound to corticosterone and coactivator peptides (SRC1-4). (A and B) Two views of the complex (rotated by 90 degrees about the vertical axis) are shown in this ribbon representation. MR is colored in *gold* and SRC1-4 peptide in *yellow.* Corticosterone, which binds MR with an affinity comparable with that of aldosterone, is shown in a *ball-and-stick* representation. Note that hormone is located in a deep pocket formed by helices 3, 5, and 7 (*H3, H5,* and *H7*), which explains the slow off-rate and high affinity. (C) Sequence alignment of the human MR LBD with other steroid hormone receptors (*GR,* glucocorticoid; *AR,* androgen; *PR,* progesterone; and *ER,* estrogen). Residues that form the steroid-binding pockets are shaded in *gray.* Key structural features for the binding of SRC peptides are noted with *stars,* and the residues that determine MR-GR hormone specificity are labeled by *arrowheads.* See Li and others[394] for further details. (From Li Y, Suino K, Daugherty J, et al. Structural and biochemical mechanisms for the specificity of hormone binding and coactivator assembly by mineralocorticoid receptor. *Mol Cell.* 2005;19:367–380.)

This accounts for the slow off-rate and high affinity of aldosterone, corticosterone, and cortisol for MR.[51] The crystal structure of the mutant (S810L) MR, in which progesterone acts as an agonist rather than an antagonist,[53] reveals that H12 is stabilized with AF2 in the active conformation.[52] The crystal structure of wild-type MR LBD also provides insight into the mechanisms underlying some forms of pseudohypoaldosteronism type I. Notably, MR/S810L has an LBD mutation in helix 5, which is predicted to disrupt interaction with the steroid ring structure,[54] whereas Q776R and L979P have been demonstrated to have markedly reduced aldosterone binding.[42] Structural analysis reveals that Q776 is located in helix H3 at the extremity of the hydrophobic ligand-binding pocket and anchors the steroid C3–ketone group.

MR binds cortisol and corticosterone with an affinity similar to that of aldosterone. 11β-HSD2 is an essential determinant of aldosterone specificity, through its effect in metabolizing glucocorticoids to their receptor-inactive keto-congeners in collecting duct principal cells, as discussed later. In tissues that do not coexpress 11β-HSD2, the physiologic ligand for MR is cortisol (corticosterone in rats and mice).[55–57] The extent to which such "unprotected" MR can be pathophysiologically activated in aldosterone excess states is discussed later (see "Disease States: Primary Aldosteronism" and "Nonepithelial Actions of Aldosterone").

#### N-TERMINAL DOMAIN

As its noncommittal name implies, the N-terminal region of MR has diverse functions, which appear to revolve primarily around protein–protein interactions and the recruitment of coactivators and corepressors. It has two potent transcriptional regulatory motifs, usually termed *AF1a* and *AF1b*.[48,58] This domain bears some functional and sequence similarity to the homologous region of GR and is capable of stimulating gene transcription when fused to an unrelated DBD.[48] Overall, however, MR and GR differ markedly in the N-terminal domain, and this region of the receptor is a central determinant of specificity.[59] Other studies have supported the idea that this domain has functional sequences that limit receptor activity through the recruitment of corepressors, in addition to transcriptional activation functions.[47,60] Its role in coactivator and corepressor recruitment is addressed further in the following section.

### MINERALOCORTICOID RECEPTOR REGULATION OF TRANSCRIPTION INITIATION: COACTIVATORS AND COREPRESSORS

The major mechanism of MR action is its effects on transcription initiation; however, there may also be effects on transcript elongation.[61,62] Much has been learned about the generation of an initiation complex and the particular roles that steroid receptors play in this process. Several review articles and book chapters have provided in-depth examinations of the biochemistry of the general transcription machinery, transcription initiation, promoter escape, and processive elongation.[63–65] Most of the coactivators identified so far interact with the C-terminal AF2 domain and include the prototypical GRIP1/TIF2 and SRC,[66,67] which sequentially recruit a series of different components of the transcriptional machinery and result in the formation of a preinitiation complex (PIC). This PIC includes all the key components of the transcription machinery, including RNA polymerase II. A detailed picture of MR-dependent PIC formation has not been determined. However, the general features are likely similar to those for ER[68] and involve the sequential recruitment by the receptor of the following: (1) chromatin-remodeling SWI/SNF and CARM1/PRTM1 proteins, which promote chromatin remodeling and initiation of complex formation; (2) histone acetylase CBP/P300 (cyclic adenosine monophosphate [cAMP]–responsive element–binding protein), which promotes an active chromatin conformation[64]; and (3) direct or indirect recruitment of the TATA-binding protein and other components of the general transcription machinery.[68]

The aforementioned mechanisms are generic and are used by many transcription factors, including all steroid receptors, through interactions with the C-terminal AF2 domain. The N-terminal region of MR, which harbors the AF1 domain, diverges from the other steroid receptors, and other studies have identified coregulators that interact selectively with this receptor domain. ELL (11-19 lysine-rich leukemia factor) is a coactivator for MR that specifically interacts with AF1b and assists in PIC formation.[61] It was originally identified as an elongation factor, and it may also affect transcript elongation. Other specific coregulators include the synergy inhibitory protein PIAS1,[60] Ubc9,[69] and p68 RNA helicase.[70] In many cases, interactions of these regulators with MR require receptor posttranslational modifications—for example, by phosphorylation, acetylation, or sumoylation.[71]

## REGULATION OF SODIUM ABSORPTION AND POTASSIUM SECRETION

### GENERAL MODEL OF ALDOSTERONE ACTION

Aldosterone enters the cell passively, binds to MR, triggers changes in gene transcription (as addressed later; see "Mechanisms of Mineralocorticoid Receptor Function and Gene Regulation"), and potentially has nongenomic effects. Aldosterone effects in the ASDN have been divided into three major phases: latent, early, and late.[1] This designation goes back to the early observations by Ganong and Mulrow that after aldosterone infusion into experimental animals, no effect was observed for at least 15 to 20 minutes.[72] A similar delay was observed in isolated epithelia.[73] The early phase, which is now known to involve primarily MR-dependent regulation of signaling mediators such as SGK1, culminates in increased apical localization—and, possibly, increased probability of the open state—of EnAc. In the late phase, aldosterone stimulates transcription of a variety of effector genes, including those that encode components of the ion transport machinery, notably the epithelial sodium channel (ENaC) and $Na^+$-$K^+$–adenosine triphosphatase ($Na^+$-$K^+$-ATPase) subunits. The major direct effect is to increase $Na^+$ reabsorption, which is accompanied variably by $Cl^-$ reabsorption and/or $K^+$ secretion and, ultimately, water reabsorption. Aldosterone's actions in the principal cells of the connecting segment and collecting duct (Fig. 12.7) are of primary significance; however, this also has been shown to influence fluid and electrolyte transport in other tubule segments, as well as in other organs. These actions of aldosterone can be surmised from the clinical features of individuals with aldosterone-secreting tumors; they have volume expansion with high blood pressure and are commonly (>50% of patients) hypokalemic.[74,75] In general, the effects of aldosterone on $Na^+$ absorption and $K^+$ secretion work together. However, there are ways whereby these actions can be separated, as discussed later.

The two basic cell processes that aldosterone regulates—$Na^+$ absorption and $K^+$ secretion—are depicted in Fig. 12.7. Most aspects of this mechanism are relevant to the various aldosterone target tissues.

$Na^+$-$K^+$-ATPase, located on the basolateral membrane (blood side), establishes the essential electrochemical gradients that drive ion transport (see Chapters 5 and 6). Importantly, it operates well below its $V_{max}$, and is seldom, if ever, the rate-limiting step in transepithelial $Na^+$ transport.[76] Rather, apical

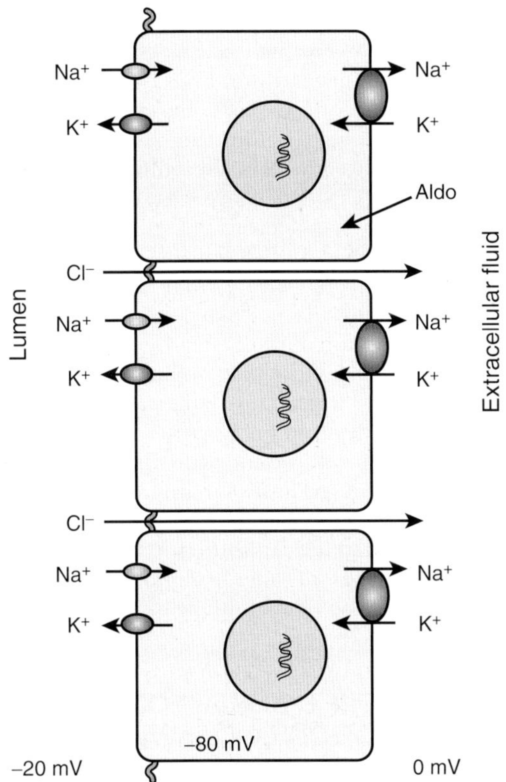


**Fig. 12.7 Schematic of principal cells in the aldosterone-sensitive distal nephron (ASDN).** The ASDN includes the distal third of the distal convoluted tubule (DCT), connecting tubule, and collecting duct. The $Na^+$-$K^+$–adenosine triphosphatase ($Na^+$-$K^+$-ATPase) establishes the gradients for passive apical entry of sodium through the epithelial sodium channel (ENaC). Transport of sodium through the ENaC creates a negative lumen potential that drives potassium secretion into the lumen. Potassium is also recycled at the basolateral surface, which facilitates potassium exchange across the $Na^+$-$K^+$-ATPase. Chloride ($Cl^-$) moves via paracellular and transcellular pathways. There is evidence to support aldosterone *(Aldo)* actions in other segments, particularly the sodium-chloride cotransporter–expressing portions of the DCT (DCT1 and DCT2).

$Na^+$ entry into the cell via the epithelial $Na^+$ channel, ENaC, is the rate-limiting step for $Na^+$ reabsorption by the ASDN and the key locus of regulation.

The discovery of the molecular composition of ENaC in 1993[77,78] opened the door to understanding how aldosterone functions to regulate this critically important ion channel. Most $Na^+$ transporters are encoded by a single gene product. In contrast, ENaC is composed of three similar but distinct subunits, each encoded by a unique gene. All three subunits come together (probably as a heterotrimer) to form an ion channel with unique biophysical characteristics, the most striking of which is the relatively long time it stays open or closed.[79] The complete loss of any one of these subunits in mice is incompatible with life,[80–82] and mutations in channel subunits cause profound disease manifestations in humans.[83] The apical entry of $Na^+$ into the cell via ENaC is the rate-limiting step in both $Na^+$ absorption and $K^+$ secretion.[84] $Na^+$ enters the cell down a steep electrochemical gradient; intracellular [$Na^+$] is approximately 10 mmol/L, and the membrane voltage is high (inside negative). Intracellular $Na^+$ is pumped out across the basolateral membrane by $Na^+$-$K^+$-ATPase, as addressed in detail in Chapter 6. Most epithelial cells have a greater density of $K^+$ channels on the basolateral membrane and thus recycle $K^+$ back into the blood. The distal nephron is unique in that it has an unusually high density of K channels on the apical membrane (primarily Kir 1.1 [renal outer medullary potassium (ROMK)] and BK channels) relative to the apical membrane of other epithelia.[85,86] This distribution of $K^+$ channels permits a large amount of $K^+$ that enters the cell via $Na^+$-$K^+$-ATPase to exit the cell into the lumen and be excreted into the urine. The vast majority of $K^+$ that appears in the urine is secreted by the distal nephron.

Much attention has been focused on the early phase of aldosterone action because it appears to be more tractable to dissection, and most changes in $Na^+$ current occur during this phase. This separation is probably somewhat artificial, however, and there is considerable overlap in events that define the early and late phases. Moreover, many efforts to manipulate mediators of the early phase (through overexpression and knockdown experiments) have been evaluated after prolonged alteration. Nevertheless, there is some heuristic value in considering the early and late phases of aldosterone action separately.

In cultured collecting duct cells deprived of corticosteroids and then exposed to high concentrations of aldosterone, an increase in ENaC-mediated $Na^+$ transport can be observed in well under 1 hour, which is consistent with animal studies.[72,87] $Na^+$ transport continues to increase for 2 to 3 hours, then plateaus for a few hours, and then gradually increases over the next several hours. After 12 hours of exposure to saturating aldosterone concentrations, the increase in ENaC activity is near maximal. The molecular basis for this increase in ENaC activity has been intensively investigated, and several key events are now apparent.

For aldosterone to increase ENaC activity, a change in gene transcription must occur. One of the earliest response genes is *SGK1*.[88–90] This serine–threonine kinase, which mediates a substantial portion of the early effects of aldosterone,[91,92] is addressed in greater detail later in this chapter, together with its major target, Nedd4-2. The genetic disease Liddle syndrome provided key first clues to ENaC, as addressed further later[93,94] and in Chapter 44.

## ALDOSTERONE AND EPITHELIAL SODIUM CHANNEL TRAFFICKING

The major action of aldosterone is to increase the number of functional ENaC units on the apical membrane. This process can involve an increase in the number of channel complexes on the surface, activation of existing complexes, or both. There is evidence to support both, although the bulk of evidence favors the idea that a change in the number of ENaC units predominates.[95–97] The redistribution of ENaC to the apical membrane can be detected in less than 2 hours after aldosterone exposure.[87]

It is less well established whether the number of channels is increased through increased insertion, decreased removal, or both. Aldosterone probably contributes to both processes. Rapid insertion of ENaC is best understood with regard to the actions of cAMP.[98] The extent to which the molecules involved in cAMP-mediated insertion are also involved in aldosterone action is uncertain, but some common mechanisms are probably used. Trafficking to the apical membrane appears to involve hsp70,[99] SNARE (soluble NEM-sensitive factor attachment protein receptor) proteins,[100] and the aldosterone-induced protein melanophilin.[101] The mitogen-activated protein kinase pathway may also be involved, because interruption of ERK phosphorylation by GILZ[102] increases ENaC surface expression.

Considerably more is known about how ENaC complexes are retrieved from the apical membrane. This understanding is the direct result of dissecting the molecular consequences of Liddle syndrome, in which mutations in the C terminus of ENaC lead to increased residence time in the apical membrane.[93,94] The missing or mutated domains in the β- or γ-subunit of ENaC in this syndrome normally bind to Nedd4-2, a ubiquitin ligase, which ultimately is responsible for initiating endocytosis and degradation.[103,104] The interaction of Sgk1 and Nedd4-2 in the actions of aldosterone is discussed later. ENaC is internalized via clathrin-coated vesicles, processed into early endosomes, and then further processed into recycling endosomes and late endosomes.[105,106] Degradation is via lysosomes or proteasomes.[107,108] The processing of ENaC by vesicular trafficking and its regulation by aldosterone has been reviewed by Butterworth et al.[109]

Phosphatidylinositol-3-kinase (PI3K)–dependent signaling is essential for epithelial $Na^+$ transport. It controls SGK1 activity (see later) and also appears to have independent effects on ENaC open probability through direct actions of 3-phosphorylated phosphoinositides, particularly phosphatidylinositol (3,4,5)-trisphosphate.[110,111] Ras-dependent signaling may also regulate ENaC and the pump in complex ways that depend on downstream signaling through Raf, MEK, and ERK, as well as through PI3K.[112–117]

The late phase of ENaC activation by aldosterone is less well understood than the early phase. A simple evaluation of the late phase is that aldosterone increases the transcription and protein abundance of the ENaC α-subunit. This idea comes from the fact that aldosterone increases the mRNA and protein abundance of α-ENaC in the kidney[96,118] after a lag of several hours.[119] Although less well studied, aldosterone appears to produce an increase in β- and γ-subunit expression in the colon.[119,120] Dietary $Na^+$ restriction, a physiologically relevant maneuver that increases aldosterone secretion, clearly increases ENaC surface expression in the renal distal nephron.[97] However, there appear to be some important differences between chronic aldosterone administration to a $Na^+$-replete animal and chronic dietary $Na^+$ restriction.[118,121] Furthermore, it should be noted that increased α-ENaC expression, in and of itself, does not increase ENaC activity in models of collecting duct and lung epithelia, although limiting its expression does restrict aldosterone stimulation.[122] It appears that increased expression of α-ENaC may be important for the consolidation of the increase, but it is not sufficient to reproduce the steroid-mediated increase in ENaC activity.

## BASOLATERAL MEMBRANE EFFECTS OF ALDOSTERONE

Over the years, research on aldosterone action has focused with varying degrees of intensity on apical effects,[123,124] basolateral effects,[125–127] and effects on metabolism.[73] There is general agreement now that the early effects of aldosterone are on apical events, primarily on ENaC, and that basolateral and metabolic effects occur later. In addition, although it is somewhat less settled whether the basolateral effects are direct or result indirectly from the enhanced entry of $Na^+$ into cells, the bulk of evidence favors the latter view. Notably, increased $Na^+$ entry has been found to control more than 80% of increased $Na^+$-$K^+$-ATPase activity and basolateral membrane density in the rat[128,129] and rabbit[129] cortical collecting tubules. Furthermore, striking increases in basolateral membrane folding and surface area occur in aldosterone-treated animals,[130] an effect that is markedly attenuated in animals fed a low-$Na^+$ diet. This result strongly suggests that apical $Na^+$ entry is required for basolateral changes to occur. However, there is good evidence for direct transcriptional stimulation of $Na^+$-$K^+$-ATPase subunit expression,[131,132] as well as reports supporting some direct effects of aldosterone in increasing basolateral pump activity[125,133] or at least in constituting the pool of latent pumps, which are then recruited to the basolateral membrane in response to a rise in intracellular $[Na^+]$.[134]

## ACTIVATION OF THE EPITHELIAL SODIUM CHANNEL BY PROTEOLYTIC CLEAVAGE

There is now clear evidence that when ENaC is delivered to the apical membrane, it can be activated by proteolytic cleavage. The first hint of this process was the demonstration that rats fed a low-Na diet or given aldosterone over the long term showed the appearance of a proteolytic fragment of the γ-ENaC subunit.[96] Subsequently, investigators have shown that both the α- and the γ- but not the β-ENaC subunits can be cleaved. Furthermore, cleavage at each site apparently initiates a degree of activation of the channel complex. ENaC complexes are activated by cleavage because specific regions of the large extracellular domain (26 residues in the α-ENaC and 46 residues in the γ-ENaC) are excised. These regions contain inhibitory sequences that when introduced exogenously, can inhibit ENaC function. Removing these regions by proteolytic cleavage releases this inhibition.[135]

Several proteases can cleave either the α- or γ-ENaC subunits. Among them are furin, prostasin, CAP2, kallikrein, elastase, matriptase, plasmin, and trypsin. It is not clear whether activation of ENaC by proteolytic cleavage can be regulated by aldosterone, but the idea certainly has attractive features. If aldosterone could regulate expression of one or more rate-limiting proteases, it would be able to regulate both the number of complexes in the apical membrane and the ability of the channel complex to be active. It appears that aldosterone may regulate the expression of prostasin.[136] Aldosterone may also regulate the expression of the protease nexin-1 (an inhibitor of prostasin) and other proteases.[137]

The discovery of ENaC activation by cleavage helps explain how aldosterone might increase ENaC activity by increasing both surface expression and the activity of a single ENaC complex. By phosphorylating Nedd4-2 via SGK1 and reducing its ability to bind to the PY domains of the ENaC subunits, aldosterone increases ENaC residence time on the apical membrane. This additional time permits proteolytic activation by one or more endogenous proteases.[138]

## POTASSIUM SECRETION AND ALDOSTERONE

One of the major effects of aldosterone is to increase $K^+$ secretion (and thus excretion). This phenomenon has been demonstrated in countless patients with aldosterone-secreting tumors and in hundreds of studies in animals given excess amounts of aldosterone. The general mechanism whereby aldosterone increases $K^+$ secretion is depicted in Fig. 12.7. The key feature of this process—with respect to the direct effects of aldosterone per se—involves the stimulation of $Na^+$ absorption via ENaC. The dependence of $K^+$ secretion on $Na^+$ absorption is the basis of the action of the so-called K-sparing diuretics, amiloride and triamterene, both of which inhibit ENaC. These drugs have no direct effect on apical $K^+$ channels.

Increasing ENaC activity produces two major secondary effects that in turn enhance $K^+$ secretion. First, the enhanced $Na^+$ conductance of the apical membrane produces depolarization and hence a more favorable electrical driving force for $K^+$ efflux into the lumen. The second effect relates to the activity of the $Na^+$-$K^+$ pump on the basolateral membrane. The more $Na^+$ that enters across the apical membrane, the more that must be extruded by the pump. Because the pump operates well below its $V_{max}$ under baseline conditions, a slight increase in intracellular $Na^+$ concentration markedly stimulates pump activity and more $K^+$ enters the cell. In isolated, perfused cortical collecting ducts, the amount of secreted $K^+$ is highly related to the amount of absorbed $Na^+$ when the stimulus for $Na^+$ absorption is mineralocorticoid hormone.[139]

Two types of $K^+$ channels are found in the apical membrane of the ASDN: small conductance (SK, 30–40 picosiemens [pS]) channels encoded by the *ROMK* gene, and large conductance (BK, 100–200 pS) channels found in many other cell types, including the apical membrane of the colon. Most of the $K^+$ channels on the apical membrane of the principal cells appear to be SK, at least as far as can be assessed by patch-clamp analysis. The activity of either channel is not directly increased by aldosterone.[140,141]

A feature of $K^+$ secretion is that although apical $K^+$ channels are abundant in the proximal portion of the ASDN (connecting tubule and cortical collecting duct), they are strikingly less abundant in the medullary collecting duct.[142–144] Because apical K channels are not regulated by aldosterone, their absence in the medullary collecting duct might uncouple aldosterone-regulated $Na^+$ reabsorption from $K^+$ secretion in this segment.

## SEPARATION OF SODIUM ABSORPTION AND POTASSIUM SECRETION BY THE ALDOSTERONE-SENSITIVE DISTAL NEPHRON

The preceding sections establish a picture that parsimoniously accounts for the effect of aldosterone to stimulate $Na^+$ reabsorption and $K^+$ secretion at the same rate. The simple stimulation of electrogenic $Na^+$ reabsorption (via ENaC) is sufficient to stimulate $K^+$ secretion, which fits well for organisms faced with a combined low-$Na^+$, high-$K^+$ diet, which was maintained most of the time through millions of years of vertebrate evolution. However, organisms do not ingest a fixed amount of $Na^+$ and $K^+$, so an inexorable linkage between $Na^+$ absorption and $K^+$ secretion by the ASDN cannot possibly occur all the time. Investigators have proposed several possibilities to explain how these processes can be separated.

### ROLE OF DISTAL TUBULE FLUID DELIVERY

A traditional view for differential $Na^+$ and $K^+$ handling stems from the differing role that aldosterone plays in potassium secretion depending on the tubular flow (and thus sodium flow) rate. Studies from adrenalectomized dogs have demonstrated that the primary regulators of potassium excretion are the serum potassium concentration and tubular flow rate. A higher serum potassium concentration yields a higher filtered load of potassium. Hyperkalemia also stimulates natriuresis from upstream segments of the nephron.[145,146] This latter effect can increase tubular flow rate, which, in turn, diminishes potassium concentration in the lumen and activates flow-stimulated BK channel–mediated potassium secretion in the collecting duct. In the setting of sufficient distal delivery of sodium, potassium loading will not yield a higher steady-state concentration of aldosterone because the two mechanisms previously mentioned are sufficient to normalize the serum potassium level.[147] However, under conditions of sodium depletion, proximal $Na^+$ reabsorption is increased, which further diminishes distal delivery of sodium and hence tubular flow rate.[148] This diminishes flow-mediated potassium secretion, so that aldosterone secretion is necessary to normalize potassium balance.

### INDEPENDENT REGULATION OF SODIUM AND POTASSIUM TRANSPORTERS

Other possible mechanisms have been suggested, which involve separate regulation of sodium and potassium transport (e.g., ENaC and ROMK) by specific stimuli, depending on the state of $Na^+$ and $K^+$ intake. With a constant $Na^+$ intake, one could envision that a high-potassium diet could enhance the activity of ROMK, whereas a low-potassium diet would reduce its activity. Such an effect would cause more or less of the $K^+$ entering the cell via the $Na^+$-$K^+$ pump to be recycled across the basolateral membrane. This mechanism, although probably very complex in its execution, is appealing in its simplicity.

### ROLE OF WNKS

Advances in understanding genetic forms of hypertension have uncovered a key functional role for a family of kinases that have potent effects on pathways regulating $Na^+$ and $K^+$ transport in the distal nephron. These kinases, called "WNKs" (*with no* lysine; *K* is the one-letter code for lysine), were initially thought to lack a conserved lysine residue in the catalytic domain, which binds adenosine triphosphate (ATP), and is essential for catalysis. Interestingly, a lysine performing the same function is indeed present, but is shifted from its canonical location in subdomain II to subdomain I to permit entry of chloride into the catalytic domain.[149] This modification contributes to the chloride regulation of WNK activity,

The spectrum of regulatory roles of WNKs is complex and remains controversial. It is clear that the $Na^+$,$Cl^-$ cotransporter (NCC) is regulated by WNK4, and it is likely that ROMK and ENaC are regulated by WNK1.[150,151] Recent evidence has also supported the idea that the chloride-binding properties of WNKs provide the basis for their functional regulation by extracellular $K^+$ concentration.[152] In the DCT, in particular, low plasma (and hence extracellular) $K^+$ concentration depolarizes the basolateral membrane via Kir4.1, which leads to a reduction in intracellular chloride, thereby activating WNK4 and SPAK (STE20/SPS1-related proline-alanine–rich kinase) and hence NCC phosphorylation.[152,153] A high plasma $K^+$ concentration has the opposite effect and inhibits NCC phosphorylation; however, the mechanism appears to be chloride-independent. Thus, through its effects to raise the plasma $K^+$ concentration, a high-$K^+$ diet has effects both locally in the kidneys and through aldosterone to stimulate $K^+$ excretion. Aldosterone acts directly in the ASDN to stimulate ENaC, which increases the driving force for $K^+$ secretion through ROMK and BK channels..[154] In conjunction, an elevated $K^+$ concentration acts directly in DCT cells to inhibit NCC phosphorylation and enhance delivery of $Na^+$ to the ENaC-expressing segments. According to this view, aldosterone does not have a direct effect on NCC-mediated electroneutral $Na^+$ transport. Further details of the mechanisms of K transport and the role of WNKs in the distal nephron are presented in Chapter 6.

## ROLE OF CHLORIDE TRANSPORT REGULATION

There is also evidence supporting the independent regulation of $Cl^-$ transport in the collecting duct. $Cl^-$ can be absorbed by the paracellular pathway (i.e., between cells) driven by the lumen-negative voltage across the epithelium. This pathway can be influenced by aldosterone.[155] $Cl^-$ can also be absorbed through the cells by specific transporters. One example of a $Cl^-$ transporter in the collecting duct is pendrin, an anion exchanger present on the apical membrane of intercalated cells. Mice that lack this transporter do not tolerate NaCl restriction as well as normal mice.[156] Its activity is dependent on $Cl^-$ delivery to the distal nephron, and it is coregulated by angiotensin II and aldosterone.[157,158,159]

As discussed in the next section, the ability of the MR in intercalated cells (but not in principal cells) to respond to aldosterone is regulated by the phosphorylation of its ligand-binding domain. It should also be noted that modulation of $Na^+$ absorption in the medullary collecting duct may also play a role in the balance of $Na^+$ reabsorption and $K^+$ secretion; this segment has little capacity to secrete $K^+$, and endogenous paracrine factors such as prostaglandins $E_2$ and transforming growth factor-β, which have potent inhibitory effects on $Na^+$ transport, are increased in response to a high-NaCl diet.[160,161]

## DIFFERENTIAL REGULATION OF INTERCALATED CELL MINERALOCORTICOID RECEPTOR

It has become increasingly clear that intercalated cell $Cl^-$ transport contributes to collecting duct NaCl absorption, and this plays an important role in allowing distinct responses to aldosterone in states of volume depletion versus hyperkalemia.[162,163] A central feature of this proposed regulation is differential phosphorylation of the MR LBD in intercalated cells, as shown schematically in Fig. 12.8. When phosphorylated at S843 in the LBD, MR cannot bind aldosterone (or cortisol) and thus cannot be activated. This phosphorylation, which is stimulated by hyperkalemia, occurs selectively in intercalated cells but not in principal cells. Angiotensin II, on the other hand, induces S843 dephosphorylation in intercalated cells, markedly increasing ligand binding and, therefore, activation. Intercalated cells are known predominantly to mediate $H^+$ transport; however, other studies have

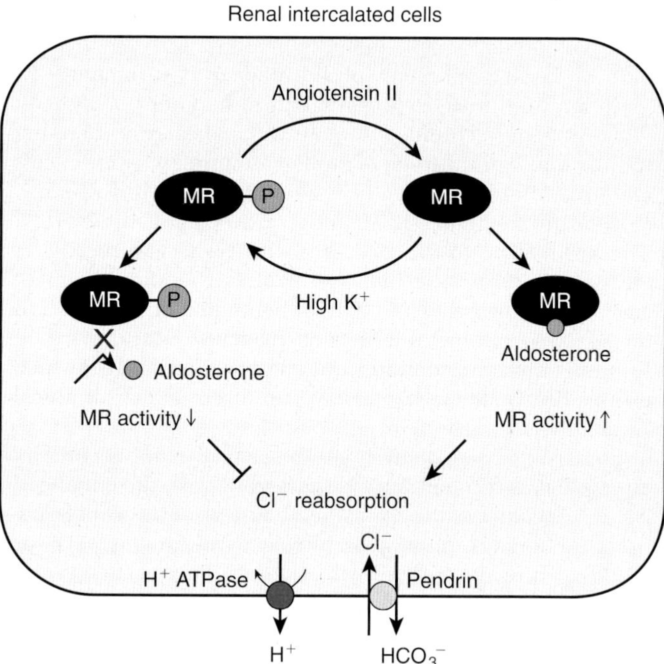


**Fig. 12.8 The role of mineralocorticoid receptor *(MR)* ligand-hormone–binding domain (LBD) phosphorylation in controlling chloride reabsorption by intercalated cells.** When phosphorylated at Ser-843 in the LBD, MR cannot bind ligand and hence cannot be activated. This phosphorylated state of MR is found only in intercalated cells, not in neighboring principal cells. In states of volume depletion, an elevated angiotensin II level decreases MR phosphorylation at Ser-843, allowing activation. In intercalated cells, MR mediates stimulation of both the proton pump and $Cl^-$-$HCO_3^-$ exchangers, thereby increasing $Cl^-$ reabsorption and promoting increased plasma volume while inhibiting $K^+$ secretion. In contrast, in states of hyperkalemia, phosphorylation of Ser-843 is increased, and hence $Cl^-$ reabsorption by intercalated cells is decreased and the principal cell–dependent $K^+$ secretion is increased. (From Shibata S, Rinehart J, Zhang J, et al. Regulated mineralocorticoid receptor phosphorylation controls ligand binding and renal response to volume depletion and hyperkalemia. *Cell Metab.* 2013;18:660–671.)

implicated them in electroneutral NaCl transport via the combined actions of the $Na^+$-dependent $Cl^-$-$HCO_3^-$ exchanger (NDCBE)[164] and the apical $Cl^-$-$HCO_3^-$ exchanger, pendrin.[165,166] Thus, when MR is active in these cells (S843 dephosphorylated), electroneutral NaCl transport occurs, without enhancing the driving force for $K^+$ secretion. Because intercalated cells lack 11β-HSD2 under these conditions, it is cortisol that binds to and activates MR. When intercalated cell MR is inactive (S843 phosphorylated), aldosterone acts in principal cells to stimulate ENaC-dependent electrogenic $Na^+$ transport, which enhances $K^+$ secretion.

## ALDOSTERONE-INDEPENDENT ENAC-MEDIATED SODIUM REABSORPTION IN THE DISTAL NEPHRON

The term "aldosterone-sensitive distal nephron" emphasizes the primacy of this key steroid in the control of ion transport in this region of the nephron. However, ENaC activity and aldosterone sensitivity exhibit axial heterogeneity from the late distal convoluted tubule (DCT2) through the connecting tubule to the cortical collecting duct and, finally, to the medullary collecting duct. In mice on a standard sodium diet, total ENaC expression increases with progression from the DCT2 to the connecting tubule,[167] although ENaC apical localization and activity are higher in the DCT2. Only under conditions of a low-sodium diet or aldosterone administration does the primacy of the connecting tubule in particular, and to a lesser extent the cortical collecting duct, emerge. The total luminal surface area in the DCT2 and connecting tubule is several-fold higher than in the cortical collecting duct,[168] and together these two segments appear to be sufficient to maintain sodium balance, even in the absence of detectable ENaC along the collecting duct. Mice lacking ENaC selectively in the collecting duct come into balance, even on a low-sodium diet.[169] Congruent with these findings, deletion of α-ENaC from the DCT2, connecting tubule, and collecting duct results in severe sodium wasting.[170] Notably, it is the connecting tubule that appears to be most important in the response to aldosterone, whereas DCT2 has the highest baseline transport in the absence of MR activation.[171] The cortical collecting duct is not as critical as was originally thought for either baseline or aldosterone-stimulated sodium reabsorption, probably due to its smaller surface area compared with the DCT2 and connecting tubule.

As we continue to traverse the nephron, further sodium reabsorption is minimal in the medullary collecting duct, on a normal sodium diet, and is not significantly stimulated by aldosterone.[139]

## SITES OF MINERALOCORTICOID RECEPTOR EXPRESSION AND LOCUS OF ACTION ALONG THE NEPHRON

### ALDOSTERONE-SENSITIVE DISTAL NEPHRON

In the kidney, MR is expressed at the highest levels in distal nephron cells extending from the last third of the DCT through the medullary collecting duct,[172] which is frequently referred to as the ASDN (Fig. 12.9).[1] This pattern of expression was first demonstrated using labeled hormone–binding studies performed before the cloning of MR[173] and has been confirmed since by several methods, including the polymerase chain reaction assay,[174] in situ hybridization,[175] and immunohistochemical analysis.[176] Effects of aldosterone on electrogenic $Na^+$ and $K^+$ transport in principal cells have been found consistently in these nephron segments,[172] which also express ENaC, and 11β-HSD2, as addressed in detail earlier.

Collecting duct intercalated cells also express MR and respond specifically to aldosterone and alter proton secretion. Aldosterone directly increases the activity of the $H^+$-ATPase in the collecting duct, and its absence results in decreased proton secretion.[177–179] Interestingly, nongenomic stimulation of $H^+$-ATPase activity in type A intercalated cells has been demonstrated in isolated murine collecting ducts.[180] Consistent with these effects, aldosterone deficiency results in distal renal tubular acidosis type 4, and excess aldosterone results in metabolic alkalosis.[181] It should be noted that aldosterone also stimulates $H^+$ secretion due to effects on principal cell $Na^+$ transport, which alter the electrical gradient. These older studies must also now be interpreted in the context of more recent data,[162] which, as noted earlier, demonstrate that the effect of aldosterone on intercalated cells depends on the genesis of the signal.

### OTHER SITES OF EXPRESSION

MR has been identified at some level in all parts of the nephron examined, including the glomerulus.[174,182–187] Its effects, at least at some of these sites, are likely to be physiologically relevant in states of volume depletion and acid–base disturbances; however, the data are not as robust and consistent as those for the ASDN.

#### Glomerulus

MR (but not 11β-HSD2) is expressed in glomerular mesangial cells, where it is thought to affect proliferation and production of reactive oxygen species[188,189] and to have profibrotic effects through SGK1.[190] These effects have been suggested to be important in the progression of renal damage, particularly in diabetic nephropathy,[191] in which glucocorticoids mimic the activity of aldosteronism in the context of tissue damage. However, the physiologic role of mesangial cell MR is uncertain.

#### Proximal Convoluted Tubule

Hierholzer and Stolte have shown, through elegant microperfusion studies, that the sodium reabsorptive capacity of the proximal convolution is decreased in adrenalectomized animals and restored by administration of aldosterone.[192] Chronic volume depletion increases sodium reabsorption in the proximal convoluted tubule, which is in part mediated by MR. The mechanisms of action in this nephron segment are controversial. Some studies have indicated an MR-dependent increase in the activity of $Na^+$-$H^+$-exchanger isoform 3, possibly through an increase in trafficking of the transporter to the membrane.[193–196] This transporter contributes to sodium and bicarbonate reabsorption. MR activation, in turn, may activate the $Na^+$-$K^+$-ATPase in the basolateral membrane of the proximal convoluted tubule to maintain a gradient for sodium reabsorption.[197–200]

#### Medullary Thick Ascending Limb

In the medullary thick ascending limb, mineralocorticoids but not glucocorticoids increase sodium and chloride reabsorption. In rodents, adrenalectomy impairs the reabsorption of NaCl in the medullary thick ascending limb, and aldosterone restores this process.[201,202] This reabsorptive defect may contribute to the urinary concentrating and diluting abnormality measured in patients with Addison disease and in mice lacking aldosterone synthase.[178,192,203] The medullary thick ascending limb also participates in the regulation of acid–base balance by reabsorbing most of the filtered $HCO_3$ that is not reabsorbed by the proximal tubule. In this context, aldosterone has been shown to stimulate the $Na^+$-$H^+$ exchanger in the amphibian thick ascending limb, possibly through a rapid nongenomic effect.[204] Other studies have also implicated regulation of the Na-K-2Cl cotransporter type 2 in the thick ascending limb—as well as the NCC in the DCT (see later)—by oxidative stress response kinase 1 (OSR1) and STE20/SPS1-related proline-alanine–rich kinase (SPAK) (OSR1/SPAK).[205,206]

#### Distal Convoluted Tubule

The studies of potassium regulation described earlier have also provided insight into the role of direct or indirect aldosterone-induced NCC transport. Aldosterone increases

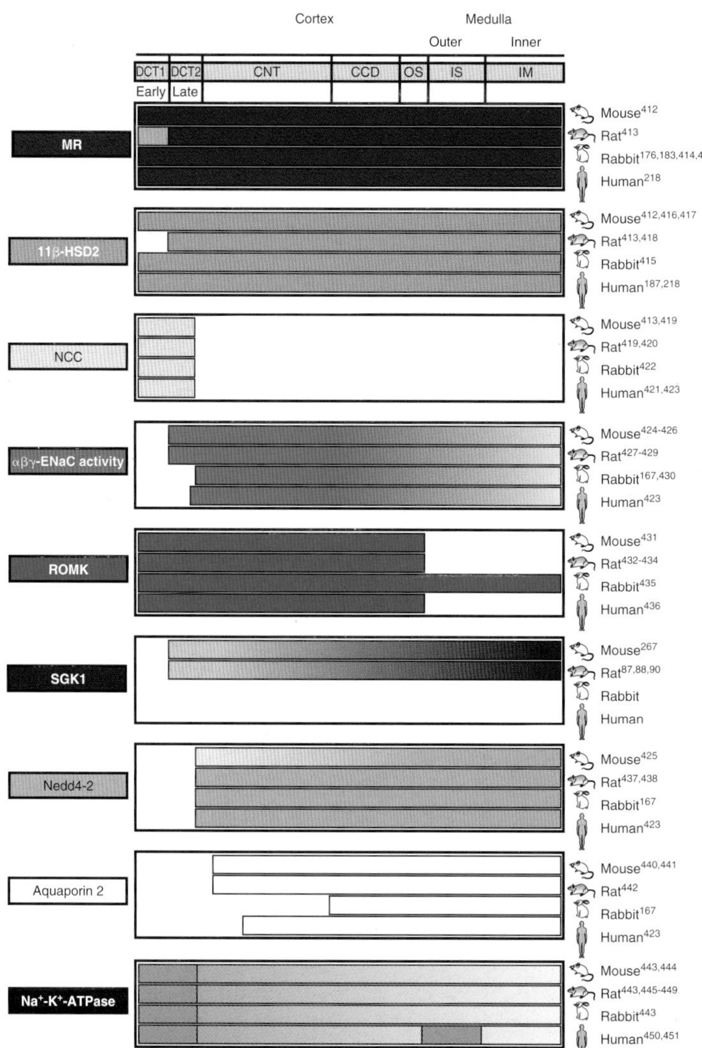


**Fig. 12.9 Expression and/or activity of the mineralocorticoid-dependent transport machinery in principal cells along the mature aldosterone-sensitive distal nephron (ASDN).** Mineralocorticoid specificity is conferred by the presence of the mineralocorticoid receptor *(MR)* and 11β-hydroxysteroid dehydrogenase type 2 *(11β-HSD2)*, beginning primarily from the latter part of the distal convoluted tubule *(DCT)*. The thiazide-sensitive sodium chloride cotransporter *(NCC)* is expressed exclusively in the DCT, but after the transition from the DCT to the connecting tubule (CNT), sodium reabsorption is distinctly determined by amiloride-sensitive sodium channel *(ENaC)* activity. ENaC activity is strongest in the CNT and decreases down to the inner medulla collecting duct. Variation in gene expression or activity along the nephron is indicated by the intensity of shading. Note that there is some variation in gene expression from mouse to human. However, the machinery for sodium reabsorption in the ASDN is predominantly conserved across species. Each nephron segment is drawn to scale, but expression of channels and transporters in intercalated cells is omitted. Expression and/or activity is based on messenger RNA, protein, and biochemical studies. *G,* Glomerulus; *PCT,* proximal convoluted tubule; *ROMK channel,* renal outer medullary potassium; *SGK1,* serum- and glucocorticoid-regulated kinase 1. (Modified from Loffing J, Korbmacher C: Regulated sodium transport in the renal connecting tubule [CNT] via the epithelial sodium channel [ENaC]. *Pflugers Archiv.* 2009;458[1]:111–135.)

NCC phosphorylation and total protein[207] abundance but, until recently, the mechanism of this upregulation was unclear. Elegant work by several groups have shown that aldosterone indirectly stimulates NCC via the activation of ENaC-mediated sodium transport and the resultant potassium secretion[208,209] and hypokalemia. In turn, a lower plasma potassium level activates NCC.[152,153] Another potential mechanism is through direct regulation by aldosterone. In rodent studies, aldosterone stimulates serum and glucocorticoid kinase 1, which inhibits the ubiquitin ligase Nedd4-2, which, in turn, can regulate WNK1 and NCC phosphorylation.[210] As discussed later, this pathway mirrors a well-known mechanism of aldosterone-mediated disinhibition of Nedd4-2 and subsequent ENaC degradation in principal cells. The specific physiologic contexts for these different direct and indirect modes of aldosterone-dependent NCC are still unknown.

## NONRENAL ALDOSTERONE-RESPONSIVE TIGHT EPITHELIA

The mineralocorticoid effects of aldosterone have predominantly been studied in the distal nephron, but do influence other—mostly ENaC-expressing—tight epithelia. ENaC is present in visceral epithelial cells of the distal colon, distal lung, salivary glands, sweat glands, and taste buds.

## COLON

Under physiologic conditions, approximately 1.3 to 1.8 L of electrolyte-rich fluid is reabsorbed per day from the colonic epithelium, which accounts for about 90% of the salt and water that enter the proximal colon from the terminal ileum. In nonmammalian vertebrates, sodium conservation by the colon plays an even more significant role.[211] This transport is regulated by several transporters and channels, including ENaC. Like the nephron, the proximal colon reabsorbs sodium via an electroneutral, ENaC-independent process. In the distal colon, electrogenic $Na^+$ absorption via ENaC channels is the predominant mode of sodium transport.[212–215] In disease states such as inflammatory bowel disease, ENaC-mediated sodium reabsorption can be reduced,[216] although in diarrheal states, elevated aldosterone levels may attenuate sodium and water loss from the colon.[217] It should be noted that in the colon, as in the distal nephron, MR signaling is aldosterone selective, reflecting the activity of 11β-HSD2.[218] Aldosterone increases electrogenic sodium absorption and potassium secretion and inhibits electroneutral absorption.[219] This is in contrast to glucocorticoids, which, at higher concentrations, activate GR to stimulate electroneutral absorption in the proximal and distal colon.[84,220] As in the distal nephron, the aldosterone response can be characterized by an early and late response. The early response gene, *SGK1,* is upregulated by aldosterone via MR.[221] However, in contrast with the kidney, aldosterone and a low-salt diet have been shown to stimulate transcription of β-ENaC but not α-ENaC in rat models.[222,223]

Aldosterone stimulates electrogenic potassium secretion from colonic epithelia. The significance of this secretion is evident in anuric patients. Potassium secretion from the colon is much higher in patients undergoing long-term hemodialysis than in patients not undergoing dialysis.[224–226] Indeed, administration of fludrocortisone, a mineralocorticoid agonist, to dialysis patients has been shown to reduce hyperkalemia in small clinical trials.[227] Low doses of the common MR antagonist spironolactone do not result in significant hyperkalemia.[228–230]

## LUNG

Vectorial transport of salt and water across the distal airway epithelium (ciliated Clara cells, nonciliated cuboidal cells) and alveoli (types I and II alveoli) primarily determines fluid clearance from the lung. ENaC is the rate-limiting step in sodium transport in the lung and plays a primary role in several physiologic and pathophysiologic conditions determined by fluid clearance.[231] At birth, the lung assumes a resorptive phenotype, and lack of functional ENaC channels leads to neonatal respiratory distress syndrome in mouse knockout models.[232] In children, lack of functional ENaC (e.g., autosomal recessive pseudohypoaldosteronism type I)[233–235] results in increased rates of recurrent infection due to increased airway liquid.[234] In the mature lung, defective ENaC channels can lead to pulmonary edema and pathologic conditions (e.g., acute respiratory distress syndrome,[236] high-altitude pulmonary edema[237]). Conversely, hyperabsorption through ENaC is emerging as an important mechanism of decreased mucus clearance in cystic fibrosis.[238]

The molecular apparatus for mineralocorticoid-stimulated liquid reabsorption via ENaC (concomitant MR and 11β-HSD2) is present in late gestational and mature adult lung in humans[218,239,240] and rats,[241] and there is some evidence for a significant physiologic role of aldosterone in ENaC-mediated sodium transport,[241] although glucocorticoids acting via GR are likely to play the predominant role in lung.[118,221,242–245] Importantly, glucocorticoids, but not mineralocorticoids, play a critical role in lung maturation in humans, and GR knockout mice, like α-ENaC knockout mice, die of respiratory insufficiency within hours of birth. In contrast, MR knockout mice demonstrate a severe salt-wasting phenotype but no significant lung phenotype.[177,246]

## EXOCRINE GLANDS AND SENSORS

ENaC-mediated sodium reabsorption is also measurable in the salivary and sweat glands.[247] The importance of these tissues for sodium and water homeostasis is underscored by rare genetic mutations that result in elevated plasma aldosterone levels and pseudohypoaldosteronism, with normal renal tubular function but significant sodium loss from salivary or sweat glands.[248,249] ENaC channels also play an important role in transduction of sodium salt taste in the anterior papillae of the tongue.[250,251] The appropriate molecular machinery for mineralocorticoid-responsive sodium reabsorption is expressed in these organs,[218,252,253] and these epithelia are model systems for the study of ENaC regulation.[247,254] As in colonic epithelia, aldosterone stimulates the expression of β- and γ-ENaC and sodium transport in glands and taste buds in animal models.[251,255] Moreover, in humans, changes in dietary sodium are inversely proportional to sodium transport across salivary epithelia.[256] Similar to the aldosterone-responsive distal nephron and distal colon, sodium uptake is coupled with potassium secretion in salivary epithelia. This effect is evident in humans with hyperaldosteronism. Such patients have a salivary $[Na^+]/[K^+]$ ratio significantly lower than that of subjects without the disorder,[257,258] although this has not been accepted as a valid means to screen for hyperaldosteronism.

# ROLE OF SERUM- AND GLUCOCORTICOID-REGULATED KINASE IN MEDIATING ALDOSTERONE EFFECTS

## INDUCTION OF SGK1 BY ALDOSTERONE

In the early to mid-1960s, primarily from the work of Edelman and colleagues, it became clear that aldosterone, like cortisol, exerted most, if not all, of its key physiologic effects by altering transcription rates of a specific subset of mRNA-encoding genes.[259] In particular, hormone-induced changes in gene transcription were shown to be essential for its effects on epithelial $Na^+$ transport.[73] Transporters involved in $Na^+$ reabsorption ($Na^+$-$K^+$-ATPase and ENaC), are regulated by aldosterone at the transcriptional level. However, these effects are manifest several hours after most of the change in $Na^+$ transport has already occurred and hence could not explain the early and greatest proportion of effects of aldosterone.[1] Considerable effort by many groups went into unbiased screening for aldosterone-regulated proteins[260] and later aldosterone-regulated mRNAs (reviewed in Verrey[1]). In 1999, SGK1 was identified as the first early-onset, aldosterone-induced gene product, which clearly stimulates ENaC-mediated sodium reabsorption in the distal nephron[221,261] without pleiotropic effects on other cellular processes. The physiologic relevance of SGK1 has now been firmly established, and investigations by numerous laboratories into its mechanism of action have revealed critical general features of the mechanism underlying hormone-regulated ion transport. It is therefore addressed in some detail here.

SGK1 mRNA levels are increased within 15 minutes, and protein levels within 30 minutes, in cultured cells on stimulation by aldosterone[262,263] and in the collecting duct by aldosterone or a low-salt diet (a physiologic stimulus for aldosterone secretion).[87,221,264] Notably, SGK1 is increased more abundantly in the kidney cortex (the connecting tubule and cortical collecting duct) than in the medulla, which is congruent with the potency of aldosterone-induced ENaC activation in these nephron segments, as noted earlier.[265,266] SGK1 is expressed in other nephron segments, including glomeruli, proximal tubule, and papillae[87,221,267]; however, its rapid induction in the ASDN appears to provide most of the basis for its role in aldosterone-regulated sodium and potassium transport. SGK1, induced by high sodium in infiltrating T cells, is also important for inflammation in the kidney and hypertension, although the specific nephron segments are unknown.[268,269]

## MOLECULAR MECHANISMS OF SGK1 ACTION IN THE ALDOSTERONE-SENSITIVE DISTAL NEPHRON

SGK1 is a serine-threonine kinase of the AGC protein kinase superfamily,[270] and its kinase activity appears to be essential for $Na^+$ transport regulation. Although it has effects on proliferation and apoptosis in kidney cells, these effects appear to be minor, and the control of ENaC and other transporters[271] predominates. SGK1 is interesting as a signaling kinase in that both its expression level and activity are highly regulated. SGK1 transcription is induced by a variety of stimuli in addition to aldosterone. As its name implies, these include serum and glucocorticoids, but also follicle-stimulating hormone, transforming growth factor-β, and osmotic stress.[272–275]

SGK1 activation is primarily regulated through phosphorylation, which is required for its stimulation of ENaC.[276–278,279,280] Like that of its close relative, Akt, SGK1 phosphorylation is stimulated by a variety of growth factors, including insulin and insulin-like growth factor-1[279–282]; these act through PI3K to trigger phosphorylation at two key residues, an activation loop (residue T256) and a hydrophobic motif (S422). Specifically, the α-isoform of the p110 subunit of PI3K stimulates PI3K-dependent kinase 1 (PDK1) to phosphorylate T256, and also stimulates mammalian target of rapamycin [mTOR] in its complex 2 variant (mTORC2, formerly called PDK2) to phosphorylate S422.[276,280,282–286] mTORC2 also uses a cofactor, SIN1, to specify activation of SGK1 rather than related family members, such as Akt.[287] In turn, the upstream kinases, PDK1 and mTORC2, phosphorylate and thereby activate SGK1 kinase, Thus, SGK1 serves as a convergence point for different classes of stimuli, which act on the one hand to control its expression (aldosterone) and on the other to control its activity (insulin and other activators), which results in the coordinate regulation of ENaC.

In the study of the physiologic and pathophysiologic roles of SGK1 in the ASDN, mice lacking SGK1 under different physiologic stimuli have provided considerable insight. Unlike MR knockout mice,[177] mice lacking SGK1 survive the neonatal period and appear normal when consuming a normal sodium diet, although circulating aldosterone is markedly elevated. When subjected to a low-sodium diet, these mice have a profound sodium-wasting phenotype, akin to pseudohypoaldosteronism type I.[288,289] Additional mouse models of SGK1 deletion have demonstrated diminished processing of ENaC subunits I.[290,291] Notably, this is a significantly milder phenotype than with deletion of MR or α-ENaC.[292] These comparisons suggest that disruption of SGK1 signaling may be insufficient to eliminate aldosterone-mediated sodium transport due to additional aldosterone-induced and aldosterone-repressed proteins, which could compensate for the lack of SGK1.

SGK1 may also play a significant role in states of aldosterone excess or upregulation of hormonal activators of SGK1 (e.g., insulin). SGK1 knockout mice are protected from the development of salt-sensitive hypertension, which accompanies the hyperinsulinemia of the metabolic syndrome.[293,294] Taken together, SGK1 is an important component of ENaC regulation to maintain both sodium and potassium homeostasis.

Despite its accepted role as a mediator of aldosterone-stimulated sodium reabsorption, the mechanisms whereby SGK1 stimulates ENaC are not fully characterized. Several mechanistic studies have demonstrated that SGK1 is rapidly induced but also rapidly degraded.[221,295,296] The N-terminus of the kinase, which distinguishes SGK1 from other kinase family members (e.g., Akt), is important for stimulation of sodium transport but is also the target for rapid degradation of the kinase via the ubiquitin-proteasome system.[297–303] The pathophysiologic implications of the N-terminus for sodium transport are unclear, but they may involve a negative feedback loop to limit sodium reabsorption in states of hypertension. The molecular mechanisms of ENaC stimulation by SGK1 can be divided into three known categories (Fig. 12.10): (1) posttranslational effects on the E3 ubiquitin ligase Nedd4-2; (2) posttranslational Nedd4-2–independent effects; and (3) transcription of gene products such as α-ENaC.

### SGK1 INHIBITS THE UBIQUITIN LIGASE NEDD4-2

Before the discovery of SGK1 as an aldosterone-induced early gene product, the E3 ubiquitin ligase known as "neural developmentally downregulated isoform 4-2" (Nedd4-2) was shown to interact with the C-terminal tails of β-ENaC and γ-ENaC[304] and decrease surface expression of the channel via channel ubiquitination, hence inhibiting the sodium current.[108,305] The genetic defect in Liddle syndrome (ENaC-mediated hypertension, hypokalemia, and metabolic alkalosis) consists of a gain-of-function mutation in the C-terminal tail of these subunits, which results in decreased inhibition by Nedd4-2 and hence increased ENaC activity.[306] Lack of Nedd4-2 in vivo results in increased ENaC activity and salt-sensitive hypertension,[307,308] recapitulating a Liddle syndrome–like phenotype. SGK1 interacts with and phosphorylates Nedd4-2[263,277] in an ENaC signaling complex[113] and enhances cell surface expression of ENaC,[262,309] a determinant of ENaC activity (see Fig. 12.10A). This interaction coordinates the phosphorylation-dependent binding of 14-3-3 proteins to inhibit Nedd4-2 and prevent the ubiquitination of ENaC.[310–313] This disinhibition of ENaC parallels a recurring theme in the regulation of ion transport in the kidney seen with the WNK kinases and NCC, other aldosterone-regulated

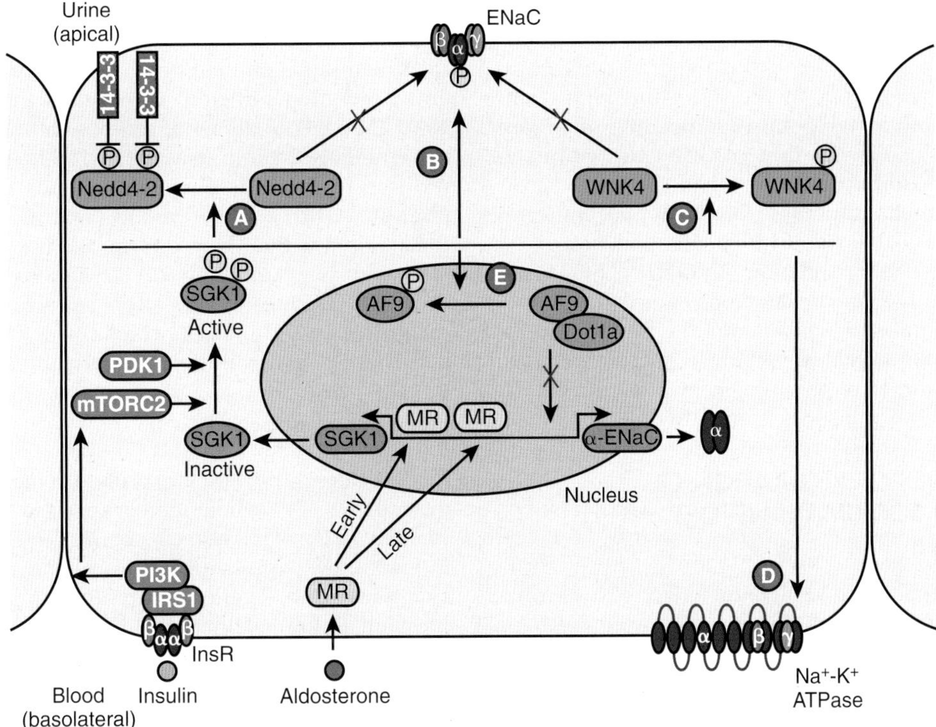


**Fig. 12.10** Mechanisms of serum- and glucocorticoid-regulated kinase 1 *(SGK1)*–mediated stimulation of the amiloride-sensitive sodium channel *(ENaC)*. Within principal cells of the mammalian kidney, SGK1 is transcriptionally upregulated as an early aldosterone-induced gene product. SGK1 is then phosphorylated twice via a phosphatidylinositol-3-kinase *(PI3K)*–dependent cascade of upstream kinases leading to active SGK1. Active SGK1 has multiple effects: it increases apical plasma membrane ENaC by inhibiting Nedd4-2 and Raf-1, and it induces transcription of the α-ENaC (thereby influencing late effects of aldosterone). (A–E, *clockwise*) Shown are the individual mechanisms that have been elucidated in principal cells. See text for details. *InsR,* Insulin receptor; *IRS1,* insulin receptor substrate 1; *MR,* mineralocorticoid receptor; *mTORC2,* mammalian target of rapamycin complex 2; *PDK1,* 3-phosphoinositide-dependent protein kinase type 1.

gene products (e.g., GILZ) and ENaC, and NHERF2 and ROMK.[270,314] Similarly, SGK1 has also been implicated in the stimulation of NCC via inhibition of Nedd4-2 and increased abundance of PY motif-containing WNK1.[210,315,316]

## SGK1 ENHANCES EPITHELIAL SODIUM CHANNEL ACTIVITY INDEPENDENTLY OF NEDD4-2

In cell culture systems, mutation of SGK1 phosphorylation sites on Nedd4-2 does not completely abolish the ability of SGK1 to stimulate ENaC.[277] Furthermore, SGK1 has been shown to stimulate ENaC channels with Liddle syndrome mutations, which are unable to bind Nedd4-2.[221,262] Consequently, other Nedd4-2–independent mechanisms of SGK1 stimulation have been proposed. SGK1 directly phosphorylates a serine residue in the intracellular C-terminal tail of α-ENaC, which directly activates channels at the cell surface (see Fig. 12.10B).[317,318] SGK1 has been implicated in the stimulation of ENaC via the phosphorylation of WNK4, a kinase mutated in pseudohypoaldosteronism type II (see Fig. 12.10C).[319] Cell surface–expressed SGK1 may also increase open probability of the channel.[318,320] In addition to showing effects on ENaC, SGK1 has been found to stimulate the activity of basolateral $Na^+$-$K^+$-ATPase, which separately increases ENaC-mediated sodium transport (see Fig. 12.10D).[321,322] The time course of these effects and their relative importance compared with Nedd4-2–dependent inhibition have not been explored.[317] The next generation of molecular studies of SGK1 will elucidate the relative importance of each of these pathways.

## SGK1 STIMULATES THE COMPONENTS OF SODIUM TRANSPORT MACHINERY

SGK1 also regulates the expression of late aldosterone-responsive genes, primarily α-ENaC.[323,324] Active SGK1 is an important mediator of aldosterone-sensitive α-ENaC transcription in vivo via inhibition of a transcriptional repression element, the disruptor of telomeric silencing alternative splice variant a (Dot1a)–ALL1–fused gene from the chromosome 9 (Af9) complex.[324] SGK1 phosphorylates Af9 and reduces the interaction between Dot1a and Af9. This releases suppression of ENaC transcription by this complex (see Fig. 12.10E). Thus, SGK1 not only acts on ENaC channels to enhance sodium channel activity rapidly through the increase of active channels at the apical surface and the increase of $Na^+$-$K^+$-ATPase at the basolateral surface, but also stimulates the transcription of elements of the machinery for sodium transport to promote a sustained response to aldosterone. SGK1 is an early-onset gene, but its effects influence both immediate- and long-term aldosterone-stimulated sodium reabsorption.

## SGK1 STIMULATES POTASSIUM SECRETION IN THE ALDOSTERONE-SENSITIVE DISTAL NEPHRON

Further evidence of a role for SGK1 in the regulation of sodium transport in the ASDN has been revealed by the study of potassium secretion. If SGK1 enhances ENaC-mediated sodium transport, the potential difference across the apical to basolateral surface of principal cells should be higher (more negative) and thus should indirectly stimulate potassium secretion. SGK1 knockout mice are unable to secrete potassium adequately in the short and long terms when challenged with a high-potassium diet, and mice with constitutive or inducible deletion of SGK1 are prone to hyperkalemia.[325–327] Moreover, the potential difference across collecting duct epithelia from these knockout mice indicates that the effect of SGK1 on potassium secretion occurs via ENaC, not through direct regulation of ROMK.[328] SGK1 also directly inhibits Nedd4-2, and deletion of Nedd4-2 predisposes low-potassium–fed mice to hypokalemia via the constitutive stimulation of ENaC-mediated sodium transport.[329] Thus, SGK1 and its effectors have physiologically relevant roles in sodium and potassium transport in the ASDN.

### ALTERNATE MODES OF REGULATION OF ENAC-MEDIATED SODIUM TRANSPORT BY ALDOSTERONE

Although SGK1 remains the best characterized aldosterone-regulated gene, other early aldosterone-induced mRNAs, including K-ras, GILZ, kidney-specific WNK1, Usp45, melanophilin, and promyelocytic leukemia zinc finger,[330–335] have also been implicated in the stimulation of ENaC. Their distinct mechanisms of action are beyond the scope of this chapter, but more recent data have suggested that micro-RNAs stimulated by aldosterone may play a prominent role in regulating both SGK1 and ENaC.

Aldosterone can upregulate or downregulate several microRNAs in cultured cells and in vivo. These micro-RNAs can then indirectly increase or decrease protein levels of intermediate regulators of ENaC-mediated transport. The first micro-RNA cluster (mmu-miR-335-3p, mmu-miR-290-5p, and mmu-miR-1983) to be described by Butterworth was downregulated by aldosterone within 24 hours and thereby released the 3′ untranslated region of ankyrin 3 to increase apical trafficking of α-ENaC.[336,337] Aldosterone also increases micro-RNAs that inhibit a negative regulator of ENaC, intersectin 2.[338] Aldosterone has also been shown to promote the rapid induction of SGK1 mRNA by decreasing micro-RNA 466g in cultured cells.[339] Taken together, SGK1 plays a prominent role in transducing the effect of aldosterone to stimulate ENaC for both regulation of blood pressure and potassium homeostasis. Additionally, there are alternate effectors of aldosterone, but the physiologic contexts of these other pathways have not been as well established.

## 11β-HYDROXYSTEROID DEHYDROGENASE TYPE 2

### ESSENTIAL DETERMINANT OF MINERALOCORTICOID SPECIFICITY

The physiologic glucocorticoid cortisol (corticosterone in rats and mice) has a high affinity for MR, equivalent to that of aldosterone and, as noted earlier, circulates at plasma free concentrations that are 100-fold or more higher than those of aldosterone. Central to the ability of MR to respond to aldosterone selectively in the ASDN is the coexpression of the enzyme 11β-HSD2.[5,6] 11β-HSD2 converts cortisol (corticosterone) to receptor-inactive 11-keto steroids (cortisone in humans, 11-dehydrocorticosterone in rats and mice), using nicotinamide adenine dinucleotide (NAD) as a cosubstrate and generating sufficient amounts of the reduced form of NAD (NADH) to alter the redox potential of the cell. This dependence sets it in contrast to 11β-HSD1, which uses the reduced form of nicotinamide adenine dinucleotide phosphate (NADPH), preferentially catalyzes the conversion of the oxidized to the reduced form, and has received substantial attention as a target for the treatment of metabolic syndrome.[340] Aldosterone has a very reactive aldehyde group at carbon 18 (see Fig. 12.1), which forms an 11,18-hemiacetal and is protected from dehydrogenation by 11β-HSD2.[5,6]

### SITES OF EXPRESSION

In the kidney, 11β-HSD2 is expressed at high levels throughout the ASDN,[175,186,341] where it is coexpressed with MR and ENaC (see Fig. 12.9).[342] It is also coexpressed in DCT with NCC.[343,344] Interestingly, expression has also been found in the thick ascending limb,[186] although expression levels appear to be substantially lower, and increase progressively in DCT. Expression is the highest in the connecting tubule and cortical collecting duct.[341,344] It is also expressed in the aldosterone-sensitive segments of the colon, particularly the distal colon, as is the case for MR, although there is species variability.[345] 11β-HSD2 expression has also been described in several nonepithelial tissues, including placenta,[346] the nucleus tractus solitarius in the brain,[347] and the vessel wall,[56] which makes all these tissues potential aldosterone target tissues.

### IMPACT ON MINERALOCORTICOID RECEPTOR ACTIVITY

The initial[5,6] and still widely held interpretation of the role of 11β-HSD2 was that of excluding active glucocorticoids from epithelial MR, which allowed aldosterone unfettered access. This is only part of the picture, however; to reduce the signal to noise ratio from 100-fold to 10% would require that 999 of every 1000 cortisol molecules entering the cell be metabolized to cortisone, a very tall order in an organ such as the kidney, which commands 20% to 25% of cardiac output. 11β-HSD2 in epithelia (and in other tissues in which it is expressed) clearly reduces glucocorticoid levels by an order of magnitude[348] but still leaves them with intracellular levels well above those of aldosterone. At the same time, although it is clear that when 11β-HSD2 is operative, glucocorticoid-occupied MR is not transcriptionally active, it is also clear that when enzyme activity is insufficient (as in apparent mineralocorticoid excess) or deficient (as in licorice abuse or by genetic mutation), cortisol can activate MR and ion transport. Although the subcellular mechanisms involved have yet to be established, it appears that glucocorticoid-MR complexes are conformationally distinct from aldosterone-MR complexes. One intriguing possibility is that these hormone-receptor complexes, in contrast to aldosterone–MR complexes, are held inactive by the obligate generation of NADH from the cosubstrate NAD, required for the operation of 11β-HSD2.[349] There is direct evidence to support the idea that redox potential affects the activity of the glucocorticoid receptor through effects on thioredoxin.[350]

## APPARENT MINERALOCORTICOID EXCESS: A DISEASE OF DEFECTIVE 11β-HYDROXYSTEROID DEHYDROGENASE TYPE 2

Apparent mineralocorticoid excess was first described by New, and the molecular mechanisms responsible were established after an intense but fruitless search for a novel mineralocorticoid.[351] The condition reflects a partial or complete deficiency of 11β-HSD2 activity, is more common in consanguinity, and manifests as severe juvenile hypertension (see also Chapters 17 and 44).[352] Confectionery licorice (or that added to chewing tobacco) contains glycyrrhizic and glycyrrhetinic acids, suicide substrates for 11β-HSD2, which thus acts as a potent inhibitor of the enzyme. Lack of functional 11β-HSD2 results in MR activation by cortisol and inappropriate mineralocorticoid-like stimulation of ENaC-mediated $Na^+$ reabsorption. This causes severe hypertension, often accompanied by hypokalemia. Plasma renin, angiotensin II, and aldosterone are suppressed. Treatment of apparent mineralocorticoid excess is the use of MR antagonists and additional antihypertensives, as required. Treatment of licorice abuse is moderation.

## ROLE IN BLOOD VESSELS

Studies of 11β-HSD2 in the human vascular wall[353] have defined the activity of aldosterone and cortisol in this physiologic aldosterone target tissue. Aldosterone at nanomolar concentrations causes a rapid rise in the intracellular pH, reflecting nongenomic activation of the $Na^+$-$H^+$ exchanger. Cortisol alone over a range of doses produced no effect, but when carbenoxolone was added to inhibit 11β-HSD2, cortisol mimicked aldosterone. Inhibitor studies have revealed that the effects of both aldosterone and cortisol are mediated by classic MR. In other studies involving tissue damage, mineralocorticoid antagonists were protective, whereas aldosterone or cortisol worsened injury. The inference from these results was that cortisol becomes an MR agonist in the context of tissue damage (or when 11β-HSD2 is pharmacologically inhibited), with alteration of reactive oxygen species generation and redox potential.[354] It is further notable that aldosterone has been shown to have both vasodilatory and vasoconstricting effects in animals and humans.[355] These contradictory results have not been fully reconciled,[356] but may well reflect a combination of direct effects on vascular smooth muscle to stimulate myosin light-chain phosphorylation through ERK activation[357,358] on the one hand, and stimulatory effects on endothelial cell nitric oxide synthase[355] on the other. Finally, it is of considerable interest that vascular smooth muscle cells express ENaC, in addition to MR, and that the channel might play a role in vascular tone.[359]

## SUMMARY OF 11β-HYDROXYSTEROID DEHYDROGENASE TYPE 2 ROLES

In summary, the enzyme 11β-HSD2 is crucial for the aldosterone-selective activation of epithelial MR and possibly of MR in other tissues, including blood vessels, nucleus of the solitary tract, and placenta. It does this in part by debulking intracellular glucocorticoids by an order of magnitude, which is not sufficient to account for its blockade of cortisol agonist activity. Current evidence supports the possibility that 11β-HSD2–mediated generation of NADH renders glucocorticoid-occupied MR inactive. Partial or complete deficiency of 11β-HSD2 results in the syndrome of apparent mineralocorticoid excess, which is mimicked by licorice abuse.

# NONGENOMIC EFFECTS OF ALDOSTERONE

The classic effects of aldosterone on ion transport are genomic, with MR acting at the nuclear level to regulate DNA-directed, RNA-mediated protein synthesis and thereby sodium transport. Such genomic effects are characterized by a lag period of 45 to 60 minutes before changes in ion transport can be measured, commensurate with a homeostatic role for aldosterone action in regulating sodium and potassium status in response to dietary intake. In other circumstances (e.g., orthostasis, acute blood volume depletion), aldosterone secretion rises rapidly, and acute nongenomic effects are an understandable response. Such rapid effects were first demonstrated over 30 years ago in the laboratory[360]; in human vascular tissues, they have been amply demonstrated both in vitro[353] and in vivo.[361] Although most of these rapid nongenomic effects appear to be mediated via activation of classic MR,[353,360] there is evidence from atomic force microscopy studies for non-MR membrane sites binding aldosterone with high affinity on cultured endothelial cells.[362] Such nongenomic effects are not unique to aldosterone, having been shown for the other recognized classes of steroid hormones[363] and reported for dehydroepiandrosterone (DHEA).[355] Genomic effects commonly have a lag period of 20 minutes or longer and are abrogated by inhibitors of transcription, such as actinomycin D. Most nongenomic effects of steroids have time courses from onset to plateau of 5 to 10 minutes and are mediated by a variety of pathways.

MR does not have a myristoylation site (e.g., unlike estrogen receptors[364]), and there is little evidence for membrane-associated classic MR. Most rapid nongenomic effects of aldosterone appear to be mediated by classic MR in that they are inhibited by the MR antagonist RU 28318. In some cases,[353] spironolactone is ineffective as an inhibitor; exclusive reliance on blockade by spironolactone has led to the assumption of a widely distributed aldosterone receptor distinct from classic MR and a long and unsuccessful search for such a membrane-bound species.[365] The physiology of nongenomic aldosterone actions has been slow to be accepted, which in part reflects the major emphasis on the clearly genomic actions of aldosterone in the kidney. The most obvious example is the conjunction of rapid secretion of aldosterone in response to orthostasis and its demonstrated rapid vascular effects.[356,366] With more interest in the pathophysiologic effects of MR activation, particularly in nonclassic aldosterone target tissues, there has been renewed interest in the rapid nongenomic effects of aldosterone (and the physiologic glucocorticoids) via classic MR. Further details of the nongenomic actions of aldosterone can be found in reports by Funder[366] and other sources.[367,368]

# DISEASE STATES

## PRIMARY ALDOSTERONISM

Clinically, the most prevalent disorder directly involving aldosterone is Conn syndrome, or primary aldosteronism.[369]

In this syndrome, aldosterone secretion is elevated and (relatively) autonomous as a result of an adrenal adenoma or, more frequently, bilateral adrenal hyperplasia and, very rarely, adrenal carcinoma or the inherited disorder glucocorticoid remediable aldosteronism (FH-1). Once considered rare (<1% of all cases of hypertension), necessarily characterized by hypokalemia and relatively benign, primary aldosteronism is now thought to account for approximately 8% to 13% of all hypertension, which reflects improved case detection and diagnosis. In contrast with previous teachings, frank hypokalemia is found in only 25% to 30% of cases, and the incidence of cardiovascular pathology (e.g., fibrosis, fibrillation, infarct, stroke) is substantially higher than in age-, gender-, and blood pressure–matched individuals with essential hypertension.[370,371]

Guidelines for the case detection, diagnosis, and management of primary aldosteronism have been published[372] as a first step in addressing what has been increasingly recognized as a major public health issue. It has long been thought and taught that the role of aldosterone in blood pressure regulation reflects its epithelial effects leading to retention of sodium, and with it water, which thus increases circulating volume. This increase, in turn, is reflected in an increased cardiac output, which is reflexively normalized by vasoconstriction and thus elevation of blood pressure (in keeping with the Guyton hypothesis[373]). Although the epithelial effects of aldosterone on vascular volume are indisputably homeostatically important, there have been compelling experimental and clinical studies to suggest a role for nonepithelial effects in mineralocorticoid-induced hypertension.[374,375] In addition to MR-mediated central nervous system and vascular effects in hypertension, roles for macrophages have been demonstrated by two groups using distinct and complementary experimental approaches.[376,377]

Other studies have suggested a role for a mutated $K^+$ channel (KCNJ5) in the pathogenesis of aldosterone-producing adrenal adenomas and in the rare condition of FH type III.[25,26] See earlier, "Aldosterone Synthesis," for additional details.

## CONGESTIVE HEART FAILURE

Aldosterone has been implicated in the pathophysiology of congestive heart failure since soon after its discovery in the mid-1950s.[378,379] Until fairly recently, most of the focus has been on the counterproductive effects of aldosterone in epithelia. More recently, the beneficial effects of MR antagonists in congestive heart failure have suggested an additional effect in myocardium itself.[380] In the Randomized Aldactone Evaluation Study (RALES),[380] addition of low-dose (mean, 26 mg/day) spironolactone to standard of care treatment in patients with progressive heart failure produced a 30% reduction in mortality and 35% fewer hospitalizations. This result is often attributed to spironolactone antagonizing the effect of aldosterone on cardiomyocyte MR, but actually reflects its antagonizing of cortisol acting as an MR agonist under ischemic conditions. Subsequently, the Eplerenone Post-Acute Myocardial Infarction Heart Failure Efficacy and Survival Study (EPHESUS) examined the effect of eplerenone, an MR antagonist with improved specificity relative to spironolactone, on heart failure due to systolic dysfunction complicating acute myocardial infarction. The study showed that adding eplerenone (25 mg/day) to conventional therapy significantly decreased mortality due to all causes (31%) and cardiovascular mortality (13%).[381] Potassium concentration was only slightly higher in the eplerenone-treated group than in the placebo-treated group (4.47 mmol/L and 4.54 mmol/L, respectively). Coupled with studies on the direct vascular effects of aldosterone addressed earlier, these data suggest that MR antagonists have a beneficial effect that cannot be accounted for by diuretic actions in the kidney alone.[382]

It is also notable that a trial (Eplerenone in Mild Patients Hospitalization And SurvIval Study in Heart Failure [EMPHASIS-HF]) examining the effect of eplerenone in New York Heart Association (NYHA) class II heart failure (milder than previously examined), was stopped early because a significant benefit was found in the treated group.[383] In summary, the pathophysiologic effects of aldosterone excess on the cardiovascular system in primary aldosteronism have been well documented, and MR also plays an important role in essential hypertension and heart failure. Importantly, MR expressed in cardiac and vascular cells may commonly be activated by cortisol rather than aldosterone, which is present in serum at levels that are higher by 100-fold or more and mimics aldosterone in the context of tissue damage.

## CHRONIC KIDNEY DISEASE

The role of MR blockade in slowing the progression of chronic kidney disease has been considered in a recent study and commentary[384,385] and in Chapter 59. The study, a double-blind, randomized, placebo-controlled trial, examined the antialbuminuric effect of the MR antagonist eplerenone in nondiabetic hypertensive patients with albuminuria.

# NONEPITHELIAL ACTIONS OF ALDOSTERONE

In addition to the classic epithelial tissues involved in ion transport—kidney, colon, sweat gland, salivary gland—there are documented effects of aldosterone in the brain, vascular wall, and possibly the placenta, as previously noted. Many other tissues and organs have been postulated as physiologic aldosterone target tissues, largely on the inadequate evidence that they express MR and can be shown in vitro to respond by some measure to aldosterone. What underpins these hypotheses is the misconception that aldosterone is the cognate ligand for MR, which is true for epithelia but not for cells not expressing 11β-HSD2, coupled with disregard for the role of cortisol. Cortisol was not only the ligand for MR in cartilaginous and bony fish, millions of years before the appearance of aldosterone synthase, but is the overwhelming occupant of MR that is not protected by 11β-HSD2 (primarily nonepithelial MR) throughout the body. It is notable that some nonepithelial MR is also protected by 11β-HSD2—for example, in the nucleus tractus solitarius.

The fact that aldosterone can activate MR under experimental conditions without 11β-HSD2 was illustrated by the work of Gómez-Sánchez and colleagues more than 2 decades ago.[386] Very low doses of aldosterone that did not affect blood pressure when infused systemically elevated blood pressure when infused into the lateral ventricle of conscious, free-living rats. That this did not reflect a physiologic role for aldosterone, however, was shown by the co-infusion of one, two, and five times the dose of corticosterone, which progressively blocked the blood pressure effect of the infused aldosterone, evidence for the absence of 11β-HSD2 in the hypothalamic nuclei involved and the overwhelming occupancy of their MR by the physiologic glucocorticoid.

The two established nonepithelial aldosterone target tissues are the vascular wall and nucleus tractus solitarius in the brain. Both these tissues express 11β-HSD2, as noted earlier, allowing aldosterone-selective MR activation; both can be reasonably envisaged as having important ancillary roles supporting the primary epithelial role of aldosterone on fluid and electrolyte homeostasis. Aldosterone vasoconstricts blood vessels, acutely and in the longer term, in response to volume depletion; similarly, it acts on the nucleus tractus solitarius to stimulate salt appetite. Both actions are thus harnessed into the physiologic role of aldosterone in maintaining fluid and electrolyte balance.

It is commonly assumed that in pathophysiologic states of high aldosterone levels, such as primary aldosteronism, the deleterious effects are mediated by aldosterone occupying and inappropriately activating nonprotected MR in cardiomyocytes, for example. It is plausible that instead of the approximately 1% physiologic occupancy (given the ≈100-fold higher levels of plasma free cortisol), aldosterone occupancy of cardiomyocyte MR might rise to 3% to 5%. Relatively minor degrees of MR occupancy have been shown to be effective for spironolactone, acting as a protective inverse agonist[387]; similarly, therefore, minor degrees of cardiomyocyte MR occupancy by aldosterone could potentially produce the deleterious effects seen.

This explanation, however, is almost certainly incorrect. Plasma aldosterone levels are as high or higher in chronic sodium deficiency (or in the effectively volume-depleted condition of secondary hyperaldosteronism), with no deleterious cardiovascular effects. In primary and secondary aldosteronism, and in chronic sodium deficiency, physiologic target tissues, both renal tubular and coronary vascular, are exposed to (and respond to) maintained high levels of aldosterone. It is thus unlikely that the cardiovascular damage in primary aldosteronism reflects increased MR activation in blood vessels, coronary and peripheral. The key difference between these circumstances is that primary aldosteronism is a state of aldosterone and sodium excess and the others of sodium and volume depletion.

A plausible but untested mechanism of aldosterone-induced damage is that it is secondary to increased renal sodium reabsorption and the action of endogenous ouabain on blood vessels. Endogenous ouabain is incompletely explored, but its levels are elevated in primary aldosteronism.[388] Like aldosterone, its secretion is elevated by ACTH and angiotensin (the latter via $AT_2R$); in stark contrast with aldosterone, it is raised (not lowered) in states of sodium excess.[389–391] It acts via $Na^+$-$K^+$-ATPase in vessel walls as a vasoconstrictor, presumably physiologically to produce a pressure natriuresis as a homeostatic response. Thus, it may be that the cardiovascular damage in primary aldosteronism reflects a combination of the effects of aldosterone plus endogenous ouabain on the vasculature; if this is the case, the source and origin of the nonepithelial effects of aldosterone remain squarely in the renal tubule and the exaggerated sodium retention therein.

## RECENT ADVANCES IN NONRENAL MINERALOCORTICOID RECEPTOR–MEDIATED DISEASE PATHOLOGY

Recent developments in the use of MR antagonists for nonrenal disease are not described in detail here. See the report by Jaisser and Farman[392] for a review. It is particularly worth noting the surprising recent use of spironolactone for the treatment of retinal diseases. MR is expressed in several retinal cell types, including glial cells, which are essential for retinal water and ion homeostasis, epithelial cells, and choroidal endothelial cells. The activation of MR has been implicated in multiple retinal pathologies, and MR antagonists, particularly spironolactone, have been shown to have therapeutic benefit.[392,393]

## ACKNOWLEDGMENTS

Our coauthor, colleague, and friend John Stokes died in 2012, just before work on the 10th edition of this textbook began. John was senior author on the chapter "Aldosterone Regulation of Ion Transport," written as a new chapter for the 9th edition of Brenner and Rector, and inspired our writing and focus for subsequent editions, including the present chapter for the 11th edition. John had a profound knowledge of aldosterone action in the renal tubules, a sharp wit, and unsurpassed work ethic. For all these reasons, he was the model coauthor and colleague. John also made enormous primary contributions to aldosterone and renal tubule research, which enriched all of us, as did his humor and enthusiasm for life. For those interested in reading more about John's inspiring life and contributions to nephrology and renal research, see the eloquent eulogy at http://www.ncbi.nlm.nih.gov/pmc/articles/PMC3715930/.

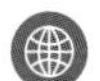 Complete reference list available at ExpertConsult.com.

## KEY REFERENCES

2. Simpson SA, Tait JF. A quantitative method for the bioassay of the effect of adrenal cortical steroids on mineral metabolism. *Endocrinology*. 1952;50(2):150–161.
3. Simpson SA, Tait JF. Physiochemical methods of detection of a previously unidentified adrenal hormone. *Mem Soc Endocrinol*. 1953;2:9–24.
4. Simpson SA, et al. Constitution of aldosterone, a new mineralocorticoid. *Experientia*. 1954;10(3):132–133.
5. Funder JW, et al. Mineralocorticoid action: target tissue specificity is enzyme, not receptor, mediated. *Science*. 1988;242(4878):583–585.
16. Lifton RP, et al. A chimaeric 11β-hydroxylase/aldosterone synthase gene causes glucocorticoid-remediable aldosteronism and human hypertension. *Nature*. 1992;355:262–265.
25. Choi M, et al. $K^+$ channel mutations in adrenal aldosterone-producing adenomas and hereditary hypertension. *Science*. 2011;331:768–772.
27. Boulkroun S, et al. Prevalence, clinical, and molecular correlates of KCNJ5 mutations in primary aldosteronism. *Hypertension*. 2012; 59(3):592–598.
29. Azizan EAB, et al. Somatic mutations in ATP1A1 and CACNA1D underlie a common subtype of adrenal hypertension. *Nat Genet*. 2013;45:1055.
36. Bhargava A, Pearce D. Mechanisms of mineralocorticoid action: determinants of receptor specificity and actions of regulated gene products. *Trends Endocrinol Metab*. 2004;15(4):147–153.
51. Li Y, et al. Structural and biochemical mechanisms for the specificity of hormone binding and coactivator assembly by mineral corticoid receptor. *Mol Cell*. 2005;19:367–380.

54. Geller DS, et al. Autosomal dominant pseudohypoaldosteronism type 1: mechanisms, evidence for neonatal lethality, and phenotypic expression in adults. *J Am Soc Nephrol.* 2006;17(5):1429–1436.
55. Krozowski ZS, Funder JW. Renal mineralocorticoid receptors and hippocampal corticosterone-binding species have identical intrinsic steroid specificity. *Proc Natl Acad Sci U. S. A.* 1983;80(19): 6056–6060.
59. Pearce D, Yamamoto KR. Mineralocorticoid and glucocorticoid receptor activities distinguished by nonreceptor factors at a composite response element. *Science.* 1993;259(5098):1161–1165.
61. Pascual-Le Tallec L, et al. The elongation factor ELL (eleven-nineteen lysine-rich leukemia) is a selective coregulator for steroid receptor functions. *Mol Endocrinol.* 2005;19(5):1158–1169.
66. Hong H, et al. GRIP1, a novel mouse protein that serves as a transcriptional coactivator in yeast for the hormone binding domains of steroid receptors. *Proc Natl Acad Sci U. S. A.* 1996;93(10):4948–4952.
67. Onate SA, et al. Sequence and characterization of a coactivator for the steroid hormone receptor superfamily. *Science.* 1995; 270(5240):1354–1357.
75. Conn JW, Knopf RF, Nesbit RM. Clinical characteristics of primary aldosteronism from an analysis of 145 cases. *Am J Surg.* 1964;107:159–172.
77. Canessa CM, et al. Amiloride-sensitive epithelial $Na^+$ channel is made of three homologous subunits. *Nature.* 1994;367(6462):463–467.
79. Garty H, Palmer LG. Epithelial sodium channels: function, structure, and regulation. *Physiol Rev.* 1997;77:359–396.
88. Chen S, et al. Epithelial sodium channel regulated by aldosterone-induced protein sgk. *Proc Natl Acad Sci U. S. A.* 1999;96:2514–2519.
97. Frindt G, Ergonul Z, Palmer LG. Surface expression of epithelial Na channel protein in rat kidney. *J Gen Physiol.* 2008;131(6): 617–627.
130. Wade JB, et al. Morphological and physiological responses to aldosterone: time course and sodium dependence. *Am J Physiol.* 1990;259(1 Pt 2):F88–F94.
138. Knight KK, et al. Liddle's syndrome mutations increase $Na^+$ transport through dual effects on epithelial $Na^+$ channel surface expression and proteolytic cleavage. *Proc Natl Acad Sci U. S. A.* 2006;103(8): 2805–2808.
139. Stokes JB. Potassium secretion by cortical collecting tubule: relation to sodium absorption, luminal sodium concentration, and transepithelial voltage. *Am J Physiol Renal Fluid Electrolyte Physiol.* 1981;241:F395–F402.
141. Estilo G, Liu W, Pastor-Soler N, et al. Effect of aldosterone on BK channel expression in mammalian cortical collecting duct. *Am J Physiol Renal Physiol.* 2008;295:F780–F788.
162. Shibata S, et al. Regulated mineralocorticoid receptor phosphorylation controls ligand binding, allowing distinct physiologic responses to aldosterone. *Cell Metab.* 2013;18(November 5):660–671.
176. Farman N, et al. Immunolocalization of gluco- and mineralocorticoid receptors in rabbit kidney. *Am J Physiol.* 1991;260(2 Pt 1):C226–C233.
177. Berger S, et al. Mineralocorticoid receptor knockout mice: pathophysiology of $Na^+$ metabolism. *Proc Natl Acad Sci U. S. A.* 1998; 95(16):9424–9429.
184. Vandewalle A, et al. Aldosterone binding along the rabbit nephron: an autoradiographic study on isolated tubules. *Am J Physiol.* 1981;240(3):F172–F179.
206. Ko B, Mistry AC, Hanson L, et al. Aldosterone acutely stimulates NCC activity via a SPAK-mediated pathway. *Am J Physiol Renal Physiol.* 2013;305:F645–F652.
217. Levitan R, Ingelfinger FJ. Effect of *d*-aldosterone on salt and water absorption from the intact human colon. *J Clin Invest.* 1965; 44:801–808.
219. Turnamian SG, Binder HJ. Regulation of active sodium and potassium transport in the distal colon of the rat: role of the aldosterone and glucocorticoid receptors. *J Clin Invest.* 1989;84(6):1924–1929.
225. Hayes CP Jr, McLeod ME, Robinson RR. An extrarenal mechanism for the maintenance of potassium balance in severe chronic renal failure. *Trans Assoc Am Physicians.* 1967;80:207–216.
226. Sandle GI, et al. Enhanced rectal potassium secretion in chronic renal insufficiency: evidence for large intestinal potassium adaptation in man. *Clin Sci.* 1986;71(4):393–401.
270. Bhalla V, et al. Disinhibitory pathways for control of sodium transport: regulation of ENaC by SGK1 and GILZ. *Am J Physiol Renal Physiol.* 2006;291(4):F714–F721.
277. Debonneville C, et al. Phosphorylation of Nedd4-2 by Sgk1 regulates epithelial Na(+) channel cell surface expression. *EMBO J.* 2001;20(24):7052–7059.
278. Snyder PM, Olson DR, Thomas BC. Serum- and glucocorticoid-regulated kinase modulates Nedd4-2-mediated inhibition of the epithelial $Na^+$ channel. *J Biol Chem.* 2002;277(1):5–8.
288. Wulff P, et al. Impaired renal Na(+) retention in the sgk1-knockout mouse. *J Clin Invest.* 2002;110(9):1263–1268.
335. Soundararajan R, et al. A novel role for glucocorticoid-induced leucine zipper protein in epithelial sodium channel-mediated sodium transport. *J Biol Chem.* 2005;280(48):39970–39981.
304. Staub O, et al. WW domains of Nedd4 bind to the proline-rich PY motifs in the epithelial $Na^+$ channel deleted in Liddle's syndrome. *EMBO J.* 1996;15(10):2371–2380.
347. Geerling JC, Loewy AD. Aldosterone in the brain. *Am J Physiol Renal Physiol.* 2009;297(3):F559–F576.
349. Funder JW. Is aldosterone bad for the heart? *Trends Endocrinol Metab.* 2004;15(4):139–142.
356. Oberleithner H. Is the vascular endothelium under the control of aldosterone? Facts and hypothesis. *Pflugers Arch.* 2007;454(2):187–193.
366. Funder JW. The nongenomic actions of aldosterone. *Endocr Rev.* 2005;26(3):313–321.
369. Young WF. Primary aldosteronism: renaissance of a syndrome. *Clin Endocrinol (Oxf).* 2007;66(5):607–618.
386. Gómez-Sánchez EP, et al. ICV infusion of corticosterone antagonizes ICV-aldosterone hypertension. *Am J Physiol.* 1990;258(4 Pt 1):E649–E653.
387. Milhailidou AS, et al. Glucocorticoids activate cardiac mineralocorticoid receptors during experimental myocardial infarction. *Hypertension.* 2009;54:1306–1312.
389. Dostanic-Larson I, et al. The highly conserved cardiac glycoside binding site of Na,K-ATPase plays a role in blood pressure regulation. *PNAS.* 2005;102(44):15845–15850.
395. McCormick JA, Yang CL, Ellison DH. WNK kinases and renal sodium transport in health and disease: an integrated view. *Hypertension.* 2008;51(3):588–596.
403. Kim GH, et al. The thiazide-sensitive Na-Cl cotransporter is an aldosterone-induced protein. *Proc Natl Acad Sci U. S. A.* 1998;95(24): 14552–14557.
404. Rozansky DJ, et al. Aldosterone mediates activation of the thiazide-sensitive Na-Cl cotransporter through an SGK1 and WNK4 signaling pathway. *J Clin Invest.* 2009;119(9):2601–2612.
415. Bonvalet JP, et al. Distribution of 11 beta-hydroxysteroid dehydrogenase along the rabbit nephron. *J Clin Invest.* 1990;86:832–837.

# 13 Arachidonic Acid Metabolites and the Kidney

Raymond C. Harris | Ming-Zhi Zhang | Richard M. Breyer

## CHAPTER OUTLINE



## KEY POINTS

- The kidney is source of eicosanoids (prostaglandins, lipoxygenase metabolies, cytochrome P450 metabolites.
- Eicosanoids derived from arachidonic acid play important roles in kidney physiology and pathophysiology.
- Prostaglandins can regulate renal hemodynamics, the renin-angiotensin system and salt and water excretion.
- Eicosanoids are important mediators of systemic blood pressure.

## CELLULAR ORIGIN OF EICOSANOIDS

Eicosanoids comprise a family of biologically active, oxygenated arachidonic acid (AA) metabolites. AA is a polyunsaturated fatty acid possessing 20 carbon atoms and four double bonds (C20:4) and is formed from linoleic acid (C18:2) by the addition of two carbons to the chain and further desaturation. In mammals, linoleic acid is derived strictly from dietary sources. Essential fatty acid deficiency occurs when dietary fatty acid precursors, including linoleic acid, are omitted, thereby depleting the hormone-responsive pool of AAs. Essential fatty acid deficiency thereby reduces the intracellular availability of AA in response to hormonal stimulation and abrogates many biologic actions of hormone-induced eicosanoid release.[1]

Of an approximate 10 g of linoleic acid ingested/day, only about 1 mg/day is eliminated as end products of AA metabolism. Following its formation, AA is esterified into cell membrane phospholipids, principally at position 2 of the phosphatidylinositol fraction (i.e., sn-2–esterified AA), the major hormone-sensitive pool of AA that is susceptible to release by phospholipases.

Multiple stimuli lead to the release of membrane-bound AA via the activation of cellular phospholipases, principally the phospholipase A2 family (PLA2).[2] This cleavage step is rate limiting in the production of biologically relevant arachidonate metabolites. In the case of PLA2 activation, membrane receptors activate guanine nucleotide-binding (G) proteins, leading to the release of AA directly from membrane phospholipids. Activation of PLC or PLD, on the other hand, releases AA via the sequential action of the phospholipase-mediated production of diacylglycerol (DAG), with the subsequent release of AA from DAG by DAG lipase.[3] This pathway may also lead to the formation of the esterified AA metabolites arachidonoylethanolamide (AEA) and 2-arachidonoylglycerol (2-AG), the endocannabinoids. These endocannabinoids can subsequently be converted to free AA by the action of monoacylglycerol lipases.[4] When considering eicosanoid formation, the physiologic significance of AA release by these other phospholipases remains uncertain because, at least in the setting of inflammation, PLA2 action appears to be essential for the generation of biologically active AA metabolites.[5]

More than 15 proteins with PLA2 activity are known to exist, including secreted (sPLA2) and cytoplasmic PLA2 (cPLA2) isoforms.[6,7] A mitogen-activated cytoplasmic PLA2 has been found to mediate AA release in a calcium-/calmodulin-dependent manner. Other hormones and growth factors, including epidermal growth factor (EGF) and platelet-derived growth factors, activate PLA2 directly through tyrosine residue kinase activity, allowing the recruitment of co-activators to the enzyme without an absolute requirement for the intermediate action of $Ca^{2+}$-calmodulin or other cellular kinases.

Following de-esterification, AA is rapidly re-esterified into membrane lipids or avidly bound by intracellular proteins, hence making AA unavailable for further metabolism. Should it escape re-esterification and protein binding, free AA becomes available as a substrate for one of three major enzymatic transformations, the common result of which is the incorporation of oxygen atoms at various sites of the fatty acid backbone, with accompanying changes in its molecular structure (e.g., ring formation).[8,9] This results in the formation of biologically active molecules, referred to as *eicosanoids*. The specific nature of the products generated is a function of the initial stimuli for AA release, as well as the metabolic enzyme available, which is determined, in part, by the cell type involved.[9,10]

These products, in turn, either mediate or modulate the biologic actions of the agonist in question. AA release may also result from nonspecific stimuli, such as cellular trauma, including ischemia and hypoxia,[11] oxygen free radicals,[12] and osmotic stress.[13] The identity of the specific AA metabolite generated in a particular cell system depends on the proximate stimulus and availability of the downstream AA metabolizing enzymes present in that cell.

Three major enzymatic pathways of free AA metabolism are present in the kidney—cyclooxygenases, lipoxygenases, and cytochrome P-450 (Fig. 13.1). The cyclooxygenase pathway mediates the formation of prostaglandins (PGs) and thromboxanes. The lipoxygenase pathway mediates the formation of mono-, di-, and trihydroxyeicosatetraenoic acids (HETEs), leukotrienes (LTs), and lipoxins (LXs). Whereas the cytochrome P-450– dependent oxygenation of AA mediates the formation of epoxyeicosatrienoic acids (EETs), their corresponding diols, HETEs, and monooxygenated AA derivatives. Fish oil diets, rich in ω-3 polyunsaturated fatty acids,[14] interfere with metabolism via all three pathways by competing with AA oxygenation, resulting in the formation of biologically inactive end products.[15] Interference with the production of proinflammatory lipids has been hypothesized to underlie the beneficial effects of fish oil in immunoglobulin A (IgA) nephropathy, and other cardiovascular diseases.[16] The following sections deal with the current understanding of the chemistry, biosynthesis, renal metabolism, mechanisms of release, receptor biology, signal transduction pathways, biologic activities, and functional significance of each of the metabolites generated by the three major routes of AA metabolism in the kidney.

## THE CYCLOOXYGENASE PATHWAY

See Fig. 13.2.

### MOLECULAR BIOLOGY

The cyclooxygenase (COX) enzyme system is the major pathway for AA metabolism in the kidney. COX (prostaglandin synthase G2/H2) is the enzyme responsible for the initial conversion of AA to prostaglandin G2 and subsequently to prostaglandin H2. The COX protein was first purified from ram seminal vesicles, and cDNA encoding COX was cloned in 1988. The protein is widely expressed, and the level of activity is not dynamically regulated. Other studies have supported the presence of a COX isoform that was dynamically regulated and responsible for increased prostanoid production in inflammation. This second inducible COX isoform was identified shortly after the cloning of the initial enzyme and designated as COX-2, whereas the initially isolated isoform is now designated as COX-1.[8,17,18] COX-1 and COX-2 are encoded by distinct genes located on different chromosomes. The human COX-1 gene (PTGS1 [prostaglandin synthase 1]) is distributed over 40 kB on 11 exons on chromosome 9, whereas COX-2 is localized on chromosome 1 and spans approximately 9 kB. The genes are also subject to dramatically different regulatory signals.

#### REGULATION OF COX GENE EXPRESSION

At the cellular level, COX-2 expression is highly regulated by several processes that alter its transcription rate, message

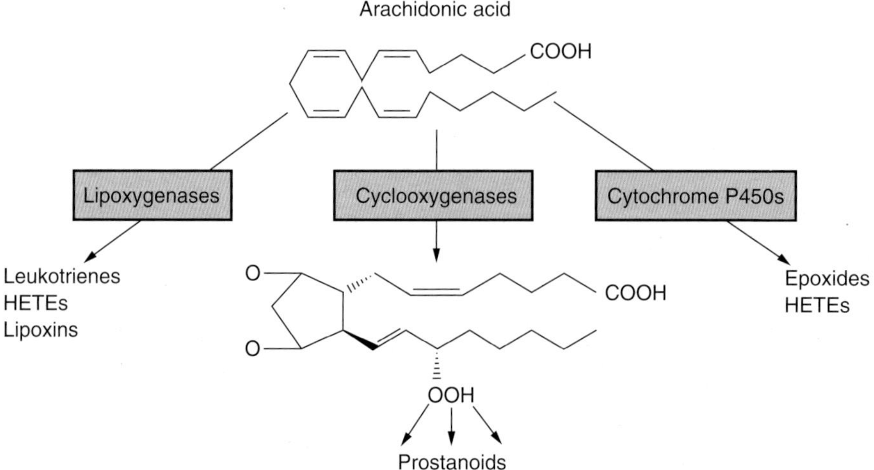


**Fig. 13.1** Pathways of enzymatically mediated arachidonic acid metabolism. Arachidonic acid can be converted into biologically active compounds by cyclooxygenase (COX), lipoxygenase (LOX), or cytochrome P450 (CYP450)–mediated metabolism. *HETE,* Hydroxyeicosatetraenoic acid.

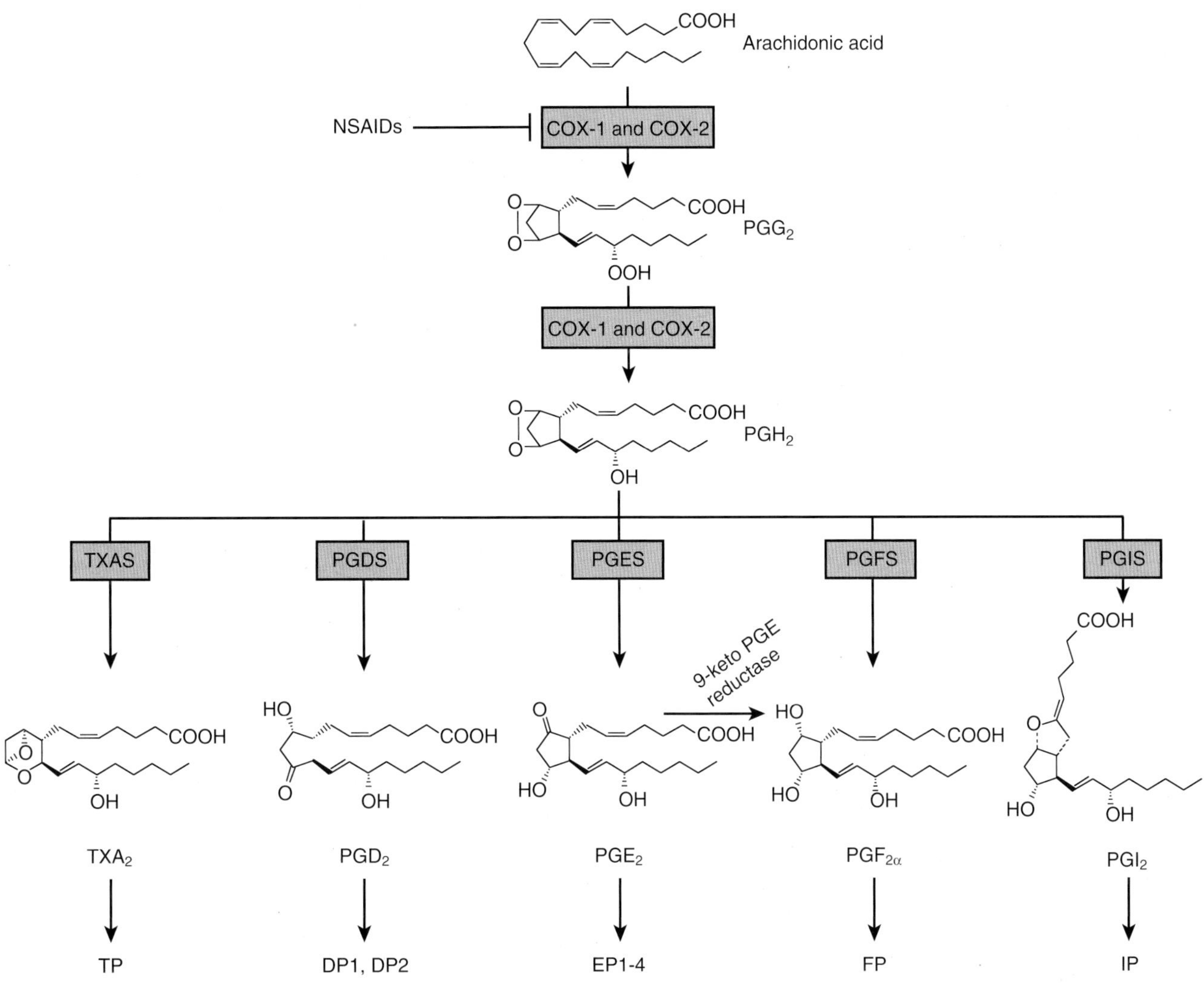


**Fig. 13.2** Cyclooxygenase (COX) metabolism of arachidonic acid (AA). Both COX-1 and COX-2 convert AA to prostaglandin (PG) H2 (PGH2), which is then acted on by specific synthases to produce prostanoids that act at G protein–coupled receptors that increase or decrease cyclic adenosine monophosphate (cAMP) or increase intracellular calcium. *NSAID,* Nonsteroidal antiinflammatory drug; *TXAS,* thromboxane synthase; *PGDS,* prostaglandin D synthase; *PGES,* prostaglandin E synthase; *PGFS,* prostaglandin F synthase; *PGIS,* prostacyclin synthase.

export from the nucleus, messenger RNA (mRNA) stability, and efficiency of mRNA translation.[19,20] These processes tightly control the expression of COX-2 in response to many of the same cellular stresses that activate arachidonate release (e.g., cell volume changes, shear stress, hypoxia),[11,21] as well as a variety of cytokines and growth factors, including tumor necrosis factor (TNF), interleukin-1ß, epidermal growth factor, and platelet-derived growth factor (PDGF). Activation of COX-2 gene transcription is mediated via the coordinated activation of several transcription factors that bind to and activate consensus sequences in the 5′ flanking region of the COX-2 gene for nuclear factor-kappa B (NF-κB), NF–IL-6/C–enhancer-binding protein (CEBP), and a cyclic adenosine monophosphate (cAMP) response element (CRE).[22] The induction of COX-2 mRNA transcription by endotoxin (lipopolysaccharide) may also involve CRE[23] and NF-κB sites.[24]

## REGULATION OF COX EXPRESSION BY ANTIINFLAMMATORY STEROIDS

A molecular basis linking the antiinflammatory effects of COX-inhibiting nonsteroidal antiinflammatory drugs (NSAIDs) and antiinflammatory glucocorticoids has long been sought. A novel mechanism for the suppression of arachidonate metabolism by corticosteroids involving the translational inhibition of COX formation had been suggested before the molecular recognition of COX-2. With the cloning of COX-2, it became well established that glucocorticoids suppress COX-2 expression and prostaglandin synthesis, an effect now viewed as central to the antiinflammatory effects of glucocorticoids. Posttranscriptional control of COX-2 expression represents another robust mechanism whereby adrenal steroids regulate COX-2 expression.[25] Accumulating evidence has suggested that COX-2 is modulated at multiple steps in addition to transcription rate, including stabilization of the mRNA and enhanced translation.[19,26] Glucocorticoids, including dexamethasone, downregulate COX-2 mRNA, in part by destabilizing the mRNA.[26] The 3′-untranslated region of the COX-2 mRNA contains 22 copies of an AUUUA motif, which are known cis-RNA sequences important in destabilizing the COX-2 message in response to dexamethasone; other 3′ sequences appear to be important for COX-2 mRNA stabilization in response to IL-1ß.[26] Effects of the 3′-untranslated region

(3′-UTR), as well as other factors regulating the efficiency of COX-2 translation, have also been suggested.[19] The factors determining the expression of COX-1 are more obscure.

## ENZYMATIC CHEMISTRY

Despite these differences, both prostaglandin (PG) synthases catalyze a similar reaction, resulting in the cyclization of C8 to C12 of the AA backbone, forming cyclic endoperoxide, accompanied by the concomitant insertion of two oxygen atoms at C15 to form PGG2 (a 15-hydroperoxide). In the presence of a reduced glutathione-dependent peroxidase, PGG2 is converted to the 15-hydroxy derivative, PGH2. The endoperoxides (PGG2 and PGH2) have very short half-lives, about 5 minutes, and are biologically active in inducing aortic contraction and platelet aggregation.[27] However, under some circumstances, the formation of these endoperoxides may be strictly limited via the self-deactivating properties of the enzyme.

The expression of recombinant enzymes and determination of the crystal structure of COX-2 have provided further insight into the observed physiologic and pharmacologic similarities to, and differences from, COX-1. It is now clear that NSAIDs work by inhibiting cyclooxygenases by sterically blocking access of AA to the heme-containing active enzymatic site.[28] Aspirin, also known as acetylsalicylic acid (ASA), predominantly targets COX-1. Particularly well conserved are COX-1 sequences surrounding the aspirin-sensitive serine residue at position 529 of COX-1, at which acetylation by aspirin irreversibly inhibits activity.[29] More recent evidence has shown that COX-1 and COX-2 are capable of forming heterodimers and sterically modulating each other's function.[30] The substrate-binding pocket of COX-2 is larger and therefore accepting of bulkier inhibitors and substrates. This difference has allowed the development and marketing of relatively and highly selective COX-2 inhibitors for clinical use as analgesics,[31] antipyretics,[32] and antiinflammatory agents.[31] In addition to its central role in inflammation, aberrantly upregulated COX-2 expression has been implicated in the pathogenesis of a number of epithelial cell carcinomas[33] and in Alzheimer disease and other degenerative neurologic conditions.[34]

## RENAL COX-1 AND COX-2 EXPRESSION

See Fig. 13.3.

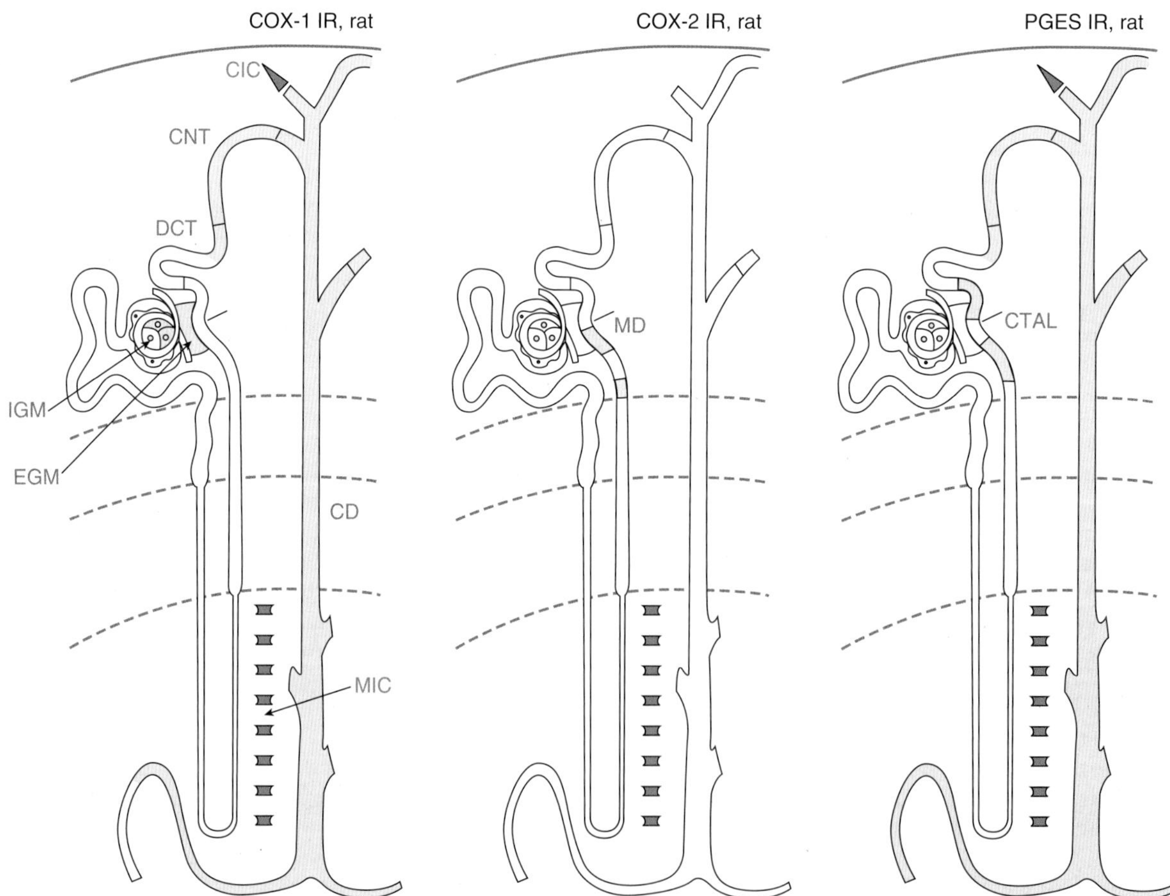


**Fig. 13.3** Localization (indicated in *blue shaded areas*) of immunoreactive (IR) cyclooxygenase 1 and 2 (COX-1, COX-2) and microsomal prostaglandin E synthase *(PGES)* along the rat nephron. Eicosanoid expression in cortical (CIC) and medullary (MIC) interstitial cells is shaded in *red*. *CD,* Collecting duct; *CNT,* connecting tubule; *CTAL,* cortical thick ascending limb; *DCT,* distal convoluted tubule; *EGM,* extraglomerular mesangium; *IGM,* intraglomerular mesangium; *MD,* macula densa. (Modified from Campean V, Theilig F, Paliege A, et al. Key enzymes for renal prostaglandin synthesis: site-specific expression in rodent kidney [rat, mouse]. *Am J Physiol Renal Physiol.* 2003;285:F19–F32.)

## COX-2 EXPRESSION

### COX-2 EXPRESSION IN THE KIDNEY

There is now definitive evidence for significant COX-2 expression in the mammalian kidney. This contrasts with the usual view that COX-2 is induced by cellular injury in other tissues, such as blood vessels. COX-2 mRNA and immunoreactive COX-2 are present at low but detectable levels in the normal adult mammalian kidney, where in situ mRNA hybridization and protein immunolocalization have demonstrated constitutive localized expression of COX-2 mRNA and immunoreactive protein in the cells of the macula densa and in a few cells in the cortical thick ascending limb (TAL) cells immediately adjacent to the macula densa.[35,36] COX-2 expression is also abundant in the lipid-laden medullary interstitial cells in the tip of the papilla.[35,37] Some investigators have reported that COX-2 may be expressed in inner medullary collecting duct cells or intercalated cells in the renal cortex in the collecting duct.[38] Nevertheless, COX-1 expression is also constitutive and clearly the most abundant isoform in the collecting duct, so the potential existence and physiologic significance of COX-2 co-expression in this segment remains uncertain.

### COX-2 EXPRESSION IN THE RENAL CORTEX

It is now well documented that COX-2 is expressed in macula densa–cortical thick ascending limb of Henle (cTALH) and in the mammalian kidney,[1,36] including the human kidney, especially in kidneys of older adults,[39,40] patients with diabetes mellitus, congestive heart failure,[41] and Bartter-like syndrome.[42]

The presence of COX-2 in the unique group of cells comprising the macula densa, points to a potential role for COX-2–derived prostanoids in regulating glomerular function.[43] Studies of the prostanoid-dependent control of the glomerular filtration rate (GFR) by the macula densa suggest effects via both dilator and constrictor effects of prostanoids contributing to tubuloglomerular feedback (TGF).[44,45] Some studies have suggested that COX-2–derived prostanoids are predominantly vasodilators.[46,47] By inhibiting the production of dilator prostanoids contributing to the patency of adjacent afferent arteriole, COX-2 inhibition may contribute to the decline in the GFR observed in patients taking NSAIDs or selective COX-2 inhibitors[48] (see later).

The volume-depleted state is typified by low NaCl delivery to the macula densa, and COX-2 expression in the macula densa is increased in states associated with volume depletion (Fig. 13.4).[35] Of note, COX-2 expression in cultured macula densa cells and cTAL cells is also increased in vitro by reducing the extracellular $Cl^-$ concentration. Studies in which cortical thick limbs and associated glomeruli were removed and perfused from rabbits pretreated with a low-salt diet to upregulate macula densa COX-2 demonstrated COX-2–dependent release of PGE2 from the macula densa in response to decreased chloride perfusate.[49] Furthermore the induction of COX-2 by low $Cl^-$ levels can be blocked by a specific p38 MAP kinase inhibitor.[50,51] Finally, in vivo, renal cortical immunoreactive pp38 expression (the active form of p38) predominantly localizes to the macula densa and cTALH and increases in response to a low-salt diet..[50] These findings point to a molecular pathway whereby enhanced COX-2 expression occurring in circumstances associated with intracellular volume depletion could result from decreased luminal chloride delivery. The carbonic anhydrase inhibitor, acetazolamide, and dopamine may both indirectly regulate macula densa COX-2 expression by inhibiting proximal reabsorption and thereby increasing luminal macula densa chloride delivery.[52,53] In mice deficient in the $Na^+$-$H^+$ exchanger subtype 2 (NHE2), the macula densa is shrunken, accompanied by increased COX-2 expression

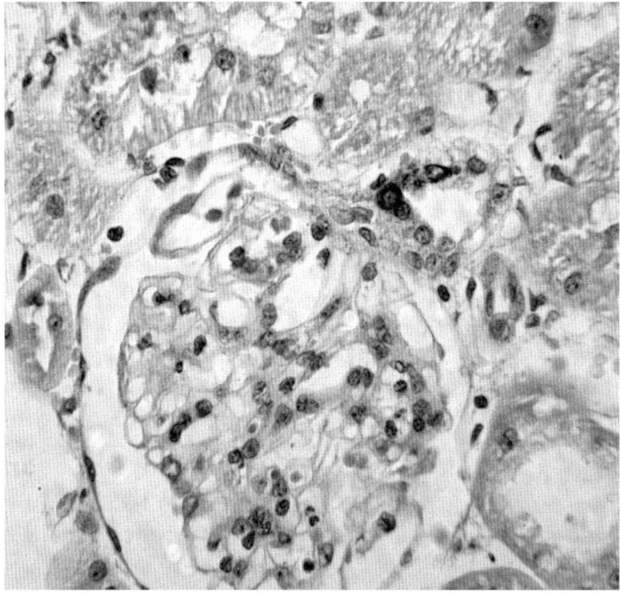

Control

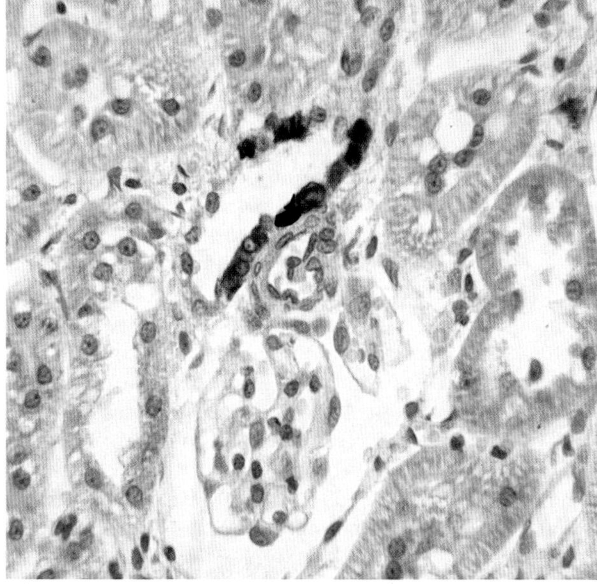

Low salt

**Fig. 13.4** Cyclooxygenase 2 (COX-2) expression is regulated in renal cortex in rats (original magnification: ×400). Under basal conditions, sparse immunoreactive COX-2 is localized to the macula densa and surrounding cortical thick ascending limb. Following chronic administration of a sodium-deficient diet, macula densa–cortical thick ascending limb COX-2 expression increases markedly.

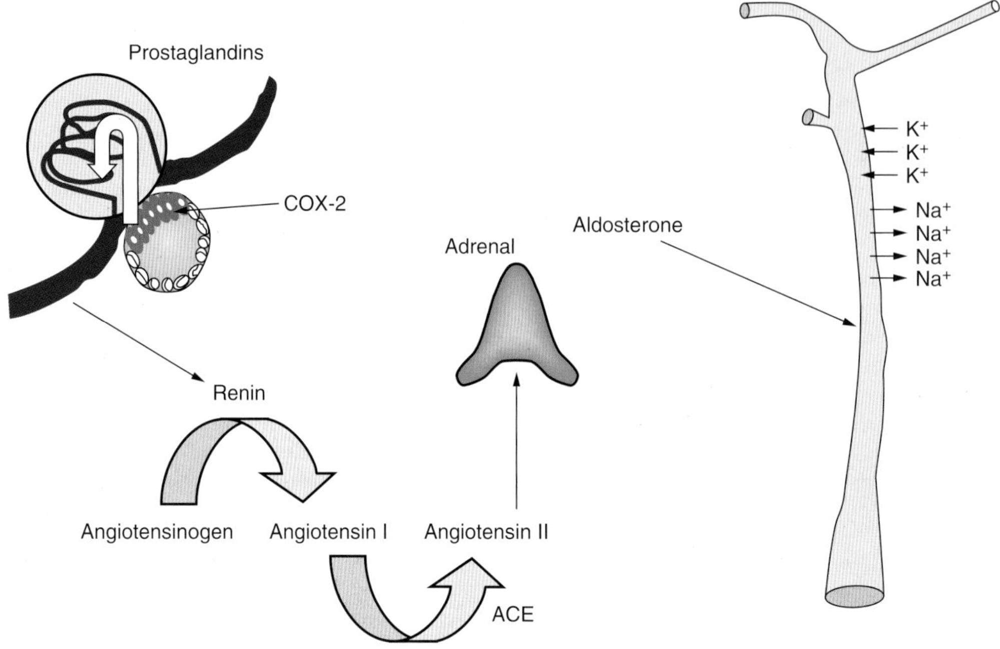


**Fig. 13.5** Proposed intrarenal roles for vasodilatory prostaglandins to regulate renal function and blood pressure control. Prostaglandins released from the macula densa and/or the afferent arteriole can vasodilate the afferent arteriole and modulate renin release from juxtaglomerular cells. *ACE,* Angiotensin-converting enzyme; *COX-2,* cyclooxygenase 2.

and juxtaglomerular renin expression, suggesting that NHE2 appears to be the major isoform associated with macula densa cell volume regulation.[54]

In the mammalian kidney, the macula densa is involved in regulating renin release by sensing alterations in luminal chloride via changes in the rate of $Na^+$-$K^+$-$2Cl^-$ cotransport (Fig. 13.5).[55] In vivo measurements in isolated perfused kidney and an isolated perfused juxtaglomerular preparation have all indicated that the administration of nonspecific COX inhibitors prevents the increases in renin release mediated by macula densa sensing of decreases in luminal NaCl.[44] Induction of a high-renin state by the imposition of a salt-deficient diet, angiotensin-converting enzyme (ACE) inhibition, diuretic administration, or experimental renovascular hypertension all significantly increase macula densa/cTALH COX-2 mRNA and immunoreactive protein levels.[43] COX-2–selective inhibitors blocked elevations in plasma renin activity, renal renin activity, and renal cortical renin mRNA in response to loop diuretics, ACE inhibitors, or a low-salt diet[43,56–58] and, in an isolated perfused juxtaglomerular preparation, increased renin release in response to lowering the perfusate NaCl concentration that was blocked by COX-2 inhibition.[59] In COX-2 knockout mice, increases in renin in response to low salt or ACE inhibitors were significantly blunted[60,61] but were unaffected in COX-1 knockout mice.[62,63] COX-2–derived PGE2, activating the type 4 (EP4) receptors on juxtaglomerular cells, has been shown to be important for the macula densa regulation of renin release.[49,64] Macula densa COX-2–derived prostanoids appear to be predominantly involved in setting tonic levels of juxtaglomerular renin expression rather than necessarily mediating acute renin release,[65,66] but PGE2 from macula densa does stimulate CD44+ mesenchymal stromal-like cells to migrate to the juxtaglomerular apparatus (JGA) and increase renin production, an effect mediated by EP4 receptors.[67] There is evidence that the effect of ACE inhibitors and angiotensin receptor blockers (ARBs) to increase macula densa COX-2 expression is mediated by feedback of angiotensin II on the macula densa, with AT1 and AT2 receptors inhibiting COX-2 expression.[56] In addition, prorenin and/or renin may stimulate macula densa COX-2 expression through activation of the prorenin receptor.[68]

COX-2 inhibitors have also been shown to decrease renin production in models of renovascular hypertension,[69,70] and studies in mice with targeted deletion of the prostacyclin receptor have suggested a predominant role for prostacyclin in mediating renin production and release in these models.[70] In a model of sepsis, COX-2 expression increased in macula densa and both cortical and medullary TAL. This increased COX-2 expression was mediated by Toll-like receptor 4 (TLR4) and, in $TLR4^{-/-}$ mice, JGA renin expression was absent.[71]

In addition to mediating juxtaglomerular renin expression, COX-2 metabolites may also modulate TGF. However, using different methodologies, investigators have reported that COX-2 metabolites predominantly modulate TGF by the production of vasodilatory prostanoids[47,72] or mediate afferent arteriolar vasoconstriction by activating thromboxane receptors through the generation of thromboxane A2 and/or PGH2.[73] Further studies will be required to reconcile these divergent results.

There is evidence that macula densa COX-2 expression is sensitive not only to alterations in intravascular volume but also to alterations in renal metabolism. Specifically, the G protein–coupled receptor, GPR91, has been shown to be a receptor for succinate, an intermediate of the citric acid cycle (Krebs cycle).[74] GPR91 is expressed in macula densa, and both GPR91 and the intrarenal production of succinate are increased in diabetes. Studies have suggested that succinate activation of GPR91 leads to increased macula densa COX-2 expression.[75,76]

## COX-2 EXPRESSION IN THE RENAL MEDULLA

The renal medulla is a major site of prostaglandin synthesis and abundant COX-1 and COX-2 expression (Fig. 13.6).[77] COX-1 and COX-2 exhibit differential compartmentalization within the medulla, with COX-1 predominating in the medullary collecting ducts and COX-2 predominating in medullary interstitial cells.[43] In the collecting duct, COX-2 has also been localized to intercalated cells but is absent in principal cells.[78] Intercalated cell COX-2 expression increases in response to angiotensin II (Ang II), and deletion exacerbates Ang II-mediated hypertension.[79] COX-2 may also be expressed in endothelial cells of the vasa recta supplying the inner medulla.

In medullary interstitial cells, dynamic regulation of COX-2 expression appears to be an important adaptive response to physiologic stresses, including water deprivation, increased dietary sodium, and exposure to endotoxins.[38,77,80,81] In contrast, COX-1 expression is unaffected by water deprivation. Although hormonal factors could also contribute to COX-2 induction, shifting cultured renal medullary interstitial cells to hypertonic media (using NaCl or mannitol) is sufficient to induce COX-2 expression directly. Because prostaglandins play an important role in maintaining renal function during volume depletion or water deprivation, induction of COX-2 by hypertonicity provides an important adaptive response.

As is the case for the macula densa, medullary interstitial cell COX-2 expression is transcriptionally regulated in response to renal extracellular salt and tonicity. Water deprivation and a high-sodium diet both induce COX-2 expression in medullary interstitial cells by activating the nuclear factor-kappa B (NF-κB) pathway.[77,81] There is also evidence that nitric oxide may modulate medullary COX-2 expression through mitogen-activated protein (MAP) kinase–dependent pathways.[82]

The mechanisms underlying the upregulation of medullary COX-2 expression in response to volume expansion are probably multifactorial. There is clear evidence that increased medullary tonicity increases medullary COX-2 expression. Different studies have indicated a role for NF-kB,[77] EGF receptor (EGFR) transactivation,[83] and mitochondria-generated reactive oxygen species (ROS).[84] Whether these represent parallel pathways or are all interrelated is not yet clear; however, it should be noted that the described EGFR transactivation is mediated by cleavage of the EGFR ligand, TGF-α, by ADAM17 (TACE), which is known to be activated by src, which can be activated by ROS. In addition to medullary COX-2, cortical COX-2 expression increases in salt-sensitive hypertension, especially in the glomerulus, and is inhibited by the superoxide dismutase mimetic, Tempol, or an ARB.[85] There is also recent evidence that COX-2 expression increases in renal macrophages in response to a high-salt diet, and selective inhibition of macrophage COX-2 expression exacerbates salt-sensitive hypertension.[86]

# COX-1 EXPRESSION

## COX-1 EXPRESSION IN THE KIDNEY

Although well-defined factors regulating COX-2 and determining the role of COX-2 expression in the kidney are coming to light, the role of renal COX-1 remains more obscure. COX-1 is constitutively expressed in platelets,[87] in the renal microvasculature, and glomerular parietal epithelial cells (Fig. 13.7). In addition, COX-1 is abundantly expressed in the collecting duct, but there is little COX-1 expressed in the

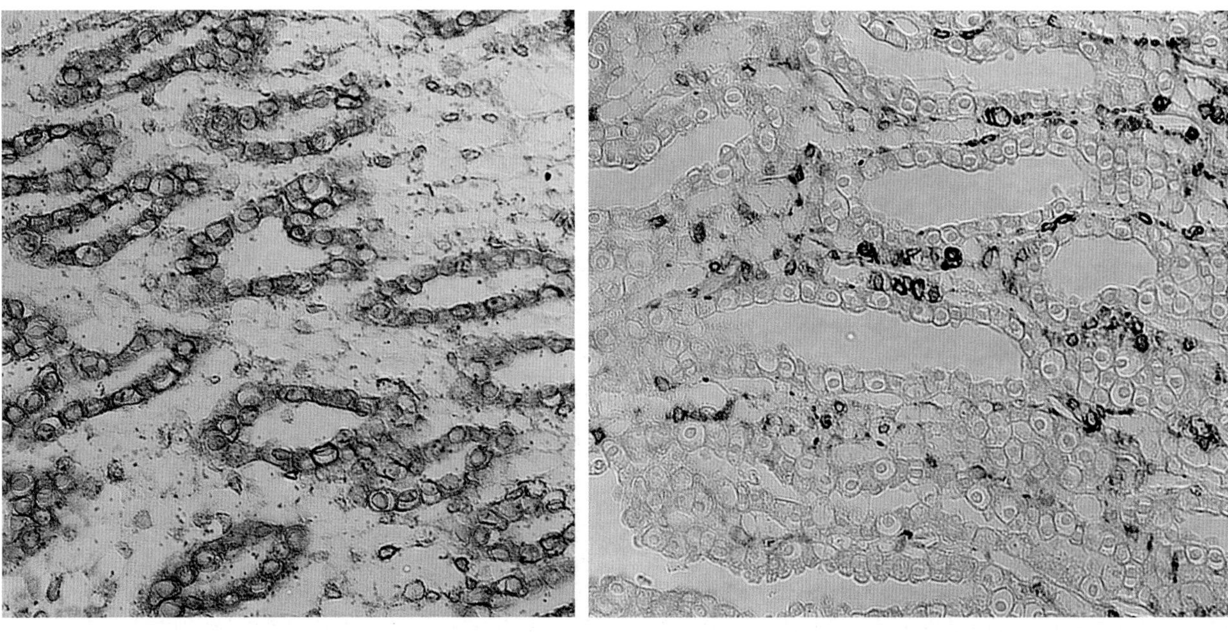


**Fig. 13.6** Differential immunolocalization of cyclooxygenase 1 (COX-1) and COX-2 in the renal medulla of rodents (original magnification ×250). COX-1 is predominantly localized to the collecting duct and is also found in a subset of medullary interstitial cells; COX-2 is predominantly localized to a subset of interstitial cells.

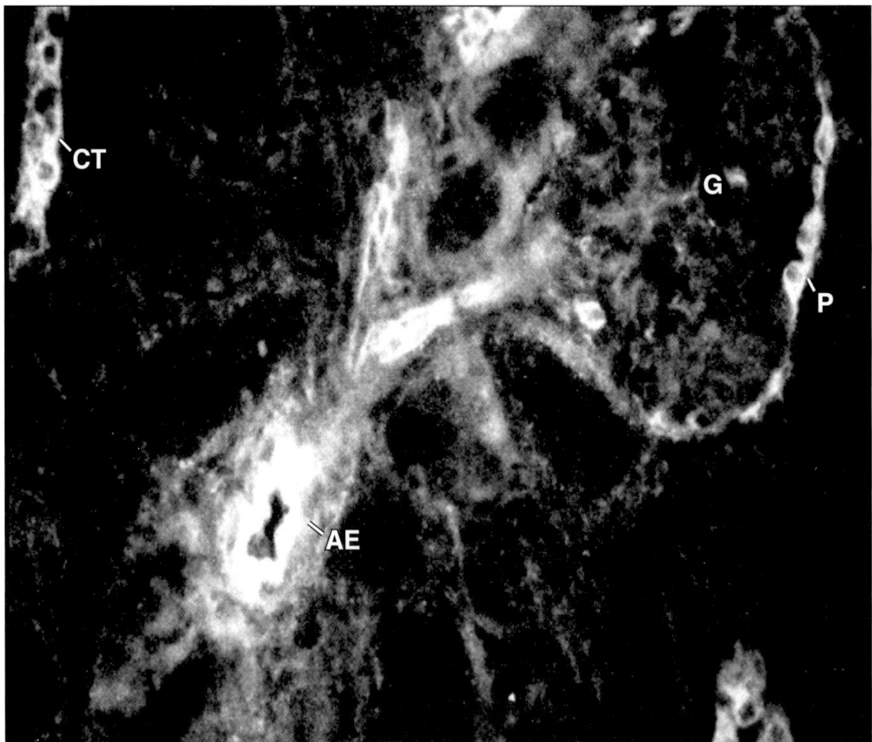


**Fig. 13.7** Renal cortical cyclooxygenase 1 (COX-1) expression. Immunoreactive COX-1 is predominantly localized to the afferent arteriole *(AE),* glomerular mesangial cells *(G),* parietal glomerular epithelial cells *(P),* and the cortical collecting tubule (CT). (Modified from Yokoyama C, Yabuki T, Shimonishi M, et al. Prostacyclin-deficient mice develop ischemic renal disorders, including nephrosclerosis and renal infarction. *Circulation.* 2002;106(18):2397–403.)

proximal tubule or TAL.[46,88] Although COX-1 expression levels do not appear to be dynamically regulated and, consistent with this observation, the COX-1 promoter does not possess a TATA box, vasopressin does increase COX-1 expression in collecting duct epithelial cells and in interstitial cells in the inner medulla.[88] The factors accounting for the tissue-specific expression of COX-1 are uncertain but may involve histone acetylation and the presence of two tandem Sp1 sites in the upstream promoter region of the gene.[89]

## RENAL COMPLICATIONS OF NONSTEROIDAL ANTIINFLAMMATORY DRUGS

### SODIUM RETENTION, EDEMA, AND HYPERTENSION

The use of nonselective NSAIDs may be complicated by the development of significant $Na^+$ retention, edema, congestive heart failure, and hypertension.[90] These complications are also apparent in patients using COX-2 selective NSAIDs. Studies with celecoxib and rofecoxib have demonstrated that like nonselective NSAIDs, these COX-2 selective NSAIDs reduce urinary sodium ($Na^+$) excretion and are associated with modest $Na^+$ retention in otherwise healthy subjects.[91,92] The evidence supporting a role for NSAID exacerbating hypertension, especially COX-2 inhibitors, continues to grow. COX-2 inhibition likely promotes salt retention via multiple mechanisms (Fig. 13.8). A reduced GFR may limit the filtered $Na^+$ load and salt excretion.[93,94] In addition, PGE2 directly inhibits $Na^+$ absorption in the TAL and collecting duct.[95] The relative abundance of COX-2 in medullary interstitial cells places this enzyme adjacent to both these nephron segments, allowing for COX-2–derived PGE2 to modulate salt absorption. COX-2 inhibitors decrease renal PGE2 production[91,96] and thereby may enhance renal sodium retention. Finally, a reduction in renal medullary blood flow by inhibition of vasodilator prostanoids may significantly reduce renal salt excretion and promote the development of edema and hypertension. COX-2–selective NSAIDs have been demonstrated to exacerbate salt-dependent hypertension.[97,98] Similarly, patients with preexisting treated hypertension commonly experience hypertensive exacerbations with COX-2–selective NSAIDs.[92] Taken together these data suggest that COX-2 selective NSAIDs have similar effects as nonselective NSAIDs with respect to salt excretion.

### HYPERKALEMIA

Nonselective NSAIDs cause hyperkalemia due to suppression of the renin-aldosterone axis. Both a decreased GFR and inhibition of renal renin release may compromise renal $K^+$ excretion. Patients on a salt-restricted diet also have decreased urinary potassium excretion when treated with a COX-2–selective inhibitor,[93,94] and COX-2–selective inhibitors may pose an equal or greater risk as nonselective NSAIDs for the development of hyperkalemia.[99]

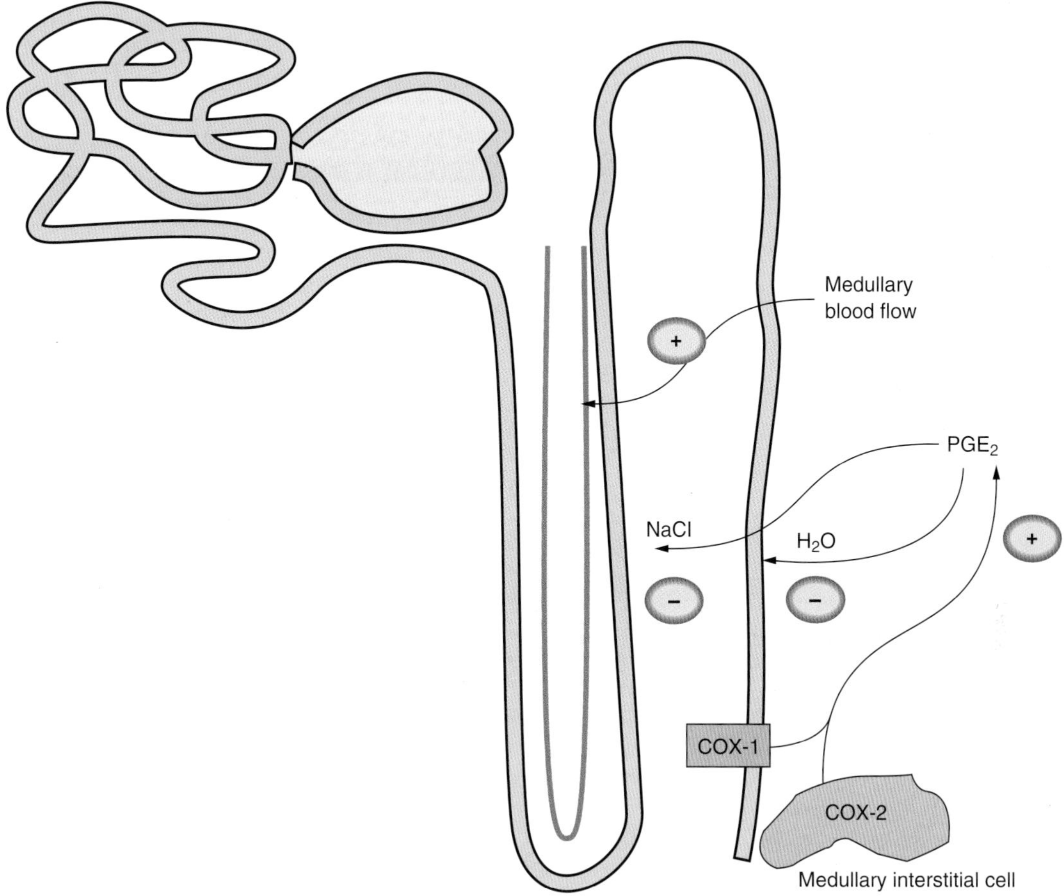


**Fig. 13.8** Integrated role of prostaglandin E2 *(PGE2)* on the regulation of salt and water excretion. PGE2 can both increase medullary blood flow and directly inhibit NaCl reabsorption in the medullary thick ascending limb (mTAL) and water reabsorption in the collecting duct. *COX-1,* Cyclooxygenase 1; *COX-2,* cyclooxygenase 2.

## PAPILLARY NECROSIS

Both acute and subacute forms of papillary necrosis have been observed with NSAID use.[100–102] Acute NSAID-associated renal papillary injury is more likely to occur in the setting of dehydration, suggesting a critical dependence of renal function on COX metabolism in this setting.[77] Long-term use of NSAIDs has been associated with papillary necrosis and progressive renal structural and functional deterioration, much like the syndrome of analgesic nephropathy observed with acetaminophen, aspirin, and caffeine combinations.[101] Experimental studies have suggested that renal medullary interstitial cells are an early target of injury in analgesic nephropathy.[103] COX-2 has been shown to be an important survival factor for cells exposed to a hypertonic medium.[37,77,104,105] The coincident localized expression of COX-2 in these interstitial cells[37,77] raises the possibility that like nonselective NSAIDs, long-term use of COX-2–selective NSAIDs may contribute to development of papillary necrosis.[106]

## ACUTE RENAL INSUFFICIENCY

Acute kidney injury (AKI) is a well-described complication of NSAID use.[90] This is generally considered to be a result of altered intrarenal microcirculation and glomerular filtration secondary to the inability to produce beneficial endogenous prostanoids when the kidney is dependent on them for normal function. Like the traditional nonselective NSAIDs, COX-2–selective NSAIDs will also reduce glomerular filtration in susceptible patients.[90] Although rare overall, NSAID-associated renal insufficiency occurs in a significant proportion of patients with underlying volume depletion, renal insufficiency, congestive heart failure, diabetes, and old age.[90] These risk factors are additive and rarely are present in patients included in study cohorts used for a safety assessment of these drugs. It is therefore relevant that the COX-2–selective inhibitors celecoxib and rofecoxib cause a slight but significant fall in the GFR rate in salt-depleted but otherwise healthy subjects.[93,94] Similar to nonselective NSAIDs, AKI can occur also secondary to COX-2–selective NSAIDs.[48,107] Preclinical studies have supported the concept that the inhibition of COX-2–derived prostanoids generated in the macula densa contributes to a fall in the GFR by reducing the diameter of the afferent arteriole. In vivo video microscopy studies have documented a reduced afferent arteriolar diameter following the administration of a COX-2 inhibitor.[47] These animal data not only support the concept that COX-2 plays an important role in regulating the GFR but also the clinical observations that COX-2–selective inhibitors can cause renal insufficiency similar to that reported with nonselective NSAIDs.

### INTERSTITIAL NEPHRITIS

The gradual development of renal insufficiency characterized by a subacute inflammatory interstitial infiltrate may occur after several months of continuous NSAID ingestion. Less commonly, the interstitial nephritis and renal failure may be fulminant. The infiltrate is typically accompanied by eosinophils; however, the clinical picture is typically much less dramatic than classic drug-induced allergic interstitial nephritis, lacking fever or rash.[108] This syndrome has also been reported with the COX-2–selective drug celecoxib.[109,110] Dysregulation of the immune system is thought to play an important role in the syndrome, which typically abates rapidly following discontinuation of the NSAID or COX-2 inhibitor.

### NEPHROTIC SYNDROME

Like interstitial nephritis, nephrotic syndrome typically occurs in patients chronically ingesting any one of a myriad of NSAIDs over the course of months.[108,111] The renal pathology is usually consistent with minimal change disease, with foot process fusion of glomerular podocytes observed on electron microscopy (EM), but membranous nephropathy has also been reported.[112] Typically, the nephrotic syndrome occurs together with the interstitial nephritis.[108] Nephrotic syndrome without interstitial nephritis may occur, as well as immune-complex glomerulopathy, in a small subset of patients receiving NSAIDs. It remains uncertain whether this syndrome results from mechanism-based COX inhibition by these drugs, an idiosyncratic immune drug reaction, or a combination of both.

### RENAL DYSGENESIS

Reports of renal dysgenesis and oligohydramnios in the offspring of women administered nonselective NSAIDs during the third trimester of pregnancy have implicated prostaglandins in the process of normal renal development.[113,114] A similar syndrome of renal dysgenesis has been reported in mice, with targeted disruption of the COX-2 gene, as well as mice treated with the specific COX-2 inhibitor SC58236.[115] Because neither COX-$1^{-/-}$ mice or mice treated with the COX-1 selective inhibitor SC58560 exhibited altered renal development, a specific role for COX-2 in nephrogenesis has been suggested.[116–118] A report of renal dysgenesis in the infant of a woman exposed to the COX-2–selective inhibitor nimesulide has suggested that COX-2 also plays a role in renal development in humans.[113]

The intrarenal expression of COX-2 in the developing kidney peaks in mice at postnatal day 4 and in the rat in the second postnatal week.[115,119] It has not yet been determined if a similar pattern of COX-2 is seen in human kidneys. Although the most intense staining is observed in a small subset of cells in the nascent macula densa and cortical TAL, expression in the papilla has also been observed.[115,119] In vitro studies have shown that exogenous PGE2 promotes renal metanephric development[120] and is a critical growth factor for renal epithelia cells; studies in zebrafish have indicated that PGE2, acting through EP2 and EP4, is a regulator of nephron formation in the zebrafish embryonic kidney.[121] Studies have indicated that angiotensin II–AT1 receptor signaling mediates COX-2–dependent postnatal development in mice.[122]

## CARDIOVASCULAR EFFECTS OF COX-2 INHIBITORS

### EFFECTS OF COX-2 INHIBITION ON VASCULAR TONE

In addition to their propensity to reduce renal salt excretion and decrease medullary blood flow, NSAIDs and selective COX-2 inhibitors have been shown to exert direct effects on systemic resistance vessels. The acute pressor effect of angiotensin infusion in human subjects was significantly increased by pretreatment with the nonselective NSAID indomethacin at all Ang II doses. The administration of selective COX-2 inhibitors or COX-2 gene knockout has been shown to accentuate the pressor effects of Ang II in mice.[46] These studies have also demonstrated that Ang II-mediated blood pressure increases are markedly reduced by the administration of a selective COX-1 inhibitor or in COX-1 gene knockout mice.[46] These findings support the conclusion that COX-1–derived prostaglandins participate in, and are integral to, the pressor activity of Ang II, whereas COX-2–derived prostaglandins are vasodilators that oppose and mitigate the pressor activity of Ang II. Other animal studies have shown more directly that that both NSAIDs and COX-2 inhibitors blunt arteriolar dilation and decrease flow through resistance vessels.[123]

### INCREASED CARDIOVASCULAR THROMBOTIC EVENTS

COX-2 is known to be induced in vascular endothelial cells in response to shear stress,[124] and selective COX-2 inhibition reduces circulating prostacyclin levels in normal human subjects.[125] Therefore, increasing evidence has indicated that COX-2–selective antagonism may carry increased thrombogenic risks due to selective inhibition of the endothelial-derived antithrombogenic prostacyclin without any inhibition of the prothrombotic platelet-derived thromboxane generated by COX-1.[126] Although animal studies have provided conflicting results about the role of COX-2 inhibition on development of atherosclerosis,[127–131] there have been recent indications that COX-2 inhibition may destabilize atherosclerotic plaques.[132] This has been suggested by studies indicating increased COX-2 expression and colocalization with microsomal PGE synthase-1 and metalloproteinases-2 and -9 in carotid plaques from individuals with symptomatic disease before endarterectomy.[133] Because of the concerns about increased cardiovascular risk, two selective COX-2 inhibitors, rofecoxib and valdecoxib, have been withdrawn from the market, and remaining coxibs and other NSAIDs have been relabeled to highlight the increased risk for cardiovascular events.

## PROSTANOIDS

### PROSTANOID SYNTHASES

Once PGH2 is formed in the cell, it can undergo a number of possible transformations, yielding biologically active prostaglandins and thromboxane A2. As seen in Fig. 13.9,

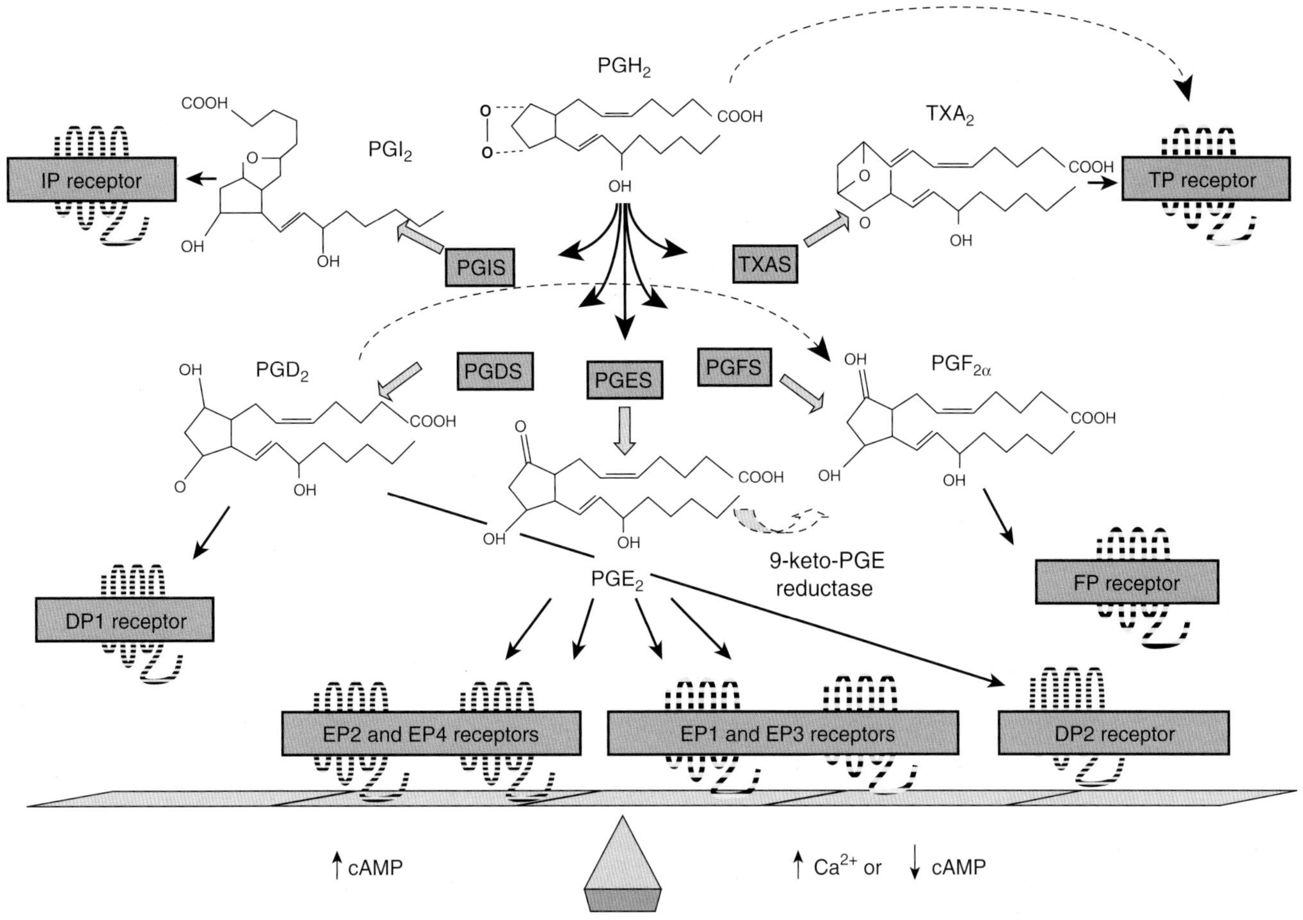


**Fig. 13.9** Prostaglandin synthases. *cAMP,* Cyclic adenosine monophosphate; *PGDS,* prostaglandin D synthase; *PGES,* prostaglandin E synthase; *PGFS,* prostaglandin F synthase; *PGIS,* prostacyclin synthase; *TXAS,* thromboxane synthase.

in the presence of isomerase and reductase enzymes, PGH2 is converted to PGE2 and PGF2α, respectively. Thromboxane synthase converts PGH2 into a bicyclic oxetane-oxane ring metabolite, thromboxane A2 (TXA2), a prominent reaction product in platelets and an established synthetic pathway in the glomerulus. Prostacyclin synthase, a 50-kDa protein located in plasma and nuclear membranes and found mostly in vascular endothelial cells, catalyzes the biosynthesis of prostacyclin (PGI2). PGD2, the major prostaglandin product in mast cells, is also derived directly from PGH2, but its role in the kidney is uncertain. The enzymatic machinery and their localization in the kidney are discussed in detail later.

## SOURCES AND NEPHRONAL DISTRIBUTION OF COX PRODUCTS

COX activity is present in arterial and arteriolar endothelial cells, including glomerular afferent and efferent arterioles.[43] The predominant metabolite from these vascular endothelial cells is PGI2.[134,135] Whole glomeruli generate PGE2, PGI2, PGF2α, and TXA2.[1] The predominant products in rat and rabbit glomeruli are PGE2, followed by PGI2 and $PGF_{2\alpha}$ and finally TXA2.

Analyses of individual cultured glomerular cell subpopulations have also provided insight into the localization of prostanoid synthesis. Cultured mesangial cells are capable of generating PGE2 and, in some cases, PGF2α and PGI2 have also been detected.[136] Other studies have suggested that mesangial cells may produce the endoperoxide PGH2 as a major COX product.[137] Glomerular epithelial cells also appear to participate in prostaglandin synthesis, but the profile of COX products generated in these cells remains controversial. Immunocytochemical studies of rabbit kidney have demonstrated intense staining for COX-1, predominantly in the parietal epithelial cells. Glomerular capillary endothelial cell PG generation profiles remain undefined but may well include prostacyclin.

The predominant synthetic site of PG synthesis along the nephron is the collecting duct (CD), particularly its medullary portion (MCT).[138] In the presence of exogenous arachidonic acid, PGE2 is the predominant PG formed in the collecting duct, the variations among the other products being insignificant.[1] PGE2 is also the major COX metabolite generated in medullary interstitial cells.[139] The role that specific prostanoid synthases may play in the generation of these products is outlined subsequently.

### Thromboxane Synthase

TXA2 is produced from PGH2 by thromboxane synthase (TXAS), a microsomal protein of 533 amino acids with a predicted molecular weight of around 60 kDa. The amino acid sequence of the enzyme exhibits homology to the cytochrome P-450s and is now classified as CYP5A1.[140] The human gene is localized on chromosome 7q and spans 180 kB. TXAS mRNA is highly expressed in hematopoietic cells, including platelets, macrophages, and leukocytes. TXAS mRNA is expressed in the thymus, kidney, lung, spleen, prostate, and placenta. Immunolocalization of TXAS demonstrates high expression in the dendritic cells of the interstitium, with lower expression in glomerular podocytes of human kidney.[141] TXA2 synthase expression is regulated by dietary salt intake.[142] Furthermore, the experimental use of ridogrel, a specific TXAS inhibitor, reduced blood pressure in spontaneously hypertensive rats.[143] The clinical use of TXA2 synthase inhibitors is complicated by the fact that its endoperoxide precursors (PGG2 and PGH2) are also capable of activating its downstream target, the TP receptor.[27]

#### Prostacyclin Synthase

The biologic effects of prostacyclin are numerous. They include nociception, antithrombosis, and vasodilator actions, which have been targeted therapeutically to treat pulmonary hypertension.

PGI2 is produced by the enzymatic conversion of PGH2 via prostacyclin synthase (PGIS). The cloned cDNA contains a 1500–base pair open reading frame that encodes a 500–amino acid protein of approximately 56 kDa. The human prostacyclin synthase gene is present as a single-copy haploid genome and is localized on chromosome 20q. Northern blot analysis shows that prostacyclin synthase mRNA is widely expressed in human tissues and is particularly abundant in the ovary, heart, skeletal muscle, lung, and prostate. PGI synthase expression exhibits segmental expression in the kidney, especially in kidney inner medulla tubules and interstitial cells.

PGI2 synthase null mice[144] have reduced PGI2 levels in the plasma, kidneys, and lungs, documenting the role of this enzyme as an in vivo source of PGI2. Blood pressure and blood urea nitrogen and creatinine levels in the PGIS knockout mice were significantly increased, and renal pathologic findings included surface irregularity, fibrosis, cysts, arterial sclerosis, and hypertrophy of vessel walls. Thickening of the thoracic aortic media and adventitia were observed in aged PGI null mice.[144] Interestingly, this is a distinct phenotype from that reported for the IP receptor knockout mouse.[145] These differences point to the presence of additional IP-independent PGI2-activated signaling pathways. Regardless, these findings demonstrate the importance of PGI2 to the maintenance of blood vessels and to the kidney.

#### Prostaglandin D Synthase

Prostaglandin D2 is derived from PGH2 via the action of specific enzymes designated as PGD synthases. Two major enzymes are capable of transforming PGH2 to $PGD_2$, including a lipocalin-type PGD synthase and a hematopoietic-type PGD synthase.[146,147] Mice lacking the lipocalin D synthase gene exhibit altered sleep and pain sensation.[148] PGD2 is the major prostanoid released from mast cells following challenge with immunoglobulin E (IgE). The kidney also appears capable of synthesizing PGD2. RNA for the lipocalin type PGD synthase has been reported to be widely expressed along the rat nephron, whereas the hematopoietic type of PGD synthase is restricted to the collecting duct.[149] Urinary excretion of lipocalin D synthase has been proposed as a biomarker predictive of renal injury,[150] and lipocalin D synthase knockout mice appear to be more prone to diabetic nephropathy.[151] However, the physiologic roles of these enzymes in the kidney remain less certain. Once synthesized, PGD2 is available to interact with the DP1 or DP2 receptors (see later) or undergo further metabolism to a PGF2α-like compound.

#### Prostaglandin F Synthesis

PGF2a is a major urinary COX product. It may be synthesized either directly from PGH2 via a PGF synthase[152] or indirectly by metabolism of PGE2 via a 9-ketoreductase.[152] Another more obscure pathway for PGF formation is by the action of a PGD2 ketoreductase, yielding a stereoisomer of PGF2α9a, 11ß-PGF2 (11epi-PGF2α).[152] This reaction, and the conversion of PGD2 into an apparently biologically active metabolite (9a,11b-PGF2α) has been documented in vivo.[153] Interestingly, this isomer can also ligate and activate the FP receptor.[154] The physiologically relevant enzymes responsible for renal PGF2α formation remain incompletely characterized.

#### Prostaglandin 9 Ketoreductase

Physiologically relevant transformations of COX products occur in the kidney via a nicotinamide adenine dinucleotide phosphate (NADPH)–dependent 9-ketoreductase, which converts PGE2 into PGF2α. This enzymatic activity is typically cytosolic[152] and may be detected in homogenates from the renal cortex, medulla, or papilla. The activity appears to be particularly robust in suspensions from the TALH. Renal PGE2 9-ketoreductase also exhibits 20α-hydroxysteroid reductase activity that could affect steroid metabolism.[152] This enzyme appears to be a member of the aldoketoreductase family 1C.[155]

Interestingly, some studies have suggested that activity of a 9-ketoreductase may be modulated by salt intake and $AT_2$ receptor activation and may play an important role in hypertension.[156] Mice deficient in the $AT_2$ receptor exhibit salt-sensitive hypertension, increased PGE2 production, and reduced production of PGF2α,[157] consistent with reduced 9-ketoreductase activity. Other studies have suggested that dietary potassium intake may also enhance the activity of conversion from PGE2 to PGF2α.[158] The intrarenal sites of expression of this enzymatic activity remain to be characterized.

#### Prostaglandin E Synthases

PGE2 is the other major product of COX-initiated AA metabolism in the kidney and is synthesized at high rates along the nephron, particularly in the collecting duct. Two membrane-associated PGE2 synthases have been identified, a 33-kDa and a 16-kDa membrane-associated enzyme.[159,160] The initial report describing the cloning of a glutathione-dependent microsomal enzyme (the 16-kDa form) that specifically converts PGH2 to PGE2[160] noted that mRNA for this enzyme is highly expressed in reproductive tissues, as well as in kidney. Genetic disruption confirms that $mPGES1^{-/-}$ mice exhibit a marked reduction in inflammatory responses compared with $mPGES1^{+/+}$[161] and indicate that mPGES1 is also critical for the induction of inflammatory fever.[162]

Intrarenal expression of mPGES1 has been demonstrated and mapped to the collecting duct, with lower expression in medullary interstitial cells and the macula densa[138,163] (see Fig. 13.3). Thus, in the kidney, this isoform colocalizes with both COX-1 and COX-2. In contrast, in inflammatory cells, this PGE synthase is co-induced with COX-2 and appears to be functionally coupled to it.[164] Notably, the kidneys of mPGES1$^{-/-}$ mice are normal and do not exhibit the renal dysgenesis observed in COX-2$^{-/-}$ mice,[117,165] nor do these mice exhibit perinatal death from a patent ductus arteriosus, which is observed with the prostaglandin EP4 receptor knockout mouse.[166]

More recently, another membrane-associated PGE synthase, with a relative mass of around 33 kDa, was purified from the heart. The recombinant enzyme was activated by several thiol (SH)-reducing reagents, including dithiothreitol, glutathione (GSH), and betamercaptoethanol. Moreover, the mRNA distribution was high in the heart and brain and was also expressed in the kidney, but the mRNA was not expressed in the seminal vesicles. The intrarenal distribution of this enzyme is, at present, uncharacterized.[159]

Other cytosolic proteins exhibit lower PGE synthase activity, including a 23-kDa glutathione S-transferase (GST) requiring cytoplasmic, PGES,[167] that is expressed in the kidney and lower genitourinary tract.[168] Some evidence has suggested that this isozyme may constitutively couple to COX-1 in inflammatory cells. In addition, several cytosolic glutathione-S-transferases have the capability to convert PGH2 to PGE2; however, their physiologic role in this process remains uncertain.[169]

## PROSTANOID RECEPTORS

See Figs. 13.10 and 13.11.

### TP RECEPTORS

The TP receptor was originally purified by chromatography using a high-affinity ligand to capture the receptor.[170] This was the first eicosanoid receptor cloned; it is a G protein–coupled transmembrane receptor capable of activating a calcium-coupled signaling mechanism. Other prostanoid receptors were cloned by finding cDNAs homologous to this TP receptor cDNA. Two alternatively spliced variants of the human thromboxane receptor have been described[171] that differ in their carboxyl-terminal tail distal to arginine (Arg). Similar patterns of alternative splicing have been described for both the EP3 and FP receptors.[172] Heterologous cAMP-mediated signaling of the thromboxane receptor may occur via its heterodimerization with the prostacyclin (IP) receptor.[173]

Either the endoperoxide, PGH2, or its metabolite, TXA2, can activate the TP receptor.[27] Competition radioligand binding studies have demonstrated a rank order of potency on the human platelet TP receptor of the ligands I-BOP—S145 > SQ29548 > $STA_2$ > U-46619.[174,175] Whereas I-BOP, $STA_2$, and U-46619 are agonists, SQ29548 and S145 are high-affinity TP receptor antagonists.[176] Studies have suggested that the TP receptor may mediate some of the biologic effects of the nonenzymatically-derived isoprostanes,[177] including modulation of tubuloglomerular feedback.[178] This latter finding may have significance in pathophysiologic conditions associated with increased oxidative stress.[179] Signal transduction studies have shown that the TP receptor activates phosphatidylinositol hydrolysis ($PIP_2$)–dependent $Ca^{2+}$ influx.[170,180] Quantitative polymerase chain reaction (PCR) analysis of mouse tissues has revealed that the highest level of TP mRNA expression is in the thymus, followed by the aorta, adrenal gland, vena cava, and spleen, with lower levels of expression in the pituitary gland, kidney, uterus, and brain.[181]

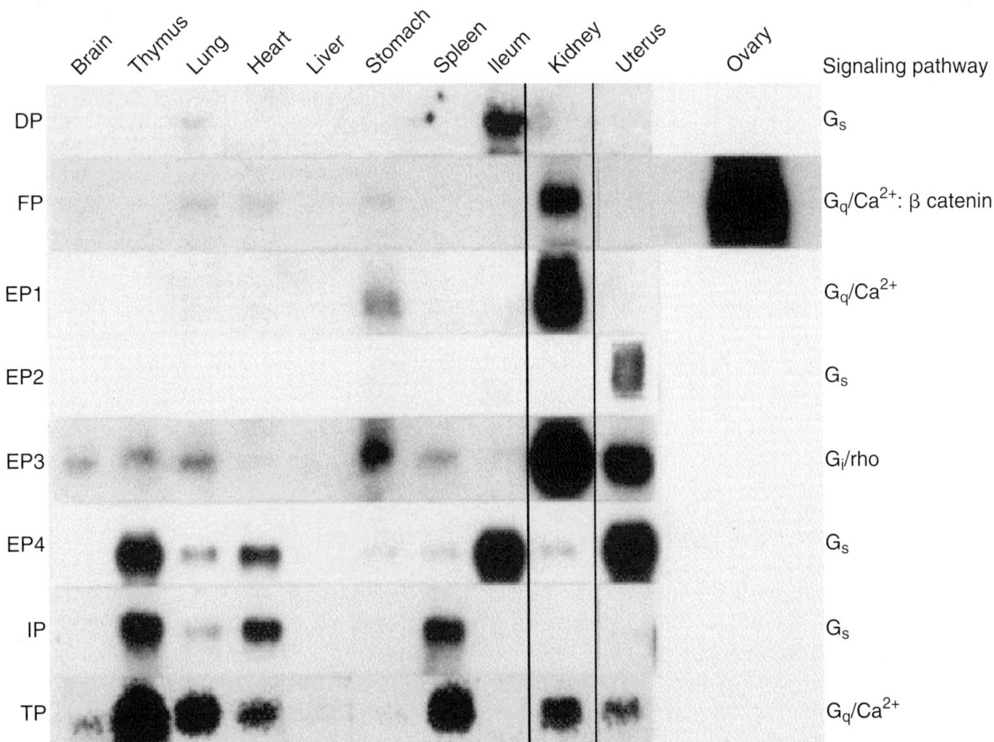


**Fig. 13.10** Tissue distribution of prostanoid receptor mRNA. (Modified from Chaudhari A, Gupta S, Kirschenbaum M. Biochemical evidence for PGI2 and PGE2 receptors in the rabbit renal preglomerular microvasculature. *Biochim Biophys Acta.* 1990;1053(2-3):156–161.)

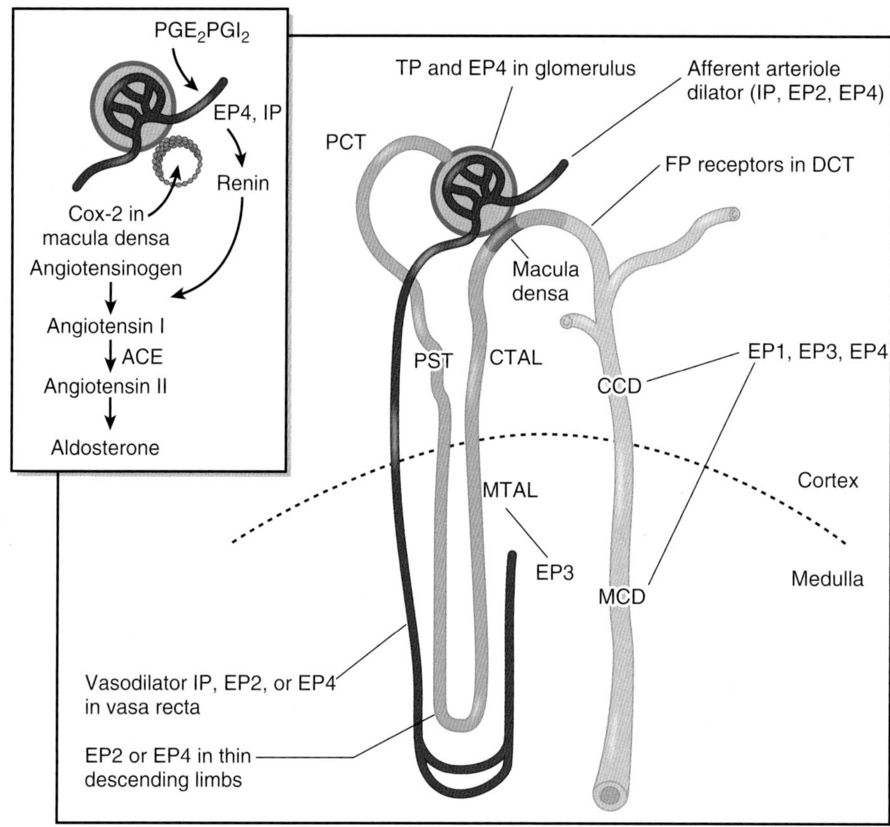


**Fig. 13.11** Intrarenal localization of prostanoid receptors. *Inset,* Prostanoid signaling in the juxtaglomerular apparatus.

**Table 13.1 Published Phenotypes of Prostanoid Receptor Knockout Mice**

| Receptor | Renal Expression | Renal Phenotype | Other Knockout Phenotypes |
|---|---|---|---|
| DP1 | Minimal? | No | Reduced allergic asthma, reduced niacin flushing |
| DP2 | Minimal? | ++ Reduced fibrosis in UUO | Decreased cutaneous inflammatory responses |
| IP | ++ Afferent arterioles | ± | Reduced inflammation, increased thrombosis |
| TP | + Glomerulus, tubules? | No | Prolonged bleeding time, platelet defect |
| FP | +++ Distal tubules | No | Failure of parturition |
| EP1 | ++++ MCD | No | Decreased Ang II hypertension |
| EP2 | ++ Interstitial stromal | ++ Salt-sensitive hypertension | Impaired female fertility |
| EP3 | ++++ TAL, MCD | + | Impaired febrile response |
| EP4 | +++ Glomerulus, + distal tubules | ++ Reduced fibrosis in UUO | Perinatal death from persistent patent ductus arteriosus |

*Ang II,* Angiotensin II; *MCD,* medullary collecting duct; *TAL,* thick ascending limb; *UUO,* unilateral ureter obstruction.

TX is a potent modulator of platelet shape change and aggregation, as well as smooth muscle contraction and proliferation. Moreover, a point mutation (Arg$^{60}$ to leucine [Leu]) in the first cytoplasmic loop of the TXA2 receptor was identified in a dominantly inherited bleeding disorder in humans, characterized by a defective platelet response to TXA2.[182] Targeted gene disruption of the murine TP receptor also resulted in prolonged bleeding times and a reduction in collagen-stimulated platelet aggregation (Table 13.1). Conversely, overexpression of the TP receptor in vascular tissue increases the severity of vascular pathology following injury.[1] Increased thromboxane synthesis has been linked to cardiovascular diseases, including acute myocardial ischemia, heart failure, and inflammatory renal diseases.[1]

In the kidney, TP receptor mRNA has been reported in the glomeruli and vasculature. Radioligand autoradiography using $^{125}$I-BOP has suggested a similar distribution of binding sites in mouse renal cortex, but additional renal medullary binding sites were observed.[183] These medullary TXA2 binding sites are absent following disruption of the TP receptor gene, suggesting that they also represent authentic TP receptors.[184] Glomerular TP receptors may participate in potent vasoconstrictor effects of TXA2 analogues on the glomerular microcirculation associated with a reduced GFR.[1] Mesangial TP receptors coupled to phosphatidylinositol hydrolysis, protein kinase C activation, and glomerular mesangial cell contraction may also contribute to these effects.[185]

An important role for TP receptors in regulating renal hemodynamics and systemic blood pressure has also been suggested. Administration of a TP receptor antagonist reduces blood pressure in spontaneously hypertensive rats (SHRs)[143] and in angiotensin-dependent hypertension.[186] The TP receptor also appears to modulate renal blood flow in Ang II–dependent hypertension[187] and in endotoxemia-induced renal failure.[188] Modulation of renal TP receptor mRNA expression and function by dietary salt intake has also been reported.[189] These studies have also suggested an important role for luminal TP receptors in the distal tubule to enhance glomerular vasoconstriction indirectly via effects on the macula densa and TGF.[190] However, other studies have revealed no significant difference in tubuloglomerular feedback between wild-type and TP receptor knockout mice.[45]

A major phenotype of TP receptor disruption in mice and humans appears to be reduced platelet aggregation and prolonged bleeding time.[184] TX may also modulate the glomerular fibrinolytic system by increasing the production of an inhibitor of plasminogen activator-1 (PAI-1) in mesangial cells, which would promote fibrin accumulation.[191] Although a specific renal phenotype in the TP receptor knockout mouse has not yet been reported, important pathogenic roles for TXA2 and glomerular TP receptors in mediating renal dysfunction in glomerulonephritis, diabetes mellitus, and sepsis seem likely.

In an Ang II-dependent mouse model of hypertension, deletion of the TP receptor gene ameliorated hypertension and reduced cardiac hypertrophy, but had no effect on proteinuria.[192] In NG-nitro-L-arginine methyl ester (L-NAME) hypertension, TP receptors again contributed to elevated blood pressure and cardiac hypertrophy. However, in this same model, TP receptors also provided unexpected protection against kidney injury—TP deletion led to an increase in worsening of histopathology and significant renal hypertrophy. This suggested that the TP receptor may play a renal protective role in some settings.[193]

## PROSTACYCLIN RECEPTORS

The cDNA for the IP receptor encodes a transmembrane protein of approximately 41 kDa. The IP receptor is selectively activated by the analogue cicaprost.[194] Iloprost and carbaprostacyclin potently activate the IP receptor but also activate the EP1 receptor. Selexipag is first in a class of long-acting IP agonists with good selectivity. Most evidence has suggested that the PGI2 receptor signals via stimulation of cAMP generation; however, at 1000-fold higher concentrations, the cloned mouse PGI2 receptor also signaled via $PIP_2$.[195] It remains unclear whether $PIP_2$ hydrolysis plays any significant role in the physiologic action of PGI2.

The IP receptor mRNA is widely expressed and is especially abundant in mouse bone marrow, vasculature, spleen, and heart[181] and in human kidney, liver, and lung.[196] In situ hybridization shows IP receptor mRNA predominantly in neurons of the dorsal root ganglia and vascular tissue, including the aorta, pulmonary artery, and renal interlobular and glomerular afferent arterioles.[197] The expression of IP receptor mRNA in the dorsal root ganglia is consistent with a role for prostacyclin in pain sensation. Mice with IP receptor gene disruption exhibit a predisposition to arterial thrombosis, diminished pain perception, and inflammatory responses.[145]

PGI2 has been demonstrated to play an important vasodilator role in the kidney,[198] including in the glomerular microvasculature,[199] as well as regulating renin release.[200,201] The capacity of PGI2 and PGE2 to stimulate cAMP generation in the glomerular microvasculature is distinct and additive,[202] demonstrating that the effects of these two prostanoids are mediated via separate receptors. IP receptor knockout mice also exhibit salt-sensitive hypertension.[203] Prostacyclin is a potent stimulus of renal renin release, and studies using $IP^{-/-}$ mice have confirmed an important role for the IP receptor in the development of renin-dependent hypertension of renal artery stenosis.[70] Selexipag has been shown to attenuate albuminuria in mouse models of diabetes in a nephrin-dependent manner.[203a]

Renal epithelial effects of PGI2 in the TAL have also been suggested,[204] and IP receptors have been reported in the collecting duct,[205] but the potential expression and role of prostacyclin in these segments are less well established. Of interest, in situ hybridization has also demonstrated significant expression of prostacyclin synthase in medullary collecting ducts,[206] consistent with a role for this metabolite in this region of the kidney. In summary, although IP receptors appear to play an important role in regulating renin release and as a vasodilator in the kidney, their role in regulating renal epithelial function seems likely.

## DP RECEPTORS

The DP1 receptor has been cloned and, like the IP and EP2/4 receptors, the DP receptor predominantly signals by increasing cAMP generation. The human DP receptor binds PGD2 with a high-affinity binding of 300 pM and a lower affinity site of 13.4 nM.[207] DP-selective PGD2 analogues include the agonist BW 245C.[208] DP receptor mRNA is highly expressed in leptomeninges, retina, and ileum but is not detected in the kidney.[209] Northern blot analysis of the human DP receptor has demonstrated mRNA expression in the small intestine and retina,[210] whereas in the mouse, the DP receptor mRNA had highest expression in the olfactory epithelium, testes, and trachea.[181] PGD2 has also been shown to affect the sleep-wake cycle,[211] pain sensation,[148] and body temperature.[212] Peripherally, PGD2 has been shown to mediate vasodilation as well as possibly inhibiting platelet aggregation. PGD2 production is especially robust in mast cells. Inconsistent with this latter finding, the DP receptor knockout mice displayed reduced inflammation in the ovalbumin model of allergic asthma.[213] PGD2 is a major mediator of niacin-induced flushing. Development of the antagonist laropiprant was undertaken to inhibit this niacin-induced vasodilation flushing response.[214] Although the kidney appears capable of synthesizing PGD2, its role in the kidney remains poorly defined. Intrarenal infusion of PGD2 resulted in a dependent increase in renal artery flow, urine output, creatinine clearance, and sodium and potassium excretion.[215]

A second DP receptor was originally cloned as an orphan chemoattractant receptor from eosinophils and T cells (TH2 subset) and designated the CRTH2 receptor.[216] This receptor, now designated as the DP2 receptor, bears no significant sequence homology to the family of prostanoid receptors discussed previously, and couples to increased cell calcium rather than increased cAMP. It binds agonists with an order of potency as follows: PGD2 = PGJ2 = 15 d PGJ2 ≫ PGF2α, PGE2 > $PGI_2$, TAX2. DP2 receptor action is blocked by the antagonist ramatroban, a drug used to treat allergic rhinitis and originally described as a TP receptor antagonist.[217] DP2 is widely expressed in a number of mouse tissues, including the kidney, and is most highly expressed in the uterus and testes.[181] Deletion of the DP2 receptor gene was protective in a mouse unilateral ureteral obstruction (UUO) model of fibrosis.[218] The recognition of this molecularly unrelated receptor allows for the possibility of the existence of a distinct and new family of prostanoid-activated membrane receptors.

## FP RECEPTORS

The cDNA encoding the PGF2α receptor (FP receptor) was cloned from a human kidney cDNA library and encodes a protein of 359 amino acid residues. The bovine and murine FP receptors, similarly cloned from the corpora lutea, encode proteins of 362 and 366 amino acid residues, respectively. Transfection of HEK293 cells with the human FP receptor cDNA conferred preferential $^3$H-P PGF2α binding with a $K_D$ of 4.3 ± 1.0 nM.[176,219] Selective activation of the FP receptor may be achieved using fluprostenol or latanoprost.[176] $^3$H-PGF2α binding was displaced by a panel of ligands with a rank order potency as follows: PGF2α = fluprostenol > PGD2 > PGE2 > U46619 > iloprost.[194] When expressed in oocytes, PGF2α or fluprostenol induced a $Ca^{2+}$-dependent $Cl^-$ current. Increased cell calcium has also been observed in fibroblasts expressing an endogenous FP receptor.[220] FP receptors may also activate protein kinase C–dependent and Rho-mediated–PKC-independent signaling pathways.[221] An alternatively spliced isoform with a shorter carboxy-terminal tail has been identified that appears to signal via a similar manner as the originally described FP receptor.[222] Studies have also suggested that these two isoforms may exhibit differential desensitization and may also activate a glycogen synthase kinase/ß-catenin–coupled signaling pathway.[223]

Tissue distribution of FP receptor mRNA shows highest expression in the ovary, followed by the heart, trachea, and kidney.[181] Expression of the FP receptor in the corpora lutea is critical for normal birth, and homozygous disruption of the murine FP receptor gene results in failure of parturition in females, apparently due to failure of the normal preterm decline in progesterone levels.[224] PGF2α is a potent constrictor of smooth muscle in the uterus, bronchi, and blood vessels; however, an endothelial FP receptor may also play a dilator role.[225] The FP receptor is also highly expressed in skin, where it may play an important role in carcinogenesis.[226] A clinically important role for the FP receptor in the eye has been demonstrated to increase uveoscleral outflow and reduce ocular pressure. The FP-selective agonist latanoprost, an ester prodrug that is activated in the cornea, has been used clinically as an effective treatment for glaucoma.[227] Bimatoprost is a structural analogue of prostaglandin F2α (PGF2α). Like other PGF2α analogues, such as latanoprost, it increases the outflow of aqueous fluid from the eye and lowers intraocular pressure. It has a curious side effect of increasing eye growth. However, in contrast to latanoprost, it does not act on the FP receptor nor on any other known prostaglandin receptor.

The role of FP receptors in regulating renal function is only partially defined. FP receptor expression has been mapped to the cortical collecting duct in mouse and rabbit kidneys.[228] FP receptor activation in the collecting duct inhibits vasopressin-stimulated water absorption via a pertussis toxin–sensitive (presumably Gi) dependent mechanism. Although PGF2α increased cell $Ca^{2+}$ levels in the cortical collecting duct, the FP-selective agonists latanoprost and fluprostenol did not increase calcium.[229] Because PGF2α can also bind to EP1 and EP3 receptors,[194,230,231] these data suggest that the calcium increase activated by PGF2α in the collecting duct may be mediated via an EP receptor. PGF2α also increases $Ca^{2+}$ in cultured glomerular mesangial cells and podocytes,[232,233] suggesting that an FP receptor may modulate glomerular contraction. In contrast to these findings, the demonstration of glomerular FP receptors at the molecular level has not been forthcoming. Other vascular effects of PGF2α have been described, including selective modulation of renal production of PGF2α by sodium or potassium loading and AT2 receptor activation.[156]

Some reports have uncovered a role of the FP receptor in regulating renin expression. Interestingly, FP agonists increased renin mRNA expression in the JGA in a dose-dependent manner but, unlike IP receptor agonists, it did not increase intracellular cAMP. Deletion of the FP receptor resulted in decreased renin levels and decreased systemic blood pressure. These data suggest that FP receptor blockade may be a novel target for the treatment of hypertension.[234]

## MULTIPLE EP RECEPTORS

Four EP receptor subtypes have been identified.[235] Although these four receptors uniformly bind PGE2 with a higher affinity than other endogenous prostanoids, the amino acid homology of each is more closely related to other prostanoid receptors that signal through similar mechanisms.[175] Thus, the relaxant cAMP-coupled EP2 receptor is more closely related to other relaxant prostanoid receptors, such as the IP and DP receptors, whereas the constrictor/$Ca^{2+}$-coupled EP1 receptor is more closely related to the other $Ca^{2+}$-coupled prostanoid receptors, such as the TP and FP receptors.[236] These receptors may also be selectively activated or antagonized by different analogues. EP receptor subtypes also exhibit differential expression along the nephron, suggesting distinct functional consequences of activating each EP receptor subtype in the kidney.[237]

### EP1 Receptors

The human EP1 receptor cDNA encodes a 402–amino acid polypeptide that signals via IP3 generation and increased cell $Ca^{2+}$ with IP3 generation. Studies of EP1 receptors may use one of several relatively selective antagonists, including ONO-871, SC19220, and SC53122. EP1 receptor mRNA has widespread expression, presumably from its vascular expression,[181] and is expressed in the kidney ≫ gastric muscularis mucosae > adrenal.[238] Renal EP1 mRNA expression determined by in situ hybridization is expressed primarily in the collecting duct and increases from the cortex to the papillae.[238] Activation of the EP1 receptor increases intracellular calcium levels and inhibits $Na^+$ and water reabsorption absorption in the collecting duct,[238] suggesting that renal EP1 receptor activation might contribute to the natriuretic and diuretic effects of PGE2.

Hemodynamic microvascular effects of EP1 receptors have also been reported. The EP1 receptor was originally described as a smooth muscle constrictor.[239] The EP1 receptor may also be present in cultured glomerular mesangial cells,[240] where it could play a role as a vasoconstrictor and a stimulus for mesangial cell proliferation. Although a constrictor PGE2 effect has been reported in the afferent arteriole of rat,[241] apparently produced by EP1 receptor activation,[242] there does not appear to be very high expression of the EP1 receptor mRNA in preglomerular vasculature or other arterial resistance vessels in mice or rabbits.[243] Other reports have suggested that EP1 receptor knockout mice exhibit hypotension and hyperreninemia, supporting a role for this receptor in maintaining blood pressure.[244]

### EP2 Receptors

Two cAMP-stimulating EP receptors, designated EP2 and EP4, have been identified. The EP2 receptor can be pharmacologically distinguished from the EP4 receptor by its sensitivity to butaprost.[245] Before 1995, the cloned EP4 receptor was designated as the EP2 receptor, but then a butaprost-sensitive EP receptor was cloned,[246] the original receptor was reclassified as the EP4 receptor and the newer butaprost sensitive protein as the EP2 receptor.[247] A pharmacologically defined EP2 receptor has now also been cloned for the mouse, rat, rabbit, dog, and cow.[248] The human EP2 receptor cDNA encodes a 358–amino acid polypeptide, which signals through increased cAMP. The EP2 receptor may also be distinguished from the EP4 receptor, the other major relaxant EP receptor, by its relative insensitivity to the EP4 agonist PGE1-OH and to the weak EP4 antagonist AH23848[245] and the high-affinity EP4 antagonists ONO-AE3-208 and L-161982.[249] The EP2 antagonist PF-04418948 has been described,[250] as has the EP2/$DP_1$ antagonist TG4-155,[251] which should greatly facilitate the characterization of EP2 versus EP4 effects in vivo.

The precise distribution of the EP2 receptor mRNA has been partially characterized. This reveals a major mRNA species of around 3.1 kb, which is most abundant in the uterus, lung, and spleen, exhibiting only low levels of expression in the kidney.[248] Studies using PCR across a range of tissue have demonstrated highest expression in the bone marrow > ovary > lung, consistent with these earlier findings.[181] EP2 mRNA is expressed at much lower levels than EP4 mRNA in most tissues.[252] There is scant evidence to suggest segmental distribution of the EP2 receptor along the nephron.[248] Interestingly, it is expressed in cultured renal interstitial cells, supporting the possibility that the EP2 receptor is predominantly expressed in this portion of the nephron.[248] Studies in knockout mice have demonstrated a critical role for the EP2 receptor role in ovulation and fertilization.[253] In addition, these studies have suggested a potential role for the EP2 receptor in salt-sensitive hypertension.[253] This latter finding supports an important role for the EP2 receptor in protecting systemic blood pressure, perhaps via its vasodilator effect or its effects on renal salt excretion. Evidence for the latter role has been revealed in studies demonstrating that a high-salt diet increases PGE2 production, and infusion of EP-selective agonists identified the EP2 receptor as mediating PGE2-evoked naturesis. Moreover, deletion of the EP2 receptor ablated the naturetic effect of PGE2.[254]

### EP3 Receptors

The EP3 receptor generally acts as a constrictor of smooth muscle.[255] Ribonuclease protection and Northern blot analysis of mRNA levels have demonstrated relatively high levels of EP3 receptor expression in several tissues, including the kidney, uterus, adrenal, and stomach, with riboprobes hybridizing to major mRNA species at around 2.4 and around 7.0 kb.[256] A metabolic pattern of expression was found by PCR with high levels of expression in the pancreas, as well as and brown fat tissue in addition to expression in the kidney.[181] This receptor is unique in that there are multiple (more than eight) alternatively spliced variants, differing only in their C-terminal cytoplasmic tails.[257–259] The EP3 splice variants bind PGE2 and the EP3 agonists MB28767 and sulprostone with similar affinity and, although they exhibit common inhibition of cAMP generation via a pertussis toxin–sensitive $G_i$-coupled mechanism, the tails may recruit different signaling pathways, including $Ca^{2+}$-dependent signaling[175,245] and the small G protein, rho.[260] A Ptx-insensitive pathway for the inhibition of cAMP generation via Gz has also been described.[261] Differences in agonist-independent activity have been observed for several of the splice variants, suggesting that they may play a role in constitutive regulation of cellular events.[262] The physiologic roles of these different C-terminal splice variants and sites of expression within the kidney remain uncertain.

In situ hybridization has demonstrated that EP3 receptor mRNA is abundant in the TAL and collecting duct.[263] This distribution has been confirmed by reverse transcriptase (RT)–PCR on microdissected rat and mouse collecting ducts and corresponds to the major binding sites for radioactive PGE2 in the kidney.[264] An important role for a $G_i$-coupled PGE receptor in regulating water and salt transport along the nephron has been recognized for many years. PGE2 directly inhibits salt and water absorption in both microperfused TALs and collecting ducts (CDs). PGE2 directly inhibits $Cl^-$ absorption in the mouse or rabbit medullary TAL from the luminal or basolateral surfaces.[265] PGE2 also inhibits hormone-stimulated cAMP generation in TAL. Good and George have demonstrated that PGE2 modulates ion transport in the rat TAL by a pertussis toxin–sensitive mechanism.[265] Interestingly, these effects also appear to involve protein kinase C activation,[266] possibly reflecting activation of a novel EP3 receptor signaling pathway and possibly corresponding to alternative signaling pathways, as described earlier.[260] Taken together, these data support a role for the EP3 receptor in regulating transport in the collecting duct and TAL.

Blockade of endogenous PGE2 synthesis by NSAIDs enhances urinary concentration. It is likely PGE2-mediated antagonism of vasopressin-stimulated salt absorption in the TAL, and water absorption in the collecting duct contributes to its diuretic effect. In the in vitro microperfused collecting duct, PGE2 inhibits both vasopressin-stimulated osmotic water absorption and vasopressin-stimulated cAMP generation.[229] Furthermore, PGE2 inhibition of water absorption and cAMP generation are both blocked by pertussis toxin, suggesting effects mediated by the inhibitory G protein, $G_i$.[229] When administered in the absence of vasopressin, PGE2 actually stimulates water absorption in the collecting duct from the luminal or basolateral side.[267] These stimulatory effects of PGE2 on transport in the collecting duct appear to be related to activation of the EP4 receptor.[267] Despite the presence of this absorption-enhancing EP receptor, in vivo studies have suggested that in the presence of vasopressin, the predominant effects of endogenous PGE2 on water transport are diuretic. Based on the preceding functional considerations, one would expect $EP3^{-/-}$ mice to exhibit an inappropriately enhanced urinary concentration. Surprisingly, $EP3^{-/-}$ mice exhibited a comparable urinary concentration following desmopressin (DDAVP), similar 24-hour water intake, and similar maximal and minimal urinary osmolality The only clear difference was that in mice allowed free access to water, indomethacin increased urinary osmolality in normal mice but not in the knockout animals. These findings raise the possibility that some of the renal actions of PGE2 normally mediated by the EP3 receptor have been co-opted by other receptors (e.g., the EP1 or FP receptor) in the EP3 knockout mouse. This remains to be formally tested.

The significance of EP3 receptor activation to animal physiology has been significantly advanced by the availability of mice with targeted disruption of this gene. Mice with targeted deletion of the EP3 receptor exhibit an impaired febrile response, suggesting that EP3 receptor antagonists could be effective antipyretic agents.[268] Other studies have suggested that the EP3 receptor plays an important vasopressor role in the peripheral circulation of mice.[243] Studies in knockout mice have also supported a potential role for the EP3 receptor as an important systemic vasopressor.[243,269] In the intrarenal circulation, the PGE2 has variable effects, acting as a vasoconstrictor in the larger proximal portion of the intralobular arteries and changing to a vasodilator effect in the smaller distal intralobular arteries and afferent arterioles.[270]

### EP4 Receptor

Although, like the EP2 receptor, the EP4 receptor signals through increased cAMP,[271] it has been found to signal through a number of other pathways as well.[272] These other pathways include arrestin-mediated signaling, PI3 kinase, signaling β-catenin, and $G_i$ coupling. The human EP4 receptor cDNA encodes a 488–amino acid polypeptide with a predicted molecular mass of ~53 kDa.[273] Note that care must be taken in reviewing the literature prior to 1995, when this receptor was generally referred to as the EP2 receptor.[247] In addition to the human receptor, EP4 receptors for the mouse, rat, rabbit, and dog have been cloned. EP4 receptors can be pharmacologically distinguished from the EP1 and EP3 receptors by insensitivity to sulprostone and from EP2 receptors by its insensitivity to butaprost and relatively selective activation by PGE1-OH.[176] EP4-selective agonists (ONO-AE1-329, ONO-4819) and antagonists (ONOAC-3208, L-161982) have been generated[245] and have been used to investigate the role of EP4 in vivo. Activation of the EP4 receptor was able to ameliorate the phenotype of a mouse model of nephrogenic diabetes insipidus.[274]

EP4 receptor mRNA is highly expressed relative to the EP2 receptor and widely distributed, with a major species of around 3.8 kb detected by Northern blot analysis in the thymus, ileum, lung, spleen, adrenal, and kidney.[252,275,275a] Dominant vasodilator effects of EP4 receptor activation have been described in venous and arterial beds.[208,255] A critical role for the EP4 receptor in regulating the perinatal closure of the pulmonary ductus arteriosus has also been suggested by studies of mice with targeted disruption of the EP4 receptor gene.[166,276] On a 129-strain background, $EP4^{-/-}$ mice had nearly 100% perinatal mortality due to persistent patent ductus arteriosus.[276] Interestingly, when bred on a mixed genetic background, only 80% of $EP4^{-/-}$ mice died, whereas around 21% underwent closure of the ductus and survived.[166] Preliminary studies in these survivors have supported an important role for the EP4 receptor as a systemic vasodepressor;[277] however, their heterogeneous genetic background complicates the interpretation of these results because survival may select for modifier genes that not only allow ductus closure but also alter other hemodynamic responses.

Other roles for the EP4 receptor in controlling blood pressure have been suggested, including the ability to stimulate aldosterone release from zona glomerulosa cells.[278] In the kidney, EP4 receptor mRNA expression is primarily in the glomerulus, where its precise function is uncharacterized,[275,279] but might contribute to the regulation of the renal microcirculation as well as renin release.[280] Studies in mice with genetic deletion of selective prostanoid receptors have indicated that $EP4^{-/-}$ mice, as well as $IP^{-/-}$ mice to a lesser extent, fail to increase renin production in response to loop diuretic administration, indicating that macula densa–derived PGE2 increases renin primarily through EP4 activation.[281] This corresponds to other studies suggesting that EP4 receptors are expressed in cultured podocytes and juxtaglomerular apparatus cells.[232,280] PGE2 may mediate increased podocyte COX-2 expression through EP4-mediated increased cAMP, which activates P38 through an independent process.[282] Finally, the EP4 receptor in the renal pelvis may participate in regulation of salt excretion by altering afferent renal nerve output.[283]

## REGULATION OF RENAL FUNCTION BY EP RECEPTORS

PGE2 exerts a number of effects in the kidney, presumably mediated by EP receptors. PGE2 not only dilates the glomerular microcirculation and vasa rectae, supplying the renal medulla,[284] but also modulates salt and water transport in the distal tubule (Fig. 13.5).[285] The maintenance of normal renal function during physiologic stress is particularly dependent on endogenous prostaglandin synthesis. In this setting, the vasoconstrictor effects of Ang II, catecholamines, and vasopressin are more effectively buffered by prostaglandins in the kidney than in other vascular beds, preserving normal renal blood flow, the GFR, and salt excretion. Administration of COX-inhibiting NSAIDs in the setting of volume depletion interferes with these dilator effects and may result in a catastrophic decline in the GFR, resulting in overt renal failure.[286]

Other evidence points to vasoconstrictor and prohypertensive effects of endogenous PGE2. PGE2 stimulates renin release from the juxtaglomerular apparatus,[287] leading to a subsequent increase in the vasoconstrictor Ang II. In conscious dogs, chronic intrarenal PGE2 infusion increases renal renin secretion, resulting in hypertension.[288] Treatment of salt-depleted rats with indomethacin not only decreases plasma renin activity, but also reduces blood pressure, suggesting that PGs support blood pressure during salt depletion via their capacity to increase renin.[289] Direct vasoconstrictor effects of PGE2 on vasculature have also been observed.[243] It is conceivable that these latter effects might predominate in circumstances where the kidney is exposed to excessively high perfusion pressures. Thus, depending on the setting, the primary effect of PGE2 may be to increase or decrease vascular tone, effects that appear to be mediated by distinct EP receptors.

### RENAL CORTICAL HEMODYNAMICS

The expression of the EP4 receptor in the glomerulus suggests that it may play an important role in regulating renal hemodynamics. PGs regulate the renal cortical microcirculation and, as suggested previously, both glomerular constrictor and dilator effects of PGs have been observed.[243,290] In the setting of volume depletion, endogenous PGE2 helps maintain the GFR by dilating the afferent arteriole.[290] Some studies have suggested roles for EP and IP receptors coupled to increased cAMP generation in mediating vasodilator effects in the preglomerular circulation.[44,280,291] PGE2 exerts a dilator effect on the afferent arteriole but not the efferent arteriole, consistent with the presence of an EP2 or EP4 receptor in the preglomerular microcirculation.

### RENIN RELEASE

Other studies have suggested that the EP4 receptor may also stimulate renin release. Soon after the introduction of NSAIDs, it was recognized that endogenous PGs play an important role in stimulating renin release.[44] Treatment of salt-depleted rats with indomethacin not only decreases plasma renin activity, but also causes blood pressure to fall, suggesting that PGs support blood pressure during salt depletion via their capacity to increase renin. Prostanoids also play a central role in the pathogenesis of renovascular hypertension, and administration of NSAIDs lowers blood pressure in animals and humans with renal artery stenosis.[292] PGE2 induces renin release in isolated preglomerular juxtaglomerular apparatus cells.[287] Like the effect of ß-adrenergic agents, this effect appears to be through a cAMP-coupled response, supporting a role for an EP4 or EP2 receptor.[287] EP4 receptor mRNA has been detected in microdissected JGAs,[293] supporting the possibility that renal EP4 receptor activation contributes to enhanced renin release. Finally, regulation of plasma renin activity and intrarenal renin mRNA does not appear to be different in wild-type and EP2 knockout mice,[294] arguing against a major role for the EP2 receptor in regulating renin release. Conversely, one report has suggested that EP3 receptor mRNA is localized to the macula densa, suggesting that this cAMP-inhibiting receptor may also contribute to the control of renin release.[279]

### RENAL MICROCIRCULATION

The EP2 receptor also appears to play an important role in regulating afferent arteriolar tone.[290] In the setting of systemic hypertension, the normal response of the kidney is to increase salt excretion, thereby mitigating the increase in blood pressure. This so-called "pressure natriuresis" plays a key role in the ability of the kidney to protect against hypertension.[295] Increased blood pressure is accompanied by increased renal perfusion pressure and enhanced urinary PGE2 excretion.[296] Inhibition of PG synthesis markedly blunts (although it does not eliminate) pressure natriuresis.[297] The mechanism whereby PGE2 contributes to pressure natriuresis may involve changes in resistance of the renal medullary microcirculation.[298] PGE2 directly dilates descending vasa recta, and increased medullary blood flow may contribute to the increased interstitial pressure observed as renal perfusion pressure increases, leading to enhanced salt excretion.[284] The identity of the dilator PGE2 receptor controlling the contractile properties of the descending vasa recta remains uncertain, but EP2 or EP4 receptors seem likely candidates.[208] Studies demonstrating salt-sensitive hypertension in mice with targeted disruption of the EP2 receptor[253] have suggested that the EP2 receptor facilitates the ability of the kidney to increase sodium excretion, thereby protecting systemic blood pressure from a high-salt diet. Given its defined role in vascular smooth muscle,[253] these effects of the EP2 receptor disruption seem more likely to relate to its effects on renal vascular tone. In particular, loss of a vasodilator effect in the renal medulla might modify pressure natriuresis and could contribute to hypertension in EP2 knockout mice. Nonetheless, a role for the EP2 or EP4 receptor in regulating renal medullary blood flow remains to be established. In conclusion, direct vasomotor effects of EP4 receptors, as well as effects on renin release, may play critical roles in regulating systemic blood pressure and renal hemodynamics.

## EFFECTS ON SALT AND WATER TRANSPORT

COX-1 and COX-2 metabolites of arachidonate have important direct epithelial effects on salt and water transport along the nephron.[299] Thus, functional effects can be observed that are thought to be independent of any hemodynamic changes produced by these compounds. Because biologically active AA metabolites are rapidly metabolized, they act predominantly in an autocrine or paracrine fashion, and thus, their locus of action will be close to their point of generation. One can expect, therefore, that direct epithelial effects of these compounds will result when they are produced by the tubule cells themselves or the neighboring interstitial cells, and the tubules possess an appropriate receptor for the ligand.

### PROXIMAL TUBULE

Neither the proximal convoluted tubule nor the proximal straight tubule appear to produce amounts of biologically active COX metabolites of arachidonic acid. As will be discussed in a subsequent section, the dominant arachidonate metabolites produced by proximal convoluted and straight tubules are metabolites of the cytochrome P-450 pathway.[300]

Early whole-animal studies have suggested that PGE2 might have an action in the proximal tubule because of its effects on urinary phosphate excretion. PGE2 blocks the phosphaturic action of calcitonin infusion in thyroparathyroidectomized rats. Nevertheless, studies using in vitro perfused proximal tubules have failed to show an effect of PGE2 on sodium chloride or phosphate transport in the proximal convoluted tubule. More recent studies have suggested that PGE2 may play a key role in the phosphaturic action of FGF-23[301] because phosphaturia in hyp mice with X-linked hyperphosphaturia is associated with markedly increased urine PGE2 excretion, and phosphaturia was normalized by indomethacin.[302] Nevertheless, there are very little data on the actions of other COX metabolites in proximal tubules and scant molecular evidence for the expression of classic G protein–coupled prostaglandin receptors in this segment of the nephron.

### LOOP OF HENLE

The nephron segments making up the loop of Henle also display limited metabolism of exogenous AA through the

COX pathway although, given the realization that COX-2 is expressed in this segment, it is of note that PGE2 was uniformly greater in the cortical segment than in the medullary TAL. The TAL has been shown to exhibit PGE2 receptors in high density.[303] Studies have also demonstrated high expression levels of mRNA for the EP3 receptor in medullary TAL of both rabbits and rats[231] (see earlier section on the EP3 receptor). Subsequent to the demonstration that PGE2 inhibits sodium chloride absorption in the medullary TAL of the rabbit TAL perfused in vitro, it was shown that PGE2 blocks antidiuretic hormone (ADH) but not cAMP-stimulated sodium chloride absorption in the medullary TAL of the mouse. It is likely that the mechanism involves activation of $G_i$ and inhibition of adenyl cyclase by PGE2, possibly via the EP3 receptors expressed in this segment.

### COLLECTING DUCT SYSTEM

In vitro perfusion studies of rabbit cortical collecting tubule have demonstrated that PGE2 directly inhibits sodium transport in the collecting duct when applied to the basolateral surface of this nephron segment. It is now apparent that PGE2 uses multiple signal transduction pathways in the cortical collecting duct, including those that modulate intracellular cAMP levels and $Ca^{2+}$. PGE2 can either stimulate or suppress cAMP accumulation. The latter may also involve stimulation of phosphodiesterase. Although modulation of cAMP levels appears to play an important role in PGE2 effects on water transport in the cortical collecting duct (see following section), it is less clear that PGE2 affects sodium transport via the modulation of cAMP levels.[229] PGE2 has been shown to increase cell calcium possibly coupled with PKC activation in in vitro perfused cortical collecting ducts.[304] This effect may be mediated by the EP1 receptor subtype coupled to phosphatidylinositol hydrolysis.[238]

### WATER TRANSPORT

Vasopressin-regulated water transport in the collecting duct is markedly influenced by COX products, especially PGs. When COX inhibitors are administered to humans, rats, or dogs, the antidiuretic action of arginine vasopressin is markedly augmented. Because vasopressin also stimulates endogenous PGE2 production by the collecting duct, these results have suggested that PGE2 participates in a negative feedback loop, whereby endogenous PGE2 production dampens the action of arginine vasopressin (AVP).[305] In agreement with this model, the early classical studies of Grantham and Orloff directly demonstrated that PGE1 blunted the water permeability response of the cortical collecting duct to vasopressin.[305a] In these early studies, the action of PGE1 appeared to be at a pre-cAMP step. Interestingly, when administered by itself, PGE1 modestly augmented basal water permeability. These earlier studies have been confirmed with respect to PGE2. PGE2 also stimulates basal hydraulic conductivity and suppresses the hydraulic conductivity response to AVP in the rabbit cortical collecting duct.[306,307] Inhibition of both AVP-stimulated cAMP generation and water permeability appears to be mediated by the EP1 and EP3 receptors, whereas the increase in basal water permeability may be mediated by the EP4 receptor.[267] In contrast, EP4 receptors may mediate vasopressin-independent water reabsorption because selective collecting duct deletion of EP4 decreases aquaporin 2 expression and leads to a urine-concentrating defect.[308]

## PROSTAGLANDINS

### METABOLISM OF PROSTAGLANDINS

#### 15-KETODEHYDROGENASE

The half-life of PGs is 3 to 5 minutes and that of TXA2 is approximately 30 seconds. The elimination of PGE2, PGF2α, and $PGI_2$ proceeds through enzymatic and nonenzymatic pathways, whereas that of TXA2 is nonenzymatic. The end products of all these degradative reactions generally possess minimal biologic activity, although this is not uniformly the case (see later). The principal enzyme involved in the transformation of PGE2, $PGI_2$, and PGF2α is 15-hydroxyprostaglandin dehydrogenase (PGDH), which converts the 15 alcohol group to a ketone.[309]

15-PGDH is an nicotinamide adenine dinucleotide ($NAD^+$)/nicotinamide adenine dinucleotide phosphate ($NADP^+$)–dependent enzyme that is 30 to 49 times more active in the kidney of the young rat (3 weeks of age) than in the adult. The $K_m$ for PGE2 is 8.4 μM and 22.6 μM for PGF2α.[309] It is mainly localized in the cortical and juxtamedullary zones,[310] with little activity detected in papillary slices. At baseline, it is found in the proximal tubule, TAL, and collecting duct. However, it was present in macula densa in COX-2 knockout mice and in the presence of a high-salt diet and in cultured macula densa cells, COX inhibition increases expression.[311] Disruption of the 15-PGDH gene in mice results in persistent patent ductus arteriosus (PDA), thought to be a result of failure of circulating PGE2 levels to fall in the immediate peripartum period.[312] Thus administration of COX-inhibiting NSAIDs rescues the knockout mice by decreasing PGs and allowing the animals to survive.

Subsequent catalysis of 15-hydroxy products by a delta-13 reductase leads to the formation of 13,14-dihydro compounds. PGI2 and TXA2 undergo rapid degradation to 6-keto-PGF1a and TXB2, respectively.[309] These stable metabolites are usually measured, and their rates of formation taken as representative of those of the parent molecules.

#### ω/ω-1-HYDROXYLATION OF PROSTAGLANDINS

Both PGA2 and PGE2 have been shown to undergo hydroxylation of the terminal or subterminal carbons by a cytochrome P450–dependent mechanism.[313] This reaction may be mediated by a CYP4A family member or CYP4F enzymes. Both CYP4A[314] and CYP4F members have been mapped along the nephron.[315] Some of these derivatives have been shown to exhibit biologic activity.

### CYCLOPENTENONE PROSTAGLANDINS

The cyclopentenone PGs include PGA2, a PGE2 derivative, and PGJ2, a derivative of PGD2. Although it remains uncertain whether these compounds are actually produced in vivo, this possibility has received increasing attention because some cyclopentenone prostanoids have been shown to be activating ligands for nuclear transcription factors, including proliferator-activated receptor (PPAR)-δ and PPARγ.[316–318] The realization that the antidiabetic thiazolidinedione drugs act through PPARγ to exert their antihyperglycemic and insulin-sensitizing effects[319] has generated intense interest in the possibility that the cyclopentenone PGs might serve as the

endogenous ligands for these receptors. Interestingly, DP2, unlike DP1 or indeed other members of the PGG protein-coupled receptor (GPCR) family, binds and is activated by PGD2 metabolites such as 15-deoxy-Δ12,14-PGJ2, which acts at nanomolar concentrations.[320] An alternative biologic activity of these compounds has been recognized in their capacity to covalently modify thiol groups, forming adducts with cysteine of several intracellular proteins, including thioredoxin 1, vimentin, actin, and tubulin.[321] Studies regarding the biologic activity of cyclopentenone prostanoids abound, and the reader is referred to several excellent sources in the literature.[322–324] Although there is evidence supporting the presence of these compounds in vivo,[325] it remains uncertain whether they can be formed enzymatically or are an unstable spontaneous dehydration product of the E and D ring PGs.[326]

## NONENZYMATIC METABOLISM OF ARACHIDONIC ACID

It has long been recognized that oxidant injury can result in the peroxidation of lipids. In 1990, Morrow and colleagues reported that a series of PG-like compounds can be produced by free radical–catalyzed peroxidation of arachidonic acid that is independent of COX activity.[327] These compounds, which are termed *isoprostanes*, have been increasingly used as a sensitive marker of oxidant injury in vitro and in vivo.[328] In addition, at least two of these compounds, 8-iso-PGF2α (15-F2-isoprostane) and 8-iso-PGE2 (15-E2-isoprostane) are potent vasoconstrictors when administered exogenously. 8-Iso-PGF2α has been shown to constrict the renal microvasculature and decrease the GFR, an effect that is prevented by thromboxane receptor antagonism.[329] However, the role of endogenous isoprostanes as mediators of biologic responses remains unclear.

## PROSTAGLANDIN TRANSPORT AND URINARY EXCRETION

It is notable that most of the PG synthetic enzymes have been localized to the intracellular compartment, yet extracellular prostaglandins are potent autacoids and paracrine factors. Thus prostanoids must be transported extracellularly to achieve efficient metabolism and termination of their signaling. Similarly, enzymes that metabolize PGE2 to inactive compounds are also intracellular, requiring uptake of the PG for its metabolic inactivation. The molecular basis of these extrusion and uptake processes are slowly being defined.

As a fatty acid, PGs may be classified as an organic anion at a physiologic pH. Early microperfusion studies have documented that basolateral PGE2 could be taken up into proximal tubules cells and actively secreted into the lumen. Furthermore, this process could be inhibited by a variety of inhibitors of organic anion transport, including Para-aminohippurate (PAH), probenecid, and indomethacin. Studies of basolateral renal membrane vesicles have also supported the notion that this transport process occurs via an electroneutral anion exchanger. These studies are of note because renal PGs enter the urine in the loop of Henle, and late proximal tubule secretion could provide an important entry mechanism.[1]

A molecule that mediates PGE2 uptake in exchange for lactate has been cloned and referred to as PGT, prostaglandin transporter.[330] PGT is a member of the SLC21/SLCO: organic anion transport family, and its cDNA encodes a transmembrane protein of 100 amino acids that exhibits broad tissue distribution (heart, placenta, brain, lung, liver, skeletal muscle, pancreas, kidney, spleen, prostate, ovary, small intestine, and colon).[331–333] Immunocytochemical studies of PGT expression in rat kidneys have suggested expression primarily in glomerular endothelial and mesangial cells, arteriolar endothelial and muscularis cells, principal cells of the collecting duct, medullary interstitial cells, medullary vasa rectae endothelia, and papillary surface epithelium.[334] PGT appears to mediate PGE2 uptake rather than release,[335] allowing target cells to metabolize this molecule and terminate signaling.[336] PGT expression is decreased with low salt and increased with high salt in the collecting duct, which may allow regulation of PG excretion by taking up more PGs excreted from the luminal surface, the site of PG transporter, thereby allowing more accumulation at the basolateral surface.[337]

Other members of the organic cation-anion-zwitterion transporter family SLC22 have also been shown to transport PGs[330] and have been suggested to mediate PG excretion into the urine. Specifically, OAT1 and OAT3 are localized on the basolateral proximal tubule membrane, where they likely participate in the urinary excretion of PGE2.[338,339] Conversely, members of the multidrug resistance protein (MRP) have been shown to transport PGs in an adenosine triphosphate (ATP)–dependent fashion.[340,341] MRP2 (also designated as ABBC2) is expressed in kidney proximal tubule brush borders and may contribute to the transport (and urinary excretion) of glutathione-conjugated PGs.[342,343] This transporter has more limited tissue expression, restricted to the kidney, liver, and small intestine, and could contribute not only to renal para-aminohippurate (PAH) excretion but also to PG excretion as well.[344]

# INVOLVEMENT OF CYCLOOXYGENASE METABOLITES IN RENAL PATHOPHYSIOLOGY

## EXPERIMENTAL AND HUMAN GLOMERULAR INJURY

### GLOMERULAR INFLAMMATORY INJURY

COX metabolites have been implicated in functional and structural alterations in glomerular and tubulointerstitial inflammatory diseases.[345] Essential fatty acid deficiency totally prevents the structural and functional consequences of the administration of nephrotoxic serum (NTS) to rats, an experimental model of antiglomerular basement membrane glomerulonephritis.[329] Changes in arteriolar tone during the course of this inflammatory lesion are mediated principally by locally released COX and lipoxygenase (LO) metabolites of AA.[329]

TXA2 release appears to play an essential role in mediating the increased renovascular resistance observed during the early phase of this disease.[1] Subsequently, increasing rates of PGE2 generation may account for the progressive dilation of renal arterioles and increases in renal blood flow (RBF) at later stages of the disease. Consistent with this hypothesis, TXA2 antagonism ameliorated the falls in RBF and GFR 2 hours post-NTS administration, but not after 24 hours. During the latter heterologous phase of NTS, COX metabolites mediate the renal vasodilation and reduction in the glomerular ultrafiltration coefficient ($K_f$) that characterize this phase.[329] The net functional result of COX inhibition during this phase of experimental glomerulonephritis, therefore would depend on the relative importance of renal perfusion versus the preservation of $K_f$ to the maintenance of the GFR. Evidence also indicates that COX metabolites are mediators of pathologic lesions and the accompanying proteinuria in this model.[1] COX-2 expression in the kidney increases in experimental anti–glomerular basement membrane (GBM) glomerulonephritis[346,347] and after the systemic administration of lipopolysaccharide.[348]

A beneficial effect of fish oil diets (enriched in eicosapentaneoic acid), with an accompanying reduction in the generation of COX products, has been demonstrated on the course of genetic murine lupus (MRL-lpr mice). In subsequent studies, enhanced renal TXA2 and PGE2 generation was demonstrated in this model, as well as in NZB mice, another genetic model of lupus.[1] In addition, studies in humans have demonstrated an inverse relation between TXA2 biosynthesis and GFR and improvement of renal function following short-term therapy with a thromboxane receptor antagonist in patients with lupus nephritis.[1] More recently, studies have indicated that in humans, as well as NZB mice, COX-2 expression is upregulated in patients with active lupus nephritis, with colocalization to infiltrating monocytes, suggesting that monocytes infiltrating the glomeruli contribute to the exaggerated local synthesis of TXA2.[349,350] COX-2 inhibition selectively decreased thromboxane production, and chronic treatment of NZB mice with a COX-2 inhibitor and mycophenolate mofetil significantly prolonged survival.[350] Taken together, these data, as well as others from animal and human studies, support a major role for the intrarenal generation of TXA2 in mediating renal vasoconstriction during inflammatory and lupus-associated glomerular injury. In contrast, an EP4-selective agonist was shown to reduce glomerular injury in a mouse model of anti-GBM disease.[351]

The demonstration of a functionally significant role for COX metabolites in experimental and human inflammatory glomerular injury has raised the question of the cellular sources of these eicosanoids in the glomerulus. In addition to infiltrating inflammatory cells, resident glomerular macrophages, glomerular mesangial cells, and glomerular epithelial cells represent likely sources for eicosanoid generation. In the anti-Thy1.1 model of mesangioproliferative glomerulonephritis, COX-1 staining was transiently increased in diseased glomeruli at day 6 and was localized mainly to proliferating mesangial cells. COX-2 expression in the macula densa region also transiently increased at day 6.[352,353] Glomerular COX-2 expression in this model has been controversial, with one group reporting increased podocyte COX-2 expression,[347] and two other groups reporting minimal, if any, glomerular COX-2 expression.[352,353] However, it is of interest that selective COX-2 inhibitors have been reported to inhibit glomerular repair in the anti-Thy1.1 model.[353] In both anti-Thy1.1 and anti-GBM models of glomerulonephritis, the nonselective COX inhibitor, indomethacin, increased monocyte chemoattractant protein-1 (MCP-1), suggesting that prostaglandins may repress the recruitment of monocytes and macrophages in experimental glomerulonephritis.[354]

A variety of cytokines has been reported to stimulate PGE2 synthesis and COX-2 expression in cultured mesangial cells. Furthermore, complement components, in particular C5b-9, which are known to be involved in the inflammatory models described previously, have been implicated in the stimulation of PGE2 synthesis in glomerular epithelial cells (GECs). Cultured GECs express predominantly COX-1, but exposure to C5b-9 significantly increases COX-2 expression[1].

## GLOMERULAR NONINFLAMMATORY INJURY

Studies have suggested that prostanoids may also mediate altered renal function and glomerular damage following subtotal renal ablation, and glomerular PG production may be altered in such conditions. Glomeruli from remnant kidneys, as well as animals fed a high-protein diet, have increased prostanoid production.[1] These studies have suggested an increase in COX enzyme activity per se rather than, or in addition to, increased substrate availability, because increases in prostanoid production were noted when excess exogenous AA was added.

Following subtotal renal ablation, there are selective increases in renal cortical and glomerular COX-2 mRNA and immunoreactive protein expression, without significant alterations in COX-1 expression.[355] This increased COX-2 expression was most prominent in the macula densa and surrounding cTALH. In addition, COX-2 immunoreactivity was also present in podocytes of remnant glomeruli, and increased PG production in isolated glomeruli from remnant kidneys was inhibited by a COX-2–selective inhibitor but was not decreased by a COX-1–selective inhibitor.[355] Of interest, in the fawn-hooded rat, which develops spontaneous glomerulosclerosis, there is increased cTALH/macula densa COX-2 and neuronal nitric oxide synthase (nNOS) and juxtaglomerular cell renin expression preceding the development of sclerotic lesions.[356] Studies have indicated that selective overexpression of COX-2 in podocytes in mice increases sensitivity to development of glomerulosclerosis, an effect that is mediated by TX receptor activation.[357–359]

When given 24 hours after subtotal renal ablation, a nonselective NSAID, indomethacin, normalized increases in renal blood flow and single-nephron GFR; similar decreases in hyperfiltration were noted when indomethacin was given acutely to rats 14 days after subtotal nephrectomy although in this latter study, the increased glomerular capillary pressure ($P_{GC}$) was not altered because both afferent and efferent arteriolar resistances increased.[1] Previous studies have also suggested that nonselective COX inhibitors may acutely decrease hyperfiltration in diabetes and inhibit proteinuria and/or structural injury[1]; more recent studies have indicated that selective COX-2 inhibitors will decrease the hyperfiltration seen in experimental diabetes or increased dietary protein.[360,361] Of note, NSAIDs have also been reported to be effective in reducing proteinuria in patients with refractory nephrotic syndrome.[1] Similarly, selective COX-2 inhibition decreased proteinuria in patients with both diabetic and nondiabetic renal disease, without alterations in blood pressure.[362]

The prostanoids involved have not yet been completely characterized, although it is presumed that vasodilatory prostanoids are involved in the mediation of the altered renal hemodynamics. Defective autoregulation of renal blood flow due to decreased myogenic tone of the afferent arteriole is seen after subtotal ablation or excessive dietary protein and is corrected by the inhibition of COX activity. In these hyperfiltering states, TGF is reset at a higher distal tubular flow rate.[1] Such a resetting dictates that afferent arteriolar vasodilation will be maintained in the face of increased distal solute delivery. It was previously shown that the alterations in TGF sensitivity after reduction in renal mass are prevented with the nonselective COX inhibitor, indomethacin.[1] An important role has been suggested for neuronal nitric oxide synthase, which is localized to the macula densa, in the vasodilatory component of TGF.[363–365] Of interest, studies by Ichihara and colleagues have determined that this nNOS-mediated vasodilation is inhibited by the selective COX-2 inhibitor, NS398, suggesting that COX-2–mediated prostanoids may be essential for arteriolar vasodilation.[47,72]

Administration of COX-2–selective inhibitors decreased proteinuria and inhibited development of glomerular sclerosis in rats with reduced functioning renal mass.[366,367] In addition, COX-2 inhibition decreased mRNA expression of TGF-$\beta_1$ and types III and IV collagen in the remnant kidney.[366] Similar protection was observed with the administration of nitroflurbiprofen (NOF), an NO-releasing NSAID without gastrointestinal toxicity.[368] Prior studies have also demonstrated that TXAS inhibitors retard the progression of glomerulosclerosis, with decreased proteinuria and glomerulosclerosis in rats with remnant kidneys and in diabetic nephropathy, in association with increased renal prostacyclin production and lower systolic blood pressure.[369] Studies in models of types 1 and 2 diabetes have indicated that COX-2–selective inhibitors retard progression of diabetic nephropathy.[370,371] Schmitz and colleagues have confirmed increases in TXB2 excretion in the remnant kidney and correlated decreased arachidonic and linoleic acid levels with increased thromboxane production because the TXAS inhibitor U63557A restores fatty acid levels and retards progressive glomerular destruction.[372]

Enhanced glomerular synthesis and/or urinary excretion of both PGE2 and TXA2 have been demonstrated in passive Heymann nephritis (PHN), and adriamycin-induced glomerulopathies in rats. Both COX-1 and COX-2 expression are increased in glomeruli with PHN.[373] Both TXAS inhibitors and selective COX-2 inhibitors also decreased proteinuria in PHN.[1]

In contrast to the putative deleterious effects of TX, the prostacyclin analogue, cicaprost, retarded renal damage in uninephrectomized dogs fed a high-sodium and high-protein diet, an effect that was not mediated by the amelioration of systemic hypertension.[374] Similarly both EP2 and EP4 agonists decreased glomerular and tubulointerstitial fibrosis in a model of subtotal renal ablation.[362] Other studies have also indicated that in models of polycystic kidney disease, there is increased COX-2 expression and increased PGE2 and TX in cyst fluid. Either COX-2 inhibition or EP2 receptor inhibition decreased cyst growth and interstitial fibrosis.[375,376]

Prostanoids have also been shown to alter extracellular matrix production by mesangial cells in culture. TXA2 stimulates matrix production by both TGF-β–dependent and TGF-β–independent pathways.[377] PGE2 has been reported to decrease steady-state mRNA levels of alpha 1(I) and alpha 1(III) procollagens, but not alpha 1(IV) procollagen and fibronectin mRNA, and to reduce the secretion of all studied collagen types into the cell culture supernatants. Of interest, this effect did not appear to be mediated by cAMP.[378] PGE2 has also been reported to increase production of matrix metalloproteinase-2 and mediate Ang II-induced increases in MMP-2.[379] Whether vasodilatory prostaglandins mediate decreased fibrillar collagen production and increased matrix degrading activity in glomeruli in vivo has not yet been studied; however, there is compelling evidence in nonrenal cells that prostanoids may mediate or modulate matrix production.[380] Cultured lung fibroblasts isolated from patients with idiopathic pulmonary fibrosis exhibit decreased ability to express COX-2 and synthesize PGE2.[381]

## ACUTE KIDNEY INJURY

When cardiac output is compromised, as in extracellular fluid volume depletion or congestive heart failure, systemic blood pressure is preserved by the action of high circulating levels of systemic vasoconstrictors (e.g., norepinephrine, Ang II, AVP). Amelioration of their effects within the renal vasculature serves to blunt the development of otherwise concomitant marked depression of renal blood flow. The intrarenal generation of vasodilator products of AA, including PGE2 and PGI2, is a central part of this protective adaptation. Increased renal vascular resistance induced by exogenously administered Ang II or renal nerve stimulation (increased adrenergic tone) is exaggerated during the concomitant inhibition of prostaglandin synthesis. Experiments in animals with volume depletion have demonstrated the existence of intrarenal AVP-prostaglandin interactions, similar to those described previously for Ang II.[1] Studies in patients with congestive heart failure have confirmed that enhanced prostaglandin synthesis is crucial in protecting kidneys from various vasoconstrictor influences in this condition.

Renal dysfunction accompanying the acute administration of endotoxin in rats is characterized by progressive reductions in RBF and GFR in the absence of hypotension. Renal histology in these animals is normal, but cortical generation of COX metabolites is markedly elevated. A number of reports have provided evidence for a role for TXA2-induced renal vasoconstriction in this model of renal dysfunction.[382] In addition, roles for PGs and TXA2 in modulating or mediating renal injury have been suggested in ischemia and reperfusion,[383] and models of toxin-mediated acute tubular injury, including those induced by uranyl nitrate,[384] amphotericin B,[385] aminoglycosides,[386] and glycerol.[387] In experimental acute renal failure, administration of vasodilator PGs has been shown to ameliorate injury.[388] Similarly, the administration of nonselective or COX-2–selective NSAIDs exacerbates experimental ischemia-reperfusion injury.[389]

COX-2 expression decreases in the kidney in response to acute ischemic injury.[390] The role of COX products in ischemia-reperfusion injury is controversial. Roles for PGs and TXA2 in modulating or mediating renal injury have been suggested in ischemia-reperfusion[383] and in models of toxin-mediated acute tubular injury, including those induced by uranyl nitrate,[384] amphotericin B,[385] aminoglycosides,[386] and glycerol.[387] Furthermore, fibrosis resulting from prolonged ischemic injury has been shown to be ameliorated by nonspecific COX inhibition.[391] In contrast, renal injury in response to ischemia-reperfusion is worsened by COX-2–selective inhibitors or in COX-2$^{-/-}$ mice,[389] and administration of vasodilator PGs has been shown to ameliorate injury,[388] possibly through a PPARα-dependent mechanism.[392]

## URINARY TRACT OBSTRUCTION

Following the induction of chronic (>24 hours) ureteral obstruction, renal PG and TXA2 synthesis are markedly enhanced, particularly in response to stimuli such as endotoxins or bradykinins. Enhanced prostanoid synthesis, especially TX, likely arises from infiltrating mononuclear cells, proliferating fibroblast-like cells, interstitial macrophages, and interstitial medullary cells.[345] Selective COX-2 inhibitors may prevent renal damage in response to unilateral ureteral obstruction.[393,394] However, PGE2 acting through the EP4 receptor can limit tubulointerstitial fibrosis resulting from UUO.[395] Prostaglandins derived from medullary COX-2 are mediators of the early phase of diuresis seen after the relief of ureteral obstruction because COX-2 inhibition prevents the acute (24-hour) phase of postobstructive diuresis. However, more persistent, chronic postobstructive diuresis is not PG-dependent but results from the downregulation of NKCC2 and decreases aquaporin-2 phosphorylation and translocation to the collecting duct membrane.[396]

## ALLOGRAFT REJECTION AND CYCLOSPORINE NEPHROTOXICITY

### ALLOGRAFT REJECTION

Acute administration of a TXA2 synthesis inhibitor is associated with significant improvement in rat renal allograft function.[397] A number of other experimental and clinical studies have also demonstrated increased TXA2 synthesis during allograft rejection,[398,399] leading some to suggest that increased urinary TXA2 excretion may be an early indicator in renal and cardiac allograft rejection.

### CALCINEURIN INHIBITOR NEPHROTOXICITY

Numerous investigators have demonstrated effects for cyclosporine A (CY-A) on renal PG and TXA2 synthesis and provided evidence for a major role for renal and leukocyte TXA2 synthesis in mediating acute and chronic CY-A nephrotoxicity in rats.[400] Fish oil–rich diets, TXA2 antagonists, or administration of CY-A in fish oil as vehicle have all been shown to reduce renal TXA2 synthesis and may therefore afford protection against nephrotoxicity. Moreover, CY-A has been reported to decrease renal COX-2 expression.[401]

## HEPATIC CIRRHOSIS AND HEPATORENAL SYNDROME

Patients with cirrhosis of the liver show an increased renal synthesis of vasodilating PGs, as indicated by the high urinary excretion of PGs and/or their metabolites. Urinary excretion of 2-3-dinor-6-keto PGF1α, an index of systemic PGI2 synthesis, is increased in patients with cirrhosis and hyperdynamic circulation, thus raising the possibility that systemic synthesis of PGI2 may contribute to the arterial vasodilation of these patients. Inhibition of COX activity in these patients may cause a profound reduction in renal blood flow and GFR, a reduction in sodium excretion, and an impairment of free water clearance.[402] The sodium-retaining properties of NSAIDs are particularly exaggerated in patients with cirrhosis of the liver, attesting to the dependence of renal salt excretion on vasodilatory PGs. In the kidneys of rats with cirrhosis, COX-2 expression increases, while COX-1 expression is unchanged; however, in these animals, selective inhibition of COX-1 leads to impaired renal hemodynamics and natriuresis, whereas COX-2 inhibition has no effect.[403,404]

Diminished renal PG synthesis has been implicated in the pathogenesis of the severe sodium retention seen in hepatorenal syndrome, as well as in the resistance to diuretic therapy.[405,406] There is reduced renal synthesis of vasodilating PGE2 in the presence of activation of endogenous vasoconstrictors and a maintained or increased renal production of TXA2.[402,407] Therefore, an imbalance between vasoconstricting systems and the renal vasodilator PGE2 has been proposed as a contributing factor to the renal failure observed in this condition. However, administration of exogenous prostanoids to patients with cirrhosis is not effective in ameliorating renal function or preventing the deleterious effect of NSAIDs.[402]

## DIABETES MELLITUS

In the streptozotocin-induced model of diabetes in rats, COX-2 expression is increased in the cTALH–macula densa region,[360,370] as well as in podocytes.[408] possibly mediated by epigenetic processes.[409] COX-2 immunoreactivity has also been detected in the macula densa region in human diabetic nephropathy.[41] Studies have suggested that COX-2 dependent vasodilator prostanoids play an important role in the hyperfiltration seen early in diabetes mellitus,[410,360,411–413] as well as in response to a high-protein diet.[414] The increased COX-2 expression appears to be mediated at least in part by increased ROS production in diabetes, because the superoxide dismutase analogue, Tempol, blocks the increased expression.[415]

It has been found that the chronic administration of a selective COX-2 inhibitor significantly decreases proteinuria and reduces extracellular matrix deposition, as indicated by decreases in immunoreactive fibronectin expression and mesangial matrix expansion.[370,416] In addition, COX-2 inhibition reduced expression of TGF-ß, PAI-1, and vascular endothelial growth factor (VEGF) in the kidneys of the diabetic hypertensive animals. Increasing intrarenal dopamine production also ameliorates diabetic nephropathy progression, at least in part by inhibiting renal cortical COX-2 expression.[417] The vasoconstrictor TXA2 may play a role in the development of albuminuria and basement membrane changes with diabetic nephropathy (DN). In addition, the administration of a selective PGE2 EP1 receptor antagonist prevented the development of experimental DN,[418] whereas EP4 receptor activation may exacerbate DN.[419] In contrast to the beneficial effect of global inhibition of COX-2, selective inhibition of renal macrophage COX-2 actually exacerbates diabetic renal injury.[420]

## PREGNANCY

Most, but not all, investigators have not reported increases in vasodilator PG synthesis or suggested an essential role for prostanoids in the mediation of the increased GFR and renal plasma flow (RPF) of normal pregnancy;[421] however, diminished synthesis of PGI2 has been demonstrated in humans and in animal models of pregnancy-induced hypertension,[422] which is associated with decreased expression of COX-2 and PGI2 synthase in placental villi.[423] In animal models, the inhibition of TXA2 synthetase has been associated with resolution of the hypertension, suggesting a possible pathophysiologic role.[424] A moderate beneficial effect of reducing TXA2 generation, while preserving PGI2 synthesis, by low-dose aspirin therapy (60–100 mg/day) has been demonstrated in patients at high risk for pregnancy-induced hypertension and preeclampsia.[425,426]

## LITHIUM NEPHROTOXICITY

Lithium chloride is a mainstay of treatment in psychiatry for bipolar illness. However, it is routinely complicated by polyuria and even frank nephrogenic diabetes insipidus. In vitro and in vivo studies have demonstrated lithium-induced renal medullary interstitial cell COX-2 protein expression via inhibition of glycogen synthase kinase-3ß (GSK-3ß). COX-2 inhibition prevented lithium-induced polyuria. COX-2 inhibition also resulted in the upregulation of aquaporin 2 (AQP2) and Na-K-2Cl co-transporter (NKCC2).[427,428]

## ROLE OF REACTIVE OXYGEN SPECIES AS MEDIATORS OF COX-2 ACTIONS

In addition to NADPH oxidase, nitric oxide synthase, and xanthine oxidase, COX-2 can also be a source of oxygen radicals.[429] COX-2 enzymatic activity is commonly accompanied by associated oxidative mechanisms (co-oxidation) and free radical production.[430] The catalytic activity of COX consists of a series of radical reactions that use molecular oxygen and generate intermediate ROS.[431] Elevated levels of COX-2 protein are associated with increased ROS production and apoptosis in cultured renal cortical cells[432] and human mesangial cells.[433] It has been suggested that COX-2–mediated lipid peroxidation, rather than PGs, can induce DNA damage via adduct formation.[434] A COX-2 specific inhibitor, NS-398, was able to reduce the oxidative activity with prevention of oxidant stress.[435]

In addition to ROS generated by COX per se, prostanoids may also activate intracellular pathways that generate ROS. Locally generated ROS may damage cell membranes, leading to lipid peroxidation and release of AA. Prostanoids released during inflammatory reactions cause rapid degenerative changes in some cultured cells, and their potential cytotoxic effect has been suggested to occur by accelerating intracellular oxidative stress. TX[436] and PGE2 acting through the EP1 receptor[437] have been reported to induce NADPH oxidase and ROS production. Of interest, PGE2 acting through the EP4 receptor inhibits macrophage oxidase activity.[438,439] As mentioned previously, there is also evidence for crosstalk between COX-2 and ROS, such that ROS may induce COX-2 expression.[434] Interestingly, during aging, there is ROS-mediated NF-κB expression, which increases COX-2 expression in the kidney.[440] Furthermore, this appears to induce a vicious cycle, because COX-2 then serves as a source of ROS. This interaction of COX-derived PG and ROS production has been posited to play a role in the development of hypertension.[441] The amount of renal ROS resulting from COX activity increases with age, so that up to 25% of total kidney ROS production in aged rat kidneys is inhibited by NSAID administration.

## THE LIPOXYGENASE PATHWAY

The lipoxygenase enzymes metabolize AA to form LTs, HETEs, and LXs (Fig. 13.12). These lipoxygenase metabolites are primarily produced by leukocytes, mast cells, and macrophages in response to inflammation and injury. There are three lipoxygenase enzymes—5-, 12-, and 15-lipoxygenase—so named for the carbon of AA where they insert an oxygen. The lipoxygenases are products of separate genes and have distinct distributions and patterns of regulation. Glomeruli, mesangial cells, cortical tubules, and vessels also produce

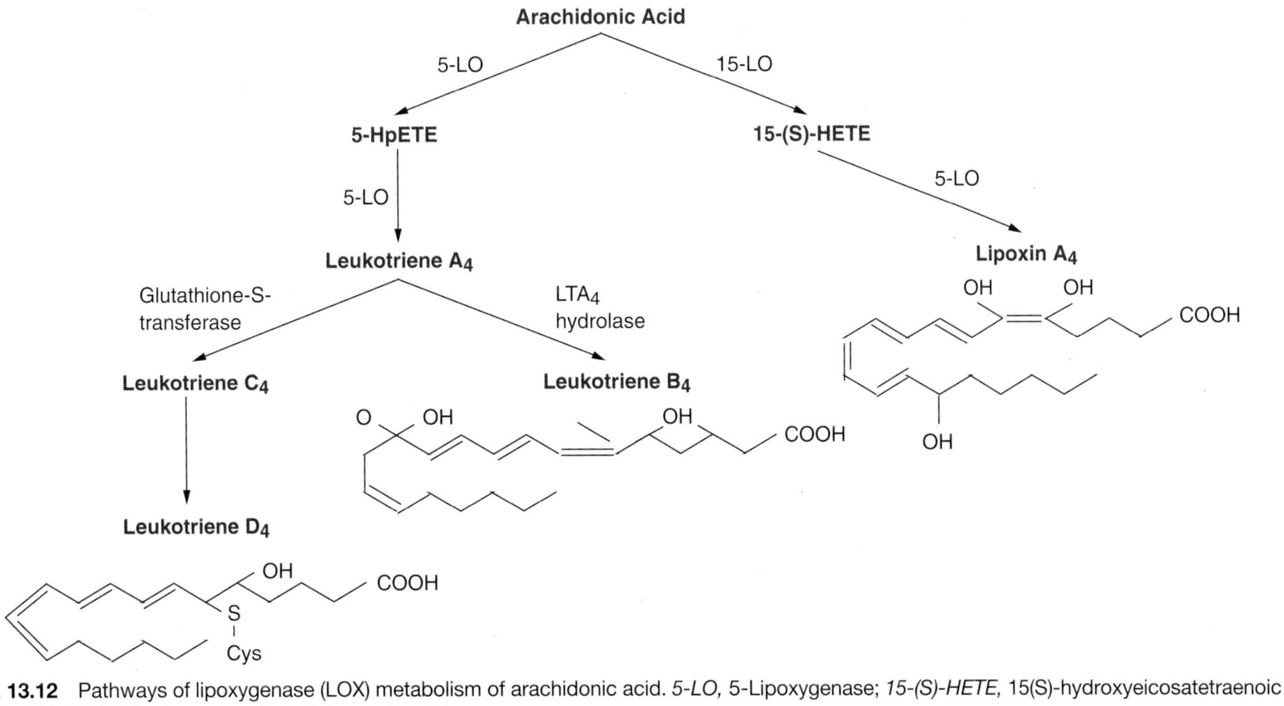

**Fig. 13.12** Pathways of lipoxygenase (LOX) metabolism of arachidonic acid. *5-LO,* 5-Lipoxygenase; *15-(S)-HETE,* 15(S)-hydroxyeicosatetraenoic acid; *5-HpETE,* 5-hydroperoxyeicosatetraenoic acid.

the 12-lipoxygenase (12-LOX) product, 12(*S*)-HETE, and the 15-LOX product, 15-HETE. Studies have localized 15-LOX mRNA primarily to the distal nephron and 12-LOX mRNA to the glomerulus. 5-LOX mRNA and 5-LOX-activating protein (FLAP) mRNA were expressed in the glomerulus and the vasa recta.[442] In polymorphonuclear leukocytes (PMNs), macrophages, and mast cells, 5-LOX mediates the formation of leukotrienes.[443] 5-LOX, which is regulated by FLAP, catalyzes the conversion of AA to 5-HpETE and then to leukotriene A4 (LTA4).[444] LTA4 is then further metabolized to the peptidyl leukotrienes (LTC4 and LTD4) by glutathione-S-transferase or to LTB4 by LTA4 hydrolase. Although glutathione-S-transferase expression is limited to inflammatory cells, LTA4 hydrolase is also expressed in glomerular mesangial cells and endothelial cells;[445] PCR analysis has actually demonstrated ubiquitous LTA4 hydrolase mRNA expression throughout the rat nephron.[442] LTC4 synthase mRNA could not be found in any nephron segment.[442]

Two cysteinyl leukotriene receptors (CysLTR) have been cloned and identified as members of the G protein–coupled superfamily of receptors. They have been localized to vascular smooth muscle and endothelium of the pulmonary vasculature.[446–448] In the kidney, the CysLTR type 1 is expressed in the glomerulus, whereas CysLTR type 2 mRNA has not been detected in any nephron segment to date.[442]

The peptidyl leukotrienes are potent mediators of inflammation and vasoconstrictors of vascular, pulmonary, and gastrointestinal smooth muscle. In addition, they increase vascular permeability and promote mucous secretion.[449] Because of the central role that peptidyl leukotrienes play in the inflammatory trigger of asthma exacerbation, effective receptor antagonists have been developed and are now an important component of asthma treatment.[450]

In the kidney, LTD4 administration has been shown to decrease RBF and GFR, and peptidyl leukotrienes are thought to be mediators of decreased RBF and GFR associated with acute glomerular inflammation. Micropuncture studies have revealed that the decreases in GFR are the result of afferent and arteriolar vasoconstriction, with more pronounced efferent vasoconstriction and a decrease in $K_f$.[1] In addition both LTC4 and LTD4 increase the proliferation of cultured mesangial cells.

The LTB4 receptor is also a seven-transmembrane G protein–coupled receptor. On PMNs, receptor activation promotes chemotaxis, aggregation, and attachment to endothelium. In the kidney LTB4, mRNA is localized to the glomerulus[442]. A second, low-affinity LTB4 receptor is also expressed,[451] which may mediate calcium influx into PMNs, thereby leading to activation. LTB4 receptor blockers lessen acute renal ischemic-reperfusion injury[452] and nephrotoxic nephritis in rats,[453] and PMN infiltration and structural and functional evidence of organ injury by ischemia and reperfusion are magnified in transgenic mice overexpressing the LTB4 receptor.[454] In addition to the activation of cell surface receptors, L TB4 has also been shown to be a ligand for the nuclear receptor PPARα.[455]

15-LOX leads to the formation of 15-S-HETE. In addition, dual oxygenation in activated PMNs and macrophages by 5- and 15-LOX leads to formation of the lipoxins. LX synthesis also can occur via transcellular metabolism of the leukocyte-generated intermediate, LTA4, by 12-LOX in platelets or adjoining cells, including glomerular endothelial cells.[456,457]

15-S-HETE is a potent vasoconstrictor in the renal microcirculation;[458] however, 15-LOX–derived metabolites antagonize proinflammatory actions of leukotrienes, both by inhibiting PMN chemotaxis, aggregation, and adherence and by counteracting the vasoconstrictive effects of the peptidyl leukotrienes.[459,460] Administration of 15-S-HETE reduced LTB4 production by glomeruli isolated from rats with acute nephrotoxic, serum-induced glomerulonephritis, and it has been proposed that 15-LOX may regulate 5-LOX activity in chronic glomerular inflammation because it is known that in experimental glomerulonephritis, lipoxin A4 (LXA4) administration increases renal blood flow and GFR, mainly by inducing afferent arteriolar vasodilation, an effect mediated in part by release of vasodilator PGs.[1] LXA4 also antagonized the effects of LTD4 to decrease the GFR, although not RBF, even though administration of LXA4 and LXB4 directly into the renal artery induced vasoconstriction. Glomerular micropuncture studies have revealed that LXA4 leads to moderate decreases in $K_f$.[459] Lipoxins signal through a specific G protein–coupled receptor denoted ALXR. This receptor is related at the nucleotide sequence level to chemokine and chemotactic peptide receptors, such as N-formyl peptide receptor.[461] It is also noteworthy that in isolated perfused canine renal arteries and veins, LTC4 and LTD4 were found to be vasodilators, which were partially dependent on an intact endothelium; this was mediated by nitric oxide production.[462]

A potential interaction between COX- and LOX-mediated pathways has been reported. Although aspirin inhibits PG formation by COX-1 and COX-2, aspirin-induced acetylation converts COX-2 to a selective generator of 15-(*S*)-HETE. This product can then be released, taken up in a transcellular route by PMNs and converted to 15-epilipoxins, which have similar biologic actions as the lipoxins.[463]

Similar to 15-HETE, 12(*S*)-HETE also potently vasoconstricts glomerular and renal vasculature.[456] 12(*S*)-HETE increases protein kinase C and depolarizes cultured vascular smooth muscle cells. Afferent arteriolar vasoconstriction and increases in smooth muscle calcium in response to 12(*S*)-HETE, were partially inhibited by voltage-gated, L-type calcium channel inhibitors.[464] 12(*S*)-HETE has also been proposed to be an angiogenic factor, because in cultured endothelial cells, 12-LOX inhibition reduces cell proliferation, and 12-LOX overexpression stimulates cell migration and endothelial tube formation.[465] 12- and 15-LOX inhibitors and elective elimination of the leukocyte 12-LOX enzyme also ameliorate the development of diabetic nephropathy in mice.[466] There is also interaction between 12- and 15-LOX pathways and TGF-ß–mediated pathways in the diabetic kidney.[467] 12(*S*)-HETE has also been proposed to be a mediator of renal vasoconstriction by Ang II, with inhibition of the 12-LOX pathway attenuating Ang II-mediated afferent arteriolar vasoconstriction and decreased renal blood flow.[468] LOX inhibition also blunted renal arcuate artery vasoconstriction by norepinephrine and KCl.[469] However, 12-LOX products have also been implicated as inhibitors of renal renin release.[470,471]

Although the major significance of LOX products in the kidney derives from their release from infiltrating leukocytes or resident cells of macrophage or monocyte origin, there is evidence to suggest that intrinsic renal cells are capable of generating LTs and LXs, either directly or through transcellular metabolism of intermediates.[472] Human and rat glomeruli can generate 12- and 15-HETE, although the cells of origin are unclear. LTB4 can be detected in supernatants of normal rat glomeruli, and its synthesis could be markedly diminished by mechanisms that deplete glomeruli of resident macrophages, such as irradiation or fatty acid deficiency. In addition, 5-,12-, and 15-HETEs were detected from pig glomeruli, and their structural identity was confirmed by mass spectrometry[1]. 12-LOX products are increased in mesangial cells exposed to hyperglycemia and in diabetic nephropathy.[473] There also appears to be crosstalk between 12- and 15-LOX and COX-2. Both are increased with diabetes or high glucose levels and, in cultured cells, 12(*S*)-HETE increases COX-2, whereas PGE2 increases 12- and 15-LOX. Knockdown of 12- and 15-LOX expression with short hairpin RNA (shRNA) decreases COX-2 expression, whereas 12- and 15-LOX overexpression increases COX-2 expression.[430]

Glomeruli subjected to immune injury release LTB4,[474] and LTB4 generation was suppressed by resident macrophage depletion. Synthesis of peptido-LTs by inflamed glomeruli has also been demonstrated,[475] but leukocytes could not be excluded because its primary source LXA4 is generated by immune-injured glomeruli.[476] Rat mesangial cells generate LXA4 when provided with LTA4 as substrate, thereby providing a potential intraglomerular source of LXs during inflammatory reactions. In nonglomerular tissue, 12-HETE production has been reported from rat cortical tubules and epithelial cells and 12- and 15-HETE from rabbit medulla[1].

## BIOLOGIC ACTIVITIES OF LIPOXYGENASE PRODUCTS IN THE KIDNEY

In early experiments, the systemic administration of LTC4 in the rat and administration of LTC4 and LTD4 in the isolated perfused kidney revealed potent renal vasoconstrictor actions of these eicosanoids. Subsequently, micropuncture measurements revealed that LTD4 exerts preferential constrictor effects on postglomerular arteriolar resistance and depresses $K_f$ and GFR. The latter is likely due to receptor-mediated contraction of glomerular mesangial cells, which has been demonstrated for LTC4 and LTD4 in vitro (see earlier). These actions of LTD4 in the kidney are consistent with its known smooth muscle contractile properties. LTB4, a potent chemotactic and leukocyte-activating agent, is devoid of constrictor action in the normal rat kidney. Lipoxin A4 dilates afferent arterioles when infused into the renal artery, without affecting efferent arteriolar tone. This results in elevations in intraglomerular pressure and plasma flow rate, thereby augmenting the GFR.[1]

## INVOLVEMENT OF LIPOXYGENASE PRODUCTS IN RENAL PATHOPHYSIOLOGY

Increased generation rates of $LTC_4$ and LTD4 have been documented in glomeruli from rats with immune complex nephritis and mice with spontaneously developing lupus nephritis.[443,476] Moreover, results from numerous physiologic studies using specific LTD4 receptor antagonists have provided strong evidence for the release of these eicosanoids during glomerular inflammation. In four animal models of glomerular immune injury (anti-GBM nephritis, anti-Thy1.1 antibody-mediated mesangiolysis, passive Heymann nephritis, and murine lupus nephritis), acute antagonism of LTD4 by receptor binding competition or inhibition of LTD4 synthesis led to highly significant increases in GFR in nephritic animals.[477] The principal mechanism underlying the improvement in GFR was reversal of the depressed values of $K_f$, which is characteristically compromised in immune-injured glomeruli. In other studies in PHN, Katoh and colleagues provided evidence that endogenous LTD4 not only mediates reductions in $K_f$ and GFR, but that LTD4-evoked increases in intraglomerular pressure underlie, to a large extent, the accompanying proteinuria.[477] Cysteinyl leukotrienes have been implicated in cyclosporine nephrotoxicity.[478] Of interest, 5- LOX deficiency accelerates renal allograft rejection.[479]

LTB4 synthesis, measured in the supernates of isolated glomeruli, is markedly enhanced early in the course of several forms of glomerular immune injury.[480] Cellular sources of LTB4 in injured glomeruli include PMNs and macrophages. All studies concur as to the transient nature of LTB4 release. LTB4 production decreases 24 hours after onset of the inflammation, which coincides with macrophage infiltration, a major source of 15-LOX activity.[481] 15-HPETE incubation decreased lipopolysaccharide-induced TNF expression in a human monocytic cell line,[482] and HVJ-liposome–mediated glomerular transfection of 15-LOX in rats decreased markers of injury (e.g., blood urea nitrogen [BUN], proteinuria) and accelerated functional (GFR, RBF) recovery in experimental glomerulonephritis (GN).[483] In addition, MK501, a FLAP antagonist, restored size selectivity and decreased glomerular permeability in acute GN.[484]

The suppression of LTB4 synthesis beyond the first 24 hours of injury is rather surprising, because both PMNs and macrophages are capable of effecting the total synthesis of LTB4; they contain the two necessary enzymes that convert AA to LTB4—namely, 5-LOX and LTA4 hydrolase. It has therefore been suggested, based on in vitro evidence, that the major route for LTB4 synthesis in inflamed glomeruli is through transcellular metabolism of leukocyte-generated LTA4 to LTB4 by LTA4 hydrolase present in glomerular mesangial, endothelial, and epithelial cells. Because the transformation of LTA4 to LTB4 is rate-limiting, regulation of LTB4 synthetic rate might relate to the regulation of LTA4 hydrolase gene expression or catalytic activity in these parenchymal cells, rather than to the number of infiltrating leukocytes. In any case, leukocytes represent an indispensable source for LTA4, the initial 5-LOX product and the precursor for LTB4, because endogenous glomerular cells do not express the 5-LOX gene.[485] Thus, it was demonstrated that the PMN cell-specific activator, N-formyl-Met-Leu-Phe, stimulated LTB4 production from isolated perfused kidneys harvested from NTS-treated rats to a significantly greater degree than from control animals treated with nonimmune rabbit serum.[486] The renal production of LTB4 correlated directly with renal myeloperoxidase activity, suggesting interdependence of LTB4 generation and PMN infiltration.

The acute and long-term significance of LTB4 generation in conditioning the extent of glomerular structural and functional deterioration has been highlighted in studies in which LTB4 was exogenously administered or in which its endogenous synthesis was inhibited. Intrarenal administration of LTB4 to rats with mild NTS-induced injury was associated with an increase in PMN infiltration, reduction in renal plasma flow rate, and marked exacerbation of the fall in the GFR, with the latter correlating strongly with the number of infiltrating PMNs and glomeruli, whereas inhibition of 5-LOX led to preservation of the GFR and abrogation of proteinuria.[486] Similarly, both 5-LOX knockout mice and wild-type mice treated with the 5-LOX inhibitor zileuton had reduced renal injury in response to ischemia and reperfusion.[487] Thus although devoid of vasoconstrictor actions in the normal kidney, increased intrarenal generation of LTB4 during early glomerular injury amplifies leukocyte-dependent reductions in glomerular perfusion and filtration rates and inflammatory injury, likely due to enhancement of PMN recruitment and activation.

12(*S*)-HETE has been reported to increase AT1 receptor (AT1R) mRNA and protein expression in cultured rat mesangial cells by stabilizing AT1R mRNA and enhancing the profibrotic effects of Ang II.[488] Ang II AT1R blockade has been shown to inhibit the development of diabetic nephropathy via the upregulation of glomerular nephrin and P-cadherin expression through inhibition of 12- and 15-LOX activation in rats.[489] Genetic or pharmacologic inhibition of 12- and 15-LOX led to decreases in 12(*S*)-HETE production, proteinuria, renal oxidative stress, and collagen deposition in type I diabetes.[490] Recently, 12(*S*)-HETE was found to increase profibrotic gene expression and enhance the permissive histone lysine modification at their promoters by upregulation of protein levels of SET7, a histone H3 lysine 4 methyltransferase, its nuclear translocation, and enhancement at profibrotic gene promoters in mesangial cells.[491]

Both LOX and leukotriene signaling pathways have been reported to be involved in the development of cisplatin-mediated acute kidney injury in Wistar albino rats.[492] Urinary 12(S)- and 15(S)-HETE levels have been shown to correlate positively with elevated serum creatinine levels after kidney transplantation.[493] In the JCR:LA-corpulent rat, a model of the metabolic syndrome, fish oil (ω-3 polyunsaturated fatty acid) supplements markedly reduced albuminuria and glomerulosclerosis in association with decreases in 5(S)-, 12(S)-, and 15(S)-HETE.[494] The nucleotide-binding oligomerization domain-like receptor containing pyrin domain 3 (NLRP3) inflammasome promotes renal inflammation and contributes to chronic kidney disease through the generation of proinflammatory cytokines IL-β and IL-18.[495] Docosahexaenoic acid (DHA, in the form of fish oil), a well-known ω-3 polyunsaturated fatty acid, inhibits inflammation and exerts a beneficial action in numerous inflammatory human diseases. Recent studies have indicated that the LOX-mediated DHA metabolite, resolving D1, attenuates podocyte injury during hyperhomocysteinemia by inhibiting NLRP3 inflammasome activation.[496]

## THE CYTOCHROME P450 PATHWAY

Following their elucidation and characterization as endogenous metabolites of AA, numerous studies have investigated the possibility that cytochrome P450 (CYP450) AA metabolites subserve physiologic and/or pathophysiologic roles in the kidney. In whole-animal physiology, these compounds have been implicated in the mediation of release of peptide hormones, regulation of vascular tone, and regulation of volume homeostasis. On the cellular level, CYP AA metabolites have been proposed to regulate ion channels and transporters and to act as mitogens. See Fig. 13.13.

CYP450 monooxygenases are mixed-function oxidases that use molecular oxygen and NADPH as cofactors[497,498] and will

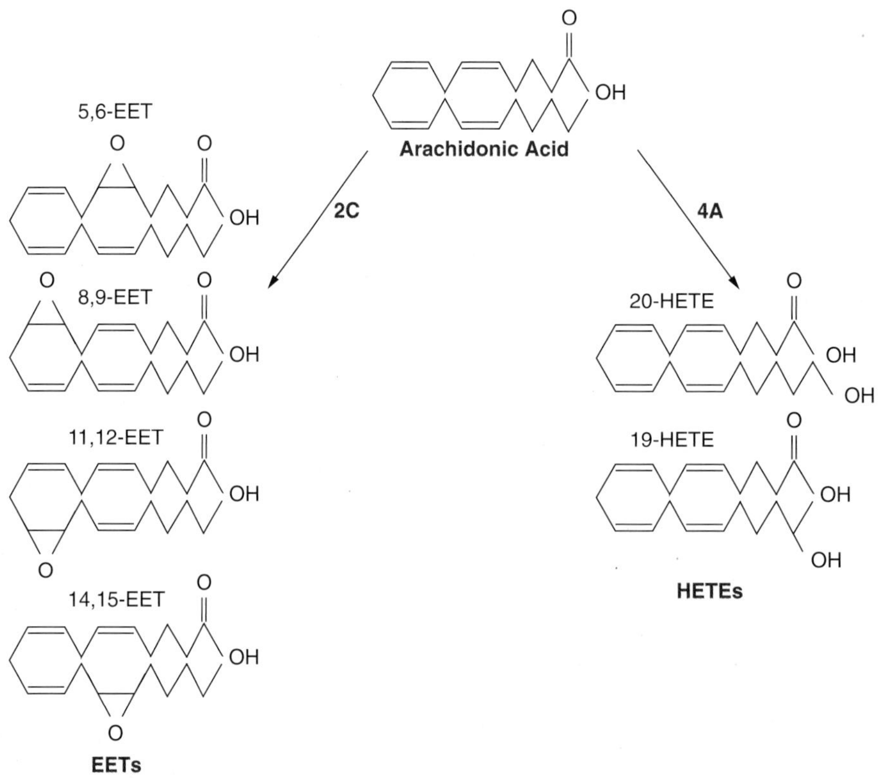

**Fig. 13.13** Pathways of CYP450 metabolism of arachidonic acid. *EET,* Epoxyeicosatrienoic acid; *HETE,* hydroxyeicosatetraenoic acid.

add an oxygen molecule to AA in a region- and stereo-specific geometry. CYP450 monooxygenase pathways metabolize AA to generate HETEs and epoxyeicosatrienoic acids (EETs); EETs can be hydrolyzed to dihydroxyeicosatrienoic acids (DHETs).[497,499,500] The kidney displays one of the highest CYP450 activities of any organ and produces CYP450 AA metabolites in significant amounts.[497,500,501] HETEs are formed primarily via CYP450 hydroxylase enzymes and EETs, and DHETs are formed primarily via CYP450 epoxygenase enzymes.[501] The CYP450 4A gene family is the major pathway for synthesis of hydroxylase metabolites, especially 20-HETE and 19-HETE,[300,501] whereas the production of epoxygenase metabolites is primarily via the 2C gene family.[497,502] A member of the 2J family that is an active epoxygenase is also expressed in the kidney.[503]

CYP450 enzymes have been localized to vasculature and tubules.[300] The 4A family of hydroxylases is expressed in preglomerular renal arterioles, glomeruli, proximal tubules, the TALH, and macula densa.[504]

The 2C and 2J families of epoxygenases are expressed at the highest levels in the proximal tubule and collecting duct.[503,505] When isolated nephron segments expressing CYP450 protein have been incubated with AA, the production of CYP450 AA metabolites can be detected. 20-HETE and EETs are both produced in the afferent arterioles,[506] glomerulus,[507] and proximal tubule.[508] 20-HETE is the predominant CYP450 AA metabolite produced by the TALH and in the pericytes surrounding vasa recta capillaries,[507] whereas EETs are the predominant CYP450 AA metabolites produced by the collecting duct.[509]

Renal production of both epoxygenase and hydroxylase metabolites has been shown to be regulated by hormones and growth factors, including Ang II, endothelin, bradykinin, parathyroid hormone, and epidermal growth factor.[300,498,502] Alterations in dietary salt intake also modulate CYP450 expression and activity.[510] Alterations in the production of CYP450 metabolites have also been reported with uninephrectomy, diabetes mellitus, and hypertension.[300,499] Glycerol-containing epoxygenase metabolites are produced endogenously and serve as high-affinity ligands for cannabinoid receptors, implicating these compounds as endocannabinoids.[511]

## VASCULATURE

### 20-TRIHYDROXYEICOSATETRAENOIC ACID

In rat and dog renal arteries and afferent arterioles, 20-HETE is a potent vasoconstrictor,[506] whereas it is a vasodilator in rabbit renal arterioles. The vasoconstriction is associated with membrane depolarization and a sustained rise in intracellular calcium. 20-HETE is produced in the smooth muscle cells, and its afferent arteriolar vasoconstrictive effects are mediated by the closure of $K_{Ca}$ channels through a tyrosine kinase- and ERK-dependent mechanism (Fig. 13.14). Recent studies have indicated that 20-HETE–induced hypertension is a mediator of kidney disease in diabetes.[512]

An interaction between CYP450 AA metabolites and nitric oxide has also been demonstrated. NO can inhibit the formation of 20-HETE in renal vascular smooth muscle (VSM) cells. A significant portion of NO's vasodilator effects in the preglomerular vasculature appear to be mediated by the inhibition of tonic 20-HETE vasoconstriction, and inhibition of 20-HETE formation attenuates the pressor response and fall in RBF seen with NO synthase inhibition.[513,514]

### EPOXIDES

Unlike CYP450 hydroxylase metabolites, epoxygenase metabolites of AA increase RBF and GFR.[300,498,502] 11,12-EET and 14,15-EET vasodilate the preglomerular arterioles

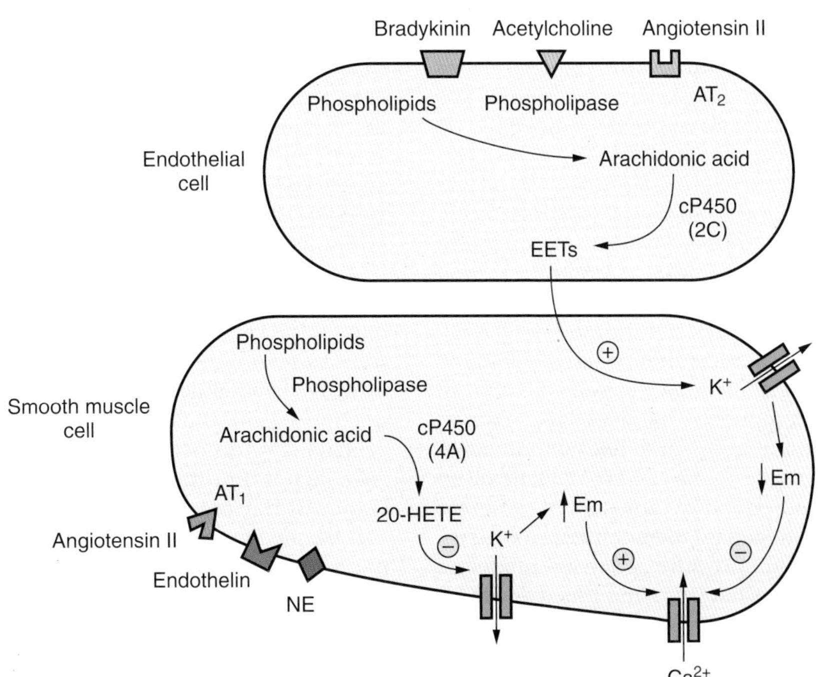


**Fig. 13.14** Proposed interactions of CYP450 arachidonic acid metabolites derived from vascular endothelial cells and smooth muscle cells to regulate vascular tone. *EET*, Epoxyeicosatrienoic acid; *HETE*, hydroxyeicosatetraenoic acid; *NE*, norepinephrine.

independently of COX activity, whereas 5,6-EET and 8,9-EET cause COX-dependent vasodilation or vasoconstriction.[515] It is possible that these COX-dependent effects are mediated by COX conversion of 5,6-EET and 8,9-EET to PG- or TX-like compounds.[516] EETs are produced primarily in the endothelial cells and exert their vasoactive effects on the adjacent smooth muscle cells. In this regard, it has been suggested that EETs, and specifically 11,12-EET, may serve as an endothelium-derived hyperpolarizing factor (EDHF) in the renal microcirculation.[502,517] EET-induced vasodilation is mediated by activation of $K_{Ca}$ channels through cAMP-dependent stimulation of protein kinase C.

CYP450 metabolites may serve as second messengers or as modulators of the actions of hormonal and paracrine agents. Vasopressin increases renal production of CYP450 metabolites,[518] and increases in intracellular calcium and proliferation in cultured renal mesangial cells are augmented by EET administration.[518] CYP450 metabolites also may serve to modulate the renal hemodynamic responses of endothelin-1, with 20-HETE as a possible mediator of the vasoconstrictive effects and EETs counteracting the vasoconstriction.[502,519] The formation of 20-HETE does not affect the ability of ET-1 to increase free intracellular calcium transient in renal vascular smooth muscle but appears to enhance the sustained elevations that represent calcium influx through voltage-sensitive channels.

CYP450 metabolites have also been implicated in mediation of renal vascular responses to Ang II. In the presence of AT1 receptor blockers, Ang II produces an endothelial-dependent vasodilation in rabbit afferent arterioles that is dependent on CYP450 epoxygenase metabolite production by AT2 receptor activation.[520] With intact AT1 receptors, Ang II increases 20-HETE release from isolated preglomerular microvessels through an endothelium-independent mechanism.[521] Ang II's vasoconstrictive effects are in part the result of 20-HETE–mediated inhibition of $K_{Ca}$, which enhances sustained increases in intracellular calcium concentration by calcium influx through voltage-sensitive channels. Inhibition of 20-HETE production reduces the vasoconstrictor response to Ang II by more than 50% in rat renal interlobular arteries in which the endothelium has been removed.[521]

## AUTOREGULATION

CYP450 metabolites of AA have been shown to be mediators of RBF autoregulatory mechanisms. When PG production was blocked in canine arcuate arteries, AA administration enhanced myogenic responsiveness, and renal blood flow autoregulation was blocked by CYP450 inhibitors.[300,500] Similarly, in the rat juxtamedullary preparation, selective blockade of 20-HETE formation significantly decreased afferent arteriolar vasoconstrictor responses to elevations in perfusion pressure, and inhibition of epoxygenase activity enhanced vasoconstriction.[522] This suggests that 20-HETE is involved in afferent arteriolar autoregulatory adjustment, whereas release of vasodilatory epoxygenase metabolites in response to increases in renal perfusion pressure acts to attenuate the vasoconstriction. In vivo studies have also implicated 20-HETE as a mediator of the autoregulatory response to increased perfusion pressure.[523] Bradykinin-induced efferent arteriolar vasodilation has been shown to be mediated in part by the direct release of EETs from this vascular segment. In addition, bradykinin-induced release of 20-HETE from the glomerulus can modulate the EET-mediated vasodilation.[524] Deficient 20-HETE production worsens ischemic kidney injury by impairing medullary blood flow.[525]

## TUBULOGLOMERULAR FEEDBACK

CYP450 metabolites may also be involved in the tubuloglomerular feedback response.[300] As noted, 20-HETE is produced by both the afferent arteriole and macula densa, and studies have suggested the possibility that HETEs may serve as a vasoconstrictive mediator of TGF released by the macula densa or as a second messenger in the afferent arteriole in response to mediators released by the macula densa, such as adenosine or ATP.[526] 20-HETE may also be a mediator of regulation of intrarenal distribution of blood flow.[527,528] In addition, there is evidence for "connecting tubule–glomerular feedback," in which increased sodium reabsorption in the connecting segment, which abuts the afferent arteriole, leads to increased AA release, leading to increased production of EETs and vasodilatory PGs. These then diffuse to the adjacent afferent arteriole and dilate it.[529]

## TUBULES

Both 20-HETE and EETs inhibit tubular sodium reabsorption.[300,498] Renal cortical interstitial infusion of the nonselective CYP450 inhibitor 17-ODYA increases papillary blood flow, renal interstitial hydrostatic pressure, and sodium excretion without affecting total RBF or GFR. High dietary salt intake in rats increases expression of the renal epoxygenase 2C23 and production and urinary excretion of EETs while decreasing 20-HETE production in the renal cortex.[497,510] 14,15-EET has also been shown to inhibit renin secretion;[530] however, clotrimazole, which is a relatively selective epoxygenase inhibitor, induced hypertension in rats fed a high-salt diet, suggesting a role in the regulation of blood pressure.[510]

### Proximal Tubule

The proximal tubule contains the highest concentration of CYP450 in the mammalian kidney and expresses minimal COX and LOX activity.[497] The 4A CYP450 family of hydroxylases that produce 19- and 20-HETE is highly expressed in the mammalian proximal tubule.[314] CYP450 enzymes of both the 2C and 2J family, which catalyze the formation of EETs, are also expressed in the proximal tubule.[497] Both EETs and 20-HETE have been shown to be produced in the proximal tubule and have been proposed to be modulators of sodium reabsorption in the proximal tubule.

Studies in isolated perfused proximal tubule have indicated that 20-HETE inhibits sodium transport, whereas 19-HETE stimulates sodium transport, suggesting that 19-HETE may serve as a competitive antagonist of 20-HETE.[508,531] Administration of EETs inhibits amiloride-sensitive sodium transport in primary cultures of proximal tubule cells[532] and in LLC-PK1 cells, a nontransformed, immortalized cell line from pig kidney with proximal tubule characteristics.[533,534]

It has been proposed that 20-HETE can be a mediator of the hormonal inhibition of proximal tubule reabsorption by parathyroid hormone (PTH), dopamine, Ang II, and EGF. Although the mechanisms of 20-HETE's inhibition have not yet been completely elucidated, there is evidence that it can inhibit $Na^+$-$K^+$-ATPase activity by phosphorylation of the $Na^+$-$K^+$-ATPase alpha subunit through a protein kinase C–dependent pathway.[535,536]

EETs may also serve as second messengers in the proximal tubule for EGF.[537] The mechanisms whereby CYPP450 AA metabolites modulate proximal tubule reabsorption have not been completely elucidated; they may involve both luminal (NHE3) and basolateral ($Na^+$-$K^+$-ATPase) transporters.[532,535] CYP450 AA metabolites may modulate the proximal tubule component of the pressure-natriuresis response.[538] Of note, intrarenal dopamine, which originates from the proximal tubule, induces the production of EETs and, if EET production is inhibited genetically, dopamine-mediated diuresis and natriuresis are inhibited.[539]

### THICK ASCENDING LIMB OF HENLE

In addition, 20-HETE serves as a second messenger to regulation transport in the TAL. It is produced in this nephron segment[504] and can inhibit net Na-K-Cl cotransport by direct inhibition of the transporter and by blocking the 70-pS apical $K^+$ channel.[540] In addition, 20-HETE has been implicated as a mediator of the inhibitory effects of Ang II[541] and bradykinin[542] on TALH transport.

### COLLECTING DUCT

In the collecting duct, EETs and/or their diol metabolites serve as inhibitors of the hydroosmotic effects of vasopressin, as well as inhibitors of sodium transport in this segment.[509,543] Patch clamp studies have indicated that the eNaC sodium channel activity in the cortical collecting duct is inhibited by 11,12-EET.[544,545] Studies using mice with selective deletion of CYP2C44, the major kidney epoxygenase, have confirmed that EETs modulate eNaC activity and that EET production is mediated in part by activation of collecting duct epidermal growth factor receptors and ERK1/2 activation.[546–549] There is also an intriguing association of 20-HETE with circadian clock sodium regulation in the collecting duct.[550]

## ROLE IN ACUTE AND CHRONIC KIDNEY DISEASE

EET-mediated increases in rat mesangial cell proliferation was the first direct evidence that CYP450 AA metabolites are cellular mitogens.[551] In cultured rabbit proximal tubule cells, CYP450 inhibitors blunted EGF-stimulated proliferation in proximal tubule cells.[537] In LLCPKcl$_4$, EETs were found to be potent mitogens, cytoprotective agents, and second messengers for EGF signaling. 14,15-EET–mediated signaling and mitogenesis are dependent on EGF receptor transactivation, which is mediated by the metalloproteinase-dependent release of heparin-binding (HB)-EGF.[552] In addition to the EETs, 20-HETE has been shown to increase thymidine incorporation in primary cultures of rat proximal tubule and LLC-PK1 cells[553] and vascular smooth muscle cells.[554] EETs are also pro-angiogenic factors.[555]

There is increasing evidence that the activation of EETs or the administration of EET analogues can protect against acute kidney injury.[556–558] Conversely, inhibition of 20-HETE is beneficial in AKI.[559]

EETs may also be protective in chronic models of renal injury, such as diabetic nephropathy, and in a 5/6 nephrectomy model.[560,561] Increasing EET levels by the inhibition of soluble epoxide hydrolase decreases the inflammation and fibrosis in a model of unilateral ureteral obstruction.[562] Similarly, an EET analogue was found to inhibit the development of radiation-induced renal fibrosis.[563]

## ROLE IN HYPERTENSION

There is increasing evidence that the renal production of CYP450 AA metabolites is altered in a variety of models of hypertension and that blockade of the formation of compounds can alter blood pressure in several of these models. CYP450 AA metabolites may have both pro- and antihypertensive properties. At the level of the renal tubule, both 20-HETE and EETs inhibit sodium transport. However, in the vasculature, 20-HETE promotes vasoconstriction and hypertension, whereas EETs are endothelial-derived vasodilators that have antihypertensive properties. Rats fed a high-salt diet increase expression of the CYP450 epoxygenase 2C23[564] and develop hypertension if treated with a relatively selective epoxygenase inhibitor. Because EETs have antihypertensive properties, efforts are underway to develop selective inhibitors of soluble epoxide hydrolase (sEH), which converts active EETs to their inactive metabolites, DHETs, and thereby increase EET levels. Studies in rats have indicated that one such sEH inhibitor, 1-cyclohexyl-3-dodecylurea, lowers blood pressure and reduces glomerular and tubulointerstitial injury in an Ang II-mediated model of hypertension in rats.[565] Furthermore, genetic deletion of CYP2C44, the major kidney epoxygenase, leads to the development of salt-sensitive hypertension.[547]

In deoxycorticosterone acetate (DOCA)-salt hypertension, the administration of a CYP450 inhibitor prevented the development of hypertension.[519,566] Ang II stimulates the formation of 20-HETE in the renal circulation,[567] and 20-HETE synthesis inhibition attenuates Ang II-mediated renal vasoconstriction[521,568] and reduces Ang II-mediated hypertension.[566]

The CYP450 4A2 gene is regulated by salt and is overexpressed in spontaneously hypertensive rats (SHRs);[569] the production of both 20-HETEs and diHETEs is increased and the production of EETs is reduced.[314,570] CYP450 inhibitors or antisense oligonucleotides directed against CYP4A1 and 4A2 lowered blood pressure in SHRs.[514,571] Conversely, studies in humans have indicated that a variant of the human CYP4A11, with reduced 20-HETE synthase activity, is associated with hypertension.[572]

In Dahl salt-sensitive rats (Dahl S), pressure natriuresis in response to salt loading is shifted so that the kidney requires a higher perfusion pressure to excrete the same amount of sodium as normotensive salt-resistant (Dahl R) rats;[300,497,498] this is because, at least in part, of increased TALH reabsorption. The production of 20-HETE and expression of CYP4A protein are reduced in the outer medulla and TALH of Dahl S rats relative to Dahl R rats, which is consistent with the observed effect of 20-HETE to inhibit TALH transport. In addition, Dahl S rats do not increase EET production in response to salt loading.

Studies have indicated that Ang II acts on AT2 receptors on renal vascular endothelial cells to release EETs that may then counteract AT1-induced renal vasoconstriction and influence pressure natriuresis.[515,573,574] AT2 receptor knockout mice develop hypertension,[575] which is associated with blunted pressure natriuresis, reduced RBF and GFR, and defects in kidney 20-HETE production.[575] There is also evidence that the natriuretic effects of dopamine are mediated by EETs and 20-HETE.[539,576]

There has been recent interest in the role of soluble epoxide hydralase (sEH), which is the major enzyme mediating the metabolism of EETs to the inactive dHETEs in the regulation of blood pressure. Ang II induces sEH in the vasculature, which may contribute to the hypertensive effects by increasing EET metabolism.[577] Progressively more selective sEH inhibitors are being developed and have been shown to be effective in reducing blood pressure in a number of experimental models of hypertension.[578]

## ACKNOWLEDGMENTS

The writing of this chapter was supported by grants from the Veterans Administration to Raymond C. Harris, National Institute of Diabetes and Digestive and Kidney Diseases (NIDDK) to Raymond C. Harris and Ming-Zhi Zhang (DK62794 and DK95785), and National Heart, Lung, and Blood Institute (NHLBI) R56HL127218 and R01HL134895 to Richard Breyer.

 Complete reference list available at ExpertConsult.com.

## KEY REFERENCES

9. Fitzpatrick FA, Soberman R. Regulated formation of eicosanoids. *J Clin Invest.* 2001;107(11):1347–1351.

35. Harris RC, McKanna JA, Akai Y, et al. Cyclooxygenase-2 is associated with the macula densa of rat kidney and increases with salt restriction. *J Clin Invest.* 1994;94(6):2504–2510.

36. Peti-Peterdi J, Harris RC. Macula densa sensing and signaling mechanisms of renin release. *J Am Soc Nephrol.* 2010;21(7):1093–1096.

79. Stegbauer J, Chen D, Herrera M, et al. Resistance to hypertension mediated by intercalated cells of the collecting duct. *JCI Insight.* 2017;2(7):e92720.

86. Zhang MZ, Yao B, Wang Y, et al. Inhibition of cyclooxygenase-2 in hematopoietic cells results in salt-sensitive hypertension. *J Clin Invest.* 2015;125(11):4281–4294.

126. Fitzgerald GA. Coxibs and cardiovascular disease. *N Engl J Med.* 2004;351(17):1709–1711.

237. Breyer MD, Breyer RM. G protein-coupled prostanoid receptors and the kidney. *Annu Rev Physiol.* 2001;63:579–605.

300. Roman RJ. P-450 metabolites of arachidonic acid in the control of cardiovascular function. *Physiol Rev.* 2002;82(1):131–185.

420. Wang X, Yao B, Wang Y, et al. Macrophage cyclooxygenase-2 protects against development of diabetic nephropathy. *Diabetes.* 2017;66(2):494–504.

464. Imig JD. Eicosanoid regulation of the renal vasculature. *Am J Physiol Renal Physiol.* 2000;279(6):F965–F981.

# SECTION II

# DISORDERS OF BODY FLUID VOLUME AND COMPOSITION

# 14 Disorders of Sodium Balance

Itzchak N. Slotki | Karl Skorecki

CHAPTER OUTLINE



Sodium ($Na^+$) and water balance and their distribution among the various body compartments are essential for the maintenance of fluid homeostasis, particularly intravascular volume. Disturbances of either or both of these components have serious medical consequences, are relatively frequent and are among the most common conditions encountered in clinical practice. In fact, abnormalities of $Na^+$ and water balance are responsible for, or associated with, a wide spectrum of medical and surgical admissions or complications. The principal disorders of $Na^+$ balance are manifested clinically as hypovolemia or hypervolemia, whereas disruption in water balance can be diagnosed only in the laboratory as hyponatremia or hypernatremia. Although disorders of $Na^+$ and water balance are often interrelated, the latter are considered separately in Chapter 15. In this chapter, the physiologic and pathophysiologic features of $Na^+$ balance are discussed. Because $Na^+$ is restricted predominantly to the extracellular compartment, this chapter also addresses perturbations of extracellular fluid (ECF) volume homeostasis.

## PHYSIOLOGY

Approximately 60% of adult body mass is composed of solute-containing fluids divided into extracellular and intracellular compartments. Because water flows freely across cell membranes in accordance with the prevailing osmotic forces on either side of the membrane, the solute/water ratios in the intracellular fluid (ICF) and ECF are almost equal. However, the solute compositions of the ICF and ECF are quite different, as shown in Fig. 14.1. The principal ECF cation is sodium; other cations are potassium ($K^+$), calcium, and magnesium. In contrast, potassium is the major ICF cation. The accompanying anions in the ECF are chloride, bicarbonate and plasma proteins (mainly albumin), whereas electroneutrality of the ICF is maintained by phosphate and the negative charges on organic molecules. The difference in cationic composition of the two compartments is maintained by a pump-leak mechanism consisting of sodium–potassium adenosine triphosphatase ($Na^+$-$K^+$-ATPase), which operates in concert with sodium and potassium conductance pathways in the cell membrane.

The free movement of water across the membrane ensures that the ECF and ICF osmolalities are the same. However, the intracellular volume is greater because the amount of potassium salts inside the cell is larger than that of sodium salts outside the cell. The movement of water is determined by the "effective osmolality," or tonicity, of each compartment, so that if tonicity of the ECF rises—for example, as a result of excess $Na^+$—water will move from the ICF to ECF to restore tonicity. On the other hand, addition of solute-free water leads to a proportionate decrease in both osmolality and tonicity of all body fluid compartments (see Chapters 10 and 15 for a detailed discussion). The restriction of $Na^+$ to the ECF compartment by the pump-leak mechanism, in combination with maintenance of the osmotic equilibrium between ECF and ICF, ensures that ECF volume is determined mainly by total body $Na^+$ content. Departures from this paradigm relate to the identification in recent years of subcutaneous $Na^+$ pools, which do not participate in movement of water in response to osmotic equilibrium, and therefore do not respond equivalently to ECF volume regulation as described below. Further departures from the classical paradigm that maintenance of osmotic balance in response to salt surfeit is mediated by increased water consumption to balance the salt load, were recently suggested by studies demonstrating that under the influence of glucocorticoid and mineralocorticoid hormone fluctuations, long-term increased sodium intake increased water retention rather than consumption in human subjects. Parallel studies in murine models attributed the water retention to increased medullary urea and urea transport.[1,2]

To maintain constancy of the ECF and ICF and thereby safeguard hemodynamic stability, even minute changes in

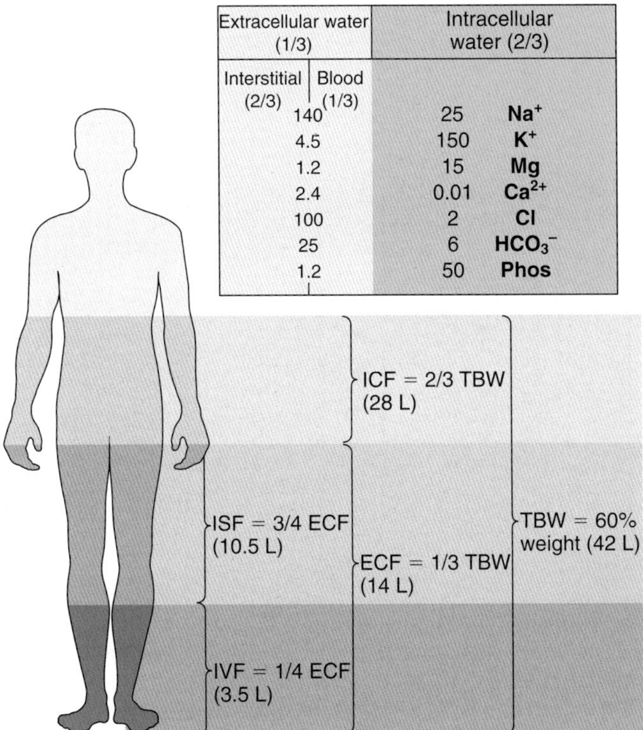


**Fig. 14.1** Composition of body fluid compartments. This is a schematic representation of electrolyte composition *(upper panel)* and volumes *(lower panel)* of the body fluid compartments in humans. In the *upper panel*, electrolyte concentrations are in millimoles per liter; intracellular concentrations are typical values obtained from muscle. In the *lower panel*, *shaded areas* depict the approximate size of each compartment as a function of body weight. In a normally built individual, the total body water content is roughly 60% of body weight. Because adipose tissue has a low concentration of water, the relative water/total body weight ratio is lower in obese individuals. Relative volumes of each compartment are shown as fractions; approximate absolute volumes of the compartments (in liters) in a 70-kg adult are shown in parentheses. *ECF*, Extracellular fluid; *ICF*, intracellular fluid; *ISF*, interstitial fluid; *IVF*, intravascular fluid; *TBW*, total body water. (From Verbalis JG. Body water osmolality. In Wilkinson B, Jamison R, editors: *Textbook of nephrology,* London: Chapman & Hall; 1997: pp 89–94. Reproduced with permission of Hodder Arnold.)

these parameters can be detected by a number of sensing mechanisms. These sensory signals lead to activation of neural and hormonal factors, which, in turn, cause appropriate adjustments in urinary $Na^+$ and water excretion (Fig. 14.2). Constancy of ECF volume ensures a high degree of circulatory stability, whereas constancy of ICF volume protects against significant brain cell swelling or shrinkage.

## SODIUM BALANCE

$Na^+$ balance is the difference between intake (diet or supplementary fluids) and output (renal, gastrointestinal, perspiratory, and respiratory). In healthy humans in steady state, dietary intake is closely matched by urinary output of $Na^+$. Thus, a person consuming a chronically low-$Na^+$ diet (20 mmol/day, or ≈1.2 g of salt/day) excretes, in the steady state, a similar quantity of $Na^+$ in the urine (minus extrarenal losses). Conversely, on a high-$Na^+$ diet (200 mmol/day, or 12 g of salt/day), approximately 200 mmol of $Na^+$ is excreted in the urine. Any perturbation of this balance leads to activation of the sensory and effector mechanisms outlined in the following discussions. In practice, any deviation in ECF volume in relation to its capacitance is sensed and translated, under the influence of neural and hormonal factors, into the appropriate change in $Na^+$ excretion, principally through the kidneys but also, to a much lesser degree, through stool and sweat.

According to the traditional two-compartmental model, body sodium balance and partitioning of extracellular fluid volume (ECFV) is based solely on exchangeable and osmotically active $Na^+$. For normal functioning of the afferent sensing and efferent effector mechanisms that regulate ECF volume, the integrity of the intravascular and extravascular subcompartments of the ECF is crucial[3] (see Fig. 14.2). Although the composition and concentration of small, noncolloid electrolyte solutes in these two subcompartments are approximately equal (slight differences are due to the Gibbs-Donnan effect), the concentration of colloid osmotic particles (mainly albumin and globulin) is higher in the intravascular compartment. The balance between transcapillary hydraulic and colloid osmotic (oncotic) gradients (Starling forces) favors the net transudation of fluid from the intravascular to interstitial compartment. However, this is countered by movement of lymphatic fluid from the interstitial to intravascular compartment via the thoracic duct. The net effect is to restore and maintain the intravascular subcompartment at 25% of the total ECF volume (corresponding to 3.5 L of plasma); the remaining 75% is contained in the interstitial space (equivalent to 10.5 L in a 70-kg man; see Fig. 14.1). The constancy of ECF volume and the appropriate partitioning of the fluid between intravascular and interstitial subcompartments are crucial for maintaining hemodynamic stability. In particular, intravascular volume in relation to overall vascular capacitance is a major determinant of left ventricular filling volume and, hence, cardiac output and mean arterial pressure (MAP).

Recently, the traditional two-compartment model of volume regulation (according to which the intravascular and interstitial spaces are in equilibrium) has been challenged. It now appears that $Na^+$ can be bound to and stored on proteoglycans in interstitial sites, where it becomes osmotically inactive; accordingly, a novel mechanism of volume regulation has been elucidated.[4–11] In rats fed a high-salt diet, this uniquely bound $Na^+$ induced a state of subcutaneous interstitial hypertonicity and systemic hypertension.[8] This hypertonicity is sensed by macrophages,[5] which then produce vascular endothelial growth factor C (VEGF-C), an angiogenic protein. In turn, VEGF-C stimulates increased numbers and density of lymphatic capillaries. In parallel, macrophages subjected to osmotic stress display activation of a transcription factor, tonicity-responsive enhancer–binding protein (TonEBP). This factor is known to activate osmoprotective genes in other hypertonic environments, such as the renal medulla.[12] Moreover, the VEGF-C promoter contains two TonEBP binding sites, which are upregulated in parallel with VEGF-C. The effect of TonEBP on VEGF-C was shown to be specific, inasmuch as small interfering RNA for TonEBP or deletion of the murine TonEBP gene, but not nonspecific small interfering RNA, inhibited the VEGF-C upregulation and increased blood pressure (BP). Furthermore, macrophage depletion or inhibition of VEGF-C signaling led to

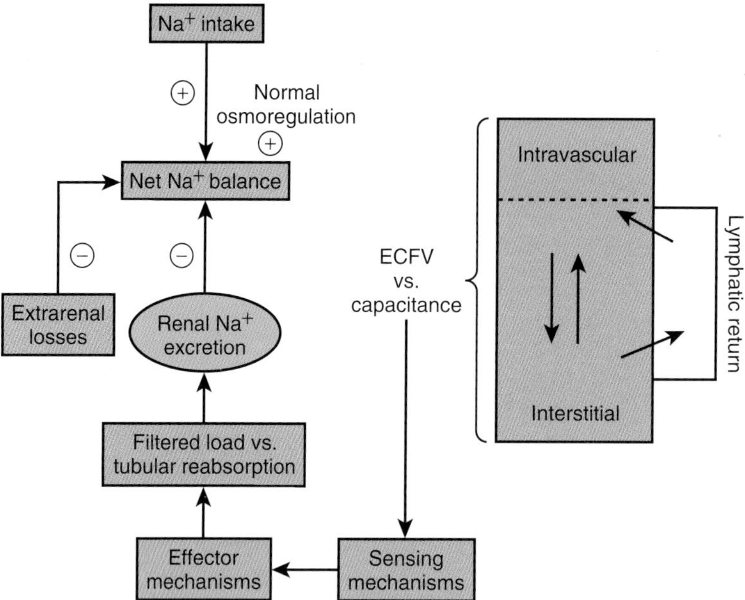


**Fig. 14.2** Traditional two-compartment scheme for body sodium balance and partitioning of extracellular fluid volume (ECFV), based on exchangeable and osmotically active $Na^+$. In the setting of normal osmoregulation, extracellular $Na^+$ content is the primary determinant of ECFV. Overall $Na^+$ homeostasis depends on the balance between losses (extrarenal and renal) and intake. Renal $Na^+$ excretion is determined by the balance between filtered load and tubule reabsorption. This latter balance is modulated under the influence of effector mechanisms, which, in turn, are responsive to sensing mechanisms that monitor the relationship between ECFV and capacitance. In rats, a high-salt diet leads to interstitial hypertonic $Na^+$ accumulation in skin, resulting in increased density and hyperplasia of the lymphatic capillary network.

exacerbation of high-salt diet–induced hypertension.[5] Also, VEGFR-3, an antibody that blocks the lymph-endothelial VEGF-C receptor, selectively inhibited macrophage-driven increases in cutaneous lymphatic capillary density, led to skin chloride ($Cl^-$) accumulation and induced salt-sensitive hypertension. Mice overexpressing soluble VEGFR-3 in epidermal keratinocytes exhibited hypoplastic cutaneous lymph capillaries and increased $Na^+$, $Cl^-$ and water retention in skin and salt-sensitive hypertension.[13] A high-salt diet also led to elevated skin osmolality above plasma levels. In addition, in humans with relatively resistant hypertension, elevated levels of VEGF-C were found,[5] and skin $Na^+$ concentration correlated with the presence of left ventricular hypertrophy in chronic kidney disease.[14] These data are consistent with a role for VEGF-C in the redistribution of excess volume to the intravascular space and exacerbation of hypertension.[15]

Interestingly, mice skin, but not muscle, arterioles isolated from animals fed a high-salt diet compared with those on a normal salt diet exhibited increased contractile sensitivity to concentrations of angiotensin II (Ang II) $\geq 10^{-10}$ M and to norepinephrine (NE) at $10^{-5}$ to $10^{-4}$ M. Finally, a unique study involving astronauts on a simulated Mars expedition, who received diets with fixed salt intake that varied between 6 and 12 g daily, each for 35 days, was recently reported (reviewed in Titze et al. [16]). At each level of salt in the diet, the astronauts reached overall equilibrium between intake and output, as measured in 24-hour urine collections, within the expected 6 days. In parallel, there were the expected early changes in body weight, ECF water and inverse relationship with the urine aldosterone level. However, changes in total body $Na^+$ only occurred after 7 days and BP reached a new steady state after 3 weeks. Moreover, on the 12-g salt diet, BP continued to rise over a further 4 weeks, with an initial rise and then subsequent fall in body weight and ECF water. During this period, urine aldosterone levels did not change, whereas total body $Na^+$ decreased back to original levels, despite the maintained high salt intake. From these data, it appears that intrinsic rhythms with a periodicity of 30 days or more exist for aldosterone and $Na^+$ retention, independent of salt intake. Taken together, all these results clearly demonstrate that the skin contains a hypertonic interstitial fluid compartment in which macrophages exert homeostatic and BP regulatory control by local organization of interstitial electrolyte clearance via TonEBP and VEGF-C/VEGFR-3–mediated modification of cutaneous lymphatic capillary function.[13] This compartment may be associated with increased vasoreactivity in precapillary arterioles, the major resistance vessel of rat skin, which could increase peripheral resistance and contribute, independently of the kidney, to higher BP in salt-sensitive individuals.[17,18]

Fig. 14.3 summarizes the novel three-compartment model of $Na^+$ balance. The reader is also referred to an excellent recent review of this fascinating subject.[16]

## EFFECTIVE ARTERIAL BLOOD VOLUME

To understand the mechanisms regulating ECF volume, it is important to appreciate that what is sensed is the effective arterial blood volume (EABV), defined as that part of the ECF in the arterial blood system that effectively perfuses the tissues. In physiologic terms, what is sensed is the threat to arterial pressure induced by the EABV[19] that perfuses the arterial baroceptors in the carotid sinus and glomerular afferent arterioles. Any change in perfusion pressure (or stretch) at these sites evokes appropriate compensatory responses. EABV is usually correlated with actual ECF volume and is proportional to total body $Na^+$. This means that the regulation of $Na^+$ balance and the maintenance of EABV are

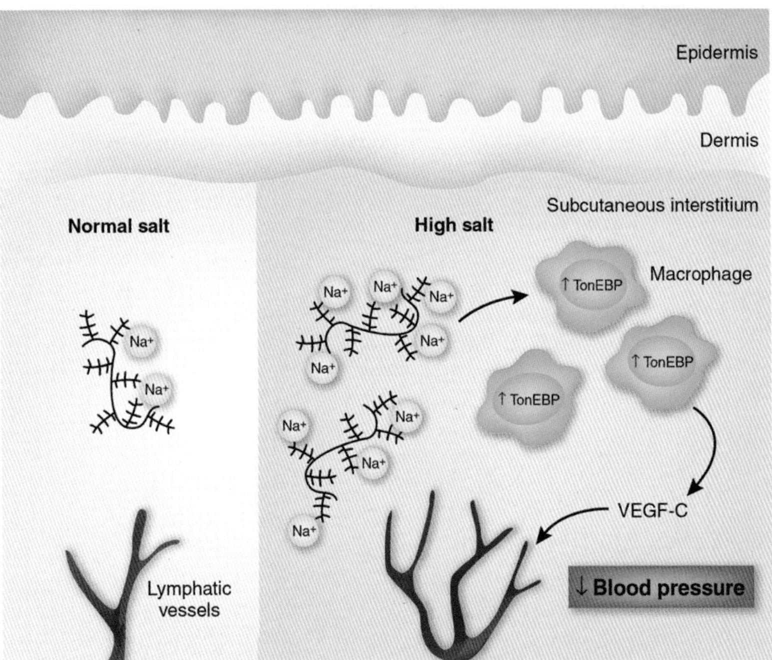


**Fig. 14.3** New model of body electrolyte balance and blood pressure homeostasis. Increased subcutaneous $Na^+$ modulates lymphangiogenesis and blood pressure. After high salt intake, osmotically inactive $Na^+$ accumulates in the skin interstitium, binding proteoglycans. Macrophages accumulate in the subcutaneous compartment, and increased interstitial tonicity activates tonicity-responsive enhancer–binding protein (TonEBP). TonEBP transactivates the *VEGFC* gene and increases vascular endothelial growth factor C secretion by macrophages. This increases lymph capillary density and attenuates the blood pressure response to high salt. (Modified from Marvar PJ, Gordon FJ, Harrison DG. Blood pressure control: salt gets under your skin. *Nature Medicine*. 2009;15:487–488.)

closely related functions. $Na^+$ loading generally leads to EABV expansion, whereas loss leads to depletion. However, in some situations, EABV and actual blood volume are not well correlated (see Table 14.5). For example, in heart failure (HF), a primary decrease in cardiac output leads to lowered perfusion pressure of the baroceptors and reduced EABV is sensed. This leads to renal $Na^+$ retention and ECF volume expansion. The net result is increased plasma and total ECF volume, in association with increased EABV. The increase in plasma volume is partially appropriate in that intraventricular filling pressure rises leading to increasing myocardial stretching and improved ventricular contractility, thereby raising cardiac output and restoring systemic BP and baroceptor perfusion. However, this response is also maladaptive in that the elevated intraarterial pressure promotes fluid movement out of the intravascular space into the tissues, which leads to peripheral and pulmonary edema.

In HF, EABV is dependent on cardiac output; in other disease settings, however, these two parameters may be dissociated. For example, in the presence of an arteriovenous fistula cardiac output rises in proportion to the blood flow through the fistula. However, the flow through the fistula shunts blood away from the capillaries perfusing the tissues and, therefore, the EABV does not rise in conjunction with the rise in cardiac output. Similarly, a fall in systemic vascular resistance (SVR)—which, together with cardiac output, is a determinant of BP—leads to reductions in BP and EABV.

Another situation in which cardiac output and EABV change in opposite directions is advanced cirrhosis with ascites. ECF volume expands because of the ascites and plasma volume is increased because of fluid accumulation in the splanchnic circulation, in which the vessels are dilated but flow is sluggish. Although cardiac output may increase modestly because of arteriovenous shunting, marked peripheral vasodilation leads to a fall in SVR, with reductions in EABV and BP. In the presence of reduced EABV, renal perfusion is impaired; under the influence of hormones, such as renin, NE, and antidiuretic hormone (or arginine vasopressin [AVP])—released in response to the perceived hypovolemia—further $Na^+$ and water retention ensue (see later section, "Efferent Limb: Effector Mechanisms for Maintaining Effective Arterial Blood Volume").

To summarize, EABV is an unmeasured index of tissue perfusion that usually, but not always, reflects actual arterial blood volume. Therefore, EABV can be viewed as a functional parameter of organ perfusion.

The diagnostic hallmark of reduced EABV is evidence of renal sodium retention, manifested as a urinary sodium ($U_{Na}$) less than 15 to 20 mmol/L. This relationship holds true with the following exceptions. If renal $Na^+$ wasting occurs because of diuretic therapy or intrinsic tubular disease or injury, then $U_{Na}$ is relatively high, despite low EABV. Conversely, the presence of selective renal or glomerular ischemia (e.g., because of bilateral renal artery stenosis or acute glomerular injury) will be misinterpreted as poor renal perfusion and is associated with renal $Na^+$ retention (low $U_{Na}$).

## REGULATION OF EFFECTIVE ARTERIAL BLOOD VOLUME

Regulation of EABV can be divided into two stages, afferent sensing and efferent effector mechanisms. A number of mechanisms for sensing low EABV exist, all of them primed to stimulate renal $Na^+$ retention.

## AFFERENT LIMB: SENSING OF EFFECTIVE ARTERIAL BLOOD VOLUME

Volume sensors are strategically situated at critical points in the circulation (Table 14.1). Each sensor reflects a specific characteristic of overall circulatory function so that atrial and ventricular sensors sense cardiac filling, arterial sensors respond to cardiac output, and renal, central nervous system (CNS) and gastrointestinal (GI) tract sensors monitor perfusion of the kidneys, brain and gut, respectively. The common mechanism whereby volume is monitored is by physical alterations in the vessel wall, such as stretch or tension. The process of mechanosensing probably is dependent on afferent sensory nerve endings in the vessel wall and activation of endothelial cells. Signal transduction mechanisms in endothelial cells include stretch-activated ion channels, cytoskeleton-associated protein kinases, integrin-cytoskeletal interactions, cytoskeletal-nuclear interactions and generation of reactive oxygen species.[20,21] In addition, mechanical stretch and tension of blood vessel walls, as well as the frictional forces of the circulation or shear stress, can lead to alterations in gene expression, mediated by specific recognition sites in the upstream promoter elements of responsive genes.[22,23] These signals induce efferent effector mechanisms that lead to modifications in renal $Na^+$ excretion, appropriate to the volume status.

### Sensors of Cardiac Filling

**Atrial Sensors.** The role of the atria in volume regulation in humans was elucidated in experiments involving head-out water immersion (HWI) and exposure to head-down tilt or nonhypotensive lower body negative pressure (LBNP). During HWI, the increased hydrostatic pressure of the water on the lower limbs leads to redistribution of the intravascular fluid from the peripheral to central circulation. The resulting increase in central blood volume causes a rise in cardiac output, which in turn produces a brisk increase in $Na^+$ and water excretion in an attempt to restore euvolemia.[24] In contrast, LBNP results in a redistribution of blood to the lower limbs, thereby reducing central venous and cardiac filling pressures without affecting arterial pressure, heart rate, or atrial diameter. The resulting retention of $Na^+$ and water occurs without any change in renal plasma flow (RPF).[25]

A second and, possibly, more dominant, mechanism of HWI-induced $Na^+$ and water dieresis involves the external hydrostatic pressure of the water reducing the hydrostatic pressure gradient across the capillary wall in the legs, leading to a net transfer of fluid from the interstitial to intravascular compartment. The resulting hemodilution causes a fall in the colloid osmotic pressure (COP).[26,27] The combination of hemodilution and central hypervolemia, through atrial stretch, induces neurohumoral changes that bring about the subsequent diuresis and natriuresis.

**Table 14.1 Mechanisms for Sensing Regional Changes in Effective Arterial Blood Volume**

| Sensors of Cardiac Filling |
|---|
| Atrial |
| Neural pathways |
| Humoral pathways |
| Ventricular |
| Pulmonary |
| **Sensors of Cardiac Output** |
| Carotid and aortic baroceptors |
| **Sensors of Organ Perfusion** |
| Renal sensors |
| CNS sensors |
| GI tract sensors |
| Hepatic receptors |
| Guanylin peptides |

*CNS*, Central nervous system; *GI*, gastrointestinal.

**Neural Pathways.** Two types of neural receptors in the atrium have been described, type A and type B. They are thought to be branching ends of small medullated fibers running in the vagus nerve. Only type B receptor activity is increased by atrial filling and stretch.[28] The signal is then thought to travel along cranial nerves IX and X to the hypothalamic and medullary centers, where a series of responses is initiated—inhibition of AVP release (left atrial signal),[29] a selective decrease in renal but not lumbar sympathetic nerve discharge,[30,31] and decreased tone in peripheral precapillary and postcapillary resistance vessels. Conversely, reduction in central venous pressure and atrial volume stimulates renal sympathetic nerve activity (RSNA).[32,33]

The effects just described occur in response to acute atrial stretch, whereas chronic atrial stretch leads to adaptation and downregulation of the neural responses.[33] Cardiac nerves appear to be essential only for the restoration of $Na^+$ balance in states of repletion, but not for the renal response to acute volume depletion.[34] For example, after human cardiac transplantation, a natural model of cardiac denervation, the expected suppression of the renin-angiotensin-aldosterone (RAAS) system in response to chronic volume expansion is not observed.[35]

**Humoral Pathways.** Even after cardiac denervation the natriuresis and diuresis induced by atrial distension is maintained, due to the presence of natriuretic peptides (NP) of cardiac origin.[36,37] The NP family is comprised of atrial NP (ANP), brain NP (BNP), C-type NP (CNP), *Dendroaspis* NP (DNP), and urodilatin. Although their structures are quite similar, each is encoded by different genes and has distinct, albeit overlapping, functions.[38–41] The actions of NPs and their interaction with other hormone systems are discussed in detail later (see section, "Efferent Limb: Effector Mechanisms for Maintaining Effective Arterial Blood Volume" and Chapter 11). This section is confined to a discussion of the afferent mechanisms of NP stimulation.

From studies in animals and humans, it is clear that acute increments in atrial stretch or pressure cause a brisk release of ANP. The process involves cleavage of the prohormone, located in preformed stores in atrial granules, to the mature 28-amino acid C-terminus peptide, in a sequence-specific manner, by corin, a transmembrane serine protease.[42] Release of the hormone appears to occur in two steps, the first a $Ca^{2+}$-sensitive $K^+$ channel-dependent release of ANP from myocytes into the intercellular space and then a $Ca^{2+}$-independent translocation of the hormone into the atrial lumen.[43] The afferent mechanism for ANP release is activated by intravascular volume expansion, supine posture, HWI, saline administration, exercise, Ang II, tachycardia and ventricular dysfunction.[44,45] Conversely, volume depletion induced by $Na^+$ restriction, furosemide administration or LNBP-mediated reduction in central venous pressure causes a fall in plasma ANP concentration.

In contrast to the effects of acute changes in atrial pressure on ANP release, the role of this peptide in the long-term regulation of plasma volume appears to be minimal. For example, although incremental oral salt loading was associated with correspondingly higher baseline plasma ANP levels, only intravenous (not oral) salt loading led to increased ANP levels.[46] Moreover, in humans given intravenous or oral salt loads, no correlation could be found between changes in ANP levels and the degree of natriuresis.[47,48] The contrasting relationships among acute and chronic $Na^+$ loading, plasma ANP levels and natriuresis have been elegantly demonstrated in ANP gene knockout mice. These mice display a reduced natriuretic response to acute ECFV expansion in comparison with their wild type counterparts. However, no differences in cumulative $Na^+$ and water excretion were observed between the knockout and wild type mice after a high- or low-$Na^+$ diet for 1 week. The only difference between the two types of mice was a significant increase in MAP. Further experiments using disruptions of the genes for ANP or its receptor, guanylate cyclase A (GC-A), have shown the importance of this system in the maintenance of normal BP and in modulating cardiac hypertrophy.[49]

In contrast to ANP, the other members of the NP family appear not to be involved in the physiologic regulation of $Na^+$ excretion.[38,50]

**Ventricular and Pulmonary Sensors.** Volume sensors have been found in the ventricles, coronary arteries, main pulmonary artery and bifurcation,[51] and juxtapulmonary capillaries in the interstitium of the lungs,[52] but not in the intrapulmonary circulation.[53] These sensors apparently mediate reflex changes in heart rate and SVR through modulation of the sympathetic nervous system (SNS) and ANP. This also appears to be true for the coronary baroceptor reflex in anesthetized dogs, by which changes in coronary artery pressure lead to alterations in lumbar and renal sympathetic discharge and a coronary artery response much slower than that of the carotid and aortic baroceptors.[54] However, ventricular and pulmonary sensors, at least in dogs, may also detect changes in blood volume through increased left ventricular pressure, which causes a reflex inhibition of plasma renin activity (PRA).[55,56]

### Sensors of Cardiac Output

The sensors described so far are situated in low-pressure sites, where they sense the fullness of the circulation and are probably more important for defending against excessive volume expansion and the consequent cardiac failure. The arterial high-pressure sensors, on the other hand, are geared more toward detecting low cardiac output or SVR, manifested as underfilling of the vascular tree (i.e., EABV depletion) threatening arterial pressure[19], and as signaling the kidneys to retain $Na^+$. These high-pressure sensors are found in the aortic arch, carotid sinus, and renal vessels.

**Carotid and Aortic Baroceptors.** The carotid baroceptor has a large content of elastic tissue in the tunica media, which makes the vessel wall highly distensible in response to changes in intraluminal pressure, thereby facilitating transmission of the stimulus intensity to sensory nerve terminals. A rise in MAP induces depolarization of these sensory endings, resulting in action potentials. Transient receptor potential vanilloid receptors may mediate this process.[57] Afferent signals from the baroceptors are integrated in the nucleus tractus solitarius (NTS) of the medulla oblongata,[58] which leads to reflex changes in systemic and renal sympathetic nerve activity and, to a lesser degree, release of AVP. Baroceptor reflex modulation in the NTS may be mediated by endocannabinoid CB(1) receptor activation, via the 5-hydroxytryptamine type 1A (5-HT1A) receptor, leading to endogenous anandamide release.[59,60,61] Conversely, hypovolemia-induced activation of NTS (A1) adenosine receptors may serve as a negative feedback regulator of sympathoinhibitory reflexes integrated in the NTS.[62] An important additional function of the carotid baroceptors is maintenance of adequate cerebral perfusion. The aortic baroceptor appears to behave in a way similar to the carotid baroceptor. Finally, there is evidence in dogs for an interaction between pulmonary arterial and carotid baroceptor reflexes.[63]

### Sensors of Organ Perfusion

**Renal Sensors.** Not only is the kidney the major effector target responding to signals that indicate the need for adjustments in $Na^+$ excretion, but also has a central role in the afferent sensing of volume homeostasis by virtue of the local sympathetic innervation. However, despite considerable knowledge concerning the mechanisms of renal sensing of EABV, the molecular identity and exact cellular location of the renal sensor(s) remains elusive.[61] The integral relationship between afferent and efferent RSNA and the central arterial baroceptors was highlighted by Kopp and colleagues.[64] They showed that a high-$Na^+$ diet increases afferent RSNA, which then decreases efferent RSNA and leads to natriuresis. Using dorsal rhizotomy to induce afferent renal denervation in rats maintained on a high-$Na^+$ diet, they demonstrated increased MAP that was dependent on impaired arterial baroreflex suppression of efferent RSNA. Animals fed a normal-$Na^+$ diet displayed no changes in arterial baroceptor function. Kopp and coworkers concluded that arterial baroreflex function contributes to increased efferent RSNA, which, in the absence of intact afferent RSNA, would eventually lead to $Na^+$ retention and hypertension. The role of RSNA in $Na^+$ regulation is discussed further later in this chapter (see section, "Neural Mechanisms: Renal Nerves and Sympathetic Nervous System").

An additional level of renal sensing depends on the close anatomic proximity of the sensor and effector limbs to one another: Volume changes may be sensed through alterations in glomerular hemodynamics and renal interstitial pressure. These alterations result simultaneously in adjustments in the physical forces governing tubular $Na^+$ handling (see section, "Efferent Limb: Effector Mechanisms for Maintaining Effective Arterial Blood Volume").

The kidneys have the ability to maintain a constant blood flow and glomerular filtration rate (GFR) at varying arterial pressures. This phenomenon, termed "autoregulation," operates over a wide range of renal perfusion pressures (RPPs).

Autoregulation of renal blood flow (RBF) occurs through three mechanisms—the myogenic response, tubuloglomerular feedback (TGF) and a third mechanism. In the myogenic response, changes in RPP are sensed by smooth muscle elements that serve as baroreceptors in the afferent glomerular arteriole and dynamically respond by adjusting transmural pressure and tension across the arteriolar wall.[65] An example of this can be seen in Ang II–infused rats on a high salt intake. These animals show reduced dynamic autoregulation of RBF, an effect mediated, at least in part, by superoxide[66] and attenuated by endothelial nitric oxide synthase (eNOS)–dependent production of nitric oxide (NO).[67]

The second mechanism, TGF, is operated by the juxtaglomerular apparatus (JGA), comprised of the afferent arteriole and, to a lesser extent, the cells of the macula densa in the early distal tubule.[65,68] The JGA is also important because of its involvement in the synthesis and release of renin,[68] which is controlled by three pathways, all driven by EABV status. First, renin release is inversely related to RPP and directly related to intrarenal tissue pressure. When RPP falls below the autoregulatory range, renin release is further enhanced. Second, renin secretion is influenced by solute delivery to the macula densa. Increased NaCl delivery past the macula densa leads to inhibition of renin release, whereas a decrease has the opposite effect. Sensing at the macula densa is mediated by NaCl entry through the $Na^+$-$K^+$-$2Cl^-$ cotransporter (NKCC2),[69,70] which leads to increased intracellular $Ca^{2+}$, production of prostaglandin $E_2$ ($PGE_2$),[71] adenosine,[72] and, subsequently, renin release. Third, changes in RSNA influence renin release. Renal nerve stimulation increases renin release through direct activation of β-adrenergic receptors on juxtaglomerular cells. This effect is independent of major changes in renal hemodynamics.[73] Sympathetic stimulation also affects intrarenal baroreceptor input, composition of the fluid delivered to the macula densa and renal actions of Ang II so that renal nerves may serve primarily to potentiate other regulatory signals.[73]

The nature of the third mechanism of RBF autoregulation is still unclear, but Seeliger and associates,[74] using a normotensive Ang II clamp in anesthetized rats, were able to abolish the resetting of autoregulation during incremental shaped RPP changes. Under control conditions, the initial TGF response was dilatory after total occlusions but constrictive after partial occlusions. The initial third mechanism response was a mirror image of TGF; it was constrictive after total occlusions but dilatory after partial occlusions. The angiotensin clamp suppressed TGF and converted the initial third mechanism response after total occlusions into dilation. Seeliger and coworkers concluded: 1. pressure-dependent renin angiotensin system (RAS) stimulation was a major factor behind hypotensive resetting of autoregulation; 2. TGF sensitivity depended strongly on pressure-dependent changes in RAS activity; 3. the third mechanism was modulated, but not mediated, by the RAS; and 4. the third mechanism acted as a counterbalance to TGF.[74] These findings may be related to feedback between the connecting tubule and glomerulus.[75] TGF is discussed later (see section, "Integration of Changes in Glomerular Filtration Rate and Tubular Reabsorption") and in detail in Chapter 3.

**Central Nervous System Sensors.** Certain areas in the CNS appear to act as sensors to detect alterations in body salt balance, at least in rats. Thus, intracerebral injection of hypertonic saline led to reduced RSNA and natriuresis,[76,77] and administration of Ang II into the cerebral ventricles and changes in dietary $Na^+$ modulated baroreflex regulation of RSNA. Stimulation of neurons in the paraventricular nucleus and in a region extending to the anteroventral third ventricle led to ANP release, inducing Ang II blockade and inhibition of salt and water intake. Conversely, disruption of these neurons, as well as of the median eminence or neural lobe, led to decreased ANP release and impaired response to volume expansion.[78] However, the exact nature, mode of operation, and relative importance of this aspect of sensing remains unclear.

**Gastrointestinal Tract Sensors.** Under normal physiologic conditions, $Na^+$ and water reach the ECF by absorption in the GI tract. Therefore, it is not surprising that sensing and regulatory mechanisms of ECF volume have been found in the GI tract itself. The evidence for this phenomenon comes from experiments that showed more rapid natriuresis after an oral salt load than after a similar intravenous load. Moreover, infusions of hypertonic saline into the portal vein led to greater natriuresis than similar infusions into the femoral vein. These findings were consistent with the presence of $Na^+$-sensing mechanisms in the splanchnic or portal circulation, or both[79] and are probably important in the pathogenesis of the hepatorenal syndrome (HRS; see later).

**Hepatoportal Receptors.** The two main neural reflexes, termed the "hepatorenal" and "hepatointestinal reflexes," originate from receptors in the hepatoportal region. They transduce portal plasma $Na^+$ concentration into hepatic afferent nerve activity; before a measurable increase in systemic $Na^+$ concentration occurs, the hepatointestinal reflex attenuates intestinal $Na^+$ absorption via the vagus nerve and the hepatorenal reflex augments $Na^+$ excretion both in humans and experimental animals.[80–82] These reflexes are impaired in the chronic bile duct ligation model of cirrhosis and portal hypertension,[83] leading to $Na^+$ retention, mediated in part by the $A_1$ adenosine receptor (A1AR)[84,85] and, possibly, also the NKCC2 cotransporter.[86] In addition, the hepatic artery shows significant autoregulatory capacity, dilating when perfusion pressure falls and constricting when pressure rises, thereby maintaining hepatic arterial blood flow over a wide range of perfusion pressures. This indicates the presence of a sensor in the hepatic artery, which responds to changes in the contribution of the portal vein to total hepatic blood flow.[87]

In addition to hepatoportal $Na^+$-sensing chemoreceptors, the liver also contains mechanoreceptors. Increased intrahepatic hydrostatic pressure, as seen in the Budd-Chiari syndrome,[88] is associated with enhanced RSNA and renal $Na^+$ retention in various experimental models,[89,90] so that hepatic volume-sensing mechanisms probably play a role in renal $Na^+$ retention (see section, "Specific Treatments Based on the Pathophysiology of Sodium Retention in Cirrhosis").

**Intestinal Natriuretic Hormones.** As described previously, the natriuretic response to a $Na^+$ load in experimental animals is more rapid when the load is delivered orally than intravenously.[73] The different responses are observed without changes in plasma aldosterone,[91] suggesting that the gut produces one or more substances that signal the kidneys to excrete excess $Na^+$. The two main candidate substances are guanylins (guanylin and uroguanylin)[92,93] and gastrin.[94]

Guanylins are small (15 to 16 amino acids), heat-stable peptides with intramolecular disulfide bridges and are found in mammals, birds, and fish.[93] Both guanylin and uroguanylin are synthesized as prepropeptides, primarily in the intestine. The former, produced mainly by the ileum through the proximal colon, circulates as proguanylin; the latter, expressed principally in the jejunum, circulates in its active form.[92] The two peptides differ in their sensitivity to proteases. Because of a tyrosine residue at the ninth amino acid, guanylin is sensitive to renal inactivation by protease digestion, whereas uroguanylin can be locally activated by the same proteases.[93] After an oral salt load, guanylin and uroguanylin released in the intestine lead to increased intestinal secretion of $Cl^-$, $HCO_3^-$ and water and to inhibition of $Na^+$ absorption. In the kidneys, $Na^+$, $K^+$, and water excretion is increased, without any change in RBF or GFR and independently of RAAS, AVP, or ANPs.[93] Guanylin signal transduction occurs via binding to and activation of the receptor guanylate cyclase C (GC-C), in the intestinal brush border and increased cGMP, which inhibits $Na^+/H^+$ exchange and activates protein kinases G II and A. These, in turn, activate the cystic fibrosis transmembrane conductance regulator (CFTR), leading to $Cl^-$ secretion, activation of the $Cl^-/HCO_3^-$ exchanger, and $HCO_3^-$ secretion.[95]

The best evidence for a link between the gut and kidneys comes from mice lacking the uroguanylin gene, which display an impaired natriuretic response to oral salt loading but not to intravenous NaCl infusion.[96] However, because plasma pro-uroguanylin levels do not rise but urinary uroguanylin levels do increase after a high-salt meal, locally released peptide by the kidneys may play a role in uroguanylin-associated natriuresis.[97,95] In the kidneys, both GC-C–dependent and GC-C–independent signaling pathways for guanylin peptides exist, inasmuch as knockout of GC-C in mice does not affect the high-salt diet–induced increase in uroguanylin.[93]

From experiments on cell lines and isolated tubules, it appears that uroguanylin acts to decrease $Na^+$ reabsorption in the proximal tubule and principal cells of the cortical collecting duct (CCD).[93] Crosstalk between guanylin peptides and ANPs may also occur in the proximal tubule.[98] In the principal cell, uroguanylin activation of a G protein–coupled receptor results in phospholipase $A_2$–dependent inhibition of the renal outer medullary potassium (ROMK) channel, which leads to depolarization and a reduced driving force for $Na^+$ reabsorption.[93] Guanylin may cause cell shrinkage in the inner medullary collecting duct (IMCD), suggestive of water secretion from this segment.[93] Together, the experimental data are highly suggestive of a role for uroguanylin as a natriuretic hormone, in response to NaCl absorbed via the GI tract.[92,93]

More recently, gastrin, secreted from the stomach and duodenum, has been proposed as a second candidate substance mediating natriuresis in response to an oral salt load. Gastrin appears to signal natiuresis via its receptor, cholecystokinin B receptor linked to a dopamine D1-like receptor.[94] However, despite all the evidence from animal studies, recent work has cast substantial doubt on the relevance of a GI renal signaling axis for $Na^+$ regulation in humans.[99]

A final point is that although multiple receptors are involved in the regulation of EABV, their functions appear to be redundant. In this regard, cardiac or renal denervation and chronic aldosterone administration in nonhuman primates do not significantly affect the maintenance of $Na^+$ balance.[100,101]

**Table 14.2 Major Renal Effector Mechanisms for Regulating Effective Arterial Blood Volume**

| |
|---|
| **Glomerular Filtration Rate and Tubular Reabsorption** |
| Tubuloglomerular feedback |
| Glomerulotubular balance |
| Peritubular capillary Starling forces |
| Luminal composition |
| Physical factors beyond proximal tubule |
| Medullary hemodynamics (pressure natriuresis) |
| **Neural Mechanisms** |
| Sympathetic nervous system |
| Renal nerves |
| **Humoral Mechanisms** |
| Renin-angiotensin-aldosterone system |
| Vasopressin |
| Prostaglandins |
| Natriuretic peptides |
| Endothelium-derived factors |
| Endothelins |
| Nitric oxide |
| Others (see text) |

## EFFERENT LIMB: EFFECTOR MECHANISMS FOR MAINTAINING EFFECTIVE ARTERIAL BLOOD VOLUME

The maintenance of $Na^+$ homeostasis is achieved by adjustments of renal $Na^+$ excretion according to the body's needs. The adjustments are made by integrated changes in GFR and tubular reabsorption, so that changes in one component lead to appropriate changes in the other to maintain $Na^+$ homeostasis. In addition, tubular reabsorption is regulated by local peritubular and luminal factors as well as by neural and humoral mechanisms (Table 14.2).

## INTEGRATION OF CHANGES IN GLOMERULAR FILTRATION RATE AND TUBULAR REABSORPTION

In humans, normal GFR leads to the delivery of approximately 24,000 mmol of $Na^+$/day to the tubules where more than 99% of the filtrate is reabsorbed. Therefore, even minute changes in the relationship between filtered load and fraction of $Na^+$ absorbed can profoundly influence net $Na^+$ balance. However, even marked perturbations in GFR are not necessarily associated with drastic alterations in $U_{Na}$ excretion and overall $Na^+$ balance is usually preserved. Such preservation results from adjustments in two important protective mechanisms—TGF, in which changes in tubular fluid $Na^+$ inversely affect GFR, and glomerulotubular balance, whereby changes in tubular flow rate resulting from changes in GFR directly affect tubular reabsorption.[68,102,103]

### Tubuloglomerular Feedback

A remarkable feature of nephron architecture is that after emerging from Bowman's capsule and descending deep into the medulla, each tubule returns to its parent glomerulus.

The functional counterpart of this anatomic relationship is TGF[104,105] (see also Chapter 3). TGF is constructed as a negative feedback loop in which an increase in NaCl concentration at the macula densa (the point of contact between the specialized tubular cells of the cortical thick ascending limb of Henle, cTALH, adjacent to the extraglomerular mesangium) leads to increases in afferent arteriolar resistance and a consequent fall in the GFR. This, in turn, leads to an increase in proximal reabsorption and a reduction in distal delivery of solute, whereby NaCl delivery to the distal nephron is maintained within narrow limits.[105]

The complexities of TGF were initially unraveled by micropuncture, imaging and electrophysiologic techniques in isolated perfused tubule/glomerulus preparations. Subsequently, the signaling mechanisms linking changes in tubular composition with altered glomerular arteriolar tone became evident through experiments in gene-manipulated mice.[105] The primary detection mechanism of TGF is uptake of salt by means of the NKCC2, located in the apical membrane of macula densa cells. The evidence comes from TGF inhibition by inhibitors of the cotransporter, furosemide and bumetanide,[106] and by deletions in mice of the A or B isoform of NKCC2, both of which are expressed in macula densa cells.[69,105] In fact, complete inactivation of the NKCC2 gene leads to the severe salt-losing phenotype of antenatal Bartter syndrome.[107] Similarly, inhibition or deletion of the ROMK channel in mice abolishes TGF.[105]

The next step in the juxtaglomerular cascade is less clear. One possibility is direct coupling of NKCC2-dependent NaCl uptake to the mediation step. Results of studies in the isolated perfused rabbit JGA have indicated that depolarization, alkalinization, and various ionic compositional changes occur after increased NaCl uptake; thus, one or more of these changes could trigger the signal.[108] A second possibility is that signal propagation is the consequence of transcellular NaCl transport and $Na^+$-$K^+$-ATPase–dependent basolateral extrusion. Experiments using double-knockout mice, in which the $\alpha_1$-subunit of $Na^+$-$K^+$-ATPase was made sensitive and the $\alpha_2$-subunit resistant to the pump inhibitor, ouabain, clearly indicate an important role for $Na^+$-$K^+$-ATPase in supporting TGF and that adenosine triphosphate (ATP) consumption is required for the process.[108]

In contrast, other studies have yielded strong evidence that ATP release and degradation, rather than consumption, may be the link connecting NaCl changes in the macula densa with alteration of glomerular arteriolar tone. According to the current working model, after NaCl uptake and transcellular transport, ATP is released from macula densa cells and undergoes stepwise hydrolysis and dephosphorylation by ecto-ATPases and nucleotidases to adenosine diphosphate, adenosine monophosphate and then adenosine. Adenosine, in a paracrine manner, then causes A1AR–dependent afferent arteriolar constriction. Although the evidence for ATP breakdown is as yet incomplete, evidence for adenosine as a mediator of TGF is very strong. For example, isolated perfused mouse afferent arterioles exposed to adenosine display vigorous vasoconstriction, an effect not seen in A1AR–deficient mice.[109,110] As shown by overexpression[111] and conditional knockout of the receptor, this A1AR effect is primarily on afferent arteriolar smooth muscle cells, although A1AR effects on extravascular, perhaps mesangial, cells appear to contribute to the TGF response.[112] The response is mediated by inhibitory G protein ($G_i$)–dependent activation of phospholipase C, release of $Ca^{2+}$ from intracellular stores and subsequent entry of $Ca^{2+}$ through L-type $Ca^{2+}$ channels.[109,113] Cellular adenosine uptake is likely to be involved in the TGF response because targeted deletion of the type 1 equilibrative nucleoside transporter (ENT1) led to significant attenuation of the response.[114] Also, vasodilatory adenosine $A_2$ receptor is more abundant than the A1AR in the renal vasculature and continuous exogenous application of adenosine to mouse kidneys is indeed vasodilatory.[115] However, the generation of adenosine in the confines of the juxtaglomerular interstitium and its exclusive delivery to the afferent arteriole, where A1AR expression predominates, ensures the appropriate response for TGF.

Other factors, both coconstrictors and modulators, appear to be involved in TGF. Ang II is an important cofactor in the vasoconstrictive action of adenosine, since deletions of the Ang II receptor or angiotensin converting enzyme (ACE) in mice were found to abolish TGF. The effect may result from nonresponsiveness to adenosine in the absence of an intact RAS.[111] By contrast, aldosterone appears to blunt TGF through superoxide-mediated activation of mineralocorticoid receptors on macula densa cells.[116,117] In turn, superoxide may also be upregulated by Ang II via the NOX2 and NOX4 isoforms of nicotinamide adenine dinucleotide phosphate (NADPH) oxidase.[118] The high levels of neuronal NO synthase (nNOS) expression in macula densa cells are thought to counterbalance Ang II–induced efferent arteriolar vasoconstriction and to modulate renin secretion by the JGA.[119–121] In contrast, chronic absence of functional nNOS in macula densa cells is associated with enhanced vasoconstriction in the subnormal flow range, probably as a result of proportional increases in preglomerular and postglomerular tone. In addition, increased delivery of fluid to the macula densa induces NO release from these cells.[120]

Inhibition of the NO system by nonselective blockers of NOS results in an exaggerated TGF response that leads to even further renal vasoconstriction, $Na^+$ and water retention, and arterial hypertension.[121] Also, TGF responses are absent in mice with concurrent deficiencies in nNOS and the A1AR, which implies that nNOS deficiency does not overcome deficient A1AR signaling. Moreover, NO modulation of TGF can be mediated by ecto 5′-nucleotidase, the enzyme responsible for adenine formation.[122] Furthermore, NO, via eNOS, modulates the afferent arteriolar myogenic response.[67] Finally, aldosterone-induced modulation of TGF appears to involve interactions between NO and superoxide.[123] Together, these data suggest that A1AR signaling is primary and that nNOS and eNOS and superoxide, play modulatory roles in TGF.

Apart from the RAAS, other hormonal systems and secondary messengers appear to be involved in TGF. For example, stimulation of the glucagon-like peptide 1 receptor leads to an increased GFR and reduced proximal tubular reabsorption.[124] Moreover, high salt intake–induced activation of AMP-activated protein kinase leads to an enhanced TGF response and increased delivery of $Na^+$ to the end of the proximal tubule.[66] Furthermore, acute saline expansion leads to an increased single-nephron glomerular filtration rate (SNGFR) and distal nephron flow rate, independently of the Ang II receptor.[125]

The afferent arteriolar A1AR may not be the sole mediator of TGF. Activation by adenosine of the low-affinity adenosine

$A_{2b}$ receptor,[115] via increased levels of eNOS,[126] has been shown to dilate mouse cortical efferent receptors. This highly specific effect occurs despite the presence of A1AR in the efferent arteriole. Apparently, therefore, the relative abundance of the various adenosine receptor subtypes in afferent and efferent arterioles ultimately allows fine-tuning of TGF by concerted changes in glomerular vascular tone.[127] On the other hand, purine receptors do not seem to be involved in TGF.[128]

Connexin 40, which plays a predominant role in the formation of gap junctions in the vasculature, also participates in the autoregulation of RBF by the afferent arteriole and, therefore, in TGF.[129] Connexin 40 knockout mice displayed impaired steady-state autoregulation to a sudden stepped increase in RPP, likely due to a marked reduction in TGF. Connexin 40–mediated RBF autoregulation occurred by paracrine signaling between tubular cells and afferent arteriolar vascular cells,[130] independently of NO.[131] Other endogenous modulators of TGF include the eicosanoid 20-hydroxyeicosatetraenoic acid (20-HETE), which modifies the myogenic afferent arteriolar and TGF responses;[132] also heme oxygenase, via carbon monoxide and cGMP generation, blocks TGF through inhibition of depolarization and $Ca^{2+}$ entry into macular densa cells.[133,134]

Sex hormones also appear to regulate TGF. Testosterone in rats leads to upregulation of TGF by generation of superoxide dismutase,[135] whereas enhanced Ang II receptor activity attenuates Ang II–dependent resetting of TGF activity in female rats.[136] A final point in the complexity of TGF is that there is evidence for three sites in addition to the macula densa that are in contact with the efferent arteriole—the terminal cTALH, the early distal tubule and the connecting tubule. In particular, perimacular cells and oscillatory cells of the early distal tubule may be involved in the intracellular $Ca^{2+}$ signaling required for adenosine-induced afferent vasoconstriction. On the other hand, the effect of the connecting tubule on the afferent arteriolar tone appears to be modulatory in that elevations in luminal NaCl and cellular $Na^+$ entry via the epithelial sodium channel (ENaC) lead to afferent arteriolar dilation[137] through the release of prostaglandins (PG) and epoxyeicosatrienoic acids.[138,139] Moreover, connecting tubule glomerular feedback has been shown to antagonize TGF,[140] at least in the acute setting.[140]

### Glomerulotubular Balance

Several factors are involved in glomerulotubular balance (GTB), which describes the ability of proximal tubular reabsorption to adapt proportionally to changes in filtered load.

**Peritubular Capillary Starling Forces.** Following acute, but probably not chronic, changes in ECFV, alterations in hydraulic and oncotic pressures (Starling forces) in the peritubular capillary seem to play an important role in the regulation of $Na^+$ and water transport, especially in the proximal nephron. The peritubular capillary network is anatomically connected in series with the capillary bed of cortical glomeruli through the efferent arteriole; thus, changes in the physical determinants of GFR critically influence Starling forces in the peritubular capillaries.

Of importance is that about 10% of glomeruli, mainly those at the corticomedullary junction, are connected in series to the vasa recta of the medulla. In the proximal tubule—whose peritubular capillaries receive 90% of blood flow from glomeruli—the relationship of hydraulic and oncotic driving forces to the transcapillary fluid flux is given by the Starling equation, as follows:

$$\text{Rate}_{abs} = K_r[(\pi_c - \pi_i) - (P_c - P_i)]$$

where $\text{Rate}_{abs}$ is the absolute rate of reabsorption of proximal tubule reabsorbate by the peritubular capillary, $K_r$ is the capillary reabsorption coefficient (the product of capillary hydraulic conductivity and absorptive surface area), $\pi_c$ and $P_c$ are the local capillary colloid osmotic (oncotic) and hydraulic pressures, respectively, and $\pi_i$ and $P_i$ are the corresponding interstitial pressures. Whereas $\pi_i$ and $P_c$ oppose fluid absorption, $\pi_c$ and $P_i$ tend to favor uptake of the reabsorbate. As a consequence of the anatomic relationship of the postglomerular efferent arteriole to the peritubular capillary, $P_c$ is significantly lower in the peritubular than in the glomerular capillary. Also, because the peritubular capillary receives blood from the glomerulus, $P_c$ is high at the outset as a result of prior filtration of protein-free fluid. It follows that the greater the GFR in relation to plasma flow rate, the higher the protein concentration in the efferent arteriolar plasma and the lower $P_c$ in the proximal peritubular capillary. Consequently, proximal fluid reabsorption is enhanced (Fig. 14.4). Therefore, in contradistinction to the glomerular and peripheral capillary, the peritubular capillary is characterized by high values of $\pi_c - \pi_i$ that greatly exceed $P_c - P_i$, which results in net reabsorption of fluid. Changes in peritubular capillary Starling forces secondary to reduced RBF, may contribute to $Na^+$-retaining and edema-forming states, such as HF (see Fig. 14.4).

From studies using micropuncture, microperfusion, and the isolated perfused tubule model,[141–145] the role of peritubular forces in the setting of increased ECF volume can be summarized as follows:

1. Acute saline expansion results in dilution of plasma proteins and reduction in efferent arteriolar $\pi_c$. SNGFR and peritubular $P_c$ may be increased as well, but the decrease in peritubular $\pi_c$ by itself results in a decreased net peritubular capillary reabsorptive force and decreased $\text{Rate}_{abs}$. GTB is disrupted because $\text{Rate}_{abs}$ falls, despite the tendency for SNGFR to rise, thereby allowing the excess $Na^+$ to be excreted and plasma volume to be restored.
2. Iso-oncotic plasma infusions tend to raise SNGFR and peritubular $P_c$ but lead to relative constancy of efferent arteriolar $\pi_c$. $\text{Rate}_{abs}$ may, therefore, decrease slightly, resulting in less disruption of GTB and less natriuresis than that observed with saline expansion.
3. Hyperoncotic expansion usually increases both SNGFR (because of volume expansion) and efferent arteriolar $\pi_c$. As a result, $\text{Rate}_{abs}$ is enhanced and GTB, therefore, tends to be better preserved than with iso-oncotic plasma or saline expansion.
4. Changes in $\pi_i$ can directly alter proximal tubular reabsorption, independently of the peritubular capillary bed.

The alterations in proximal peritubular Starling forces that modulate fluid and solute movement across the peritubular basement membrane into the surrounding capillary bed appear to be accompanied by corresponding changes in

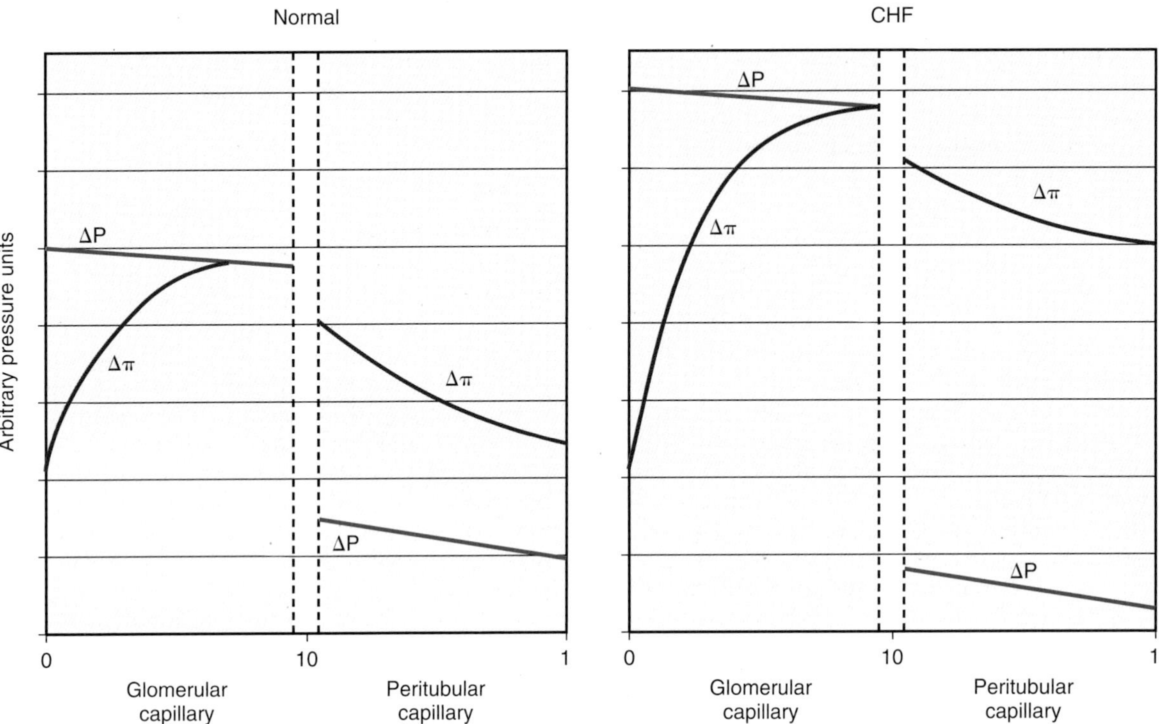


**Fig. 14.4** The glomerular and peritubular microcirculations. *Left,* Approximate transcapillary pressure profiles for the glomerular and peritubular capillaries in normal humans. Vessel lengths are given in normalized nondimensional terms, with 0 being the most proximal portion of the capillary bed and 1 the most distal portion. Thus, for the glomerulus, 0 corresponds to the afferent arteriolar end of the capillary bed and 1 corresponds to the efferent arteriolar end. The transcapillary hydraulic pressure difference ($\Delta P$) is relatively constant with distance along the glomerular capillary and the net driving force for ultrafiltration ($\Delta P - \Delta\pi$) diminishes primarily as a consequence of the increase in the opposing COP difference ($\Delta\pi$), the latter resulting from the formation of an essentially protein-free ultrafiltrate. As a result of the drop in pressure along the efferent arteriole, the net driving pressure in the peritubular capillaries ($\Delta P - \Delta\pi$, in which $\Delta\pi$ is the change in transcapillary oncotic pressure) becomes negative, favoring reabsorption. *Right,* Hemodynamic alterations in the renal microcirculation in congestive heart failure (CHF). The fall in renal plasma flow (RPF) rate in heart failure is associated with a compensatory increase in $\Delta P$ for the glomerular capillary, which is conducive to a greater than normal rise in the plasma protein concentration and, hence, in $\Delta\pi$ along the glomerular capillary. This increase in $\Delta\pi$ by the distal end of the glomerular capillary also translates to an increase in $\Delta\pi$ in the peritubular capillaries, resulting in an increased net driving pressure for enhanced proximal tubule fluid absorption, believed to take place in heart failure. The increased peritubular capillary absorptive force in heart failure also probably results from the decline in $\Delta P$, a presumed consequence of the rise in renal vascular resistance. (From Humes HD, Gottlieb M, Brenner BM. *The kidney in congestive heart failure: contemporary issues in nephrology*. Vol 1, New York: Churchill Livingstone 1978: pp 51–72.)

structure of the peritubular interstitial compartment. Ultrastructural data from rats have suggested that the peritubular capillary wall is in tight apposition to the tubule basement membrane for about 60% of the tubule basolateral surface. However, over the other 40%, irregularly shaped wide portions of peritubular interstitium intercede between the tubule and peritubular capillaries. Alterations in the physical properties of the interstitial compartment could conceivably modulate net fluid transport in the proximal tubule via changes in $P_i$. Also, Starling forces in the peritubular capillary are thought to regulate the rate of fluid entry from the peritubular interstitium into the capillary. Any change in this rate of flux could also lead to changes in Pi that secondarily modify proximal tubule solute transport. This formulation could explain why raising $P_i$ (e.g., by infusion of renal vasodilators, renal venous constriction, renal lymph ligation) were associated with a natriuretic response, whereas the opposite effect was seen with renal decapsulation, which lowers $P_i$ (see section, "Medullary Hemodynamics and Interstitial Pressure in the Control of Sodium Excretion: Pressure Natriuresis").

Because of the relatively high permeability of the proximal tubule, changes in interstitial Starling forces are likely to be transduced mainly through alterations in passive bidirectional paracellular flux through the tight junctions.[146] These changes might be mediated by the claudin family of adhesion molecules present in the tight junctions.[147–149] Among the 24 known mammalian claudin family members, at least two—claudin-2 and claudin-10—are located in the proximal nephron of the mouse.[148,150] In particular, claudin-2 is selectively expressed in the proximal nephron.[151,152] However, the exact role of claudins in the influence of Starling forces on fluid reabsorption remains to be elucidated.[152]

**Luminal Composition.** Even when the native peritubular environment is kept constant while the rate of perfusion of proximal tubular segments with native tubular fluid is changed, GTB can still be fully expressed.[153] A transtubular anion gradient, normally present in the late portion of the proximal nephron, is necessary for this flow dependence to occur.[154] Establishment of this anion gradient depends on

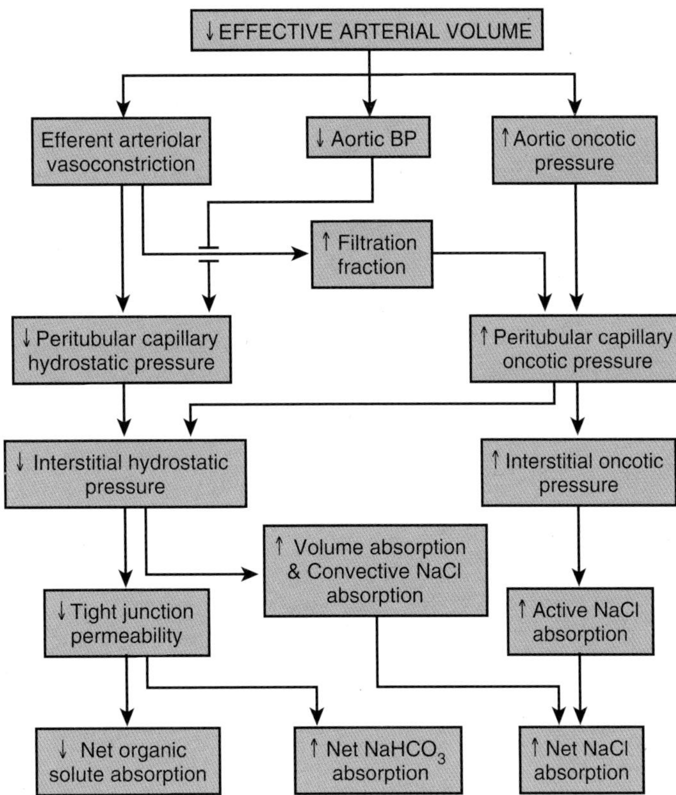


**Fig. 14.5** Effects of hemodynamic changes on proximal tubule solute transport. *BP*, Blood pressure. (From Seldin DW, Preisig PA, Alpern RJ. Regulation of proximal reabsorption by effective arterial blood volume. *Semin Nephrol.* 1991;11:212–219.)

the close coupling of $Na^+$ transport with the cotransport of glucose, amino acids and other organic solutes. The increased delivery of organic solutes that accompanies increases in GFR, together with the preferential reabsorption of $Na^+$ with bicarbonate in the early proximal tubule, would lead to increased delivery of both $Cl^-$ and organic solutes to the late proximal tubule. The resulting transtubular anion gradient would then facilitate the "passive" reabsorption of the organic solutes and NaCl in this segment, although overall net reabsorption would be reduced.

In summary, regardless of the exact mechanism, ECFV expansion impairs the integrity of GTB, allowing increased delivery of salt and fluid to more distal parts of the nephron. The major factors acting on the proximal nephron during a decrease in ECF and effective arterial circulating volume are outlined schematically in Fig. 14.5.

**Physical Factors Beyond the Proximal Tubule.** The final urinary excretion of $Na^+$, in response to volume expansion or depletion, can be dissociated from the amount delivered out of the superficial proximal nephron. This is achieved by appropriate modulation of $Na^+$ and water excretion in the loop of Henle, distal tubule, cortical and papillary collecting ducts. However, direct evidence that these transport processes are mediated by changes in Starling forces per se is lacking (see Jamison et al.[155] for a detailed review of experimental evidence).

In summary, if ECFV is held relatively constant, an increase in GFR leads to little or no increase in salt excretion because of a close coupling between GFR and intrarenal physical forces acting at the peritubular capillary to control $Rate_{abs}$. In addition, changes in the filtered load of small organic solutes and perhaps other, as yet uncharacterized, substances in tubular fluid may influence $Rate_{abs}$. Any changes in the $Na^+$ load delivered to more distal segments are accompanied by parallel changes in distal reabsorptive rates, thereby ensuring a high overall degree of GTB. Conversely, ECFV expansion leads to large increases in $Na^+$ excretion, even in the presence of a reduced GFR. Changes in $Na^+$ reabsorption in the proximal tubule partially account for this natriuresis, but suppression of more distal $Na^+$ reabsorption is also likely.

**Medullary Hemodynamics and Interstitial Pressure in the Control of Sodium Excretion: Pressure Natriuresis.** First proposed in the 1960s and elucidated in the 1970s and 1980s,[156,157] ECFV expansion (or elevation in systemic BP) was shown to elicit an increase in RPP that is transmitted as enhanced medullary plasma flow; this leads to a subsequent loss of medullary hypertonicity, elimination of the medullary osmotic gradient ("medullary washout"), thereby, decreasing water reabsorption in the thin descending loop of Henle. This decrease in water reabsorption lowers the $Na^+$ concentration in the fluid entering the ascending loop of Henle, thus decreasing the transepithelial driving force for salt transport in this nephron segment, particularly in juxtamedullary nephrons. The result is an increase in $Na^+$ and water excretion, thereby decreasing circulating blood volume and restoring arterial pressure.[158,159] The phenomenon, known as "pressure natriuresis,"[158–162] occurred in the absence of changes in total RBF, GFR, or filtered load of $Na^+$ and seems to be triggered by changes in medullary and papillary circulation.[156,161,163–165]

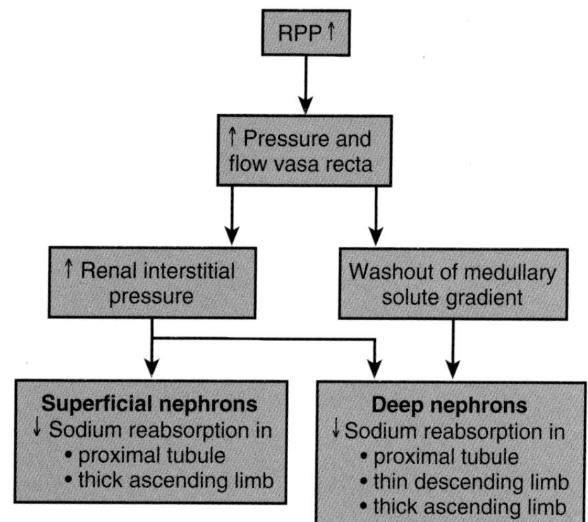


**Fig. 14.6** Role of the renal medulla in modulating tubular reabsorption of sodium in response to changes in renal perfusion pressure (RPP). (Modified from Cowley AW, Jr. Role of the renal medulla in volume and arterial pressure regulation. *Am J Physiol.* 1997;273:R1–R15.)

An increase in medullary plasma flow leads not only to medullary washout and a consequent reduction in $Na^+$ reabsorption in the ascending loop of Henle but also to a rise in $P_i$. In fact, increasing $P_i$ by ECFV expansion by infusion of renal vasodilatory agents, long-term mineralocorticoid escape, or hilar lymph ligation results in a significant increase in $Na^+$ excretion.[166,167] Prevention of the increase in $P_i$ by removal of the renal capsule attenuates, but does not completely block, the natriuretic response to elevations in RPP. Thus as depicted in Fig. 14.6, elevation in RPP is associated with an increase in medullary plasma flow and increased vasa recta capillary pressure, which results in an increase in medullary $P_i$. This increase of $P_i$ is thought to be transmitted to the renal cortex in the encapsulated kidneys and to provide a signal that inhibits $Na^+$ reabsorption along the nephron. In that regard, the renal medulla may be viewed as a sensor that detects changes in RPP and initiates pressure natriuresis.

To explain how changes in systemic BP are transmitted to the medulla in the presence of efficient RBF and GFR autoregulation, it has been suggested that shunt pathways connect preglomerular vessels of juxtamedullary nephrons directly to the postglomerular capillaries of the vasa recta.[156] Alternatively, autoregulation of RBF might lead to increased shear stress in the preglomerular vasculature, triggering the release of NO and perhaps cytochrome P450 products of arachidonic acid metabolism (see later), thereby driving the cascade of events that inhibit $Na^+$ reabsorption.[168,169] The mechanisms by which changes in $P_i$ decrease tubular $Na^+$ reabsorption and increase $U_{Na}$ excretion, as well as the nephron sites responding to the alterations in $P_i$, have not been fully clarified.[167] As noted earlier, elevations in $P_i$ may increase passive backleak or paracellular pathway hydraulic conductivity, with a resultant increase in back flux of $Na^+$ through this pathway.[166] However, the absolute changes in $P_i$, in the range of 3 to 8 mm Hg in response to increments of about 50 to 90 mm Hg in RPP, are probably not sufficient to account for the decrease in $Na^+$ reabsorption, even in the proximal tubule, the nephron segment with the highest transepithelial hydraulic conductivity.[160] The decreased proximal tubular $Na^+$ reabsorption may also be explained by redistribution of the apical $Na^+/H^+$ exchanger from the brush border into intracellular compartments and concomitantly decreased basolateral $Na^+$-$K^+$-ATPase activity in response to increased RPP.[170] The reduction in proximal fluid reabsorption is especially marked in deep nephrons, leading to enhanced delivery to the loop of Henle, inhibition of $Na^+$ reabsorption in the thin descending limb and reduced blood flow in the vasa recta.[166] Pressure-induced changes in tubular reabsorption may also occur in the ascending loop of Henle, distal tubule, and collecting duct.[171]

The demonstration of pressure natriuresis in states of volume expansion and renal vasodilation and its significant attenuation in states of volume depletion[166] suggested that changes in $P_i$ may be amplified by hemodynamic, hormonal and paracrine factors.[156,161,163,166] For example, RAAS inhibition potentiates whereas cyclooxygenase inhibitors attenuate the pressure natriuretic response.[166,172] Moreover, blockade of the Ang II type 2 receptor allows the same amount of $Na^+$ to be excreted at lower arterial pressure.[173] However, RAAS blockade does not completely eliminate pressure natriuresis, which indicates that the RAAS act as modulators and not as mediators of the phenomenon.

Pressure natriuresis is also modulated by endothelium-derived NO and P450 eicosanoids.[174–176] NO, generated in large amounts in the renal medulla, plays a critical role in the regulation of medullary blood flow and $Na^+$ excretion.[174–176] In this regard, inhibition of intrarenal NO production reduces $Na^+$ excretion and markedly suppresses pressure natriuresis,[177] whereas administration of an NO agonist normalizes the defect in the pressure natriuresis response in Dahl salt-sensitive rats.[178] Similarly, a positive correlation between urinary excretion of nitrites and nitrates (metabolites of NO) and changes in renal arterial pressure or $U_{Na}$ excretion was observed both in dogs[174,179,180] and rats.[174] Hydrogen peroxide ($H_2O_2$) has also been invoked in the mediation of RPP-induced changes in outer medullary blood flow and natriuresis. The response appears to be localized to the medullary thick ascending limb of Henle (mTALH), in contrast to the NO effect, which occurs in the vasa recta.[174] Other factors involved in the regulation of medullary blood flow and pressure natriuresis include superoxide, heme oxygenase,[175,180] and the cytochrome P450 eicosanoid 20-HETE.[168,169,181,182]

One mechanism by which acute elevations in RPP in the autoregulatory range lead to increased endothelial release of NO and reactive oxygen species could be via increased blood flow velocity and shear stress. Enhanced renal production of these molecules may then increase $U_{Na}$ excretion by acting directly on tubular $Na^+$ reabsorption or through a renal vasodilatory effect. ATP is another paracrine factor involved in pressure natriuresis by inhibiting salt and water reabsorption. ATP release appears to be mediated by mechanosensitive connexin 30 hemichannels.[183] The mechanisms of these cellular events have not been fully elucidated, but they may be related directly to changes in $P_i$ or to changes in the intrarenal paracrine agents described previously.

A major assumption of the pressure natriuresis theory is that changes in systemic and RPP mediate the natriuretic response by the kidneys. As noted in comprehensive reviews, acute regulatory changes in renal salt excretion may occur without measurable elevation in arterial BP.[48,184–186] In many of these studies, natriuresis was accompanied by a decrease in the activity of the RAAS, without changes in plasma ANP levels.[48,74,185,186] Thus, whereas increases in arterial BP can drive renal $Na^+$ excretion, other pressure-independent control mechanisms must also operate to mediate the natriuresis.[48]

### Neural Mechanisms: Renal Nerves and Symphathetic Nervous System

Extensive sympathetic innervation, predominantly adrenergic, occurs at all segments of the renal vasculature and tubule.[187] Only the basolateral membrane separates the nerve endings from the tubular cells. The greatest innervation is found at the level of the afferent arterioles, followed by the efferent arterioles and outer medullary descending vasa recta.[188] However, high-density tubular innervation is found in the ascending limb of the loop of Henle, with the lowest density in the collecting duct, inner medullary vascular elements and papilla.[189,190] The magnitude of the tubular response to renal nerve activation may thus be proportional to the differential density of innervation.

In accordance with these anatomic observations, stimulation of the renal nerve results in vasoconstriction of afferent and efferent arterioles[190,191] mediated by activation of postjunctional $\alpha_1$-adrenoreceptors.[192] With respect to tubular function, $\alpha_1$-adrenergic receptors and most $\alpha_2$-adrenergic receptors are localized in the basolateral membranes of the proximal tubule.[193] In the rat, $\beta_1$-adrenoreceptors have been found in the cTALH.[194] The predominant neurotransmitters in renal sympathetic nerves are noradrenaline and, to a lesser extent, dopamine and acetylcholine.[190] Consistent with their location, changes in RSNA play an important role in controlling body fluid homeostasis and BP.[73,187,191] Renal sympathetic nerve activity can influence renal function and $Na^+$ excretion through several mechanisms: 1. changes in renal and glomerular hemodynamics; 2. effect on renin release from juxtaglomerular cells, with increased formation of Ang II; and 3. direct effect on renal tubular fluid and electrolyte reabsorption.[73] Graded direct electrical stimulation of renal nerves produces frequency-dependent changes in RBF and GFR, reabsorption of renal tubular $Na^+$ and water and secretion of renin.[73,187] The lowest frequency (0.5–1.0 Hz) stimulates renin secretion and frequencies of 1.0 to 2.5 Hz increase renal tubule $Na^+$ and water reabsorption. Increasing the frequency of stimulation to 2.5 Hz and higher results in decreased RBF and GFR.[73,191]

The decrease in SNGFR in response to enhanced RSNA results from a combination of increases in afferent and efferent glomerular resistance, as well as decreases in glomerular capillary hydrostatic pressure ($\Delta P$) and ultrafiltration coefficient (Kf).[187,191] In Munich-Wistar rats, renal nerve stimulation at different frequencies revealed that the effector loci for vasomotor control by renal nerves were in the afferent and efferent arteriole. In addition, although urine flow and $Na^+$ excretion declined with renal nerve stimulation, there was no change in absolute proximal fluid reabsorption rate, which suggests that reabsorption is increased in the more distal segments of the nephron.

The SNS also has a role in regulating the renal response to varying $Na^+$ loads. In response to isotonic saline volume expansion and furosemide-induced volume contraction, a low-$Na^+$ diet resulted in a reduction in right atrial pressure and an increase in RSNA. Conversely, a high-$Na^+$ diet resulted in increased right atrial pressure and a reduction in RSNA.[191] Other studies using HWI and left atrial balloon inflation have similarly yielded evidence of the importance of reflex regulation of RSNA.[73]

Collectively, these studies demonstrated the reciprocal relationship between ECFV and RSNA and the role of central cardiopulmonary mechanoreceptors governing RSNA. Moreover, efferent RSNA is of special significance during conditions of dietary $Na^+$ restriction, when the need for renal $Na^+$ conservation is maximal. Indeed, when the linkage between the renal SNS and excretory renal function is defective, abnormalities in the regulation of ECF volume and BP may develop.[187,195] Thus, in euvolemic animals, acute denervation of the kidneys is associated with increased urine flow and $Na^+$ excretion, but without alteration in any of the determinants of SNGFR. However, absolute proximal reabsorption was significantly reduced in the absence of changes in peritubular capillary oncotic pressure, hydraulic pressure and renal interstitial pressure. $Na^+$ and water reabsorption was also reduced in the loop of Henle and more distal segments.[191] In rats with HF, in contrast, denervation ameliorated both renal vasoconstriction, by decreasing afferent and efferent arteriolar resistance and natriuresis, by reduced $Na^+$ reabsorption.[191]

Human studies, using the renal NE spillover technique, have confirmed that a true increase of efferent RSNA and a fall in $U_{Na}$ excretion occurs secondary to $Na^+$ restriction, with no change in cardiac NE uptake.[196] Similarly, low-dose NE in salt-replete volunteers resulted in antinatriuresis with a significant decline in lithium ($Li^+$) clearance, indicating enhanced proximal tubule reabsorption. The reduced $Na^+$ excretion occurred without change in GFR.[197]

The cellular mechanisms mediating the tubular actions of NE include stimulation of $Na^+$-$K^+$-ATPase activity and $Na^+/H^+$ exchange in proximal tubular epithelium.[191] This occurs via $\alpha_1$-adrenoreceptor stimulation, mediated by phospholipase C, causing an increase in intracellular $Ca^{2+}$ that activates the $Ca^{2+}$ calmodulin-dependent calcineurin phosphatase. Calcineurin converts $Na^+$-$K^+$-ATPase from its inactive phosphorylated form to its active dephosphorylated form.[198] The stimulatory effect of renal nerves on $Na^+/H^+$ exchange is mediated through the $\alpha_2$-adrenoreceptor.[191]

In addition to the direct action of $Na^+$ on epithelial cell transport and renal hemodynamics, interactions of renal nerve input with other effector mechanisms may contribute to the regulation of renal handling of $Na^+$. Efferent sympathetic nerve activity influences the rate of renal renin secretion both directly and via the macula densa and vascular baroreceptors.[191] The increase in renin secretion is mediated primarily by $\beta_1$-adrenergic receptors located on juxtaglomerular granular cells and is augmented during RPP reduction.[191] Intrarenal generation of Ang II facilitates NE release during renal nerve stimulation,[191] but the physiologic significance of this remains unclear.[199]

Sympathetic activity is also a stimulus for the production and release of renal PG, coupled to adrenergic-mediated renal vasoconstriction.[191] Renal vasodilatory PG attenuate the renal hemodynamic vasoconstrictive response to renal adrenergic activation.[191] The primary factor responsible for the reduction in glomerular Kf during renal nerve stimulation may be Ang II rather than NE and endogenously produced

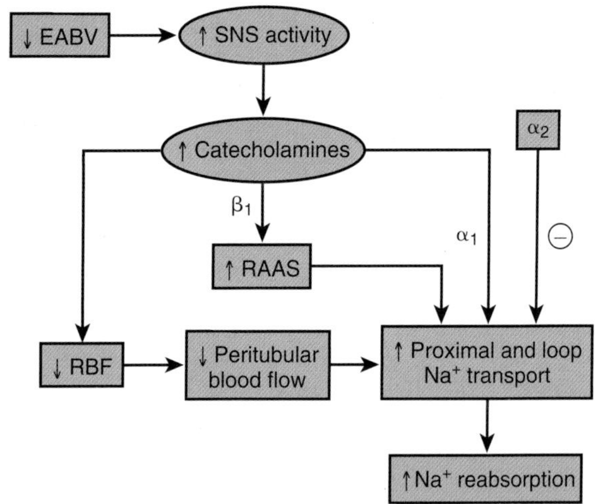


**Fig. 14.7** Sympathetic nervous system (SNS)–mediated effects of decreased effective arterial blood volume (EABV) on the kidneys. $\alpha_1$, $\alpha_2$, $\beta_1$, $\alpha_1$-, $\alpha_2$-and $\beta_1$-Adrenergic receptors, respectively. *RAAS*, Renin-angiotensin-aldosterone system; *RBF*, renal blood flow; –, inhibitory effect.

PG neutralize the vasoconstrictive effects of renal nerve stimulation at the intraglomerular rather than arteriolar level.

The renal SNS also interacts with AVP, which exerts a dose-related effect on the arterial baroreflex. Low doses of AVP sensitize the central baroreflex neurons to afferent input, whereas higher doses cause direct excitation of these neurons, resulting in reduced renal sympathetic outflow.[191] This response depends on the number of afferent inputs from baroreceptors.[207] Conversely, renal nerve stimulation results in elevated plasma AVP levels and arterial pressure in conscious, baroreceptor-intact rats.[200] Many studies have demonstrated in normal and pathologic situations that increased RSNA can antagonize the natriuretic/diuretic response to ANP and that removal of the influence of sympathetic activity enhances the natriuretic action of the peptide.[191] Conversely, renal denervation in Wistar rats increased ANP receptors and cGMP generation in glomeruli, resulting in increased Kf after ANP infusion.[201]

In summary, renal sympathetic nerves regulate $U_{Na}$ and water excretion by changing renal vascular resistance, by influencing renin release from the juxtaglomerular granular cell and through a direct effect on tubular epithelial cells (Fig. 14.7). These effects may be modulated by other hormonal systems, including ANP, PG, and AVP.

### Humoral Mechanisms

**Renin-Angiotensin-Aldosterone System.** The RAAS plays a central role in the regulation of ECF volume, $Na^+$ homeostasis and cardiac function.[202] The system is activated in situations that compromise hemodynamic stability, such as blood loss, reduced EABV, low $Na^+$ intake, hypotension and increase in sympathetic nerve activity. The RAAS is comprised of a coordinated hormonal cascade whose synthesis is initiated by the release of renin from the JGA in response to reduced renal perfusion or decrease in arterial pressure.[203] Renin acts on its circulating substrate, angiotensinogen, which is produced and secreted mainly by the liver, but also by the kidneys.[202] ACE1, which cleaves Ang I to Ang II, exists in large amounts in the microvasculature of the lungs but also on endothelial cells of other vascular beds and cell membranes of the proximal nephron brush border, heart, and brain.[202] Ang II is the principal effector of the RAAS, although other smaller metabolic products of Ang II also have biologic activities.[204,205] Nonrenin (cathepsin G, plasminogen-activating factor, tonin) and non-ACE pathways (chymase, cathepsin G) also exist in these tissues and may contribute to tissue Ang II synthesis.[202]

In addition to its important function as a circulating hormone, Ang II produced locally acts as a paracrine growth-promoting agent in the cardiovascular system and kidneys.[202] For example, proximal tubular epithelial cells, which abundantly express the mRNA for angiotensinogen, synthesize and secrete Ang II into the lumen;[206] this leads to approximately 1000 times higher local concentrations in proximal tubular fluid, as well as higher levels in interstitial fluid and medulla than in the plasma.[207] Moreover, the mechanisms regulating intrarenal levels of Ang II appear to be dissociated from those controlling the systemic concentrations of the peptide.[206]

The biologic actions of Ang II are mediated through activation of $AT_1$ and $AT_2$ receptors, encoded by different genes residing on different chromosomes.[208,209] Both receptors are G protein–coupled, seven-transmembrane polypeptides containing approximately 360 amino acids.[202,210] The $AT_1$ receptor mediates most of the biologic activities of Ang II, whereas the $AT_2$ receptor appears to have a vasodilatory and antiproliferative effect.[204,211] $AT_1$ is expressed in the vascular poles of glomeruli, JGA and mesangial cells, whereas the quantitatively lower expression of $AT_2$ is confined to renal arteries and tubular structures.[209] In addition to their functional distinction, the two receptor types use different downstream pathways. Stimulation of the $AT_1$ receptor activates phospholipases $A_2$, C and D, resulting in increased cytosolic $Ca^{2+}$ and inositol triphosphate and inhibition of adenylate cyclase. In contrast, activation of the $AT_2$ receptor results in increases in NO and bradykinin levels, which lead to elevation in cGMP concentrations and vasodilation.[208]

In addition to being an important source of several components of the RAAS, the kidney is a major target organ for Ang II and aldosterone. The direct effect of Ang II is mediated via $AT_1$ receptors to induce renal vasoconstriction, stimulation of tubular epithelial $Na^+$ reabsorption, augmentation of TGF sensitivity, modulation of pressure natriuresis, and stimulation of mitogenic pathways.[202] Moreover, circulating levels of Ang II in the picomolar range are highly effective in modulating renal hemodynamic and tubular function, in comparison with the 10- to 100-fold higher concentrations required for its extrarenal effects. Thus the kidneys appear to be uniquely sensitive to the actions of Ang II. Furthermore, the synergistic interactions between the renal vascular and tubular actions of Ang II significantly amplify the influence of Ang II on $Na^+$ excretion.[206] Ang II elicits a dose-dependent decrease in RBF but slightly augments GFR as a result of its preferential vasoconstrictive effect on the efferent arteriole, thereby increasing filtration fraction. In turn, this may further modulate peritubular Starling forces, possibly by decreasing interstitial hydraulic and increasing COP. These peritubular changes eventually lead to enhanced proximal $Na^+$ and water reabsorption. Of importance, however, is that changes in preglomerular resistance have also been described during

Ang II infusion or blockade.[212] These may be secondary to changes in systemic arterial pressure (myogenic reflex) or to increased sensitivity of TGF because Ang II does not alter preglomerular resistance when RPP is clamped or adjustments in TGF are prevented.[212]

In addition, Ang II may affect GFR by reducing Kf, thereby altering the filtered load of $Na^+$.[213] This effect is likely mediated by mesangial cell contractility and increasing permeability to macromolecules.[212] Finally, Ang II leads to reduced cortical and medullary blood flow and decreased $Na^+$ and water excretion.[212,214] As noted earlier, changes in medullary blood flow may affect medullary tonicity, which determines the magnitude of passive salt reabsorption in the loop of Henle and may also modulate pressure natriuresis through alterations in renal interstitial pressure.[214]

The other well-characterized renal effect of Ang II is a direct action on proximal tubular epithelial transport, independently of changes in renal or systemic hemodynamics.[202,215] Ang II exerts a dose-dependent biphasic effect on proximal $Na^+$ reabsorption. Peritubular capillary infusion with solutions containing low concentrations of Ang II ($10^{-12}$ to $10^{-10}$ mol) stimulate, whereas higher concentrations ($>10^{-7}$ mol) inhibit proximal $Na^+$ reabsorption. Addition of ACE inhibitors (ACEIs) or angiotensin II receptor blockers (ARB) directly into the luminal fluid results in a significant decrease in proximal $Na^+$ reabsorption, indicative of tonic regulation of proximal tubule transport by endogenous Ang II.[216]

The specific mechanisms by which Ang II influences proximal tubule transport include increases in reabsorption of $Na^+$ and $HCO_3^-$ by stimulation of the apical $Na^+$-$H^+$ antiporter, $Na^+/H^+$-exchanger isoform 3 (NHE3), basolateral $Na^+$-$3HCO_3^-$ symporter and $Na^+$-$K^+$-ATPase.[217,218] Thus, Ang II can affect NaCl absorption by two mechanisms:

1. Activation of NHE3 can directly increase NaCl absorption.
2. Increasing the rate of $NaHCO_3$ absorption can stimulate passive NaCl absorption by increasing the concentration gradient for passive $Cl^-$ diffusion.[219]

$Na^+$ reabsorption is further promoted by the action of Ang II on NHE3 and $Na^+$-$K^+$-ATPase in the mTALH.[202]

In the early and late portions of the distal tubule, as well as the connecting tubule, Ang II regulates $Na^+$ and $HCO_3^-$ reabsorption by stimulating NHE3 and the amiloride-sensitive $Na^+$ channel.[220–222] Two additional mechanisms may amplify the antinatriuretic effects of Ang II. The first concerns the increased sensitivity of TGF in the presence of Ang II and the second is related to the effect of Ang II on pressure natriuresis. The decrease in distal delivery produced by the action of Ang II on renal hemodynamics and proximal fluid reabsorption could elicit afferent arteriolar vasodilation by means of the TGF mechanism, which, in turn, could antagonize the Ang II–mediated increase in proximal reabsorption. This effect, however, is minimized because Ang II increases the responsiveness of the TGF mechanism, thus maintaining GFR at a lower delivery rate to the macula densa.[75] The second mechanism by which the antinatriuretic effects of Ang II may be amplified is blunting of the pressure natriuresis mechanism so that higher pressures are needed to induce a given amount of $Na^+$ excretion.[168,202] This shift to the right in the pressure natriuresis curve may be an important $Na^+$-conserving mechanism in situations of elevated arterial pressure.

As already stated, most of the known intrarenal effects of Ang II in the regulation of renal hemodynamics and proximal tubule reabsorption of $Na^+$ and $HCO_3^-$ are mediated by the $AT_1$ receptor.[209] However, activation of the $AT_2$ receptor may play a counterregulatory protective role against the $AT_1$ receptor–mediated antinatriuretic and pressor actions of Ang II.[209]

Ang I is converted not only to Ang II but also to angiotensin-(1–7) (Ang 1–7)[223] either directly by the homolog of ACE, ACE2, or indirectly, via angiotensin-(1–9), followed by ACE-mediated conversion to Ang 1–7.[223] Ang 1–7, through its G protein–coupled receptor, Mas, may play a significant role as a regulator of cardiovascular and renal function by opposing the effects of Ang II, through vasodilation, diuresis, and an antihypertrophic action.[223] Thus, the RAAS can currently be envisioned as a dual-function system in which the vasoconstrictor/proliferative or vasodilator/antiproliferative actions are driven primarily by the ACE/ACE2 balance. According to this model, an increased ACE/ACE2 activity ratio leads to increased generation of Ang II and increased catabolism of Ang 1–7, which is conducive to vasoconstriction; conversely, a decreased ACE/ACE2 ratio reduces Ang II and increases Ang 1–7 levels, facilitating vasodilation. The additional effect of Ang 1–7/Mas to antagonize the actions of Ang II directly adds a further level of counterregulation.[223]

The final component of the RAAS, aldosterone, is produced via Ang II stimulation of the adrenal cortex and also plays an important physiologic role in the maintenance of ECFV and $Na^+$ homeostasis.[224] The primary sites of aldosterone action are the principal cells of the cortical collecting tubule and distal convoluted tubule, in which the hormone promotes the reabsorption of $Na^+$ and the secretion of $K^+$ and protons.[224,225] Aldosterone may also enhance electrogenic $Na^+$ transport, but not $K^+$ secretion, in the IMCD[226] and proximal tubule.[227] Aldosterone exerts its effects by increasing the number of open $Na^+$ and $K^+$ channels in the luminal membrane and the activity of $Na^+$-$K^+$-ATPase in the basolateral membrane.[228] The effect of aldosterone on $Na^+$ permeability appears to be the primary event because blockade of the ENaC with amiloride prevents the initial increase in $Na^+$ permeability and $Na^+$-$K^+$-ATPase activity.[228] This effect on $Na^+$ permeability is mediated by changes in intracellular $Ca^{2+}$, intracellular pH,[229] trafficking via protein kinase D1-phosphatidylinositol 4-kinaseIIIβ trans Golgi signaling,[230] and methylation of channel proteins, thus increasing the mean open probability of ENaC.[229] However, the long-term effect of aldosterone on $Na^+$-$K^+$-ATPase activity involves de novo protein synthesis, which is regulated at the transcriptional level by serum- and glucocorticoid-induced kinase-1.[229]

Aldosterone specifically regulates the α-subunit of ENaC and changes in expression of a variety of genes are important intermediates in this process. Microarray analysis in a mouse IMCD line showed that the most prominent transcript induced acutely by aldosterone was period homolog 1 (Per1), an important component of the circadian clock and that disruption of the Per1 gene led to attenuated expression of mRNA encoding for the α-subunit and increased $U_{Na}$ excretion. mRNA encoded by the α-subunit was also expressed in an apparent circadian pattern that was dramatically altered in mice lacking functional Per1 genes.[231] These results imply that the circadian clock has a role in the control of $Na^+$ balance and provide molecular insight into how the circadian cycle directly affects $Na^+$ homeostasis.

The $Na^+$-retaining effect of aldosterone in the collecting tubule induces an increase in the transepithelial potential difference, which is conducive to $K^+$ excretion. In terms of overall body fluid homeostasis, the actions of aldosterone in the defense of ECF result from the net loss of an osmotically active particle confined primarily to the intracellular compartment ($K^+$) and its replacement with a corresponding particle confined primarily to the ECF ($Na^+$). The effect of a given circulating level of aldosterone on overall $Na^+$ excretion depends on the volume of filtrate reaching the collecting duct and the composition of luminal and intracellular fluids. As noted earlier, this delivery of filtrate is, in turn, determined by other effector mechanisms (Ang II, sympathetic nerve activity and peritubular physical forces) acting at more proximal nephron sites.

$Na^+$ balance can be regulated over a wide range of intake, even in subjects without adrenal glands and despite fixed low or high supplemental doses of mineralocorticoids. Under these circumstances, other effector mechanisms predominate in controlling urinary $Na^+$ excretion, although often in a setting of altered ECF volume or $K^+$ concentration. In this regard, how renal $Na^+$ reabsorption and $K^+$ excretion are coordinately regulated by aldosterone has long been a puzzle. In states of EABV depletion, aldosterone release stimulated by Ang II induces maximal $Na^+$ reabsorption without significantly affecting plasma $K^+$ levels. Conversely, hyperkalemia-induced aldosterone secretion stimulates maximum $K^+$ excretion without major effects on renal $Na^+$ handling.

Elegant studies on the intracellular signaling pathways involved in renal $Na^+$ and $K^+$ transport have shed light on this puzzle. The key elements in this transport regulation are the Ste20/SPS1-related proline/alanine-rich kinase (SPAK), oxidative stress-related kinase (OSR1) the with-no-lysine kinases (WNKs) and their effectors, the thiazide-sensitive NaCl cotransporter and the $K^+$ secretory channel ROMK. According to the proposed model, when EABV is reduced or dietary salt intake is low, Ang II, mediated by the $AT_1$ receptor, leads to phosphorylation of WNK4, which stimulates phosphorylation of SPAK and OSR1. In turn, SPAK and OSR1 phosphorylate the NaCl cotransporter, inducing $Na^+$ transport and conservation. Simultaneous phosphorylation of the full-length isoform of WNK1, WNK1-L, causes endocytosis of the ROMK channel, thereby enabling $K^+$ conservation, despite high aldosterone levels. In contrast, in the presence of hyperkalemia or low dietary salt, Ang II levels are low so that WNK4 cannot be activated, SPAK, OSR1 and the NaCl cotransporter are not phosphorylated and NaCl cotransporter trafficking to the apical membrane is inhibited. At the same time, $K^+$-induced kidney-specific WNK1 leads to suppression of WNK1-L, which allows ROMK trafficking to the apical membrane and maximal $K^+$ secretion.[232] For further details, the reader is referred to Chapter 6.

For BP maintenance, systemic vasoconstriction—another major extrarenal action of Ang II—is the appropriate response to perceived ECF volume contraction. As mentioned previously, higher concentrations of Ang II are needed to elicit this response than those governing the antinatriuretic actions of Ang II. Transition from an antinatriuretic to a natriuretic action of Ang II at high infusion rates is almost entirely due to a concomitant BP rise.[233]

In addition to the adrenal glomerulosa, aldosterone, similar to Ang II, is also produced by the heart and vasculature, exerting powerful mitogenic and fibrogenic effects on blood vessels, independently of regulation of salt and water balance.[234] It directly increases the expression and production of transforming growth factor-β (TGF- β) and thus is involved in the development of glomerulosclerosis, hypertension and cardiac injury/hypertrophy.[202,224,235]

In summary, Ang II, the principal effector of the RAAS, regulates extracellular volume and renal $Na^+$ excretion through intrarenal and extrarenal mechanisms. The intrarenal hemodynamic and tubular actions of the peptide and its main extrarenal actions (systemic vasoconstriction and aldosterone release) act in concert to adjust $U_{Na}$ excretion under a variety of circumstances associated with alterations in ECF volume. Many of these mechanisms are synergistic and tend to amplify the overall influence of the RAAS. However, additional counterregulatory mechanisms, induced directly or indirectly by Ang II, provide a buffer against the unopposed actions of the primary components of the RAAS.

**Vasopressin.** AVP is a nonapeptide hormone, synthesized in the paraventricular and supraoptic nuclei of the hypothalamus and secreted from the posterior pituitary gland into the circulation in response to an increase in plasma osmolality (through osmoreceptor stimulation) or a decrease in EABV and BP (through baroreceptor stimulation).[236] AVP acts through at least three different G protein–coupled receptors. Two of these, $V_{1A}$ and $V_2$, are abundantly expressed in the cardiovascular system and the kidneys; $V_{1B}$ receptors are expressed on the surfaces of corticotropic cells of the anterior pituitary gland, in the pancreas and adrenal medulla. $V_{1A}$ and $V_2$ receptors mediate the two main biologic actions of the hormone, vasoconstriction and increased water reabsorption by the kidneys, respectively. $V_{1A}$ and $V_{1B}$ receptors operate through the phosphoinositide signaling pathway, causing release of intracellular $Ca^{2+}$. The $V_{1A}$ receptor, found in vascular smooth muscle cells (VSMC), hepatocytes and platelets, mediates vasoconstriction, glycogenolysis and platelet aggregation, respectively. The $V_2$ receptor, found mainly in renal collecting duct epithelial cells, is linked to the adenylate cyclase/cAMP pathway. A $V_3$ receptor is not involved in the regulation of ECFV and is not discussed further.[237]

Under physiologic conditions, AVP functions primarily to regulate body water content by adjusting reabsorption in the collecting duct according to plasma tonicity. A change in plasma tonicity by as little as 1% causes a parallel change in AVP release. AVP activates $V_2$ receptors in the basolateral membrane of the principal cells, leading to increased cytosolic cAMP, which stimulates the activity of protein kinase A. The latter triggers a series of phosphorylation events that promotes the translocation of AQP2 from intracellular stores to the apical membrane,[238] as well as the synthesis of AQP2 mRNA and protein;[239] this allows the reabsorption of water from lumen to cells. Water then exits the cell to the hypertonic interstitium via aquaporin-3 and aquaporin-4 channels at the basolateral membrane.[240] (See Chapter 10 for further details).

The second major effect of AVP on the collecting duct is to increase the permeability of the IMCD to urea through activation of the urea transporter UT-A1, enabling the accumulation of urea in the interstitium; there, along with $Na^+$, it contributes to the hypertonicity of the medullary interstitium, a prerequisite for maximum urine concentration and water reabsorption.[241] AVP also mediates an increase in $Na^+$ reabsorption from the mTAL, distal and connecting tubule and collecting duct, by activation of the segment-specific $Na^+$ transporters; this effect is important for maintenance of the axial corticomedullary osmotic gradient necessary for maximal water reabsorption (see reviews in Kortenoeven et al.[236] and Knepper et al.[242]).

In addition, AVP, via the $V_{1A}$ receptor, reduces RBF, especially to the inner medulla, an effect modulated by local release of NO and PG.[243] At higher concentrations, AVP may also decrease total RBF and GFR as part of the generalized vasoconstrictor effect.[239,244] Experiments in $V_{1A}$ receptor–deficient ($V_{1A}R^{-/-}$) mice have shown decreases in plasma volume, BP, GFR, $U_{Na}$ excretion, AVP-dependent cAMP generation, levels of $V_2$ receptor and renal AQP2 expression with concomitantly increased urine volume compared with wild type mice; the data imply impaired urinary concentration in $V_{1A}R^{-/-}$ mice. Moreover, plasma renin and Ang II levels were decreased, as was renin expression in granule cells. In addition, the expression of renin stimulators such as nNOS and cyclooxygenase-2 (COX-2) in macula densa cells, where $V_{1A}R$ is specifically expressed, was decreased in $V_{1A}R^{-/-}$ mice. Thus, AVP regulates body fluid homeostasis and GFR through the $V_{1A}R$ in macula densa cells by activating the RAAS and subsequently the $V_2$ receptor–AQP2 system.[244,245]

In addition to its renal effects, AVP also regulates extrarenal vascular tone through the $V_{1A}$ receptor. Stimulation of this receptor by AVP results in a potent arteriolar vasoconstriction in various vascular beds, with a significant increase in SVR.[242] However, physiologic increases in AVP do not usually cause a significant increase in BP because AVP also potentiates the sinoaortic baroreflexes that subsequently reduce heart rate and cardiac output.[246] Nevertheless, at supraphysiologic concentrations, such as those seen when EABV is severely compromised (e.g., in shock or HF), AVP plays an important role in supporting arterial pressure and maintaining adequate perfusion to vital organs such as the brain and myocardium. AVP also has a direct, $V_1$ receptor–mediated, inotropic effect in the isolated heart, but, in vivo, leads to decreased myocardial function; this effect is attributed to AVP-induced cardioinhibitory reflexes or coronary vasoconstriction.[247] Of more importance is that AVP, similar to Ang II and catecholamines, has been shown to stimulate cardiomyocyte hypertrophy and protein synthesis in neonatal rat cardiomyocytes and intact myocardium through a $V_1$-dependent mechanism.[247] This effect may contribute to the induction of cardiac hypertrophy and remodeling in HF.[247]

To summarize, regardless of the effects of AVP on $Na^+$ excretion, the predominant influence of the hormone is indirectly through water accumulation or vasoconstriction. In fact, the vasoconstrictive $V_1$ receptor effect of AVP overrides the osmotically driven effect in the presence of an ECF volume deficit of 20% or more (see Chapters 10 and 15). Nevertheless, the vasoconstrictive and water-retaining effects of AVP are modulated, respectively, by concomitant increases in baroreflex-mediated sympathoinhibition or $PGE_2$ and direct or $PGE_2$-mediated suppression of $V_2$ receptor activation.[248]

**Prostaglandins.** Prostaglandins (see also Chapter 16), or cyclooxygenase–derived prostanoids, possess diverse regulatory functions in the kidneys, including hemodynamic, renin secretion, growth response, tubular transport, and immune responses.[249,250] Two principal isoforms of cyclooxygenase, COX-1 and COX-2, catalyze the synthesis of prostaglandin $H_2$ ($PGH_2$) from arachidonic acid, released from membrane phospholipids. $PGH_2$ is then metabolized to the five major prostanoids—$PGE_2$, $PGD_2$, $PGF_2\alpha$, and thromboxane $A_2$ ($TXA_2$)—through specific synthases (see also Chapter 16).

Prostanoids are rapidly degraded, so their effect is localized strictly to their site of synthesis, which accounts for their predominant autocrine and paracrine modes of action. Each prostanoid has a location-specific cell surface G protein–coupled receptor that determines the function of the PG in the given cell type.[250] The major sites for PG production (and hence for local actions) are the renal arteries, arterioles, and glomeruli in the cortex and interstitial cells in the medulla, with additional contributions from epithelial cells of the cortical and medullary collecting tubules.[251,252] COX-1 is constitutively and abundantly expressed in the kidneys, especially in the collecting duct but also in medullary interstitial, mesangial, and arteriolar endothelial cells.[250] In contrast, COX-2 is inducible, cell type–specific, and prominently expressed in cells of the medullary interstitium, cTALH and macula densa, in which expression is regulated in response to salt intake.[250] $PGE_2$ and $PGI_2$ are the main products in the cortex of normal kidneys, whereas $PGE_2$ predominates in the medulla.[250] $PGF_2$ and $TXA_2$ are also produced in smaller amounts.[250] In addition, the metabolism of arachidonic acid by other pathways (e.g., lipoxygenase, epoxygenase) leads to products involved in crosstalk with COX.[249]

The two major roles for PG in volume homeostasis are modulation of 1. RBF and GFR and 2. tubular handling of salt and water. $PGI_2$ and $PGE_2$ have predominantly vasodilating and natriuretic activities, modulate the action of AVP and tend to stimulate renin secretion. $TXA_2$ causes vasoconstriction, although the importance of the physiologic effects of $TXA_2$ on the kidneys is still controversial. The end results of the stimulation of renal PG secretion in the kidneys are vasodilation, increased renal perfusion, natriuresis, and facilitation of water excretion.

The cellular targets of vasodilatory PG are the afferent and efferent arteriolar VSMC, glomerular mesangial cells peritubular capillaries, and vasa recta to modulate renal vascular resistance and glomerular function. Intrarenal infusions of $PGE_2$ and $PGI_2$ cause vasodilation and increased RBF.[251] In isolated renal microvessels, $PGE_2$ and $PGE_1$ attenuate Ang II–induced afferent and $PGI_2$ antagonizes Ang II–induced efferent arteriolar vasoconstriction.[253] Similarly, $PGE_2$ can counteract renal nerve stimulation[254] and Ang II–induced contraction of isolated glomeruli and cultured mesangial cells.[255] Furthermore, in volume-contracted states, COX-2 expression and $PGE_2$ release in the macula densa and cTALH dramatically increases in response to decreased luminal $Cl^-$ delivery. In addition to its direct vasodilatory effect on afferent arterioles, $PGE_2$ leads to increased renin release from the macula densa.[250] The resulting rise in Ang II and consequent efferent arteriolar constriction also ensures maintenance of GFR.

In volume-replete states, the renal vasoconstrictive influences of Ang II and NE are mitigated by their simultaneous stimulation of vasodilatory renal PG, so that RBF and GFR are maintained.[256] However, in the setting of heightened vasoconstrictor input from the RAAS, SNS and AVP, as in states of EABV depletion, the vasorelaxant action of $PGE_2$ and $PGI_2$ is overwhelmed, with the concomitant risk for the development of acute kidney injury.[250] Similarly, when this PG-mediated counterregulatory mechanism is suppressed by nonselective or COX-2–selective inhibitors, the unopposed actions of Ang II and NE can lead to a rapid deterioration in renal function.[257] Moreover, COX-2–derived prostanoids also promote natriuresis and stimulate renin secretion.[250] Therefore, during states of volume depletion, low $Na^+$ intake or the use of loop diuretics, COX-2 inhibitors and nonselective COX inhibitors can cause $Na^+$ and $K^+$ retention, edema, HF and hypertension.[252]

Besides modulating glomerular vasoreactivity, $PGE_2$-induced renal vasodilation affects $U_{Na}$ excretion, by inducing medullary interstitial solute washout.[251] The natriuretic response to $PGE_2$ may also be attenuated by preventing an increase in renal interstitial hydraulic pressure, even in the presence of a persistent increase in RBF.[258] In addition, the natriuresis accompanying direct expansion of renal interstitial volume is significantly attenuated by inhibition of PG synthesis.[258] $PGE_2$ also affects $U_{Na}$ excretion by direct effects on epithelial transport processes.[251] In the mTALH and collecting tubule, $PGE_2$ causes a decrease in the reabsorption of water, $Na^+$ and $Cl^-$ which correlates with reduced $Na^+$-$K^+$-ATPase activity. In contrast, in the distal convoluted tubule, $PGE_2$ causes increased $Na^+$-$K^+$-ATPase activity.[259] The net effect of PG on tubular $Na^+$ handling is probably inhibitory because complete blockade of PG synthesis by indomethacin in rats receiving a normal or salt-loaded diet increases fractional $Na^+$ reabsorption and enhances medullary $Na^+$-$K^+$-ATPase activity.[260] In addition, $PGE_2$ inhibits AVP-stimulated NaCl reabsorption in the mTALH and AVP-stimulated water reabsorption in the collecting duct.[261,262] Both these effects tend to antagonize the overall hydroosmotic response to AVP. However, the cTALH, which can augment NaCl reabsorption in response to an increased delivered load, is not affected by PG; also, the effects of PG on solute transport in the collecting tubule remain unresolved. Therefore, the contribution of direct epithelial effects of PG to overall $Na^+$ excretion is unclear.[261]

Not only does renal COX expression influence salt handling, but also changes in $Na^+$ intake affect the renal expression of these enzymes. COX-2 expression in the macula densa and TALH is increased by a low-salt diet, RAAS inhibition and renal hypoperfusion. Conversely, a high-salt diet leads to decreased COX-2, but unchanged COX-1, expression in the renal cortex.[249,250] In the medulla, whereas a low-salt diet downregulated both COX-1 and COX-2, a high-salt diet enhanced their expression.[249,250] High osmolarity of the medium of cultured IMCD cells induced COX-2 expression whereas infusion of a selective COX-2 inhibitor into anesthetized dogs on a normal $Na^+$ diet reduced $U_{Na}$ excretion and urine flow rate, without affecting renal hemodynamics or systemic BP.[252]

Collectively, the differential regulation of COX-2 in the renal cortex and medulla can be integrated into a physiologically relevant model in which upregulation of COX-2 in the cTALH and macula densa is induced in a volume-contracted or vasoconstrictor state. In the cTALH, the effect is by direct inhibition of $Na^+$ excretion, whereas in the macula densa, COX-2 stimulates renin release, which leads to Ang II–mediated $Na^+$ retention. In contrast, medullary COX-2 is induced by a high-salt diet, which leads to net $Na^+$ excretion.[250]

Finally, in addition to their hemodynamic and direct epithelial effects, PG may mediate the physiologic responses to other hormonal agents. The intermediacy of PG in renin release responses has already been cited. As another example, some, but not all, of the physiologic effects of bradykinin are mediated by PG production (e.g., inhibition of AVP-stimulated osmotic water permeability in the cortical collecting tubule).[261] In addition, the renal and systemic actions of Ang II appear to be differentially regulated by COX-1 and COX-2. For example, COX-2 deficiency in mice, induced by inhibitors or gene knockout, dramatically augmented the systemic pressor effect of Ang II, whereas COX-1 deficiency abolished this effect. Similarly, Ang II infusion reduced medullary blood flow in COX-2–deficient, but not COX-1–deficient animals, which suggests that COX-2–dependent vasodilators are synthesized in the renal medulla. Moreover, the diuretic and natriuretic effects of Ang II were absent in COX-2–deficient but remained in COX-1–deficient animals. Thus, COX-1 and COX-2 seem to exert opposite effects on systemic BP and renal function.[263]

**Natriuretic Peptides.** There are four NPs: ANP, BNP, CNP, and DNP.[264] Although encoded by different genes, their structures, gene regulation and degradation pathways are very similar, and they exert various actions on renal, cardiac, and vascular tissues.[265] ANP, a 28-amino acid peptide, plays an important role in BP and volume homeostasis through its natriuretic/diuretic and vasodilatory responses.[264,265] BNP has an amino acid sequence similar to that of ANP, with an extended $NH_2$-terminus. In humans, BNP is produced from pro–brain NP (proBNP), which contains 108 amino acids and, by proteolysis, releases a mature, 32–amino acid molecule and N-terminal fragment into the circulation. Although BNP was originally cloned from the brain, it is now considered a circulating hormone produced mainly in the cardiac ventricles.[266,267] CNP, produced mostly by endothelial cells, shares the ring structure common to all NP members; however, it lacks the C-terminal tail. DNP is released by the kidney and is a more effective activator of renal functions than ANP.[268]

The biologic effects of the natriuretic peptides (NPs) are mediated by binding to specific membrane receptors localized to numerous tissues, including the vasculature, renal arteries, glomerular mesangial and epithelial cells, collecting ducts, adrenal zona glomerulosa, and CNS.[264] At least three different, subtypes of NP receptors have been identified—NP-A, NP-B and NP-C. NP-A and NP-B, single-transmembrane proteins with molecular weights of approximately 120 to 140 kDa, mediate most of the biologic effects of NPs. Both are coupled to guanylate cyclase (GC) in their intracellular portions.[269] After binding to their receptors, all three NP isoforms markedly increase cGMP in target tissues and plasma. Therefore analogs of cGMP or inhibitors of its degradation mimic the vasorelaxant and renal effects of NPs. NP-C (molecular weight, 60 to 70 kDa), the most abundant NP receptor in many key target organs, is believed to be a clearance receptor because it is not coupled to any known second-messenger system.[270]

Two additional routes for the removal of NPs should be noted. The first is the enzymatic degradation by neutral endopeptidase (NEP) 24.11, a metalloproteinase located mainly in the lungs and the kidneys.[270] Extensive research into this pathway culminated in the development of a specific NEP inhibitor, which leads to enhanced NP activity and improved HF outcomes (see section, "Specific Treatments Based on the Pathophysiology of Congestive Heart Failure"). The second route involves the negative regulation of ANP by microRNA-425 (miRNA-425). In this context, carriers of the rs5068 minor G allele of the gene encoding ANP, *NPPA,* have ANP levels 50% higher than those with two copies of the major A allele and have a 15% lower risk of hypertension. miRNA-425, expressed in human atria and ventricles, is predicted to bind the sequence spanning rs5068 in the 3′ untranslated region of the A, but not G, allele. Only the A allele was silenced by miRNA-425, whereas possession of the G allele conferred resistance to miR-425. The results raise the possibility that miR-425 antagonists could be used to treat disorders of salt overload, such as hypertension and HF.[271]

**Atrial Natriuretic Peptide.** Studies in humans and experimental animals have established the role of ANP in the regulation of ECFV and BP by acting on all organs and tissues involved in the homeostasis of $Na^+$ and BP (Table 14.3).[267] Therefore, it is not surprising that ANP and $NH_2$-terminal ANP levels are increased in: 1. conditions associated with enhanced atrial pressure; 2. systolic or diastolic cardiac dysfunction; 3. cardiac hypertrophy/remodeling; and 4. severe myocardial infarction.[38] In the kidneys, ANP exerts hemodynamic/glomerular effects that increase $Na^+$ and water delivery to the tubule and inhibits tubular $Na^+$ and water reabsorption, leading to significant natriuresis and diuresis.[267]

In addition, ANP relaxes vascular smooth muscle and leads to vasodilation by antagonizing the concomitant vasoconstrictive influences of Ang II, endothelin (ET), AVP, and $\alpha_1$-adrenergic input.[267] This vasodilation reduces preload, resulting in a fall in cardiac output.[267] ANP also reduces cardiac output by shifting fluid from the intravascular to extravascular compartment, an effect mediated by increased capillary hydraulic conductivity.[272] Studies in endothelial-restricted, GC-A knockout mice have found that ANP, through GC-A, enhances albumin permeability in the microcirculation of the skin and skeletal muscle. This effect is mediated by caveolae[273] and is critically involved in the hypovolemic and hypotensive actions of ANP in vivo.[274]

ANP also inhibits proliferation of cultured mesangial, vascular smooth muscle and endothelial cells.[275] ANP causes afferent vasodilation, efferent vasoconstriction and mesangial relaxation, which leads to increased glomerular capillary pressure, GFR and filtration fraction.[267] In combination with increased medullary blood flow, these hemodynamic effects enhance diuresis and natriuresis, although the natriuretic effect of ANP infusion does not usually require these changes in glomerular function. In the tubules, ANP inhibits the stimulatory effect of Ang II on the luminal $Na^+/H^+$ exchanger of the proximal tubule, the thiazide-sensitive NaCl cotransporter in the distal tubule, ENaC and AVP-induced AQP2 incorporation into the apical membrane of the collecting duct (see Table 14.3).[267]

**Table 14.3 Physiologic Actions of the Natriuretic Peptides**

| Target Organ | Biologic Effects |
|---|---|
| Kidney | Increased GFR |
| | Afferent arteriolar vasodilation |
| | Efferent arteriolar vasoconstriction |
| | Natriuresis |
| | Inhibition of $Na^+/H^+$ exchanger (proximal tubule) |
| | Inhibition of $Na^+$-$Cl^-$ cotransporter (distal tubule) |
| | Inhibition of $Na^+$ channels (collecting duct) |
| | Diuresis |
| | Inhibition of AVP-induced AQP2 incorporation into CD-AM |
| Cardiac | Reduction in preload, leading to reduced cardiac output |
| | Inhibition of cardiac remodeling |
| Hemodynamic | Vasorelaxation |
| | Elevation of capillary hydraulic conductivity |
| | Decreased cardiac preload and afterload |
| Endocrine | Suppression of RAAS |
| | Suppression of sympathetic outflow |
| | Suppression of AVP |
| | Suppression of endothelin |
| Mitogenesis | Inhibition of mitogenesis in VSMC |
| | Inhibition of growth factor–mediated hypertrophy of cardiac fibroblasts |

*AQP2*, Aquaporin 2; *AVP*, arginine vasopressin; *CD-AM*, collecting duct apical membrane; *GFR*, glomerular filtration rate; *RAAS*, renin-angiotensin-aldosterone system.

**Brain Natriuretic Peptide.** BNP is produced by activated satellite cells in ischemic skeletal muscle or by cardiomyocytes, mainly by the ventricles but also, in small amounts, by the atrium, in response to volume or pressure load, as seen in HF and hypertension. BNP, like ANP, induces natriuretic, endocrine, and hemodynamic responses.[267] BNP levels rise with age, more than doubling from age 55 to 64 years to 75 years and older. However, in HF and other chronic volume-expanded conditions much greater elevations occur in BNP levels.[276]

Studies in animals and humans have demonstrated the natriuretic effects of pharmacologic doses of BNP. The combination with ANP produced no further effect.[267] Moreover, like ANP, BNP exerts a hypotensive effect in animals and humans. For example, transgenic mice, overexpressing either the BNP or ANP gene exhibit lifelong hypotension.[267] Therefore, it is clear that BNP induces its biologic actions through mechanisms similar to those of ANP.[267]

This notion is supported by several findings: 1. both ANP and BNP act through the same receptors and induce similar renal, cardiovascular and endocrine actions in association with an increase in cGMP production (see Table 14.3); and 2. BNP suppresses ACTH-induced aldosterone generation both in cell culture and following infusion. The latter action may be attributed to inhibition of renin secretion in dogs, although apparently not in humans.[267] At high, but not low, doses, BNP caused a profound fall in systolic BP in humans.[267] In the clinical setting, the effects of BNP are used routinely to monitor volume overload in HF (see section, "Specific Treatments Based on the Pathophysiology of Congestive Heart Failure").

**C-Type Natriuretic Peptide.** Although CNP is considered a neurotransmitter in the CNS, considerable amounts are produced by endothelial cells, where it plays a role in the local regulation of vascular tone.[270] Smaller amounts of CNP are produced by the kidneys, heart ventricles and intestines[270] and can be detected in human plasma.[277] CNP is produced in response to hypoxia, cytokines, shear stress, and fibrotic growth factors[278] and enhanced expression of CNP mRNA has been reported after volume overload.[270] Infusion of CNP decreases BP, cardiac output, urinary volume and $Na^+$ excretion; the effects are less pronounced than those of ANP and BNP, despite strong stimulation of cGMP and inhibition of vascular smooth muscle cell proliferation.

All three NPs inhibit the RAAS, although CNP does not induce significant changes in cardiac output, BP or plasma volume in sheep.[270] This finding supports the widely-accepted concept that ANP and BNP are the major circulating NPs, whereas CNP is a local regulator of vascular structure and tone.

**D-Type Natriuretic Peptide.** DNP infused into rabbits increased urine volume and electrolyte excretion. The effects were more pronounced than those of ANP, possibly because of DNP resistance to degradation by endogenous peptidases. DNP, via the NP-A receptor, preferentially induced cGMP production in glomeruli compared with cortical, outer medullary and inner medullary tubules. Thus, DNP may play a regulatory role in the kidney, via specific NP receptors with a GC domain.[268]

Together, the various biologic actions of NPs lead to reduction of EABV, in response to perceived overfilling of the central intrathoracic circulation. Furthermore, all NPs counteract the adverse effects of the RAAS, suggesting that the two systems act in opposite directions in the regulation of body fluid and cardiovascular homeostasis.

**Endothelial-Derived Factors.** The endothelium is a major source of factors that regulate vascular tone in health and disease.[300] These factors regulate the perfusion pressure of multiple organ systems involved in water and $Na^+$ balance, such as the kidneys, heart and vasculature. This section summarizes some concepts regarding actions of ET and NO relevant to volume homeostasis.

**Endothelin.** The ET system consists of three vasoactive peptides—endothelin 1 (ET-1), endothelin 2 (ET-2) and endothelin 3 (ET-3), which act in a paracrine and autocrine manner.[279] Endothelins are synthesized by proteolytic cleavage from specific preproendothelins that are further cleaved to form 37- to 39-amino acid precursors called "big ET". Big ET is then converted into the biologically active 21-amino acid peptide by a highly specific endothelin-converting enzyme (ECE), a phosphoramidon-sensitive, membrane-bound metalloprotease. There are two main isoforms of ECE, ECE-1 and ECE-2. ECE-1 itself has four isoforms.[279] ECE-2 is localized mainly to VSMC and is probably intracellular. Both chymase[280] and carboxypeptidase A[281] are also involved in mature ET production.

Endothelins bind to two distinct receptors, types A and B (ET-A and ET-B).[279] The ET-A receptor shows a higher affinity for ET-1 than for ET-2 or ET-3. The ET-B receptor shows equal affinity for all three ETs. ET-A receptors are found mainly on VSMC, on which their activation leads to vasoconstriction through an increase in cytosolic $Ca^{2+}$. ET-B receptors are also found on VSMC, where they can mediate vasoconstriction, but are found predominantly on vascular endothelium, where their activation results in vasodilation through prostacyclin and NO.[279] Endothelin is detectable in the plasma of humans and experimental animals and, therefore, can also act as a circulating vasoactive hormone.[279]

Selective ET-A receptor antagonism is associated with vasodilation and a reduction in BP, whereas selective ET-B antagonism is accompanied by vasoconstriction and a rise in BP.[279] These data suggest complementary roles for the ET receptor subtypes in the maintenance of vascular tone. In addition to its vasoconstrictive action, ET has a variety of renal effects.[282–284] The kidney (mainly the inner medulla) is both a source and target of ET. ET-1, the principal subtype involved in renal functional regulation, is synthesized by vascular endothelial cells, whereas ET-1 and ET-3 are produced by various renal cell types, but at a rate one to two orders of magnitude lower than ET-1.[279]

In relation to volume homeostasis, ET-1 acts in a paracrine or autocrine manner to regulate: 1. renal and intrarenal blood flow; 2. glomerular hemodynamics; and 3. tubular salt and water transport. Both ET-A and ET-B receptors are present in the glomerulus, renal vessels and tubular epithelial cells, but most ET-B receptors are found in the medulla.[285] The renal vasculature is exquisitely sensitive to the vasoconstrictor action of ET-1. Infusion of ET-1 into the renal artery of anesthetized rabbits was found to decrease RBF, GFR, natriuresis, and urine volume.[286] ET-1 increases afferent and efferent arteriolar resistance (afferent > efferent), which results in reduced glomerular plasma flow. In addition, Kf is reduced because of mesangial cell contraction, resulting in a diminished SNGFR.

The profound reduction of RBF and concomitant lesser reduction in GFR should result in a rise in filtration fraction, but this is not evident in all models. Infusion of ET-1 for 8 days into conscious dogs increased plasma levels of ET by two- to threefold and resulted in increased renal vascular resistance and decreased GFR and RBF.[287] Interestingly, the effect of ET on regional intrarenal blood flow is not homogeneous. As measured by laser Doppler flowmetry, administration of ET-1 to rats produced sustained cortical vasoconstriction but only transient medullary vasodilation.[288] These results are in line with the medullary predominance of ET-B receptors and the high density of ET-A-binding sites in the cortex.[279]

The effect of ET on $Na^+$ and water excretion varies, depending on the dose and source of ET. Systemic infusion of ET in high doses results in profound antinatriuresis and antidiuresis, apparently secondary to a decrease in GFR and RBF. However, in low doses, or when produced locally in tubular epithelial cells, ET decreases salt and water reabsorption, consistent with tubular ET-1 target sites.[289] Also, administration of big ET has been shown to cause natriuresis, supporting the notion of direct autocrine inhibition of ET on tubular salt reabsorption.[290]

The natriuretic and diuretic actions of big ET-1 are significantly reduced by ET-B–specific blockade.[291] Furthermore, ET-B knockout rats have salt-sensitive hypertension reversed by luminal ENaC blockade with amiloride, by a $Ca^{2+}$-dependent effect, which suggests that collecting duct ET-B tonically inhibits ENaC activity.[292] Similarly, mice with collecting duct–specific knockout of the ET-1 gene have impaired $Na^+$ excretion in response to $Na^+$ load and develop hypertension with a high salt intake.[279] These mice also have heightened sensitivity to AVP and reduced ability to excrete an acute water load. These findings are in line with observations that ET-B mediates the inhibitory effects of ET-1 on $Na^+$ and water transport in the collecting duct and TALH.[283] Thus if vascular and mesangial ET exert a greater physiologic effect than tubule-derived ET, then RBF is diminished and net fluid retention occurs. Whereas if the tubule-derived ET effect predominates, salt and water excretion are increased.

Renal endothelin production is regulated differently than in the vasculature. Whereas vascular (and mesangial) ET generation is controlled by thrombin, Ang II and TGF–β, tubular ET production seems to particularly depend on medullary tonicity. For example, a high-salt diet, by raising medullary tonicity, stimulates ET-1 release, which in turn leads to increased eNOS (NOS3) expression and natriuresis.[293] (see "Nitric Oxide" section, later). The signaling mechanisms for these phenomena, as well other renal actions of ET-1, continue to be a subject of intensive research and the interested reader is referred to a recent review summarizing the current state of knowledge.[279]

**Nitric Oxide.** Nitric oxide (NO) is a diffusible gaseous molecule produced from L-arginine by the enzyme NOS, which exists in three distinct isoforms—nNOS (NOS1), inducible NOS (iNOS, or NOS2) and eNOS (NOS3).[291] NOS is expressed in renal vascular endothelial cells (mainly eNOS), tubular epithelial and mesangial cells and macula densa (mainly nNOS). There is controversy regarding iNOS expression in normal kidneys, but upregulation is clearly seen in pathologic conditions such as ischemia-reperfusion injury.[294]

Selective NOS inhibitors and NOS knockout mice have been used to elucidate the role of NOS isoforms in the regulation of renal function.[294] The action of NO is mediated by activation of a soluble GC, thereby increasing intracellular levels of cGMP.[295] In the kidneys, the physiologic roles of NO include the regulation of glomerular hemodynamics, attenuation of TGF, mediation of pressure natriuresis, maintenance of medullary perfusion, inhibition of tubular $Na^+$ reabsorption and modulation of RSNA.[291,296] Renal NOS activity is regulated by several factors, such as Ang II (see earlier section, "Tubuloglomerular Feedback") and salt intake.[120]

The role of NO in the regulation of renal hemodynamics and excretory function is best illustrated by the fact that inhibition of intrarenal NO production results in increased BP and impaired renal function.[294] Infusion of the NOS inhibitor, $N^G$-monomethyl-L-arginine (L-NMMA), into one kidney in anesthetized dogs resulted in a dose-dependent decrease in urinary cGMP levels, decreases in RBF and GFR, $Na^+$ and water retention in the ipsilateral compared with the contralateral kidney.[297] In addition, acute NO blockade amplified the renal vasoconstrictive action of Ang II in isolated microperfused rabbit afferent arterioles and in conscious rats.[120,294] Also L-NMMA–induced vasoconstriction led to decreased RBF and Kf, effects reversed by RAAS blockade. Thus, a major effect of NO is to counterbalance the efferent vasoconstrictive action of Ang II as well as modulate renin secretion by the JGA (see section, "Tubuloglomerular Feedback").

The involvement of NO in promoting diuresis and natriuresis in normal and increased salt intake/volume-expanded states is well characterized.[291] In conscious dogs on a normal $Na^+$ diet, NO inhibition induced a significant decrease in natriuresis and diuresis with no change in arterial pressure. On a high-$Na^+$ diet, treatment with the NO inhibitor, $N^G$-nitro-L-arginine methyl ester (L-NAME), increased arterial pressure and cumulative $Na^+$ balance.[298] Similarly, rats on a high salt intake for 2 weeks had increased $Na^+$ excretion and proportionally elevated urinary concentrations of the NO metabolites, $NO_2$ and $NO_3$. The increase in urinary NO metabolites is attributed to enhanced expression of all three NOS isoforms in the renal medulla.[121]

NO exerts a vasodilatory effect on the renal medullary circulation and promotes $Na^+$ excretion.[164] Consistent with these data are the high levels of eNOS in the renal medulla and the inhibitory effect of NO on collecting duct $Na^+$-$K^+$-ATPase.[298] In contrast, in salt-sensitive hypertension, NOS activity (mainly nNOS) is significantly lower in salt-sensitive than salt-resistant rats maintained on a high-salt diet.[299,300] Also, L-arginine-induced NO production prevented the development of salt-induced hypertension in Dahl salt-sensitive rats.[301] These findings suggest that nNOS plays an important role in $Na^+$ handling and decreased nNOS activity may be involved in the mechanism of salt-sensitive hypertension.

The involvement of NO in salt retention and subsequent hypertension could result from an inadequate direct effect on proximal and distal tubular $Na^+$ reabsorption. However, attenuated NO inhibition of renin secretion and TGF may also contribute. In this context, macula densa-derived NO could blunt the TGF-mediated vasoconstriction during high salt intake in salt-resistant but not salt-sensitive rats.[302] As noted, the medullary and other effects of NO occur in response to local ET production.[291] For example, the inhibition of NOS by L-NAME or the highly selective ET-B antagonist A-192621 abolished the diuretic and natriuretic effects of big ET-1 in anesthetized rat kidneys.[303] In addition, ET-1 acutely activated eNOS in the isolated mTALH and nNOS in isolated IMCD cells, via ET-B activation, an effect dependent on increased NOS protein, but not mRNA, expression.[291] These data suggest that nNOS and eNOS activation occur by posttranscriptional pathways. NO also reduces $Cl^-$ absorption in CCD through an ENaC-dependent mechanism.[304]

Activation of eNOS, by a paracrine effect in the IMCD, where the highest renal NOS activity is found,[305] is also associated with inhibition of $Na^+$ reabsorption in the mTALH through phosphatidylinositol-3-kinase (PI3K)–stimulated Akt activity, leading to eNOS phosphorylation at Ser1177.[305] However, the functional corollary of nNOS activation in the IMCD remains to be determined. NO also reduces paracellular $Na^+$ reabsorption in the mTALH, and the magnitude of this effect is equal to that due to NO inhibition of transcellular transport.[306] A further action of NO is inhibition of AVP-enhanced $Na^+$ reabsorption and hydroosmotic water permeability of the CCD.[307] A mouse model of specific collecting duct NOS1 gene deletion should be a valuable tool to study the signaling mechanisms involved in the NO effects on AVP-enhanced $Na^+$ reabsorption, as well as salt-dependent BP mechanisms.[296] The role of NO in pressure natriuresis and RSNA has been discussed in the relevant sections.

**Kinins.** The kallikrein-kinin system (KKS) is a complex cascade responsible for the generation and release of vasoactive kinins. The active peptides bradykinin (BK) and kallidin are formed from precursors (kininogens) that are cleaved by tissue and circulatory kinin-forming enzymes.[229] Kinins are produced by many cell types and can be detected in urine, saliva, sweat, interstitial fluid and, rarely, venous blood. Circulating BK is almost undetectable because of rapid metabolism by kininases, particularly kininase II/ACE1. The renal KKS can produce local BK concentrations much higher than those in blood. In the kidney, bradykinin is metabolized by NEP.[308]

Kinins play an important role in hemodynamic and excretory processes through their G protein–coupled receptors, BK-$B_1$ and BK-$B_2$. BK-$B_2$ receptors mediate most of the actions of kinins and are located mainly in the kidneys, although they are also detectable in the heart, lungs, brain, uterus and testes.[308] Activation of BK-$B_2$ receptors results in vasodilation, probably through an NO– or arachidonic acid metabolite–dependent mechanism.[309] BK selectively increases medullary perfusion, especially to the inner layer, via activation of NO and $Ca^{2+}$-activated $K^+$ channels.[310] BK also has multiple effects on the cardiovascular system, particularly vasodilation and plasma extravasation.[309]

In the kidney, kinins induce diuresis and natriuresis through activation of BK-$B_2$ receptors, increased RBF and secondary inhibition of $Na^+$ and water reabsorption via ENaC in the distal nephron.[229] Unlike many vasodilators, BK increases RBF without significantly affecting GFR or proximal tubular $Na^+$ reabsorption.

Studies with transgenic animals have elaborated the physiologic role of kinins and the interaction between the KKS and the RAAS.[309] In the kidney, $Na^+$ depletion-induced Ang II, acting via the $AT_2$ receptor, stimulates a vasodilator cascade of BK, NO and cGMP.[297] In the absence of the $AT_2$ receptor, pressor and antinatriuretic hypersensitivity to Ang II is associated with BK and NO deficiency.[297] Furthermore, renal kinins are involved in pressure natriuresis.[311] BK also mediates Ang 1–7–mediated diuresis and natriuresis, as shown in rats transgenic for the kallikrein gene.[312] Because ACE is involved in kinin degradation, ACE inhibitors not only attenuate Ang II formation but may also lead to kinin accumulation. The latter effect may be responsible in part for the beneficial effects of ACE inhibitors in HF, but also for their troublesome side effect of cough.[313] In summary, the KKS seems to play a pivotal role as a counterregulatory modulator of vasoconstrictor and $Na^+$-retaining mechanisms.

**Adrenomedullin.** Human adrenomedullin (AM) is a 52-amino acid peptide, discovered in 1993 in extracts of human pheochromocytoma cells and approximately 30% homologous in structure with calcitonin gene–related peptide and amylin.[314] AM is produced from a 185–amino acid preprohormone that contains a unique $NH_2$-terminus 20–amino acid sequence, "proadrenomedullin $NH_2$-terminal 20 peptide," with biologic activity similar to that of AM. AM mRNA is expressed in endothelial cells, glomeruli, distal and medullary collecting tubules. Synthesis and secretion of AM are stimulated by Ang II, NE, ET, bradykinin, and shear stress.[314] AM acts through a 395–amino acid G protein-like–coupled receptor, belonging to the calcitonin receptor–like receptor and a family of receptor activity–modifying proteins.[314] Receptor activation in VSMC increases intracellular cAMP and calcium-activated potassium channel activity,[314] leading to prolonged dose-dependent generalized vasodilation and hypotension, accompanied by increases in heart rate and cardiac output caused by positive inotropic effects.[314] The vasodilating effect of AM is also stimulated by calcium-dependent NO synthesis in endothelial cells.[314]

In addition to its hypotensive action, AM increases RBF through preglomerular and postglomerular arteriolar vasodilation,[315,316] accompanied by dose-dependent diuresis and natriuresis.[316,317] These effects result from a decrease in tubular $Na^+$ reabsorption, despite the AM-induced hyperfiltration[315] and may be mediated partially by locally released NO[318,319] and PG.[320] In addition, NEP inhibition potentiates exogenous AM-induced natriuresis without affecting GFR.[321] Like NPs, AM suppresses aldosterone secretion in response to Ang II and high potassium levels.[317] Furthermore, in cultured VSMC, AM inhibits ET production induced by various stimuli.[317] In the hypothalamus, AM inhibits AVP secretion, which may also contribute to its diuretic and natriuretic actions.[317]

Two other members of the AM family, AM-2 (intermedin) and AM-5, have cardiovascular effects similar to those of AM-1. AM-2, but not AM-5, also has renal effects similar to those of AM-1.[322,323]

Together, these findings show that AM may be involved in the physiologic control of vascular tone and cardiac function; in the kidney, AM may modulate sodium and water excretion in a paracrine fashion.[324]

**Urotensin.** Urotensin II (UT II) is a highly-conserved peptide that binds to the human orphan G protein–coupled receptor GPR14, or UT II receptor. The parent peptide, prepro–UT II, is widely expressed in human tissues, including the kidney where it can be detected in tubular epithelial cells, especially of the distal tubule, and endothelial cells of renal capillaries.[325] The C-terminus of the prohormone is cleaved to produce UT II, an 11–amino acid residue peptide. Human UT II includes a cyclic hexapeptide sequence fundamental for the action of the peptide. Substantial local UT II has been demonstrated in the heart, liver, and kidneys.[326]

Infusion of UT II leads to local forearm vasoconstriction, no effect, or cutaneous vasodilation, according to species variation, site and modality of injection, dose, vascular bed and experimental model.[327] The vasoconstrictive action is probably direct, whereas the vasodilatory response is likely mediated by factors such as cyclooxygenase products and NO.

The involvement of the UT II system in the regulation of renal function in mammals is unclear and the data are as contradictory as those for vascular tone. In normal rats, intravenous boluses in the nanomolar range caused minor reductions in GFR and no effect on $Na^+$ excretion.[325] However, bolus injections in the picomolar range produced a dose-dependent decrease in GFR associated with reduced urine flow and $Na^+$ excretion.[328] In contrast, continuous infusion of UT II in the picomolar range elicited increases in GFR and NO–dependent diuresis and natriuresis.[325] Thus, the effect of UT II on renal function seems dependent on the mode of administration and experimental condition.

The variability in renal and vascular responses to UT II may also depend on regulation at the receptor level. The binding density of UT II is correlated with vasoconstrictor response in rats and small changes in receptor density may result in pathophysiologic effects. Under normal conditions, most UT II receptors are already occupied by UT II. Changes in unoccupied receptor reserve—perhaps in response to alterations in UT II levels in experimental models or in disease states—might explain, at least in part, the observed variability in renal and vascular actions.[325]

Selective UT II receptor antagonists have been developed and, in normal rats, can increase GFR, urine flow and $Na^+$ excretion.[329] However, in light of the complex renal effects of UT II, it is unlikely that these antagonists will have a role in the management of sodium disorders.[325]

**Digitalis-Like Factors.** The existence of endogenous digitalis-like factors was hypothesized in the 1960s and initially reported in the late 1970s.[330] Among these factors, also known as endogenous cardiotonic steroids, two have been characterized extensively in humans, cardenolide (or ouabain) and bufadienolide (marinobufagenin). The main site of synthesis of these compounds is the adrenal cortex.[331] Cardiotonic steroids act by inhibiting $Na^+$-$K^+$-ATPase, leading to attenuation of tubular $Na^+$ transport and increased vascular resistance via enhanced cytosolic $Ca^{2+}$ in VSMC.[330] The latter mechanism has been implicated in the pathogenesis of hypertension.[330]

**Neuropeptide Y.** Neuropeptide Y (NPY), a 36–residue peptide, is a sympathetic cotransmitter stored and released together with NE by adrenergic nerve terminals of the SNS.[332,333] Although originally isolated from the brain and highly expressed in the CNS, the peptide exhibits a wide spectrum of biologic activities in the cardiovascular system, GI tract and kidneys through multiple $G_{i/o}$ protein–coupled receptors.[333,334] Experimentally, NPY can reduce RBF and increase renal vascular resistance without significantly affecting GFR in various species, including humans.[333] Similarly, the peptide may exert a natriuretic or antinatriuretic action, depending on experimental conditions and species studied.[333] However, overall, NPY appears to have no significant role in the physiological regulation of sodium.

**Apelin.** Apelin is the endogenous ligand of the APJ receptor, a G protein–coupled receptor involved in water homeostasis, regulation of cardiovascular tone and cardiac contractility.[335] Apelin and its receptor are widely expressed in the CNS, endothelial cells (systemic and renal), VSMC of glomerular arterioles and, to a lesser extent, in other nephron segments.[336]

AJP activation leads to inhibition of cAMP production and activation of the $Na^+/H^+$ exchanger type 1 (NHE1). Through the former pathway, apelin enhances vascular dilation via induction of eNOS, whereas NHE1 activation in cardiomyocytes leads to a dose-dependent increase in myocardial contractility.[336] With regard to the renal effects of apelin, direct injection into the hypothalamus of lactating rats inhibited AVP release and reduced circulating AVP. Conversely, water deprivation led to increased systemic AVP and decreased apelin levels.[335] Moreover, APJ expression in the rat collecting duct occurs near the vasopressin $V_2$ receptor and apelin directly counteracts the $V_2$ receptor-mediated antidiuretic effect of AVP.[337] Thus, AVP and apelin have a reciprocal relationship in controlling water diuresis.

With respect to vascular tone, the apelin/APJ system acts as a counterregulator of the RAS. For example, intravenous apelin caused an NO–dependent fall in arterial pressure, whereas apelin receptor knockout mice displayed an enhanced vasopressor response to systemic Ang II.[336] Intravenous injection of apelin also induced vasorelaxation of Ang II–preconstricted efferent and afferent arterioles, as well as a significant diuresis.[338] Activation of endothelial apelin receptors caused release of NO, which inhibited the Ang II–induced rise in intracellular $Ca^{2+}$ levels.[336] Furthermore, apelin had a direct receptor-mediated vasoconstrictive effect on vascular smooth muscle.[336] These results indicate that apelin has complex effects on the preglomerular and postglomerular microvasculature regulating renal hemodynamics.

### Glucagon-Like Peptide-1

The incretin hormone glucagon-like peptide-1 (GLP-1) is released from the gut in response to fat or carbohydrate and contributes to negative feedback control of blood glucose by stimulating insulin secretion, inhibiting glucagon and slowing gastric emptying. GLP-1 receptors (GLP-1Rs) are also expressed in the proximal tubule and the GLP-1 agonist, exenatide, has natriuretic effects by inhibiting NHE-3, thereby reducing proximal tubular $Na^+$ reabsorption; this effect may be mediated by Ang II inhibition.[339] Exenatide also increased SNGFR by 33% to 50%, doubled early distal flow rate and increased urine flow rate sixfold without altering GTB, TGF responsiveness, or the tonic influence of TGF. This implies that exenatide is a proximal diuretic and a renal vasodilator.[339] Because the natural agonist for the GLP-1 receptor is regulated by intake of fat and carbohydrate, but not by salt or fluid, the control of salt excretion by the GLP-1R system departs from the usual negative-feedback paradigm for regulating salt balance.[340]

### Novel Factors

A novel intrarenal paracrine mechanism for sodium regulation in mice was recently described. Early studies showed that changes in dietary acid-base load could reverse the direction of apical transport of the tricarboxylic acid intermediate, α-ketoglutarate (α-KG), in the proximal tubule and loop of Henle from reabsorption following an acid load to secretion following a base load.[341] Work on isolated microperfused CCDs from *Oxgr1*$^{-}$/$^{-}$ mice indicated that the concentration of α-KG is sensed by the α-KG receptor, OXGR1, expressed in type B and non-A, non-B intercalated cells of the connecting tubule and CCD. Addition of 1 mM α-KG to the tubular lumen strongly stimulated Cl-dependent $HCO_3^-$ secretion and electroneutral NaCl reabsorption in tubules of wild type but not *Oxgr1*$^{-}$/$^{-}$ mice. *Oxgr1*$^{-}$/$^{-}$ mice also displayed significantly increased ENaC activity, without changes in plasma aldosterone.[341] In contrast, α-KG inhibited amiloride-sensitive sodium reabsorption in principal cells independently of OXGR1 activation. This effect is possibly related to increased ATP production, inducing autocrine activation of P2Y2 receptors and, thereby, inhibition of ENaC.[342] It appears that receptor-dependent and receptor-independent effects of α-KG converge to compensate for an alkalosis-induced decrease in proximal tubular reabsorption of NaCl by favoring NaCl reabsorption over $Na^+/K^+$ exchange along the connecting tubule and CCD.[341] Taken together, the data indicate that α-KG acts as a paracrine mediator involved in the functional coordination of proximal and distal parts of the tubule in the adaptive regulation of $HCO_3^-$ secretion and NaCl reabsorption in the presence of acid-base disturbances.[341]

Members of the epidermal growth factor (EGF) family have been shown to be important for maintaining transepithelial $Na^+$ transport. For example, a high salt diet was shown to decrease cortical EGF levels promoting ENaC-mediated $Na^+$ reabsorption in the collecting duct and the development of hypertension. Conversely, intravenous EGF decreased ENaC activity, prevented the development of hypertension and attenuated glomerular and renal tubular damage in the Dahl salt-sensitive rat.[343] The inhibitory effect of EGF on ENaC-dependent $Na^+$ absorption appears to be mediated via the H-Ras/c-Raf, MEK/ERK signaling pathway, and Cav-1 is an essential component of this EGF-activated signaling mechanism.[344] The physiological implications of these observations are eagerly awaited.

The role of obesity in the pathogenesis of hypertension and renal dysfunction has led to the exploration of appetite-related hormones in salt and water retention. In this context, the orexigenic hormone, ghrelin, secreted by the stomach, has been shown to stimulate $Na^+$ absorption through cAMP-dependent trafficking of ENaC in the CCD.[345] The effect appears to be mediated via ghrelin receptor upregulation of Sirt-1 and was also shown in rats fed a low-salt diet.[346] These data indicate that the ghrelin-Sirt1 system may participate in regulating sodium reabsorption in the distal nephron, but its physiologic and pathologic roles in sodium homeostasis remain to be clarified.[347]

Another novel development is the growing interest in the circadian rhythmicity of many basic physiologic functions. These functional rhythms are driven, in part, by the circadian clock, a ubiquitous molecular mechanism allowing cells and tissues to anticipate and prepare for regular environmental events. This clock has been shown to play a role in the regulation and maintenance of RPF, GFR, tubular reabsorption, and secretion of $Na^+$, $Cl^-$ and $K^+$.[348] Studies in clock-deficient mice have identified the 20-HETE synthesis pathway as one of the clock's principal renal targets to mediate $Na^+$ excretion.[349] By exerting dynamic control over renal sodium handling, the circadian clock could affect BP, at least in part.

Rhythmicity of salt regulation seems to occur not only at the circadian level but also on a longer periodic basis (so-called infradian rhythms). In a fascinating study on men involved in space flight simulations, Rakova and colleagues[350] have shown that even on fixed salt diets (6, 9, or 12 g/day), daily $Na^+$ excretion exhibited aldosterone-dependent, weekly (circaseptan) rhythms, resulting in periodic $Na^+$ storage. Changes in total-body $Na^+$ (±200 to 400 mmol) exhibited monthly or longer period lengths, without parallel changes in body weight and extracellular water. These changes were directly related to urinary aldosterone excretion and inversely to urinary cortisol, suggesting rhythmic hormonal control. These findings suggest the existence of rhythmic $Na^+$ excretory and retention patterns independent of BP or body water and irrespective of salt intake.[350]

# SODIUM BALANCE DISORDERS

## HYPOVOLEMIA

### DEFINITION

Hypovolemia is the condition in which the volume of the ECF compartment is reduced in relation to its capacitance. As noted, the reduction may be absolute or relative. In states of absolute hypovolemia, $Na^+$ balance is truly negative, reflecting past or ongoing losses. Hypovolemia is described as "relative" when there is no $Na^+$ deficit but the capacitance of the ECF compartment is increased. In this situation of reduced EABV, the ECF intravascular and extravascular (interstitial) compartments may vary in the same or opposite directions. ICF volume, reflected by measurements of plasma $Na^+$ or osmolality, may or may not be concomitantly disturbed; thus, hypovolemia may be classified as normonatremic, hyponatremic or hypernatremic.

### ETIOLOGY

The causes of hypovolemia are summarized in Table 14.4. Absolute and relative hypovolemia, in turn, can have extrarenal or renal causes. Absolute hypovolemia results from massive blood loss or fluid loss from the skin, GI or respiratory

**Table 14.4 Causes of Absolute and Relative Hypovolemia**

| |
|---|
| **Absolute** |
| **Extrarenal** |
| Gastrointestinal fluid loss |
| Bleeding |
| Skin fluid loss |
| Respiratory fluid loss |
| Extracorporeal ultrafiltration |
| **Renal** |
| Diuretics |
| Obstructive uropathy/postobstructive diuresis |
| Hormone deficiency |
|   Hypoaldosteronism |
|   Adrenal insufficiency |
| $Na^+$ wasting tubulopathies |
|   Genetic |
|   Acquired tubulointerstitial disease |
| **Relative** |
| **Extrarenal** |
| Edematous states |
|   Heart failure |
|   Cirrhosis |
| Generalized vasodilation |
|   Sepsis |
|   Drugs |
|   Pregnancy |
| Third-space loss |
| **Renal** |
| Severe nephrotic syndrome |

system, or kidneys. Relative hypovolemia results from states of vasodilation, generalized edema or third-space loss. In both absolute and relative hypovolemia, the perceived reduction in EABV prompts the compensatory hemodynamic changes and renal responses described earlier (see section, "Physiology").

## PATHOPHYSIOLOGY

### Absolute Hypovolemia

**Extrarenal.** The commonest causes of absolute hypovolemia are persistent diarrhea, vomiting and massive bleeding, either gastrointestinal or as a result of trauma. The reduction in ECF volume is isotonic inasmuch as there is a proportionate loss of water and plasma. The consequent fall in systemic BP leads to compensatory tachycardia and vasoconstriction and the ensuing altered transcapillary Starling hydraulic forces enable a shift of fluid from the interstitial to intravascular compartment. In addition, the neural and hormonal responses to hypovolemia (see section, "Physiology") result in renal $Na^+$ and water retention, with the aim of restoring intravascular volume and hemodynamic stability.

Similar compensatory mechanisms become activated after fluid losses from the skin, GI system and respiratory system. Because of the large surface area of the skin, large amounts of fluid can be lost from this tissue as a result of burns or excessive perspiration. Severe burns allow the loss of large volumes of plasma and interstitial fluid and can lead rapidly to profound hypovolemia. Without medical intervention, hemoconcentration and hypoalbuminemia supervene. As occurs after massive bleeding, the fluid loss is isotonic, so plasma $Na^+$ concentration and osmolality remain normal. In contrast, excessive sweating, induced by exertion in a hot environment, leads to hypotonic fluid loss as a result of the relatively low $Na^+$ concentration (20 to 50 mmol/L) in sweat. The resulting hypovolemia may therefore be accompanied by hypernatremia and hyperosmolality and the type of fluid replacement must be tailored accordingly (see Chapter 15).

In addition to oral intake, the GI tract is characterized by the entry of approximately 7 L of isotonic fluid, the overwhelming majority of which is reabsorbed in the large intestine. Hence, in normal conditions, fecal fluid loss is minimal. However, in the presence of pathologic conditions, such as vomiting, diarrhea, colostomy and ileostomy secretions, especially those caused by infection, considerable or even massive fluid loss may occur. The ionic composition, osmolality and pH of secretions vary according to the part of the GI tract involved; therefore, the resulting hypovolemia is associated with a large spectrum of electrolyte and acid–base abnormalities (see Chapters 16 and 17 for further discussion).

In contrast to the massive losses that can occur from the skin and GI system, fluid loss from the respiratory tract—as occurs in febrile states and in patients who receive mechanical ventilation with inadequate humidification—is usually modest and hypovolemia ensues only in the presence of accompanying causes. Finally, a special situation in which hypovolemia can occur is after excessive ultrafiltration in dialysis patients (see Chapter 63).

**Renal.** Even when GFR is markedly impaired, the amount of filtered $Na^+$ far exceeds the dietary intake, and all but 1% of the filtered load is reabsorbed. However, if one or more of the tubular reabsorptive mechanisms is impaired, serious $Na^+$ deficit and absolute volume depletion can occur. The causes of absolute renal $Na^+$ losses include pharmacologic agents and renal structural, endocrine, and systemic disorders (see Table 14.4). All diuretics used to treat hypervolemic states may induce hypovolemia if administered in excess or inappropriately. Particularly, the powerful loop diuretics, furosemide, bumetanide, torsemide, and ethacrynic acid, are often given in combination with diuretics acting on other tubular segments (e.g., thiazides, aldosterone antagonists, distal ENaC blockers, and carbonic anhydrase inhibitors). Patients receiving these combinations need to be carefully monitored and fluid balance scrupulously adjusted to prevent hypovolemia. Patients commonly at risk are those with HF or underlying hypertension who develop intercurrent infections.

In patients with hypertension, diuretic treatment appreciably increases the risk of volume depletion. Osmotic diuretics, endogenous or exogenous, may also reduce tubular $Na^+$ reabsorption. Endogenous agents include urea, the principal molecule involved in the polyuric recovery phase of acute kidney injury and postobstructive diuresis, and glucose in hyperglycemia. In patients with increased intracranial pressure, exogenous agents, such as mannitol or glycerol, may be used to induce translocation of fluid from the ICF to the ECF compartment and decrease brain swelling. The resulting polyuria may be associated with electrolyte and acid-base disturbances, the nature of which depends on the complex interplay between fluid intake and intercompartmental fluid shifts.

$Na^+$ reabsorption may also be disrupted in inherited and acquired tubular disorders. Inherited disorders of the proximal tubules (e.g., Fanconi syndrome) and distal tubules (e.g., Bartter and Gitelman syndromes) may lead to salt-wasting states in association with other electrolyte or acid-base disturbances. Acquired disorders of $Na^+$ reabsorption may be acute, as in nonoliguric acute kidney injury, the period immediately after renal transplantation, the polyuric recovery phase of acute kidney injury and postobstructive diuresis (see relevant chapters for further details), or they may be chronic as a result of tubulointerstitial diseases with a propensity for salt wasting. Chronic kidney disease stages 3 to 5 of any cause is associated with heightened vulnerability to $Na^+$ losses because the ability to match tubular reabsorption with the sum of filtered load minus dietary intake is impaired.

In addition to intrinsic tubular disorders, endocrine and other systemic disturbances may lead to impaired $Na^+$ reabsorption. The principal endocrine causes are mineralocorticoid deficiency and resistance states. A controversial cause is the systemic disturbance known as cerebral salt wasting (CSW). In this condition, salt wasting is thought to occur in response to an as yet unidentified factor released in the setting of acute head injury or intracranial hemorrhage.[351,352] CSW is usually diagnosed because of concomitant hyponatremia and signs of volume depletion in contrast to the normovolemia characteristic of the syndrome of inappropriate antidiuresis.[353] However, CSW remains an enigmatic and not universally accepted clinical entity.[354]

An underappreciated, but not uncommon, clinical setting for renal $Na^+$ loss is after the administration of large volumes of intravenous saline to patients over several days after surgery or after trauma. In this situation, tubular reabsorption of $Na^+$ is downregulated. If intravenous fluids are stopped before full reabsorptive capacity is restored, volume depletion may ensue. The phenomenon can be minimized by graded reduction in the infusion rate, which allows $Na^+$ reabsorptive pathways to be restored gradually.

In the context of volume depletion, diabetes insipidus should be mentioned. However, because this results from a deficiency of or tubular resistance to AVP, water loss is the main consequence and the impact on ECF volume is only minor. AVP-related disorders are considered in Chapter 15

### Relative Hypovolemia

**Extrarenal.** As outlined previously, the principal causes of relative hypovolemia are edematous states, vasodilation and third-space loss (see Table 14.4). Vasodilation may be physiologic, as in normal pregnancy, or induced by drugs (hypotensive agents, such as hydralazine or minoxidil, that cause arteriolar vasodilation), or it may occur in sepsis during the phase of peripheral vasodilation and consequent low SVR.[355]

Edematous states in which the EABV and, hence, tissue perfusion, are reduced include HF, decompensated cirrhosis with ascites and nephrotic syndrome. In severe HF, low cardiac output and resulting low systemic BP lead to a fall in RPP. As in absolute hypovolemia, the kidneys respond by retaining $Na^+$. Because the increased venous return cannot raise the cardiac output, a vicious cycle is created in which edema is further exacerbated and the persistently reduced cardiac output leads to further $Na^+$ retention. In decompensated cirrhosis, splanchnic venous pooling leads to decreased venous return, a consequent fall in cardiac output and compensatory renal $Na^+$ retention. The pathophysiology of edematous states is discussed later (see section, "Hypervolemia"). Third-space loss occurs when fluid is sequestered into compartments not normally perfused with fluids, as in states of GI obstruction, after trauma, burns, or in pancreatitis, peritonitis, or malignant ascites. The result is that, even though total body $Na^+$ is markedly increased, the EABV is severely reduced.

**Renal.** Approximately 10% of patients with the nephrotic syndrome—especially children with minimal change disease, but also any patient with a serum albumin level lower than 2 g/dL—manifest clinical signs of hypovolemia. The low plasma oncotic pressure is conducive to movement of fluid from the ECF compartment to the interstitial space, thereby leading to reduced EABV.[356]

## CLINICAL MANIFESTATIONS

The clinical manifestations of hypovolemia depend on the magnitude and rate of volume loss, solute composition of the net fluid loss (i.e., the difference between input and output) and vascular and renal responses. The clinical features are related to the underlying pathophysiologic process, hemodynamic consequences and electrolyte and acid-base disturbances accompanying the renal response to hypovolemia. A detailed history usually reveals the cause of volume depletion (bleeding, vomiting, diarrhea, polyuria, diaphoresis, medications).

The symptoms and physical signs of hypovolemia appear only when intravascular volume is decreased by 5% to 15% and are often related to tissue hypoperfusion. Symptoms include generalized weakness, muscle cramps, and postural light-headedness. Thirst is prominent if concomitant hypertonicity is present (hypertonic hypovolemia). Physical signs are related to the hemodynamic consequences of hypovolemia and include tachycardia, hypotension (postural, absolute or relative to the usual BP) and low central or jugular venous pressure. Elevated jugular venous pressure, however, does not rule out hypovolemia, because of the possible confounding effects of underlying HF or lung disease. When volume depletion exceeds 10% to 20%, circulatory collapse is liable to occur, with severe supine hypotension, peripheral cyanosis, cold extremities and impaired consciousness, extending even to coma. This is especially likely if fluid loss is rapid or occurs against a background of comorbid conditions. When the source of volume loss is extrarenal, oliguria also occurs. The traditional signs—reduced skin turgor, sunken eyes, and dry mucous membranes—are inconstant findings and their absence does not rule out hypovolemia. Reduction in the EABV, as manifested by relative hypotension, may also be observed in generalized edematous states, even though there is an overall excess of $Na^+$ and water; however, this excess is maldistributed between the extracellular and interstitial spaces.

## DIAGNOSIS

The diagnosis of hypovolemia is based essentially on the clinical findings. Nevertheless, when these are equivocal, various laboratory parameters may be helpful for confirming the diagnosis or for elucidating other changes that may be associated with volume depletion.

### Laboratory Findings

**Hemoglobin and Plasma Albumin.** Hemoglobin may decrease if significant bleeding has occurred or is ongoing, but the change, which is caused by hemodilution owing to fluid translocation from the interstitial to intravascular compartment, may take up to 24 hours. Therefore, stable hemoglobin does not rule out significant bleeding. Moreover, the adaptive response of hemodilution may moderate the severity of hemodynamic compromise and resulting physical signs. In hypovolemic situations that do not arise from bleeding, hemoconcentration is often, but not universally, seen, inasmuch as underlying anemia of chronic disease may mask the differential loss of plasma.

Hemoconcentration may also be manifested as a rise in plasma albumin concentration if albumin-free fluid is lost from the skin, GI tract, or kidneys. On the other hand, when albumin is lost, either in parallel with other extracellular fluids (as in proteinuria, hepatic disease, protein-losing enteropathy, or catabolic states) or in protein-rich fluid (third-space sequestration, burns), significant hypoalbuminemia is observed.

**Plasma $Na^+$ Concentration.** This may be low, normal, or high, depending on the solute composition of the fluid lost and the replacement solution administered by the patient or physician. For example, the hypovolemic stimulus for AVP release may lead to preferential water retention and hyponatremia, especially if hypotonic replacement fluid is used. In contrast, the fluid content of diarrhea may be hypotonic or hypertonic, resulting in hypernatremia or hyponatremia, respectively. The plasma $Na^+$ concentration reflects the tonicity of plasma and provides no direct information about volume status, which is a clinical diagnosis.

**Plasma $K^+$ and Acid-Base Parameters.** These can also change in hypovolemic conditions. After vomiting and after some forms of diarrhea, loss of $K^+$ and $Cl^-$ may lead to alkalosis. More often, the principal anion lost in diarrhea is bicarbonate, which leads to hyperchloremic (nonanion gap) acidosis. When diuretics or Bartter and Gitelman syndromes (the inherited tubulopathies; see Chapter 44) are the cause of hypovolemia, hypokalemic alkalosis is again typically seen. On the other hand, $U_{Na}$ loss that occurs in adrenal insufficiency or due to aldosterone hyporesponsiveness is accompanied by a tendency for hyperkalemia and metabolic acidosis. Finally, when hypovolemia is sufficiently severe to impair tissue perfusion, high anion gap acidosis caused by lactic acid accumulation may be observed.

**Blood Urea and Creatinine Levels.** These frequently rise in hypovolemic states and reflect impaired renal perfusion. If tubular integrity is preserved, then the rise in urea levels is typically disproportionate to that of creatinine, so-called prerenal azotemia (see Chapter 28). This results mainly from AVP-enhanced urea reabsorption in the medullary collecting duct (MCD), but also from augmented proximal tubular reabsorption due to increased filtration fraction.[357] In critically ill patients, an increased urea generation rate (from exogenous or endogenous protein catabolism) or low creatinine generation rate due to muscle wasting may lead to an erroneous diagnosis of prerenal azotemia.[358] In the presence of severe hypovolemia, acute kidney injury may ensue, leading to loss of the differential rise in urea level. Proportional rises in urea and creatinine are also observed when hypovolemia occurs against a background of underlying renal functional impairment, as in chronic kidney disease, stages 3 to 5.

**Urine Biochemical Parameters.** In hypovolemia due to extrarenal fluid losses, the intact kidney will respond to hypoperfusion by enhanced tubular reabsorption of $Na^+$ and water. The ensuing oliguria will be characterized by urine-specific gravity greater than 1.020, $Na^+$ concentration less than 10 mmol/L and osmolality greater than 400 mOsm/kg. When urine $Na^+$ concentration is 20 to 40 mmol/L, the finding of a fractional excretion of $Na^+$ $\frac{\text{urine Na}^+ \times \text{plasma creatinine}}{\text{plasma Na}^+ \times \text{urine creatinine}} \times 100$ of less than 1%, in the presence of oliguria, may be helpful. However, in a patient on previous diuretic therapy, especially with loop diuretics, these indices may merely reflect $U_{Na}$ losses. In that case, fractional excretion of urea of less than 30% to 35% may help in the diagnosis of hypovolemia, although the specificity of this test is rather low.[359,360]

**Other Laboratory Parameters.** When hypovolemia occurs in the presence of arterial vasodilation, as observed in sepsis, some, but not all, of the clinical manifestations of hypovolemia are observed. Thus, tachycardia and hypotension are usually present, but the extremities are warm, suggesting that perfusion is maintained. This finding is misleading because vital organs, particularly the brain and kidneys, are underperfused as a result of the hypotension. The presence of lactic acidosis helps establish the correct diagnosis.

## TREATMENT

### Absolute Hypovolemia

**General Principles.** The goals of treatment of hypovolemia are to restore normal hemodynamic status and tissue perfusion. These goals are achieved by reversal of the clinical symptoms and signs, described previously. Treatment can be divided into three stages: 1. initial replacement of the immediate fluid deficit; 2. maintenance of the restored ECF volume in the presence of ongoing losses; and 3. treatment of the underlying cause, whenever possible. The main strategies to be addressed by the clinician are the route, volume, rate of administration, and composition of the replacement and maintenance fluids. These are liable to change according to the patient's response.

In general, when hypovolemia is associated with a significant hemodynamic disturbance, intravenous rehydration is required. (The use of oral electrolyte solutions in the management of infants and children is discussed in Chapter 73.) The volume of fluid and rate of administration should be determined on the basis of the urgency of the threat to circulatory integrity, adequacy of the clinical response, and underlying cardiac function. Older patients are especially vulnerable to aggressive fluid challenge and careful monitoring is required, particularly to prevent acute left ventricular failure and pulmonary edema from overzealous correction.

Sometimes the clinical signs do not point unequivocally to the diagnosis of hypovolemia, even though the history is strongly suggestive. Invasive monitoring of central venous and pulmonary venous pressures has not been shown to improve outcomes in this situation[361,362]; monitoring preload by stroke volume variation may improve outcomes, at least after major abdominal surgery.[363] However, in case of doubt, a diagnostic fluid challenge should be performed. If the patient improves clinically, BP and urine output increase and no overt signs of HF appear over the succeeding 6 to 12 hours, then the diagnosis is substantiated, and fluid therapy can be cautiously continued. Conversely, if overt signs of fluid overload appear, the fluid challenge can be stopped, and diuretic therapy reinstituted.

The initial calculations for replacing the fluid deficit are based on hemodynamic status. These deficits are notoriously difficult to calculate; therefore, good clinical judgment is necessary for successful management. Patients with life-threatening circulatory collapse and hypovolemic shock require rapid intravenous replacement through the cannula with the widest bore possible. Replacement should continue until BP and tissue perfusion are restored. In the second stage, the rate of fluid replacement should be reduced to maintain BP and tissue perfusion. In older patients and those with underlying cardiac dysfunction, the risk of overrapid correction and precipitating pulmonary edema is heightened; therefore slower treatment is preferable, to allow gradual filling of the ECF volume rather than causing pulmonary edema and the threat of mechanical ventilation associated with adverse outcomes.[364]

**Composition of Replacement Fluids.** The composition of replacement fluid may also affect outcomes. The two main categories of replacement solution are crystalloid and colloid solutions. Crystalloid solutions are based largely on NaCl of varying tonicity or dextrose. Isotonic (0.9%) saline, containing 154 mmol of $Na^+$/L, is the mainstay of volume replacement therapy being confined to the ECF compartment in the absence of deviations in $Na^+$ concentration. One L of isotonic saline increases plasma volume by approximately 300 mL; the rest is distributed to the interstitial compartment. In contrast, 1 L of 5% dextrose in water ($D_5W$), which is also isosmotic (277 mOsm/L), is eventually distributed throughout all the body fluid compartments so that only 10% to 15% (100 to 150 mL) remains in the ECF. Therefore, $D_5W$ should not be used for volume replacement.

Administration of 1 L of .45% saline (77 mmol of $Na^+$/L) in $D_5W$ is equivalent to giving 500 mL of isotonic saline and the same volume of solute-free water. The distribution of the solute-free compartment throughout all the fluid compartments would result in plasma dilution and reduction in the plasma $Na^+$. Therefore, this solution should be reserved for the management of hypernatremic hypovolemia. Even in that situation, it must be remembered that volume replacement is less efficient than with isotonic saline and, early in the treatment course, may cause plasma tonicity to fall too rapidly.

When hypovolemia is accompanied by severe metabolic acidosis (pH <7.10; plasma $HCO_3^-$ <10 mmol/L), bicarbonate supplementation may be indicated. (For a discussion of bicarbonate balance, see Chapter 16.) Because this anion is manufactured as 8.4% sodium bicarbonate (1000 mmol/L) for use in cardiac resuscitation, appropriate dilution is required for the treatment of acidosis associated with hypovolemia. Two convenient methods are suggested. Either 75 mL (75 mmol) of 8.4% $NaHCO_3^-$ can be added to 1 L of .45% saline, or 150 mL of concentrated bicarbonate can be added to 1 L of $D_5W$. Although the latter is hypertonic in the short term, it is unlikely to be harmful.

In the presence of accompanying hypokalemia, especially if metabolic alkalosis is also present, volume replacement solutions should be supplemented with $K^+$. Commercially available 1-L solutions of isotonic saline supplemented with 10 or 20 mmol of KCl make this option safe and convenient. (For details, see Chapter 17.) On the other hand, newer, commercially available crystalloid solutions containing lactate (converted by the liver to bicarbonate) and low concentrations of KCl may offer advantages over isotonic saline. In a recent large prospective observational study performed in the intensive care unit setting, two periods were compared; in the control period, all patients received isotonic saline as fluid replacement, whereas during the intervention period, Hartmann solution (lactate-containing), Plasma-Lyte 148 (a balanced salt solution), or chloride-poor 20% albumin solution was administered. The chloride-poor solutions were associated with a significantly lower risk of subsequent acute kidney injury, even after adjustment for covariates.[365] Clearly, these provocative results indicate the need for randomized controlled trials comparing chloride-rich with more balanced salt solutions for fluid resuscitation.[366,367]

Colloid solutions include plasma, albumin and high-molecular-weight carbohydrate molecules, such as hydroxyethyl starch and dextrans, at concentrations that exert COPs equal to or greater than that of plasma. Because the transcapillary barrier is impermeable to these large molecules, in theory they expand the intravascular compartment more rapidly and efficiently than crystalloid solutions. Colloid solutions may be useful in the management of burns and severe trauma when plasma protein losses are substantial and rapid plasma expansion with relatively small volumes is efficacious. However, when capillary permeability is increased, as in states of multiorgan failure or the systemic inflammatory response syndrome, colloid administration is ineffective. Moreover, randomized controlled studies, in which crystalloid solutions were compared with colloid solutions, have shown no survival benefit and even harm with some colloid solutions, particularly hydroxyethyl starch.[367] Therefore, the much cheaper and more readily available crystalloid solutions should remain the mainstay of therapy.

#### Relative Hypovolemia

Treatment of relative hypovolemia is more difficult than that of absolute hypovolemia because there is no real fluid deficit. If the relative hypovolemia is caused by peripheral vasodilation, as in sepsis, it may be necessary to administer cautiously a crystalloid solution, such as isotonic saline, to maintain ECF volume until the SVR and venous capacitance return to normal; the excess volume administered can then be excreted by the kidneys. When vasodilation is more severe, vasoconstrictor agents may be needed to maintain systemic BP. In severe HF, advanced cirrhosis with portal hypertension and severe nephrotic syndrome, when EABV is low but there is an overall excess of $Na^+$ and water, treatment may be extremely challenging. Crystalloid solution will, likely, lead to worsening interstitial edema without significantly affecting EABV. In these situations, prognosis is determined by whether the underlying condition can be reversed.

## HYPERVOLEMIA

### DEFINITION

Hypervolemia occurs when the volume of the ECF compartment is expanded relative to its capacitance. Normally, increments in $Na^+$ intake are matched by corresponding changes in $Na^+$ excretion as elaborated earlier (see section, "Physiology"). However, in the approximately 20% of the population who are salt sensitive, the upward shift in ECF volume induced by high salt intake leads to a persistent rise in systemic arterial pressure, albeit without other signs of fluid retention (see Chapter 46). Here, the discussion is confined to hypervolemia, in which $Na^+$ retention is ongoing and inappropriate for the prevailing ECF volume, with the appearance of clinical signs of volume overload.

### ETIOLOGY

Hypervolemia may result from either primary renal $Na^+$ retention or can be secondary to disease in other major organs (Table 14.5).

#### Primary Renal $Na^+$ Retention

This can be subclassified as caused by intrinsic kidney disease or primary mineralocorticoid excess. Of the primary renal diseases causing $Na^+$ retention, oliguric renal failure limits the ability to excrete $Na^+$ and water and affected patients are at risk for rapidly developing ECF volume overload (see Chapter 28). In contrast, in chronic kidney disease, renal tubular adaptation to salt intake is usually efficient until late

**Table 14.5 Causes of Renal Sodium Retention**

| Primary |
|---|
| Oliguric acute kidney injury |
| Chronic kidney disease |
| Glomerular disease |
| Severe bilateral renal artery stenosis |
| $Na^+$-retaining tubulopathies (genetic) |
| Mineralocorticoid excess |
| **Secondary** |
| Heart failure |
| Cirrhosis |
| Idiopathic edema |

stage 4 and stage 5. However, in some primary glomerular diseases, especially in the presence of nephrotic range proteinuria, significant $Na^+$ retention may occur, even when GFR is close to normal (see section, "Pathophysiology," and Chapter 30). Primary mineralocorticoid excess leads to transient $Na^+$ retention. However, because of "mineralocorticoid escape," the dominant clinical feature is hypertension (see Chapters 12 and 46).

### Secondary Renal $Na^+$ Retention

This occurs in low- and high-output cardiac failure with systolic and/or diastolic dysfunction. Nephrotic syndrome and hepatic cirrhosis with portal hypertension are also accompanied by renal $Na^+$ retention. In this chapter, only HF and cirrhosis are considered. Nephrotic syndrome is discussed in Chapter 28.

## PATHOPHYSIOLOGY

Primary renal $Na^+$ retention is caused by disruption of normal renal function. In contrast, secondary renal $Na^+$ retention occurs because of reduced EABV in the presence of total ECF volume expansion or in response to factors secreted by the heart or liver that signal the kidneys to retain $Na^+$ (Fig. 14.8). In secondary $Na^+$ retention, the renal effector mechanisms that normally operate to conserve $Na^+$ and protect against a $Na^+$ deficit are exaggerated and maintained, despite subtle or overt ECF volume expansion. The pathophysiology of hypervolemia involves local mechanisms of edema formation and stimulation of renal $Na^+$ retention by reduced EABV either directly or indirectly, via abnormalities of the afferent volume sensing mechanisms.

### Local Mechanisms of Edema Formation

Peripheral interstitial fluid accumulation, which is common to all conditions causing hypervolemia, results from disruption of the normal balance of transcapillary Starling forces. Transcapillary fluid and solute transport consists of both convective and diffusive flow. Bulk water movement occurs via convective transport induced by hydraulic and osmotic pressure gradients. Capillary hydraulic pressure ($P_c$) is under the influence of several factors, including systemic arterial and venous BPs, local blood flow and precapillary and postcapillary resistance. Systemic arterial BP, in turn, is determined by cardiac output, intravascular volume and SVR; systemic venous pressure is determined by right atrial pressure, intravascular volume and venous capacitance. $Na^+$ balance is a key determinant of these latter hemodynamic parameters. Also, massive accumulation of fluid in the peripheral interstitial compartment (anasarca) can itself diminish venous compliance and, thereby, alter overall cardiovascular performance.[368]

The balance of Starling forces prevailing at the arteriolar end of the capillary ($\Delta P > \Delta\pi$, in which $\Delta\pi$ is the change in transcapillary oncotic pressure) favors net filtration of fluid into the interstitium. Net outward movement of fluid along the length of the capillary is associated with an axial decrease in $P_c$ and an increase in $\pi_c$. Nevertheless, the local $\Delta P$ continues to exceed the opposing $\Delta\pi$ throughout the length of the capillary bed in several tissues; thus, filtration occurs along its entire length.[369] In such capillary beds, a substantial volume of filtered fluid must, therefore, return to the circulation via lymphatic vessels. Hence, to minimize edema formation, the lymphatic vessels must be able to expand and proliferate and lymphatic flow increase in response to increased interstitial fluid formation.

Several other mechanisms for minimizing edema formation have been identified. First, precapillary vasoconstriction tends to lower $P_c$ and diminish the filtering surface area in a given capillary bed. Indeed, in the absence of appropriate regulation of the microcirculatory myogenic reflex, as occurs with some $Ca^{2+}$ channel blockers, excessive precapillary vasodilation may lead to lower extremity interstitial edema.[370] Second, increased net filtration itself is associated with dissipation of $P_c$, dilution of interstitial fluid protein concentration and a corresponding rise in intracapillary plasma protein concentration. The resulting change in the balance of Starling forces will tend to mitigate further interstitial fluid accumulation.[371] Finally, interstitial fluid hydraulic pressure ($P_i$) is normally subatmospheric; however, even small increases in interstitial fluid volume tend to augment $P_i$, again opposing further transudation of fluid into the interstitial space.[372] The appearance of generalized edema in association with expansion of the ECF volume therefore implies the presence of one or more disturbances in microcirculatory hemodynamics—increased venous pressure transmitted to the capillary, unfavorable adjustments in precapillary and postcapillary resistances, and/or inadequacy of lymphatic flow for draining the interstitial and replenishing the intravascular compartment.

For the clinical detection of generalized edema, the volume of accumulated interstitial fluid required (>2 to 3 L) necessitates expansion of ECF volume and, hence, body exchangeable $Na^+$ content. Since continued net accumulation of interstitial fluid without renal $Na^+$ retention might result in serious intravascular volume contraction and cessation of interstitial fluid formation, generalized edema must indicate substantial renal $Na^+$ retention.

### Systemic Factors Stimulating Renal Sodium Retention

**Reduced Effective Arterial Blood Volume.** Renal $Na^+$ (and water retention) in edematous disorders occurs due to reduced EABV, despite an increase in total blood and ECF volumes and normal intrinsic renal function.[19] If the underlying stimulus for hypervolemia is removed, as dramatically seen after heart[373] or liver transplantation,[374] $Na^+$ excretion is restored to normal. Conversely, when kidneys from patients with end-stage liver disease are transplanted into patients with normal liver function, $Na^+$ retention no longer occurs.[374]

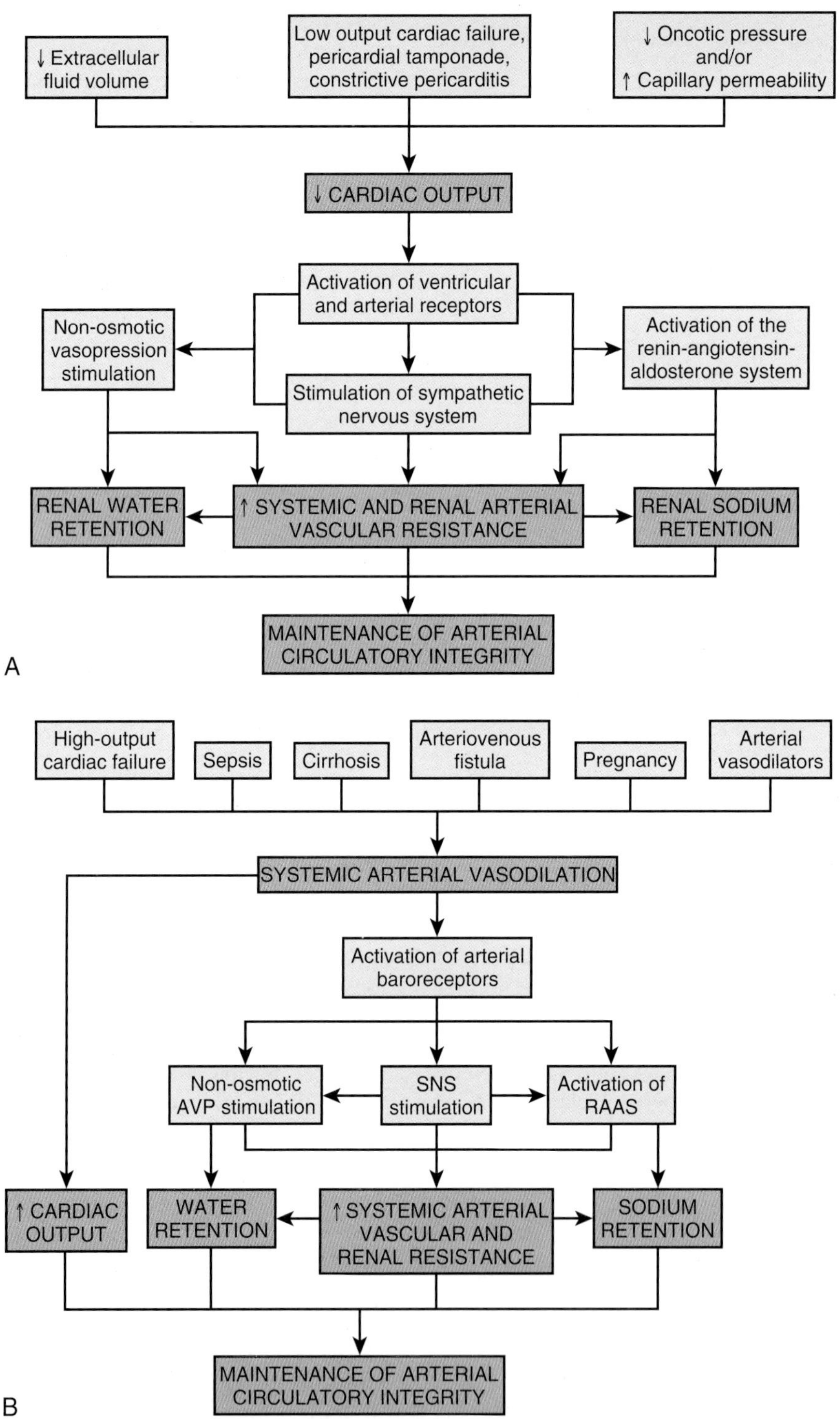


**Fig. 14.8** Sensing mechanisms that initiate and maintain renal sodium and water retention in various clinical conditions in which arterial underfilling, with resultant neurohumoral activation and renal sodium and water retention, is caused by a decrease in cardiac output (A) and by systemic arterial vasodilation (B). In addition to activating the neurohumoral axis, adrenergic stimulation causes renal vasoconstriction and enhances sodium and fluid transport by the proximal tubule epithelium. (From Schrier RW. Decreased effective blood volume in edematous disorders: what does this mean? *J Am Soc Nephrol*. 2007;18:2028–2031.)

Because 85% of blood circulates in the venous compartment, expansion of that compartment leads to overall ECF volume excess that could occur concurrently with arterial underfilling. The latter could result from low cardiac output, peripheral arterial vasodilation, or a combination of the two. In turn, low cardiac output could result from true ECF volume depletion (see earlier discussion), cardiac failure, or decreased $\pi_c$, with or without increased capillary permeability. All these stimuli would cause activation of ventricular and arterial sensors. Similarly, conditions such as high-output cardiac failure, sepsis, cirrhosis and normal pregnancy lead to peripheral arterial vasodilation and activation of arterial baroceptors. Activation of these afferent mechanisms would then induce the neurohumoral mechanisms that result in renal $Na^+$ and water retention (see Fig. 14.8).[375]

Although the mechanisms leading to $Na^+$ retention in HF and cirrhosis are similar, specific differences between the two conditions have been observed and are discussed separately in the following sections.

### Renal Sodium Retention in Heart Failure

**Abnormalities of Sensing Mechanisms in Heart Failure.** Both the cardiopulmonary and baroceptor reflexes are blunted in HF, so that they cannot exert an adequate tonic inhibitory effect on sympathetic outflow.[376] The resulting SNS activation triggers renal $Na^+$ retention, as already described. A variety of models of HF have shown marked attenuation of atrial receptor firing and loss of nerve ending arborization in HF.[377] Similarly, altering central cardiac filling pressures in response to postural stimuli (e.g., head-up tilt, LBNP) in HF patients, in contrast to normal subjects, usually do not demonstrate significant alterations in limb blood flow, circulating catecholamines, AVP, or renin activity.[378,379] This diminished reflex responsiveness is proportionate to the severity of ventricular dysfunction.

Arterial baroceptor reflex impairment has been observed in HF. High baseline values of muscle sympathetic activity were found in patients with HF who failed to respond to activation and deactivation of arterial baroreceptors by infusion of phenylephrine and $Na^+$ nitroprusside, respectively.[377] Carotid and aortic baroreceptor function were also depressed in experimental models of HF.[377] These changes were associated with upward resetting of receptor threshold and a reduced range of pressures over which the receptors functioned.

Multiple abnormalities have been described in cardiopulmonary and arterial baroreceptor control of RSNA in HF. Thus, rats with coronary ligation displayed an increased basal level of efferent RSNA that failed to decrease normally during volume expansion.[73,254] Similarly, in sinoaortic denervated dogs with pacing-induced HF, or following left atrial baroreceptor stimulation, the cardiopulmonary baroreflex control of efferent RSNA was markedly attenuated.[380]

The abnormal regulation of efferent RSNA was caused by impaired function of aortic and cardiopulmonary baroreflexes; the latter defect was functionally more important.[254] Mechanisms implicated in the pathogenesis of these abnormal baroreflexes include loss of compliance in the dilated hearts, gross changes in receptor structure and augmented $Na^+$-$K^+$-ATPase activity in the baroreceptor membranes.[377] Increased activity of Ang II through the $AT_1$ receptor also contributes to depressed baroreflex sensitivity. Thus RAAS inhibition in rats or rabbits with HF significantly improved arterial baroreflex control of RSNA or heart rate, respectively.[377,380] This effect of Ang II could also be blocked by central $\alpha_1$-adrenoreceptor stimulation.[381]

More recent studies have indicated that Ang II in the paraventricular nucleus potentiates—and $AT_1$ receptor antisense mRNA normalizes—the enhanced cardiac sympathetic afferent reflex in rats with chronic HF.[377] $AT_1$ receptors in the nucleus tractus solitarii are thought to mediate the interaction between the baroreflex and cardiac sympathetic afferent reflex.[382] Consistent with this notion, Ang II generation is enhanced and its degradation reduced in central sympathoregulatory neurons, as shown by upregulation of ACE1 and downregulation of ACE2.[383] $AT_2$ receptors in the rostral ventrolateral medulla inhibited sympathetic outflow, an effect mediated at least partly by an arachidonic acid metabolic pathway.[384] These studies indicated that a downregulation in the $AT_2$ receptor was a contributory factor in the sympathetic neural excitation in HF.[377]

Together, these data provide evidence of the role of high endogenous levels of Ang II, acting through the $AT_1$ receptor in concert with downregulation of the $AT_2$ receptor, in the impaired baroreflex sensitivity observed in HF, both in the afferent limb of the reflex arch and at more central sites. The central effect may be mediated through a central $\alpha_1$-adrenoreceptor. The blunted cardiopulmonary and arterial baroreceptor sensitivity in HF may also lead to an increase in AVP release and renin secretion.[377]

The disturbances in sensing mechanisms that initiate and maintain renal $Na^+$ retention in HF are summarized in Fig. 14.8A. As indicated, a decrease in cardiac output or a diversion of systemic blood flow diminishes the blood flow to the critical sites of the arterial circuit with pressure- and flow-sensing capabilities. The responses to diminished blood flow culminate in renal $Na^+$ retention, mediated by the effector mechanisms. An increase in systemic venous pressure promotes the transudation of fluid from the intravascular to interstitial compartment by increasing the peripheral transcapillary $\Delta P$. These processes augment the perceived loss of volume and flow in the arterial circuit. In addition, distortion of the pressure-volume relationships as a result of chronic dilation in the cardiac atria attenuates the normal natriuretic response to central venous congestion. This attenuation is manifested predominantly as a diminished neural suppressive response to atrial stretch, which results in increased sympathetic nerve activity and augmented release of renin and AVP.

**Abnormalities of Effector Mechanisms in Heart Failure.** The adaptive changes in the efferent limb of the volume control system in HF are generally similar to those seen in states of true $Na^+$ depletion. These include adjustments in glomerular hemodynamics and tubular transport, brought about by alterations in the neural, humoral and paracrine systems. However, in contrast to true $Na^+$ depletion, HF is also associated with activation of vasodilatory/natriuretic agents, which tend to oppose the effects of the vasoconstrictor/antinatriuretic systems. The final effect on urinary $Na^+$ excretion is determined by the dynamic balance among these antagonistic effector systems.

### Alterations in Glomerular Hemodynamics

HF is characterized not only by increased renal vascular resistance and reduced GFR, but also by an even greater reduction in RPF, so that the filtration fraction is increased.[385] As shown in rat models of HF, these changes seem to result from diminished Kf and elevated afferent and efferent arteriolar resistances. The rise in filtration fraction is probably caused by a disproportionate increase in efferent arteriolar resistance.[385]

In Fig. 14.9, a comparison of the glomerular capillary hemodynamic profile in the normal versus the HF state is illustrated on the left graph of each panel. First, $\Delta P$ declines

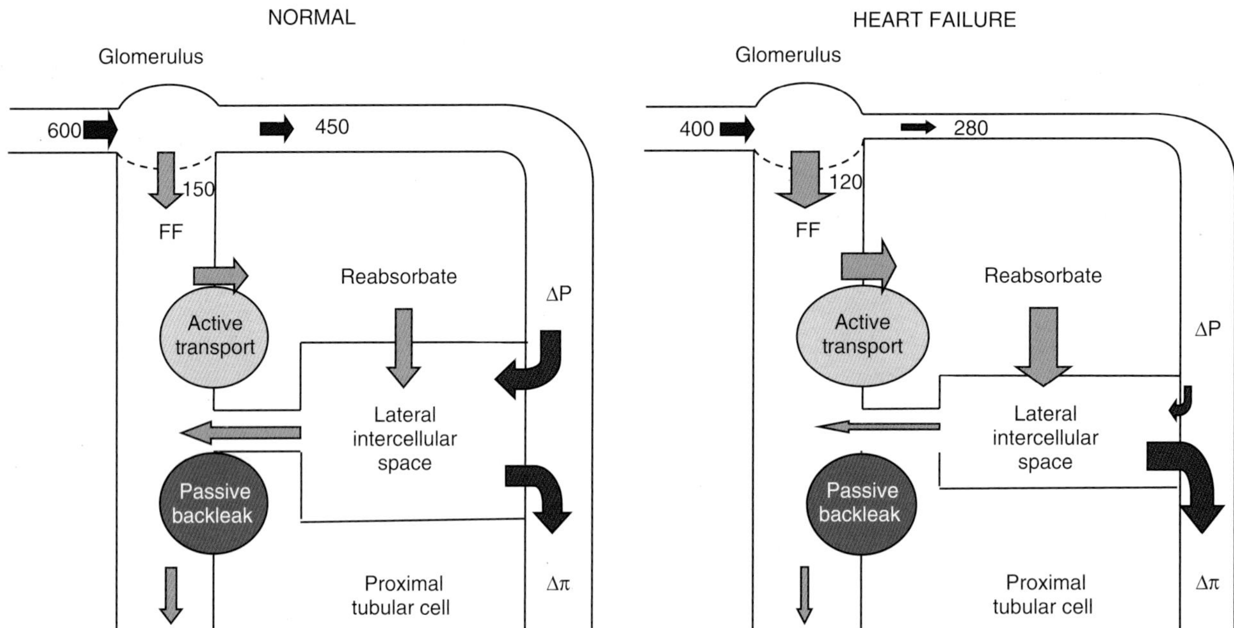


**Fig. 14.9** Peritubular control of proximal tubule fluid reabsorption. Fluid reabsorption in the normal state *(left)* and in patients with heart failure *(right)* is shown. Increased postglomerular arteriolar resistance in heart failure is depicted as narrowing. The thickness and font size of the *block arrows* depict relative magnitude of effect. The increase in filtration fraction (FF) in heart failure causes $\Delta\pi$ to rise. The increase in renal vascular resistance in heart failure is believed to reduce $\Delta P$. Both the increase in $\Delta\pi$ and the fall in $\Delta P$ enhance peritubular capillary uptake of proximal reabsorbate and thus increase absolute $Na^+$ reabsorption by the proximal tubule. Numbers and *red block arrows* depict blood flow in preglomerular and postglomerular capillaries; $\Delta P$ and $\Delta\pi$ are the transcapillary hydraulic and oncotic pressure differences across the peritubular capillary, respectively; *yellow block arrows* indicate transtubular transport; *purple block arrows* represent the effect of peritubular capillary Starling forces on uptake of proximal reabsorbate. (Modified from Humes HD, Gottlieb M, Brenner BM. *The kidney in congestive heart failure: contemporary issues in nephrology*. Vol 1. New York; Churchill Livingstone; 1978, pp 51–72.)

along the length of the glomerular capillary in normal and HF states, but much more so in HF because of the increased efferent arteriolar resistance. Second, $\Delta\pi$ increases over the length of the glomerular capillary in both states as fluid is filtered into Bowman's space, but again to a greater extent in HF because of the increased filtration fraction. As outlined below (see section, "Renin-Angiotensin-Aldosterone System"), the preferential increase in efferent arteriolar resistance is mediated principally by Ang II and is critical for the preservation of GFR in the presence of reduced RPF. Because of the intense efferent arteriolar vasoconstriction, further compensation is not possible if RPP falls as a result of systemic hypotension, causing a sharp decline in GFR. This phenomenon is dramatically illustrated by HF patients whose Ang II drive is removed by RAAS inhibitors, particularly those with preexisting renal failure, massive diuretic treatment and limited cardiac reserve.[385] In these patients, BP may fall below the level necessary to maintain renal perfusion.

**Enhanced Tubular Reabsorption of Sodium.** A direct consequence of the glomerular hemodynamic alterations and augmented single-nephron filtration fraction is an increase in the fractional reabsorption of filtered $Na^+$ in the proximal tubule. In Fig. 14.9, the peritubular capillary hemodynamic profile of the normal state is compared with that of HF on the right graph of each panel. In HF, in comparison with the normal state, the average value of $\Delta\pi$ along the peritubular capillary is increased and that of $\Delta P$ is decreased. These values favor fluid movement into the capillary and may also help reduce paracellular backleak of fluid into the tubule, promoting overall net reabsorption.

The peritubular control of proximal fluid reabsorption in normal and HF states is illustrated schematically in Fig. 14.9. A critical mediator of the enhanced tubular reabsorption of $Na^+$ is Ang II, which, by increasing efferent arteriolar resistance, increases the filtration fraction and augments proximal epithelial transporter activities directly, thereby amplifying the overall increase in proximal $Na^+$ reabsorption. This is clearly illustrated by the favorable effects of RAAS blockers in HF to modulate single-nephron filtration fraction and normalize proximal peritubular capillary Starling forces and $Na^+$ reabsorption.[385]

Enhanced reabsorption of $Na^+$ in HF has been shown in the loop of Henle, probably due to altered renal hemodynamics, as in the proximal tubule.[156] In the distal tubule and collecting duct, elevated Ang II and aldosterone levels, respectively, enhance activities of the NaCl cotransporter and ENaC.[386]

**Neurohumoral Mediators.** The primary vasoconstrictor/antinatriuretic (and antidiuretic) systems mediating $Na^+$ and water retention in HF include the RAAS, SNS, AVP, and ETs. The antagonistic vasodilator/natriuretic substances include NO, PG, AM, UT II, and NPY. The development of positive $Na^+$ balance and edema in HF occurs at the point when the vasoconstrictor/antinatriuretic forces predominate (Fig. 14.10). The dominant activity of $Na^+$-retaining systems in HF is clinically important, as it is associated with globally-impaired

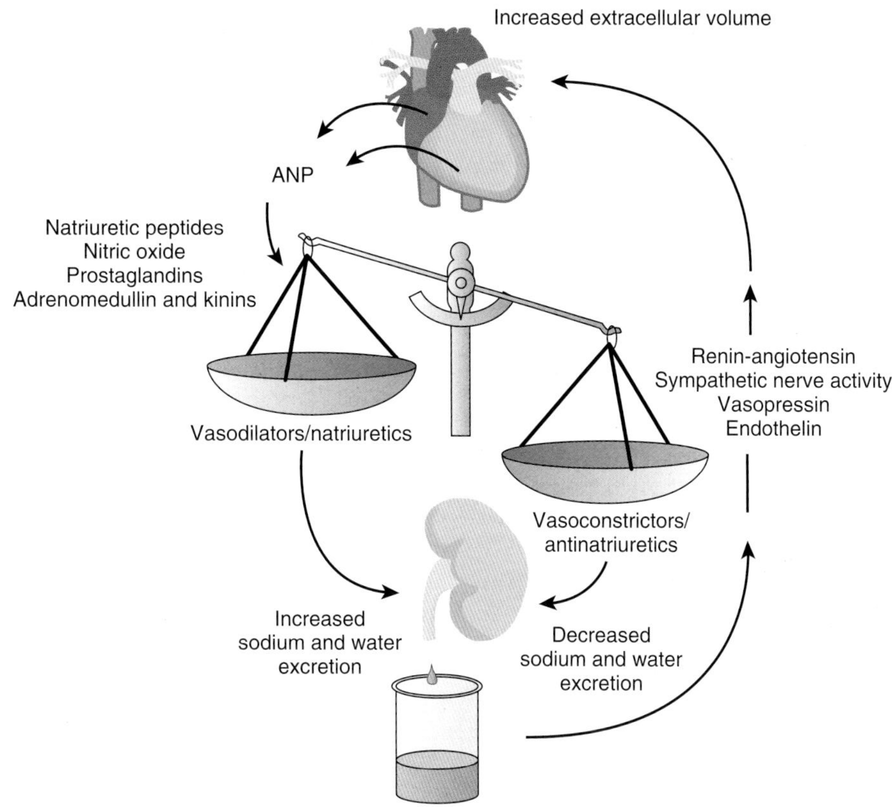


**Fig. 14.10** Efferent limb of extracellular fluid volume control in heart failure. Volume homeostasis in heart failure is determined by the balance between natriuretic and antinatriuretic forces. In decompensated heart failure, enhanced activities of the $Na^+$-retaining systems overwhelm the effects of the vasodilatory/natriuretic systems, which leads to a net reduction in $Na^+$ excretion and an increase in ECF volume. ANP, Atrial natriuretic peptide. (Modified from Winaver J, Hoffman A, Abassi Z, et al. Does the heart's hormone, ANP, help in congestive heart failure? *News Physiol Sci*. 1995;10:247–253.)

renal function, a strong predictor of mortality[385]; moreover, reversal of neurohumoral impairment is associated with improved outcomes.[385]

## VASOCONSTRICTOR/ANTINATRIURETIC (ANTIDIURETIC) SYSTEMS

### Renin-Angiotensin-Aldosterone System

The activity of the RAAS is enhanced in most patients with HF in correlation with the severity of cardiac dysfunction[234] and provides a prognostic index for HF patients. Initially, RAAS activation is beneficial by inducing direct systemic vasoconstriction and activating other neurohormonal systems such as AVP, which contribute to maintaining adequate intravascular volume.[234] However, numerous studies in patients and in experimental models of HF have established that continued activation of the RAAS leads to maladaptive myocardial remodeling[234] and progression of cardiovascular and renal dysfunction.[364]

The kidneys in particular are highly sensitive to the action of Ang II, and a decrease in RPF and SNGFR, as well as elevations in efferent arteriolar resistance and filtration fraction, are observed in both clinical and experimental HF. These changes are completely reversed by ACE inhibitors, as well as a low-salt diet.[387]

Activation of Ang II in response to the decreased pumping capacity of the failing myocardium also promotes systemic vasoconstriction and mesangial cell contraction.[202] In addition, Ang II reduces renal cortical circulation in rats with HF and increases tubular $Na^+$ reabsorption directly and by augmenting aldosterone release.[202]

Local RAAS in the heart and kidney is also important in maintaining $Na^+$ retention in HF. The phenomenon explains the presence of positive $Na^+$ balance as well as the maintained efficacy of RAAS inhibition in chronic HF, in the absence of elevated systemic levels of the component hormones.[388] In general, it appears that systemic RAAS activation is most pronounced in acute decompensated HF, whereas local renal RAAS activation may dominate in chronic stable HF.

In the heart, local RAAS activation has a number of effects. In addition to the mechanical stress exerted on the myocardium due to systemic Ang II–mediated increased afterload, pressure overload activates local Ang II production as a result of upregulation of angiotensinogen and tissue ACE.[389] Local Ang II acts through $AT_1$ in a paracrine/autocrine manner, leading to cell swelling and cardiac hypertrophy, remodeling and fibrosis (mediated by TGF-β) and reduced coronary flow, hallmarks of severe HF.[388] These observations explain the improved cardiac function, prolonged survival, prevention of end-organ damage, and prevention or regression of cardiac hypertrophy in HF treated with RAAS inhibitors.[203,389] In addition, these drugs may improve endothelial dysfunction, vascular remodeling and potentiation of the vasodilatory effects of kinins.[309]

Like Ang II, aldosterone is produced locally by and acts directly on the myocardium in HF, inducing structural remodeling of the interstitial collagen matrix.[390] These adverse effects of aldosterone were elegantly illustrated using eplerenone, a specific aldosterone antagonist, which prevented progressive left ventricular systolic and diastolic dysfunction by reducing interstitial fibrosis, cardiomyocyte hypertrophy and left ventricular chamber sphericity in dogs with HF. Similarly, eplerenone attenuated ventricular remodeling and reactive (but not reparative) fibrosis after myocardial infarction in rats.[391,392] These findings have been translated into the now routine clinical use of aldosterone antagonists in HF (see section, "Specific Treatments Based on the Pathophysiology of Heart Failure").[393]

As noted, in addition to its renal and cardiovascular hemodynamic effects, the RAAS is involved directly in the exaggerated tubular $Na^+$ reabsorption in HF. Ang II, produced systemically and locally, directly stimulates proximal tubular $Na^+$ reabsorption.[394] In contrast, in the cortical and MCD, enhanced $Na^+$ reabsorption is mediated largely by aldosterone, as outlined previously. The pivotal role of aldosterone in HF is amply illustrated by elevated plasma and urine levels and the natriuretic effects of aldosterone antagonists in HF, despite further activation of other antinatriuretic systems.[395]

The importance of RAAS action in the $Na^+$ retention of HF varies with the stage and severity of disease and, in more severe HF, positive $Na^+$ balance is associated with blunted renal and hemodynamic responses to ANP; this response to ANP is restored by RAAS inhibition (for further details, see later section, "Natriuretic Peptides").[396] Also, despite low plasma osmolality, patients with HF display increased thirst, probably because of the high Ang II concentrations, which stimulate thirst center cells in the hypothalamus.[397] This phenomenon may contribute to the positive water balance and hyponatremia often seen in advanced HF (see section, "Arginine Vasopressin").

#### Sympathetic Nervous System

As mentioned earlier, patients with HF experience progressive activation of the SNS with declining cardiac function[234,376] and the adverse influence of sympathetic overactivity on the progression and outcome of patients with HF is abundantly clear.[398,399] Thus, plasma NE levels are frequently elevated and correlate with increased neural traffic. SNS activity is also significantly correlated with intracardiac pressures, cardiac hypertrophy and left ventricular ejection fraction (LVEF).[398,399] Activation of the SNS not only precedes the appearance of congestive symptoms but also is preferentially directed toward the heart and kidneys, as seen in patients with mild HF who have higher NE levels in the coronary sinus than in the renal veins.[399] In early HF, increased SNS activity ameliorates the hemodynamic abnormalities, including hypoperfusion, diminished plasma volume and impaired cardiac function, via vasoconstriction and avid $Na^+$ reabsorption.[376] However, chronic SNS activation induces several long-term adverse myocardial effects, including apoptosis and hypertrophy, with overall reduction in cardiac contractility. Some of these effects may be mediated by RAAS activation which, in turn, can augment sympathetic activity and create a vicious cycle.[234]

Basal sympathetic outflow to the kidneys is significantly increased in patients with HF[376] and increased efferent RSNA contributes to the increased renal vasoconstriction, avid $Na^+$ and water retention, renin secretion, and attenuation of the renal actions of ANP.[264] In rats with experimental HF caused by coronary artery ligation, renal denervation resulted in increased RPF and SNGFR and decreased afferent and efferent arteriolar resistance.[398] In the same model, the decrease in RSNA in response to an acute saline load was less than that of control rats.[254] Conversely, bilateral renal denervation restored the natriuretic response to volume expansion. Similarly, in dogs with low cardiac output induced by vena caval constriction, administration of a ganglion blocker resulted in a marked increase in $Na^+$ excretion.[398] Also, in dogs with high-output HF induced by aortocaval fistula, total postprandial urinary $Na^+$ excretion was approximately twofold higher in dogs with renal denervation than in those with intact nerves.[398] In line with these observations, administration of the $\alpha$-adrenoreceptor blocker dibenamine to patients with HF caused an increase in fractional $Na^+$ excretion, without a change in RPF or GFR. Treatment with ibopamine, an oral dopamine analog, resulted in vasodilation and positive inotropic and diuretic effects in these patients.[400] Moreover, for a given degree of cardiac dysfunction, the concentration of NE is significantly higher in patients with abnormal than in those with preserved renal function.[401] These findings suggest that the association between renal function and prognosis in patients with HF is linked by both systemic and CNS neurohormonal activation.

RSNA may also affect renal hemodynamics and $Na^+$ excretion in HF by an antagonistic interaction with ANP. On the one hand, ANP has sympathoinhibitory effects;[402,403] on the other, the SNS-induced salt and water retention in HF may reduce renal responsiveness to ANP. For example, the blunted diuretic/natriuretic response to ANP in rats with HF could be restored by prior renal denervation[404] or clonidine,[405] a centrally acting $\alpha_2$-adrenoreceptor agonist, which decreases RSNA in HF. These examples illustrate the complexity of interactions between the SNS and other humoral factors involved in the pathogenesis of $Na^+$ retention in HF.

In summary, the SNS plays an important role in the regulation of $Na^+$ excretion and glomerular hemodynamics in HF, either by a direct renal action or by a complex interplay between the SNS itself and other neurohumoral mechanisms that act on the glomeruli and renal tubules. The recent introduction of renal denervation as a potential therapeutic treatment for HF should facilitate further elucidation of these neurohumoral interactions.

#### Vasopressin

Numerous studies have demonstrated elevated plasma levels of AVP in HF, mostly in advanced HF with hyponatremia, but also in asymptomatic patients with left ventricular dysfunction.[406] These high levels are related to nonosmotic factors such as attenuated left atrial compliance, hypotension and RAAS activation, and are reversed by RAAS inhibition or $\alpha$-blockade (prazosin).[407]

The high circulating levels of AVP adversely affect the kidneys and cardiovascular system. In fact, raised levels of the C-terminal portion of the AVP prohormone (copeptin) at the time of diagnosis of acute decompensated HF are highly predictive of 1-year mortality.[408] The prognostic power of an increased copeptin level in HF is similar to that of BNP levels (see section, "Brain Natriuretic Peptide"). The most recognized renal effect of AVP in HF is the development of hyponatremia, especially in advanced stages of the disease, which most probably results from impaired solute-free water excretion, independent of plasma osmolality. In accordance with this notion, animal models of HF have demonstrated increased collecting duct expression of AQP2.[409] In addition, administration of specific $V_2$ receptor antagonists (VRAs) is associated with improvement in plasma $Na^+$ levels in animals and patients with hyponatremia.[410,411] The improvement is associated with correction of the impaired urinary dilution in response to acute water load,[412] increased plasma osmolarity and downregulation of renal AQP2 expression, but with no effect on RBF, GFR or $Na^+$ excretion.[413]

The adverse effects of AVP on cardiac function[414] occur through its $V_{1A}$ receptor to increase SVR (i.e., cardiac afterload), as well as by $V_2$-receptor–mediated water retention, which leads to systemic and pulmonary congestion (increased preload). In addition, AVP, through its $V_{1A}$ receptor, causes a direct rise in cardiomyocyte intracellular $Ca^{2+}$ and activation of mitogen-activated kinases and protein kinase C. These signaling mechanisms appear to mediate the observed cardiac remodeling, dilation and hypertrophy. The remodeling might be further exacerbated by the abnormalities in preload and afterload.

In summary, the data suggest that AVP is involved in the pathogenesis of water retention and hyponatremia that characterize HF; and that AVP receptor antagonists result in remarkable diuresis in experimental and clinical models of HF. Treatment of HF with VRA will be discussed further (see section, "Specific Treatments Based on the Pathophysiology of Heart Failure").

### Endothelin

ET-1 is involved in both the development and progression of HF as well as in the associated reduced renal function by inducing renal remodeling, interstitial fibrosis, glomerulosclerosis, hypoperfusion, hypofiltration and positive salt and water balance.[279] The pathophysiologic role of ET-1 in HF is supported by two major lines of evidence: 1. The ET system is activated in HF; and 2. ET-1 receptor antagonists modify this pathophysiologic process.[279] The first line of evidence is based on elevated plasma ET-1 and big ET-1 concentrations in clinical HF and experimental models of HF; these levels correlate with hemodynamic severity and symptoms.[415] Also, the degree of pulmonary hypertension was the strongest predictor of plasma ET-1 level in patients with HF.[416] Moreover, plasma levels of big ET and ET-1 are especially high in patients with moderate to severe HF and are independent markers of mortality and morbidity.[415] The increase in plasma ET-1 levels may be the result of enhanced synthesis in the lungs, heart and circulation by stimuli such as Ang II and thrombin or decreased pulmonary clearance.[416] In parallel to ET-1 levels, ET-A receptors are upregulated, whereas ET-B receptors are downregulated in the failing human heart.[417]

A cause-and-effect relationship between these hemodynamic abnormalities and ET-1 in HF was demonstrated using selective and highly specific ET receptor antagonists.[416] In this regard, acute administration of the mixed ET-A/ET-B receptor antagonists, bosentan and tezosentan significantly improved renal cortical perfusion, reversed the profoundly increased renal vascular resistance and increased RBF and $Na^+$ excretion in rats with severe decompensated HF.[418] In addition, chronic blockade of ET-A by selective or dual ET-A/ET-B receptor antagonists attenuated the magnitude of $Na^+$ retention and prevented the decline in GFR in experimental HF.[419] These data are in line with earlier observations that rats with decompensated HF, as compared with normal rats, displayed severely blunted cortical vasoconstriction but significantly prolonged medullary vasodilation in response to ET-1 infusion. These effects could have resulted from activation of vasodilatory systems such as PG and NO, as exemplified by higher medullary immunoreactive eNOS levels in rats with HF than controls.[420] Taken together, the data indicate a role for ET in the pathogenesis of renal cortical vasoconstriction and $Na^+$ retention in HF.

## VASODILATORY/NATRIURETIC SYSTEMS

### Natriuretic Peptides

In decompensated HF, renal $Na^+$ and water retention occur, despite ECF volume expansion, even when the NP system is activated. Many clinical and experimental studies have implicated both ANP and BNP in the pathophysiology of the deranged cardiorenal axis in HF.

**Atrial Natriuretic Peptide.** Plasma levels of ANP and $NH_2$-terminal ANP are frequently elevated in HF and are correlated positively with the severity of cardiac failure, elevated atrial pressure and left ventricular dysfunction.[264] Hence, circulating ANP level was proposed as a diagnostic marker of cardiac dysfunction and as a predictor of survival in HF.[44] However, in this context, ANP has since been superseded by BNP. There is also evidence that midregional (MR) proANP may perform similarly to BNP as a biomarker of ADHF (see section, "Brain Natriuretic Peptide").[473]

The high plasma ANP levels are attributed to increased production rather than to decreased clearance. Although volume-induced atrial stretch is the main source for the elevated circulating ANP levels in HF, enhanced synthesis and release of the hormone by ventricular tissue in response to Ang II and ET also contribute to the elevated levels.[264] Despite the high levels, patients and experimental animals with HF retain salt and water because renal responsiveness to NPs is attenuated.[421] However, infusion of ANP to patients with HF does lead to hemodynamic improvement and inhibition of activated neurohumoral systems. These data are in line with findings that ANP is a weak counterregulator of the vasoconstriction mediated by the SNS, RAAS, and AVP.[422] However, despite the blunted renal response to ANP in HF, elimination of ANP production by atrial appendectomy in dogs with HF aggravated the activation of the vasoconstrictive factors and resulted in marked $Na^+$ and water retention.[423] These data suggest that ANP plays a critical role in suppressing $Na^+$-retaining systems and as an important adaptive or compensatory mechanism aimed at reducing pulmonary vascular resistance and hypervolemia.

**Brain Natriuretic Peptide.** Plasma levels of BNP and N-terminal (NT)–proBNP are elevated in severe HF in proportion to the degree of myocardial systolic and diastolic dysfunction and New York Heart Association (NYHA) classification.[264,424] The extreme elevation of plasma BNP in severe HF stems mainly from increased synthesis by the hypertrophied ventricular tissue, but the atria also contribute.[264,424]

Although echocardiography remains the gold standard for the evaluation of left ventricular dysfunction, plasma levels of BNP and NT-proBNP are reliable markers and, in fact, superior to ANP and NT-proANP for the diagnosis and prognosis of HF.[276] NT-proBNP in particular has high sensitivity, specificity and negative predictive value in patients with an ejection fraction less than 35%. Similar high predictive values are found in patients with concomitant left ventricular hypertrophy, either in the absence of or after myocardial infarction.[276] The added presence of renal dysfunction appears to enhance these predictive values,[425,426] and graded increases in mortality throughout each quartile of BNP levels have been shown in several clinical trials.[276] In addition, elevated plasma BNP (or NT-proBNP) levels and LVEF lower than 40% are complementary independent predictors of death, HF and new myocardial infarction at 3 years after a first infarction. Moreover, risk stratification with the combination of LVEF lower than 40% and high levels of NT-proBNP is substantially better than that provided by either alone.[427] However, even though BNP levels tend to be lower in patients with preserved LVEF than in HF patients with reduced LVEF, the prognosis in patients with preserved LVEF is as poor as in those with reduced LVEF for a given BNP level.[427]

In asymptomatic patients with preserved LVEF, elevated BNP levels are correlated with diastolic abnormalities on Doppler studies. Conversely, a reduction in BNP levels with treatment is associated with a reduction in left ventricular filling pressures, lower readmission rates and a better prognosis; thus, monitoring of BNP levels may provide valuable information regarding treatment efficacy and expected patient outcomes.[428]

Another diagnostic role for BNP is in the distinction of dyspnea caused by HF from that caused by noncardiac diseases. Using specific cut points, NT-proBNP levels are highly sensitive and specific for the diagnosis of acute HF. Levels lower than 300 pg/mL rule out acute HF, with a negative predictive value of 99%. An increased level of NT-proBNP is the strongest independent predictor of a final diagnosis of acute HF. NT-proBNP testing alone was superior to clinical judgment, the National Health and Nutrition Examination score and Framingham clinical parameters alone for diagnosing acute HF; NT-proBNP plus clinical judgment was superior to NT-proBNP or clinical judgment alone.[276]

There is also evidence, albeit of rather low quality, that circulating BNP and NT-proBNP levels can be useful as a guide to therapeutic efficacy of drugs typically prescribed in HF, including RAAS inhibitors, diuretics, digitalis and β-blockers.[429,430] Also, BNP, but not NT-proBNP, levels at 24 and 48 hours after admission for acute decompensated HF (ADHF) predicted both 30-day and 1-year mortality. Predischarge levels of both peptides were predictive of 30-day and 1-year mortality but not 1-year readmission due to HF.[431] In contrast, BNP levels were not helpful in reducing length of hospital stay and costs.[429]

Together, these findings suggest that a simple and rapid determination of plasma levels of BNP or NT-proBNP in HF patients, together with clinical and echocardiographic measures, can be used to assess cardiac dysfunction, serve as a diagnostic and prognostic marker and possibly assist in titrating relevant therapy.[276] However, it should be emphasized that plasma NP levels are affected by age, salt intake, gender, obesity, hemodynamic status and renal function leading to considerable overlap among diagnostic groups.[276,432] Measurement of a panel may enhance the ability of biomarkers to distinguish between cardiac and noncardiac causes of dyspnea.[433]

**C-Type Natriuretic Peptide.** Like those of ANP and BNP, plasma CNP levels are increased in HF and are directly correlated with NYHA classification, levels of BNP, ET-1, and AM and with pulmonary capillary wedge pressure, ejection fraction, and left ventricular end-diastolic diameter.[434] CNP is synthesized mainly in the kidney,[278] but it is also processed by the myocardium. Overexpression of CNP in the myocardium during HF may be involved in counteracting cardiac remodeling.[434] On the other hand, renal CNP secretion is blunted in HF.[435] In contrast to the diminished physiologic responses to ANP and BNP in animals with HF, CNP elicited twice as much sGC activity as ANP, due to dramatic reductions in NP receptor A (NPR-A) but not NPR-B activity.[434] These findings imply a significant role for NPR-B–mediated NP activity in HF and may explain the modest effects of the NPR-A–selective nesiritide (BNP) treatment in HF.[436]

Overall, current evidence points to a role of CNP either in the peripheral vascular compensatory response in HF or in mitigating the cardiac remodeling characteristic of HF. Elaboration of the exact role of CNP in HF appears crucial for the design of more effective NP analogs than those currently available for the management of HF.

### Overall Relationship Between Natriuretic and Antinatriuretic Factors in Heart Failure

The maintenance of $Na^+$ balance in the initial compensated phase of HF is at least in part due to the elevated ANP and BNP levels.[264] This notion is supported by the findings that, in experimental HF, inhibition of NP receptors by specific antibodies increased renal vascular resistance and decreased GFR, RBF, urine flow, $Na^+$ excretion and RAAS activation.[437] In addition, NPs inhibited the Ang II–induced systemic vasoconstriction, proximal tubule $Na^+$ reabsorption, and secretion of aldosterone and ET.[438]

In view of the remarkable activation and ability of NPs to counter the vasoconstrictor/antinatriuretic neurohormonal effects, why then do salt and water retention occur in overt HF? Several mechanisms could explain this paradox:

1. Appearance of abnormal circulating peptides and inadequate secretory reserves in comparison with the degree of HF. Using an extremely sensitive mass spectrometry–based method, altered processing of proBNP1-108 and/or BNP1-32 has been demonstrated, resulting in very low levels of BNP1-32, despite markedly elevated levels of immunoreactive (i.e., total) BNP.[439] Moreover, proBNP1-108 has a lower affinity for the GC-A receptor, which would reduce effector function of BNP.[440]
2. Decreased availability of NPs by downregulation of corin[441] or upregulation of NEP and clearance receptors.[437] With respect to corin, lower plasma levels have been observed in HF patients in parallel with elevated levels of proANP. On the other hand, circulating cGMP levels are elevated in HF, implying enhanced activity of NPs. These apparently contradictory findings could be reconciled by the demonstration of low intracardiac corin levels in an experimental model of HF caused by dilated cardiomyopathy. Moreover,

transfection of the gene encoding for corin into these animals led to a reduction in cardiac fibrosis, improvement in contractility and reduced mortality.[441] Regarding clearance receptors, there is no convincing evidence to date of upregulation in the renal tissue of HF animals or patients, although increased abundance of clearance receptors for NPs in platelets of patients with advanced HF has been reported.[442] In contrast, enhanced expression and activity of NEP in experimental HF is well documented[264] and NEP inhibitors improve the vascular and renal response to NPs in HF (see section, "Specific Treatments Based on the Pathophysiology of Heart Failure").

3. Activation of vasoconstrictor/antinatriuretic factors and renal hyporesponsiveness to ANP. Renal resistance to ANP may be present, even in the early presymptomatic stage of the disease and progresses proportionately as HF worsens.[437] In advanced HF, when RPF is markedly impaired, the ability of NPs to antagonize the renal effects of the maximally activated RAAS is limited.[264] The mechanisms underlying the attenuated renal effects of ANP in HF include Ang II–induced afferent and efferent vasoconstriction, mesangial cell contraction, activation of cGMP phosphodiesterases that attenuate the accumulation of the second messenger of NPs in target organs and stimulation of $Na^+$-$H^+$-exchanger and $Na^+$ channels in the proximal tubule and collecting duct, respectively.[443]
4. Activation of the SNS also can overwhelm the renal effects of ANP. As described earlier, overactivity of the SNS leads to vasoconstriction of the peripheral circulation and of the afferent and efferent arterioles, which causes reduction of RPF and GFR. These actions, together with the direct stimulatory effects of SNS on $Na^+$ reabsorption in the proximal tubule and loop of Henle, contribute to the attenuated renal responsiveness to ANP in HF. Moreover, the SNS-induced renal hypoperfusion/hypofiltration stimulates renin secretion, thereby aggravating the positive $Na^+$ and water balance. In rat models of HF, the natriuretic responses to ANP were increased after sympathetic inhibition by low-dose clonidine[405] or bilateral renal denervation.[444] The beneficial effects of renal denervation could be attributed to upregulation of NP receptors and cGMP production.[201]

In summary, the development of renal hyporesponsiveness to NPs is paralleled closely by overreactivity of the RAAS and SNS and represents a critical point in the development of positive salt balance and edema formation in advanced HF.

#### Nitric Oxide

NO is implicated in the increased vascular resistance and impaired endothelium-dependent vascular responses characteristic of HF.[445,446] The impaired activity is mediated by reduced shear stress associated with the decreased cardiac output, downregulation or uncoupling of eNOS, decreased availability of the NO precursor L-arginine caused by increased activity of arginase and increased levels of the endogenous NOS inhibitor asymmetric dimethyl arginine (ADMA). In addition, inactivation of NO by superoxide ion and alteration of the redox state of sGC through oxidative stress lead to reduced levels of the NO-sensitive form of sGC and, thereby, of its second messenger cGMP.[445,446] Oxidative stress may be further exacerbated by overactivity of counterregulatory neurohumoral systems, such as the RAAS and the release of proinflammatory messengers.[445,446]

Altered activity of the NO-sGC-cGMP system also underlies the regional vasomotor dysregulation of the renal circulation in HF and Ang II may be involved in mediating the impaired NO–dependent renal vasodilation.[447] The resulting imbalance between NO and excessive activation of the RAAS and ET systems could explain some of the beneficial effects of RAAS inhibition.[448] Support for this imbalance concept came from a model of experimental HF in rats overexpressing eNOS in the renal medulla and, to a lesser extent, in the cortex.[420] This eNOS might play a role in the preservation of intact medullary perfusion and could attenuate the severe cortical vasoconstriction. Accumulation of ADMA as exemplified by elevated plasma levels in normotensive HF could also account for the impaired renal hemodynamics in HF. In fact, in a multiple regression analysis, ADMA levels independently predicted reduced RBF.[449]

Locally generated NO by the myocardium is also believed to modulate cardiac function and, thereby, lead to the impaired renal function in HF.[445,446] Alterations in the expression of cardiac NOS isoforms in HF are complex and the functional consequences of these changes depend on a balance among various factors, including disruption of the unique subcellular localization of each isoform and nitroso-redox imbalance.[445,446]

In summary, endothelium-dependent vasodilation is attenuated in various vascular beds in HF. This attenuation may occur as a result of decreased NO levels and downregulation or inhibition of downstream NO signal transduction pathways. These effects may occur directly or via counterregulatory vasoconstrictor neurohumoral mechanisms.

#### Protaglandins

PG play an important role in maintaining renal function in the setting of the impaired RBF in HF. Renal hypoperfusion, directly or by RAAS activation, stimulates the release of PG that exert a vasodilatory effect, predominantly on the afferent arteriole, and promote $Na^+$ excretion by inhibiting reabsorption in the TALH and the MCD.[450,451] Evidence for the compensatory role of PG in experimental and clinical HF comes from two sources. First, plasma levels of $PGE_2$, $PGE_2$ metabolites, and 6-keto-$PGF_1$ were higher in HF patients than in normal subjects.[452] Moreover, in both experimental and human HF there is a direct relationship between PRA/Ang II and plasma and urinary $PGE_2$ and $PGI_2$ metabolite concentrations.[453] This correlation probably reflects both Ang II–induced stimulation of PG synthesis and PG-mediated increased renin release. A similar counterregulatory role of PG regarding the other vasoconstrictors (e.g., catecholamines, AVP) may also be inferred.

The second approach, which established the protective role of renal and vascular PG in HF, was by using nonsteroidal antiinflammatory drugs (NSAIDs) to inhibit PG synthesis. In various experimental models of HF, this maneuver was associated with elevated urinary $PGE_2$ excretion, increase in body weight and renal vascular resistance with resultant decrease in RBF, mainly due to afferent arteriolar constriction.[452,454] Urine flow rate declined significantly and serum creatinine and urea rose.[454] Similarly, in patients with HF and hyponatremia, in whom extreme activation of the SNS and RAAS occurred, significant decreases in RBF and GFR accompanied by reduced urinary $Na^+$ excretion, followed NSAID treatment.[452,455] These effects were prevented by intravenous $PGE_2$. Moreover, pretreatment with indomethacin attenuated the captopril-induced increase in RBF.[455] Thus ACEI-associated improvement in renal hemodynamics is mediated in part by increased PG synthesis.

Selective COX-2 inhibitors also lead to a significant worsening of chronic HF and renal function, especially in older patients taking diuretics.[456–458] These deleterious effects are predictable given the relative abundance of COX-2 in renal tissue and, to a lesser extent, in the myocardium of HF patients.[450,459]

In summary, HF can be viewed as a PG-dependent state, in which elevated Ang II levels and enhanced RSNA stimulate renal synthesis of $PGE_2$ and $PGI_2$, to counteract the vasoconstrictor neurohumoral stimuli and maintain GFR and RBF. Both COX-2 and nonselective COX inhibitors should be avoided in HF, as they leave the vasoconstrictor systems unopposed, leading to hypoperfusion, hypofiltration, and $Na^+$ and water retention.[450]

### Adrenomedullin

AM seems to play a role in the pathophysiology of HF. HF patients have up to fivefold elevations in plasma levels of AM, in proportion to the severity of cardiac, hemodynamic, and neurohumoral derangements, including pulmonary arterial and capillary wedge pressure, NE, ANP, BNP levels, and PRA.[317,460] Plasma levels of AM decreased with effective anti-HF treatment, such as carvedilol.[461] High levels of midregional proAM are also strong predictors of mortality in HF.[462–464] The origin of the increased circulating AM appears to be the failing ventricular and, to a lesser extent, atrial myocardium.[461,465]

Not only cardiac but also renal AM levels are significantly increased in some, although not all, experimental models of HF.[466,467] The renal upregulation is consistent with the favorable acute and more prolonged (4 days) effects of AM on creatinine clearance, $Na^+$ and water excretion, as well as on the hemodynamic abnormalities of experimental HF.[461] In contrast, acute administration of AM to HF patients increased forearm blood flow but less so than in normal subjects. Stroke index and dilation of resistance arteries were increased, and plasma aldosterone reduced, but $Na^+$ and water excretion were unaffected.[461] Collectively, the data suggest that AM acts to balance the elevation in SVR and volume expansion in HF.[317]

Because the favorable effects of AM alone are rather modest, combination therapy with other vasodilatory/natriuretic substances has been attempted. Combinations with BNP, ACEIs, NEP inhibitors and epinephrine resulted in hemodynamic and renal benefits greater than those achieved by each agent alone.[461,468] A small long-term clinical trial of combined ANP and AM in acute decompensated HF demonstrated a significant increase in cardiac output, reductions in MAP, pulmonary arterial pressure, systemic and pulmonary vascular resistance without changing heart rate. In addition, levels of aldosterone, BNP and free radical metabolites fell and $Na^+$ and water excretion rose.[469]

With the advent of NEP inhibitors, which enhance the activities of vasodilatory/natriuretic peptides, including AM, HF outcomes have been significantly improved. (See section "Specific treatments based on the pathophysiology of HF".)

### Urotensin

A role for UT II and its receptor, GPR14, in the pathogenesis of HF has been suggested. First, some, but not all, studies revealed that plasma levels of UT II are elevated in patients with HF in correlation with levels of other markers, such as NT-proBNP and ET-1.[470] Second, strong myocardial expression of UT II in end-stage HF correlates with the degree of cardiac impairment.[470] The upregulated UT II in HF may also have a role in the regulation of renal function in HF. In rat models of HF, UT II acted primarily as a renal vasodilator, apparently by an NO–dependent mechanism.[325] RPF and GFR, but not urinary $Na^+$ excretion, were also increased. On the other hand, UT II in control rats led to intense renal vasoconstriction, a fall in GFR and $Na^+$ retention.[325] In light of the contradictory effects of UT II in different conditions, the clinical application of these data will be challenging.

### Neuropeptides

Because NPY co-localizes and is released with adrenergic neurotransmitters, high circulating NE levels in HF are accompanied by excessive co-release of NPY and plasma levels are correlated with disease severity in HF patients.[334] In contrast, local myocardial levels, like those of NE, were lower than normal in association with decreased Y1 and increased Y2 receptor expression.[334] Because Y1 receptor activation is associated with cardiomyocyte hypertrophy and Y2 receptor activation with angiogenesis, the data in this model suggest that NPY may simultaneously attenuate the maladaptive cardiac remodeling observed in HF and stimulate angiogenesis in the ischemic heart.[334] Similar patterns of receptor expression change were observed in the kidneys and these were proportional to the degree of renal failure and $Na^+$ retention.[334] In contrast, administration of NPY in experimental models of HF led to diuresis and natriuresis, probably by increasing ANP release and inhibiting the RAAS.[471] Therefore, in HF, the higher circulating levels, together with the reduced tissue levels of NPY, could be a counterregulatory mechanism to modulate the vasoconstrictive and $Na^+$ retaining, as well as the cardiac remodeling, effects of the RAAS and SNS. In addition, the downregulation of Y1 receptors, by reducing vasoconstriction, could contribute to reduced coronary and renal vascular resistance. However, once the stage of decompensated HF is reached, the RAAS and SNS effects likely dominate, thereby overwhelming any favorable effects of NPY.

Levels of other neuropeptides, such as catestatin, may be elevated in HF and have been investigated as potential biomarkers, but did not improve diagnostic accuracy over BNP.[471] In summary, laboratory data on neuropeptides in HF have not translated into clinical application.

### Apelin

The expression of apelin and its receptor in the kidney and heart and the involvement of the system in the maintenance of water balance suggested a potential role in HF. Circulating levels rise in early HF but decline in later stages of the disease.[472,473] However, this decline correlates poorly with severity of HF, making apelin not useful as a biomarker of HF progression.[474]

The fact that activation of the apelin receptor induces aquaresis, vasodilation and a positive inotropic effect suggested the receptor as a potential therapeutic target in HF. Along these lines, acute IV injection of apelin to rats with HF following induced myocardial function led to improved systolic and diastolic function. Moreover, more chronic infusion (3 weeks) decreased Ang II–induced cardiac fibrosis and remodeling.[472] In HF patients, acute intravenous apelin increased cardiac output, reduced BP and vascular resistance.[472] No data are yet available on the direct renal effects of apelin in HF, although, by reducing AVP levels and improving the renal microcirculation, apelin might increase aquaresis. In addition, the favorable effects on cardiac function are likely to increase renal perfusion and hence promote diuresis.[475] Stable apelin analogs are currently in development.[476]

#### Peroxisome Proliferator-Activated Receptors

Peroxisome proliferator–activated receptors (PPARs) are nutrient-sensing nuclear transcription factors, of which PPARγ is of special interest in the context of $Na^+$ and water retention because of its ligands, the thiazolidinediones (TZD). TZD, by increasing insulin sensitivity, are used for the management of type 2 diabetes mellitus. TZD also decrease circulating free fatty acids and triglycerides, lower BP, reduce levels of inflammatory markers and reduce atherosclerosis. Moreover, they have a beneficial effect on cardiac remodeling in myocardial ischemia.[477] However, a troubling side effect of TZD is fluid retention mainly resulting from PPARγ-induced $Na^+$ reabsorption mediated by increased ENaC expression in collecting duct epithelium.[478] However, TZD may also augment proximal tubular $Na^+$ reabsorption by upregulation of apical NEH3, basolateral $Na^+$-$HCO_3^-$ cotransporter, and $Na^+$-$K^+$-ATPase. These effects are mediated by PPARγ-induced nongenomic transactivation of the epidermal growth factor receptor and downstream extracellular signal-regulated kinases.[479] Moreover, by reducing SVR, TZD might lead to higher capillary perfusion pressures and fluid extravasation[478];TZD are also potent VEGF inducers, leading to increased vascular permeability. In clinical terms, the $Na^+$-retaining effect of TZD translates into an increased incidence of HF[478] and, therefore, they are contraindicated in advanced HF.

Because of the $Na^+$-retaining and fluid-retaining effects, as well as other concerns related to increased cardiovascular events on the one hand and favorable effects on the myocardium on the other, the exact role of TZD in HF remains a hotly debated subject.[480]

In summary, alterations in the efferent limb of volume regulation in HF include both enhanced activities of vasoconstrictor/$Na^+$-retaining systems and counterregulatory vasodilatory/natriuretic systems. The magnitude of $Na^+$ excretion by the kidneys and, therefore, the disturbance in volume homeostasis in HF are largely determined by the balance between these antagonistic systems. In the early stages of HF, the vasodilatory/natriuretic systems are important in the maintenance of circulatory and renal function. However, with the progression of HF, the balance shifts toward dysfunction of the vasodilatory/natriuretic systems and enhanced activation of the vasoconstrictor/antinatriuretic systems. The net result is renal circulatory and tubular alterations that result in avid retention of salt and water, and edema formation.

**Renal Sodium Retention in Cirrhosis With Portal Hypertension.** Avid $Na^+$ and water retention commonly occurs in cirrhosis with portal hypertension, leading eventually to ascites, a major cause of morbidity and mortality, with the occurrence of spontaneous bacterial peritonitis, variceal bleeding, and development of the HRS.[481,482] As in HF, the pathogenesis of renal $Na^+$ and water retention in cirrhosis is related to extrarenal regulation of renal $Na^+$ and water handling.

A *sine qua non* for the $Na^+$ and water retention in cirrhosis is the development of intrasinusoidal portal hypertension, with values of portal pressure above 12 mm Hg generally being required. In contrast, presinusoidal hypertension alone, as observed in portal vein thrombosis, is not associated with fluid retention. The hallmark of fluid retention in cirrhosis is peripheral arterial vasodilation, in association with renal vasoconstriction. In the early stages of cirrhosis, vasodilation occurs in the splanchnic vascular bed, with arterial pressure maintained through increases in plasma volume and cardiac output, leading to the so-called "hyperdynamic circulation" (overfilling). At this stage, renal $Na^+$ and water retention is already evident and aids in the maintenance of EABV.[483] However, as cirrhosis progresses, vasodilation in the systemic and pulmonary circulations becomes prominent and cardiac output can no longer compensate for the progressive decrease in SVR.[484] The resulting relative arterial underfilling[483] and reduced EABV leads to unloading of the arterial high-pressure baroreceptors and other volume receptors, in turn, stimulating the classical compensatory neurohumoral response. This response manifests itself as renal, brachial, femoral, and cerebral vasoconstriction and further $Na^+$ and fluid retention.[485]

**Peripheral Arterial Vasodilation.** The initial trigger for splanchnic arterial vasodilation is hepatic tissue damage itself, which leads to venous outflow obstruction, reduced portal venous and increased hepatic arterial blood flow. Moreover, the lower the portal venous flow, the higher the hepatic arterial flow (Fig. 14.11A). These changes lead to increased intrahepatic vascular resistance and sinusoidal pressure.[483] Increased hepatic resistance to portal flow causes the gradual development of portal hypertension, collateral vein formation and shunting of blood to the systemic circulation. As portal hypertension develops, local production of vasodilators—mainly NO, but also carbon monoxide, glucagon, prostacyclin, AM, and endogenous opiates—increases, leading to splanchnic vasodilation.[485] Other contributing factors to splanchnic vasodilation include intestinal bacterial translocation, proinflammatory cytokines and mesenteric angiogenesis.[486,487]

The decreases in SVR associated with low arterial BP and high cardiac output account for the well-known clinical manifestations of the hyperdynamic circulation commonly seen in patients with cirrhosis. These include warm extremities, cutaneous vascular spiders, wide pulse pressure, capillary pulsations in the nail bed[488] and pulmonary vasodilation, associated with the hepatopulmonary syndrome.[489]

**Abnormalities of Sensing Mechanisms in Cirrhosis**

***Nitric Oxide.*** The NO system is integrally involved in the pathogenesis of the hyperdynamic circulation and $Na^+$ and water retention in cirrhosis, as well as in hepatic encephalopathy, hepatopulmonary syndrome, and cirrhotic cardiomyopathy.[490] NO is produced in excess by the vasculature of different animal models of portal hypertension, as well as in cirrhotic patients.[490] In animal models, the increased production of NO can be detected at the onset of $Na^+$ retention

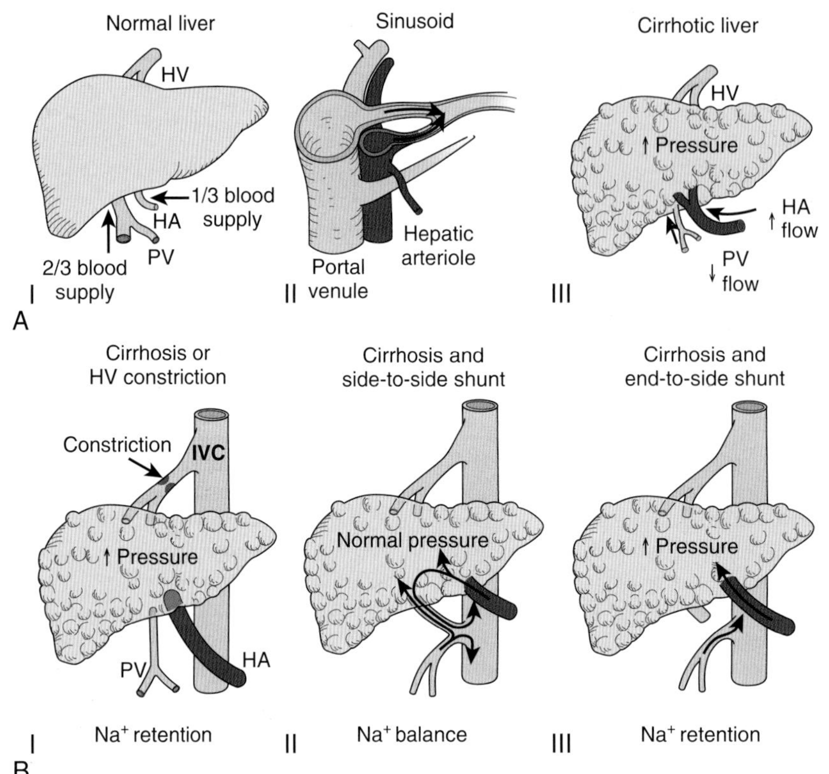


**Fig. 14.11** Characteristics of hepatic blood flow. A, Hepatic circulation. I, The normal liver receives two thirds of its blood flow from the portal vein (PV) and the remaining third from the hepatic artery (HA). II, Both the portal venules and hepatic arterioles drain into hepatic sinusoids, but the exact arrangement that allows forward flow of the mixed venous and arterial blood remains unclear. III, Cirrhosis increases intrahepatic vascular resistance and sinusoidal pressure. In addition, PV flow is markedly decreased, and HA flow is unchanged or increased. B, Hepatic vascular hemodynamics and sodium balance. I, Cirrhosis or restriction of HV flow increases intrahepatic vascular resistance and sinusoidal pressure, markedly decreasing PV flow and increasing HA flow. Changes in the physical forces or in the composition of the hepatic blood trigger $Na^+$ retention and edema formation. II, Insertion of a side-to-side portocaval shunt decreases sinusoidal pressure and maintains mixing of PV and HA blood, irrigating the liver. Under these conditions and despite cirrhosis, there is no $Na^+$ retention. III, Insertion of an end-to-side portocaval shunt only partially decreases the elevated sinusoidal pressure and prevents mixing of PV and HA blood supplies, inasmuch as the PV blood is diverted to the inferior vena cava (IVC). Under these conditions and, despite normalization of PV pressure, $Na^+$ retention continues unabated. (Modified from Oliver JA, Verna EC. Afferent mechanisms of sodium retention in cirrhosis and HRS. *Kidney Int*. 2010;77:669–680.)

and before the appearance of ascites and NO has been implicated in the impaired vascular responsiveness to vasoconstrictors.[491] Moreover, removal of the vascular endothelial layer abolishes the difference in vascular reactivity between cirrhotic and control vessels.[488]

Inhibition of NOS has beneficial effects in experimental models of cirrhosis and in cirrhotic patients. By reducing the high NO production to control levels, the hyperdynamic circulation in cirrhotic rats with ascites was corrected and accompanied by a marked increase in $Na^+$ and water excretion and regression of ascites. Concomitant decreases in PRA, aldosterone and vasopressin concentrations were also observed.[492,493] In cirrhotic patients, the vascular hyporesponsiveness of the forearm circulation to NE could be reversed by NOS inhibition.[494] Inhibition of NO production also corrected the hypotension and hyperdynamic circulation, led to improved renal function and $Na^+$ excretion and to a decrease in plasma NE levels in these patients. However, in patients with established ascites, NOS inhibition did not improve renal function.[495]

The main enzymatic isoform responsible for the increased systemic vascular NO generation in cirrhosis appears to be eNOS in the systemic and splanchnic circulations.[490] Upregulation of eNOS appears, at least in part, to be caused by increased shear stress as a result of portal venous hypertension with increased splanchnic blood flow.[490] Increased NO release, as well as eNOS upregulation, in the superior mesenteric arteries was found to precede the development of the hyperdynamic splanchnic circulation.[490] In accord with this concept, upregulation of hepatic eNOS (or nNOS) expression in rats with experimental cirrhosis was associated with a decrease in portal hypertension.[496] However, mice with targeted deletion of eNOS alone or combined deletions of eNOS and iNOS, can still develop a hyperdynamic circulation in association with portal hypertension.[493] This suggests that activation of other vasodilatory agents such as $PGI_2$, endothelium-derived hyperpolarizing factor, carbon monoxide, and AM may participate in the pathogenesis of the hyperdynamic circulation in experimental cirrhosis.[491]

In addition to eNOS, other isoforms may be involved in the generation of the hyperdynamic circulation and fluid retention in experimental cirrhosis. Increased expression of nNOS in mesenteric nerves may compensate partially for eNOS deficiency in eNOS knockout mice and reduce intrahepatic venous resistance and portal hypertension.[496] Also, splanchnic vasodilation is modestly promoted, possibly by modulating neurogenic NE release.[496] In contrast, the role of iNOS remains controversial; some researchers have shown increased iNOS in the superior mesenteric arteries of animals with experimental biliary cirrhosis but not in other forms of experimental cirrhosis.[496] Specific iNOS inhibition led to peripheral vasoconstriction, but had no effect on portal hypertension.[496] iNOS is primarily regulated at the transcription level by many proinflammatory factors, principally nuclear factor-kappaB (NF-κB), which could be induced by endotoxin, from translocated intestinal bacteria. Interestingly, there is also an interaction between eNOS and iNOS in the vasculature in cirrhosis. Overexpression of eNOS in large arteries results in systemic hypotension and increased blood flow. These effects can be abrogated by activated iNOS in the small splanchnic vessels.[496] Thus, overall, available data indicate a predominant role for eNOS deficiency, with possible modulation by both nNOS and iNOS.

In marked contrast to the increased NO generation in the splanchnic and systemic circulation, NO production and endothelial function in the intrahepatic microcirculation are impaired in cirrhotic rats.[496] The resulting paradoxical increase in intrahepatic vascular resistance is likely to result from contraction of myofibroblasts and stellate cells and mechanical distortion of the vasculature by fibrosis.[496] A second mechanism for the increased intrahepatic vascular resistance could be that the locally decreased NO production shifts the balance in favor of local vasoconstrictors (ET, leukotrienes, $TXA_2$, Ang II).[497] The increased vascular resistance may also play a role in the pathogenesis of intrahepatic thrombosis and collagen synthesis in cirrhosis.[497]

Several cellular mechanisms have been implicated in the upregulation of splanchnic eNOS and in the downregulation of intrahepatic eNOS. Elevation in shear stress as a result of the hyperdynamic circulation and portal hypertension has already been mentioned and is generally consistent with this well-documented mechanism for upregulating eNOS gene transcription. However, eNOS activity is not only regulated transcriptionally, but also posttranscriptionally, by tetrahydrobiopterin ($THB_4$) and direct phosphorylation of eNOS protein.[496] Furthermore, circulating endotoxins may increase the enzymatic production of $THB_4$, thereby enhancing mesenteric vascular eNOS activity.[496]

Potential contributors to intrahepatic eNOS downregulation include interactions with caveolin, calmodulin, heat shock protein 90, eNOS trafficking inducer,[496] disorders of GC activity,[498] and increased levels of the NO inhibitor, ADMA.[498] In fact, ADMA levels correlate with the severity of portal hypertension during hepatic inflammation and levels are higher in patients with decompensated than compensated cirrhosis.[499] Raised ADMA levels have been linked to reduced activity of dimethylarginine dimethylaminohydrolases (DDAHs) that metabolize ADMA to citrulline.[500] Similarly, patients with alcoholic cirrhosis and superimposed alcoholic hepatitis have higher plasma and tissue levels of ADMA, higher portal venous pressures and decreased DDAH expression.[499] However, attempts at pharmacological or genetic upregulation of DDAH to reduce ADMA levels and increase NO in experimental cirrhosis have not translated into improved management of decompensated portal hypertension.[501]

In the final analysis, the relative importance of the various mechanisms involved in the reduced intrahepatic and increased splanchnic and systemic NOS activity in cirrhosis remains to be determined.

***Endocannabinoids.*** Endogenous cannabinoids are lipid-signaling molecules that mimic the activity of Δ9-tetrahydrocannabinol, the main psychotropic constituent of marijuana. *N*-arachidonoylethanolamide (anandamide) and 2-arachidonoylglycerol are the most widely studied endocannabinoids that bind the two specific receptors, $CB_1$ and $CB_2$. Anandamide also interacts with the vanilloid receptor.[502]

In animal models of cirrhosis, both $CB_1$ and $CB_2$ receptors and endocannabinoid production are greatly upregulated and anandamide caused a dose-dependent increase in intrahepatic vascular resistance, especially in the isolated perfused cirrhotic liver. The effect appeared to be mediated by $CB_1$ receptor-enhanced production of COX-derived vasoconstrictive eicosanoids. Also, the $CB_1$ receptor antagonist, rimonabant, in cirrhotic rats reversed arterial hypotension, increased hepatic vascular resistance, decreased mesenteric arterial blood flow and portal venous pressure, and prevented ascites formation. The reduction in splanchnic blood flow was enhanced by the vanilloid receptor antagonist, capsazepine. These findings indicate that the transient receptor potential vanilloid type 1 protein and the $CB_1$ receptor have a dual role in the splanchnic vasodilation characteristic of cirrhosis.[502]

Endotoxin was found to be a major stimulus for endocannabinoid generation in monocytes and platelets of cirrhotic animals. This pathway could operate in patients with advanced cirrhosis in whom elevated circulating endotoxin levels are frequently found. Endocannabinoid production could then trigger splanchnic and peripheral vasodilation, arterial hypotension, and intrahepatic vasoconstriction through activation of $CB_1$ receptors in the vascular wall and perivascular nerves.[502] The potentially favorable effect of $CB_1$ receptor blockade on $Na^+$ excretion opens the possibility of pharmacologic modification of human HRS.

In summary, afferent sensing of volume in cirrhosis is characterized by increased intrahepatic vascular resistance and sinusoidal pressure, decreased portal venous blood flow, and increased hepatic arterial flow. Either changes in intrahepatic physical forces or in the composition of the mixed intrahepatic blood could initiate abnormal $Na^+$ retention and edema formation (see Fig. 14.11B). Side-to-side portocaval shunt (currently performed by transjugular intrahepatic portovenous shunt insertion) prevents (if inserted before induction of cirrhosis) or corrects (if inserted after induction of cirrhosis) renal $Na^+$ retention. This outcome could result from decreases in sinusoidal pressure or maintenance of the mixing of portal venous and hepatic arterial blood perfusing the liver. In contrast, it diverts blood to the inferior vena cava (IVC), but only partially decreases sinusoidal pressure and prevents mixing of portal venous and arterial hepatic blood supplies. Although portal venous pressure is normalized, $Na^+$ retention continues unabated (see Fig. 14.11B). Consequently, end-to-side shunting is no longer used clinically.

***Afferent Sensing of Intrahepatic Hypertension.*** Available data are most consistent with the view that the putative EABV sensor(s) in the hepatic circulation is pathologically activated in cirrhosis, failing to respond to the expanded ECF volume.[87]

The sensing mechanisms likely respond specifically to elevated hepatic venous pressure with increased hepatic afferent nerve activity. The relays for these impulses consist of two autonomic nerve plexuses, surrounding the hepatic artery and portal vein, respectively.[503] These neural networks connect hepatic venous congestion to enhanced renal and cardiopulmonary sympathetic activity.

Occlusion of the IVC at the diaphragm was associated with increases in hepatic, portal and renal venous pressures and resulted in markedly increased hepatic afferent nerve traffic and renal and cardiopulmonary sympathetic efferent nerve activity. Section of the anterior hepatic nerves eliminated the reflex increase in renal efferent nerve activity[503] and hepatic denervation in dogs with IVC constriction increased urinary $Na^+$ excretion.[89] This effect of hepatic denervation was shown to be mediated by the adenosine A1 receptor in cirrhotic rats.[504]

Apart from the adenosine-mediated hepatorenal reflex, other currently undefined humoral pathways could provide an anatomic or physiologic basis for the primary effects of alterations in intrahepatic hemodynamics on renal function. Despite the wealth of information on hepatic volume sensing, the molecular identity, cellular location of the sensor, and what is sensed remain elusive.

***Arterial Underfilling.*** Several mechanisms have been proposed to account for the development of relative hypovolemia. The first is disruption in normal Starling relationships governing fluid movement in the hepatic sinusoids. Unlike other capillaries, these are highly permeable to plasma proteins. As a result, partitioning of ECF between the intravascular (intrasinusoidal) and interstitial (space of Disse) and lymphatic compartments of the liver is determined predominantly by the $\Delta P$ along the length of the hepatic sinusoids. Obstruction of hepatic venous outflow promotes enhanced efflux of a protein-rich filtrate into the space of Disse and results in augmented hepatic lymph formation.[486,505] In parallel, vastly increased hepatic lymph formation is accompanied by increased flow through the thoracic duct.[506] When the rate of enhanced hepatic lymph formation exceeds the capacity for return to the intravascular compartment via the thoracic duct, hepatic lymph accumulates as ascites and the intravascular compartment is further compromised. As liver disease progresses, fibrosis around Kupffer cells lining the sinusoids renders the sinusoids less permeable to serum proteins. Under such circumstances, termed "capillarization of sinusoids," a decrease in oncotic pressure also promotes transudation of ECF within the hepatic lymph space, as in other vascular beds.[507]

Another consequence of intrahepatic hypertension is transmission of elevated intrasinusoidal pressures to the portal vein. This leads to expansion of the splanchnic venous system, collateral vein formation and portosystemic shunting, resulting in increased vascular capacitance and diversion of blood flow from the arterial circuit.[508] Not only splanchnic but also systemic vasodilation occurs and this has been attributed to refractoriness to the vasoconstrictive effects of hormones such as Ang II and catecholamines, although the mechanism remains unknown.[509] Along with diminished hepatic reticuloendothelial cell function, portosystemic shunting allows various products of intestinal metabolism and absorption to bypass the liver and escape hepatic elimination. Among these products, endotoxins are thought to contribute to perturbations in renal function in cirrhosis, either due to intestinal bacterial translocation, stimulating the release of proinflammatory cytokines (e.g., tumor necrosis factor-$\alpha$ [TNF-$\alpha$] and interleukin-6), secondary to the hemodynamic consequences of endotoxemia, or through direct renal effects.[486]

Levels of conjugated bilirubin and bile acids may become elevated as a result of intrahepatic cholestasis or extrahepatic biliary obstruction. Bile acids directly decrease proximal tubular reabsorption of $Na^+$, tending to promote natriuresis.[510] This diuretic effect might contribute to the underfilling state in advanced cirrhosis.[510,511]

Hypoalbuminemia in advanced cirrhosis, either as a result of decreased synthesis by the liver or dilution caused by ECF volume expansion, could also contribute to the development of hypovolemia by diminishing COP in the systemic capillaries and hepatic sinusoids.[507] In addition, tense ascites might reduce venous return (preload) to the heart, leading to reduced cardiac output and diminished arterial BP.[484]

Other factors that may also adversely affect cardiac performance include diminished $\beta$-adrenergic receptor signal transduction, cardiomyocyte cellular plasma membrane dysfunction, and increased activity or levels of cardiodepressants, such as cytokines, endocannabinoids, and NO. Although the cardiac dysfunction, termed "cirrhotic cardiomyopathy," usually is clinically mild or silent, overt HF can be precipitated by stresses such as liver transplantation or transjugular intrahepatic portosystemic shunt (TIPS) insertion.[484] Finally, intravascular volume depletion in cirrhotic patients may be aggravated by vomiting, occult variceal bleeding and excessive diuretic use, leading to cardiovascular collapse.

Table 14.6 summarizes the various causative factors contributing to underfilling of the circulation in patients with advanced liver disease. In summary, the early stages of compensated cirrhosis are characterized by increased plasma volume, which frequently antedates ascites formation.[512] However, as cirrhosis progresses, EABV decreases, leading to increased neurohumoral activity (RAAS, SNS, and AVP) and severe $Na^+$ and water retention.

**Abnormalities of Effector Mechanisms in Cirrhosis.** The efferent limb of volume regulation in cirrhosis is similar to that in HF, consisting of adjustments in glomerular hemodynamics and tubular transport mediated by vasoconstrictor/antinatriuretic forces (RAAS, SNS, AVP, and ET) and

**Table 14.6 Factors Causing Underfilling of the Circulation in Cirrhosis**

| |
|---|
| Peripheral vasodilation and blunted vasoconstrictor response to reflex, chemical and hormonal influences |
| Arteriovenous shunts, particularly in portal circulation |
| Increased vascular capacity of portal and systemic circulation |
| Hypoalbuminemia |
| Impaired left ventricular function, so-called cirrhotic cardiomyopathy |
| Diminished venous return secondary to advanced tense ascites |
| Occult gastrointestinal bleeding from ulcers, gastritis, or varices |
| Volume losses caused by vomiting and excessive use of diuretics |

counterbalanced by vasodilator/natriuretic systems (NPs and PG). Tilting the balance toward $Na^+$ retaining forces leads to renal $Na^+$ and water retention, as in HF.[485]

## VASOCONSTRICTOR AND ANTINATIURETIC (ANTIDIURETIC) SYSTEMS

### Renin-Angiotensin-Aldosterone System

As in HF, the RAAS plays a central role in mediating renal $Na^+$ retention in cirrhosis. Although positive $Na^+$ balance may already be evident in the preascitic phase of the disease, PRA and aldosterone levels remain within the normal range or may even be depressed at this stage.[513] With progression of the disease, RAAS activation increases in parallel and aldosterone levels are inversely correlated with renal $Na^+$ excretion in preascitic cirrhotic patients, particularly in the upright position.[513] Moreover, treatment with the ARB, losartan, at a dosage that did not affect systemic and renal hemodynamics or GFR, was associated with a significant natriuresis,[514] likely due to inhibition of the local intrarenal RAAS.[513,514] Indeed, activation of the intrarenal RAAS may precede systemic activation.[515] In addition, losartan caused a decrease in portal venous pressure in cirrhotic patients with portal hypertension.[516] The postural-induced RAAS activation and the beneficial effects of low-dose losartan treatment in preascitic cirrhosis may be explained by splanchnic venous compartmentalization of the expanded blood volume on standing and translocation toward the central and arterial circulatory beds during recumbency.[513]

In contrast, in $Na^+$-retaining cirrhotic patients with ascites, Ang II inhibition, even at low doses, resulted in decreased GFR and $Na^+$ excretion.[517] At this stage of the disease, RAAS activation serves to maintain arterial pressure and adequate circulation. Therefore, RAAS blockade may lead to a profound decrease in RPP. This scenario might be important in the pathogenesis of the HRS, which is regularly preceded by $Na^+$ retention and may be precipitated by a hypovolemic insult. Abnormalities of the renal circulation in HRS include marked diminution of RPF with renal cortical ischemia and increased renal vascular resistance, abnormalities consistent with the known actions of Ang II on the renal microcirculation.[518] In this regard, RAAS activation correlates with worsening hepatic hemodynamics and decreased survival in patients with cirrhosis.[519] Therefore ACEIs and ARBs should be avoided in patients with cirrhosis and ascites.

Evolving knowledge on the ACE2, Ang 1–7, Mas receptor pathway has shed new light on the role of the RAAS in the pathogenesis of $Na^+$ retention in cirrhosis. In this regard, exogenous Ang 1–7 elicited a marked NO-dependent vasodilatory effect on the Ang-II-evoked vasoconstrictive response in the portal vein of isolated perfused cirrhotic rat liver.[520,521] The data raise the possibility of reducing intrahepatic resistance and portal pressure by targeted upregulation of the alternate RAAS pathway in the liver.[522]

### Sympathetic Nervous System

Activation of the SNS is characteristic of cirrhosis and ascites.[523] Circulating NE levels, as well as urinary excretion of catecholamines and their metabolites, are elevated in patients with cirrhosis and usually are correlated with the severity of the disease. Moreover, high levels of plasma NE in patients with decompensated cirrhosis are predictive of increased mortality.[523] The increased NE levels stem from enhanced SNS activity, rather than reduced dissipation, with nerve terminal spillover from hepatic, cardiac, renal, muscular, and cutaneous innervation.[524] Elevated plasma NE levels were correlated closely with $Na^+$ and water retention in cirrhotic patients.[525] In addition, increased efferent renal sympathetic tone, perhaps due to defective arterial and cardiopulmonary baroreflex control, was observed in experimental cirrhosis.[526,527] This scenario could explain why volume expansion does not suppress enhanced RSNA in cirrhosis.

Concomitant with the increase in NE release, cardiovascular responsiveness to reflex autonomic stimulation may be impaired in patients with cirrhosis.[525] This impairment could be explained partially by increased occupancy of endogenous catecholamine receptors, downregulation of adrenergic receptors, or a defect in postreceptor signaling.[524] Excessive NO-dependent vasodilation alone could, in fact, account for the vascular hyporesponsiveness in cirrhosis.[528,529] Also, enhanced release of NPY may be a compensatory mechanism to counteract splanchnic vasodilation by restoring the vasoconstrictor efficacy of endogenous catecholamines.[524]

The increase in RSNA and plasma NE levels could contribute to the antinatriuresis of cirrhosis by decreasing total RBF, or its intrarenal distribution, or by acting directly on the tubular epithelium to enhance $Na^+$ reabsorption. Patients with compensated cirrhosis may have decreased RBF and, as the disease progresses, RBF tends to decline further, concomitantly with increased sympathetic activity.[523] Indeed, SNS activation in cirrhotic patients is associated with a rightward and downward shift of the RBF-RPP autoregulatory curve such that RBF becomes critically dependent on RPP. This phenomenon was found to contribute to the development of the HRS. Furthermore, insertion of TIPS to reduce portal venous pressure in patients with HRS leads to a fall in plasma NE levels and to an upward shift in the RBF-RPP curve.[530]

Reflex activation of the splenic afferent and renal sympathetic nerves also controls renal microvascular tone. In portal hypertension, the splenorenal reflex–mediated reduction in renal vascular conductance exacerbates $Na^+$ and water retention and may eventually contribute to renal dysfunction. Also increased splenic venous outflow pressure resulting from, but independent of, portal hypertension, reflexly activates adrenergic-angiotensinergic and vasodilator mesenteric nerves, and the RAAS. Finally, the spleen itself may be the source of a vasoactive factor.[531,532]

The centrality of SNS overactivity in cirrhosis has been illustrated by the finding that in patients with cirrhosis and increased SNS activity, addition of clonidine or guanfacine to diuretic treatment induces an earlier and enhanced diuretic response, with fewer complications.[533,534] In advanced cirrhosis, increased SNS activity parallels increases in RAAS and AVP activities.[534] This marked neurohumoral activation probably reflects a shift toward decompensation, characterized by a severe decrease in EABV depletion.[535] Overall, the three pressor systems might be activated by the same mechanisms and operate in concert to counteract the low arterial BP and decrease in EABV.[483]

### Arginine Vasopressin

Impaired water excretion as a result of nonosmotic release of AVP secondary to decreased EABV is frequent in advanced cirrhosis, leading to water retention with hyponatremia.[536]

Affected patients also have higher PRA and aldosterone levels and lower urinary $Na^+$ excretion.[483] In rats with experimental cirrhosis, plasma levels of AVP were elevated in association with overexpression of hypothalamic AVP mRNA and diminished pituitary AVP content.[537] Concomitantly increased expression of AQP2, the AVP-regulated water channel in the collecting duct, was significantly diminished by the AVP receptor antagonist, terlipressin, indicating the important role of AQP2 in the water retention associated with hepatic cirrhosis.[538]

As noted earlier, AVP supports arterial BP through its action on the $V_1$ receptors on VSMC, whereas the $V_2$ receptor is responsible for water transport in the collecting duct.[539] The availability of selective blockers of these receptors has provided clear evidence for the dual roles of AVP in pathogenesis of cirrhosis.[412,539] Thus, administration of a $V_2$ receptor antagonist to cirrhotic patients, as well as to rats with experimental cirrhosis, increases urine volume, decreases urine osmolality, and corrects hyponatremia[412,539] (see further discussion in section, "Specific Treatments Based on the Pathophysiology of Sodium Retention in Cirrhosis").

AVP also increases the synthesis of the vasodilatory $PGE_2$ and $PGI_2$ in renal and other vascular beds, as well as in the collecting duct. This increase may offset the vasoconstrictive, as well as the hydroosmotic effect of AVP in cirrhosis.[540]

#### Endothelin

Levels of ET-1 and big ET-1 in plasma, splanchnic, and renal venous beds are markedly elevated in patients with cirrhosis and ascites, as well as in the HRS.[541,542] Levels correlate positively with portal venous pressure and cardiac output and inversely with central blood volume.[542] The rise in ET-1 is accompanied by a reduction in ET-3 levels and the consequently elevated ET-1/ET-3 ratio is associated with a poor outcome of portal hypertension.[543] In animal models of cirrhosis with portal hypertension, ET-A receptor activation and attenuated ET-B receptor repression on the portal vein has been reported.[544] ET-B receptor blockade led to sinusoidal constriction and hepatotoxicity,[545] whereas the dual ET-A and B receptor blocker, tezosentan, had no effect on hepatic blood flow.[546]

In humans with HRS, ET-1 and big ET-1 levels were significantly reduced in portal and renal veins 1 to 2 months after TIPS insertion, with a parallel increase in creatinine clearance and urinary $Na^+$ excretion.[541] Similar improvements have been observed within 1 week after successful orthotopic liver transplantation.[547] Conversely, temporary occlusion of TIPS by angioplasty balloon inflation led to a transient increase in portal venous pressure, increased plasma ET-1, marked reduction of RPF, and increased intrarenal generation of ET-1.[548]

The importance of the intrarenal ET system has been demonstrated in a rat model of HRS.[549] Plasma ET-1 increased twofold after the onset of liver and renal failure and the ET-A receptor was upregulated in the renal cortex. Bosentan, a nonselective ET receptor antagonist, prevented the development of renal failure when given before or 24 hours after onset of liver injury.[549]

Increased intrahepatic production of ET probably also contributes to the development of portal (and pulmonary) hypertension in cirrhosis through contraction of the stellate cells and a concomitant decrease in sinusoidal blood flow.[550] To summarize, the hemodynamic changes in cirrhosis with refractory ascites could be related to local ET-1 production by the splanchnic and renal vascular beds. After TIPS and orthotopic liver transplantation, there are improvements in both ET and other vasoconstrictive factors (e.g., RAAS and vasopressin).[551] Therefore, the contribution of the intrarenal ET system relative to other vasoconstrictor hormones in the pathogenesis of the HRS remains speculative.

#### Apelin

The possible involvement of apelin in the pathogenesis of cirrhosis was suggested by the raised plasma levels[552] and enhanced expression of its receptor in proliferated arterial capillaries directly connected with sinusoids.[553,554] In addition, an apelin receptor antagonist led to a reduction in the raised cardiac index, reversal of the increased total peripheral resistance, and improvement in $Na^+$ and water excretion in rats with experimental cirrhosis.[552] However, to date no therapeutic role of apelin antagonism in the management of severe HRS has been elucidated, possibly owing to the complex effects of apelin on glomerular hemodynamics.[338]

### VASODILATORS/NATIURETICS

Apart from their role in the hyperdynamic circulation characteristic of advanced cirrhosis, vasodilators play an important part in the pathogenesis of renal $Na^+$ retention. The principal vasodilators involved are NPs and PGs.

#### Natriuretic Peptides

**Atrial Natriuretic Peptide.** In recent years, measurements of BNP and NT-proBNP have largely superseded ANP as a biomarker of cirrhosis and portal hypertension. Nevertheless, the role of NPs in the pathogenesis of HRS was largely elucidated through studies on ANP and these are summarized here. Plasma ANP is elevated in cirrhosis at all stages, irrespective of the EABV.[555,556] In the preascitic stage, increased plasma ANP may be important for the maintenance of $Na^+$ homeostasis, but with progression of the disease, resistance to the natriuretic action of the peptide develops.[555,556] The high levels of ANP mostly reflect increased cardiac release rather than impaired clearance.[557] The stimulus for increased cardiac ANP synthesis and release in early cirrhosis is likely increased left atrial size caused by overfilling of the circulation, secondary to intrahepatic hypertension–related renal $Na^+$ retention.[558]

In addition to elevated ANP, preascitic patients also had significantly elevated left and right pulmonary volumes, despite normal BP, PRA, aldosterone, and NE levels.[559] High $Na^+$ intake in these patients resulted in weight gain and positive $Na^+$ balance for 3 weeks, followed by a return to normal $Na^+$ balance, thereby preventing fluid retention and the development of ascites.[560] The factors responsible for maintaining relatively high levels of ANP during the later stages of cirrhosis, in association with arterial underfilling, may be related to a futile cycle of mutual interactions between vasoconstrictor/$Na^+$-retaining and vasodilatory/natriuretic forces. The fact that ANP levels do not increase further as patients proceed from early to late decompensated stages of cirrhosis would be consistent with this explanation. Furthermore, infusion of Ang II mimicked the nonresponder state by causing patients with cirrhosis, who still responded to ANP, to become unresponsive.[561] This Ang II effect occurred at proximal (decreased distal delivery of $Na^+$) and distal nephron sites to abrogate ANP-induced natriuresis and was reversible. The importance of distal solute delivery was confirmed using mannitol, which also resulted in an improved natriuretic response to ANP in responders but not nonresponders.[562,563] ANP resistance was also ameliorated by endopeptidase inhibitors, renal sympathetic denervation, peritoneovenous shunting and orthotopic liver transplantation.[564–567]

To summarize, ANP resistance is best explained by an effect of decreased delivery of $Na^+$ to ANP-responsive distal nephron sites (glomerulotubular imbalance caused by abnormal systemic hemodynamics and activation of the RAAS) combined with an overriding effect of more powerful antinatriuretic factors to overcome the natriuretic action of ANP in the medullary collecting tubule.[568] The latter effect could result from decreased delivery as well as permissive paracrine/autocrine cofactors, such as PGs and kinins.

**Brain Natriuretic Peptide and C-Type Natriuretic Peptide.** BNP levels are also elevated in cirrhosis with ascites and, like ANP, its natriuretic effect is blunted in these patients.[569–572] Plasma BNP levels may be correlated with cardiac dysfunction[570] and severity of disease and may be of prognostic value in the progression of cirrhosis.[572,573] Plasma CNP levels in cirrhotic preascitic patients, although normal, were directly correlated with natriuresis and urine volume[574] and inversely correlated with arterial compliance but not SVR.[575] These data suggested that compensatory downregulation of CNP occurs in cirrhosis when vasodilation persists and that regulation of large and small arteries by CNP may differ.

In contrast with the preascitic stage, patients with more advanced disease and impaired renal function had lower plasma and higher urinary CNP levels than those with intact renal function. Moreover, urinary CNP was correlated inversely with urinary $Na^+$ excretion. In patients with refractory ascites or HRS treated with terlipressin infusion or TIPS (see later section, "Specific Treatments Based on the Pathophysiology of Sodium Retention in Cirrhosis"), urinary CNP declined and urinary $Na^+$ excretion increased 1 week later.[574,665] Thus CNP may have a significant role in renal $Na^+$ handling in cirrhosis.

Finally, *Dendroaspis* NP levels were found to be increased in cirrhotic patients with ascites, but not in those without and levels were correlated with disease severity.[576] The significance of these findings remains unknown.

#### Prostaglandins

As noted, PG modulate the hydroosmotic effect of AVP and protect RPF and GFR when the activity of endogenous vasoconstrictor systems is increased. These properties of PG appear to be critical in decompensated cirrhosis with ascites but no renal failure. Such patients excrete more vasodilatory PG than healthy subjects, suggesting that renal production of PG is increased.[577] Similarly, in experimental cirrhosis, there is increased synthesis and activity of renal and vascular PG as well as upregulation of COX-2.[577,578] $PGE_2$ upregulation in the thick ascending limb of preascitic cirrhotic rats is mediated by downregulation of calcium-sensing receptors (CaSRs). This maneuver resulted in increased expression of the NKCC2, increased $Na^+$ reabsorption in this segment, and augmented free water reabsorption in the collecting duct. The effects were reversed by the CaSR agonist poly-L-arginine.[579]

Not surprisingly, nonselective COX inhibitors resulted in a significant decrease in GFR and RPF in cirrhotic patients, with or without ascites. The decrement in renal hemodynamics varied directly with the degree of $Na^+$ retention and neurohumoral activation, so that patients with high PRA and NE levels were particularly sensitive to these adverse effects.[577,578] These negative effects of COX- inhibition appear to be solely COX-1-dependent because selective COX-2 antagonists spare renal function in both human and experimental cirrhosis, even with ascites.[577,578] The favorable renal effect of selective COX-2 antagonists may be indirect and related to hepatic upregulation of COX-2 in that celecoxib can ameliorate portal hypertension by hepatic anti-angiogenic and antifibrotic actions.[580]

In contrast with nonazotemic patients with cirrhosis and ascites, patients with HRS have reduced renal synthesis of vasodilatory PG.[581] However, treatment with intravenous $PGE_2$ or its oral analogue, misoprostol, did not improve renal function in HRS patients.[582] This $PGE_2$ resistance may be related to overwhelming neurohumoral vasoconstrictive/antinatriuretic effects and may be crucial in the pathogenesis of HRS.[577]

#### Integrated View of the Pathogenesis of Sodium Retention in Cirrhosis

Portal hypertension leads to increased intestinal permeability, bacterial translocation, endotoxemia and exposure to bacterial DNA. In turn, hepatic NO and PG increase, leading to splanchnic, then systemic vasodilation, with increased cardiac output, decreased SVR, and arterial pressure ("hyperdynamic circulation"). The resulting imbalance between vascular capacity and plasma volume induces baroceptor and subsequent neurohumoral activation (RAAS, SNS) leading to systemic and renal vasoconstriction, $Na^+$ retention, and maintained circulation (compensated cirrhosis). In addition, a yet elusive hepatic-derived factor may also act directly to induce renal $Na^+$ retention (overflow theory). If there is enough compensatory increase in systemic natriuretic factors and renal synthesis of PG and NO, renal function is also maintained. However, as cirrhosis advances and portal hypertension worsens, features of the HRS appear: EABV falls (underfilling), vasoconstrictive/antinatriuretic factors dominate over vasodilatory/natriuretic factors, GFR declines, and $Na^+$ retention is further exacerbated leading to edema and ascites. Also, at this stage nonosmotic release of AVP becomes prominent, leading to impaired water excretion and hyponatremia.

## CLINICAL MANIFESTATIONS OF HYPERVOLEMIA

Apart from the clinical manifestations of the underlying disease, the symptoms and signs of hypervolemia per se depend on the amount and relative distribution of fluid between the intravascular and interstitial spaces. Arterial volume overload is manifested as hypertension, whereas venous overload is characterized by raised jugular venous pressure (JVP). Interstitial fluid accumulation appears as peripheral edema, effusions in the pleural or peritoneal cavity (ascites) or in the alveolar space (pulmonary edema), or a combination of these. If cardiac and hepatic functions are normal and transcapillary Starling forces intact, the excess volume is distributed proportionately throughout the ECF compartments. In this situation, the signs of hypervolemia will be hypertension and raised JVP. Peripheral edema appears only when interstitial volume overload exceeds 3 L, usually due to ongoing renal $Na^+$ retention.

When cardiac systolic function is impaired, as a result of myocardial, valvular, or pericardial disease, pulmonary and systemic venous hypertension predominate, and systemic BP may be low as a result of disproportionate fluid accumulation in the venous rather than the arterial circulation. Disruption in transcapillary Starling forces, as found in advanced cardiac and hepatic disease, may lead to fluid transudation into the pleural and peritoneal spaces, manifested as pleural effusions and ascites, respectively.

As already mentioned, advanced cirrhosis or fulminant hepatic failure lead to ascites and oliguric renal failure in the absence of diuretics, nephrotoxins, shock, and without evidence of significant intrarenal pathology. This is referred to as hepatorenal syndrome (HRS). Two subtypes of HRS have been defined. Type 1 is characterized by a rapid decline in renal function (doubling of serum creatinine level to >2.5 mg/dL, or 50% reduction in creatinine clearance to <20 mL/min) over a 2-week period. Typically, an acute precipitating factor can be identified. Type 2 develops spontaneously and progressively over months (serum creatinine level >1.5 mg/dL, or creatinine clearance <40 mL/min). More recently the International Club of Ascites has adopted the AKIN criteria for AKI, a rise of 0.3 mg/dL and/or 50% or more rise from baseline for the diagnosis of HRS. This more sensitive definition allows the possibility for earlier treatment of HRS but has yet to be tested in terms of prognostic significance.[483,535] HRS is discussed in detail in Chapter 28.

## DIAGNOSIS

The diagnosis of hypervolemia is usually evident from the clinical history and physical examination. Any combination of peripheral edema, raised JVP, pulmonary crepitations, and pleural effusions is likely to be diagnostic. In the presence of these findings, high BP would suggest renal failure as the cause of hypervolemia, whereas relatively low BP would point to severe HF or advanced cirrhosis as the precipitating factor. In more enigmatic cases, in which dyspnea is the sole complaint and clinical findings are minimal, measurement of plasma biomarkers such as BNP, NTproBNP, and MR-proANP may help distinguish between cardiac and pulmonary causes of the dyspnea.[583,584]

Simple laboratory tests may aid in confirming the clinical diagnosis. An elevated cardiac troponin level is consistent with myocardial damage and high levels may be observed in acute decompensated HF.[585,586] Transaminase levels may be raised in hepatic disease and hypoalbuminemia would be consistent with hepatic cirrhosis or nephrotic-range proteinuria caused by glomerular disease. The latter, of course, is confirmed by appropriate urine testing.

When BP is low, evidence of prerenal azotemia (increased ratio of blood urea nitrogen [BUN] to creatinine) may be found, as in advanced cardiac or hepatic failure (cardiorenal syndrome and HRS, respectively); intrinsic renal failure—proportionate increases in BUN and creatinine—may also ensue (see Chapter 28 for detailed discussion). Low EABV in the presence of hypervolemia is confirmed by a low urine $Na^+$ concentration or low fractional excretion of $Na^+$, indicative of secondary renal $Na^+$ retention.

## TREATMENT

Therapy for volume overload can be divided into management of the volume overload itself and prevention or minimization of its recurrence and associated morbidity and mortality. The critical first step is recognition and treatment of the underlying cause of hypervolemia. Thus, when the EABV is significantly reduced, as in cardiac and hepatic failure (or severe nephrotic syndrome), hemodynamic parameters should be optimized. Otherwise, therapy to induce negative $Na^+$ balance is associated with an enhanced risk for worsening hemodynamic compromise.

Once the EABV is restored, negative $Na^+$ balance can be induced by dietary $Na^+$ restriction, diuretics, and extracorporeal ultrafiltration. The degree of hypervolemia and the clinical urgency for $Na^+$ removal determine which modality should be used. Therefore, in a patient with life-threatening pulmonary edema, immediate intravenous loop diuretics are indicated; if high doses of these drugs do not induce significant diuresis, then extracorporeal ultrafiltration may be life-saving. At the other extreme, a hypertensive patient with mild volume overload and preserved renal function may require only dietary salt restriction and a thiazide diuretic.

Once acute hypervolemia has been controlled, therapy is directed toward the prevention or minimization of further acute episodes and improvement in prognosis. In addition to maintenance diuretic treatment, several strategies, based on the pathophysiologic process of $Na^+$ retention, are available clinically or are under experimental development.

### Sodium Restriction

Until recently, the prevailing belief was that effective management of hypervolemia of any cause must include $Na^+$ restriction. Without this intervention, the success of diuretic therapy was thought to be limited because the relative hypovolemia induced by diuretics led to compensatory $Na^+$ retention, increased diuretic dosage, further reduction in EABV and still more renal $Na^+$ retention. However, this view was challenged by a randomized controlled trial in patients with acute decompensated HF. In this study, no difference in weight loss or clinical stability was observed at 3 days between the group restricted to 800 mg sodium/day and those with a more liberal sodium intake. Moreover, those on the severely sodium-restricted diet were significantly thirstier than their less restricted counterparts.[587] In light of these new data, a reasonable goal is to restrict $Na^+$ intake to 50 to 80 mmol (approximately 3 to 5 g of salt/day).[588] Because of the generally poor palatability of salt-restricted diets, salt substitutes may be used; however, these preparations usually contain high concentrations of potassium and must be used with caution by patients with renal impairment or those taking potassium-retaining RAAS antagonists.

In hospitalized patients, extra attention must be paid to amounts and types of intravenous fluids administered. A frequent scenario encountered by nephrologists consulted in internal medicine departments is a patient receiving intravenous saline together with high-dose diuretics. The usual rationale offered for this combination is that the saline will expand the intravascular volume while the diuretic will mobilize excess interstitial volume. This logic has no sound physiologic or therapeutic basis, since both modalities operate principally on the intravascular space. Moreover, the combination of saline and furosemide in HF is associated with adverse outcomes.[589] Furthermore, water restriction is also inappropriate, except in the presence of accompanying hyponatremia (plasma $Na^+$ <135 mmol/L). On the other hand, intravenous infusion of small volumes of hypertonic saline during diuretic dosing and liberalizing dietary salt intake while continuing to limit water consumption may improve fluid removal in HF patients. Furthermore, less deterioration in renal function, shorter hospitalizations, reduced readmission rates, and even reductions in mortality have been observed.[590,591]

### Diuretics

Diuretics are classified according to their sites of action along the nephron and are discussed in detail in Chapter 50. The reader is also referred to a comprehensive review.[592] Diuretics are described briefly here in relation to the treatment of hypervolemia.

**Proximal Tubule Diuretics.** The prototype proximal tubular diuretic is acetazolamide, a carbonic anhydrase inhibitor that inhibits the reabsorption of sodium bicarbonate. Prolonged use may cause hyperchloremic metabolic acidosis and the drug is usually used in the management of chronic glaucoma rather than for reducing volume overload. Another proximally acting diuretic is the thiazide-like metolazone, which also inhibits the NaCl cotransporter in the distal tubule. The proximal action of metolazone may be associated with phosphate loss greater than that seen with traditional thiazides.[593] In general, metolazone is used as an adjunct to loop diuretics in resistant HF.[594] Mannitol, which also inhibits proximal tubular reabsorption,[595] can be used in combination with furosemide for the management of acute decompensated HF.[596]

**Loop Diuretics.** This group includes the most powerful diuretics, furosemide, bumetanide, torsemide, and ethacrynic acid. They act by inhibiting transport via the NKCC2 in the apical membrane of the thick ascending limb of the loop of Henle (see Chapter 6).[592] They are used for the treatment of severe hypervolemia and hypertension, especially in stages 4 and 5 of chronic kidney disease. Loop diuretics may lead to hypokalemia, intravascular volume depletion, and worsening prerenal azotemia, especially in older patients and those with reduced EABV. They are also hypercalciuric.[597]

**Distal Tubule Diuretics.** Diuretics in this segment block the apical NaCl cotransporter and include hydrochlorothiazide, chlorthalidone and metolazone (see also earlier section, "Proximal Tubule Diuretics"). They are typically used as adjuncts to loop diuretics in resistant HF, particularly metolazone. Inhibition of $Na^+$ reabsorption by diuretics in the proximal tubule (except for carbonic anhydrase inhibitors), loop of Henle, and distal tubule leads to increased solute delivery to the collecting duct. Consequently, potassium and proton secretion are enhanced, which may lead to hypokalemia and metabolic alkalosis.[598] Thiazides are also hypocalciuric.[597]

**Collecting Duct Diuretics.** Collecting duct ($K^+$-sparing) diuretics operate by competing with aldosterone for occupation of the mineralocorticoid receptor (spironolactone, eplerenone) or by direct inhibition of the ENaC (amiloride and triamterene).[592] As their alternative name implies, important side effects of this group are hyperkalemia and metabolic acidosis, resulting from concomitant suppression of $K^+$ and proton secretion. Therefore, they are widely used in combination with thiazide and loop diuretics to minimize hypokalemia. Aldosterone antagonists are especially useful in the management of disorders characterized by secondary hyperaldosteronism, such as cirrhosis with ascites. Moreover, these drugs are cardioprotective and renoprotective via nonepithelial mineralocorticoid receptor blockade (see sections, "Pathophysiology" and "Specific Treatments Based on the Pathophysiology of Heart Failure" in this chapter; also see Chapter 12).

**Diuretic Resistance.** As noted, when $Na^+$ retention is severe and resistant to conventional doses of loop diuretics, combinations of diuretics acting at different nephron sites may produce effective natriuresis. Another method for overcoming diuretic resistance is the administration of a bolus dose of loop diuretic to yield a high plasma level, followed by high-dose continuous infusion. Alternately, high doses given intermittently may be successful in reversing diuretic resistance. There appears to be no difference between continuous infusion and repeated bolus administration of high or low doses of furosemide in improvement of shortness of breath or volume of diuresis at 72 hours after admission for acute decompensated HF.[599]

Whichever method is used to treat diuretic resistant hypervolemia, plasma $Na^+$, $K^+$, $Mg^{2+}$, $Ca^{2+}$, phosphate, BUN, and creatinine should be monitored carefully, and any deviations appropriately corrected. Rarer side effects of diuretics include cutaneous allergic reactions, acute interstitial nephritis (see Chapter 28), pancreatitis, and, rarely, blood dyscrasias.[600]

### Extracorpreal Ultrafiltration

On occasion, extreme resistance to diuretics occurs, often accompanied by renal functional impairment. In such cases, effective removal of volume excess may be achieved by ultrafiltration using hemofiltration, hemodialysis, peritoneal dialysis (see Chapter 65), or small devices designed for isolated ultrafiltration (UF).[599] Chronic ambulatory peritoneal dialysis may also reduce hospitalization rates in patients with resistant HF who are not candidates for surgical intervention.[601] However, a randomized controlled trial comparing intensive diuretic therapy with UF for the management of acute decompensated HF with worsened renal function (CARRESS-HF) was halted early because of lack of benefit of UF and an excess of early and late (60 days) adverse events.[602] Moreover, UF was inferior to diuretic therapy in terms of the bivariate primary endpoint of body weight and rise in serum creatinine level at 96 hours after commencement of therapy. Therefore, UF should currently be reserved for those patients with unequivocal diuretic resistance and as part of an algorithmic stepped approach to HF management.[599]

## SPECIFIC TREATMENTS BASED ON THE PATHOPHYSIOLOGY OF HEART FAILURE

Because the clinical situation of an HF patient at any given time depends on the delicate balance between vasoconstrictor/antinatriuretic and vasodilator/natriuretic factors, any treatment that can tip the balance in favor of the latter should be efficacious. Thus, treatment is aimed at either pharmacologically increasing natriuretic or reducing antinatriuretic mechanisms. The principal approaches include reducing RAAS or SNS activity or increasing NP activity.

## INHIBITION OF THE RENIN-ANGIOTENSIN-ALDOSTERONE SYSTEM

Based on the maladaptive actions of locally produced or circulatory Ang II, numerous studies have shown that ACE inhibition and ARBs improve renal function, cardiac performance and life expectancy of HF patients.[234,603] A small decline in GFR is occasionally observed as a result of blockade of Ang II–induced preferential efferent arteriolar constriction, which leads to a sharp fall in glomerular capillary pressure, but this is usually not clinically significant. Because patients with HF cannot overcome the $Na^+$-retaining action of aldosterone, blockade of the latter by spironolactone or eplerenone induces substantial natriuresis in these patients.[603]

Overall, the effect of RAAS inhibition on renal function in HF depends on a multiplicity of interacting factors. On the one hand, RBF may improve as a result of lower efferent arteriolar resistance. Systemic vasodilation may be associated with a rise in cardiac output. Under such circumstances, reversal of the hemodynamically mediated effects of Ang II on $Na^+$ reabsorption would promote natriuresis. Moreover, RAAS inhibition could facilitate the action of NPs to improve GFR and enhance $Na^+$ excretion. On the other hand, Ang II–induced elevation of the single-nephron filtration fraction facilitates preservation of GFR in the presence of diminished RPF. In patients with precarious renal hemodynamics, a fall in systemic arterial pressure below the autoregulatory range, combined with removal of the Ang II effect on glomerular hemodynamics, may cause severe deterioration of renal function. The net result depends on the integrated sum of these physiologic effects, which, in turn, depends on the severity of HF (Table 14.7).

**Table 14.7 Renal Effects of Renin-Angiotensin-Aldosterone System Inhibition in Heart Failure**

| |
|---|
| **Factors Favoring Improvement in Renal Function** |
| Maintenance of $Na^+$ balance |
| Reduction in diuretic dosage |
| Increase in $Na^+$ intake |
| Mean arterial pressure >80 mm Hg |
| Minimal neurohumoral activation |
| Intact counterregulatory mechanisms |
| **Factors Favoring Deterioration in Renal Function** |
| Evidence of $Na^+$ depletion or poor renal perfusion |
| Large doses of diuretics |
| Increased urea/creatinine ratio |
| Mean arterial pressure <80 mm Hg |
| Evidence of maximal neurohumoral activation |
| AVP-induced hyponatremia |
| Interruption of counterregulatory mechanisms |
| Coadministration of prostaglandin inhibitors |
| Adrenergic dysfunction (e.g., diabetes mellitus) |

*AVP*, Arginine vasopressin.

In addition to promoting $Na^+$ retention, the RAAS contributes to vascular and cardiac remodeling by inducing perivascular and interstitial fibrosis in HF.[234,604] In accordance with this mechanism, the addition of small doses of aldosterone inhibitors to standard therapy, including ACEIs or ARBs, substantially reduces mortality rate and morbidity in HF patients.[234,603] In contrast, combinations of ACEI and ARB are not useful and, often, are detrimental, owing to increased risk of hypotension, AKI, and hyperkalemia.[604] However, the combination of RAAS inhibitor, aldosterone inhibitor β-blocker, and low-dose loop diuretics is associated with a better prognosis than chronic use of increasing loop-diuretic dose alone.[605]

Finally, all patients receiving one or more RAAS inhibitors require careful follow-up for detection and management of hyperkalemia, particularly those with renal dysfunction.[604]

## β-BLOCKADE

Insofar as β-blockade is now the standard of care in the management of HF, this review would not be complete without mention of these drugs. However, because their effect in HF is not directly related to $Na^+$ and water, this important therapy is not elaborated further in this chapter. The reader is referred to a recent meta-analysis for up-to-date information.[606]

## NITRIC OXIDE DONOR AND REACTIVE OXYGEN SPECIES/PEROXYNITRATE SCAVENGERS

Because NO signaling is disrupted in HF, achieving NO balance by NO donors or selective NOS inhibitors could be important for correcting the pathophysiologic process of HF.[607] In this regard, the beneficial effects of combined isosorbide dinitrate (NO donor) and hydralazine (reactive oxygen species and peroxynitrite scavenger) therapy, particularly in African-American patients, are well-established.[608] Newer methods for enhancing NO activity include NOS and GC stimulators and inhibitors of GC breakdown.[607] Relaxin-mediated and waon-mediated NOS stimulation, in particular, are currently being tested in a phase 3 clinical trial. Relaxin mediates NO production both immediately via stimulation of eNOS and chronically via increased expression of iNOS. Treatment of acute HF with serelaxin, recombinant relaxin-2, was associated with dyspnea relief and reduced 180-day but had no effect on hospital readmission. Serelaxin treatment was well tolerated and safe.[609] Further trials are in the pipeline.

Waon or "soothing warm" therapy, which causes vasodilation via eNOS stimulation, is a thermal treatment developed in Japan and shown in a recent clinical trial to improve NYHA class and exercise tolerance in chronic HF.[610] Waon also enhanced the favorable actions of RAAS inhibition and reduced SNS activity.[611]

An additional strategy exploits upregulation of nNOS in the paraventricular nucleus and a reduction in sympathetic outflow. This observation raised the potential for nNOS upregulation by ACE2 therapy in HF.[612,613]

## ENDOTHELIN ANTAGONISTS

Acute ET nonselective antagonists decrease vascular resistance and increase cardiac index and cardiac output in HF. However, both short- and long-term clinical trials with ET-A receptor antagonists have demonstrated no benefits, but serious adverse events, including fluid retention, increased need for hospitalization, hepatic dysfunction, and mortality in HF patients.[614] These disappointing results may be explained by the observation that ET-A receptor antagonism in experimental HF further activates the RAAS in association with sustained $Na^+$ retention.[279] Moreover, the increased cardiac, pulmonary, and renal ET-1 production in HF, together with the marked vasoconstrictor and mitogenic properties of the molecule, suggest that ET-1 exacerbates $Na^+$ retention directly and indirectly by aggravating renal and cardiac functions, respectively.[279] In addition, nonspecific ET-B receptor blockade could have exacerbated cardiac remodeling. Given the antiproliferative effect of ET-B1–receptor activation and the detrimental vasoconstrictor effect of ET-B2 stimulation, combined ET-B1 stimulation and ET-B2 blockade was recently proposed for control of the remodeling associated with postischemic HF.[417] Concomitant ET-A blockade would help to prevent the undesired effects of unopposed ET-1 activity and exploit the established therapeutic effects of ET-A antagonists.[417] In this regard, a recent report that dual ET-A/ET-B receptor inhibition improves echocardiographic parameters in a mouse model of HF with preserved ejection fraction (HfpEF) is encouraging.[615] The favorable effects occurred by abrogating adverse cardiac remodeling and reducing stiffness. Additional studies on the role of dual ET-1 receptor antagonists in patients with HfpEF are eagerly awaited.

## NATRIURETIC PEPTIDES

As noted previously, circulating NP levels are elevated in HF in proportion to disease severity, but renal actions of NPs are attenuated in severe HF. Nevertheless, elimination of NP action using NPR-A blockers or surgical removal of the atrium disrupted renal function and cardiac performance in experimental HF.[616] Conversely, increasing circulating levels of NPs (BNP > ANP) by intravenous administration improved general clinical status,[617] reduced pulmonary arterial and capillary wedge pressures, right atrial pressure and SVR, with improved cardiac output, systemic BP and diuresis. In parallel, plasma NE and aldosterone levels were suppressed.[618] However, these beneficial effects have not translated into clinical efficacy, with several controlled studies showing minimal natriuretic effects of BNP (nesiritide) compared with placebo.[264] Furthermore, serious adverse events of nesiritide treatment were seen, including dose-related hypotension, worsening renal function, and possible increased risk of death.[264] Finally, in a randomized controlled trial comparing nesiritide or low-dose dopamine as add-on therapy to intravenous furosemide in patients with HF and renal dysfunction, no improvement in decongestion or renal function was observed with either combination therapy over furosemide alone.[619] Similarly, ularitide, the pharmacological equivalent of the NP, urodilatin, as add-on therapy did not affect a clinical composite endpoint or reduce long-term cardiovascular mortality, despite significant reductions in NT-proBNP levels (TRUE-AHF trial). Therefore, the therapeutic role of NP in HF remains unclear and novel approaches are being explored. These include strategies to convert the prohormone into its active form might be efficacious, CNP analogs and designer chimeric peptides such as CD-NP, consisting of CNP and part of DNP.[620]

## NEUTRAL ENDOPEPTIDASE INHIBITORS AND VASOPEPTIDASE INHIBITORS

Correcting the imbalance between the RAAS and NP systems can also be achieved by inhibiting the enzymatic degradation of NPs by NEP. In both experimental models and clinical trials NEP inhibitors enhanced plasma ANP and BNP levels in association with vasodilation, natriuresis, diuresis, reduced cardiac preload and afterload.[439] However, initial favorable hemodynamic, neurohormonal, and renal effects of NEP inhibitors in HF patients[621,622] were not confirmed in later studies. These showed enhanced RAAS activation, increased ET-1 levels and attenuated renal and hemodynamic improvement.[439] On the basis of these findings, combined RAAS and NEP (vasopeptidase) inhibitors were designed and, indeed, initially shown to have more favorable hemodynamic and renal effects, such as preserved GFR, than each treatment alone.[439]

However, randomized clinical trials indicated that neither vasopeptidase inhibitors nor NEP inhibitors as add-on therapy to RAAS inhibition were more effective than RAAS inhibitors alone in the treatment of HF. Furthermore, the combination was associated with a significantly increased incidence of severe angioedema.[439] Possible reasons for the failure of NEP inhibitors include disproportionate increase in RAAS and ET activity over time, the development of tolerance with chronic treatment and downregulation of NP receptors in response to degradation of NEP inhibitors. The increased incidence of angioedema with vasopeptidase inhibition may result from excessive accumulation of bradykinin or inhibition of aminopeptidase P.[439]

The challenge of preventing angioedema led to the development of combined ARB-NEP inhibition since ARBs do not disrupt bradykinin metabolism. Three trials in HF with reduced EF, IMPRESS, OVERTURE and PARADIGM-HF, compared combined NEP/RAS inhibition with RAS inhibition alone and reported clinical outcomes. The pooled hazard ratio (HR) for all-cause death or HF hospitalization and all-cause mortality was significantly reduced in patients receiving combined NEP/RAS inhibition in all three trials. Combined NEP/RAS inhibition compared with ACE inhibition was associated with more hypotension, but less renal dysfunction and hyperkalaemia.[623] These results pave the way for a paradigm shift in the management of severe HF.[624]

## VASOPRESSIN RECEPTOR ANTAGONISTS

AVP receptor antagonists (vaptans) are small, orally active, nonpeptide molecules that lack agonist effects and display high affinity for and specificity to their corresponding receptors.[412,625] Highly selective and potent antagonists for the $V_{1A}$, $V_2$, and $V_{1B}$ receptor subtypes and mixed $V_{1A}/V_2$ receptor antagonists are now available.[412] In clinical trials and experimental models of compensated and decompensated HF with hyponatremia, $V_2$ receptor–specific vaptans produced hemodynamic improvement, with transient decrease in SVR and increased cardiac output. Water diuresis caused decreases in body weight and edema, hyponatremia was corrected, and RBF and renal function stabilized.[412,625] Dyspnea lessened in some but not all patients. Both tolvaptan, a $V_2$ selective receptor antagonist, and conivaptan, a nonselective $V_{1A}/V_2$ receptor antagonist (both US Food and Drug Administration [FDA]-approved for use in HF) induced these favorable effects after treatment for up to 60 days. Similar results were reported for tolvaptan in stable class II or III HF.[626,627] Positive effects were observed, regardless of whether LVEF was less or greater than 40%.[412,625] In patients with LVEF less than 40%, a single dose of conivaptan reduced pulmonary capillary wedge and right atrial pressure in comparison with placebo; cardiac index, pulmonary arterial pressure, systemic, and pulmonary vascular resistance, systemic arterial pressure and heart rate were unaffected. Urine output rose and osmolarity fell significantly.[628,629] However, functional capacity, exercise tolerance, and overall quality of life were unchanged.[627]

The effect of vaptans on survival is unclear. In one study, mortality rate two months after discharge was halved in patients treated with tolvaptan who had an increase in serum $Na^+$ of 2 mmol/L or more, compared with those with no increase in serum $Na^+$.[630] In contrast, in the other trial, tolvaptan given for 60 days had no effect on survival after 9 months of follow-up.[627] Lixivaptan, another $V_2$ selective antagonist, was associated with an excessive mortality rate, despite favorable clinical and laboratory effects similar to those of tolvaptan.[631] Hence, the FDA did not approve lixivaptan for use in HF.[632]

Tolvaptan did not adversely affect cardiac remodeling or LVEF after 1 year of treatment in patients receiving optimal, background therapies for HF (RAAS and β-blockers).[633] In contrast, in a murine model of HF, tolavaptan was associated with increased remodeling and mortality, which was prevented by concomitant furosemide therapy.[634] Therefore, vigilance will need to be exercised in the long-term use of tolvaptan in HF.

In view of the impressive diuretic effect of vaptans, there is considerable interest in a potential loop diuretic–sparing effect, as mentioned previously. To summarize results to date, tolvaptan compared with furosemide alone or in combination, was not associated with improvement in dyspnea 24 hours after admission for acute HF, with or without preserved LVEF, despite greater diuresis and weight loss.[635–638] Tolvaptan was associated with better preserved renal function and serum electrolytes.[635–637] A Japanese multicenter clinical effectiveness of tolvaptan in patients with acute decompensated heart failure and renal failure (AQUAMARINE) study, in which tolvaptan is being compared with standard furosemide therapy in HF patients with renal impairment is ongoing (University Medical Information Network [UMIN] clinical trial registry number, UMIN000007109).[639]

The adverse effects of vaptans appear to be relatively few and, overall, minor. Thirst and dry mouth are not unexpected; hypokalemia occurs in less than 10% of recipients similar to loop diuretics. In the largest study to date, involving more than 4000 patients, there was a small but significant increase in strokes but a small but significant reduction in myocardial infarctions.[406]

In summary, AVP receptor antagonists appear to have important short-term benefits in the treatment of advanced HF. However, the question of improvement in longer term prognosis, especially the high mortality among HF patients already receiving optimal treatment with RAAS inhibitors (±NEP inhibition) and β-blockers remains open.[640]

## SODIUM-GLUCOSE TRANSPORTER-2 INHIBITORS

Sodium-glucose transporter-2 (SGLT-2) inhibitors decrease proximal tubular $Na^+$ and $Cl^-$ reabsorption, leading to a reset of TGF. This induces plasma volume contraction without activation of the SNS, decreases glomerular hyperfiltration leading to better long-term renal preservation, and improves diuretic and natriuretic responses to other diuretics. Moreover, SGLT-2 inhibitors might improve the efficiency of myocardial energetics by offering β-hydroxybutyrate as an attractive fuel for oxidation and increase hematocrit improving oxygen transport. Finally, decreased vascular stiffness and improved endothelial function are observed with the use of SGLT-2 inhibitors in diabetes. These multiple nonglycemic effects make SGLT-2 inhibitors preferred glucose-lowering drugs in diabetic patients with HF and raise the possibility for use in HF without diabetes.[641]

## SPECIFIC TREATMENTS BASED ON THE PATHOPHYSIOLOGY OF SODIUM RETENTION IN CIRRHOSIS

The prognosis of type 1 HRS is dismal. The mortality rate, which rises with increased AKI stage, is as high as 80% in the first 2 weeks and only 10% of patients survive longer than 3 months. Therefore specific aggressive therapy in these patients is usually indicated in preparation for liver transplantation.[483,535] Type 2 HRS has a better prognosis. Median survival is approximately 6 months.[483,535] Aggressive management for HRS includes pharmacologic therapy, TIPS insertion, renal replacement therapy (RRT), and liver transplantation. The management of precipitating factors is discussed elsewhere.

### PHARMACOLOGIC TREATMENT

The goals of pharmacologic therapy are to reverse the functional renal failure and serve as a bridge to liver transplantation. Earlier attempts to reverse renal vasoconstriction with low-dose dopamine, the $PGE_1$ analog misoprostol, RAAS and ET inhibitors were unsuccessful and even detrimental.[483,485,519] Therefore current treatment is based on reversal of splanchnic and systemic arterial vasodilation, AVP-induced water retention and hyponatremia.

#### SYSTEMIC VASOCONSTRICTORS

Three groups of vasoconstrictors have been studied—vasopressin $V_1$ receptor analogs, a somatostatin analog, and α-adrenergic agonists.[483,535]

##### Vasopressin $V_1$ Receptor Analogs

These agents cause marked vasoconstriction through their action on $V_1$ receptors in the arterial smooth muscle wall. They are used for the management of acute variceal bleeding in cirrhosis and portal hypertension. Ornipressin infusion in combination with volume expansion led to a remarkable increase in RPF, GFR, and $Na^+$ excretion in almost 50% of treated patients. However, significant ischemic adverse effects in 30% of patients led to the abandonment of this drug.[642]

Terlipressin, without significant adverse ischemic reactions, is now the vasoconstrictor drug of choice. Terlipressin and albumin in type 1 HRS is associated with a significant improvement in GFR, increase in arterial pressure, near-normalization of neurohumoral levels, and reduction of serum creatinine level in 40% to 50% of cases.[483,535,643] Response rates to terlipressin in type 2 HRS are better than those in type 1, with more than 80% survival at 3 months.[481,538] Despite relapses in 50% of cases, reintroduction of therapy produces a further response.[481,538]

The results of several randomized controlled trials, 2 meta-analyses and several Cochrane reviews, have shown that the combination of terlipressin and albumin is clearly superior to albumin or terlipressin alone in improving renal function and survival in both types 1 and 2 HRS.[644–647] No difference in efficacy between boluses and infusions was found, although the latter was associated with fewer adverse effects.[648] The optimum duration of terlipressin therapy is not clear, but it is usually given until serum creatinine levels decrease to less than 1.5 mg/dL or for a maximum of 15 days. Whether extending therapy beyond 15 days will add any benefit is unknown. A key prognostic target after combined terlipressin-albumin therapy may be a rise in MAP of 10 mm Hg or more; these patients required less dialysis and were more likely to attain liver transplantation than those with smaller responses in MAP. This response was associated with better short-term, long-term, and transplant-free survival.[649] Moreover, pretransplantation normalization of renal function by terlipressin resulted in similar posttransplantation outcomes to those of patients with normal renal function.[650]

In patients with HRS undergoing living related donor liver transplantation, terlipressin intra- and postoperatively is associated with significant increases in MAP, SVR, and renal function. Significantly decreased heart rate, cardiac output, hepatic and renal arterial resistive indices, portal venous blood flow, and use of vasoconstrictor drugs were seen during reperfusion.[651,652] To summarize, terlipressin and albumin infusion may be appropriate only for patients awaiting or already undergoing liver transplantation and a favorable hemodynamic response is associated with a better overall prognosis both before and after liver transplantation.

Unfortunately, terlipressin is currently unavailable in the United States and Canada and the results of a phase 3 clinical trial, comparing terlipressin with placebo (mannitol) in these countries, are, therefore, eagerly awaited (CONFIRM study, ClincialTrials.gov NCT 02770716).

### Somatostatin Analogs and α-Adrenergic Agonists

Octreotide is an α-adrenergic agonist that inhibits the release of glucagon and other vasodilator peptides. Octreotide with albumin infusion or midodrine had no effect on renal function in HRS. However, both agents in combination with albumin infusion led to a significant improvement in renal function and survival in types 1 and 2 HRS in comparison with controls.[653–655] However, no effect of this combination on outcomes of subsequent liver transplantation was observed.[656] Attempts to prevent relapse of type 2 HRS with midodrine after terlipressin-induced improvement were also unsuccessful.[657] Moreover, terlipressin plus albumin was significantly more effective than octreotide, midodrine and albumin, in terms of improved renal function, complete reversal of HRS and 90-day survival.[658] Finally, NE was compared with terlipressin in the treatment of type 1 HRS in three randomized controlled trials. Responses to both agents were similar in terms of MAP and renal function. Cumulative survival and adverse event rates were not significantly different between the two drugs. NE is less expensive than terlipressin, but, unlike terlipressin, NE administration requires cardiac monitoring. Therefore, total costs might be similar for the two therapies.[483,535]

### VASOPRESSIN $V_2$ RECEPTOR ANTAGONISTS

As noted, hyponatremia, caused by persistent nonosmotic AVP-induced water retention, is often seen in HRS and is a marker of poor prognosis.[659] Therefore, attaining a water diuresis and reversing hyponatremia using $V_2$ receptor antagonists are potentially important therapeutic goals. Several controlled studies, using lixivaptan, tolvaptan, and satavaptan have shown modest improvements in serum $Na^+$, but without effect on mortality or adverse events.[659–661] Satavaptan in combination with diuretics was associated with a higher mortality rate than either agent alone, leading to early termination of one study.[662] The specific role of satavaptan in the increased mortality was uncertain, given that most deaths were due to complications of cirrhosis. Overall, the effects of vaptans in HRS appear to be modest; this may be explained by avid proximal tubular solute reabsorption leading to reduced distal delivery or by $V_2$ receptor–independent pathways of water retention.[410]

## TRANSJUGULAR INTRAHEPATIC PORTOSYSTEMIC SHUNT

The efficacy of TIPS in the reduction of portal venous pressure in patients with cirrhosis and refractory ascites with type 1 or 2 HRS has been demonstrated in several small cohort and controlled studies.[481,663] Significant improvement in renal hemodynamics, GFR, and vasoconstrictive neurohumoral factors were observed in most patients.[519] Liver transplant-free survival also was markedly improved[663] and might be better than that reported for terlipressin and albumin infusion.[664] Some patients who were dialysis dependent were able to discontinue this treatment after TIPS insertion. Moreover, liver transplantation was performed in two patients when the medical condition that precluded transplantation had resolved after TIPS insertion.[665] However, TIPS seems to increase wait-time for liver transplantation and days in hospital after transplantation, although without effect on 30-day mortality.[666]

TIPS appears to exert its favorable effects by reducing sinusoidal hypertension with suppression of the putative hepatorenal reflex (see earlier), improvement of EABV by shunting portal venous blood into the systemic circulation, or amelioration of cardiac dysfunction.[551]

TIPS is currently recommended in the setting of refractory ascites, particularly in type-2 HRS, but is contraindicated in severe liver failure, severe intrinsic renal failure (serum creatinine >3 mg/dL), HF, severe porto-pulmonary hypertension, recurrent or persistent severe hepatic encephalopathy despite adequate treatment, and uncontrolled sepsis.[667]

## RENAL AND LIVER REPLACEMENT THERAPY

The benefits of conventional hemodialysis and continuous RRT, in terms of prolonging survival, are dubious,[668] and morbidity resulting from these therapies is high.[669] In oliguric patients awaiting liver transplantation who do not respond to vasoconstrictors or TIPS and who develop diuretic-resistant volume overload, hyperkalemia, or intractable metabolic acidosis, RRT may be considered. In view of the dismal prognosis of HRS, especially type 1, RRT should probably be used solely as a bridge to transplantation.

In contrast with conventional RRT, albumin-dialysis offers the potential advantage of removing albumin-bound, water-soluble vasoactive agents, toxins, and proinflammatory cytokines. Molecules relevant to the pathogenesis of advanced cirrhosis include bile acids, TNF-α, interleukin-6, and NO.[485] Three albumin dialysis systems, molecular adsorbent recirculating system (MARS), fractionated plasma separation, adsorption and hemodialysis (Prometheus system), and single-pass albumin dialysis, have been examined in randomized trials for supportive treatment of liver failure. These therapies enable partial recovery of hepatic function and provide simultaneous RRT. They lead to a decrease in renal vascular resistance and improvement in the splenic resistance index, a parameter related to portal resistance. The hemodynamic effects are thought to be mediated by clearance of vasoactive substances.[670] Bilirubin levels, encephalopathy grade, serum creatinine, and serum $Na^+$ all improved.[671] In a recent meta-analysis, albumin dialysis achieved a significant net decrease in serum total bilirubin level relative to standard medical therapy but not in serum ammonia or bile acids. Albumin dialysis achieved an improvement in hepatic encephalopathy relative to standard medical therapy but had no effect on survival. Bearing in mind the limited reporting of adverse events, no major safety concerns were detected. Extracorporeal nonbiologic liver support system should at present probably be considered only as a bridge to transplantation.[672]

## LIVER TRANSPLANTATION

Liver transplantation is the treatment of choice for HRS because it offers a cure for the liver disease and renal dysfunction. Large case series indicate that survival is significantly lower in transplant recipients with HRS (types 1 and 2) both immediately postoperatively and long-term than in those without the syndrome (3-year survival rates of 60% vs. 70% to 80%) but may be improved by the bridging therapies described previously.[673,674]

With respect to renal function after transplantation in patients with HRS, GFR decreases in the first month owing to the stress of surgery, infections, immunosuppressive therapy, and other factors. Despite the prompt correction of hemodynamic and neurohumoral parameters, GFR recovers incompletely (30 to 40 mL/min at 1 to 2 months) and often remains impaired over the long term. Although dialysis requirement in the first month is greater in patients with HRS than without HRS (35% vs. 5%), duration of dialysis pretransplantation does not influence renal recovery posttransplantation. Predictors of renal recovery included younger recipient and donor, nonalcoholic liver disease, and low posttransplantation serum bilirubin.[675] Overall, the rate of posttransplantation reversal of HRS has been estimated to be no greater than 58%.

Unsurprisingly, the 5-year risk of ESRD posttransplantation in patients with HRS is significantly higher than in those without HRS. Moreover, combined simultaneous liver and kidney transplantation (SLKT) apparently offers no greater benefit over liver transplantation alone with respect to early posttransplantation kidney function. However, better 5-year survival rates are more likely after SLKT than after liver transplantation alone in patients with pretransplantation serum creatinine levels greater than 2.2 mg/dL, irrespective of dialysis requirement.[674] More studies are needed to enable a rational decision about who should receive SLKT, rather than liver transplants alone. At present, SLKT should probably be reserved for patients who are dialysis dependent for 8 weeks or more pretransplantation.[485,674,676]

The introduction of Model of End-stage Liver Disease (MELD) scores for the allocation of livers has increased the number of transplantations in patients with impaired renal function, but more SLKTs are also being performed.[677] On the other hand, a favorable response to vasoactive therapy reduces the MELD score and may lead to a paradoxical delay in liver transplantation.[678] Therefore, only pretreatment MELD scores should be used to predict potential outcomes of liver transplantation in HRS.[481] A further paradox is that patients with type 2 HRS have lower MELD scores than those with type 1 HRS, resulting in the former being ascribed a lower priority for transplantation and a longer time on the waiting list. This delay is associated with higher mortality, especially in the presence of hyponatremia and persistent ascites.[677] Therefore, the criteria for donor allocation need to be modified to incorporate these factors into the final score for prioritization.[481]

For a general summary of all aspects of liver transplantation, the reader is referred to several excellent recent reviews.[679,680]

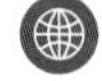 Complete reference list available at ExpertConsult.com.

# Disorders of Water Balance

# 15

Joseph G. Verbalis

CHAPTER OUTLINE



Disorders of body fluids are among the most commonly encountered problems in clinical medicine. This is, in large part, because many different disease states can disrupt the finely balanced mechanisms that control the intake and output of water and solute. Because body water is the primary determinant of the osmolality of the extracellular fluid, disorders of water metabolism can be broadly divided into hyperosmolar disorders, in which there is a deficiency of body water relative to body solute, and hypoosmolar disorders, in which there is an excess of body water relative to body solute. Because sodium is the main constituent of plasma osmolality, these disorders are typically characterized by hypernatremia and hyponatremia, respectively. Before discussing specific aspects of these disorders, this chapter will first review the regulatory mechanisms underlying water metabolism, which, in concert with sodium metabolism, maintains body fluid homeostasis.

## BODY FLUIDS: COMPARTMENTALIZATION, COMPOSITION, AND TURNOVER

Water constitutes approximately 55% to 65% of body weight, varying with age, gender, and amount of body fat, and therefore constitutes the largest single constituent of the body. Total body water (TBW) is distributed between the intracellular fluid (ICF) and extracellular fluid (ECF) compartments. Estimates of the relative sizes of these two pools differ significantly, depending on the tracer used to measure the ECF volume, but most studies in animals and humans have indicated that 55% to 65% of TBW resides in the ICF, and 35% to 45% is in the ECF. Approximately 75% of the ECF compartment is interstitial fluid, and only 25% is intravascular fluid (blood volume).[1,2] Fig. 15.1 summarizes the estimated body fluid spaces of an average weight adult.

The solute composition of the ICF and ECF differs considerably because most cell membranes possess multiple transport systems that actively accumulate or expel specific solutes. Thus, membrane-bound $Na^+$-$K^+$-ATPase maintains $Na^+$ in a primarily extracellular location and $K^+$ in a primarily intracellular location.[3] Similar transporters effectively result in confining $Cl^-$ largely to the ECF, and $Mg^{2+}$, organic acids, and phosphates to the ICF. Glucose, which requires an insulin-activated transport system to enter most cells, is present in significant amounts only in the ECF because it is rapidly converted intracellularly to glycogen or metabolites. $HCO_3^-$ is present in both compartments but is approximately three times more concentrated in the ECF. Urea is unique among the major naturally occurring solutes in that it diffuses freely across most cell membranes[4]; therefore, it is present in similar concentrations in almost all body fluids, except in the renal medulla, where it is concentrated by urea transporters (see Chapter 10).

Despite very different solute compositions, both the ICF and ECF have an equivalent osmotic pressure,[5] which is a function of the total concentration of all solutes in a fluid compartment. This is because most biologic membranes are semipermeable (i.e., freely permeable to water but not to all aqueous solutes). Thus, water will flow across membranes into a compartment with a higher solute concentration until a steady state is reached and the osmotic pressures have equalized on both sides of the cell membrane.[6] An important consequence of this thermodynamic law is that the volume of distribution of body $Na^+$ and $K^+$ is actually the TBW rather than just the ECF or ICF volume, respectively.[7] For example, any increase in ECF sodium concentration ($[Na^+]$) will cause water to shift from the ICF to ECF until the ICF and ECF osmotic pressures are equal, thereby effectively distributing the $Na^+$ across extracellular and intracellular water.

Osmolality is defined as the concentration of all of the solutes in a given weight of fluid. The total solute

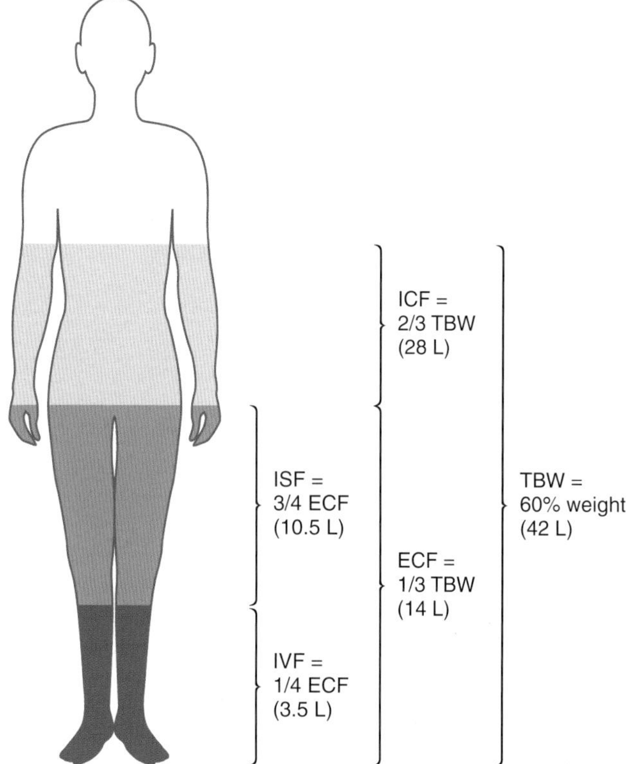


**Fig. 15.1** Schematic representation of body fluid compartments in humans. The *shaded areas* depict the approximate size of each compartment as a function of body weight. The *numbers* indicate the relative sizes of the various fluid compartments and the approximate absolute volumes of the compartments (in liters) in a 70-kg adult. *ECF,* Extracellular fluid; *ICF,* intracellular fluid; *ISF,* interstitial fluid; *IVF,* intravascular fluid; *TBW,* total body water. (From Verbalis JG: Body water and osmolality. In Wilkinson B, Jamison R, eds. *Textbook of Nephrology.* London: Chapman & Hall; 1997:89–94.)

concentration of a fluid can be determined and expressed in several different ways. The most common method is to measure its freezing point or vapor pressure because these are colligative properties of the number of free solute particles in a volume of fluid.[8] The result is expressed relative to a standard solution of known concentration using units of osmolality (milliosmoles of solute per kilogram of water, mOsm/kg $H_2O$), or osmolarity (milliosmoles of solute per liter of water, mOsm/L $H_2O$). Plasma osmolality ($P_{osm}$) can be measured directly, as described earlier, or can be calculated by summing the concentrations of the major solutes present in the plasma:

$$P_{osm}\,(\text{mOsm/kg } H_2O) = 2 \times \text{plasma [Na+] (mEq/L)} + \frac{\text{glucose (mg/dL)}}{18} + \frac{\text{BUN (mg/dL)}}{2.8}$$

where BUN = blood urea nitrogen.

Both methods produce comparable results under most conditions (the value obtained using this formula is generally within 1% to 2% of that obtained by direct osmometry), as will simply doubling the plasma [$Na^+$], because sodium and its accompanying anions are the predominant solutes present in plasma. However, the total osmolality of plasma is not always equivalent to the effective osmolality, often referred to as the "tonicity of the plasma," because the latter is a function of the relative solute permeability properties of the membranes separating the two compartments. Solutes that are impermeable to cell membranes (e.g., $Na^+$, mannitol) are restricted to the ECF compartment. They are effective solutes because they create osmotic pressure gradients across cell membranes, leading to the osmotic movement of water from the ICF to ECF compartments. Solutes that are permeable to cell membranes (e.g., urea, ethanol, methanol) are ineffective solutes because they do not create osmotic pressure gradients across cell membranes and therefore are not associated with such water shifts.[9] Glucose is a unique solute because, at normal physiologic plasma concentrations, it is taken up by cells via active transport mechanisms and therefore acts as an ineffective solute but, under conditions of impaired cellular uptake (e.g., insulin deficiency), it becomes an effective extracellular solute.[10]

The importance of this distinction between total and effective osmolality is that only the effective solutes in plasma are determinants of whether clinically significant hyperosmolality or hypoosmolality is present. An example of this is uremia; a patient with BUN concentration that has increased by 56 mg/dL will have a corresponding 20-mOsm/kg $H_2O$ elevation in plasma osmolality, but the effective osmolality will remain normal because the increased urea is proportionally distributed across the ECF and ICF. In contrast, a patient whose plasma [$Na^+$] has increased by 10 mEq/L will also have a 20-mOsm/kg $H_2O$ elevation of plasma osmolality because the increased cation must be balanced by an equivalent increase in plasma anions. However, in this case, the effective osmolality will also be elevated by 20 mOsm/kg $H_2O$ because the $Na^+$ and accompanying anions will largely remain restricted to the ECF due to the relative impermeability of cell membranes to $Na^+$ and other ions. Thus, elevations of solutes such as urea, unlike elevations of sodium, do not cause cellular dehydration and consequently do not activate mechanisms that defend body fluid homeostasis by increasing body water stores.

Both body water and solutes are in a state of continuous exchange with the environment. The magnitude of the turnover varies considerably, depending on physical, social, and environmental factors, but, in healthy adults, it averages 5% to 10% of the total body content each day. For the most part, daily intake of water and electrolytes is not determined by physiologic requirements but is more a function of dietary preferences and cultural influences. Healthy adults have an average daily fluid ingestion of approximately 2 to 3 L, but with considerable individual variation; approximately one-third of this is derived from food or the metabolism of fat and the rest from discretionary ingestion of fluids. Similarly, of the 1000 mOsm of solute ingested or generated by the metabolism of nutrients each day, nearly 40% is intrinsic to food, another 35% is added to food as a preservative or flavoring, and the rest is mostly urea. In contrast to the largely unregulated nature of basal intakes, the urinary excretion of water and solute is highly regulated to preserve body fluid homeostasis. Thus, under normal circumstances, almost all ingested $Na^+$, $Cl^-$, and $K^+$, as well as ingested and metabolically generated urea, are excreted in the urine under the control of specific regulatory mechanisms. Other ingested solutes, such as divalent minerals, are excreted primarily by the gastrointestinal tract. Urinary excretion of water is also tightly regulated by the secretion and renal effects of arginine vasopressin (AVP; vasopressin, antidiuretic hormone), discussed in greater detail in Chapter 10 and in the following section ("Water Metabolism").

## WATER METABOLISM

Water metabolism is responsible for the balance between the intake and excretion of water. Each side of this balance equation can be considered to consist of a regulated and unregulated component, the magnitudes of which can vary markedly under different physiologic and pathophysiologic conditions. The unregulated component of water intake consists of the intrinsic water content of ingested foods, consumption of beverages primarily for reasons of palatability or desired secondary effects (e.g., caffeine), or for social or habitual reasons (e.g., alcoholic beverages), whereas the regulated component of water intake consists of fluids consumed in response to a perceived sensation of thirst. Studies of middle-aged subjects have shown mean fluid intakes of 2.1 L/24 hours, and analyses of the fluids consumed have indicated that the vast majority of the fluid ingested is determined by influences such as meal-associated fluid intake, taste, or psychosocial factors, rather than by true thirst.[11]

The unregulated component of water excretion occurs via insensible water losses from a variety of sources (e.g., cutaneous losses from sweating, evaporative losses in exhaled air, gastrointestinal losses), as well as the obligate amount of water that the kidneys must excrete to eliminate solutes generated by body metabolism, whereas the regulated component of water excretion is comprised of the renal excretion of free water in excess of the obligate amount necessary to excrete metabolic solutes. Unlike solutes, a relatively large proportion of body water is excreted by evaporation from the skin and lungs. This amount varies markedly, depending on several factors, including dress, humidity, temperature, and exercise.[12] Under the sedentary and temperature-controlled indoor conditions typical of modern urban life, daily insensible water loss in healthy adults is minimal, approximately 8 to 10 mL/kg body weight (BW; ≈0.5–0.7 L in a 70-kg adult man or woman). However, insensible losses can increase to twice this level (20 mL/kg BW) simply under conditions of increased activity and temperature and, if environmental temperature or activity is even higher, such as in an arid environment, the rate of insensible water loss can even approximate the maximal rate of free water excretion by the kidney.[12] Thus, in quantitative terms, insensible loss and the factors that influence it can be just as important to body fluid homeostasis as regulated urine output.

Another major determinant of unregulated water loss is the rate of urine solute excretion, which cannot be reduced below a minimal obligatory level required to excrete the solute load. The volume of urine required depends not only on the solute load, but also on the degree of antidiuresis. At a typical basal level of urinary concentration (urine osmolality = 600 mOsm/kg $H_2O$) and a typical solute load of 900 to 1200 mOsm/day, a 70-kg adult would require a total urine volume of 1.5 to 2.0 L (21–29 mL/kg BW) to excrete the solute load. However, under conditions of maximal antidiuresis (urine osmolality = 1200 mOsm/kg $H_2O$), the same solute load would require a minimal obligatory urine output of only 0.75 to 1.0 L/day and, conversely, a decrease in urine concentration to minimal levels (urine osmolality = 60 mOsm/kg $H_2O$) would obligate a proportionately larger urine volume of 15 to 20 L/day to excrete the same solute load.

The earlier discussion emphasizes that water intake and water excretion have very substantial unregulated components, and these can vary tremendously as a result of factors unrelated to the maintenance of body fluid homeostasis. In effect, the regulated components of water metabolism are those that act to maintain body fluid homeostasis by compensating for whatever perturbations have resulted from unregulated water losses or gains. Within this framework, the major mechanisms responsible for regulating water metabolism are pituitary secretion and the renal effects of vasopressin and thirst, each of which will be discussed in greater detail in the following sections.

### VASOPRESSIN SYNTHESIS AND SECRETION

The primary determinant of free water excretion in animals and humans is the regulation of urinary water excretion by circulating levels of AVP in plasma. The renal effects of AVP are covered extensively in Chapter 10. This chapter will focus on the regulation of AVP synthesis and secretion.

#### STRUCTURE AND SYNTHESIS

Before AVP was biochemically characterized, early studies used the general term "antidiuretic hormone" (ADH) to describe this substance. Now that AVP is known to be the only naturally occurring antidiuretic substance, it is more appropriate to refer to it by its correct hormonal designation. AVP is a nine–amino acid peptide that is synthesized in the hypothalamus. It is composed of a six–amino acid, ringlike structure formed by a disulfide bridge, with a three–amino acid tail, at the end of which the terminal carboxyl group is amidated. Substitution of lysine for arginine in position 8 yields lysine vasopressin, the antidiuretic hormone found in pigs and other members of the suborder Suina. Substitution of isoleucine for phenylalanine at position 3 and of leucine for arginine at position 8 yields oxytocin (OT), a hormone found in all mammals and in many submammalian species.[13] OT has weak antidiuretic activity[14] but is a potent constrictor of smooth muscle in mammary glands and uterus. As implied by their names, arginine and lysine vasopressin also cause the constriction of blood vessels, which was the property that led to their original discovery in the late 19th century,[15] but this pressor effect occurs only at concentrations many times higher than those required to produce antidiuresis. This is probably of little physiologic or pathologic importance in humans except under conditions of severe hypotension and hypovolemia, where it acts to supplement the vasoconstrictive actions of angiotensin II (Ang II) and the sympathetic nervous system.[16] The multiple actions of AVP are mediated by different G protein–coupled receptors, designated $V_{1a}$, $V_{1b}$, and $V_2$[17] (see Chapter 10).

AVP and OT are produced by the neurohypophysis, often referred to as the "posterior pituitary gland," because the neural lobe is located centrally and posterior to the adenohypophysis, or anterior pituitary gland, in the sella turcica. However, it is important to understand that the posterior pituitary gland consists only of the distal axons of the

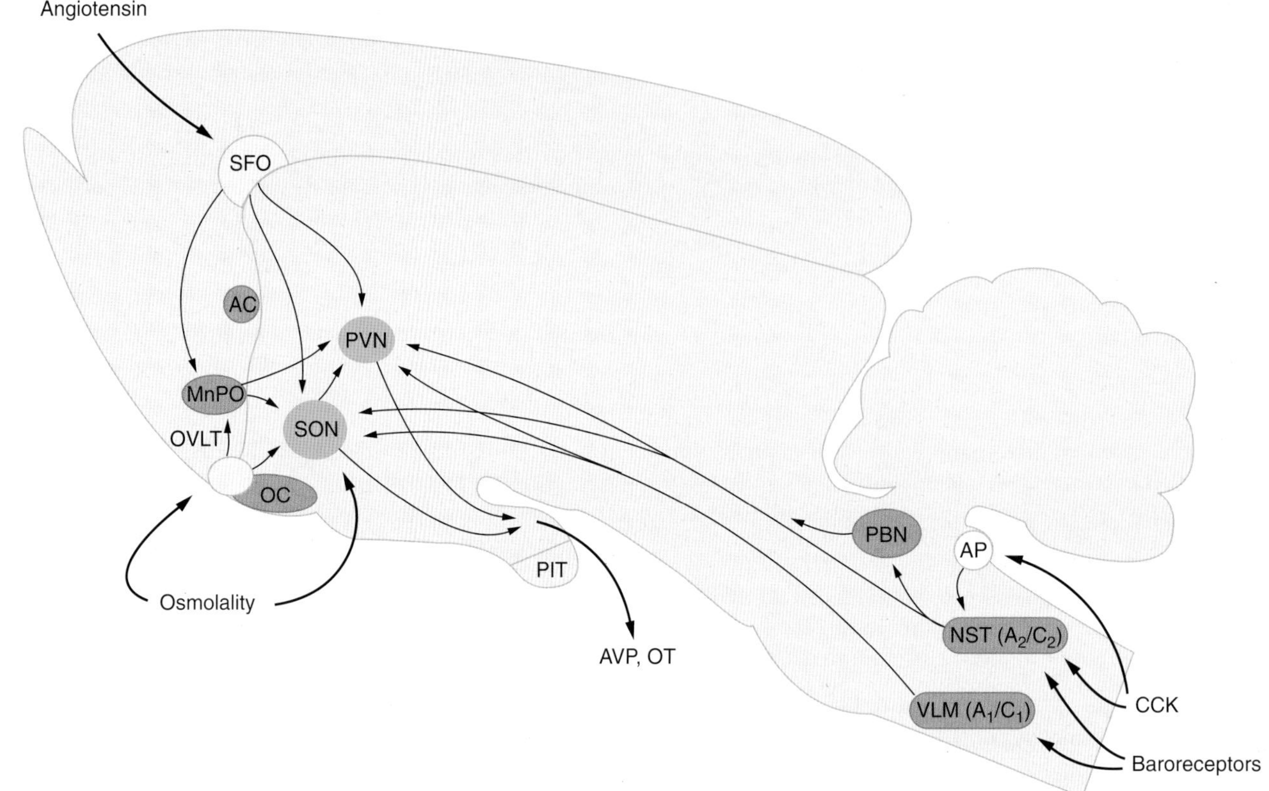


**Fig. 15.2** Summary of the main anterior hypothalamic pathways that mediate secretion of arginine vasopressin (AVP) and oxytocin (OT). The vascular organ of the lamina terminalis (OVLT) is especially sensitive to hyperosmolality. Hyperosmolality also activates other neurons in the anterior hypothalamus, such as those in the subfornical organ (SFO) and median preoptic nucleus (MnPO), and magnocellular neurons, which are intrinsically osmosensitive. Circulating angiotensin II (Ang II) activates neurons of the SFO, an essential site of Ang II action, as well as cells throughout the lamina terminalis and MnPO. In response to hyperosmolality or Ang II, projections from the SFO and OVLT to the MnPO activate excitatory and inhibitory interneurons that project to the supraoptic nucleus (SON) and paraventricular nucleus (PVN) to modulate direct inputs to these areas from the circumventricular organs. Cholecystokinin (CCK) acts primarily on gastric vagal afferents that terminate in the nucleus of the solitary tract (NST) but, at higher doses, it can also act at the area postrema (AP). Although neurons are apparently activated in the ventrolateral medulla (VLM) and NST, most neurohypophyseal secretion appears to be stimulated by monosynaptic projections from $A_2$-$C_2$ cells, and possibly also noncatecholaminergic somatostatin-inhibin B cells, of the NST. Baroreceptor-mediated stimuli, such as hypovolemia and hypotension, are more complex. The major projection to magnocellular AVP neurons appears to arise from $A_1$ cells of the VLM that are activated by excitatory interneurons from the NST. Other areas, such as the parabrachial nucleus (PBN), may contribute multisynaptic projections. Cranial nerves IX and X, which terminate in the NST, also contribute input to magnocellular AVP neurons. *AC,* Anterior commissure; *OC,* optic chiasm; *PIT,* anterior pituitary. (From Stricker EM, Verbalis JG: Water intake and body fluids. In Squire LR, Bloom FE, McConnell SK, et al, eds. *Fundamental Neuroscience,* San Diego: Academic Press; 2003:1011–1029.)

magnocellular neurons that comprise the neurohypophysis. The cell bodies of these axons are located in specialized (magnocellular) neural cells located in two discrete areas of the hypothalamus, the paired supraoptic nuclei (SON) and paraventricular nuclei (PVN; Fig. 15.2). In adults, the posterior pituitary is connected to the brain by a short stalk through the diaphragm sellae. The neurohypophysis is supplied with blood by branches of the superior and inferior hypophysial arteries, which arise from the posterior communicating and intracavernous portion of the internal carotid artery. In the posterior pituitary, the arterioles break up into localized capillary networks that drain directly into the jugular vein via the sellar, cavernous, and lateral venous sinuses. Many of the neurosecretory neurons that terminate higher in the infundibulum and median eminence originate in parvicellular neurons in the PVN; they are functionally distinct from the magnocellular neurons that terminate in the posterior pituitary because they primarily enhance secretion of adrenocorticotropic hormone (ACTH) from the anterior pituitary. AVP-containing neurons also project from parvicellular neurons of the PVN to other areas of the brain, including the limbic system, nucleus tractus solitarius, and lateral gray matter of the spinal cord. The full extent of the functions of these extrahypophysial projections are still under study.

The genes encoding the AVP and OT precursors are located in close proximity on chromosome 20, but are expressed in mutually exclusive populations of neurohypophyseal neurons.[18] The AVP gene consists of approximately 2000 base pairs and contains three exons separated by two intervening sequences or introns (Fig. 15.3). Each exon encodes one of the three functional domains of the preprohormone, although small parts of the nonconserved sequences of neurophysin are located in the first and third exons that code for AVP and the C-terminal glycoprotein, called copeptin, respectively. The untranslated 5′-flanking genomic region, which regulates expression of the gene, shows extensive sequence homology

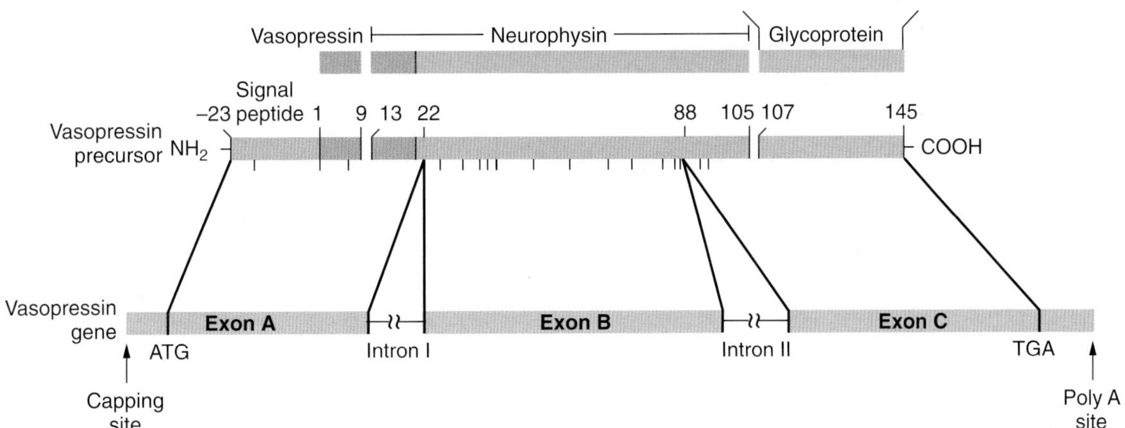


**Fig. 15.3** The arginine vasopressin (AVP) gene and its protein products. The three exons encode a 145–amino acid prohormone with an $NH_2$-terminal signal peptide. The prohormone is packaged into neurosecretory granules of magnocellular neurons. During axonal transport of the granules from the hypothalamus to the posterior pituitary, enzymatic cleavage of the prohormone generates the final products—AVP, neurophysin, and a COOH-terminal glycoprotein called copeptin. When afferent stimulation depolarizes the AVP-containing neurons, the three products are released into capillaries of the posterior pituitary in equimolar amounts. (Adapted from Richter D, Schmale H: The structure of the precursor to arginine vasopressin, a model preprohormone. *Prog Brain Res.* 1983;60:227–233.)

across several species but is markedly different from the otherwise closely related gene for OT. This regulatory or promoter region of the AVP gene in the rat contains several putative regulatory elements, including a glucocorticoid response element, cyclic adenosine monophosphate (cAMP) response element, and four activating protein-2 (AP-2) binding sites.[19] Experimental studies have suggested that the DNA sequences between the AVP and OT genes, the intergenic region, may contain critical sites for cell-specific expression of these two hormones.[20]

The gene for AVP is also expressed in a number of other neurons, including but not limited to the parvicellular neurons of the PVN and SON. AVP and OT genes are also expressed in several peripheral tissues, including the adrenal medulla, ovary, testis, thymus, and certain sensory ganglia.[21] However, the AVP mRNA in these tissues appears to be shorter (620 bases) than its hypothalamic counterpart (720 bases), apparently because of tissue-specific differences in the length of the polyA tails. More importantly, the levels of AVP in peripheral tissues are generally two or three orders of magnitude lower than in the neurohypophysis, suggesting that AVP in these tissues likely has paracrine rather than endocrine functions. This is consistent with the observation that destruction of the neurohypophysis essentially eliminates AVP from the plasma, despite the presence of these multiple peripheral sites of AVP synthesis.

The secretion of AVP and its associated neurophysin and copeptin peptide fragments occurs by a calcium-dependent exocytotic process, similar to that described for other neurosecretory systems. Secretion is triggered by propagation of an electrical impulse along the axon that causes depolarization of the cell membrane, an influx of $Ca^{2+}$, fusion of secretory granules with the cell membrane, and extrusion of their contents. This view is supported by the observation that AVP, neurophysin, and the glycoprotein copeptin are released simultaneously by many stimuli.[22] However, at the physiologic pH of plasma, there is no binding of AVP or OT to their respective neurophysins so, after secretion, each peptide circulates independently in the bloodstream.[23]

Stimuli for secretion of AVP or OT also stimulate transcription and increase the mRNA content of both prohormones in the magnocellular neurons. This has been well documented in rats, in which dehydration, which stimulates secretion of AVP, accelerates transcription and increases the levels of AVP (and OT) mRNA,[24,25] and hypoosmolality, which inhibits the secretion of AVP, produces a decrease in the content of AVP mRNA.[26] These and other studies have indicated that the major control of AVP synthesis most likely resides at the level of transcription.[27]

Antidiuresis occurs via interaction of the circulating hormone with AVP $V_2$ receptors in the kidney, which results in increased water permeability of the collecting duct through the insertion of the aquaporin-2 (AQP2) water channel into the apical membranes of collecting tubule principal cells (see Chapter 10). The importance of AVP for maintaining water balance is underscored by the fact that the normal pituitary stores of this hormone are very large, allowing more than 1 week's supply of hormone for maximal antidiuresis under conditions of sustained dehydration.[27] Knowledge of the different conditions that stimulate pituitary AVP release in humans is therefore essential for understanding water metabolism.

## OSMOTIC REGULATION

AVP secretion is influenced by many different stimuli, but since the pioneering studies of ADH secretion by Ernest Basil Verney, it has been clear that the most important stimulus under physiologic conditions is the osmotic pressure of plasma. With further refinement of radioimmunoassays for AVP, the unique sensitivity of this hormone to small changes in osmolality, as well as the corresponding sensitivity of the kidney to small changes in plasma AVP levels, have become apparent. Although the magnocellular neurons themselves have been found to have intrinsic osmoreceptive properties,[28] research over the last several decades has clearly shown that the most sensitive osmoreceptive cells that can sense small changes in plasma osmolality and transduce these changes into AVP secretion are located in the anterior hypothalamus, likely in or near the circumventricular organ termed the "organum vasculosum of the lamina terminalis" (OVLT; see Fig. 15.2).[29] Perhaps the strongest evidence for location of the primary osmoreceptors in this area of the brain are the multiple studies that have demonstrated that destruction of this area disrupts osmotically stimulated AVP secretion and thirst, without affecting the neurohypophysis or its response to nonosmotic stimuli.[30,31]

Although some debate still exists with regard to the exact pattern of osmotically stimulated AVP secretion, most studies to date have supported the concept of a discrete osmotic threshold for AVP secretion, above which there is a linear relationship between plasma osmolality and AVP levels (Fig. 15.4).[32] At plasma osmolalities below a threshold level, AVP secretion is suppressed to low or undetectable levels; above this point, AVP secretion increases linearly in direct proportion to plasma osmolality. The slope of the regression line relating AVP secretion to plasma osmolality can vary significantly across individual human subjects, in part because of genetic factors,[33] but also in relation to other factors. In general, each 1-mOsm/kg $H_2O$ increase in plasma osmolality causes an increase in the plasma AVP level, ranging from 0.4 to 1.0 pg/mL. The renal response to circulating AVP is similarly linear, with urinary concentration that is directly proportional to AVP levels from 0.5 to 4 to 5 pg/mL, after which urinary osmolality is maximal and cannot increase further, despite additional increases in AVP levels (Fig. 15.5). Thus, changes of as little as 1% in plasma osmolality are sufficient to cause significant increases in plasma AVP levels, with proportional increases in urine concentration, and maximal antidiuresis is achieved after increases in plasma osmolality of only 5 to 10 mOsm/kg $H_2O$ (2%–4%) above the threshold for AVP secretion.

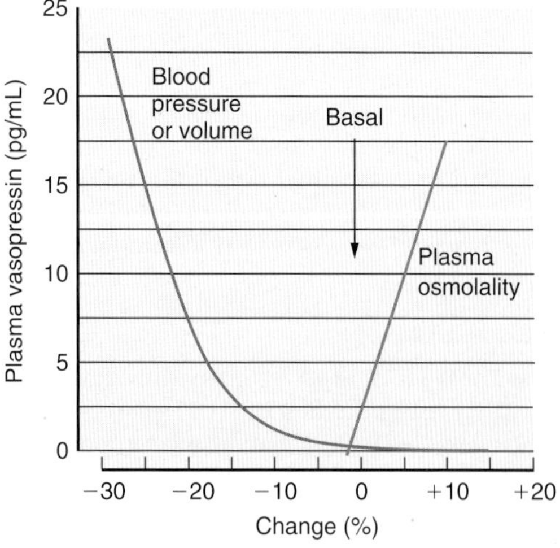


**Fig. 15.4** Comparative sensitivity of arginine vasopressin (AVP) secretion in response to increases in plasma osmolality versus decreases in blood volume or blood pressure in human subjects. The *arrow* indicates the low plasma AVP concentrations found at basal plasma osmolality. Note that AVP secretion is much more sensitive to small changes in blood osmolality than to small changes in volume or pressure. (Adapted from Robertson GL: Posterior pituitary. In Felig P, Baxter J, Frohman LA, eds. *Endocrinology and Metabolism,* New York: McGraw-Hill; 1986:338–386.)

However, even this analysis underestimates the sensitivity of this system to regulate free water excretion. Urinary osmolality is directly proportional to plasma AVP levels as a consequence of the fall in urine flow induced by the AVP, but urine volume is inversely related to urine osmolality (see Fig. 15.5). An increase in plasma AVP concentration from 0.5 to 2 pg/mL has a much greater relative effect to decrease urine flow than a subsequent increase in AVP concentration from 2 to 5 pg/mL, thereby magnifying the physiologic effects of small changes in lower plasma AVP levels. Furthermore, the rapid response of AVP secretion to changes in plasma osmolality, coupled with the short half-life of AVP in human plasma (10–20 minutes), allows the kidneys to respond to changes in plasma osmolality on a minute to minute basis. The net result is a finely tuned osmoregulatory system that adjusts the rate of free water excretion accurately to the ambient plasma osmolality, primarily via changes in pituitary AVP secretion.

The set point of the osmoregulatory system also varies from person to person. In healthy adults, the osmotic threshold for AVP secretion ranges from 275 to 290 mOsm/kg $H_2O$ (averaging ≈280–285 mOsm/kg $H_2O$). Similar to sensitivity, individual differences in the set point of the osmoregulatory system are relatively constant over time and appear to be genetically determined.[33] However, multiple factors can alter the sensitivity and/or set point of the osmoregulatory system for AVP secretion, in addition to genetic influences.[33] Foremost among these are acute changes in blood pressure, effective blood volume, or both (discussed in the following section). Aging has been found to increase the sensitivity of the osmoregulatory system in multiple studies.[34,35] Metabolic factors, such as serum $Ca^{2+}$ levels and various drugs, can alter the slope of the plasma AVP-osmolality relationship as well.[36] Lesser degrees of shifting of the osmosensitivity and set point for AVP secretion have been noted with alterations in gonadal hormones. Some studies have found increased osmosensitivity in women, particularly during the luteal phase of the menstrual cycle,[37] and in estrogen-treated men,[38] but these effects were relatively minor, and others have found no significant gender differences.[33] The set point of the osmoregulatory system is reduced more dramatically and reproducibly during pregnancy.[39] Evidence has suggested the possible involvement of the placental hormone relaxin,[40] rather than gonadal steroids or human chorionic gonadotropin hormone in pregnancy-associated resetting of the osmostat for AVP secretion. Both the changes in volume and in osmolality have been reproduced by the infusion of relaxin into virgin female and normal rats and reversed in pregnant rats by immunoneutralization of relaxin.[41] Increased nitric oxide (NO) production by relaxin has been reported to increase vasodilation, and estrogens also increase NO synthesis.[42] That multiple factors can influence the set point and sensitivity of osmotically regulated AVP secretion is not surprising because AVP secretion reflects a balance of bimodal inputs—inhibitory and stimulatory[43]—from multiple different afferent inputs to the neurohypophysis (Fig. 15.6).[44]

Understanding the osmoregulatory mechanism also requires addressing the observation that AVP secretion is not equally sensitive to all plasma solutes. Sodium and its anions, which normally contribute more than 95% of the osmotic pressure of plasma, are the most potent solutes in terms of their capacity to stimulate AVP secretion and thirst, although certain

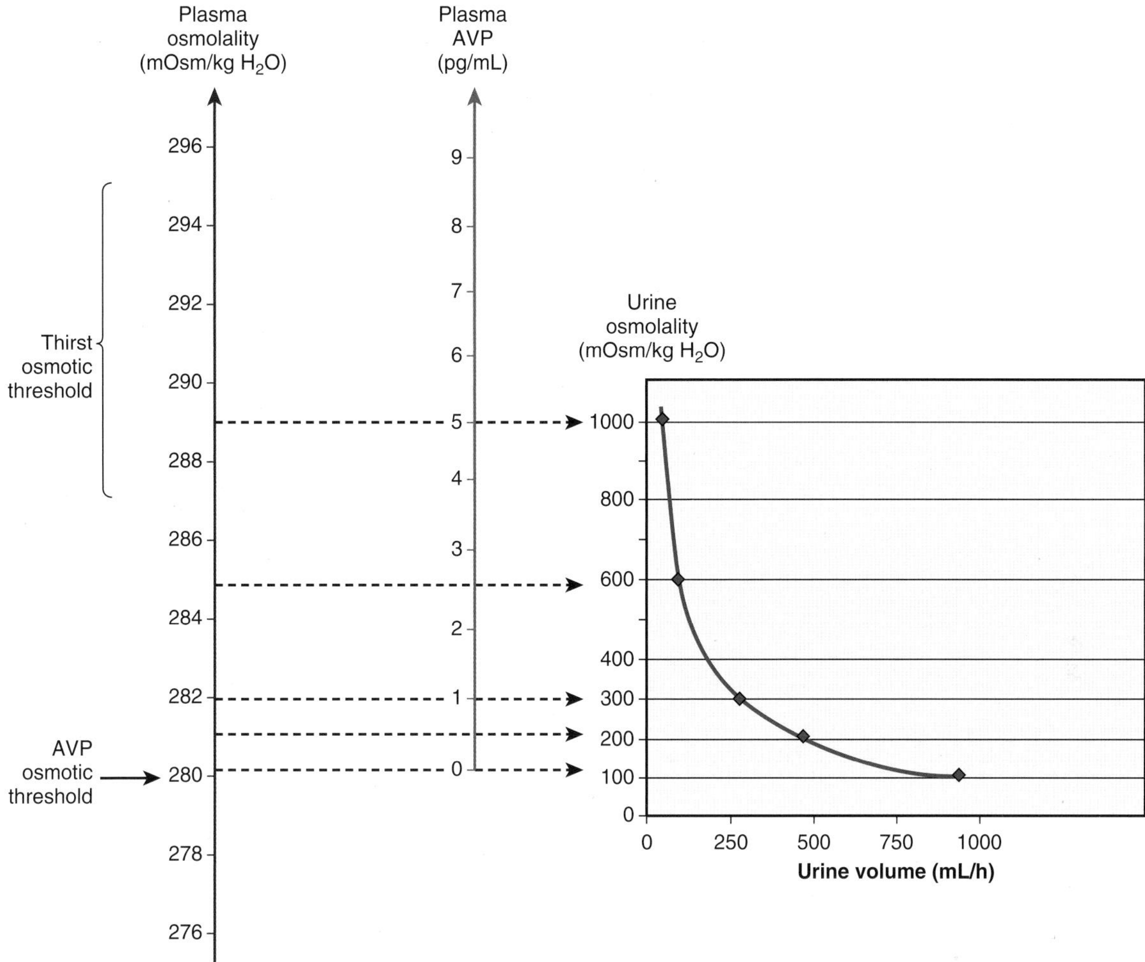


**Fig. 15.5** Relationship of plasma osmolality, plasma arginine vasopressin (AVP) concentrations, urine osmolality, and urine volume in humans. The osmotic threshold for AVP secretion defines the point at which urine concentration begins to increase, but the osmotic threshold for thirst is significantly higher and approximates the point at which maximal urine concentration has already been achieved. Note also that because of the inverse relation between urine osmolality and urine volume, changes in plasma AVP concentrations have much larger effects on urine volume at low plasma AVP concentrations than at high plasma AVP concentrations. (Adapted from Robinson AG: Disorders of antidiuretic hormone secretion. *J Clin Endocrinol Metab.* 1985;14:55–88.)

sugars such as mannitol and sucrose are also equally effective when infused intravenously.[9] In contrast, increases in plasma osmolality caused by noneffective solutes such as urea or glucose result in little or no increase in plasma AVP levels in nondiabetic humans or animals.[9,45] These differences in response to various plasma solutes are independent of any recognized nonosmotic influence, indicating that they are a property of the osmoregulatory mechanism itself. According to current concepts, the osmoreceptor neuron is stimulated by osmotically induced changes in its water content. In this case, the stimulatory potency of any given solute would be an inverse function of the rate at which it moves from the plasma to the inside of the osmoreceptor neuron. Solutes that penetrate slowly, or not at all, create an osmotic gradient that causes an efflux of water from the osmoreceptor, and the resultant shrinkage of the osmoreceptor neuron activates a stretch-inactivated, noncationic channel that initiates depolarization and firing of the neuron.[46] Conversely, solutes that penetrate the cell readily create no gradient and thus have no effect on the water content and cell volume of the osmoreceptors. This mechanism agrees well with the observed relationship between the effect of certain solutes on AVP secretion, such as $Na^+$, mannitol, and glucose, and the rate at which they penetrate the blood-brain barrier.[29]

Many neurotransmitters have been implicated in mediating the actions of the osmoreceptors on the neurohypophysis. The supraoptic nucleus is richly innervated by multiple pathways, including acetylcholine, catecholamines, glutamate, gamma-aminobutyric acid (GABA), histamine, opioids, Ang II, and dopamine.[47] Studies have supported a potential role for all of these and others in the regulation of AVP secretion, as has local secretion of AVP into the hypothalamus from dendrites of the AVP-secreting neurons.[48] Although it remains unclear which of these are involved in the normal physiologic control of AVP secretion, in view of the likelihood that the osmoregulatory system is bimodal and integrated with multiple different afferent pathways (see Fig. 15.6), it seems likely that magnocellular AVP neurons are influenced by a very complex mixture of neurotransmitter systems, rather than only a few.

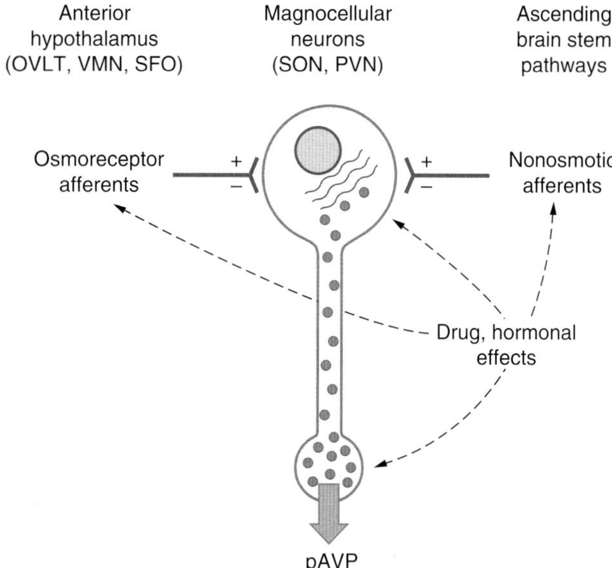


**Fig. 15.6** Schematic model of the regulatory control of the neurohypophysis. The secretory activity of individual magnocellular neurons is determined by an integration of the activities of excitatory and inhibitory osmotic and nonosmotic afferent inputs. Superimposed on this are the effects of hormones and drugs, which can act at multiple levels to modulate the output of the system. *OVLT,* Organum vasculosum of the lamina terminalis; *PVN,* paraventricular nucleus; *SFO,* subfornical organ; *SON,* supraoptic nucleus; *VMN,* ventromedial nucleus. (Adapted from Verbalis JG: Osmotic inhibition of neurohypophyseal secretion. *Ann N Y Acad Sci.* 1983;689:227–233.)

Exactly how cells sense volume changes is a critical step for all the mechanisms activated to achieve osmoregulation. Some of the most exciting new data have come from studies of brain osmoreceptors.[29] The cellular osmosensing mechanism used by the OVLT cells is an intrinsic depolarizing receptor potential. This potential is generated in these cells via a molecular transduction complex. Studies have suggested that this likely includes members of the transient receptor potential vanilloid (TRPV) family of cation channel proteins. These channels are generally activated by cell membrane stretch to cause a nonselective conductance of cations, with a preference for $Ca^{2+}$. Multiple studies have characterized various members of the TRPV family as cellular mechanoreceptors in different tissues.[49] Both in vitro and in vivo studies of the TRPV family of cation channel proteins have provided evidence supporting the roles of TRPV1, TRPV2, and TRPV4 proteins in the transduction of osmotic stimuli in mammals that are important for sensing cell volume.[50] Moreover, genetic variation in the TRPV4 gene affects TRPV4 function and may influence water balance on a population-wide basis.[51] The details of exactly how and where various members of the TRPV family of cation channel proteins participate in osmoregulation in different species remains to be ascertained by additional studies. However, a strong case can already be made for their involvement in the transduction of osmotic stimuli in the neural cells in the OVLT and surrounding hypothalamus that regulate osmotic homeostasis, which appears to have been highly conserved throughout evolution.[50]

## NONOSMOTIC REGULATION

### Hemodynamic Stimuli

Not surprisingly, hypovolemia also is a potent stimulus for AVP secretion in humans[32,52] because an appropriate response to volume depletion should include renal water conservation. In humans and many animal species, lowering blood pressure suddenly by any of several methods increases plasma AVP levels by an amount proportional to the degree of hypotension achieved.[32,53] This stimulus-response relationship follows an exponential pattern, so that small reductions in blood pressure, of the order of 5% to 10%, usually have only small effects on plasma AVP levels, whereas blood pressure decreases of 20% to 30% result in hormone levels many times higher than those required to produce maximal antidiuresis (see Fig. 15.4). The AVP response to acute reductions in blood volume appears to be quantitatively and qualitatively similar to the response to blood pressure. In rats, plasma AVP increases as an exponential function of the degree of hypovolemia. Thus, little increase in plasma AVP can be detected until blood volume falls by 5% to 8%; beyond that point, plasma AVP increases at an exponential rate in relation to the degree of hypovolemia and usually reaches levels 20 to 30 times normal when blood volume is reduced by 20% to 40%.[54,55] The volume-AVP relationship has not been as thoroughly characterized in other species, but it appears to follow a similar pattern to that in humans.[56] Conversely, acute increases in blood volume or pressure suppress AVP secretion. This response has been characterized less well than that of hypotension or hypovolemia but seems to have a similar quantitative relationship (i.e., relatively large changes, ≈10%–15%, are required to alter hormone secretion appreciably).[57]

The minimal to absent effect of small changes in blood volume and pressure on AVP secretion contrasts sharply with the extraordinary sensitivity of the osmoregulatory system (see Fig. 15.4). Recognition of this difference is essential for understanding the relative contribution of each system to control AVP secretion under physiologic and pathologic conditions. Because daily variations of total body water rarely exceed 2% to 3%, their effect on AVP secretion must be mediated largely, if not exclusively, by the osmoregulatory system. Nonetheless, modest changes in blood volume and pressure do, in fact, influence AVP secretion indirectly, even though they are weak stimuli by themselves. This occurs via shifting the sensitivity of AVP secretion to osmotic stimuli so that a given increase in osmolality will cause a greater secretion of AVP during hypovolemic conditions than during euvolemic states (Fig. 15.7).[58,59] In the presence of a negative hemodynamic stimulus, plasma AVP continues to respond appropriately to small changes in plasma osmolality and can still be fully suppressed if the osmolality falls below the new (lower) set point. The retention of the threshold function is a vital aspect of the interaction because it ensures that the capability to regulate the osmolality of body fluids is not lost, even in the presence of significant hypovolemia or hypotension. Consequently, it is reasonable to conclude that the major effect of moderate degrees of hypovolemia on AVP secretion and thirst is to modulate the gain of the osmoregulatory responses, with direct effects on thirst and AVP secretion occurring only during more severe degrees of hypovolemia (e.g., >10% to 20% reduction in blood pressure or volume).

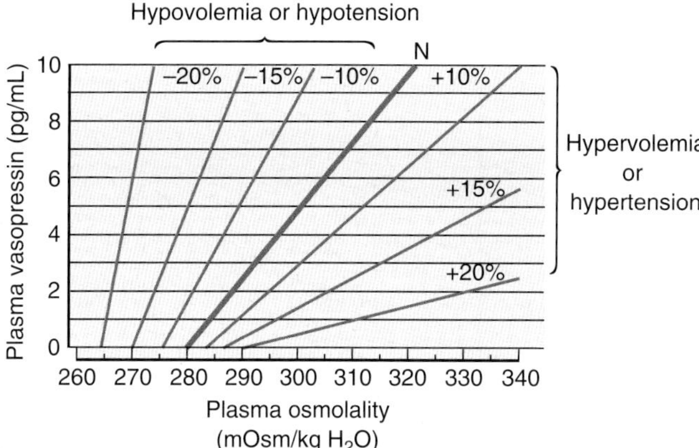


**Fig. 15.7** The relationship between the osmolality of plasma and concentration of arginine vasopressin (AVP) in plasma is modulated by blood volume and pressure. The line labeled *N* shows plasma AVP concentration across a range of plasma osmolalities in an adult with normal intravascular volume (i.e., euvolemic) and normal blood pressure (i.e., normotensive). The lines to the left of *N* show the relationship between plasma AVP concentration and plasma osmolality in adults whose low intravascular volume (i.e., hypovolemia) or blood pressure (i.e., hypotension) is 10%, 15%, and 20% below normal, respectively. Lines to the right of *N* indicate volumes and blood pressures 10%, 15%, and 20% above normal, respectively. Note that hemodynamic influences do not disrupt the osmoregulation of AVP but rather raise or lower the set point, and possibly also the sensitivity, of AVP secretion in proportion to the magnitude of the change in blood volume or pressure. (Adapted from Robertson GL, Athar S, Shelton RL: Osmotic control of vasopressin function. In Andreoli TE, Grantham JJ, Rector FC, Jr, eds. *Disturbances in Body Fluid Osmolality,* Bethesda, MD: *Am Physiol Soc* 1977: 125.)

These hemodynamic influences on AVP secretion are mediated, at least in part, by neural pathways that originate in stretch-sensitive receptors, generally termed "baroreceptors," in the cardiac atria, aorta, and carotid sinus (see Fig. 15.2; reviewed in detail in Chapter 14). Afferent nerve fibers from these receptors ascend in the vagus and glossopharyngeal nerves to the nuclei of the tractus solitarius (NTS) in the brain stem.[60] A variety of postsynaptic pathways from the NTS then project, directly and indirectly via the ventrolateral medulla and lateral parabrachial nucleus, to the PVN and SON in the hypothalamus.[61] Early studies have suggested that the input from these pathways is predominantly inhibitory under basal conditions because interrupting them acutely results in large increases in plasma AVP levels, as well as in arterial blood pressure.[62] However, as for most neural systems, including the neurohypophysis, innervation is complex and consists of excitatory and inhibitory inputs. Consequently, different effects have been observed under different experimental conditions.

The baroreceptor mechanism also appears to mediate a large number of pharmacologic and pathologic effectors of AVP secretion (Table 15.1). Among them are diuretics, isoproterenol, nicotine, prostaglandins, nitroprusside, trimethaphan, histamine, morphine, and bradykinin, all of which stimulate AVP, at least in part by lowering blood volume or pressure,[52] and norepinephrine, which suppresses AVP by raising blood pressure.[63] In addition, an upright posture, sodium depletion, congestive heart failure, cirrhosis, and

**Table 15.1 Drugs and Hormones That Affect Vasopressin Secretion**

| Stimulatory | Inhibitory |
|---|---|
| Acetylcholine | Norepinephrine |
| Nicotine | Fluphenazine |
| Apomorphine | Haloperidol |
| Morphine (high doses) | Promethazine |
| Epinephrine | Oxilorphan |
| Isoproterenol | Butorphanol |
| Histamine | Opioid agonists |
| Bradykinin | Morphine (low doses) |
| Prostaglandin | Ethanol |
| β-Endorphin | Carbamazepine |
| Cyclophosphamide IV | Glucocorticoids |
| Vincristine | Clonidine |
| Insulin | Muscimol |
| 2-Deoxyglucose | Phencyclidine |
| Angiotensin II | Phenytoin |
| Lithium | |
| Corticotropin-releasing factor | |
| Naloxone | |
| Cholecystokinin | |

nephrosis likely stimulate AVP secretion by reducing the effective circulating blood volume.[64,65] Symptomatic orthostatic hypotension, vasovagal reactions, and other forms of syncope stimulate AVP secretion more markedly via greater and more acute decreases in blood pressure, with the exception of the orthostatic hypotension associated with the loss of afferent baroregulatory function.[66] Almost every hormone, drug, or condition that affects blood volume or pressure will also affect AVP secretion but, in most cases, the degree of change of blood pressure or volume is modest and will result in a shift of the set point and/or sensitivity of the osmoregulatory response, rather than marked stimulation of AVP secretion (see Fig. 15.7).

### Drinking

Peripheral neural sensors other than baroreceptors also can affect AVP secretion. In humans, as well as dogs, drinking lowers plasma AVP before there is any appreciable decrease in plasma osmolality or serum [$Na^+$]. This is clearly a response to the act of drinking itself because it occurs independently of the composition of the fluid ingested,[67,68] although it may be influenced by the temperature of the fluid because the degree of suppression appears to be greater in response to colder fluids.[69] The pathways responsible for this effect have not been delineated, but likely include sensory afferents originating in the oropharynx and transmitted centrally via the glossopharyngeal nerve.

### Nausea

Among other nonosmotic stimuli to AVP secretion in humans, nausea is the most prominent. The sensation of nausea, with or without vomiting, is the most potent stimulus to AVP secretion known in humans. Although 20% increases in osmolality will typically elevate plasma AVP levels to the range of 5 to 20 pg/mL, and 20% decreases in blood pressure to 10 to 100 pg/mL, nausea has been described to cause AVP elevations in excess of 200 to 400 pg/mL.[70] The pathway

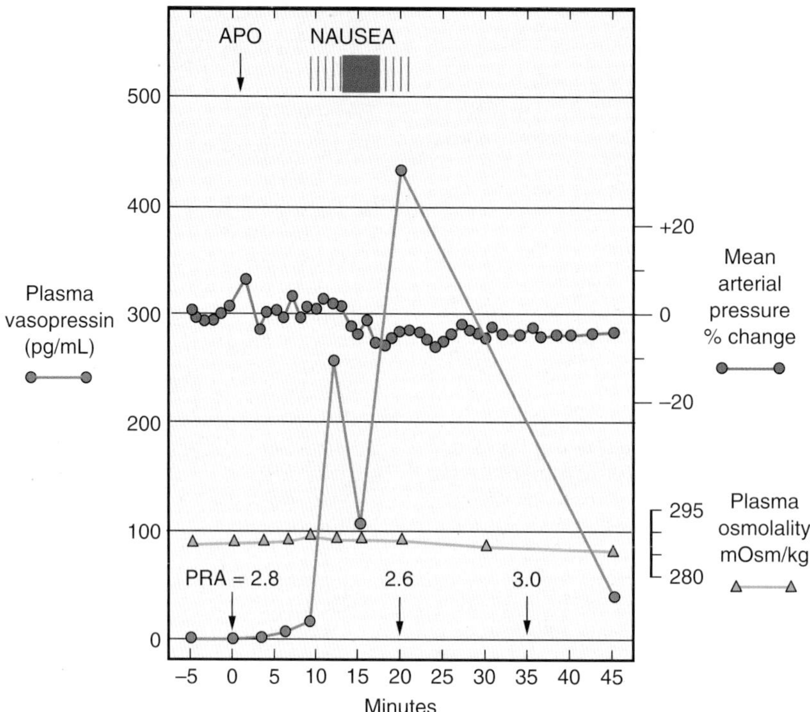


**Fig. 15.8** Effect of nausea on arginine vasopressin (AVP) secretion. Apomorphine (APO) was injected at the point indicated by the *vertical arrow*. Note that the rise in plasma AVP coincided with the occurrence of nausea and was not associated with detectable changes in plasma osmolality or blood pressure. *PRA,* Plasma renin activity. (Adapted from Robertson GL: The regulation of vasopressin function in health and disease. *Recent Prog Horm Res.* 1977; 33:333–385.)

mediating this effect has been mapped to the chemoreceptor zone in the area postrema of the brain stem in animal studies (see Fig. 15.2). It can be activated by a variety of drugs and conditions, including apomorphine, morphine, nicotine, alcohol, and motion sickness. Its effect on AVP is instantaneous and extremely potent (Fig. 15.8), even when the nausea is transient and not accompanied by vomiting or changes in blood pressure. Pretreatment with fluphenazine, haloperidol, or promethazine in doses sufficient to prevent nausea completely abolishes the AVP response. The inhibitory effect of these dopamine antagonists is specific for emetic stimuli because they do not alter the AVP response to osmotic and hemodynamic stimuli. Water loading blunts, but does not abolish, the effect of nausea on AVP release, suggesting that osmotic and emetic influences interact in a manner similar to that for osmotic and hemodynamic pathways. Species differences also affect emetic stimuli. Whereas dogs and cats appear to be even more sensitive than humans to the emetic stimulation of AVP release, rodents have little or no AVP response but release large amounts of OT instead.[71]

The emetic response probably mediates many pharmacologic and pathologic effects on AVP secretion. In addition to the drugs and conditions already noted, it may be responsible at least in part for the increase in AVP secretion that has been observed with vasovagal reactions, diabetic ketoacidosis, acute hypoxia, and motion sickness. Because nausea and vomiting are frequent side effects of many other drugs and diseases, many additional situations likely occur as well. The reason for this profound stimulation is not known (although it has been speculated that the AVP response assists evacuation of stomach contents via the contractions of gastric smooth muscle, AVP is not necessary for vomiting to occur), but it is responsible for the intense vasoconstriction that produces the pallor often associated with nausea.

### Hypoglycemia

Acute hypoglycemia is a less potent but reasonably consistent stimulus for AVP secretion.[72,73] The receptor and pathway that mediate this effect are unknown; however, they appear separate from those of other recognized stimuli because hypoglycemia stimulates AVP secretion, even in patients who have selectively lost the capacity to respond to hypernatremia, hypotension, or nausea.[73] The factor that actually triggers the release of AVP is likely intracellular deficiency of glucose or ATP because 2-deoxyglucose is also an effective stimulus to AVP secretion.[74] Generally, more than 20% decreases in glucose are required to increase plasma AVP levels significantly; the rate of decrease in the glucose level is probably the critical stimulus, however, because the rise in plasma AVP is not sustained with persistent hypoglycemia.[72] However, glucopenic stimuli are of unlikely importance in the physiology or pathology of AVP secretion because there are probably few drugs or conditions that lower plasma glucose rapidly enough to stimulate release of the hormone and because this effect is transient.

### Renin-Angiotensin-Aldosterone System

The renin-angiotensin-aldosterone system (RAAS) has also been intimately implicated in the control of AVP secretion.[75] Animal studies have indicated dual sites of action. Bloodborne Ang II stimulates AVP secretion by acting in the brain at the circumventricular subfornical organ (SFO),[76] a small structure located in the dorsal portion of the third cerebral ventricle (see Fig. 15.2). Because circumventricular organs lack a blood-brain barrier, the densely expressed Ang II receptor type 1 ($AT_1R$) of the SFO can detect very small increases in blood levels of Ang II.[77] Neural pathways from the SFO to the hypothalamic SON and PVN mediate AVP secretion and also appear to use Ang II as a neurotransmitter.[78] This accounts for the observation that the most sensitive site for angiotensin-mediated AVP secretion and thirst is intracerebroventricular injection into the cerebrospinal fluid. Further evidence in support of Ang II as a neurotransmitter is that the intraventricular administration of angiotensin receptor antagonists inhibits the AVP response to osmotic and hemodynamic stimuli.[79] The level of plasma Ang II required to stimulate AVP release is quite high, leading some to argue that this stimulus is active only under pharmacologic conditions. This is consistent with observations that even pressor doses of Ang II increase plasma AVP only about two- to fourfold[75] and may account for the failure of some investigators to demonstrate stimulation of thirst by exogenous angiotensin. However, this procedure may underestimate the physiologic effects of angiotensin because the increased blood pressure caused by exogenously administered Ang II appears to blunt the thirst induced via activation of inhibitory baroreceptive pathways.[80]

### Stress

Nonspecific stress caused by factors such as pain, emotion, or physical exercise has long been thought to cause AVP secretion, but it has never been determined whether this effect is mediated by a specific pathway or is secondary to the hypotension or nausea that often accompanies stress-induced vasovagal reactions. In rats[81] and humans,[82] a variety of noxious stimuli capable of activating the pituitary-adrenal axis and sympathetic nervous system do not stimulate AVP secretion unless they also lower blood pressure or alter blood volume. The marked rise in plasma AVP levels elicited by the manipulation of the abdominal viscera in anesthetized dogs has been attributed to nociceptive influences,[83] but mediation by emetic pathways cannot be excluded in this setting. Endotoxin-induced fever stimulates AVP secretion in rats, and studies have supported the possible mediation of this effect by circulating cytokines, such as interleukin-1 (IL-1) and IL-6.[84] Clarification of the possible role of nociceptive and thermal influences on AVP secretion is particularly important in view of the frequency with which painful or febrile illnesses are associated with osmotically inappropriate secretion of antidiuretic hormone.

### Hypoxia and Hypercapnia

Acute hypoxia and hypercapnia also stimulate AVP secretion.[85,86] In conscious humans, however, the stimulatory effect of moderate hypoxia (arterial partial pressure of oxygen [$PaO_2$] > 35 mm Hg) is inconsistent and seems to occur mainly in subjects who develop nausea or hypotension. In conscious dogs, more severe hypoxia ($PaO_2$ < 35 mm Hg) consistently increases AVP secretion without concomitant reductions in arterial pressure.[87] Studies of anesthetized dogs have supported these studies and suggested that the AVP response to acute hypoxia depends on the level of hypoxemia achieved. At a $PaO_2$ of 35 mm Hg or lower, plasma AVP increases markedly, even though there is no change or even an increase in arterial pressure, but less severe hypoxia ($PaO_2$ > 40 mm Hg) has no effect on AVP levels.[88] These results indicate that there is likely a hypoxemic threshold for AVP secretion and suggest that severe hypoxemia alone may also stimulate AVP secretion in humans. If so, it may be responsible, at least in part, for the osmotically inappropriate AVP elevations noted in some patients with acute respiratory failure.[89] In conscious or anesthetized dogs, acute hypercapnia, independent of hypoxia or hypotension, also increases AVP secretion.[87,88] It has not been determined whether this response also exhibits threshold characteristics or otherwise depends on the degree of hypercapnia, nor is it known whether hypercapnia has similar effects on AVP secretion in humans or other animals. The mechanisms whereby hypoxia and hypercapnia release AVP remain undefined, but they likely involve peripheral chemoreceptors and/or baroreceptors because cervical vagotomy abolishes the response to hypoxemia in dogs.[90]

### Drugs

As will be discussed more extensively in the section on clinical disorders, a variety of drugs also stimulates AVP secretion, including nicotine (see Table 15.1). Drugs and hormones can potentially affect AVP secretion at many different sites. As already discussed, many excitatory stimulants such as isoproterenol, nicotine, high doses of morphine, and cholecystokinin act, at least in part, by lowering blood pressure and/or producing nausea. Others, such as substance P, prostaglandin, endorphin, and other opioids, have not been studied sufficiently to define their mechanism of action, but they may also work by one or both of the same mechanisms. Inhibitory stimuli similarly have multiple modes of action. Vasopressor drugs such as norepinephrine inhibit AVP secretion indirectly by raising the arterial pressure. In low doses, a variety of opioids of all subtypes, including morphine, met-enkephalin, and κ-agonists, inhibit AVP secretion in rats and humans.[91] Endogenous opioid peptides interact with the magnocellular neurosecretory system at several levels to inhibit basal and stimulated secretion of AVP and oxytocin. Opioid inhibition of AVP secretion has been found to occur in isolated posterior pituitary tissue, and the action of morphine and of several opioid agonists such as butorphanol and oxilorphan likely occurs via activation of κ-opioid receptors located on nerve terminals of the posterior pituitary.[92] The well-known inhibitory effect of ethanol on AVP secretion may be mediated, at least in part, by endogenous opiates because it is due to an elevation in the osmotic threshold for AVP release[93] and can be partially blocked by treatment with naloxone.[94] Carbamazepine inhibits AVP secretion by diminishing the sensitivity of the osmoregulatory system; this effect occurs independently of changes in blood volume, blood pressure, and/or blood glucose levels.[95] Other drugs that inhibit AVP secretion include clonidine, which appears to act via central and peripheral adrenoreceptors[96]; muscimol,[97] which acts as a GABA antagonist; and phencyclidine,[98] which probably acts by raising blood pressure. However, despite the importance of these stimuli during pathologic conditions, none of them is a significant determinant of the physiologic regulation of AVP secretion in humans.

## DISTRIBUTION AND CLEARANCE

Plasma AVP concentration is determined by the difference between the rates of secretion from the posterior pituitary gland and removal of the hormone from the vascular compartment via metabolism and urinary clearance. In healthy adults, intravenously injected AVP distributes rapidly into a space equivalent in size to the ECF compartment. This initial, or mixing, phase has a half-life of 4 to 8 minutes and is virtually complete in 10 to 15 minutes. The rapid mixing phase is followed by a second slower decline that corresponds to the metabolic clearance of AVP. Most studies of this phase have yielded mean values of 10 to 20 minutes by steady-state and non–steady-state techniques,[32] consistent with the observed rates of change in urine osmolality after water loading and injection of AVP, which also support a short half-life.[99] In pregnant women, the metabolic clearance rate of AVP increases nearly fourfold,[100] which becomes significant in the pathophysiology of gestational diabetes insipidus (see later discussion). Smaller animals such as rats clear AVP much more rapidly than humans because their cardiac output is higher relative to their BW and surface area.[99]

Although many tissues have the capacity to inactivate AVP, metabolism in vivo appears to occur largely in the liver and kidney.[99] The enzymatic processes whereby the liver and kidney inactivate AVP involve an initial reduction of the disulfide bridge, followed by aminopeptidase cleavage of the bond between amino acid residues 1 and 2 and cleavage of the C-terminal glycinamide residue. Some AVP is excreted intact in the urine, but there is disagreement about the amount and factors that affect it. For example, in healthy, normally hydrated adults, the urinary clearance of AVP ranges from 0.1 to 0.6 mL/kg/min under basal conditions and has never been found to exceed 2 mL/kg/min, even in the presence of solute diuresis.[32] The mechanisms involved in the excretion of AVP have not been defined with certainty, but the hormone is probably filtered at the glomerulus and variably reabsorbed at sites along the nephron. The latter process may be linked to the reabsorption of $Na^+$ or other solutes in the proximal nephron because the urinary clearance of AVP has been found to vary by as much as 20-fold in direct relation to the solute clearance.[32] Consequently, measurements of urinary AVP excretion in humans do not provide a consistently reliable index of changes in plasma AVP and should be interpreted cautiously when glomerular filtration or solute clearance is inconstant or abnormal.

## THIRST

Thirst is the body's defense mechanism to increase water consumption in response to perceived deficits of body fluids. It can be most easily defined as a consciously perceived desire for water. True thirst must be distinguished from other determinants of fluid intake such as taste, dietary preferences, and social customs, as discussed previously. Thirst can be stimulated in animals and humans by intracellular dehydration caused by increases in the effective osmolality of the ECF or by intravascular hypovolemia caused by losses of ECF.[101,102] As would be expected, these are many of the same variables that provoke AVP secretion. Of these, hypertonicity is clearly the most potent. Similar to AVP secretion, substantial evidence to date has supported mediation of osmotic thirst by osmoreceptors located in the anterior hypothalamus of the brain,[30,31] whereas hypovolemic thirst appears to be stimulated via activation of low- and/or high-pressure baroreceptors[103] and circulating Ang II.[104] Regardless of the origin of the stimulus to thirst, the actual perception of thirst occurs in higher brain centers, specifically the anterior cingulate cortex (ACC) and insular cortex (IC), which receive information from circumventricular organs such as the organum OVLT and SFO (see Fig. 15.2) via relay nuclei in the thalamus.[105]

### OSMOTIC THIRST

In healthy adults, an increase in effective plasma osmolality of only 2% to 3% above basal levels produces a strong desire to drink.[106] This response is not dependent on changes in ECF or plasma volume because it occurs similarly whether plasma osmolality is raised by the infusion of hypertonic solutions or by water deprivation. The absolute level of plasma osmolality at which a person develops a conscious urge to seek and drink water is termed the "osmotic thirst threshold." It varies appreciably among individuals, likely as a result of genetic factors,[33] but in healthy adults it averages approximately 295 mOsm/kg $H_2O$. Of physiologic significance is the fact that this level is above the osmotic threshold for AVP release and approximates the plasma osmolality at which maximal concentration of the urine is normally achieved (see Fig. 15.5).

The brain pathways that mediate osmotic thirst have not been well defined, but it is clear that the initiation of drinking requires osmoreceptors located in the anteroventral hypothalamus and OVLT in the same area as the osmoreceptors that control osmotic AVP secretion.[30,31] Whether the osmoreceptors for AVP and thirst are the same cells or are simply located in the same general area remains unknown.[29] However, the properties of the osmoreceptors are very similar. Ineffective plasma solutes such as urea and glucose, which have little or no effect on AVP secretion, are equally ineffective at stimulating thirst, whereas effective solutes such as NaCl and mannitol can stimulate thirst.[9,107] The sensitivities of the thirst and AVP osmoreceptors cannot be compared precisely, but they are also probably similar. Thus, in healthy adults, the intensity of thirst increases rapidly in direct proportion to serum [$Na^+$] or plasma osmolality and generally becomes intolerable at levels only 3% to 5% above the threshold level.[108] Water consumption also appears to be proportional to the intensity of thirst in humans and animals and, under conditions of maximal osmotic stimulation, can reach rates as high as 20 to 25 L/day. The dilution of body fluids by ingested water complements the retention of water that occurs during AVP-induced antidiuresis, and both responses occur concurrently when drinking water is available.

As with AVP secretion, the osmoregulation of thirst appears to be bimodal because a modest decline in plasma osmolality induces a sense of satiation and reduces the basal rate of spontaneous fluid intake.[108,109] This effect is sufficient to prevent hypotonic overhydration, even when antidiuresis is fixed at maximal levels for prolonged periods, suggesting that osmotically inappropriate secretion of AVP (syndrome of inappropriate antidiuretic hormone secretion [SIADH]) should not result in the development of hyponatremia unless the satiety mechanism is impaired or fluid intake is inappropriately high for some other reason, such as the unregulated components of fluid intake discussed earlier.[109] Also similar to AVP secretion, thirst can be influenced by oropharyngeal or upper gastrointestinal receptors that respond to the act of drinking itself.[68] In humans, however, the rapid relief of thirst provided by this mechanism lasts only a matter of minutes, and thirst quickly recurs until enough water is absorbed to lower plasma osmolality to normal. Therefore, although local oropharyngeal sensations may have a significant short-term influence on thirst, it is the hypothalamic osmoreceptors that ultimately determine the volume of water intake in response to dehydration.

### HYPOVOLEMIC THIRST

In contrast, the threshold for producing hypovolemic or extracellular thirst is significantly higher in animals and humans. Studies in several species have shown that sustained decreases in plasma volume or blood pressure of at least 4% to 8%, and in some species 10% to 15%, are necessary to stimulate drinking consistently.[110,111] In humans, the degree of hypovolemia or hypotension required to produce thirst has not been precisely defined, but it has been difficult to demonstrate any effects of mild to moderate hypovolemia to stimulate thirst independently of osmotic changes occurring with dehydration. This blunted sensitivity to changes in ECF volume or blood pressure in humans probably represents an adaptation that occurred as a result of the erect posture of primates, which predisposes them to wider fluctuations in blood and atrial filling pressures as a result of the orthostatic pooling of blood in the lower body. Stimulation of thirst (and AVP secretion) by such transient postural changes in blood pressure might lead to overdrinking and inappropriate antidiuresis in situations in which the ECF volume was actually normal but only transiently maldistributed. Consistent with a blunted response to baroreceptor activation, studies have also shown that the systemic infusion of Ang II to pharmacologic levels is a much less potent stimulus to thirst in humans than in animals,[112] in whom it is one of the most potent dipsogens known. Nonetheless, this response is not completely absent in humans, as demonstrated by rare cases of polydipsia in patients with pathologic causes of hyperreninemia.[113] The pathways whereby hypovolemia or hypotension produces thirst have not been well defined, but probably involve the same brain stem baroreceptive pathways that mediate hemodynamic effects on AVP secretion,[103] as well as a likely contribution from circulating levels of Ang II in some species.[114]

### ANTICIPATORY THIRST

Recent studies of the neural circuitry underlying drinking behavior have identified a new type of thirst that precedes physiological challenges to osmotic and volume homeostasis, which has been termed "anticipatory thirst." The best studied example of this is the increase in drinking that occurs in animals a few hours at the end of their awake period, which serves to maintain hydration during the sleep period when there is no fluid intake. This drinking behavior appears to be mediated by vasopressin-containing neurons in the suprachiasmatic nucleus (SCN), which is the brain nucleus that controls diurnal rhythms. SCN vasopressin neurons project to the OVLT, where they excite thirst-activating neurons, thereby enabling maintenance of osmotic homeostasis during sleep.[115]

### INTEGRATION OF VASOPRESSIN SECRETION AND THIRST

A synthesis of what is presently known about the regulation of AVP secretion and thirst in humans leads to a relatively simple but elegant system to maintain water balance. Under normal physiologic conditions, the sensitivity of the osmoregulatory system for AVP secretion accounts for the maintenance of plasma osmolality within narrow limits by adjusting renal water excretion to small changes in osmolality. Stimulated thirst does not represent a major regulatory mechanism under these conditions, and unregulated fluid ingestion supplies adequate water in excess of true "need," which is then excreted in relation to osmoregulated pituitary AVP secretion. However, when unregulated water intake cannot adequately supply body needs in the presence of plasma AVP levels sufficient to produce maximal antidiuresis, plasma osmolality rises to levels that stimulate thirst (see Fig. 15.5), and water intake increases proportionally to the elevation of osmolality above this thirst threshold.

In such a system, thirst essentially represents a backup mechanism that becomes active when pituitary and renal mechanisms prove insufficient to maintain plasma osmolality within a few percentage points of basal levels. This arrangement has the advantage of freeing humans from frequent episodes of thirst. These would require a diversion of activities toward behavior oriented to seeking water when water deficiency is sufficiently mild to be compensated for by renal water conservation, but would stimulate water ingestion once water deficiency reaches potentially harmful levels. Stimulation of AVP secretion at plasma osmolalities below the threshold for subjective thirst acts to maintain an excess of body water sufficient to eliminate the need to drink whenever slight elevations in plasma osmolality occur. This system of differential effective thresholds for thirst and AVP secretion nicely complements many studies that have demonstrated excess unregulated (or need-free) drinking in humans and animals. Only when this mechanism becomes inadequate to maintain body fluid homeostasis does thirst-induced regulated fluid intake become the predominant defense mechanism for the prevention of severe dehydration.

## DISORDERS OF INSUFFICIENT VASOPRESSIN OR VASOPRESSIN EFFECT

Disorders of insufficient AVP or AVP effect are associated with inadequate urine concentration and increased urine output, termed "polyuria." If thirst mechanisms are intact, this is accompanied by compensatory increases in fluid intake ("polydipsia") as a result of stimulated thirst to preserve body fluid homeostasis. The net result is polyuria and polydipsia, with preservation of normal plasma osmolality and serum electrolyte concentrations. However, if thirst is impaired, or if fluid intake is insufficient for any reason to compensate for the increased urine excretion, then hyperosmolality and hypernatremia can result, with the consequent complications associated with these disorders. The quintessential disorder of insufficient AVP is diabetes insipidus (DI), which is a clinical syndrome characterized by excretion of abnormally large volumes of urine (diabetes) that is dilute (hypotonic) and devoid of taste from dissolved solutes (e.g., insipid), in contrast to the hypertonic, sweet-tasting urine characteristic of diabetes mellitus (from the Greek, meaning honey).

Several different pathophysiologic mechanisms can cause hypotonic polyuria (Box 15.1). Central DI (also called hypothalamic, neurogenic, or neurohypophyseal DI) is due to inadequate secretion and usually deficient synthesis of

### Box 15.1 Causes of Hypotonic Polyuria

**Central (Neurogenic) Diabetes Insipidus**

Congenital (congenital malformations; autosomal dominant, arginine vasopressin [AVP] neurophysin gene mutations)
Drug- or toxin-induced (ethanol, diphenylhydantoin, snake venom)
Granulomatous (histiocytosis, sarcoidosis)
Neoplastic (craniopharyngioma, germinoma, lymphoma, leukemia, meningioma, pituitary tumor; metastases)
Infectious (meningitis, tuberculosis, encephalitis)
Inflammatory, autoimmune (lymphocytic infundibuloneurohypophysitis)
Traumatic (neurosurgery, deceleration injury)
Vascular (cerebral hemorrhage or infarction, brain death)
Idiopathic

**Osmoreceptor Dysfunction**

Granulomatous (histiocytosis, sarcoidosis)
Neoplastic (craniopharyngioma, pinealoma, meningioma, metastases)
Vascular (anterior communicating artery aneurysm or ligation, intrahypothalamic hemorrhage)
Other (hydrocephalus, ventricular or suprasellar cyst, trauma, degenerative diseases)
Idiopathic

**Increased AVP Metabolism**

Pregnancy

**Nephrogenic Diabetes Insipidus**

Congenital (X-linked recessive, AVP $V_2$ receptor gene mutations; autosomal recessive or dominant, aquaporin-2 water channel gene mutations)
Drug-induced (demeclocycline, lithium, cisplatin, methoxyflurane)
Hypercalcemia
Hypokalemia
Infiltrating lesions (sarcoidosis, amyloidosis)
Vascular (sickle cell anemia)
Mechanical (polycystic kidney disease, bilateral ureteral obstruction)
Solute diuresis (glucose, mannitol, sodium, radiocontrast dyes)
Idiopathic

**Primary Polydipsia**

Psychogenic (schizophrenia, obsessive-compulsive behaviors)
Dipsogenic (downward resetting of thirst threshold, idiopathic or similar lesions, as with central DI)

AVP in the hypothalamic neurohypophyseal system. Lack of AVP-stimulated activation of the $V_2$ subtype of AVP receptors in the kidney collecting tubules (see Chapter 10) causes the excretion of large volumes of dilute urine. In most cases, thirst mechanisms are intact, leading to compensatory polydipsia. However, in a variant of central DI, osmoreceptor dysfunction, thirst is also impaired, leading to hypodipsia. DI of pregnancy is a transient disorder due to an accelerated metabolism of AVP as a result of increased activity of the enzyme oxytocinase or vasopressinase in the serum of pregnant women, again leading to polyuria and polydipsia. Accelerated metabolism of AVP during pregnancy may also cause a patient with subclinical DI from other causes to shift from a relatively asymptomatic state to a symptomatic state as a result of the more rapid AVP degradation. Nephrogenic DI is due to inappropriate renal responses to AVP. This produces excretion of dilute urine, despite normal pituitary AVP secretion and secondary polydipsia, similar to central DI. The final cause of hypotonic polyuria, primary polydipsia, differs significantly from the other causes because it is not due to deficient AVP secretion or impaired renal responses to AVP, but rather to excessive ingestion of fluids. This can result from an abnormality in the thirst mechanism, in which case it is sometimes called "dipsogenic DI," or from psychiatric disorders, in which case it is generally referred to as "psychogenic polydipsia."

## CENTRAL DIABETES INSIPIDUS

### CAUSES

Central diabetes insipidus (CDI) is caused by inadequate secretion of AVP from the posterior pituitary in response to osmotic stimulation. In most cases, this is due to destruction of the neurohypophysis by a variety of acquired or congenital anatomic lesions that destroy or damage the neurohypophysis by pressure or infiltration (see Box 15.1). The severity of the resulting hypotonic diuresis depends on the degree of destruction of the neurohypophysis, leading to complete or partial deficiency of AVP secretion.

Despite the wide variety of lesions that can potentially cause CDI, it is much more common not to have CDI in the presence of such lesions than actually to produce the syndrome. This apparent inconsistency can be understood by considering several common principles of neurohypophyseal physiology and pathophysiology that are relevant to all these causes.

First, the synthesis of AVP occurs in the hypothalamus (see Fig. 15.2); the posterior pituitary simply represents the site of storage and secretion of the neurosecretory granules that contain AVP. Consequently, lesions contained within the sella turcica that destroy only the posterior pituitary generally do not cause CDI because the cell bodies of the magnocellular neurons that synthesize AVP remain intact, and the site of release of AVP shifts more superiorly, typically into the blood vessels of the median eminence at the base of the brain. Perhaps the best examples of this phenomenon are large pituitary macroadenomas that completely destroy the anterior and posterior pituitary. DI is a distinctly unusual presentation for such pituitary adenomas because destruction of the posterior pituitary by such slowly enlarging intrasellar lesions merely destroys the nerve terminals, but not the cell bodies, of the AVP neurons. As this occurs, the site of release of AVP shifts more superiorly to the pituitary stalk and median eminence. Sometimes this can be detected on noncontrast magnetic resonance imaging (MRI) scans as a shift of the pituitary bright spot more superiorly to the level of the infundibulum or median eminence,[116] but this process is often too diffuse to be detected in this manner. The development of DI from a pituitary adenoma is so uncommon, even with macroadenomas that completely obliterate sellar contents sufficiently to cause panhypopituitarism, that its presence should lead to consideration of alternative diagnoses, such as craniopharyngioma. This often causes damage to the median eminence because of adherence of the capsule to the base of the hypothalamus, more rapidly enlarging sellar or suprasellar masses that do not allow sufficient time for shifting the site of AVP release more superiorly (e.g., metastatic lesions, acute hemorrhage), or granulomatous disease, with more diffuse hypothalamic involvement (e.g., sarcoidosis, histiocytosis). With very large pituitary adenomas that produce ACTH deficiency, it is actually more likely that patients will present with hypoosmolality from an SIADH-like picture as a result of the impaired free water excretion that accompanies hypocortisolism, as will be discussed later.

A second general principle is that the capacity of the neurohypophysis to synthesize AVP is greatly in excess of the body's daily needs for the maintenance of water homeostasis. Carefully controlled studies of surgical section of the pituitary stalk in dogs have clearly demonstrated that destruction of 80% to 90% of the magnocellular neurons in the hypothalamus is required to produce polyuria and polydipsia in these species.[117] Thus, even lesions that cause destruction of the AVP magnocellular neuron cell bodies must result in a large degree of destruction to produce DI. The most illustrative example of this is surgical section of the pituitary stalk in humans. Necropsy studies of these patients have revealed atrophy of the posterior pituitary and loss of the magnocellular neurons in the hypothalamus.[118] This loss of magnocellular cells presumably results from the retrograde degeneration of neurons whose axons were cut during surgery. As is generally true for all neurons, the likelihood of retrograde neuronal degeneration depends on the proximity of the axotomy, in this case section of the pituitary stalk, to the cell body of the neuron. This was shown clearly in studies of human subjects in whom section of the pituitary stalk at the level of the diaphragm sellae (a low stalk section) produced transient but not permanent DI, whereas section at the level of the infundibulum (a high stalk section) was required to cause permanent DI in most cases.[119]

Several genetic causes of AVP deficiency have also been characterized. Prior to the application of techniques for the amplification of genomic DNA, the only experimental model to study the mechanism of hereditary hypothalamic DI was the Brattleboro rat, a strain that was found serendipitously to have CDI.[120] In this animal, the disease demonstrates a classic pattern of autosomal recessive inheritance in which DI is expressed only in the homozygotes. The hereditary basis of the disease has been found to be a single base deletion producing a translational frameshift beginning in the third portion of the neurophysin coding sequence. Because the gene lacks a stop codon, there is a modified neurophysin, no glycopeptide, and a long polylysine tail.[121] Although the mutant prohormone accumulates in the endoplasmic reticulum, sufficient AVP is produced by the normal allele that the heterozygotes are asymptomatic. In contrast, almost all families with genetic CDI in humans that have been described to date demonstrate an autosomal dominant mode of inheritance.[122–124] In these cases, DI is expressed, despite the expression of one normal allele, which is sufficient to prevent the disease in the heterozygous Brattleboro rats. Numerous studies have been directed at understanding this apparent anomaly. Two potentially important clues about the cause of the DI in familial genetic CDI are the following:

1. Severe to partial deficiencies of AVP and overt signs of DI do not develop in these patients until several months to several years after birth and then gradually progress over the ensuing decades,[122,125] suggesting adequate initial function of the normal allele, with later decompensation.
2. A limited number of autopsy studies have suggested that some of these cases are associated with gliosis and a marked loss of magnocellular AVP neurons in the hypothalamus,[126] although other studies have shown normal neurons, with decreased expression of AVP or no hypothalamic abnormality. In most of these cases, the hyperintense signal normally emitted by the neurohypophysis in T1-weighted MRI scans (see later discussion) is also absent, although some exceptions have been reported.[127]

Another interesting, but as yet unexplained, observation is that some adults in these families have been described in whom DI was clinically apparent during childhood but who went into remission as adults, without evidence that their remissions could be attributed to renal or adrenal insufficiency or to increased AVP synthesis.[128]

The autosomal dominant form of familial CDI is caused by diverse mutations in the gene that codes for the AVP-neurophysin precursor (Fig. 15.9). All the mutations identified to date have been in the coding region of the gene and affect only one allele. They are located in all three exons and are predicted to alter or delete amino acid residues in the signal peptide, AVP, and neurophysin moieties of the precursor. Only the C-terminus glycopeptide, or copeptin moiety, has not been found to be affected. Most are missense mutations, but nonsense mutations (premature stop codons) and deletions also occur.[129] One feature shared by all the mutations is that they are predicted to alter or delete one or more amino acids known, or reasonably presumed, to be crucial for processing, folding, and oligomerization of the precursor protein in the endoplasmic reticulum.[122,124] Because of the related functional effects of the mutations, the common clinical characteristics of the disease, the dominant-negative mode of transmission, and the autopsy and hormonal evidence of postnatal neurohypophyseal degeneration, it has been postulated that all the mutations act by causing the production of an abnormal precursor protein that accumulates and eventually kills the neurons because it cannot be correctly processed, folded, and transported out of the endoplasmic reticulum. Expression studies of mutant DNA from several human mutations in cultured neuroblastoma cells have supported this misfolding-neurotoxicity hypothesis by demonstrating abnormal trafficking and accumulation of mutant prohormone in the endoplasmic reticulum with low or absent expression in the Golgi apparatus, suggesting difficulty with packaging into neurosecretory granules.[130] However, cell death may not be necessary to decrease available AVP. Normally, proteins retained in the endoplasmic reticulum are selectively degraded but, if excess mutant is produced and the selective normal degradative process is overwhelmed, an alternate, nonselective, degradative system (autophagy) is activated. As more and more mutant precursor builds up in the endoplasmic reticulum, the normal wild-type protein becomes trapped with the mutant protein and degraded by the activated nonspecific degradative system. In this case, the amount of AVP that matures and is packaged would be markedly reduced.[131,132] This explanation is consistent with

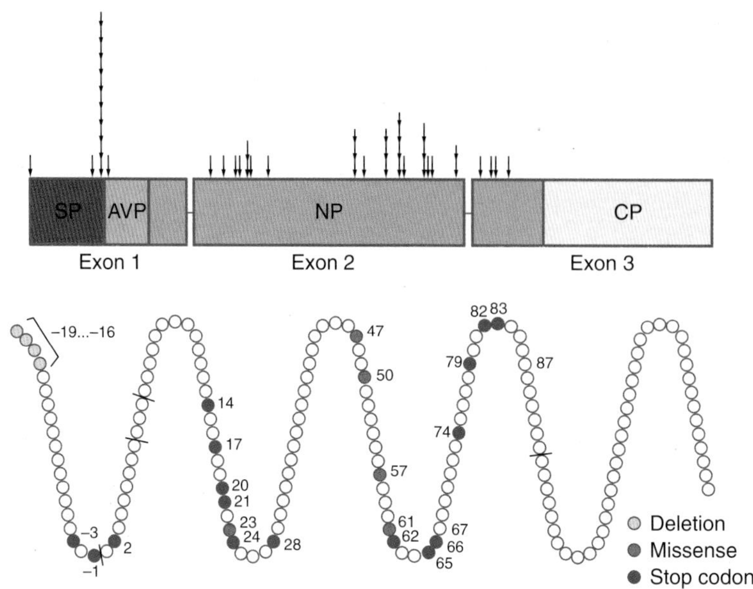


**Fig. 15.9** Location and type of mutations in the gene that codes for the arginine vasopressin (AVP)–neurophysin precursor in kindreds with the autosomal dominant form of familial central diabetes insipidus (CDI). The location of the mutation in a different kindred is indicated by the *arrows.* The various portions of the precursor protein are designated by AVP (vasopressin), CP (copeptin), NP (neurophysin), and SP (signal peptide). Deletion and missense mutations are those expected to remove or replace one or more amino acid residues in the precursor. Those designated stop codons are expected to cause premature termination of the precursor. Note that none of the mutations causes a frameshift or affects the part of the gene that encodes the copeptin moiety, all the stop codons are in the distal part of the neurophysin moiety, and only one of the mutations affects the AVP moiety. All these findings are consistent with the concept that a mutant precursor is produced but cannot be folded properly because of interference with the binding of AVP to neurophysin, formation of intrachain disulfide bonds, or extreme flexibility or rigidity normally required at crucial places in the protein. (Adapted from Rittig S, Robertson GL, Siggaard C, et al: Identification of 13 new mutations in the vasopressin-neurophysin gene in 17 kindreds with familial autosomal dominant neurohypophyseal DI. *Am J Hum Genet.* 1996;58:107–117; and Hansen LK, Rittig S, Robertson GL: Genetic basis of familial neurohypophyseal diabetes insipidus. *Trends Endocrinol Metab.* 1997;8:363–372.)

cases in which little pathology is found in the magnocellular neurons and also with DI in which a small amount of AVP can still be detected.

Wolfram syndrome is a rare autosomal recessive disease with DI, diabetes mellitus, optic atrophy, and deafness (DIDMOAD). The genetic defect is the protein wolframin, which is found in the endoplasmic reticulum and is important for folding proteins.[133] Wolframin is involved in beta cell proliferation, intracellular protein processing, and calcium homeostasis, producing a wide spectrum of endocrine and central nervous system (CNS) disorders. DI is usually a late manifestation associated with decreased magnocellular neurons in the paraventricular and supraoptic nuclei.[134]

Idiopathic forms of AVP deficiency represent a large pathogenic category in adults and children. A study in children has revealed that over half (54%) of all cases of CDI were classified as idiopathic.[135] These patients do not have historic or clinical evidence of any injury or disease that can be linked to their DI, and MRI of the pituitary-hypothalamic area generally reveals no abnormality other than the absence of the posterior pituitary bright spot and sometimes varying degrees of thickening of the pituitary stalk. Several lines of evidence have suggested that many of these patients may have had an autoimmune destruction of the neurohypophysis to account for their DI. First, the entity of lymphocytic infundibuloneurohypophysitis has been documented to be present in a subset of patients with idiopathic DI.[136] Lymphocytic infiltration of the anterior pituitary, lymphocytic hypophysitis, has been recognized as a cause of anterior pituitary deficiency for many years, but it was not until an autopsy called attention to a similar finding in the posterior pituitary of a patient with DI that this pathology was recognized to occur in the neurohypophysis as well.[137] Since that initial report, a number of similar cases have been described, including cases in the postpartum period, which is characteristic of lymphocytic hypophysitis.[138] With the advent of MRI, lymphocytic infundibuloneurohypophysitis has been diagnosed based on the appearance of a thickened stalk and/or enlargement of the posterior pituitary, mimicking a pituitary tumor. In these cases, the characteristic bright spot on MRI T1-weighted images is lost. The enlargement of the stalk can mimic a neoplastic process, resulting in some of these patients undergoing surgery based on the suspicion of a pituitary tumor.

Since then, a number of patients with a suspicion of infundibuloneurohypophysitis and no other obvious cause of DI have been followed and have shown regression of the thickened pituitary stalk over time.[135,136,139] Several cases have been reported with the coexistence of CDI and adenohypophysitis; these presumably represent cases of combined lymphocytic infundibuloneurohypophysitis and hypophysitis.[140–143] A second line of evidence supporting an autoimmune cause in many cases of idiopathic DI is based on the finding of AVP antibodies in the serum of as many as one-third of patients with idiopathic DI and two-thirds of those with Langerhans cell histiocytosis X, but not in patients with DI caused by tumors.[144] A recently recognized form of infundibuloneurohypophysitis occurs in middle-aged to older men and is associated with immunoglobulin G4 (IgG4)–related systemic disease.[145,146] Various organs, especially the pancreas, are infiltrated with IgG4 plasma cells, and neurohypophysitis is only one manifestation of a multiorgan disease that may include other endocrine glands. This cause should be considered as a cause of DI based on age and gender at presentation and evidence of other systemic disease. The diagnosis can be established by elevated serum IgG4 levels and characteristic histology of biopsies. Response to steroids or other immunosuppressive drugs is characteristic.

## PATHOPHYSIOLOGY

The normal inverse, and nonlinear, relationship between urine volume and urine osmolality (see Fig. 15.5) means that initial decreases in maximal AVP secretion will not cause an increase in urine volume sufficient to be detected clinically by polyuria. In general, basal AVP secretion must fall to less than 10% to 20% of normal before basal urine osmolality decreases to less than 300 mOsm/kg $H_2O$ and urine flow increases to symptomatic levels (i.e., >50 mL/kg BW/day). This resulting loss of body water produces a slight rise in plasma osmolality that stimulates thirst and induces a compensatory polydipsia. The resultant increase in water intake restores balance with urine output and stabilizes the osmolality of body fluids at a new, slightly higher but still normal level. As the AVP deficit increases, this new steady-state level of plasma osmolality approximates the osmotic threshold for thirst (see Fig. 15.5). It is important to recognize that the deficiency of AVP need not be complete for polyuria and polydipsia to occur; it is only necessary that the maximal plasma AVP concentration achievable at or below the osmotic threshold for thirst is inadequate to concentrate the urine.[147] The degree of neurohypophyseal destruction at which such failure occurs varies considerably from person to person, largely because of individual differences in the set point and sensitivity of the osmoregulatory system.[33] In general, functional tests of AVP levels in patients with DI of variable severity, duration, and cause have indicated that AVP secretory capacity must be reduced by at least 75% to 80% for significant polyuria to occur. This also agrees with neuroanatomic studies of cell loss in the supraoptic nuclei of dogs with experimental pituitary stalk section[117] and of patients who had undergone pituitary surgery.[118]

Because renal mechanisms for sodium conservation are normal in patients with impaired or absent AVP secretion, there is no accompanying sodium deficiency. Although untreated DI can lead to hyperosmolality and volume depletion, until the water losses become severe, volume depletion is minimized by osmotic shifts of water from the ICF compartment to the more osmotically concentrated ECF compartment. This phenomenon is not as evident following increases in ECF [$Na^+$] because such osmotic shifts result in a slower increase in the serum [$Na^+$] than would otherwise occur. However, when non–sodium solutes such as mannitol are infused, this effect is more obvious due to the progressive dilutional decrease in serum [$Na^+$] caused by the translocation of intracellular water to the ECF compartment. Because patients with DI do not have impaired urine $Na^+$ conservation, the ECF volume is generally not markedly decreased, and regulatory mechanisms for the maintenance of osmotic homeostasis are primarily activated—stimulation of thirst and

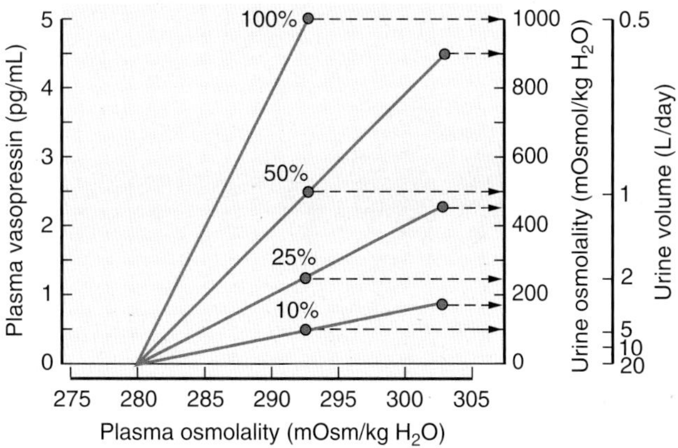


**Fig. 15.10** Relationship between plasma arginine vasopressin (AVP) levels, urine osmolality, and plasma osmolality in subjects with normal posterior pituitary function (100%) compared with patients with graded reductions in AVP-secreting neurons (to 50%, 25%, and 10% of normal). Note that the patient with a 50% secretory capacity can achieve only half the plasma AVP level and half the urine osmolality of normal subjects at a plasma osmolality of 293 mOsm/kg $H_2O$. However, with increasing plasma osmolality, this patient can nonetheless eventually stimulate sufficient AVP secretion to reach a near-maximal urine osmolality. In contrast, patients with more severe degrees of AVP-secreting neuron deficits are unable to reach maximal urine osmolalities at any level of plasma osmolality. (Adapted from Robertson GL: Posterior pituitary. In Felig P, Baxter J, Frohman LA, eds. *Endocrinology and Metabolism.* New York: McGraw-Hill; 1986:338–386.)

AVP secretion (to whatever degree the neurohypophysis is still able to secrete AVP). In cases in which AVP secretion is totally absent (complete DI), patients are dependent entirely on water intake for the maintenance of water balance. However, in cases in which some residual capacity to secrete AVP remains (partial DI), plasma osmolality can eventually reach levels that allow for moderate degrees of urinary concentration (Fig. 15.10).

The development of DI following surgical or traumatic injury to the neurohypophysis represents a unique situation and can follow any of several different, well-defined patterns. In some patients, polyuria develops 1 to 4 days after injury and resolves spontaneously. Less often, the DI is permanent and continues indefinitely (see previous discussion on the relationship between the level of pituitary stalk section and development of permanent DI). Most interestingly, a triphasic response can occur as a result of pituitary stalk transection (Fig. 15.11).[119] The initial DI (first phase) is due to axon shock and lack of function of the damaged neurons. This phase lasts from several hours to several days and is followed by an antidiuretic phase (second phase) that is the result of the uncontrolled release of AVP from the disconnected and degenerating posterior pituitary or from the remaining severed neurons.[148] Overly aggressive administration of fluids during this second phase does not suppress the AVP secretion and can lead to hyponatremia. The antidiuresis can last from 2 to 14 days, after which DI recurs following depletion of the AVP from the degenerating posterior pituitary gland (third phase).[149]

Transient hyponatremia without preceding or subsequent DI has been reported following transsphenoidal surgery for pituitary microadenomas,[150] which generally occurs 5 to 10

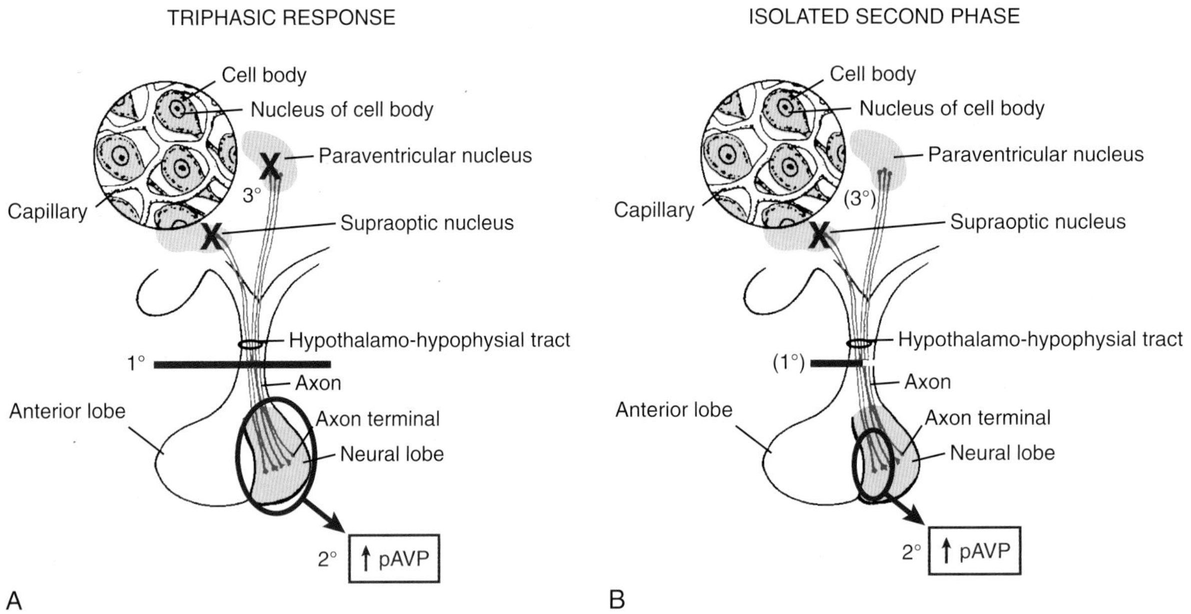

**Fig. 15.11** Mechanisms underlying the pathophysiology of the triphasic pattern of diabetes insipidus (DI) and the isolated second phase. (A) In the triphasic response, the first phase of DI is initiated following a partial or complete pituitary stalk section, which severs the connections between the AVP neuronal cell bodies in the hypothalamus and nerve terminals in the posterior pituitary gland, thus preventing stimulated AVP secretion (1 degree). This is followed in several days by the second phase of syndrome of inappropriate antidiuretic hormone secretion (SIADH), which is caused by uncontrolled release of AVP into the bloodstream from the degenerating nerve terminals in the posterior pituitary (2 degrees). After all the AVP stored in the posterior pituitary gland has been released, the third phase of DI returns if more than 80% to 90% of the AVP neuronal cell bodies in the hypothalamus have undergone retrograde degeneration (3 degrees). (B) In the isolated second phase, the pituitary stalk is injured, but not completely cut. Although the maximum AVP secretory response will be diminished as a result of the stalk injury, DI will not result if the injury leaves intact at least 10% to 20% of the nerve fibers connecting the AVP neuronal cell bodies in the hypothalamus to the nerve terminals in the posterior pituitary gland (1 degree). However, this is still followed in several days by the second phase of SIADH, which is caused by the uncontrolled release of AVP from the degenerating nerve terminals of the posterior pituitary gland that have been injured or severed (2 degrees). Because a smaller portion of the posterior pituitary is denervated, the magnitude of AVP released as the pituitary degenerates will be smaller and of shorter duration than with a complete triphasic response. After all the AVP stored in the damaged part of the posterior pituitary gland has been released, the second phase ceases, but clinical DI will not occur if less than 80% to 90% of the AVP neuronal cell bodies in the hypothalamus undergo retrograde degeneration (3 degrees). (From Loh JA, Verbalis JG: Disorders of water and salt metabolism associated with pituitary disease. *Endocrinol Metab Clin North Am*. 2008;37:213–234.)

days postoperatively. The incidence may be as high as 30% when these patients are carefully followed, although most cases are mild and self-limited.[151,152] This is due to inappropriate AVP secretion via the same mechanism as in the triphasic response, except that in these cases only the second phase occurs (isolated second phase) because the initial neural lobe or pituitary stalk damage is not sufficient to impair AVP secretion enough to produce clinical manifestations of DI (see Fig. 15.11).[153]

Once a deficiency of AVP secretion has been present for more than a few weeks, it rarely improves, even if the underlying cause of the neurohypophyseal destruction is eliminated. The major exception to this is in patients with postoperative DI, for whom spontaneous resolution is the rule. Although recovery from DI that persists more than several weeks postoperatively is less common, well-documented cases of long-term recovery have nonetheless been reported.[149] The reason for amelioration and resolution is apparent from the pathologic and histologic examination of neurohypophyseal tissue following pituitary stalk section.[154,155] Neurohypophyseal neurons that have intact perikarya are able to regenerate axons and form new nerve terminal endings capable of releasing AVP into nearby capillaries. In animals, this may be accompanied by a bulbous growth at the end of the severed stalk, which represents a new, albeit small, neural lobe. In humans, the regeneration process appears to proceed more slowly, and formation of a new neural lobe has not been noted. Nonetheless, histologic examination of a severed human stalk from a patient 18 months after hypophysectomy has demonstrated reorganization of neurohypophyseal fibers, with neurosecretory granules in close proximity to nearby blood vessels, closely resembling the histology of a normal posterior pituitary.[155]

Recognition of the fact that almost all patients with CDI retain a limited capacity to secrete some AVP allows for an understanding of some otherwise perplexing features of the disorder. For example, in many patients, restricting water intake long enough to raise plasma osmolality by only 1% to 2% induces sufficient AVP secretion to concentrate the urine (Fig. 15.12). As the plasma osmolality increases further, some patients with partial DI can even secrete enough AVP to achieve near-maximal urine osmolality (see Fig. 15.10). However, this should not cause confusion about the diagnosis of DI because, in these patients, the urine osmolality will still be inappropriately low at a plasma osmolality within a normal range, and they will respond to exogenous AVP administration with further increases in urine osmolality. These responses to dehydration illustrate the relative nature

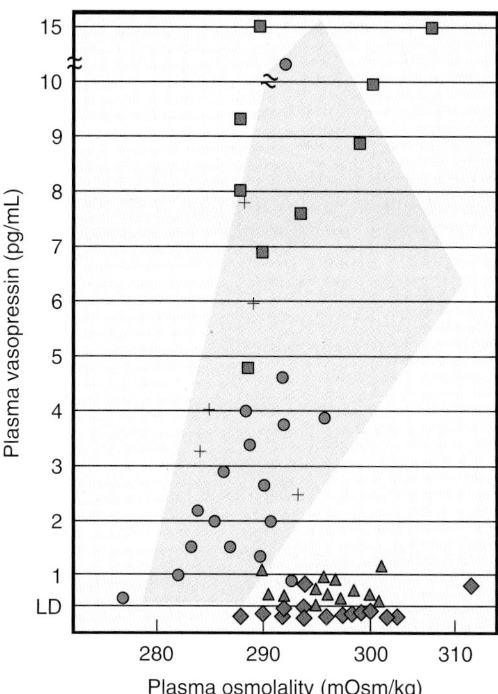


**Fig. 15.12** Relationship between plasma arginine vasopressin (AVP) and concurrent plasma osmolality in patients with polyuria of diverse causes. All measurements were made at the end of a standard dehydration test. *Shaded area,* Range of normal. In patients with severe (◆) or partial (▲) central diabetes insipidus (DI), plasma AVP was almost always subnormal relative to plasma osmolality. In contrast, the values from patients with primary polydipsia (●) or nephrogenic DI (■) were consistently within or above the normal range. (From Robertson GL: Diagnosis of diabetes insipidus. In Czernichow AP, Robinson A, eds. *Diabetes Insipidus in Man: Frontiers of Hormone Research.* Basel, Switzerland: S. Karger; 1985:176.)

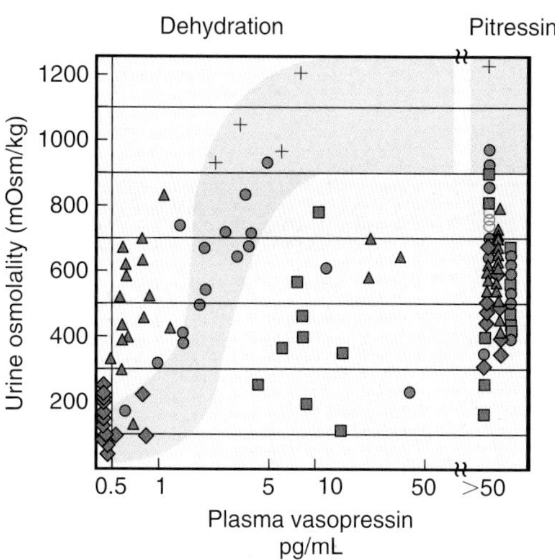


**Fig. 15.13** Relationship between urine osmolality and concurrent plasma arginine vasopressin (AVP) in patients with polyuria of diverse causes. All measurements were made at the end of a standard dehydration test. *Shaded area,* Range of normal. In patients with severe (◆) or partial (▲) central diabetes insipidus (DI), urine osmolality is normal or supranormal relative to plasma AVP when the latter is submaximal. In patients with nephrogenic DI (■), urine osmolality is always subnormal for plasma AVP. In patients with primary polydipsia (●), the relationship is normal at submaximal levels of plasma AVP but usually subnormal when plasma AVP is high. (From Robertson GL: Diagnosis of diabetes insipidus. In Czernichow AP, Robinson A, eds. *Diabetes Insipidus in Man: Frontiers of Hormone Research.* Basel, Switzerland: S. Karger; 1985:176.)

of the AVP deficiency in most cases and underscore the importance of the thirst mechanism to restrict the use of residual secretory capacity under basal conditions of ad libitum water intake.

CDI is also associated with changes in the renal response to AVP. The most obvious change is a reduction in maximal concentrating capacity, which has been attributed to washout of the medullary concentration gradient caused by the chronic polyuria in combination with decreased synthesis of AQP2 in the renal collecting duct principal cells. The severity of this defect is proportional to the magnitude of the polyuria and is independent of its cause.[147] Because of this, the level of urinary concentration achieved at maximally effective levels of plasma AVP is reduced in all types of DI. In patients with CDI, this concentrating abnormality is offset to some extent by an apparent increase in renal sensitivity to low levels of plasma AVP (Fig. 15.13). The cause of this supersensitivity is unknown, but it may reflect upward regulation of AVP $V_2$ receptor expression or function secondary to a chronic deficiency of the hormone.[156]

## OSMORECEPTOR DYSFUNCTION

### CAUSES

There is extensive literature in animals indicating that the primary osmoreceptors controlling AVP secretion and thirst are located in the anterior hypothalamus; lesions of this region in animals, called the "AV3V area," cause hyperosmolality through a combination of impaired thirst and impaired osmotically stimulated AVP secretion.[30,31] Initial reports in humans described this syndrome as essential hypernatremia,[157] and subsequent studies used the term "adipsic hypernatremia" in recognition of the profound thirst deficits found in most of the patients.[158] Based on the known pathophysiology, all these syndromes can be grouped together, termed "disorders of osmoreceptor dysfunction."[159] Although the pathologies responsible for this condition can be quite varied, all the cases reported to date have been due to various degrees of osmoreceptor destruction associated with a variety of different brain lesions, as summarized in Box 15.1. Many of these are the same types of lesions that can cause CDI but, in contrast to CDI, these lesions usually occur more rostrally in the hypothalamus, consistent with the anterior hypothalamic location of the primary osmoreceptor cells (see Fig. 15.2). One lesion that is unique to this disorder is an anterior communicating cerebral artery aneurysm. Because the small arterioles that feed the anterior wall of the third ventricle originate from the anterior communicating cerebral artery, an aneurysm in this region[160]—but more often following surgical repair of such an aneurysm that typically involves ligation of the anterior communicating artery[161]—produces infarction of the part of the hypothalamus containing the osmoreceptor cells.

### PATHOPHYSIOLOGY

The cardinal defect of patients with this disorder is lack of the osmoreceptors that regulate thirst. With rare exceptions, osmoregulation of AVP is also impaired, although the

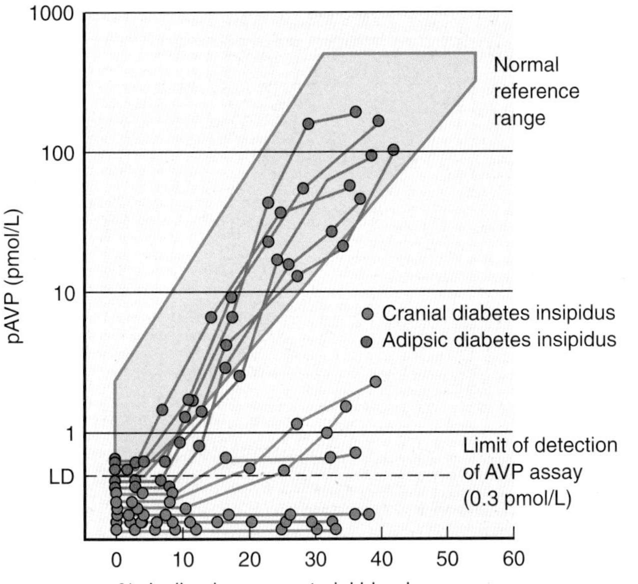


**Fig. 15.14** Plasma arginine vasopressin (AVP) responses to arterial hypotension produced by the infusion of trimethaphan in patients with central DI (cranial diabetes insipidus) and osmoreceptor dysfunction (adipsic diabetes insipidus). Normal responses in healthy volunteers are shown by the *shaded area.* Note that despite absent or markedly blunted AVP responses to hyperosmolality, patients with osmoreceptor dysfunction respond normally to baroreceptor stimulation induced by hypotension. (From Baylis PH, Thompson CJ: Diabetes insipidus and hyperosmolar syndromes. In Becker KL, ed. *Principles and Practice of Endocrinology and Metabolism,* Philadelphia: JB Lippincott; 1995:257.)

hormonal response to nonosmotic stimuli remains intact (Fig. 15.14).[162,163] Four major patterns of osmoreceptor dysfunction have been described, and each is characterized by defects in thirst and/or AVP secretory responses, as follows: (1) upward resetting of the osmostat for both thirst and AVP secretion (normal AVP and thirst responses but at an abnormally high plasma osmolality); (2) partial osmoreceptor destruction (blunted AVP and thirst responses at all plasma osmolalities); (3) total osmoreceptor destruction (absent AVP secretion and thirst, regardless of plasma osmolality); and (4) selective dysfunction of thirst osmoregulation with intact AVP secretion.[159] Regardless of the actual pattern, the hallmark of this disorder is an abnormal thirst response in addition to variable defects in AVP secretion. Thus, such patients fail to drink sufficiently as their plasma osmolality rises and, as a result, the new set point for plasma osmolality rises far above the normal thirst threshold. Unlike patients with CDI, whose polydipsia maintains their plasma osmolality within a normal range, patients with osmoreceptor dysfunction typically have osmolality in the range of 300 to 340 mOsm/kg $H_2O$. This again underscores the critical role played by normal thirst mechanisms in maintaining body fluid homeostasis; intact renal function alone is insufficient to maintain plasma osmolality within normal limits in such cases.

The rate of the development and severity of hyperosmolality and hypertonic dehydration in patients with osmoreceptor dysfunction is influenced by a number of factors. First is the ability to maintain some degree of osmotically stimulated thirst and AVP secretion, which will determine the new set point for plasma osmolality. Second are environmental influences that affect the rate of water output. When physical activity is minimal, and the ambient temperature is not elevated, the overall rates of renal and insensible water loss are low, and the patient's diet may be sufficient to maintain a relatively normal balance for long periods of time. Anything that increases perspiration, respiration, or urine output greatly accelerates the rate of water loss and thereby uncovers the patient's inability to mount an appropriate compensatory increase in water intake.[12] Under these conditions, severe and even fatal hypernatremia can develop relatively quickly. When the dehydration is only moderate (plasma osmolality = 300 to 330 mOsm/kg $H_2O$), the patient is usually asymptomatic, and signs of volume depletion are minimal, but if the dehydration becomes severe, the patient can exhibit symptoms and signs of hypovolemia, including weakness, postural dizziness, paralysis, confusion, coma, azotemia, hypokalemia, hyperglycemia, and secondary hyperaldosteronism (see later, "Clinical Manifestations of Diabetes Insipidus"). In severe cases, there may also be rhabdomyolysis, with marked serum elevations in muscle enzyme levels and occasionally acute renal failure.

However, a third factor also influences the degree of hyperosmolality and dehydration present in these patients. For all cases of osmoreceptor dysfunction, it is important to remember that afferent pathways from the brain stem to the hypothalamus remain intact; therefore, these patients will usually have normal AVP and renal concentrating responses to baroreceptor-mediated stimuli, such as hypovolemia and hypotension (see Fig. 15.14),[163] or to other nonosmotic stimuli, such as nausea (see Fig. 15.8).[158,162] This has the effect of preventing severe dehydration because, as hypovolemia develops, this will stimulate AVP secretion via baroreceptive pathways through the brain stem (see Fig. 15.2). Although protective, this effect often causes confusion, because sometimes these patients appear to have DI yet at other times they can concentrate their urine quite normally. Nonetheless, the presence of refractory hyperosmolality with absent or inappropriate thirst should alert clinicians to the presence of osmoreceptor dysfunction, regardless of occasional apparent normal urine concentration.

In a few patients with osmoreceptor dysfunction, forced hydration has been found to lead to hyponatremia in association with inappropriate urine concentration.[157,158] This paradoxic defect resembles that seen in SIADH and has been postulated to be caused by two different pathogenic mechanisms. One is continuous or fixed secretion of AVP because of loss of the capacity for osmotic inhibition and stimulation of hormone secretion. These observations, as well as electrophysiologic data,[43] have strongly suggested that the osmoregulatory system is bimodal (i.e., it is composed of inhibitory and stimulatory input to the neurohypophysis; see Fig. 15.6). The other cause of the diluting defect appears to be hypersensitivity to the antidiuretic effects of AVP because, in some patients, urine osmolality may remain elevated, even when the hormone is undetectable.[158]

Hypodipsia is also a common occurrence in older adults in the absence of any overt hypothalamic lesion.[164] In such cases, it is not clear whether the defect is in the hypothalamic osmoreceptors, in their projections to the cortex, or in some other regulatory mechanism. However, in most cases, the osmoreceptor is likely not involved because basal and stimulated plasma AVP levels have been found to be normal, or even hyperresponsive, in relation to plasma osmolality in older adults, with the exception of only a few studies that showed decreased plasma levels of AVP relative to plasma osmolality.[165]

## GESTATIONAL DIABETES INSIPIDUS

### CAUSES

A relative deficiency of plasma AVP can also result from an increase in the rate of AVP metabolism.[100,166] This condition has been observed only in pregnancy and therefore is generally termed "gestational diabetes insipidus."[167,168] It is due to the action of a circulating enzyme called cysteine aminopeptidase (oxytocinase or vasopressinase) that is normally produced by the placenta to degrade circulating oxytocin and prevent premature uterine contractions.[169] Because of the close structural similarity between AVP and OT, this enzyme degrades both peptides.[170] There are two types of gestational diabetes insipidus.[169] In the first type, the activity of cysteine aminopeptidase is extremely and abnormally elevated. This syndrome has been referred to as vasopressin-resistant diabetes insipidus of pregnancy.[171] It can occur in association with preeclampsia, acute fatty liver, and coagulopathies (e.g., HELLP syndrome [*h*emolysis, *e*levated *l*iver enzymes, and *l*ow *p*latelet count]). These patients have decreased metabolism of vasopressinase by the liver.[172] Usually, in subsequent pregnancies, these women have neither diabetes insipidus nor acute fatty liver. In the second type, the accelerated metabolic clearance of vasopressin produces DI in a patient with borderline vasopressin function from a specific disease (e.g., mild nephrogenic DI or partial CDI). AVP is rapidly destroyed, and the neurohypophysis is unable to keep up with the increased demand. Labor and parturition usually proceed normally, and patients have no trouble with lactation. Severe dehydration can occur if DI is unrecognized, which may pose a threat to a pregnant woman and her fetus. The relationship of this disorder to the transient nephrogenic DI (NDI) of pregnancy is not clear.[171]

### PATHOPHYSIOLOGY

The pathophysiology of gestational DI is similar to that of CDI. The only exception is that the polyuria is usually not corrected by the administration of AVP because this is rapidly degraded, just as is endogenous AVP, but it can be controlled by treatment with desmopressin, the AVP $V_2$ receptor agonist that is more resistant to degradation by oxytocinase or vasopressinase.[169] It should be remembered that patients with partial CDI in whom only low levels of AVP can be maintained, or patients with compensated NDI in whom the lack of response of the kidney to AVP may not be absolute, can be relatively asymptomatic with regard to polyuria. However, with accelerated destruction of AVP during pregnancy, the underlying DI may become manifest. Consequently, patients presenting with gestational DI should not be assumed simply to have excess oxytocinase or vasopressinase; rather, these patients should be evaluated for other possible underlying pathologic diagnoses (see Box 15.1).[173]

## NEPHROGENIC DIABETES INSIPIDUS

### CAUSES

Resistance to the antidiuretic action of AVP is usually due to some defect within the kidney, and is commonly referred to as "nephrogenic diabetes insipidus" (NDI). It was first recognized in 1945 in several patients with the familial, sex-linked form of the disorder. Subsequently, additional kindreds with the X-linked form of familial NDI were identified. Clinical studies of NDI have indicated that symptomatic polyuria is present from birth, plasma AVP levels are normal or elevated, resistance to the antidiuretic effect of AVP can be partial or almost complete, and the disease affects mostly males and is usually, although not always,[174] mild or absent in carrier females. More than 90% of cases of congenital NDI are caused by mutations of the AVP $V_2$ receptor[175,176] (see Chapter 44). Most mutations occur in the part of the receptor that is highly conserved among species and/or is conserved among similar receptors, such as homologies with AVP $V_{1A}$ or OT receptors. The effect of some of these mutations on receptor synthesis, processing, trafficking, and function has been studied by in vitro expression.[177,178]

These types of studies have shown that the various mutations cause several different defects in cellular processing and function of the receptor but can be classified into four general categories based on differences in transport to the cell surface and AVP binding and/or stimulation of adenylyl cyclase, as follows: (1) the mutant receptor is not inserted in the membrane; (2) the mutant receptor is inserted in the membrane but does not bind or respond to AVP; (3) the mutant receptor is inserted in the membrane and binds AVP but does not activate adenylyl cyclase; or (4) the mutant protein is inserted into the membrane and binds AVP but responds subnormally in terms of adenylyl cyclase activation. Two studies have shown a relationship between the clinical phenotype and genotype and/or cellular phenotype.[177,179] Approximately 10% of the $V_2$ receptor defects causing congenital NDI are thought to be de novo. This high incidence of de novo cases, coupled with the large number of mutations that have been identified, hinders the clinical use of genetic identification because it is necessary to sequence the entire open reading frame of the receptor gene rather than short sequences of DNA. Nonetheless, the use of automated gene sequencing techniques in selected families has been shown to identify mutations in patients with clinical disease and in asymptomatic carriers.[180] Although most female carriers of the X-linked $V_2$ receptors defect have no clinical disease, some have been reported with symptomatic NDI.[174] Carriers can have a decreased maximum urine osmolality in response to plasma AVP levels, but are generally asymptomatic because of the absence of overt polyuria. In one study, a girl manifested severe NDI due to a $V_2$ receptor mutation, which was likely due to skewed inactivation of the normal X chromosome.[181]

Congenital NDI can also result from mutations of the autosomal gene that codes for AQP2, the protein that forms the water channels in renal medullary collecting tubules. When the proband is a girl, it is likely the defect is a mutation of the *AQP2* gene on chromosome 12, region q12-q13.[182] More than 25 different mutations of the *AQP2* gene have been described[183] (see Chapter 44). The patients may be heterozygous for two different recessive mutations[184] or homozygous for the same abnormality from both parents.[185] Because most of these mutations are recessive, the patients usually do not present with a family history of DI unless consanguinity is present. Functional expression studies of these mutations have shown that all of them result in varying degrees of reduced water transport because the mutant aquaporins are not expressed in normal amounts, are retained in various cellular organelles, or simply do not function as effectively as water channels. Regardless of the type of mutation, the renal phenotype of NDI from AQP2 mutations is identical to that produced by $V_2$ receptor mutations. Of interest, and sometimes helpful clinically, an AVP $V_2$ receptor agonist still stimulates the release of von Willebrand factor (vWF) from the Weibel-Palade bodies of endothelial cells in patients with AQP2 mutations. Some of the defects in cellular routing and water transport can be reversed by treatment with chemicals that act like chaperones,[186] suggesting that misfolding of the mutant AQP2 may be responsible for misrouting. Similar salutary effects of chaperones have been found to reverse defects in cell surface expression and function of selected mutations of the AVP $V_2$ receptor.[187]

NDI can also be caused by a variety of drugs, diseases, and metabolic disturbances, including lithium, hypokalemia, and hypercalcemia (see Box 15.1). Some of these disorders (e.g., polycystic kidney disease) act to distort the normal architecture of the kidney and interfere with the normal urine concentration process. However, experimental studies in animal models have suggested that many have in common a downregulation of AQP2 expression in the renal collecting tubules (Fig. 15.15; see also Chapter 10).[188,189] The polyuria associated with potassium deficiency develops in parallel with decreased expression of kidney AQP2, and repletion of potassium reestablishes the normal urinary concentrating mechanism and normalizes the renal expression of AQP2.[190] Similarly, hypercalcemia has also been found to be associated with downregulation of AQP2.[191] A low-protein diet diminishes the ability to concentrate the urine, primarily by a decreased delivery of urea to the inner medulla, thus decreasing the medullary concentration gradient, but rats on a low- protein diet also appear to downregulate AQP2, which could be an additional component of the decreased ability to concentrate the urine.[192] Bilateral urinary tract obstruction causes an inability to produce a maximum concentration of the urine, and rat models have demonstrated a downregulation of AQP2, which persists for several days after release of the obstruction.[193] However, it is not yet clear which of these effects on AQP2 expression are primary or secondary and which cellular mechanism(s) are responsible for the downregulation of AQP2 expression.

The administration of lithium to treat psychiatric disorders is the most common cause of drug-induced NDI and illustrates the multiple mechanisms likely involved in producing this disorder. As many as 10% to 20% of patients on chronic lithium therapy develop some degree of NDI.[194] Lithium is known to interfere with the production of cAMP[195] and produces a dramatic (95%) reduction in kidney AQP2 levels in animals.[196] The defect of aquaporins is slow to correct in experimental animals and humans and, in some cases, it can be permanent,[197] in association with glomerular or tubulointerstitial nephropathy.[198] Several other drugs that are known to induce renal concentrating defects have also been associated with abnormalities of AQP2 synthesis.[199]

## PATHOPHYSIOLOGY

Similar to CDI, renal insensitivity to the antidiuretic effect of AVP also results in the excretion of an increased volume of dilute urine, decrease in body water, and rise in plasma osmolality, which by stimulating thirst induces a compensatory increase in water intake. As a consequence, the osmolality of body fluid stabilizes at a slightly higher level, which approximates the osmotic threshold for thirst. As in patients with CDI, the magnitude of polyuria and polydipsia varies greatly depending on a number of factors, including the degree of renal insensitivity to AVP, individual differences in the set points and sensitivity of thirst and AVP secretion, and total solute load. It is important to note that the renal insensitivity to AVP need not be complete for polyuria to occur; it is only necessary that the defect is great enough to prevent the concentration of the urine at plasma AVP levels achievable under ordinary conditions of ad libitum water intake (i.e., at plasma osmolalities near the osmotic threshold for thirst). Calculations similar to those used for states of AVP deficiency indicate that this requirement is not met until the renal sensitivity to AVP is reduced by more than

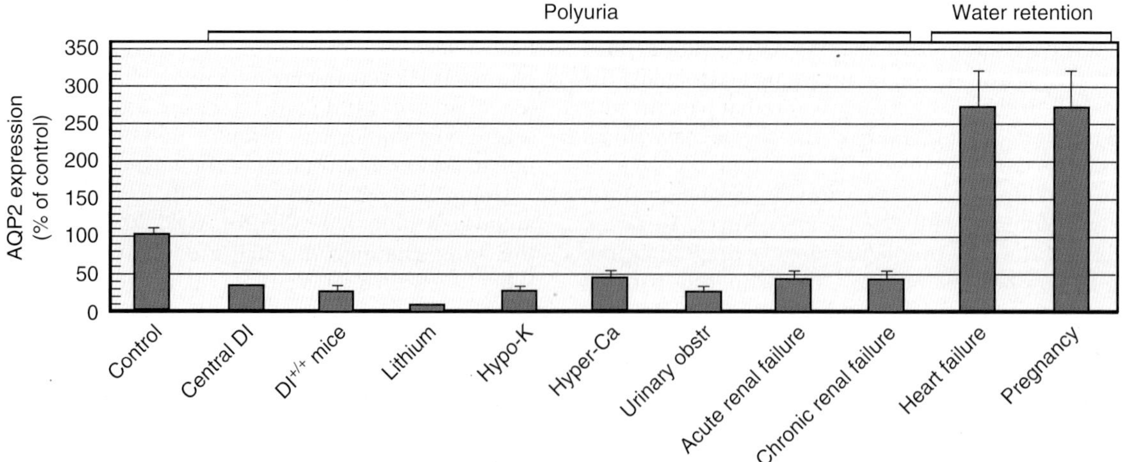


**Fig. 15.15** Kidney expression of the water channel aquaporin-2 in various animal models of polyuria and water retention. Note that kidney aquaporin-2 expression is uniformly downregulated relative to levels in controls in all animal models of polyuria, but upregulated in animal models of inappropriate antidiuresis. *DI*$^{+/+}$, Genetic diabetes insipidus; *Hyper-Ca,* hypercalcemia; *Hypo-K,* hypokalemia; *Urinary obstr,* ureteral obstruction. (From Nielsen S, Kwon TH, Christensen BM, et al: Physiology and pathophysiology of renal aquaporins. *J Am Soc Nephrol.* 1999;10:647–663.)

10-fold. Because renal insensitivity to the hormone is often incomplete, especially in cases of acquired rather than congenital NDI, many patients with NDI are able to concentrate their urine to varying degrees when they are deprived of water or given large doses of desmopressin.

Information about the renal concentration mechanism from studies of AQP2 expression in experimental animals (see Chapter 10) has suggested that a form of NDI is likely associated with all types of DI, as well as with primary polydipsia. Brattleboro rats have been found to have low levels of kidney AQP2 expression compared with Long-Evans control rats; AQP2 levels are corrected by treatment with AVP or desmopressin, but this process takes 3 to 5 days, during which time urine concentration remains subnormal, despite pharmacologic concentrations of AVP.[200] Similarly, physiologic suppression of AVP by chronic overadministration of water produces a downregulation of AQP2 in the renal collecting duct.[200] Clinically, it is well known that patients with both CDI and primary polydipsia often fail to achieve maximally concentrated urine when they are given desmopressin during a water deprivation test to differentiate among the various causes of DI. This effect has long been attributed to a washout of the medullary concentration gradient as a result of the high urine flow rates in polyuric patients; however, based on the results of animal studies, it seems certain that at least part of the decreased response to AVP is due to a downregulation of kidney AQP2 expression. This also explains why it takes time, typically several days, to restore normal urinary concentration after patients with primary polydipsia and CDI are treated with water restriction or antidiuretic therapy.[201]

## PRIMARY POLYDIPSIA

### CAUSES

Excessive fluid intake also causes hypotonic polyuria and, by definition, polydipsia. Consequently, this disorder must be differentiated from the various causes of DI. Furthermore, it is apparent that despite normal pituitary and kidney function, patients with this disorder share many characteristics of both CDI (AVP secretion is suppressed as a result of the decreased plasma osmolality) and NDI (kidney AQP2 expression is decreased as a result of the suppressed plasma AVP levels). Many different names have been used to describe patients with excessive fluid intake, but the term "primary polydipsia" remains the best descriptor because it does not presume any particular cause for the increased fluid intake. Primary polydipsia is often due to a severe mental illness, such as schizophrenia, mania, or an obsessive-compulsive disorder,[202] in which case it is termed "psychogenic polydipsia." These patients usually deny true thirst and attribute their polydipsia to bizarre motives, such as a need to cleanse their body of poisons. Studies of a series of polydipsic patients in a psychiatric hospital have shown an incidence as high as 42% of patients with some form of polydipsia and, in most reported cases, there was no obvious explanation for the polydipsia.[203]

However, primary polydipsia can also be caused by an abnormality in the osmoregulatory control of thirst, in which case it has been termed "dipsogenic diabetes insipidus."[204] These patients have no overt psychiatric illness and invariably attribute their polydipsia to a nearly constant thirst. Dipsogenic DI is usually idiopathic but can also be secondary to organic structural lesions in the hypothalamus identical to any of the disorders described as causes of CDI, such as neurosarcoidosis of the hypothalamus, tuberculous meningitis, multiple sclerosis, or trauma. Consequently, all polydipsic patients should be evaluated with an MRI scan of the brain before concluding that excessive water intake has an idiopathic or psychiatric cause. Primary polydipsia can also be produced by drugs that cause a dry mouth or by any peripheral disorder causing pathologic elevations of renin and/or angiotensin levels.[113]

Finally, primary polydipsia is sometimes caused by physicians, nurses, or the lay press who advise a high fluid intake for valid (e.g., recurrent nephrolithiasis) or unsubstantiated reasons of health.[205] These patients lack overt signs of mental illness but also deny thirst and usually attribute their polydipsia to habits acquired from years of adherence to their drinking regimen.

### PATHOPHYSIOLOGY

The pathophysiology of primary polydipsia is essentially the reverse of that in CDI—the excessive intake of water expands and slightly dilutes body fluids, suppresses AVP secretion, and dilutes the urine. The resultant increase in the rate of water excretion balances the increase in intake, and the osmolality of body water stabilizes at a new, slightly lower level that approximates the osmotic threshold for AVP secretion. The magnitude of the polyuria and polydipsia vary considerably, depending on the nature or intensity of the stimulus to drink. In patients with abnormal thirst, the polydipsia and polyuria are relatively constant from day to day. However, in patients with psychogenic polydipsia, water intake and urine output tend to fluctuate widely and, at times, can be quite large.

Occasionally, fluid intake rises to such extraordinary levels that the excretory capacity of the kidneys is exceeded, and dilutional hyponatremia develops.[206] There is little question that excessive water intake alone can sometimes be sufficient to override renal excretory capacity and produce severe hyponatremia. Although the water excretion rate of normal adult kidneys can generally exceed 20 L/day, maximum hourly rates rarely exceed 1000 mL/h. Because many psychiatric patients drink predominantly during the day or during intense drinking binges,[207] they can transiently achieve symptomatic levels of hyponatremia, with the total daily volume of water intake less than 20 L if ingested rapidly enough. This likely accounts for many of the patients who present with maximally dilute urine, accounting for as many as 50% of patients in some studies, and are corrected quickly via free water diuresis.[208] The prevalence of this disorder, based on hospital admissions for acute symptomatic hyponatremia, may have been underestimated because studies of polydipsic psychiatric patients have shown a marked diurnal variation in serum [$Na^+$], from 141 mEq/L at 7 AM to 130 mEq/L at 4 PM, suggesting that many such patients drink excessively during the daytime but then correct themselves via water diuresis at night.[209] This and other considerations have led to defining this disorder as the "psychosis, intermittent hyponatremia, and polydipsia" (PIP) syndrome.[207]

However, many other cases of hyponatremia with psychogenic polydipsia have been found to meet the criteria for a diagnosis of SIADH, suggesting the presence of nonosmotically stimulated AVP secretion. As might be expected, in the presence of much higher than normal water intake, almost any impairment of urinary dilution and water excretion can exacerbate the development of a positive water balance and thereby produce hypo-osmolality. Acute psychosis itself can also cause AVP secretion,[210] which often appears to take the form of a reset osmostat.[202] It is therefore apparent that no single mechanism can completely explain the occurrence of hyponatremia in polydipsic psychiatric patients, but the combination of higher than normal water intake plus modest elevations of plasma AVP levels from a variety of potential sources appears to account for a significant portion of these cases.

## CLINICAL MANIFESTATIONS OF DIABETES INSIPIDUS

The characteristic clinical symptoms of DI are the polyuria and polydipsia that result from the underlying impairment of urine-concentrating mechanisms, which have been described earlier in the sections on the pathophysiology of specific types of DI. Interestingly, patients with DI typically describe a craving for cold water, which appears to quench their thirst better.[69] Patients with CDI also typically describe a precipitous onset of their polyuria and polydipsia, which simply reflects the fact that urinary concentration can be maintained fairly well until the number of AVP-producing neurons in the hypothalamus decreases to 10% to 15% of normal, after which plasma AVP levels decrease to the range at which urine output increases dramatically.

However, patients with DI, particularly those with osmoreceptor dysfunction syndromes, can also present with varying degrees of hyperosmolality and dehydration, depending on their overall hydration status. It is therefore also important to be aware of the clinical manifestations of hyperosmolality. These can be divided into the signs and symptoms produced by dehydration, which are largely cardiovascular, and those caused by the hyperosmolality itself, which are predominantly neurologic and reflect brain dehydration as a result of osmotic water shifts out of the CNS. Cardiovascular manifestations of hypertonic dehydration include hypotension, azotemia, acute tubular necrosis secondary to renal hypoperfusion or rhabdomyolysis, and shock.[211,212] Neurologic manifestations range from nonspecific symptoms, such as irritability and cognitive dysfunction, to more severe manifestations of hypertonic encephalopathy, such as disorientation, decreased level of consciousness, obtundation, chorea, seizures, coma, focal neurologic deficits, subarachnoid hemorrhage, and cerebral infarction.[211,213] One study has also suggested an increased incidence of deep venous thrombosis in hyperosmolar patients.[214]

The severity of symptoms can be roughly correlated with the degree of hyperosmolality, but individual variability is marked and, for any single patient, the level of serum [$Na^+$] at which symptoms will appear cannot be accurately predicted. Similar to hypoosmolar syndromes, the length of time over which hyperosmolality develops can markedly affect the clinical symptomatology. The rapid development of severe hyperosmolality is frequently associated with marked neurologic symptoms, whereas gradual development over several days or weeks generally causes milder symptoms.[211,215] In this case, the brain counteracts osmotic shrinkage by increasing the intracellular content of solutes. These include electrolytes such as potassium and a variety of organic osmolytes, which previously had been termed "idiogenic osmoles"; for the most part, these are the same organic osmolytes that are lost from the brain during adaptation to hypoosmolality.[216] The net effect of this process is to protect the brain against excessive shrinkage during sustained hyperosmolality. However, once the brain has adapted by increasing its solute content, rapid correction of the hyperosmolality can produce brain edema because it takes a finite length of time (24–48 hours in animal studies) to dissipate the accumulated solutes and, until this process has been completed, the brain will accumulate excess water as plasma osmolality is normalized.[217] This effect is usually seen in dehydrated pediatric patients who can develop seizures with rapid rehydration,[218] but has been described only rarely in adults, including the most severely hyperosmolar patients with nonketotic hyperglycemic hyperosmolar coma.

## DIFFERENTIAL DIAGNOSIS OF POLYURIA

Before beginning involved diagnostic testing to differentiate among the various forms of DI and primary polydipsia, the presence of true hypotonic polyuria should be established by measurement of a 24-hour urine for volume and osmolality. Generally accepted standards are that the 24-hour urine volume should exceed 50 mL/kg BW, with an osmolality lower than 300 mOsm/kg $H_2O$.[219] Simultaneously, there should be a determination of whether the polyuria is due to an osmotic agent such as glucose or intrinsic renal disease. Routine laboratory studies and the clinical setting will usually distinguish these disorders; diabetes mellitus and other forms of solute diuresis usually can be excluded by the history, routine urinalysis for glucose, and/or measurement of the solute excretion rate (urine osmolality × 24-hour urine volume [in liters] > 15 mOsm/kg BW/day). There is general agreement that the diagnosis of DI requires stimulating AVP secretion osmotically and then measuring the adequacy of the secretion by direct measurement of plasma AVP levels or indirect assessment by urine osmolality.

In a patient who is already hyperosmolar, with submaximally concentrated urine (i.e., urine osmolality < 800 mOsm/kg $H_2O$), the diagnosis is straightforward and simple; primary polydipsia is ruled out by the presence of hyperosmolality,[219] confirming a diagnosis of DI. CDI can then be distinguished from NDI by evaluating the response to the administration of AVP (5 units subcutaneously) or, preferably, of the AVP $V_2$ receptor agonist desmopressin (1-deamino-8-D-arginine vasopressin [DDAVP], 1–2 μg subcutaneously or intravenously). A significant increase in urine osmolality within 1 to 2 hours after injection indicates insufficient endogenous AVP secretion, and therefore CDI, whereas an absent response indicates renal resistance to AVP effects, and therefore NDI. Although conceptually simple, interpretational difficulties can arise because the water diuresis produced by AVP deficiency in CDI produces a washout of the renal medullary concentrating gradient and downregulation of the kidney AQP2 water channels (see earlier), so that initial increases in urine osmolality in response to administered AVP or desmopressin are not as great as would be expected. Generally, increases of urine osmolality of more than 50% reliably indicate CDI, and responses of less than 10% indicate NDI, but responses between 10% and 50% are indeterminate.[147] Therefore, plasma AVP levels should be measured to aid in this distinction; hyperosmolar patients with NDI will have clearly elevated plasma AVP levels, whereas those with CDI will have absent (complete) or blunted (partial) AVP responses relative to their plasma osmolality (see Fig. 15.11). Because it will not be known beforehand which patients will have diagnostic versus indeterminate responses to AVP or desmopressin, a plasma AVP level should be determined prior to AVP or desmopressin administration in patients with hyperosmolality and inadequately concentrated urine without a solute diuresis.

Patients with DI have intact thirst mechanisms, so they usually do not present with hyperosmolality, but rather with a normal plasma osmolality and serum [Na$^+$] and symptoms of polyuria and polydipsia. In these cases, it is most appropriate to perform a fluid deprivation test. The relative merits of the indirect fluid deprivation test (Miller-Moses test[220]) versus direct measurement of plasma AVP levels after a period of fluid deprivation[147] has been debated in literature, with substantial pros and cons in support of each of these tests. On the one hand, the standard indirect test has a long track record of making an appropriate diagnosis in the large majority of cases, generally yields interpretable results by the end of the test, and does not require sensitive assays for the notoriously difficult measurement of plasma AVP levels.[221,222] However, maximum urine-concentrating capacity is well known to be variably reduced in all forms of DI, as well as primary polydipsia[147] and, as a result, the absolute levels of urine osmolality achieved during fluid deprivation and after AVP administration are reduced to overlapping degrees in patients with partial CDI, partial NDI, and primary polydipsia.

Measurements of basal plasma osmolality or serum [Na$^+$] are of little use because they also overlap considerably among these disorders.[219] Although association with certain diseases, surgical procedures, or family history often helps differentiate among these disorders, sometimes the clinical setting may not be helpful because certain disorders (e.g., sarcoidosis, tuberculous meningitis, other hypothalamic pathologies) can cause more than one type of DI (see Box 15.1). Consequently, a simpler approach that has been proposed is to measure plasma or urine AVP before and during a suitable osmotic stimulus, such as fluid restriction or hypertonic NaCl infusion, and plot the results as a function of the concurrent plasma osmolality or plasma [Na$^+$] (see Figs. 15.12 and 15.13).[223,224]

Using a highly sensitive and validated research assay for plasma AVP determinations, this approach has been shown to provide a definitive diagnosis in most cases, provided that the final level of plasma osmolality or sodium achieved is above the normal range (>295 mOsm/kg $H_2O$ or 145 mmol/L, respectively). The diagnostic effectiveness of this approach derives from the fact that the magnitude of the AVP response to osmotic stimulation is not appreciably diminished by chronic overhydration[202] or dehydration. Hence, the relationship of plasma AVP to plasma osmolality is usually within or above normal limits in NDI and primary polydipsia. In most cases, these two disorders can then be distinguished by measuring urine osmolality before and after the dehydration test and relating these values to the concurrent plasma AVP concentration (see Fig. 15.12). However, because maximal concentrating capacity can be severely blunted in patients with primary polydipsia, it is often better to analyze the relationship under basal nondehydrated conditions, when the plasma AVP level is not elevated. Because of the solute diuresis that often ensues following infusion of hypertonic NaCl, measurements of urine osmolality or AVP excretion are unreliable indicators of changes in hormone secretion and are of little or no diagnostic value when this procedure is used to increase osmolality to more than 295 mOsm/kg $H_2O$. Given the proven usefulness of the indirect and direct approaches, a combined fluid deprivation test that synthesizes the crucial aspects of both tests can easily be performed (Box 15.2). In many cases, this will allow interpretation of the plasma AVP levels and response to an AVP challenge.

Because measurement of vasopressin in plasma is difficult, recent studies have suggested that the C-terminal fragment of the vasopressin prohormone copeptin (see Fig. 15.3) may

**Box 15.2 Fluid Deprivation Test for the Diagnosis of Diabetes Insipidus (DI)**

**Procedure**

1. Initiation of the deprivation period depends on the severity of the DI; in routine cases, the patient should be made NPO after dinner, whereas in patients with more severe polyuria and polydipsia, this may be too long a period without fluids, and the water deprivation should be started early on the morning (e.g., 6 AM) of the test.
2. Obtain plasma and urine osmolality and serum electrolyte and plasma AVP or copeptin levels at the start of the test.
3. Measure urine volume and osmolality hourly or with each voided urine.
4. Stop the test when body weight decreases by ≥3%, the patient develops orthostatic blood pressure changes, the urine osmolality reaches a plateau (i.e., <10% change over two or three consecutive measurements), or the serum Na$^+$ > 145 mmol/L.
5. Obtain plasma and urine osmolality and serum electrolyte and plasma AVP or copeptin levels at the end of the test, when the plasma osmolality is elevated, preferably >300 mOsm/kg $H_2O$.
6. If serum Na$^+$ < 146 mmol/L or plasma osmolality < 300 mOsm/kg $H_2O$ when the test is stopped, then consider a short infusion of hypertonic saline (3% NaCl at a rate of 0.1 mL/kg/min for 1 to 2 hours) to reach these end points.
7. If hypertonic saline infusion is not required to achieve hyperosmolality, administer AVP (5 U) or desmopressin (DDAVP; 1 µg) subcutaneously and continue following urine osmolality and volume for an additional 2 hours.

**Interpretation**

1. An unequivocal urine concentration after AVP or DDAVP (>50% increase) indicates central diabetes insipidus (CDI); an unequivocal absence of urine concentration (<10%) strongly suggests nephrogenic DI (NDI) or primary polydipsia (PP).
2. Differentiating between NDI and PP, as well as cases in which the increase in urine osmolality after AVP or DDAVP administration is more equivocal (e.g., 10%–50%), is best done using the relationship between plasma AVP or copeptin levels and plasma osmolality obtained at the end of the dehydration period and/or hypertonic saline infusion and the relationship between plasma AVP levels and urine osmolality determined under basal conditions (see Figs. 15.12, 15.13, and 15.16).

be a reliable and more convenient surrogate measure of vasopressin secretion.[225] Copeptin is released with AVP in a 1 : 1 stoichiometric ratio because both peptides are part of the same prohormone, and several studies have demonstrated high correlations between plasma AVP and copeptin levels (Fig. 15.16).[226] This has led to studies that indicate a higher accuracy of the correct diagnosis of the cause of polyuria using plasma copeptin levels at the end of water deprivation than by indirect measurement of the urine osmolality response to AVP or desmopressin.[227,228] Consequently, it seems likely that the measurement of copeptin will replace the measurement of AVP to establish a diagnosis of DI in the future, although successful interpretation of either measure will require measurement during hyperosmolality via water deprivation or hypertonic saline challenge.[229]

With use of the fluid deprivation test for plasma AVP or copeptin determinations, most cases of polyuria and polydipsia can be diagnosed accurately. A useful approach in the remaining indeterminate cases is to conduct a closely monitored trial with standard therapeutic doses of desmopressin. If this treatment abolishes thirst and polydipsia, as well as polyuria, for 48 to 72 hours without producing water intoxication, the patient most likely has uncomplicated CDI. On the other hand, if the treatment abolishes the polyuria but has no or a lesser effect on thirst or polydipsia and results in the development of hyponatremia, it is more likely that the patient has some form of primary polydipsia. If desmopressin has no effect over this time interval, even when given by injection, it is almost certain that the patient has some form of NDI. However, if this approach is used, serum sodium levels must be checked within several days to avoid the development of severe hyponatremia in patients with primary polydipsia.

MRI has also proved to be useful for diagnosing DI. In normal subjects, the posterior pituitary produces a characteristic bright signal in the posterior part of the sella turcica that is similar on T1-weighted images, usually best seen in sagittal views.[230] This was originally thought to represent fatty tissue, but more recent evidence has indicated that the bright spot is actually due to the stored hormone in neurosecretory granules.[231] An experimental study done in rabbits subjected to dehydration for varying periods of time has shown a linear correlation between pituitary AVP content and the signal intensity of the posterior pituitary by MRI.[232] As might be expected from the fact that destruction of more than 85% to 90% of the neurohypophysis is necessary to produce clinical symptomatology of DI, this signal has been found to be almost always absent in patients with CDI in multiple studies.[233]

However, as with any diagnostic test, its clinical usefulness is dependent on the sensitivity and specificity of the test. Although earlier studies using small numbers of subjects demonstrated the presence of the bright spot in all normal subjects, subsequent larger studies reported an age-related absence of a pituitary bright spot in up to 20% of normal subjects.[234] Conversely, some studies have reported the presence of a bright spot in patients with clinical evidence of DI.[235] This may be because some patients with partial CDI have not yet progressed to the point of depletion of all neurohypophyseal reserves of AVP, or because a persistent bright spot in patients with DI might be due to the pituitary content of OT rather than AVP. In support of this, it is known that oxytocinergic neurons are more resistant to destruction by trauma than vasopressinergic neurons in rats[236] and in humans.[22] The presence of a positive posterior pituitary bright spot has been variably reported in other polyuric disorders. In primary polydipsia, the bright spot is usually seen,[233] consistent with studies in animals in which even prolonged lack of secretion of AVP caused by hyponatremia did not cause a decreased content of AVP in the posterior pituitary.[26] In NDI, the bright spot has been reported to be absent in some patients, but present in others.[127] Consequently, specificity is lacking in regard to using MRI routinely as a diagnostic screening test for DI. Nonetheless, the sensitivity is sufficient to allow a high probability that a patient with a bright spot on MRI does not have CDI. Thus, MRI is more useful for ruling out than for ruling in a diagnosis of CDI.

Additional useful information can be gained through MRI via assessment of the pituitary stalk. Enlargement of the stalk beyond 2 to 3 mm is generally considered to be pathologic[237] and can be caused by multiple disease processes.[238] Consequently, when MRI scans reveal thickening of the stalk, especially with absence of the posterior pituitary bright spot, systemic diseases should be searched for diligently, including cerebrospinal fluid (CSF), plasma β-human chorionic gonadotropin (β-hCG), and alpha-fetoprotein measurements for the evaluation of suprasellar germinoma, chest imaging and CSF and plasma angiotensin-converting enzyme (ACE) levels for the evaluation of sarcoidosis, and bone and skin surveys for the evaluation of histiocytosis. When a diagnosis is still in doubt, MRI should be repeated every 3 to 6 months. Continued enlargement, especially in children over the first 3 years of follow-up, suggests a germinoma and mandates a biopsy, whereas a decrease in the size of the stalk over time is more indicative of an inflammatory process, such as lymphocytic infundibuloneurohypophysitis.[239]

## TREATMENT OF DIABETES INSIPIDUS

The general goals of treatment of all forms of DI are a correction of any preexisting water deficits and a reduction in the ongoing excessive urinary water losses. The specific therapy required (Box 15.3) will vary according to the type of DI present and clinical situation. Awake ambulatory patients with normal thirst have relatively little body water deficit, but benefit greatly by alleviation of the polyuria and polydipsia that disrupt their normal daily activities. In contrast, comatose patients with acute DI after head trauma are unable to drink in response to thirst and, in these patients, progressive hyperosmolality can be life-threatening.

**Box 15.3 Therapies for the Treatment of Diabetes Insipidus**

Water
Antidiuretic agents
Arginine vasopressin (Pitressin)
1-Deamino-8-D-arginine vasopressin (desmopressin; DDAVP)
Antidiuresis-enhancing agents
Chlorpropamide
Prostaglandin synthetase inhibitors (e.g., indomethacin, ibuprofen, tolmetin)
Natriuretic agents
Thiazide diuretics
Amiloride

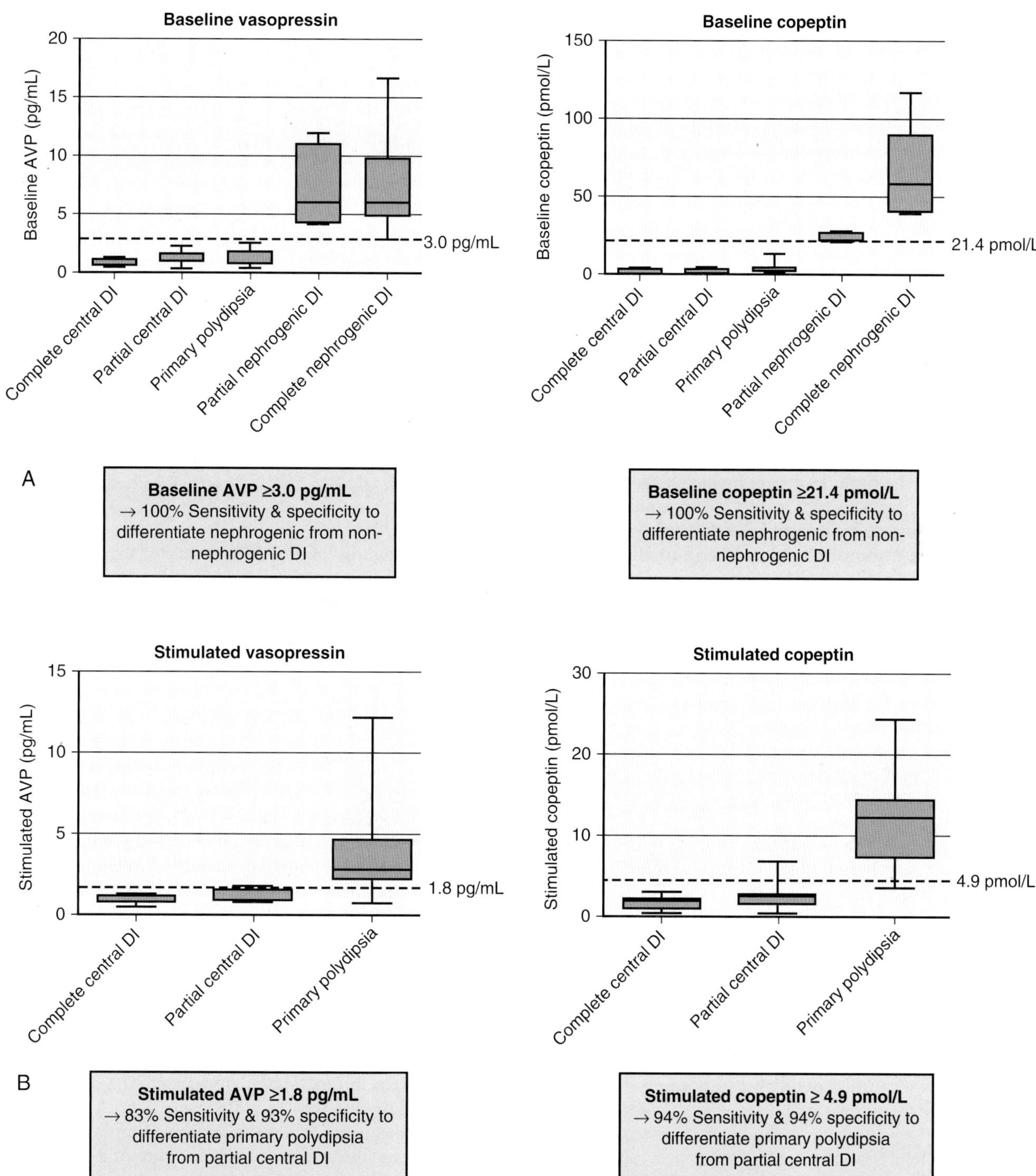


**Fig. 15.16** (A) Baseline arginine vasopressin (AVP) and copeptin plasma levels in the differential diagnosis of the polyuria and polydipsia. Box plots depict interquartile ranges, with medians and whiskers depicting minimal and maximal values for baseline AVP and copeptin levels without prior thirsting in patients with complete and partial central diabetes insipidus (DI), primary polydipsia, and complete and partial nephrogenic diabetes insipidus. Cutoffs for best discrimination between nephrogenic versus nonnephrogenic diabetes insipidus for AVP and copeptin are shown. (B) Osmotically stimulated AVP and copeptin plasma levels in the differential diagnosis of polyuria and polydipsia. Box and whisker plots with medians and minimal and maximal values for stimulated AVP and copeptin plasma values at a plasma sodium level >147 mmol/L are depicted for patients with complete and partial central diabetes insipidus and for patients with primary polydipsia. Osmotic stimulation was provided by a combined water deprivation and saline infusion test. The cutoffs for best discrimination between primary polydipsia versus central diabetes insipidus for AVP and copeptin are depicted. *DI,* Diabetes insipidus; *PP,* primary polydipsia. (From Christ-Crain M, Moganthaler NG, Fenske W: Copeptin as a biomarker and a diagnostic tool in the evaluation of patients with polyuria-polydipsia and hyponatremia. *Best Pract Res Clin Endocrinol Metab.* 2016;30:235–247.)

The total body water deficit in a hyperosmolar patient can be estimated using the following formula:

$$\text{Total body water deficit} = (0.6 \times \text{premorbid weight}) \times (1 - 140/[\text{Na}^+])$$

where $[Na^+]$ is the serum sodium concentration in millimoles per liter and weight is in kilograms. This formula is dependent on three assumptions: (1) total body water is approximately 60% of the premorbid body weight; (2) no body solute was lost as the hyperosmolality developed; and (3) the premorbid serum $[Na^+]$ was 140 mEq/L.

To reduce the risk of CNS damage from protracted exposure to severe hyperosmolality, in most cases the plasma osmolality should be rapidly lowered in the first 24 hours to the range of 320 to 330 mOsm/kg $H_2O$, or by approximately 50%. Plasma osmolality may be most easily estimated as twice the serum $[Na^+]$ if there is no hyperglycemia, and measured osmolality may be substituted if azotemia is not present. As discussed earlier, the brain increases intracellular osmolality by increasing the content of a variety of organic osmolytes as protection against excessive shrinkage during hyperosmolality.[216] Because these osmolytes cannot be immediately dissipated, further correction to a normal plasma osmolality should be spread over the next 24 to 72 hours to avoid producing cerebral edema during treatment.[217] This is especially important in children,[240] in whom several studies have indicated that limiting correction of hypernatremia to a maximal rate of no greater than 0.5 mmol/L/h prevents the occurrence of symptomatic cerebral edema with seizures.[218,241] In addition, the possibility of associated thyroid or adrenal insufficiency should also be kept in mind because patients with CDI caused by hypothalamic masses can have associated deficiencies of anterior pituitary function.

The earlier formula does not take into account ongoing water losses and is, at best, a rough estimate. Frequent serum and urine electrolyte determinations should be made, and the administration rate of oral water, or IV 5% dextrose in water, should be adjusted accordingly. Note, for example, that the estimated deficit of a 70-kg patient whose serum $[Na^+]$ is 160 mEq/L is 5.25 L of water. In such an individual, administration of water at a rate greater than 200 mL/h would be required simply to correct the established deficit over 24 hours. Additional fluid would be needed to keep up with ongoing losses until a definitive response to treatment has occurred.

## THERAPEUTIC AGENTS

The therapeutic agents available for the treatment of DI are shown in Box 15.3. Water should be considered a therapeutic agent because, when ingested or infused in sufficient quantity, there is no abnormality of body fluid volume or composition.

As noted previously, in most patients with DI, thirst remains intact, and the patient will drink sufficient fluid to maintain a relatively normal fluid balance. A patient with known DI should therefore be treated to decrease the polyuria and polydipsia to acceptable levels that allow him or her to maintain a normal lifestyle. Because the major goal of therapy is improvement in symptomatology, the therapeutic regimen prescribed should be individually tailored to each patient to accommodate his or her needs. The safety of the prescribed agent and use of a regimen that avoids potential detrimental effects of overtreatment are primary considerations because of the relatively benign course of DI in most cases and the potential adverse consequences of hyponatremia. Available treatments are summarized later; their use is discussed separately for different types of DI.

### Arginine Vasopressin

Arginine vasopressin (Pitressin) is a synthetic form of naturally occurring human AVP. The aqueous solution contains 20 units/mL. Because of the drug's relatively short half-life (2- to 4-hour duration of antidiuretic effect) and propensity to cause acute increases in blood pressure when given as an IV bolus, this route of administration should generally be avoided. This agent is mainly used for acute situations, such as postoperative DI. However, repeated dosing is required unless a continuous infusion is used, and the frequency of dosing or infusion rate must be titrated to achieve the desired reduction in urine output (see subsequent discussion of postoperative DI).

### Desmopressin

DDAVP is an agonist of the AVP $V_2$ receptor that was developed for therapeutic use because it has a significantly longer half-life than AVP (8- to 20-hour duration of antidiuretic effect) and is devoid of the latter's pressor activity because of the absence of activation of AVP $V_{1A}$ receptors on vascular smooth muscle.[242] As a result of these advantages, it is the drug of choice for acute and chronic administration in patients with CDI.[243] Several different preparations are available. The intranasal form is provided as an aqueous solution containing 100 μg/mL in a bottle with a calibrated rhinal tube, which requires specialized training to use appropriately, or as a nasal spray delivering a metered dose of 10 μg in 0.1 mL. An oral preparation is also available in doses of 0.1 or 0.2 mg. Rather recently, a sublingual preparation, called Minirin Melt, has been introduced in doses of 60 to 120 μg.[244]

Neither the intranasal or oral preparations should be used in an acute emergency setting, in which it is essential that the patient achieve a therapeutic dose of the drug. In this case, the parenteral form should always be used. This is supplied as a solution containing 4 μg/mL and may be given by the intravenous, intramuscular, or subcutaneous route. The parenteral form is approximately 5 to 10 times more potent than the intranasal preparation, and the recommended dosage of DDAVP is 1 to 2 μg every 8 to 12 hours. For intranasal and parenteral preparations, increasing the dose generally has the effect of prolonging the duration of antidiuresis for several hours rather than increasing its magnitude; consequently, altering the dose can be useful to reduce the required frequency of administration.

### Chlorpropamide

Chlorpropamide (Diabinese) is primarily used as an oral hypoglycemic agent; this sulfonylurea also potentiates the hydroosmotic effect of AVP in the kidney. Chlorpropamide has been reported to reduce polyuria by 25% to 75% in patients with CDI. This effect appears to be independent of the severity of the disease and is associated with a proportional rise in urine osmolality, correction of dehydration, and elimination of the polydipsia, similar to that caused by small doses of AVP or desmopressin.[219]

The major site of action of chlorpropamide appears to be at the renal tubule to potentiate the hydroosmotic action of circulating AVP, but there is also evidence of a pituitary effect to increase the release of AVP; the latter effect may account for the observation that chlorpropamide can produce significant antidiuresis, even in patients with severe CDI and presumed near-total AVP deficiency.[219] The usual dose is 250 to 500 mg/day, with a response noted in 1 or 2 days and a maximum antidiuresis in 4 days. It should be remembered that this is an off-label use of chlorpropamide; it should not be used in pregnant women or in children, it should never be used in an acute emergency setting in which achieving rapid antidiuresis is necessary, and it should be avoided in patients with concurrent hypopituitarism because of the increased risk of hypoglycemia. Other sulfonylureas share chlorpropamide's effect but generally are less potent. In particular, the newer generation of oral hypoglycemic agents, such as glipizide and glyburide, are almost devoid of any AVP-potentiating effects.

#### Prostaglandin Synthase Inhibitors

Prostaglandins have complex effects in the CNS and kidney, many of which are still incompletely understood due to the variety of different prostaglandins and their multiplicity of cellular effects. In the brain, intracerebroventricular infusion of E prostaglandins stimulates AVP secretion,[245] and administration of prostaglandin synthase inhibitors attenuates osmotically stimulated AVP secretion.[246] However, in the kidney, prostaglandin E2 (PGE2) has been reported to inhibit AVP-stimulated generation of cAMP in the cortical collecting tubule by interacting with inhibitory G protein ($G_i$).[247] Thus, the effect of prostaglandin synthase inhibitors to sensitize AVP effects in the kidney likely result from enhanced cAMP generation on AVP binding to the $V_2$ receptor. The predominant renal effects of these agents has been demonstrated by the fact that clinically these agents successfully reduce urine volume and free water clearance, even in patients with NDI of different causes.[248]

#### Natriuretic Agents

Thiazide diuretics have a paradoxic antidiuretic effect in patients with CDI.[249] However, given that better antidiuretic agents are available for the treatment of CDI, its main therapeutic use is in NDI. Hydrochlorothiazide at doses of 50 to 100 mg/day usually reduces urine output by approximately 50%, and its efficacy can be further enhanced by restricting sodium intake. Unlike desmopressin or the other antidiuresis-enhancing drugs, these agents are equally effective for treating most forms of NDI (see later).

## TREATMENT OF DIFFERENT TYPES OF DIABETES INSIPIDUS

### Central Diabetes Insipidus

Patients with CDI should generally be treated with intranasal or oral desmopressin. Unless the hypothalamic thirst center is also affected by the primary lesion causing superimposed osmoreceptor dysfunction, these patients will develop thirst when the plasma osmolality increases by only 2% to 3%.[219] Severe hyperosmolality is therefore not a risk in the patient who is alert, ambulatory, and able to drink in response to perceived thirst. Polyuria and polydipsia are thus inconvenient and disruptive, but not life-threatening. However, hypo-osmolality is largely asymptomatic and may be progressive if water intake continues during a period of continuous antidiuresis. Therefore, treatment must be designed to minimize polyuria and polydipsia but without an undue risk of hyponatremia from overtreatment.

Treatment should be individualized to determine optimal dosage and dosing intervals. Although tablets offer greater convenience and are generally preferred by patients, it is useful to start with the nasal spray initially because of the greater consistency of absorption and physiologic effect, and then switch to oral tablets only after the patient is comfortable with use of the intranasal preparation to produce antidiuresis. Having tried both preparations, the patient can then choose which she or he prefers for long-term usage. Because of variability in response among patients, it is desirable to determine the duration of action of individual doses in each patient.[250] A satisfactory schedule can generally be determined using modest doses, and the maximum dose of desmopressin needed is rarely above 0.2 μg orally or 10 μg (one nasal spray) given two or occasionally three times daily.[251] These doses generally produce plasma desmopressin levels many times more than those required to produce maximum antidiuresis but obviate the need for more frequent treatment. Rarely, once-daily dosing suffices. In a few patients, the effect of intranasal or oral desmopressin is erratic, probably as a result of variable interference with absorption from the gastrointestinal tract or nasal mucosa. This variability can be reduced and the duration of action prolonged by administering the oral agent on an empty stomach[252] or use of the intranasal preparation after thorough cleansing of the nostrils. Resistance caused by antibody production has not been reported.

Hyponatremia is the major complication of desmopressin therapy, and 27% incidences of mild hyponatremia (131–134 mmol/L) and 15% incidences of more severe hyponatremia (≤130 mmol/L) have been reported with long-term follow-up of patients with chronic CDI.[253] This generally occurs if the patient is continually antidiuretic while maintaining a fluid intake sufficient to become volume-expanded and natriuretic.[254] There have been reports of hyponatremia in patients with normal AVP function, and presumably normal thirst, when they are given desmopressin to treat hemophilia and von Willebrand disease[255] and in children treated with desmopressin for primary enuresis.[256] In these cases, the hyponatremia can develop rapidly and is often first noted by the onset of convulsions and coma.[257] Severe hyponatremia in patients with DI who are being treated with desmopressin can be avoided by monitoring serum electrolyte levels frequently during the initiation of therapy. Patients who show a tendency to develop a low serum [$Na^+$] and do not respond to recommended decreases in fluid intake should then be instructed to delay a scheduled dose of desmopressin once or twice weekly so that polyuria recurs, thereby allowing any excess retained fluid to be excreted.[220]

Acute postsurgical DI occurs relatively frequently following surgery that involves the suprasellar hypothalamic area,[258] but several confounding factors must be considered. These patients often receive stress doses of glucocorticoids, and the resulting hyperglycemia with glucosuria may confuse a diagnosis of DI. Thus, the blood glucose level must first be brought under control to eliminate an osmotic diuresis as the cause of the polyuria. In addition, excess fluids administered intravenously may be retained perioperatively but then excreted normally postoperatively. If this large output is matched with continued intravenous input, an incorrect diagnosis of DI may be made based on the resulting polyuria. Therefore, if the serum [$Na^+$] is not elevated concomitantly with the polyuria, the rate of parenterally administered fluid should be slowed, with careful monitoring of serum [$Na^+$] and urine output to establish the diagnosis.

Once a diagnosis of DI is confirmed, the only acceptable pharmacologic therapy is an antidiuretic agent. However, because many neurosurgeons fear water overload and brain edema after this type of surgery, the patient is sometimes treated only with intravenous fluid replacement for a considerable time before the institution of antidiuretic hormone therapy (see the potential benefits of this approach later). If the patient is awake and able to respond to thirst, he or she can be treated with an antidiuretic hormone, and the patient's thirst can then be the guide for water replacement. However, if the patient is unable to respond to thirst because of a decreased level of consciousness or from hypothalamic damage to the thirst center, fluid balance must be maintained by administering fluid intravenously. The urine osmolality and serum [$Na^+$] must be checked every several hours during the initial therapy and then at least daily until stabilization or resolution of the DI. Caution must also be exercised regarding the volume of water replacement because excess water administered during the continued administration of AVP or desmopressin can create a syndrome of inappropriate antidiuresis and potentially severe hyponatremia. Studies in experimental animals have indicated that desmopressin-induced hyponatremia markedly impairs the survival of AVP neurons after pituitary stalk compression,[236] suggesting that overhydration with subsequent decreased stimulation of the neurohypophysis may also increase the likelihood of permanent DI.

Postoperatively, desmopressin may be given parenterally in a dose of 1 to 2 µg subcutaneously, intramuscularly, or intravenously. The intravenous route is preferable because it obviates any concern about absorption, is not associated with significant pressor activity, and has the same total duration of action as the other parenteral routes. A prompt reduction in urine output should occur; the duration of the antidiuretic effect is generally 6 to 12 hours. Usually, the patient is hypernatremic, with relatively dilute urine when therapy is started. One should monitor the urine osmolality and urine volume to be certain that the dose was effective, and check the serum [$Na^+$] at frequent intervals to ensure some improvement of hypernatremia. It is generally advisable to allow some return of the polyuria before the administration of subsequent doses of desmopressin because postoperative DI is often transient, and return of endogenous AVP secretion will become apparent by a lack of return of the polyuria. Also, in some cases, transient postoperative DI is part of a triphasic pattern that has been well described following pituitary stalk transection (see previous discussion and Fig. 15.11). Because of this possibility, allowing a return of polyuria before redosing with desmopressin will allow for the earlier detection of a potential second phase of inappropriate antidiuresis and decrease the likelihood of producing symptomatic hyponatremia by continuing antidiuretic therapy and intravenous fluid administration when it is not required.

Some clinicians have recommended using a continuous intravenous infusion of a dilute solution of AVP to control DI postoperatively. Algorithms for continuous AVP infusion in postoperative and posttraumatic DI in pediatric patients have begun at infusion rates of 0.25 to 1.0 mU/kg/h and titrated the rate using urine specific gravity (goal of 1.010–1.020) and urine volume (goal of 2–3 mL/kg/h) as a guide to the adequacy of the antidiuresis.[259] Although pressor effects have not been reported at these infusion rates, and the antidiuretic effects are quickly reversible in 2 to 3 hours, it should be remembered that use of continuous infusions versus intermittent dosing will not allow assessing when the patient has recovered from transient DI or entered the second phase of a triphasic response. If DI persists, the patient should eventually be switched to maintenance therapy with intranasal or oral preparations of desmopressin for the treatment of chronic DI.

Acute traumatic DI can occur after injuries to the head, usually a motor vehicle accident. DI is more common with deceleration injuries that result in a shearing action on the pituitary stalk and/or cause hemorrhagic ischemia of the hypothalamus and/or posterior pituitary.[260] Similar to the onset of postsurgical DI, posttraumatic DI is usually recognized by hypotonic polyuria in the presence of increased plasma osmolality. The clinical management is similar to that for postsurgical DI, as outlined earlier, except that the possibility of anterior pituitary insufficiency must also be considered in these cases, and the patient should be given stress doses of glucocorticoids (e.g., hydrocortisone, 50–100 mg intravenously every 8 hours) until anterior pituitary function can be definitively evaluated.

### Osmoreceptor Dysfunction

Acutely, patients with hypernatremia due to osmoreceptor dysfunction should be treated the same as any hyperosmolar patient by replacing the underlying free water deficit, as described at the beginning of this section. The long-term management of osmoreceptor dysfunction syndromes requires a thorough search for potentially treatable causes (see Box 15.1) in conjunction with the use of measures to prevent recurrence of dehydration. Because the hypodipsia cannot be cured, and rarely if ever improves spontaneously, the mainstay of management is education of the patient and family about the importance of continuously regulating her or his fluid intake in accordance with the hydration status.[261] This is never accomplished easily in such patients, but can be done most efficaciously by establishing a daily schedule of water intake based on changes in BW, regardless of the patient's thirst.[262] In effect, a prescription for daily fluid intake must be written for these patients because they will not drink spontaneously. In addition, if the patient has polyuria, desmopressin should also be given, as for any patient with DI. The success of this regimen should be monitored periodically (weekly at first and later every month, depending on the stability of the patient) by measuring the serum [$Na^+$]. In addition, the target weight (at which hydration status and the serum [$Na^+$] concentration are normal) may need to be recalculated periodically to allow for growth in children or changes in body fat in adults.

### Gestational Diabetes Insipidus

The polyuria of gestational DI is usually not corrected by the administration of AVP itself because this is rapidly degraded by high circulating levels of oxytocinase or vasopressinase, just as endogenous AVP is degraded by these enzymes. The treatment of choice is desmopressin because this synthetic AVP $V_2$ receptor agonist is not destroyed by the cysteine aminopeptidase (oxytocinase or vasopressinase) in the plasma of pregnant women[263] and, to date, appears to be safe for both the mother and child.[264,265] Desmopressin has only 2% to 5% the oxytocic activity of AVP[243] and can be used with minimal stimulation of the OT receptors in the uterus. Doses should be titrated to individual patients because higher doses and more frequent dosing intervals are sometimes required as a result of the increased degradation of the peptide. However, physicians should remember that the naturally occurring volume expansion and reset osmostat that occurs in pregnancy maintains the serum [$Na^+$] at a lower level during pregnancy.[39] During delivery, these patients can maintain adequate oral intake and continued administration of desmopressin. However, physicians should be cautious about the overadministration of fluid parenterally during delivery because these patients will not be able to excrete the fluid and will be susceptible to the development of water intoxication and hyponatremia. After delivery, oxytocinase and vasopressinase levels decrease in the plasma within several days and, depending on the cause of the DI, the disorder may disappear or the patient may become asymptomatic with regard to fluid intake and urine volume.[266]

### Nephrogenic Diabetes Insipidus

By definition, patients with NDI are resistant to the effects of AVP. Some patients with NDI can be treated by eliminating the drug (e.g., lithium) or disease (e.g., hypercalcemia) responsible for the disorder. For many others, however, including those with the genetic forms, the only practical form of treatment at present is to restrict sodium intake and administer a thiazide diuretic alone[249] or in combination with a prostaglandin synthetase inhibitor or amiloride.[267–269] The natriuretic effect of the thiazide class of diuretics is conferred by their ability to block sodium absorption in the renal cortical diluting site. When combined with dietary sodium restriction, these drugs cause modest hypovolemia. This stimulates isotonic proximal tubular solute reabsorption and diminishes solute delivery to the more distal diluting site, at which experimental studies have indicated that thiazides also act to enhance water reabsorption in the inner medullary collecting duct independently of AVP.[270] Together, these effects diminish renal diluting ability and free water clearance, also independently of any action of AVP. Thus, agents of this class are the mainstay of therapy for NDI. Monitoring for hypokalemia is recommended, and potassium supplementation is occasionally required. Any drug of the thiazide class may be used with equal potential for benefit, and clinicians should use the one with which they are most familiar from use in other conditions. Care must be exercised when treating patients taking lithium with diuretics because the induced contraction of plasma volume may increase lithium concentrations and worsen potential toxic effects of the therapy. In the acute setting, diuretics are of no use in NDI, and only free water administration can reverse hyperosmolality.

Indomethacin, tolmetin, and ibuprofen have been used in this setting,[267,271,272] although ibuprofen may be less effective than the others. The combination of thiazides and a nonsteroidal antiinflammatory drug (NSAID) will not increase urinary osmolality above that of plasma, but lessening of the polyuria is nonetheless beneficial to patients. In many cases, the combination of thiazides with the potassium-sparing diuretic amiloride is preferred to lessen the potential side effects associated with long-term use of NSAIDs.[268,269] Amiloride also has the advantage of decreasing lithium entrance into cells in the distal tubule and, because of this, may have a preferable action for the treatment of lithium-induced NDI.[273,274]

Although desmopressin is generally not effective in NDI, a few patients may have receptor mutations that allow partial responses to AVP or desmopressin,[275] with increases in urine osmolality following much higher doses of these agents than those typically used to treat CDI (e.g., 6–10 μg intravenously). It is generally worth a trial of desmopressin at these doses to ascertain whether this is a potential useful therapy in selected patients in whom the responsivity of other affected family members is not already known. Potential therapies involving the administration of chaperones to bypass defects in cellular routing of misfolded aquaporin[186] and AVP $V_2$ receptor proteins[187] is an exciting, future possibility.[175]

### Primary Polydipsia

At present, there is no completely satisfactory treatment for primary polydipsia. Fluid restriction would seem to be the obvious treatment of choice. However, patients with a reset thirst threshold will be resistant to fluid restriction because of the resulting thirst from stimulation of brain thirst centers at higher plasma osmolalities.[276] In some cases, the use of alternative methods to ameliorate the sensation of thirst (e.g., wetting the mouth with ice chips, using sour candies to increase salivary flow) can help reduce fluid intake. Fluid intake in patients with a psychogenic cause of polydipsia is driven by psychiatric factors that have responded variably to behavioral modification and pharmacologic therapy. Several reports have suggested limited efficacy of the antipsychotic drug clozapine as an agent to reduce polydipsia and prevent recurrent hyponatremia in at least a subset of these patients.[277] Administration of any antidiuretic hormone or thiazide to decrease polyuria is hazardous because they invariably produce water intoxication.[219,278] Therefore, if the diagnosis of DI is uncertain, any trial of antidiuretic therapy should be conducted with close monitoring, preferably in the hospital, with frequent evaluation of fluid balance and serum electrolyte levels.

## DISORDERS OF EXCESS VASOPRESSIN OR VASOPRESSIN EFFECT

The disorders of the renal concentrating mechanism described in the previous section can lead to water depletion, sometimes in association with hyperosmolality and hypernatremia. In contrast, disorders of the renal diluting mechanism usually present as hyponatremia and hypoosmolality. Hyponatremia is among the most common electrolyte disorders encountered in clinical medicine, with an incidence of 0.97% and a prevalence of 2.48% in hospitalized adult patients when the serum [$Na^+$] less than 130 mEq/L is the diagnostic criterion[279] and as high as 15% to 30% if the serum [$Na^+$] less than 135 mEq/L is used as the diagnostic criterion.[280] The prevalence may be somewhat lower in the hospitalized pediatric population but, conversely, the prevalence is higher than originally recognized in the geriatric population.[280–282]

## RELATIONSHIP BETWEEN HYPOOSMOLALITY AND HYPONATREMIA

Because plasma osmolality is usually measured to help evaluate hyponatremic disorders, it is useful to bear in mind the basic relationship of plasma osmolality to the plasma or serum [$Na^+$]. As reviewed in the introduction to this chapter, $Na^+$ and its associated anions account for almost all the osmotic activity of plasma. Therefore, changes in serum [$Na^+$] are usually associated with comparable changes in plasma osmolality. The osmolality calculated from the concentrations of $Na^+$, urea, and glucose is usually in close agreement with that obtained from a measurement of osmolality.[283] When the measured osmolality exceeds the calculated osmolality by more than 10 mOsm/kg $H_2O$, an osmolar gap is present.[283] This occurs in two circumstances: (1) with a decrease in the water content of the serum; and (2) with the addition of a solute other than urea or glucose to the serum.

A decrease in the water content of serum is usually due to its displacement by excessive amounts of protein or lipids, which can occur in severe hyperlipidemia or hyperglobulinemia. Normally, 92% to 94% plasma volume is water, with the remaining 6% to 8% being lipids and protein. Because of its ionic nature, $Na^+$ dissolves only in the water phase of plasma. Thus, when a greater than normal proportion of plasma is accounted for by solids, the concentration of $Na^+$ in plasma water remains normal, but the concentration in the total volume, as measured by flame photometry, is artificially low. Such a discrepancy can be avoided if [$Na^+$] is measured with an ion-selective electrode.[284] However, the sample needs to remain undiluted (direct potentiometry) for accurate measurement of the serum [$Na^+$]. Whereas the flame photometer measures the concentration of $Na^+$ in the total plasma volume, the ion-selective electrode measures it only in the plasma water. Normally, this difference is only 3 mEq/L but, in the settings under discussion, the difference can be much greater. Because the large lipid and protein molecules contribute only minimally to the total osmolality, the measurement of osmolality by freezing point depression remains normal in these patients.

Hyponatremia associated with normal osmolality has been termed "factitious hyponatremia" or "pseudohyponatremia." The most common causes of pseudohyponatremia are primary or secondary hyperlipidemic disorders. The serum need not appear lipemic because increments in cholesterol alone can cause the same discrepancy.[284] Plasma protein level elevations above 10 g/dL, as seen in multiple myeloma or macroglobulinemia, can also cause pseudohyponatremia. The administration of intravenous immune globulin has been reported to be associated with hyponatremia without hypoosmolality in several patients.[285]

The second setting in which an osmolar gap occurs is the presence in plasma of an exogenous low-molecular-weight substance such as ethanol, methanol, ethylene glycol, or mannitol.[286] Undialyzed patients with chronic renal failure, as well as critically ill patients,[287] also have an increment in the osmolar gap of unknown cause. Whereas all these exogenous substances, as well as glucose and urea, elevate measured osmolality, the effect that they have on the serum [$Na^+$] and intracellular hydration depends on the solute in question. As noted, in the presence of relative insulin deficiency, glucose does not penetrate cells readily and remains in the ECF. As a consequence, water is drawn osmotically from the ICF compartment, causing cell shrinkage, and this translocation of water commensurately decreases the [$Na^+$] in the ECF. In this setting, therefore, the serum [$Na^+$] can be low while plasma osmolality is normal or high. It is generally estimated that for every 100-mg/dL rise in serum glucose, the osmotic shift of water causes serum [$Na^+$] to fall by 1.6 mEq/L. However, it has been suggested that this may represent an underestimate of the decrease caused by more severe degrees of hyperglycemia, and a 2.4-mEq/L correction factor is recommended in such cases.[288]

Similar "translocational" hyponatremia occurs with mannitol or maltose or with the absorption of glycine during transurethral prostate resection, as well as in gynecologic and orthopedic procedures. A potential toxicity for glycine in this setting also requires consideration.[289] The recent introduction of bipolar retroscopes, which allow for the use of NaCl as an irrigant, should result in the disappearance of this clinical entity. When the plasma solute is readily permeable (e.g., urea, ethylene glycol, methanol, ethanol), it enters cells and so does not establish an osmotic gradient for water movement. There is no cellular dehydration, despite the hyperosmolar state, so the serum [$Na^+$] remains unchanged. The relationship among plasma osmolality, plasma tonicity, and serum [$Na^+$] in the presence of various solutes is summarized in Table 15.2.

**Table 15.2 Relationship Between Serum Tonicity and Sodium Concentration in the Presence of Other Substances**

| Condition or Substance | Serum Osmolality | Serum Tonicity | Serum [$Na^+$] |
|---|---|---|---|
| Hyperglycemia | ↑ | ↑ | ↓ |
| Mannitol, maltose, glycine | ↑ | ↑ | ↓ |
| Azotemia (high blood urea) | ↑ | ↔ | ↔ |
| Ingestion of ethanol, methanol, ethylene glycol | ↑ | ↔ | ↔ |
| Elevated serum lipid or protein | ↔ | ↔ | ↓ |

↑, Increased; ↓, decreased; ↔, unchanged.

## VARIABLES THAT INFLUENCE RENAL WATER EXCRETION

In considering clinical disorders that result from excessive or inappropriate secretion of AVP, it is important to remember the many other variables that also influence renal water excretion. These factors fall into four broad categories.

### Fluid Delivery From the Proximal Tubule

In spite of the fact that proximal fluid reabsorption is isoosmotic and therefore does not contribute directly to urine dilution, the volume of tubular fluid that is delivered to the distal nephron largely determines the volume of dilute urine that can be excreted. Thus, if glomerular filtration is decreased or proximal tubule reabsorption is greatly enhanced, the resulting diminution in the amount of fluid delivered to the distal tubule itself limits the rate of renal water excretion, even if other components of the diluting mechanism are intact.

### Dilution of Tubular Fluid

The excretion of urine that is hypotonic to plasma requires that some segment of the nephron reabsorb solute in excess of water. The water impermeability of the entire ascending limb of Henle, as well as the capacity of its thick segment to reabsorb NaCl, actively endows this segment of the nephron with the characteristics required by the diluting process. Thus, the transport of NaCl by the $Na^+$-$K^+$-$2Cl^-$ cotransporter converts the hypertonic tubule fluid delivered from the descending limb of the loop of Henle to a distinctly hypotonic fluid. Likewise, the distal convoluted tubule is impermeable to water, and reabsorption of NaCl by the thiazide-sensitive NaCl cotransporter further dilutes the luminal fluid (down to an osmolality of ≈100 mOsm/kg $H_2O$). Interference with the reabsorption of $Na^+$ and $Cl^-$ in these segments, as occurs with loop and thiazide diuretics, will therefore impair urine dilution.

### Water Impermeability of the Collecting Duct

The excretion of urine that is more dilute than the fluid that is delivered to the distal convoluted tubule requires continued solute reabsorption and minimal water reabsorption in the terminal segments of the nephron. Because the water permeability of the collecting duct epithelium is primarily dependent on the presence or absence of AVP, this hormone plays a pivotal role in determining the fate of the fluid delivered to the collecting duct and thus the concentration or dilution of the final urine (see Chapter 10). In the absence of AVP, the collecting duct remains essentially impermeable to water, even though some water is still reabsorbed. The continued reabsorption of solute then results in the excretion of a maximally dilute urine (≈50 mOsm/kg $H_2O$). Because the medullary interstitium is always hypertonic, the absence of circulating AVP, which renders the collecting duct impermeable to water, is critical to the normal diluting process. This diluting mechanism allows for the intake and subsequent excretion of large volumes of water, without major alterations in the tonicity of body water.[290] Rarely, this limit can be exceeded, causing water intoxication. Much more commonly, however, hyponatremia occurs at lower rates of water intake because of an intrarenal defect in urine dilution or the persistent secretion of AVP in the circulation. Because hypoosmolality normally suppresses AVP secretion,[291] the hypoosmolar state frequently reflects the persistent secretion of AVP in response to hemodynamic or other nonosmotic stimuli.[291]

### Solute Excretion Rate

At any fixed urine osmolality, the total osmolar load that needs to be excreted each day determines the daily urine volume and hence the volume of free water that can be excreted.[292] This osmolar load is made up predominantly of salt and urea and is therefore dependent on dietary protein intake. This explains why patients with a very low protein intake can develop hyponatremia,[293] and why increasing the intake of protein, or administration of urea, can correct chronic hyponatremia.

## PATHOGENESIS AND CAUSES OF HYPONATREMIA

The plasma or serum [$Na^+$] is determined by the body's total content of sodium, potassium, and water, as shown by the following equation:

$$\text{Serum }[Na^+] = (\text{total body exchangeable } Na^+ + \text{total body exchangeable }[K^+])/\text{total BW}$$

This formula has been simplified from the observations made by Edelman in the 1950s, which introduced some errors in the prediction of changes in serum [$Na^+$] and has been subject to reinterpretation by Nguyen and Kurtz.[294] Although this revision of the formula is more accurate, there are so many inaccuracies in the measurements of sodium, potassium, and water losses, as well as intake, that there is no substitute for frequent measurements of the serum [$Na^+$] in rapidly changing clinical settings.[295] As the previous relationship depicts, hyponatremia can therefore occur by an increase in TBW, a decrease in body solutes ($Na^+$ or $K^+$), or any combination of these. In most cases, more than one of these mechanisms is operant. Therefore, a classification system to separate the various causes of hyponatremia should be based on factors other than the level of serum [$Na^+$] itself. In approaching the hyponatremic patient, the physician's first task is to ensure that hyponatremia actually reflects a hypoosmolar state and is not a consequence of pseudohyponatremia or translocational hyponatremia, as discussed earlier. Thereafter, an assessment of ECF volume (Fig. 15.17) provides the most useful working classification of the cause of the hyponatremia because a low serum [$Na^+$] can be associated with a decreased, normal, or high total body sodium content.[296,297]

### HYPONATREMIA WITH EXTRACELLULAR FLUID VOLUME DEPLETION

Patients with hyponatremia who have ECF volume depletion have sustained a deficit in total body $Na^+$ that exceeds the deficit in TBW. The decrease in ECF volume is manifested by physical findings such as flat neck veins, decreased skin turgor, dry mucous membranes, orthostatic hypotension, and tachycardia. If sufficiently severe, volume depletion is a potent stimulus to AVP secretion. When the osmoreceptors and volume receptors receive opposing stimuli, the former remains active but the set point of the system is lowered (see Fig. 15.7). Thus, in the presence of hypovolemia, AVP is secreted and water is retained, despite hypoosmolality. Whereas the hyponatremia in this setting clearly involves a depletion of body solutes, the concomitant AVP-mediated retention of water is critical to the pathologic process producing hyponatremia.

As depicted in the flow chart in Fig. 15.17, measurement of the urine [$Na^+$] concentration is helpful in assessing whether the fluid losses are renal or extrarenal in origin. A urine [$Na^+$] of less than 30 mEq/L reflects a normal renal response to volume depletion and indicates an extrarenal source of fluid loss. This is usually seen in patients with gastrointestinal disease with vomiting or diarrhea. Other causes include loss of fluid into a third space, such as the abdominal cavity in pancreatitis or the bowel lumen with

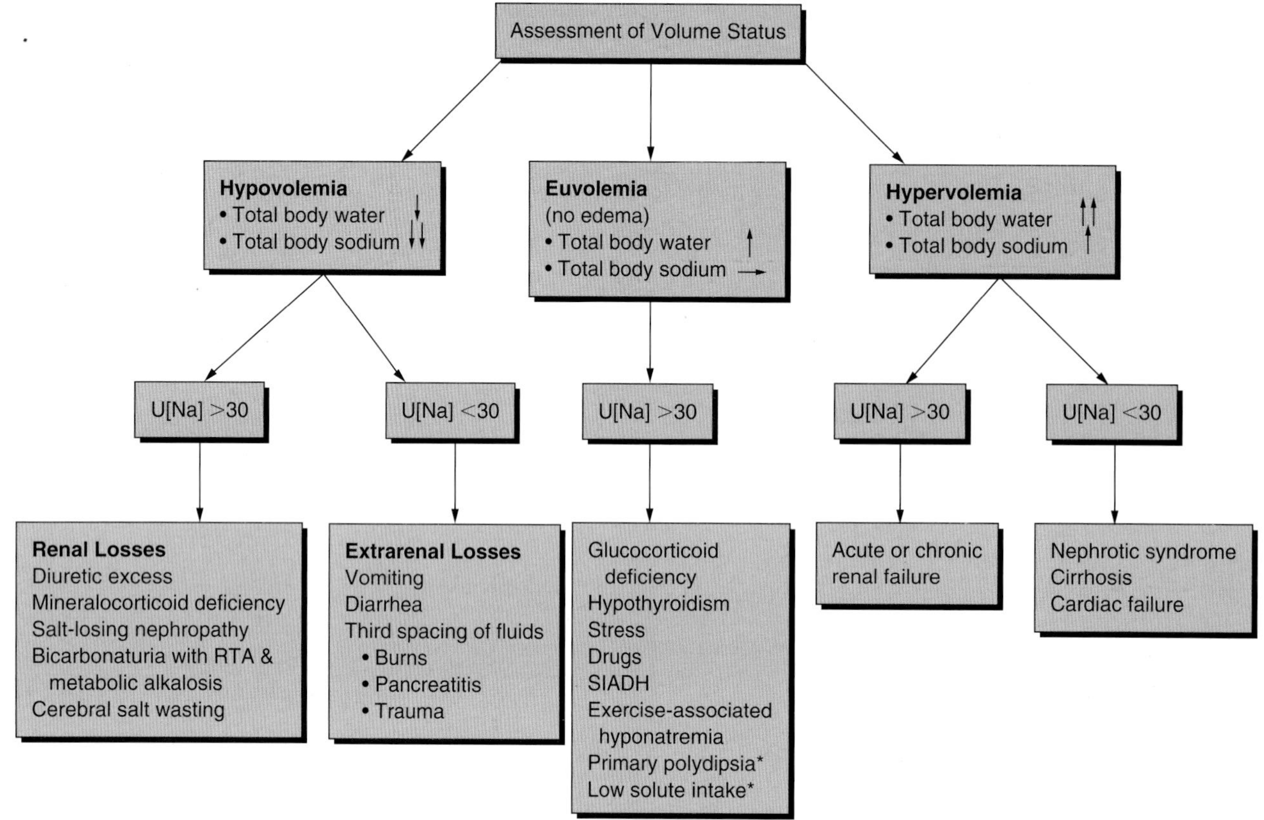


**Fig. 15.17** Diagnostic approach to the hyponatremic patient. *SIADH,* Syndrome of inappropriate antidiuretic hormone secretion; *U[Na],* urinary [$Na^+$]. (Modified from Halterman R, Berl T: Therapy of dysnatremic disorders. In Brady H, Wilcox C, eds. *Therapy in Nephrology and Hypertension,* Philadelphia: WB Saunders; 1999:256.)

ileus. Burns and muscle trauma can also be associated with large fluid and electrolyte losses. Because many of these pathologic states are associated with increased thirst, an increase in orally ingested or parenterally infused free water can lead to hyponatremia.

Hypovolemic hyponatremia in patients whose urine [$Na^+$] is higher than 30 mEq/L indicates the kidney as the source of the fluid losses. Diuretic-induced hyponatremia, a commonly observed clinical entity, accounts for a significant proportion of symptomatic hyponatremia in hospitalized patients. It occurs almost exclusively with thiazide rather than loop diuretics. This is most likely because, whereas both classes of diuretics can impair urine diluting ability, loop diuretics also impair the generation of the medullary interstitial concentrating gradient, thus limiting the maximal urinary concentration that can be achieved. The hyponatremia is usually evident within 14 days in most patients, but occasionally can occur as late as 2 years after the initiation of therapy.[298] Underweight women appear to be particularly prone to this complication, and advanced age has been found to be a risk factor in some, but not all, studies.[298–300] A careful study of diluting ability in older adults has revealed that thiazide diuretics exaggerate the already slower recovery from hyponatremia induced by water ingestion in this population.[301]

Diuretics can cause hyponatremia by several mechanisms: (1) volume depletion, which results in impaired water excretion by enhanced AVP release and decreased tubular fluid delivery to the diluting segment; (2) a direct effect on the diluting function of the thick ascending limb or distal convoluted tubule; and (3) $K^+$ depletion that frequently accompanies diuretic use, which contributes to the loss of total body exchangeable solute ($Na^+ + K^+$).[302] The concomitant administration of potassium-sparing diuretics does not prevent the development of hyponatremia. Although the diagnosis of diuretic-induced hyponatremia is frequently obvious, surreptitious diuretic abuse should always be considered in patients in whom other electrolyte abnormalities and high urinary $Cl^-$ excretion suggest this possibility. Recent genetic and phenotyping studies have suggested that an inherited defect in PGE2 uptake in the collecting duct may confer an increased risk of thiazide-induced hyponatremia, which raises the possibility that patients at risk of this adverse effect of thiazides may be able to be identified before exposure to the drug.[303,304]

Salt-losing nephropathy occurs in some patients with advanced renal insufficiency. In most of these patients, the $Na^+$-wasting tendency is not one that manifests itself at normal rates of sodium intake; however, some patients with interstitial nephropathy, medullary cystic disease, polycystic kidney disease, or partial urinary obstruction develop sufficient $Na^+$ wasting to exhibit hypovolemic hyponatremia.[305] Patients with proximal renal tubular acidosis exhibit renal $Na^+$ and $K^+$ wasting, despite modest renal insufficiency, because bicarbonaturia obligates these cation losses.

It has long been recognized that adrenal insufficiency is associated with impaired renal water excretion and hyponatremia. This diagnosis should be considered in the volume-contracted hyponatremic patient whose urine [$Na^+$] is not low, particularly when the serum [$K^+$], urea, and creatinine levels are elevated. Separate mechanisms for mineralocorticoid and glucocorticoid deficiency have been defined.[306] Observations in glucocorticoid-replete adrenalectomized experimental animals have provided evidence to support a role of mineralocorticoid deficiency in the abnormal water excretion. Conscious adrenalectomized dogs given physiologic doses of glucocorticoids develop hyponatremia. Saline or physiologic doses of mineralocorticoids corrected the defect in association with ECF volume repletion and improvement in renal hemodynamics. Immunoassayable AVP levels were elevated in a similarly treated group of mineralocorticoid-deficient dogs, despite hypoosmolality.[307] The decreased ECF volume thus provides a nonosmotic stimulus of AVP release. More direct evidence for the role of AVP has been provided in studies using an AVP receptor antagonist. When glucocorticoid-replete, adrenally insufficient rats were given an AVP antagonist, minimal urine osmolality was significantly lowered but urine dilution was not fully corrected, in contrast to the mineralocorticoid-replete rats, thereby supporting a role for an AVP-independent mechanism.[308] This is in agreement with studies of adrenalectomized homozygous Brattleboro rats, which also have a defect in water excretion that can be partially corrected by mineralocorticoids or by the normalization of volume. In summary, therefore, the mechanism of the defect in water excretion associated with mineralocorticoid deficiency is mediated by AVP and by AVP-independent intrarenal factors, both of which are activated by decrements of ECF volume, more so than by a deficiency of the hormone per se.

The presence in the urine of an osmotically active, nonreabsorbable or poorly reabsorbable solute causes the renal excretion of $Na^+$ and culminates in volume depletion. Glycosuria secondary to uncontrolled diabetes mellitus, mannitol infusion, or urea diuresis after relief of obstruction are common causes of this disorder. In patients with diabetes, the $Na^+$ wasting caused by the glycosuria can be aggravated by ketonuria because hydroxybutyrate and acetoacetate also cause urinary electrolyte losses. In fact, ketonuria can contribute to the renal $Na^+$ wasting and hyponatremia seen in states of starvation and alcoholic ketoacidosis. $Na^+$ and water excretion are also increased when a nonreabsorbable anion appears in the urine. This is observed principally with the metabolic alkalosis and bicarbonaturia that accompany severe vomiting or nasogastric suction. In these patients, the excretion of $HCO_3^-$ requires the concomitant excretion of cations, including $Na^+$ and $K^+$, to maintain electroneutrality. Whereas the renal losses in such clinical settings is often hypotonic, the volume contraction–stimulated thirst and water intake can result in the development of hyponatremia.

Cerebral salt wasting is a rare syndrome described primarily in patients with subarachnoid hemorrhage, but also with other types of CNS lesions, which can lead to renal salt wasting and volume contraction.[309] Although hyponatremia is frequently reported in these patients, true cerebral salt wasting is probably less common than reported.[310] One critical review has found no conclusive evidence for volume contraction or renal salt wasting in any of these patients,[311] as has a more recent study of patients with subarachnoid hemorrhage.[312] The mechanism of this natriuresis is unknown, but an increased release of brain natriuretic peptides has been suggested.[313]

## HYPONATREMIA WITH EXCESS EXTRACELLULAR FLUID VOLUME

In advanced stages, the edematous states listed in Fig. 15.17 are associated with a decrease in serum [$Na^+$]. Patients generally have an increase in total body $Na^+$ content, but the rise in TBW exceeds that of $Na^+$. With the exception of renal failure, these states are characterized by avid $Na^+$ retention (urine $Na^+$ concentration often < 10 mEq/L). This avid retention may be obscured by the concomitant use of diuretics, which are frequently used in treating these patients.

## CONGESTIVE HEART FAILURE

The common association between congestive heart failure and $Na^+$ and water retention is well established. A mechanism mediated by decreased delivery of tubule fluid to the distal nephron and/or increased release of AVP has been proposed. In an experimental model of low cardiac output, both AVP and diminished delivery to the diluting segment were found to be important in mediating the abnormality in water excretion. It thus appears that the decrement in effective blood volume and decrease in arterial filling are sensed by aortic and carotid sinus baroreceptors, which stimulate AVP secretion.[314]

This stimulation must supersede the inhibition of AVP release that accompanies acute distention of the left atrium. In fact, there is evidence that chronic distention of the atria blunts the sensitivity of this baroreceptor, so high-pressure baroreceptors can act in an uninhibited manner to stimulate AVP release. The importance of AVP in the abnormal dilution in experimental models of heart failure has been underscored by correction of the water excretory defect by an AVP antagonist in rats with inferior vena cava constriction.[315]

High plasma AVP levels have been demonstrated in patients with congestive heart failure in the presence and absence of diuretics.[316] Similarly, the hypothalamic mRNA message for the AVP preprohormone is elevated in rats with chronic cardiac failure.[317] Although these studies did not exclude a role for intrarenal factors in the pathogenesis of the abnormal water retention, they complement the experimental observations that demonstrate a critical role for AVP in the pathologic process. It is most likely that nonosmotic pathways, whose activation is suggested by the increase in sympathetic activity seen in congestive heart failure,[318] are the mediators of AVP secretion in edema-forming states. These neurohumoral factors further contribute to the hyponatremia by decreasing the glomerular filtration rate (GFR) and enhancing tubular $Na^+$ reabsorption, thereby decreasing fluid delivery to the distal diluting segments of the nephron. The degree of neurohumoral activation correlates with the clinical severity of left ventricular dysfunction.[319] Hyponatremia is a powerful prognostic factor in these patients.[320]

The role of the AVP-regulated water channel (AQP2) has also been examined in heart failure. Two studies have described an upregulation of this water channel in rats with heart failure.[321,322] In the latter study, the nonpeptide $V_2$ receptor antagonist OPC31260 reversed the upregulation, suggesting that a receptor-mediated function, most likely enhanced cAMP generation, is responsible for the process.[321] Consistent with these observations, a selective $V_2$ receptor antagonist decreased AQP2 excretion and increased urine flow in patients with heart failure.[323]

## HEPATIC FAILURE

Patients with advanced cirrhosis and ascites frequently present with hyponatremia as a consequence of their inability to excrete a water load.[324] The classic view suggests that a decrement in effective arterial blood volume leads to avid $Na^+$ and water retention in an attempt to restore volume toward normal. In this regard, a number of the pathologic derangements in cirrhosis, including splanchnic venous pooling, diminished plasma oncotic pressure secondary to hypoalbuminemia, and decrease in peripheral resistance, could all contribute to a decrease in effective arterial blood volume.[325] This theory was challenged by observations that suggested primary renal $Na^+$ retention, termed the "overflow hypothesis."[326] A proposal that unifies these views has been presented—that is, $Na^+$ retention occurs early in the pathologic process, but is a consequence of the severe vasodilation-mediated arterial underfilling.[327]

As with cardiac failure, the relative roles of intrarenal versus extrarenal factors in impaired water excretion has been a matter of some controversy. The observation that expansion of intravascular volume with saline, mannitol, ascites fluid, water immersion, or peritoneovenous shunting improves water excretion in cirrhosis could be interpreted as implicating an intrarenal mechanism in the impaired water excretion. This is because these maneuvers increase the GFR and improve distal delivery. Such maneuvers could also suppress baroreceptor-mediated AVP release and cause an osmotic diuresis, which would also improve water excretion.[323] Experimental models of deranged liver function, including acute portal hypertension by vein constriction, bile duct ligation, and chronic cirrhosis produced by the administration of carbon tetrachloride, have demonstrated a predominant role for AVP secretion in the pathogenesis of the disorder. In this latter model, an increment in hypothalamic AVP mRNA has also been demonstrated.[328] A study using an AVP antagonist also has indicated a central role for AVP in the process.[329] As was the case in heart failure, increased expression of AQP2 has also been reported in the cirrhotic rat,[330] but dysregulation of AQP1 and AQP3 is also present in carbon tetrachloride ($CCl_4$)–induced cirrhosis.[331] In contrast, in the common bile duct model of cirrhosis, no increase in AQP2 was observed.[332]

Although patients with cirrhosis who have no edema or ascites excrete a water load normally, those with ascites usually do not. Several studies have demonstrated elevated AVP levels in these patients.[324] Patients who had a defect in water excretion had higher levels of AVP, plasma renin activity, plasma aldosterone, and norepinephrine,[333] as well as lower rates of PGE2 production. Similarly, their serum albumin level was lower, as was their urinary excretion of $Na^+$, all suggesting a decrease in effective arterial blood volume. As is the case in heart failure, sympathetic tone is high in cirrhosis.[334] In fact, the plasma concentration of norepinephrine, a good index of baroreceptor activity in humans, appears to correlate well with the levels of AVP and excretion of water. These studies, therefore, offer strong support for the view that effective arterial blood volume is contracted, rather than expanded, in decompensated cirrhosis.[327] This concept is further strengthened by observations of subjects during head-out water immersion. This maneuver, which translocates fluid to the central blood volume, caused a decrease in AVP levels and improved water excretion[335] but, in this study, peripheral resistance decreased further. By combining head-out water immersion with norepinephrine administration in an effort to increase systemic pressure and peripheral resistance, water excretion was completely normalized.[336] Such observations underline the critical role of peripheral vasodilation in the pathologic process. The observation that the inhibition of nitric oxide corrects the arterial hyporesponsiveness to vasodilators and the abnormal water excretion in cirrhotic rats provides strong evidence of a role for nitric oxide in the vasodilation.[337–339]

## NEPHROTIC SYNDROME

The incidence of hyponatremia in the nephrotic syndrome is lower than in congestive heart failure or cirrhosis, most likely as a consequence of the higher blood pressure, higher GFR, and more modest impairments in $Na^+$ and water excretion than in the other groups of patients.[340] Because lipid levels are frequently elevated, a direct measurement of plasma osmolality should always be done. Diminished excretion of free water was first noted in children with the nephrotic syndrome and, since then, other investigators[341] have noted elevated plasma levels of AVP in these patients. In view of the alterations in Starling forces that accompany hypoalbuminemia and allow the transudation of salt and water across capillary membranes to the interstitial space, patients with the nephrotic syndrome are thought to have intravascular volume contraction. Increased levels of neurohumoral markers of decreased effective arterial blood volume also support this underfilling theory.[342] The possibility that this nonosmotic pathway stimulates AVP release has been suggested by studies in which head-out water immersion and blood volume expansion[342] increases water excretion in nephrotic subjects. However, these pathogenic events may not be applicable to all patients with the disorder. Some patients with the nephrotic syndrome have increased plasma volumes, with suppressed plasma renin activity and aldosterone levels.[343] The cause of these discrepancies is not immediately evident, but this overfill view has been subject to some criticism.[344] It is most likely that the underfilling mechanism is operant in patients with a normal GFR and with the histologic lesion of minimal change disease, and that hypervolemia may be more prevalent in patients with underlying glomerular pathology and decreased renal function. In such patients, an intrarenal mechanism probably causes $Na^+$ retention, as has been described in an experimental model of nephrotic syndrome.[345] Also, in contrast to the increase in AQP2 found in the previously described $Na^+$- and water-retaining states, the expression of AQP2 was decreased in two models of nephrotic syndrome induced with puromycin aminonucleoside[346] or doxorubicin.[347] The animals were not hyponatremic and most likely had expanded ECF volumes to explain the discrepancy.

## RENAL FAILURE

Hyponatremia with edema can occur with acute or chronic renal failure. It is clear that in the setting of experimental or human renal disease, the ability to excrete free water is maintained better than the ability to reabsorb water. Nonetheless, the patient's GFR still determines the maximal rate of free water formation. Thus, if minimal urine osmolality is limited to 150 to 250 mOsm/kg $H_2O$ and fractional water excretion approaches 20% to 30% of the filtered load, a uremic patient with a GFR of 2 mL/min/1.73 $m^2$ is estimated to excrete only ~300 mL of free water/day. Intake of more fluid than this will result in hyponatremia. Thus, in most cases, a decrement in GFR with an increase in thirst underlies the hyponatremia of patients with renal insufficiency.[348]

## HYPONATREMIA WITH NORMAL EXTRACELLULAR FLUID VOLUME

Fig. 15.17 lists the clinical entities that have to be considered in patients with hyponatremia whose volume is neither contracted nor expanded and who are, at least by clinical assessment, euvolemic. These are considered individually here.

### SYNDROME OF INAPPROPRIATE ANTIDIURETIC HORMONE SECRETION

SIADH is the most common cause of hyponatremia in hospitalized patients.[279] As first described by Schwartz and associates[349] in two patients with bronchogenic carcinoma, and later characterized further by Bartter and Schwartz,[350] patients with this syndrome have serum hypoosmolality when excreting urine that is less than maximally dilute (>100 mOsm/kg $H_2O$). Thus, a diagnostic criterion for this syndrome is the presence of inappropriate urine concentration. The development of hyponatremia with a dilute urine (<100 mOsm/kg $H_2O$) should raise suspicion of a primary polydipsic disorder. Although large volumes of fluid need to be ingested to overwhelm the normal water excretory ability, this volume need not be excessively high if there are concomitant decreases in solute intake.[293] In SIADH, the urinary $Na^+$ concentration is dependent on intake, because $Na^+$ balance is well maintained. As such, urinary $Na^+$ concentration is usually high, but it may be low in patients with the syndrome who are receiving a low-sodium diet. The presence of $Na^+$ in the urine is helpful in excluding extrarenal causes of hypovolemic hyponatremia, but a low urinary $Na^+$ concentration does not exclude SIADH. Before the diagnosis of SIADH is made, other causes for a decreased diluting capacity, such as renal, pituitary, adrenal, thyroid, cardiac, or hepatic disease, must be excluded. In addition, nonosmotic stimuli for AVP release, particularly hemodynamic derangements (e.g., caused by hypotension, nausea, or drugs), need to be ruled out.

Another clue to the presence of SIADH is the finding of hypouricemia. In one study, 16 of 17 patients with a diagnosis of SIADH had levels below 4 mg/dL, whereas in 13 patients with hyponatremia of other causes, the level was higher than 5 mg/dL. Hypouricemia appears to occur as a consequence of increased urate clearance.[351] Measurement of an elevated level of AVP can confirm the clinical diagnosis, but is not necessary. It should be noted that most patients with SIADH have AVP levels in the normal range (2–10 pg/mL); the presence of any measurable AVP is, however, abnormal in the hypoosmolar state. Plasma AVP levels have never been a requirement for the diagnosis of SIADH, in part because they are elevated in states of hypovolemic hyponatremia as well as SIADH, and therefore have little differential diagnostic value. For similar reasons, the measurement of copeptin levels has been found to be of little diagnostic value in the differential diagnosis of hyponatremia.[352] Because the presence of hyponatremia is itself evidence for abnormal dilution, a formal urine-diluting test need not be performed in most cases. The water loading test is helpful in determining whether an abnormality remains in a patient whose serum [$Na^+$] has been corrected by water restriction. Because Brattleboro rats receiving AVP[353] have displayed upregulation of AQP2 expression, the excretion of AQP2 has been investigated as a marker for the persistent secretion of AVP. The excretion of the water channel remains elevated in patients with SIADH, but this is not specific to this entity because a similar pattern was observed in patients with hyponatremia due to hypopituitarism.[354]

#### Pathophysiology

In 1953, Leaf and associates[355] described the effects of chronic AVP administration on $Na^+$ and water balance. They noted that high-volume water intake was required for the development of hyponatremia. Concomitant with the water retention, an increment in urinary $Na^+$ excretion was observed. The relative contributions of the water retention and $Na^+$ loss to the development of hyponatremia were subsequently investigated. Acute water loading causes transient natriuresis but, when water intake is increased more slowly, no significant negative $Na^+$ loss can be documented. These studies have clearly demonstrated that the hyponatremia is mainly a consequence of water retention; however, it must be noted that the net increase in water balance fails to account entirely for the decrement in serum [$Na^+$].[355]

In a carefully studied model of SIADH in rats, the retained water was found to be distributed in the intracellular space and in equilibrium with the tonicity of the ECF.[356] The natriuresis and kaliuresis that occur early in the development of this model contribute to a decrement of body solutes and, in part, account for the observed hyponatremia.[357] Studies involving analysis of whole-body water and electrolyte content have demonstrated that the relative contributions of water retention and solute losses vary with the duration of induced hyponatremia; the former is central to the process but, with more prolonged hyponatremia, $Na^+$ depletion becomes predominant.[358] In this regard, it has even been suggested that the natriuresis and volume contraction are important components of the syndrome that maintains the secretion of AVP,[359] with atrial natriuretic peptide as a potential mediator of the $Na^+$ loss.[360] Therefore, although natriuresis frequently accompanies the syndrome, nonosmotically stimulated AVP secretion is essential. Finally, patients with the syndrome must also have abnormal thirst regulation, whereby the osmotic inhibition of water intake is not operant. The mechanism of this failure to suppress thirst is not fully understood, but may simply reflect the continued ingestion of beverages for reasons other than true thirst.

After the initial retention of water, loss of $Na^+$, and development of hyponatremia, continued administration of AVP is accompanied by reestablishment of $Na^+$ balance and a decline in the hydroosmotic effect of the hormone. The integrity of renal regulation of $Na^+$ balance is manifested by the ability to conserve $Na^+$ during $Na^+$ restriction and by the normal excretion of a $Na^+$ load. Thus, the mechanisms that regulate $Na^+$ excretion are intact. Loss of the hydroosmotic effect of AVP, albeit to varying degrees, has been evident in many studies[355,357] because urine flow increases and urine osmolality decreases, despite continued administration of the hormone. This effect has been termed "vasopressin escape."[361] Several studies have demonstrated that hypotonic ECF volume expansion, rather than chronic administration of AVP per se, is needed for escape to occur because the escape phenomenon is seen only when a positive water balance is achieved.[361]

The cellular mechanisms responsible for vasopressin escape have been the subject of some investigation. Studies of broken epithelial cell preparations of the toad urinary bladder have revealed downregulation of AVP receptors,[362] as well as vasopressin binding in the inner medulla.[363] Post-cAMP mechanisms are probably also operant. In this regard, a decrease in the expression of AQP2 has been reported in the process of escape from desmopressin-induced antidiuresis, without a concomitant change in basolateral AQP3 and AQP4.[364,365] The decrement in AQP2 was associated with decreased $V_2$ responsiveness.[364] The distal tubule also has an increase in sodium transporters, including the alpha and gamma subunits of the epithelial sodium channel and the thiazide-sensitive $Na^+$-$Cl^-$ cotransporter.[366] In addition to a renal mechanism, it appears that chronic hyponatremia causes a decrement in hypothalamic mRNA production, a process that could ameliorate the syndrome in the clinical setting.[27]

### Clinical Settings

It is now apparent that the previously described pathophysiologic sequence occurs in a variety of clinical settings characterized by persistent AVP secretion. Since the original report of Schwartz and coworkers,[349] the syndrome has been described in an increasing number of clinical settings (Table 15.3). These fall into four general categories[367]: (1) malignancies; (2) pulmonary disease; (3) CNS disorders; and (4) drug effects. In addition, an increasing number of patients with acquired immunodeficiency syndrome have been reported to have hyponatremia. The frequency may be as high as 35% of hospitalized patients with the disease and, in as many as two-thirds, SIADH may be the underlying cause.[368] As noted previously, hyponatremia caused by excessive water repletion can occur after moderate and severe exercise.[369–372] Finally, it has been increasingly recognized that an idiopathic form is common in older adults.[373–376] In one study, as many as 25% of older patients admitted to a rehabilitation center had a serum $[Na^+]$ lower than 135 mEq/L.[374] In a significant proportion of these patients, no underlying cause was discovered.

A material with antidiuretic properties has been extracted from some of the tumors or metastases of patients with malignancy-associated SIADH. However, not all patients with the syndrome have AVP in their tumors. Of the tumors that cause SIADH secretion, bronchogenic carcinoma, and particularly small cell lung cancer, is the most common, with a reported incidence of 11%.[377] It appears that patients with bronchogenic carcinoma have higher plasma AVP levels in relation to plasma osmolality, even if they do not manifest full-blown SIADH; however, in patients with the syndrome, levels of the hormone are higher. The possibility that the hormone could serve as a marker of bronchogenic carcinoma has been suggested, and SIADH has been reported occasionally to precede diagnosis of the tumor by several months.[378] Recent epidemiologic analyses have strongly implicated hyponatremia as a predictor of subsequent malignancies. Among 625,114 Danish subjects, all-cause mortality was increased in mild, moderate, and severe hyponatremia compared with normonatremic individuals. Of special note, the incident rate ratio of a subsequent diagnosis of head and neck or pulmonary cancer was markedly increased in patients at all levels of hyponatremia; 1893 of 14,517 of all hyponatremic patients (13%) subsequently had a diagnosis

**Table 15.3 Disorders Associated With Syndrome of Inappropriate Antidiuretic Hormone Secretion**

| Carcinomas | Pulmonary Disorders | Central Nervous System Disorders | Other Disorders |
|---|---|---|---|
| Bronchogenic carcinoma | Viral pneumonia | Encephalitis (viral or bacterial) | AIDS |
| Carcinoma of the duodenum | Bacterial pneumonia | Meningitis (viral, bacterial, tuberculous, fungal) | Prolonged exercise |
| Carcinoma of the ureter | Pulmonary abscess | Head trauma | Idiopathic (in older adults) |
| Carcinoma of the pancreas | Tuberculosis | Brain abscess | Nephrogenic |
| Thymoma | Aspergillosis | Guillain-Barré syndrome | Acute intermittent porphyria |
| Carcinoma of the stomach | Positive pressure breathing | Subarachnoid hemorrhage or subdural hematoma | |
| Lymphoma | Asthma | Cerebellar and cerebral atrophy | |
| Ewing sarcoma | Pneumothorax | Cavernous sinus thrombosis | |
| Carcinoma of the bladder | Mesothelioma | Neonatal hypoxia | |
| Prostatic carcinoma | Cystic fibrosis | Shy-Drager syndrome | |
| Oropharyngeal tumor | | Rocky Mountain spotted fever | |
| | | Delirium tremens | |
| | | Cerebrovascular accident (cerebral thrombosis or hemorrhage) | |
| | | Acute psychosis | |
| | | Peripheral neuropathy | |
| | | Multiple sclerosis | |

Adapted from Berl T, Schrier RW: Disorders of water metabolism. In Schrier RW, ed. *Renal and Electrolyte Disorders.* 6th ed. Philadelphia: Lippincott Williams & Wilkins; 2003.

of cancer, leading to the conclusion that hyponatremia is linked to an increased risk of being subsequently diagnosed with any cancer, particularly pulmonary and head and neck cancers.[379] In view of the potential to treat patients with this tumor, it is important that patients with unexplained SIADH be fully investigated and evaluated for the presence of this malignancy. Head and neck malignancies are the second most common tumors associated with SIADH, which occurs in approximately 3% of these patients.

The mechanism whereby AVP is produced in other pulmonary disorders is not known, but the associated abnormalities in blood gases could act as mediators of the effect. Antidiuretic activity has also been assayed in tuberculous lung tissue. The syndrome can also occur in the setting of miliary rather than only lung-limited tuberculosis.[380] In CNS disorders, AVP is most likely released from the neurohypophysis. Studies of monkeys have shown that elevations of intracranial pressure cause AVP secretion, which may be the mechanism that mediates the syndrome in at least some CNS disorders. The magnocellular AVP-secreting cells in the hypothalamus are subject to numerous excitatory inputs (see Fig. 15.6), and therefore it is conceivable that a large variety of neurologic disorders can stimulate the secretion of AVP.

Although SIADH as typically described is associated with inappropriate secretion of AVP, hyponatremia has been described in two infants who met all the criteria for a diagnosis of SIADH but had undetectable AVP levels. Genetic analysis revealed a gain-of-function mutation at the X-linked AVP $V_2$ receptor, where in codon 137 a missense mutation resulted in the change from arginine to cysteine or leucine. The authors termed this "nephrogenic syndrome of inappropriate antidiuresis" (NSIAD).[381]

Zebra and colleagues have studied the osmoregulation of AVP secretion in a large group of patients with SIADH.[382] In the great majority, the plasma AVP concentration was inadequately suppressed relative to the hypotonicity present. In most patients, the plasma AVP concentration ranged from 1 to 10 pg/mL, the same range as in normally hydrated healthy adults. Inappropriate secretion, therefore, can often be demonstrated only by measuring AVP under hypotonic conditions. Even with this approach, however, abnormalities in plasma AVP were not apparent in almost 10% of patients with clinical evidence of SIADH. To define the nature of the osmoregulatory defect in these patients better, plasma AVP was measured during infusion of hypertonic saline. When this method of analysis was applied to 25 patients with SIADH, four different types of osmoregulatory defects were identified.

As shown in Fig. 15.18, infusion of hypertonic saline in the type A osmoregulatory defect was associated with large and erratic fluctuations in plasma AVP, which bore no relation to the rise in plasma osmolality. This pattern was found in 6 of 25 patients studied who had acute respiratory failure, bronchogenic carcinoma, pulmonary tuberculosis, schizophrenia, or rheumatoid arthritis. This pattern indicates that the secretion of AVP had been totally divorced from osmoreceptor control or was responding to some periodic nonosmotic stimulus.

A completely different type of osmoregulatory defect is exemplified by the type B response (see Fig. 15.18). The infusion of hypertonic saline resulted in prompt and progressive rises in plasma osmolality. Regression analyses have shown that the precision and sensitivity of this response are essentially

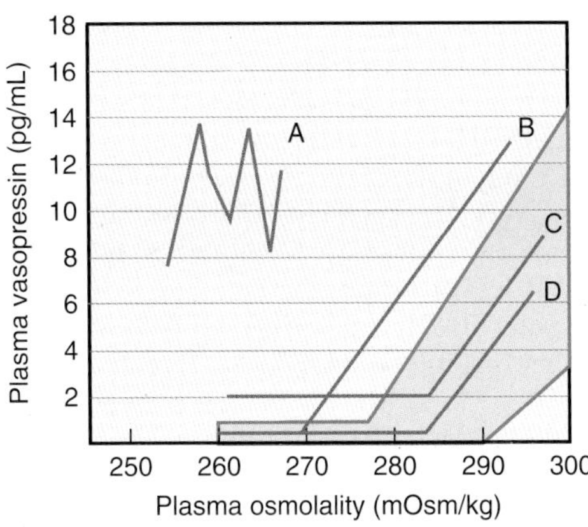


**Fig. 15.18** Plasma vasopressin as a function of plasma osmolality during the infusion of hypertonic saline in four groups of patients with the clinical syndrome of inappropriate antidiuretic hormone (SIADH). *Shaded area,* Range of normal values. See text for description of each group. (From Zerbe R, Stropes L, Robertson G: Vasopressin function in the syndrome of inappropriate antidiuresis. *Annu Rev Med.* 1980;31:315–327.)

the same as those in healthy subjects, except that the intercept or threshold value at 253 mOsm/kg is well below the normal range. This pattern, which reflects the resetting of the osmoreceptor, was found in 9 of 25 patients who had a diagnosis of bronchogenic carcinoma, cerebrovascular disease, tuberculous meningitis, acute respiratory disease, or carcinoma of the pharynx. Another patient was reported with hyponatremia and acute idiopathic polyneuritis who reacted in an identical manner to the hypertonic saline infusion and was determined to have had resetting of the osmoreceptor. Because their threshold function is retained when they receive a water load, this patient and others with reset osmostats have been able to dilute their urine maximally and sustain a urine flow sufficient to prevent a further increase in body water. Thus, an abnormality in AVP regulation can exist, in spite of the ability to dilute the urine maximally and excrete a water load at some lower level of plasma osmolality.

In the type C response (see Fig. 15.18), plasma AVP was elevated initially but did not change during the infusion of hypertonic saline until plasma osmolality reached the normal range. At that point, plasma AVP began to rise appropriately, indicating a normally functioning osmoreceptor mechanism. This response was found in 8 of 25 patients with the diagnosis of CNS disease, bronchogenic carcinoma, carcinoma of the pharynx, pulmonary tuberculosis, or schizophrenia. Its pathogenesis is unknown, but the authors speculated that it may be due to a constant, nonsuppressible leak of AVP, despite otherwise normal osmoregulatory function.[382] Unlike type B, the resetting type of defect, the type C response results in impaired urine dilution and water excretion at all levels of plasma osmolality.

In the type D response (see Fig. 15.18), the osmoregulation of AVP appears to be completely normal, despite a marked inability to excrete a water load. The plasma AVP is appropriately suppressed under hypotonic conditions and does not rise until plasma osmolality reaches the normal threshold level. When this procedure is reversed by water loading, plasma osmolality and plasma AVP again fall normally, but urine dilution does not occur, and the water load is not excreted. This defect was present in 2 of 25 patients diagnosed with bronchogenic carcinoma, indicating that in these patients, the antidiuretic defect is caused by some abnormality other than SIADH. It could be due to increased renal tubule sensitivity to AVP or the presence of an antidiuretic substance other than AVP. Alternatively, it is possible that currently available assays are not sensitive enough to detect significant levels of AVP. It is intriguing to speculate that some of these subjects have NSIAD, as described previously,[381] but only a small number of adult kindreds with this diagnosis have been described.[383]

It is of interest that patients with bronchogenic carcinoma, which was generally believed to be associated with ectopic production of AVP, manifest every category of osmoregulatory defect, including the reset osmostat. It has been suggested that many of these tumors probably cause SIADH secretion not by producing the hormone ectopically, but by interfering with the normal osmoregulation of AVP secretion from the neurohypophysis through direct invasion of the vagus nerve, metastatic implants in the hypothalamus, or some other more generalized neuropathic change.

## GLUCOCORTICOID DEFICIENCY

Considerable evidence exists for an important role for glucocorticoids in the abnormal water excretion of adrenal insufficiency.[384] The water excretory defect of anterior pituitary insufficiency, and particularly ACTH deficiency, is associated with elevated AVP levels[385,386] and corrected by physiologic doses of glucocorticoids. Similarly, adrenalectomized dogs receiving replacement of mineralocorticoids still have abnormal water excretion. The relative importance of intrarenal factors and AVP in defective water excretion has been a matter of controversy. Studies using a sensitive radioimmunoassay for plasma AVP and the Brattleboro rat with hypothalamic DI have provided evidence that both factors are involved. Support for a role for AVP has been obtained in studies of conscious adrenalectomized, mineralocorticoid-replaced dogs[387] and rats[388] and with the use of an inhibitor of the hydroosmotic effect of AVP.[308] Because the plasma AVP level was elevated despite a fall in plasma osmolality, the hormone's release was likely nonosmotically mediated. Although ECF volume was normal in both these studies, a decrease in systemic pressure and cardiac function[387,388] could have provided the hemodynamic stimulus for AVP release. In addition, there may be a direct effect of glucocorticoids that inhibits AVP secretion. In this regard, AVP gene expression is increased in glucocorticoid-deficient rats.[389] The presence of a glucocorticoid-responsive element on the AVP gene promoter may be responsible for the inhibition of AVP gene transcription by glucocorticoids.[390] Also, glucocorticoid receptors are present in magnocellular neurons and are increased during hypoosmolality.[391]

A role for AVP-independent intrarenal factors was defined in the antidiuretic-deficient, adrenalectomized Brattleboro rat[388] and with the use of AVP receptor antagonists.[308] It appears that prolonged glucocorticoid deficiency (14–17 days) is accompanied by decreases in renal hemodynamics that impair water excretion. A direct effect of glucocorticoid deficiency that enhances water permeability of the collecting duct has been proposed, but such a concept has not been supported by studies of anuran membranes, suggesting that glucocorticoids enhance rather than inhibit water transport. Also, in vitro perfusion studies of the collecting duct of adrenalectomized rabbits have shown an impaired rather than an enhanced AVP response,[392] a defect that may be related to enhanced cAMP metabolism.[393] AQP2 and AQP3 abundance appears not to be sensitive to glucocorticoids.[394]

In summary, the defect in glucocorticoid deficiency is primarily AVP-dependent, but an AVP-independent mechanism becomes evident with more prolonged hormone deficiency. It appears likely that alterations in systemic hemodynamics account for the nonosmotic release of AVP, but a direct effect of glucocorticoid hormone on AVP release has not been entirely excluded. The AVP-independent renal mechanism is probably caused by alterations in renal hemodynamics and not by a direct increase in collecting duct permeability. It should be remembered that secondary hypoadrenalism, as occurs in hypopituitarism, can also be associated with hyponatremia.[395,396]

## HYPOTHYROIDISM

Patients and experimental animals with hypothyroidism often have impaired water excretion and sometimes develop hyponatremia.[384,397] The dilution defect is reversed by treatment with thyroid hormone. Decreased delivery of filtrate to the diluting segment and persistent secretion of AVP, alone or in combination, have been proposed as mechanisms responsible for the defect.

Hypothyroidism has been shown to be associated with decreases in GFR and renal plasma flow.[397] In the AVP-deficient Brattleboro rat, the decrement in maximal free water excretion can be entirely accounted for by the decrease in GFR. The osmotic threshold for AVP release appears not to be altered in hypothyroidism.[398] The normal suppression of AVP release with water loading and the normal response to hypertonic saline,[399] coupled with the failure to observe upregulation of hypothalamic AVP gene expression in hypothyroid rats,[400] supports an AVP-independent mechanism. There is, however, also evidence for a role of AVP in impairing water excretion in hypothyroidism. In experimental animals[401] and humans with advanced hypothyroidism,[397] elevated AVP levels were measured in the basal state and after a water load. Although increased sensitivity to AVP in hypothyroidism has been proposed, experimental evidence has suggested the contrary because urine osmolality is relatively low for the circulating levels of the hormone,[401] and AVP-stimulated cyclase is impaired in the renal medulla of hypothyroid rats,[402] possibly leading to decreased AQP2 expression.[403] However, the predominant defect is one of water excretion with increased AQP2 expression and reversal with a $V_2$ receptor antagonist.[404] It appears, therefore, that diminished distal fluid delivery and persistent AVP release mediate the impaired water excretion in this disorder, but the relative contributions of these two factors remain undefined and may depend on the severity of the endocrine disorder.

## PRIMARY POLYDIPSIA

It has long been recognized that patients with psychiatric disease demonstrate increased water intake. Although such polydipsia is normally not associated with hyponatremia, it has been observed that these patients are at increased risk of developing hyponatremia when they are acutely psychotic.[405] Most of these patients have schizophrenia, but some have psychotic depression. The frequency of hyponatremia in this population of patients is unknown, but in a survey conducted in one large psychiatric hospital, 20 polydipsic patients with a serum [$Na^+$] lower than 124 mEq/L were reported,[406] and another survey found hyponatremia in 8 of 239 patients.[407] Elucidation of the mechanism of the impaired water excretion has been confounded by antipsychotic drug treatment (see later). The relative contributions of the pharmacologic agent and the psychosis are therefore difficult to define, because thiazides and carbamazepine are also frequently implicated.[408] Nonetheless, there have been reports of psychotic patients who suffered water intoxication, even when free of medication.[409]

The mechanism responsible for the hyponatremia in psychosis appears to be multifactorial. In a comprehensive study of water metabolism in eight psychotic hyponatremic patients and seven psychotic, normonatremic control subjects, no unifying defect emerged. The investigators found a small defect in osmoregulation that caused AVP to be secreted at plasma osmolalities somewhat lower than those of the control group, but they did not observe a true resetting of the osmostat. Also, the hyponatremic patients had a mild urine dilution defect, even in the absence of AVP. When AVP was present, the renal response was somewhat enhanced, suggesting increased renal sensitivity to the hormone. Psychotic exacerbations appear to be associated with increased AVP levels in schizophrenic patients with hyponatremia.[410] Finally, thirst perception is also increased, because excessive water intake that exceeds excretory capacity is responsible for most episodes of hyponatremia in these patients. However, concurrent nausea caused increased AVP levels in some of the subjects.[411] Although each of these derangements by itself would remain clinically unimportant, it is possible that during exacerbation of the psychosis the defects are more pronounced, and that in combination they can culminate in hyponatremia.[412]

Hyponatremia occurs in beer drinkers (so-called "beer potomania"). Although this has been ascribed to an increase in fluid intake in the setting of very low solute intake,[413] such patients may also have sustained significant solute losses.[414] A similar presentation can occur in patients who do not drink beer excessively, but have very low solute intake, either due to patient preference for a specific diet (e.g., ovolacto-vegetarian), poor appetite, or limited access to food ("tea and toast" diet).[293]

## POSTOPERATIVE HYPONATREMIA

The incidence of hospital-acquired hyponatremia is high in adults[214] and children[415] and is particularly prevalent in the postoperative stage[416,417] (incidence ≅ 4%). Most affected patients appear clinically euvolemic and have measurable levels of AVP in their circulation.[416,418] Although this occurs primarily as a consequence of administration of hypotonic fluids,[419] a decrease in serum [$Na^+$] can occur in this high-AVP state, even when isotonic fluids are given.[420] Hyponatremia has also been reported following cardiac catheterization in patients receiving hypotonic fluids.[421] Although the presence of hyponatremia is a marker for poor outcomes, this is likely a consequence not of the hyponatremia per se but of the severe underlying disease associated with it. There is, however, a subgroup of postoperative hyponatremic patients, almost always premenstrual women, who develop catastrophic neurologic events, frequently accompanied by seizures and hypoxia.[422,423]

## ENDURANCE EXERCISE

There has been increasing recognition that strenuous endurance exercise, such as military training[424] and marathons and triathlons,[369] can cause hyponatremia that is frequently symptomatic (often referred to as "exercise-associated hyponatremia"). A prospective study of 488 runners in the Boston Marathon revealed that 13% of the runners had a serum [$Na^+$] lower than 130 mEq/L. A multivariate analysis has revealed that weight gain, presumably related to excessive fluid intake, is the strongest single predictor of the hyponatremia. Longer racing times and a very low body mass index (BMI) were also predictors.[425] Composition of the fluids consumed and use of NSAIDs was not predictive. Symptomatic hyponatremia is even more frequent in ultraendurance events.[426] In addition to excessive intake of hypotonic fluids, patients with exercise-associated hyponatremia generally have inappropriately elevated AVP levels, suggesting that nonosmotic AVP secretion contributes to its pathogenesis.[427]

## PHARMACOLOGIC AGENTS

Many drugs have been associated with water retention. Some of the more clinically important agents are discussed here.

### Desmopressin

Because desmopressin is a selective agonist of the AVP $V_2$ receptors, it would be expected that patients treated with desmopressin are at increased risk of developing hyponatremia. The reported incidence in patients treated with desmopressin for DI is relatively low because they generally do not drink excessive amounts of fluid. However, a recent study has reported a 27% incidence of mild hyponatremia (131–134 mmol/L) and a 15% incidence of more severe hyponatremia (≤130 mmol/L) with long-term follow-up of patients with chronic CDI.[226] Patients who receive desmopressin at higher doses for indications such as von Willebrand disease,[428] or older patients with decreased renal function who receive desmopressin for nocturnal enuresis,[429,430] are also at risk to develop symptomatic hyponatremia.

### Chlorpropamide

The incidence of mild hyponatremia in patients taking chlorpropamide may be as high as 7%, but severe hyponatremia (<130 mEq/L) occurs in 2% of patients so treated.[431] As noted earlier, the drug exerts its action primarily by potentiating the renal action of AVP.[432] Studies of the toad urinary bladder have demonstrated that although chlorpropamide alone has no effect, it enhances AVP- and theophylline-stimulated water flow but decreases cAMP-mediated flow. The enhanced response may be due to the upregulation of AVP $V_2$ receptors.[433] Alternatively, studies of chlorpropamide-treated animals have suggested that the drug enhances solute reabsorption in the medullary ascending limb (thereby increasing interstitial tonicity and the osmotic drive for water reabsorption), rather than a cAMP- mediated alteration in collecting duct water permeability.[434]

### Antiepileptic Drugs

The anticonvulsant drug carbamazepine is well known to have antidiuretic properties. The incidence of hyponatremia in carbamazepine-treated patients was believed to be as high as 21%, but a survey of patients with mental retardation has reported a lower incidence of 5%.[435] Cases continue to be reported.[436] The antiepileptics oxcarbazepine and eslicarbazapine, both of the same class as carbamazepine, have been reported to cause hyponatremia at even higher rates than carbamazepine (43% and 33% vs. 16% incidences).[437] Evidence exists for a mechanism mediated by AVP secretion and for renal enhancement of the hormone's action[438] to explain carbamazepine's antidiuretic effect. The drug also appears to decrease the sensitivity of the AVP response to osmotic stimulation.[439]

### Psychotropic Drugs

An increasing number of psychotropic drugs have been associated with hyponatremia, and they are frequently implicated to explain the water intoxication in psychotic patients. Among the agents implicated are the phenothiazines, the butyrophenone haloperidol, and the tricyclic antidepressants.[440–442] An increasing number of cases of amphetamine (ecstasy)-related hyponatremia have been described.[443,444] Similarly, the widely used antidepressants fluoxetine,[445] sertraline,[446] and paroxetine[447] have been associated with hyponatremia. In this latter study, involving 75 patients, 12% developed hyponatremia (serum [$Na^+$] < 135 mmol/L). Older adults appear to be particularly susceptible, with an incidence as high as 22% to 28%.[448–451] The tendency for these drugs to cause hyponatremia is further compounded by their anticholinergic effects; by drying the mucous membranes, they can stimulate water intake. The role of these drugs in impaired water excretion has not, in most cases, been dissociated from the role of the underlying disorder for which the drug was given. Furthermore, evaluation of the effect of the drugs on AVP secretion has frequently revealed a failure to increase levels of the hormone, particularly if the mean arterial pressure remained unaltered. Therefore, although a clinical association between antipsychotic drugs and hyponatremia is frequently encountered, the pharmacologic agents themselves may not be the principal factors responsible for the water retention.

### Antineoplastic Drugs

Several drugs used in cancer therapy cause antidiuresis. The effect of vincristine may be mediated by the drug's neurotoxic effect on the hypothalamic microtubule system, which then alters normal osmoreceptor control of AVP release.[452] A retrospective survey has suggested that this may be more common in Asians who were given the drug.[453] Cyclophosphamide administration also causes hyponatremia. The mechanism of the diluting defect that results from cyclophosphamide is not fully understood. It may act, at least in part, to enhance action, because the drug does not increase hormone levels.[454] It is known that the antidiuresis has its onset 4 to 12 hours after injection of the drug, lasts as long as 12 hours, and seems to be temporally related to excretion of a metabolite. The importance of anticipating potentially severe hyponatremia in cyclophosphamide-treated patients who are vigorously hydrated to prevent urologic complications cannot be overstated. The synthetic analogue of cyclophosphamide, ifosfamide, has also been associated with hyponatremia and AVP secretion.[455]

### Narcotics

Since the 1940s, it has been known that the administration of opioid agonists, such as morphine, reduces urine flow by causing the release of an antidiuretic substance. The possibility that endogenous opioids could serve as potential neurotransmitters has been suggested by the finding of enkephalins in nerve fibers projecting from the hypothalamus to the neurohypophysis. However, the reported effects vary; they range from stimulation to no change and even to inhibition of AVP secretion. The reasons for these diverse observations may be that the opiates and their receptors are widely distributed in the brain, implying that the site of action of the opiate can differ markedly, depending on the route of administration. Also, there are multiple opiate peptides and receptor types. It has now been determined that agonists of μ-receptors have antidiuretic properties, whereas δ-receptors have the opposite effect.

### Miscellaneous Agents

Several case reports have suggested an association between the use of ACE inhibitors and hyponatremia.[456–458] Of interest is that all three reported patients were women in their 60s. The use of ACE inhibition was also a concomitant risk factor for the development of hyponatremia in a survey of veterans who received chlorpropamide.[431] However, given the widespread use of these agents, the true incidence of hyponatremia must be vanishingly low. Similarly, an association with angiotensin receptor blockers has not been reported to date. Rare patients have been reported to develop hyponatremia during amiodarone loading.[459] There have been increasing reports of hyponatremia associated with the use of tacrolimus, mostly in patients after organ transplantation.[460,461] This seems to be more frequent with tacrolimus than cyclosporin, suggesting that it is not a class effect of calcineurin inhibitors.[462,463]

## HYPONATREMIA: SYMPTOMS, MORBIDITY, AND MORTALITY

Symptoms of hyponatremia correlate with the degree of decrease in the serum [$Na^+$] and with the chronicity of the hyponatremia. Most clinical manifestations of hyponatremia usually begin at a serum [$Na^+$] lower than 130 mEq/L, but mild neurocognitive symptoms can begin at any sodium level that is low (Table 15.4). Although gastrointestinal complaints often occur early, most of the manifestations of hyponatremia are neurologic, including lethargy, confusion, disorientation, obtundation, and seizures, designated as "hyponatremic encephalopathy."[464] Many of the more marked symptoms of hyponatremic encephalopathy are caused by cerebral edema, which may, at least in part, be mediated by AQP4.[465] In its most severe form, the cerebral edema can lead to tentorial herniation; in such cases, death can occur as a result of brainstem compression with respiratory arrest. The cerebral edema can also cause a neurogenic pulmonary edema and hypoxemia,[466] which can in turn increase the severity of brain swelling.[467] The most severe life-threatening clinical features of hyponatremic encephalopathy are generally seen in cases of acute hyponatremia, currently defined as shorter than 48 hours in duration. A few acutely hyponatremic patients have been reported to develop rhabdomyolysis as well.[359]

The development of neurologic symptoms depends on the age, gender, and magnitude and acuteness of the process. Older persons and young children with hyponatremia are most likely to develop symptoms. Neurologic complications

**Table 15.4 Classification of Hyponatremia According to Severity of Presenting Symptoms**

| Severity | Serum Sodium Level | Neurologic Symptoms | Typical Duration of Hyponatremia |
|---|---|---|---|
| Severe | Generally <125 mmol/L | Vomiting, seizures, obtundation, respiratory distress, coma | Acute (<24–48 hours) |
| Moderate | Generally <130 mmol/L | Nausea, confusion, disorientation, altered mental status, unstable gait, falls | Intermediate or chronic (>24–48 hours) |
| Mild | <135 mmol/L | Headache, irritability, difficulty concentrating, altered mood, depression | Chronic (several days to many weeks or months) |

From Verbalis JG: Emergency management of acute and chronic hyponatremia. In Matfin G, ed. *Endocrine and metabolic emergencies,* Washington DC: Endocrine Press; 2014:352.

may occur more frequently in menstruating women. In a case-control study, Ayus and colleagues have noted that despite an approximately equal incidence of postoperative hyponatremia in males and females, 97% of those with permanent brain damage were women, and 75% of them were menstruating.[423] However, this view is not universally held, because others have not found increased postoperative hyponatremia in this population.[468]

The degree of clinical impairment is not as much related to the absolute measured level of lowered serum [$Na^+$] as it is to the rate and extent of the decrease in ECF osmolality. In a survey of hospitalized hyponatremic patients (serum [$Na^+$] < 128 mEq/L), 46% had CNS symptoms, and 54% were asymptomatic.[469] It is notable, however, that the authors thought that the hyponatremia was the cause of the symptoms in only 31% of the symptomatic patients. In this subgroup of symptomatic patients, the mortality was no different from that of asymptomatic patients (9%–10%). In contrast, the mortality of patients whose CNS symptoms were not caused by hyponatremia was high (64%), suggesting that the mortality of these patients is more often due to the associated comorbidity than to the electrolyte disorder itself. This is in agreement with an earlier study of Anderson,[279] which noted a 60-fold increase in mortality in hyponatremic patients over that of normonatremic control subjects. However, in the hyponatremic patients death frequently occurred after the plasma [$Na^+$] was returned to normal and was generally thought to be due to the progression of severe underlying disease. These studies suggested that hyponatremia is an indicator of severe underlying disease and poor prognosis rather than a cause of the observed increased mortality of such patients. In contrast to this point of view, a recent meta-analysis of studies in which some patients had correction of their hyponatremia indicated that improvement in serum [$Na^+$] was associated with a 50% reduction in mortality of the corrected groups compared with patients in whom the hyponatremia remained uncorrected, suggesting that hyponatremia may, in fact, be causally related to increased mortality.[470]

Other studies have further indicated that even mild hyponatremia is an independent predictor of higher mortality across a wide variety of disorders, including patients with acute ST-elevation myocardial infarction, heart failure, and liver disease.[471,472] A large study of more than 55,000 electronic heath records from a single Boston hospital has shown that the association of hyponatremia with inpatient mortality is significant across all levels of hyponatremia and even began at serum [$Na^+$] levels in the lower part of the normal range.[473] These findings were corroborated in studies of 249,000 Danish patients hospitalized over a 5-year period that showed increased 30-day and 1-year mortality associated with all levels of hyponatremia, including the range of 130 to 134.9 mmol/L,[474] and analyses of 2.3 million hospitalized patients enrolled in the Cerner Health Facts database.[475] The mortality associated with chronic hyponatremia is much less well studied, but results of the Rotterdam Longitudinal Aging Study noted significantly decreased survival of older patients with hyponatremia over a 12-year period of observation.[476]

The observed severe CNS symptoms are most likely related to the cellular swelling and cerebral edema that result from acute lowering of ECF osmolality, which leads to the movement of water into cells. In fact, such cerebral edema occasionally causes herniation, as has been noted in postmortem examinations of humans and experimental animals. The increase in brain water is, however, much less marked than would be predicted from the decrease in tonicity were the brain to operate as a passive osmometer. The volume regulatory responses that protect against cerebral edema, and which probably occur throughout the body, have been extensively studied and reviewed.[477] Studies of rats have demonstrated a prompt loss of solutes from cells, both electrolytes and organic osmolytes, after the onset of hyponatremia.[478] Some of the solute losses occur very quickly within 24 hours[479] and, in experimental animals, most of the brain solute loss is completed by 48 hours (Fig. 15.19).

The rate at which the brain restores the lost electrolytes and osmolytes when hyponatremia is corrected is also of pathophysiologic importance. $Na^+$, $K^+$, and $Cl^-$ recover quickly and even overshoot normal brain contents.[480] However, the reaccumulation of organic osmolytes is considerably delayed (see Fig. 15.19). This process is likely to account for the more marked cerebral dehydration that accompanies the correction in previously adapted animals,[481] which predisposes them to the development of myelinolysis as a result of disruption of the blood-brain barrier.[482,483] It has been observed that urea may prevent the myelinolysis associated with this pathology. This may be due to the more rapid reaccumulation of organic osmolytes, particularly inositol in the azotemic state,[484] and is consistent with a dearth of reports of the osmotic demyelination syndrome (OSD) in patients with chronic kidney disease, despite wide swings in serum [$Na^+$] during dialysis.

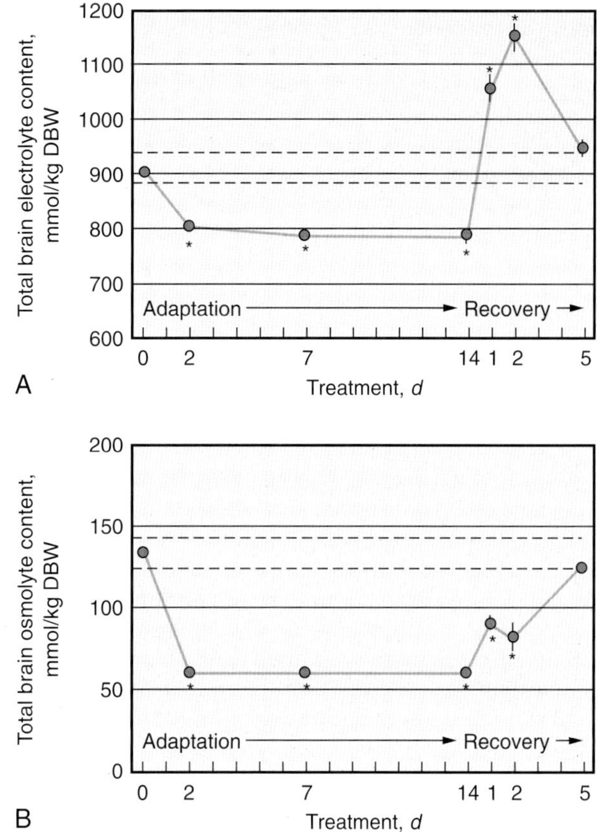


**Fig. 15.19** Comparison of changes in brain electrolyte (A) and organic osmolyte (B) content during adaptation to hyponatremia and after rapid correction of hyponatremia in rats. Electrolytes and organic osmolytes are lost quickly after the induction of hyponatremia, beginning on day (d) 0. The brain content of both solutes remains depressed during maintenance of hyponatremia from days 2 through 14. After rapid correction of the hyponatremia on day 14, electrolytes reaccumulate rapidly and overshoot normal brain contents on the first 2 days after correction, before returning to normal levels by the fifth day after correction. In contrast, brain organic osmolytes recover much more slowly and do not return to normal brain contents until the fifth day after correction. The *dashed lines* indicate ± SEM (standard error of mean) from the mean values of normonatremic rats on day 0; $P < .01$ compared with brain contents of normonatremic rats. *DBW,* Dry brain weight. (Data from Verbalis JG, Gullans SR: Hyponatremia causes large sustained reductions in brain content of multiple organic osmolytes in rats. *Brain Res.* 1991;567:274–282; and Verbalis JG, Gullans SR: Rapid correction of hyponatremia produces differential effects on brain osmolyte and electrolyte re-accumulation in rats. *Brain Res.* 1993;606:19–27.)

In contrast to acute hyponatremia, chronic hyponatremia is much less symptomatic. The reason for the profound differences between the symptoms of acute and chronic hyponatremia is now well understood to be caused by the process of brain volume regulation, described earlier.[485] Despite this powerful adaptation process, chronic hyponatremia is frequently associated with neurologic symptomatology, albeit milder and more subtle in nature (see Table 15.4). One report has found a fairly high incidence of symptoms in 223 patients with chronic hyponatremia as a result of thiazide administration—49% had malaise-lethargy, 47% had dizzy spells, 35% had vomiting, 17% had confusion-obtundation, 17% experienced falls, 6% had headaches, and 0.9% had seizures.[486] Although dizziness can potentially be attributed to a diuretic-induced hypovolemia, symptoms such as confusion, obtundation, and seizures are more consistent with hyponatremic symptomatology. Because thiazide-induced hyponatremia can be readily corrected by stopping the thiazide and/or administering sodium, this represents an ideal situation in which to assess improvement in hyponatremia symptomatology with normalization of the serum [Na$^+$]; in this study, all these symptoms improved with correction of the hyponatremia. This represents one of the best examples demonstrating reversal of the symptoms associated with chronic hyponatremia by correction of the hyponatremia because the patients in this study did not in general have severe underlying comorbidities that might complicate interpretation of their symptoms, as is often the case in patients with SIADH.

Even in patients adjudged to be "asymptomatic" by virtue of a normal neurologic examination, accumulating evidence has suggested that there may be previously unrecognized adverse effects as a result of chronic hyponatremia. In one study, 16 patients with hyponatremia secondary to SIADH, in the range of 124 to 130 mmol/L, demonstrated a significant gait instability that normalized after correction of the hyponatremia to a normal range.[487] The functional significance of the gait instability was illustrated in a study of 122 Belgian patients with a variety of levels of hyponatremia, all judged to be asymptomatic at the time of visiting an emergency department (ED). These patients were compared with 244 age-, gender-, and disease-matched controls also presenting to the ED during the same time period. Researchers found that 21% of the hyponatremic patients came to the ED because of a recent fall, compared with only 5% of the controls; this difference was highly significant and remained so after multivariable adjustment.[487] Analogous results were found in a study of admissions to a US hospital geriatric trauma unit over a 3-year period; when patients admitted because of a fall ($n = 1841$) were analyzed for risk factors associated with falls, the odds ratio for serum [Na$^+$] < 135 mmol/L was 1.81 ($P < .001$), which was greater than all other risk factors except age older than 85 years.[488] Consequently, these studies have clearly documented an increased incidence of falls in so-called asymptomatic hyponatremic patients. Recent studies in both experimental animals[489] and humans[490] have demonstrated decreases in nerve conduction associated with hyponatremia as a potential cause of gait disturbances.

The clinical significance of the gait instability and fall data have been indicated by multiple independent international studies that have demonstrated increased rates of bone fractures in patients with hyponatremia.[491–494] Other studies have shown that hyponatremia is associated with increased bone loss in experimental animals and with a significantly increased odds ratio for osteoporosis of the femoral neck in those older than 50 years in the Third National Health and Nutrition Examination Survey (NHANES III) database.[495] These findings have been corroborated by multiple epidemiologic studies that demonstrated decreased bone mineral density in human subjects.[496,497] In the largest epidemiologic analysis to date (2.9 million independent electronic health records), the odds ratios for osteoporosis and fractures were significantly greater for hyponatremia (3.99 and 3.05, respectively) than for any other diseases or medications associated with increased bone loss and fracture risk.[498] Of particular note, the odds ratios for both osteoporosis and fractures were the highest in patients with chronic persistent hyponatremia, indicating that the duration of hyponatremia represents an important risk factor for bone disease and fractures.[498] These findings were supported by a subsequent clinical study of hip fractures in Argentina.[499]

Recent studies of a cohort of 5435 community-dwelling men older than 65 years of age in the in the United States have found that hyponatremia is independently associated with greater cognitive impairment and cognitive decline in this population,[500] and a retrospective study of 4900 hyponatremic patient in Taiwan has found that the hyponatremic patients have a 2.36-fold higher hazard ratio of developing dementias compared with matched controls, which increased to a hazard ratio of 4.29 for patients with more severe hyponatremia. Thus, the major clinical significance of chronic hyponatremia may lie in the increased morbidity and mortality associated with falls, fractures, neurocognitive impairments, and dementias in our older population, as well as potential adverse effects not yet studied in humans.[501]

## HYPONATREMIA TREATMENT

Correction of hyponatremia is associated with markedly improved neurologic outcomes in patients with severely symptomatic hyponatremia. In a retrospective review of patients who presented with severe neurologic symptoms and a serum [$Na^+$] lower than 125 mmol/L, prompt therapy with isotonic or hypertonic saline resulted in a correction of approximately 20 mEq/L over several days and neurologic recovery in almost all cases. In contrast, in patients who were treated with fluid restriction alone, there was very little correction over the study period (<5 mEq/L over 72 hours), and the neurologic outcomes were much worse, with most of these patients dying or entering a persistent vegetative state.[502] Consequently, based on this and many similar retrospective analyses, prompt therapy to increase the serum [$Na^+$] rapidly represents the standard of care for treatment of patients presenting with severe life-threatening symptoms of hyponatremia.

Brain herniation, the most dreaded complication of hyponatremia, is seen almost exclusively in patients with acute hyponatremia (usually <24 hours) or in patients with intracranial pathology.[503–505] In postoperative patients, and in patients with self-induced water intoxication associated with marathon running, psychosis, or use of ecstasy (3,4-methylenedioxymethamphetamine [MDMA]), nonspecific symptoms such as headache, nausea and vomiting, or confusion can rapidly progress to seizures, respiratory arrest, and ultimately death or to a permanent vegetative state as a complication of severe cerebral edema.[506] Hypoxia from noncardiogenic pulmonary edema and/or hypoventilation can exacerbate brain swelling caused by the low serum [$Na^+$].[466,467] Seizures can complicate severe chronic hyponatremia and acute hyponatremia. Although usually self-limited, hyponatremic seizures may be refractory to anticonvulsants.

As discussed earlier, chronic hyponatremia is much less symptomatic as a result of the process of brain volume regulation. Because of this adaptation process, chronic hyponatremia is arguably a condition that clinicians think they may not need to be as concerned about, which has been reinforced by common usage of the descriptor "asymptomatic hyponatremia" for many of these patients. However, as noted, it is clear that many such patients very often do have neurologic symptoms, even if milder and more subtle in nature, including headaches, nausea, mood disturbances, depression, difficulty concentrating, slowed reaction times, unstable gait, increased falls, confusion, and disorientation.[487] Consequently, all patients with hyponatremia who manifest any neurologic symptoms that could possibly be related to the hyponatremia should be considered as candidates for treatment, regardless of the chronicity of the hyponatremia or the level of serum [$Na^+$]. An additional reason for treating even asymptomatic hyponatremia effectively is to prevent a lowering of the serum [$Na^+$] to more symptomatic and dangerous levels during treatment of underlying conditions (e.g., increased fluid administration via parenteral nutrition, treatment of heart failure with loop diuretics).

### CURRENT THERAPIES

Conventional management strategies for hyponatremia range from saline infusion and fluid restriction to pharmacologic measures to adjust fluid balance. Although there are many available treatments for hyponatremia, some are not appropriate for the correction of symptomatic hyponatremia because they work too slowly or inconsistently to be effective in hospitalized patients (e.g., demeclocycline, mineralocorticoids). Consideration of treatment options should always include an evaluation of the benefits and potential toxicities of any therapy and must be individualized for each patient.[507] It should always be remembered that sometimes simply stopping treatment with an agent associated with hyponatremia is sufficient to correct a low serum [$Na^+$], which is especially true for thiazide-induced hyponatremia.[508]

#### HYPERTONIC SALINE

Acute hyponatremia presenting with severe neurologic symptoms is life-threatening and should be treated promptly with hypertonic solutions, typically 3% NaCl ([$Na^+$] = 513 mmol/L), because this represents the most reliable method to raise the serum [$Na^+$] quickly. A continuous infusion of hypertonic NaCl is generally used in inpatient settings. Various formulas have been suggested for calculating the initial rate of infusion of hypertonic solutions,[503] but there has been no consensus regarding optimal infusion rates of 3% NaCl. One of the simplest methods to estimate an initial 3% NaCl infusion rate uses the following relationship[507]:

$$\text{Patient's weight (in kg)} \times \text{desired correction rate (in mEq/L/h)} = \text{infusion rate of 3\% NaCl (in mL/h)}$$

This may not achieve the desired correction rate, but frequent monitoring of the serum [$Na^+$] will inform the clinician about whether the rate should be increased or decreased, similar to using the measurement of the serum glucose level to guide the infusion rate of insulin drips. Depending on individual hospital policies, the administration of a hypertonic solution may require special considerations (e.g., placement in the intensive care unit [ICU], sign-off by a consultant), which each clinician needs to be aware of to optimize patient care. One barrier to the use of hypertonic saline that appears to be overstated and unfounded is the frequent requirement for a central intravenous catheter for chronic infusion. A recent study has demonstrated a low rate of complications using peripheral infusions of 3% NaCl (6% infiltration and 3% thrombophlebitis) and concluded that the peripheral administration of 3% NaCl carries a low risk of minor, nonlimb, or life-threatening complications.[509]

An alternative option for more emergent situations is the administration of a 100-mL bolus of 3% NaCl, repeated once if there is no clinical improvement in 30 minutes. This was recommended by a consensus conference organized to develop guidelines for the prevention and treatment of exercise-induced hyponatremia, an acute and potentially lethal condition,[510] and adopted as a general recommendation by an expert panel.[511] Injecting this amount of hypertonic saline intravenously raises the serum [Na$^+$] by an average of 2 to 4 mmol/L, which is well below the recommended maximal daily rate of change of 10 to 12 mmol/24 hours or 18 mmol/48 hours.[512] Because the brain can only accommodate an average increase of approximately 8% to 10% in brain volume before herniation occurs, quickly increasing the serum [Na$^+$] by as little as 2 to 4 mmol/L in acute hyponatremia can effectively reduce brain swelling and intracranial pressure.[513]

## ISOTONIC SALINE

The treatment of choice for depletional hyponatremia (hypovolemic hyponatremia) is isotonic saline ([Na$^+$] = 154 mmol/L) to restore ECF volume and ensure adequate organ perfusion. This initial therapy is appropriate for patients who have clinical signs of hypovolemia or in whom a spot urine [Na$^+$] is lower than 20 to 30 mEq/L.[511] However, this therapy is usually ineffective for dilutional hyponatremias such as SIADH,[514] and continued inappropriate administration of isotonic saline to a euvolemic patient may worsen the hyponatremia[515] and/or cause fluid overload. Although isotonic saline may improve the serum [Na$^+$] in some patients with hypervolemic hyponatremia, their volume status will generally worsen with this therapy, so unless the hyponatremia is profound, isotonic saline should be avoided.

## FLUID RESTRICTION

For patients with chronic hyponatremia, fluid restriction has been the most popular and most widely accepted treatment. When SIADH is present, fluids should generally be limited to 500 to 1000 mL/24 hours. Because fluid restriction increases the serum [Na$^+$] largely by underreplacing the excretion of fluid by the kidneys, some have advocated an initial restriction to 500 mL less than the 24-hour urine output.[516] When instituting a fluid restriction, it is important for the nursing staff and patient to understand that this includes all fluids that are consumed, not just water (Box 15.4). Generally, the water content of ingested food is not included in the restriction because this is balanced by insensible water losses (e.g., perspiration, exhaled air, feces), but caution should be exercised with foods that have a high fluid concentration (e.g., fruits, soups). Restricting fluid intake can be effective when properly applied and managed in select patients, but the serum [Na$^+$] is generally increased only slowly (1–2 mmol/L/day), even with severe fluid restriction.[514] In addition, this therapy is often poorly tolerated because of an associated increase in thirst, leading to poor compliance with long-term therapy. However, it is economically favorable, and some patients do respond well to this option.

### Box 15.4 General Recommendations for Using Fluid Restriction and Predictors of Its Increased Likelihood of Failure

**General Recommendations**

- Restrict all intake that is consumed by drinking, not just water.
- Aim for a fluid restriction that is 500 mL/day below the 24-hour urine volume.
- Do not restrict sodium or protein intake unless indicated.

**Predictors of Likely Failure of Fluid Restriction**

- High urine osmolality (>500 mOsm/kg $H_2O$)
- Sum of urine Na$^+$ and K$^+$ concentrations exceeds serum Na$^+$ concentration
- 24-hour urine volume < 1500 mL/day
- Increase in serum Na$^+$ sodium concentration < 2 mmol/L/day in 24 hours on fluid restriction ≤ 1 L/day

From Verbalis JG, Goldsmith SR, Greenberg A, et al: Diagnosis, evaluation, and treatment of hyponatremia: expert panel recommendations. *Am J Med.* 2013;126(Suppl 1):S1–S42.

Fluid restriction should not be used with hypovolemic patients and is particularly difficult to maintain in hospitalized patients with very elevated urine osmolalities secondary to high AVP levels (e.g., >500 mOsm/kg $H_2O$) because urine solute-free water excretion is very low. Also, if the sum of the urine Na$^+$ and K$^+$ concentrations exceeds the serum [Na$^+$], most patients will not respond to a fluid restriction because an electrolyte-free water clearance will be difficult to achieve.[292,517,518] These and other predictors of failure of fluid restriction have been confirmed in clinical studies[519–521] and are summarized in Box 15.4. The presence of any of these factors in hospitalized patients with symptomatic hyponatremia makes this less than ideal as an initial therapy. In addition, fluid restriction is not practical for some patients, particularly patients in an ICU setting who often require the administration of significant volumes of fluids as part of their therapy. Consequently, such patients are candidates for more effective pharmacologic or saline treatment strategies.

## ARGININE VASOPRESSIN RECEPTOR ANTAGONISTS

Conventional therapies for hyponatremia, although effective in specific circumstances, are suboptimal for many different reasons, including variable efficacy, slow responses, intolerable side effects, and serious toxicities. However, perhaps the most striking deficiency of most conventional therapies is that most of these therapies do not directly target the underlying cause of most dilutional hyponatremias—namely, inappropriately elevated plasma AVP levels. A newer class of pharmacologic agents, vasopressin receptor antagonists, also known as vaptans, which directly block AVP-mediated receptor activation, have been approved for the treatment of euvolemic hyponatremia (in the United States and European Union) and hypervolemic hyponatremia (in the United States).[522]

Conivaptan has been approved by the US Food and Drug Administration (FDA) for euvolemic and hypervolemic hyponatremia in hospitalized patients. It is available only as

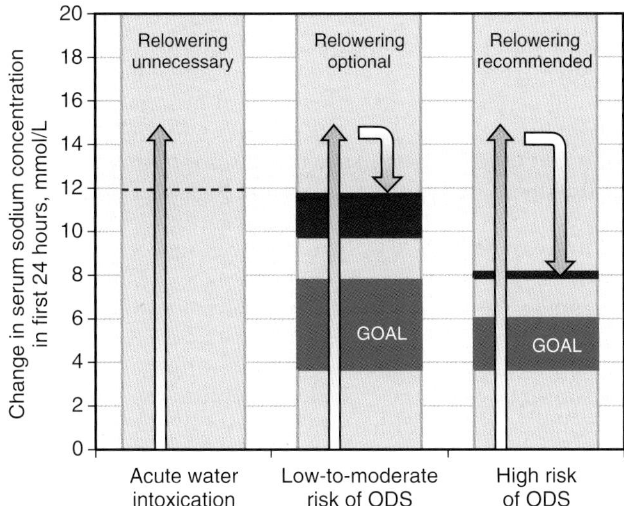


**Fig. 15.20** Recommended goals *(green)* and limits *(red)* for correction of hyponatremia based on the risk of producing osmotic demyelination syndrome (ODS). Also shown are recommendations for relowering of the serum [Na$^+$] to goals for patients presenting with serum [Na$^+$] < 120 mmol/L who exceed the recommended limits of correction in the first 24 hours. (From Verbalis JG, Goldsmith SR, Greenberg A, et al: Diagnosis, evaluation, and treatment of hyponatremia: expert panel recommendations. *Am J Med.* 2013;126(Suppl 1):S1–S42.)

an intravenous preparation and is given as a 20-mg loading dose over 30 minutes, followed by a continuous infusion of 20 or 40 mg/day.[523] Generally, the 20-mg continuous infusion is used for the first 24 hours to gauge the initial response. If the correction of serum [Na$^+$] is thought to be inadequate (e.g., <5 mmol/L), the infusion rate can be increased to 40 mg/day. Some clinical studies have supported the efficacy of bolus infusions of conivaptan rather than continuous infusions.[524] Therapy is limited to a maximum duration of 4 days because of drug interaction effects with other agents metabolized by the CYP3A4 hepatic isoenzyme.

Importantly, for conivaptan and all other vaptans, it is critical that the serum [Na$^+$] be measured frequently during the active phase of correction of the hyponatremia, a minimum of every 6 to 8 hours for conivaptan but more frequently in patients with risk factors for OSD.[507] If the correction exceeds 10 to 12 mmol/L in the first 24 hours, the infusion should be stopped and the patient monitored closely. Consideration should be given to administering sufficient water, orally or as intravenous 5% dextrose in water, to avoid a correction of more than 12 mmol/L/day. The maximum correction limit should be reduced to 8 mmol/L over the first 24 hours in patients with risk factors for ODS[511] (Fig. 15.20; Box 15.5). The most common side effects of conivaptan include headache, thirst, and hypokalemia.[525,526]

Tolvaptan, an oral vasopressin receptor antagonist, is also FDA-approved for the treatment of euvolemic and hypervolemic hyponatremia. In contrast to conivaptan, the availability of tolvaptan in tablet form allows short- and long-term use.[527] Similar to conivaptan, tolvaptan treatment must be initiated in the hospital so that the rate of correction can be monitored carefully. In the United States, patients with a serum [Na$^+$] lower than 125 mmol/L are eligible for therapy with tolvaptan as primary therapy; if the serum [Na$^+$] is 125 mmol/L or higher, tolvaptan therapy is only indicated if the patient has symptoms that could be attributable to the hyponatremia, and the patient is resistant to attempts at fluid restriction.[528] In the European Union, tolvaptan is approved only for the treatment of euvolemic hyponatremia, but any symptomatic euvolemic patient is eligible for tolvaptan therapy, regardless of the level of hyponatremia or response to previous fluid restriction. The starting dose of tolvaptan is 15 mg on the first day although, in clinical practice, some clinicians recommend starting with a lower dose of 7.5 mg,[529] and the dose can be titrated to 30 and 60 mg at 24-hour intervals if the serum [Na$^+$] remains lower than 135 mmol/L or the increase in serum [Na$^+$] has been less than 5 mmol/L in the previous 24 hours. As with conivaptan, it is essential that the serum [Na$^+$] be measured frequently during the active phase of correction of the hyponatremia at a minimum of every 6 to 8 hours, particularly in patients with risk factors for ODS. Goals and limits for the safe correction of hyponatremia and methods to compensate for overly rapid corrections are the same as described previously for conivaptan (see Fig. 15.20). One additional factor that helps avoid overly rapid correction with tolvaptan is the recommendation that fluid restriction not be used during the active phase of correction, thereby allowing the patient's thirst to compensate for an overly vigorous aquaresis. Common side effects of tolvaptan include dry mouth, thirst, increased urinary frequency, dizziness, nausea, and orthostatic hypotension.[527,528]

Vaptans are not needed for the treatment of hypovolemic hyponatremia because simple volume expansion would be expected to abolish the nonosmotic stimulus to AVP secretion and lead to a prompt aquaresis. Furthermore, inducing increased renal fluid excretion via diuresis or aquaresis can cause or worsen hypotension in these patients. This possibility has resulted in the labeling of these drugs as contraindicated for hypovolemic hyponatremia.[507] Importantly, clinically significant hypotension was not observed in the conivaptan or tolvaptan clinical trials in euvolemic and hypervolemic hyponatremic patients. Although vaptans are not contraindicated with decreased renal function, these agents generally will not be effective if the serum creatinine level is more than 3.0 mg/dL.

**Box 15.5 Factors Increasing Risk of Osmotic Demyelination Syndrome[a]**

- Serum sodium concentration ≤ 105 mmol/L
- Hypokalemia[b]
- Alcoholism[b]
- Malnutrition[b]
- Advanced liver disease[b]

[a]Requiring slower correction of chronic hyponatremia.
[b]Unlike the rate of increase in serum [Na$^+$], neither the precise level of the serum potassium concentration nor the degree of alcoholism, malnutrition, or liver disease that alters the brain's tolerance to an acute osmotic stress have been rigorously defined.

From Verbalis JG, Goldsmith SR, Greenberg A, et al: Diagnosis, evaluation, and treatment of hyponatremia: expert panel recommendations. *Am J Med.* 2013;126(Suppl 1):S1–S42.

The FDA has issued a caution about hepatic injury[530] that was noted in patients who received tolvaptan in a 3-year clinical trial examining the effect of tolvaptan on autosomal dominant polycystic kidney disease, the Tolvaptan Efficacy and Safety in Management of Autosomal Dominant Polycystic Kidney Disease and Its Outcomes (TEMPO) study.[531] An external panel of liver experts found that three cases of reversible jaundice and increased transaminase levels in this trial were probably or highly likely caused by tolvaptan. Additionally, 4.4% of autosomal dominant polycystic kidney disease (ADPKD) patients on tolvaptan (42 of 958) exhibited elevations of alanine aminotransferase (ALT) levels more than three times that of the upper limit of normal (ULN) compared with 1.0% of patients (5 of 484) on placebo.

These findings indicate that tolvaptan has the potential to cause irreversible and potentially fatal liver injury. The doses used in the TEMPO study were up to twice the maximum dose approved for hyponatremia (tolvaptan, 120 mg/day). Also, in clinical trials of tolvaptan at doses approved by the FDA for treatment of clinically significant euvolemic or hypervolemic hyponatremia, liver damage was not reported, including long-term trials longer than 30 days (e.g., SALT-WATER, EVEREST [Efficacy of Vasopressin Antagonism in Heart Failure: Outcome Study with Tolvaptan]).[532,533] Of note, meta-analyses of studies involving vasopressin antagonist use for the treatment of hyponatremia have confirmed increased drug-related adverse events, including rapid sodium level correction, constipation, dry mouth, thirst, and phlebitis in vasopressin antagonist-treated patients, but found no differences in the total number of AEs, discontinuations due to AEs, serious AEs, death, headache, hypotension, nausea, anemia, hypernatremia, urinary tract infection, renal failure, pyrexia, upper gastrointestinal bleeding, diarrhea, vomiting, peripheral edema, and dizziness between the vasopressin antagonist-treated and control groups.[534]

Based largely on the hepatic injury noted in the TEMPO trial, the FDA, on April 30, 2013, recommended that "Samsca [tolvaptan] treatment should be stopped if the patient develops signs of liver disease. Treatment duration should be limited to 30 days or less, and use should be avoided in patients with underlying liver disease, including cirrhosis."[530] The European Medicines Agency (EMA) has approved the use of tolvaptan for SIADH but not for hyponatremia due to heart failure or cirrhosis. Based on the TEMPO trial results, the EMA also issued a warning about the possible occurrence of hepatic injury in patients treated with tolvaptan, but did not recommend any restrictions on the duration of treatment of SIADH patients with tolvaptan.[535]

Accordingly, appropriate caution should be exercised in patients treated with tolvaptan for hyponatremia for extended periods (e.g., >30 days), but this decision should be based on the clinical judgment of the treating physician. Patients who are refractory to or unable to tolerate or obtain other therapies for hyponatremia, and for whom the benefits of tolvaptan treatment outweigh the risks, remain candidates for long-term therapy with tolvaptan. In these patients, liver function tests should be monitored carefully and serially (i.e., every 3 months) and the drug discontinued in the event of significant changes in liver function test results (i.e., twice the ULN of ALT).[510] With rare exceptions, tolvaptan should not be used for patients with underlying liver disease, given the difficulty of attributing causation to any observed deterioration of hepatic function. Such an exception may be hyponatremic patients with end-stage liver disease awaiting imminent liver transplantation who are at little risk of added hepatic injury and will benefit from the correction of hyponatremia prior to surgery to decrease the risk of ODS postoperatively.[536]

An additional barrier to the use of vasopressin antagonists for treatment of hyponatremia is the high cost of the drug. This is true in the United States and European Union, but not in Asian countries. Despite this pronounced geographic disparity, many economic analyses have confirmed the increased economic burden of hyponatremia, which is largely driven by longer hospital and ICU stays.[537,538] An economic analysis of use of tolvaptan compared with fluid restriction has shown favorable cost savings that offset the high cost of tolvaptan, suggesting that selective use of these agents in appropriate inpatients may, in fact, be cost-effective.[539]

## UREA

Urea has been described as an alternative oral treatment for SIADH and other hyponatremic disorders. The mode of action is to correct hypoosmolality not only by increasing solute-free water excretion but also by decreasing urinary sodium excretion. Dosages of 15 to 60 g/day are generally effective; the dose can be titrated in increments of 15 g/day at weekly intervals as necessary to achieve normalization of the serum [$Na^+$]. It is advisable to dissolve the urea in orange juice or some other strongly flavored liquid to camouflage the bitter taste. Even if completely normal water balance is not achieved, it is often possible to allow the patient to maintain a less strict regimen of fluid restriction while receiving urea. The disadvantages associated with the use of urea include poor palatability (although some clinicians believe that this has been exaggerated), the development of azotemia at higher doses, and the unavailability until recently of a convenient or FDA-approved form of the agent. Evidence has suggested that blood urea concentrations may double during treatment,[540] but it is important to remember that this does not represent renal impairment. There is now a product available in the United States (Ure-Na) that has been approved by the FDA as a medical food for the management of euvolemic and hypervolemic hyponatremia.

Reports from retrospective uncontrolled studies have suggested that the use of urea has been effective in treating SIADH in patients with hyponatremia due to subarachnoid hemorrhage and in critical care patients,[541] and case reports have documented success in infants with chronic SIADH[542] and NSIAD.[543] Evidence from a short study in a small cohort of SIADH patients has suggested that urea may have a comparable efficacy to vaptans in reversing hyponatremia due to chronic SIADH.[544] Although these reports suggest that urea might be an acceptable alternative for treatment of chronic hyponatremia, data regarding the efficacy and safety of long-term urea treatment of hyponatremia are lacking at this time.[545]

In patients with hyponatremia caused or exacerbated by low protein ingestion, increasing dietary protein intake may have a similar effect as urea and improve the serum sodium concentration.[293]

## FUROSEMIDE AND NACL

The use of furosemide (20 to 40 mg/day), coupled with a high salt intake (e.g., 200 mEq/day, often administered as salt tablets), which represents an extension of the treatment of acute symptomatic hyponatremia[546] to the chronic management of euvolemic hyponatremia, has also been reported to be successful in select cases.[547] However, the efficacy of this approach to correct symptomatic hyponatremia promptly and within accepted goals limits (see Fig. 15.20) is unknown.

## EFFICACY OF DIFFERENT TREATMENTS FOR HYPONATREMIA DUE TO SYNDROME OF INAPPROPRIATE ANTIDIURETIC HORMONE SECRETION

There have been no adequately powered, randomized controlled trials to compare the efficacy and safety of different treatments used to correct hyponatremia. However, results of a prospective observational study in a large number of hospitalized patients in the United States and European Union have provided useful data about the success rates of different therapies when used as monotherapy in patients with SIADH (Table 15.5).[519,548] In this study, "success" was defined by three different criteria: (1) the least stringent was an increase in serum [$Na^+$] of at least 5 mmol/L; (2) the next was correction to a serum [$Na^+$] of 130 mmol/L or higher; and (3) the most stringent was correction to a normal serum [$Na^+$] of 135 mmol/L or higher. As seen in Table 15.5, only 3% NaCl and tolvaptan had success rates significantly higher than 50% for the least stringent criterion, and only tolvaptan achieved this level for the next most stringent criteria and a significantly higher rate for the most stringent criteria of normalization of the serum [$Na^+$]. Of particular note, fluid restriction alone, the most frequently prescribed therapy in the Hyponatremia Registry patients, achieved a correction of serum [$Na^+$] in only 44% of patients treated with this therapy and isotonic saline in only 36% of patients. These data underscore the importance of carefully selecting therapy for individual patients to meet predefined goals for the correction of serum [$Na^+$].

**Table 15.5 Efficacy of Different Treatments Used as Monotherapy for Syndrome of Inappropriate Antidiuretic Hormone Secretion From the Hyponatremia Registry (%)**

| Treatment | δ [$Na^+$] ≥ 5 mmol/L | [$Na^+$] ≥ 130 mmol/L | [$Na^+$] ≥ 135 mmol/L |
|---|---|---|---|
| No treatment (*n* = 168) | 41 | 45 | 20 |
| Fluid restriction (*n* = 625) | 44 | 29 | 10 |
| Isotonic saline (*n* = 384) | 36 | 20 | 4 |
| Tolvaptan (*n* = 183) | 78 | 74 | 40 |
| 3% NaCl (*n* =78) | 60 | 25 | 13 |

From Verbalis JG, et al: Diagnosing and treating the syndrome of inappropriate antidiuretic hormone secretion. *Am J Med.* 2016;129:537.e9–537.e23.

## HYPONATREMIA TREATMENT GUIDELINES

Although many authors have published recommendations on the treatment of hyponatremia,[503,505,507,511,549–553] no standardized treatment algorithms have yet been universally accepted, and there are still some major differences between the various guidelines and expert recommendations.[554,555] For almost all treatment recommendations, the initial evaluation includes an assessment of the ECF volume status of the patient because treatment recommendations differ for hypovolemic, euvolemic, and hypervolemic hyponatremic patients. Recommendations for hypovolemic and hypervolemic patients have been updated rather recently.[511] Euvolemic patients, mainly including those with SIADH, represent a unique challenge because of the multiplicity of causes and presentations of patients with SIADH. A synthesis of recommendations for the treatment of hyponatremia is illustrated in Fig. 15.21. This algorithm is based primarily on the neurologic symptomatology of hyponatremic patients rather than the serum [$Na^+$] or the chronicity of the hyponatremia, because the latter is often difficult to ascertain accurately.

### LEVELS OF SYMPTOMS

A careful neurologic history and assessment should always be done to identify potential causes for the patient's symptoms other than hyponatremia. However, it will not always be possible to exclude an additive contribution from the hyponatremia to an underlying neurologic condition. In this algorithm, patients are divided into three major groups based on their presenting symptoms (see Table 15.4).

#### Severe Symptoms

Coma, obtundation, seizures, respiratory distress or arrest, and unexplained vomiting usually imply a more acute onset or worsening of hyponatremia that requires immediate active treatment. Therapies that will quickly raise the serum [$Na^+$] are necessary to reduce cerebral edema and decrease the risk of potentially fatal brain herniation.

#### Moderate Symptoms

Altered mental status, disorientation, confusion, unexplained nausea, gait instability, and falls generally indicate some degree of brain volume regulation and absence of clinically significant cerebral edema. These symptoms can be chronic or acute, but allow more time to elaborate a deliberate approach to the choice of therapies.

#### Mild or Absent Symptoms

Minimal symptoms, such as difficulty concentrating, irritability, altered mood, depression, or unexplained headache, or a virtual absence of discernible symptoms, indicate that the patient may have chronic or slowly evolving hyponatremia. These symptoms necessitate a cautious approach, especially when patients have underlying comorbidities, to prevent worsening of the hyponatremia and overly rapid correction with the production of ODS.

Patients with severe neurologic symptoms should be treated with hypertonic (3%) NaCl as first-line therapy, followed after 24 to 48 hours by fluid restriction and/or vaptan therapy. Because overly rapid correction of the serum [$Na^+$] occurs in more than 10% of patients treated with hypertonic NaCl,[556] such patients are at risk for ODS unless carefully monitored.

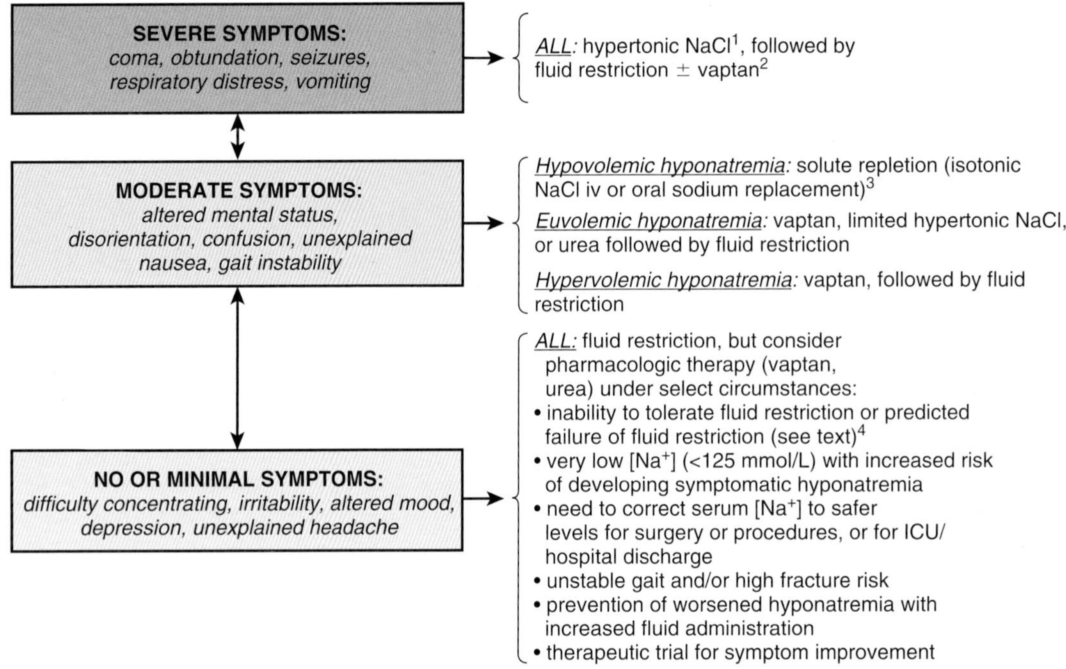

SEVERE SYMPTOMS:
coma, obtundation, seizures, respiratory distress, vomiting
ALL: hypertonic NaCl1, followed by fluid restriction ± vaptan2
MODERATE SYMPTOMS:
altered mental status, disorientation, confusion, unexplained nausea, gait instability
Hypovolemic hyponatremia: solute repletion (isotonic NaCl iv or oral sodium replacement)3
Euvolemic hyponatremia: vaptan, limited hypertonic NaCl, or urea followed by fluid restriction
Hypervolemic hyponatremia: vaptan, followed by fluid restriction
NO OR MINIMAL SYMPTOMS:
difficulty concentrating, irritability, altered mood, depression, unexplained headache
ALL: fluid restriction, but consider pharmacologic therapy (vaptan, urea) under select circumstances:
• inability to tolerate fluid restriction or predicted failure of fluid restriction (see text)4
• very low [Na+] (<125 mmol/L) with increased risk of developing symptomatic hyponatremia
• need to correct serum [Na+] to safer levels for surgery or procedures, or for ICU/ hospital discharge
• unstable gait and/or high fracture risk
• prevention of worsened hyponatremia with increased fluid administration
• therapeutic trial for symptom improvement


1. Some authors recommend simultaneous treatment with desmopressin to limit speed of correction.
2. No active therapy should be started within 24 hours of hypertonic saline to decrease the risk of overly rapid correction of [$Na^+$] and risk of ODS.
3. With isotonic NaCl infusion, serum [$Na^+$] must be followed closely to prevent overly rapid correction and risk of ODS due to secondary water diuresis.

**Fig. 15.21** Algorithm for the treatment of patients with euvolemic hyponatremia based on their presenting symptoms. The *arrows* between the symptom boxes indicate movement of patients between different symptom levels. *ALL,* All types of hypotonic hyponatremia; *ICU,* intensive care unit; *iv,* intravenous; *ODS,* osmotic demyelination syndrome. (Modified from Verbalis JG: Emergency management of acute and chronic hyponatremia. In Matfin G, ed. *Endocrine and Metabolic Emergencies.* Washington, DC: Endocrine Press; 2014:359.)

For this reason, some authors have proposed simultaneous treatment with desmopressin to reduce the rate of correction to only that produced by the hypertonic NaCl infusion itself.[557,558] Whether sufficient clinical data eventually prove that this approach is effective and safe in larger numbers of patients remains to be determined.[559,560] Only one case of ODS has been reported in a patient receiving vaptan monotherapy,[561] and two abstracts have reported ODS when vaptans were used directly following hypertonic saline administration within the same 24-hour period.[511] Consequently, no additional active hyponatremia therapy should be administered until at least 24 hours following successful increases in the serum [$Na^+$] using hypertonic NaCl.

The choice of treatment for patients with moderate symptoms will depend on their ECF volume status (see Fig. 15.21). Hypovolemic patients should be treated with solute repletion via isotonic NaCl infusion or oral sodium replacement.[511] Euvolemic patients, typically with SIADH, will benefit from vaptan therapy, limited hypertonic saline administration or, in some cases, urea, where available. This can be followed by fluid restriction or long-term vaptan therapy when the cause of the SIADH is expected to be chronic.[511] In hypervolemic patients with heart failure, vaptans are usually the best choice because fluid restriction is rarely successful in this group,[562] saline administration can cause fluid retention with increased edema, and urea can lead to ammonia buildup in the gastrointestinal tract if hepatic function is impaired. Although moderate neurologic symptoms can indicate that a patient is in an early stage of acute hyponatremia, they more often indicate a chronically hyponatremic state with sufficient brain volume adaptation to prevent marked symptomatology from cerebral edema. Most patients with moderate hyponatremic symptoms have a more chronic form of hyponatremia, so guidelines for goals and limits of correction should be followed closely (see Fig. 15.20), and close monitoring of these patients in a hospital setting is warranted until their symptoms improve or stabilize.

Patients with no or minimal symptoms should be managed initially with fluid restriction, although treatment with pharmacologic therapy, such as vaptans or urea, may be appropriate for a wide range of specific clinical conditions (see Fig. 15.21). Foremost of these is a failure to improve the serum [$Na^+$], despite reasonable attempts at fluid restriction, or the presence of clinical characteristics associated with poor responses to fluid restriction (see Box 15.5).

A special case is when spontaneous correction of hyponatremia occurs at an undesirably rapid rate because of the onset of water diuresis. This can occur following cessation of desmopressin therapy in a patient who has become hyponatremic, replacement of glucocorticoids in a patient with adrenal insufficiency, replacement of solutes in a patient with hypovolemia, cessation of thiazides in diuretic-induced hyponatremia, or spontaneous resolution of transient SIADH. Brain damage from ODS can clearly ensue in this setting if the preceding period of hyponatremia has been long enough (usually, ≥48 hours) to allow brain volume regulation to occur. If the correction parameters discussed earlier have been exceeded, and the correction is proceeding more rapidly than planned (usually because of continued excretion of hypotonic urine), the pathologic events leading to demyelination can be reversed by the administration of hypotonic fluids, with or without desmopressin. The efficacy of this approach has been suggested from animal studies[563] and case reports in humans,[505,564] even when patients are overtly symptomatic.[565] However, relowering the serum [Na+] after an initial, overly rapid correction is only strongly recommended for patients at high risk of ODS (see Box 15.5). It is considered optional for patients with a low to moderate risk of ODS and unnecessary for patients with acute water intoxication (see Fig. 15.20).

Although this classification is based on presenting symptoms at the time of initial evaluation, it should be remembered that in some cases, patients initially exhibit more moderate symptoms because they are in the early stages of hyponatremia. In addition, some patients with minimal symptoms are prone to develop more symptomatic hyponatremia during periods of increased fluid ingestion. In support of this, approximately 70% of 31 patients presenting to a university hospital with symptomatic hyponatremia and a mean serum [Na+] of 119 mmol/L had preexisting asymptomatic hyponatremia as the most common risk factor identified.[566] Consequently, therapy for chronic hyponatremia should also be considered to prevent progression from a lower to higher level of symptomatic hyponatremia, particularly in patients with a past history of repeated presentations for symptomatic hyponatremia.

## MONITORING SERUM SODIUM CONCENTRATION IN HYPONATREMIC PATIENTS

The frequency of serum [Na+] monitoring is dependent on the severity of the hyponatremia and therapy chosen. In all hyponatremic patients, neurologic symptomatology should be carefully assessed very early in the diagnostic evaluation to assess the symptomatic severity of the hyponatremia and determine whether the patient requires more urgent therapy. All patients undergoing active treatment with hypertonic saline for symptomatic hyponatremia should have frequent monitoring of their serum [Na+] and ECF volume status (every 1–4 hours) to ensure that the serum [Na+] does not exceed the limits of safe correction during the active phase of correction,[507] because overly rapid correction of serum sodium will increase the risk of ODS.[567] Patients treated with vaptans for mild to moderate symptoms should have their serum [Na+] monitored every 6 to 8 hours during the active phase of correction, which will generally be the first 24 to 48 hours of therapy. Active treatment with hypertonic saline or vaptans should be stopped when the patient's symptoms are no longer present, a safe serum [Na+] has been achieved (usually, >120 mmol/L), or the rate of correction has reached maximum limits of 12 mmol/L within 24 hours or 18 mmol/L within 48 hours[507,512] or 8 mmol/L over any 24-hour period in patients at high risk of ODS (see Box 15.5). In patients with a stable level of serum [Na+] treated with fluid restriction or therapy other than hypertonic saline, measurement of the serum [Na+] daily is generally sufficient because levels will not change that quickly in the absence of active therapy or large changes in fluid intake or administration.

## LONG-TERM TREATMENT OF CHRONIC HYPONATREMIA

Some patients will benefit from continued treatment of hyponatremia following discharge from the hospital. In many cases, this will consist of continued fluid restriction. However, as discussed, long-term compliance with this therapy is poor because of the increased thirst that occurs with more severe degrees of fluid restriction. Thus, for select patients who have responded to tolvaptan in the hospital, consideration should be given to continuing the treatment as an outpatient after discharge. In patients with established chronic hyponatremia, tolvaptan has shown to be effective for maintaining a normal [Na+] for as long as 3 years of continued daily therapy.[568] However, many patients with inpatient hyponatremia have a transient form of SIADH, without the need for long-term therapy. In the conivaptan open-label study, approximately 70% of patients treated as an inpatient for 4 days had normal serum [Na+] concentrations 7 and 30 days after the cessation of the vaptan therapy in the absence of chronic therapy for hyponatremia. Selection of which patients with inpatient hyponatremia are candidates for long-term therapy should be based on the cause of the SIADH. Fig. 15.22 shows estimates of the relative probability that patients with different causes of SIADH will have persistent hyponatremia that may benefit from long-term treatment with tolvaptan following hospital discharge. Nonetheless, for any individual patient, this simply represents an estimate of the likelihood of requiring long-term therapy. In all cases, consideration should be given to a trial of stopping the drug 2 to 4 weeks after discharge to determine if hyponatremia is still present. A reasonable period of tolvaptan cessation to evaluate the presence of continued SIADH is 7 days, because this period was found to be sufficient for demonstration of a recurrence of hyponatremia in the tolvaptan SALT trials.[568,569] The serum [Na+] should be monitored every 2 to 3 days following the cessation of tolvaptan so that the drug can be resumed as quickly as possible in patients with recurrent hyponatremia; the longer the patient is hyponatremic, the greater the risk of subsequent ODS with overly rapid correction of the low serum [Na+].

Findings of hepatotoxicity in a small number of patients on high doses of tolvaptan in a clinical trial of polycystic kidney disease have led to a recent FDA recommendation that tolvaptan not be used for longer than 30 days.[530] This decision should be based on a risk-benefit analysis individualized for specific patients; if tolvaptan is used for longer than 30 days, liver function should be assessed at regular intervals (e.g., every 3 months).[511]

## FUTURE OF HYPONATREMIA TREATMENT

Despite the many advances made in understanding the manifestations and consequences of hyponatremia, and the availability of effective pharmacologic therapies for the treatment of hyponatremia, it is obvious that we do not yet have a uniformly accepted consensus on how and when this disorder should be treated. In particular, indications for the use of vasopressin receptor antagonists by regulatory agencies

| Etiology of SIADH | Likely duration of SIADH* | Relative risk of chronic SIADH |
|---|---|---|
| Tumors producing vasopressin ectopically (small-cell lung carcinoma, head and neck carcinoma) | Indefinite | High |
| Drug-induced, with continuation of offending agent (carbamazepine, SSRI) | Duration of drug therapy | |
| Brain tumors | Indefinite | |
| Idiopathic (senile) | Indefinite | |
| Subarachnoid hemorrhage | 1–4 weeks | |
| Stroke | 1–2 weeks | |
| Inflammatory brain lesions | Dependent on response to therapy | Medium |
| Respiratory failure (chronic obstructive lung disease) | Dependent on response to therapy | |
| HIV infection | Dependent on response to therapy | |
| Traumatic brain injury | 2–7 days to indefinite | |
| Drug-induced, with cessation of offending agent | Duration of drug therapy | |
| Pneumonia | 2–5 days | |
| Nausea, pain, prolonged exercise | Variable, depending on cause | |
| Postoperative hyponatremia | 2–3 days postoperatively | Low |

*Time frames are based on clinical experience.

**Fig. 15.22** Estimated probability of need for long-term treatment of SIADH, depending on underlying cause.

differ substantially worldwide, and various treatment guidelines published to date also differ substantially in regard to appropriate hyponatremia management.[511,570,571] There are many reasons for this failure to achieve consensus and, until this occurs via further clinical research studies, physicians must recognize the primary role that clinical judgment must continue to play in making decisions about the management of hyponatremia in individual patients. Their recommendations should take into account appropriate appraisals of evidence by authoritative experts in the field, the decisions of regulatory agencies based on critical reviews of the efficacy and safety data for approved treatments for hyponatremia and, most importantly, the specialized needs of individual hyponatremic patients.[571]

In the meantime, clinical trials using vasopressin receptor antagonists will enable investigators to answer some long-standing questions about the role of vasopressin $V_2$ receptor activation in various physiologic conditions (e.g., regulation of sweat production),[572] pathophysiologic states (e.g., hyponatremic patients without measurable vasopressin levels), and especially the potential reversibility of long-term adverse effects associated with hyponatremia, such as falls, bone loss, and fractures. This may, in part, account for the increased mortality and morbidity in hyponatremic patients across multiple different comorbidities, as well as in older, community-dwelling subjects without known underlying diseases.

Complete reference list available at ExpertConsult.com.

## KEY REFERENCES

1. Edelman IS, Leibman J. Anatomy of body water and electrolytes. *Am J Med.* 1959;27:256–277.
17. Thibonnier M, Conarty DM, Preston JA, et al. Molecular pharmacology of human vasopressin receptors. *Adv Exp Med Biol.* 1998;449:251–276.
26. Robinson AG, Roberts MM, Evron WA, et al. Hyponatremia in rats induces downregulation of vasopressin synthesis. *J Clin Invest.* 1990;86:1023–1029.
32. Robertson GL. The regulation of vasopressin function in health and disease. *Recent Prog Horm Res.* 1976;33:333–385.
43. Leng G, Brown CH, Bull PM, et al. Responses of magnocellular neurons to osmotic stimulation involves coactivation of excitatory and inhibitory input: an experimental and theoretical analysis. *J Neurosci.* 2001;21:6967–6977.
46. Bourque CW, Voisin DL, Chakfe Y. Stretch-inactivated cation channels: cellular targets for modulation of osmosensitivity in supraoptic neurons. *Prog Brain Res.* 2002;139:85–94.
50. Liedtke W. Role of TRPV ion channels in sensory transduction of osmotic stimuli in mammals. *Exp Physiol.* 2007;92:507–512.
54. Dunn FL, Brennan TJ, Nelson AE, et al. The role of blood osmolality and volume in regulating vasopressin secretion in the rat. *J Clin Invest.* 1973;52:3212–3219.
64. Schrier RW. Pathogenesis of sodium and water retention in high-output and low-output cardiac failure, nephrotic syndrome, cirrhosis, and pregnancy. *N Engl J Med.* 1988;319:1065–1072.
106. Phillips PA, Rolls BJ, Ledingham JG, et al. Osmotic thirst and vasopressin release in humans: a double-blind crossover study. *Am J Physiol.* 1985;248(Pt 2):R645–R650.

135. Maghnie M, Cosi G, Genovese E, et al. Central diabetes insipidus in children and young adults. *N Engl J Med.* 2000;343:998–1007.
136. Imura H, Nakao K, Shimatsu A, et al. Lymphocytic infundibuloneurohypophysitis as a cause of central diabetes insipidus. *N Engl J Med.* 1993;329:683–689.
147. Zerbe RL, Robertson GL. A comparison of plasma vasopressin measurements with a standard indirect test in the differential diagnosis of polyuria. *N Engl J Med.* 1981;305:1539–1546.
152. Olson BR, Gumowski J, Rubino D, et al. Pathophysiology of hyponatremia after transsphenoidal pituitary surgery. *J Neurosurg.* 1997;87:499–507.
162. DeRubertis FR, Michelis MF, Beck N, et al. "Essential" hypernatremia due to ineffective osmotic and intact volume regulation of vasopressin secretion. *J Clin Invest.* 1971;50:97–111.
166. Durr JA, Hoggard JG, Hunt JM, et al. Diabetes insipidus in pregnancy associated with abnormally high circulating vasopressinase activity. *N Engl J Med.* 1987;316:1070–1074.
175. Morello JP, Bichet DG. Nephrogenic diabetes insipidus. *Annu Rev Physiol.* 2001;63:607–630.
182. Deen PM, Knoers NV. Vasopressin type-2 receptor and aquaporin-2 water channel mutants in nephrogenic diabetes insipidus. *Am J Med Sci.* 1998;316:300–309.
189. Nielsen S, Kwon TH, Christensen BM, et al. Physiology and pathophysiology of renal aquaporins. *J Am Soc Nephrol.* 1999;10:647–663.
210. Goldman MB, Robertson GL, Luchins DJ, et al. Psychotic exacerbations and enhanced vasopressin secretion in schizophrenic patients with hyponatremia and polydipsia. *Arch Gen Psychiatry.* 1997;54:443–449.
216. Gullans SR, Verbalis JG. Control of brain volume during hyperosmolar and hypoosmolar conditions. *Annu Rev Med.* 1993;44:289–301.
219. Robertson GL. Diabetes insipidus. *Endocrinol Metab Clin North Am.* 1995;24:549–572.
244. Oiso Y, Robertson GL, Norgaard JP, et al. Clinical review: treatment of neurohypophyseal diabetes insipidus. *J Clin Endocrinol Metab.* 2013;98:3958–3967.
250. Richardson DW, Robinson AG. Desmopressin. *Ann Intern Med.* 1985;103:228–239.
280. Hawkins RC. Age and gender as risk factors for hyponatremia and hypernatremia. *Clin Chim Acta.* 2003;337:169–172.
297. Androgue HJ, Madias NE. Hyponatremia. *N Engl J Med.* 2000;342:1581–1589.
349. Schwartz WB, Bennett W, Curelop S, et al. A syndrome of renal sodium loss and hyponatremia probably resulting from inappropriate secretion of antidiuretic hormone. *Am J Med.* 1957;23:529–542.
350. Bartter FE, Schwartz WB. The syndrome of inappropriate secretion of antidiuretic hormone. *Am J Med.* 1967;42:790–806.
355. Leaf A, Bartter FC, Santos RF, et al. Evidence in humans that urine electrolyte loss induced by pitressin is a function of water retention. *J Clin Invest.* 1953;32:868–878.
357. Verbalis JG, Drutarosky M. Adaptation to chronic hypo-osmolality in rats. *Kidney Int.* 1988;34:351–360.
365. Ecelbarger C, Nielsen S, Olson BR, et al. Role of renal aquaporins in escape from vasopressin antidiuresis in rat. *J Clin Invest.* 1997;99:1852–1863.
375. Hirshberg B, Ben-Yehuda A. The syndrome of inappropriate antidiuretic hormone secretion in the elderly. *Am J Med.* 1997;103:270–273.
381. Feldman BJ, Rosenthal SM, Vargas GA, et al. Nephrogenic syndrome of inappropriate antidiuresis. *N Engl J Med.* 2005;352:1884–1890.
386. Oelkers W. Hyponatremia and inappropriate secretion of vasopressin in patients with hypopituitarism. *N Engl J Med.* 1989;321:492–496.
418. Anderson RJ, Chung H-M, Kluge R, et al. Hyponatremia: a prospective analysis of its epidemiology and the pathogenetic role of vasopressin. *Ann Intern Med.* 1985;102:164–168.
425. Almond CS, Shin AY, Fortescue EB, et al. Hyponatremia among runners in the Boston Marathon. *N Engl J Med.* 2005;352:1550–1556.
471. Upadhyay A, Jaber BL, Madias NE. Incidence and prevalence of hyponatremia. *Am J Med.* 2006;119(suppl 1):S30–S35.
487. Renneboog B, Musch W, Vandemergel X, et al. Mild chronic hyponatremia is associated with falls, unsteadiness, and attention deficits. *Am J Med.* 2006;119:71.
493. Kinsella S, Moran S, Sullivan MO, et al. Hyponatremia independent of osteoporosis is associated with fracture occurrence. *Clin J Am Soc Nephrol.* 2010;5:275–280.
494. Hoorn EJ, Rivadeneira F, van Meurs JB, et al. Mild hyponatremia as a risk factor for fractures: the Rotterdam Study. *J Bone Miner Res.* 2011;26:1822–1828.
495. Verbalis JG, Barsony J, Sugimura Y, et al. Hyponatremia-induced osteoporosis. *J Bone Miner Res.* 2010;25:554–563.
511. Verbalis JG, Goldsmith SR, Greenberg A, et al. Diagnosis, evaluation, and treatment of hyponatremia: expert panel recommendations. *Am J Med.* 2013;126(suppl 1):S1–S42.
517. Furst H, Hallows KR, Post J, et al. The urine/plasma electrolyte ratio: a predictive guide to water restriction. *Am J Med Sci.* 2000;319:240–244.
522. Greenberg A, Verbalis JG. Vasopressin receptor antagonists. *Kidney Int.* 2006;69:2124–2130.
527. Schrier RW, Gross P, Gheorghiade M, et al. Tolvaptan, a selective oral vasopressin V2-receptor antagonist, for hyponatremia. *N Engl J Med.* 2006;355:2099–2112.
532. Berl T, Quittnat-Pelletier F, Verbalis JG, et al. Oral tolvaptan is safe and effective in chronic hyponatremia. *J Am Soc Nephrol.* 2010;21:705–712.
533. Konstam MA, Gheorghiade M, Burnett JC Jr, et al. Effects of oral tolvaptan in patients hospitalized for worsening heart failure: the EVEREST Outcome Trial. *JAMA.* 2007;297:1319–1331.
549. Ellison DH, Berl T. Clinical practice. The syndrome of inappropriate antidiuresis. *N Engl J Med.* 2007;356:2064–2072.
558. Sterns RH, Hix JK, Silver S. Treating profound hyponatremia: a strategy for controlled correction. *Am J Kidney Dis.* 2010;56:774–779.
567. Sterns RH, Riggs JE, Schochet SS Jr. Osmotic demyelination syndrome following correction of hyponatremia. *N Engl J Med.* 1986;314:1535–1542.

# 16 Disorders of Acid-Base Balance

L. Lee Hamm | Thomas D. DuBose, Jr.

CHAPTER OUTLINE



Acid-base homeostasis is critical for normal health. However, a variety of both acute and chronic conditions commonly alter acid-base homeostasis and blood pH. This chapter will review normal acid-base homeostasis and various conditions causing disorders. The approach to acid-base homeostasis in this chapter uses measurements of arterial pH, $PCO_2$, and $[HCO_3^-]$ plus an analysis of the electrolytes and anion gap. This is the most widely used and generally accepted approach used clinically by nephrologists, and the easiest model to understand.[1] Other approaches, such as that using "base excess" or "strong ion difference", are used by some groups but will not be used here.

## ACID-BASE HOMEOSTASIS

Acid-base homeostasis normally maintains systemic arterial pH within a narrow range, certainly between 7.35 and 7.45 pH units. This tight regulation is accomplished through 1) chemical buffering in each of the body fluid compartments and 2) control of $CO_2$ and $HCO_3^-$ by the lungs and kidneys, respectively. These processes efficiently dispose of the physiologic daily load of acid in the forms of $CO_2$ (forming carbonic acid $H_2CO_3$) and nonvolatile acids, mainly derived from metabolism and dietary protein intake, and defend against the occasional addition of pathologic quantities of acid and alkali.

The intracellular $H^+$ concentration ($[H^+]_i$), or $pH_i$, is also regulated at a relatively stable value, usually less than plasma. Both cellular ion exchange mechanisms and intracellular buffers (hemoglobin, tissue proteins, organophosphate complexes, and bone apatite) participate in the blunting of changes in both $[H^+]_i$ and $[H^+]_e$. Extracellular and intracellular buffers provide the *first line of defense* against the addition of acid or base to the body. As a brief review, the relationship between an undissociated acid (HA) and its conjugate, disassociated base (A–) may be represented as follows:

$$HA \leftrightarrow H^+ + A^- \tag{16.1}$$

Weak acids and their conjugate bases, and also weak bases and their conjugate acids, represent buffer pairs that are most effective when the pair are at the same concentration, e.g., HA = $A^-$; this occurs at a certain H+ concentration or pH (pH = $-\log_{10}[H^+]$). This $H^+$ concentration also equals the equilibrium constant $K_a$ of the reaction above:

$$K_a = \frac{[H^+][A^-]}{[HA]} \tag{16.2}$$

Buffer systems are critical to the physiology and pathophysiology of acid-base homeostasis because they attenuate the pH change in a solution or tissue by reversibly combining with or releasing $H^+$. Thus, the pH change of a solution during the addition of acid or base equivalents is smaller in the presence of a buffer system than would have occurred if no buffer systems were present. The major buffer system in the body is the $CO_2/HCO_3^-$ system represented by the reversible reactions below, catalyzed by carbonic anhydrase:

$$H_2O + CO_2 \xleftrightarrow[\text{Anhydrase}]{\text{Carbonic}} H_2CO_3 \leftrightarrow H^+ + HCO_3^- \tag{16.3}$$

This system is effective because of its abundance and especially because $CO_2$ and $HCO_3^-$ can be independently modified by the lungs and kidneys, respectively. Note that because the reaction is reversible, changes in $[H^+]$ or pH can result from either an addition of an acid, e.g. $H^+$, or loss of $[HCO_3^-]$ (or base), which would "pull" the reaction to the right. Physiologically, for pH considerations, gain of an acid is equivalent to the loss of a base or alkali.

Because the concentration of $H_2CO_3$ is low and proportional to the concentration of dissolved $CO_2$, one can condense the equations above to:

$$CO_2 + H_2O \leftrightarrow H^+ + HCO_3^- \quad (16.4)$$

and then derive:

$$K = \frac{[H^+][HCO_3]}{[CO_2][H_2O]} \quad (16.5)$$

The familiar Henderson-Hasselbach equation then can be derived and results when the solubility of $CO_2$ is considered (dissolved $CO_2$ in mmol/L = 0.03 x $PCO_2$ in mm Hg) and the pK of 6.1 is used:

$$pH = pK' + \log_{10}\frac{[HCO_3^-]}{\alpha_{CO2}PCO_2} \quad (16.6)$$

Note that this equation illustrates that pH is a complex function of the ratio of $HCO_3^-$ concentration to $PCO_2$, and therefore pH can be altered by changes in either $HCO_3^-$ or $PCO_2$. However, if the $HCO_3^-$ or $PCO_2$ changes, the ratio and pH can be returned toward or to normal by a similarly directed change in the other. For instance, if $HCO_3^-$ is decreased by 50%, pH decreases; but then if $PCO_2$ decreases by 50% then pH is returned to normal.

If buffers, including the $HCO_3^-/CO_2$ system, are conceptualized as the first line of immediate defense of pH, the second line of defense can be conceptualized as the respiratory system. Pulmonary participation in acid-base homeostasis relies on the excretion of $CO_2$ by the lungs. Large amounts of $CO_2$ accumulate as metabolic end products of tissue metabolism (10 to 12 mmol/day). This $CO_2$ load is transported in the blood to the lungs as hemoglobin-generated $HCO_3^-$ and hemoglobin-bound carbamino groups.[2] Because, under most circumstances, $CO_2$ excretion and $CO_2$ production are matched, the usual steady-state arterial $PCO_2$, $Paco_2$, is maintained at 40 mm Hg. Underexcretion of $CO_2$ produces hypercapnia, and overexcretion produces hypocapnia. $Paco_2$ is regulated primarily by neurorespiratory factors and is not subject to regulation by the rate of metabolic $CO_2$ production. Increases or decreases in $PCO_2$ represent derangements of control of neurorespiratory regulation or can result from compensatory changes in response to a primary alteration in the plasma $HCO_3^-$ concentration. The respiratory response to acidemia or alkalemia blunts the change in blood pH that would occur otherwise. Such respiratory alterations that adjust blood pH toward normal are referred to as *secondary* or *compensatory* alterations, because they occur in response to primary metabolic changes (or changes in $HCO_3^-$ discussed below). Ventilation can change within minutes of systemic pH changes and compensate for acid or base loads by adjustments in $Paco_2$. Complete respiratory compensation can take hours. Primary changes in $Paco_2$ can also occur and result in acidosis or alkalosis, depending on whether $CO_2$ is elevated above or depressed below the normal value: 40 mm Hg. Such disorders are termed *respiratory acidosis* and *respiratory alkalosis*, respectively.

The third component of pH protection can be conceptualized as the plasma $HCO_3^-$ concentration, which can be modulated by both metabolic and renal regulatory mechanisms. When discussed as a protective mechanism, renal induced changes in $HCO_3^-$ can compensate for primary respiratory acid-base disorders (primary changes in $PCO_2$) or in response to a "metabolic" acid or base load. "Metabolic" here refers to "non-volatile" acids or bases, namely non-$CO_2$ acids. As discussed below, the kidneys can regulate plasma $HCO_3^-$.

Metabolism generates a daily load of relatively strong acids (lactate, citrate, acetate, and pyruvate), which must be removed by other metabolic reactions. The oxidation of these organic acids in the Krebs cycle, for example, generates $CO_2$, which must be excreted by the lungs. Nevertheless, the complete combustion of carbon involves the intermediate generation and metabolism of relatively strong organic acids, such as lactic acids, tricarboxylic acids, ketoacids, or other acids, depending on the type of fuel consumed. These organic acids do not accumulate in the body under most circumstances, with concentrations remaining in the low millimolar range. If production and consumption rates become mismatched, however, these organic acids can accumulate (e.g., lactic acid accumulation with strenuous exertion). Correspondingly, the $HCO_3^-$ in the extracellular fluid (ECF) will decline as the organic acid concentration increases. During recovery, the organic acids reenter metabolic pathways to $CO_2$ production, removal of $H^+$, and generation of $HCO_3^-$. Nevertheless, if the organic anions are excreted (e.g., ketonuria), these entities are no longer available for regeneration of $HCO_3^-$. Considered in this way, metabolizable organic anion may be viewed as "potential bicarbonate". The metabolism of some body constituents such as proteins, nucleic acids, and small fractions of lipids and certain carbohydrates generate specific organic acids that cannot be burned to $CO_2$ (e.g., uric, oxalic, glucuronic, hippuric acids). In addition, the inorganic acids $H_2SO_4$ and $H_3PO_4$, derived respectively from sulfur-containing dietary amino acids and organophosphates, must be excreted by the kidneys or the gastrointestinal tract. Persons eating a typical Western diet have a daily acid challenge, typically 0.5-1 mEq/kg body weight. The amount of net nonvolatile acid produced by diet and metabolism is defined as *endogenous acid production.* Net endogenous acid production is, therefore, dependent in part on diet, especially the relative amount of animal-derived dietary protein.[3]

Metabolic *regulation* of $HCO_3^-$ is of minor importance in terms of overall physiologic regulation of acid-base balance. Nevertheless, regulatory enzymes, whose activity may be pH sensitive, may catalyze metabolic reactions that either generate or consume organic acids. Such a process constitutes a negative feedback regulatory system. The best example is phosphofructokinase, the pivotal enzyme in the glycolytic pathway. Phosphofructokinase is a kinase enzyme that phosphorylates fructose 6-phosphate in glycolysis. The activity of phosphofructokinase is inhibited by low pH and enhanced by high pH. Thus, an increase in $pH_i$ accelerates glycolysis and generates pyruvate and lactate. It follows, therefore, that the generation of lactic acid in patients with lactic acidosis, and the generation of ketoacids in patients with ketoacidosis, are impeded by acidemia. Conversely, generation of lactic acid in patients with lactic acidosis, and the generation of ketoacids in patients with ketoacidosis, are augmented by reversal of acidemia.

## RENAL REGULATION

Although temporary relief from changes in the pH of body fluids may be accomplished by chemical buffering or respiratory compensation, the ultimate defense against the addition of nonvolatile acid or of alkali is the responsibility of the kidneys. The addition of a strong acid (HA) to the ECF titrates or consumes plasma $HCO_3^-$:

$$HA + NaHCO_3 \leftrightarrow NA + H_2O + CO_2 \quad (16.7)$$

The $CO_2$ is expired by the lungs, and body $HCO_3^-$ buffer stores are diminished. This process occurs constantly as endogenous metabolic acids are generated. To maintain a normal plasma $HCO_3^-$ in the face of constant production of metabolic acids, predominantly as a result of dietary protein metabolism, the kidneys must 1) reabsorb virtually all of the $HCO_3^-$ present in glomerular filtrate, and 2) regenerate the $HCO_3^-$ consumed by reaction with metabolic acids (Equation 16.7). The first process ($HCO_3^-$ reabsorption) is accomplished predominantly in the proximal tubule, with an additional contribution by the loop of Henle and a lesser, but critical, contribution by more distal nephron segments (Fig. 16.1). Under most circumstances, the filtered load of $HCO_3^-$ is absorbed almost completely, especially during an acid load. "Acid production" in biologic systems is represented by the milliequivalents (mEq) of protons ($H^+$) added to body fluids. Ordinarily on a Western diet, especially animal-based proteins, there is a net daily endogenous acid load which consumes $HCO_3^-$. Conversely, base addition to the extracellular fluid via the GI tract is derived primarily from dietary fruits and vegetables. If less acid is generated or when, in the face of an alkali load, the plasma $HCO_3^-$ concentration increases above the normal value of 25 mEq/L, $HCO_3^-$ will be excreted into the urine. Therefore, the kidney must efficiently excrete any excess in alkali added to the ECF as well as regenerate the bicarbonate lost when net endogenous acid production is significant. The difference between endogenous acid production and the input of alkali absorbed by the gastrointestinal system, i.e. the difference in acid production and base generation, is known as *net endogenous acid production.* Since a Western diet is high in animal-based protein, net endogenous production is positive and consumes bicarbonate; therefore, the kidney must regenerate the bicarbonate consumed by dietary protein intake.

The process of $HCO_3^-$ regeneration, is represented by the renal output of acid or *net acid excretion*:

$$\text{Net Acid Excretion} = NH_4^+ + \text{Titratable Acid} - HCO_3^- \quad (16.8)$$

The mechanisms of net acid excretion are discussed below, but include two components: titratable acid and ammonium $NH_4^+$ (Fig. 16.2). Titratable acid (TA) is the acid added to tubular fluid along the nephron to lower fluid pH to that of the final urine. The final pH of urine will depend on the amount of urinary buffer, principally phosphate, and the amount of acid added. TA can be measured by titrating urine (after removing ammonia) back to plasma pH or can be calculated using the urine and plasma pH and the buffer concentration (as a first approximation phosphate) and its pKa. $NH_4^+$ represents acid excretion since, as described in another chapter, for each $NH_4^+$ produced *and* excreted the carbon skeleton of glutamine from which it derives has been converted to $HCO_3^-$ (Fig. 16.3).

On balance, each milliequivalent of net acid excreted corresponds to 1 mEq of $HCO_3^-$ returned to the ECF (i.e., regeneration of $HCO_3^-$. This process of $HCO_3^-$ regeneration is necessary to replace the $HCO_3^-$ lost by the endogenous acid entry into the ECF or, less commonly, the $HCO_3^-$ excreted in stool or urine. Because a typical Western diet, rich in animal-based proteins, generates fixed acids at 35 to 70 mEq/day, net acid excretion must approximate 35 to 70 mEq/day to match net acid production, and avoid metabolic acidosis.

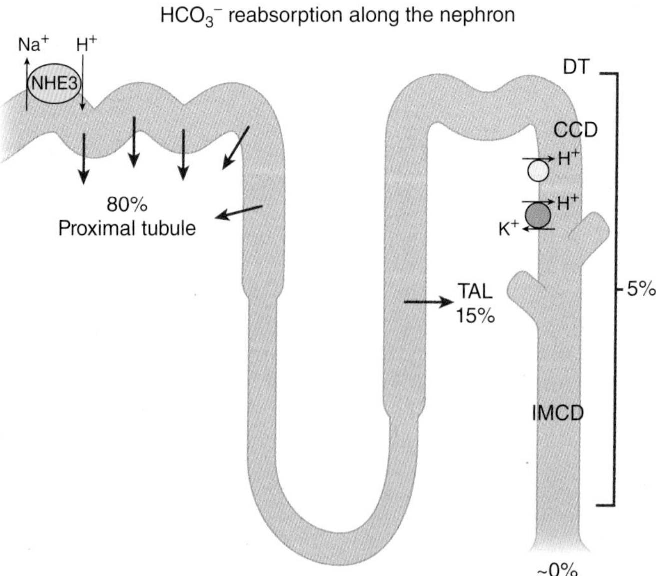


**Fig. 16.1** $HCO_3^-$ reabsorption along the nephron. The proximal tubule reabsorbs approximately 80% of the filtered $HCO_3^-$. Substantial amounts are also reabsorbed in the thick ascending limb. The remaining amounts (~ 5%) are reabsorbed in the collecting duct, which is critical for final regulation of acid excretion. The mechanisms are described in another chapter but the main apical transporters (Na-H exchange and $H^+$-ATPase) are illustrated. Little $HCO_3^-$ (~0 %) remains in the final urine.

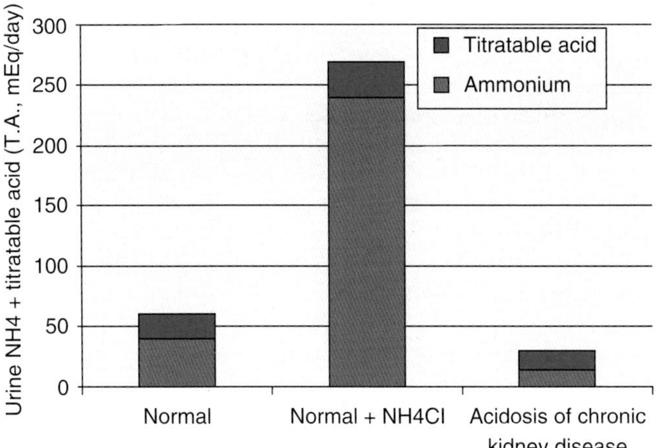


**Fig. 16.2** Net acid excretion with typical Western diets, with acid loading, and with acidosis in chronic kidney disease (CKD). Ammonium excretion has the capability for the most increase in acidosis, and is also the component that is most compromised in CKD. *T.A.,* Urine titratable acidity. (From Gauthier P, Simon EE, Lemann J, Jr. Acidosis of Chronic Renal Failure. In: DuBose TD, Hamm LL, editors. *Acid-Base And Electrolyte Disorders.* Philadelphia: Saunders; 2002. pp. 207-216.)

## SYSTEMIC RESPONSE TO RESPIRATORY ACIDOSIS OR ALKALOSIS

### ACUTE RESPONSE: GENERATION OF RESPIRATORY ACIDOSIS OR ALKALOSIS

Some conditions independent of pH stimulate a primary increase in ventilation, which lowers systemic $Pa_{CO_2}$, and thus raises pH – respiratory alkalosis. These conditions include hypoxemia, fever, anxiety, central nervous system disease, acute cardiopulmonary processes, septicemia, liver failure, pregnancy, and drugs (e.g., salicylates).[4] Conversely, $Pa_{CO_2}$ increases if the respiratory system is depressed by suppression of the respiratory control center or of the respiratory apparatus itself (neuromuscular, parenchymal, and airway components[5]) – pH is lowered, respiratory acidosis. In both kinds of acute respiratory disorders, $CO_2$ is added to or subtracted from the body until the $Pa_{CO_2}$ assumes a new steady state so that pulmonary $CO_2$ excretion equals $CO_2$ production. The acute accumulation or loss of $CO_2$ causes changes in blood pH within minutes. The plasma $HCO_3^-$ decreases slightly as the $Pa_{CO_2}$ is reduced in acute respiratory alkalosis and increases slightly in acute respiratory acidosis.[2,4–6] The small changes in $HCO_3^-$ concentration are due to buffering by nonbicarbonate buffers.[2,4–6] The estimated change in blood $HCO_3^-$ concentration is approximately equal to 0.1 mEq/L of [$HCO_3^-$] increase for each millimeter of mercury (mm Hg) increase in $PCO_2$ and 0.25 mEq/L decrease for each mm Hg decrease in $PCO_2$.[5] Acute alterations in $PCO_2$ in either direction within the physiologic range do not acutely

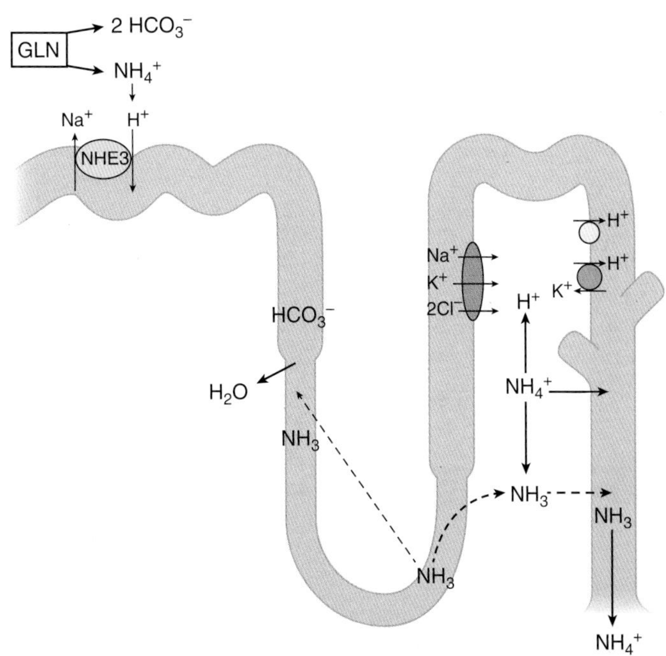


**Fig. 16.3** Synchrony of regulation of ammonium production (from glutamine [GLN] precursors, and excretion). Process allows generation of "new" $HCO_3^-$ by the kidney. $NH_4^+$ excretion is regulated in response to changes in systemic acid-base and $K^+$ balance. Contributing segments include the proximal convoluted tubule, proximal straight tubule, thin descending limb, thick ascending limb, and medullary collecting duct. Upregulated by acidosis and hypokalemia. Inhibited by hyperkalemia.

change the blood $HCO_3^-$ concentration by more than a total of about 4 to 5 mEq/L from normal.

## CHRONIC RESPONSE

Although the blood pH is relatively poorly defended during acute changes in $Paco_2$, during chronic changes, the kidneys excrete or retain $HCO_3^-$ and return blood pH toward normal. The persistence of hypocapnia reduces renal $HCO_3^-$ absorption to achieve a further decrease in the plasma $HCO_3^-$ concentration. Hypocapnia decreases renal $HCO_3^-$ reabsorption[4] by inhibiting acidification in both the proximal[6] and the distal nephrons. The resulting decrease in plasma $HCO_3^-$ concentration is equal to about 0.4 to 0.5 mEq/L for each mm Hg decrease in $PCO_2$.[6] Thus the arterial pH falls toward but not completely back to normal.

With chronic hypocapnia, several hours to days are required for full expression of the renal response,[5,6] which includes a reduction in the rate of $H^+$ secretion, an increase in urine pH, a decrease in $NH_4^+$ and titratable acid excretion, and a modest bicarbonaturia. An increase in blood $Cl^-$ concentration occurs simultaneously by means of several mechanisms: a shift of $Cl^-$ out of red blood cells, ECF volume contraction, and enhanced $Cl^-$ reabsorption.

During chronic hypercapnia, the increase in generation of $HCO_3^-$ by the kidney takes several days for completion. The mechanism of $HCO_3^-$ retention involves increased $H^+$ secretion by both proximal and distal nephron segments, regardless of sodium bicarbonate or sodium chloride intake, mineralocorticoid levels, or $K^+$ depletion.[2,5–7] Chronic hypercapnia results in sustained increases in renal cortical $PCO_2$, and the increase in renal cortical $PCO_2$ that occurs with chronic hypercapnia stimulates acidification.[6] The increased $PCO_2$ enhances distal $H^+$ secretion so that increased $NH_4^+$ excretion occurs even with a low-salt diet or with hypoxemia. These responses are blunted in AKI or chronic kidney disease (CKD). For instance, if hyperkalemia ensues or is present initially, the renal adaptation to chronic hypercapnia is blunted significantly.[7] With time, an adaptation occurs in the proximal nephron: $HCO_3^-$ reabsorption is stimulated after several days of hypercapnia.[8] In summary, although primary alterations in systemic $Paco_2$ cause relatively marked changes in blood pH, renal homeostatic mechanisms allow the blood pH to return toward normal over a sufficient period. The renal response to chronic hypercapnia is manifest primarily by an increase in net acid excretion and $HCO_3^-$ absorption, which is accomplished by augmented $H^+$ secretion in both proximal and distal nephron segments.[9] In chronic hypercapnia, the blood $HCO_3^-$ concentration increases about 0.25 to 0.50 mEq/L for each mm Hg elevation in $Paco_2$.[5,6]

# SYSTEMIC RESPONSE TO ADDITION OF METABOLIC ACIDS

In addition to generating large quantities of $CO_2$, the metabolic processes of the body produce a smaller quantity of nonvolatile acids or metabolic acids. The lungs readily excrete $CO_2$, and this process can respond rapidly to changes in production. In contrast, the kidneys must excrete nonvolatile acids through a much slower adaptive response, taking a few days for full effect.

## SOURCES OF ENDOGENOUS ACIDS

Pathologically, acid loads may be derived from endogenous acid production (e.g., generation of ketoacids and lactic acids) or loss of base (e.g., diarrhea) or from exogenous sources (e.g., ammonium chloride or toxin ingestion). Under normal physiologic circumstances, a daily input of acid derived from the diet and metabolism confronts the body with an acid challenge. The net result of these processes amounts to the entry of about 0.5 to 1.0 mEq of new $H^+$ per kilogram per day into the ECF.[2,6]

Sulfuric acid is formed when organic sulfur from methionine and cysteine residues of proteins are oxidized to $SO_4^{2}$–. The metabolism of sulfur-containing amino acids is the primary source of acid in the usual Western diet, especially animal-derived proteins, accounting for approximately 50%. The quantity of sulfuric acid generated is equal to the $SO_4^{2}$– excreted in the urine.

Organic acids are derived from intermediary metabolites formed by partial combustion of dietary carbohydrates, fats, and proteins as well as from nucleic acids (uric acid). Organic acid generation contributes to net endogenous acid production when the conjugate bases are excreted in the urine as organic anions. If full oxidation of these acids can occur, however, $H^+$ is reclaimed and eliminated as $CO_2$ and water. The net amount of $H^+$ added to the body from this source can be estimated by the quantity of organic anions excreted in the urine.

Phosphoric acid can be derived from hydrolysis of $PO_4^{3}$– esters in proteins and nucleic acids if it is not neutralized by mineral cations (e.g., $Na^+$, $K^+$, and $Mg^{2+}$). The contribution of dietary phosphates to acid production is dependent on the kind of protein ingested. Some proteins generate phosphoric acid, whereas others generate only neutral phosphate salts.[2,6]

Potential sources of bases are also found in the diet (e.g., acetate, lactate, citrate), primarily from fruits and vegetables, and can be absorbed to neutralize partially the $H^+$ loads from the three sources just mentioned. These potential base equivalents may be estimated by subtracting the unmeasured anions in the stool ($Na^+ + K^+ + Ca^{2+} + Mg^{2+} - Cl^- - 1.8\ P$) from those measured in the diet. The net base absorbed by the gastrointestinal tract is derived from the anion gap (AG) of the diet minus that of the stool.

In summary, diets contain many sources of acids and bases. The usual North American diet, which is replete in animal-derived proteins, represents a daily source of acid generation for which the body must compensate constantly.

## HEPATIC AND RENAL ROLES IN ACID-BASE HOMEOSTASIS

The generation of acid by protein catabolism is balanced by the generation of new $HCO_3^-$ through renal $NH_4^+$ and titratable acid excretion (or, in sum, net acid excretion). Hepatic catabolism of proteins, with the exception of sulfur- and $PO_4^{3}$—containing amino acids, can be considered a neutral process. The products of these neutral reactions are $HCO_3^-$ and $NH_4^+$. Most of the $NH_4^+$ produced by metabolism of amino acids reacts with $HCO_3^-$ and forms urea and thus has no impact on acid-base balance. A portion of this $NH_4^+$ is diverted to glutamine synthesis, the amount of which is regulated by pH. Acidemia promotes and alkalemia inhibits glutamine synthesis. Glutamine enters the circulation and reaches the kidney, where it is deaminated to form glutamate initially; glutamate can also be deaminated, releasing another $NH_4^+$ and forming α-ketoglutarate. Renal glutamine deamination results in $NH_4^+$ production and initiates a metabolic process that generates new $HCO_3^-$ through α-ketoglutarate. Glutamine deamination in the kidney is also highly regulated by systemic pH, so that acidemia augments and alkalemia inhibits $NH_4^+$ and $HCO_3^-$ production. The ultimate control, however, resides in the renal excretion of $NH_4^+$, because the $NH_4^+$ must be excreted to escape entry into the hepatic urea synthetic pool. Hepatic urea synthesis would negate the new $HCO_3^-$ realized from α-ketoglutarate in the kidney. Hepatic regulation of $NH_4^+$ metabolic pathways appears to facilitate glutamine production when $NH_4^+$ excretion is stimulated by acidemia or, conversely, blunts glutamine production when excretion is inhibited by alkalemia.[10]

## RESPIRATORY RESPONSE TO ACIDEMIA

A critically important response to an acid load is the control of ventilation. A fall in systemic arterial pH is sensed by the chemoreceptors that stimulate ventilation and, therefore, reduce $Pa{CO_2}$. The fall in blood pH that would otherwise occur in uncompensated metabolic acidosis is therefore blunted. The pH is not restored to normal; however, with normal lungs $Pa{CO_2}$ declines by an average of 1.25 mm Hg for each 1.0 mEq/L drop in $HCO_3^-$ concentration. The clinical features are hyperpnea (increased tidal volume) and tachypnea (increased respiratory rate), which is termed Kussmaul respiration. The appropriate $Pa{CO_2}$ in steady-state metabolic acidosis can be estimated from the prevailing $HCO_3^-$ concentration according to the following expression[11]:

$$PaCO_2 = 1.5\,[HCO_3^-] + 8\ (\pm 2\ \text{mm Hg}) \qquad (16.9)$$

Other formulas to predict respiratory compensation are also available. Because the $Pa{CO_2}$ cannot fall below about 10 to 12 mm Hg, the blood pH is less well defended by respiration after very large reductions in the plasma $HCO_3^-$ concentration (Table 16.1). Approximately 12 to 24 hours is required to achieve full respiratory compensation for metabolic acidosis (see Fig. 16.4).

## RENAL EXCRETION

As already discussed, the kidneys eliminate the acid that is produced daily by metabolism and diet and have the capacity to increase urinary net acid excretion (and, hence, $HCO_3^-$ generation) in response to endogenous or exogenous acid loads. Acidosis enhances proximal $HCO_3^-$ absorption, decreasing delivery of $HCO_3^-$ out of the proximal tubule, and enhances distal acidification. The enhanced distal acidification serves to reabsorb any remaining $HCO_3^-$ and facilitate titratable acid excretion and $NH_4^+$ excretion. Increased $HCO_3^-$ reabsorption per se in the proximal tubule does not facilitate acid excretion since little $HCO_3^-$ is excreted into the urine even in normal circumstances. Net acid excretion is increased by stimulation of $NH_4^+$ production and excretion. Renal excretion of acid is usually matched to the net production of metabolic and dietary acids, often about 35 to 70 mEq/day, so little disturbance in systemic pH or $HCO_3^-$ concentration occurs.

As an acid load is incurred, the kidneys respond to restore balance primarily by increasing $NH_4^+$ excretion

**Table 16.1 Acid-Base Abnormalities and Appropriate Compensatory Responses for Simple Disorders**

| Primary Acid-Base Disorders | Primary Defect | Effect on pH | Compensatory Response | Expected Range of Compensation | Limits of Compensation |
|---|---|---|---|---|---|
| Respiratory acidosis | ↑ $PCO_2^-$<br>Alveolar hypoventilation | ↓ | $HCO_3^-$ ↑<br>Chronic: ↑ Renal reabsorption & production $HCO_3^-$ | Acute<br>Δ $[HCO_3^-]$ = +1 mEq/L for each ↑ Δ$PCO_2$ of 10 mm Hg<br>Chronic<br>Δ $[HCO_3^-]$ = +4 mEq/L for each ↑ Δ$PCO_2$ of 10 mm Hg | Acute<br>$[HCO_3^-]$ = 38 mEq/L<br>Chronic<br>$[HCO_3^-]$ = 45 mEq/L |
| Respiratory alkalosis | ↓ $PCO_2$<br>Alveolar hyperventilation | ↑ | $HCO_3^-$ ↓<br>Chronic: ↓ Renal $HCO_3^-$ reabsorption | Acute<br>Δ $[HCO_3^-]$ = -2 mEq/L for each ↓ Δ$PCO_2$ of 10 mm Hg<br>Chronic<br>Δ $[HCO_3^-]$ = -5 mEq/L for each ↓ Δ$PCO_2$ of 10 mm Hg | Acute<br>$[HCO_3^-]$ = 18 mEq/L<br>Chronic<br>$[HCO_3^-]$ = 15 mEq/L |
| Metabolic acidosis | ↓ $HCO_3^-$<br>Loss of $HCO_3^-$ or gain of $H^+$ | ↓ | ↓ $PCO_2$<br>Alveolar hyperventilation | $PCO_2$ = 1.5$[HCO_3^-]$ + 8 ± 2<br>$PCO_2$ = last 2 digits of pH x 100<br>$PCO_2$ = 15 + $[HCO_3^-]$ | $[PCO_2]$ = 15 mm Hg |
| Metabolic alkalosis | ↑ $HCO_3^-$<br>Gain of $HCO_3^-$ or loss of $H^+$ | ↑ | ↑ $PCO_2$<br>Alveolar hypoventilation | $PCO_2$ = +0.6 mm Hg for Δ $[HCO_3^-]$ of 1 mEq/L<br>$PCO_2$ = 15 + $[HCO_3^-]$ | $[PCO_2]$ = 55 mm Hg |

*$PCO_2$*, Carbon dioxide pressure.

Adapted from Bidani A, Tauzon DM, Heming TA. Regulation of whole body acid-base balance. In DuBose TD, Hamm LL, editors: *Acid-base and electrolyte disorders: a companion to Brenner and Rector's the kidney*, Philadelphia: Saunders; 2002, pp 1-2.

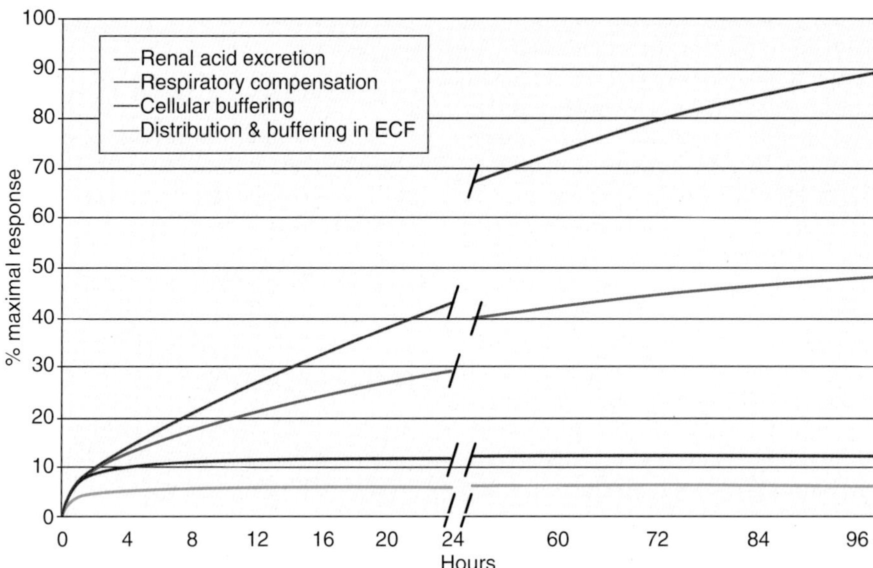


**Fig. 16.4** Conceptual illustration of time course of acid-base compensatory mechanisms in response to a metabolic acid load. Component processes include rapid distribution and extracellular buffering mechanisms and cellular buffering events. But these most rapid mechanisms have limited capacity. Slower are respiratory and renal regulatory processes. *ECF,* Extracellular fluid.

since titratable acid excretion has limited capacity for upregulation (Fig. 16.2). With continued acid loading, renal net acid excretion increases over the course of 3 to 5 days (see Fig. 16.4). Thus, the renal response to an acid load requires 1) reabsorption of the filtered $HCO_3^-$ by the proximal tubule, and 2) augmentation of $NH_4^+$ production and excretion by the distal nephron. In this way, the kidneys efficiently retain all filtered base and attempt to generate enough new base to restore the arterial pH toward normal.

There is some controversy about whether the kidneys *completely* excrete higher than usual acid loads, particularly in patients with CKD. Certainly patients with reduced plasma $HCO_3^-$ have a chronic metabolic acidosis. But some patients with CKD and normal plasma $HCO_3^-$ levels may have positive acid balance (e.g., acid retention), perhaps buffered by bone carbonate and reflected in an acid renal interstitium.[3,12] There is also growing evidence (discussed more below) that not only does acidosis accelerate progression of CKD but that higher ammonium production and excretion may be harmful.[13] On the other hand, in some studies higher urinary acid and ammonia excretion may be beneficial and/or be present in patients with slower progression.[14] Both the mechanistic understandings and clinical implications are under active investigation. Certainly, current recommendations are to maintain plasma $[HCO_3^-] > 22$ mEq/L in patients with CKD with either alkali supplements (see below) or diets with less acid and more fruits and vegetables (more plant-based proteins versus animal-based proteins). Whether to treat patients with CKD with normal plasma $HCO_3^-$ levels is currently under consideration.

## SYSTEMIC RESPONSE TO GAIN OF ALKALI

Base or alkali loads are somewhat less common but rely on the same three systems outlined for defense of an acid challenge, namely, cellular buffering and distribution within the ECF, respiratory compensation, and renal excretion.

### DISTRIBUTION AND CELLULAR BUFFERING

Ninety-five percent of a base load in the form of $HCO_3^-$ is distributed in the ECF within about 25 minutes[2,6,10,15] (see Fig. 16.4). The cellular buffering over the next few hours against an alkaline load is somewhat less effective than the defense against an acid load. There is also poorer stabilization of intracellular pH in the alkaline than in the acid range.[2,15]

### RESPIRATORY COMPENSATION

The pulmonary response to an acute increase in $HCO_3^-$ concentration is biphasic. Neutralization of sodium bicarbonate by buffers ($H^+$ buffer–) results in $CO_2$ liberation and an increase in $PCO_2$:

$$Na^+HCO_3^- + Hbuffer^- \leftrightarrow Na^+buffer^- + H_2CO_3 \leftrightarrow H_2O + CO_2 \quad (16.10)$$

A clinical corollary would be the acute increase in $PCO_2$ observed in patients given intravenous $NaHCO_3$ infusions. The increased $PCO_2$ stimulates ventilation acutely to return $PCO_2$ toward normal. If the pulmonary system is compromised or the ventilation rate is controlled artificially, increased $CO_2$ production from infused sodium bicarbonate can lead to hazardous hypercapnia.[2,6,15]

About an hour after an abrupt increment in the $HCO_3^-$ concentration, when the increased generation of $CO_2$ subsides, stimulation of respiration is transformed into suppression of respiration by elevated pH, and $PCO_2$ increases. This secondary hypercapnic response takes several hours and partially compensates for the elevated $HCO_3^-$ concentration so that arterial pH is returned toward (although not completely to) normal (see Fig. 16.4).

The hypercapnic response to metabolic alkalosis is more difficult to reliably predict than other acid-base disturbances.

Most studies have found that an increase in $PCO_2$ regularly occurs in response to alkalosis. The hypoventilatory response can lead to borderline or even frank hypoxemia in patients with chronic lung disease.[15] In general, the increase in $Paco_2$ can be predicted to equal 0.75 mm Hg per 1.0 mEq/L increase in plasma $HCO_3^-$; or more simply, add the value of 15 to the measured plasma $[HCO_3^-]$[16] to predict the expected $Paco_2$ (see Table 16.1).

## RENAL EXCRETION

### WITH EXTRACELLULAR VOLUME EXPANSION

The addition of sodium bicarbonate to the body results in prompt cellular buffering and respiratory compensation. However, as with an acid load, the kidneys have the ultimate responsibility for the disposal of base and restoration of base stores to normal. The speed and efficiency with which $HCO_3^-$ can be excreted by the kidneys are such that it is difficult to render a patient with normal renal function more than mildly alkalotic on a long-term basis, even when as much as 24 mEq/kg/day of sodium bicarbonate is ingested for several weeks.[15] This efficiency results from the fact that ordinarily the kidneys actively reabsorb some 4000 mEq of $HCO_3^-$ per day; to excrete excess $HCO_3^-$, the kidneys only need to reabsorb less.

The proximal tubule is responsible principally for $HCO_3^-$ excretion when the blood $HCO_3^-$ concentration increases. Absolute proximal $HCO_3^-$ reabsorption does not increase in proportion to $HCO_3^-$ load because of suppression of proximal acidification by alkalemia so that $HCO_3^-$ delivery to the distal nephron increases. The limited capacity of the distal nephron to secrete $H^+$ can be overwhelmed easily, and bicarbonaturia increases progressively. $NH_4^+$ and titratable acid excretion decline in response to the increasing systemic and urine pH.[7,16]

The type B intercalated cell in the collecting tubule also secretes $HCO_3^-$ through the activity of the $HCO_3^-/Cl^-$ exchanger pendrin. In the face of an alkaline systemic pH this exchanger is responsible for net bicarbonate secretion. Accordingly, $HCO_3^-$ secretion by the type B intercalated cell prevents a more severe alkalosis and participates in the $HCO_3^-$ excretory response.

In summary, when kidney function and ECF volume are both normal, an acute base load is excreted entirely, and the blood $HCO_3^-$ concentration is returned to normal within 12 to 24 hours because of depression of fractional proximal $HCO_3^-$ reabsorption. In addition to suppression of reabsorption of the filtered $HCO_3^-$ load, direct $HCO_3^-$ secretion in the cortical collecting tubule (CCT) has been proposed as another mechanism for mediating $HCO_3^-$ disposal during metabolic alkalosis.[16]

The increased delivery of $HCO_3^-$ out of the proximal tubule in response to an increased blood $HCO_3^-$ concentration (and, hence, filtered $HCO_3^-$ load) in the setting of ECF expansion facilitates $HCO_3^-$ excretion and the return of blood pH toward normal. However, other factors may independently enhance distal $H^+$ secretion sufficiently to prevent $HCO_3^-$ excretion and thus counterbalance the suppressed proximal $HCO_3^-$ reabsorption. Under these circumstances, the alkalosis is maintained. For example, in the setting of primary hyperaldosteronism, despite the expanded ECF, a stable mild alkalotic condition persists because of augmented collecting duct $H^+$ secretion.[16] In such cases, concurrent hypokalemia facilitates the generation and maintenance of metabolic alkalosis by enhancing $NH_4^+$ production and excretion.[7,16] Moreover, chronic hypokalemia dramatically enhances the abundance and functionality of the $H^+$–$K^+$–adenosine triphosphatase ($H^+$-$K^+$-ATPase) in the medullary collecting tubule, thus increasing rather than decreasing distal bicarbonate absorption.[16–19]

### WITH EXTRACELLULAR VOLUME CONTRACTION AND POTASSIUM DEFICIENCY

The renal response to an increase in plasma $HCO_3^-$ concentration can be modified significantly in the presence of ECF contraction and $K^+$ depletion. $Na^+$, $Cl^-$, and ECF volume depletion are almost always present together and for most clinical purposes are nearly synonymous. Effective ECF and $K^+$ stores are critical in modifying net $HCO_3^-$ reabsorption. Deficiency of both $Cl^-$ and $K^+$ is common in metabolic alkalosis because of renal and/or gastrointestinal losses that occur concurrently with the generation of the alkalosis.[18,20] With $Cl^-$ depletion alone, the normal bicarbonaturic response to an increase in plasma $HCO_3^-$ is prevented and metabolic alkalosis can develop. $K^+$ depletion, even without mineralocorticoid administration, can cause metabolic alkalosis. When $Cl^-$ and $K^+$ depletion coexist, severe metabolic alkalosis may develop.

Two general mechanisms serve to maintain increased plasma $HCO_3^-$ in the setting of $Cl^-$ and $K^+$ depletion: 1) decreased glomerular filtration rate (GFR) and therefore diminished $HCO_3^-$ filtration, and 2) increased $HCO_3^-$ reabsorption and increased new $HCO_3^-$ generation by acid excretion.[16–19,21] That extracellular and plasma volume depletion decrease GFR is well documented. GFR can also be decreased by $K^+$ depletion, possibly the result of increased production of the vasoconstrictors angiotensin II and thromboxane $B_2$.[17,19] By reducing filtered $HCO_3^-$ (compared to what it would be with elevated plasma $HCO_3^-$ in metabolic alkalosis), all of the filtered $HCO_3^-$ can be reabsorbed without any increase in proximal or distal $HCO_3^-$ reabsorption. But as to the second mechanism, $Cl^-$ deficiency and/or $K^+$ deficiency do increase overall renal $HCO_3^-$ reabsorption in the setting of a normal GFR and high filtered $HCO_3^-$ load. Overall renal $HCO_3^-$ reabsorption and, therefore, acidification is increased. An increase in renal acidification occurs as a result of an increase in $H^+$ secretion by the proximal and the distal nephron.[16–18] The increase in $HCO_3^-$ absorption in the proximal tubule is due, at least in part, to an increase in the delivered load of $HCO_3^-$. The augmented $HCO_3^-$ absorption in distal nephron segments appears to be due to a primary increase in $H^+$ secretion that is independent of the $HCO_3^-$ load delivered. Chronic hypokalemia dramatically enhances the abundance and function of the $H^+$, $K^+$-ATPase in the medullary collecting tubule. Therefore, upregulation of the $H^+$, $K^+$-ATPase by hypokalemia may be a significant factor in the maintenance of chronic metabolic alkalosis.[17,22,23]

The maintenance of a high plasma $HCO_3^-$ concentration by the kidney can be repaired by repletion of $Cl^-$.[24] The mechanism by which $Cl^-$ repairs metabolic alkalosis may include normalization of the low GFR that was induced by ECF repletion. In addition, $Cl^-$ repletion results in a decrease in proximal $HCO_3^-$ reabsorption and an increase in $HCO_3^-$ secretion by the distal nephron.

In summary, the normal physiologic response by the kidney to a base load associated with volume *expansion* is to excrete the base. In the setting of $K^+$ and/or $Cl^-$ deficiency, base is instead retained by a decreased GFR, an increased proximal $HCO_3^-$ reabsorption, and enhanced distal $HCO_3^-$ reabsorption, acid excretion.

## STEPWISE APPROACH TO THE DIAGNOSIS OF ACID-BASE DISORDERS

Acid-base derangements are important for their own physiologic consequences but also as indicators of underlying processes, which sometimes may not be otherwise apparent. Therefore, analysis of acid-base status is important in many clinical circumstances, particularly in the critically ill. An acid-base disorder may be suspected from the clinical circumstance, from an abnormal arterial blood gas (ABG; i.e, abnormal pH, $Paco_2$, or $HCO_3^-$ concentration), or from abnormal electrolytes even in the absence of a blood gas. It is important to stress that relying only on serial oxygen saturation levels in a critically ill patient is inadequate when assessing the acid-base status of a patient.

The four simple acid-base disorders and the predicted compensatory responses are summarized in Table 16.1. The complete diagnosis can best be determined by a stepwise approach presented below (Table 16.2).[25] Before initiating direct examination of acid-base parameters, certain parameters such as history and other electrolytes should be considered.

### CLINICAL AND LABORATORY PARAMETERS IN ACID-BASE DISORDERS

For correct diagnosis of a simple or mixed acid-base disorder, it is imperative that a careful history be obtained. Patients with pneumonia, sepsis, or cardiac failure frequently have a respiratory alkalosis, and patients with chronic obstructive pulmonary disease or a sedative drug overdose often display respiratory acidosis. *The clinical setting of an acid-base disorder may be much more revealing than complex formulas.* The patient's drug history assumes importance because patients taking loop or thiazide diuretics may have metabolic alkalosis and patients receiving acetazolamide frequently have metabolic acidosis. Physical findings are often helpful as well. Tetany may occur with alkalemia, cyanosis with respiratory acidosis, and volume contraction with metabolic alkalosis.

**Table 16.2 Systematic Method for Diagnosis of Simple and Mixed Acid-Base Disorders**

1. Measure arterial blood gas and electrolyte concentrations simultaneously.
2. Determine whether the compensation is appropriate for a simple acid-base disorder; if inappropriate, a mixed acid-base disorder is present (see Table 16.1 and Fig. 16.5).
3. Calculate the anion gap (corrected for albumin) to determine the presence of a high AG metabolic acidosis.
   Appreciate the four major categories of high anion gap acidoses: ketoacidosis, lactic acidosis, renal failure acidosis, toxin- or poison-induced acidosis
   Appreciate the two major causes of non—AG acidoses: gastrointestinal loss of $HCO_3^-$, renal loss of $HCO_3^-$
4. Compare the relative changes of $HCO_3^-$ and AG ($\Delta HCO_3^-$ and $\Delta$AG, respectively) to look for mixed disorders (see text).

The plasma $K^+$ value is often useful but should be considered only in conjunction with the $HCO_3^-$ concentration and blood pH. It is generally appreciated that the serum $K^+$ value can be altered by primary acid-base disturbances as a result of shifts of $K^+$ either into the extracellular compartment or into the intracellular compartment.[26] Metabolic acidosis frequently leads to hyperkalemia. Some suggest that for each decrease in blood pH of 0.10 pH unit, the $K^+$ concentration should increase by 0.6 mEq/L. Thus, a patient with a pH of 7.20 would be expected to have a plasma $K^+$ value of 5.2 mEq/L. However, considerable variation in this relationship has been reported in several conditions due to endogenous acid production, especially diabetic ketoacidosis (DKA) and lactic acidosis, which are often associated with $K^+$ depletion. The lack of correlation between the degree of acidemia and the plasma $K^+$ level is a result of several factors, including the nature and cellular permeability of the accompanying anion, the magnitude of the osmotic diuresis, the level of renal function, the presence or absence of preexisting changes in $K^+$ homeostasis, and the degree of catabolism. It is important to appreciate that the relationship between arterial blood pH and plasma $K^+$ is complex and therefore often variable. Nevertheless, the failure of a patient with severe acidosis to exhibit hyperkalemia or, conversely, the failure of a patient with severe metabolic alkalosis to exhibit hypokalemia raises the possibility of a significant derangement of body $K^+$ homeostasis. The combination of a low plasma $K^+$ and elevated $HCO_3^-$ suggests metabolic alkalosis (or the action of aldosterone or the like, see below), whereas the combination of an elevated plasma $K^+$ and low $HCO_3^-$ suggests metabolic acidosis.

It is helpful to compare the serum $Cl^-$ concentration with the $Na^+$ concentration. In the absence of an exogenous source of concentrated sodium (e.g. hypertonic saline or $NaHCO_3$), the serum $Na^+$ concentration changes only as a result of changes in hydration or total body water. The Cl– concentration changes for two reasons: 1) changes in hydration and 2) changes in acid-base balance. Thus, changes in $Cl^-$ not reflected by proportional changes in $Na^+$ suggest the presence of an acid-base disorder. For example, consider a patient with a history of vomiting, volume depletion, a $Cl^-$ concentration of 85 mEq/L, and an $Na^+$ concentration of 130 mEq/L. In this case, both $Na^+$ and $Cl^-$ are reduced, but the reduction in Cl– is proportionally greater (15% versus 7%). A disproportionate decrease in $Cl^-$ suggests metabolic alkalosis or respiratory acidosis, and a disproportionate increase in $Cl^-$ suggests metabolic acidosis or respiratory alkalosis.

The four simple acid-base disorders and the predicted compensatory responses are summarized in Table 16.1. The complete diagnosis, including the possibility of complex mixed disturbances, can best be determined by a stepwise approach (Table 16.2).

## STEP 1: MEASURE ARTERIAL BLOOD GAS AND ELECTROLYTE VALUES

For a complete diagnosis of acid-base disorders, one needs both an ABG and a simultaneous set of electrolytes. For a simple single disorder, the diagnosis is easy: if the pH is low, a respiratory acidosis (with high $PCO_2$ and somewhat high $HCO_3^-$) or metabolic acidosis (with low $HCO_3^-$ and secondarily low $PCO_2$) is present. The opposite situations occur with high pH. Or with electrolytes, if the $HCO_3^-$ concentration is low and the $Cl^-$ concentration is high, either chronic respiratory alkalosis or hyperchloremic metabolic acidosis is present. The ABG determination serves to differentiate the two conditions. Although both have a decreased $Pa{CO_2}$, the pH is high with a primary respiratory alkalosis and low in a metabolic acidosis. Chronic respiratory acidosis and metabolic alkalosis are both associated with high $HCO_3^-$ and low $Cl^-$ concentration in plasma. Again, a pH measurement distinguishes the two conditions.

But neither ABG nor electrolytes alone can necessarily give a complete picture. For instance, an ABG alone may miss mixed disorders, which are only revealed by an analysis of the anion gap (see later discussion). And while electrolyte abnormalities may suggest an acid-base disorder (e.g., high anion gap metabolic acidosis), the actual pH and the complete diagnosis with compensatory response requires an ABG. Of note, the calculated value for $HCO_3^-$ or (total $CO_2$) reported with the ABG should be within ±2 mEq/L of the measured $HCO_3^-$ concentration (total $CO_2$) obtained on the electrolyte panel. A greater difference may imply a laboratory error or non-simultaneous measurements.

## STEP 2: DETERMINE THE COMPENSATION TO DISTINGUISH SIMPLE FROM MIXED ACID-BASE DISORDERS

In many clinical situations, a mixture of acid-base disorders may exist. Diagnosis of these disturbances requires additional information and a more complex analysis of data.

A convenient, but not always reliable, approach is an acid-base map, such as the one displayed in Fig. 16.5, which defines the 95% confidence limits of simple acid-base disorders.[26,27] If the arterial acid-base values fall within one of the blue bands in Fig. 16.3, one may assume that a simple acid-base disturbance is present, and a tentative diagnostic category can be assigned. There can be complex exceptions. Values that fall outside the blue areas imply, but do not prove, that a mixed disorder exists.

The two broad types of acid-base disorders are metabolic and respiratory. Metabolic acidosis and alkalosis are disorders characterized by primary disturbances in the concentration of $HCO_3^-$ in plasma, whereas respiratory disorders involve primarily alteration of $Pa{CO_2}$. The most commonly encountered clinical disturbances are simple acid-base disorders, that is, one of the four cardinal acid-base disturbances—metabolic acidosis, metabolic alkalosis, respiratory acidosis, or respiratory alkalosis—occurring in a pure or simple form. More complicated clinical situations, especially in severely ill patients, may give rise to *mixed acid-base disturbances.*[27]

To appreciate and recognize a mixed acid-base disturbance, it is important to understand the physiologic compensatory responses that occur in the simple acid-base disorders. Primary respiratory disturbances invoke secondary metabolic responses, and primary metabolic disturbances evoke a predictable respiratory response (see Table 16.1 and Fig. 16.3). *These predictable compensations are defined as being part of the primary simple acid-base disorder.* To illustrate, metabolic acidosis as a result of gain of endogenous acids (e.g., lactic acid or ketoacidosis) lowers the concentration of $HCO_3^-$ in the ECF and thus extracellular pH. As a result of *acidemia,* the medullary chemoreceptors are stimulated and invoke an increase in ventilation. As a result of the hypocapnic response, the ratio of $HCO_3^-$ to $Pa{CO_2}$ and the subsequent pH are returned

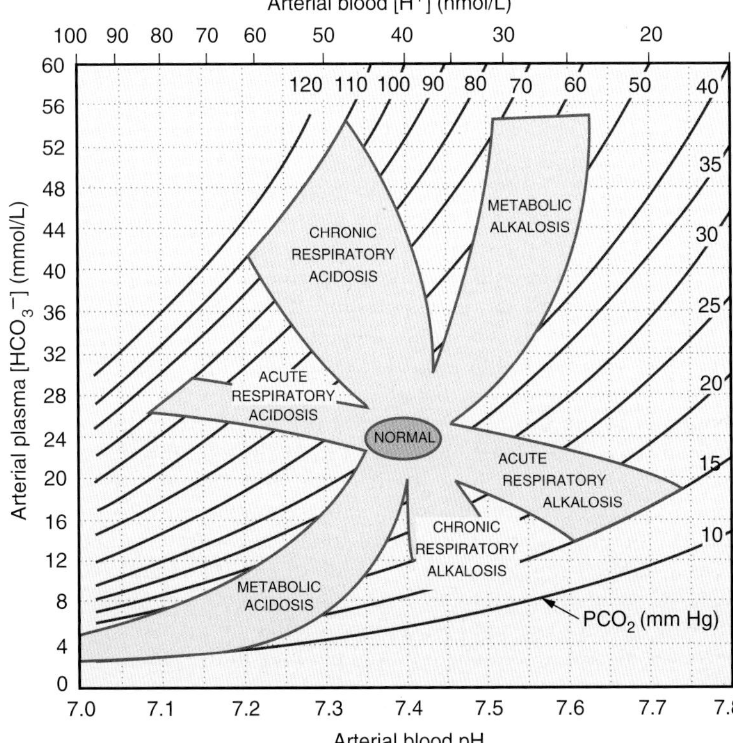


**Fig. 16.5** Acid-base nomogram (map). *Shaded areas* represent the 95% confidence limits of the normal respiratory and metabolic compensations for primary acid-base disturbances. Data falling *outside the shaded areas* denote a mixed disorder if a laboratory error is not present (see text).

toward, but not completely to, normal. Thus, a patient with metabolic acidosis and a plasma $HCO_3^-$ concentration of 12 mEq/L would be expected to have a $Paco_2$ between 24 and 28 mm Hg. Values of $Paco_2$ below 24 or higher than 28 mm Hg define a *mixed metabolic-respiratory disturbance* (metabolic acidosis and respiratory alkalosis or metabolic acidosis and respiratory acidosis, respectively). Therefore, by definition, an inappropriate compensation, too little or too much, identifies one form of a mixed acid-base disturbance.

*Compensation is a predictable physiologic consequence of the primary disturbance and does not represent a secondary acidosis or alkalosis* (see Fig. 16.5 and Table 16.1). The recognition of mixed disturbances may alert one to an additional clinical disorder that may require immediate attention or additional therapy (e.g., inadequate respiratory response to metabolic acidosis defining a respiratory acidosis).

The limits of compensation should also be recognized (see Table 16.1). For example, the plasma $HCO_3^-$ concentration rarely falls below 12 to 15 mEq/L as a result of compensation for respiratory alkalosis and rarely exceeds 45 mEq/L as a result of compensation for respiratory acidosis.[27]

## STEP 3: CALCULATE THE ANION GAP TO DETERMINE THE PRESENCE OF A HIGH AG METABOLIC ACIDOSIS

All evaluations of acid-base disorders should include a simple calculation of the AG since an elevated AG usually implies a metabolic acidosis. The AG is calculated from the serum electrolytes and is defined as follows:

$$AG = Na^+ - (Cl^- + HCO_3^-) = 10 \pm 2 \text{ mEq/L} \qquad (16.11)$$

The AG represents the unmeasured anions normally present in plasma and unaccounted for by the serum electrolytes exclusive of $K^+$ that are measured on the electrolyte panel. Normal values for AG vary with the laboratory and analyte measurement techniques, but in general have declined with more precise measurement of serum electrolytes by ion selective electrodes. The normal value for AG ranges from 8-12 mEq/L, but the clinician should know the normal value for the AG in clinical laboratories used in their practice. Because of this range of normal values for the AG and for convenience, the following computations will use the value of 10 mEq/L as the "normal" anion gap. The unmeasured anions that contribute to this value are normally present in serum and include anionic proteins (principally albumin and, to lesser extent, α- and β-globulins), $PO_4^{3}$–, $SO_4^{2}$–, and organic anions. As already emphasized, interpretation of the anion gap requires either a normal serum albumin, or correction of the AG to a normal plasma albumin. In general, reduction in the serum albumin level by 1 g/dL from the normal value of 4.5 g/dL decreases the AG by 2.5 mEq/L. When acid anions, such as acetoacetate and lactate, are produced endogenously in excess and accumulate in ECF, the AG increases above the normal value. This is referred to as a *high anion gap* acidosis.[27,28] Additionally, in a simple high AG metabolic acidosis, for each milliequivalent per liter increase in the corrected AG, there should be an equal decrease, measured as milliequivalent per liter, in the plasma $HCO_3^-$ concentration.

A number of conditions other than metabolic acidosis can occasionally change the AG up or down (Table 16.3). An increase in the AG may be due to a decrease in unmeasured cations or an increase in unmeasured anions. Combined severe hypocalcemia and hypomagnesemia represent a decrease in the contribution of unmeasured cations. In addition, the AG may increase secondary to an increase in anionic albumin, as a consequence of either an increased albumin concentration or alkalemia.[27,28] The increased AG in severe alkalemia can be explained in part by the effect of alkaline pH on the electrical charge of albumin.

A decrease in the AG can be generated by an increase in unmeasured cations or a decrease in unmeasured anions (see Table 16.3). A decrease in the AG can result from 1) an increase in unmeasured cations ($Ca^{2+}$, $Mg^{2+}$, $K^+$), or 2) the addition to the blood of abnormal cations, such as $Li^+$ ($Li^+$ intoxication) or cationic immunoglobulins (immunoglobulin G as in plasma cell dyscrasias). Because albumin is the major unmeasured anion, the AG will also decrease if the quantity of albumin is low (e.g., nephrotic syndrome, protein malnutrition, capillary leak).[29] Since with each decline in the serum albumin level by 1 g/dL from the normal value of 4.5 g/dL, the AG will decline by 2.5 mEq/L. When hypoalbuminemia exists, it is possible to underestimate the AG and even miss an increased AG unless correction for the low albumin and its effect on the AG is taken into account. For example, in a patient with an albumin level of 1.5 g/dL

**Table 16.3 Anion Gap = $Na^+ - (Cl^- + HCO_3^-) = 9 \pm 3$ mEq/L (Assumes Normal Albumin)[a]**

| Increased Anion Gap | Decreased Anion Gap |
|---|---|
| **Increased Anions (Not $Cl^-$ or $HCO_3^-$)** | **Increased Cations (Not $Na^+$)** |
| ↑ **Albumin** | ↑ $Ca^{2+}$, $Mg^{2+}$ |
| Alkalosis | ↑ $Li^+$ |
| ↑ Inorganic anions | ↑ Immunoglobulin G |
| Phosphate | |
| Sulfate | **Decreased Anions (Not $Cl^-$ or $HCO_3^-$)** |
| ↑ **Organic anions** | |
| **L-Lactate** | **Hypoalbuminemia**[a] |
| D-Lactate | Acidosis |
| **Ketones** | |
| **Uremic** | **Laboratory Error** |
| ↑ Exogenously supplied anions | Hyperviscosity |
| **Salicylate** | Bromism |
| Paraldehyde | |
| **Ethylene glycol** | |
| Propylene glycol | |
| **Methanol** | |
| Toluene | |
| Pyroglutamic acid (5-oxyprolene) | |
| Other toxins | |
| **Uremic** | |
| Hyperosmolar, nonketotic states | |
| Myoglobinuric acute renal failure | |
| **Decreased Cations (Not $Na^+$)** | |
| ↓ $Ca^{2+}$, $Mg^{2+}$ | |

[a]For each decline in albumin by 1 g/dL from normal (4.5 g/dL), the anion gap decreases by 2.5 mEq/L.

**The items in bold are most common or notable.**

and an uncorrected AG of 10 mEq/L, the "corrected" AG is 17.5 mEq/L.

Laboratory errors can create a falsely low AG. Hyperviscosity and hyperlipidemia lead to an underestimation of the true $Na^+$ concentration, and bromide ($Br^-$) intoxication causes an overestimation of the true $Cl^-$ concentration.[27]

In the presence of a normal serum albumin level, elevation of unmeasured anions is usually due to addition of non–$Cl^-$-containing acid anion (e.g., lactate). *Thus, in most clinical circumstances, a high AG indicates that a metabolic acidosis is present.* The anions accompanying such acids include inorganic ($PO_4^{3}$–, $SO_4^{2}$–), organic (ketoacids, lactate, uremic organic anions), exogenous (salicylate or ingested toxins with organic acid production), or unidentified anions.[27] The preexisting $Cl^-$ concentration is unchanged when the new acid anion is added to the blood. Therefore, the high AG acidoses exhibit normochloremia as well as a high gap. If the kidney does not excrete the anion, the magnitude of the decrement in $HCO_3^-$ concentration will match the increment in the AG. If the retained anion can be metabolized to $HCO_3^-$ directly or indirectly (e.g., ketones or lactate, after successful treatment), normal acid-base balance is restored as the AG returns toward the normal value. Alternatively, if the anion is excreted, hyperchloremic acidosis may emerge as the anion is excreted and the AG disappears.

The presence of a significant elevation of the AG (unexplained by laboratory error or the unusual conditions noted) implies the presence of a metabolic acidosis process whether or not acidemia (low pH) exists.[30] For instance, a coexisting respiratory alkalosis or metabolic alkalosis could dominate the net pH even in the presence of a metabolic acidosis.

Utility of identifying an elevated AG derives from knowledge of the four causes of a high AG metabolic acidosis: 1) ketoacidosis, 2) lactic acidosis, 3) renal failure acidosis, and 4) toxin-induced metabolic acidosis (Table 16.4). In contrast, if the AG is normal in the face of metabolic acidosis, a hyperchloremic or non-AG acidosis exists. The specific causes of hyperchloremic acidosis that must be appreciated are outlined in a later section. Table 16.4 displays the directional changes in pH, $PCO_2$, and $HCO_3^-$ for the four simple acid-base disorders. With this stepwise approach, in subsequent sections, the specific causes of the major types of acid-base disorders are reviewed in detail.

**Table 16.4 Clinical Causes of High Anion Gap and Normal Anion Gap Acidosis**

| High Anion Gap Acidosis | Non-Anion Gap Acidosis |
|---|---|
| Ketoacidosis | Gastrointestinal loss of $HCO_3^-$ (negative urine anion gap) |
| **Diabetic ketoacidosis** | **Diarrhea** |
| **Alcoholic ketoacidosis** | External fistula |
| Starvation ketoacidosis | **Renal loss of $HCO_3^-$ or failure to excrete NH4⁺** |
| Lactic acidosis | Positive urine anion gap = low net acid excretion |
| **L-Lactic acidosis (types A and B)** | Proximal renal tubular acidosis (RTA) (low serum $K^+$) |
| D-Lactic acidosis | Classical distal renal tubular acidosis (low serum $K^+$) |
| **Renal failure acidosis** | **Generalized distal renal tubular defect (high serum $K^+$)** |
| Toxin-induced acidosis | **Drugs that cause RTA** |
| **Ethylene glycol** | Carbonic anhydrase inhibitors (mixed proximal-distal RTA) |
| **Methyl alcohol** | Amphotericin B ("gradient" classical distal RTA) |
| **Salicylate** | **Miscellaneous** |
| Propylene glycol | NH4Cl ingestion |
| Pyroglutamic acid (5-oxyprolene) | Sulfur ingestion |
| | Dilutional acidosis |

*RTA,* Renal tubular acidosis.
**The items in bold are most common or notable.**

## STEP 4: COMPARE RELATIVE CHANGES OF $HCO_3^-$ AND AG (DELTA/DELTA)

By definition, a high AG acidosis has two identifying features: a low $HCO_3^-$ concentration and an elevated AG. The elevated AG will remain present even if another disorder coincides to modify the $HCO_3^-$ concentration independently. Simultaneous metabolic acidosis of the high AG variety plus either metabolic alkalosis or chronic respiratory acidosis is an example of such a situation. The resulting $HCO_3^-$ concentration may be normal or even high in such a setting. However, the AG will be high, and the $Cl^-$ concentration relatively depressed. Consider a patient with chronic obstructive pulmonary disease with compensated respiratory acidosis ($Paco_2$ of 65 mm Hg and $HCO_3^-$ concentration of 40 mEq/L initially) in whom acute bronchopneumonia and respiratory decompensation develop. If this patient has an $HCO_3^-$ concentration of 24 mEq/L, $Na^+$ of 145 mEq/L, $K^+$ of 4.8 mEq/L, and $Cl^-$ of 96 mEq/L, it would be incorrect to assume that this "normal" $HCO_3^-$ concentration represents improvement in acid-base status toward normal. Indeed, the arterial pH would probably be low (7.19), as a result of a more serious degree of hypercapnia than observed previously (e.g., if the $PCO_2$ increased from 65 to 80 mm Hg as a result of pneumonia). Even without blood gas measurements, prompt recognition that the AG was elevated to 25 mEq/L should suggest that a life-threatening lactic acidosis is superimposed on a preexisting chronic respiratory acidosis, which necessitates immediate therapy. In this example, the change in AG, frequently referred to as ΔAG, is computed as 25–10, or patient's calculated AG minus the normal AG, and is equal to 15 mEq/L.

Similarly, a normal arterial $HCO_3^-$ concentration, $Paco_2$, and pH do not ensure the absence of an acid-base disturbance. For example, an alcoholic patient who has been vomiting may develop a metabolic alkalosis with a pH of 7.55, $HCO_3^-$ concentration of 40 mEq/L, $PCO_2$ of 48 mm Hg, $Na^+$ of 135 mEq/L, $Cl^-$ of 80 mEq/L, and $K^+$ of 2.8 mEq/L. If such a patient were then to develop a superimposed alcoholic ketoacidosis (AKA) with a β-hydroxybutyrate concentration of 15 mmol/L, the arterial pH would fall to 7.40, $HCO_3^-$ concentration to 25 mEq/L, and $PCO_2$ to 40 mm Hg. Although the blood gas values are normal, the AG (assuming no change in $Na^+$ or $Cl^-$) is elevated (25 mEq/L), and the ΔAG is 15 mEq/L, which indicates the existence of a mixed metabolic acid-base disorder (mixed metabolic alkalosis and metabolic acidosis). The combination of metabolic acidosis and metabolic alkalosis is not uncommon and is most easily recognized, as in this case, when the ΔAG is elevated, but the $HCO_3^-$ concentration and pH are near normal (ΔAG > $ΔHCO_3^-$, or 15 vs. 0 mEq/L).

Although a variety of formulaic approaches have been proposed to compare the ΔAG and $ΔHCO_3^-$, a conceptual approach as above with attention to the clinical ingredients is most useful. With an elevated AG, if the $HCO_3^-$ is higher than expected based on the ΔAG, then suspect a coexisting metabolic alkalosis or chronic respiratory acidosis (which also elevates the $HCO_3^-$). With an elevated AG, if the $HCO_3^-$ is lower than expected (or Cl-higher) based on the ΔAG, suspect a coexisting hyperchloremic metabolic acidosis or chronic respiratory alkalosis.

### MIXED ACID-BASE DISORDERS

Mixed acid-base disorders—defined as independently coexisting disorders, not merely compensatory responses—are often seen in patients in critical care units and can lead to dangerous extremes of pH. Patients with underlying pulmonary disease may not respond to metabolic acidosis with an appropriate ventilatory response because of insufficient respiratory reserve. Such imposition of respiratory acidosis on metabolic acidosis can lead to severe acidemia and a poor outcome. Note that failure of an appropriate ventilator response to metabolic acidosis represents a combined metabolic acidosis and respiratory acidosis. A patient with DKA (metabolic acidosis) may develop an independent respiratory problem, leading to respiratory acidosis or alkalosis. When metabolic acidosis and metabolic alkalosis coexist in the same patient, the pH may be normal or near normal. When the pH is normal, an elevated AG denotes the presence of a metabolic acidosis. A discrepancy in the ΔAG (prevailing minus normal AG of 10 mEq/L) and the $ΔHCO_3^-$ (normal, 25 mEq/L, minus prevailing $HCO_3^-$) indicates the presence of a mixed high gap acidosis–metabolic alkalosis (see example later).

Even more complex are triple acid-base disturbances. For example, patients with metabolic acidosis due to alcoholic ketoacidosis may develop metabolic alkalosis due to vomiting and superimposed respiratory alkalosis due to the hyperventilation of hepatic dysfunction or alcohol withdrawal. Conversely, when hyperchloremic acidosis and metabolic alkalosis occur concomitantly, the increase in $Cl^-$ is out of proportion to the change in $HCO_3^-$ concentration ($ΔCl^- > ΔHCO_3^-$).[27]

In summary, an AG exceeding that expected for a patient's albumin concentration, i.e. > 10 mEq/L, denotes the existence of either a simple high AG metabolic acidosis or a complex acid-base disorder in which an organic acidosis is superimposed on another acid-base disorder.

## RESPIRATORY DISORDERS

### RESPIRATORY ACIDOSIS

Respiratory acidosis occurs as the result of severe pulmonary disease, respiratory muscle disorders, or depression in ventilatory control. An increase in $Paco_2$ owing to reduced alveolar ventilation is the primary abnormality leading to acidemia. In acute respiratory acidosis, there is an immediate small compensatory elevation in $HCO_3^-$ (due to cellular buffering mechanisms) of 1 mEq/L for every 10 mm Hg increase in $Paco_2$. In chronic respiratory acidosis (>24 hours), renal adaption is achieved and the $HCO_3^-$ increases by 4 mEq/L for every 10 mm Hg increase in $Paco_2$. The serum bicarbonate concentration usually does not increase above 38 mEq/L, however.

The clinical features of respiratory acidosis vary according to the underlying disease, the severity, duration, and presence or absence of accompanying hypoxemia. A rapid increase in $Paco_2$ may result in anxiety, dyspnea, confusion, psychosis, and hallucinations and may progress to coma. More subtle dysfunction in chronic hypercapnia may include sleep disturbances, loss of memory, daytime somnolence, and personality changes. Coordination may be impaired, and motor disturbances such as tremor, myoclonic jerks, and asterixis may develop. The sensitivity of the cerebral vasculature to the vasodilating effects of $CO_2$ can cause headaches and other signs that mimic increased intracranial pressure, such as papilledema, abnormal reflexes, and focal muscle weakness.

Causes of respiratory acidosis are listed in Table 16.5. A reduction in ventilatory drive from depression of the respiratory center by a variety of drugs, injury, or disease can produce respiratory acidosis. Acutely, this may occur with general anesthetics, sedatives, narcotics, alcohol, and head trauma. Chronic causes of respiratory center depression include sedatives, alcohol, intracranial tumors, and the syndromes of sleep-disordered breathing, including the primary alveolar and obesity-hypoventilation syndromes. Neuromuscular disorders involving abnormalities or disease in the motor neurons, neuromuscular junction, and skeletal muscle can cause hypoventilation. Although a number of diseases should be considered in the differential diagnosis, drugs and electrolyte disorders should always be ruled out.

Mechanical ventilation, may result in respiratory acidosis when not properly adjusted and supervised or when complicated by barotrauma or displacement of the endotracheal tube. This occurs if carbon dioxide production rises (e.g., fever, agitation, sepsis, overfeeding) or if alveolar ventilation falls because of worsening pulmonary function. High levels of positive end-expiratory pressure in the presence of reduced cardiac output may cause hypercapnia as a result of large increases in alveolar dead space.

Permissive hypercapnia may be utilized in the critical care setting since lower tidal volumes may reduce the incidence of the barotrauma associated with high airway pressure and peak airway pressures in mechanically ventilated patients with respiratory distress syndrome.[31] Acute hypercapnia of any cause can lead to severe acidemia, neurologic dysfunction, and death. However, when $CO_2$ levels are allowed to increase gradually, the resulting acidosis is less severe, and the elevation in arterial $PCO_2$ is tolerated more readily. Although the resulting hypercapnia is not the goal of this approach, but secondary to the attempt to limit airway pressures, the arterial pH will decline. The magnitude of the acidemia associated with permissive hypercapnia may be augmented if superimposed on metabolic acidosis, such as lactic acidosis. This combination is not uncommon in the critical care unit. Bicarbonate infusion may be indicated with mixed metabolic acidosis–respiratory acidosis, but the goal of therapy with alkali is to not increase the bicarbonate and pH to normal. With low tidal volume ventilation, a reasonable therapeutic

**Table 16.5 Respiratory Acid-Base Disorders**

| Alkalosis |
|---|
| Central nervous system stimulation |
| Pain |
| Anxiety |
| Psychosis |
| Fever |
| Cerebrovascular accident |
| Meningitis |
| Encephalitis |
| Tumor |
| Trauma |
| Hypoxemia or tissue hypoxia |
| High-altitude acclimatization |
| Pneumonia, Pulmonary edema |
| Aspiration |
| Severe anemia |
| Drugs or hormones |
| Pregnancy (progesterone) |
| Salicylates |
| Nikethamide |
| Stimulation of chest receptors |
| Hemothorax |
| Flail chest |
| Cardiac failure |
| Pulmonary embolism |
| Miscellaneous |
| Septicemia |
| Hepatic failure |
| Mechanical hyperventilation |
| Heat exposure |
| Recovery from metabolic acidosis |
| **Acidosis** |
| Central nervous system depression |
| Drugs (anesthetics, morphine, sedatives) |
| Stroke |
| Infection |
| Airway obstruction |
| Asthma |
| Parenchyma disease |
| Emphysema/chronic obstructive pulmonary disease |
| Pneumoconiosis |
| Bronchitis |
| Adult respiratory distress syndrome |
| Barotrauma |
| Mechanical ventilation |
| Hypoventilation |
| Permissive hypercapnia |
| Neuromuscular |
| Poliomyelitis |
| Kyphoscoliosis |
| Myasthenia gravis |
| Muscular dystrophies |
| Multiple sclerosis |
| Miscellaneous |
| Obesity |
| Hypoventilation |

target for arterial pH is approximately 7.25.[31] Moreover, with hypercapnia in the range of 60 mm Hg, a larger amount of bicarbonate will be necessary to achieve this goal. Bicarbonate administration will further increase the $PCO_2$, especially in patients with fixed rates of ventilation, and will add to the magnitude of the hypercapnia. Use of a continuous bicarbonate infusion in this setting may be necessary, but frequent monitoring of arterial blood gases, electrolytes, and the volume status of the patient is necessary.

Disease and obstruction of the airways, when severe or long-standing, causes respiratory acidosis. Acute hypercapnia follows sudden occlusion of the upper airway or the more generalized bronchospasm that occurs with severe asthma, anaphylaxis, and inhalational burn or toxin injury. Chronic hypercapnia and respiratory acidosis occur in end-stage obstructive lung disease.[5] Restrictive disorders involving either the chest wall or the lungs can cause acute and chronic hypercapnia. Rapidly progressing restrictive processes in the lung can lead to respiratory acidosis, because the high cost of breathing causes ventilatory muscle fatigue. Intrapulmonary and extrapulmonary restrictive defects present as chronic respiratory acidosis in their most advanced stages.

The diagnosis of respiratory acidosis requires, by definition, the measurement of arterial $Paco_2$ and pH. Detailed history and physical examination often provide important diagnostic clues to the nature and duration of the acidosis. When a diagnosis of respiratory acidosis is made, its cause should be investigated. Chest radiography is an initial step. Pulmonary function studies, including spirometry, diffusion capacity, lung volumes, and arterial $Paco_2$ and oxygen saturation usually provide adequate assessment of whether respiratory acidosis is secondary to lung disease. Workup for nonpulmonary causes should include a detailed drug history, measurement of hematocrit, and assessment of upper airway, chest wall, pleura, and neuromuscular function.[4,5]

The treatment of respiratory acidosis depends on the underlying disease, the severity and rate of onset. Acute respiratory acidosis can be life-threatening, and measures to reverse the underlying cause should be undertaken simultaneously with restoration of adequate alveolar ventilation to relieve severe hypoxemia and acidemia. Temporarily, this may necessitate tracheal intubation and assisted mechanical ventilation. Oxygen level should be carefully titrated in patients with severe chronic obstructive pulmonary disease and chronic $CO_2$ retention who are breathing spontaneously. When oxygen is used injudiciously, these patients may experience progression of the respiratory acidosis when ventilation is driven by oxygen pressure ($Pao_2$) and not the normal parameters of $Paco_2$ and pH. Aggressive and rapid correction of hypercapnia should be avoided, because the falling $Paco_2$ may provoke the same complications noted with acute respiratory alkalosis (i.e., cardiac arrhythmias, reduced cerebral perfusion, and seizures). It is advisable to lower the $Paco_2$ gradually in chronic respiratory acidosis, with the aim of restoring the $Paco_2$ to baseline levels while at the same time providing sufficient chloride and potassium to enhance the renal excretion of bicarbonate.[5]

Chronic respiratory acidosis is frequently difficult to correct, but general measures aimed at maximizing lung function, including cessation of smoking; use of oxygen, bronchodilators, corticosteroids, etc. and/or diuretics; and physiotherapy can help some patients and can forestall further deterioration.

Various respiratory stimulants used in the past are seldom utilized presently.

## RESPIRATORY ALKALOSIS

Alveolar hyperventilation decreases the $Pa{CO_2}$ and increases the $HCO_3^-/Pa{CO_2}$ ratio, thus increasing pH (alkalemia). Nonbicarbonate cellular buffers respond by titrating $HCO_3^-$ down. Hypocapnia develops whenever a sufficiently strong ventilatory stimulus causes $CO_2$ output in the lungs to exceed the metabolic production of $CO_2$ by tissues. Plasma pH and $HCO_3^-$ concentration vary approximately proportionately with $Pa{CO_2}$ over a range from 40 to 15 mm Hg. The arterial $[HCO_3^-]$ will decrease acutely approximately 2 mEq/L for each 10 mm Hg decrease in $PCO_2$. The relationship between pH and $Pa{CO_2}$ is about 0.01 pH unit/mm Hg.[4]

Beyond 2 to 6 hours, sustained hypocapnia is further compensated by renal response, a decrease in renal ammonium and titratable acid excretion and a reduction in filtered $HCO_3^-$ reabsorption. The full expression of renal adaptation may take several days and depends on a normal volume status and renal function. The kidneys appear to respond directly to the lowered $Pa{CO_2}$ rather than to the alkalemia per se, although both pH and $PCO_2$ may be factors. With chronic respiratory alkalosis, a 1 mm Hg fall in $Pa{CO_2}$ causes a 0.4 to 0.5 mEq/L drop in $HCO_3^-$ and a 0.003 unit rise in pH, or the $[HCO_3^-]$ will decrease 4 mEq/L for each 10 mm Hg decrease in $Pa{CO_2}$.[4] Chronic respiratory alkalosis is an exception to the general rule that physiologic compensation is never 100% efficient, since some patients with this acid-base disorder may exhibit a normal arterial pH and are, therefore, fully compensated.

The effects of respiratory alkalosis vary according to its duration and severity and the underlying disease. Acute respiratory alkalosis causes intracellular shifts of sodium, potassium, and phosphate and reduces ionized calcium by increasing the protein-bound fraction of calcium based on the acute pH changes. A rapid decline in $Pa{CO_2}$ may cause dizziness, mental confusion, and seizures, even in the absence of hypoxemia, as a consequence of reduced cerebral blood flow. The cardiovascular effects of acute hypocapnia in the awake human are generally minimal, but in the anesthetized or mechanically ventilated patient, cardiac output and blood pressure may fall because of the depressant effects of anesthesia and positive pressure ventilation on heart rate, systemic resistance, and venous return. Cardiac rhythm disturbances may occur in patients with coronary artery disease as a result of changes in oxygen unloading by blood from a left shift in the hemoglobin-oxygen dissociation curve (Bohr effect). Hypocapnia-induced hypokalemia is usually minor.[4]

Respiratory alkalosis is among the most common acid-base disturbances in critically ill patients (often as a component of a mixed disorder) and, when severe, portends a poor prognosis. Many cardiopulmonary disorders manifest respiratory alkalosis in the early to intermediate stages. Hyperventilation usually results in hypocapnia. Respiratory alkalosis is a common occurrence during mechanical ventilation. In those with respiratory disorders or distress, the finding of normocapnia (particularly after prior hypocapnia) and increasing hypoxemia may herald the onset of rapid respiratory failure and should prompt an assessment to determine whether the patient is becoming fatigued.

The causes of respiratory alkalosis are summarized in Table 16.5. The hyperventilation syndrome may mimic a number of serious conditions and may be disabling. Paresthesias, circumoral numbness, chest wall tightness or pain, dizziness, inability to take an adequate breath, and, rarely, tetany may be themselves sufficiently stressful to perpetuate a vicious circle. ABG analysis demonstrates an acute or chronic respiratory alkalosis, often with hypocapnia in the range of 15 to 30 mm Hg and no hypoxemia. Central nervous system diseases or injury can produce several patterns of hyperventilation with sustained arterial $Pa{CO_2}$ levels of 20 to 30 mm Hg. Salicylates, the most common cause of drug-induced respiratory alkalosis, stimulate the medullary chemoreceptor directly. The methylxanthine drugs theophylline and aminophylline stimulate ventilation and increase the ventilatory response to $CO_2$. High progesterone levels increase ventilation and decrease the arterial $Pa{CO_2}$ by as much as 5 to 10 mm Hg. Thus, chronic respiratory alkalosis is an expected feature of pregnancy. Respiratory alkalosis is a prominent feature in liver failure, and its severity correlates well with the degree of hepatic insufficiency and mortality. Respiratory alkalosis is common in patients with gram-negative septicemia, and it is often an early finding, before fever, hypoxemia, and hypotension develop. It is presumed that some bacterial product or toxin acts as a respiratory center stimulant, but the precise mechanism remains unknown.

The diagnosis of respiratory alkalosis requires measurement of arterial pH and $Pa{CO_2}$ (higher and lower than normal, respectively). The plasma $K^+$ concentration is often reduced, and the serum Cl– concentration increased. In the acute phase, respiratory alkalosis is not associated with increased renal $HCO_3^-$ excretion, but within hours, net acid excretion is reduced. In general, the $HCO_3^-$ concentration falls by 2.0 mEq/L for each 10 mm Hg decrease in $Pa{CO_2}$ acutely. Chronic hypocapnia reduces the serum bicarbonate concentration by 4 to 5 mEq/L for each 10 mm Hg decrease in $Pa{CO_2}$. It is unusual to observe a plasma bicarbonate concentration below 12 mEq/L as a result of a pure respiratory alkalosis. When a diagnosis of hyperventilation or respiratory alkalosis is made, the cause should be investigated. The diagnosis of hyperventilation syndrome is made by exclusion. In some cases, it may be important to rule out other conditions such as pulmonary embolism, coronary artery disease, pneumothorax, and hyperthyroidism.

The treatment of respiratory alkalosis is primarily directed toward alleviation of the underlying disorder. Respiratory alkalosis is rarely life-threatening. Direct measures to correct respiratory alkalosis will be unsuccessful if the underlying stimulus remains unchecked. If respiratory alkalosis complicates ventilator management, changes in dead space, tidal volume, and frequency can minimize the hypocapnia. Patients with hyperventilation syndrome may benefit from reassurance, rebreathing into a paper bag (with oxygenation monitoring) during symptomatic attacks, and attention to underlying psychologic stress. Antidepressants and sedatives are not recommended, although in a few patients, β-adrenergic blockers may help to ameliorate distressing peripheral manifestations of the hyperadrenergic state. The relationship of (and treatment of) recurrent hyperventilation syndrome and psychological disorders and panic attacks can be explored.

# METABOLIC DISORDERS

## METABOLIC ACIDOSIS

Metabolic acidosis occurs mechanistically as a result of : 1) a marked increase in endogenous production of acid (such as L-lactic acid and ketoacids) such that the ability of the kidneys to respond is exceeded, 2) loss of $HCO_3^-$ or potential $HCO_3^-$ salts (diarrhea or renal tubular acidosis [RTA]), or 3) inability of the kidneys to excrete acid resulting in progressive accumulation of endogenous acids. However, empirically for diagnostic purposes, metabolic acidosis is frequently classified according to the anion gap (AG): high anion gap metabolic acidosis or non-anion gap acidosis (or probably more appropriately, hyperchloremic metabolic acidosis). The AG, which can be corrected for the prevailing albumin concentration,[27] serves a useful role in the diagnosis of the metabolic acidoses and should always be considered. Metabolic acidosis with a normal AG (hyperchloremic or non-AG acidosis) suggests that $HCO_3^-$ has been effectively replaced by $Cl^-$. Thus, the AG does not change.

In contrast, a high anion gap usually indicates accumulation of an anion other than hydrochloric acid in the ECF. Metabolic acidosis with a high AG (see Table 16.3) reflects that an anion replaces titrated $HCO_3^-$ without disturbing the $Cl^-$ concentration. Hence, the acidosis is normochloremic and the AG increases. In some cases, a disease process may cause an acidosis that is either hyperchloremic (non-anion gap) or high-anion gap; early CKD and diabetic ketoacidosis in well-hydrated persons are the best examples. The excretion rate of the accompanying anion (e.g., acetoacetate in ketoacidosis) is the determining factor in which type acidosis is found in a given person.[24,28]

## HYPERCHLOREMIC (NON-ANION GAP) METABOLIC ACIDOSES

The diverse clinical disorders that may result in hyperchloremic or non-gap metabolic acidosis are outlined in Table 16.6. Because a reduced plasma $HCO_3^-$ and elevated $Cl^-$ concentration may also occur in chronic respiratory alkalosis, it is often important to confirm the acidemia by measuring arterial pH. Normal anion gap metabolic acidosis occurs most often as a result of loss of $HCO_3^-$ from the gastrointestinal tract (diarrhea) or as a result of a renal acidification defect. The majority of disorders in this category can be attributed to one of two major causes: 1) loss of bicarbonate from the gastrointestinal tract (diarrhea) or from the kidney (proximal RTA), or 2) inappropriately low renal acid excretion (classical distal RTA [cDRTA], type 4 RTA, or renal failure). Hypokalemia may accompany both gastrointestinal loss of $HCO_3^-$ and proximal RTA and cDRTA. Therefore, a major challenge in some cases is distinguishing these causes to be able to determine whether the response of renal tubular function to the prevailing acidosis is appropriate (gastrointestinal origin) or inappropriate (renal origin).

*Diarrhea* results in the loss of large quantities of $HCO_3^-$ or potential $HCO_3^-$ (organic acid anions such as propionate and butyrate which could be metabolized to $HCO_3^-$) and therefore, metabolic acidosis frequently results. Volume depletion and hypokalemia often coexist due to sodium and $K^+$ losses. Hypokalemia is additionally from volume depletion causing secondary hyperaldosteronism, which enhances renal $K^+$ secretion by the collecting duct.

Although a low urine pH may be found with diarrhea, consistent with metabolic acidosis and appropriate renal response, in some cases a urine pH of 6.0 or more may be found. This occurs because chronic metabolic acidosis and hypokalemia increase renal $NH_4^+$ synthesis and excretion,

**Table 16.6 Differential Diagnosis of Non-Anion Gap (Hyperchloremic) Metabolic Acidosis**

| |
|---|
| **Gastrointestinal Bicarbonate Loss** |
| Diarrhea |
| External pancreatic or small bowel drainage |
| Uterosigmoidostomy, jejunal loop |
| Drugs |
| Calcium chloride (acidifying agent) |
| Magnesium sulfate (diarrhea) |
| Cholestyramine (bile acid diarrhea) |
| **Renal Acidosis** |
| Hypokalemia |
| Proximal RTA (type 2) |
| Distal (classical) RTA (type 1) |
| Drug-induced acidosis |
| Acetazolamide and topiramate (proximal RTA) |
| Amphotericin B (distal RTA) |
| Ifosfamide |
| Hyperkalemia |
| **Generalized distal nephron dysfunction (type 4 RTA)** |
| Mineralocorticoid deficiency (e.g., **low renin/aldosterone in diabetic nephropathy**) |
| Mineralocorticoid resistance (PHA-1 autosomal dominant) |
| Voltage defects (PHA-1, autosomal recessive) |
| PHA-2 |
| ↓ $Na^+$ delivery to distal nephron |
| Tubulointerstitial disease |
| **Drug-induced acidosis** |
| Potassium-sparing diuretics (amiloride, triamterene, spironolactone) |
| Trimethoprim |
| Pentamidine |
| Angiotensin-converting enzyme inhibitors |
| Angiotensin II receptor blockers |
| Nonsteroidal antiinflammatory drugs |
| Cyclosporine, Tacrolimus |
| Normokalemia |
| **Chronic kidney disease (stage 3-4)** |
| Other |
| Acid loads (ammonium chloride, hyperalimentation) |
| Loss of potential bicarbonate: ketosis with ketone excretion |
| Dilution acidosis (rapid saline administration) |
| Hippurate |
| Cation exchange resins |

*PHA,* Pseudohypoaldosteronism; *RTA,* renal tubular acidosis.
**Bold = common in adults.**

which can increase urine pH. Therefore, the urine pH, when 6.0 or higher, may erroneously suggest a renal cause of acidosis. Nevertheless, metabolic acidosis caused by gastrointestinal losses with a high urine pH can be differentiated from renal causes by measuring or estimating urinary NH4$^+$, as described below. Urinary $NH_4^+$ excretion is typically low in patients with renal causes of acidosis and high in patients with diarrhea.[32,33] Urine acidification and pH may also be low with marked volume depletion, which impairs delivery of distal sodium delivery which in turn limits distal acidification.

The level of urinary $NH_4^+$ excretion (not usually measured by clinical laboratories) in metabolic acidosis can be assessed indirectly[34] by calculating the urine anion gap (UAG) or urine osmolal gap. The UAG is:

$$UAG = [Na^+ + K^+]_u - [Cl^-]_u \quad (16.12)$$

where $u$ denotes the urine concentration of these electrolytes. The rationale for using the UAG as a surrogate for ammonium excretion is that, in chronic metabolic acidosis, ammonium excretion should be elevated if renal tubular function is intact. Because ammonium is a cation, it should balance part of the negative charge of chloride in the previous expression, assuming there is not a lot of $HCO_3^-$ in the urine as in an alkaline urine. Therefore, the UAG should become progressively negative as the rate of ammonium excretion increases in response to acidosis or to acid loading.[24,32] $NH_4^+$ can be assumed to be present if the sum of the major cations ($Na^+$ + $K^+$) is less than the concentration of $Cl^-$ in urine. A negative UAG (more than –20 mEq/L) implies that appropriate $NH_4^+$ is present in the urine with the acidosis, as might occur with an extrarenal origin of the hyperchloremic acidosis, e.g., diarrhea. Conversely, urine estimated to contain little or no $NH_4^+$ has more $Na^+$ + $K^+$ than $Cl^-$ (UAG is positive),[32] which indicates a renal mechanism for the hyperchloremic acidosis, such as in cDRTA (with hypokalemia) or hypoaldosteronism with hyperkalemia. Note that this qualitative test is useful only in the differential diagnosis of a non-gap metabolic acidosis. If the patient has ketonuria, drug anions (penicillins or aspirin), or toluene metabolites in the urine, the test is not reliable and should not be used. And the test is controversial in the sense that its reliability and utility remain in question.

The urinary ammonium ($U_{NH4+}$) may also be estimated more reliably from the urine osmolal gap, which is the difference in measured urine osmolality ($U_{osm}$), and the urine osmolality calculated from the urine [$Na^+$ + $K^+$] and the urine urea and glucose (all expressed in mmol/L):

$$U_{NH4+} = 0.5\,(U_{osm} - [2\,Na^+ + K^+]_u + urea_u + glucose_u) \quad (16.13)$$

Urinary ammonium concentrations of 75 mEq/L or more would be anticipated if renal tubular function is intact and the kidney is responding to a prevailing metabolic acidosis by increasing ammonium production and excretion. Conversely, values below 25 mEq/L in the presence of acidosis denote inappropriately low urinary ammonium concentrations. In addition to the UAG and osmolal gap, the fractional excretion of $Na^+$ may be helpful and would be expected to be low (<1% to 2%) in patients with $HCO_3^-$ loss from the gastrointestinal tract but usually exceeds 2% to 3% in patients with RTA.[33,35]

Gastrointestinal $HCO_3^-$ loss, as well as proximal RTA (type 2) and cDRTA (type 1), results in ECF contraction and stimulation of the renin-aldosterone system, which leads typically to hypokalemia. The serum $K^+$ concentration therefore serves to distinguish the previous disorders, which have a low $K^+$, from either generalized distal nephron dysfunction (e.g., type 4 RTA), in which the renin–aldosterone–distal nephron axis is abnormal and hyperkalemia exists, or the acidosis of progressive chronic kidney disease, in which normokalemia or mild hyperkalemia is common (see later).

In addition to gastrointestinal tract $HCO_3^-$ loss, external loss of pancreatic and biliary secretions, as well as cholestyramine, calcium chloride, and magnesium sulfate ingestion can all cause a non-gap acidosis (see Table 16.6), especially in patients with renal insufficiency. Coexistent lactic acidosis is common in severe diarrheal illnesses and noted by an increase in the AG.

Severe non-gap or hyperchloremic metabolic acidosis with hypokalemia may occur in patients with ureteral diversion procedures. Because the ileum and the colon are both endowed with $Cl^-/HCO_3^-$ exchangers, when the Cl– from the urine enters the gut, or pouch, the $HCO_3^-$ concentration increases as a result of the exchange process.[24] Moreover, $K^+$ secretion is stimulated, which, together with $HCO_3^-$ loss, can result in a hyperchloremic hypokalemic metabolic acidosis. This defect is particularly common in patients with ureterosigmoidostomies and is more common with this type of diversion because of the prolonged transit time of urine caused by stasis in the colonic segment.

Dilutional acidosis, acidosis caused by exogenous acid loads and the posthypocapnic state, can usually be excluded by the history. When isotonic saline is infused rapidly, particularly in patients with temporary or permanent renal functional impairment, the serum $HCO_3^-$ declines reciprocally in relation to $Cl^-$,[24] in part due the dilutional effect of the fluid. Hyperchloremic acidosis can also be caused by administration of acid or acid equivalents such as infusion of arginine or lysine hydrochloride during parenteral hyperalimentation or ingestion of ammonium chloride.

Hyperchloremic metabolic acidosis may also occur in some settings of ketoacidosis. In mild, chronic ketoacidosis if GFR is maintained with adequate ECFV expansion and renal ketone excretion is high, the continued titration of $HCO_3^-$ with $Cl^-$ retention and excretion of potential base (ketones) may result in hyperchloremic acidosis. A similar situation could contribute to continued acidosis during recovery from typical high anion gap ketoacidosis when the sodium salts of ketones may be excreted and lost as potential $HCO_3^-$.[36] A similar mechanism for hyperchloremic acidosis in early CKD may occur with metabolism of sulfur to sulfuric acid and excretion of $SO_4 2^-$ with $Cl^-$ retention.

Loss of functioning renal parenchyma in progressive kidney disease is known to be associated with metabolic acidosis. Typically, the acidosis is a hyperchloremic, non-gap type when the GFR is between 20 and 50 mL/min but may convert to the typical high AG acidosis of uremia with more advanced renal failure, that is, when the GFR is less than 20 mL/min.[37] It is generally assumed that such progression is observed more commonly in patients with tubulointerstitial forms of renal disease, but non-anion gap metabolic acidosis can also occur with advanced glomerular disease. The acidoses of CKD with an anion gap and hyperkalemic, hyperchloremic metabolic acidosis are discussed subsequently below. The principal defect in acidification of advanced renal failure is that ammoniagenesis is reduced in proportion to the loss of functional renal mass. In addition, medullary $NH_4^+$ accumulation and trapping in the outer medullary collecting tubule may be impaired.[37] Because of adaptive increases in $K^+$ secretion by the collecting duct and colon, the acidosis of chronic renal insufficiency is typically normokalemic.[37]

Non-anion gap metabolic acidosis accompanied by hyperkalemia is almost always associated with a generalized dysfunction of the distal nephron.[33,35] However, $K^+$-sparing diuretics (amiloride, triamterene), as well as pentamidine, cyclosporine, tacrolimus, nonsteroidal antiinflammatory drugs (NSAIDs), angiotensin-converting enzyme (ACE) inhibitors, angiotensin II receptor blockers (ARBs), beta-blockers, and heparin may mimic or cause this disorder, resulting in hyperkalemia and a non-gap metabolic acidosis.[33,35] Because hyperkalemia augments the development of acidosis by suppressing urinary net acid excretion, discontinuing these agents while reducing the serum $K^+$ allows ammonium production and excretion to increase, which will help repair the acidosis.

## PROXIMAL RENAL TUBULAR ACIDOSIS

### Physiology

The proximal tubule reabsorbs 80% of the large amount of filtered $HCO_3^-$ so that defects in the proximal tubule cause initial profound loss of $HCO_3^-$ into the urine.[6] When $HCO_3^-$ that is not absorbed floods the distal nephron, the $HCO_3^-$ delivery exceeds the distal nephron's capacity to reabsorb $HCO_3^-$, and bicarbonaturia ensues. Enhanced $Cl^-$ reabsorption, stimulated by ECF volume contraction, also results in a hyperchloremic metabolic acidosis. As serum $HCO_3^-$ levels fall, less will be filtered, eventually reaching a level of distal delivery of $HCO_3^-$ such that the distal nephron can reabsorb the remaining $HCO_3^-$, and the distal nephron can acidify the urine (to pH < 5.5) (Fig. 16.1). A steady state with lower serum $HCO_3^-$ is reached in which acid excretion is normal. The serum $HCO_3^-$ concentration usually reaches a nadir of 15 to 18 mEq/L, so that systemic acidosis is not progressive. With bicarbonate administration, the amount of bicarbonate in the urine increases dramatically when blood levels increase with the fractional excretion of bicarbonate ($FE_{HCO3}-$) rising to 10% to 15%, and the urine pH becomes alkaline.[33]

## PATHOGENESIS – INHERITED AND ACQUIRED FORMS

Proximal RTA can present in one of three ways: isolated $HCO_3^-$ defect, generalized proximal tubule defect, and as a part of a mixed proximal/distal RTA (type 3). Inheritance patterns for isolated proximal RTA include autosomal recessive and autosomal dominant. Isolated, recessive proximal RTA with accompanying ocular abnormalities has been most studied and has been attributed to missense mutations of the gene *SLCA4* that encodes for the basolateral transporter, NBCe1. A rare variant, inherited as an autosomal dominant trait with short stature, has been described and appears to be a mutation of the gene that encodes the apical $Na^+/H^+$ exchanger, NHE-3.

Familial disorders associated with proximal RTA and generalized proximal defects, referred to as Fanconi's syndrome, include cystinosis, tyrosinemia, hereditary fructose intolerance, galactosemia, glycogen storage disease type 1, Wilson's disease, and Lowe's syndrome. These have defects in reabsorption of many substances reabsorbed in the proximal tubule: glucose, amino acids, phosphate, uric acid, citrate. These substances spill into the urine. Numerous defects of the proximal tubule have been proposed and verified experimentally as feasible. Certain drugs (e.g., aminoglycosides, cisplatin, ifosfamide, tenofovir, valproic acid), heavy metal intoxications, and myeloma proteins can also cause Fanconi's syndrome.

Development of Fanconi's syndrome by intracellular $PO_4^{3-}$ depletion has also been proposed in hereditary fructose intolerance, in which ingestion of fructose leads to accumulation of fructose 1-phosphate in the proximal tubule. Because these patients lack the enzyme fructose 1-phosphate aldolase, fructose 1-phosphate cannot be further metabolized, and intracellular $PO_4^{3-}$ is sequestered in this form.[33,38]

Vitamin D deficiency and proximal RTA with aminoaciduria and urinary phosphate wasting are also associated. Correction of vitamin D deficiency has allowed correction of the proximal tubule dysfunction.[39] Similar results have been obtained in patients with vitamin D–dependent and vitamin D–resistant rickets treated with dihydrotachysterol.[33] The mechanisms involved in the proximal tubule dysfunction are not yet clear.

Additionally, features of both proximal RTA (bicarbonate wasting), and distal acidification abnormalities are evident in patients with autosomal recessive RTA (mixed proximal and distal, or type 3 RTA) that has been attributed to a defect in CA2 that encodes for carbonic anhydrase II (CAII), an intracellular form of the enzyme distributed to the proximal tubule, TALH, DCT, CCD, and MCD.[33] The phenotype includes osteopetrosis, cerebral calcifications, and ocular abnormalities (Guibaud-Vainsel syndrome). Sly and associates, who worked out much of the pathophysiology, found no other evidence for proximal tubule dysfunction, and intact carbonic anhydrase IV.[40] Carbonic anhydrase II is present in the cytoplasm of renal cells, and thus an acidification defect occurring in association with its deficiency is not unexpected.

### Clinical Spectrum

In general, proximal RTA is more common in children due to the genetic diseases noted above. In adults, the most common causes of acquired proximal RTA are multiple myeloma, in which increased excretion of immunoglobulin light chains injures the proximal tubule epithelium, and chemotherapeutic drug injury of the proximal tubule (e.g., ifosfamide). The light chains that cause injury in multiple myeloma often have a variable domain that is resistant to degradation by proteases in lysosomes in proximal tubule cells. Accumulation of the variable domain fragments may be responsible for the impairment in tubular function. Carbonic anhydrase inhibitors cause pure bicarbonate wasting but not Fanconi's syndrome. A comprehensive list of the disorders associated with proximal RTA is presented in Table 16.7.[33] Some of the entities on this list are no longer seen and are of only historic interest. For example, application of sulfanilamide to the skin of patients with large-surface-area burns is no longer practiced in most centers, but sulfanilamide, a carbonic anhydrase inhibitor, is absorbed from burned skin. Topiramate, widely used in the prevention of migraine headaches and treatment of seizure disorders, is a potent carbonic anhydrase inhibitor and an important cause of non-gap metabolic acidosis. As many as 15% to 25% of patients on topiramate will manifest a stable non-gap metabolic acidosis. Since the enzyme carbonic

**Table 16.7 Proximal Renal Tubular Acidosis**

**Isolated Pure Bicarbonate Wasting (Unassociated With Fanconi's Syndrome)**

Primary
Inherited autosomal recessive with ocular abnormalities (missense mutations of *SLC4A4*)
Autosomal dominant with short stature (mutation of *SLC9A3/NHE3*)
Carbonic anhydrase deficiency, inhibition, or alteration
  Drugs: acetazolamide, topiramate, sulfanilamide, mafenide acetate
  Carbonic anhydrase II deficiency with osteopetrosis (mixed proximal and distal RTA –type 3)

**Generalized (Associated With Fanconi's Syndrome)**

Primary (without associated systemic disease)
  Genetic
  Sporadic
Genetically transmitted systemic diseases
  Cystinosis
  Lowe's syndrome
  Wilson's syndrome
  Tyrosinemia
  Galactosemia
  Hereditary fructose intolerance (during fructose ingestion)
  Metachromatic leukodystrophy
  Pyruvate carboxylase deficiency
  Methylmalonic acidemia
Dysproteinemic states
  Multiple myeloma, monoclonal gammopathy
Secondary hyperparathyroidism with chronic hypocalcemia
  Vitamin D deficiency or resistance, vitamin D dependency
Drugs or toxins
  Ifosfamide, lead, outdated tetracycline, 3-methylchromone, streptozotocin, amphotericin B (historic)
Tubulointerstitial diseases
  Sjögren's syndrome
  Medullary cystic disease
  Renal transplantation
Other renal and miscellaneous diseases
  Nephrotic syndrome, amyloidosis, paroxysmal nocturnal hemoglobinuria

anhydrase II is present in both the proximal and distal tubules, topiramate appears to cause a mixed form of renal tubular acidosis (RTA), having features of both proximal and distal RTA (type 3 RTA). This manifestation subsides when topiramate is discontinued. Pharmaceutical manufacturing techniques have improved, and outdated tetracycline is no longer associated with proximal RTA. Some of the agents and disorders on this list—such as ifosfamide, Sjögren's syndrome, renal transplantation, and amyloidosis—also appear as causes of distal RTA (see Table 16.7).

### Diagnosis

The diagnosis of proximal RTA relies initially on the documentation of a chronic hyperchloremic metabolic acidosis. In the steady state these patients generally show chronic metabolic acidosis, an acid urine pH (< 5.5), and a low fractional excretion of $HCO_3^-$ (when plasma levels are low). With alkali therapy or slow infusion of sodium bicarbonate intravenously, bicarbonaturia ensues, and the urine becomes alkaline. When the plasma bicarbonate concentration is increased with an intravenous infusion of sodium bicarbonate at a rate of 0.5 to 1.0 mEq/kg/hr, the urine pH, even if initially acid, will increase once the reabsorptive threshold for bicarbonate has been exceeded. Thus, the urine pH may exceed 7.5 and $FE_{HCO_3^-}$ will increase dramatically to 15% to 20%, making it very difficult to increase serum $HCO_3^-$ levels to the normal range.

Hypokalemia is usually present. If bicarbonate administration has been high in an attempt to repair the acidosis, the bicarbonaturia will drive kaliuresis and the hypokalemia may be severe.[33] Patients with proximal tubule dysfunction exhibit intact distal nephron function (generate steep urine pH gradients and titrate luminal buffers) when the serum $HCO_3^-$ concentration and hence distal $HCO_3^-$ delivery are sufficiently reduced. A low $HCO_3^-$ threshold exists. Below this plasma $HCO_3^-$ concentration, distal acidification can compensate for defective proximal acidification, although at the expense of systemic metabolic acidosis. When the plasma $HCO_3^-$ concentration is raised to normal values, a large fraction of the filtered $HCO_3^-$ is inappropriately excreted because the limited reabsorptive capacity of the distal nephron cannot compensate for the reduced proximal nephron reabsorption.

### Associated Clinical Features

$K^+$ excretion is typically high in patients with proximal RTA, especially during $NaHCO_3$ administration.[33] Kaliuresis is promoted by the increased delivery of a relatively impermeant anion, $HCO_3^-$, to the distal nephron in the setting of secondary hyperaldosteronism, which is due to mild volume depletion. Therefore, correction of acidosis in such patients leads to an exaggeration of the kaliuresis and $K^+$ deficiency.

If the acidification defect is part of a generalized proximal tubule dysfunction (Fanconi's syndrome), such patients will have hypophosphatemia, hyperphosphaturia, hypouricemia, hyperuricosuria, glycosuria, aminoaciduria, hypercitraturia, hypercalciuria, and proteinuria.

Although $Ca^{2+}$ excretion may be high in patients with proximal RTA, nephrocalcinosis and renal calculi are rare. This may be related to the high rate of citrate excretion in patients with proximal RTA compared with that of most patients with acidosis from other causes. Osteomalacia, rickets, abnormal gut $Ca^{2+}$ and phosphorus absorption, and abnormal vitamin D metabolism in children are common, although not invariantly present. Adults tend to have osteopenia without pseudofractures.[33]

The proximal reabsorption of filtered low-molecular-weight proteins may also be abnormal in proximal RTA. Lysozymuria and increased urinary excretion of immunoglobulin light chains can occur.[33]

### Treatment

The magnitude of the bicarbonaturia (>10% of the filtered load) at a normal $HCO_3^-$ concentration requires that large amounts of $HCO_3^-$ be administered for treatment. At least 10 to 30 mEq/kg/day of $HCO_3^-$ or its metabolic equivalent (citrate) is required to maintain plasma $HCO_3^-$ concentration at normal levels. Correcting the $HCO_3^-$ to near normal values (22 to 24 mEq/L) is desirable in children to reestablish normal growth. Correction to this level is less desirable in adults. Large supplements of $K^+$ are often necessary because of the kaliuresis induced by high distal $HCO_3^-$ delivery when the plasma $HCO_3^-$ concentration is normalized. Thiazides have proved useful in diminishing therapeutic requirements for $HCO_3^-$ supplementation by causing ECF contraction to stimulate proximal absorption. However, $K^+$ wasting continues to be a problem, often requiring the addition of a $K^+$-sparing diuretic.[33] Vitamin D and $PO_4^{3-}$ may be supplemented and in some patients even improve the acidification defect. Fructose should be restricted in patients with fructose intolerance.[38]

## DISTAL RENAL TUBULE ACIDOSIS (CLASSIC WITH HYPOKALEMIA)

### Pathophysiology

The mechanisms involved in the pathogenesis of hypokalemic distal RTA, or classic distal RTA, cDRTA (type 1 RTA) have been established for many cases by modern genetic and molecular methods. The inherited forms of cDRTA can be due to defects in the basolateral $HCO_3^-/Cl^-$ exchanger (SLC4A1), or subunits of the $H^+$-ATPase (ATP6V1B1 and ATP6V0a4).

Defects in these transport pathways and an increase in apical membrane permeability are displayed in Fig. 16.6, which depicts acid-base transporters of a type A intercalated cell in the medullary collecting duct and the possible abnormalities causing cDRTA. Although the classical feature of this entity is an inability to acidify the urine maximally (to a pH of <5.5) in the face of systemic acidosis, attention to urine ammonium excretion rather than urine pH alone is necessary to diagnose this disorder.[32,33] The pathogenesis of the acidification defect in most patients has been shown previously by the response of the urine $PCO_2$ to sodium bicarbonate infusion. When normal subjects are given large infusions of sodium bicarbonate to produce a high $HCO_3^-$ excretion, distal nephron $H^+$ secretion leads to the generation of a high $PCO_2$ in the renal medulla and final urine.[41] The magnitude of the urinary $PCO_2$ (often referred to as the *urine minus blood $PCO_2$* or *U – B $PCO_2$*) has been and can be used as an index of distal nephron $H^+$ secretory capacity.[39,42] The U – B $PCO_2$ is generally subnormal in classical hypokalemic distal RTA, with the notable exception of amphotericin B–induced distal RTA, which remains the most common example of the "gradient" or permeability defect.[41–43] A leakage defect independent of amphotericin B has been reported or postulated in rare patients with cDRTA without exposure to the antibiotic, but has never been documented unequivocally.[44]

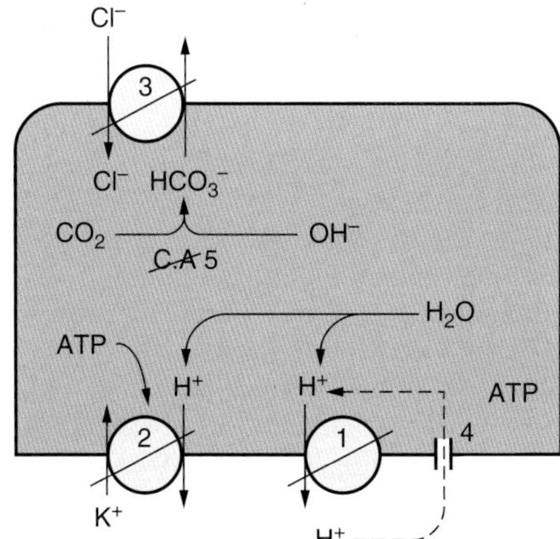


**Fig. 16.6** Type A intercalated cell of the collecting duct displaying five pathophysiologic defects that could result in classical distal renal tubular acidosis: defective $H^+$-ATPase, defective $H^+$-$K^+$-ATPase, defective $HCO_3^-/Cl^-$ exchanger, $H^+$ leak pathway, and defective intracellular carbonic anhydrase (type II). *ATP,* Adenosine triphosphate.

Patients with impaired collecting duct $H^+$ secretion and cDRTA also exhibit uniformly low excretory rates of $NH_4^+$ when the degree of systemic acidosis is taken into account.[7,32,33] Low $NH_4^+$ excretion equates with inappropriately low renal regeneration of $HCO_3^-$, which indicates that the kidney is responsible for causing or perpetuating the chronic metabolic acidosis. Low $NH_4^+$ excretion in classical hypokalemic distal RTA occurs because of the failure to trap $NH_4^+$ in the medullary collecting duct as a result of higher than normal tubule fluid pH in this segment and loss of the disequilibrium pH (pH > 6.0).[45] The high urine pH indicates impaired $H^+$ secretion.

**Inherited and Acquired Defects in Type A Intercalated Cell Acid-Base Transporters Responsible for cDRTA.** Recessive cDRTA with deafness is caused by loss-of-function mutations in either of two subunits of the $H^+$-ATPase of type A intercalated cells (the B1 subunit of the V1 cytoplasmic ATPase, and the a4 subunit of the V0 transmembrane complex). Dominant and recessive forms of cDRTA are also caused by loss-of-function mutations in the basolateral membrane AE1 $Cl^-/HCO_3^-$ exchanger of type A intercalated cells. Depending on the type, associated erythroid changes may be mild or severe.[46,47] Karet and colleagues[48] have described two different mutations in the *ATP6VIB1* gene encoding the B1 subunit of $H^+$-ATPase. One defect is associated with sensorineural deafness (*rdRTA1*) and the other with normal hearing (*rdRTA2*).[49] The former recessive disorder is manifest in the first year of life as a failure to thrive; bilateral sensorineural hearing deficits; hyperchloremic, hypokalemic metabolic acidosis; severe nephrolithiasis; nephrocalcinosis; and osteodystrophy. The $H^+$-ATPase is critical for maintaining pH in the cochlea and endolymph, and its loss in this disorder explains the hearing deficit as well as the renal tubule acidification defect. An autosomal recessive form that is much less commonly associated with deafness is due to a defect in the *ATP6V0a4* gene that encodes for the $H^+$-ATPase a4 subunit.[50,51] The genetic and molecular basis of distal RTA is outlined in Table 16.8.

Acquired defects of $H^+$-ATPase have been demonstrated in renal biopsy specimens of patients with Sjögren's syndrome with evidence of classical hypokalemic distal RTA.[33] These biopsy specimens revealed an absence of $H^+$-ATPase protein in the apical membrane of type A intercalated cells.

Theoretically, abnormalities in $H^+$, $K^+$-ATPase could also result in both hypokalemia and metabolic acidosis. This has been experimentally supported by rat studies using vanadate. Of note, an unusually high incidence of hypokalemic distal RTA (endemic RTA) has been observed in northeastern Thailand.[52] To date, no genetic linkages between $H^+$-$K^+$-ATPase genes and inherited forms of cDRTA have been documented. Nevertheless, such an abnormality has been suggested in an infant with severe metabolic acidosis and hypokalemia.[33]

**Table 16.8 Genetic and Molecular Bases of Distal Renal Tubular Acidoses (RTA)**

| | |
|---|---|
| **Classical Distal RTA** | |
| **Inherited** | |
| Autosomal dominant | Defect in AE1 gene encodes for missense mutation in the $HCO_3^-/Cl^-$ exchanger (band 3 protein)<br>Transporter may be mistargeted to apical membrane |
| Autosomal recessive With deafness | Mutations in ATP6V1B1 encoding B1-subunit of the apical $H^+$-ATPase in distal tubule (rdRTA1) |
| With normal hearing | Mutations in ATP6V0a4 (rdRTA2) |
| Carbonic anhydrase II | Defect in CA II in red blood cells, bone, kidney |
| Endemic (northeastern Thailand) | Possible abnormality in $H^+,K^+$-ATPase |
| Acquired | Reduced apical expression of $H^+$-ATPase (Sjögren's syndrome) |
| **Generalized Distal Nephron Dysfunction** | |
| Pseudohypoaldosteronism type 1 | |
| Autosomal recessive | Loss-of-function mutations of ENaC; mutations of genes encoding three subunits of ENaC |
| Autosomal dominant | Heterozygous mutations of mineralocorticoid receptor gene |
| Pseudohypoaldosteronism type 2 | Mutations in WNK1 and WNK4, and in cullin-RING ligase (CRL) proteins cullin 3 (Cul3) 4 and kelch-like 3 (KLHL3) constitutively activate NCCT, increasing NaCl absorption in distal convoluted tubule |

*ENaC,* Epithelial sodium channel.

### Clinical Spectrum and Associated Features

The phenotypic hallmark of classical hypokalemic distal RTA, when fully expressed, is the inability to acidify the urine appropriately during spontaneous or chemically induced metabolic acidosis, and is a disease of type A intercalated cells of the collecting duct. The defect in acidification by the collecting duct secondarily impairs $NH_4^+$ and titratable acid excretion and results in positive acid balance, hyperchloremic metabolic acidosis, and volume depletion.[33,53–55] Moreover, medullary interstitial disease, which commonly occurs in conjunction with distal RTA, may impair $NH_4^+$ excretion by interrupting the medullary countercurrent system for $NH_4^+$.[32,33,53,54] The complete form of classical distal RTA is manifest by a non-anion gap metabolic acidosis. The clinical spectrum of complete cDRTA may include stunted growth, hypercalciuria, hypocitrituria, osteopenia, nephrolithiasis, and nephrocalcinosis, all as direct consequence of the chronic non-gap metabolic acidosis. The dissolution of bone is due to calcium resorption and mobilization from bone in response to the acidosis[33] and through activation of the pH sensitive G-protein coupled receptor, OGR1 or *GPR68*, which resides in bone.[56] Interestingly OGR1/*GPR68* is also a pH- and shear stress-sensor on vascular endothelial cells. Other common electrolyte abnormalities, not due to acidosis include hypokalemia, hypernatremia and salt wasting, and polyuria due to nephrogenic diabetes insipidus. The hypokalemia, previously attributed to volume depletion and activation of the renin-angiotensin-aldosteronism system, may be due to a signaling pathway involving activation and release of PGE2 by beta intercalated cells that directly communicate to enhance sodium absorption and potassium secretion by activation of the epithelial sodium channel (ENaC) in collecting duct principal cells. Because chronic metabolic acidosis also increases proximal tubule reabsorption of citrate,[7,32,33] the resulting hypocitraturia in combination with hypercalciuria creates an environment favorable for urinary stone formation and nephrocalcinosis. Nephrocalcinosis appears to be a reliable marker for cDRTA because nephrocalcinosis does not occur in proximal RTA or with generalized dysfunction of the nephron associated with hyperkalemia.[32,33] Nephrocalcinosis probably aggravates further the reduction in net acid excretion by impairing the transfer of ammonia from the loop of Henle into the collecting duct. Pyelonephritis is a common complication of distal RTA, especially in the presence of nephrocalcinosis, and eradication of the causative organism may be difficult.[33] Distal RTA occurs frequently in patients with Sjögren's syndrome.[57]

The clinical spectrum of cDRTA is outlined in detail in Table 16.9.[32,33,55,57]

**Treatment.** Correction of chronic metabolic acidosis can usually be achieved readily in patients with cDRTA by administration of alkali in an amount sufficient to neutralize the production of metabolic acids derived from the diet and metabolism.[33] The goal is to correct the plasma $HCO_3^-$ concentration to normal (25 mEq/L) and should be monitored frequently. In adult patients with distal RTA, this amount may be equal to no more than 1 to 3 mEq/kg/day.[58] In growing children, endogenous acid production is usually between 2 and 3 mEq/kg/day but may, on occasion, exceed 5 mEq/kg/day. Larger amounts of bicarbonate must be administered to fully correct the acidosis and maintain normal growth.[32,33] The various forms of alkali replacement are outlined in Table 16.10.

In adult patients with distal RTA, correction of acidosis with alkali therapy reduces urinary $K^+$ excretion and typically corrects the hypokalemia and $Na^+$ depletion.[33] Therefore, in most adult patients with distal RTA, $K^+$ supplementation is usually not necessary once potassium has been corrected initially. Frank wasting of $K^+$ may occur in a minority of adult patients and in some children in association with secondary hyperaldosteronism despite correction of the acidosis by alkali therapy, so that $K^+$ supplementation is needed. If required, potassium can be administered as potassium bicarbonate (K-Lyte 25 or 50 mEq), potassium citrate (Urocit-K), or potassium citrate combination products (PolyCitra, K-Shohl's solution).[32,33] Maintenance of a normal serum bicarbonate concentration with alkali therapy also raises urinary citrate level, reduces urinary calcium excretion, lowers the frequency of nephrolithiasis, and tends to correct bone disease and restore normal growth in children.[58,59] Therefore, every

**Table 16.9 Classical Distal Renal Tubular Acidosis**

**Primary**

**Familial**

Autosomal dominant
- AE1 gene

Autosomal recessive
- With deafness (rdRTA1 or ATP6V1B1 gene)
- Without deafness (rdRTA2 or ATP6V0A4)

Sporadic

**Endemic**

Northeastern Thailand

**Secondary to Systemic Disorders**

**Autoimmune Diseases**: **Sjögren's syndrome**: Hyperglobulinemic purpura, cryoglobulinemia, thyroiditis, human immunodeficiency syndrome nephropathy, fibrosing alveolitis, chronic active hepatitis, primary biliary cirrhosis, polyarthritis nodosa

**Hypercalciuria and Nephrocalcinosis**: Primary hyperparathyroidism, vitamin D intoxication, hyperthyroidism, idiopathic hypercalciuria, medullary sponge kidney, Wilson's disease, Fabry's disease, hereditary fructose intolerance, X-linked hypophosphatemia

**Drug- and Toxin-Induced Disease:** Amphotericin B, toluene, cyclamate, mercury, hepatic cirrhosis, vanadate, ifosfamide, **lithium,** classical analgesic nephropathy, foscarnet

**Tubulointerstitial Diseases:** Balkan nephropathy, kidney transplantation, chronic pyelonephritis, leprosy, obstructive uropathy, jejunoileal bypass with hyperoxaluria, vesicoureteral reflux

**Associated with Genetically Transmitted Diseases:** Ehlers-Danlos syndrome, hereditary elliptocytosis, sickle cell anemia, Marfan's syndrome, medullary cystic disease, jejunal bypass with hyperoxaluria, hereditary sensorineural deafness, carnitine palmitoyltransferase deficiency, osteopetrosis with carbonic anhydrase II deficiency (mixed proximal-distal RTA - type 3)

**Table 16.10 Forms of Alkali Replacement**

| | |
|---|---|
| Shohl's Solution: $Na^+$ epithelial sodium channel citrate 500 mg, citric acid 334 mg/5 mL | Each 1 mL contains 1 mEq sodium and is equivalent to 1 mEq of bicarbonate |
| $NaHCO_3$ tablets | 3.9 mEq/tablet (325 mg)<br>7.8 mEq/tablet (650 mg) |
| Baking soda | 60 mEq/teaspoon |
| K-Lyte | 25-50 mEq/tablet |
| $Na^+$ citrate and $K^+$ citrate (Virtrate-2 or Cytra-3) $Na^+$ citrate 500 mg, and $K^+$ citrate 550 mg/5 mL | Each 1 mL contains 1 mEq potassium and 1 mEq sodium and is equivalent to 2 mEq bicarbonate |
| $K^+$ citrate 550 mg, citric acid 334 mg/5 mL | |
| Polycitra-K crystals $K^+$ citrate 3300 mg, citric acid 1002 mg/packet | Each packet contains 30 mEq potassium and is equivalent to 30 mEq bicarbonate |
| Urocit-K tablets, $K^+$ citrate | 5 or 10 mEq/tablet |

attempt should be made to correct and maintain a near-normal serum [$HCO_3^-$] in all patients with cDRTA.

Severe hypokalemia with flaccid paralysis, metabolic acidosis, and hypocalcemia may occur in some patients under extreme circumstances and require immediate therapy. Initial increasing systemic pH with alkali therapy may worsen the hypokalemia, potentially resulting in respiratory failure from respiratory muscle paralysis. Therefore, immediate intravenous potassium replacement should be achieved prior to alkali administration.

## HYPERKALEMIC RENAL TUBULAR ACIDOSIS, GENERALIZED DISTAL NEPHRON DYSFUNCTION (TYPE 4 RTA)

The coexistence of hyperkalemia and hyperchloremic (non-gap) metabolic acidosis often indicates a generalized dysfunction in the cortical and medullary collecting tubules. In the differential diagnosis, it is important to evaluate the functional status of the renin-aldosterone system and ECF volume. The specific disorders causing hyperkalemic hyperchloremic metabolic acidosis are outlined in detail in Table 16.11.[32,33] The classification of these disorders varies with some experts including both the frequent hyporeninemic hypoaldosteronism (e.g., in diabetics with mild to moderate CKD) and so-called voltage defects in type 4 RTA; other experts separate the voltage defect disorders as separate from type 4 RTA. All of these disorders have hyperkalemia and hyperchloremic metabolic acidosis that is disproportionate to any decreased GFR.

The regulation of potassium excretion is primarily the result of regulation of potassium secretion, which responds to hyperkalemia, aldosterone, sodium delivery, acid-base status, and nonreabsorbable anions in the CCD. Therefore, a clinical estimate of $K^+$ transfer into that segment can be helpful to recognize hyperkalemia of renal origin. An abnormally low excretion of potassium in the face of hyperkalemia implies hyperkalemia of renal origin. Calculation of the transtubular potassium gradient (TTKG) can be helpful in this regard. When the TTKG is low (<5), or the fractional excretion of potassium ($FE_{K+}$) is less than 25%, in a hyperkalemic patient, it reveals that the collecting tubule is not responding appropriately to the prevailing hyperkalemia and that potassium secretion is impaired. In contrast, in hyperkalemia of nonrenal origin, the kidney should respond by increasing $K^+$ secretion, as evidenced by a sharp increase in the TTKG. The TTKG calculation assumes that there is no significant net addition or absorption of $K^+$ between the CCD and the final urine, that CCD tubular fluid osmolality is approximately the same as plasma osmolality, that "osmoles" are not extracted between CCD and the final urine, and that plasma [$K^+$] approximates peritubular fluid [$K^+$]. It is important to note that under certain clinical conditions, some or none of these assumptions may be entirely correct. With high urine flow rates, for example, the TTKG underestimates $K^+$ secretory capacity in the hyperkalemic patient.

Hyperkalemia should also be regarded as an important mediator of the renal response to acid-base balance. Potassium status can affect distal nephron acidification by both direct and indirect mechanisms. First, the level of potassium in systemic blood is an important determinant of aldosterone

**Table 16.11 Disorders With Dysfunction of Renal Acidification—Generalized Abnormality of Distal Nephron With Hyperkalemia**

**Mineralocorticoid Deficiency**

**Primary Mineralocorticoid Deficiency**

Combined deficiency of aldosterone, deoxycorticosterone, and cortisol
- Addison's disease, bilateral adrenalectomy, bilateral adrenal destruction, hemorrhage, or carcinoma

Congenital enzymatic defects
- 21-hydroxylase deficiency, 3β-hydroxydehydrogenase deficiency, Desmolase deficiency

Isolated (selective) aldosterone deficiency
- Chronic idiopathic hypoaldosteronism, heparin (low-molecular weight or unfractionated) administration in critically ill patient, familial hypoaldosteronism, corticosterone methyl oxidase deficiency types 1 and 2, primary zona glomerulosa defect, transient hypoaldosteronism of infancy, persistent hypotension, and/or hypoxemia

Angiotensin II converting enzyme inhibition
- Endogenous, **Angiotensin-converting enzyme inhibitors and angiotensin II receptor antagonists**

**Secondary Mineralocorticoid Deficiency**

Hyporeninemic hypoaldosteronism
- **Diabetic nephropathy, tubulointerstitial nephropathies, nephrosclerosis, nonsteroidal antiinflammatory agents**, acquired immunodeficiency syndrome, immunoglobulin M monoclonal gammopathy, **obstructive uropathy**

**Mineralocorticoid Resistance**

PHA-1—autosomal dominant (human mineralocorticoid receptor defect)

**Renal Tubular Dysfunction (Voltage Defect)**

PHA-1—autosomal recessive

PHA-2—autosomal dominant

Drugs that interfere with $Na^+$ channel function in the CCT
- **Amiloride, triamterene, Trimethoprim**, pentamidine

Drugs that interfere with $Na^+$-$K^+$-ATPase in the CCT
- **Cyclosporine, tacrolimus**

Drugs that inhibit aldosterone effect on the CCT
- **Spironolactone, epleronone**

Disorders associated with tubulointerstitial nephritis and renal insufficiency
- Lupus nephritis, methicillin nephrotoxicity, obstructive nephropathy, kidney transplant rejection, sickle cell disease, Williams' syndrome with uric acid nephrolithiasis

elaboration, which is also an important determinant of distal $H^+$ secretion. Chronic hyperkalemia can suppress ammoniagenesis.[60,61] These changes in ammonium production may also affect medullary interstitial ammonium concentration and buffer availability.[61] Hyperkalemia has no effect on ammonium transport in the superficial proximal tubule but markedly impairs ammonium absorption in the thick ascending limb of the loop of Henle (TAL), reducing inner medullary concentrations of total ammonia and decreasing secretion of $NH_3$ into the inner medullary collecting duct. Hyperkalemia may also decrease entry of $NH_4^+$ into the medullary collecting duct through competition of $NH_4^+$ and $K^+$ for the $K^+$-secretory site on the basolateral membrane Na-K-ATPase (Figs. 16.7 and 16.8).[26,62]

**Table 16.12 Effects of Hyperkalemia on Ammonium Excretion**

Decrease in $NH4^+$ production
Decrease in $NH4^+$ absorption in thick ascending limb of loop of Henle
Decrease in interstitial $NH4^+$ concentration
Impaired countercurrent multiplication
Decrease in NH3/ $NH4^+$ secretion into outer and inner medullary collecting ducts

In summary, hyperkalemia may have a dramatic impact on ammonium production and excretion (Table 16.12). Chronic hyperkalemia decreases ammonium production in the proximal tubule and whole kidney, inhibits absorption of $NH_4^+$ in the mTAL, reduces medullary interstitial concentrations of $NH_4^+$ and $NH_3$, and decreases entry of $NH_4^+$ and $NH_3$ into the medullary collecting duct. This same series of events leads, in the final analysis, to a marked reduction in urinary ammonium excretion. The potential for development of a hyperchloremic metabolic acidosis is greatly augmented when a reduction in functional renal mass (GFR of <60 mL/min) coexists with hyperkalemia or when aldosterone deficiency or resistance is present.

### Clinical Disorders

Type 4 RTA with a generalized distal nephron dysfunction is manifest as a hyperchloremic (non-gap), hyperkalemic metabolic acidosis in which urinary ammonium excretion is invariably depressed and renal function is often compromised. Although all patients with CKD may have some tendency to acidosis and hyperkalemia, these abnormalities are not usually severe, particularly in the early stages of CKD. Patients with type 4 RTA often have marked hyperkalemia (>5.5 mEq/L) that is disproportionate to the reduction in the GFR. The TTKG and/or the fractional excretion of $K^+$ ($FE_K{}^+$) is usually low in patients with this disorder. In such patients, often with diabetic nephropathy or tubulointerstitial disease, a unique dysfunction of potassium and acid secretion by the collecting tubule coexists and can be attributed to either mineralocorticoid deficiency, resistance to mineralocorticoid, or a specific type of renal tubular dysfunction (voltage defects). The clinical spectrum of generalized abnormalities in the distal nephron is summarized in Table 16.11.

### Primary Mineralocorticoid Deficiency

Angiotensin II and plasma $K^+$ are the principal determinants of production and secretion of aldosterone. Adrenocorticotropic hormone (ACTH), endothelin, dopamine, acetylcholine, epinephrine, nitric oxide, renin, and plasma $Mg^{2+}$ can also have some influence. Destruction of the adrenal cortex by hemorrhage, infection, ischemia, invasion by tumors, amyloid or autoimmune processes results in Addison's disease. This disorder is manifest by combined glucocorticoid and mineralocorticoid deficiency and is recognized clinically by hypoglycemia, anorexia, weakness, hyperpigmentation, and a

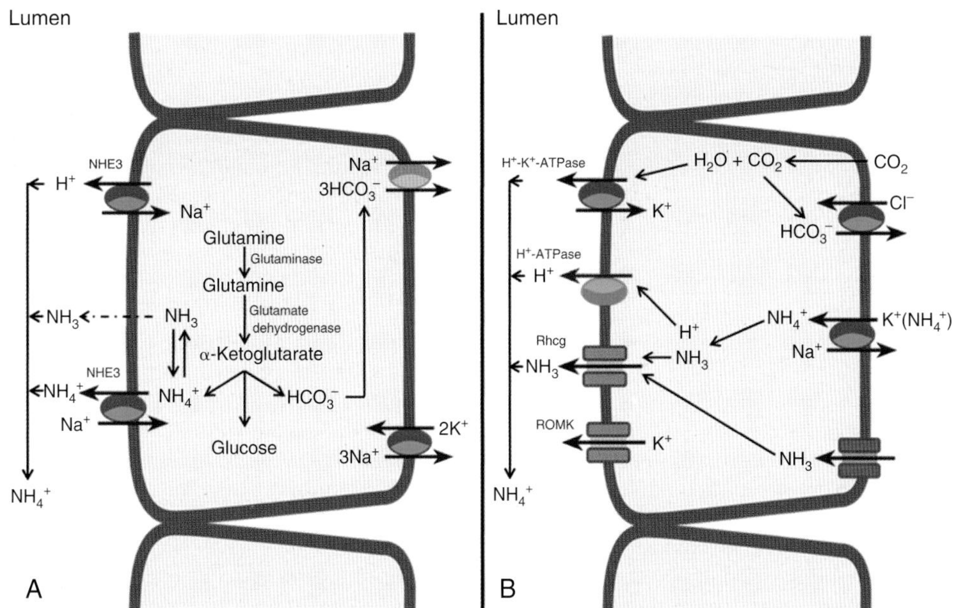


**Fig. 16.7** Cell models of ammonia synthesis and excretion pathways. **A,** Proximal convoluted tubule. Ammonia is derived from glutamine precursors to produce two $NH_4^+$ and two $HCO_3^-$ molecules through an enzymatic pathway activated by acidemia and hypokalemia and inhibited by alkalemia and hyperkalemia. **B,** Type A intercalated cell in collecting tubule. Ammonium entry across basolateral membrane through substitution of $NH_4^+$ for $K^+$ on $K^+$ conductance and secreted across apical membrane via ROMK or RhCG (see text). In both **A** and **B,** $NH_3$ diffusion coupled with $H^+$ secretion traps $NH_4^+$ in the tubule lumen.

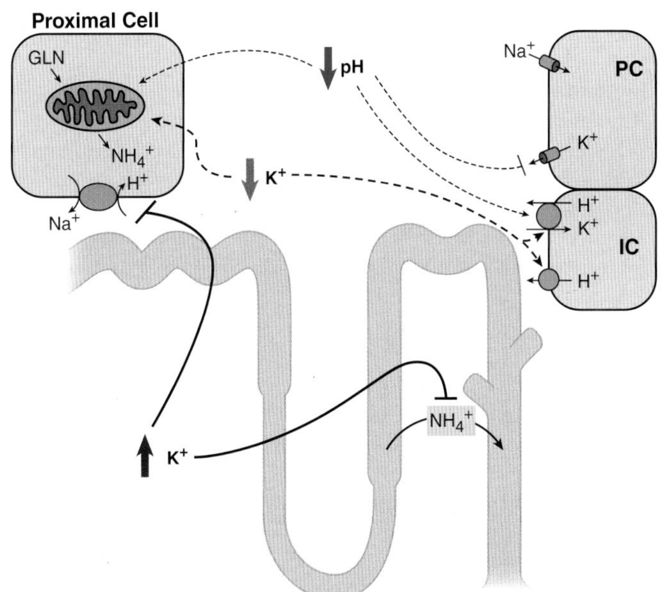


**Fig. 16.8 Diagram of some of the renal interactions of acid-base status and K⁺.** Proximal tubule cell, and a collecting duct principal cell (PC) and intercalated cell (IC) are shown. Acidosis (↓ pH) causes renal potassium retention by several actions including inhibiting secretory $K^+$ channels, stimulating $H^+$-$K^+$-ATPase which reabsorbs $K^+$, and increasing ammoniagenesis which may have secondary actions that block $K^+$ secretion. Alkalosis can have the reverse effects. The effects also work in the other direction: potassium depletion (↓ $K^+$) stimulates ammoniagenesis and $H^+$ secretion/bicarbonate reabsorption, and also distal acid secretion – all of which may cause metabolic alkalosis. Hyperkalemia can have some of the opposite effects; such as inhibiting thick ascending limb ammonium transport, inhibiting urinary ammonium excretion, an effect which may cause acidosis. (From Hamm LL, Hering-Smith KS, Nakhoul NL. Acid-base and potassium homeostasis. *Semin Nephrol.* 2013;333:257-64.)

failure to respond to stress. These defects can occur in association with renal salt wasting and hyponatremia, hyperkalemia, and metabolic acidosis, all associated with mineralocorticoid deficiency alone. The most common congenital adrenal defect in steroid biosynthesis is 21-hydroxylase deficiency, which is associated with salt wasting, hyperkalemia, and metabolic acidosis in a fraction of patients. Causes of Addison's disease include tuberculosis, autoimmune adrenal failure, fungal infections, adrenal hemorrhage, metastasis, lymphoma, acquired immunodeficiency syndrome (AIDS), amyloidosis, and drug toxicity (ketoconazole, fluconazole, phenytoin, rifampin, and barbiturates). These disorders are associated with low plasma aldosterone levels and high levels of plasma renin activity.[33] The metabolic acidosis of mineralocorticoid deficiency results from a decrease in hydrogen ion secretion in the collecting duct secondary to decreased $H^+$-ATPase activity. The accompanying hyperkalemia of mineralocorticoid deficiency decreases ammonium production and excretion.

### Hyporeninemic Hypoaldosteronism

In contrast to patients with primary adrenal disorders, patients with hyporeninemic hypoaldosteronism exhibit low plasma renin activity, are usually older (mean age 65 years), and frequently have mild to moderate renal insufficiency (70%) and acidosis (50%) in association with chronic hyperkalemia in the range of 5.5 to 6.5 mEq/L (Table 16.13).[33] In this relatively common disorder, the metabolic acidosis and the hyperkalemia are out of proportion to the level of reduction in GFR. The most frequently associated renal diseases are diabetic nephropathy and tubulointerstitial disease. Additional disorders associated with hyporeninemic hypoaldosteronism include obstructive uropathy, systemic lupus erythematosus, and human immunodeficiency virus (HIV) infection. For 80% to 85% of such patients, there is a reduction in plasma renin activity that does not respond to the usual physiologic

**Table 16.13 Hyporeninemic Hypoaldosteronism: Typical Clinical Features**

| |
|---|
| Mean age 65 yrs |
| Asymptomatic hyperkalemia (75%) |
| Hyperchloremic metabolic acidosis (>50%) |
| Renal insufficiency (70%) |
| Diabetes mellitus (50%) |
| Hypertension (75%) |
| Weakness (25%) |
| Arrhythmia (25%) |
| Congestive heart failure (50%) |

maneuvers. Because approximately 30% of patients with hyporeninemic hypoaldosteronism are hypertensive, the finding of a low plasma renin activity in such patients suggests a volume-dependent form of hypertension with physiologic suppression of renin elaboration. The mechanism(s) of renin suppression is not firmly established for all cases but possibilities include volume expansion, atrial natriuretic peptides, and direct effects of the various renal diseases.

Impaired ammonium excretion is the combined result of hyperkalemia, impaired ammoniagenesis, a reduction in nephron mass, reduced proton secretion, and impaired transport of ammonium by nephron segments in the inner medulla.[32,33,63] Hyperchloremic metabolic acidosis occurs in approximately 50% of patients with hyporeninemic hypoaldosteronism but is often less of a clinical issue than the hyperkalemia. Drugs that may result in similar manifestations are reviewed later.

### Isolated Hypoaldosteronism in Critically Ill Patients

Isolated hypoaldosteronism, which may occur in critically ill patients, particularly in the setting of severe sepsis or cardiogenic shock, is manifest by markedly elevated ACTH and cortisol levels in concert with a decrease in aldosterone elaboration in response to angiotensin II. This may be secondary to selective inhibition of aldosterone synthase as a result of hypoxia or in response to cytokines such as tumor necrosis factor-α or interleukin-1 or, alternatively, as a result of high circulating levels of atrial natriuretic peptide (ANP).[32,33,64] ANP, a powerful suppressor of aldosterone secretion, may be elevated in congestive heart failure (CHF), with atrial arrhythmias, in subclinical cardiac disease, and in volume expansion. The tendency to manifest the features of hypoaldosteronism, including hyperkalemia and metabolic acidosis, is often potentiated by the administration of potassium-sparing diuretics, potassium loads in parenteral nutrition solutions, or heparin. The latter (both unfractionated and low molecular weight heparin) can suppress aldosterone synthesis in the critically ill patient.

### Resistance to Mineralocorticoid and Voltage Defects: Hyperkalemic Distal Renal Tubular Acidosis

A generalized defect in distal tubule secretory function that results in hyperkalemic hyperchloremic metabolic acidosis has been designated as *hyperkalemic distal RTA* because of the coexistence of hyperkalemia, and an inability to acidify the urine (urine pH of >5.5) during spontaneous acidosis or following an acid load. The hyperkalemia is the result of impaired renal $K^+$ secretion, and the TTKG or $FE_{K^+}$ is invariably lower than expected for non-renal hyperkalemia. Urine ammonium excretion is reduced, but aldosterone levels may be low, normal, or even increased. Hyperkalemic distal RTA can be distinguished from selective hypoaldosteronism because plasma renin and aldosterone levels are usually high or normal. In selective hypoaldosteronism, the urine pH is typically low and the defect in urinary acid excretion can be attributed to the decrease in ammonium excretion.

### Drug-Induced Renal Tubular Secretory Defects

**Impaired Renin-Aldosterone Elaboration.** Drugs may impair renin or aldosterone elaboration or cause mineralocorticoid resistance and produce effects that mimic the clinical manifestations of the acidification defect seen in the generalized form of distal RTA with hyperkalemia. COX inhibitors (NSAIDs or COX-2 inhibitors) can generate hyperkalemia and metabolic acidosis as a result of inhibition of renin release.[65] β-adrenergic antagonists cause hyperkalemia by altering potassium distribution and by interfering with the renin-aldosterone system. Heparin impairs aldosterone synthesis as a result of direct toxicity to the zona glomerulosa and inhibition of aldosterone synthase. ACE inhibitors and ARBs interrupt the renin-aldosterone system and result in hypoaldosteronism with hyperkalemia and acidosis, particularly in patients with advanced renal insufficiency or in patients with a tendency to develop hyporeninemic hypoaldosteronism (diabetic nephropathy). The combination of potassium-sparing diuretics and ACE inhibitors should be avoided in diabetic patients.

**Inhibitors of Potassium Secretion in the Collecting Duct.** Spironolactone and eplerenone act as competitive inhibitors of aldosterone and inhibit aldosterone action. These drugs may cause hyperkalemia and metabolic acidosis when administered to patients with significant renal insufficiency, patients with advanced liver disease, or patients with unrecognized renal hemodynamic compromise. Similarly, amiloride and triamterene may be associated with hyperkalemia, but through an entirely different mechanism. Both potassium-sparing diuretics occupy and thus block the apical $Na^+$-selective channel (ENaC) in the collecting duct principal cell. Occupation of ENaC inhibits $Na^+$ absorption and reduces the negative transepithelial voltage, which alters the driving force for $K^+$ secretion.

Trimethoprim (TMP) and pentamidine are related structurally to amiloride and triamterene and inhibit ENaC.[66–68] Hyperkalemia has been observed in 20% to 50% of HIV-infected patients receiving high-dose trimethoprim-sulfamethoxazole (TMP-SMX) or TMP-dapsone for the treatment of opportunistic infections and as many as 100% of patients with AIDS-associated infections (due to *Pneumocystis jiroveci*) receiving pentamidine for longer than 6 days.[68] Because both TMP and pentamidine decrease the electrochemical driving force for both $K^+$ and $H^+$ secretion in the CCT, metabolic acidosis may accompany the hyperkalemia even in the absence of severe renal failure, adrenal insufficiency, tubulointerstitial disease, or hypoaldosteronism. Whereas it has been assumed that such a "voltage" defect could explain the decrease in $H^+$ secretion, it is likely that, in addition, hyperkalemia plays a significant role in the development of metabolic acidosis by inhibition of ammonium production and excretion (see Fig. 16.8 and Table 16.12).

The calcineurin inhibitors cyclosporine A and tacrolimus may be associated with hyperkalemia in transplant recipients as a result of inhibition of the basolateral $Na^+$-$K^+$-ATPase and the consequent decrease in intracellular $[K^+]$ and the transepithelial potential, which together reduce the driving force for $K^+$ secretion.[65] Additionally, studies indicate that calcineurin inhibitors may also inhibit $K^+$ secretion by directly interfering with the ROMK $K^+$ channel.[69] An additional explanation for the association of hyperkalemia, volume expansion and hypertension, a syndrome that resembles the phenotype of familial hyperkalemic hypertension or PHA-2, is enhanced activity of NCC in the DCT.[70]

### Secondary Renal Diseases Associated With Acquired Voltage Defects

Hyperkalemia that is out of proportion to the degree of renal insufficiency can also be observed in the nephropathies associated with sickle cell disease, HIV infection, systemic lupus erythematosus, obstructive uropathy, acute and chronic renal allograph rejection, hypoaldosteronism, multiple myeloma, and amyloidosis.[33,71] Tubulointerstitial disease with hyperkalemia and hyperchloremic metabolic acidosis with or without salt wasting may be associated with analgesic abuse, nephrolithiasis, nephrocalcinosis, and hyperuricemia.[33]

A variety of familial disorders are associated with hyperkalemia and hyperchloremic metabolic acidosis. Autosomal dominant pseudohypoaldosteronism type 1 (PHA-1) is an example of a voltage defect in the collecting tubule resulting from aldosterone resistance. This disorder, which is clinically less severe than the autosomal recessive form discussed later, is associated with hyperkalemia from impaired potassium secretion, renal salt wasting, elevated levels of renin and aldosterone, and relative hypotension. Physiologic mineralocorticoid replacement therapy does not correct the hyperkalemia. The autosomal dominant disorder has been shown to be the result of a mutation in the intracellular mineralocorticoid receptor in the collecting tubule.[72] In contrast to the autosomal recessive disorder, this defect is not expressed in organs other than the kidney and becomes less severe with advancing age. Because of the decrease in mineralocorticoid actions, apical $Na^+$ absorption and the transepithelial voltage difference are reduced and $K^+$ secretion is secondarily impaired. Four hours after administration of fludrocortisone (0.1 mg orally) to patients with autosomal dominant PHA-1, the TTKG will *not* increase, which demonstrates that resistance to mineralocorticoid causes the hyperkalemia.

Autosomal recessive PHA-1 is a prototypical voltage defect in the CCT. This disorder is the result of a loss-of-function mutation of the gene that encodes one of the $\alpha$-, $\beta$-, or $\gamma$-subunits of the ENaC.[73–77] Children with this disorder have severe hyperkalemia and renal salt wasting because of impaired sodium absorption in principal cells of the CCT. In addition, the hyperchloremic metabolic acidosis may be severe and is associated with hypotension and marked elevations of plasma renin and aldosterone. These children also manifest vomiting, hyponatremia, failure to thrive, and respiratory distress. The latter is due to involvement of ENaC in the alveolus, which prevents $Na^+$ and water absorption in the lungs.[76–78] Patients with this disease respond to a high salt intake and correction of the hyperkalemia. Unlike the autosomal dominant form, autosomal recessive PHA-1 persists throughout life.

**Familial Hyperkalemic Hypertension.** A number of additional adult patients have been reported with a rare form of autosomal dominant low-renin hypertension that is invariably associated with hyperkalemia, hyperchloremic metabolic acidosis, mild volume expansion, normal renal function, and low aldosterone levels. The acidosis in these patients is mild and can be accounted for by the hyperkalemia; the acidosis and renal potassium excretion are resistant to mineralocorticoid administration. Thiazide diuretics consistently correct the hyperkalemia and metabolic acidosis, as well as the hypertension, plasma aldosterone level, and plasma renin level. This syndrome has been recently designated *familial hyperkalemic hypertension* (FHH) but is also known as *pseudohypoaldosteronism type 2* (PHA-2)[79] or *Gordon's syndrome.*[80,81] Both genes encode members of the WNK (*w*ith *n*o lysine [*K*]) family of serine-threonine kinases. These kinases signal via serine/threonine protein kinase 39 (SPAK; STK39) and oxidative stress-response 1 (OxSR1 or OSR1; OXSR1), which phosphorylate and activate the thiazide sensitive Na-Cl cotransporter (NCC) in the distal convoluted tubule, among other transporters affected.[81–83] Cul3 is part of an E3 ubiquitin ligase complex that regulates protein degradation. Loss of regulation of NCC by WNK4 results in a gain in NCC function, which, through enhanced absorption of $Na^+$ and $Cl^-$, causes volume expansion, decreased more distal delivery of $Na^+$ and therefore reduced $K^+$ secretion particularly in the connecting tubule.[81,84] More recent studies have revealed that FHH is more commonly caused by mutations in the cullin-RING ligase (CRL) proteins cullin 3 (Cul3)[4] and kelch-like 3 (KLHL3).[85,86] Loss of inhibition of NCC by WNK4 results in a gain in NCC function, which, through enhanced absorption of $Na^+$ and $Cl^-$, causes volume expansion, decreased distal delivery of $Na^+$ and therefore reduced $K^+$ secretion, particularly in the connecting tubule.[87]

**Treatment.** In patients with hyperkalemic hyperchloremic metabolic acidosis, ideally treatment follows delineation of the underlying cause. However, in certain clinical situations the cause can be easily surmised and treatment begun. For instance, hyporeninemic hypoaldosteronism is common in patients with diabetes and mild to moderate CKD; and certain drugs commonly cause hyperkalemic, hyperchloremic metabolic acidosis. A good history and assessment of the clinical setting are crucial. Contributing or precipitating factors should be considered, including low urine flow or decreased distal $Na^+$ delivery, a rapid decline in GFR (especially in AKI superimposed on chronic renal failure), hyperglycemia or hyperosmolality, and sources of exogenous $K^+$ intake. Assessment of the blood pressure and volume status is important. In cases in which aldosterone is low or suspected to be low, consideration and/or exclusion of combined cortisol deficiency (Addison's disease) is crucial. The workup may include evaluation of the TTKG or the fractional excretion of potassium and an estimate of renal ammonium excretion (UAG or urine osmolar gap, and urine pH).[1]

---

[1]The urine pH may be assessed under stimulated conditions with dietary salt restriction and furosemide-induced volume depletion, and measurement of the response of potassium excretion to furosemide and fludrocortisone. An increase in the TTKG to a value of more than 6 measured 4 hours after a single oral dose of fludrocortisone (0.05 mg) suggests that mineralocorticoid deficiency, but not resistance, is causative.

Since acidosis and hyperkalemia are frequently interrelated, treatment of one may aid the other. Treatment options are given in Table 16.14. The severity of the hyperkalemia often drives the treatment. Reduction in the serum potassium level will often improve the metabolic acidosis by increasing ammonium excretion. In hyporeninemic hypoaldosteronism, loop diuretics may improve volume status, blood pressure, potassium and acidosis. Correction of hyperkalemia with oral agents (ZS-9, patiromir) that act as gastrointestinal cation exchangers may be useful. In the past, sodium polystyrene was used but reports of intestinal necrosis have limited its use. Presently patiromer and sodium zirconium cyclosilicate (ZS-9) are used for this purpose. Alkali therapy may be useful not only for the acidosis, but indirectly to help the potassium. In hyporeninemic hypoaldosteronism, exogenous mineralocorticoids are frequently not a first-line treatment because of the coexistent hypertension and volume overload. Patients with combined glucocorticoid and mineralocorticoid deficiency should receive both adrenal steroids in replacement dosages. Volume depletion should be avoided unless the patient is volume overexpanded or hypertensive. Infants with autosomal recessive or dominant PHA-1 should receive salt supplements in amounts sufficient to correct the volume depletion, hypotension, and other features of the syndrome and to allow normal growth. In contrast, patients with PHA-2 should receive thiazide diuretics along with dietary salt restriction.

In drug-induced disorders, obviously discontinuing the offending agent is ideal. In some cases, this may not always be feasible such as in patients with life-threatening disorders, for example, during TMP-SMX or pentamidine therapy in AIDS patients with *Pneumocystis jiroveci* pneumonia. Based on the previous discussion, other mechanisms to increase distal potassium secretion or gastrointestinal exchangers can be tried.

**Table 16.14 Treatment of Generalized Dysfunction of the Nephron With Hyperkalemia**

Loop diuretic (furosemide, bumetanide)
Alkali therapy (Shohl's solution or NaHCO3 tablets)
$K^+$ binding resin
Low-potassium diet
Fludrocortisone (0.1-0.3 mg/day)
  Avoid in hypertension, volume expansion, heart failure
  Combine with loop diuretic
Avoid drugs associated with hyperkalemia, herbs and over-the-counter preparations containing potassium
In pseudohypoaldosteronism type 1, add NaCl tablets

**Distinguishing the Types of Renal Tubular Acidosis.** The contrasting findings and diagnostic features of the three types of RTA discussed in this chapter are summarized in Table 16.15.

**Acidosis of Chronic Kidney Disease.** Chronic kidney disease has long been known to be associated with acidosis.[88,89] Acidosis is usually recognized with a GFR below 40 mL/min,[90] but is present in only some patients, not all. But recent evidence suggests that acid may be retained in at least some patients with CKD who do not have typical manifestations of acidosis such as reduced plasma $HCO_3^-$.[91,92] Bone buffering may account for the relative stability of the plasma $HCO_3^-$.[3] The metabolic acidosis when present is initially hyperchloremic but may convert to the high AG metabolic acidosis as GFR falls below 15 mL/min.[37,93] The principal defect in net acid excretion in patients with reduced GFR is an inability to excrete $NH_4^+$ sufficiently to match net endogenous acid production. Endogenous acid production in adults is usually about 1 mEq per kg body weight (2-3 mEq/kg in children) but varies with diet such that low protein and high fruits and vegetables will lower the amount. Unlike patients with distal RTA, most patients with CKD can lower urine pH and excrete titratable acid normally.[37]

The numerous consequences of chronic positive acid balance in CKD and certainly acidosis include progression of CKD at a faster rate[91]and, dissolution of bone,[35] impaired hydroxylation of 25-hydroxycholecalciferol, and renal osteodystrophy[37,94] sarcopenia from enhanced skeletal muscle protein degradation, loss of muscle strength, and insulin resistance. Acidosis has also been associated with increased mortality in CKD.[95,96] The mechanisms whereby acidosis worsens progression of CKD are not totally understood but may include 1) increased fibrosis from activation of complement from increased interstitial $NH4^+$ and 2) increased hormones such as endothelin, angiotensin II, and aldosterone.

Corresponding with the findings that acidosis worsens progression of CKD, several studies at this point have shown that treatment of acidosis can improve the course of CKD. Interestingly, patients with stage 2 and 3 CKD even without overt clinical metabolic acidosis, when given oral alkali progress more slowly (i.e., GFR declines less rapidly) and exhibit a significant reduction in net acid excretion.[91,97]

**Table 16.15 Contrasting Features and Diagnostic Studies in Renal Tubular Acidosis**

| | Type of Renal Tubular Acidosis | | |
|---|---|---|---|
| Finding | Proximal | Classical Distal | Generalized Distal Dysfunction |
| Plasma [$K^+$] | Low | Low | High |
| Urine pH with acidosis | <5.5 | >5.5 | <5.5 or >5.5 |
| Fanconi's lesion | Present with acquired PRTA | Absent | Absent |
| Fractional bicarbonate excretion | 10%-15% during alkali therapy | 2%-5% | 5%-10% |
| Associated features | Fanconi's syndrome | Nephrocalcinosis/Hyperglobulinemia | Renal insufficiency |

Moreover, a recent study in patients with stage 4 CKD found that a diet emphasizing fruits and vegetables had as beneficial an effect on slowing progression of CKD and compared favorably to $NaHCO_3$ therapy.[98] Note that neither approach, alkali supplementation, or additional fruits and vegetables in the diet require dietary protein restriction.

Alkali therapy not only slows progression of CKD but also helps to reverse the deleterious effects of chronic acidosis on bone and skeletal muscle.[97] An amount of alkali slightly in excess (1 to 2 mEq/kg/day) of dietary metabolic acid production, typically restores the $[HCO_3^-]$ to recommended levels (> 22 mEq/L; see below).[35] The clinical guidelines endorsed by the National Kidney Foundation Kidney Disease Outcomes Quality Initiative (KDOQI) recommend monitoring of total $CO_2$ in patients with chronic kidney disease with a goal of maintaining the $[HCO_3^-]$ above 22 mEq/L.[99] Alkali therapy may consist of $NaHCO_3$ tablets or modified Shohl's (Citric Acid – Sodium Citrate) Solution. Addition of alkali even in the form of $NaHCO_3$ does not lead to salt retention or worsened hypertension. There is some concern that plasma $HCO_3^-$ could be raised to a higher level than desired, which has been associated in epidemiologic studies to worsen outcomes.[88]

During the treatment of more advanced CKD patients, phosphate binders are usually prescribed. Sevelamer hydrochloride has been a widely used phosphate binder since it does not contain calcium; however, it is associated with an acid load.[100,101] Use of sevelamer carbonate, the more recent formulation of sevelamer, avoids this issue.

As kidney disease progresses below a GFR of 15 mL/min, the non-AG acidosis typically evolves into the usual high AG acidosis of end-stage renal disease. An increased anion gap may be seen earlier when the anion gap is fully adjusted for albumin etc.[102] The anions that account for the elevated anion gap include phosphate, sulfate, urate, etc.

**High Anion Gap Acidoses.** When the non-Cl– anion of an acid load is not excreted rapidly, a high AG acidosis results, with a normal plasma $Cl^-$. The normo-chloremic acidosis is maintained as long as the anion that was part of the original acid load remains in the blood. High AG acidosis is caused by the accumulation of organic acids such as lactate or ketoacids. This may occur if the anion does not undergo glomerular filtration (e.g., uremic acid anions), if the anion is filtered but is readily reabsorbed, or if, because of alteration in metabolic pathways (ketoacidosis, L-lactic acidosis), the anion cannot be utilized in the body sufficiently rapidly. Conceptually, an acid such as lactic acid or ketoacid will react with plasma $HCO_3^-$, "consuming" the $HCO_3^-$ or converting it to $CO_2$ which will be exhaled, replacing that $HCO_3^-$ anion with the acid anion such as $lactate^-$ or ketoacid anion.

Theoretically, with a pure AG acidosis, the increment in the AG ($\Delta AG$) above the normal value of approximately 10 mEq/L should conceptually equal the decrease in bicarbonate concentration ($\Delta HCO_3^-$) below the normal value of 25 mEq/L. In some cases, the increment in AG may be the leading indicator of the existence of the high AG acidosis, not a decrement in pH or $HCO_3^-$. For example, with a mixed metabolic alkalosis and high AG acidosis, the $HCO_3^-$ and pH may not fully reflect the metabolic acidosis, but the AG should. Such findings are not unusual when uremia or ketoacidosis leads to vomiting, for example.

Identification of the underlying cause of a high AG acidosis is facilitated by consideration of the clinical setting and associated laboratory values. The common causes are outlined in Table 16.16 and include 1) lactic acidosis (e.g., L-lactic acidosis and D-lactic acidosis), 2) ketoacidosis (e.g., diabetic, alcoholic, and starvation ketoacidoses), 3) toxin- or poison-induced acidosis (e.g., ethylene glycol, methyl alcohol, propylene glycol, or pyroglutamic acidosis), and 4) uremic acidosis.

Initial screening to differentiate the high AG acidoses should focus on 1) a history or other evidence of drug or toxin ingestion and ABG measurement to detect coexistent respiratory alkalosis (as with salicylates), 2) historical evidence of diabetes mellitus (diabetic ketoacidosis; DKA), 3) evidence of alcoholism or increased levels of β-hydroxybutyrate (alcoholic ketoacidosis; AKA), 4) observation for clinical signs of uremia and determination of the blood urea and creatinine

**Table 16.16 Metabolic Acidosis With High Anion Gap**

| |
|---|
| **Conditions Associated with Type A Lactic Acidosis** |
| Hypovolemic shock |
| Cholera |
| Septic shock |
| Cardiogenic shock |
| Regional hypoperfusion |
| Severe hypoxia |
| Severe asthma |
| Carbon monoxide poisoning |
| Severe anemia |
| **Conditions Associated with Type B Lactic Acidosis** |
| Liver disease |
| Diabetes mellitus |
| **Metformin** |
| Catecholamine excess |
| Thiamine deficiency |
| Intracellular inorganic phosphate depletion |
| Intravenous fructose, xylose, or sorbitol |
| Alcohols and other ingested compounds metabolized by alcohol dehydrogenase |
| Ethanol, methanol, ethylene glycol, propylene glycol |
| Mitochondrial toxins |
| **Salicylates**, cyanide, 2,4-dinitrophenol, **Nonnucleoside anti–reverse transcriptase drugs** |
| Other drugs (propofol, linezolid) |
| Metastatic tumors (large tumors with regional hypoxemia or liver metastasis) |
| **Seizures** |
| Inborn errors of metabolism |
| **D-Lactic Acidosis** |
| Short bowel syndrome, ischemic bowel, Small-bowel obstruction |
| **Ketoacidosis** |
| Diabetic |
| Alcoholic |
| **Intoxications** |
| Salicylates |
| Ethylene glycol |
| Methanol |
| Pyroglutamic acid |
| **Uremia (Late Renal Failure)** |

levels (uremic acidosis), 5) inspection of the urine for oxalate crystals (ethylene glycol), and, finally, 6) recognition of the numerous settings in which lactic acid levels may be increased (hypotension, sepsis, cardiac failure, ischemic bowel, intestinal obstruction and bacterial overgrowth, leukemia, cancer, and exposure to certain drugs).

### Lactic Acidosis

***Physiology.*** Lactic acid can exist in two forms: L-lactic acid and D-lactic acid. In mammals, only the L stereoisomer is a product of metabolism and most lactic acidosis is therefore L-lactic acidosis. L-lactic acidosis is one of the most common forms of a high AG acidosis.

Lactate usually derives from pyruvate in the cytosolic reaction of lactate dehydrogenase:

$$\text{Pyruvate}^- + \text{NADH} + \text{H}^+ \leftrightarrow \text{Lactate}^- + \text{NAD}^+ \qquad (16.14)$$

Pyruvate is generated with the metabolism of glucose by cytosolic anaerobic glycolysis. Pyruvate in aerobic conditions will be further metabolized in mitochondria in the Krebs or tricarboxylic acid cycle. But in the cytosol, the equation above is a near equilibrium reaction such that the lactate to pyruvate ratio (usually about 10) is governed by the $H^+$ concentration or pH and the NADH: $NAD^+$ ratio, or the oxidation-reduction potential (or redox potential) of the cell.

After rearranging the mass action equation, the ratio of lactate concentration to pyruvate concentration may be expressed as

$$\frac{[\text{Lactate}^-]}{[\text{Pyruvate}^-]} = K_{eq}[\text{H}^+]\frac{[\text{NADH}]}{[\text{NAD}^+]} \qquad (16.15)$$

The NADH/$NAD^+$ ratio is also involved in many other metabolic redox reactions.[103] Moreover, the steady-state concentrations of all these redox reactants are related to one another. Important in other considerations of acid-base pathophysiology are the redox pairs β-hydroxybutyrate–acetoacetate and ethanol-acetaldehyde, discussed below. In clinical practice, these considerations can be of practical importance in assessing diabetic and alcoholic ketoacidosis (discussed below).

Normally, the rates of lactate entry and exit from the blood are in balance, so that net lactate accumulation is zero. This dynamic aspect of lactate metabolism in which lactate is converted back to glucose in the liver is termed the *Cori cycle.* In conditions of lactic acidosis either net overproduction of lactic acid from glucose by some tissues or underutilization by other tissues results in net addition of L-lactic acid to the blood. Ischemia accelerates lactate production and simultaneously decreases lactate utilization.

The production of lactic acid has been estimated to be about 15 to 20 mEq/kg/day in normal humans.[35] This enormous quantity contrasts with total ECF buffer base stores of only about 10 to 15 mEq/kg, so that with enhanced production, lactic acid can accumulate. The quantitative aspects of normal lactate production and consumption in the Cori cycle demonstrate that the development of lactic acidosis can be the most rapid and devastating form of metabolic acidosis.[103,104] The rate of lactic acid production can be increased by ischemia, seizures, extreme exercise, catecholamines, leukemia, and alkalosis.[103] The increase in production occurs principally through enhanced phosphofructokinase activity.

Decreased lactate consumption may also lead to L-lactic acidosis, and probably plays an important role in most clinical lactic acidosis. The principal organs for lactate removal during rest are the liver and kidneys. Both the liver and the kidneys and perhaps muscle have the capacity for increased lactate removal under the stress of increased lactate loads.[103] Hepatic utilization of lactate can be impeded by several factors: poor perfusion of the liver; defective active transport of lactate into cells; and inadequate metabolic conversion of lactate into pyruvate because of altered intracellular pH, redox state, or enzyme activity. Examples of states causing impaired hepatic lactate removal include primary diseases of the liver, enzymatic defects, tissue anoxia or ischemia, severe acidosis, and altered redox states, as occurs with alcohol intoxication, fructose consumption by fructose-intolerant individuals, or administration of nucleoside (analog) reverse transcriptase inhibitors (NRTIs) such as zidovudine and stavudine in patients with HIV infection[103,105,106] or biguanides such as metformin.[103,107,108] Deaths have been reported due to refractory lactic acidosis secondary to thiamine deficiency in patients receiving parenteral nutrition formulations without thiamine.[109] Thiamine is a cofactor for pyruvate dehydrogenase that catalyzes the oxidative decarboxylation of pyruvate to acetyl–coenzyme A under aerobic conditions. Pyruvate cannot be metabolized in this manner in the presence of thiamine deficiency, so that excess pyruvate is converted to hydrogen ions and lactate.

***Diagnosis.*** Because lactic acid has a $pK_a$ of 3.8, addition of lactic acid to the blood leads to a reduction in blood $HCO_3^-$ concentration and an equivalent elevation in lactate concentration, which is associated with an increase in the AG. Lactate concentrations are mildly increased in various nonpathologic states (e.g., exercise), but the magnitude of the elevation is generally small. In practical terms, a lactate concentration greater than 4 mmol/L (normal is 0.67 to 1.8 mmol/L) is generally accepted as evidence that the metabolic acidosis is due to net lactic acid accumulation.

***Clinical Spectrum.*** In the classical classification of the L-lactic acidoses (see Table 16.16), type A L-lactic acidosis is due to tissue hypoperfusion or acute hypoxia, whereas type B L-lactic acidosis is less common but associated with some common diseases, drugs and toxins, and hereditary and miscellaneous disorders.[103]

Tissue underperfusion and acute tissue hypoxia are the most common causes of type A lactic acidosis. Severe arterial hypoxemia even in the absence of decreased perfusion can generate L-lactic acidosis. Inadequate cardiac output, of either the low-output or the high-output variety, is the common pathogenetic factor. Among the most common causes of L-lactic acidosis is bowel ischemia and infarction in patients in the medical intensive care unit. The prognosis is related directly to the increment in plasma L-lactate and the severity of the acidemia.[103,104]

Numerous medical conditions (without tissue hypoxia) predispose to type B L-lactic acidosis (see Table 16.16). Hepatic failure reduces hepatic lactate metabolism, and leukemia increases lactate production. Catecholamines stimulate glycolysis and lactate production. Severe anemia, especially as a result of iron deficiency or methemoglobulinemia, may cause lactic acidosis. Malignant cells produce more lactate than normal cells even under aerobic conditions. This phenomenon is magnified if the tumor expands rapidly and outstrips the blood supply. Therefore, exceptionally large tumors may be associated with severe L-lactic acidosis. Seizures, extreme exertion, heat stroke, and tumor lysis syndrome may all cause L-lactic acidosis. Lactic acidosis with seizures is transient and self-limited, as the lactate that is produced can be rapidly metabolized.

Several drugs and toxins predispose to L-lactic acidosis (see Table 16.16). Of these, metformin and other biguanides (such as phenformin) are the most widely reported to have this effect.[103,107,108] The occurrence of phenformin-induced lactic acidosis prompted the withdrawal of the drug from U.S. markets in 1977. Although much less frequent than phenformin-induced lactic acidosis, metformin-induced lactic acidosis is at higher risk in patients with CKD (and is contraindicated when the serum creatinine exceeds 1.4 mg/dL), and whenever there is hypoperfusion, hypotension, or chronic metabolic acidosis. Metformin should be discontinued several days before contrast dye administration. Although rare, metformin-induced lactic acidosis is the most frequent cause of lactic acidosis in diabetic patients and is associated with a mortality of up to 50%. Carbon monoxide poisoning frequently produces lactic acidosis by reduction of the oxygen-carrying capacity of hemoglobin. Cyanide binds cytochrome $a$ and $a_3$ and blocks the flow of electrons to oxygen. In patients with HIV infection nucleoside analogs can induce toxic effects on mitochondria by inhibiting DNA polymerase-γ. Hyperlactatemia is common with NRTI therapy, especially stavudine and zidovudine, but the serum L-lactate level is usually only mildly elevated and compensated.[103,106,110] This combination carries a high mortality.

***Associated Clinical Features.*** Hyperventilation, abdominal pain, and disturbances in consciousness are frequently present, as are signs of inadequate cardiopulmonary function in type A L-lactic acidosis. Leukocytosis, hyperphosphatemia, and hyperuricemia are common, and hypoglycemia may occur.[103] Hyperkalemia may or may not accompany acute lactic acidosis.

***Treatment of L-Lactic Acidosis: General Supportive Care.*** The overall mortality of patients with L-lactic acidosis is approximately 60%, but increases in those with coexisting hypotension.[103] The basic principle and only effective form of therapy for L-lactic acidosis is first to correct the underlying condition(s) initiating the disruption in normal lactate metabolism. In type A L-lactic acidosis, cessation of acid production by improvement of tissue oxygenation, restoration of the circulating fluid volume, improvement or augmentation of cardiac function, resection of ischemic tissue, and amelioration of sepsis are necessary in many cases. Septic shock requires control of the underlying infection and volume resuscitation in hypovolemic shock. Lactate levels are often followed as an indicator of tissue perfusion. Sodium bicarbonate administration is of little value in this setting.

***Alkali Therapy.*** Alkali therapy is generally advocated only for acute, severe acidemia (pH of <7.1) to improve the detrimental hemodynamic consequences of the acidosis: decreased inotropy, venoconstriction, arterial vasodilation, and decreased catecholamine responsiveness. The only exception in milder acidosis may be with coexistent severe acute kidney injury.[111] However, in experimental models and clinical examples of lactic acidosis, $NaHCO_3$ therapy in large amounts may depress cardiac performance and exacerbate the acidemia. Paradoxically, bicarbonate therapy activates phosphofructokinase, which is regulated by intracellular pH, thereby increasing lactate production. The use of alkali in states of moderate L-lactic acidemia is therefore controversial, and it is generally agreed that attempts to normalize the pH or $HCO_3^-$ concentration by intravenous $NaHCO_3$ therapy is both potentially deleterious and practically impossible. Thus, raising the plasma $HCO_3^-$ to approximately 15 mEq/L (not to the normal value) and the pH to between 7.2 to 7.25 is a reasonable goal to improve tissue pH. Constant infusion of hypertonic bicarbonate has many disadvantages and is discouraged. Fluid overload occurs rapidly with $NaHCO_3$ administration because of the massive amounts required in some cases. With rapid infusions of $HCO_3^-$, $PCO_2$ may increase, ionized calcium decrease, and hypernatremia develop. In addition, central venoconstriction and decreased cardiac output are common. The accumulation of lactic acid may be relentless and may necessitate administration of diuretics, ultrafiltration, or dialysis. Hemodialysis can simultaneously deliver $HCO_3^-$, remove lactate, remove excess ECF volume, and correct electrolyte abnormalities. The use of continuous renal replacement therapy (CRRT) as a means of lactate removal and simultaneous alkali addition is a promising adjunctive treatment in critically ill patients with L-lactic acidosis but has not consistently proved to be beneficial. It is important to note that CRRT also removes lactate in the dialysate and can confound interpretation of serial measurements of lactate concentrations.

If the underlying cause of the L-lactic acidosis can be remedied, blood lactate will be reconverted to $HCO_3^-$. $HCO_3^-$ derived from lactate conversion and any new $HCO_3^-$ generated by renal mechanisms during acidosis and from exogenous alkali therapy are additive and may result in an overshoot alkalosis.

***Other Agents.*** Dichloroacetate (an activator of pyruvate dehydrogenase), methylene blue, THAM (0.3 mol/L tromethamine), and Tribonat (a mixture of THAM, acetate, $NaHCO_3$, and phosphate) have all been advocated with experimental support in the past, but none has been proved to be effective clinically.[112,113] Lactated Ringer's solution and lactate-containing peritoneal dialysis solutions should be avoided. These solutions contain racemic mixtures of both L- and D-lactate.

***D-Lactic Acidosis.*** D-lactic acidosis is a rare cause of high AG acidosis. D-lactate can accumulate in some individuals as a by-product of metabolism by bacteria, which accumulate and overgrow in the gastrointestinal tract with jejunal bypass or short bowel syndrome. The diagnosis can be especially difficult since hospital laboratories routinely only measure L-lactic acid levels using stereospecific enzymatic assays, which do not detect D-lactic acid.

The manifestations of D-lactate acidosis are typically episodic encephalopathy and high AG acidosis in association with short bowel syndrome. Features include slurred speech, confusion, cognitive impairment, clumsiness, ataxia, hallucinations, and behavioral disturbances. D-Lactic acidosis has been described in patients with bowel obstruction, jejunal bypass, short bowel, or ischemic bowel disease. These disorders have in common ileus or stasis associated with overgrowth of flora in the gastrointestinal tract, which is exacerbated by a high-carbohydrate diet.[103] D-lactate acidosis occurs when fermentation by colonic bacteria in the intestine causes D-lactate to accumulate so that it can be absorbed into the circulation. The disorder should be suspected in patients with an unexplained AG acidosis and some of the typical features noted previously. While results of specific testing are pending, the patient should not receive oral nutrition. Serum D-lactate levels of greater than 3 mmol/L confirm the diagnosis. Treatment with a low-carbohydrate diet and antibiotics (neomycin, vancomycin, or metronidazole) is often effective.[114–117]

D lactate levels are also elevated in diabetic ketoacidosis[118] and in some cases with infusions of drugs dissolved in propylene glycol.

***Diabetic Ketoacidosis.*** Diabetic ketoacidosis (DKA) is due to increased fatty acid metabolism and the accumulation of ketoacid anions (acetoacetate and β-hydroxybutyrate) as a result of insulin deficiency or resistance, in association with elevated glucagon levels. There is also frequently increased secretion of catecholamines, cortisol, and growth hormone contributing to the pathogenesis. Insulin deficiency and/or resistance (as from high catecholamine levels) increases lipolysis releasing free fatty acids and glycerol. With high delivery of fatty acids to mitochondria in the setting of low insulin and high glucagon, acetyl-CoA entry into the Krebs cycle is limited and instead is converted to the ketoacid acetoacetic acid. Acetoacetic acid may then be reduced to beta-hydroxybutyric acid.

DKA is usually seen in insulin-dependent diabetes mellitus upon cessation of insulin therapy or during an intercurrent illness, such as an infection, gastroenteritis, pancreatitis, or myocardial infarction, which increases insulin requirements acutely. The accumulation of the anions of the ketoacids accounts for the increment in the AG, which is accompanied, most often, by evidence of hyperglycemia (glucose level of >300 mg/dL). In comparison to patients with AKA, described later, patients with DKA have metabolic profiles characterized by a higher plasma glucose level and lower β-hydroxybutyrate/acetoacetate and lactate/pyruvate ratios.[117,119,120]

Atypical instances of DKA with euglycemia has been reported in patients with both type 1 and type 2 diabetes taking sodium glucose cotransporter 2 (SGLT2) inhibitors.[121] These drugs are only approved in type 2 diabetes but have been used some in type 1 patients. The drugs are not only effective in lowering glucose but also have cardio- and possibly renal protective effects. Suppressed insulin and elevated glucagon are implicated in the pathogenesis of the ketoacidosis.

The extent of the acidosis and the rise in the anion gap in DKA will depend not only on the rate of net ketoacid production but also the loss of ketoacid anions in the urine and the rate of acid excretion by the kidneys. Patients with good kidney function that are well hydrated may excrete large amounts of the ketoacid anions in the urine and even present with a hyperchloremic metabolic acidosis rather than a high AG acidosis.[36] As discussed above, some portion of the usual elevation in AG may be D lactate.

In assessing the levels of ketoacids, coexistent lactic acidosis and the redox state discussed above can be important considerations. If lactate levels are increased as a result of lactic acidosis concurrently with ketone overproduction as a result of diabetic acidosis, the ketones exist primarily in the form of β-hydroxybutyrate. The results of certain tests for ketones that measure only acetoacetate (such as the nitroprusside reaction, e.g., Acetest tablets and reagent sticks), therefore may be misleadingly low or even negative despite high total ketone concentrations. Some hospital laboratories no longer use the nitroprusside reaction to estimate total ketones, and measurement of β-hydroxybutyrate and acetoacetate are the preferred tests.

***Treatment.*** The treatment of DKA has been well studied and recommendations standardized for most patients.[122,123] The treatment usually requires volume repletion, insulin administration, and potassium repletion at the appropriate time. As discussed below, the acidosis may correct without specific treatment other than for the issues above.

Most, if not all, patients with DKA require correction of the volume depletion that almost invariably accompanies the osmotic diuresis of DKA. Several consensus algorithms have been published.[122,123] Initially, fluid replacement is given as isotonic saline and later changed to 0.45% sodium chloride.[117,119] Fluid therapy not only hopefully stabilizes cardiovascular function but also reduces stress hormone levels (including various vasoconstrictors) and improves renal function. Fluid therapy not only hopefully stabilizes cardiovascular function but also reduces stress hormone levels (including various vasoconstrictors) and improves renal function.

Total body $K^+$ depletion is usually present in DKA, although the $K^+$ level on admission may be elevated or normal. A normal or reduced $K^+$ value on admission indicates severe $K^+$ depletion and should be approached with caution. Administration of fluid, insulin, and alkali may cause the $K^+$ level to plummet. When urine output has been established, 20 to 30 mEq of potassium chloride should be administered in each liter of fluid as long as the $K^+$ value is less than 4.0 mEq/L. Equal caution should be exercised in the presence of hyperkalemia, especially if the patient has renal insufficiency, because the usual therapy does not always correct hyperkalemia. Never administer potassium chloride empirically.

For the acidosis per se, most experts only advise giving $HCO_3^-$ if arterial pH is less than 6.9.[122,123] There is no evidence to support the use of exogenous $HCO_3^-$ administration when the pH is above 6.9. With extremely low pH, (pH < 6.9), giving $HCO_3^-$ may improve cardiac contractility, lessen arterial vasodilatation, improve tissue perfusion, and drive $K^+$ into cells. $HCO_3^-$ has several potential disadvantages: reducing ventilatory drive (and theoretically and paradoxically reducing central nervous system [CNS] pH), worsening ketogenesis, and inducing a post-treatment alkalosis when ketones are metabolized to $HCO_3^-$.

The AG should be followed closely during therapy because it is expected to decline as ketones are cleared from the plasma and precedes an increase in plasma $HCO_3^-$ as the acidosis is repaired. It is not usually necessary to monitor blood ketone levels continuously.[117,119,120]

As patients are treated with fluids, more ketoacid anions (beta-hydroxybutryrate and acetoacetate) may be excreted into the urine lowering the AG, but not necessarily changing the pH or $HCO_3^-$. However, the excreted anions represent loss of "potential $HCO_3^-$" because the anions if retained could be metabolized to yield $HCO_3^-$. Therefore, the urinary excretion of ketoacid anions alone may not change the acidosis itself or the plasma $HCO_3^-$, but simply shift the acidosis to a hyperchloremic acidosis.[124] Almost all patients with DKA treated with isotonic saline (a hyperchloremic solution) will evolve to a hyperchloremic metabolic acidosis during treatment. With time, as plasma ketoacid anions are metabolized to $HCO_3^-$ and as the kidneys excrete sufficient acid (simultaneously producing "new" $HCO_3^-$), the acidosis will correct to normal.

***Alcoholic Ketoacidosis (AKA).*** Some patients with chronic alcoholism, especially binge drinkers who discontinue solid food intake while continuing alcohol consumption, develop the alcoholic form of ketoacidosis when alcohol ingestion is curtailed abruptly. Usually the onset of vomiting and abdominal pain with dehydration leads to cessation of alcohol consumption before the patient comes to the hospital.[119,120] The metabolic acidosis may be severe but is accompanied by only modestly abnormal glucose levels, which are usually low but may be slightly elevated. Typically, insulin levels are low and levels of triglyceride, cortisol, epinephrine, glucagon, and growth hormone are increased.[125] The net result of this deranged metabolic state is ketosis. The acidosis is primarily due to elevated levels of ketones, which exist predominantly in the form of β-hydroxybutyrate because of the altered redox state induced by the metabolism of alcohol. The altered redox state will also produce higher lactate concentrations. Compared with patients with DKA, patients with AKA have lower plasma glucose concentrations and higher β-hydroxybutyrate/acetoacetate and lactate/pyruvate ratios.[119,120] Qualitative ketone tests such as nitroprusside, which are more sensitive to acetoacetate, may be only trace positive or negative in AKA, despite markedly increased β-hydroxybutyrate levels. The metabolic acidosis may be severe but is accompanied by only modestly abnormal glucose levels, which are usually low but may be slightly elevated. Typically, insulin levels are low and levels of triglyceride, cortisol, epinephrine, glucagon, and growth hormone are increased.[125] The net result of this deranged metabolic state is ketosis. The acidosis is primarily due to elevated levels of ketones, which exist predominantly in the form of β-hydroxybutyrate because of the altered redox state induced by the metabolism of alcohol. The altered redox state will also produce higher lactate concentrations. Compared with patients with DKA, patients with AKA have lower plasma glucose concentrations and higher β-hydroxybutyrate/acetoacetate and lactate/pyruvate ratios.[119,120] Qualitative ketone tests such as nitroprusside that are more sensitive to acetoacetate may be only trace positive or negative in AKA, despite markedly increased β-hydroxybutyrate levels.

This disorder is not rare and is underdiagnosed. The clinical presentation in AKA may be complex, and is often underdiagnosed. The typical high anion gap acidosis is often mixed with metabolic alkalosis (vomiting), respiratory alkalosis (alcoholic liver disease), lactic acidosis (hypoperfusion), and/or hyperchloremic acidosis (renal excretion of ketoacids). Finally, the elevation in the osmolar gap is usually accounted for by an increased blood alcohol level, but the differential diagnosis should always include ethylene glycol and/or methanol intoxication.

***Treatment.*** Therapy includes intravenous glucose and saline administration, but insulin should be avoided. $K^+$, $PO_4^{3-}$, $Mg^{2+}$, and vitamin supplementation (especially thiamine) are frequently necessary. Glucose in isotonic saline, not saline alone, is the mainstay of therapy. Because of superimposed starvation, patients with AKA often develop hypophosphatemia within 12 to 18 hours of admission. Treatment with glucose-containing intravenous fluids increases the risk of severe hypophosphatemia. Levels should be checked on admission and at 4, 6, 12, and 18 hours. Profound hypophosphatemia may provoke aspiration, platelet dysfunction, hemolysis, and rhabdomyolysis. Therefore, phosphate replacement should be provided promptly when indicated. Hypokalemia and hypomagnesemia are also common and should not be overlooked.[119,120]

***Starvation Ketoacidosis.*** Fasting alone can increase ketoacid levels, although not usually above 10 mEq/L. Ketosis occurs within the first 24 to 48 hours of fasting, is accentuated by exercise and pregnancy, and is rapidly reversible by glucose or insulin administration. Frank ketoacidosis of more than a moderate extent is unusual. Low carbohydrate diets have also been implicated but ketogenic diets do not routinely cause frank acidosis.[126] Starvation-induced hypoinsulinemia and accentuated hepatic ketone production have been linked pathogenically.[119,120]

***Drug- and Toxin-Induced Acidosis: Salicylate.*** Intoxication with salicylates is more common in children than in adults and may result in the development of a high AG metabolic acidosis, but the acid-base abnormality most commonly associated with salicylate intoxication in adults is respiratory alkalosis due to direct stimulation of the respiratory center by salicylates.[117] Adult patients with salicylate intoxication usually have pure respiratory alkalosis or mixed respiratory alkalosis–metabolic acidosis.[117] Metabolic acidosis when it occurs is due to uncoupling of oxidative phosphorylation, and hence the usual high AG acidosis is mostly due to lactic acid and ketoacids. Only part of the increase in the AG is due to the increase in plasma salicylate concentration; for instance, a toxic salicylate level of 100 mg/dL would account for an increase in the AG of only 7 mEq/L. High ketone concentrations have been reported to be present in as many as 40% of adult salicylate-intoxicated patients, sometimes as a result of salicylate-induced hypoglycemia.[127] L-Lactic acid production is also often increased, partly as a direct drug effect[117] and partly as a result of the hyperventilation induced by salicylate. Acidosis enhances the transit of salicylates into the central nervous system since the protonated form of salicylate preferentially crosses the blood-brain barrier. Pulmonary edema and acute lung injury may also occur during salicylate intoxication. Adult patients with salicylate intoxication usually have pure respiratory alkalosis or mixed respiratory alkalosis–metabolic acidosis.[117] Metabolic acidosis when it occurs is due to uncoupling of oxidative phosphorylation, and hence the usual high AG acidosis is mostly due to lactic acid and ketoacids. Only part of the increase in the AG is due to the increase in plasma salicylate concentration; for instance, a toxic salicylate level of 100 mg/dL would account for an increase in the AG of only 7 mEq/L. High ketone concentrations have been reported to be present in as many as 40% of adult salicylate-intoxicated patients, sometimes as a result of salicylate-induced hypoglycemia.[127] L-Lactic acid production is also often increased, partly as a direct drug effect[117] and partly as a result of the hyperventilation induced by salicylate. Acidosis enhances the transit of salicylates into the central nervous system since the protonated form of salicylate preferentially crosses the blood brain barrier. Pulmonary edema and acute lung injury may also occur during salicylate intoxication.

***Treatment.*** General treatment should always consist of initial vigorous gastric lavage with isotonic saline followed by administration of activated charcoal via nasogastric tube. Treatment of the metabolic acidosis can be helpful because acidosis can enhance the entry of salicylate into the CNS. An alkaline diuresis will aid renal excretion of salicylate, so

$NaHCO_3$ is usually given cautiously, avoiding pH > 7.6 (and hypokalemia) with coexisting respiratory alkalosis. Acetazolamide is not recommended. Hemodialysis may be necessary in severe poisoning, especially if renal failure coexists; it is preferred in cases of severe intoxication and is superior to hemofiltration, which does not correct the acid-base abnormality.[117,127]

***Toxins: The Osmolar Gap in Toxin-Induced Acidosis.*** The so-called "osmolar gap" can indicate the presence of certain toxins. Under most physiologic conditions, $Na^+$ (and its accompanying anions), urea, and glucose generate much of the osmotic pressure of blood. Serum osmolality is calculated according to the following expression:

$$\text{Osmolality} = 2\,[\text{Na}^+] + \frac{\text{BUN}}{2.8} + \frac{\text{Glucose (mg/dL)}}{18} \qquad (16.16)$$

The calculated and determined osmolalities usually agree within 10 mOsm/kg. When the measured osmolality exceeds the calculated osmolality by more than 10 mOsm/kg, one of two possibilities usually exists. First, the serum $Na^+$ may be spuriously low, as occurs with hyperlipidemia or hyperproteinemia (pseudohyponatremia). Second, osmolytes other than sodium salts, glucose, or urea may have accumulated in plasma. Examples are infused mannitol, radiocontrast media, or other solutes, including the alcohols, ethylene glycol, and acetone, which can increase the osmolality in plasma. For these examples, the difference between the osmolality and the measured osmolality is proportional to the concentration of the unmeasured solute. Such differences in these clinical circumstances have been referred to as the *osmolar gap*. In the presence of an appropriate clinical history and index of suspicion, the osmolar gap becomes a very reliable and helpful screening tool in assessing for toxin-associated high AG acidosis. An increase in the osmolar gap can be associated with AKA and lactic acidosis as discussed in the previous section, but in general, ethanol intoxication per se does not cause a high AG acidosis, although it can cause an elevated osmolar gap. Isopropyl alcohol (rubbing alcohol) poisoning similarly is not metabolized to a strong acid and does not elevate the AG, although the osmolar gap can be elevated and there can be a positive nitroprusside reaction from the metabolism to acetone.

***Ethylene Glycol.*** Ingestion of ethylene glycol (EG), used in antifreeze, leads to a high AG metabolic acidosis[117,128,129] in addition to severe CNS, cardiopulmonary, and renal damage.[125] A disparity between the measured and calculated blood osmolality (high osmolar gap) is often present, especially in the first few hours after ingestion. Typically over time, as EG is metabolized, the osmolar gap begins to fall and the anion gap begins to rise so that in advanced EG intoxication, the AG will be very high but the osmolar gap will close. The high AG is attributable to ethylene glycol metabolites, especially oxalic acid, glycolic acid, and other incompletely identified organic acids in addition to severe CNS, cardiopulmonary, and renal damage.[125] L-Lactic acid production also increases as a result of a toxic depression in the reaction rates of the citric acid cycle and altered intracellular redox state.[129] Recognition of oxalate crystals in the urine facilitates diagnosis. L-Lactic acid production also increases as a result of a toxic depression in the reaction rates of the citric acid cycle and altered intracellular redox state. Fluorescence of the urine by Wood's light (if the ingested ethylene glycol contains a fluorescent vehicle) has been suggested as a diagnostic indicator but is neither specific nor sensitive.[128,129] The Wood's lamp also may detect the fluorescent vehicle on the shirt or blouse of the patient who has ingested the agent. Fluorescence of the urine by Wood's light (if the ingested ethylene glycol contains a fluorescent vehicle) has been suggested as a diagnostic indicator but is neither specific nor sensitive.[128,129] Treatment includes prompt institution of osmotic diuresis, thiamine and pyridoxine supplementation, administration of 4-methylpyrazole (fomepizole),[130] or ethyl alcohol administration and dialysis.[117,128,130] Do not induce vomiting. Intravenous fomepizole is the drug of choice. Both ethanol and fomepizole are competitive inhibitors of alcohol dehydrogenase and delay the conversion of ethylene glycol into its more toxic metabolites. Competitive inhibition of alcohol dehydrogenase with either fomepizole or ethyl alcohol is absolutely necessary in all patients to lessen toxicity, because ethanol and fomepizole compete for metabolic conversion of ethylene glycol and alter the cellular redox state. Fomepizole (initiated as a loading dose of 15 mg/kg, followed by 10 mg/kg every 12 hours), offers several advantages including set dosing and a predictable decline in ethylene glycol levels without the adverse effect of excessive obtundation, as seen with ethyl alcohol infusion. When these measures have been accomplished, hemodialysis may be initiated to remove the ethylene glycol metabolites. If intravenous ethanol is the only inhibitor of alcohol dehydrogenase available, its infusion should be increased during hemodialysis to allow maintenance of the blood alcohol level in the range of 100 to 150 mg/dL or more than 22 mmol/L. Ethanol can even be added to the dialysate bath. Importantly, hemodialysis can remove fomepizole. The usual indications for hemodialysis include 1) arterial pH of less than 7.3, 2) $HCO_3^-$ concentration of less than 20 mEq/L, 3) osmolal gap of more than 10 mOsm/kg, and 4) oxalate crystalluria.[128]

***Methanol.*** Methanol has wide application in commercially available solvents and is used for industrial and automotive purposes. Sources include windshield wiper fluid, paint remover or thinner, deicing fluid, canned heating sources, varnish and shellac. Ingestion of methanol (wood alcohol) causes metabolic acidosis in addition to severe optic nerve and central nervous system manifestations resulting from its metabolism to formic acid from formaldehyde.[117,128] Lactic acids and ketoacids as well as other unidentified organic acids may contribute to the acidosis. Because of the low molecular mass of methanol (32 Da), an osmolar gap is usually present early in the course but declines as the anion gap increases, the latter reflecting the metabolism of methanol. Therapy is generally similar to that for ethylene glycol intoxication, including general supportive measures, fomepizole administration, folate administration, and usually hemodialysis.[125,130] Lactic acids and ketoacids as well as other unidentified organic acids may contribute to the acidosis. Because of the low molecular mass of methanol (32 Da), an osmolar gap is usually present early in the course but declines as the anion gap increases, the latter reflecting the metabolism of methanol. Therapy is generally similar to that for ethylene glycol intoxication, including general supportive measures, fomepizole administration, folate administration, and usually hemodialysis.[125,130]

***Paraldehyde.*** Intoxication with paraldehyde is very rare but is of historic interest. It is a result of the accumulation of acetic acid, the metabolic product of the drug from acetaldehyde, and other organic acids. Unmetabolized paraldehyde is exhaled through the respiratory system.

***Pyroglutamic Acid.*** Pyroglutamic acid, or 5-oxoproline, is an intermediate in the γ-glutamyl cycle for the synthesis of glutathione. Acetaminophen ingestion can, in rare cases, deplete intracellular glutathione. This results in increased formation of γ-glutamyl cysteine, which is metabolized to pyroglutamic acid.[131] Accumulation of this intermediate, first appreciated in the rare patients with congenital glutathione synthetase deficiency, has been reported in critically ill patients taking acetaminophen. Many cases now appear to be in chronically ill, malnourished women taking acetaminophen chronically.[132] Such patients have severe high AG acidosis and often alterations in mental status.[131,132] All had elevated blood levels of pyroglutamic acid, which increased in proportion to the increase in the AG. Unfortunately, the assay is not widely available. It is conceivable that the heterozygote state for glutathione synthetase deficiency could predispose to pyroglutamic acidosis, because only a minority of critically ill patients receiving acetaminophen develop this form of metabolic acidosis.[131]

***Propylene Glycol.*** Propylene glycol is used as a vehicle for some intravenous medications and some cosmetics and is metabolized to lactic acid in the liver by alcohol dehydrogenase. Patients can have an elevated osmolar gap, an elevated AG, and an acidosis.[133] Numerous intravenous preparations contain propylene glycol as the vehicle (lorazepam, diazepam, pentobarbital, phenytoin, nitroglycerin, and TMP-SMX). Propylene glycol may accumulate and cause a high AG, high osmolar gap acidosis in patients receiving continuous infusion or higher dosages of these agents, especially in the presence of chronic kidney disease, chronic liver disease, alcohol abuse, or pregnancy. The acidosis is the result of accumulation of L-lactic acid, D-lactic acid, and L-acetaldehyde. The acidosis typically abates with cessation of the offending agent and supportive care; occasionally dialysis is used and fomepizole can be considered.[125]

***Uremia.*** Advanced CKD usually eventually converts the non-gap metabolic acidosis discussed earlier to the typical high AG acidosis, or "uremic acidosis"[37,89] reduced rate of $NH_4^+$ production and excretion because of cumulative and significant loss of renal mass[37] reduced rate of $NH_4^+$ production and excretion because of cumulative and significant loss of renal mass.[37] Usually, acidosis does not occur until a major portion of the total functional nephron population (>75%) has been compromised, because of the adaptation by surviving nephrons to increase ammoniagenesis. Eventually, however, there is a decrease in total renal ammonia excretion as renal mass is reduced to a level at which the GFR is 20 mL/min or less. $PO_4^{3-}$ balance is maintained until late stage CKD as a result of both hyperparathyroidism, which decreases proximal $PO_4^{3-}$ absorption, and an increase in plasma $PO_4^{3-}$ as GFR declines. However, protein restriction and the administration of phosphate binders reduce the availability of $PO_4^{3-}$.

***Treatment of Acidosis of Chronic Renal Failure.*** The uremic acidosis of renal failure can be treated with oral alkali replacement to maintain the $HCO_3^-$ concentration above 22 mEq/L. This can be accomplished with relatively modest amounts of alkali (1.0 to 1.5 mEq/kg/day). Shohl's solution or sodium bicarbonate tablets (650-mg tablets) are equally effective. It is assumed that alkali replacement serves to prevent the harmful effects of prolonged positive $H^+$ balance, especially progressive catabolism of muscle and loss of bone. Because sodium citrate (Shohl's solution) has been shown to enhance the absorption of aluminum from the gastrointestinal tract, it should never be administered to patients receiving aluminum-containing antacids because of the risk of aluminum intoxication. When hyperkalemia is present, furosemide (60-80 mg/day in divided doses usually) can be added. Occasionally a patient may require long-term treatment with potassium binding or exchange resins as discussed above.

***Metabolic Alkalosis: Diagnosis of Simple and Mixed Forms of Metabolic Alkalosis.*** Metabolic alkalosis is a primary acid-base disturbance that is manifest in the most pure or simple form as alkalemia (elevated arterial pH) and an increase in $Pa{CO_2}$ as a result of compensatory alveolar hypoventilation. Metabolic alkalosis is one of the more common acid-base disturbances in hospitalized patients and can be manifest as either a simple and a mixed acid-base disorder. A patient with a high plasma $HCO_3^-$ concentration and a low plasma $Cl^-$ concentration has either metabolic alkalosis or chronic respiratory acidosis. The arterial pH establishes the diagnosis, because it is increased in metabolic alkalosis and decreased in respiratory acidosis. Modest increases in the $Pa{CO_2}$ are expected in metabolic alkalosis. A combination of the two disorders is not unusual, because many patients with chronic obstructive lung disease are treated with diuretics, which promote ECF contraction, hypokalemia, and metabolic alkalosis. Metabolic alkalosis is also frequently observed not as a pure or simple acid-base disturbance, but in association with other disorders such as respiratory acidosis, respiratory alkalosis, and metabolic acidosis (*mixed disorders*). *Mixed metabolic alkalosis–metabolic acidosis can be only be detected by laboratory parameters if the accompanying metabolic acidosis is a high AG acidosis.* The mixed disorder can be appreciated by comparison of the change in the AG above the normal value of 10 mEq/L (ΔAG = patient's AG – 10) with the decrement in the [$HCO_3^-$] below the normal value of 25 mEq/L ($\Delta HCO_3^-$ = 25 – patient's $HCO_3^-$). In a pure high AG metabolic acidosis the increase in the AG (or ΔAG) should approximate the decrease in $HCO_3^-$ ($\Delta$ $HCO_3^-$). A mixed metabolic alkalosis–high AG metabolic acidosis is recognized because the delta values are not similar. Often, there is no bicarbonate deficit, yet the AG is significantly elevated. Thus, in a patient with an AG of 20 but a near-normal $HCO_3^-$ concentration, mixed metabolic alkalosis–metabolic acidosis should be strongly considered. Common examples include renal failure acidosis (uremic) with vomiting or DKA with vomiting.

Respiratory compensation for metabolic alkalosis is less predictable than that for metabolic acidosis. In general, the anticipated $PCO_2$ can be estimated by adding 15 to the patient's serum [$HCO_3^-$] in the range of $HCO_3^-$ from 25 to 40 mEq/L. Further elevation in $PCO_2$ is limited by hypoxemia and, to some extent, hypokalemia, which often accompany metabolic alkalosis. Nevertheless, if a patient has a $PCO_2$ of only 40 mm Hg while the [$HCO_3^-$], is frankly elevated (e.g., 35 mEq/L) and the pH is in the alkalemic range, then respiratory compensation is inadequate and a mixed metabolic alkalosis–respiratory alkalosis exists.

In assessing a patient with metabolic alkalosis, two questions must be considered: 1) What is the source of alkali gain (or acid loss) that *generated* the alkalosis? and 2) What renal mechanisms are operating to prevent urinary excretion of excess $HCO_3^-$, thereby *maintaining*, rather than correcting, the alkalosis? This second question is critical because under normal conditions and renal function, a patient should be able to excrete excess $HCO_3^-$ just by reabsorbing less of the large amounts filtered. In the following discussion, the entities responsible for *generating* alkalosis are discussed individually and reference is made to the mechanisms necessary to sustain the increase in blood $HCO_3^-$ concentration in each case. The general mechanisms responsible for the *maintenance of alkalosis* have been discussed in detail earlier in this chapter, and are often a result of the combined effects of a reduction in GFR as well as chloride, ECF volume, and potassium depletion (Fig. 16.9).

Hypokalemia is often an important component of the maintenance phase of metabolic alkalosis and has selective effects on 1) $H^+$ secretion and 2) ammonium excretion. The former is a result, in part, of stimulation of the $H^+$-$K^+$-ATPase in type A intercalated cells of the collecting duct by hypokalemia. The latter, ammonium excretion, is a direct result of enhanced ammoniagenesis and ammonium transport (proximal convoluted tubule, TAL, medullary collecting duct) in response to hypokalemia. Finally, hyperaldosteronism (primary or secondary) participates in sustaining the alkalosis by increasing activity of the $H^+$-ATPase and $H^+$-$K^+$-ATPase in type A intercalated cells as well as the ENaC and the $Na^+$-$K^+$-ATPase in collecting duct principal cells. The net result of the latter process is to stimulate $K^+$ secretion through $K^+$-selective channels in this same cell, which thus maintains the hypokalemia and alkalosis.[16]

Under normal circumstances, the kidneys display an impressive capacity to excrete $HCO_3^-$. Thus, *the development of metabolic alkalosis represents a failure of the kidneys to eliminate $HCO_3^-$ at the normal capacity.* The kidneys retain, rather than excrete, the excess alkali and maintain the alkalosis if one of several mechanisms is operative (see Fig. 16.9):

1. $Cl^-$ deficiency (ECF volume contraction) exists concurrently with $K^+$ deficiency to decrease GFR and/or enhance proximal and distal $HCO_3^-$ absorption. This combination of disorders evokes secondary hyperreninemic hyperaldosteronism and stimulates $H^+$ secretion in the collecting duct. Hypokalemia independently stimulates ammoniagenesis and net acid excretion, thereby, adding additional or "new" bicarbonate to the systemic circulation. Repair of the alkalosis may be accomplished by saline and $K^+$ administration. These cases are sometimes referred to as chloride or saline responsive. This is usually indicated by a low urinary $Cl^-$ once any effect of a diuretic has gone.
2. Increased mineralocorticoids (e.g., aldosterone) and hypokalemia are induced in other cases by autonomous factors unresponsive to increased ECF. The stimulation of distal $H^+$ secretion is then sufficient to reabsorb the increased filtered $HCO_3^-$ load and to overcome the decreased proximal $HCO_3^-$ reabsorption caused by ECF expansion. Repair of the alkalosis in this case rests with removal of the excess autonomous mineralocorticoid and potassium repletion; saline administration is ineffective. These cases are sometimes referred to as chloride resistant or saline resistant. Such conditions are usually indicated by a higher urinary $Cl^-$.

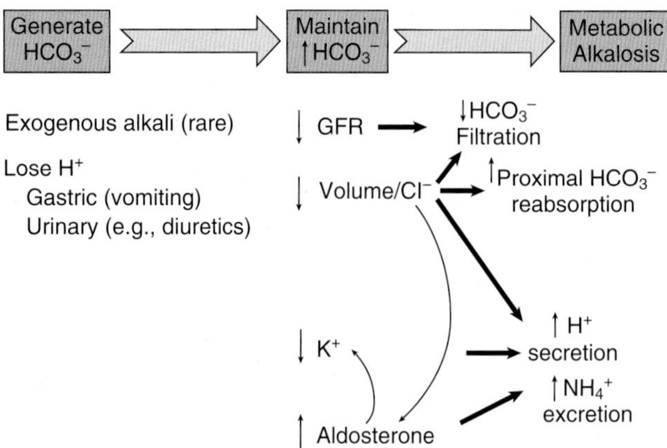


**Fig. 16.9** Pathophysiologic basis of the generation and maintenance of chronic metabolic alkalosis. Paradoxical stimulation of bicarbonate absorption ($H^+$ secretion) and $NH_4^+$ production and excretion is the combined result of $Cl^-$ deficiency (with reduction in GFR), $K^+$ deficiency, and secondary hyperaldosteronism. *GFR,* Glomerular filtration rate.

The various causes of metabolic alkalosis are summarized in Table 16.17. In attempting to establish the cause of metabolic alkalosis, one must assess the clinical circumstance (e.g., diuretics, vomiting) and the status of the ECF volume, blood pressure, serum $K^+$ concentration, and in some cases the renin-aldosterone system. Urine electrolyte determinations and urine screening for diuretics are helpful diagnostic tools (Table 16.18). A diagnostic approach to metabolic alkalosis is summarized in the flow diagram in Fig. 16.10 but the clinical circumstance may be the best starting point – history of gastric fluid losses, diuretics, hypertension, etc. In the absence of historical clues, the presence or absence of hypertension differentiates those conditions with primary sodium chloride retention (e.g., primary hyperaldosteronism, Cushing's syndrome) versus those with excess losses (e.g., Bartter's or Gitelman's syndrome).

***Exogenous Bicarbonate Loads.*** Long-term administration of alkali to individuals with normal renal function results in minimal, if any, alkalosis, since excess $HCO_3^-$ is easily excreted normally. In patients with chronic renal insufficiency, however, overt alkalosis can develop after alkali administration, presumably because the capacity to excrete $HCO_3^-$ is exceeded or because coexistent hemodynamic disturbances have caused enhanced $HCO_3^-$ reabsorption.

***Bicarbonate and Bicarbonate-Precursor Administration.*** The propensity of patients who have ECF contraction or renal disease plus alkali loads to develop alkalosis is exemplified by patients who receive oral or intravenous $HCO_3^-$, acetate loads in parenteral hyperalimentation solutions, sodium citrate loads (via regional anticoagulation, transfusions, plasma exchange anticoagulant, or infant formula), or antacids plus cation exchange resins. The use of trisodium citrate solution for regional anticoagulation has been reported to be a cause of metabolic alkalosis in patients receiving continuous renal replacement therapy.[134–136] Citrate metabolism consumes a hydrogen ion and thereby generates $HCO_3^-$ in liver and skeletal muscle.[136] Citrate metabolism consumes a hydrogen ion and thereby generates $HCO_3^-$ in liver and skeletal muscle.

**Table 16.17 Causes of Metabolic Alkalosis**

**Exogenous $HCO_3^-$ Loads**
Acute alkali administration
**Milk-alkali syndrome**
**Effective ECV Contraction, Normotension, $K^+$ Deficiency, and Secondary Hyperreninemic Hyperaldosteronism**
Gastrointestinal origin
- **Vomiting**
- **Gastric aspiration**
- Congenital chloridorrhea
- Villous adenoma

Renal origin
- **Diuretics (especially thiazides and loop diuretics)**
- **Edematous states**
- Post-hypercapnic state
- Hypercalcemia-hypoparathyroidism
- Recovery from lactic acidosis or ketoacidosis
- Nonreabsorbable anions such as penicillin, carbenicillin
- $Mg^{2+}$ deficiency
- **$K^+$ depletion**
- Bartter's syndrome (loss of function mutations in thick ascending limb of Henle)
- Gitelman's syndrome (loss-of-function of $Na^+/Cl^-$ cotransporter - DCT)
- Carbohydrate refeeding after starvation

**ECV Expansion, Hypertension, $K^+$ Deficiency, and Hypermineralocorticoidism**
Associated with high renin level
- Renal artery stenosis
- Accelerated hypertension
- Renin-secreting tumor
- Estrogen therapy

Associated with low renin level
- **Primary aldosteronism**
- Adrenal adenoma
- Hyperplasia
- Carcinoma
- Glucocorticoid suppressible

Adrenal enzymatic defects
- 11β-hydroxylase deficiency
- 17α-hydroxylase deficiency

Cushing's syndrome or disease
- Ectopic corticotrophin
- Adrenal carcinoma
- Adrenal adenoma
- Primary pituitary

Other
- Licorice
- Carbenoxolone
- Smokeless (chewing) tobacco
- Lydia Pinkham tablets

**Gain-of-Function Mutation of ENaC with ECV Expansion, Hypertension, $K^+$ Deficiency, and Hyporeninemic Hyperaldosteronism**
- Liddle's syndrome

Another setting whereby exogenous alkali can cause a temporary metabolic alkalosis is *after* treatment of an organic acidosis such as lactic acidosis or ketoacidosis. In such disorders, there are two sources of $HCO_3^-$, first administered $HCO_3^-$ used to treat the acidosis, and second, metabolized organic anion which can be converted to $HCO_3^-$ as the disorder is treated (e.g., improved systemic circulation in lactic acidosis or insulin in DKA). Any metabolic alkalosis will correct spontaneously unless maintained by volume / $Cl^-$ depletion (perhaps caused in part by the acidosis) and/or $K^+$ deficiency.

**Table 16.18 Diagnosis of Metabolic Alkalosis**

| Saline-Responsive Alkalosis | Saline-Unresponsive Alkalosis |
|---|---|
| Low Urinary [$Cl^-$] (<10 mEq/L) | High or Normal Urinary [$Cl^-$] (>15-20 mEq/L) |
| Normotensive | Hypertensive |
| Vomiting | Primary aldosteronism |
| Nasogastric aspiration | Cushing's syndrome |
| Diuretic use (distant) | Renal artery stenosis |
| Post-hypercapnia | Renal failure plus alkali therapy |
| Villous adenoma | Liddle's syndrome |
| Bicarbonate treatment of organic acidosis | Normotensive |
| $K^+$ deficiency | $Mg^{2+}$ deficiency |
| | Severe $K^+$ deficiency |
| | Bartter's syndrome |
| | Gitelman's syndrome |
| | Diuretic use (recent) |

***Milk-Alkali Syndrome.*** Another cause of metabolic alkalosis historically was excessive ingestion of milk and antacids. Patients have hypercalcemia, metabolic alkalosis, and renal insufficiency. The syndrome is now seen mainly because of the use of calcium supplementation (e.g., for osteoporosis) with other alkali (e.g., calcium carbonate). Older women with poor dietary intake ("tea and toasters") are especially prone. In Asia, betel nut chewing is a cause because the nut is often wrapped in calcium hydroxide. Both hypercalcemia and vitamin D excess have been suggested to increase renal $HCO_3^-$ reabsorption. Patients with these disorders are prone to develop nephrocalcinosis, renal insufficiency, and metabolic alkalosis.[16] Renal insufficiency is a clear part of the syndrome and involved in the pathogenesis, limiting the excretion of $HCO_3^-$. Discontinuation of alkali ingestion is usually sufficient to repair the alkalosis.

***Loss of Acid: Vomiting and Gastric Aspiration.*** Gastrointestinal loss of $H^+$ results in production of $HCO_3^-$ in the body fluids. As discussed above, loss of an acid is the same as the gain of alkali in terms of pH. Increased $H^+$ loss through gastric secretions can be caused by vomiting due to physical or psychiatric reasons, nasogastric tube aspiration, or a gastric fistula (see Table 16.17).[16]

The fluid and sodium chloride loss in vomitus or in nasogastric suction results in ECF contraction with an increase in plasma renin activity, aldosterone, and other antinatriuretic factors.[16] These factors decrease GFR and also enhance the capacity of the renal tubule to reabsorb $HCO_3^-$.[15] During the active phase of vomiting, there is continued addition of $HCO_3^-$ to plasma in exchange for $Cl^-$. The plasma $HCO_3^-$ concentration increases to a level that exceeds the reabsorptive capacity of the proximal tubule. The excess sodium bicarbonate enters the distal tubule, where, under the influence of the increased level of aldosterone, $K^+$ and $H^+$ secretion is stimulated. Because of ECF contraction and hypochloremia,

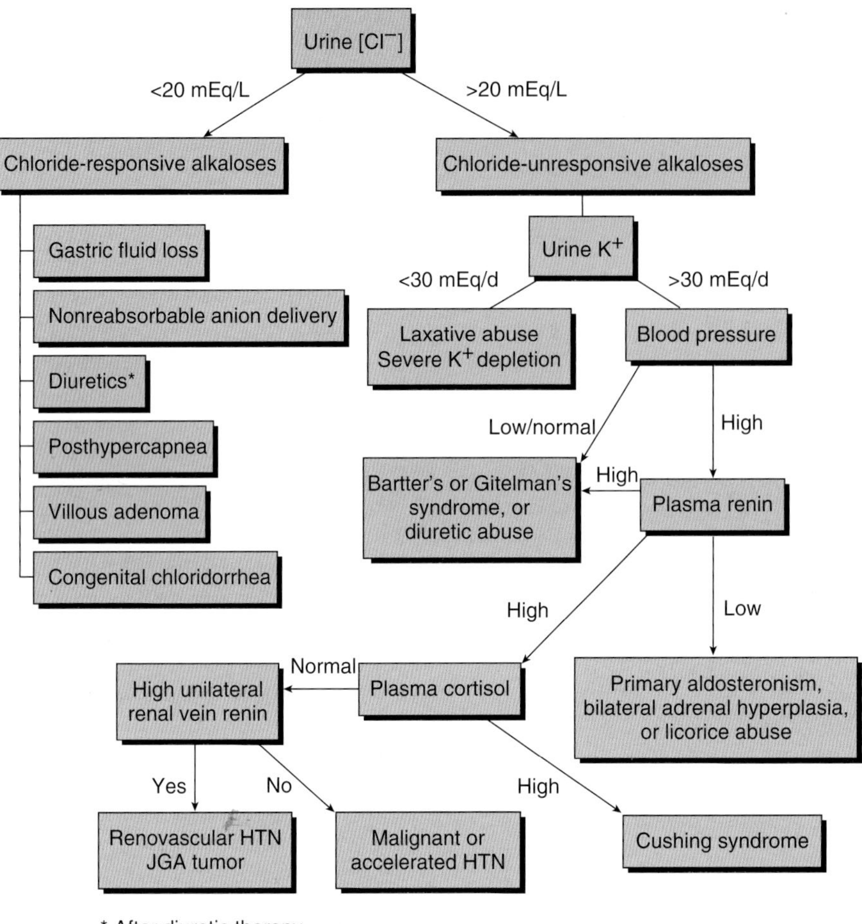


**Fig. 16.10** Diagnostic algorithm for metabolic alkalosis, based on the spot urine $Cl^-$ and $K^+$ concentrations. *HTN,* Hypertension; *JGA,* juxtaglomerular apparatus.

the kidney avidly conserves $Cl^-$. Consequently, in this disequilibrium state generated by active vomiting, the urine contains large quantities of $K^+$, but has a low concentration of $Cl^-$. On cessation of vomiting, the plasma $HCO_3^-$ concentration falls to the $HCO_3^-$ reabsorptive capacity, which is markedly elevated by the continued effects of ECF contraction, hypokalemia, and hyperaldosteronism. The alkalosis is maintained at a slightly lower level than during the phase of active vomiting, and the urine is now relatively acidic with low concentrations of $Na^+$, $HCO_3^-$, and $Cl^-$.

Correction of the ECF contraction with sodium chloride may be sufficient to reverse these events, with restoration of normal blood pH even without repair of $K^+$ deficits.[15] Good clinical practice, however, dictates $K^+$ repletion as well.[16] Good clinical practice, however, dictates $K^+$ repletion as well.[16]

***Unusual Causes of Diarrhea: Villous Adenoma and Congenital Chloridorrhea.*** Most stool is alkaline and most forms of diarrhea cause metabolic acidosis. However, some unusual forms of diarrhea can cause metabolic alkalosis. Metabolic alkalosis has been described in cases of villous adenoma and is ascribed to high adenoma-derived $K^+$ secretory rates. $K^+$ and volume depletion likely cause the alkalosis. Congenital chloridorrhea is a rare autosomal recessive disorder associated with severe diarrhea, fecal acid loss, and $HCO_3^-$ retention. The pathogenesis is loss of the normal ileal $HCO_3^-/Cl^-$ anion exchange mechanism so that $Cl^-$ cannot be normally reabsorbed. This is usually the result of mutations in the gene SLC26A3, also known as downregulated in adenoma (DRA).[137] The parallel $Na^+/H^+$ ion exchanger remains functional, which allows $Na^+$ to be reabsorbed and $H^+$ to be secreted. Subsequently, net $H^+$ and $Cl^-$ exit in the stool, which causes $Na^+$ and $HCO_3^-$ retention in the ECF.[15,16] Alkalosis results and is sustained by concomitant ECF contraction with hyperaldosteronism and $K^+$ deficiency. Therapy consists of oral supplements of sodium and potassium chloride. The use of proton pump inhibitors has been advanced as a means of reducing chloride secretion by the parietal cells and thus reducing the diarrhea.[138] Alkalosis results and is sustained by concomitant ECF contraction with hyperaldosteronism and $K^+$ deficiency. Therapy consists of oral supplements of sodium and potassium chloride. The use of proton pump inhibitors has been advanced as a means of reducing chloride secretion by the parietal cells and thus reducing the diarrhea.[138]

***Renal Loss of Acid: Diuretics.*** Drugs that induce chloruresis without bicarbonaturia, such as thiazides and loop diuretics (furosemide, bumetanide, and torsemide), acutely diminish ECF volume without altering the total body $HCO_3^-$ content. The $HCO_3^-$ concentration in the blood and ECF increases. The $PCO_2$ does not increase commensurately, and a "contraction" alkalosis results.[16] The degree of alkalosis is usually small, however, because of cellular and non-$HCO_3^-$ ECF buffering processes.[15,16] Administration of diuretics long term tends to generate an alkalosis by increasing distal salt delivery, so that both $K^+$ and $H^+$ secretion are stimulated. Diuretics, by blocking $Cl^-$ reabsorption in the distal tubule or by increasing $H^+$ pump activity, may also stimulate distal $H^+$ secretion and increase net acid excretion. Maintenance of alkalosis is ensured by the persistence of ECF contraction, secondary hyperaldosteronism, $K^+$ deficiency, enhanced ammonium production, stimulation of the apical $H^+$- and $H^+$-$K^+$-ATPases, which persists for as long as diuretic administration continues. Repair of the alkalosis is achieved by cessation of diuretic administration and by providing $Cl^-$ to normalize the ECF deficit.

***Edematous States.*** In diseases associated with edema formation (CHF, nephrotic syndrome, cirrhosis), effective arterial blood volume is diminished, although total ECF is increased. Common to these diseases is often diminished renal plasma flow and GFR with limited distal $Na^+$ delivery. Net acid excretion is usually normal, and alkalosis does not develop, even with an enhanced proximal $HCO_3^-$ reabsorptive capacity. However, the distal $H^+$ secretory mechanism is primed by hyperaldosteronism to excrete excessive net acid if GFR can be increased to enhance distal $Na^+$ delivery or if $K^+$ deficiency or diuretic administration supervenes.

***Posthypercapnia.*** Prolonged $CO_2$ retention with chronic respiratory acidosis enhances renal $HCO_3^-$ absorption and the generation of new $HCO_3^-$ (increased net acid excretion). If the $PCO_2$ is returned to normal as with mechanical ventilation, metabolic alkalosis, caused by the persistently elevated $HCO_3^-$ concentration, emerges. Normally there may be a brisk loss of urine $HCO_3^-$ proportional to the change in $PCO_2$, and a return to normal acid-base status. But often there are other factors that cause retention of excess $HCO_3^-$ and therefore a metabolic alkalosis. Associated ECF contraction, secondary hyperaldosteronism, diuretics, or $K^+$ deficiency may help maintain the metabolic alkalosis.

***Bartter's Syndrome.*** Bartter's syndrome and Gitelman's syndrome described next are distal nephron salt losing disorders characterized by hypokalemia, metabolic alkalosis, high renin and aldosterone, and often high prostaglandin E2.[139] As noted below, there are multiple genes involved resulting in heterogeneity in specific phenotypes.[139] Both classic Bartter's syndrome and antenatal Bartter's syndrome are inherited as autosomal recessive disorders and involve impaired TAL salt absorption, which results in salt wasting, volume depletion, and activation of the renin-angiotensin system.[140] These manifestations are the result of loss-of-function mutations of one of the genes that encode three transporters or regulatory proteins involved in NaCl absorption in the TAL.[139] The most prevalent disorder is the inheritance from both parents of mutations of the gene *NKCC2* that encodes the bumetanide-sensitive $Na^+$-2Cl—$K^+$ cotransporter on the apical membrane. Other mutations have also been described in rare families. For example, a mutation has been discovered in the gene *KCNJ1* that encodes the ATP-sensitive apical $K^+$ conductance channel (ROMK) that operates in parallel with the $Na^+$-2Cl—$K^+$ transporter to recycle $K^+$. Both defects can be associated with classic Bartter's syndrome. A third mutation of the *CLCNKb* gene encoding the voltage-gated basolateral chloride channel (ClC-Kb) is associated only with classic Bartter's syndrome and is milder and rarely associated with nephrocalcinosis. All three defects above have the same net effect, loss of $Cl^-$ transport in the TAL.[141] Antenatal Bartter's syndrome has been observed in consanguineous families in association with sensorineural deafness. The responsible gene, *BSND,* encodes the associated subunit, Barttin, that co-localizes with the ClC-Kb channel in both the TAL and K-secreting epithelial cells in the inner ear. Barttin appears to be necessary for the function of the voltage-gated chloride channel. Expression of ClC-Kb is lost when coexpressed with mutant Barttins. Thus, mutations in *BSND* represent a fourth category of patients with Bartter syndrome.[142] With the exception of the deafness, the electrolyte and acid-base abnormalities are similar to the other forms of Bartter syndrome.

Two groups of investigators have reported features of Bartter's syndrome in patients with tetany who inherit autosomal dominant hypocalcemia as a result of activating mutations in the calcium-sensing receptor (CaSR).[143] Gain-of-function mutations of the gene encoding CaSR on the basolateral surface of the TAL cell inhibits the function of ROMK. Thus, mutations in CaSR appear to represent a fifth gene associated with Bartter's syndrome.[139] Acquired forms of Bartter's syndrome, usually characterized by hypokalemic metabolic alkalosis, hypomagnesemia, hypocalcemia and normal kidney function, have been reported in children and adults in association with aminoglycoside toxicity including gentamicin, amikacin, netilmicin, capreomycin, viomycin, colistin, and neomycin. Similarily, cisplatin and cyclosporine have also been implicated. Although the cellular mechanism of this association has not been clearly elucidated, *in vitro* studies suggest an effect on the CaSR.

Therefore, these defects, when considered collectively, lead to ECF contraction, hyperreninemic hyperaldosteronism, and increased delivery of $Na^+$ to the distal nephron and, thus, alkalosis and renal $K^+$ wasting and hypokalemia. Secondary overproduction of prostaglandins, juxtaglomerular apparatus hypertrophy, and vascular pressor unresponsiveness would then ensue. Most patients have hypercalciuria and normal serum magnesium levels, which distinguishes this disorder from Gitelman's syndrome.

Distinction from surreptitious vomiting, surreptitious diuretic use, and laxative abuse is necessary to make the diagnosis of Bartter's syndrome. The finding of a low urinary $Cl^-$ concentration is helpful in identifying the vomiting patient. The urinary $Cl^-$ concentration in Bartter's syndrome would be expected to be normal or increased, rather than depressed. Bartter-like manifestations have been reported in sporadic cases associated with chronic intermittent diuretic and laxative abuse, cystic fibrosis, and congenital chloride diarrhea.

The treatment of Bartter's syndrome will generally include $K^+$ supplementation and nonsteroidal antiinflammatory drugs (NSAIDs) to block prostaglandin production, and also amiloride or spironolactone to lessen distal $K^+$ secretion. ACE inhibitors have been used with limited success.

***Gitelman's Syndrome.*** Patients with Gitelman's syndrome have a phenotype resembling that of Bartter's syndrome in that an autosomal recessive chloride-resistant metabolic alkalosis is associated with hypokalemia, normal to low blood pressure, volume depletion with secondary hyperreninemic hyperaldosteronism, and juxtaglomerular hyperplasia.[141,144] However, hypocalciuria and symptomatic hypomagnesemia are usually useful in distinguishing Gitelman's syndrome from

Bartter's syndrome on clinical grounds.[139,144] These unique features mimic the effect of long-term thiazide diuretic administration. In contrast, in most patients with Bartter's syndrome, the urine calcium level is elevated. However, hypocalciuria and symptomatic hypomagnesemia are usually useful in distinguishing Gitelman's syndrome from Bartter's syndrome on clinical grounds.[139,144] These unique features mimic the effect of long-term thiazide diuretic administration. In contrast, in most patients with Bartter's syndrome, the urine calcium level is elevated.

A number of missense mutations in the gene *SLC12A3,* which encodes the thiazide-sensitive sodium-chloride cotransporter NCC in the distal convoluted tubule, have been described and account for the spectrum of clinical features, including the classical finding of hypocalciuria.[145] Symptoms may include salt craving, nocturia, cramps, and fatigue.[146]

Treatment of Gitelman's syndrome, as of Bartter's syndrome, consists of potassium supplementation (KCl 40 mEq, three or four times daily, or more), but also magnesium supplementation in most patients. Amiloride (5 to 10 mg twice daily) is more effective than spironolactone. ACE inhibitors or ARBs in very low dose have been suggested as helpful in selected patients but may cause symptomatic hypotension. NSAIDs may be useful.

***Nonreabsorbable Anions and Magnesium Deficiency.*** Administration of large amounts of nonreabsorbable anions, such as penicillin or carbenicillin, can enhance distal acidification and $K^+$ excretion by increasing the luminal potential difference attained or possibly by allowing $Na^+$ delivery to the CCT without $Cl^-$, which favors $H^+$ secretion without $Cl^-$–dependent $HCO_3^-$ secretion.[16] $Mg^{2+}$ deficiency can also result in hypokalemic alkalosis, perhaps by causing $K^+$ deficiency or by enhancing distal acidification through stimulation of renin and hence aldosterone secretion.

***Potassium Depletion.*** Isolated $K^+$ depletion can occasionally cause metabolic alkalosis, although generally of only modest severity. In most cases of metabolic alkalosis, $K^+$ depletion or hypokalemia is one of several contributing factors including volume or Cl- depletion or mineralocorticoid excess. $K^+$ deficiency is known in various experimental models to cause 1) an intracellular acidosis, 2) activate $H^+$ secretion in proximal and distal nephron segments, and 3) increase ammonium production and excretion.[26] Activation of the renal $H^+$, $K^+$-ATPase in the collecting duct by chronic hypokalemia likely plays a role in maintenance of alkalosis associated with $K^+$ depletion. The alkalosis associated with severe $K^+$ depletion is resistant to salt administration and repair of the $K^+$ deficiency is necessary to correct the alkalosis.

***Excess Mineralocorticoid Activity (see Table 16.17).*** As previously discussed, excess mineralocorticoids increase net acid excretion and tend to cause metabolic alkalosis in combination with volume expansion and hypertension. The degree of alkalosis is augmented by the simultaneous increase in $K^+$ excretion, which leads to $K^+$ deficiency and hypokalemia. Salt intake for sufficient distal $Na^+$ delivery is a prerequisite for the development of both the hypokalemia and the alkalosis. Hypertension develops partly as a result of ECF expansion from salt retention. The alkalosis is not progressive and is generally mild and not associated with edema, partly as a result of mechanisms referred to as "aldosterone escape". Volume expansion tends to antagonize the decrease in GFR through increases in natriuretic peptides (e.g. atrial natriuretic peptide) and/or increase in tubule acidification induced by hypermineralocorticoidism and $K^+$ deficiency. Increased mineralocorticoid levels may be the result of autonomous primary adrenal overproduction of mineralocorticoids or of secondary aldosterone release by primary renal overproduction of renin. In both cases, the normal feedback by ECF on net mineralocorticoid production is disrupted and volume retention results in hypertension.

***High Renin Levels, Secondary Hyperaldosteronism.*** States accompanied by inappropriately high renin levels may be associated with hyperaldosteronism and alkalosis. Renin levels are elevated because of primary elaboration of renin or, secondarily, by diminished effective circulating blood volume. Total ECF may not be diminished. Examples of high-renin hypertension include renovascular, accelerated, and malignant hypertension. Estrogens increase renin substrate and hence angiotensin II formation. Primary tumor overproduction of renin is another rare cause of hyperreninemic hyperaldosterone–induced metabolic alkalosis.[16]

***Low Renin Levels, Primary Increased Mineralocorticoids.*** In some disorders, primary adrenal overproduction of mineralocorticoid suppresses renin elaboration. Hypertension occurs as the result of mineralocorticoid excess with volume overexpansion.

***Primary Aldosteronism.*** Tumor involvement (adenoma or, rarely, carcinoma) or hyperplasia of the adrenal gland is associated with aldosterone overproduction. Mineralocorticoid administration or excess production (primary aldosteronism of Cushing's syndrome and adrenal cortical enzyme defects) increases net acid excretion and may result in metabolic alkalosis, which may be worsened by associated $K^+$ deficiency. ECF volume expansion from salt retention causes hypertension and antagonizes the reduction in GFR and/or increases tubule acidification induced by aldosterone and by $K^+$ deficiency. The kaliuresis may persist and cause continued $K^+$ depletion with polydipsia, inability to concentrate the urine, and polyuria.

***Glucocorticoid-Remediable Hyperaldosteronism.*** Glucocorticoid-remediable hyperaldosteronism is an autosomal dominant form of hypertension, the features of which resemble those of primary aldosteronism (hypokalemic metabolic alkalosis and volume-dependent hypertension). In this disorder, however, glucocorticoid administration corrects the hypertension as well as the excessive excretion of 18-hydroxysteroid in the urine. Dluhy and associates have demonstrated that this disorder results from unequal crossing over between two genes located in close proximity on chromosome 8.[147] This region contains the glucocorticoid-responsive promoter region of the gene encoding 11β-hydroxylase (*CYP11B1*) where it is joined to the structural portion of the *CYP11B2* gene encoding aldosterone synthase.[147] The chimeric gene produces excess amounts of aldosterone synthase, unresponsive to serum potassium or renin levels, but suppressed by glucocorticoid administration. Although a rare cause of primary aldosteronism, the syndrome is important to distinguish because treatment differs and it can be associated with severe hypertension, stroke, and accelerated hypertension during pregnancy. This region contains the glucocorticoid-responsive promoter region of the gene encoding 11β-hydroxylase (*CYP11B1*) where it is joined to the structural portion of the *CYP11B2* gene encoding aldosterone synthase.[147] The chimeric gene produces excess amounts of aldosterone synthase, unresponsive to serum potassium or renin levels, but suppressed by glucocorticoid administration.

Although a rare cause of primary aldosteronism, the syndrome is important to distinguish because treatment differs and it can be associated with severe hypertension, stroke, and accelerated hypertension during pregnancy.

***Cushing's Disease or Syndrome.*** Abnormally high glucocorticoid production caused by adrenal adenoma or carcinoma or ectopic corticotropin production causes metabolic alkalosis. The alkalosis may be ascribed to coexisting mineralocorticoid (deoxycorticosterone and corticosterone) hypersecretion or by direct effects of the glucocorticoids. Glucocorticoids also have the ability to enhance net acid secretion and $NH_4^+$ production by occupancy of mineralocorticoid receptors.

***Liddle's Syndrome (Low Renin, Low Aldosterone).*** Liddle's syndrome is associated with severe hypertension often presenting in childhood, and is frequently accompanied by hypokalemic metabolic alkalosis. These features resemble those of primary hyperaldosteronism, but the renin and aldosterone levels are suppressed (pseudohyperaldosteronism). The defect is constitutive activation of the ENaC at the apical membrane of principal cells in the CCD. Liddle originally described patients with low renin and low aldosterone levels that did not respond to spironolactone. The defect in Liddle's syndrome is inherited as an autosomal dominant form of monogenic hypertension. This disorder has been attributed to an inherited gain of function abnormality in the genes that encodes the β- or the γ-subunit of renal ENaC, resulting in certain abnormalities of the cytoplasmic tails of the β- or γ-subunit. The C termini contain PY amino acid motifs that are highly conserved, and essentially all mutations in Liddle's syndrome patients involve disruption or deletion of this motif. These PY motifs are important in regulating the number of sodium channels in the luminal membrane by binding to the WW domains of the Nedd4 (neural developmentally downregulated isoform 4)–like family of ubiquitin-protein ligases.[148] Disruption of the PY motif dramatically increases the surface localization of ENaC complex, because these channels are not internalized or degraded (Nedd4 pathway), but remain activated on the cell surface.[148] Persistent $Na^+$ absorption results in volume expansion, hypertension, hypokalemia, and metabolic alkalosis.

***Apparent Mineralocorticoid Excess and Related Conditions.*** The syndrome of apparent mineralocorticoid excess is a rare autosomal recessive form of hypertension resulting from a defective enzyme 11-beta-hydroxysteroid dehydrogenase type 2 isoform (11-beta-HSD2), which is the kidney isoform of 11-beta-HSD.[149] This enzyme in the collecting duct normally converts cortisol to cortisone which does not activate the mineralocorticoid receptor, in contrast to cortisol which does. Thus, with a defective enzyme, circulating levels of cortisol will activate collecting duct mineralocorticoid receptors causing all the features of mineralocorticoid excess: volume expansion, low renin level, low aldosterone level, and a salt-sensitive form of hypertension, which may include metabolic alkalosis and hypokalemia. Ingestion of certain licorice products or chewing tobacco can also cause a typical pattern of hypermineralocorticoidism due to the presence of carbenoxolone or glycyrrhetinic acid. These substances inhibit 11β-hydroxysteroid dehydrogenase. The hypertension in these conditions responds to thiazides and spironolactone.

***Symptoms.*** Symptoms of metabolic alkalosis can include changes in central and peripheral nervous system function similar to those in hypocalcemia: mental confusion, obtundation, and a predisposition to seizures, as well as paresthesias, muscular cramping, and even tetany. Aggravation of arrhythmias and hypoxemia in chronic obstructive pulmonary disease is also a potential problem. Related electrolyte abnormalities, including hypokalemia and hypophosphatemia, are common, and patients may show symptoms of these deficiencies.

***Treatment.*** The maintenance of metabolic alkalosis represents a failure of the kidney to excrete $HCO_3^-$ sufficiently because of chloride or potassium deficiency or continuous mineralocorticoid activity or both. Treatment is primarily directed at correcting the underlying stimulus for $HCO_3^-$ generation and at restoring the ability of the kidney to excrete the excess $HCO_3^-$. The diagnosis can be aided by assessing the urinary chloride concentration, systemic blood pressure, and the volume status of the patient (particularly the presence or absence of orthostasis) (see Fig. 16.10). Particularly helpful in the history is the presence or absence of vomiting, diuretic use, or alkali therapy. A high urine chloride level and hypertension suggest that mineralocorticoid excess is present. If primary aldosteronism is present, correction of the underlying cause (adenoma, bilateral hyperplasia, Cushing's syndrome) will reverse the alkalosis. Patients with bilateral adrenal hyperplasia may respond to spironolactone. Normotensive patients with a high urine chloride concentration may have Bartter's or Gitelman's syndrome, if diuretic use or vomiting can be excluded. A low urine chloride level and relative hypotension suggests a chloride-responsive metabolic alkalosis such as vomiting or nasogastric suction. $[H^+]$ loss by the stomach or kidneys can be mitigated by the use of proton pump inhibitors or the discontinuation of diuretics. The second aspect of treatment is to remove the factors that sustain $HCO_3^-$ reabsorption, such as ECF volume contraction or $K^+$ deficiency.

Patients with CHF or unexplained volume overexpansion represent special challenges in the critical care setting. Patients with a low urine chloride concentration, usually indicative of a "chloride-responsive" form of metabolic alkalosis, may not tolerate normal saline infusion. Renal $HCO_3^-$ loss can be accelerated by administration of acetazolamide (250 to 500 mg intravenously), a carbonic anhydrase inhibitor, if associated conditions that preclude infusion of saline (e.g., elevated pulmonary capillary wedge pressure, or evidence of CHF) are present.[16] Acetazolamide is usually very effective in patients with adequate renal function, but can exacerbate urinary $K^+$ losses. Hypokalemia should be expected following acetazolamide IV in alkalotic patients and must be treated promptly. Dilute hydrochloric acid (0.1 normal HCl) is also effective but must be infused slowly in a central line because of severe hemolysis and is difficult to titrate. If 0.1 N HCl is used, the goal should not be to restore the pH to normal, but to reduce the pH to approximately 7.50. Patients receiving continuous renal replacement therapy in the intensive care unit typically develop metabolic alkalosis when high-bicarbonate dialysate is used or when citrate regional anticoagulation is employed. Therapy should include reduction of alkali loads via dialysis by reducing the bicarbonate concentration in the dialysate when possible. If not effective, 0.1 N HCl IV may be necessary in this setting.

 Complete reference list available at ExpertConsult.com.

## KEY REFERENCES


1. Adrogue HJ, Gennari FJ, Galla JH, et al. Assessing acid-base disorders. *Kidney Int.* 2009;76(12):1239–1247.
2. Bidani A, Tuazon D, Heming T. Regulation of whole body acid-base balance. In: DuBose TD, Hamm LL, eds. *Acid-Base and Electrolyte Disorders: A Companion to Brenner and Rector's The Kidney*. Philadelphia: Saunders; 2002:1–21.
3. Lemann J Jr, Bushinsky DA, Hamm LL. Bone buffering of acid and base in humans. *Am J Physiol Renal Physiol.* 2003;285(5):F811–F832.
4. Madias N, Adrogué H. Respiratory alkalosis. In: DuBose TD, Hamm LL, eds. *Acid-Base and Electrolyte Disorders: A Companion to Brenner and Rector's The Kidney*. Philadelphia: Saunders; 2002:147–164.
5. Madias NE. Renal acidification responses to respiratory acid-base disorders. *J Nephrol.* 2010;23(suppl 16):S85–S91.
7. DuBose TD Jr, Good DW. Effects of diuretics on renal acid-base transport. *Semin Nephrol.* 1988;8(3):282–294.
12. Goraya N, Simoni J, Sager LN, et al. Acid retention in chronic kidney disease is inversely related to GFR. *Am J Physiol Renal Physiol.* 2018;314(5):F985–F991.
13. Nath KA, Hostetter MK, Hostetter TH. Pathophysiology of chronic tubulo-interstitial disease in rats. Interactions of dietary acid load, ammonia, and complement component C3. *J Clin Invest.* 1985; 76(2):667–675.
14. Scialla JJ. The balance of the evidence on acid-base homeostasis and progression of chronic kidney disease. *Kidney Int.* 2015;88(1):9–11.
15. Gennari FJ. Pathophysiology of metabolic alkalosis: a new classification based on the centrality of stimulated collecting duct ion transport. *Am J Kidney Dis.* 2011;58(4):626–636.
16. DuBose TD. Metabolic alkalosis. In: Gilbert S, Weiner DE, eds. *National Kidney Foundation Primer on Kidney Diseases.* 6th ed. Philadelphia: Elseiver; 2013:137–143.
25. Hamm LL. Mixed acid-base disorders. In: Kokko JP, Tannen R, eds. *Fluid and Electrolytes.* 3rd ed. Philadelphia: Saunders; 1996.
26. Hamm LL, Hering-Smith KS, Nakhoul NL. Acid-base and potassium homeostasis. *Semin Nephrol.* 2013;33(3):257–264.
27. Emmett M. Diagnosis of simple and mixed disorders. In: DuBose TD, Hamm LL, eds. *Acid-Base and Electrolyte Disorders: A Companion to Brenner and Rector's The Kidney.* Philadelphia: Saunders; 2002:41–53.
28. Oh MS, Carroll HJ. The anion gap. *N Engl J Med.* 1977;297(15):814–817.
30. Gabow PA, Kaehny WD, Fennessey PV, et al. Diagnostic importance of an increased serum anion gap. *N Engl J Med.* 1980;303(15):854–858.
32. DuBose TD, Goode AK. Renal tubular acidosis. In: Coffma TM, Falk RJ, Molitoris BA, et al, eds. *Schrier's Diseases of The Kidney.* Philadelphia: Lippincott Williams & Wilkins; 2013:587–614.
33. DuBose TD, Alpern RJ. *Renal Tubular Acidosis. The Metabolic and Molecular Bases of Inherited Disease.* New York: McGraw-Hill; 2001.
35. DuBose TD, McDonald GA. Renal tubular acidosis. In: DuBose TD, Hamm LL, eds. *Acid-Base and Electrolyte Disorders: A Companion to Brenner and Rector's The Kidney.* Philadelphia: Saunders; 2002:189–206.
36. Adrogue HJ, Wilson H, Boyd AE 3rd, et al. Plasma acid-base patterns in diabetic ketoacidosis. *N Engl J Med.* 1982;307(26):1603–1610.
37. Kraut JA, Kurtz I. Metabolic acidosis of CKD: diagnosis, clinical characteristics, and treatment. *Am J Kidney Dis.* 2005;45(6):978–993.
43. Batlle D, Haque SK. Genetic causes and mechanisms of distal renal tubular acidosis. *Nephrol Dial Transplant.* 2012;27(10):3691–3704.
55. Laing CM, Toye AM, Capasso G, et al. Renal tubular acidosis: developments in our understanding of the molecular basis. *Int J Biochem Cell Biol.* 2005;37(6):1151–1161.
67. Kleyman TR, Roberts C, Ling BN. A mechanism for pentamidine-induced hyperkalemia: inhibition of distal nephron sodium transport. *Ann Intern Med.* 1995;122(2):103–106.
70. Hoorn EJ, Walsh SB, McCormick JA, et al. The calcineurin inhibitor tacrolimus activates the renal sodium chloride cotransporter to cause hypertension. *Nat Med.* 2011;17(10):1304–1309.
80. Wilson FH, Disse-Nicodeme S, Choate KA, et al. Human hypertension caused by mutations in WNK kinases. *Science.* 2001;293(5532): 1107–1112.
82. Hadchouel J, Ellison DH, Gamba G. Regulation of renal electrolyte transport by WNK and SPAK-OSR1 kinases. *Annu Rev Physiol.* 2016;78:367–389.
83. Murthy M, Kurz T, O'Shaughnessy KM. WNK signalling pathways in blood pressure regulation. *Cell Mol Life Sci.* 2017;74(7):1261–1280.
84. Boyden LM, Choi M, Choate KA, et al. Mutations in kelch-like 3 and cullin 3 cause hypertension and electrolyte abnormalities. *Nature.* 2012;482(7383):98–102.
88. Kraut JA, Madias NE. Metabolic acidosis of CKD: an update. *Am J Kidney Dis.* 2016;67(2):307–317.
89. Nagami GT, Hamm LL. Regulation of acid-base balance in chronic kidney disease. *Adv Chronic Kidney Dis.* 2017;24(5):274–279.
90. Chen W, Abramowitz MK. Epidemiology of acid-base derangements in CKD. *Adv Chronic Kidney Dis.* 2017;24(5):280–288.
91. Wesson DE, Simoni J, Broglio K, et al. Acid retention accompanies reduced GFR in humans and increases plasma levels of endothelin and aldosterone. *Am J Physiol Renal Physiol.* 2011;300(4):F830–F837.
92. Vallet M, Metzger M, Haymann JP, et al. Urinary ammonia and long-term outcomes in chronic kidney disease. *Kidney Int.* 2015; 88(1):137–145.
93. Abramowitz MK, Melamed ML, Bauer C, et al. Effects of oral sodium bicarbonate in patients with CKD. *Clin J Am Soc Nephrol.* 2013.
94. Gauthier P, Simon EE, Lemann J Jr. Acidosis of chronic renal failure. In: DuBose TD, Hamm LL, eds. *Acid-Base and Electrolyte Disorders.* Philadelphia: Saunders; 2002:207–216.
95. Menon V, Tighiouart H, Vaughn NS, et al. Serum bicarbonate and long-term outcomes in CKD. *Am J Kidney Dis.* 2010;56(5):907–914.
96. Navaneethan SD, Schold JD, Arrigain S, et al. Serum bicarbonate and mortality in stage 3 and stage 4 chronic kidney disease. *Clin J Am Soc Nephrol.* 2011;6(10):2395–2402.
97. Loniewski I, Wesson DE. Bicarbonate therapy for prevention of chronic kidney disease progression. *Kidney Int.* 2014;85(3):529–535.
98. Goraya N, Simoni J, Jo CH, et al. A comparison of treating metabolic acidosis in CKD stage 4 hypertensive kidney disease with fruits and vegetables or sodium bicarbonate. *Clin J Am Soc Nephrol.* 2013; 8(3):371–381.
103. Laski ME, Wesson DE. Lactic acidosis. In: DuBose TD, Hamm LL, eds. *Acid-Base and Electrolyte Disorders: A Companion to Brenner and Rector's The Kidney.* Philadelphia: Saunders; 2002.
117. Whitney GM, Szerlip HM. Acid-base disorders in the critical care setting. In: DuBose TD, Hamm LL, eds. *Acid-Base and Electrolyte Disorders: A Companion to Brenner and Rector's The Kidney.* Philadelphia: Saunders; 2002:165–187.
119. Halperin ML, Kamel KS, Cherney DZ. Ketoacidosis. In: DuBose TD, Hamm LL, eds. *Acid-Base and Electrolyte Disorders: A Companion to Brenner and Rector's The Kidney.* Philadelphia: Saunders; 2002: 67–82.
121. Peters AL, Buschur EO, Buse JB, et al. Euglycemic diabetic ketoacidosis: a potential complication of treatment with sodium-glucose cotransporter 2 inhibition. *Diabetes Care.* 2015;38(9):1687–1693.
125. Kraut JA, Kurtz I. Toxic alcohol ingestions: clinical features, diagnosis, and management. *Clin J Am Soc Nephrol.* 2008;3(1):208–225.
128. Brent J. Fomepizole for ethylene glycol and methanol poisoning. *N Engl J Med.* 2009;360(21):2216–2223.
139. Seyberth HW, Weber S, Komhoff M. Bartter's and Gitelman's syndrome. *Curr Opin Pediatr.* 2017;29(2):179–186.
144. Shaer AJ. Inherited primary renal tubular hypokalemic alkalosis: a review of Gitelman and Bartter syndromes. *Am J Med Sci.* 2001;322(6):316–332.
149. Funder JW. Apparent mineralocorticoid excess. *J Steroid Biochem Mol Biol.* 2017;165(Pt A):151–153.

# Disorders of Potassium Balance

17

David B. Mount

CHAPTER OUTLINE



## POTASSIUM DISORDERS

The diagnosis and management of potassium disorders are central skills in clinical nephrology, relevant not only to consultative nephrology but also to dialysis and renal transplantation. An understanding of the underlying physiology is critical to the diagnostic and management approach to hyper- and hypokalemic patients. This chapter reviews those aspects of the physiology of potassium homeostasis judged to be relevant to the understanding of potassium disorders; a more detailed review of renal potassium transport is provided in Chapter 6.

The pathophysiology of potassium disorders continues to evolve. The expanding list of drugs with a potential to affect the plasma potassium concentration ($K^+$) has made clinical management more complex, yet has provided the opportunity to new insight into potassium homeostasis. The evolving molecular understanding of both common and rare disorders affecting plasma $K^+$ continues to uncover novel pathways of regulation.[1–8] These advances can be incorporated into an increasingly mechanistic, molecular understanding of potassium disorders.

## NORMAL POTASSIUM BALANCE

The dietary intake of potassium ranges from less than 35 to more than 110 mmol/day in US men and women. Despite this widespread variation in intake, homeostatic mechanisms serve to maintain plasma $K^+$ precisely between 3.5 and 5.0 mmol/L. In a healthy individual at steady state, the entire daily intake of potassium is excreted, approximately 90% in the urine and 10% in the stool. More than 98% of total body potassium is intracellular, chiefly in muscle (Fig. 17.1). Buffering of extracellular $K^+$ by this large intracellular pool plays a crucial role in the regulation of plasma $K^+$.[9] Thus, within 60 minutes of an intravenous load of 0.5 mmol/kg of $K^+$-$Cl^-$, only 41% appears in the urine, yet the serum $K^+$ level rises by no more than 0.6 mmol/L.[9] Adding the equivalent 35 mmol exclusively to the extracellular space of a 70-kg man would be expected to raise the serum $K^+$ level by ~2.5 mmol/L.[10] Changes in cellular distribution also serve to defend plasma $K^+$ during $K^+$ depletion. For example, military recruits have been shown to maintain a normal serum $K^+$ level after 11 days of basic training in hot environments, despite a profound $K^+$ deficit generated by renal and extrarenal losses.[11] The rapid exchange of intracellular $K^+$ with extracellular $K^+$ plays a crucial role in maintaining plasma $K^+$ within such a narrow range; this is accomplished by overlapping and synergistic[12] regulation of a number of renal and extrarenal transport pathways.

### POTASSIUM TRANSPORT MECHANISMS

The intracellular accumulation of $K^+$ against its electrochemical gradient is an energy-consuming process, mediated by the ubiquitous $Na^+/K^+$-ATPase enzyme. The $Na^+/K^+$-ATPase functions as an electrogenic pump, because the stoichiometry of transport is three intracellular $Na^+$ ions to two extracellular $K^+$ ions. The enzyme complex is made up of a tissue-specific combination of multiple alpha, beta, and gamma subunits, which are further subject to tissue-specific patterns of regulation.[13] The $Na^+/K^+$-ATPase proteins share significant homology with the corresponding subunits of the $H^+/K^+$-ATPase enzymes (see "Potassium Transport in the Distal Nephron"). Cardiac glycosides, such as digoxin and ouabain, bind to the alpha subunits of $Na^+/K^+$-ATPase at an exposed extracellular hairpin loop that also contains the major binding sites for extracellular $K^+$.[14] The binding of digoxin and $K^+$ to the $Na^+/K^+$-ATPase complex is thus mutually antagonistic, explaining in part the potentiation of digoxin toxicity by hypokalemia.[15] Although the four alpha subunits have equivalent affinity for ouabain, they differ significantly in intrinsic $K^+$–ouabain antagonism.[16] Ouabain binding to isozymes containing the ubiquitous alpha-1 subunit is relatively insensitive to $K^+$ concentrations within the physiologic range, such that this isozyme is protected from digoxin under conditions wherein cardiac alpha-2 and alpha-3 subunits, the probable therapeutic targets,[17] are inhibited.[16] Genetic reduction in cardiac alpha-1

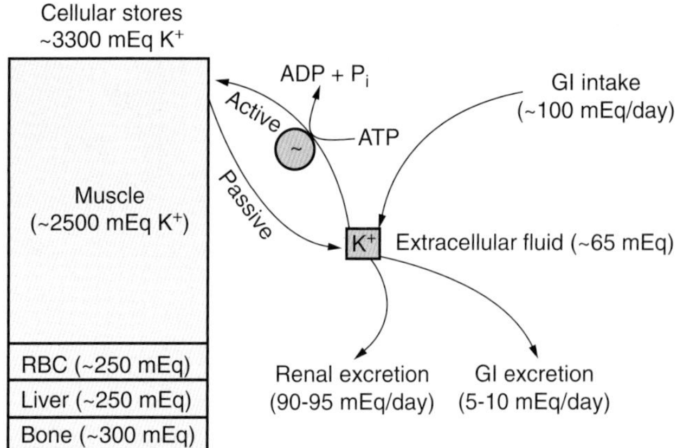


**Fig. 17.1** Body $K^+$ distribution and cellular $K^+$ flux. *ADP,* Adenosine diphosphate; *ATP,* adenosine triphosphate; *GI,* gastrointestinal; *RBC,* red blood cell. (From Wingo CS, Weiner ID. Disorders of potassium balance. In Brenner BM ed. *The Kidney.* ed 6. Philadelphia: WB Saunders; 2000:998–1035.)

content has a negative ionotropic effect,[17] such that the relative resistance of this subunit to digoxin at physiologic plasma $K^+$ has an additional cardioprotective effect. Notably, the digoxin-ouabain binding site of alpha subunits is highly conserved, suggesting a potential role in the physiologic response to endogenous ouabain–digoxin-like compounds. Mice that express alpha-2 subunits with engineered resistance to ouabain are strikingly resistant to ouabain-induced hypertension and to adrenocorticotropic hormone (ACTH)-dependent hypertension,[18] the latter known to involve an increase in circulating ouabain-like glycosides. These provocative data lend credence to the controversial role of such ouabain-like molecules in hypertension and cardiovascular disease. Furthermore, modulation of the $K^+$-dependent binding of circulating ouabain-like compounds to $Na^+/K^+$-ATPase may underlie at least some of cardiovascular complications of hypokalemia[19] (see "Effects of Hypokalemia").

Skeletal muscle contains as much as 75% of body potassium (see Fig. 17.1) and exerts considerable influence on extracellular $K^+$. Exercise is thus a well-described cause of transient hyperkalemia; interstitial $K^+$ in human muscle can reach levels as high as 10 mM after fatiguing exercise.[20] Not surprisingly, therefore, changes in skeletal muscle $Na^+/K^+$-ATPase activity and abundance are major determinants of the capacity for extrarenal $K^+$ homeostasis. Hypokalemia induces a marked decrease in muscle $K^+$ content and $Na^+/K^+$-ATPase activity,[21] an altruistic[22] mechanism to regulate plasma $K^+$. This is primarily as a result of dramatic decreases in the protein abundance of the alpha-2 subunit of $Na^+/K^+$-ATPase.[23] In contrast, hyperkalemia caused by potassium loading is associated with adaptive increases in muscle $K^+$ content and $Na^+/K^+$-ATPase activity.[24] These interactions are reflected in the relationship between physical activity and the ability to regulate extracellular $K^+$ during exercise.[25] For example, exercise training is associated with increases in muscle $Na^+/K^+$-ATPase concentration and activity, with reduced interstitial $K^+$ in trained muscles[26] and an enhanced recovery of plasma $K^+$ after defined amounts of exercise.[25]

Potassium can also accumulate in cells by coupling to the gradient for $Na^+$ entry, entering via the electroneutral $Na^+$-$K^+$-$2Cl^-$ cotransporters NKCC1 and NKCC2. The NKCC2 protein is found only at the apical membrane of the thick ascending limb (TAL) and macula densa cells (Fig. 17.2; see Fig. 17.10), where it functions in transepithelial salt transport and tubular regulation of renin release.[27] In contrast, NKCC1 is widely expressed in multiple tissues,[27] including muscle.[28] The cotransport of $K^+$-$Cl^-$ by the four $K^+$-$Cl^-$ cotransporters (KCC1-4) can also function in the transfer of $K^+$ across membranes; although the KCCs typically function as efflux pathways, they can mediate influx when extracellular $K^+$ increases.[27]

The efflux of $K^+$ out of cells is largely accomplished by $K^+$ channels, which comprise the largest family of ion channels in the human genome. There are three major subclasses of mammalian $K^+$ channels—the six-transmembrane domain (TMD) family, which encompasses both the voltage-sensitive and $Ca^{2+}$-activated $K^+$ channels; the two-pore, four TMD family; and the two TMD family of inward rectifying $K^+$ (Kir) channels.[29] There is tremendous genomic variety in human $K^+$ channels, with at least 26 separate genes encoding principal subunits of the voltage-gated Kv channels and 17 genes encoding the principal Kir subunits. Further complexity is generated by the presence of multiple accessory subunits and alternative patterns of mRNA splicing. Not surprisingly, an increasing number and variety of $K^+$ channels have been implicated in the control of $K^+$ homeostasis and the membrane potential of excitable cells such as muscle and heart, with important, evolving roles in the pathophysiology of potassium disorders.[2,30–32]

## FACTORS AFFECTING INTERNAL DISTRIBUTION OF POTASSIUM

A number of hormones and physiologic conditions have acute effects on the distribution of $K^+$ between the intracellular and extracellular space (Table 17.1). Some of these factors are of particular clinical relevance and are therefore reviewed here in detail.

### INSULIN

The hypokalemic effect of insulin has been known since the early 20th century.[33] The impact of insulin on plasma $K^+$ and plasma glucose is separable at multiple levels, suggesting independent mechanisms.[21,34,35] For example, despite impaired glucose uptake, peripheral $K^+$ uptake is not impaired in humans with type 2 diabetes.[35] Notably, the hypokalemic effect of insulin is not renal-dependent.[36] Insulin and $K^+$ appear to form a feedback loop of sorts, in that increases in plasma $K^+$ have a marked stimulatory effect on insulin levels.[21,37] Insulin-stimulated $K^+$ uptake, measured in rats using a $K^+$ clamp technique, is rapidly reduced by 2 days of $K^+$ depletion, before a modest drop in plasma $K^+$,[38] and in the absence of a change in plasma $K^+$ in rats subject to a lesser $K^+$ restriction for 14 days.[12] Insulin-mediated $K^+$ uptake is thus modulated by the factors that serve to preserve plasma $K^+$ in the setting of $K^+$ deprivation (see also "Control of Potassium Secretion: Effect of Potassium Intake"). Inhibition of basal insulin secretion in normal subjects by somatostatin infusion increases serum $K^+$ by up to 0.5 mmol/L, in the absence of a change in urinary excretion, emphasizing the crucial role of circulating insulin in the regulation of plasma $K^+$.[39] Clinically, inhibition of insulin secretion by the

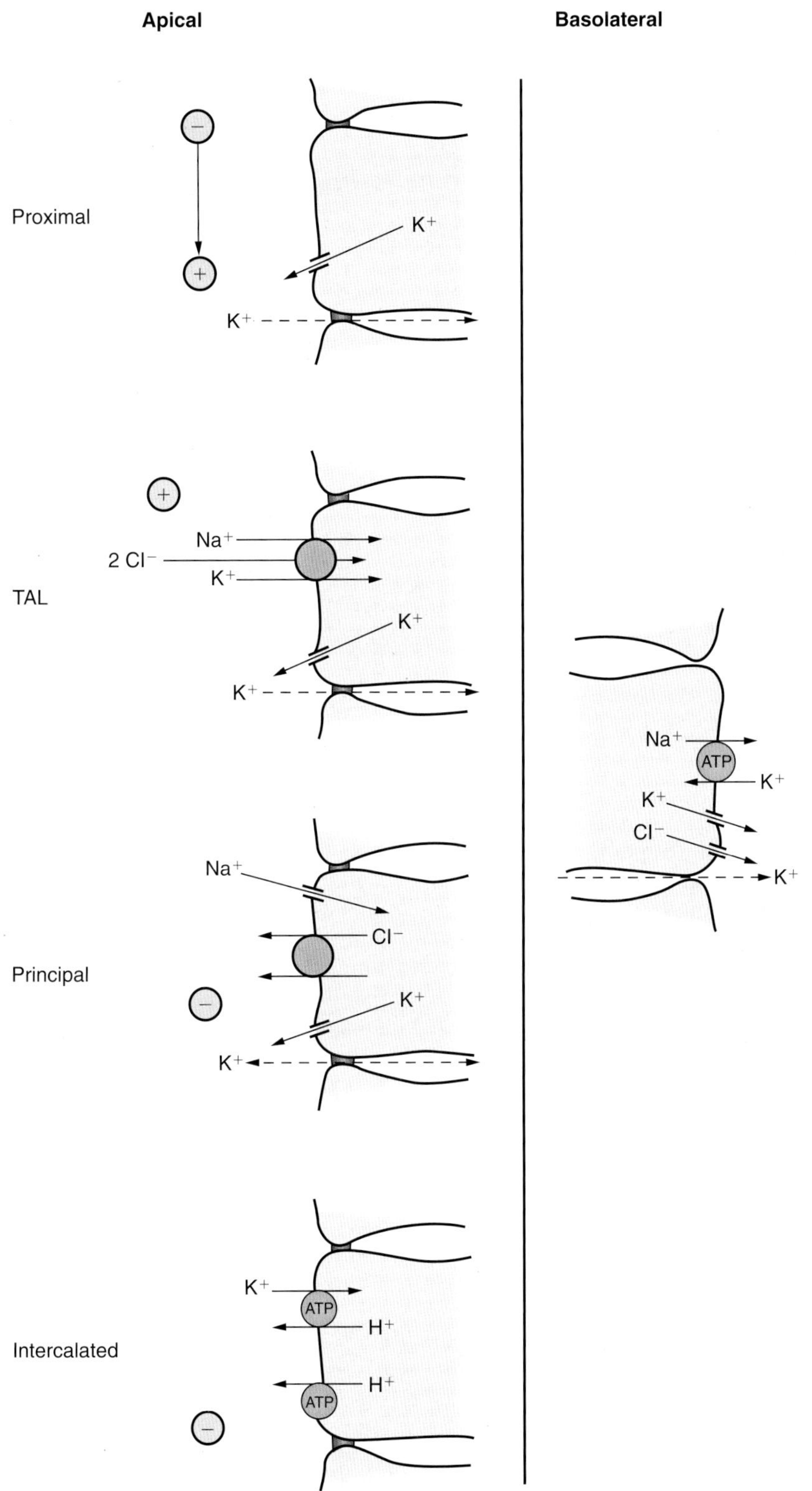


**Fig. 17.2** Schematic cell models of potassium transport along the nephron. Cell types are as specified; Note the differences in luminal potential difference along the nephron. *ATP*, Adenosine triphosphate; *TAL*, thick ascending limb. (From Giebisch G. Renal potassium transport: mechanisms and regulation. *Am J Physiol.* 1998;274:F817–F833.)

somatostatin agonist octreotide can cause significant hyperkalemia in both anephric patients[40] and patients with normal renal function.[41]

Insulin stimulates the uptake of $K^+$ by several tissues, most prominently liver, skeletal muscle, cardiac muscle, and fat.[21,42] It does so by activating several $K^+$ transport pathways, with particularly well-documented effects on the $Na^+/K^+$-ATPase.[43] Insulin activates $Na^+$-$H^+$ exchange and/or $Na^+$-$K^+$-$2Cl^-$ cotransport in several tissues. Although the ensuing increase in intracellular $Na^+$ was postulated to have a secondary activating

**Table 17.1 Factors Affecting Distribution of Potassium Between Intracellular and Extracellular Compartments**

| Factor | Effect |
|---|---|
| **Acute: Effect on Potassium** | |
| Insulin | Enhanced cell uptake |
| • β-Catecholamines | Enhanced cell uptake |
| • α-Catecholamines | Impaired cell uptake |
| Acidosis | Impaired cell uptake |
| Alkalosis | Enhanced cell uptake |
| External potassium balance | Loose correlation |
| Cell damage | Impaired cell uptake |
| Hyperosmolality | Enhanced cell efflux |
| **Chronic: Effect on ATP Pump Density** | |
| Thyroid | Enhanced |
| Adrenal steroids | Enhanced |
| Exercise (training) | Enhanced |
| Growth | Enhanced |
| Diabetes | Impaired |
| Potassium deficiency | Impaired |
| Chronic renal failure | Impaired |

From Giebisch G: Renal potassium transport: mechanisms and regulation. *Am J Physiol.* 1998;274:F817-F833.

**Table 17.2 Sustained Effects of β- and α-Adrenergic Agonists and Antagonists on Serum Potassium Concentration**

| Catecholamine Specificity | Sustained Effect on Serum $K^+$ |
|---|---|
| Beta-1 + beta-2 agonist (e.g., epinephrine, isoproterenol) | Decreased |
| Pure beta-1 agonist (e.g., ITP) | None |
| Pure beta-2 agonist (e.g., salbutamol, soterenol, terbutaline | Decreased |
| Beta-1 + beta-2 antagonist (e.g., propranolol, sotalol) | Increased; blocks the effect of beta agonists |
| Beta-1 antagonist (e.g., practolol, metoprolol, atenolol) | None; does not block effect of beta agonists |
| Beta-2 antagonist (e.g., butoxamine, H 35/25) | Blocks hypokalemic effect of beta agonists |
| Alpha agonist (e.g., phenylephrine) | Increased |
| Alpha antagonist (e.g., phenoxybenzamine) | None; blocks effect of alpha agonists |

*ITP,* Isopropylamino-3-(2-thiazoloxy)-2-propanol.
From Giebisch G: Renal potassium transport: mechanisms and regulation. *Am J Physiol.* 1998;274:F817-F833.

effect on $Na^+/K^+$-ATPase,[29] it is clear that this is not the primary mechanism in most cell types.[44] Insulin induces translocation of the $Na^+/K^+$-ATPase alpha-2 subunit to the plasma membrane of skeletal muscle cells, with a lesser effect on the alpha-1 subunit.[45] This translocation is dependent on the activity of phosphoinositide-3 (PI-3) kinase,[45] which itself also binds to a proline-rich motif in the N-terminus of the alpha subunit.[46] The activation of PI3 kinase by insulin thus induces phosphatase enzymes to dephosphorylate a specific serine residue adjacent to the PI3 kinase binding domain. Trafficking of $Na^+/K^+$-ATPase to the cell surface also appears to require the phosphorylation of an adjacent tyrosine residue, perhaps catalyzed by the tyrosine kinase activity of the insulin receptor itself.[47] Finally, the serum and glucocorticoid-induced kinase-1 (SGK1) plays a critical role in insulin-stimulated $K^+$ uptake, presumably via the known stimulatory effects of this kinase on $Na^+/K^+$-ATPase activity and/or $Na^+$-$K^+$-$2Cl^-$ cotransport.[48] The hypokalemic effect of insulin plus glucose is blunted in SGK1 knockout mice, with a marked reduction in hepatic insulin-stimulated $K^+$ uptake.[48]

## SYMPATHETIC NERVOUS SYSTEM

The sympathetic nervous system plays a prominent role in regulating the balance between extracellular and intracellular $K^+$. Again, as is the case for insulin, the effect of catecholamines on plasma $K^+$ has been known for some time[49]; however, a complicating issue is the differential effect of stimulating α- and β-adrenergic receptors (Table 17.2). Uptake of $K^+$ by liver and muscle, with resultant hypokalemia, is stimulated via beta-2 receptors.[29] The hypokalemic effect of catecholamines appears to be largely independent of changes in circulating insulin[29] and has been reported in nephrectomized animals.[50] The cellular mechanisms whereby catecholamines induce $K^+$ uptake in muscle include an activation of the $Na^+/K^+$-ATPase,[51] likely via increases in cyclic adenosine monophosphate (cAMP).[52] However, beta-adrenergic receptors in skeletal muscle also activate the inwardly directed $Na^+$-$K^+$-$2Cl^-$ cotransporter NKCC1, which may account for as much as one-third of the uptake response to catecholamines.[21,28]

In contrast to beta-adrenergic stimulation, alpha-adrenergic agonists impair the ability to buffer increases in $K^+$ induced via intravenous loading or by exercise[53]; the cellular mechanisms whereby this occurs are not known. It is thought that beta-adrenergic stimulation increases $K^+$ uptake during exercise to avoid hyperkalemia, whereas alpha-adrenergic mechanisms help blunt the ensuing postexercise nadir.[53] The clinical consequences of the sympathetic control of extrarenal $K^+$ homeostasis are reviewed elsewhere in this chapter.

## ACID-BASE STATUS

The association between changes in pH and plasma $K^+$ was observed some time ago.[54] It has long been thought that acute disturbances in acid-base equilibrium result in changes in serum $K^+$ such that alkalemia shifts $K^+$ into cells, whereas acidemia is associated with $K^+$ release.[55,56] It is believed that this apparent $K^+$-$H^+$ exchange and/or $K^+$-$HCO_3^-$ cotransport helps maintain extracellular pH.[57] Several different transport mechanisms together result in the net exchange of $K^+$ with $H^+$, including functional coupling between $Na^+$-$H^+$ exchangers with the $Na^+/K^+$-ATPase, coupling between $Na^+$-$2HCO_3^-$ cotransport with the $Na^+/K^+$-ATPase, and coupling between $Cl^-$-$HCO_3^-$ exchange and $K^+$-$Cl^-$ cotransporters.[57]

Rather limited data exist for the durable concept that a change of 0.1 unit in serum pH will result in a 0.6-mmol/L change in serum $K^+$ in the opposite direction.[58] However, despite the complexities of changes in $K^+$ homeostasis associated with various acid-base disorders, a few general observations can be made. The induction of metabolic acidosis by the infusion of mineral acids ($NH_4^+$-$Cl^-$ or $H^+$-$Cl^-$) consistently increases serum $K^+$,[55,56,58–60] whereas organic acidosis generally fails to increase serum $K^+$.[56,59,61,62] Notably, a more recent report failed to detect an increase in serum $K^+$ in normal human subjects with acute acidosis secondary to duodenal $NH_4^+$-$Cl^-$ infusion, in which a modest acidosis was accompanied by an increase in circulating insulin.[63] However, as noted by Adrogué and Madias,[64] the concomitant infusion of 350 mL of dextrose 5% in water (D5W) in these fasting subjects may have served to increase circulating insulin, thus blunting the potential hyperkalemic response to $NH_4^+$-$Cl^-$. Clinically, use of the oral phosphate binder sevelamer hydrochloride in patients with end-stage kidney disease (ESKD) is associated with acidosis caused by effective gastrointestinal absorption of $H^+$-$Cl^-$; in hemodialysis patients, this acidosis has been associated with an increase in serum $K^+$, which is ameliorated by an increase in dialysis bicarbonate concentration.[65] Of note, hyperkalemia is not an expected complication of sevelamer carbonate, which has started to supplant sevelamer hydrochloride as a phosphate binder.

Metabolic alkalosis induced by sodium bicarbonate infusion usually results in a modest reduction in serum $K^+$.[55,56,58,60,66] Respiratory alkalosis reduces plasma $K^+$ by a magnitude comparable to that of metabolic alkalosis.[55,56,58,66] Finally, acute respiratory acidosis increases plasma $K^+$; the absolute increase is smaller than that induced by metabolic acidosis secondary to inorganic acids.[55,56,58] Again, however, some studies have failed to show a change in serum $K^+$ following acute respiratory acidosis.[56,67] The smaller increments in serum $K^+$ with respiratory acidosis are explained in part by the elevated serum $HCO_3^-$ levels in respiratory acidosis, which blunt pH effects on the $Na^+$-$2HCO_3^-$ cotransporter, resulting in lesser apparent $K^+$-$H^+$ exchange than in metabolic acidosis.[57]

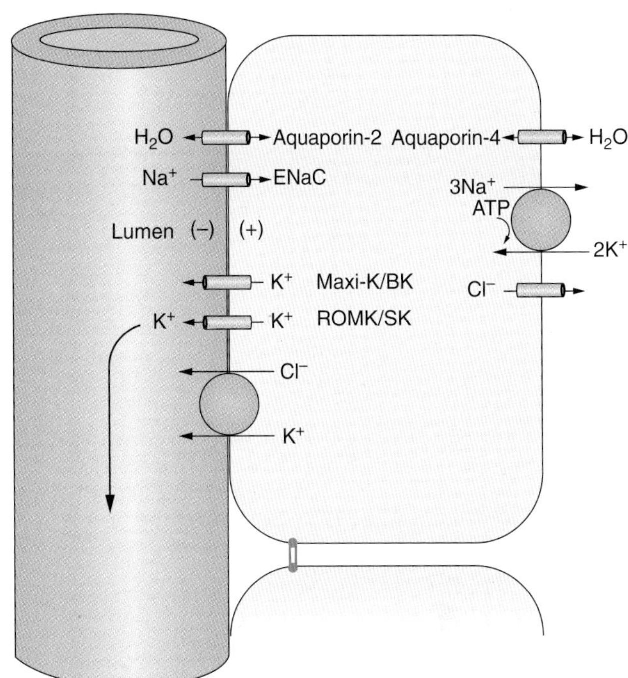


**Fig. 17.3** $K^+$ secretory pathways in principal cells of the connecting segment and cortical collecting duct. The absorption of $Na^+$ via the amiloride-sensitive epithelial sodium channel *(ENaC)* generates a lumen-negative potential difference, which drives $K^+$ excretion through the apical secretory $K^+$ channel ROMK. Flow-dependent $K^+$ secretion is mediated by an apical voltage-gated, calcium-sensitive BK channel. Chloride-dependent, electroneutral $K^+$ secretion is likely mediated by a $K^+$-$Cl^-$ cotransporter. Water transport in principal cells occurs via aquaporin-2 (Aqp-2) and aquaporins-3/4 (Aqp-3/4). *ATP,* Adenosine triphosphate.

## RENAL POTASSIUM EXCRETION

### POTASSIUM TRANSPORT IN THE DISTAL NEPHRON

The proximal tubule and loop of Henle mediate the bulk of potassium reabsorption, such that a considerable fraction of filtered potassium is reabsorbed before entry into the superficial distal tubules.[68] Renal potassium excretion is primarily determined by regulated secretion in the distal nephron, specifically within the connecting segment (CNT) and cortical collecting duct (CCD). The principal cells of the CNT and CCD play a dominant role in $K^+$ secretion; the relevant transport pathways are shown in Fig. 17.3 (see Fig. 17.2). Apical $Na^+$ entry via the amiloride-sensitive epithelial $Na^+$ channel (ENaC)[69] results in the generation of a lumen-negative potential difference in the CNT and CCD, which drives passive $K^+$ exit through apical $K^+$ channels. A critical, clinically relevant consequence of this relationship is that $K^+$ secretion is dependent on the delivery of adequate luminal $Na^+$ to the CNT and CCD;[70,71] $K^+$ secretion by the CCD essentially ceases as the luminal $Na^+$ drops below 8 mmol/L.[72] Selective increases in thiazide-sensitive $Na^+$-$Cl^-$ cotransporter in the distal convoluted tubule (DCT), as seen in familial hyperkalemia with hypertension (FHHt; see "Hereditary Tubular Defects and Potassium Excretion"), reduce $Na^+$ delivery to principal cells in the downstream CNT and CCD, leading to hyperkalemia.[73] Dietary $Na^+$ intake also influences $K^+$ excretion, such that excretion is enhanced by excess $Na^+$ intake and reduced by $Na^+$ restriction (see Fig. 17.4).[70,71] Basolateral exchange of $Na^+$ and $K^+$ is mediated by the $Na^+$/$K^+$-ATPase, providing the driving force for both $Na^+$ entry and $K^+$ exit at the apical membrane (see Figs. 17.2 and 17.3).

Under basal conditions of high $Na^+$-$Cl^-$ and low $K^+$ intake, the bulk of aldosterone-stimulated $Na^+$ and $K^+$ transport occurs in the CNT, before the entry of tubular fluid into the CCD.[74] The density of both $Na^+$ and $K^+$ channels is considerably greater in the CNT than in the CCD.[75,76] Thus, in the setting of replete $Na^+$-$Cl^-$ intake, the capacity of the CNT for $Na^+$ reabsorption may be as much as 10 times greater than that of the CCD.[76] The recruitment of ENaC subunits in response to dietary $Na^+$ restriction begins in the CNT, with the progressive recruitment of subunits to the apical membrane of the CCD at lower levels of dietary $Na^+$.[78] The activity of the secretory $K^+$ channels in the CNT is also influenced by changes in dietary $K^+$[79]; again, this is consistent with progressive axial recruitment of transport capacity for the absorption of $Na^+$ and secretion of $K^+$ along the distal nephron.

Electrophysiologic characterization has documented the presence of several subpopulations of apical $K^+$ channels in

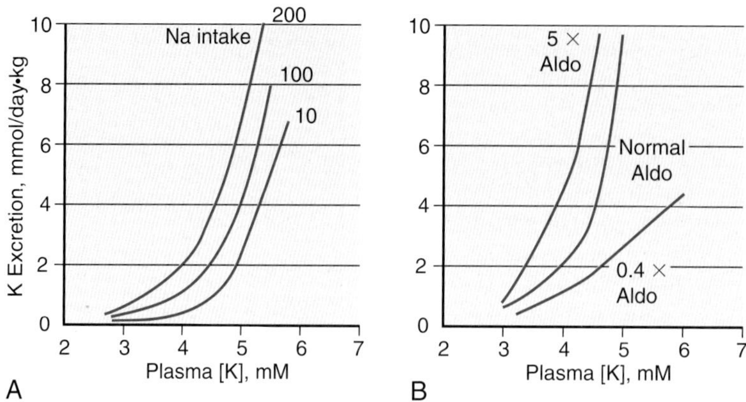


**Fig. 17.4** (A) Relationship between steady-state plasma K$^+$ and urinary K$^+$ excretion in the dog, as a function of dietary Na$^+$ intake (mmol/day). Animals were adrenalectomized and replaced with aldosterone, dietary K$^+$ and Na$^+$ content were varied as specified. (B) Relationship between steady-state plasma K$^+$ and urinary K$^+$ excretion as a function of circulating aldosterone. Animals were adrenalectomized and variably replaced with aldosterone *(Aldo)*; dietary K$^+$ content was varied. (A from Young DB, Jackson TE, Tipayamontri U, Scott RC. Effects of sodium intake on steady-state potassium excretion. *Am J Physiol.* 1984;246:F772–F778; B from Young DB. Quantitative analysis of aldosterone's role in potassium regulation. *Am J Physiol.* 1988;255:F811–F822.)

the CCD and CNT, most prominently a small-conductance (SK) 30-picosiemens (pS) channel[75,77] and a large-conductance, Ca$^{2+}$-activated 150-pS (BK) channel[75,78] (see Fig. 17.3). The SK channel is thought to mediate K$^+$ secretion under baseline conditions—hence, its designation as the "secretory" K$^+$ channel. SK channel activity is mediated by the ROMK (*r*enal *o*uter *m*edullary *K*$^+$ channel) protein, encoded by the *Kcnj1* gene; targeted deletion of this gene in mice results in complete loss of SK activity within the CCD.[78] Increased distal flow has a significant stimulatory effect on K$^+$ secretion, due in part to both enhanced delivery and absorption of Na$^+$ and to increased removal of secreted K$^+$.[71,72] The apical Ca$^{2+}$-activated BK channel plays a critical role in flow-dependent K$^+$ secretion by the CNT and CCD.[77] BK channels have a heteromeric structure, with alpha subunits that form the ion channel pore and modulatory beta subunits.[77] The beta-1 subunits of BK channels are restricted to principal cells within the CNT,[77,79] whereas beta-4 subunits are detectable at the apical membranes of the TAL, DCT, and intercalated cells.[79] Flow-dependent K$^+$ secretion is reduced in mice with targeted deletion of the alpha-1 and beta-1 subunits,[77,80,81] consistent with a dominant role for BK channels. The Ca$^{2+}$-permeable TRPV4 channel increases intracellular Ca$^{2+}$ concentrations in response to tubular flow, resulting in the activation of BK channels.[82]

In addition to apical K$^+$ channels, considerable evidence implicates apical K$^+$-Cl$^-$ cotransport in distal K$^+$ secretion.[70,83,84] Pharmacologic studies of perfused tubules are consistent with K$^+$-Cl$^-$ cotransport mediated by the KCC proteins.[83] A particularly provocative study has underlined the importance of ENaC-independent K$^+$ excretion, whether it is mediated by apical K$^+$-Cl$^-$ cotransport and/or by other mechanisms.[85] Rats were infused with amiloride via osmotic minipumps, generating urinary concentrations considered sufficient to inhibit more than 98% of ENaC activity. Whereas amiloride almost abolished K$^+$ excretion in rats on a normal K$^+$ intake, acute and long-term high-K$^+$ diets led to an increasing fraction of K$^+$ excretion that was independent of ENaC activity (~50% after 7–9 days on a high-K$^+$ diet).[85] Therefore, increased K$^+$ intake induces a K$^+$ excretion pathway that is independent of ENaC activity.

In addition to secretion, the distal nephron is capable of considerable reabsorption of K$^+$, particularly during restriction of dietary K$^+$.[21,68,86,87] This reabsorption is accomplished primarily by intercalated cells in the outer medullary collecting duct (OMCD), via the activity of apical H$^+$/K$^+$-ATPase pumps (see Fig. 17.2). Therefore, decreased K$^+$ intake induces a K$^+$ reabsorption pathway that is independent of ENaC activity.

## CONTROL OF POTASSIUM SECRETION: ALDOSTERONE

Aldosterone is well established as an important regulatory factor in K$^+$ excretion, and increases in plasma K$^+$ are an important stimulus for aldosterone secretion (see also "Regulation of Renal Renin and Adrenal Aldosterone"). However, an important principle is that aldosterone plays a permissive, synergistic, but not essential role in K$^+$ homeostasis.[88–90] This is reflected clinically in the frequent absence of hyper- or hypokalemia in disorders associated with a deficiency or an overabundance of circulating aldosterone, respectively (see "Hyperaldosteronism" and "Hypoaldosteronism"). Regardless, it is clear that aldosterone and downstream effectors of this hormone have clinically relevant effects on plasma K$^+$ levels and that the ability to excrete K$^+$ is modulated by systemic aldosterone levels (Fig. 17.4).

Aldosterone has no effect on the density of apical SK channels in the CCD or CNT; rather, the hormone induces a marked increase in the density of apical Na$^+$ channels,[91] thus increasing the driving force for apical K$^+$ excretion. The apical amiloride-sensitive epithelial Na$^+$ channel (ENaC) is comprised of three subunits, alpha, beta, and gamma, that assemble together to traffic to the cell membrane synergistically and mediate Na$^+$ transport. Aldosterone activates ENaC channel complexes by multiple mechanisms. First, it induces transcription of the alpha-ENaC subunit,[92,93] increasing the availability for co-assembly with the more abundant beta and gamma subunits.[94] Second, aldosterone and dietary Na$^+$-Cl$^-$ restriction stimulate a significant redistribution of ENaC subunits in the CNT and early CCD, from a largely cytoplasmic location during dietary $Na^+$-$Cl^-$ excess to a purely apical distribution after aldosterone administration or $Na^+$-$Cl^-$ restriction.[95–97] Third, aldosterone induces the expression of SGK1[98]; coexpression of SGK1 with ENaC subunits results in increased expression at the plasma membrane.[96] SGK1 modulates membrane expression of ENaC by interfering with regulated endocytosis of its channel subunits. Specifically, the kinase interferes with interactions between ENaC subunits and the ubiquitin ligase Nedd4-2.[94] The so-called PPxY domains in the C-termini of all three ENaC subunits bind to WW domains of Nedd4-2[99]; these PPxY domains are deleted, truncated, or mutated in patients with Liddle syndrome[100] (see "Liddle Syndrome"), leading to a gain of function in channel activity.[101] Nedd4-2 ubiquitinates ENaC subunits, thus inducing removal of channel subunits from the cell membrane followed by degradation in lysosomes and the proteosome.[94] A PPxY domain in SGK1 also binds to Nedd4-2, which is a phosphorylation substrate for the kinase; phosphorylation of Nedd4-2 by SGK1 abrogates the inhibitory effect of this ubiquitin ligase on ENaC subunits[3] (Fig. 17.5).

The importance of SGK1 in $K^+$ and $Na^+$ homeostasis is illustrated by the phenotype of SGK1 knockout mice.[102,103] On a normal diet, homozygous SGK1$^{-/-}$ mice exhibit normal blood pressure and a normal plasma $K^+$, with only a mild elevation of circulating aldosterone. However, dietary $Na^+$-$Cl^-$ restriction of these mice results in relative $Na^+$ wasting and hypotension, marked weight loss, and a drop in the glomerular filtration rate (GFR), despite considerable increases in circulating aldosterone.[103] In addition, dietary $K^+$ loading over 6 days leads to a 1.5-mmol/L increase in serum $K^+$, also accompanied by a considerable increase in circulating aldosterone (~fivefold greater than that of wild-type littermate controls).[102] This hyperkalemia occurs despite evident increases in apical ROMK expression, compared with the normokalemic littermate controls. The amiloride-sensitive, lumen-negative potential difference generated by ENaC is reduced in these SGK1 knockout mice,[102] resulting in a decreased driving force for distal $K^+$ secretion and the observed susceptibility to hyperkalemia. Notably, however, a more recent characterization of this same knockout strain failed to detect a reduction in the increase in ENaC activity induced by dietary potassium loading, suggesting that the hyperkalemia in these mice is caused by a defect in ENaC-independent $K^+$ excretion.[104]

Another mechanism whereby aldosterone activates ENaC involves proteolytic cleavage of the channel proteins by serine proteases. A so-called channel-activating protease that increases channel activity of ENaC was initially identified in *Xenopus laevis* A6 cells.[105] The mammalian ortholog, denoted CAP1 (channel-activating protease-1), or prostasin, is an aldosterone-induced protein in principal cells.[106] Urinary excretion of CAP1 is increased in hyperaldosteronism, with a reduction after adrenalectomy.[106] CAP1 is membrane-associated, via a glycosylphosphatidylinositol (GPI) linkage[105]; mammalian principal cells also express two transmembrane proteases, denoted CAP2 and CAP3, with homology to CAP1.[107] These and other proteases (e.g., furin, plasmin) activate ENaC by excising extracellular inhibitory domains from the alpha and gamma subunits, increasing the open probability of channels at the plasma membrane.[107,108] This proteolytic cleavage of ENaC appears to activate the channel by removing the self-inhibitory effect of external $Na^+$[109]; in the case of furin-mediated proteolysis of α-ENaC, this appears to involve the removal of an inhibitory domain from within the extracellular loop.[110] Extracellular $Na^+$ appears to interact with a specific acidic cleft in the cleaved extracellular loop of α-ENaC, causing inhibition of the channel.[111] Because SGK1 increases channel expression at the cell surface,[96] one would expect synergistic activation by coexpressed CAP1–3 and SGK; this is indeed the case.[107] Therefore, aldosterone activates ENaC by at least three separate synergistic mechanisms; induction of α-ENaC, induction of SGK1 and repression of Nedd4-2, and induction of channel-activating proteases. Clinically, the inhibition of channel-activating proteases by the protease inhibitor nafamostat causes hyperkalemia as a result of the inhibition of ENaC activity.[112,113] Nafamostat has been used as a regional anticoagulant for hemodialysis in patients at high risk for bleeding. In contrast with heparin, nafamostat prolongs clotting times only in the extracorporeal circuit.

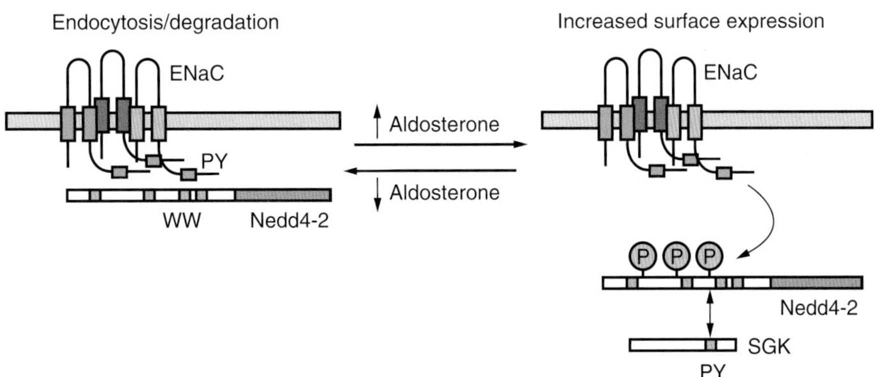


**Fig. 17.5** Coordinated regulation of the epithelial sodium channel *(ENaC)* by the aldosterone-induced SGK kinase and the ubiquitin ligase Nedd4-2. Nedd4-2 binds via its WW domains to ENaC subunits via their PPXY domains (denoted *PY* here), ubiquitinating the channel subunits and targeting them for removal from the cell membrane and destruction in the proteasome. Aldosterone induces the SGK kinase, which phosphorylates and inactivates Nedd4-2, thus increasing the surface expression of ENaC channels. Mutations that cause Liddle syndrome affect the interaction between ENaC and Nedd4-2. (From Snyder PM, Olson DR, Thomas BC. Serum and glucocorticoid-regulated kinase modulates Nedd4-2-mediated inhibition of the epithelial Na+ channel. *J Biol Chem.* 2002;277:5–8.)

## CONTROL OF POTASSIUM SECRETION: EFFECT OF POTASSIUM INTAKE

Changes in $K^+$ intake strongly modulate $K^+$ channel activity in the CNT and CCD (secretory capacity) in addition to $H^+/K^+$-ATPase activity in the OMCD (reabsorptive capacity). Increased dietary $K^+$ rapidly increases the activity of SK channels in the CCD and CNT,[114,115] along with a modest increase in $Na^+$ channel (ENaC) activity[91]; this is associated with an increase in apical expression of the ROMK channel protein.[116] The increase in ENaC and SK channel density in the CCD occurs within hours of assuming a high-$K^+$ diet, with a minimal associated increase in circulating aldosterone.[115] BK channels in the CNT and CCD are also activated by dietary $K^+$ loading. Trafficking of BK subunits is thus affected by dietary $K^+$, with largely intracellular distribution of alpha subunits in $K^+$-restricted rats and prominent apical expression in $K^+$-loaded rats.[117] Again, aldosterone does not directly contribute to the regulation of BK channel activity or expression in response to a high-$K^+$ diet.[118] However, aldosterone does participate in marked upregulation of the TRPV4 channel in response to a high-$K^+$ diet; $Ca^{2+}$ entry via TRPV4 increases intracellular $Ca^{2+}$ concentrations in response to tubular flow, thus activating BK channels.[82] TRPV4 knockout mice demonstrate an impaired adaptation to high-$K^+$ diet.[82]

A complex synergistic mix of signaling pathways regulates $K^+$ channel activity in response to changes in dietary $K^+$. In particular, the WNK (*with no* lysine) *k*inases play a critical role in modulating distal $K^+$ secretion. WNK1 and WNK4 were initially identified as the causative genes for FHHt (see also "Hyperkalemia: Hereditary Tubular Defects and Potassium Excretion"). ROMK expression at the membrane of *Xenopus* oocytes is reduced by coexpression of WNK4; FHHt-associated mutations increase this effect, suggesting a direction inhibition of SK channels in FHHt.[119] Transcription of the WNK1 gene generates several different isoforms; the predominant intrarenal WNK1 isoform is generated by a distal nephron transcriptional site that bypasses the N-terminal exons that encode the kinase domain, yielding a kinase-deficient short isoform[120] (WNK1-S). Full-length WNK1 (WNK1-L) inhibits ROMK by inducing endocytosis of the channel protein; the shorter, kinase-deficient WNK1-S isoform inhibits this effect of WNK1-L,[121,122] and ROMK activity is impaired in WNK1-S knockout mice.[123] The ratio of WNK1-S to WNK1-L transcripts is reduced by $K^+$ restriction (greater endocytosis of ROMK)[122,124] and increased by $K^+$ loading (reduced endocytosis of ROMK),[121,124] suggesting that this ratio between WNK1-S and WNK1-L functions as a molecular switch to regulate distal $K^+$ secretion. The BK channel is also regulated by the WNK kinases.[125–127]

The membrane trafficking of ROMK is also modulated by tyrosine phosphorylation of the channel protein such that tyrosine phosphorylation stimulates endocytosis, and tyrosine dephosphorylation induces exocytosis.[128,129] Intrarenal activity of the cytoplasmic tyrosine kinases c-src and c-yes is inversely related to dietary $K^+$ intake, with a decrease under high-$K^+$ conditions and a marked increase after several days of $K^+$ restriction.[130,131] Several studies have implicated the intrarenal generation of superoxide anions in the activation of cytoplasmic tyrosine kinases by $K^+$ depletion.[132–134] Potential candidates for the upstream hormonal signals include angiotensin II (Ang II) and growth factors such as insulin-like growth factor-1 (IGF-1).[132] In particular, Ang II inhibits ROMK activity in $K^+$-restricted rats, but not rats on a normal $K^+$ diet.[135] This inhibition by Ang II involves downstream activation of superoxide production and c-src activity, such that the induction of Ang II by a low-$K^+$ diet appears to play a major role in reducing distal tubular $K^+$ secretion.[136]

## INTEGRATED REGULATION OF DISTAL SODIUM ABSORPTION AND POTASSIUM SECRETION

Under certain physiologic conditions associated with marked induction of aldosterone, such as dietary sodium restriction, $Na^+$ balance can be maintained without significant effects on $K^+$ excretion. Yet, by activating ENaC and generating a more lumen-negative potential difference, increases in aldosterone should lead to an obligatory kaliuresis; how is this physiologic consequence avoided? The mechanisms that underlie this so-called aldosterone paradox, the independent regulation of $Na^+$ and $K^+$ handling by the aldosterone-sensitive distal nephron, have been elucidated. The major factors that allow for integrated but independent control of $Na^+$ and $K^+$ transport appear to include electroneutral thiazide-sensitive $Na^+$-$Cl^-$ transport within the CCD,[137–139] ENaC-independent $K^+$ excretion within the distal nephron,[85] and the differential regulation of various signaling pathways by aldosterone, Ang II, and dietary $K^+$ [141,142] (see also Chapter 6).

Electroneutral $Na^+$-$Cl^-$ transport in the CCD and ENaC-independent $K^+$ secretion may play important roles in disconnecting $Na^+$ and $K^+$ transport within the distal nephron. Electroneutral, thiazide-sensitive, and amiloride-resistant $Na^+$-$Cl^-$ transport within the CCD[137–139] is mediated by the combined activity of the $Na^+$-dependent SLC4A8 $Cl^-$-$HCO_3^-$ exchanger and the SLC26A4 $Cl^-$-$HCO_3^-$ exchanger[139] (see also Chapter 6). This transport mechanism is apparently responsible for as much 50% of $Na^+$-$Cl^-$ transport in mineralocorticoid-stimulated rat CCD,[137,138] allowing for ENaC-independent, electroneutral $Na^+$ absorption that will not directly affect $K^+$ secretion. The converse effect emerges after dietary $K^+$ loading, which increases the fraction of ENaC-independent, amiloride-resistant $K^+$ excretion to about 50%.[85]

NCC, the thiazide-sensitive $Na^+$-$Cl^-$ cotransporter in the DCT, plays a key role in $K^+$ homeostasis. Selective increases in DCT NCC activity, as seen in FHHt, reduce $Na^+$ delivery to principal cells in the downstream CNT and CCD, leading to hyperkalemia.[73] The DCT also clearly functions as a potassium sensor, directly responding to changes in circulating potassium. Reduction in potassium intake and/or hypokalemia thus lead to reduced basolateral $[K^+]$ in the DCT; the subsequent hyperpolarization is dependent on basolateral KIR4.1-containing $K^+$ channels.[4] Hyperpolarization leads to chloride exit, via basolateral CLC-NKB chloride channels, and a reduction in intracellular chloride; the reduction in intracellular chloride activates the WNK cascade, resulting in phosphorylation of NCC and activation of the transporter.[4] Ang II also activates NCC via WNK-dependent activation of the SPAK kinase and phosphorylation of the transporter protein,[140,141] reducing delivery of $Na^+$ to the CNT and limiting $K^+$ secretion. In contrast, Ang II inhibits ROMK activity via several mechanisms, including downstream activation of c-src tyrosine kinases (see previously).[134–136] Whereas $K^+$ restriction induces renin and circulating Ang II levels (see "Effects of Hypokalemia"), increases in dietary $K^+$ are suppressive.[136,142]

A high-$K^+$ diet also inactivates NCC[143] as a result of the associated decrease in Ang II, in addition to the increase in the ratio of WNK1-S to WNK1-L isoforms that occurs with increased $K^+$ intake.[121,122,124] WNK1-S antagonizes the effect of WNK1-L on NCC, leading to the inhibition of NCC in conditions with a relative excess of WNK1-S.[144] Nedd4-2 also negatively regulates NCC and WNK1, in addition to ENaC; mice with homozygous deletion of the Nedd4-2 gene develop severe hypokalemia during $K^+$ restriction, indicating a key role in renal adaptation.[145]

Finally, in principal cells, increases in aldosterone induce the SGK1 kinase, which phosphorylates WNK4 and attenuates the effect of WNK4 on ROMK,[146] while activating ENaC.[94,96,98] However, when dietary $K^+$ intake is reduced, c-src tyrosine kinase activity increases under the influence of increased Ang II, causing direction inhibition of ROMK activity via tyrosine phosphorylation of the channel.[128,147,148] The increase in c-src tyrosine kinase activity also abrogates the inhibitory effect of SGK1 on WNK4[149]; src family tyrosine kinases also directly phosphorylate WNK4 and modulate its effects on ROMK.[150] Again, Ang II appears to mediate part of its inhibitory effect on ROMK through the activation of c-src,[136] such that c-src serves as an important component of the switch that regulates $K^+$ secretion in response to changes in dietary $K^+$.

To summarize these important physiologic principles, the differential effects of $K^+$ intake on Ang II versus aldosterone appear to be critical in resolving the aldosterone paradox; so too are the differential effects of $K^+$ intake on NCC-dependent $Na^+$-$Cl^-$ transport in the DCT and on secretory $K^+$ channels in the downstream CNT and CCD (Fig. 17.6). Under conditions of low $Na^+$ intake but moderate $K^+$ intake, Ang II and aldosterone are both strongly induced, leading to enhanced $Na^+$-$Cl^-$ transport via NCC, increased ENaC activity, and decreased secretory $K^+$ channel activity. Although ENaC is activated, the relative inhibition of ROMK by the increased Ang II prevents excessive kaliuresis. Ang II-dependent activation of c-src kinases has direct inhibitory effects on ROMK trafficking and also abrogates the inhibitory effect of SGK1 on WNK4,[149] leading to unopposed inhibition of ROMK by WNK4. In addition, the aldosterone-dependent induction of electroneutral $Na^+$-$Cl^-$ transport within the CCD[137–139] increases $Na^+$-$Cl^-$ reabsorption but blunts the effect on the lumen-negative potential as a result of increased ENaC activity, thus limiting kaliuresis. When dietary $K^+$ increases,

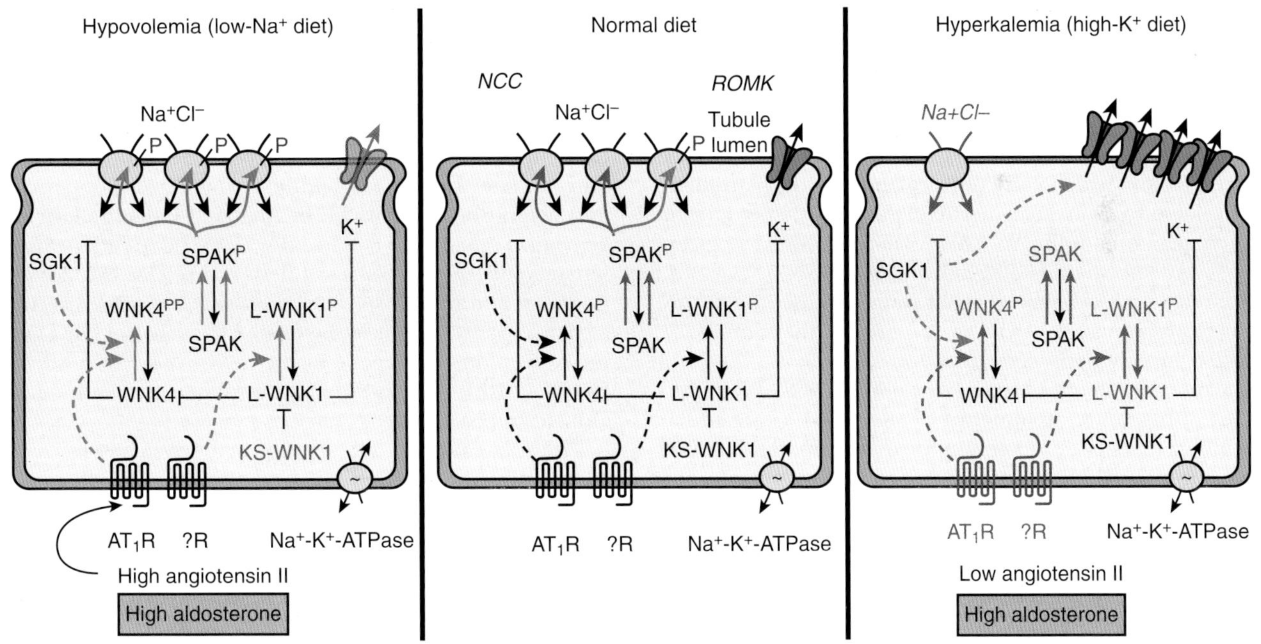


**Fig. 17.6** Integrated regulation of $Na^+$-$Cl^-$ and $K^+$ transport in the distal convoluted tubule (DCT), connecting segment (CNT), and cortical collecting duct (CCD) (*green arrowheads,* activating pathways; *red blunt end,* inhibitory pathway). *Left,* Pathway in the setting of a low-$Na^+$ diet, wherein angiotensin II (Ang II) and SGK1 signaling leads to phosphorylation of WNK4. This stimulates the phosphorylation of SPAK, which in turn phosphorylates and activates thiazide-sensitive $Na^+$-$Cl^-$ cotransport in the DCT via the NCC. Stimulation of unknown receptors is hypothesized to cause phosphorylation of L-WNK1, which can also stimulate SPAK phosphorylation. L-WNK1 also has other functions: (1) It blocks the NCC inhibitory form of WNK4, thus activating NCC. (2) It inhibits the secretion of $K^+$ via ROMK channels. *Center,* Normal diet. *Right,* Pathway in the setting of high dietary $K^+$ intake, wherein aldosterone is stimulated and Ang II is low. In the absence of sufficient Ang II, the $AT_1$ receptor ($AT_1R$) cannot activate WNK4. This reduces SPAK activation and NCC phosphorylation. Dietary potassium loading also increases the level of the KS-WNK1 isoform to suppress the activity of L-WNK1. In consequence, the inhibitory effect of WNK4 on NCC dominates, blocking traffic of NCC to the apical membrane and thereby reducing NCC activity. KS-WNK1 also blocks the effect of L-WNK1 on ROMK endocytosis, causing ROMK to increase at the apical membrane. The net effect is that $K^+$ secretion in the DCT, CNT, and CCD is maximized, whereas NCC is suppressed. Aldosterone stimulation of ENaC (not shown) offsets the decreased $Na^+$ reabsorption by NCC, allowing robust potassium secretion without changes in sodium balance. The roles of WNK3, SGK1, and c-src cytoplasmic tyrosine kinases are not shown in the interest of clarity; see text for further details. *NCC,* NaCl cotransporter; *ROMK,* renal outer medullary $K^+$ channel; *SPAK,* STE20/SPS1-related proline–alanine-rich kinase; *WNK,* with no (lysine) kinase. (From Welling PA, Chang YP, Delpire E, Wade JB. Multigene kinase network, kidney transport, and salt in essential hypertension. *Kidney Int.* 2010;77:1063–1069.)

circulating aldosterone is moderately induced but Ang II is suppressed. This leads to the inhibition of NCC and increased downstream delivery of $Na^+$ to principal cells in the CNT and CCD, where ENaC activity is increased and ROMK and BK channels are significantly activated. ENaC-independent $K^+$ secretion is also strongly induced by increased dietary $K^+$ intake,[85] contributing significantly to the ability to excrete $K^+$ in the urine.

## REGULATION OF RENAL RENIN AND ADRENAL ALDOSTERONE

Modulation of the renin-angiotensin-aldosterone system (RAAS) axis has profound clinical effects on $K^+$ homeostasis. Although multiple tissues are capable of renin secretion, renin of renal origin has a dominant physiologic impact. Renin secretion by juxtaglomerular cells in the afferent arteriole is initiated in response to a signal from the macula densa,[151] specifically a decrease in luminal chloride[152] transported through the $Na^+$-$K^+$-$2Cl^-$ cotransporter (NKCC2) at the apical membrane of macula densa cells.[27] In addition to this macula densa signal, decreased renal perfusion pressure and renal sympathetic tone stimulate renal renin secretion.[153] The various inhibitors of renin release include Ang II, nitric oxide, aldosterone, endothelin,[154] adenosine,[155] atrial natriuretic peptide (ANP),[156] tumor necrosis factor-α (TNF-α),[157] and active vitamin D.[158] The cyclic guanosine monophosphate (cGMP)-dependent protein kinase type II (cGKII) tonically inhibits renin secretion, in that renin secretion in response to several stimuli is exaggerated in homozygous *cGKII* knockout mice.[159] Activation of cGKII by ANP and/or nitric oxide has a marked inhibitory effect on the release of renin from juxtaglomerular cells.[156] Local factors that stimulate renin release from juxtaglomerular cells include prostaglandins,[160] adrenomedullin,[161] catecholamines (beta-1 receptors),[162] and succinate (GPR91 receptor).[163]

The relationship between renal renin release, the RAAS, and cyclooxygenase-2 (COX-2) is particularly complex.[160] COX-2 is heavily expressed in the macula densa,[160] with a significant recruitment of COX-2$^{(+)}$ cells seen with salt restriction or furosemide treatment.[21,160] Reduced intracellular chloride in macula densa cells appears to stimulate COX-2 expression via p38 MAP kinase,[164] whereas both aldosterone and Ang II reduce its expression.[160] Prostaglandins derived from COX-2 in the macula densa play a dominant role in the stimulation of renal renin release by salt restriction, furosemide, renal artery occlusion, or angiotensin-converting enzyme (ACE) inhibition.[21,165] Specifically, COX-2–derived prostaglandins appear to play a role in the tonic expression of renin in juxtaglomerular (JG) cells via the modulation of intracellular cAMP and calcium, rather than functioning in the acute regulation of renin release.[160] Prostaglandins generated by the macula densa also participate in the recruitment during salt restriction of $CD44^+$ mesenchymal stromal cells, which differentiate into renin-producing cells.[166]

Renin released from the kidney ultimately stimulates aldosterone release from the adrenal via Ang II. Hyperkalemia per se is also an independent and synergistic stimulus (Fig. 17.7) for aldosterone release from the adrenal gland,[21,167] although dietary $K^+$ loading is less potent than dietary $Na^+$-$Cl^-$ restriction in increasing circulating aldosterone.[88] The resting membrane potential of adrenal glomerulosa cells is hyperpolarized as a result of the activity of the "leak" $K^+$

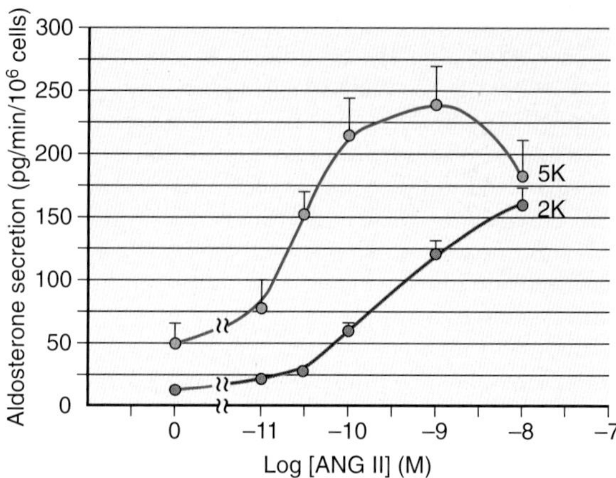


**Fig. 17.7** Synergistic effect of increased extracellular $K^+$ and angiotensin II *(ANG-II)* in inducing aldosterone release from bovine adrenal glomerulosa cells. Dose response curves for ANG-II were performed at an extracellular $K^+$ of 2 mmol/L *(red •)* and 5 mmol/L *(blue •)*. (From Chen XL, Bayliss DA, Fern RJ, Barrett PQ. A role for T-type $Ca^{2+}$ channels in the synergistic control of aldosterone production by ANG II and $K^+$. *Am J Physiol.* 1999;276:F674–F683.)

channels TASK-1 and TASK-3; combined deletion of genes encoding these channels leads to baseline depolarization of adrenal glomerulosa cells and an increase in serum aldosterone that is resistant to dietary sodium loading.[168] Ang II and $K^+$ both activate $Ca^{2+}$ entry in glomerulosa cells via voltage-sensitive, T-type $Ca^{2+}$ channels,[21,169] primarily Cav3.2.[170] Elevations in extracellular $K^+$ thus depolarize glomerulosa cells and activate these $Ca^{2+}$ channels, which are independently and synergistically activated by Ang II.[169] Calcium-dependent activation of calcium calmodulin (CaM)-dependent protein kinase in turn activates the synthesis and release of aldosterone via induction of aldosterone synthase.[171] $K^+$ and Ang II also enhance transcription of the Cav3.2 $Ca^{2+}$ channel by abrogating repression of this gene by the neuron restrictive silencing factor (NRS); this ultimately amplifies the induction of aldosterone synthase.[170]

The role of adrenal $K^+$ sensing in aldosterone release has been dramatically underlined by the reports of both germline and somatic mutations, in aldosterone-producing adenomas, of transport proteins that control membrane excitability of adrenal zona glomerulosa cells (see also "Hyperaldosteronism"). For example, somatic mutations in the adrenal $K^+$ channel KCNJ5 (GIRK4) can be detected in about 40% of aldosterone-producing adrenal adenomas[172]; these mutations endow the channel with a novel $Na^+$ conductance, leading to adrenal glomerulosa cell depolarization, $Ca^{2+}$ influx, and aldosterone release.

The adrenal release of aldosterone caused by increased $K^+$ is dependent on an intact adrenal renin-angiotensin system,[173] particularly during $Na^+$ restriction. ACE inhibitors and angiotensin-receptor blockers (ARBs) thus completely abrogate the effect of high $K^+$ on salt-restricted adrenals.[174] Direct, G-protein–dependent activation of the TASK-1 and/or TASK-3 $K^+$ channels by Ang II $AT_{1A}$ or $AT_{1B}$ receptors is thought to underlie the effect of Ang II on adrenal aldosterone release,[168] with abrogation of this effect by ARBs or ACE inhibitors. Other clinically relevant activators of adrenal aldosterone release include prostaglandins[175] and catecholamines[176] via increases in cAMP.[177,178] Finally, ANP exerts a potent negative effect on aldosterone release induced by $K^+$ and other stimuli,[179] at least in part by inhibiting early events in aldosterone synthesis.[180] ANP is therefore capable of inhibiting both renal renin release and adrenal aldosterone release, functions that may be central to the pathophysiology of hyporeninemic hypoaldosteronism.

### URINARY INDICES OF POTASSIUM EXCRETION

A bedside test to measure distal tubular $K^+$ secretion in humans directly would be ideal; however, for obvious reasons this is not technically feasible. A widely used surrogate is the transtubular $K^+$ gradient (TTKG), which is defined as follows:

$$TTKG = ([K^+]_{urine} \times Osm_{blood})/([K^+]blood \times Osm_{urine})$$

The expected values of the TTKG are largely based on historical data and are less than 3 to 4 in the presence of hypokalemia and more than 6 to 7 in the presence of hyperkalemia. Varying opinions regarding the physiologically appropriate TTKG in hyperkalemia have been reviewed multiple times.[181] Clearly, water absorption in the CCD and medullary collecting duct is an important determinant of the absolute $K^+$ concentration in the final urine—hence, the use of a ratio of urine-to-plasma osmolality. Indeed, water absorption may, in large part, determine the TTKG, such that it far exceeds the limiting $K^+$ gradient.[182] More recently, the originators of the TTKG have suggested that it fails to incorporate the putative effects of distal tubular urea reabsorption in $K^+$ excretion; however, neither urea transporter knockout mice nor rats treated with a urea transporter inhibitor[183] have demonstrated abnormalities in $K^+$ homeostasis. The TTKG may be less useful in patients ingesting diets of changing $K^+$ and mineralocorticoid intake.[184] There is, however, a linear relationship between plasma aldosterone and the TTKG, suggesting that it provides a rough approximation of the ability to respond to aldosterone with a kaliuresis.[185] The response of the TTKG to mineralocorticoid administration, typically fludrocortisone, can thus be used in the diagnostic approach to hyperkalemia.[181] In hypokalemic patients, a TTKG of less than 2 to 3 separates patients with redistributive hypokalemia from those with hypokalemia caused by renal potassium wasting, who will have TTKG values that are more than 4.[186]

An alternative to the TTKG in hypokalemic patients is the measurement of the urine $K^+$-to-creatinine ratio. This ratio is usually less than 13 mEq/g creatinine (1.5 mEq/mmol creatinine) when hypokalemia is caused by poor dietary intake, transcellular potassium shifts, gastrointestinal losses, or previous use of diuretics.[186] Higher values are indicative of ongoing renal potassium wasting. The utility of the $K^+$-to-creatinine ratio has been evaluated in a study of 43 patients with severe hypokalemia (range, 1.5–2.6 mmol/L) associated with paralysis.[186] The urine $K^+$-to-creatinine ratio reliably distinguished between the 30 patients with hypokalemic periodic paralysis and the 13 patients with hypokalemia due mostly to renal potassium wasting. The $K^+$-to-creatinine ratio was thus significantly lower in the patients with periodic paralysis (11 vs. 36 mEq/g creatinine; 1.3 vs. 4.1 mEq/mmol creatinine). The cutoff value was approximately 22 mEq/g creatinine (2.5 mEq/mmol).

The determination of urinary electrolytes for calculation of the TTKG or urine $K^+$-to-creatinine ratio provides the opportunity to measure the urinary $Na^+$, which will determine whether significant prerenal stimuli are limiting distal $Na^+$ delivery and thus $K^+$ excretion (see Fig. 17.4). Urinary electrolytes also afford the opportunity to calculate the urinary anion gap, an indirect index of urinary $NH_4^+$ content and thus indicating the ability to respond to an acidemia.[187]

## CONSEQUENCES OF HYPERKALEMIA AND HYPOKALEMIA

Hyperkalemia and hypokalemia have a number of effects, as discussed here.

### EFFECTS OF HYPOKALEMIA

#### EXCITABLE TISSUES: MUSCLE AND HEART

Hypokalemia is a well-described risk factor for both ventricular and atrial arrhythmias.[29,188] For example, in patients undergoing cardiac surgery, a serum $K^+$ level of less than 3.5 mmol/L is a predictor of serious intraoperative arrhythmia, perioperative arrhythmia, and postoperative atrial fibrillation.[189] Moderate hypokalemia does not, however, appear to increase the risk of serious arrhythmia during exercise stress testing.[190] Electrocardiographic changes in hypokalemia include broad flat T waves, ST depression, and QT prolongation; these are most marked when the serum $K^+$ level is less than 2.7 mmol/L.[191] Hypokalemia, often accompanied by hypomagnesemia, is an important cause of the long QT syndrome (LQTS) and torsades de pointes, either alone[192] or in combination with drug toxicity[193] or with LQTS-associated mutations in cardiac $K^+$ and $Na^+$ channels.[194] Hypokalemia accelerates the clathrin-dependent internalization and degradation of the cardiac HERG (human ether-a-go-go) $K^+$ channel protein.[31] HERG encodes pore-forming subunits of the cardiac rapidly activating, delayed rectifier $K^+$ channel ($I_{Kr}$); $I_{Kr}$ is largely responsible for potassium efflux during phases 2 and 3 of the cardiac action potential.[195] Loss-of-function mutations in HERG reduce $I_{Kr}$ and cause type II LQTS[31]; downregulation of HERG and $I_{Kr}$ by hypokalemia provides an elegant explanation for the association with LQTS and torsades de pointes.

In accordance with the Nernst equation, the resting membrane potential is related to the ratio of the intracellular to extracellular potassium concentration. In skeletal muscle, a reduction in plasma $K^+$ will increase this ratio and therefore hyperpolarize the cell membrane (i.e., make the resting potential more electronegative); this impairs the ability of the muscle to depolarize and contract, leading to weakness. However, in some human cardiac cells, particularly Purkinje fibers in the conducting system, hypokalemia results in a paradoxic depolarization[196]; this paradoxic depolarization plays an important role in the genesis of hypokalemic cardiac arrhythmias.[196,197] The resting membrane potential in excitable cells is largely determined by a large family of K2P1 $K^+$ channels, so-named because of the presence of two pore-forming (P) loop domains in each subunit. Hypokalemia causes K2P1 channels, which are normally selective for potassium, to transport sodium suddenly into cells, causing the paradoxic depolarization.[198] Notably, rodent cardiac cells respond to hypokalemia with a Nernst equation–predicted hyperpolarization and, unlike human cardiomyocytes, do not express the K2P1 channel TWIK-1. Genetic manipulation has indicated that TWIK-1 expression confers this paradoxic depolarization behavior on human and mouse cardiomyocytes.[198]

Another important mechanism for hypokalemia-induced arrhythmia involves downregulation of cardiac $Na^+/K^+$-ATPase activity.[199,200] The resulting increase in intracellular $Na^+$, which impedes removal of intracellular $Ca^{2+}$ by the $Na^+$-$Ca^{2+}$ exchanger and other mechanisms, leads to intracellular calcium overload. The ensuing increase in calmodulin kinase II activity reduces repolarization reserve by activating late $Na^+$ and $Ca^{2+}$ currents.[201] This, in turn, predisposes the heart to early afterdepolarization-associated arrhythmias, such as torsades de pointes and polymorphic ventricular tachycardia (PVT).[201]

In skeletal muscle, hypokalemia causes hyperpolarization, thus impairing the capacity to depolarize and contract. Weakness and paralysis are therefore not infrequent consequences of hypokalemia of diverse causes.[202,203] On a historical note, the realization in 1946 that $K^+$ replacement reversed the hypokalemic diaphragmatic paralysis induced by treatment of diabetic ketoacidosis (DKA) was a milestone in diabetes care.[204] Pathologically, muscle biopsies in hypokalemic myopathy demonstrate phagocytosis of degenerating muscle fibers, fiber regeneration, and atrophy of type 2 fibers.[205] Most patients with significant myopathy will have elevations in creatine kinase levels, and hypokalemia of diverse causes predisposes to rhabdomyolysis with acute renal failure.

### RENAL CONSEQUENCES

Hypokalemia causes a host of structural and functional changes in the kidney, which are reviewed in detail elsewhere.[206] In humans, the renal pathology includes a relatively specific proximal tubular vacuolization,[206–208] interstitial nephritis,[209] and renal cysts.[210] Hypokalemic nephropathy can cause ESKD, mostly in patients with long-standing hypokalemia because of eating disorders and/or laxative abuse[211]; acute renal failure with proximal tubular vasculopathy has also been described.[212] In animal models, hypokalemia increases susceptibility to acute renal failure induced by ischemia, gentamicin, and amphotericin.[21] Potassium restriction in rats induces cortical Ang II and medullary endothelin-1 expression, with an ischemic pattern of renal injury.[213] Hypokalemic nephropathy in rats is associated with progressive capillary loss, with reduced angiogenesis because of reduced vascular endothelial growth factor (VEGF) expression.[214]

The prominent functional changes in renal physiology that are induced by hypokalemia include $Na^+$-$Cl^-$ retention, polyuria,[207] phosphaturia,[29] hypocitraturia,[215] and increased ammoniagenesis.[206] $K^+$ depletion in rats causes proximal tubular hyperabsorption of $Na^+$-$Cl^-$ in association with an upregulation of Ang II,[213] $AT_1$ receptor,[29] and $\alpha_2$-adrenergic receptor[29] in this nephron segment. NHE3, the dominant apical $Na^+$ entry site in the proximal tubule, is massively (>700%) upregulated in $K^+$-deficient rats,[216] which is consistent with the observed hyperabsorption of both $Na^+$-$Cl^-$ and bicarbonate.[206] Polyuria in hypokalemia is caused by polydipsia[217] and to a vasopressin-resistant defect in urinary concentrating ability.[206] This renal concentrating defect is multifactorial, with evidence for both a reduced hydroosmotic response to vasopressin in the collecting duct[206] and decreased $Na^+$-$Cl^-$ absorption by the TAL.[29] $K^+$ restriction has been shown to result in a rapid reversible decrease in the expression of aquaporin-2 in the collecting duct,[218] beginning in the CCD and extending to the medullary collecting duct within the first 24 hours.[219] Downregulation of aquaporin-2 and several other proteins in hypokalemic nephrogenic diabetes insipidus appears to occur via authophagy.[220] In the TAL, the marked reductions seen during $K^+$ restriction in both the apical $K^+$ channel ROMK and the apical $Na^+$-$K^+$-$2Cl^-$ cotransporter NKCC2[216] reduce $Na^+$-$Cl^-$ absorption and thus inhibit countercurrent multiplication and the driving force for water absorption by the collecting duct.

### CARDIOVASCULAR CONSEQUENCES

A large body of experimental and epidemiologic evidence has implicated hypokalemia and/or reduced dietary $K^+$ in the genesis or worsening of hypertension, heart failure, and stroke.[221] $K^+$ depletion in young rats induces hypertension,[222] with a salt sensitivity that persists after $K^+$ levels are normalized; presumably this salt sensitivity is as a result of the significant tubulointerstitial injury induced by $K^+$ restriction.[213] Hypokalemia has also recently been linked to vascular calcification and arterial stiffness via induction of autophagy and promotion of vascular smooth muscle calcification.[223] Elevated autophagy and cAMP response element–binding protein (CREB) signaling were demonstrated in calcified arteries from mice fed a low-potassium diet, as well as arteries exposed to low potassium ex vivo. This novel insight may prove to be a causative effect of dietary potassium intake on atherosclerotic vascular calcification and stiffness. Short-term $K^+$ restriction in healthy humans and patients with essential hypertension also induces $Na^+$-$Cl^-$ retention and hypertension,[29] and abundant epidemiological data has linked dietary $K^+$ deficiency and/or hypokalemia with hypertension.[221,224] Correction of hypokalemia is particularly important in hypertensive patients treated with diuretics; blood pressure in this setting is improved with the establishment of normokalemia,[225] and the cardiovascular benefits of diuretic agents are blunted by hypokalemia.[29,226] Hypokalemia reduces insulin secretion; this mechanism may play an important role in thiazide-associated diabetes.[227] Finally, $K^+$ depletion may play important roles in the pathophysiology and progression of heart failure.[221]

## CONSEQUENCES OF HYPERKALEMIA

### EXCITABLE TISSUES: MUSCLE AND HEART

Hyperkalemia constitutes a medical emergency, primarily because of its effect on the heart. In skeletal muscle, a reduction in plasma $K^+$ will hyperpolarize the cell membrane. Furthermore, as noted, in Purkinje fibers of the human conducting system, hypokalemia results in a paradoxic depolarization. In contrast, hyperkalemia depolarizes cardiac myocytes, reducing the membrane potential from −90 mV to about −80 mV. This brings the membrane potential closer to the threshold for generation of an action potential; mild and/or rapid onset hyperkalemia will initially increase cardiac excitability because a lesser depolarizing stimulus is required to generate an action potential. Mild increases in extracellular $K^+$ also affect the repolarization phase of the cardiac action potential via increases in $I_{Kr}$; as discussed earlier (see "Effects of Hypokalemia"), $I_{Kr}$ is highly sensitive to changes in extracellular $K^+$.[31] This effect on repolarization is thought to underlie the early signs of hyperkalemia,[228] including ST-T segment depression, peaked T waves, and Q-T interval shortening.[195]

Persistent and increasing depolarization inactivates cardiac sodium channels, thus reducing the rate of phase 0 of the action potential ($V_{max}$); the decrease in $V_{max}$ results in a reduction in myocardial conduction, with progressive prolongation of the P wave, PR interval, and QRS complex.[195] Severe hyperkalemia results in loss of the P wave and a progressive widening of the QRS complex; fusion with T waves causes a sine wave sinoventricular rhythm.

Cardiac arrhythmias associated with hyperkalemia include sinus bradycardia, sinus arrest, slow idioventricular rhythms, ventricular tachycardia, ventricular fibrillation, and asystole[228,229]; a multitude of mechanisms are involved.[201] The differential diagnosis and treatment of a wide-complex tachycardia in hyperkalemia can be particularly problematic; moreover, hyperkalemia potentiates the blocking effect of lidocaine on the cardiac $Na^+$ channel, so that use of this agent may precipitate asystole or ventricular fibrillation in this setting.[230] Hyperkalemia can also cause a type I Brugada pattern in the electrocardiogram (ECG), with a pseudo–right bundle branch block (RBBB) and persistent "coved" ST segment elevation in at least two precordial leads. This hyperkalemic Brugada sign occurs in critically ill patients with significant hyperkalemia (serum $K^+$ >7 mmol/L), and can be differentiated from genetic Brugada syndrome by an absence of P waves, marked QRS widening, and an abnormal QRS axis.[231]

Classically, the electrocardiographic manifestations in hyperkalemia progress as shown in Table 17.3. However, these changes are notoriously insensitive, so that only 55% of patients with serum $K^+$ more than 6.8 mmol/L in one case series manifested peaked T waves.[232] There is large interpatient variability in the absolute potassium level leading to electrocardiographic changes and cardiac toxicity of hyperkalemia. Relevant variables include the rapidity of the onset of hyperkalemia[233,234] and the presence or absence of concomitant hypocalcemia, acidemia, and/or hyponatremia.[235,236] Hemodialysis patients[236] and patients with chronic renal failure,[237] in particular, may not demonstrate electrocardiographic changes. Care should also be taken to distinguish the symmetrically peaked, church steeple T waves induced by hyperkalemia adequately from T wave changes because of other causes.[238] The ratio of the precordial T wave to R wave amplitude (T:R ratio) may be a more specific sign of hyperkalemia than T wave tenting.[239]

**Table 17.3 Approximate Relationship Between Hyperkalemic Electrocardiographic Changes and Serum Potassium Concentration**

| Serum $K^+$ Concentration (mmol/L) | Electrocardiographic Abnormality |
|---|---|
| 5.5–6.5 | Tall peaked T waves with narrow base, best seen in precordial leads |
| 6.5–8.0 | Peaked T waves; prolonged PR interval; decreased amplitude of P waves; widening of QRS complex |
| >8.0 | Absence of P waves; Intraventricular blocks, fascicular blocks, bundle branch blocks, QRS axis shift; progressive widening of the QRS complex; sine wave pattern (sinoventricular rhythm), ventricular fibrillation, asystole |

From Mattu A, Brady WJ, Robinson DA: Electrocardiographic manifestations of hyperkalemia. *Am J Emerg Med.* 2000; 18:721–729.

Hyperkalemia can also rarely present with ascending paralysis,[21] denoted "secondary hyperkalemic paralysis" to differentiate it from familial hyperkalemic periodic paralysis (HYPP). This presentation of hyperkalemia can mimic Guillain-Barré syndrome and may include diaphragmatic paralysis and respiratory failure.[240] Hyperkalemia from a diversity of causes can cause paralysis, as reviewed by Evers and associates.[241] The mechanism is not entirely clear; however, nerve conduction studies in one case have suggested a neurogenic mechanism, rather than a direct effect on muscle excitability.[241]

In contrast with secondary hyperkalemic paralysis, HYPP is a primary myopathy. Patients with HYPP develop myopathic weakness during hyperkalemia induced by increased $K^+$ intake or rest after heavy exercise.[242] The hyperkalemic trigger in HYPP serves to differentiate this syndrome from hypokalemic periodic paralysis (HOKP); a further distinguishing feature is the presence of myotonia in HYPP.[242] Depolarization of skeletal muscle by hyperkalemia unmasks an inactivation defect in a tetrodotoxin-sensitive $Na^+$ channel in patients with HYPP, and autosomal dominant mutations in the *SCN4A* gene encoding this channel cause most forms of the disease.[243] Mild muscle depolarization (5–10 mV) in HYPP results in a persistent inward $Na^+$ current through the mutant channel; the normal, allelic SCN4 channels quickly recover from inactivation and can then be reactivated, resulting in myotonia. When muscle depolarization is more marked—that is, 20 to 30 mV—all the $Na^+$ channels are inactivated, rendering the muscle inexcitable and causing weakness (Fig. 17.8). Related disorders because of mutations within the large SCN4A channel protein include HOKP type II,[244] paramyotonia congenita,[243] and $K^+$-aggravated myopathy.[243] American quarter horses have a high incidence (4.4%) of HYPP due a mutation in equine *SCN4A* traced to the sire "Impressive" (see Fig. 17.8).[243] Finally, loss-of-function mutations in the muscle-specific $K^+$ channel subunit called "MinK-related peptide 2" (MiRP2) have also been shown to cause HYPP; MiRP2 and the associated Kv3.4 $K^+$ channel play a role in setting the resting membrane potential of skeletal muscle.[245]

## RENAL CONSEQUENCES

Hyperkalemia has a significant effect on the ability to excrete an acid urine because of interference with the urinary excretion of ammonium ($NH_4^+$). Potassium loading in humans results in modest reduction in urinary $NH_4^+$ excretion and an impaired response to acid loading.[246] In rats, chronic potassium loading leads to hyperkalemia and a metabolic acidosis because of a 40% reduction in urinary $NH_4^+$ excretion.[247] Proximal tubular ammonia generation falls, but without a significant effect on proximal tubular secretion of $NH_4^+$.[248] The TAL absorbs $NH_4^+$ from the tubular lumen, followed by countercurrent multiplication and ultimately excretion from the medullary interstitium.[248] Hyperkalemia appears to inhibit renal acid excretion by competing with

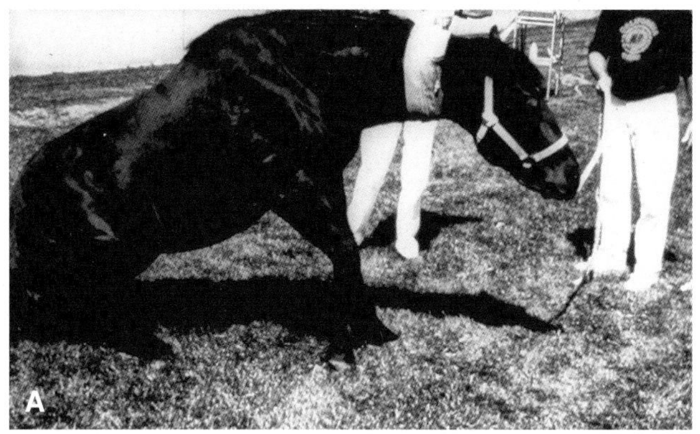


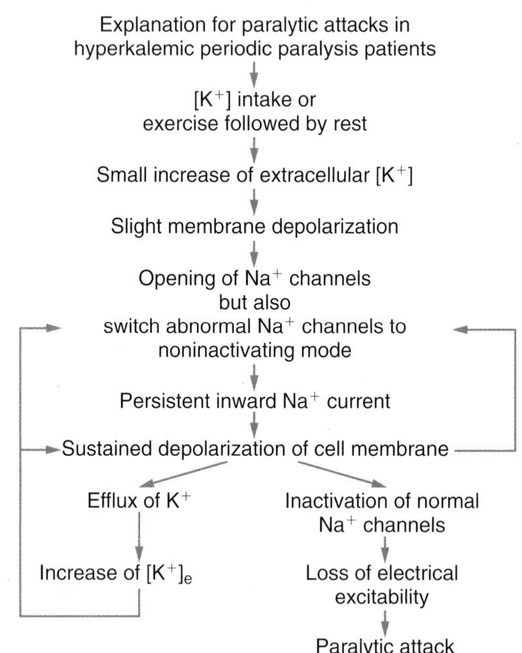


**Fig. 17.8** Hyperkalemic periodic paralysis (HYPP) caused by mutations in the voltage-gated $Na^+$ channel of skeletal muscle. (A) This disorder is particularly common in thoroughbred quarter horses; an affected horse is shown during a paralytic attack, triggered by rest after heavy exercise. (B) Mechanistic explanation for muscle paralysis in HYPP. (A, courtesy Dr. Eric Hoffman; B from Lehmann-Horn F, Jurkat-Rott K. Voltage-gated ion channels and hereditary disease. *Physiol Rev.* 1999;79:1317–1372.)

$NH_4^+$ for reabsorption by the TAL, thus preventing augmented $NH_4^+$ levels in the medullary interstitium.[249]

The $NH_4^+$ ion has the same ionic radius as $K^+$ and can be transported in lieu of $K^+$ by NKCC2,[250] the apical $Na^+$-$K^+$/$NH_4^+$-$2Cl^-$ cotransporter of the TAL; $NH_4^+$ exits the TAL via the basolateral $Na^+/H^+$ exchanger NHE4.[251] As is the case for other cations, countercurrent multiplication of $NH_4^+$ by the TAL greatly increases the concentration of $NH_4^+/NH_3$ available for secretion in the collecting duct. The $NH_4^+$ produced by the proximal tubule in response to acidosis is thus reabsorbed across the TAL, concentrated by countercurrent multiplication in the medullary interstitium and secreted in the collecting duct. The capacity of the TAL to reabsorb $NH_4^+$ is increased during acidosis because of an induction of NKCC2[250] and NHE4 expression.[251] Hyperkalemia induces acidosis in rats by reducing the $NH_4^+$ between the vasa recta (surrogate for interstitial fluid) and collecting duct[249] caused by interference by $K^+$ with absorption of $NH_4^+$ by the TAL.

More recently, in a mouse model for hyporeninemic hypoaldosteronism with prominent, treatable hyperkalemic acidosis, hyperkalemia was correlated with reduced expression of ammonia-generating enzymes in the proximal tubule, combined with upregulation of the ammonia-recycling enzyme glutamine synthetase.[252] Hyperkalemia did not affect the expression of NKCC2 or NHE3. However, these mice demonstrated decreased expression of the ammonia transporter family member Rhcg and decreased apical polarization of $H^+$-ATPase in the inner stripe of the OMCD, further compromising urinary $NH_4^+$ excretion. These various changes in enzyme and transporter expression were reversed by correcting the hyperkalemia.[252]

Clinically, patients with hyperkalemic acidosis caused by hyporeninemic hypoaldosteronism demonstrate an increase in urinary $NH_4^+$ excretion in response to normalization of plasma $K^+$ with cation exchange resins,[253,254] indicating a significant role for hyperkalemia in the generation of the acidosis.

# HYPOKALEMIA

## CAUSES OF HYPOKALEMIA

A number of causative factors are involved in the development of hypokalemia.

### EPIDEMIOLOGY

Hypokalemia is a relatively common finding in both outpatients and inpatients, perhaps the most common electrolyte abnormality encountered in clinical practice.[255] When defined as a serum $K^+$ of less than 3.6 mmol/L, it is found in approximately 20% of hospitalized patients[256,257]; defined as a serum $K^+$ of less than 3.4 mmol/L, it occurs in 16.8% of first-time hospital admissions.[258] Hypokalemia is usually mild, with $K^+$ levels in the 3.0 to 3.5 mmol/L range, but in up to 25% of hypokalemic patients it can be moderate to severe (<3.0 mmol/L).[256,259] The most common causative factors in hospitalized patients with hypokalemia are gastrointestinal losses of potassium, diuretic therapy, and hypomagnesemia.[260] It is a particularly prominent problem in patients receiving thiazide diuretics for hypertension, with an incidence of up to 48% (average, 15%–30%).[29,261] The thiazide-type diuretic metolazone is frequently used for the management of heart failure refractory to loop diuretics alone, causing moderate ($K^+ \leq 3.0$ mmol/L) or severe ($K^+ \leq 2.5$ mmol/L) hypokalemia in approximately 40% and 10% of patients, respectively.[262] Hypokalemia is also a common finding in patients undergoing peritoneal dialysis, with 10% to 20% requiring potassium supplementation.[263] Hypokalemia per se can increase the in-hospital mortality rate up to tenfold,[258,259] likely caused by the profound effects on arrhythmogenesis, blood pressure, and cardiovascular morbidity.[221,264]

### SPURIOUS HYPOKALEMIA

Delayed sample analysis is a well-recognized cause of spurious hypokalemia as a result of increased cellular uptake; this may become clinically relevant if the ambient temperature is increased.[29,265,266] Very rarely, patients with profound leukocytosis caused by acute leukemia present with artifactual hypokalemia caused by the time-dependent uptake of $K^+$ by the large white cell mass.[265] Such patients do not develop clinical or electrocardiographic complications of hypokalemia, and the plasma $K^+$ level is normal if measured immediately after venipuncture.

## REDISTRIBUTION AND HYPOKALEMIA

Manipulation of the factors affecting internal distribution of $K^+$ (see "Factors Affecting Internal Distribution of Potassium") can cause hypokalemia as a result of redistribution of $K^+$ between the extracellular and intracellular compartments. Endogenous insulin is rarely a cause of hypokalemia; however, administered insulin is a frequent cause of iatrogenic hypokalemia[256] and may be a factor in the so-called *dead in bed syndrome* associated with aggressive glycemic control.[267] Insulin also may play a significant role in the hypokalemia associated with refeeding syndrome.[268] Alterations in the activity of the endogenous sympathetic nervous system can cause hypokalemia in several settings, including alcohol withdrawal,[269] acute myocardial infarction,[221,270] and head injury.[271,272] Redistributive hypokalemia after severe head injury can be truly profound, with reported serum $K^+$ levels of 1.2 mmol/L[271] and 1.9 mmol/L[272] and marked rebound hyperkalemia after repletion.

Because of their ability to activate both $Na^+/K^+$-ATPase[51] and the $Na^+$-$K^+$-$2Cl^-$ cotransporter NKCC1,[21,28] beta-2 agonists are powerful activators of cellular $K^+$ uptake. These agents are chiefly encountered in the therapy of asthma; however, tocolytics such as ritodrine, can induce hypokalemia and arrhythmias during maternal labor.[273] The long-acting beta-2 agonist clenbuterol, not approved for medical use in the United States, has caused hypokalemia in poisonings, including outbreaks of toxicity from clenbuterol-adulterated heroin.[274] Occult sources of sympathomimetics, such as pseudoephedrine and ephedrine in cough syrup[203] or dieting agents,[275] can be overlooked causes of hypokalemia. Finally, downstream activation of cAMP by xanthines such as theophylline[21,276] and dietary caffeine[277] may induce hypokalemia and may synergize in this respect with beta-2 agonists.[278]

Whereas beta-2 agonists activate $K^+$ uptake via the $Na^+/K^+$-ATPase, one would expect that inhibition of passive $K^+$ efflux would also lead to hypokalemia; this is accomplished by barium, a potent inhibitor of inward-rectifying $K^+$ channels.[279] This rare cause of hypokalemia is usually because of ingestion of the rodenticide (colloquially known as rat poison) barium carbonate, either unintentionally or during a suicide attempt.[280] Suicidal ingestion of barium-containing shaving powder[281] and hair remover[282] has also been described. Barium salts are widely used in industry, and poisoning has been described by various mechanisms in industrial accidents.[21,283] Patients have a particularly prominent U wave, likely because of direct inhibition of cardiac inward-rectifying $K^+$ channels.[279] Muscle paralysis can also occur[279] because of inhibition of muscle KIR channels. Treatment of barium poisoning with $K^+$ serves to increase plasma $K^+$ and displace barium from affected $K^+$ channels[280]; hemodialysis is also an effective treatment.[284]

Cesium also inhibits multiple $K^+$ channels and can provoke hypokalemia and associated arrhythmias, with inappropriate kaliuresis presumably because of the inhibition of ROMK and BK secretory channels.[285] Hypokalemia is also common with chloroquine toxicity or overdose,[286] although the mechanism is not entirely clear.

## HYPOKALEMIC PERIODIC PARALYSIS

The periodic paralyses have both genetic and acquired causes, and are further subdivided into hyper- and hypokalemic forms.[21,242–244] The genetic and secondary forms of hyperkalemic paralysis are discussed previously (see "Consequences of Hyperkalemia"). Autosomal dominant mutations in the *CACNA1S* gene encoding the alpha-1 subunit of L-type calcium channels are the most common genetic cause of hypokalemic periodic paralysis (HOKP type I), whereas type II HOKP is because of mutations in the *SCN4A* gene encoding the skeletal $Na^+$ channel.[287] In Andersen syndrome, autosomal dominant mutations in the *KCNJ2* gene encoding the inwardly rectifying $K^+$ channel Kir2.1 cause periodic paralysis, cardiac arrhythmias, and dysmorphic features.[288] Paralysis in Andersen syndrome can be normokalemic, hypokalemic, or hyperkalemic; however, the symptomatic trigger is consistent within individual kindreds.[288]

The pathophysiology of HOKP is complex. Structurally, about 90% of the HOKP-associated mutations result in loss of positively charged arginine residues in the S4, voltage sensor domains of L-type calcium channels and the skeletal $Na^+$ channel.[244] This generates a so-called "gating current," generated by a cation leak through an aberrant pore; this abnormal cation leak may directly lead to $K^+$-dependent paradoxic depolarization and hypokalemic weakness.[289] Muscles of an $Na^+$ channel knock-in mutant mouse ($Na_v$1.4-R669H) also exhibit an anomalous inward current at hyperpolarized potentials, attributed to this gating pore current.[290]

Abnormalities in insulin-sensitive transport events may also contribute to the hypokalemic weakness in HOKP. Reversible attacks of paralysis with hypokalemia in HOKP are typically precipitated by rest after exercise and/or meals rich in carbohydrates.[244] Although the induction of endogenous insulin by carbohydrate meals is thought to reduce plasma $K^+$, thus triggering weakness, insulin can precipitate paralysis in HOKP in the absence of significant hypokalemia.[291] The generation of action potentials and muscle contraction are reduced in types I and II HOKP muscle fibers exposed to insulin in vitro[287,292]; this effect is seen at an extracellular $K^+$ of 4.0 mmol/L and is potentiated as $K^+$ decreases.[292] Type I HOKP muscles have a reduced activity of ATP-sensitive, inward rectifying $K^+$ channels ($K_{ATP}$),[293,294] which likely contributes to hypokalemia because of the resultant unopposed activity of muscle $Na^+/K^+$-ATPase.[295] Insulin inhibits the remaining $K_{ATP}$ activity in muscle fibers of both type I HOKP patients[292] and hypokalemic rats,[296] resulting in a depolarizing shift toward the equilibrium potential for the $Cl^-$ ion (≈50 mV); at this potential, voltage-dependent $Na^+$ channels are largely inactivated, resulting in paralysis.

Paralysis is associated with multiple other causes of hypokalemia, both acquired and genetic.[202,203,297] Renal causes of hypokalemia with paralysis include Fanconi syndrome,[298] Gitelman syndrome,[297] and the various causes of hypokalemic distal renal tubular acidosis.[29,299] The activity and regulation of skeletal muscle $K_{ATP}$ channels are aberrant in animal models of hypokalemia, suggesting a parallel muscle physiology to that of genetic HOKP (see previously). However, the pathophysiology of thyrotoxic periodic paralysis (TPP), a particularly important cause of hypokalemic paralysis, is distinctly different from that of HOKP; for example, despite the clinical similarities between the two syndromes, thyroxine has no effect on HOKP.

TPP is classically seen in patients of Asian origin, but also occurs at higher frequencies in Hispanic patients.[300] This shared predisposition has been linked to genetic variation in the *KCNJ18* gene encoding Kir2.6, a muscle-specific, thyroid hormone– responsive $K^+$ channel.[30] Genome-wide association studies have also implicated variations in the *KCNJ2* gene, which encodes a related muscle $K^+$ channel, Kir 2.1, with a predisposition to TPP.[301] Patients typically present with weakness of the extremities and limb girdles, with attacks occurring most frequently between 1 and 6 AM. As in HOKP, paralytic attacks in TPP may be precipitated by rest and/or by carbohydrate-rich meals. Clinical signs and symptoms of hyperthyroidism are not invariably present.[300,302] Hypokalemia is profound, ranging between 1.1 and 3.4 mol/L, and is frequently accompanied by hypophosphatemia and hypomagnesemia[300]; all three abnormalities presumably contribute to the associated weakness. Diagnostically, a TTKG of less than 2 to 3 or urine $K^+$-to-creatinine ratio of less than 2.5 mmol/mmol separates patients with TPP from those with hypokalemia because of renal potassium wasting, who will have TTKG values that are higher than 4.[186] This distinction is of considerable therapeutic relevance; patients with large potassium deficits require aggressive repletion with $K^+$-$Cl^-$, which has a significant risk of rebound hyperkalemia in TPP and related disorders.[186,303]

The hypokalemia in TPP is most likely because of both direct and indirect activation of the $Na^+/K^+$-ATPase, given the evidence for increased activity in erythrocytes and platelets in TPP patients.[29,304] Thyroid hormone clearly induces expression of multiple subunits of the $Na^+/K^+$-ATPase in skeletal muscle.[305] Increases in the β-adrenergic response because of hyperthyroidism also play an important role because high-dose propranolol (3 mg/kg) rapidly reverses the hypokalemia, hypophosphatemia, and paralysis seen in acute attacks.[306,307] Of particular importance, no rebound hyperkalemia is associated with this treatment, whereas aggressive $K^+$ replacement in TPP is associated with an incidence of about 25%[303]; repletion-associated rebound hyperkalemia in TPP can be fatal.[308]

Outward-directed, inward-rectifying $K^+$ current, mediated by KIR channels (primarily Kir2.1 and Kir2.2 tetramers), is also reduced in skeletal muscles of patients with TPP,[294] providing an additional mechanism for hypokalemia. Together with increased $Na^+/K^+$-ATPase activity and increased circulating insulin, this reduced KIR current may trigger a feed-forward cycle of hypokalemia, leading to inactivation of muscle $Na^+$ channels, paradoxic depolarization, and paralysis.[309] The role of TPP-associated sequence variants in the *KCNJ18* gene that encodes Kir 2.6 is not entirely clear at this point, given that some genetic studies have failed to find a convincing association.[310] As noted, the muscle Kir channel is largely formed by tetramers of Kir 2.1 with Kir 2.2 proteins, with robust expression of these channel proteins at the plasma membrane and T tubules of skeletal muscle.[311] In contrast, wild-type Kir 2.6 protein appears to be restricted primarily to the endoplasmic reticulum (ER), with a dominant negative effect on expression and function of Kir 2.1 and Kir 2.2 subunits.[311] It remains unclear how TPP-associated sequence variants, perhaps induced by high levels of thyroid hormone,[30] explain the proposed predisposition to TPP.

## NONRENAL POTASSIUM LOSS

The loss of $K^+$ from skin is typically low, with the exception of extremes in physical exertion.[11] Direct gastric loss of $K^+$ because of vomiting or nasogastric suctioning is also typically minimal; however, the ensuing hypochloremic alkalosis results in persistent kaliuresis caused by secondary hyperaldosteronism and bicarbonaturia.[312,313] Intestinal loss of $K^+$ as a result of diarrhea is a quantitatively important cause of hypokalemia, given the worldwide prevalence of diarrheal disease, and may be associated with acute complications such as myopathy and flaccid paralysis.[314] The presence of a non–anion gap metabolic acidosis with a negative urinary anion gap[187] (consistent with an intact ability to increase $NH_4^+$ excretion) should strongly suggest diarrhea as a cause of hypokalemia. Polyethylene glycol–based bowel preparation regimens for colonoscopy can also lead to hypokalemia in older patients[315] and/or patients on diuretics.[316] Noninfectious gastrointestinal processes such as celiac disease,[317] ileostomy, and chronic laxative abuse can present with acute hypokalemic syndromes or with chronic complications such as ESKD.[21]

There has been an appreciation of the role of intestinal BK $K^+$ channels in hypokalemia associated with intestinal disease. Three reports initially identified a novel association between colonic pseudo-obstruction (Ogilvie syndrome) and hypokalemia as a result of secretory diarrhea with an abnormally high $K^+$ content.[318–320] In one patient with concomitant ESKD, immunohistochemistry revealed massive upregulation of the apical BK channel throughout the surface crypt axes[318]; colonic BK channels may play a significant role in intestinal $K^+$ secretion in a variety of pathologies, including ESKD.[321] Several hypotheses for the association between Ogilvie syndrome and enhanced intestinal $K^+$ secretion have been postulated, including active stimulation by catecholamines induced by colonic pseudo-obstruction[320]; BK channels appear to mediate adrenaline-induced colonic $K^+$ secretion.[322] Notably, aldosterone also induces colonic BK channel expression and activity[323]; consistent with a role for aldosterone, a dramatic response to spironolactone in Ogilvie syndrome–associated diarrhea and hypokalemia was recently reported.[324]

Increased fecal loss of $K^+$ may play a broader role in hypokalemia associated with diarrhea.[321] Recruitment of colonic BK channels along intestinal crypts, similar to that seen in Ogilvie syndrome, has thus been demonstrated as a consistent feature of colonic biopsies in ulcerative colitis.[325] Direct enhancement of intestinal $K^+$ excretion has also been demonstrated in a hypokalemic patient with Crohn disease following treatment with budesonide.[326]

## RENAL POTASSIUM LOSS

### Drugs

Diuretics are an especially important cause of hypokalemia because of their ability to increase distal flow rate and distal delivery of $Na^+$. Thiazides generally cause more hypokalemia[21,225,261] than loop diuretics, despite their lower natriuretic efficacy. One potential explanation is the differential effect of loop diuretics and thiazides on calcium excretion. Whereas thiazides and loss-of-function mutations in the $Na^+$-$Cl^-$ cotransporter decrease $Ca^{2+}$ excretion,[327] loop diuretics cause a significant calciuresis.[328] Increases in luminal $Ca^{2+}$ in the distal nephron serve to reduce the lumen-negative driving force for $K^+$ excretion,[329] perhaps by direct inhibition of ENaC in principal cells. A mechanistic explanation is provided by the presence of an apical calcium-sensing receptor (CaSR) in the collecting duct.[330] Analogous to the evident decrease in the apical trafficking of aquaporin-2 induced by luminal $Ca^{2+}$, tubular $Ca^{2+}$ may stimulate endocytosis of ENaC via the CaSR and thus limit generation of the lumen-negative potential difference that is so critical for distal $K^+$ excretion. Regardless of the underlying mechanism, the increase in distal delivery of $Ca^{2+}$ induced by loop diuretics may serve to blunt kaliuresis; such a mechanism would not occur with thiazides, which reduce distal delivery of $Ca^{2+}$, with unopposed activity of ENaC and increased kaliuresis.

A substantial and growing body of evidence has indicated a key role for the NCC in $K^+$ homeostasis, the thiazide-sensitive $Na^+$-$Cl^-$ cotransporter in the DCT, so that it is not surprising that thiazide treatment has such potent effects on serum $K^+$. Selective increases in DCT NCC activity, as seen in FHHt, reduce $Na^+$ delivery to principal cells in the downstream CNT and CCD, leading to hyperkalemia.[73] The DCT also clearly functions as a potassium sensor, directly responding to changes in circulating potassium.[4] A high-$K^+$ diet also inactivates NCC, whereas NCC is activated in hypokalemia.[143]

Other drugs associated with hypokalemia because of kaliuresis include toxic levels of acetaminophen, which causes dose-dependent hypokalemia.[331] High doses of penicillin-related antibiotics are another important cause of hypokalemia, increasing obligatory $K^+$ excretion by acting as nonreabsorbable anions in the distal nephron. In addition to penicillin, implicated antibiotics include nafcillin, dicloxacillin, ticarcillin, oxacillin, and carbenecillin.[332] Increased distal delivery of other anions such as $SO_4^{2-}$ and $HCO_3^-$ also induces a kaliuresis. The usual explanation is that $K^+$ excretion increases so as to balance the negative charge of these nonreabsorbable anions. However, increased delivery of such anions will also increase the electrochemical gradient for $K^+$-$Cl^-$ exit via apical $K^+$-$Cl^-$ cotransport or parallel $K^+$-$H^+$ and $Cl^-$-$HCO_3^-$ exchange[70,83,84] (see also "Potassium Transport in the Distal Nephron"). Drugs are also an important cause of Fanconi syndrome,[333] which is often associated with significant hypokalemia (see "Renal Tubular Acidosis").

Several tubular toxins result in both $K^+$ and magnesium wasting. These include gentamicin, which can cause tubular toxicity with hypokalemia that can masquerade as Bartter syndrome.[334] Other drugs that can cause mixed magnesium and $K^+$ wasting include amphotericin, foscarnet,[335] cisplatin,[21,336] and ifosfamide.[337] One intriguing cause of hypomagnesemia and hypokalemia is cetuximab, a humanized monoclonal antibody specific for the receptor for epidermal growth factor (EGF)[338], and often used in metastatic colorectal carcinoma. Paracrine EGF stimulates magnesium transport via the apical TRPM6 cation channel in the DCT, with magnesium wasting and hypomagnesemia in patients treated with cetuximab.[339] Aggressive replacement of magnesium is obligatory in the treatment of combined hypokalemia and hypomagnesemia because successful $K^+$ replacement depends on treatment of the hypomagnesemia (see "Hypomagnesemia").

Finally, a handful of drugs lead to hypokalemia through the inhibition of 11β-hydroxysteroid dehydrogenase-2 (11β-HSD-2), resulting in unopposed mineralocorticoid activity of circulating cortisol. The classic 11β-HSD-2 inhibitor is licorice through the active components glycyrrhetinic, glycyrrhizinic acid, and carbenoxolone. More recently, the antifungals itraconazole and posaconazole have been shown to inhibit 11β-HSD-2,[340] with several reports of hypertension and hypokalemia in patients treated with these agents[341,342] (see "Syndromes of Apparent Mineralocorticoid Excess").

### Hyperaldosteronism

Increases in circulating aldosterone (hyperaldosteronism) may be primary or secondary. Increased levels of circulating renin in secondary forms of hyperaldosteronism leads to increased Ang II and thus aldosterone and can be associated with hypokalemia. Causes include renal artery stenosis,[343] Page kidney (renal compression by a subcapsular mass or hematoma, with hyperreninemia),[344] a paraneoplastic process,[345] or renin-secreting renal tumors.[346] The incidence of hypokalemia in renal artery stenosis is thought to be less than 20%.[343] An unusual presentation of renal artery stenosis and renal ischemia is the hyponatremic hypertensive syndrome, in which concurrent hypokalemia may be profound.[347]

Primary hyperaldosteronism (PA) may have a hereditary, genetic cause. Hypertension and hypokalemia, generally attributed to increases in circulating 11-deoxycorticosterone,[348] are seen in patients with congenital adrenal hyperplasia because of defects in either steroid 11β-hydroxylase[348] or steroid 17α-hydroxylase.[349] Deficient 11β-hydroxylase results in virilization and other signs of androgen excess,[348] whereas reduced sex steroids in 17α-hydroxylase deficiency result in hypogonadism.[349]

The two major hereditary forms of isolated PA are denoted familial hyperaldosteronism type I (FH-I, also known as glucocorticoid-remediable hyperaldosteronism [GRA])[350] and familial hyperaldosteronism type II (FH-II), in which aldosterone production is not repressible by exogenous glucocorticoids. Patients with FH-II are clinically indistinguishable from sporadic forms of PA because of bilateral adrenal hyperplasia; a gene has been localized to chromosome 7p22 by linkage analysis, but has yet to be characterized.[351] A third form of familial hyperaldosteronism (FH-III) was initially described in 2008, with hyporeninemia, hyperaldosteronism resistant to dexamethasone, and very high levels of 18-oxocortisol and 18-hydroxycortisol.[352] FH-III is caused by somatic mutations in the adrenal $K^+$ channel KCNJ5, which endow the channel with a novel $Na^+$ conductance and activate adrenal glomerulosa proliferation and aldosterone release.[2] Somatic mutations in KCNJ5 are also found in spontaneous adrenal adenomas (see later). More recently, a fourth form of familial hyperaldosteronism (FH-IV), caused by autosomal dominant gain-of-function mutations in the *CACNA1H* gene, which encodes the CaV3.2 calcium channel.[353,354] The CaV3.2 calcium channel protein is expressed in human adrenal glomerulosa cells,[353] and the mutant channels demonstrate gain-of-function phenotypes, leading to increased induction of aldosterone synthase in cultured adrenal cells.[354] The clinical characteristics of patients with FH-IV has not been fully described; however, the index patients had developed PA in childhood, and one subject had a multiplex developmental disorder.[353,354]

Patients with FH-I/GRA are generally hypertensive, typically presenting at an early age; the severity of hypertension is, however, variable, so that some genetically affected individuals are actually normotensive.[350] Aldosterone levels are modestly elevated and regulated solely by ACTH. The diagnosis can be biochemically confirmed by a dexamethasone suppression test, with a suppression of aldosterone to less than 4 ng/dL, consistent with the diagnosis.[355] Patients also have high levels of abnormal hybrid 18-hydroxylated steroids, generated by the transformation of steroids typically formed in the zona fasciculata by aldosterone synthase, an enzyme that is normally expressed in the zona glomerulosa.[356,357] FH-I has been shown to be caused by a chimeric gene duplication between the homologous 11β-hydroxylase (*CYP11B1*) and aldosterone synthase (*CYP11B2*) genes, fusing the ACTH-responsive 11β-hydroxylase promoter to the coding region of aldosterone synthase. This chimeric gene is thus under the control of ACTH and is expressed in a glucocorticoid-repressible fashion.[356] Ectopic expression of the hybrid *CYP11B1-CYP11B2* gene in the zona fasciculata has been reported in a single case where adrenal tissue became available for molecular analysis.[358] Direct genetic testing for the hybrid *CYP11B1-CYP11B2* has largely supplanted biochemical screening for FH-I. Genetic testing for FH-I should be pursued in patients with PA and a family history of PA and/or of strokes at a young age, or in young patients with PA (<20 years of age).[359] For reasons that are unclear, patients with FH-I have a high frequency of hemorrhagic stroke caused by cerebral aneurysms, roughly equivalent to the frequency in autosomal polycystic kidney disease.[360]

Although the initial patients reported with FH-I were hypokalemic, most were normokalemic,[357,361] albeit perhaps with a propensity to develop hypokalemia while on thiazide diuretics.[357] Patients with FH-I are able to increase $K^+$ excretion appropriately in response to $K^+$ loading or fludrocortisone, but fail to increase plasma aldosterone in response to hyperkalemia.[362] This may reflect the ectopic expression of the chimeric aldosterone synthase in the adrenal fasciculata, which likely lack the appropriate constellation of ion channels to respond to increases in extracellular $K^+$ with an increase in aldosterone secretion.

Acquired causes of PA classically include aldosterone-producing adenomas (APAs; 35% of cases), primary or unilateral adrenal hyperplasia (PAH; 2% of cases), idiopathic hyperaldosteronism (IHA) caused by bilateral adrenal hyperplasia (60% of cases), and adrenal carcinoma (<1% of cases).[363] A rare case involving paraneoplastic overexpression of aldosterone synthase in lymphoma has also been described.[364]

The molecular characterization of adrenal adenomas with whole-genome sequencing and related techniques has been remarkably fruitful. In particular, acquired somatic mutations of the adrenal $K^+$ channel *KCNJ5* gene can be detected in about 40% of aldosterone-producing adrenal adenomas.[172] As in FH-III (see previously), these somatic mutations endow the channel with a novel $Na^+$ conductance, leading to adrenal glomerulosa cell depolarization, $Ca^{2+}$ influx, and aldosterone release. Clinically, patients with adrenal *KCNJ5* mutations have a higher preoperative aldosterone level[172] and higher lateralization index in adrenal vein sampling,[365] without affecting the surgical response to adrenalectomy.[172] Less frequently, somatic mutations in adrenal adenomas can be detected in the calcium channel *CACNA1D*[366] or in a subunit (*ATP2B3*) of the $Ca^{2+}$-ATPase pump,[367] predicted also to lead to increased $Ca^{2+}$ influx and aldosterone release.[366] Acquired mutations in the $ATP_{1A}$ alpha-1 subunit of the $Na^+/K^+$-ATPase are, in turn, thought to generate chronic depolarization, leading also to exaggerated aldosterone release.[367] A common consequence of the mutations in these so-called aldosterone driver genes is that they ultimately increase aldosterone production through increased expression of aldosterone synthase (*CYP11B2*).[368]

Recently, other pathways separate from aldosterone signaling have been implicated in the genesis of APAs. Mutations in the *CTNNB1* gene encoding β-catenin have also been described in APAs.[369,370] The mutations described appear to stabilize β-catenin, suggesting a role in WNT signaling, which has previously been implicated in adrenal development and adrenal adenomas.[369]

Landmark studies with monoclonal antibodies to CYP11B2 (aldosterone synthase) and CYP11B1 (steroid 11β-hydroxylase, which catalyzes the terminal step in cortisol production) have provided a molecular definition of the zonation of human adrenal cortices.[368,371] Whereas CYP11B1 expression is uniformly expressed throughout the zona fasciculata, there is only sporadic expression of CYP11B2 in the zona glomerulosa of normal human adrenal glands.[371] However, a subcortical population of nonneoplastic clusters of cells can also be detected; given the coexpression of other steroidogenic enzymes that are required for aldosterone synthesis, these CYP11B2+ clusters have been designated "aldosterone-producing cell clusters" (APCCs).[368,371,372] APCCs have also been demonstrated in adrenal tissues adjacent to APAs, suggesting that APCCs are a precursor to APA.[368,371] Consistent with this hypothesis, mutations in the known aldosterone-driver genes can be seen in about 35% of APCCs in normal adrenal glands.[372]

Immunochemical characterization of APAs also indicates expression of cortisol-producing enzymes CYP17A1 and CYP11B1,[371,373] providing a molecular explanation for the hypercortisolism associated with hyperaldosteronism.[373,374] In hyperaldosteronism as a result of both bilateral adrenal hyperplasia and aldosterone-producing adenomas, there is significant urinary excretion of cortisol and other glucocorticoid metabolites, exceeded only in patients with clinically overt Cushing syndrome.[374] Glucocorticoid excretion in primary aldosteronism appears to correlate better with metabolic risk (type 2 diabetes, osteoporosis, metabolic syndrome) than aldosterone excretion.[374] To the extent that hypercortisolism is not affected by mineralocorticoid antagonists, these findings tend to underscore the preference for adrenalectomy in APAs. Increasing utilization of the plasma aldosterone (PAC)/plasma renin activity (PRA) ratio in hypertension clinics has led to reports of a much higher incidence of PA than previously appreciated, with incidence rates in hypertension ranging from 0% to 72%.[375] However, the prevalence was 3.2% in a large multicenter study of patients with mild to moderate hypertension without hypokalemia.[376]

It should be noted that recent studies have revealed that there is a continuum in renin-independent hyperaldosteronism between normotensive individuals with suppressed renin and inappropriately "normal" or high aldosterone levels, individuals with unrecognized but biochemically overt PA, and individuals with severe hypertensive PA.[377,378] The presumed pathophysiology behind this continuum of increasing autonomous aldosterone secretion is the age-dependent development of APCCs, the evident precursor to APAs.[368,371,372] Regardless, the PAC:PRA ratio is a screening tool, which classically must be confirmed by aldosterone suppression testing, measuring

PAC or aldosterone secretion after loading with or salt or intravenous saline.[379] After controlling hypertension and hypokalemia (serum $K^+ \geq 4.0$ mEq/L),[379] oral salt loading over 3 days is followed by measurement of 24-hour urine aldosterone, sodium, and creatinine excretion. The 24-hour sodium excretion should exceed 200 mmol/day for adequate suppression, and a urinary aldosterone level of more than 33 nmol/day (12 µg/day) is consistent with PA. Alternatively, in the saline infusion test, recumbent patients are infused with 2 L of isotonic saline over 4 hours, followed by measurement of PAC. In patients without PA, the measured PAC after saline infusion should decrease to less than 139 pmol/L. The measured PAC in patients with PA usually does not suppress to less than 277 pmol/L; indeterminate values between 139 and 277 pmol/L can be seen in patients with IHA.[363] Patients with high probability features (hypokalemia, hypertension, high PAC:PRA ratio, abnormalities) may not necessarily require confirmatory testing, proceeding instead directly to imaging and adrenal venous sampling.[380]

Because surgery can be curative in APA, adequate differentiation of APA from IHA is critical; this requires both adrenal imaging and adrenal venous sampling (Fig. 17.9). Contemporary reports and recommendations have thus emphasized the continued importance of adrenal vein sampling in subtype differentiation.[379] Laparoscopic adrenalectomy is increasingly the preferred surgical management for APA or PAH.[379] Radiofrequency ablation appears to be an effective alternative in patients judged to be inappropriate for surgery.[381] Mineralocorticoid receptor antagonists are indicated for medical therapy of PA, with carefully monitored use of glucocorticoid to suppress ACTH in some patients with FH-I/GRA.[379]

The true incidence of hypokalemia in patients with acquired forms of PA remains difficult to evaluate because of a variety of factors:

1. Historically, patients have only been screened for hyperaldosteronism when hypokalemia is present; hence, even recent case series from clinics with such a referral pattern may suffer from a selection bias. Other recent series have concentrated on hypertensive patients, also a selection bias.

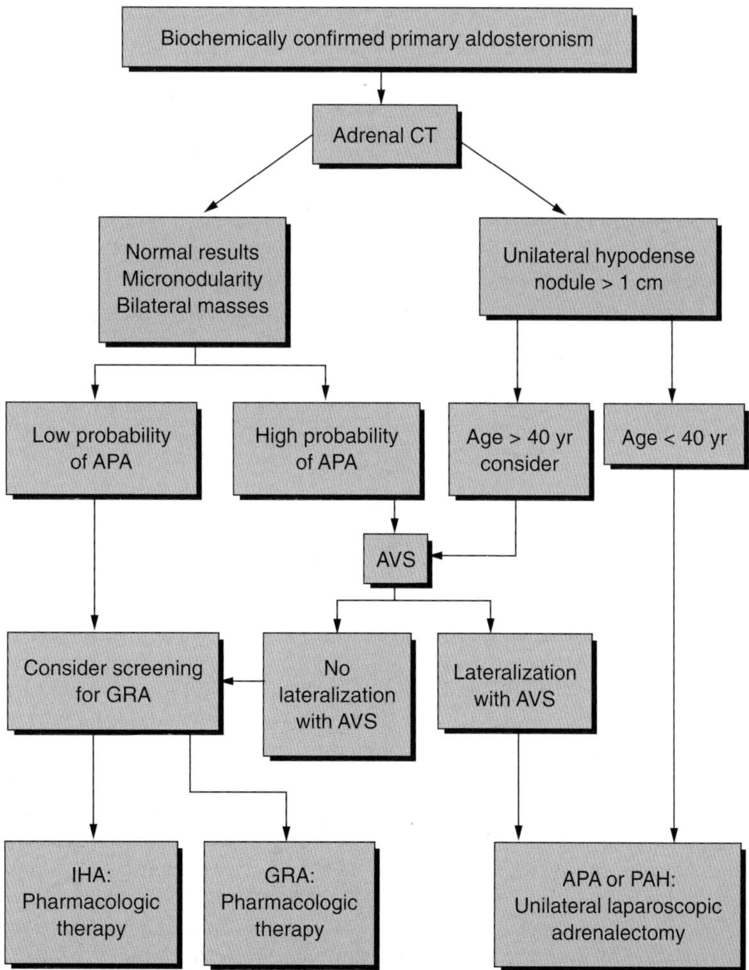


**Fig. 17.9** Diagnostic algorithm in patients with primary hyperaldosteronism. Adrenal adenoma *(APA)* must be distinguished from glucocorticoid remediable hyperaldosteronism (FH-I *[or GRA]*), primary or unilateral adrenal hyperplasia *(PAH),* and idiopathic hyperaldosteronism *(IHA)*. This requires computed axial tomography *(CT)*, adrenal venous sampling *(AVS)*, and the relevant diagnostic biochemical and hormonal assays (see text). (From Young WF Jr. Adrenalectomy for primary aldosteronism. *Ann Intern Med.* 2003:138(2):157–159.)

2. The incidence of hypokalemia is higher in adrenal adenomas than in IHA, likely because of higher average levels of aldosterone.[382]
3. Because increased kaliuresis in hyperaldosteronism can be induced by dietary $Na^+$-$Cl^-$ loading or diuretics, dietary factors and/or medications may play a role in the incidence of hypokalemia at presentation.
4. As noted earlier, there is a continuum in renin-independent hyperaldosteronism between normotensive individuals with suppressed renin and inappropriately "normal" or high aldosterone levels, individuals with unrecognized but biochemically overt PA, and individuals with severe hypertensive PA.[377,378]

Nevertheless, it is clear that hypokalemia is not a universal feature of PA; this is perhaps not unexpected, because aldosterone does not appear to affect the hypokalemic response of $H^+/K^+$-ATPase,[383] the major reabsorptive pathway for $K^+$ in the distal nephron. A related issue is whether PA is underdiagnosed when hypokalemia is used as a criterion for further investigation.

Finally, hypokalemia may also occur with systemic increases in glucocorticoids.[384,385] In actual Cushing syndrome caused by increases in pituitary ACTH, the incidence of hypokalemia is only 10%, whereas it is 57% to 100% in patients with ectopic ACTH,[384,385] despite a similar incidence of hypertension. Ectopic ACTH expression is associated primarily with neuroendocrine malignancies, most commonly bronchial carcinoid tumors, small lung cancer, and other neuroendocrine tumors.[386] Indirect evidence has suggested that the activity of renal 11β-HSD-2 is reduced in patients with ectopic ACTH compared with Cushing syndrome,[387] resulting in a syndrome of apparent mineralocorticoid excess (see later). Whether this reflects a greater degree of saturation of the enzyme by circulating cortisol or direct inhibition of 11β-HSD-2 by ACTH is not entirely clear, and there is evidence for both mechanisms.[385] However, indirect indices of 11β-HSD-2 activity in patients with ectopic ACTH expression correlate with hypokalemia and other measures of mineralocorticoid activity.[388] Similar mechanisms likely underlie the severe hypokalemia reported in patients with familial glucocorticoid resistance, in which loss-of-function mutations in the glucocorticoid receptor result in marked hypercortisolism without cushingoid features, accompanied by very high ACTH levels.[389]

### Syndromes of Apparent Mineralocorticoid Excess

The syndromes of apparent mineralocorticoid excess (AME) have a self-explanatory label. In the classic form of AME, recessive loss-of-function mutations in the 11β-HSD-2 gene (*11β-HSD-2*) cause a defect in the peripheral conversion of cortisol to the inactive glucocorticoid cortisone; the resulting increase in the half-life of cortisol is associated with a marked decrease in synthesis, so that plasma levels of cortisol are normal and patients are not cushingoid.[390] The 11β-HSD-2 protein is expressed in epithelial cells that are targets for aldosterone; in the kidney, these include cells of the DCT, CNT, and CCD.[391] Because the mineralocorticoid receptor (MR) has equivalent affinity for aldosterone and cortisol, generation of cortisone by 11β-HSD-2 serves to protect mineralocorticoid-responsive cells from illicit activation by cortisol.[392] In patients with AME, the unregulated mineralocorticoid effect of glucocorticoids results in hypertension, hypokalemia, and metabolic alkalosis, with suppressed PRA and aldosterone.[390] Biochemical diagnosis entails measuring the urinary-free cortisol to the urinary free cortisone ratio on a 24-hour urine collection. Biochemical studies of mutant enzymes usually indicate a complete loss of function; lesser enzymatic defects in patients with AME are associated with altered ratios of urinary cortisone/cortisol metabolites,[393] lesser impairment in the peripheral conversion of cortisol to cortisone,[394] and/or older age at presentation.[395]

Mice with a homozygous targeted deletion of *11β-HSD-2* exhibit hypertension, hypokalemia, and polyuria; the polyuria is likely secondary to the hypokalemia (see "Hypokalemia: Renal Consequences"), which reaches 2.4 mmol/mL in 11β-HSD-2–null mice.[396] As expected, both PRA and plasma aldosterone in the *11β-HSD-2*-null mice are profoundly suppressed, with a decreased urinary $Na^+$:$K^+$ ratio that is increased by dexamethasone (given to suppress endogenous cortisol). These knockout mice have significant nephromegaly because of a massive hypertrophy and hyperplasia of DCTs. The relative effect of genotype on the morphology of cells in the DCT, CNT, and CCD has not been determined by the appropriate phenotypic studies[397]; however, it is known that both the DCT and CCD are target cells for aldosterone,[398,399] and both cell types express 11β-HSD-2. The induction of ENaC activity by unregulated glucocorticoid, now having mineralocorticoid-like activity, causes the $Na^+$ retention and the marked increase in $K^+$ excretion in *11β-HSD-2*-null mice; distal tubular micropuncture studies in rats treated with a systemic inhibitor of 11β-HSD-2 are consistent with such a mechanism.[400] In addition, the cellular gain of function in the DCT would be expected to be associated with hypercalciuria, given the phenotype of pseudohypoaldosteronism type II and Gitelman syndrome (see "Hereditary Tubular Defects and Potassium Excretion" and "Familial Hypokalemic Alkalosis: Gitelman Syndrome"). Indeed, patients with AME are reported to exhibit nephrocalcinosis.[390]

Pharmacologic inhibition of 11β-HSD-2 is also associated with hypokalemia and AME. The most infamous offender is licorice, in its multiple guises (e.g., licorice root, tea, candies, herbal remedies). The early observations that licorice required small amounts of cortisol to exert its kaliuretic effect, in the addisonian absence of endogenous glucocorticoid,[401] presaged the observations that its active ingredients (glycyrrhetinic, glycyrrhizinic acid, and carbenoxolone) inhibit 11β-HSD-2 and related enzymes.[390] Licorice intake remains considerable in European countries, particularly Iceland, the Netherlands, and Scandinavia.[402] Pontefract cakes, eaten both as a sweet and a laxative, are a continued source of licorice in England,[402] whereas it is an ingredient in several popular sweeteners and preservatives in Malaysia.[403] Glycyrrhizinic acid is also a component of Chinese herbal remedies, prescribed for disorders such as for allergic rhinitis.[404] Pharmacologic inhibition of 11β-HSD-2 has also been tested in patients with ESKD as a novel mechanism to control hyperkalemia (see "Management of Hyperkalemia").[405] Carbenoxolone is, in turn, used in some countries in the management of peptic ulcer disease.[390] More recently, the antifungals itraconazole and posaconazole have been shown to inhibit 11β-HSD-2,[340] with several reports of hypertension and hypokalemia in patients treated with these agents[341,342]

Finally, a mechanistically distinct form of AME has been reported, because of a gain-of-function mutation in the MR.[406]

A single kindred was thus described with autosomal dominant inheritance of severe hypertension and hypokalemia; the causative mutation involved a serine residue that is conserved in the MR from multiple species, yet differs from other nuclear steroid receptors. This mutation results in constitutive activation of the MR in the absence of ligand, also with significant affinity for progesterone.[406] The MR is thus constitutively "on" in these patients, with a marked stimulation by progesterone. Of interest, pregnancies in affected female members of the family have been complicated by severe hypertension caused by marked increases in plasma progesterone levels induced by the gravid state.[406]

### Liddle Syndrome

Liddle syndrome constitutes an autosomal dominant gain in function of ENaC, the amiloride-sensitive $Na^+$ channel of the CNT and CCD.[407] Patients manifest severe hypertension with hypokalemia, unresponsive to spironolactone yet sensitive to triamterene and amiloride. Liddle syndrome could therefore also be classified as a syndrome of apparent mineralocorticoid excess. Both hypertension and hypokalemia are variable aspects of the Liddle phenotype; consistent features include a blunted aldosterone response to ACTH and reduced urinary aldosterone excretion.[100,408] The differential diagnosis for Liddle syndrome, as a cause of hereditary hypertension with hypokalemia and suppressed aldosterone, includes AME because of deficient 11β-HSD-2; however, whereas the Liddle syndrome phenotype is resistant to blockade of the mineralocorticoid receptor with spironolactone and sensitive to amiloride, AME patients are sensitive to both drugs. Commercial genetic testing for both syndromes is available in the United States.

The vast majority of mutations target the C-terminus of either the beta or gamma ENaC subunit, with a very small minority of mutations in α-ENaC. ENaC channels containing Liddle syndrome mutations are constitutively overexpressed at the cell membrane[101,409]; unlike wild-type ENaC channels, they are not sensitive to inhibition by intracellular $Na^+$,[410] an important regulator of endogenous channel activity in the CCD.[411] The mechanism whereby mutations in the C-terminus of ENaC subunits lead to this channel phenotype are discussed earlier in this chapter (see Fig. 17.5 and "Control of Potassium Secretion: Aldosterone"). In addition to effects on interaction with Nedd4-2–dependent retrieval from the plasma membrane, Liddle-associated mutations increase proteolytic cleavage of ENaC at the cell membrane[412]; aldosterone-induced "channel-activating proteases" activate ENaC channels at the plasma membrane. This important result provides a mechanistic explanation for the long-standing observation that Liddle-associated mutations in ENaC appear to have a dual activating effect on both the open probability of the channel (i.e., on channel activity) and on expression at the cell membrane.[101]

Given the overlapping and synergistic mechanisms that regulate ENaC activity, it stands to reason that mutations in ENaC that give rise to Liddle syndrome might do so by a variety of means. Indeed, mutation of a residue within the extracellular domain of γ-ENaC, versus the usual C-terminal site of mutations in Liddle syndrome, increases open probability of the channel without changing surface expression; the patient with this mutation has a typical Liddle syndrome phenotype.[413] More recently, a missense mutation in the extracellular domain of α-ENaC has also been described in a Liddle kindred, increasing the open probability of the channel without increasing susceptibility to activation by proteases.[414] Extensive searches for more common mutations and polymorphisms in ENaC subunits that correlate with blood pressure in the general population have essentially been negative, despite characterization of specific gain-of-function variants.[415] However, there are a few genetic studies that correlate specific variants in ENaC subunits with biochemical evidence of greater in vivo activity of the channel—that is, a suppressed PRA and aldosterone level and/or to-increased ratios of urinary $K^+$-to-aldosterone/PRA.[416,417]

### Familial Hypokalemic Alkalosis: Bartter Syndrome

Bartter and Gitelman syndromes are the two major variants of familial hypokalemic alkalosis; Gitelman syndrome is a much more common cause of hypokalemia than Bartter.[418] Whereas a clinical subdivision of these syndromes has been used in the past, a genetic classification is increasingly in use, due in part to phenotypic overlap. Patients with classic Bartter syndrome (BS) typically suffer from polyuria and polydipsia and manifest a hypokalemic, hypochloremic alkalosis. They may have an increase in urinary calcium ($Ca^{2+}$) excretion, and 20% are hypomagnesemic.[419] Other features include marked elevation of plasma Ang II, plasma aldosterone, and plasma renin levels. Patients with antenatal BS present earlier in life with a severe systemic disorder characterized by marked electrolyte wasting, polyhydramnios, and significant hypercalciuria with nephrocalcinosis. Prostaglandin synthesis and excretion are significantly increased and may account for many of the systemic symptoms. Decreasing prostaglandin synthesis by COX inhibition can improve polyuria in patients with BS by reducing the amplifying inhibition of urinary concentrating mechanisms by prostaglandins. Indomethacin also increases plasma $K^+$ and decreases plasma renin activity, but does not correct the basic tubular defect; it does, however, appear to help increase the growth of BS patients.[420] Of interest, COX-2 immunoreactivity is increased in the TAL and macula densa of patients with BS,[421] and reports have indicated a clinical benefit of COX-2 inhibitors.[422]

Early studies in Bartter syndrome have suggested that these patients have a defect in the function of the TAL.[423] Many of the clinical features are mimicked by the administration of loop diuretics, to which at least a subset of patients with antenatal BS do not respond.[424] The apical $Na^+$-$K^+$-$2Cl^-$ cotransporter (NKCC2, SLC12A1) of the mammalian TAL[27] (see Fig. 17.10) was thus an early candidate gene. In 1996, disease-associated mutations were found in the human NKCC2 gene in four kindreds with antenatal BS[425]; in the genetic classification of BS, these patients are considered to have BS type I. Although the functional consequences of disease-associated NKCC2 mutations have not been comprehensively studied, the first[425] and subsequent reports[29] have included patients with frameshift mutations and premature stop codons that predict the absence of a functional NKCC2 protein.

BS is a genetically heterogeneous disease. Given the role of apical $K^+$ permeability in the TAL, encoded at least in part by ROMK,[78,426] this $K^+$ channel was another early candidate gene. $K^+$ recycling via the $Na^+$-$K^+$-$2Cl^-$ cotransporter and apical $K^+$ channels generates a lumen-positive potential difference in the TAL, which drives the paracellular transport of $Na^+$ and other cations[427] (see also Fig. 17.10). Multiple disease-associated

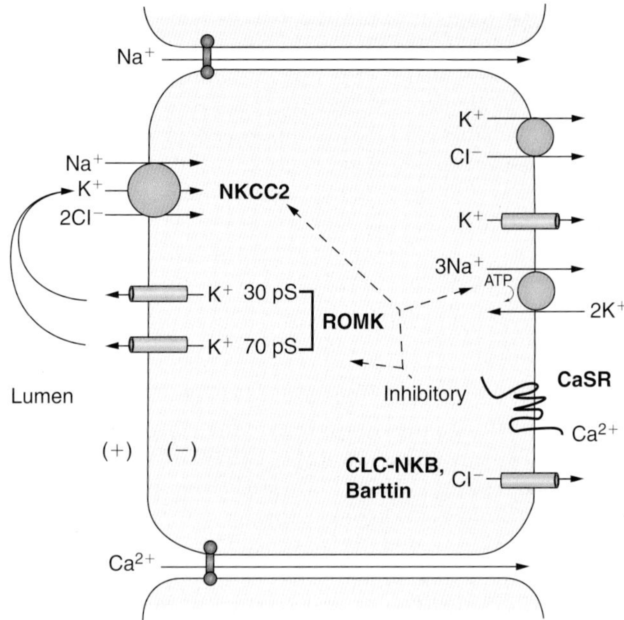


**Fig. 17.10** Bartter syndrome and the thick ascending limb. Bartter syndrome can result from loss-of-function mutations in the $Na^+$-$K^+$-$2Cl^-$ cotransporter NKCC2, the $K^+$ channel subunit ROMK, or the $Cl^-$ channel subunits CLC-NKB and Barttin (Bartter syndrome, types I–IV, respectively). Gain-of-function mutations in the calcium-sensing receptor (CaSR) can also cause a Bartter syndrome phenotype (type V); the CaSR has an inhibitory effect on salt transport by the thick ascending limb, targeting several transport pathways. ROMK encodes the low-conductance, 30-pS $K^+$ channel in the apical membrane and also appears to function as a critical subunit of the higher conductance 70-pS channel. The loss of $K^+$ channel activity Bartter syndrome type II leads to reduced apical $K^+$ recycling and reduced $Na^+$-$K^+$-$2Cl^-$ cotransport. Decreased apical $K^+$ channels also lead to a decrease in the lumen-positive potential difference, which drives paracellular $Na^+$, $Ca^{2+}$, and $Mg^{2+}$ transport. *ROMK,* Renal outer medullary $K^+$ channel.

mutations in ROMK have been reported in patients with BS type II, most of whom exhibit the antenatal phenotype.[420,428] Finally, mutations in BS type III have been reported in the chloride channel CLC-NKB,[429] which is expressed at the basolateral membrane of at least the TAL and DCT.[430] In a significant fraction of patients with BS, the NKCC2, ROMK, and CLC-NKB genes are not involved.[429] For example, a subset of patients with associated sensorineural deafness exhibit linkage to chromosome 1p31[29]; the gene for this syndrome, denoted Barttin, is an obligatory subunit for the CLC-NKB chloride channel.[431] The occurrence of deafness in these patients suggests that Barttin functions in the regulation or function of $Cl^-$ channels in the inner ear. Notably, the CLC-NKB gene is immediately adjacent to another epithelial $Cl^-$ channel, denoted CLC-NKA; inactivation of both genes was described in two siblings with deafness and BS,[432] suggesting that CLC-NKA plays an important role in Barttin-dependent $Cl^-$ transport in the inner ear.

Patients with activating mutations in the CaSR have been described with autosomal dominant hypocalcemia and hypokalemic alkalosis.[433,434] The CaSR is heavily expressed at the basolateral membrane of the TAL,[435] where it is thought to play an important inhibitory role in regulating the transcellular transport of both $Na^+$-$Cl^-$ and $Ca^{2+}$. For example, activation of the basolateral CaSR in the TAL is known to reduce apical $K^+$ channel activity,[436] which would induce a Bartter-like syndrome (see Fig. 17.10). Coexpression of NKCC2 with a Bartter syndrome gain-of-function mutant in the CaSR reveals reduced phosphorylation and reduced activity of NKCC2, dependent on the generation of inhibitory arachidonic acid–derived metabolites known to inhibit TAL function.[437] Genetic activation of the CaSR by these mutations is also expected to increase urinary $Ca^{2+}$ excretion by inhibiting the generation of the lumen-positive potential difference that drives paracellular $Ca^{2+}$ transport in the TAL. In addition, the set point of the CaSR response to $Ca^{2+}$ in the parathyroid is shifted to the left, inhibiting parathyroid hormone (PTH) secretion by this gland. No doubt the positional cloning of other BS genes will have a considerable impact on our mechanistic understanding of the TAL.

Despite the reasonable correlation between the disease gene involved and the associated subtype of familial alkalosis, there is significant phenotypic overlap and phenotypic variability in hereditary hypokalemic alkalosis. For example, patients with mutations in CLC-NKB most frequently (44.5%) exhibit classic BS, but can present with a more severe antenatal phenotype (29.5%) or even with a phenotype similar to GS (26.0%).[29,438,439] With respect to BS because of mutations in NKCC2, a number of patients have been described with variant presentations, including an absence of hypokalemia.[29] Two brothers were described with a late onset of mild BS; they were found to be compound heterozygotes for a mutant form of NKCC2 that exhibits partial function, with a loss-of-function mutation on the other NKCC2 allele.[440] Further genetic heterogeneity has also recently emerged, with the description of patients with hypokalemic alkalosis because of mutations in claudin 10, which presumably disrupt paracellular cation transport by the TAL.[441] Notably, the genetic heterogeneity in BS, GS, and related disorders is arguably not a major clinical issue in contemporary clinical practice; most commercial genetic analyses of patients with hereditary hypokalemic alkalosis now involve testing an extensive panel of relevant genes, rather than testing single genes.

BS type II is particularly relevant to $K^+$ homeostasis, given that ROMK is the SK secretory channel of the CNT and CCD (see "Potassium Transport in the Distal Nephron"). Patients with BS type II typically have slightly higher serum $K^+$ level than the other genetic forms of BS[428,438]; patients with severe (9.0 mmol/L), transient, neonatal hyperkalemia have also been described.[442] It is likely that this reflects a transient developmental deficit in the other $K^+$ channels involved in distal $K^+$ secretion, including the apical maxi-K channel responsible for flow-dependent $K^+$ secretion in the distal nephron.[77,443] Distal $K^+$ secretion in ROMK knockout mice is primarily mediated by maxi-K–BK channel activity[444] so that developmental deficits in this channel would indeed lead to hyperkalemia in BS type II. The mammalian TAL has two major apical $K^+$ conductances, the 30-pS channel corresponding to ROMK and a 70-pS channel[445]; both are thought to play a role in transepithelial salt transport by the TAL. ROMK is evidently a subunit of the 70-pS channel, given the absence of this conductance in TAL segments of ROMK knockout mice.[446] The identity of the other putative subunit of this 70-pS channel is not as yet known; one would assume that deficiencies in this gene would also be a cause of BS.

Finally, BS must be clinically differentiated from the various causes of "pseudo-Bartter" syndrome; these commonly include laxative abuse, furosemide abuse, and bulimia (see "Clinical Approach to Hypokalemia"). Other reported causes include gentamicin nephrotoxicity,[334] Sjögren syndrome,[29] and cystic fibrosis (CF).[29,447] Augmented $Na^+$-$Cl^-$ loss in sweat is likely the dominant predisposing factor for hypokalemic alkalosis in patients with CF; patients with this presentation generally respond promptly to intravenous fluids and electrolyte replacement. However, the cystic fibrosis transmembrane conductance regulator (CFTR) protein co-associates with ROMK in the TAL and confers sensitivity to both ATP and glibenclamide to apical $K^+$ channels in this nephron segment.[448] Lu and coworkers have proposed that this interaction serves to modulate the response of ROMK to cAMP and vasopressin, so that $K^+$ excretion in CFTR deficiency would not be appropriately reduced during water diuresis, thus predisposing such patients to the development of hypokalemic alkalosis.[448]

### Familial Hypokalemic Alkalosis: Gitelman Syndrome

A major advance in the understanding of hereditary alkaloses was the realization that a subset of patients exhibit marked hypocalciuria, rather than the hypercalciuria typically seen in BS; patients in this hypocalciuric subset are universally hypomagnesemic.[327] Such patients are now clinically classified as suffering from Gitelman syndrome.[449] Although plasma renin activity may be increased, renal prostaglandin excretion is not elevated in these hypocalciuric patients,[450] another distinguishing feature between Bartter and Gitelman syndromes. Gitelman syndrome (GS) is a milder disorder than BS; however, patients do report significant morbidity, mostly related to muscular symptoms and fatigue.[449,451] The QT interval is frequently prolonged in GS, suggesting an increased risk of cardiac arrhythmia[452]; however, a more exhaustive cardiac evaluation of a large group of patients has failed to detect significant abnormalities of cardiac structure or rhythm.[453] However, presyncope and/or ventricular tachycardia has been observed in at least two patients with GS,[29,194] one with concomitant long QT syndrome because of a mutation in the cardiac KCNQ1 $K^+$ channel.[194]

The hypocalciuria detected in GS was an expected consequence of inactivating the thiazide-sensitive $Na^+$-$Cl^-$ cotransporter NCC (SLC12A2), and loss-of-function mutations in the human gene have been reported[454]; many of these mutations lead to a defect in cellular trafficking when introduced into the human NCC protein.[455] GS is genetically homogeneous, except for patients with mutations in CLC-NKB and an overlapping phenotype.[29,194,438,439] Loss-of-function mutations in the *KCNJ10* encoding the basolateral Kir 4.1 $K^+$ channel in the DCT have been implicated in a related syndrome of hypokalemic metabolic alkalosis with hypomagnesemia accompanied by seizures, sensorineural deafness, ataxia, and mental retardation (SeSAME or EAST syndrome).[32,456] In Kir 4.1-deficient, *KCNJ10* knockout mice, the loss of basolateral $K^+$ conductance reduces basolateral $Cl^-$ conductance, leading to reduced expression of SPAK kinase and reduced apical NCC expression.[150] Notably, the genetic heterogeneity in GS and related disorders is arguably not a major clinical issue in contemporary clinical practice; most commercial genetic analyses of patients with hereditary hypokalemic alkalosis now involve testing an extensive panel of relevant genes, rather than testing for mutations in single candidate genes.

The NCC protein is localized to the apical membrane of epithelial cells in the DCT and CNT. A mouse strain with targeted deletion of the *Slc12a2* gene encoding NCC exhibits hypocalciuria and hypomagnesemia, with a mild alkalosis and marked increase in circulating aldosterone.[457] These knockout mice exhibit marked morphologic defects in the early DCT,[457] with both a reduction in absolute number of DCT cells and changes in ultrastructural appearance. That GS is a disorder of cellular development and/or cellular apoptosis should perhaps not be a surprise, given the observation that thiazide treatment promotes marked apoptosis of this nephron segment.[458] This cellular deficit leads to downregulation of the DCT magnesium channel TRPM6,[459] resulting in the magnesium wasting and hypomagnesemia seen in GS. The downstream CNT tubules are hypertrophied in NCC-deficient mice,[457] reminiscent of the hypertrophic DCT and CNT segments seen in furosemide-treated animals.[29] These CNT cells also exhibit an increased expression of ENaC at their apical membranes versus littermate controls[457]; this is likely because of activation of SGK1-dependent trafficking of ENaC by the increase in circulating aldosterone (see "Control of Potassium Secretion: Aldosterone").

Hypokalemia does not occur in $NCC^{-/-}$ mice on a standard rodent diet, but emerges on a $K^+$-restricted diet; plasma $K^+$ levels of these mice are about 1 mM lower than in $K^+$-restricted littermate controls.[460] Several mechanisms account for the hypokalemia seen in GS and $NCC^{-/-}$ mice. The distal delivery of both $Na^+$ and fluid is decreased in $NCC^{-/-}$ mice, at least on a normal diet; however, the increased circulating aldosterone and CNT hypertrophy likely compensate, leading to increased kaliuresis. As discussed previously for thiazides, decreased luminal $Ca^{2+}$ in NCC deficiency may augment baseline ENaC activity,[329] further exacerbating the kaliuresis. Of particular interest, NCC-deficient mice develop considerable polydipsia and polyuria on a $K^+$-restricted diet[460]; this is reminiscent perhaps of the polydipsia that has been implicated in thiazide-associated hyponatremia.[461]

Hypocalciuria in GS is not accompanied by changes in plasma calcium, phosphate, vitamin D, or PTH levels,[462] suggesting a direct effect on renal calcium transport. The late DCT is morphologically intact in NCC-deficient mice, with preserved expression of the epithelial calcium channel (ECAC1, or TRPV5) and the basolateral $Na^+$-$Ca^{2+}$ exchanger.[457] Furthermore, the hypocalciuric effect of thiazides persists in mice deficient in TRPV5,[459] arguing against the putative effects of this drug on distal $Ca^{2+}$ absorption. Rather, several lines of evidence have argued that the hypocalciuria of GS and thiazide treatment is because of increased absorption of $Na^+$ by the proximal tubule,[457,459] with secondary increases in proximal $Ca^{2+}$ absorption. Regardless, reminiscent of the clinical effect of thiazides on bone, there are clear differences in bone density between affected and unaffected members of specific Gitelman kindreds. Thus, homozygous patients have much higher bone densities than unaffected wild type family members, whereas heterozygotes have intermediate values for both bone density and calcium excretion.[462] An interesting association has repeatedly been described between chondrocalcinosis, the abnormal deposition of calcium pyrophosphate dihydrate (CPPD) in joint cartilage, and GS.[463]

Patients have also been reported with ocular choroidal calcification.[464]

Treatment of GS encompasses liberalization of salt intake and lifelong supplementation with oral magnesium and potassium. Reasonable targets for serum potassium and serum magnesium are 3.0 mEq/L and 0.6 mmol/L (1.46 mg/dL), respectively.[449] Organic anion salts of magnesium are preferred over magnesium chloride, magnesium hydroxide, or magnesium oxide. Patients with refractory hypokalemia may require treatment with potassium-sparing diuretics, RAAS inhibitors, and/or nonsteroidal inflammatory drugs (NSAIDs).[449]

Finally, as in BS, there have been reports of acquired tubular defects that mimic GS. These include patients with hypokalemic alkalosis, hypomagnesemia, and hypocalciuria after chemotherapy with cisplatin.[465] Patients have also been described with acquired GS caused by Sjögren syndrome and tubulointerstitial nephritis,[29,466] with a documented absence of coding sequence mutations in NCC.[466]

### Renal Tubular Acidosis

Renal tubular acidosis (RTA) and related tubular defects can be associated with hypokalemia. Proximal RTA is characterized by a reduction in proximal bicarbonate absorption, with a reduced plasma bicarbonate concentration. Isolated proximal RTA is quite rare; genetic causes include loss of function by mutations in the basolateral $Na^+$-bicarbonate transporter. More commonly, proximal RTA occurs in the context of multiple proximal tubular transport defects, encompassing the Fanconi syndrome.[333] The cardinal features of Fanconi syndrome include hyperaminoaciduria, glycosuria with a normal plasma glucose concentration, and phosphate wasting. The finding of severe hypophosphatemia with metabolic acidosis should alert clinicians to this possibility, especially if acute kidney injury is also present. Associated defects include the proximal RTA, hypouricemia, hypercalciuria, hypokalemia, salt wasting, and increased excretion of low-molecular-weight proteins. Fanconi syndrome is usually drug-associated; currently, important causes include aristolochic acid, ifosfamide, and the acyclic nucleoside phosphonates (e.g., tenofovir, cidofovir, adefovir).[333] Before treatment with bicarbonate, patients with a proximal RTA will typically demonstrate mild hypokalemia, due primarily to baseline hyperaldosteronism[467]; patients have, however, been described with profound hypokalemia on presentation before treatment.[468] Regardless, treatment with oral sodium bicarbonate will markedly increase distal tubular $Na^+$ and $HCO_3^-$ delivery, causing a marked increase in renal potassium wasting.[467] Patients will often require mixed base replacement with oral citrate and bicarbonate in addition to aggressive $K^+$-$Cl^-$ supplementation.

Hypokalemia is also associated with distal RTA, the so-called *type I RTA*. Hypokalemic distal RTA is usually caused by a secretory defect, with reduced $H^+$-ATPase activity and decreased ability to acidify the urine. For example, hereditary defects in subunits of the $H^+$-ATPase are associated with profound hypokalemia, in addition to acidosis and hypercalciuria.[469] The pathophysiology of the associated hypokalemia is multifactorial because of the loss of electrogenic $H^+$ secretion (with enhanced $K^+$ secretion to maintain electroneutrality in the distal nephron), loss of resorptive $H^+/K^+$-ATPase activity, and increases in aldosterone.[470,471] Notably, in hereditary distal RTA, hypokalemia is more common in those with $H^+$-ATPase defects than in patients with mutations in the basolateral $Cl^-$-$HCO_3^-$ exchanger.[472] Sjögren syndrome is perhaps the most common cause of hypokalemic distal RTA in adults; the associated hypokalemia can be truly profound, often resulting in marked weakness and respiratory arrest.[471]

### Magnesium Deficiency

Magnesium deficiency results in refractory hypokalemia, particularly if the plasma $Mg^{2+}$ level is less than 0.5 mmol/L[256]; hypomagnesemic patients are thus refractory to $K^+$ replacement in the absence of $Mg^{2+}$ repletion.[473,474] Magnesium deficiency is also a common concomitant of hypokalemia, in part because associated tubular disorders (e.g., aminoglycoside nephrotoxicity) may cause both a kaliuresis and magnesium wasting. Plasma $Mg^{2+}$ levels must thus be checked on a routine basis in hypokalemia.[255,475]

Several mechanisms appear to contribute to the effect of magnesium depletion on plasma $K^+$ levels. Magnesium depletion has inhibitory effects on muscle $Na^+/K^+$-ATPase activity,[476] resulting in significant efflux from muscle and a secondary kaliuresis. Distal $K^+$ secretion also appears to be enhanced because of a reduction in the normal physiologic inward rectification of ROMK secretory $K^+$ channels, with a subsequent increase in outward conductance.[477] ROMK and other KIR channels are inward rectifying—that is, $K^+$ flows inward more readily than outward, even though outward conductance is usually less than inward conductance, $K^+$ efflux predominates in the CNT and CCD because the membrane potential is more positive than the equilibrium potential for $K^+$. Intracellular $Mg^{2+}$ plays a key role in inward rectification, binding and blocking the pore of the channel from the cytoplasmic side.[477] The hypomagnesemia-associated reduction in cytoplasmic $Mg^{2+}$ in principal cells reduces inward rectification of ROMK, increasing outward conductance and increasing $K^+$ secretion; this has been confirmed in vivo.[478] Finally, it has been suggested that the repletion of intracellular $K^+$ is impaired in hypomagnesemia, even in normokalemic patients.[475] Decreased intracellular $Mg^{2+}$ enhances $K^+$ efflux from the cytoplasm of cardiac and perhaps skeletal myocytes, likely because of reduced intracellular blockade of inward rectifying $K^+$ channels (increased efflux) and inhibition of the $Na^+/K^+$-ATPase (decreased influx). Plasma $K^+$ levels thus remain normal at the expense of intracellular $K^+$.[21,475,479] This phenomenon is particularly important in patients with cardiac disease taking both diuretics and digoxin. In such patients, hypokalemia and arrhythmias will respond to correction of magnesium deficiency and potassium supplementation.[21,475]

## CLINICAL APPROACH TO HYPOKALEMIA

The initial priority in the evaluation of hypokalemia is an assessment for signs and/or symptoms (e.g., muscle weakness, electrocardiographic changes) suggestive of an impending emergency that requires immediate treatment. The cause of hypokalemia is usually obvious from history, physical examination, and/or basic laboratory tests. However, persistent hypokalemia despite appropriate initial intervention requires a more rigorous workup; in most cases, a systematic approach reveals the underlying cause (Fig. 17.11).

The history should focus on medications (e.g., diuretics, laxatives, antibiotics, herbal medications), diet and dietary supplements (e.g., licorice), and associated symptoms (e.g.,

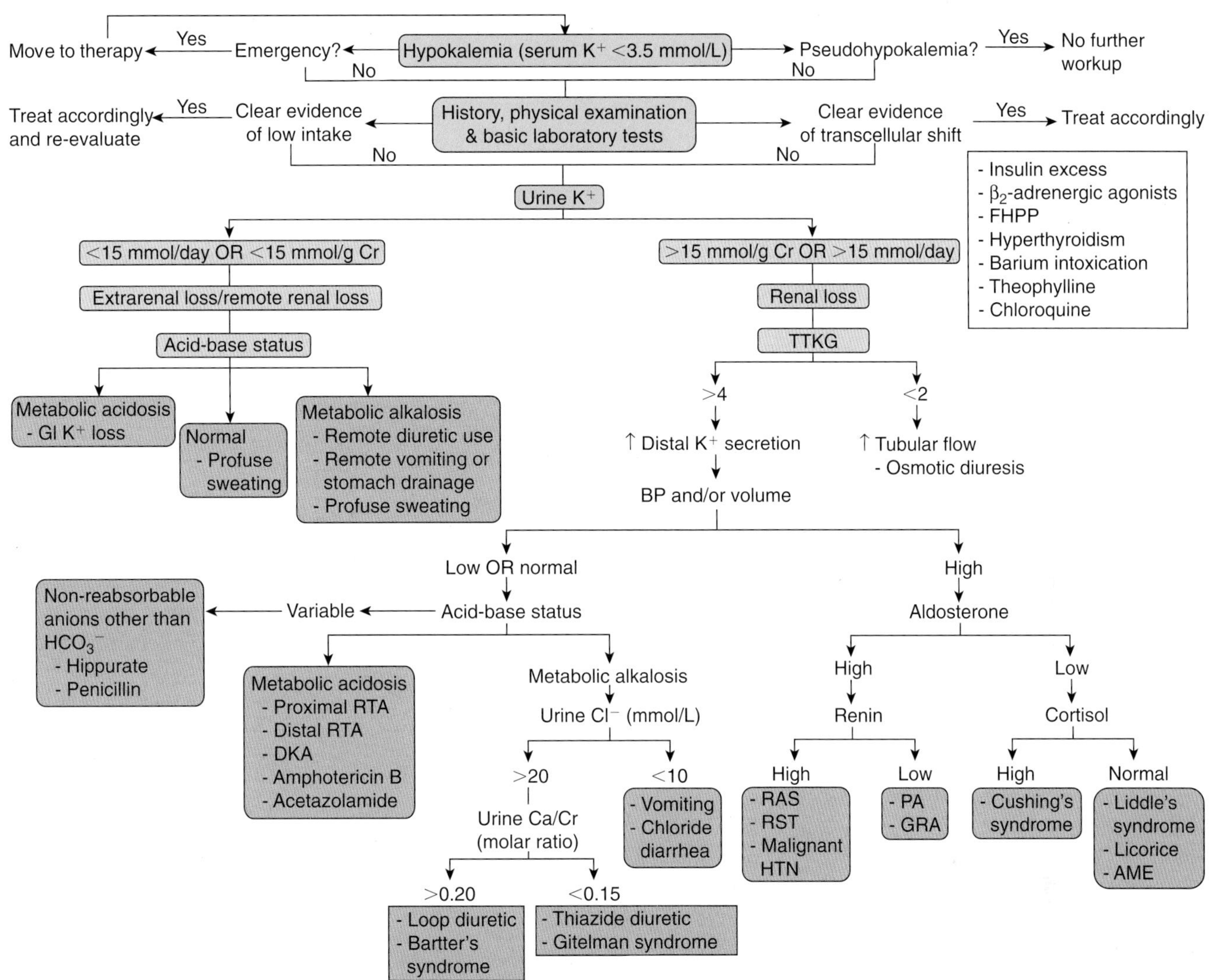


**Fig. 17.11** The clinical approach to hypokalemia. See text for details. *AME,* Apparent mineralocorticoid excess; *BP,* blood pressure; *CCD,* cortical collecting duct; *DKA,* diabetic ketoacidosis; *FHPP,* familial hypokalemic periodic paralysis; *GI,* gastrointestinal; *GRA,* glucocorticoid-remediable aldosteronism; *HTN,* hypertension; *PA,* primary aldosteronism; *RAS,* renal artery stenosis; *RST,* renin-secreting tumor; *RTA,* renal tubular acidosis; *TTKG,* transtubular potassium gradient.

diarrhea). During the physical examination, particular attention should be paid to blood pressure, volume status, and signs suggestive of specific disorders associated with hypokalemia (e.g., hyperthyroidism, Cushing syndrome). Initial laboratory tests should include electrolytes, urea, creatinine, plasma osmolality, $Mg^{2+}$, and $Ca^{2+}$, a complete blood count, and urinary pH, osmolality, creatinine, and electrolytes. Plasma and urine osmolality are required for calculation of the TTKG[181] and urinary $K^+$-to-creatinine ratio (see "Urinary Indices of Potassium Excretion"). A TTKG of less than 2 to 3 separates patients with redistributive hypokalemia from those with hypokalemia because of renal potassium wasting, who will have TTKG values that are more than 4.[186] Further tests such as urinary $Mg^{2+}$ and $Ca^{2+}$ and plasma renin and aldosterone levels may be necessary in specific cases (see Fig. 17.11). The timing and evolution of hypokalemia are also helpful in differentiating the cause, particularly in hospitalized patients—for example, hypokalemia because of transcellular shift usually occurs in a matter of hours.[480]

The most common causes of chronic, diagnosis-resistant hypokalemia are GS, surreptitious vomiting, and diuretic abuse.[481] Alternatively, an associated acidosis would suggest the diagnosis of hypokalemic distal or proximal renal tubular acidosis. Hypokalemia occurred in 5.5% of patients with eating disorders in an American study from the mid-1990s,[482] mostly in those with surreptitious vomiting (bulimia) or laxative abuse (the purging[313] subtype of anorexia nervosa). These patients may have a constellation of associated symptoms and signs, including dental erosion and depression.[483] Hypokalemic patients with bulimia will have an associated metabolic alkalosis, with an obligatory natriuresis accompanying the loss of bicarbonate; urinary $Cl^-$ is typically less than 10 mmol/L, and this clue can often yield the diagnosis.[481,484] Urinary electrolyte levels are, however, generally unremarkable in unselected, mostly normokalemic patients with bulimia.[483] Urinary excretion of $Na^+$, $K^+$, and $Cl^-$ is high in patients who abuse diuretics, albeit not to the levels seen in GS. Marked variability in urinary electrolyte levels is an important clue for diuretic abuse, which can be verified with urinary drug screens.

Clinically, nephrocalcinosis is very common in furosemide abuse because of the increase in urinary calcium excretion.[485] Differentiation of GS from BS requires a 24-hour urine test to assess calcium excretion because hypocalciuria is a distinguishing feature for the former[327]; patients with GS are also invariably hypomagnesemic. BS must be differentiated from "pseudo-Bartter" syndrome because of gentamicin toxicity,[334,486] mutations in CFTR, the cystic fibrosis gene,[447,487] or Sjögren syndrome with tubulointerstitial nephritis.[488] Acquired forms of GS have, in turn, been reported after cisplatin therapy[465] and in patients with Sjögren syndrome.[29,466] Finally, although laxative abuse is perhaps a less common cause of chronic hypokalemia, an accompanying metabolic acidosis with a negative urinary anion gap should raise the diagnostic suspicion of this cause.[187]

## TREATMENT OF HYPOKALEMIA

The goals of therapy in hypokalemia are to prevent life-threatening conditions (e.g., diaphragmatic weakness, rhabdomyolysis, cardiac arrhythmias), replace any $K^+$ deficit, and diagnose and correct the underlying cause. The urgency of therapy depends on the severity of hypokalemia, associated conditions and settings (e.g., a patient with heart failure on digoxin, or a patient with hepatic encephalopathy), and the rate of decline in plasma $K^+$. A rapid drop to less than 2.5 mmol/L poses a high risk of cardiac arrhythmias and calls for urgent replacement.[489] Although replacement is usually limited to patients with a true deficit, it should be considered in patients with hypokalemia caused by redistribution (e.g., hypokalemic periodic paralysis) when serious complications such as muscle weakness, rhabdomyolysis, and cardiac arrhythmias are present or imminent.[490] The risk of arrhythmia from hypokalemia is highest in older patients, patients with evidence of organic heart disease, and patients on digoxin or antiarrhythmic drugs.[255] In these high-risk patients, an increased incidence of arrhythmias may occur at even mild to modest degrees of hypokalemia. The American Heart Association guidelines on the use of hospital telemetry have recommended monitoring in patients with hypokalemia and a prolonged QT interval.[491]

It is also crucial to diagnose and eliminate the underlying cause to tailor therapy to the pathophysiology involved. For example, the risk of overcorrection or rebound hyperkalemia in hypokalemia caused by redistribution is particularly high, with the potential for fatal hyperkalemic arrhythmias.[256,271,308,490,492] When increased sympathetic tone or increased sympathetic response is thought to play a dominant role in the hypokalemia, the use of nonspecific β-adrenergic blockade with short-lived propranolol generally avoids this complication and should be considered. The relevant causes of hypokalemia include thyrotoxic periodic paralysis,[306] theophylline overdose,[493] and acute head injury.[271]

$K^+$ replacement is the mainstay of therapy in hypokalemia. However, hypomagnesemic patients can be refractory to $K^+$ replacement alone[474] so that concomitant $Mg^{2+}$ deficiency should always be addressed with oral or parenteral repletion. To prevent hyperkalemia caused by excessive supplementation, the deficit and the rate of correction should be estimated as accurately as possible. Renal function, medications, and comorbid conditions such as diabetes (with a risk of both insulinopenia and autonomic neuropathy) should also be considered to gauge the risk of overcorrection. Arbitrary adjustments in the dose of administered $K^+$-$Cl^-$ replacement based on the estimated GFR can potentially reduce the risk of hyperkalemia.[494] The goal is to raise the plasma $K^+$ to a safe range rapidly and then replace the remaining deficit at a slower rate, over days to weeks.[255,256,490] In the absence of abnormal $K^+$ redistribution, the total deficit correlates with serum $K^+$,[257,491,496] so that serum $K^+$ drops by approximately 0.27 mmol/L for every 100-mmol reduction in total-body stores. Loss of 400 to 800 mmol of body $K^+$ results in a reduction in serum $K^+$ by approximately 2.0 mmol/L[495]; these parameters can be used to estimate replacement goals. However, such estimates are just an approximation of the amount of $K^+$ replacement required to normalize plasma $K^+$, with as much as a 1 in 6 risk of overreplacement[260]; serum $K^+$ should also be closely monitored during replacement, withdrawing or adjusting $K^+$ replacement if necessary.

Although the treatment of asymptomatic patients with borderline or low normal serum $K^+$ remains controversial, supplementation is recommended in patients with a serum $K^+$ lower than 3 mmol/L. In high-risk patients (e.g., those with heart failure, cardiac arrhythmias, myocardial infarction, ischemic heart disease, or taking digoxin), the serum $K^+$ level should be maintained at 4.0 mmol/L or higher[255] or even 4.5 mmol/L or more.[264] Patients with severe hepatic disease may not be able to tolerate mild to moderate hypokalemia because of the associated augmentation in ammoniagenesis, so the serum $K^+$ should be maintained at approximately 4.0 mmol/L.[496,497] In asymptomatic patients with mild to moderate hypertension, an attempt should be made to maintain serum $K^+$ above 4.0 mmol/L,[255] and potassium supplementation should be considered when serum $K^+$ falls below 3.5 mmol/L.[255] Notably, prospective studies have shown an inverse relationship between dietary potassium intake and both fatal and nonfatal stroke, independent of the associated antihypertensive effect.[255,498,499]

Potassium is available in the form of potassium chloride, potassium phosphate, potassium bicarbonate or its precursors (potassium citrate, potassium acetate), and potassium gluconate.[255,256,490] Potassium phosphate is indicated when a phosphate deficit accompanies $K^+$ depletion (e.g., in diabetic ketoacidosis).[490] Potassium bicarbonate (or its precursors) should be considered in patients with hypokalemia and metabolic acidosis.[255,490] Potassium chloride should otherwise be the default salt of choice in most patients, for several reasons. First, metabolic alkalosis typically accompanies chloride loss from a renal (e.g., diuretics) or upper gastrointestinal route (e.g., vomiting) and contributes significantly to renal $K^+$ wasting.[256] In this setting, replacing chloride along with $K^+$ is essential in treating the alkalosis and preventing further kaliuresis; because dietary $K^+$ is mainly in the form of potassium phosphate or potassium citrate, it usually does not suffice. Second, potassium bicarbonate may offset the benefits of $K^+$ administration by aggravating concomitant alkalosis. Third, potassium chloride raises serum $K^+$ at a faster rate than potassium bicarbonate, a factor that is crucial in patients with marked hypokalemia and related symptoms. In all likelihood, this faster rise in plasma $K^+$ occurs because $Cl^-$ is mainly an extracellular fluid anion that does not enter cells to the same extent as bicarbonate, keeping the $K^+$ in the extracellular fluid compartment.[500]

Parenteral (intravenous) $K^+$ administration should be limited to patients unable to use the enteral route or when the patient is experiencing associated signs and symptoms. However, rapid correction of hypokalemia through oral supplementation is possible and may be faster than intravenous $K^+$ supplementation because of limitations in the rapidity of intravenous $K^+$ infusion. For example, serum $K^+$ can be increased by 1 to 1.4 mmol/L in 60 to 90 minutes, following the oral intake of 75 mmol of $K^+$[501]; the ingestion of approximately 125 to 165 mmol of $K^+$ as a single oral dose can increase serum $K^+$ by approximately 2.5 to 3.5 mmol/L in 60 to 120 minutes.[502] The oral route is thus both effective and appropriate in patients with asymptomatic severe hypokalemia. If the patient is experiencing life-threatening signs and symptoms of hypokalemia, however, the maximum possible IV infusion of $K^+$ should be administered acutely for symptom control, followed by rapid oral supplementation.

The usual intravenous dose is 20 to 40 mmol of $K^+$-$Cl^-$ in 1 L of vehicle solution.[490] The vehicle solution should be dextrose-free to prevent a transient reduction in the serum $K^+$ level of 0.2 to 1.4 mmol/L because of an enhanced endogenous insulin secretion induced by the dextrose.[503] Higher concentrations of $K^+$-$Cl^-$ (up to 400 mmol/L, as 40 mmol in 100 mL of normal saline) have been used in life-threatening conditions.[504,505] In these cases, the amount of $K^+$ per intravenous bag should be limited (e.g., 20 mmol in 100 mL of saline solution) to prevent inadvertent infusion of a large dose.[505,506] These solutions are best given through a large central vein. Femoral veins are preferable because infusion through upper body central lines can acutely increase the local concentration of $K^+$, with deleterious effects on cardiac conduction.[505,506] As a general rule, and to avoid venous pain, irritation, and sclerosis, concentrations of more than 60 mmol/L should not be given through a peripheral vein.[490]

Although the recommended rate of administration is 10 to 20 mmol/hour, rates of 40 to 100 mmol/hour or even higher (for a short period) have been used in patients with life-threatening conditions.[504,506–508] However, a rapid increase in serum $K^+$ associated with electrocardiographic changes may occur with higher rates of infusion (e.g., ≥80 mmol/hour).[509] Intravenous administration of $K^+$ at a rate of more than 10 mmol/hour requires continuous electrocardiographic monitoring.[490] In patients receiving $K^+$ at such a high infusion rate, close monitoring of the appropriate physiologic consequences of hypokalemia is essential; after these effects have abated, the rate of infusion should be decreased to the standard dose of 10 to 20 mmol/hour.[506] It is important to remember that volume expansion in patients with moderate to severe hypokalemia and $Cl^-$-responsive metabolic alkalosis should be performed cautiously and with close follow-up of serum $K^+$ because bicarbonaturia associated with volume expansion may aggravate renal $K^+$ wasting and hypokalemia.[489] In patients with combined severe hypokalemia and hypophosphatemia (e.g., diabetic ketoacidosis), intravenous $K^+$ phosphate can be used. However, this solution should be infused at a rate of less than 50 mmol over 8 hours to prevent the risk of hypocalcemia and metastatic calcification.[489] A combination of potassium phosphate and potassium chloride may be necessary to correct hypokalemia effectively in these patients.

The easiest and most straightforward method of oral $K^+$ supplementation is to increase the dietary intake of potassium-rich foods[256] (Box 17.1). One study has compared the effectiveness of diet versus medication supplementation in cardiac surgery patients receiving diuretics in hospital and found no difference between the two groups in respect to the maintenance of serum $K^+$. However, limitations of this study included a small number of subjects, relatively short duration, and lack of information on acid-base status, making it less than conclusive and not generalizable.[510]

Nevertheless, dietary $K^+$ is mainly in the form of potassium phosphate or potassium citrate and is inadequate in most patients who have combined $K^+$ and $Cl^-$ deficiency.[511] For example, bananas contain only 2 mEq of potassium/inch, with a dominance of nonchloride anions.[511] Most patients will therefore need to combine a high-$K^+$ diet with a prescribed dose of $K^+$-$Cl^-$.[256] Salt substitutes are an inexpensive and potent source of $K^+$-$Cl^-$; each gram contains 10 to 13 mmol of $K^+$[513]; however, patients, particularly those with an impaired ability to excrete potassium, need to be counseled regarding the

**Box 17.1 Foods With High Potassium Content**

**Highest Content (>1000 mg [25 mmol]/100 g)**

- Dried figs
- Molasses
- Seaweed

**Very High Content (>500 mg [12.5 mmol]/100 g)**

- Dried fruits (dates, prunes)
- Nuts
- Avocados
- Bran cereals
- Wheat germ
- Lima beans

**High Content (>250 mg [6.2 mmol]/100 g)**

- Vegetables
  - Spinach
  - Tomatoes
  - Broccoli
  - Winter squash
  - Beets
  - Carrots
  - Cauliflower
  - Potatoes
- Fruits
  - Bananas
  - Cantaloupe
  - Kiwis
  - Oranges
  - Mangos
- Meats
  - Ground beef
  - Steak
  - Pork
  - Veal
  - Lamb

From Gennari FJ: Hypokalemia. *N Engl J Med.* 1998;339:451–458.

**Table 17.4 Oral Preparations of Potassium Chloride**

| Supplement | Characteristics |
|---|---|
| Controlled-release microencapsulated tablets | Disintegrate better in stomach than encapsulated microparticles; less adherent and less cohesive |
| Encapsulated, controlled-release, microencapsulated particles | Fewer gastrointestinal tract erosions than with wax matrix tablets |
| Potassium chloride elixir | Inexpensive, tastes bad, poor patient adherence; few gastrointestinal tract erosions; immediate effect |
| Potassium chloride (effervescent tablets) for solution | Convenient, but more expensive than elixir; immediate effect |
| Wax matrix extended-release tablets | Easier to swallow; more gastrointestinal tract erosions than with microencapsulated formulas |

From Cohn JN, Kowey PR, Whelton PK, et al: New guidelines for potassium replacement in clinical practice: a contemporary review by the National Council on Potassium in Clinical Practice. *Arch Intern Med.* 2000;160:2429–2436.

appropriate amount and the potential for hyperkalemia.[512] Potassium chloride is also available in liquid or tablet form (Table 17.4).[255] In general, the available preparations are well absorbed.[256] Liquid forms are less expensive but are less well tolerated. Slow-release forms are more palatable and better tolerated; however, they have been associated with gastrointestinal ulceration and bleeding, ascribed to local accumulation of high concentrations of $K^+$.[257,507] Notably, this risk is rather low and is lower still with the microencapsulated forms.[256] The chance of overdose and hyperkalemia is higher with slow-release formulations; unlike the immediate-release forms, these tablets are less irritating to the stomach and less likely to induce vomiting.[513] The usual dose is 40 to 100 mmol of $K^+$ (as $K^+$-$Cl^-$)/day, bid or tid, in patients taking diuretics[256] ($K^+$-$Cl^-$ can be toxic in doses > 2 mmol/Kg).[513] This dose is effective in maintaining serum $K^+$ in up to 90% of patients; however, in the 10% of patients who remain hypokalemic, increasing the oral dose or adding a $K^+$-sparing diuretic is an appropriate choice.[256]

In addition to potassium supplementation, strategies to minimize $K^+$ losses should be considered. These measures may include minimizing the dose of non–$K^+$-sparing diuretics, restricting $Na^+$ intake, and using a combination of non–$K^+$-sparing and $K^+$-sparing medications (e.g., ACE inhibitors, ARBs, $K^+$-sparing diuretics, beta-blockers).[225,255] The use of a $K^+$-sparing diuretic is of particular importance in hypokalemia resulting from primary hyperaldosteronism and related disorders, such as Liddle syndrome and AME; $K^+$ supplementation alone may be ineffective in these settings.[514–516] In patients with hypokalemia caused by loss through upper gastrointestinal secretion (e.g., with continuous nasogastric tube suction, continuous or self-induced vomiting), proton pump inhibitors are reportedly useful in helping correct the metabolic alkalosis and reduce hypokalemia.[517]

## HYPERKALEMIA

### EPIDEMIOLOGY

Hyperkalemia is usually defined as a potassium level of 5.5 mmol/L or higher,[518,519] although in some studies 5.0 to 5.4 mmol/L qualifies for the diagnosis.[520] Hyperkalemia has been reported in 1.1% to 10% of all hospitalized patients,[232,518–521] with approximately 1.0% of patients (8%–10% of hyperkalemic patients) having significant hyperkalemia (≥6.0 mmol/L).[518] Hyperkalemia has been associated with a higher mortality rate (14.3%–41%),[29,518,519] accounting for approximately 1 death/1000 patients in one case series from the mid-1980s.[522] In most hospitalized patients, the pathophysiology of hyperkalemia is multifactorial, with reduced renal function, medications, older age (≥60 years), and hyperglycemia being the most common contributing factors.[232,518,519]

In patients with ESKD, the prevalence of hyperkalemia is 5% to 10%.[523–525] Data from the NephroTest cohort have indicated that the prevalence of hyperkalemia increases from 2% to 42% as the GFR decreases from 60 to 90 to less than 20 mL/min/1.73 $m^2$.[2,25,26] The risk of hyperkalemia is increased in males with chronic kidney disease (CKD) and tripled by treatment with ACE inhibitors or ARBs.[526] Hyperkalemia accounts for or contributes to 1.9% to 5% of deaths among patients with ESKD.[232,525] Notably, however, the risk of death from hyperkalemia is reduced as CKD progresses, presumably caused by as yet uncharacterized cardiac adaptation to chronic hyperkalemia.[527] However, multiple studies have implicated hyperkalemia with increased risk of death in ESKD, as managed by both hemodialysis[528] and peritoneal dialysis.[529] Hyperkalemia is the reason for emergency hemodialysis in 24% of patients with ESKD on hemodialysis,[525] and renal failure is the most common cause of hyperkalemia diagnosed in the emergency room.[523] The prevalence of marked hyperkalemia ($K^+$ ≥5.8 mmol/L) is approximately 1% in a general medicine outpatient setting. Alarmingly, the management of outpatient hyperkalemia is often suboptimal, with approximately 25% of patients lacking any follow-up, ECGs performed in only 36% of cases, and frequent delays in repeating serum $K^+$.[530]

### PSEUDOHYPERKALEMIA

Factitious or pseudohyperkalemia is an artifactual increase in the serum $K^+$ caused by the release of $K^+$ during or after venipuncture. There are several potential causes for pseudohyperkalemia[531]:

1. Forearm contraction,[532] fist clenching,[21] or tourniquet use[531] may increase $K^+$ efflux from local muscle and thus raise the measured serum $K^+$.
2. Thrombocytosis,[533] leukocytosis,[534] and/or erythrocytosis[535] may also cause pseudohyperkalemia because of release from these cellular elements.
3. Acute anxiety during venipuncture may provoke a respiratory alkalosis and hyperkalemia because of redistribution.[55,56,58,66]

This hyperkalemic response is mediated by enhanced α-adrenergic activity and counterregulated, in part, by β-adrenergic stimulation. Increased catecholamine concentrations may be as a result of the decrease in plasma bicarbonate.

4. Sample contamination with $K^+$ EDTA, used as a sample anticoagulant for some laboratory assays, can cause spurious hyperkalemia.[536]

   There are several mechanisms for sample contamination with $K^+$ EDTA during blood draws or sample handling.[536] Gross contamination with $K^+$ EDTA usually results in spurious hypocalcemia and hypomagnesemia; lesser contamination is less obvious, leading to the practice in some laboratories to perform EDTA assays on samples with a plasma $K^+$ of more than 6 mmol/L with $K^+$ EDTA.

5. Mechanical and physical factors may induce pseudohyperkalemia after blood has been drawn.

   For example, pneumatic tube transport has been shown to induce pseudohyperkalemia in one patient with leukemia and massive leukocytosis.[537] Cooling of blood before the separation of cells from serum or plasma is also a well-recognized cause of artifactual hyperkalemia.[538] The converse is the risk of increased uptake of $K^+$ by cells at high ambient temperatures, leading to normal values for hyperkalemic patients and/or to spurious hypokalemia in patients who are normokalemic.[29,266] This issue is particularly important for outpatient primary practice samples that are transported off site and analyzed at a central facility[29]; this phenomenon leads to "seasonal pseudohyperkalemia and hypokalemia,"[29,539] with fluctuations of outpatient samples as a function of season and ambient temperature.

6. There are several hereditary subtypes of pseudohyperkalemia, caused by increase in passive $K^+$ permeability of erythrocytes.

Abnormal red cell morphology, varying degrees of hemolysis, and/or perinatal edema can accompany hereditary pseudohyperkalemia, whereas in many kindreds there are no overt hematologic consequences. Serum $K^+$ increases in pseudohyperkalemic patient samples that have been left at room temperature because of abnormal $K^+$ permeability of erythrocytes. Several subtypes have been defined, based on differences in the temperature dependence curve of this red cell leak pathway.[29,540] The disorder is genetically heterogeneous, with characterized genes on chromosome 17q21 (SLC4A1), 16q23-ter (*PIEZO1*), and 2q35-36 (*ABCB6*).[29,541] Initially, 11 pedigrees of patients with autosomal dominant hemolysis, pseudohyperkalemia, and temperature-dependent loss of red cell $K^+$ were found to have heterozygous mutations in the *SLC4A1* gene on chromosome 17q21, which encodes the band 3 anion exchanger, AE1.[540] The mutations that were detected all cluster within exon 17 of the gene,[540] between transmembrane domains 8 and 10 of the AE1 protein. These mutations reduce anion transport in both red cells and *Xenopus* oocytes injected with AE1, with the novel acquisition of a nonselective transport pathway for both $Na^+$ and $K^+$. Pseudohyperkalemia in these patients thus results from a genetic event that endows AE1 with the ability to transport $K^+$; the fact that single point mutations can convert an anion exchanger to a nonselective cation channel serves to underline the narrow boundaries that separate exchangers and transporters from ion channels.[540] Notably, however, other reports have suggested that these mutations in *SLC4A1* induce cation fluxes that are independent of the AE1 anion exchanger protein—that is, mediated by other transport pathways.[542,543]

In another study, mutations in the red cell Rh-associated glycoprotein (RhAG) have been linked to the monovalent cation leak associated with overhydrated hereditary stomatocytosis.[544] These mutations cause an exaggerated cation leak in the RhAG, thought to function as an $NH_3$ or $NH_4^+$ transporter RhAG. Exaggerated red cell cation leaks are also implicated in stomatocytosis because of mutations in the mechanically activated cation channel PIEZO1[545]; disease-associated mutations give rise to mechanically activated currents that inactivate more slowly than the wild-type channel. Physiologically, calcium influx via the PIEZO1 channel collaborates with the calcium-activated Gardos $K^+$ channel (encoded by *KCNN4*) in controlling red cell volume.[541] Not surprisingly, mutations in the KCNN4 that increase the calcium sensitivity of the Gardos channel are associated with stomatocytosis.[546] Finally, mutations in the gene encoding the ATP-binding cassette family member 6 (ABCB6) transporter have also been associated with familial pseudohyperkalemia.[541]

## EXCESS INTAKE OF POTASSIUM AND TISSUE NECROSIS

Increased intake of even small amounts of $K^+$ may provoke severe hyperkalemia in patients with predisposing factors. For example, the oral administration of 32 millimoles to a diabetic patient with hyporeninemic hypoaldosteronism resulted in an increase in serum $K^+$ from 4.9 mmol/L to a peak of 7.3 mmol/L, within 3 hours.[547] Increased intake or changes in intake of dietary sources rich in $K^+$ (Box 17.1) may also provoke hyperkalemia in susceptible patients. Very rarely, marked intake of $K^+$—for example in sports beverages[548] —may provoke severe hyperkalemia in individuals free of predisposing factors. Other occult sources of $K^+$ must also be considered, including salt substitutes,[549] alternative medicines,[550] and alternative diets.[551] Geophagia with ingestion of $K^+$-rich clay[29] and cautopyreiophagia[552] (ingestion of burnt matchsticks) are two forms of pica that have been reported to cause hyperkalemia in dialysis patients. Sustained-release $K^+$-$Cl^-$ tablets can cause hyperkalemia in suicidal overdoses.[513] Such pills are radiopaque and may thus be seen on radiographs; whole-bowel irrigation should be used for gastrointestinal decontamination.[513] Iatrogenic causes include simple overreplacement with $K^+$-$Cl^-$, as can occur commonly in hypokalemic patients,[260] or administration of a potassium-containing medication, such as $K^+$ penicillin,[553] to a susceptible patient.

Red cell transfusion is a well-described cause of hyperkalemia, typically seen in children or in those receiving a massive transfusion. Risk factors for transfusion-related hyperkalemia include the rate and volume of the transfusion, use of a central venous infusion and/or pressure pumping, use of irradiated blood, and age of the blood infused.[21,554] Whereas 7-day-old blood has a free $K^+$ concentration of about 23 mmol/L, this rises to the 50-mmol/L range in 42-day-old blood.[555] Hyperkalemia is a common occurrence in patients with severe trauma, with a period prevalence of 29% in massively traumatized patients at a US military combat support hospital in Iraq.[556] Although red cell and/or blood product transfusion plays an important role, this and other studies have indicated a complex pathophysiology for resuscitative hyperkalemia, with low cardiac output, acidosis, hypocalcemia, and other factors contributing to the risk of hyperkalemia in patients with severe trauma.[554,556]

Tissue necrosis is an important cause of hyperkalemia. Hyperkalemia because of rhabdomyolysis is particularly common due the enormous store of $K^+$ in muscle (see Fig. 17.1). In many cases, volume depletion, medications (statins in particular), and a metabolic predisposition contribute to the genesis of rhabdomyolysis. Hypokalemia is an important metabolic predisposing factor in rhabdomyolysis (see "Effects of Hypokalemia"); others include hypophosphatemia, hypernatremia and hyponatremia, and hyperglycemia. Patients with hypokalemia-associated rhabdomyolysis in whom redistribution is the cause of hypokalemia are at particular risk of subsequent hyperkalemia as rhabdomyolysis evolves and renal function worsens.[21,282] Finally, massive release of $K^+$ and other intracellular contents may occur as a result of acute tumor lysis.[547]

## REDISTRIBUTION AND HYPERKALEMIA

Several different mechanisms can induce an efflux of intracellular $K^+$, resulting in hyperkalemia. The infusion of hypertonic mannitol or saline, but not hypertonic bicarbonate, generates an increase in serum $K^+$.[557] Potential mechanisms include a dilutional acidosis with a subsequent shift in $K^+$, increased passive exit of $K^+$ because of an increase in intracellular $K^+$ activity from intracellular water loss, acute hemolysis, and a solvent drag effect as water exits cells.[558,559] Regardless, severe hyperkalemia, typically with an acute dilutional hyponatremia, is a well-described complication of mannitol for the treatment or prevention of cerebral edema.[559–561] Diabetics are prone to severe hyperkalemia in response to intravenous hypertonic glucose in the absence of adequate coadministered insulin because of a similar osmotic effect.[562,563] Finally, a retrospective report has documented considerable increases in serum $K^+$ after IV contrast dye in five patients with CKD, four on dialysis and one with stage IV CKD[564]; again, the acute osmolar load was the likely cause of the acute hyperkalemia in these patients. The implications of this provocative study are not entirely clear; however, one would expect the development or worsening of hyperkalemia in dialysis patients exposed to large volumes of hyperosmolar contrast dye.

Several reports have appeared regarding the risk of hyperkalemia with epsilon-aminocaproic acid (Amicar),[565–567] a cationic amino acid that is structurally similar to lysine and arginine. Cationic but not anionic amino acids induce an efflux of $K^+$ from cells, although the transport pathways involved are unknown.[21] A recent resurgence in the use of cationic amino acid infusions during endoradiotherapy has served to emphasize this risk, with the development of significant hyperkalemic acidosis.[568]

Muscle plays a dominant role in extrarenal $K^+$ homeostasis, primarily via regulated uptake by the $Na^+/K^+$-ATPase. Although exercise is a well-described cause of acute hyperkalemia, this effect is usually transient, and the clinical relevance is difficult to judge. ESKD patients on dialysis do not have an exaggerated increase in plasma $K^+$ with maximal exercise, perhaps because of greater insulin, catecholamine, and aldosterone responses to exercise and/or to their preexisting hyperkalemia.[569] The results and design of this and other studies of exercise-associated hyperkalemia in ESKD have been criticized by a more recent report, which linked abnormal extrarenal $K^+$ homeostasis to increased fatigue in ESKD patients.[570] Regardless, however, exercise-associated hyperkalemia is not a major clinical cause of hyperkalemia. Dialysis patients are, however, susceptible to modest increases in plasma $K^+$ after prolonged fasting as a result of the relative insulinopenia in this setting.[571] This may be clinically relevant in preoperative ESKD patients, for whom intravenous glucose infusions with or without insulin are appropriate preventive measures for the development of hyperkalemia.[571]

Insulin stimulates the uptake of $K^+$ by several tissues, primarily via stimulation of $Na^+/K^+$-ATPase activity.[29,43,45,48] Reduction in circulating insulin is thus an important factor or cofactor in the generation of hyperkalemia in diabetic patients. Patients with DKA typically present with serum $K^+$ levels that are within normal limits or moderately elevated, but with profound whole-body potassium deficits. However, significant hyperkalemia (serum $K^+ > 6$–$6.5$ mmol/L) is not uncommon in DKA[572,573] because of a variety of potential factors—insulinopenia, renal dysfunction, and the hyperosmolar effect of severe hyperglycemia.[572–574] Inhibition of insulin secretion by the somatostatin agonist octreotide can also cause significant hyperkalemia in both anephric patients[40] and patients with normal renal function.[41]

Digoxin inhibits $Na^+/K^+$-ATPase and thus impairs the uptake of $K^+$ by skeletal muscle (see "Factors Affecting Internal Distribution of Potassium") so that digoxin overdose can result in hyperkalemia. The skin and venom gland of the cane toad *Bufo marinus* contains high concentrations of bufadienolide, structurally similar to a glycoside. The direct ingestion of such toads[575] or toad extracts can result in fatal hyperkalemia. In particular, certain herbal aphrodisiac pills contain appreciable amounts of toad venom and have led to several case reports in the United States.[21,576] Patients may have detectable plasma levels using standard digoxin assays because bufadienolide is immunologically similar to digoxin. Moreover, treatment with a digoxin-specific Fab fragment, indicated for treatment of digoxin overdoses, may be effective and lifesaving in bufadienolide toxicity.[21,576] Finally, fluoride ions also inhibit $Na^+/K^+$-ATPase so that fluoride poisoning is typically associated with hyperkalemia.[577]

Succinylcholine depolarizes muscle cells, resulting in the efflux of $K^+$ through acetylcholine receptors (AChRs) and a rapid, but usually transient, hyperkalemia. The use of this agent is contraindicated in patients who have sustained thermal trauma, neuromuscular injury (upper or lower motor neuron), disuse atrophy, mucositis, or prolonged immobilization in an intensive care unit (ICU) setting; the efflux of $K^+$ induced by succinylcholine is enhanced in these patients and can result in significant hyperkalemia.[578] These disorders share a 2- to 100-fold upregulation of AChRs at the plasma membrane of muscle cells, with loss of the normal clustering at the neuromuscular junction.[578] Depolarization of these upregulated AChRs by succinylcholine results in an exaggerated efflux of $K^+$ through the receptor-associated cation channels that are spread throughout the muscle cell membrane (Fig. 17.12). Concomitant upregulation of the neuronal $\alpha_7$-AChR subunit has also been observed in denervated muscle; the $\alpha_7$-containing AChR is a homomeric, pentameric channel that depolarizes in response to both succinylcholine and choline, its metabolite.[578] Depolarization $\alpha$7-AChRs in response to choline is furthermore not subject to desensitization, and

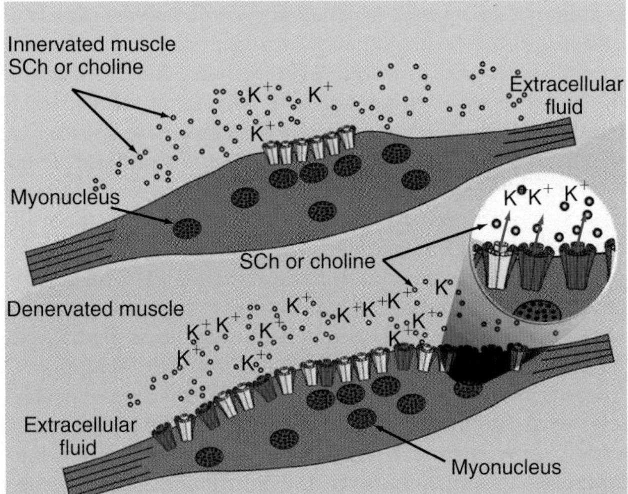


**Fig. 17.12** Succinylcholine-induced efflux of potassium is increased in denervated muscle. In innervated muscle, succinylcholine *(SCh)* interacts with the entire plasma membrane, but depolarizes only the junctional ($\alpha_1$, $\beta_1$, $\delta$, and $\varepsilon$; *multicolored*) acetylcholine receptors (AChRs); this leads to a modest transient hyperkalemia. With denervation, there is a considerable upregulation of muscle AChRs, with increased extrajunctional AChRs ($\alpha_1$, $\beta_1$, $\delta$, and $\varepsilon$; *multicolored*) and acquisition of homomeric, neuronal-type $\alpha_7$-AChRs. Depolarization of denervated muscle leads to an exaggerated $K^+$ efflux as a result of the upregulation and redistribution of these AChRs. In addition, choline generated from metabolism of succinylcholine maintains the depolarization mediated via $\alpha_7$-AChRs, thus enhancing and prolonging the $K^+$ efflux after paralysis has subsided. (From Martyn JA, Richtsfeld M. Succinylcholine-induced hyperkalemia in acquired pathologic states: etiologic factors and molecular mechanisms. *Anesthesiology.* 2006;104:158–169.)

may explain in part the hyperkalemic effect that persists in some patients well after the paralytic effect of succinylcholine has subsided.[578] Perhaps consistent with this neuromuscular pathophysiology, patients with renal failure do not appear to have an increased risk of succinylcholine-associated hyperkalemia.[579]

A report of three patients has suggested the possibility that drugs that share the ability to open $K_{ATP}$ channels may have an underappreciated propensity to cause hyperkalemia in critically ill patients. The implicated drugs included cyclosporine, isoflurane, and nicorandil.[580] These patients exhibited hyperkalemia that resisted usual therapies (insulin/dextrose ± hemofiltration), with a temporal hypokalemic response to the $K_{ATP}$ inhibitor glibenclamide (glyburide). The daring, off-label use of glibenclamide was presumably instigated by the senior author's observation that cyclosporine activates $K_{ATP}$ channels in vascular smooth muscle.[581] $K_{ATP}$ channels are widely distributed, including in skeletal muscle, so that activation of these channels is a plausible cause of acute hyperkalemia. Other case reports have emerged of nicorandil-associated hyperkalemia.[582,583]

Finally, beta-blockers cause hyperkalemia, in part by inhibiting cellular uptake, but also through hyporeninemic hypoaldosteronism induced by effects of these drugs on both renal renin release and adrenal aldosterone release (see "Regulation of Renal Renin and Adrenal Aldosterone"). Labetalol, a combined alpha and beta-blocker, is a particularly common cause of hyperkalemia in susceptible patients.[21,584] However, both nonspecific and cardiospecific beta-blockers have been shown to reduce PRA, Ang II, and aldosterone,[585] so that beta blockade in general will increase susceptibility to hyperkalemia.

## REDUCED RENAL EXCRETION OF POTASSIUM

### Hypoaldosteronism

Aldosterone promotes kaliuresis by activating apical amiloride-sensitive $Na^+$ currents in the CNT and CCD, thus increasing the lumen-negative driving force for $K^+$ excretion (see "Control of Potassium Excretion"). Aldosterone release from the adrenals may be reduced by hyporeninemic hypoaldosteronism and its multiple causes, by medications, or because of an isolated deficiency of ACTH. The isolated loss in pituitary secretion of ACTH leads to a deficit in circulating cortisol; variable defects in other pituitary hormones are likely secondary to this reduction in cortisol.[586] Concomitant hyporeninemic hypoaldosteronism is frequent[29]; however, hyperkalemia is perhaps less common in secondary hypoaldosteronism than in Addison disease.[586]

Primary hypoaldosteronism may be genetic or acquired.[587] The X-linked disorder adrenal hypoplasia congenita is caused by loss-of-function mutations in the transcriptional repressor Dax-1. Patients with adrenal hypoplasia congenita present with primary adrenal failure and hyperkalemia either shortly after birth or much later in childhood.[588] This bimodal presentation pattern does not appear to be influenced by *Dax-1* genotype; rather, if patients survive the early neonatal period, they will then miss being diagnosed until much later in life, presenting with delayed puberty (see later) or with an adrenal crisis. The steroidogenic factor-1 (SF-1), a functional partner for *Dax-1*, is also required for adrenal development in mice and humans. Both genes are involved in gonadal development, with *Dax-1* deficiency leading to hypogonadotropic hypogonadism[588] and *SF-1* deficiency causing male to female sex reversal in addition to adrenal insufficiency.

Reduced steroidogenesis causes two other important forms of primary hypoaldosteronism.[587] Congenital lipoid adrenal hyperplasia (lipoid CAH) is a severe autosomal recessive syndrome characterized by impaired synthesis of mineralocorticoids, glucocorticoids, and gonadal steroids.[21] Patients present in early infancy with adrenal crisis, including severe hyperkalemia.[589] Genotypically male 46,XY patients with lipoid CAH have female external genitalia because of the developmental absence of testosterone. Lipoid CAH is caused by loss-of-function mutations in steroidogenic acute regulatory protein, a small mitochondrial protein that helps shuttle cholesterol from the outer to the inner mitochondrial membrane, thus initiating steroidogenesis[590]; some patients may alternatively have mutations in the side chain cleavage P450 enzyme.[591] The classic, salt-wasting form of CAH because of 21-hydroxlase deficiency is associated with marked reductions in both cortisol and aldosterone, leading to adrenal insufficiency.[592] Concomitant overproduction of androgenic steroids results in virilization in female patients with this form of CAH.

Isolated deficits in aldosterone synthesis with hyperreninemia are caused by loss-of-function mutations in aldosterone synthase, although genetic heterogeneity has been reported.[593] Patients typically present in childhood with volume depletion and hyperkalemia.[594] Much like pseudohypoaldosteronism because of loss-of-function mutations in the MR (see later), patients tend to become asymptomatic in adulthood. Acquired hyperreninemic hypoaldosteronism has been described in critical illness,[21] type 2 diabetes,[595] amyloidosis because of familial Mediterranean fever,[596] and after metastasis of carcinoma to the adrenal gland.[21] Finally, aldosterone synthesis is selectively reduced by heparin, with a 7% incidence of hyperkalemia associated with heparin therapy.[597] Both unfractionated[597] and low-molecular-weight[21,598] heparin can cause hyperkalemia. Hyperkalemia because of prophylactic subcutaneous unfractionated heparin (5000 U bid) has also been reported.[599] Heparin reduces the adrenal aldosterone response to Ang II and hyperkalemia, resulting in hyperreninemic hyperaldosteronism. Histologic findings in experimental animals include a marked diminution in size of the zona glomerulosa and an attenuated hyperplastic response to salt depletion.[597]

Most primary adrenal insufficiency is as a result of autoimmunity in Addison disease or in the context of a polyglandular endocrinopathy.[587,600] Adrenal insufficiency can be seen following adrenalectomy for primary hyperaldosteronism, with 14% developing postoperative hyperkalemia and 5% developing long-term insufficiency requiring fludrocortisone.[601] The antiphospholipid syndrome may also cause bilateral adrenal hemorrhage and adrenal insufficiency.[602] Another renal syndrome in which there should be a high index of suspicion for adrenal insufficiency is renal amyloidosis.[603] Finally, HIV is a particularly important infectious cause of adrenal insufficiency. The most common cause of adrenalitis in HIV disease is cytomegalovirus (CMV); however, a long list of infectious, degenerative, and infiltrative processes may involve the adrenal glands in these patients.[604] Although the adrenal involvement in HIV is usually subclinical, adrenal insufficiency may be precipitated by stress, drugs such as ketoconazole that inhibit steroidogenesis, or the acute withdrawal of steroid agents such as megestrol.

Current estimates of the risk of hyperkalemia with Addison disease are lacking, but the incidence is likely 50% to 60%.[21] The interaction between dietary $Na^+$ and $K^+$ intake and sweat $Na^+$ loss is especially clinically relevant in physically active individuals with Addison disease in humid environments. Mineralocorticoid supplementation may be necessary in these active individuals. The absence of hyperkalemia in such a high percentage of typical hypoadrenal patients underscores the importance of aldosterone-independent modulation of $K^+$ excretion by the distal nephron. A high-$K^+$ diet and high peritubular $K^+$ serves to increase apical $Na^+$ reabsorption and $K^+$ secretion in the CNT and CCD (see "Control of Potassium Excretion"). In most patients with reductions in circulating aldosterone, this homeostatic mechanism would appear to be sufficient to regulate plasma $K^+$ to within normal limits.

### Hyporeninemic Hypoaldosteronism

Hyporeninemic hypoaldosteronism[605] is a very common predisposing factor in several large, overlapping subsets of hyperkalemic patients—diabetics,[606] older adults,[21,179,607] and patients with renal insufficiency.[21] Hyporeninemic hypoaldosteronism has also been described in systemic lupus erythematosus (SLE),[21,608] multiple myeloma,[29] and acute glomerulonephritis.[29] Classically, patients should have suppressed plasma renin activity (PRA) and aldosterone, which cannot be activated by typical maneuvers such as furosemide or sodium restriction.[605] Approximately 50% have an associated acidosis, with a reduced renal excretion of $NH_4^+$, a positive urinary anion gap, and urine pH less than 5.5.[187,254] Although the generation of this acidosis is clearly multifactorial,[609] strong clinical[253,254,610] and experimental[249] evidence has suggested that hyperkalemia per se is the dominant factor as a result of competitive inhibition of $NH_4^+$ transport in the TAL and reduced distal excretion of $NH_4^+$.[611] (See also "Consequences of Hyperkalemia.")

Several factors account for the reduced PRA in diabetic patients with hyporeninemic hypoaldosteronism.[606] First, many patients have an associated autonomic neuropathy, with impaired release of renin during orthostatic challenges.[21] Failure to respond to isoproterenol with an increase in PRA, despite an adequate cardiovascular response, suggests a postreceptor defect in the ability of the juxtaglomerular apparatus to respond to β-adrenergic stimuli[21] (see also "Regulation of Renal Renin and Adrenal Aldosterone"). Second, the conversion of prorenin to active renin is impaired in some diabetics,[606] despite adequate release of prorenin in response to furosemide[21]; this suggests a defect in the normal processing of prorenin. Third, as is the case with perhaps all patients with hyporeninemic hypoaldosteronism (see later), many diabetic patients appear to be volume-expanded, with subsequent suppression of PRA.

The most attractive unifying hypothesis for the suppression of PRA in hyporeninemic hypoaldosteronism is that primary volume expansion increases circulating ANP levels, which then exerts a negative effect on renal renin and adrenal aldosterone release (see also "Regulation of Renal Renin and Adrenal Aldosterone"). There is evidence that these patients are volume-expanded, and many will respond to $Na^+$-$Cl^-$ restriction or to furosemide with an increased PRA—that is, renin is physiologically rather than pathologically suppressed.[612–614] Patients with hyporeninemic hypoaldosteronism caused by a diversity of underlying causes have elevated ANP levels,[21,29,179,613,615] which is also an indicator of their underlying volume expansion. Patients who respond to furosemide with an increase in PRA exhibit a concomitant decrease in ANP.[613] Furthermore, the infusion of exogenous ANP can suppress the adrenal aldosterone response to hyperkalemia[179] and dietary $Na^+$-$Cl^-$ depletion.[616]

### Acquired Tubular Defects and Potassium Excretion

Unlike hyporeninemic hypoaldosteronism, hyperkalemic distal renal tubular acidosis is associated with a normal or increased aldosterone and/or PRA. Urine pH in these patients is more than 5.5, and they are unable to increase acid or $K^+$ excretion in response to furosemide, $Na^+$-$SO_4^{2-}$, or fludrocortisone.[617–619] Classic causes include SLE,[617] sickle cell anemia,[21,619] and amyloidosis.[21]

### Hereditary Tubular Defects and Potassium Excretion

Hereditary tubular causes of hyperkalemia have overlapping clinical features with hypoaldosteronism—hence, the shared label pseudohypoaldosteronism (PHA). PHA-I has both an autosomal recessive and autosomal dominant form. The autosomal dominant form is caused by loss-of-function mutations in the mineralocorticoid receptor.[620] These patients require aggressive salt supplementation during early childhood; however, similar to the hypoaldosteronism caused by mutations in aldosterone synthase, they typically become asymptomatic in adulthood.[407] Of interest, the lifelong increases in circulating aldosterone, Ang II, and renin seen in this syndrome do not appear to have untoward cardiovascular consequences.[620]

The recessive form of PHA-I is caused by various combinations of mutations in all three subunits of ENaC, resulting in impairment in its channel activity.[407] Patients with this syndrome present with severe neonatal salt wasting, hypotension, and hyperkalemia; in contrast to the autosomal dominant form of PHA-I, the syndrome does not improve in adulthood.[407] One unexpected result in the physiologic characterization of ENaC was that mice with a targeted deletion of the α-ENaC subunit were found to die within 40 hours of birth caused by pulmonary edema.[29] Patients with recessive PHA-I may have pulmonary symptoms, which can occasionally be very severe.[621] However, it appears that unlike in ENaC-deficient mice, the modest residual activity associated with heteromeric PHA-I channels is generally sufficient to mediate pulmonary $Na^+$ and fluid clearance in humans with loss-of-function mutations in ENaC.[622]

Pseudohypoaldosteronism type II (PHA-II) (also known as Gordon syndrome and, more recently, as FHHt) is in every respect the mirror image of GS; the clinical phenotype includes hypertension, hyperkalemia, hyperchloremic metabolic acidosis, suppressed PRA and aldosterone, hypercalciuria, and reduced bone density.[623] FHHt behaves like a gain of function in the thiazide-sensitive $Na^+$-$Cl^-$ cotransporter NCC, and treatment with thiazides typically results in resolution of the entire clinical picture.[623] FHHt is an extreme form of hyporeninemic hypoaldosteronism caused by volume expansion; aggressive salt restriction decreases ANP levels and increases PRA, with resolution of the hypertension, hyperkalemia, and metabolic acidosis.[615]

FHHt is an autosomal dominant syndrome, with four genetic loci. In an initial landmark paper, mutations in two related serine-threonine kinases were detected in various kindreds with FHHt.[624] The catalytic sites of these kinases lack specific catalytic lysines conserved in other kinases—hence, the designation WNK. Whereas FHHt mutations in WNK4 affect the C-terminus of the coding sequence, large intronic deletions in the WNK1 gene result in increased expression. Both kinases are expressed in the distal nephron, in both DCT and CCD cells; whereas WNK1 localizes to the cytoplasm and basolateral membrane, WNK4 protein is found at the apical tight junctions.[624] WNK-dependent phosphorylation and activation of the downstream SPAK (STE20/SPS1-related proline/alanine-rich kinase) and OSR1 (oxidative stress-responsive kinase 1) kinases lead to phosphorylation of a cluster of N-terminal threonines in NCC, resulting in an activation of $Na^+$-$Cl^-$ cotransport[144] (see also Fig. 17.6). However, coexpression of WNK4 with NCC reveals an additional inhibitory influence of the kinase on NCC, effects that are blocked by FHHt-associated point mutations in the kinase.[625] In particular, the inhibitory effects of WNK4 appear to dominate in mouse models with overexpression of wild-type versus FHHt mutant WNK4.[73] Mutations in the *Cullin 3* and *kelch-like 3* (*KLHL3*) genes also cause FHHt; the proteins encoded by these genes are part of a ubiquitin ligase complex that regulates the WNK1 and WNK4 kinase proteins. Autosomal dominant mutations in both *Cullin 3* and *KLHL3* act through dominant negative effects.[626,627]

A key insight from the mechanistic study of FHHt is that the activation of NCC in the DCT in this syndrome serves to reduce $Na^+$ delivery to principal cells in the downstream CNT and CCD, leading to hyperkalemia.[73] This and other effects of the WNK pathways on distal $K^+$ secretion are discussed earlier in this chapter (see "Control of Potassium Secretion: Effect of Potassium Intake").

## MEDICATION-RELATED HYPERKALEMIA

### Cyclooxygenase Inhibitors

Hyperkalemia is a well-recognized complication of NSAIDs that inhibit cyclooxygenases. NSAIDs cause hyperkalemia by a variety of mechanisms, as would be predicted from the relevant physiology. By decreasing the GFR and increasing sodium retention, they decrease distal delivery of $Na^+$ and reduce the distal flow rate. Moreover, the flow-activated apical maxi-K channel in the CNT and CCD is activated by prostaglandins[628]; hence, NSAIDs will reduce its activity and the flow-dependent component of $K^+$ excretion.[77,443] NSAIDs are also a classic cause of hyporeninemic hypoaldosteronism.[629,630] The administration of indomethacin to normal volunteers thus attenuates furosemide-induced increases in PRA.[165,631] Finally, NSAIDs would not cause hyperkalemia with such regularity if they did not also blunt the adrenal response to hyperkalemia, which is at least partially dependent on prostaglandins acting through prostaglandin EP2 receptors and cAMP.[178]

The physiology reviewed earlier in this chapter (see "Regulation of Renal Renin and Adrenal Aldosterone") would suggest that COX-2 inhibitors are equally likely to cause hyperkalemia. Indeed, COX-2 inhibitors can clearly cause sodium retention and a decrease in the GFR,[632,633] suggesting NSAID-like effects on renal pathophysiology. COX-2–derived prostaglandins stimulate renal renin release,[21] and COX-2 inhibitors reduce PRA in both dogs[29] and humans.[165] Salt restriction potentiates the hyperkalemia seen in dogs treated with COX-2 inhibitors[29] so that hypovolemic patients may be particularly prone to hyperkalemia in this setting. The COX-2 inhibitor celecoxib and the nonselective NSAID ibuprofen have equivalent negative effects on $K^+$ excretion after a defined oral load.[634] Not surprisingly, hyperkalemia and acute kidney injury are associated with COX-2 inhibitors.[21,635,636] Where the data have been reported, circulating PRA and/or aldosterone levels have been reduced in hyperkalemia associated with COX-2 inhibitors.[29,636]

### Cyclosporine and Tacrolimus

Both cyclosporine[637] (CsA) and tacrolimus[638] cause hyperkalemia; the risk of sustained hyperkalemia may be higher in renal transplant patients treated with tacrolimus than in those treated with CsA.[639] CsA is perhaps the most versatile of all drugs in the variety of mechanisms whereby it causes hyperkalemia. It causes hyporeninemic hypoaldosteronism,[640] due in part to its inhibitory effect on COX-2 expression in the macula densa.[641] CsA inhibits apical SK secretory $K^+$ channels in the distal nephron[642] in addition to basolateral $Na^+$-$K^+$-ATPase.[21] Finally, CsA causes redistribution of $K^+$ and hyperkalemia, particularly when used in combination with beta-blockers.[643] A provocative but preliminary report has linked acute hyperkalemia secondary to CsA to indirect activation of $K_{ATP}$ channels (also see earlier).[580]

### Epithelial $Na^+$ Channel Inhibition

Inhibition of apical ENaC activity in the distal nephron by amiloride and other $K^+$-sparing diuretics predictably results in hyperkalemia. Amiloride is structurally similar to the antibiotics TMP and pentamidine, which can also inhibit ENaC.[644–646] TMP thus inhibits $Na^+$ reabsorption and $K^+$ secretion in perfused CCDs.[647] Both TMP-SMX (Bactrim) and pentamidine were reported to cause hyperkalemia during high-dose treatment of *Pneumocystis* pneumonia in HIV patients,[21,646] who are otherwise predisposed to hyperkalemia. However, this side effect is not restricted to high-dose intravenous therapy. In a study of hospitalized patients treated with standard doses of TMP, significant hyperkalemia occurred in more than 50%, with severe hyperkalemia (>5.5 mmol/L) in 21%.[648] Risk factors for hyperkalemia because of normal-dose TMP include renal insufficiency,[648] hyporeninemic hypoaldosteronism,[649] and concomitant use of ACE inhibitors and ARBs.[650] This is not a trivial association, in that TMP-SMX administration increases the risk of sudden death in patients treated with ACE inhibitors, ARBs, or spironolactone.[651]

Whereas TMP and pentamidine directly inhibit ENaC, a novel indirect mechanism for ENaC inhibition–associated hyperkalemia has also been reported.[21,112] Aldosterone induces expression of the membrane-associated proteases CAP1–3 (see "Control of Potassium Excretion"). Nafamostat, a protease inhibitor that is used for pancreatitis, especially in Japan, and during hemodialysis as an anticoagulant to prevent the proteolysis of fibrinogen into fibrin, is known to cause hyperkalemia.[112] Indirect evidence has suggested that the mechanism involves inhibition of amiloride-sensitive $Na^+$ channels in the CCD.[21] Treatment of rats with nafamostat was also shown to reduce the urinary excretion of CAP1/prostasin, in contrast to the reported effect of aldosterone.[106] Thus, inhibition of the protease activity of CAP1 by nafamostat appears to abrogate its activating effect on ENaC (Fig. 17.13) and may reduce expression of the protein in the CCD.[113]

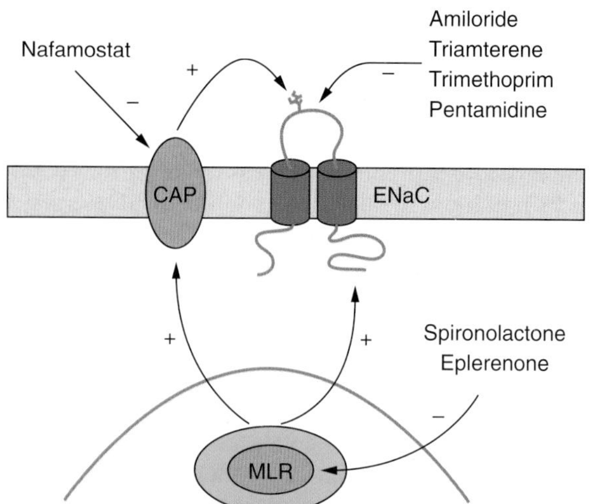


**Fig. 17.13** Pharmacologic inhibition of the epithelial $Na^+$ channel *(ENaC)*. Whereas amiloride and related compounds directly inhibit the channel, the protease inhibitor nafamostat inhibits membrane-associated proteases such as channel-activating protease *(CAP)*, thus indirectly inhibiting the channel. Spironolactone and related drugs inhibit the mineralocorticoid receptor *(MLR)*, thus reducing transcription of the alpha subunit of ENaC, the ENaC-activating kinase SGK, and several other target genes (see text for details).

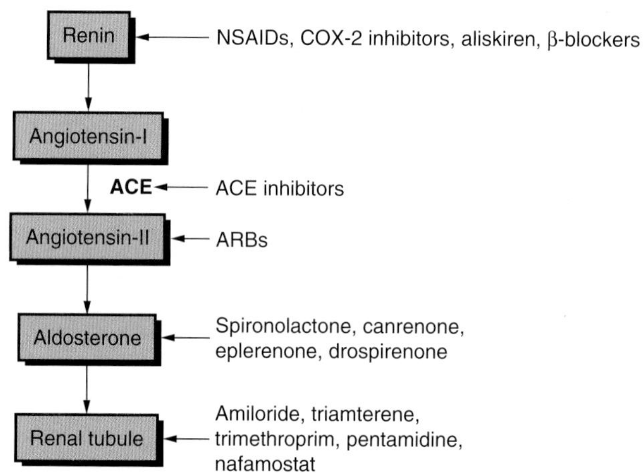


**Fig. 17.14** Medications that target the renin-angiotensin-aldosterone axis are common causes of hyperkalemia, as are drugs that inhibit epithelial $Na^+$ channels (ENaC) in the renal tubule (connecting segment [CNT] or cortical collecting duct [CCD]). *ACE,* Angiotensin-converting enzyme; *ARB,* angiotensin-receptor blocker; *COX-2,* cyclooxygenase-2; *NSAIDs,* nonsteroidal inflammatory drugs.

### Angiotensin-Converting Enzyme Inhibitors and Mineralocorticoid and Angiotensin Antagonists

Hyperkalemia is a predictable and common effect of ACE inhibition, direct renin inhibition, and antagonism of the mineralocorticoid and angiotensin receptors[652] (Fig. 17.14). The oral contraceptive agent Yasmin-28 and related products contain the progestin drospirenone, which inhibits the mineralocorticoid receptor[653] and can potentially cause hyperkalemia in susceptible patients. As with many other causes of hyperkalemia, that induced by pharmacologic targeting of the RAAS axis depends on concomitant inhibition of the adrenal aldosterone release by hyperkalemia. The adrenal release of aldosterone because of increased $K^+$ is clearly dependent on an intact adrenal RAAS, such that this response is abrogated by systemic ACE inhibitors and ARBs[173] (see "Regulation of Renal Renin and Adrenal Aldosterone"). Dual treatment with lisinopril and spironolactone in subjects with CKD is also associated with a reduction in extrarenal potassium disposition, given that reduced $K^+$ excretion alone does not explain the substantial increase in serum $K^+$ after a defined oral potassium load.[654] Similarly, the addition of spironolactone to losartan in the treatment of diabetic nephropathy causes a significant increase in serum $K^+$ without significant changes in urinary $K^+$ excretion.[655] ACE inhibitors and ARBs have the additional potential to cause acute renal failure and acute hyperkalemia in patients with an angiotensin-dependent GFR; the renin inhibitor aliskiren has also been reported to cause acute renal failure with acute hyperkalemia, albeit in conjunction with spironolactone.[656]

RAAS inhibitors are an increasingly important cause of hyperkalemia, given the indications to combine spironolactone with ACE inhibitors and/or ARBs in renal and cardiac disease,[657] in addition to the emergence of mineralocorticoid receptor antagonists with perhaps a greater potential for hyperkalemia.[658] Hyperkalemia can occur within 1 week of starting angiotensin receptor blockade.[659] Heart failure, diabetes, and CKD increase the risk of hyperkalemia from these agents.[652,660,661] The prevalence of hyperkalemia associated with the combined use of mineralocorticoid receptor antagonists and ACE inhibitors/ARBs appears to be much higher in clinical practice (~10%[662]) than what has been reported in large clinical trials,[652] in part because of the use of higher than recommended doses.[21] Notably, Juurlink and colleagues have studied the correlation between the rate of spironolactone prescription for Canadian patients with heart failure on ACE inhibitors following the publication of the Randomized Aldactone Evaluation Study (RALES), with hyperkalemia and associated morbidity.[663,664] This provocative study found an abrupt increase in the rate of prescribing for spironolactone after the release of RALES, with a temporal correlation to increases in the rate of admissions with hyperkalemia.[664] The association remained statistically significant for admissions where hyperkalemia was the primary diagnosis.[665] However, a study from the United Kingdom found a similar increase in spironolactone use after the publication of RALES, but without an increase in hyperkalemia or hyperkalemia-associated admissions to hospital.[666] It should also be emphasized that the development of hyperkalemia, or for that matter the presence of predisposing factors for hyperkalemia, does not appear to mitigate the mortality benefits of eplerenone in heart failure.[661]

Given the mounting evidence supporting the combined use of ACE inhibitors, ARBs, and/or mineralocorticoid receptor antagonists, it is prudent to adhere systematically to measures that will minimize the chance of associated hyperkalemia, therefore allowing patients to benefit from the cardiovascular and renal effects of these agents. The patients at risk for the development of hyperkalemia in response to drugs that target the RAAS axis, singly or in combination therapy, are those in whom the ability of kidneys to excrete the potassium load is markedly diminished because of one or a combination of the following: (1) decreased delivery of sodium to the CCD (e.g., as in congestive heart failure, volume depletion); (2) decreased circulating aldosterone (e.g., hyporeninemic hypoaldosteronism, drugs such as heparin or ketoconazole); (3) inhibition of amiloride-sensitive $Na^+$ channels in the CNT and CCD by coadministration of TMP-SMX, pentamidine, or amiloride; (4) chronic tubulointerstitial disease, with associated dysfunction of the distal nephron; and (5) increased potassium intake (e.g., salt substitutes, diet). Overall, patients with diabetes, heart failure, and/or CKD are at particular risk for hyperkalemia from RAAS inhibition.[652,660,661] In these susceptible patients, the following approach is recommended to prevent or minimize the occurrence of hyperkalemia in response to medications that interfere with the RAAS[29,667]:

1. Estimate the GFR using the MDRD and/or related equations.
2. Inquire about diet and dietary supplements (e.g., salt substitutes, licorice) and prescribe a low-potassium diet, preferably with the assistance of a nutritionist.
3. Inquire about medications, particularly those that can interfere with renal $K^+$ excretion (e.g., NSAIDs, COX-2 inhibitors, $K^+$-sparing diuretics) and, if appropriate, discontinue these agents.
4. Continue or initiate loop or thiazide-like diuretics, if otherwise appropriate (e.g., hypertension, edema).
5. Correct acidosis with sodium bicarbonate.
6. Initiate treatment with a low dose of only one of the agents(e.g., ACE inhibitor, ARB, mineralocorticoid receptor antagonist).
7. Check serum $K^+$ 3 to 5 days after initiation of therapy and each dose increment, at most within 1 week,[659] followed by another measurement 1 week later.
8. If the serum $K^+$ is more than 5.6 mmol/L, ACE inhibitors, ARBs, and/or mineralocorticoid receptor blockers should be stopped and the patient should be treated for hyperkalemia.
9. If the serum $K^+$ is increased but less than 5.6 mmol/L, reduce the dose and reassess the possible contributing factors. If the patient is on a combination of ACE inhibitors, ARBs, and/or mineralocorticoid receptor blockers, all but one should be stopped and the potassium level rechecked.
10. A combination of a mineralocorticoid receptor blocker and an ACE inhibitor or ARB should be used with extreme caution in patients with CKD stage IV or V (eGFR < 30 mL/min/1.73 m$^2$).
11. The dose of spironolactone in combination with ACE inhibitors or ARBs should be no more than 25 mg/day.

## CLINICAL APPROACH TO HYPERKALEMIA

The first priority in the management of hyperkalemia is to assess the need for emergency treatment (electrocardiographic changes, $K^+ \geq 6.5$ mmol/L). This should be followed by a comprehensive workup to determine the cause (Fig. 17.15). The history and physical examination should focus on medications (e.g., ACE inhibitors, NSAIDs, TMP-SMX), diet and dietary supplements (e.g., salt substitute), risk factors for kidney failure, reduction in urine output, blood pressure, and volume status. Initial laboratory tests should include electrolytes, urea, creatinine, plasma osmolality, $Mg^{2+}$, and $Ca^{2+}$, a complete blood count, and urinary pH, osmolality, creatinine, and electrolytes. Plasma and urine osmolality are required for calculation of the TTKG. The determination of urinary electrolytes for calculation of the TTKG or urine $K^+$-to-creatinine ratio also provides the opportunity for the measurement of urinary $Na^+$, which will determine whether significant prerenal stimuli are limiting distal $Na^+$ delivery and thus $K^+$ excretion (see "Urinary Indices of Potassium Excretion"). Plasma renin activity, plasma aldosterone, and assessing the response in TTKG or urinary $K^+$-to-creatinine ratio to fludrocortisone, after a few hours, may be necessary to determine the specific cause of an inappropriately low TTKG in hyperkalemia.

## MANAGEMENT OF HYPERKALEMIA

Indications for the hospitalization of patients with hyperkalemia are poorly defined, in part because there is no universally accepted definition for mild, moderate, or severe hyperkalemia. The clinical sequelae of hyperkalemia, which are primarily cardiac and neuromuscular, depend on many other variables (e.g., plasma calcium level, acid-base status, plasma $K^+$ rate of change[234-237]), in addition to the absolute value of the serum $K^+$;[521,668] these issues are likely to influence management decisions. Severe hyperkalemia (serum $K^+ \geq 8.0$ mmol/L), electrocardiographic changes other than peaked T waves,

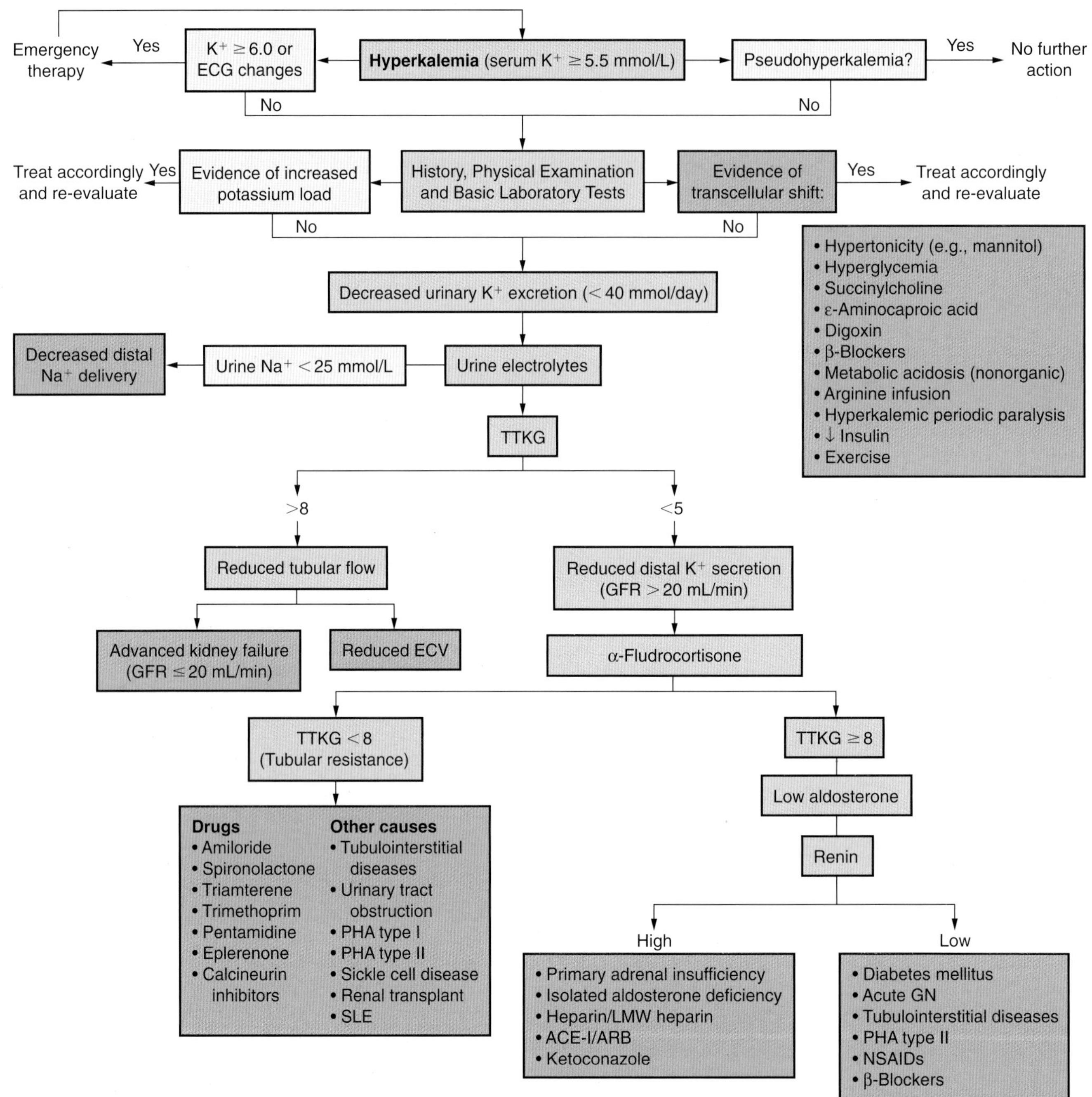


**Fig. 17.15** The clinical approach to hyperkalemia. See text for details. *ACE-I,* Angiotensin-converting enzyme inhibitor; *ARB,* angiotensin-receptor blocker; *ECG,* electrocardiogram; *ECV,* effective circulatory volume; *GFR,* glomerular filtration rate; acute *GN,* acute glomerulonephritis; *LMW heparin,* low-molecular-weight heparin; *NSAIDs,* nonsteroidal antiinflammatory drugs; *PHA,* pseudohypoaldosteronism; *SLE,* systemic lupus erythematosus; *TTKG,* transtubular potassium gradient.

acute deterioration of renal function, and the existence of additional medical problems have been suggested as appropriate criteria for hospitalization.[521] However, hyperkalemia in patients with any electrocardiographic manifestation should be considered a true medical emergency and treated urgently[229,520,669,670]; adequate management and serial monitoring of serum $K^+$ will generally require admission. Given the limitations of electrocardiographic changes as a predictor of cardiac toxicity (see "Consequences of Hyperkalemia"), patients with severe hyperkalemia ($K^+$ ≥6.5–7.0 mmol/L) in the absence of electrocardiographic changes should be aggressively managed.[195,229,520,670–672]

Urgent management of hyperkalemia constitutes a 12-lead ECG, admission to the hospital, continuous electrocardiographic monitoring, and immediate treatment. The treatment of hyperkalemia is generally divided into three categories: (1) antagonism of the cardiac effects of hyperkalemia; (2) rapid reduction in $K^+$ by redistribution into cells; and (3) removal of $K^+$ from the body. The necessary measures to treat the underlying conditions causing hyperkalemia should be undertaken to minimize the factors that are contributing to hyperkalemia and to prevent future episodes.[229] Dietary restriction (usually 60 mEq/day) with emphasis on $K^+$ content of total parenteral nutrition (TPN) solutions and enteral feeding products (typically 25–50 mmol/L) and adjustment of medications and intravenous fluids are necessary; hidden sources of $K^+$, such as intravenous antibiotics,[553] should not be overlooked.

## ANTAGONISM OF CARDIAC EFFECTS

Intravenous calcium is the first-line drug in the emergency management of hyperkalemia, even in patients with normal calcium levels. The mutually antagonistic effects of calcium and $K^+$ on the myocardium and the protective role of $Ca^{2+}$ in hyperkalemia have long been known.[673] Calcium raises the action potential threshold to a less negative value, without changing the resting membrane potential; by restoring the usual 15-mV difference between resting and threshold potentials, myocyte excitability is reduced.[195,674] Administration of calcium also alters the relationship between $V_{max}$ and the resting membrane potential, maintaining a more normal $V_{max}$ at less negative resting membrane potentials and thus restoring myocardial conduction.[195]

Calcium is available as calcium chloride or calcium gluconate (10-mL ampules of 10% solutions) for intravenous infusion. Each milliliter of 10% calcium gluconate or calcium chloride has 8.9 mg (0.22 mmol) and 27.2 mg (0.68 mmol) of elemental calcium, respectively.[675] Calcium gluconate[676] is less irritating to the veins and can be used through a peripheral intravenous (IV) line; calcium chloride can cause tissue necrosis if it extravasates and requires a central line. The efficacy and onset of action are equivalent for calcium chloride and calcium gluconate, despite the higher molar calcium concentration of calcium chloride ampules.[677] A study of patients undergoing cardiac surgery with extracorporeal perfusion (with concomitant high gluconate infusion) has suggested that the increase in the ionized calcium level is significantly lower with calcium gluconate.[678] This finding was attributed to a requirement for hepatic metabolism in the release of ionized calcium from calcium gluconate, so that less ionized calcium would be bioavailable in cases of liver failure or diminished hepatic perfusion.[678] However, further in vitro studies in animals, in humans with normal hepatic function, and during the anhepatic stage of liver transplantation have shown equal and rapid dissociation of ionized calcium from equal doses of calcium chloride and calcium gluconate, indicating that the release of ionized calcium from calcium gluconate is independent of hepatic metabolism.[29,677]

The recommended dose is 10 mL of 10% calcium gluconate (3–4 mL of calcium chloride), infused intravenously over 2 to 3 minutes and under continuous electrocardiographic monitoring. The effect of the infusion starts in 1 to 3 minutes and lasts 30 to 60 minutes.[525,672] The dose should be repeated if there is no change in electrocardiographic findings or if they recur after initial improvement.[525,672,677] However, calcium should be used with extreme caution in patients taking digitalis because hypercalcemia potentiates the toxic effects of digitalis on the myocardium.[676] In this case, 10 mL of 10% calcium gluconate should be added to 100 mL of D5W and infused over 20 to 30 minutes to avoid hypercalcemia and allow for an even distribution of calcium in the extracellular compartment.[523,671,674] To prevent the precipitation of calcium carbonate, calcium should not be administered in solutions containing bicarbonate.

## REDISTRIBUTION OF $K^+$ INTO CELLS

Sodium bicarbonate, beta-2 agonists, and insulin with glucose are all used in the treatment of hyperkalemia to induce a redistribution of $K^+$. Of these treatments, insulin with glucose is the most constant and reliable, whereas bicarbonate is the most controversial. However, they are all temporary measures and should not be substituted for the definitive therapy of hyperkalemia, which is removal of $K^+$ from the body.

### Insulin and Glucose

Insulin has the ability to lower the plasma $K^+$ level by shifting $K^+$ into cells, particularly into skeletal myocytes and hepatocytes (see "Factors Affecting Internal Distribution of Potassium"). This effect is reliable, reproducible, dose-dependent,[525] and effective, even in patients with CKD and ESKD[679–681] and in the anhepatic stage of liver transplantation.[682] The effect of insulin on plasma $K^+$ levels is independent of age, adrenergic activity,[683] and its hypoglycemic effect, which may be impaired in patients with CKD and/or ESKD.[29]

Insulin can be administered with glucose as a constant infusion or as a bolus injection.[680,681] One recommended dose for insulin with glucose infusion is 10 U of regular insulin in 500 mL of 10% dextrose, given over 60 minutes (there is no further drop in plasma $K^+$ after 90 minutes of insulin infusion).[674,683] However, a bolus injection is easier to administer, particularly under emergency conditions.[229] The recommended dose is 10 U of regular insulin administered intravenously followed immediately by 50 mL of 50% dextrose (25 g of glucose).[669,680,684,685] The effect of insulin on the $K^+$ level begins in 10 to 20 minutes, peaks at 30 to 60 minutes, and lasts for 4 to 6 hours.[525,671,680,686] In almost all patients, the serum $K^+$ drops by 0.5 to 1.2 mmol/L after this treatment.[681,682,685,686] The dose can be repeated as necessary.

Despite glucose administration, hypoglycemia may occur in up to 75% of patients treated with the bolus regimen described previously, typically 1 hour after the infusion.[680] The likelihood of hypoglycemia is greater when the dose of glucose given is less than 30 g.[523] To prevent this, infusion of 10% dextrose at 50 to 75 mL/hour and close monitoring of the blood glucose levels is recommended.[669,684] Administration of glucose without insulin is not recommended because the endogenous insulin release may be variable.[571] Glucose in the absence of insulin may increase the plasma $K^+$ by increasing plasma osmolality.[562,563,684] In hyperglycemic patients with glucose levels of 200 to 250 mg/dL or more, insulin should be administered without glucose and with close monitoring of the plasma glucose level.[674] Combined treatment with beta-2 agonists, in addition to their synergism with insulin in lowering plasma $K^+$, may reduce the level of hypoglycemia.[680] Of note, the combined regimen may increase the heart rate by $15.1 \pm 6.0$ beats per minute.[680]

There are theoretic reasons to consider the use of newer, rapid-acting forms of insulin that do not form insulin hexamers, particularly in patients with renal insufficiency.[687] At present, however, in the absence of rigorous clinical trials that directly compare different regimens,[688] there is no perceived need to alter the "typical" recommended dose of

10 U of regular insulin administered intravenously followed immediately by 50 mL of 50% dextrose (25 g of glucose).

### $\beta_2$-Adrenergic Agonists

$\beta_2$-Agonists are an important but underused group of agents for the acute management of hyperkalemia. They exert their effect by activating $Na^+/K^+$-ATPase and the NKCC1 $Na^+$-$K^+$-$2Cl^-$ cotransporter, shifting $K^+$ into hepatocytes and skeletal myocytes (see also "Factors Affecting Internal Distribution of Potassium"). Albuterol (Salbutamol), a selective beta-2 agonist, is the most widely studied and used. It is available in oral, inhaled, and intravenous forms; both the intravenous and inhaled or nebulized forms are effective.[689]

The recommended dose for intravenous administration, which is not available in the United States, is 0.5 mg of albuterol in 100 mL of 5% dextrose, given over 10 to 15 minutes.[674,689,690] Its $K^+$-lowering effect starts in a few minutes, is maximal at about 30 to 40 minutes,[689,690] and lasts for 2 to 6 hours.[523] It reduces serum $K^+$ levels by approximately 0.9 to 1.4 mmol/L.[523]

The recommended dose for inhaled albuterol, also known as salbutamol, is 10 to 20 mg of nebulized albuterol in 4 mL of normal saline, inhaled over 10 minutes[680] (nebulized levalbuterol is as effective as albuterol).[691] This dose is distinct from the 100-µg dose administered by each puffer spray. Its kaliopenic effect starts at about 30 minutes, reaches its peak at about 90 minutes,[680,689] and lasts for 2 to 6 hours.[523,689] Inhaled albuterol reduces serum $K^+$ levels by approximately 0.5 to 1.0 mmol/L[523]; albuterol administered by a metered-dose inhaler with spacer reduces serum $K^+$ level by approximately 0.4 mmol/L.[692] Albuterol (in inhaled or parenteral form) and insulin with glucose have an additive effect on reducing serum $K^+$ levels by approximately 1.2 to 1.5 mmol/L in total.[523,680,686] However, a subset of patients with ESKD (~20%–40%) are not responsive to the $K^+$-lowering effect of albuterol ($\Delta K \leq 0.4$ mmol/L); albuterol (or other beta-2 agonists) should not be used as a single agent in the treatment of hyperkalemia.[525,571] In an attempt to reduce pharmacokinetic variability, one study tested the effects of weight-based dosing on serum $K^+$ levels, using 7 µg/kg of subcutaneous terbutaline (a beta-2 agonist) in a group of ESKD patients.[693] The results showed a significant decline in serum $K^+$ levels in almost all patients (mean, $1.31 \pm 0.5$ mmol/L; range, 0.5 to 2.3 mmol/L) in 30 to 90 minutes; of note, the heart rate increased by an average of $25.8 \pm 10.5$ beats per minute (range, 6.5–48 beats per minute).[693]

Treatment with albuterol may result in an increase in plasma glucose (~2–3 mmol/L) and heart rate. The increase in heart rate is more pronounced with the intravenous form (~20 beats per minute) than with the inhaled form (~6–10 beats per minute).[571,689] There is no significant increase in systolic or diastolic blood pressure with nebulized or intravenous administration of albuterol.[689] However, it is prudent to use these agents with caution in patients with ischemic heart disease.[523]

### Sodium Bicarbonate

Bicarbonate has prevailed as a preferred treatment modality of hyperkalemia for decades. For example, in a survey of nephrology training program directors in 1989, it was ranked as the second-line treatment, after $Ca^{2+}$.[694] Its use to treat acute hyperkalemia was mainly based on small, older, uncontrolled clinical studies with a very limited number of patients,[58,695,696] in which bicarbonate was typically administered as a long infusion over many hours (contrary to an IV push, which later became the routine).[697] One of these studies, which is frequently quoted, concluded that the $K^+$-lowering effect of bicarbonate is independent of changes in pH.[695] However, confounding variables included the duration of infusion, use of glucose-containing solutions, and infrequent monitoring of serum $K^+$.[695,698]

The role of bicarbonate in the acute treatment of hyperkalemia has been challenged.[681,697,699] Blumberg and colleagues have compared different $K^+$-lowering modalities (Fig. 17.16) and showed that bicarbonate infusion (isotonic or hypertonic) for up to 60 minutes has no effect on serum $K^+$ in their cohort of ESKD patients on hemodialysis[681]; there is, however, an effect of isotonic bicarbonate at 4 to 6 hours (see later).[697] These observations were later confirmed by others, who failed to show any acute (60–20 minutes) $K^+$-lowering effects for bicarbonate.[697–699] A few studies have shown that metabolic acidosis may attenuate the physiologic responses to insulin and beta-2 agonists.[525,699] The combined effect of bicarbonate and insulin with glucose has been studied, with conflicting results.[699] In addition, bicarbonate and albuterol coadministration failed to show any additional benefit over albuterol alone.[699]

In summary, bicarbonate administration, especially as a single agent without dilution, has no role in the contemporary treatment of acute hyperkalemia. Prolonged infusion of isotonic bicarbonate in ESKD patients does, however, reduce serum $K^+$ at 5 to 6 hours by up to 0.7 mmol/L; approximately half of this effect can be attributed to volume expansion.[697] Regardless of the mechanism, bicarbonate

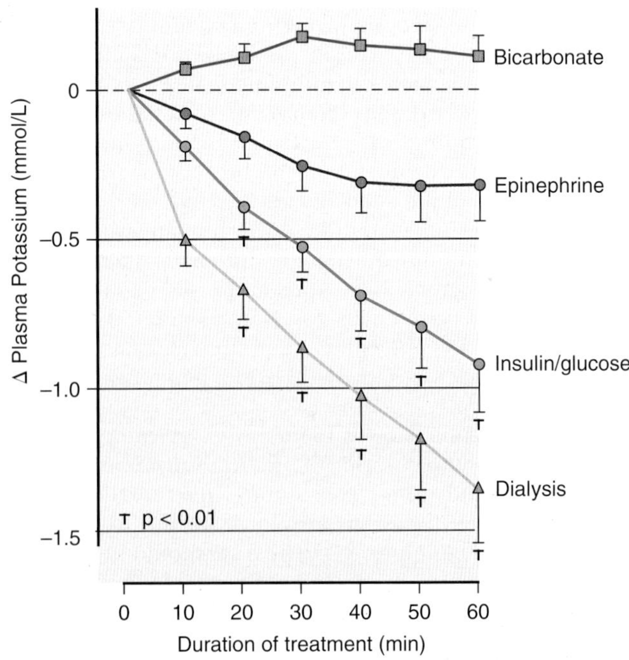


**Fig. 17.16** Changes in serum $K^+$ during intravenous infusion of bicarbonate, epinephrine, or insulin in glucose and during hemodialysis. (From Blumberg A, Weidmann P, Shaw S, Gnadinger M. Effect of various therapeutic approaches on plasma potassium and major regulating factors in terminal renal failure. *Am J Med.* 1988;85:507–512.)

infusion may thus have a limited role in the subacute control of hyperkalemia—for example in the nondialytic management of patients with severe hyperkalemia.[700] The acute effect of bicarbonate infusion on serum $K^+$ in severely acidemic patients is not clear; however, it may be of some benefit in this setting.[229,669] Of note, the infusion of sodium bicarbonate may reduce serum ionized calcium levels and cause volume overload, issues of relevance in acidemic patients with renal failure.[525,671] When bicarbonate administration is used for hyperkalemia, we recommend isotonic infusion of sodium bicarbonate; although hypertonic sodium bicarbonate does not increase the serum $K^+$ level,[558] it has been reported to cause hypernatremia.[681]

### Removal of Potassium

**Diuretics.** Diuretics have a relatively modest effect on urinary $K^+$ excretion in patients with CKD,[701] particularly in an acute setting.[672] However, diuretics are reasonable therapy for hyperkalemia in patients who have sufficient residual renal function to respond with an increase in urine output, particularly if successful control of serum $K^+$ may avoid the need for dialysis. In patients with impaired renal function, use of the following agents is recommended for acute control of serum $K^+$: (1) oral diuretics with the highest bioavailability (e.g., torsemide) and the least renal metabolism, (e.g., torsemide, bumetanide) to minimize the chance of accumulation and toxicity; (2) intravenous agents (short-term treatment) with the least hepatic metabolism (e.g., furosemide rather than bumetanide); (3) combinations of loop and thiazide-like diuretics for better efficacy, although this may decrease the GFR because of activation of tubuloglomerular feedback[702]; and (4) the maximal effective "ceiling" dose.[701,702] To avoid causing hypovolemia, it may be necessary to increase the rate of IV hydration with normal saline or isotonic bicarbonate. This will also serve to help increase distal tubular delivery of $Na^+$, augmenting $K^+$ excretion.

For the chronic management of hyperkalemia, diuretic therapy is not recommended in patients who are euvolemic or who otherwise lack indications for diuretic therapy, given the potential for inducing hypovolemia. However, with liberalization of fluid and salt intake, if appropriate, diuretics can be useful for correcting hyperkalemia in patients with the syndrome of hyporeninemic hypoaldosteronism[703] and selective renal $K^+$ secretory problems (e.g., after transplantation or administration of TMP).[704,705]

**Mineralocorticoids.** Limited data are available on the role of mineralocorticoids in the management of acute hyperkalemia.[29,706] However, these agents have been used to treat chronic hyperkalemia in patients with hypoaldosteronism, with or without hyporeninism, those with SLE,[707] kidney transplant patients on cyclosporine,[708] and ESKD patients on hemodialysis with interdialytic hyperkalemia.[709,710] The recommended dose is 0.1 to 0.3 mg/day of fludrocortisone, a synthetic glucocorticoid with potent mineralocorticoid activity and modest glucocorticoid activity (0.3 mg of fludrocortisone is equal to 1 mg of prednisone with regard to glucocorticoid activity).[29,708–710] In patients with ESKD on hemodialysis, this regimen reduces serum $K^+$ by 0.5 to 0.7 mmol/L and has not been associated with significant changes in blood pressure or weight (as a surrogate for fluid retention).[709] However, other studies of 0.1 mg/day of fludrocortisone in patients on chronic hemodialysis have resulted in statistically significant but clinically inconsequential effects on serum $K^+$.[711,712] The long-term safety of fludrocortisone in ESKD has not been established and, given the minimal effect on serum $K^+$, I do not recommend its use for the management of interdialytic hyperkalemia.

Pharmacologic inhibition of 11β-HSD-2 with glycyrrhetinic acid (GA) has also been tested as a novel mechanism to control hyperkalemia in ESKD.[405] As in other aldosterone-sensitive epithelia, the 11β-HSD-2 enzyme protects colonic epithelial cells from illicit activation of the mineralocorticoid receptor by cortisol. Hypothesizing that GA would activate extrarenal potassium secretion by the colon and other tissues, Farese and associates have tested the effect of the drug in a double-blind, placebo-controlled trial in 10 ESKD patients. Treatment with GA significantly increased the serum ratio of cortisol to cortisone, consistent with successful inhibition of 11β-HSD-2. This effect was associated with a significant reduction in mean serum $K^+$, with 70% of predialysis values in the normal range (3.5–4.7 mmol/L) in the GA phase of the trial, versus 24% in the placebo phase.[405] Plasma renin activity and aldosterone levels also dropped, perhaps because of the lower median plasma $K^+$ level. GA is thus a promising agent for long-term management of plasma $K^+$ in ESKD; clearly, however, more extensive clinical testing is required before widespread use.

**Cation Exchange Resins.** Ion exchange resins are cross-linked polymers containing acidic or basic structural units that can exchange r anions or cations on contact with a solution. They are capable of binding to a variety of monovalent and divalent cations. Cation exchange resins are classified based on the cation (e.g., hydrogen, ammonium, sodium, potassium, calcium) that is cycled during the synthesis of the resin to saturate sulfonic or carboxylic groups. In 1950, Elkinton and colleagues successfully used a carboxylic resin in the ammonium cycle in three patients with hyperkalemia.[713] However, hydrogen- or ammonium-cycled resins were associated with metabolic acidosis[714] and mouth ulcers,[715] making the sodium-cycled resins preferable.[716] Calcium-cycled resins may have other potential benefits, including a phosphate-lowering effect; however, this requires large, potentially toxic, doses of resin[717]; moreover, these resins have been associated with hypercalcemia.[718] The dominant resin clinically available in the United States is sodium polystyrene sulfonate (SPS).

SPS exchanges $Na^+$ for $K^+$ in the gastrointestinal tract, mainly in the colon,[669,715,719] and has been shown to increase the fecal excretion of $K^+$.[715] Occasional constipation easily controlled with enema or cathartics has been reported with the oral administration of SPS in water.[715] To prevent constipation and facilitate the passage of the resin through the gastrointestinal tract, Flinn and coworkers added sorbitol to the resin,[720] despite an absence of prior constipation or impaction in the relevant, cited reference.[716] It has since become routine to administer SPS with sorbitol, with approximately 5 million annual doses administered in the United States alone.[721] Notably, although SPS is used herein to denote sodium polystyrene sulfonate, SPS is a brand name for sodium polystyrene sulfonate in sorbitol, illustrating the frequency with which these agents are administered together.[670]

The effect of ingested SPS on serum $K^+$ is slow; it may take from 4 to 24 hours to see a significant effect on the serum

$K^+$.[672,673,715] The oral dose is usually 15 to 30 g, which can be repeated every 4 to 6 hours. Each gram of resin binds 0.5 to 1.2 mEq of $K^+$ in exchange for 2 to 3 mEq of $Na^+$.[673,715,722,723] The discrepancy is caused, in part, by the binding of small amounts of other cations.[715] The hypokalemic effect may be as a result of the coadministered laxative. One study of healthy subjects has compared the rate of fecal excretion of $K^+$ by different laxatives, with or without SPS, and found that the combination of phenolphthalein-docusate with resin produced greater fecal excretion of $K^+$ (49 mmol in 12 hours) than did phenolphthalein/docusate alone (37 mmol in 12 hours) or other laxative-resin combinations.[722]

Earlier studies with SPS, mostly before the era of chronic hemodialysis, used multiple doses of the exchange resin orally or rectally as an enema and were associated with declines in the serum $K^+$ of 1 mmol/L and 0.8 mmol/L in 24 hours, respectively.[715] However, with the advent of routine hemodialysis, it has become common to order only a single dose of resin cathartic in the management of acute hyperkalemia. One study has addressed the efficacy of this practice, evaluating the effect of four single-dose resin cathartic regimens on serum $K^+$ levels of six patients with CKD on maintenance hemodialysis; none of the regimens used reduced the serum $K^+$ below the initial baseline.[723] Notably, the subjects in this study were normokalemic. Regardless, if SPS is judged to be appropriate in the management of hyperkalemia (see later), repeated doses are usually required for an adequate effect.

SPS can be administered rectally as a retention enema in patients unable to take or tolerate the oral form. The recommended dose is 30 to 50 g of resin as an emulsion in 100 mL of an aqueous vehicle (e.g., 20% dextrose in water) every 6 hours. It should be administered warm (body temperature), after a cleansing enema with body temperature tap water, through a rubber tube placed at about 20 cm from the rectum, with the tip well into the sigmoid colon. The emulsion should be introduced by gravity, flushed with an additional 50 to 100 mL of non–sodium-containing fluid, retained for at least 30 to 60 minutes, and followed by a cleansing enema (250–1000 mL of body temperature tap water).[724] SPS in sorbitol should not be used for enemas, given the risk of colonic necrosis.[672,725]

An increasing concern with SPS in sorbitol is intestinal necrosis because of the administration of this preparation[721,725–728]; this is frequently a fatal complication.[721,725,727] Studies in experimental animals have suggested that sorbitol is required for the intestinal injury[725]; however, a recent animal study has indicated that SPS alone can cause intestinal necrosis, with no requirement for sorbitol.[729] Additionally, SPS crystals can often be detected in human pathologic specimens, adherent to the injured mucosa.[727,728] Several cases of colonic necrosis following oral SPS alone, without sorbitol, have also been reported,[730,731] directly implicating SPS in the intestinal injury. The risk of intestinal necrosis appears to be greatest when SPS is given with sorbitol within the first week after surgery. For example, of 117 patients who received SPS with sorbitol within 2 weeks of surgery, two patients developed intestinal necrosis.[726] Notably, however, in a case series of SPS in sorbitol-associated intestinal necrosis, only 2 of 11 confirmed cases occurred in the postoperative setting.[727] Although most cases of intestinal necrosis have occurred in patients receiving SPS in 70% sorbitol, this has also been reported in patients receiving SPS in 33% sorbitol.[721]

In response to these reports, the US Food and Drug Administration (FDA) removed recommendations for the concomitant or postdosing use of sorbitol from the labeling of SPS in 2005.[721] However, the FDA allowed continuous marketing of the most frequently used ready-made SPS in sorbitol suspension, given that it contained only 33% sorbitol. Subsequently, more cases of intestinal necrosis were reported, with some reportedly associated with SPS in 33% sorbitol.[721] As a result, in September 2009, the FDA changed safety labeling for SPS powder, stating that concomitant administration of sorbitol is no longer recommended.[721] As noted, several cases of colonic necrosis following oral SPS alone have also been reported.[730,731]

Given these serious concerns, clinicians must carefully consider whether emergency treatment with SPS is actually necessary for the treatment of hyperkalemia.[670,721,732] Additionally, patiromer and ZS-9, newly available alternatives, should be used in preference to SPS. There are minimal data on the efficacy of SPS within the first 24 hours of administration for hyperkalemia[721]; at best, the effect occurs within 4 to 6 hours of administration.[671,672,715] This temporal limitation should be taken into consideration when deciding whether or not to administer SPS in acute hyperkalemia. In patients with intact renal function, alternative measures such as hydration, to increase distal tubular delivery of $Na^+$ and distal tubular flow rate, and/or diuretics are often sufficient for potassium removal. In patients with advanced renal failure, the use of SPS is reasonable as a temporizing maneuver while awaiting hemodialysis but, if hemodialysis is available within 1 to 4 hours, the need for SPS should be questioned, given the delayed hypokalemic response and the risk of potentially fatal intestinal necrosis. Furthermore, if a patient has an existing vascular access for hemodialysis, the risk of intestinal necrosis outweighs that of the dialysis procedure.

If SPS is administered, the preparation should ideally not contain sorbitol; SPS without sorbitol is typically available as a powder that must be reconstituted with water. If a laxative other than sorbitol is coadministered, it should not contain potassium or other cations such as magnesium or calcium, which can compete with potassium for binding to the resin. In patients with renal insufficiency, the laxative should not contain phosphorus. Reasonable laxatives for this purpose include lactulose and some preparations of polyethylene glycol 3350. However, data demonstrating the efficacy and safety of these laxatives with SPS are not available.[670] It should also be noted that administering SPS without sorbitol might not eliminate the risk of intestinal necrosis, given the role for the SPS resin itself in this complication.[727,728,730,731] Note that SPS without sorbitol is rarely available in the United States; many pharmacies and hospitals only stock SPS premixed with sorbitol.[721] Although there are indications that SPS preparations with 33% sorbitol have a lesser risk, cases of intestinal necrosis have also been described with this preparation. Clinicians will have to weigh the relative risk of using this preparation in the management of acute hyperkalemia.[721] Regardless, SPS with sorbitol should not be used in patients at higher risk for intestinal necrosis, including postoperative patients, patients with a history of bowel obstruction, patients with slow intestinal transit, patients with ischemic bowel disease, and renal transplant recipients.

Finally, oral SPS with sorbitol can also injure the upper gastrointestinal tract, although the clinical significance of these findings is not known.[733] Other potential complications include reduction of serum calcium levels,[734] volume overload,[714] interference with lithium absorption,[735] and iatrogenic hypokalemia.[724]

**Novel Intestinal Potassium Binders.** Two new $K^+$ binders, patiromer and ZS-9, have recently become available for the treatment of hyperkalemia. Given the clinical need and serious limitations of SPS, there is considerable interest in these drugs. At this time, the drugs are expensive and limited in availability at many US-based hospital settings.

Patiromer is a nonabsorbed polymer, provided as a powder for suspension, which binds $K^+$ in exchange for $Ca^{2+}$. In a study of 237 patients with CKD and hyperkalemia, the mean change in serum $K^+$ after treatment with patiromer was −1.01 ± 0.03 mM.[736] Approximately 75% of patients achieved the target serum $K^+$ level of 3.8 to 5.0 mEq/L. The 107 patients whose baseline serum $K^+$ was 5.5 mEq/L or higher and who achieved the target serum $K^+$ during the initial 4-week treatment period were randomly assigned to patiromer or placebo for another 8 weeks. Serum $K^+$ remained the same in patients who continued on patiromer and increased by 0.7 mEq/L in those assigned placebo. The incidence of hyperkalemia (≥5.5 mEq/L) was significantly higher in the placebo group (60% vs. 15%). Serious adverse events were rare. However, a serum magnesium level less than 1.4 mg/dL occurred in 8 patients (3%) during the initial phase, and 9 patients were initiated on magnesium replacement, suggesting that impaired intestinal absorption of magnesium may be a limitation in long-term use. Patiromer also binds to ingested medications, with characterized interactions with ciprofloxacin, thyroxine, and metformin; these three drugs need to be administered more than 3 hours before or after patiromer.[737]

Sodium zirconium cyclosilicate (ZS-9) is an inorganic, nonabsorbable crystalline compound that exchanges sodium and hydrogen ions for $K^+$ and $NH_4^+$ in the intestine. The binding of $K^+$ to ZS-9 has some similarity to the selectivity filter of $K^+$ channels, with a more than 25-fold selectivity for $K^+$ over $Ca^{2+}$ and $Mg^{2+}$.[738] The efficacy of ZS-9 in hyperkalemic outpatients was evaluated in two nearly identical phase III, randomized, placebo-controlled trials.

In the Hyperkalemia Randomized Intervention Multidose ZS-9 Maintenance (HARMONIZE) study, 258 adult patients with persistent hyperkalemia entered a 48-hour, open-label, run-in during which they received 10 g of ZS-9 tid.[739] Of the 258 patients who entered the open-label run-in, 237 (92%) achieved a normal serum $K^+$ (3.5–5.0 mEq/L) at 48 hours and were then randomly assigned to placebo or 5, 10, or 15 g of ZS-9 once daily for 4 weeks. During randomized therapy, the mean serum $K^+$ was significantly lower with ZS-9 (4.8, 4.5, and 4.4 mEq/L with 5-, 10-, and 15-g dosing, respectively) as compared with placebo (5.1 mEq/L). Similarly, the proportion of normokalemic patients at the end of the study was significantly greater with ZS-9 (71%–85% as compared with 48% with placebo). Serious adverse events were uncommon and were not significantly increased with ZS-9. However, edema was more common with the 10-g and 15-g doses compared with placebo, as was hypokalemia.

In a second ZS-9 trial,[740] 753 adult patients with a serum $K^+$ of 5.0 to 6.5 mM were randomly assigned to receive 1.25, 2.5, 5, or 10 g of ZS-9 tid daily for 48 hours. A normal serum $K^+$ (3.5–4.9 mEq/L) at 48 hours was attained by 543 patients (72%), and they were then reassigned to receive placebo or 1.25, 2.5, 5, or 10 g of ZS-9 once daily for 2 weeks. The serum potassium level at 2 weeks was significantly lower in patients receiving 5 and 10 g doses of ZS-9 as compared with placebo (by ≈0.3 and 0.5 mEq/L, respectively), but not with 1.25- and 2.5-g doses. Adverse events were similar with placebo and ZS-9.

In these trials, the steepest decline in serum potassium with ZS-9 occurred during the first 4 hours of therapy.[739,740] This suggests an acute effect on intestinal potassium secretion, rather than simply a reduction in intestinal potassium absorption.

**Dialysis.** All modes of acute renal replacement therapies are effective in removing $K^+$. Continuous hemodiafiltration has been increasingly used in the management of critically ill and hemodynamically unstable patients.[741] Peritoneal dialysis, although not very effective in an acute setting, has been used effectively in cardiac arrest complicating acute hyperkalemia.[742] Peritoneal dialysis is capable of removing significant amounts of $K^+$ (5 mmol/hour [or 240 mmol in 48 hours]) using 2-L exchanges, with each exchange taking almost 1 hour.[674] However, hemodialysis is the preferred mode when rapid correction of a hyperkalemic episode is desired.[743]

An average 3- to 5-hour hemodialysis session removes approximately 40 to 120 mmol of $K^+$.[29,743-750] Approximately 15% of the total $K^+$ removal results from ultrafiltration, with the remaining clearance from dialysis.[744,745] Of the total $K^+$ removed, about 40% is from extracellular spaces, and the remainder is from intracellular compartments.[744,746,747] In most patients, the greatest decline in serum $K^+$ (1.2–1.5 mmol/L) and the largest amount of $K^+$ removed occur during the first hour; the serum $K^+$ usually reaches its nadir at about 3 hours. Despite a relatively constant serum $K^+$, $K^+$ removal continues until the end of the hemodialysis session, although at a significantly lower rate.[29,744,748]

The amount of $K^+$ removed depends primarily on the type and surface area of the dialyzer used, blood flow rate, dialysate flow rate, dialysis duration, and serum-to-dialysate $K^+$ gradient. However, about 40% of the difference in removal cannot be explained by the abovementioned factors and may instead be related to the relative distribution of $K^+$ between the intracellular and extracellular spaces.[746] Glucose-free dialysates are more efficient in removing $K^+$.[745,748] This effect may be caused by alterations in endogenous insulin levels, with concomitant intracellular shift of $K^+$; the insulin level is 50% lower when glucose-free dialysates are used.[746] Furthermore, these findings imply that $K^+$ removal may be greater if hemodialysis is performed with the patient in a fasting state.[745] Treatment with beta-2 agonists also reduces the total $K^+$ removal by approximately 40%.[743] The change in pH during dialysis has been thought to have no significant effect on $K^+$ removal.[743,745] One study evaluated this issue in detail, examining the effect of dialysate bicarbonate concentration on both serum $K^+$ and $K^+$ removal. Dialysates with a bicarbonate concentration of 39 mmol/L (high), 35 mmol/L (standard), and 27 mmol/L (low) were used. The use of a high concentration of bicarbonate was associated with a more rapid decline in serum $K^+$; this was statistically significant for high versus standard and low-bicarbonate dialysates, at 60 and 240 minutes, respectively. However, the total amount of $K^+$ removed was higher with the low-bicarbonate dialysate (116.4 ±

21.6 mmol/dialysis) in comparison to standard (73.2 ± 12.8 mmol/dialysis) and high (80.9 ± 15.4 mmol/dialysis) bicarbonate dialysates, all statistically insignificant.[749] Therefore, whereas high-bicarbonate dialysis *may acutely* have a more rapid effect on serum $K^+$, this advantage is potentially mitigated by a lesser total removal of the ion over the course of a typical treatment session.

One of the major determinants of total $K^+$ removal is the $K^+$ gradient between the plasma and dialysate. Dialysates with a lower $K^+$ concentration are more effective at reducing plasma $K^+$.[746,750] Many nephrologists use the so-called rule of 7s to set the dialysate $K^+$ concentration; the plasma $K^+$ plus the dialysate $K^+$ should equal approximately 7. However, this then entails dialysis with a 0- or 1.0-mEq/L $K^+$ dialysate (0 K and 1 K bath) in patients with serum potassium concentrations that exceed 6 to 7.0 mmol/L. However, a rapid decline in plasma $K^+$ caused by 0 K or 1 K dialysates can be deleterious because of several mechanisms. First, an acute decrease in plasma $K^+$ can be associated with rebound hypertension (i.e., a significant increase in blood pressure 1 hour after dialysis),[750] which is attributed in part to the peripheral vasoconstriction that is a direct result of the change in plasma $K^+$.[744] Second, a low plasma $K^+$ can alter the rate of tissue metabolism, the so-called Solandt effect,[751] and decrease tissue oxygen consumption, promoting arteriolar constriction.[750] This vasoconstriction, in turn, may reduce the efficiency of dialysis[29]; a randomized, prospective study did not, however, confirm this finding.[748] The difference may have been as a result of the glucose content of the dialysate (i.e., 200 mg/dL in the former and 0 mg/dL in the latter study); differences in circulating insulin may have had additional, unrelated effects on muscle blood flow.[752] Finally, dialysates with a very low $K^+$ concentration may increase the risk of significant arrhythmia and sudden cardiac death.[753–756]

Several studies have found an increased incidence of significant arrhythmia with hemodialysis, occurring during and immediately after treatment[755,757,758]; an incidence of up to 76% has been reported.[759] In addition to ventricular arrhythmias, hemodialysis can provoke atrial fibrillation, particularly in patients with a lower dialysate $K^+$ concentration.[760] Historically, some investigators did not consider the hemodialysis procedure to be significantly arrhythmogenic,[761–763] whereas others had suggested that a relationship exists among decreases in $K^+$, dialysate $K^+$, and the incidence of significant arrhythmias.[755] Given the more recent data,[754,756] it seems prudent to recommend that dialysates with a very low $K^+$ (0 or 1 mmol/L) be used cautiously, if at all. Higher risk patients include patients receiving digoxin, those with a history of arrhythmia, coronary artery disease, left ventricular hypertrophy, or high systolic blood pressure, and those of an advanced age. Continuous cardiac monitoring for all patients dialyzed against a 0 or 1 mmol/L $K^+$ bath is strongly recommended.[525]

Given the risk of inducing arrhythmias with very low potassium dialysates, an alternative approach has been proposed for the treatment of significant hyperkalemia.[525,764] In this regimen, dialysis is initiated with a 3 to 4 mEq/L potassium bath, which will immediately lower the plasma potassium concentration in a slower and perhaps safer manner.[755] The potassium concentration in the dialysate may then be lowered in a stepwise fashion with each subsequent hour. A more sophisticated approach uses potassium profiling to maintain a constant potassium gradient during dialysis.[764–766] Potassium profiling results in a more sustained, even removal of potassium[765] than dialysis against a fixed-potassium bath (2.5 mEq/L), with less effect on ventricular ectopy.[764–766]

For the management of severe hyperkalemia (serum $K^+$ ≥7.0 mEq/L), I favor the use of stepped reduction or potassium profiling of dialysate potassium concentrations. I rarely encounter the need to use 0- or 1-K dialysate baths, which I also avoid at the beginning of dialysis sessions for acute hyperkalemia. I recommend restricting the up-front use of these low-potassium baths to patients with life-threatening hyperkalemic arrhythmias and/or life-threatening conduction abnormalities.

A rebound increase in plasma $K^+$ can occur after hemodialysis. This phenomenon can be especially marked in cases of massive release from devitalized tissues (e.g., tumor lysis, rhabdomyolysis), requiring frequent monitoring of serum $K^+$ and further hemodialysis. However, a rebound increase may also occur in ESKD patients during regular maintenance hemodialysis, despite technically adequate treatment,[744] particularly in those patients with a high predialysis $K^+$. Factors attenuating $K^+$ removal and thus increasing the risk and magnitude of postdialysis rebound include pretreatment with beta-2 agonists,[743] pretreatment with insulin and glucose, eating early during the dialysis treatment,[745] a high predialysis plasma $K^+$,[747] and higher dialysate $Na^+$ concentrations.[767] Notably, a recent study of emergency hemodialysis treatments for hyperkalemia has failed to detect an association among the predialysis $K^+$, administration of pretreatment expected to cause a shift in serum $K^+$, and either recurrent hyperkalemia or the need for repeat dialysis within 24 hours.[768]

Complete reference list available at ExpertConsult.com.

## KEY REFERENCES


4. Terker AS, et al. Potassium modulates electrolyte balance and blood pressure through effects on distal cell voltage and chloride. *Cell Metab.* 2015;21:39–50.
22. McDonough AA, Thompson CB, Youn JH. Skeletal muscle regulates extracellular potassium. *Am J Physiol Renal Physiol.* 2002;282:F967–F974.
31. Guo J, et al. Extracellular K+ concentration controls cell surface density of IKr in rabbit hearts and of the HERG channel in human cell lines. *J Clin Invest.* 2009;119:2745–2757.
57. Aronson PS, Giebisch G. Effects of pH on potassium: new explanations for old observations. *J Am Soc Nephrol.* 2011;22:1981–1989.
73. Lalioti MD, et al. Wnk4 controls blood pressure and potassium homeostasis via regulation of mass and activity of the distal convoluted tubule. *Nat Genet.* 2006;38:1124–1132.
82. Mamenko MV, et al. The renal TRPV4 channel is essential for adaptation to increased dietary potassium. *Kidney Int.* 2017;91:1398–1409.
114. Frindt G, Shah A, Edvinsson J, et al. Dietary K regulates ROMK channels in connecting tubule and cortical collecting duct of rat kidney. *Am J Physiol Renal Physiol.* 2009;296:F347–F354.
108. Kleyman TR, Carattino MD, Hughey RP. ENaC at the cutting edge: regulation of epithelial sodium channels by proteases. *J Biol Chem.* 2009;284:20447–20451.
115. Palmer LG, Frindt G. Regulation of apical K channels in rat cortical collecting tubule during changes in dietary K intake. *Am J Physiol.* 1999;277:F805–F812.
143. Vallon V, Schroth J, Lang F, et al. Expression and phosphorylation of the Na+-Cl− cotransporter NCC in vivo is regulated by dietary salt, potassium, and SGK1. *Am J Physiol Renal Physiol.* 2009;297:F704–F712.
174. Mazzocchi G, Malendowicz LK, Markowska A, et al. Role of adrenal renin-angiotensin system in the control of aldosterone secretion in sodium-restricted rats. *Am J Physiol Endocrinol Metab.* 2000;278:E1027–E1030.

179. Clark BA, Brown RS, Epstein FH. Effect of atrial natriuretic peptide on potassium-stimulated aldosterone secretion: potential relevance to hypoaldosteronism in man. *J Clin Endocrinol Metab.* 1992;75:399–403.
186. Lin SH, et al. Laboratory tests to determine the cause of hypokalemia and paralysis. *Arch Intern Med.* 2004;164:1561–1566.
187. Batlle DC, Hizon M, Cohen E, et al. The use of the urinary anion gap in the diagnosis of hyperchloremic metabolic acidosis. *N Engl J Med.* 1988;594-599.
195. Parham WA, Mehdirad AA, Biermann KM, et al. Hyperkalemia revisited. *Tex Heart Inst J.* 2006;33:40–47.
197. Goldstein SA. K2P potassium channels, mysterious and paradoxically exciting. *Sci Signal.* 2011;4:pe35.
222. Ray PE, Suga S, Liu XH, et al. Chronic potassium depletion induces renal injury, salt sensitivity, and hypertension in young rats. *Kidney Int.* 2001;59:1850–1858.
223. Sun Y, et al. Dietary potassium regulates vascular calcification and arterial stiffness. *JCI Insight.* 2017;2.
241. Evers S, Engelien A, Karsch V, et al. Secondary hyperkalaemic paralysis. *J Neurol Neurosurg Psychiatry.* 1998;64:249–252.
249. DuBose TD Jr, Good DW. Chronic hyperkalemia impairs ammonium transport and accumulation in the inner medulla of the rat. *J Clin Invest.* 1992;90:1443–1449.
272. Tse HF, Yeung CK. From profound hypokalemia to fatal rhabdomyolysis after severe head injury. *Am J Med.* 2000;109:599–600.
294. Puwanant A, Ruff RL. INa and IKir are reduced in Type 1 hypokalemic and thyrotoxic periodic paralysis. *Muscle Nerve.* 2010;42:315–327.
319. Blondon H, Bechade D, Desrame J, et al. Secretory diarrhoea with high faecal potassium concentrations: a new mechanism of diarrhoea associated with colonic pseudo-obstruction? Report of five patients. *Gastroenterol Clin Biol.* 2008;32:401–404.
340. Beck KR, et al. Inhibition of 11beta-hydroxysteroid dehydrogenase 2 by the fungicides itraconazole and posaconazole. *Biochem Pharmacol.* 2017;130:93–103.
368. Nanba K, Vaidya A, Rainey WE. Aging and adrenal aldosterone production. *Hypertension.* 2018;71:218–223.
396. Kotelevtsev Y, et al. Hypertension in mice lacking 11beta-hydroxysteroid dehydrogenase type 2. *J Clin Invest.* 1999;103:683–689.
437. Carmosino M, et al. NKCC2 activity is inhibited by the Bartter's syndrome type 5 gain-of-function CaR-A843E mutant in renal cells. *Biol Cell.* 2015;107:98–110.
439. Seys E, et al. Clinical and genetic spectrum of Bartter syndrome type 3. *J Am Soc Nephrol.* 2017;28:2540–2552.
441. Bongers E, et al. A novel Hypokalemic-alkalotic salt-losing tubulopathy in patients with CLDN10 mutations. *J Am Soc Nephrol.* 2017;28:3118–3128.
449. Blanchard A, et al. Gitelman syndrome: consensus and guidance from a Kidney Disease: improving Global Outcomes (KDIGO) Controversies Conference. *Kidney Int.* 2017;91:24–33.
456. Bockenhauer D, et al. Epilepsy, ataxia, sensorineural deafness, tubulopathy, and KCNJ10 mutations. *N Engl J Med.* 2009;360:1960–1970.
471. Comer DM, Droogan AG, Young IS, et al. Hypokalaemic paralysis precipitated by distal renal tubular acidosis secondary to Sjogren's syndrome. *Ann Clin Biochem.* 2008;45:221–225.
478. Yang L, Frindt G, Palmer LG. Magnesium modulates ROMK channel-mediated potassium secretion. *J Am Soc Nephrol.* 2010;21:2109–2116.
481. Reimann D, Gross P. Chronic, diagnosis-resistant hypokalaemia. *Nephrol Dial Transplant.* 1999;14:2957–2961.
495. Sterns RH, Cox M, Feig PU, et al. Internal potassium balance and the control of the plasma potassium concentration. *Medicine (Baltimore).* 1981;60:339–354.
501. Nicolis GL, Kahn T, Sanchez A, et al. Glucose-induced hyperkalemia in diabetic subjects. *Arch Intern Med.* 1981;141:49–53.
503. Kunin AS, Surawicz B, Sims EAH. Decrease in serum potassium concentrations and appearance of cardiac arrhythmias during infusion of potassium with glucose in potassium-depleted patients. *N Engl J Med.* 1962;266:228–233.
526. Moranne O, et al. Timing of onset of CKD-related metabolic complications. *J Am Soc Nephrol.* 2009;20:164–171.
528. Kovesdy CP, et al. Serum and dialysate potassium concentrations and survival in hemodialysis patients. *Clin J Am Soc Nephrol.* 2007;2:999–1007.
562. Goldfarb S, Strunk B, Singer I, et al. Paradoxical glucose-induced hyperkalemia. Combined aldosterone-insulin deficiency. *Am J Med.* 1975;59:744–750.
565. Perazella MA, Biswas P. Acute hyperkalemia associated with intravenous epsilon-aminocaproic acid therapy. *Am J Kidney Dis.* 1999;33:782–785.
578. Martyn JA, Richtsfeld M. Succinylcholine-induced hyperkalemia in acquired pathologic states: etiologic factors and molecular mechanisms. *Anesthesiology.* 2006;104:158–169.
597. Oster JR, Singer I, Fishman LM. Heparin-induced aldosterone suppression and hyperkalemia. *Am J Med.* 1995;98:575–586.
605. Schambelan M, Stockigt JR, Biglieri EG. Isolated hypoaldosteronism in adults. A renin-deficiency syndrome. *N Engl J Med.* 1972;287:573–578.
630. Tan SY, Shapiro R, Franco R, et al. Indomethacin-induced prostaglandin inhibition with hyperkalemia. A reversible cause of hyporeninemic hypoaldosteronism. *Ann Intern Med.* 1979;90:783–785.
646. Velazquez H, Perazella MA, Wright FS, et al. Renal mechanism of trimethoprim-induced hyperkalemia. *Ann Intern Med.* 1993;119:296–301.
680. Allon M, Copkney C. Albuterol and insulin for treatment of hyperkalemia in hemodialysis patients. *Kidney Int.* 1990;38:869–872.
681. Blumberg A, Weidmann P, Shaw S, et al. Effect of various therapeutic approaches on plasma potassium and major regulating factors in terminal renal failure. *Am J Med.* 1988;85:507–512.
697. Blumberg A, Weidmann P, Ferrari P. Effect of prolonged bicarbonate administration on plasma potassium in terminal renal failure. *Kidney Int.* 1992;41:369–374.
729. Ayoub I, et al. Colon necrosis due to sodium polystyrene sulfonate with and without sorbitol: an experimental study in rats. *PLoS ONE.* 2015;10:e0137636.
739. Kosiborod M, et al. Effect of sodium zirconium cyclosilicate on potassium lowering for 28 days among outpatients with hyperkalemia: the HARMONIZE randomized clinical trial. *JAMA.* 2014;312:2223–2233.
754. Hung AM, Hakim RM. Dialysate and serum potassium in hemodialysis. *Am J Kidney Dis.* 2015;66:125–132.
765. Santoro A, et al. Patients with complex arrhythmias during and after haemodialysis suffer from different regimens of potassium removal. *Nephrol Dial Transplant.* 2008;23:1415–1421.

# 18 Disorders of Calcium, Magnesium, and Phosphate Balance

Michel Chonchol | Miroslaw J. Smogorzewski | Jason R. Stubbs | Alan S.L. Yu

CHAPTER OUTLINE



## DISORDERS OF CALCIUM HOMEOSTASIS

The extracellular fluid (ECF) calcium concentration in the human body is tightly regulated by a complex process. Three organs—skeleton, kidney, and intestine—are involved in this process through their direct or indirect interaction with parathyroid hormone (PTH), parathyroid hormone–related peptide (PTHrP), vitamin D, and calcitonin. Phosphatonins such as fibroblast growth factor 23 (FGF-23), although they participate in phosphate and vitamin D homeostasis, do not directly modify extracellular calcium.

This homeostatic system is modulated by dietary and environmental factors, including vitamins, hormones, medications, and mobility. Disorders of extracellular calcium homeostasis may be regarded as perturbations of this homeostatic system, either at the level of the genes controlling this system (e.g., as in familial hypocalciuric hypercalcemia, pseudohypoparathyroidism, or vitamin D–dependent rickets) or perturbations of this system induced by nongenetic means (e.g., as in lithium toxicity or postsurgical hypoparathyroidism).

Calcium fluxes between the ECF and one of the organs (skeleton, kidney, intestine) or their combination, as well as abnormal binding of the calcium to serum protein, can cause hypercalcemia. PTH directly protects against hypocalcemia by augmenting calcium mobilization from bone, increasing kidney tubular reabsorption of calcium, and enhancing intestinal absorption of calcium. PTH also indirectly protects against hypocalcemia through its effect on vitamin D metabolism. The phosphate mobilization from bone that is induced by PTH is countered by PTH-mediated decreases in kidney tubular reabsorption of phosphate. States with excess PTH may cause hypercalcemia, whereas PTH deficiency is associated with hypocalcemia. Similarly, PTHrP promotes bone resorption, enhances kidney reabsorption of calcium, and decreases kidney tubular reabsorption of phosphate. Excess of this hormone is responsible for the hypercalcemia of malignancy. Vitamin D and its metabolites increase intestinal absorption of calcium and cause bone resorption; therefore, excess vitamin D would induce hypercalcemia. Calcitonin inhibits bone resorption, but its physiologic role in the protection against hypercalcemia in humans is not proven.

### WHOLE-BODY CALCIUM HOMEOSTASIS

An adult human body contains approximately 1000 to 1300 g of calcium, with 99.3% in bone and teeth as hydroxyapatite crystal, 0.6% in soft tissues, and 0.1% in ECF, including 0.03% in plasma.[1] Intracellular concentrations of free calcium are very low (~100 nM) compared with extracellular concentrations of free calcium (~1 mM). Indeed, a 10,000-fold gradient is present. Maintenance of normal calcium balance and serum calcium levels depends on the integrated regulation of calcium absorption and secretion by the intestinal tract, excretion of calcium by the kidney, and calcium release from and deposition into bone. In young adults, calcium balance is neutral. Approximately 1000 mg of calcium is ingested per day, 200 mg absorbed by the gut, mainly the duodenum, and 800 mg excreted via the gut. Of 10 g of calcium filtered by the kidney daily, only approximately 200 mg is excreted in the urine. At the same time, 500 mg of calcium is released from bone, and the same amount is deposited with new bone formation. PTH, by stimulating bone resorption and distal tubular calcium reabsorption in the kidney and by activating kidney hydroxylation of $25(OH)D_3$ to $1,25(OH)D_3$, increases serum calcium levels. Depression in serum levels of calcium, by itself, stimulates, through the calcium-sensing receptor (CaSR) in the parathyroid gland, the secretion of preformed

PTH from the parathyroid gland within seconds. Subsequently, PTH biosynthesis by the parathyroid gland increases over 24 to 48 hours and, if sustained chronically, is followed by parathyroid gland hypertrophy and hyperplasia. Vitamin D metabolites, serum phosphorus, and FGF-23 levels also regulate PTH levels in blood.

The values for total serum calcium concentration in adults vary among clinical laboratories, depending on the methods of measurement, with the normal range being between 8.6 and 10.3 mg/dL (2.15–2.57 mmol/L).[2,3] Variations in serum calcium levels occur, depending on age and gender, with a general trend for a lower serum calcium level with aging.[4]

Calcium in blood exists in three distinct fractions—protein-bound calcium (40%), free (ionized) calcium (48%), and calcium complexed to various anions, such as phosphate, lactate, citrate, and bicarbonate (12%).[5] The latter two forms, complexed calcium and free calcium ion, together comprise the fraction of plasma calcium that can be filtered. Plasma albumin is responsible for 90% and globulins for 10% of protein-bound calcium. Free calcium is the physiologically active component of extracellular calcium with regard to CaSR signaling, cardiac myocyte contractility, neuromuscular activity, bone mineralization, and other calcium-dependent processes. It is measured in most hospitals using ion-selective electrodes; values in adults range from 4.65 to 5.28 mg/dL (1.16–1.32 mmol/L).[4,6] Total calcium reflects the levels of free calcium if plasma levels of protein, pH, and anions are normal.

The relationship between calcium ion and the concentration of protein in the serum is represented by a simple mass action expression:

$$([\text{Ionized Ca}^{2+}]\times[\text{protein}])/(\text{calcium proteinate}) = K$$

where [protein] equals the concentration of serum proteins, primarily albumin. Because K is a constant, the numerator and denominator must change proportionately in any physiologic or pathologic state. A change in the concentration of total serum calcium will occur after a change in the concentration of serum proteins or alterations in their binding properties and after a primary change in the concentration of calcium ion. A fall in the serum albumin level reduces the protein and calcium proteinate levels proportionately, resulting in a fall in the total serum calcium level, with the free calcium ion concentration remaining normal. If plasma levels of albumin are low, an adjustment of the measured serum levels of calcium should be made (commonly but erroneously referred to as a "correction"). For the routine clinical interpretation of serum calcium needed for appropriate care of patients, a simple formula for adjustment of the total serum calcium concentration for changes in plasma albumin concentration is used by clinicians.

In conventional units:

$$\text{Adjusted total calcium (mg/dL)} = \text{total calcium (mg/dL)} + 0.8(4 - \text{albumin [g/dL]})$$

In SI units:

$$\text{Adjusted total calcium (mmol/L)} = \text{total calcium (mmol/L)} + 0.002(40 - \text{albumin [g/dL]})$$

This formula was endorsed in 1977 by an editorial in the *British Medical Journal*[7]; the correction factor of 0.02 (in SI units) was chosen arbitrarily for simplicity from the range available in the literature at that time (0.018– 0.025). This adjustment can also correct for errors in measurement of total calcium related to the hemoconcentration of a blood sample because of the prolonged use of a tourniquet or because of hemodilution when blood is drawn in hospitalized patients in a supine position.[3] Other formulas have been developed, particularly for chronic kidney disease (CKD) patients, that have a slightly better (although not statistically significant) discriminatory ability to make the diagnosis of hypocalcemia or hypercalcemia, as established from the measurement of free calcium.[8,9] Also, a fall in pH of 0.1 unit will cause approximately a 0.1-mEq/L rise in the concentration of ionized calcium, because hydrogen ion displaces calcium from albumin, whereas alkalosis decreases free calcium by enhancing the binding of calcium to albumin.[4] There is no correction for this effect of pH in the previous formula, which also limits its accuracy.

Calcium binding to globulin is low (1.0 g of globulin binds 0.2–0.3 mg of calcium), and it is unusual to see a change in the total concentration of serum calcium as a result of alterations in the globulin levels in blood. However, in cases in which the globulin concentration in serum is extremely high (>8.0 g/dL), such as in multiple myeloma, a mild to moderate hypercalcemia may be seen because of an elevation of the globulin-bound calcium. In addition, immunoglobulin G (IgG) myeloma proteins may have increased calcium-binding properties, and an elevation in the total level of serum calcium could occur, even with a moderate increase in serum levels of globulins. In these cases, the ionized calcium in serum is normal; therefore, this type of hypercalcemia would not require treatment.

Unfortunately, calcium status will be incorrectly predicted by this formula in 20% to 30% of subjects,[10] and the agreement between corrected and free calcium is only fair.[11] Thus, free calcium should be assessed, particularly in critically ill patients with acid-base disturbances, in patients exposed to large amounts of citrated blood, and in those with severe blood protein disorders. Patients with CKD and those treated with dialysis may also benefit from free calcium measurements in an evaluation of their mineral bone metabolism status.[12] It is important to recognize that free calcium results in blood are affected by factors related to the handling of specimens, including duration of cellular metabolism, loss of $CO_2$, and use of anticoagulants.[2]

## HYPERCALCEMIA

Hypercalcemia is relatively common and frequently overlooked, with an annual incidence estimated to be about 0.1% to 0.2% and a prevalence of 0.17% to 2.92% in a hospital population and 1.07% to 3.9% in a normal population.[13]

Hypercalcemia results from an alteration in the net fluxes of calcium to and from four compartments—bone, gut, kidney, and serum-binding proteins (Box 18.1). Usually, the hypercalcemia is caused by net calcium movement from the skeleton into ECF through increased osteoclastic bone resorption, as in hyperparathyroidism (HPT) or excess PTHrP production in malignancy. PTH acts via the PTH receptor 1 on the osteoblasts. PTH receptor 1 is encoded by the *PTH1R* gene. It activates cyclic adenosine monophosphate (cAMP) signaling in osteoblasts and upregulates the expression of receptor activator for nuclear factor-kappa B (RANK) ligand (RANKL)

**Box 18.1 Causes of Hypercalcemia**

Malignancy-associated hypercalcemia
- Humoral hypercalcemia of malignancy (HHM) with secretion of parathyroid hormone (PTH)–related protein by the tumor
- Local osteolytic hypercalcemia (LOH)
- Tumor (lymphoma, germinoma) generation of 1,25$(OH)_2D$
- Ectopic PTH secretion from tumor

Primary hyperparathyroidism
- Adenoma, hyperplasia, carcinoma
- Multiple endocrine neoplasia types 1 and 2a

Familial hypocalciuric hypercalcemia

Neonatal severe hyperparathyroidism

Other endocrine disorders
- Hyperthyroidism
- Acromegaly
- Pheochromocytoma
- Acute adrenal insufficiency

Granulomatous disorders
- Sarcoidosis
- Tuberculosis
- Berylliosis
- Disseminated coccidioidomycosis or candidiasis
- Histoplasmosis
- Leprosy
- Granulomatous lipoid pneumonia
- Silicone-induced granuloma
- Eosinophilic granuloma
- Farmer's lung

Vitamin overdoses
- Vitamin D
- Vitamin A

Immobilization

Kidney disease
- Diuretic phase of acute kidney injury, especially resulting from rhabdomyolysis
- Chronic kidney disease
- After kidney transplantation

Medications
- Milk-alkali syndrome
- Thiazide diuretics
- Lithium
- Foscarnet
- Growth hormone
- Recombinant human PTH (1-34; teriparatide)
- Theophylline and aminophylline toxicity
- Estrogen and selective estrogen receptor modulators (SERMs)
- Vasoactive intestinal polypeptide
- Hyperalimentation regimens

Idiopathic hypercalcemia of infancy

Increased serum protein level
- Hemoconcentration
- Hyperglobulinemia due to multiple myeloma

in osteoblasts. RANKL binds to RANK on osteoclasts. RANK activation on osteoclasts through the RANK-RANKL interaction causes recruitment, proliferation, and activation of osteoclasts for bone resorption. Therefore, it is somewhat curious that PTH exerts a direct effect on osteoblasts and an indirect effect on osteoclasts. An increase in the bone resorption rate without an increase in the bone formation rate will cause hypercalcemia.

Myeloma cells may induce multiple osteoclastogenic factors such as RANKL in nonosteoblastic stromal cells or decrease production of osteoprotegerin, a decoy receptor for RANKL. As with PTH, excess, circulating 1,25-dihydroxyvitamin D (1,25$[OH]_2D$) from various causes also activates osteoclastic bone resorption indirectly through osteoblasts. Increased intestinal calcium absorption may lead to the development of hypercalcemia, as in vitamin D overdose or milk-alkali syndrome. In general, the kidney does not contribute to hypercalcemia; rather, it defends against the development of hypercalcemia. Typically, hypercalciuria precedes hypercalcemia. Extracellular calcium itself appears to have a calciuric effect on the kidney tubule by its direct action on the CaSR of the thick ascending limb (TAL). Thus, in most hypercalcemic states, kidney calcium handling is subject to competing influences; excess PTH or PTHrP acts on the PTH-PTHrP receptor to promote kidney calcium reabsorption, and excess calcium acts on the calcium receptor to promote calcium excretion.[14]

In rare cases, the kidney can actively contribute to the development of hypercalcemia. As opposed to primary HPT and humoral hypercalcemia of malignancy, in which increases in kidney calcium excretion are observed, kidney calcium excretion is not elevated in familial hypocalciuric hypercalcemia because of a defective kidney response to calcium itself. The hypercalcemia associated with thiazide use is also mediated by the kidney; in both thiazide use and its genetic counterpart, Gitelman syndrome, kidney calcium excretion is decreased.

## SIGNS AND SYMPTOMS

Hypercalcemia adversely affects the function of almost all organ systems, but in particular the kidney, central nervous system, and cardiovascular system. The clinical manifestations of hypercalcemia relate more to the degree of hypercalcemia and rate of increase than to the underlying cause. Hypercalcemia may be classified based on the level of total serum calcium:[15]

- Mild: [Ca] = 10.4 to 11.9 mg/dL
- Moderate: [Ca] = 12.0 to 13.9 mg/dL
- Severe (hypercalcemic crisis): [Ca] = 14.0 to 16 mg/dL

Much higher levels are occasionally observed. Signs and symptoms and complications of hypercalcemia are summarized in Box 18.2.

As many as 10% of patients with elevated levels of serum calcium are detected by a routine screening test of blood chemistry and are considered to have so-called asymptomatic hypercalcemia. However, even very mild hypercalcemia may be of clinical significance in as much as some studies have suggested an increased cardiovascular risk from mild but prolonged calcium level elevations.[16]

In symptomatic patients, the spectrum of the clinical presentation is varied and could be nonspecific. Mild hypercalcemia may present with malaise, weakness, minor joint pain, and other vague symptoms. In patients with severe hypercalcemia, the major symptoms are more likely to be nausea, vomiting, constipation, polyuria, and mental disturbances, ranging from headache and lethargy to coma. Recent loss of memory could be prominent and may be a presenting symptom.

**Box 18.2 Clinical Features of Hypercalcemia**

**General**

Malaise, tiredness, weakness

**Neuropsychiatric**

Impaired concentration, loss of memory, headache, drowsiness, lethargy, disorientation, confusion, irritability, depression, paranoia, hallucinations, ataxia, speech defects, visual disturbances, deafness (calcification of eardrum), pruritus, mental retardation (infants), stupor, coma

**Neuromuscular**

Muscle weakness, hyporeflexia or absent reflexes, hypotonia, myalgia, arthralgia, bone pain, joint effusion, chondrocalcinosis, dwarfism (infants)

**Gastrointestinal**

Loss of appetite, dry mouth, thirst, polydipsia, nausea, vomiting, constipation, abdominal pain, weight loss, acute pancreatitis (calcifying), peptic ulcer, acute gastric dilation

**Kidney**

Polyuria, nocturia, nephrocalcinosis, nephrolithiasis, interstitial nephritis, acute kidney injury and chronic kidney disease

**Cardiovascular**

Arrhythmia, bradycardia, first-degree heart block, short Q-T interval, bundle branch block, arrest (rare), hypertension, vascular calcification

**Metastatic Calcification**

Band keratopathy, red eye syndrome, conjunctival calcification nephrocalcinosis, vascular calcification, pruritus

Hypercalciuria induced by hypercalcemia causes nephrogenic diabetes insipidus, with polyuria and polydipsia leading to ECF volume depletion and a decreased glomerular filtration rate (GFR) and causing further increases in the serum calcium level. The effect of hypercalcemia on urinary concentration is mediated through CaSR activation, which decreases vasopressin-dependent aquaporin-2 (AQP2) water channels trafficking in the inner medullary collecting duct.[17] Nephrolithiasis and nephrocalcinosis are common complications of hypercalcemia, seen in 15% to 20% of cases of primary HPT, respectively.

## LABORATORY FINDINGS

Laboratory findings in patients with hypercalcemia include abnormalities related to the underlying disease causing the hypercalcemia, which are beyond the scope of this chapter. Alterations in the electrocardiogram (ECG) and electroencephalogram (EEG) occur in hypercalcemic patients, independently of the cause of the hypercalcemia. The ECG shows a shortened ST segment and therefore a reduced QT interval as a result of an increased rate of cardiac repolarization. In patients with severe hypercalcemia (>16 mg/dL), there is a widening of the T waves, resulting in an increase in the QT interval. Bradycardia and first-degree heart block may be present in the ECGs of patients with acute and severe hypercalcemia. The EEG displays slowing and other nonspecific changes.

## DIAGNOSIS

A careful history, physical examination, and routine laboratory tests will, in most patients, lead to the correct diagnosis in hypercalcemia. A flow diagram for the evaluation of hypercalcemia is shown in Fig. 18.1. Primary HPT (PHPT) and malignancy-associated hypercalcemia together are responsible for 90% of cases of hypercalcemia, with malignancy being the most common cause in hospitalized patients and PHPT being the most common cause in the outpatient clinic.[15,18–20]

It is generally easy to differentiate these two entities. Hypercalcemia is only rarely an early finding in occult malignancy. PTH levels are essential in the diagnosis of hypercalcemia. There are two types of assay for PTH, depending on which epitopes of 1-84 PTH are recognized by the antibodies in the assay. Second-generation assays, the immunoradiometric assay (IRMA) and immunochemiluminometric assay (IMCA), use antibodies against amino acid 7-34 and 39-84 epitopes of 1-84 PTH. Despite their being called "intact PTH assays," implying that they measure only the biologically active PTH, they also detect large carboxy-terminal fragments of PTH, such as PTH (7-84). Thus, they may overestimate the amount of bioactive hormone in serum, especially in CKD patients. The third-generation, whole or biointact PTH assays, use antibodies against amino acid 1-5 and C-terminal epitopes and detect biologically active intact PTH. The normal levels of PTH measured by various assays range from 8 to 80 Pg/mL (1–9 pmol/L).[2,21] Intraoperative PTH measurements are frequently used to assess the adequacy of parathyroidectomy. There is no cross-reactivity between PTH and PTHrP assays. In PHPT, levels of PTH can be frankly elevated but can also be in the middle or upper range of normal, particularly in younger individuals (Fig. 18.2).

The differential diagnosis of patients with hypercalcemia and elevated PTH level includes HPT due to thiazide diuretics or lithium, familial hypocalciuric hypercalcemia (FHH), and the tertiary HPT associated with chronic dialysis and kidney transplantation. Patients with FHH have a positive family history, onset of hypercalcemia at a young age, very low urinary calcium excretion, and specific gene abnormalities. In malignancy-associated hypercalcemia and in hypercalcemia of most other causes, PTH levels are low. The diagnosis of humoral hypercalcemia of malignancy (HHM) frequently can be made on clinical grounds. In addition, PTHrP can now be assayed by commercial clinical laboratories to support HHM or when the cause of hypercalcemia is obscure.

Approximately 10% of cases of hypercalcemia are due to other causes. Of particular importance in the evaluation of a hypercalcemic patient are the family history (because of familial syndromes, including multiple endocrine neoplasia type 1 [MEN1], MEN2, and familial hypocalciuric hypercalcemia), medication history (because of the several medication-induced forms of hypercalcemia), and presence of other disease (e.g., granulomatous or malignant disease). Plasma 1,25$(OH)_2$D levels should be measured when granulomatous disorders or 1,25$(OH)_2$D lymphoma syndrome is considered. Very high 1,25$(OH)_2$D levels may suggest vitamin D intoxication as a cause of hypercalcemia. However, this condition is rare.

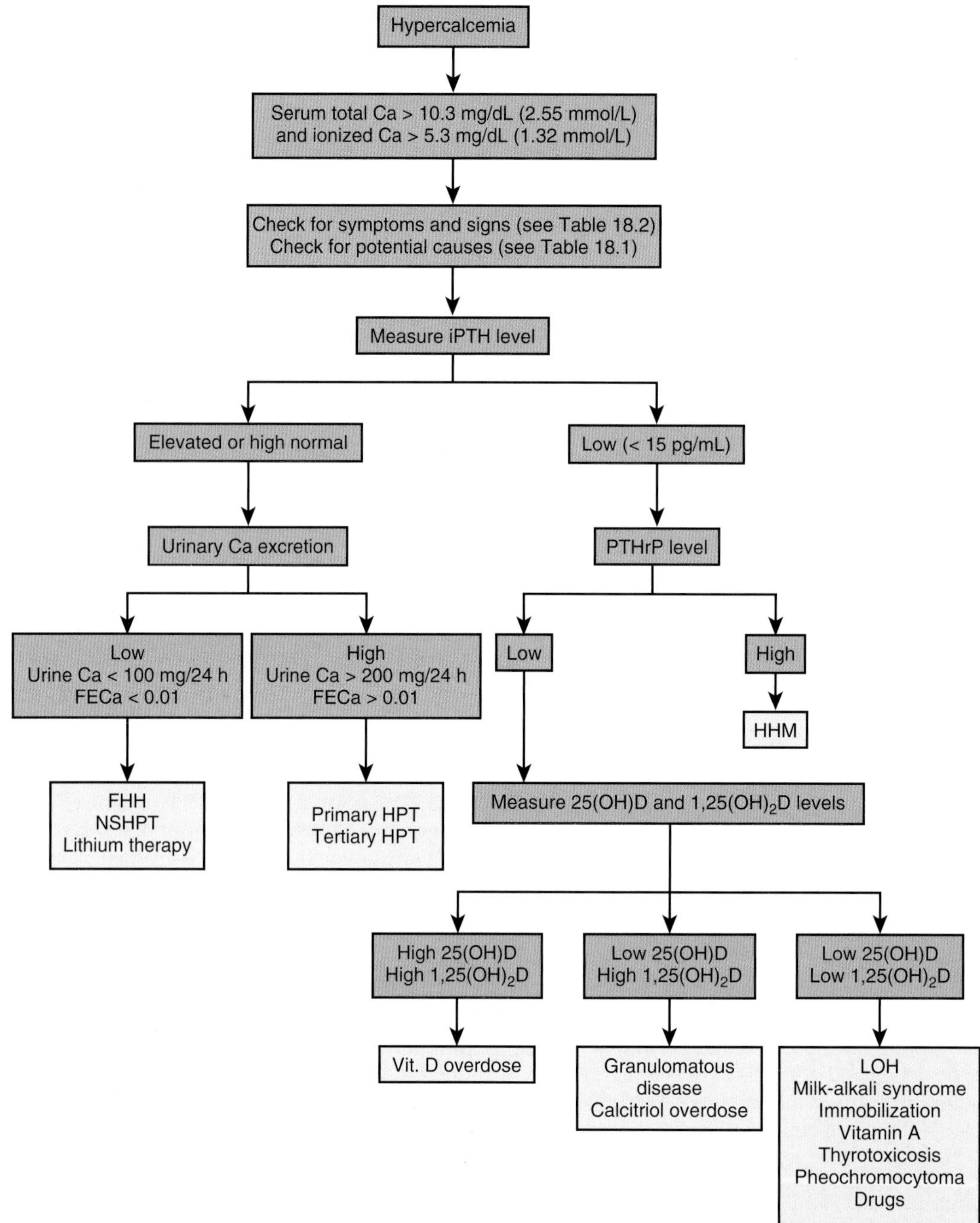


**Fig. 18.1** Algorithm for the evaluation of hypercalcemia. *FECa,* Fractional excretion of calcium; *FHH,* familial hypocalciuric hypercalcemia; *HHM,* humoral hypercalcemia of malignancy; *HPT,* hyperparathyroidism; *iPTH,* intact parathyroid hormone; *LOH,* localized osteolytic hypercalcemia; *NSHPT,* neonatal severe hyperparathyroidism; *PTHrP,* parathyroid hormone–related peptide.

## CAUSES

### Primary Hyperparathyroidism

PHPT is caused by excessive and incompletely regulated secretion of PTH, with consequent hypercalcemia and hypophosphatemia (see Box 18.1). It is the underlying cause of approximately 50% of hypercalcemic cases in the general population. The estimated prevalence of PHPT is about 1%, but may be as high as 2% in postmenopausal women.[22,23] The annual incidence is approximately 0.03% to 0.04%.[22–24]

A single enlarged parathyroid gland (adenoma) is the cause of PHPT in 80% to 85% of cases. These adenomas are benign clonal neoplasms of parathyroid chief cells, which lose their normal sensitivity to calcium. In about 15% to 20% of patients with PHPT, all four parathyroid glands are hyperplastic. This occurs in sporadic PHPT or in conjunction with MEN1 or MEN2.[19] In diffuse hyperplasia, the set point for calcium is not changed in any given parathyroid cell, but the increased number of cells causes excess PTH production and hypercalcemia. Parathyroid carcinoma is seen in no more than 0.5% to 1% of patients with PHPT.[25]

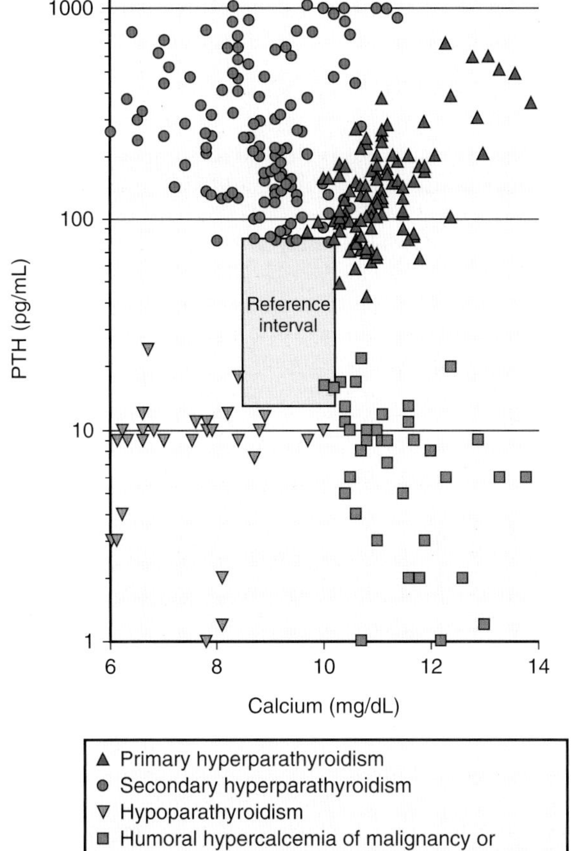


**Fig. 18.2** Relationship between total serum calcium and intact parathyroid hormone *(PTH)* concentrations. Values for patients with known primary hyperparathyroidism, secondary hyperparathyroidism, humoral hypercalcemia of malignancy, or other PTH-independent cause of hypercalcemia, and hypoparathyroidism are plotted. The *rectangle* represents the normal reference range for the assays. (From O'Neill S, Gordon C, Guo R, et al. Multivariate analysis of clinical, demographic, and laboratory data for classification of patients with disorders of calcium homeostasis. *Am J Clin Pathol.* 2011;135:100–107.)

PHPT occurs at all ages but is most common in older individuals; peak incidence is in the sixth decade of life. After age 50 years, women are about three times more frequently affected than men. Sporadic PHPT is the most common. External neck irradiation during childhood is recognized as a risk factor for PHPT. The genetic alterations underlying parathyroid adenomas have been partially elucidated.[26] Rearrangements and overexpression of the PRAD-1–cyclin D1 oncogene have been observed in about 20% of parathyroid adenomas.[27,28] The MEN1 tumor suppressor gene is inactivated in about 15% of adenomas.[29,30] Other chromosomal regions may also harbor parathyroid tumor suppressor genes.

PHPT typically presents in one of three ways. In 60% to 80% of cases, there are minimal or no symptoms, and mild hypercalcemia is usually discovered during routine laboratory examination. Another 20% to 25% of patients have a chronic course manifested by mild or intermittent hypercalcemia, recurrent kidney stones, and complications of nephrolithiasis; in these patients, the parathyroid tumor is small (<1.0 g) and slow-growing. In 5% to 10% of patients, there is severe and symptomatic hypercalcemia and overt osteitis fibrosa cystica; in these patients, the parathyroid tumor is usually large (>5.0 g). Patients with parathyroid carcinoma typically have severe hypercalcemia, with classic kidney and bone involvement.[26]

The diagnosis of PHPT is now usually suggested by the incidental finding of hypercalcemia rather than by any of the sequelae of PTH excess, such as skeletal and kidney complications or symptomatic hypercalcemia.[18] Hypercalcemia may be mild and intermittent. Hypercalciuria was noted in 40% of PHPT, nephrolithiasis in 19%, and classic bone disease and osteitis fibrosa cystica only in 2% of studies performed between 1984 and 2000 in the United States.[16] However, even in individuals with mild PHPT, there is also progressive bone loss, as measured by bone mineral densitometry over 15 years of observation.[31]

The diagnosis of PHPT is established by laboratory tests showing hypercalcemia, inappropriately normal or elevated blood levels of PTH, hypercalciuria, hypophosphatemia, phosphaturia, and increased urinary excretion of cAMP. Hyperchloremic acidosis may be present, and the ratio of serum chloride to phosphorus is elevated. The serum levels of alkaline phosphatase and uric acid may be also elevated. The serum concentration of magnesium is usually normal but may be low or high.

Some controversy surrounds the potential relationship between PHPT and increased mortality.[15] A number of studies have shown that PHPT may be associated with hypertension, dyslipidemia, diabetes, increased thickness of the carotid artery,[3] and increased mortality, primarily from cardiovascular disease.[20,32] The morbidity from PHPT can also be substantial, especially in symptomatic patients with severe hypercalcemia and a late diagnosis.

The classic bone lesion in PHPT, osteitis fibrosa cystica, is now rarely seen. Diffuse osteopenia is more common.[20,32] Even in asymptomatic patients, increased rates of bone turnover are always present.[20,32]

Surgery is still standard therapy for PHPT.[18,32,33] It is generally agreed that parathyroidectomy is indicated for all patients with biochemically confirmed PHPT who have specific symptoms or signs of disease, such as a history of life-threatening hypercalcemia, CKD, and/or kidney stones. In 2013, a Fourth International Workshop on Hyperparathyroidism updated the guidelines for the management of asymptomatic HPT.[33] Surgery is advised for asymptomatic disease in patients with serum calcium levels greater than 1 mg/dL above normal, reduced bone mass (T-score < −2.5 at lumbar spine, total hip, femoral neck, or distal third of the radius), creatinine clearance less than 60 mL/min, or age younger than 50 years. Hypercalciuria (>400 mg calcium/24 hours) with increased stone risk by biochemical stone risk analysis and the presence of nephrolithiasis or nephrocalcinosis by imaging techniques are currently considered an indication for parathyroid surgery. Patients older than 50 years with no obvious symptoms should receive close follow-up, including measurements of bone density every 1 to 2 years and serum creatinine and calcium levels annually. All monitored patients should be repleted with vitamin D to achieve a 25-hydroxyvitamin D (25[OH]) D level above 20 ng/dL and should maintain calcium intake the same as individuals without PHPT.

Preoperative localization of the parathyroid glands has generally been considered unnecessary in uncomplicated patients undergoing surgery for the first time with bilateral neck exploration. However, imaging studies are recommended to be used in complicated cases and if minimally invasive surgery is planned.[34] Sestamibi scanning is the most popular and sensitive technique to localize PTH glands, with accuracy rates up to 94%, followed by ultrasound of the neck.[32,35] If a single adenoma is visualized, minimally invasive parathyroidectomy may be an option, with a cure rate of 95% to 98%: this procedure requires the surgeon to visualize only one gland as long as resection results in a substantial intraoperative decline in PTH level. Otherwise, all four parathyroid glands should be surgically identified. Recurrence of HPT is rare after identification and removal of one enlarged gland.[36] If the initial exploration fails, and hypercalcemia persists or recurs, more extensive preoperative parathyroid localization should be performed.[18,32,35] Complications are greater with reexploration of the neck than after the initial operation.

Although parathyroidectomy remains the definitive treatment of PHPT, patients refusing surgery, those with contraindications for surgery, or those who do not meet current operative guidelines can be treated pharmacologically. There are four classes of medications that can be useful—calcimimetics, bisphosphonates, estrogens, and selective estrogen receptor modulators.[32,37] There are insufficient long-term data to recommend any of these medications as alternatives to surgery. The CaSR agonist, cinacalcet, has been approved in some European countries for PHPT and in the United States for severe hypercalcemia in adult patients with PHPT who are unable to undergo parathyroidectomy. Cinacalcet therapy in PHPT patients reduced plasma PTH levels, normalized serum calcium levels in the short and long terms, and preserved bone mineral density (BMD).[37–40] Bisphosphonates and hormone replacement therapy decreased bone turnover and increased BMD in PHPT patients without change in serum calcium levels.[37]

Parathyroid carcinoma probably accounts for less than 1% of PHPT cases.[25] The diagnosis of parathyroid carcinoma may be difficult to make in the absence of metastases because the histologic appearance may be similar to that of atypical adenomas.[41] In general, parathyroid carcinomas are typically large (3 cm), irregular, hard tumors with a low degree of aggressive growth, and survival is common if the entire gland can be removed.[25,42] Cinacalcet is approved for patients with inoperable parathyroid cancer to control hypercalcemia.

### Malignancy

Hypercalcemia occurs in approximately 10% to 25% of patients with some cancer, especially during the last 4 to 6 weeks of their life. It can be classified into four categories—HHM, local osteolytic hypercalcemia (LOH), 1,25 $(OH)_2$ vitamin D–induced hypercalcemia, and ectopic secretion of authentic PTH.[43,44]

HHM from secretion of PTHrP by a malignant tumor accounts for approximately 80% of cases. Numerous types of malignancies are associated with HHM, including squamous cell cancer (e.g., head and neck, esophagus, cervix, lung) and renal cell carcinoma, breast cancer, and ovarian carcinoma. Lymphomas associated with human T-lymphotropic virus type 1 (HTLV-1) infection may cause PTHrP-mediated HHM, and other non-Hodgkin lymphomas may also be associated with PTHrP-mediated hypercalcemia.[44,45] PTHrP is a large protein encoded by a gene on chromosome 12; it is similar to PTH only at the $NH_2$ terminus, where the initial eight amino acids are identical.[45] PTHrP is widely expressed in a variety of tissues, including keratinocytes, mammary gland, placenta, cartilage, nervous system, vascular smooth muscle, and various endocrine sites.[46] Injection of PTHrP produces hypercalcemia in rats[47] and essentially reproduces the entire clinical syndrome of HHM, but other circulating factors such as cytokines may also be important. Normal circulating levels of PTHrP are negligible; these are probably unimportant in normal calcium homeostasis. However, mice with a targeted disruption in the PTHrP gene have shown a lethal defect in bone development,[48–50] thus demonstrating its importance in normal development.

Circulating PTHrP interacts with the PTH/PTHrP receptor in bone and the kidney tubule. It activates bone resorption and suppresses osteoblastic bone formation, thus causing flux of calcium (up to 700–1000 mg/day) from bone into ECF. The reason for this uncoupling of bone formation from bone resorption remains unclear.[45] One possible explanation is a difference in the affinity of PTH versus that of PTHrP for the PTH receptor on osteoblasts.[49] PTHrP mimics the anticalciuric effect of PTH on the kidney, which exacerbates hypercalcemia. Other effects of PTHrP include phosphaturia, hypophosphatemia, and increased cAMP excretion by the kidney.

HHM is associated with a reduction in $1,25(OH)_2D$ levels (in contrast to PHPT), which may limit intestinal calcium absorption. Patients are hypercalcemic and hypophosphatemic and demonstrate increased osteoclastic bone resorption, increased urinary cAMP levels, and hypercalciuria.

Local osteolytic hypercalcemia (LOH) accounts for 20% of patients with malignancy-associated hypercalcemia. LOH-producing tumors include breast and prostate cancers and hematologic neoplasms (e.g., multiple myeloma, lymphoma, leukemia). LOH is caused by locally produced osteoclast-activating cytokines, which include PTHrP, interleukin-1 (IL-1), IL-6, and IL-8. PTHrP increases RANKL expression in osteoblasts and RANK-mediated osteoclast bone resorption. The resorbing bone releases transforming growth factor-β (TGF-β), which in turn stimulates PTHrP expression on tumor cells.[50,51] The bone metastases can be classified as osteolytic, osteoblastic, or mixed. Osteolytic lesions are caused by osteoclast activation by malignant cells and appear as areas of increased radiolucency on radiographs. LOH leads to predictable pathophysiologic events, which include hypercalcemia, suppression of circulating PTH and $1,25(OH)_2D$, hyperphosphatemia, and hypercalciuria. Bone metastases may produce severe pain and pathologic fractures.

Hypercalcemia in breast cancer is associated with the presence of extensive osteolytic metastases and HHM.[50,51] Extensive osteolytic bone destruction is seen in multiple myeloma.[52] Although bone lesions develop in all patients with myeloma, hypercalcemia occurs only in 15% to 20% of patients in later stages of disease and with impaired kidney function. The degree of hypercalcemia and bone destruction has not been not well correlated.[53] Treatment with bisphosphonates appears to protect against the development of skeletal complications (including hypercalcemia) in patients with myeloma and lytic bone lesions.[54]

Hypercalcemia caused by $1,25(OH)_2$ vitamin D production by malignant lymphomas has been reported.[55,56] All types of lymphoma can cause this syndrome. The malignant cells or adjacent cells overexpress the enzyme 1α-hydroxylase, which converts 25(OH)D to 1,25(OH)$_2$D. Hypercalcemia is mainly secondary to increased intestinal calcium, although decreased kidney clearance and bone resorption may also develop. In addition, increased osteoclastic activity mediated through activation of the RANKL pathway by 1,25(OH)$_2$D– augmented hypercalcemia. Ectopic production of authentic PTH by a nonparathyroid tumor may occur, but is very rare.[57]

### Familial Primary Hyperparathyroidism Syndromes

Familial primary HPT syndromes are defined by a combination of hypercalcemia and elevated or nonsuppressed serum PTH levels.

**Familial Hypocalciuric Hypercalcemia and Neonatal Severe Hyperparathyroidism.** FHH (benign) is a rare disease (estimated prevalence, 1/78,000), with autosomal dominant inheritance, high penetrance for hypercalcemia, and relative hypocalciuria.[58–60] FHH was first described in 1966 by Jackson and Boonstra and in 1972 by Foley and colleagues.[61,62] The hypercalcemia is typically mild to moderate (10.5–12 mg/dL), and affected patients do not exhibit the typical complications associated with elevated serum calcium concentrations. Both total and ionized calcium concentrations are elevated, but the PTH level is generally inappropriately normal, although mild elevations in approximately 15% to 20% of cases have been reported. Urinary calcium excretion is not elevated, as would be expected in hypercalcemia of other causes. The fractional excretion of calcium is usually less than 1%.[59] The serum magnesium level is commonly mildly elevated, and the serum phosphate level is decreased. Bone mineral density is normal, as are vitamin D levels. The finding of a right-shifted set point for $Ca^{2+}$-regulated PTH release in FHH has indicated the role of CaSR in FHH.[63]

Most families have FHH type 1, which is caused by autosomal dominant loss-of-function mutations in the CaSR gene located on chromosome 3q, which encodes for the CaSR. FHH types 2 and 3 are much rarer and are caused by heterozygous mutations in the GNA11 (guanidine nucleotide-binding protein alpha-11) gene or the AP2S1 (adaptor-related protein complex 2, sigma 1 subunit) gene, respectively.[64,65] Both genes localize on chromosome 19q13, and their mutations render the CaSR less sensitive to extracellular calcium.

The fact that relative hypocalciuria persists, even after parathyroidectomy in FHH patients, confirms the role of CaSR in regulating kidney calcium handling.[66] More than 257 mutations have been described for the CaSR, most of which are inactivating and missense mutations, found throughout the large predicted structure of the CaSR protein.[63,67,68] Expression studies of mutant CaSRs have shown great variability in their effect on calcium responsiveness. In some cases, CaSR mutations only slightly shift the set point for calcium; other mutations appear to render the receptor largely inactive.[69–71] CaSR mutation analysis has an occasional role in the diagnosis of FHH in cases in which biochemical test results remain inconclusive, and the distinction of FHH from mild primary HPT is unclear. It is critically important to make an accurate diagnosis because the hypercalcemia in FHH is benign and does not respond to subtotal parathyroidectomy.

Hypercalcemia in FHH has a generally benign course and is resistant to medications, but it has been successfully treated with cinacalcet in some patients.[72] A potential benefit of calcimimetic agents in FHH has been supported by in vitro studies with human CaSR mutants, which have shown that the calcimimetic agent R-568 enhances the potency of extracellular calcium toward the mutants.[73]

Patients who inherit two copies of CaSR alleles bearing inactivating mutations develop neonatal severe HPT (NSHPT). NSHPT is an extremely rare disorder that is often reported in the offspring of consanguineous FHH parents; it is characterized by severe hyperparathyroid hyperplasia, PTH elevation, severe hyperparathyroid bone disease, and elevated extracellular calcium levels.[58,63,74,75] In a few affected infants, only one defective allele has been found, but it is unclear whether this finding is due to the presence of an undetected defect in the other CaSR allele. Treatment is total parathyroidectomy, followed by vitamin D and calcium supplementation. This disease is usually lethal without surgical intervention.

**Multiple Endocrine Neoplasia.** MEN1 is a rare, autosomal dominant disorder with an estimated prevalence of two to three cases/100,000, characterized by endocrine tumors in at least two of three main tissues—parathyroid gland, pituitary gland, and enteropancreatic tissue. It is the most common form of familial PHPT. PHPT is present in 87% to 97% of patients, whereas pancreatic and pituitary tumors are more likely to be absent.[18,76] The responsible gene, MEN1,[77] encodes a nuclear protein, menin, of 610 amino acids, which functions in cell division, genome stability, and transcription regulation.[78]

MEN2A is a syndrome of heritable predisposition to medullary thyroid carcinoma, pheochromocytoma, and PHPT. Mutations in the RET proto-oncogene, which encodes a tyrosine kinase receptor, are responsible for MEN2A.[79] The biochemical diagnoses and indications for surgery for patients with PHPT in association with MEN1 or MEN2A are similar to those for sporadic PHPT.[80]

**Hyperparathyroidism–Jaw Tumor Syndrome.** Hyperparathyroidism–jaw tumor (HPT-JT) syndrome is a rare autosomal dominant disorder characterized by severe hypercalcemia, parathyroid adenoma, and fibro-osseous tumors of mandible or maxilla.[81] Kidney manifestations include cysts, hamartomas, and Wilms' tumor. Mutations in the *HRPT2* (hyperparathyroidism 2) gene, and elimination of its product, parafibromin, which has tumor suppressor activity, are responsible for HPT-JT.[82] If biochemical changes consistent with PHPT are present, parathyroidectomy is indicated.

### Nonparathyroid Endocrinopathies

Hypercalcemia may occur in patients with other endocrine diseases. Mild hypercalcemia is present in up to 20% of patients with hyperthyroidism, but severe hypercalcemia is uncommon.[83,84] Thyroid hormones (e.g., thyroxine, triiodothyronine) increase bone resorption and lead to hypercalcemia and/or hypercalciuria when bone resorption exceeds bone formation significantly.[85] Because of a possible increased association between hyperthyroidism and parathyroid adenoma, the latter must be ruled out in patients with thyrotoxicosis and hypercalcemia. Furthermore, the hypercalcemia in a patient with thyrotoxicosis should be attributed to this disease only if it resolves after achieving an euthyroid state.

Pheochromocytoma may be associated with hypercalcemia[86]; it is usually caused by coincident PHPT and MEN2A. In some patients, hypercalcemia disappears after removal of the adrenal tumor, and some of these tumors produce PTHrP.[87] Acute adrenal insufficiency is a rare cause of hypercalcemia.[88] Because these patients may be dehydrated and have hemoconcentration, a rise in the serum albumin concentration and increased binding of calcium to serum albumin secondary to hyponatremia may contribute to the increase in serum calcium levels. In addition, isolated adrenocorticotropic hormone (ACTH) deficiency can result in hypercalcemia.[89]

Growth hormone administration[90] and acromegaly[91] have both been associated with hypercalcemia. Acromegaly is often (15%–20% of cases) accompanied by mild hypercalcemia, which results from enhanced intestinal calcium absorption and augmented bone resorption.[92,93] In acromegalic patients with hypercalcemia, the serum levels of PTH are normal but may be inappropriately high for the levels of serum calcium.

### Vitamin D–Mediated Hypercalcemia

Vitamin D is naturally generated in skin under exposure to ultraviolet B (UVB) light or is acquired from the diet and medical supplements. Excess of vitamin D or its metabolites can cause hypercalcemia and hypercalciuria. The mechanism of hypercalcemia is a combination of increased intestinal calcium absorption and bone resorption induced by vitamin D and decreased kidney calcium clearance resulting from dehydration. The effect of toxic amounts of vitamin D is due to an increase in total plasma 25(OH)D, well in excess of 100 ng/mL, which exceeds the binding capacity of vitamin D–binding protein (DBP) for 25(OH)D. The resulting increase in free circulating 25(OH)D may activate the vitamin D nuclear receptor (VDR). Vitamin D metabolites may also displace $1\alpha,25(OH)_2D$ from DBP, increasing free $1\alpha,25(OH)_2D$ levels and thus increasing signal transduction.[94]

Hypercalcemia has been reported in accidental overdoses of vitamin D from fortified cow's milk,[95,96] consumption by children of a fish oil with manufacturing error that caused an excess of vitamin D, and over-the-counter supplements.[97] Serum 25(OH)D levels were elevated, $1,25(OH)_2D$ levels were normal, and PTH levels were depressed or normal in these settings. However, vitamin D well in excess of the tolerable upper intake of 2000 IU/day is required for this form of hypercalcemia to develop.[98] Polymorphism in genes that regulate vitamin D metabolism may predispose certain individuals to develop toxicity, even with exposure to small vitamin D doses.[96] The diagnosis is made by the history and detection of elevated 25(OH)D levels. In the syndrome of idiopathic infantile hypercalcemia, a defect in degradation of $1,25(OH)_2D$ to $24,25(OH)_2D$ caused by a CYP24A1 loss-of-function mutation is responsible for extremely high levels of $1,25(OH)_2D$ and hypercalcemia. Vitamin D analogues, including $1,25(OH)_2D$ used in the treatment of HPT and metabolic bone disease in CKD patients, can also cause hypercalcemia.[99]

### Medications

Hypercalcemia and HPT is a long-recognized, well-described consequence of lithium therapy.[100–103] The prevalence of lithium-associated hypercalcemia has been estimated to be 4% to 6%.[101,104] Lithium probably interferes with signal transduction elicited by the CaSR, which increases the set point for extracellular calcium to inhibit PTH secretion.[103–105] This leads to parathyroid hyperplasia or adenoma.[106] The spectrum of lithium-induced calcium disorders is wide and includes patients with overt HPT and mild or severe hypercalcemia, with or without elevated PTH levels. Hypocalciuria is common, although hypercalciuria was reported in a few case series. Hypercalcemia can be reversible after a few weeks of discontinuing lithium in most patients with short lithium treatment (<5 years). The CaSR agonist cinacalcet was also used with good results in those patients when cessation of lithium therapy was not an option.[107] Symptomatic patients with HPT should be treated with parathyroidectomy.[102,103]

Vitamin A intake in doses exceeding the recommended daily allowance over prolonged periods, especially in older adults and patients with impaired kidney function, may cause hypercalcemia, with increased alkaline phosphatase levels, presumably from increased osteoclast-mediated bone resorption.[108–110] The hypercalcemia is accompanied by high retinol plasma levels, and discontinuation of vitamin A caused normalization of plasma calcium levels. Vitamin A analogues, used in the management of dermatologic and hematologic malignant diseases, have also been reported to cause hypercalcemia.[111,112]

Estrogens and selective estrogen receptor modifiers (e.g., tamoxifen) used in the management of breast cancer may cause hypercalcemia early during treatment, even in the presence of bone metastasis.[113]

The incidence of thiazide-associated hypercalcemia increased after 1997 and peaked in 2006, with an annual incidence of 20 cases/100,000, compared with an overall rate of 12 cases/100,000 in 1992–2010 in the population of Olmsted County, Minnesota.[114,115] A reduction in urinary calcium excretion, volume contraction, and metabolic alkalosis are the major reasons for thiazide-induced hypercalcemia. Also, thiazides may increase intestinal calcium absorption and reveal PHPT.[115–117] Hypercalcemia is usually mild and asymptomatic. Subjects with unsuppressed PTH levels, despite hypercalcemia or with severe and continued hypercalcemia, may have PHPT.

Many other medications occasionally cause hypercalcemia, including theophylline, foscarnet, growth hormone, parenteral nutrition, and manganese in toxic doses.

### Milk-Alkali Syndrome

Milk-alkali syndrome was originally described in patients with duodenal ulcers receiving therapy with sodium bicarbonate and large amounts of milk. These patients have hypercalcemia, hyperphosphatemia, hypocalciuria, and CKD, together with kidney and other soft tissue calcifications.[118] During the last 20 years, calcium supplements in the form of calcium carbonate for the prevention and treatment of osteoporosis have become the main cause of this syndrome.[119,120] In the most recent literature, the name "calcium-alkali syndrome" was proposed.[121] In some studies, milk-alkali syndrome was the third most common cause of hypercalcemia in non–end-stage kidney disease (ESKD) hospitalized patients.[122] The pathogenesis of milk-alkali syndrome can be divided into two phases, the generation of hypercalcemia by the intake of calcium and the maintenance phase. Usually, oral intake of more than 4g of elemental calcium/day has been reported, but even 2 g of calcium/day, especially if taken together with vitamin D, may induce this syndrome. Hypercalcemia activates the kidney CaSR, causing natriuresis and water diuresis, with volume depletion and a decrease in the GFR. Increased tubular reabsorption of calcium as a result of metabolic alkalosis and volume depletion contribute to the maintenance of hypercalcemia.[120] The diagnosis is made largely by the history and may not be obvious because of atypical dietary sources of calcium and alkali. Hypercalcemia can be corrected, but kidney damage may be permanent.

#### Immobilization

Immobilization, especially in high bone turnover states (e.g., in young people and in those with hyperparathyroidism, breast cancer with bone involvement, Paget disease), suppresses osteoblastic bone formation and increases osteoclastic bone resorption, leading to uncoupling of these two processes, with subsequent release of calcium from the bone and hypercalcemia.[123,124] Typically, it takes from 10 days to a few weeks for the development of immobilization hypercalcemia. Increased sclerostin production by osteocytes during mechanical unloading and disuse of the bone is implicated in the pathogenesis of hypercalcemia.[125] Sclerostin is a glycoprotein that inhibits Wnt/β catenin signaling in the osteoblast and decreases bone formation.[126] It is of interest that antisclerostin antibodies are being studied for the treatment of osteoporosis. Bisphosphonates may help decrease hypercalcemia and osteopenia in the setting of immobilization-induced hypercalcemia.[127] There are case reports showing that denosumab also can correct hypercalcemia of immobilization. Denosumab is a fully humanized monoclonal antibody that prevents the binding of RANK to RANKL, thereby reducing the formation, function, and survival of osteoclasts. Mobilization remains the ultimate cure for immobilization-associated hypercalcemia.

#### Granulomatous Disease

A variety of granulomatous diseases are associated with hypercalcemia. The most common is sarcoidosis—prevalence of hypercalcemia and hypercalciuria of 10% and 20%, respectively—but tuberculosis, berylliosis, histoplasmosis, coccidioidomycosis, pneumocystosis, leprosy, histiocytosis X, eosinophilic granulomatosis, and inflammatory bowel disease may present with hypercalcemia.[89,128–130] Hypercalcemia is more common in chronic and disseminated granulomatous diseases. Sun exposure, or even small doses of vitamin D supplementation, may precipitate or worsen this syndrome. The hypercalcemia, which has been best studied in sarcoidosis, is caused by inappropriate extrarenal production of $1,25(OH)_2D$ by activated macrophages with increased 1α-hydroxylase activity.[131,132] Elevated circulating $1,25(OH)_2D$ levels have been described in most granulomatous diseases during hypercalcemia, except in coccidioidomycosis. The $1,25(OH)_2D$ in turn leads to intestinal hyperabsorption of calcium, hypercalciuria, and hypercalcemia. Osteopontin, highly expressed by histiocytes in granulomas, may contribute to hypercalcemia via osteoclast activation and bone resorption. Bone mineral content tends to be reduced in these patients. Hypercalciuria may precede hypercalcemia and may be an early indicator of this complication.

Standard treatment consists of administration of glucocorticoids, which decreases the abnormal $1,25(OH)_2D$ production.[133] Chloroquine and ketoconazole, which also decrease $1,25(OH)_2D$ production by competitive inhibition of CYP450-dependent 1α-hydroxylase, have also been shown to be efficacious.[134,135]

#### Liver Disease

Hypercalcemia has been reported in patients with end-stage liver disease with hyperbilirubinemia who are awaiting liver transplantation in the absence of HPT or hypervitaminosis D.[136]

#### Acute and Chronic Kidney Disease

Hypercalcemia may be observed in patients with certain forms of acute and chronic kidney disease and in kidney transplant recipients. These conditions are discussed in detail in Chapter 55.

### MANAGEMENT OF HYPERCALCEMIA

The optimal therapy for hypercalcemia must be tailored to the severity of hypercalcemia, clinical condition, and underlying cause (Table 18.1).[15] Theoretically, a decrease in serum calcium levels can be achieved by enhancing its urinary excretion, augmenting net movement of calcium into bone, inhibiting bone resorption, reducing intestinal absorption of calcium, and/or removing calcium from the ECF by other means. Patients with mild hypercalcemia (<12 mg/dL) do not require immediate treatment. They should discontinue any medications implicated in causing hypercalcemia, avoid volume depletion and physical inactivity, and maintain adequate hydration. Moderate hypercalcemia (12–14 mg/dL), especially if acute and symptomatic, requires more aggressive therapy. Patients with severe hypercalcemia (>14 mg/dL), even without symptoms, should be treated intensively.

#### Volume Repletion and Loop Diuretics

Correction of the ECF volume is the first and most important step in the treatment of severe hypercalcemia from any causes. It can be achieved with a normal isotonic saline infusion at 200 to 500 mL/hour, adjusted to obtain a urine output of 150 to 200 mL/hour and with appropriate hemodynamic monitoring.[15,137,138] Volume repletion can lower the calcium concentration by approximately 1 to 3 mg/dL by increasing GFR and decreasing sodium and calcium reabsorption in the proximal and distal tubules.

Once volume expansion is achieved, loop diuretics can be given concurrently with saline to increase the calciuresis by blocking the $Na^+$-$K^+$-$2Cl^-$ cotransporter in the TAL.[137] Usually, furosemide is given at a dose of 40 to 80 mg every 6 hours and this, together with saline therapy, may decrease the serum calcium concentration by 2 to 4 mg/dL. Urinary losses of fluid, potassium, and magnesium should be evaluated at intervals of 2 to 4 hours and quantitatively replaced to prevent dehydration, hypokalemia, and hypomagnesemia. Usually, 20 to 40 mEq of KCl and 15 to 30 mg of magnesium ion/L of saline infusion are adequate to replenish the urinary losses of these electrolytes. Care must be taken to monitor the patient's volume status closely during the administration of large amounts of saline and diuretic, particularly in hospitalized patients with cardiac or pulmonary disease. It must be noted that the use of loop diuretics for hypercalcemia is not supported by any randomized controlled studies and has

**Table 18.1 Pharmacologic Therapy for Hypercalcemia[a]**

| Intervention | Dose | Adverse Effects |
|---|---|---|
| **Hydration or Calciuresis** | | |
| Intravenous saline | 200–500 mL/h, depending on patient's cardiovascular and kidney status | Congestive heart failure |
| Furosemide | 20–40 mg IV (after rehydration has been achieved) | Dehydration, hypokalemia, hypomagnesemia |
| **First-Line Medications** | | |
| IV bisphosphonates[b] | | |
| Pamidronate | 60–90 mg IV over 2 hours in 50–200 mL saline solution or 5% dextrose in water[d] | Acute kidney injury, transient flulike syndrome with aches, chills, and fever |
| Zoledronate | 4 mg IV over 15 minutes in 50 mL of saline solution or 5% dextrose in water | Acute kidney injury, transient flulike syndrome with aches, chills, and fever |
| **Second-Line Medications** | | |
| Glucocorticoids[c] | Example: prednisone, 60 mg orally daily, for 10 days | Potential interference with chemotherapy; hypokalemia, hyperglycemia, hypertension, Cushing syndrome, immunosuppression |
| Mithramycin | Single dose of 25 μg/kg of body weight over 4–6 hours in saline | Thrombocytopenia, platelet aggregation defect, anemia, leukopenia, hepatitis, kidney failure[e] |
| Calcitonin | 4–8 U/kg subcutaneously or intramuscularly every 12 hours | Flushing, nausea, escape phenomenon |
| Gallium nitrate | 100–200 mg/m$^2$ of body surface area IV given continuously over 24 hours for 5 days | Acute kidney injury |
| Denosumab[f] | 120 mg on days 1, 8, 15, and 29 and every 4 weeks | Hypocalcemia, hypophosphatemia, osteonecrosis of the jaw, atypical femoral fractures |

[a]Many recommendations in this table are based on historical precedent and common practice rather than on randomized clinical trials. There are data from randomized trials comparing bisphosphonates to the other agents listed and to one another.
[b]Pamidronate and zoledronate are approved by the US Food and Drug Administration (FDA). Ibandronate and clodronate are available in continental Europe, the United Kingdom, and elsewhere. Bisphosphonates should be used with caution, if at all, when the serum creatinine level exceeds 2.5 to 3.0 mg/dL (221.0–265.2 μmol/L).
[c]Pamidronate is generally used at a dose of 90 mg, but the 60-mg dose may be used to treat patients of small stature or those with kidney impairment or mild hypercalcemia.
[d]These drugs have a slow onset of action, as compared with bisphosphonates; approximately 4 to 10 days are required for a response.
[e]These effects have been reported in association with higher dose regimens used to treat testicular cancer (50 μg/kg body weight/day over a period of 5 days) and in patients receiving multiple doses of 25 μg/kg; they are not expected to occur with a single dose of 25 μg/kg unless preexisting liver, kidney, or hematologic disease is present.
[f]Approved by the FDA for the prevention of skeletal-related events in patients with bone metastasis from solid tumor; used in an open-label fashion as a rescue therapy if bisphosphonates are not effective.
Modified from Stewart AF. Clinical practice. Hypercalcemia associated with cancer. *N Engl J Med.* 2005;352:373–379. With permission.

been criticized for this reason.[138] However, in our opinion, loop diuretics still remain an important tool in the management of hypercalcemia, especially for patients at risk of volume overload.

### Inhibition of Bone Resorption

The increase in bone resorption, as the most common pathology leading to hypercalcemia, must be addressed concurrently with volume expansion and hydration. Bisphosphonates are currently the agents of choice in the treatment of mild to severe hypercalcemia, especially that associated with cancer and vitamin D toxicity.[96] They are pyrophosphate analogues with a high affinity for hydroxyapatite and inhibit osteoclast function in areas of high bone turnover.[15] The US Food and Drug Administration (FDA) has approved two bisphosphonates for the treatment of hypercalcemia, zoledronate (4 mg intravenous [IV] over 15 minutes or longer) and pamidronate (60–90 mg IV over 2–24 hours). The clinical response takes 48 to 96 hours and is sustained for up to 3 weeks. Doses can be repeated no sooner than every 7 days. Both agents are effective in lowering calcium levels. Zoledronate was slightly more efficacious than pamidronate in a randomized clinical trial.[139] In Europe, other bisphosphonates, such as clodronate and ibandronate, have also been approved.

Fever is observed in about 20% of patients taking bisphosphonates; rare side effects include acute kidney injury, collapsing glomerulopathy, and osteonecrosis of the jaw. Ibandronate seems to have minimal to no kidney toxicity. The dose of bisphosphonates should be adjusted in patients with preexisting kidney disease.[140] The kidney component of hypercalcemia, which includes increased distal tubular calcium reabsorption driven by PTH-PTHrP, does not respond to bisphosphonates.

Calcitonin is also an effective inhibitor of osteoclast bone resorption. It has a rapid onset (within 12 hours), its effect is transient, and it has minimal toxicity.[141–145] Calcitonin is usually given as 4 to 8 U/kg subcutaneously every 6 to 12 hours.[141,142] Its role is mainly in the initial treatment of severe hypercalcemia while waiting for the more sustained effect of bisphosphonates.

Gallium nitrate inhibits bone resorption by increasing the solubility of hydroxyapatite crystals. The usual dose is 200 mg/$m^2$ IV over 24 hours, with adequate hydration for 5 consecutive days; the hypocalcemic effect is not generally observed until the end of this period. Gallium nitrate is effective, but can be nephrotoxic.[143,144]

Denosumab, is a fully humanized monoclonal antibody that binds to RANKL and inhibits osteoclasts. Denosumab inhibits the maturation of preosteoclasts to osteoclasts by binding to and inhibiting RANKL. In 2010, denosumab was approved by the FDA for postmenopausal women at risk for osteoporosis.[145] It was also approved for the prevention of skeleton-related events in patients with bone metastasis from a solid tumor. It has also been approved for the treatment of hypercalcemia of malignancy not corrected by bisphosphonates.[145,146]

Plicamycin (Mithramycin), 25 μg/kg IV, every 5 to 7 days, may be used in patients with advanced kidney disease. Other therapies for hypercalcemia, such as chelation with ethylenediaminetetraacetic acid (EDTA) and IV phosphate, have adverse side effect profiles and are no longer recommended.

Glucocorticoids are useful therapy for hypercalcemia in a specific subset of causes. They are most effective in hematologic malignancies (e.g., multiple myeloma, Hodgkin disease) and disorders of vitamin D metabolism (e.g., granulomatous disease, vitamin D toxicity).[128,133]

In severely hypercalcemic patients who are comatose with changes in the ECG, in severe acute kidney injury, or who cannot receive aggressive hydration, hemodialysis with a low- or no-calcium dialysate is an effective treatment.[147] Continuous kidney replacement therapy can also be used to treat severe hypercalcemia.[148] The effect of dialysis is transitory and needs to be followed by other measures.

As discussed previously, cinacalcet, an allosteric activator of CaSR, is approved for patients with inoperable parathyroid cancer to control hypercalcemia. The off-label use of cinacalcet has been reported in patients with PHPT who have mild disease, failed parathyroid surgery, or contraindications to surgery.[32,37,39,40] Other hypercalcemic disorders, such as FHH[72] and lithium-induced HPT, have also been treated with cinacalcet.[104,107]

## HYPOCALCEMIA

Hypocalcemia is usually defined as a total serum calcium concentration, corrected for protein, of less than 8.4 mg/dL and/or an ionized calcium level less 1.16 mmol/L, although these values may vary slightly, depending on the laboratory. Estimation of the ionized calcium concentration based on the total serum calcium corrected for albumin is encumbered with errors, as discussed in the introduction. Thus, ionized calcium should be directly measured before a major workup for the causes of hypocalcemia is undertaken.

Hypocalcemia is highly prevalent in hospitalized patients (10%–18%) and is particularly common in the intensive care unit (70%–80%).[149,150]

### SIGNS AND SYMPTOMS

Acute hypocalcemia can result in severe clinical symptoms that need rapid correction, whereas chronic hypocalcemia may be an asymptomatic laboratory finding. The clinical features of hypocalcemia are summarized in Box 18.3. Their presentation reflects the absolute calcium concentration and the rapidity of its fall. The threshold for overt symptoms depends also on serum pH and the severity of any concurrent hypomagnesemia, hyponatremia, or hypokalemia. The classic symptoms of hypocalcemia include neuromuscular excitability in the form of numbness, circumoral tingling, feeling of pins and needles in the feet and hands, muscle cramps, carpopedal spasms, laryngeal stridor, and frank tetany. Tapping over the facial nerve anterior to the ear can induce facial muscle spasm (Chvostek sign). However, a Chvostek sign may occur in 10% of normal people, and it was negative in 29% of patients with mild hypocalcemia. A Trousseau sign of *main d'accoucheur,* (French for "hand of the obstetrician"), elicited by inflation of a sphygmomanometer cuff placed on the upper arm to 10 mm Hg above systolic blood pressure for 3 minutes, has greater than 90% sensitivity and specificity.[151] Patients with hypocalcemia may experience emotional disturbances, irritability, impairment of memory, confusion, delusion, hallucination, paranoia, and depression. Epileptic seizures, often Jacksonian, may occur but are usually not associated with aura, loss of consciousness, and incontinence. Patients with chronic hypocalcemia, including those with idiopathic and postsurgical hypoparathyroidism and those with pseudohypoparathyroidism, may have papilledema, elevated cerebrospinal fluid pressure, and neurologic signs simulating those of a cerebral tumor.

**Box 18.3 Clinical Features of Hypocalcemia**

**Neuromuscular Irritability**

General fatigability and muscle weakness
Paresthesia, numbness
Circumoral and peripheral extremity tingling
Muscle twitching and cramping
Tetany, carpopedal spasms
Chvostek sign, Trousseau sign
Laryngeal and bronchial spasms

**Altered Central Nervous System Function**

Emotional disturbances—irritability, depression
Altered mental status, coma
Tonic-clonic seizures
Papilledema, pseudotumor cerebri
Cerebral calcifications

**Cardiovascular**

Lengthening of the QTc interval
Dysrhythmias
Hypotension
Congestive heart failure

**Dermatologic and Ocular**

Dry skin, coarse hair, brittle nails
Cataracts

Bilateral cataracts affecting the anterior and posterior subcapsular areas of the cortical portions of the lens may develop after 1 year of hypocalcemia. The cataracts do not resolve after correction of the hypocalcemia. In patients with idiopathic hypoparathyroidism, the skin could be dry and scaly, eczema and psoriasis may worsen, and candidiasis can occur. The eyelashes and eyebrows may be scanty, and axillary and pubic hair may be absent. Because some forms of this disease have an autoimmune cause, manifestations of other autoimmune diseases, such as adrenal, thyroid, and gonadal insufficiency, diabetes mellitus, pernicious anemia, vitiligo, and alopecia areata may be present and should be sought.

Long-lasting hypocalcemia in children and adults can result in congestive heart failure caused by cardiomyopathy, which is reversible with correction of the calcium.[152–154] Prolongation of the QTc interval on the ECG is a well-known effect of hypocalcemia on heart conduction.

Hypoparathyroidism in children often causes teeth abnormalities, such as defective enamel and root formation, dental hypoplasia, or failure of adult teeth to erupt. Severe skeletal mineralization may occur in the fetus of untreated pregnant women with hypoparathyroidism and hypocalcemia.

## LABORATORY FINDINGS

It is important to establish the diagnosis of hypocalcemia, based not only on the measurement of total calcium with proper adjustment to albumin and pH levels, but with evidence that ionized calcium is low. The alterations in serum PTH and serum and urinary electrolyte levels in various hypocalcemic states depend on the mechanisms responsible for the hypocalcemia (see Fig. 18.2), and knowledge of these changes aids in the differential diagnosis of these disorders.

An x-ray examination of the skull or computed tomography (CT) scanning of the brain may reveal intracranial calcifications, especially of the basal ganglia.[155] These have been noted in up to 20% of hypocalcemic patients with idiopathic hypoparathyroidism but are less common in postsurgical hypoparathyroidism unless the disease is long-standing. Such calcifications are also encountered in patients with pseudohypoparathyroidism. Bone disease may be observed, but its findings differ in the various causes of hypocalcemia (see later).

## DIAGNOSIS

The most common causes of hypocalcemia in the nonacute setting are hypoparathyroidism, hypomagnesemia, CKD, and vitamin D deficiencies (Box 18.4). These entities should be considered early in the diagnosis of hypocalcemic individuals. It is conceptually and clinically useful to subclassify hypocalcemic individuals into those with elevated PTH levels and those with subnormal or inappropriately normal PTH concentrations, as in primary hypoparathyroidism (Fig. 18.3). A thorough medical history and physical examination are diagnostically important because hypocalcemia can be caused by postsurgical, pharmacologic, inherited, developmental, and nutritional problems, in addition to being part of complex syndromes.

## CAUSES

The causes of hypocalcemia are summarized in Box 18.4. They can be broadly classified into one of three

### Box 18.4 Causes of Hypocalcemia

Inherited and genetic syndromes with hypoparathyroidism
- PTH gene mutations, isolated congenital hypoparathyroidism
- Autosomal dominant hypoparathyroidism with activating mutation of the CaSR (OMIM 146200)
- DiGeorge syndrome (OMIM 188400)
- Other forms of familial hypoparathyroidism

Inherited and genetic syndromes with resistance to PTH action
- Pseudohypoparathyroidism, types 1a, 1b, and 2
- Hypomagnesemic syndromes

Acquired hypoparathyroidism, inadequate PTH production
- Damage or destruction of the parathyroid glands
  - Postsurgical
  - Autoimmune—isolated or with multiple endocrine dysfunction
    - Acquired antibodies against CaSR
    - Polyglandular failure syndrome type I (OMIM 240300 and 607358)
  - Irradiation
  - Metastatic and infiltrative diseases
  - Deposition of heavy metals—iron overload, copper overload
- Reversible impairment of PTH secretion
  - Severe hypomagnesemia
  - Hypermagnesemia

Inadequate vitamin D production
  - Vitamin D deficiency—nutritional, lack of sunlight exposure
  - Malabsorption
  - End-stage liver disease and cirrhosis
  - Chronic kidney disease

Vitamin D resistance
  - Pseudovitamin D deficiency rickets (vitamin D–dependent rickets type 1)
  - Vitamin D–resistant rickets (vitamin D–dependent rickets type 2)

Miscellaneous causes
  - Hyperphosphatemia
  - Phosphate retention caused by acute or chronic kidney disease
  - Excess phosphate absorption caused by enemas, oral supplements
  - Massive phosphate release caused by tumor lysis or crush injury

Drugs
  - Foscarnet
  - Bisphosphonate therapy (especially in patients with vitamin D deficiency)
  - Denosumab

Rapid transfusion of large volumes of citrate-containing blood

Acute critical illness (multiple contributing causes)

Hungry bone syndrome, recalcification tetany
  - Postthyroidectomy for Graves disease
  - Postparathyroidectomy

Osteoblastic metastases

Acute pancreatitis

Rhabdomyolysis

Substances interfering with the laboratory assay for total calcium
  - Gadolinium salts in contrast agents given during MRI, MRA

*CaSR,* Calcium-sensing receptor; *OMIM,* Online Mendelian Inheritance in Man; *MRI,* magnetic resonance imaging; *MRA,* magnetic resonance angiography; *PTH,* parathyroid hormone.

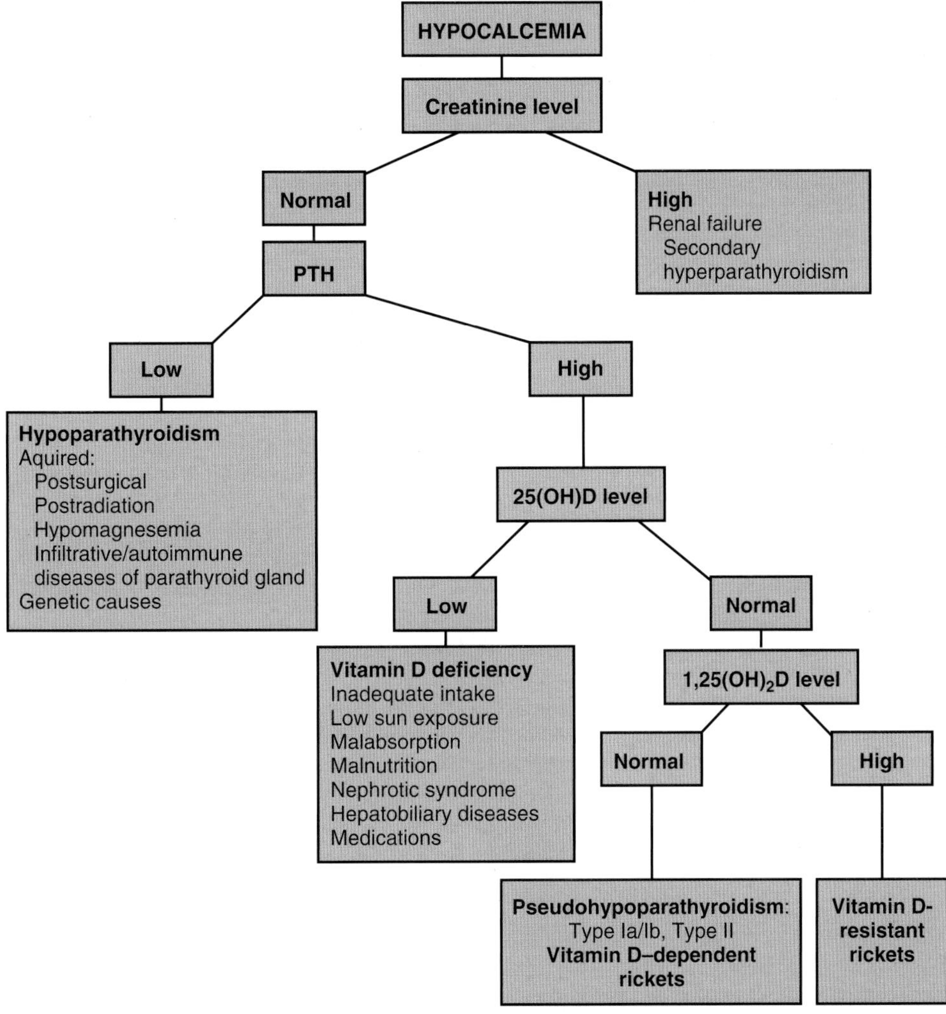


**Fig. 18.3** Algorithm for the evaluation of hypocalcemia. *PTH*, Parathyroid hormone.

categories—PTH-related (hypoparathyroidism and pseudohypoparathyroidism), vitamin D–related (low production, vitamin D resistance), and miscellaneous causes.

### Parathyroid Hormone–Related Disorders: Hypoparathyroidism and Pseudohypoparathyroidism

This group of disorders presents with hypocalcemia and hyperphosphatemia caused by failure of the parathyroid gland to secrete adequate amounts of biologically active PTH or resistance to PTH action at the tissue level. Both can be inherited or acquired. The levels of PTH are low or absent in hypoparathyroidism (HP) due to lack of PTH production, but elevated in pseudohypoparathyroidism (PHP) due to a secondary or adaptive increase in PTH secretion. The fractional calcium excretion is elevated in HP and low in PHP. Insufficient 1,25(OH)$_2$D is generated for efficient intestinal calcium absorption because of decreased activity of 1$\alpha$-hydroxylase in the proximal tubules. Skeletal response in both categories is appropriate to the levels of circulating PTH, with low bone turnover in HP and excessive bone remodeling in PHP.[156,157] Hypoparathyroidism is a rare disorder. One study from Japan has found the prevalence to be 7.2 cases/million people.[158]

**Genetic Causes of Hypoparathyroidism.** At least four different mutations affecting the PTH gene(s) involved in parathyroid development have been identified as a cause of familial isolated HP (Table 18.2). All these conditions present during the neonatal period with severe hypocalcemia without any other organ involvement and respond well to therapy with vitamin D analogues.

Heterozygous gain-of-function mutations in the CaSR can activate CaSR or cause CaSR to be hyperresponsive to extracellular calcium.[163] The phenotype seen is essentially the opposite of FHH and has been termed "autosomal dominant hypoparathyroidism" or "familiar hypocalcemia with hypercalciuria." Patients present with mild hypocalcemia, hypomagnesemia and hypercalciuria, with low or inappropriately normal PTH levels. The set point for PTH secretion is shifted to the left. Treatment with calcium supplements and vitamin D is warranted only for patients with severe symptomatic hypocalcemia. The goal should be to increase the calcium level to render the patient asymptomatic, not necessarily to a normocalcemic level. Kidney calcium excretion requires monitoring because these patients may develop frank hypercalciuria and nephrocalcinosis.[168,169] Thiazide diuretics or injectable PTH can be used to decrease calciuria at any given level of serum calcium.[170,171]

**Table 18.2 Genetic Syndromes With Hypoparathyroidism**

| Reference | Syndrome | Other Clinical Features | Process Affected | Inheritance | Gene Mutated | Syndrome OMIM No. |
|---|---|---|---|---|---|---|
| Ding et al[159] | Familial isolated hypoparathyroidism | None | Parathyroid gland development | AR | *GCM2* | 146200 |
| Bowl et al[160] | | | | X-linked | *SOX3?* | 307700 |
| Parkinson and Thakker[161] | | | PTH gene mutation affecting its synthesis | AR | Prepro-PTH splice site | |
| Arnold et al[162] | | | | AD | Prepro-PTH signal peptide | |
| Pollak et al[163] | Autosomal dominant hypoparathyroidism | Hypocalcemia, hypomagnesemia, hypercalciuria | Calcium sensing | AD | *CaSR* | 146200 601298 |
| Yagi et al[164] | DiGeorge, CATCH22 | Cardiac anomalies, abnormal facies, thymic aplasia, cleft palate | Defective third and fourth branchial pouch development | Sporadic or AD | Chromosome 22q11 deletions (including TBX1) | 188400 |
| Van Esch et al[165] | HDR | Hypoparathyroidism, deafness, kidney anomalies | Parathyroid development | AD | *GATA3* transcription factor | 146255 |
| Parvari et al[166] | Kenny-Caffey, Sanjad-Sakati | Microcephaly, mental retardation, growth failure ± osteosclerosis | | AR | *TBCE* (chaperone for tubulin folding) | 241410 244460 |
| Neufeld et al[167] | Autoimmune polyendocrinopathy—candidiasis—ectodermal dystrophy (APECED) | Chronic mucocutaneous candidiasis, Addison disease | Immune tolerance | AR | *AIRE* (autoimmune transcriptional regulator) | 240300 |

*AD,* Autosomal dominant; AR, autosomal recessive; *CaSR,* calcium-sensing receptor; *OMIM,* Online Mendelian Inheritance in Man; *PTH,* parathyroid hormone.

A number of rare congenital syndromes with multiple developmental abnormalities can also be associated with familial hypoparathyroidism, including DiGeorge syndrome, hypoparathyroid, deafness, and renal anomalies (HDR), autoimmune polyendocrinopathy—candidiasis—ectodermal dystrophy (APECED), and mitochondrial disorders (see Table 18.2).

**Genetic Syndromes With Resistance to Parathyroid Hormone Action.** Individuals with PHP are hypocalcemic and hyperphosphatemic but have elevated PTH levels. This condition, reported in 1942 by Albright, was the first described example of a hormone resistance disease.[172] The patients exhibited a pattern of features of Albright hereditary osteodystrophy (AHO) that included short stature, round face, mental retardation, brachydactyly, and the lack of a phosphaturic response to parathyroid extract. PHP is now recognized as a heterogeneous group of related disorders.[173,174] It may be inherited or sporadic.

PHP is subdivided into two types, depending on the kidney tubular response to infused exogenous PTH. PHP type 1 (PHP-1) refers to complete resistance to the effects of PTH, as demonstrated by the failure of patients to increase serum calcium, urinary cAMP, and phosphate levels in response to PTH infusion.[175,176] PHP-1 is subdivided into PHP type 1a (PHP-1a), with AHO, and PHP type1b (PHP-1b), without AHO. The presence of AHO without hypocalcemia and endocrine dysfunction has been termed "pseudopseudohypoparathyroidism" (PPHP).

PHP-1a and PPHP result from loss-of-function mutations of the GNAS1 gene, which encodes the stimulatory G protein $\alpha$-subunit ($G_{\alpha s}$) that couples the type 1 PTH/PTHrP receptor (PTH1R) to the adenylyl cyclase pathway.[177] Patients with the GNAS1 gene mutation also have resistance to thyroid-stimulating hormone (TSH), gonadotropins, glucagons, calcitonin, and gonadotropin-releasing hormone (GnRH) because the same $G_{\alpha s}$ pathway is used by these hormones. Promoter-specific genomic imprinting of GNAS1 has been established and provides the probable explanation for the complex phenotypic expression of the dominantly inherited genetic defect. Maternal transmission of the mutation causes PHP-1a; paternal transmission leads to PPHP.[178]

PHP-1b appears to be caused by mutations that affect the regulatory elements of GNAS1, mainly in the proximal tubules.[179,180] Patients with PHP-1c exhibit the features of PHP-1, but without defective $G_{\alpha s}$ activity.

PHP-2 is a heterogeneous group of disorders characterized by a reduced phosphaturic response to PTH but a normal increase in urinary cAMP levels.[181] The cause is unclear but may be caused by a defect in the intracellular response to cAMP or some other component of the PTH signaling pathway. It does not appear to follow a clear familial pattern.

### Hypomagnesemic Syndromes

Impaired PTH secretion and inadequate PTH response to hypocalcemia are typically observed in hypomagnesemic patients. This is corrected by magnesium replacement. Congenital defects leading to hypomagnesemia and hypocalcemia are discussed later (see "Magnesium Disorders") and in Chapters 44 and 73.

### Acquired Hypoparathyroidism and Inadequate Parathyroid Hormone Production

**Postsurgical Causes.** The most common cause of acquired hypoparathyroidism in adults is surgical removal of or damage to the parathyroid glands. Transient hypocalcemia after thyroid surgery has been observed in 2% to 23% of cases, whereas permanent hypocalcemia occurred in approximately 1% to 2% of cases.[171,182–184] Hypocalcemia was more likely to occur after total thyroidectomy for cancer, Graves' disease, radical neck dissection for other cancers, and repeated operations for parathyroid adenoma removal. Hypoparathyroidism may result from inadvertent removal of the parathyroids, damage from bleeding, or devascularization-infarction. Removal of a single hyperfunctioning parathyroid adenoma can result in transient hypocalcemia because of hypercalcemia-induced suppression of PTH secretion from the normal glands. Surgical experience and use of appropriate surgical technique may reduce the frequency of hypothyroidism.[184]

The so-called hungry bone or recalcification syndrome represents an important cause of prolonged hypocalcemia after parathyroidectomy or thyroidectomy for any form of HPT or hyperthyroidism, respectively.[185] Postoperative withdrawal of PTH decreases osteoclastic bone resorption, presumably mediated be decreased RANKL release from osteoblasts, without affecting osteoblastic bone formation activity, which leads to increased bone uptake of calcium, phosphate, and magnesium. Risk factors for the development of this hungry bone syndrome include large parathyroid adenomas, age older than 60 years, and high preoperative levels of serum PTH, calcium, and alkaline phosphatase. There have been reports that bisphosphonate therapy for Paget disease and cinacalcet use for secondary HPT can also cause a medical hungry bone syndrome.[186,187]

Acquired HP from nonsurgical causes is rare, with the exception of autoimmune disorders and magnesium deficiency. Although metal overload diseases (e.g., hemochromatosis, Wilson disease),[188,189] granulomatous diseases, miliary tuberculosis, amyloidosis, or neoplastic infiltrate are often mentioned as causes of hypoparathyroidism, these entities are rare. Alcohol consumption has been reported to cause transient hypocalcemia.[190]

**Magnesium Disorders.** Both magnesium excess and deficiency can produce generally mild hypocalcemia and reversible HP. Acute infusion of magnesium or hypermagnesemia inhibits PTH secretion.[191] Magnesium is an extracellular CaSR agonist, although less potent than calcium. Hypermagnesemia, when severe enough, as observed in patients with CKD or who have received acute high doses of IV magnesium sulfate (used in obstetrics), can activate the CaSR and inhibit PTH secretion.[192]

Hypomagnesemic patients typically have low or inappropriately normal PTH levels for the degree of hypocalcemia observed.[193] Moderate hypomagnesemia (serum magnesium levels = 0.8–1 mg/dL) primarily causes PTH resistance at the level of target organ,[194] whereas severe hypomagnesemia, in addition, decreases PTH secretion.[195] The effect of chronic severe hypomagnesemia is not from an extracellular effect on CaSR but from intracellular magnesium depletion, which leads to $G_{\alpha s}$ activation, enhanced CaSR signaling and, hence, blunted PTH secretion.[195] The appropriate therapy is magnesium repletion; in the absence of adequate magnesium repletion, the hypocalcemia is resistant to PTH and vitamin D therapy.

**Autoimmune Disease.** Autoimmune HP can present as an isolated finding or as part of the polyendocrinopathy type 1 syndrome (APS1). APS1 can be sporadic or familial (also referred to as APECED; see Table 18.2).[196] Autoantibodies against parathyroid tissue have been reported in a significant percentage of cases of hypoparathyroidism, but the causative role of these antibodies is unclear. The CaSR has been identified as a possible autoantigen in some cases of autoimmune HP (isolated or polyglandular).[197]

### Vitamin D–Related Disorders

**Low Vitamin D Production.** Inherited and acquired disorders of vitamin D and its metabolites can be associated with hypocalcemia.[198] Vitamin D is a fat-soluble vitamin that is produced in the skin under UVB radiation from 7-dehydrocholesterol or absorbed in the gastrointestinal tract from external sources. Vitamin D is present naturally in a few foods, is artificially added to others, and is available as a food supplement or drug.[199]

Despite routine dietary supplementation in milk and other foods, vitamin D deficiency is common in certain populations,[198,199] such as breastfeeding infants, older adults, people with dark skin and limited sun exposure, people with fat malabsorption,[199] and patients after gastric bypass surgery.[200] A study of hospitalized patients has found a high prevalence of vitamin D deficiency, even in younger patients without risk factors who were consuming the recommended daily allowance of vitamin $D_3$.[201] Fat malabsorption syndromes, common in liver diseases, sprue, and Whipple and Crohn diseases, may result in malabsorption of vitamin D.[202,203] Liver diseases may impair the hydroxylation of vitamin D to 25(OH) D (calcidiol), and drugs such as phenytoin and barbiturates stimulate the conversion of 25(OH)D to inactive metabolites.[204] Therapy of hepatic osteodystrophy with vitamin D and calcium is not fully effective.[205]

Deficiency of 1α-hydroxylase, as observed in advanced CKD, leads to a deficiency of $1,25(OH)_2D$ (calcitriol), the most important biologic form for maintaining calcium and phosphorus homeostasis. Vitamin D deficiency with hypocalcemia is commonly seen in patients with kidney disease (see Chapter 55). Patients with nephrotic syndrome may also have decreased 25(OH)D levels as a result of urinary loss, leading to hypocalcemia and secondary HPT.[206]

The serum level of 25(OH)D is the best indicator of vitamin D status. Levels of $1,25(OH)_2D$ do not decrease until vitamin D deficiency is severe. Prolonged vitamin D deficiency causes rickets in children (a disorder of mineralization of growing bone) and osteomalacia in adults (a disorder of mineralization of formed bone). The combination of calcium deficiency and vitamin D deficiency accelerates skeletal abnormalities and the development of hypocalcemia. The diagnosis of vitamin D deficiency is confirmed by measurement of the serum 25(OH)D levels. Hypocalcemia can be observed only in severe vitamin D deficiency—25(OH)D levels less than 10 ng/mL—and when skeletal stores of calcium are depleted; otherwise, the compensatory rise of PTH would be able to mobilize calcium from bone.[198,199,207,208] The 24-hour urinary calcium excretion is low to very low. Hypophosphatemia and increased alkaline phosphatase and normal FGF-23 levels are typically seen with vitamin D deficiency.[198]

**Vitamin D Resistance.** The observation that some forms of rickets cannot be cured by regular doses of vitamin D has led to the discovery of rare inherited abnormalities in vitamin D metabolism or the vitamin D receptor. Vitamin D–dependent rickets type 1 (VDDR-1; Online Mendelian Inheritance in Man [OMIM database] 264700) is characterized by autosomal recessive, childhood-onset rickets, hypocalcemia, secondary HPT, and aminoaciduria. The biochemical abnormality is defective 1α-hydroxylation of 25(OH)D, caused by mutations in the gene for the 25(OH)D–1α-hydroxylase.[209] Therapy with calcitriol or 1α(OH)D (alfacalcidol) restores serum $1,25(OH)_2D$ and must be continued for life.

VDDR-2 (also called "hereditary vitamin D–resistant rickets") is an autosomal recessive disorder (OMIM 277440). Affected patients have extreme elevations in $1,25(OH)_2D$ levels, in addition to alopecia and the abnormalities seen in VDDR-1.[210] Biochemically, the disorder results from end-organ resistance to $1,25(OH)_2D$. A number of different mutations have been found in the vitamin D receptor gene of affected individuals.[211] High-dose calcium intake and calcium infusion may be the only way to treat hypocalcemia and rickets in these children.

### Miscellaneous Causes

**Medications.** Medication-induced hypocalcemia is a relatively common cause of hypocalcemia, particularly in hospitalized patients.[212,213] Some of the gadolinium-based contrast agents (e.g., gadodiamide, gadoversetamide) used in magnetic resonance imaging (MRI) studies cause pseudohypocalcemia by interference with colorimetric assays for calcium. Calcium readings can be as low as 6 mg/dL, but with no symptoms or signs of hypocalcemia.[212,213] Propofol and IV contrast agents may also complex calcium.

Drug-induced hypomagnesemia (e.g., cisplatin, aminoglycoside, amphotericin, diuretics) and hypermagnesemia (e.g., magnesium sulfate infusion, magnesium-containing antacids) can cause hypocalcemia. Inhibitors of bone resorption (e.g., bisphosphonates, denosumab, calcimimetics, mithramycin, calcitonin) may depress serum calcium to subnormal levels.[212] Proton pump inhibitors and histamine-2 antagonists may reduce calcium absorption, provoke hypocalcemia, and/or inhibit bone resorption.[214] Regional citrate anticoagulation for continuous kidney replacement therapy (CRRT) and for plasmapheresis can chelate calcium and cause hypocalcemia.[215,216] Transfusions of citrated blood rarely cause significant hypocalcemia, but it may occur in the course of a massive transfusion.[217]

Foscarnet (trisodium phosphonoformate), an antiviral medication used to treat herpes viruses, is a structural mimic of the pyrophosphate anion. Foscarnet can cause hypocalcemia through the chelation of extracellular calcium ions, so normal total calcium measurements may not reflect ionized hypocalcemia.[218] Magnesium losses by the kidney may exaggerate hypocalcemia. Patients treated with foscarnet should undergo total calcium and ionized calcium measurements. As noted, anticonvulsants, particularly phenytoin and phenobarbital, can induce the hepatic CYP3A4 enzyme, which shortens vitamin D half-life and causes vitamin D deficiency.[213] Fluoride overdose is an exceedingly rare cause of hypocalcemia. Oral sodium phosphate–induced hyperphosphatemia may cause hypocalcemia, particularly in patients with CKD.[212,219] Other drugs associated with hypocalcemia include antiinfectious (e.g., pentamidine, ketoconazole) and chemotherapeutic agents (e.g., asparaginase, cisplatin, doxorubicin).

**Critical Illness.** In complicated, critically ill patients, total calcium measurements may be poor indicators of the ionized calcium concentration because many factors that could interfere with or alter calcium and protein binding may be present (e.g., albumin infusion, citrate, IV fluids, acid-base disturbances, dialysis therapy, propofol infusion). Thus, it is particularly important to measure ionized calcium in this setting. Hypocalcemia is frequently noted in gram-negative sepsis and toxic shock syndrome.[150,220] This entity is multifactorial; the primary cause is unclear, but a direct effect of IL-1 on parathyroid function may be partly responsible.[221]

**Other Causes.** Hypocalcemia is common in acute pancreatitis and is a poor prognostic indicator. It is probably due to calcium chelation by free fatty acids generated by the action of pancreatic lipase, although some animal studies have challenged this hypothesis.[222] Massive tumor lysis, particularly from rapidly growing hematologic malignancies, may cause hyperphosphatemia, hyperuricemia, and hypocalcemia.[223] The early phase of rhabdomyolysis may include severe hyperphosphatemia and associated hypocalcemia, in contrast to the recovery phase, when hypercalcemia is common. In hemodialysis patients, hypocalcemia is common and may result, at least in part, from reduced kidney phosphate clearance and consequent hyperphosphatemia and reduced $1,25(OH)_2D$ production (see Chapter 55).

## MANAGEMENT OF HYPOCALCEMIA

The optimal management of hypocalcemia has not been examined in clinical trials, but there are accepted practices. The treatment depends on the speed of onset and severity of clinical and laboratory features. Oral calcium supplementation may be sufficient treatment for mild hypocalcemia. Patients with acute, severe symptomatic hypocalcemia (Ca level <7–7.5 mg/dL; ionized $Ca^{2+}$ < 0.8 mmol/L), such as after parathyroidectomy, with evidence of neuromuscular effects or tetany, should be treated promptly with IV calcium. The preferred calcium salt is calcium gluconate (10 mL of 10% calcium gluconate contains 93 mg of elemental calcium). Initially, 1 to 2 g (93–186 mg of elemental Ca) of IV calcium gluconate in 50 mL of 5% dextrose is given over a period of 10 to 20 minutes, followed by slow infusion at a rate of 0.3 to 1.0 mg elemental Ca/kg per hour.[194] The dose can be adjusted to maintain the serum calcium level at the lower end of normal values.

Moderate asymptomatic hypocalcemia (ionized $Ca^{2+}$ >0.8 mmol/L) can be treated by repeated doses of 1 to 2 g calcium gluconate IV every 4 hours, without continuous infusion. Ionized Ca should be measured every 4 to 6 hours initially.

The infusion solution should not contain phosphates or bicarbonates. IV infusion may be needed until the patient is stabilized, and oral calcium and calcitriol therapy begin to take effect. Correction of hypomagnesemia and hyperphosphatemia should also be undertaken, when present. Dialysis may be appropriate if hyperphosphatemia is also present.

Treatment of chronic hypocalcemia depends on the underlying cause. For example, underlying hypomagnesemia or vitamin D deficiency should be corrected. The principal therapy for primary parathyroid dysfunction or PTH resistance is dietary calcium supplementation and vitamin D therapy. Oral calcium supplementation, beginning with 500 to 1000 mg of elemental calcium daily and increasing up to a maximum of 2000 mg daily, is a good strategy. Correction of the serum calcium level to the low-normal range is generally advised; correction to normal levels may lead to frank hypercalciuria. Several preparations of vitamin D are available for the treatment of hypocalcemia. The role of vitamin D therapy in CKD is discussed separately.

Replacement therapy using synthetic human parathyroid hormone, PTH (1-34) (teriparatide, 20 μg subcutaneously once daily) has been FDA-approved for the treatment of osteoporosis. Teriparatide has also been used as hormone replacement therapy in patients with hypoparathyroidism in a dose of 20 μg subcutaneously, twice daily.[224] More recently, PTH (1-84) (100 μg every other day) was studied in 30 hypoparathyroid patients for 24 months.[225] Improvement or normalization of the serum calcium level was observed with both hormone preparations.

## DISORDERS OF MAGNESIUM HOMEOSTASIS

### HYPOMAGNESEMIA AND MAGNESIUM DEFICIENCY

The terms "hypomagnesemia" and "magnesium deficiency" tend to be used interchangeably. In marked contrast with the distribution of calcium, extracellular fluid magnesium accounts for only 1% of total body magnesium, so serum magnesium concentrations have been found to correlate poorly with overall magnesium status. In patients with magnesium deficiency, serum magnesium concentrations may be normal or may seriously underestimate the severity of the magnesium deficit.[226] Approximately 50% to 60% of magnesium is in the skeleton, and most of the remaining 40% to 50% is intracellular. No satisfactory clinical test to assay body magnesium stores is available.[227]

The magnesium tolerance test has been proposed to be the best test of overall magnesium status.[227] It is based on the observation that magnesium-deficient patients tend to retain a greater proportion of a parenterally administered magnesium load and excrete less in the urine than normal individuals.[228] Clinical studies have indicated that the results of a magnesium tolerance test correlate well with magnesium status, as assessed by skeletal muscle magnesium content and exchangeable magnesium pools. However, the test is invalid in patients who have impaired kidney function or a kidney magnesium-wasting syndrome or in patients taking diuretics or other medications that induce kidney magnesium wasting. Thus, and also because of the time and effort required to perform the magnesium tolerance test, it is used primarily as a research tool.

The serum magnesium concentration, although an insensitive measure of magnesium deficit, remains the only practical test of magnesium status in widespread use. Surveys of serum magnesium levels in hospitalized patients have indicated a high incidence of hypomagnesemia (presumably an underestimate of the true incidence of magnesium deficiency), ranging from 11% in general inpatients[229] to 60% in patients admitted to intensive care units (ICUs).[230,231] Furthermore, in ICU patients, hypomagnesemia was associated with increased mortality when compared with normomagnesemic patients.[230]

The functionally important value is believed to be the ionized $Mg^{2+}$ concentration, which is less than total serum magnesium due to protein binding. Measurements with ion-selective electrodes have found ionized $Mg^{2+}$ concentrations that are approximately 70% of the total serum magnesium, a proportion that is fairly constant in the general population.[227] However, in critically ill patients, there is a poor correlation between total and ionized serum magnesium levels.[231] It is surprising that we rarely measure ionized serum magnesium.

### CAUSES

Magnesium deficiency may be caused by decreased intake or intestinal absorption, increased losses via the gastrointestinal tract, kidneys, or skin or, rarely, sequestration in the bone compartment (Fig. 18.4). It is often helpful to distinguish between kidney magnesium wasting and extrarenal causes of magnesium deficiency by assessing urinary magnesium excretion. In the setting of magnesium deficiency, a urine magnesium excretion rate greater than 24 mg/day is abnormal and is usually suggestive of kidney magnesium wasting.[232] If a 24-hour urine collection is unavailable, the fractional excretion of magnesium ($F_EMg$) can be calculated from a random urine specimen as follows:

$$F_EMg = \text{urine Mg concentration} \times \text{plasma Cr} / ([0.7 \times \text{plasma total Mg concentration}] \times \text{urine Cr concentration})$$

where Cr is creatinine. Note that a correction factor of 0.7 is applied to the plasma total magnesium concentration to estimate the free magnesium concentration. In general, a $F_EMg$ value of more than 3% to 4% in an individual with a normal GFR is indicative of inappropriate urinary magnesium loss.[193] If kidney magnesium wasting has been excluded, the losses must be extrarenal in origin, and the underlying cause can usually be identified from the case history.

#### Extrarenal Causes

**Nutritional Deficiency.** Development of magnesium deficiency due to dietary deficiency in normal individuals is unusual because almost all foods contain significant amounts of magnesium, and kidney adaptation to conserve magnesium is very efficient. Thus, magnesium deficiency of nutritional origin is observed primarily in two clinical settings—alcoholism and parenteral feeding.

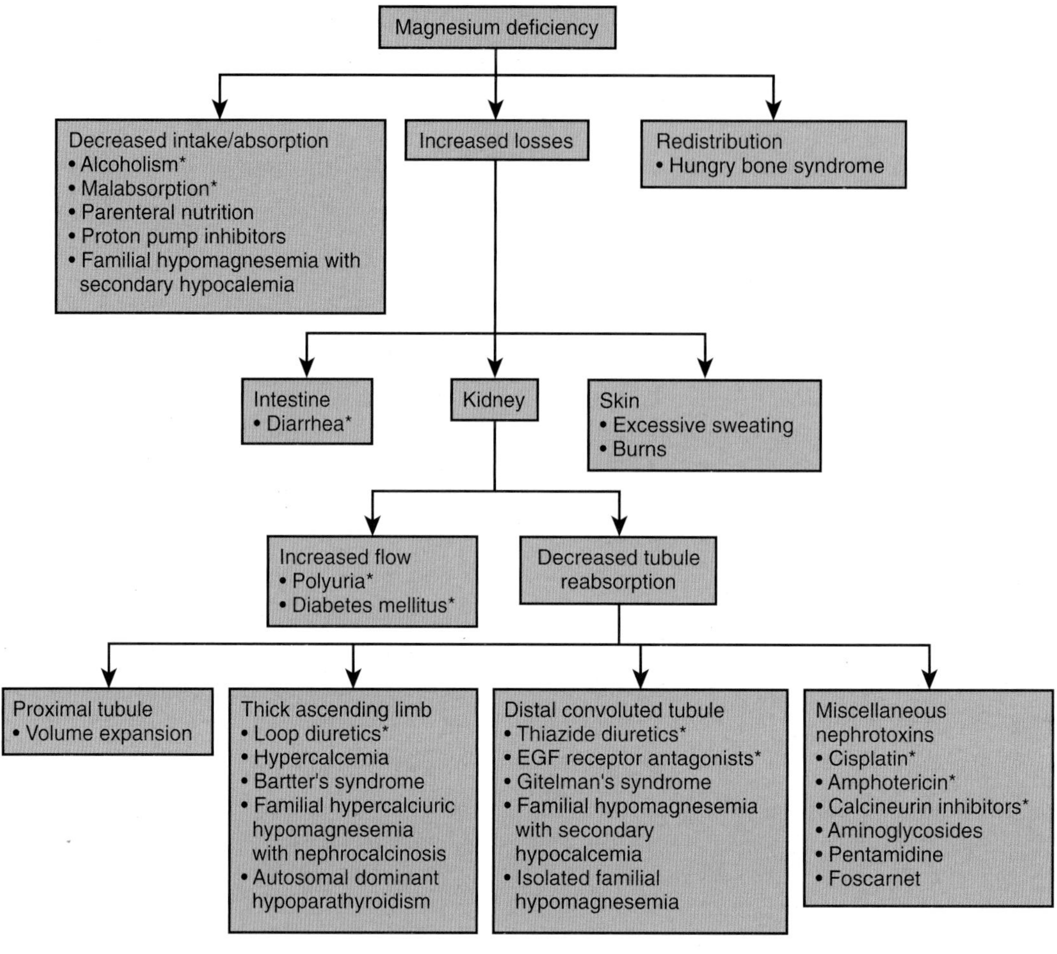


**Fig. 18.4** Causes of magnesium deficiency. *EGF*, Epidermal growth factor.

In chronic alcoholics, the intake of ethanol substitutes for the intake of important nutrients.[233] Approximately 20% to 25% of alcoholics are frankly hypomagnesemic, and most can be shown to be magnesium-deficient with the magnesium tolerance test.[228] Alcohol also impairs kidney magnesium reabsorption.[234]

Patients receiving parenteral nutrition may also develop hypomagnesemia.[235] In general, these patients are sicker than the average inpatient and are more likely to have other conditions associated with a magnesium deficit and ongoing magnesium losses.

Hypomagnesemia may also be a consequence of the refeeding syndrome.[236] In this condition, overzealous parenteral feeding of severely malnourished patients causes hyperinsulinemia, as well as a rapid cellular uptake of glucose and water, together with phosphorus, potassium, and magnesium.

**Intestinal Malabsorption.** Generalized malabsorption syndromes caused by conditions such as celiac disease, Whipple disease, and inflammatory bowel disease are frequently associated with intestinal magnesium wasting and magnesium deficiency.[237] In fat malabsorption with concomitant steatorrhea, free fatty acids in the intestinal lumen may combine with magnesium to form nonabsorbable soaps, a process termed "saponification," thus contributing to impaired magnesium absorption. The severity of hypomagnesemia in patients with malabsorption syndrome correlates with the fecal fat excretion rate and, in rare patients, reduction of dietary fat intake alone, which reduces steatorrhea, can correct the hypomagnesemia. Previous intestinal resection, particularly of the distal part of the small intestine, is also an important cause of magnesium malabsorption.[238] Magnesium deficiency was a common complication of bariatric surgery by jejunoileal bypass,[239] but fortunately does not occur with the modern technique of gastric bypass.[240]

Proton pump inhibitors (PPIs) have been reported to cause hypomagnesemia due to intestinal magnesium malabsorption.[241] Among patients admitted to an ICU, concurrent use of PPIs with diuretics has been associated with a significant increase of hypomagnesemia (odds ratio [OR], 1.54) and a 0.03-mg/dL lower serum magnesium concentration compared with patients taking diuretics alone, whereas patients taking PPI alone did not have an increased risk of hypomagnesemia.[242] Interestingly, in a recent case-control study of hospitalized patients, hypomagnesemia at the time of hospital admission was not associated with out of hospital use of PPI.[243] However, most of these patients were not taking diuretics. A rare mutation of the TRPM6 magnesium transport channel can also lead to intestinal magnesium malabsorption, along with kidney magnesium wasting, causing hypomagnesemia with secondary hypocalcemia.[244]

**Diarrhea and Gastrointestinal Fistula.** The magnesium concentration of diarrheal fluid is high and ranges from 1 to 16 mg/dL,[238] so magnesium deficiency may occur in patients with chronic diarrhea of any cause, even in the absence of concomitant malabsorption.[226] It also occurs in patients who abuse laxatives. By contrast, secretions from the upper gastrointestinal tract are low in magnesium content, and significant magnesium deficiency is, therefore, rarely observed in patients with an intestinal, biliary, or pancreatic fistula, ileostomy, or prolonged gastric drainage (except as a consequence of malnutrition).[238]

**Cutaneous Losses.** Hypomagnesemia may be observed after prolonged intense exertion. For example, serum magnesium concentrations fall 20% on average after a marathon run.[245] About 25% of the decrease in the serum magnesium level can be accounted for by losses in sweat, which can contain up to 0.5 mg/dL of magnesium; the remainder is most likely due to transient redistribution into the intracellular space. Magnesium supplements may be indicated in a number of sports, especially if the athlete is on a suboptimal magnesium diet.[246]

Hypomagnesemia occurs in 40% of patients with severe burn injuries during the early period of recovery. The major cause is loss of magnesium in the cutaneous exudate, which can exceed 1 g/day.[247]

**Redistribution to Bone Compartment.** Hypomagnesemia may occasionally accompany the profound hypocalcemia of hungry bone syndrome observed in some patients with HPT and severe bone disease immediately after parathyroidectomy.[248] In such cases, there is high bone turnover, and sudden removal of excess PTH is believed to result in virtual cessation of bone resorption, with a continued high rate of bone formation and consequent sequestration of calcium and magnesium into bone mineral.

**Diabetes Mellitus.** Hypomagnesemia is common in patients with diabetes mellitus and has been reported to occur in 13.5% to 47.7% of nonhospitalized patients with type 2 diabetes.[249] The cause is thought to be multifactorial; contributing factors include decreased oral intake of magnesium-rich foods, poor intestinal absorption due to diabetic autonomic neuropathy, and increased kidney excretion. The latter could, in turn, be caused by glomerular hyperfiltration, osmotic diuresis, or decreased TAL and distal tubule magnesium reabsorption caused by functional insulin deficiency.[250,251] In addition, some studies have suggested that magnesium deficiency might itself impair glucose tolerance, thus partly explaining the association. Conversely, genetic variants in the magnesium transport channels, TRPM6 and TRPM7, may increase the risk of type 2 diabetes mellitus in women on a diet with less than 250 mg/day of magnesium.[252]

### Renal Magnesium Wasting

The diagnosis of kidney magnesium wasting is made by demonstrating an inappropriately high rate of kidney magnesium excretion in the face of hypomagnesemia, as described earlier. The causes are summarized in Fig. 18.4.

**Polyuria.** Increased urine output from any cause is often accompanied by increased kidney losses of magnesium. Kidney magnesium wasting occurs with osmotic diuresis—for example, in hyperglycemic crises in diabetics.[253,254] Hypermagnesuria also occurs during the polyuric phase of recovery from acute kidney injuty (AKI) in a native kidney, during recovery from ischemic injury in a transplanted kidney, and in postobstructive diuresis. In such cases, it is likely that residual tubule reabsorptive defects persisting from the primary kidney injury play as important a role as polyuria itself in inducing kidney magnesium wasting.[255]

**Extracellular Fluid Volume Expansion.** In the proximal tubule, magnesium reabsorption is passive and driven by the reabsorption of sodium and water in this segment. Extracellular volume expansion, which decreases proximal sodium and water reabsorption, also increases urinary magnesium excretion. Thus chronic therapy with magnesium-free parenteral fluids, crystalloid or hyperalimentation,[256] can cause kidney magnesium wasting, as can hyperaldosteronism.[257]

**Diuretics.** Loop diuretics inhibit the apical membrane $Na^+$-$K^+$-2Cl– cotransporter of the TAL and abolish the transepithelial potential difference, thereby inhibiting paracellular magnesium reabsorption. Hypomagnesemia is, therefore, a frequent finding in patients undergoing chronic loop diuretic therapy.[258] Chronic treatment with thiazide diuretics, which inhibit the NaCl cotransporter (NCC), also causes kidney magnesium wasting. Thiazide diuretics or knockout of NCC in mice causes downregulation of expression of the apical magnesium entry channel in the distal convoluted tubule, TRPM6, which may explain the mechanism of the magnesuria.[259]

**Epidermal Growth Factor Receptor Blockers.** Hypomagnesemia is common in patients receiving cetuximab[260] and panitumumab,[261] which are monoclonal blocking antibodies of the epidermal growth factor (EGF) receptor used in the treatment of metastatic colorectal cancer. The incidence of hypomagnesemia increases with increasing duration of therapy, reaching almost 50% in patients treated for longer than 6 months.[262] The median time to onset of hypomagnesemia after beginning treatment is 99 days, and it generally reverses 1 to 3 months after discontinuing therapy.[263] $F_EMg$ is inappropriately elevated, suggesting a defect in kidney magnesium reabsorption.[264] Studies have suggested that the EGF receptor is located basolaterally in the distal convoluted tubule (DCT).[264] Autocrine or paracrine activation of the receptor stimulates redistribution of TRPM6 to the apical membrane via a Rac1-dependent signaling pathway[265] and presumably increases transepithelial magnesium reabsorption. Thus EGF receptor blockade likely causes kidney magnesium wasting by antagonizing this pathway.

**Hypercalcemia.** Elevated serum ionized $Ca^{2+}$ levels—for example, in patients with malignant bone metastases—directly induce kidney magnesium wasting and hypomagnesemia,[266] probably by stimulating the basolateral CaSR in the TAL of Henle. In HPT, the situation is more complicated because the hypercalcemia-induced tendency to Mg wasting is counteracted by the action of PTH to stimulate magnesium reabsorption; thus, kidney magnesium handling is usually normal, and magnesium deficiency is rare.[267]

**Tubule Nephrotoxins.** Cisplatin, a widely used chemotherapeutic agent for solid tumors, frequently causes kidney magnesium wasting. Hypomagnesemia is almost universal at a monthly dose of 50 mg/m$^2$.[268] The occurrence of Mg wasting does not appear to correlate with the incidence of cisplatin-induced AKI.[269] Kidney magnesuria continues after cessation of the drug for a mean of 4 to 5 months, but can persist for years.[269] Although the nephrotoxic effects of cisplatin are manifested histologically as acute tubular necrosis confined to the S3 segment of the proximal tubule, the magnesuria does not correlate temporally with the clinical development of AKI secondary to acute tubular necrosis. Furthermore, patients who become hypomagnesemic are also subject to the development of hypocalciuria, thus suggesting that the reabsorption defect may actually be in the DCT. Mouse studies have also suggested that cisplatin may reduce the expression of transport proteins in the DCT.[270] Cisplatin may also impair intestinal magnesium absorption.[271] Carboplatin, an analogue of cisplatin, is considerably less nephrotoxic, and only rarely causes AKI or hypomagnesemia.[272]

Amphotericin B is a well-recognized tubule nephrotoxin that can cause kidney potassium wasting, distal kidney tubular acidosis, and AKI, with tubule necrosis and calcium deposition noted in the DCT and TAL on kidney biopsy.[273] Amphotericin B causes kidney magnesium wasting and hypomagnesemia related to the cumulative dose administered, but these effects may be observed after as little as a 200-mg total dose.[274] Interestingly, the amphotericin-induced magnesuria is accompanied by the reciprocal development of hypocalciuria so, as with cisplatin, the serum calcium concentration is usually preserved, again suggesting that the functional tubule defect resides in the DCT.

Aminoglycosides cause a syndrome of kidney magnesium and potassium wasting with hypomagnesemia, hypokalemia, hypocalcemia, and tetany. Hypomagnesemia may occur, despite levels in the appropriate therapeutic range.[275] Most patients have reported that they had delayed onset of hypomagnesemia occurring after at least 2 weeks of therapy, and received total doses in excess of 8 g, thus suggesting that it is the cumulative dose of aminoglycoside that is the key predictor of toxicity. In addition, no correlation was found between the occurrence of aminoglycoside-induced acute tubular necrosis and hypomagnesemia. Magnesium wasting persists after cessation of the aminoglycoside, often for several months. All aminoglycosides in clinical use have been implicated, including gentamicin, tobramycin, and amikacin, as well as neomycin when administered topically for extensive burn injuries. This form of symptomatic aminoglycoside-induced kidney magnesium wasting is now relatively uncommon because of heightened general awareness of its toxicity. However, asymptomatic hypomagnesemia can be observed in one-third of those treated with a single course of an aminoglycoside at standard doses (3–5 mg/kg/day, for a mean of 10 days). In these cases, the hypomagnesemia occurs on average 3 to 4 days after the start of therapy and readily reverses after cessation of therapy.[276]

IV pentamidine causes hypomagnesemia as a result of kidney magnesium wasting in most patients, typically in association with hypocalcemia.[277] The average onset of symptomatic hypomagnesemia occurs after 9 days of therapy, and the defect persists for at least 1 to 2 months after the discontinuation of pentamidine. Hypomagnesemia is also observed in two- thirds of AIDS patients with cytomegalovirus retinitis treated intravenously with the pyrophosphate analogue foscarnet.[278] As with aminoglycosides and pentamidine, foscarnet-induced hypomagnesemia is often associated with significant hypocalcemia.

The calcineurin inhibitors cyclosporine and tacrolimus cause kidney magnesium wasting and hypomagnesemia in patients after organ transplantation.[279] The mechanism is thought to be downregulation of the distal tubule magnesium channel, TRPM6.[280]

**Tubulointerstitial Nephropathies.** Kidney Mg wasting has occasionally been reported in patients with acute or chronic tubulointerstitial nephritis that is not caused by nephrotoxic drugs—for example, in chronic pyelonephritis and acute kidney allograft rejection. Other manifestations of tubule dysfunction, such as salt wasting, hypokalemia, kidney tubular acidosis, and Fanconi syndrome, may also be present and provide clues to the diagnosis.[255]

#### Inherited Kidney Magnesium-Wasting Disorders

***Primary Magnesium-Wasting Disorders.*** Primary magnesium-wasting disorders are rare. Patients can be broadly classified into distinct clinical syndromes, depending on whether the hypomagnesemia is isolated, occurs together with hypocalcemia, or is associated with hypercalciuria and nephrocalcinosis.[281] The pathogenesis and clinical features of these syndromes, which generally present in childhood, are discussed in detail in Chapter 73.

***Bartter and Gitelman Syndromes.*** Bartter syndrome is an autosomal recessive disorder characterized by Na wasting, hypokalemic metabolic alkalosis, and hypercalciuria that usually occurs in infancy or early childhood (see also Chapter 44).[282] All Bartter syndrome patients are by definition hypercalciuric and, in addition, one-third have hypomagnesemia with inappropriate magnesuria, consistent with loss of the TAL transepithelial potential difference that drives paracellular divalent cation reabsorption. Thus the physiology of Bartter syndrome is essentially identical to that of chronic loop diuretic therapy. Gitelman syndrome is a variant of Bartter syndrome distinguished primarily by hypocalciuria.[283] Patients with Gitelman syndrome are identified later in life, usually after the age of 6 years, and have milder symptoms. The genetic defect in these families is caused by inactivating mutations in the DCT electroneutral thiazide-sensitive NCC and therefore resembles chronic thiazide diuretic therapy. Kidney magnesium wasting and hypomagnesemia are universally found in patients with Gitelman syndrome.

***Calcium-Sensing Disorders.*** In FHH, the hypercalcemia is due to inactivating mutations in CaSR (discussed earlier). As a consequence of the inactivated CaSR, the normal magnesuric response to hypercalcemia is impaired,[284] so these patients are paradoxically mildly hypermagnesemic. Activating mutations in CaSR cause the opposite syndrome, autosomal dominant hypoparathyroidism. As might be expected, most of these patients are mildly hypomagnesemic, presumably because of TAL magnesium wasting.[168]

## CLINICAL MANIFESTATIONS

Hypomagnesemia may cause symptoms and signs of disordered cardiac, neuromuscular, and central nervous system function. It is also associated with an imbalance of other electrolytes, such as potassium and calcium. Many of the cardiac and neurologic manifestations attributed to magnesium deficiency may be explained by the frequent coexistence of hypokalemia and hypocalcemia in the same patient. Patients with mild hypomagnesemia or who are magnesium-deficient with normal serum magnesium levels may be completely asymptomatic.[285] Thus, the clinical importance of mild to moderate magnesium depletion remains controversial, although it has been associated with a number of disorders, such as hypertension and osteoporosis (see later).

### Cardiovascular System

Magnesium has protean and complex effects on myocardial ion fluxes. Because magnesium is an obligate cofactor in all reactions that require ATP, it is essential for the activity of $Na^+$-$K^+$-ATPase.[286] During magnesium deficiency, $Na^+$-$K^+$-ATPase function is impaired. The intracellular potassium concentration falls, which may potentially result in a relatively depolarized resting membrane potential and predispose to ectopic excitation and tachyarrhythmias.[287] Furthermore, the magnitude of the outward potassium gradient is decreased, thereby reducing the driving force for the potassium efflux needed to terminate the cardiac action potential and, as a result, repolarization is delayed. Changes in the ECG may be observed with isolated hypomagnesemia and usually reflect abnormal cardiac repolarization, including bifid T waves and other nonspecific abnormalities in T wave morphology, U waves, prolongation of the QT or QU interval and, rarely, electrical alternation of the T or U wave.[288]

Numerous anecdotal reports have indicated that hypomagnesemia alone can predispose to cardiac tachyarrhythmias, particularly of ventricular origin, including torsades de pointes, monomorphic ventricular tachycardia, and ventricular fibrillation, which may be resistant to standard therapy and respond only to magnesium repletion.[288] Many of the reported patients also had a prolonged QT interval, an abnormality known to predispose to torsades de pointes, and may also increase the period of vulnerability to the R-on-T phenomenon. In the setting of exaggerated cardiac excitability, hypomagnesemia may be the trigger for other types of ventricular tachyarrhythmias.[288] In addition, hypomagnesemia, like hypokalemia, facilitates the development of digoxin cardiotoxicity.[289] Because cardiac glycosides and magnesium depletion inhibit $Na^+$-$K^+$-ATPase, their additive effects on intracellular potassium depletion may account for their enhanced toxicity in combination.

It is clear that patients with underlying cardiac disease who have severe hypomagnesemia, particularly in combination with hypokalemia, may develop arrhythmias. The issue of whether mild isolated hypomagnesemia and magnesium depletion in individuals without overt heart disease carries the same risk has been controversial.[290] In one small prospective study, low dietary magnesium appeared to increase the risk for supraventricular and ventricular ectopy, despite the absence of frank hypomagnesemia, hypokalemia, and hypocalcemia.[291] In the Framingham Offspring Study, lower levels of serum magnesium were associated with a higher prevalence of ventricular premature complexes.[292] A low serum magnesium level is also associated with the development of atrial fibrillation.[293] In the Framingham Offspring Study, individuals in the lowest quartile of serum magnesium were, after up to 20 years of follow-up, approximately 50% more likely to develop atrial fibrillation compared with those in the upper quartiles.

Several large population-based studies have shown a strong association between low serum magnesium levels and increased cardiovascular and all-cause mortality.[294–296] Higher magnesium intake is associated with reduced risk of coronary heart disease and cardiac death, stroke, and coronary calcification.[297–302]

An inverse relationship between dietary magnesium intake and blood pressure has also been observed.[303–306] Hypomagnesemia and/or reduction of intracellular magnesium have also been inversely correlated with blood pressure. This may be especially important in diabetes mellitus.[307] Patients with essential hypertension were found to have reduced free magnesium concentrations in red blood cells. The magnesium levels were inversely related to systolic and diastolic blood pressures. Intervention studies with magnesium therapy in hypertension have led to conflicting results. Several have shown a positive blood pressure–lowering effect of supplements, but others have not. Other dietary factors may also play a role. In the DASH study, a diet rich in fruits and vegetables, which increased magnesium intake from 176 to 423 mg/day (along with an increase in potassium), significantly lowered blood pressure.[308] The mechanism whereby magnesium deficit may affect blood pressure is not clear, but magnesium does regulate vascular tone and reactivity and attenuates agonist-induced vasoconstriction. Magnesium depletion may involve decreased production of prostacyclin, increased production of thromboxane A2, and enhanced vasoconstrictive effects of angiotensin II and norepinephrine. Importantly, in none of these studies has magnesium therapy been rigorously studied, whether as a therapy for blood pressure reduction or prophylaxis against cardiovascular disease, arrhythmias, or stroke.

The only setting in which the role of magnesium deficiency and clinical utility of adjunctive magnesium therapy has been studied extensively is in acute myocardial infarction (AMI). Magnesium deficiency may be a risk factor because it has been shown to play a role in systemic and coronary vascular tone, in cardiac dysrhythmias (see earlier), and in the inhibition of steps in the coagulation process and platelet aggregation. Although several small controlled trials have suggested that adjunctive magnesium therapy reduces mortality from AMI by 50%, three major trials have defined our understanding of magnesium therapy in AMI.[309] The LIMIT-2 study was the first study involving large numbers of participants. Magnesium treatment showed an approximately 25% lower mortality rate. In the Fourth International Study of Infarct, unlike LIMIT-2, the mortality rate in the magnesium-treated group was not significantly different from that in the control group. The most recently published Magnesium in Coronaries (MAGIC) trial was designed to address early intervention in higher risk patients.[309] Over a 3-year period, 6213 participants were studied. The magnesium-treated group mortality at 30 days was not significantly different from that of those given placebo. The overall evidence from clinical trials does not support the routine application of adjunctive magnesium therapy in patients with AMI at this time.

### Neuromuscular System

Symptoms and signs of neuromuscular irritability, including tremor, muscle twitching, Trousseau and Chvostek signs, and frank tetany, may develop in patients with isolated hypomagnesemia[310] and in patients with concomitant hypocalcemia. Hypomagnesemia is also frequently manifested as seizures, which may be generalized and tonic-clonic in nature or may be multifocal motor seizures, and they are sometimes triggered by loud noises.[310] Interestingly, noise-induced seizures and sudden death are also characteristic of mice made hypomagnesemic by dietary magnesium deprivation. The effects of magnesium deficiency on brain neuronal excitability are thought to be mediated by *N*-methyl-D-aspartate (NMDA)–type glutamate receptors.[311] Glutamate is the principal excitatory neurotransmitter in the brain; it acts as an agonist at NMDA receptors and opens a cation conductance channel that depolarizes the postsynaptic membrane. Extracellular magnesium normally blocks NMDA receptors, so hypomagnesemia may release the inhibition of glutamate-activated depolarization of the postsynaptic membrane and thereby trigger epileptiform electrical activity.[312] Vertical nystagmus is a rare but diagnostically useful neurologic sign of severe hypomagnesemia.[313] In the absence of a structural lesion of the cerebellar or vestibular pathways, the only recognized metabolic causes are Wernicke encephalopathy and severe magnesium deficiency.[313]

### Skeletal System

Dietary magnesium depletion in animals has been shown to lead to a decrease in skeletal growth and increased skeletal fragility.[314] A decrease in osteoblastic bone formation and an increase in osteoclastic bone resorption are implicated as the cause of decreased bone mass. In humans, epidemiologic studies have suggested a correlation between bone mass and dietary magnesium intake.[315] Few studies have been conducted assessing magnesium status in patients with osteoporosis. Low serum and red blood cell (RBC) magnesium concentrations, as well as high retention of parenterally administered magnesium, have suggested a deficit. Low skeletal magnesium content has been observed in some, but not all, studies. The effect of supplements on bone mass has generally led to an increase in bone mineral density, although study design limits useful information. Larger long-term, placebo-controlled, double-blind investigations are required.

There are several potential mechanisms that may account for a decrease in bone mass in magnesium deficiency. Magnesium is mitogenic for bone cell growth; therefore, deficiency may directly result in a decrease in bone formation. It also affects crystal formation—a lack results in a larger, more perfect crystal, which may affect bone strength. Magnesium deficiency may result in a fall in serum PTH and 1,25 $(OH)_2$ vitamin D levels (see earlier). Because both hormones are trophic for bone, impaired secretion or skeletal resistance may result in osteoporosis. A low serum 1,25 $(OH)_2$ vitamin D level may also result in decreased intestinal calcium absorption. An observed increased release of inflammatory cytokines in bone may result in the activation of osteoclasts and increased bone resorption in rodents.[314,316]

### Electrolyte Homeostasis

Patients with hypomagnesemia are frequently also hypokalemic. Many of the conditions associated with hypomagnesemia that have been outlined earlier can cause simultaneous magnesium and potassium loss. However, hypomagnesemia by itself can induce hypokalemia in humans and experimental animals, and such patients are often refractory to potassium repletion until their magnesium deficit is corrected.[317] The cause of the hypokalemia appears to be increased secretion in the distal nephron.[318] The mechanism has been attributed to cytosolic magnesium depletion, which would release intracellular block of the apical secretory potassium channel, ROMK.[319]

Hypocalcemia is present in approximately 50% of patients with hypomagnesemia.[285] The major cause is impairment of PTH secretion by magnesium deficiency, which is reversed within 24 hours by magnesium repletion.[194] In addition, hypomagnesemic patients also have low circulating 1,25$(OH)_2$D levels and end-organ resistance to PTH and vitamin D.[194]

### Other Disorders

Magnesium depletion has also been associated with several other disorders, such as insulin resistance and the metabolic syndrome in type 2 diabetes mellitus.[307,320] Magnesium deficiency has been associated with migraine headache, and magnesium therapy has been reported to be effective in the treatment of migraine.[321] Because magnesium deficiency results in smooth muscle spasm, it has also been implicated in asthma, and magnesium therapy has been effective in asthma in some studies.[322,323] Finally, a high dietary magnesium intake has been associated with a reduced risk of colon cancer.[324,325]

## TREATMENT

Magnesium deficiency can sometimes be prevented. Individuals whose dietary intake has been reduced or who are being maintained by parenteral nutrition should receive magnesium supplementation. The recommended daily allowance of magnesium for adults is 420 mg (35 mEq) for men and 320 mg (27 mEq) for women.[326] Thus, in the absence of dietary magnesium intake, an appropriate supplement would therefore be one 140-mg tablet of magnesium oxide four to five times daily or the equivalent dose of an alternative oral magnesium-containing salt. Because the oral bioavailability of magnesium is approximately 33% in patients with normal intestinal function, the equivalent parenteral maintenance requirement of magnesium would be 10 mEq daily.

Once symptomatic magnesium deficiency develops, patients should clearly be repleted with magnesium. However, the importance of treating asymptomatic magnesium deficiency remains controversial. Given the clinical manifestations outlined earlier, it seems prudent to replete all magnesium-deficient patients with a significant underlying cardiac or seizure disorder, patients with concurrent severe hypocalcemia or hypokalemia, and patients with isolated asymptomatic hypomagnesemia, if it is severe ($<$1.4 mg/dL).

### Intravenous Replacement

In the inpatient setting, the IV route of administration of magnesium is favored because it is highly effective and inexpensive, and is usually well tolerated. The standard preparation is $MgSO_4 \bullet 7H_2O$. The initial rate of repletion depends on the urgency of the clinical situation. In a patient who is actively seizing or who has a cardiac arrhythmia, 8 to 16 mEq (1–2 g) may be administered IV over a 2- to 4-minute period; otherwise, a slower rate of repletion is safer. Because the added extracellular magnesium equilibrates slowly with the intracellular compartment, and because kidney excretion of extracellular magnesium exhibits a threshold effect, approximately 50% of parenterally administered magnesium is excreted into urine.[327]

A slower rate and prolonged course of repletion would be expected to decrease these urinary losses and therefore be much more efficient and effective at replenishing body magnesium stores. The magnitude of the magnesium deficit is difficult to gauge clinically and cannot be readily deduced from the serum magnesium concentration. In general, however, the average deficit can be assumed to be 1 to 2 mEq/kg body weight.[327] A simple regimen for nonemergency magnesium repletion is to administer 64 mEq (8 g) of $MgSO_4$ over the first 24 hours and then 32 mEq (4 g) daily for the next 2 to 6 days. It is important to remember that serum magnesium levels rise early, whereas intracellular stores take longer to replete, so magnesium repletion should continue for at least 1 to 2 days after the serum magnesium level normalizes. In patients with kidney magnesium wasting, additional magnesium may be needed to replace ongoing losses. In patients with a reduced GFR, the rate of repletion should be reduced by 25% to 50%,[327] the patient should be carefully monitored for signs of hypermagnesemia, and the serum magnesium level should be checked frequently.

The main adverse effects of magnesium repletion are due to hypermagnesemia as a consequence of an excessive rate or amount of magnesium administered. These effects include facial flushing, loss of deep tendon reflexes, hypotension, and atrioventricular block. Monitoring the tendon reflexes is a useful bedside test to detect magnesium overdose. In addition, IV administration of large amounts of $MgSO_4$ results in an acute decrease in the serum ionized $Ca^{2+}$ level,[328] which is related to increased urinary calcium excretion and complexing of calcium by sulfate. Thus, in an asymptomatic patient who is already hypocalcemic, administration of $MgSO_4$ may further lower the ionized $Ca^{2+}$ level and thereby precipitate tetany.[329]

#### Oral Replacement

Oral magnesium administration is used initially for the repletion of mild cases of hypomagnesemia or for continued replacement of ongoing losses in the outpatient setting after an initial course of IV repletion. A number of oral magnesium salts are available that vary in their content of elemental magnesium and their oral bioavailability, but little is known about their relative efficacy. Importantly, all of them cause diarrhea, which limits the dose that can be used. Magnesium hydroxide and magnesium oxide are alkalinizing salts with the potential to cause systemic alkalosis, whereas the sulfate and gluconate salts, which present nonreabsorbable anions to the collecting duct, may potentially exacerbate potassium wasting.

A typical daily dose in a patient with normal kidney function and severe hypomagnesemia is 10 to 40 mmol of elemental magnesium in divided doses. Half of this may be sufficient in cases of mild hypomagnesemia, whereas in patients with intestinal magnesium malabsorption, the dose may need to be increased twofold to fourfold. Sustained-release preparations, such as magnesium chloride (Mag-Delay, Slow-Mag) and magnesium L-lactate sustained release (Mag-Tab SR) have the advantage that they are slowly absorbed and thereby minimize kidney excretion of the administered magnesium. By allowing the use of lower doses, these preparations minimize diarrhea.

#### Potassium-Sparing Diuretics

In patients with inappropriate kidney magnesium wasting, potassium-sparing diuretics that block the distal tubule epithelial sodium channel, such as amiloride and triamterene, may reduce kidney magnesium losses.[330] These drugs may be particularly useful in patients who are refractory to oral repletion or who require such high doses of oral magnesium that diarrhea develops. In rats, amiloride and triamterene have been demonstrated to reduce kidney magnesium clearance at baseline and after induction of magnesium diuresis by furosemide, but the mechanism is unknown. One possibility is that these drugs, by reducing luminal sodium uptake and inhibiting the development of a negative luminal transepithelial potential difference, may favor passive reabsorption of magnesium in the late distal tubule or collecting duct.[331]

## HYPERMAGNESEMIA

### CAUSES

In states of body magnesium excess, the kidney has a very large capacity for magnesium excretion. Once the apparent kidney threshold is exceeded, most of the excess filtered magnesium is excreted unchanged into the final urine; the serum magnesium concentration is then determined by the GFR. Thus, hypermagnesemia generally occurs only in two clinical settings, compromised kidney function and excessive magnesium intake.

#### Kidney Disease

In CKD, the remaining nephrons adapt to the decreased filtered load of magnesium by markedly increasing their fractional excretion of magnesium.[332] As a consequence, serum magnesium levels are usually well maintained until the creatinine clearance falls below about 20 mL/min.[332] Even in advanced kidney disease, significant hypermagnesemia is rare unless the patient has received exogenous magnesium in the form of antacids, cathartics, or enemas. Increasing age is an important risk factor for hypermagnesemia in individuals with apparently normal kidney function; it presumably reflects the decline in GFR that normally accompanies older age.[333]

#### Excessive Magnesium Intake

Hypermagnesemia can occur in individuals with a normal GFR when the rate of magnesium intake exceeds the kidney excretory capacity. It has been reported with excessive oral ingestion of magnesium-containing antacids[334] and cathartics,[335] with the use of rectal magnesium sulfate enemas,[336] and is common with large parenteral doses of magnesium, such as those given for preeclampsia. Toxicity from enterally administered magnesium salts is particularly common in patients with inflammatory disease, obstruction,[334] or perforation of the gastrointestinal tract, presumably because magnesium absorption is enhanced.

#### Miscellaneous Causes

Modest elevations in serum magnesium levels have occasionally been described in patients receiving lithium therapy, as well as in postoperative patients and in those with bone metastases, milk-alkali syndrome, familial hypocalciuric hypercalcemia,[284] hypothyroidism, pituitary dwarfism, and Addison disease. In most cases, however, the mechanism is unknown.

## CLINICAL MANIFESTATIONS

Magnesium toxicity is a serious and potentially fatal condition. Progressive hypermagnesemia is usually associated with a predictable sequence of symptoms and signs.[337] Initial manifestations, observed once the serum magnesium level exceeds 4 to 6 mg/dL, are hypotension, nausea, vomiting, facial flushing, urinary retention, and ileus. If untreated, it may progress to flaccid skeletal muscular paralysis and hyporeflexia, bradycardia and bradyarrhythmias, respiratory depression, coma, and cardiac arrest. An abnormally low (or even negative) serum anion gap may be a clue to hypermagnesemia,[333] but it is not consistently observed and probably depends on the nature of the anion that accompanies the excess body magnesium.

### Cardiovascular System

Hypotension is one of the earliest manifestations of hypermagnesemia,[338] is often accompanied by cutaneous flushing, and is thought to be due to the vasodilation of vascular smooth muscle and inhibition of norepinephrine release by sympathetic postganglionic nerves. Electrocardiographic changes are common but nonspecific.[338] Sinus or junctional bradycardia may develop, as well as varying degrees of sinoatrial, atrioventricular, and His bundle conduction block. Cardiac arrest as a result of asystole is often the terminal event.

### Nervous System

High levels of extracellular magnesium inhibit acetylcholine release from the neuromuscular end plate,[339] leading to the development of flaccid skeletal muscle paralysis and hyporeflexia when the serum magnesium level exceeds 8 to 12 mg/dL. Respiratory depression is a serious complication of advanced magnesium toxicity.[338] Smooth muscle paralysis also occurs and is manifested as urinary retention, intestinal ileus, and pupillary dilation. Signs of central nervous system depression, including lethargy, drowsiness, and eventually coma, have been well described in cases of severe hypermagnesemia, but may also be entirely absent.

### Treatment

Mild cases of magnesium toxicity in individuals with good kidney function may require no treatment other than cessation of magnesium supplements because kidney magnesium clearance is usually quite rapid. The normal half-life of serum magnesium is approximately 28 hours. In the event of serious toxicity, particularly cardiac toxicity, temporary antagonism of the effect of magnesium may be achieved by the administration of IV calcium (1 g of calcium chloride infused into a central vein over a period of 2 to 5 minutes, or calcium gluconate infused through a peripheral vein, repeated after 5 minutes if necessary).[337] Kidney excretion of magnesium can be enhanced by saline diuresis and the administration of furosemide, which inhibits tubular reabsorption of magnesium in the medullary TAL.

In patients with ESKD, the only way to clear the excess magnesium may be by dialysis or hemofiltration. The typical dialysate for hemodialysis contains 0.6 to 1.2 mg/dL of magnesium, but magnesium-free dialysate can also be used and is generally well tolerated, except for muscle cramps.[340] Hemodialysis is extremely effective at removing excess magnesium and can achieve clearances of up to 100 mL/min.[340] As a rough rule of thumb, the expected change in the serum magnesium level after a 3- to 4-hour dialysis session with a high-efficiency membrane is approximately one-third to one-half the difference between the dialysate $Mg^{2+}$ concentration and predialysis serum ultrafilterable magnesium (estimated at 70% of total serum magnesium).[340] Note that when hemodialysis is performed using a bath with the same total concentration of magnesium as in serum, the net transfer of magnesium into the patient occurs because the ultrafilterable (and therefore free) magnesium concentration in serum is less than the total concentration; thus, the gradient of free $Mg^{2+}$ is directed from the dialysate to blood.

## DISORDERS OF PHOSPHATE HOMEOSTASIS

Body phosphate metabolism is regulated through plasma inorganic phosphorus (Pi) concentration. Of the total body phosphorus content (500–800 g), 85% is in the skeleton, 14% in soft tissues, and the rest is distributed between other tissues and ECF. Of the Pi contained in bone, roughly 200 mg is recycled daily.[1] Two-thirds of the phosphorus in blood exists as organic phosphates (mainly phospholipids) and one-third as Pi. Pi in blood, for practical purposes, involves two orthophosphates, $H_2PO_4^-$ and $HPO_4^{2-}$. At a plasma pH of 7.4, there are four divalent $HPO_4^{2-}$ ions for every one monovalent $H_2PO_4^-$ ion, so the composite valence is 1.8 (i.e., 1 mmol Pi = 1.8 mEq). Thus, Pi in plasma circulates as phosphates, but is measured in the laboratory as phosphorus (normal values, 2.5–4.5 mg/dL). There are great variations in the normal range of plasma Pi levels with age, from up to 7.4 mg/dL in infants and up to 5.8 mg/dL in children between 1 and 2 years of age.[4,341] Even in adults, there is a gradual decline in plasma Pi with age, although postmenopausal women, in general, tend to have slightly higher plasma Pi levels compared with their male counterparts.[342] Between 85% and 90% of plasma phosphorus is filterable by the kidneys (50% as ionized Pi and 40% complexed with cations), and the remainder is bound to plasma proteins.

The average daily phosphorus intake varies from 800 to 1500 mg, mostly as Pi. Approximately 60% of this is absorbed by the intestine through active transport and paracellular diffusion. The active transport of intestinal phosphate is primarily through type IIb sodium-phosphate cotransporters (NaPi-IIb) and, to a lesser extent, type III transporters (Pit1 and Pit2).[343] Systemic $1,25(OH)_2D$ levels and dietary phosphorus are important physiologic regulators of intestinal phosphate absorption, with high $1,25(OH)_2D$ and low dietary phosphate levels promoting the intestinal uptake of phosphate. However, the discovery of several novel phosphatonins, combined with other studies suggesting the existence of a poorly defined intestine-kidney signaling axis,[344] has implied that this process may be more complex than originally appreciated. In addition to its absorption from the small intestine, approximately 150 to 200 mg of phosphorus is secreted daily by the colon.[1]

As discussed in detail in Chapter 7, the kidney is the major organ regulating phosphate homeostasis. The net kidney excretion of Pi under steady-state conditions is the same as Pi absorbed by the gastrointestinal tract. Up to 80% of kidney reabsorption of phosphate occurs in the proximal tubule by means of the NaPi cotransporter family of proteins, type IIa (NaPi-IIa) and type IIc (NaPi-IIc) in the luminal brush border membrane.[345] The rest of the urinary phosphate is reabsorbed in the distal tubules or excreted in the urine. PTH increases Pi excretion by decreasing the abundance of NaPi-IIa and NaPi-IIc in the brush border membrane. FGF-23 possesses similar actions as those of PTH to limit phosphate reabsorption in the proximal tubule; however, unlike PTH, FGF-23 blocks kidney $1{,}25(OH)_2D$ production by suppressing 1α-hydroxylase activity and stimulating 24-hydroxylation. A low serum phosphate level stimulates kidney NaPi cotransporters and hence phosphate reabsorption.[345] Urinary phosphate excretion can be quantified directly from a 24-hour urine collection or can be estimated by calculating the fractional excretion of filtered phosphate ($FE_{Pi}$) or the kidney tubular maximum reabsorption of phosphate (TmP) to the GFR ratio[346] (in mg/dL):

$$\text{TmP/GFRCr} = \text{serum Pi} - (\text{urine Pi} \times [\text{serum Cr/urine Cr}])$$

The latter method is preferred because the TmP/GFR ratio is independent of kidney function. The normal range for TmP/GFR is 2.6 to 4.4 mg/dL[347]; lower values indicate a decreased maximum kidney phosphate reabsorption threshold and hence excessive urinary phosphate loss. Of note, similar to plasma phosphate levels, TmP/GFR appears to steadily decline with age but, again, slightly increases in women around the time of menopause.[342]

## HYPERPHOSPHATEMIA

Hyperphosphatemia is generally defined as a serum phosphate level elevated above 5 mg/dL. For children, the upper range of normal is 6 mg/dL. In infants, phosphorus levels as high as 7.4 mg/dL are considered normal.[341] The serum phosphorus level usually exhibits diurnal variation, with the lowest levels typically being observed in the later morning and peak levels occurring in the first morning hours.[348] In CKD, the lowest concentration occurs at 0800 and highest at 1600 and 0400 hours. The circadian pattern in CKD is modifiable by phosphate intake.

The clinical causes of hyperphosphatemia[349] can be broadly classified into one of four groups—reduced kidney excretion of phosphate, exogenous phosphate load, acute extracellular shift of phosphorus, or pseudohyperphosphatemia (Box 18.5).

### Box 18.5 Causes of Hyperphosphatemia

**Decreased Kidney Excretion of Phosphorus**

Chronic kidney disease stages 3–5
Acute kidney injury
Hypoparathyroidism, pseudohypoparathyroidism
Acromegaly
Tumoral calcinosis
- Fibroblast growth factor 23 (FGF-23) inactivating gene mutation
- *GALNT3* mutation with aberrant FGF-23 glycosylation
- *KLOTHO* inactivating mutation with FGF-23 resistance
- Bisphosphonates

**Exogenous Phosphorus Administration**

Ingestion of phosphate, phosphate-containing enemas
Intravenous phosphate delivery

**Redistribution of Phosphorus (Intracellular to Extracellular Shift)**

Respiratory acidosis, metabolic acidosis
Tumor lysis syndrome
Rhabdomyolysis
Hemolytic anemia
Catabolic state

**Pseudohyperphosphatemia**

Hyperglobulinemia
Hyperlipidemia
Hyperbilirubinemia
Medications
- Liposomal amphotericin B
- Rec tissue plasma activator
- Heparin

Hemolysis of blood specimen

## CAUSES

### Decreased Kidney Phosphate Excretion

**Reduced Glomerular Filtration Rate.** Both AKI and CKD can lead to hyperphosphatemia. In the early stages of kidney injury, elevations in PTH and FGF-23 levels increase the urinary fractional excretion of phosphate to compensate for the declining GFR, thus maintaining plasma Pi levels in the normal range. With further decrements in GFR (as in severe AKI or CKD, stage 4 or 5), the reduced functional nephron mass is insufficient to maintain maximal Pi excretion, resulting in hyperphosphatemia. A detailed discussion of hyperphosphatemia caused by decreased kidney function is not provided here; this topic is extensively reviewed in Chapter 55 in the context of chronic kidney disease–mineral bone disorder.

**Hypoparathyroidism and Pseudohypoparathyroidism.** Deficient secretion of PTH (hypoparathyroidism) or kidney resistance to PTH (pseudohypoparathyroidism) decrease the kidney excretion of phosphate, leading to hyperphosphatemia. In these entities, circulating phosphorus generally reaches a higher than normal steady-state level (6–7 mg/dL) and is accompanied by hypocalcemia due to decreased bone resorption and urine calcium losses. Hypoparathyroidism and pseudohypoparathyroidism have been discussed extensively (see earlier).

**Acromegaly.** Some patients with acromegaly demonstrate hyperphosphatemia. Parathyroid function is usually normal or slightly increased in acromegaly.[91] The hyperphosphatemia observed appears to result from increased proximal tubule phosphate reabsorption. Growth hormone and insulin-like growth factor-1 directly stimulate proximal tubule phosphorus reabsorption and increase the TmP/GFR.[350]

**Familial Tumoral Calcinosis.** Familial tumoral calcinosis (FTC; OMIM 211900) is a rare autosomal recessive disorder characterized by hyperphosphatemia and the progressive deposition of calcium phosphate crystals in periarticular and soft tissues. The hyperphosphatemia in this disease results from increased proximal tubular reabsorption of phosphate, usually due to loss-of-function mutations in the *N*-acetyl-α-D-galactosamine gene *(GALNT3)*,[351] which encodes a glycosyltransferase that is thought to prevent the degradation of intact FGF-23.[352,353] Additional gene mutations have been linked to tumoral calcinosis, including deactivating mutations in the FGF-23 gene,[354,355] and in the *KLOTHO* gene, which encodes a cofactor necessary for FGF-23 binding to its receptor.[356] FTC has been described mainly in families of African and Mediterranean descent.

The unifying pathogenic mechanism in FTC is abrogation of the phosphaturic effect of FGF-23. As such, missense mutations in FGF-23 inhibit its secretion, mutations in *GALNT3* cause aberrant glycosylation and premature degradation of FGF-23,[352] and mutations in *KLOTHO* lead to end-organ resistance to FGF-23. Similar to humans, mice lacking FGF-23 or *KLOTHO* expression exhibit severe hyperphosphatemia associated with extensive soft tissue calcification.[357] Thus, FTC may be the phenotypic opposite of X-linked and autosomal dominant hypophosphatemic rickets (see later discussion).

PTH, alkaline phosphatase, and calcium levels in FTC are commonly in the normal range. On the other hand, serum $1,25(OH)_2D$ levels are often increased.[358] Together, a normal serum calcium concentration and increased serum phosphorus level lead to an elevated calcium-phosphate product and the slow tissue deposition of calcium phosphate crystals. Decreasing the intestinal absorption of phosphate, either by decreasing dietary phosphorus intake or adding phosphate binders such as sevelamer, is standard therapy for FTC. Additional studies have indicated that the chronic use of acetazolamide may increase urinary phosphate wasting and reduce calcium-phosphate deposits in these patients.[359]

**Bisphosphonates.** Bisphosphonates generally cause mild hyperphosphatemia by altering systemic phosphate distribution and decreasing urinary phosphate excretion.[360,361] The levels of PTH and response with urinary excretion of cAMP to exogenous PTH are normal in patients receiving bisphosphonates.

### Exogenous Phosphate Load

Severe hyperphosphatemia has been recognized for at least a half-century as a complication of sodium phosphate taken orally as a cathartic agent or as a sodium phosphate monobasic or dibasic rectal enema (Fleet enema).[349] Acute kidney injury, hypocalcemia, severe electrolyte disturbances, and death have been described in response to high-dose sodium phosphate administration. Despite these reports, sodium phosphate preparations remain widely used for bowel preparation prior to colonoscopy. Although the risk for hyperphosphatemia is most pronounced in patients with underlying CKD, even healthy individuals can experience a substantial rise in serum Pi levels (up to 9.6 mg/dL in one prospective study) following sodium phosphate therapy.[362] Over the last 10 years, numerous case reports and case series have described an association between the use of oral sodium phosphate for bowel cleansing and phosphate nephropathy. The typical presentation of phosphate nephropathy involves an acute deterioration in kidney function days to weeks following a colonoscopy. Kidney biopsy shows acute and chronic tubular injury, with calcium phosphate deposits (tubular calcifications).[363,364] Most patients will not recover kidney function fully, and some progress to end-stage disease. Overall, such adverse kidney effects are uncommon in patients treated with sodium phosphate but, for those select few who are affected, consequences may be serious. The risk factors for developing phosphate nephropathy are advanced age, female gender, impaired kidney function, volume contraction, ulceration of bowel mucosa, bowel obstruction or ileus, hypertension, and use of angiotensin-converting enzyme inhibitors (ACEIs), angiotensin receptor blockers (ARBs), and nonsteroidal antiinflammatory drugs (NSAIDs).[363,365] Alternative methods of bowel preparation should be considered for patients with these risk factors.

Less commonly, hyperphosphatemia can be observed in the ICU setting when an excessive amount of IV phosphate is given for hyperalimentation, particularly in patients with ESKD. Similarly, the administration of high-dose fosphenytoin for seizure treatment in the setting of kidney dysfunction has been associated with hyperphosphatemia because phosphate is one of the major metabolites of this drug.[366] Finally, vitamin D intoxication can result in hyperphosphatemia, largely because of the simultaneous suppression of PTH production and stimulation of intestinal absorption of phosphate.

### Intracellular to Extracellular Shift of Phosphorus

**Respiratory Acidosis and Metabolic Acidosis.** Respiratory acidosis can lead to hyperphosphatemia, kidney resistance to the effects of PTH, and hypocalcemia.[367] The effect is more pronounced in acute respiratory acidosis than in the chronic form. Respiratory acidosis does not appear to alter the kidney handling of phosphorus significantly. Rather, efflux of phosphate from cells into the extracellular space is probably responsible for the hyperphosphatemia of respiratory acidosis.[368]

Lactic acidosis and, to lesser extent, diabetic ketoacidosis also cause hyperphosphatemia.[369,370] Metabolic acidosis in general reduces glycolysis and Pi utilization. In lactic acidosis, this effect is intensified by tissue hypoxia and intracellular Pi release. Patients with uncontrolled diabetes mellitus are intracellularly phosphate-depleted, despite hyperphosphatemia, an abnormality that becomes unmasked once insulin therapy is initiated.

**Tumor Lysis and Rhabdomyolysis.** Because phosphate is predominantly stored intracellularly, clinical conditions associated with increased catabolism and tissue destruction, such as rhabdomyolysis, fulminant hepatitis, hemolytic anemia, severe hyperthermia, and tumor lysis syndrome, often result in hyperphosphatemia. The severity of the hyperphosphatemia may be exacerbated by the development of AKI.

Tumor lysis syndrome is a constellation of metabolic abnormalities such as hyperuricemia, hyperkalemia, and hyperphosphatemia caused by rapid and massive breakdown of tumor cells.[371,372] Clinical consequences may include AKI, pulmonary edema, cardiac arrhythmia, and seizures. The syndrome typically occurs from 3 days before to 7 days after the initiation of chemotherapy. Hyperphosphatemia is an extremely common clinical finding following treatment for Burkitt lymphoma, especially in patients with preexisting kidney disease; it is also seen in other forms of lymphoma, lymphoblastic and myelogenous leukemias and in patients with solid cancers characterized by a high tumor burden. Malignant lymphoid cells may contain up to four times more intracellular phosphorus compared with mature lymphoid cells, which explains the high prevalence of hyperphosphatemia following chemotherapy in patients with lymphoid malignancies. The lactate dehydrogenase level before the initiation of therapy appears to correlate with the development of hyperphosphatemia and azotemia in these patients.[373] Phosphate nephropathy with tubular calcifications has been reported in tumor lysis syndrome cases exhibiting extremely high serum Pi levels.[371]

To prevent tumor lysis syndrome, intensive volume expansion is generally recommended before chemotherapy to induce a high urine output (120–150 mL/hour) and phosphate and uric acid excretion.[374] The usefulness of urine alkalinization (pH >7) with bicarbonate infusion and/or acetazolamide is unclear, and its practice is controversial. Alkalinization may increase uric acid solubility in the tubules but requires caution; nephrocalcinosis can occur with aggressive alkalinization of the urine because calcium phosphate crystals usually precipitate in alkaline urine. Phosphate binders can be used to decrease the intestinal absorption of phosphate in patients who maintain their oral intake during chemotherapy, but the utility of these drugs is limited in this setting. In severe cases of tumor lysis syndrome, hemodialysis may be necessary to control severe hyperphosphatemia and associated metabolic derangements, with CRRT being most efficacious for maintaining phosphate homeostasis.

#### Pseudohyperphosphatemia

Spurious measurements of high plasma phosphorus levels may occur under certain conditions as a result of interference with the analytic method used. This problem is most common in the case of paraproteinemia (as occurs in multiple myeloma or Waldenström macroglobulinemia).[375] This phenomenon can also be observed in patients being treated with liposomal amphotericin B,[376] recombinant tissue plasminogen activator,[377] or heparin therapy.[378] Spurious phosphate readings can also occur in hemolyzed specimens or in samples from patients with severe hyperlipidemia or hyperbilirubinemia.

### CLINICAL MANIFESTATIONS AND TREATMENT

Most of the acute clinical manifestations of hyperphosphatemia stem from hypocalcemia, discussed earlier in this chapter. Chronic hyperphosphatemia of CKD and its metabolic consequences are discussed in Chapter 55. Little is known about the effects of chronic hyperphosphatemia in the absence of CKD because this is very rarely observed.

Treatment of chronic hyperphosphatemia is generally accomplished through dietary phosphate restriction, oral phosphate binders, and kidney replacement therapy. Acute hyperphosphatemia in association with hypocalcemia requires rapid attention. Discontinuation of supplemental phosphates and initiation of hydration are indicated for patients with acute exogenous Pi overload and intact kidney function. Volume expansion can significantly increase urinary phosphate excretion, but plasma calcium levels must be followed closely because further hypocalcemia may occur due to hemodilution. Acetazolamide administration may also increase urinary phosphate excretion.[379–381] Severe hyperphosphatemia in patients with reduced kidney function or AKI, particularly in those with tumor lysis syndrome, may require kidney replacement therapy. In patients with respiratory or metabolic acidosis, treatment of the underlying acidosis corrects the phosphate derangement. Similarly, in diabetic ketoacidosis, treatment with insulin and correction of metabolic acidosis rapidly reverses the hyperphosphatemia.

## HYPOPHOSPHATEMIA

Hypophosphatemia is a decrease in the concentration of Pi in plasma, and phosphate depletion is a decrease in the total body content of phosphorus. Hypophosphatemia can occur in the presence of a low, normal, or high total body phosphorus content. Similarly, total body phosphate depletion may exist with low, normal, or high plasma Pi levels. The incidence of hypophosphatemia is from 0.2% to 2.2% in hospitalized populations but may be present in up to 30% of chronic alcoholics, 28% to 34% of ICU patients, and 65% to 80% of patients with sepsis.[382,383] There is an association between hypophosphatemia and in-hospital mortality among hospitalized patients[384] and all-cause mortality in the dialysis population.[385] It is unclear if hypophosphatemia is a direct contributor to these outcomes.

### CLINICAL MANIFESTATIONS

Moderate hypophosphatemia (plasma Pi, 1.0–2.5 mg/dL) usually occurs without significant phosphate depletion and without specific signs or symptoms. In severe hypophosphatemia (plasma Pi < 1.0 mg/dL), phosphate depletion is typically present and can have significant clinical consequences.

The clinical manifestations of hypophosphatemia and phosphate depletion generally result from a decrease in intracellular ATP levels. In addition, erythrocytes experience a decrease in 2,3-diphosphoglycerate levels, which increases hemoglobin-oxygen affinity and prevents efficient oxygen delivery to tissues.[386] Hypophosphatemia causes a rise in intracellular cytosolic calcium in cells such as leukocytes, pancreatic islets, and synaptosomes isolated from phosphate-depleted animals. These elevated cytosolic calcium levels have been associated with decreased ATP levels and impaired cell response to stimuli.[387]

Hematologic consequences include a predisposition to hemolysis, thought to result from increased red cell rigidity.[388,389] Spontaneous hemolysis is rarely observed with hypophosphatemia alone, but hypophosphatemia can predispose to red cell lysis in the presence of other risk factors. Phagocytosis and chemotaxis of polymorphonuclear cells are diminished because impaired ATP production decreases the phagocytic capability of these cells.[390]

Severe hypophosphatemia can result in numerous neuromuscular and skeletal abnormalities, including proximal myopathy, bone pain,[382,391] and rhabdomyolysis.[392] Because cell breakdown may lead to the release of intracellular phosphate, normophosphatemia or hyperphosphatemia in this setting may mask the existence of true phosphate depletion. Overt heart failure and respiratory failure as a result of decreased muscle performance may also be observed.[393,394] Correction of the Pi level leads to improvement of myocardial and pulmonary function.[395,396] Neurologic manifestations of severe hypophosphatemia include paresthesia, tremor, and encephalopathy; these also improve with phosphate replacement.[382] Chronic phosphate depletion alters bone metabolism, leading to increased bone resorption and severe mineralization defects that impair bone structure and strength (e.g., osteomalacia, rickets).

Chronic hypophosphatemia can also lead to proximal and distal kidney tubule defects resulting in water diuresis, glucosuria, bicarbonaturia, hypercalciuria, and hypermagnesuria.[397] The hypercalciuria is not solely the result of altered kidney calcium handling but also reflects increased calcium release from bone, consequent to phosphate mobilization, and increased intestinal calcium absorption in response to the accompanying elevation in plasma $1,25(OH)_2D$ levels.[398] Metabolic consequences of hypophosphatemia include insulin resistance, diminished gluconeogenesis, hypoparathyroidism, and metabolic acidosis, with reduced $H^+$ excretion and ammonia generation. Hypophosphatemia is also a potent stimulator of $1\alpha$-hydroxylation to convert 25(OH)D to $1,25(OH)_2D$.

## DIAGNOSIS

The cause of hypophosphatemia can often be delineated from the clinical history or physical examination alone. Shifts of phosphorus from the extracellular to intracellular space usually occur in the setting of an acute illness or treatment (e.g., respiratory alkalosis, treatment of diabetic ketoacidosis). Thus, hypophosphatemia in hospitalized patients typically results from shifts of phosphorus into the intracellular compartment as opposed to kidney losses of phosphorus.[399]

In situations in which the underlying diagnosis is not immediately apparent, it can be clinically useful to determine the rate of urine phosphate excretion by quantification in a 24-hour urine collection or by calculation of the $FE_{Pi}$ or TmP/GFR. A 24-hour urine phosphate greater than 100 mg, $FE_{Pi}$ greater than 5%, or TmP/GFR less than 2.5 mg/100 mL indicates inappropriate urinary phosphate wasting.[347] A high urine phosphate level in the presence of hypophosphatemia results from an acquired defect (e.g., PHPT) or genetic defect (e.g., X-linked hypophosphatemic rickets) in phosphate reabsorption by the proximal tubule.

## CAUSES

Hypophosphatemia may be due to increased kidney phosphate excretion, decreased intestinal absorption, shift of phosphate from extracellular to intracellular fluid, or a combination of these mechanisms (Box 18.6).

### Box 18.6 Causes of Hypophosphatemia

**Increased Urinary Phosphate Excretion**

Increased production or activity of fibroblast growth factor 23 (FGF-23)
- Inherited disorders
  - X-linked hypophosphatemia (*PHEX* mutations)
  - Autosomal dominant hypophosphatemic rickets (FGF-23 mutations)
  - Autosomal recessive hypophosphatemic rickets (*DMP1* and *ENPP1* mutations)
- Acquired disorder
  - Tumor-induced osteomalacia

Disorders of proximal tubule Pi reabsorption
- Hereditary hypophosphatemic rickets with hypercalciuria (*SLC34A3* mutations)
- Autosomal recessive kidney phosphate wasting (*SLC34A1* mutations)
- *NHERF*1 mutations
- *KLOTHO* mutations
- Fanconi syndrome
- Primary and secondary hyperparathyroidism
- Postkidney transplantation
- Medications—acetazolamide, calcitonin, glucocorticoids, diuretics, bicarbonate, acetaminophen, iron (intravenous), antineoplastics, antiretrovirals, aminoglycosides, anticonvulsants
- Acute tubular necrosis recovery, posturinary obstruction
- Miscellaneous—posthepatectomy, colorectal surgery, volume expansion, osmotic diuresis

**Decreased Intestinal Absorption of Phosphate**

Malnutrition with low phosphate intake, anorexia, starvation
Malabsorption of phosphate—chronic diarrhea, gastrointestinal tract diseases
Intake of phosphate-binding agents
Vitamin D deficiency or vitamin D resistance
- Nutritional deficiency—low dietary intake, low sun exposure
- Malabsorption
- Chronic kidney disease
- Chronic liver disease
- Vitamin D synthesis and vitamin D receptor defects

**Altered Phosphorus Distribution, Intracellular Shift**

Acute respiratory alkalosis
Refeeding of malnourished patients, alcoholics
Hungry bone syndrome (postparathyroidectomy)

**Hypophosphatemia Resulting From Multiple Mechanisms**

Alcoholism
Diabetic ketoacidosis, insulin therapy
Miscellaneous
- Tumor consumption of phosphate—leukemia blast crisis, lymphoma
- Sepsis
- Heat stroke and hyperthermia

### Increased Kidney Phosphate Excretion

Hypophosphatemia caused by increased urinary phosphate excretion is generally the result of excess PTH, increased production or activity of FGF-23 from normal or dysplastic bone, or a disorder of kidney phosphate handling in the proximal tubule. The recent discovery of several inherited disorders of renal phosphate wasting has contributed to the elucidation of the underlying mechanisms (Fig. 18.5).

**Hyperparathyroidism.** Both primary and secondary HPT may lead to hyperphosphaturia and hypophosphatemia. PHPT has been discussed earlier in this chapter. The degree of hypophosphatemia observed is usually mild to moderate in severity; increased urinary phosphate excretion is balanced by the mobilization of Pi from the bone and enhanced intestinal absorption of Pi. Secondary HPT resulting from vitamin D deficiency causes hypophosphatemia, not only through the promotion of urinary phosphate wasting by PTH, but also through decreased intestinal absorption of phosphate from low vitamin D levels. The secondary HPT observed in patients with CKD is typically associated with hyperphosphatemia because of a decreased ability of the kidney to excrete phosphorus.

**Increased Production or Activity of Phosphatonins.** There are several rare syndromes of kidney phosphate wasting

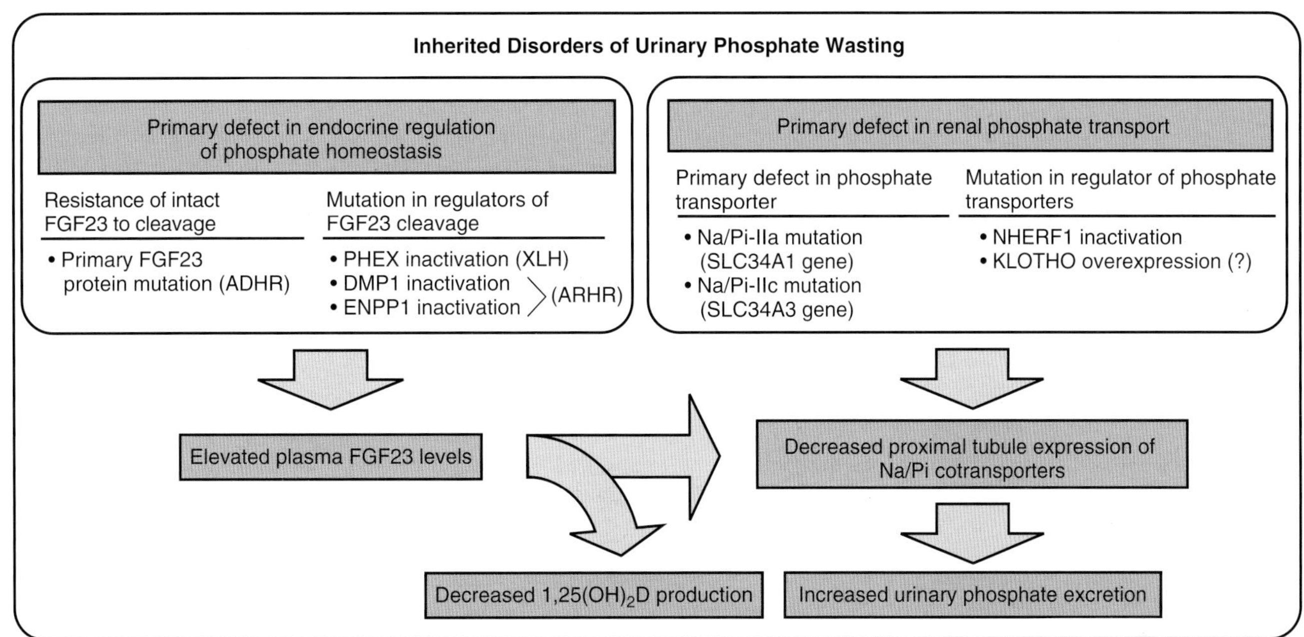


**Fig. 18.5** Summary of the inherited disorders of urinary phosphate wasting. Inherited diseases characterized by phosphaturia and hypophosphatemia can occur from a defect in endocrine pathways involved in the systemic regulation of phosphate homeostasis or from a direct mutation in local regulators of renal phosphate transport. *ADHR,* Autosomal dominant hypophosphatemic rickets; *ARHR,* autosomal recessive hypophosphatemic rickets; *DMP1,* dentin matrix protein 1; *ENPP1,* ectonucleotide pyrophosphatase/phosphodiesterase 1; *FGF23,* fibroblast growth factor 23; *Na/Pi-IIa,* type IIa sodium-phosphate cotransporter; *Na/Pi-IIc,* type IIc sodium-phosphate cotransporter; *NHERF1,* sodium-hydrogen exchanger regulatory factor; *PHEX,* phosphate-regulating gene with homology to endopeptidases on the X chromosome; *XLH,* X-linked hypophosphatemic rickets.

associated with rickets or osteomalacia that result from increased production or activity of FGF-23 or other phosphatonins (see Fig. 18.4).[400]

**X-Linked Hypophosphatemia.** X-linked hypophosphatemia (XLH; OMIM 307800) is a rare X-linked dominant disorder characterized by hypophosphatemia, rickets and osteomalacia, growth retardation, decreased intestinal calcium and phosphate absorption, and decreased kidney phosphate reabsorption. Because it is an X-linked dominant disorder, only one copy of the defective gene is sufficient to cause the disorder when inherited from a parent who has the disorder. Serum 1,25(OH)D levels are inappropriately normal or low, and calcium and PTH levels are normal in patients with XLH. It differs from most cases of rickets in that vitamin D supplementation does not cure it. The prevalence of the disease is 1 : 20,000, penetrance is high, and both females and males are affected.[401]

The gene responsible for this disorder, a phosphate-regulating gene with homology to endopeptidases on the X chromosome *(PHEX),* was identified by positional cloning.[402] Binding of *PHEX* to another bone-derived protein, dentin matrix protein 1 (DMP1), appears to be critical for the suppression of osteocyte production of FGF-23 in bone.[403] Inactivating mutations in *PHEX* or DMP1 result in higher circulating levels of FGF-23 and resultant phosphate wasting.[402,404,405] Abnormal synthesis of $1,25(OH)_2D$ in XLH can be explained by increased levels of FGF-23, which suppress kidney $1\alpha$-hydroxylase activity.[406]

Treatment of XLH patients with oral phosphate and calcitriol improves their growth rate; however, these therapies do not reduce kidney phosphate excretion. As a result, the major goal of therapy in these patients has been to allow normal growth and reduce bone pain.[407] In 2018, the FDA approved burosumab, a human anti-FGF23 monoclonal antibody that appears to be effective for treatment of XLH in children 1 year and older. Burosumab offers a more effective therapeutic strategy, with limited side effects. Studies of burosumab for tumor-induced osteomalacia are in progress.[408] Thus, FGF23-neutralizing antibodies hold considerable promise as a future treatment for XLH patients.

**Autosomal Dominant Hypophosphatemic Rickets.** Autosomal dominant hypophosphatemic rickets (ADHR, OMIM 193100) is an extremely rare disorder of phosphate wasting, with a clinical phenotype similar to that of XLH. Some individuals initially present in childhood with hypophosphatemia associated with lower extremity deformities, whereas others present in adolescence or adulthood with bone pain, weakness, and phosphate wasting. In some individuals with early-onset disease, the phosphate wasting returns to normal after puberty.

The ADHR locus has been mapped to chromosome 12p13.3 and identified as FGF-23. Missense mutations of FGF-23 appear to interfere with its proteolytic cleavage by furin or other subtilisin-like proprotein convertases,[409–411] causing prolonged or enhanced FGF-23 action on the kidney. Treatment is with phosphate replacement and calcitriol, similar to that for patients with XLH.

**Autosomal Recessive Hypophosphatemic Rickets.** Reports describing families with autosomal recessive forms of hypophosphatemic rickets have also emerged. As noted, inactivating mutations in the gene encoding DMP1 lead to a hypophosphatemic syndrome in humans.[412] Similarly, a more recently described mutation in ectonucleotide pyrophosphatase/phosphodiesterase 1 (ENPP1), a protein responsible for the conversion of extracellular ATP into inorganic pyrophosphate,[413] has also been demonstrated to result in a phosphate-wasting syndrome in humans.[414] Interestingly, the deletion of ENPP1 in mice not only leads to increased FGF-23 production by bone and associated urinary phosphate wasting, but also to defective bone mineralization and soft tissue calcification.[415] To date, no studies have elucidated how ENPP1 or pyrophosphate may regulate FGF-23 production.

**Tumor-Induced Osteomalacia.** Tumor-induced osteomalacia (TIO), or oncogenic osteomalacia, is an acquired paraneoplastic syndrome of kidney phosphate wasting. Usually this syndrome presents in older adults, with a protracted course. Hypophosphatemia with normal serum calcium and PTH levels, kidney Pi wasting, low calcitriol levels, and decreased bone mineralization are the hallmarks of TIO.[416] It is caused by mesenchymal tumors that express and secrete FGF-23.[417] In addition to FGF-23, other phosphaturic factors are often secreted by these tumors, including matrix extracellular phosphoglycoprotein (MEPE), frizzled-related protein 4 (FRP-4), and FGF-7.[418]

The definitive treatment of TIO is complete resection of the inciting tumor; however, these mesenchymal tumors are often small and difficult to localize. Medical treatment with phosphate supplementation and calcitriol is frequently necessary to improve bone healing in patients for whom tumor localization or resection is unsuccessful. Cinacalcet has also been used to induce hypoparathyroidism and decrease phosphate wasting, with good response,[419] although hypocalcemia is always a concern when using this therapy in patients with normal kidney function.

### Disorders of Proximal Tubule Inorganic Phosphorus Reabsorption

**Hereditary Hypophosphatemic Rickets With Hypercalciuria.** Hereditary hypophosphatemic rickets with hypercalciuria (HHRH; OMIM 241530) is a rare autosomal recessive syndrome characterized by rickets, short stature, kidney phosphate wasting, and hypercalciuria. HHRH is caused by mutations in *SLC34A3*, the gene encoding the kidney sodium-phosphate cotransporter NaPi-2c.[420] Patients have an appropriate elevation in 1,25$(OH)_2$D levels, which results in hypercalciuria. They are treated with phosphorus supplementation.

A similar autosomal recessive disorder has been described in two patients with loss-of-function mutations in the *SLC34A1* gene, which encodes the NaPi-IIa sodium phosphate cotransporter. However, unlike HHRH, these patients also had Fanconi syndrome (see later).[421]

More recently, gene mutations in the sodium-hydrogen exchanger regulatory factor 1 (NHERF1) have been described in patients with hypophosphatemia and nephrolithiasis from kidney phosphate wasting.[422] NHERF1 is a protein that plays an essential role in the delivery of sodium phosphate cotransporters to the apical membrane in the proximal tubule.[423] Similarly, a de novo translocation mutation in the *KLOTHO* gene has also been linked to a syndrome characterized by elevated plasma α-klotho levels, hypophosphatemia, and HPT.[424] The membrane-bound form of klotho is expressed locally in the kidney in the proximal and distal tubules; prior studies have suggested that klotho has an independent role in kidney phosphate transport.[425] However, the exact mechanisms responsible for the clinical phenotype in this patient exhibiting a translocation mutation of the *KLOTHO* gene remain undetermined.

**Fanconi Syndrome.** Fanconi syndrome is a disorder characterized by generalized proximal tubule dysfunction leading to defects in the reabsorption of glucose, phosphate, calcium, amino acids, bicarbonate, uric acid, and other organic compounds.[426] This syndrome can be genetic or acquired. Inherited causes of Fanconi syndrome include cystinosis, tyrosinemia, and Wilson disease. Acquired causes include monoclonal gammopathies, amyloidosis, collagen vascular diseases, kidney transplant rejection, and many drugs or toxins, such as heavy metals, antineoplastic agents, antiretroviral agents, aminoglycosides, and anticonvulsants.[427,428] Over time, severe hypophosphatemia in Fanconi syndrome can lead to defective bone mineralization, with increased fracture risk. Of interest, a recessive loss-of-function mutation in the *SLC34A1* gene encoding the NaPi-IIa proximal tubule transporter was shown to cause Fanconi syndrome, including phosphaturia and hypophosphatemia and other perturbations in proximal tubule transport, perhaps arising from the accumulation of the misfolded gene product and consequent endoplasmic reticulum–associated stress response.[429]

**Kidney Transplantation.** Hypophosphatemia is observed in up to 90% of patients after kidney transplantation.[430,431] It is typically mild to moderate and mostly occurs during the first weeks after surgery, but may persist for months to years.[430] These patients have phosphaturia and decreased TmP/GFR, with a well-preserved GFR. The causes of posttransplantation hypophosphatemia include persistent (tertiary) HPT,[430] excess of FGF-23 in the posttransplantation period,[432] 25(OH)D and 1,25$(OH)_2$D deficiency, and immunosuppressive medication.[433] Pretransplantation levels of PTH and FGF-23 predict the severity of hypophosphatemia, and both hormones may act synergistically to increase phosphaturia in this setting.[434] Cinacalcet has been shown to correct urinary phosphate wasting and normalize plasma Pi in posttransplantation patients by decreasing PTH levels without an impact on high levels of FGF-23.[435] The major consequence of posttransplantation hypophosphatemia is progressive bone loss and osteomalacia. Management of posttransplantation hypophosphatemia includes replacement of phosphate, correction of vitamin D deficiency, and treatment of HPT.

**Drug-Induced Hypophosphatemia.** There is an extensive and growing list of medications that can cause hypophosphatemia and phosphate urinary losses as part of Fanconi syndrome, as discussed previously, or by affecting only NaPi transporters in the kidney. Diuretics, including acetazolamide, loop diuretics, and some thiazides with carbonic anhydrase activity, such as metolazone, can increase phosphaturia. The volume contraction that accompanies the use of diuretics usually stimulates proximal tubular NaPi reabsorption and prevents the development of severe hypophosphatemia. Conversely, volume expansion with saline can cause phosphaturia and hypophosphatemia.[436] Corticosteroids decrease intestinal phosphorus absorption and increase kidney phosphorus excretion and thus may cause mild to moderate hypophosphatemia.[437] Hypophosphatemia has been reported in patients treated for malignancies with many of the novel tyrosine kinase inhibitors, including imatinib (50%),[438] sorafenib (13%),[439] and nilotinib.[440] The mechanism is thought to be due to inhibition of calcium and Pi resorption from bone, together with secondary HPT, leading to phosphaturia,[441] or may be caused by the development of a partial Fanconi syndrome.[442] Administration of parenteral iron formulations containing carbohydrate moieties has been associated with hypophosphatemia, phosphate wasting, and inhibition of 1α-hydroxylation of vitamin D,[443,444] which was found to be mediated by an increase in circulating levels of intact FGF-23.[445] Hypophosphatemia has also been reported in acetaminophen toxicity; the mechanism for this association is likely multifactorial, but appears at least partially to result from urinary phosphate wasting.[446] Finally, the administration of large doses of estrogens in patients with metastatic prostate carcinoma can also produce hypophosphatemia.[447]

**Miscellaneous Causes.** Significant urinary losses of phosphate may lead to hypophosphatemia during recovery from acute tubular necrosis and from obstructive uropathy. Postoperative hypophosphatemia has been reported after liver resection, colorectal surgery, aortic bypass, and cardiothoracic surgery.[448–450] Posthepatectomy hypophosphatemia appears to be due to a transient increase in kidney fractional excretion of phosphate rather than to increased metabolic demand by the regenerative liver.[451]

### Decreased Intestinal Absorption

**Malnutrition.** Malnutrition with a low phosphate intake is not a common cause of hypophosphatemia. Increased kidney reabsorption of phosphorus can compensate for all but the most severe decreases in oral phosphate intake. However, if phosphate deprivation is prolonged and severe (<100 mg/day), or if it coexists with diarrhea, the continued colonic secretion of phosphate can lead to hypophosphatemia. Hypophosphatemia seen in children with protein malnutrition and kwashiorkor correlates with increased mortality.[452]

**Malabsorption.** More common is hypophosphatemia resulting from malabsorption. Most phosphorus absorption occurs in the duodenum and jejunum, and intestinal disorders affecting the small intestine may lead to hypophosphatemia.[453] Phosphate-binding cations such as aluminum, calcium, magnesium, and iron form complexes with phosphorus in the gastrointestinal tract, resulting in decreased phosphate absorption. Hypophosphatemia can develop quickly, even in patients given a relatively moderate but sustained dosage of phosphate binders. When combined with poor nutritional intake or extensive dialysis, this therapy may result in so-called overshoot hypophosphatemia. Prolonged use of phosphate-binding antacids can lead to clinically significant osteomalacia.[454]

**Vitamin D–Mediated Disorders.** Vitamin D is critical for the normal control of phosphorus. Deficiency of vitamin D leads to decreased intestinal absorption of phosphorus and to hypocalcemia, HPT, and a consequent PTH-mediated increase in kidney phosphorus excretion. Syndromes of vitamin D deficiency or resistance characterized by hypophosphatemia, hypocalcemia, and bone disease are discussed in an earlier section of this chapter that discusses hypocalcemia.

**Redistribution of Phosphate.** Redistribution of phosphate from the extracellular space into cells is a common cause of hypophosphatemia in hospitalized patients. This shift of phosphate occurs by various mechanisms, including elevated levels of insulin, glucose, and catecholamines, respiratory alkalosis, increased cell proliferation (leukemia blast crisis, lymphoma), and rapid bone mineralization (hungry bone syndrome).

**Respiratory Alkalosis.** The fall in carbon dioxide during acute respiratory alkalosis causes carbon dioxide diffusion from the intracellular space, increases intracellular pH, and stimulates glycolysis. The consequent increase in the formation of phosphorylated carbohydrates leads to a decrease in extracellular phosphorus levels.[455] When the alkalosis is prolonged and severe, phosphorus levels can drop below 1 mg/dL.[456] Mild hypophosphatemia may occur during the increased ventilation after treatment of an asthma attack[457] and in patients with panic disorders with intermittent hypocapnia. Hypophosphatemia is common in mechanically ventilated patients, particularly if they are also receiving glucose infusions. The urinary phosphate excretion can drop to undetectable levels, indicating maximal urinary Pi reabsorption.

**Refeeding Syndrome.** In chronically malnourished individuals, rapid refeeding can result in significant hypophosphatemia. The incidence of refeeding-related hypophosphatemia is high in hospitalized patients receiving parenteral nutrition, as high as one in three in one series.[458,459]

Risk factors for refeeding syndrome include eating disorders, chronic alcoholism, kwashiorkor, cancer, and diabetes mellitus.[458] Refeeding after even very short periods of starvation can lead to hypophosphatemia.[459] The mechanism is related to an insulin-induced increase in cellular phosphate uptake and utilization. The maintenance of serum Pi in the normal range is essential in the management of refeeding syndrome. Adequate phosphate (20–30 mmol of Pi/L) in the parenteral nutrition formulation generally prevents this complication. Even higher amounts may be required for patients with diabetes or chronic alcoholism.

### Hypophosphatemia Resulting From Multiple Mechanisms

**Alcoholism.** Hypophosphatemia and phosphate depletion are particularly common and often a severe problem in alcoholic patients with poor intake, vitamin D deficiency, and heavy use of phosphate-binding antacids.[460] Alcohol-induced proximal tubule dysfunction also contributes to phosphate depletion.[234] Alcoholics frequently develop acute respiratory alkalosis due to alcohol withdrawal, sepsis, or cirrhosis. Phosphorus deficiency is often not manifested as hypophosphatemia at the initial evaluation for medical care. Typically, refeeding, administration of IV glucose, or both in this patient population stimulates shifts of phosphorus into cells and thereby uncovers severe hypophosphatemia. Hypophosphatemic alcoholics are at high risk for the development of rhabdomyolysis.[392]

**Diabetic Ketoacidosis.** In uncontrolled diabetes, phosphate is released from cells and ultimately appears in the urine because of concomitant glycosuria, ketonuria, acidosis, and osmotic diuresis. which all increase urinary phosphate excretion.[461] Although serum phosphate levels may be normal, total body phosphate stores are usually low. During treatment of diabetic ketoacidosis, the development of hypophosphatemia is extremely common.[462] Administration of insulin stimulates the cellular uptake of phosphorus, and thus the serum phosphate level can fall dramatically with treatment.[370] However, routine administration of phosphate in this setting, before the development of hypophosphatemia, is discouraged because it may lead to significant hypocalcemia.[463] Phosphate depletion can itself be a cause of insulin resistance, and a decrease in insulin requirements has been observed after phosphate replacement therapy.[464,465]

**Miscellaneous Disorders.** Moderate, and at times severe, hypophosphatemia may be observed in acute leukemia in the leukemic phase of lymphomas[466] and during hematopoietic reconstitution after stem cell transplantation.[467] Rapid cell growth, with consequent phosphorus utilization, is very likely responsible for the decrease in extracellular phosphorus. Hypophosphatemia has been observed in a woman with toxic shock syndrome[468] and is commonly observed in sepsis,[469] but the complicated clinical picture in septic patients makes it difficult to delineate a specific mechanism. Rapid volume expansion diminishes proximal tubule sodium phosphate reabsorption and may lead to transient hypophosphatemia.[436] Hypophosphatemia is seen in patients with heat stroke, as well as hyperthermia, mainly due to increased kidney phosphorus excretion.

## TREATMENT

The first step in the management of hypophosphatemia is to establish the cause of the low Pi, followed by a determination of whether Pi replacement is necessary. There is little evidence that mild hypophosphatemia (Pi = 2.0–2.5 mg/dL) has significant clinical consequences in humans or that aggressive Pi replacement is needed. This is particularly true when the Pi shift is the major cause of the hypophosphatemia.

Patients with symptomatic hypophosphatemia and phosphate depletion do require replacement therapy. Those with severe hypophosphatemia, with a plasma Pi level less than 1 mg/dL, even in the absence of phosphate depletion, will need IV phosphate therapy. Because the serum level of phosphorus may not be an accurate reflection of total body stores, it is essentially impossible to predict the amount of phosphorus necessary to correct phosphorus deficiency and hypophosphatemia.[470] In chronically malnourished patients (e.g., anorectics, alcoholics), significant phosphorus repletion will be necessary, whereas in patients who are hypophosphatemic from other causes (e.g., antacid ingestion, acetazolamide use), correction of the underlying problem may be sufficient.

Phosphate can be administered orally or parenterally. In mild or moderate hypophosphatemia, oral repletion with low-fat milk (containing 0.9 mg Pi/mL) is well tolerated and effective. Alternatively, oral tablets containing 250 mg (8 mmol) of phosphorus from a combination of sodium phosphate and potassium phosphate salts can be prescribed. A typical patient with moderate to severe hypophosphatemia would probably need 1000 to 2000 mg (32–64 mmol) of phosphorus/day to have body stores repleted within 7 to 10 days. Side effects include diarrhea, hyperkalemia, and volume overload.

IV phosphorus repletion is generally reserved for individuals with severe hypophosphatemia (Pi <1 mg/dL). Various regimens are used in clinical practice, all based on uncontrolled observational studies. Some are more conservative in the amount of phosphate delivered to avoid side effects, which may include kidney failure, hypocalcemic tetany, and hyperphosphatemia. One standard regimen is to administer 2.5 mg/kg body mass of elemental phosphorus (0.08 mmol/kg of phosphate over a 6-hour period for severe asymptomatic hypophosphatemia; 5 mg/kg body mass of elemental phosphorus [0.16 mmol/kg of phosphate] over a 6-hour period for severe symptomatic hypophosphatemia).[471] Others have used a more intensive regimen of 10 mg/kg body mass (0.32 mmol/kg of phosphate) administered over 12 hours.[472] However, even with these higher doses, only 58% of treated patients achieved serum Pi levels above 2 mg/dL. A graded dosing scheme for IV phosphate replacement (0.16 mmol/kg over 4 to 6 hours, 0.32 mmol/kg over 4 to 6 hours, and 0.64 mmol/kg over 6 to 8 hours for serum Pi levels of 2.3–3.0, 1.6–2.2, and <1.5 mg/dL, respectively) has been used effectively in ICU patients without kidney dysfunction and hypercalcemia.[473] Other intensive phosphate replacement regimens have been reported and found to be effective and safe in the ICU for select patients with severe hypophosphatemia.[384]

Complete reference list available at ExpertConsult.com.

## KEY REFERENCES


4. Portale AA. Blood calcium, phosphorus, and magnesium. In: Favus MJ, ed. *Primer on the Metabolic Bone Diseases and Disorders of Mineral Metabolism.* Philadelphia: Lippincott Williams & Wilkins; 1999:115–118.
5. Moore EW. Ionized calcium in normal serum, ultrafiltrates, and whole blood determined by ion-exchange electrodes. *J Clin Invest.* 1970;49:318–334.
11. Gauci C, Moranne O, Fouqueray B, et al. Pitfalls of measuring total blood calcium in patients with CKD. *J Am Soc Nephrol.* 2008; 19:1592–1598.
31. Rubin MR, Bilezikian JP, McMahon DJ, et al. The natural history of primary hyperparathyroidism with or without parathyroid surgery after 15 years. *J Clin Endocrinol Metab.* 2008;93:3462–3470.
45. Mundy GR, Edwards JR. PTH-related peptide (PTHrP) in hypercalcemia. *J Am Soc Nephrol.* 2008;19:672–675.
52. Edwards CM, Zhuang J, Mundy GR. The pathogenesis of the bone disease of multiple myeloma. *Bone.* 2008;42:1007–1013.
57. Nussbaum SR, Gaz RD, Arnold A. Hypercalcemia and ectopic secretion of parathyroid hormone by an ovarian carcinoma with rearrangement of the gene for parathyroid hormone. *N Engl J Med.* 1990;323:1324–1328.
59. Marx SJ, Attie MF, Levine MA, et al. The hypocalciuric or benign variant of familial hypercalcemia: clinical and biochemical features in fifteen kindreds. *Medicine (Baltimore).* 1981;60:397–412.
63. Egbuna OI, Brown EM. Hypercalcaemic and hypocalcaemic conditions due to calcium-sensing receptor mutations. *Best Pract Res Clin Rheumatol.* 2008;22:129–148.
64. Nesbit MA, Hannan FM, Howles SA, et al. Mutations affecting G-protein subunit alpha11 in hypercalcemia and hypocalcemia. *N Engl J Med.* 2013;368:2476–2486.
74. Pollak MR, Brown EM, Chou YH, et al. Mutations in the human Ca(2+)-sensing receptor gene cause familial hypocalciuric hypercalcemia and neonatal severe hyperparathyroidism. *Cell.* 1993;75: 1297–1303.

89. Jacobs TP, Bilezikian JP. Clinical review: rare causes of hypercalcemia. *J Clin Endocrinol Metab.* 2005;90:6316–6322.
96. Vagiatzi MG, Jackobson-Dickman E, DeBoer MD, et al. Vitamin D supplementation and risk of toxicity in pediatrics: a review of current literature. *J Clin Endocrinol Metab.* 2014;99:1132–1141.
103. Khairallah W, Fawaz A, Brown EM, et al. Hypercalcemia and diabetes insipidus in a patient previously treated with lithium. *Nat Clin Pract Nephrol.* 2007;3:397–404.
119. Felsenfeld AJ, Levine BS. Milk alkali syndrome and the dynamics of calcium homeostasis. *Clin J Am Soc Nephrol.* 2006;1:641–654.
123. Stewart AF, Adler M, Byers CM, et al. Calcium homeostasis in immobilization: an example of resorptive hypercalciuria. *N Engl J Med.* 1982;306:1136–1140.
125. Gaudio A, Pennisi P, Bratengeier C, et al. Increased sclerostin serum levels associated with bone formation and resorption markers in patients with immobilization-induced bone loss. *J Clin Endocrinol Metab.* 2010;95:2248–2253.
137. Suki WN, Yium JJ, Von Minden M, et al. Acute treatment of hypercalcemia with furosemide. *N Engl J Med.* 1970;283:836–840.
146. Hu MI, Glezerman I, Leboulleux S, et al. Denosumab for patients with persistent or relapsed hypercalcemia of malignancy despite recent bisphosphonate treatment. *J Natl Cancer Inst.* 2013;105:1417–1420.
147. Camus C, Charasse C, Jouannic-Montier I, et al. Calcium-free hemodialysis: experience in the treatment of 33 patients with severe hypercalcemia. *Intensive Care Med.* 1996;22:116–121.
163. Pollak MR, Brown EM, Estep HL, et al. Autosomal dominant hypocalcaemia caused by a Ca(2+)-sensing receptor gene mutation. *Nat Genet.* 1994;8:303–307.
171. Bilezikian JP, Khan A, Potts JT Jr, et al. Hypoparathyroidism in the adult: epidemiology, diagnosis, pathophysiology, target-organ involvement, treatment, and challenges for future research. *J Bone Miner Res.* 2011;26:2317–2337.
174. Ringel MD, Schwindinger WF, Levine MA. Clinical implications of genetic defects in G proteins. The molecular basis of McCune-Albright syndrome and Albright hereditary osteodystrophy. *Medicine (Baltimore).* 1996;75:171–184.
191. Cholst IN, Steinberg SF, Tropper PJ, et al. The influence of hypermagnesemia on serum calcium and parathyroid hormone levels in human subjects. *N Engl J Med.* 1984;310:1221–1225.
209. Kitanaka S, Takeyama K, Murayama A, et al. Inactivating mutations in the 25-hydroxyvitamin D3 1alpha-hydroxylase gene in patients with pseudovitamin D-deficiency rickets. *N Engl J Med.* 1998;338: 653–661.
212. Liamis G, Milionis HJ, Elisaf M. A review of drug-induced hypocalcemia. *J Bone Miner Metab.* 2009;27:635–642.
213. Kelly A, Levine MA. Hypocalcemia in the critically ill patient. *J Intensive Care Med.* 2013;28:166–177.
230. Tong GM, Rude RK. Magnesium deficiency in critical illness. *J Intensive Care Med.* 2005;20:3–17.
241. Cundy T, Dissanayake A. Severe hypomagnesaemia in long-term users of proton-pump inhibitors. *Clin Endocrinol (Oxf).* 2008;69:338–341.
242. Danziger J, William JH, Scott DJ, et al. Proton-pump inhibitor use is associated with low serum magnesium concentrations. *Kidney Int.* 2013;83:692–699.
244. Schlingmann KP, Weber S, Peters M, et al. Hypomagnesemia with secondary hypocalcemia is caused by mutations in TRPM6, a new member of the TRPM gene family. *Nat Genet.* 2002;31:166–170.
249. Pham PC, Pham PM, Pham SV, et al. Hypomagnesemia in patients with type 2 diabetes. *Clin J Am Soc Nephrol.* 2007;2:366–373.
259. Nijenhuis T, Vallon V, van der Kemp AW, et al. Enhanced passive $Ca2^{2+}$ reabsorption and reduced $Mg^{2+}$ channel abundance explains thiazide-induced hypocalciuria and hypomagnesemia. *J Clin Invest.* 2005;115:1651–1658.
260. Schrag D, Chung KY, Flombaum C, et al. Cetuximab therapy and symptomatic hypomagnesemia. *J Natl Cancer Inst.* 2005;97:1221–1224.
264. Groenestege WM, Thebault S, van der Wijst J, et al. Impaired basolateral sorting of pro-EGF causes isolated recessive kidney hypomagnesemia. *J Clin Invest.* 2007;117:2260–2267.
270. van Angelen AA, Glaudemans B, van der Kemp AW, et al. Cisplatin-induced injury of the kidney distal convoluted tubule is associated with hypomagnesaemia in mice. *Nephrol Dial Transplant.* 2013;28:879–889.
280. Nijenhuis T, Hoenderop JG, Bindels RJ. Downregulation of Ca(2+) and Mg(2+) transport proteins in the kidney explains tacrolimus (FK506)-induced hypercalciuria and hypomagnesemia. *J Am Soc Nephrol.* 2004;15:549–557.
293. Khan AM, Lubitz SA, Sullivan LM, et al. Low serum magnesium and the development of atrial fibrillation in the community: the Framingham Heart Study. *Circulation.* 2013;127:33–38.
299. Chiuve SE, Sun Q, Curhan GC, et al. Dietary and plasma magnesium and risk of coronary heart disease among women. *J Am Heart Assoc.* 2013;2:e000114.
309. Magnesium in Coronaries (MAGIC) Trial Investigators. Early administration of intravenous magnesium to high-risk patients with acute myocardial infarction in the Magnesium in Coronaries (MAGIC) trial: a randomised controlled trial. *Lancet.* 2002;360:1189–1196.
342. Cirillo M, Ciacci C, De Santo NG. Age, kidney tubular phosphate reabsorption, and serum phosphate levels in adults. *N Engl J Med.* 2008;359:864–866.
343. Marks J, Debnam ES, Unwin RJ. Phosphate homeostasis and the kidney-gastrointestinal axis. *Am J Physiol Renal Physiol.* 2010;299: F285–F296.
345. Murer H, Hernando N, Forster I, et al. Proximal tubular phosphate reabsorption: molecular mechanisms. *Physiol Rev.* 2000;80:1373–1409.
353. Ichikawa S, Sorenson AH, Austin AM, et al. Ablation of the Galnt3 gene leads to low-circulating intact fibroblast growth factor 23 (Fgf23) concentrations and hyperphosphatemia despite increased Fgf23 expression. *Endocrinology.* 2009;150:2543–2550.
357. Shimada T, Kakitani M, Yamazaki Y, et al. Targeted ablation of FGF23 demonstrates an essential physiological role of FGF23 in phosphate and vitamin D metabolism. *J Clin Invest.* 2004;113:561–568.
384. Brunelli SM, Goldfarb S. Hypophosphatemia: clinical consequences and management. *J Am Soc Nephrol.* 2007;18:1999–2003.
398. Shimada T, Hasegawa H, Yamazaki Y, et al. FGF-23 is a potent regulator of vitamin D metabolism and phosphate homeostasis. *J Bone Miner Res.* 2004;19:429–435.
402. A gene (PEX) with homologies to endopeptidases is mutated in patients with X-linked hypophosphatemic rickets. The HYP Consortium. *Nat Genet.* 1995;11:130–136.
406. Shimada T, Mizutani S, Muto T, et al. Cloning and characterization of FGF23 as a causative factor of tumor-induced osteomalacia. *Proc Natl Acad Sci USA.* 2001;98:6500–6505.
426. Roth KS, Foreman JW, Segal S. The Fanconi syndrome and mechanisms of tubular transport dysfunction. *Kidney Int.* 1981;20:705–716.

# EPIDEMIOLOGY AND RISK FACTORS IN KIDNEY DISEASE

SECTION III

# 19 Epidemiology of Kidney Disease

Morgan E. Grams | Andrew S. Levey | Josef Coresh

**CHAPTER OUTLINE**



**KEY POINTS**

- The chronic kidney disease (CKD) definition has remained stable since 2002, with staging now including cause, glomerular filtration rate, and proteinuria categories.
- The prevalence of CKD globally is approximately 10%, with a suggestion of higher and rising prevalence in low- and middle-income countries.
- Risk factors for CKD incidence and progression provide a foundation for prevention.
- Genetic susceptibility to CKD is now better understood, including a large effect by the *APOL1* susceptibility locus in populations of African descent.
- The incidence of end-stage kidney disease (ESKD) has stabilized at a high level in the United States and a number of other high-income countries but enormous racial and ethnic disparities exist globally, with rates increasing in low- and middle-income countries.
- Kidney transplantation provides the best treatment for ESKD and, despite a limited supply of organs, the prevalence of transplant recipients is increasing markedly, forming an important subset of patients with CKD.
- Acute kidney injury is both a consequence of CKD and a cause of further CKD progression.

## INTRODUCTION

There has been growing interest in the epidemiology of kidney disease in recent decades, fueled by the rising prevalence of kidney failure and observations of disproportionate disease burden by region, race, and clinical characteristics. Kidney disease epidemiology, the study of disease incidence, distribution, and determinants, has enabled substantial progress in the field. Notable developments over the past decade include the issuance of guidelines for acute and chronic kidney disease (CKD), with consensus definitions based on widely used clinical measures, the effective use of disease registries and electronic health records to identify and address areas of unmet need, the discovery of genetic variants that increase kidney disease risk, and the application of innovative technologies for the discovery of biomarkers of kidney disease.

### CONSENSUS DEFINITIONS, CONCEPTUAL MODELS, AND CLASSIFICATION OF CHRONIC AND ACUTE KIDNEY DISEASE

The terms to describe chronic and acute kidney disease have evolved over the years. Consensus definitions were first provided in clinical practice guidelines in the early 2000s, a critical step to allow the clinical translation of epidemiologic research. The definition and classification for CKD was proposed by the U.S. National Kidney Foundation (NKF) Kidney Disease Outcome Quality Initiative (KDOQI) in 2002,[1] adopted by the international guideline group Kidney Disease Improving Global Outcomes (KDIGO) in 2005,[2] and updated by KDIGO in 2012.[3] The definition and classification of acute kidney injury (AKI) were proposed by the Acute Dialysis Quality Initiative (ADQI) in 2004,[4] modified by the Acute Kidney Injury Network (AKIN) in 2007,[5] and harmonized

**Table 19.1 Definitions and Classification of Chronic Kidney Disease (CKD) and Acute Kidney Injury (AKI)**

| Parameter | CKD | AKI |
|---|---|---|
| **Definition** | | |
| Functional criteria | GFR < 60 mL/min/1.73 m$^2$ | Increase in serum creatinine level (SCr) by 50% within 7 days *or*<br>Increase in SCr by 0.3 mg/dL within 2 days, *or*<br>Oliguria (urine output <0.5 mL/kg/h for >6 hours) |
| Structural criteria | Kidney damage | None |
| Duration | >3 months | ≤1 week |
| **Classification** | | |
| Cause | Presence or absence of systemic disease and location in the kidney of pathologic–anatomic abnormalities (e.g., glomerular, tubulointerstitial, vascular, cystic) | Pathophysiology (decreased kidney perfusion, obstruction of the urinary tract, parenchymal kidney disease other than acute tubular necrosis, and acute tubular necrosis) |
| Severity (stage) | Stages based on GFR (G) and albuminuria (A) categories, and related terms[a]:<br>G1 ≥90: Normal or high<br>G2 60–89: Mildly decreased[b]<br>G3a 45–59: Mildly to moderately decreased<br>G3b 30–44: Moderately to severely decreased<br>G4 15–29: Severely decreased<br>G5 <15 or KRT (kidney failure)<br>A1 <0: Normal to mildly increased<br>A2 30–300: Moderately increased[b]<br>A3 >300: Severely increased[b] | Stages based on SCr or urine output:<br>1. SCr ≥1.5–1.9 times baseline *or* >0.3-mg/dL increase *or* urine output <0.5 ml/kg/h for 6–12 hours<br>2. SCr ≥2.0–2.9 times baseline *or* urine output <0.5 mL/kg/h for ≥12 hours<br>3. SCr ≥3.0 times baseline *or* to ≥4.0 mg/dL *or* KRT<br>In patients aged <18 years, decrease in eGFR to <35 mL/min/1.73 m$^2$ *or* urine output <0.3 mL/kg/h for ≥24 hours *or* anuria for ≥12 hours |
| Risk categories | Moderate (G1–G2, A2; G3a, A1)<br>High (G1–G2, A3; G3a, A2; G3b, A1)<br>Very high (G3a, A3; G3b, A2–A3; G4, A1–A3; G5, A1–A3) | Not specified separately |
| Treatment | KRT included in stage 5, defined as ESKD | KRT included in stage 3 |

[a]Units for GFR, mL/min/1.73 m$^2$; units for albuminuria categories, AER mg/day, ACR mg/g. In the absence of evidence of kidney damage, GFR category G1 or G2 does not fulfill the criteria for CKD. In the absence of GFR < 60, albuminuria category A1 does not fulfill the criteria for CKD.

[b]Terms for categories G2 and A2 are relative to young adult levels. Category A3 includes nephrotic syndrome (albumin excretion usually >2200 mg/day [ACR >2220 mg/g; >220 mg/mmol]).

*ACR,* Albumin-to-creatinine ratio; *AER,* albumin excretion rate; *CKD,* chronic kidney disease; *ESKD,* end-stage kidney disease; *GFR,* glomerular filtration rate; *KRT,* kidney replacement therapy; *SCr,* serum creatinine concentration.

Adapted from Kidney Disease: Improving the Improving Global Outcomes (KDIGO) Acute Kidney Work Group. KDIGO clinical practice guideline for acute kidney injury. *Kidney Int Suppl.* 2012,2:1–138; and Kidney Disease: Improving Global Outcomes (KDIGO) CKD Work Group. KDIGO 2012 clinical practice guideline for the evaluation and management of chronic kidney disease. *Kidney Int Suppl.* 2013;3:1–150.

by KDIGO in 2011, which also provided a definition for acute kidney diseases and disorders (AKDs).[6] The definitions and staging systems for CKD and AKI are based on kidney measures that are frequently obtained in clinical practice and population studies (Table 19.1).

The conceptual models for the development, progression, and complications of chronic and acute kidney diseases are similar.[3,6] They include antecedents associated with an increased risk for the development of kidney disease, stages of disease, and complications of disease, including death (Fig. 19.1). Risks for the development of kidney disease may be categorized as susceptibility due to demographic and genetic factors or exposure to factors that might initiate kidney disease. Kidney disease is defined by abnormalities in structure or function, with abnormalities in kidney structure (damage) often, but not always, preceding abnormalities in function. Markers of kidney damage include pathologic findings on biopsy, abnormalities in urine sediment or imaging, proteinuria, and alterations in tubular function. Kidney function is best measured by the glomerular filtration rate (GFR). A GFR < 60 mL/min/1.73 m$^2$ is considered moderately decreased kidney function, and a GFR < 15 mL/min/1.73 m$^2$ is defined as kidney failure. Complications include conditions that occur more often in people with compared with people without kidney disease. In addition to metabolic and hormonal disorders associated with uremia (e.g., anemia, mineral and bone disease, malnutrition, neuropathy), complications include cardiovascular disease (CVD), drug toxicity, and a wide variety of other conditions, such as infections, cognitive impairment, and frailty. Death may result from kidney failure or complications.

Kidney disease is classified according to its duration, severity, cause, and prognosis (Fig. 19.2).[3] Duration of kidney disease longer than 3 months is defined as CKD, whereas duration less than or equal to 3 months is defined as AKD, of which AKI is the subset of cases that occur within 7 days. Criteria

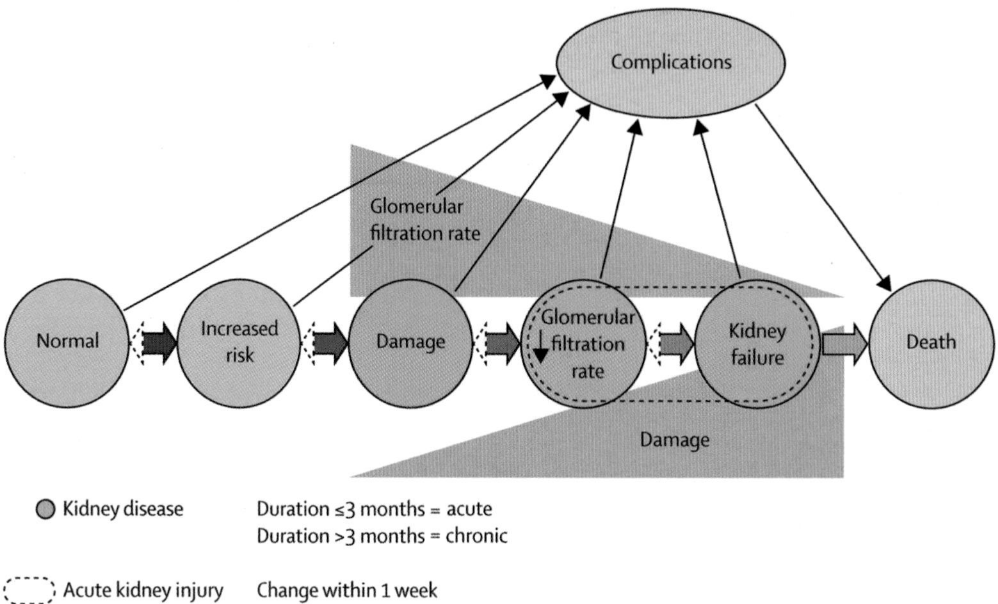


**Fig. 19.1** Factors associated with increased risk of kidney disease *(blue),* stages of disease *(green),* and complications (including death; *purple*). (From Eckardt KU, Coresh J, Devuyst O, et al. Evolving importance of kidney disease: from subspecialty to global health burden. *Lancet*. 2013;382[9887]:158–169.)

**Prognosis of CKD by GFR and albuminuria categories: KDIGO 2012**

| | | | | **Persistent albuminuria categories Description and range** | | |
|---|---|---|---|---|---|---|
| | | | | **A1** | **A2** | **A3** |
| | | | | Normal to mildly increased | Moderately increased | Severely increased |
| | | | | <30 mg/g <3 mg/mmol | 30-300 mg/g 3-30 mg/mmol | >300 mg/g >30 mg/mmol |
| **GFR categories (ml/min/ 1.73 m²) Description and range** | **G1** | Normal or high | ≥90 | | | |
| | **G2** | Mildly decreased | 60-89 | | | |
| | **G3a** | Mildly to moderately decreased | 45-59 | | | |
| | **G3b** | Moderately to severely decreased | 30-44 | | | |
| | **G4** | Severely decreased | 15-29 | | | |
| | **G5** | Kidney failure | <15 | | | |

**Fig. 19.2** Chronic kidney disease staging. Classification is based on the identification of cause (C), glomerular filtration rate *(GFR)* category *(G)*, and albuminuria *(A)*. This is collectively known as "CGA staging." (From Kidney Disease: Improving Global Outcomes [KDIGO] CKD Work Group. Clinical practice guideline for the evaluation and management of chronic kidney disease. *Kidney Int Suppl*. 2013;3:1–150.)

for CKD include GFR < 60 mL/min/1.73 $m^2$ or markers of kidney damage. The severity of CKD is assessed by the level of GFR (stages G1–G5) and albuminuria (stages A1–A3), with end-stage kidney disease (ESKD) as the subset of stage G5 treated by dialysis and transplantation, collectively known as "kidney replacement therapy" (KRT). Causes of CKD are classified according to the presence or absence of systemic disease and location of pathologic and anatomic abnormalities within the kidney. Prognosis is determined based on G and A staging and categorized as moderate, high, and very high risk.

Criteria for AKI include a rise in the serum creatinine level or oliguria, and severity is staged according to peak value for the serum creatinine level or nadir value for urine output. Patients requiring acute KRT are classified as stage 3, the most severe stage. Causes of AKI are classified by pathophysiology as decreased kidney perfusion, obstruction of the urinary tract, and parenchymal kidney diseases (including acute tubular necrosis); all may occur in people with or without underlying CKD. Incomplete recovery of AKD can lead to new-onset CKD in those without underlying CKD or progression of CKD in those with underlying CKD. In addition, there is overlap among the risk factors, causes, and complications between AKD and CKD.

## PRINCIPLES OF EPIDEMIOLOGY AND USE IN KIDNEY DISEASE RESEARCH

This chapter focuses on the prevalence, incidence, outcomes, and risk factors for kidney disease. Disease prevalence is the proportion of individuals in a given population with disease; disease incidence is the number of new cases that develop among individuals without prevalent disease over a given period of time. Disease prevalence thus depends not only on disease incidence, but also on survival and how long the disease persists. Outcomes refer to events of interest that may occur with greater frequency among affected individuals, and risk factors refer to characteristics that precede the onset of disease or outcome. It should be noted that much of the epidemiologic literature is observational, and thus observed associations among risk factors, kidney disease, and outcomes may be causal or noncausal. The Bradford Hill criteria provide guidelines for inferring causation and specify the minimal conditions that need to be met to support a causal relationship between the risk factor (exposure) and disease (outcome; Table 19.2).[7] Trends refer to changes in disease incidence, prevalence, or outcomes over time and may be due to changes in population demographics, risk factor distribution, risk factor control, or availability and effectiveness of treatment. The latter explanation is particularly relevant for trends in ESKD, which is defined by treatment with KRT.

**Table 19.2 Bradford Hill Criteria for Causation**

| Criteria | Explanation |
|---|---|
| Strength of association | The stronger the association, the more likely the relationship is causal. |
| Consistency | A casual association is consistent when replicated in different populations and studies. |
| Specificity | A single putative cause produces a single effect. |
| Temporality | Exposure precedes outcome; that is, risk factor predates disease. |
| Biologic gradient | Increasing exposure to a risk factor increases risk of the disease, and reduction in exposure reduces risk. |
| Plausibility | The observed association is consistent with biologic mechanisms of disease processes. |
| Coherence | The observed association is compatible with existing theory and knowledge within a given field. |
| Experimental evidence | The factor under investigation is amenable to modification by an appropriate experimental approach. |
| Analogy | An established cause and effect relationship exists for a similar exposure or disease. |

Adapted from Hill AB. The environment and disease: association or causation? *Proc R Soc Med.* 1965;58:295–300.

## RECENT CONTRIBUTIONS OF EPIDEMIOLOGY TO NEPHROLOGY

Epidemiologic studies underlie many of the important advances in kidney disease in the past 2 decades. The development of GFR-estimating equations and recognition of albuminuria as a risk factor for adverse outcomes were central to the definition and staging of CKD, which in turn enabled studies of the prevalence of CKD, identification of CKD as a risk factor for CVD, and recognition of CKD as a global public health problem. In addition, estimated GFR (eGFR) and albuminuria are now widely used as prognostic markers in clinical practice and as surrogate markers of kidney disease outcomes in clinical trials of treatment for kidney disease.[8] Advances in genetic epidemiology have revolutionized our understanding of both common and uncommon diseases.[9] Common variations among individuals of African ancestry in a single gene encoding apolipoprotein L1 (APOL1) are now recognized to increase the risk for ESKD.[10–13] Similarly, large cohort studies have demonstrated that the presence of sickle cell trait increases the risk for both CKD and ESKD, increasing our understanding of racial disparities in kidney disease.[14,15] Genome-wide association studies in membranous and immunoglobulin A (IgA) nephropathy have provided strong evidence of heritability and a role for the immune system in the development of disease.[16–20] Rare genetic variants have been identified as the cause of several monogenic diseases, such as polycystic kidney disease, familial nephrotic syndrome, and congenital anomalies of the kidney and urinary tract (CAKUT).[21,22] Global collaboration, coupled with the increasing availability of large databases with rigorously defined clinical characteristics, frequent ascertainment of kidney measures, and genomic, proteomic, and metabolomic data will allow continued advances in research, clinical practice, and public health.

# CHRONIC KIDNEY DISEASE

## EPIDEMIOLOGY

Obtaining accurate and comparable estimates of CKD burden across world regions is difficult for several reasons. Identification of disease requires testing for kidney disease measures (e.g., serum creatinine or cystatin C for eGFR, urine albumin, urine total protein), which are not uniformly performed. Differences across populations may reflect differences in laboratory testing practice, because CKD in its early stages is often asymptomatic, with low awareness of disease.[23,24] For example, if only eGFR is ascertained, prevalence estimates reflect CKD stages G3–G5 and will be lower than if albuminuria is also ascertained, enabling prevalence estimates of CKD stages G1–G5 and A1–A3. Two populations with equal proportions of CKD also may have very different prevalence estimates if one performs near-universal laboratory testing and the other screens only high-risk individuals. In addition, because CKD is defined using kidney disease measures, assays must be standardized to derive comparable estimates. In the United States, standardization of creatinine assays was achieved in the past decade[25]; however, standardization of cystatin C and urine albumin assays are still ongoing. Finally, estimating equations for GFR are not consistently applied, and there is known variation in CKD prevalence when, for example, the Modification of Diet in Renal Disease (MDRD) or Chronic Kidney Disease Epidemiology Collaboration (CKD-EPI) equations are used.[26,27] Progress in CKD awareness, testing, definitions, and measurement should enable substantial progress in the field in the coming decade.

## PREVALENCE

Estimates of the prevalence of CKD worldwide vary, but generally range between 8% and 16%.[28] The most accurate CKD prevalence estimates come from nationally representative surveys, such as the National Health and Nutritional Examination Survey (NHANES) in the United States. In this sampling design, people are selected from the general population and undergo detailed physical and laboratory examinations. Estimates of disease prevalence are obtained by weighting sample proportions by inverse probability of selection from the general population. In NHANES 2011–2012, the estimate of U.S. prevalence of CKD was based on a one-time measurement of eGFR creatinine (Cr) and the urine albumin-to-creatinine (ACR) ratio, was 14.2%, representing 7.3% for stages G1 and G2 and 6.9% for stage G3 or G4.[29] It should be noted that this study did not assess the chronicity of abnormalities of these measures and thus may have slightly overestimated their prevalence. However, other considerations suggested an underestimation of prevalence of CKD. Markers of kidney damage other than albuminuria were not assessed. People with CKD, stage G5—those undergoing KRT and those with an eGFR < 15 mL/min/1.73 $m^2$—were not included in the NHANES estimates. In addition, NHANES does not include people living in institutionalized settings or who are involved in the military.

Despite the relatively high prevalence of CKD in the United States, the recent NHANES study did report some encouraging trends.[29] An earlier study of NHANES showed an increasing prevalence of CKD over time (from 10.0%–13.1% from 1988–1994 to 1999–2004, using a definition that adjusted for short-term variability in the urine ACR).[30] Since that time, however, a recent study has suggested that the prevalence of the CKD remained unchanged (14.0% in 2003–2004 to 14.2% in 2011–2012), which is all the more encouraging when one considers the significant increases in the prevalence of diabetes mellitus and obesity.[31,32] Similarly, the prevalence of CKD stages G3 and G4 was stable when participants were stratified by age, gender, and diabetes status (Fig. 19.3). In

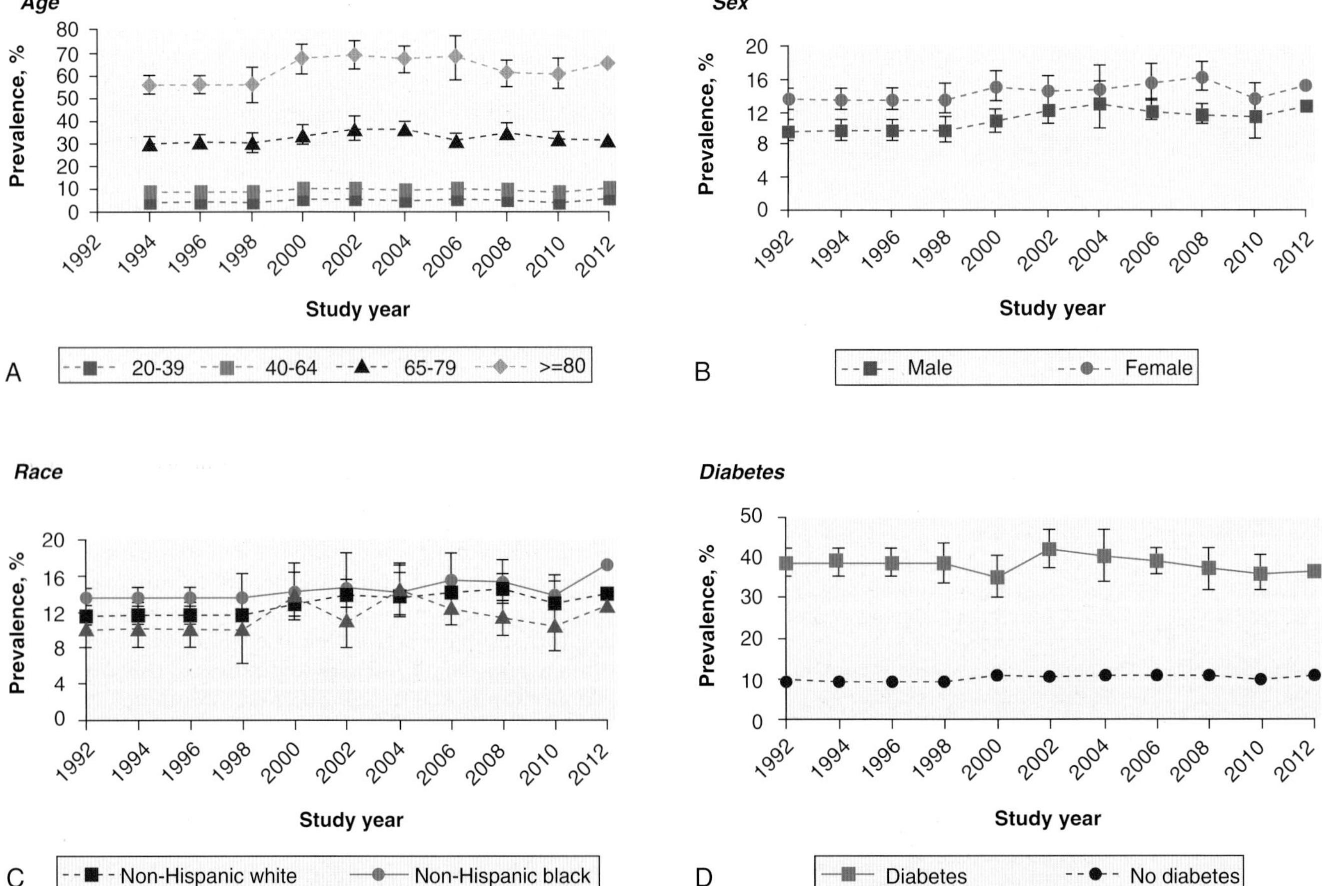


**Fig. 19.3** Adjusted prevalence of chronic kidney disease (CKD) stages 3 and 4 (estimated glomerular filtration rate of 15–59 mL/min/1.73 $m^2$, calculated with the Chronic Kidney Disease Epidemiology Collaboration equation [CKD-EPI]; see text[26,27]) in U.S. adults by age (A), sex (B), race and ethnicity (C), and presence or absence of diabetes (D), NHANES 1988–1994 through 2011–2012. Each subgroup is adjusted for the other three subgroup variables (e.g., age-specific prevalence is adjusted for gender, race and ethnicity, and diabetes status). *NHANES,* National Health and Nutrition Examination Survey. (Adapted from Murphy D, McCulloch CE, Lin F, et al. Trends in prevalence of chronic kidney disease in the United States. *Ann Intern Med.* 2016;165:473–481.)

fact, the only subgroup tested in which crude prevalence meaningfully increased from 2003–2004 to 2011–2012 was non-Hispanic blacks (4.9% in 2003–2004 to 6.2% in 2011–2012). Given the already disproportionate burden of CKD among black people, these results are worrisome, and additional efforts are needed to address racial disparities in CKD. Subsequent phases of NHANES will confirm whether these trends persist.

In Europe, no multinational survey data exist, so a study combined data from 19 general population studies in 13 European countries to estimate age- and gender-adjusted CKD prevalence.[33] There was large heterogeneity by country, even when stratified by diabetes, hypertension, and obesity status, with lower rates of CKD stages G3–G5 in central Italy (1%) but higher in northeast Germany (5.9%). Similarly, the prevalence of CKD stages G1–G5 ranged from 3.3% in Norway to 17.3% in northeast Germany. Fig. 19.4 indicates the differences by region in the population aged 45 to 74 years, and highlights the relatively localized source populations, which may not be representative of all of Europe. Other limitations noted by the authors included the heterogeneity in laboratory methods, with not all assays being isotope dilution mass spectrometry (IDMS)-standardized, and differences in dietary habits, with certain high-protein diets typical of northern Germany known to influence serum creatinine (Cr), resulting in an underestimate of eGFRcr.

Global estimates of CKD are also heterogeneous (Table 19.3; see also Chapter 75).[34,35] A systematic analysis of 33 studies from 32 countries (nearly 50% of the world's population) has found the crude prevalence of CKD stages G1–G5 ranges in men from 4.5% in South Korea to 25.7% in El Salvador, and in women from 4.1% in Saudi Arabia to 16.0% in Singapore.[34] In addition to 17 studies that were included which were derived from a regional or multisite source population and thus not necessarily generalizable to the nation as a whole, underlying studies differed in the creatinine measurement method, the eGFR Cr equation used, and the protocol for assessing albuminuria. Noting these caveats, the authors estimated the age-standardized global prevalence of CKD in 2010 as 10.4% in men and 11.8% in women. They also reported substantial differences by gross national product, with high-income countries estimated to have lower CKD prevalence (8.6% and 9.6% in men and women, respectively) than low- and middle-income countries (10.6% and 12.5%).

Diabetes and hypertension are considered the major causes of CKD globally.[28] In the U.S. population with diabetes mellitus, an estimated 39.4% had CKD in 2011–2014; in the population with hypertension, an estimated 32.1% had CKD, and in the population with obesity, an estimated 17.6% had CKD.[24] Interestingly, measures of kidney disease varied slightly within each comorbidity—47% of the CKD within the diabetes group was manifest by albuminuria only, 27% by decreased GFR only, and 26% by both, compared with 36%, 45%, and 19%, respectively, for hypertension and 30%, 55%, and 15%, respectively, for obesity (Fig. 19.5). The prevalence of CKD by specific cause is difficult to estimate, but if the prevalence of diabetes mellitus in the United States is approximately 10%,[34] and over one-third of people with diabetes mellitus have CKD,[36] then the prevalence of diabetic kidney disease in the U.S. population may be close to 3% to 4%, or one-third of all prevalent CKD cases. In contrast to trends in the prevalence of kidney disease in those with diabetes mellitus, which has been estimated to be fairly flat,[29] trends in the prevalence of diabetic kidney disease in the general population have been reported to follow the increasing trends in the prevalence of diabetes.[37]

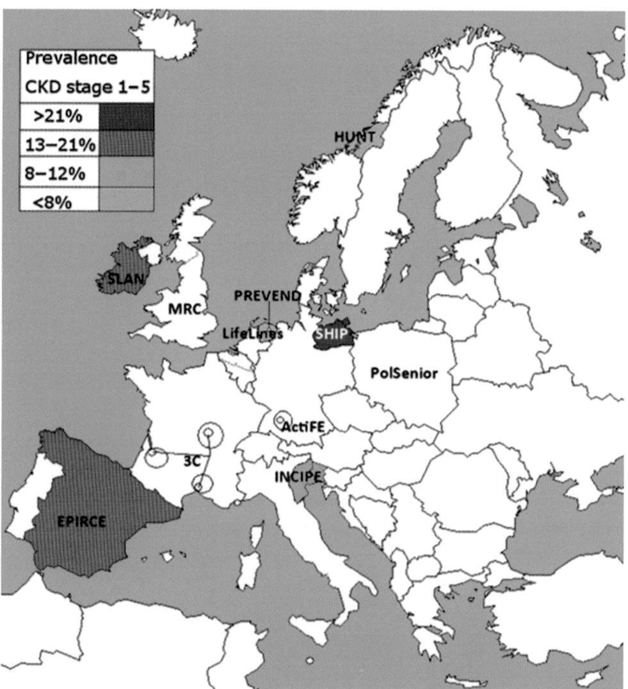


**Fig. 19.4** Adjusted prevalence of chronic kidney disease (CKD) stages 1–5 in the population aged 45–74 years, in isotope dilution mass spectrometry (IDMS) studies. Prevalence was age- and gender-adjusted to the EU27 population of 2005. The study names in the uncolored regions are studies that used non-IDMS-standardized creatinine or studies that recruited subjects aged 50+ years. *IDMS*, Isotope dilution mass spectrometry. (From Brück K, VS, Gambaro G, et al. CKD prevalence varies across the European general population. *J Am Soc Nephrol.* 2016;27:2135–2147.)

## INCIDENCE

Compared with estimates of CKD prevalence, information on the incidence of CKD is relatively sparse. Calculation of the incidence—the development of new cases of CKD—requires a population-representative sample, longitudinal follow-up, and regular and comparable ascertainment of kidney measures in each individual. The incidence of disease stemming from clinical populations may not be valid, because higher-risk individuals are more likely to receive testing. On the other hand, the incidence of disease stemming from population-based cohorts may underestimate CKD incidence due to loss to follow-up and relatively infrequent study visits (e.g., visits every 3 or 5 years).

In the United States, a few long-running prospective cohorts have provided estimates of incident CKD, but the frequency of assessment of kidney measures differed. The Atherosclerosis Risk in Communities (ARIC) study, a cohort of middle-aged black and white individuals aged 45 to 65 years of age, from 4 U.S. communities, estimated an incidence of 10.4 cases of CKD stages G3–G5/1000 years of follow-up, or a 7.3% incidence over 8.8 years when eGFRcr was assessed every 3 years.[38] The Framingham study, a community-based study of

**Table 19.3 Global Estimates of Chronic Kidney Disease[a]**

| | High-Income Countries | | | | Low- and Middle-Income Countries | | | |
|---|---|---|---|---|---|---|---|---|
| | CKD Stages 1–5 | | CKD Stages 3–5 | | CKD Stages 1–5 | | CKD Stages 3–5 | |
| **Age (Years)** | *Men* | *Women* | *Men* | *Women* | *Men* | *Women* | *Men* | *Women* |
| **Prevalence, % (95% CI)** | | | | | | | | |
| 20–29 | 3.7 (2.7–5.1) | 5.3 (3.8–6.3) | 0.7 (0.3–1.4) | 0.9 (0.4–1.6) | 7.3 (6.4–9.0) | 6.6 (6.2–7.3) | 3.0 (1.7–5.4) | 2.0 (1.4–3.3) |
| 30–39 | 5.0 (4.0–6.0) | 5.9 (4.4–6.9) | 1.3 (0.7–2.1) | 1.6 (0.9–2.6) | 8.1 (6.8–10.3) | 9.0 (8.6–9.7) | 3.1 (1.9–5.0) | 3.1 (2.1–5.1) |
| 40–49 | 6.8 (5.5–8.2) | 7.7 (5.9–9.0) | 2.1 (1.4–3.1) | 3.2 (2.0–4.8) | 10.2 (9.0–12.6) | 11.5 (11.0–12.7) | 3.0 (1.8–6.2) | 4.0 (2.5–7.7) |
| 50–59 | 10.2 (8.6–12.2) | 11.1 (8.6–13.8) | 4.6 (3.2–6.7) | 7.4 (5.2–10.2) | 12.0 (10.4–15.1) | 15.7 (14.7–17.8) | 4.9 (3.5–8.1) | 6.7 (4.5–11.7) |
| 60–69 | 16.0 (13.6–18.1) | 15.6 (12.6–18.9) | 9.4 (7.8–11.6) | 12.2 (9.6–15.8) | 16.3 (14.7–20.0) | 21.3 (19.6–24.9) | 9.7 (6.1–15.6) | 13.1 (9.5–19.7) |
| ≥70 | 28.1 (23.4–33.0) | 28.9 (22.7–34.3) | 22.7 (20.0–26.4) | 28.5 (26.1–31.5) | 20.6 (19.4–24.1) | 28.4 (26.3–32.7) | 11.8 (9.0–17.6) | 17.3 (12.6–27.2) |
| Total | 10.1 (8.8–11.1) | 12.1 (9.9–13.7) | 5.4 (4.6–6.5) | 8.6 (6.9–10.7) | 10.2 (9.1–12.4) | 12.1 (11.6–13.3) | 4.3 (2.9–7.1) | 5.3 (3.8–8.2) |
| Age-standardized | 8.6 (7.3–9.8) | 9.6 (7.7–11.1) | 4.3 (3.5–5.2) | 5.7 (4.4–7.6) | 10.6 (9.4–13.1) | 12.5 (11.8–14.0) | 4.6 (3.1–7.7) | 5.6 (3.9–9.2) |
| **Absolute Numbers (in Thousands; 95% CI)** | | | | | | | | |
| 20–29 | 3453 (2485–4718) | 4647 (3307–5500) | 694 (288–1275) | 800 (307–1570) | 37,121 (32,209–45,651) | 32,054 (30,213–35,932) | 14,998 (8471–27,644) | 9863 (6746–16,328) |
| 30–39 | 4699 (3802–5684) | 5298 (4000–6235) | 1221 (659–1957) | 1440 (712–2514) | 33,274 (27,740–42,285) | 35,920 (34,256–38,727) | 12,499 (7803–20,591) | 12,265 (8185–20,402) |
| 40–49 | 6326 (5158–7691) | 7120 (5519–8386) | 2004 (1290–2934) | 2990 (1731–4700) | 35,322 (31,190–43,673) | 39,012 (37,165–43,201) | 10,253 (6328–21,335) | 13,495 (8579–26,111) |
| 50–59 | 8531 (7149–10,157) | 9752 (7541–12,136) | 3874 (2625–5549) | 6485 (4218–9418) | 29,618 (25,640–37,287) | 38,337 (35,959–43,651) | 12,167 (8612–19,988) | 16,355 (10,900–28,611) |
| 60–69 | 9579 (8155–10,849) | 10,425 (8411–12,690) | 5608 (4694–6963) | 8291 (6329–11,264) | 22,434 (20,338–27,637) | 31,136 (28,731–36,396) | 13,420 (8430–21,497) | 19,232 (13,883–28,848) |
| ≥ 70 | 15,699 (13,066–18,416) | 24,426 (19,150–29,003) | 12,690 (11,136–14,745) | 24,065 (21,769–27,161) | 19,606 (18,459–22,925) | 33,637 (31,150–38,706) | 11,176 (8541–16,673) | 20,509 (14,912–32,240) |
| Total | 48,285 (42,349–53,284) | 61,669 (50,394–69,929) | 26,091 (22,014–31,078) | 44,071 (35,296–54,831) | 177,375 (159,157–215,924) | 210,096 (200,787–231,704) | 74,513 (50,324–123,460) | 91,719 (66,697–143,121) |

[a]Age-specific and age-standardized prevalence estimates and absolute numbers of men and women with CKD in high-, low-, and middle-income countries.
*CI,* Confidence interval; *CKD,* chronic kidney disease.
From Mills KT, Xu Y, Zhang W, et al. A systematic analysis of worldwide population-based data on the global burden of chronic kidney disease in 2010. *Kidney Int.* 2015;88(5):950–957.

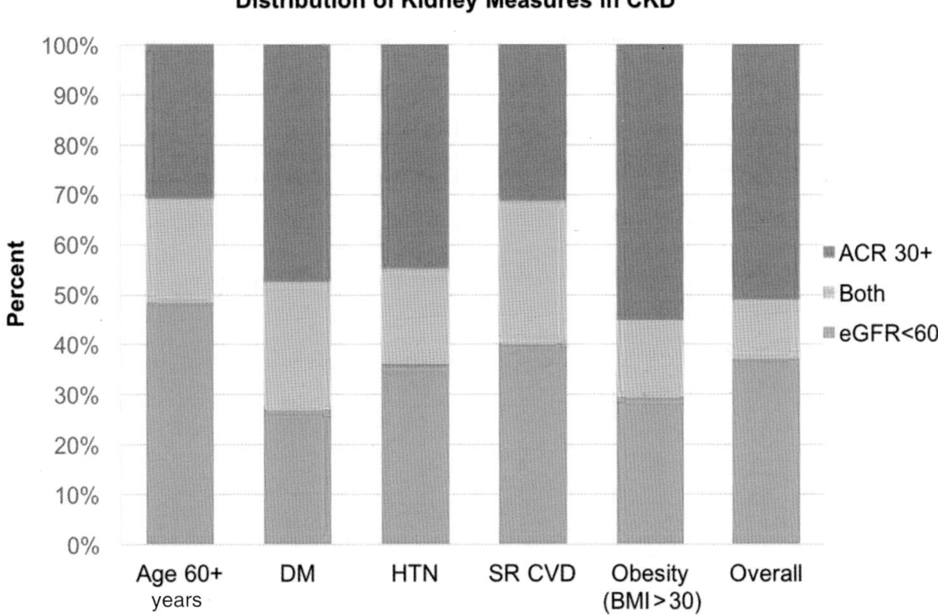


**Fig. 19.5** Distribution of kidney measures in NHANES participants with chronic kidney disease (CKD) older than 60 years and those with diabetes mellitus *(DM)*, hypertension *(HTN)*, self-reported cardiovascular disease *(SR CVD)*, obesity (BMI > 30), and overall. Single-sample estimates of eGFR and ACR; eGFR calculated using the Chronic Kidney Disease Epidemiology Collaboration equation (CKD-EPI) equation. *ACR,* Urine albumin-to-creatinine ratio; *BMI,* body mass index; *eGFR,* estimated glomerular filtration rate; *NHANES,* National Health and Nutrition Examination Survey. (Adapted from United States Renal Data System. 2016 USRDS annual data report: epidemiology of kidney disease in the United States. https://www.ajkd.org/article/ S0272-6386(16)30703-X/fulltext.)

predominantly white individuals with a relatively low rate of diabetes (2.7% vs. 11.4% in the ARIC study), and a mean age of 43 years, reported 9.4% of 2585 individuals developed CKD stages G3–G5 in a subsequent visit 18.5 years later.[39] In the Cardiovascular Health Study, a community-based longitudinal study of older adults with a mean age of 72 years, 10% developed CKD stages G3–G5 by year 7 when assessed using eGFRVt, and 19% developed CKD stages G3–G5 when assessed using eGFRcys.[40] In each of these studies, the rate of incident CKD was higher with older age. Notably, none assessed the incidence of albuminuria, so they likely underestimated the incidence of CKD.

Racial differences in incident CKD also exist. In the Coronary Artery Risk Development in Young Adults cohort, a study of black and white individuals aged 18–30 years, the risk of developing CKD stages G3–G5 (in this study, assessed from eGFRcr and requiring an accompanied 25% decline in eGFR) at 10, 15, or 20 years after baseline was 2.6 times higher in blacks than whites.[41] Similarly, there were large racial disparities in the Multi-Ethnic Study of Arteriosclerosis (mean age, 60 years), in which blacks had more than threefold higher risk of developing CKD stages G3–G5 (in this study, assessed from eGFRcys and required a ≥1 mL/min/1.73 $m^2$ decline in eGFR) compared with whites in a population with baseline eGFR > 90 mL/min/1.73 $m^2$ (3.4 cases/1000 years vs. 0.9 cases/1000 years).[42] Incidence rates were higher among participants with eGFR between 60 and 90 mL/min/1.73 $m^2$, and racial differences persisted, albeit slightly attenuated (26.3 cases/1000 years vs. 18.5 cases/1000 years in blacks and whites, respectively). When modeled as incidence over a lifetime using NHANES and registry data, racial disparities again were present, with African Americans projected to develop CKD stages G3–G5 at younger ages and greater disparities in the incidence of more severe disease (Fig. 19.6).[43]

In Europe, the incidence of CKD assessed using eGFRcr and urine albumin excretion >30 mg/day has been reported in the PREVEND cohort, a population-based cohort that oversampled for people with urine albumin concentrations ≥10 mg/L on a first morning void urine sample.[44] Participants were followed over 10 years at 5 separate visits. The incidence of developing CKD stages G1–G5 was 18.6/1000 person-years; the incidence of developing albuminuria was 13.4/1000 person-years, and the incidence of developing decreased GFR was 5.8/1000 person-years. In an administrative cohort, the incidence of serum creatinine ≥1.7 mg/dL (eGFR ranging from 37–57 mL/min/1.73 $m^2$ for men and 28–43 mL/min/1.73 $m^2$ for women) was 1701 cases/million population in Southampton, United Kingdom, with much higher rates of CKD among older compared with younger inhabitants.[45]

## OUTCOMES

CKD has been increasingly recognized as a top public health priority due to its strong association with adverse outcomes. In some areas of the world, CKD is one of the top five causes of death.[46] Lower GFR and higher albuminuria levels result in a significantly diminished life expectancy at all ages (Fig. 19.7).[24] Part of this increase in mortality is exerted through the higher risk of kidney failure, both untreated and treated by dialysis or transplantation.[47] In addition, earlier stages of CKD are associated with increased risk of death, AKI, CKD progression, CVD, heart failure, and even some types of cancer.[48–52] For AKI as well as other adverse outcomes, risk

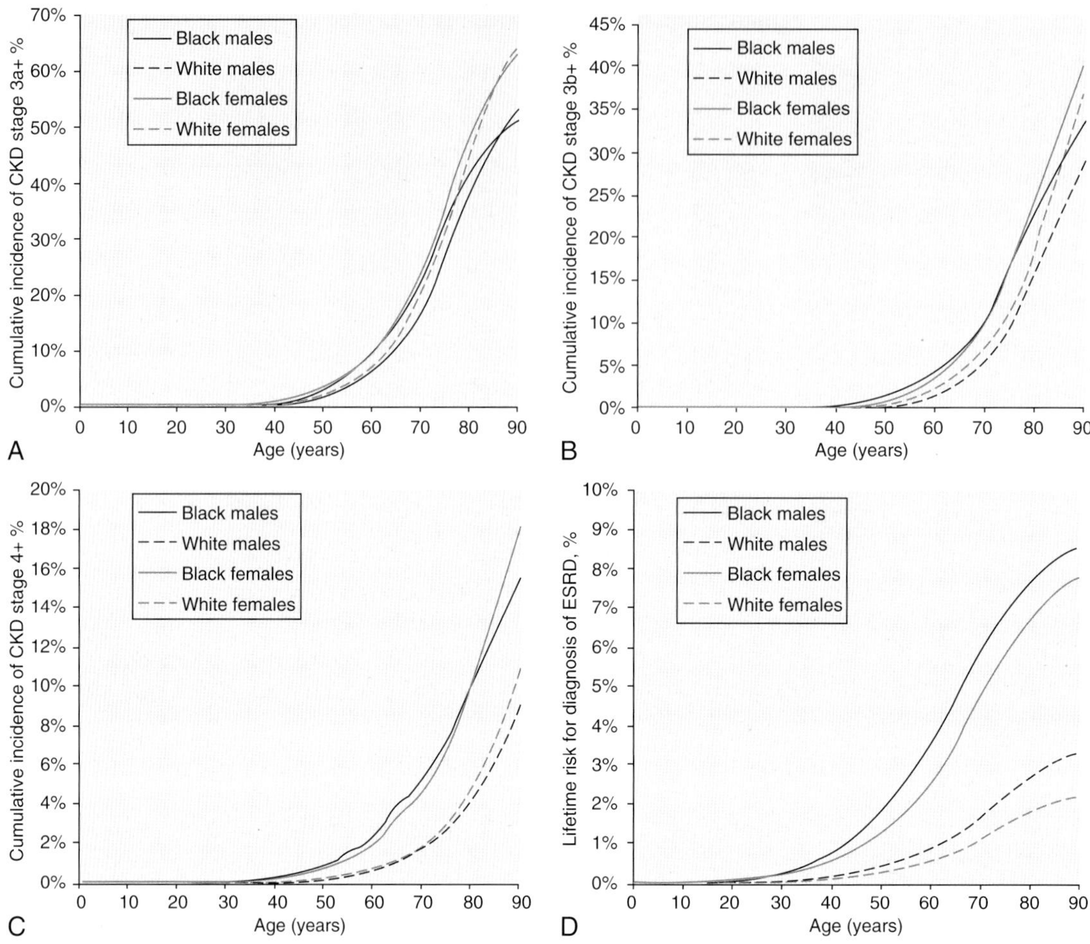


**Fig. 19.6** Cumulative incidence from birth by race and gender of chronic kidney disease *(CKD)* stage 3a (A), 3b (B), 4 (C), and end-stage renal disease *(ESKD;* D). (From Grams ME, Chow EK, Segev DL, et al. Lifetime incidence of CKD stages 3–5 in the United States. *Am J Kidney Dis.* 2013;62:245–252.)

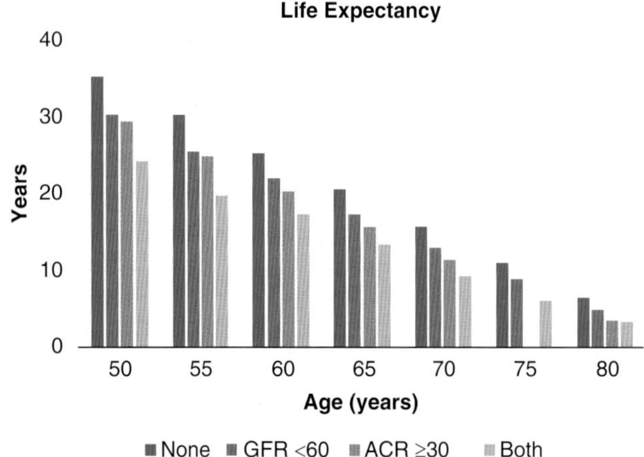


**Fig. 19.7** Life expectancy of NHANES participants with or without abnormalities in chronic kidney disease (CKD) measures, 1999–2011. GFR < 60 mL/min/1.73 m$^2$ or ACR ≥30 mg/g indicate CKD. ACR, urine albumin-to-creatinine ratio; GFR, estimated glomerular filtration rate; *NHANES,* National Health and Nutrition Examination Survey. (Adapted from U.S. Renal Data System. 2016 USRDS annual data report: epidemiology of kidney disease in the united states. https://www.ajkd.org/article/S0272-6386(16)30703-X/fulltext.)

increases with lower GFR and higher albuminuria are generally independent, with each parameter carrying risk, and higher risk with higher stages of disease (Fig. 19.8).[53,54] Risk relationships have been observed in low-risk as well as high-risk groups for ESKD and mortality.[55–58]

There is intense interest in defining earlier outcomes of CKD progression, with the goal of enhancing drug development and clinical prevention.[59–61] Provided that there are no acute effects on eGFR, decline in eGFR by 30% to 40% is now accepted by the U.S. Food and Drug Administration (FDA) as a surrogate outcome for CKD progression, previously assessed by doubling of the serum creatinine level (equivalent to a 57% decline in eGFR) or the development of ESKD.[8] Changes in albuminuria are also associated with ESKD and death,[62] and remission of the nephrotic syndrome is used as a surrogate endpoint in trials of some glomerular diseases.

Kidney measures are not the only risk factors for adverse outcomes, and there is a growing literature on the use of other factors to explain variations in the risk of progression to ESKD within stages of CKD.[63–65] For a given level of GFR or albuminuria, older adults are less likely to experience ESKD than their younger counterparts, possibly due to treatment preference (e.g., refusal of dialysis or transplantation as a therapy) or because of the competing event of death

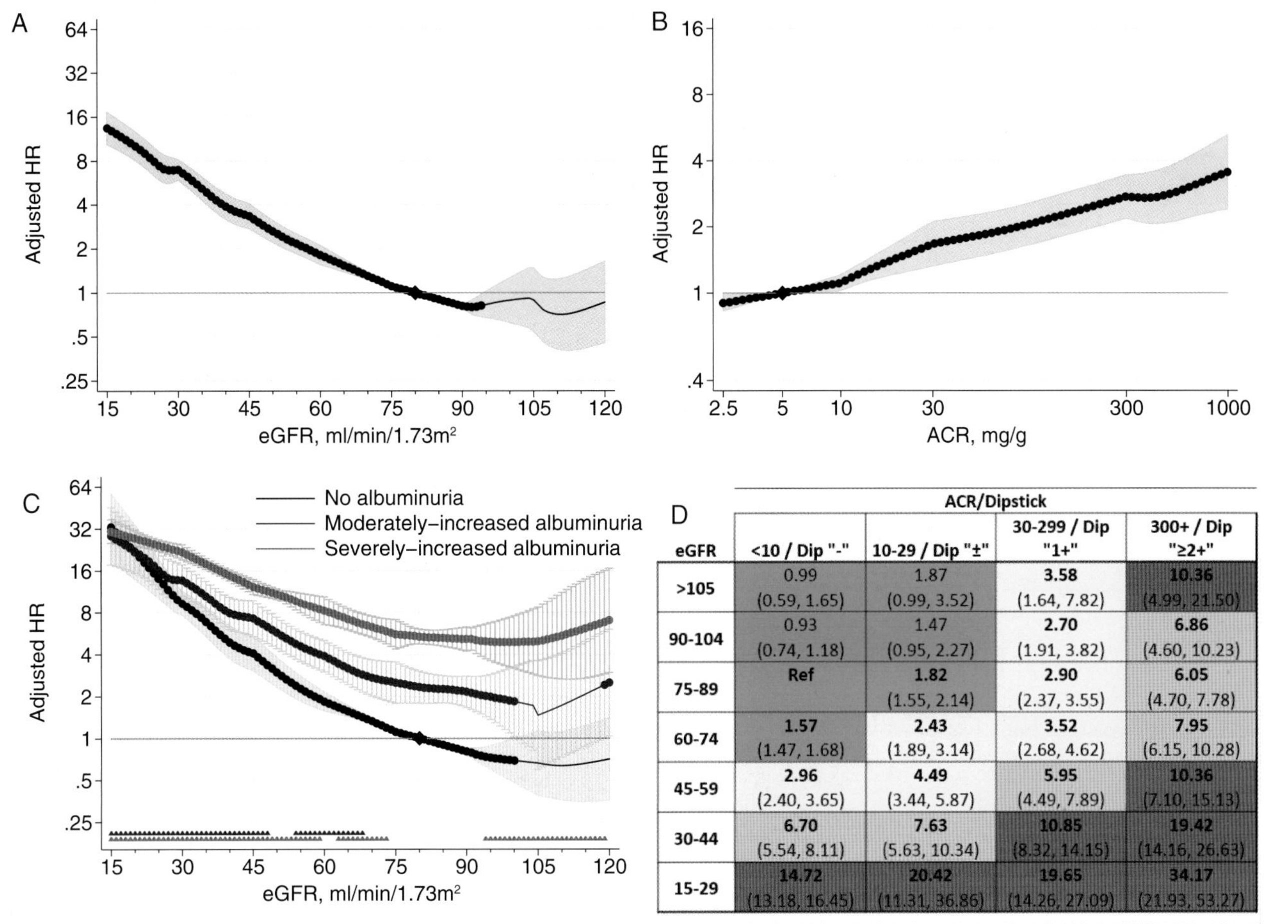


| eGFR | ACR/Dipstick <10 / Dip "-" | 10-29 / Dip "±" | 30-299 / Dip "1+" | 300+ / Dip "≥2+" |
|---|---|---|---|---|
| >105 | 0.99 (0.59, 1.65) | 1.87 (0.99, 3.52) | **3.58** (1.64, 7.82) | **10.36** (4.99, 21.50) |
| 90-104 | 0.93 (0.74, 1.18) | 1.47 (0.95, 2.27) | **2.70** (1.91, 3.82) | **6.86** (4.60, 10.23) |
| 75-89 | **Ref** | **1.82** (1.55, 2.14) | **2.90** (2.37, 3.55) | **6.05** (4.70, 7.78) |
| 60-74 | **1.57** (1.47, 1.68) | **2.43** (1.89, 3.14) | **3.52** (2.68, 4.62) | **7.95** (6.15, 10.28) |
| 45-59 | **2.96** (2.40, 3.65) | **4.49** (3.44, 5.87) | **5.95** (4.49, 7.89) | **10.36** (7.10, 15.13) |
| 30-44 | **6.70** (5.54, 8.11) | **7.63** (5.63, 10.34) | **10.85** (8.32, 14.15) | **19.42** (14.16, 26.63) |
| 15-29 | **14.72** (13.18, 16.45) | **20.42** (11.31, 36.86) | **19.65** (14.26, 27.09) | **34.17** (21.93, 53.27) |

**Fig. 19.8** Adjusted hazard ratios *(HRs)* of acute kidney injury in the general population cohorts by level of estimated glomerular filtration rate *(eGFR)* and albuminuria in continuous (A, B, C) and categoric (D) analysis. (C) *Thick lines* indicate statistical significance compared with the reference (*black diamond*) at eGFR of 80 mL/min/1.73 m$^2$ in the no-albuminuria group, defined as urine albumin-to-creatinine ratio *(ACR)* <30 mg/g or urine protein dipstick <1+. Stars along the *x*-axis represent significant pointwise directions: the relative risks associated with a particular category of albuminuria compared with the no-albuminuria category at that value of eGFR is significantly different than the corresponding relative risk seen at eGFR of 90 mL/min/1.73 m$^2$. A graph without stars would reflect parallel risk associations. HRs were derived from meta-analyses of the general population cohorts and are adjusted for gender, race, body mass index, systolic blood pressure, total cholesterol, history of cardiovascular disease, diabetes, and smoking status. The table represents adjusted HRs derived from categoric analyses of the general population cohorts, with *bold font* representing statistical significance and color coding by risk quartile. (From Grams ME, Sang Y, Ballew SH, et al. A meta-analysis of the association of estimated GFR, albuminuria, age, race, and sex with acute kidney injury. *Am J Kidney Dis.* 2015;66:591–601.)

(i.e., older adults with a given level of GFR or albuminuria are relatively more likely to die than progress to ESKD).[66] Moreover, the absolute risks of ESKD and death may vary based on indications for selection into a study population; research study populations often report higher risk of ESKD than death, whereas clinical population information drawn from medical records data often show a higher risk of death than ESKD.[67,68] Regional variation in the absolute risk of progression to ESKD has also been reported. A validated risk calculator designed to estimate the probability of ESKD in the subsequent 2 to 5 years among patients with CKD stages G3–G5 has incorporated a regional calibration factor to account for the fact that adjusted ESKD risk was higher in North America compared with other countries (Fig. 19.9).[64] Some of this risk differential may be due to the resources allotted to providing treatment rather than underlying characteristics of the countries themselves.[69]

A lower GFR has also been associated with concomitant bone, metabolic, endocrine, and hematologic abnormalities.[70] Well-known pathophysiologic mechanisms underlie the associations of hyperphosphatemia, hyperparathyroidism, metabolic acidosis, and anemia with a lower GFR.[71] The relationship between these abnormalities and albuminuria is less consistent, but the presence of albuminuria does appear to impart a higher risk of hyperparathyroidism and anemia over and above the GFR level.

## RISK FACTORS

Age is one of the strongest risk factors for the development of CKD. The prevalence of CKD stages G1–G5 has been reported as nearly 40% in those older than 70 years and over 50% in those 75 years and older in the United Kingdom.[72] Although some have dismissed age as a risk factor, suggesting

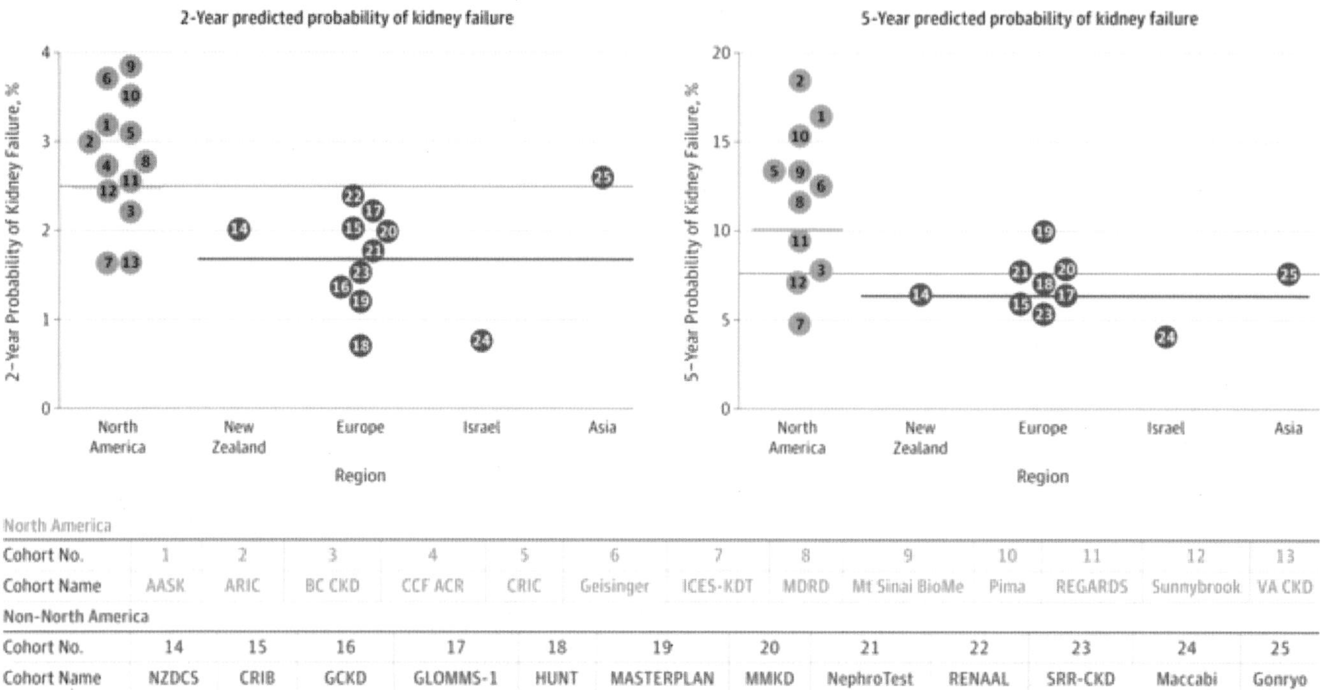


**Fig. 19.9** Refit baseline hazard of original four-variable equation at 2 and 5 years in individual cohorts stratified by region. Horizontal *gray line* represents the centered baseline hazard for the original four-variable kidney failure risk equation (age, 70 years; male, 56%; eGFR, 36 mL/min/1.73 m$^2$; urine albumin-to-creatinine ratio *(ACR)*, 170 mg/g); the *orange* and *blue horizontal lines* represent the weighted mean refit baseline hazard within each region (North America and non–North America). The 25 cohorts included represent studies with available ACR values. Studies with dipstick proteinuria were not included in the calculation. *AASK,* African American Study of Kidney Disease and Hypertension; *ARIC,* Atherosclerosis Risk in Communities; *BC CKD,* British Columbia Chronic Kidney Disease; *CCF,* Cleveland Clinic Foundation; *CRIB,* Chronic Renal Impairment in Birmingham; *CRIC,* Chronic Renal Insufficiency Cohort; eGFR, estimated glomerular filtration rate; GCKD, German CKD; GLOMMS, Grampian Laboratory Outcomes, Morbidity and Mortality Studies; *HUNT,* Nord Trøndelag Health Study; *ICES-KDT,* Institute for Clinical Evaluative Sciences, Provincial Kidney, Dialysis, and Transplantation; *MASTERPLAN,* Multifactorial Approach and Superior Treatment Efficacy in Renal Patients With the Aid of a Nurse Practitioner; *MDRD,* Modification of Diet in Renal Disease; *MMKD,* mild to moderate kidney disease; *NZDCS,* New Zealand Diabetes Cohort Study; *REGARDS,* Reasons for Geographic and Racial Differences in Stroke Study; *RENAAL,* Reduction of Endpoints in Non–insulin Dependent Diabetes Mellitus With the Angiotensin II Antagonist Losartan; *SRR-CKD,* Swedish Renal Registry CKD; *VA CKD,* Veterans Administration CKD. (From Tangri N, Grams ME, Levey AS, et al. Multinational assessment of accuracy of equations for predicting risk of kidney failure: a meta-analysis. *JAMA.* 2016;315:164–174.)

that nephron loss is a normal part of aging,[73,74] associations between a lower GFR and higher albuminuria and adverse outcomes, including both death and ESKD, persisted in all subgroups of age in an individual-level meta-analysis of 2 million participants from 46 cohort studies.[58] On the other hand, among people with stages G3–G5 CKD, older age is negatively associated with risk for ESKD, which may be due to the higher risk of mortality, both overall and attributable to CKD at an older age (Fig. 19.10).[63,64]

Gender is also a risk factor for CKD, although the relationships are a bit nuanced. Women are at a slightly higher risk for the development of CKD stage G3; however, later stages of CKD are more common in men, suggesting that men may be at higher risk for CKD progression.[43,75] The relationship between eGFR and albuminuria and adverse outcomes was examined by gender in an individual-level meta-analysis of 2 million participants. Men had a higher absolute risk of ESKD, death, and cardiovascular mortality at all levels of eGFR and albuminuria, but the relationship between eGFR and albuminuria and adverse outcomes was similar between the genders.[76]

Compared with Americans of primarily European ancestry, African Americans have a much higher risk of later-stage CKD and CKD progression. These racial differences are only partially explained by differences in socioeconomic or clinical risk factors.[77–80] Interestingly, some studies have suggested that the prevalence and incidence of earlier stages of CKD are similar by race, with only the later stages demonstrating a higher burden among African Americans.[81] For example, in a nationally representative cohort of adults older than 45 years, the prevalence of an eGFR of 50–59 mL/min/1.73 m$^2$ was 18.9% among black individuals and 31.1% among white individuals, and only at an eGFR < 30 mL/min/1.73 m$^2$ was there a higher prevalence among blacks compared with whites.[81]

Advances in explaining the racial disparities in CKD include the identification of *APOL1* high-risk alleles, a genetic variant that when present in two copies confers approximately a twofold higher risk of CKD progression and ESKD.[10,12,82,83] The gene variants provide resistance to infection with *Trypanosoma brucei rhodesiense,* a parasite endemic to Africa (Fig. 19.11).[84] The mechanism for increased kidney risk remains uncertain,[85] and *APOL1* high-risk status—present in about 12% of African Americans but less than 1% of whites in population-based studies in the US[86]—explains some but not all of the racial disparities in CKD. The presence of sickle

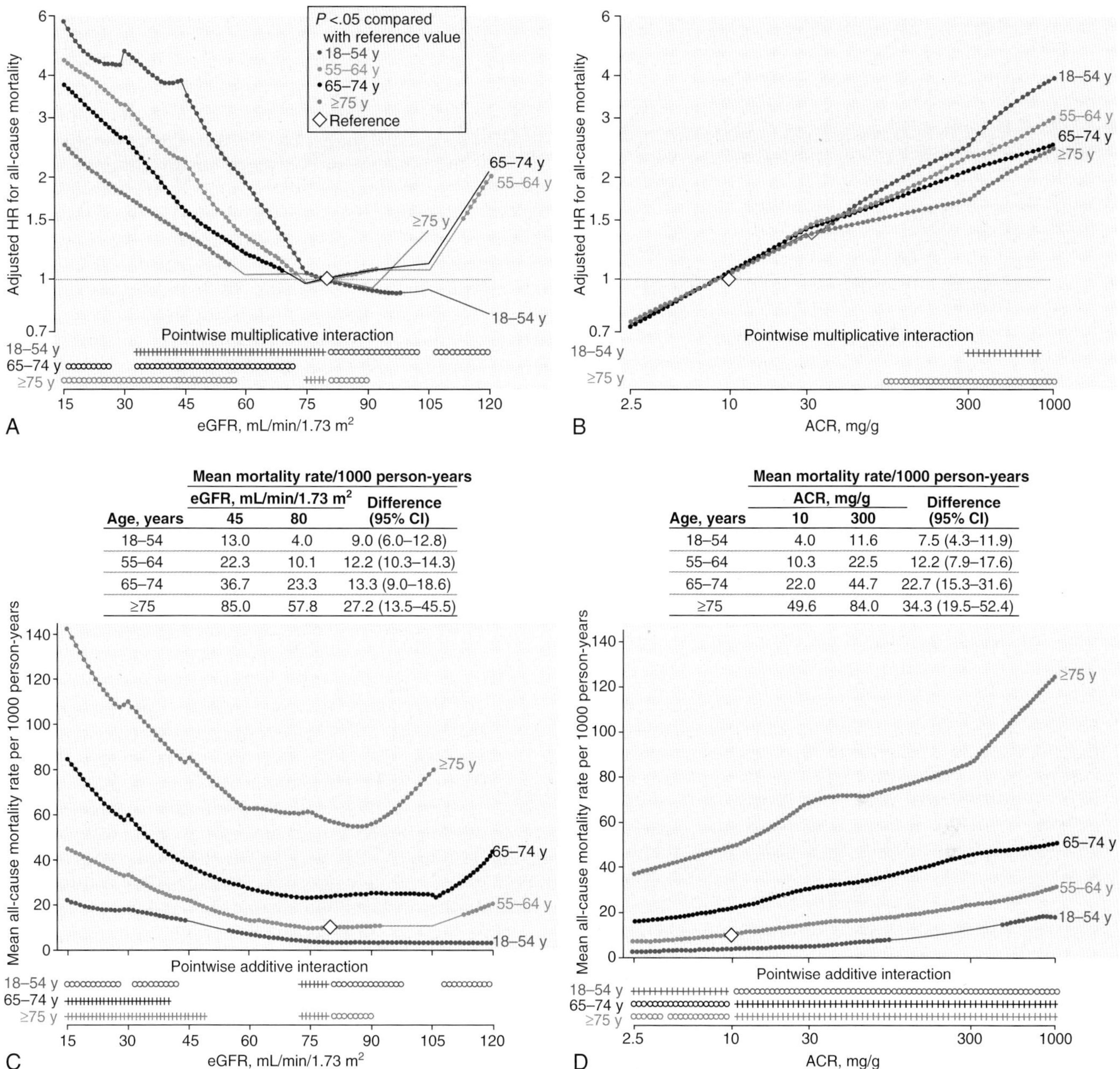


| Age, years | eGFR, mL/min/1.73 m² 45 | eGFR 80 | Difference (95% CI) |
|---|---|---|---|
| 18–54 | 13.0 | 4.0 | 9.0 (6.0–12.8) |
| 55–64 | 22.3 | 10.1 | 12.2 (10.3–14.3) |
| 65–74 | 36.7 | 23.3 | 13.3 (9.0–18.6) |
| ≥75 | 85.0 | 57.8 | 27.2 (13.5–45.5) |

Mean mortality rate/1000 person-years

| Age, years | ACR, mg/g 10 | ACR 300 | Difference (95% CI) |
|---|---|---|---|
| 18–54 | 4.0 | 11.6 | 7.5 (4.3–11.9) |
| 55–64 | 10.3 | 22.5 | 12.2 (7.9–17.6) |
| 65–74 | 22.0 | 44.7 | 22.7 (15.3–31.6) |
| ≥75 | 49.6 | 84.0 | 34.3 (19.5–52.4) |

Mean mortality rate/1000 person-years

**Fig. 19.10** Adjusted hazard ratios *(HRs)* for all-cause mortality and mean mortality rates according to estimated glomerular filtration rate *(eGFR)* and albumin-creatinine ratio *(ACR)* within each age category. *Solid circles* denote statistical significance ($P < .05$) compared with the reference *(diamond)* eGFR of 80 mL/min/1.73 m², or ACR of 10 mg/g within each age category in (A) and (B) and compared with the age category of 55 to 64 years in (C) and (D). *Plus signs* and *open circles* at the bottom of each graph represent significantly positive (greater effect size) and negative (smaller effect size) pointwise interactions ($P < .05$), respectively, compared with age 55 to 64 years. Gaps indicate no significant pointwise interaction. Models are meta-analyses of general population and high-risk cohorts adjusted for gender, race, body mass index, systolic blood pressure, total cholesterol, history of cardiovascular disease, diabetes, smoking status, and albuminuria (A and C) or eGFR (B and D). (From Hallan SI, Matsushita K, Sang Y, et al. Age and association of kidney measures with mortality and end-stage renal disease. *JAMA.* 2012;308:2349–2360.)

cell trait, present in 7% of African Americans but virtually absent in whites, also confers up to a twofold higher risk of ESKD, although less reliably across studies.[14,15] Both *APOL1* high-risk status and sickle cell trait are present in greater proportions in the ESKD population than in the general population.[87,88]

Other discovered genetic variants may also have effects on the development and progression of CKD, but they have generally had much smaller population prevalences or effect sizes than *APOL1* risk alleles and the sickle cell trait.[89–92] For example, genetic variation in *UMOD,* the gene coding for uromodulin, expressed in the thick ascending limb of the loop of Henle, may play a role in CKD. Uromodulin is the most commonly found protein in normal urine and likely affects renal salt handling.[93,94] Common variants in the promoter region of *UMOD* have been associated with increased risk of CKD, CKD progression, ESKD, and hypertension in genome-wide association studies, albeit with a difference in

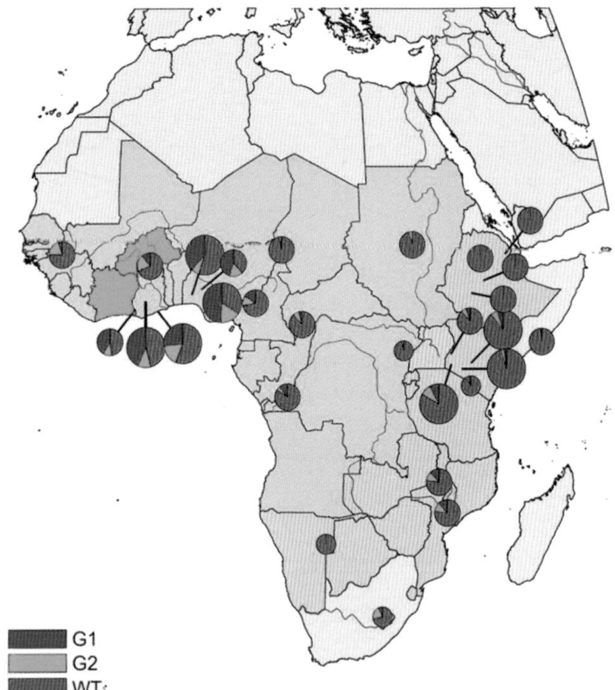


**Fig. 19.11** Distribution of the G1 and G2 *APOL1* variants across Africa. Allele frequencies of the G1 and G2 variants are indicated as *blue* and *green wedges*, respectively. Circle size reflects the number of individuals genotyped: small, <10 individuals/20 chromosomes; medium, 10–100 individuals/20–200 chromosomes; large, >100 individuals/200 chromosomes. Countries are shaded according to the subspecies of *Trypanosoma brucei* that cause African sleeping sickness. *Darker green,* gambiense types 1 and 2; *light green,* gambiense type 1; *pink,* both rhodesiense and gambiense type 1; *purple,* rhodesiense. (From Thomson R, Genovese G, Canon C, et al. Evolution of the primate trypanolytic factor APOL1. *Proc Natl Acad Sci U S A.* 2014;111:E2130–E2139.)

the rate of eGFR decline in the range of 0.15 mL/min/1.73 $m^2$ per year.[91,95–101] Genome-wide association studies have also identified genomic regions associated with more specific disease types, such as IgA nephropathy and idiopathic membranous nephropathy.[20,102] Many genetic variants underlying monogenic disease have also been determined, such as variants in *PKD1* or *PKD2* causing autosomal dominant polycystic kidney disease and more than 20 genes involved in syndromic and nonsyndromic CAKUT (a leading cause of kidney disease in children), but most of these genotypes are rare (<1 in 1000 for dominant diseases and <1 in 40,000 for recessive diseases).[22,103,104]

Among clinical risk factors, the presence of diabetes mellitus and hypertension appear to be the most robustly associated with CKD. The presence of diabetes mellitus was a risk factor for the development of CKD after full or partial nephrectomy[105] and also in several community-based studies.[106,107] Diabetes has also been linked to the development of kidney failure,[108] and diabetes is considered the most common cause of ESKD in the world today.[24] Evidence that tight glycemic control helps forestall the development of mild to moderate albuminuria in clinical trials further advances the notion that the presence of diabetes mellitus is on the causal pathway for the development and progression of many types of CKD.[109] Interestingly, among people with CKD, diabetes is a weaker risk factor for ESKD once the GFR and albuminuria are accounted for.[64]

In contrast to the well-accepted role of diabetes in the development of CKD, there is ongoing debate as to whether hypertension is a cause or merely a consequence of CKD. Many observational studies have linked higher blood pressure to the development and progression of CKD,[39,108,110] but evidence from randomized controlled trials that lowering blood pressure helps forestall CKD progression is inconsistent.[111–113] The MDRD study ($N$ = 840) showed no benefit of the lower blood pressure goal on GFR decline during the trial period (mean, 2.2 years) but a beneficial effect on ESKD during longer follow-up. The African American Study of Kidney Disease and Hypertension ($N$= 1094) showed no benefit of the lower blood pressure goal on GFR decline over a mean of 4 years or on ESKD during longer follow-up.[111] However, both these studies suggested a larger benefit of the lower blood pressure goal in patients with higher proteinuria.[114,115] The REIN-2 trial did not show a difference in progression to ESKD with a lower blood pressure goal, but this study achieved the lower blood pressure goal using a calcium channel blocker, which increases proteinuria, which may have blunted any beneficial effect.[99] In PKD, the HALT-PKD study showed a beneficial effect of a lower blood pressure goal on enlargement in total kidney volume but not on eGFR decline.[116] In SPRINT, a lower blood pressure goal appeared to result in a lower eGFR over the first 18 months, but eGFR trajectories remained relatively stable after that time, with a large beneficial effect of lower blood pressure on death and CVD, despite the higher risk of incident CKD.[117]

Another increasingly prevalent risk factor for CKD is obesity.[32] In a study of 320,252 participants in a U.S. health plan, obesity was associated with more than a threefold risk of developing ESKD over a mean of 26 years of follow-up. Contemporary studies with shorter follow-up have shown slightly more modest risks of CKD stages G4–G5 associated with obesity, such as one in the United Kingdom, which estimated a twofold risk associated with body mass index (BMI) between 30 and 35 kg/$m^2$.[118] Similarly, a meta-analysis of ESKD risk among over 4 million potential kidney donor candidates showed a 1.16 times higher risk per 5 kg/$m^2$ higher BMI over 30 kg/$m^2$.[119] The risk of CKD progression associated with obesity may be smaller still; in one cohort of Swedish people with CKD stages G4–G5, BMI was unrelated to subsequent ESKD. On the other hand, weight loss achieved by lifestyle modification or bariatric surgery has been associated with a reduction in albuminuria and preservation of eGFR.[120–122] For example, in Look AHEAD, a clinical trial in 5145 participants with diabetes, an intensive lifestyle intervention resulted in 4 kg of weight loss compared with the control arm and a 31% reduction in the development of CKD in very high-risk categories, as defined by KDIGO. Obesity may contribute to CKD as a risk factor mediated by the development of diabetes and hypertension or with independent causal effects. In animal models, obesity results in glomerular hypertension and hyperfiltration, a proinflammatory milieu, and reduced adiponectin levels, all of which may contribute to CKD risk.[123]

There have been localized epidemics of kidney disease, such as Balkan nephropathy, those due to Chinese herbal supplements (now attributed to aristolochic acid[124]), and the more recent Mesoamerican nephropathy,[125] which point to environmental factors that may additionally alter the risk of ESKD in populations.

# END-STAGE KIDNEY DISEASE

## EPIDEMIOLOGY

In the United States, data regarding ESKD are generally excellent due to the establishment of comprehensive and well-maintained kidney disease registries by the National Institutes of Health in 1989.[126] Today, the Annual Data Reports of the U.S. Renal Data System (USRDS) and the Scientific Registry of Transplant Recipients (SRTR) provide extensive epidemiologic information on incident and prevalent ESKD based on required reporting by providers of dialysis and transplantation services. As such, the epidemiology of ESKD reflects the clinical practice of initiation of KRT as well as the progression of CKD to kidney failure. Information on untreated kidney failure—GFR < 15 mL/min/1.73 m$^2$ not treated by KRT—is not captured by the USRDS or SRTR. Some data sources have suggested that untreated kidney failure could represent a substantial number of kidney failure cases, particularly among the very old.[47,66] Causes of kidney disease among those with ESKD are ascertained from the Centers for Medicare & Medicaid Services Form 2728, but are frequently missing and have not been validated.[127] Because dialysis is the predominant mode of KRT, the epidemiology of ESKD largely reflects the epidemiology of dialysis. Specific topics related to the epidemiology of kidney transplantation are covered in a separate section.

## PREVALENCE

As of December 31, 2014, there were 678,383 prevalent cases of ESKD in the United States, or a rate of 2067/million population.[24] Both figures increased over the preceding year (3.5% and 2.6%, respectively). For reference, in 1996, the number of cases of ESKD was 303,311, or 1095 cases/million population (Fig. 19.12). Much of the growth in prevalence was attributable to the aging of the population (ESKD is more common in older populations) and growth in ESKD in those aged 75 years and older, in whom the sex- and race-adjusted prevalence of ESKD increased from 2989/million population in 1996 to 6243/million population in 2014. The growth in prevalence is also partly due to a decline in mortality, which decreased from 186/1000 patient-years to 137 deaths/1000 patient-years over the corresponding time period.

In the United States, approximately 70% of prevalent ESKD cases were treated by dialysis, either hemodialysis (63.1%) or peritoneal dialysis (6.9%). Most ESKD cases were attributed to diabetes or hypertension (37.8% and 25.3% of the age-, gender-, and race-adjusted prevalence, respectively), followed by glomerulonephritis (16.4%) and cystic kidney disease (3.8%).

In 2014, the USRDS collected ESKD data from 60 different countries, enabling comparisons of both the absolute counts of ESKD cases as well as the prevalence per million population. In total, there were 2,217,350 patients with ESKD counted globally. Patients in the United States accounted for 30% of the total, followed by Japan (14%) and Brazil (7%). The prevalence of ESKD within the population varied substantially across the participating country, ranging from 113/million population in Bangladesh to 3219 cases/million population in Taiwan. Japan had the second highest prevalence, 2505/million population. All countries providing annual data since 2001 ($N = 32$) showed increases in prevalence (median, 48%). The increase was greatest in the Philippines and Thailand, where the percentage changes from 2001 to 2014 were 1092% and 902%, respectively.

Large variations also existed among countries with respect to the distribution of KRT modality (Fig. 19.13). In Norway, 72% of prevalent ESKD patients are treated with a functioning

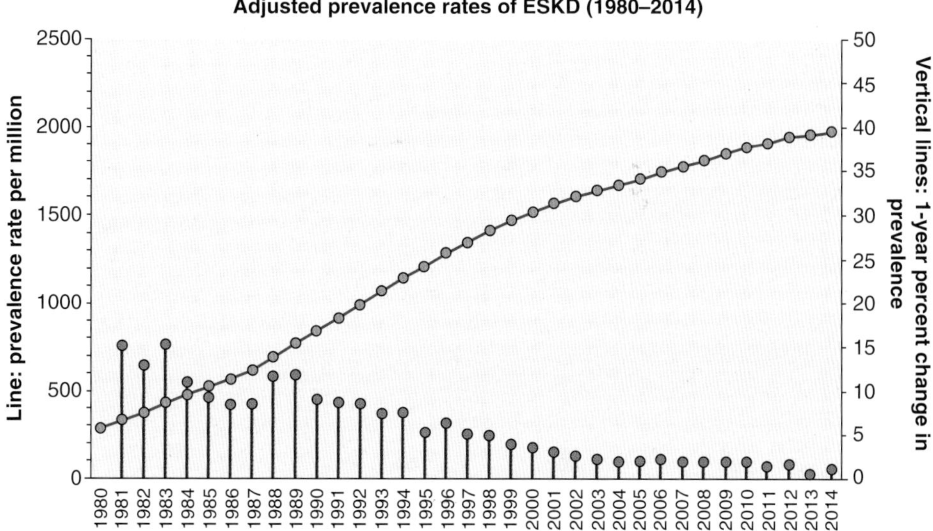


**Fig. 19.12** Trends in adjusted* ESKD prevalence (per million; trend lines; scale on left), and annual percentage (%) change in adjusted* prevalence of ESKD (*vertical lines;* scale on right) in the U.S. population, 1980–2014, adjusted for age, gender, race, and ethnicity. The standard population was the U.S. population in 2011. (Data from U.S. Renal Data System. 2014 USRDS annual data report: epidemiology of kidney disease in the United States. https://www.ajkd.org/article/S0272-6386(15)00744-1/fulltext; and U.S. Renal Data System. 2016 USRDS annual data report: epidemiology of kidney disease in the United States. https://www.ajkd.org/article/S0272-6386(16)30703-X/fulltext.)

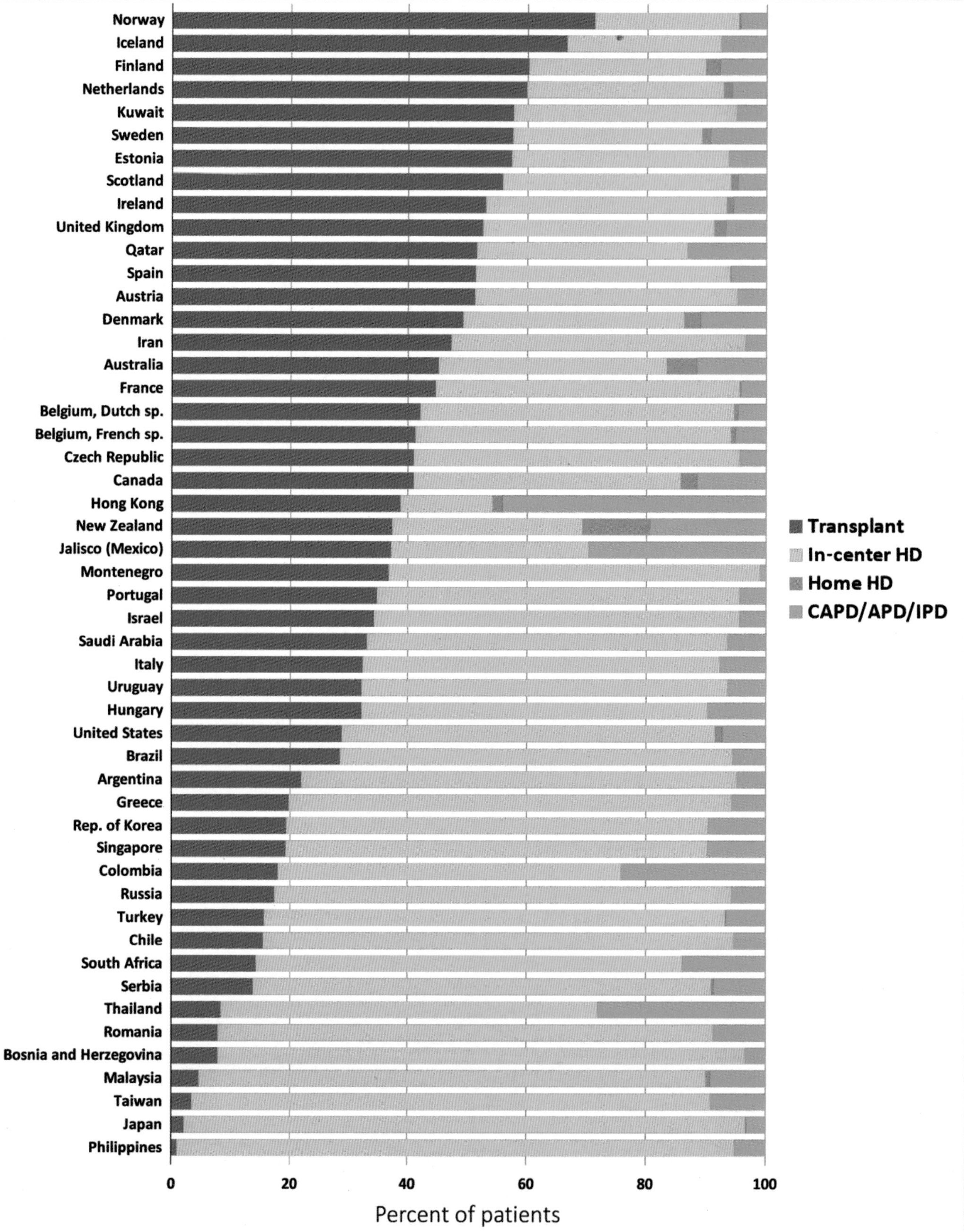


**Fig. 19.13** Percentage distribution of type of kidney replacement therapy modality used by patients with end-stage kidney disease. By country, in 2014. (From U.S. Renal Data System. 2016 USRDS annual data report: epidemiology of kidney disease in the United States. https://www.ajkd.org/article/S0272-6386(16)30703-X/fulltext.)

transplant, 24% receive in-center hemodialysis, and 4% receive peritoneal dialysis. Peritoneal dialysis is most common in Mexico, where 44% receive peritoneal dialysis, 39% have a functioning transplant, and 17% receive in-center or home hemodialysis. In contrast, in-center hemodialysis consitutes 94% of ESKD in both Japan and the Philippines. Additional information on differences in hemodialysis practice by country was collected by the Dialysis Outcomes and Practice Patterns Study (DOPPS) between June 1996 and March 2012.[128] Interestingly, in the population of 35,964 hemodialysis patients sampled from 12 countries, the proportion of women was much lower than that of the general population. This appeared attributable to a greater incidence of ESKD among men rather than better survival, because the male-to-female mortality ratio was close to 1.

There is evidence to suggest that the variation in ESKD prevalence has much to do with the resources available to provide KRT. A recent study has suggested that the gap between people worldwide who require KRT and those who undergo KRT was at least 2.3 million in 2010.[69] The authors estimated the prevalence of ESKD undergoing KRT to be 1839 cases/million people in North America, followed by 719 cases/million people in Europe, 686 cases/million in Oceania, and 626 cases/million in Latin America. Asia, which was reported to have an ESKD prevalence of 232 cases/million population, was estimated to have the highest absolute number of people with ESKD, at nearly 1 million cases in 2010. Gross national product was highly associated with prevalence, with the highest-income countries reporting a much higher prevalence of patients undergoing KRT. Interestingly, this relationship was much stronger than the relationship between the prevalence of diabetes and the prevalence of patients undergoing KRT (Fig. 19.14).

## INCIDENCE

The incidence, or rate of new cases, of ESKD is also reported annually by the USRDS.[24] In the United States, the number of incident cases of ESKD in 2014 was 120,688, or an incidence rate of 370/million per year. These figures are 2.2% and 1.1% increases, respectively, over the prior year. In 1996, the number of incident cases of ESKD was 77,018, or 278 cases/million population. Much of this increase in incidence rates can be attributed to the aging of the U.S. population and the increase in incidence of ESKD among those older than 75 years, for whom the race- and gender-adjusted incidence rate increased from 1203 cases/million population in 1996 to 1556 cases/million population in 2014.

Most of the new ESKD cases initiated KRT using hemodialysis (87.9%), whereas 9.3% used peritoneal dialysis and 2.6% received a kidney transplant without prior dialysis. These proportions have remained relatively stable over the past decade. The adjusted incidences of ESKD due to diabetes, hypertension, and cystic disease have remained relatively consistent with respect to each other; the adjusted incidence of glomerulonephritis declined slightly. The adjusted incidence rate ratios for blacks versus whites in 2014 was 3.1; for Native Americans and Asians, the ratio versus whites was 1.2.

When extended to estimate the lifetime incidence of ESKD, racial and ethnic disparities remain.[43,129,130] One study using 2013 USRDS data has suggested that the lifetime incidence of ESKD is 3.1% for a non-Hispanic white man, 6.2% for a Hispanic man, and 8.0% for a non-Hispanic black man.[129] Furthermore, these disparities changed very little over the previous decade.

When compared with other countries, the incidence of ESKD in the United States was among the highest, trailing only Taiwan and the Jalisco region of Mexico in 2014 (Fig. 19.15).[24] Other high-ESKD incidence countries included Thailand, Singapore, Japan, Korea, and Malaysia. Among the countries represented, the lowest incidence rate/million population per year was in Bangladesh, with 49 ESKD cases/million per year; Iceland, with 58 cases/million per year; and Russia, with 60 cases/million per year. Trends in the incidence of ESKD varied by country, with many of the Northern European countries experiencing a lower ESKD incidence over time. In contrast, there were large increases in incidence rates in many of the developing countries (Fig. 19.16).

Interestingly, the proportion of new cases attributed to diabetes also varied by country. In Asia, Latin America, and the United States, most countries reported over 40% of the new cases as attributable to diabetes. In contrast, many of the European countries reported only 20% of the new cases as being attributed to diabetes (Fig. 19.17). In addition, in all countries, there was a disparity in new ESKD by gender. Men had higher rates of new ESKD than women, sometimes even twofold higher.

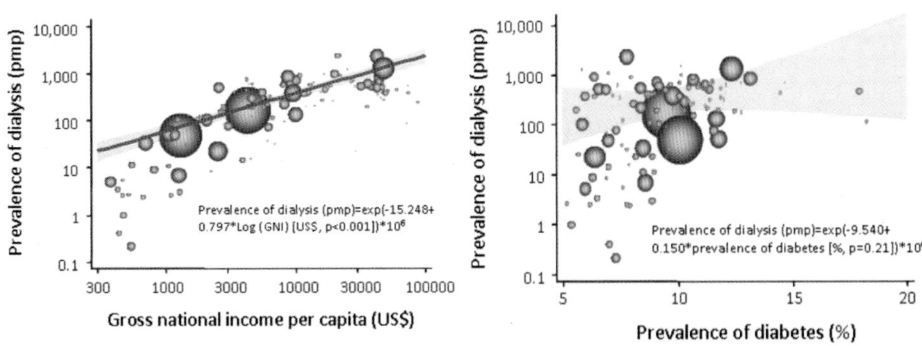


**Fig. 19.14** Association between prevalence of end-stage kidney disease (ESKD) treated by dialysis in 123 countries and (gross national income per capita [left], prevalence of diabetes [right]). In both graphs, China and India are represented by the largest and second largest circles, respectively. (From Liyanage T, Ninomiya T, Jha V, et al. Worldwide access to treatment for end-stage kidney disease: a systematic review. *Lancet.* 2015;385[9981]:1975–1982.)

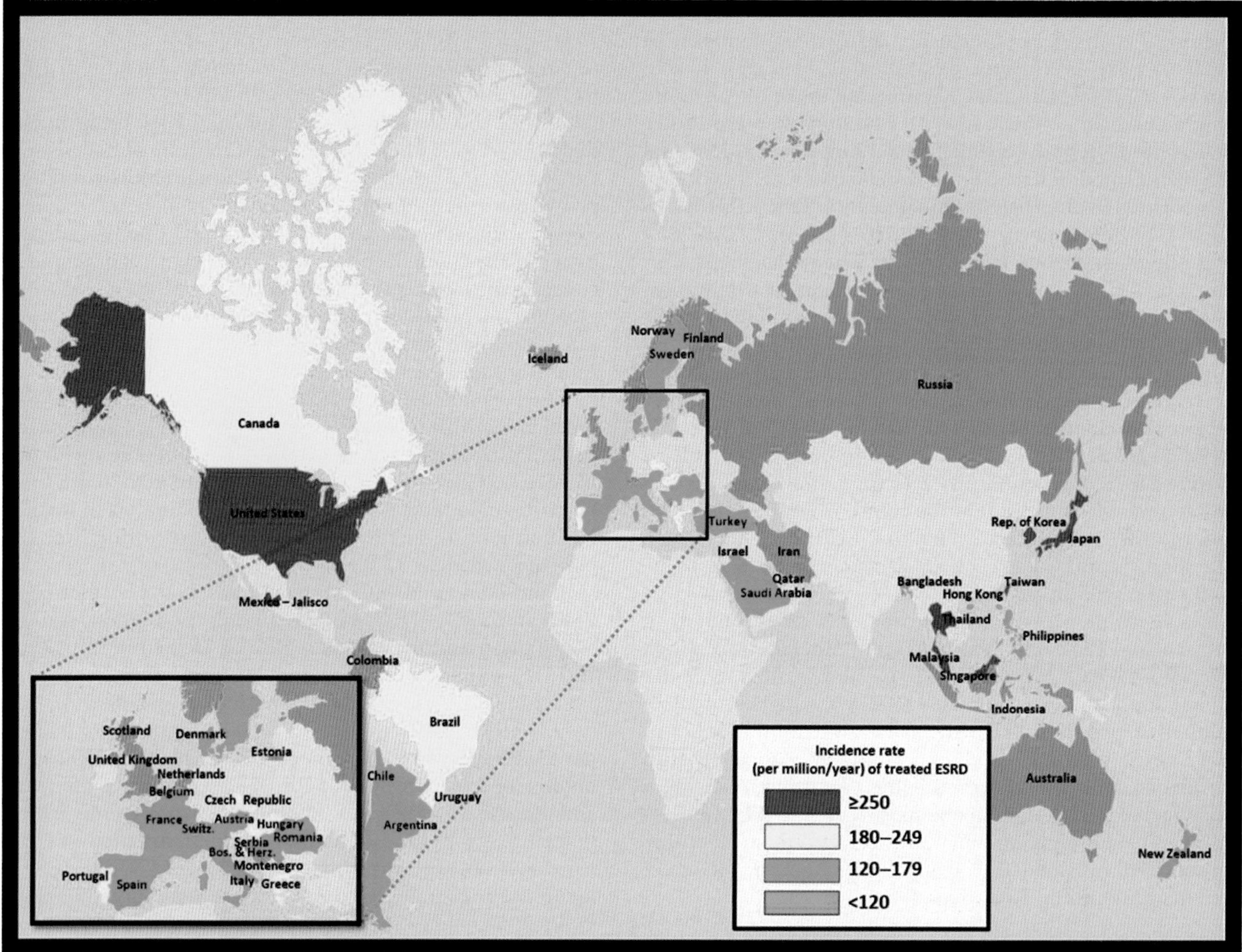


**Fig. 19.15** Geographic variations in the incidence rate of treated end-stage kidney disease (*ESKD;* per million population/year), by country, 2014. (From U.S. Renal Data System. 2016 USRDS annual data report: epidemiology of kidney disease in the United States. https://www.ajkd.org/article/S0272-6386(16)30703-X/fulltext.)

## OUTCOMES

Age-adjusted mortality in ESKD is much higher than in the general population.[24,131,132] In 2014, the USRDS reported that the adjusted mortality rate for ESKD was 136 deaths/1000 patient years. For patients receiving hemodialysis, adjusted mortality rates were 169 deaths/1000 patient-years; for peritoneal dialysis, the rate was 157 deaths/1000 patient-years. In the year after dialysis initiation, the risk of death peaked at 2 months for patients receiving hemodialysis and increased slowly over the year for patients receiving peritoneal dialysis. Approximately 41% of all deaths among dialysis patients in 2012 were attributed to CVD.

Mortality rates in incident dialysis patients vary by age and underlying comorbid conditions. Early mortality is more common among people with lower serum albumin and phosphorus levels, as well as those with congestive heart failure and cancer.[133] Although racial differences in dialysis mortality have been noted, particularly in older age groups, they may be due in part to differences in the rate of transplantation, the level of residual kidney function at dialysis initiation, and the presence and severity of comorbid conditions.[134]

Mortality rates in incident dialysis patients also vary by country. In patients selected for the DOPPS, the mortality rate ranged from 17 deaths/100 patient-years in the first 120 days in Japan to 33.5 deaths/100 patient-years in the first 120 days in Belgium.[131] Long-term mortality was even more disparate: after the first year on dialysis, there were 5.2 deaths/100 patient-years in Japan compared with 19.9 deaths/100 patient-years in Belgium. It should be noted that the proportion of patients 75 years of age and older was smaller in Japan; however, adjusted mortality rates were also lower in Japan than in any other included countries. In general, European and North American long-term mortality rates were fairly similar, with the United States reporting the highest adjusted mortality rates (Fig. 19.18).

It should also be noted that mortality on dialysis is sometimes related to withdrawal of therapy. In Australia and New Zealand, nearly 40% of deaths within the first 120 days were coded as being due to withdrawal from care, compared

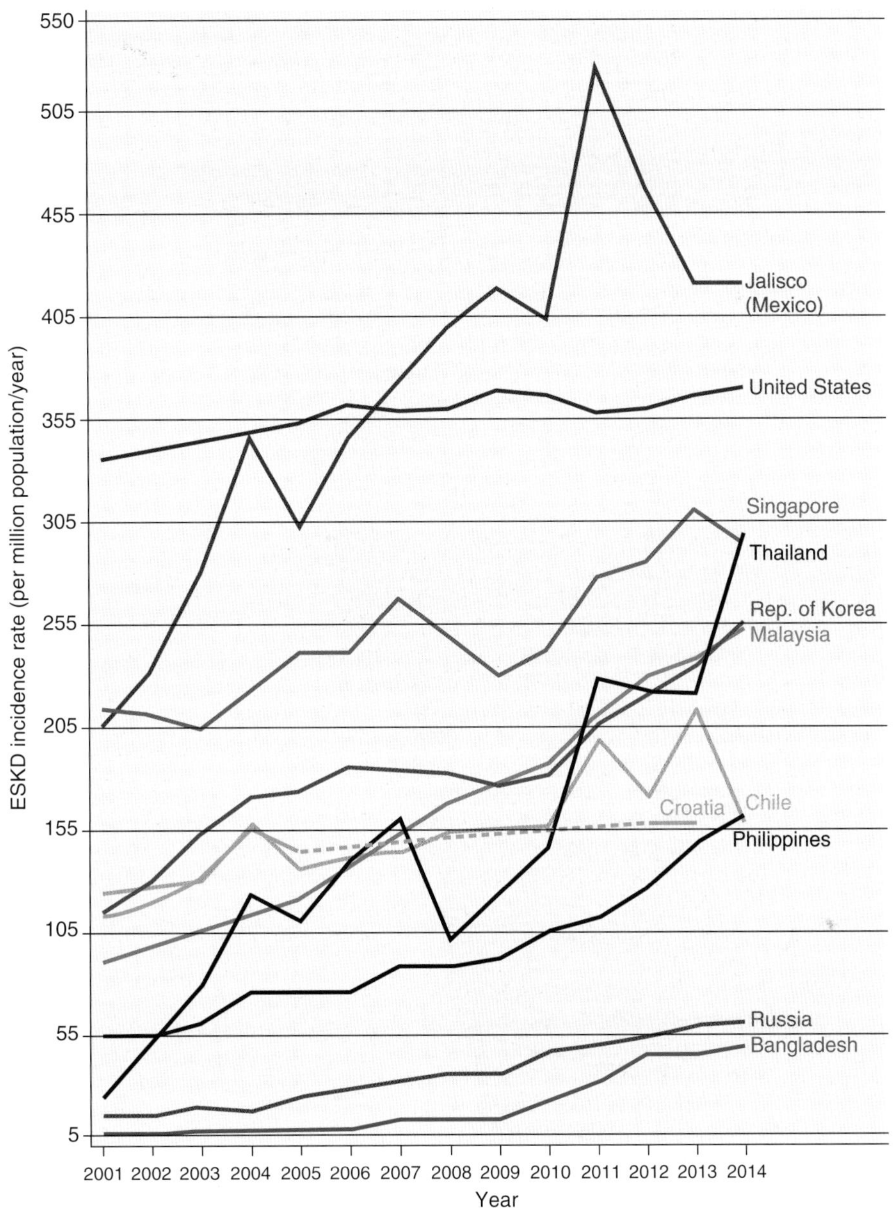


**Fig. 19.16** Trends in the incidence rate of treated end-stage kidney disease (*ESKD;* per million population/year), by country, 2001– 2014. The 10 countries with the highest percentage rise in ESKD incidence rate in 2001–2002 versus that in 2013–2014, plus the United States. (From U.S. Renal Data System. 2016 USRDS Annual data report: epidemiology of kidney disease in the United States. https://www.ajkd.org/article/S0272-6386(16)30703-X/fulltext.)

with much lower rates in regions such as Italy, France, and Germany.[131]

Trends in mortality have suggested that dialysis patients in the United States are living longer compared with previous decades, with the overall mortality rate decreasing by 32% since 1996. Although there have been numerous improvements in dialysis treatment, their relative contribution to the trend toward lower mortality is uncertain. With the exception of antihypertensive treatment, controlled trials evaluating single interventions have not shown an effect on all-cause mortality in dialysis patients.[135–143] In our view, this may be due in part to the difficulty of showing a reduction in all-cause mortality with interventions targeting a single risk factor. The adoption of multiple interventions in practice may achieve this goal.

## RISK FACTORS

Risk factors for the development of ESKD demonstrate some notable differences from those that portend a higher risk of incidence of earlier stages of CKD. Most notably, age has often demonstrated an inverse association with ESKD risk, adjusted for other factors.[65,144,145] Given the strong association between older age and incidence of CKD, the reverse association is somewhat surprising. Possible explanations are that the competing event of mortality becomes much more common in

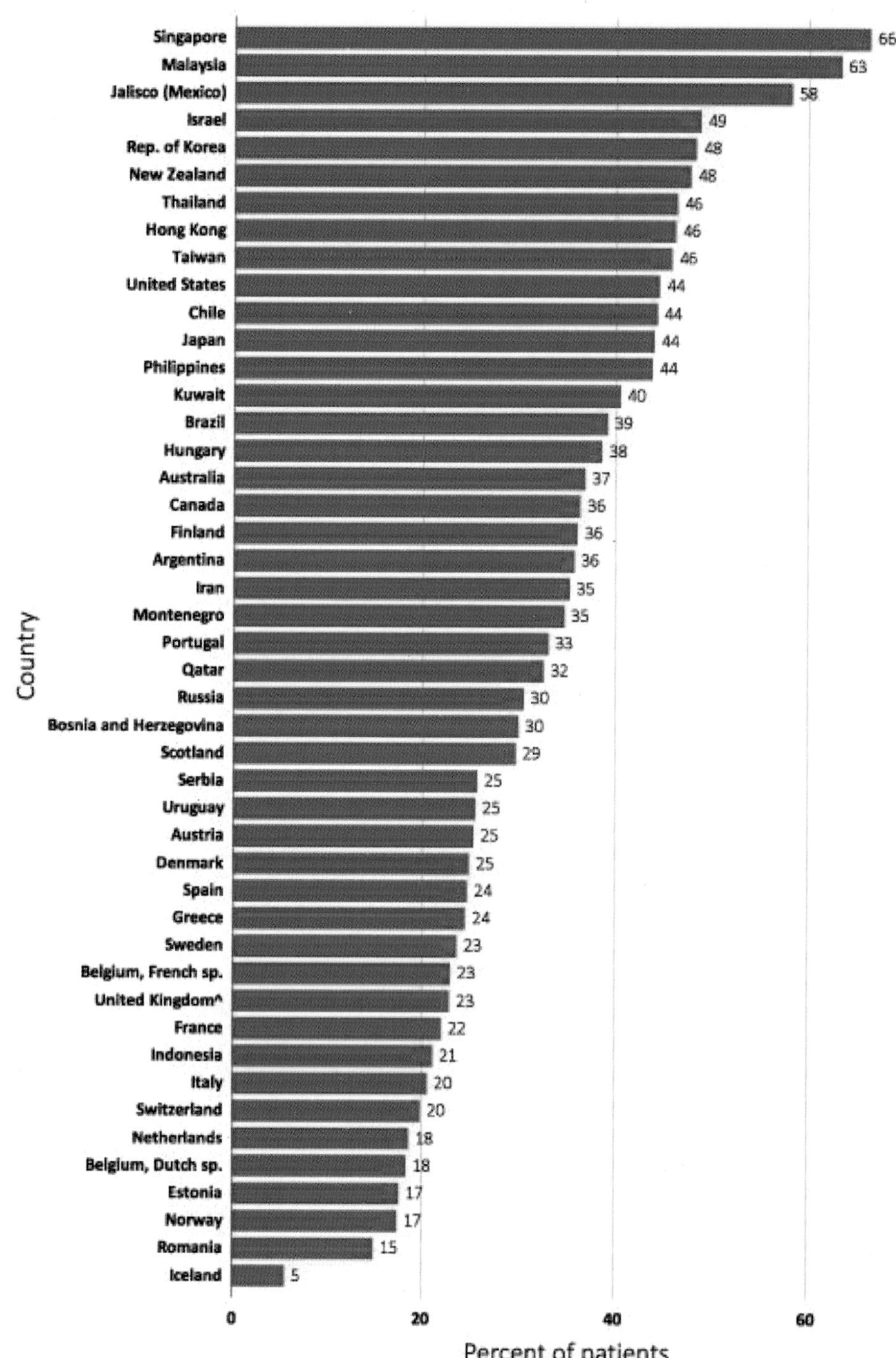


**Fig. 19.17** Proportions of incident end-stage kidney disease (ESKD) due to diabetes, by country, 2014. (From U.S. Renal Data System. 2016 USRDS annual data report: epidemiology of kidney disease in the United States. https://www.ajkd.org/article/S0272-6386(16)30703-X/fulltext.)

older adults, and many older adults may choose not to initiate dialysis. Indeed, in Canada, people who were 85 years or older with an eGFR from 15 to 29 mL/min/1.73 $m^2$ experienced 20 cases of untreated kidney failure/1000 patient-years and 1.5 cases/1000 patient-years of treated kidney failure (i.e., undergoing dialysis or transplantation).[66] In contrast, for people ages 18 to 44 years with a similar eGFR, the rates were 3.5 cases/1000 person-years and 17 cases/1000 person-years of untreated and treated kidney failure, respectively. Similar observations have been demonstrated in the United States.[47] Finally, it is possible that eGFR decline is slower among older compared with younger individuals.[146]

Gender and race are additional risk factors that display somewhat disparate associations with the incidence of earlier stages of CKD compared with ESKD. For example, although women may be at a slightly higher risk for eGFR < 60 mL/min/1.73 $m^2$,[147] men make up a greater proportion of incident and prevalent ESKD patients.[24] The higher risk of ESKD among men persists, even after adjusting for demographic and clinical factors. Reasons for ESKD differences by gender may

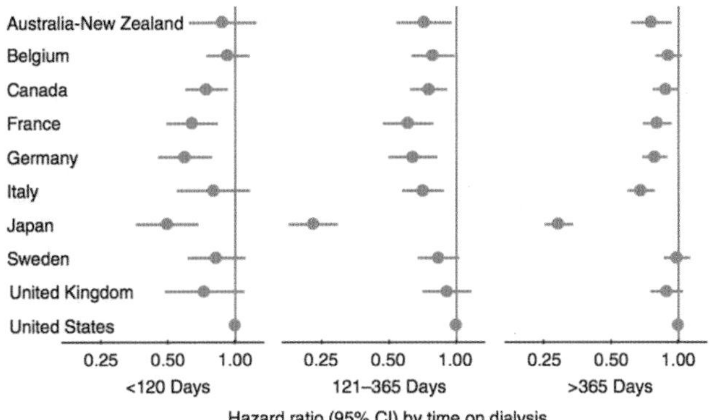


**Fig. 19.18** Mortality in each DOPPS (Dialysis Outcomes and Practice Patterns Study) country versus the United States by time on hemodialysis (HD). Model adjusted for age, gender, race, and diabetes as the cause of end-stage kidney disease, stratified by study phase (*N* = 86,886 HD patients from DOPPS census [2002–2008]). *CI*, Confidence interval. (From Robinson BM, Zhang J, Morgenstern H, et al. Worldwide, mortality risk is high soon after initiation of hemodialysis. *Kidney Int.* 2014;85:158–165.)

stem from hormonal differences[148] or simply from differences in care delivery and preference. For example, women tend to start dialysis at a lower eGFR than men.[149] In contrast, despite later initiation of dialysis among African Americans, African Americans have nearly a fourfold higher ESKD risk than Caucasians.[24,43,149] These disparities persist after adjustment for socioeconomic status, clinical characteristics, and access to health care.[77,150,151] The age- and gender-adjusted incidence of ESKD among African Americans was 876.7 cases/million per year in 2014, compared with 357.3 cases/million among Asians, 331.1 cases/million among Native Americans, and 286.3/million among U.S. whites.

As discussed previously, diabetes mellitus is considered to be the major cause of ESKD worldwide, in part due its growing incidence and prevalence.[24,152] In Singapore, 66% of incident ESKD cases in 2014 were attributed to diabetes; the corresponding figure in the United States was 46%. In a USRDS survey of 46 world regions, only 6 reported that less than 20% of ESKD cases were due to diabetes (the Netherlands, Dutch-speaking Belgium, Estonia, Norway, Romania, and Iceland).[24] Furthermore, diabetes mellitus can be considered as a risk factor for both CKD incidence and disease progression. Diabetic CKD is frequently characterized by the presence of albuminuria, which is also a risk factor for CKD progression to ESKD.[63,64] The second most common listed cause for ESKD in the United States is hypertension, although it is believed that many of the cases ascribed to hypertension may be due to other factors, such as *APOL1* risk alleles or parenchymal disease.[153] Obesity has also variably been associated with increased ESKD risk, with older studies with longer follow-up demonstrating stronger associations than more contemporary studies.[119,154]

Geographic region accounts for some of the differences in ESKD risk as well. In a validation of a kidney failure risk equation calculator in 31 international cohorts, only the region of cohort was observed to improve calibration for a model that included age, gender, eGFR, and albuminuria.[63] Therefore, a regional calibration factor was introduced that incorporated a lower baseline risk by 32.9% at 2 years and 16.5% at 5 years for countries outside North America (see kidneyfailurerisk.com). The use of a calibration factor for geographical region is consistent with a recent systematic review, which reported differences in ESKD prevalence by region. In that study North America had the highest prevalence, at 1839 cases/million people, followed by Europe, at 719 cases/million people.[69] These differences appeared driven in large part by income of the country, with an estimated 74-fold difference in prevalence between high-income and low-income countries.

## KIDNEY TRANSPLANTATION

### PREVALENCE

In the United States, approximately 30% of prevalent ESKD cases have a functioning kidney transplant, corresponding to 200,907 people in 2014.[24] The number of prevalent cases has more than doubled over the past 2 decades, from 83,199 in 1996. The prevalence is currently one of the highest in the world, at 630 people with a functioning kidney transplant/million population in the United States, but other countries such as Norway (657 cases/million) and Portugal (642 cases/million) also have a high prevalence. In general, the prevalence of those with functioning kidney transplants is highest in North America and Europe and lowest in South America and parts of Asia. Prevalence in all assessed countries has increased over the past decade. As a proportion of prevalent ESKD cases, patients living with a functioning transplant was fairly stable in most countries. The highest proportions were generally found in Northern Europe, where more than 50% of ESKD patients were living with a functional kidney transplant.

### INCIDENCE

In the United States, there are approximately 18,000 transplantations/year, a number that has remained relatively stable over the past decade, despite a growing prevalence of patients with ESKD (Fig. 19.19).[24] In 2014, the proportion of transplanted organs that originated from a deceased donor was 69%, a figure that has increased slightly over the years, with a concomitant decline in living donor transplants.[155] Approximately 30% of living donor transplant procedures were performed prior to the initiation of dialysis.[156] The median waiting time for transplantation was 3.4 years in 2009 for both living and deceased donor transplants combined. Waiting time was significantly different by blood type, panel-reactive antibodies (PRA), and region. Using 2014 data, kidney transplantation rates/1000 dialysis patient-years also varied—highest among people aged 21 years and younger (321) and lowest among those aged 75 years and older (4). On average, women had slightly lower transplantation rates than men (32 vs. 39/1000 dialysis patient-years) as did black patients compared with other races (25 vs. 41, 27, and 42 for white, Native American, and Asian dialysis patients, respectively).

Internationally, there is even greater variation in kidney transplantation rates, due in part to differences in health care systems, availability of organs, and cultural beliefs. In 2014, the highest transplantation rates/1000 dialysis patients were seen in Northern Europe, with Norway and the Netherlands the highest, at 205 and 154 transplants/1000 dialysis

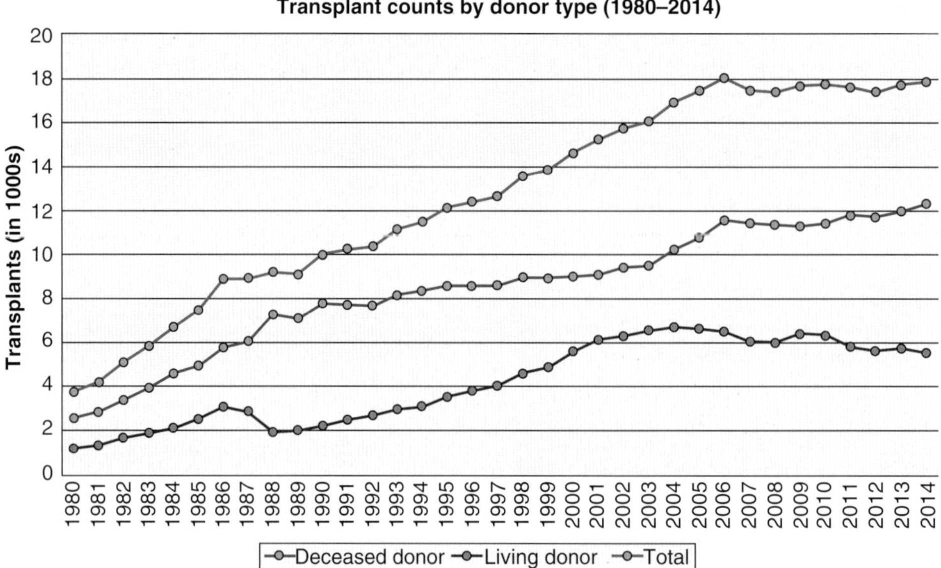


**Fig. 19.19** Number of kidney transplants by donor type, 1980-2014. (Data from U.S. Renal Data System. 2013 Annual data report: atlas of chronic kidney disease and end-stage renal disease in the United States. https://www.ajkd.org/article/S0272-6386(13)01544-8/pdf; and U.S. Renal Data System. 2016 USRDS annual data report: epidemiology of kidney disease in the United States. https://www.ajkd.org/article/S0272-6386(16)30703-X/fulltext.)

patients, respectively. In Norway, nearly all patients younger than 65 years and most patients older than 65 years received transplants within 4 years of initiating KRT.[157]

## OUTCOMES

Randomized controlled trials have not been performed, but kidney transplantation is generally accepted as the preferred KRT modality, with lower mortality and better quality of life compared with hemodialysis or peritoneal dialysis.[158] These benefits are thought to extend to recipients of both living and deceased donor organs, including those who receive organs with so-called marginal characteristics.[159–161] Benefits of transplantation are also seen in older recipients; for example, patients older than 70 years who received transplants had a 41% lower risk of death compared with wait-listed counterparts in adjusted analysis.[162] Whereas cardiovascular mortality increases with dialysis vintage, there is no such increase in cardiovascular events with kidney transplantation vintage, suggesting that some of the mortality benefit seen with transplantation may be a reduction in the development of CVD.[163]

On the other hand, kidney transplantation is not without risk. The leading cause of death is CVD. Among risk factors for CVD, new-onset diabetes mellitus after transplantation is of particular relevance because it may be increased by the calcineurin inhibitor tacrolimus, a commonly used agent for immunosuppression. New-onset diabetes is variably captured but has been reported in as many as 50% of transplant recipients, with a higher risk among older recipients.[164] Infections are the second leading cause of death in transplant recipients, and the infection rate in the first 3 years after transplantation is estimated at 45 infections/100 recipient-years of follow-up.[165,166] Cancer is the third leading cause of death, with the incidence of cancer mortality two- to threefold higher than the general population.[167,168]

## DISPARITIES IN KIDNEY TRANSPLANTATION

Several international studies have suggested disparities in rates of kidney transplantation by socioeconomic status and race, particularly for living donor kidney transplants.[169,170] In the United States, disparities have been documented in transplant referral, recipient candidate approval, placement on the waiting list, time on the waiting list, and allograft survival.[170–175] It has been estimated that eligible African American transplant candidates receive 35% fewer transplants than eligible Caucasian transplant candidates.[176] A study in Australia has found that recipients from socioeconomically advantaged areas were more likely to receive a living kidney donor transplant than those of lower socioeconomic status, although rates of deceased donor transplantation were similar.[177] Some of the disparities in living donor transplantation may be due to increased risk of CKD in family members due to the presence of genetic risk variants. Similarly, the presence of the *APOL1* high-risk genotype in the allograft (but, interestingly, not the recipient), is a risk factor for shortened allograft survival.[178]

# ACUTE KIDNEY INJURY

## EPIDEMIOLOGY

There are many similarities in the epidemiology of AKI and CKD, in part because the definitions for both include a criterion based on a measure of GFR (see Table 19.1). The urine output criterion is unique to the definition of AKI, but it is also relatively recent, not captured in much of the previous literature, and has been criticized for both logistic and theoretic reasons.[179,180] Studies of AKI typically capture disease by changes in creatinine level (with a wide range of definitions) or by relying on billing codes, such as those classified in the *International Classification of Disease, Ninth Clinical Modification.*[179] Studies using diagnostic codes to identify AKI events are particularly problematic, because labeling an event as AKI depends on the provider's perception of what constitutes AKI. Using a creatinine-based definition of AKI, the sensitivity of diagnostic codes has been shown to vary by era and patient age.[181]

## INCIDENCE

By definition, AKI is a transient disease; kidney disease lasting longer than 3 months is defined as CKD.[3,6] Thus, AKI can be described only through incidence rather than prevalence. One study of community-dwelling people in Northern California has estimated the incidence rate to be 522.4 cases of AKI/100,000 person-years and 29.5 cases of dialysis-requiring AKI/100,000 person-years.[182] A population-based study from Scotland has estimated the AKI and AKI requiring dialysis rates as 214.7 and 18.3 cases/100,000 patient-years, respectively.[183] In a Canadian cohort of patients with both creatinine and urine protein measurements, incidence rates were much higher, ranging from 100 to 11,700 cases of hospitalized AKI/100,000 person-years, depending on the level of GFR and proteinuria.[184] In patients with Medicare insurance and older than 65 years, 4.0% had a hospitalization with AKI over the course of 1 year, as identified by a billing code for AKI.[24]

In a hospitalized population, the rate of AKI may be even higher. A meta-analysis of hospitalized patients worldwide has estimated that almost 25% had AKI ascertained using the KDIGO definition; approximately 10% of cases required KRT.[185] A similar estimate was derived from U.S. Department of Veterans Affairs patients and, notably, only 49% of those with AKI ascertained by the serum creatinine criterion had an associated AKI billing code.[24] Rates of AKI have also been defined in certain hospital settings, such as after major surgery. Estimates using Veterans Affairs data have suggested that the 7-day incidence of AKI after major surgery ranges from 4.1% after ear, nose, and throat surgery to 18.7% after cardiac surgery (Fig. 19.20).[186] Causes of AKI are rarely assessed in large studies, but some studies have suggested that among hospitalized patients, approximately two-thirds of AKI episodes were community-acquired and one-third were hospital-acquired.[187]

## OUTCOMES

The study of AKI has been prioritized in both clinical and basic science research because of the recognition that outcomes, including development and progression of CKD, are worse among patients who experience even a small increase in serum creatinine level compared with those with stable values. In addition, studies have suggest that oliguria, even when not accompanied by a rise in serum creatinine level sufficient to meet the AKI criterion, may confer higher risk.[181,188] The incidence of CKD, decline in eGFR, ESKD, and death are all higher in patients who experience AKI, with higher AKI stage conferring higher risk.[179,189–193] For example, in one U.S. study, the risk of developing stage G4 or G5 CKD was 28 times higher after surviving an episode of KRT-requiring AKI.[194] Even modest changes in serum creatinine level have been associated with higher costs and length of stay. One 2005 study has estimated that an increase in serum creatinine level of 0.5 mg/dL or higher was associated with 3.5 additional hospital days and $7500 in excess costs.[195] The absolute risk of adverse outcomes varies based on underlying characteristics and stage of AKI, but many of those with AKI severe enough to require KRT never recover kidney function fully.[190,194,196] Controversial is whether the adverse outcomes are caused by AKI or simply due to shared risk factors.[197,198] There are no trials that have definitively proven causation due to the lack of effective therapy for AKI prevention and the need for very large sample sizes and long-term follow-up.[199]

## RISK FACTORS

Risk factors for AKI are similar to those for CKD: older age, male gender and, variably, black race.[53] Racial disparities in AKI may be confounded by differences in socioeconomic

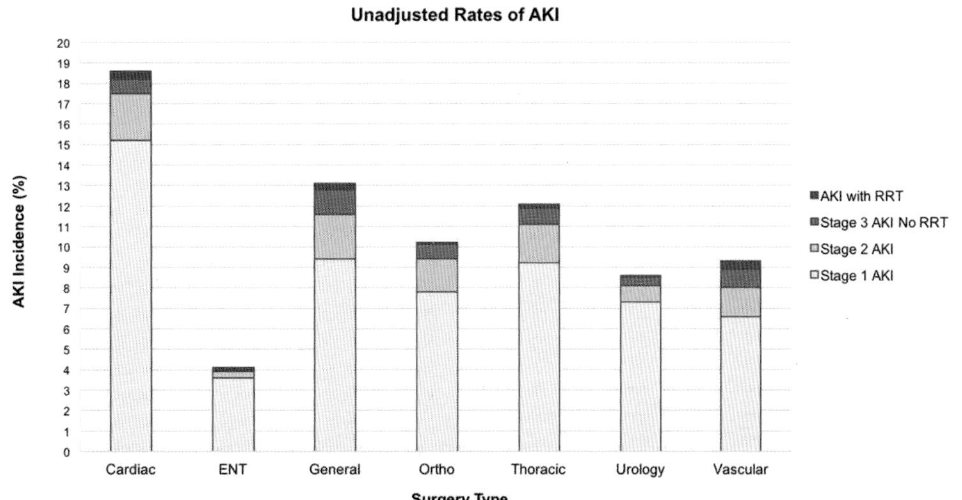


**Fig. 19.20** Unadjusted rates of acute kidney injury, by surgery type and stage. *AKI,* Acute kidney injury; *ENT,* ear, nose, throat; *RRT,* renal replacement therapy. (Adapted from Grams ME, Sang Y, Coresh J, et al. Acute kidney injury after major surgery: a retrospective analysis of Veterans Health Administration data. *Am J Kidney Dis.* 2016;67[6]:872–880.)

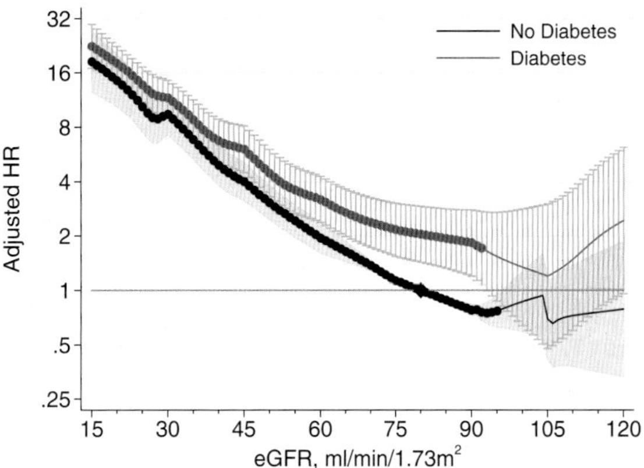


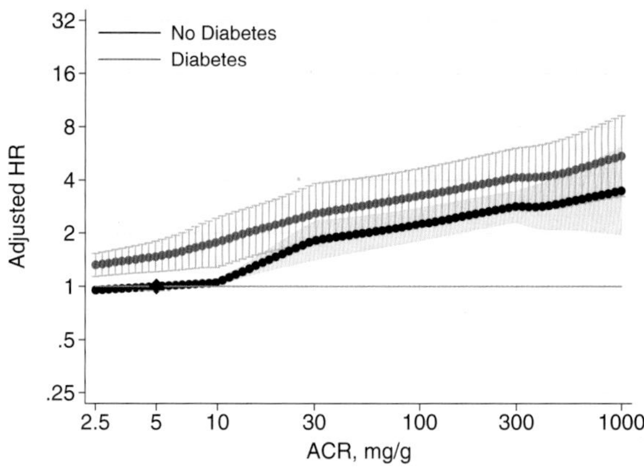


**Fig. 19.21** Acute kidney injury risk by estimated glomerular filtration rate *(eGFR)* and urine albumin-to-creatinine ratio *(ACR),* stratified by diabetes status. Hazard ratios (*HRs;* with 95% CI [confidence interval]) of acute kidney injury, using common referent group without diabetes, according to eGFR (reference, 80 mL/min/1.73 m$^2$ without diabetes, left) and ACR (reference, 5 mg/g without diabetes; right) in individuals with and without diabetes in general population cohorts. (From James MT, Grams ME, Woodward M, et al. A meta-analysis of the association of estimated GFR, albuminuria, diabetes mellitus, and hypertension with acute kidney injury. *Am J Kidney Dis.* 2015;66:602–612.)

status—itself a risk factor for AKI—and, in a small study, were not explained by differences in kidney risk variants in APOL1.[200] Diabetes also confers an increased risk for AKI, with odds of AKI from 1.5- to 2.5-fold higher among persons with diabetes.[54,201] The strongest risk factors, however, appear to be lower eGFR and higher albuminuria, with each conferring a higher risk in a graded fashion, and little difference with the presence or absence of diabetes mellitus or hypertension (Fig. 19.21).

## EVIDENCE GAPS AND LIMITATIONS OF THE LITERATURE

The literature of the epidemiology of kidney disease has important gaps:

1. Studies of the onset of disease are limited by the timing of and indication for ascertainment of kidney disease measures. Serum creatinine level is frequently measured during health encounters for acute and chronic illness. Markers of kidney damage are measured less frequently than serum creatinine level in clinical practice, and thus AKD and CKD are often underestimated. In research cohorts, measurements of serum creatinine levels are general not frequent enough to distinguish AKI, AKD, and CKD.
2. Factors other than GFR can affect serum concentrations of creatinine and cystatin C.
3. Many identified risk factors do not meet all the criteria for causality outlined by Bradford Hill.[7]
4. There are no uniform definitions for cause of kidney disease, and the clinical information necessary for ascertaining cause of disease is generally not available in research studies and clinical populations.
5. ESKD is defined by a therapy for which the indications for initiation are not uniform. Symptoms of kidney failure are poorly defined and ascertained, and the availability of KRT varies widely among countries, limiting inferences about kidney failure from ESKD studies.
6. Laboratory methods for the assessment of kidney measures can differ. Guidelines have improved comparability across studies by recommending standardization of assays for serum creatinine and cystatin C levels and routine reporting of eGFR, as well as measurement of urine albumin rather than total protein, but additional work is needed.

## CONCLUSION

In conclusion, kidney disease is now recognized as a pressing global health concern. Over 10% of the world's population has CKD, and nearly 25% of the global hospitalized population experiences AKI. Enormous disparities exist in access to treatment, and millions of people are undertreated or untreated. Kidney disease epidemiology plays a critical role in providing evidence for the issuance of guideline definitions and recommendations, harmonization of research, development of trial endpoints, and success of global initiatives, such as those of the International Society of Nephrology, which seek to define global needs in CKD and eliminate preventable deaths from AKI by 2025.

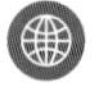 Complete reference list available at ExpertConsult.com.

### KEY REFERENCES


3. Kidney Disease: Improving Global Outcomes (KDIGO) CKD Work Group. KDIGO 2012 clinical practice guideline for the evaluation and management of chronic kidney disease. *Kidney Int Suppl.* 2013;3:1–150.
6. Kellum JA, Lameire N. KDIGO AKI Guideline Work Group. Diagnosis, evaluation, and management of acute kidney injury: a KDIGO summary (Part 1). *Crit Care.* 2013;17:204.
8. Levey AS, Inker LA, Matsushita K, et al. GFR decline as an end point for clinical trials in CKD: a scientific workshop sponsored by the National Kidney Foundation and the US Food and Drug Administration. *Am J Kidney Dis.* 2014;64:821–835.
9. Wuttke M, Kottgen A. Insights into kidney diseases from genome-wide association studies. *Nat Rev Nephrol.* 2016;12:549–562.
12. Genovese G, Friedman DJ, Ross MD, et al. Association of trypanolytic ApoL1 variants with kidney disease in African Americans. *Science.* 2010;329:841–845.

14. Naik RP, Derebail VK, Grams ME, et al. Association of sickle cell trait with chronic kidney disease and albuminuria in African Americans. *JAMA*. 2014;312:2115–2125.
22. Eckardt KU, Coresh J, Devuyst O, et al. Evolving importance of kidney disease: from subspecialty to global health burden. *Lancet*. 2013;382:158–169.
25. Myers GL, Miller WG, Coresh J, et al. Recommendations for improving serum creatinine measurement: a report from the Laboratory Working Group of the National Kidney Disease Education Program. *Clin Chem*. 2006;52:5–18.
26. Levey AS, Bosch JP, Lewis JB, et al. A more accurate method to estimate glomerular filtration rate from serum creatinine: a new prediction equation. Modification of Diet in Renal Disease Study Group. *Ann Intern Med*. 1999;130:461–470.
27. Levey AS, Stevens LA, Schmid CH, et al. A new equation to estimate glomerular filtration rate. *Ann Intern Med*. 2009;150:604–612.
28. Jha V, Garcia-Garcia G, Iseki K, et al. Chronic kidney disease: global dimension and perspectives. *Lancet*. 2013;382:260–272.
29. Murphy D, McCulloch CE, Lin F, et al. Trends in prevalence of chronic kidney disease in the United States. *Ann Intern Med*. 2016;165(7):473–481.
30. Coresh J, Selvin E, Stevens LA, et al. Prevalence of chronic kidney disease in the United States. *JAMA*. 2007;298:2038–2047.
33. Bruck K, Stel VS, Gambaro G, et al. CKD prevalence varies across the European general population. *J Am Soc Nephrol*. 2016;27:2135–2147.
34. Mills KT, Xu Y, Zhang W, et al. A systematic analysis of worldwide population-based data on the global burden of chronic kidney disease in 2010. *Kidney Int*. 2015;88:950–957.
35. Matsushita K, Mahmoodi BK, Woodward M, et al. Comparison of risk prediction using the CKD-EPI equation and the MDRD study equation for estimated glomerular filtration rate. *JAMA*. 2012;307:1941–1951.
37. de Boer IH, Rue TC, Hall YN, et al. Temporal trends in the prevalence of diabetic kidney disease in the United States. *JAMA*. 2011;305:2532–2539.
42. Peralta CA, Katz R, DeBoer I, et al. Racial and ethnic differences in kidney function decline among persons without chronic kidney disease. *J Am Soc Nephrol*. 2011;22:1327–1334.
49. Matsushita K, van der Velde M, Astor BC, et al. Association of estimated glomerular filtration rate and albuminuria with all-cause and cardiovascular mortality in general population cohorts: a collaborative meta-analysis. *Lancet*. 2010;375:2073–2081.
53. Grams ME, Sang Y, Ballew SH, et al. A meta-analysis of the association of estimated GFR, albuminuria, age, race, and sex with acute kidney injury. *Am J Kidney Dis*. 2015;66(4):591–601.
54. James MT, Grams ME, Woodward M, et al. A meta-analysis of the association of estimated GFR, albuminuria, diabetes mellitus, and hypertension with acute kidney injury. *Am J Kidney Dis*. 2015;66(4):602–612.
58. Hallan SI, Matsushita K, Sang Y, et al. Age and association of kidney measures with mortality and end-stage renal disease. *JAMA*. 2012;2349–2360.
59. Coresh J, Turin TC, Matsushita K, et al. Decline in estimated glomerular filtration rate and subsequent risk of end-stage renal disease and mortality. *JAMA*. 2014;311:2518–2531.
60. Kovesdy CP, Coresh J, Ballew SH, et al. Past decline versus current eGFR and subsequent ESRD risk. *J Am Soc Nephrol*. 2016;27:2447–2455.
62. Carrero JJ, Grams ME, Sang Y, et al. Albuminuria changes are associated with subsequent risk of end-stage renal disease and mortality. *Kidney Int*. 2017;91:244–251.
63. Tangri N, Grams ME, Levey AS, et al. Multinational assessment of accuracy of equations for predicting risk of kidney failure: a meta-analysis. *JAMA*. 2016;315:164–174.
65. Grams ME, Yang W, Rebholz CM, et al. Risks of adverse events in advanced CKD: the Chronic Renal Insufficiency Cohort (CRIC) study. *Am J Kidney Dis*. 2017.
66. Hemmelgarn BR, James MT, Manns BJ, et al. Rates of treated and untreated kidney failure in older vs younger adults. *JAMA*. 2012;307:2507–2515.
69. Liyanage T, Ninomiya T, Jha V, et al. Worldwide access to treatment for end-stage kidney disease: a systematic review. *Lancet*. 2015;385:1975–1982.
70. Inker LA, Coresh J, Levey AS, et al. Estimated GFR, albuminuria, and complications of chronic kidney disease. *J Am Soc Nephrol*. 2011;22:2322–2331.
82. Parsa A, Kao WH, Xie D, et al. APOL1 risk variants, race, and progression of chronic kidney disease. *N Engl J Med*. 2013;369:2183–2196.
89. O'Seaghdha CM, Yang Q, Wu H, et al. Performance of a genetic risk score for CKD stage 3 in the general population. *Am J Kidney Dis*. 2012;59:19–24.
101. Gorski M, Tin A, Garnaas M, et al. Genome-wide association study of kidney function decline in individuals of European descent. *Kidney Int*. 2015;87:1017–1029.
103. Nicolaou N, Renkema KY, Bongers EM, et al. Genetic, environmental, and epigenetic factors involved in CAKUT. *Nat Rev Nephrol*. 2015;11:720–731.
106. Hsu CY, Bates DW, Kuperman GJ, et al. Diabetes, hemoglobin A(1c), cholesterol, and the risk of moderate chronic renal insufficiency in an ambulatory population. *Am J Kidney Dis*. 2000;36:272–281.
112. Ruggenenti P, Perna A, Loriga G, et al. Blood-pressure control for renoprotection in patients with non-diabetic chronic renal disease (REIN-2): multicentre, randomised controlled trial. *Lancet*. 2005;365:939–946.
113. Klahr S, Levey AS, Beck GJ, et al. The effects of dietary protein restriction and blood-pressure control on the progression of chronic renal disease. Modification of Diet in Renal Disease Study Group. *N Engl J Med*. 1994;330:877–884.
114. Appel LJ, Wright JT Jr, Greene T, et al. Intensive blood-pressure control in hypertensive chronic kidney disease. *N Engl J Med*. 2010;363:918–929.
117. Beddhu S, Rocco MV, Toto R, et al. Effects of intensive systolic blood pressure control on kidney and cardiovascular outcomes in persons without kidney disease: a secondary analysis of a randomized trial. *Ann Intern Med*. 2017;167:375–383.
119. Grams ME, Sang Y, Levey AS, et al. Kidney failure risk projection for the living kidney-donor candidate. *N Engl J Med*. 2016;374:411–421.
134. Kucirka LM, Grams ME, Lessler J, et al. Association of race and age with survival among patients undergoing dialysis. *JAMA*. 2011;306:620–626.
135. Cooper BA, Branley P, Bulfone L, et al. A randomized, controlled trial of early versus late initiation of dialysis. *N Engl J Med*. 2010;363:609–619.
136. Eknoyan G, Beck GJ, Cheung AK, et al. Effect of dialysis dose and membrane flux in maintenance hemodialysis. *N Engl J Med*. 2002;347:2010–2019.
138. Baigent C, Landray MJ, Reith C, et al. The effects of lowering LDL cholesterol with simvastatin plus ezetimibe in patients with chronic kidney disease (Study of Heart and Renal Protection): a randomised placebo-controlled trial. *Lancet*. 2011.
152. Tuttle KR, Bakris GL, Bilous RW, et al. Diabetic kidney disease: a report from an ADA Consensus Conference. *Am J Kidney Dis*. 2014;64:510–533.
171. Purnell TS, Luo X, Kucirka LM, et al. Reduced racial disparity in kidney transplant outcomes in the United States from 1990 to 2012. *J Am Soc Nephrol*. 2016;27:2511–2518.
182. Hsu CY, McCulloch CE, Fan D, et al. Community-based incidence of acute renal failure. *Kidney Int*. 2007;72:208–212.
184. James MT, Hemmelgarn BR, Wiebe N, et al. Glomerular filtration rate, proteinuria, and the incidence and consequences of acute kidney injury: a cohort study. *Lancet*. 2010;376:2096–2103.
186. Grams ME, Sang Y, Coresh J, et al. Acute kidney injury after major surgery: a retrospective analysis of Veterans Health Administration Data. *Am J Kidney Dis*. 2016;67(6):872–880.
196. Wald R, Quinn RR, Luo J, et al. Chronic dialysis and death among survivors of acute kidney injury requiring dialysis. *JAMA*. 2009;302:1179–1185.

# 20 Risk Prediction in Chronic Kidney Disease

Kelsey Connelly | Maarten W. Taal | Navdeep Tangri

CHAPTER OUTLINE



KEY POINTS

- Because of a large variance in chronic kidney disease (CKD) progression, there is a need to develop methods for risk stratification within CKD to identify the relatively small subgroup of patients who are at risk of progression to end-stage kidney disease (ESKD) and who may benefit from intervention.
- The combination of risk factors (age, gender, ethnicity, etc.) and biomarkers (proteinuria, anemia, fibroblast growth factor 23, etc.) can be useful in risk stratification of patients with CKD.
- In a similar manner to the Framingham risk score for prediction of cardiovascular risk, renal risk scores such as the kidney failure risk equation (KFRE) have allowed for the accurate prediction of CKD progression.
- Equations such as the KFRE are externally validated and ready to be implemented in a clinical setting.

Chronic kidney disease (CKD) currently affects more than 26 million Americans[1] and a meta-analysis of studies from around the globe has reported a prevalence for CKD stages 1–5 among adults of 8.7% to 18.4% with a global mean prevalence of 13.4% [95% confidence interval (95% CI), 11.7% to 15.1%].[2] The large number of people known to be affected by CKD has major implications for the provision of health care – in particular, nephrology services. In the past two decades, nephrology has moved from a position where it provided highly specialized services to a relatively small number of patients with specific and relatively rare kidney disease or advanced CKD, to one where it must concern itself with the care of less-advanced CKD in a substantial proportion of the general population. Furthermore, early stage CKD is largely asymptomatic, and detection therefore requires a screening process. Studies have indicated that screening whole populations is not cost-effective,[3] and a means of identifying high-risk subgroups for targeted screening is therefore required. Successful screening programs are likely to identify large numbers of patients with previously undiagnosed CKD; however, in most countries, nephrology services are unable to provide long-term care to all CKD patients, and the associated costs would be prohibitive. A solution to this problem was suggested by studies showing that there is substantial heterogeneity among patients who meet the diagnostic criteria for CKD, with most being at relatively low risk of ever progressing to end-stage kidney disease (ESKD). One reason for this heterogeneity is the use of an estimated glomerular filtration rate (eGFR) < 60 mL/min/1.73 $m^2$ as the standard of CKD diagnosis in clinical practice.[4] This provides susceptibility to both overdiagnosis and underdiagnosis of CKD as any given level of eGFR will have a large variation in the risk for progression to kidney failure.[5] As a result, there will be situations in which low-risk patients are overrecognized and receive unnecessary treatment or, conversely, high-risk patients being under-recognized and receiving less-than-optimal treatment with regard to CKD progression.[6] The Kidney Disease Outcomes and Quality Initiative (K/DOQI) classification system for CKD was widely adopted and proved valuable, particularly for identifying the prevalence of different stages of CKD in epidemiologic studies.[7] It was noted, however, that the classification provided little information on the future risk of decline in renal function.[8] The Kidney Disease Improving Global Outcomes (KDIGO) classification system therefore modified the K/DOQI system so that categories defined by eGFR and albuminuria do correlate with risk,[9] but this does not provide accurate, individual risk prediction. Previous studies identified a wide range of rates of decline in GFR among patients with CKD, and up to 15% may even show an increase over time.[10]

In a retrospective cohort study done by O'Hare et al. using patients with advanced CKD from the United States Renal Data System and Veterans Affairs databases, the following trajectories were discovered: 1. consistently low eGFR < 30 mL/min/1.73 $m^2$ with a mean yearly decrease of 7.8 mL/min/1.73 $m^2$, 2. progressive loss of initial eGFR at stage 3 CKD (eGFR of 30–59 mL/min/1.73 $m^2$) with a mean yearly decrease of 16.3 mL/min/1.73 $m^2$, 3. accelerated loss of initial eGFR > 60 mL/min/1.73 $m^2$ with a mean yearly decrease of 32.3 mL/min/1.73 $m^2$, and 4. dramatic loss of initial eGFR > 60 mL/min/1.73 $m^2$ in 6 months or less, with a mean yearly decrease of 50.7 mL/min/1.73 $m^2$.[11] In a similar study, Li et al. also found distinct patterns of CKD progression, this time using patients from the African American Study of Kidney Disease and Hypertension (AASK), which included 846 patients that were followed over a 3-year period. The patterns of progression included 1. stable or increasing eGFR, defined as less than 2 mL/min/1.73 $m^2$ decrease per year, 2. rapid decrease in eGFR, defined as a loss of more than 4 mL/min/1.73 $m^2$ per year, and 3. alternating combinations of the previously mentioned categories. It was determined that a stable or increasing eGFR was the most common pattern of CKD progression, with 58% of participants following such a trajectory.[12] Due to such a variance in progression of CKD, there is a need to develop methods for risk stratification within CKD to identify the relatively small subgroup of patients who are at risk of progression to ESKD and who may benefit from specialist intervention to slow or halt disease progression. Such risk stratification would be equally important for identifying individuals who are at low risk for progression who could be reassured and spared unnecessary referral to a nephrologist.

Another important aspect of CKD is its association with a substantially increased risk of future cardiovascular events (CVEs) that in most patients with mild CKD substantially exceeds the risk of ESKD.[13] Whereas CKD is associated with a high prevalence of many traditional risk factors for cardiovascular disease (CVD), such as hypertension and dyslipidemia, risk prediction tools such as the Framingham risk score substantially underestimate cardiovascular risk in patients with CKD.[14] It has been proposed that this observation is due to the role of several nontraditional cardiovascular risk factors that are specific to CKD.

From the aforementioned discussion, it is clear that there is a need to identify and understand factors associated with an increased risk of developing CKD and, once diagnosed, factors associated with an increased risk of progression to ESKD and CVE. In this chapter, we will review current knowledge of these risk factors and the methods being applied to predict risk in CKD patients. Risk factors for CVD in patients with CKD, many of which overlap with risk factors for CKD progression, are discussed in Chapter 54.

## DEFINITION OF A RISK FACTOR

A risk factor is a variable that has a causal association with a disease or disease process such that the presence of said variable in an individual is associated with an increased risk of the disease being present or developing in the future. Thus risk factors are a useful tool for identifying subjects with increased risk for a disease or particular outcome due to a disease process. In the course of epidemiologic research, many variables may show associations with a disease of interest but these may be chance associations, noncausal associations, or causal associations (true risk factors). The Bradford Hill criteria provide minimum requirements to be fulfilled to identify a causal relationship between a putative risk factor (exposure) and a disease (outcome; Table 20.1). In complex diseases such as CKD that result from the combined effects of multiple factors, it is likely that many risk factors will not fulfill all the criteria. Nevertheless, they do provide a useful framework for assessing the strength of a proposed causal relationship between risk factor and disease.

## RISK FACTORS AND MECHANISMS OF CHRONIC KIDNEY DISEASE PROGRESSION

It has been appreciated for several decades that once GFR has decreased to below a critical level, it tends to progress relentlessly toward ESKD. This observation suggests that loss of a critical number of nephrons provokes a vicious cycle of further nephron loss. Detailed studies have elucidated a number of interrelated mechanisms that together contribute to CKD progression, including glomerular hemodynamic responses to nephron loss [raised glomerular capillary

**Table 20.1 Bradford Hill Criteria of Causality**

| Parameter | Explanation |
|---|---|
| Strength of association | The stronger the association, the more likely the relationship is causal. |
| Consistency | A causal association is consistent when replicated in different populations and studies. |
| Specificity | A single putative cause produces a single effect. |
| Temporality | Exposure precedes outcome (i.e., risk factor predates disease). |
| Biological gradient | Increasing exposure to risk factor increases risk of disease, and reduction in exposure reduces risk. |
| Plausibility | The observed association is consistent with biologic mechanisms of disease processes. |
| Coherence | The observed association is compatible with existing theory and knowledge in a given field. |
| Experimental evidence | The factor under investigation is amenable to modification by an appropriate experimental approach. |
| Analogy | An established cause-and-effect relationship exists for a similar exposure or disease. |

Modified from Hill AB. The environment and disease: association or causation? *Proc R Soc Med.* 1965;58: 295–300.

hydraulic pressure and single-nephron GFR (SNGFR)], proteinuria, and proinflammatory responses. A generally good prognosis after unilateral nephrectomy[15] attests to the fact that a single pathogenic factor may be insufficient to initiate progressive CKD, but the multihit hypothesis proposes that multiple factors interact to overcome renal reserve and provoke progressive nephron loss.[16] To meet the Bradford Hill criteria of plausibility and coherence, a putative risk factor should therefore somehow affect known mechanisms of CKD progression (see Chapter 51 for further details). Fig. 20.1 shows how risk factors may interact with pathophysiologic mechanisms to initiate or accelerate CKD progression.

Based on our understanding of the mechanisms underlying the pathogenesis of CKD and its progression, risk factors may be divided into susceptibility factors, initiation factors, and progression factors (Table 20.2). First, susceptibility includes risk factors associated with an increased risk of an individual developing CKD after exposure to a factor that has potential to cause renal damage. An example is a reduced nephron number after uninephrectomy, which is associated with an increased risk of developing diabetic nephropathy if the individual develops diabetes.[17] Initiation factors directly cause or initiate kidney damage in a susceptible individual. Examples include exposure to nephrotoxic drugs, urinary tract obstruction, or primary glomerulopathies that may provoke CKD in some (but not all) exposed individuals. Finally, progression factors are those that contribute to the progression of kidney damage once CKD has developed. An

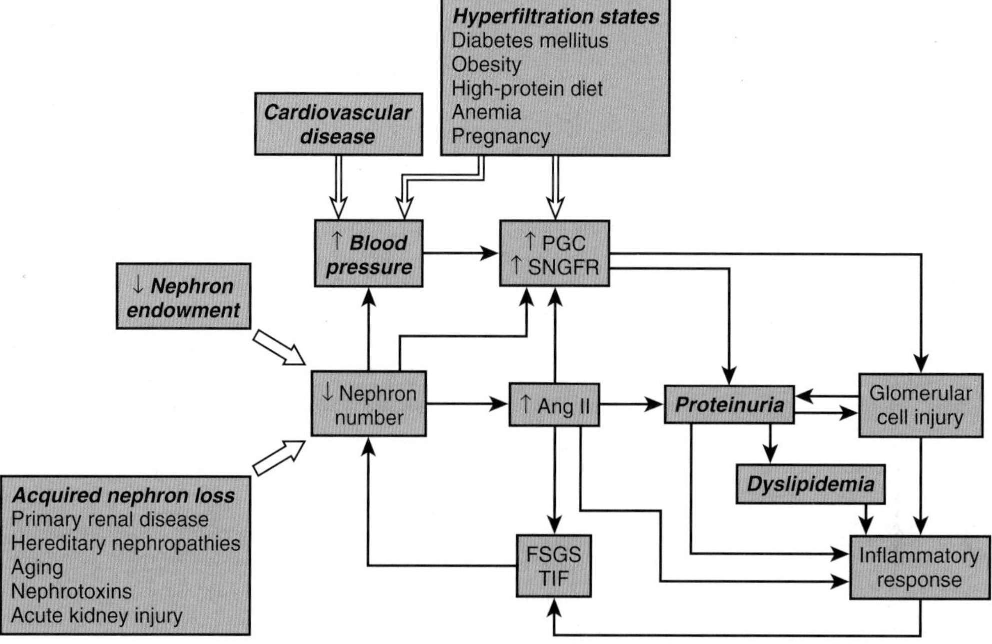


**Fig. 20.1** Schematic representation showing the interaction of risk factors for chronic kidney disease progression with pathophysiologic mechanisms that contribute to a vicious cycle of progressive nephron loss. *Ang II,* Angiotensin II; *FSGS,* focal segmental glomerulosclerosis; *PGC,* glomerular capillary hydraulic pressure; *SNGFR,* single-nephron glomerular filtration rate; *TIF,* tubulointerstitial fibrosis. (Adapted from Taal MW, Brenner BM. Predicting initiation and progression of chronic kidney disease: developing renal risk scores. *Kidney Int.* 2006;70:1694–1705.)

**Table 20.2 Risk Factors for Chronic Kidney Disease**

| Risk Factor | Susceptibility | Initiating | Progression |
|---|---|---|---|
| Older age | + | | |
| Gender | + | | |
| Ethnicity | + | | + |
| Family history of chronic kidney disease | + | | |
| Metabolic syndrome | + | | |
| Hemodynamic factors | | | |
| Low nephron number | + | | + |
| Diabetes mellitus | + | + | + |
| Hypertension | + | | + |
| Obesity | + | | + |
| High protein intake | + | | + |
| Pregnancy | | + | + |
| Primary renal disease | | + | |
| Genetic renal disease | | + | |
| Urologic disorders | | + | |
| Acute kidney injury | | + | + |
| Cardiovascular disease | + | | + |
| Albuminuria | | | + |
| Hypoalbuminemia | | | + |
| Anemia | + | | + |
| Dyslipidemia | + | | + |
| Hyperuricemia | + | | + |
| ↑ Asymmetric dimethylarginine | | | + |
| Hyperphosphatemia | | | + |
| Low serum bicarbonate | | | + |
| Smoking | + | | + |
| Nephrotoxins | | + | + |

example is hypertension, which exacerbates raised intraglomerular hydraulic pressure and therefore accelerates glomerular damage. Studies investigating progression factors should recruit subjects with relatively early stage CKD in a cohort study design. Nevertheless, distinguishing among these categories may in some cases be difficult because some factors [e.g., diabetes mellitus (DM)] may act in all three ways and, in some studies, it may be impossible to separate susceptibility factors from progression factors due to inadequate characterization of participants at study entry.

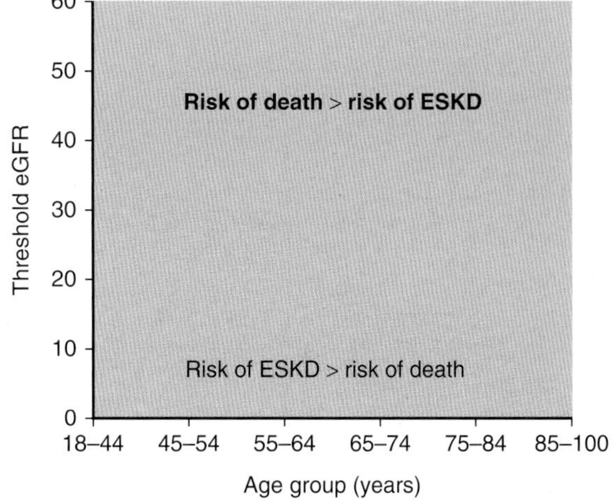


**Fig. 20.2** Baseline estimated glomerular filtration rate (eGFR) threshold. Below this the risk for end-stage kidney disease (ESKD) exceeded the risk for death in each age group among 209,622 US veterans with chronic kidney disease stages 3 to 5 followed for a mean of 3.2 years. (From O'Hare AM, Choi AI, Bertenthal D, et al. Age affects outcomes in chronic kidney disease. *J Am Soc Nephrol.* 2007;18:2758–2765.)

## DEMOGRAPHIC VARIABLES

### AGE

The prevalence of CKD increases with age and is reported to be as high as 56% in those 75 years or older.[18] Longitudinal studies of subjects without kidney disease have observed a decline in GFR with increasing age in some subjects, implying that nephron loss may be regarded as part of normal aging.[19] By contrast, aging is associated with an increase in several other risk factors for CKD, including hypertension, obesity, and CVD, which may contribute to the rise in CKD prevalence. Several population-based studies have found a higher incidence of proteinuria and CKD[20–22] as well as ESKD with increasing age.[23] Similarly, the incidence of a decline in renal function over 5 years was greater among older patients with hypertension.[24] One study reported that advanced age is a negative predictor of ESKD among patients with CKD, although older age was associated with a greater rate of decline in GFR.[25] This apparent contradiction is most likely explained by the competing risks of death and ESKD in older patients, illustrated by the observation from one longitudinal study that for patients 65 years and older, the risk of ESKD exceeded the risk of death only when the GFR was ≤15 mL/min/1.73 m$^2$ (Fig. 20.2).[26] By contrast, it has been found that a more rapid decrease of eGFR was associated with CKD in persons of a younger age, which in turn is associated with an increase in the 1-year mortality rate.[11]

A large individual-level meta-analysis that included data from 2,051,244 participants in 46 cohort studies has provided robust data regarding the effect of age on the risks associated with CKD. In the general population and high cardiovascular risk cohorts, the increase in relative risk of mortality associated with lower GFR declined with increasing age, but the increase in absolute risk of death was higher in older age groups. Similar trends were observed for the mortality risks associated with albuminuria. By contrast, the relative increase in risk of mortality did not decrease with increasing age in data from CKD cohorts. Furthermore, there was no attenuation of the risk of ESKD with increasing age in any of the cohort categories.[27]

Thus older age is a susceptibility factor for CKD, and the associated increase in risk of death and ESKD is observed at all ages. These observations suggest that targeted screening for CKD in older subjects would be a cost-effective strategy, but further studies are required to investigate the extent to which the risks associated with CKD in older adults may be attenuated by intervention. For further discussion of CKD in older age groups, see Chapters 22 and 84.

## GENDER

Data regarding the effect of gender on the risk of CKD and progression are somewhat contradictory. Studies have reported a higher incidence of proteinuria and CKD among men in the general population and an increased risk of ESKD or death associated with CKD,[20,23,28] a higher risk of decline in renal function in male hypertensive patients,[24] a lower risk of ESKD in female patients with CKD stage 3,[25] and a shorter time to renal replacement therapy (RRT) in male patients with CKD stage 4 or 5.[29] In addition, most national registries, including the US Renal Data Service (USRDS), have reported a substantially higher incidence of ESKD in males [413 per million population (pmp) in 2003] versus females (280 pmp).[30] Previous meta-analyses have, however, yielded conflicting results, with one reporting a higher rate of decline in GFR in men[31] and another reporting a higher risk of doubling of the serum creatinine level or ESKD in women after adjustment for baseline variables, including blood pressure and urinary protein excretion.[32]

The largest metaanalysis to date included data from studies of 2,051,158 participants investigating the impact of gender on CKD-related outcomes. Whereas the risk of all-cause and cardiovascular mortality was higher in men than women, the relative risk of mortality increased with lower GFR and higher albuminuria in both, and the slope of increase in risk was steeper in women than men. Importantly, the relative risk of ESKD increased with lower GFR and higher albuminuria in both sexes and there was no evidence of a difference in the increase in risk between men and women (Fig. 20.3).[33] One limitation of many of the studies quoted is that menopausal status of the women was not documented. Nevertheless, it is clear from the most robust data published that CKD is associated with at least the same relative increase in risk of death and ESKD in women as in men. The reasons for the higher absolute incidence of RRT in men versus women require further investigation, and may be related to treatment preferences for RRT rather than biological differences in disease progression. For further discussion of the impact of gender on CKD, see Chapters 19, 21, and 51.

## ETHNICITY

African Americans are overrepresented in the US dialysis population, suggesting that ethnicity is a strong risk factor for the progression of CKD to ESKD. Population-based studies have found a higher incidence of ESKD among African Americans that was attributable only in part to socioeconomic and other known risk factors.[7,23,34,35] Similarly, the risk of early renal function decline (increase in serum creatinine ≥ 0.4 mg/dL) was approximately threefold higher [odds ratio (OR), 3.15; 95% CI, 1.86 to 5.33] among black versus white diabetic adults, but 82% of this excess risk was attributable to socioeconomic and other known risk factors.[36] The risk of renal function decline over 5 years among hypertensive patients was greater in African Americans,[24] and African ancestry was independently associated with a greater rate of GFR decline in the Modification of Diet in Renal Disease (MDRD) study.[10] Interestingly, data from the Reasons for Geographic and Racial Differences in Stroke (REGARDS) Cohort Study have shown a lower prevalence of eGFR (50 to 59 mL/min/1.73 $m^2$) among African Americans but a higher prevalence of eGFR (10 to 19 mL/min/1.73 $m^2$) among white subjects[37] suggesting that African-American ethnicity acts as a progression factor but not as a susceptibility factor. A 2012 report from the USRDS showed a substantially higher incidence of ESKD in African Americans (3.3 times higher than whites), Hispanics (1.5 times higher than non-Hispanics), and Native Americans (1.5 times higher than whites).[38] Similarly, the prevalence of ESKD in 2012 was higher among minority groups: African Americans, 5671 pmp; Native Americans, 2600 pmp; Hispanics, 2932 pmp; Asians, 2272 pmp; and whites, 1432 pmp.[38] CKD and ESKD have also been reported to be more prevalent in other ethnic groups, including Asians,[39] Hispanics,[40] Native Americans,[41] Mexican Americans,[42] and Aboriginal Australians.[43] A large meta-analysis that included data from 940,366 participants in 25 general population cohort studies investigated the impact of ethnicity on the risks associated with CKD in blacks, whites, and Asians. The absolute risk of all-cause or cardiovascular mortality (after adjustment for age) and ESKD was higher in black versus white versus Asian participants. However, the relative risk of all-cause or cardiovascular mortality and ESKD increased to a similar degree with lower GFR or greater albuminuria in all the ethnic groups.[44]

Thus the risk between lower GFR or greater albuminuria and mortality or ESKD was not modified by ethnicity. The mechanisms underlying the associations between ethnicity and CKD remain to be elucidated, but possible explanations include genetic factors (see the "Hereditary Factors" section); increased prevalence of DM; lower nephron endowment; increased susceptibility to salt-sensitive hypertension; and environmental, lifestyle, and socioeconomic differences. Ethnicity and CKD are discussed further in Chapters 19, 21, and 51.

# HEREDITARY FACTORS

Hereditary renal diseases resulting from a single gene defect, such as autosomal dominant polycystic kidney disease (PKD),

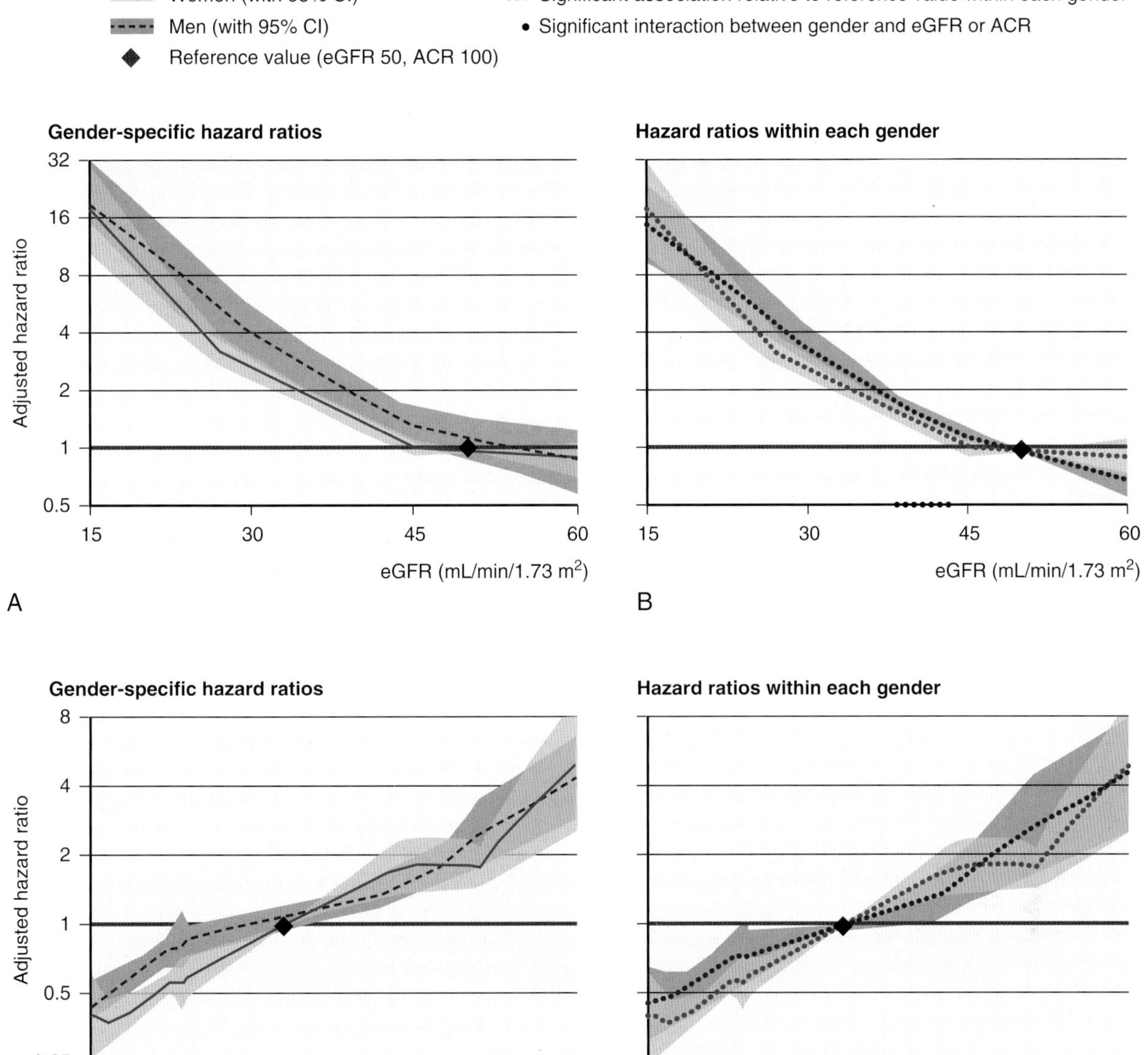


**Fig. 20.3** (A and B) Hazard ratios of end-stage kidney disease according to estimated glomerular filtration rate (eGFR). (C and D) Urinary albumin-to-creatinine ratio (ACR) in men versus women in chronic kidney disease cohorts. (A and C) Gender-specific hazard ratios, including a main effect for male gender at the reference point. (B and D) Hazard ratios in each gender, thus visually removing the baseline difference between men and women. Hazard ratios were adjusted for age, gender, race, smoking status, systolic blood pressure, history of cardiovascular disease, diabetes, serum total cholesterol concentration, body mass index, and estimated glomerular filtration rate splines or albuminuria. *CI,* Confidence interval. (Adapted from Nitsch D, Grams M, Sang Y, et al. Associations of estimated glomerular filtration rate and albuminuria with mortality and renal failure by sex: a meta-analysis. *BMJ* 2013;346:f324.)

Alport disease, Fabry disease, and congenital nephrotic syndrome, account for a relatively small yet clinically important proportion of all patients with CKD. Nevertheless, evidence is rapidly accumulating that genetic factors account for familial clustering of many other forms of CKD with multifactorial causes. Among 25,883 incident ESKD patients, 22.8% reported a family history of ESKD,[45] and screening of the relatives of patients with ESKD revealed evidence of CKD in 49.3%.[46] In another case–control study, including 689 patients with ESKD and 361 controls, having one first-degree relative with CKD increased the risk of ESKD by 30% [hazards ratio (HR), 1.3; 95% CI, 0.7 to 2.6] and having two such relatives increased it tenfold (HR, 10.4; 95% CI, 2.7 to 40.2) after controlling for multiple known risk factors, including diabetes and hypertension.[47] Similarly, a case–control study of 103 US white patients with ESKD reported a 3.5-fold increase in risk of ESKD (95% CI, 1.5 to 8.4) with the presence of a first-, second-, or third-degree relative with ESKD.[48] A genetic explanation for the high incidence of ESKD observed in African Americans was provided by groundbreaking research that identified strong associations between ESKD and two coding variants in the apolipoprotein L1 (*APOL1*) gene. These gene variants confer resistance to infection with *Trypanosoma brucei rhodesiense*, which causes sleeping sickness. This observation explains how selection likely resulted in a high prevalence of these variants in the population. Subsequent studies have identified associations between *APOL1* risk variants and several renal pathologies, including focal segmental glomerulosclerosis (FSGS), human immunodeficiency virus (HIV)-associated nephropathy (HIVAN), sickle cell kidney disease, and severe lupus nephritis.[49] Moreover, cohort studies have reported associations between *APOL1* risk variants and risk of progression to ESKD. Risk of progression was the lowest in European Americans (with no risk variants), intermediate in African Americans (with no or one risk variant), and highest in African Americans (with two risk variants).[50] It is estimated that *APOL1* variants account for 40% of disease burden due to CKD in African Americans.

Despite the strong association between inheritance of two *APOL1* risk variants and ESKD, only a minority of people with this genotype actually develop kidney disease, suggesting that the action of a second factor is required to cause disease in genetically susceptible individuals. HIV is one example of such a second hit, but it has been proposed that other viruses and other gene variants may also be important.[49]

Other studies have suggested that genetic factors also increase susceptibility to early manifestations of CKD. In a study of 169 families with one type 2 diabetic proband, the diabetic siblings of probands with microalbuminuria had a significantly increased risk of also having microalbuminuria, after adjustment for confounding risk factors (OR, 3.94; 95% CI, 1.93 to 9.01), than the diabetic siblings of probands without microalbuminuria.[51] Furthermore, the nondiabetic siblings of diabetic probands with microalbuminuria had a significantly higher urinary albumin excretion rate (within the normal range) than the nondiabetic siblings of normoalbuminuric diabetic probands.

Genome-wide association studies (GWASs) have identified multiple novel loci that are significantly associated with serum creatinine levels or CKD.[52–54] Furthermore, a recent GWAS meta-analysis conducted in 63,558 participants of European descent identified significant associations between GFR decline over time and three gene loci – uromodulin (*UMOD*) (previously associated with CKD and ESKD), *GALNTL5/GALNT11,* and *CDH23*. It was estimated that the heritability of GFR decline in this population was 38%.[55] Further studies have investigated the role of epigenetic factors (heritable changes in the pattern of gene expression not attributable to changes in the primary nucleotide sequence) that may affect the risk of CKD progression. One study compared the genome-wide DNA methylation profile in 20 people from the Chronic Renal Insufficiency Cohort (CRIC) study with the most rapid decline in GFR and 20 with the most stable GFR. Results identified differences in the methylation of several genes associated with epithelial-to-mesenchymal transition and inflammation that may be involved in the mechanisms of CKD progression.[56]

From this discussion, it is clear that genetic factors may act as susceptibility factors in some subjects, initiating factors in those with CKD due to a single gene defect, or progression factors in others. The rapid growth in knowledge of genetic aspects of CKD will likely result in genetic risk factors becoming increasingly important in risk prediction for patients with CKD. For a more detailed discussion of genetic aspects of kidney disease, see Chapters 43–45.

## HEMODYNAMIC FACTORS

Experimental studies have shown that glomerular hemodynamic responses (e.g., glomerular capillary hypertension and hyperfiltration) to nephron loss[57] and chronic hyperglycemia[58] are critical factors in establishing the vicious cycle of nephron loss characteristic of CKD. In addition, any factor that further increases glomerular hypertension and/or hyperfiltration may be expected to exacerbate glomerular damage and accelerate the progression of CKD (see Fig. 20.1).

### DECREASED NEPHRON NUMBER

#### NEPHRON ENDOWMENT

Autopsy studies have revealed that the number of nephrons per kidney varies widely in humans, from 210,332 to 2,702,079 in one series.[59] Multiple factors have been shown to influence nephron endowment, including those that affect the feto-maternal environment as well as genetic factors.[60] A substantial body of evidence supports the hypothesis that low nephron endowment predisposes individuals to CKD by provoking an increase in SNGFR and, therefore, a reduction in renal reserve. The ascertainment of nephron number in living human subjects is currently not possible, but autopsy studies have shown an association between reduced nephron number and hypertension,[61] as well as glomerulosclerosis.[62] In human autopsy studies, low birth weight is directly associated with reduced nephron number,[63,64] and birth weight may therefore serve as a marker of nephron endowment. Low birth weight is also a risk factor for later-life hypertension and DM, both of which further increase the risk of CKD.[65] One meta-analysis of 32 studies, which included data from >2 million subjects, reported a significantly increased risk of albuminuria (OR, 1.81; 95% CI, 1.19 to 2.77) and ESKD (OR, 1.58; 95% CI, 1.33 to 1.88) associated with low birth weight.[66] Thus low birth weight, acting as a marker of reduced nephron endowment, may be regarded as a susceptibility and progression risk factor for CKD. Factors affecting nephron endowment and the consequences of reduced nephron endowment are discussed in more detail in Chapter 21.

#### ACQUIRED NEPHRON DEFICIT

In experimental models of acquired nephron deficit, severe nephron loss (5/6 nephrectomy) alone initiates a cycle of progressive injury in the remaining glomeruli, mediated primarily through glomerular hypertension and hyperfiltration.[57] In 14 patients subjected to similarly large reductions in nephron number following partial resection of a single kidney, two developed ESKD and nine developed proteinuria, the extent of which was inversely correlated with the amount of renal tissue remaining.[67] Lesser degrees of acquired nephron loss, such as removal of one of two previously normal kidneys (uninephrectomy), may not be sufficient to cause CKD in most subjects.[15,68,69] However, nephrectomy for renal cell carcinoma is associated with an increased risk of developing CKD that is greater after radical nephrectomy than partial nephrectomy, suggesting that in the presence of subclinical kidney damage, acquired nephron loss may provoke CKD, and that the risk is proportional to the number of nephrons removed.[70]

Nephron loss may also predispose individuals to CKD if they are also exposed to other risk factors. This is perhaps best illustrated by the observation that uninephrectomy exacerbates renal injury in experimental diabetic nephropathy[71] and, in persons with diabetes, uninephrectomy increases the risk of developing diabetic nephropathy.[17]

The interaction between nephron loss and other risk factors is further illustrated by the observation that in a study of 488 people who had surgery for renal cell carcinoma, radical nephrectomy (compared with partial nephrectomy), diabetes, and increased age were each independently associated with an increased risk of developing CKD at least 6 months after surgery. In those who had a partial nephrectomy but no additional risk factors, only 7% developed CKD, but this increased to 24%, 30%, and 42% in those 60 years or older, those with hypertension, and diabetes, respectively.[72]

In most forms of CKD, initial nephron loss due to primary renal disease, multisystem disorders that involve the kidney, or exposure to nephrotoxins is focal, but hemodynamic adaptations in the remaining glomeruli are thought to contribute to nephron loss by provoking further glomerulosclerosis (see Chapter 51). Several epidemiologic studies have supported this hypothesis by showing that patients with a reduced GFR are at increased risk of a further decline in renal function. Two large meta-analyses of cohort studies identified baseline GFR as a strong predictor of ESKD. Among 845,125 participants from the general population, the eGFR was independently associated with an increased risk of developing ESKD when it fell below 75 mL/min/1.73 m$^2$. For groups of patients with average eGFRs of 60, 45, and 15 mL/min/1.73 m$^2$, the hazard ratios for developing ESKD were 4, 29, and 454, respectively, when compared with a reference group with an eGFR of 95 mL/min/1.73 m$^2$. Similar findings were reported in a further 173,892 participants selected for being at increased risk of developing CKD (Fig. 20.4).[73] Among 21,688 patients selected for having CKD, a lower eGFR was an independent risk factor for ESKD, such that a fall of 15 mL/min/1.73 m$^2$ below a threshold of 45 mL/min/1.73 m$^2$ was associated with a pooled hazard ratio of 6.24.[74] Further analyses by the CKD Prognosis Consortium have confirmed that the association between reduced GFR and increased risk of ESKD persists independently of gender,[33] age,[27] ethnicity,[44] diabetes,[75] and hypertension.[76] In addition, analysis of data from 1,530,648 participants has shown that change in GFR over time is strongly predictive of future risk

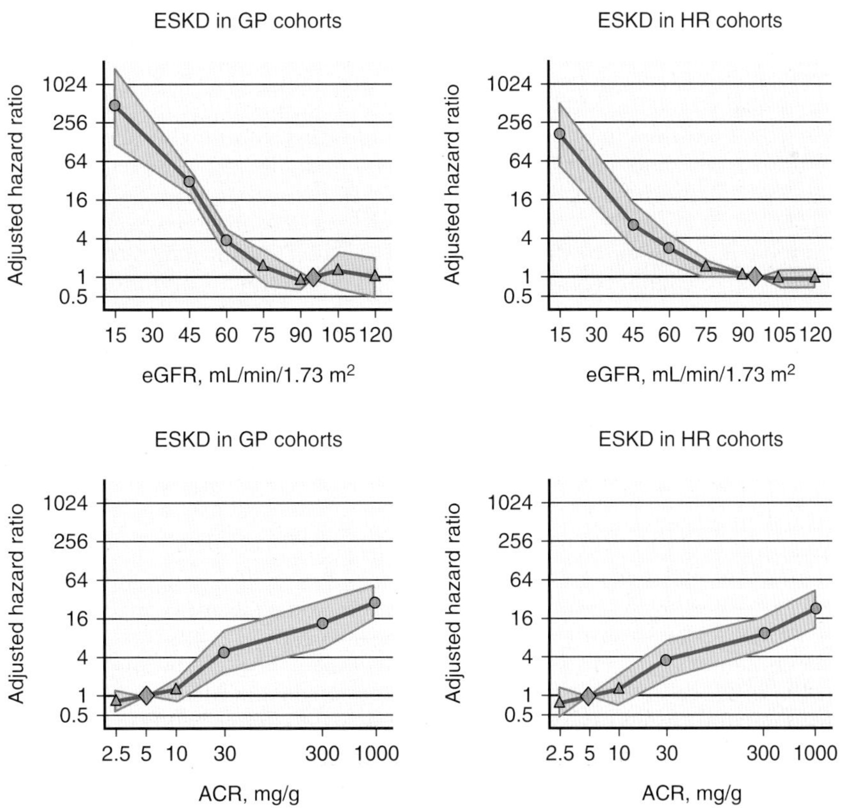


**Fig. 20.4** Pooled hazard ratios (95% confidence interval) for end-stage kidney disease (ESKD) according to spline estimated glomerular filtration rate (eGFR) *(upper panels)* and albumin-to-creatinine ratio *(lower panels),* adjusted for each other and for age, gender, and cardiovascular risk factors (continuous analyses). Reference categories are eGFR of 95 mL/min/1.73 m$^2$ and albumin-to-creatinine ratio of 5 mg/g or dipstick negative or trace. *(Left panels)* Results for general population cohorts. *(Right panels)* High-risk cohorts. Dots represent statistical significance, triangles represent nonsignificance, and shaded areas are 95% confidence interval. *ACR,* Albumin-to-creatinine ratio; *GP,* general population; *HR,* high risk. (From Gansevoort RT, Matsushita K, van der Velde M, et al. Chronic Kidney Disease Prognosis Consortium: lower estimated GFR and higher albuminuria are associated with adverse kidney outcomes in both general and high-risk populations. A collaborative meta-analysis of general and high-risk population cohorts. *Kidney Int.* 2011;79:1341–1352.)

of ESKD (and mortality), suggesting that a GFR decline of 30% may be useful as a surrogate marker of CKD progression in clinical trials.[77] Thus, in different contexts, acquired nephron deficit may be regarded as a susceptibility factor (e.g., after donor nephrectomy in a healthy kidney donor), initiation factor (when severe nephron loss provokes glomerulosclerosis in remaining previously normal glomeruli), or progression factor (when nephron loss accelerates preexisting damage in remaining glomeruli).

The importance of GFR as a risk factor has emphasized the need for more accurate methods to estimate it. Adoption of the MDRD equation improved detection of CKD and made possible much of the epidemiologic research on CKD, but it was recognized from the outset that the MDRD equation was imperfect and, in particular, tended to underestimate true GFR at values >60 mL/min/1.73 $m^2$. This is important because this is the threshold below which CKD may be diagnosed without other evidence of kidney damage. Several other equations have been developed to estimate GFR from serum creatinine concentration, culminating in a recommendation by KDIGO that the MDRD equation should be replaced by the Chronic Kidney Disease Epidemiology Collaboration (CKD-EPI) equation, which is more accurate than the MDRD equation and results in less bias, particularly at GFR values >60 mL/min/1.73 $m^2$. Further analysis by the CKD Prognosis Consortium found that the eGFR determined by the CKD-EPI equation results in a lower prevalence of CKD stages 3 to 5 (8.7% vs. 6.3%) and affords better risk prediction than the MDRD equation. Among those classified as having an eGFR of 59 to 45 mL/min/1.73 $m^2$ by the MDRD equation, 34.7% were reclassified by the CKD-EPI as having an eGFR of 89 to 60 mL/min/1.73 $m^2$, and those reclassified had a lower incidence of adverse outcomes versus those not reclassified (e.g., incidence of all-cause mortality 9.9 vs. 34.5/1000 person-years).[78]

The limitations of creatinine as a marker of GFR due to nonrenal factors that affect serum creatinine concentration, including muscle mass and diet, have prompted a search for alternatives. Cystatin C, a peptide produced by all nucleated cells and therefore not affected by muscle mass, has emerged as the most promising alternative. The production of reference material to standardize cystatin C assays has greatly improved the potential for clinical application, and equations have been developed to estimate the GFR from the serum cystatin C concentration or from creatinine and cystatin C levels together. The combined equation and CKD-EPI (creatinine) equation have similar bias, but the combined equation yields better precision and accuracy.[79] Further work by the CKD Prognosis Consortium has reported that when cystatin C is used to estimate GFR, reclassification to a higher GFR category (higher than that assigned by eGFR creatinine) is associated with a lower risk of all-cause mortality, cardiovascular mortality, and ESKD.[80] It should be noted, however, that in this analysis, CKD was defined by a single eGFR value. In one analysis that included 1741 persons with CKD recruited from primary care on the basis of two abnormal eGFR results, the use of cystatin C resulted in reclassification of only 7.7% as not having CKD and a large proportion (59%) were reclassified as having a more advanced stage of CKD with no improvement in risk prediction.[81] Further studies are warranted to further evaluate the potential benefits of using cystatin C for estimating GFR.

## ACUTE KIDNEY INJURY

Despite previous perceptions that patients who recover from acute kidney injury (AKI) regain normal renal function and have a good prognosis, several cohort studies have reported that recovery from AKI is associated with a substantially increased risk of CKD and death. Among 3769 adults who required dialysis for AKI and survived dialysis free for at least 30 days, the incidence rate for chronic dialysis was 2.63/100 versus 0.91/100 person-years in 13,598 matched controls (adjusted HR, 3.23; 95% CI, 2.70 to 3.86).[82] The relative risk was particularly high for those with no previous diagnosis of CKD (adjusted HR, 15.54; 95% CI, 9.65 to 25.03). There was no difference in survival between the groups. In another study of similar design, outcomes were investigated in 343 patients with a preadmission eGFR > 45 mL/min/1.73 $m^2$ who required dialysis for AKI but survived for at least 30 days after discharge without dialysis. After controlling for potential confounders, AKI that required dialysis was associated with a 28-fold increase in the risk of developing CKD stage 4 or 5 (adjusted HR, 28.1; 95% CI, 21.1 to 37.6) and more than double the risk of death (adjusted HR, 2.3; 95% CI, 1.8 to 3.0) versus 555,660 adult patients hospitalized during the same period but without AKI.[83]

Analysis of data from a cohort of 233,803 Medicare beneficiaries 67 years or older who were hospitalized in 2000 reported a substantially increased risk of developing ESKD in those who developed AKI on a background of CKD (HR, 41.2; 95% CI, 34.6 to 49.1) or without previous CKD (HR, 13.0; 95% CI, 10.6 to 16.0) versus those who did not develop AKI. The importance of AKI as a risk factor for CKD initiation was further illustrated by the observation that among patients who had AKI without preexisting CKD ($N = 4730$), 72.1% developed CKD within 2 years of the AKI episode. Furthermore, 25.2% of those who developed ESKD had a history of AKI.[84] In a similar study, a cohort of 113,272 patients hospitalized with a primary diagnosis of acute tubular necrosis (ATN), AKI, pneumonia, or myocardial infarction (control group) was studied. Overall, 11.4% progressed to CKD stage 4 during follow-up, including 20.0% of those with ATN, 13.2% of those with AKI, 24.7% of those with preexisting CKD, and 3.3% of the control patients. After controlling for other variables, having a diagnosis of AKI, ATN, or CKD increased the risk of developing CKD stage 4 by 303%, 564%, and 550%, respectively, versus controls. After controlling for covariates, AKI and CKD were associated with an increased risk of death of 12% and 20%, respectively, versus controls.[85]

The multiplicative effect of AKI on CKD progression is further illustrated by a study of 39,805 patients with an eGFR < 45 mL/min/1.73 $m^2$ prior to hospitalization. Those who survived an episode of dialysis-requiring AKI had a very high risk of developing ESKD within 30 days of hospital discharge (i.e., nonrecovery of AKI) that was related to the preadmission eGFR. For an eGFR of 30 to 44 mL/min/1.73 $m^2$, the incidence of ESKD was 42%, and for an eGFR of 15 to 29 mL/min/1.73 $m^2$, it was as high as 63%, whereas the incidence of ESKD was only 1.5% in those who did not have dialysis-requiring AKI. In patients who survived longer than 30 days after hospital discharge without ESKD, the incidence of ESKD and death at 6 months was 12.7% and 19.7%, respectively, versus 1.7% and 7.4% in the comparator group with CKD but no AKI. After adjustment for multiple risk factors, AKI was associated with a 30% increase in long-term risk for death or ESKD (adjusted HR, 1.30; 95% CI, 1.04 to 1.64).[86]

Consistent with the findings of individual studies, a meta-analysis of 13 cohort studies reported a significantly increased risk of developing CKD and ESKD in patients who had survived an episode of AKI versus participants without AKI (pooled adjusted HR for CKD, 8.8; 95% CI, 3.1 to 25.5; pooled HR for ESKD, 3.1; 95% CI, 1.9 to 5.0).[87] Taken together, these data show that AKI should be regarded as an important risk factor for CKD initiation and progression. The mechanisms responsible for these observations require further elucidation, but have been proposed to include nephron loss, loss of peritubular capillaries, cell cycle arrest, cell senescence, pericyte and myofibroblast activation, fibrogenic cytokine production, and interstitial fibrosis.[88,89]

The incidence of AKI has increased, and it is likely to become an increasingly important risk factor for CKD among older patients.

## HYPERTENSION

Hypertension, which is defined as an increased systolic blood pressure >140 mm Hg and/or diastolic blood pressure >90 mm Hg, or the need for pharmacologic therapy to achieve BP targets, is an almost universal consequence of reduced renal function.[90] From a CKD-focused standpoint, this is due to sodium retention, hypervolemia, and neurohormonal activation associated with progressive decrease in GFR.[91–93] However, hypertension itself is also known to be an important factor in the progression of CKD toward ESKD. In the hypothesis of CKD progression presented in Fig. 20.1, it is clear that elevated systemic blood pressure transmitted to the glomerulus would contribute to glomerular hypertension and thus accelerate glomerular damage. Hypertension has been shown to be predictive of ESKD risk in several large population-based studies.[20,21,28,94] Furthermore, a close association between the magnitude of increased risk and level of blood pressure has been reported in several studies, so that even elevations in blood pressure below the threshold for the diagnosis of hypertension were associated with increased risk of ESKD.[20,28,95]

Among patients with CKD in the MDRD study, higher baseline mean arterial pressure (MAP) independently predicted a greater rate of GFR decline.[10] These observations have led to the suggestion that blood pressure be viewed as a continuous rather than dichotomous risk factor for CKD, with less emphasis on traditional definitions of hypertension and normotension.[96] Whereas the primary analysis of data from the MDRD study found no significant difference between the rate of decline in GFR between patients randomized to intensive blood pressure control (target MAP < 92 mm Hg, equivalent to <125/75 mm Hg) and standard blood pressure control (target MAP < 107 mm Hg, equivalent to 140/90 mm Hg), a secondary analysis did show benefit associated with the low blood pressure target in patients with higher levels of baseline proteinuria.[97] Further secondary analysis showed that the lower achieved blood pressure was also associated with a slower GFR decline, an effect that was more marked in patients with higher baseline proteinuria.[98] Thus the MDRD study results suggest a significant interaction between blood pressure and proteinuria as risk factors for CKD progression.

The Systolic Blood Pressure Intervention Trial, which randomized >9000 subjects, including about one-third with nondiabetic CKD, was able to determine that targeting systolic blood pressure of <120 mm Hg, as compared with <140 mm Hg, in high-risk CVD patients without diabetes resulted in fewer fatal and nonfatal CVEs and death.[99] A subgroup analysis of the 2646 participants with CKD showed no difference in the primary renal outcome of ≥50% decline in GFR or ESKD, though there was a greater decrease in GFR after 6 months (−0.47 versus −0.32 mL/min/1.73 $m^2$ per year) associated with the lower BP target. The risks of all-cause mortality (HR, 0.72; 95% CI, 0.53 to 0.99) and CVE (HR, 0.81; 95% CI, 0.63 to 1.05) were lower in the low BP target group and there was no overall increase in serious adverse events, though AKI, hypokalemia, and hyperkalemia were increased in the low BP target group.[100] In the HALT Progression of Polycystic Kidney Disease (HALT-PKD) study, targeting of a blood pressure of ≤120/70 mm Hg in patients with autosomal dominant polycystic kidney disease (ADPKD) through use of lisinopril and telmisartan allowed for a slower increase in total kidney volume, no overall change in eGFR, a greater decline in left ventricular mass index, and a greater reduction in albuminuria.[101]

Taken together, there is convincing evidence that elevated blood pressure is an important risk factor for progression of CKD, although unequivocal evidence from randomized controlled trials is lacking, and some uncertainty remains regarding optimal treatment targets.

## OBESITY AND METABOLIC SYNDROME

In experimental models, obesity is associated with hypertension, proteinuria, and progressive renal disease. Micropuncture studies have confirmed that obesity is another cause of glomerular hyperfiltration and glomerular hypertension that can be predicted to exacerbate the progression of CKD.[102,103] Furthermore, several other factors associated with obesity and the metabolic syndrome may contribute to renal damage, including hormones and proinflammatory molecules produced by adipocytes,[104] increased mineralocorticoid levels and/or mineralocorticoid receptor activation by cortisol,[105] and reduced adiponectin levels.[106] In humans, severe obesity is associated with increased renal plasma flow, glomerular hyperfiltration, and albuminuria, abnormalities that are reversed by weight loss.[107] Obesity, as defined by increased body mass index (BMI), has been associated with increased risk of developing CKD in several large population-based studies.[21,108,109] Furthermore, one study has found a progressive increase in relative risk of developing ESKD associated with increasing BMI (relative risk, 3.57; 95% CI, 3.05 to 4.18 for BMI of 30.0 to 34.9 kg/$m^2$ vs. BMI of 18.5 to 24.9 kg/$m^3$) among 320,252 subjects confirmed to have no evidence of CKD at initial screening.[110]

There is evidence that obesity may directly cause a specific form of glomerulopathy characterized by proteinuria and histologic features of focal and segmental glomerulosclerosis,[111,112] but it is likely that it also acts as a risk factor in the development of several other forms of renal disease. One study has identified childhood obesity as a risk factor for CKD in adulthood. Among 4340 participants born in one week in 1946, pubertal-onset obesity and obesity throughout childhood were associated with an increased risk of CKD (defined by eGFR < 60 mL/min/1.73 $m^2$ or albuminuria) at age 60 to 64 years.[113] Interest has also focused on the role of the metabolic syndrome (insulin resistance), as defined by the presence of abdominal obesity, dyslipidemia, hypertension, and fasting hyperglycemia, in the development of CKD. An analysis of data from the Third National Health and Nutrition Examination Survey (NHANES III) data found a significantly increased risk of CKD and microalbuminuria in subjects with the metabolic syndrome as well as a progressive increase in risk associated with the number of components of the metabolic syndrome present.[114] Furthermore, a large longitudinal study of 10,096 patients without diabetes or CKD at baseline identified metabolic syndrome as an independent risk factor for the development of CKD over 9 years (adjusted OR, 1.43; 95% CI, 1.18 to 1.73). Again, there was a progressive increase in risk associated with the number of traits of the metabolic syndrome present (OR, 1.13; 95% CI, 0.89 to 1.45 for one trait vs. OR, 2.45; 95% CI, 1.32 to 4.54 for five traits).[115] In another study, patient hip-to-waist ratio, a marker of insulin resistance, was independently associated with impaired renal function, even in lean individuals (BMI < 25 kg/$m^3$), among a population-based cohort of 7676 subjects.[116]

It is widely recognized that weight loss is difficult to achieve in obese individuals, but surgical intervention in the form of gastric banding or bypass appears to offer the most effective long-term outcomes. Beneficial renoprotective effects of weight loss have been reported in a meta-analysis of observational studies that found an association between weight loss and reduction in proteinuria independent of blood pressure,[117] as well as smaller studies that reported improvement or stabilization of renal function[118] or reduction in proteinuria[119] following bariatric surgery in subjects with CKD.

The best method for assessing obesity in CKD remains to be determined. A further systematic review analyzed the effects of weight loss achieved by bariatric surgery, medication, or diet in 31 studies and found that in most studies, weight loss was associated with reductions in proteinuria. In people with glomerular hyperfiltration, the GFR tended to decrease with weight loss, and in those with a reduced GFR, it tended to increase.[120] BMI is the most widely applied method but does not take body composition into account. One study has reported a high sensitivity but relatively low specificity of BMI to detect obesity in subjects with CKD.[121]

## HIGH DIETARY PROTEIN INTAKE

Consistent with the hypothesis that the glomerular hemodynamic changes associated with hyperfiltration accelerate glomerular injury, experimental studies have reported that a high-protein diet accelerates renal disease progression, whereas dietary protein restriction[122,123] results in normalization of glomerular capillary hydraulic pressure as well as SNGFR and marked attenuation of glomerular damage.[57] Observational studies in humans have reported an increased risk of microalbuminuria associated with higher dietary protein intake in subjects with diabetes and hypertension (OR, 3.3; 95% CI, 1.4 to 7.8), but not in healthy subjects or those with isolated diabetes or hypertension,[124] again illustrating the interaction between risk factors for CKD. In another study, high intake of protein, particularly nondairy animal protein, was associated with a greater rate of GFR decline among women with an eGFR of 80 to 55 mL/min/1.73 $m^2$ but not in those with an eGFR of >80 mL/min/1.73 $m^2$.[125] Randomized trials investigating the effects of high-protein diet are lacking, but several studies have sought to examine the potential renoprotective effects of dietary protein restriction. In the MDRD study, primary analysis revealed no significant difference in the mean rate of GFR decline in subjects randomized to low- or very-low-protein diets,[97] but secondary analysis of outcomes according to achieved dietary protein intake indicated that a reduction in protein intake of 0.2 g/kg/day correlated with a 1.15-mL/min/year reduction in the rate of GFR decline, equivalent to a 29% reduction in the mean rate of GFR decline.[126] By contrast, long-term follow-up of participants in study 2 of the MDRD trial found no renoprotective benefit among those randomized to very-low-protein diet in the original study, but did report a higher risk of death in this group (HR, 1.92; 95% CI, 1.15 to 3.20).[127] As such, dietary protein restriction cannot be routinely recommended for patients with CKD. Additional discussion on the role of dietary protein restriction in the management of CKD is available in Chapters 51 and 60.

## PREGNANCY AND PREECLAMPSIA

Physiologic adaptations during pregnancy provoke glomerular hyperfiltration that usually does not cause renal damage. In the context of preexisting CKD, however, the glomerular hyperfiltration of pregnancy can be predicted to exacerbate proteinuria and glomerular injury. Several studies have shown an increased risk of CKD progression during pregnancy, particularly when the pregestational serum creatinine is ≥1.4 mg/dL (≥124 μmol/L). In one study of 82 pregnancies in 67 women with primary renal disease and serum creatinine level of ≥1.4 mg/dL, blood pressure, serum creatinine, and proteinuria increased during pregnancy. In 70 pregnancies with postpartum data available, persistent loss of maternal renal function at 6 months was reported in 31%, and by 12 months eight women had progressed to ESKD. Adverse obstetric outcomes included preterm delivery in 59% and low birth weight in 37%, although fetal survival was 93%.[128]

In a more recent series of 49 women with CKD stage 3 to 5 before pregnancy, the mean GFR declined during pregnancy (from 35 ± 12.2 to 30 ± 13.8 mL/min/1.73 $m^2$), but there was no change in the mean postpartum rate of GFR decline. Nevertheless, a pregestational GFR < 40 mL/min/1.73 $m^2$, combined with proteinuria of >1 g/day, was associated with a more rapid postpartum GFR decline and a shorter time to ESKD or halving of GFR and low birth weight.[129] Although earlier reports suggested good outcomes, one recent study has reported adverse effects associated even with early stage CKD. In 91 pregnancies with predominantly CKD stages 1 and 2, modest increases in hypertension, serum creatinine, and proteinuria were observed.[130] An increase in adverse obstetric outcomes, including preterm delivery, lower birth weight, and admission to a neonatal intensive care unit versus low-risk pregnancy controls was also reported; this remained true, even when only those with CKD stage 1 were considered, although there were no perinatal deaths. By contrast, pregnancy was not associated with a more rapid decline in the GFR over 5 years in a cohort of 245 women of childbearing age with IgA nephropathy and serum creatinine level of ≤1.2 mg/dL (in the majority).[131]

Complications of pregnancy and, in particular, hypertension and preeclampsia, may also cause renal damage. In one large population-based study, renal outcomes were assessed in 570,433 women who had had at least one singleton pregnancy. Only 477 women developed ESKD at a mean of 17 ± 9 years after the first pregnancy (overall rate, 3.7/100,000 women/year), but preeclampsia was associated with a significant increase in the risk of ESKD, ranging from a relative risk of 4.7 for preeclampsia in a single pregnancy (95% CI, 3.6 to 6.1) to a relative risk of 15.5 for preeclampsia in two or three pregnancies (95% CI, 7.8 to 30.8). The risk was further increased if the pregnancy resulted in a low-birth-weight or preterm infant. Causes of ESKD were glomerulonephritis in 35%, hereditary or congenital disease in 21%, diabetic nephropathy in 14%, and interstitial nephritis in 12%.[132] Similarly, in women with diabetes prior to pregnancy, preeclampsia and preterm birth were associated with significantly increased risks of ESKD and death, illustrating how different risk factors for CKD may interact to increase risk.[133]

A large cohort study reported an increased risk of multiple adverse health outcomes after hypertension during pregnancy, including CVD, DM, and CKD (HR, 1.91; 95% CI, 1.18 to 3.09).[134] Similarly, a very large case–control study found that hypertension during pregnancy was associated with a substantially increased risk of subsequent CKD (HR, 9.38; 95% CI, 7.09 to 12.4) or ESKD (HR, 12.4; 95% CI, 8.53 to 18.0).[135] In both these studies, the risks of CKD were substantially higher if preeclampsia developed during the pregnancy. Possible explanations for these observations include the presence of pathogenic factors common to CKD and preeclampsia, including obesity, hypertension, insulin resistance, and endothelial dysfunction; exacerbation by preeclampsia of preexisting subclinical CKD; and effects of preeclampsia on the kidney that increase the risk of CKD later in life.[136] That preeclampsia may provoke renal damage has been suggested by several studies showing an increased incidence of microalbuminuria after preeclampsia. A meta-analysis of seven of these studies reported a 31% prevalence of microalbuminuria at a weighted mean of 7.1 years after preeclampsia versus 7% in a control group with uncomplicated pregnancies.[137] Further research is required to identify which mechanisms are most relevant but, even without further information, preeclampsia should be regarded as a risk factor for the development and progression of CKD.

## MULTISYSTEM DISORDERS

### DIABETES MELLITUS

Diabetic nephropathy has rapidly become the single most common cause of ESKD worldwide. Diabetes was associated with a substantially increased risk of ESKD or death associated with CKD in one population-based study of 23,534 subjects (HR, 7.5; 95% CI, 4.8 to 11.7),[28] as well as an increased risk of moderate CKD (estimated creatinine clearance < 50 mL/min) in another study of 1428 subjects with an estimated creatinine clearance of >70 mL/min at baseline.[138] Evidence that glycemic control is a key risk factor for the development of diabetic nephropathy has been shown in randomized trials that found a reduced risk of developing nephropathy in subjects with type 1[139] and type 2[140] diabetes randomized to tight glycemic control. The pathogenesis of diabetic nephropathy is complex and involves multiple mechanisms, including glomerular hemodynamic factors,[58,141] advanced glycation end product formation, generation of reactive oxygen species, and upregulation of profibrotic growth factors and cytokines.[142,143] In at least one study, diabetic nephropathy was associated with more rapid progression to ESKD than other causes of CKD.[29,144,145] Thus diabetes may be regarded as a susceptibility, initiation, and progression risk factor for CKD. For further discussion of the pathogenesis of diabetic nephropathy, see Chapter 39.

## PRIMARY RENAL DISEASE

Whereas substantial variation in the rate of GFR decline has been observed among subjects with a common cause of CKD, there is also evidence that some forms of CKD may provoke more rapid progression than others. In the MDRD study[10] and the Chronic Renal Insufficiency Standards Implementation Study (CRISIS),[144] a diagnosis of ADPKD was an independent predictor of a greater rate of GFR decline. In several cohort studies, diabetic nephropathy was associated with shorter time to ESKD[29] or a more rapid GFR decline than other diagnoses.[144,145]

## CARDIORENAL SYNDROME

Multiple studies have reported that CKD is associated with a substantial increase in the risk of CVD,[146] and it is therefore not surprising that CVD is also associated with an increased risk of CKD. Among hospitalized Medicare beneficiaries, the prevalence of CKD stage 3 or worse was 60.4% for those with heart failure and 51.7% for those with myocardial infarction. The presence of CKD in addition to heart disease was associated with a significantly increased risk of death and progression to ESKD.[147] These observations may in part be explained by the fact that CVD and CKD share many risk factors, including obesity, metabolic syndrome, hypertension, DM, dyslipidemia, and smoking. In addition, CVD may exert effects on the kidneys that promote the initiation and progression of CKD, including decreased renal perfusion in heart failure and atherosclerosis of the renal arteries. This is a phenomenon known as cardiorenal syndrome (CRS), which is an acute or chronic dysfunction in one organ system leading to dysfunction in the other, specifically in the cardiovascular and renal systems. Mechanisms that lead to the development of CRS include neurohormonal activation, altered renal blood flow, renal congestion, and right ventricular dysfunction.[148] A typical example of CRS is seen in renal atherosclerosis, which was detected in 39% of patients (≥70% stenosis in 7.3%) undergoing elective coronary angiography.[149] Furthermore, arterial stiffness may result in greater transmission of an elevated systemic blood pressure to glomerular capillaries and exacerbate glomerular hypertension. In one study, pulse wave velocity (PWV) and augmentation index (AI), markers of arterial stiffness, were identified as independent risk factors for progression to ESKD among subjects with CKD stage 4 or 5[150]; in another study, AI was an independent determinant of rate of creatinine clearance decline among subjects with CKD stage 3.[151] By contrast, neither PWV nor AI was a predictor of the rate of GFR decline in a cohort of subjects with CKD stages 2 to 4.[152] In two relatively small cohort studies of those with CKD, a diagnosis of CVD was associated with an increased risk of progression to ESKD[153,154] but, in the CRIC study, a history of any CVD at baseline was not associated with an increased risk of the primary endpoint of ESKD or 50% GFR reduction among 3939 participants. Conversely, in the same study, a history of heart failure was independently associated with a 29% higher risk of the primary outcome.[155] For further discussion of CVD in patients with CKD, see Chapter 54.

## CONVENTIONAL BIOMARKERS

Biomarkers are parameters that are measured and evaluated to differentiate between normal and abnormal biological processes or predict adverse outcomes. For CKD, biomarkers may be considered a reflection of renal function impairment. Some of the standard biomarkers indicated in CKD progression include proteinuria and several routine serum biomarkers that are essential for evaluation of persons with reduced GFR.[99] The more novel biomarkers, which will be further discussed in Chapter 27, are serum and urinary substances that allow for more targeted risk prediction in CKD.[148]

### PROTEINURIA

Proteinuria is an indicator of dysfunction in the glomerular filtration barrier and is therefore a marker of glomerulopathy and an index of disease severity. Proteinuria is often a result of glomerular injury and is associated with hyperfiltration, intraglomerular hypertension, glomerular hypertrophy, and glomerulosclerosis.[148] Experimental evidence has suggested that proteinuria may also contribute to progressive renal damage in CKD (see Chapter 30). A large body of evidence attests to a strong association between proteinuria and the risk of CKD progression, a relationship mediated through several mechanisms including tubular injury, inflammation, and fibrosis, as well as cardiovascular and all-cause mortality. Mass screening of a general population of 107,192 participants by dipstick urinalysis identified proteinuria as the most powerful predictor of ESKD risk over 10 years (OR, 14.9; 95% CI, 10.9 to 20.2).[20]

Similarly, among 12,866 middle-aged men enrolled in the Multiple Risk Factor Intervention Trial (MRFIT), proteinuria detected by dipstick test was associated with a significantly increased risk of developing ESKD over 25 years (HR for 1+ proteinuria, 3.1; 95% CI, 1.8 to 3.8; HR for ≥2+ proteinuria, 15.7; 95% CI, 10.3 to 23.9). Furthermore, detection of 2+ proteinuria or more increased the hazard ratio for ESKD associated with an eGFR < 60 mL/min/1.73 $m^2$ from 2.4 without proteinuria (95% CI, 1.5 to 3.8) to 41 with proteinuria (95% CI, 15.2 to 71.1).[156] Similar associations have been reported for measurements of urinary albumin in the general population. In the Nord-Trøndelag Health (HUNT 2) study, which included 65,589 adults, microalbuminuria and macroalbuminuria were independent predictors of ESKD after 10.3 years (HR, 13.0 and 47.2, respectively) and combining reduced eGFR with albuminuria substantially improved the prediction of ESKD.[157]

Among patients selected for having CKD from a wide variety of causes, baseline proteinuria has consistently predicted renal outcomes.[158–160] In three large prospective studies that included patients with nondiabetic CKD [MDRD study, Ramipril Efficacy In Nephropathy (REIN) study, and AASK], higher baseline proteinuria was strongly associated with a more rapid decline in GFR.[10,98,161,162] Similarly, among patients with diabetic nephropathy, the baseline urinary albumin-to-creatinine ratio (ACR) was a strong independent predictor of ESKD in the Reduction of Endpoints in NIDDM with the Angiotensin II Antagonist Losartan (RENAAL) study and Irbesartan in Diabetic Nephropathy Trial (IDNT).[163,164] The findings of these individual studies have been confirmed by two large meta-analyses. In one analysis, which included nine general population cohorts ($N$ = 845,125) and eight cohorts with increased risk of developing CKD ($N$ = 173,892), urine ACRs of >30, 300, and 1000 mg/g were independently associated with progressive increases in the risk of ESKD, progressive CKD, and AKI, respectively (Fig. 20.4).[73] Among 21,688 patients known to have CKD from 13 studies, an eightfold higher urine ACR or protein-to-creatinine ratio (PCR) was associated with increased all-cause mortality (pooled HR, 1.40) and risk of ESKD (pooled HR, 3.04).[74] Further meta-analyses by the CKD Prognosis Consortium have shown that the magnitude of proteinuria remains a risk factor for ESKD independent of gender,[33] ethnicity,[44] age,[27] diabetes,[75] or hypertension.[76]

Recognition of the importance of proteinuria as a risk factor in CKD prompted the addition of an albuminuria category (A1 to A3) to the CKD classification proposed by KDIGO.[9] These important observations raise the question of how best to measure proteinuria. As discussed, all measurements of proteinuria have been reported to predict renal outcomes, including dipstick urinalysis, spot urine ACR, or PCR, ideally using the patient's first morning voids or, less frequently, using 24-hour urine collections. A secondary analysis of data from the RENAAL trial found that urine ACR measured on the first morning void was better than 24-hour urinary protein or albumin concentration as a predictor of time to doubling of the serum creatinine level or ESKD among patients with diabetes and CKD.[165] By contrast, retrospective analysis of data from 5586 patients with CKD reported similar HRs associated with urinary ACR and PCR for the outcomes of all-cause mortality, start of RRT, or doubling of serum creatinine.[166] Further analysis of these data identified a cohort of patients with a normal urine ACR, but elevated urine PCR in whom the risk of ESKD or death was intermediate between the groups with both urine ACR and PCR abnormal or normal.[167] Analysis of data from the CRIC study also reported that urine ACR and PCR had similar associations with complications of CKD.[168] Together, these data imply that any measure of proteinuria is better than no measurement. If the goal is to detect and monitor low levels of albuminuria (category A1 and A2), the urine ACR measured on the first morning void is best. For patients with CKD, urine ACR or PCR may be used, and there is some evidence that there may be added information gained by requesting both.[169]

### SERUM ALBUMIN

Serum albumin levels are widely regarded as a marker of nutritional status but may also be reduced due to proteinuria or inflammation. Several studies have identified lower serum albumin levels as a risk factor for CKD progression. In the MDRD study, higher baseline serum albumin was associated with slower subsequent rate of GFR decline but, in a multivariable analysis, this was displaced by a similar correlation with baseline serum transferrin levels, another marker of protein nutrition.[10] Three studies have found associations between serum albumin and renal outcomes in patients with type 2 diabetes and CKD. Among 182 patients with a mean serum creatinine of 1.5 mg/dL at baseline, hypoalbuminemia was an independent risk factor for ESKD.[170] In a long-term follow-up of 343 patients, lower baseline serum albumin was an independent predictor of CKD progression and,[171] in the RENAAL study, lower serum albumin was an independent predictor of ESKD.[163] Similar observations have been reported in other forms of CKD. In a large cohort of patients with IgA nephropathy ($N$ = 2269), lower serum total protein (composed largely of albumin) was an independent risk factor for ESKD.[172] In these studies, the predictive value of serum albumin was independent of and additional to that of proteinuria, indicating that it was not merely acting as a marker of albuminuria.

## ANEMIA

Chronic anemia due to inherited hemoglobinopathy is associated with increased renal plasma flow, glomerular hyperfiltration, and subsequent development of proteinuria, hypertension, and ESKD.[173,174] Anemia is a common complication of CKD from any cause, and several studies have shown that it is also an independent predictor of CKD progression. In the RENAAL study, baseline hemoglobin was a significant independent predictor of ESKD among diabetic patients – each 1-g/dL decrease in hemoglobin was associated with an 11% increase in the risk of ESKD.[175] Baseline hemoglobin was also one of four variables included in the renal risk score developed from the RENAAL data.[163] Similarly, a higher hemoglobin level was independently associated with lower risk of progression to ESKD (halving of GFR or need for dialysis) or death among 131 patients with all forms of CKD (HR, 0.778; 95% CI, 0.639 to 0.948 for each 1-g/dL increase).[160] Furthermore, time-averaged hemoglobin of <12 g/dL was associated with a significantly increased risk of ESKD among 853 male veterans with CKD stages 3 to 5 (HR, 0.74; 95% CI, 0.65 to 0.84 for each 1-g/dL increase in hemoglobin).[176]

Consistent with the hypothesis that anemia contributes directly to CKD progression, two small randomized studies have reported a renoprotective benefit associated with erythropoietin therapy. Among patients with serum creatinine of 2 to 4 mg/dL and hematocrit < 30%, erythropoietin treatment was associated with significantly improved renal survival.[177] In nondiabetic patients with serum creatinine of 2 to 6 mg/dL, early treatment (started when hemoglobin < 11.6 g/dL) with erythropoietin alpha was associated with a 60% reduction in the risk of doubling the serum creatinine level, ESKD, or death versus delayed treatment (started when hemoglobin < 9.0 g/dL).[178] By contrast, two other studies that had left ventricular mass as their primary endpoint[179,180] and the Trial to Reduce Cardiovascular Events with Aranesp Therapy (TREAT)[181] found no effect of a high versus low hemoglobin target on the rate of decline in the GFR. Several studies have, however, reported adverse outcomes associated with normalization of hemoglobin in patients with CKD. In the Cardiovascular Risk Reduction by Early Anemia Treatment with Epoetin Beta (CREATE) study, randomization to a higher hemoglobin target (13 to 15 mg/dL) was associated with a shorter time to initiation of dialysis than a lower target (10.5 to 11.5 mg/dL).[182] In TREAT, randomization to a higher hemoglobin target was associated with an increased risk of stroke[181] and, in the Correction of Hemoglobin and Outcomes in Renal Insufficiency (CHOIR) study, a higher hemoglobin target was associated with an increased incidence of the combined endpoint of all-cause mortality, myocardial infarction, or hospitalization for congestive cardiac failure.[183]

## DYSLIPIDEMIA

Lipid abnormalities are common in patients with CKD, and several studies have identified dyslipidemia as a susceptibility and progression factor for CKD. In population-based studies, several lipid profile abnormalities have been associated with an increased risk of developing CKD, including an elevated low-density lipoprotein (LDL)–to–high-density lipoprotein (HDL) cholesterol ratio,[184] higher triglyceride and lower HDL cholesterol levels,[185] lower HDL cholesterol levels[21] and elevated total cholesterol, low HDL cholesterol, and elevated total cholesterol-to-HDL cholesterol ratio.[186] In the MDRD study, lower HDL cholesterol levels independently predicted a more rapid decline in GFR[10]; in a smaller study of patients with CKD, total cholesterol, LDL cholesterol, and apolipoprotein B levels were all associated with a more rapid decline in the GFR.[187] Among 223 patients with IgA nephropathy, hypertriglyceridemia was independently predictive of CKD progression.[188] Hypercholesterolemia was reported to predict loss of renal function in patients with type 1 or 2 diabetes[189,190] and, among nondiabetic patients, CKD advanced more rapidly in those with hypercholesterolemia and hypertriglyceridemia.[191]

Randomized controlled trials of lipid lowering have produced mixed results with respect to renal outcomes. Subgroup analysis of a prospective randomized trial of pravastatin treatment in patients with previous myocardial infarction found that pravastatin slowed the rate of decline in patients with an eGFR < 40 mL/min/1.73 $m^2$, an effect that was also more pronounced in those with proteinuria.[192] Similarly, in the Heart Protection Study, patients with previous CVD or diabetes randomized to simvastatin treatment had a smaller increase in serum creatinine than those who received placebo.[193] In a placebo-controlled, open-label study, atorvastatin treatment in patients with CKD, proteinuria, and hypercholesterolemia was associated with preservation of creatinine clearance, whereas it declined in those receiving placebo.[194] By contrast, lipid lowering with fibrates was not associated with renoprotection in two studies,[184,195] although one study did show a reduced incidence of microalbuminuria in patients with type 2 diabetes receiving fenofibrate.[196]

Analysis of data from a relatively small subgroup of studies with renal endpoints recorded in a meta-analysis found that statin therapy was associated with a reduction in proteinuria but with no improvement in creatinine clearance in participants with CKD.[197] Furthermore, analysis of data from 3939 participants in the CRIC study found no association between total or LDL cholesterol and the risk of ESKD or 50% reduction in eGFR. Indeed, among participants with proteinuria of <0.2 g/day, higher LDL and total cholesterol were associated with a lower risk of reaching this endpoint.[198] The Study of Heart and Renal Protection (SHARP) is the largest randomized controlled trial to investigate the cardiovascular and renoprotective effects of lipid lowering in CKD. Patients with CKD or undergoing dialysis were randomized to treatment with simvastatin and ezetimibe or placebo. In 6245 participants with CKD not requiring dialysis, treatment resulted in an average reduction in LDL cholesterol of 0.96 mmol/L but was not associated with a reduction in the primary outcome of ESKD or secondary outcome of ESKD or creatinine doubling.[199] Together, evidence that dyslipidemia is a risk factor for CKD progression remains mixed, with the most recent studies indicating no association. Mechanisms whereby dyslipidemia may contribute to CKD progression are discussed in Chapter 51.

### SERUM URIC ACID

Hyperuricemia is a common consequence of chronic renal failure and may also contribute to CKD progression. Most but not all population-based studies have identified hyperuricemia as an independent risk factor for the development of incident CKD. Similarly, most cohort studies that included people with CKD have identified a higher serum uric acid level as a risk factor for CKD progression. Possible mechanisms whereby hyperuricemia may contribute to CKD progression are exacerbation of glomerular hypertension,[200,201] endothelial dysfunction,[202,203] and proinflammatory effects.[204] By contrast, it is possible that an elevated uric acid concentration is acting as a marker of reduced kidney function or oxidative stress – uric acid is produced by xanthine oxidase, which also generates reactive oxygen species.

To date, only small studies investigating the effect of uric acid–lowering therapy on CKD progression have been published. A meta-analysis of eight trials found no difference in the eGFR among participants treated with allopurinol versus those with no treatment or placebo in five trials, whereas three trials that reported only serum creatinine reported benefit in favor of allopurinol. In five trials that measured proteinuria, no benefit was observed.[205] Together, published evidence suggests that an elevated serum uric acid level may act as a susceptibility and progression risk factor in CKD, but large randomized trials are still required to determine whether treatment of hyperuricemia is beneficial for slowing CKD progression.

### METABOLIC ACIDOSIS

Metabolic acidosis commonly occurs in CKD patients and is the result of a decrease in functional nephron mass. As a result, there is a subsequent elevation of cortical ammonia levels, renin–angiotensin–aldosterone system activation, complement cascade activation, endothelial/aldosterone activation, inflammation, all of which lead to impaired renal acid clearance.[206] At least five studies have investigated metabolic acidosis as a risk factor in human CKD. In all except the MDRD study,[207] lower serum bicarbonate levels, even within the normal range, were independently associated with an increased risk of CKD progression.[208–211] Two small randomized trials have reported slowing of CKD progression with bicarbonate supplementation,[212,213] and another trial found that correction of acidosis with oral sodium bicarbonate or a diet rich in fruits and vegetables was associated with a lower rate of GFR decline.[214] Several randomized controlled trials have also indicated that correction of acidosis with bicarbonate supplementation has minimal sodium loading and impact on hypertension.[212,214] Bicarbonate supplementation is already recommended for patients with levels <22 mEq/L, but several studies are underway to investigate further whether it is beneficial in the setting of less severe acidosis.[215]

## NOVEL BIOMARKERS

### PLASMA ASYMMETRIC DIMETHYLARGININE

Asymmetric dimethylarginine (ADMA) is formed by the breakdown of arginine-methylated proteins and acts as an endogenous inhibitor of nitric oxide synthase to reduce nitric oxide production. The increased ADMA levels observed with a reduced GFR have been proposed as one mechanism for the endothelial dysfunction associated with CKD. Elevated ADMA levels are associated with CVD and cardiovascular mortality in patients with CKD.[216] In animal models, administration of ADMA was associated with the development of hypertension, increased deposition of collagen I and III and fibronectin in glomeruli and blood vessels, and rarefaction of peritubular capillaries.[217] Conversely, the overexpression of dimethylarginine dimethylaminohydrolase, the enzyme responsible for degradation of ADMA, was associated with reduced ADMA levels and amelioration of renal injury in rats after 5/6 nephrectomy, implying that ADMA may also promote CKD progression.[218]

Among 131 patients with CKD, a higher plasma ADMA level was an independent risk factor for ESKD or death (HR, 1.20; 95% CI, 1.07 to 1.35 for each 0.1-μmol/L increase).[160] In 227 relatively young patients with mild-to-moderate nondiabetic CKD, higher ADMA levels predicted progression to the combined endpoint of creatinine doubling or ESKD (HR, 1.47; 95% CI, 1.12 to 1.93 for each 0.1-μmol/L increase).[219] Finally, retrospective analysis of data from 109 patients with IgA nephropathy showed associations between ADMA levels and glomerular and tubulointerstitial injury. Furthermore, the plasma ADMA level was an independent determinant of annual GFR reduction rate.[220]

### SERUM PHOSPHATE AND FGF23

When rats were fed a high-phosphate diet after uninephrectomy, renal calcium and phosphate deposition, as well as tubulointerstitial injury, were observed within 5 weeks.[221] Furthermore, in animals and humans with CKD, dietary phosphate restriction or treatment with oral phosphate binders was associated with reductions in proteinuria and glomerulosclerosis and attenuation of CKD progression.[222–225] Together, these data suggest that phosphate loading and/or hyperphosphatemia exacerbate renal injury in CKD. Three cohort studies of patients with CKD have identified higher serum phosphate levels as an independent risk factor for progression.[208,226,227] By contrast, the largest study to date, which included 10,672 participants with CKD, found no independent association between higher serum phosphate and risk of progression.[228] It should be noted, however, that the number of ESKD events was low, and the study therefore had limited power to detect a moderate association between serum phosphate levels and CKD progression.[229] In addition, higher levels of the phosphatonin, fibroblast growth factor 23 (FGF23), which is a hormone involved in calcium and phosphate regulation through decreasing serum phosphate and 1,25-dihydroxyvitamin $D_3$, have been identified as an independent predictor of CKD progression.[230,231] Along with adverse renal effects, higher levels of FGF23 are associated with CVEs and related surrogate outcomes in patients with CKD.[232–234] In the CRIC study, higher levels of FGF23 were determined to be an independent risk factor for ESKD, but only in patients with a higher baseline eGFR (HR, 1.3; 95% CI, 1.04–1.6 if the eGFR was 30–44 mL/min/1.73 $m^2$; and HR, 1.7; 95% CI, 1.1–2.4 if the eGFR was >45 mL/min/1.73 $m^2$).[232] A recent meta-analysis confirmed the association between elevated FGF23 and CVE as well as all-cause mortality but suggested that the relationship was not causal due to lack of an exposure–response relationship.[234] Currently, the exact clinical significance of FGF23 is uncertain but there appears to be potential for its use as an important biomarker, specifically in CKD and ESRD patients.[148]

## NEUTROPHIL GELATINASE-ASSOCIATED LIPOCALIN

Neutrophil gelatinase-associated lipocalin (NGAL) is an iron-carrying protein expressed throughout the distal tubule epithelium and is overexpressed in response to AKI.[235] While it is known mostly for its role in AKI, the role of urinary NGAL in CKD progression is currently a point of interest in nephrology.[236] The Atherosclerosis Risk in Communities (ARIC) study found that baseline urinary NGAL was highest in those patients with incident CKD (OR, 2.1; 95% CI, 0.96–4.6).[237] In the CRIC study, urinary NGAL was determined to be an independent risk factor for ESRD (HR, 1.7; 95% CI, 1.2–2.5), but added no significant improvement in prediction of CKD progression beyond eGFR decline and proteinuria.[238]

## KIDNEY INJURY MOLECULE-1

Kidney injury molecule-1 (KIM-1) is a transmembrane glycoprotein typically undetected in a normal kidney, but is detected in patients with AKI and CKD.[239] One cohort study found that serum KIM-1 levels increased with the stage of CKD, and were predictive of eGFR decrease and ESRD.[240] The Multi-Ethnic Study of Atherosclerosis determined that doubling of urinary KIM-1 levels was associated with CKD and rapid eGFR decrease >3 mL/min/1.73 $m^2$ per year (OR, 1.2; 95% CI, 1.02–1.3).[241]

## SOLUBLE UROKINASE-TYPE PLASMINOGEN ACTIVATOR RECEPTOR

Soluble urokinase-type plasminogen activator receptor (suPAR) is a protein involved in cell adhesion and migration of endothelial and immune cells. Increased suPAR levels have been detected in patients with glomerular disease, specifically glomerulosclerosis, as well as adverse CVEs.[148] One study done by Hayek et al. using 2292 patients from the Emory Cardiovascular Bank found that higher baseline suPAR levels were associated with CKD (eGFR < 60 mL/min/1.73 $m^2$). This relationship was further validated using a sample of 347 patients in the Women's Interagency Human Immunodeficiency Virus Study, where again a higher baseline suPAR level was associated with greater incidence of CKD. Despite this, caution must be exercised because results may be misleading. For example, 30% of patients with an eGFR > 90 mL/min/1.73 $m^2$ also had an increase in baseline suPAR levels, indicating that levels may be linked to inflammation in addition to kidney function.[242] These results emphasize the need for further validation in other studies.

## UROMODULIN

Uromodulin (UMOD) is a kidney-specific glycoprotein synthesized by epithelial cells found in the ascending loop of Henle. While its exact function is currently unknown, one proposed role has been in protection against urinary tract infections, innate immunity activation, and kidney stone prevention. GWASs indicated that single-nucleotide polymorphism (SNP) variants of the *UMOD* gene were associated with a decrease in eGFR and development of CKD in European cohorts.[243,244] One GWAS using 3203 Icelandic patients with CKD found an association between CKD and creatinine with a variant adjacent to the *UMOD* gene on chromosome 16p12, which was strengthened with age. For clinical purposes, however, there have been conflicting results with regard to the use of UMOD as a biomarker in CKD progression. A meta-analysis of GWAS for UMOD including six studies and 10,884 patients found that two loci located around the *UMOD* gene were associated with increased UMOD levels.[245] However, Shlipak et al. found that among 879 individuals of the Heart and Soul Study, UMOD SNP variants influenced UMOD levels, but did not affect incident CKD risk.[246] These conflicting results indicate that further investigation is required before clinical implementation of UMOD as a CKD biomarker.[148]

## PROTEOMIC APPROACHES

Proteomics assess low-molecular-weight proteins using electrophoresis and mass spectrophotometry in both targeted (known pathophysiology) and nontargeted (unknown pathophysiology) approaches.[247] However, this approach poses several challenges given biosampling variability due to age, sex, diet, exercise, and other limitations. Using proteomics in a Scottish cohort with type II DM, investigators for the Innovative Diabetes Tools study were able to identify at least 62 of 207 serum protein biomarkers that were associated with rapid progression of CKD (>40% baseline eGFR loss in 3.5 years). The use of a 14-biomarker panel (including FGF23 and KIM-1) in risk prediction models allowed for an increase in the area under the receiver operating characteristic curve (AUROC) from 0.706 to 0.868.[248] Another study, which used capillary electrophoresis with mass spectrophotometry, looked at the utility of urinary proteomics in validating previously established biomarkers of CKD. The study used a general population cohort of 223 healthy individuals and 1767 patients with CKD (defined as eGFR < 90 mL/min/1.73 $m^2$ or urine albumin excretion > 30 mg/L), finding that the proteome performed better in detection and prediction of CKD progression, improving the AUROC based on baseline eGFR and albuminuria from 0.758 to 0.83.[249] The use of novel serum or urinary biomarkers will likely be of value in the future risk prediction models through enhancing discrimination beyond traditional risk predictors including GFR and proteinuria. Given the interplaying mechanisms that may result in any given patients with CKD, it is unlikely that any one single novel biomarker will have a large effect on risk prediction models. However, the development of biomarker panels through the use of proteomics shows potential in discriminating between disease and nondisease states as well as risk prediction, and its future role in the clinical setting is promising.[148]

### OTHER BIOMARKERS

A number of other biomarkers are currently being investigated as risk factors in CKD. Although many have been reported to be associated with adverse outcomes, the challenge is to identify biomarkers that add to the predictive power of established risk factors. For a detailed review of biomarkers in kidney disease, see Chapter 27.

## ENVIRONMENTAL RISK FACTORS

### SMOKING

Population-based studies have identified cigarette smoking as an independent risk factor for various manifestations of CKD, including proteinuria,[250] elevated serum creatinine levels,[251] decreased eGFR,[21,252] and development of ESKD or death associated with CKD (HR, 2.6; 95% CI, 1.8 to 3.7).[28] In the latter study, 31% of the attributable risk of CKD was associated with smoking. In a longitudinal study of 10,118 middle-aged Japanese workers, smoking was associated with an increased risk of developing glomerular hyperfiltration (eGFR ≥ 117 mL/min/1.73 m$^2$; OR, 1.32 vs. nonsmokers) as well as proteinuria (OR, 1.51 vs. nonsmokers).[253] Two other similar longitudinal studies from Japan have confirmed that smoking is associated with an increased risk of developing proteinuria but with a higher mean eGFR than in nonsmokers.[254,255] In one study, smoking was associated with a reduced risk of developing CKD stage 3.[255] Smoking has been shown to increase the risk of progression of CKD due to diabetes,[256,257] hypertensive nephropathy,[258] glomerulonephritis,[259] lupus nephritis,[260] IgA nephropathy,[261] and adult PKD.[261] Randomized trials of the effect of smoking cessation on CKD progression are lacking but, in one observational study, smoking cessation was associated with less progression to macroalbuminuria and a slower rate of GFR decline than continued smoking in patients with diabetes.[262] Similarly, in the CRIC study, nonsmoking was associated with a reduced risk of CKD progression (HR, 0.68; 95% CI, 0.55 to 0.84), atherosclerotic CVEs (HR, 0.55; 95% CI, 0.40 to 0.75), and mortality (HR, 0.45; 95% CI, 0.34 to 0.60).[263] Among 9270 participants with CKD in the SHARP, current smoking was associated with an increased risk of all-cause mortality, CVE, and cancer but was not associated with risk of ESRD or rate of GFR decline in 6245 participants not receiving dialysis at baseline.[264] Possible mechanisms whereby cigarette smoking may contribute to renal damage include sympathetic nervous system activation, glomerular capillary hypertension, endothelial cell injury, and direct tubulotoxocity.[265]

### ALCOHOL

The role of alcohol consumption as a potential risk factor for CKD remains unclear. One case–control study found a significant association between ESKD and consumption of more than two alcoholic drinks daily,[266] whereas another similar study found no association (with the exception of moonshine).[267] Some population-based studies have found that alcohol consumption is not related to CKD risk,[268–270] but one study found a significant association of heavy alcohol intake (more than four drinks daily) and prevalent CKD, as well as the risk of developing CKD in participants with a normal GFR.[252] Furthermore, heavy alcohol intake substantially increased the risk of CKD progression associated with smoking, such that participants who smoked and drank heavily had an almost fivefold increased risk of developing CKD.[252]

Conversely, several large cohort studies have reported an inverse relationship between alcohol consumption and the risk of developing CKD[271,272] or ESKD.[273] Another study found that moderate-to-heavy alcohol consumption was associated with an increased risk of developing albuminuria but decreased risk of eGFR < 60 mL/min/1.73 m$^2$.[274] The most rigorous study published to date investigated the incidence of CKD defined by an eGFR determined using the combined cystatin C and creatinine equation or albuminuria > 30 mg/day based on two consecutive 24-hour urine collections. The risk of developing CKD over a mean of 10.2 years decreased progressively with increasing alcohol consumption: HR of 0.85 (95% CI, 0.69 to 1.04) for occasional alcohol consumption (<10 g/week), HR of 0.82 (95% CI, 0.69 to 0.98) for light alcohol consumption (10 to 69.9 g/week), HR of 0.71 (95% CI, 0.58 to 0.88) for moderate alcohol consumption (70 to 210 g/week), and HR of 0.60 (95% CI, 0.42 to 0.86) for heavier alcohol consumption (>210 g/week).[275]

### RECREATIONAL DRUGS

The role of recreational drugs as a risk factor for CKD has not been widely studied, but one case–control study reported a positive association between heroin, cocaine, or psychedelic drug use and ESKD.[276] Following reports of a specific renal lesion characterized by proteinuria and FSGS, termed "heroin nephropathy," other investigators reported a wide range of renal lesions in patients with a history of heroin abuse. It is unclear whether the observed renal lesions resulted from direct effects of heroin or were attributable to impurities in the drug or associated blood-borne virus infections and endocarditis. An association with renal amyloidosis, possibly due to chronic skin infections, has also been reported.[277] Interestingly, heroin abuse was not associated with an increased risk of mild CKD in 647 hypertensive patients who showed an association between illicit drug abuse and CKD.[278] Cocaine exerts several adverse effects that may induce renal injury, including rhabdomyolysis, vasoconstriction, activation of the renin–angiotensin–aldosterone system, oxidative stress, and increased collagen synthesis.[277] Furthermore, chronic administration of cocaine to rats resulted in multiple renal lesions, including glomerular atrophy and sclerosis, tubule cell necrosis, and areas of interstitial necrosis.[279] Among 647 patients attending a hypertension clinic, a history of any illicit drug use was independently associated with a relative risk of 2.3 (95% CI, 1.0 to 5.1) for mild CKD, whereas cocaine and psychedelic drug use were associated with relative risks of 3.0 (95% CI, 1.1 to 8.0) and 3.9 (95% CI, 1.1 to 14.4), respectively.[278] In one prospective cohort study using 2286 participants of the Life Span study, use of opiates and cocaine were both found to have an association with greater OR of reduced eGFR (<60 mL/min/1.73 m$^2$; OR, 2.71 and 95% CI, 1.50–4.89 for opiates; OR, 1.40 and 95% CI, 0.87–2.24 for cocaine) and were associated with greater OR of albuminuria (ACR > 30 mg/g; OR, 1.20 and 95% CI, 0.83–1.73 for opiates; OR, 1.80 and 95% CI, 1.29–2.51 for cocaine).[280]

## ANALGESICS

Analgesic nephropathy has been well described as a cause of CKD and ESKD resulting from abuse of combination analgesics containing aspirin and phenacetin; this was prevalent in Australia and Switzerland until the sale of these products was restricted[281] (see Chapter 81). Cohort studies of participants without CKD at baseline have, however, not reported strong associations between analgesic use and the development of CKD. Among 1697 women in the Nurses Health Study, consumption of >3000 g of acetaminophen was associated with an increased risk of a GFR decline of >30 mL/min/1.73 m$^2$ over 11 years (HR, 2.04; 95% CI, 1.28 to 3.24), but greater use of aspirin or nonsteroidal antiinflammatory drugs (NSAIDs) was not associated with increased risk.[282] Among 4494 male physicians, there was no association between occasional-to-moderate use of aspirin, acetaminophen, and NSAIDs and GFR decline over 14 years.[283] By contrast, analgesic use may exacerbate the progression of established CKD. In one large study of 19,163 patients with newly diagnosed CKD, use of aspirin, acetaminophen, or NSAIDs was associated with an increased risk of progression to ESKD in a dose-dependent manner. Among cyclooxygenase 2 inhibitors, use of rofecoxib but not celecoxib was associated with increased risk of ESKD.[284] In a cohort study of 4101 people with rheumatoid arthritis, chronic use of NSAIDs was not associated with a more rapid GFR decline in the entire study population, but NSAID use was independently associated with more rapid GFR decline in a small minority of patients with CKD stage 4 or 5 ($N$= 17).[285] A meta-analysis of three studies that included data from 54,663 participants with CKD stages 3 to 5 found no association between regular NSAID use and accelerated GFR decline (defined as ≥15 mL/min over 2 years) but did report an association with high-dose NSAID use (defined as 90th percentile or above in one study and not defined in the other) in two studies.[286] The use of single-compound acetaminophen or aspirin was reported not to accelerate progression among patients with CKD stage 4 or 5,[287] but a systematic review of the safety of paracetamol treatment reported an increased risk of renal adverse events in three of four observational studies – in addition to an increased risk of all-cause mortality and cardiovascular and gastrointestinal adverse events in other studies.[288]

As the authors noted, these results must be interpreted with some caution due to the possibility of "confounding by indication" resulting from associations between the indication for prescribing analgesia and adverse outcomes.

## HEAT STRESS

An epidemic of CKD has been reported in Central American farmworkers, fittingly termed Mesoamerican nephropathy (MeN). The disease itself has been most prominent in El Salvadorian sugarcane cutters, but has been reported in areas ranging from southern Mexico to Costa Rica. MeN is usually asymptomatic and is not associated with proteinuria and the usual CKD-related comorbidities, such as diabetes or hypertension, but it does have a high risk of progressing to ESRD. While the exact pathology causing MeN has been debated, varying from side effects of pesticides to medication use, the currently accepted hypothesis is that it is linked to heat-induced dehydration.[289–291] A recent population-based study done by García-Trabanino et al. looked at the renal effects of dehydration after a single shift in the sugarcane fields of El Salvador.[291a] Using 168 male sugarcane cutters, aged 18–49 years, who worked a mean (SD) shift time of 4 (1.4–11) hours, they found significant changes between preshift and postshift assessments of renal biomarkers. Specifically, there was a consistent increase in mean urine specific gravity, urine osmolality, and creatinine, and a decrease in urinary pH. The study also looked at the prevalence of reduced eGFR (<60 mL/min/1.73 m$^2$) in the sample, noting that 14% of these workers had signs of potential CKD. Recent findings have also indicated that the Mesoamerican demographic in which MeN is occurring also has a higher exposure to nephrotoxins, high fructose intake, and higher use of NSAIDs than other populations, a combination of which may further exacerbate the risk of CKD.[292] CKD with similar characteristics has been identified in other tropical areas of the world and an alternative term, CKD of unknown etiology (CKDu), has been proposed.[293]

## HEAVY METALS

Chronic exposure and subsequent toxicity of heavy metals, specifically lead and cadmium, has been known to result in well-recognized instances of nephropathy. Overt lead toxicity results in the well-recognized entity of lead nephropathy, characterized by chronic interstitial nephritis and an association with gout. In addition, epidemiologic studies have reported that mild elevations in blood lead levels are associated with moderate reductions in GFR and/or hypertension in the general population.[294,295] Furthermore, a prospective study has identified elevations in blood lead levels and body lead burden (BLB) within the normal range as important risk factors for progression in patients with CKD.[296] Similarly, BLB was a risk factor for progression among 108 patients with low-normal BLB values and no history of lead exposure.[297] Furthermore, randomization to chelation therapy was associated with a modest improvement in GFR over 24 months versus a small decline in those randomized to control (+6.6 ± 10.7 versus −4.6 ± 4.3 mL/min/1.73 m$^2$; $P$ < .001).[297]

Like lead, chronic exposure to cadmium is also associated with a distinctive nephropathy, which is characterized by proximal tubule damage and low-molecular-weight proteinuria.[298] Furthermore, low-level cadmium exposure resulting from environmental contamination was associated with tubular proteinuria[299]; and analysis of data from 14,778 participants in NHANES showed an independent increased risk of albuminuria, reduced GFR, or both between the highest and lowest quartiles of blood cadmium levels.[300] Comparison of the lowest and highest quartiles for blood cadmium and lead levels showed an even greater increased risk of albuminuria, reduced GFR, or both.[300] In another NHANES study, blood and urine cadmium levels were positively correlated with the urine ACR and negatively associated with GFR. Higher blood and urine cadmium levels were independently associated with albuminuria, and higher blood cadmium levels were associated with albuminuria and a reduced GFR.[298] Occupational or low-level environmental exposure to cadmium was associated with an increased risk of ESKD in a population-based study from Sweden.[301]

## RENAL RISK SCORES

The focus on investigating risk factors that predict the development and/or progression of CKD in diverse populations has led to the observation that a relatively small group of risk factors appears to be common to different forms of CKD. This supports the notion of a common pathway of mechanisms that underlie the progression of CKD. It has also led to the proposal that these common risk factors could be combined to develop a renal risk score to predict the development and future risk of progression of CKD in a manner analogous to the Framingham risk score for predicting cardiovascular risk in the general population.[302] The revised classification system for CKD proposed by KDIGO has in part addressed this need by incorporating the evidence that a reduced GFR and albuminuria are powerful risk factors to incorporate into a system in which CKD categories correspond to risk categories.[9]

In addition, considerable progress has been made in developing renal risk scores to facilitate more accurate risk prediction. These may conveniently be divided into two groups – those that apply to the general population (i.e., without CKD as baseline) and those that predict the risk of progression in patients already diagnosed with CKD. In addition, one study has developed a risk score to predict the development of CKD after an episode of AKI.

### METHODS OF RENAL RISK SCORE DEVELOPMENT

Prior to clinical implementation, renal risk scores must first hold both internal and external validity, improvement over the current risk classification system, and must be easily integrated into clinical setting. The presence of internal validity indicates that the prediction model has been developed from a sample that accurately reflects the relationships between the variables used in the prediction model and the outcome of interest. These predictor variables must have clear definitions and must be measured in each patient well before the final outcome is reached. The outcome itself, in order to avoid bias, must also be clearly defined and assessed equally in all patients, blind to the status of the predictor variable.[208] In order to develop such a risk model, appropriate statistical approaches must be taken. If censoring of the variable is negligible and the follow-up period is clearly defined, logistic regression is used. However, if there is significant censoring present, the Cox proportional hazards model is preferred.[303,304] In addition to the general validation issues discussed earlier, several metrics specific to performance of the prediction model are used in order to assess internal validity.

### METRICS OF MODEL PERFORMANCE

#### DISCRIMINATION

Discrimination is used as a method in determining the model's ability to accurately assign higher probabilities to patients in whom the event of interest occurs, compared with those in whom it does not. The concordance or C-statistic, which is the most commonly used tool of discrimination, is defined as the proportion of times the prediction model correctly discriminates between a randomly selected pair of individuals (case and control), and can be considered identical to the "area under the receiver operator curve" (AUROC). Like the AUROC, a C-statistic of 0.50 indicates that the model performance is essentially no better than chance; a C-statistic of 0.70–0.80 indicates that the model has a good performance in discrimination; and a C-statistic of >0.80 indicates excellent discriminatory performance. The comparison of C-statistics is a frequently used method for comparing the discrimination of multiple prediction models in order to determine which one is superior in risk prediction).[305–308] However, as the value of the C-statistic approaches 1, it becomes difficult to appreciate a significant difference in the values of different models and a more sensitive method, such as the Integrated Discrimination Index (IDI), must be used. The IDI looks at the difference in the discrimination slopes of the two separate models and describes it on an absolute and relative scale, achieving an effective comparison of discrimination values when the C-statistics are no longer sufficient.[309,310]

#### CALIBRATION

Model calibration is another metric of model performance, referring to how well the predictions made from the model align with actual data. For logistic regression models, the Hosmer–Lemeshow chi square statistic is the most commonly used method for such assessments. This method ranks participants based on predicted probability into deciles and the mean probability of each decile is then compared with the actual frequency of outcomes among participants in each decile. A chi square is then used to assess for significant discrepancies between the predicted and actual probabilities. Chi square statistics that are said to be significant indicate that the model calibration is suboptimal.[311] The metric of calibration is important for clinical risk prediction models because a poorly calibrated model will result in either underprediction or overprediction of risk, which is problematic when clinical decision-making is dependent on such prediction models.[208]

#### RECLASSIFICATION

It is standard for clinical treatments and tests to be selected based on the predicted risk of having an event. In the development of a new prediction model, it is essential to consider whether or not it reclassifies patients into more appropriate risk categories than was the case in the old prediction model. If a patient has an event and the new model had assigned the said patient to an appropriately higher-risk category, the new model will be considered a success. Similarly, for patients who do not have an event, the new model is successful if it reclassifies the patient to lower-risk category than the previous model. However, if the new prediction model reassigns the patient to a risk category that is opposite of the actual outcome, the new model is considered unsuccessful and is not superior to the previous model. This success or failure can be quantified by the Net Reclassification Index, values for which range from −2.0 to +2.0, with positive values indicating successful reclassification and negative values indicating unsuccessful reclassification).[309,310]

### CLINICAL UTILITY

Even the best risk prediction model is unusable in a clinical setting if it cannot be rapidly and efficiently implemented. As previously indicated, prediction models are derived through a series of complex logistic or proportional hazards models that cannot be easily applied to patients using simple calculations. This means that the model, once validated, needs to be translated into a simpler clinically useful bedside tool. However, in simplifying the scoring system, there is some inevitable loss of precision, discrimination, and calibration. Recently, the advent of rapid access to Web-based calculators or smartphone apps has allowed for complex prediction models to be applied in their original form via a simplified user interface, and without the need for complex calculations by the user.[312–315]

### EXTERNAL VALIDITY

External validity, unlike internal validity, addresses whether or not the results of the study sample can be applied to the general population. The external validity of a prediction model can never be assumed, because it is likely that a model generated from one set of data (derivation cohort) will not perform exactly the same in other cohorts. This is likely due to underlying biological factors, including differences in disease or physiology of the cohorts and false associations between predictors and outcomes in the original derivation cohort. Attempts to minimize errors between cohorts can be achieved by careful selection of cohorts that are representative of the clinical condition, and by choosing predictor variables based on clinical relevance rather than statistical associations.[308]

## MODELS PREDICTING INCIDENT CHRONIC KIDNEY DISEASE

Risk scores have been proposed to assess the risk of developing CKD in the general population and, in some cases, its subsequent progression. These are summarized in Table 20.3 and have been assessed in a systematic review.[316] In the first study, data from 8530 adults included in NHANES were used to identify risk factors for prevalent CKD (defined as eGFR < 60 mL/min/1.73 m$^2$). The authors proposed a risk score that included age, female gender, hypertension, anemia, diabetes, peripheral vascular disease, history of CVD, congestive heart failure, and proteinuria. The AUROC was high at 0.88, and a score of ≥4 resulted in a sensitivity of 92% and specificity of 68%. The positive predictive value was low at 18%, but the negative predictive value was 99%. External validation using data from the ARIC study gave an AUROC value of 0.71.[317] This was a cross-sectional study, and the risk score therefore did not predict the risk of future CKD. Rather, it identified individuals at increased risk of having current undiagnosed CKD. As such, it would be useful for guiding efforts to screen populations for CKD, but gives no information about the future risk of CKD progression. The applicability of the score to general populations is somewhat weakened by the inclusion of two variables that require prior laboratory testing: anemia and proteinuria. Furthermore, the presence of significant proteinuria is sufficient to diagnose CKD in the absence of any reduction in GFR.

Another risk score was developed to predict the risk of incident CKD using combined data from 14,155 participants in the ARIC study and Cardiovascular Health Study (CHS; ≥45 years) with baseline eGFR > 60 mL/min/1.73 m$^2$. After identifying 10 predictors of incident CKD (defined as eGFR < 60 mL/min/1.73 m$^2$ during follow-up for up to 9 years), they proposed a simplified model based on eight variables: age, anemia, female gender, hypertension, DM, peripheral vascular disease, and history of congestive heart failure or CVD. This gave an AUROC value of 0.69, and a score of ≥3 resulted in a sensitivity of 69% and specificity of 58% but the positive predictive value was low, only 17%.[318] A similar study used data from 2490 participants in the Framingham Heart Study to produce a risk score for incident CKD, defined as eGFR < 60 mL/min/1.73 m$^2$. The final model included age, diabetes, hypertension, baseline eGFR, and albuminuria and gave an AUC value of 0.813. External validation was performed with data from the ARIC study (AUROC = 0.79 and 0.75 in whites and blacks, respectively).[319] One further study developed a risk score for incident CKD (eGFR < 60 mL/min/1.73 m$^2$) in 5168 Chinese participants. Age, BMI, diastolic blood pressure, type 2 diabetes, previous stroke, serum uric acid, postprandial blood glucose, hemoglobin $A_{1c}$ levels, and proteinuria > 100 mg/dL were included in two risk scores (one using clinical variables only and a second with all variables) that gave an AUROC value of 0.77. The study was limited by relatively short follow-up (median, 2.2 years) and a low AUROC value of 0.67 for external validation data.[320]

These scores are useful to identify individuals at higher risk of developing CKD for monitoring or intervention to reduce risk, but do not distinguish the minority who are at risk of progressing to ESKD from the majority who are at low risk. In an attempt to identify only high-risk individuals, another group used data from persons (775,091 women and 799,658 men aged 35 to 74 years, without a recorded diagnosis of CKD) in 368 primary care practices in the United Kingdom to develop a risk score. Two outcomes were studied over a period of up to 7 years – moderate-to-severe CKD (defined as kidney transplantation, dialysis, diagnosis of nephropathy, proteinuria, or eGFR < 45 mL/min/1.73 m$^2$) and ESKD (defined as kidney transplantation, dialysis, or eGFR < 15 mL/min/1.73 m$^2$); separate risk scores were developed for men and women. The final model for moderate-to-severe CKD included age, ethnicity, social deprivation, smoking, BMI, systolic blood pressure, diabetes, rheumatoid arthritis, CVD, treated hypertension, congestive cardiac failure, peripheral vascular disease, use of NSAIDs, and family history of kidney disease. In women, it also included systemic lupus erythematosus and history of kidney stones. The model for ESKD was similar but did not include NSAID use. Internal and external validation was performed, giving AUROC values of 0.818 to 0.878.[321]

One important limitation of this study is that it was observational and therefore likely to be subject to significant

**Table 20.3 Renal Risk Scores for the General Population**

| | Study | | | | | |
|---|---|---|---|---|---|---|
| **Parameter** | SCORED[317] | SCORED2[318] | Chinese[320] | Framingham[319] | QKIDNEY[321] | PREVEND[322] |
| Population | NHANES | CHS + ARIC | General population | FHS | QResearch | eGFR > 45 |
| Outcome | eGFR < 60 mL/min/1.73 m$^2$ (prevalent) | eGFR < 60 mL/min/1.73 m$^2$ (incident) | eGFR < 60 mL/min/1.73 m$^2$ (incident) | eGFR < 60 mL/min/1.73 m$^2$ (incident) | CKD, ESKD | Rapid ↓ GFR |
| Factor | Age | Age | Age | Age | Age | Age |
| | Female | Female | | | | |
| | | | | | Ethnicity | |
| | | | | | Deprivation | |
| | | | | | Family history | |
| | | | | | Smoking | |
| | | | BMI | | | |
| | HT | HT | | HT | HT | HT |
| | DM | DM | Type 2 DM | DM | DM | |
| | PVD | PVD | | | PVD | |
| | CVD | CVD | Stroke | | CVD | |
| | CCF | CCF | | | CCF | |
| | | | | | RA | |
| | Anemia | Anemia | | | | |
| | | | DBP | | SBP | SBP |
| | | | | | BMI | |
| | | | | eGFR | | eGFR |
| | Proteinuria | | Proteinuria | Albuminuria | | Albuminuria |
| | | | | | | CRP |
| | | | Uric acid | | | |
| | | | $HbA_{1c}$ | | | |
| | | | Glucose | | | |
| | | | | | NSAIDs | |
| AUC | 0.88 | 0.69 | 0.77 | 0.81 | 0.88 | 0.84 |
| Validation | ARIC | CHS + ARIC | General population | ARIC | THIN | Internal |

*ARIC*, Atherosclerosis Risk in Communities; *AUC*, area under the concentration–time curve; *BMI*, body mass index; *CCF*, congestive cardiac failure; *CHS*, Cardiovascular Health Study; *CKD*, chronic kidney disease; *CRP*, C-reactive protein; *CVD*, cardiovascular disease; *DBP*, diastolic blood pressure; *DM*, diabetes mellitus; *eGFR*, estimated glomerular filtration rate; *ESKD*, end-stage kidney disease; *FHS*, Framingham Heart Study; *$HbA_{1c}$*, hemoglobin $A_{1c}$; *HT*, hypertension; *NHANES*, National Health and Nutrition Examination Survey; *NSAIDs*, nonsteroidal antiinflammatory drugs; *PREVEND*, Prevention of Renal and Vascular End-stage Disease; *PVD*, peripheral vascular disease; *RA*, rheumatoid arthritis; *SBP*, systolic blood pressure; *THIN*, the Health Improvement Network.

bias. Furthermore, only 56% of participants had a serum creatinine level recorded at inclusion, and it is therefore probable that several had undiagnosed CKD. The composite outcome of moderate-to-severe CKD was composed of several disparate variables and is therefore not clinically useful, but the ESKD outcome is relevant because it identified only the minority at increased risk of severe progression. This study also illustrates the utility of a risk score that could be programmed into primary care computer systems to alert family practitioners to patients who are at risk of progression to ESKD.

Another study used data from 6809 participants in the Prevention of Renal and Vascular End-stage Disease (PREVEND) study to develop a risk score with the primary outcome of progressive CKD over 6.4 years, defined as the 20% of participants with the most rapid decline in GFR and eGFR < 60 mL/min/1.73 m$^2$. The final risk score included baseline eGFR, age, albuminuria, systolic blood pressure, C-reactive protein, and known hypertension. The AUROC value was 0.84, and internal validation was performed using a bootstrapping procedure.[322] Despite this, the risk score has a relatively low sensitivity and positive predictive value. The proposed threshold score of ≥27 identified 2.1% of the population as high risk, but with a sensitivity of only 15.7% and a positive predictive value of 28.1%. The specificity and negative predictive value were high at 98.4% and 96.7%, respectively. Thus a low score is useful to identify low-risk individuals but a high score does not identify most high-risk individuals. Selecting a lower threshold would improve sensitivity with some reduction in specificity and could be used to identify a group at intermediate risk for closer monitoring. Limitations of this study are that it was performed in a white population and was not validated externally. External validation in other populations is therefore required before it can be considered for clinical use.

## MODELS PREDICTING KIDNEY FAILURE

Several risk scores have been developed for patients with diagnosed CKD in a variety of study populations and are summarized in Table 20.4 and in systematic reviews.[316,323]

**Table 20.4 Renal Risk Scores for Patients With Chronic Kidney Disease (CKD)**

| | Study | | | | | |
|---|---|---|---|---|---|---|
| **Parameter** | RENAAL[163] | AIPRD[324] | IGAN[172] | KPC[325] | CRIB[226] | SHC[208] |
| Disease studied | DN | CKD | IgAN | CKD, stage 3 or 4 | CKD, stages 3 to 5 | CKD, stages 3 to 5 |
| Variables | | Age | Age | Age | | Age |
| | | | Male | Male | Female | Male |
| | Creatinine | Creatinine | 1/creatinine | eGFR | Creatinine | eGFR |
| | UACR | UPE | Proteinuria | N/A | UACR | UACR |
| | | SBP | SBP | HT | | |
| | | | | DM | | |
| | Alb | | TP | | | Alb |
| | Hb | | | Anemia | | |
| | | | | | | Calcium |
| | | | | | Phos | Phos |
| | | | | | | Bicarb |
| | | | Histol | | | |
| | | | Hematuria | | | |
| Outcome | ESKD | ESKD or doubling of serum creatinine level | ESKD | RRT | ESKD | ESKD |
| AUC | | | 0.939 | 0.89 | 0.873 | 0.917 |
| Validation | No | No | No | No | Yes | Yes |

*AIPRD,* ACE Inhibition in Progressive Renal Disease study; *Alb,* serum albumin; *AUC,* area under the concentration–time curve; *Bicarb,* serum bicarbonate; *CRIB,* Chronic Renal Impairment in Birmingham study; *DM,* diabetes mellitus; *DN,* diabetic nephropathy; *eGFR,* estimated glomerular filtration rate; *ESKD,* end-stage kidney disease; *Hb,* hemoglobin; *Histol,* histologic grade; *HT,* hypertension; *IgAN,* IgA nephropathy; *KPC,* Kaiser Permanente Cohort; *N/A,* not available; *Phos,* serum phosphate; *Proteinuria,* urine dipstick proteinuria; *RENAAL,* Reduction of Endpoints in NIDDM with the Angiotensin II Antagonist Losartan study; *RRT,* renal replacement therapy; *SBP,* systolic blood pressure; *SHC,* Sunnybrook Hospital cohort; *TP,* serum total protein; *UACR,* urine albumin-to-creatinine ratio; *UPE,* 24-hour urinary protein excretion.

Analysis of data from 1513 patients with diabetic nephropathy included in the RENAAL study identified urine ACR, serum albumin, serum creatinine, and hemoglobin as independent risk factors for ESKD. A risk score was derived from the coefficients of these variables in the Cox proportional hazards model, which successfully separated the participants into quartiles of ESKD risk (Fig. 20.5), with a marked difference in risk between the first and last quartiles (6.7 vs. 257.2/1000 patient-years).[163]

Among 1860 patients with nondiabetic CKD from a combined database of 11 clinical trials, Cox proportional hazards analysis identified age, serum creatinine, proteinuria, and systolic blood pressure as independent risk factors for the combined endpoint of time to ESKD or creatinine doubling. Using similar methodology as the previous study, a risk model based on these variables was developed to stratify patients into quartiles of risk. The annual incidence of the combined endpoint was 0.4% versus 28.7% in the lowest versus highest quartile for patients in the control group and 0.2% versus 19.7% in those randomized to angiotensin-converting enzyme inhibitor treatment.[324] Analysis of data from 2269 patients with IgA nephropathy identified systolic blood pressure, proteinuria (assessed with urine dipstick test), serum total protein, 1/serum creatinine, and histologic grade at initial biopsy as predictors of time to ESKD. Age, gender, and severity of hematuria were added to these variables to develop a scoring system for estimating 4- and 7-year cumulative incidence of ESKD. There was close agreement between estimated and observed risks (AUROC value = 0.939).[172]

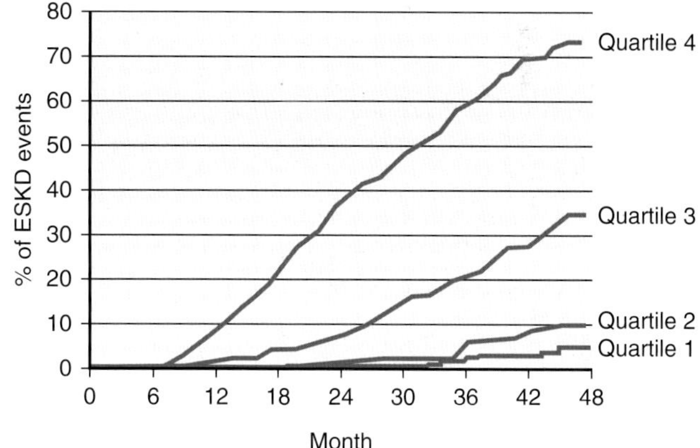


**Fig. 20.5** Kaplan–Meier curve for the end-stage kidney disease (ESKD) endpoint stratified by quartile of risk score in 1513 patients with diabetic nephropathy from the Reduction of Endpoints in NIDDM with the Angiotensin II Antagonist Losartan (RENAAL) study. *NIDDM,* Non–insulin-dependent diabetes mellitus. (From Keane WF, Zhang Z, Lyle PA, et al. Risk scores for predicting outcomes in patients with type 2 diabetes and nephropathy: the RENAAL study. *Clin J Am Soc Nephrol.* 2006;1:761–767.)

In a retrospective study, data from 9782 patients with CKD stages 3 to 4 were analyzed with regard to a primary outcome of onset of RRT (dialysis or transplantation). Six independent risk factors were identified—age, male gender, eGFR, hypertension, diabetes, and anemia—and were incorporated into a risk score that stratified participants into quintiles of risk.

The risk of progression to RRT was 19% in the highest risk quintile versus 0.2% in the lowest. The AUROC value was 0.89, and observed risk differed from predicted by <1%.[325] One limitation of this study, apart from its retrospective design, was the lack of data regarding proteinuria.

Among 382 patients with CKD stages 3 to 5 from the Chronic Renal Impairment in Birmingham (CRIB) study, independent risk factors for progression to ESKD during a mean of 4.1 years' follow-up were female gender, serum creatinine, serum phosphate, and urine ACR. A risk score was derived from these variables (AUROC value = 0.873) and externally validated in a similar cohort of patients with CKD stages 3 to 5 (East Kent cohort), giving an AUROC value of 0.91, even though the urine ACR was not available in the validation cohort.[226]

## KIDNEY FAILURE RISK EQUATIONS

The kidney failure risk equations (KFREs) for predicting ESKD were developed by Tangri and colleagues using data from a cohort of 3449 Canadian patients with CKD stages 3 to 5 (Sunnybrook Hospital cohort).[208] It included age, male gender, eGFR, albuminuria, serum calcium, serum phosphate, serum bicarbonate, and serum albumin (AUROC value = 0.917). External validation was performed with data from a separate cohort of 4942 patients with CKD stages 3 to 5 (British Columbia CKD Registry), giving an AUROC value of 0.841. There was close agreement between predicted and observed risk in the validation cohort (Fig. 20.6). Simpler three-variable (age, gender, and eGFR) and four-variable models (age, gender, eGFR, and albuminuria) also performed well [C-statistic (equivalent to AUROC) of 0.89 and 0.91, respectively, in the development cohort; Table 20.5], but the eight-variable equation (C statistics 0.92) performed better in the validation cohort with respect to discrimination (C-statistic, 0.79 and 0.83, respectively, for the three- and four-variable equations), calibration, and reclassification. The authors facilitated clinical application of this risk score by producing an electronic risk calculator and a smartphone

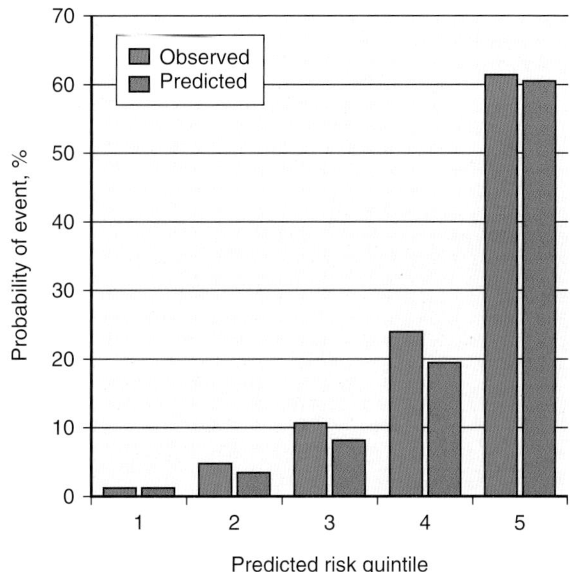


**Fig. 20.6** Renal risk score predicted versus observed risk of developing end-stage kidney disease at 3 years in a validation cohort of patients with chronic kidney disease stages 3 to 5. (From Tangri N, Stevens LA, Griffith J, et al. A predictive model for progression of chronic kidney disease to kidney failure. *JAMA* 2011;305:1553–1559.)

**Table 20.5 Hazard Ratios and Goodness of Fit for Sequential Models in the Development Data Set for Three-, Four-, and Eight-Variable Kidney Failure Risk Equations**

| Variable | Three-Variable Model | Four-Variable Model | Eight-Variable Model |
|---|---|---|---|
| **Hazard Ratio for Kidney Failure (Censored for Mortality)** | | | |
| Baseline GFR, per 5 mL/min/1.73 m$^2$ | 0.54 | 0.57 | 0.61 |
| Age, per 10 year | 0.75 | 0.8 | 0.82 |
| Male sex | 1.46 | 1.26 | 1.16 |
| Log spot urine ACR[a] | | 1.60 | 1.42 |
| Serum albumin, per 0.5 g/dL | | | 0.84 |
| Serum phosphate, per 1.0 mg/dL | | | 1.27 |
| Serum bicarbonate, per 1.0 mEq/L | | | 0.92 |
| Serum calcium, per mg/dL | | | 0.81 |
| **Goodness of Fit Metrics** | | | |
| C-statistics | 0.89 | 0.91 | 0.92 |
| Akaike information criterion[b] | 4834 | 4520 | 4432 |
| *P* value[c] | <.001 | <.001 | <.001 |

[a]Hazard ratio for ACR represents a 1.0 point higher ACR on the natural log scale. For the average patient with 20 mg/g of albuminuria, this represents an increase to 55 mg/g.

[b]Null values for C-statistic and Akaike information criterion are 0.50 and 5569, respectively. Higher values for C-statistic and lower values for Akaike information criterion indicate better models.

[c]*P* values are for comparison of C-statistics between sequential models.

*ACR,* Albumin-to-creatinine ratio; *GFR,* glomerular filtration rate.

From Tangri N, Stevens LA, Griffith J, et al. A predictive model for progression of chronic kidney disease to kidney failure. *JAMA* 2011;305:1553–1559.

app (available for no charge at www.qxmd.com/calculate-online/nephrology/kidney-failure-risk-equation) that report an estimated risk of ESKD at 2 and 5 years. Further external validation of this risk equation has been reported by independent investigators from the MASTERPLAN (Multifactorial Approach and Superior Treatment Efficacy in Renal Patients with the Aid of Nurse practitioners) study, a cohort of 595 people from the Netherlands with CKD stages 3 to 5. The model again performed well with the eight-variable equation, giving an AUROC value of 0.89.[326] A further advantage of the Tangri risk score is that it includes variables that are all available to a biochemistry laboratory, making it possible for laboratories to automate reporting of a risk score with each eGFR.

In order to determine if KFREs could be implemented clinically on a global scale, a multinational validation study of the equations was performed in 35 cohorts consisting of 720,000 patients with CKD (stages 3–5) from 23 countries across four continents.[327] After a 4-year follow-up, 23,829 cases of kidney failure were observed in the cohorts. The KFRE was able to achieve excellent discrimination through all cohorts (C-statistic, 0.90; 95% CI, 0.89–0.92 at 2 years; C-statistic, 0.88; 95% CI, 0.86–0.90 at 5 years). Calibration was adequate in North American cohorts, but the original risk equations overestimated risk in some non-North American cohorts. However, through use of a simple calibration factor for non-North American populations, which lowered the baseline risk by 32.9% at 2 years and 16.5% at 5 years, calibration was improved in 12 of 15 and 10 of 13 non-North American cohorts at 2 and 5 years, respectively ($P = .04$ and $P = .02$). This indicated that the KFREs were consistently accurate in predicting progression to ESKD throughout each of the 35 cohorts with discrimination being independent of age, sex, race, or diabetic status. Moreover, the simplified four-variable equation produced similar discrimination to the eight-variable equation (at 2 years C-statistics were 0.89 vs. 0.90 and at 5 years 0.86 vs. 0.88, respectively). An online risk calculator has been produced that utilizes the four-variable equation and incorporates the correction for persons outside of North America (http://kidneyfailurerisk.com/). These findings were a strong indicator that the KFREs would be ready for clinical implementation in the near future.

> ***Clinical Relevance***
>
> **Kidney Failure Risk Equations**
>
> Patients with chronic kidney disease (CKD) are at risk of kidney failure, cardiovascular events, and early mortality. In moderate to severe CKD, estimated glomerular filtration rate (eGFR) and albuminuria are important functional, diagnostic, and prognostic biomarkers, and can be combined in risk equations to estimate the risk of adverse events. The kidney failure risk equations have been developed using eGFR, albuminuria, and readily available demographic and laboratory variables, and predict the risk of kidney failure requiring dialysis or transplant with accuracy. The equations can be used to determine need for nephrology referral, intensity of care, timing of dialysis education, access formation, and preemptive transplantation. Studies evaluating the use of the risk equation in clinical settings are needed.

## MODELS PREDICTING DEATH AND CARDIOVASCULAR DISEASE

As mentioned before, patients with CKD progression also evidence an increased risk of death and CVD as they carry a burden of both traditional and nontraditional risk factors for CVD. Existing risk scores have shown poor prediction model metrics in patients with CKD, with no successful attempts in development of a clinically useful model for determining risk of CVD.[328] However one such prediction model developed by Bansal et al. showed promise in assessing 5-year risk of mortality. The risk prediction model, which was developed in a cohort of 828 older adults (mean age 80 ± 5.6 years) from the CHS, included the predictor variables of age, sex, race, eGFR, urine ACR, smoking, DM, and history of heart failure and stroke (C-statistic = 0.72; 95% CI, 0.68 to 0.74). The model was externally validated in 789 participants from the Health, Aging and Body Composition Study (C-statistic = 0.69; 95% CI, 0.64 to 0.74). However, patients with advanced CKD (stages 4–5) in the CHS were underrepresented, and hence the findings would require further validation before clinical implementation. Nevertheless, this model provides a very important starting point for future models to be developed in prediction of all-cause mortality in patients with CKD.[329]

## MODELS PREDICTING CHRONIC KIDNEY DISEASE AFTER ACUTE KIDNEY INJURY

A growing appreciation of the risk of CKD and progression to ESKD following an episode of AKI has prompted efforts to develop a risk score for identifying those at highest risk. Three risk prediction models were developed in one study population of 5351 predominantly male veterans with a primary admission diagnosis of AKI to predict the risk of progression to CKD stage 4. Risk factors that entered the models included increased age, low serum albumin, diabetes, lower baseline eGFR, higher mean serum creatinine levels during hospitalization, and severity of AKI as assessed by the RIFLE score (**r**isk, **i**njury, **f**ailure, **l**oss, and **e**nd-stage kidney disease) or need for dialysis, non–African-American ethnicity, and time at risk. The AUROC value was 0.77 to 0.82 for the three models. Sensitivity at the optimal cut-point was 0.71 to 0.77, and specificity was 0.64 to 0.74. External validation was performed on a control population of 11,589 patients admitted for pneumonia or myocardial infarction and yielded good prediction accuracy (AUROC value = 0.81 to 0.82). Sensitivity at the optimal cut-point was 0.66 to 0.71, and specificity was 0.61 to 0.70).[330]

Further validation in other populations that include a more representative proportion of women is required before these risk models can be applied. A validated risk score for patients recovering from AKI may prove very important for identifying high-risk patients for closer follow-up and interventions to reduce the risk of progressive CKD, although further trials are required to evaluate the impact of renoprotective interventions in this setting.

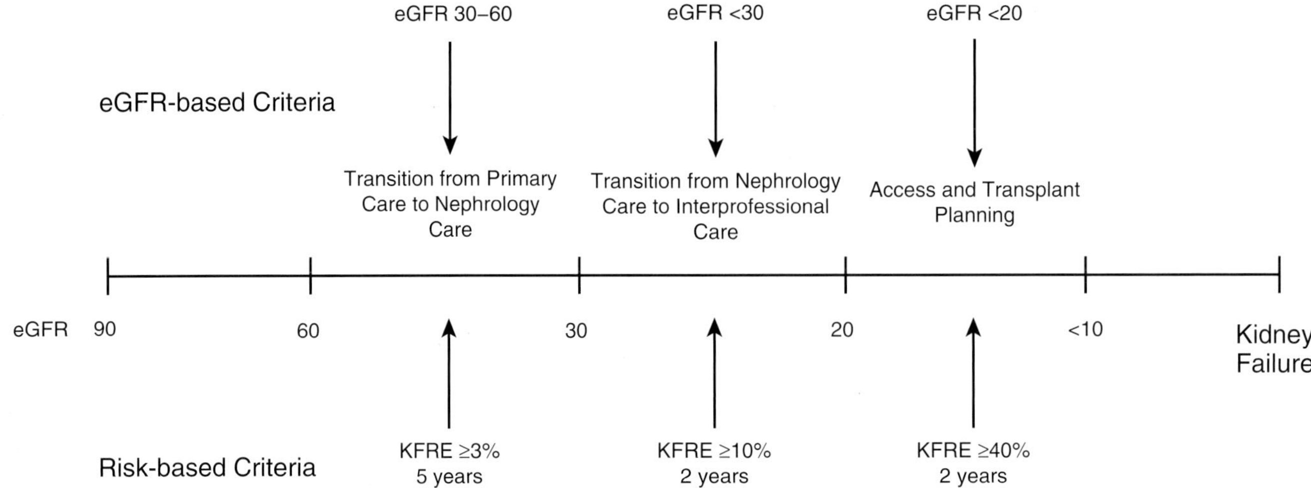


**Fig. 20.7** A risk-based versus estimated glomerular filtration rate (eGFR)-based approach to clinical decision-making in patients with chronic kidney disease (CKD). *KFRE,* Kidney failure risk equation. (Reproduced with permission from Tangri N, Ferguson T, Komenda P. Pro: risk scores for chronic kidney disease progression are robust, powerful and ready for implementation. *Nephrol Dial Transplant.* 2017;32:748–751.)

## CLINICAL IMPLEMENTATION OF RISK MODELS

Clinical implementation of risk-based care requires the interaction of both a validated risk prediction model and absolute risk thresholds to guide therapy decision. Through the simultaneous use of risk equations and previously set thresholds, an optimal and cost-effective management plan can be provided to the patient. This is currently exemplified by an approach using the KFREs with risk thresholds to prompt transition from one stage of care to the next (Fig. 20.7).[64,331]

### PRIMARY CARE TO NEPHROLOGY TRANSITION

In the initial stages of CKD, patients often develop salt and water retention, hypertension, and anemia.[332] Primary care physicians are able to manage these symptoms and provide optimal care for these patients, avoiding both unnecessary spending and treatments. However, when patients exhibit a high risk of CKD progression, referral to a nephrology service and subsequent access to interdisciplinary care teams is necessary in to order to delay CKD progression, prevent suboptimal dialysis initiation, and reduce the chances of early mortality.[6,333] The use of risk equations and risk thresholds may allow physicians to be better informed about when such a referral should be considered. This approach may also prevent low-risk CKD patients from exposure to unnecessary treatments and the anxiety associated with referral.[334] Integrating risk prediction models into clinical care can also be potentially useful in the planning of follow-up. Patients with a high risk of CKD progression but only moderately reduced eGFR can be followed at 3- or 6-month intervals, whereas those with lower risk can be assessed on an annual basis.[335]

### INTERDISCIPLINARY CARE

The use of an interdisciplinary nephrology team, which involves a nurse, pharmacist, and dietician, may improve concordance with treatment, reduce suboptimal dialysis initiation, and could even reduce mortality for high-risk CKD patients. As with most specialized clinical services, inclusion of too many patients with a low risk of CKD progression can saturate interdisciplinary resources with minimal benefits.[331] This was a major issue in Ontario, Canada, where health-care administrators struggled with excess demand for interdisciplinary care with a limited health-care budget. As a result, in 2016 the Ontario Renal Network, which is responsible for administering the provinces renal health resources, adopted a risk-based cutoff for eligibility of clinical resources. Patients with a KFRE-calculated 2-year risk of ESRD exceeding 10% or an eGFR < 15 mL/min/1.73 m$^2$ were eligible for interdisciplinary care. This drastically lowered the number of patients eligible for interdisciplinary care as the previous threshold for such treatment was an eGFR < 30 mL/min/1.73 m$^2$, irrespective of risk. It was determined using the KFREs that only two-thirds of patients that fit this previous criteria had a 2-year risk >10%. Also from implementation of these new criteria, a small proportion of patients with an eGFR between 30 and 45 mL/min/1.73 m$^2$ were determined at very high risk of CKD progression and were now eligible for interdisciplinary care. This reallocation of resources led to cost savings of approximately 6 million Canadian dollars annually and has allowed high-risk patients with an eGFR > 30 mL/min/1.73 m$^2$ earlier access to interdisciplinary care.[336]

### DIALYSIS ACCESS AND MODALITY PLANNING

Current clinical practice guidelines recommend dialysis modality planning for patients with an eGFR < 30 mL/

min/1.73 m$^2$. However the majority of these patients, particularly the elderly, may never actually progress to ESKD.[337] For these patients, the prospect of dialysis creates unnecessary anxiety, and results in unnecessary treatment planning. In particular, the risk–benefit balance for arteriovenous fistula (AVF) insertion is important. While AVF is the standard form of dialysis access for patients on hemodialysis, the benefits may be reduced in the elderly. These individuals suffer from a higher likelihood of primary AVF failure and adverse events including heart failure and steal syndrome. Older people at low risk of developing ESRD also tend to have a higher risk of competing morbidities, thereby making preemptive AVF formation both futile and costly.[338] The use of a risk prediction model to guide the timing of AVF formation can overcome some of these limitations and provide more optimal treatment plans. Patients with low-risk CKD progression will adopt a monitoring-based approach, whereas those with the highest risk of progression can be recommended for access placement for dialysis. In 2014, a Markov model was developed for assessing the implementation of the KFREs on simulated CKD progression in the Sunnybrook hospital cohort. The goal was to determine if the KFREs could select, with the highest accuracy, those patents in need of access for dialysis, while simultaneously avoiding creation of access in patents who either died before ESRD or who did not progress to dialysis within 2 years of access insertion. It was found the KFRE-based threshold of 20% annual risk was superior to eGFR-based thresholds in predicting the need for dialysis and AVF formation.[339]

## FUTURE CONSIDERATIONS

Considerable progress has been made since 2000 in identifying risk factors that predict the progression of CKD in diverse cohorts from the general population and nephrology clinics. There is some variation among studies, likely due to differences in the populations and variables studied. Remarkably, a relatively small group of risk factors appears common to many studies, and much progress has been made in developing risk scores based on these variables to predict CKD progression.

Future studies will likely focus on the use of novel biomarkers and genetic factors as risk factors (see Chapter 27) and variables in risk scores, although measurement of such markers is likely to be associated with greater cost than the simple risk factors used to date. Accurate risk scores can align risk and resources while allowing for the most personalized care for persons with CKD. As a result, now is the time to implement these risk scores into clinical care to help patients and clinicians navigate the transition from CKD to dialysis. Further studies are also required to develop risk scores to predict cardiovascular risk in patients with CKD that take into account the close association between CKD and CVD.

Complete reference list available at ExpertConsult.com.

## KEY REFERENCES


4. Matsushita K, Mahmoodi BK, Woodward M, et al. Comparison of risk prediction using the CKD-EPI equation and the MDRD study equation for estimated glomerular filtration rate. *JAMA*. 2012;307(18):1941–1951.
9. Stevens PE, Levin A. Evaluation and management of chronic kidney disease: synopsis of the kidney disease: improving global outcomes 2012 clinical practice guideline. *Ann Intern Med*. 2013;158:825–830.
10. Hunsicker LG, Adler S, Caggiula A, et al. Predictors of the progression of renal disease in the Modification of Diet in Renal Disease Study. *Kidney Int*. 1997;51:1908–1919.
11. O'Hare AM, Batten A, Burrows NR, et al. Trajectories of kidney function decline in the 2 years before initiation of long-term dialysis. *Am J Kidney Dis*. 2012;59(4):513–522.
15. Ibrahim HN, Foley R, Tan L, et al. Long-term consequences of kidney donation. *N Engl J Med*. 2009;360:459–469.
17. Jeon HG, Jeong IG, Lee JW, et al. Prognostic factors for chronic kidney disease after curative surgery in patients with small renal tumors. *Urology*. 2009;74:1064–1068.
20. Iseki K, Iseki C, Ikemiya Y, et al. Risk of developing end-stage renal disease in a cohort of mass screening. *Kidney Int*. 1996;49:800–805.
21. Fox CS, Larson MG, Leip EP, et al. Predictors of new-onset kidney disease in a community-based population. *JAMA*. 2004;291:844–850.
23. Weller JM, Wu SC, Ferguson CW, et al. End-stage renal disease in Michigan. Incidence, underlying causes, prevalence, and modalities of treatment. *Am J Nephrol*. 1985;5:84–95.
24. Shulman NB, Ford CE, Hall WD, et al. Prognostic value of serum creatinine and effect of treatment of hypertension on renal function. Results from the hypertension detection and follow-up program. The Hypertension Detection and Follow-up Program Cooperative Group. *Hypertension*. 1989;13:I80–I93.
25. Eriksen BO, Ingebretsen OC. The progression of chronic kidney disease: a 10-year population-based study of the effects of gender and age. *Kidney Int*. 2006;69:375–382.
26. O'Hare AM, Choi AI, Bertenthal D, et al. Age affects outcomes in chronic kidney disease. *J Am Soc Nephrol*. 2007;18:2758–2765.
27. Hallan SI, Matsushita K, Sang Y, et al. Age and association of kidney measures with mortality and end-stage renal disease. *JAMA*. 2012;308:2349–2360.
28. Haroun MK, Jaar BG, Hoffman SC, et al. Risk factors for chronic kidney disease: a prospective study of 23,534 men and women in Washington County, Maryland. *J Am Soc Nephrol*. 2003;14:2934–2941.
29. Evans M, Fryzek JP, Elinder CG, et al. The natural history of chronic renal failure: results from an unselected, population-based, inception cohort in Sweden. *Am J Kidney Dis*. 2005;46:863–870.
33. Nitsch D, Grams M, Sang Y, et al. Associations of estimated glomerular filtration rate and albuminuria with mortality and renal failure by sex: a meta-analysis. *BMJ*. 2013;346:f324.
44. Wen CP, Matsushita K, Coresh J, et al. Relative risks of chronic kidney disease for mortality and end-stage renal disease across races are similar. *Kidney Int*. 2014;86:819–827.
54. Kottgen A, Pattaro C, Boger CA, et al. New loci associated with kidney function and chronic kidney disease. *Nat Genet*. 2010;42:376–384.
57. Hostetter TH, Olson JL, Rennke HG, et al. Hyperfiltration in remnant nephrons: a potentially adverse response to renal ablation. *J Am Soc Nephrol*. 2001;12:1315–1325.
73. Gansevoort RT, Matsushita K, van der Velde M, et al. Lower estimated GFR and higher albuminuria are associated with adverse kidney outcomes in both general and high-risk populations. A collaborative meta-analysis of general and high-risk population cohorts. *Kidney Int*. 2011;80:93–104.
74. Astor BC, Matsushita K, Gansevoort RT, et al. Lower estimated glomerular filtration rate and higher albuminuria are associated with mortality and end-stage renal disease. A collaborative meta-analysis of kidney disease population cohorts. *Kidney Int*. 2011;79:1331–1340.
75. Fox CS, Matsushita K, Woodward M, et al. Associations of kidney disease measures with mortality and end-stage renal disease in individuals with and without diabetes: a meta-analysis. *Lancet*. 2012;380:1662–1673.
76. Mahmoodi BK, Matsushita K, Woodward M, et al. Associations of kidney disease measures with mortality and end-stage renal disease in individuals with and without hypertension: a meta-analysis. *Lancet*. 2012;380:1649–1661.
79. Inker LA, Schmid CH, Tighiouart H, et al. Estimating glomerular filtration rate from serum creatinine and cystatin C. *N Engl J Med*. 2012;367:20–29.
97. Klahr S, Levey AS, Beck GJ, et al. The effects of dietary protein restriction and blood-pressure control on the progression of chronic

renal disease. Modification of Diet in Renal Disease Study Group. *N Engl J Med.* 1994;330:877–884.
99. SPRINT Research Group, Wright JT, Williamson JD, et al. A randomized trial of intensive versus standard blood-pressure control. *N Engl J Med.* 2015;373(22):2103–2116.
139. The effect of intensive treatment of diabetes on the development and progression of long-term complications in insulin-dependent diabetes mellitus. *N Engl J Med.* 1993;329:977–986.
148. Collister D, Ferguson T, Komenda P, et al. The patterns, risk factors, and prediction of progression in chronic kidney disease: a narrative review. *Semin Nephrol.* 2016;36(4):273–282.
160. Ravani P, Tripepi G, Malberti F, et al. Asymmetrical dimethylarginine predicts progression to dialysis and death in patients with chronic kidney disease: a competing risks modeling approach. *J Am Soc Nephrol.* 2005;16:2449–2455.
163. Keane WF, Zhang Z, Lyle PA, et al. Risk scores for predicting outcomes in patients with type 2 diabetes and nephropathy: the RENAAL Study. *Clin J Am Soc Nephrol.* 2006;1:761–767.
169. McIntyre NJ, Taal MW. How to measure proteinuria? *Curr Opin Nephrol Hypertens.* 2008;17:600–603.
172. Wakai K, Kawamura T, Endoh M, et al. A scoring system to predict renal outcome in IgA nephropathy: from a nationwide prospective study. *Nephrol Dial Transplant.* 2006;21:2800–2808.
181. Pfeffer MA, Burdmann EA, Chen CY, et al. A trial of darbepoetin alfa in type 2 diabetes and chronic kidney disease. *N Engl J Med.* 2009;361:2019–2032.
208. Tangri N, Stevens LA, Griffith J, et al. A predictive model for progression of chronic kidney disease to kidney failure. *JAMA.* 2011;305:1553–1559.
212. de Brito-Ashurst I, Varagunam M, Raftery MJ, et al. Bicarbonate supplementation slows progression of CKD and improves nutritional status. *J Am Soc Nephrol.* 2009;20:2075–2084.
226. Landray MJ, Emberson JR, Blackwell L, et al. Prediction of ESRD and death among people with CKD: the Chronic Renal Impairment in Birmingham (CRIB) prospective cohort study. *Am J Kidney Dis.* 2010;56:1082–1094.
232. Isakova T, Xie H, Yang W, et al. Fibroblast growth factor 23 and risks of mortality and end-stage renal disease in patients with chronic kidney disease. *JAMA.* 2011;305(23):2432–2439.
252. Shankar A, Klein R, Klein BE. The association among smoking, heavy drinking, and chronic kidney disease. *Am J Epidemiol.* 2006; 164:263–271.
292. Madero M, García-Arroyo FE, Sánchez-Lozada L-G. Pathophysiologic insight into MesoAmerican nephropathy. *Curr Opin Nephrol Hypertens.* 2017;26(4):296–302.
304. Tangri N, Ansell D, Naimark D. Predicting technique survival in peritoneal dialysis patients: comparing artificial neural networks and logistic regression. *Nephrol Dial Transplant.* 2008;23(9):2972–2981.
307. Cook NR. Use and misuse of the receiver operating characteristic curve in risk prediction. *Circulation.* 2007;115(7):928–935.
308. Steyerberg EW, Vickers AJ, Cook NR, et al. Assessing the performance of prediction models: a framework for some traditional and novel measures. *Epidemiology.* 2010;21(1):128–138.
323. Tangri N, Kitsios GD, Inker LA, et al. Risk prediction models for patients with chronic kidney disease: a systematic review. *Ann Intern Med.* 2013;158:596–603.
324. Kent DM, Jafar TH, Hayward RA, et al. Progression risk, urinary protein excretion, and treatment effects of angiotensin-converting enzyme inhibitors in nondiabetic kidney disease. *J Am Soc Nephrol.* 2007;18:1959–1965.
327. Tangri N, Grams ME, Levey AS, et al. Multinational assessment of accuracy of equations for predicting risk of kidney failure: a meta-analysis. *JAMA.* 2016;315(2):164–174.
328. Lerner B, Desrochers S, Tangri N. Risk prediction models in CKD. *Semin Nephrol.* 2017;37(2):144–150.
329. Bansal N, Katz R, De Boer IH, et al. Development and validation of a model to predict 5-year risk of death without ESRD among older adults with CKD. *Clin J Am Soc Nephrol.* 2015;10(3):363–371.
331. Tangri N, Ferguson T, Komenda P. Pro: risk scores for chronic kidney disease progression are robust, powerful and ready for implementation. *Nephrol Dial Transplant.* 2017;32(5):748–751.
333. Collister D, Rigatto C, Hildebrand A, et al. Creating a model for improved chronic kidney disease care: designing parameters in quality, efficiency and accountability. *Nephrol Dial Transplant.* 2010;25(11):3623–3630.
338. Drew DA, Lok CE, Cohen JT, et al. Vascular access choice in incident hemodialysis patients: a decision analysis. *J Am Soc Nephrol.* 2015;26(1):183–191.

21

# Developmental Programming of Blood Pressure and Renal Function Through the Life Course

Valérie A. Luyckx | Karen M. Moritz | John F. Bertram

CHAPTER OUTLINE



The large variation in individual susceptibility to kidney disease and other chronic diseases is not easily explained.[1] Genetic factors are important determinants of development and function of major organ systems as well as of susceptibility to disease. Rare genetic and congenital abnormalities leading to abnormal kidney development are associated with the occurrence of subsequent renal dysfunction, often manifest very early in life.[2,3] Most renal disease in the general population, however, is not ascribable to genetic mutations, with the most common etiologic associations with end-stage kidney disease (ESKD) worldwide being the polygenic disorders of diabetes and hypertension. Of note here is the association between mutations in the apolipoprotein-1 (*APOL1*) gene in people of African descent with increased predisposition to the development of HIV-associated nephropathy and focal and segmental glomerulosclerosis (FSGS). However, searches for other specific gene polymorphisms or mutations have not implicated specific genes but instead point to a likely complex interplay between polygenic predisposition and environmental factors in the development of hypertension, diabetes, and renal disease.[4–9] Hypertension and renal disease prevalence vary between populations from different ethnic backgrounds, with very high rates observed among Aboriginal Australians, Native Americans, and people of African descent.[10–12] It is well established that lifestyle and socioeconomic factors pose significant risk for the development and persistence of hypertension and diabetes in the general population, with obesity becoming an increasing concern, especially in the developing world.[7,13] However, more and more evidence is pointing also to the far-reaching effects of the intrauterine environment and early postnatal growth on organ development, organ function, and subsequent susceptibility to adult disease.[14–16] Stresses experienced during fetal life (for which low birth weight, being small for gestational age, preterm birth, or high birth weight may be surrogate markers), such as maternal malnutrition, ill health, preeclampsia, or gestational diabetes, or those experienced in early childhood, such as poor early nutrition, infections, and environmental exposures, may "program" long-term organ function and may be the first in a succession of challenges or "hits" that ultimately manifest in overt disease. This chapter outlines the effects of fetal and early-life programming on renal development (particularly nephrogenesis), nephron endowment, and the risks of hypertension and kidney disease throughout the life course. Major congenital renal anomalies are discussed elsewhere in this book (see Chapter 72). In addition, it must be borne in mind that low birth weight and preterm birth also predict later-life diabetes, cardiovascular disease, metabolic syndrome, and preeclampsia; therefore, renal function may be additionally impacted through developmental programming of these disorders and in turn may impact outcomes of these diseases, the discussion of which is beyond the scope of the current chapter.[16–20]

## DEVELOPMENTAL PROGRAMMING

The process through which an environmental insult experienced early in life can predispose to adult disease is known as "developmental programming," which refers to the observation that an environmental stimulus experienced during a critical period of development in utero or early postbirth can induce long-term structural and functional effects in the organism.[15,21] This phenomenon, often termed "developmental origins of health and disease," can have far-reaching implications in that the effects can be perpetuated across generations.[22,23] The association between adverse intrauterine events and subsequent cardiovascular disease has long been recognized.[15,21,24,25] In early studies, adults of low birth weight were found to have higher cardiovascular morbidity and mortality than those of normal birth weight.[26] Subsequently, evidence from diverse populations has confirmed these findings and expanded them to include other conditions, such as hypertension, impaired glucose tolerance, type 2 diabetes, obesity, preeclampsia, and chronic kidney disease (CKD).[21,27–33] Of these, the associations between low birth weight and preterm birth and subsequent hypertension have been the most studied.[34–37] Until recently, attention has largely focused on preterm birth and low birth weight as markers for developmental programming of hypertension and renal disease, but being small for gestational age or having a high birth weight, often as a result of a diabetic pregnancy or maternal obesity, are also emerging as risk factors.[38–41] Currently, birth weight and preterm birth are the best available surrogates for an adverse intrauterine environment, but some intrauterine stresses may not manifest as such and therefore may not be recognized. Ongoing work is required to develop more sensitive measures of developmental stress. Table 21.1 outlines the definitions of birth weight and gestational age categories, which are referred to throughout this chapter. Globally, the respective incidences of low birth weight and preterm birth are around 15%–20% and 11%.[42,43] Importantly, as shown in Fig. 21.1, a large proportion of babies born small for gestational age have a birth weight above 2.5 kg, highlighting the need to identify all small-for-gestational-age infants who are also at risk of programming effects.[44] The global incidence of high birth weight is rising, ranging from 5%–20% in high-income and 0.5%–15% in lower-income countries.[40] A significant number of infants born yearly therefore likely undergo developmental programming and are at risk for chronic disease later in life.

**Table 21.1 Definitions of Birth Weight and Prematurity Categories**

| Category | Definition |
|---|---|
| **Birth Weight Categories** | |
| Normal birth weight | >2500 g and <4000 g (usually) |
| Large for gestational age | >2 standard deviations above the mean birth weight for gestational age |
| Low birth weight | <2500 g |
| Very low birth weight | <1500 g |
| Appropriate for gestational age | Within ±2 standard deviations of the mean birth weight for gestational age |
| Small for gestational age | >2 standard deviations below the mean birth weight for gestational age |
| Intrauterine growth restriction | Evidence of fetal malnutrition and growth restriction at any time during gestation |
| **Gestational Categories** | |
| Extremely preterm | <28 weeks of gestation |
| Very preterm | <32 and >28 weeks of gestation |
| Moderately preterm | <34 and >32 weeks of gestation |
| Late preterm | <37 and >34 weeks of gestation |
| Full term | >37 weeks of gestation |

Taken from Abitbol CL, Rodriguez MM. The long-term renal and cardiovascular consequences of prematurity. *Nat Rev Nephrol.* 2012;8:265–274.

## DEVELOPMENTAL PROGRAMMING IN THE KIDNEY

The kidney is the organ central to the development of hypertension. The relationship between renal sodium handling, intravascular volume homeostasis, and hypertension is well accepted.[45,46] That factors intrinsic to the kidney itself affect blood pressure has been demonstrated clinically in kidney transplantation in which the blood pressure in the recipient after transplantation has been shown to be related to the blood pressure or hypertension risk factors of the donor: that is, hypertension "follows" the kidney.[47] In 1988, Brenner and colleagues[48] proposed that congenital (programmed) low nephron number may explain why some individuals are susceptible to hypertension and renal injury, whereas others may seem relatively resistant under similar circumstances (e.g., sodium excess or diabetes mellitus). Low nephron number and low whole-kidney glomerular surface area would result in reduced sodium excretory capacity, enhancing susceptibility to hypertension, and a relatively reduced renal reserve capacity, limiting compensation for renal injury. This hypothesis was attractive in that an association between low nephron number and low birth weight, for example, could explain differences in hypertension and renal disease prevalence observed in populations of different ethnicity, among whom those who tend to have lower birth weights often have a greater prevalence of hypertension and renal disease.[49–52]

### PLAUSIBILITY OF THE NEPHRON NUMBER HYPOTHESIS

An obstacle to investigation of the nephron number hypothesis has been the difficulty of accurately counting or estimating the total number of nephrons in a kidney.[53] Review of early studies shows that humans were believed to have an average of approximately 1 million nephrons per kidney.[54] This was the nephron number published in textbooks for decades, and implied that there is little variability in human nephron number and therefore likely little relationship with adult disease risk. Such studies, however, were performed using

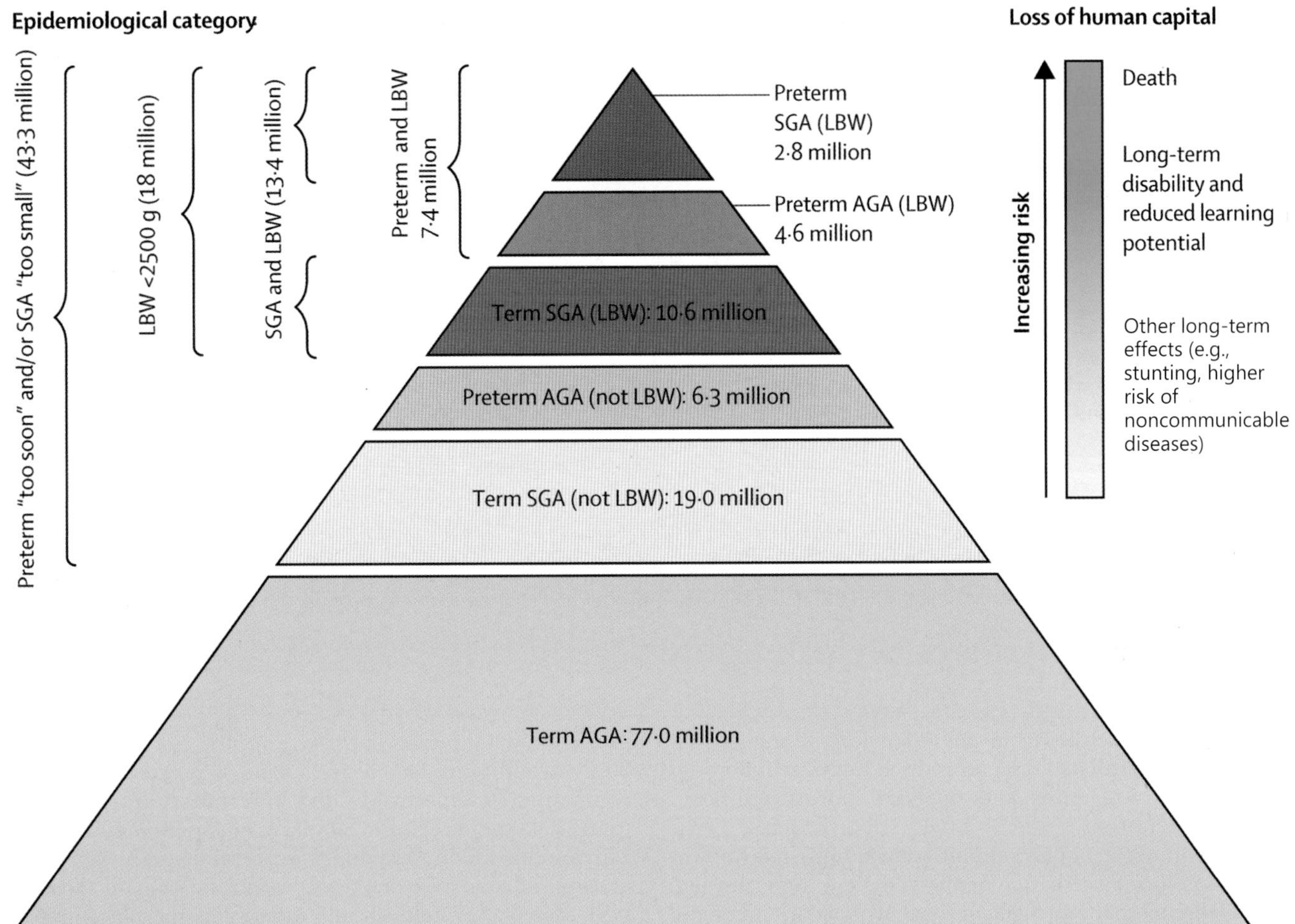


**Fig. 21.1** Public health implications of the burden of preterm and SGA births for 120 million births in countries of low and middle income in 2010. *AGA*, Appropriate for gestational age; *LBW*, low birth weight; *SGA*, small for gestational age. (From Lee AC, Katz J, Blencowe H, et al. National and regional estimates of term and preterm babies born small for gestational age in 138 low-income and middle-income countries in 2010. *Lancet Glob Health*.)

techniques such as acid maceration or traditional model-based stereologic approaches, which are prone to bias because of required assumptions, extrapolations, and operator sensitivity.[53–55] Moreover, many of the early studies analyzed only a handful of kidneys, and therefore, population variability in nephron number was not observed.

Over the past 25 years, the design-based (often termed "unbiased") dissector/fractionator method has emerged as the gold standard method for estimating total glomerular, and thereby nephron, number because it generates accurate (no bias) and precise (low-variance) estimates.[53–55] With this approach, the dissector principle[56] is used to sample glomeruli in representative histologic samples of the three-dimensional renal cortex with equal probability (regardless of their size, shape, and location), and then these sampled glomeruli are counted. Glomeruli are counted in a "known" fraction of kidney tissue, allowing simple algebraic estimation of the total number of glomeruli in the whole kidney.

As the dissector/fractionator method requires sampling from a whole kidney, all studies to date with this technique have been performed on autopsy samples. For 37 normal Danish adults, the average glomerular (nephron) number was reported to be 617,000 per kidney (range: 331,000–1,424,000).[54] A positive correlation was noted between glomerular number and kidney weight, but this has not been the case in all studies.[57] The large variation in nephron number in Danes has subsequently been reported in several other populations (Table 21.2), with the largest range to date being a 13-fold variation in the largest sample yet investigated (African Americans; 159 subjects; 210,332 to 2,702,079 per kidney).[58] This previously unappreciated variability in total nephron number in subjects without kidney disease, apart from age-associated changes, may influence susceptibility to hypertension and kidney disease.[54,58,59]

In general, numbers of viable glomeruli are reduced in kidneys from older subjects, owing to age-related glomerulosclerosis and obsolescence.[54,60] Recently, Denic et al.[61] estimated glomerular number in 1638 living donor kidneys using a method combining computed tomographic (CT) estimation of renal cortical volume (prior to donation) with stereologic estimation of glomerular numerical density (number per unit volume of cortex) obtained on biopsies at the time of donation. Multiplication of these two estimates provided an estimate of total glomerular number. Separate estimates of nonsclerotic and sclerotic glomeruli were obtained. A striking decrease in numbers of nonsclerotic glomeruli was observed between 18–29-year-olds and donors aged 70–75 years. Moreover, the total number of sclerotic and nonsclerotic

**Table 21.2 Variability of Nephron Number Per Kidney in Humans**

| Population | Sample Size | Mean | Range | Fold[a] | Reference |
|---|---|---|---|---|---|
| Danish | 37 | 617,000 | 331,000–1,424,000 | 4.3 | 54 |
| French | 28 | 1,107,000 | 655,000–1,554,000 | 2.4 | 534 |
| German (all) | 20 | 1,074,414 | 531,140–1,959,914 | 3.7 | 59 |
| German hypertensive | 10 | 702,379 | 531,140–954,893 | 1.8 | |
| German normotensive | 10 | 1,429,200 | 884,458–1,959,914 | 2.2 | |
| African-American | 105 | 884,938 | 210,332–2,026,541 | 9.6 | 292 |
| White American | 84 | 843,106 | 227,327–1,660,232 | 7.3 | |
| Australian non-Aborigines | 24 | 861,541 | 380,517–1,493,665 | 3.9 | 220 |
| Australian Aborigines | 19 | 713,209 | 364,161–1,129,223 | 3.1 | |
| Senegalese | 47 | 992,353 | 536,171–1,764,421 | 3.3 | 291, 535 |
| African and white Americans, Australian Aborigines and non-Aborigines and Senegalese | 420 | 901,902 | 210,332–2,702,079 | 12.8 | 536 |
| Japanese males (all) | 18 | 544,819 | 306,092–960,756 | 3.1 | 221 |
| Japanese Hypertensive (males) | 9 | 423,498 | 306,092–550,222 | 1.8 | |
| Japanese Normotensive (males) | 9 | 666,140 | 419,282–960,756 | 2.3 | |
| Kidney donors | 1638 | 873,696 | | | 61 |

[a]Fold change from lowest to highest nephron number.

Adapted from Puelles VG, Hoy WE, Hughson MD, et al. Glomerular number and size variability and risk for kidney disease. *Curr Opin Nephrol Hypertens.* 2011;20:7–15.

glomeruli was much lower in the older donors, suggesting that many glomeruli had disappeared without trace following global glomerulosclerosis, and/or older donors were born with fewer nephrons.

In support of the nephron number hypothesis, it is known that persons born with severe nephron deficits, for example, unilateral renal agenesis, bilateral renal hypoplasia, and oligomeganephronia, develop progressive proteinuria, glomerulosclerosis, and renal dysfunction with time.[3,62] Analogously, therefore, people born with nephron numbers at or below the median level may be more susceptible to superimposed postnatal factors that act as subsequent "hits"; thus, a significant proportion of the population may be at risk for the development of hypertension and renal disease, given that some 30% of the world's adult population is hypertensive.[7,14]

The counterargument to the nephron number hypothesis is that in experimental animals and in humans, removal of one kidney (presumed reduction in nephron number by 50%) under varying circumstances may be associated with higher blood pressures or low-grade proteinuria but does not always lead to hypertension and renal disease.[55,63,64] Of interest, however, uninephrectomy on postnatal day 1 in rats or fetal uninephrectomy in sheep, that is, loss of nephrons at a time when nephrogenesis is not yet completed, does lead to adult hypertension prior to any evidence of renal injury.[65–67] These data support the hypothesis that congenitally acquired low nephron number may be associated with different compensatory mechanisms in the developing and growing kidney, or with a reduced compensatory capacity compared with later nephron loss, resulting in increased risk of hypertension. Consistent with this, kidneys from rats that underwent unilateral nephrectomy at 3 days of age showed a similar total glomerular number but a significantly reduced number of mature glomeruli in the remaining kidney compared with those that underwent nephrectomy at 120 days of age.[68] Furthermore, the mean glomerular volume in the remaining kidney of rats following unilateral nephrectomy in the neonatal period increased by 59% as compared with 20% in adult rats, likely indicating a greater burden of compensatory hypertrophy and hyperfiltration in response to neonatal nephrectomy. Similarly, rats spontaneously born with a solitary kidney are highly susceptible to the induction of hypertension (via deoxycorticosterone acetate (DOCA) salt), as well as proteinuria and reduced glomerular filtration rate (GFR) compared with rats that underwent a uninephrectomy 8 weeks after birth.[69] Nephrons in mice born with low nephron endowment were found to be less capable of coping with a stress such as unilateral ureteral obstruction than mice with the normal nephron complement.[70]

In potential contrast, however, a study of 97 subjects with a radiologically normal single kidney, aged 2.5–25 years, found that renal function declined faster over time in those with acquired single kidneys (surgical removal of the other kidney) versus congenital single kidneys, although blood pressures and proteinuria were not different.[71] These findings may be confounded by indication for nephrectomy, however, as approximately 25% of the nephrectomies were performed for obstruction, which may impact nephron development in the contralateral kidney as will be discussed later.[72,73] In addition, unilateral in utero nephrectomy in sheep was associated with significant renal hypertrophy and a 45% increase in nephron number in the remaining kidney, indicating that a congenital solitary kidney may have a higher than normal nephron endowment and therefore be relatively protected compared with an acquired single kidney.[74,75] Thus, timing of nephron loss is likely a crucial factor in determining the compensatory capacity of remaining nephrons.

## ESTIMATING NEPHRON NUMBER

Until recently, most estimates of glomerular number were obtained using acid maceration of kidneys obtained at autopsy or model-based or design-based stereological analysis of histological samples obtained at autopsy. While useful, reliance on autopsy samples precludes studies in living animals and

**Table 21.3 Glomerular Characteristics by Birth Weight in Humans**

| Birth Weight Mean (Range), kg | *N* | Number of Glomeruli[a] | Mean Glomerular Tuft Volume ($\mu m^3 \times 10^6$) | Total Glomerular Tuft Volume ($cm^3$) |
|---|---|---|---|---|
| 2.65 (1.81–3.12) | 29 | 770,860 (658,757–882,963) | 9.2 | 6.7 |
| 3.27 (3.18–3.38) | 28 | 965,729 (885,714–1,075,744) | 7.2 | 6.8 |
| 3.93 (3.41–4.94) | 30 | 1,005,356 (900,094–1,110,599) | 6.9 | 6.6 |

[a]Adjusted for age, gender, race, body surface area.
From Hoy WE, Hughson MD, Bertram JF, et al. Nephron number, hypertension, renal disease, and renal failure. *J Am Soc Nephrol.* 2005;16:2557–2264.

patients, as well as longitudinal studies. In recent years, we have seen the development of several new approaches for imaging, counting, and sizing glomeruli, some of which do not require autopsy tissue. For example, the methods of Denic et al.[61,76] and of Fulladosa et al.,[77] which use CT or magnetic resonance imaging (MRI) estimation of cortical volume and estimation of glomerular numerical density in biopsies, do not require autopsy tissue. The number of functional (nonsclerotic) glomeruli has also been estimated by dividing the whole kidney ultrafiltration coefficient ($K_f$; calculated from renal plasma flow from para-amino-hippurate clearance) by single-nephron $K_f$ estimated from electron microscopic measurements of the glomerular filtration barrier using kidney biopsies.[78,79]

An MRI technique using cationic ferritin to label glomeruli shows promise,[80,81] but to date, studies have been ex vivo. Cationic ferritin is injected intravenously into animals or into ex vivo human kidneys via the renal artery and binds to anionic charges on the glomerular basement membrane. With this approach, all glomeruli in whole rat,[82,83] mouse,[84] and human[80] kidneys are imaged, counted, and sized, providing, for the first time, the glomerular volume distribution for whole kidneys. New tissue-clearing approaches also facilitate imaging (using light sheet microscopy), counting, and sizing of all glomeruli in ex vivo rodent kidneys,[85] but whether modifications to this approach can be safely used in vivo appears unlikely at this time. With these recent advances in glomerular imaging and counting, we can hope that in vivo glomerular imaging and quantitation will be possible in the not-too-distant future.

## NEPHRON NUMBER AND GLOMERULAR VOLUME

Human glomeruli have been reported to increase in size up to sevenfold from infancy to adulthood.[86–88] This can be considered normal physiological growth. Glomerular size also increases in adulthood in people without overt renal disease and is associated with increasing age, increasing body size, and lower birth weight.[89] Mean glomerular volume has also been consistently noted to vary inversely with total glomerular number, although the correlation appears stronger among Caucasians and Australian Aboriginals than in people of African origin.[59,90–92] This relationship suggests that larger glomeruli may reflect compensatory hyperfiltration and hypertrophy in subjects with fewer nephrons and may therefore be a surrogate marker for a reduced nephron number.[60,91] In fact, Hoy and coworkers[90] found that, although mean glomerular volume was increased in subjects with reduced nephron number, total renal glomerular tuft volume (a surrogate for total renal filtration surface area) was not different among groups with different nephron numbers (Table 21.3). This suggests that total renal filtration surface area may initially be maintained in the setting of a low or reduced nephron number but at the expense of glomerular hypertension and hypertrophy, which are maladaptive and predictors of poor outcomes.[93–95] Consistent with this possibility, glomerulomegaly is common in renal biopsies from Australian Aborigines, a population with high rates of low birth weight and renal disease, and has also been associated with faster rate of decline of GFR in Pima Indians.[96–98] Furthermore, in a study of donor kidneys, maximal planar area of glomeruli was found to be higher in kidneys from African Americans compared with whites and a predictor of poorer transplant function.[94] Among 111 adult males from four ethnic groups, mean glomerular volume and variability were highest among African Americans and Aboriginal Australians, likely associated with susceptibility to hypertension and renal disease.[99] In populations at high risk of kidney failure, therefore, large glomeruli are a common finding at early stages of renal disease and may reflect programmed reductions in nephron number in these populations in which access to prenatal and subsequent health care is often suboptimal.[100–102] An increase in glomerular volume, however, is not always associated with lower glomerular number, and individual glomerular volume varies considerably within kidneys.[92] Overall, however, glomerulomegaly and greater intrasubject variability in glomerular volume were associated with older age, fewer nephrons, lower birth weight, hypertension, obesity, and severity of cardiovascular disease.[99]

# EVIDENCE FOR PROGRAMMING IN THE KIDNEY

## DEVELOPMENTAL PROGRAMMING OF NEPHRON ENDOWMENT

### EXPERIMENTAL EVIDENCE FOR PROGRAMMING OF NEPHRON ENDOWMENT

Developmental programming of nephron number has been the most rigorously studied link to later-life hypertension and kidney disease so far. Numerous animal models have demonstrated the association between low birth weight (induced by gestational exposure to low-protein or low-calorie diets, uterine ischemia, dexamethasone, vitamin A deprivation, alcohol) with subsequent hypertension.[103–110] The link between

**Table 21.4 Associations of Nephron Number and Renal Size With Blood Pressure and Renal Function**

**Experimental Evidence**

**Reduction in Nephron Number**

| *Experimental Model* | *Animal* | *Glomerular Number (% change)* | *Birth Weight* | *Blood Pressure* | *Renal Function* |
|---|---|---|---|---|---|
| Maternal calorie restriction[174,537,538] | Rat | ↓ 20–40 | ↓ | ↑ | ↓ GFR proteinuria |
| Uterine artery ligation[112,302,402] | Rat | ↓ 20–30 | ↓ | ↑ | Impaired proteinuria |
| Low-protein diet during gestation[108,115,539–541] | Rat | ↓ 25 | | | ↓ GFR |
| | | ↓ 17 | ↓/↔ | ↑ | proteinuria |
| | | ↓ 16 | | | ↓Longevity |
| Postnatal nutrient restriction[406] | Rat | ↓ 27 | Normal | ↑ | NA |
| Iron deficiency[322] | Rat | ↓ 22 | ↓ | ↑ | NA |
| Vitamin A deficiency[115,326] | Rat | ↓ 20 | ↔ | NA | NA |
| Zinc deficiency[324] | Rat | ↓ 25 | NA | ↑ | ↓ GFR proteinuria |
| Ethanol[379,381] | Sheep | ↓ 11 | ↔ | NA | NA |
| | Rat | | ↓ | ↑ | ↓ GFR (females) ↑ GFR (males) |
| Hypoxia[542] | Rats | ↓ 26–52 | ↓ | NA | NA |
| Cigarette smoke[543] | Mouse | NA | ↓ | NA | ↓ Kidney mass |
| Ureteral obstruction, neonatal[73] | Rat | ↓ 50 | NA | ↑ | ↓ GFR ↓ Renal growth postrelief of obstruction |
| Prematurity[113] | Mouse | ↓ 17–24 | ↓ | ↑ | ↓ GFR ↑ Albuminuria |
| Glucocorticoids[103,107,356,544] | Rat | ↓ 20 | ↓/↔ | ↑ | Glomerulosclerosis |
| | Sheep | ↓ 38 | ↔ | ↑ | ↑ Collagen deposition |
| Maternal diabetes[148,341] | Rat | ↓ 10–35 | ↔ | ↑ | Salt sensitivity |
| Gentamicin[370,372] | Rat | ↓ 10–20 | ↓ | NA | NA |
| β-Lactams[374] | Rat | ↓ 5–10 | ↔ | NA | Tubular dilatation Interstitial inflammation |
| Cyclosporine[176,545] | Rabbits | ↓ 25–33 | ↓/↔ | ↑ | ↓ GFR ↑ RVR proteinuria |
| Dahl salt sensitive[48] | Rat | ↓ 15 | | ↑ with Na intake | Accelerated FSGS |
| Munich-Wistar-Frömter[48,546] | Rat | ↓ 40 | | ↑ with age | ↑ SNGFR FSGS |
| Milan hypertensive[48] | Rat | ↓ 17 | | ↑ | NA |
| PVG/c[48] | Rat | ↑ 122 | | Resistant | Resistant to FSGS |
| PAX2 mutations[306,396,400] | Mouse Human | ↓ 22 | | NA | Renal coloboma syndrome in humans, small kidneys |
| GDNF heterozygote[392,547] | Mouse | ↓ 30 | ↔ | ↑ | Normal GFR Enlarged glomeruli |
| c-ret null mutant[297] | Mouse | ↓ | NA | NA | Severe renal dysplasia |
| hIGFBP-1 overexpression[339] | Mouse | ↓ 18–25 | ↓ | NA | Glomerulosclerosis |
| Bcl-2 deficiency[397] | Mouse | ↓ | NA | NA | ↑BUN and creatinine |
| p53 transgenic[401] | Mouse | ↓ 50 | NA | NA | Glomerular hypertrophy Renal failure |
| COX2 null mutant[548] | Mouse | NA | ↔ | ↔ | ↓GFR |
| Fibroblast growth factor (FGF) 7 null mutant[115] | Mouse | ↓ 30 | NA | NA | Reduced ureteric branching |
| **Augmentation of Nephron Number** | | | | | |
| Vitamin A supplementation (with low-protein diet)[419] | Rat | Normalized | NA | NA | NA |
| Amino acid (glycine, urea, or alanine) supplementation to maternal low protein diet[549] | Rat | Normalized | NA | Normalized with glycine only | NA |
| Restoration of postnatal nutrition postintrauterine growth restriction[112] | Rat | Normalized | ↓ | Normalized | NA |

**Table 21.4 Associations of Nephron Number and Renal Size With Blood Pressure and Renal Function (Cont'd)**

| *Experimental Model* | *Animal* | *Glomerular Number (% change)* | *Birth Weight* | *Blood Pressure* | *Renal Function* |
|---|---|---|---|---|---|
| Iron supplementation to iron-deficient mothers[323] | Rat | Partial rescue | NA | NA | NA |
| Ouabain administration (with low-protein diet)[415] | Mouse | Prevented ↓ | NA | NA | NA |
| Maternal uninephrectomy prior to gestation[420] | Rat | ↑ | NA | NA | NA |
| Postnatal overfeeding, normal birth weight[137] | Rat | ↑ 20 | ↔ | ↑ | Glomerulosclerosis |
| Maternal high-fat diet prior to and during pregnancy and lactation[350] | Mouse | ↑ 20–25 | ↔ | NA | NA |

**Human Evidence**

| *Clinical Circumstance* | *Population/ Age* | *Glomerular Number/ Kidney Volume[a] (% change)* | *Birth Weight* | *Blood Pressure* | *Renal Function* |
|---|---|---|---|---|---|
| Low birth weight[91,124] | Human 0–1 year | ↓ 13–35 | ↓ | NA | NA |
| Preterm birth[122] | Human | ↓ Correlated with gestational age | ↓ | NA | NA |
| Females vs. males[285] | Human | ↓ 12 | NA | Variable | Variable |
| Hypertensive vs. normotensive Caucasian[59,120] | Human 35–59 years | ↓ 19–50 | NA | ↑ | No ↑ Glomerulosclerosis |
| Hypertensive vs. normotensive African American[120] | Human 35–59 years | NS ↓ | NA | ↑ | No ↑ Glomerulosclerosis |
| Aboriginal Australians vs. Caucasian Australians[55] | Human 0–85 years | ↓ 23 | ↓ | NA | |
| Senegalese Africans[535,550] | Human 5–70 years | NA | NA | NA | ↑ Variability of glomerular size with ↓ glomerular numbers |
| Maternal vitamin A deficiency[460] | Indian vs. Canadian newborns | ↓ Newborn renal volume | NA | NA | NA |
| Genetic polymorphisms: | | | | | |
| *RET(1476A)* polymorphism[121] | Newborns | ↓ 10[a] | NA | NA | NA |
| *PAX2 AAA* haplotype[306] | Newborns | ↓ 10[a] | NA | NA | NA |
| Combined *RET(1476A)* polymorphism and *PAX2 AAA* haplotype[121] | Newborns | ↓ 23[a] | NA | NA | NA |
| *I/D ACE* polymorphism[551] | Newborns | ↓ 8[a] | NA | NA | NA |
| *BMPR1A*$^{rs7922846}$ polymorphism[307] | Newborns | ↓ 13[a] | NA | NA | NA |
| *OSR1*$^{rs12329305(T)}$ polymorphism[310] | Newborns | ↓ 12[a] | NA | NA | NA |
| Combined *OSR1* and *RET* polymorphisms[310] | Newborns | ↓ 22[a] | NA | NA | NA |
| Combined *OSR1* and *PAX2* polymorphisms[310] | Newborns | ↓ 27[a] | NA | NA | NA |
| *ALDH1A2*$^{rs7169289(G)}$ polymorphism[308] | Newborns | ↑ 22[a] | NA | NA | NA |

[a]Numbers relate to kidney volume and not to glomerular number.

*BUN*, Blood urea nitrogen; *FSGS*, focal segmental glomerulosclerosis; *GDNF*, glial cell line-derived neurotrophic factor; *GFR*, glomerular filtration rate; *NA*, not assessed; *NS*, nonsignificant; *RVR*, renal vascular resistance; *SNGFR*, single-nephron GFR.

Adapted from Luyckx VA, Bertram JF, Brenner BM, et al. Effect of fetal and child health on kidney development and long-term risk of hypertension and kidney disease. *Lancet.* 2013;382:273–283; Brenner BM, Garcia DL, Anderson S. Glomeruli and blood pressure. Less of one, more the other? *Am J Hypertens.* 1988;1:335–347; Kett MM, Bertram JF. Nephron endowment and blood pressure: what do we really know? *Curr Hypertens Rep.* 2004;6:133–139; Clark AT, Bertram JF. Molecular regulation of nephron endowment. *Am J Physiol.* 1999;276:F485–F497; Moritz KM, Wintour EM, Black MJ, et al. Factors influencing mammalian kidney development: implications for health in adult life. *Adv Anat Embryol Cell Biol.* 2008;196:1–78.

adult hypertension and low birth weight in these animal models appears to be mediated, at least in part, by an associated congenital nephron deficit.[103,107,108] Corresponding blood pressures and nephron numbers associated with various programming models are outlined in Table 21.4. As shown, the association between birth weight, nephron numbers, and blood pressures varies between models, as discussed in detail later, underscoring the complexity of developmental programming and the need for better markers than birth weight.

Vehaskari and colleagues[108] demonstrated an almost 30% lower glomerular number in offspring of pregnant rats fed a low-protein diet compared with a normal-protein diet during pregnancy (see Fig. 21.2A). As shown in Fig. 21.2B, the low-protein offspring had tail-cuff systolic blood pressures that were around 40 mm Hg higher by 8 weeks of age.[108] Similarly, prenatal administration of dexamethasone was associated with low birth weight and fewer glomeruli than controls.[103] In these nephron-deficient rats, GFR was reduced, albuminuria was increased, and urinary sodium excretion was lower than those with a normal nephron complement.[103] Uteroplacental insufficiency, induced by maternal uterine artery ligation late in gestation, also results in low nephron number and was associated with increased profibrotic renal gene expression with age, although hypertension developed only in males.[111,112] Conversely, adequate postnatal nutrition, by cross-fostering onto normal lactating females at birth, restored nephron number and prevented subsequent hypertension in growth-restricted male rats.[112] In a study of the impact of preterm birth, mice delivered 1–2 days early (normal mouse gestation, 21 days) had lower nephron numbers, lower GFR, and higher blood pressures and albuminuria than mice born at term.[113] Interestingly, nephron numbers were lower in mice delivered 2 days compared with 1 day early, suggesting the degree of preterm birth is important in determining final nephron endowment, even though nephrogenesis continues for about 5 days after birth in the normal mouse. Not surprisingly, in animal studies, timing of the gestational insult has been found to be crucial in renal programming, with the greatest impact on nephron number occurring during periods of most active nephrogenesis.[114]

The complexity of the effects of perturbations to the feto-maternal environment and genetic variants on kidney development was recently highlighted in two studies. Sampogna et al.[115] compared the effects of vitamin A deficiency,

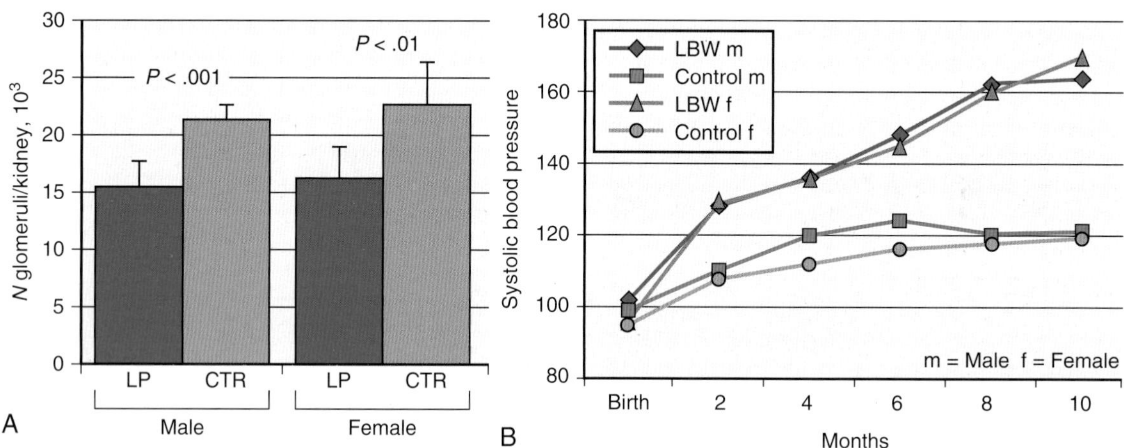


**Fig. 21.2** Fetal programming of hypertension in low-birth-weight rats (induced by maternal low-protein diet). (A) Total number of glomeruli per kidney at 8 weeks of age, and (B) systolic blood pressure throughout life, in male ($n$ = 7) and female ($n$ = 6) offspring from low-protein pregnancies and in male ($n$ = 7) and female ($n$ = 7) control rats *(Control)*. *LBW*, Low birth weight. (Adapted from Vehaskari VM, Aviles DH, Manning J. Prenatal programming of adult hypertension in the rat. *Kidney Int.* 2001;59:238–245.)

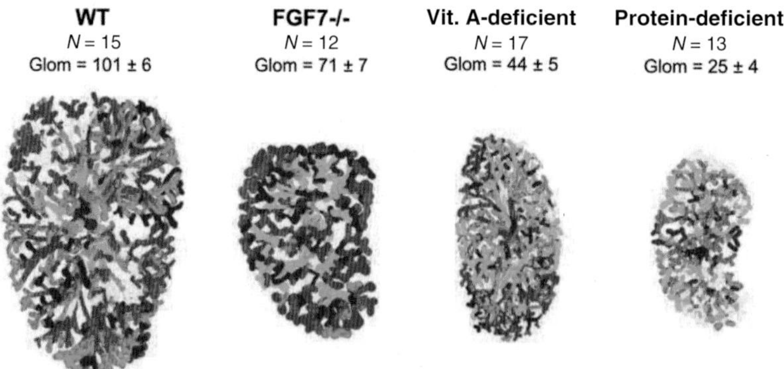


**Fig. 21.3** Architecture of wild type *(WT)*, FGF7 null mutant, vitamin A–deficient, and protein-deficient mouse kidneys. Embryonic day 15.5 ureteric tree tracings for each condition (to scale). *N* is the maximum branching generation number, and *Glom* represents the mean glomerular count (minimum of three kidneys studied per condition). In each case, glomerular count is reduced compared with the wild type. The number of branching generations is specific to each condition. (From Sampogna RV, Schneider L, Al-Awqati Q. Developmental program- ming of branching morphogenesis in the kidney. *J Am Soc Nephrol.* 2015;26(10):2414–2422.)

protein deficiency, and FGF7 deletion on kidney development and nephron endowment in mice (Fig. 21.3). Perturbations to kidney development included developmental delay, defects in nephron induction, changes in the growth axis, and alterations in ureteric branching morphogenesis. These produced up to a threefold decrease in glomerular number and a twofold decrease in total branching events. Boubred et al.[116] carefully compared the effects of two perturbations to the feto-maternal environment on nephron number and adult renal physiology in rats. Maternal gestational low-protein diet and betamethasone both led to a similar level of growth restriction, but nephron numbers were lower in betamethasone than the low-protein-diet offspring. Betamethasone offspring had impaired GFR, increased blood pressure, and glomerulosclerosis, whereas renal function and structure were unaltered in low-protein-diet offspring at 22 months of age. These findings suggest that the degree of reduction in nephron number is a risk factor for cardiovascular and renal disease. In summary, the available evidence suggests that the effect of a suboptimal feto-maternal environment on offspring nephron endowment and adult health may be influenced by species, the nature, timing, duration and severity of the perturbation, gender, and the postnatal nutritional environment (including lactation, infant nutrition, and subsequent growth).

## PROGRAMMING OF NEPHRON NUMBER IN HUMANS

As noted earlier, total nephron number varies widely in the normal human population (see Table 21.2).[58,117] A significant proportion of the interindividual variability in nephron number appears to be already present perinatally, demonstrating a strong developmental effect.[118,119] Overall, the data support a direct relationship between nephron number and birth weight and an inverse relationship between nephron number and glomerular volume.[87,91,120,121] Hughson and colleagues[87] reported a linear relationship between glomerular number and birth weight, and calculated a regression coefficient predicting an increase of 257,426 glomeruli per increase in birth weight, although the generalizability of the regression coefficient to populations in which the distribution of nephron number appears bimodal, such as among African Americans, may not be valid.

In recent years, glomerular loss associated with aging in healthy human kidneys has come to be better appreciated. Rates of loss of glomeruli per year have been variously reported as approximately 6750 glomeruli per year after the age of 18 years,[60] 4500 glomeruli per year,[90] and 6200 glomeruli per year.[61] Specifically, the number of nonsclerotic functional glomeruli per kidney was found to decrease by almost 50% from young adulthood (aged 18–29 years: 990,661 glomeruli) to old age (aged 70–75 years: 520,410 glomeruli).[61] Glomerular number tends to be lower in women than in men.[60,61] A kidney starting with a lower nephron number, therefore, would conceivably reach a critical reduction of nephron mass, either with age or in response to a renal insult, earlier than a kidney with a greater nephron complement, predisposing to hypertension and/or renal dysfunction.

Nephrogenesis in humans begins during the 9th week of gestation and continues until the 34th to 36th week.[90] Nephron number at birth is therefore largely dependent on the intrauterine environment and gestational age. It is generally believed that no new nephrons are formed in humans after term birth. To investigate whether glomerulogenesis does continue postnatally in preterm infants, Rodriguez and colleagues[122] studied kidneys at autopsy from 56 extremely preterm infants compared with 10 full-term infants as controls. The radial glomerular counts (an estimate of glomerular number based on the number of layers of glomeruli in the cortex) were lower in preterm versus full-term infants and correlated with gestational age. Furthermore, evidence of active glomerulogenesis, indicated by the presence of S-shaped bodies immediately under the renal capsule, was seen in preterm infants who died before 40 days, but was absent in those who died after 40 days of life, suggesting that nephrogenesis may continue for up to 40 days after preterm birth. These authors also stratified their cases by presence or absence of renal failure.[122] Among infants surviving longer than 40 days, those with renal failure (serum creatinine >2.0 mg/dL) had significantly fewer glomeruli than those without renal failure. This cross-sectional observation may suggest that renal failure inhibited glomerulogenesis or, conversely, that fewer glomeruli lowered the threshold to develop renal failure in these infants. Those preterm infants surviving longer than 40 days without renal failure exhibited glomerulomegaly, which may reflect, at least in the short term, a compensatory renoprotective response. Faa and colleagues[118] also reported evidence of active glomerulogenesis in kidneys of preterm infants and two term infants who died at birth, but not in a child who died at age 3 months, suggesting that glomerular maturation may continue even after term birth for a short period.

In contrast, Hinchliffe and associates[123,124] studied nephron number in preterm or full-term stillbirths or infants who died at 1 year of age and who were born with either appropriate weight for gestational age or small-for-gestational age. At both time points, growth-restricted infants had fewer nephrons than controls. In addition, the number of nephrons in growth-restricted infants dying at 1 year of age had not increased compared with the growth-restricted stillbirths, demonstrating a lack of postnatal nephrogenesis (Fig. 21.4A). Manalich and coworkers[91] examined the kidneys of neonates dying within 2 weeks of birth in relation to their birth weights (see Fig. 21.4B). A significant direct correlation was found between glomerular number and birth weight, and a strong inverse correlation between glomerular volume and glomerular number, independent of sex and race. These studies all support the hypothesis that an adverse intrauterine environment, which may manifest as low birth weight, small-for-gestational age, or preterm birth, is associated with a congenital reduction in nephron endowment and an early, compensatory increase in glomerular volume.

In a population of 140 adults aged 18 to 65 years who died of various causes, a significant correlation was also observed between birth weight and glomerular number.[120] Glomerular volume was inversely correlated with glomerular number. Total glomerular number did not differ statistically between African-American and white subjects, although the distribution among African Americans appeared bimodal. The range of nephron number was greatest in African Americans. Significantly, however, none of the subjects in this study had been of low birth weight; therefore, no conclusion can be drawn as to whether an association with low birth weight and nephron number existed in either population group.[120] It may be argued that as low birth weight is more

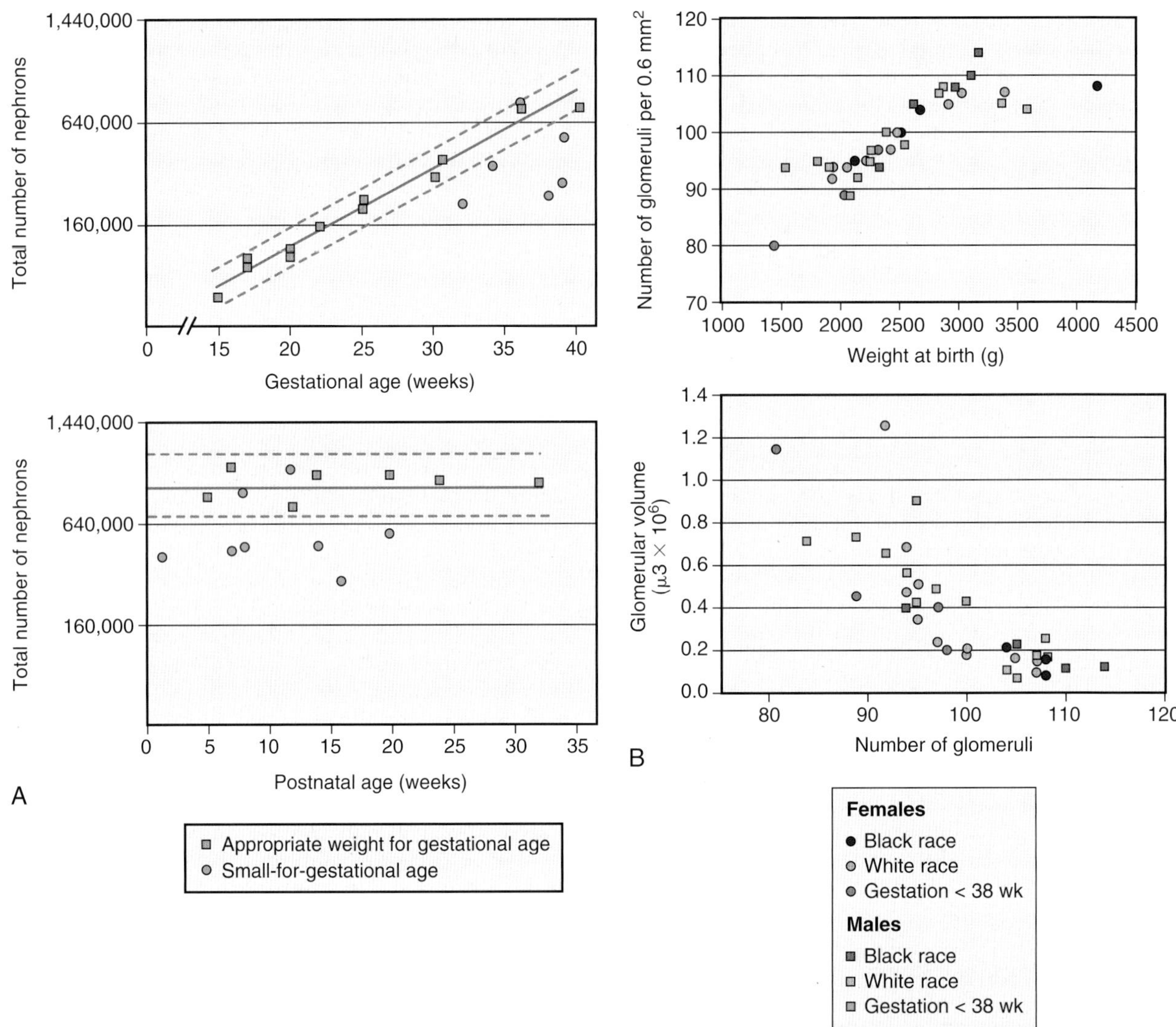


**Fig. 21.4** Effect of intrauterine grown restriction (IUGR) on nephron number in humans. (A) Nephron number at birth in relation to gestational age (*upper panel*), and lack of postnatal catch-up in nephron number (*lower panel*). (From Hinchliffe SA, Lynch MR, Sargent PH, et al. The effect of intrauterine growth retardation on the development of renal nephrons. *Br J Obstet Gynaecol.* 1992;99:296–301.) (B) Relationship between birth weight and glomerular number (*upper panel*), and between glomerular number and glomerular volume (*lower panel*) in neonates. (From Manalich R, Reyes L, Herrera M, et al. Relationship between weight at birth and the number and size of renal glomeruli in humans: a histomorphometric study. *Kidney Int.* 2000;58:770–773.)

prevalent among African Americans, this cohort was more representative of the general white population than the general black population, having included only subjects of normal birth weight.[125] In a European study, among 26 subjects with non–insulin-dependent diabetes compared with 19 age-matched nondiabetic controls, no difference in glomerular number was found, but again, all subjects had birth weights above 3 kg; therefore, the impact of low birth weight on nephron number could not be assessed.[126]

### Kidney Size as a Correlate for Nephron Number

Analysis of the relationship between kidney weight and nephron endowment in infants younger than 3 months of age (a time at which compensatory hypertrophy has likely not yet occurred) revealed a direct relationship (Fig. 21.5).[121] Regression analysis predicted an increase of 23,459 nephrons per gram of kidney weight.[121] Renal mass is therefore proportional to nephron number in the early postnatal period, and renal volume is proportional to renal mass; therefore, renal volume has been used as a surrogate for nephron endowment in infants in vivo.[54] Ultrasound evaluation of fetal renal function in utero revealed a reduction in hourly urine volume, higher prevalence of oligohydramnios, reduced renal perfusion, and reduced renal volume in growth-restricted fetuses.[127–129] These findings may represent reduced fetal perfusion in situations of uterine compromise, however, and do not necessarily reflect altered renal development. Similarly, among preterm infants, kidney volume at a corrected age of 38 weeks was significantly lower than in term infants and was associated with a significantly lower GFR estimated from serum cystatin C.[130] Analysis of kidney size and postnatal growth measured by ultrasound in 178 children born preterm or small for gestational age compared with 717 mature children with appropriate weight for gestational age at 0, 3, and 18 months found that weight for gestational age was positively associated with kidney volume at all three time points.[131] Slight

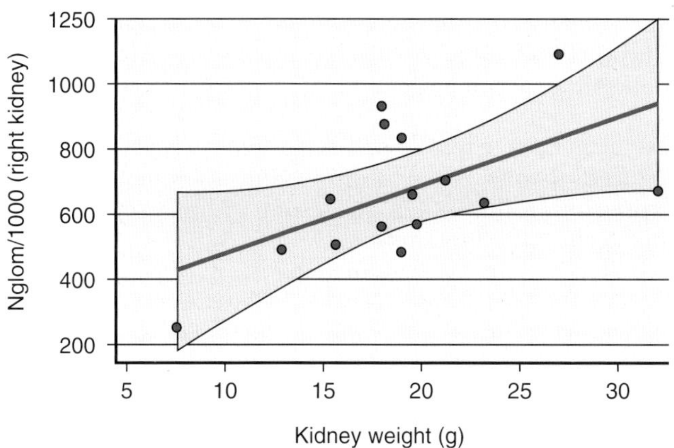


**Fig. 21.5** Relationship between nephron number and mass of the right kidney in Caucasian infants aged ≤3 months who died within the first 3 months of life. *Nglom/1000,* Number of glomeruli per kidney in 1000s. (From Zhang Z, Quinlan J, Hoy WE, et al. A common RET variant is associated with reduced newborn kidney size and function. *J Am Soc Nephrol.* 2008;19:2027–2034.)

catch-up in kidney growth was observed in growth-restricted infants but not in preterm infants. Similarly, in a South Indian population, kidney volumes were lower in low-birth-weight and small-for-gestational-age neonates compared with those of normal and appropriate-for-gestational-age birth weights.[132] Kidneys in the low-birth-weight and small-for-gestational-age infants remained small and grew more slowly than kidneys of normal-birth-weight or appropriate birth-weight-for-gestational-age infants during the first 2 years of life. In a study of multiethnic children in the Netherlands, lower fetal weight gain and lower early infant weight gain led to smaller kidneys at 6 years of age.[133] However, only lower fetal weight gain, not postnatal weight gain, was associated with lower estimated GFR (eGFR). These findings suggest that suboptimal early growth affects kidney function in later life.

Among term neonates, renal parenchymal thickness, proposed as a more accurate screening tool than renal volume estimation, was significantly reduced in those with low compared with normal birth weights.[134] In Australian Aboriginal children, low birth weight was also found to be associated with lower renal volumes on ultrasound.[135] Comparison of renal volume between children aged 9–12 years born preterm, at either small or appropriate weight for gestational age, and controls, found that kidneys were smallest in those who had been preterm and small for gestational age, but when adjusted for body surface area (BSA), there were no significant differences between the groups.[136] A smaller kidney size, therefore, may be a surrogate marker for a reduced nephron endowment, but importantly, growth in kidney size on ultrasound cannot distinguish between normal growth with age and renal hypertrophy. In contrast to the situation in infants and children, in adults, kidney size is not a reliable marker of nephron number tautology. Findings from six studies in adults in which kidney size was reported and nephron number had been estimated using the dissector/fractionator combination were analyzed.[57] Only data from subjects aged 18–60 years without renal disease were included. Although an association between renal size and nephron number was found, only about 5% of the variation in nephron numbers was explained by differences in renal size.

**Table 21.5 Developmentally Programmed Changes Observed in the Kidney**

- Nephron number
- Glomerular volume
- Accelerated maturation of glomeruli
- Tubular sodium transporter expression and/or activity
- Altered renal vascular reactivity
- Alterations in renin-angiotensin system
- Alterations in sympathetic nervous system activity
- Accelerated senescence, especially after catch-up growth
- Predisposition to inflammation and fibrosis
- Kidney size

## EVIDENCE OF ADDITIONAL PROGRAMMING EFFECTS IN THE KIDNEY

Taken together, there is no doubt that nephron endowment varies widely in human kidneys and that a range of perturbations to the feto-maternal environment in animal models can dramatically influence nephron endowment. Once nephrogenesis ends, no new nephrons can form, and therefore, any deficit in nephron number is permanent. Nephron endowment is likely an independent factor determining susceptibility to essential hypertension and subsequent renal injury. However, low nephron number alone does not account for all observed programmed hypertension (see Table 21.4). Supplementation of a low-protein diet during gestation with glycine, urea, or alanine resulted in a normalization of nephron number in rat offspring, but blood pressure only normalized in those supplemented with glycine.[34] Likewise, augmentation of nephron number by postnatal hypernutrition resulted in a 20% increase in nephron number but also obesity, hypertension, and glomerulosclerosis with age.[137] These findings suggest that additional factors also contribute to developmental programming of hypertension. Recent evidence has shown alterations in renal tubular sodium handling and vascular function in developmentally programmed kidneys that likely also contribute to later-life blood pressure and renal functional changes, as outlined in Table 21.5.[114,138]

### Altered Sodium Handling by the Kidney

The pressure–natriuresis curve is shifted to the right in most forms of hypertension. A low total renal filtration surface area associated with a low nephron number is one plausible hypothesis to explain the associated higher blood pressures. Consistent with this, salt sensitivity has been reported in several animal models associated with low birth weight and low nephron number.[35,139–143] Some authors have reported the presence of salt-sensitive hypertension in rats in which low birth weight was induced by maternal uterine artery ligation, whereas others report no salt sensitivity in rats in which low birth weight was induced by maternal protein restriction, although timing of dietary intervention and age at study appear to play a role.[140,144,145] Elevations in blood pressure in response to a high-salt diet have been more consistently observed in aging rather than young rats, suggesting an early adaptive mechanism that may decline with age or worsening salt sensitivity as nephron number declines with age.[146] In young rats, however, despite no change in blood pressure, an increase in plasma volume was observed, consistent with sodium retention.[147] Similar salt sensitivity was observed in adult rat offspring exposed to maternal gestational diabetes, a model also associated with low nephron number.[148]

The effect of nephron "dose" and total renal filtration surface area on salt sensitivity was examined in glial cell line–derived neurotrophic factor (GDNF) heterozygous mice that have either 1 kidney (HET1K) and 65% few nephrons than wild type littermates, or two kidneys (HET2K) and 25% fewer nephrons than GDNF wild type mice.[149] Given the accompanying glomerular hypertrophy, total glomerular surface area was normal in HET2K but remained reduced in HET1K mice at 48–52 weeks of age. At baseline, the mice did not have elevated blood pressures; however, both heterozygous groups became hypertensive in response to high-sodium feeding. A gradient of increasing blood pressure was observed from GDNF wild type to HET2K to HET1K, suggesting dependence on nephron number and filtration surface area, given that no change in expression of tubular sodium transporters was observed.[149] In contrast, transforming growth factor-β2 (TGF-β2) heterozygous mice, which have 30% more nephrons than TGF-β2 wild type mice, were relatively protected against developing high blood pressures on a chronic high-salt diet compared with wild type mice.[150] Surprisingly, however, these mice did develop increased blood pressures in response to an acute sodium load, suggesting that the benefit conferred by the higher nephron number requires time for adaptation to occur. Early change in sodium diet in itself has been found to have a long-term impact on programming of hypertension in low-birth-weight rats. Short-term feeding of a low-salt diet from weaning to 6 weeks of age abrogated, whereas high-salt feeding exacerbated hypertension at 10 and 51 weeks despite reinstitution of normal salt diet at 6 weeks.[139,151] The role of sodium intake on long-term renal programming requires further study.

Salt sensitivity, therefore, does appear to be developmentally programmed. From the GDNF mouse data, total renal filtration surface area may be crucial in determining salt sensitivity, but as discussed earlier, it is often not reduced in the setting of low nephron number due to concomitant glomerular hypertrophy. Expression and activity of renal tubule sodium transporters have therefore been investigated. Expression of the Na-K-2Cl (NKCC2) and Na-Cl (NCC) transporters were significantly increased in prehypertensive offspring of rats fed a protein-restricted diet during gestation compared with controls, although expression of the sodium–hydrogen exchanger type III (NHE3) and epithelial sodium channel (ENaC) were not changed (Fig. 21.6A).[152] Increased activity of NKCC2 was shown by increases in chloride transport and lumen positive transepithelial potential difference in the medullary thick ascending limb in offspring of protein-restricted or dexamethasone-treated mothers (Fig. 21.6B).[153] Furthermore, after development of hypertension, furosemide administration reduced blood pressure, supporting increased NKCC2 activity as a mediator of hypertension in the protein restriction model.[153] Expression of the glucocorticoid receptor and the glucocorticoid responsive α1- and β1-subunits of Na-K-ATPase were increased in offspring of pregnant rats fed a low-protein diet.[154] In rats suckled by low protein–fed mothers during lactation, expression of Na-K-ATPase was increased by 40%, but Na-K-ATPase activity was increased by 300%, demonstrating that expression levels may not fully reflect activity levels.[155] Prenatal dexamethasone administration was associated with increased expression of proximal tubular NHE3, as well as the more distal NKCC2 and NCC, but no change in ENaC expression.[156] Interestingly, renal denervation reduced systolic blood pressure and sodium transporter expression in this model, suggesting indirect regulation of these genes via sympathetic nerve activity.[156] In rats subjected to maternal diabetes, baseline expression of β and γ ENaC, but not α ENaC, as well as Na-K-ATPase, were significantly increased compared with controls.[148] Despite several studies showing no change in ENaC expression in programmed animals, an enhanced natriuretic response to the ENaC inhibitor benzamil demonstrated increased ENaC activity in offspring of mothers fed a low-protein diet (Fig. 21.6C).[157] Taken together, despite differences among models, the data suggest increased sodium transport in all segments of the renal tubule. Whether a reduced nephron number contributes indirectly to increased sodium transport through increased single-nephron GFR (SNGFR), necessitating glomerulotubular balance, or sodium transporter activity is independently programmed, has not yet been elucidated.

### Renin–Angiotensin System

All components of the renin–angiotensin–aldosterone system (RAAS) are expressed in the developing kidney.[158] Alterations in the renal RAAS have been studied in various programming models, and a common, though not universal, finding has been inhibition of the system during the period of active nephrogenesis with an upregulation in adulthood, often associated with changes in blood pressure.[159] For example, expression of angiotensinogen and renin mRNA was decreased in neonatal kidneys of rats subjected to uterine ischemia but increased in mouse offspring of diabetic mothers.[160,161] Outcomes likely reflect species differences, differences in timing of intervention, timing of study, and so on, as summarized in Table 21.6.[75] The importance of angiotensin II in nephrogenesis was demonstrated by the administration of the angiotensin II subtype 1 receptor (AT1R) blocker, losartan, to normal rats during the first 12 days of life (while nephrogenesis is proceeding), which resulted in a low final nephron number and subsequent development of hypertension.[162,163] Angiotensin II can stimulate the expression of Pax-2 (an antiapoptotic factor) through AT2R.[164] AT2R expression, therefore, is likely to affect nephrogenesis and kidney development, but its role in programming is still unclear. Administration of an angiotensin-converting enzyme inhibitor (ACEI), captopril, or losartan to low-birth-weight rats from 2 to 4 weeks of age abrogated the development of adult hypertension.[21,112,160,165] Similarly, administration of angiotensin II or ACEI to adult rats subjected to a low-protein diet in utero resulted in a more exaggerated hypertensive or hypotensive response, respectively, than in control rats.[21,166–168] However, a recent study in aged offspring born growth restricted demonstrated that AT1 receptor blockade could not prevent hypertension, suggesting lesser dependence on the RAAS with age.[169] Differential regulation of the RAAS by sex hormones during development is thought to contribute to the observation that the effects of developmental programming are often less severe in young females.[159,170] Overall, programmed suppression of the intrarenal RAAS during nephrogenesis is likely to contribute to low nephron number

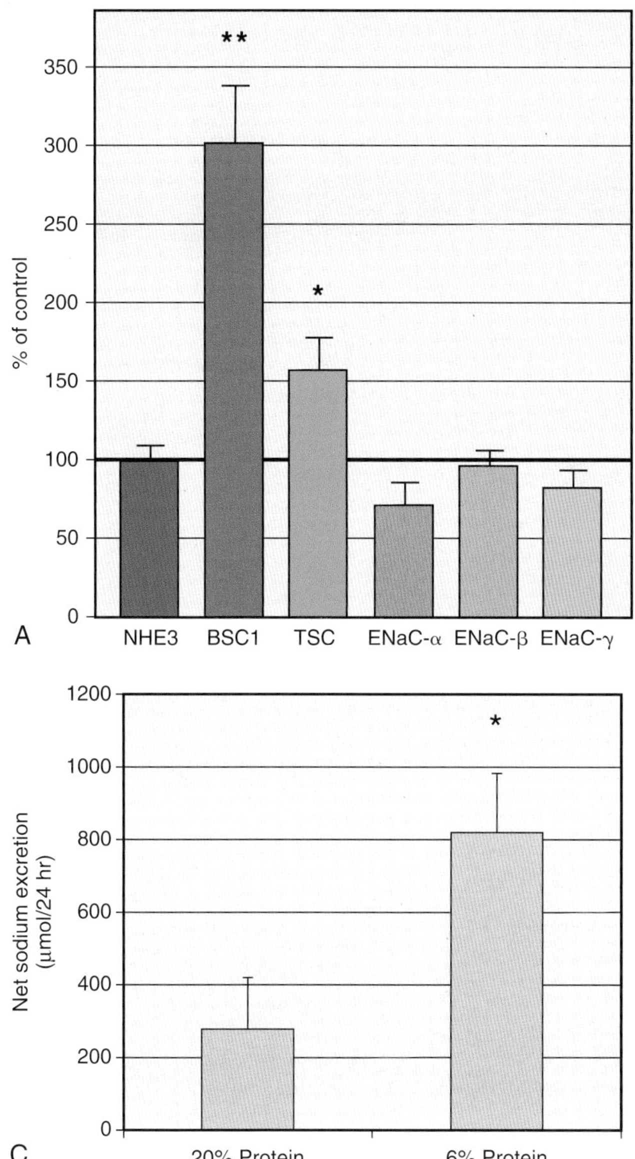


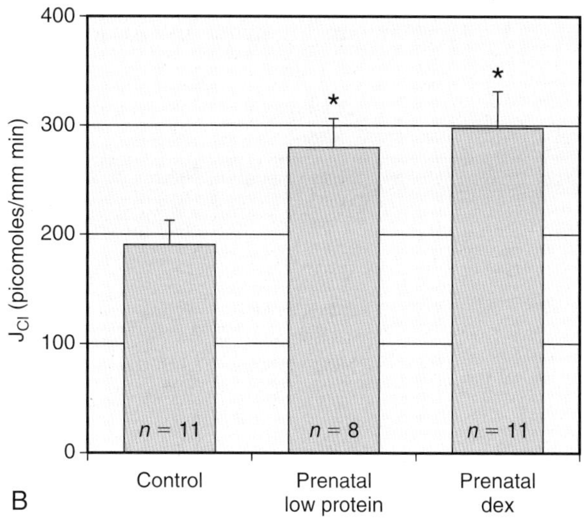


**Fig. 21.6** (A) Apical renal sodium transporter expression, quantified by immunoblotting, in 4-week-old rat offspring from maternal low-protein diet. $^*P < .05$; $^{**}P < .001$. *BSC*, Bumetanide-sensitive cotransporter (NKCC2); *ENac*, epithelial sodium channel *TSC*, thiazide-sensitive cotransporter (NCC); *NHE3*, Na/H exchanger isoform 3. (From Vehaskari VM, Woods LL. Prenatal programming of hypertension: lessons from experimental models. *J Am Soc Nephrol.* 2005;16:2545–2556.) (B) Increased rate of medullary thick ascending limb (mTAL) chloride transport ($J_{Cl}$) in in vitro perfused mTAL from 6-week-old rat offspring of mothers given a prenatal low-protein diet or prenatal dexamethasone. $^*P < .05$ versus control. (From Dagan A, Habib S, Gattineni J, et al. Prenatal programming of rat thick ascending limb chloride transport by low-protein diet and dexamethasone. *Am J Physiol Regul Integr Comp Physiol.* 2009;297:R93–R99.) (C) Net increase in urine sodium excretion after administration of ENaC inhibitor, benzamil, in adult rat offspring of mothers fed a low-protein (6%) or normal-protein (20%) diet during gestation. Data are expressed as means ± standard error. $^*P < .05$. (From Cheng CJ, Lozano G, Baum M. Prenatal programming of rat cortical collecting tubule sodium transport. *Am J Physiol Renal Physiol.* 2012;302:F674–F678.)

under adverse circumstances, and postnatal upregulation of the AT1R, possibly mediated by an increase in glucocorticoid activity or sensitivity, may contribute to the subsequent development of hypertension and glomerular hyperfiltration as reviewed in detail elsewhere.[75,159]

Underscoring the relevance of the RAAS in developmental programming of blood pressure, angiotensin-converting enzyme (ACE) activity was significantly elevated in children of low birth weight compared with normal birth weight, and there was a greater frequency of the ACE gene DD genotype among low-birth-weight children with highest blood pressures, suggesting that the programming effect of blood pressure may be in part modulated by ACE gene polymorphisms.[171]

### The Sympathetic Nervous System and Renal Vascular Reactivity

Within the kidney, the sympathetic nervous system modulates activity of the RAAS, sodium transport, and vascular function and thereby contributes to blood pressure through regulation of vascular tone and volume status.[75] Development of the renal sympathetic nervous system and how this may be programmed during nephrogenesis, and modulated by the RAAS, is expertly reviewed by Kett and Denton.[75] Renal denervation has been shown to abrogate development of adult hypertension and alter sodium transporter expression in the prenatal dexamethasone and uterine ischemia programming models, as well as the age-associated hypertension that develops in growth-restricted female rats.[156,172,173] Consistent with the whole animal findings, within the kidney, an increase in baseline renal vascular resistance has been described in several programming models.[174–176] For example, renal arterial responses to β-adrenergic stimulation and sensitivity to adenylyl cyclase were increased in 21-day-old growth-restricted offspring subjected to placental insufficiency.[177] Although the renal expression of β2-adrenoreceptor mRNA was increased in these pups, there was also evidence of adaptations

**Table 21.6 Programming Effects on the Renin–Angiotensin System**

| Model | Species | Timing of Insult | Age and Sex of Offspring at Study | mRNA or Protein Expression | Physiologic Response | Reference(s) |
|---|---|---|---|---|---|---|
| Glucocorticoids | Sheep | Early gestation | 40 mo ♀ | ↔ Plasma renin, ANG II, or Aogen | ↑ Basal MAP, females only | 116 |
| | Rat | | 6–7 mo ♂♀ | ↔ Renal Aogen<br>↑ PRA, plasma Aogen in females only | ↑ Basal TBP, females only | 108 |
| | Rat | Mid- to late gestation | 6 mo | ↑ Renal ACE and renin in males and females | ND | 159 |
| | Rat | Mid- to late gestation | 4 and 8 wk ♂ | ↔ PRA, plasma ANG II, and renal ANG II levels<br>↑ Urine ANG II at 4 and 8 wk | ↑ Basal TBP at 8 but not 4 wk of age | 27 |
| Maternal nutrient restriction or low-protein diet | Sheep | Early- to midgestation | 9 mo old | ↑ Renal cortical ACE protein<br>↔ AT1R in the renal cortex and medulla<br>↔ Renal cortical but ↑ renal medulla AT2R | ↑ Basal MAP | 47 |
| | Rat | Mid- to late gestation | 4–12 wk ♂♀ | ↑ PRA | ↑ Basal TBP from 8 wk of age | 11 |
| | Rat | Throughout gestation | 1–5 days and 22 wk ♂ | ↓ Renal renin mRNA and ANG II levels at 1 to 5 days of age | ↑ Basal MAP at 22 wk of age<br>↔ No change GFR or RBF | 154, 155 |
| | Rat | Throughout gestation | 16 wk ♂ | ↓ Renal AT1R and AT2R protein | ↑ Basal TBP, ↓ sodium excretion, ↔ GFR | 99 |
| | Rat | Throughout gestation | 4 wk ♂ | ↑ Renal AT1R protein<br>↓ Renal AT2R protein<br>↑ Ang II receptor binding<br>↔ Renal renin and Ang II tissue levels | ↑ Basal MAP (anesthetized)<br>↑ Basal renal vascular resistance<br>↔ No change GFR or RBF | 125, 126 |
| | Rat | Mid- to late gestation | 1 to 11 mo ♂♀: | | ↑ Basal TBP at 8 wk of age | 94, 95, 146, 147 |
| | | | 1–2 mo | ↓ PRA<br>↓ Renal AT1R protein and mRNA<br>↓ Renal AT2R protein, ↑ AT2R mRNA | Salt-sensitive TBP<br>TBP normalized by ACE inhibition and low-salt diet<br>Urinary protein/creatinine ratio increased in males only | |
| | | | 6 to 11 mo | ↑ PRA<br>↔ Plasma or renal ANG I and ANG II<br>↑ AT1R protein and mRNA<br>↑ AT2R protein, ↔ AT2R mRNA | | |
| Placental insufficiency | Rat | Late gestation | 0 to 16 wk ♂ | | | 53, 110 |
| | | | Newborn: | ↓ renal renin and aogen | ↑ Basal MAP that was abolished by ACEi treatment | |
| | | | 16 wk: | ↑ Renal renin and aogen mRNA, ↑ ACE activity<br>↔ Renal $AT_1R$ and ANG II, ↔ PRA and plasma ACE | ↑ Pressor response to ANG II in presence of ACEi<br>↓ GFR | |
| Maternal renal hypertension | Rabbit | Throughout gestation | 10–45 wk, ♂ ♀ | ↓ PRA–5 and 10 wk<br>↔ PRA 30 and 45 wk | ↑ Basal MAP at 30 and 45 wk | 31, 32, 92 |

*ACE*, Angiotensin-converting enzyme; *ACEi*, angiotensin-converting enzyme inhibition; *Aogen*, angiotensinogen; *AT1R*, angiotensin receptor type 1; *GFR*, glomerular filtration rate; *MAP*, mean arterial pressure; *ND*, not done; *PRA*, plasma renin activity; *RBF*, renal blood flow; *TBP*, tail artery pressure.

Taken from Kett MM, Denton KM. Renal programming: cause for concern? *Am J Physiol Regul Integr Comp Physiol.* 2011;300:R791–R803.

to the signal transduction pathway contributing to the β-adrenergic hyperresponsiveness.[177] Intriguingly, these findings were much more marked in the right compared with the left kidney, an observation that remains unexplained but that is not without precedent: asymmetry of renal blood flow was found in 51% of a cohort of hypertensives without renovascular disease.[177,178] In this study, the growth-restricted rats had low glomerular number, glomerular hyperfiltration, and hyperperfusion, and had significantly increased proteinuria compared with controls, suggesting alteration in glomerular pressures likely mediated by renal vasoreactivity. Interestingly, in a cohort of white and black U.S. subjects, the effect of birth weight on subsequent blood pressures was significantly modified by β-adrenergic receptor genotype, further underscoring a relationship between birth weight, sympathetic activity, and blood pressure.[179]

## PROGRAMMING OF RENAL FUNCTION AND DISEASE

In contrast to preterm infants or those of low birth weight in whom nephron numbers have been shown to be reduced, in adults, there are no data on nephron number, specifically in those born with low birth weight. The association between nephron number and birth weight and preterm birth, however, is a consistent finding in infants, so it seems reasonable to extrapolate that nephron numbers would remain reduced in adults of low birth weight.[87] The determination of nephron number in vivo is not yet possible; therefore, the most used in vivo surrogate markers at present are birth weight and preterm birth. Importantly, however, in some animal models, low nephron numbers have also been observed in the setting of normal birth weight (see Table 21.4). Therefore, in humans, if birth weight is the only surrogate marker used, the impact of renal programming on any outcome is likely to be underestimated.[180] Other clinical surrogates for an adverse intrauterine environment and low nephron numbers are outlined in Table 21.7.

### EXPERIMENTAL EVIDENCE

Glomerulomegaly is consistently observed in the setting of low nephron number (see Fig. 21.4B). In rats in which low birth weight was induced by maternal protein restriction, GFR was reduced by 10%, although nephron number was reduced by 25%, implying some degree of compensatory hyperfunction per nephron.[35] Although this may be a compensatory mechanism to restore filtration surface area, it is conceivable that renal reserve in these kidneys is reduced.[90] If this is the case, these kidneys may be expected to be less able to compensate further in the setting of additional renal insults and to begin to manifest signs of renal dysfunction (i.e., proteinuria, elevations in serum creatinine, and hypertension). To investigate this hypothesis, diabetes was induced by streptozotocin injection in subgroups of low-birth-weight (induced by maternal protein restriction) and normal-birth-weight rats.[181] Low-birth-weight rats had reduced nephron numbers and higher blood pressures compared with those of normal birth weight. Among those rendered diabetic, there was a greater proportional increase in renal size and glomerular hypertrophy in the low-birth-weight rats compared with normal-birth-weight controls after 1 week (Fig. 21.7).[181] This study demonstrates that the renal response to injury in the setting of a reduced nephron number may be exaggerated and could lead to accelerated loss of renal function.

Subsequently, the same authors published outcomes in low-birth-weight versus normal-birth-weight diabetic rats at 40 weeks.[182] Histologically, the podocyte density was reduced and the average area covered by each podocyte was greater in the low-birth-weight diabetic rats than in the normal-birth-weight controls. These findings correlated with urine albumin excretion rate, which was higher in low-birth-weight diabetic rats, although this did not reach statistical significance. In support of the role of altered podocyte physiology in renal disease progression, similar findings were observed in the Munich Wistar-Frömter rat, a strain that has congenitally reduced nephron numbers and develops spontaneous renal disease.[183] Whether these podocyte changes are secondary to an increase in glomerular pressure in the setting of reduced nephron numbers or a primary programmed structural change leading to glomerular injury is not yet known. The podocyte depletion hypothesis has emerged as a potentially unifying concept in glomerular pathology in recent years, with podocyte depletion defined as either loss of podocytes, decreased podocyte density due to glomerular hypertrophy, or a change in podocyte phenotype.[184] Given that podocytes have little or no capacity to increase their numbers in adulthood, it will be important to determine if those feto-maternal environmental factors that result in low nephron endowment also produce low podocyte endowment. Humans and animals born with both a low nephron endowment and low podocyte endowment could be expected to be at further risk of developing CKD.

Of interest, in contrast, in low-birth-weight rats exposed to prenatal dexamethasone and subsequently fed a high-protein diet, GFR was similar to that in normal-birth-weight controls.[185] Nephron numbers were reduced by 13% in only the male low-birth-weight rats. This finding suggests that there is a threshold reduction in nephron number, above which compensation is adequate or that the high-protein diet–induced supranormal GFRs in both groups, masking subtle differences in baseline GFR. Another study that measured GFR in low-birth-weight rats, induced by placental insufficiency, also failed to demonstrate lower GFRs in low-birth-weight rats, but the low-birth-weight offspring were hypertensive compared with normal-birth-weight controls.[110] Conceivably, in this study, the higher intraglomerular pressure due to elevated blood pressure and reduced nephron mass in low-birth-weight rats

**Table 21.7 Clinical Surrogates for Programmed Low Nephron Number in Humans**

- Low birth weight[91,122,124]
- Preterm birth[122,124]
- Low kidney mass[54,121]
- Reduced kidney volume[131,135]
- Glomerulomegaly[87,91,124]
- Female sex[285]
- Ethnicity: Australian Aboriginal[285]
- Older age[61]

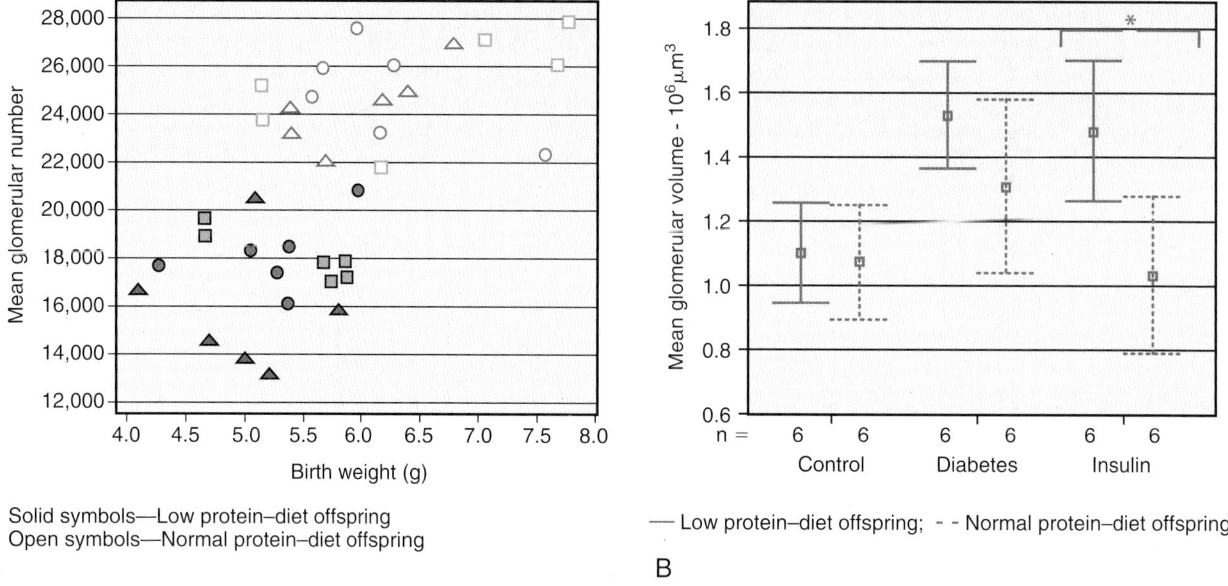


**Fig. 21.7** Influence of glomerular number on adaptation to diabetes in rats. (A) Scatterplot of mean glomerular number and birth weight in rats on low-protein diet *(solid symbols)* and normal protein diet *(open symbols)*; control groups *(triangles)*; diabetes *(circles)*; diabetes treated with insulin *(squares)*. (B) Plot of glomerular volume in rats on low-protein diet *(solid lines)* and normal-protein diet *(dotted lines)*. Error bars represent 95% confidence intervals. **P* = .015. (From Jones SE, Bilous RW, Flyvbjerg A, et al. Intra-uterine environment influences glomerular number and the acute renal adaptation to experimental diabetes. *Diabetologia* 2001;44:721–728.)

may have led to a compensatory increase in SNGFR and, thus, normalization of whole-kidney GFR.

The definitive pathophysiologic impact of a reduction in nephron number in the development of renal dysfunction is difficult to elucidate from the existing literature comprising very varied experimental conditions. Overall, however, it is possible that, although whole-kidney GFR may not change, SNGFR is likely to be increased in the setting of a reduced nephron number and exacerbated in the face of renal injury. Interestingly, SNGFR was found to be significantly elevated in the Munich-Wistar-Frömter rat, which has reduced nephron numbers and is known to develop spontaneous progressive glomerular injury, compared with the control Wistar rat strain.[183] Renal dysfunction may also result from a programmed predisposition to inflammation and scarring, which may be independent of glomerular pressures. In a glomerulonephritis model, anti–Thy-1 antibody injection in low-birth-weight rats resulted in significant upregulation of inflammatory markers and development of sclerotic lesions by day 14, but with no difference in blood pressure or proteinuria compared with normal-birth-weight controls.[186]

## HUMAN EVIDENCE

Most human data rely on the surrogates of birth weight and preterm birth and kidney size to reflect likelihood of renal programming. Although there is no direct proven relationship between renal risk and nephron number in humans, the consistency of the data is strongly suggestive of a programming effect.

### BIRTH WEIGHT, PRETERM BIRTH, AND BLOOD PRESSURE

Two meta-analyses and systematic reviews have shown consistent associations with lower birth weight and preterm birth and higher blood pressures in later life.[36,37] Meta-analysis of 27 studies investigating the relationship between birth weight and blood pressure found that systolic blood pressures were 2.28 mm Hg (95% confidence interval 1.24–3.33 mm Hg) higher in subjects with birth weights below, compared with higher 2.5 kg (Fig. 21.8A).[37] Many studies do not discriminate between low birth weight occurring as a result of growth restriction (a marker of intrauterine stress) at any gestational age or as a result of preterm birth with an appropriate (low) weight for gestational age. Therefore the relative impact of growth restriction and preterm birth on subsequent blood pressures is not always easy to dissect.[187] To investigate this question, a study of 50-year-old subjects all born at term, but with or without growth restriction, reported an odds ratio (OR) of 1.9 (95% confidence interval [CI]: 1.1 to 3.3) for hypertension among those who had experienced growth restriction compared with those who had normal birth weights.[188] Growth restriction before birth per se, therefore, is associated with subsequent higher blood pressure.

A systematic review of 10 studies comparing preterm or very low–birth-weight subjects versus those born at term found that the preterm subjects, having a mean gestational age of 30.2 weeks and a mean birth weight of 1280 g, had 2.5 mm Hg higher (95% CI: 1.7 to 3.3 mm Hg) systolic blood pressures in later life compared with those born at term (see Fig. 21.8B).[36] Preterm birth, therefore, is also independently associated with higher blood pressure, which, in some studies, meets the definition of hypertension by 1–2 years of age.[189–191] Whether the risk of higher blood pressure is greater among preterm subjects who were born small for gestational age (growth restricted) versus appropriate for gestational age, however, is not yet clear, with some studies suggesting an additional effect of growth restriction, whereas others do not.[192–195] Ultimately, the importance of dissecting the risk from low birth weight "versus" preterm birth may lie in the

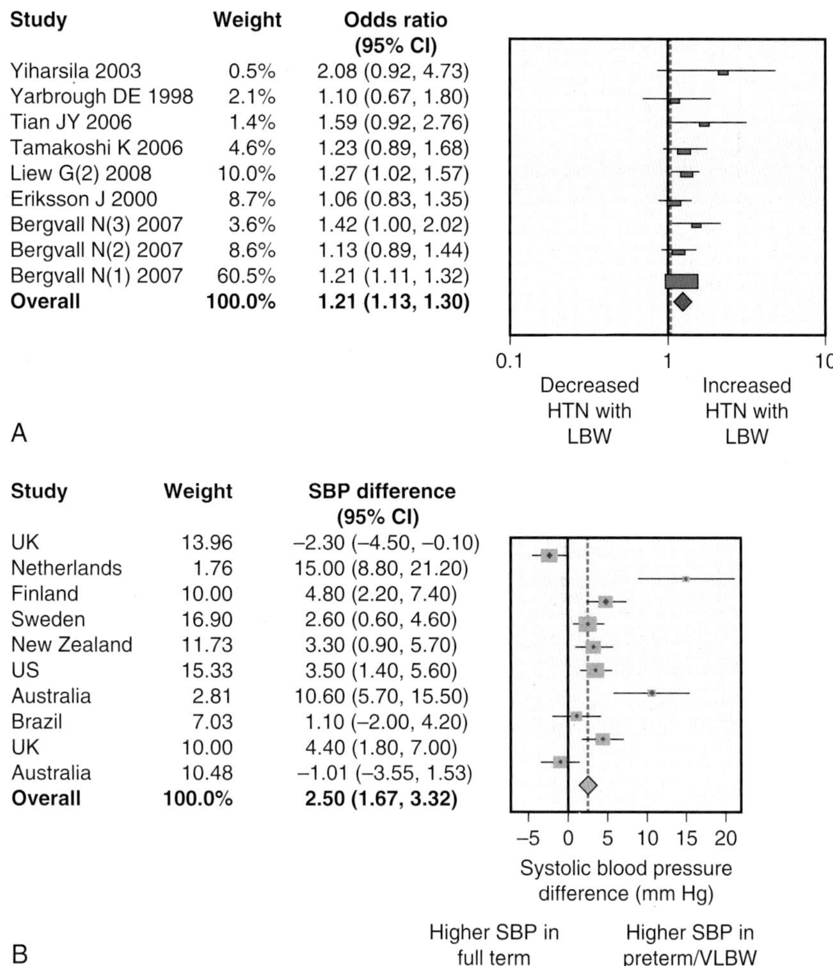


**Fig. 21.8** Relationship between birth weight, preterm birth, and blood pressure. (A) Meta-analysis of odds for hypertension *(HTN)* in individuals with birth weights below 2500 g (low birth weight *[LBW]*) compared with birth weights above 2500 g. The pooled odds ratio is shown as a *diamond*. (From Mu M, Wang SF, Sheng J, et al. Birth weight and subsequent blood pressure: a meta-analysis. *Arch Cardiovasc Dis.* 2012;105:99–113; see original paper for full references). (B) Meta-analysis of difference in systolic blood pressure *(SBP)* between individuals born preterm or very low birth weight *(VLBW)* compared with full term. Pooled SBP difference is indicated by the *diamond* and *dashed vertical line*. (From de Jong F, Monuteaux MC, van Elburg RM, et al. Systematic review and metaanalysis of preterm birth and later systolic blood pressure. *Hypertension.* 2012;59:226–234; see original paper for full references).

future potential for prevention, but, given that effect estimates for risk of higher blood pressures were similar in the meta-analyses and systematic reviews cited earlier, at present, both events must be deemed important risk factors for subsequent high blood pressure.

Importantly, blood pressures of low- and normal-birth-weight subjects, although different, may still be within the normal range in childhood, but differences become amplified with age, such that adults who had been of low birth weight often develop overt hypertension, which increases with age.[196] Although the majority of studies have been conducted in Caucasian populations, generally consistent data are accumulating in other populations.[197] An association of higher blood pressure with lower birth weight in African-American children has been reported in some studies, but not all, suggesting additional factors may contribute to the greater severity of blood pressure in those of African origin.[197–202] An important effect modifier of the association with low birth weight or preterm birth and blood pressure, noted in diverse populations, is current body mass index, which may override an effect of birth weight, especially in children at different stages of growth.[197,203] Furthermore, in most populations, blood pressures are highest in those born preterm or of low birth weight who "catch up" fastest in postnatal weight (i.e., rapid upward crossing of weight centiles), highlighting the importance of early postnatal nutrition in developmental programming.[204–208]

Elevated blood pressure associated with low birth weight was recently reported in a multiethnic cohort of adolescents.[209] From the National Health and Nutrition Examination Survey (NHANES) study, 5352 participants aged 12–15 years were classified as low birth weight, very low birth weight, or normal birth weight by parental/proxy recall. Low/very low-birth-weight adolescents had a greater odds of having a blood pressure ≥95th percentile for age, height, and sex [Low birth weight: OR: 2.90; 95% CI: 1.48 to 5.71; very low birth weight: OR 5.23; 95% CI: 1.11 to 24.74]. Whether preterm birth and/or small for gestational age contributed to the low birth weight in the population was not known.

Associations between blood pressure and other markers of potential developmental stresses have also been reported.

A meta-analysis of 31 studies found that blood pressures were also higher in children who had high birth weights; however, blood pressures tended to be lower in high-birth-weight adults, suggesting that age may modify this risk differently compared with that in low-birth-weight subjects in whom it increases with age (Table 21.8).[39,210] Additionally, a systematic review and meta-analysis investigating the impact of a diabetic pregnancy on blood pressure found an overall association with higher blood pressure in offspring aged 2–20 years, but this effect was only seen in males (Table 21.8).[211] The authors did not discuss the potential impact of birth weight in this study, however, and whether these effects may have been modified by offspring of high birth weight was not reported. Another potential risk factor for higher offspring blood pressure is maternal gestational hypertension or preeclampsia.[212,213] Indeed, in a systematic review of 18 studies among children and young adults, systolic blood pressures were 2.39 mm Hg (95% CI: 1.74 to 3.05) higher in young adults who had been exposed to preeclampsia compared with those not exposed (Table 21.8).[214] Whether the effect is mediated by the often accompanying fetal growth restriction or preterm birth or may be associated with circulating antiangiogenic factors or other humoral changes in preeclampsia requires further investigation. In a recent study of young adults (males and females) born preterm, soluble endoglin and soluble fms-like tyrosine kinase-1 (sflt-1) levels were significantly elevated ($P < .001$ for both) compared with controls born at term, and proportional to current systolic blood pressures, suggesting a programming effect of preterm birth on angiogenesis and blood pressure.[215] Interestingly, sflt-1 levels in this study were even further elevated in those who had been preterm and exposed to a hypertensive pregnancy ($P < .002$), suggesting an additional impact of preeclampsia. Having been born small for gestational age or preterm, in turn, are risk factors for a woman subsequently developing preeclampsia in her own pregnancies, emphasizing the intergenerational effects of developmental programming.[33,190] Whether the programmed risk for preeclampsia is mediated by elevated circulating antiangiogenic factors and/or the programmed risk of higher blood pressures and renal dysfunction resulting from a mother's own low birth weight or preterm birth status is not known.

Gender differences in programming effects on blood pressure have been inconsistently reported. In some studies, programming effects appear more pronounced in males, and in others, the differential effects of gender are modified by age, ethnicity, and body mass index.[197] In a meta-regression of 20 Nordic cohorts, including 183,026 males and 14,928 women, a linear inverse association between birth weight and systolic blood pressure was present across all birth weights in males, which strengthened with age, whereas the relationship was U-shaped in women, with increasing risk also observed with birth weights above 4 kg.[216] Potential mechanisms whereby developmental programming may be expressed differently in males and females will be discussed later and are reviewed in detail elsewhere.[159,170]

The relative importance of genetics and environmental factors in programming of blood pressure has been studied in twins.[217-219] In a large Swedish cohort of 16,265 twins, the overall adjusted OR for hypertension was 1.42 (95% CI: 1.25 to 1.62) for each 500-g decrease in birth weight. Within like-sexed twin pairs, the ORs were 1.43 (95% CI: 1.07 to 1.69) and 1.74 (95% CI: 1.13 to 2.70) for dizygotic and monozygotic pairs, respectively, suggesting that environmental factors that contributed to differences in birth weight had a greater impact than genetics in this cohort, consistent with a developmental programming effect.[217]

### Nephron Number and Blood Pressure

In support of the potential association between nephron number and hypertension, a study of Caucasians aged 35 to 59 years who died in accidents found that in 10 subjects with a history of essential hypertension, the number of glomeruli per kidney was significantly lower and glomerular volume significantly higher than in 10 normotensive-matched controls (Fig. 21.9).[59] Birth weights were not reported in this study, but the authors concluded that a reduced nephron number is associated with susceptibility to essential hypertension. Similarly, kidneys of Australian Aborigines with a history of hypertension contained approximately 30% fewer nephrons than Aborigines with no history of hypertension.[220] Although the sample size was small and birth weights were not available, this is a population with high rates of socioeconomic disadvantage and low birth weight. Kanzaki et al.[221] also recently reported that kidneys from Japanese men with a history of hypertension contained approximately 40% fewer nephrons than age-matched normotensive men. The data therefore seem consistent across several populations that higher blood

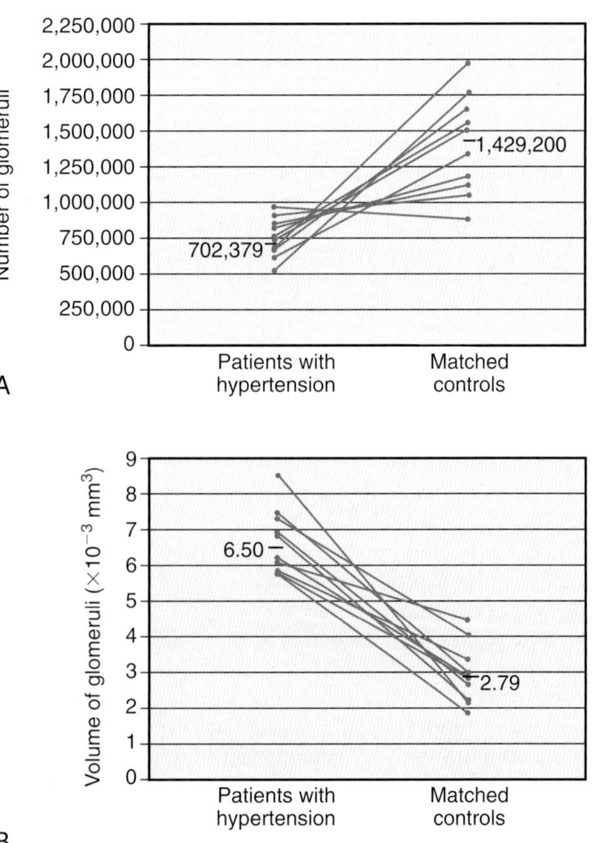


**Fig. 21.9** (A) Nephron number, and (B) glomerular volume in Caucasian subjects with primary hypertension compared with controls. (From Keller G, Zimmer G, Mall G, et al. Nephron number in patients with primary hypertension. *N Engl J Med.* 2003;348:101–108.)

**Table 21.8 Systematic Reviews, Metaanalyses, and Population-Based Studies of Developmentally Programmed Associations With Blood Pressure and Kidney Disease**

| Reference | Condition | Age | Number Included in the Analysis | Study Type | Outcome | Risk (95% CI) |
|---|---|---|---|---|---|---|
| **Programmed Associations With Blood Pressure** | | | | | | |
| 36 | Preterm birth[a] | 17.8 years | 3080 subjects | Systematic review and meta-analysis | SBP | Increase by 2.5 mm Hg (1.7–3.3 mm Hg) vs. term birth |
| 37 | Low birth weight | 4–84 years | 20 studies | Meta-analysis | Hypertension | OR 1.21 (1.13–1.3) |
| | | | | | SBP | Increase by 2.28 mm Hg (1.24–3.33 mm Hg) for BW <2500 g vs. BW >2500 g |
| | High birth weight | | | | SBP | Decrease by 2.08 mm Hg (−2.98 to −1.17 mm Hg) for BW >4000 g vs. BW <4000 g |
| 39 | High birth weight | 4–83 years | 31 studies | Meta-analysis | Hypertension, children | RR 1.18 (95% CI 1.05–1.32) |
| | | | | | Hypertension, adult | RR 0.97 (95% CI 0.86–0.97) |
| | | | | | Overall | RR 1.0 (95% CI 0.93–1.06) |
| 552 | Birth weight | 0–84 years | 444,000 subjects | Systematic review | SBP | Decrease by 2 mm Hg per kg increase in BW |
| | Catch-up growth | | | | SBP | Increase with catch-up growth<br>Highest blood pressure values in LBW after catch-up |
| 214 | Offspring of pregnancy complicated by preeclampsia | Children, young adult | 45,249 subjects | Systematic review | SBP | Increase by 2.39 mm Hg (1.74–3.05 mm Hg) |
| | | | | | DBP | Increase by 1.35 mm Hg (0.9–1.8 mm Hg) |
| | | | | | BMI | Increase by 0.62 kg/m$^2$ |
| | | | | | SBP | |
| 211 | Pregnancy complicated by diabetes | 2–17 years | 61,852 individuals | Systematic review and meta-analysis | SBP | Increase (0.47–3.28 mm Hg) in ODM<br>(only statistically significant in males when stratified by sex) |
| 217 | Genes vs. environment | Birth years 1926–1958 | 16,265 subjects | Same-sex twin study, all | Hypertension | OR 1.42 (1.25–1.69) per 500-g decrease |
| | | | 595 subjects | Dizygotic pairs[b] | Hypertension | OR 1.34 (1.07–1.69) per 500-g decrease |
| | | | 250 subjects | Monozygotic pairs[b] | Hypertension | OR 1.74 (1.13–2.70) per 500-g decrease |
| 293 | Fetal and/or infant exposure to famine | 37– 43 years | 1,339 subjects | Cohort, Biafra famine, Nigeria (1967–1970) | SBP | Increase in exposure |
| | | | | | Hypertension | OR 2.87 (1.9–4.34) in exposure |
| 295 | | 59 years | 971 subjects | Cohort, Dutch famine (1944–1945) | SBP | Increase (0.25–5.30 mm Hg) after ≥10 weeks' exposure |
| | | | | | DBP | Not significant |
| | | | | | Hypertension | OR 1.44 (1.04–2.00) after ≥10 weeks' exposure |
| 238 | | 48–53 years | 724 subjects | Cohort, Dutch famine (1944–1945) | Albuminuria | OR 3.2 (1.4–7.7) for exposure to famine in midgestation |
| | | | | | SBP, DBP | Not significant |
| 553 | | 52–53 years | 549 subjects | Cohort, siege of Leningrad (1941–1944) | SBP | Not significant |
| | | | | | Albuminuria | Not significant |

*Continued on following page*

**Table 21.8 Systematic Reviews, Metaanalyses, and Population-Based Studies of Developmentally Programmed Associations With Blood Pressure and Kidney Disease (Cont'd)**

| Reference | Condition | Age | Number Included in the Analysis | Study Type | Outcome | Risk (95% CI) |
|---|---|---|---|---|---|---|
| **Programmed Associations With Kidney Disease** | | | | | | |
| 32 | Low birth weight | 12–75 years | 46,249 subjects | Systematic review | Chronic kidney disease | OR 1.73 (1.44–2.08) |
| | | | | | End-stage renal disease | OR 1.58 (1.33–1.88) |
| | | | | | Albuminuria | OR 1.81 (1.19–2.77) |
| | | | | | Reduced glomerular filtration rate | OR 1.79 (1.31–2.45) |
| 274 | Low birth weight | <21 years | 1994 cases | Case–control study | Childhood chronic kidney disease[c] | OR 2.88 (2.28–3.63) |
| | Maternal GDM | | 20,032 controls | | | OR 1.54 (1.13–2.09) |
| | Maternal overweight | | | | | OR 1.24 (1.05–1.48) |
| | Maternal obesity | | | | | OR 1.26 (1.05–1.52) |
| | High birth weight | | | | | Not significant |

[a]Mean gestational age 30.2 weeks, mean birth weight 1280 g.
[b]Twin pairs discordant for hypertension.
[c]Chronic kidney disease definition included reduced renal function, renal dysplasia and/or aplasia, and obstructive uropathy.
*BMI*, Body mass index; *CI*, confidence interval; *DBP*, diastolic blood pressure; *GDM*, gestational diabetes mellitus; *ODM*, offspring of diabetic mother; *OR*, odds ratio; *RR*, relative risk; *SBP*, systolic blood pressure.
From Luyckx VA, Brenner BM. Birth weight, malnutrition and kidney-associated outcomes—a global concern. *Nat Rev Nephrol.* 2015;11:135–149.

pressures are associated with lower nephron numbers. These studies attempted to exclude loss of nephrons due to hypertension as a potential confounder of the association in the absence of birth weight data.

Interestingly, among a subset of 63 subjects in whom mean arterial pressures and birth weights were available, Hughson and coworkers[120] reported a significant correlation between birth weight and glomerular number, mean arterial pressure, and glomerular number as well as mean arterial pressure and birth weight among Caucasian but not African American subjects. Among African Americans having nephron numbers below the mean, however, twice as many were hypertensive as normotensive, suggesting a possible contribution of lower nephron number in this group as well.[120] The relationship of low birth weight and nephron number was similar in a cohort of black and white Cuban neonates; therefore, it is expected that a similar relationship between low birth weight and low nephron number exists in the black population.[91] Glomerular volumes were found to be higher among the hypertensive African American subjects than the hypertensive whites.[120] The consistent finding of larger glomeruli among African Americans may suggest a greater prevalence of low nephron number in this population as a result of the known higher prevalence of low birth weight, or may reflect independent or additional programming of glomerular size. This topic warrants further research.

Consistent with an association between nephron number and blood pressure in humans, salt sensitivity has been found to correlate inversely with birth weight and inversely with kidney size in adults and children (Fig. 21.10).[142,143] In both studies, salt-induced changes were independent of GFR, excluding confounding by renal function. Among 1512 subjects aged 62 years, investigators found an inverse association between birth weight and blood pressure among those with birth weights below 3050 g, with a progressive 2.48-mm Hg (95% CI: 0.4 to 4.52 mm Hg) increase in blood pressure for every 1-g rise in daily salt intake until 10 g/d.[222] Interestingly, above this threshold birth weight, there was no association between blood pressure and salt intake, potentially suggesting protection against salt sensitivity with higher birth weights.

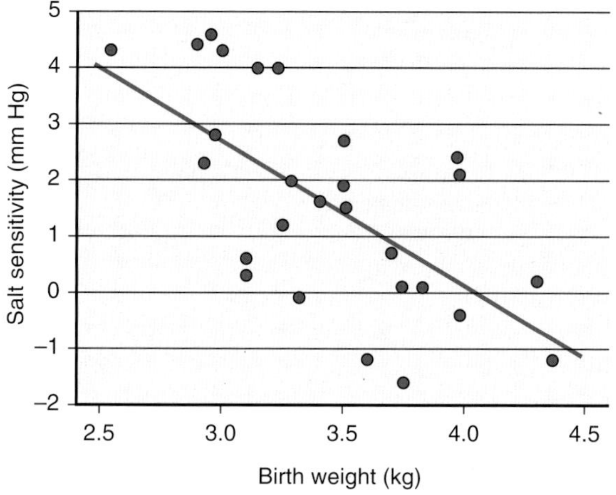


**Fig. 21.10** Correlation between birth weight and salt sensitivity in 27 normotensive adults. Salt sensitivity of blood pressure was defined as the difference of mean arterial pressure on high-salt diet (200 mmol/d) compared with low-salt diet (60 mmol/d). $R = -0.06$; $P = .002$. (From de Boer MP, Ijzerman RP, de Jongh RT, et al. Birth weight relates to salt sensitivity of blood pressure in healthy adults. *Hypertension* 51:928–932, 2008.)

## BIRTH WEIGHT, PRETERM BIRTH, AND KIDNEY FUNCTION

As with blood pressure, programmed changes in renal function that occur, at least in the early stages, may not be outside of normal limits. With time or exposure to additional insults, however, these changes may manifest as kidney disease.

### Glomerular Filtration Rate

The GFR, in the absence of compensatory hyperfiltration, should reflect the filtration surface area and, therefore, nephron number. Compensatory hyperfiltration is thought not to occur in the immediate neonatal period, and therefore, measurement of neonatal GFR may be a good proxy for nephron endowment. Consistent with this, amikacin clearance on day 1 of life, measured as a correlate for neonatal GFR, was found to be significantly lower in low-birth-weight and preterm neonates than in term controls.[223] Similarly, in a cohort of very preterm children aged 7.6 years, although still within the normal range, GFR measured by inulin clearance was significantly lower among those who had been growth restricted compared with non–growth restricted perinatally.[224] Importantly, the GFR was lower among children who had been growth restricted before (in utero) or in the first weeks after birth (in intensive care), pointing also to the role of postnatal nutrition in renal programming. Several studies in children found similar associations of decreased GFR in low-birth-weight or preterm children; however, studies using creatinine-based formulas may underestimate the impact of birth weight on GFR, suggesting a need to validate measures of renal function in low-birth-weight and preterm subjects, whose body composition may remain different over time.[223,225–231] The relationship between birth weight and eGFR appears to track with time, suggesting consistency of the associations. Among 5352 adolescents from the NHANES study, eGFRs were lower in low-birth-weight (OR: 1.49; 95% CI: 1.06 to 2.10) and very low–birth-weight (OR: 2.49; 95% CI: 1.20 to 5.18) subjects compared with those with normal birth weight.[209] As discussed earlier, this study is the first population-based assessment among adolescents of multiple ethnicities permitting an estimation of the population-attributable fraction of birth weight to blood pressures and eGFR: 1 in 13 low-birth-weight or 1 in 5 very low–birth-weight adolescents had systolic blood pressures ≥95th percentile and/or eGFR < 90 mL/min/1.73 m$^2$.[209]

Overall, a recent metaanalysis found an OR of 1.79 (95% CI: 1.31 to 2.45) for a reduced GFR with low birth weight (see Table 21.8).[32] Linear regression analysis in a cohort of 2192 British adults aged 60–64 years revealed that for each 1-kg decrease in birth weight, adult GFR estimated using cystatin C was reduced by 2.25 mL/min per 1.73 m$^2$ (95% CI: 0.69 to 3.58 mL/min per 1.73 m$^2$).[232] Taken together, these findings are consistent with low birth weight and preterm birth being risk factors for a reduced GFR. The relative contributions of genetics and the fetal environment on programming of renal function were investigated in 653 twins.[233] Creatinine clearance was significantly lower in low-birth-weight compared with normal-birth-weight twins. Furthermore, intrapair birth weight differences were positively correlated with GFR in both monozygotic and dizygotic twin pairs, suggesting that feto-placental factors have a greater impact than genetic factors on adult renal function.

To approach an understanding of the mechanism of the reduced GFR in low-birth-weight and preterm individuals, renal functional reserve, determined by measuring GFR and effective renal plasma flow (ERPF) before and after low-dose dopamine infusion or an oral amino acid load, was studied in 20-year-old subjects who had been preterm and either small or appropriate for gestational age, versus controls, born full term and normal birth weight.[192] After renal stimulation, the relative increase in GFR tended to be lower in small-for-gestational-age compared with appropriate-for-gestational-age and control subjects, and ERPF was lower in both groups of preterm subjects, although statistical significance was not reached, likely because of small numbers. Reduced renal functional reserve was also observed among young adults with type 1 diabetic mothers, who had been exposed to diabetes during gestation, but not those with diabetic fathers, again suggesting a programming rather than genetic effect.[72] A reduced renal reserve capacity in these subjects may be consistent with a programmed reduction in nephron number.

### Proteinuria

One of the earliest signs of hyperfiltration, which would be expected in the setting of a reduced nephron number and filtration surface area, is microalbuminuria, which may progress to overt proteinuria with ongoing renal injury and worsening hyperfiltration. Consistent with this hypothesis, Aboriginal Australians who had low birth weights evidenced an OR for macroalbuminuria of 2.8 (95% CI: 1.26 to 6.31) compared with those who had normal birth weights, and this increased with age.[234] Importantly, proteinuria was also associated with a higher rate of cardiovascular and renal deaths, underscoring its clinical relevance.[97] A meta-analysis including eight additional studies reported an OR of 1.81 (95% CI: 1.19 to 2.77) for albuminuria with low birth weight (see Table 21.8).[32] More recently, the Australian group reported that low birth weight, childhood poststreptococcal glomerulonephritis, and current body mass were all independent predictors of albumin to creatinine levels in young Aboriginal adults.[235,236] These findings are compatible with the "multihit" model of CKD, of which nephron endowment at birth may be the first "hit" increasing susceptibility to kidney disease throughout the life course.

As with blood pressure, whether preterm birth modifies the association of birth weight with proteinuria is not always easy to dissect, although studies of preterm children and adolescents show consistent findings. Among children aged 4 years who had been preterm, albuminuria was higher in both boys and girls who had reached normal height (presumably caught up in growth), and among 19-year-olds who had been very preterm, albuminuria was higher among those who had been growth restricted, again highlighting the interplay between preterm birth, growth restriction, and catch-up growth on later risk of disease.[230,237] In contrast, however, among 12- to 15-year-old NHANES participants, despite there being significant differences in blood pressure and eGFRs, there was no difference in the albumin/creatinine ratio between adolescents born with low birth weight, very low birth weight, or normal birth weight.[209] This unexpected finding might be due to the fact that albuminuria was determined on a single random, nonsupine sample, which may lack the specificity needed to distinguish patients with true kidney disease.

Analysis of 724 subjects aged 48 to 53 years who had been subjected to malnutrition in midgestation during the Dutch famine revealed an increased prevalence of microalbuminuria (12%) when compared with those subjected to malnutrition during early gestation (9%), late gestation (7%), or not exposed to famine (4%–8%) (see Table 21.8).[238] Size at birth was not associated with the observed increase in microalbuminuria, however, suggesting that renal development may have been irreversibly affected in midgestation, although in later gestation, whole-body growth was able to catch up with restoration of more normal nutrition. This observation again emphasizes the need for surrogate markers in addition to birth weight in order to identify individuals at risk for renal programming.

A U-shaped association between birth weight and proteinuria was described among Pima Indians, showing that the risk increased for birth weights below 2.5 kg and above 4.5 kg.[12] The strongest predictor of proteinuria among high-birth-weight subjects in this study was exposure to gestational diabetes, raising the question of whether gestational diabetes exposure, rather than birth weight per se, was the predominant programming risk factor.[12] In a Canadian study, urine albumin/creatinine ratios were lower in infants of diabetic mothers compared with nondiabetic mothers at 1 year of age, but were higher at 3 years, although independent of birth weight.[239] The authors interpret these findings to reflect abnormal renal programming in offspring of diabetic mothers; however, the effects of gestational diabetes and high birth weight on renal programming require much more study.

### Neonatal Acute Kidney Injury

Preterm birth is an important risk factor for acute kidney injury (AKI) in neonates, estimated to occur in between 12.5% and 71%, depending on the population studied.[240,241] In turn, AKI in very low–birth-weight infants is an independent predictor of longer hospital stays, mortality, and subsequent CKD.[187,242] A retrospective analysis of preoperative renal volume in neonates undergoing congenital heart surgery found higher peak postoperative creatinine values and, therefore, potentially increased risk of AKI in infants with a renal volume ≤ 17 $cm^3$.[243] High creatinine values were associated with lower gestational age and lower birth weight *z*-score. Neonates in intensive care are particularly susceptible to renal dysfunction, not only because of potentially programmed risk and low nephron number but also because of critical illness and frequent nephrotoxin exposure such as aminoglycosides and nonsteroidal antiinflammatory drugs.[122,241,244–248] Medications administered during pregnancy or prior to delivery, such as tocolytics and antibiotics, may also impact fetal nephrogenesis and increase the risk of neonatal AKI.[249–251] These factors all likely adversely impact any postnatal nephrogenesis, which may occur under optimal circumstances for several weeks following preterm birth.[122]

The actual risk of AKI with exposure to nephrotoxins among preterm infants is not well described. Among 269 infants perinatally exposed to potential nephrotoxic medication (i.e., in late pregnancy or within the first 7 days postbirth), ibuprofen exposure was associated with an OR of 2.6 (95% CI: 1.2 to 5.3) for a reduced GFR on day 7 of life, which persisted over the first month.[250] Other authors found that exposure to aminoglycosides was associated with higher serum creatinine in preterm infants born small for gestational age at 2 months.[252] Neonatologists are working to raise awareness of the renal risk; however, the definition of renal failure in this population remains a challenge. Creatinine cutoff values have been proposed according to gestational age.[227] Serum creatinine in the neonate reflects maternal creatinine early on, however; therefore, urinary biomarkers and cystatin C have been proposed as superior markers to detect AKI early.[244,253] More recently, the Neonatal Kidney Disease: Improving Global Outcomes Classification has been proposed for more consistency in the definition.[244] The risk and significant adverse consequences of AKI associated with preterm birth therefore highlight the need for long-term follow-up of preterm infants.[240] Studies are emerging linking perinatal AKI to the long-term risk of CKD, which is significantly increased among those who subsequently become obese.[187,254–257] Prevention of perinatal AKI may therefore be important to reduce the risk of later-life CKD, and long-term follow-up of infants who develop AKI is required to appropriately modify this risk.[242,258]

### Chronic Kidney Disease and End-Stage Kidney Disease

A case series of six patients, aged 15–52 years, who had been born preterm with very low birth weight, described findings consistent with secondary FSGS, associated with glomerulomegaly in all biopsies.[259] The authors suggest a susceptibility to hyperfiltration and glomerulosclerosis associated with preterm birth and low birth weight. Similar histologic findings have been reported in several Japanese individuals who had very low birth weights and developed early renal dysfunction or proteinuria.[260,261] These individuals responded well to ACEI therapy, supporting the pathophysiologic role of hyperfiltration in developmental programming of renal disease. Consistent with these findings, a variety of generally small studies have reported a greater severity of renal disease and more rapid progression of diverse renal diseases, including immunoglobulin A (IgA) nephropathy, membranous nephropathy, minimal change disease, chronic pyelonephritis, Alport syndrome, and polycystic kidney disease among children and adults who had been of low birth weight.[41,262–270] A handful of studies have examined the relationship between birth weight and diabetic nephropathy and found an increased susceptibility among subjects who had been growth restricted, although not invariably.[12,265,271,272]

Strong associations have recently been reported between both low birth weight (defined as <2.5 kg) and gestational age with the development of CKD in Japanese and North American children attending pediatric CKD clinics.[273,274] In the U.S. population, low birth weight, maternal gestational diabetes, and maternal overweight and obesity were all significantly associated with an increased risk of childhood CKD (see Table 21.8).[274] In addition, a significant association was found between low birth weight and maternal pregestational diabetes and real dysplasia/aplasia, and between low birth weight, maternal gestational diabetes, and maternal overweight or obesity and congenital obstruction. In the Japanese population, the association remained highly significant, even after exclusion of children with congenital anomalies of the kidney and urinary tract (CAKUT), with an estimated population attributable fraction of pediatric CKD being 21.1% (95% CI: 16.0% to 26.1%) for low birth weight and 18.2% (95% CI: 16.5 to 25.6%) for preterm birth.[273]

**Table 21.9 Risk of End-Stage Renal Disease According to Birth Weight and Gestational Age Category[a]**

| | LBW (BW <10th percentile) | LBW (<2.5 kg) | SGA (<37 weeks) | Preterm (<37 weeks) | Term LBW | Preterm LBW | Term SGA | Preterm AGA | Preterm SGA |
|---|---|---|---|---|---|---|---|---|---|
| All ages | 1.63 (1.29–2.06) | 2.25 (1.59–3.19) | 1.67 (1.3–2.07) | 1.36 (0.94–1.99) | 1.56 (1.18–2.07) | 1.89 (1.25–2.86) | 1.54 (1.2–1.96) | 1.09 (0.69–1.73) | 4.03 (2.08–7.80) |
| 1–18 y | 2.72 (1.88–3.92) | | 1.93 (1.28–2.91) | | | | | | |
| 18–42 y | 1.23 (0.9–1.68) | | 1.53 (1.15–2.03) | | | 1.42 (0.82–2.48) | 1.41 (1.05–1.90) | | 4.02 (1.79–9.03) |

[a]All comparisons for term birth, LBW term, AGA term as relevant. Data expressed as hazard ratios (95% confidence intervals).
*AGA*, Appropriate for gestational age; *BW*, birth weight; *LBW*, low birth weight; *SGA*, small for gestational age.
Reproduced from Low Birth Weight and Nephron Number Working Group. The impact of kidney development on the life course: a consensus document for action. *Nephron.* 2017;136:3–49.
Derived from Ruggajo P, Skrunes R, Svarstad E, et al. Familial factors, Low birth weight, and development of ESRD: a nationwide registry study. *Am J Kidney Dis.* 2016;67(4):601–608.

Taken together, most observations suggest that low birth weight and preterm birth are risk factors for renal disease. Consistent with this notion, a meta-analysis of 18 studies reported an OR for CKD of 1.73 (95% CI: 1.44 to 2.08) with low birth weight (see Table 21.8).[32] Similarly, in retrospective analysis of a cohort of over 2 million white children, the relative risk of developing ESKD was 1.7 (95% CI: 1.4 to 2.2) in those with birth weights <10th percentile.[31] In a follow-up study, these investigators showed a stronger relationship between low birth weight and ESKD in individuals under 18 years (OR: 2.72; 95% CI: 1.88 to 3.92) compared with 18–42 years of age (OR: 1.23; 95% CI: 1.15 to 2.03), again demonstrating the likely impact of CAKUT in the younger population (Table 21.9).[41] Overall in this study, both low birth weight and being small for gestational age were associated with a progressively increasing risk of ESKD (Fig. 21.11). There was no evidence for modulation of these associations by familial factors, again emphasizing the strong impact of environmental exposures in renal programming.[41] In a dialysis-based study, low birth weight was also associated with increased risk of ESKD, but the OR for diabetic ESKD was also increased among those having birth weights greater than 4000 g (OR 2.4; 95% CI: 1.3 to 4.2).[50] The relevance of high birth weight was also highlighted by a U-shaped association of renal disease with birth weight found in two large population-based studies, although effects differed between males and females in both studies, again reflecting potential effect modification by gender under conditions as yet not fully elucidated.[30,31] Whether high birth weight in these studies was associated with intrauterine exposure to diabetes is not known.

Among 1850 Pima Indians younger than 45 years with diabetes, the incidence rate ratio of developing ESKD was 4.12 (95% CI: 1.54 to 11.02) among those who had been exposed to diabetes in utero compared with those without exposure.[275] Interestingly, this effect disappeared after controlling for duration of diabetes in this relatively young cohort, suggesting the ESKD risk may be mediated predominantly by a programmed risk for earlier-onset diabetes among those exposed to diabetes in utero. This study emphasizes that programming of renal risk may be indirect as a consequence of programming of other disorders such as diabetes, underscoring the need for a holistic and life-course approach to understand and tackle programming of renal disease.

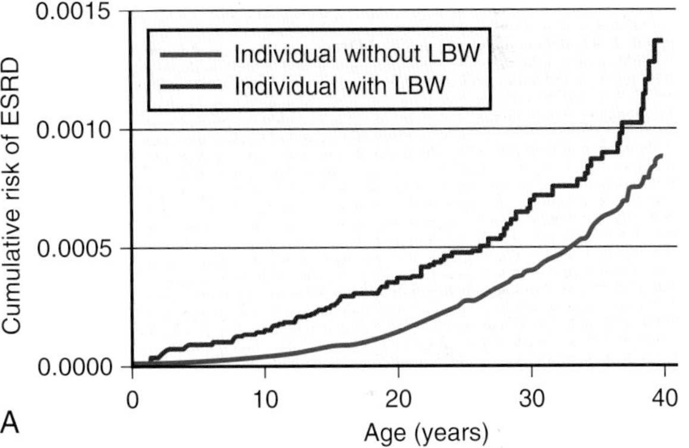


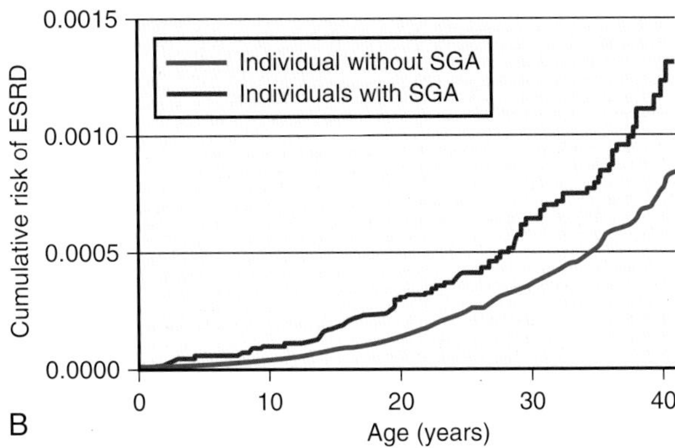


**Fig. 21.11** Cumulative risk for end-stage renal disease *(ESRD)* in individuals with age, according to whether the individual was (A) low birth weight *(LBW)* or (B) small for gestational age *(SGA)*. From Ruggajo P, Skrunes R, Svarstad E, et al. Low birth weight, and development of ESRD: a nationwide registry study. *Am J Kidney Dis.* 2016;67:601–608.

It is likely too simplistic to assume that altered kidney development associated with low birth weight, preterm birth, or other developmental stresses itself is enough to cause renal disease, but exposure to additional "hits" (e.g., nephrotoxin exposure, AKI, glomerulonephritis), or superimposed developmental programming of conditions that are themselves risk factors for kidney disease (i.e., diabetes, cardiovascular disease, metabolic syndrome, obesity), all likely exacerbate renal risk.[16,19,187,235,275,276] Overall, combined meta-analysis of 31 studies, including over 2 million subjects, concluded that individuals of low birth weight have a 70% increased risk of developing CKD, including albuminuria, reduced GFR, and renal failure in later life.[32] Clinical associations of developmental programming in the kidney are outlined in Table 21.10.

## RELATIVE IMPACT OF BEING BORN SMALL OR PRETERM ON RENAL PROGRAMMING

As illustrated in Fig. 21.1, a low birth weight may be the result of preterm birth and/or growth restriction. Most studies have not differentiated between these two occurrences, so the relative impact of each has remained unclear. A recent Norwegian population study including data from >1.8 million subjects under age 40 years has examined these effects, using the following definitions: low birth weight <10th percentile for Norway (<2800 g), small for gestational age <10th percentile for gestational age (determined by ultrasonography in gestational weeks 17–20), and preterm birth <37 weeks' gestation (see Table 21.9).[41] Overall, the hazard ratio (HR) for ESKD was 1.56 (95% CI: 1.18 to 2.07) for low-birth-weight term births, 1.89 (95% CI: 1.25 to 2.86) for low-birth-weight preterm births, 1.54 (95% CI: 1.20 to 1.96) for term small-for-gestational-age births, and 4.03 (95% CI: 2.08 to 7.80) for preterm small-for-gestational-age births (Fig. 21.11).[41] Preterm birth with appropriate weight for gestational age was not associated with an increased risk of ESKD in this study. Being born small for gestational age was therefore the strongest predictor of ESKD risk. Subsequently, the same authors reported that being small for gestational age and low birth weight were associated with an increased risk of ESKD among a cohort of young adults with IgA nephropathy.[277] The IgA subgroup was chosen because it is a common disease and unlikely to be directly impacted by programming (in contrast to CAKUT or diabetic nephropathy). Low birth weight and small for gestational age were associated with increased risk of progression to ESKD in IgA nephropathy.[41] This study again points to developmental programming being a first "hit" leading to accelerated progression of a primary renal disease. Again, in this study, the highest risk for ESKD was conferred by a small birth weight for gestational age (HR: 2.2; 95% CI: 1.1 to 4.2); however, this effect was only significant in males. Patients who were both low birth weight and small for gestational age had the highest risk (HR: 3.2; 95%: CI 1.5 to 6.8), suggesting a greater impact at lower birth weights, likely reflecting more adverse intrauterine exposures.

## POTENTIAL IMPACT OF ETHNICITY ON RENAL PROGRAMMING

The nephron number hypothesis was initially put forward as a potential explanation for the disproportionately higher risks of hypertension and kidney disease among disadvantaged populations.[48] Hypertension, CKD, and ESKD prevalences tend to be highest among Aboriginal Australians, Native Americans, people of African origin, and ethnic minorities in developed countries.[10,12,50,278] The incidence of birth circumstances and maternal risk factors for renal programming are high across low- and middle-income countries, as highlighted in Table 21.11, suggesting a potentially significant population impact. Most studies regarding programming of blood pressure and kidney disease have thus far been conducted in western Caucasian populations and may not be generalizable to all populations. In the Norwegian population, for example, only 3.3% of subjects had birth weights below 2.5 kg, whereas around 13%–15% of babies in sub-Saharan Africa have low birth weights.[41,279] Furthermore, the causes of low birth weight or preterm birth differ across regions, with maternal nutrition, poverty, and infections being important in lower-income regions and advanced maternal age, multiple gestations, and use of assisted reproduction technology predominating in high-income regions.[280–282] How such differences may modulate programming risk across populations is not known.[283–286]

Kidney size, as measured by ultrasound at birth, among 715 South Asians (Pakistani, Indian, and Bangladeshi origin) from the Born in Bradford (United Kingdom) cohort study was smaller than that among 872 white babies, and the difference persisted after adjustment for potential confounders, including birth weight.[287] Total kidney volume was also found to be lower in low-birth-weight and preterm Australian Aborigines at 32 and 38 weeks of gestation and at term compared within nonindigenous Australians, suggesting a lower nephron number in the indigenous children.[288] However, in this study, calculated GFR (serum cystatin C) was similar in Aboriginal and nonindigenous neonates, suggesting SNGFR was increased in the Aborigines. In a study comparing eGFR in 152 African and white American children at a mean age of 1.5 years, the eGFR was found to be significantly lower among African American children (82 vs. 95 mL/min/1.73 m$^2$).[289] Birth weight was significantly and positively associated with eGFR in African American but not white children, suggesting that some of the racial disparities in adult CKD may have origins in the prenatal period.

Nephron numbers have thus far been counted only in small cohorts of Caucasians, African Americans, Australian Aboriginals, Senegalese Africans, and Japanese males, in many of whom birth weights were not available. Therefore, the relationship between birth weight and nephron number remains unknown in most populations. A recent study on nephron number and hypertension among older Japanese males found the nephron count in the normotensive subjects was one of the lowest reported to date (~640,000 nephrons), suggesting that Japanese people may be especially vulnerable to adult hypertension and CKD, particularly if a "second hit" occurs.[221] This hypothesis would be consistent with the fact that Japan has the second-highest incidence of ESKD in the world.[290] Low birth weight is strongly associated with reduced nephron numbers and susceptibility to kidney disease among Australian Aboriginals, a population that is also significantly disadvantaged compared with their white counterparts.[96,97] The association between nephron number and birth weight does appear to be consistent among subjects of African origin as in Caucasian subjects.[87,91,291,292] The relationship between low nephron numbers and higher blood pressures seen in Aboriginal Australians and Caucasians, however, was not as consistent among African Americans.[285] Similarly, the association of low birth weight with blood pressure is also less consistently reported among African-American compared with Caucasian children; therefore, additional factors likely augment blood pressure risk in the African-origin population.[198,289]

Evidence for developmental programming of blood pressure in an African population has, however, been shown among

**Table 21.10 Clinical Associations of Renal Programming**

| | Low Birth Weight | Small for Gestational Age | Preterm Birth | High Birth Weight | Gestational Diabetes Exposure | Exposure to Preeclampsia/ Eclampsia | Maternal Overweight/ Obesity | Maternal Vitamin A Deficiency | Rapid Catch-Up Growth/ Overweight | Low Nephron Number | Smaller Kidney Size/ Weight | Increased Glomerular Volume |
|---|---|---|---|---|---|---|---|---|---|---|---|---|
| Increased blood pressure | ✓ | | ✓ | ✓ | ✓ | ✓ | ✓ | | ✓ | ✓ | ✓ | ✓ |
| Salt sensitivity | ✓ | | | | a | | | | | a | ✓ | |
| Reduced GFR | ✓ | ✓ | ✓ | | a | | | | ✓ | a | ✓ | |
| Reduced renal functional reserve | | ✓ | ✓ | | ✓ | | | | | | | |
| Proteinuria | ✓ | | ✓ | ✓ | ✓ | | | | ✓ | a | ✓ | |
| Acute kidney injury (neonates) | | | ✓ | | | | | | | ✓ | ✓ | |
| Chronic kidney disease | ✓ | ✓ | ✓ | | ✓ | ✓ | ✓ | | ✓ | a | ✓ | ✓ |
| End-stage renal disease | ✓ | | | ✓ | ✓ | | | | | | | |
| Transplant outcomes | ✓ | | | | | | | | | | ✓ | ✓ |
| Death | ✓ | | | | | | | | | | | |
| Increased glomerular volume | ✓ | | ✓ | | a | | | | ✓ | ✓ | | |
| Smaller kidney size/weight | ✓ | ✓ | ✓ | | | | | ✓ | | ✓ | | |
| Congenital obstruction | ✓ | | | NS | ✓ | | ✓ | | | a | | |
| Renal dysplasia/ aplasia | ✓ | | | NS | ✓ | | NS | | | ✓ | | ✓ |

✓, Evidence from human studies; *a*, evidence from animal studies only; *NS*, not significant.
Modified from prior Table 23.8, readapted from Luyckx, 2015, 2002.

**Table 21.11 Prevalence of LBW, Preterm Birth, Maternal Diabetes, and Obesity in Low- and Middle-Income Countries[a]**

| | LBW (2010) | Preterm Birth (2010) | HBW (2004-2008) | Gestational Diabetes[a] (2013) | Maternal Overweight (2003–2009) | Maternal Obesity (2003–2009) | Chronic Hypertension/ Preeclampsia/ Eclampsia |
|---|---|---|---|---|---|---|---|
| Proportions in LMICs (country *n*) | 15% (138) | 11.3% (138) | 0.5%–14.9% (23) | 0.4%–24.3% (15) | 13.7% (27 Sub-Saharan countries) | 5.3% (27 sub-Saharan countries) | 2.3% (17) |

[a]Variable rates in part related to differences in cut-off values for diagnosis.

*HBW*, High birth weight; *LBW*, low birth weight; *LMIC*, low- and middle-income countries.

Adapted from Low Birth Weight and Nephron Number Working Group. The impact of kidney development on the life course: a consensus document for action. *Nephron.* 2017;136:3–49. Compiled from Koyanagi A, Zhang J, Dagvadorj A, et al. Macrosomia in 23 developing countries: an analysis of a multicountry, facility-based, cross-sectional survey. *Lancet.* 2013;381:476–483; Lee AC, Katz J, Blencowe H, et al. National and regional estimates of term and preterm babies born small for gestational age in 138 low-income and middle-income countries in 2010. *Lancet Glob Health.* 2013;1:e26–e36; Cresswell JA, Campbell OM, De Silva MJ, et al. Effect of maternal obesity on neonatal death in sub-Saharan Africa: multivariable analysis of 27 national datasets. *Lancet.* 2012;380:1325–1330; (Kanguru L, Bezawada N, Hussein J, et al. The burden of diabetes mellitus during pregnancy in low- and middle-income countries: a systematic review. *Glob Health Action.* 2014;1;7:23987; and Abalos E, Cuesta C, Carroli G, et al. Pre-eclampsia, eclampsia and adverse maternal and perinatal outcomes: a secondary analysis of the world health organization multicountry survey on maternal and newborn health. *BJOG.* 2014;121(suppl 1):14–24.).

Nigerian adults exposed to the Biafran famine (1967–1970) during fetal life and early childhood.[293] Consistent with observations among Caucasians exposed to the Dutch famine (1944–1945), blood pressures were elevated in adult Nigerians exposed to the famine.[293–295] Interestingly, however, blood pressures in Biafran subjects were elevated 15 to 20 years earlier than among the Dutch subjects (see Table 21.8), potentially again suggesting aggravating factors present in African-origin subjects.[293,295] In addition, in both populations, exposure to famine was also associated with increased risks of glucose intolerance and obesity, again underscoring the multisystem consequences of developmental programming.[293,294]

Variants in the *APOL1* gene have been strongly linked to risk of CKD in African Americans and in West Africans.[4,9] The relationship between *APOL1* genotype and nephron number was recently investigated.[296] Glomerular number was not reduced, and glomerular size was not increased among African Americans with one or two *APOL1* variant alleles, but there was evidence of more accelerated loss of nephrons after the age of 38 years, which was exacerbated by obesity.[296] A programming interaction with *APOL1* genotype, therefore, has not yet been established; however, age-related loss of glomeruli appears accelerated.

## PROPOSED MECHANISMS OF DEVELOPMENTAL PROGRAMMING IN THE KIDNEY

Kidney development is a complex process involving tightly controlled expression of many genes and constant remodeling.[111,297–301] The molecular regulation of kidney development is exhaustively reviewed elsewhere (see Chapter 1).[298–301] Many experimental models, as discussed earlier and outlined in Table 21.4, have been shown to result in a reduced nephron number, and these have been used to gain insight into potential mechanisms contributing to programmed disease outcomes. In many of the experimental models of programming, reduced nephron number has been shown to be associated with low birth weight and subsequent hypertension and renal injury. Interestingly, in normal rat litters, those pups with naturally occurring low birth weight (i.e., birth weights < −2 standard deviations [SDs] from the mean) were found to have a 13% reduction in nephron number, which was associated with glomerulomegaly and proteinuria.[302] Low birth weight in rodents, therefore, may be associated with a low nephron number, even under nonexperimental conditions. Maternal factors that affect birth weight and preterm birth in humans may also directly affect nephrogenesis, as illustrated in Table 21.12, and some of these factors may compound the effect of low birth weight or preterm birth.[90,303] In humans, nephrogenesis begins in week 9 of gestation and continues until about 36 weeks. Approximately two-thirds of the nephrons develop during the last trimester, making this the window of greatest susceptibility to adverse effects, although earlier insults can also impact nephrogenesis.[123,304] In rodents, nephrogenesis continues for up to 10 days after birth but is most active mid- to late gestation when studies show the most impact from manipulation of environmental factors.[304]

Our current understanding highlights three processes that are considered to play critical roles in determining nephron endowment at the conclusion of nephrogenesis: branching of the ureteric tree, condensation of metanephric mesenchymal cells at the ureteric branch tips, and conversion of these mesenchymal condensates into nephron epithelium.[298–301] It has been estimated that a 2% decrease in ureteric tree branching efficiency would result in a 50% reduction in final nephron complement after 20 generations of branching.[305] The specific molecular mechanisms whereby nephron numbers may be affected and/or function altered, however, are not yet completely understood. Perturbations to the feto-maternal environment that result in reduced nephron endowment are summarized in Table 21.13 and discussed later.

**Table 21.12 Potential Renal Programming Effects of Risk Factors for Preterm Delivery**

| | Animal | | Human | | |
|---|---|---|---|---|---|
| **Maternal Risk Factor for Preterm Birth** | BP | Nephron Number/ Kidney Size | BP | Nephron Number/ Kidney Size[a] | Kidney Function |
| Vitamin D deficiency | ↑ | ↑ Immature glomeruli | ND | ND | ND |
| Anemia/iron deficiency | ↑ | ↓ | ND | ND | ND |
| Smoking | ND | ↓ | ↑ | ↓ | ↓ |
| Alcohol intake | ND | ↓ | ND | ND | ND |
| Antibiotic use (UTI) | ND | ↓ | ND | ND | ND |
| Chorioamnionitis | ND | ↓ | ND | ND | ND |
| Steroids | ↑ | ↓ | Normal | Not different | Unknown |
| Cyclosporine/tacrolimus (maternal transplant) | ↑ | ↓ | ND | ND | Possibly normal |
| Maternal dialysis | ND | ND | ND | ND | Some ↓ |
| Maternal diabetes | ↑ | ↓ | ↑ | ND | ↓ |
| Preeclampsia | ND | ND | ↑ | ND | ND |

[a]Kidney size generally determined by ultrasound.
*BP*, Blood pressure; *ND*, not determined; *UTI*, urinary tract infection; ↑, increased; ↓, decreased.
Compiled from references 176, 246, 322, 330, 356, 362, 363, 374, 379, 465, 466, 543, and 555–559.
Reprinted with permission from Luyckx VA. Preterm birth and its impact on renal health. *Semin Nephrol.* 2017;37:311–319.

## GENETIC VARIANTS ASSOCIATED WITH KIDNEY SIZE AND NEPHRON NUMBER IN HUMANS

Rare genetic and CAKUT contribute to about 40% of all childhood ESKD (NAPRTCS Report 2014). The common pathology linking these malformations involves a disturbance of the normal interaction between the ureteric bud and the pool of renal progenitor cells.[383] Of the >25 mutant genes associated with monogenic forms of CAKUT, most encode transcription factors (e.g., *PAX2, GATA3*) and growth factor receptors (e.g., *RET*) expressed in ureteric bud/tree cells during branching morphogenesis or in intermediate mesoderm (e.g., *SIX2, EYA1, ROBO*), where they set the fate of renal progenitor cells and regulate interactions with the ureteric bud.

Completely dysfunctional alleles for crucial developmental genes are rare, because they produce malformations with a major disadvantage. However, there is some evidence that mild mutations of these same genes exert subtler effects on renal mesenchyme/ureteric bud interactions and may be fairly common in the normal population (see Table 21.4). For example, heterozygous null alleles of the *PAX2* gene cause the rare autosomal dominant renal coloboma syndrome, characterized by decreased ureteric branching during fetal life, sharply reduced nephron number at birth, and progressive renal failure in childhood. *PAX2* is highly expressed in the ureteric bud, where it suppresses apoptosis and optimizes the extent of branching. Interestingly, an intronic *PAX2* polymorphism, which reduces *PAX* transcript levels from the mutant allele by only 50%, is found in 18.5% of Canadians and is associated with a subtle (10%) reduction in newborn kidney size.[306] Ureteric branching morphogenesis is also highly dependent on *GDNF* signaling from the metanephric mesenchyme to the ureteric bud via the *RET* tyrosine kinase receptor on ureteric tip cells. Although no common hypomorphic variants of the human *GDNF* gene have been shown to affect kidney size, a polymorphic variant of the *GDNF* receptor, *RET(1476A)*, was associated with a 10% reduction in kidney volume at birth compared with the wild type (*RET 1476G*) allele.[121] In this study, newborn kidney volume was shown to be proportional to nephron number, suggesting that the modest renal hypoplasia seen with somewhat dysfunctional *PAX2* and *RET* polymorphisms represents a reduction in congenital nephron number.[121] Newborn kidney size was reduced by 13% among Polish babies with a common variant of the *BMPR1A* gene, encoding a bone morphogenetic protein receptor on ureteric epithelial cells.[307] Conversely, 22% of Canadian newborns inherit a variant of the *ALHD1A2* gene *(rs7169289)* associated with increased production of all-*trans* retinoic acid metabolism in fetal tissues; this retinoid is known to enhance RET expression in the ureteric epithelium, and newborns with the G allele were shown to have a 22% increase in newborn kidney size compared with the wild type allele.[308]

Although final nephron number is clearly affected by genes regulating the extent of ureteric branching, animal studies also indicate that the size of the renal progenitor cell pool may also be rate limiting. One of the earliest transcription factors marking the nephron progenitor cells of intermediate mesoderm is *OSR1*; Osr1 knockout mice lack nephrogenic mesenchyme and are anephric at birth.[309] A variant of the human *OSR1* gene that interferes with mRNA splicing was identified in about 6% of normal Caucasians.[310] This *OSR1rs12329305(T)* variant was associated with a 12% reduction in newborn kidney size. Taken together, these observations suggest that final nephron endowment may represent a complex polygenic trait determined by the additive effects of multiple genes regulating either the extent of ureteric branching or the renal progenitor cell pool during fetal life. As reviewed by Walker and Bertram,[301] full or partial deletion of more than 25 genes has been shown to result in kidney hypoplasia, and deletion of several of these genes results in low nephron endowment. Not all have been studied in humans; therefore, the impact of genetic variation on nephron endowment alone and in the context of developmental stresses and the risk of later-life hypertension and renal disease requires further study.

**Table 21.13 Proposed Mechanisms of Developmental Programming in the Kidney**

| Experimental Model | Possible Mechanism of Nephron Number Reduction | References |
|---|---|---|
| Maternal low-protein diet | ↑ Apoptosis in metanephros and postnatal kidney<br>Altered gene expression in developing kidney<br>Altered gene methylation<br>↓ Placental 11-β HSD2 expression → increased fetal exposure to glucocorticoids | 313, 315, 320, 488 |
| Maternal vitamin A restriction | ↓ Branching of ureteric bud<br>? Maintenance of spatial orientation of vascular development<br>↓ c-ret expression | 326 |
| Maternal iron restriction | ? Reduced oxygen delivery<br>? Altered glucocorticoid responsiveness<br>? Altered micronutrient availability<br>↑ Inflammation<br>? Tissue hypoxia | 322, 323 |
| Maternal zinc deficiency | ↑ Apoptosis<br>↓ Antioxidant activity | 324 |
| Gestational glucocorticoid exposure | ↑ Fetal glucocorticoid exposure<br>? Enhanced tissue maturation<br>↑ Glucocorticoid receptor expression<br>↑ Na-K-ATPase, $\alpha_1$ and $\beta_2$ subunit expression<br>↓ Renal and adrenal 11-β HSD2 expression | 154, 356, 361, 560 |
| Uterine artery ligation/ embolization | ↑ Proapoptotic gene expression in developing kidney: caspase-3, Bax, p53<br>↓ Antiapoptotic gene expression: PAX2, bcl-2<br>Altered gene methylation<br>Altered renin–angiotensin gene expression | 160, 402 |
| Maternal diabetes/ hyperglycemia | ↓ IGF-2/mannose-6-phosphate receptor expression<br>Altered IGF-2 activity/bioavailability<br>Activation of NF-κB<br>Altered ureteric branching morphogenesis | 161, 338, 342, 345 |
| Gestational drug exposure | | 176, 372, 374, 376 |
| • Gentamicin | ↓ Branching morphogenesis | |
| • β-lactams | ↑ Mesenchymal apoptosis | |
| • Cyclosporine | Arrest of nephron formation | |
| • Ethanol | ? Via reduced vitamin A levels | |
| • COX2 inhibitors | Affects prostaglandins | |
| Maternal hypoxia | ? Affects expression of retinoid receptors<br>? Increased expression of glucocorticoid receptors<br>? Increased expression of angiopoietin-2<br>Accelerated aging | 542 |
| Ureteral obstruction: postnatal | ↓ Cell proliferation<br>↑ Apoptosis of tubular cells<br>Delayed maturation of interstitial fibroblasts → interstitial fibrosis<br>? Alteration of postinductive processes | 73 |
| Preterm birth | Abnormal maturation of glomeruli<br>? Factors associated with shift from intrauterine to extrauterine environment<br>? Loss of progenitor cell populations | 113, 561 |

## MATERNAL NUTRITION

### UNDERNUTRITION

Suboptimal maternal nutrition during pregnancy has long been thought to be the basis of programmed deficits in offspring.[311] In humans, maternal malnutrition, as measured by hemoglobin, triceps skinfold thickness, or lower weight gain during later pregnancy, were all associated with higher offspring blood pressures, suggesting a programming effect.[312] Longitudinal study of people conceived or born during the Dutch Hunger Winter of 1944–1945 has demonstrated that periods of severe undernourishment can result in hypertension[295] and albuminuria,[238] even in the absence of overt fetal growth restriction. Experimental alterations in maternal dietary composition at different stages of gestation have been shown to program kidney gene expression early in the course of gestation, which later affects nephron number (Table 21.13).[313] Maternal "protein and calorie restriction" during all or the later stages of pregnancy have been the most widely studied models of low birth weight and reduced nephron number since as early as 1968.[314] Not all low-protein diets have the same programming effects, however. It has been proposed that the source of carbohydrate and the relative deficiencies of specific amino acids—methionine or glycine, for example—may have a greater impact on organ development than total protein restriction per se, potentially through epigenetic modulation of gene expression.[34,315] Effects are also dependent on the degree of protein restriction and the sex of the fetus, with a more severe restriction required to impair kidney development and program hypertension in female rats than males.[141,316] Fetal nutrient supply is also affected by alterations in placental development that affect uteroplacental blood flow and transfer of nutrients to the fetus. Placental insufficiency is the most common cause of fetal growth restriction in the Western world, and as recently reviewed,[317] the placental phenotype most likely underpins the developmental programming of chronic disease in the offspring. Similarly, in the rat, uterine ischemia in late pregnancy resulted in a nephron deficit and hypertension in male offspring, but interestingly, restoration of good fetal nutrition postnatally, during ongoing nephrogenesis, resulted in restoration of nephron number.[112]

Increased fetal exposure to glucocorticoids and alterations to the RAAS have been proposed as mechanisms whereby low-protein diet reduces nephron number, both of which are discussed later.[318] Other potential mechanisms include reduced renal angiogenesis, associated with reduced VEGF expression, observed in offspring of mothers exposed to 50% calorie restriction during gestation[319]; global downregulation of gene expression, as seen in fetal kidneys of microswine exposed to low-protein diet in late gestation/early lactation[320]; and altered epigenetic DNA methylation, which may affect gene expression, described in livers of offspring of protein-restricted mothers.[321]

In terms of micronutrients, maternal "iron restriction" during pregnancy also leads to a reduction in birth weight and nephron number and the development of hypertension in rat offspring.[322] In another study, offspring of iron-deficient dams had reduced radial glomerular counts and increased tubulointerstitial fibrosis, which were rescued with iron supplementation during gestation.[323] Conceivably, fetal anemia may result in reduced tissue oxygen delivery, altered fetal kidney glucocorticoid sensitivity, or altered availability of other micronutrients that may affect nephrogenesis.[322] Similarly, pre- or postweaning "zinc deficiency" was also associated with decreased nephron number, reduced GFR, and higher blood pressures in rats, potentially mediated by reduction in the antioxidant antiapoptotic effects of zinc.[324] As yet, there is no evidence for programmed renal outcomes in children of iron- or zinc-deficient mothers, although in a population with a high prevalence of anemia, iron supplementation resulted in an increase in birth weight.[325]

Maternal "vitamin A restriction" has also been associated with a reduction in nephron number in rat offspring.[106,326] Severe vitamin A deficiency during pregnancy is associated with congenital malformations and renal defects in the offspring. Vitamin A and all-*trans* retinoic acid have been shown to stimulate nephrogenesis through modulation of branching capacity in ureteric epithelial cell culture and in maintenance of spatial organization of blood vessel development in cultured renal cortical explants.[326] Analysis of 21-day-old fetal rats (just before birth) revealed a direct correlation between plasma retinol concentration and nephron number, as shown in Fig. 21.12.[326] The reduction in nephron number in the setting of vitamin A deficiency is likely mediated, at least in part, by modulation of genes regulating branching morphogenesis.[326] In vivo, a vitamin A–deficient diet sufficient to reduce circulating vitamin A levels by 50% in pregnant rats resulted in a 25% reduction in nephron endowment in the offspring, whereas supplementation of vitamin A increased nephron endowment.[326] In contrast, supplemental retinoic acid was studied as a means

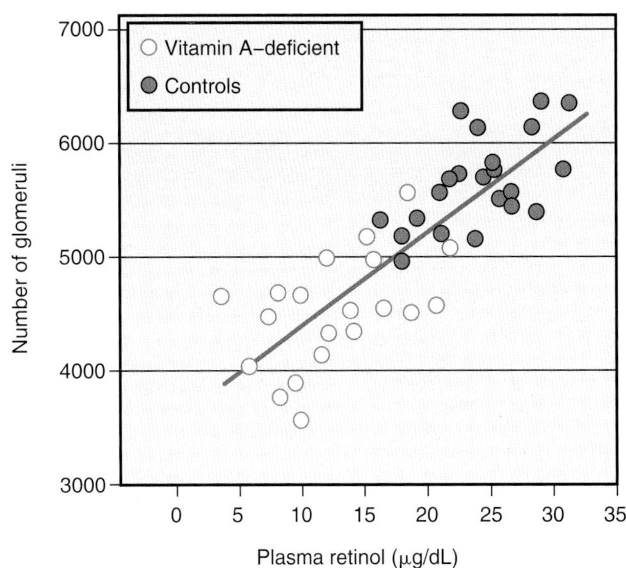


**Fig. 21.12** Relationship between nephron number (number of glomeruli) and plasma retinol concentration in term rat fetuses. $P < .001$; $R = 0.829$. (From Merlet-Benichou C. Influence of fetal environment on kidney development. *Int J Dev Biol.* 1999;43:453–456.)

to stimulate nephrogenesis in postnatal preterm baboons, but no effect was observed, suggesting a more proximal window where vitamin A may be most critical.[327]

It is interesting to note that smoking and alcohol intake may be associated with reduced levels of circulating vitamin A, and both, as discussed later, are associated with low birth weight and programming of disease outcomes. Subtle differences in vitamin A level during pregnancy, therefore, may be a significant factor contributing to the wide distribution of nephron number in the general population.[90]

Emerging evidence also suggests "vitamin D deficiency" during pregnancy can alter kidney development; in animal models, offspring from vitamin D–deficient dams had delayed glomerular development and altered renal function.[328–330] In humans, severe 25-hydroxy Vitamin D (25OHD) deficiency is associated with low birth weight and gestational age at delivery, both of which are known to influence kidney development.[329]

Recognizing the importance of nutrition during pregnancy and after birth, maternal and neonatal replacement of micronutrients has been implemented as a public health policy in several countries (Table 21.14).[331] From a global review, the incidence of low birth weight was reduced by 19% with iron and folate supplementation and by 11%–13% with multimicronutrient supplements, and balanced energy supplementation increased birth weights by a mean of 73 g and reduced the risk of being small for gestational age by 34%.[331,332] Vitamin A supplementation alone did not affect birth weight but did improve child mortality.[331,333,334] Interestingly, children of mothers who received folate or a preparation containing folate + iron + zinc during pregnancy in addition to vitamin A supplementation in early postpartum in Nepal had a lower risk of low birth weight but no change in later blood pressure.[334,335] Microalbuminuria was less frequent, however, suggesting a potential programming effect of these micronutrients.[335] Very high doses of vitamin A have been

**Table 21.14 Impact of Nutritional Interventions on Birth Weight and Preterm Birth and Programming of Blood Pressure and Kidney Disease**

| | LBW/SGA | Preterm Birth | Preeclampsia/ Eclampsia | HBW/LGA | Child Blood Pressure | Child GFR | Child Microalbuminuria |
|---|---|---|---|---|---|---|---|
| Iron and folate supplementation | ↓ | ↓ | | | ↓ | ↑ | |
| Micronutrient supplementation | ↓ | | | | ↑ or ↓ (No effect vs. iron/folate) | | |
| Calcium supplementation | | ↓ | ↓ | | ↓ | | |
| Protein supplementation | ↓ | | | | No effect | | |
| Vitamin A supplementation | No effect/↓ | | | | Possible ↓ | | |
| Folate supplementation | | | | | | | ↓ |
| Zinc supplementation | | ↓ | | | No effect | | |
| Iodine supplementation | ↓ | | | | | | |
| Malaria prevention and Rx | ↓ | | | | | | |
| Rx of genital infections | ↓ | ↓ | | | | | |
| Rx asymptomatic bacteriuria | ↓ | | | | | | |
| Magnesium sulphate | | | ↓ | | | | |
| Antiplatelet agents | ↓ | ↓ | ↓ | | | | |
| Diabetes education | | | | ↓ | | | |
| Smoking cessation | ↓ | ↓ | | | | | |

*GFR*, Glomerular filtration rate; *HBW*, high birth weight; *LBW*, low birth weight, *LGA*, large for gestational age; *SGA*, small for gestational age.
Compiled from references 461, 457, 334, 335, 562, and 577–583.
Reproduced from Low Birth Weight and Nephron Number Working Group. The impact of kidney development on the life course: a consensus document for action. *Nephron.* 2017;136:3–49.

shown to be teratogenic and reduce nephrogenesis; therefore, vitamin A supplementation as a strategy to rescue nephron number should target normalization of vitamin A levels and avoid excess.[336] Folate is not known to impact renal development; however, it does affect gene methylation, and deficiencies may program epigenetic effects.[321] Diastolic blood pressures appeared marginally lower (0.78 mm Hg; 95% CI: 0.16 to 1.28) in 4.5-year-old children whose mothers had received early prenatal food supplements in Bangladesh, but were marginally higher (0.87 mm Hg: 95% CI: 0.18 to 1.56) among those whose mothers received a multimicronutrient supplement.[337] GFRs were 4.98 mL/min per 1.73 $m^2$ higher in children whose mothers had received higher-dose iron supplementation, however.[337] Potential confounders or effect modifiers in these cohorts include baseline vitamin A supplementation, which may have an overriding renal programming effect in all subjects, as well as frequent persistent malnutrition and stunting. Long-term follow-up of children of mothers who received supplements during pregnancy is sparse and thus far does not consistently suggest a positive impact on renal programming. The effects should become clearer as cohorts of children age and more data emerges.[331,337]

## OVERNUTRITION: EXPOSURE TO MATERNAL DIABETES AND OBESITY

Focus on long-term programming effects of maternal diet has more recently moved to consider the effects of overnutrition, including the consequences for offspring born to diabetic women and obese women. As discussed earlier, in some populations high birth weight is associated with an increased susceptibility to proteinuria and renal disease.[12,38,50] High birth weight is a complication of gestational hyperglycemia and diabetes and may therefore also be a surrogate marker of abnormal intrauterine programming. Human offspring of diabetic pregnancies have a higher incidence of congenital malformations, resulting from defects in early organogenesis and have an increased risk of CKD (see Table 21.8).[274,338] It is known that expression and bioavailability of the insulin-like growth factors (IGFs) are altered in diabetic pregnancies and that IGFs and their binding proteins are important regulators of fetal development.[338] The impact of maternal diabetes on metanephric expression of IGFs and their receptors was studied in rats in which diabetes was induced by streptozotocin compared with gestational age–matched normal controls.[338] There was no significant difference in IGF-1 or IGF-2 or insulin receptor expression at any stage, but in offspring of diabetic mothers, there was a significantly increased expression of the IGF-2/mannose-6-phosphate receptor. This receptor tightly regulates the action of IGF-2, and an increase in expression would lead to reduced IGF-2 bioavailability.[338] IGF-2 is a critical player in renal development. The same investigators examined the role of IGF binding protein-1 (IGFBP-1) on nephrogenesis in genetically modified mice.[339] Offspring of females overexpressing human IGFBP-1 were growth restricted and had an 18% to 25% reduction in nephron number, depending on whether human IGFBP-1 was overexpressed in the mother only, fetus only, or both. When metanephroi from these mice were cultured in the presence of IGF-I or IGF-II, only IGF-2 increased nephron numbers by 25% to 40% in a concentration-dependent manner.[339] Interestingly, in a cohort of preterm infants, diastolic blood pressure at age 4 years was found to correlate positively with IGFBP-1 levels measured at postnatal weeks 32.6–34.6, potentially suggesting a programming effect of this pathway in humans.[340]

In offspring of rats rendered hyperglycemic during pregnancy either by inducing diabetes mellitus with streptozotocin

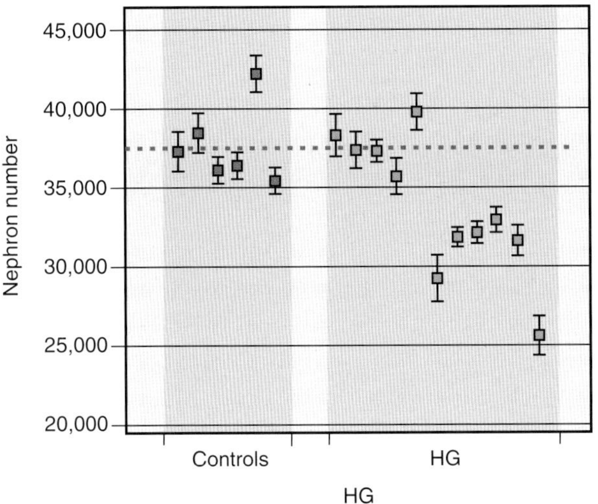


**Fig. 21.13** Effects of maternal hyperglycemia on nephron number in rat offspring. *Dotted line* represents mean value in control group. *HG*, Hyperglycemia. (From Amri K, Freund N, Vilar J, et al. Adverse effects of hyperglycemia on kidney development in rats: in vivo and in vitro studies. *Diabetes* 1999;48:2240–2245.)

or by infusing glucose from gestational days 12 to 16, nephron numbers were reduced by 10% to 35%, correlating with the degree of maternal hyperglycemia (Fig. 21.13).[341] Furthermore, culture of metanephroi in varying glucose concentrations demonstrated that tight glucose control is necessary for optimal metanephric growth and differentiation. In mice, offspring of diabetic mothers had fewer nephrons, associated with increased evidence of apoptosis in tubules and podocytes, potentially mediated via increased renal angiotensinogen and renin mRNA expression and NF-κB activation.[161] Other authors suggest altered branching morphogenesis, increased asymmetric dimethylarginine, and reduced nitric oxide levels as potential mediators of reduced nephron numbers in offspring of diabetic mothers.[342,343] These offspring developed higher blood pressures and renal hypertrophy and had greater tubulointerstitial injury compared with controls, and these changes were abrogated by normalization of asymmetric dimethyl arginine (ADMA) levels achieved by maternal supplementation with L-citrulline.[343] Multiple pathways are therefore likely implicated in hyperglycemia-induced renal programming. Functionally, study of adult rat offspring of diabetic mothers revealed glomerular hypertrophy, reduced GFR and renal plasma flow, hypertension, and decreased endothelium-mediated vasodilation.[344,345]

Maternal obesity and associated pregnancy complications, including gestational diabetes, maternal hypertension, and sleep apnea, are now thought to present the greatest risk for in utero programming of adult disease. Pregnancies in overweight and obese mothers can result in both low- and high-weight infants, suggesting that programming of offspring by maternal obesity may be multifactorial.[346] Feeding animals a high-fat (+/− high carbohydrate) diet prior to and throughout pregnancy can result in programmed outcomes. Exposure to a high-fat diet for 10 days prior to pregnancy until weaning resulted in rat female offspring with hypertension but no change in nephron endowment, although renal renin and Na/K-ATPase activity were altered.[347] Rat dams fed an obesogenic diet for a more sustained period (a high-fat/high-fructose diet from 6 weeks prior to mating) resulted in offspring with albuminuria, which was further exacerbated by a postnatal high-fat diet.[348] A similar model also caused increased renal norepinephrine and renin expression in offspring.[349] Conversely, in mice, a maternal high-fat diet caused an increase in offspring nephron number, with no consequences for renal function.[350] Dams in that study were glucose intolerant prior to mating but had normal glucose tolerance during pregnancy, suggesting complex interactions between maternal obesity and diabetes. These data suggest that it may not be the high-fat diet per se causing changes in renal development but rather the resultant maternal hyperglycemia. Of note, many calorie-dense foods are also deficient in essential micronutrients.[279]

## MATERNAL AND FETAL EXPOSURE TO GLUCOCORTICOIDS

Elevated maternal glucocorticoids due to stress or glucocorticoid therapy may impact fetal growth and renal development. Under normal circumstances, the fetus is protected, at least in part, from exposure to excess endogenous maternal corticosteroids by the placental enzyme 11β-hydroxysteroid dehydrogenase type 2 (11β-HSD2), which metabolizes corticosterone to the inert 11-dehydrocorticosterone.[21] However, this barrier is not complete, and administration of high physiologic concentrations of cortisol (in sheep) or corticosterone (in rats and mice) all resulted in offspring with low nephron number.[351–353] Offspring of these models developed hypertension and impairment of renal function, including albuminuria, that was, in all cases, associated with changes in the renal renin–angiotensin system (discussed later).[351,354,355] These outcomes occurred even following very short-term exposure (48–60 hours) that did not affect birth weight in sheep and mice.[353,356] Prenatal administration of dexamethasone, a steroid not metabolized by 11β-HSD2, lead to fetal growth restriction, 20% to 60% lower nephron number, glomerulomegaly, and subsequent hypertension in rats and sheep.[103,107,185,356] Metanephric organ culture experiments have demonstrated that dexamethasone can cause a dose-dependent inhibition of branching morphogenesis in part through regulation of *GDNF* gene expression.[357] Rats and humans with mutations in the *11β-HSD2* gene have low levels of placental *11β-HSD2* and give birth to low birth weight offspring in whom hypertension develops prematurely.[358,359] Maternal low-protein diet during gestation has been shown to result in decreased placental expression of *11β-HSD2*, therefore likely increasing exposure of the fetus to maternal corticosteroids.[34,154] Treatment of pregnant rats fed a low-protein diet with an inhibitor of steroid synthesis ameliorates the programming of hypertension and increases nephron numbers in the offspring.[21,34,360] Although this rescue was not complete, these data strongly implicate glucocorticoids as modulators of nephrogenesis in the setting of maternal low-protein diet.[360] Excessive fetal steroid exposure may drive inappropriate gene expression and affect growth and nephrogenesis, potentially through more rapid maturation of tissues.[34] Furthermore, expression of steroid-responsive receptors, including the corticosteroid responsive renal Na/K-ATPase $\alpha_1$- and $\beta_1$-subunits, was found to be significantly increased in offspring of rats fed a low-protein diet during gestation.[154] In another study, prenatal dexamethasone was associated with increased proximal tubule sodium transport, in part related to increased activity of the tubular NHE3.[361] These changes may contribute to hypertension.

In humans, there has been concern about perinatal exposure to corticosteroids; however, follow-up of subjects whose mothers participated in a randomized placebo-controlled study of antenatal betamethasone did not find any difference in blood pressure or other cardiovascular risk factors at age 30 years in exposed compared with unexposed individuals.[362] Although no effect on blood pressure or renal function was noted among preterm infants who had received antenatal steroids within the first 2 years of life compared with those who did not, recent evidence, however, highlights glucocorticoid therapy may have lasting effects on the brain and result in increased mental disorders at age 8 years.[191,363,364] Longitudinal examination of the consequences of sustained glucocorticoid therapy (e.g., throughout pregnancy) has not been performed.

## MATERNAL AND FETAL HYPOXIA

In addition to maternal iron deficiency (resulting in anemia) and placental insufficiency discussed earlier, a range of conditions, including high altitude, maternal smoking, and sleep apnea, can result in fetal hypoxia. These conditions have all been shown to result in low birth weight in humans, but as yet, there is little evidence to suggest long-term effects on kidney function. In mice, a short-term severe, hypoxic insult (5.5%–7.5% maternal oxygen) from E9.5–10.5 caused a CAKUT phenotype, whereas mild hypoxia in midpregnancy (12% from E12.5–14.5) resulted in low nephron endowment mediated in part through suppression of β-catenin signaling.[365] A similar mild hypoxia in late gestation resulted in fetal growth restriction, low nephron number in male but not female offspring, and hypertension in both sexes.[366] In a mouse model of cigarette smoke exposure, male offspring had fewer nephrons and increased albumin/creatinine ratio.[367] Short-term cord occlusion in fetal sheep did not cause overt long-term renal damage, highlighting that the timing and duration of hypoxia are important in mediating renal outcomes.[368]

## FETAL DRUG AND ALCOHOL EXPOSURE

Several medications commonly used during pregnancy or in the early postnatal period have been studied for their effects on birth weight and nephrogenesis. Among 397 pregnant women, antibiotic use was associated with a 138-g lower offspring birth weight compared with nonantibiotic use.[369] Furthermore, analysis of methylation levels of imprinted genes showed antibiotic use to be associated with methylation at five differentially mediated regions, although methylation at only one region was associated with birth weight.[369] The aminoglycoside antibiotic gentamicin administered to pregnant rats results in a permanent nephron deficit in offspring.[370] Significantly lower numbers of ureteric branch points and nephrons were observed in metanephric explants cultured in the presence of gentamicin.[371,372] In contrast, however, other investigators did not find a reduction in nephron number in rat pups administered gentamicin intraperitoneally from birth to 14 days of age.[373] The β-lactams have also been shown to result in impaired nephrogenesis.[374] Administration of ampicillin to pregnant rats leads to an 11% average reduction in nephron endowment in offspring, as well as evidence of focal cystic tubule dilatation and interstitial inflammation. Administration of ceftriaxone in vivo did not result in a nephron deficit, but histologically, there was evidence of renal interstitial inflammation. The penicillins were also found to inhibit nephrogenesis in cultured metanephroi in a dose-dependent fashion, an effect that was less evident with ceftriaxone. Importantly, nephrogenesis was affected even at therapeutic doses of penicillins in the rat. The mechanism whereby the β-lactams reduce nephron endowment is likely through an increase in apoptosis in the induced mesenchyme.[106] Overall, antibiotic use during pregnancy may reduce nephron endowment. Further research on those antibiotics that are frequently used in human pregnancy and preterm infants in warranted.

The immunosuppressive medication cyclosporine is a known nephrotoxin in humans that crosses the placenta. Women treated with cyclosporine may have successful pregnancies, although infants tend to have birth weights in the low range, and its effect on the fetal kidney is not well described.[375] Cyclosporine administration in varying doses and at different stages of gestation was evaluated in pregnant rabbits compared with rabbits receiving either vehicle or no drug.[375] Cyclosporine administration in the later, but not the earlier, period of gestation resulted in smaller litters and growth-restricted pups. All pups exposed to cyclosporine in utero had a 25% to 33% lower nephron number than controls. The reduction in nephron number was accompanied by glomerulomegaly and was independent of birth weight. At 1 month of age, these kidneys also demonstrated foci of glomerulosclerosis. Subsequent functional evaluation of the kidneys of rabbits exposed to cyclosporine in utero demonstrated lower GFR at 18 and 35 weeks of age and an increase in proteinuria at 11, 18, and 35 weeks of age.[176] Rabbits exposed to cyclosporine in utero developed spontaneous hypertension by 11 weeks of age, which worsened progressively with time.[176] In the presence of cyclosporine, nephron formation was found to be arrested, potentially due to inhibition of conversion of metanephric mesenchyme to epithelium.[106]

Nonsteroidal antiinflammatory drugs are sometimes used in preterm children postnatally. Administration of a cyclooxygenase 2 inhibitor, but not a cyclooxygenase 1 inhibitor, postnatally in rats and mice resulted in reduced cortical volume, impairment of nephrogenesis, and reduced glomerular diameter.[376] Administration of indomethacin or ibuprofen postnatally did not affect nephron number in rats.[373] In the preterm baboon kidney, early postnatal administration of five doses of ibuprofen (consistent with recommended dosing in preterm infants with patent ductus arteriosus) was associated with a reduction in width of the nephrogenic zone, suggesting premature termination of nephrogenesis.[377] The impact of these medications on human nephrogenesis is not known.

Maternal alcohol consumption: Renal malformations have been reported in children with fetal alcohol syndrome.[378] In sheep, repeated ethanol exposure during the second half of pregnancy resulted in an 11% reduction in nephron number and impaired vascular function in late pregnancy, although offspring outcomes were not examined.[379,380] In rats, exposure to 2 days of a high dose of alcohol in mid–late pregnancy resulted in a low nephron number and offspring with hypertension and sex-dependent impairments in GFR.[381] Using metanephric organ culture, alcohol was found to cause dose-dependent decreases in branching morphogenesis, which were prevented by retinoic acid supplementation.[382] An abstract has reported an impact of maternal alcohol ingestion on kidney development in children, but it is not known whether the effects were mediated by associated vitamin A deficiency or other mechanisms.[90]

## OBSTRUCTION OF THE DEVELOPING KIDNEY

Around one-half of all pediatric kidney transplants are required as a result of CAKUT, predominantly obstructive nephropathy, and hypoplasia/dysplasia.[383] Being small for gestational age was associated with a higher risk of ESKD (OR: 2.5; 95% CI: 1.6 to 3.7) compared with normal birth weight, suggesting that nephron number acquired at birth may be an important modulator of this risk.[31] Most cases of CAKUT result from multiple genetic, epigenetic, and fetal developmental factors such as exposure to maternal diabetes, as discussed earlier (see Table 21.8).[274] As recently reviewed, many developmental abnormalities of the urinary tract are associated with impaired nephrogenesis, which, in turn, is compounded by obstructive injury.[384,385] From animal studies, it has become clear that perinatal urinary obstruction may lead to reduced nephron numbers, which may exacerbate the impact of other programming factors.[70,386] In rats, unilateral ureteral obstruction (UUO) on postnatal day 1 and relieved on day 5, or on postnatal day 14 and relieved on day 19, reduced nephron number by 50% in both groups.[73] Similar intervention in adult rats did not affect nephron number or tubular development. A follow-up study using this model of early-life UUO demonstrated that renin was decreased and glomerulotubular maturation was delayed.[387] These studies demonstrate that urinary obstruction in a normal developing kidney can impact not only nephrogenesis but also tubular development, which may have long-term impacts on renal solute handling. Importantly, temporary neonatal urinary obstruction was also associated with histologic scarring and loss of function of the contralateral kidney in 1-year-old rats, suggesting consequent programming in the contralateral kidney as well.[388] Developing and neonatal kidneys therefore appear to be highly susceptible to obstructive injury, suggesting that early relief of urinary tract obstruction may be important to preserve nephron number.

## MOLECULAR PATHWAYS AFFECTED IN FETAL PROGRAMMING OF THE KIDNEY

The molecular regulation of kidney development, particularly in the mouse, has been comprehensively described elsewhere.[298] In a number of animal models of developmental programming, changes in expression levels of genes regulating branching morphogenesis, apoptosis, and renal growth have been described (for a review, see Wang and Garrett[389]), and studies have applied microarray or deep-sequencing techniques to determine the effects of a maternal perturbation on the whole genome.[299,313,390] Epigenetic changes are now thought to play a role in programming of disease across generations, but as yet, the evidence for epigenetic changes within the kidney is limited.[391]

### URETERIC BRANCHING MORPHOGENESIS

GDNF signaling through its receptor-tyrosine kinase Ret is a key ligand–receptor interaction driving ureteric budding and branching. The *c-ret* receptor is expressed on the tips of the ureteric bud branches, and knockout of this receptor in mice leads to severe renal dysplasia and reduction in nephron number.[297] Homozygous *GDNF*-null mutant mice have complete renal agenesis and die shortly after birth.[392] Heterozygous *GDNF* mice, as described earlier, have reduced nephron numbers, develop glomerulomegaly, and are susceptible to hypertension.[149] Polymorphisms in *RET*, but not *GDNF*, are associated with newborn renal size in humans.[121,393] As described earlier, maternal dietary vitamin A has a significant impact on nephrogenesis (Fig. 12.12). In cultured metanephroi, the expression of *c-ret* was found to be regulated by retinoic acid supplementation in a dose-dependent manner.[326] *GDNF* expression was not affected by vitamin A fluctuations. Modulation of *c-ret* expression is therefore likely to be a significant pathway through which vitamin A availability regulates nephrogenesis and nephron endowment. Expression of *GDNF* has also been shown to be decreased following maternal glucocorticoid exposure[357] and maternal alcohol consumption,[381] which may contribute to a reduction in branching morphogenesis and lower nephron endowment.

Further evidence for impairments in ureteric branching comes from a mouse model of maternal diabetes during pregnancy, where optical projection tomography was used to demonstrate a reduction in branch number and length within the developing kidney.[342] In another mouse model of diabetes, changes in TGF-β1 signaling were disrupted due to increased expression of a hedgehog interacting protein.[394] This protein was localized to differentiated metanephric mesenchyme and the ureteric epithelium during early kidney development and then was found in maturing glomerular endothelial and tubulointerstitial cells. Increased expression of this protein due to high glucose-impaired branching morphogenesis resulted in neonates with small kidneys.

### APOPTOSIS

To evaluate at which stage of development a low-protein diet impacts nephrogenesis, embryonic rat metanephroi were studied at different time points.[313] At embryonic day 13, the metanephros has just formed, the ureteric bud has branched once, branch tips are surrounded by condensed mesenchyme that later transforms into tubule epithelium, and the ureteric stalk is surrounded by loose stromal mesenchyme.[313] By day 15, multiple branching cycles have occurred, and primitive nephrons begin to be formed.[313] At embryonic day 13, there was no difference in the number of cells in metanephroi from embryos whose mothers received low- or normal-protein diets, but by day 15, there were significantly fewer cells per metanephros in the low-protein group. In contrast, a significant increase in the number of apoptotic cells was observed in the low-protein group at day 13 but not at day 15, suggesting that increased apoptosis on day 13 likely contributed to the reduced cell numbers on day 15.[313] On postnatal day 1 in kidneys from offspring of mothers exposed to 50% calorie restriction, apoptosis was most evident in the nephrogenic zone, colocalizing to the mesenchyme and peritubular aggregates, suggesting a role in modulation of nephrogenesis.[395] In 8-week-old hypertensive low-birth-weight rat offspring of mothers subjected to a low-protein diet, the kidneys were histologically normal but also showed evidence of increased apoptosis, without an increase in proliferation, compared with normal-birth-weight controls.[108] The increase in apoptotic activity observed in the kidney in these studies suggests possible successive waves of apoptosis at different stages of nephrogenesis in programmed rats that may impact nephron endowment.

Several studies have suggested that altered regulation of apoptosis in the developing kidney may be due to downregulation of antiapoptotic factors (e.g., Pax-2 or Bcl-2) and/or upregulation of proapoptotic factors in response to environmental or other stimuli (e.g., Bax, p53, Fas receptor, caspase 3 and 9).[395–399] Humans with haploinsufficiency of *PAX2* have renal coloboma syndrome, and those with certain *PAX2* polymorphisms have smaller neonatal kidney size as discussed earlier.[306,396,400] *PAX2* is an antiapoptotic transcriptional regulator that is highly expressed in the branching ureteric tree as well as in foci of induced nephrogenic mesenchyme during kidney development.[396] Heterozygous mice with *Pax2* mutations were very small at birth and had significant reductions in nephron number. In addition, there was a significant increase in apoptotic cell death in the developing kidneys. Subsequently, the same group[400] demonstrated that loss of *Pax2* antiapoptotic activity reduced ureteric branching and increased ureteric apoptosis. Similarly, loss of the antiapoptotic factor *Bcl-2* or gain of function of the proapoptotic factor p53 are both associated with a significant reduction in nephron number, associated with increased apoptosis in metanephric blastemas, in *Bcl-2* knockout mice and *p53* transgenic mice.[397,401]

Mutant mouse models, although providing evidence that an increase in apoptosis results in reduced nephron numbers, do not, however, address the impact of environmental factors on renal development. Pham and associates[402] examined gene expression in the kidneys of offspring of rats subjected to uterine artery ligation during gestation. These authors found a 25% reduction in glomerular number was associated with increased evidence of apoptosis and increased proapoptotic caspase-3 activity in the kidney at birth. Furthermore, they found evidence of increased mRNA expression of the proapoptotic genes *Bax* and *p53* and decreased expression of the antiapoptotic gene *Bcl-2*. These authors also found evidence of hypomethylation of the *p53* gene, which, in addition to a decrease in *Bcl-2* expression, would lead to an increase in *p53* activity, suggesting epigenetic programming of a proapoptotic milieu as a potential modulator of nephron endowment. Increased apoptosis was also observed in a similar rat model during late gestation (E20) and 1 week after birth (PN7), suggesting inappropriate apoptosis even after birth.[403] Of great interest in that study, the growth-restricted offspring, but not control offspring, had evidence of ongoing nephrogenesis at PN7, suggesting a delay in kidney development in the growth-restricted group. Gene microarray studies in rodent models of maternal iron deficiency[390] and diabetes[404] have also identified apoptotic signaling pathways in fetal kidneys.

### IMPACT OF SEX

In some experimental models and human studies, although not all, programming effects on blood pressure and kidney function appear to be different between males and females, especially at young ages. In female rats with similar programmed reductions in nephron numbers, blood pressures are often not as high or increase much later than in males.[108,405] Often a secondary challenge such as pregnancy, however, will "unmask" a disease phenotype in females. For example, males but not females born small as a result of bilateral uterine vessel ligation develop hypertension and insulin resistance.[111,406,407] However, growth-restricted females develop glucose intolerance during pregnancy.[408] Sex hormones may, in part, explain these differences. Growth-restricted males (induced by uterine artery ligation) have elevated testosterone levels compared with controls, and hypertension can be abrogated by castration.[405] Such changes are not observed in male offspring of protein-restricted mothers, however, pointing to the intricacies of the programming models. In female rats growth restricted by placental insufficiency, hypertension only develops late, but onset can be accelerated by ovariectomy.[405] These data suggest that in the uterine ischemia programming model, testosterone exacerbates and estrogen protects against hypertension. Sex differences in relative expression of components of the RAAS appear to participate in programming of hypertension, potentially differentially altering the balance between vasoconstriction and vasodilation and sodium handling.[159,405] Furthermore, growth-restricted male rats exhibit increased markers of renal oxidative stress compared with controls, which are absent in similarly programmed females, and antioxidant treatment normalized blood pressure in the male rats.[170,409] Multiple other suggested mechanisms underlying these gender differences have been reviewed by Ojeda et al., as outlined in Fig. 21.14.[170,405]

Sex differences may also originate in utero due to differences in growth of male and female fetuses and sex-specific placental responses to maternal perturbations (reviewed in Kalisch-Smith et al.[410]). In particular, the placenta has an important role in preventing excess maternal glucocorticoids from reaching the fetus via the activity of placental 11β-HSD2. This enzyme has the ability to convert the active glucocorticoid into an inactive form, as discussed earlier. The placenta of female fetuses is known to have higher levels of this enzyme compared with males,[411] and as such, the male fetus is likely to be exposed to more glucocorticoids. Furthermore, in women treated with synthetic glucocorticoids when threatening to deliver preterm, placental 11β-HSD2 was elevated more in placentas of females than males.[412] The sex of the fetus has not always been taken into account when performing studies on renal development; however, a recent metaanalysis demonstrated the adult human kidney showed sex-specific expression of more than 200 genes.[413]

## POTENTIAL FOR RESCUE OF NEPHRON NUMBER

Given the evidence for developmental programming of hypertension and kidney disease and the associations with birth weight, preterm birth, other intrauterine exposures, and the impact of nutrition in early childhood, it is possible that interventions could be designed to modulate developmentally programmed changes in the kidney and reduce long-term disease risk. Optimization of maternal health and nutrition prior to and during pregnancy to attenuate any risk factors for low birth weight and preterm birth is the most obvious

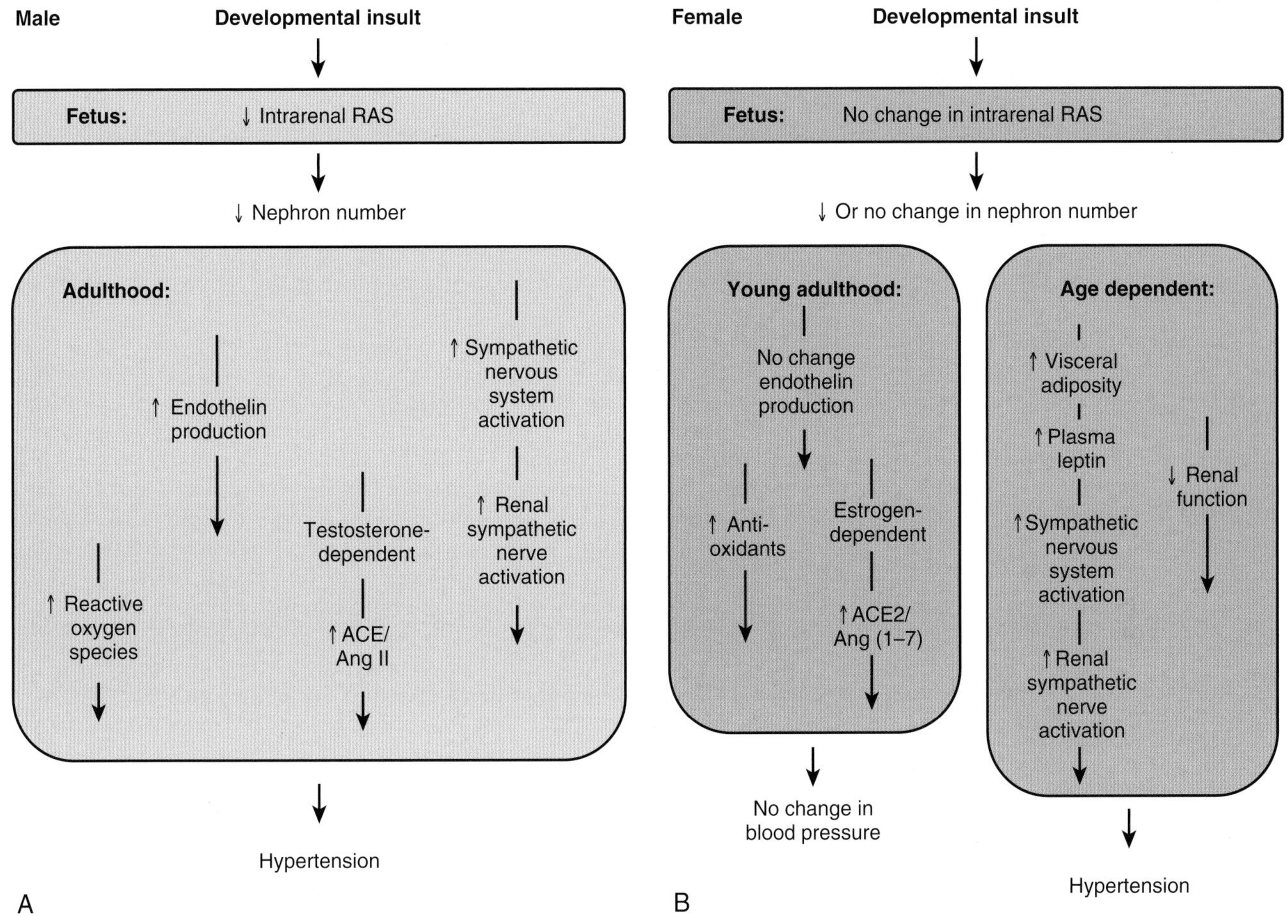


**Fig. 21.14** Potential differing mechanisms impacting developmental programming of blood pressure in (A) males, and (B) females. These mechanisms may be due to the influence of the hormonal milieu on the renin–angiotensin system *(RAS)* due to innate sex differences in production of reactive oxygen species or endothelin, or impacted by increased susceptibility that occurs with age and the development of age-dependent increases in adiposity leading to activation of the sympathetic renal nerves (females). The fetus also exhibits innate sex differences in expression of the intrarenal RAS, which may or may not (as in females) reduce nephron number. *ACE*, Angiotensin-converting enzyme; *Ang*, angiotensin. (From Ojeda NB, Intapad S, Alexander BT. Sex differences in the developmental programming of hypertension. *Acta Physiol (Oxf)*. 2014;210:307–316.)

intervention, as it has been estimated that intrauterine factors determine around 60% of the variation in birth weight.[414] In addition, minimization of nephrotoxin exposure and attention to neonatal nutrition in preterm infants are important to permit optimal nephrogenesis after birth. Specific interventions that may augment nephron number per se have been investigated, some of which are clinically feasible, while others are still in research stages (see Table 21.4). Interventions to modulate other aspects of developmental programming in the kidney have not yet been reported, but the assumption would be that the impact may be similar to those affecting nephrogenesis.

Prevention is likely more realistic than rescue of low nephron number. Ouabain is a highly specific ligand for Na/K-ATPase, the activity of which is known to be reduced in erythrocytes of low-birth-weight young men.[415,416] Na/K-ATPase is a ubiquitously expressed plasma membrane protein that regulates the release of calcium waves and thereby is an important regulator of early development.[415] In vitro addition of ouabain to the medium of metanephroi in culture was found to abrogate the effect of serum starvation on ureteric branching.[415] Similarly, in vivo, ouabain administration throughout pregnancy prevented the reduction in nephron number in rats subjected to maternal low-protein diet.[415] Whether ouabain can rescue nephron number if given late in pregnancy was not addressed in this study. Supplementation of glycine, urea, or alanine to a maternal low-protein diet prevented development of low nephron numbers in rat offspring, but only glycine supplementation prevented subsequent hypertension.[34] Intriguingly, water restriction of rat mothers during gestation resulted in augmentation of normal nephron number but also induced hypertension in the offspring. The authors implicate vasopressin as a mediator of this programming effect.[417]

Vitamin A deficiency is common among women in poorer nations and in animals is associated with reduced nephron number as discussed earlier.[326,418] In rats exposed to maternal low-protein diet, nephron number was restored to normal by one dose of retinoic acid given to the pregnant dams during early nephrogenesis.[419] In preterm baboons, however, administration of retinoic acid postnatally did not rescue nephron number, suggesting that vitamin A is likely necessary earlier in gestation.[327] These baboons also received postnatal antibiotics, which may have confounded the effect of the vitamin A.

Postnatal nutrition is an important modulator of kidney development, especially in preterm infants. Restoration of normal protein intake by cross-fostering growth-restricted pups onto normal mothers after birth reduced nephron number and prevented hypertension compared with those fed by protein-deficient mothers.[112]

A maternal single kidney may impact fetal kidney development. In offspring of rats that had undergone nephrectomy prior to pregnancy, nephron numbers were increased at birth, although not at 6 weeks.[420,421] A circulating renotrophic factor in the mother may therefore accelerate nephrogenesis but does not appear to affect final nephron endowment. How these observations would apply in humans is difficult to extrapolate, as outcomes may be different depending on maternal age, whether she has a congenital or acquired single kidney, or a kidney transplant with the attendant required medications, which, in turn, may affect nephrogenesis.

Modulation of regression of nephron number, although still hypothetical, has been suggested as a potential pathway to augment final nephron number.[422] Glomerular number was evaluated from postnatal days 7 to 28 in normal mice. Maximal nephron number was seen at day 7, with a subsequent regression and plateau at day 18. Such a time course would need to be studied in growth-restricted animals before any potential intervention to inhibit this regression could be tested.

## CATCH-UP GROWTH

Postnatal nutrition is important for infant growth, especially in the setting of preterm birth or growth restriction, and can impact nephron number and long-term renal function, as discussed earlier.[187,224] Cross-fostering of growth-restricted newborn rats (induced by placental insufficiency) onto normal mothers permitted restoration of normal nephron number and prevented subsequent hypertension, demonstrating the potential "rescue" effect of adequate postnatal nutrition.[112] Postnatal overfeeding of low-birth-weight rats, induced by reduction of litter size to three pups, however, did not augment low nephron numbers, and with aging, rats became obese and hypertensive and developed renal injury.[423] In this model, despite the mother being switched to a normal-protein diet at time of delivery, the pups may remain somewhat protein deficient despite consuming larger quantities of milk, as opposed to cross-fostering, which provides normal milk immediately, which may explain why nephron number remained low and underscores the importance of diet composition. In contrast, overfeeding of normal-birth-weight rats led to higher than normal nephron numbers, despite which high blood pressure and renal injury developed over time.[137] These animal data suggest that restoration of normal dietary components after growth restriction may permit some reversal of programmed changes, but overfeeding appears harmful.

In diverse populations worldwide, rapid "catch-up" growth (defined as upward crossing of weight centiles), or an increase in body mass index, even in children of normal birth weight, is associated with higher blood pressures and increased cardiovascular risk.[424–426] On the other hand, catch-up growth has been advocated in poorer countries to improve child survival from infectious diseases and reduce stunting and malnutrition.[427] Among 7-year-old children who had been preterm, GFRs were reduced in those who had experienced either intrauterine or extrauterine growth restriction (i.e., inadequate growth early postbirth), highlighting the importance of adequate early postnatal nutrition for kidney development.[224] Nutrition in preterm infants is challenging, and balancing benefits and risks of rapid growth must be considered, including optimizing neurodevelopment and metabolic outcomes.[428]

The timing of catch-up growth in early infancy and childhood, which tends to occur rapidly in low-birth-weight children when adequate nutrition is available, appears a crucial factor in determining this long-term risk.[426,427,429,430] The importance of birth weight and catch-up growth was examined in a cohort of British 22-year-olds, in whom systolic blood pressure was observed to increase by 1.3 mm Hg (95% CI: 0.3 to 2.3 mm Hg) for each SD decrease in birth weight and to increase by 1.6 mm Hg (95% CI: 0.6 to 2.7 mm Hg) for each SD increase in weight gain between the ages of 1 and 10 years.[431] Such observations have been reproduced in several populations, together with evidence of increased arterial stiffness and greater prevalence of cardiovascular risk factors in early childhood after rapid growth, with children who had been of low birth weight but became overweight being at highest risk.[208,424,429] The consequences of catch-up growth may, however, differ if growth is linear (i.e., growth in height) or in weight, and may differ between developed and developing countries where health priorities differ.[432] Thus far, it appears that among those born with low birth weight or preterm, the development of overweight or obesity is the predominant risk factor.[208,426,429,430,433] Low birth weight independently predicted both proteinuria and obesity in a rural Canadian cohort, demonstrating likely simultaneous programming of multiple risk factors for kidney disease.[434] Risk factors for childhood overweight and obesity also include high birth weight and exposure to gestational diabetes.[435] Obesity, in turn, is a risk factor for renal disease.[436,437] Finding the balance where postnatal nutrition is optimized to improve short-term survival and reduce long-term risk of chronic disease requires further study. In general, avoidance of overweight through diet and exercise are safe principles.[438,439]

### IMPACT OF EARLY GROWTH ON KIDNEY FUNCTION

Grijalva-Eternod[440] and colleagues developed a model to test whether "mismatch" between a small kidney and a (relatively) larger body, as would occur with catch-up growth and overweight after being born small, is associated with hypertension. Birth weight was presumed to reflect the homeostatic metabolic capacity of the kidney and childhood body composition to reflect the metabolic load. When applied to a birth cohort of children, the model found that a high metabolic load, relative to innate metabolic capacity, was associated with higher blood pressures (Fig. 21.15). Consistent with this hypothesis, proteinuric renal disease progressed faster in children who had been born prematurely and became obese compared with those who were not obese.[441] In this study, all obese children, whether born at term or preterm, were found to have glomerulomegaly, although kidney size remained small in all those born preterm, even among the obese. Similarly, excessive weight gain was a predictor of worse renal function at age 7.5 years in a cohort of very low–birth-weight preterm infants who had experienced AKI.[442]

Accelerated senescence has been proposed as a potential mechanism whereby catch-up growth may increase the risk of

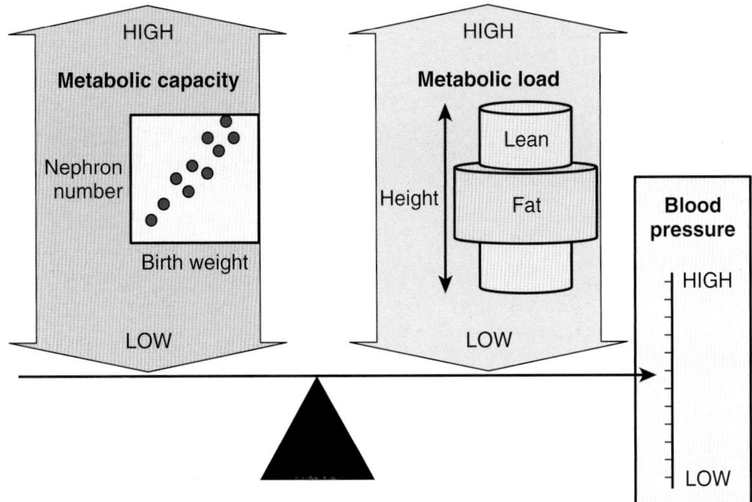


**Fig. 21.15** Diagram illustrating the concepts of metabolic capacity and metabolic load in relation to blood pressure. Metabolic capacity, meaning the capacity to maintain normal metabolic homeostasis, is dependent on nephron number, which scales positively with birth weight. Metabolic load, meaning the demand placed on homeostatic systems, is dependent on body size and adiposity, and hence on height, lean mass, and fat mass. Here they are portrayed using a cylinder model in which cylinder lengths are proportional to height, and the volumes are proportional to the masses of lean and fat mass. A high load and low capacity are each predicted to increase blood pressure. (From Grijalva-Eternod CS, Lawlor DA, Wells JC. Testing a capacity-load model for hypertension: disentangling early and late growth effects on childhood blood pressure in a prospective birth cohort. *PLoS One.* 2013;8:e56078.)

cardiovascular and renal disease.[443] Senescence is a state of cellular growth arrest that naturally occurs with age but may be accelerated in the face of stress, mediated by upregulation of cell cycle inhibitors (p53, p21, and p16INK4a) and progressive shortening of telomeres.[444] Increased expression of senescence markers has been observed in diseased human kidneys.[445] In animals, rapid weight gain in growth-restricted animals was associated with evidence of accelerated senescence in the kidney and cardiovascular system and premature death, consistent with accelerated aging.[443,446,447] Senescence markers are not more highly expressed at birth in growth-restricted versus normal birth weight animals but increase more rapidly as the animals age.[446] Hyperfiltration in a small kidney, exacerbated by high metabolic demand from increasing body size, likely contributes to ongoing injury and progressive senescence.[445,446] Senescence markers have not been studied in low-birth-weight human kidneys, but leukocyte telomere length was found to be significantly shorter among 5-year-old Bangladeshi children who had been of low birth weight compared with those of normal birth weight, lending support to this hypothesis.[448,449] Oxidative stress is a driver of senescence, and in small-for-gestational-age children, markers of oxidative stress were higher in those who experienced catch-up growth compared with controls, suggesting oxidative stress as a possible initiator of accelerated senescence.[450] A programmed link between low nephron number, catch-up growth, and accelerated senescence as a potential mediator of hypertension and renal disease in humans has yet to be proven.

Given the normal age-related loss of nephrons and potential for accelerated senescence in the kidney, it could be expected that the impact of prenatal programming would be compounded by age.[41] This has not yet been extensively studied; however, a single Japanese study found that among elderly subjects with ESKD, diabetic nephropathy was more common among those who had had a low birth weight.[451] This observation may suggest a programming effect of diabetes, kidney disease, or both and requires further study.[275]

## MATERNAL HEALTH AND INTERGENERATIONAL EFFECTS OF PROGRAMMING

Maternal health and nutrition are crucial determinants of a healthy pregnancy, offspring birth weight, and fetal kidney development.[279] Socioeconomic and structural factors are important determinants of maternal health and thereby the health of future generations.[1] Maternal prepregnancy underweight is associated with a higher odds of having a small-for-gestational-age (OR: 1.81; 95% CI: 1.76 to 1.87) or low-birth-weight infant (OR: 1.47; 95% CI: 1.27 to 1.71), as well as a higher risk of preterm birth.[452,453] In contrast, being overweight before pregnancy increases the risk of high birth weight compared with nonobese women (OR: 1.67; 95% CI: 1.42 to 1.97).[453] The risks of gestational diabetes and preeclampsia double with prepregnancy maternal overweight.[452] Preconception care and weight loss may positively impact these adverse outcomes, although around two-thirds of preterm births remain unexplained.[452,454–456]

Maternal risk factors for low birth weight or preterm birth are highlighted in Table 21.15, and global prevalences of some of these factors are outlined in Table 21.16.[1] Short maternal stature, maternal underweight, or iron deficiency are risk factors for offspring low birth weight.[284,457–459] Maternal vitamin A levels are associated with newborn kidney size and nephron number.[460] Supplementation of various nutrients in pregnant women has been shown to reduce the risks of low birth weight or preterm birth, but the long-term impact on childhood or later blood pressure and kidney function are not yet clear (see Table 21.14).[1,457,461] Maternal smoking, alcohol, and caffeine consumption during pregnancy may also increase

**Table 21.15 Maternal Factors Associated With Birth Weight and Preterm Delivery**

| Maternal Factor | |
|---|---|
| Developmental | Maternal birth weight <2.5 kg or >4.0 kg |
| | Short stature, stunting (height <145 cm) |
| Behavioral | Cigarette smoking |
| | Alcohol consumption |
| | Substance and/or drug abuse |
| Demographic | Age <18 years or >40 years |
| | Ethnicity |
| Health-related | Undernutrition, low maternal BMI |
| | Iron deficiency |
| | Malaria |
| | Diabetes or gestational diabetes mellitus |
| | Hypertension |
| | Preeclampsia, eclampsia |
| | Chronic kidney disease, transplant, dialysis |
| | Birth before term |
| | Multiple gestations |
| | Multiparous (≥3) |
| | Assisted reproduction |
| | Infections |
| | Obesity |
| Social | Highly active antiretroviral therapy for HIV |
| | Prenatal care |
| | Unplanned pregnancy, birth spacing |
| | Teenage pregnancy |
| | Marriage during childhood |
| | Conflict, war, stress |
| | Environmental conditions |
| | Education level |
| | Poverty |
| Environmental | Seasonal variations in nutrient availability |
| | Toxin or pollutant exposure |

*BMI*, Body mass index.

From Luyckx VA, Brenner BM. Birth weight, malnutrition and kidney-associated outcomes—a global concern. *Nat Rev Nephrol.* 2015;11:135–149, Box 2.

the risk of low birth weight and preterm birth and have been associated with changes in childhood blood pressures and kidney size and function.[462–467] Infections during pregnancy or chronic maternal illness all increase the risks of adverse pregnancy outcomes (Table 21.15).[303,468,469] Acute infections such as malaria are highly prevalent in lower-income regions and may contribute to a large number of low-birth-weight or preterm births annually.[470] In high-income countries, delays in pregnancy, use of assisted reproduction, or chronic maternal illness are increasingly common, ranging from 3%–20% in different studies.[471,472] Maternal chronic disease increases the risk of having a preterm birth or small-for-gestational-age infant; therefore, planning of pregnancies in such women is important to minimize these risks.[456,473] Specifically, pregnant women with CKD have a higher risk of low birth weight, small for gestational age, and preterm birth.[474,475] CKD is also a major risk factor for preeclampsia, in addition to maternal preexisting hypertension, diabetes, anemia, heart disease, and urinary tract infections/pyelonephritis.[476] Teenage pregnancies are at higher risk of preeclampsia, low birth weight, and preterm birth.[454,477,478] These factors therefore may all impact fetal programming.

In a population-based cohort of women, the odds of pregnancy-associated gestational diabetes or gestational hypertension (including preeclampsia or eclampsia) among those who had been born preterm were significantly increased and were higher with lower gestational age, suggesting a "dose–response" relationship with degree of maternal prematurity (OR: 1.95; 95% CI: 1.54 to 2.47 if mother born at <32 weeks; OR: 1.14; 95% CI: 1.03 to 1.25 if mother born at 32–36 weeks).[190] Gestational hypertension and preeclampsia, in turn, are risk factors for low birth weight and preterm birth, and gestational diabetes is a risk factor for high birth weight; therefore, the offspring of these pregnancies are likely at risk for programmed hypertension and renal dysfunction, including gestational hypertension.[476] The programming cycle could therefore continue across generations. Maternal low birth weight or preterm birth are also risk factors for having low-birth-weight or preterm infants.[1,479,480] A direct intergenerational programming effect of maternal preterm birth on subsequent offspring preterm birth is supported by the observed increasing risk of preterm birth with lower maternal gestational age and the absence of risk if the father was born preterm.[481] Maternal obesity and gestational diabetes are increasing worldwide and are established risk factors for both low and high birth weight.[482–484] Obesity in pregnant women who had themselves been born with low birth weight was associated with a 3.65-fold increased risk of preterm delivery compared with those who were not obese.[480] Maternal low or high birth weight is also associated with a higher risk of developing gestational diabetes.[485] Maternal birth circumstances and subsequent obesity therefore affect risk of adverse pregnancy outcomes and may program the health of their offspring. The mechanisms, however, remain unclear.[391,408,486,487]

In rats, maternal protein restriction results in transgenerational programming persisting into the F2 generation.[488] These effects have been proposed to be mediated largely by changes in DNA methylation, determined by amino acid availability, resulting in epigenetic changes in gene expression.[21] Whether these epigenetic changes can be transmitted through the germline and persist in the offspring, or whether a mother who had been subjected to adverse intrauterine events may experience changes in renal function and blood pressure during pregnancy that may, in turn, de novo impact the development of her offspring is still a point of debate.[391,408,486] The latter hypothesis seems more likely.

## IMPACT OF NEPHRON ENDOWMENT IN TRANSPLANTATION

Nephron endowment in transplantation is relevant for both the donor and the recipient. Removal of a kidney in a healthy donor implies loss of 50% of original nephron endowment, and gain of a kidney in a recipient may provide more or less than half of the recipient's original nephron endowment, depending on relative sizes of donor and recipient, periprocedural nephron loss, and other factors. Consideration of nephron endowment prior to transplantation could impact long-term renal health in both donors and recipients.

**Table 21.16 Global Incidence/Prevalence of Programming Risk Factors**

| Maternal Risk Factors | Global Incidence/Prevalence (%) | Reference |
|---|---|---|
| Undernutrition women 20–49 years (BMI <18) | 12 | 280, 457 |
| Short stature women of reproductive age (<155 cm) | 19.7–68.5 | 457, 459 |
| Malaria during pregnancy | 41.2 (LMIC) | 470 |
| Hepatitis B infection (sAg) in women of childbearing age | 1.5–8.5 (2005) | 563 |
| Anemia in pregnant women (Hb <110 g/L) | 38.2 (95 CI: 34.3–42.0) | 331, 457 |
| Iron deficiency in pregnant women | 19.2 (95 CI: 17.1–21.5) | |
| Vitamin A deficiency in pregnant women (night blindness) | 7.8 (95 CI: 6.5–9.1) | |
| Zinc deficiency (general population) | 17.3 (95 CI: 15.9–18.8) | |
| Preeclampsia | 4.6 (95 CI: 2.7–8.2) | 564 |
| Eclampsia | 1.4 (95 CI: 1.0–2.0) | |
| Hyperglycemia in pregnancy women 20–49 years (diabetes/gestational diabetes) | 16.9 | 565 |
| Maternal chronic illness | 15.8 (Denmark, 2013) | 471 |
| Maternal overweight (BMI 25–29.9 kg/m$^2$) | 30 | 457, 566, 567 |
| Maternal obesity (BMI ≥30 kg/m$^2$) | 11 | 457, 482 |
| Maternal smoking | 9–16 HIC<br>2.6 (LMIC) | 568, 569 |
| Assisted reproduction technology | 2–3 annual births HIC | 570, 571 |
| Teenage pregnancy (<19 years) | 15 million per year | 478, 572, 573 |
| **Infant/Child Risk Factors** | | |
| Low birth weight | 15 | 44 |
| Preterm birth | 11.1 | 44, 574 |
| Small for gestational age (<10th percentile) | 12.1 | 44 |
| High birth weight (>4 kg) | 0.5–14.9 (LMIC) | 40 |
| Not weighed at birth | 48 | 43 |
| Child <5 years of age Overweight/obesity, 2016 | 6.0 (95 CI: 5.1, 7.1) | 575 |
| Childhood stunting (2016) | 22.9 (95 CI: 21.1, 24.7) | |

*BMI*, Body mass index; *HIC*, high-income country; *LMIC*, low- and middle-income country; *sAg*, surface antigen–positive hepatitis B.

## IMPLICATIONS OF NEPHRON ENDOWMENT FOR THE DONOR

Living donation, after appropriate donor screening, has generally been presumed to be safe, although recent studies have described some risk of ESKD after kidney donation, highlighting the urgent need to better understand predictors of renal function postdonation in living donors.[489–492] In predominantly Caucasian cohorts, hypertension and proteinuria do increase over time in living donors, but renal function remains generally well preserved over the first decades.[64,493,494] In a cross-sectional retrospective study of donors followed for up to 40 years, however, donor GFRs were found to decline after 15–17 years postdonation; therefore, duration of follow-up is important to fully understand potential associations with risk.[495] Obesity significantly increases this risk over time.[496] There are donor groups, including the young and obese, the older donor, and some ethnic groups, that may be at increased risk of long-term renal dysfunction but have not been well represented in the current literature.[489,497] A recent analysis of the U.S. donor population estimated the risk of ESKD among average donors to be 34 cases per 10,000 donors; however, this risk increased to 256 cases per 10,000 in higher-risk donors and was associated with black race, elevated body mass index, donation to a first-degree relative, and with age among nonblack donors.[497] Black race was associated with the greatest risk of ESKD (HR: 2.96; 95% CI: 2.25 to 3.89).[497] Whether developmental programming of nephron number in a prospective donor may impact these risks has not been studied. Among African Americans, we now know that many donors may carry *APOL1* risk genotypes; therefore, this risk may be multifactorial. In support of a programmed risk of accelerated loss of renal function postdonation, Aboriginal Australian donors were found to have a significantly increased risk of hypertension, renal dysfunction, and ESKD at a median of 16 years postdonation compared with Caucasians (Table 21.17).[498] Similarly, hypertension and proteinuria were much more prevalent among Aboriginal compared with Caucasian Canadian donors at 20 years of follow-up, and African Americans as well as Hispanics had more hypertension and CKD after donation than white Americans (Table 21.17).[499–501] These data are troubling because the donors were screened prior to donation; therefore, donor nephrectomy can be implicated in the disease process. Importantly, African Americans and Aboriginal Australian populations have lower birth weights than their Caucasian counterparts, and Canadian Aboriginals have higher birth weights; therefore, developmental programming of the kidney may be a risk factor contributing to poorer outcomes postdonation.[502] Given the increasing need for donors worldwide, better understanding of renal risk in these populations is urgently needed.

**Table 21.17 Hypertension and Renal Function in Living Kidney Donors at Risk of Adverse Renal Programming**

| | **United States** | | **Australia** | | **Canada** | | **Germany** | |
|---|---|---|---|---|---|---|---|---|
| **Population** | Black Donor | White Donor | Indigenous Donors | Nonindigenous Donors | Aboriginal Donors | White Donors | BW ≤2.5 kg | BW >2.5 kg |
| Donor number | 12,387 | 71,769 | 22 | 28 | 38 | 76 | 18 | 73 |
| Programmed risk | LBW prematurity | ref | LBW | ref | HBW (offspring of DM pregnancies) | ref | LBW | ref |
| HT | – | – | 50% | 6% | 42% | 19% | 39% | 15% |
| Proteinuria | – | – | 81% | 6% | 21% | 4% | 81% | 35% |
| ↓ GFR | – | – | 81% | 38% | Not different | | Not different | |
| ESKD | 74.4 per 10,000 vs. 23.9 per 10,000 in nondonors | 22.7 per 10,000 vs. 0.0 per 10,000 in nondonors | 19% | 0% | 1 | 0 | 0 | 0 |
| Follow-up (years) | 7.6 (IQR 3.9–11.5) | | 16.1 (1.27–20.2) | 6.37 (2.54–21.2) | 14.6 ± 9.3 | 13.4 ± 9.5 | ≥5 | ≥1–3 |
| Reference | 490 | | 498 | | 501 | | 503 | |

*BW*, Body weight; *DM*, diabetes mellitus; *ESKD*, end-stage kidney disease; *GFR*, glomerular filtration rate; *HBW*, high birth rate; *IQR*, interquartile range; *LBW*, low birth weight.

Reproduced from Low Birth Weight and Nephron Number Working Group. The impact of kidney development on the life course: a consensus document for action. *Nephron.* 2017;136:3–49.

A study from Germany found that GFRs were lower and proteinuria and hypertension were more frequent at 5 years postdonation among donors with birth weights <2.5 kg (see Table 21.17).[503] A group of potential donors that has not been studied is women who have had preeclampsia, who are known to be at an increased, albeit small, risk of ESKD.[504] As discussed earlier, the risk of preeclampsia is increased in women who had been of low birth weight or preterm; therefore, a proportion of women with preeclampsia were likely at risk of renal programming.[190] The risk of gestational hypertension and preeclampsia is also increased among female donors, suggesting that a reduced nephron mass may be a risk factor.[505] Caution should therefore be advised in considering women with a history of preeclampsia, low birth weight, or having been born preterm as kidney donors, as each of these factors may be a marker for programmed renal risk.[1]

## IMPLICATIONS OF NEPHRON ENDOWMENT FOR THE RECIPIENT

Prescription of donor kidneys is largely based on immunologic matching. In animal experiments of renal transplantation, however, the impact of transplanted nephron mass, independent of immunologic factors, on the subsequent development of chronic allograft nephropathy has been demonstrated.[506–510] Despite such evidence, prescription of kidneys on the basis of the physiologic capacity of the donor organ to meet the metabolic needs of the recipient has not generally been considered.[511] More and more data are accumulating, however, suggesting a significant impact of transplanted renal mass on long-term posttransplantation outcomes.

Demographic and anthropomorphic factors associated with late renal allograft loss include donor age, sex, and race, as well as recipient BSA.[512–514] In general, kidneys from older, female, and African American donors fare worse.[54,77,95,515] Indirectly, these observations suggest that the intrinsic nephron endowment of the transplanted kidney is likely to play a role in the development of chronic allograft nephropathy. As nephron numbers are not yet measurable in vivo, several investigators have compared recipient and donor BSA as surrogates for metabolic demand and kidney size; others have used kidney weights or renal volumetric measurements by ultrasound as surrogates for nephron mass.[516–520] Importantly, although kidney mass and kidney volume have been thought to be proportional to nephron number, and measures of body size tend to be proportional to kidney size, these relationships do vary in strength of association[57]; therefore, these data should be interpreted cautiously. In general, however, the preponderance of evidence does support the hypothesis that small kidneys perform less well when transplanted into larger recipients.[516–520]

A retrospective analysis of 32,083 patients who received a first cadaver kidney found that large recipients of kidneys from small donors had a 43% increased risk of late allograft failure compared with medium-sized recipients receiving kidneys from medium-sized donors.[519] Outcomes were best in small recipients receiving kidneys from large donors. Subsequently, among 69,737 deceased donor kidney transplants, a severe recipient/donor size mismatch (BSA ratio >1.38) was associated with higher 10-year graft loss compared with closer matches, and the risk was doubled in the case of extended criteria donors with severe mismatches (22% vs. 10%, respectively).[521] Similar findings were seen among recipients of older (>60 years) versus younger kidneys.[522] These data suggest that donor and recipient size should be considered in organ allocation decisions, especially if the donor kidney is known to be "suboptimal." Smaller studies have not consistently found similar results, however, potentially reflecting lack of statistical power.[518,519]

Kidney size, however, may not always be directly proportional to BSA; therefore, ratios of donor to recipient BSA may not be an ideal method of estimating nephron mass to recipient mismatch. Kidney weight may be a better surrogate for nephron mass.[54,523] Using this parameter, Kim and associates[524] analyzed the ratio of donor kidney weight to recipient body weight (DKW/RBW) in 259 live-donor transplants. These authors found that a higher DKW/RBW of greater than 4.5 g/kg was significantly associated with improved allograft function at 3 years compared with a ratio of less than 3.0 g/kg. A similar study including 964 recipients of cadaveric kidneys, in whom proteinuria and Cockroft-Gault creatinine clearances were also calculated, found that 10% of the subjects were "strongly" mismatched, having a DKW/RBW ratio of less than 2 g/kg.[515] The DKW/RBW ratio was lowest when male recipients received kidneys from female donors. The risk of having proteinuria higher than 0.5 g/24 h was significantly greater, and developed earlier, in those with DKW/RBW below 2 g/kg as compared with those with higher ratios. Proteinuria was present in 50% of those with DKW/RBW less than 2 g/kg, 33% of those with DKW/RBW of 2 to 4 g/kg, and 23% in those with DKW/RBW of 4 g/kg or greater. At 5 years follow-up, however, there was no difference in graft survival among the three DKW/RBW groups, but the authors conceded that longer follow-up was needed.[515] Subsequent analysis of the same cohort 5 years later showed that GFR declined more rapidly after 7 years in the low versus the high DKW/RBW group, suggesting that the smaller kidneys were likely hyperfiltering early on, which initiated the cycle of progressive nephron loss (see Fig. 21.16).[525]

In an attempt to more accurately reflect transplanted nephron mass, other investigators have used renal ultrasonography to measure cadaveric transplant kidney (Tx) cross-sectional area in relation to recipient body weight (W) to calculate a "nephron dose index," Tx/W.[526] These authors found that during the first 5 years after transplantation, serum creatinine was significantly lower in patients with a high Tx/W compared with those with lower values, with a trend toward better graft survival. A similar analysis using renal volume determined by CT angiographic volumetry (done pretransplant in living donors) to recipient BSA found that posttransplant GFRs during the first year correlated with recipient GFR, more significantly among those with a donor/recipient BSA ratio of 1 or less.[527] A small kidney transplanted into a large recipient may not have an adequate capacity to meet the metabolic needs of the recipient without imposing glomerular hyperfiltration, which ultimately leads to nephron loss and eventual allograft failure.[528,529]

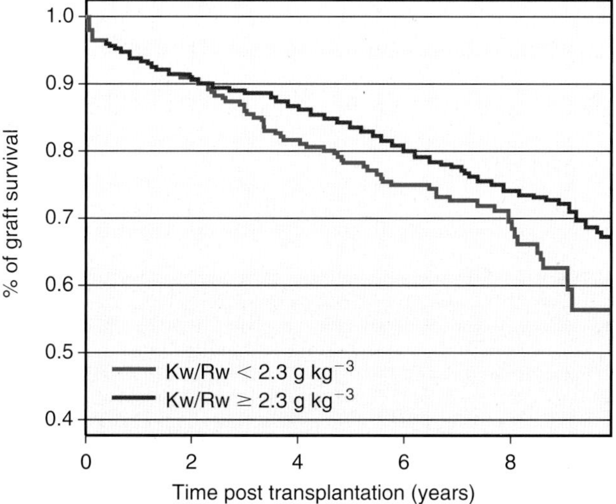


**Fig. 21.16** Correlation between kidney weight *(Kw)*–to–recipient weight *(Rw)* ratio and long-term graft survival in renal transplantation. Graft survival declines faster with a Kw/Rw <2.3 g/kg ($P = .016$). (From Giral M, Foucher Y, Karam G, et al. Kidney and recipient weight incompatibility reduces long-term graft survival. *J Am Soc Nephrol.* 2010;21:1022–1029.)

Transplanted nephron mass may be a function of congenital endowment and attrition of nephrons with age but is also impacted by peritransplant renal injury (i.e., donor hypotension, prolonged cold and warm ischemia, nephrotoxic immunosuppressive drugs). All of these factors must be closely considered, in addition to immunologic matching, in selection of appropriate recipients in whom the allograft is likely to function for the longest time and therefore provide best possible improvement in quality of life.

## GLOBAL HEALTH RELEVANCE OF RENAL PROGRAMMING

The known risk factors—low birth weight, small for gestational age, preterm birth, high birth weight—are prevalent worldwide, in both low- and high-income settings, although underlying causes may differ (see Table 21.16). Millions of infants born each year are at risk, therefore, of future hypertension and kidney disease as well as other programmed conditions. How much developmental programming contributes to the growing burden of chronic noncommunicable diseases worldwide is unknown but may be significant, especially in regions where access to preventive health care is limited. In the current era of sustainable development goals, it may be possible to reduce the impact of developmental programming on future generations through a multisectoral approach encompassing not only the health system but education, infrastructure, and reducing social inequities. Strategies to reduce the impact of developmental programming in individual infants should be simple to implement and, as reviewed in depth elsewhere,[1] include documentation of birth weight and gestational age in each child to identify those at risk; heightened awareness of the risk of neonatal AKI in preterm infants and implementation of strategies to reduce these risks; and education of parents about healthy lifestyle choices to prevent obesity and stunting, low birth weight, small for gestational age, and preterm. Children born to mothers with preeclampsia, diabetes, or obesity should be screened for hypertension and proteinuria, especially if they become overweight; as adults these individuals require long-term screening, early intervention with renoprotective strategies, and strong emphasis on healthy lifestyles.

## CONCLUSION

The association between an adverse fetal environment and subsequent hypertension as well as kidney disease in later life is now quite compelling and appears to be mediated, at least in part, by impaired nephrogenesis and suboptimal

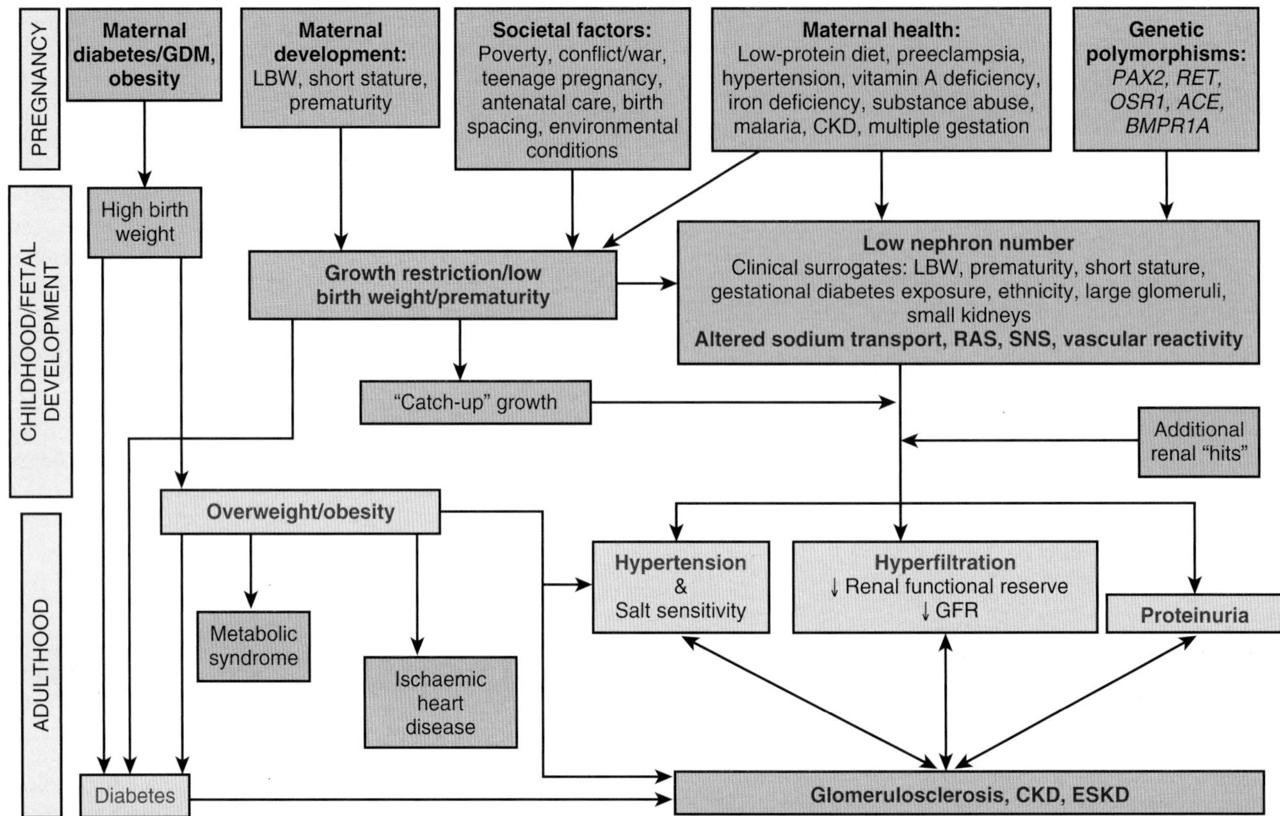


**Fig. 21.17** Proposed mechanisms of fetal programming of hypertension and renal disease. *CKD*, Chronic kidney disease; *ESKD*, end-stage kidney disease; *GDM*, gestational diabetes mellitus; *GFR*, glomerulat filtration rate; *LBW*, low birth weight; *RAS*, renin–angiotensin system; *SNS*, sympathetic nervous system. (Adapted from Luyckx VA, Bertram JF, Brenner BM, et al. Effect of fetal and child health on kidney development and long-term risk of hypertension and kidney disease. *Lancet* 2013;382:273–283.)

nephron endowment (Fig. 21.17). Concomitant glomerular hypertrophy and altered expression of sodium transporters in the programmed kidney also contribute to the vicious circle of glomerular hypertension, glomerular injury, and sclerosis, leading to worsening hypertension and ongoing renal injury. In addition, numerous other factors, such as increased oxidative stress, renal inflammation, accelerated senescence, and catch-up body growth, are all likely contributors to ongoing nephron loss and eventual renal disease.[284,530–533] The number of nephrons in humans without kidney disease varies widely, suggesting that a significant proportion of the general population, especially in areas where high or low birth weights are prevalent, may be at increased risk of developing later-life hypertension and renal dysfunction. Measurement of nephron number in vivo remains an obstacle, with the best surrogate markers thus far being a low birth weight, high birth weight, preterm birth, being small for gestational age, and, in the absence of other known renal diseases, a reduced kidney volume on ultrasound, especially in children, and glomerular enlargement on kidney biopsy. A kidney with a reduced complement of nephrons would have less renal reserve to adapt to dietary excesses or to compensate for renal injury. The molecular mechanisms through which fetal programming exerts its effects on nephrogenesis are varied and likely complementary and intertwined. Although in some animal studies, nephron number and blood pressure can be "rescued" by good postnatal nutrition or vitamin A supplementation, applicability of these findings to humans requires further study. The fact that even seemingly minor influences, such as composition of maternal diet during fetal life, can have major consequences on renal development in the offspring underscores the critical importance of optimization of perinatal care and early nutrition, which could have a major impact on population health in the future.

 Complete reference list available at ExpertConsult.com.

## KEY REFERENCES

1. Low Birth W, Nephron Number Working G. The impact of kidney development on the life course: a consensus document for action. *Nephron*. 2017;136(1):3–49.
15. Barker DJ. Developmental origins of adult health and disease. *J Epidemiol Community Health*. 2004;58(2):114–115.
26. Barker DJ, Hales CN, Fall CH, et al. Type 2 (non-insulin-dependent) diabetes mellitus, hypertension and hyperlipidaemia (syndrome X): relation to reduced fetal growth. *Diabetologia*. 1993;36(1):62–67.
32. White SL, Perkovic V, Cass A, et al. Is low birth weight an antecedent of CKD in later life? A systematic review of observational studies. *Am J Kidney Dis*. 2009;54(2):248–261.
34. Langley-Evans S, Langley-Evans A, Marchand M. Nutritional programming of blood pressure and renal morphology. *Arch Physiol Biochem*. 2003;111(1):8–16.
36. de Jong F, Monuteaux MC, van Elburg RM, et al. Systematic review and meta-analysis of preterm birth and later systolic blood pressure. *Hypertension*. 2012;59(2):226–234.
37. Mu M, Wang SF, Sheng J, et al. Birth weight and subsequent blood pressure: a meta-analysis. *Arch Cardiovasc Dis*. 2012;105(2):99–113.

38. Nelson RG, Morgenstern H, Bennett PH. Intrauterine diabetes exposure and the risk of renal disease in diabetic pima Indians. *Diabetes.* 1998;47(9):1489–1493.
48. Brenner BM, Garcia DL, Anderson S. Glomeruli and blood pressure. Less of one, more the other? *Am J Hypertens.* 1988;1(4 Pt 1):335–347.
58. Puelles VG, Hoy WE, Hughson MD, et al. Glomerular number and size variability and risk for kidney disease. *Curr Opin Nephrol Hypertens.* 2011;20(1):7–15.
75. Kett MM, Denton KM. Renal programming: cause for concern? *Am J Physiol Regul Integr Comp Physiol.* 2011;300(4):R791–R803.
87. Hughson M, Farris AB, Douglas-Denton R, et al. Glomerular number and size in autopsy kidneys: the relationship to birth weight. *Kidney Int.* 2003;63(6):2113–2122.
99. Hoy WE, Hughson MD, Diouf B, et al. Distribution of volumes of individual glomeruli in kidneys at autopsy: association with physical and clinical characteristics and with ethnic group. *Am J Nephrol.* 2011;33(suppl 1):15–20.
108. Vehaskari VM, Aviles DH, Manning J. Prenatal programming of adult hypertension in the rat. *Kidney Int.* 2001;59(1):238–245.
112. Wlodek ME, Mibus A, Tan A, et al. Normal lactational environment restores nephron endowment and prevents hypertension after placental restriction in the rat. *J Am Soc Nephrol.* 2007;18(6):1688–1696.
114. Baum M. Role of the kidney in the prenatal and early postnatal programming of hypertension. *Am J Physiol Renal Physiol.* 2010;298(2):F235–F247.
121. Zhang Z, Quinlan J, Hoy W, et al. A common RET variant is associated with reduced newborn kidney size and function. *J Am Soc Nephrol.* 2008;19(10):2027–2034.
122. Rodriguez MM, Gomez AH, Abitbol CL, et al. Histomorphometric analysis of postnatal glomerulogenesis in extremely preterm infants. *Pediatr Dev Pathol.* 2004;7(1):17–25.
159. Moritz KM, Cuffe JS, Wilson LB, et al. Review: sex specific programming: a critical role for the renal renin-angiotensin system. *Placenta.* 2010;31(suppl):S40–S46.
170. Ojeda NB, Intapad S, Alexander BT. Sex differences in the developmental programming of hypertension. *Acta physiologica.* 2014;210(2):307–316.
181. Jones SE, Bilous RW, Flyvbjerg A, et al. Intra-uterine environment influences glomerular number and the acute renal adaptation to experimental diabetes. *Diabetologia.* 2001;44(6):721–728.
187. Abitbol CL, Rodriguez MM. The long-term renal and cardiovascular consequences of prematurity. *Nat Rev Nephrol.* 2012;8(5):265–274.
190. Boivin A, Luo ZC, Audibert F, et al. Pregnancy complications among women born preterm. *CMAJ.* 2012;184(16):1777–1784.
209. Khalsa DD, Beydoun HA, Carmody JB. Prevalence of chronic kidney disease risk factors among low birth weight adolescents. *Pediatr Nephrol.* 2016;31(9):1509–1516.
217. Bergvall N, Iliadou A, Johansson S, et al. Genetic and shared environmental factors do not confound the association between birth weight and hypertension: a study among Swedish twins. *Circulation.* 2007;115(23):2931–2938.
223. Schreuder MF, Wilhelm AJ, Bokenkamp A, et al. Impact of gestational age and birth weight on amikacin clearance on day 1 of life. *Clin J Am Soc Nephrol.* 2009;4(11):1774–1778.
224. Bacchetta J, Harambat J, Dubourg L, et al. Both extrauterine and intrauterine growth restriction impair renal function in children born very preterm. *Kidney Int.* 2009;76(4):445–452.
230. Keijzer-Veen MG, Schrevel M, Finken MJ, et al. Microalbuminuria and lower glomerular filtration rate at young adult age in subjects born very premature and after intrauterine growth retardation. *J Am Soc Nephrol.* 2005;16(9):2762–2768.
235. Hoy WE, White AV, Tipiloura B, et al. The multideterminant model of renal disease in a remote Australian aboriginal population in the context of early life risk factors: lower birth weight, childhood post-streptococcal glomerulonephritis, and current body mass index influence levels of albuminuria in young aboriginal adults. *Clin Nephrol.* 2015;83(7 suppl 1):75–81.
244. Selewski DT, Charlton JR, Jetton JG, et al. Neonatal acute kidney injury. *Pediatrics.* 2015;136(2):e463–e473.
246. Sutherland M, Ryan D, Black MJ, et al. Long-term renal consequences of preterm birth. *Clin Perinatol.* 2014;41(3):561–573.
274. Hsu CW, Yamamoto KT, Henry RK, et al. Prenatal risk factors for childhood CKD. *J Am Soc Nephrol.* 2014;25(9):2105–2111.
276. Hanson M, Gluckman P. Developmental origins of noncommunicable disease: population and public health implications. *Am J Clin Nutr.* 2011;94(6 suppl):1754S–1758S.
284. Luyckx VA, Brenner BM. Birth weight, malnutrition and kidney-associated outcomes—a global concern. *Nat Rev Nephrol.* 2015;11(3): 135–149.
299. Little MH, McMahon AP. Mammalian kidney development: principles, progress, and projections. *Cold Spring Harb Perspect Biol.* 2012; 4(5).
300. Moritz KM, Wintour EM, Black MJ, et al. Factors influencing mammalian kidney development: implications for health in adult life. *Adv Anat Embryol Cell Biol.* 2008;196:1–78.
303. Luyckx VA. Preterm birth and its impact on renal health. *Semin Nephrol.* 2017;37(4):311–319.
315. Langley-Evans SC. Nutritional programming of disease: unravelling the mechanism. *J Anat.* 2009;215(1):36–51.
341. Amri K, Freund N, Vilar J, et al. Adverse effects of hyperglycemia on kidney development in rats: in vivo and in vitro studies. *Diabetes.* 1999;48(11):2240–2245.
348. Jackson CM, Alexander BT, Roach L, et al. Exposure to maternal overnutrition and a high-fat diet during early postnatal development increases susceptibility to renal and metabolic injury later in life. *Am J Physiol Renal Physiol.* 2012;302(6):F774–F783.
385. Chevalier RL. Congenital urinary tract obstruction: the long view. *Adv Chronic Kidney Dis.* 2015;22(4):312–319.
391. O'Sullivan L, Combes AN, Little MH, et al. Epigenetics and developmental programming of adult onset diseases. *Pediatr Nephrol.* 2012;27(12):2175–2182.
405. Ojeda NB. Prenatal programming of hypertension: role of sympathetic response to physical stress. *Hypertension.* 2013;61(1):16–17.
427. Jain V, Singhal A. Catch up growth in low birth weight infants: striking a healthy balance. *Rev Endocr Metab Disord.* 2012;13(2): 141–147.
440. Grijalva-Eternod CS, Lawlor DA, Wells JC. Testing a capacity-load model for hypertension: disentangling early and late growth effects on childhood blood pressure in a prospective birth cohort. *PLoS ONE.* 2013;8(2):e56078.
441. Abitbol CL, Chandar J, Rodriguez MM, et al. Obesity and preterm birth: additive risks in the progression of kidney disease in children. *Pediatr Nephrol.* 2009;24(7):1363–1370.
442. Abitbol CL, Bauer CR, Montane B, et al. Long-term follow-up of extremely low birth weight infants with neonatal renal failure. *Pediatr Nephrol.* 2003;18(9):887–893.
479. Boivin A, Luo ZC, Audibert F, et al. Risk for preterm and very preterm delivery in women who were born preterm. *Obstet Gynecol.* 2015;125(5):1177–1184.
486. Aiken CE, Ozanne SE. Transgenerational developmental programming. *Hum Reprod Update.* 2014;20(1):63–75.
489. Mueller TF, Luyckx VA. The natural history of residual renal function in transplant donors. *J Am Soc Nephrol.* 2012;23(9):1462–1466.
525. Giral M, Foucher Y, Karam G, et al. Kidney and recipient weight incompatibility reduces long-term graft survival. *J Am Soc Nephrol.* 2010;21(6):1022–1029.

22

# The Physiology and Pathophysiology of the Kidneys in Aging

Richard J. Glassock | Aleksandar Denic | Andrew D. Rule

CHAPTER OUTLINE



## GENERAL OVERVIEW OF THE BIOLOGY OF AGING

All, or nearly all, biologic organisms exhibit the phenomenon of aging. The few exceptions are scientific curiosities.[1] Many speculations and hypotheses concerning the biologic basis of aging have been advanced, but as yet none have provided a universal explanation for the aging process.[2] The life span of humans is regarded as limited at some maximum term that few approach.[1–3] Aging is an inevitable consequence of life. The rate of aging varies considerably, even among identical members of the same species,[1] an indication of the relatively minor role of heredity per se in determination of the life span of species. It has been estimated, from studies of monozygotic twins, that only 20% to 35% of the life span can be attributed to heredity (chromosomal or mitochondrial).[4] Thus, most theories of aging consider heredity, the environment, and chance to play variable roles in determination of the observed life span.[1] Metabolic rates and the balance of energy demand and supply appear to have a strong influence on life span.[5]

The fundamental biologic pathways accounting for the diverse manifestations of aging have been the subject of intense investigation for many decades. Much progress has been made; however, many gaps in our knowledge of this process still remain,[6–31] including the process of renal aging. It is generally regarded that aging is a composite effect of disordered gene function, environmental influences, and chance.[1] At the cellular level, degeneration and faulty gene repair are core mechanisms of aging.[1] The net result is cellular and organ senescence. The rate of aging appears to be partially controlled by genetic pathways and biochemical processes. The explanation for the conservation of these processes that occur after maximal reproductive success is largely lacking.[1,3,4] As such, it is possible that many aspects of the aging process have not been evolutionarily conserved. Because of these factors, it seems likely that the biologic events responsible for aging may differ among species, complicating the study of aging enormously—studies of aging in experimental animals may therefore have limited relevance to human aging.

The major hallmarks of aging are genomic instability, epigenetic alterations, mitochondrial dysfunction, dysregulated nutrient sensing, telomere attrition, loss of protein homeostasis, stem cell exhaustion, accumulation of senescent cells, oxidation and glycation of tissue proteins, and altered intercellular communication (reviewed by Sturmlechner and coworkers[27] and López-Otín and associates[32]).

A detailed description of these processes underlying aging is beyond the scope of this brief introductory review. Age-dependent accumulation of stochastic damage to critical molecular pathways seems to be a dominant driver of aging.[1] The generation of ATP to provide energy to sustain cellular function is key for life, and this process is systematically altered in aging.[33]

Energy production, via mitochondrial dysfunction, regularly declines with age,[1,33] possibly due to stochastic damage to mitochondrial DNA and inefficient repair. Oxidative damage to DNA has been postulated to be one of the root causes of aging.[5,34] Mitochondrial inefficiency can lead to impaired cellular autophagy and cellular senescence.[35–38] Alternate hypotheses of defects in oxidative metabolism leading to a shift from aerobic to anaerobic metabolism are also possible.[5] A mismatch occurs in aging between lowered energy demand and excess supply. Caloric restriction has been found to be one of the most powerful experimental means of retarding the aging process.[32,39] Sirtuins, nicotinamide adenine dinucleotide ($NAD^+$)-dependent proteins, which deacetylate crucial enzymes in the oxidative metabolic pathway, may be responsible for this effect.[10,11,32,40,41] Sirtuin production diminishes with age and promotion of sirtuin production, as by the administration of mammalian target of rapamycin (mTOR) inhibitors, which mimic caloric restriction, can prolong life span.[32] This is known as the "bioenergetic theory of aging."[2] Whether a genetic program (the aging clock) defines the decline in bioenergetics with aging is unclear.[42] However, as stated above, it is well known that the rate of aging varies considerably, even among genetically identical humans and other species.[1] Epigenetic alterations and DNA methylation may account for some of these variations.[43]

Aging is also associated with shortening of the telomeres in nuclear DNA due to changes in the activity of telomerase, an enzyme essential for maintaining telomere length in dividing cells.[2,44,45] Gradual loss of telomeres leads to cessation of cell division after a maximum number of cell divisions, known as the *Hayflick limit*, and induces senescence, ultimately leading to cell death.[46] Attrition of telomeres with aging may explain in part the association of a higher risk for cancer in older people. Diseases of premature aging, such as progeria or Cockayne syndrome, can be caused by specific mutations (laminin in progeria), and are associated with marked telomere shortening or defects in DNA repair.[47,48] Indeed, telomere length and urinary 8-oxo-7,8-dihydroguanosine excretion are good biomarkers of aging.[49]

The individual organ systems of the human body exhibit phenomena connected to the overall aging process, also at variable rates. These organ-based manifestations of aging include loss of skin elasticity, decreases in hair pigmentation, slowing of nerve impulses, decreased mineral density of bone, decreased compliance of major vessels, decreased forced expiratory lung volume, decreased muscle mass, reduced metabolic rate, and many others. The kidneys share in these inevitable biologic consequences of aging, as will be detailed in this chapter. Numerous reviews and treatises covering the general topic of renal aging have been published over the past 4 decades. They represent a rich source of collateral reading on this fascinating subject.[6–31] It seems likely that the complex processes operating in aging at the organism level also play important roles in the manifestations of organ-based senescence, such as that displayed the kidneys.

The genetic component of renal aging has been analyzed by genome-wide association studies and transcriptomics,[50–52] and several candidate loci and factors have been identified. Increased oxidative or glycative stress,[53,54] reduced Klotho generation,[15,55–58] enhanced fibrosis,[59,60] increased capillary rarefaction,[9] and increased activation of the angiotensin II type 1 receptor[61–63] may all play important roles in renal aging. Klotho deficiency promotes inflammation.[55,56] Toxins such as D-serine[64] might be involved in the development of fibrosis in aging. Experimental evidence (in mice) has suggested that the level of fructokinase activity may be essential for renal aging.[65] In addition, endostatin and transglutaminase activity might also be involved in the renal fibrosis of aging according to studies in mice, but both these effects might be species specific.[66] The factors postulated to be involved in renal aging are summarized in Box 22.1.

**Box 22.1 Some Factors Postulated to be Involved in Renal Aging**

↓Sirtuin 1/6 (a histone deacetylase enzyme)
↓Klotho expression (and Wnt signaling)
↓Antioxidant production, ↑oxidant activity
↓ Energy demand: ↑energy supply (mitochondrial dysfunction)
↑Telomere shortening
↑ DNA damage repair
↑ DNA methylation
↑Angiotensin II receptor signaling (via Wnt)
↑Cell cycle arrest (GI, via P16ink)
↓Autophagy
↑Fibrosis (transforming growth factor beta [TGF-β]–mediated)
↓Elimination of senescent cells
↓Insulin-like growth factor 1 (IGF-1) signaling
↓Proliferator-activated receptor-γ (PPARγ) activity
↑Capillary rarefaction
↑Podocyte apoptosis or detachment (podocytopenia—absolute and/or relative to capillary surface area)
↑Vascular sclerosis and glomerular ischemia
↑Advanced glycation end products
↑D-Serine toxicity
↑ Endostatin, transglutaminase activation

*GI*, Gastrointestinal.

## HEALTHY AGING AND AGE-RELATED COMORBIDITY

The aging process not only leads to subtle and cumulative alterations in cellular and organ function, but it also predisposes an individual to certain age-related diseases, such as atherosclerosis, hypertension, diabetes, cancer, osteoporosis, and dementia. Disentanglement of these disease states from phenomena that might be called "healthy" aging can be very challenging. Healthy aging might be defined as the state that is universal, or nearly so, in all aging subjects, whereas age-related comorbidities affect only some of the aging population and involve processes that are disease-specific. For example, a decline in bone density or forced expiratory lung volume is characteristic of aging; defining a threshold for a disease-associated decline in these functions requires comparison with the expected changes with healthy aging. Type 2 diabetes prevalence increases with aging, and the aging process leads to beta cell exhaustion in the pancreatic islet cells. Therefore, aging per se predisposes some older subjects to develop overt diabetes.[67] The best examples of healthy aging are individuals selected for the donation of one kidney for renal transplantation, but even this healthiest of the healthy may not be entirely normal because they also may be mildly obese, have treated mild hypertension, or have covert diseases not easily identifiable, even in an exhaustive clinical, laboratory, and imaging-based pretransplantation evaluation. Studies of older apparently healthy adults in the community are inevitably an admixture of healthy aging and aging with comorbidity, sometimes clinically unrecognized.[68] In this context, proteomic analyses of low-molecular-weight proteins in urine obtained from supposedly healthy subjects have suggested resemblances between healthy aging and chronic kidney disease (CKD), but these findings might be the consequence of overlapping comorbidities (covert and overt) with aging per se.[69] In this chapter, we will use the healthy adult living kidney donor as the prototype for normal aging, recognizing some of the pitfalls in this assumption. A detailed discussion on the approach to management of the kidney disease in older adults can be found in Chapter 84.

## DIFFERENCES BETWEEN HUMANS AND OTHER ANIMALS

Although many of the fundamental cellular processes of biologic aging are evolutionarily conserved, disparities at the organ system level may exist between species concerning the anatomic and functional consequences of aging. For example, many animal species (e.g., murine species) continue to grow throughout their life span, whereas humans cease growing after attaining maturity. The growth regulatory genetic program might be evolutionarily conserved among mammals, but the pace of growth is modulated in larger animals, including humans.[70] Metabolic demand may therefore differ among aging humans and aging experimental animals. Such differences can have profound effects on the organ-based manifestations of aging, including the kidneys. Thus, one needs to be cautious about inferring mechanisms of organ aging in humans from studies of experimental animals or lower organisms. The circumstances of birth, unique to humans, and in utero organogenesis can also have effects later in life, as will be discussed later.[71]

## ANATOMIC CHANGES OF THE KIDNEYS WITH AGING

### MACROSCOPIC CHANGES

As presently understood, aging is a universal and inevitable biologic process that is associated with macroscopic and microscopic structural changes in the kidneys, likely to be a causal association. Advances in the understanding of macroscopic structural changes have been made, first using ultrasound and more recently using computed tomography (CT) and magnetic resonance imaging (MRI).

#### KIDNEY SIZE AND VOLUME

Older studies that investigated kidney size with one- or two-dimensional measurements of kidney length or area have noted some degree of decrease with age.[72,73] Emamian and colleagues obtained ultrasound measurements of the kidney in 665 adult volunteers between 30 and 70 years of age and found that smaller kidney volumes correlated with older age.[74] Gourtsoyiannis and colleagues analyzed CT scans from 360 patients with no kidney disease to estimate kidney parenchymal thickness.[75] They found that for each decade of older age, kidney parenchymal thickness decreased about 10%. Another CT study in 1040 asymptomatic adults found that the factors associated with larger kidney size were male gender, taller height, and larger body mass index (BMI); whereas age and renal artery stenosis were associated with smaller kidney size.[76] Another study of 1056 patients showed similar findings and provided evidence that atherosclerosis accelerated the kidney size decline with older age.[77] However, a study of 225 adult healthy potential kidney donors did not find a statistically significant decrease in kidney size with older age, although the findings may have been limited by the age range and sample size of the study.[78]

A large MRI study assessed total kidney volume in 1852 subjects from the Framingham Heart Study.[79] The authors reported that the average decline in the total kidney volume in both genders was 16.3 $cm^3$/decade, with a stronger decline beyond 60 years of age, and a stronger decline in men than in women. In addition, using a subset of 196 healthy women and 112 apparently healthy men, this study determined the gender-specific upper and lower 10th percentile thresholds for the total kidney volume. In the multivariable models, the kidney volume above the 90th percentile was associated with younger age (odds ratio [OR], 0.67), whereas kidney volume below the 10th percentile was associated with older age (OR, 1.67).

#### KIDNEY CORTEX AND MEDULLA

Wang and colleagues have studied the CT scans of 1344 potential living kidney donors up to 75 years of age. They found a stable kidney parenchymal volume in those up to 50 years of age and a decline thereafter.[80] This study also obtained the volumes of the kidney cortex (average, 73% of parenchymal volume) and medulla (average, 27% of parenchymal volume) separately. An increasing medullary volume with age seems to attenuate some of the loss of total kidney parenchymal volume with age due to decreasing cortical volume (Fig. 22.1). Besides increased medullary volume, with age masking some of the kidney volume decline with age,

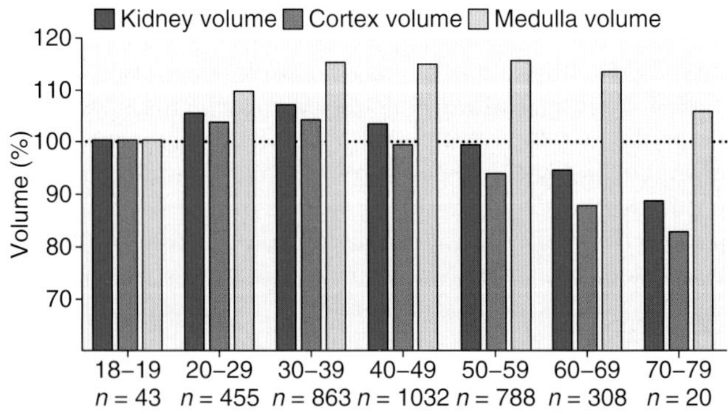


**Fig. 22.1** Total kidney, cortical, and medullary volumes among 3509 potential kidney donors in the Aging Kidney Anatomy study (expansion of previously reported findings). Among all donors, older than 40 years, cortical volume decreases and medullary volume increases, making total kidney volume relatively constant until 50 years of age. Beyond that, medullary volume no longer increases, leading to a decrease in total kidney volume from the decreasing cortical volume. Findings were compared proportional to the respective volumes in the youngest age group (18–19 years). (From Wang X, Vrtiska TJ, Avula RT, et al. Age, kidney function, and risk factors associate differently with cortical and medullary volumes of the kidney. *Kidney Int.* 2014;85:677–685.)

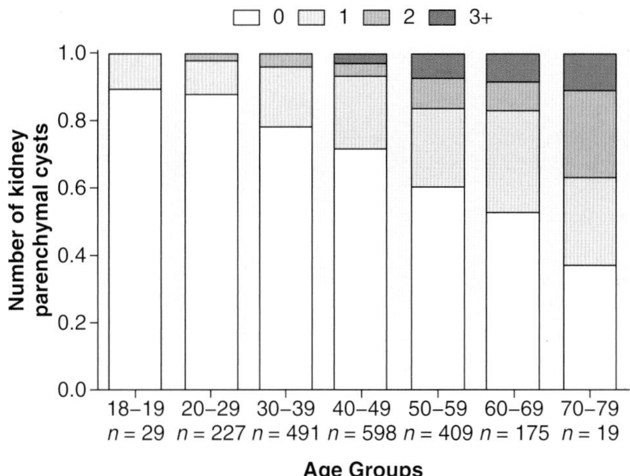


**Fig. 22.2** Number of cortical and medullary simple cysts 5 mm or more by age among 1948 potential living kidney donors. In the figure fraction, *white* represents no cysts, whereas *dark purple* represents the fraction of three or more cysts. Intermediate fractions on a *light purple* scale represent the presence of one or two cysts.

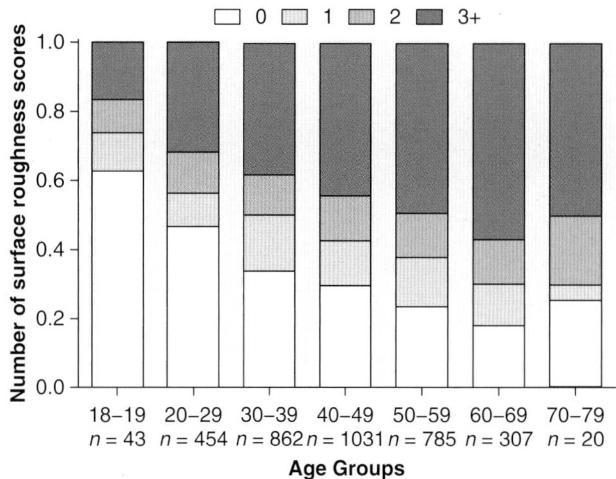


**Fig. 22.3** Kidney surface roughness increasing with age among 3502 potential kidney donors in the Aging Kidney Anatomy study (expansion of previously reported findings). Based on the involved proportion of kidney surface with roughness (lumpy irregular rather than smooth surface), scores were given from 0 to 3 for each kidney and then averaged between kidneys. A score of 0 indicates no roughness; 1, roughness up to 25%; 2, roughness of 26% to 50%; and 3, roughness >50% of the kidney surface. (From Denic A, Alexander MP, Kaushik V, et al. Detection and clinical patterns of nephron hypertrophy and nephrosclerosis among apparently healthy adults. *Am J Kidney Dis.* 2016; 68:58–67.)

other studies have also suggested that an increase in renal sinus fat with age also masks some of the observed total kidney volume decline with older age.[74,75]

## KIDNEY CYSTS

Kidney cysts are relatively common, of tubular diverticuli origin,[81] and their frequency and size increase with older age (Fig. 22.2).[82,83] There has been increased detection of cysts due to technologic advancements with imaging modalities, so it is important to consider cyst size thresholds when counting cysts.[82] A study of 1948 potential kidney donors demonstrated that even in this predominantly healthy population, cortical and medullary cysts larger than or equal to 5 mm were more frequent in older men and were associated with larger body surface area, albuminuria, and hypertension.[82] Moreover, this study generated upper reference limits (97.5th percentile) for the number of cysts in both genders by age. The upper reference limit for the number of cysts in both kidneys of 18 to 29-year-olds is one for both men and women, but increases to ten in men and four in women older than 60 years. Besides simple kidney cysts, parapelvic cysts, hyperdense cysts, angiomyolipomas, and cysts or tumors suspicious for cancer are also more frequent with older age.[82] Parapelvic cysts are thought to have a lymphatic origin[84] and increase with age, but are not associated with hypertension or albuminuria.

## OTHER STRUCTURAL CHANGES

Other kidney parenchymal changes that become more prevalent with older age in ostensibly healthy adults include calcifications, focal cortical scars, fibromuscular dysplasia, and renal artery atherosclerosis without stenosis.[85] Of these, the two findings most strongly associated with age are atherosclerosis of renal arteries and focal cortical scarring. In donors younger than 30 years, the prevalence of atherosclerosis and focal scarring were 0.4% and 1.5%, respectively. However, in donors older than 60 years, the prevalence of atherosclerosis was nearly 25%, and the prevalence of focal scarring was 8%. Focal scarring also contributes to an increase in a kidney surface roughness with age (Fig. 22.3).[86]

# MICROSCOPIC CHANGES

## GLOMERULI

### Number of Glomeruli

Several different approaches have been used to count the total number of glomeruli per kidney, with similar findings. On average, humans have 900,000 glomeruli/kidney, but with significant variability, ranging from as low as 200,000 up to 2.7 million glomeruli/kidney.[87,88] Lower glomerular number counts are likely the result of both the reduction in nephrogenesis stemming from intrauterine events and the progressive loss of glomeruli with age. Counts of the glomerular number have been obtained from autopsy studies, where complete sectioning of the kidney can be performed.[89] However, many autopsy studies have not distinguished normal nonsclerotic glomeruli from globally sclerotic glomeruli in their counts. Furthermore, the comorbid state in autopsy studies (often unknown, with sudden unexpected deaths) may increase global glomerulosclerosis beyond that expected from aging alone.

Living kidney donors provide a unique opportunity to determine how the glomerular number relates to aging. A study in 1638 living kidney donors who were carefully screened to confirm health estimated numbers of nonsclerotic and globally sclerotic glomeruli using the predonation CT scan and the implantation biopsy.[88] The youngest kidney donors (18–29 years of age) had a mean number of nonsclerotic glomeruli of about 990,000 and 17,000 globally sclerotic glomeruli/kidney. The oldest kidney donors (70–75 years) had about 520,000 nonsclerotic glomeruli and 142,000 globally

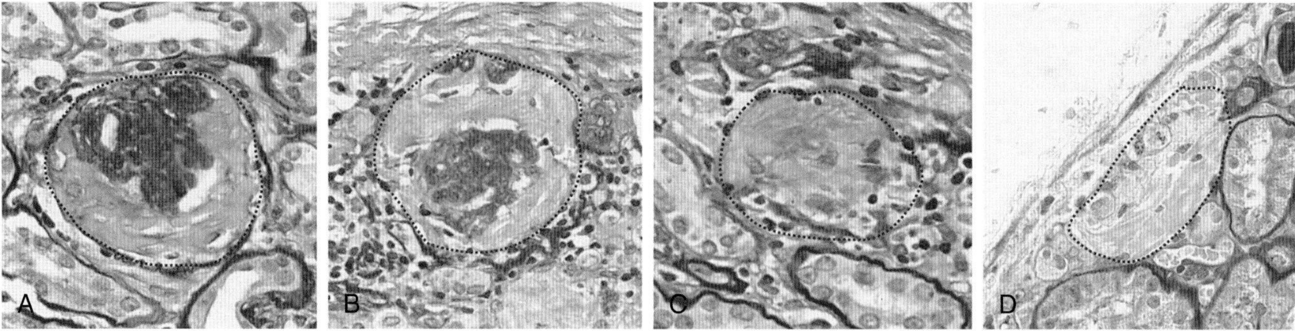


**Fig. 22.4** Examples of globally sclerosed glomeruli (GSG) in different stages of their involution. (A, B) GSG are easily discernible in the biopsy sample. (C, D) GSG that may be overlooked because they progressively atrophy and lose a discernible capsule. All GSG are traced with a *black dashed line.*

sclerotic glomeruli per kidney. The 48% loss in nonsclerotic glomeruli, with only a 15% increase in globally sclerotic glomeruli numbers, supports the hypothesis that globally sclerotic glomeruli are eventually completely reabsorbed or significantly atrophied so that they can no longer be clearly detected on tissue sections examined by light microscopy (Fig. 22.4). This is in agreement with an older study by Hayman and associates, who postulated that "scars of destroyed glomeruli disappear without leaving recognizable traces."[90] The concept of missing or reabsorbed glomeruli is very important because a regular pathology report of the percentage of glomerulosclerosis on a renal biopsy may substantially underappreciate the true age-related loss of glomeruli.

**Table 22.1 Expected Number of Globally Sclerotic Glomeruli per Biopsy Section[a]**

| Age Group (years) | Total Number of Glomeruli Found per Biopsy Section | | | | | | | |
|---|---|---|---|---|---|---|---|---|
| | 1 | 2 | 3–4 | 5–8 | 9–16 | 17–32 | 33–48 | 49–64 |
| 18–29 | 0.5 | 0.5 | 0.5 | 0.5 | 1 | 1 | 1 | 1 |
| 30–34 | 0.5 | 0.5 | 0.5 | 0.5 | 1 | 1 | 1 | 1.5 |
| 35–39 | 0.5 | 0.5 | 0.5 | 0.5 | 1 | 1.5 | 2 | 2 |
| 40–44 | 0.5 | 0.5 | 0.5 | 1 | 1 | 2 | 2.5 | 3 |
| 45–49 | 0.5 | 0.5 | 1 | 1 | 1.5 | 2 | 3 | 4 |
| 50–54 | 1 | 1 | 1 | 1.5 | 2 | 3 | 5 | 5 |
| 55–59 | 1 | 1 | 1.5 | 1.5 | 2 | 3.5 | 4.5 | 6 |
| 60–64 | 1 | 1.5 | 1.5 | 2 | 2.5 | 4 | 5.5 | 7 |
| 65–69 | 1 | 2 | 2 | 2.5 | 3 | 4.5 | 6.5 | 8 |
| 70–74 | 1 | 2 | 2.5 | 3 | 4 | 5.5 | 7.5 | 9 |
| 75–77 | 1 | 2 | 2.5 | 3 | 4 | 6 | 8 | 9.5 |

[a]As predicted by the total number of glomeruli and age from the Aging Kidney Anatomy study.

Adapted from Kremers WK, Denic A, Lieske JC, et al. Distinguishing age-related from disease-related glomerulosclerosis on kidney biopsy: the Aging Kidney Anatomy study. *Nephrol Dial Transplant.* 2015;30:2034–2039.

*Clinical Relevance 1*

The reabsorption of globally sclerosed glomeruli with age may lead to an underappreciation of the older kidneys according to renal biopsy assessment.

Despite significant methodologic differences, studies have reported strikingly similar rates of glomerular loss per kidney per year—6200 in living kidney donors[88] and 6800 in autopsy studies.[89]

## Glomerulosclerosis

An increasing percentage of global glomerulosclerosis is a feature of an aging kidney that has been demonstrated in autopsy and living kidney donor studies.[89,91,92] An autopsy study of 58 kidneys (48 from adults) from a mixed population of Australian Aborigines and non-Aborigines, US Caucasians, and African-Americans has shown a range of 0% to 23% with global glomerulosclerosis and a strong association with older age.[89] A study of 1203 living kidney donors has confirmed these findings and showed an increasing prevalence of focal and global glomerulosclerosis (FGGS), but not focal and segmental glomerulosclerosis (FSGS) with older age.[91] Whereas the prevalence of any global glomerulosclerosis was only 19% in the youngest kidney donors (age 18–29 years), the prevalence was 82% among the 11 oldest donors (70–77 years of age). In a study of 1847 of 2052 living kidney donors who were normotensive across three centers, the upper 95th percentile reference limit of glomerulosclerosis expected for age was determined (Table 22.1).[93] For example, for a 25-year-old who has a biopsy with 24 glomeruli, up to one globally sclerotic glomeruli on biopsy would be reasonable before suspecting glomerulosclerosis from disease. However, for a 76-year-old who has a biopsy with 24 glomeruli, up to six globally sclerotic glomeruli on biopsy would be reasonable before suspecting glomerulosclerosis from disease. In this study, among the 5% of donors in whom the number of globally sclerotic glomeruli was higher than the 95th percentile expected for age, a greater prevalence of hypertension and interstitial fibrosis and a higher percentage of ischemic-appearing glomeruli (pericapsular fibrosis, capsular thickening, and capillary loop wrinkling) on a biopsy were observed.[93] The association between the abnormal number of globally sclerotic glomeruli for age and ischemic glomeruli remained, even after hypertensive donors were excluded. Interestingly, use of these age-specific reference limits for globally sclerotic glomeruli helps identify which patients with nephrotic syndrome will develop progressive CKD.[94]

Certain morphologic findings of globally sclerotic glomeruli should also be taken into consideration; for example, solidification forms of glomerulosclerosis are always pathologic and are never simply an age-related finding.[95–97]

> *Clinical Relevance 2*
> Glomerulosclerosis associated with aging is focal and global, in contrast to focal, segmental, and solidification forms of glomerulosclerosis occurring with disease.

The obsolescent type of morphology of global glomerulosclerosis is characterized by the filling of Bowman's space with collagenous material, accompanied by retraction of the capillary tuft. This is the type of global glomerulosclerosis obsereved in normal aging kidneys. Alternatively, the solidified type of glomerulosceroisis is assocated with and commonly seen in hypertensive nephrosclerosis found in black people, with or without high-risk alleles on the APOL1 locus.[98] The obsolescent-type global glomerulosclerosis is presumed to reflect an ischemic process. FSGS is not associated with healthy aging in humans, unlike murine species. The lesion of FSGS in growing rats is likely to be mediated by podocyte injury and detachment. FSGS lesions in humans, therefore almost always indicates an underlying pathologic disease process and not simple renal senescence.[95–97]The possession of two risk alleles for APOL1 appears to enhance age-related global glomerulosclerosis in individuals of (West) African ancestry.[99,100] This phenomenon might help explain in part the higher risk of black people for the development of hypertension and GFR decline at an earlier age among black people compared with white people.[101]

### Glomerular Hypertrophy

Entire nephrons hypertrophy in diabetes and obesity,[102–105] conditions that often become more prevalent with older age. Nephron hypertrophy is also seen in subjects with low nephron endowment at birth.[106] Although hypertrophy occurs in the glomerular and tubular segments of a nephron unit,[107] glomerulomegaly is much easier to appreciate on visual inspection of a kidney biopsy than tubular enlargement. The relationship between glomerular size and older age needs to account for the underlying study population (e.g., age-related comorbidites such as diabetes and obesity or nephron endowement at birth) and whether glomerular size was estimated from only nonsclerotic glomeruli or both nonsclerosed and the smaller globally sclerosed glomeruli that become more common with age.

Many studies have reported conflicting results, likely related to these issues, with some showing an increase in glomerular size with age[108–110] and others showing a decrease in glomerular size with age.[111,112] Studies that were limited to carefully screened healthy living kidney donors and only studied nonsclerosed glomeruli have found no change in glomerular size with aging.[86,88,113] Nonsclerosed glomerular volume in patients with renal tumors who underwent radical nephrectomy was stable until 75 years of age, similar to findings in living kidney donors.[114] However, beyond 75 years of age, nonsclerosed glomerular volume decreased due to a higher proportion of smaller, ischemic-appearing glomeruli. Given this lack of increase in glomerular volume, albuminuria would not be expected with aging alone in humans because albuminuria occurs with glomerular hypertrophy via a disorganized glomerular structure that is unable to prevent protein leaking efficiently.[110] Glomerular enlargement is also observed in blacks with two risk alleles at the APOL1 locus, which rather suggests low nephron endowment (see later) and/or accelerated loss of nephrons with aging.[99–101] Increased glomerular volume (glomerular hypertrophy) and glomerulosclerosis in aging subjects is predicted by comorbidity, such as obesity, diabetes, hypertension, and proteinuria. Such hypertrophy is also associated with male gender, taller height, and a family history of end-stage kidney disease (ESKD).[105,113]

## TUBULES

### Tubular Hypertrophy

Notably, glomeruli only comprise about 4% of the total cortical volume.[88] The remaining parenchymal volume is largely comprised of renal tubules and tubular enlargement.[107–115] Although glomerulomegaly most likely does not occur with healthy aging (or in the absence of APOL1 risk alleles in individuals of African origin), in humans tubular enlargement with older age is evident with increased area of tubular profiles.[86] Increase in tubular size as well as atrophy and disappearance of globally sclerotic glomeruli disperses the remaining glomeruli further apart from each other, thereby decreasing glomerular density with aging.[116] However, the relationship between glomerular (nonsclerosed and globally sclerosed) density varies, depending on how much global glomerulosclerosis is present in the section biopsied. In biopsy sections with less than 10% global glomerulosclerosis, the glomerular density is decreased with age, whereas in biopsy sections with more than 10% global glomerulosclerosis, the glomerular density is increased with age.[116] In regions of the renal cortex without significant glomerulosclerosis, age-related tubular enlargement disperses glomeruli further apart, decreasing their density. However, in regions with significant glomerulosclerosis, the overall atrophy of tubules and glomeruli brings the glomeruli closer together, thereby increasing their density (Fig. 22.5).

### Tubular Diverticuli

Darmady and colleagues found in an autopsy study that tubular diverticuli increase with older age.[110] This finding parallels two other age-related findings in healthy adults. First, simple parenchymal cysts, which likely originate from these diverticuli,[81] become more frequent with older age. Second, the mean profile tubular area increases with older age.[86] Enlargement of tubules, with upregulation of growth factors, may contribute to the development of diverticuli, with the eventual formation of cysts.[117,118]

## ARTERIES AND ARTERIOLES

Arteriosclerosis and arteriolar hyalinosis are two common findings in the kidney biopsy of normal adults that become

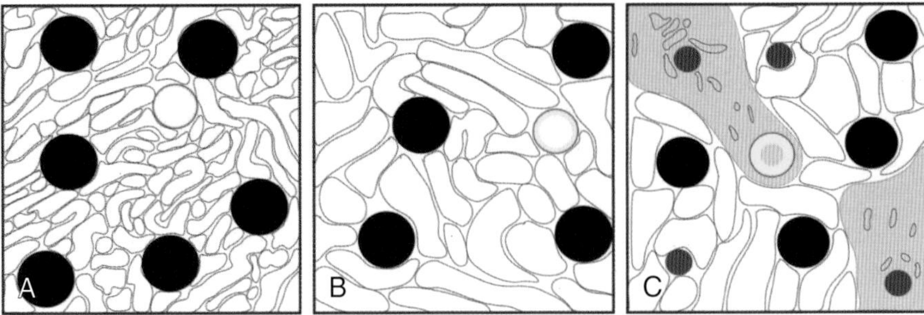


**Fig. 22.5** Schematic illustration of how the percentage of glomerulosclerosis influences glomerular density. (A) Example of a young individual with a certain glomerular density *(blue solid circle)*, normal tubules and normal artery *(orange circle),* with minimal to no intimal thickening *(yellow circle).* (B) In an older person in whom the biopsy shows less than 10% glomerulosclerosis, tubules become larger and disperse the glomeruli apart, and their density decreases. (C) In older persons in whom there is more than 10% glomerulosclerosis *(pink solid circles)*, the associated interstitial fibrosis and tubular atrophy *(light pink areas)* bring the glomeruli closer together, thus increasing their density. Arteriosclerosis with intimal thickening *(thicker yellow line)* is also pronounced in these regions in older adults.

more prevalent with age.[86] Arteriosclerosis (luminal stenosis by intimal thickening) with aging may cause ischemic injury, leading to a lower cortical to medullary volume ratio, even in healthy adults.[86] Arteriolar hyalinosis increases with age and is associated with renal artery atherosclerosis in healthy adults, consistent with studies that associate arterolar hyalinosis with renal atherosclerosis in hypertensive patients.[119–121] Older age and hypertension may lead to global glomerulosclerosis and nephrosclerosis via reduced blood flow due to ischemic injury from the narrowing of small arteries and arterioles.[122] Notably, lower total nephron number/kidney is associated with arteriosclerosis, even after adjusting for age and gender.[88]

## NEPHROSCLEROSIS AND INTERSTITIAL FIBROSIS

The term *nephrosclerosis* describes a microstructural biopsy pattern of global glomerulosclerosis, arteriosclerosis, and interstitial fibrosis with tubular atrophy. Nephrosclerosis is notably seen with hypertension,[123] but is also described in healthy older kidney donors without hypertension or only mild hypertension.[91] The nephrosclerosis appearance is thought to be due to increased intimal thickening of small arteries in the kidneys (arteriosclerosis, arteriolosclerosis), leading to glomerular ischemia, with the wrinkling of capillary tufts, thickening of the basement membrane, and progressive pericapsular fibrosis.[123,124] Simultaneously, proteinaceous material accumulates in Bowman's space, likely due to a combination of a disturbed balance between formation and breakdown of the glomerular extracellular matrix[125] and podocyte depletion,[91,109,125] probably due to perturbations in local mechanical forces.[126] Eventually, ischemic glomerular tufts fully collapse, forming globally sclerosed glomeruli. As a consequence of glomerulosclerosis, accompanying tubules atrophy, with an accumulation of surrounding interstitial fibrosis.

All four features of nephrosclerosis—global glomerulosclerosis, arteriosclerosis, interstitial fibrosis, and tubular atrophy—increase with older age and, when combined together (at equal weighting) they represent a so-called nephrosclerosis score (Fig. 22.6).[91] If we define the nephrosclerosis as presence of at least two of the previously mentioned abnormalities, then from Fig. 22.6 we can see that the youngest donors (18–19 years of age) do not have detectable nephrosclerosis. The prevalence of nephrosclerosis

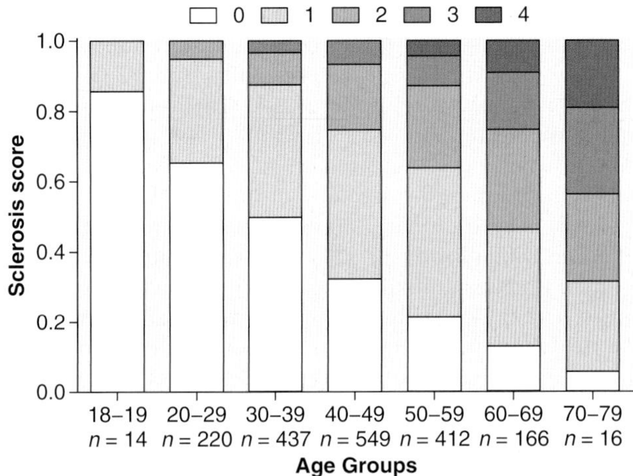


**Fig. 22.6** The nephrosclerosis score increases with age among 1814 living kidney donors from the Aging Kidney Anatomy study (expansion of previously reported findings). The total nephrosclerosis score is obtained by adding the individual scores of histologic abnormalities: any global glomerulosclerosis, any arteriosclerosis, interstitial fibrosis greater than 5%, and any tubular atrophy. *White bars* in all age groups represent a score of 0 (no abnormalities present), and a *dark purple bar* represents a score of 4 (presence of all four pathologic abnormalities). Three intermediate scores are presented with different shades of *purple color*. (From Rule AD, Amer H, Cornell LD, et al. The association between age and nephrosclerosis on renal biopsy among healthy adults. *Ann Intern Med.* 2010;152:561–567.)

in 20- to 29-year-old donors is 5% and rises to 69% among the oldest donors.

Thus, the number and size of the nephrons are the primary determinants of the kidney cortical volume. A combination of age-related glomerulosclerosis with corresponding interstitial fibrosis and tubular atrophy is responsible for the observed loss of cortical volume with healthy aging seen in living kidney donors. This nephrosclerosis typically starts in glomeruli in the superficial cortical zones. Because the corresponding tubules of these superficial glomeruli contribute more to the cortical volume, their atrophy with age-related nephrosclerosis leads to a decrease in cortical volume with aging. At the same time, there is tubular hypertrophy of the remaining nephrons, particularly those in the medulla. This observation explains why, despite a 48% decrease in nephron number from ages 18 to 76 years, there is only a 17% decrease in cortical volume and only a 12% decrease in kidney volume.[74,75]

One might expect that with age-related nephrosclerosis, there would be compensatory hypertrophy of the remaining, still functional glomeruli. However, studies in living kidney donors have not confimed this hypothesis.[116] A possible explanation may be that with healthy human aging, there is a decreased metabolic demand for glomerular function, so that the loss of glomeruli does not cause the enlargement of the remaining glomeruli. Notably, comorbidities that can become more prevalent in old age, such as obesity and diabetes, with albuminuria, do associate with glomerular hypertrophy.[116] Also, low nephron endowment at birth, or disorders that accelarate nephron loss with advancing age, can contibute to the glomerulomegaly observed in adulthood.

## FUNCTIONAL CHANGES OF THE KIDNEYS WITH AGING

These include changes in the GFR and other functional changes.

### GLOMERULAR FILTRATION RATE

#### WHOLE-KIDNEY GLOMERULAR FILTRATION RATE

In a series of pioneering studies begun over 60 years ago, Davies and Shock examined 70 healthy adults between the ages of 24 and 89 years and, in a cross-sectional analysis, showed (by urinary inulin clearance) a linear GFR decline in subjects older than 30 years.[127] The GFR in the oldest group was found to be 46% less as compared with the GFR in the youngest group. Several decades later, Lindeman and colleagues carried out a longitudinal study (the first of its kind) by following 254 mostly healthy adult individuals, although some had diabetes, for up to 14 years.[128] They found that the mean annual decline in GFR, estimated by 24-hour urinary creatinine clearance, was 7.5 mL/min per decade; however, one-third of the subjects had no decrease in kidney function, and a small subset actually had an increase. In addition to measurement error explaining this finding, a rise in GFR with age might also be explained by hyperfiltration due to the comorbidities (e.g., obesity, diabetes) that become more common with aging.[129] This longitudinal rate of GFR decline is similar to the cross-sectional decline of 6.3 mL/min per decade obtained from a study of potential kidney donors (GFR measured by iothalamate clearance).[91] Among 4500 potential kidney donors in the expanded analysis from the Aging Kidney Anatomy study (Fig. 22.7), the average decline per decade for estimated GFR was 7.4 mL/min, whereas for measured GFR (iothalamate clearance) it was 6.1 mL/min/1.73 m$^2$. The estimated GFR by the Chronic Kidney Disease Epidemiology Collaboration (CKD-EPI) equation underestimates the GFR in healthy populations, such as potential kidney donors, because it was developed using mostly CKD patients.[130,131]

Although Fig. 22.7 shows mean estimated GFR (eGFR) and measured GFR, there is variability within each age group (Table 22.2).[132] It can be appreciated that both upper and lower reference limits also decline with aging. Similar findings

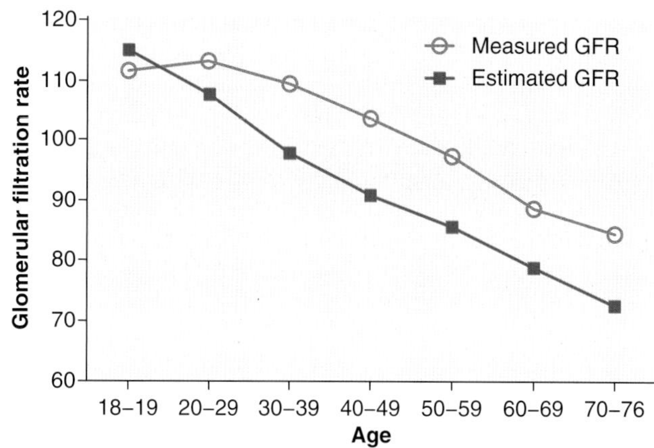


**Fig. 22.7** Age-related glomerular filtration rate (*GFR*; mean values) decline among 4500 potential kidney donors in the Aging Kidney Anatomy study (expansion of previously reported findings). Decline in the estimated GFR (CKD-EPI study equation; see text) is calculated to be 7.4 mL/min/decade and 6.1 mL/min/decade for the measured GFR. (From Rule AD, Amer H, Cornell LD, et al. The association between age and nephrosclerosis on renal biopsy among healthy adults. *Ann Intern Med.* 2010;152:561–567.)

**Table 22.2 Reference Values for Estimated and Measured Glomerular Filtration Rate in Potential Kidney Donors[a]**

| Age Group (years) | No. | Estimated Glomerular Filtration Rate (GFR) (Measured GFR) Fifth Percentile | Median | Mean | 95th Percentile |
|---|---|---|---|---|---|
| 18–19 | 46 | 88 (87) | 114 (107) | 115 (111) | 145 (144) |
| 20–29 | 584 | 81 (84) | 108 (111) | 108 (113) | 130 (149) |
| 30–39 | 1090 | 75 (82) | 98 (106) | 98 (109) | 118 (147) |
| 40–49 | 1364 | 69 (77) | 91 (102) | 91 (104) | 110 (135) |
| 50–59 | 1001 | 65 (72) | 85 (94) | 85 (97) | 103 (133) |
| 60–69 | 379 | 61 (64) | 78 (87) | 79 (88) | 97 (118) |
| 70–76 | 36 | 55 (57) | 71 (85) | 73 (84) | 91 (113) |

[a]Expansion of previously reported findings.

From Murata K, Baumann NA, Saenger AK, et al. Relative performance of the MDRD and CKD-EPI equations for estimating glomerular filtration rate among patients with varied clinical presentations. *Clin J Am Soc Nephrol.* 2011;6:1963–1972.

in healthy donors have been reported by Pottel and colleagues.[133] Other longitudinal studies of the decline in renal function (GFR or creatinine clearance) with aging have shown generally similar findings to those of Lindeman and associates,[128] including the relative stability of renal function for extended periods in some otherwise healthy aging subjects.[134–136] In addition, in these studies, the rate of decline of renal function appeared to increase with each passing decade in those older than about 30 to 40 years.

#### SINGLE-NEPHRON GLOMERULAR FILTRATION RATE

Several studies have found that a higher whole-kidney GFR correlates with larger kidneys or kidney cortical volume.[79,80,86] A study of 1520 healthy living kidney donors also investigated how the whole-kidney GFR correlated with the microstructural components of cortical volume. After age and gender adjustments, a higher whole-kidney GFR was associated with larger nephrons (larger glomeruli and tubules), whereas a lower whole-kidney GFR did not associate with any measure of nephrosclerosis, including global glomerulosclerosis, interstitial fibrosis with tubular atrophy, and arteriosclerosis.[86] The age-related nephron loss due to increased nephrosclerosis is followed by a parallel whole-kidney GFR decline.[88] To disentangle whole-kidney GFR from the nephron number, further single-nephron GFR (snGFR) studies are required.

Although in vivo measurements of snGFR through micropuncture are possible and have been done in animal studies,[137,138] a direct measure of snGFR (by micropuncture) is not feasible or safe in humans. However, dividing the whole-kidney GFR by the number of functional (nonsclerosed) glomeruli in both kidneys allows for an estimation of the mean snGFR.[139] The snGFR remains stable with age because the loss of nephrons parallels the loss in the total GFR.[88] Thus, the effect of age on snGFR is minimal, consistent with other physiologic characteristics, including height and gender, whereas obesity, family history of ESKD, and nephrosclerosis exceeding that expected for age are associated with an increased snGFR.[139,140] There may be higher snGFR among the oldest donors (70–75 years of age), but this finding may be confounded by donor selection factors (e.g., the requirement of whole-kidney GFR >80 mL/min/1.73 $m^2$) in this age group, which may only allow those with some degree of hyperfiltration to donate and be available to study with a kidney biopsy.[139,140]

Although other studies of snGFR in living human subjects are lacking, there have been studies assessing the single-nephron ultrafiltration coefficient ($snK_f$) in individuals similar to living kidney donors.[141–143] The $snK_f$ represents the filtering capacity of the glomerulus, as determined by the surface area and permeability of the glomerular filtration barrier. In these studies, $snK_f$ was estimated from electron microscopy measures of the glomeruli on kidney biopsy.[141] The snGFR could be calculated by multiplying $snK_f$ by the perfusion pressure across the glomerular filtration barrier.[144] Thus, it is possible that the relationship of clinical characteristics to snGFR may be similar to that of $snK_f$. Consistent with the findings of a relatively stable snGFR across the age spectrum described above, $snK_f$ did not show significant differences between younger and older living kidney donors.[141,145] Adaptive hyperfiltration does occur in the aging kidney following unilateral nephrectomy[146]; however, either due to an increase in Kf, glomerular capillary filtration pressure, or increased glomerular plasma flow or some combination of the three, the extent of the increase in snGFR (and whole-kidney GFR [wkGFR]) is reduced compared with younger persons. The definition of hyperfiltration based on measurements of the whole-kidney GFR is best determined by an age-adapted measured GFR (not eGFR), uncorrected for body surface area. However, such definitions do not distinguish between a higher snGFR and higher nephron number.[147]

## OTHER FUNCTIONAL CHANGES

### RENAL PLASMA FLOW

Renal plasma flow (RPF) represents the volume of plasma delivered to both kidneys per unit of time. The RPF can be calculated from the amount of plasma that is cleared of para-aminohippurate (PAH) per unit of time. PAH is a compound with a nearly 100% extraction through the kidneys. A Swedish study of 122 potential kidney donors, ages 21 to 67, has shown that similar to the GFR, the RPF declines with older age.[140] Older age influences the degree of renal blood flow change as a response to exercise,[148,149] attenuates the renal hemodynamic response to atrial natriuretic peptide[150] and the degree of vasodilation.[151] One study has postulated that higher levels of the endogenous nitric oxide (NO) inhibitor asymmetric dimethylarginine (ADMA) lead to a reduced RPF and hypertension with older age.[152] Animal studies have provided some evidence that ADMA is associated with tubulointerstitial ischemia and fibrosis,[153] glomerular capillary loss, and glomerulosclerosis.[154] In a study of 19 healthy individuals, divided into three age groups—young, middle-aged, and older—an infusion of dopamine and amino acids was used to test the effects of maximal vasodilation on RPF and NO levels. Whereas both RPF and NO levels increased in young and middle-aged individuals, they did not change in the older group.[155] This suggests that due to advanced age-related vascular changes in older adults, renal blood vessels are less responsive to maximal vasodilation.

### FILTRATION FRACTION

The filtration fraction (FF) represents the proportion of fluid entering the kidneys that reaches into the renal tubules—that is, it is a ratio between the GFR and RPF. Normally, the value for FF is about 20%. However, in older age, atherosclerosis and arteriosclerosis of the arteries and arterioles reduces blood flow to kidneys. Thus, the FF may increase, particularly in those of very advanced age.[140]

### RENAL RESERVE IN AGING

The phenomenon of renal reserve refers to an acute increase in GFR (usually by 20% or more from basal values) when subjects are fed oral protein loads (typically cooked red meat) or infused intravenously with certain amino acids.[155–159] The mechanisms underlying such physiologic changes is not fully understood, but appears to be a consequence of vasodilatation, an increase in glomerular plasma flow, and an increase in the snGFR.[160] See Chapter 3. Growth hormone may be involved, but this is controversial[155–157] The efficiency of renal reserve is blunted to some degree by aging per se, most often in the very older.[155] Renal functional reserve is well maintained up to about age 80 years in otherwise healthy men and women.[161] Diminished levels of sex hormones may play a role in the diminished renal reserve seen with aging (see later). The diurnal variation in GFR is also blunted with aging.[162]

Aging in indigenous Kuna Indians (Panama), who subsist on a low-protein, high–dark chocolate diet and remain largely free of hypertension and cardiovascular disease (CVD), even at an advanced age, is associated with a steady decline in GFR and RFP with aging, similar to that observed in westernized countries.[163] These findings are not consistent with a hypothesis that rising blood pressures (hypertension) are causally related to the decline in GFR with aging.

### SEXUAL DIMORPHISM IN AGING

In a series of studies, mainly focused in murine species, Baylis and coworkers developed the concept of sexual dimorphism in renal aging[164–168] (also see review by Gava and associates[169]). Females develop less age-related decline in renal function, perhaps due to a renoprotective action of estrogens. In contrast, males have a greater loss of renal function with age, perhaps due to the adverse effects of androgens. The mechanisms involved are complex, but seem to implicate disturbances of the NO synthesis pathways, and a lower rate of NO production might be influenced by sex steroids.[165,166] A role for the renin-angiotensin-aldosterone system (RAAS) has also been described.[168] Interestingly, in aging experimental animals, there was no observed rise in glomerular capillary pressure or glomerulomegaly in males or females, castrated or not. This suggests that the age-dependent sexually dimorphic loss of renal function does not appear to be dependent on hemodynamic changes or glomerular hypertrophy, similar to that observed in humans.[168] Age-dependent sexual dimorphic effects on renal function might be related to increased body size in males and therefore may be conditional to a disparity between energy demand and supply.

### Pathophysiologic Explanations for Aging-Associated Nephrosclerosis

**Podocentric Versus Ischemic Hypotheses (Animal and Human Studies).** As stated earlier, it has been shown that renal blood flow declines with older age.[170] Studies in rats have shown that in addition to the reduction in blood flow, renal arterioles in older rats have altered sensitivity to NO[171] and angiotensin II.[172] However, the main limitation of animal studies is the virtual absence of arteriosclerosis, thus limiting studies of age-related ischemic changes. Studies in human kidneys have demonstrated that age-related arteriolosclerosis and intimal and medial hypertrophy in intrarenal arteries resemble those observed in extrarenal arteries.[173,174] These pathologic changes are especially common in interlobular arteries and are frequently observed in renal biopsies from normal individuals without cardiovascular disease. Although it is unclear what causes the vascular changes in intrarenal arteries, Martin and Sheaff have postulated that they are directly linked to global glomerulosclerosis, which occurs first in the superficial cortical layers and is followed by local interstitial fibrosis and tubular atrophy.[124] Subsequently, as a compensatory mechanism, the deeper glomeruli hypertrophy and, over time, undergo hyperfiltration injury, ultimately developing glomerulosclerosis. More recently, studies in healthy living kidney donors have corroborated the hypothesis of Martin and Sheaff that age-related glomerulosclerosis is primarily of vascular origin due to observed ischemic changes in the glomeruli, intracapsular fibrosis,[175] and increased prevalence of arteriosclerosis.[91] Moreover, implantation renal biopsies of healthy kidney donors can also be ischemic appearing, presumably still functional glomeruli, with a wrinkling of capillary loops, thickened basement membrane, and mild intracapsular fibrosis. All these described findings may be associated with ischemia and gradually lead to progressive shrinkage of the glomerular tufts and collagen deposition in Bowman's space, finally ending with complete global glomerulosclerosis.

Alternatively, podocyte depletion can also give rise to the glomerulosclerosis of aging. The podocytes are highly differentiated and specialized epithelial cells in a glomerulus, with limited capacity for cell division and turnover.[176,177] The two main reasons that lead to podocyte depletion, in absolute or relative terms, are actual loss of podocytes (cell death or detachment from the tuft) and glomerulomegaly—each podocyte subsequently has to cover the increased filtration surface area. The notion that podocyte dysbiosis may be the culprit for glomerulosclerosis is not new. Three decades ago, Kriz and colleagues[178] postulated that podocyte depletion and a subsequent bare glomerular basement membrane is the first step that leads to focal and segmental glomerulosclerosis. Studies in rats have provided evidence that reduced numbers of podocytes lead to glomerulosclerosis.[179,180] Using puromycin aminonucleoside (PAN) treatment as a model for podocyte oxidative injury, one study has linked glomerulosclerosis and podocyte number depletion.[179] Others have shown increased glomerulosclerosis (usually of the focal and segmental variety) when podocytes fail to follow glomerular growth as a result of molecular growth signalling[180] or may be due to podocyte hypertrophic stress associated with glomerulomegaly in rats without calorie restriction.[181] Interestingly, calorie restriction abolished glomerulomegaly, podocyte hypertrophy/stress and pydocyte loss with resulting glomerulosclerosis.[181] Using a transgenic approach in rats, the same group has also developed evidence that the reduced number of podocytes alone is sufficient to cause glomerulosclerosis.[182]

Taken together, all these animal (murine) studies favor the concept that acquired or congenital podocytopenia (absolute or relative) is a critical driving force for the development of glomerulosclerosis, particularly of the focal and segmental variety (see review by Kriz and associates[178]). However, the biology of aging in experimental animals differs from that of humans (see above), and these differences must be taken into account when translating pathophysiologic concepts from animals to humans.

More recently, human kidney biopsies have been used to study podocytes; these have found that the pattern of global glomerulosclerosis with aging is somewhat different in studies not limited to living kidney donors.[108] A study of 89 kidney biopsies from living kidney donors, deceased kidney donors, and normal poles of radical nephrectomy specimens performed for tumor, found that podocyte depletion is identified as a potential culprit for age-related glomerulosclerosis.[108] The authors counted podocytes, measured their size and density, and demonstrated a decline in podocyte density with older age due to a reduced count of podocytes per glomerulus and larger glomerular volume. In particular, younger individuals had more than a threefold higher podocyte density compared with individuals older than 70 years (>300 podocytes/$10^6$ $\mu m^3$ vs. <100 podocytes/$10^6$ $\mu m^3$). In the older individuals, not only was the podocyte density lower, but their detachment rate was much higher, and podocytes showed molecular evidence of cell stress. Moreover, in some glomeruli with significant podocyte detachment, the authors observed binucleated podocytes as evidence of failed mitotic attempts and glomerular capillary wrinkling, tuft collapse, and pericapsular fibrosis. All these findings led the authors to propose a hypothesis (the podocentric hypothesis) for the glomerular natural history with aging, extending from glomerular hypertrophy to tuft collapse to glomerulosclerosis.[108] However, studies limited to living donors did not show glomerular hypertrophy with aging,[86] suggesting that age-related comorbidities rather than aging alone may explain these findings. In addition, it is noteworthy that increasing albuminuria is not a feature of normal healthy aging.[91] Thus, the podocentric hypothesis may not be relevant to human renal aging.

## CONTRIBUTION OF COMORBIDITIES TO RENAL AGING

Aging is commonly accompanied by comorbidities that can have an independent impact on renal structure and function. These include obesity, diabetes, and nephron endowment at birth. For example, obesity and/or diabetes (type 2) can lead to glomerulomegaly, glomerular hyperfiltration, and albuminuria (see Chapter 51). In part, these comorbidities contribute to the rising prevalence of increased albuminuria with aging seen in cross-sectional epidemiologic studies.[68] Hypertension, commonly seen in older adults, can also modify the underlying normal pattern of renal senescence seen with aging, as discussed earlier.

It also seems likely that nephron endowment at birth will have a modifying effect on the pace of normal physiologic renal aging. Nephron underendowment at birth, due to fetal dysmaturity, will be accompanied by early single-nephron hyperfiltration and glomerular enlargement, which can lead to maladaptive glomerular injury, podocytopenia, glomerulosclerosis and perhaps an acceleration of the normal rate of nephron loss.[183] The combination of glomerulopenia (low nephron endowment at birth) and physiologic renal senescence could, at least theoretically, lead to features of CKD (reduced GFR and/or albuminuria) observed in later life. This postulated phenomenon has not been well studied, so these effects are largely speculative. Reduced glomerular density and glomerular hypertrophy are signs of nephron underendowment and have been shown to have an adverse effect on the progression of many renal diseases, including some that may affect older adults.[184,185] Low birth weight, fetal dysmaturity, and impaired nephrogenesis can contribute to the burden of kidney disease globally, especially in older adults and in subjects with primary or secondary glomerular diseases (see Chapter 21).[185]

## FLUID, ELECTROLYTE, AND ACID-BASE HOMEOSTASIS IN AGING

### SODIUM HOMEOSTASIS

A study in 89 healthy subjects has demonstrated that older age significantly affects the kidney's capacity to reabsorb filtered sodium. Following the initiation of sodium restriction, subjects older than 60 years needed nearly twice as much time to reduce sodium excretion than subjects younger than 30 years (31 vs. 17.6 hours, respectively).[186] The observed difference may be due to the significantly reduced sodium reabsorption in the distal tubules, which was found to be nearly 30% less in older people versus younger controls.[187] Sodium homeostasis can also be influenced by age-related changes in levels and responses to renin and aldosterone, hormones that regulate sodium conservation (discussed further in Chapter 14). Although plasma renin activity and aldosterone levels are lower in older adults, they are not associated with changes in fluid or electrolyte metabolism.[188] These changes increase older adults' susceptibility to sodium retention in disease states or with the use of medications that alter renin release. More recently, the slower response to sodium restriction observed in older adults was reproduced by using angiotensin-converting enzyme (ACE) inhibitors and blocking the RAAS.[189]

One group studied the natriuretic response in normal individuals of different ages after volume expansion and volume contraction. In the 24-hour period following a 2-L infusion of normal saline, the natriuresis was slower in older individuals.[190] It has been hypothesized that the higher prevalence of hypertension in older subjects may be due in part to this attenuated natriuretic response with aging. There is also a reduction in the natriuretic response to saline loading in older versus younger kidney donors after donation.[189]

Atrial natriuretic peptide (ANP) is a hormone secreted by atrial myocytes, and one of its many functions is to control sodium excretion at the tubular level. With older age, the tubular response to ANP is reduced. ANP inhibits sodium reabsorption from the luminal side and induces hyperfiltration and suppression of renin release, all of which together lead to natriuresis, diuresis, and lowering of blood pressure. Normally, ANP is cleared rapidly from plasma; however, if degradation enzymes or clearance receptors are blocked, the half-life can be prolonged.[191] Studies have shown that the plasma ANP levels are several times higher in older individuals, and this may be a compensatory effect of the reduced response at the receptor level. This hypothesis is in agreement with two studies in which sodium excretion plateaued after an ANP infusion in older subjects,[192,193] whereas in younger subjects sodium excretion continued to increase with increasing ANP dose.[192] Of importance, it appears that ANP production does not change with older age; therefore the observed increase of ANP levels in older adults results from reduced metabolic clearance.[194,195] Moreover, others have shown that in response to a saline load, plasma levels of ANP increase more robustly in older compared with younger individuals.[196,197]

The role of altered renal sodium handling in the pathogenesis of age-related elevation of systemic arterial pressure is a topic of great contemporary interest (see also Chapter 46; reviewed by Frame and Wainford[198]). Clearly vascular factors, such as reduced compliance of major arterial vessels, and neurohumoral alterations, such as increased sympathetic nervous system activity, play important roles in the elevation of systolic blood pressure with aging. The sensitivity of blood pressure changes consequent to salt administration increases with age.[199] Animal studies have also suggested increased intrarenal angiotensin II signaling in age-related blood pressure increases.[200] Experimental studies in rodents has also shown decreased expression of the sodium potassium chloride cotransporter (NKCC2) in the loop of Henle with aging[201]; the activity of the thiazide-sensitive sodium chloride cotransporter (NCC) in the distal tubule may be altered in aging, but this is controversial.[198]

The expression of the epithelial sodium channel (ENaC) can be reduced in aging rodents.[202] These studies collectively indicate that dysregulation of sodium handling by the aging nephron can be involved in age-related blood pressure elevation. Integration of this knowledge into the complex array of biologic factors in systems affecting blood pressure (e.g., aortic compliance, sympathetic nervous system activity, RAAS) will be challenging.[198] The role of reduced nephron mass (glomerulopenia) that accompanies physiologic aging cannot be ignored as a participant in blood pressure changes with aging.

## POTASSIUM HOMEOSTASIS

Potassium homeostasis is regulated by several different mechanisms; specifically, in the kidney, the potassium excretion rate is altered depending on the intake. The role of the kidney in potassium homeostasis is very important because normally around 90% of the dietary potassium intake is excreted in the urine and only around 10% in the gastrointestinal tract. The normal internal potassium distribution is also regulated by hormones, such as insulin, catecholamines, and aldosterone. In general, after filtering through the glomerulus, potassium is primarily reabsorbed via the proximal tubule and thick ascending limb of Henle such that only a small amount should normally reach the distal tubules (discussed further in Chapter 17).[203]

Total body potassium (TBK) declines with older age with a reduction in intracellular stores that accompany the decline in muscle mass (sarcopenia) seen with normal aging. A study of 188 healthy volunteers has shown that the annual rate of TBK decline is 7.2 mg/kg in women and 9.2 mg/kg in men,[204] which increases in both genders after 60 years of age.[205] The observed decline in TBK may also be explained by the lower renin and aldosterone levels,[206] as well as the blunted response to aldosterone in older adults (see later).[207] A study of 43 healthy older individuals demonstrated a relative decrease in fractional potassium excretion in relation to creatinine clearance.[208] This finding is consistent with animal studies in which potassium excretion was less efficient in old rats fed a high-potassium diet.[209] The same group subsequently showed that the transtubular potassium gradient is reduced in older compared with young subjects, implying reduced efficiency in potassium excretion in older adults.[210] Insulin-mediated potassium homeostasis in human subjects is not influenced by the age of the subject.[211]

Older age is usually accompanied by comorbidities, and older adults often take medications that interfere with potassium excretion. Examples are potassium-sparing diuretics, renin inhibitors, ACE inhibitors, angiotensin receptor blockers, heparin, calcineurin inhibitors, sodium channel blockers, and nonsteroidal antiinflammatory drugs (NSAIDs). Care is needed when starting these medications for older patients, given their increased propensity to develop hyperkalemia.

> ***Clinical Relevance 3***
> Older adults are at increased risk of hyperkalemia, even given their reduced total body potassium stores and altered tubular potassium transport.

## MAGNESIUM HOMEOSTASIS

It is estimated that about 99% of magnesium is stored in cells, predominantly in bones and muscles, and only about 1% is in extracellular fluid, including plasma. Normally, the kidneys reabsorb 96% of filtered magnesium[212] and regulate magnesium homeostasis (see Chapter 18).

Because plasma and intracellular magnesium homeostasis are very finely regulated,[213] total plasma magnesium is maintained remarkably stable with increasing age in healthy individuals.[214,215] However, a study of 36 healthy older individuals has demonstrated a significant subclinical deficit of magnesium that was not detected by serum magnesium levels.[216] Another more recent study has confirmed this finding, and older subjects (>65 years) had significantly reduced serum levels of both ionized and total magnesium.[214]

The published literature is scarce with regard to normal age-related changes in magnesium homeostasis in the kidneys. Changes in magnesium homeostasis are likely due to diseases that frequently occur in older age, use of therapeutic agents that alter its metabolism, and previously discussed age-related kidney functional decline.[214] The microstructural changes that lead to functional decline in older kidneys may also result in reduced tubular reabsorption of magnesium, thus causing hypomagnesemia. In addition to the age-related changes in the kidney, other comorbidities and drugs (e.g., loop diuretics, digitalis) in older adults can further worsen the magnesium deficiency.[214] On the other hand, hypermagnesemia occurs very rarely, even in the disease setting, including in those with severe acute kidney injury (AKI), CKD, or ESKD.[217] Interestingly, low dietary magnesium intake in older adults may also contribute to a faster rate of decline in the GFR, potentially exacerbating a proinflammatory milieu, endothelial dysfunction, and promotion of vascular calcification.[218]

## CALCIUM HOMEOSTASIS

In normal adults, every day approximately 10 g of calcium is filtered through the glomeruli, and 98% to 99% is reabsorbed, so that net calcium excretion during a 24-hour period ranges from 100 to 200 mg. Most filtered calcium reabsorption (≈60%–70%) occurs in the proximal tubules, around 20% in the loop of Henle (thick ascending limb), around 5% to 10% in the distal convoluted tubule, and only around 5% in the collecting ducts (see also Chapter 18).

There have been several studies of calcium homeostasis with aging. A study of rats in three different age groups has shown that calcium excretion and reabsorption are equally maintained in all three groups, which may be linked to observed age-related renal hypertrophy in older rats.[219] However, other animal studies and studies in humans have shown that there are age-related changes in renal calcium homeostasis, such as decreased tubular reabsorption and/or the renal response to parathyroid hormone (PTH).[220–223] Renal and intestinal calbindins are proteins with a critical role in active transcellular calcium transport, and their expression decreases with age.[224–226] There is also an age-related decrease in the capacity of 1,25-dihydroxyvitamin $D_3$ (1,25-$(OH)_2D_3$) to stimulate calcium reabsorption, increasing PTH levels in both rats and humans.[227,228] A study in mice has found that an age-related reduction in TRPV5 and TRPV6 (renal and duodenal calcium intracellular transporters, respectively) lead to impaired renal and duodenal calcium reabsorption, consistent with the increased calciuria observed in older mice.[229] Alpha-Klotho (α-Klotho) is a gene associated with accelerated aging when mutated.[230] It encodes a protein that is predominantly expressed in tissues involved with calcium homeostasis. A study in mice has demonstrated that alpha-klotho binds to a subunit of sodium-potassium adenosine triphosphatase ($Na^+$-$K^+$-ATPase),[231] suggesting that the age-related decline in klotho protein could contribute to reduced sodium potassium ATPase sensing of low calcium levels. Serum-soluble α-Klotho (sKlotho) levels decline with advancing age in humans, independent of the GFR.[55]

There is also an age-related decrease in intestinal calcium reabsorption, which is linked with reduced 1α-hydroxylase activity, 1,25-$(OH)_2D_3$ levels, and increased basal PTH levels. A study of 22 healthy men has found that older individuals have a twofold higher serum PTH level, with no difference in blood ionized calcium. Moreover, older men also had a higher threshold for PTH release; however, this was not associated with a decrease in blood ionized calcium or 1,25-$(OH)_2D_3$.[232] This finding suggests that the relationship between PTH and calcium in older age is changed so that regardless of calcium concentrations, PTH levels are higher. An interesting study has compared healthy older individuals (≥75 years of age) to patients with CKD and a similar GFR and found that CKD patients have higher serum levels and fractional excretion of calcium, suggesting greater calcium wasting in these patients.[233] Concentrations of vitamin D–dependent calcium-binding proteins also decrease with older age, which is associated with the change in intestinal calcium absorption.[209,224] Another study of healthy young and older men sought to determine whether older age affects renal responsiveness to PTH infusion. The authors found that the renal response to PTH infusion and renal vitamin D levels were equivalent in both groups, with the only difference being that the production of vitamin D is somewhat delayed in older adults.[234]

## PHOSPHORUS HOMEOSTASIS

More than 99% of body phosphorus is stored in the bones and less than 1% is in the serum in the form of inorganic phosphate (Pi). The maintenance of a narrow range of serum Pi levels is critical for numerous cellular functions, including energy metabolism and bone formation, or as a constituent of phospholipids and nucleic acids. Decline in the GFR with older age leads to reduced levels of non–protein-bound (free) serum calcium, but increased levels of serum phosphate.[235] In response to this, PTH synthesis increases, which in turn decreases the number of sodium phosphate cotransporters in the proximal tubules, thus leading to increased phosphaturia. High serum phosphate levels also stimulate the production of fibroblast growth factor 23 (FGF23), which has been suggested to be involved in regulating normal serum phosphate levels during kidney functional decline and suppressing 1,25 $(OH)_2D_3$ formation. FGF23 levels have been found to increase with declining GFR but not with age per se.[55]

In addition to the hormonal regulation of phosphate levels in aging, animal studies have demonstrated a PTH-independent reduction in the intrinsic tubular capacity to reabsorb phosphate.[236] In this study, kidneys of older thyroparathyroidectomized animals responded to pharmacologic dose of PTH to a lesser extent than younger animals.[236] Others have demonstrated that kidneys in aged animals show impaired phosphate transport in renal tubules in response to a low-phosphate diet.[237,238] It has been proposed that the reason for this impaired phosphate transport is decreased fluidity of a luminal brush border membrane due to the age-related increase in cholesterol and sphingomyelin,[238] which then negatively affects sodium phosphate cotransporter activity directly.[239] The same group later showed that acute and chronic changes in cholesterol differentially affected sodium phosphate cotransporter activity.[240] Whereas acute changes in cholesterol modulate the apical membrane expression of sodium phosphate cotransporter (posttranslational regulation), chronic changes modulate the abundance of this cotransporter (translational regulation).[240] Consistent with in vivo studies, an in vitro study of cultured renal tubular cells harvested from young and adult rats has shown reduced phosphate uptake and adaptation to a phosphate-free medium only in the adult renal cells.[241] Another study has revealed that the reason for the age-related decline in tubular phosphate reabsorption and tubular adaptation to a low dietary phosphate is the lower expression of the renal sodium phosphate cotransporters on the apical brush border membrane.[242]

## VITAMIN D HOMEOSTASIS

Older persons commonly exhibit vitamin D insufficiency or deficiency, often in association with a subtle state of chronic inflammation. Serum levels of 25-hydroxyvitamin D (25- [OH]D) are inversely associated with biomarkers of inflammation in older adults, such as C-reactive protein and interleukin 6 (IL-6).[243] It is not known whether these changes are due to primary changes in vitamin D metabolism or to a secondary effect of inflammation. Vitamin D absorption from dietary sources may not be impaired with aging, but reduced dietary intake can contribute to low serum 25-(OH) D levels in aging individuals.[244] The reduced production of 7-deoxyhydrocholestrol in the aging epidermis with ultraviolet exposure is likely involved in the decreased production of pre–vitamin $D_3$ (cholecalciferol) in older adults.[245] Serum 1,25-$(OH)_2D$ (calcitriol) levels decline in aging, at least in part due to the decline in the GFR and impaired hydroxylation of 25-(OH)D mentioned above.[244] Changes in vitamin D sufficiency or insufficiency in older subjects can modulate left ventricular geometry and participate in the risk of left ventricular hypertrophy in hypertensive older subjects.[246]

It is important to keep in mind the age-related changes of 1,25-$(OH)_2D$ metabolism on intestinal phosphate absorption (described earlier), because several studies have shown that dietary vitamin D supplementation improves renal and intestinal phosphate absorption in vitamin D–deficient animals.[247–249] Regarding the previously mentioned role of cholesterol in the fluidity of the apical brush membrane, it appears that deprivation or administration of vitamin D alters the levels of several fatty acids in this membrane.[250] Therefore, age-related changes in 1,25-$(OH)_2D$ production may potentially have an effect on phosphate reabsorption by modulating lipid content in the apical brush membrane.

Thus, aging has diverse effects on calcium, phosphorus, and vitamin D metabolism. These include a decrease in intestinal absorption of calcium, impaired vitamin D production in the skin, dietary vitamin D deficiency, impaired production of 1,25-$(OH)_2D_3$, increased PTH secretion, lower serum Klotho levels, higher FGF23 levels, and alterations in renal tubular handling of calcium and phosphorus.

## ACID-BASE HOMEOSTASIS

The kidneys also play a major role in the regulation of acid-base homeostasis. Normally, during the 24-hour period, kidneys reabsorb around 4500 mmol of filtered bicarbonate. Kidneys have a large capacity to excrete the endogenously generated proton ($H^+$) by generating ammonia ($NH_3$) and its excretion ($NH_4^+$; see Chapter 16). Older adults are more prone to develop acid-base dysregulation for several reasons. First, age-related structural and functional changes in the kidney lead to reduced adaptive responsiveness to dietary and/or environmental changes. Second, the age-related decline in the GFR reduces the capacity of the kidney to buffer metabolic changes and excrete the excess $H^+$ load.[251] Along with age-related kidney functional decline, there is also a reduced capacity for bicarbonate conservation and generation, which, combined with the stable endogenous $H^+$ production, may lead to metabolic acidosis. This process is enhanced and worrisome in patients with concomitant CKD.[252] A community-based observational study of healthy subjects aged 6 to 75 years has found that the capacity for $H^+$ excretion is similar from childhood to young adulthood, but is significantly reduced in older age.[253]

Ammonium excretion decreases with age. Administration of an acute acid load in 26 healthy men of various ages has demonstrated that despite a prompt increase in acid excretion in all of them, the older subjects excreted a much lower percentage of ingested acid.[254] Interestingly, because reduced acid excretion was equivalent to reduced inulin clearance, acid excretion normalized per the GFR was similar in both young and old subjects. Additional studies in four young and four older subjects who, in addition to acid load, received glutamine, showed equivalent responses of young and old kidneys to glutamine.[254] Taken together, it has been suggested that the age-related decrease in $H^+$ excretion is due to reduced renal tubular mass, rather than tubular dysfunction.[254] A study of young and old rats who received an acid load was consistent with the human study.[255] After rats received the acid load, total $H^+$ excretion was reduced in older rats—50% the first day and 25% the second day. Additional insights from this study were the increased activity of the sodium-hydrogen exchanger and decreased phosphate transport in isolated proximal tubules in both age groups.[255]

Overall, these studies suggest that older age appears not to alter the physiologic regulation of acid-base homeostasis but does lead to reduced and diminished responses. The age-related perturbations of acid-base homeostasis seem to influence electrolyte balance. A Swedish study of 85 healthy older individuals has shown an association between net acid excretion and potassium-adjusted magnesuria, irrespective of magnesium intake.[256] Another study of 384 older individuals, followed over 3 years, found that a potassium-rich, alkaline residue (vegetable-rich) diet, which results in increased potassium excretion, was associated with a higher percentage of lean body mass.[257] The protective effect of an alkaline residue diet on muscle mass in older adults is consistent with the opposing effect of an acid residue (red meat-rich) diet. A study of nearly 10,000 participants in the general population has found that a higher dietary acid load is associated with lower serum bicarbonate concentrations; the association is much stronger in middle-aged and older than younger individuals.[258] Consistent with this, a study of older patients with CKD has found that oral sodium bicarbonate supplementation corrects metabolic acidosis, improves serum albumin levels, and decreases whole-body protein degradation.[259] Potassium bicarbonate supplementation in postmenopausal women neutralized the endogenous acid, improved calcium and phosphate balance, and reduced bone reabsorption.[260] This was confirmed in a more recent double-blind study of older men and women—in which particularly bicarbonate and not potassium—had a protective effect on bone reabsorption and calcium excretion.[261] Another recent randomized, double-blind, placebo-controlled study of 52 healthy older men and women has found that oral potassium citrate neutralizes the dietary acid load and has a long-lasting effect to reduce calciuria, without affecting gastrointestinal calcium absorption.[262] Taken together, the results of several studies are consistent with the hypothesis that a higher alkaline residue (vegetarian) diet prevents bone loss in older individuals.

## WATER HOMEOSTASIS

Water homeostasis is regulated by a high-gain feedback mechanism that involves the hypothalamus, neurohypophysis, and kidneys.[263,264] In kidneys, the water and sodium from the glomerular filtrate are reabsorbed in tubules through water channel aquaporins (AQPs) and sodium cotransporters.[265–267] The tubular reabsorption of water primarily depends on the driving force (high interstitial osmolality in the deeper medullary zones) and osmotic equilibrium of water across the tubular epithelia (high osmotic water permeability of the membrane). The large majority of glomerular filtrate is reabsorbed in the proximal tubules and descending thin limbs of the loop of Henle.[266,268] The next tubular segments (thin and thick ascending limbs and distal convoluted tubules) are relatively water-impermeable.[269,270] Finally, the main parts of the nephron where vasopressin-based regulation of body water homeostasis occurs are the connecting tubule and collecting duct[271–273] (see also Chapter 15). Both maximum urinary concentration and diluting capacity are decreased by aging,[274] leading to a higher risk for hypernatremia and hyponatremia, respectively.

Findley has proposed an age-related dysfunction of the hypothalamic-renal axis based on clinical observations of increased vasopressin secretion in older age.[275] With older age, maximal urine concentrating ability is particularly reduced.[274] Compared with younger individuals, older adults have about a 50% reduced capacity to conserve water and solutes. Due to the combined effect of age-related changes in body composition, progressive microstructural changes in the kidney, and changes in plasma osmolality and fluid volume, some older adults are more prone to developing disturbances in water homeostasis. One of the major changes in body composition is an increase in total fraction of body fat by 5% to 10% and an equivalent decrease in total body water, so that an older man on average has 7 to 8 fewer liters of total body water than a young man with the same body weight.[276] The obvious consequence is that in the event of acute loss, or overload of body water, a more severe change in osmolality will occur in older men. A study comparing plasma osmolality in older and younger individuals before and after a similar extent of water deprivation has confirmed this presumption.[277] Alterations in water and sodium balance frequently lead to hypo- or hypernatremia associated with hypo- or hypervolemia in older adults.[278,279] In addition, dysfunction in water homeostasis may also occur due to abnormal expression and trafficking of AQPs and solute transporters. For example, an animal study has shown that the AQP2 transporter involved in urine-concentrating ability is downregulated in the medulla of older rats.[280] This molecular mechanism is consistent with a reduced urine-concentrating ability in older adults. Water homeostasis is also influenced by the previously described microstructural changes that occur with the aging kidney. These changes occurring with healthy aging do not pose an acute threat or have an impact while an individual is healthy. However, in the event of stress, acute disease, volume load, or dehydration, the combined effects of age-related loss of renal mass (i.e., functional reserve) and the change in body composition may cause a significant disruption in water and solute homeostasis.[281,282]

One of the consequences of the age-related GFR decline is an increase in filtrate reabsorption in the proximal tubules and decreased fluid delivery to the distal diluting tubules, resulting in a reduced diluting capacity of the kidney.[283] This is evidenced by a reduced ability to excrete a free water load[277] or reduced maximal free water clearance in older adults.[283] In addition to the reduced diluting capacity, older kidneys also lose the capacity to conserve water during states of dehydration.[284] Interestingly, another study has demonstrated that the reduced capacity of water conservation occurs regardless of high plasma vasopressin levels; thus, this is most likely due to intrinsic renal factors.[285] Taken together, therefore, these age-related changes may have significant clinical implications, such as worsening of dehydration in older adults in the setting of vomiting, diarrhea, or reduced water and food intake.

Vasopressin secretion, the renal response to vasopressin, and thirst control are also affected by aging. Vasopressin secretion in the hypothalamus is under the delicate control of osmoreceptors in and around the organum vasculosum of the lamina terminalis and the anterior wall of the third ventricle in the brain. Most studies have found that basal vasopressin concentrations in the healthy older are usually higher than in younger controls.[276] One study has reported no age-related differences in basal vasopressin levels,[286] whereas another study has found that basal vasopressin may actually be lower in older individuals.[287] Nevertheless, most studies about water homeostasis in aging have shown that compared with younger individuals, older adults have a greater increase of vasopressin secretion per unit change in plasma osmolality, and this is consistent with the higher osmoreceptor sensitivity in older adults.[288]

Vasopressin regulates renal water excretion by controlling the abundance of the water channel AQP2 and its insertion into the apical membrane of epithelial cells in the distal nephron and collecting tubules.[289] In the membrane, AQP2 proteins form channels that allow reabsorption of water molecules from the lumen of the collecting ducts into the medullary interstitium driven by the medullary osmotic gradient. Given that vasopressin levels are mostly found to be higher in older adults, a potential secretory defect in the pituitary gland is improbable and cannot explain the age-related reduced renal response to vasopressin. Animal studies have offered potential explanations for the reduced renal response to vasopressin, which include reduced expression of vasopressin receptors in the collecting ducts and impaired second messenger response to vasopressin receptor signaling. One study has demonstrated that despite a normal vasopressin secretory response, there is an age-related reduction in renal concentrating ability after moderate water restriction.[290] This occurred due to the lower expression of AQP2 water channels in older rats and an impaired ability to upregulate AQP2 production. Other animal studies have proposed that reduced vasopressin receptor signaling significantly hinders the medullary concentrating gradient required for urine concentration.[289,290]

Normally, stimulation of thirst osmoreceptors in the hypothalamus signals the higher cerebral cortex to develop a conscious perception of thirst and water-seeking behavior. Aging also affects thirst control.[291] One study has demonstrated that water-deprived older men do not show a subjective thirst increase or mouth dryness.[287] Moreover, when access to water was allowed, compared with younger participants, older adults consumed less water and were unable to restore serum and plasma osmolality to predeprivation levels.[287] This finding suggests that older adults have a reduced thirst response to osmotic changes. It has been proposed that they may have a higher osmolal set point for thirst—that is, for a given plasma osmolality, older adults have a reduced degree of perceived thirst, thus leading to less water intake.[292] Maximum diluting capacity is mildly impaired in older adults, largely a reflection of the reduced GFR.[293] The minimum urinary osmolality (Uosm) after a water load averages about 90 mOsm/kg $H_2O$ in subjects older than 70 years, whereas in younger subjects the value is about 50 mOsm/kg $H_2O$. If solute excretion is reduced (e.g., with protein or salt restriction), the mild impairment of diluting capacity can expose older patients to water excess syndromes (hyponatremia), with only modest intakes of free water. For example, at a Uosm of 90 mOsm/kg $H_2O$ (maximum dilution in older adults) and a daily osmolal excretion of 360 mOsm/day (about half of normal levels), the maximal electrolyte free water intake would be about 4 L/day. Any free water intake in excess of this value would lead to dilutional hyponatremia.

Thus, aging undoubtedly influences water homeostasis in many different ways. Water conservation (urinary concentrating ability) is primarily affected, although a mild form of impaired diluting capacity may also be present. This is important to keep in mind, not only during the diagnostic process, but also while taking care of older adults and planning for different clinical, surgical, or pharmacologic interventions. Alterations in solute intake (e.g., protein or sodium) in older adults can also have profound effects on water homeostasis.

## RENAL ENDOCRINE CHANGES WITH AGING

### RENIN-ANGIOTENSIN-ALDOSTERONE SYSTEM

Aging is associated with a decline in plasma renin activity (PRA), serum aldosterone levels, and urinary aldosterone excretion rates, accompanied by reduced responses to actions that stimulate the RAAS, such as upright posture or salt depletion.[62,63] This state is known as *aging-associated hyporeninemic hypoaldosteronism*. Both renal renin formation and release are reduced in aging.[294] In addition, activity of the RAAS has been linked to aging phenomena in a pathogenic fashion.[295] Defects in renal NO generation can be linked to reduced activity of the RAAS in aging.[10] The activity of the RAAS can also be linked to canonical Wnt signaling,[10] and both can be dysregulated in the aging process.[8] Although a decline in activity of the RAAS regularly occurs with aging (independently of gender), neither a change in renal perfusion pressure or delivery of solute to the macula densa appears to be involved.[10] Increased ANP levels, reduced sympathetic nervous system activity, or both can be seen with aging and might be involved in the perturbations of the RAAS seen with aging.[10] Reduced renal renin generation with aging appears to be a posttranslational phenomenon due to impaired release of stored renin.[10] Trivial changes in ACE activity and angiotensinogen conversion occur in aging.[10] The sensitivity of the glomerular afferent and efferent vessels to angiotensin II appear to increase with aging.[10] Treatment of animals (rats) with an age-dependent decline in renal function and proteinuria can reduce proteinuria and glomerulosclerosis, but this does not have any effect on glomerulomegaly or the snGFR.[8,10] Distinguishing the effects of aging per se and superimposed disease states (e.g., low nephron endowment) on the RAAS can be very difficult.

Aldosterone production and serum and urinary aldosterone levels are lower in older adults compared with younger persons,[296] and there may also be reduced aldosterone responsivity to elevations in serum potassium levels.[297] In addition, there are age-related changes in adrenal aldosterone synthetase–producing cells, causing islands or clusters of aldosterone-producing cells in the adrenal cortex of aging humans. These may be precursors of aldosterone-secreting adenomas in some cases.[296]

## ERYTHROPOIETIN

Serum levels of erythropoietin (EPO) levels tend to increase with age, even in nonanemic subjects.[297,298] This might be in compensation for increased (subclinical) blood loss, accelerated red blood cell turnover (decreased erythrocyte half-life), or increased resistance of red cell precursors to the effect of EPO.[298] Testosterone deficiency might be involved in the latter phenomenon.[299] A mild anemia (hemoglobin <12 g/dL) is fairly common in aging, but this varies by geography.[300] In about one-third of these subjects, a nutritional deficiency (e.g., iron, folate, vitamin $B_{12}$) is responsible, in one-third, a concomitant chronic disease is the culprit (e.g., CKD, cancer, infection), but in one-third no precise cause can be determined.[300] Independent of anemia, high spontaneous EPO levels in older adults are associated with an increased risk of congestive heart failure, but not myocardial infarction or progressive CKD.[301] The mechanisms responsible for this association are not well understood, but could be due to tissue hypoxia in low-perfusion states associated with heart failure.

# IMPLICATIONS OF NORMAL PHYSIOLOGY ON RENAL FUNCTION

This has effects on the diagnosis and prognosis of chronic kidney disease in aging adults.

## DIAGNOSIS

The diagnosis of CKD has been codified by the Kidney Disease Outcomes Quality Initiative (KDOQI) and Kidney Disease: Improving Global Outcomes (KDIGO) clinical practice guideline initiatives,[302,303] published in 2002 and 2013, respectively, as well as others from more regional formulations, such as NICE in the United Kingdom and CARI in Australia.[304,305] These classification and categorization recommendations rely principally on the GFR (estimated or measured, in mL/min/1.73 m$^2$) and albuminuria (usually the urinary albumin-to-creatinine ratio [uACR], in mg/g or mg/mmol] in spot urine samples; see also Chapters 23 and 30). However, other signs of renal injury, such as abnormal urinalyses (e.g., hematuria), imaging, or renal biopsy findings could lead to a diagnosis of CKD, even with a normal GFR (even adjusted for age) or uACR. Abnormalities in these biomarkers must persist for at least 3 months to qualify as a valid indicator of CKD, a requirement that is frequently not met in many epidemiologic studies that are carried out only once. When these classification schemes were developed, it was arbitrarily decided that any adult subject, 20 years of age or older, with a persisting GFR of less than 60 mL/min/1.73 m$^2$, could be classified as having CKD (category 3A, 3B, 4, or 5), irrespective of any other signs of renal injury, including abnormal urinalysis, albuminuria, imaging, or renal pathology. Thus, a persisting GFR of 45 to 59 mL/min/1.73$^2$ could lead to a diagnosis of CKD (category 3A) in an adult. This guideline created a conundrum because values of the GFR in this range can also be observed in healthy older adults. The lower limit of normal for the measured GFR (mGFR) in a healthy adult 60 to 69 years of age is about 55 mL/min/1.73 m$^2$ and, for an adult 70 to 79 years of age, it is about 49 mL/min/1.73 m$^2$.[133] Significant overlap is present between the threshold for classifying CKD (independent of age) and the normal values for GFR in older adults. The lower value for the GFR in older adults is a manifestation of a physiologic process of nephron loss unaccompanied by compensatory hyperfiltration in the residual nephrons (see above), so it is difficult to conflate these findings as a disease. Not surprisingly, a substantial and continuing debate has arisen concerning the utility of an absolute threshold for defining CKD, based on the GFR alone, without any modification for age.[306–310] Because abnormal albuminuria is not consistent with normal, healthy human aging, this controversy largely focuses on possible overdiagnosis in older adults of the G3A/a1 category of CKD (GFR, 45 to 59 mL/min/1.73 m$^2$ and uACR of <30 mg/g [3 mg/mmol]) according to KDIGO.[311] The GFR may fall below 45 mL/min/1.73 m$^2$ in subjects older than 80 years, but it can be very difficult to determine if such subjects are entirely healthy because they frequently have concomitant disorders, such as cancer, heart failure, dietary protein deficiency, and sarcopenia. This can complicate evaluation of the GFR (mGFR or eGFR). In addition, significant comorbidity and biochemical abnormalities are commonly observed in individuals older than 60 years of age, compounding the difficulty of ascertaining kidney health based on the GFR alone.[312,313]

Typically, the GFR values used in categorizing CKD are estimates rather than measured values. This use of estimating formulas for the GFR (eGFR) results in another conundrum in the diagnosis of CKD in aging—namely, the imprecision and variability in eGFR formulas for evaluating the true GFR in older adults[312] (discussed further in Chapters 59 and 84). In a population-wide study of community-living adults, Ebert and coworkers[312] found the prevalence of CKD categories 3, 4, and 5 (eGFR <60 mL/min/1.73 m$^2$) in subjects 70 to 79 years of age to range between 16% and 52%, depending on the formula used to estimate the GFR. The corresponding value for subjects 80 to 89 years of age were 42% to 84%.

The lowest values for CKD prevalence were found using the CKD-EPI creatinine equation; the highest values were found using the Berlin Initiative Study (BIS)-1 creatinine equation.[312] In subjects older than 70 years of age, the BIS-1 creatine equation is a more precise estimate of mGFR compared with the CKD-EPI equation, at least in a European, largely white population.[314] Estimating formulas for GFR when applied at the population level generally give high values for CKD prevalence (≈11%– 14%),[315] especially when the formulas were derived from a largely CKD cohort. Much lower values for CKD are observed when eGFR formulas are derived from a normal healthy cohort[316]

The use of cystatin C–based GFR estimating equations (alone or in combination with creatinine-based equations) has been advanced as a tool to aid in the diagnosis of CKD. In 2012, KDIGO suggested measuring eGFR-creatinine-cystatin C and eGFR-cystatin C in adults (including older adults) when the eGFR-creatinine is 45 to 59 mL/min/1.73 $m^2$ (and no other markers of CKD are present). If eGFR-cystatin C or eGFR-creatinine-cystatin C are less than 60 mL/min/1.73 $m^2$, the diagnosis of CKD is confirmed.[303] The degree to which these suggestions specifically apply to older adults has not been rigorously tested and may depend on the form of the eGFR-cystatin C or eGFR-creatinine-cystatin C equation. For example, in older adults, the BIS-2 cystatin C equation is a more accurate estimate of mGFR than the CKD-EPI-cystatin C equation.[314] Other eGFR equations, such as the FAS-creatinine, FAS-cystatin C equation, or Lund-Malmo creatinine equation need further evaluation for improving the precision and accuracy of the diagnosis of CKD in older adults using the eGFR alone, but early studies have shown great promise for the utility of these equations in an older population.[317]

It must also be recalled that cystatin C is a mid-molecular-weight (13.3 kD) serine proteinase inhibitor involved in the inflammatory response.[318] It is normally filtered and then completely destroyed by tubular reabsorption and degradation. Very little cystatin C is present in normal urine. Thus, production rates of cystatin C are difficult to assess and can vary in many states (e.g., obesity, diabetes, thyroid disease, inflammation) commonly found in older adults. Like creatinine, there are many non-GFR determinants of its serum concentration, the variable used in calculation of the eGFR.[319,320] In older adults, loss of muscle mass (sarcopenia) may lower serum creatinine values relative to the measured GFR and give rise to an overestimate of mGFR by eGFR creatinine equations. However, serum cystatin C levels tend not be affected greatly by muscle mass or gender, and not at all by ancestry. In contrast, in older adults with chronic inflammation (of any cause), obesity, diabetes, and the metabolic syndrome may alter cystatin C production, leading to underestimation of the mGFR. The combination of eGFR-creatinine-cystatin C may give a slightly more accurate assessment of the true GFR in population-based studies,[321] but there will still be much individual variation.[322–324] Tracking eGFR-cystatin C with metabolic factors that can contribute to CVD complicates its suitability as a biomarker for CVD risk related to the GFR in older adults.[325] In addition, endothelial injury consequent to inflammation or capillary hypertension might further impair the transglomerular permeability coefficient for cystatin C (the shrunken pore theory),[326] giving rise to reduced cystatin C eGFR values relative to the inulin or iohexol mGFR.[326] Furthermore, a low serum albumin level (perhaps reflecting subtle degrees of chronic inflammation) is associated with reduced eGFR-creatinine in older frail subjects.[327]

Direct comparisons of a gold standard method of measuring the GFR and estimating formulas for the GFR in aging subjects are relatively uncommon, but both the BIS[314] and Reykjavik older cohort studies[322] have provided much valuable information. In the latter study, the Lund-Malmo and full age spectrum (FAS) creatinine equation have somewhat higher accuracy than the CKD-EPI-creatinine formula. The CKD-EPI, Lund-Malmo, and FAS creatinine-based equations were roughly equivalent for the detection of a mGFR less than 60 mL/min/1.73 $m^2$. All formulas incorporating a cystatin C measurement exhibited consistent improvements in accuracy compared with the corresponding creatinine-based equations. The relevance of these findings to the diagnosis of CKD in individual older subjects needs further study, but they clearly demonstrate some of the pitfalls in using creatinine-based eGFR formulas for the older adult population.

Thus, the effects of physiologic renal aging on the GFR confound its use as the defining characteristic of CKD in older adults because CKD is a diagnosis made most frequently in older adults with category 3A CKD (GFR, 45–59 mL/min/1.73 $m^2$), usually with normal albuminuria (category A1; uACR <30 mg/g [3 mg/mmol]). This conundrum raises an issue of possible overdiagnosis and mislabeling of CKD, both at the individual and population-wide level, that distorts evaluation of the true societal burden of CKD. When added to the false-positive identification of CKD in single epidemiologic studies (see above), this leads to the possibility that CKD is not as common as it is alleged to be, and calls for revising the definition of CKD in older adults should be taken seriously. The vagaries of estimating equations for the GFR in older adults cannot be ignored.[328]

## PROGNOSIS

In the KDIGO classification of CKD, the prognosis for adverse events (all-cause mortality, ESKD, doubling of serum creatinine level, CVD [e.g., ischemic heart disease, congestive heart failure, stroke]) is the third dimension of the scheme. This is usually displayed as a multicolored heat map of the rising risk of events—green, no added risk; red, high risk—often determined from large-scale epidemiologic studies.[302,303] The risk values are usually stated as relative risk or odds ratio compared with some arbitrary control group, often those with eGFR greater than 60 mL/min/1.73 $m^2$ and no signs of renal injury (e.g., normal uACR). These prognosis- based heat maps are commonly assembled from data acquired from single time point epidemiologic studies, so that the persistence of the CKD-defining abnormality (eGFR, uACR, or both) is not confirmed. When a more rigorous assessment of chronicity is pursued, it has been noted that such single time point studies commonly overestimate the prevalence of CKD by as much as 30% due to false-positives.[329]

The use of the eGFR to evaluate prognosis is also confounded by the fact that an age variable is included in all adult estimating formulas to adjust for the effects of age per se on the synthesis and production biomarker (creatinine or cystatin C). The age coefficients in these formulas are optimized for estimating the mGFR, not prognostication for all-cause mortality or ESKD risk. However, when the values obtained by such estimates are applied to prognostication, the age variable becomes important, because age, independent of the GFR, has a marked influence on some of the risks evaluated, such as mortality. If an estimating equation using one or more biomarkers that accurately assess GFR, without a requirement for the age variable, were developed, the accuracy of the risk prediction might be improved and made comparable to that found with the true GFR. It should be stressed that although the number and size of studies using the mGFR as the dependent variable in prognostic evaluation are relatively small in comparison to the large-scale, eGFR-based epidemiologic studies, the patterns linking the GFR to outcome are similar. These studies describe a pattern of a threshold (nonlinear) relationship, in which the threshold varies according to age.[330] With albuminuria, the risks varies in a log-linear fashion with the uACR, independent of age, and without a threshold (above normal values). When one compares the relative risk of all-cause mortality using a reference value for the GFR that approximates the normal young adult mean value (≈107 mL/min/1.73 $m^2$), then the minimum relative risk for an all-cause mortality event is above an eGFR of 75 mL/min/1.73 $m^2$ for subjects 18 to 54 years of age, but above 45 mL/min/1.73 $m^2$ for those older than 75 years.[331] The relative risk of all-cause mortality relative to a declining eGFR is blunted by advancing age, but the absolute rates of all-cause mortality remain high with aging. This analysis strongly suggests that with a prognosis-dominated matrix for creating a GFR threshold for CKD, an age-stratified approach is desirable. It is noteworthy that the remaining life expectancy at any age older than about 35 years is not materially affected until the eGFR falls below about 45 mL/min/1.73 $m^2$.[332–334] Adding an age stratification to the existing scheme for identifying true CKD and its associated risks has proven to be a challenging task. Simple adjustments, such as altering the threshold of eGFR to <45 mL/min/1.73 $m^2$ for subjects without abnormal albuminuria who are older than 65 years, may be useful, but result in unintended consequences, like the so-called birthday paradox (when a 64-year-old reaches a 65th birthday, CKD is "cured").

Other methods of age stratification for CKD diagnosis have been advanced that may have greater practicality in large health care systems for improved triage.[335] Creation of multiple age-stratified heat maps using the eGFR and estimates of prognosis for all-cause mortality may also be helpful.[336] Whatever the solution may be to this ongoing conundrum of defining CKD and its risks in aging subjects, it is imperative also to recognize that the specific formula for identifying the eGFR as the variable introduces a complexity of its own due to the variability of bias, precision, and accuracy among the numerous estimating formulas and biomarkers used, especially when applied to older adults. For example, the eGFR-creatinine formulas do not add much to the prediction of CVD (and thereby all-cause mortality) risk in older adults, whereas eGFR-cystatin C formulas do, despite not being superior to eGFR-creatinine for estimating the mGFR.[325] Both formulas can incrementally increase the accuracy of CVD risk prediction (see later).

## CARDIOVASCULAR DISEASE AND DECLINE IN THE GLOMERULAR FILTRATION RATE WITH AGING

There is little doubt that a progressive decline in the GFR is associated with an increased risk of fatal or nonfatal CVD, including atherosclerotic CVD and congestive heart failure (CHF), sudden cardiac death, nonvalvular atrial fibrillation, stroke, and peripheral vascular disease. Cross-sectional, population-based epidemiologic studies cannot easily determine whether these associations are causal or not. In fact, the existence of CVD may itself result in a decline in the GFR (e.g., severe CHF, atherosclerotic renovascular diseases, ischemic nephropathy), thus confounding the directional nature of the observed associations. Aging itself can be a mechanism for some of the associations between a decline in the GFR and CVD, but this can be adjusted for by examining the CVD prevalence in older subjects with a better-preserved GFR. However, the fact that the GFR declines regularly with aging requires that the comparator group used for such adjustments have GFR values (on average) similar to those predicted for by normal physiologic aging. Teasing out age-related GFR decline from pathologic GFR decline in an aging individual can be difficult, but the demonstration of other biomarkers of renal injury, such as the presence of abnormal albuminuria or abnormal imaging, can be very helpful (abnormal albuminuria does not occur with healthy aging).[91] The threshold for a GFR-related augmentation of CVD risk is likely to be age-dependent. In studies of older individuals, the risk of excess CVD events seem to appear at an eGFR less than 45 mL/min/1.73 $m^2$ (category 3B CKD),[333] but this will likely be modified by the nature and severity of comorbidities present, such as dyslipidemia, diabetes, or long-standing hypertension. A decreased GFR can influence the risk of CVD, independent of the traditional risk factors (e.g., obesity, smoking, dyslipidemia, diabetes, hypertension), but the magnitude of the additional risk for CVD events imposed by a reduced GFR in the range of 45 to 59 mL/min/1.73 $m^2$ is small in older adults. For this reason, a reduced GFR is not commonly included in CVD risk prediction scoring systems (e.g., Framingham Risk Score, American College of Cardiology/American Heart Association [ACC/AHA] pooled risk prediction model).[337]

As discussed in detail in other chapters (see Chapters 40 and 54), more advanced forms of CKD can augment the CVD risk by numerous mechanisms, including endothelial cell or vascular wall injury from uremic toxins, vascular ossification, myocardial hypertrophy and pathologic remodeling, chronic volume expansion, chronic inflammation, uremic dyslipidemia (proatherogenic high-density lipoprotein [HDL], hypertriglyceridemia), arterial hypertension, and thrombotic microangiopathy. The fundamental phenomenon of aging can interact with these pathologic processes in numerous ways that are very difficult to disentangle unambiguously.

## END-STAGE RENAL DISEASE AND AGING

A requirement for treatment by renal replacement modalities (renal replacement therapy [RRT]; dialysis and/or transplantation) is not uncommon in older adults. According to the US Renal Data System (USRDS) Annual Report in 2017, the age-specific annual incidence rate for RRT for subjects 75 years of age or older was about 1600 per million population (pmp) and, for those 65 to 74 years of age, was about 1250 pmp in 2015 (www.usrds.org). Both these values have been slowly declining (for uncertain reasons) since about 2010 but are still well above the average (all-age) RRT incident rate of 378 pmp/year. As has been the case for many years, males outnumber females for incident counts of RRT by about 20% to 30%. For pre-ESKD CKD, the male-to-female ratio is exactly the opposite (www.usrds.org). However, this may in part be artifactual due to the gender coefficient in eGFR creatinine equations, which give women lower eGFR values, and the lower muscle mass in women than men, which increases their ACR. The precursors of ESKD are the earlier stages (categories) of CKD, some of which progress, at varying rates, to ESKD. An important consideration of the development of RRT requiring ESKD is the competing risk of death, usually from a CVD or neoplasia event. This risk is magnified in older adults so that at an advanced age, any patient with CKD category 3 (eGFR, 30–59 mL/min/1.73 m$^2$) is more likely to die before reaching ESKD.[338]

In a landmark study, Eriksen and Ingebretsen conducted a 10-year, population- based study in Tromso, Norway, including subjects (median age, 75 years; interquartile range [IQR], 67.7–80.4 years) with confirmed CKD category 3.[340] About 70% of the subjects experienced some decline in the eGFR over time, somewhat slower in females than in males. The 10-year cumulative risk of reaching treated ESKD was 4% (greater in men than in women), whereas the cumulative risk of death was 51% (greater in men than in women). The prognosis of CKD and the eventual likelihood of requiring RRT was highly gender-dependent and greatly influenced by the competing risk of death. In another key study, O'Hare and coworkers[338] studied 209,622 US veterans (97% male; mean age, 73 ± 9 years) with category 3 to 5 CKD followed for a mean of 3.2 years. Although the rates of death and ESKD were inversely related to the eGFR value at baseline irrespective of age, at comparable levels of eGFR, older age was associated with higher death rates and a lower rate of ESKD treatment. The threshold of eGFR below which the rate of ESKD exceeded the risk of death was about 15 mL/min/1.73 m$^2$ for subjects 65 to 84 years of age. As with the Eriksen and Ingebretsen study,[340] the rate of decline of the eGFR was slower in the older subjects. The effect of gender could not be examined in this study. Nevertheless, both these studies clearly indicated that both age and gender are important modifying factors for the transition from CKD (category 3–5) to treated ESKD.

The impact of age on the association of eGFR and albuminuria on outcomes of mortality and treated ESKD were also studied in an exhaustive analysis of 2,051,244 participants from 33 general population or high-risk CVD cohorts and 13 CKD cohorts by Hallan and colleagues in the CKD Prognosis Consortium.[330] In most of these cohorts, the eGFR values were determined only once, and CKD was not confirmed by the duration criteria, leading to the possibility of a high false-positive rate for the identification of CKD. In addition, the analysis used a single reference value of 80 mL/min/1.73 m$^2$ for the eGFR. The study showed a roughly comparable hazard ratio for the risk of ESKD with declining eGFR at all ages, but the average absolute rate of ESKD declined substantially with age as a function of the declining eGFR, consistent with the observations discussed above. The relative and absolute risks for ESKD both increased as the uACR rose above 10 mg/g, but the magnitude of these risks were somewhat blunted in much older adults (>75 years). Although a threshold of about 60 mL/min/1.73 m$^2$ was noted for defining an increased relative risk of ESKD at all ages, the choice of a single reference comparator of 80 mL/min/1.73 m$^2$ (rather than the lowest risk group for age as the reference comparator) might have influenced the findings, as discussed above in relationship to the impact of the eGFR on all-cause mortality at varying ages). It is noteworthy that the absolute rate of ESKD in the very old (>75 years) did not increase above baseline values until the eGFR was well below 45 mL/min/1.73 m$^2$.

In a longitudinal study conducted by Shardlow and colleagues[341,342] in the United Kingdom, older subjects (mean age, 73 years) with category 3 CKD (mean eGFR, 53 mL/min/1.73 m$^2$) had a low prevalence of abnormal albuminuria (16%). After 5 years of additional follow-up, they had a low prevalence of ESKD (0.2%), progression to a higher stage of CKD occurred in 17.7%, remissions of CKD developed in 19.3%, and stable renal function was observed in 34.1%. Albuminuria at diagnosis was a key risk factor for progression. In this study, 14.2% died before the 5-year follow-up and 14.8% were lost to follow-up.

## ACUTE KIDNEY INJURY AND DISEASES OF THE KIDNEY AND URINARY TRACT IN AGING

A strong relationship exists between the incidence and prevalence of AKI and age.[343] The pathophysiologic mechanisms underlying this association are complex and multifactorial (discussed further in Chapter 28). The physiologic reduction of nephron number and GFR with advancing age, discussed above, alters the pharmacokinetics of many water-soluble drugs. This can lead to an accumulation of nephrotoxic levels of agents in body fluids, leading to AKI.[344] Dosage modifications, primarily in the interval between dosing, rather than in loading dosage, are required to minimize such risks.[198] Agents that affect glomerular hemodynamics, such as NSAIDs or RAAS inhibitors, can cause a reduction in the GFR in aging subjects that is more profound than in younger subjects, particularly when combined with some degree of extracellular volume depletion. Older subjects also may have a comorbidity that exposes them to an episode of AKI, such as CHF, diabetes, urosepsis, and cancer, and require more interventions that may predispose to AKI, such as surgery and angiography. As discussed later, aging is also associated with an increased prevalence of diseases of the kidney and urinary tract that may directly cause AKI.

### DISEASES OF THE KIDNEY AND URINARY TRACT IN AGING

The occurrence of specific diseases of the kidneys and urinary tract can be influenced markedly by the age of a subject. These diseases are discussed in detail in Chapters 36, 37, and 41 and will not be elaborated further here. Certain glomerular and vascular diseases have a predilection to affect older adults (Box 22.2).[31,345–347] Benign prostatic hypertrophy is common in older men and can result in lower urinary tract obstruction and CKD, sometimes irreversible. Obstructive uropathy can also be the consequence of ureteric involvement in gynecologic cancer in older women and bladder dysfunction associated with neurologic diseases and diabetes.

**Box 22.2 Kidney and Urinary Tract Diseases That Occur More Commonly in Older Adults**

**Glomerular and Vascular Diseases**

Crescentic glomerulonephritis due to systemic or renal-limited antineutrophil cytoplasmic autoantibody (ANCA)–associated vasculitis
Membranous nephropathy (primary and cancer-related)
Monoclonal immunoglobulin deposition diseases (AL amyloidosis and nonamyloid types)
Diabetic nephropathy
Fibrillary glomerulonephritis
Anti–glomerular basement membrane (GBM) disease (mainly females)
Atheroembolic disease
Atheromatous renovascular stenosis

**Tubulointerstitial Diseases**

Acute kidney injury (toxic or ischemic cause)
Lymphomatous infiltration
Renal cell cancer

**Urinary Tract Disorders**

Lower urinary tract obstruction due to prostate disease
Ureteric obstruction from cancer (cervical cancer in females)
Transitional cell carcinoma of the bladder
Prostate cancer

## CAN RENAL AGING BE MODIFIED?

As the molecular mechanisms of organ senescence are gradually revealed, it is natural to ask about their potential for modification.[348–351] This is a difficult question because the biologic processes are so complex and are active over an extended time period. In addition, it is necessary to make a clear distinction between the effects of interventions directed at diseases associated with aging (e.g., better glycemic control in diabetes, avoidance of obesity, control of hypertension) and the modification of the fundamental aging process itself. So far, no elixir of life or "fountain of youth" has been discovered, but several promising avenues have been identified. Caloric restriction, mTOR inhibition, and RAAS blockade all retard aging across many animal species,[352] but their effects in humans are less well understood for obvious reasons. It is possible that all three of these approaches converge on mitochondrial energy production to slow aging. The angiotensin II type I receptor may play a pivotal role in renal senility,[352] independent of angiotensin II, perhaps via a sirtuin-linked mechanism.[352,353] However, because normal healthy aging, with the steady attrition of glomeruli, is not usually accompanied by albuminuria or a rise in the snGFR (see above), the prospects of RAAS inhibition as a means of retarding the rate of renal aging are not promising. Caloric restriction seems to cause a reduction in renal fibrosis (via mTOR inhibition and 5'-adenosine monophosphate-activated protein kinase [AMPK] activation).[35,353] Calorie restriction and mTOR inhibition activates sirtuin 1, which has antiaging properties. Other agents, such as the biguanide metformin, may also have antiaging effects via an action on the AMPK/mTOR pathway.[354] Telomere shortening can be modulated by telomerase activity, but whether the manipulation of telomere length will be safe and effective in delaying organ senescence is unknown. Modulating Klotho expression pharmacologically might have beneficial effects, via reduced oxidative stress. Elimination of senescent cells (senolytic therapy) by targeting apoptosis of senescent cells (TASCs) via disruption of the FOX04 peptide-p53 interaction, shows great promise in improving renal function in aging mice.[355,356] Resveratrol, a polyphenol present in many pigmented vegetables and fruits, can ameliorate aging as a calorie restriction mimetic, possibly by improving the metabolic profile and inhibiting cyclic adenosine monophosphate (cAMP) phosphodiesterases and the AMPK pathway.[357] Because an imbalance of energy demand and energy supply may underlie aging, a reprogramming of metabolism from anaerobic glycolysis to aerobic glycolysis might be an effective strategy.[5] Antifibrosis regimens, such as with the transforming growth factor beta (TGF-β)/smad pathway inhibition, BMP-7 administration, or the use of other agents, represents a promising avenue of research,[339,358] especially in the domain of renal aging. Translating studies carried out in lower animals (e.g., *Caenorhabditis elegans*, mice, rats) to the human organism will be tedious, time-consuming, and fraught with obstacles. Armed with new tools, however, such as nephron number quantification, it may be possible to test some of the most promising strategies directly in humans. Hopefully, in the not too distant future, renal aging will not be inevitable, even though immortality will of course continue to be an elusive goal.

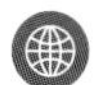
Complete reference list available at ExpertConsult.com.

## KEY REFERENCES


2. Robert L, Fulop T. Aging: facts and theories. *Interdiscip Top Gerontol.* 2014;39:1–215.
7. Epstein M. Aging and the kidney. *J Am Soc Nephrol.* 1996;7(8):1106–1122. Review.
23. Bitzer M, Wiggins J. Aging biology in the kidney. *Adv Chronic Kidney Dis.* 2016;23(1):12–18. doi:10.1053/j.ackd.2015.11.005. Review.
30. Choudhury D, Levi M. Aging and kidney Disease. In: *Brenner and Rector, the Kidney.* 10th ed. New York: Elsevier; 2015:727–751.
60. Yang HC, Fogo AB. Fibrosis and renal aging. *Kidney Int Suppl (2011).* 2014;4(1):75–78. Review.
63. Conti S, Cassis P, Benigni A. Aging and the renin-angiotensin system. *Hypertension.* 2012;60(4):878–883. [Epub 2012 Aug 27]; Review.
68. Inker LA, Okparavero A, Tighiouart H, et al. Midlife blood pressure and late-life GFR and albuminuria: an elderly general population cohort. *Am J Kidney Dis.* 2015;66(2):240–248. doi:10.1053/j.ajkd.2015.03.030. [Epub 2015 May 16].
71. Luyckx VA, Brenner BM. Birth weight, malnutrition and kidney-associated outcomes–a global concern. *Nat Rev Nephrol.* 2015;11(3):135–149. doi:10.1038/nrneph.2014.251. [Epub 2015 Jan 20]; Review.
86. Denic A, Alexander MP, Kaushik V, et al. Detection and clinical patterns of nephron hypertrophy and nephrosclerosis among apparently healthy adults. *Am J Kidney Dis.* 2016;68:58–67.
88. Denic A, Lieske JC, Chakkera HA, et al. The substantial loss of nephrons in healthy human kidneys with aging. *J Am Soc Nephrol.* 2017;28:313–320.
91. Rule AD, Amer H, Cornell LD, et al. The association between age and nephrosclerosis on renal biopsy among healthy adults. *Ann Intern Med.* 2010;152:561–567.
106. Thomson SC, Vallon V, Blantz RC. Kidney function in early diabetes: the tubular hypothesis of glomerular filtration. *Am J Physiol Renal Physiol.* 2004;286:F8–F15.
109. Hodgin JB, Bitzer M, Wickman L, et al. Glomerular aging and focal global glomerulosclerosis: a podometric perspective. *J Am Soc Nephrol.* 2015;26:3162–3178.

114. Denic A, Mathew J, Nagineni VV, et al. Clinical and pathology findings associate consistently with larger glomerular volume. *J Am Soc Nephrol.* 2018;29(7):1960–1969. [Epub 2018 May 22]; Erratum in: *J Am Soc Nephrol.* 2018;29(9):2445.
116. Rule AD, Semret MH, Amer H, et al. Association of kidney function and metabolic risk factors with density of glomeruli on renal biopsy samples from living donors. *Mayo Clin Proc.* 2011;86:282–290.
124. Martin JE, Sheaff MT. Renal ageing. *J Pathol.* 2007;211:198–205.
128. Lindeman RD, Tobin J, Shock NW. Longitudinal studies on the rate of decline in renal function with age. *J Am Geriatr Soc.* 1985;33:278–285.
133. Pottel H, Delanaye P, Weekers L, et al. Age-dependent reference intervals for estimated and measured glomerular filtration rate. *Clin Kidney J.* 2017;10(4):545–551. doi:10.1093/ckj/sfx026. [Epub 2017 Apr 28].
135. Cohen E, Nardi Y, Krause I, et al. A longitudinal assessment of the natural rate of decline in renal function with age. *J Nephrol.* 2014;27(6):635–641.
139. Denic A, Mathew J, Lerman LO, et al. Single-nephron glomerular filtration rate in healthy adults. *N Engl J Med.* 2017;376:2349–2357.
145. Hoang K, Tan JC, Derby G, et al. Determinants of glomerular hypofiltration in aging humans. *Kidney Int.* 2003;64(4):1417–1424.
147. Chakkera HA, Denic A, Kremers WK, et al. Comparison of high glomerular filtration rate thresholds for identifying hyperfiltration. *Nephrol Dial Transplant.* 2018;doi:10.1093/ndt/gfy332. [Epub ahead of print].
160. De Moor B, Vanwalleghem JF, Swennen Q, et al. Haemodynamic or metabolic stimulation tests to reveal the renal functional response: requiem or revival? *Clin Kidney J.* 2018;11(5):623–654.
164. Reckelhoff JF, Samsell L, Dey R, et al. The effect of aging on glomerular hemodynamics in the rat. *Am J Kidney Dis.* 1992;20(1):70–75.
175. Glassock RJ, Rule AD. The implications of anatomical and functional changes of the aging kidney: with an emphasis on the glomeruli. *Kidney Int.* 2012;82:270–277.
198. Frame AA, Wainford RD. Mechanisms of altered renal sodium handling in age-related hypertension. *Am J Physiol Renal Physiol.* 2018;315(1):F1–F6.
205. Kyle UG, Genton L, Hans D, et al. Age-related differences in fat-free mass, skeletal muscle, body cell mass and fat mass between 18 and 94 years. *Eur J Clin Nutr.* 2001;55:663–672.
230. Kuro-o M, Matsumura Y, Aizawa H, et al. Mutation of the mouse klotho gene leads to a syndrome resembling ageing. *Nature.* 1997; 390:45–51.
233. Musso CG, Juarez R, Vilas M, et al. Renal calcium, phosphorus, magnesium and uric acid handling: comparison between stage III chronic kidney disease patients and healthy oldest old. *Int Urol Nephrol.* 2012;44:1559–1562.
246. Ameri P, Canepa M, Milaneschi Y, et al. Relationship between vitamin D status and left ventricular geometry in a healthy population: results from the Baltimore Longitudinal Study of Aging. *J Intern Med.* 2013;273(3):253–262.
258. Amodu A, Abramowitz MK. Dietary acid, age, and serum bicarbonate levels among adults in the United States. *Clin J Am Soc Nephrol.* 2013;8:2034–2042.
274. Sands JM. Urine concentrating and diluting ability during aging. *J Gerontol A Biol Sci Med Sci.* 2012;67:1352–1357.
281. Beck LH. The aging kidney. Defending a delicate balance of fluid and electrolytes. *Geriatrics.* 2000;55:26–28, 31–32.
297. Mulkerrin E, Epstein FH, Clark BA. Aldosterone responses to hyperkalemia in healthy older humans. *J Am Soc Nephrol.* 1995;6(5): 1459–1462.
298. Ershler WB, Sheng S, McKelvey J, et al. Serum erythropoietin and aging: a longitudinal analysis. *J Am Geriatr Soc.* 2005;53(8):1360–1365.
307. Glassock R, Delanaye P, El Nahas M. An age-calibrated classification of chronic kidney disease. *JAMA.* 2015;314(6):559–560.
308. Levey AS, Inker LA, Coresh J. Chronic kidney disease in older people. *JAMA.* 2015;314(6):557–558.
312. Ebert N, Jakob O, Gaedeke J, et al. Prevalence of reduced kidney function and albuminuria in older adults: the Berlin Initiative Study. *Nephrol Dial Transplant.* 2017;32(6):997–1005.
315. Glassock RJ, Warnock DG, Delanaye P. The global burden of chronic kidney disease: estimates, variability and pitfalls. *Nat Rev Nephrol.* 2017;13(2):104–114.
317. Pottel H, Delanaye P, Schaeffner E, et al. Estimating glomerular filtration rate for the full age spectrum from serum creatinine and cystatin C. *Nephrol Dial Transplant.* 2017;32(3):497–507.
323. Meeusen JW, Rule AD, Voskoboev N, et al. Performance of cystatin C- and creatinine-based estimated glomerular filtration rate equations depends on patient characteristics. *Clin Chem.* 2015;61(10):1265–1272.
324. Fan L, Levey AS, Gudnason V, et al. Comparing GFR estimating equations using cystatin C and creatinine in older individuals. *J Am Soc Nephrol.* 2015;26(8):1982–1989.
325. Nerpin E, Ingelsson E, Risérus U, et al. The combined contribution of albuminuria and glomerular filtration rate to the prediction of cardiovascular mortality in older men. *Nephrol Dial Transplant.* 2011;26(9):2820–2827.
326. Grubb A, Lindström V, Jonsson M, et al. Reduction in glomerular pore size is not restricted to pregnant women. Evidence for a new syndrome: 'Shrunken pore syndrome'. *Scand J Clin Lab Invest.* 2015;75(4):333–340.
330. Hallan SI, Matsushita K, Sang Y, et al. Age and association of kidney measures with mortality and end-stage renal disease. *JAMA.* 2012;308(22):2349–2360.
331. Denic A, Glassock RJ, Rule AD. Structural and functional changes with the aging kidney. *Adv Chronic Kidney Dis.* 2016;23(1):19–28.
332. Gansevoort RT, Correa-Rotter R, Hemmelgarn BR, et al. Chronic kidney disease and cardiovascular risk: epidemiology, mechanisms, and prevention. *Lancet.* 2013;382(9889):339–352.
336. Warnock DG, Delanaye P, Glassock RJ. Risks for all-cause mortality: stratified by age, estimated glomerular filtration rate and albuminuria. *Nephron.* 2017;136(4):292–297.
338. O'Hare AM, Choi AI, Bertenthal D, et al. Age affects outcomes in chronic kidney disease. *J Am Soc Nephrol.* 2007;18(10):2758–2765.
341. Shardlow A, McIntyre NJ, Fluck RJ, et al. Chronic kidney disease in primary care: outcomes after five years in a prospective cohort study. *PLoS Med.* 2016;13(9):e1002128.
346. Jin B, Zeng C, Ge Y, et al. The spectrum of biopsy-proven kidney diseases in elderly Chinese patients. *Nephrol Dial Transplant.* 2014;29(12):2251–2259.
351. Kanasaki K, Kitada M, Koya D. Pathophysiology of the aging kidney and therapeutic interventions. *Hypertens Res.* 2012;35(12):1121–1128.

# EVALUATION OF THE PATIENT WITH KIDNEY DISEASE

SECTION IV

23

# Laboratory Assessment of Kidney Disease: Glomerular Filtration Rate, Urinalysis, and Proteinuria

Anoushka Krishnan | Adeera Levin

## CHAPTER OUTLINE



## KEY POINTS

- The glomerular filtration rate (GFR) is the amount of fluid filtered into the Bowman space per unit of time and is dependent on the porosity and the surface area of the glomerular membrane as well as the hydraulic pressure and oncotic pressure on the capillary side and in the Bowman space. Normal GFR is > 90 mL/min/1.73 $m^2$. There is a gradual decline in GFR with age, but the effect of age is variable.
- GFR measurement is cumbersome, as it needs the measurement of clearance of an exogenous filtration marker such as inulin. Hence, estimated GFRs (eGFRs) are calculated using the values of plasma creatinine. The most commonly used methods include the Cockcroft–Gault (CG) equation, the Modification of Diet in Renal Disease (MDRD) study equation, and more recently the Chronic Kidney Disease Epidemiology Collaboration (CKD-EPI) equation. The CKD-EPI equation is more accurate than the MDRD equation and both are more accurate than the CG equation.
- Special formulae may need to be used for children and the elderly, but the full age spectrum method of eGFR calculation may help circumnavigate this problem. Other unique groups include pregnant women, renal transplant recipients, and those with unusual body habitus or muscle mass.
- The main use of eGFR equations is in the detection, monitoring, and prognostication of CKD, which is largely asymptomatic. These equations have been derived from populations with stable CKD and are therefore not useful in the acute setting.
- Creatinine is a widely used marker of renal function. Many factors affect creatinine levels, such as muscle mass/injury, diet, age, gender, physical activity, and race. Creatinine is insensitive to even significant declines in GFR at the upper limit of normal due to the nonlinear relationship between creatinine and GFR. This is due to compensatory hyperfiltration of remaining functioning nephrons.
- Creatinine clearance (CrCl) is measured by collecting the patient's urine for 24 hours and measuring the total amount of excreted creatinine and the volume of urine. CrCl usually tends to overestimate eGFR.
- Proteinuria is one of the earliest markers of renal disease, occurring before a reduction in eGFR is noticed. It imparts diagnostic and prognostic information and is now a part of the Kidney Disease Improving Global Outcomes criteria for stratification of CKD.
- Casts are cylindrical bodies of renal origin that form from the aggregation of fibrils of Tamm–Horsfall glycoprotein (uromodulin). Red cell casts are always pathologic and indicate significant glomerular pathology.

An appreciation of the components of laboratory assessment of kidney disease is essential to the practicing clinician. This chapter describes three key aspects of laboratory assessment: the glomerular filtration rate (GFR), urinalysis, and proteinuria. Issues related to measurement tools, precision, bias, and interpretation are addressed for each of these variables, so that the reader may better appreciate the role of the laboratory in the diagnosis, follow-up, and management of kidney disease. Understanding the physiology of kidney function is essential to the interpretation of laboratory measurements and is highlighted within each section.

GFR is the single best measure of kidney function. Large studies consistently demonstrate the relationship of GFR to outcomes in general and renal populations, and the Kidney Disease Improving Global Outcomes (KDIGO) classification system uses GFR as one of the key dimensions in the diagnosis of chronic kidney disease (CKD). Urinary abnormalities may indicate acute or chronic conditions and isolated kidney or systemic diseases, and can be used to monitor both kidney and systemic diseases. Proteinuria is similarly an important marker of kidney disease and can also be seen in acute or chronic kidney conditions. In patients with CKD, the magnitude of albuminuria is proposed as a second dimension for the classification of severity in the KDIGO classification system because it affects prognosis.

The laboratory assessment of kidney disease can be used to diagnose, prognosticate, and measure progression of disease or response to therapy. CKD is increasingly recognized as an important public health problem, so accurate and appropriate use of laboratory testing is important. This chapter facilitates understanding and interpretation of key tests used in the assessment of kidney disease, both acute and chronic.

## GLOMERULAR FILTRATION RATE

"Glomerular filtration rate" describes one of the key roles of the kidney: to filter plasma so as to excrete waste products and produce urine (an ultrafiltrate of plasma). In clinical practice, estimates of GFR are obtained using equations, and direct measurement is reserved for specific circumstances. This section reviews normal physiology, use of various filtration markers, the development and use of equations, and special circumstances in which GFR interpretation needs to be contextualized.

### NORMAL PHYSIOLOGY

Separation of an ultrafiltrate of plasma across the barrier composed of the capillary wall, glomerular basement membrane, and podocyte is the first step in the production of urine and multiple functions of the kidney. The amount of fluid filtered into the Bowman space per unit of time is the GFR. Fluid movement is governed by Starling forces and so the glomerular filtrate that is produced is dependent on the following determinants:

- Porosity of the membrane (p)
- Surface area of the membrane (K)
- Hydraulic pressure and oncotic pressure on the capillary side ($P_{GC}$ and $\pi_{GC}$)

**Table 23.1 Factors That May Alter Determinants of Glomerular Filtration Rate**

| | |
|---|---|
| p | Generally less important than other factors |
| K | ↑ by relaxation of mesangial cells<br>↓ in glomerulonephritis and glomerulosclerosis |
| $P_{GC}$ | ↑ by afferent arteriole dilatation and efferent arteriole constriction |
| $P_{BS}$ | ↑ by raised intratubular pressure due to obstruction |
| $\pi_{GC}$ | ↑ by raised systemic oncotic pressure or decreased renal plasma flow |
| $\pi_{BS}$ | Minimal impact |

*K*, Surface area of the membrane; *p*, porosity of the glomerular membrane; $P_{BS}$, hydraulic pressure in the Bowman space; $P_{GC}$, glomerular capillary hydraulic pressure; $\pi_{BS}$, oncotic pressure in the Bowman space; $\pi_{GC}$, glomerular capillary oncotic pressure.

- Hydraulic pressure and oncotic pressure in the Bowman space ($P_{BS}$ and $\pi_{BS}$)

GFR can be calculated using the following equation:

$$GFR = p \times [(P_{GC} - P_{BS}) - K(\pi_{GC} - \pi_{BS})]$$

Factors that may alter these determinants of GFR are shown in Table 23.1. For further discussion of the physiology of glomerular ultrafiltration, please see Chapter 3.

The kidney filters approximately 180 L of plasma per day, which is equivalent to 125 mL/min. Kidney function is proportional to kidney size, which in turn is proportional to body surface area (BSA). Normal GFR is > 90 mL/min/1.73 $m^2$. In young adults GFR is approximately 120 to 130 mL/min/1.73 $m^2$. There is a gradual decline in GFR with age, but the effect of age is variable, in that some elderly patients have no change in renal function (see Chapter 22).

Protein intake and hyperglycemia can raise GFR by increasing renal plasma flow; the mechanism by which this occurs is unclear but may be activation of the intrarenal renin–angiotensin system.

### MEASUREMENT OF GFR

GFR can be measured provided that the concentration of a substance that is freely filtered at the glomerulus and neither reabsorbed nor secreted in the renal tubule is measured in the plasma and in a timed urine collection. GFR is equivalent to the "clearance rate" of this substance or filtration marker, which can be calculated as follows:

$$GFR = \frac{\text{Urine concentration of marker} \times \text{urine volume}}{\text{Plasma concentration of marker} \times \text{duration of urine collection}}$$

Filtration markers may be endogenous (e.g., creatinine, cystatin C) or exogenous (e.g., inulin, iohexol). GFR can be expressed as normalized to BSA to reflect physiologic matching of GFR to kidney size and in turn to BSA (mL/min/1.73 $m^2$), or as an absolute value (mL/min). An absolute value of GFR is useful in the setting of drug dosing, which is discussed further later. As an alternative to direct measurement of the clearance of a filtration marker, GFR can be estimated using an equation based on the plasma concentration of a filtration marker in steady state.

The most appropriate method for measurement of GFR depends on the purpose for which kidney function is being monitored. Direct measurement of GFR is time-consuming and may require medical supervision or the patient's presence at the hospital, so it is not usually performed as part of everyday practice. An exact value of the GFR is not required for most clinical settings. Understanding the trend within an individual patient's renal function is often what is needed. As a result, plasma urea and creatinine and estimated GFR (eGFR) calculations based on plasma creatinine are most often used. Alternatively, accuracy in the measurement of GFR is important for drug dosing of medications with narrow therapeutic windows (e.g., chemotherapy drugs) and is vital for appropriate selection and approval of live donors for kidney transplantation.

## GLOMERULAR FILTRATION MARKERS

The ideal glomerular filtration marker probably does not exist. Such a marker would have the following characteristics:

- Distributed freely and instantaneously throughout the extracellular space
- Not bound to plasma proteins
- Freely filtered at the glomerulus
- Not secreted or reabsorbed at the tubules
- Eliminated wholly by the kidney
- Resistant to degradation
- Easy and inexpensive to measure

An understanding of the limitations of each filtration marker is important to be able to interpret results. Given that kidney disease is often asymptomatic and dependent on the accuracy of laboratory tests, it is imperative that the clinician knows the advantages and disadvantages of each specific test before making clinical decisions.

### ENDOGENOUS GLOMERULAR FILTRATION MARKERS

#### Urea

Urea is not an accurate filtration marker because it is subject to a number of influences in addition to glomerular filtration. The liver produces urea in the urea cycle as a waste product of the digestion of protein. Therefore increased plasma levels may be due to factors independent of renal function, such as increased production in high protein intake, gastrointestinal bleeding due to absorption of amino acids from blood in the gastrointestinal tract, and high catabolic states such as those associated with glucocorticoid therapy.

Low urea levels are seen in decreased protein intake and chronic liver disease due to reduced synthesis of urea.

Urea is readily reabsorbed in the proximal tubule, particularly at low urinary flow rates. As a filtration marker, urea therefore has limited use because, although it is freely filtered, significant reabsorption means that the amount that is excreted is not what was filtered. High levels of urea may not necessarily indicate poor renal function but could instead reflect hypovolemia and renal hypoperfusion.

#### Serum Creatinine

Creatinine is a product of normal muscle metabolism. Phosphocreatine is a source for replenishment of phosphate when adenosine triphosphate is used by muscle cells. Creatine and phosphocreatine are nonenzymatically converted at an almost steady rate (approximately 2% of total creatine per day) to creatinine. Creatinine is not bound to plasma proteins, being freely filtered by the kidney, but it is unfortunately secreted by the tubules, making it an imperfect filtration marker. Despite its many limitations, however, its measurement is still the test most widely used by physicians to gauge renal function.

Serum creatinine level does not measure GFR but varies inversely with GFR and so is an indirect marker of GFR. The serum creatinine level can be used in estimation equations for GFR, and urinary creatinine clearance (CrCl) can be used to approximate GFR.

Factors affecting creatinine levels unrelated to renal function include muscle mass and/or injury and consumption of meat or creatine. Factors affecting muscle mass, such as age, sex, race, and physical activity, can in turn affect creatinine levels. Women, for example, have lower creatinine levels than men at the same level of GFR. Rhabdomyolysis has also been suggested to cause a greater rise in serum creatinine than other causes of acute kidney injury (AKI), because of the release of preformed creatine and phosphocreatine that is converted into creatinine.

Secretion of creatinine by the renal tubule is affected by

*Drugs (decrease secretion):* For example, trimethoprim, cimetidine, pyrimethamine, dapsone.

*Decreased renal function:* Each tubule excretes a higher proportion of creatinine as renal function declines. This secretory process is saturated when the serum creatinine level exceeds 1.5 to 2 mg/dL (132–176 μmol/L).

Extrarenal degradation of creatinine in the gut also rises as renal function declines due to bacterial overgrowth in the intestines leading to increased bacterial creatininase activity.[1] This extrarenal clearance may be as much as two-thirds of total daily creatinine excretion.

**Sources of Error in Measurement of Creatinine.** Clinicians may be unaware of the intricacies and complexities of creatinine measurement and how they may be relevant to day-to-day practice.

Laboratory methods to measure serum creatinine include

- Alkaline picrate (Jaffe method)
- Enzymatic methods
- Isotope dilution mass spectrometry (IDMS)
- High-performance liquid chromatography (HPLC)

There is wide variation in measured creatinine concentration, depending on the laboratory method and the instruments used. In 2003, the College of American Pathologists conducted a survey of 5624 participating laboratories that showed a bias from the reference value of between −0.06 and 0.31 mg/dL or −7% and 34%.[2] This bias was thought to be predominantly due to differences in instrument calibration among manufacturers. As a result, a creatinine standard reference material was prepared by the National Institute of Standards and

Technology, which is currently being used by almost all major manufacturers for calibration. The method of analysis (Jaffe or enzymatic) should also have minimal bias in comparison with the IDMS reference methodology.

Measurement of creatinine obviously affects measured CrCl and calculation of estimated CrCl or GFR, and therefore it has been recommended as part of the KDIGO initiative guidelines that all creatinine results be traceable to reference materials and methods listed on the Joint Committee for Traceability in Laboratory Medicine database.

The Jaffe method measures creatinine by complexing creatinine with alkaline picrate, followed by measurement with a colorimetric technique. This colorimetric assay may falsely measure normal plasma constituents such as glucose and plasma proteins as creatinine. As a result, the measured creatinine result may be falsely high. The Jaffe method may also report falsely low creatinine levels if there are very high serum bilirubin levels. Modified Jaffe methods attempt to take this into account by removing these interfering chromogens before analysis. This inference is sometimes corrected for by some manufacturers by deducting an estimated value based on average bias from measured results. Currently, the techniques used in most laboratories are modified alkaline picrate and enzymatic methods, but it is recommended that the enzymatic method be adopted because this is more specific.

Although serum creatinine concentration is widely used as a marker of renal function, it is insensitive to even significant declines in GFR at the upper limit of normal due to the nonlinear relationship between creatinine and GFR (Fig. 23.1). This is due to compensatory hyperfiltration of remaining functioning nephrons, secretion of creatinine, and extrarenal elimination of creatinine as the GFR declines. It is consequently a poor screening tool for early kidney disease.

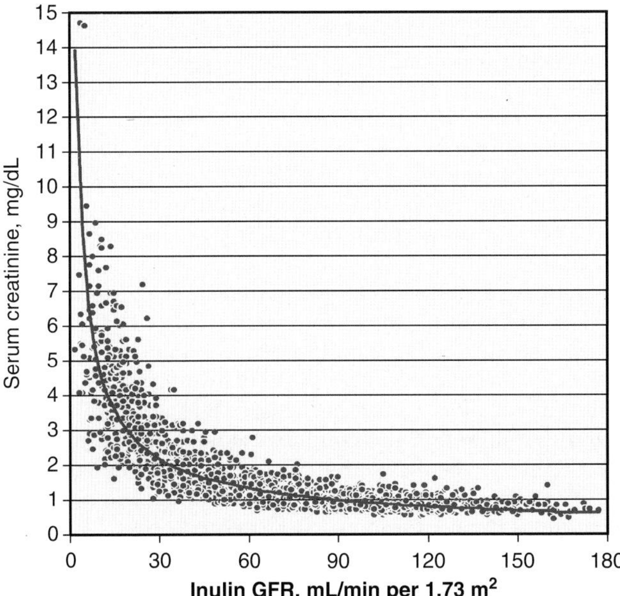


**Fig. 23.1** Relationship between plasma creatinine and glomerular filtration rate (GFR). (From Botev R, Mallie JP, Couchoud C, et al. Estimating glomerular filtration rate: Cockcroft-Gault and Modification of Diet in Renal Disease formulas compared to renal inulin clearance. *Clin J Am Soc.* 2009;4:899–906.)

Within-person variability of creatinine is also significant, at 8%; therefore significant change in serum creatinine is generally defined as at least 10%, which at early stages of kidney disease may represent a significant decline in GFR.

Serum creatinine results should be interpreted in the clinical context. The same serum creatinine concentration may correspond to a vastly different GFR in patients of different body composition. Volume status should also be taken into account because dilution of creatinine leads to an apparently low result.

**Creatinine Clearance.** CrCl is measured by collecting the patient's urine for 24 hours and measuring the total amount of excreted creatinine and the volume of urine. With the equation discussed earlier to calculate clearance of a filtration marker, CrCl is calculated as follows:

For example, for a patient with a serum creatinine value of 100 μmol/L, a urine creatinine value of 10,000 μmol/L, and a urine volume of 1.44 L, CrCl would be calculated as follows:

$$\text{CrCl} = \frac{\text{urine creatinine concentration} \times \text{urine volume}}{\text{plasma creatinine concentration} \times \text{duration of urine collection}}$$
$$= 144\ \text{L}/24\ \text{h} = 100\ \text{mL/min}$$

If this result is adjusted for BSA in a small person (height = 160 cm, weight = 50 kg, BSA 1.5 m), then the CrCl would be

$$\frac{\text{CrCl} \times 1.73}{\text{BSA}} = \frac{100 \times 1.73}{1.5} = 115\ \text{mL/min}/1.73\ \text{m}^2$$

For a larger person with a BSA of 2.0 m (height = 180 cm, weight = 80 kg), the adjusted CrCl would be 86.5 mL/min/1.73 m$^2$.

Although the clearance of an ideal substance would be equivalent to GFR, CrCl tends to exceed true GFR by approximately 10% to 20% because of the secretion of creatinine by the tubules. This error was previously compensated for by errors in the Jaffe assay that would overestimate serum creatinine value. Now that creatinine measurement has been standardized CrCl will consistently overestimate true GFR.

The main problem with CrCl is its reliance on timed urine collection, which is often inaccurate. Furthermore, tubular secretion of creatinine increases with decreased renal function, thus masking a true drop in GFR. In addition, the practical difficulties of conducting a 24-h urine collection for patients and the challenges of handling large volumes of urine for laboratories have resulted in this method being used only infrequently.

### Cystatin C

Cystatin C is a low-molecular-weight (LMW; 13-kD) basic protein that is produced at a constant rate by all nucleated cells. It is freely filtered by the glomerulus and is not secreted; proximal tubule cells reabsorb and catabolize the filtered cystatin C so that little is normally excreted in the urine. Therefore although plasma cystatin C levels are used in estimating GFR, cystatin C measurement cannot be used as a conventional urinary excretory marker for GFR. Rather, cystatin C has been regarded as one of several available novel markers of kidney injury.

Plasma cystatin C levels are highest in the first days of life and stabilize after 1 year of age, with levels approximating those of adults. Polymorphic variants in the *CST3* gene encoding cystatin C appear to affect production, and interindividual variations in cystatin C values account for 25% of its biologic variability, in comparison with 93% for creatinine. Within-person variation of cystatin C values is 6.8%.[3]

Cystatin C levels were reported to be independent of sex, muscle mass, and age after 12 months, but there is a growing body of evidence that this may not be the case. Cystatin C levels may be affected by factors independent of renal function, such as corticosteroids, thyroid dysfunction, obesity, diabetes, smoking, and high C-reactive protein value. This is problematic as, for example, cystatin C may not be useful in renal transplant patients because they have subclinical inflammation and commonly use long-term corticosteroids.

A meta-analysis published in 2002 showed that serum cystatin C measured with an immunonephelometric assay is more accurate than serum creatinine as a marker of GFR.[4,5] However, as noted previously, the cystatin C value, like the creatinine value, may be affected by a number of factors other than the GFR.

Laboratory techniques to measure cystatin C include latex immunoassays, such as automated particle-enhanced turbidimetric immunoassay and nephelometric immunoassay. Other techniques are radioimmunoassay, fluorescent techniques, and enzymatic immunoassays. Most of these assays are more expensive than the measurement of serum creatinine and although the International Federation of Clinical Chemists has developed a reference material for standardization of cystatin C, international standardization remains in process.[6–8]

A number of equations utilizing cystatin C have been developed to estimate GFR. The 2008 Chronic Kidney Disease Epidemiology Collaboration (CKD-EPI) cystatin C and CKD-EPI creatinine–cystatin C equations were developed in a preliminary study to assess the impact of cystatin C level on eGFR in individuals with CKD prior to the standardization of the cystatin C assay.[9] The 2012 CKD-EPI cystatin C and the CKD-EPI cystatin C–creatinine equations were developed from a diverse group of 5352 individuals from 13 studies. These equations were then validated in 1119 participants from 5 different studies in which GFR had been measured. The creatinine–cystatin C equation was found to perform better than equations that used creatinine or cystatin C alone—it produced an eGFR that was within 20% of the measured GFR (mGFR) in a significantly higher proportion of participants. Bias with the new, combined creatinine–cystatin C equation and with the average of the new cystatin C equation and the creatinine equation was similar to that with the individual creatinine and cystatin C equations, but they had greater precision and accuracy and resulted in more accurate classification of GFR as < 60 mL/min/1.73 $m^2$, the threshold for the diagnosis of CKD.[10] This was found to hold true even in individuals with low body mass index (a subgroup in which creatinine-based GFR estimates are known to be less accurate) and was less subject to the effects of age, sex, and race.

Other equations have been reported since the development of the CKD-EPI cystatin C and creatinine–cystatin C equations, which perform as well or better than the CKD-EPI cystatin C equation in some subgroups but do not perform better than the CKD-EPI equation in a diverse population.[11–14]

It has been proposed that cystatin C–based equations may be more accurate in populations with lower creatinine production, such as in children, the elderly, or cirrhotic patients,[15–17] although whether cystatin C correlates better with GFR than serum creatinine in patients with diabetic nephropathy is unclear.[18] In addition, steroids may affect cystatin C levels, thus making its utility in transplant recipients unclear.[15]

The 2012 KDIGO guidelines recommend using serum creatinine and a GFR estimating equation for initial assessment and to use additional testing such as cystatin C or a clearance measurement for confirmatory testing if eGFR based on serum creatinine is less accurate. For reporting $eGFR_{cys}$ and $eGFR_{cr-cys}$ in adults, the guideline recommended using the 2012 CKD-EPI cystatin C equations or another cystatin C–based GFR estimating equation if it has demonstrated improved accuracy of GFR estimates compared with these CKD-EPI cystatin C equations. The guideline recommends measuring cystatin C in adults with $eGFR_{cr}$ of 45–59 mL/min/1.73 $m^2$ without markers of kidney damage if CKD confirmation is required. If $eGFR_{cys}/eGFR_{cr-cys}$ is also < 60 mL/min/1.73 $m^2$, the CKD diagnosis is confirmed. If $eGFR_{cys}/eGFR_{cr-cys}$ is ≥ 60 mL/min/1.73 $m^2$, the CKD diagnosis is not confirmed.[19] While this might help in risk stratification, the guidelines do leave a number of questions unanswered, such as how to incorporate cystatin-based GFR estimates into routine clinical practice and use this equation for longitudinal follow-up of patients. The NKF-KDOQI commentary on the KDIGO guideline concurred with their recommendations for GFR evaluation but recommended against widespread use of cystatin C because of concerns regarding incomplete understanding of its non-GFR determinants, higher costs, and incomplete standardization of assays.[20]

### Novel Endogenous Filtration Markers

Several alternative novel endogenous substances are under investigation as potential markers that could be used aside from urea, creatinine, and cystatin C. They are beta-trace protein (BTP), $\beta_2$-microglobulin (B2M), and symmetrical dimethylarginine.

BTP is a 23–29-kDa protein, larger isoforms of which are found in the serum and urine. In late 2000s, the White and Pöge equations were developed, using BTP alone or in combination with urea or creatinine to determine eGFR. However, they were not felt to offer any significant benefit over the Modification of Diet in Renal Disease (MDRD) equation.[21,22]

B2M is a 11.8-kDa protein commonly used as a prognostic marker for multiple myeloma. It is freely filtered by the glomerulus and is extensively reabsorbed and metabolized in the proximal tubule.[23] The CKD-EPI investigators attempted to develop eGFR equations using both BTP and B2M.[24] They found that although the combined equation was similar to the CKD-EPI creatinine and cystatin C–based equations, it did not offer an improvement over either, nor was it as accurate as the combined CKD-EPI equation.

Interestingly, both BTP and B2M were subsequently found to be strong predictors for CKD progression, cardiovascular disease, and mortality.[25,26]

Used alone, these markers have a number of shortcomings, such as lack of standardization of assays, lack of certified reference materials, and a number of non-GFR determinants (such as male gender, markers of inflammation, and body mass index). They do, however, hold promise as potential endogenous filtration markers that could not only improve GFR estimation in combination with other measurements (by reducing bias and improving accuracy), but also potentially predict the risk of ESKD and mortality. The future of GFR measurement will likely involve the use of kidney metabolomics, looking to use several plasma-based markers to give a better estimate of GFR, predict risk, and reduce the impact of individual non-GFR determinants.[27]

### Equations for Estimating GFR

Because direct measurement of GFR is not practical in clinical practice, estimation equations have been developed to aid clinicians in interpretation of serum creatinine, given the limitations previously cited.

A multitude of equations (Table 23.2) derived for the estimation of GFR are available. They all attempt to transform the serum concentration of a filtration marker into a value approximating the GFR, usually with the addition of other factors, such as age, sex, weight, and height, in part because the main filtration marker that is used is creatinine, which is known to be affected by these factors.

The main use of eGFR equations is in the detection, monitoring, and prognostication of CKD, which is largely asymptomatic. These equations have been derived from populations with stable CKD and are therefore not useful in the acute setting. Translating creatinine values, especially at the upper limit of normal (which as previously discussed do not reflect significant declines in GFR), into an eGFR has heightened the awareness of CKD. Estimation equations

**Table 23.2 Most Commonly Used Equations for Estimating Glomerular Filtration Rate**

| Equation Name | Equation | Derivation Population |
|---|---|---|
| Cockcroft–Gault (1976) | (140 – age) × wt (kg)/creatinine (μmol/L) × 0.81<br>Female: × 0.85<br>(140 – age) × lean body weight (kg)/Cr (mg/dL) × 72 | 249 male veterans<br>Median GFR 34 |
| MDRD equation (1999) | $175 \times SCr^{-1.154} \times age^{-0.26} \times 0.742$ (if female) × 1.212 (if black) | 1628 patients enrolled in the MDRD Study (mean age, 50.6 years) |
| MDRD equation without ethnicity factor[a] | $175 \times SCr^{2190} \times age^{-0.26} \times 0.742$ (if female) | Mean GFR 39.8 mL/min/1.73 $m^2$ |
| CKD-EPI equation (2009) | $141 \times \min(SCr/\kappa, 1)^{\alpha} \times \max(SCr/\kappa, 1)^{-1.209} \times 0.993^{Age} \times 1.018$ (if female) × 1.159 (if black),<br>where<br>κ is 0.7 for females and 0.9 for males<br>α is –0.329 for females and –0.411 for males<br>min indicates the minimum of SCr/κ or 1<br>max indicates the maximum of SCr/κ or 1 | 8254 participants from 6 research studies and 4 clinical populations (mean age, 47 years)<br>Mean GFR 68 mL/min/1.73 $m^2$ |
| CKD-EPI cystatin C (2012) | $133 \times \min(SCysC/0.8, 1)^{-0.499} \times \max(SCysC/0.8, 1)^{-1.328} \times 0.996^{Age} \times 0.932$ (if female),<br>where<br>min indicates the minimum of SCysC/0.8 or 1<br>max indicates the maximum of SCysC/0.8 or 1 | 5352 participants from 13 studies (mean age, 47 years)<br>Mean GFR 68 mL/min/1.73 $m^2$ |
| CKD-EPI creatinine–cystatin C (2012) | $135 \times \min(SCr/\kappa, 1)^{\alpha} \times \max(SCr/\kappa, 1)^{-0.601} \times \min(SCysC/0.8, 1)^{-0.375} \times \max(SCysC/0.8, 1)^{-0.711} \times 0.995^{Age} \times 0.969$ (if female) × 1.08 (if black),<br>where<br>α is –0.248 for females and –0.207 for males<br>κ is 0.7 for females and 0.9 for males<br>min(SCr/κ,1) indicates the minimum of SCr/k or 1 and<br>max(SCr/κ,1) indicates the maximum of SCr/k or 1<br>min(SCysC/0.8,1) indicates the minimum of SCysC/0.8 or 1 and<br>max(SCysC/0.8,1) indicates the maximum of SCysC/0.8 or 1 | 34 mL/min |
| BIS equation<br>BIS1: creatinine<br>BIS2: creatinine and cystatin C (2012) | $BIS1 = 3736 \times creatinine^{-0.123} \times age^{-0.131} \times 0.82$ (if female)<br>$BIS2 = 767 \times cystatin\ C^{-0.98} \times creatinine^{-0.77} \times age^{-0.94} \times 0.87$ (if female) | 610 individuals over 70 years of age<br>Mean age: 78.5 years |
| FAS equation: normalized serum creatinine (SCr/Q) (2016) | eGFR = 107.3 × / [Scr/Q] for 2 years < age ≤ 40 years<br>eGFR = 107.3 × 0.988(age – 40)/[Scr/Q] for age >40 years | 6870 individuals spanning all age groups (<18 to >70 years) |

[a]African-American coefficient of the MDRD study equation.

*BIS*, Berlin Initiative Study; *CKD-EPI*, Chronic Kidney Disease Epidemiology Collaboration; *Cr*, creatinine; *eGFR*, estimated glomerular filtration rate; FAS, full age spectrum; *GFR*, glomerular filtration rate; *MDRD*, Modification of Diet in Renal Disease; *SCr*, serum creatinine; *SCr/Q*, normalized serum creatinine, where Q is the median serum creatinine from healthy populations to account for age and gender; *SCysC*, serum cystatin C; *wt*, weight.

Adapted from Tables 12 and 16 in Kidney Disease: Improving Global Outcomes (KDIGO) CKD Work Group. KDIGO 2012 clinical practice guideline for the evaluation and management of chronic kidney disease. *Kidney Int Suppl.* 2013;3:1–150.

also appear to be reasonably accurate for following changes in GFR over time.[28,29]

**Bias, Precision, and Accuracy.** The performance of estimation equations is assessed by measurements of bias, precision, and accuracy.

- "Bias" results from the systematic underestimation or overestimation of the GFR in a population due to an error within the equation itself. It is calculated as the mean or median difference between the mGFR and eGFR values.
- "Precision" refers to the reliability and reproducibility of repeated measurements with one another. In the case of eGFR, it is usually expressed as the standard deviation or interquartile range of differences between eGFR and mGFR values.
- "Accuracy" combines bias and precision and is the most useful assessment of an estimation equation. It is measured as the percentage of GFR estimations within a particular percentage range (usually 30%) from their respective GFR measurements.

The problem of bias with eGFR equations can potentially be overcome with derivation of the equation from larger sample sizes and use of filtration markers such as cystatin C, which are less subject to interference by other factors. Accuracy, however, is difficult to achieve in a heterogeneous population. Even the latest Chronic Kidney Disease Epidemiology Collaboration (CKD-EPI) equation using creatinine, which is being adopted widely, has accuracy such that 80.6% of eGFR values are within 30% of mGFR (Fig. 23.2). This means that one in five values of eGFR in the general population is incorrect. Again, in day-to-day clinical practice, accuracy may not be necessary, and establishing an eGFR trend within an individual patient with CKD is probably more important.

**Modification of Diet in Renal Disease and Chronic Kidney Disease Epidemiology Collaboration Equations.** Although a number of GFR estimation equations have been developed, two equations are most widely used in clinical practice.

***MDRD.*** The MDRD study equation was initially derived in 1999 from a population of 1628 individuals who had participated in the MDRD study, using creatinine measured by a modified Jaffe method.[30] A new MDRD equation was expressed in 2004 for IDMS-traceable creatinine values. The MDRD equation was compared against a gold standard, urinary clearance of iothalamate. The performance of the MDRD equation was evaluated in a number of populations because it was initially derived from a primarily Caucasian American population. A number of coefficients have been derived to compensate for differences in body mass and diet in populations of different ethnicity with varying degrees of performance.

The MDRD equation was widely adopted in the United States, Europe, and Australia, where eGFR is now routinely reported with serum creatinine results. It is gradually being replaced by the CKD-EPI equation.

The limitations of the MDRD equation are mainly its tendency to underestimate the GFR and its relatively low accuracy at higher GFR values.

***CKD-EPI.*** The CKD-EPI equation was derived in 2009 in 8254 patients (a further 3896 patients pooled from 16 studies were used for validation), with urinary clearance of iothalamate again used as the gold standard.[31] It has less bias and greater accuracy than the MDRD equation, especially at higher GFR. A meta-analysis involving 1.1 million adults showed that the CKD-EPI equation reclassified a significant number of patients (24.4%) into a higher GFR range[32]; 34.7% of patients who were classified as having stage 3A CKD (eGFR 45–59 mL/min/1.73 m$^2$) with the MDRD equation did not have GFRs < 60 mL/min/1.73 m$^2$ with the CKD-EPI equation

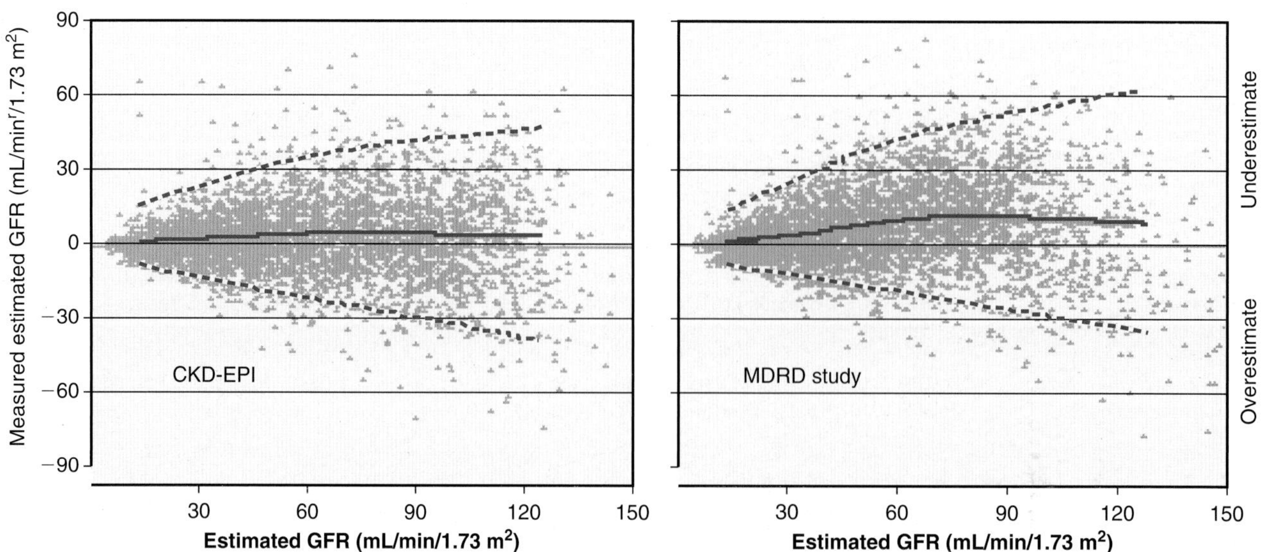


**Fig. 23.2** Difference between measured and estimated glomerular filtration rate (GFR) using the Modification of Diet in Renal Disease (MDRD) and Chronic Kidney Disease Epidemiology Collaboration (CKD-EPI) estimation equations. Shown are smoothed regression lines and hashed 95% confidence interval lines. Although both the MDRD and CKD-EPI equations tend to underestimate the GFR, the CKD-EPI equation does so to a lesser degree, particularly at higher GFR. Therefore the CKD-EPI equation has less bias. (From Levey AS, Stevens LA, Schmid CH, et al. A new equation to estimate glomerular filtration rate. *Ann Intern Med.* 2009;150:604–612.)

and were therefore no longer regarded as having CKD according to the newest definition. The precision of the CKD-EPI and MDRD equations is still suboptimal, however, because eGFR and mGFR values varied by at least 16.6 and 18.3 mL/min/1.73 $m^2$ (the interquartile range of differences for patients across the range of GFR), respectively.

CKD-EPI equations have also been derived for cystatin C and a combination of cystatin C and creatinine. Cystatin C measurement in the derivation of these equations was traceable to the standard reference material for cystatin C, although cystatin C measurement is not uniformly standardized, as noted previously. GFR estimation using cystatin C and creatinine in combination has been shown to be more accurate than either marker alone, but eGFR using cystatin C is not superior to eGFR using creatinine.[33] The KDIGO 2012 guidelines recommend initial GFR evaluation using serum creatinine and a GFR estimating equation and confirmatory testing using tests such as serum cystatin C or a clearance measurement in certain circumstances if $eGFR_{cr}$ is less accurate. For confirmatory testing using a clearance measurement, the recommendations include using plasma or urinary clearance of an exogenous filtration marker rather than CrCl. Recommendations to clinical laboratories included using assays for creatinine and cystatin C that are traceable to reference standards, and reporting eGFR using the CKD-EPI equations, or alternative equations if they are superior.[19]

Risk Stratification of CKD with eGFR: eGFR equations transform the creatinine or cystatin C measurement into a value that approximates the mGFR. This value can also be used to classify the patient according to the stage of CKD. Decreasing values of GFR in patients with CKD have been associated with increasing risk for metabolic complications of CKD, end-stage kidney disease (ESKD), cardiovascular disease, and death.[34] The many eGFR equations have performed variably in their ability to predict certain outcomes in different populations. This difference in ability to risk stratify is due to the different degrees of importance placed on factors such as age and sex, which also affect prognosis, in these equations. The importance of accuracy in measuring GFR versus stratification of risk as a result of decreased GFR is a matter of ongoing debate and beyond the scope of this text. For further discussion of risk factors in CKD, please see Chapter 20.

**Cockcroft–Gault Equation.** The Cockcroft–Gault (CG) equation estimates CrCl rather than the GFR. This equation was developed in 1976 from a cohort of 249 men, and the creatinine assay method that was used to derive this equation was not standardized.[35] The equation is

$$\text{CrCl (mL/min)} = \frac{(140 - \text{age}) \times \text{lean body weight (kg)}}{\text{Cr (mg/dL)} \times 72}$$

The CG equation has not been re-expressed since the adoption of new assay methods for estimation of creatinine. For these reasons, the CG equation systematically overestimates GFR and should not be used without an understanding of its limitations, although it is currently still often used to guide drug dosing including drug research. There is especially a risk of overdosing drugs that have a narrow therapeutic index with the CG equation.

## EXOGENOUS GLOMERULAR FILTRATION MARKERS

### Inulin

Inulin remains the gold standard filtration marker but its use is impractical for routine clinical purposes. Inulin is a polymer of fructose found in tubers such as the Jerusalem artichoke and chicory. It distributes in extracellular fluid, does not bind to plasma proteins, is freely filtered at the glomerulus, and is neither reabsorbed nor secreted by the renal tubules.

Inulin is intravenously infused at a constant rate while blood and urine are sampled frequently over several hours, ideally following insertion of a bladder catheter. The patient takes an oral water load and must continue consuming water throughout the test to ensure a high urine output.

### Clearance Methods for Other Exogenous Glomerular Filtration Markers

Owing to the difficulty and expense of using inulin, new reference standard filtration markers have been introduced as alternatives and have been widely used since the 1990s. Urinary iothalamate and iohexol have now been adopted now been adopted as the reference standard for measurement of GFR. Clearance of these filtration markers can be measured in the urine or in blood or with nuclear imaging in the case of radiolabeled markers to avoid problems with urine collection.[36]

GFR is calculated from plasma clearance after a bolus intravenous injection of an exogenous filtration marker, with clearance being calculated from the amount of the marker administered divided by the area under the curve of plasma concentration over time. The decline in serum concentration is due initially to the disappearance of the marker from the plasma into its volume of distribution (fast component) and then subsequently to renal excretion (slow component). It is best estimated using a two-compartment model that requires blood sampling early (usually two or three time points until 60 min) and late (one to three time points from 120 min onward). GFR can also be measured by counting a radioactive exogenous filtration marker over the kidneys and bladder areas; however, this technique is thought to be generally less accurate.

These methods are not perfect and are subject to imprecision, albeit at a much lower level than that of equations that estimate GFR.

### Radiolabeled Markers

Radiolabeled iothalamate, ethylenediaminetetraacetic acid (EDTA), and diethylenetriaminepentaacetic acid (DTPA) are all used as glomerular filtration markers.

Iothalamate may be labeled with iodide I 125 ($^{125}I$) or used unlabeled. EDTA is commonly used in Europe, whereas DTPA is widely used in the United States. EDTA is usually labeled with chromium Cr 51 ($^{51}Cr$), but EDTA may be reabsorbed by the tubules, leading to underestimation of GFR. DTPA is labeled with technetium Tc 9m ($^{99m}Tc$), and the major limitation of its use is the potential for an unpredictable dissociation of $^{99m}Tc$ from DTPA and binding to plasma proteins, resulting in underestimation of GFR.

### Unlabeled Radiocontrast Agents

Because of concerns about exposure to radiation, storage, and disposal of radionuclide markers, techniques have been developed to measure low levels of iodine in urine and plasma. Iothalamate and iohexol concentrations have been measured using HPLC, but the main disadvantage of this approach is the complexity of the HPLC assay. X-ray fluorescence of samples may also be used to measure iodine levels but requires a higher dose of contrast agent.

Iohexol is a nonionic, low-osmolar contrast agent. It is not reabsorbed, metabolized, or secreted by the kidney and is excreted completely unmetabolized in the urine. It has low toxicity and is usually used in doses 10 to 50 times higher in radiologic procedures than those used for GFR determination.

Urinary clearances of iothalamate and iohexol closely correlate with urinary inulin clearance, and are therefore the methods most commonly used to measure GFR.

## SPECIFIC CIRCUMSTANCES OR POPULATIONS

### CHILDREN

Adult GFR equations such as the MDRD have been shown to be inappropriate in children aged ≤9 years (see also Chapter 72). Multiple equations (Table 23.3) have been derived for estimation of GFR in children, but the most popular is the Schwartz equation, which was devised in 1976[37]

$$eGFR = \frac{k \times L}{SCr}$$

where k depends on the age of the child, L is length or height, and SCr is serum creatinine. Like the CG equation, the Schwartz equation has now been shown to systematically overestimate GFR. The reasons are the creatinine assay technique and measurement factors specific to children. As previously mentioned, the Jaffe method can be interfered with by plasma proteins, and the correction factor that is deducted to account for this interference is estimated by taking an average bias from measured results. In children, who have lower levels of plasma proteins, this correction factor may be too high, resulting in an erroneously low creatinine value. Because of the low muscle mass of children, the influence of a measurement error is also proportionately larger than an error of the same magnitude in an adult sample.

The simple bedside Schwartz equation—eGFR = 0.413 × (height [cm]/serum creatinine [mg/dL])—was developed using standardized creatinine methods in 2009.[38] This equation provides good approximation of a more complicated Schwartz eGFR formula, using creatinine, urea, and cystatin C as well as height.[38] Cystatin C has been suggested to be more accurate than creatinine as an indirect marker of renal function in children.[39]

A limitation is that the equation was derived from a cohort of 600 children with CKD who had abnormal growth. Therefore this GFR estimation equation may not be accurate for children who have less impairment of renal function and normal skeletal growth (Table 23.3).

### ELDERLY POPULATION

Elderly individuals were either not included or were poorly represented in the study populations used to develop the CG, MDRD, and CKD-EPI equations. The Berlin Initiative Study (BIS) attempted to develop an equation based on serum creatinine concentration, gender, and age using a study population that included 610 individuals aged >70 years. The equation was compared with a gold standard iohexol plasma clearance measurement, three creatinine-based equations

**Table 23.3 Equations Using Serum Biomarkers for Estimating GFR in Children and Adolescents**

| | | Derivation Population | | |
|---|---|---|---|---|
| Equation Name | Equation | No. Children | Age (Years) | GFR Range or Median (mL/min) |
| **Creatinine Based** | | | | |
| Schwartz, 1976 | $0.55 \times Ht/Scr$ | 77 | 1–21 | 3–220 |
| Counahan, 1976 | $0.43 \times Ht/Scr$ | 103 | 0.2–14 | 4–200 |
| Leger, 2002 | $(0.641 \times Wt)/Scr + (0.00131 \times Ht^3)/Scr$ | 97 | 1–21 | 97 |
| Schwartz, 2009 | $0.413 \times Ht/Scr$<br>$40.7 \times (HT/Scr)^{0.640} \times (30/BUN)^{0.25}$ | 349 | 1–17 | 41 |
| **Cystatin C Based** | | | | |
| Filler, 2003 | $91.62 \times (cysC)^{-1.123}$ | 85 | 1–18 | 103 |
| Grubb, 2005 | $84.69 \times (cysC)^{-1.680} \times 1.384$ if <14 years | 85 | 3–17 | 108 |
| Zappitelli, 2006 | $75.94 \times (cysC)^{-1.17} \times 1.2$ if Tx | 103 | 1–18 | 74 |
| **Creatinine and Cystatin C Based** | | | | |
| Bouvet, 2006 | $63.2 \times (Scr/1.086)^{-0.19} \times (cysC/1.2)^{-0.93} \times (Wt/45)^{0.68} \times (years/14)^{0.77}$ | 100 | 1–23 | 92 |
| Zappitelli, 2006 | $43.82 \times e^{0.004} \times Ht \times (cysC)^{-0.635} \times (Scr)^{-0.547}$ | 103 | 1–18 | 74 |
| Schwartz, 2009 | $39.1 \times (HT/Scr)^{0.516} \times (1.8/cysC)^{0.294} \times (30/BUN)^{0.40} \times (1.099)$ if male $\times (HT/1.4)^{0.9}$ | 349 | 1–17 | 41 |

*BUN,* Blood urea nitrogen; *cysC,* cystatin C; *GFR,* glomerular filtration rate; *Ht/HT,* height; *Scr,* serum creatinine; *Tx,* transplant; *Wt,* weight.
Adapted from Table 3 in Schwartz GJ, Work DF. Measurement and estimation of GFR in children and adolescents. *Clin J Am Soc Nephrol.* 2009;4:1832–1843.

(CG, MDRD, and CKD-EPI), and three equations based on cystatin C and was shown to produce less bias than any of its counterparts. Four variables were taken into account—namely, age, sex, serum creatinine, and serum cystatin C—but not ethnicity as the cohort consisted of Germans of Caucasian origin. Two equations were derived—the BIS1 using serum creatinine only and BIS2 using serum creatinine and serum cystatin C (Table 23.2). These formulae showed better precision and agreement with mGFR, especially in a population with eGFR > 30 mL/min/1.73 $m^2$. The BIS equations appear to provide a more accurate estimation of GFR in the elderly and improve identification of individuals with CKD.[11] The BIS1 equation was subsequently shown to be useful in a Chinese group of 332 elderly subjects as well as in a different Caucasian cohort of 224 subjects.[40,41]

## PREGNANCY

It is well known that there a physiologic increase in GFR, increased effective renal plasma flow, and a drop in serum creatinine occur in pregnancy. Serum creatinine decreases because of a real increase in GFR but also because of physiologic hemodilution.

Estimation equations are inappropriate for measuring GFR in pregnant women because they were not derived from this population. Most pregnant women have GFRs > 60 mL/min/1.73 $m^2$, which is above the range at which the MDRD or CKD-EPI equations are known to be accurate in any case. The 24-h urine collection for CrCl therefore remains the best method in pregnancy.[42]

Nevertheless, eGFR has been used to study midterm renal hyperfiltration, a hemodynamic phenomenon that occurs early in pregnancy and persists until delivery.[43] This is regarded as a marker of renal functional reserve in pregnancy. Recently, Park et al. described a retrospective study looking at 1931 singleton pregnancies with midterm serum creatinine data between 2001 and 2015 in South Korea, using the CKD-EPI equation. Midterm hyperfiltration was defined as > 120 mL/min. They demonstrated a nonlinear U-shaped relationship between midterm eGFR and adverse outcomes, with values between 120 and 150 mL/min/1.73 $m^2$ being associated with the lowest incidence of adverse pregnancy outcomes (defined by preterm birth, low birth weight, or preeclampsia as well as the composite of these three features). There are several limitations to this study, but the data suggest that further research is needed to understand the pathophysiology of intrarenal hemodynamic dysfunction in pregnancy and how this may contribute to adverse outcomes.[44,45]

## ACUTE KIDNEY INJURY

Measurement of GFR in patients with AKI is difficult as it is constantly changing, and measurements or estimates that depend on a steady state are not readily applicable. Serum creatinine is the most commonly used marker of GFR in this setting, but creatinine is slow to rise in response to a decrease in GFR and is subject to the influence of dilution by fluid given as part of treatment for AKI.[46,47] As previously mentioned, creatinine is also insensitive to substantial decreases in GFR. Estimation equations for GFR in patients with AKI are inaccurate because these equations have been derived from stable patients, in whom the creatinine is at a steady state, and are not applicable to the diverse AKI patient population. A kinetic GFR estimation equation has been developed but has not yet been validated.[48]

Accurate measurement of GFR in this population can be achieved by calculation of the elimination kinetics after a single bolus injection of a glomerular filtration marker. Alternatively, brief-duration measurements of GFR, such as short-duration urinary CrCl, can be performed, assuming that a patient's creatinine does not increase rapidly over 2 to 8 hours.[49] These tests are not widely performed and are probably impractical in many centers. This situation has led to extensive research into a biomarker that is more sensitive in demonstrating early stages of AKI to facilitate more timely intervention.

## DRUG DOSING

The CG equation, despite its limitations, is still used regularly in many jurisdictions for drug dose adjustment in patients with renal impairment. Historically this equation has been used to enroll subjects in renal impairment categories for pharmacokinetic studies. The U.S. Food and Drug Administration (FDA) in its "Guidance for Industry Pharmacokinetics in Patients with Impaired Renal Function" suggested using either the MDRD equation or the CG equation for this purpose in new drug development,[50] although one should be cautious as this does not imply that CrCl is equivalent to eGFR. The FDA guidance has not been updated since the KDIGO and KDOQI have recommended that the CKD-EPI equation replace the MDRD equation in routine clinical practice. Because the CKD-EPI and MDRD study equations perform similarly at GFR < 60 mL/min/1.73 $m^2$, it would be reasonable to use eGFR computed using the CKD-EPI equation or the MDRD study equation for pharmacokinetic studies and drug dosing.[51]

A large simulation study comparing drug dosages administered to patients through the use of the MDRD and CG equations showed that the concordance figures of the two equations' GFR estimates with mGFR was similar.[52] Because the majority of FDA-approved drug dosing labels use the CG equation, which expresses CrCl in mL/min, the eGFR value corrected for BSA must be converted to units of mL/min by multiplying by the individual's BSA and dividing by 1.73 $m^2$. The stimulation study concluded that either equation can be used for drug dosing but that caution should be exercised in patients in whom the creatinine value may be inaccurate. This caution is particularly relevant in sick or hospitalized patients, in whom low body weight or changes in body weight are present, in the elderly, and in amputees. The CG equation in these cases tends to give a lower estimate of renal function,[53] leading to a dose reduction.[54] The lower estimate results from the greater effect of age and weight on the CG equation. The use of the CG equation may lead to drug dosing errors that are due to "underdosing," thus minimizing exposure to toxicity. By contrast, in the elderly patients, the MDRD and CKD-EPI equations have been shown to overestimate the GFR in some studies but to be reliable in others.[55,56] The elderly patients are more likely to experience side effects and to be subject to the dangers of polypharmacy, so using the CG equation in these patients may be more appropriate.[53]

Ultimately the importance of drug dosage adjustment depends on the purpose of the medication as well as the therapeutic range and toxicity of the drug. In cases in which a medication has a narrow therapeutic window, such as chemotherapy, all estimation equations may have an unacceptable degree of error, and accurate measurement of GFR using an exogenous filtration marker should be performed.

The CG equation should not be completely abandoned in favor of the MDRD equation, especially because recommendations for drug dosages of existing medications were based on the CG equation. The CKD-EPI equation has not yet been considered in this context.

### FULL AGE SPECTRUM METHOD OF EGFR ESTIMATION

Owing to the methods by which various equations were developed for different populations, there can be a discontinuity when switching from pediatric equations to adult equations or from adult to older-adult equations. The full age spectrum (FAS) equation, developed in 2016, tries to correct for this disparity by deriving a single (age-knotted) eGFR equation that is applicable to all ages by normalizing serum creatinine for age (for children and adolescents) and sex (for adolescents and adults). A normalized serum creatinine (SCr/Q) is used, where Q is the median serum creatinine from healthy populations to account for age and gender (see Table 23.2).

Validation was performed in a total of 6870 healthy and kidney disease–affected white individuals including 735 children (<18 years of age), 4371 adults (aged between 18 and 70 years), and 1764 older adults (>70 years of age) with mGFR (inulin, iohexol, and iothalamate clearance) and IDMS-equivalent serum creatinine. Bias, precision, and accuracy were tested. The equation was found to be less biased and more accurate than the Schwartz equation for children and adolescents, less biased and as accurate as the CKD-EPI for young and middle-aged adults, and more accurate and less biased than CKD-EPI for older adults. The equation may not need further changes for age and gender but may need validation in other ethnicities and derivation of Q values for different populations. External validation in a large population suggested that the FAS equation might perform better than the Schwartz and CKD-EPI equations. There was better accuracy and precision for older adults with mGFR > 60 mL/min/1.73 $m^2$. As the FAS is based on SCr/Q values for a healthy population, it is expected that this will work better for a healthy and general population rather than in patients with CKD; however, in the validation population subgroups with mGFR < 60 mL/min/1.73 $m^2$ the FAS equation was not found to perform worse than the CKD-EPI equation.[57]

### RENAL TRANSPLANT RECIPIENTS

Currently, renal transplant function is monitored using the endogenous marker serum creatinine along with eGFR. Serum creatinine, however, is affected by a number of drugs used in transplant medicine. For instance, corticosteroids are shown to increase eGFR in animal models as well as in humans; glomerular micropuncture studies have shown that corticosteroids vasodilate both the afferent and efferent arterioles, resulting in increased plasma flow and hence a higher eGFR. Chronic steroid administration has also been shown to increase prostaglandin synthesis in some species.[58] Paradoxically, steroids also increase serum creatinine by about 10%. This is presumably due to steroid-induced hypercatabolic state with associated protein wasting and muscle loss. In addition, muscle mass in transplant recipients may differ from the general population and those with other clinical conditions due to a chronic inflammatory state from chronic illness, infection, and episodes of rejection.[59–61] In addition, trimethoprim used for *Pneumocystis jirovecii* prophylaxis can cause elevated creatinine by blocking its tubular secretion. As discussed earlier, eGFR can decrease substantially before there is an evident increase in serum creatinine levels; thus calcineurin inhibitor toxicity and rejection may not be detected early enough.

Serum creatinine tends to be used in renal transplant recipients to detect rejection, infection, or drug toxicity and eGFR is infrequently used to guide management decisions due to concerns that the equations may be less reliable in transplant recipients than other populations. Nevertheless, in a systematic review of 3622 solid-organ transplant recipients, Shaffi et al. demonstrated that the CKD-EPI and the four-variable MDRD study equations were more accurate than alternative equations (even those developed in populations of transplant recipients only) and as accurate as observed in other clinical populations. CKD-EPI performed better at higher GFRs and MDRD performed better at lower GFRs. However, these equations were still inaccurate (different from mGFR by more than 30%) in one of five patients.[62,63]

## URINALYSIS

Urinalysis may be used in the assessment of acute kidney disease or CKD, workup for kidney stones, or the evaluation of systemic conditions with potential renal involvement, such as systemic lupus erythematosus. There are three ways to obtain a urine specimen: spontaneous voiding, uretheral catheterization, and percutaneous bladder puncture. Technique is important in collecting a sample to avoid contamination. For spontaneously voided urine, a midstream sample should be collected after cleaning of the external genitalia. If a patient has an indwelling catheter, a fresh specimen should be submitted for analysis; samples that have been stagnant in the catheter tubing or bag may have undergone degradation. Suprapubic needle aspiration of the bladder is used when urine cannot easily be obtained by other means, most commonly in infants. Whatever the collection method, it is recommended that a sample be analyzed within 2 to 4 hours of the time of collection to prevent cell lysis and precipitation of solutes.[64] There are numerous techniques for examining urine; this section focuses on methods commonly used for assessment of chemical content and microscopy.

### COLOR

The color of urine is determined by chemical content, concentration, and pH (Table 23.4). Urine may be almost colorless if the output is high and the osmolality is low. Abnormal color changes can be due to drugs, foods, and pathologic conditions. Cloudy urine is most commonly due to leukocytes and bacteria. The most common cause of red urine is hemoglobin. Red urine in the absence of red blood cells in the sediment usually indicates either free hemoglobin or myoglobin. In the latter case, the patient's serum is not pink. Red urine with red sediment indicates hemoglobin. By contrast, red urine with clear sediment is most often the result of myoglobin but may also be seen in some porphyrias,

**Table 23.4 Main Causes of Abnormal Color Changes in Urine**

| | Cause | Color |
|---|---|---|
| Pathologic conditions | Gross hematuria, hemoglobinuria, myoglobinuria | Pink, red, brown, black |
| | Jaundice | Yellow to brown |
| | Chyluria | White milky urine |
| | Massive uric acid crystalluria | Pink |
| | Porphyrinuria, alkaptonuria | Red to black; increases after urine left to stand |
| Medications | Rifampin | Yellow-orange to red |
| | Propofol | White |
| | Phenytoin, phenazopyridine | Red |
| | Chloroquine, nitrofurantoin | Brown |
| | Triamterene, blue dyes of enteral feeds | Green |
| | Metronidazole, methyldopa, imipenem–cilastatin | Darkening after urine left to stand |
| Foods | Beetroot | Red |
| | Senna rhubarb | Yellow to brown red |

From Fogazzi GB, Verdesca S, Garigali G. Urinalysis: core curriculum 2008. *Am J Kidney Dis.* 2008;51:1052–1067; and Davsion A. *Urinalysis.* 3rd ed. Oxford: Oxford University Press; 2005.

or with the use of some medications or the ingestion of beets in some individuals.[65]

## ODOR

The most common cause of abnormal urine odor is infection and in this case the abnormal odor is caused by the production of ammonia by bacteria. Ketones may cause a fruity or sweet odor. Some rare pathologic conditions may confer a specific odor to the urine. Examples are maple syrup urine disease (maple syrup odor), phenylketonuria (mousy odor), isovaleric acidemia (sweaty feet odor), and hypermethioninemia (fishy odor).[64]

## RELATIVE DENSITY

The concentration, or relative density, of urine can be assessed by either specific gravity or osmolality. "Specific gravity" is defined as the weight of a solution relative to that of an equal volume of water. It is determined by the number and size of particles in the urine. Specific gravity is traditionally measured by a urinometer, which is a weighted float marked with a scale from 1.000 to 1.060. This method is simple but outdated owing to the need for a larger volume of urine than with other methods and the potential for inaccuracy in reading the device. Today, specific gravity is commonly measured by refractometry or dry chemistry methods. Refractometry measures specific gravity using the refractive index of a solution, which is a function of the weight of solute per unit volume. It requires only a drop of urine.

Dry chemistry techniques are used in reagent strips. An indirect method is used to determine specific gravity, relying on the fact that there is generally a linear relationship between urine's ionic strength and its specific gravity. The reagent strip contains a polyionic polymer that has binding sites that are saturated with hydrogen ions, and an indicator substance. The release of hydrogen ions when they are competitively replaced with urinary cations causes a change in the pH-sensitive indicator dye. Specific gravity values measured by dipstick tend to be falsely high if the urine pH is <6 and falsely low if the pH is >7. The effects of nonionized molecules such as glucose and urea on osmolality are not reflected by changes in the dipstick specific gravity. Dry chemistry measurements of specific gravity therefore tend to correlate poorly with refractometry and osmolality.[64]

"Osmolality," the gold standard for relative density, is defined as the number of osmoles of solute per kilogram of solvent. It is measured directly with an osmometer. It depends on the number of particles in solution and is not influenced by their size or temperature. High-glucose solutions significantly increase osmolality (10 g/L glucose = 55.5 mOsmol/L).[64] Urine specific gravity is generally proportional to the osmolality and rises by approximately 0.001 for every 35- to 40-mOsmol/kg increase in urine osmolality.[66] A urine osmolality of 280 mOsmol/kg (which is isosmotic to normal plasma) is usually associated with a urine specific gravity of 1.008 or 1.009. Specific gravity is affected by protein, mannitol, dextrans, and radiographic contrast media. In these settings, specific gravity can be increased disproportionately to the osmolality, falsely suggesting highly concentrated urine. There are no causes of a falsely low urine specific gravity value, and thus a specific gravity ≤1.003 measured by refractometry always indicates a maximally dilute urine (≤100 mOsmol/kg).

## URINE PH

Urine pH is usually measured with a reagent test strip. Most commonly, the double indicators methyl red and bromothymol blue are used in the reagent strips to give a broad range of colors at different pH values. The normal range for urine pH is 4.5 to 7.8. Significant deviations from true pH occur with values <5.5 or >7.5 with reagent strip methods.[52,56] Urine pH can be useful in diagnosing systemic acid–base disorders when used in conjunction with other investigations, although in isolation it provides little useful diagnostic information. A very alkaline urine (pH > 7.0) is suggestive of infection with a urea-splitting organism, such as *Proteus mirabilis.* Prolonged storage can lead to overgrowth of urea-splitting bacteria and the laboratory measurement of a high urine pH. Diuretic therapy, vomiting, gastric suction, and alkali therapy can also cause a high urine pH. Acidic urine (pH < 5.0) is seen most commonly in metabolic acidosis. A urine pH > 5 in the setting of metabolic acidosis may indicate one of the forms of renal tubular acidosis, though there are forms of renal acidosis in which the urine pH is low despite a defect in the total kidney ability to excrete acid and generate bicarbonate (see also Chapters 16 and 24).[65]

## BILIRUBIN AND UROBILINOGEN

Only conjugated bilirubin is passed into the urine. Thus the result of a reagent test for bilirubin is typically positive in patients with obstructive or hepatocellular jaundice, whereas it is usually negative in patients with jaundice due to hemolysis. In patients with hemolysis, the urine urobilinogen result is often positive. Reagent test strips are very sensitive to bilirubin, detecting as little as 0.05 mg/dL. However, the measurement of bilirubin in the urine is not very sensitive for detecting liver disease. Prolonged storage and exposure to light can lead to false-negative results.[65] False-positive test results for urine bilirubin can occur if the urine is contaminated with stool.

## LEUKOCYTE ESTERASE AND NITRITES

The esterase method relies on the fact that esterases are released from lysed urine granulocytes (leukocytes). These esterases liberate 3-hydroxy-5-phenylpyrrole after substrate hydrolysis. The pyrrole reacts with a diazonium salt in the test strip, yielding a pink to purple color. The result is usually interpreted as negative, trace, small, moderate, or large. Factors that may increase leukocyte lysis include allowing urine to stand for long periods, low pH, and low relative density. In these settings, there may be a positive dipstick result for leukocyte esterase with no leukocytes seen on microscopy. High levels of glucose, albumin, ascorbic acid, tetracycline, cephalexin, or cephalothin or large amounts of oxalic acid may inhibit the reaction and cause false-negative results.[67]

Urinary nitrites indicate the presence of nitrate-reducing bacteria. In the reagent strip test, nitrite reacts with a *p*-arsanilic acid to form a diazonium compound; further reaction with 1,2,3,4-tetrahydrobenzo(h)quinolin-3-ol results in a pink color endpoint. Results are usually interpreted as positive or negative. High specific gravity and ascorbic acid may interfere with the test. False-negative results are common and may be due to prolonged sample storage or low dietary intake. It may take up to 4 hours to convert nitrate to nitrite, so inadequate bladder retention time can also give false-negative results.[67]

## GLUCOSE

Glycosuria due to hyperglycemia may occur at blood glucose levels >10 mmol/L (180 mg/dL) in subjects with normal renal function. Less commonly, glycosuria indicates failure of proximal renal tubular reabsorption in tubular disorders such as Fanconi syndrome. Most reagent strips use an oxidase–peroxidase method to measure glucose. Glucose is first oxidized to form glucuronic acid and hydrogen peroxide. Hydrogen peroxide then reacts via a peroxidase with a reduced chromogen to form a colored product.[64] This test is sensitive to glucose concentrations between 0.5 and 20 g/L.[64] Large quantities of ketones, ascorbate, and phenazopyridine hydrochloride (Pyridium) metabolites may interfere with the color reaction, causing false-negative results. Oxidizing agents and hydrochloric acid may cause false-positive results.[67] Enzymatic methods such as a hexokinase give more precise quantification of urinary glucose levels.[64]

## KETONES

Ketones (acetoacetate and acetone) are generally detected with the nitroprusside reaction.[67] Ascorbic acid and phenazopyridine can give false-positive reactions. It is important to appreciate that β-hydroxybutyrate (often 80% of total serum ketones in ketosis) is not normally detected by the nitroprusside reaction. Ketones may appear in the urine, but not in serum, with prolonged fasting or starvation. Ketones may also be detected in the urine in alcoholic or diabetic ketoacidosis.

## HEMOGLOBIN AND MYOGLOBIN

Reagent strips use the peroxidase-like activity of the heme moiety of hemoglobin to catalyze the reaction between a peroxide and a chromogen, giving a colored product. This test is very sensitive for the presence of heme in the urine. False-negative results are uncommon but may be caused by ascorbic acid, a strong reducing agent. False-positive results may occur because of oxidizing contaminants, povidone-iodine, semen, or a high concentration of bacteria with pseudoperoxidase activity (such as Enterobacteriaceae, staphylococci, and *Streptococcus* spp).[64] Normally, haptoglobin binds circulating heme-containing substances, such as hemoglobin and myoglobin. When these substances are produced in large quantities, as occurs in hemolysis or rhabdomyolysis, the capacity for binding is overwhelmed and they appear in the urine. A positive dipstick test result for hemoglobin in the absence of red blood cells in the urine sediment therefore suggests either hemolysis or rhabdomyolysis.

# PROTEINURIA

Proteinuria (see also Chapter 30) is an important sign of kidney disease, imparting powerful diagnostic and prognostic information. It is a cornerstone of the workup for CKD, AKI, hematuria, and preeclampsia. It is often the earliest marker of glomerular diseases, occurring before a reduction in GFR. Proteinuria is associated with hypertension, obesity, and vascular disease. It can be used to predict risks of CKD progression, cardiovascular disease, and all-cause mortality in general population[68] cohorts and patients with diabetes[69] and CKD.[70] Proteinuria-lowering therapies may be renoprotective,[71] and monitoring proteinuria is a key aspect of assessing treatment response in a variety of kidney diseases, including diabetes[72] and nondiabetic glomerulopathies.[19] In addition, filtered protein probably contributes to the pathogenesis of renal injury and disease progression rather than just being a marker of it.[73] Although measurement of urinary protein has long been recommended in clinical practice guidelines, recommendations regarding this practice vary substantially.[74] This section reviews the normal physiology of proteinuria as well as strengths, limitations, and applications of the different measurement techniques.

## NORMAL PHYSIOLOGY

In humans, on the basis of a GFR of 100 mL/min, 180 L of primary urine is produced per day from plasma that contains about 10 kg of protein. However, only about 0.01% or 1 g of protein passes through the glomerular filtration barrier into the filtrate.[75] The glomerular filtration barrier acts as a size-, shape-, and charge-dependent permselective molecular sieve, the unique properties of which are still incompletely understood. It restricts the passage of macromolecules, such as albumin and globulin, and enables the excretion of an almost protein-free ultrafiltrate containing water and small solvents.[76]

The glomerular filtration barrier acts to minimize diffusion of large molecules (with a Stokes–Einstein radius >1.5 nm)[77] that would otherwise occur down a concentration gradient from the plasma to the filtrate (see also Chapter 3). It is composed of three major layers—endothelial cells, the glomerular basement membrane, and podocytes, which cover the basement membrane on the side of the urinary space. Podocytes are highly specialized epithelial cells with long, interdigitated foot processes that wrap around the glomerular capillaries, forming 40-nm wide gaps, known as filtration slits, between adjacent processes (see also Chapter 4).[78] The slit diaphragm is a cell-to-cell contact that inserts laterally into the podocyte cell membrane, bridging the filtration slit. The podocyte plays a central role in integrating the components of the glomerular filtration barrier by interacting with the glomerular basement membrane and signaling at the slit diaphragm.[79] To date, at least 26 podocyte-specific gene defects, such as those encoding for the podocyte proteins nephrin and podocin, have been identified in hereditary causes of nephrotic syndrome.[80–82] In response to signals from the podocytes and mesangium, the endothelial cells acquire a highly fenestrated phenotype, with small pores covering about 20% of their surfaces.[78] This phenotype facilitates high-flux transport of fluid and small solutes. Normally, large quantities of high-molecular-weight (HMW) plasma proteins traverse the glomerular capillaries, mesangium, or both without entering the urinary space. Damage to any one of the three layers of the glomerular filtration barrier allows proteins through, resulting in abnormal, "glomerular" proteinuria.

Albumin, the dominant HMW protein in plasma, is a negatively charged, approximately 67-kDa protein.[76] Size selectivity restricts the passage of albumin through the glomerular filtration barrier. Charge selectivity, in which the negatively charged proteoglycans and heparan sulfates in the glomerular basement membrane repel albumin molecules, is a theory seeking to explain the low glomerular sieving coefficient of albumin in relation to other molecules of its size.[83] However, experimental data have called the role of basement membrane charge in permselectivity into question.[84–86] Some albumin filtration across the capillary wall does occur, after which it is resorbed by the proximal tubule cells.[87,88]

LMW proteins (<20,000 Da) pass readily across the glomerular capillary wall. Because the plasma concentration of these proteins is much lower than that of albumin and globulins, however, the filtered load is small. Moreover, LMW proteins are normally reabsorbed by the proximal tubule. Thus proteins such as $\alpha_2$-microglobulin, apoproteins, enzymes, and peptide hormones are normally excreted in only very small amounts in the urine.[65]

A small amount of protein that normally appears in the urine is the result of normal tubular secretion. Tamm–Horsfall protein is an HMW glycoprotein ($23 \times 10^6$ Da) that is formed on the epithelial surfaces of the thick ascending limb of the loop of Henle and early distal convoluted tubule. Immunoglobulin A (IgA) and urokinase are also secreted by the renal tubule and appear in the urine in small amounts.[65]

## TYPES OF PROTEINURIA

The types of proteinuria are as follows:

Glomerular: Increased filtration of macromolecules across the glomerular filtration barrier may occur from a loss of charge and size selectivity. Unlike the other types listed here, glomerular proteinuria often results in urinary protein loss >1 g/day.

Tubular: Tubular damage or dysfunction may inhibit the normal resorptive capacity of the proximal tubule, resulting in higher amounts of mostly LMW proteins in the urine. A degree of tubular proteinuria often occurs with glomerular proteinuria. Classic causes of tubular proteinuria in isolation are Fanconi syndrome and Dent disease.

Overflow: Normal or abnormal plasma proteins produced in increased amounts may be filtered at the glomerulus and may overwhelm the resorptive capacity of the proximal tubule. This occurs particularly with small or positively charged proteins and is of clinical importance principally in plasma cell dyscrasias (e.g., myeloma). It may also occur with myoglobin in rhabdomyolysis and with hemoglobin in severe intravascular hemolysis.

Postrenal: Small amounts of protein, usually nonalbumin IgG or IgA, may be excreted in the urinary tract in the setting of infection or stones. Leukocytes are also commonly present in the urine sediment.

## NORMAL LEVELS OF PROTEINURIA

As previously described, two main groups of proteins are present in the urine: plasma proteins, predominately albumin, that cross the filtration barrier, and nonplasma proteins, predominantly Tamm–Horsfall protein, that originate in renal tubules or the urinary tract. In normal physiologic conditions, about half of the excreted protein is Tamm–Horsfall protein, and <30 mg of albumin is excreted per day.[74] At normal levels of protein loss, albumin accounts for approximately 20% of total protein. As protein loss increases, albumin becomes the most significant single protein present.[89]

## CATEGORIZATION OF PROTEINURIA

The persistent excretion of abnormal levels of urinary albumin, equivalent to between 30 and 300 mg/day, that is below the level that can be detected by a standard urine protein dipstick is now termed "moderately increased albuminuria" (historically termed "microalbuminuria") and corresponds to the KDIGO albuminuria category A2. Albumin excretion of >300 mg/day is now considered as "overt

**Table 23.5 Kidney Disease: Improving Global Outcomes (KDIGO) Guideline: Categories of Proteinuria[a]**

| | Normal to Mildly Increased (KDIGO A1) | Moderately Increased (KDIGO A2) | Severely Increased (KDIGO A3) |
|---|---|---|---|
| AER (mg/24 h) | <30 | 30–300 | >300 |
| PER (mg/24 h) | <150 | 150–500 | >500 |
| ACR: | | | |
| mg/mmol | <3 | 3–30 | >30 |
| mg/g | <30 | 30–300 | >300 |
| PCR: | | | |
| mg/mmol | <15 | 15–50 | >50 |
| mg/g | <150 | 150–500 | >500 |
| Protein reagent strip | Negative to trace | Trace to + | + or greater |

[a]Relationships between AER and ACR and between PER and PCR are based on the assumption that average creatinine excretion rate is 1.0 g/day or 10 mmol/day (conversions are rounded for pragmatic reasons).

*ACR,* Albumin-to-creatinine ratio; *AER,* albumin excretion rate; *PCR,* protein-to-creatinine ratio; *PER,* protein excretion rate.

From Kidney Disease: Improving Global Outcomes (KDIGO) CKD Work Group. KDIGO 2012 clinical practice guideline for the evaluation and management of chronic kidney disease. *Kidney Int Suppl.* 2013;3:1–150.

proteinuria or severely increased albuminuria" (KDIGO albuminuria category A3, historically termed "macroalbuminuria") and can be detected by a standard urine dipstick. "Nephrotic-range proteinuria" is protein excretion of >3.5 g/24 hours and is usually indicative of glomerular pathology. The 2012 KDIGO guidelines discourage the use of the term "microalbuminuria," instead suggesting that the term "albuminuria" be used and the level subsequently quantified (Table 23.5).[19] This recommendation has been sanctioned by the Association of Laboratory Physicians and Clinical Chemists in different jurisdictions. The presence of proteinuria or albuminuria strongly predicts outcomes of CKD progression as well as of cardiovascular and all-cause mortality in the population with CKD. The risk rises continuously as albuminuria increases.[90] The 2012 KDIGO guidelines added a category for albuminuria to the classification of CKD to improve risk stratification.[19]

## SOURCES OF ERROR IN MEASUREMENT

The 24-hour urine collection for protein measurement is considered the gold standard for measuring protein or albumin (Tables 23.6 and 23.7). Methods such as reagent strips, random measurement of protein or albumin concentrations, and albumin- or protein-to-creatinine ratios (ACRs or PCRs) aim to estimate a 24-hour protein measure. A positive result from a semiquantitative test, such as a urinary dipstick test, should prompt further evaluation with a quantitative test. Both preanalytical factors and factors intrinsic to the analysis itself can be sources of error in protein measurement. In the assessment of the quality of a test, both accuracy and precision need to be taken into account. Although a test may give reproducible results, it may not accurately measure all clinically significant types of proteinuria. The heterogeneous types of protein and the different molecular forms of proteins (such as albumin) that may be present in urine make for a challenge to both accuracy and precision of measurement. Using a consistent form of measurement with a consistent assay to monitor proteinuria, and using multiple measurements to confirm findings, is therefore advisable.

**Table 23.6 Patient Factors That May Increase Urinary Protein or Albumin**

- Posture (postural proteinuria)
- Urinary tract infection
- Hematuria
- High dietary protein intake
- High-intensity exercise
- Congestive cardiac failure
- Menstruation or vaginal discharge
- Drugs (e.g., nonsteroidal antiinflammatory drugs)

Adapted from Johnson DW, Jones GR, Mathew TH, et al. Chronic kidney disease and measurement of albuminuria or proteinuria: a position statement. *Med J Aust.* 2012;197:224–225; and Miller WG, Bruns DE, Hortin GL, et al. Current issues in measurement and reporting of urinary albumin excretion [article in French]. *Ann Biol Clin (Paris).* 2010;68:9–25.

**Table 23.7 Factors Influencing Accuracy of Proteinuria Measurement**

| Preanalysis Phase | Analysis Phase |
|---|---|
| Collection type | Total protein or albumin measurement |
| Timed or random | |
| timing of random measurement | |
| Degradation of protein or albumin | Assay type |
| during storage | |
| adsorption to plastic | |
| Storage temperature | |

Adapted from Miller WG, Bruns DE, Hortin GL, et al. Current issues in measurement and reporting of urinary albumin excretion [article in French]. *Ann Biol Clin (Paris).* 2010;68:9–25; and Martin H. Laboratory measurement of urine albumin and urine total protein in screening for proteinuria in chronic kidney disease. *Clin Biochem Rev.* 2011;32:97–102.

## ADVANTAGES OF URINARY ALBUMIN OVER TOTAL PROTEIN MEASUREMENTS

Either albumin or total protein can be measured in urine. Many current guidelines recommend the measurement of urine albumin on the basis of a need to detect lower levels of protein than were previously thought to be clinically significant. Multiple studies have shown that the presence of small amounts of albumin in the urine—between 30 and 300 mg/day—have prognostic significance; increasing amounts of albuminuria are associated with continuous increases in risk of all-cause and cardiovascular mortality, AKI, and ESKD in the general population,[91] with decline in eGFR,[92,93] and with adverse outcomes in CKD.[94] Measures of total protein are imprecise at low levels of protein and are insensitive at detecting clinically important changes in albuminuria.[74] Relatively large increases in urinary albumin excretion can occur without causing a measurable increase in urinary total protein.[95] Urine albumin measurements are more specific and more sensitive for changes in glomerular permeability than are measures of urinary total protein.[19,74,95–97] In addition, because a single protein is being measured, standardization of albumin measurement is simpler than standardization of total protein measurements.[98]

## CONSIDERATIONS REGARDING MEASURING URINARY ALBUMIN RATHER THAN TOTAL PROTEIN

### EVIDENCE FOR CKD PROGRESSION RISK AND INTERVENTIONS

Much evidence on the natural history and progression of CKD has centered on measurement of 24-hour total protein.[98] In general, studies of diabetic patients have used measurements of urinary albumin, but studies of interventions and outcomes for glomerular diseases, preeclampsia, and in children have used proteinuria measurements. One difficulty with the implementation of albumin as a replacement for total protein is the lack of a constant numerical relationship between the two that would enable clinicians to translate the existing evidence base from one to the other.[74]

### MISSED TUBULAR PROTEINURIA

Relying on measurement of urinary albumin risks missing "tubular" and "overflow" proteinuria, in which nonalbumin proteins predominate. However, total protein assays are generally more sensitive to albumin than to LMW proteins, and many also have poor sensitivity for detecting tubular proteinuria.[99] Although "tubular" disorders are characterized by a relative increase in the proportion of LMW protein to albumin, albumin generally still constitutes a significant portion of total protein, probably because of failure of tubular resorption of protein.[100] In the AusDiab study, random urine samples from >10,000 people in the Australian adult population were tested, using cutoff values of 3.45 mg/mmol for ACR and 22.6 mg/mmol for PCR. Of patients who screened positive for albuminuria, 68% had negative results for proteinuria. Albuminuria performed well as a screening test for proteinuria: sensitivity was 91.7%, specificity 95.3%, and negative predictive value 99.8%. However, among those with proteinuria, 8% excreted albumin within the normal range. The investigators postulated that these individuals may have had light-chain proteinuria or interstitial nephropathies.[89] In a study of 23 patients with Dent disease, a rare but classic tubular disorder, only 2 patients had no significant urinary albumin loss in addition to losses of LMW proteins. In these two patients, the levels of LMW proteinuria were low enough that they would probably also have been missed by a total protein measurement approach.[101]

Overall, the significance of this issue in both the CKD and general populations is difficult to estimate with the currently available data. If tubular proteinuria is suspected, it is best assessed with immunoassays directed at a specific tubular protein, such as $\alpha_1$-microglobulin or monoclonal heavy or light chains.[19,74] One study that attempted to identify the proteins composing tubular proteinuria in elderly people with mild proteinuria was unable to consistently identify proteins using electrophoresis, and the researchers suggested that the elevated urinary protein measurements were due to artifact.[102]

## DIAGNOSTIC UTILITY OF PROTEIN TYPE

Simultaneous measurement of different types of urinary protein may be a useful tool in differentiating between glomerular and tubulointerstitial diseases. Several studies using gel electrophoretic techniques to separate proteins on the basis of molecular size have shown that larger proteins such as albumin predominate in glomerular disease and that the ratio of LMW proteins is increased in tubulointerstitial disorders.[103] Higher albumin-to-total protein ratios, obtained from simultaneous measurement of ACR and PCR, have been shown to be significantly associated with glomerular rather than nonglomerular pathology on renal biopsy in patients with kidney disease.[104]

## METHODS TO MEASURE URINARY TOTAL PROTEIN

Total protein in urine has been measured by chemical, turbidimetric, and dye binding (colorimetric) methods (Table 23.8). These methods are prone to interference by inorganic ions and nonprotein substances in the urine.[74] Falsely high results may occur as result of interference by aminoglycoside antibiotics,[105] plasma expanders,[106] and other substances. There is large sample-to-sample variation in the type and composition of proteins present, making accurate measurement difficult. Turbidimetric methods, which are commonly used, are imprecise, with a coefficient of variation as high as 20%.[107] Currently there is no reference measurement procedure or standardized reference material for urinary protein. Each of the different methods in use has differing sensitivity and specificity for the diverse range of proteins found in urine, potentially leading to divergent results. The range of methods and calibrants in use means that between-laboratory variation is unavoidable. Most laboratories currently use turbidimetric or colorimetric measures, which tend to react more strongly with albumin than with globulin and other nonalbumin proteins.[108]

## METHODS TO MEASURE URINARY ALBUMIN

Urinary albumin can be measured in a number of ways. An antibody binding method, in particular immunoturbidimetry,

**Table 23.8 Methods of Proteinuria Measurement**

| Method | Description | Detection Limit (mg/L) | Protein Types | Causes of Falsely Increased Results | Causes of Falsely Decreased Results |
|---|---|---|---|---|---|
| Chemical: Biuret | Copper reagent, measures peptide bonds | 50 | — | — | Tubular/LMW proteins |
| Kjeldahl | Precipitated nitrogen | | | | |
| Turbidimetric (sulfosalicylic acid, trichloroacetic acid) | Addition of precipitant denatures protein; suspension's turbidity is read in a densitometer | 50–100 | Many, including γ-globulin light chains and albumin<br>More sensitive to albumin than to globulins and nonalbumin proteins | Tolmetin sodium (Tolectin), tolbutamide, antibiotics (penicillin, nafcillin, oxacillin), radiocontrast agents | Tubular/LMW proteins |
| Dye binding (e.g., Coomassie Brilliant Blue, pyrogallol red) | Indicator changes color in presence of protein | 50–100 | More sensitive to albumin than to globulins and nonalbumin proteins (pyrogallol red improves this shortcoming) | Pyrogallol red: aminoglycoside, gelatin solutions such as plasma expanders | Tubular/LMW proteins |

*LMW,* Low molecular weight.
Adapted from Cameron JS. The patient with proteinuria and or hematuria. In: Davison A, ed. *Oxford Textbook of Clinical Nephrology.* 3rd ed. Oxford: Oxford University Press; 2005:389–411.

is most commonly used.[74,108] Because a single protein is being measured, performance of albumin assays tend to be superior to total protein assays, at least at low concentrations of protein.[108] However, the urine of healthy individuals contains a range of albumin molecules. Albumin may be immunoreactive, nonimmunoreactive, fragmented, or biochemically modified[109] and the proportions of these different types of albumin molecules in normal urine are variable.

Albumin fragments may be generated during proteolysis of albumin in renal tubules or plasma and may account for a significant proportion of total urinary albumin. A study in subjects with type 1 diabetes found that 99% of albumin was excreted as fragments <10 kDa. Another study showed that albumin fragments constituted up to 30% of total urinary protein in patients with nephrotic syndrome.[110] Intact albumin has at least five antigenic sites.[111] Routine clinical methods use both polyclonal and monoclonal antibodies, which have different sensitivities for the detection of altered forms of albumin.[98] Nonimmunoreactive forms of albumin also exist; these are either fragments that do not contain the binding sites for the antibody in use in a particular assay or intact albumin in which the epitopes have undergone conformational change.[112]

HPLC detects both immunoreactive and nonimmunoreactive albumin. Higher values for urinary albumin are generally seen in HPLC than in immunologic detection methods. This observation led to a hypothesis that there are clinically significant amounts of nonimmunoreactive albumin in urine. In a study exploring this issue, differences in urinary albumin were detected by four immunoassays and HPLC. However, the higher values seen in HPLC techniques may also represent the detection of nonalbumin macromolecules.[113] Conformational change in albumin molecules may be induced by changes in urinary pH, urea, glucose, and ascorbate concentrations. Bilirubin usually occupies a small proportion of albumin molecules, but in severe hyperbilirubinemia it may bind to >50% of albumin.[98]

## DIFFERENT LABORATORY METHODS TO MEASURE ALBUMIN IN THE URINE

The laboratory methods for measuring urinary albumin are as follows:

Immunoturbidimetric technique: Albumin in a sample of urine reacts with a specific antibody. The turbidity is measured with a spectrophotometer, and the absorbency is proportional to the albumin concentration.[114]

Double-antibody radioimmunoassay: Albumin in a urine sample competes with a known amount of radiolabeled albumin for fixed binding sites of antialbumin antibodies. Free albumin can be separated from bound albumin by immunoabsorption of the (albumin-bound) antibody. Albumin concentration in the resulting sample of albumin-bound antibody is inversely proportional to its radioactivity, which is measured against a standard curve.[115] This is a sensitive assay, but its use is limited by its expense and the need that it is to be performed in a laboratory that can manage radioactive substances.[109]

Nephelometry: Albumin in the urine sample reacts with a specific antialbumin antibody, forming light-scattering antigen–antibody complexes that can be measured with a laser nephelometer. The amount of albumin is directly proportional to scatter in the signal.[116]

Size-exclusion HPLC (SE-HPLC): Chromatographic techniques are used to measure both immunoreactive and nonimmunoreactive albumin. Proteins of different sizes are separated as they pass at different speeds through a column containing size-selective gel.[117] SE-HPLC is more sensitive for the detection of albumin than the immune-based methods, but its specificity is limited by an inability to discriminate between albumin and other proteins of the same size, such as globulins.[109]

Although the correlation among results obtained using most of these quantitative assays is very good,[96] a good correlation indicates only precision, a strong linear relationship, but not accuracy in quantifying all clinically significant proteins present. Results obtained by radioimmunoassay, immunoturbidimetry, nephelometry, and HPLC may vary significantly.[109] Therefore, ideally, the same assay should be used when albuminuria results are compared over time for a given patient. The choice of assay used to measure albuminuria is largely determined by issues of accuracy, cost, and convenience. Currently, there is no standardized procedure for measuring urine albumin and reporting results in standardized units; however, considering the recommendations for using ACRs as the standard measure for urinary protein, a number of professional bodies have moved toward establishing standard laboratory collection, measuring, and reporting procedures.[98] Standardization for measurement of albumin requires a reference material and reference measurement procedure. Using purified albumin as the reference material would not reflect the various molecular forms that may be present in the urine but may be the most practical approach to standardization. Most routine methods for urinary albumin measurement are currently calibrated against dilutions of CRM 470, a higher-order serum protein reference material with an albumin concentration of 39.7 g/L.[98,108] Other issues that would need to be addressed to standardize the measurement of urinary albumin include clarification of the molecular forms of albumin in freshly voided urine, the degree of degradation that occurs during storage and freezing, and the appropriate upper limits of normal in different age and sex groups.[98]

## TIMED VERSUS RANDOM COLLECTION FOR PROTEINURIA ASSESSMENT

Random "spot" specimens for urinary protein, expressed as a concentration, are often inaccurate for estimation of 24-hour levels because of the impact of patient hydration status on urine concentration. There is also variation in protein excretion, which can occur throughout the day (especially resulting from exercise and posture) and from day to day.[118] Methods to improve the accuracy of spot urine testing include corrections for urine creatinine and specific gravity.[119]

Protein or albumin measurement in 24-hour urine collection is generally considered the gold standard for measuring protein excretion. However, it can also be inaccurate, primarily through inaccurate urine collection. Urine creatinine can be measured to judge the adequacy of the 24-hour collection. If creatinine excretion is similar to that in previous 24-hour samples, the collection is likely to be reasonably accurate. If no other collections are available for comparison, the adequacy of collection can be judged from the expected normal range of creatinine excretion. For hospitalized men aged 20 to 50 years, this range was found to be 18.5 to 25.0 mg/kg of body weight per day, and for women of the same age, 16.5 to 22.4 mg/kg per day. These values declined with age, so that for men aged 50 to 70 years, creatinine excretion was 15.7 to 20.2 mg/kg per day, and for women, 11.8 to 16.1 mg/kg per day.[65] Factors influencing the daily creatinine excretion include determinants of muscle mass, such as gender, race, age, and BSA.[97]

## TRANSLATING URINE PCR AND ACR VALUES INTO TOTAL DAILY PROTEIN MEASUREMENTS

Urine ACR and PCR are obtained by dividing the urine protein concentrations by the urine creatinine concentration and expressing the result as mg/mmol or mg/g. Both enzymatic and Jaffe assays are used for the measurement of creatinine in urine.[19] The ratio-based tests aim to correct for the effects of urine concentration on protein measurements. Overall, these tests have shown greater accuracy and less intraindividual variability than concentrations measured in random samples[98,119,120] and are more acceptable to patients than 24-hour protein measurements. Intraindividual variability is further reduced by using a first void rather than a daytime collection specimen to measure ACR. However, there remains substantial day-to-day variability in both PCR and ACR.[98] A positive result should be followed with a second measurement, ideally in an early morning sample, to confirm the result.[19,97]

Clinicians commonly use these tests as estimations of the 24-hour protein in milligrams by multiplying the PCR in mg/mmol or ACR in mg/mmol by 10 (given an average daily creatinine excretion of 10 mmol) or using the value as given if measured in mg/g. (Although the PCR or ACR in mg/g should be multiplied by 8.8 to get an exact value in mg/mmol, these are estimates of 24-hour levels only.) Despite the reasonable performance of the ratio-based tests to estimate 24-hour protein measurements, their ability to predict the true 24-hour protein for an individual is limited by two major factors. The first is variability in the total daily creatinine excretion, in and between individuals, which affects the ratio. The second is the fluctuations in protein excretion that occur throughout the day. An understanding of the factors that may make a urine ACR or PCR value inaccurate is important for clinicians using these tests.

## CORRELATION BETWEEN RATIOS AND 24-HOUR URINE PROTEIN

Summary tables of studies comparing urine ACR and PCR with timed collections for urinary albumin and protein can be found in the 2012 KDIGO-CKD guideline. There is a relatively high degree of correlation between 24-hour urine protein excretion and PCR in random, single-voided urine samples in healthy controls[121] and in patients with a variety of kidney diseases.[122–125] The correlation has been shown in studies in patients with glomerulonephritis[126] and with type 1 diabetes mellitus (DM),[127] and in renal transplant recipients.[128,129] In some studies, the correlation between PCR and 24-hour protein measurements was less robust when proteinuria was in the nephrotic range and above.[124,127]

The urine ACR has been shown to correlate well with 24-hour urinary albumin measurements in a number of studies in people with diabetes.[130] However, a large study evaluating the correlation between ACR and 24-hour albumin excretion in 1186 subjects with type 1 DM enrolled in the Diabetes Control and Complications Trial and its follow-up study, Epidemiology of Diabetes Interventions and Complications, showed that ACR systematically underestimated albumin excretion, particularly in men.[131] Another study in the diabetic population showed that ACR increased relative to 24-hour albumin excretion with increasing age.[132] These studies highlight the fact that variability in creatinine excretion in certain groups alters the ratio. Individuals with lower muscle mass, such as females and elderly patients, would be expected to have higher ACRs than those with higher muscle mass for the same level of urinary albumin excretion.

## VARIABILITY IN CREATININE EXCRETION

Under normal circumstances, a steady rate of creatinine excretion occurs throughout the day.[133] The accuracy of the ratio-based variables depends on a constant excretion rate. This drawback limits their usefulness in the setting of rapidly changing renal function such as AKI, in which creatinine excretion is reduced, increasing the ratio for the same amount of protein excretion.

Creatinine excretion rises with increasing muscle mass, so ACR and PCR are reduced for a given level of protein excretion in groups with higher muscle mass, such as men, younger people, and certain population ancestry groups.[134,135] The fact that the average urinary creatinine excretion is 40% to 50% higher in men than in women[131,132] has led some guidelines to recommend gender-specific cutoff values for ACRs, with lower thresholds for men than women. Commonly used urine ACR thresholds for diabetic nephropathy are 25 mg/g (2.5 mg/mmol) for males and 35 mg/g (3.5 mg/mmol) for females.[97] However, the 2012 KDIGO guidelines recommend an ACR threshold of 3.0 mg/mmol for both sexes, reflecting that the ACR is an estimation with a variety of other variables, such as age and population ancestry, that are not corrected for.[19]

## FLUCTUATIONS IN PROTEIN EXCRETION

Factors that may cause transient increases in urinary protein excretion include exercise, urinary tract infections, and upright posture. High-intensity exercise may cause transient proteinuria lasting for 24 to 48 hours in healthy subjects.[136,137] Patients with CKD or diabetes have been shown to have higher levels of urinary protein or albumin excretion after exercise than control subjects.[138–140] Some guidelines have recommended screening for urinary tract infection if proteinuria is detected. However, a review of available studies suggested that asymptomatic urinary tract infection was unlikely to cause proteinuria and that screening may be unnecessary.[141]

Upright posture can cause an increase in urine protein excretion in otherwise healthy young adults.[142] Postural proteinuria is usually diagnosed by detecting proteinuria in a random sample taken while that subject has been upright that is absent in a first morning void specimen. It usually does not exceed 1 g in 24 hours. Kidney histologic examination in patients with postural proteinuria generally yields normal or nonspecific findings,[142,143] and patients with postural proteinuria have been shown to have an excellent long-term prognosis.[144] An increased urine protein excretion found on a random sample in a young person should prompt a testing of an early morning specimen to exclude postural proteinuria.[98]

Diurnal variation in protein excretion occurs in healthy individuals and patients with CKD. Overnight urinary protein excretion is lower, and the amount less variable, than in the daytime.[145,146] Thus timing of urine collection is likely to influence the sensitivity and specificity of screening tests for urine protein or albumin excretion. Samples taken at first void are most likely to accurately quantify 24-hour protein or albumin excretion,[147,148] and first void specimens are therefore regarded as preferable by a number of guidelines.[19,72,97]

## URINARY ACR VERSUS PCR

Because the relationship between albumin excretion and total protein excretion is nonlinear,[149] an ACR cannot be derived from a PCR, and vice versa. The ACR, rather than PCR, has been recommended by a number of guidelines because of an improved ability to standardize urinary albumin versus total protein measurement and the fact that albumin is the predominant protein lost in the urine.[19,97] These advantages have already been outlined. ACR has not been shown to be superior to PCR in determining prognosis or detecting CKD in nondiabetic subjects.[97] A retrospective cohort study comparing urine PCR, ACR, and 24-hour protein at a single center showed that the three were equal in predictive utility for doubling of serum creatinine, commencement of renal replacement therapy, and all-cause mortality.[149]

## REAGENT STRIP TESTING

Multireagent dipstick urinalysis has been used widely as an initial screening tool for the evaluation of proteinuria because of its low cost, availability, and ability to provide rapid point-of-care information to clinicians. Most dipstick reagents are semiquantitative, containing a pH-sensitive colorimetric indicator that changes color when negatively charged proteins bind to it. Dipstick testing for protein has limited sensitivity for nonalbumin and positively charged proteins[64,150–152] and therefore often has false-negative results in the presence of predominantly LMW (tubular or overflow) proteinuria.[109] Albumin-specific dipsticks may also be used.

The dipstick tests protein or albumin concentration, rather than an excretion rate, so it is strongly affected by changes in urine concentration. Very dilute urine may give false-negative results, and concentrated urine may give false-positive results. Measuring specific gravity concurrently with urinary protein on a dipstick can thus help with interpretation of a urine dipstick result.[153] A very high urine pH (>7.0) can give false-positive results, as can contamination of the urine with blood. Operator-dependent differences may also occur with manual reading of dipsticks, decreasing reproducibility.[147,151] The use of automated reader devices improves interoperator variability.

### ALBUMIN-SPECIFIC DIPSTICKS

In addition to dipsticks that are designed to measure total protein, albumin-specific dipsticks are in use. Many of these use dye binding methods[154–156] but antibody-based detection methods are also available.[157] Several studies have examined the sensitivity and specificity of the newer reagent strips that measure very low concentrations of urine albumin. Most of these investigations studied patients with diabetes, and most examined the Micral-Test[155,158–161] (Boehringer Mannheim, Mannheim, Germany), the Micro-Bumintest[155,162] (Ames

Division, Miles Laboratories, Elkhart, Indiana), or both. In general, these albumin reagent strip tests are more sensitive than standard dipstick tests, but they also have a relatively high rate of false-positive results.

### NEW DEVICES FOR POINT-OF-CARE PROTEIN TESTING

New systems with a creatinine test pad can report ACRs in the range previously classified as "microalbuminuria" (corresponding to <300 mg/g) or total PCRs. They overcome some of the error inherent in measuring urinary protein concentrations rather than protein excretion rates. The CLINITEK system (CLINITEK microalbumin, Siemens Medical Solutions Diagnostics, Mishawaka, Indiana) uses a reagent strip with two pads, using a dye binding method for albumin measurement and a creatinine assay based on the peroxidase-like activity of a copper creatinine complex. The reagent strips are used in combination with an analyzer to give a semiquantitative assessment of ACR.[163,164]

### ROLE OF POINT-OF-CARE AND REAGENT STRIP TESTING

The role of urinary reagent strip testing, using either protein or albumin-specific dipsticks, in the general and high-risk population is the subject of debate. Most guidelines do not recommend the use of the urine dipstick as an initial screening test for proteinuria.[74] However, reagent strip testing may be of particular use in settings where laboratory access is limited. Newer point-of-care devices that can measure low levels of albuminuria and provide ACRs may have a role to play in population screening, but this role has not yet been defined by large studies.[19]

#### General Population

Observational studies have shown that reagent strip–proven proteinuria is associated with progression to ESKD and mortality in the general population.[68,70] However, general population screening could lead to unnecessary investigations, possible harm, and excess costs.[165–168] As with all diagnostic tests, the positive and negative predictive values of the urinary reagent strips and point-of-care devices depend on the setting in which they are used as well as their sensitivity and specificity.[169,170] A study comparing urinary ACRs with protein dipsticks (Bayer Multistix) using data from the previously mentioned AusDiab study showed that positive predictive values varied greatly across low- and high-risk subgroups. The dipstick test showed a good ability to rule out proteinuria, with a reagent strip result of less than trace having a negative predictive value of 97.6% for ACR values of 30 mg/g or higher and a negative predictive value of 100% for ACR values of 300 mg/g or higher.[171] The investigators concluded that urine reagent strip testing is a reasonable "rule-out" test for proteinuria. However, an analysis by Samal and Linder argues that the rate of false-positive results, which was as high as 53% using an ACR cutoff of 30 mg/g or higher, makes urinary reagent strip testing unacceptable in the general population owing to the cost, anxiety, and workload generated by false-positive results.[168] Because of the high rate of false-positive results, a positive reagent strip test result mandates confirmation with a quantitative test. This is a factor that significantly limits the cost-effectiveness of reagent strip testing for population screening.[166,168]

Screening of schoolchildren with urinary reagent strips in Japan, Taiwan, and Korea can detect asymptomatic renal disease at an early stage.[172–174] However, there are no data to show that this policy results in improved outcomes or has benefits from a health economics perspective. Several studies have used models to assess the benefits of general population screening with urinary reagent strips, followed by angiotensin-converting enzyme inhibitor or angiotensin-receptor blocker use in the proteinuric population. One such study, assessing the utility of general practitioner–led general population screening for proteinuria in Australia in 2002, concluded that there was insufficient evidence to support this practice.[166] A study that assessed this practice in a nondiabetic, nonhypertensive U.S. population using cost per quality-adjusted life year concluded that it was cost-effective only if selectively directed toward high-risk groups (aged >60 years or with hypertension) or conducted at long intervals (10 years).[167]

#### High-Risk Populations

In contrast to general population screening, there are several studies showing the cost-effectiveness of high-risk population screening for proteinuria with urinary dipstick testing[167,175,176] and subsequent antiproteinuric therapy. A model based on screening of a hypertensive, diabetic U.S. population cohort with Micral-II semiquantitative reagent strips for albumin and initiating irbesartan treatment in patients who had microalbuminuria (estimated 24-hour urinary albumin excretion >20 μg/min) or higher levels of urinary albumin showed a 44% reduced incidence in the cumulative incidence of ESKD and was likely to be cost-effective.[175] Screening high-risk populations, such as patients with diabetes, hypertension, or known vascular disease, for microalbuminuria is recommended in most guidelines,[19,177,178] although the frequency at which testing should occur is either not specified or inconsistent. Guidelines generally advise the use of laboratory rather than reagent strip testing in the high-risk population.[179] Studies using newer devices such as the CLINITEK system have shown good negative predictive values, making it an effective rule-out test.[180–182] The CLINITEK system has shown good performance in diabetic, general population,[163] and CKD cohorts.[183] However, the usefulness and cost-effectiveness of these newer devices are yet to be confirmed by large studies.

## PROTEINURIA MEASUREMENT IN SPECIFIC POPULATIONS

### PREGNANT PATIENTS

Proteinuria is generally defined as ≥300 mg/24 hours for the diagnosis of preeclampsia. The roughly equivalent urine PCR of 300 mg/g (30 mg/mmol) showed reasonable performance in estimating 24-hour protein excretion and as a rule-out test in two systematic reviews of studies in this setting, although there were no data on PCR for predicting outcomes. Currently, there is insufficient evidence to substitute urine albumin measurement for total protein in pregnant women with hypertension or suspected preeclampsia.[184,185]

### CHILDREN

Normal levels of protein excretion in children are <10 mg/$m^2$/day, or <4 mg/$m^2$/h.[186] Nephrotic-range proteinuria is defined as 1000 mg/$m^2$/day, or 40 mg/$m^2$/h, or higher.

Urine PCR has been shown to have reasonable accuracy in reflecting 24-hour levels of protein excretion in a small study of 15 children.[187] PCR has been shown to predict an increased rate of GFR decline in children.[188–190] There is currently insufficient evidence linking elevated urine ACR with adverse outcomes to recommend the use of ACR in a pediatric population.[191] A number of studies have shown contradictory data with regard to the relationship of urinary albumin excretion in healthy children and various conditions, such as obesity, hypertension, fasting glucose, and insulin resistance.[192]

### KIDNEY TRANSPLANT RECIPIENTS

Proteinuria predicts allograft loss, cardiovascular risk, and death in kidney transplant recipients.[193] One study showed that 24-hour urinary albumin measurement was superior to total protein measurement in predicting graft loss[194]; another using urine ACR and PCR showed equivalent performances.[195]

## URINE MICROSCOPY

Examination of the urine by microscopy has been performed systematically at least since the 19th century[196] and remains a vital investigation that is often considered a component of the physical examination of a patient in whom kidney disease is suspected.

### PREPARATION AND METHOD

Formed elements in urine degrade rapidly and so urine microscopy is best performed on a fresh urine sample within 2 hours of collection. Urine preservation is not a routinely applied technique but has been performed successfully by some institutions. Traditionally, ethanol is used to preserve uroepithelial cells for cytology but this does not prevent lysis of red and white blood cells.[197] Formaldehyde-based solutions have been used to preserve urine sediment for up to 3 months, and commercial preservatives such as buffered boric acid are also available.

The first urine of the morning specimen has been recommended in the past for urine microscopy because it is acidic and concentrated, but a midstream specimen of the second urine of the morning is favored owing to the lysis of urine particles after prolonged storage of urine in the bladder overnight. Specimens should preferably not be refrigerated because this may cause precipitation of crystals. High urine pH and dilute urine lead to more degradation of formed elements.

A guideline provided by the European Confederation of Laboratory Medicine suggests standardization of preparation of the urine sediment for microscopy.[198] A sample of 5–12 mL of urine should be centrifuged at 400 g or 2000 rpm for 5 minutes, a defined volume of supernatant removed by suction rather than arbitrary decanting, and the pellet resuspended by gentle agitation. A drop of urine should be placed on a slide under a coverslip, and it should be examined ideally with phase-contrast microscopy rather than usual brightfield microscopy, at low power (×160) then at high power (×400). Staining or polarized light may also be useful to identify certain substances.

### CELLS OF THE URINARY SEDIMENT

#### ERYTHROCYTES

"Hematuria" is defined as three or more erythrocytes per high-power field. Transient hematuria is common and may be due to strenuous exercise. Persistent hematuria on three repeated urine samples warrants investigation. Studies show great variation in the prevalence of microscopic hematuria from as low as 0.18% to as high as 16.1%.[199] A study of more than a million Israeli military recruits showed an incidence of persistent hematuria of 0.3%.[200] This finding was associated with an increased risk of subsequent ESKD (hazard ratio = 19.5) although the absolute risk of ESKD was low, at 34.0 per 100,000 person-years.

Even when the urine appears red the sediment should be examined to determine whether red blood cells are present because a red appearance may be due to other causes, such as hemoglobinuria and myoglobinuria. Macroscopic hematuria is much more likely to be due to malignancy. Isomorphic red blood cells, which look similar to the erythrocytes found in the bloodstream, are thought to be nonglomerular in origin. Dysmorphic red blood cells (Fig. 23.3) are erythrocytes from the glomerular capillary, and their irregular appearance is a consequence of damage due to pH and osmolality changes as the cells travel through the tubule. Glomerular hematuria is defined by some institutions in terms of percentage of dysmorphic red blood cells, but the threshold at which this value is believed to be significant is not standardized. Glomerular hematuria is variously defined as more than 10% to 80% dysmorphic red blood cells or more than 2% to 5% acanthocytes, which are a subtype of dysmorphic red blood cells with protruding blebs.

Automated methods of examining for glomerular or nonglomerular hematuria have been developed in an attempt to overcome the problems with reliability and reproducibility of urine microscopy. These methods function by measuring the mean corpuscular volume (MCV) of the red cells. An MCV smaller or larger than the normal range (50–80 fL) is recorded as dysmorphic. The role of urinary red blood cell MCV in diagnosis was reviewed in a meta-analysis,[201] which concluded that the diagnostic value of this test is limited and that the urinary MCV test was not reliable in cases of low-grade hematuria because of interfering debris.

Causes of hematuria are listed in Table 23.9. Although anticoagulation often unmasks another underlying etiology for hematuria, over-anticoagulation itself may cause glomerular bleeding, as in the case of the relatively newly recognized condition warfarin-induced nephropathy, in which obstruction of tubules by red blood cell casts may cause AKI.[202]

#### URINE CYTOLOGY

Cytology is usually performed and is recommended as part of the investigation for nonglomerular hematuria. Although it is the realm of urologists, nephrologists may frequently encounter patients with nonglomerular hematuria as part of the investigative process for asymptomatic microscopic hematuria. A number of studies have suggested that the value of routine urine cytology as part of the workup for nonglomerular hematuria is limited if other investigations such as imaging and flexible cystoscopy are performed. For example, in a study of 2778 patients[203] who presented to a

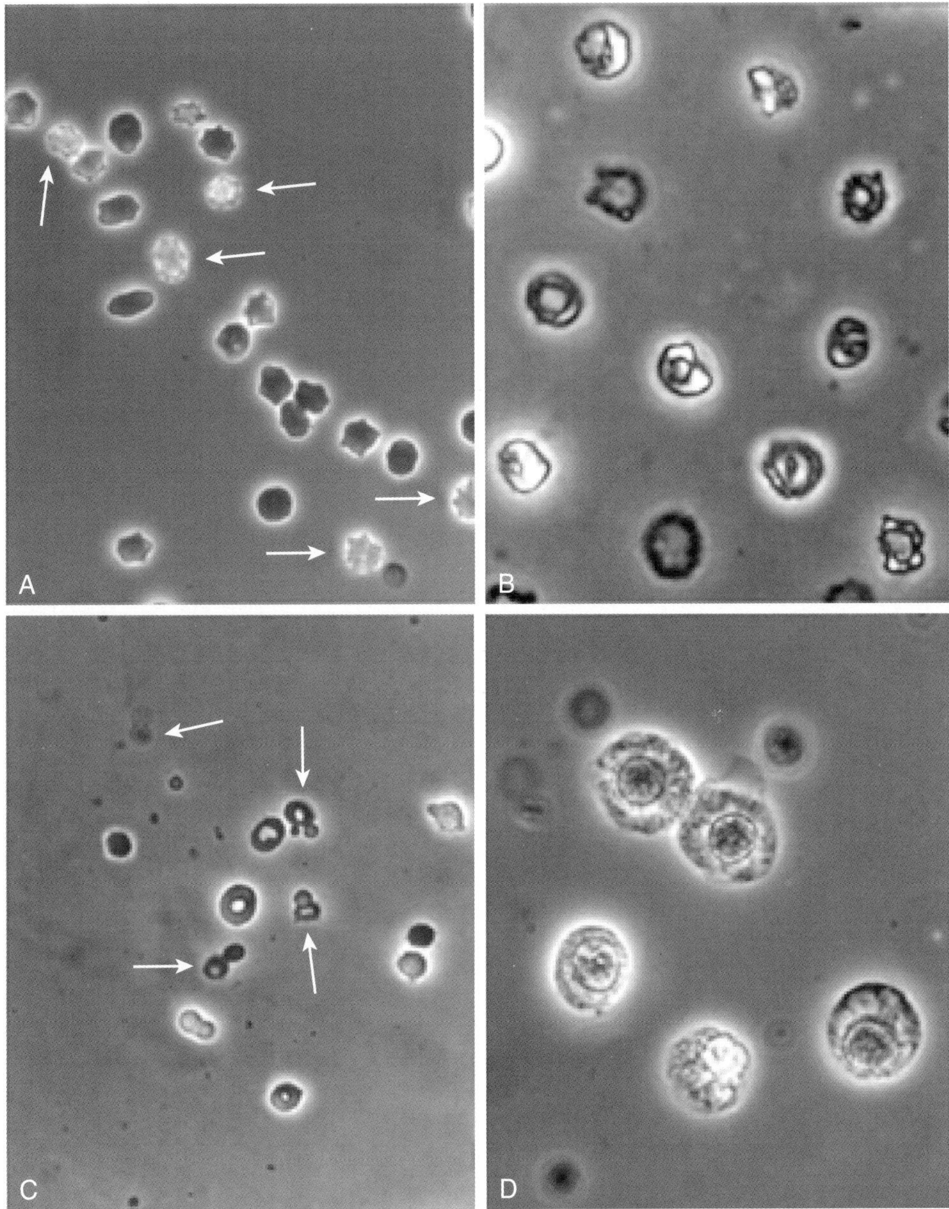


**Fig. 23.3** Erythrocytes in urine. (A) Isomorphic erythrocytes, some with a "crenated" appearance *(arrows)*. (B) Different types of dysmorphic erythrocytes. (C) Acanthocytes *(arrows)*. (D) Proximal renal tubule cells. (From Fogazzi GB, Verdesca S, Garigali G. Urinalysis: core curriculum 2008. *Am J Kidney Dis.* 2008;51:1052–1067.)

hospital hematuria clinic in the United Kingdom, 974 patients had "nonvisible" or microscopic hematuria. Of the patients with microscopic hematuria, 4.6% had a urothelial malignancy, which in 93% was a bladder tumor. Urothelial cancer cytology demonstrated only 45.5% sensitivity and 89.5% specificity. Only two patients with abnormal urine cytology as the only positive finding had urothelial malignancy on further investigation.

## LEUKOCYTES

The most common leukocytes found in the urine, neutrophils, are usually an indication of infection or contamination. Eosinophils are detectable with Wright stain or Hansel stain. Hansel stain has improved sensitivity, especially because a urine pH of <7 inhibits Wright stain. Although eosinophiluria was initially associated with drug-induced hypersensitivity, the list of diseases that may be associated with eosinophiluria is diverse and includes renal cholesterol embolism, rapidly progressive glomerulonephritis, and prostatitis.

The diagnostic value of the presence of other leukocytes, such as lymphocytes and macrophages, is currently limited, although lymphocytes have been indicative of transplant rejection, and macrophages may be found in glomerulonephritis.

## OTHER CELLS

"Squamous cells," the largest cells of the urinary sediment, derive from the urethra or external genitalia. "Renal tubule

**Table 23.9 Causes of Hematuria[a]**

| Glomerular Hematuria |
|---|
| **Glomerular Lesions** |
| Thin basement membrane nephropathy |
| Mesangial immunoglobulin A (IgA) glomerulonephritis |
| Focal and segmental hyalinosis and sclerosis (focal glomerulosclerosis) |
| Lupus glomerulonephritis |
| Crescentic glomerulonephritis, including Wegener granulomatosis, microscopic polyangiitis, and Goodpasture syndrome |
| Membranous glomerulonephritis |
| Mesangiocapillary glomerulonephritis |
| Dense deposit disease |
| Poststreptococcal glomerulonephritis |
| **Nonglomerular Disease** |
| Autosomal dominant polycystic kidney disease |
| Exercise hematuria |
| Bleeding diathesis |
| Drugs, including anticoagulants |
| **Nonglomerular Hematuria** |
| Urinary tract infection |
| Urinary tract calculi |
| Hypercalciuria and hyperuricosuria |
| Autosomal dominant polycystic kidney disease |
| Benign prostatic hypertrophy |
| Transitional cell carcinoma |
| Renal cell carcinoma |
| Prostatic carcinoma |
| Exercise hematuria |
| Trauma |
| Bleeding diathesis and anticoagulants |
| Drugs |
| Renal papillary necrosis |
| Sickle cell disease |

[a]Unknown whether glomerular or nonglomerular hematuria after percutaneous coronary artery angioplasty.

From Kincaid Smith P, Fairley K. The investigation of haematuria. *Semin Nephrol.* 2005;25:127–135.

**Table 23.10 Common Casts**

| Cast | Main Clinical Association(s) |
|---|---|
| Hyaline | Normal and in renal disease |
| Granular | Renal disease of any cause |
| Waxy | Renal disease of any cause |
| Fatty | Heavy proteinuria |
| Red blood cell | Proliferative glomerulonephritis, glomerular bleeding |
| White blood cell | Acute interstitial nephritis, acute pyelonephritis |
| Tubular epithelial cell | Acute tubular necrosis ("muddy brown" casts), acute interstitial nephritis, proliferative glomerulonephritis |

From Fogazzi GB, Verdesca S, Garigali G. Urinalysis: core curriculum 2008. *Am J Kidney Dis.* 2008;51:1052–1067.

**Table 23.11 Common Crystals and Their Appearance**

| Crystal | Appearance |
|---|---|
| Uric acid | Usually lozenges but varying shape, yellow-tinged |
| Calcium oxalate | Monohydrate: ovoid or dumbbell-shaped, biconcave disks<br>Dihydrate: bipyramidal |
| Calcium phosphate | Prisms, star-like particles or needles of various sizes |
| Triple phosphate (struvite) | Coffin lids |
| Cholesterol | Transparent thin plates |
| Cystine | Hexagonal plates with irregular sides |

From Fogazzi GB, Verdesca S, Garigali G. Urinalysis: core curriculum 2008. *Am J Kidney Dis.* 2008;51:1052–1067.

epithelial cells" may be present in tubular injury. "Urothelial cells" may be seen in urologic diseases such as malignancy.

## OTHER ELEMENTS

### LIPIDS

Lipids appear as spherical, translucent drops of varying size. They may also be within the cytoplasm of cells as "oval fat bodies." Under polarized light, lipid droplets look like Maltese crosses. Lipiduria is usually associated with heavy proteinuria but may also be present in Fabry disease.

### CASTS

"Casts" (Fig. 23.4) are cylindrical bodies of renal origin that form from the aggregation of fibrils of Tamm–Horsfall glycoprotein (uromodulin), which is secreted by cells of the thick ascending limb of the loop of Henle. Trapping of various particles within the cast matrix, as well as degenerative processes, results in casts with different appearances and clinical significance (Table 23.10). Hyaline casts are nonspecific and may be present normally. Granular casts are nonspecific and contain protein aggregates or degenerated cellular elements. Waxy casts are also nonspecific and result from degeneration of other casts. Broad casts are wider waxy casts that are seen in chronic renal failure in which there is dilation of the tubule. Renal tubule epithelial cell casts are formed from the aggregation of desquamated cells of the tubule lining. Because the epithelial cells still appear intact, this finding is usually the result of an acute disease process such as acute tubular necrosis. Red blood cell casts are always pathologic and indicate significant glomerular bleeding, which is often due to rapidly progressive glomerulonephritis.

### CRYSTALS

A large variety of crystals can be seen in the urine that may be of diagnostic value (Table 23.11). However, uric acid, calcium oxalate, and calcium phosphate crystals are common and may have little clinical significance because they may precipitate as a result of transient supersaturation of urine

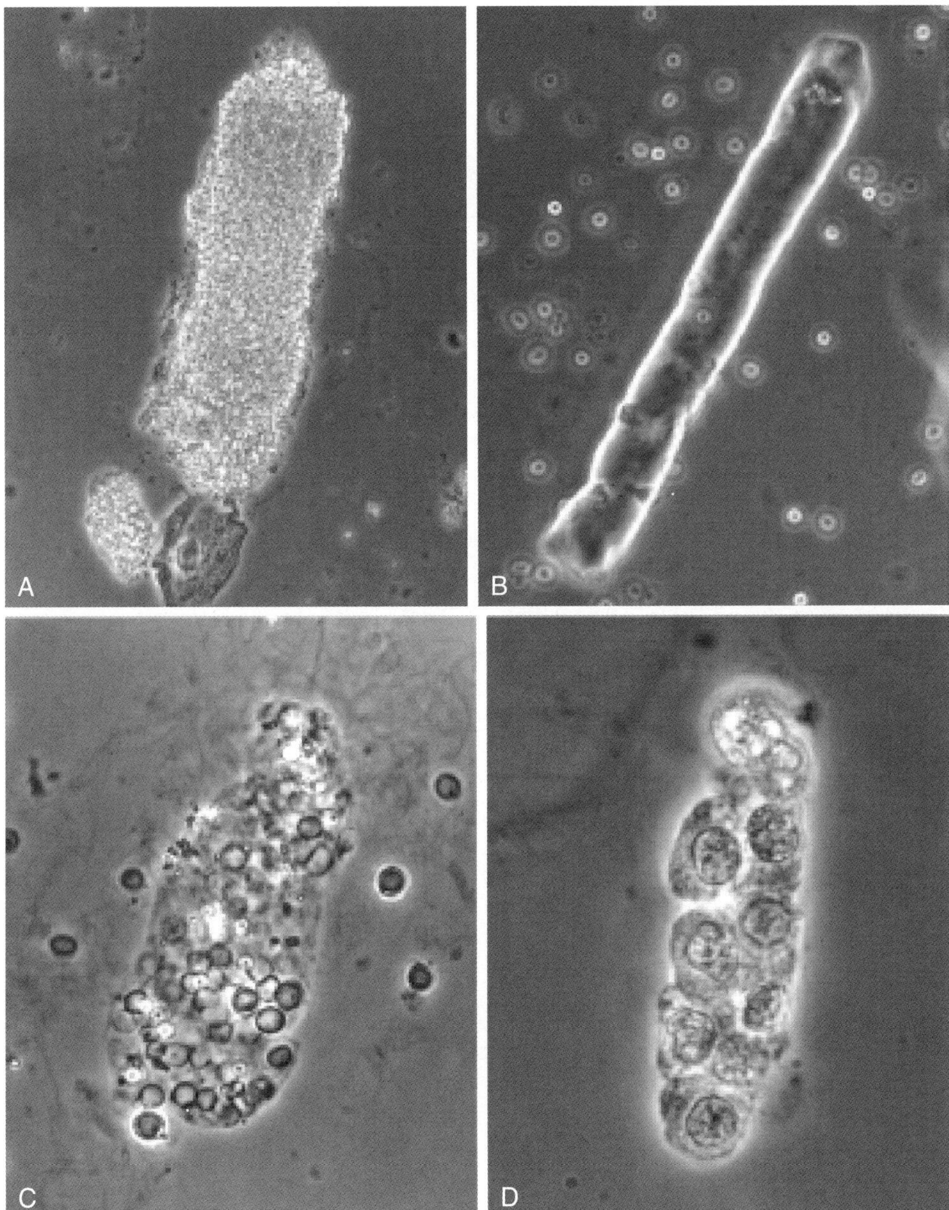


**Fig. 23.4** Urinary casts. (A) A finely granular cast. (B) Waxy cast with the typical "melted wax" appearance. (C) A red blood cell cast. (D) A renal tubule epithelial cell cast. (From Stevens LA, Nolin TD, Richardson MM, et al. Comparison of drug dosing recommendations based on measured GFR and kidney function estimating equations. *Am J Kidney Dis.* 2009;54:33–42.)

due to dehydration or cooling of the sample. Of course, depending on the clinical setting, uric acid crystals may be highly significant because they are present in acute uric acid nephropathy as part of tumor lysis syndrome, and calcium oxalate crystals may indicate ethylene glycol poisoning or hyperoxaluria.

A growing list of drugs, beginning with acyclovir and indinavir, may cause crystals in the urine that commonly have unusual shapes.

### MICROORGANISMS

Bacteria are commonly seen because of contamination or infection. Fungi such as *Candida*, protozoa such as *Trichomonas*, and parasites such as *Schistosoma* may also be seen.

## LIMITATIONS

Urine microscopy depends on expertise and has poor interobserver reliability. In a study involving 10 nephrologists, agreement for various elements in urine microscopy ranged from 31.4% to 79.1% and interobserver agreement was not associated with seniority.[204] Despite this limitation, urinary microscopy is still a vital component of the laboratory assessment of renal disease because its findings may crucially influence management of a patient. For example, identification of dysmorphic red blood cells and red blood cell casts in a patient with AKI may prompt empirical treatment with immunosuppressive therapy in advance of results of serology or renal biopsy.

## SUMMARY

Despite advances in the field of laboratory assessment of kidney disease, this domain continues to be an evolving science with future research aiming to derive tests and equations that will not only reduce bias but also improve precision and accuracy. There is an ongoing need for better understanding of the intricacies of these tests by physicians and clinical chemists to appropriately diagnose and prognosticate patients and guide their management.

Complete reference list available at ExpertConsult.com.

## KEY REFERENCES


2. Miller WG, Myers GL, Ashwood ER, et al. Creatinine measurement: state of the art in accuracy and interlaboratory harmonization. *Arch Pathol Lab Med.* 2005;129(3):297–304.
5. Dharnidharka VR, Kwon C, Stevens G. Serum cystatin C is superior to serum creatinine as a marker of kidney function: a meta-analysis. *Am J Kidney Dis.* 2002;40(2):221–226.
19. Kidney Disease: Improving Global Outcomes (KDIGO) CKD Work Group. KDIGO 2012 clinical practice guideline for the evaluation and management of chronic kidney disease. *Kidney Int Suppl.* 2013;3:1–150.
30. Levey AS, Bosch JP, Lewis JB, et al. A more accurate method to estimate glomerular filtration rate from serum creatinine: a new prediction equation. Modification of Diet in Renal Disease Study Group. *Ann Intern Med.* 2009;130(6):461–470.
31. Levey AS, Stevens LA, Schmid CH, et al. A new equation to estimate glomerular filtration rate. *Ann Intern Med.* 2009;150:604–612.
32. Matsushita K, Mahmoodi BK, Woodward M, et al. Comparison of risk prediction using the CKD-EPI equation and the MDRD study equation for estimated glomerular filtration rate. *JAMA.* 2012;307(18):1941–1951.
33. Eriksen BO, Mathisen UD, Melsom T, et al. The role of cystatin C in improving GFR estimation in the general population. *Am J Kidney Dis.* 2012;59(1):32–40.
35. Cockcroft DW, Gault MH. Prediction of creatinine clearance from serum creatinine. *Nephron.* 2012;16(1):31–41.
37. Schwartz GJ, Haycock GB, Edelmann CM, et al. A simple estimate of glomerular filtration rate in children derived from body length and plasma creatinine. *Pediatrics.* 1976;58(2):259–263.
38. Schwartz GJ, Muñoz A, Schneider MF, et al. New equations to estimate GFR in children with CKD. *J Am Soc Nephrol.* 1976;20(3):629–637.
39. Schwartz GJ, Work DF. Measurement and estimation of GFR in children and adolescents. *Clin J Am Soc Nephrol.* 2009;4(11):1832–1843.
48. Chen S. Retooling the creatinine clearance equation to estimate kinetic GFR when the plasma creatinine is changing acutely. *J Am Soc Nephrol.* 2013;24(6):877–888.
49. Endre ZH, Pickering JW, Walker RJ. Clearance and beyond: the complementary roles of GFR measurement and injury biomarkers in acute kidney injury (AKI). *Am J Physiol Renal Physiol.* 2013;301(4):F697–F707.
52. Stevens LA, Nolin TD, Richardson MM, et al. Comparison of drug dosing recommendations based on measured GFR and kidney function estimating equations. *Am J Kidney Dis.* 2009;54(1):33–42.
55. Kilbride HS, Stevens PE, Eaglestone G, et al. Accuracy of the MDRD (Modification of Diet in Renal Disease) study and CKD-EPI (CKD Epidemiology Collaboration) equations for estimation of GFR in the elderly. *Am J Kidney Dis.* 2013;61(1):57–66.
64. Fogazzi GB, Verdesca S, Garigali G. Urinalysis: core curriculum 2008. *Am J Kidney Dis.* 2008;51(6):1052–1067.
65. Israni A, Kasiske B, et al. Laboratory assessment of kidney disease: glomerular filtration rate, urinalysis, and proteinuria. In: Taal M, Chertow G, Marsden P, eds. *Brenner and Rector's the Kidney.* 9th ed. Philadelphia: Saunders; 2011:868–892.
67. Jacobs D, De Mott WR, Willie GR, et al. Urinalysis and clinical microscopy. In: Jacobs D, Kasten BL, De Mott WR, eds. *Laboratory Test Handbook.* Baltimore: Williams & Wilkins; 1990:906–909.
68. Kannel WB, Stampfer MJ, Castelli WP, et al. The prognostic significance of proteinuria: the Framingham study. *Am Heart J.* 1984;108(5):1347–1352.
72. KDOQI. KDOQI clinical practice guidelines and clinical practice recommendations for diabetes and chronic kidney disease. *Am J Kidney Dis.* 2007;49(2 suppl 2):S12–S154.
74. Lamb EJ, MacKenzie F, Stevens PE. How should proteinuria be detected and measured? *Ann Clin Biochem.* 2009;46(Pt 3):205–217.
77. Cameron JS. The patient with proteinuria and or hematuria. In: Davison A, ed. *Oxford Textbook of Clinical Nephrology.* 3rd ed. Oxford: Oxford University Press; 2005:389–411.
78. Brinkkoetter PT, Ising C, Benzing T. The role of the podocyte in albumin filtration. *Nat Rev Nephrol.* 2013;9(6):328–336.
87. Russo LM, Bakris GL, Comper WD. Renal handling of albumin: a critical review of basic concepts and perspective. *Am J Kidney Dis.* 2002;39(5):899–919.
89. Atkins RC, Briganti EM, Zimmet PZ, et al. Association between albuminuria and proteinuria in the general population: the AusDiab study. *Nephrol Dial Transplant.* 2003;18(10):2170–2174.
91. Hillege HL, Fidler V, Diercks GF, et al. Urinary albumin excretion predicts cardiovascular and noncardiovascular mortality in general population. *Circulation.* 2002;106(14):1777–1782.
97. Johnson DW, Jones GR, Mathew TH, et al. Chronic kidney disease and measurement of albuminuria or proteinuria: a position statement. *Med J Aust.* 2012;197(4):224–225.
98. Miller WG, Bruns DE, Hortin GL, et al. Current issues in measurement and reporting of urinary albumin excretion. *Ann Biol Clin (Paris).* 2010;68(1):9–25.
108. Martin H. Laboratory measurement of urine albumin and urine total protein in screening for proteinuria in chronic kidney disease. *Clin Biochem Rev.* 2011;32(2):97–102.
109. Viswanathan G, Upadhyay A. Assessment of proteinuria. *Adv Chronic Kidney Dis.* 2011;18(4):243–248.
111. Sviridov D, Drake SK, Hortin GL. Reactivity of urinary albumin (microalbumin) assays with fragmented or modified albumin. *Clin Chem.* 2008;54(1):61–68.
118. Naresh CN, Hayen A, Craig JC, et al. Day-to-day variability in spot urine protein-creatinine ratio measurements. *Am J Kidney Dis.* 2012;60(4):561–566.
119. Newman DJ, Pugia MJ, Lott JA, et al. Urinary protein and albumin excretion corrected by creatinine and specific gravity. *Clin Chim Acta.* 2000;294(1–2):139–155.
124. Ruggenenti P, Gaspari F, Perna A, et al. Cross sectional longitudinal study of spot morning urine protein:creatinine ratio, 24 hour urine protein excretion rate, glomerular filtration rate, and end stage renal failure in chronic renal disease in patients without diabetes. *BMJ.* 1998;316(7130):504–509.
125. Price CP, Newall RG, Boyd JC. Use of protein:creatinine ratio measurements on random urine samples for prediction of significant proteinuria: a systematic review. *Clin Chem.* 2005;51(9):1577–1586.
142. Robinson RR. Isolated proteinuria in asymptomatic patients. *Kidney Int.* 1980;18:395–406.
148. Witte EC, Lambers Heerspink HJ, de Zeeuw D, et al. First morning voids are more reliable than spot urine samples to assess microalbuminuria. *J Am Soc Nephrol.* 2009;20(2):436–443.
149. Methven S, Macgregor MS, Traynor JP, et al. Comparison of urinary albumin and urinary total protein as predictors of patient outcomes in CKD. *Am J Kidney Dis.* 2011;57(1):21–28.
165. Iseki K, Kinjo K, Iseki C, et al. Relationship between predicted creatinine clearance and proteinuria and the risk of developing ESRD in Okinawa, Japan. *Am J Kidney Dis.* 2004;44(5):806–814.
166. Craig JC, Barratt A, Cumming R, et al. Feasibility study of the early detection and treatment of renal disease by mass screening. *Intern Med J.* 2002;32(1–2):6–14.
167. Boulware LE, Jaar BG, Tarver-Carr ME, et al. Screening for proteinuria in US adults: a cost-effectiveness analysis. *JAMA.* 2003;290(23):3101–3114.
168. Samal L, Linder JA. The primary care perspective on routine urine dipstick screening to identify patients with albuminuria. *Clin J Am Soc Nephrol.* 2013;8(1):131–135.
186. Hogg RJ, Portman RJ, Milliner D, et al. Evaluation and management of proteinuria and nephrotic syndrome in children: recommendations from a pediatric nephrology panel established at the National Kidney Foundation Conference on proteinuria, albuminuria, risk, assessment, detection, and elimination (PARADE). *Pediatrics.* 2000;105(6):1242–1249.

195. Panek R, Lawen T, Kiberd BA. Screening for proteinuria in kidney transplant recipients. *Nephrol Dial Transplant.* 2011;26(4): 1385–1387.
200. Vivante A, Afek A, Frenkel-Nir Y, et al. Persistent asymptomatic isolated microscopic hematuria in Israeli adolescents and young adults and risk for end-stage renal disease. *JAMA.* 2011;306(7): 729–736.
201. Offringa M, Benbassat J. The value of urinary red cell shape in the diagnosis of glomerular and post-glomerular haematuria. A meta-analysis. *Postgrad Med J.* 1992;68(802):648–654.
203. Mishriki SF, Aboumarzouk O, Vint R, et al. Routine urine cytology has no role in hematuria investigations. *J Urol.* 2013;189(4):1255–1258.
204. Wald R, Bell CM, Nisenbaum R, et al. Interobserver reliability of urine sediment interpretation. *Clin J Am Soc Nephrol.* 2009;4(3):567–571.

# 24 Interpretation of Electrolyte and Acid-Base Parameters in Blood and Urine

Kamel S. Kamel | Mitchell L. Halperin

**CHAPTER OUTLINE**



An analysis of laboratory data from samples of blood and urine is essential to make accurate diagnoses and to design optimal therapy for patients with disturbances of water, sodium ($Na^+$), potassium ($K^+$), and acid-base homeostasis.[1] Our clinical approach and interpretation of these tests rely heavily on an understanding of the basic concepts of the physiology of the renal regulation of water, electrolyte, and acid-base homeostasis. Hence, each section in this chapter begins with a discussion of physiologic concepts that help focus on the important factor(s) in the regulation of the homeostasis of the substances in question.

Based on this understanding of physiology, we discuss the laboratory data used to help determine the underlying pathophysiology of the disturbance. This information is then used to construct our approach to patients with each of these disorders. At the end of each section, clinical cases are presented succinctly to illustrate how this approach is used at the bedside.

We emphasize that there are no normal values for the urinary excretion of water and electrolytes because subjects in the steady state excrete all ions that are consumed and not lost by nonrenal routes. Hence, data should be interpreted in the context of the prevailing stimulus and the expected renal response.

## WATER AND SODIUM

In this section, we illustrate how we use information about the volume and composition of the urine in the clinical approach to patients with disorders causing polyuria, those causing a decreased effective arterial blood volume (EABV), and those causing hyponatremia.

### POLYURIA

There are two definitions of polyuria. The conventional definition of polyuria is a urine volume that is more than 2.5 L/day. This is an arbitrary definition based on comparing the 24-hour urine volume in the patient with the usual values of 24-hour urine volumes observed in individuals who consume a typical Western diet.

We prefer a physiology-based definition. Polyuria is present if the urine flow rate is higher than what is expected in a specific setting. In the presence of vasopressin action, urine volume is determined by the rate of excretion of effective osmoles and the effective osmolality of the medullary interstitial compartment. Hence, polyuria is present if the urine volume is higher than what is expected for the rate of excretion of effective osmoles, even if the urine volume does not exceed 2.5 L/day. In contrast, if the concentration of $Na^+$ in plasma ($P_{Na}$) is less than 135 mmol/L, the release of vasopressin should be inhibited, and the urine flow rate could be as high as 10 to 15 mL/min in an adult subject (which extrapolates to around 14 to 22 L/day). A lower urine volume in this setting, although still higher than 2.5 L/day, represents oliguria and not polyuria.

There are two categories of polyuria, a water diuresis and an osmotic diuresis.

### WATER DIURESIS

#### Concept 1

To move water across a membrane, there must be a channel that allows water to cross that membrane (an aquaporin [AQP]) and a driving force for the movement of water—a difference in the concentrations of effective osmoles or a difference in the hydrostatic pressures across that membrane.

**Water Channels.** There are two critically important aquaporin water channels in the luminal membranes of cells in the kidney, AQP1 and AQP2 (Fig. 24.1). AQP1 channels are nonregulated water channels that are constitutively present in the luminal membrane of proximal tubule (PT) cells. AQP1 channels are also constitutively present in the luminal membrane of the descending thin limbs of the loop of Henle

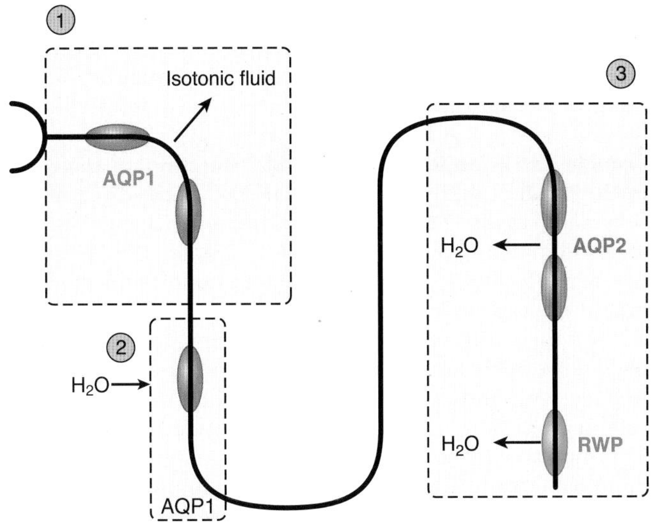


**Fig. 24.1** Functional units of the nephron based on presence of aquaporins AQP1 and AQP2. The *solid line* represents a nephron; AQP1 is represented as a *small pink ovals* and AQP2 as *blue ovals*. With regard to water excretion, we divide the nephron into three functional units (delineated by rectangles with dashed lines) on the basis of the presence of AQP1 or AQP2. AQP1 is always present in the proximal tubule cells—the first functional nephron unit **(1)**. AQP1 is also present in the descending thin limb of the loop of Henle (DtL) of the juxtamedullary nephrons, which constitute about 15% of the total nephrons—the second functional nephron unit **(2)**. Vasopressin causes the insertion of AQP2 into the luminal membrane of principal cells in the cortical collecting duct (CCD) and the medullary collecting duct (MCD); together, these nephron segments constitute the final or third functional unit **(3)**. Even in the absence of vasopressin, there seems to be a small degree of water permeability in the inner MCD, which is called residual water permeability (RWP). (Modified from Halperin ML, Kamel KS, Goldstein MB. *Fluid, Electrolyte, and Acid-Base Physiology; A Problem-Based Approach.* ed 4. Philadelphia: Elsevier; 2012.)

(DtLs) of the juxtamedullary nephrons, which constitute about 15% of the total number of nephrons. Of note, AQP1 channels are not present in the luminal membrane of the DtLs of the superficial nephrons; thus, the entire loop of Henle of these nephrons (i.e., 85% of all the nephrons) is relatively impermeable to water.[2]

Vasopressin causes the insertion of AQP2 channels into the luminal membrane of principal cells in the cortical collecting duct (CCD), and the medullary collecting duct (MCD). Notwithstanding, even in the absence of vasopressin action, there seems to be a small degree of water permeability in the inner MCD, called basal or residual water permeability (RWP).

**Driving Force.** Water is drawn from a compartment with a lower effective osmolality to one with a higher effective osmolality. Effective osmoles are osmoles that have a difference in their concentrations between two compartments. The magnitude of this driving force could be very large, because a difference of 1 mOsmol/kg $H_2O$ generates a pressure of 19.3 mm Hg. Vasopressin causes the insertion of AQP2 in the luminal membrane of principal cells in the CCD and MCD. Hence, as soon as water reaches a nephron segment that has AQP2 in the luminal membrane of its cells, water will be reabsorbed until the effective osmolality in the luminal fluid is nearly equal to the effective osmolality in the surrounding interstitial fluid compartment.

Because vasopressin causes the insertion of urea transporters in the luminal membrane of cells in the inner MCD, the concentration of urea in the interstitial fluid in the inner medulla becomes nearly equal to its concentration in the lumen in the inner MCD. Hence, at the usual rate of urea excretion, which does not exceed the transport capacity of the urea transporters, urea is not an effective urine osmole (i.e., the excretion of urea does not obligate the excretion of $H_2O$).

## Concept 2

The urine volume during a water diuresis is determined by the volume of distal delivery of filtrate and the volume of filtrate that is reabsorbed in the inner MCD via its RWP.[3]

**Distal Delivery of Filtrate.** The volume of distal delivery of filtrate is the volume of glomerular filtration minus the volume of filtrate that is reabsorbed in the nephron segments prior to the CCD. There are data to suggest that AQP1 channels are not present in the luminal membranes of the DtLs of the superficial nephrons, which constitute 85% of the total number of nephrons.[2] If that is the case, then the entire loop of Henle of most of the nephrons is impermeable to water. Hence, the volume of distal delivery of filtrate should be approximately equal to the volume of glomerular filtration minus the volume that is reabsorbed by PT.

It was thought that about 66% of the glomerular filtration rate (GFR) is reabsorbed along the entire PT. This was based on the measured ratio of the concentration of inulin in fluid samples obtained from the lumen of the PT (TF) and its concentration in simultaneous plasma (P) samples—$(TF/P)_{inulin}$—in micropuncture studies in rats. Because inulin is freely filtered at the glomerulus and is not reabsorbed or secreted in the PT, a $(TF/P)_{inulin}$ value of around 3 has suggested that approximately 66% of the filtrate is reabsorbed in the PT. However, these micropuncture measurements underestimate the volume of fluid that is actually reabsorbed in the PT because these measurements were made at the last accessible portion of the PT at the surface of the renal cortex, and hence did not take into account that additional volume may be reabsorbed in the deeper part of the PT, including its pars recta portion.

If the entire loop of Henle of most nephrons can be assumed to lack AQP1 and thereby be largely impermeable to water, the volume of filtrate that enters the loop of Henle can be deduced from the minimum value for the $(TF/P)_{inulin}$ obtained using the micropuncture technique from the early distal convoluted tubule (DCT), which has been done in rats. Because this value is around 6, a reasonable estimate of the proportion of filtrate that is reabsorbed in the rat PTs is close to five-sixths (83%). This value is close to the estimate of fractional reabsorption in the PT obtained with measurement of lithium clearance, which is thought to be a marker for fractional reabsorption in PT in human subjects.

If these findings can be extrapolated to humans with GFR values of 180 L/day, only about 30 L of filtrate/day (180 ÷ 6) would be delivered to the early DCT if all nephrons were superficial nephrons. This value of the volume of filtrate delivered to the DCT needs to be adjusted downward because juxtamedullary nephrons have AQP1 along their DtLs and, hence, are permeable to water. If these nephrons constitute 15% of the total number of nephrons and therefore receive 27 L of glomerular filtrate/day (15% of 180 L/day), and if five-sixths of the glomerular filtrate of these nephrons is reabsorbed along their PTs, around 4.5 L/ day reach their DtLs. Because the interstitial osmolality rises threefold (from 300 to 900 mOsmol/kg $H_2O$) in the outer medulla, two-thirds, or 3 L of the 4.5 L/day, are reabsorbed in the DtLs of these nephrons. Therefore, the volume of filtrate delivered to DCTs is likely to be around 27 L/day (around 30 L/day exit the PTs minus around 3 L/day that are reabsorbed in DtLs of the juxtamedullary nephrons).

**Residual Water Permeability.** There are two pathways for transport of water in the inner MCD, a vasopressin-responsive system via AQP2 and a vasopressin-independent system, RWP. Two factors may affect the volume of water reabsorbed via RWP. First, the driving force is the enormous difference in osmotic pressure between the luminal and interstitial fluid compartments in the inner MCD during a water diuresis. Second, the contraction of the renal pelvis, because each time the renal pelvis contracts, some of the fluid in the renal pelvis travels in a retrograde direction up toward the inner MCD, and some of that fluid may be reabsorbed via RWP after it reenters the inner MCD for a second (or maybe a third) time.

As calculated above, around 27 L/day are delivered to the distal nephron in a normal subject. The observed urine flow rate during maximum water diuresis is around 10 to 15 mL/ min (around 14–22 L/day). If this maximum water diuresis could be maintained for 24 hours, then somewhat more than 5 L of water would be reabsorbed per day in the inner MCD via its RWP during water diuresis.

### Concept 3

Another component of the physiology of water diuresis is the formation of electrolyte-free water. This process of desalination occurs in nephron segments that can reabsorb $Na^+$ but are impermeable to water because they lack AQPs (i.e., the cortical and medullary thick ascending limbs (TALs) of the loop of Henle and the DCT).

Regulation of the reabsorption of $Na^+$ and $Cl^-$ in the medullary TAL (mTAL) seems to occur via dilution of the concentration of an inhibitor of this process in the medullary interstitial compartment (possibly ionized calcium) by water reabsorption from the water-permeable nephron segments in the renal medulla (i.e., the MCD and DtLs of the juxtamedullary nephrons).[4] During water diuresis, reabsorption of $H_2O$ in inner MCD via its RWP may serve the purpose of diluting the concentration of this inhibitor of the reabsorption of $Na^+$ and $Cl^-$ in the mTAL, hence allowing desalination of the luminal fluid and the formation of electrolyte-free water to occur in this nephron segment.

### Tools for Assessing Water Diuresis

**Urine Flow Rate.** The observed urine flow rate during peak water diuresis in normal adult subjects is around 10 to 15 mL/ min (extrapolated to around 14–22 L/day). Notwithstanding, this high urine flow rate will not be sustained because the volume of distal delivery of filtrate will ultimately fall.

The urine flow rate declines when desmopressin (DDAVP) is given to a patient with central diabetes insipidus (DI). The urine flow rate, however, will be higher than that observed in response to DDAVP in a normal subject who consumes a typical Western diet. The reason is that the medullary interstitial osmolality is likely to be lower owing to a prior medullary washout during the water diuresis.

**Osmole Excretion Rate.** The osmole excretion rate is equal to the product of the urine osmolality ($U_{osm}$) and the urine flow rate (see Eq. 24.1). In subjects eating a typical Western diet, the rate of excretion of osmoles is 600 to 900 mOsmol/ day, with electrolytes and urea each accounting for close to half of the total urine osmoles. During a water diuresis due to the absence of vasopressin action, the rate of excretion of osmoles does not directly affect the urine volume because AQP2 are not present in the luminal membrane of principal cells in the CCD and MCD. Nevertheless, the rate of excretion of osmoles must be calculated in the patient with a water diuresis because, if high, polyuria due to an osmotic diuresis may be unmasked after there is a renal response to the administration of DDAVP.

$$\text{Osmole excretion rate} = U_{osm} \times \text{urine flow} \quad (24.1)$$

**Urine Osmolality.** The $U_{osm}$ is equal to the number of excreted osmoles divided by the urine volume. Therefore during a water diuresis, a change in the $U_{osm}$ could reflect a change in the osmole excretion rate and/or in the volume of filtrate delivered to the distal nephron, which is the major factor that determines the urine volume during a water diuresis. For example, if the rate of excretion of osmoles is 800 mOsmol/ day, the $U_{osm}$ will be 50 mOsmol/kg $H_2O$ if the 24-hour urine volume is 16 L and 100 mOsmol/kg $H_2O$ if the 24-hour urine volume is 8 L. This higher urine osmolality does not reflect a better urine concentrating ability, but a lower volume of distal delivery of filtrate.

**Electrolyte-Free Water Balance.** Tonicity is a term used to describe the effective osmolality of a solution. For plasma water, this can be approximated (in the absence of hyperglycemia) by the total concentration of cations ($Na^+ + K^+$) and their accompanying anions. The basis of the calculation of electrolyte-free water balance is the determination of how much water needs to be added to or subtracted from a solution with a given total amount of $Na^+ + K^+$ to make its tonicity equal to the normal plasma tonicity—that is, 150 mmol of cations plus an equal concentration of anions in 1 L of water. This calculation is used to determine the basis of a change in plasma $Na^+$ concentration ($P_{Na}$), and the appropriate therapy to achieve normonatremia. To calculate the electrolyte-free water balance, one must know the volume and concentrations of $Na^+ + K^+$ in the input and the output (mainly the urine).

For example, consider a patient who receives 3 L of 0.9% saline ($Na^+$ concentration = 150 mmol/L) and excretes 3 L of urine with a concentration of $Na^+ + K^+$ of 50 mmol/L. There is no electrolyte-free water in the input because it has the same tonicity as the plasma water (150 mmol/L cations, plus an equal concentration of anions). With regard to the output, this patient excreted the equivalent of 1 L of isotonic salt solution and 2 L of electrolyte-free water. Hence, the patient has a negative electrolyte-free water balance of 2 L, and the $P_{Na}$ would be expected to rise. Another patient receives 3 L of 0.9% saline but excretes 3 L of urine with a concentration of $Na^+ + K^+$ of 200 mmol/L. As in the first example,

**Table 24.1 Comparison of a Tonicity Balance and Electrolyte-Free Water Balance in a Patient With Hypernatremia[a]**

| Parameter | $Na^+ + K^+$ (mmol) | Water (L) | Electrolyte-Free Water Balance (L) |
|---|---|---|---|
| **Infusion of 3 L of Isotonic Saline** | | | |
| • Input | 450 | 3 | 0 |
| • Output | 150 | 3 | 2 |
| • **Balance** | **+300** | **0** | **−2** |
| **Infusion of 4 L of Isotonic Saline** | | | |
| • Input | 600 | 4 | 0 |
| • Output | 150 | 3 | 2 |
| • **Balance** | **+450** | **+1** | **−2** |
| **No Intravenous Fluid Infusion** | | | |
| • Input | 0 | 0 | 0 |
| • Output | 150 | 3 | 2 |
| • **Balance** | **−150** | **−3** | **−2** |

[a]Three case examples are described, in each patient the $P_{Na}$ rose from 140 to 150 mmol/L. In all three examples, the urine volume was 3 L with a concentration of $Na^+ + K^+$ of 50 mmol/L. The only difference is the volume of isotonic saline infused in each case example. Note that although the balances for $Na^+ + K^+$ and for water are very different in these three examples, the calculation of electrolyte-free water balance shows a negative balance of 2 L in all of them. Calculation of tonicity balance however, reveals that the patient in the first example has a positive balance of 300 mmol of $Na^+ + K^+$, while the patient in the second example has a positive balance of 450 mmol of $Na^+ + K^+$ and a positive balance of 1 L of water, and the patient in the third example has a negative balance of 150 mmol of $Na^+ + K^+$ and a negative balance of 3 L of water. The goals for therapy—to correct the hypernatremia and to return the volume and composition of the extracellular and intracellular fluid compartments to their normal values—are clear only after a tonicity balance is calculated.

there is no electrolyte-free water in the input. With regard to the output, because this patient would have needed to excrete 4 L (and not 3 L) of urine to make this total of 600 mmol of $Na^+ + K^+$ (with 600 mmol of accompanying anions) into an isotonic solution, the patient has a positive electrolyte-free water balance of 1 L; hence, the $P_{Na}$ will fall (i.e., 1 L of body water lost 150 mmol of $Na^+ + K^+$ with 150 mmol of accompanying anions and hence, became 1 L electrolyte-free water). Calculation of the electrolyte-free water balance however, although it correctly predicts the change in $P_{Na}$, does not reveal whether its basis is a change in water balance or in fact a change in $Na^+ + K^+$ balance. An example of this is shown in Table 24.1. Although the balances for $Na^+ + K^+$ and for water are very different in the three examples used, calculation of the electrolyte-free water balance provided the same answer in all of them, a negative balance of 2 L of electrolyte-free water. Hence, calculation of the electrolyte-free water balance is not helpful to design the therapy needed to return the volume and composition of the extracellular fluid (ECF) and intracellular fluid (ICF) compartments to their normal values.

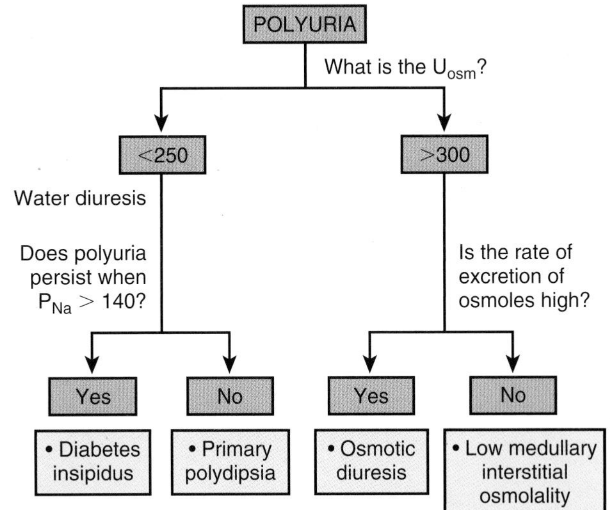


**Flow Chart 24.1** (From Kamel KS, Halperin ML. *Fluid, Electrolyte, and Acid-Base Physiology; A Problem-Based Approach.* ed 5. Philadelphia: Elsevier; 2017.)

**Tonicity Balance.** To determine the basis for a change in the $P_{Na}$ and to define the proper therapy to return the volume and composition of the ECF and ICF compartments to their normal values, we calculate the tonicity balance. A tonicity balance refers to the balance of water and the balance of electrolytes that determine body tonicity (i.e., $Na^+ + K^+$).[5] To calculate a tonicity balance, one must examine the input and output volumes and the quantity of $Na^+$ and $K^+$ infused and the quantity of $Na^+ + K^+$ excreted over the time period during which the $P_{Na}$ changed (see Table 24.1). In practical terms, a tonicity balance can be calculated only in a hospital setting, where inputs and outputs are accurately recorded. In a febrile patient, balance calculations will not be as accurate because sweat losses are not measured. Nevertheless, restricting analysis of the output to the urine data would be sufficient in an acute setting if the changes in $P_{Na}$ occurred over a relatively short period of time.

Even if measurements of the concentrations of $Na^+$ and $K^+$ in the urine are not available, if the $P_{Na}$ at the beginning and end of a certain period, volume of the urine, and volume and amount of $Na^+ + K^+$ in the fluid infused during that period are known, the clinician can use these data together with an estimation of total body water (TBW) to calculate the quantity of $Na^+ + K^+$ excreted in the urine. Hence, the basis for the change in $P_{Na}$ can be determined.

## CLINICAL APPROACH TO THE PATIENT WITH POLYURIA

The steps to take to determine the diagnosis in a patient with polyuria are outlined in Flow Charts 24.1 and 24.2.

### Step 1: What Is the Urine Osmolality?

A value of the $U_{osm}$ that is less than 250 mOsmol/kg $H_2O$ indicates that the polyuria is due to a water diuresis. If the $P_{Na}$ is less than 135 mmol/L, the polyuria is due to primary polydipsia. Once the $P_{Na}$ has returned to the normal range, the urine flow rate should decrease, and the $U_{osm}$ should rise to a value that is at least higher than the $P_{osm}$. Note that the prior water diuresis may have caused a lower

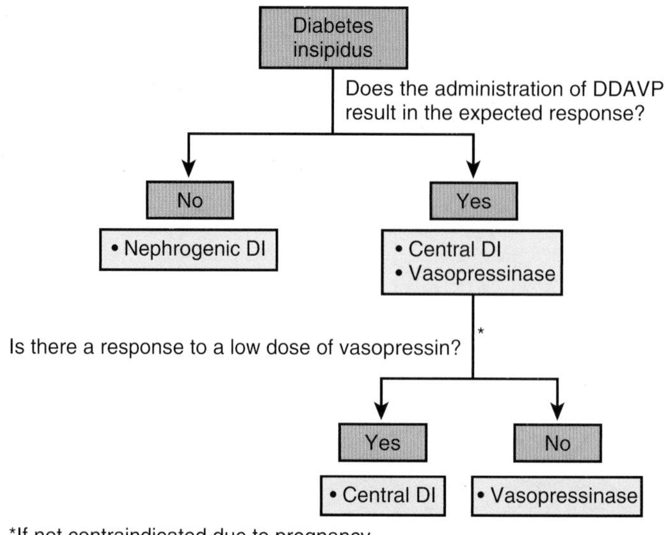


**Flow Chart 24.2** *DI,* Diabetes insipidus; *DDAVP,* desmopressin. (From Kamel KS, Halperin ML. *Fluid, Electrolyte, and Acid-Base Physiology; A Problem-Based Approach.* ed 5. Philadelphia: Elsevier; 2017.)

medullary interstitial osmolality due to medullary washout, so the maximal urine-concentrating ability may not be achieved initially. In contrast, if the water diuresis persists when the $P_{Na}$ is higher than 140 mmol/L, the cause of polyuria is DI.

If the $U_{osm}$ is greater than 300 mOsmol/kg $H_2O$, calculate the osmole excretion rate (see Eq. 24.1). The usual value is close to 0.6 mOsmol/min (600–900 mOsmol/day) in subjects consuming a typical Western diet. If the osmole excretion rate is appreciably increased, then the polyuria is due to an osmotic diuresis. Conversely, if the osmole excretion rate is not increased, then the cause of the polyuria is a defect that leads to a lower medullary interstitial osmolality.

### Step 2: Examine the Renal Response to Vasopressin or Desmopressin

See Flow Chart 24.2.

If the cause of the polyuria is DI, this could be due to a lesion in the hypothalamic–posterior pituitary axis, which controls the production and release of vasopressin (central DI), the presence of a circulating vasopressinase that breaks down vasopressin, or a renal lesion that prevents the binding of vasopressin to its V2 receptor (V2R) or interferes with vasopressin effect to cause the insertion of AQP2 in the luminal membrane of principal cells in the CCD and MCD (nephrogenic DI).

In the diagnostic approach to the patient with a water diuresis, DDAVP should only be administered if the patient continues to have a water diuresis, despite $P_{Na}$ greater than 140 mmol/L. In normal subjects consuming a typical Western diet, the expected urine flow rate in response to the administration of DDAVP is around 0.5 mL/min. This is because the inner medullary interstitial effective osmolality (nonurea osmolality) is around 450 mOsmol/kg $H_2O$, and the rate of excretion of effective osmoles (electrolytes) is around 450 mOsmol/day; hence, the expected urine flow rate is 450/450 = 1 L/day, or 0.7 mL/min. In a patient with central DI, the urine flow rate is expected to fall in response to the administration of DDAVP but, because of medullary washout by the water diuresis, the urine flow rate is likely to be higher than 0.7 mL/min, perhaps around 1 mL/min if the effective inner medullary interstitial osmolality has fallen to say around 300 mOsmol/kg $H_2O$. The urine flow rate will be even higher if there is an appreciable increase in the rate of excretion of effective osmoles (e.g., because of prior expansion of the effective arterial blood volume with excessive administration of saline). In a patient with central DI, the $U_{osm}$ should rise to a value that is at least higher than $P_{osm}$ in response to the administration of DDAVP.

Similar responses in terms of a fall in urine flow rate and a rise in $U_{osm}$ are also observed in patients with water diuresis caused by hydrolysis of vasopressin by circulating vasopressinase(s), because DDAVP is resistant to degradation by these enzymes. One could, in theory, examine the response to the administration of vasopressin after the effect of DDAVP has worn off, and the patient is having a water diuresis again. In contrast to the response to the administration of DDAVP, a patient in whom a vasopressinase has been released will not respond to the administration of a small dose of vasopressin. However, this should not be attempted in pregnant women because of the oxytocic effect of vasopressin.

If the urine osmolality and flow rate do not respond appropriately to DDAVP, then the diagnosis is nephrogenic diabetes insipidus.

### Step 3: Establish the Basis for Central Diabetes Insipidus

Central DI results from decreased release of vasopressin because of an inborn error (hereditary central DI) or because of a variety of infiltrative, neoplastic, vascular, or traumatic lesions that may involve the osmostat, the site where vasopressin is synthesized (the hypothalamic paraventricular and supraoptic nuclei), the tracts connecting these nuclei to the posterior pituitary, and/or a lesion involving the posterior pituitary (Fig. 24.2; see also Chapter 15). In a patient with hypernatremia, the absence of thirst suggests that the lesion involves the osmostat.

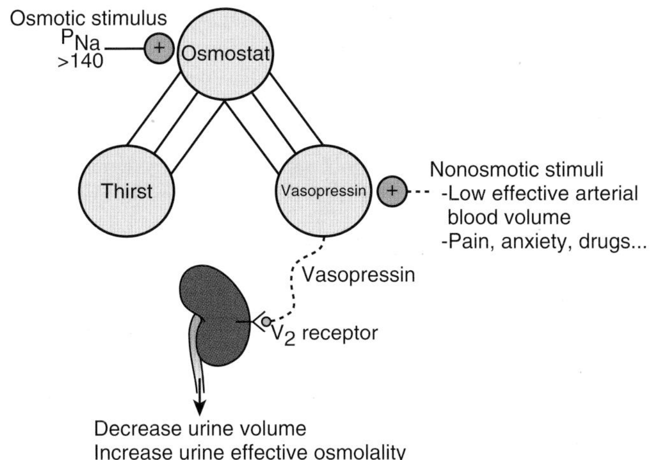


**Fig. 24.2** Water control system. The sensor is the osmostat or the tonicity stat *(top circle)*, which detects a change in $P_{Na}$ via an effect on the volume of its cells. The osmostat is linked to the thirst center *(left circle)* and to the vasopressin release center *(right circle)*. Nonosmotic stimuli (e.g., certain drugs, nausea, pain, anxiety) also influence the release of vasopressin. Vasopressin release is also stimulated when there is a large decrease in the effective arterial blood volume. (From Kamel KS, Halperin ML. *Fluid, Electrolyte, and Acid-Base Physiology; A Problem-Based Approach.* ed 5. Philadelphia: Elsevier; 2017.)

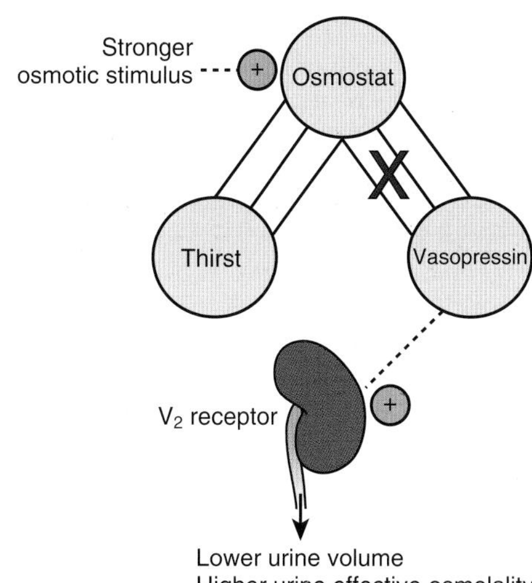


**Fig. 24.3** Lesion causing partial central diabetes insipidus. The *top circle* represents the osmostat or the tonicity stat, which is the sensor, the *left circle* represents the thirst center, and the *right circle* is the vasopressin release center. The X symbol represents a hypothetic lesion that causes the severing of some but not all the fibers connecting the osmostat to the vasopressin release center. A stronger osmotic stimulus can overcome the defect and stimulate sufficient vasopressin release to concentrate the urine. (From Kamel KS, Halperin ML. *Fluid, Electrolyte, and Acid-Base Physiology; A Problem-Based Approach.* ed 5. Philadelphia: Elsevier; 2017.)

### Step 4: Establish the Basis for Nephrogenic Diabetes Insipidus

If DDAVP fails to cause a rise in $U_{osm}$ to a value that is equal to or higher than $P_{osm}$, the diagnosis is nephrogenic DI. Nephrogenic DI results from a lesion that prevents the binding of vasopressin to V2R or one that interferes with its effect to cause the insertion of AQP2 into the luminal membrane of principal cells in the collecting ducts. Hereditary nephrogenic DI could be due to an X-linked recessive V2R mutation (more common), or autosomal recessive or dominant AQP2 mutations. The most common cause of nonhereditary nephrogenic DI in an adult is the ingestion of lithium (see Chapter 15).

Patients with classic nephrogenic DI need to be distinguished from patients with a defect that leads to a lower medullary interstitial osmolality (e.g., due to a medullary interstitial disease). From a pathophysiologic perspective, these are two different disorders. Furthermore, in patients with classic nephrogenic DI, the urine flow rate is largely determined by the volume of distal delivery of filtrate and the volume reabsorbed via RWP in the inner MCD. In contrast, in patients with low medullary interstitial osmolality, the urine flow rate is determined by the rate of excretion of effective osmoles.

## CLINICAL CASE 1: WHAT IS "PARTIAL" ABOUT PARTIAL CENTRAL DIABETES INSIPIDUS?

A 32-year-old previously healthy man had a recent basal skull fracture. Since his head injury, his urine output had been consistently about 4 L/day, and his $U_{osm}$ around 200 mOsmol/kg $H_2O$ in multiple 24-hour urine collections. Vasopressin was not detected in his plasma when his $P_{Na}$ was around 140 mmol/L. During the daytime, his $U_{osm}$ was consistently around 90 mOsmol/kg $H_2O$, and his $P_{Na}$ was around 137 mmol/L. When he was given DDAVP, his urine flow rate decreased to 0.5 mL/min, and the $U_{osm}$ rose to 900 mOsmol/kg $H_2O$. Interestingly, it was noted that if he stopped drinking water after supper, his sleep was not interrupted by a need to void, and his $U_{osm}$ was around 425 mOsmol/kg $H_2O$ in his first voided urine samples in the morning. His urine flow rate fell to 0.5 mL/min, and his $U_{osm}$ rose to 900 mOsmol/kg $H_2O$, after an infusion of hypertonic saline.

### Questions and Discussion

Is this a water diuresis? Because the patient's urine volume was around 4 L/day and his $U_{osm}$ was around 200 mOsmol/kg $H_2O$, the cause of his polyuria was a water diuresis (see Flow Chart 24.1). His osmole excretion rate was 800 mOsmol/day, which is within the usual rate of excretion of osmoles in a subject consuming a typical Western diet. In response to the administration of DDAVP, his urine flow rate decreased to 0.5 mL/min, and the $U_{osm}$ rose to 900 mOsmol/kg $H_2O$. Hence, the diagnosis was central DI. Because his urine volume was only 4 L/day and not 10 to 15 L/day, he was thought to have partial central DI.

*Central diabetes insipidus.* The diagnosis of central DI was straightforward. Because he complained of thirst, his osmostat and his thirst center, as well as the fibers connecting them, appeared to be functionally intact (see Fig. 24.2). Interesting to note that the $U_{osm}$ was greater than the $P_{osm}$ in the first-voided morning urine ($U_{osm}$ = 425 mOsmol/kg $H_2O$) when he stopped drinking water several hours before he went to sleep. This suggests that the vasopressin release center seems to function but only when there is a strong stimulus for the release of this hormone, presumably a higher $P_{Na}$. In keeping with this hypothesis is the fact that his urine flow rate fell to 0.5 mL/min and $U_{osm}$ rose to 900 mOsmol/kg $H_2O$ after an infusion of hypertonic saline. Therefore, a possible site for the lesion is destruction of some but not of all the fibers linking the osmostat to the vasopressin release center (Fig. 24.3).

Such a lesion might explain why polyuria was not present overnight if the patient stopped water intake several hours prior to going to sleep, because he might develop a negative water balance sufficient to cause his $P_{Na}$ to rise to a level high enough to cause the release of vasopressin. This clinical case provides insights into the pathophysiology of partial central DI.[6]

*Primary polydipsia.* If the patient's $P_{Na}$ was high enough early in the morning to stimulate the release of vasopressin, whereas during the daytime, when his $P_{Na}$ was 137 mmol/L, his $U_{osm}$ was consistently around 90 mOsmol/kg $H_2O$, this suggests that primary polydipsia was present while he was awake. Its basis probably was a learned behavior to avoid the uncomfortable feeling of thirst. This interpretation provides insights into understanding the pathophysiology of the polyuria in this patient and, importantly, to determine the options for therapy to decrease his urine volume.

What are the best options for therapy? The major point here is that a higher $P_{Na}$ could stimulate the release of vasopressin in this patient. A rise in $P_{Na}$ may be induced by a positive balance for $Na^+$ or a negative balance for water. The patient chose to use oral NaCl tablets to raise his $P_{Na}$ to control his daytime polyuria. This therapy would avoid the risk of acute hyponatremia, which might occur if he were given DDAVP and drank an excessive quantity of water by habit. In contrast, he selected water deprivation starting several hours before going to bed to raise his $P_{Na}$ overnight, which seemed to permit him to have undisturbed sleep.

## CLINICAL CASE 2: IN A PATIENT WITH CENTRAL DIABETES INSIPIDUS, WHY DID POLYURIA PERSIST AFTER THE ADMINISTRATION OF DESMOPRESSIN?

A 16-year-old male (weight, 50 kg; total body water, 30 L) underwent craniopharyngioma resection. We are asked to see the patient because of polyuria and hypernatremia. His urine output was 3 L over 5 hours (urine flow rate = 10 mL/min), and his $P_{Na}$ rose from 140 to 150 mmol/L. During this time period, he received 3 L of isotonic saline. His $U_{osm}$ was 120 mOsmol/kg $H_2O$, and the urine [$Na^+ + K^+$] concentration was 50 mmol/L. To confirm the diagnosis of central DI, he was given DDAVP, and the urine flow rate fell to 6 mL/min, the $U_{osm}$ rose to 375 mOsmol/kg $H_2O$, and the urine [$Na^+ + K^+$] concentration rose to 175 mmol/L.

### Questions and Discussion

Does the drop in the patient's urine flow rate to 6 mL/min represent a partial response to DDAVP? When DDAVP acts, the urine flow rate is directly proportional to the osmole excretion rate and inversely proportional to the medullary interstitial osmolality. The expected urine flow rate in response to DDAVP can be calculated by considering several factors. First, the usual rate of excretion of osmoles in an adult subject consuming a typical Western diet is about 900 mOsmol/day; approximately half are urea osmoles and half are electrolyte osmoles. As will be detailed later, at its usual rate of excretion, urea is not an effective osmole in the lumen of the inner MCD. Therefore, around 450 effective mOsmol are excreted each day. Interstitial osmolality in the inner medulla is around 900 mOsmol/kg $H_2O$. If half of this is due to urea osmoles and half is due to electrolyte osmoles, the effective osmolality of the interstitium in the inner medulla is therefore around 450 mOsmol/kg $H_2O$. When DDAVP acts, the effective osmolality of the fluid exiting the inner medulla will be equal to the effective osmolality of the interstitium in the inner medulla—in other words, 450 mOsmol/kg $H_2O$. The 450 mOsmol of effective (electrolyte) osmoles will therefore bring 1 L of urine with them each day. This is a flow rate of 1000 mL/1440 min, or 0.7 mL/min. The osmole excretion rate in this patient before the administration of DDAVP was 1.2 mOsmol/min ($U_{osm}$ = 120 mOsmol/kg $H_2O \times$ urine flow rate = 10 mL/min). This value is double the usual osmole excretion rate (900 mOsmol/1440 min = 0.6 mOsmol/min) in subjects consuming a typical Western diet. Another point merits emphasis with regard to the nature of the excreted osmoles. Prior to the administration of DDAVP, the concentration of $Na^+ + K^+$ in the urine was 50 mmol/L. Hence, the vast majority of the osmoles excreted in the urine (100 osmoles—50 × 2 to account for the accompanying anions—out of each 120 osmoles) were electrolyte osmoles, which are effective osmoles that obligate the excretion of $H_2O$ when DDAVP acts. In this case, the likely source of this was the NaCl infusion that the patient was receiving concurrently.

It is also important to recognize that because of a prior water diuresis, there would be a degree of washout of the renal medulla. Hence, the maximum $U_{osm}$ in response to the administration of DDAVP would be significantly lower than that observed in normal subjects. This may explain why this patient's $U_{osm}$ rose to only 375 mOsmol/kg $H_2O$ following the administration of DDAVP.

Therefore, the drop in the patient's urine flow rate to only about 6 mL/min does not represent a partial response to DDAVP but, rather, the expected response because of the high rate of excretion of effective osmoles (osmotic diuresis) and the low effective medullary interstitial osmolality (urinary concentrating defect due to medullary washout).

Why did the $P_{Na}$ rise from 140 to 150 mmol/L during this large water diuresis? Although the tendency here is to assume that this patient's hypernatremia was due to a water deficit because he had a large water diuresis, the actual basis of the rise in his $P_{Na}$ can be determined with a calculation of the tonicity balance.

*Water balance.* The patient received 3 L of isotonic saline, and hence had an input of 3 L of water. He excreted 3 L of urine, so there is a neutral balance of water.

*$Na^+ + K^+$ balance.* The patient received 450 mmol of $Na^+$ (3 L × 150 mmol $Na^+$/L) and excreted only 150 mmol of $Na^+ + K^+$ (3 L urine × 50 mmol $Na^+ + K^+$/L). Hence, he had a positive balance of 300 mmol of $Na^+ + K^+$. When one divides this surplus of $Na^+ + K^+$ by the total body water (60% of body weight of 50 kg = 30 L), the rise in $P_{Na}$ of 10 mmol/L is largely due to a positive balance of $Na^+$ rather than a deficit of water. The proper treatment to restore body tonicity and the volume and composition of the ECF and ICF compartments in this patient was to induce a negative balance of 300 mmol of $Na^+ + K^+$.

## OSMOTIC DIURESIS

### Concept 4

When vasopressin acts, it causes the insertion of AQP2 into the luminal membrane of principal cells in the CCD and

MCD. Water is reabsorbed until the concentration of effective osmoles in the lumen of the CCD and MCD is nearly equal to their concentration in the surrounding cortical and medullary interstitial fluid, respectively. The volume of urine during an osmotic diuresis is directly proportional to the rate of excretion of effective osmoles and indirectly proportional to effective osmolality of the interstitial fluid in the inner medulla.

Because cells in the inner MCD have urea transporters in their luminal membranes when vasopressin acts, urea is usually an ineffective osmole—the concentration of urea is nearly equal in the interstitial fluid in the inner medulla and in the lumen of the inner MCD. Thus, urea does not obligate the excretion of water. The net result of excreting some extra urea is a higher $U_{osm}$ but not a higher urine flow rate. Therefore, it is more correct to say that the urine flow rate is directly proportional to the number of nonurea or effective osmoles in the lumen of the inner MCD and is inversely proportional to the concentration of nonurea or effective osmoles in the interstitial fluid in the inner medulla.

Urea, however, may be an effective urine osmole when the rate of excretion of urea rises by a large amount because urea might not be absorbed fast enough to achieve equal concentrations in the lumen of the inner MCD and in the interstitial fluid in the inner medulla.

#### Concept 5

The medullary interstitial osmolality falls during an osmotic diuresis because of medullary washout. During an osmotic diuresis, a larger number of liters of fluid is delivered to and is reabsorbed in the MCD during an osmotic diuresis than during antidiuresis. Hence, medullary washout occurs, and medullary interstitial osmolality falls. The $U_{osm}$ is usually close to 600 mOsmol/kg $H_2O$ during an osmotic diuresis. Lower values of the $U_{osm}$ that are even close to $P_{osm}$ may be observed when there is a large rate of excretion of osmoles.

### Tools for Evaluation of Osmotic Diuresis

**Urine Osmolality.** In a patient who has an osmotic diuresis, the $U_{osm}$ should be higher than the $P_{osm}$.

**Osmole Excretion Rate.** In an adult during an osmotic diuresis, the rate of excretion of osmoles should be much greater than 1000 mOsmol/day (>0.7 mOsmol/min).

**Nature of the Urine Osmoles.** The nature of the urine osmoles should be determined by measuring the rate of excretion of the individual osmoles in the urine. One can deduce which solute is likely to be responsible for the osmotic diuresis by measuring the concentration in plasma (e.g., glucose, urea). A large amount of mannitol is not commonly given; hence, it is unlikely to be the sole cause of a large and sustained osmotic diuresis. A saline-induced osmotic diuresis may occur if the EABV was overly expanded with the infusion of a large amount of saline, or if the patient has cerebral or renal salt wasting. For diagnosis of a state of salt wasting, there must be an appreciable excretion of $Na^+$ when the EABV is definitely contracted.

**Sources of the Urine Osmoles.** In a patient with a glucose- or a urea-induced osmotic diuresis, it is important to determine whether these osmoles were derived from an exogenous source or from catabolism of endogenous proteins.

**Source of Urea.** Urea appearance rate. The rate of appearance of urea can be determined from the amount of urea that is retained in the body plus the amount that is excreted in the urine over a given period of time. The former can be calculated from the rise in the concentration of urea in plasma ($P_{urea}$) and by assuming a volume of distribution of urea that is equal to total body water (~60% of body weight).

One can use the following calculation to determine whether the source of urea was the breakdown of exogenous or endogenous proteins if the intake of proteins is known. Close to 16% of the weight of protein is nitrogen. Therefore if 100 g of protein were oxidized, 16 g of nitrogen would be formed. The molecular weight of nitrogen is 14, so about 1140 mmol of nitrogen would be produced. Because each molecule of urea contains two atoms of nitrogen, about 570 mmol of urea would be produced from the oxidation of 100 g of protein (or 5.7 mmol of urea/1 g protein). Because each kilogram of lean body mass has around 180 g of protein, the breakdown of 1 kg of lean body mass will produce about 1026 mmol of urea (5.7 mmol of urea/1 g protein × 180 g of protein).

**Source of Glucose.** The production of glucose from endogenous sources is relatively small. In more detail, only 60% of the weight of protein can be converted to glucose. Hence, to produce enough glucose from protein to induce 1 L of osmotic diuresis, which requires the excretion of around 300 mmol of glucose, one would need the catabolism of 90 g of protein (equivalent to the catabolism of about 0.5 kg of lean body mass). Therefore, if there is a large glucose-induced osmotic diuresis, the glucose must be from an exogenous source (e.g., the ingestion of large volumes of fruit juice or sugar-containing soft drinks in a patient who lacks insulin actions).

## CLINICAL APPROACH TO THE PATIENT WITH AN OSMOTIC DIURESIS

The steps in the clinical approach to the patient with osmotic diuresis are illustrated in Flow Chart 24.3.

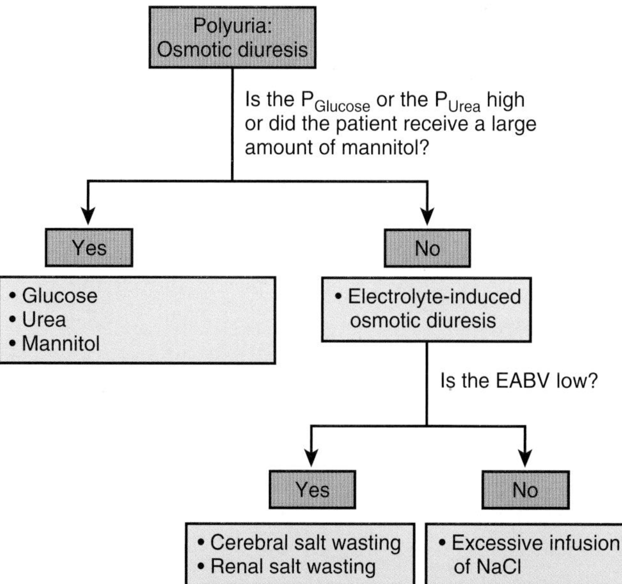


**Flow Chart 24.3** *EABV,* Effective arterial blood volume. (From Kamel KS, Halperin ML. *Fluid, Electrolyte, and Acid-Base Physiology; A Problem-Based Approach.* ed 5. Philadelphia: Elsevier; 2017.)

### Step 1: Calculate the Osmole Excretion Rate

If the $U_{osm}$ is greater than the $P_{osm}$, and the osmole excretion rate significantly exceeds 1000 mOsmol/day (0.7 mOsmol/min), an osmotic diuresis is likely to be present.

### Step 2: Define the Nature of the Excreted Osmoles

One can make a reasonable assessment of the likelihood that a solute will cause polyuria if its concentration in plasma is measured, the GFR is estimated, and the renal handling of that solute is known. One should also determine whether enough mannitol was administered to cause the observed degree of polyuria. Osmotic diuresis could be due to a saline diuresis if $Na^+$ and $Cl^-$ are excreted at high rates and represent the majority of the urine osmoles.

### Step 3: Identify the Source of the Osmoles in the Urine

In a patient with a glucose- or urea-induced osmotic diuresis, it is important to decide whether these osmoles were derived from an exogenous source or from catabolism of endogenous proteins. The clinician should also be aware of the possibility of a large amount of glucose in the lumen of the gastrointestinal tract because when it is absorbed it may contribute to the osmotic diuresis.

In a patient with a saline-induced osmotic diuresis, one must determine why so much NaCl is being excreted. Some potential causes are prior excessive saline administration (a common situation in hospitalized patients), administration of a loop diuretic in a patient with marked degree of peripheral edema, cerebral salt wasting, or renal salt wasting.

## CLINICAL CASE 3: UNUSUALLY LARGE OSMOTIC DIURESIS IN A PATIENT WITH DIABETES MELLITUS

A 50-kg, 14-year-old female had a long history of type 1 diabetes mellitus, which was poorly controlled because she did not take insulin regularly. In the past 48 hours, she was thirsty, drank large volumes of fruit juice, and noted that her urine volume was very high. On physical examination, her EABV was not appreciably contracted. The urine flow rate was 10 mL/min over a 100-min period while she was in the emergency room. Other laboratory data included the following: pH = 7.33, plasma bicarbonate ($HCO_3^-$) concentration ($P_{HCO_3}$) = 24 mmol/L, plasma anion gap ($P_{anion\ gap}$) = 16 mEq/L, plasma $K^+$ concentration ($P_K$) = 4.8 mmol/L, plasma creatinine concentration ($P_{Cr}$) = was close to her usual values of 1.0 mg/dL (88 µmol/L), blood urea nitrogen (BUN) = 22 mg/dL ($P_{urea}$ = 8 mmol/L), and hematocrit = 0.50. Of note, there was no decrease in her plasma glucose concentration ($P_{Glu}$) over that time period, despite the excretion of a large amount of glucose in her urine. The following results were also reported:

| | *Admission* | | *After 100 min* | |
|---|---|---|---|---|
| *Parameter* | *Plasma* | *Urine* | *Plasma* | *Urine* |
| Glucose, mg/dL (mmol/L) | 1260 (70) | 5400 (300) | 1260 (70) | 5400 (300) |
| $Na^+$, mmol/L | 125 | 50 | 123 | 50 |
| Osmolality, mOsmol/kg $H_2O$ | 320 | 450 | 316 | 450 |

### Questions and Discussion

What is the basis of the polyuria?

*$U_{osm}$.* The $U_{osm}$ of 450 mOsmol/kg $H_2O$ indicates that this polyuria was due to an osmotic diuresis. The $U_{osm}$ was lower than the expected value during an osmotic diuresis, probably reflecting the very high osmole excretion rate, which caused a larger fall in the patient's medullary interstitial osmolality due to medullary washout as a result of the reabsorption of a large volume of water in her MCD.

*Osmole excretion rate.* The product of her $U_{osm}$ (450 mOsmol/L) and urine flow rate (10 mL/min) yielded an osmole excretion rate of 4.5 mOsmol/min, a value that is sevenfold higher than the usual value in an adult subject consuming a typical Western diet (≈0.6 mOsmol/min).

*Nature of the urine osmoles.* Because the patient's GFR was not low and her $P_{Glu}$ was extremely high (1260 mg/dL, 70 mmol/L), the filtered load of glucose was markedly higher than the maximum tubular capacity for its reabsorption. Hence, this was a glucose-induced osmotic diuresis, confirmed by the finding of a $U_{Glu}$ of about 300 mmol/L.

*Sources of the urine osmoles.* Of special emphasis, this patient's $P_{Glu}$ did not decline despite such a high rate of excretion of glucose. In quantitative terms, the total content of glucose in her ECF compartment was 126 g—1260 mg/dL × 10 to convert to mg/L × 10 L ECFV ÷ 1000. During this 100-minute period, she excreted 54 g of glucose—5400 mg/dL × 10 to convert to mg/L × 1 L ÷ 1000. Therefore, although she excreted close to half of the content of glucose in her entire ECF compartment, there was no change in her $P_{Glu}$. Accordingly, to maintain this degree of hyperglycemia, she needed a large input of glucose over a short period of time. The only likely source of such a large amount of glucose was glucose that was retained in her stomach. As a reference, 1 L of apple juice contains about 135 g of glucose. Although the usual effect of hyperglycemia is to slow gastric emptying, this did not seem to be the case in this patient because she seemed to have had a rapid rate of exit of fluid from her stomach, with its subsequent absorption in her intestine.[7]

What dangers do you anticipate in this patient?

*Cerebral edema.* Brain cell swelling might occur if there were a significant fall in her effective $P_{osm}$ (Eq. 24.2).[8] A fall in her effective $P_{osm}$ may occur if the absorbed glucose and water from the gastrointestinal (GI) tract were retained in the body and glucose was subsequently metabolized; hence, there would be a gain of electrolyte-free water in the body.

$$\text{Effective } P_{osm} = 2(P_{Na} + P_{Glu})\ \text{(all values in mmol/L)} \qquad (24.2)$$

## DECREASED EFFECTIVE ARTERIAL BLOOD VOLUME

Principles governing the regulation of EABV are briefly discussed here and in more detail in Chapter 14.

### Concept 6

Water crosses cell membranes rapidly through AQP channels to achieve osmotic equilibrium. Hence, the numbers of effective osmoles in the ECF and ICF compartments determine their respective volumes. The effective osmoles in the ECF compartment are primarily $Na^+$ and its attendant anions ($Cl^-$ and $HCO_3^-$); their content in the ECF compartment determines its volume.

### Concept 7

The hydrostatic pressure and the oncotic pressure across the capillary membrane are the major forces that determine the distribution of the ECF compartment volume between its intravascular and interstitial spaces.

The major driving force for outward movement of an ultrafiltrate of plasma across the capillary membrane is the hydrostatic pressure difference. The hydrostatic pressure at the venous end of the capillary is higher under conditions that lead to venous hypertension (e.g., venous obstruction, congestive heart failure).

The major driving force for inward fluid movement from the interstitial space to the intravascular space is the colloidal osmotic pressure difference. This is largely due to the higher concentration of albumin in the intravascular space (40 g/L) than in the interstitial space (10 g/L). Fluid accumulates in the interstitial space in patients with hypoalbuminemia (e.g., patients with nephrotic syndrome). Thus, the ECF volume (ECFV) in these patients may be increased but their EABV may be decreased.

### Concept 8

Control mechanisms for $Na^+$ homeostasis are set to defend the EABV rather than the ECFV. EABV can be defined as the part of the ECFV that is located in the arterial blood system and that effectively perfuses tissues. Changes in the EABV are sensed by baroreceptors located in the large blood vessels (the carotid sinus and the aortic arch) and the afferent glomerular arterioles. These are stretch receptors that detect changes in the filling of these vessels.

## TOOLS FOR EVALUATING DECREASED EFFECTIVE ARTERIAL BLOOD VOLUME

### Quantitative Assessment of the Extracellular Fluid Volume

The physical examination, the plasma concentrations of $HCO_3^-$, creatinine, urea, and urate, as well as the fractional excretions of $Na^+$, $Cl^-$, urea, and urate are useful at times to suggest that the EABV is contracted. Nevertheless, they do not provide a quantitative estimate of the ECFV. A quantitative assessment of the ECFV can be obtained using the hematocrit (Table 24.2) or the concentration of total proteins in plasma, assuming that their values were normal to begin with.[9] The hematocrit is the ratio of red blood cells (RBCs) volume to blood volume, as given in the following formula:

$$\text{Hematocrit} = \text{RBC volume}/(\text{RBC volume} + \text{plasma volume}) \quad (24.3)$$

Blood volume in an adult subject is around 70 mL/kg body weight (i.e., around 5 L in a 70-kg subject). With a blood volume of 5 L and a hematocrit of 0.40, the RBC volume is 2 L and the plasma volume is 3 L (Eq. 24.3). When the hematocrit is 0.50, and assuming no change in the RBC volume (2 L), the blood volume is 4 L. Hence, the plasma volume is 2 L (i.e., reduced by one-third from its normal value of 3 L). If one ignores changes in Starling forces for simplicity, the ECFV should have declined by approximately one-third of its normal volume (see Table 24.2).

**Table 24.2 Use of the Hematocrit to Estimate the Extracellular Fluid Volume[a]**

| Hematocrit | % Change ECFV |
|---|---|
| 0.40 | 0 |
| 0.50 | −33 |
| 0.60 | −60 |

[a]The assumptions made when using this calculation are that the patient does not have anemia or erythrocytosis, that the red blood cell (RBC) volume is 2 L, and that the plasma volume is 3 L (blood volume 5 L). The formula is:
Hematocrit = RBC volume/(RBC volume + plasma volume)
Values between those listed can be deduced by interpolation.
*ECFV,* Extracellular fluid volume.

**Table 24.3 Urine Electrolyte Values in a Patient With a Contracted Effective Arterial Blood Volume[a]**

| Condition | Urine $Na^+$ | Urine $Cl^-$ |
|---|---|---|
| **Vomiting** | | |
| Recent | High | Low |
| Remote | Low | Low |
| **Diuretics** | | |
| Recent | High | High |
| Remote | Low | Low |
| Diarrhea or laxative abuse | Low | High |
| Bartter syndrome or Gitelman syndrome | High | High |

[a]Values of the urine electrolyte concentration must be adjusted when polyuria is present. Urine $Cl^-$ is high in patients with diarrhea or laxative abuse if they have a high rate of excretion of $NH_4^+$. *High,* Urine concentration >15 mmol/L; *low,* urine concentration <15 mmol/L.

### Urinary Tests for Low Effective Arterial Blood Volume

The expected response to a low EABV is to excrete as little $Na^+$ and $Cl^-$ as possible in the urine. Because 24-hour urine collections to calculate rates of excretion of $Na^+$ and $Cl^-$ are usually not practical in clinical circumstances in which a quick assessment is required, clinicians use the urinary concentrations of $Na^+$ ($U_{Na}$) and $Cl^-$ ($U_{Cl}$) in a spot urine sample (Table 24.3) to assess the renal response to the presence of a low EABV. These, however, are concentration terms, which may not necessarily reflect low rates of excretion if the urine flow rate is high. To avoid this type of error, the $U_{Na}$ and $U_{Cl}$ should be related to the concentration of creatinine in the urine ($U_{Cr}$) because the rate of excretion of creatinine is relatively constant throughout the day; its 24-hour excretion rate can be estimated based on assessment of the patient's muscle mass. There are some caveats in using the urine $Na^+$ and $Cl^-$ excretion rates to assess EABV.[10]

**Low Rate of Excretion of Sodium and Chloride.** A low rate of excretion of $Na^+$ and $Cl^-$ in a patient with a decreased EABV suggests either a loss of NaCl via nonrenal routes (e.g., sweat, GI tract) or that there was a prior renal loss of $Na^+$ and $Cl^-$ (e.g., remote use of diuretics). In the absence of a low EABV, a low rate of excretion of $Na^+$ and $Cl^-$ may reflect a low intake of NaCl.

**High Rate of Excretion of Sodium but Little Excretion of Chloride.** In a patient with a low EABV, a high rate of excretion of $Na^+$ but not $Cl^-$ suggests that there is an anion other than $Cl^-$ being excreted with $Na^+$. If the anion is $HCO_3^-$ (the urine pH is alkaline), suspect recent vomiting. The anion could also be one that was ingested or administered (e.g., penicillinate anion), in which case the urine pH would be close to 6.

**High Rate of Excretion of Chloride but Little Excretion of Sodium.** In a patient with a low EABV, a high rate of excretion of $Cl^-$ but not $Na^+$ suggests that a cation other than $Na^+$ is being excreted with $Cl^-$. Most often the cation is $NH_4^+$, and the setting is diarrhea or laxative abuse, causing hyperchloremic metabolic acidosis.

**Excretions of Sodium and Chloride Are Not Low.** In a patient who has a low EABV, a high rate of excretion of both $Na^+$ and $Cl^-$ suggests the absence of a stimulator of the reabsorption of $Na^+$ and $Cl^-$ (e.g., aldosterone deficiency), the presence of an inhibitor of their reabsorption (e.g., a diuretic), or an intrinsic renal lesion that has effects similar to those of a diuretic (e.g., Bartter syndrome or Gitelman syndrome). The pattern of excretion of electrolytes in multiple spot urine samples throughout the day can provide a helpful clue to the cause of the loss of NaCl. For example, the use of diuretics is suspected if $U_{Na}$ and $U_{Cl}$ in spot urine samples are very low at times but high at others. By contrast, in a patient with Bartter syndrome or Gitelman syndrome, these rates of excretion are persistently high.

### Fractional Excretion of Sodium or Chloride

Calculation of the fractional excretion of $Na^+$ ($FE_{Na}$) or $Cl^-$ ($FE_{Cl}$) expresses the amount of $Na^+$ or $Cl^-$ that is excreted in the urine as a percentage of the amount that is filtered. For example, adults consuming a typical Western diet excrete about 150 mmol/day each of $Na^+$ and $Cl^-$. Because a normal GFR is about 180 L/day, the kidney filters about 27,000 mmol of $Na^+$ and about 20,000 mmol of $Cl^-$ per day ($P_{Na}$ or $P_{Cl} \times$ GFR). Hence, $FE_{Na}$ is about 0.5%, and $FE_{Cl}$ is about 0.75%. (The formula for this calculation is shown in Eq. 24.4.)

$$FE_{Na} = 100 \times ([U_{Na}/P_{Na}]/[U_{Cr}/P_{Cr}]) \qquad (24.4)$$

Note that $U_{Na}$ or $U_{Cl}$ and $P_{Na}$ or $P_{Cl}$ must be in the same units (generally mmol/L), and $U_{Cr}$ and $P_{Cr}$ must be in the same units (e.g., either both in mg/dL or both in mmol/L).

One should bear in mind three practical points when using the $FE_{Na}$ or $FE_{Cl}$:

1. The excretions of $Na^+$ and $Cl^-$ are directly related to the dietary intake of NaCl.
   Hence, a low $FE_{Na}$ or $FE_{Cl}$ may represent a low intake of NaCl rather than a low EABV.
2. The numeric values for $FE_{Na}$ and $FE_{Cl}$ will be twice as high, at steady state, in a euvolemic subject who consumes 150 mmol of NaCl daily whose GFR is reduced by 50% as in another subject who consumes the same amount of NaCl and has a normal GFR.
   Hence, the numeric values of $FE_{Na}$ and $FE_{Cl}$ must be interpreted in the context of the GFR at the time the measurements are made.
3. As is the case with the use of $U_{Na}$ or $U_{Cl}$, the $FE_{Na}$ may be high in a patient with a low EABV when there is an unusually large excretion of another anion (e.g., $HCO_3^-$) in the urine, and the $FE_{Cl}$ may be high in a patient with a low EABV when there is an unusually large excretion of another cation (e.g., $NH_4^+$) in the urine.
   Calculations of $FE_{Na}$ and $FE_{Cl}$ are commonly used in patients with acute kidney injury in the differential diagnosis of prerenal azotemia versus acute tubular necrosis (in the absence of diuretics).[11] The advantage of using fractional excretion in this setting over the urinary $Na^+$ and $Cl^-$ concentrations is that the use of $FE_{Na}$ and $FE_{Cl}$ adjusts these concentration terms for water reabsorption in the nephron.

### Determining the Nephron Site Where There Is a Defect in Reabsorption of Sodium

If another compound or an ion that should have been reabsorbed in a given nephron segment is being excreted, one has presumptive evidence for a defect in that nephron segment. For example, if the defect is in the PT, one might find glucosuria in the absence of hyperglycemia (e.g., Fanconi syndrome).

The presence of hypokalemia may suggest a defect in the TAL of the loop of Henle or in the DCT with enhanced rate of $K^+$ secretion in the aldosterone-sensitive distal nephron (ASDN, which includes the second portion of the DCT [DCT2], the connecting segment, and the CCD) due to both increased distal delivery of $Na^+$ and increased aldosterone levels because of decreased EABV. The presence of hypocalciuria would suggest that the site of the lesion is in the DCT (e.g., Gitelman syndrome, thiazide diuretics), whereas hypercalciuria suggests a lesion in the TAL (e.g., Bartter syndrome or use of loop diuretics). The presence of hyperkalemia suggests a lesion in the ASDN (e.g., Addison disease, use of potassium-sparing diuretics such as spironolactone).

## CLINICAL CASE 4: ASSESSMENT OF THE EFFECTIVE ARTERIAL BLOOD VOLUME

A 25-year-old woman was assessed by her family physician because she was feeling weak. Although she admitted to being concerned about her body image, she denied vomiting and the intake of diuretics. Her blood pressure was 90/60 mm Hg, her pulse rate was 110 beats/min, and her jugular venous pressure was low. Measurements in a venous blood sample showed $P_{HCO_3} = 24$ mmol/L, $P_{anion\ gap} = 17$ mEq/L, $P_K = 2.9$ mmol/L, hematocrit = 0.50, and plasma albumin concentration ($P_{Alb}$) = 5.0 g/dL (50 g/L). The urine electrolyte values were $U_{Na}$ less than 5 mmol/L, $U_{Cl}$ = 42 mmol/L, urinary $K^+$ concentration ($U_K$) = 10 mmol/L, and $U_{Cr}$ = 7 mmol/L.

### Questions and Discussion

How severe is the degree of this patient's ECFV contraction? The elevated value for the hematocrit (0.50) provides quantitative information about her ECFV (see Table 24.2), as does the elevated $P_{Alb}$. Based on a hematocrit of 0.50, her ECFV was reduced by around 33%. If she had prior anemia, the degree of her ECFV contraction might be even greater.

What is the cause of her low EABV? The low $U_{Na}$ implies that her EABV was low. The high $U_{Cl}$ (42 mmol/L), which exceeded the sum of her $U_{Na}$ + $U_K$, indicates that there was another cation in that urine, most likely $NH_4^+$.

*Interpretation.* Calculating the content of $HCO_3^-$ in this patient's ECF compartment ($P_{HCO_3}$ × her current ECFV) revealed that she had a deficit of $NaHCO_3$. Loss of NaCl plus $NaHCO_3$ via the GI tract was suspected as the cause of contracted EABV. The patient later admitted to the frequent use of a laxative. Hypokalemia could be explained by the loss of $K^+$ via the GI tract because her low $U_K/U_{Cr}$ ratio suggests that the loss of $K^+$ was extrarenal (see section on potassium). Hypokalemia is associated with acidosis in PT cells, which stimulates ammoniagenesis. The increased rate of excretion of the cation $NH_4^+$ obligates the excretion of $Cl^-$, despite the presence of a low EABV.

## HYPONATREMIA

*Hyponatremia* is defined as a $P_{Na}$ less than 135 mmol/L.

### Concept 9

Because water moves across cell membranes to achieve osmotic equilibrium, acute hyponatremia is associated with the swelling of brain cells. Brain cells adapt by exporting effective osmoles, mainly $K^+$ (and an anion from their ICF) and a number of organic solutes (e.g., taurine, myoinositol).

If hyponatremia is present for more than 48 hours, these adaptive changes have proceeded sufficiently to return brain cells back close to their normal volume. In this setting, a rapid increase in the $P_{Na}$ shrinks cerebral vascular endothelial cells, leading to opening of the blood-brain barrier, allowing lymphocytes, complement, and cytokines to enter the brain, damage oligodendrocytes, and cause demyelination. Microglial activation also plays a role in this process. This has important implications for the management of patients with hyponatremia (see Chapter 15).

### Concept 10

Chronic hyponatremia is usually due to a defect in the renal excretion of water. There are two causes for diminished renal excretion of water, low distal delivery of filtrate and the actions of vasopressin.

Hyponatremia is not a specific disease; rather, it is a diagnostic category with many different causes. The traditional approach to the pathophysiology of hyponatremia centers on a reduced electrolyte-free water excretion due to the actions of vasopressin. In some clinical settings, release of vasopressin is thought to be due to a diminished EABV. Nevertheless, at least in some patients with hyponatremia, the degree of decrease in EABV does not seem to be large enough to cause the release of vasopressin. We suggest that hyponatremia may develop in some patients in the absence of vasopressin actions. Two factors are important in this context, the volume of filtrate that is delivered to the distal nephron and the volume of water that is reabsorbed in the inner MCD through its RWP.[3]

The volume of distal delivery of filtrate is reduced if the GFR is decreased or the fractional reabsorption of NaCl in the PT is increased.

The fractional reabsorption of NaCl in the PT is increased in response to a decreased EABV. Decreased EABV can be due to a total body deficit of NaCl (e.g., diuretic use in a patient who consumes little salt, NaCl loss in diarrhea fluid or sweat) or to a disorder that causes a low cardiac output. Because there is an obligatory minimal loss of $Na^+$ in each liter of urine during a large water diuresis, a deficit of $Na^+$ can be created during the polyuria induced by a large intake of water in a subject who consumes little NaCl (e.g., a patient with beer potomania).

The driving force for water reabsorption via RWP is the osmotic pressure gradient generated by the difference in osmolality between the luminal fluid in the inner MCD and that in the medullary interstitium. As discussed previously, we estimate that somewhat more than 5 L of water is reabsorbed per day in the inner MCD by RWP during water diuresis.

In some patients, hyponatremia is caused by reduced electrolyte-free water excretion due to actions of vasopressin, but the release of vasopressin is not caused by a decreased EABV. This category is called the syndrome of the inappropriate secretion of antidiuretic hormone (SIADH). SIADH, however, is a diagnosis of exclusion; it cannot be made if the patient has a condition that may lead to a low distal delivery of filtrate. A rare cause of SIADH is a mutation in the gene encoding V2R, causing V2R to be constitutively active. This disorder is called "nephrogenic syndrome of inappropriate antidiuresis," and it is suspected in a patient with SIADH of undetermined cause in whom the vasopressin level is undetectable and who does not respond to the administration of a V2R antagonist (e.g., tolvaptan) with a water diuresis.

### TOOLS FOR EVALUATING HYPONATREMIA

#### Measurement of Plasma Sodium Concentration

Pseudohyponatremia is present when the $P_{Na}$ measured by the laboratory is lower than the actual ratio of $Na^+$ to plasma water in the patient. This occurs when the method used requires dilution of the plasma sample. This is because 7% of the plasma volume is a nonaqueous volume (i.e., lipids and proteins), which is not taken into account when adjusting for the volume of the diluent. Hence, although the concentration of $Na^+$ in plasma water is 150 mmol/L, the measured value by flame photometry is 140 mmol/L, and lower values will be obtained by this method if the nonaqueous volume in plasma is larger ( e.g., in a patient with hypertriglyceridemia or hyperparaproteinemia) because the same volume of diluent is added to a smaller volume of plasma water. With the use of an ion-selective electrode, the activity of $Na^+$ in the aqueous plasma volume is measured; nevertheless, because of the use of automatic aspirators and dilutors to prepare the plasma samples, pseudohyponatremia remains an issue. This error in the measurement of $P_{Na}$ is detected by the finding of a normal $P_{osm}$ value in the absence of high concentration of other osmoles, such as urea, glucose, or alcohol.[12]

**Hyponatremia Due to Hyperglycemia.** In the absence of actions of insulin, glucose is an effective osmole for skeletal muscle and, if hyperglycemia is associated with a rise in plasma effective osmolality, there will be a shift of water out of skeletal muscle. Although a number of formulas have been proposed to predict the fall in $P_{Na}$ based on a given rise in $P_{Glu}$, these formulas are based on theoretic calculations with the addition of glucose without water to the ECF compartment. Different correction factors have been proposed based on assumptions made about ECFV and the volume of distribution of glucose in the absence of insulin actions. Moreover, because patients with hyperglycemia have variable fluid intake and variable loss of water and $Na^+$ in the urine, one cannot assume a fixed relationship between the rise in $P_{Glu}$ and the fall in $P_{Na}$.

### Detection of a Low Effective Arterial Blood Volume

A difficulty in making the diagnosis of SIADH is that patients may have a mild to modest degree of EABV contraction, causing a low distal delivery of filtrate that cannot always be detected by the physical examination. The following laboratory tests may provide helpful clues to detect the presence of EABV contraction. At times, however, EABV expansion with the infusion of saline may be required to rule out low distal delivery of filtrate as the cause of hyponatremia. Absence of water diuresis despite EABV expansion confirms the diagnosis of SIADH.

**Concentrations of Sodium and Chloride in Urine.** The assessment of $U_{Na}$ and $U_{Cl}$ are helpful to detect the presence of a low EABV, and they may also provide clues about its cause. In the absence of the caveats noted above, a $U_{Na}$ and $U_{Cl}$ higher than 30 mmol/L is thought to be in keeping with euvolemia and the diagnostic category of SIADH.

**Concentrations of Urea and Urate in Plasma.** Expansion of the EABV diminishes the rate of reabsorption of urea and urate in PT, resulting in higher rates of their fractional excretions and lower levels of their plasma concentrations. Because patients with SIADH are likely to have an expanded EABV, a $P_{Urea}$ less than 3.6 mmol/L (BUN < 21.6 mg/dL), a plasma urate level less than 0.24 mmol/L (<4 mg/dL), a fractional excretion of urea greater than 55 %, and a fractional excretion of urate greater than 12% are thought to be more in keeping with the diagnostic category of SIADH. The fractional excretions of urea and urate, however, are not reliable markers in patients who are thought to have cerebral salt wasting and decreased EABV because the defect in $Na^+$ reabsorption in these patients seems to involve the PT. Therefore, these patients will have a high fractional excretion of urea and urate despite decreased EABV.

Because the reabsorption of urea in PT is strongly influenced by the EABV, the relative rise in $P_{Urea}$ is usually larger than the rise in $P_{Creatinine}$ in patients with low EABV. A ratio of $P_{Urea}/P_{Creatinine}$ (where both are in mmol/L units) greater than 100, or BUN/$P_{Creatinine}$ ( where both are in mg/dL units) greater than 20, suggests a low EABV. This, however, may not be the case if protein intake is low.

**Other Tests.** A rise in the $P_{Cr}$ and a low or a high $P_{HCO_3}$ level may suggest that the EABV is low.

The clinical approach to the diagnosis of the cause of chronic hyponatremia is illustrated in Flow Chart 24.4.

## CLINICAL CASE 5: HYPONATREMIA WITH BROWN SPOTS

A 22-year-old woman had myasthenia gravis. In the previous 6 months, she noted a marked decline in her energy and weight loss (down from 50 to 47 kg). She often felt faint when standing up quickly. On physical examination, her blood pressure was 80/50 mm Hg, pulse rate was 126 beats/min, jugular venous pressure was below the level of the sternal angle, and there was no peripheral edema. Brown pigmented spots were evident in her buccal mucosa. The biochemistry data are as follows.

| *Findings* | *Plasma* | *Urine* |
|---|---|---|
| $Na^+$, mmol/L | 112 | 130 |
| $K^+$, mmol/L | 5.5 | 24 |
| Urea | BUN: 28 mg/dL (10 mmol/L) | Urea: 130 mmol/L |
| Creatinine | 1.7 mg/dL (150 µmol/L) | 6.0 mmol/L |
| Osmolality, mOsmol/kg $H_2O$ | 240 | 438 |

### Questions and Discussion

What is the most likely basis for the very low EABV? The very contracted EABV (manifested by the low blood pressure and tachycardia), the low $P_{Na}$, the high $P_K$ of 5.5 mmol/L, and the renal salt wasting strongly suggest that the most likely diagnosis is adrenal insufficiency. This is likely due to autoimmune adrenalitis because the patient also had myasthenia gravis. The low EABV was due to renal salt wasting because of lack of aldosterone and was also caused in part by a lower degree of contraction of venous capacitance vessels because of glucocorticoid deficiency.

What dangers to the patient are present on presentation? Two potential emergencies dominate the initial management, a very contracted EABV and the lack of cortisol. To deal with the former and restore hemodynamic stability, the initial intravenous infusion can be given as 0.9% saline. Once the patient is hemodynamically stable, to expand her EABV further without changing her $P_{Na}$, the intravenous fluid should be changed to one that is isotonic to the patient. The second potential danger is related to the lack of cortisol and is dealt with by administering cortisol.

It did not seem that the patient had an acute component of hyponatremia requiring the induction of a rapid initial rise in her $P_{Na}$ because she did not have significant symptoms that could be related to increased intracranial pressure and she also denied a recent large water intake.

What dangers should be anticipated during therapy, and how can they be avoided? Re-expansion of the patient's EABV could lead to an increased excretion of water due to an increased distal delivery of filtrate and suppression of the release of vasopressin. In addition, the administration of cortisol would improve her hemodynamic state and also inhibit the release of corticotropin-releasing hormone and, hence, of vasopressin. The net result of this therapy would be to cause water diuresis and thereby a dangerous rise in the $P_{Na}$. Because the patient had a small muscle mass (and therefore a small total body water volume), the excretion of a relatively small volume of electrolyte-free water could lead to too rapid a rise in $P_{Na}$. In addition, because of her poor nutritional state (which becomes even more evident if one interprets her weight loss in conjunction with a large gain of water in her cells, hence her loss of muscle mass was larger than revealed by her weight loss), she was at high risk for osmotic demyelination if her $P_{Na}$ were to rise rapidly. The

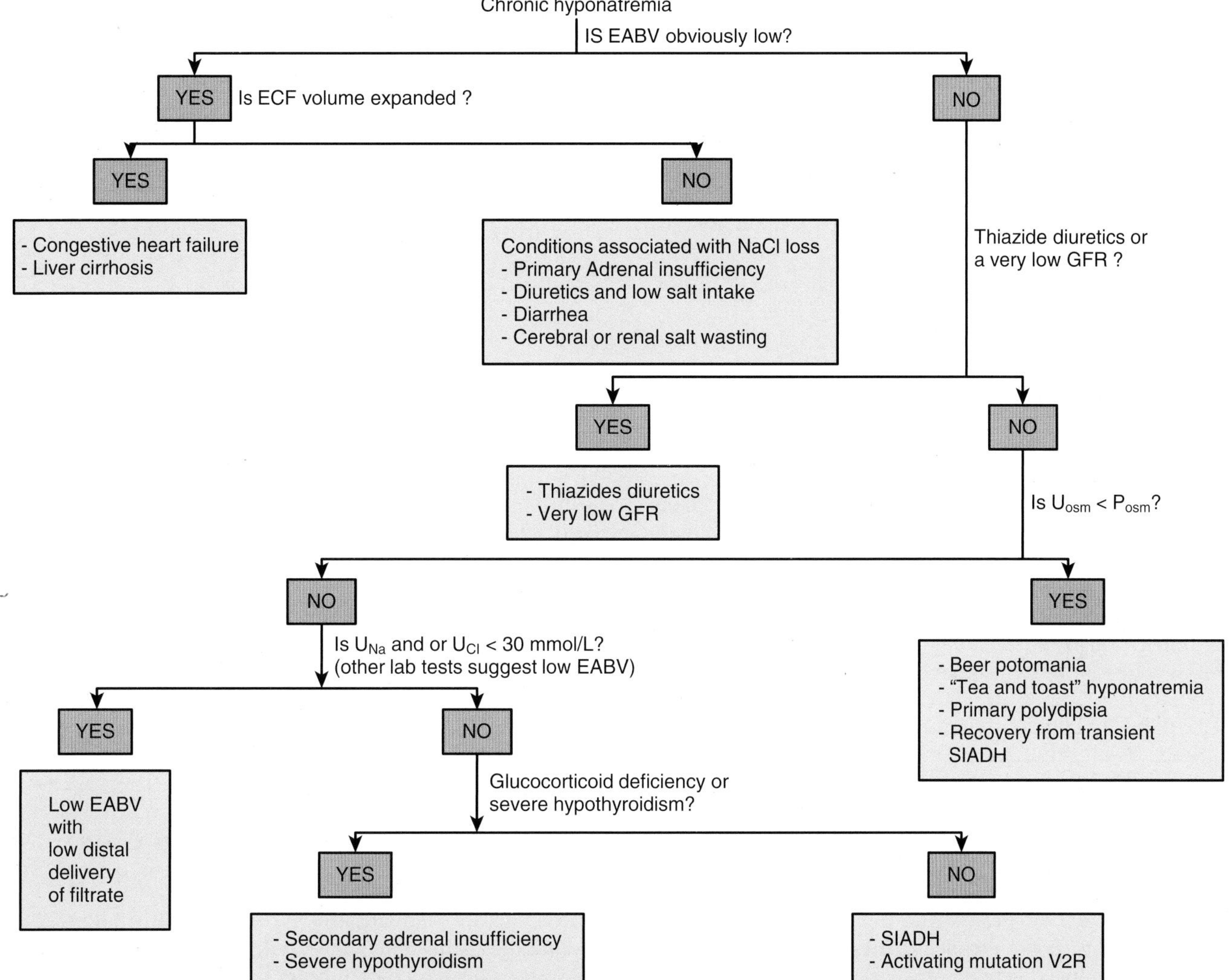


**Flow Chart 24.4** *EABV,* Effective arterial blood volume; *ECF,* extracellular fluid; *GFR,* glomerular filtration rate; *SIADH,* syndrome of inappropriate diuretic hormone secretion. (From Kamel KS, Halperin ML. *Fluid, Electrolyte, and Acid-Base Physiology; A Problem-Based Approach.* ed 5. Philadelphia: Elsevier; 2017.)

rise in her $P_{Na}$ should not exceed a maximum of 4 to 6 mmol/L/24 hours. Accordingly, we would administer DDAVP early in therapy to prevent water diuresis.

## CLINICAL CASE 6: HYPONATREMIA IN A PATIENT ON THIAZIDE DIURETIC THERAPY

A 71-year-old woman was prescribed a thiazide diuretic for the treatment of hypertension. She had chronic kidney disease (CKD) due to ischemic nephropathy, with an estimated GFR of 28 mL/min/1.73 m$^2$ (around 40 L/day). She consumed a low-salt, low-protein diet and drank several large cups of water and tea a day following the advice to remain hydrated. A month later, she presented to her family doctor feeling unwell. Her blood pressure was 130/80 mm Hg, her heart rate was 80 beats/min, there were no postural changes in her blood pressure or heart rate, and her jugular venous pressure was about 1 cm below the level of the sternal angle. Her $P_{Na}$ was 112 mmol/L. Other laboratory results are as follows.

| *Findings* | *Plasma* | *Urine* |
|---|---|---|
| $Na^+$, mmol/L | 112 | 22 |
| $K^+$, mmol/L | 3.6 | 10 |
| $HCO_3^-$, mmol/L | 28 | 0 |
| Urea, mmol/L | 8 | 241 |
| Creatinine, µmol/L (mg/dL) | 145 (1.3) | |
| Creatinine mmol/L (g/L) | | 6.1 (0.7) |
| Osmolality mOsmol/kg $H_2O$ | 240 | 325 |

### Questions and Discussion

What is the most likely basis for the chronic hyponatremia in this patient? Although the patient was taking a thiazide diuretic, the degree of decrease in her EABV did not seem to be large enough to cause the release of vasopressin. The patient had a low baseline estimated GFR of 28 mL/min/1.73 m$^2$ (around 40 L/day). The use of diuretics and the low-salt diet led to a deficit of $Na^+$ and a mild reduction in the EABV. Even a relatively small decrease in EABV leads to increased release of catecholamines, and activation of the renin angiotensin aldosterone system by β-adrenergic stimulation, both of which increase the reabsorption of sodium and water in the PT. If the patient were to reabsorb 90% of her GFR of 40 L/day (which may be even lower because of the mild reduction in her EABV) in the PT, instead of 83% (as discussed previously, this is the percentage of the filtrate that is usually reabsorbed in the PT in the absence of low EABV), less than 4 L/day of filtrate would be delivered distally. This is the maximum volume of urine she could excrete. This volume exceeds the usual daily intake of water, but hyponatremia might still develop in such a patient because there is water reabsorption by RWP along the inner MCD, even in the absence of vasopressin action.

The ability to generate electrolyte- free water is also diminished by the effect of thiazide diuretics to inhibit the reabsorption of NaCl (without water) in DCT. With regard to the volume of water that may be reabsorbed in her inner MCD, the driving force is the difference in osmolalality between the luminal fluid and the interstitial fluid in the inner MCD. Because of the low rate of excretion of osmoles, and because the volume of filtrate delivered to the inner MCD in the absence of vasopressin is larger than during antidiuresis, the osmolality of fluid in the lumen of the inner MCD will be low. If the osmole excretion rate in this patient is 300 mOsmol/day, and if 4 L are delivered to the inner MCD, the osmolality of the luminal fluid in the inner MCD would be 75 mOsmol/kg $H_2O$. Even if the medullary interstitial osmolality is substantially lower than normal—for example, 375 mOsmol/kg $H_2O$—there is still an enormous osmotic driving force for water reabsorption along the inner MCD because a difference of 1 mOsmol/kg $H_2O$ generates a pressure of about 19.3 mm Hg.

A recent study suggested another mechanism for the decreased ability to excrete electrolyte-free water in patients with thiazide-induced hyponatremia, that is also independent of vasopressin. This study showed that nearly half the patients with thiazide-induced hyponatremia carry a single-nucleotide polymorphism in the prostaglandin transporter (PGT) encoded by *SLCO2A1*. Under normal conditions, the effect of vasopressin to cause the insertion of AQP2 into the luminal membrane of principal cells is counterbalanced by increased renal prostaglandin E2 (PGE2) production. PGE2 is directed to the basolateral side of the collecting duct by this prostaglandin transporter, where binding of PGE2 to its basolateral EP1 and EP3 receptors sends out signals for the retrieval of AQP2 from the apical membrane. Administration of a thiazide diuretic leads to increased PGE2 production, although the mechanism is not clear. In some patients with the SLCO2A1 variant, because of the decreased transport capacity of PGT, the concentration of PGE2 in the tubular lumen increases. Binding of PGE2 to its luminal EP4 receptors has the opposite effect and signals for the insertion of AQP2 into the apical membrane of principal cells. This results in increased water reabsorption, independently of vasopressin.[13]

What dangers should be anticipated during therapy, and how can they be avoided? Understanding this pathophysiology has clinical implications for the management of the patient with hyponatremia. Initially, this patient's hyponatremia was thought to be caused by stimulation of vasopressin release due to decreased EABV owing to her intake of a thiazide diuretic; hence, she was given isotonic saline to re-expand her EABV. Even a relatively small volume of saline (especially if it were given as a bolus) might be sufficient to reduce the fractional reabsorption of filtrate in the PT and increase its distal delivery. If the fractional reabsorption in PT were decreased to 83% of the GFR of 40 L/day, distal delivery of filtrate would increase to about 7 L/day. This may exceed the capacity for water reabsorption by RWP (or via the PGE2/EP4–mediated insertion of AQP2 into the luminal membrane of principal cells), so water diuresis would ensue. Because of the patient's small muscle mass, even a modest water diuresis might be large enough to cause a rapid rise in $P_{Na}$ and increase the risk of osmotic demyelination syndrome, especially if she were malnourished or potassium-depleted.

# POTASSIUM

Hypokalemia and hyperkalemia are common electrolyte disorders in clinical practice that may cause life-threatening cardiac arrhythmias. The analysis of the urine composition provides essential information to establish the underlying pathophysiology and plan therapy.

The regulation of $K^+$ homeostasis has two main aspects:

1. Control of the transcellular distribution of $K^+$, which is vital for survival because it limits acute changes in the $P_K$.
2. Regulation of $K^+$ excretion by the kidney, which maintains whole-body $K^+$ balance; this is, however, a much slower process.

## TRANSCELLULAR DISTRIBUTION OF POTASSIUM

### Concept 11

Three factors regulate the movement of $K^+$ across cell membranes—the concentration difference for $K^+$, the electrical voltage across cell membranes, and the presence of open $K^+$ channels in cell membranes.

*Approximately 98% of $K^+$ in the body is in cells.* Although the concentration difference would favor the movement of $K^+$ out of cells via $K^+$ channels in the cell membrane, $K^+$ ions are retained inside the cells by an electrical force because the cell interior has a negative voltage caused by the negatively charged intracellular organic phosphates. These chemical and electrical forces eventually come into balance, and the equilibrium potential for $K^+$ ($E_K$) is achieved. Because cell membranes have much higher permeability to $K^+$ ions than to $Na^+$ ions, the resting membrane potential (RMP) of cells is close to $E_K$.

*The shift of $K^+$ into cells requires an increase in cell interior negative voltage.* This can be achieved by increasing flux via the $Na^+$-$K^+$ adenosine triphosphatase pump ($Na^+$-$K^+$-ATPase). This is because $Na^+$-$K^+$-ATPase is an electrogenic pump that exports three $Na^+$ ions out of the cell while importing only two $K^+$ ions into the cell. Hence, activation of $Na^+$-$K^+$-ATPase leads to the net export of positive charges out of the cell. There are three ways to increase ion pumping acutely by the $Na^+$-$K^+$-ATPase:

1. A rise in the concentration of its limiting substrate—intracellular $Na^+$
2. An increase in the affinity (lower $K_m$ [concentration for half-maximal activation]) for $Na^+$ and $K^+$ or an increase

in the $V_{max}$ (maximal pump turnover rate) of the $Na^+$-$K^+$-ATPase units in cell membranes

3. An increase in the number of active $Na^+$-$K^+$-ATPase pump units in the cell membrane through the recruitment of new units

A long-term increase in $Na^+$-$K^+$-ATPase pump activity requires the synthesis of new pump units, as occurs with exercise training, excess thyroid hormones, or high dietary $K^+$ intake.

Insulin causes a shift of $K^+$ into cells as it promotes the translocation of $Na^+$-$K^+$-ATPase units from an intracellular pool to the cell membrane. Insulin causes the phosphorylation of FXYD1 (phospholemann) via atypical protein kinase C, which increases the $V_{max}$ of $Na^+$-$K^+$-ATPase. Insulin also activates the $Na^+$-$H^+$ exchanger isoform 1 (NHE1) and hence increases the electroneutral entry of $Na^+$ into cells. $\beta_2$-Adrenergic agonists induce the phosphorylation of FXYD1 via cyclic adenosine monophosphate (cAMP)–mediated activation of protein kinase A. NHE1 is also activated by a rise in the intracellular $H^+$ concentration. Monocarboxylic acids (e.g., L-lactic acid, ketoacids) do not cause hyperkalemia. This is because they enter cells on the monocarboxylic acid cotransporter (MCT). An increase in intracellular $H^+$ concentration in the submembrane area where NHE1 is located may activate NHE1,which leads to an increase in the electroneutral entry of $Na^+$ into cells and, in the presence of insulin, a shift of $K^+$ into cells (Fig. 24.4).[14] A shift of $K^+$ out of cells may occur in patents with metabolic acidosis due to the gain of inorganic acids, which are not transported by the MCT (e.g., in patients with diarrhea causing the loss of $NaHCO_3$ [gain of HCl]).

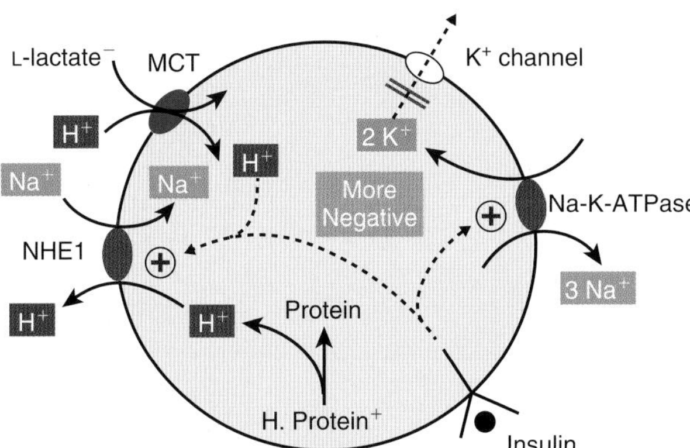


**Fig. 24.4** Possible mechanism for how monocarboxylic acids may cause a shift of $K^+$ into cells. The *circle* represents a cell. The $Na^+$-$H^+$ exchanger isoform 1 *(NHE1)* in cell membranes is activated by insulin and by a high concentration of $H^+$ in the cell interior because $H^+$ binds to the modifier site of NHE1. The concentration of $H^+$ near NHE1 could rise when monocarboxylic acids (lactic acid in this example) enter cells on the monocarboxylic acid cotransporter *(MCT)* and their $H^+$ ions are released close to NHE1. In the presence of insulin, which activates the $Na^+$-$K^+$-ATPase and NHE1 in cell membranes, electroneutral entry of $Na^+$ into cells is increased. The subsequent transport of $Na^+$ out of cells via the electrogenic $Na^+$-$K^+$-ATPase increases the cell interior negative voltage and causes the retention of $K^+$ in cells. The source of bulk of $H^+$ ions transported out of the cell is $H^+$ ions that were bound to intracellular proteins (shown as H. Proteins$^+$) (From Kamel KS, Halperin ML. *Fluid, Electrolyte, and Acid-Base Physiology; A Problem-Based Approach.* ed 5. Philadelphia: Elsevier; 2017.)

## RENAL EXCRETION OF POTASSIUM

Renal $K^+$ excretion. Control of $K^+$ secretion occurs primarily in the ASDN, which includes the DCT2, the connecting segment, and the CCD (see Chapter 6 for a detailed discussion). Two factors influence the rate of excretion of $K^+$—the net secretion of $K^+$ by principal cells in the ASDN, and the flow rate in the ASDN.

### $K^+$ Secretion in the Aldosterone-Sensitive Distal Nephron

The process for secretion of $K^+$ by principal cells in the ASDN requires two elements.[15] First, a lumen-negative transepithelial voltage must be generated by the electrogenic reabsorption of $Na^+$ (i.e., reabsorption of $Na^+$ via the amiloride-sensitive sodium channel, ENaC, without an accompanying anion, which is usually $Cl^-$). Second, a sufficient number of open renal outer medullary $K^+$ (ROMK) channels in the luminal membranes of principal cells must be present.

Aldosterone actions lead to an increase in the number of open ENaC units in the luminal membranes of principal cells in the ASDN.

It was thought that the paracellular pathway plays an important role in the reabsorption of $Cl^-$ in the ASDN, but the large peritubular-luminal concentration difference for $Cl^-$ and the relatively small luminal-peritubular electrical driving force make this mechanism unlikely. An electroneutral, thiazide-sensitive, and amiloride-resistant NaCl transport process has been identified in the luminal membrane of β-intercalated cells of the CCD in mice. This seems to be mediated by the parallel activity of the $Na^+$-independent $Cl^-/HCO_3^-$exchanger (pendrin) and the $Na^+$-dependent $Cl^-/HCO_3^-$ exchanger (NDCBE), resulting in electroneutral NaCl reabsorption.[16]

An increase in luminal fluid concentration of $HCO_3^-$ and/or an alkaline luminal fluid pH seem to increase the amount of $K^+$ secreted in the ASDN.[17] It has been suggested that this effect might be due to a decrease in the paracellular permeability of $Cl^-$. A different mechanism for the effect of luminal $HCO_3^-$ may be that because a gradient for $HCO_3^-$ is needed to increase flux through the $Cl^-/HCO_3^-$ exchanger; pendrin, an increase in luminal $HCO_3^-$ concentration may inhibit flux through pendrin, and hence NDCBE, thereby decreasing the rate of electroneutral NaCl reabsorption, and in turn increasing the rate of electrogenic reabsorption of $Na^+$ and hence the secretion of $K^+$.

ROMK channels are the most important $K^+$ channels for the secretion of $K^+$ in the ASDN. Big $K^+$ conductance—BK or maxi-$K^+$—channels seem to play an important role in flow-dependent $K^+$ secretion, but their role in the physiologic regulation of renal excretion of $K^+$ and its disorders is not clear.[18]

A complex network of with-no-lysine (WNK) kinases, WNK4 and WNK1, via effects on the thiazide-sensitive NaCl cotransporter (NCC) in the DCT1 and ROMK in the ASDN, may function as a switch to change the aldosterone response of the kidney to conserve $Na^+$ or excrete $K^+$.[19] WNK4, and a full-length, kinase-active form of WNK1 (L-WNK1), can increase the activity of NCC, thereby diminishing the delivery of NaCl to the ASDN and hence the rate of electrogenic reabsorption of $Na^+$ and the ability to generate a large negative luminal voltage. Increasing delivery of $Na^+$ and hence the flow rate in the ASDN may also increase $K^+$ secretion via the flow -activated BK channels. Both WNK4 and L-WNK1 also induce endocytosis of ROMK.[20] See Chapter 6 for a detailed discussion of this complex and rapidly evolving field.

### Concept 12

When vasopressin acts, the flow rate in the ASDN is determined by the number of effective osmoles present in luminal fluid. Vasopressin causes the insertion of AQP2 channels into the luminal membranes of principal cells, the osmolality of fluid in the terminal CCD becomes equal to the $P_{osm}$ and hence is relatively fixed. Therefore the number of osmoles present in the luminal fluid in the terminal CCD determines the number of liters of fluid that exit the terminal CCD. These osmoles are largely urea, $Na^+$, $Cl^-$, and $K^+$, with an accompanying anion. Owing to the process of intrarenal urea recycling, the largest fraction of the osmoles delivered to the ASDN is urea osmoles. In subjects eating a typical Western diet, the amount of urea that recycles would be approximately 600 mmol/day. This process of urea recycling adds an extra 2 L to the flow rate in the terminal CCD (600 mOsmol divided by a luminal fluid osmolality that is equal to plasma osmolality—that is, ≈300 mOsmol/kg $H_2O$).

In a quantitative analysis, Kamel and Halperin have illustrated that even in patients with a large defect in the ability to generate a lumen-negative voltage in the ASDN, a significant degree of hyperkalemia is not likely to develop with a usual $K^+$ intake unless there is decreased flow rate in the ASDN. Restricting protein intake may decrease the amount of urea that recycles and hence the rate of flow in the ASDN.[21]

### Concept 13

There is no normal rate of $K^+$ excretion in the urine because normal subjects in a steady state excrete all the $K^+$ they eat and absorb from the GI tract. To assess the renal response to hypokalemia, we use the observed rate of excretion of $K^+$ in patients who developed hypokalemia due to a nonrenal cause. In subjects who became $K^+$-depleted because of low dietary $K^+$ intake, the rate of $K^+$ excretion fell to 10 to 15 mmol/day. In normal subjects given a large load of $K^+$ (>200 mmol/day) on a chronic basis, the rate of renal excretion of $K^+$ rose to match their intake, with only a modest rise in their $P_K$. Hence, the development of chronic hyperkalemia requires a defect in renal $K^+$ excretion.

## TOOLS FOR EVALUATING A PATIENT WITH A DYSKALEMIA

### Assess the Rate of Excretion of Potassium in the Urine

A 24-hour urine collection is not necessary to assess the daily rate of excretion of $K^+$. Taking advantage of the fact that creatinine is excreted at a near-constant rate throughout the day, we use the ratio of the concentration of $K^+$ in the urine ($U_K$) to the concentration of creatinine in the urine ($U_{Cr}$)—$U_K/U_{Cr}$. This approach has the following advantages. The data can be available in a short time period, and more relevant information is gathered if one knows the stimulus, the $P_K$, that influences the rate of excretion of $K^+$ during that time frame. The limitation is that there is a diurnal variation in $K^+$ excretion, but this does not negate the advantages. The expected $U_K/U_{Cr}$ in patients with hypokalemia due to an intracellular shift of $K^+$ and in those with chronic hypokalemia due to extrarenal loss of $K^+$ is less than 18 mmol $K^+$/g creatinine or less than 2 mmol $K^+$/mmol creatinine. The expected ratio in a patient with hyperkalemia and a normal renal response is more than 200 mmol $K^+$/g creatinine or more than 20 mmol $K^+$/mmol creatinine. To develop *chronic* hyperkalemia, however, one must have a defect in the renal excretion of $K^+$; hence, $U_K/U_{Cr}$ does not provide clinically useful information in that situation. Because of diurnal variation in $K^+$ excretion, a 24-hour urine collection, rather than a random $U_K/U_{Cr}$, may be needed to assess the contribution of dietary $K^+$ intake to the degree of hyperkalemia.

### Transtubular Potassium Concentration Gradient

The transtubular potassium concentration gradient (TTKG) was developed to provide a semiquantitative reflection of the driving force for $K^+$ secretion in the ASDN. The rationale behind this calculation was to adjust $U_K$ for the amount of water that was reabsorbed in downstream nephron segments (i.e., the MCD) to estimate the concentration of $K^+$ in the luminal fluid in the terminal CCD ($K_{CCD}$) .To calculate the [$K_{CCD}$], we suggested dividing the $U_K$ by the ratio of $U_{osm}$ to the $P_{osm}$ ($U_{osm}/P_{osm}$) because the osmolality in the luminal fluid in the terminal CCD should be equal to $P_{osm}$ when vasopressin causes the insertion of AQP2 into the luminal membranes of principal cells in the CCD.

The assumption made with use of the $U_{osm}/P_{osm}$ ratio is that most of the osmoles delivered to the MCD are not reabsorbed in this nephron segment, and therefore the rise in osmolality from its value in the terminal CCD and its value in the urine reflects water reabsorption in the MCD. Although the amount of electrolytes reabsorbed in the MCD should not pose a problem, this is not true for urea because of intrarenal urea recycling. We estimated that in subjects eating a typical Western diet, almost 600 mmol of urea is reabsorbed downstream from the CCD/day. It follows that the calculated $K_{CCD}$ obtained from ($U_K \div [U_{osm}/P_{osm}]$) is likely to be appreciably higher than the actual value in vivo.[21] Therefore we no longer use the TTKG in the clinical assessment of patients with dyskalemia. Rather, we use the $U_K/U_{Cr}$ ratio to provide the information needed to assess the renal response in these patients.

**Establishing the Basis for the Abnormal Rate of Excretion of Potassium.** In a patient with hypokalemia, a higher than expected rate of excretion of $K^+$ implies that there is a higher lumen-negative voltage in the ASDN, and that open ROMK channels are present in the luminal membranes of principal cells. The higher lumen-negative voltage is due to a higher rate of electrogenic $Na^+$ reabsorption in the ASDN. The converse is true in a patient with hyperkalemia, in whom there is a lower than expected rate of excretion of $K^+$.

The clinical indices that help in the differential diagnosis of the pathophysiology of the abnormal rate of electrogenic reabsorption of $Na^+$ in the ASDN are an assessment of the EABV and the presence or absence of hypertension. The measurement of the plasma renin concentration or activity ($P_{Renin}$) and the plasma aldosterone concentration ($P_{Aldo}$) are helpful in in this differential diagnosis (Table 24.4).

**Table 24.4 Use of Plasma Renin and Plasma Aldosterone Values to Assess the Basis of Hypokalemia or Hyperkalemia**

| Parameter | Renin Value | Aldosterone Value |
|---|---|---|
| **Lesions That Cause Hypokalemia** | | |
| Adrenal Gland | | |
| • Primary hyperaldosteronism | Low | High |
| • Glucocorticoid-remediable hyperaldosteronism | Low | High |
| Kidney | | |
| • Renal artery stenosis | High | High |
| • Malignant hypertension | High | High |
| • Renin-secreting tumor | High | High |
| • Liddle syndrome | Low | Low |
| • Disorders involving 11β-hydroxysteroid dehydrogenase-2 | Low | Low |
| **Lesions That Cause Hyperkalemia** | | |
| Adrenal Gland | | |
| Addison disease | High | Low |
| Kidney | | |
| Pseudohypoaldosteronism type 1 | High | High |
| Hyporeninemic hypoaldosteronism | Low | Low |

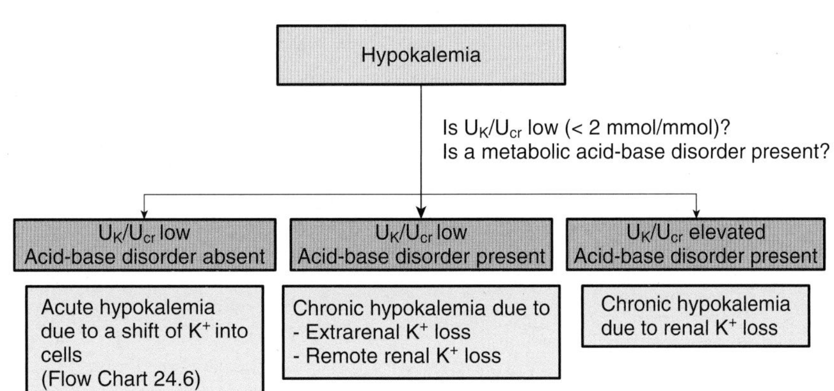


**Flow Chart 24.5** (From Kamel KS, Halperin ML. *Fluid, Electrolyte, and Acid-Base Physiology; A Problem-Based Approach.* ed 5. Philadelphia: Elsevier; 2017.)

## CLINICAL APPROACH TO THE PATIENT WITH HYPOKALEMIA

### Step 1. Deal With Medical Emergencies That May Be Present on Presentation, and Anticipate and Prevent Risks That May Arise During Therapy

The major emergencies related to hypokalemia are cardiac arrhythmias and respiratory muscle weakness leading to respiratory failure. Patients with chronic hyponatremia and hypokalemia are also at a high risk for the development of osmotic demyelination, with a rapid rise in $P_{Na}$. Administration of KCl may lead to a rapid rise in $P_{Na}$[22] because $K^+$ ions enter and $Na^+$ ions leave muscle cells. This movement of $Na^+$ ions into the ECF compartment may also expand the EABV, leading to an increase in distal delivery of filtrate, resulting in water diuresis.

### Step 2. Determine Whether the Basis for Hypokalemia Is an Acute Shift of Potassium Into Cells

A low rate of excretion of $K^+$ ($U_K/U_{Cr}$ <18 mmol of $K^+$/g of creatinine or <2 mmol of $K^+$/mmol of creatinine) and the absence of a metabolic acid-base disorder suggest that the major basis of hypokalemia is an acute shift of $K^+$ into cells (Flow Chart 24.5).[23]

Having established that the major pathophysiology of the hypokalemia is an acute shift of $K^+$ into cells, the next step is to determine whether an adrenergic surge may have caused this shift of $K^+$ (Flow Chart 24.6). In these settings, tachycardia, a wide pulse pressure, and systolic hypertension are often present. It is very important to recognize patients with these features because the administration of nonspecific beta-blockers can lead to a very rapid recovery without the

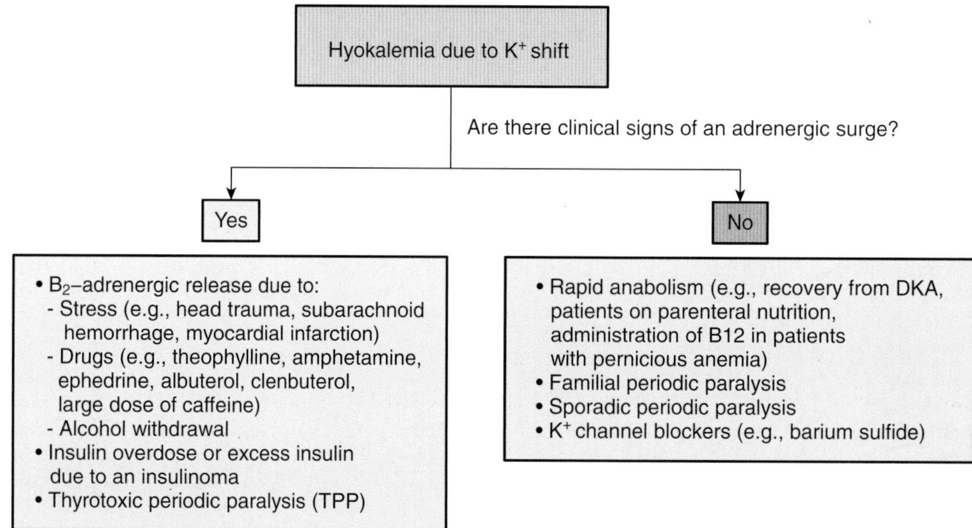


**Flow Chart 24.6** *DKA,* Diabetic ketoacidosis. (From Kamel KS, Halperin ML. *Fluid, Electrolyte, and Acid-Base Physiology; A Problem-Based Approach.* ed 5. Philadelphia: Elsevier; 2017.)

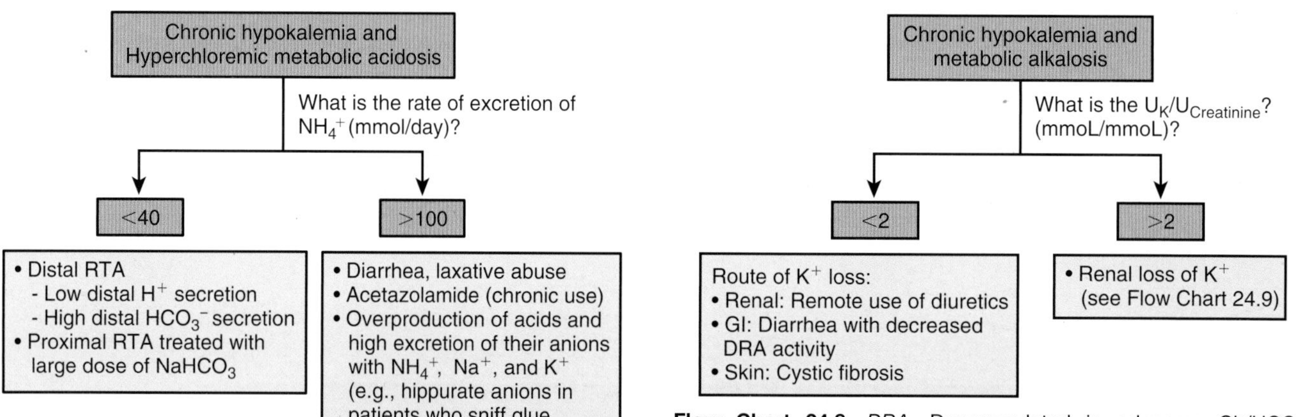


**Flow Chart 24.7** *DKA,* Diabetic ketoacidosis; *RTA,* renal tubular acidosis. (From Kamel KS, Halperin ML. *Fluid, Electrolyte, and Acid-Base Physiology; A Problem-Based Approach.* ed 5. Philadelphia: Elsevier; 2017.)

**Flow Chart 24.8** *DRA,* Downregulated in adenoma $Cl^-/HCO_3^-$ exchanger; *GI,* gastrointestinal. (From Kamel KS, Halperin ML. *Fluid, Electrolyte, and Acid-Base Physiology; A Problem-Based Approach.* ed 5. Philadelphia: Elsevier; 2017.)

administration of a large amount of KCl and hence avoid the risk of the development of rebound hyperkalemia when the stimulus for shift of $K^+$ ions abates.[24]

### Step 3. Examine the Acid-Basis Status in the Patient With Chronic Hypokalemia

In the patient with chronic hypokalemia, the first step is to examine the acid-base status in plasma.

**Subgroup With Metabolic Acidosis.** The group of patients with metabolic acidosis (usually hyperchloremic metabolic acidosis) can be divided into two categories according to the rate of excretion of $NH_4^+$ in the urine (Flow Chart 24.7). The rate of excretion of $NH_4^+$ can be estimated with use of the urine osmolal gap (see discussion of metabolic acidosis).

**Subgroup With Metabolic Alkalosis.** The first step in the patient with metabolic alkalosis is to determine whether the site of loss of $K^+$ is renal or extrarenal on the basis of the assessment of the rate of renal excretion of $K^+$ using the $U_K/U_{Cr}$ (Flow Chart 24.8). Patients with a low value for this ratio (i.e., <18 mmol of $K^+$/g of creatinine or <2 mmol of $K^+$/mmol of creatinine) have conditions with loss of $K^+$ via nonrenal routes, such as in sweat (e.g., patients with cystic fibrosis) or via the GI tract (e.g., patients with diarrhea associated with decreased activity of the colonic luminal $Cl^-/HCO_3^-$ exchanger, DRA, such as congenital chloridorrhea, villous adenoma, and some patients with laxative abuse). On the other hand, patients in whom the $U_K/U_{Cr}$ is higher than these values have a condition associated with a renal loss of $K^+$.[24a] The steps to take to determine the underlying pathophysiology in this latter group of patients are outlined in Flow Chart 24.9.

In essence, we are trying to determine the cause of a higher rate of electrogenic reabsorption of $Na^+$ in the ASDN. The

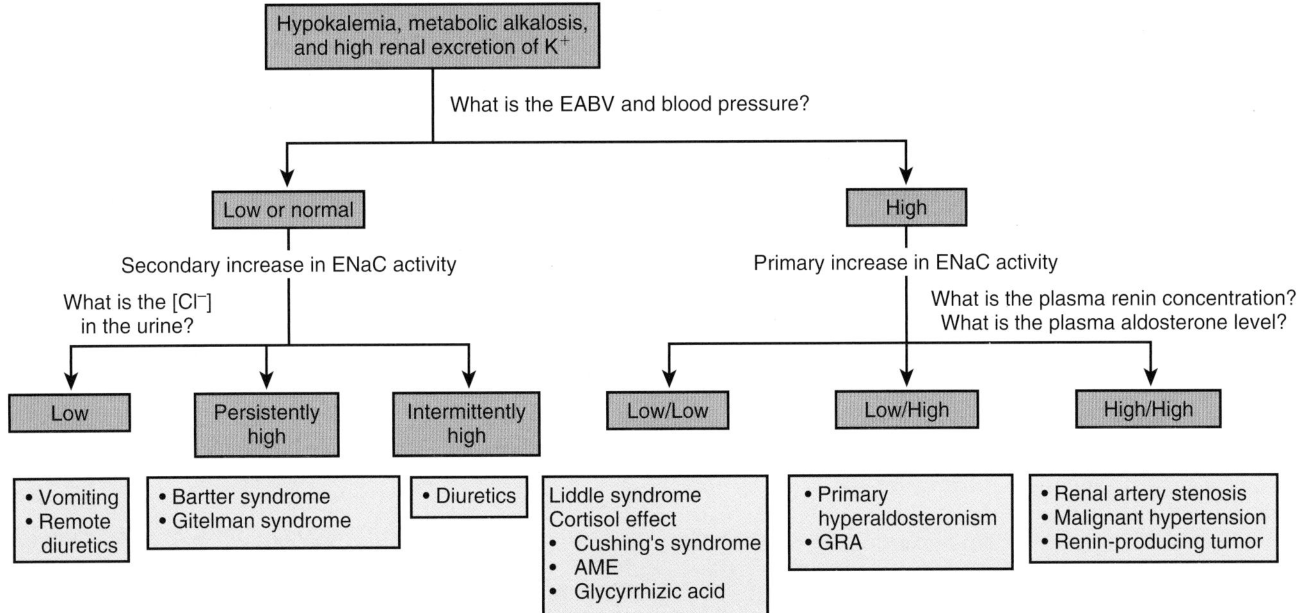


**Flow Chart 24.9** *AME,* Apparent mineralocorticoid excess syndrome; *EABV,* effective arterial blood volume; *GRA,* glucocorticide remediable aldosteronism. (From Kamel KS, Halperin ML. *Fluid, Electrolyte, and Acid-Base Physiology; A Problem-Based Approach.* ed 5. Philadelphia: Elsevier; 2017.)

primary reason is an increased number of open ENaC units in the luminal membranes of principal cells in the ASDN. This increase could be due to two groups of disorders.

The first group involves a secondary increase in ENaC activity due to the release of aldosterone in response to a low EABV. Patients with these disorders are not likely to have high blood pressure. The most common causes are vomiting and the use of diuretic agents. In some patients, the diuretic effect may be due to an inherited disorder affecting NaCl reabsorption in the medullary TAL (i.e., Bartter syndrome) or in the DCT (i.e., Gitelman syndrome). Ligands that occupy the calcium-sensing receptor in the medullary TAL (e.g., ionized calcium in a patient with hypercalcemia), drugs (e.g., gentamicin, cisplatin), and possibly cationic proteins (e.g., cationic monoclonal immunoglobulins in a patient with multiple myeloma) could potentially mimic Bartter syndrome. The use of urine electrolyte values in the differential diagnosis of hypokalemia in a patient with a contracted EABV is summarized in Table 24.3. It is currently recommended that hypertensive patients who develop hypokalemia while taking diuretics be screened for primary hyperaldosteronism.

The second group of disorders involves conditions that are associated with a primary increase in ENaC activity (e.g., primary hyperreninemic hyperaldosteronism, primary hyperaldosteronism, disorders in which cortisol acts as a mineralocorticoid in the ASDN, or a constitutively active ENaC in the luminal membrane of principal cells in the ASDN). The EABV in these patients is not low, and the blood pressure is commonly high.

In some patients a decreased rate of electroneutral $Na^+$ reabsorption may contribute to the increased rate of electrogenic $Na^+$ reabsorption and enhanced kaliuresis. This may be the case when $Na^+$ is delivered to the ASDN with little $Cl^-$ (e.g., delivery of $Na^+$ with $HCO_3^-$ in a patient with recent vomiting or with an anion of a drug such as penicillin).

Magnesium ($Mg^{2+}$) deficiency is frequently associated with hypokalemia. This relationship is largely due to the underlying disorders that cause losses of both $Mg^{2+}$ and $K^+$ (e.g., diarrhea, diuretic therapy, Gitelman syndrome). $K^+$ secretion in the ASDN is mediated by ROMK, a process that is inhibited by intracellular $Mg^{2+}$. A decrease in intracellular $Mg^{2+}$, caused by $Mg^{2+}$ deficiency, releases the $Mg^{2+}$-mediated inhibition of ROMK. $Mg^{2+}$ deficiency alone, however, does not necessarily cause hypokalemia, because an increase in the rate of electrogenic reabsorption of $Na^+$ is required to enhance the rate of secretion of $K^+$.

## CLINICAL CASE 7: HYPOKALEMIA AND A LOW RATE OF POTASSIUM EXCRETION

A 28-year-old Asian woman presented with sudden onset of generalized muscle weakness and inability to ambulate on awakening one morning. She had lost 7 kg of body weight in the last 2 months but denied nausea, vomiting, diarrhea, or the use of diuretics, laxatives, exogenous thyroid hormone, herbal medications, or illicit drugs. The attack was not preceded by strenuous exercise or the consumption of a carbohydrate-rich meal. She had no family history of hypokalemia, periodic paralysis, or hyperthyroidism. On physical examination, she was alert and oriented; blood pressure was 150/70 mm Hg, heart rate was 116 beats/min, and respiratory rate was 18 breaths/min. The thyroid gland was not obviously enlarged, and there was no exophthalmos. Symmetric flaccid paralysis with areflexia was present in all four limbs. The remainder of the physical examination was unremarkable. The pH and $P_{CO_2}$ values shown in the following table of laboratory findings were from an arterial blood sample, whereas all other blood data were from a venous blood sample. The electrocardiogram (ECG) showed sinus tachycardia and prominent U waves.

| *Findings* | *Blood* | *Urine* |
|---|---|---|
| $K^+$, mmol/L | 1.8 | 12 |
| Creatinine | 0.7 mg/dL (62 μmol/L) | 1.9 g/L (16.8 mmol/L) |
| $Na^+$, mmol/L | 140 | 179 |
| $Cl^-$, mmol/L | 108 | 184 |
| pH | 7.41 | — |
| $P_{CO_2}$, mm Hg | 36 | — |
| $HCO_3^-$, mmol/L | 23 | — |
| Glucose, mg/dL | 112 | 0 |

### Questions and Discussion

Is there a medical emergency? Because the ECG did not show changes due to hypokalemia other than U waves, and because respiratory muscle weakness causing hypoventilation was not present, as assessed from the arterial $P_{CO_2}$, there were no emergencies related to hypokalemia at this time.

What is the basis of the hypokalemia? A $U_K/U_{Cr}$ ratio less than 1 (mmol/mmol) and the absence of a metabolic acid-base disorder on presentation suggest that the basis of the severe hypokalemia in this patient was an acute shift of $K^+$ into cells.

Possible reasons for potassium shift into cells: The presence of tachycardia, systolic hypertension, and wide pulse pressure suggest that an adrenergic surge was the cause of the acute shift of $K^+$ into cells. On further laboratory testing, she was found to have hyperthyroidism, so the diagnosis was thyrotoxic periodic paralysis (TPP). Patients with TPP often have only subtle signs and symptoms of thyrotoxicosis. In contrast to standard teaching, most patients with TPP do not have clear precipitating factors such as strenuous exercise or the consumption of a carbohydrate-rich meal. Increased $Na^+$-$K^+$-ATPase activity has traditionally been implicated in the pathogenesis of TPP. Studies have shown that susceptibility to TPP can be conferred by mutations in the skeletal muscle–specific, inward-rectifying $K^+$ (Kir) channel, Kir2.6.

What are the options for therapy? The patient received intravenous KCl at a rate of 10 mmol/hour by the administration of a solution of 0.9% saline with 40 mEq/L KCl at a rate of 250 mL/hour. In a patient with severe hypokalemia, one should not use a dextrose-containing solution because this may cause the release of insulin, which could induce a further shift of $K^+$ into cells and aggravate the severity of hypokalemia. Although she received only 80 mmol of KCl, rebound hyperkalemia ($P_K$, 5.7 mmol/L) developed; the $P_K$ returned to normal 6 hours later. Studies have suggested that hypokalemia in patients with TPP can be rapidly corrected without the risk of rebound hyperkalemia by the administration of a nonselective beta-blocker and only a small dose of KCl.

## CLINICAL CASE 8: HYPOKALEMIA AND HIGH RATE OF POTASSIUM EXCRETION

Progressive muscle weakness developed over the last 6 hours in a 76-year-old Asian man that became so severe that he was unable to move. He reported that he exercised that morning and ate a large carbohydrate meal for breakfast, which he usually does after he has a good exercise session. He had no other neurologic symptoms. He denied vomiting, or diarrhea, or the use of diuretics or laxatives. Hypokalemia ($P_K$, 3.3 mmol/L) and hypertension had been noted 1 year ago but had not been investigated further. On this admission, his blood pressure was 160/96 mm Hg and his heart rate was 70 beats/min. A neurologic examination revealed symmetric flaccid paralysis with areflexia but no other findings. The laboratory data prior to therapy are shown in the following table. The pH and $P_{CO_2}$ values are from an arterial blood sample. Results of measurement of the $P_{Renin}$ and $P_{Aldo}$, which became available later, showed that both levels were low. The plasma cortisol value was in the normal range.

| *Findings* | *Blood* | *Urine* |
|---|---|---|
| $K^+$, mmol/L | 1.8 | 26 |
| $Na^+$, mmol/L | 147 | 132 |
| $Cl^-$, mmol/L | 90 | 138 |
| Creatinine | 0.8 mg/dL (70 μmol/L) | 0.6 g/L (5.3 mmol/L) |
| pH | 7.55 | |
| $P_{CO_2}$, mm Hg | 40 | — |
| $HCO_3^-$, mmol/L | 45 | 0 |
| Osmolality, mOsm/kg $H_2O$ | 302 | 482 |

### Questions and Discussion

What is the cause of hypokalemia in this patient? In the presence of hypokalemia, the $U_K/U_{Cr}$ was 5 (mmol/mmol), and metabolic alkalosis was also present. Hence, the hypokalemia was largely due to a disorder that caused excessive loss of $K^+$ in the urine. The acute presentation with extreme weakness was likely due to an acute shift of $K^+$ into cells in conjunction with a chronic disorder that caused the loss of $K^+$. This component, of an acute shift of $K^+$ into cells, was attributed to the predominant $\beta_2$-adrenergic effect during rest after vigorous exercise, and the release of insulin due to the large carbohydrate intake during breakfast prior to the onset of symptoms.

On clinical assessment, the patient's EABV volume was thought not to be contracted, and he had hypertension. Therefore, the increased electrogenic reabsorption of $Na^+$ in the ASDN was due to a primary increase in ENaC activity. The differential diagnosis was guided by measurements of the $P_{Renin}$ and $P_{Aldo}$ (see Table 24.4). Because both the $P_{Aldo}$ and $P_{Renin}$ were suppressed, the differential diagnosis was between disorders in which cortisol acts as mineralocorticoid and those with constitutively active ENaC in the luminal membranes of principal cells in the ASDN. Inherited disorders in which ENaC is constitutively active (Liddle syndrome) seemed unlikely, considering the patient's age. Plasma cortisol values were not elevated. Computed tomography of the chest did not show a lung mass. Although the patient denied consuming licorice or chewing tobacco, it turned out that he used an herbal preparation containing large amounts of glycyrrhizic acid (the active ingredient in licorice) to sweeten his tea. The patient was treated initially with intravenous KCl; the weakness improved when the $P_K$ reached 2.5 mmol/L. Oral KCl supplementation was continued. Two weeks later, $P_K$ and blood pressure values returned to normal levels, and his body weight had decreased from 78 to 74 kg as a result of natriuresis after stopping the glycyrrhizic acid–containing herbal preparation.

## CLINICAL APPROACH TO THE PATIENT WITH HYPERKALEMIA

### Step 1. Address Emergencies

Hyperkalemia constitutes a medical emergency, primarily because of its effect on the heart, which may lead to cardiac conduction abnormalities, arrhythmias and, ultimately, asystole.

### Step 2. Determine Whether the Cause of the Hyperkalemia Is an Acute Shift of Potassium Out of Cells in vivo or Pseudohyperkalemia

Flow Chart 24.10 illustrates the initial approach for determining the cause of the hyperkalemia. If the time course for the development of hyperkalemia was short and/or the hyperkalemia developed while the intake of $K^+$ was low, then the following three categories should be considered.

**Destruction of Cells in the Body.** Cell destruction could be due, for example, to rhabdomyolysis or tumor lysis syndrome.

**Shift of $K^+$ Out of Cells in the Body.** Shift of $K^+$ out of cells in the body may occur in conditions in which there is a less negative voltage in cells. Such conditions include lack of a stimulus for $Na^+$-$K^+$-ATPase (e.g., lack of insulin in patients with diabetic ketoacidosis [DKA], $\beta_2$-adrenergic blockade), and conditions in which there is an $\alpha$-adrenergic surge causing inhibition of the release of insulin or directly causing a shift of $K^+$ out of hepatic cells. Digoxin inhibits $Na^+$-$K^+$-ATPase, so digoxin overdose can result in hyperkalemia. A shift of $K^+$ may also occur in conditions with metabolic acidosis due to nonmonocarboxylic acids—that is, acids that cannot be transported on the MCT (e.g., metabolic acidosis due to a gain of HCl from loss of $NaHCO_3$ in a patient with diarrhea, ingestion of citric acid). Acute hyperkalemia may occur during exhaustive exercise or in patients with status epilepticus. Severe hyperkalemia has been described as a complication of the administration of mannitol for the treatment or prevention of cerebral edema. This is because a rise in effective osmolality in the interstitial fluid causes the movement of water out of cells via AQP channels in cell membranes, which raises the concentration of $K^+$ in the ICF and provides a chemical driving force for the movement of $K^+$ out of cells. Succinylcholine depolarizes muscle cells, resulting in the efflux of $K^+$ through acetylcholine receptors in conditions that may lead to the upregulation of acetylcholine receptors (e.g., burns, neuromuscular injury [upper or lower motor neuron], disuse atrophy, prolonged immobilization). Fluoride can open the $Ca^{2+}$-sensitive $K^+$ channels; as a result, fluoride intoxication can lead to fatal hyperkalemia. A positive family history for acute hyperkalemia suggests that there may be a molecular basis for this disorder (e.g., hyperkalemic periodic paralysis).

**Pseudohyperkalemia May Be Present.** The presence of changes in the ECG related to hyperkalemia rules out pseudohyperkalemia as the sole cause of the hyperkalemia. Pseudohyperkalemia is caused by the release of $K^+$ during or after venipuncture. Excessive fist clenching during blood sampling may increase $K^+$ release from local muscle and thus may raise the measured $P_K$ by as much as 1 mmol/L. Pseudohyperkalemia can be present in cachectic patients in whom the normal T tubule architecture in skeletal muscle may be disturbed. Mechanical trauma to red blood cells

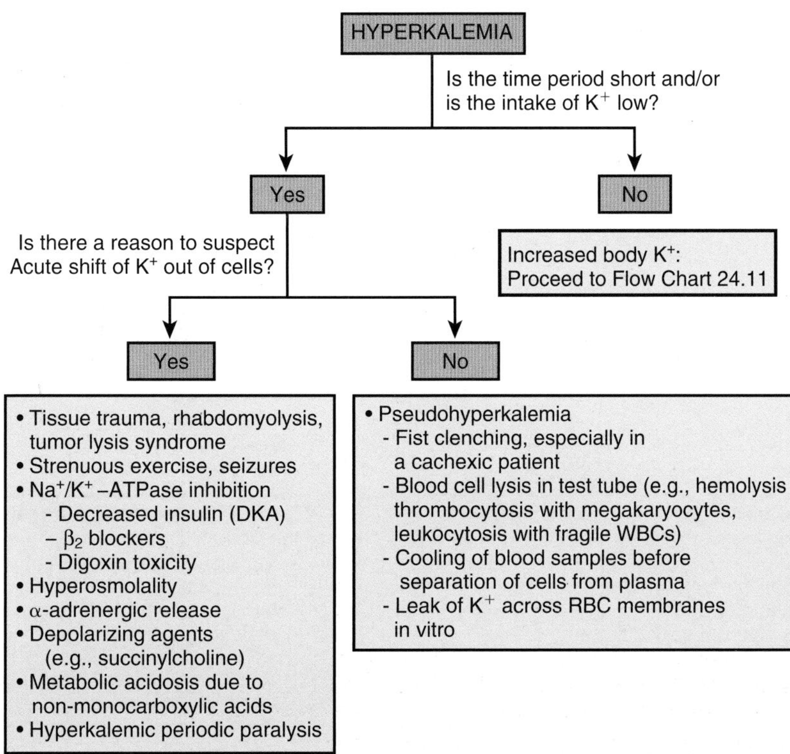


**Flow Chart 24.10** *DKA,* Diabetic ketoacidosis; *RBC,* red blood cells; *WBC,* white blood cells. (From Kamel KS, Halperin ML. *Fluid, Electrolyte, and Acid-Base Physiology; A Problem-Based Approach.* ed 5. Philadelphia: Elsevier; 2017.)

during venipuncture, due for example to the use of a very small-gauge needle, can result in their hemolysis and the release of $K^+$ in the test tube. $K^+$ ions are normally released from platelets during blood clotting, so pseudohyperkalemia may be noted in patients with thrombocytosis (especially with megakaryocytosis). Pseudohyperkalemia may also be present in patients with severe leukocytosis, especially due to fragile leukemia cells, because of the breakdown of cells during venipuncture, when shaken by pneumatic transport, or during centrifugation. Cooling of blood prior to the separation of cells from plasma is another cause of pseudohyperkalemia. There are several hereditary subtypes of pseudohyperkalemia caused by an increase in passive $K^+$ permeability of erythrocytes. The $P_K$ increases in blood samples from patients with this disorder when left at room temperature.

### Step 3. What Is the Rate of Potassium Excretion?

In a patient with chronic hyperkalemia, pseudohyperkalemia should be ruled out first. In normal subjects, a $K^+$ load can augment the rate of excretion of $K^+$ to more than 200 mmol/day, with only a modest increase in $P_K$. Thus, patients with chronic hyperkalemia generally have some defect in renal $K^+$ excretion. In a steady state, they excrete what they eat (minus the amount of $K^+$ lost in stool), but at the expense of maintaining hyperkalemia. Therefore, the value of assessing the rate of $K^+$ excretion is primarily to determine the contribution of $K^+$ intake to the degree of hyperkalemia. A 24-hour urine collection is necessary for this purpose, rather than determination of $U_K/U_{Cr}$ in a spot urine sample, because of the diurnal variation in $K^+$ excretion.

### Step 4. What Is the Basis for the Defect in Renal Potassium Excretion?

The clinical approach to determine the basis for the renal defect in $K^+$ excretion is illustrated in Flow Chart 24.11. More than one cause may be present in a single patient (e.g., intake of a drug that blocks the renin-angiotensin-aldosterone system [RAAS] in a patient with chronic renal insufficiency).

**Does the Patient Have Advanced Chronic Renal Failure?** The estimated GFR is generally less than 15 ml/minute if this is the sole cause of hyperkalemia.

**Is the patient taking drugs that interfere with the renal excretion of potassium?** Drugs that may interfere with the renal excretion of $K^+$ include inhibitors of the RAAS axis, inhibitors of ENaC (including amiloride, trimethoprim, and

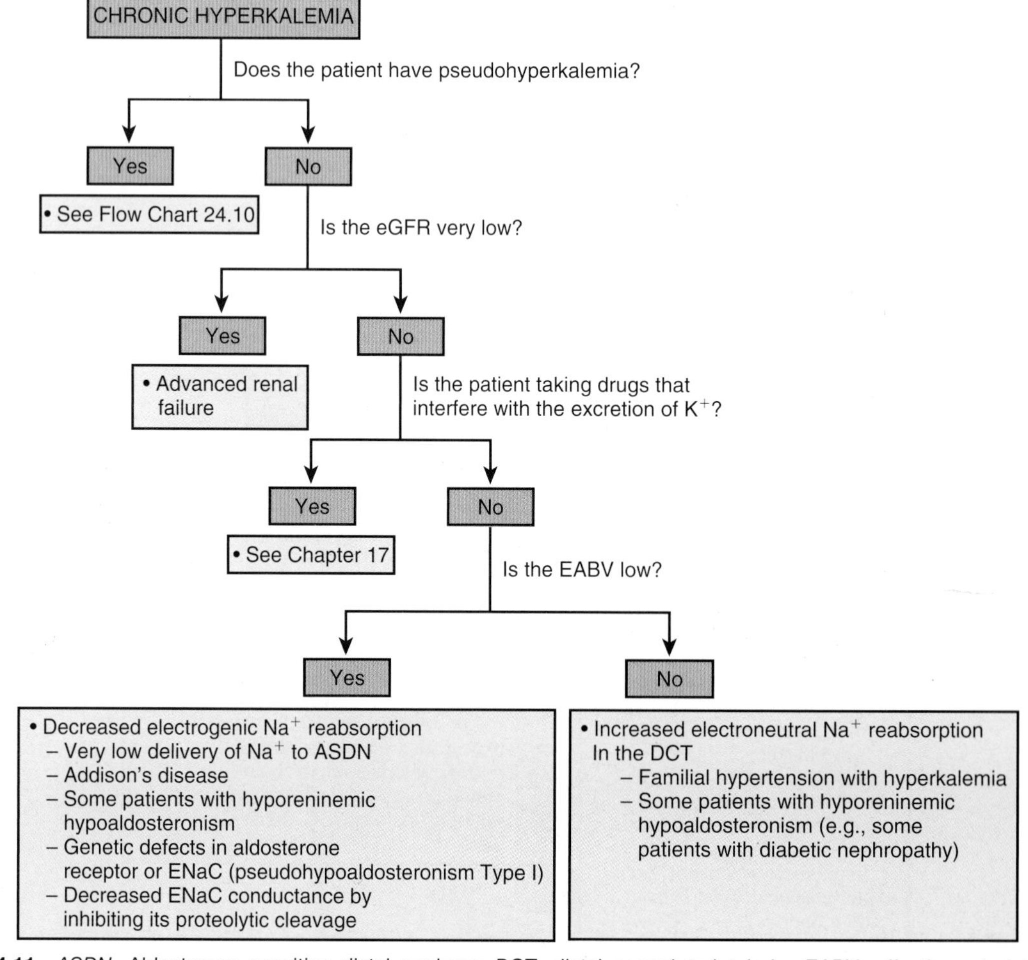


**Flow Chart 24.11** *ASDN,* Aldosterone sensitive distal nephron; *DCT,* distal convoluted tubule; *EABV,* effective arterial blood volume; *eGFR,* estimated glomerular filtration rate; *ENaC,* epithelial sodium channel. (From Kamel KS, Halperin ML. *Fluid, Electrolyte, and Acid-Base Physiology; A Problem-Based Approach.* ed 5. Philadelphia: Elsevier; 2017.)

pentamidine), and serine protease inhibitors that interfere with activation of ENaC via proteolytic cleavage (nafamostat). See Chapter 17 for further discussion.

**Does the Patient Have a Disorder That Leads to Diminished Reabsorption of Sodium via ENaC in the ASDN?** One subgroup of patients may have a very low delivery of $Na^+$ to the ASDN due to marked decrease in the EABV. A second subgroup consists of patients who have lesions that lead to a diminished number of open ENaC units in the luminal membranes of principal cells in the ASDN. This includes patients who have hypoaldosteronism (e.g., adrenal insufficiency) and those with molecular defects that involve the aldosterone receptor or ENaC. Patients in this subgroup have a low EABV, higher than expected rates of excretion of $Na^+$ and $Cl^-$ in a setting of low EABV and a high $P_{Renin}$. The $P_{Aldo}$ is helpful to determine the reason for this diminished $Na^+$ reabsorption via ENaC in the ASDN.

A subset of patients with hypoaldosteronism has low $P_{Renin}$ (hyporeninemic hypoaldosteronism) and a low EABV. Their lesions may be destruction of or a biosynthetic defect in the juxtaglomerular apparatus, leading to a low $P_{Renin}$ and thereby a low $P_{Aldo}$. Patients with such disorders are expected to have a significant rise in $U_K/U_{Cr}$ with the administration of exogenous mineralocorticoids for several days.

**Does the Patient Have a Disorder That Increases Electroneutral Sodium Reabsorption in the Distal Convoluted Tubule?** In this group of patients, the site of the lesion is the DCT1, where there is increased reabsorption of $Na^+$ and $Cl^-$ via NCC, due to its activation by WNK4 or L-WNK1. Suppression of release of aldosterone by an expanded EABV leads to a diminished number of open ENaC units in the luminal membranes of principal cells in the ASDN. This, together with decreased delivery of $Na^+$ from the DCT lumen to the ASDN, and also a decreased flow rate, abrogates electrogenic $Na^+$ reabsorption and flow-induced K secretion (see Chapter 6). These kinases also cause endocytosis of ROMK from the luminal membranes of principal cells in the ASDN. Such patients tend to have an expanded EABV, hypertension, and suppressed $P_{Renin}$ and $P_{Aldo}$ (hyporeninemic hypoaldosteronism). Patients with this pathophysiology are expected to show a good response to the administration of thiazide diuretics in terms of lowering of blood pressure and correction of hyperkalemia.

The clinical picture in patients with the syndrome of familial hyperkalemia with hypertension (also known as pseudohypoaldosteronism type II or Gordon syndrome) resembles that of a gain-of-function in the thiazide-sensitive NCC. Major deletions in the gene encoding for WNK1 and missense mutations in the gene encoding for WNK4 have been reported in these patients.[25] A set of clinical findings similar to those in patients with familial hyperkalemia with hypertension may occur in other patients, most commonly those with diabetic nephropathy.[20] Support for the hypothesis that suppression of renin release in these patients is the result of EABV expansion are the findings that circulating atrial natriuretic peptide blood levels are elevated in these patients and many show response to NaCl restriction or furosemide therapy with an increased $P_{Renin}$. Another example of this pathophysiology is the hyperkalemia in patients treated with calcineurin inhibitors.[26]

**Does the Patient Have a Disorder That Increases Electroneutral Reabsorption of Sodium in the Cortical Collecting Duct?** We hypothesize that the pathophysiology of the hyperkalemia in some patients may be due to increased electroneutral $Na^+$ reabsorption in the CCD via parallel increases in the transport activity of pendrin and the NDCBE. This may be the pathophysiology for what used to be thought of as chloride shunt disorder.[27] These patients will also have an expanded EABV and suppressed $P_{Renin}$ and $P_{Aldo}$ (hyporeninemic hypoaldosteronism). Increasing the concentration of $HCO_3^-$ in the luminal fluid in the CCD my diminish flux through pendrin and thereby NDCBE. Hence we speculate that this subset of patients may be more responsive, in terms of increasing $K^+$ excretion, to the induction of bicarbonaturia by the administration of the carbonic anhydrase inhibitor acetazolamide than to the administration of thiazide diuretics. This speculation, however, needs to be examined in a clinical study.

### Step 5. Is a Low Flow Rate in the ASDN Contributing to Hyperkalemia?

Because of the process of intrarenal urea recycling, a large fraction of the osmoles delivered to the ASDN is urea osmoles. A low protein intake may decrease the amount of urea that recycles and hence the rate of flow in the ASDN. The usual rate of excretion of urea in subjects consuming a typical Western diet is about 400 mmol/day. If the rate of excretion of urea is appreciably lower than that, a low flow rate in the ASDN may be a contributing factor to the degree of hyperkalemia.

## CLINICAL CASE 9: HYPERKALEMIA IN A PATIENT TAKING TRIMETHOPRIM

*Pneumocystis jiroveci* pneumonia (PJP) developed in a 35-year-old cachectic man with human immunodeficiency virus (HIV) infection. On admission, he was febrile, there were no physical findings indicating contraction of his EABV volume, and all plasma electrolyte values were in a normal range. He was treated with cotrimoxazole (sulfamethoxazole and trimethoprim). Three days later, he was noted to have low blood pressure, his EABV was low, and his $P_K$ rose to 6.8 mmol/L. An ECG showed tall, peaked, narrow-based T waves. The urine volume was 0.8 L/day, and the $U_{osm}$ value was 350 mOsmol/kg $H_2O$; other laboratory findings were as follows.

| *Findings* | *Blood* | *Urine* |
|---|---|---|
| $K^+$, mmol/L | 6.8 | 14 |
| $Na^+$, mmol/L | 130 | 60 |
| $Cl^-$, mmol/L | 105 | 43 |
| Creatinine | 0.9 mg/dL | 0.8 g/L |
| pH | 7.30 | — |
| $P_{CO_2}$, mm Hg | 30 | — |
| $HCO_3^-$, mmol/L | 15 | 0 |
| Urea | BUN: 14 mg/dL | Urea concentration: 280 mmol/L |

### Questions and Discussion

What is the cause of hyperkalemia in this patient? The steps to follow are provided in Flow Charts 24.10 and 24.11. Although an element of pseudohyperkalemia could have been present because of repeated fist clenching during venipuncture in this cachectic patient, the ECG changes indicated that he had true hyperkalemia.

Is the time course for the development of hyperkalemia short and/or did hyperkalemia develop while the intake of $K^+$ was low? The $U_K$ was 14 mmol/L, and his rate of excretion of $K^+$ was extremely low in the presence of hyperkalemia ($U_K/U_{Cr}$ of 17.5 [mmol $K^+$/g creatinine]), so one might conclude that the major basis for the hyperkalemia is the low rate of $K^+$ excretion. This severe degree of hyperkalemia developed over a relatively short period of time, and while the patient was consuming very little $K^+$. Therefore, a shift of $K^+$ from cells rather than a large positive external balance for $K^+$ is likely the major cause of hyperkalemia. The cause of this exit of $K^+$ from cells could be inhibition of the release of insulin by the α-adrenergic effect of adrenaline released in response to the low EABV. Nevertheless, he also had a large defect in renal $K^+$ excretion. Because the EABV was low and $U_{Na}$ and $U_{Cl}$ were inappropriately high in the presence of a contracted EABV, the low $U_K/U_{Cr}$ was due to diminished reabsorption of $Na^+$ in the ASDN (see Flow Chart 24.11). The initial diagnosis was adrenal insufficiency due to an infection in a patient with HIV. However, plasma cortisol was measured and was appropriately high. In addition, there was no increase in $U_K/U_{cr}$ in response to the administration of an exogenous mineralocorticoid. It was concluded that the diminished $Na^+$ reabsorption in the ASDN was due to inhibition of ENaC by the trimethoprim that was used to treat the PJP. Both the $P_{Renin}$ and $P_{Aldo}$ were high (results became available later), as expected in this setting (see Table 24.4).

*Interpretation.* Renal salt wasting due to blockade of ENaC by trimethoprim led to the development of a contracted EABV. The major cause of hyperkalemia was a shift of $K^+$ out of cells, probably because of inhibition of insulin release by the binding of catecholamines, released in response to the low EABV, to pancreatic islet cell α-adrenergic receptors. Blockade of ENaC by trimethoprim diminished the rate of electrogenic $Na^+$ reabsorption in the ASDN and the generation of lumen-negative voltage for $K^+$ secretion. Because of the low EABV and the low intake of proteins, there was a low rate of flow in the ASDN. This, in addition to diminishing the rate of $K^+$ excretion, caused the concentration of trimethoprim to be higher in the lumen of the ASDN; hence, trimethoprim became a more effective blocker of ENaC.

What are the implications of the pathophysiology of hyperkalemia for the choice of treatment in this patient? Because of the presence of changes in the ECG related to hyperkalemia, insulin (with glucose to prevent hypoglycemia) was given to induce a shift of $K^+$ into cells. The patient was given saline to expand his EABV, which would also suppress the release of catecholamines and remove the α-adrenergic inhibition of insulin release. Because the basis of hyperkalemia in this patient is a shift of $K^+$ out of cells, inducing a large loss of $K^+$ is not needed because there is no total body $K^+$ surplus. The question arose, thereafter, as to whether trimethoprim should be discontinued. Because the drug was needed to treat the PJP, a means to remove its renal ENaC-blocking effect was sought. The concentration of trimethoprim would fall in the lumen of the ASDN if the flow rate in the ASDN were to rise through an increase in the number of osmoles delivered to this nephron segment. To achieve this aim, one could increase the delivery of NaCl to the ASDN by inhibiting the reabsorption of $Na^+$ and $Cl^-$ in the TAL of the loop of Henle using a loop diuretic, plus the infusion of enough NaCl to prevent EABV contraction. Because it is the cationic form of trimethoprim that blocks ENaC, increasing the delivery of $HCO_3^-$ to the ASDN by inhibiting its reabsorption in the PT with administration of the carbonic anhydrase IV inhibitor acetazolamide could also be considered to lower the concentration of $H^+$ in the luminal fluid in the ASDN and thereby the concentration of the cationic form of the drug. Enough $NaHCO_3$ should be given to prevent the development of metabolic acidosis.

## CLINICAL CASE 10: CHRONIC HYPERKALEMIA IN A PATIENT WITH TYPE 2 DIABETES MELLITUS

A 50-year-old man with a history of type 2 diabetes mellitus was referred for investigation of hyperkalemia; his $P_K$ ranged from 5.5 to 6 mmol/L in a number of measurements that were done over the last several weeks. He was previously taking an angiotensin-converting enzyme (ACE) inhibitor for the treatment of hypertension, this medication was discontinued but hyperkalemia persisted. He is currently taking amlodipine, 10 mg, once a day. He was noted to have microalbuminuria but no other history of macrovascular or microvascular disease related to diabetes mellitus. On physical examination, his blood pressure was 160/90 mm Hg, his jugular venous pressure was about 2 cm above the level of the sternal angle, and he had pitting edema of the ankles bilaterally. Results of laboratory investigations were as follows:

| *Parameter* | *Findings* |
|---|---|
| $P_{Na}$, mmol/L | 140 |
| $P_K$, mmol/L | 5.7 |
| $P_{Cl}$, mmol/L | 108 |
| $P_{Renin}$, ng/L | 4.50 (range, 9.30–43.4) |
| $P_{Ald}$, pmol/L | 321 (range 111–860) |
| $P_{HCO_3}$, mmol/L | 19 |
| $P_{Alb}$, g/L (mg/dL) | 40 (4.0) |
| $P_{Cr}$, µmol/L (mg/dL) | 100 (1.2) |

### Questions and Discussion

What is the cause of hyperkalemia in this patient? The first step is to rule out pseudohyperkalemia. The presence of hyperchloremic metabolic acidosis (HCMA) would suggest true hyperkalemia. Hyperkalemia is associated with an alkaline PT cell pH, which leads to the inhibition of ammoniagenesis. $K^+$ ions compete with $NH_4^+$ for transport on the $Na^+$-$K^+$-$2Cl^-$ cotransporter in the TAL of the loop of Henle, which leads to decreased medullary interstitial availability of $NH_3$. Studies have suggested that hyperkalemia is also associated with decreased expression of the ammonia transporter Rh type C glycoprotein in the collecting duct.[28]

The patient did not have advanced renal dysfunction and was not currently taking drugs that might interfere with renal excretion of $K^+$. The $P_{Renin}$ was decreased and $P_{Aldo}$ was suppressed compared with what is expected in a patient with hyperkalemia. He was then thought to have hyporeninemic hypoaldosteronism, commonly labeled as type IV renal tubular acidosis (RTA). This disorder is traditionally thought to be the result of destruction of, or a biosynthetic defect in, the juxtaglomerular apparatus (JGA), leading to low $P_{Renin}$ and thereby to low $P_{Aldo}$. If this were the pathophysiology, one would expect the patient to have renal salt wasting with a decreased EABV and the absence of hypertension. These features are not found in many patients with this disorder. Another hypothesis is that suppression of renin release in patients with this disorder is the result of EABV expansion because levels of atrial natriuretic peptide in the blood are elevated, and many cases respond to NaCl restriction or the administration of furosemide with an increased $P_{Renin}$. The basis of the disorder remains to be established. It is possible that the reabsorption of $Na^+$ and $Cl^-$ may be augmented in the DCT as in patients with familial hyperkalemia with hypertension. Of interest in regard to patients with type 2 diabetes mellitus, who may have hyperinsulinemia and the metabolic syndrome, is the finding that long-term insulin infusion in rats is associated with the retention of NaCl owing to its enhanced reabsorption in different nephron segments, including the DCT.[20] Studies in hyperinsulinemic db/db mice have suggested that the phosphatidylinositol-3-kinase (PI3K)/Akt signaling pathway activates the WNK-NCC phosphorylation cascade.[29]

Differentiation between these two groups of patients with hyporeninemic hypoaldosteronism—those with a JGA defect or destruction and those with excessive $Na^+$ and $Cl^-$ reabsorption in the DCT—has implications for therapy. The use of exogenous mineralocorticoids (e.g., 9α-fludrocortisone) is of benefit for the first group because it results in both a kaliuresis and re-expansion of the EABV. Diuretic therapy would pose a threat to these patients because it would cause a more severe degree of EABV contraction. In contrast, mineralocorticoids may aggravate the hypertension in patients with excessive reabsorption of $Na^+$ and $Cl^-$ in the DCT. In this group, the administration of thiazide diuretics to inhibit NCC should lead to both kaliuresis and lowering of the blood pressure.

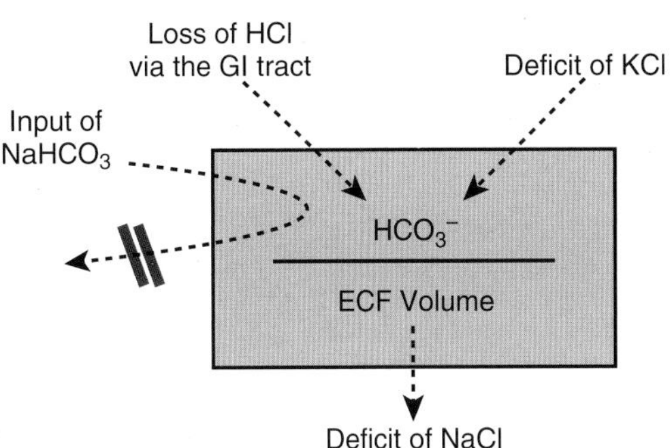


**Fig. 24.5** Basis for a high concentration of $HCO_3^-$ in the extracellular fluid *(ECF)* compartment. The *rectangle* represents the ECF compartment. The concentration of $HCO_3^-$ is the ratio of the content of $HCO_3^-$ in the ECF compartment (numerator) and the ECF volume (ECFV) (denominator). The major causes for a rise in the content of $HCO_3^-$ in the ECF compartment are a deficit of HCl and a deficit of KCl (the latter leads increased excretion of $NH_4Cl$ and diminished excretion of organic anions in the urine). The major cause for a fall in the ECFV is a deficit of NaCl. An intake of $NaHCO_3$ is not sufficient on its own to cause a sustained increase in the content of $HCO_3^-$ in the ECF compartment unless there is also reduced renal output of $NaHCO_3$ (indicated by the double red lines on the arrow on the left side of the figure) due to marked reduction in the glomerular filtration rate or there is another lesion that leads to maintaining the stimuli for the reabsorption of $NaHCO_3$ in the proximal convoluted tubule. *Double red lines* on the arrow on the left portion of the figure indicate the reduced renal output of $NaHCO_3$. *GI,* Gastrointestinal. (From Kamel KS, Halperin ML. *Fluid, Electrolyte, and Acid-Base Physiology; A Problem-Based Approach.* ed 5. Philadelphia: Elsevier; 2017.)

## METABOLIC ALKALOSIS

Metabolic alkalosis is an electrolyte disorder that is accompanied by an elevated $P_{HCO_3}$ and a high plasma pH. Most patients with metabolic alkalosis have a deficit of NaCl, KCl, and/or HCl, any of which may lead to a higher $P_{HCO_3}$.

### Concept 14

The concentration of $HCO_3^-$ in the ECF compartment (assessed by the measurement of the concentration of $HCO_3^-$ in plasma), is the ratio of the content of $HCO_3^-$ in the ECF compartment (numerator) and the ECFV (denominator), as shown in Eq. 24.5.

$$[HCO_3^-] \text{ in ECF} = \text{quantity of } HCO_3^- \text{ in ECF/ECFV} \quad (24.5)$$

A rise in the concentration of $HCO_3^-$ in the ECF compartment might be due to an increase in its numerator (positive balance of $HCO_3^-$) and/or a decrease in its denominator (low ECFV) (Fig. 24.5; see Eq. 24.5). A quantitative assessment of the ECFV is critical to estimate the quantity of $HCO_3^-$ in the ECF compartment and thereby to determine the basis of the metabolic alkalosis.

### Concept 15

Electroneutrality must be present in every body compartment and in the urine. We do not use the term $Cl^-$ depletion alkalosis because it does not provide an adequate description of the pathophysiology of metabolic alkalosis. The deficit of $Cl^-$ must be defined as being due to a deficit of HCl, KCl, and/or NaCl to determine why the $P_{HCO_3}$ level has gone up, what changes have occurred in the composition of the ECF and ICF compartments, and what is the appropriate therapy.[30] Although balance data are not available in clinical settings, with a quantitative assessment of the ECFV, tentative conclusions about the contribution of deficits of each of the different $Cl^-$-containing compounds to the development of metabolic alkalosis can be deduced (Flow Chart 24.12; see also discussion of Clinical Case 11).

### Concept 16

There is no tubular maximum for renal $HCO_3^-$ reabsorption. Central to understanding the pathophysiology of metabolic alkalosis is that contrary to the widely held view, there is no tubular maximum for the reabsorption of $HCO_3^-$. If there were a tubular maximum for the reabsorption of $HCO_3^-$, then if the filtered load of $HCO_3^-$ were to exceed this maximum, the excess $HCO_3^-$ would be spilled out in the urine. Therefore, maintaining a high concentration of $HCO_3^-$ in the ECF compartments requires a marked reduction in the GFR or a derangement in the tubular handling of $HCO_3^-$ that increases the reabsorption of $HCO_3^-$ above this tubular maximum. The vast majority of $HCO_3^-$ reabsorption occurs in the PT via $H^+$ secretion, mediated by the $Na^+/H^+$ exchanger 3 (NHE3). The usual circulating levels of angiotensin II (Ang II), the usual concentration of $H^+$ in PT cells, provide sufficient stimuli to NHE3 for the reabsorption of most of the filtered $HCO_3^-$. Experiments in which a tubular maximum for the reabsorption of $HCO_3^-$ was demonstrated were carried out with the

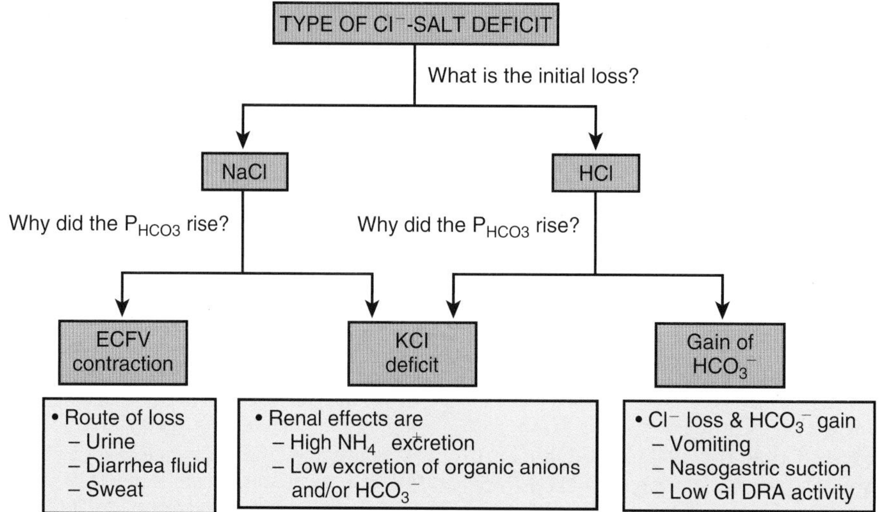


**Flow Chart 24.12** *DRA,* Downregulated in adenoma $Cl^-/HCO_3^-$ exchanger; *ECFV,* extracellular fluid volume; *GI,* gastrointestinal. (From Kamel KS, Halperin ML. *Fluid, Electrolyte, and Acid-Base Physiology; A Problem-Based Approach.* ed 5. Philadelphia: Elsevier; 2017.)

administration of a load of $NaHCO_3$. This, however, may have resulted in removal of the two stimuli for $HCO_3^-$ reabsorption in PT because the $Na^+$ load expands the EABV, causing suppression of the release of Ang II, and the administered $HCO_3^-$ load would increase the $HCO_3^-$ concentration in the peritubular capillaries in the PT, causing inhibition of the reabsorption of $HCO_3^-$. In other experimental studies, in which a large increase in $P_{HCO_3}$ was achieved without expanding the EABV, no bicarbonaturia was observed, in keeping with the notion that there is no tubular maximum for $HCO_3^-$ reabsorption.[31,32] Filtered $HCO_3^-$ ions are reabsorbed and retained in the ECF compartment as long as the abovementioned stimuli for their reabsorption are maintained.

A deficit of NaCl or HCl may cause a higher $P_{HCO_3}$ and may also lead to a secondary deficit of $K^+$ and hypokalemia. A deficit of $K^+$ may be associated with an acidified PT cell pH, which can then both initiate and sustain a high $P_{HCO_3}$ as a result of new renal $HCO_3^-$ generation (higher rate of excretion of $NH_4^+$) and enhanced reabsorption of $HCO_3^-$ and organic anions (which are metabolized to produce $HCO_3^-$) in the PT (see Flow Chart 24.12).

## TOOLS FOR ASSESSMENT OF METABOLIC ALKALOSIS

### QUANTITATIVE ESTIMATE OF THE EXTRACELLULAR FLUID VOLUME

It is critical to have a quantitative estimate of the ECFV to determine its content of $HCO_3^-$ and thereby why the $P_{HCO_3}$ rose. As discussed earlier in this chapter, we use the hematocrit for this purpose, provided that anemia or polycythemia are not present (see Table 24.2).

### BALANCE DATA FOR SODIUM, POTASSIUM, AND CHLORIDE

Balance data for $Na^+$, $K^+$, and $Cl^-$ are rarely available in clinical medicine. Nevertheless, they can be deduced if one has a quantitative estimate of the ECFV and measurements of the $P_{Na}$, $P_{Cl}$, and $P_{HCO_3}$. One cannot know the balances for $K^+$ from these calculations, but its rough magnitude can be deduced by comparing the differences in the content of $Na^+$ versus that of $Cl^-$ and $HCO_3^-$ in the ECF compartment (see Clinical Case 11).

### CLINICAL APPROACH TO THE PATIENT WITH METABOLIC AKALOSIS

Our clinical approach to a patient with metabolic alkalosis is outlined in Flow Chart 24.13. The first step is to rule out the common causes of metabolic alkalosis—namely, vomiting and the use of diuretics. Some patients may deny vomiting or the use of diuretics; measuring urine electrolyte levels may provide helpful clues if one of these diagnoses is suspected (see Table 24.3).

A very useful initial test to detect the cause of metabolic alkalosis is to examine the $U_{Cl}$. A very low $U_{Cl}$ (<20 mmol/L) is expected when there is a deficit of HCl and/or NaCl. The $U_{Cl}$ may not be low if there is recent intake of diuretics (see Table 24.3). If the $U_{Cl}$ is not low, assessment of the EABV and blood pressure helps identify patients with disorders of primary high ENaC activity in the ASDN (see Flow Chart 24.9; the EABV is not low, hypertension is present) and distinguish them from patients with recent use of diuretics and those with Bartter syndrome or Gitelman syndrome (EABV is low, absence of hypertension). Measurements of $U_{Cl}$ in multiple spot urine samples are helpful to separate patients with Bartter or Gitelman syndrome (persistent high $U_{Cl}$) from those with diuretic abuse ($U_{Cl}$ is high only while the diuretic is acting).

### CLINICAL CASE 11: METABOLIC ALKALOSIS WITHOUT VOMITING OR USE OF DIURETICS

After a forced 6-hour intense training exercise in the desert in the heat of the day, an elite corps soldier was the only one in his squad who collapsed. He perspired profusely during the training exercise and drank a large volume of water and sugar-containing fluids. He denied vomiting or the intake of any medications. Physical examination revealed a markedly contracted EABV. Initial laboratory data are shown in the

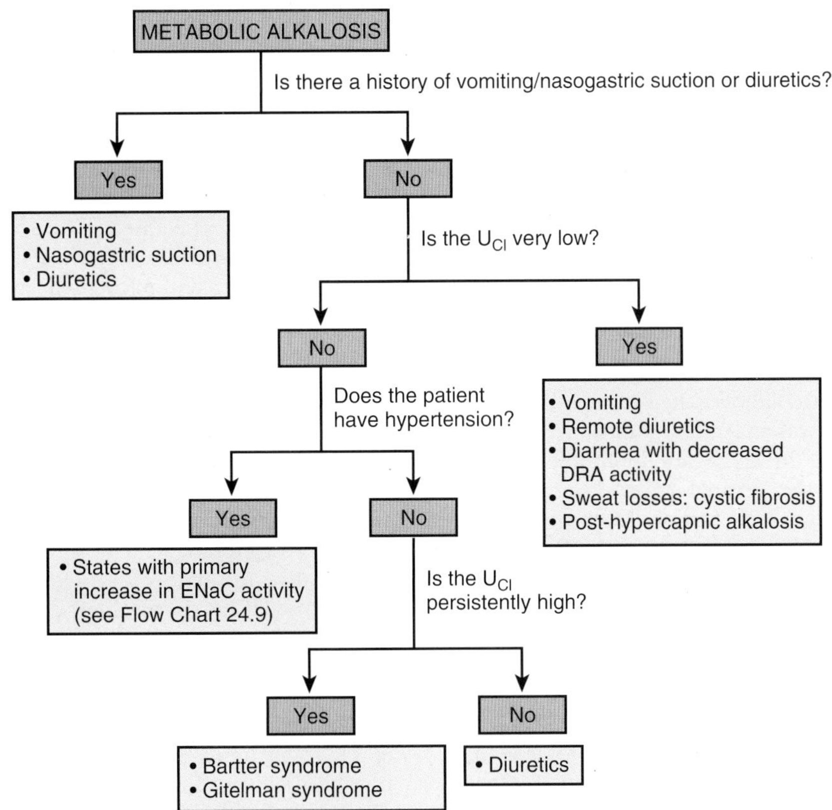


**Flow Chart 24.13** *DRA,* Downregulated in adenoma $Cl^-/HCO_3^-$ exchanger; *ENaC,* epithelial sodium channel. (From Kamel KS, Halperin ML. *Fluid, Electrolyte, and Acid-Base Physiology; A Problem-Based Approach.* ed 5. Philadelphia: Elsevier; 2017.)

table. The pH and $P_{CO_2}$ values are from an arterial blood sample; all other findings are from a venous blood sample.

| *Parameter* | *Findings* |
|---|---|
| $P_{Na}$, mmol/L | 125 |
| $P_K$, mmol/L | 2.7 |
| $P_{Cl}$, mmol/L | 70 |
| Hematocrit | 0.50 |
| pH | 7.50 |
| $P_{HCO_3}$, mmol/L | 38 |
| $P_{CO_2}$, mm Hg | 47 |

## Questions and Discussion

What are the major threats to the patient, and how should they dictate therapy?

*Acute hyponatremia.* The danger is brain herniation due to increased intracranial pressure from swelling of brain cells.

Basis of hyponatremia. The patient weighed 80 kg and had a muscular build, so his initial total body water (TBW) was about 50 L (ECFV ≈ 15 L; ICF volume ≈ 35 L). Because he had hyponatremia, his ICF volume was expanded because of a water gain. The percentage expansion of ICF volume is close to the percentage fall in $P_{Na}$ (i.e., ≈ 11%). Hence, he had a water gain in his ICF compartment of about 4 L. With a hematocrit of 0.50, his ECFV was decreased by one-third from its normal value of about 15 L to about 10 L; accordingly, he lost 5 L of ECFV. This represents the loss of 5 L of water and 700 mmol of $Na^+$ (5 L × $P_{Na}$ 140 mmol/L). In addition, as the $P_{Na}$ decreased from 140 to 125 mmol/L, each of the remaining 10 L of ECVF had a loss of 15 mmol of $Na^+$. Hence, his total $Na^+$ loss was 850 mmol. In total body balance terms, he had a loss of 850 mmol of $Na^+$ and 1 L of water—a loss of 5 L of water from the ECF compartment and a gain of 4 L of water in the ICF compartment. Therefore, the primary basis of his hyponatremia was $Na^+$ loss.

*Hemodynamic instability.* An infusion of isotonic saline was started in the field, and the patient was hemodynamically stable on arrival at the emergency department. After it was recognized that his $P_{Na}$ was 125 mmol/L, intravenous therapy was changed from isotonic saline to 3% hypertonic saline. The goal of therapy was to raise the $P_{Na}$ to 130 mmol/L. Because the hyponatremia was acute, there was little if any risk of osmotic demyelination from rapidly raising the $P_{Na}$ to 130 mmol/L.

*Hypokalemia.* The hypokalemia did not represent an emergency because he did not have a cardiac arrhythmia or respiratory muscle weakness. An intravenous infusion of isotonic saline supplemented with 40 mmol/L of KCl was started. The $P_K$ was followed closely.

What is the basis for metabolic alkalosis? To distinguish between HCl, KCl, and NaCl deficits, a quantitative analysis of the degree of contraction of the ECFV is needed. As mentioned previously, with a hematocrit of 0.50, this patient's

ECFV was decreased by one-third, from its normal value of 15 L to about 10 L, so he had lost 5 L of ECFV.

*Deficit of HCl.* There was no history of vomiting, so an HCl deficit is a very unlikely basis for the metabolic alkalosis.

*Deficit of NaCl.* The decrease in his ECFV was about 5 L. One can now calculate how much this degree of ECFV contraction would raise the $P_{HCO_3}$ (divide the normal content of $HCO_3^-$ in the ECF compartment (15 L × 25 mmol/L, or 375 mmol) by the new ECFV (10 L), and the result is 37.5 mmol/L. This value is remarkably close to the measured $P_{HCO_3}$, 38 mmol/L, suggesting that the major reason for the rise in the $P_{HCO_3}$ is the fall in his ECFV.

$Na^+$ deficit. As calculated above, the deficit of $Na^+$ in the ECF compartment was about 850 mmol.

$Cl^-$ deficit. Multiplying the $P_{Cl}$ before the training exercise (103 mmol/L) by the normal ECFV (15 L) yields a $Cl^-$ content of about 1545 mmol. After the training exercise, the $P_{Cl}$ was 70 mmol/L, and the ECF volume was 10 L, so the ECF $Cl^-$ content was 700 mmol. Accordingly, the deficit of $Cl^-$ was about 840 mmol, a value close to the deficit of $Na^+$.

*Deficit of KCl.* There was little difference between the deficits of $Na^+$ and $Cl^-$, so there was no appreciable deficit of KCl to account for a drop in the $P_K$ to 2.7 mmol/L. Especially in this muscular elite soldier, the loss of $K^+$ would have to be very large to account for this degree of hypokalemia. Accordingly, the major mechanism for the hypokalemia is likely to be a shift of $K^+$ into cells due to a $\beta_2$-adrenergic surge and possibly the alkalemia.

Routes for NaCl loss. The next issue is to examine possible routes for a large loss of NaCl in such a short time. Because diarrhea and polyuria were not present, the only route for a large NaCl loss was via sweat. To have a high electrolyte concentration in sweat and a large sweat volume, the likely underlying lesion would be cystic fibrosis. The diagnosis of cystic fibrosis was confirmed later by molecular studies.

What is the therapy for metabolic alkalosis in this patient? Because the basis for the metabolic alkalosis was largely an acute deficit of NaCl, the patient required a positive balance of about 850 mmol of NaCl to replace the deficit. He was initially given hypertonic saline to raise his $P_{Na}$ to 130 mmol/L. If all of this deficit of NaCl were replaced with 3% hypertonic saline, which would also give him about 1.5 L of $H_2O$, his new total body $Na^+$ will be around 6975 mmol (initial TBW 49 L × initial $P_{Na}$ 125 mmol/L = 6975 mmol; to that add 850 mmol = 7825 mmol), his new TBW will be around 50.5 L, and the $P_{Na}$ would rise to about 138 mmol/L. He might, however, still have a large volume of water in the GI tract that could be absorbed later and cause the $P_{Na}$ to drop. Hence, the $P_{Na}$ should be followed closely. After the administration of only 40 mmol of KCl, the patient's $P_K$ rose to 3.8 mmol/L, adding support to our conclusion that the major cause of the hypokalemia was an acute shift of $K^+$ into cells.

## METABOLIC ACIDOSIS

Metabolic acidosis is a process that causes a drop in the $P_{HCO_3}$ and a rise in the concentration of $H^+$ in plasma. Metabolic acidosis represents a diagnostic category with many different causes (see Chapter 16). The risks for the patient depend on the underlying disorder that caused the metabolic acidosis, the ill effects of the binding of $H^+$ to intracellular proteins in vital organs (e.g., the brain and the heart), and possible dangers associated with the anions that accompanied the $H^+$ load (e.g., chelation of ionized calcium by citrate in a patient with metabolic acidosis due to ingestion of citric acid).[33]

As previously articulated in Concept 14, the concentration of $HCO_3^-$ in the ECF compartment is equal to the ratio of the content of $HCO_3^-$ in the ECF compartment to the ECFV. It is important to distinguish between acidemia and acidosis. The term acidemia simply describes an elevation in the concentration of $H^+$ in plasma. Acidemia may not be present in a patient who has metabolic acidosis if there is, for example, a large decrease in the ECFV, which may sufficiently raise the $P_{HCO_3}$, even though there is a decreased content of $HCO_3^-$ in the ECF compartment (e.g., in the patient with severe diarrhea[34] and in some patients with DKA). For a diagnosis of metabolic acidosis to be made in this setting, a quantitative estimate of the ECFV is needed to assess its content of $HCO_3^-$ in the ECF compartment.

**Concept 17**

$H^+$ ions must be removed by the bicarbonate buffer system (BBS) to avoid their binding to intracellular proteins. Binding of $H^+$ to proteins could change their charge, shape, and possibly their functions. The bulk of BBS is in the ICF compartment and the interstitial spaces of skeletal muscles.[35]

### TOOLS FOR ASSESSMENT OF METABOLIC ACIDOSIS

The tools for assessing metabolic acidosis are listed in Table 24.5.

#### QUANTITATIVE ASSESSMENT OF THE EXTRACELLULAR FLUID VOLUME

As discussed earlier in this chapter, we use the hematocrit to obtain a quantitative assessment of the ECFV, provided that anemia or polycythemia were not present (see Table 24.2).

#### Tools to Assess the Removal of Hydrogen by the Bicarbonate Buffer System

As shown in Eq. 24.6, the BBS is driven by pull—that is, by a lower $P_{CO_2}$. Effective buffering of $H^+$ by the BBS requires a low $P_{CO_2}$ primarily in the interstitial space and ICF of skeletal muscles.

$$H^+ + HCO_3^- \leftrightarrow H_2CO_3 + CO_2 \quad (24.6)$$

Acidemia stimulates the respiratory center, leading to a fall in arterial $P_{CO_2}$. Although the arterial $P_{CO_2}$ sets the lower limit on the $P_{CO_2}$ in capillaries, it does not guarantee that the capillary $P_{CO_2}$ in skeletal muscles will be low enough to ensure effective buffering of $H^+$ by the BBS. Because the free-flowing brachial venous $P_{CO_2}$ reflects the $P_{CO_2}$ in capillary blood of skeletal muscles in its drainage pool, it should provide a means of assessing the effectiveness of the BBS in patients with metabolic acidosis. The capillary $P_{CO_2}$ in skeletal muscles will be higher if the rate of blood flow to muscles is low—for example, as a result of a decreased EABV. If muscle oxygen consumption in this setting remains unchanged, more oxygen

**Table 24.5 Laboratory Tests for Diagnosis of Metabolic Acidosis**

| Question | Parameter(s) Assessed | Tool(s) to Use |
|---|---|---|
| Is the total amount of $HCO_3^-$ in the ECF compartment low? | ECFV | Hematocrit or total plasma proteins |
| Is metabolic acidosis due to overproduction of organic acids? | Appearance of new anions in the body or the urine | Plasma anion gap<br>Urine anion gap |
| Is metabolic acidosis due to ingestion of alcohol? | Presence of alcohols as unmeasured osmoles | Plasma osmolal gap |
| Is effective bicarbonate buffering in skeletal muscle available? | Adequacy of tissue perfusion and $CO_2$ clearance from muscle, enabling buffering of $H^+$ by $HCO_3^-$ in interstitial fluid and intracellular fluid compartments | Brachial venous $PCO_2$ |
| Is the renal response to chronic acidemia adequate? | Examine the rate of excretion of $NH_4^+$ | Urine osmolal gap |
| If $NH_4^+$ excretion is high, which anion is excreted with $NH_4^+$? | Gastrointestinal loss of $NaHCO_3$<br>Acid added, but the anion is excreted in the urine | Urine $Cl^-$<br>Urine anion gap |
| What is the basis for a low excretion of $NH_4^+$? | Low distal $H^+$ secretion<br>Low $NH_3$ availability<br>Both defects | Urine pH >7.0<br>Urine pH ≈ 5.0<br>Urine pH ≈ 6.0 |
| Where is the defect in $H^+$ secretion? | Distal $H^+$ secretion<br>Proximal $H^+$ secretion | $PCO_2$ in alkaline urine<br>Fractional excretion of $HCO_3$, urine citrate excretion |

*ECF,* Extracellular fluid; *ECFV,* extracellular fluid volume.
From Kamel KS, Halperin ML. Fluid, electrolytes and acid-base physiology. A problem-based approach, ed 5. Philadelphia: Elsevier; 2017.

will be extracted from, and more $CO_2$ will be added to, each liter of blood. The higher $PCO_2$ in muscle capillaries will diminish the effectiveness of the BBS to remove extra $H^+$. Hence, the circulating $H^+$ concentration rises, and a larger burden of $H^+$ will be titrated by intracellular proteins in muscle, as well as by other organs, including the brain. Notwithstanding this, because of autoregulation of cerebral blood flow, it is likely that the $PCO_2$ in brain capillary blood will change minimally unless there is a severe degree of contraction of the EABV and failure of autoregulation of cerebral blood flow. Hence, the BBS in the brain will continue to titrate much of this large $H^+$ load. Considering, however, the limited amount of $HCO_3^-$ in the brain, and that the brain receives a relatively larger proportion of the cardiac output (and of the $H^+$ load), there is a risk of more $H^+$ binding to intracellular proteins in the brain, further compromising their function (Fig. 24.6).[36] At usual rates of blood flow and metabolic work at rest, the brachial venous $PCO_2$ is about 6 mm Hg greater than arterial $PCO_2$. If the blood flow rate to muscles is low, their venous $PCO_2$ will be more than 6 mm Hg greater than the arterial $PCO_2$. Enough saline should be administered to increase this blood flow rate to muscle to achieve a brachial venous $PCO_2$ that is no more than 6 mm Hg higher than the arterial $PCO_2$.

## CLINICAL APPROACH: INITIAL STEPS

The initial steps in the clinical approach to a patient with metabolic acidosis are summarized in Flow Chart 24.14.

1. Identify threats for that patient and anticipate and prevent dangers that may arise during therapy.
2. Determine if effective buffering of $H^+$ by the BBS in skeletal muscles is available.

## METABOLIC ACIDOSIS DUE TO ADDED ACIDS

### Concept 18

Addition of acids can by detected by the appearance of new anions. These new anions may remain in the body or may be excreted (e.g., in the urine or diarrhea fluid).

### TOOLS FOR ASSESSING METABOLIC ACIDOSIS DUE TO ADDED ACIDS

Tools for assessment of metabolic acidosis due to added acids are summarized in Table 24.5.

#### Detect New Anions in Plasma

The accumulation of new anions in plasma can be detected from a calculation of the plasma anion gap ($P_{anion\ gap}$).[37,38] The major cation in plasma is $Na^+$, and the major anions are $Cl^-$ and $HCO_3^-$. The difference between $P_{Na}$ and ($P_{Cl}$ + $PHCO_3$) reflects the other negative charges in plasma, which are predominantly due to the negative charge on albumin. Although it is commonly said that the normal value of the $P_{anion\ gap}$ is 12 ± 2 mEq/L, the mean value of a normal $P_{anion\ gap}$ varies greatly among clinical laboratories because of different laboratory methods, and the range of normal values is wide. When using the calculation of the $P_{anion\ gap}$ to detect the presence of new anions in plasma, one must adjust the baseline value of the $P_{anion\ gap}$ for the $P_{Alb}$. As a rough estimate, the baseline value for the $P_{anion\ gap}$ falls (or rises) by 2.5 mEq/L for every 10-g/L or 1-g/dL fall (or rise) in the $P_{Alb}$.[39] Even with this adjustment, it seems that net negative valence on albumin is increased if there is an appreciable decrease in the EABV.[40]

Stewart has recommended another approach to detect new anions in plasma, the strong ion difference (SID).[41] This

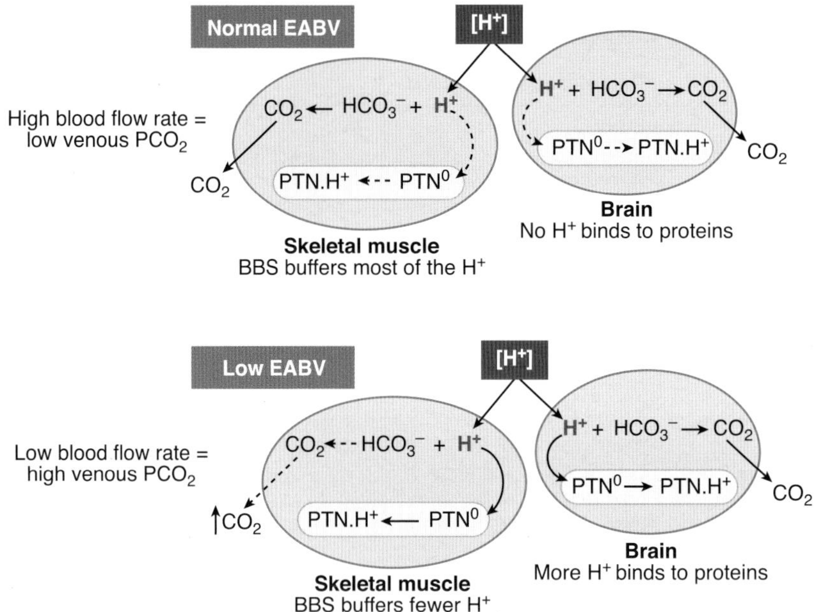


**Fig. 24.6** Buffering of $H^+$ in the brain in a patient with metabolic acidemia and a contracted effective arterial blood volume (EABV). *Top,* Buffering of $H^+$ in a patient with a normal EABV and thereby a low muscle venous $P_{CO_2}$. The vast majority of $H^+$ removal occurs by the bicarbonate buffer system (BBS) in the interstitial space and in cells of skeletal muscles. *Bottom,* Buffering of an $H^+$ load in a patient with a contracted EABV and thereby a high muscle venous $P_{CO_2}$ values. A high muscle venous $P_{CO_2}$ prevents $H^+$ removal by muscle BBS. As a result, the degree of acidemia may become more pronounced, and more $H^+$ may bind to proteins (PTN·$H^+$) in other organs, including the brain. (From Kamel KS, Halperin ML. *Fluid, Electrolyte, and Acid-Base Physiology; A Problem-Based Approach.* ed 5. Philadelphia: Elsevier; 2017.)

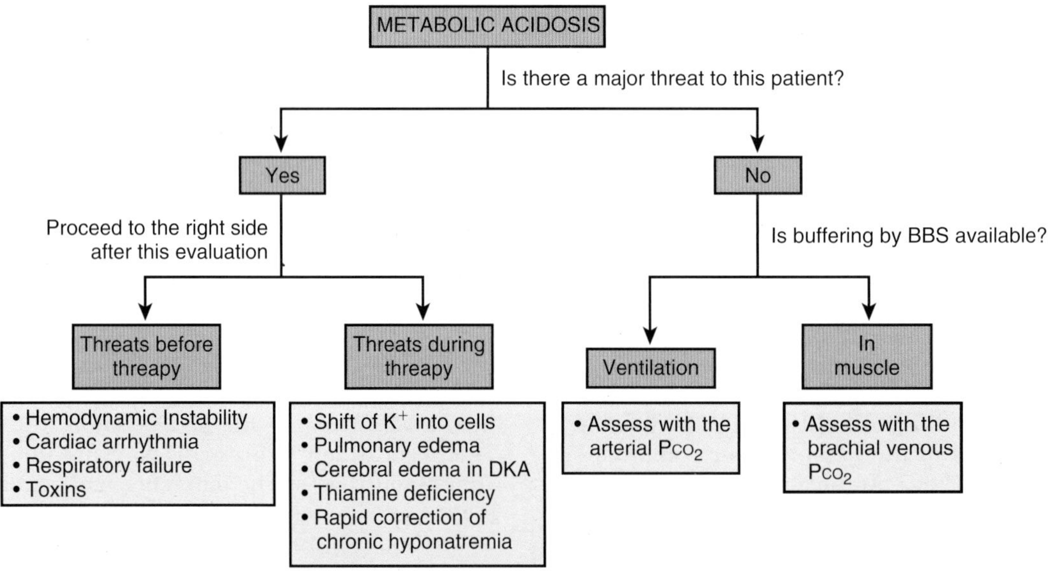


**Flow Chart 24.14** *BBS,* Bicarbonate buffer system; *DKA,* diabetic ketoacidosis. (From Kamel KS, Halperin ML. *Fluid, Electrolyte, and Acid-Base Physiology; A Problem-Based Approach.* ed 5. Philadelphia: Elsevier; 2017.)

approach is rather complex and offers only a minor advantage over the $P_{anion\ gap}$ in that it includes a correction for the net negative charge on $P_{Alb}$.[42]

**Use of the Delta Plasma Anion Gap/Delta Plasma $HCO_3^-$.** The relationship between the rise in the $P_{anion\ gap}$ and the fall in the $P_{HCO_3}$ (or the delta $P_{anion\ gap}$/delta $P_{HCO_3}$) is used to detect the presence of coexisting metabolic alkalosis (the rise in $P_{anion\ gap}$ is larger than the fall in $P_{HCO_3}$) or the presence of both an "acid overproduction" type and an "$NaHCO_3$ loss" type of metabolic acidosis (the rise in the $P_{anion\ gap}$ is smaller than the fall in the $P_{HCO_3}$).

There are several pitfalls in using this relationship. One is failure to adjust for changes in the ECFV.[43] Consider, for example, a patient with DKA who has a fall in $P_{HCO_3}$ by 15 mmol/L, from 25 to 10 mmol/L, and the "expected" 1:1 ratio of a rise in $P_{anion\ gap}$ from a normal value of 12 mEq/L to 27 mEq/L. The patient had a normal ECFV of 10 L before

DKA developed but, as a result of the glucose-induced osmotic diuresis and natriuresis, the current ECFV is only 8 L. Although the fall in the $P_{HCO_3}$ and the rise in the concentration of ketoacid anions (as judged from the rise in the $P_{anion\ gap}$) are equal, the deficit of $HCO_3^-$ and the amount of ketoacids added to the ECF compartment are not. The sum of the content of $HCO_3^-$ and ketoacid anions in the ECF compartment prior to the development of DKA is 250 mmol ([25 + 0 mmol/L] × 10 L). Their sum in the ECF compartment after DKA developed, however, is only 200 mmol ([10 + 15] mmol/L × 8 L). The deficit of $HCO_3^-$ in this example is 170 mmol, but the quantity of new anions in the ECF is only 120 mmol. This is because there is another component of the loss of $HCO_3^-$ that occurred when ketoacids were added that is not detected by an increase in the $P_{anion\ gap}$. Some of the ketoacid anions were excreted in the urine with $Na^+$ and/or $K^+$, an indirect form of $NaHCO_3$ loss. Hence the rise in the $P_{anion\ gap}$ underestimated the actual quantity of net production of ketoacids, and the fall in $P_{HCO3}$ underestimated the actual magnitude of the deficit of $HCO_3^-$. When the ECFV is re-expanded with saline, the degree of deficit of $HCO_3^-$ will become evident. In addition, the fall in the $P_{anion\ gap}$ will not be matched by a rise in the $P_{HCO_3}$ because some ketoacid anions will be lost in urine when their filtered load is increased with the rise in GFR.

Another pitfall in the use of the delta $P_{anion\ gap}$/delta $P_{HCO_3}$ is the failure to correct for the net negative valence attributable to $P_{Alb}$. When calculating the $P_{anion\ gap}$, one must adjust the base value for changes in the charge on the most abundant unmeasured anion in plasma, which is albumin. We emphasize that adjustments should be made for a decrease or an increase in $P_{Alb}$.

### Detect New Anions in the Urine

New anions can be detected with the calculation of the urine anion gap ($U_{anion\ gap}$; Eq. 24.7).

$$U_{anion\ gap} = (U_{Na} + U_K + U_{NH4}) - U_{Cl} \quad (24.7)$$

The concentration of $NH_4^+$ in the urine ($U_{NH4}$) is estimated from the urine osmolal gap ($U_{osm\ gap}$), as discussed in the next section. The nature of these new anions may sometimes be deduced by comparing their filtered load with their excretion rate. For example, when there is a very large quantity of the new anion in the urine in comparison with the rise in $P_{anion\ gap}$, one should suspect that this anion is secreted in the PT (e.g., hippurate anion from the metabolism of toluene) or is freely filtered and poorly reabsorbed by the PT (e.g., reabsorption of ketoacid anions may be inhibited by salicylate anions, D-lactate anions). On the other hand, a very low rate of excretion of new anions suggests that they are avidly reabsorbed in the PT (e.g., L-lactate anions).

### Detect Toxic Alcohols

The presence of alcohols in plasma can be detected by calculating the plasma osmolal gap ($P_{osm\ gap}$; Eq. 24.8). This occurs because alcohols are uncharged compounds, have a low molecular weight, and usually large quantities are ingested.

$$P_{osm\ gap} = \text{measured } P_{osm} - (2 \times P_{Na} + P_{Glu} + P_{Urea}) \quad (24.8)$$

In Eq. 24.8, all terms are in mmol/L. If $P_{Glu}$ is in mg/dL, divide by 180, and if $P_{Urea}$ is expressed as mg/dL of urea nitrogen, divide by 2.8 to obtain units in mmol/L.

## CLINICAL APPROACH TO THE PATIENT WITH METABOLIC ACIDOSIS DUE TO ADDED ACIDS

The steps in the clinical approach to the patient with metabolic acidosis due to added acids are shown in Flow Chart 24.15. If metabolic acidosis develops over a short period, the likely causes are overproduction of L-lactic acid (e.g., hypoxic L-lactic acidosis, ingestion of alcohol in a patient with thiamine deficiency) or ingestion of acids (e.g., metabolic acidosis due to ingestion of citric acid). Measurement of plasma levels of L-lactate and β-hydroxybutyrate confirms the diagnosis of L-lactic acidosis or ketoacidosis respectively. If suspected, measurements of blood levels levels of methanol, ethylene glycol, acetaminophen or acetylsalicylic acid should be obtained. Acetaminophen overdose may be associated with L-lactic acidosis or pyroglutamic acidosis. A detailed discussion of the various causes of metabolic acidosis due to added acids is provided in Chapter 16.

## CLINICAL CASE 12: SEVERE METABOLIC ACIDOSIS IN A PATIENT WITH CHRONIC ALCOHOLISM

A 52-year-old man presented to the emergency department with abdominal pain, visual disturbances, and shortness of breath.[44] He had a history of drinking excessive amounts of alcohol on a regular basis. He admitted to drinking approximately 1 L of vodka the day before hospital admission but denied ingesting any other substances. During the 24 hours before admission, he had not eaten at all. In the 5 hours before his admission, he had had several bouts of vomiting and did not drink any alcohol. His dietary intake had been generally very poor over the last several months because he had diminished appetite.

On physical examination, he was fully conscious and oriented. His respiration rate was rapid (40 breaths/min). His pulse rate was also rapid (150 beats/min), and his blood pressure was 120/58 mm Hg. Neurologic examination was unremarkable.

The patient's urine tested strongly positive for ketones. His initial laboratory results on admission to the emergency department are shown in the following table. The pH and $P_{CO_2}$ are from an arterial blood sample, whereas all other findings are from a venous blood sample.

| *Parameter* | *Findings* |
|---|---|
| $P_{Na}$, mmol/L | 132 |
| $P_K$, mmol/L | 5.4 |
| $P_{Cl}$, mmol/L | 85 |
| $P_{HCO3}$, mmol/L | 3.3 |
| $P_{anion\ gap}$ mEq/L | 44 |
| $P_{osm}$, mOsmol/kg $H_2O$ | 325 |
| Hematocrit | 0.46 |
| pH | 6.78 |
| $P_{CO_2}$, mm Hg | 23 |
| $P_{Glu}$, mmol/L | 3.0 |
| $P_{Alb}$, g/L | 36 |
| $P_{osm\ gap}$, mOsmol/kg $H_2O$ | 42 |

### Questions and Discussion

What dangers may be present on admission or may arise during therapy?

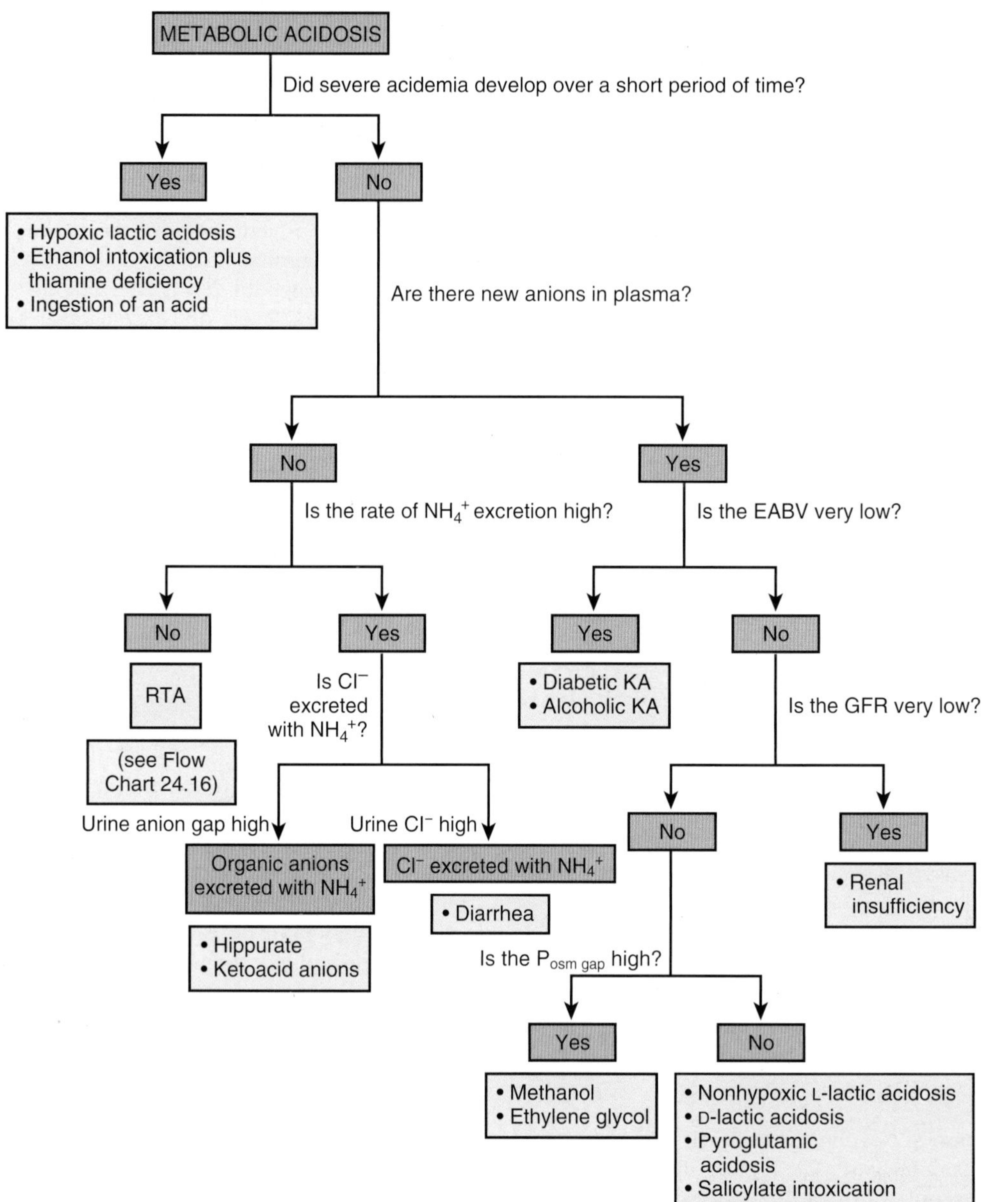


**Flow Chart 24.15** *RTA,* Renal tubular acidosis; *KA,* ketoacidosis; *GFR,* glomerular filtration rate; *Posm gap,* plasma osmolal gap. (From Kamel KS, Halperin ML. Fluid, electrolytes, and acid-base physiology. A problem based approach, ed 5. Philadelphia: Elsevier, 2017.)

*Severe acidemia.* The patient had a severe degree of acidemia with a large increase in the $P_{anion\ gap}$, indicating overproduction of acids. For the time being, he is hemodynamically stable, but a quantitatively small additional $H^+$ load would produce a disproportionately large fall in the $P_{HCO_3}$ and plasma pH. For example, halving the $P_{HCO_3}$ would cause the arterial pH to drop by 0.30 unit if the arterial $P_{CO_2}$ has not changed. By the same token, doubling of the $P_{HCO_3}$ would raise the plasma pH by 0.30 unit. A large dose of $NaHCO_3$ would be needed to achieve this because the administered $NaHCO_3$ might lead to back titration of some of the large $H^+$ load that is bound to the patient's intracellular proteins and, in addition, he might still have ongoing production of acids.

*Toxic alcohol ingestion.* Because the patient had a severe degree of metabolic acidemia with a large $P_{osm\ gap}$, ingestion of methanol or ethylene glycol was suspected. Aldehydes produced from the metabolism of these alcohols by the enzyme alcohol dehydrogenase in the liver are the major cause of toxicity because they rapidly bind to tissue proteins. Although the patient ingested a large amount of ethanol, which could have caused the large $P_{osm\ gap}$, and his urine was strongly positive for ketones, such a severe degree of acidemia is not usual in patients with alcoholic ketoacidosis. Because of the strong clinical suspicion of toxic alcohol ingestion, the patient was started on fomepizole (an inhibitor of alcohol dehydrogenase) while waiting for the determination of the level of these toxic alcohols in his blood.

*Thiamine deficiency.* Malnourished patients who present with alcoholic ketoacidosis are at risk for the development of encephalopathy due to thiamine deficiency. Ketoacids, when available, are the preferred brain fuel because they are derived from storage fat and, hence, proteins from lean body mass are spared as a source of glucose for the brain during prolonged starvation. After successful treatment of alcoholic ketoacidosis, ketoacids are no longer available as a brain fuel, so the brain must regenerate most of its ATP from the oxidation of glucose. Thiamine (vitamin $B_1$) is a key cofactor for pyruvate dehydrogenase (PDH). The activity of PDH is diminished by the lack of thiamine, so the rate of regeneration of ATP in brain cells will not be sufficient for their biologic work. Therefore, glycolysis will be stimulated in the brain to make ATP. As a result, there will be a sudden rise in the production of $H^+$ and L-lactate anions in areas of the brain where the metabolic rate is the most rapid and/or areas that have the lowest reserve of thiamine. Thiamine must be administered early in therapy in such patients.

More information. Two hours after presentation, additional laboratory results became available. The patient's plasma L-lactate level was 23 mmol/L, and the assays for methanol and ethylene glycol were negative.

What is the cause of the severe degree of L-lactic acidosis in this patient? A rise in the concentration of L-lactate anions and $H^+$ can be caused by an increased rate of production and/or a decreased rate of removal of L-lactic acid. The rapid development and severity of L-lactic acidosis in this patient suggest that the L-lactic acidosis is largely due to overproduction of L-lactic acid.

The degree of L-lactic acidosis in patients presenting with alcohol intoxication is usually mild (plasma L-lactate level is usually <5 mmol/L) because it is due to the increased nicotinamide adenine dinucleotide, reduced form ($NADH.H^+$)/nicotinamide adenine dinucleotide ($NAD^+$) ratio owing to the ongoing production of $NADH.H^+$ through ethanol metabolism, which is largely restricted to the liver where the enzymes alcohol dehydrogenase and aldehyde dehydrogenase are expressed. Other organs in the body are capable of oxidizing the L-lactate produced by the liver and, hence, the degree of L-lactic acidosis is usually mild.

$$\text{Pyruvate}^- + \text{NADH.H}^+ \leftrightarrow \text{L-lactate}^- + \text{NAD}^+ \quad (24.9)$$

However, a severe degree of L-lactic acidosis may develop rapidly if there is a large intake of alcohol in a patient who is thiamine-deficient. The site of L-lactic acid production is likely to be the liver because there will be both accumulation of pyruvate (owing to diminished activity of PDH) and a high $NADH.H^+/NAD^+$ ratio (due to metabolism of ethanol). There is also diminished removal of L-lactic acid by other organs due to diminished activity of PDH.

## HYPERCHLOREMIC METABOLIC ACIDOSIS

Hyperchloremic metabolic acidosis is characterized by the absence of a rise in the $P_{\text{anion gap}}$; hence, it is often also called non–anion gap metabolic acidosis. There are two major groups of causes for this type of metabolic acidosis, the direct loss of $NaHCO_3$ and the indirect loss of $NaHCO_3$. The direct loss of $NaHCO_3$ may occur via the GI tract—for example, in patients with diarrhea or through the urine in patients at the early phase of a disease process that causes proximal renal tubular acidosis (pRTA). The indirect loss of $NaHCO_3$ may be due to a low rate of excretion of $NH_4^+$ that is insufficient to match the daily rate of production of sulfuric acid from the metabolism of sulfur-containing amino acids (e.g., in patients with chronic renal failure or patients with distal renal tubular acidosis [dRTA], or patients with pRTA in the steady state). Indirect loss of $NaHCO_3$ may also be due to an overproduction of an acid (e.g., hippuric acid formed during the metabolism of toluene, ketoacids), with the excretion of its conjugate base (e.g., hippurate anions, ketoacids anions) in the urine at a rate that exceeds the rate of excretion of $NH_4^+$.

### Concept 19

The expected renal response to chronic metabolic acidosis is a high rate of excretion of $NH_4^+$. Based on findings in normal subjects given an acid load of ammonium chloride for several days, the expected normal renal response in a patient with chronic metabolic acidosis, is the excretion of close to 200 mmol of $NH_4^+$/day.[45] There is a lag period of a few days, however, before high rates of excretion of $NH_4^+$ can be achieved. Patients with a hyperchloremic metabolic acidosis that have an appropriately high rate of $NH_4^+$ excretion generally have diarrhea or an added organic acid the anion of which is excreted in the urine at a rapid rate. These two disorders can be differentiated by assessing the urine anion gap and urine chloride concentration (see Flow Chart 24.15).

### Concept 20

A low rate of excretion of $NH_4^+$ in a patient with hyperchloremic metabolic acidosis could be due to a decreased medullary interstitial availability of $NH_3$ or a decreased net $H^+$ secretion in the distal nephron.[46]

A low rate of ammoniagenesis has several possible causes. One is intracellular alkalinization of PT cells due to hyperkalemia or a genetic or an acquired disorder that compromises proximal $H^+$ secretion or $HCO_3^-$ exit from PT cells (also causing a reduced capacity to reabsorb $HCO_3^-$ [i.e., pRTA]). The other involves a reduction in the GFR, which diminishes the filtered load of $Na^+$ because less work is performed in PT cells; thus, the availability of ADP is decreased and the rate of oxidation of glutamine in PT cells is reduced.

The other main cause of a low rate of excretion of $NH_4^+$ is a low net secretion of $H^+$ in the distal nephron. This could be due to an $H^+$-ATPase defect (e.g., autoimmune and hypergammaglobulinemic disorders, including Sjögren syndrome), backleak of $H^+$ (e.g., due to drugs such as amphotericin B), or a disorder associated with the distal secretion of $HCO_3^-$ (e.g., in some patients with Southeast Asian ovalocytosis [SAO]). Patients with medullary interstitial disease (e.g., due to infections, drugs, infiltrations, precipitations, inflammatory disorders, sickle cell disease) may have a low rate of excretion of $NH_4^+$ because of both diminished accumulation of $NH_4^+$ in the medullary interstitium and a decreased rate of $H^+$ secretion in the MCD.

### TOOLS FOR ASSESSING HYPERCHLOREMIC METABOLIC ACIDOSIS

Table 24.5 summarizes the steps for the assessment of patients with hyperchloremic metabolic acidosis.

### Assess the Rate of Excretion of $NH_4^+$ in the Urine

**Urine Osmolal Gap.** A direct assay for urine $NH_4^+$ is not often available in clinical settings. In our opinion, calculation of the $U_{osm\ gap}$ provides the best indirect estimate of the $U_{NH4}$ (Eq. 24.10) because it detects all $NH_4^+$ salts in the urine (Fig. 24.7).[47,48]

$$\begin{aligned} &U_{osm\ gap} = \text{measured } U_{osm} - \text{calculated } U_{osm} \\ &\text{Calculated } U_{osm} = 2\,(U_{Na} + U_K) + U_{Urea} + U_{Glu} \\ &\text{All values are in mmol/L.} \\ &\text{Urinary concentration of } NH_4 = U_{osm\ gap}/2 \end{aligned} \qquad (24.10)$$

We use the $U_{NH4}/U_{Cr}$ ratio in a spot urine sample to assess the rate of excretion of $NH_4^+$. The rationale is that the rate of excretion of creatinine is relatively constant over a 24-hour period. In a patient with chronic metabolic acidosis, the expected normal renal response is a $U_{NH4}/U_{Cr}$ ratio higher than 150 mmol $NH_4^+$/g creatinine (higher than 15 if creatinine is measured in mmol).

There are two issues in using the urine net charge ( or urine anion gap) to assess the rate of excretion of $NH_4^+$ that, in our opinion, limit its utility. First, the calculation of the urine net charge detects high rates of excretion of $NH_4^+$ in the urine only when the anion excreted with $NH_4^+$ is $Cl^-$. Second, the equation that describes the relationship between $U_{NH4}$ and the urine net charge, which was based on values obtained from 24 hour urine collection, is shown below (Eq. 24.11).

$$U_{NH4} = -0.8 \text{ (urine anion gap)} + 82 \qquad (24.11)$$

where 82 is the difference between the usual rates of excretion of other unmeasured anions and other unmeasured cations in the urine in subjects described as consuming normal diet.[48a] This value however may have large variations depending on dietary intake.

### Determine Why the Rate of Excretion of $NH_4^+$ Is Low

**Urine pH.** The urine pH is not a reliable indicator for the rate of excretion of $NH_4^+$ (Fig. 24.8).[49] On the other hand, the basis for the low rate of excretion of $NH_4^+$ may be deduced from the urine pH. A urine pH about 5 suggests that the primary basis for a low rate of excretion of $NH_4^+$ is decreased availability of $NH_3$ in the medullary interstitial compartment due to a defect in $NH_4^+$ production or its transfer in the mTAL of the loop of Henle. A urine pH higher than 7.0 suggests that $NH_4^+$ excretion is low because there is a defect in net $H^+$ secretion in the distal nephron. Conversely, a urine pH about 6 would suggest a medullary interstitial disease that diminishes both accumulation of $NH_4^+$ in the medullary interstitium and $H^+$ secretion in the MCD.[50]

**Assess Distal Hydrogen Secretion.** $H^+$ secretion in the distal nephron can be evaluated using the measurement of the $PCO_2$ in an alkaline urine ($UPCO_2$) during bicarbonate loading (Fig. 24.9).[51] The patient is given a load of $NaHCO_3$ to increase the filtered load of $HCO_3^-$ and its delivery to the distal nephron; the urine must be freshly collected under mineral oil to minimize diffusion of $CO_2$ and must be analyzed immediately. A $PCO_2$ that is about 70 mm Hg in a second-voided alkaline urine implies that $H^+$ secretion in the distal nephron is likely to be normal, whereas much lower $UPCO_2$ values suggest that distal $H^+$ secretion is impaired. Some patients with low net distal $H^+$ secretion have a high $UPCO_2$. This occurs if there is a lesion causing a backleak of $H^+$ from the lumen of the collecting ducts (e.g., due to the use of amphotericin B)[52] or distal secretion of $HCO_3^-$ (as in some

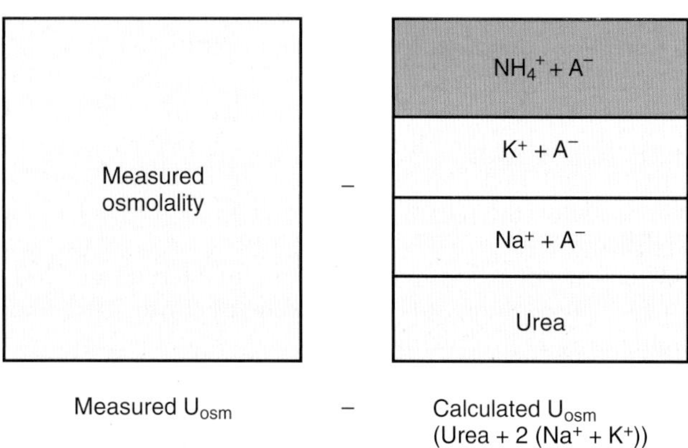


**Fig. 24.7** Indirect assessment of the concentration of $NH_4^+$ in the urine using the urine osmolal gap. The essence of the test is that a high concentration of $NH_4^+$ (shown in the *red shaded region* on the *right*) is detected in the urine from its contribution to the urine osmolality. The urine osmolal gap is the difference between the measured urine osmolality and the urine osmolality calculated from the concentrations (in mmol/L) of the principal usual urine osmoles; urea, double the concentrations of $Na^+$ + $K^+$ (to account for the concentrations of the usual monovalent anions in the urine) and glucose in a patient with hyperglycemia. The concentration of $NH_4^+$ in the urine is the urine osmolal gap divided by 2. *A*⁻, Anion. (From Kamel KS, Halperin ML. *Fluid, Electrolyte, and Acid-Base Physiology; A Problem-Based Approach.* ed 5. Philadelphia: Elsevier; 2017.)

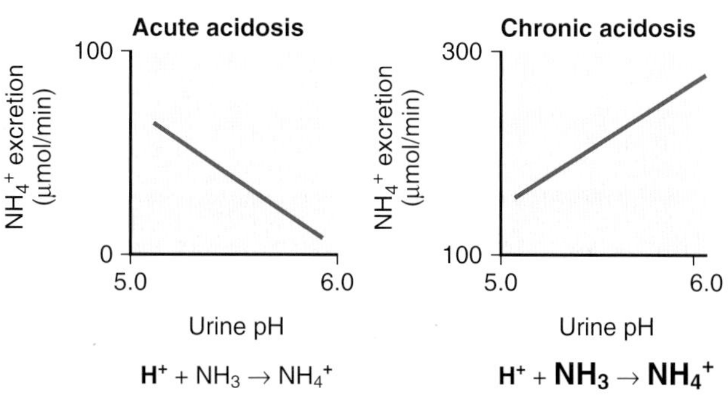


**Fig. 24.8** The urine pH is not a reliable indicator for the rate of excretion of $NH_4^+$. *Left,* During acute metabolic acidosis, the rate of excretion of $NH_4^+$ is only modestly higher, and the urine pH is low. This is because distal $H^+$ secretion is enhanced, and there is a time lag before the rate of renal production of $NH_4^+$ and the availabilty of $NH_3$ in the medullary interstitial compartment are augmented. *Right,* In contrast, during chronic metabolic acidosis, the rate of renal production of $NH_4^+$ is so high that the availability of $NH_3$ in the medullary interstitial compartment provides more $NH_3$ in the lumen of the medullary collecting duct than $H^+$ secretion in this nephron segment. Note the much higher $NH_4^+$ excretion rate at a urine pH of 6. Note also the different scales on the *y*-axes. (From Kamel KS, Halperin ML. *Fluid, Electrolyte, and Acid-Base Physiology; A Problem-Based Approach.* ed 5. Philadelphia: Elsevier; 2017.)

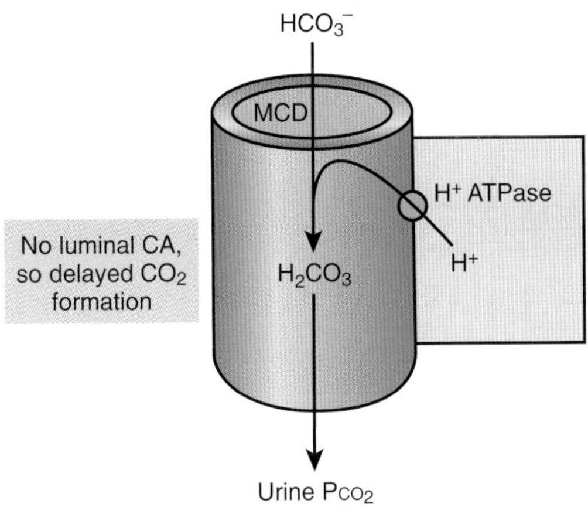


**Fig. 24.9** Use of the $PCO_2$ in alkaline urine to assess the distal secretion of $H^+$. The cylinder represents the medullary collecting duct *(MCD)* and the rectangle on its right side represents an alpha-intercalated cell, which contains an $H^+$-ATPase pump. There are two requirements for using the urine $PCO_2$ in alkaline urine to reflect the capacity to secrete $H^+$. First, enough $NaHCO_3$ is administered to achieve a second voided-urine sample with a pH >7.0. Second, because the luminal membranes of the MCD lack carbonic anhydrase *(CA)*, the carbonic acid formed is delivered to the lower urinary tract, where it decomposes to $CO_2$ and $H_2O$ and thereby elevates the urine $PCO_2$. A high $PCO_2$ in alkaline urine (usually to ≈70 mm Hg) suggests that there is no major defect in $H^+$ secretory capacity in this nephron segment. (From Kamel KS, Halperin ML. *Fluid, Electrolyte, and Acid-Base Physiology; A Problem-Based Approach.* ed 5. Philadelphia: Elsevier; 2017.)

patients with SAO who have a mutation in the $HCO_3^-/Cl^-$ anion exchanger that leads to its mistargeting to the luminal membranes of α-intercalated cells).[53]

### Assessment of Proximal Cell pH

*Fractional excretion of $HCO_3^-$.* In patients suspected of having a disorder that leads to a reduced capacity for the reabsorption of $HCO_3^-$ in the PT (pRTA), some clinicians would measure the fractional excretion of $HCO_3^-$ after infusing $NaHCO_3$ to confirm this diagnosis. In our opinion, this evaluation is not needed. These disorders are recognized clinically by failure to correct the metabolic acidemia after the administration of large amounts of $NaHCO_3$. The defect in $NaHCO_3$ reabsorption in the PT may be an isolated defect or part of a generalized PT cell dysfunction (i.e., Fanconi syndrome), in which other $Na^+$-linked transport functions of PT are affected, leading to renal glucosuria, aminoaciduria, and increased rates of excretion of phosphate, urate, and citrate. The most common cause of Fanconi syndrome in the pediatric population is cystinosis, whereas common causes in the adult population are paraproteinemias and use of drugs such as tenofovir and ifosfamide.

*Rate of citrate excretion.* The rate of excretion of citrate is a marker of pH in cells of the PT.[54] The rate of excretion of citrate in children and adults consuming their usual diet is about 400 mg/day (≈2.1 mmol/day). The rate of excretion of citrate is very low during most forms of metabolic acidosis because of the effect of intracellular acidosis in PT cells to stimulate the reabsorption of citrate. The absence of hypocitraturia would suggest that the pathophysiology of the defect in proximal $H^+$ secretion is due to a disorder causing an alkaline PT cell pH, such as conditions associated with pRTA or carbonic anhydrase II deficiency (which also impairs distal $H^+$ secretion).

## CLINICAL APPROACH TO THE PATIENT WITH HYPERCHLOREMIC METABOLIC ACIDOSIS

The steps in the clinical approach to the patient with hyperchloremic metabolic acidosis are shown in Flow Chart 24.15 and Flow Chart 24.16.

## CLINICAL CASE 13: DOES THIS PATIENT HAVE DISTAL RTA?

A 28-year-old man had been intermittently sniffing glue for the last number of years. Over the past 3 days, he became profoundly weak and had a very unsteady gait. On physical examination, his blood pressure was 100/60 mm Hg and his pulse rate was 110 beats/min when he was lying flat. When he sat up, his blood pressure fell to 80/50 mm Hg and his pulse rate rose to 130 beats/min. Arterial blood pH was 7.20, arterial $PCO_2$ was 25 mm Hg, and $PHCO_3$ was 10 mmol/L. Venous blood and urine laboratory values were as follows.

| *Parameter* | *Venous Blood* | *Urine* |
|---|---|---|
| pH | 7.0 | 6.0 |
| $PCO_2$, mm Hg | 60 | — |
| $HCO_3^-$, mmol/L | 12 | — |
| $Na^+$, mmol/L | 120 | 50 |
| $K^+$, mmol/L | 2.3 | 30 |
| $Cl^-$, mmol/L | 90 | 5 |
| Creatinine | 1.7 mg/dL (150 μmol/L) | 3.0 mmol/L |
| Glucose | 63 mg/dL (3.5 mmol/L) | 0 |
| Urea | BUN: 14 mg/dL (5.0 mmol/L) | 150 mmol/L |
| Albumin | 60 g/L: (6 g/dL) | — |
| Osmolality, mOsm/kg $H_2O$ | 260 | 400 |

#### Questions and Discussion

What dangers were present on admission?

*Hemodynamic instability.* The patient had a marked degree of EABV contraction.

*Severe degree of hypokalemia.* The dangers of a severe degree of hypokalemia are cardiac arrhythmias and respiratory muscle weakness. However, this patient's ECG demonstrated only prominent U waves. Analysis of arterial blood gases showed that the patient had an arterial $PCO_2$ of 25 mm Hg, which was appropriate for the fall in $PHCO_3$; hence, there is no superimposed respiratory acidosis. Therefore, although he had a severe degree of hypokalemia that would require aggressive $K^+$ therapy, he did not have an emergency related to hypokalemia on admission.

*Hyponatremia.* Hyponatremia was likely chronic because there were no symptoms that would strongly suggest an appreciable acute component to the hyponatremia nor was there a history of a recent large water intake.

*Binding of $H^+$ to proteins in cells.* Because the brachial venous $PCO_2$ (60 mm Hg) was considerably higher than the arterial

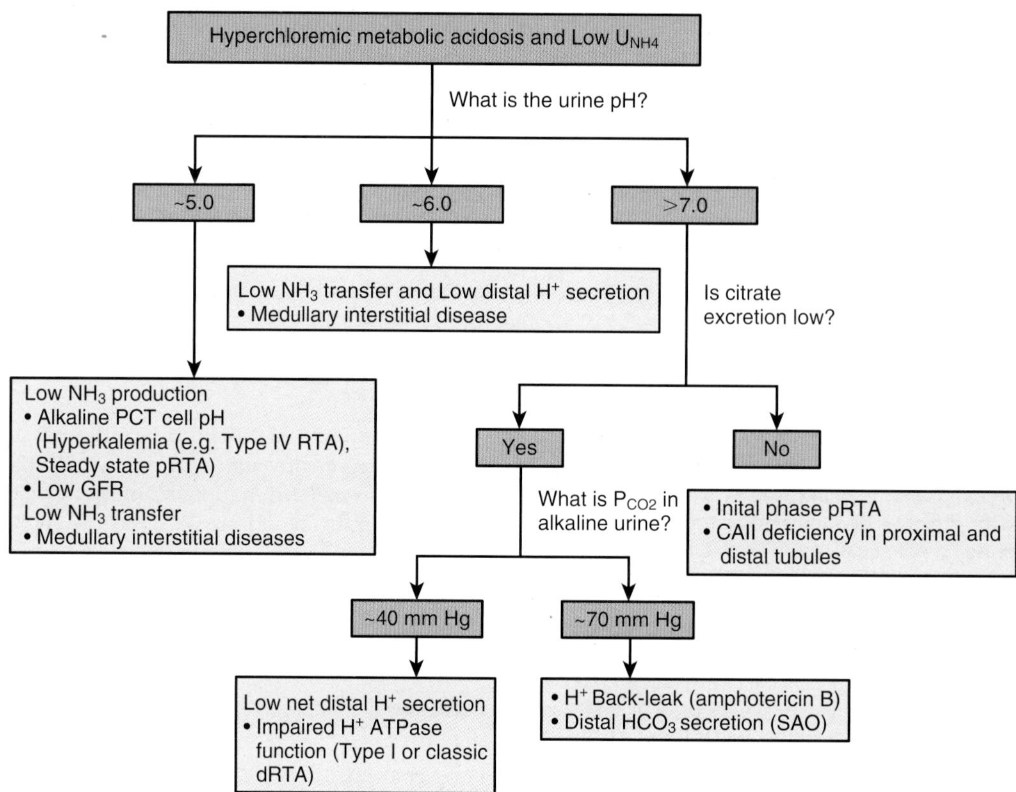


**Flow Chart 24.16** *pRTA,* Proximal renal tubular acidosis; *GFR,* glomerular filtration rate; *CA II,* carbonic anhydrase type II; *dRTA,* distal RTA; *SAO,* South Asain ovalocytosis. (From Kamel KS, Halperin ML. Fluid, electrolytes and acid-base physiology. A problem based approach, ed 5. Philadelphia: Elsevier, 2017.)

$P_{CO_2}$ (25 mm Hg), buffering of $H^+$ by the BBS in muscle was compromised, and there was a risk of more $H^+$ binding to proteins in cells of vital organs (e.g., the heart and brain; see Fig. 24.6).

What dangers should be anticipated during therapy?

*A more severe degree of hypokalemia.* Re-expansion of the EABV with the administration of saline can lead to decreased levels of catecholamines. This removes the inhibition of the release of insulin by the binding of catecholamines to pancreatic islet cells α-adrenergic receptors. The release of insluin could result in a shift of $K^+$ into cells, with worsening hypokalemia. Administration of $NaHCO_3$ to correct the metabolic acidemia may also cause a shift of $K^+$ into cells and a more severe degree of hypokalemia.

*Rapid rise in $P_{Na}$.* The $P_{Na}$ may rise rapidly if water diuresis occurs with re-expansion of the EABV. As $K^+$ is administered, there will be a shift of $K^+$ into muscle cells in exchange for $Na^+$, which will also lead to a rise in $P_{Na}$. Patients who are malnourished and/or hypokalemic are at high risk of osmotic demyelination with a rapid rise in $P_{Na}$. It is our opinion that the maximum rise in $P_{Na}$ in high-risk patients should not exceed 4 to 6 mmol/L in the first 24 hours.

*Further fall in $P_{HCO_3}$.* Expansion of the EABV with rapid administration of saline may also lead to a further fall in $P_{HCO_3}$. First, there is a dilution effect. Second, with improved blood flow to muscles and the fall in capillary $P_{CO_2}$, there will be titration of $HCO_3^-$ by $H^+$ ions that are bound to intracellular proteins. The need to give $NaHCO_3$, however, must be balanced by the danger of creating more severe hypokalemia. We would not administer $NaHCO_3$ unless there is hemodynamic instability that is not responsive to the usual maneuvers to restore blood pressure and, with a central venous line in place, to give a sufficient amount of KCl rapidly if needed.

Plan for initial therapy. On arrival to the emergency department, the patient was given 1 L of intravenous isotonic saline. To correct the hypokalemia while also avoiding a rapid rise in $P_{Na}$, the intravenous solution was changed to 0.45% NaCl (77 mmol/L) to which KCl, 40 mmol/L, was added. The concentration of effective cation osmoles of this solution (77 + 40 = 117 mmol/L) is close to his $P_{Na}$, and thus should not itself lead to a rapid rise in $P_{Na}$. The danger of a rapid rise in $P_{Na}$ due to enhanced delivery of filtrate to the distal nephron and/or due to eliminating decreased EABV-mediated release of vasopressin is still present. Therefore, the patient was given DDAVP to prevent a water diuresis, and water restriction was imposed. Hemodynamic status, $P_K$, $P_{Na}$, arterial pH, arterial $P_{CO_2}$, brachial venous $P_{CO_2}$, and $P_{HCO_3}$ were monitored closely.

What is the basis for the metabolic acidosis? Because the $P_{anion\ gap}$ was not increased, despite the high value for the $P_{Alb}$, the metabolic acidosis was judged not to be due to a gain of acids. In fact, the initial diagnosis was type I or classic dRTA which was thought to explain the metabolic acidemia, urine pH of 6.0, and hypokalemia. Calculation of the $U_{osm\ gap}$ (90 mOsmol/kg $H_2O$), however, revealed a high urinary concentration of $NH_4^+$ (45 mmol/L). Furthermore, the $U_{NH4}/U_{Cr}$ was about 15 (mmol/mmol) and the rate of excretion of creatinine in this patient was estimated to be 10 mmol/day (based on his body weight); hence, the rate of excretion of $NH_4^+$ was estimated to be around 150 mmol/day. Therefore, the basis for the patient's hyperchloremic metabolic acidosis was not dRTA.

The anion that was excreted with $NH_4^+$ was not $Cl^-$, so diarrhea was not the cause of the hyperchloremic metabolic acidosis. Hence, the patient had an acid gain–type of metabolic acidosis, with a high rate of excretion of its anion in the urine. Because the $P_{anion\ gap}$ was not elevated, these new anions were more likely to have entered the urine via secretion in the PT, akin to *p*-aminohippurate anions. The major chemical in glue is toluene; it is converted to benzoic acid by cytochrome P450 in the liver, and benzoic acid is in turn conjugated to the amino acid glycine to form hippuric acid.[55] $H^+$ titrate $HCO_3^-$ resulting in metabolic acidosis, whereas the hippurate anions are actively secreted by PT, so their concentration is very low in plasma and very high in the urine. The rate of excretion of hippurate anions exceeds the rate of excretion of $NH_4^+$ in the urine because a limited amount of $NH_4^+$ can be made in the PT, so hippurate anions are excreted along with $Na^+$, resulting in the indirect loss of $NaHCO_3$ ($HCO_3^-$ loss due to titration by added $H^+$; $Na^+$ loss due to excretion in the urine with hippurate anions) and contraction of the EABV. The low EABV, via activation of the RAAS, leads to high levels of aldosterone in plasma, causing electrogenic reabsorption of $Na^+$ in the ASDN and thereby a high rate of secretion of $K^+$, leading to hypokalemia.

## CLINICAL CASE 14: DETERMINE THE CAUSE OF HYPERCHLOREMIC METABOLIC ACIDOSIS

A 23-year-old woman with SAO was referred for assessment of hypokalemia. Her physical examination was unremarkable. The laboratory results in plasma and a spot urine sample are summarized in the following table. The pH and $P_{CO_2}$ are from an arterial blood sample, whereas all other blood findings are from a venous plasma sample. The urine was glucose-free.

| *Parameter* | *Blood* | *Urine* |
|---|---|---|
| Arterial pH | 7.35 | 6.8 |
| Arterial $P_{CO_2}$, mm Hg | 30 | — |
| $Na^+$, mmol/L | 140 | 75 |
| $K^+$, mmol/L | 3.1 | 35 |
| $Cl^-$, mmol/L | 113 | 95 |
| $HCO_3^-$, mmol/L | 15 | 10 |
| Anion gap, mEq/L | 12 | 5 |
| Osmolality, mOsm/kg $H_2O$ | 290 | 450 |
| Creatinine, mg/dL | 0.7 | 6.0 mmol/L |
| Urea (mmol/L) | | 220 |
| Citrate | — | Low |

### Questions and Discussion

What is the basis for the hyperchloremic metabolic acidosis? The patient had a low $U_{NH_4}$ because the measured $U_{osm}$ (450 mOsmol/kg $H_2O$) was very similar to the calculated $U_{osm}$, 440 mOsmol/kg $H_2O$—that is, $2(U_{Na}$ [75 mmol/L] + $U_K$ [35 mmol/L]) + $U_{urea}$ (220 mmol/L) + $U_{Glu}$ (0). The rate of excretion of $NH_4^+$ was low because the $U_{NH_4}/U_{Cr}$ was very low. Hence, the diagnosis was RTA.

What is the cause of the low rate of excretion of $NH_4^+$?

*Urine pH.* Because the urine pH is 6.8, and urine citrate was low, the basis for the low rate of $NH_4^+$ excretion is a low net secretion of $H^+$ in the distal nephron (see Flow Chart 24.16).

*Assessment of distal $H^+$ secretion.* After hypokalemia was corrected, $H^+$ secretion in the distal nephron could be evaluated using $U_{PCO_2}$ during bicarbonate loading. The $U_{PCO_2}$ in alkaline urine was 70 mm Hg (see Flow Chart 24.16). Because the $U_{PCO_2}$ was unexpectedly high and a backleak of an $H^+$-type of defect was unlikely, it was suggested that the defect may be one of increased distal $HCO_3^-$ secretion. In some patients with SAO, another mutation in the $Cl^-/HCO_3^-$ exchanger causes it to be targeted abnormally to the luminal membranes of α-intercalated cells. The $U_{PCO_2}$ would be high with bicarbonate loading due to the distal secretion of $HCO_3^-$ by alkaline intercalated cells, which increases the luminal fluid pH resulting in release of $H^+$ from monovalent phosphate ($H_2PO_4^-$) in the luminal fluid, the formation of $H_2CO_3$, which then dissociates to $CO_2$ and $H_2O$.

Complete reference list available at ExpertConsult.com.

## KEY REFERENCES

1. Kamel KS, Halperin ML. *Fluid, Electrolyte, and Acid-Base Physiology; a Problem-Based Approach.* 5th ed. Philadelphia: Elsevier; 2017.
2. Zhai XY, Fenton RA, Andreasen A, et al. Aquaporin-1 is not expressed in descending thin limbs of short-loop nephrons. *J Am Soc Nephrol.* 2007;18:2937–2944.
3. Kamel KS, Halperin ML. The importance of distal delivery of filtrate and residual water permeability in the pathophysiology of hyponatremia. *Nephrol Dial Transplant.* 2012;27:872–875.
5. Carlotti AP, Bohn D, Mallie JP, et al. Tonicity balance, and not electrolyte-free water calculations, more accurately guides therapy for acute changes in natremia. *Intensive Care Med.* 2001;27:921–924.
9. Napolova O, Urbach S, Davids MR, et al. Assessing the degree of extracellular fluid volume contraction in a patient with a severe degree of hyperglycaemia. *Nephrol Dial Transplant.* 2003;18:2674–2677.
15. Kamel KS, Schrieber M, Halperin ML. Renal potassium physiology: integration of the renal response to dietary potassium depletion. *Kidney Int.* 2018;93:41–53.
21. Kamel KS, Halperin ML. Intrarenal urea recycling leads to a higher rate of renal excretion of potassium: an hypothesis with clinical implications. *Curr Opin Nephrol Hypertens.* 2011;20:547–554.
25. Wilson FH, Disse-Nicodeme S, Choate KA, et al. Human hypertension caused by mutations in WNK kinases. *Science.* 2001;293:1107–1112.
30. Halperin ML, Scheich A. Should we continue to recommend that a deficit of KCl be treated with NaCl? A fresh look at chloride-depletion metabolic alkalosis. *Nephron.* 1994;67:263–269.
35. Gowrishankar M, Kamel KS, Halperin ML. Buffering of a $H^+$ load; A "brain-protein-centered" view. *J Am Soc Nephrol.* 2007;18:2278–2280.
37. Kraut JA, Madias NE. Serum anion gap: its uses and limitations in clinical medicine. *Clin J Am Soc Nephrol.* 2007;2:162–174.
43. Kamel KS, Halperin ML. Acid-base problems in diabetic ketoacidosis. *N Engl J Med meant.* 2015;372:546–554.
47. Dyck R, Asthana S, Kalra J, et al. A modification of the urine osmolal gap: an improved method for estimating urine ammonium. *Am J Nephrol.* 1990;10:359–362.
48. Kamel KS, Halperin ML. An improved approach to the patient with metabolic acidosis: a need for four amendments. *J Nephrol.* 2006;65:S76–S85.
50. Kamel KS, Briceno LF, Santos MI, et al. A new classification for renal defects in net acid excretion. *Am J Kidney Dis.* 1997;29:136–146.

# 25 Diagnostic Kidney Imaging

Vinay A. Duddalwar | Hossein Jadvar | Suzanne L. Palmer

CHAPTER OUTLINE



KEY POINTS

- Imaging tests are tailored to answer specific clinical scenarios and are often modified to address specific clinical questions.
- Positron emission tomography with a number of different radiotracers may allow for imaging characterization of the underlying tumor biology in renal cell carcinoma.
- Contrast enhanced ultrasound is an additional imaging technique to consider using especially in the presence of abnormal renal function.
- The development of multiple radiation dose reduction techniques and the development of dual energy CT scans have made an impact in the imaging strategy of patients requiring follow-up imaging.
- Techniques such as dynamic contrast media-enhanced MR renography, diffusion-weighted imaging (DWI), and blood oxygen level-dependent (BOLD) MRI can help evaluate various aspects of renal function.

Medical imaging has made major strides over the past century since the discovery of x-rays by Wilhelm Roentgen. Imaging tools now include sophisticated systems that can noninvasively interrogate structure, function, and metabolism in health and disease states of all organ systems, including the urinary system. X-ray studies primarily provide anatomic information and include plain radiography, intravenous urography (IVU), antegrade and retrograde pyelography, and computed tomography (CT). Ultrasonography (US), which does not have ionizing radiation, involves the use of high-frequency sound waves. The development of additional techniques in US such as Doppler US, elastography, and contrast-enhanced US has led to an expansion of the role of US in the evaluation of the kidney. Magnetic resonance imaging (MRI) uses the phenomenon of nuclear magnetic resonance and yields primarily anatomic information but also can provide some functional information. Nuclear medicine studies, including planar and single-photon computed tomography (SPECT) techniques, contribute primarily functional information; positron emission tomography (PET) and integrated PET-CT and PET-MRI, in conjunction with a number of current and novel radiotracers, provide means for a quantitative assessment of a variety of physiologic parameters. In addition, there have been significant changes in image processing and visualization technology that have led to an increase in the imaging applications for the kidney. Understanding the diagnostic utility and limitation of each imaging modality facilitates the proper evaluation of patients in various specific clinical settings.

## IMAGING TECHNIQUES

### PLAIN RADIOGRAPH OF THE ABDOMEN

Historically, plain radiography of the abdomen was used as the starting point in the evaluation of the kidneys, as well as the rest of the abdomen. Relative to more advanced technology, radiography of the kidneys, ureters, and bladder (KUB) (Fig. 25.1) yields little significant information on its own and if used at all, should be the starting point for further evaluation of the kidneys, such as the scout film for IVU.

### INTRAVENOUS UROGRAPHY

Previously IVU (also known as intravenous pyelography) was used as the primary means of evaluating the kidneys and urinary tract[1,2]; however, CT has supplanted IVU for routine imaging. An IVU is now seldom performed and usually only when specific clinical questions need to be answered.[3] A scout film (KUB) is performed before any contrast material is injected intravenously. Timed sequential images of the kidneys and the remainder of the genitourinary system are then obtained.[4,5] The nephrogram demonstrates the size and

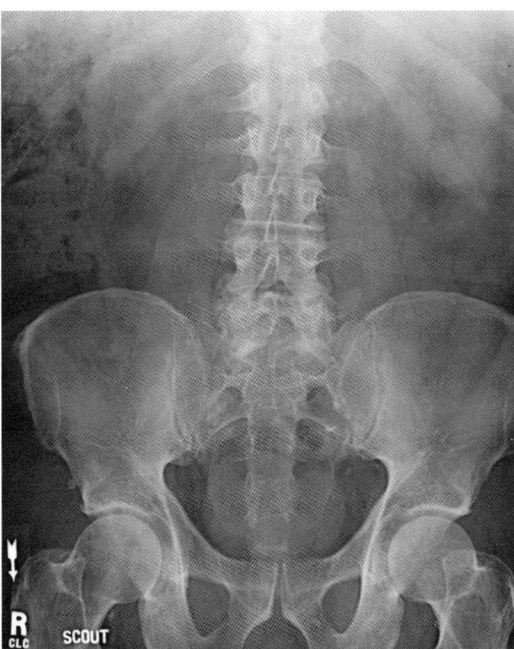


**Fig. 25.1** Plain radiograph of the abdomen: kidneys, ureters, and bladder. The kidneys lie posteriorly in the retroperitoneum in the upper abdomen. They are surrounded by fat. The ribs overlie the kidney, and bowel gas is visible in the right upper quadrant. The psoas muscles are also well visible because retroperitoneal fat abuts them.

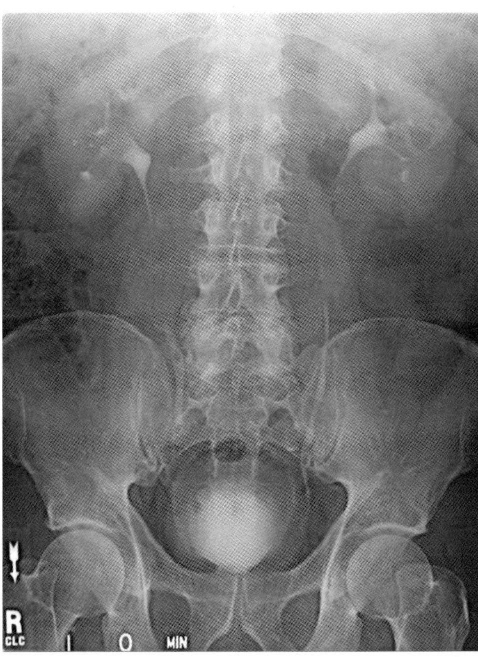


**Fig. 25.2** Intravenous urography: excretory phase. This image was obtained 10 minutes after the injection of the contrast material. The kidneys are well visualized; contrast material outlines the calyces, pelvis, ureters, and bladder.

shape of the kidney while anatomic depiction of the calyces, infundibula, and pelvis is best displayed on subsequent images by 5 to 10 minutes after injection. Imaging of the ureters is usually accomplished 10 to 15 minutes after injection[6] (Fig. 25.2).

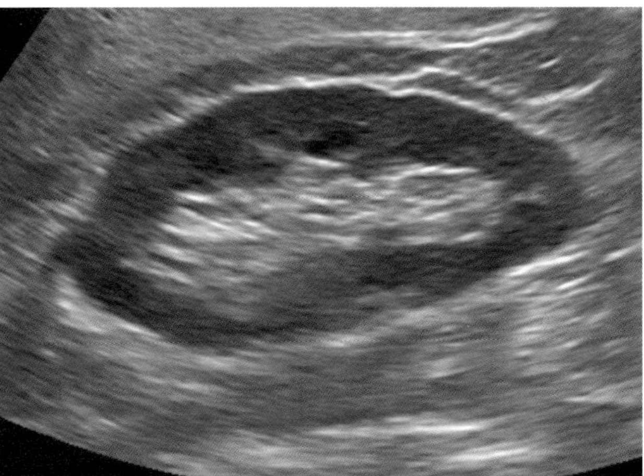

**Fig. 25.3** Renal ultrasonography: normal kidney. The central echogenic structure represents the vascular elements, calyces, and renal sinus fat. The peripheral cortex is noted to be smooth and regular. Renal pyramids may be depicted as hypoechoic structures between the central echo complex and the cortex.

## ULTRASONOGRAPHY

US is the most frequently used diagnostic examination for the evaluation of the kidneys and urinary tract.[7] It is noninvasive, uses no ionizing radiation, and requires minimal patient preparation. It is the first-line examination in azotemic patients to assess renal size and the presence or absence of hydronephrosis and obstruction. It is used to assess the vasculature of native and transplanted kidneys. US is also used to evaluate renal structure and to characterize renal masses. It is the primary modality of imaging for evaluation of a transplanted kidney. It is also the most commonly used modality for imaging guidance for a kidney biopsy.

Diagnostic US is an outgrowth of sound navigation and ranging (sonar) technology. In medical US, high-frequency sound waves are used to evaluate various organs. In the abdomen and, more particularly, the kidneys, 2.5- to 4.0-mHz sound waves are generally employed.

The US unit consists of a transducer, which sends and receives the sound waves; a microprocessor or computer, which obtains and processes the returning signal; and an image display system or monitor, which displays the processed images. The piezoelectric transducer converts electrical energy into high-frequency sound waves that are transmitted through the patient's body. It converts the returning reflected sound waves back into electrical energy that can be processed by a computer. Sound travels as a waveform through the tissues being imaged. The speed of the sound wave depends on the tissue through which it is traveling.

Different tissues and the interface between these tissues have different acoustic impedance. As the sound wave travels through different tissues, part of the wave is reflected back to the transducer. The depth of the tissue interface is measured by the time the sound wave takes to return to the transducer. A gray-scale image is produced by the measured reflected sound, in which the intensity of the pixels (picture elements) is proportional to the intensities of the reflected sound (Fig. 25.3). When the acoustic interfaces are quite large, strong echoes result. These are known as *specular reflectors* and are visible from the renal capsule and bladder wall.

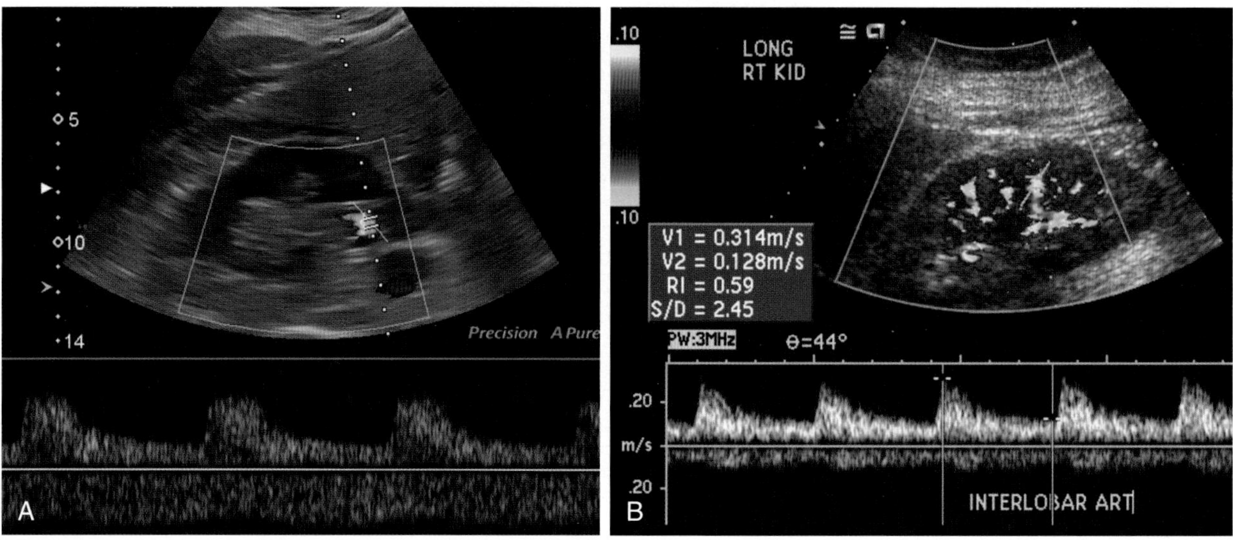


**Fig. 25.4** Spectral Doppler ultrasound of the normal kidney. **A,** Normal waveform. **B,** Calculation of the resistive index (RI). *V1*, peak systolic velocity (S); *V2*, end diastolic velocity (D). RI = (S-D)/S.

Nonspecular reflectors generate echoes of lower amplitude and are visible in the renal parenchyma. Strong reflection of sound by bone and air results in little or no information from the tissues beneath; this appearance is known as *shadowing*. Lack of acoustic impedance as observed in fluid-filled structures, such as the urinary bladder and renal cysts, allows the sound waves to penetrate further, which results in a relative increase in intensity distal to the structures; this is known as *increased through transmission*. All of these features are used to help characterize various lesions. Real-time US, which provides sequential images at a rapid frame rate, allows the demonstration of motion of organs and pulsation of vessels.

Doppler US, based on the Doppler frequency shift of the sound wave caused by moving objects, can be used to assess venous and arterial blood flow.[8,9] The movement of blood cells in blood vessels is used to generate Doppler information, and this is used to derive diagnostic information. Spectral Doppler is a technique that displays the blood flow measurements graphically, displaying flow velocities over time. This can be in the form of a continuous wave (CW) Doppler or pulsed wave (PW) Doppler. CW Doppler permits measurement of flow along the line of evaluation whereas the PW technique allows evaluation of flow at a particular location. In clinical practice a combination of the two techniques is used together for evaluation. In a technique called pulsed wave Doppler US, quantification of this flow and assessment of the waveforms can be used in evaluating various organ systems (Fig. 25.4A). With Doppler color-flow US, the image is encoded with colors assigned to the pixels representing the direction and volume of flow within vessels (Fig. 25.5). In power Doppler US, the amplitude of the signal, without any directional information, is used to produce a color map of the intrarenal vasculature and flow within the kidneys (Fig. 25.6).

Resistive index is a measure of the resistance to blood flow caused by the microvascular bed distally. This serves as a nonspecific indicator of disease in both native and transplanted kidneys. In general, a normal resistive index is 0.70 or less (see Fig. 25.4B). An increased resistive index is a

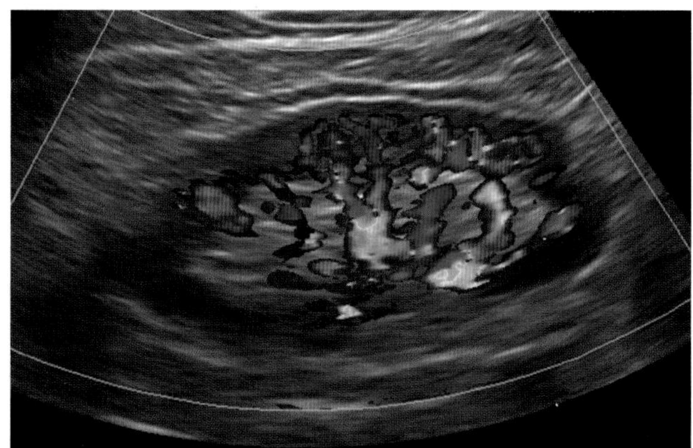

**Fig. 25.5** Doppler color-flow ultrasonography: normal kidney. The red echogenic areas represent arterial flow (flow toward the transducer), and blue echogenic areas represent venous flow (flow away from the transducer).

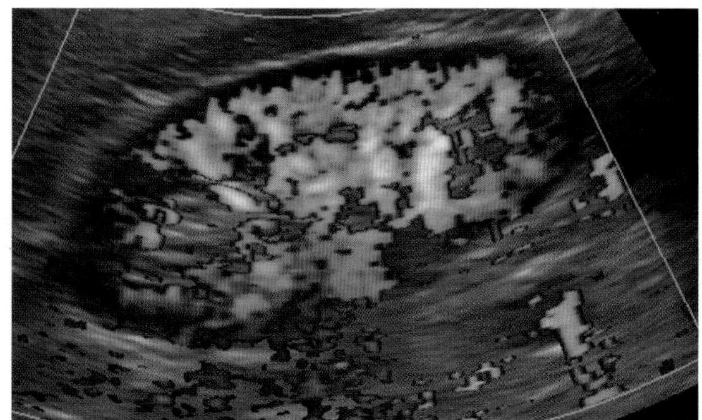

**Fig. 25.6** Power Doppler ultrasonography: normal kidney. The color image represents a summation of all flow—arterial and venous—within the kidney.

nonspecific indicator of disease and a sign of increased peripheral vascular resistance.[8–10]

Elastography is another technique by which the mechanical properties of a target tissue are assessed. It is a measure of the stiffness in a tissue, and its role in the evaluation of chronic parenchymal disease is being evaluated. The change in the elasticity of a particular tissue is assessed by changes in the propagation velocity of ultrasound waves.[11] Elastography techniques are the focus of interest in evaluating both native kidneys in chronic kidney disease as well as evaluating transplant kidneys.

There has been an increase in the use of intravenous contrast agents with US for the evaluation of the kidneys and renal masses, a technique called contrast-enhanced ultrasound (CEUS).[12] The contrast agents are microbubbles of a high-molecular-weight gas such as perfluorocarbons that are stabilized by a thin capsule of lipid or protein. They are of the same size as blood cells and therefore are not filtered out in the lungs or the kidneys. The advantage of these agents is that they are excreted by pulmonary ventilation, and therefore they can be used in patients with very poor renal function. They remain in the vascular system (acting as blood pool agents) and can provide another method of providing information on organ perfusion and vascularity. These contrast agents have expanded the role of US and have given an additional option in the imaging of patients with compromised renal function. The development of these US-specific contrast agents enables the display of microvasculature and dynamic enhancement patterns which are not visible using other methodologies.

Imaging after injection of these contrast agents is performed using contrast-specific ultrasonographic modes using a low mechanical index technique. These are based on the cancellation of linear ultrasound signals from tissue and using a nonlinear response from microbubbles.

Uses for CEUS in the kidney include the following: (1) characterization of focal renal lesions: accurate characterization of complex renal cysts into different Bosniak groups, increase in diagnostic confidence in the evaluation of focal renal masses, permits differentiation of variant normal anatomy, including conditions such as a hypertrophied column of Bertin[13]; (2) evaluation of transplanted kidney: CEUS can help identify vascular complications such as arterial and venous thrombosis and ischemia; and (3) follow-up of renal trauma.[14] CEUS can also identify and characterize post-intervention complications.[15]

US is the most common imaging technique in guiding a renal biopsy. Its advantages include the lack of radiation and mobility, thus allowing bedside procedures. US guidance is also used for other interventional procedures such as percutaneous nephrostomy placement and renal mass ablations. In addition, US along with Doppler US is very commonly used for mapping and assessment of access sites in both arteriovenous (AV) shunts and fistulas in a patient undergoing dialysis.

### ULTRASONOGRAPHY: NORMAL ANATOMY

US images of the kidneys are generally obtained in the longitudinal, transverse, and parasagittal planes.[16] The appearance of the perinephric fat varies from slightly less echogenic to highly echogenic in comparison with the renal cortex. The renal capsule is visible as an echogenic line surrounding the kidney. The centrally located renal sinus and hilum, containing renal sinus fat, vessels, and the collecting system, are usually echogenic because of the presence of fat (see Fig. 25.3). The amount of renal sinus fat generally increases with age. Tubular structures corresponding to vessels and the collecting system may be visible in the renal hilum. Doppler color-flow US may be used to differentiate the vessels from the collecting system.

The normal renal cortex is less echogenic (i.e., it appears darker) than the liver and spleen. The renal medullary pyramids are hypoechoic, and their triangular shape points to the renal hilum. The renal cortex lies peripherally, and its separation from the medulla is usually demarcated by an echogenic focus attributable to the arcuate arteries along the corticomedullary junction. Columns of Bertin have the same echogenicity as the renal cortex and separate the renal pyramids. On occasion, a large column of Bertin may simulate a mass. Even when a column of Bertin is large or prominent, its echogenicity is the same as the remainder of the cortex, and the vascular pattern observed on power Doppler images is also the same.

Renal size is accurately measured by US. Normal kidneys range from 8.5 to 13 cm, depending on the age, sex, and body habitus of the patient. The contours of the kidneys should be smooth; occasionally some slight nodularity is present as a result of developmental fetal lobulation. The renal arteries and veins may be visible extending from the renal hilum to the aorta and inferior vena cava (IVC). The veins lie anterior to the arteries. The renal arterial branching pattern within the kidneys may be visible on Doppler color-flow US (see Fig. 25.5).[17] The resistive indices of the main, intralobar, and arcuate vessels may be calculated (see Fig. 25.4B). With power Doppler US, the intrarenal vasculature may be assessed; it demonstrates an overall increased pattern in the cortex in relation to the medulla, which corresponds to the normal arterial flow to the kidney (see Fig. 25.6).[18,19] The renal calyces and collecting systems are not typically visible with US unless distension caused by diuresis or obstruction is present. When visible, the collecting systems are anechoic structures in the renal sinus fat, connecting together at the renal pelvis. The urinary bladder is visible in the pelvis as a fluid-filled anechoic structure. The entrance of the ureters into the bladder at the trigone may be visualized on Doppler color-flow US as ureteral jets (Fig. 25.7).

When a kidney is not identified in its normal location, the remainder of the abdomen and pelvis should be assessed. Ectopic kidneys may lie lower in the abdomen or within the pelvis and may also be located on the opposite side; the kidneys may even be fused (e.g., horseshoe kidneys). Horseshoe kidneys tend to lie lower in the retroperitoneum, and their axes may be different from those of normal kidneys.

## COMPUTED TOMOGRAPHY

CT has become an essential imaging tool for diagnosis in all areas of the body. In the genitourinary tract, it has supplanted IVU, especially for the evaluation of flank pain, hematuria, renal masses, and trauma. Even in areas in which US is the first-line imaging modality, CT offers a complementary and sometimes superior means of imaging. CT is now the first examination to be performed in patients with renal colic, renal stone disease, renal trauma, renal infection and abscess, renal mass, hematuria, and urothelial abnormalities.

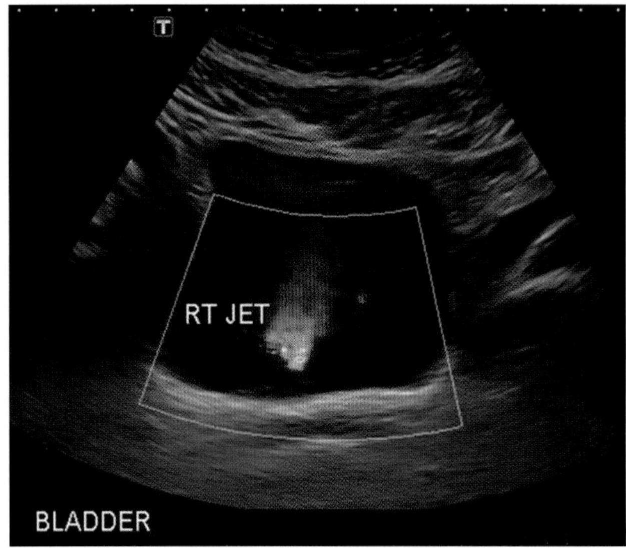


**Fig. 25.7** Ureteral jet. Color-flow image of urine entering the bladder.

After CT was first developed in 1970, it evolved rapidly with new technical innovations, image processing, and visualization methods.[20] In addition, over the last decade, concerted efforts have resulted in the reduction of the radiation absorbed by patients during a CT scan.

CT is the computer reconstruction of a radiographically generated image that depicts a slice through the area being studied in the body. The x-ray tube produces a highly collimated fan beam and is mounted opposite an array of electronic detectors. This system rotates in tandem around the patient. The detector system collects hundreds of thousands of samples representing the attenuation of the x-ray along the line formed from the x-ray source to the detector as the rotation occurs. This data set is transferred to a computer, where the image is reconstructed. The CT image is made up of pixels (picture elements), each corresponding to a CT density number (Hounsfield unit [HU]) that represents the number of x-rays absorbed by the patient at a particular point in the cross-sectional image. These pixels represent a two-dimensional display of a three-dimensional object or volume element (voxel). The third dimension is the slice thickness or depth. Thus the HU is the average attenuation of x-rays of all the tissues within a specific voxel, which is then used to create the individual image. The images are then displayed on a computer monitor for reviewing and analysis.

The HU of water is 0. Tissues that attenuate more x-rays than water have positive HU, and those with less x-ray attenuation than water have negative HU. Different shades of gray on a scale of white to black are assigned to HU (the highest number is depicted as white, the lowest as black). The image of each slice is thus created on a display monitor, and this image may be manipulated on viewing monitors to accentuate the regions being imaged. The advantage of this digital image set is that by using various tools such as window levels and widths and different summation and reconstruction techniques, images can be optimized to evaluate a particular organ or region.

The initial CT scanners were relatively slow because the technology required a point-and-shoot process. This initial generation of body CT scanner led to a scan of the abdomen that took up to 2 to 4 minutes or more to complete. In 1990, helical/spiral technology was introduced in which the x-ray tube and detector system continuously rotated around the patient, and the patient moved continuously through the gantry. Scan time through the abdomen was significantly reduced. After helical/spiral CT, a two-detector system was introduced that produced two slices for every 360-degree rotation of the x-ray tube and detector system. Multidetector CT (MDCT) systems with 640 detectors are in use primarily for advanced applications, such as computed tomographic angiography (CTA) for the coronary arteries. Most commonly today, MDCT systems varying from 64 to 320 detectors are used in abdominal and pelvic scanning. With MDCT, each 360-degree rotation results in the number of slices equal to the number of detectors (i.e., a 64-detector system produces 64 slices in one 360-degree rotation). These technologic advances have led to a dramatic increase in the speed of scans (4–10 seconds), a routine use of thin slices or collimation (1–2 mm thick), and a marked improvement in spatial resolution (ability to display small objects clearly).[21]

As a result of the faster scanning times, the use of enhancement by intravenous contrast material has improved and become more widely used.[22] For example, the kidneys can be scanned in the arterial, corticomedullary, nephrographic, and delayed phases, which allows for a more complete assessment. Current, state-of-the-art MDCT acquires data as a volumetric study, and the slice thickness has been reduced to the point that sagittal, coronal, oblique, and off-axis images may be displayed with no loss of resolution. The data acquisition may also be displayed as a three-dimensional volumetric display with the regions of interest highlighted.[21] The kidneys are well suited for assessment with MDCT.[22–26]

More recent technical developments include dual-energy and spectral-energy scanners that offer the ability to image an organ at different energy strengths.[27] Tissues behave differently at different energies, and this fact is used in techniques such as characterization of calculi and obtaining virtual unenhanced images and iodine maps in different organs (Fig. 25.8).

## COMPUTED TOMOGRAPHY TECHNIQUE, INCLUDING UROGRAPHY

Most clinical questions require the use of intravenous contrast and a tailored CT urography (CTU) is a way to provide a comprehensive examination of the genitourinary tract. CTU may be used to assess the kidney as a whole (anatomic), the vascular tree (function and perfusion), and the excretory (urothelial) patterns.[28] Noncontrast scans enable assessment of renal calculi, high-density cysts, and contour abnormalities.[29] Early-phase scans (12–15 seconds) enable arterial assessment, for example, the evaluation for renal artery stenosis (RAS). Scanning at 25 to 30 seconds (corticomedullary phase) results in clear corticomedullary differentiation, recommended for renal mass evaluation. At 90 to 100 seconds, true nephrographic-phase imaging of the kidneys is obtained.[22] Delayed imaging, typically at 5 to 10 minutes, enables the evaluation of the urothelium (calyces, renal pelvis, ureters, and bladder) in the excretory phase.[30] Axial images, multiplanar reconstructions, maximum-intensity projection images, and three-dimensional volumetric displays complement each other in CTU. CTU is superior to IVU.[31–34] Not all the phases are required for all clinical situations; therefore the examination should be tailored to a specific clinical question. Urothelial lesions can often be evaluated by combining the nephrographic and delayed phases into a single phase by

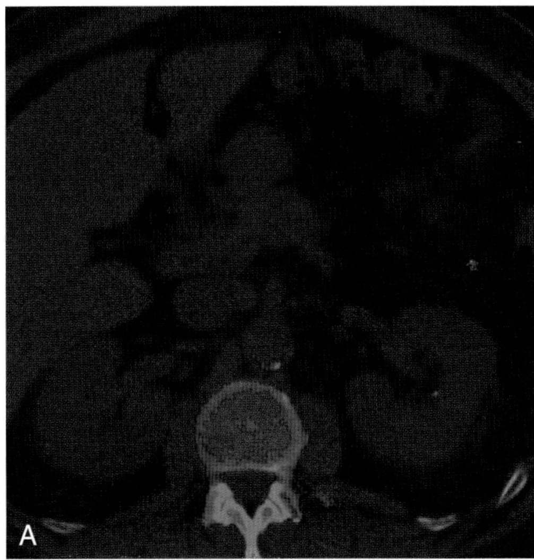
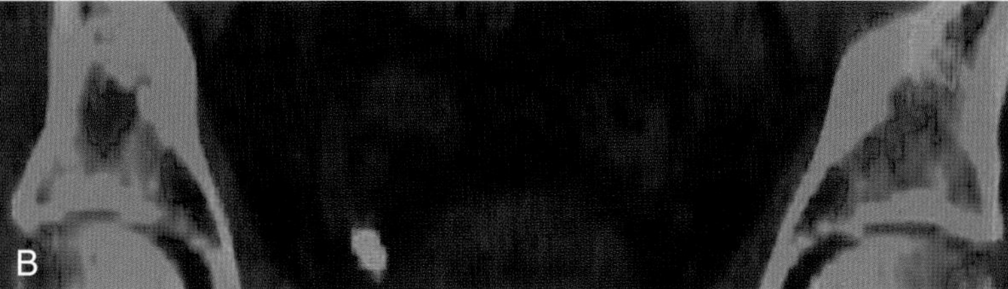

**Fig. 25.8** Dual-energy computed tomography (CT) for stone characterization in two different patients. **A,** Postprocessed color-coded axial CT image in a 54-year-old patient obtained after dual-energy CT scanning shows a left renal calculus coded blue, indicating a nonuric acid stone. **B,** Postprocessed color-coded coronal CT image in a 66-year-old patient obtained after dual-energy CT scanning shows a right distal ureteric calculus color-coded red, indicating a uric acid stone. Technique: An initial routine stone protocol multidetector CT scan is performed for detection and localization of the calculi along the renal pelvicalyceal system. Subsequently, a focused dual-source CT scan is performed in the region of the stone. Dual-energy CT is performed on the dual-source CT scanner (Somatom Definition) with the following technique: 80 kV/350–380 mAs and 140 kV/80-98 mAs, 14 × 1.2 mm/64 × 0.6 mm. The postprocessing is performed using a three-material decomposition algorithm on the dual-energy software on the scanner console (Syngo.via). (Image courtesy Avinash Kambadakone, MD, Massachusetts General Hospital, Boston, MA.)

using a split–contrast bolus technique. This involves giving the iodinated contrast intravenously in two separate boluses but scanning only once.

Another technical innovation is the development of spectral CT or multienergy CT.[27] This involves the ability to scan a particular tissue with two or more different energies. Knowing how a target tissue attenuates at different energies can provide further details of the tissue composition. For example, spectral CT can help in differentiating types of renal calculi and characterizing renal masses. It also provides the ability to generate virtual unenhanced data sets, as well as increasing detection rates of iodine-containing tissues.

Work on reducing radiation exposure is also being aggressively pursued. Because of the development of new reconstruction algorithms such as iterative reconstruction and model-based reconstruction, there has been a significant (50%–70%) reduction in the resultant radiation dose without any change in the quality of the study. Further advances in technology will result in incremental reductions of dose.

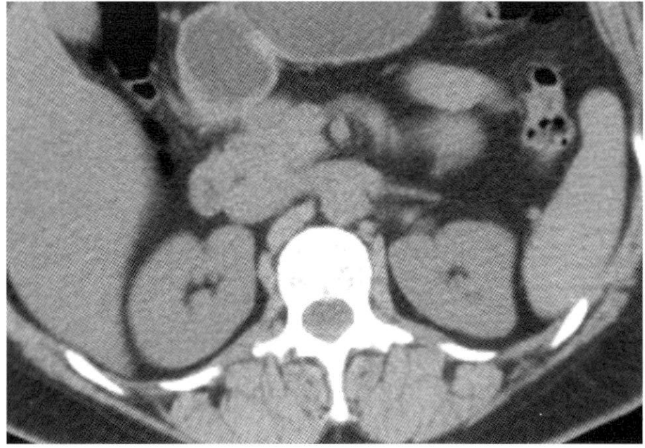

**Fig. 25.9** Noncontrast computed tomographic scan through the midportion of normal kidneys. The kidneys lie in the retroperitoneum with the lumbar spine and psoas muscles more centrally. The liver is anterolateral to the right kidney, and the spleen anterolateral to the left kidney.

## COMPUTED TOMOGRAPHY: NORMAL ANATOMY

The retroperitoneal anatomy is easily viewed with CT (Figs. 25.9 to 25.14). The kidneys lie in the retroperitoneum, surrounded by Gerota's fascia in the perinephric space. Perinephric fat surrounds the kidneys with the liver anterosuperior on the right, the spleen superior on the left, and the spine, aorta, and IVC central to each kidney. The abdominal intraperitoneal contents lie anteriorly. The renal arteries are easily seen on both arterial and venous phases, generally located posterior to the venous structures. The adrenal glands are found in a location superior to the upper poles of the kidneys. In corticomedullary phase imaging, it is easy to distinguish the renal cortex from the medulla. Cortical thickness and medullary appearance may be readily assessed. The nephrographic phase should demonstrate symmetric enhancement of each kidney.[22] At 7 to 10 minutes in the excretory phase, the calyces should be well depicted with sharp fornices, a cupped central section, and a narrow, smooth infundibulum leading to the renal pelvis.[30] Coronal images in slab maximum-intensity projection three-dimensional volumetric reformations help in displaying the anatomic details.[33] The excretory phase images delineate the ureters from the renal pelvis to the bladder. A curved reformatted series of images or three-dimensional display is needed to display the ureters in their entirety. Proper tailoring of the examination to the diagnostic problem provides guidance for the correct imaging acquisition.[23,25,34]

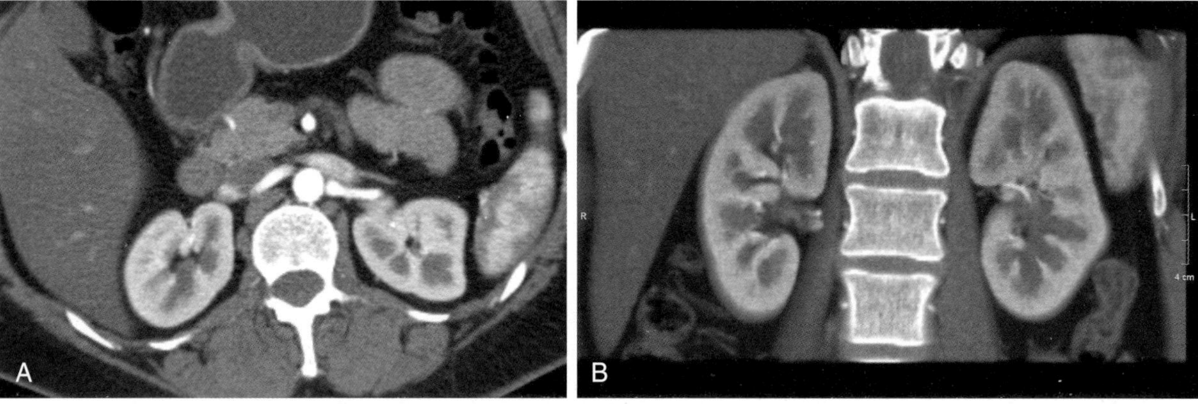


**Fig. 25.10** Computed tomographic scan: normal corticomedullary phase. Axial slice **(A)** and coronal image **(B)** demonstrate the dense enhancement of the cortex in relation to the medulla containing the renal pyramids.

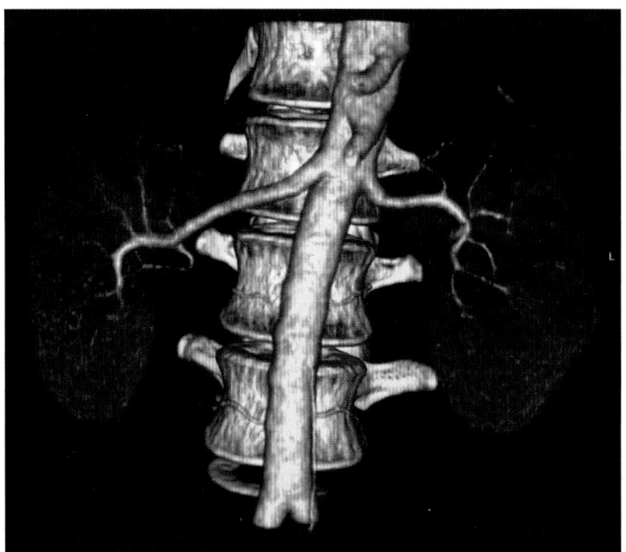

**Fig. 25.11** Renal computed tomographic angiogram: normal findings. The aorta and the exiting renal arteries on the right and left are visible in this volume rendered reconstruction. The kidneys are visible peripherally with the branching renal arteries.

## IODINATED CONTRAST MEDIA

Over the years, many different intravascular contrast media have been employed.[35] Since the mid-2000s, virtually all studies involving intravascular injection of contrast material have been performed with low osmolar (LOCM) or isoosmolar (IOCM) contrast media.

Contrast material has a plasma half-life of 1 to 2 hours in patients with normal renal function. Virtually all contrast material is excreted by the kidneys within 24 hours. In patients with renal failure, contrast media may be excreted via other routes, including the biliary system or gastrointestinal tract. All iodinated contrast agents are dialyzable.

Reactions to the injection of any of the contrast agents may occur; however, these reactions are not "allergic" responses in the sense of an antigen-antibody reaction and are referred to as idiosyncratic.[36] The exact causative mechanism is unclear but is likely as a result of complex effects on various vasoactive mediators such as histamine, complement and the kinin chain. Although the majority of these reactions are mild or minor, severe reactions and deaths do occur. With ionic high osmolar contrast media (HOCM) the reaction rate in the general population is 5% to 6%.[37] The rates of reactions to LOCM and IOCM agents are much lower, in the range of 1% to 2%.[38–40] Serious reactions are rare with a historical rate of 0.04%. Mild reactions consist of flushing, nausea, and vomiting, and treatment is not required. Mild dermal reactions, primarily urticaria, do occur and may or may not necessitate treatment. Moderate and severe reactions, which occur considerably less frequently, include bronchospasm, laryngeal edema, seizures, arrhythmias, syncope, shock, and cardiac arrest. All moderate and severe reactions necessitate treatment.

Because the reaction that occurs in patients after injection of contrast material is not antigen-antibody mediated, pretesting plays no role.[41] Neither the rate of injection nor the dose of contrast material has been clearly established as a determinant in the occurrence of contrast material–related reactions.[38,42] The only regimen that has proven to reduce the incidence of contrast-induced reactions is the modified Greenberger protocol[17]:

> ***Clinical Relevance***
>
> The only regimens proven to reduce the incidence of contrast-induced reactions to include pretreatment with glucocorticoids and antihistamines.
>
> Two frequently used regimens are as follows: (1) prednisone—50 mg orally at 13 hours, 7 hours, and 1 hour before contrast injection, plus diphenhydramine 50 mg intravenously, intramuscularly, or orally 1 hour before contrast medium.[42] (2) Methylprednisolone—32 mg orally 12 hours and 2 hours before contrast media injection.[43] An antihistamine (as in option 1) can also be added to this regimen. An alternative that may be used in specific clinical circumstances, although less desirable than the 13-hour protocol is a 5-hour protocol consisting of methyl prednisolone 40 mg intravenously or hydrocortisone 200 mg IV immediately and every 4 hours before contrast injection plus diphenhydramine 50 mg IV 1 hour before admission.[44]

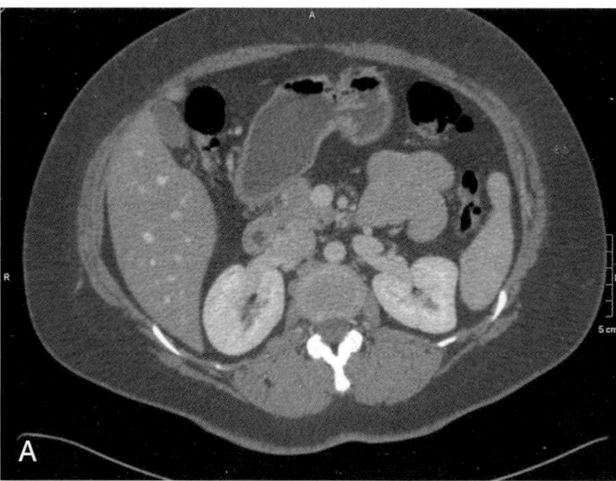

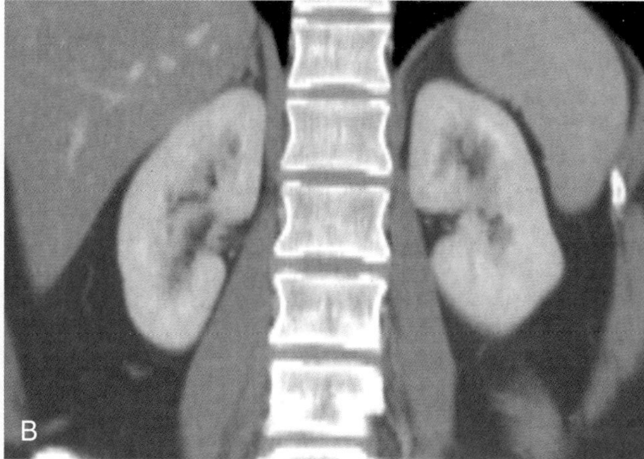

**Fig. 25.12** Computed tomographic scan: normal nephrographic phase. The axial image **(A)** and the coronal image **(B)** demonstrate the homogeneous appearance of the kidneys, with the cortex and medulla no longer differentially enhanced. These images are typically obtained 80 to 120 seconds after the injection of contrast material.

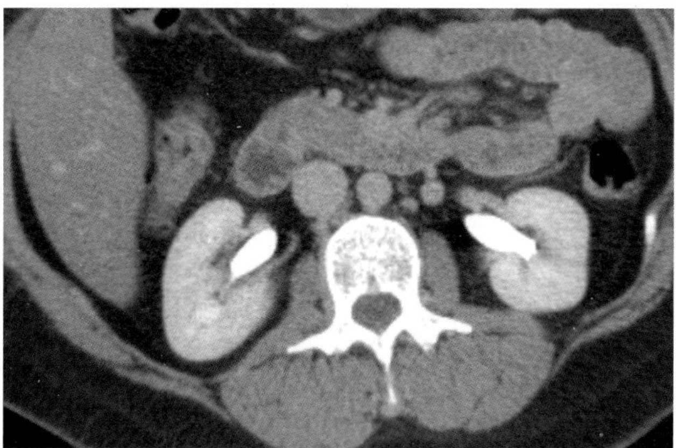

**Fig. 25.13** Computed tomographic scan: normal excretory phase. The calyces and renal pelvis are now easily noted because they are opacified by the excreted contrast material. This scan is obtained 5 to 10 minutes after the injection of contrast material.

Currently, the success rate of this accelerated protocol is based on a large single trial which showed a noninferior result. The overall goal of the premedication strategy is to reduce the risk of contrast reactions through standardized protocols and recognizing that contrast reactions may still happen despite premedication (breakthrough reactions). Most experts believe that the likelihood of a reaction is reduced in patients who are premedicated.[45]

## POSTCONTRAST ACUTE KIDNEY INJURY (PC-AKI) AND CONTRAST-INDUCED NEPHROPATHY (CIN)

There is an ongoing debate around occurrence, causes, screening strategies and management of PC-AKI. Please see Chapters 28 and 29 for a discussion of this topic in the context of the pathophysiology and management of AKI. For clarification, we describe the terms as in the American College of Radiology Manual on contrast media.[45] (v.10.3, https://www.acr.org/-/media/ACR/Files/Clinical-Resources/Contrast_Media.pdf)

PC-AKI.: a deterioration in renal function occurring within 48 hours following intravascular administration of iodinated contrast, regardless of the cause of the worsening of renal function. PC-AKI is a correlative diagnosis.

CIN: a subset of PC-AKI in which the intravascularly administered contrast is the cause of the deterioration of renal function. CIN is a causative diagnosis and is a subgroup of PC-AKI.

Contrast media–induced nephropathy (CIN) is most often qualitatively defined as acute kidney injury (AKI) occurring within 48 hours of exposure to intravascular radiographic contrast material that is not attributable to other causes. However, there is no universally accepted quantitative definition of CIN. The most commonly used definition is a 25% increase in serum creatinine from baseline value or an absolute increase of at least 0.5 mg/dL that appears within 48 hours after contrast administration and is maintained for 2 to 5 days.[46] Importantly, these definitions do not follow the Acute Kidney Injury Network (AKIN)[47] or Kidney Disease: Improving Global Outcomes (KDIGO)[48] definitions of AKI. Lack of uniformity in definition has contributed to significant variation in incidence of CIN reported in the literature. The American College of Radiology therefore proposed using AKIN/KDIGO criteria for a definition of AKI related to intravascular CIN:

The diagnosis of PC-AKI is made if any of the following occurs within 48 hours of contrast injection:

1. Absolute increase in serum creatinine level of 0.3 mg/dL or higher and more than 26.4 μmol/L
2. A percentage increase in serum creatinine level of 50% or higher (1.5-fold above baseline), or
3. Urine output reduced to 0.5 mL/kg/h or less for at least 6 hours

The concept that contrast agents pose serious risks has become a dogma with far-reaching consequences. Yet this belief stems from clinical studies with significant limitations. Inclusion of highly selected patient populations (e.g., those undergoing angiography), poor study design (i.e., uncontrolled case studies), larger volumes of contrast, especially hyperosmolar contrast and use of inconsistent definitions of CIN call into question to what extent the risk for CIN is applicable to the vast majority of people undergoing diagnostic

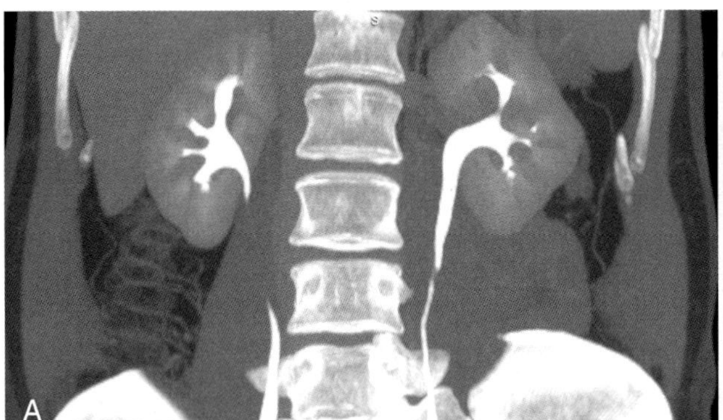

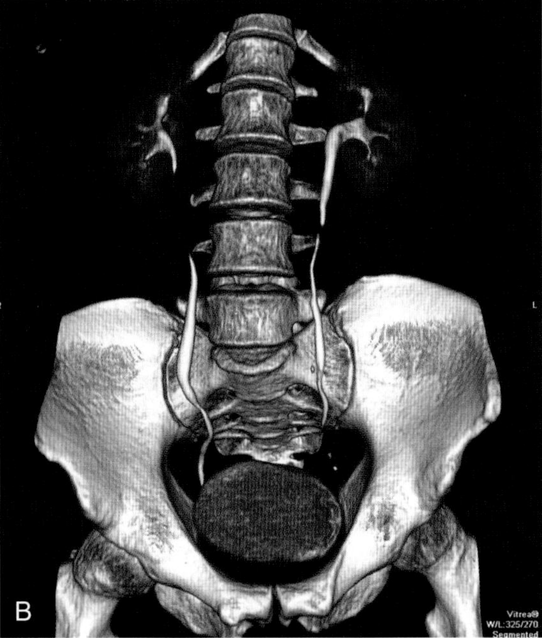

**Fig. 25.14** Computed tomographic urogram: normal findings. The maximum-intensity projection (MIP) image **(A)** and the volume-rendered image **(B)** demonstrate the calyces, renal pelvis, ureters, and bladder. The MIP image is a slab, 15-mm thick, in the coronal plane. The volume-rendered image was taken as the extraneous tissues adjacent to the kidneys were removed, and it highlights the genitourinary tract.

radiology studies.[49] In addition, increased awareness in the last 15 years has led to optimized use of contrast in high-risk individuals. Another factor that has led to confounding data is that a lot of the studies may have referred to two distinct populations—those undergoing cardiac angiography and those undergoing contrast-enhanced CT. The patients undergoing angiography should be assessed separately as the contrast is administered differently. It is injected directly into the arterial system by a catheter which could potentially dislodge thromboemboli. In addition, the contrast bolus to the kidneys is more likely to be concentrated as well as abrupt compared with a peripheral intravenous injection of contrast.[50–52]

There is a relative paucity of controlled studies to evaluate the incidence and causality of CIN. Although these studies are a significant improvement over noncontrolled studies, bias in control group selection within the studies may also have introduced error. Two studies by Davenport et al, and McDonald et al, used prospective propensity matching to correct for potential bias introduced by assigning patients to contrast or noncontrast groups on the basis of factors such as age and the presence of a preexisting low eGFR, other than those which the experiment was designed to test.[53,54] Davenport et al, found that patients with a serum creatinine less than 1.5 mg/dL before CT scan were not at risk for nephropathy.[53] As creatinine levels increased, the risk for AKI after CT scan increased for both groups (contrast group and noncontrast group), but contrast medium administration remained an independent risk factor. In contrast, McDonald et al, concluded that intravenous contrast medium was not associated with increased risk for nephrotoxicity, even in those with preexisting chronic kidney disease (CKD).[54]

The clinical course of patients with PC-AKI and CIN depend on a number of factors including the baseline renal function, coexisting risk factors, medication, and hydration. The usual clinical course (which may be asymptomatic in PC-AKI) is of a transient elevation of serum creatinine within 24 hours of contrast administration, peaking within 96 hours and returning to baseline within 7 to 10 days.[55,56] Although in the vast majority of patients this is transient, many studies have reported that patients with PC-AKI have longer hospital stays, higher mortality and higher incidences of cardiac and neurologic events. However, these studies did not include control groups and some of the mortality and morbidity attributed to CIN in the past may be due to factors not associated with contrast administration.[45]

Because current data cannot definitely refute the existence of CIN, many professional society guidelines advise a conservative approach, and this fact in itself may have contributed to the reduction in observed incidence of CIN in recent years. The European Society of Urogenital Radiology guidelines identify an estimated glomerular filtration rate (eGFR) of 45 mL/min/1.73 $m^2$ as a threshold below which contrast medium poses a risk.[57,58] The Canadian Association of Radiologists suggests that nephropathy risk begins to increase at an eGFR of 45 mL/min/1.73 $m^2$ and increases significantly when the eGFR reaches 30 mL/min/1.73 $m^2$.[59]

The following section provides the protocols used at the University of Southern California Keck School of Medicine for administration of intravenous contrast in adults. These practices were developed based on consensus developed by a department clinical committee and based on review of multiple guidelines from national and international radiology organizations, practices at other academic institutions and advice from colleagues in nephrology and laboratory medicine.

Each patient referral should be considered on an individual basis within the context of this background information, and strict adherence to these guidelines in all cases is discouraged. Physician judgment is paramount.

## SCREENING/EVALUATION OF RISK FACTORS

There have been a number of attempts to identify and isolate risk factors for CIN. These include patient age older than 60 years, history of renal disease (including dialysis, transplant, renal surgery), history of diabetes, hypertension and heart failure; however, volume depletion or renal hypoperfusion are the most significant risk factors.[59–61]

## CONTRAST ADMINISTRATION IN PATIENTS WITH ELEVATED CREATININE LEVEL

The decision to proceed with contrast administration in patients with an eGFR below 45 mL/min/1.73 $m^2$ should always be a matter of clinical judgment. If contrast administration is considered essential, the following options should be considered:

HYDRATION or VOLUME EXPANSION is one of the most important methods for decreasing the incidence of CIN. Broad consensus exists that volume expansion reduces the risk for CIN. Adequate volume expansion improves renal blood flow, induces diuresis with dilution of contrast material within the tubules, reduces the activation of the renin angiotensin aldosterone system, suppresses the secretion of antidiuretic hormone, and minimizes reductions in the renal production of endogenous vasodilators such as nitric oxide and prostacyclin. The hydration protocol is not as important as the fact that some form of hydration is administered; however, controversy exists about the route of hydration and the composition. For example, intravenous hydration has not been proven superior to oral hydration and the use of intravenous sodium chloride versus sodium bicarbonate are also debated. In addition, the practicality of routine use of parenteral hydration protocols in an outpatient setting is questionable.

ORAL VERSUS INTRAVENOUS HYDRATION: Studies directly comparing intravenous with oral hydration are sparse because most of the hydration studies used intravenous hydration and included other forms of therapy for prevention of CIN. One study, Preparation for Angiography in Renal Dysfunction (PREPARED), showed no significant difference between outpatient oral hydration and inpatient intravenous hydration.[62] However, another study by Trivedi et al, favored intravenous hydration over oral hydration.[63] This study was limited by lack of an objective measurement of oral volume intake in the unrestricted oral hydration group. A study comparing oral fluids (1100 mL) versus intravenous fluids showed no difference in the incidence of CIN in patients with mild CKD.[64] KDIGO 2012 recommends volume expansion with intravenous fluids because there are currently not many studies showing oral volume expansion is as effective as intravenous volume expansion.[65] Because intravenous administration allows certainty of volume of hydration and may be achieved more rapidly, intravenous hydration is suggested when practical.[66]

SODIUM BICARBONATE VERSUS SALINE: The use of sodium bicarbonate instead of sodium chloride has been advocated as the resulting urinary alkalinization reduces the generation of harmful free radicals and may also increase urine flow. Several clinical trials and meta-analyses suggest that sodium bicarbonate provides equal or superior protection to isotonic saline.[67–70] However, these results have been subsequently challenged and the recently completed PRESERVE trial concluded that there was no benefit of using sodium bicarbonate in reducing PC-AKI. The 2018 American College of Radiology (ACR) guidelines do not recommend using sodium bicarbonate as a prophylactic measure to reduce the incidence of PC-AKI.[71]

VOLUME EXPANSION PROTOCOLS: The rationale of volume expansion before contrast administration is to reduce the possible risk of CIN, although the ideal route and volume of hydration is uncertain.[45] Studies have recommended that optimal hydration with intravenous normal saline is 1 to 1.5 mL/kg/h for at least 6 hours before and after contrast, in patients who are not at risk for volume overload. Although these protocols are impractical in the outpatient setting, they should be implemented for inpatients after discussion with the referring clinician, with particular attention to volume load and cardiac function. An alternative proposed intravenous volume expansion protocol (using either isotonic saline or sodium bicarbonate) is 3 mL/kg/h for 1 hour or 1 mL/kg/h for 6 hours before the procedure followed by 1 mL/kg/h for 6 hours after the procedure. Additional studies are required to assess whether a single bolus of sodium bicarbonate administered just before contrast medium administration is effective, as Tamura et al, suggested, because this protocol would be extremely useful in daily practice.[72] Due to the logistical complications of performing hydration protocols in an outpatient setting, the following regimen is suggested for outpatients with an eGFR of less than 45 mL/min/1.73 $m^2$: Oral hydration should be strongly encouraged in all such patients and if the patient can tolerate hydration, isotonic saline should be administered before and after the examination, adjusted according to cardiac status. In patients at risk of heart failure, but not in florid heart failure, a safer alternative to active hydration may be to withhold diuretics of the day prior to and/or the day of the contrast examination. If a patient is in overt heart failure it is preferable to delay contrast administration until heart failure is recompensated. Clinical judgment is always required.

USE OF LOW OSMOLAR CONTRAST MEDIA: Iopamidol (Isovue) and iohexol (Omnipaque) are LOCM. Most centers no longer use intravascular HOCM because of the higher incidence of various adverse effects associated with their use. Studies have failed, however, to show a clear advantage of the intravenous isoosmolar agent, iodixanol, over intravenous LOCM with regard to CIN.[71]

DECREASE TOTAL AMOUNT OF CONTRAST ADMINISTERED: It should be noted that robust data supporting a dose-toxicity relationship for intravenous iodinated contrast media administration are lacking. However, limiting volume of contrast injection and frequency in a short period of time is prudent clinical practice.[73]

INCREASE THE AMOUNT OF TIME BETWEEN CONTRAST-ENHANCED STUDIES: It takes approximately 24 hours for the entire administered dose of contrast media to be excreted by the kidneys (if the GFR is normal), so it has long been recommended to avoid intervals of less than 24 hours between studies except in urgent situations. For example, it has been recommended that patients should not receive more than 300 mL of contrast media within 24 hours unless the benefits clearly outweigh the risks.

Little solid data support this recommendation. A 2009 paper from Massachusetts General Hospital, although criticized by some authorities for methodologic issues, supports checking a repeat creatinine level before performing a second contrast media-enhanced CT (CE-CT) examination within 24 hours of a prior CE-CT scan.[68] The 2017 ACR guidelines, however, find there is insufficient evidence to justify this recommendation.[74]

### Nephroprotective Strategies

N-ACETYLCYSTEINE: Multiple randomized controlled trials and meta-analyses have shown conflicting results regarding the utility of acetylcysteine to prevent CIN. It is controversial whether it is truly nephroprotective or simply lowers the serum creatinine level without preventing renal damage. Given the heterogeneity of data, it is difficult to support the administration of acetylcysteine as a proven and effective means by which to prevent CIN.[73,75] More recently, however, there is increasing literature on different pharmacologic measures including ascorbic acid, statins, fenoldopam, and others which require further study.[76]

DISCONTINUE CONCURRENT NEPHROTOXIC DRUGS, IF POSSIBLE

CORRECT ANY UNDERLYING CLINICAL CONDITIONS THAT MAY AFFECT RENAL PERFUSION

## MAGNETIC RESONANCE IMAGING

Like CT, MRI is a computer-based, multiplanar imaging modality. Instead of ionizing radiation, however, electromagnetic radiation is used in MRI. MRI is an alternative to CE-CT, especially in patients with allergy to iodinated contrast material and in patients for whom reduction of radiation exposure is desired, such as pregnant women and children. MRI routinely allows detailed tissue characterization of the kidney and surrounding structures. The properties of physics underlying MRI are complex and are addressed only briefly.

Clinical MRI is based on the interaction of hydrogen ions (protons) and radiofrequency waves in the presence of a strong magnetic field.[77–79] The strong magnetic field, called the *external magnetic field,* is generated by a large-bore, high-field strength magnet. Most magnets in clinical use are superconducting magnets. The magnet strength is measured in teslas (T) and can range from 0.2 to 3 T for clinical imaging and up to 15 T for animal research. Renal imaging is performed best on high-field magnets (1.5–3 T) that allow for higher spatial resolution and faster imaging.

Images of the patient are obtained through a multistep process of energy transfer and signal transmission. When a patient is placed in the magnet, the mobile protons associated with fat and water molecules align longitudinal to the external magnetic field. No signal is obtained unless a resonant radiofrequency pulse is applied to the patient. The radiofrequency pulse causes the mobile protons within the patient to move from a lower, stable energy state to a higher, unstable energy state *(excitation).* When the radiofrequency pulse is removed, the protons return to the lower-energy steady state while emitting frequency transmissions or signals *(relaxation).* In radiologic terms, an external radiofrequency pulse "excites" the protons, causing them to "flip" to a higher energy state. When the radiofrequency pulse is removed, the protons "relax" with emission of a "radio signal." The signals produced during proton relaxation are separated from one another with applied magnetic field gradients. The emitted signals are captured by a receiving coil and reconstructed into images through a complex computerized algorithm: the Fourier transform.[77–79]

Different tissues have different relaxation rates that lead to different levels of signal production or signal intensity. The signal intensity of each tissue is determined by three characteristics:

1. *Proton density of the tissue.* The greater the number of mobile protons, the greater the signal produced by the tissue. For example, a volume of urine has more mobile protons than does the same volume of renal tissue; therefore, urine produces more signal than do the kidneys. Stones have far fewer mobile protons per unit volume and therefore produce little signal.
2. *T1 relaxation time.* The T1 time is how quickly a proton returns to the preexcitation energy state. The shortest T1 times (rapid relaxation) produce the strongest signal.
3. *T2 relaxation time.* The T2 time is how quickly the proton signal decays as a result of nonuniformity of the magnetic field. A nonuniform field accelerates signal decay and leads to signal loss.[77–79]

In MRI, multiple pulse sequences are obtained. A pulse sequence is a set of defined radiofrequency pulses and timing parameters used to obtain image data. These sequences include, but are not limited to, spin echo, gradient echo, inversion recovery, and steady-state free precession. The data are obtained in volumes (voxels), reconstructed as two-dimensional pixels, and displayed in relation to variations in tissue signal intensity (tissue contrast). Tissue contrast, like signal intensity, is determined by proton density and relaxation times. T1 weighting is related to the rate of T1 relaxation and the time allowed for relaxation, also known as the *pulse repetition time* (TR). T2 weighting is related to the rate of T2 relaxation and the time at which the "radio signal" is sampled by the receiver coil, also known as the *echo time* (TE). TR and TE are programmable parameters that can be altered to accentuate T1 and T2 weighting with contrast media.[77–79] For the general observer, T1-weighted sequences have short TR and TE and show simple fluid as black. T2-weighted sequences have long TR and TE and show simple fluid as white (Fig. 25.15).

Many programmable parameters other than TR and TE are used to optimize imaging. These include, but are not limited to, choice of pulse sequence, coil types and gradients, slice orientation and thickness, field of view and matrix, gating to reduce motion, and use of intravenous contrast material. Although many pulse sequences are used in clinical MRI, ultrafast sequences are preferred for renal imaging. These fast sequences can be obtained in less than 30 seconds while the patients hold their breath. The benefits of rapid acquisition include improvement in image quality, as a result of reduction of motion artifact, reduction of total scan time, and the ability to perform dynamic imaging.[80]

MRI is not possible for patients who have certain implanted medical devices, such as most pacemakers, ferromagnetic aneurysm clips, and ferromagnetic stapedial implants. Not all implants or devices cause problems, but knowledge of the type of device is crucial for determining whether the

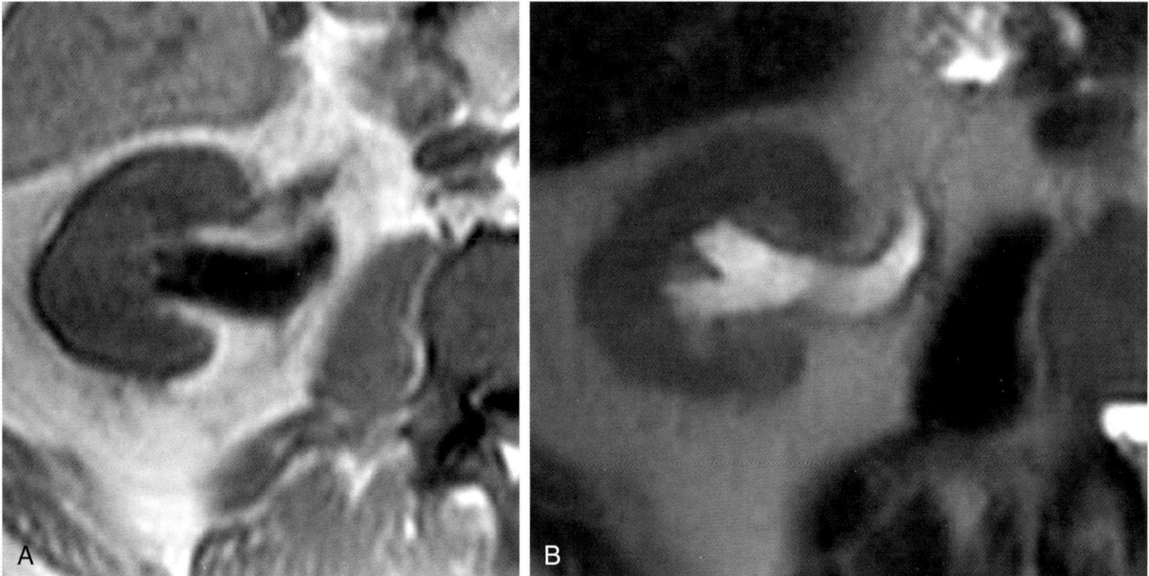


**Fig. 25.15** Normal signal characteristics of simple fluids on magnetic resonance imaging. Urine appears dark on T1-weighted sequences **(A)** and bright on T2-weighted sequences **(B).**

patient can safely enter the magnet.[81] Regularly updated information regarding patient safety and the compatibility of a medical device in the MRI environment may be found at Shellock's MRIsafety.com.[82]

## GADOLINIUM-BASED CONTRAST AGENTS (GBCA) AND NEPHROGENIC SYSTEMIC FIBROSIS

Intravenous contrast material is used routinely in renal imaging because it improves lesion detection and diagnostic accuracy. Gadolinium is a paramagnetic substance that shortens the T1 and T2 relaxation times, resulting in increased signal intensity on T1-weighted images and decreased signal intensity on T2-weighted sequences. The pharmacokinetics and enhancement patterns of intravenous gadolinium-based contrast agents (GBCA) used in renal imaging are similar to those of iodinated contrast agents used for IVU and CT examinations, with GBCA typically eliminated by the kidneys. There are a few agents with some amount of liver excretion. Unlike iodinated contrast agents, the dose response to GBCA is nonlinear; the signal intensity increases at low concentrations and then decreases at higher concentrations. Hence, the collecting systems, ureters, and bladder first brighten and then darken on T1-weighted sequences as the gadolinium concentration within the urine increases.

GBCA have been approved for parenteral use since the 1980s and are generally well tolerated with a good safety profile. Although most GBCA are clinically interchangeable, they can be differentiated on the basis of molecular stability, viscosity, and osmolality. GBCA can be divided into three categories based on molecular configuration: nonionic linear, ionic linear, and macrocyclic (Table 25.1). Macrocyclic agents have the greatest kinetic stability. Adverse reactions occur in approximately 0.07% to 2.4% of cases.[83] Minor reactions include coldness, warmth or pain at the injection site, nausea, vomiting, headache, paresthesia, dizziness, and itching. Rash, hives, or urticaria occurs in 0.004% to 0.07% of cases; and severe, life-threatening reactions occur in approximately 0.001% to 0.01%. Risk factors for adverse reactions include a history of prior reaction to GBCA, where rates are at an eightfold higher risk, and asthma, as well as other allergies, where rates are reported as high as 3.7%.[84] If a patient has had a prior adverse reaction to GBCA, premedication with antihistamines and corticosteroids is recommended (same premedication regimen as discussed for iodinated contrast media).

**Table 25.1 Classification of Gadolinium-Based Contrast Agents Relative to Risk of Nephrogenic Systemic Fibrosis**

|  |  |
|---|---|
| Group I: associated with greatest number of nephrogenic systemic fibrosis (NSF) cases | Gadodiamide (Omniscan®)<br>Gadopentetate dimeglumine (Magnevist®)<br>Gadoversetamide (OptiMARK®) |
| Group II: associated with few/none unconfounded NSF cases | Gadobenate dimeglumine (MultiHance®) Gadoteridol (ProHance®)<br>Gadobutrol (Gadavist®/Gadovist)<br>Gadoterate acid (Dotarem®) |
| Group III: data remain limited regarding NSF risk | Gadoxetic acid (Eovist®/Primovis) |

Modified from the ACR contrast manual 10.3, https://www.acr.org/Clinical-Resources/Contrast-Manual

GBCA are considered to have no nephrotoxicity at the approved doses used for clinical MRI.[85–88] Because there have been some case reports of nephrotoxicity with high doses of intravenous GBCA in populations at high risk (moderate to severe kidney injury), the use of GBCA in conventional angiography is not recommended.[89,90] GBCA may interfere with serum calcium and magnesium measurements, especially in patients with renal insufficiency.[91] GBCA do not cause an actual reduction in serum calcium level; GBCA interfere with standard colorimetric methods of measuring serum calcium. As with iodinated contrast material, hemodialysis filters GBCA effectively, and dialysis is therefore recommended immediately after use of contrast material in patients already on hemodialysis.[92]

It is now widely accepted that there is an association between exposure to GBCA and nephrogenic systemic fibrosis (NSF), a rare, multiorgan, fibrosing condition that involves primarily the skin and subcutaneous tissues, including development of symmetric, dark red patches or papules on the skin, swelling of extremities, and thickening of skin that sometimes is described as "woody" and like an "orange peel"[93] (see also Chapter 58). Skin thickening can inhibit motion of joints, leading to contractures and immobility. Burning, itching, or severe pain in involved areas or "deep bone pain" in hips and ribs have been described. Other structures affected include the lungs, esophagus, skeletal muscles, and heart leading to restriction of function, and although NSF is not by itself a cause of death, the resulting restriction of function may contribute to death.[94] Symptoms may develop over a period of days to months; however, in approximately 5% of patients, the course may be rapidly progressive.[94] Diagnosis is confirmed by full-thickness skin biopsy, which reveals thickened collagen bundles, mucin deposition, and proliferation of fibroblasts and elastic fibers without signs of inflammation. There appears to be no predilection for gender or ethnicity. Although no treatment is known to be consistently successful, improving renal function appears to slow or stop the progression of NSF.[94]

NSF was first described in 1997. In 2006 several groups presented a possible causal relationship between the use of GBCA in patients with advanced renal disease and NSF.[95–97] This was quickly followed by published warnings and restrictive guidelines from the U.S. Food and Drug Administration (FDA), European Medicines Agency (EMA), and the ACR. These restrictive guidelines have resulted in a drastic reduction in the number of reported cases. Since 1988, more than 300 million patients have been exposed to GBCA; however, less than 600 cases of NSF have been reported in the literature. The patients at highest risk are those with severely impaired renal function, both acute and chronic. Based on data prior to the institution of restrictive use recommendations, the risk for developing NSF in patients with end-stage and severe chronic kidney disease was estimated to be from 1% to 7%, and higher with acute kidney injury.[74,98–100] The duration and underlying cause of the kidney disease appears to be irrelevant. The FDA, EMA, and ACR continue to update recommendations for the use of all classes of GBCA in high-risk patients as new information and products become available.[45,57,94,101,102]

Recently, residual gadolinium has been found in neural tissue of patients who have received multiple doses of GBCA over their lifetimes. To date, no known adverse clinical consequences have been found[103–107]; however, because the clinical significance and health implications of neural tissue deposition are unknown and relatively undefined, rigorous investigation has been initiated. Emerging data indicate that the amount of accumulated gadolinium varies with chelate stability, gadolinium deposition in the brain may be dose dependent, and gadolinium deposition has been found in patients with no evidence of kidney or liver disease.[105–109]

The most current 2018 recommendations for the use of GDCA are as follows[45,104]:

1. There are no absolute contraindications to the use of GBCA intravenously. Therefore there should be careful consideration of the clinical benefit of using GBCA for the diagnosis and treatment against the potential risks, known and unknown, especially if the patient may undergo multiple contrast-enhanced examinations over their lifetime or if the patient has acute kidney injury.
2. Screen for renal disease before the use of a GBCA. Patients who may be at high risk include those with a history of renal disease (prior dialysis, renal transplant, single kidney, kidney surgery, renal cancer), diabetes, and/or hypertension requiring medical therapy. If an outpatient is high risk for renal disease and has no prior eGFR, eGFR should be obtained. If the patient has eGFR obtained within 6 weeks of the exam, eGFR does not need to be repeated, unless the prior result was less than 45 mL/min/1.73m.[2] Outpatients with known eGFR values less than 45 mL/min/1.73 $m^2$ and inpatients should have eGFR obtained within two days of the MRI study. Estimated GFR is not helpful in patients on dialysis (any type) or in patients with acute kidney injury; therefore eGFR may not be necessary to obtain prior to the MRI study.
3. Severe renal impairment (eGFR ≤30 mL/min/1.73 $m^2$): There is a possibility that NSF may occur in this patient population; therefore contrast should be used in these patients only after careful consideration, including consideration of alternative imaging. If contrast is deemed necessary, Group II agents are recommended (see Table 25.1). Group I agents are contraindicated. Informed consent for contrast administration is not mandatory but may be obtained at the discretion of individual centers.
4. If a patient is on dialysis, determine whether the patient is a candidate for contrast-enhanced (CE) CT rather than GBCA-enhanced MRI. If MRI is to be performed, group II agents should be used because group I agents are contraindicated. Elective GBCA-enhanced MRI examinations should be performed as closely before hemodialysis as possible. Although GBCA are effectively removed with hemodialysis, no published report has proved that early dialysis prevents the development of NSF.[102] It is not recommended to start hemodialysis on patients not already on hemodialysis for the prevention of NSF. Peritoneal dialysis has not been adequately studied; however, switching to hemodialysis is not recommended after GBCA-enhanced MRI in these patients.
5. Patients with stable CKD 3 and patients with CDK 1 or 2 (stable eGFR >30 mL/min/1.73 $m^2$) do not require special precautions and may receive GBCA per routine protocol.
6. All contrast material should be avoided in patients with AKI due to increased risk for developing NSF. Group II GBCA should be administered only if absolutely necessary. Group 1 agents are contraindicated.

For further information regarding the different FDA-approved Gd-C agents, including their properties, how these properties may affect safety profiles, and updated recommendations to clinical practice, please refer to "ACR manual on contrast media, Version 10.3",[45] the "ACR Guidance Document for

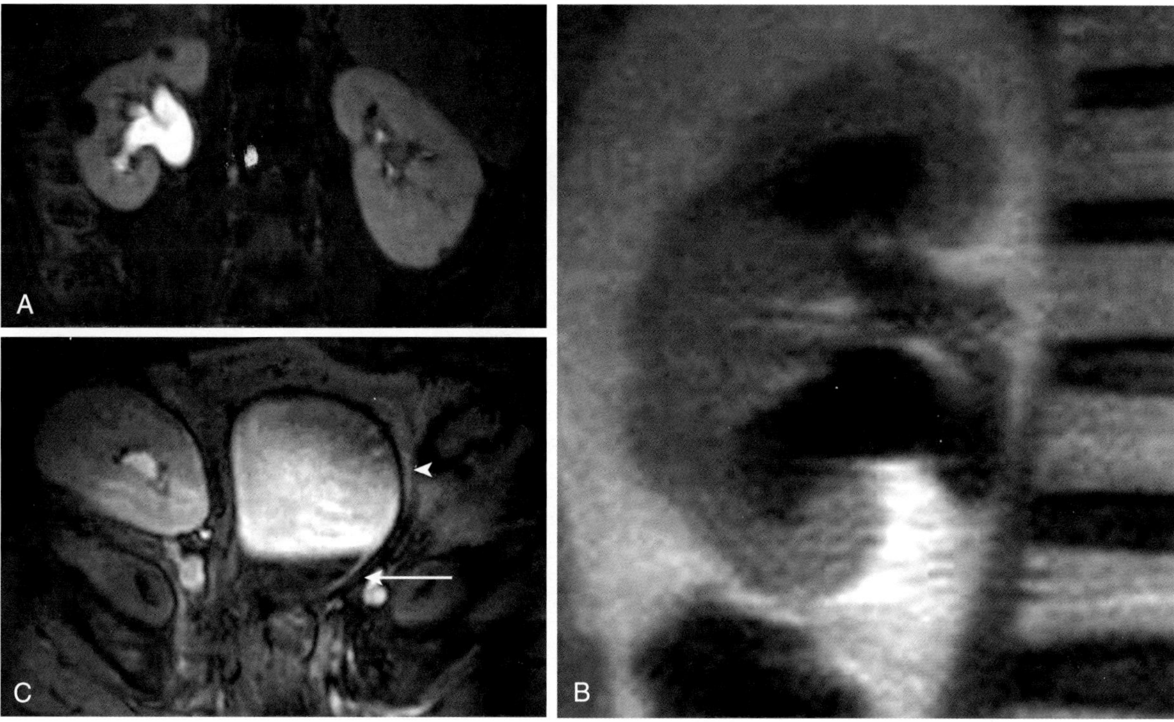

**Fig. 25.16** Paramagnetic effects of gadolinium on urine. **A,** Coronal T1-weighted image from a magnetic resonance urogram (MRU) demonstrates enhancement of the urine in the collection system. **B,** Coronal T2-weighted image from an MRU demonstrates low signal intensity of urine in the collecting system secondary to effects of gadolinium. **C,** Axial T1-weighted, delayed image after contrast medium enhancement demonstrates layering of contrast material. The denser, more concentrated gadolinium is dark *(arrow).* The less concentrated gadolinium is brighter and layers above *(arrowhead).*

Safe MR Practices,"[101] and the FDA Drug Safety website (https://www.fda.gov/Drugs/DrugSafety).

## DIAGNOSTIC MAGNETIC RESONANCE IMAGING TECHNIQUE

Routine MRI evaluation of the kidneys includes axial and coronal T1-weighted and T2-weighted sequences. Dynamic contrast media-enhanced T1-weighted sequences with fat suppression are also routinely obtained. Due to excellent tissue differentiation provided by MRI, the renal cortex and medullary pyramids are easily differentiated on sequences that are not enhanced by contrast media. On T1-weighted sequences the renal cortex has higher signal intensity than do the medullary pyramids. On T2-weighted sequences the renal cortex has lower signal intensity than do the medullary pyramids (Fig. 25.16). With kidney injury, this corticomedullary differentiation disappears.[45,110] Urine, like water, normally appears black on T1-weighted sequences and white on T2-weighted sequences (Fig. 25.15 and Fig. 25.17).

CE-MRI allows for dynamic evaluation of the kidneys and surrounding structures. Serial acquisitions are obtained after bolus injection of Gd-C (0.1–0.2 mmol per kilogram of body weight) at 2 mL/sec.[111,112] The injection should be administered by means of an automatic, MRI-compatible power injector to ensure accuracy of the timed bolus, including volume and rate of injection.[112,113] The corticomedullary-arterial phase (approximately 20 seconds after injection) is best for evaluating the arterial structures and corticomedullary differentiation. In the nephrographic phase (70–90 seconds after injection), tumor detection is maximized, and the renal veins and surrounding structures are best demonstrated (Fig. 25.18). Imaging can be performed in any plane, but the coronal plane is used most frequently for dynamic imaging because it allows imaging of the kidneys, ureters, vessels, and surrounding structures in the fewest number of images. The characteristics of parenchymal enhancement are similar to those observed on CE-CT.

The blood vessels can be variable in signal intensity on routine MRI that is not enhanced by contrast media, ranging from white to black. This is due to many factors, including, but not limited to, flow-related parameters, location and orientation of the imaged vessel, and choice of pulse sequence. By taking advantage of some of these factors, diagnostic angiography and venography may be performed without the use of intravenous contrast; these sequences are sometimes called "bright-blood" sequences. Although contrast media-enhanced magnetic resonance angiography (CE-MRA) remains the preferred method of vascular imaging, high-quality MRA that is not enhanced by contrast media has regained popularity because of the advancement in MR hardware and imaging sequences, as well as the risk of NSF in patients with poor renal function. MRA not enhanced by contrast media is particularly attractive for evaluating the renal arteries in patients with severe renal dysfunction or those with a relative contraindication for CE-CMA. The most robust sequences are based on inversion recovery, and balanced steady-state free precession techniques.[114,115] Older, less robust techniques include time-of-flight MRA, which is based on flow-related enhancement, and phase-contrast MRA, which is based on velocity and direction of flow. Phase-contrast

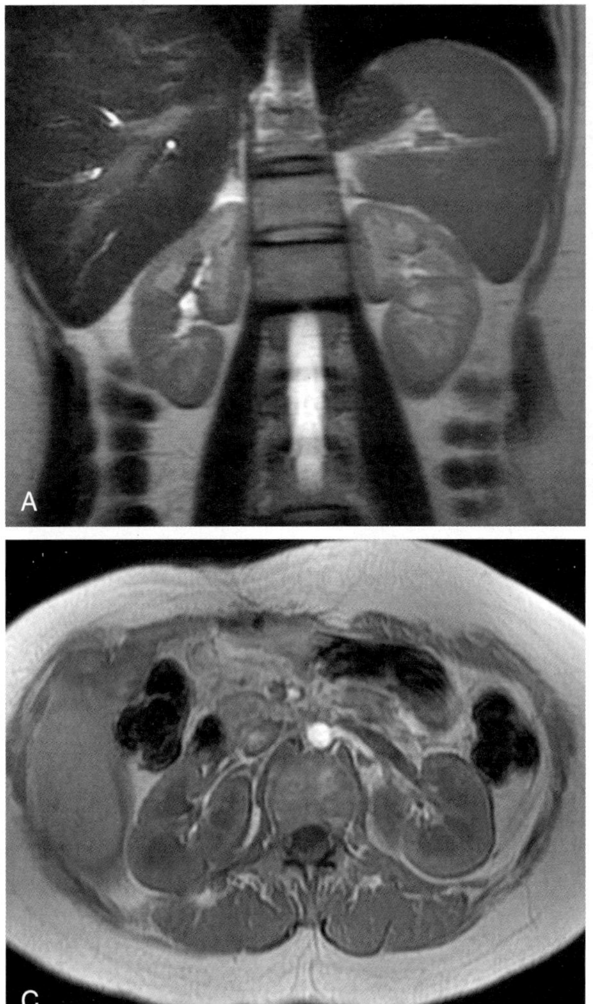


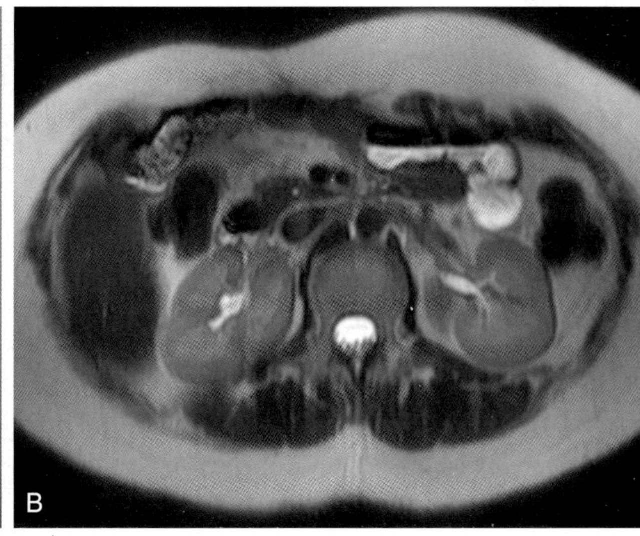


**Fig. 25.17** Normal appearance of corticomedullary differentiation on magnetic resonance imaging. Coronal **(A)** and axial **(B)** T2-weighted images demonstrate decreased signal intensity of the renal cortex in relation to the medullary pyramids. Axial T1-weighted image (**C**) demonstrates increased signal intensity of the renal cortex in relation to the medullary pyramids.

MRA can be used in conjunction with CE-MRA to detect turbulent flow and high velocities associated with stenoses. Unlike MRA that is not enhanced by contrast media, CE-MRA minimizes flow-related enhancement and motion. The success of CE-MRA depends on the T1-shortening properties of gadolinium, which allow for faster imaging, increased coverage, and improved resolution.[77,116] Accurate timing of the bolus injection is critical in CE-MRA. The time at which the bolus arrives at the renal arteries may be determined with a bolus injection of 1 mL of Gd-C, followed by a saline flush. A three-dimensional T1-weighted gradient-echo MRI pulse sequence is then obtained in the coronal plane during the injection of approximately 15 to 20 mL of Gd-C at 2 mL/sec, timed to capture the arterial phase.[111,112] Sequential three-dimensional sequences are obtained to capture the venous phase (magnetic resonance venography). The data sets can be postprocessed into multiple formats, improving ease and accuracy of interpretation (Fig. 25.19).[117–119]

Magnetic resonance urography (MRU) consists of protocols tailored to the evaluation of the renal collecting system and the disease found there. MRU can be performed with heavily T2-weighted sequences, in which urine provides the intrinsic contrast, or with contrast media-enhanced T1-weighted sequences, which mimic conventional IVU and CTU. Heavily T2-weighted sequences are most useful in patients with dilated collecting systems, in whom all water-filled structures are bright (Fig. 25.20), and in patients with impaired renal excretion, in whom contrast media-enhanced urography is most limited. Unfortunately, without adequate distension of the collecting system, T2-weighted evaluation is limited. Although a good morphologic examination, T2-weighted urography is ultimately limited by a lack of functional information. For example, T2-weighted urography cannot reliably differentiate between an obstructed system and an ectatic collecting system (Fig. 25.21).[120] Contrast media-enhanced T1-weighted urography in the excretory phase is superior to T2-weighted urography because both structure and function can be evaluated.[120–122]

T2-weighted and contrast media-enhanced T1-weighted sequences are complementary and are frequently obtained together as part of a complete MRU examination. In patients with nondilated systems, both techniques require hydration and furosemide for adequate distension of the renal collecting system.[120,123] Typical MRU starts with a coronal, heavily T2-weighted sequence in which simple fluid (urine, cerebrospinal fluid, ascites) is bright and all other tissues are dark (see Fig. 25.20). This rapid breath-hold sequence takes less than 5 seconds to obtain and is presented as a urogram-like image. The T2-weighted sequence is used as an initial survey of fluid within the collecting system. Low-dose

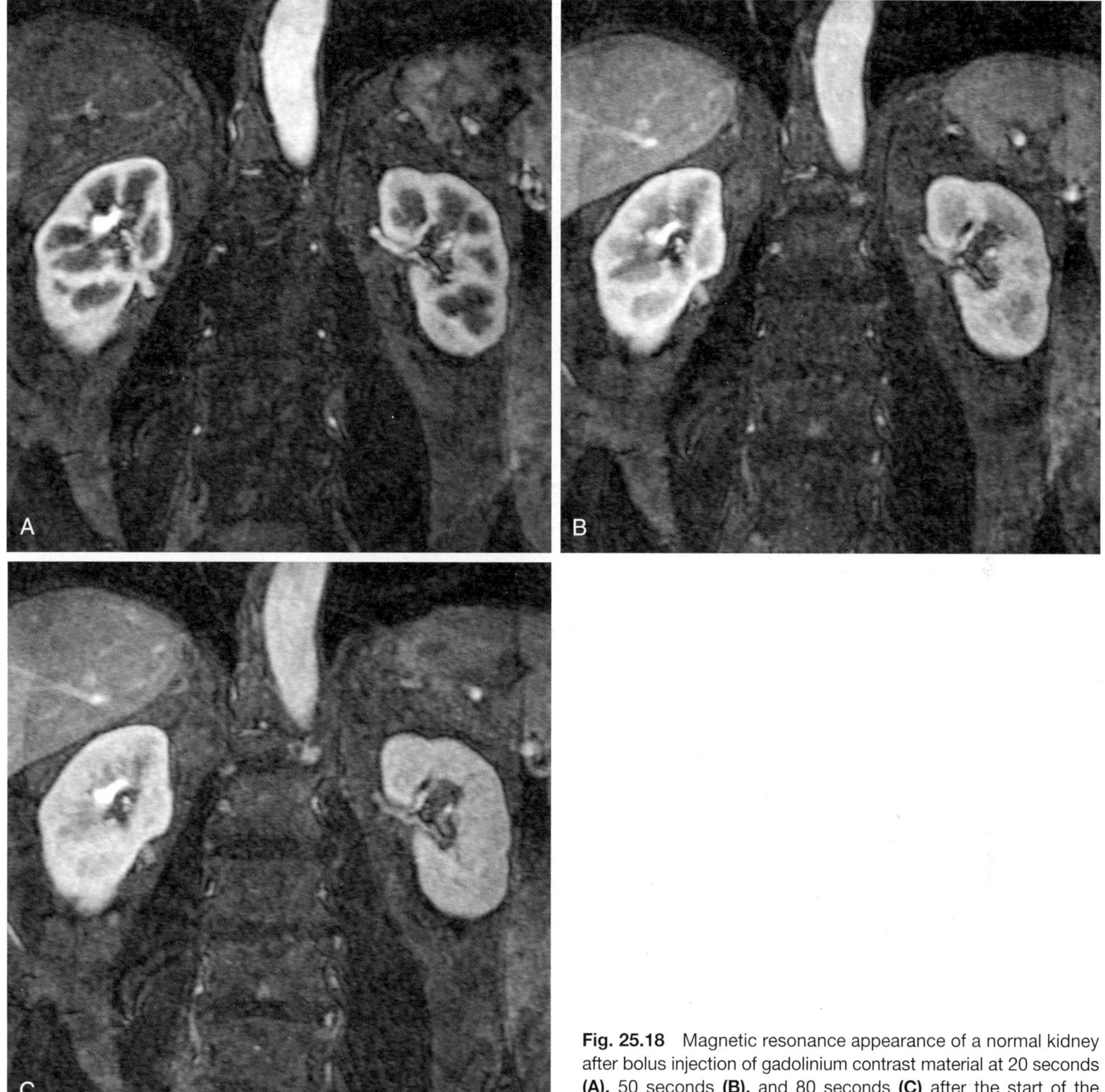


**Fig. 25.18** Magnetic resonance appearance of a normal kidney after bolus injection of gadolinium contrast material at 20 seconds **(A),** 50 seconds **(B),** and 80 seconds **(C)** after the start of the injection.

furosemide (0.1 mg per kilogram of body weight; maximum dose, 10 mg) may be administered intravenously in selected cases, 30 to 60 seconds before the intravenous administration of Gd-C (0.1 mmol/kg).[121,122] Furosemide is given to increase urine volume and dilute the Gd-C within the collecting system.[121,123] Coronal, three-dimensional, contrast media-enhanced T1-weighted sequences are obtained with the same technique as in renal CE-MRA, in the corticomedullary-arterial phase, nephrographic phase, and excretory phase (see Fig. 25.20).[122] Additional sequences may be obtained in any plane to better evaluate suspected pathologic conditions.

By combining renal MRI and MRU, the clinician can obtain a comprehensive morphologic and functional evaluation of the urinary tract. MRU helps to accurately evaluate the upper urinary tract and is useful in the evaluation of anatomic anomalies, including duplications, ureteropelvic obstruction, anomalous crossing vessels, and ureteroceles[123,124] (Fig. 25.22). Obstructive disease is well evaluated regardless of whether the cause is intrinsic or extrinsic to the collecting system.

## FUNCTIONAL MAGNETIC RESONANCE IMAGING OF THE KIDNEY

MRI is suited for measurement of various aspects of renal function, given the role of the kidney in fluid regulation. Techniques for the evaluation of renal function include dynamic contrast media-enhanced MR renography, diffusion-weighted imaging (DWI), and blood oxygen level-dependent (BOLD) MRI. Dynamic contrast media-enhanced MR renography is a contrast media-enhanced sequence in which dynamic images are obtained during the 7 to 10 minutes after administration of intravenous contrast material; tissue signal intensities are converted to tissue gadolinium concentrations, and these

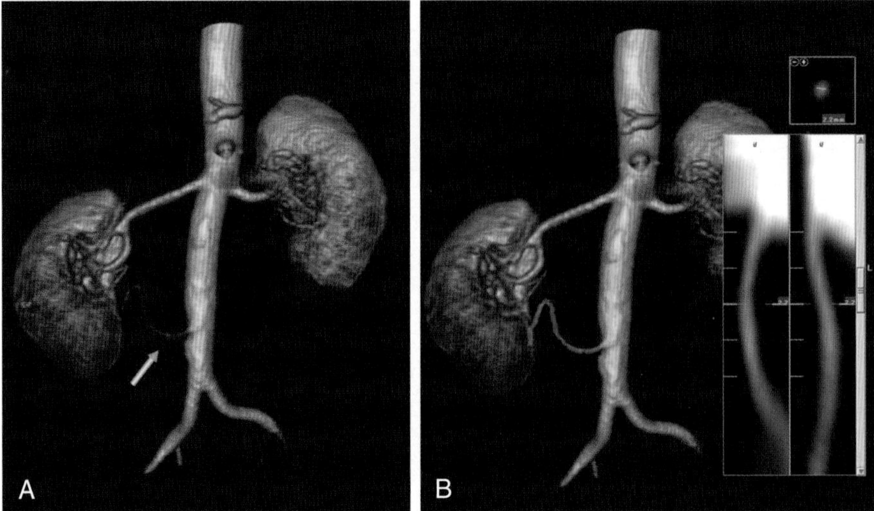


**Fig. 25.19** Magnetic resonance angiogram reconstructed with three-dimensional software. **A,** Visualization of a small accessory right renal artery *(arrow)* is excellent. **B,** The accessory artery is depicted in a way to make more accurate luminal measurements.

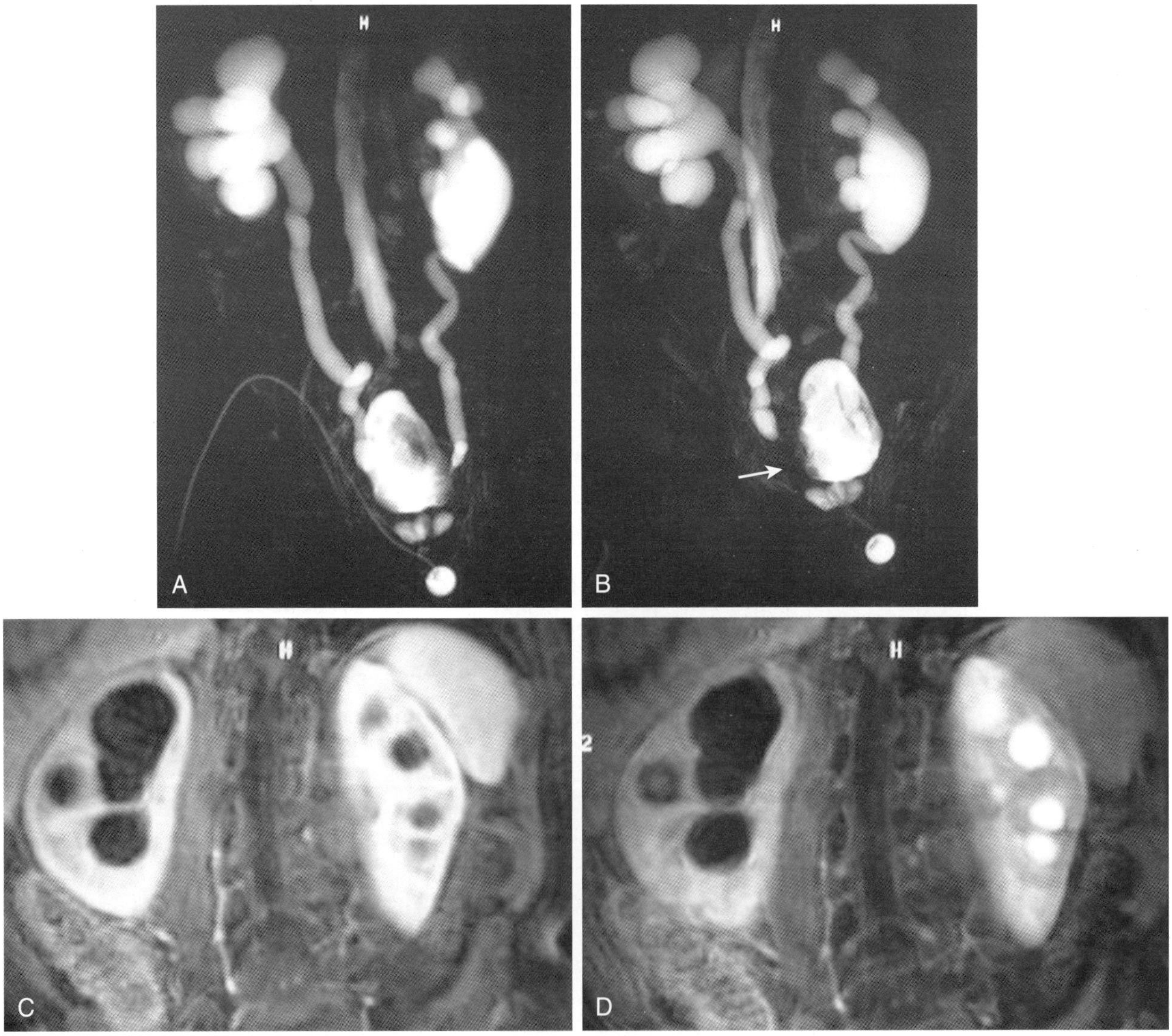

**Fig. 25.20** Bilateral hydronephrosis secondary to bladder tumor. **A** and **B,** Heavily T2-weighted magnetic resonance urograms (MRUs) demonstrate bilateral hydronephrosis and hydroureter caused by bladder mass *(arrow).* **C,** Contrast medium-enhanced MRU in the nephrographic phase demonstrates asymmetric enhancement of the kidneys. **D,** MRU in the excretory phase demonstrates asymmetric excretion of gadolinium. There is no excretion on the right as demonstrated by unenhanced (dark) urine within the collecting system.

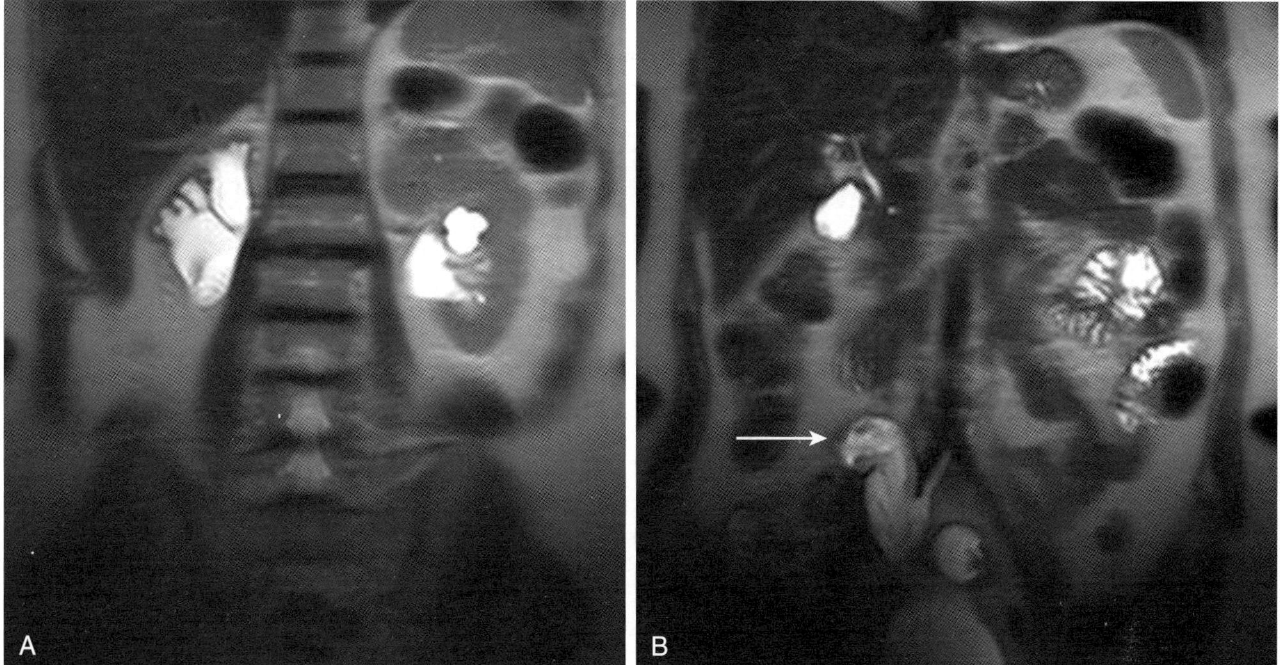


**Fig. 25.21** **A** and **B,** Coronal T2-weighted images demonstrate right renal atrophy and dilation of the right collecting system in a patient who had undergone bladder resection and ilioconduit reconstruction *(arrow)*. On these static images, it is difficult to differentiate between an obstructed system and a nonobstructed system. The patient had pelvocaliectasis without obstruction, demonstrated on the contrast medium-enhanced portion of the examination.

values are plotted against time. Current clinical applications include the evaluation of the renal artery stenosis, both with and without the use of angiotensin-converting enzyme (ACE) inhibitors, functional urinary obstruction, and the evaluation of early postoperative renal transplant dysfunction, to distinguish acute rejection from acute tubular necrosis. What prevents widespread clinical use, however, is the lack of consensus on optimal imaging technique and methods of data analysis.[125]

DWI is based on the Brownian motion of water molecules in tissue and is a noncontrast MRI technique that is used for both structural and functional imaging. Initial experience with DWI has yielded reproducible information on renal function, with the possibility of determining the degree of dysfunction.[126] No large studies have been performed, and further research is required before the usefulness of DWI is confirmed. Animal research is being performed with the hope of using noninvasive DWI as a tool for monitoring early renal graft rejection after transplantation.[127]

BOLD MRI is a noninvasive technique to estimate intrarenal oxygenation.[125] Various researchers use this technique to explore renal artery stenosis, renal transplant dysfunction, and diabetic nephropathy. Sadowski et al,[128] demonstrated the feasibility of using BOLD MRI to evaluate the oxygen status of renal transplants and to detect the presence of acute rejection. They concluded that BOLD MRI may differentiate acute rejection from normal function and acute tubular necrosis, but further research is required.

## NUCLEAR MEDICINE

Scintigraphy offers imaging-based diagnostic information on renal structure and function.[129] Many single-photon radiotracers have long been in routine clinical use in renal scintigraphy; they are tailored to provide physiologic information complementing the primarily anatomic and structural-based imaging modalities, such as US, CT, and MRI. With the rapid expansion of PET and hybrid structural-functional imaging systems such as PET-CT, additional unprecedented opportunities have developed for quantitative imaging evaluation of renal diseases in clinical medicine and research.[127] Scintigraphy, including PET, makes a unique contribution to the imaging evaluation of renal structure and function. The common radiopharmaceuticals used in renal scintigraphy are described first.

## RADIOPHARMACEUTICALS

### Technetium 99M-Labeled Diethylenetriaminepentaacetic Acid

Technetium 99m-labeled diethylenetriaminepentaacetic acid ($^{99m}$Tc-DTPA) is a common agent for assessing GFR. The ideal agent for measuring GFR would be cleared only by glomerular filtration and would not be secreted or reabsorbed. $^{99m}$Tc-DTPA satisfies the first requirement but has variable degrees of protein binding, which deviate its kinetics from an ideal agent such as inulin. For a 20-mCi (740-MBq) dose, the radiation exposures of the kidneys and the urinary bladder are 1.8 and 2.3 rad, respectively.[130]

### Iodine 131-Labeled Ortho-Iodohippurate

The mechanisms underlying renal clearance of iodine 131-labeled ortho-iodohippurate ($^{131}$I-ortho-iodohippurate) are GFR (approximately 20%) and tubular secretion (approximately 80%). $^{131}$I-ortho-iodohippurate is an acceptable alternative to *p*-aminohippuric acid (PAH) for determining

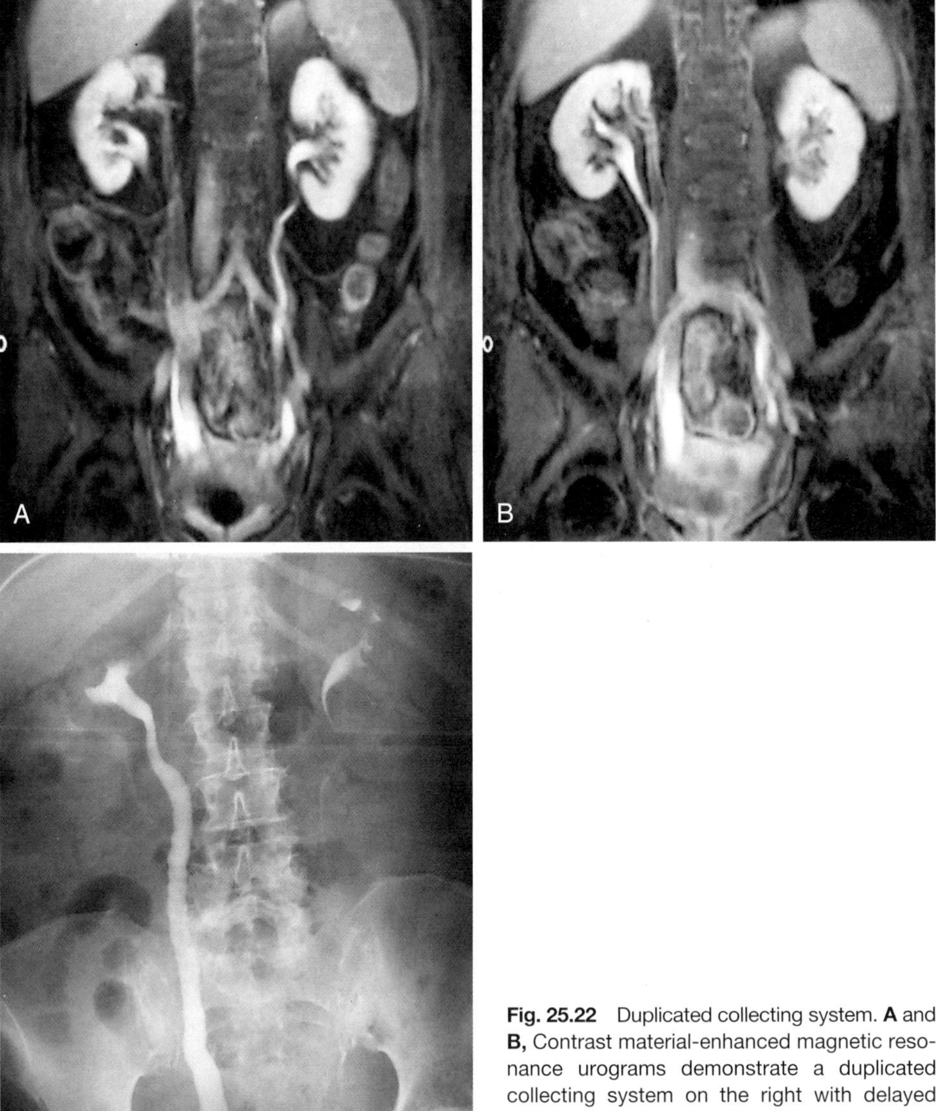


**Fig. 25.22** Duplicated collecting system. **A** and **B,** Contrast material-enhanced magnetic resonance urograms demonstrate a duplicated collecting system on the right with delayed excretion of the upper pole moiety. **C,** Obstruction of the upper pole moiety is confirmed on intravenous urogram.

renal plasma flow (RPF), although the amount cleared is 15% lower than that of PAH. PAH is not entirely cleared by the kidneys; approximately 10% of arterial PAH remains in the renal venous blood. Therefore $^{131}$I-ortho-iodohippurate helps measure effective RPF. The efficiency of tubular extraction of $^{131}$I-ortho-iodohippurate is 90%, and there is no hepatobiliary excretion. Ortho-iodohippurate may also be labeled with iodine 123, which not only provides urinary kinetics equivalent to those provided by iodine 131 but also enables improved image quality because the administered dose is typically larger, in view of its more favorable profile of radiation exposure. For a 300-μCi (11.1-MBq) dose of $^{131}$I-ortho-iodohippurate, the radiation exposures of the kidneys and the urinary bladder are 0.02 and 1.4 rad, respectively. A few drops of nonradioactive iodine (e.g., saturated solution of potassium iodide) administered orally help minimize the thyroid uptake of free iodine 131.[130]

### Technetium 99M-Labeled Mercaptoacetyltriglycine

Technetium 99m-labeled mercaptoacetyltriglycine ($^{99m}$Tc-MAG3) has properties similar to those of $^{131}$I-ortho-iodohippurate but has significant advantages of better image quality and less radiation exposure. The tubular extraction fraction of $^{99m}$Tc-MAG3 is lower than that of $^{131}$I-ortho-iodohippurate, at approximately 60% to 70%. Also, hepatobiliary excretion is approximately 3%, which increases with renal insufficiency. Despite these features, however, $^{99m}$Tc-MAG3 is commonly used in scintigraphic evaluation of renal function. For a 10-mCi (370-MBq) dose, the radiation exposures of the kidneys and the urinary bladder are 0.15 and 4.4 rad, respectively.[130]

### Technetium 99M-Labeled Dimercaptosuccinic Acid

Technetium 99m-labeled dimercaptosuccinic acid ($^{99m}$Tc-DMSA) localizes to the renal cortex at high concentration and has a slow urinary excretion rate. Approximately 50%

of the injected dose accumulates in the renal cortex in 1 hour. The tracer is bound to the renal proximal tubular cells. In view of the high retention of $^{99m}$Tc-DMSA in the renal cortex, it has become useful for imaging of the renal parenchyma. For a 6-mCi (222-MBq) dose, the radiation exposures of the kidneys and the urinary bladder are 3.78 and 0.42 rad, respectively.[130]

#### Fluorine 18 2-Fluoro-2-Deoxy-D-Glucose

Fluorine 18 2-fluoro-2-deoxy-D-glucose (FDG) is the most common positron-labeled radiotracer in PET. FDG is a modified form of glucose in which the hydroxyl group in the 2′ position is replaced by the fluorine 18 positron emitter. FDG accumulates in cells in proportion to glucose metabolism. Cell membrane glucose transporters facilitate the transport of glucose and FDG across the cell membrane. Both glucose and FDG are phosphorylated in the 6′ position by the hexokinase. The conversion of glucose-6-phosphate or FDG-6-phosphate back to glucose or FDG, respectively, is affected by the enzyme phosphatase. In most tissues, including cancer cells, there is little phosphatase activity. FDG-6-phosphate cannot undergo further conversions and is therefore trapped in the cell.

FDG is excreted in the urine. The typical FDG dose is 0.144 mCi/kg (minimum, 1 mCi; maximum, 20 mCi). The urinary bladder wall receives the highest radiation dose from FDG.[128,131] The radiation dose depends on the excretion rate, the varying size of the bladder, the bladder volume at the time of FDG administration, and an activity curve of estimated bladder time. For a typical 15-mCi dose of FDG and voiding at 1 hour after tracer injection, the average estimated radiation dose absorbed by the adult bladder wall is 3.3 rad (0.22 rad/mCi).[132] The doses absorbed by other organs are between 0.75 and 1.28 rad (0.050–0.085 rad/mCi); the average dose absorbed is 1.0 rad.[133] Renal failure may alter the FDG biodistribution, which may necessitate reduction of dose or image acquisition time after tracer administration, or both.[134] Specifically, in patients with suspected renal failure (blood serum creatinine level in excess of 1.1 mg/dL), the FDG accumulation in the brain may decrease, whereas the blood pool activity is increased.[135]

## IMAGING IN CLINICAL NEPHROLOGY

### NORMAL RENAL FUNCTION

GFR and effective RPF may be assessed by means of dynamic quantitative nuclear imaging techniques. The GFR quantifies the amount of filtrate formed per minute (normal, 125 mL/min in adults). Only 20% of RPF is filtered through the semipermeable membrane of the glomerulus. The filtrate is protein free and almost completely reabsorbed in the tubules. Filtration is maintained over a range of arterial pressures with autoregulation. The ideal agent for the determination of GFR is inulin, which is only filtered but is neither secreted nor reabsorbed.[131,136]

In these studies, $^{99m}$Tc-DTPA is often used to demonstrate renal perfusion and assess glomerular filtration, although 5% to 10% of injected $^{99m}$Tc-DTPA is protein bound and 5% remains in the kidneys after 4 hours. A typical imaging protocol includes posterior 5-second flow images for 1 minute, followed by 1-minute-per-frame images for 20 minutes. The GFR may be obtained through the Gates method, in which images of renal uptake are obtained during the second and third minutes after $^{99m}$Tc-DTPA administration. Regions of interest are drawn over the kidneys, and background activity correction is applied. A standard dose is counted by the gamma camera for normalization. Depth photon attenuation is corrected according to a formula relating body weight and height. A split GFR can be obtained for each kidney, which is not possible with the creatinine clearance method.[131,136]

The effective RPF (normal, 585 mL/min in adults) can be obtained with $^{131}$I-ortho-iodohippurate and $^{99m}$Tc-MAG3 imaging.[137] However, $^{131}$I-ortho-iodohippurate has been largely replaced by $^{99}$Tc-MAG3 because MAG3 has better imaging characteristics and dosimetry (when radiolabeled with $^{99m}$Tc). Currently $^{99}$Tc-MAG3 is the renal imaging agent of choice primarily because of the combined renal clearance of $^{99}$Tc-MAG3 by both filtration and tubular extraction, which enables clinicians to obtain relatively high-quality images even in patients with impaired renal function. The imaging protocol includes posterior 1-second images for 60 seconds (flow study), followed by 1-minute images for 5 minutes and then 5-minute images for 30 minutes. The relative tubular function may be obtained by drawing renal regions of interest, corrected for background activity.[138,139] A renogram is constructed to depict the renal tracer uptake over time. The first portion of the renogram has a sharp upward slope occurring approximately 6 seconds after peak aortic activity (phase I); the upward slope represents perfusion. This is followed by extension to the peak value, which represents both renal perfusion and early renal clearance (phase II), which can be dependent on body position.[140] The next phase (phase III) is depicted by a downward slope, which represents excretion. Normal perfusion of the kidneys is symmetric (50% ± 5%). The peak of the renogram occurs at approximately 2 to 3 minutes (vs. 3–5 minutes with DTPA) in normal adults, and by 30 minutes, more than 70% of the tracer is cleared and present in the urinary bladder (Fig. 25.23).[120,126,131,136,141] Assessment of renal function is further discussed in Chapter 23.

Renal cortical structure can be imaged with $^{99m}$Tc-DMSA; the appearance of these images is strongly correlated with differential GFR and differential renal blood flow. Imaging is started 90 to 120 minutes after administration of the tracer and can be obtained up to 4 hours later. Planar images are obtained in the anterior, posterior, left anterior oblique/right anterior oblique, and right posterior oblique/left posterior oblique projections. SPECT is also often performed. In a scan with normal results, renal cortical uptake is evenly distributed. Normal variations include dromedary hump (splenic impression on the left kidney), fetal lobulation, horseshoe kidney, crossed fused ectopy, and hypertrophied column of Bertin. The renal images also allow accurate assessment of the relative renal size, position, and axis.[131,136]

### KIDNEY INJURY: ACUTE AND CHRONIC

When a patient presents with previously undiagnosed renal failure, the question is whether the kidney disease is acute or chronic. US is the most helpful initial imaging study for evaluating the patient with an elevated creatinine level of unknown duration. US can help separate chronic, end-stage kidney disease (ESKD) from potentially reversible AKI or

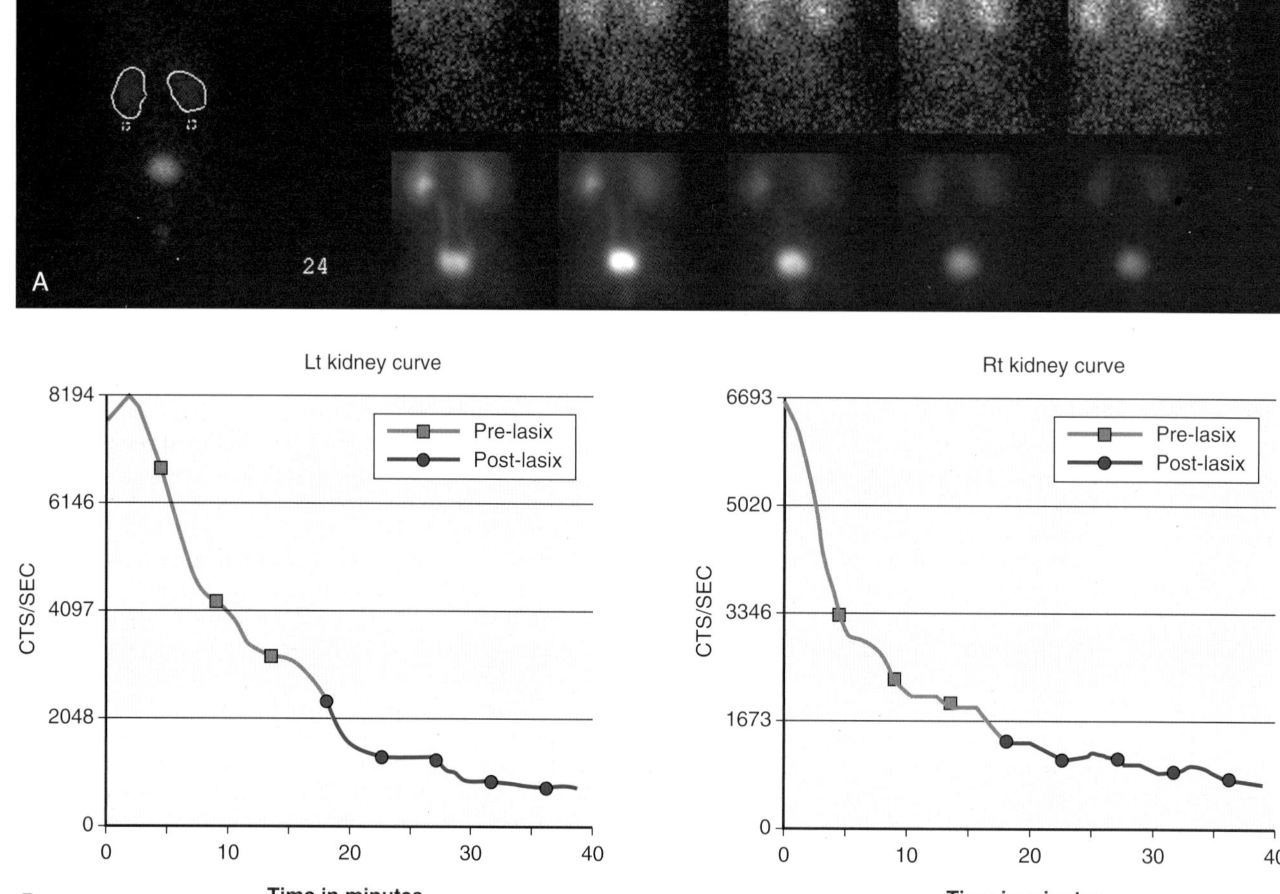


**Fig. 25.23.** Normal-appearing renogram with technetium 99m-labeled mercaptoacetyltriglycine (MAG3). **A**, Planar posterior images. *Left:* Static image with whole kidney regions of interest (ROI; *white outlines*), and background ROIs *(circular dashed lines)* inferiorly. *Right upper series:* Sequential flow images at 5-second intervals show prompt symmetric uptake of tracer in both kidneys. *Right lower series:* Sequential functional images at 1-minute intervals show normal excretion of tracer with visualization of the ureters and urinary bladder. **B,** Time-activity curves for each kidney, corrected for background, collected from the ROIs in A., showing the excretory phase. Less than 30% of peak activity is retained in each kidney after 20 minutes, which is normal. At 20 minutes, intravenous furosemide (Lasix) was given to demonstrate normal washout. *CTS/SEC*, Radioactivity counts per second.

CKD by defining renal size, echogenicity, and presence or absence of hydronephrosis and cystic disease. This is easily achieved using gray-scale US.[142] A thin rim of decreased echogenicity may surround the kidneys in patients experiencing kidney injury, also known as renal sweat.[143] Small, echogenic kidneys indicate preexisting CKD; however, acute reversible components must still be searched for. Acute, reversible components that can be diagnosed on imaging are few but include hydronephrosis and hypertension caused by renal artery stenosis. If no acute process is found on US, no further imaging workup is necessary (according to the ACR appropriateness criteria for elevated Cr of unknown duration).[144] Normal renal size, with or without increased echogenicity, typically requires more extensive evaluation for acute causes because gray-scale US may not be accurate in the minimally dilated obstructive situation.

Many causes of AKI are encountered in the hospital setting. Prerenal and renal causes include hypotension or dehydration resulting in hypoperfusion of the kidneys and nephrotoxic drugs[145] and account for more than 90% of all cases. Typically, prerenal and renal causes are diagnosed clinically, not with imaging. Although postrenal causes for AKI are less common, when they are identified and treated, the AKI is often rapidly reversible.

US is more than 95% accurate in detecting hydronephrosis (i.e., dilation of the collecting systems and renal pelvis)[144,146]; however, the cause of the hydronephrosis may not be seen. If US cannot determine the cause of obstruction, CT or MRI that is not enhanced by contrast media is the appropriate next imaging study.[147] The typical US findings of hydronephrosis are a dilated, anechoic, fluid-filled renal pelvis and calyces. Hydronephrosis is generally graded according to the extent of calyceal dilation and the degree of cortical thinning.[133,144,148] In mild (grade I) hydronephrosis the pelvicalyceal system is filled with fluid, which causes slight separation of the central renal sinus fat (Fig. 25.24). The calyces are not distorted, and the thickness of the renal cortex appears normal. In moderate (grade II) hydronephrosis the pelvicalyceal system appears more distended with greater separation of the central echo complex. The contour of the calyces is rounded, but the cortical thickness is unaltered (Fig. 25.25). With moderate-to-severe (grade III) hydronephrosis the calyces are more distended, and cortical thinning is recognized. In severe (grade IV) hydronephrosis the calyceal system is markedly dilated (Fig. 25.26). The calyces appear as large, ballooned, fluid-filled structures with a dilated renal pelvis of variable size. Cortical loss is evident, with the dilated calyces approaching or reaching the renal capsule. In general, the length and overall size of a hydronephrotic kidney is increased. Long-standing obstruction may, however, result in renal parenchymal atrophy, and the kidney may be somewhat small, with marked cortical thinning. The degree of hydronephrosis is not always correlated with the amount of obstruction.

Although hydronephrosis is usually easily diagnosed with US, it must not be confused with renal cystic disease. In hydronephrosis the dilated calyces have a visibly direct communication with the renal pelvis, which is also dilated.[16] In cystic disease the round fluid-filled cysts have walls, and no direct communication is evident between each calyx and the renal pelvis. Cases of peripelvic cysts are frequently misdiagnosed as a dilated renal pelvis. Renal artery aneurysm may also be confused with a dilated renal pelvis but can be diagnosed correctly with added Doppler color-flow US.

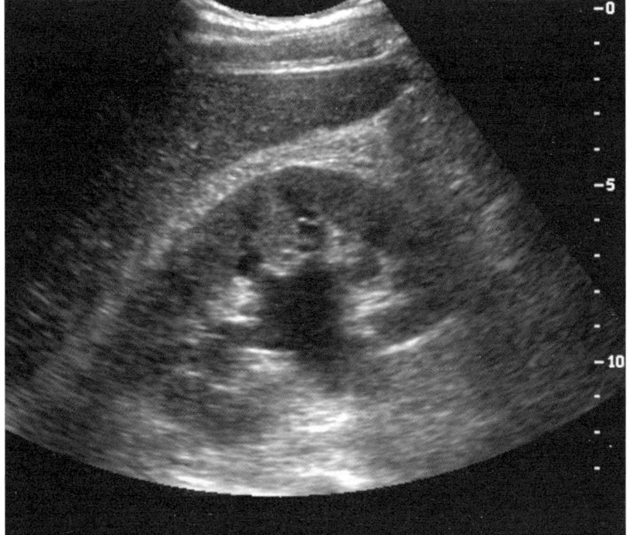

Fig. 25.24 Mild (grade I) hydronephrosis: ultrasonography. The central echo complex is separated by the mildly distended calyces and renal pelvis. Notice the connection between the calyces and the renal pelvis. The thickness of the cortex is preserved, and the renal border remains smooth.

The presence of hydronephrosis on US does not always indicate obstruction.[149,150] Grade I hydronephrosis and possibly more severe grades may be observed in patients in whom no obstructive cause is found. Nonobstructive causes of hydronephrosis include increased urine production and flow, acute and chronic infection, vesicoureteral reflux, papillary necrosis, congenital megacalyces, overdistended bladder, and postobstructive dilation.[151] In patients with repeated episodes of intermittent or partial obstruction, the calyces become quite distensible or compliant, which causes the appearance of hydronephrosis to vary, depending on the state of hydration and urine production. Patients with vesicoureteral reflux also demonstrate distensible pelvicalyceal systems. Doppler color-flow US has been suggested as an additive means of differentiating obstructive from nonobstructive hydronephrosis.[152,153] The measurement of resistive indices has been investigated as a means of diagnosing acute renal obstruction as well; the acutely obstructed kidney has an elevated resistive index, and the nonobstructed kidney has a normal resistive index of less than 0.70.[154,155] The results have been variable, and thus no consistent recommendation is available[155,156]

US is also used in patients with CKD. Cortical echogenicity may be increased in both acute and chronic renal parenchymal disease (Fig. 25.27).[157] The pattern should be bilateral in CKD, and the degree of cortical echogenicity is correlated with the severity of the interstitial fibrosis, global sclerosis, focal tubular atrophy, and number of hyaline casts per glomerulus.[10] Similar correlation is observed with decreasing renal size. These findings, however, are nonspecific, and kidney biopsy may be required for diagnosis. The normal corticomedullary differentiation is lost with increasing cortical echogenicity.[148] Cortical echogenicity may also be increased

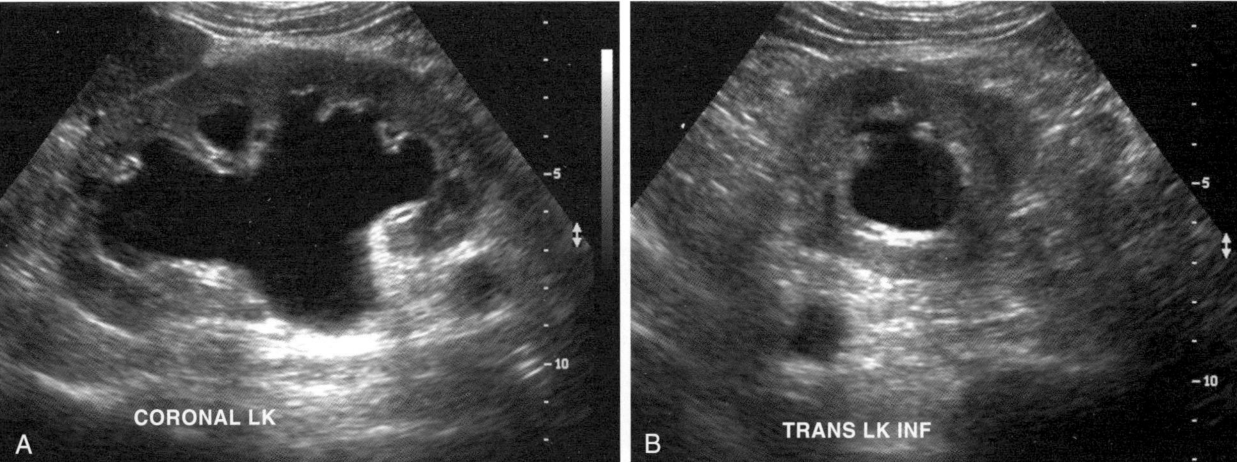


Fig. 25.25 Moderate (grade II) hydronephrosis: ultrasonography. Longitudinal image **(A)** and transverse image **(B)**. The dilated calyces are rounded and filled with urine. The renal pelvis is dilated as well. Again, note the connection between the calyces and the renal pelvis. The cortex remains relatively normal in thickness, and the renal border is smooth.

in some patients with AKI, as in glomerulonephritis and lupus nephritis. Sequential studies over time may be used to assess the progression of disease by monitoring the renal size and cortical echogenicity.

The key to the diagnosis of renal parenchymal disease is renal core biopsy and resulting histopathologic study.[157] US facilitates the performance of kidney biopsy by demonstrating the kidney and the proper location for biopsy. US may also be used to evaluate for complications associated with kidney biopsy, such as perirenal hematoma and arteriovenous fistula.

When US evaluation demonstrates hydronephrosis, but not the cause, it is usually followed by CT. Noncontrast CT will demonstrate the dilated pelvicalyceal systems in the kidney. The parenchymal thickness can be visualized in relation to the dilated collecting systems; the urine-filled calyces and pelvis are less dense than the surrounding parenchyma. The course of the dilated ureters may be followed distally to the bladder and prostate to establish the site of obstruction. The cause of obstruction is frequently visible and may include pelvic tumors, distal ureteral stones, and retroperitoneal adenopathy or mass. For patients in whom chronic long-standing obstruction is the cause of kidney injury, CT generally demonstrates large, fluid-containing kidneys with little or no cortex remaining.

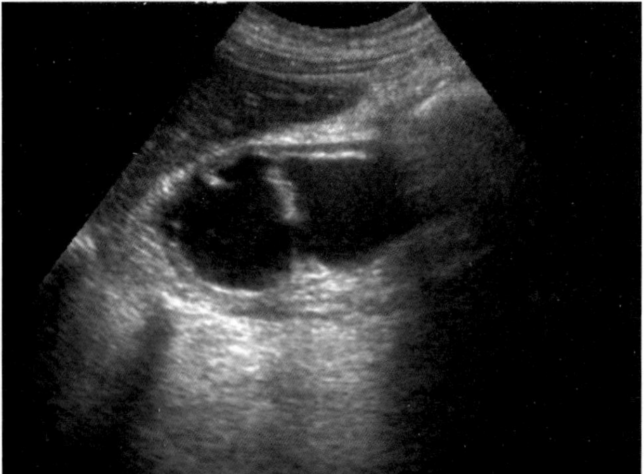

**Fig. 25.26** Severe (grade IV) hydronephrosis: ultrasonography. Longitudinal image of the right kidney demonstrates a large fluid-filled sac; no normal elements of the kidney remain visible. The cortex is almost gone, but the outer border of the kidney remains smooth.

In CKD without obstruction, CT typically demonstrates small, contracted kidneys, which may also show evidence of adulthood-acquired polycystic disease if the patient is on dialysis (Fig. 25.28). In general, the overall size and thickness of the renal parenchyma appear to decrease with age.[158] Other causes for CKD may be demonstrated on imaging, including autosomal dominant polycystic kidney disease (Fig. 25.29); the kidneys are enlarged and contain innumerable cysts. Frequently some of the cyst walls may contain thin rims of calcification. The density of the internal contents of the cysts may also vary as a result of hemorrhage or proteinaceous debris. For patients undergoing regular dialysis, iodinated contrast may be given if necessary for CT scans because the material is dialyzable.

Like CT, MRI is accurate in demonstrating renal structure, as well as prerenal and postrenal causes of kidney injury. MRI is sensitive for the detection of renal parenchymal disease, but the renal parenchymal causes of injury have nonspecific features, and biopsy is generally required.[159] Noncontrast MRI routinely allows for detailed tissue characterization of the kidney and surrounding structures. Both iodinated contrast and Gd-C should be avoided if possible in patients with AKI and CKD stage 4 and 5. Newer MRI sequences, such as diffusion-weighted and bright blood techniques, provide a way to increase the detection of neoplastic and vascular causes of renal failure without the use of intravenous contrast agents.[102,160]

In kidney injury, glomerular and tubular dysfunctions are reflected by abnormal findings on renal scintigraphy and renography. Renal uptake of $^{99m}$Tc-MAG3 is prolonged, with tubular tracer stasis and little or no excretion. In patients with AKI, if $^{99m}$Tc-MAG3 has more renal activity than hepatic activity 1 to 3 minutes after injection, recovery is likely, whereas when renal uptake is less than the hepatic uptake, dialysis may be needed.[161] In CKD, renal perfusion, cortical tracer extraction, and tracer excretion are diminished. However, this imaging pattern is nonspecific and must be interpreted in the clinical context.[131]

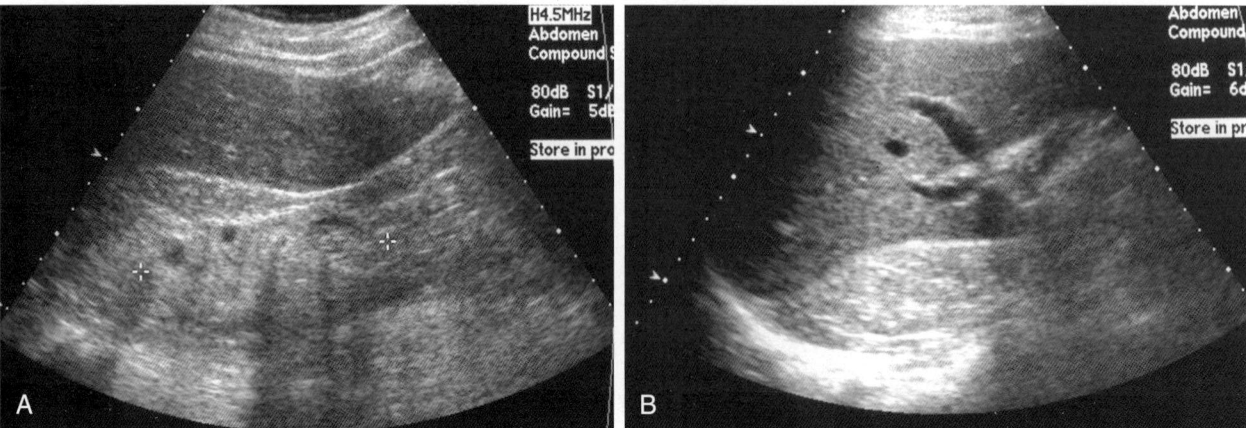


**Fig. 25.27** End-stage kidney disease: ultrasonography. **A** and **B,** The kidneys are highly echogenic in relation to the adjacent liver. No normal renal structures are visible, but the kidneys remain smooth in overall contour. Note the two small hypoechoic renal cysts in the surface in **A.**

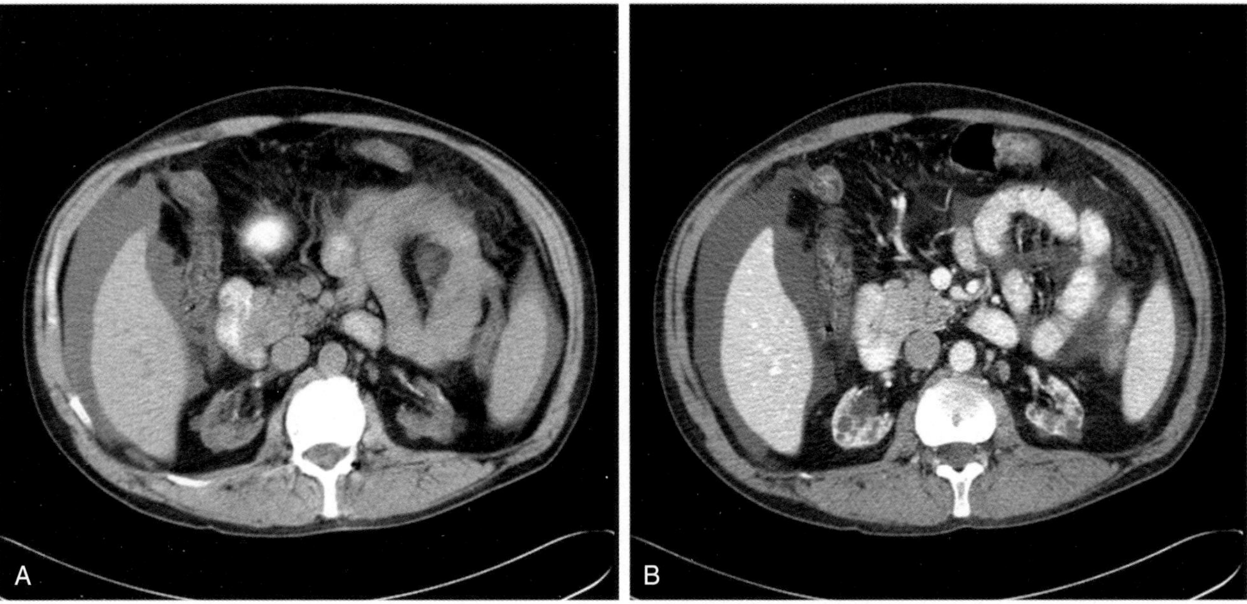


**Fig. 25.28** Adulthood-acquired polycystic kidney disease: computed tomographic scan, axial image without contrast material **(A)** and axial image after administration of contrast material **(B).** The kidneys are small bilaterally with multiple 1-cm cysts primarily in the cortex.

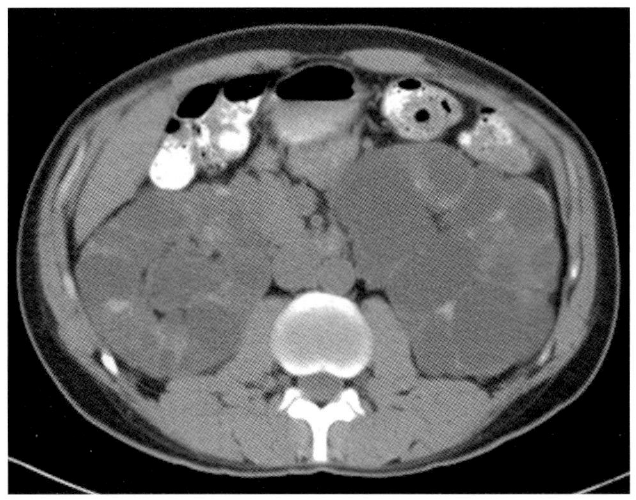

**Fig. 25.29** Autosomal dominant polycystic kidney disease: computed tomographic (CT) scan without contrast material. This CT image demonstrates the markedly enlarged kidney bilaterally with multiple low-density cysts throughout both kidneys. The little remaining renal parenchyma is noted by the sparse, higher density material squeezed by the cysts.

## UNILATERAL OBSTRUCTION

If US cannot determine the cause of obstruction, CT is the next imaging modality of choice due to rapid speed of acquisition and accuracy.[147] IVU and antegrade or retrograde pyelography may be used if CT is not available.[144] With IVU the site of obstruction may be visible, but the cause may be only inferred; this is also true with antegrade and retrograde pyelography.

CE-CT and, more specifically, CTU are most useful in assessing the patient with unilateral obstruction.[26] Small differences in the enhancement pattern of the kidneys are well demonstrated with CE-CT (Fig. 25.30). Differences in the excretion patterns by the kidneys are also sensitively depicted on CE-CT.[25,26] The urine-filled or contrast material-filled ureters point to the obstruction with demonstration of both intraureteral and extraureteral causes of the obstruction (Fig. 25.31). MRI demonstrates similar findings and may be used when CE-CT is contraindicated.

Nuclear medicine assessment by means of diuretic renography may also be used to evaluate for obstructive uropathy. Scintigraphy with $^{99m}$Tc-MAG3 is often employed. Furosemide (Lasix) is administered intravenously (1 mg/kg; higher dose in cases of renal insufficiency) when the renal pelvis and ureter are maximally distended.[162] Regions of interest are drawn around each renal pelvis, with the background regions as crescent shapes lateral to each kidney. After furosemide administration, in cases of dilation without obstruction, the collecting system empties rapidly, with a subsequent steep decline in the renogram curve. Obstruction can be ruled out if the clearance half-time of the renal pelvic emptying is less than 10 minutes. A curve that reaches a plateau or continues to rise after administration of furosemide is indicative of obstruction, with a clearance half-time of more than 20 minutes (Fig. 25.32). A slow downward slope after furosemide administration may be indicative of partial obstruction. An apparent poor response to furosemide may also occur in patients with severe pelvic dilation (reservoir effect). Other pitfalls include poor injection technique of either the diuretic or the radiotracer, impaired renal function, and dehydration, in which delayed tracer transit and excretion may not be overcome by the effect of a diuretic. Kidneys in neonates (<1 month of age) may be too immature to respond to furosemide, and neonates are thus not suitable candidates for diuretic renal scintigraphy.[131,163]

Various protocols in relation to the timing of furosemide administration have also been reported. In the F0 method, furosemide is injected simultaneously with $^{99m}$Tc-MAG3 administration. A 17-year clinical experience at one institution

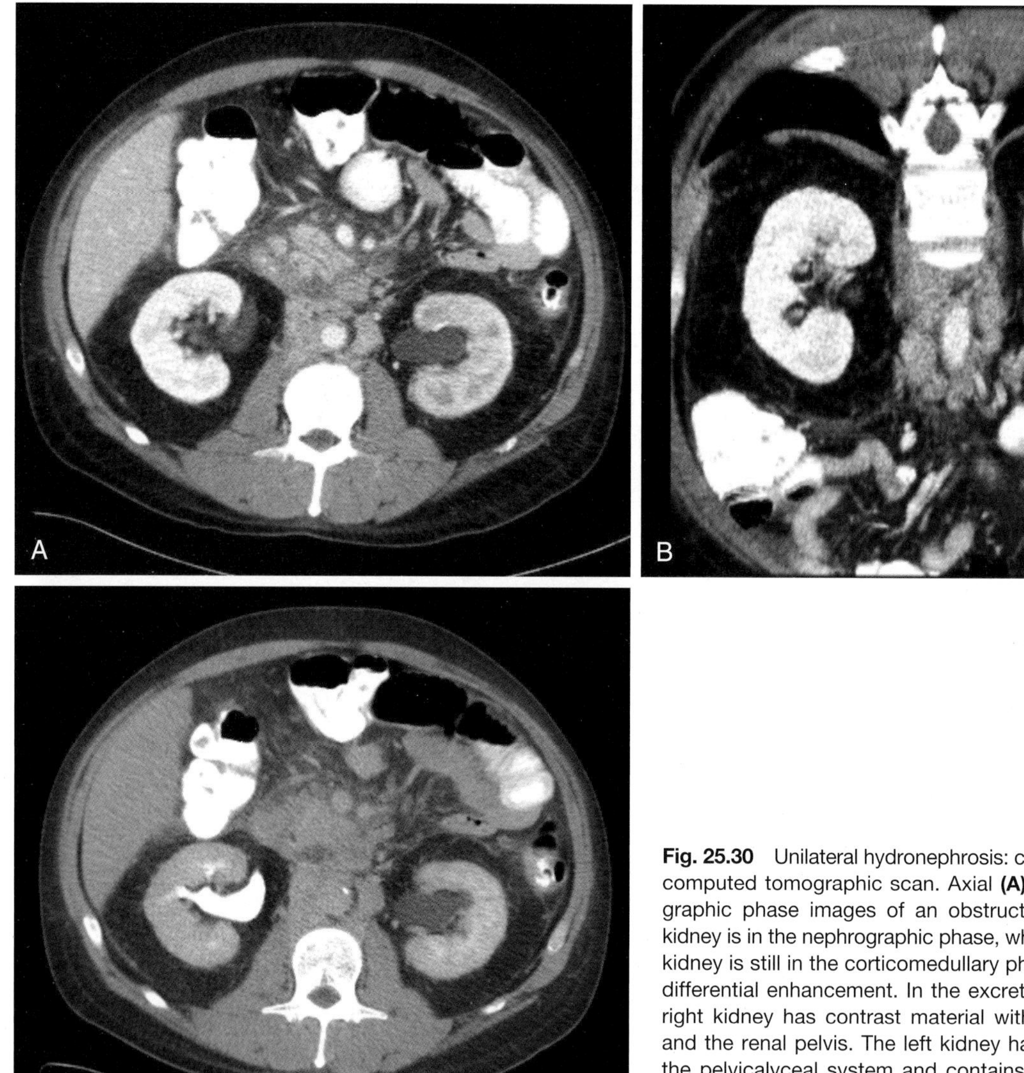


**Fig. 25.30** Unilateral hydronephrosis: contrast material-enhanced computed tomographic scan. Axial **(A)** and coronal **(B)** nephrographic phase images of an obstructed left kidney. The right kidney is in the nephrographic phase, whereas the left (obstructed) kidney is still in the corticomedullary phase; this is apparent with differential enhancement. In the excretory phase image **(C),** the right kidney has contrast material within the collecting system and the renal pelvis. The left kidney has no contrast material in the pelvicalyceal system and contains only nonopacified urine. The patient had lymphoma with retroperitoneal lymph nodes, which caused the obstruction more distally.

proved that this protocol is useful for patients of all ages and for all indications.[164] Taghavi et al compared diuresis renographic protocols with injection of furosemide 15 minutes before (F−15) and 20 minutes after (F+20) administration of $^{99m}$Tc-MAG3.[165] In this comparative study of 21 patients with dilation of the pelvicalyceal system, the F−15 protocol produced fewer equivocal results than did the F+20 method and therefore was considered the preferable protocol. Further experience is needed to determine the most optimal timing interval between furosemide and $^{99m}$Tc-MAG3 injections in diuresis renography.

## RENAL CALCIFICATIONS AND RENAL STONE DISEASE

Calcifications may occur in many regions of the kidney.[166] Nephrolithiasis or renal calculi are the most common and occur in the pelvicalyceal system. Nephrocalcinosis refers to diffuse or punctate renal parenchymal calcification occurring in either the medulla or cortex, usually bilaterally. Some patients with nephrocalcinosis may also develop nephrolithiasis. Calcifications also occur in vascular structures, particularly in patients with diabetes and advanced atherosclerotic disease. Rimlike calcifications may occur in simple renal cysts and polycystic disease. Patients with renal carcinomas may exhibit variable calcifications as well. All types of calcification are best demonstrated on noncontrast CT.

Cortical calcification is most often associated with cortical necrosis from any cause.[166] The calcifications are dystrophic and tend to resemble tram tracks and to be circumferential. Other entities in which cortical calcification are found include hyperoxaluria, Alport's syndrome, and, in rare cases, chronic glomerulonephritis. The stippled calcifications of hyperoxaluria may be found in both the cortex and the medulla, as well as in other organs, such as the heart. In Alport's syndrome, only cortical calcifications are found.

Calcifications in the medulla are much more common than cortical calcifications.[166] The most common cause of medullary nephrocalcinosis is primary hyperparathyroidism. The distribution appears to be within the renal pyramid and may be either focal or diffuse and either unilateral or bilateral. Nephrocalcinosis occurs in other diseases in which

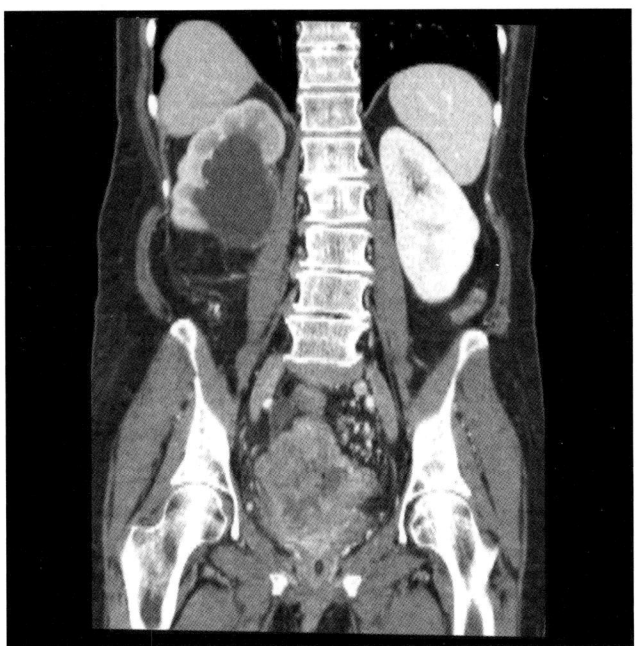

**Fig. 25.31** Unilateral obstruction: contrast material-enhanced computed tomographic scan. The coronal image demonstrates the difference in enhancement between the two kidneys, with the moderately dilated renal pelvis and calyces on the right. The large heterogeneous pelvis mass is the source of the obstruction: recurrent rectal carcinoma.

hypercalcemia or hypercalciuria occur, such as hyperthyroidism, sarcoidosis, hypervitaminosis D, immobilization, multiple myeloma, and metastatic neoplasms. These calcifications are nonspecific and punctate in appearance and are usually medullary in location.

In 70% to 75% of cases of renal tubular acidosis, there is evidence of nephrocalcinosis. The calcifications tend to be uniform and distributed throughout the renal pyramids bilaterally. With medullary sponge kidney and renal tubular ectasia, small calculi form in the distal collecting tubules, probably because of stasis. The appearance varies from involvement of only a single calyx to involvement of both kidneys throughout. The calcifications are small, round, and within the peak of the pyramid adjacent to the calyx. Medullary sponge kidney is also associated with nephrolithiasis, because the small calculi in the distal collecting tubules may pass into the collecting systems and ureters, resulting in renal colic.[165]

The calcifications that occur in renal tuberculosis are typically medullary in location and may mimic other forms of nephrocalcinosis.[169] Calcification occurs in the pyramids as part of the healing process. With overwhelming involvement of the kidney, the entire kidney may be destroyed; this results in diffuse, heavy calcification throughout the entire kidney, which becomes small and scarred. Medullary calcifications are also visible in patients with renal papillary necrosis. With necrosis of the papilla, the material is sloughed into the calyces. Retained tissue fragments may calcify and have the appearance of medullary nephrocalcinosis.

Nephrolithiasis is a common clinical entity. The lifetime risk for developing renal calculi is 12%, with males being two to three times more at risk than females.[167] Most urinary tract stones are composed of calcium salts of either oxalate or phosphate or a combination of the two.[168–171] This composition accounts for the dense appearance on imaging. Stasis contributes to the formation of stones in the urinary tract. Renal colic or flank pain is the most common presenting symptom. Most patients also have hematuria, although it may be absent if a ureter is completely obstructed by the stone. The pain that occurs with a passing renal stone is probably caused by the distension of the tubular system and renal capsule of the kidney and by the peristalsis associated with ureteral contractions as the stone moves distally.

Most urinary calculi that are 4 mm or smaller pass with conservative treatment.[172] The larger the stone, the more likely other measures will be necessary to treat the stone and associated obstruction.

Plain radiograph of the abdomen yields little significant information on its own and should not be used to diagnose stone disease.[173] The KUB is useful for following stone disease only when a stone is densely calcified and large enough to be visible (Fig. 25.33). For years, IVU was the method of choice for the assessment of patients with renal colic[174,175]; however, it has been supplanted by CT that is not enhanced by contrast media, which is a more rapid examination and more accurate than IVU.[173] In addition, a CT examination would also permit evaluation of nonurinary tract causes of pain.

Ultrasonographic assessment has also been used in the evaluation of renal colic.[176] This is a quick and usually easily performed examination. Unilateral hydronephrosis may be observed, although the examination results may be normal early in the passage of a renal stone. Renal stones may be visualized within the kidney as hyperechoic foci with distal acoustic shadowing or reverberation artifacts (Fig. 25.34).[176] Ureteral stones are rarely seen because of overlying bowel gas. Distal ureteral stones near the ureterovesical junction may be visualized through the urine-filled bladder transabdominally. US may demonstrate an absent ureteral jet in the bladder on the side in which a stone is being passed. Doppler US and assessment of the peripheral vasculature resistance may occasionally be helpful in pointing to the affected kidney, but the study results have been variable.[154]

Noncontrast CT scanning of the abdomen and pelvis has emerged as the standard evaluation in patients with renal colic.[177–181] The sensitivities for CT are 96% to 100%, the specificities are 95% to 100%, and the accuracy rates are 96% to 98%; for this reason, nonenhanced CT has supplanted plain radiography, IVU, and US.[178,182–184] In comparisons of nonenhanced CT and IVU, CT is much more useful, with 94% to 100% sensitivity and 92% to 100% specificity; IVU has 64% to 97% sensitivity and 92% to 94% specificity.[178] Also, when noncontrast CT was used as the reference standard in comparison with US, 24% sensitivity and 90% specificity were found for US.[185,186] An alternative diagnosis is made in patients with "renal colic" in 9% to 29% of cases in which noncontrast CT is used for evaluation.[187]

Nonenhanced CT is performed from the top of the kidneys to below the pubic symphysis. No preparation is needed. Intravenous contrast material is rarely needed. The studies are performed with 3-mm collimation or less, and the slices are reconstructed to be contiguous or slightly overlapping.[188–190] Virtually all renal stones are denser than the adjacent soft tissues (Fig. 25.35)[191]; exceptions are renal stones associated with indinavir (a protease inhibitor used in the management of acquired immunodeficiency syndrome (AIDS) and very

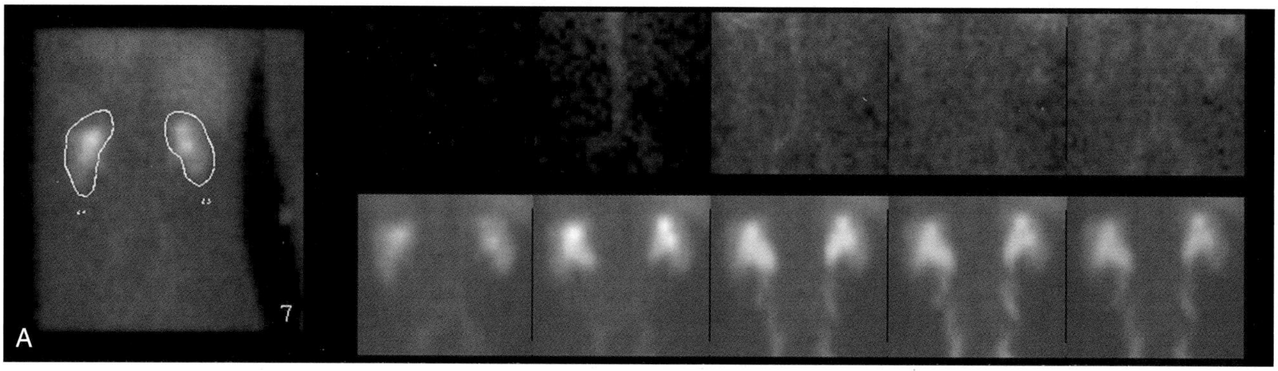

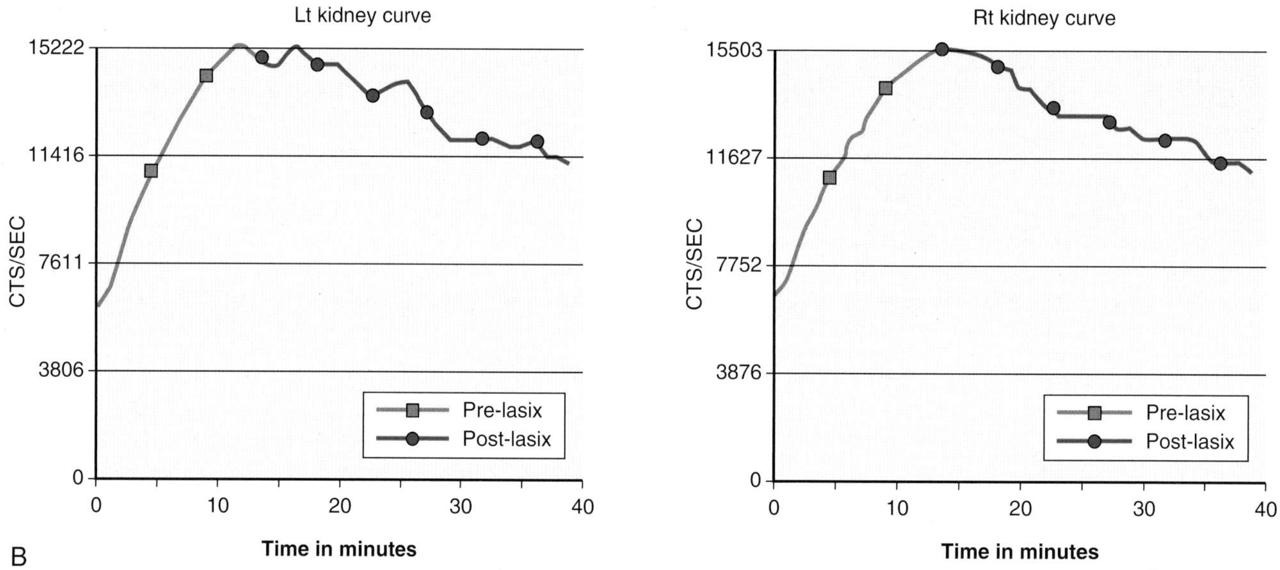

**Fig. 25.32** Abnormal findings on renogram with technetium 99m-labeled mercaptoacetyltriglycine, demonstrating obstructive urinary kinetics with a poor response to furosemide. **A,** Static and timed images in the same format as in Fig. 25.23A. **B,** Individual time-activity curves for each kidney. Intravenous furosemide (Lasix) was given at 15 minutes. *CTS/SEC*, radioactivity counts per second.

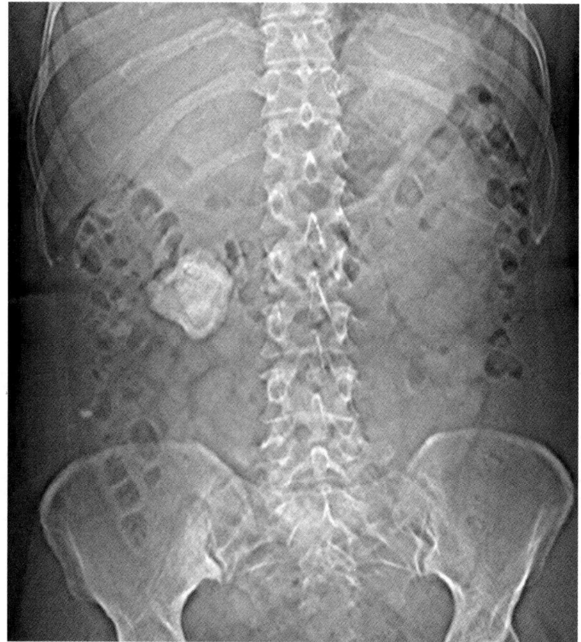

**Fig. 25.33** Renal stone: plain radiograph of the kidneys, ureters, and bladder. A large laminated stone is visible in the renal pelvis of the right kidney. The outline of the normal left kidney can be seen with no calcifications overlying it. The right kidney outline cannot be seen.

small uric acid stones (<1–2 mm in diameter).[192,193] As expected, calcium oxalate and calcium phosphate stones are the most dense.[168,169] Matrix stones, which are rare, may also be relatively low in density, but they usually contain calcium impurities that make them visible.[168,171]

For detecting stones, low-dose scanning has been shown to be as effective as CT with standard techniques.[194,195] The radiation dose is usually 20% to 25% of the standard dose. The development of iterative reconstruction techniques has also reduced radiation doses. Dual-energy imaging with CT has demonstrated the ability to distinguish different types of stones[187,196] (see Fig. 25.8).

Calculi may be visible in all parts of the collecting system and the urinary tract. Small punctate calcifications (≈1 mm) are occasionally observed just at the tip of the renal pyramid. These may represent the calcification noted in Randall plaques.[197] Obstruction occurs most commonly at the ureteropelvic junction, at the pelvic brim, where the ureters cross over the iliac vessels, and at the ureterovesical junction. The diagnosis is made on the noncontrast CT scan by demonstrating the calcified stone within the urine-filled ureters (Fig. 25.36).[188] Secondary signs may be present to assist in the diagnosis.[182] Hydronephrosis and hydroureter to the point of the stone may be visible. Asymmetric perinephric and periureteral stranding may also be related to forniceal rupture and urine leak (Fig. 25.37).[198] The involved

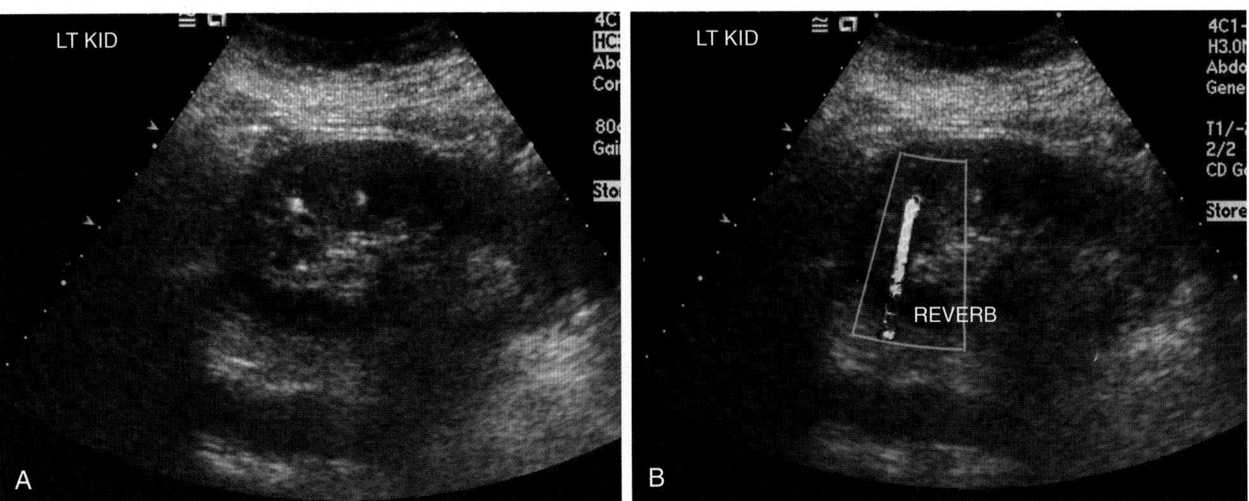


**Fig. 25.34** Renal stone: ultrasonography. Longitudinal image **(A)** and Doppler color-flow image **(B)** demonstrate an echogenic focus at the corticomedullary junction. Not all stones show shadowing, but in this case, reverberation artifact (REVERB) is visible on the Doppler color-flow image, which helps establish the diagnosis.

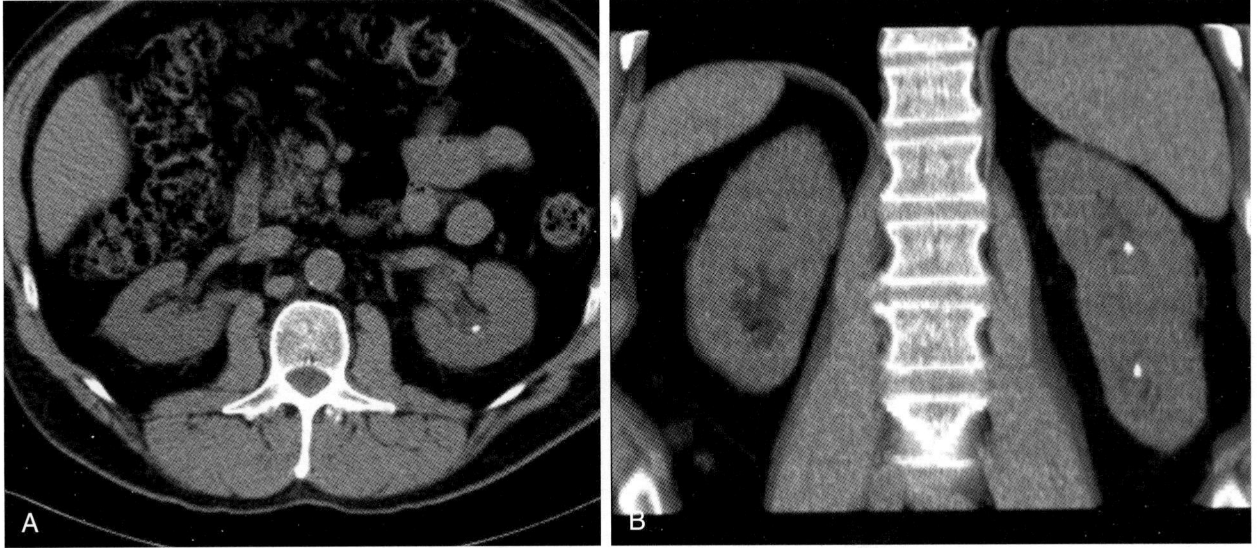


**Fig. 25.35** Renal stones: noncontrast computed tomographic scan. Axial image **(A)** and coronal image **(B)** demonstrate 4- to 5-mm stones in the upper and lower poles of the left kidney. There are no signs of obstruction.

kidney may be less dense than the normal kidney because of increased interstitial fluid and edema.[199,200] The affected kidney may also be larger than the normal kidney. At the point of obstruction, the stone may be visible within the ureter, with soft tissue thickening of the ureteral wall at that level. This thickening is probably caused by edema and inflammation associated with the passage of the stone.

Noncontrast CT has the additional advantage of assessing the overall stone burden of the patient, not just the passing stone. Also, the size may be accurately measured, which enables clinicians to make treatment decisions.[173,201,202] Distal ureteral stones are occasionally confused with phleboliths, which are common in the pelvis (see Fig. 25.37). Images reconstructed in the coronal plane along the course of the ureters down to the level of the stone may be helpful.[203] Also, close inspection of phleboliths frequently reveals a small, soft tissue tag leading to the calcification: the "comet tail" sign.[204] Enhancement with contrast material is occasionally necessary in confusing or difficult cases. Also, CE-CT may be used in complicated cases in which the patient is febrile and pyelonephritis or pyohydronephrosis is suspected.[170]

In the evaluation of acute stone disease, MRI or MRU is not the examination of first choice, but it is a suitable alternative for selected patients, especially those in whom reduction of radiation exposure is desired (pediatric and pregnant patients).[205] Stones are difficult to identify in nondilated systems, even in retrospect. When stones are observed on MRI, they are visible as black foci on both T1- and T2-weighted sequences. Stones become more conspicuous in a dilated collecting system (Fig. 25.38); however, a nonenhanced filling defect is a nonspecific finding. Blood, air, or debris may have the same appearance. If stones or other calcifications are a concern, noncontrast CT is the examination of choice for improved conspicuity.

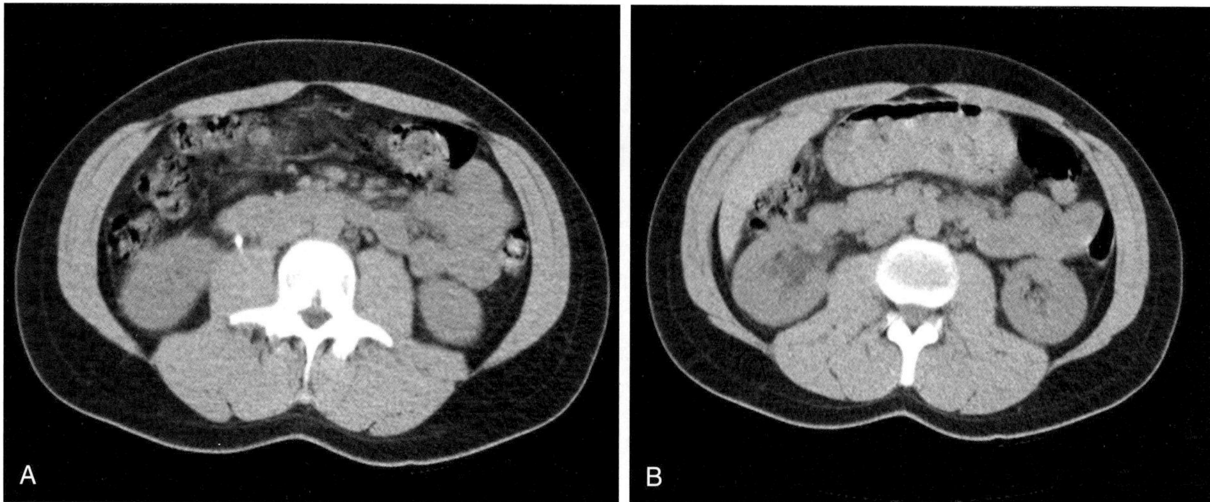


**Fig. 25.36** Ureteral stone: noncontrast computed tomographic scan. **A,** A 5- to 6-mm stone is noted in the midportion of the right ureter. **B,** Axial image of the midportion of the kidneys reveals the urine-filled right renal pelvis and a right kidney that is slightly less dense than the left. These are signs of obstruction.

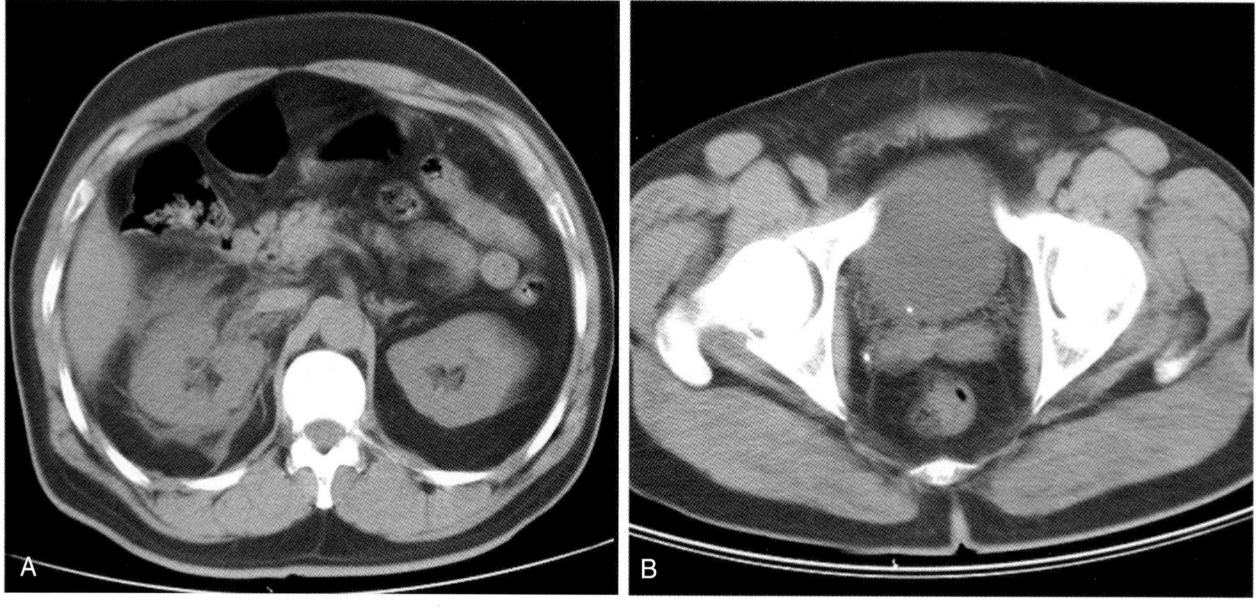


**Fig. 25.37** Ureteral stone: noncontrast computed tomographic scan. Axial images of the kidneys show perinephric and peripelvic stranding and fluid on the right **(A)** caused by forniceal rupture and leakage of urine as a result of the distal obstructing stone at the right ureterovesical junction **(B)**. Note the phlebolith on the right posterior to the bladder and lateral to the seminal vesicle; phleboliths are commonly confused with distal ureteral stones.

When the use of iodinated contrast material is contraindicated, or when reduction of radiation exposure is desired, MRU can be used to determine the cause and location of an obstructing process (Fig. 25.39). MRU is highly accurate in demonstrating obstruction, regardless of whether the process is acute or chronic.[205] Acute obstruction may be associated with perinephric fluid, which is well demonstrated on T2-weighted sequences.[205,206] However, perinephric fluid is a nonspecific finding and can be found in association with other renal disease. MRI is useful in evaluating the patient who has recently undergone surgery for renal stone disease. MRI has been reported as being more accurate than CT in differentiating perirenal and intrarenal hematomas (Figs. 25.40 and 25.41).[207] CE-MRI can also demonstrate damage to the collecting system and areas of ischemia without the risk for nephrotoxicity. Stone disease is discussed further in Chapter 38.

## RENAL INFECTION

Acute pyelonephritis is typically a diagnosis made clinically.[208] Most cases of acute pyelonephritis occur by the ascending

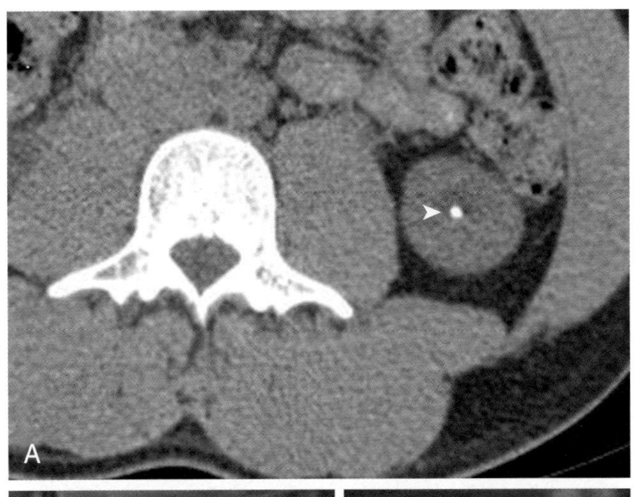


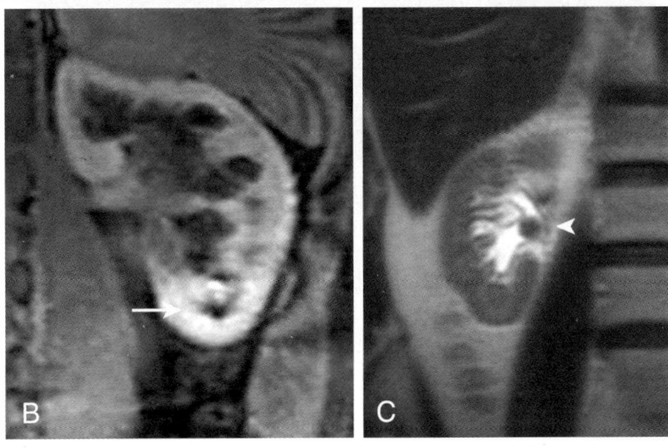


**Fig. 25.38** Renal stones. Calcification *(arrowhead)* well viewed on computed tomography **(A)** is difficult to demonstrate on magnetic resonance imaging **(B)** *(arrow)*, even in retrospect. **C,** A stone *(arrowhead)* is more conspicuous when it is located within a mildly dilated collection system.

route from the bladder and are caused by gram-negative bacteria.[209] Vesicoureteral reflux may contribute, although the ascent of the bacteria up the ureter also occurs in its absence. This is due to the presence of the adhesin P fimbriae and powerful endotoxins that appear to inhibit ureteral peristalsis creating a functional obstruction.[210] The bacteria are transported to the renal pelvis, where intrarenal reflux occurs and the bacteria traverse the calyceal system to the ducts and tubules within the renal pyramid. Enzyme release results in destruction of tubular cells with subsequent bacterial invasion of the interstitium. As the infection progresses, it spreads throughout the pyramid and to the adjacent parenchyma. The inflammatory response leads to focal or more diffuse swelling of the kidney. Without adequate treatment, necrosis of the involved regions and microabscess formation occur. These microabscesses may coalesce into larger macroabscesses, which tend to be surrounded by a rim of granulation tissue.[211] Perinephric abscess results from the rupture of an intrarenal abscess through the renal capsule or the leak from an infected and obstructed kidney (pyonephrosis). The overall distribution in the kidney is usually patchy or lobar, but sometimes it is diffuse.[209] Subsequent scarring of the kidney after treatment reflects the magnitude of the infection and tissue destruction that occurred.

Pyelonephritis may also occur by hematogenous spread of bacteria to the cortex of the kidney and eventual involvement of the medulla. The pattern of involvement is usually round, peripheral, and frequently multiple. Blood-borne infection is less common than ascending infection and is usually observed in intravenous drug abusers, immunocompromised patients, or patients with a source of infection outside the kidney, such as heart valves or teeth.

Imaging is rarely used or needed in uncomplicated pyelonephritis, and most patients respond to therapy within 72 hours. Imaging should be reserved for patients who are not responding to conventional antibiotic treatment, patients with an unclear diagnosis, patients with coexisting stone disease and possible obstruction, patients with diabetes and poor antibiotic response, and patients who are immunocompromised. Imaging is used to assess complications of acute pyelonephritis, including renal and perinephric abscess, emphysematous pyelonephritis, and xanthogranulomatous pyelonephritis.[212–214] All of these entities are imaged best with cross-sectional imaging techniques, specifically CT.

US results are normal in the majority of patients with acute pyelonephritis. When the examination results are abnormal, the findings are often nonspecific. US is performed to look for a cause for acute pyelonephritis, such as obstruction or renal calculi, and to search for complications. Altered parenchymal echogenicity is the most frequent finding with loss of the normal corticomedullary differentiation. The echogenicity is usually decreased or heterogeneous in the affected area (Fig. 25.42). There may be focal or generalized swelling of the kidney. Power Doppler imaging may improve sensitivity in demonstrating focal hypoperfusion, but this is nonspecific. Tissue harmonic US imaging may be more sensitive in demonstrating focal or segmental, patchy, hypoechoic areas extending from the medulla to the renal capsule.[215]

CE-CT is the most sensitive and specific imaging study in the patient with acute pyelonephritis.[216,217] The nephrographic phase of CT is best for imaging in patients with acute pyelonephritis (Fig. 25.43). Wedge-shaped areas of decreased density extending from the renal pyramid to the cortex are most characteristic.[216] The nephrogram may be streaky or striated in either a focal or global manner (Fig. 25.44).[218] There may be focal or diffuse swelling of the kidney.[219] The areas of involvement may appear almost mass-like (see Fig. 25.43). The changes in the nephrogram are related to decreased concentration of contrast media in the tubules with focal ischemia. Tubular destruction and obstruction with debris are also present. There is usually a sharp demarcation between diseased tissue and the normal parenchyma, which continues to enhance normally in the nephrographic phase. Soft tissue stranding and thickening of Gerota's fascia are caused by the adjacent inflammatory process (see Fig. 25.44).[211] The walls of the renal pelvis and proximal ureter may be thickened. The calyces and renal pelvis may be effaced. Mild dilation is also occasionally noted. With hematogenous-related pyelonephritis, the early findings tend to be multiple, round cortical regions of hypodensity that become more confluent and involve the medulla with time.[219] These findings may persist for weeks despite successful treatment with antibiotics.

MRI is comparable with CE-CT for the evaluation of pyelonephritis.[220] The enhancement characteristics of acute pyelonephritis on MRI are similar to those on CT. On

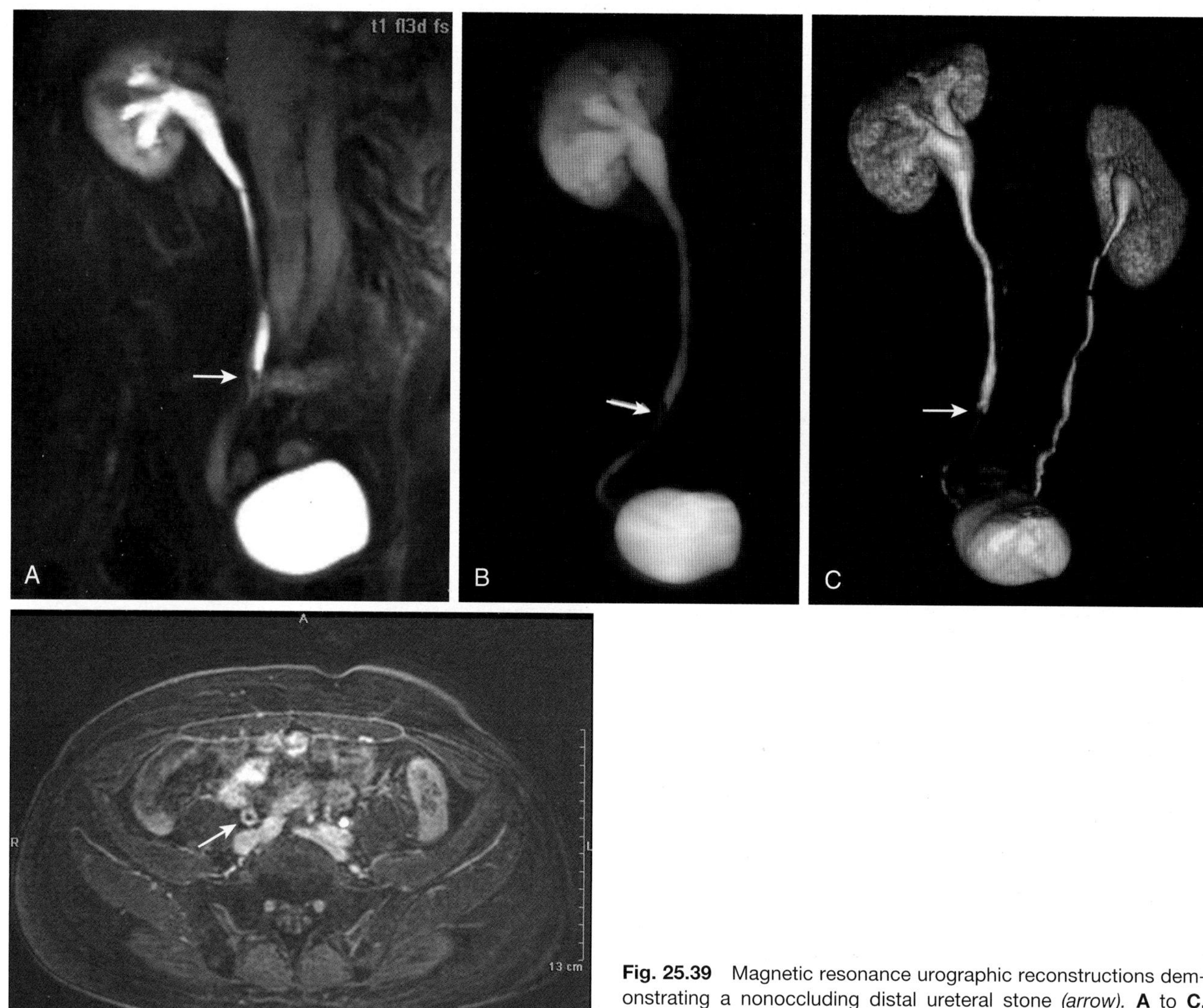


**Fig. 25.39** Magnetic resonance urographic reconstructions demonstrating a nonoccluding distal ureteral stone *(arrow).* **A** to **C,** Three-dimensional postrenal processing techniques are used to mimic intravenous urography. **D,** Postcontrast axial imaging demonstrates a stone within the lumen of the distal ureters.

noncontrast sequences, the affected area has increased T2 signal intensity and decreased T1 signal intensity in relation to the normal renal parenchyma.

Other modalities do not have a significant role in evaluating acute pyelonephritis, unless CT is unavailable. IVU findings may appear normal in up to 75% of cases[211,216]; IVU has been shown to be noncontributory to clinical care in 90% of patients with pyelonephritis.[209,217] Radiolabeled leukocyte scans (e.g., indium 111-labeled white blood cells) and gallium 67 citrate scans can identify acute pyelonephritis. However, these methods have the drawbacks of extended imaging time (more than 24 hours) and higher radiation exposure. Cortical imaging with $^{99m}$Tc-DMSA has been shown to be highly sensitive for detecting acute pyelonephritis in the appropriate clinical setting.[221,222] In acute pyelonephritis, segmental regions of decreased tracer uptake are demonstrated in oval, round, or wedge patterns. There may also be diffuse generalized decrease in renal uptake, which, in association with a normal or slightly enlarged kidney, is suggestive of an acute infectious process. The pathophysiologic basis for decline in $^{99m}$Tc-DMSA cortical uptake in infection is related to diminished delivery of the tracer to the infected area and to direct infectious injury to the tubular cells, which compromises their function and tracer uptake. A wedge-shaped cortical defect with regional decrease in renal size is compatible with postinfectious scarring. Renal infarcts may also have similar appearance.[131,136] Attention to $^{99m}$Tc-DMSA image processing and quality is paramount to achieving high interreader agreement.[223,224] There may also be a role for FDG PET-CT in the imaging evaluation of renal infection.[225]

Renal abscess results from severe pyelonephritis and occurs two to three times more frequently in patients with diabetes.[213] Abscesses are more common with hematogenous infection than with ascending infection.[208] CE-CT characteristics of renal abscess include a reasonably well-defined mass with a low-density central region and a thick, irregular wall or

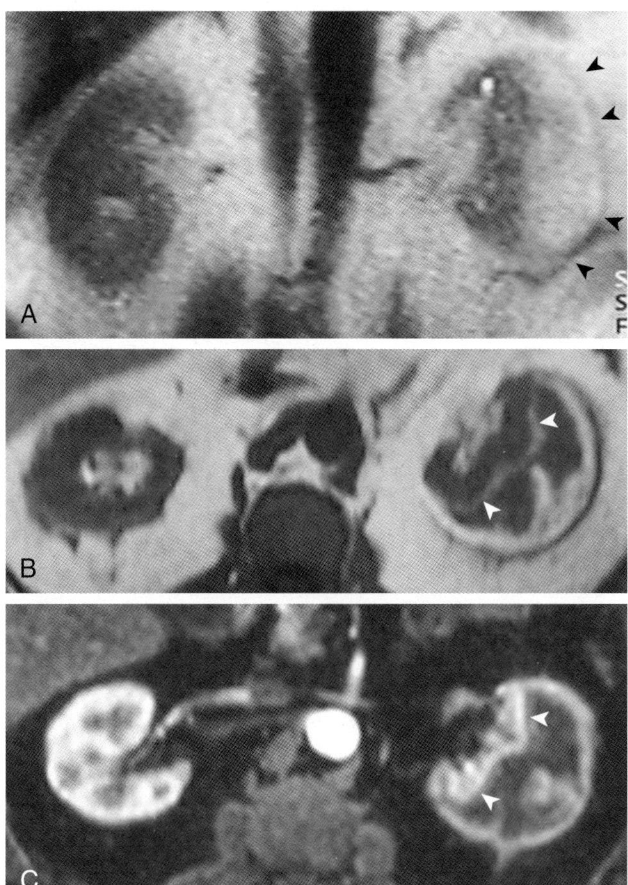

**Fig. 25.40** Subcapsular hematoma after lithotripsy. Coronal T2-weighted sequence **(A)** demonstrates high-signal intensity blood contained by left renal capsule *(arrowheads)*. Axial T1-weighted image **(B)** and gadolinium-enhanced T1-weighted image **(C)** show mass effect on left kidney *(arrowheads)* caused by a subcapsular hematoma. The signal intensity is consistent with the presence of intracellular methemoglobin.

pseudocapsule (Fig. 25.45).[216] Enhancement adjacent to the abscess is variable, depending on the amount of inflammation. Mature abscesses may demonstrate a more sharply demarcated border with peripheral rim enhancement. Gas may be visible within the abscess. MRI is comparable with CE-CT for the evaluation of renal abscess.[220] The central region of the abscess can have a variable appearance, but generally it is of decreased T1 and increased T2 signal intensity. The wall enhancement characteristics are also similar to those on CE-CT (Fig. 25.46).

Renal parenchymal infections can extend into the perinephric space with resulting abscess formation.[219] CT and MRI best reveal the involvement of the perinephric and paranephric spaces within the retroperitoneum. In general, inflammatory changes and heterogeneous fluid-density or signal intensity collections may be identified. Associated gas is best identified on CT.

In patients with preexisting cystic disease, suspected infection can be best evaluated using US, CT, or MRI. The presence of enhancement and documentation of changes compared with prior imaging is crucial.

Emphysematous pyelonephritis is a severe necrotizing infection of the renal parenchyma, usually caused by gram-negative bacteria (*Escherichia coli, Klebsiella pneumoniae, Proteus mirabilis*).[216] Of patients with emphysematous pyelonephritis, 90% have uncontrolled diabetes.[213] Emphysematous pyelonephritis is characterized by severe acute pyelonephritis, urosepsis, and hypotension. The gas found in the renal parenchyma is believed to form as a result of the high levels of glucose in the tissue by fermentation with the production of $CO_2$. The gas may also be observed in the pelvicalyceal system or perinephric space (or both). If the gas is extensive enough, it may be visible on plain radiographs or KUB images. The gas is usually mottled, bubbly, or streaky in appearance and may be observed in the areas over the kidneys. US may suggest the diagnosis of emphysematous pyelonephritis by demonstrating gas within the kidney.[226] With gas present, there is acoustic shadowing in the involved region. CT is the most specific and sensitive modality for the identification of renal gas.[227] The gas dissects through the parenchyma in a linear focal or global manner, radiating along the pyramid to the cortex. It may extend into the perinephric space. There is generally extensive parenchymal destruction with streaks or mottled collections of gas within the kidney (Fig. 25.47). Little or no fluid is seen. Emphysematous pyelitis represents gas within the pelvicalyceal system without parenchymal gas.[228] The distinction is important because emphysematous pyelitis carries a less grave prognosis.

Xanthogranulomatous pyelonephritis is an end-stage condition resulting from chronic obstruction with long-standing infection, usually with *Proteus* species or *E. coli*.[218] The renal parenchyma is destroyed and replaced by vast amounts of lipid-laden macrophages. The kidney is usually barely functional or nonfunctional. The destruction is typically global, but it may involve only a portion of the kidney. A staghorn calculus may be seen on KUB. On US the kidney appears enlarged with loss of identifiable landmarks. A large calculus or staghorn calculus usually fills the renal pelvis, with debris filling adjacent hypoechoic regions (Fig. 25.48). CT defines the extent and adjacent organ involvement best. The findings on CT include an enlarged but generally reniform mass filling the perinephric space.[214,229] Calcification is found in 75% of cases, excretion is absent or markedly decreased in 85% of cases, and the involved region appears as a mass in more than 85% of cases.[214] The process is focal in fewer than 15% of cases. There is frequent perinephric extension. Fistulas may occur in adjacent structures, with adenopathy noted in the retroperitoneum. MRI may show many similar findings when compared with CT, although calcifications are less conspicuous (Fig. 25.49).

Malacoplakia is a rare inflammatory condition that most commonly involves the bladder but may also involve the ureter and kidney. Typically, the kidney is affected by obstruction from the lower urinary tract. When the kidney is directly involved, it is a multifocal process that may appear similar to xanthogranulomatous pyelonephritis on imaging.

Renal tuberculosis occurs by hematogenous spread. The genitourinary tract is the second most common extrapulmonary site of involvement.[230] Evidence of previous pulmonary tuberculosis is found in fewer than 50% of patients with genitourinary tuberculosis.[231] Only 5% may have active tuberculosis. Renal involvement is bilateral; the findings are determined by the extent of the infection, the stage of the

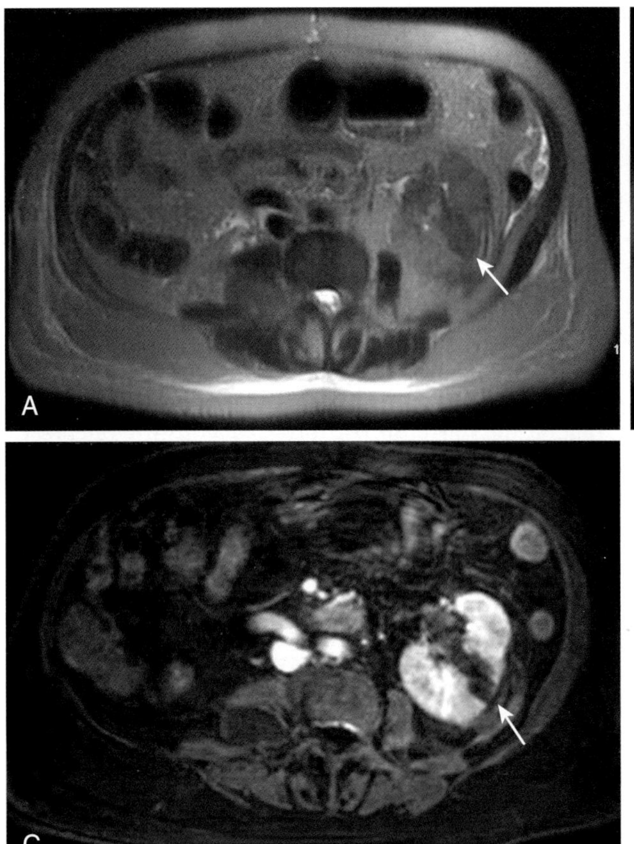


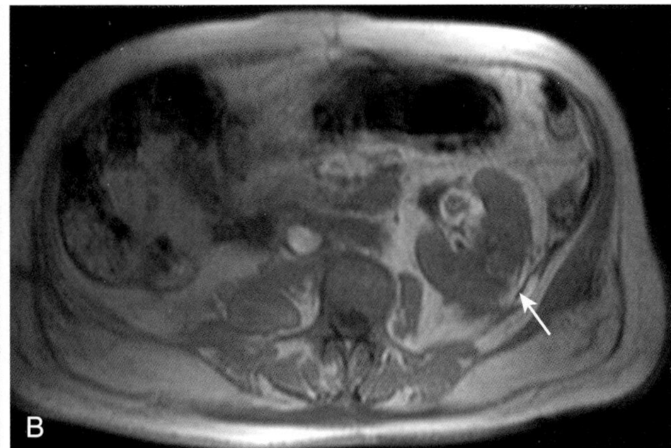


**Fig. 25.41** Hematoma status after surgical removal of staghorn calculus. T2-weighted axial image **(A)**, T1-weighted axial image **(B)**, and postcontrast T1-weighted axial image **(C)** show an intrarenal hematoma (*arrows*) at the site of incision plane. This extends into the renal pelvis. No urine extravasation was demonstrated.

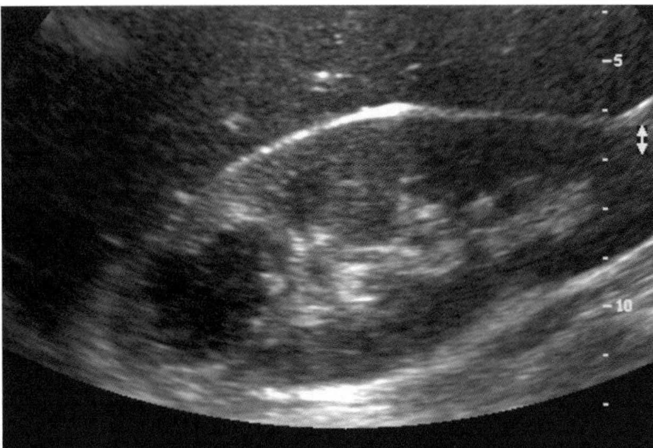

**Fig. 25.42** Acute pyelonephritis: renal ultrasonography. The hypoechoic region in the upper pole represents an area affected by acute pyelonephritis. The surrounding parenchyma is somewhat distorted, with loss of the normal corticomedullary junction.

infection, and the host's response. Calcified granuloma may be found within the cortex or medulla, papillary necrosis may be visible (Fig. 25.50), and hydrocalyx with infundibular strictures may develop (Fig. 25.51). The kidney may become focally or globally scarred as the disease progresses. There may be areas of nonfunction with dystrophic calcifications. In the end stage, the kidney may be small and scarred with bizarre calcifications; this condition is the so-called autonephrectomy.[164,232]

Chronic pyelonephritis is usually associated with vesicoureteral reflux that occurs in childhood.[232] One or both kidneys may be involved. An affected kidney has focal scars that are associated with calyceal dilation. The scarring is often separated by normal regions of the kidney and normal-appearing calyces. When involvement is global, the kidney may be small. IVU demonstrates dilated or ballooned calyces that extend to the cortical surface, which is thinned. The outline of the affected kidney is distorted. With US the kidneys have irregular outlines with regions of cortical loss. Underlying dilated calyces may be visible. The regions of scarring may be echogenic in comparison with the adjacent normal kidney. CT and MRI demonstrate the abnormal architecture of the affected kidney.[219,220] Nephrographic phase images reveal the regions of cortical loss; the involved dilated calyces extend to the capsular surface. Dilation of the calyces is variable. Chronic pyelonephritis may be unilateral or bilateral. Excretory phase images best delineate the extent of involvement, especially in the coronal format.

In the patient with AIDS, urinary tract infections are quite common.[233,234] The infections are frequently hematogenous with unusual organisms such as *Pneumocystis jiroveci*, cytomegalovirus, and *Mycobacterium avium-intracellulare.* The infections may also be seen in other abdominal organs—liver, spleen, and adrenals.[235,236] In patients with AIDS, renal

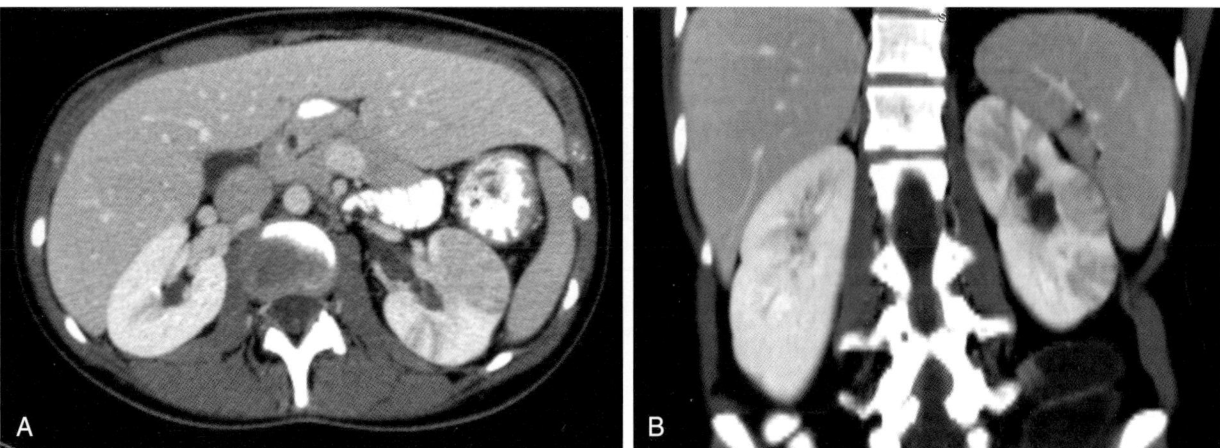


**Fig. 25.43** Acute pyelonephritis: contrast material-enhanced computed tomographic scan, axial **(A)** and coronal **(B)** images. The left kidney shows multiple areas of involvement. The hypodense region in the midportion of the kidney appears almost mass-like (**A** and **B**). A nephrogram is striated in the region of involvement in the upper pole **(B)**.

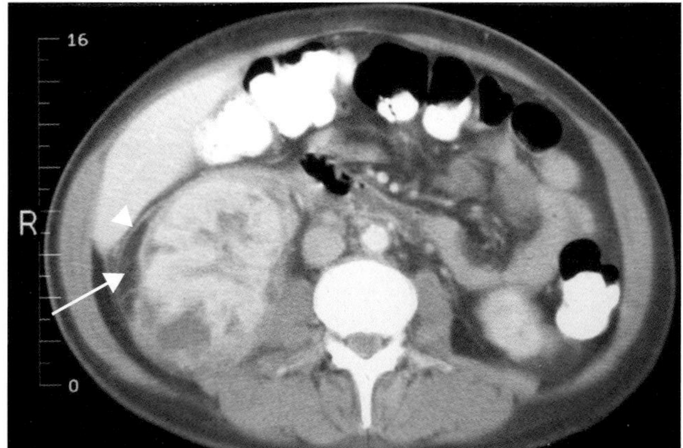


**Fig. 25.44** Acute pyelonephritis: contrast material-enhanced computed tomographic (CT) scan. The heterogeneous CT nephrogram shows the diffuse involvement of the right kidney. Stranding and some fluid are visible in the perinephric space *(arrow)* with thickening of Gerota's fascia (*arrowhead*).

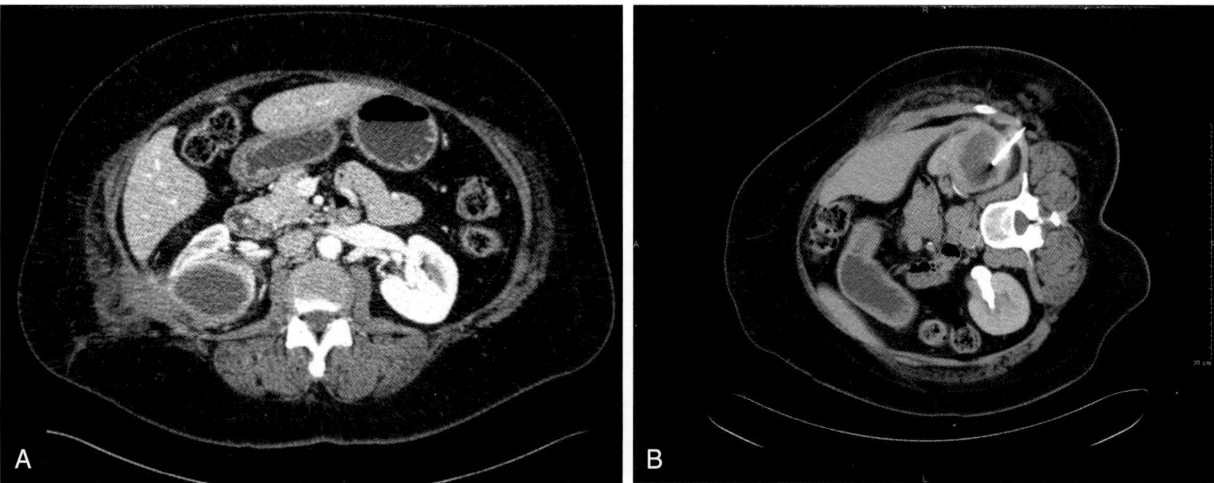


**Fig. 25.45** Renal abscess: contrast material-enhanced computed tomographic scan. **A,** Axial image demonstrates the hypodense abscess in the right kidney with extension into the perinephric space and the right flank. **B,** Axial image with the patient in the decubitus position reveals the method of diagnosis: needle aspiration. A drainage catheter was subsequently placed for treatment.

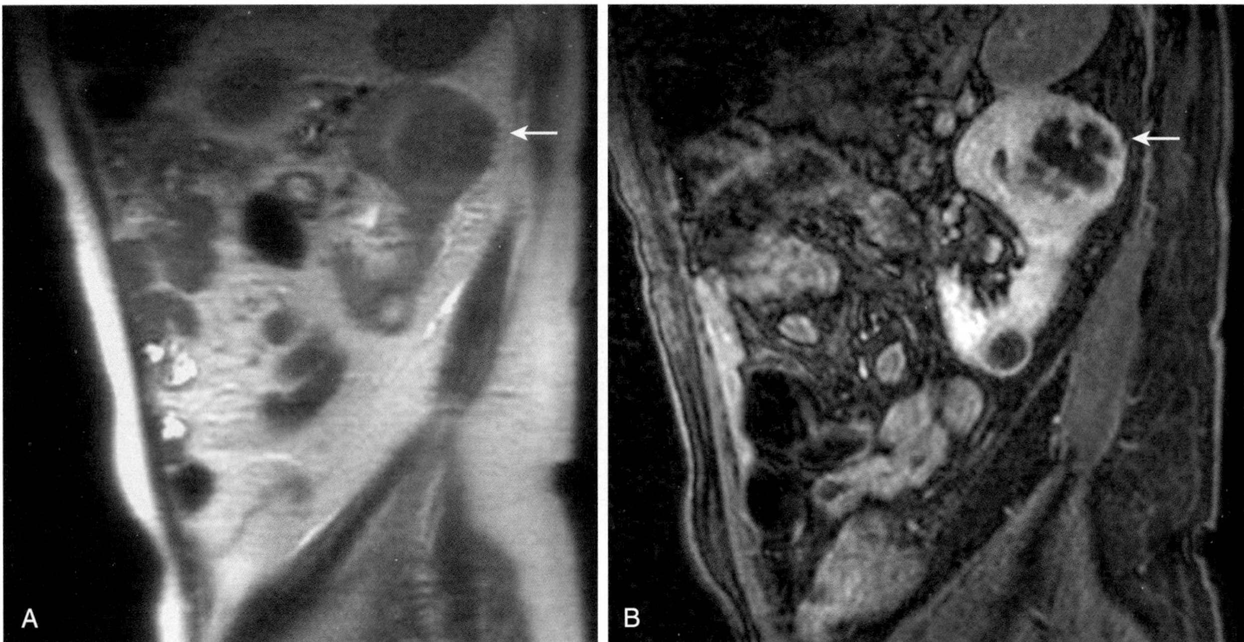


**Fig. 25.46** Renal abscess. A mass in the upper pole of the left kidney demonstrates intermediate to low signal intensity *(arrow)* on the sagittal T2-weighted image **(A)** and heterogeneous but predominantly peripheral enhancement *(arrow)* on the sagittal postcontrast T1-weighted image **(B).** On biopsy, this mass was found to be *Aspergillus* infection.

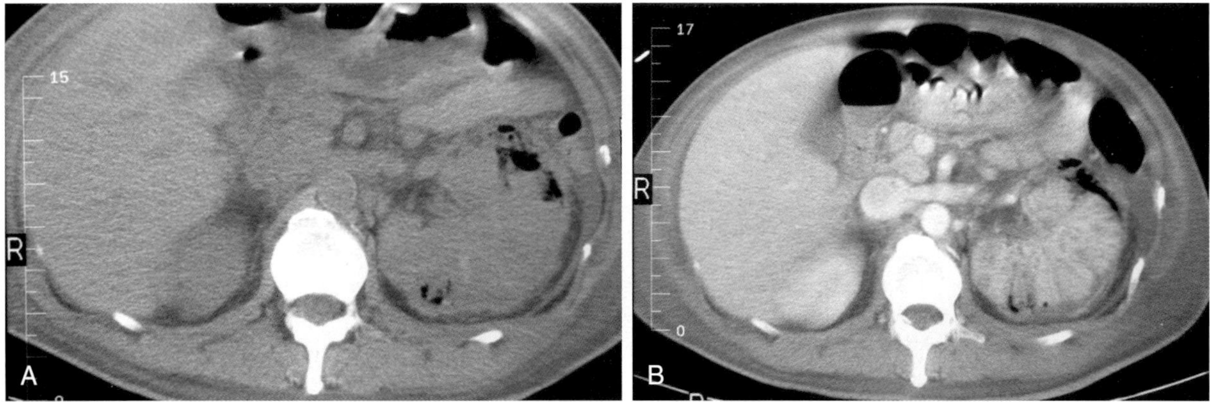


**Fig. 25.47** Emphysematous pyelonephritis: contrast material-enhanced computed tomographic scan. A noncontrast image **(A)** and a contrast material-enhanced image **(B)** demonstrate gas in the left renal parenchyma with extension into the perinephric space. The nephrogram is striated throughout. Global involvement of the kidney is frequent.

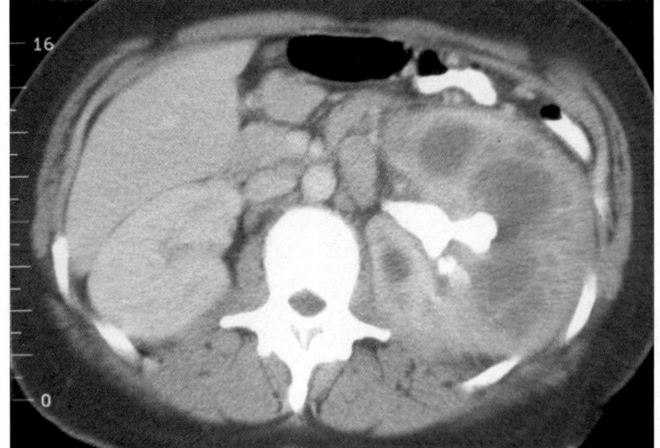


**Fig. 25.48** Xanthogranulomatous pyelonephritis: contrast material-enhanced computed tomographic scan. A large staghorn calculus fills the renal pelvis and collecting systems in the left kidney. Much of the remainder of the kidney is replaced by hypodense material—the xanthogranulomatous infection—within the calyces and parenchyma; some minimal enhancement of the cortex remains.

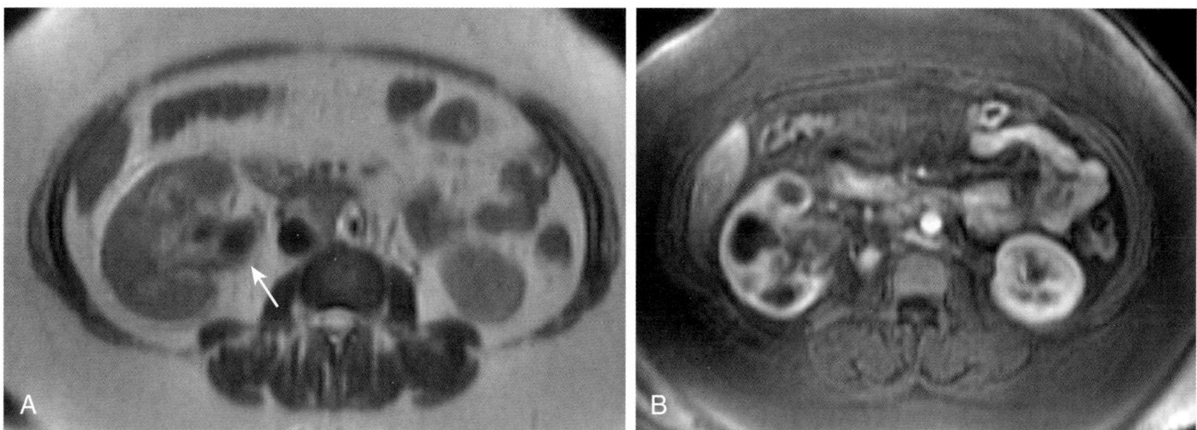

**Fig. 25.49** Xanthogranulomatous pyelonephritis with staghorn calculus. **A,** Axial T2-weighted image demonstrates a stone of low signal intensity within the right renal pelvis *(arrow)* that is associated with increased renal size and replacement of the medullary pyramids and calyces with material of high signal intensity. **B,** Axial postcontrast T1-weighted image demonstrates asymmetric enhancement and hydronephrosis.

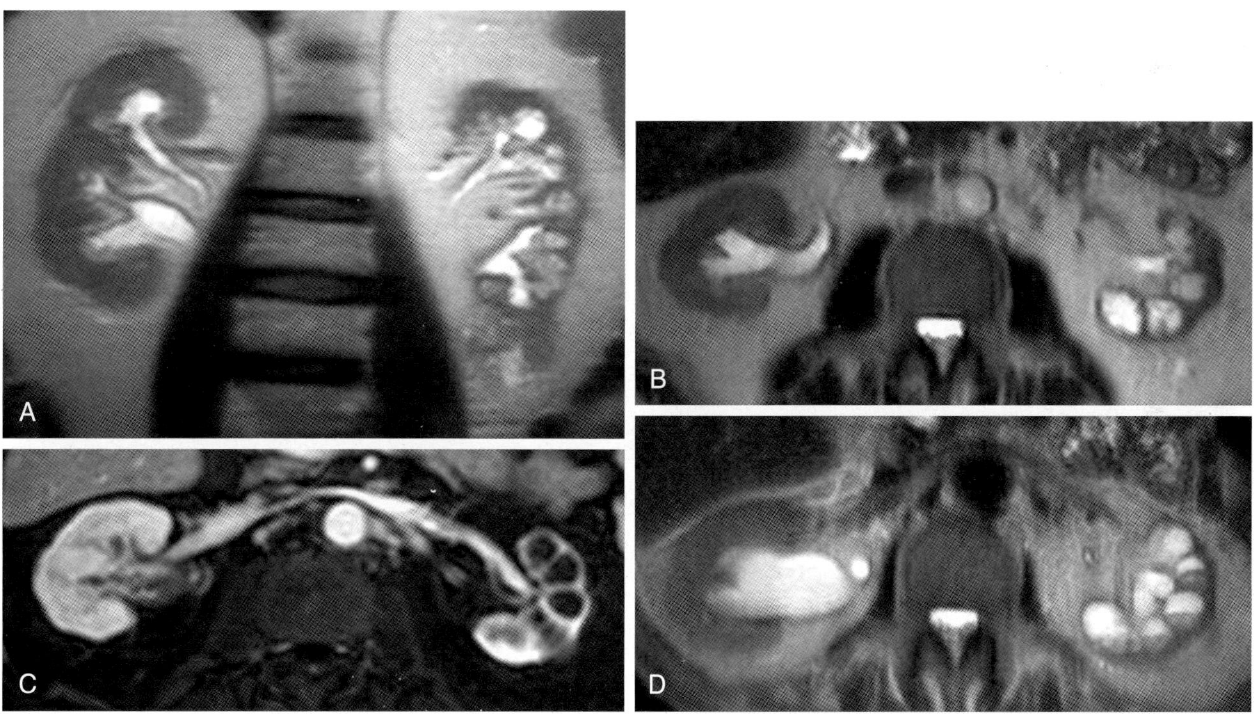

**Fig. 25.50** Renal tuberculosis. **A** and **B,** T2-weighted images demonstrate asymmetric cortical thinning and focal areas of increased signal intensity in the distribution of the medullary pyramids. **C,** Postcontrast T1-weighted image shows absence of enhancement, which is consistent with the presence of granulomas with caseous necrosis. **D,** T2-weighted image after treatment shows distorted, dilated calyces containing debris. Right-sided hydronephrosis is present as a result of a distal ureteral stricture.

involvement may be detected in US demonstrating increased cortical echogenicity and loss of the corticomedullary differentiation (Fig. 25.52).[236] Renal size is also increased, and it is a bilateral process. Infections of the urinary tract are discussed further in Chapter 36.

## RENAL MASS: CYSTS TO RENAL CELL CARCINOMA

Most renal masses are simple cysts, frequently found incidentally on US, CT, and MRI. They rarely occur in individuals younger than 25 years of age, but are found in more than 50% of patients older than 50 years of age. Typically, renal cysts are asymptomatic and cortical in location; they may be single or multiple. Their cause is unknown, although tubular obstruction has been postulated to be a necessary element.

Renal masses produce variable findings on imaging studies, depending on their location. For years IVU was the imaging modality of choice for detection of renal masses; however, the findings on IVU are frequently nonspecific, and further imaging is necessary to characterize most abnormalities found (Fig. 25.53). Studies have shown that IVU has low sensitivity

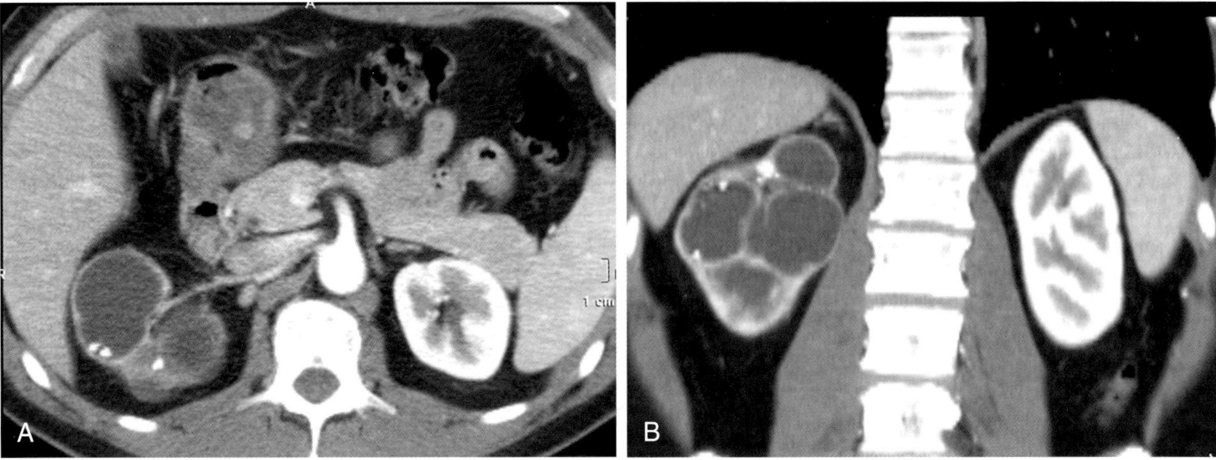


**Fig. 25.51** Renal tuberculosis: contrast material-enhanced computed tomographic scan. Axial **(A)** and coronal **(B)** images show the destruction of the right kidney as a result of renal tuberculosis. Parenchymal calcifications are present with dilated calyces as a result of the attenuation and truncation of the renal pelvis and ureter.

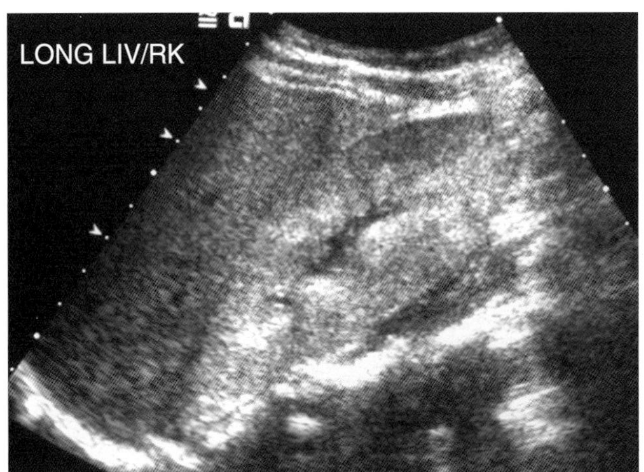


**Fig. 25.52** Acquired immunodeficiency syndrome-related nephropathy: ultrasonography. Longitudinal image of the right kidney. The size of the kidney is normal to slightly increased. The corticomedullary distinction is lost with diffuse increased cortical echogenicity.

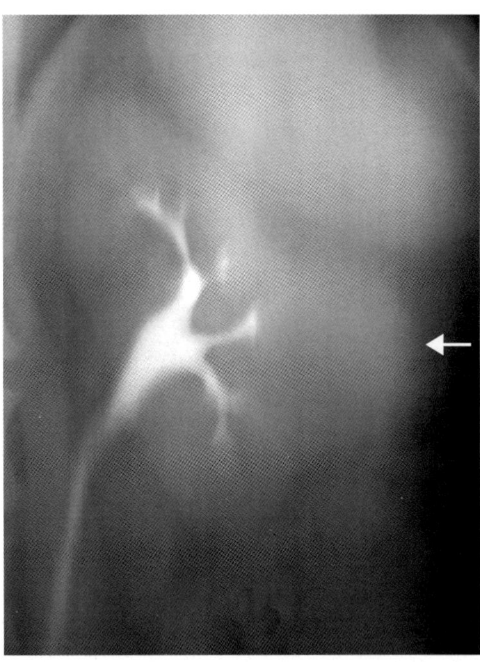

**Fig. 25.53** Renal mass: nephrotomogram. A slightly hypodense mass projects off the lateral border of the left kidney (*arrow*). Subsequent imaging proved this to be a renal cyst.

for detection of renal masses, especially those smaller than 3 cm in diameter.[237] With CT as the gold standard, IVU detected 10% of masses smaller than 1 cm in diameter, 21% of masses 1 to 2 cm in diameter, 52% of masses 2 to 3 cm in diameter, and 85% of masses larger than 3 cm in diameter.[237] US fared better than IVU but detected only 26% of masses smaller than 1 cm, 60% of those 1 to 2 cm, 82% of those 2 to 3 cm, and 85% of those larger than 3 cm.[237]

The findings on IVU are nonspecific, and US, CT, and MRI are used to characterize the renal mass, differentiating solid from cystic.

US is an excellent means of diagnosing a simple renal cyst if all imaging criteria are met.[16] The lesion in the kidney must be round or oval and anechoic (Fig. 25.54); it must be well circumscribed with a smooth wall, and there must be enhanced through-transmission with a sharp interface between the wall and adjacent renal parenchyma. Thin septa may be visible within the cyst, but no nodules should be visible (Fig. 25.55). If all these criteria are met, the diagnosis of cyst is established. If there is any deviation from these criteria, further imaging with CT or MRI is necessary.

CE-CT is the method of choice for characterizing and differentiating renal masses.[238–240] A simple renal cyst appears as a well-circumscribed, round, water-density lesion with no measurable wall (Fig. 25.56). The contents should not enhance after the injection of contrast media. The contents may vary slightly from water density, but no more than 10 to 15 HU. The interface with the adjacent parenchyma is sharp. The margins are smooth with no perceptible nodules. Thin rim-like calcification may be visible. "High-density" cysts may be encountered with density ranging from 50 to 80 HU; these are cysts containing hemorrhagic or proteinaceous debris. Like simple cysts, they should demonstrate no wall nodularity

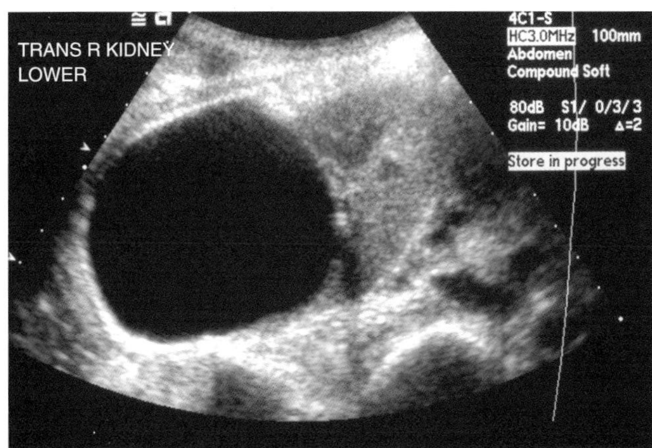


**Fig. 25.54** Renal cyst: ultrasonography. A large, anechoic renal mass projects off the lateral border of the right kidney. The features of the cyst include a well-circumscribed lesion with a sharp back wall and increased through-transmission. There are no internal echoes or nodularity, and the wall is smooth. There is a clear interface with the kidney.

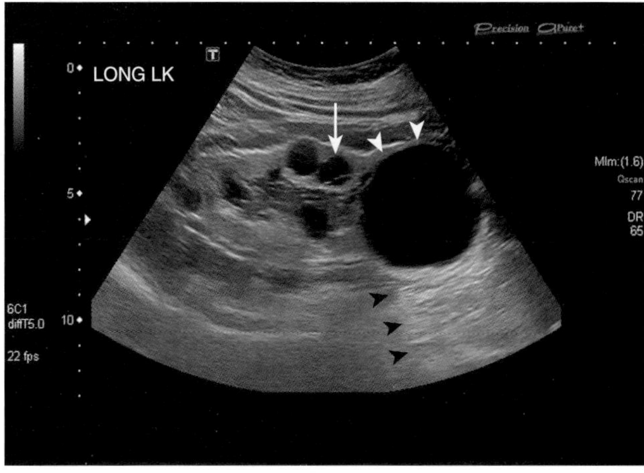


**Fig. 25.55** Gray-scale ultrasonographic longitudinal image reveals a cyst *(white arrowheads)* that is completely anechoic, and there are no septations in it. The appearance of posterior acoustic enhancement *(black arrowheads)* further confirms that the lesion is a cyst. The small, more superficial lesion *(small white arrow)* has a single thin septation, thus representing a Bosniak category II cyst.

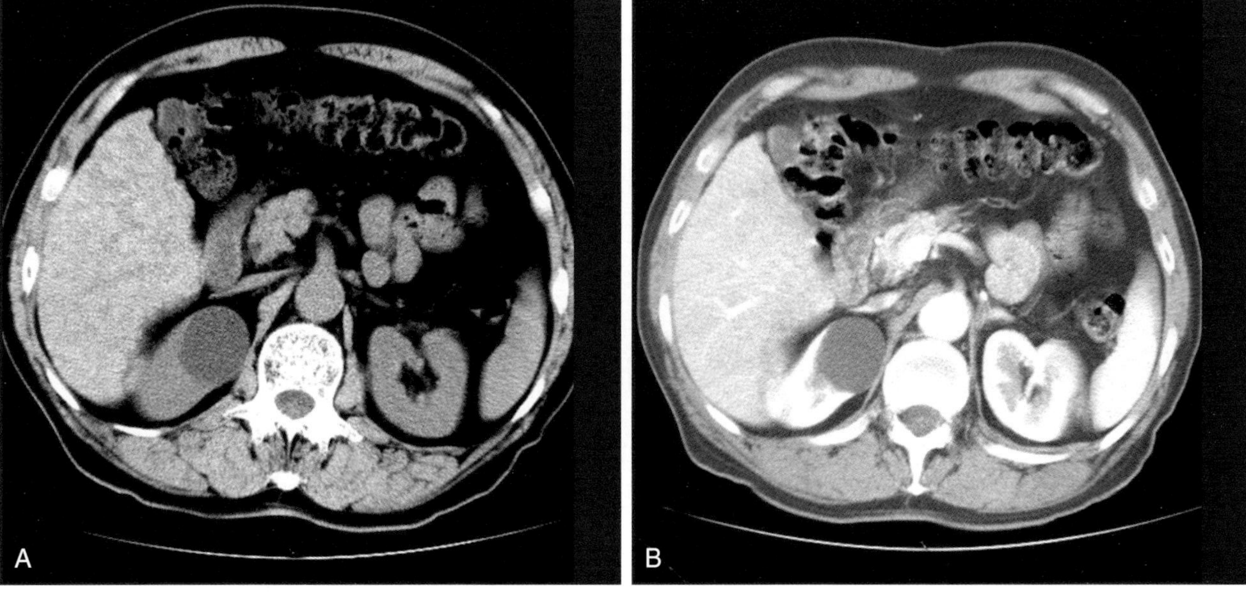


**Fig. 25.56** Renal cyst: computed tomographic (CT) scan. Noncontrast **(A)** and postcontrast **(B)** axial images. The cyst is well circumscribed with no enhancement. It displays water density with CT numbers of 0 to 5. There is a sharp interface with the kidney and no perceptible wall. No nodules are visible, and the cyst is uniform throughout.

and have no significant enhancement after injection of contrast material. High-density cysts are common in polycystic or multicystic kidneys. Cysts are well demonstrated on MRI because of excellent soft tissue contrast. On MRI, simple cysts are well-circumscribed, thin-walled structures containing fluid that appears dark on T1-weighted sequences and bright on T2-weighted sequences (Fig. 25.57). Complex cysts contain proteinaceous or hemorrhagic fluid and may have septations and calcification. The T1 signal intensity of the fluid is higher than expected for simple fluid, ranging from isointense to hyperintense. T2 signal intensity is lower than expected for simple fluid and may be black, depending on the blood content. Cysts do not enhance. In comparison with CE-CT, CE-MRI has been found to have higher contrast material resolution, which allows for better visualization of septa.[241,242] MRI also better characterizes blood products and is more sensitive to subtle enhancement, especially when subtraction techniques are used. This makes MRI superior to CT in differentiating a complex cyst from a cystic neoplasm[241–243] (Figs. 25.58 and 25.59).

Polycystic renal disease is classified as infantile, adult, or acquired. The infantile form is inherited as an autosomal recessive disorder.[244] It has a variable manifestation: severe kidney injury is found in the neonatal period, and CHF and hepatic failure manifest in older children. Organomegaly is common, with bilateral symmetric renal enlargement. IVU yields poor visualization of the kidneys because of renal impairment, and the nephrogram is prolonged and mottled

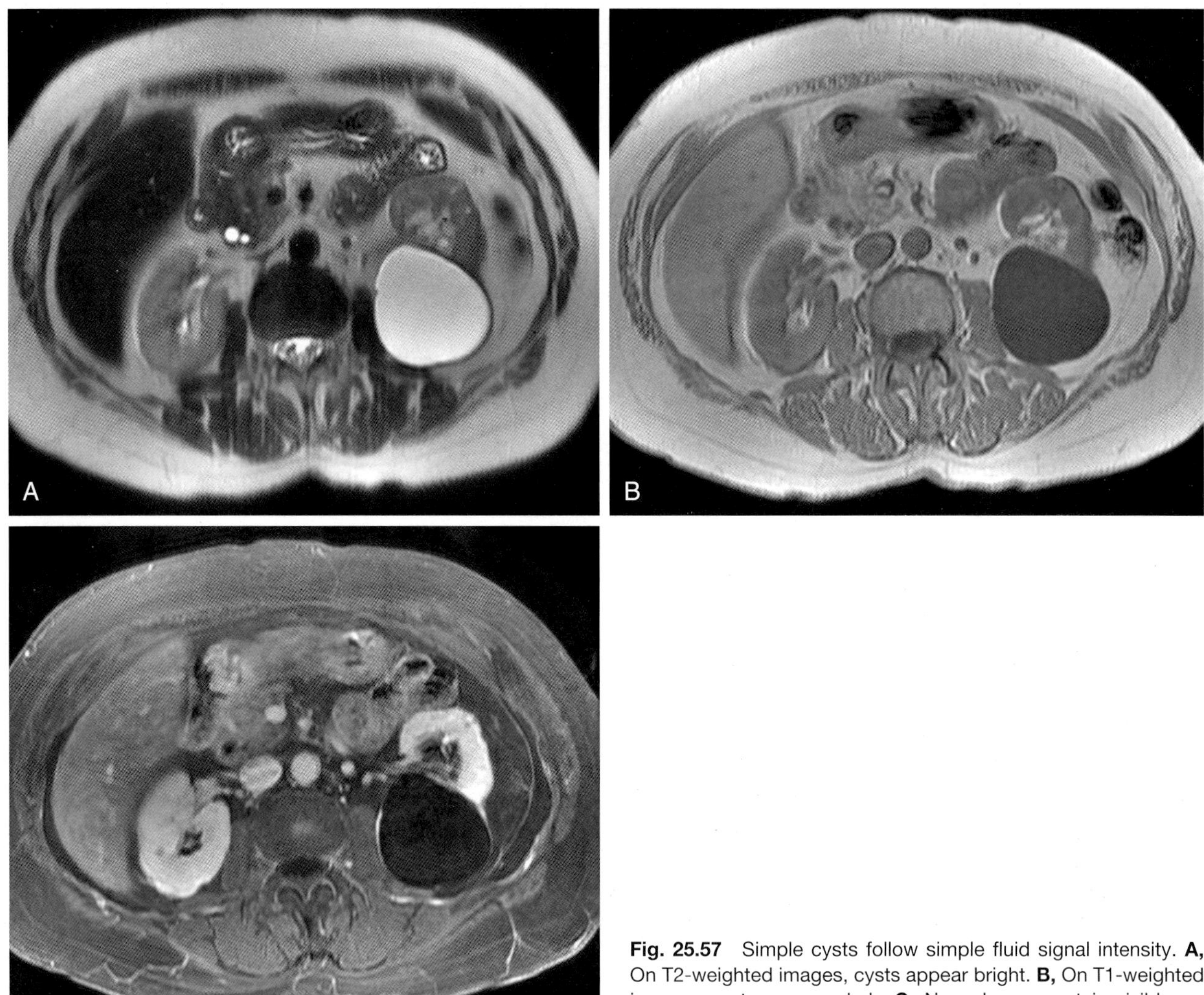


**Fig. 25.57** Simple cysts follow simple fluid signal intensity. **A,** On T2-weighted images, cysts appear bright. **B,** On T1-weighted images, cysts appear dark. **C,** No enhancement is visible on gadolinium-enhanced T1-weighted images.

with a striated or streaky appearance. US reveals enlarged, diffusely hyperechoic kidneys as a result of dilated, ectatic collecting tubules.[245] There is loss of the corticomedullary differentiation as well. Because the diagnosis is made clinically with the associated US findings, CT and MRI are rarely used in this condition.

Autosomal dominant polycystic kidney disease (ADPKD) is the adult form.[246] There is no role for KUB or IVU in the evaluation for ADPKD. US reveals bilateral enlargement of the kidneys, which are markedly lobulated and contain multiple anechoic areas of varying size throughout.[247]

CT and MRI in ADPKD depict enlarged, lobulated kidneys with cysts of varying size throughout (Fig. 25.60). One kidney may be more involved than the other. The cysts may have calcifications with the wall. It is not uncommon to encounter cysts with varying density or signal intensity as a result of episodes of hemorrhage that occur within the cysts (Fig. 25.61). A fluid level may be visible as a result of the presence of debris or hemorrhage within some of the cysts. In the excretory phase, there is marked distortion of the calyces. The extent of renal involvement by ADPKD is better appreciated on CT and MRI than on US. Cysts may be found in the liver, spleen, and pancreas as well.

Adult-acquired polycystic kidney disease occurs in patients with kidney injury who are undergoing continuous peritoneal dialysis or hemodialysis[248] (Fig. 25.62). The longer the patient has undergone dialysis, the more likely the patient is to develop adult-acquired polycystic kidney disease.[249,250] The cysts are generally quite small (0.5–2 cm in most patients). Calcification may occur in the wall. Plain radiographs and IVU play no role in evaluation because renal function is impaired. US reveals small, shrunken kidneys with anechoic or hypoechoic regions that represent the cysts. The findings are usually bilateral. CT or MRI shows the small bilateral kidneys with cysts of size that varies, but usually in the range of 1 to 2 cm (Fig. 25.63; see Fig. 25.28).[251,252] These cysts must be closely evaluated for solid components because carcinomas and adenomas occur with increased frequency in these patients. Solid lesions smaller than 3 cm in diameter may represent either adenomas or renal cell carcinomas, whereas most lesions larger than 3 cm are renal cell carcinomas.[253,254] Screening for adult-acquired polycystic kidney disease is usually done with US every 6 months; CT or MRI is reserved for patients with questionable or solid lesions.[255]

Medullary sponge kidney, or renal tubular ectasia, is a nonhereditary developmental disorder with ectasia and cystic

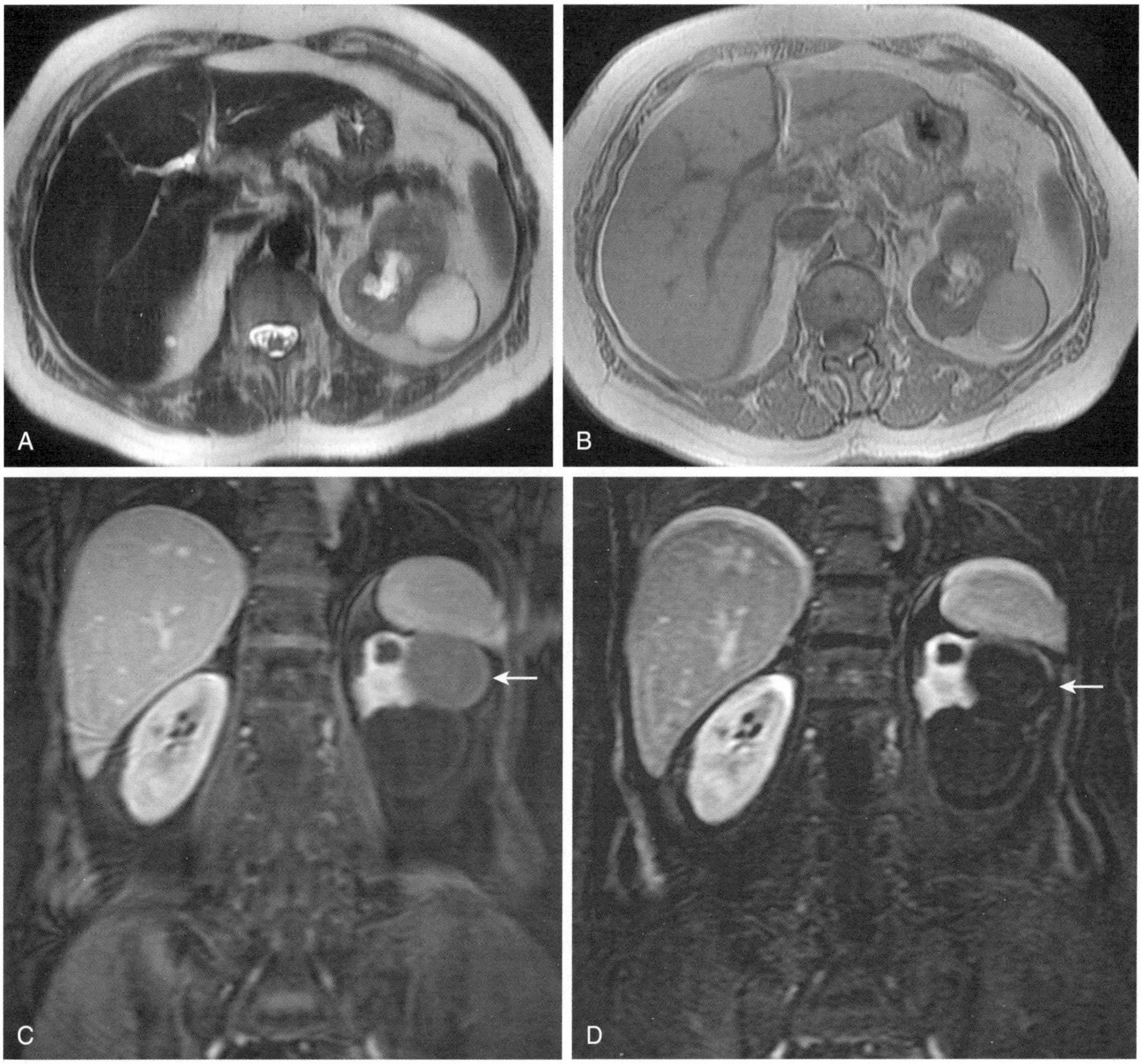

**Fig. 25.58** Complex cyst confirmed by magnetic resonance imaging with image subtraction. **A,** T2-weighted axial image shows a bright left upper pole structure. **B,** T1-weighted axial image shows the same structure as intermediate in signal intensity. The cyst has internal debris that is visible on both sequences. Because the postcontrast T1-weighted coronal image **(C)** shows higher signal intensity than expected for a cyst *(arrow),* postcontrast subtraction images **(D)** are needed to confirm absence of enhancement *(arrow).*

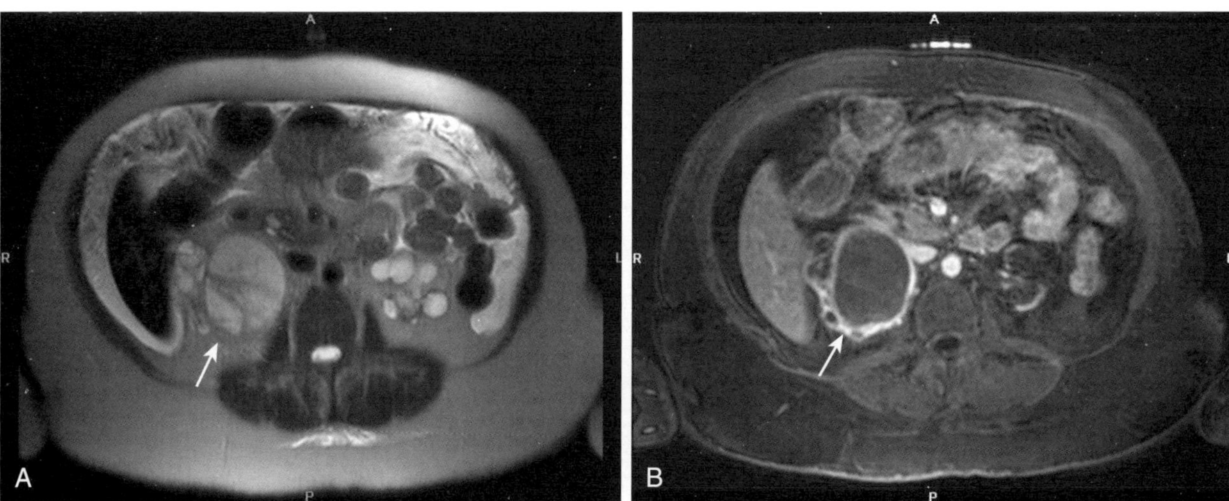

**Fig. 25.59** Complex hemorrhagic cyst. **A,** T1-weighted axial images show a complex right renal structure, bright on both sequences and with internal septations *(arrow).* **B,** Gadolinium on T1-weighted images produced no enhancement *(arrow).* This structure was diagnosed on fine-needle aspiration as a hemorrhagic cyst.

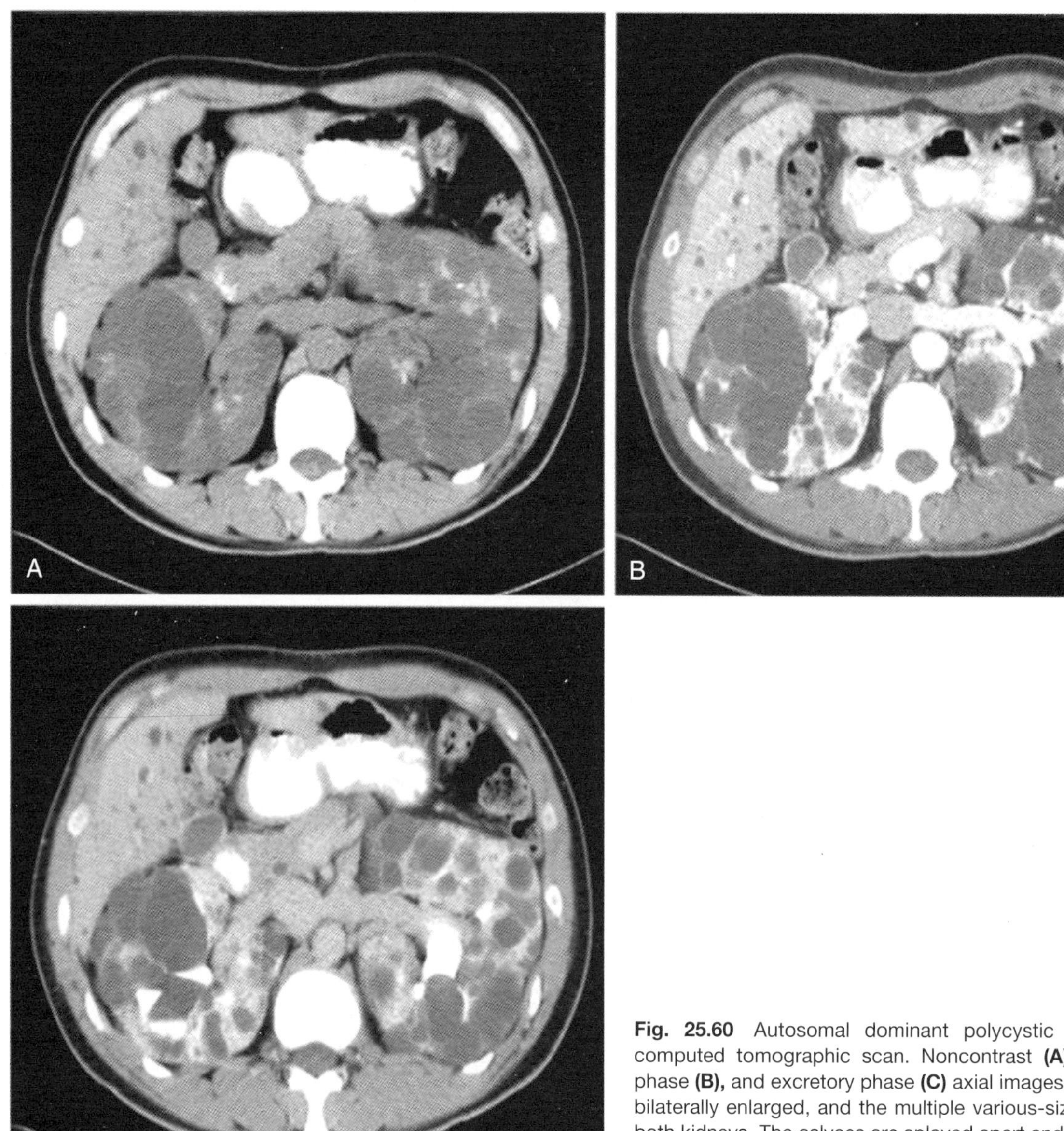


**Fig. 25.60** Autosomal dominant polycystic kidney disease: computed tomographic scan. Noncontrast **(A),** nephrographic phase **(B),** and excretory phase **(C)** axial images. The kidneys are bilaterally enlarged, and the multiple various-sized cysts involve both kidneys. The calyces are splayed apart and appear distorted in the excretory phase image **(C).** Note the multiple small cysts also present in the involved liver.

dilation of the distal collecting tubules. The cystic spaces predispose to stasis, which leads to stone formation and potential infection. Involvement is usually bilateral, although not always symmetric, with as few as one calyx involved. The kidneys are typically normal sized with an appearance of medullary nephrocalcinosis when small stones are present.[165] IVU reveals linear or round collections of contrast material extending from the calyceal border, forming parallel brush-like striations. With more severe involvement, the cystic dilations may appear grape-like or bead-like. CT is an excellent method for demonstrating the calculi, although the striations or cystic dilation may be difficult to visualize even with thin-section excretory phase imaging.

Multicystic dysplastic kidney is an uncommon, congenital, nonhereditary condition. It is usually unilateral and affects the entire kidney. In rare cases only a portion of the kidney is involved. US reveals multiple anechoic cystic structures of varying size replacing the kidney, with no normal parenchyma. Calcification in the wall of the cystic spaces may be visible. CT demonstrates multiple fluid-filled structures filling the renal fossa. Septa and some rim-like calcifications may be visible. The density of the fluid is usually the same as or slightly higher than water. The kidney does not enhance after the injection of intravenous contrast material, and the renal artery on the affected side is not visible. It may be difficult to differentiate this condition from severe hydronephrosis if no cyst walls or septa are visible.

Small cortical cysts may occur in some hereditary syndromes (e.g., tuberous sclerosis) and in acquired conditions (e.g., lithium nephropathy; Fig. 25.63). These cysts are typically multiple and very small (millimeters). They are viewed best with MRI but may also be viewed on CT if the cysts are slightly larger.[256] Cortical cysts may be larger in hereditary disorders, such as von Hippel–Lindau disease (Fig. 25.64).[257] Pyelogenic cysts or calyceal diverticula are small cystic structures that connect with a portion of the pelvicalyceal system. On contrast

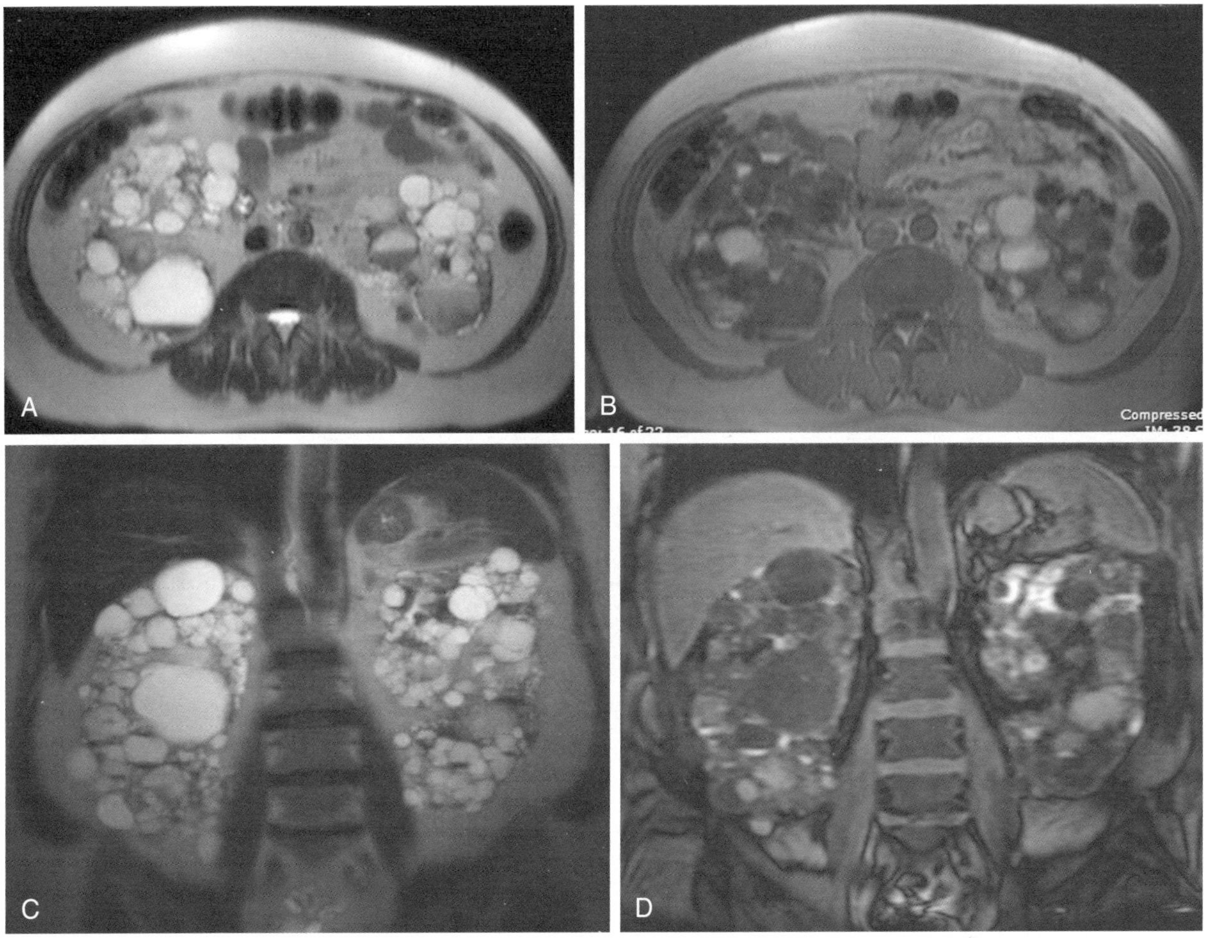

**Fig. 25.61** Autosomal dominant polycystic kidney disease. Axial **(A)** and coronal **(C)** T2-weighted images show bilateral renal cortical atrophy and multiple cysts, most of which are bright. Axial T1-weighted image **(B)** shows multiple bright and dark structures that are not enhanced after gadolinium injection; this appearance was confirmed with subtraction image **(D)** and is therefore consistent with cysts.

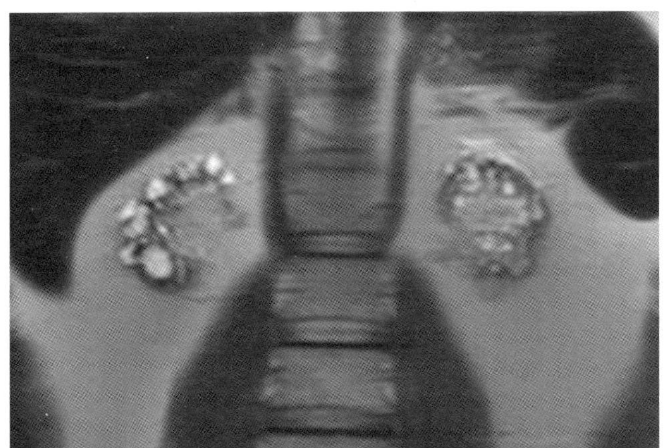

**Fig. 25.62** End-stage kidney disease. T2-weighted coronal image shows diffuse atrophy and multiple acquired cysts in a patient on chronic dialysis.

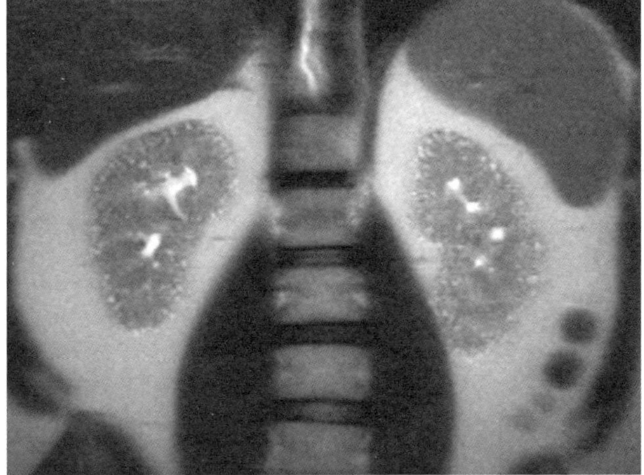

**Fig. 25.63** Lithium toxicity. Coronal T2-weighted image demonstrates innumerable small renal cortical cysts, characteristic of lithium toxicity.

material-enhanced studies a calyceal diverticulum appears as a small round or oval collection of contrast material connected to the fornix of the calyx. As stasis occurs within the diverticulum, renal stone formation may occur.

Cystic renal masses present a diagnostic problem in that not all are benign.[258] In 1986, Bosniak developed a classification system based on CT imaging characteristics to help guide the clinical management of cystic renal masses.[256–263] Category I lesions are simple, benign cysts (see Fig. 25.56). Category II cysts are benign with thin septa, fine rim-like calcification, or they are uniform high-density cysts less than 3 cm in diameter that do not enhance (Fig. 25.65). Category IIF represents more

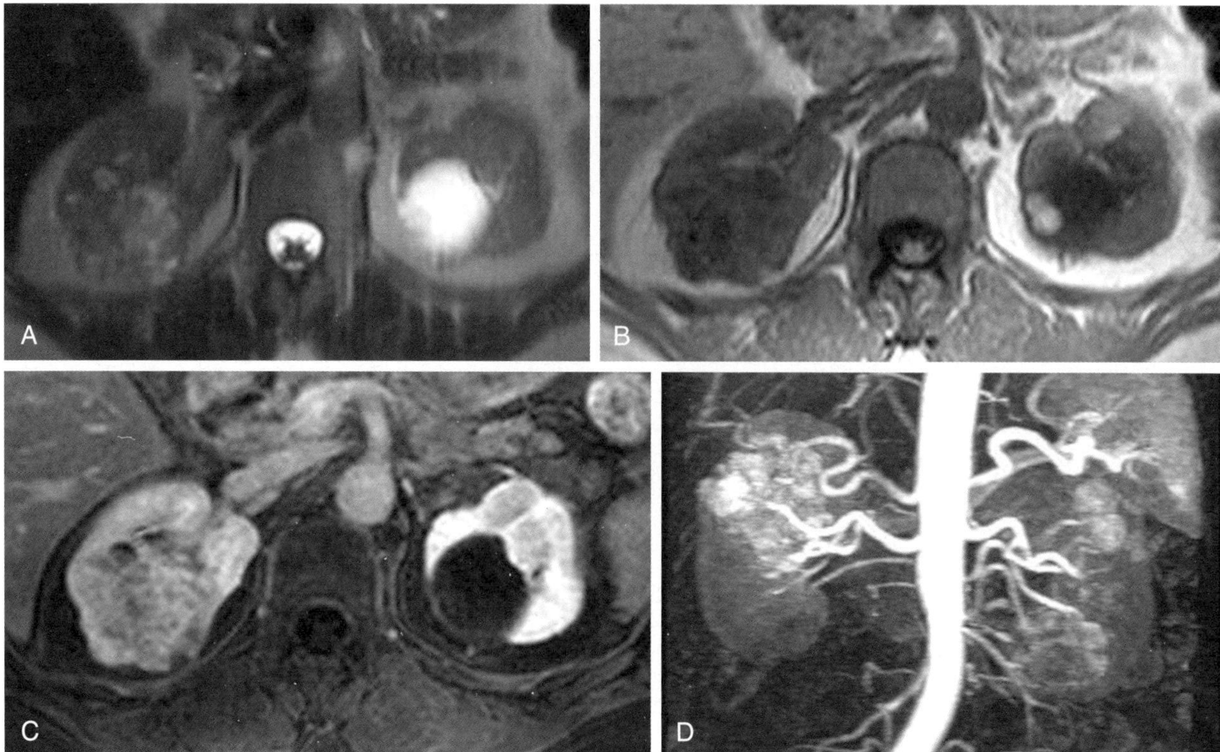


**Fig. 25.64** Bilateral clear cell carcinoma in von Hippel-Lindau syndrome. Bilateral heterogeneous renal masses and left renal cyst are visible on T2-weighted image **(A)** and T1-weighted image **(B)**. **C,** The larger right renal mass demonstrates heterogeneous enhancement, and two smaller left renal masses demonstrate more homogeneous enhancement. **D,** Maximum-intensity projection depicts the multiple renal masses in angiographic format.

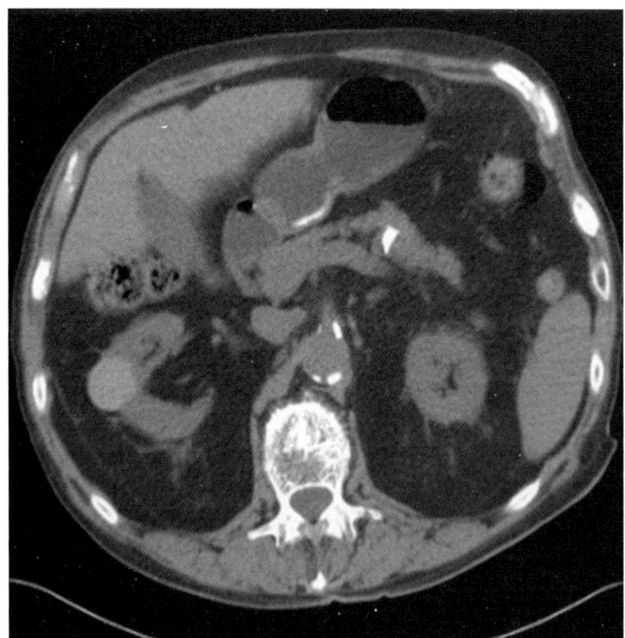

**Fig. 25.65** Hyperdense renal cyst: computed tomographic scan, axial noncontrast image. A single well-circumscribed hyperdense mass is visible in the right kidney. This represents a Bosniak category II renal cyst. It is sharply defined and less than 3 cm in diameter, and it will demonstrate no enhancement on the contrast material-enhanced scan.

indeterminate category II lesions that necessitate follow-up, usually at 6 to 12 months, to prove benignity (Fig. 25.66).[262] These cystic lesions may have multiple septa, or an area of thick or nodular calcification, or they may be high-density cysts larger than 3 cm in diameter. Category III cystic lesions have thickened, irregular walls, which demonstrate some enhancement. Dense irregular calcification may also be visible. In these cases, clinical history may be helpful in determining whether they are renal abscesses or infected cysts. Although some of these lesions are benign, surgery may be necessary for diagnosis and treatment.[263] Biopsy has been advocated by some authorities.[264–267] Category IV cystic masses are clearly malignant and demonstrate distinct enhanced soft tissue masses or nodules within the cyst (Fig. 25.67).[268] Nephrectomy is required for these lesions, although if they are not larger than 5 to 6 cm and are in proper locations, a nephron-sparing procedure may be performed. Cystic diseases of the kidney are further discussed in Chapter 45.

CE-CT is the imaging modality of choice for the characterization of all solid masses, suspected solid masses, or masses that do not meet US criteria for a true renal cyst.[259,266,269] MRI has sensitivities and specificities similar to those of CT but is generally reserved for cases in which the patient has a contraindication to iodinated contrast medium or in which radiation dose must be limited. MRI may be helpful in cases of renal masses for which CT yielded indeterminate findings, in cases with venous involvement, and in distinguishing vessels from retroperitoneal lymph nodes. CEUS is now an additional technique that can be used especially in patients with compromised renal function (Fig. 25.68).

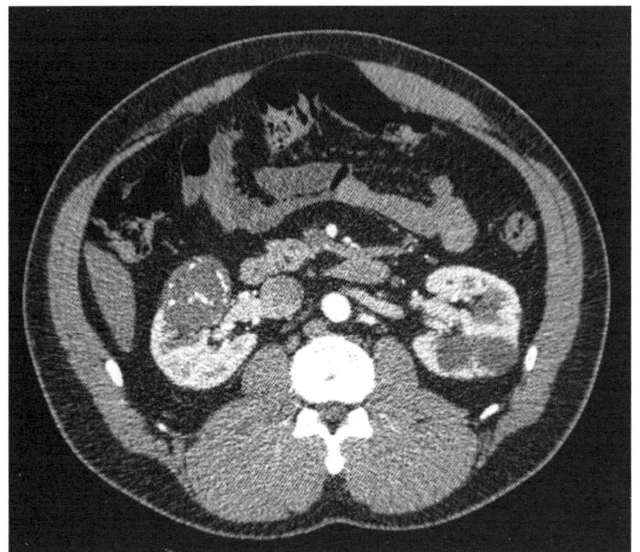

**Fig. 25.66** Bosniak category IIF renal cyst: computed tomographic (CT) scan, axial nephrographic phase image. A cystic lesion in the right kidney also demonstrates large clumps of calcification on the outer wall and on internal septa. There was no change in the CT numbers between the noncontrast scan and the enhanced images. This cyst necessitates follow-up. Note the Bosniak category I cysts in the left kidney.

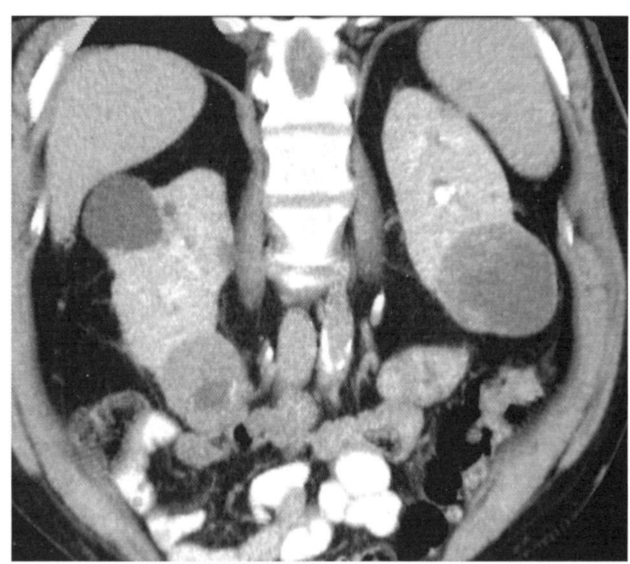

**Fig. 25.67** Bosniak category IV left renal cyst: computed tomographic scan, coronal nephrographic phase image. A cystic mass is visible in the left kidney with an internal solid component in the lower pole. In the lower pole of the right kidney, there is a solid mass with central necrosis, which represents a renal cell carcinoma. Note the Bosniak category I cysts in the upper pole of the right kidney. A renal calculus is also present in the midportion of the left kidney. The left lower pole cystic lesion proved to be a renal cell carcinoma, papillary type.

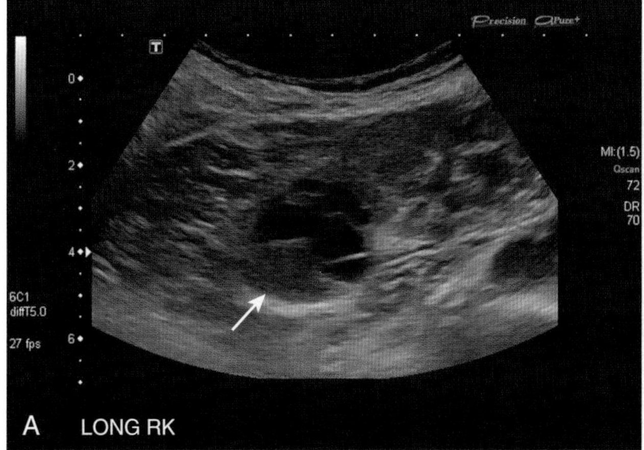


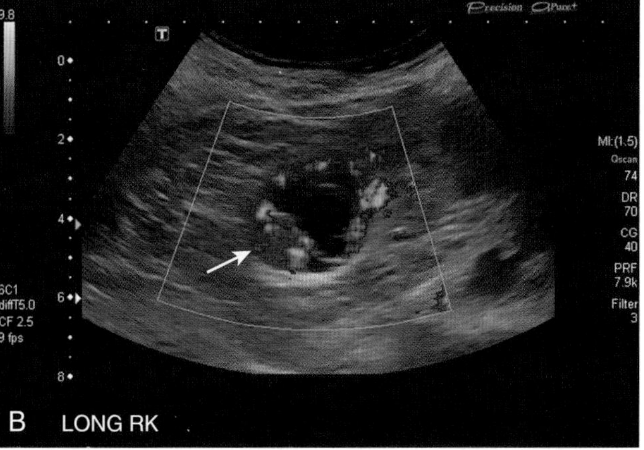


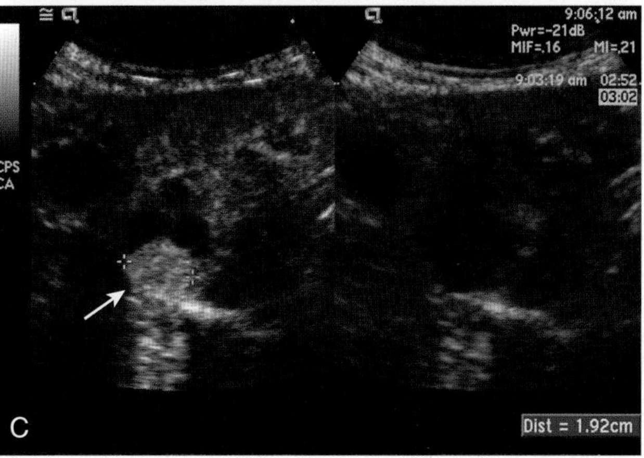


**Fig. 25.68** A Bosniak category IV cyst in a 58-year-old woman. **A,** Gray-scale ultrasonogram reveals a complex cyst with a solid nodular component *(arrow)*. **B,** Power Doppler image reveals flow within the nodular component of the lesion *(arrow),* confirming its vascularized nature. **C,** Composite image including a contrast material–enhanced image on the left and a gray-scale image on the right. The nodule *(arrow)* reveals dense arterial phase enhancement with heterogeneous washout. The findings were consistent with a neoplastic cyst. The lesion was subsequently resected and was found to be a clear cell carcinoma, Fuhrman grade 2.

Renal neoplasms may arise from either the renal parenchyma or the urothelium of the pelvicalyceal system. With the increased use of cross-sectional imaging techniques, more small neoplasms are discovered incidentally.[270,271] Renal adenoma is the most common benign neoplasm; it almost always is less than 2 to 3 cm in size and has no characteristic radiologic features to distinguish it from other solid tumors. Typically, renal adenomas are corticomedullary in location, appear solid on US, and demonstrate uniform enhancement on CE-CT.

Renal hamartomas, known as angiomyolipomas (AMLs), are benign renal tumors composed of different tissues, including fat, muscle, vascular elements, and even cartilage. It is the fat component that makes AML distinguishable radiologically (Fig. 25.69).[272,273] On US the mass is solid and hyperechoic due to the presence of fat.[274,275] On CT the diagnosis of AML can be made with ease, because most AML have a large amount of fat that exhibits low attenuation (<–10 HU). In uncommon cases, only a minimal amount of fat is present, and it must be searched for diligently.[276–279] MRI with fat-suppressed and opposed-phase chemical shift sequences can be used to make an accurate diagnosis.[280] Signal intensity of fat is high on both T1- and T2-weighted sequences. Macroscopic fat in AML has decreased signal intensity with fat-suppression sequences. Opposed-phase chemical shift sequences cause an "India ink" outline of the tumor at its interface with normal renal parenchyma. The enhancement pattern of AML may be variable, depending on the composition of the lesion. Fat should be searched for in all solid lesions in the kidney; if present, the diagnosis of AML is virtually ensured.[281–283] Most AMLs measuring 4 cm in diameter or smaller are monitored; surgery is reserved for larger ones, especially with hemorrhage.[284,285] Multiple, bilateral AMLs may be found in patients with tuberous sclerosis.

Oncocytoma is an uncommon benign tumor originating in the epithelium of the proximal collecting tubule. Radiologically, its features include a solid mass with homogeneous enhancement, a central stellate scar that may be visible on US, CE-CT, or MRI, and a spoked-wheel pattern on angiography.[286–288] These findings are nonspecific, however, and histologic confirmation is needed.[289,290] Oncocytic renal cell carcinomas also occur, and surgery is generally needed for the correct diagnosis.

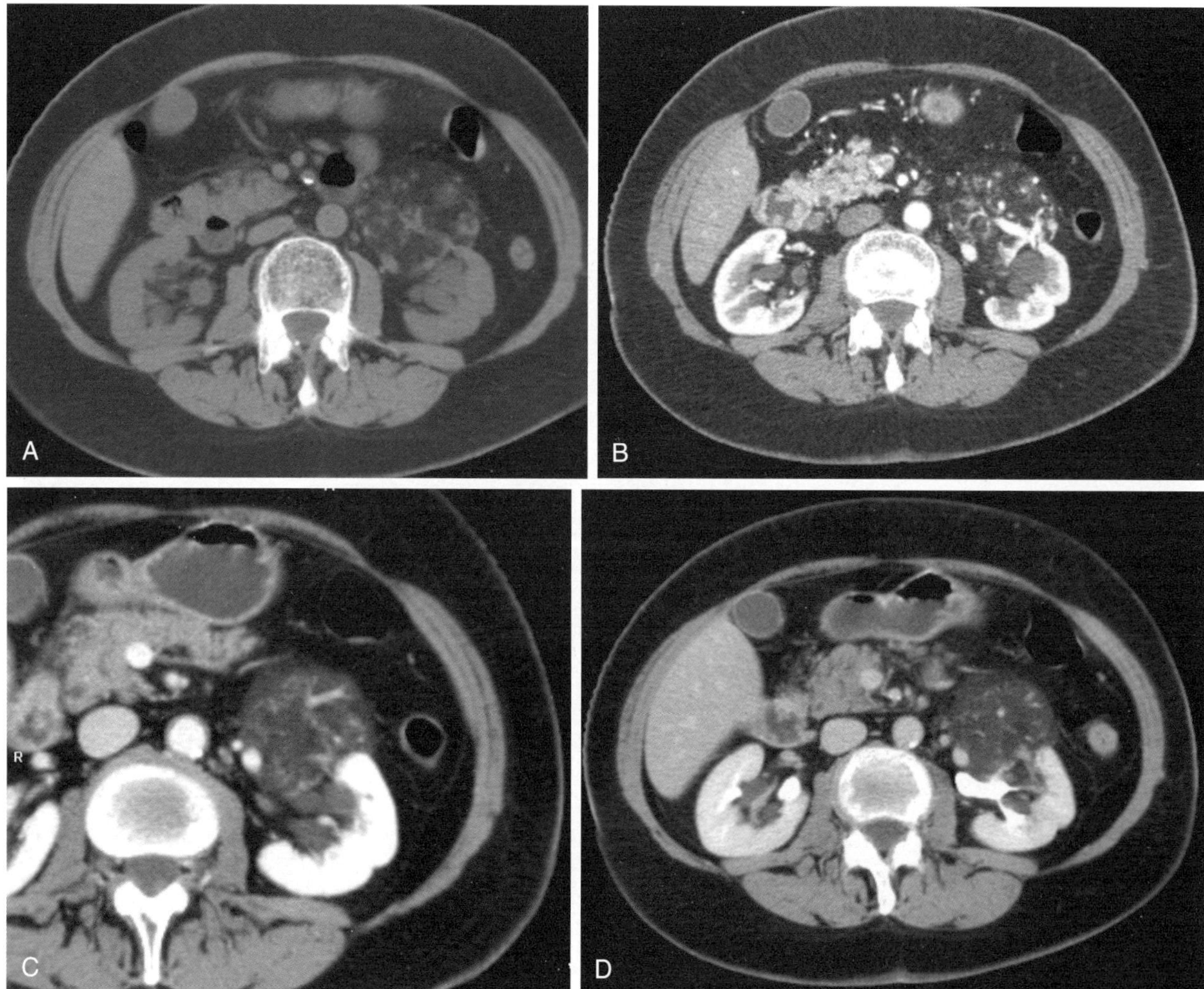


**Fig. 25.69** Angiomyolipoma: computed tomographic scan, noncontrast **(A)**, corticomedullary phase **(B)**, nephrographic phase **(C)**, and excretory phase **(D)** axial images. The fat-containing mass is visible projecting anteriorly from the left kidney. The internal structure in this very vascular benign tumor demonstrates enhancement.

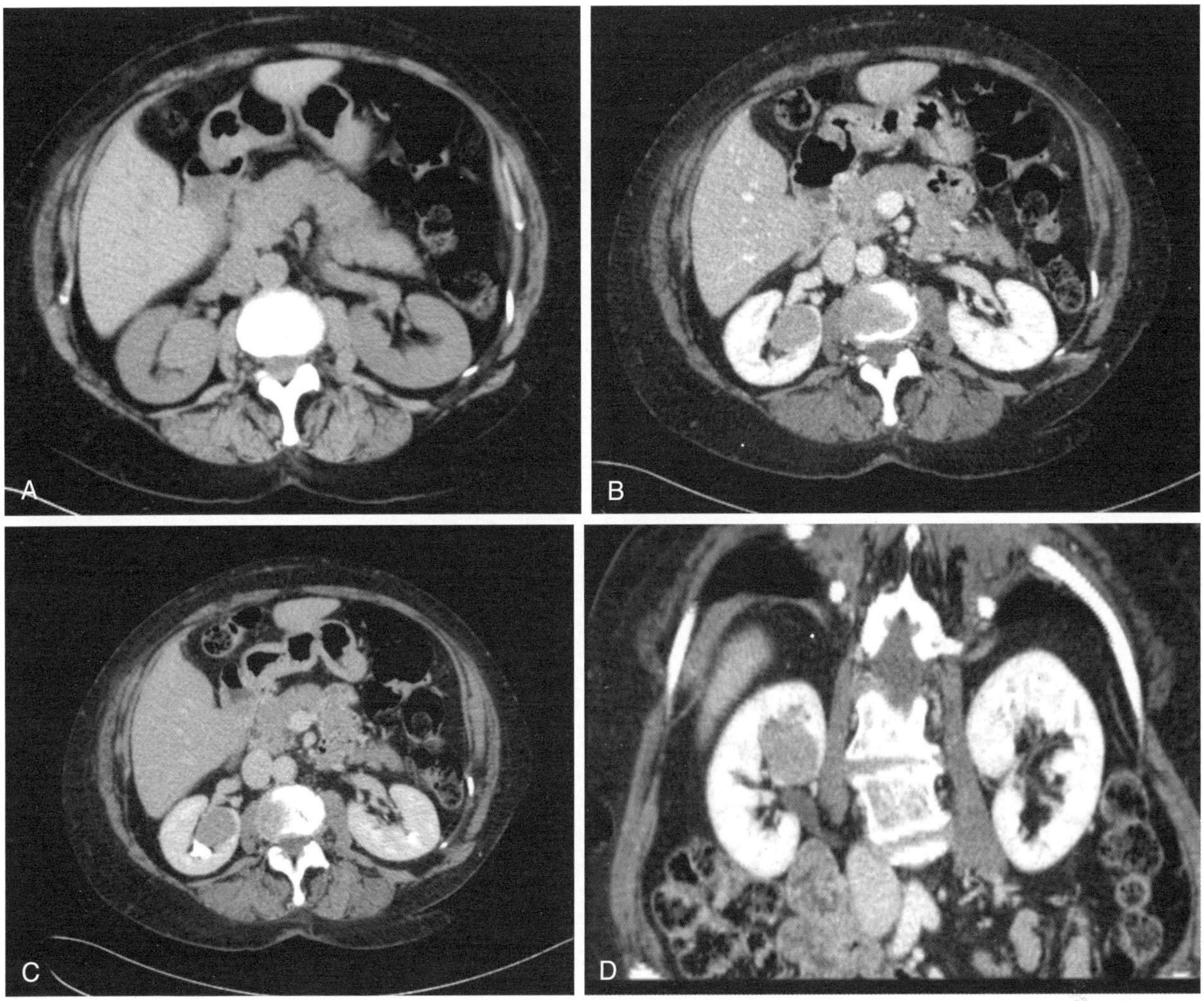

**Fig. 25.70** Renal cell carcinoma: computed tomographic scan. Noncontrast **(A)**, nephrographic phase **(B)**, and excretory phase **(C)** axial images combined with a coronal nephrographic phase image **(D)**. On the noncontrast scan **(A)**, the right renal mass appears slightly hyperdense in relation to the rest of the kidney. Contrast material-enhanced scans (**B**, **C**, and **D**) show the enhanced structure surrounded by the normal renal parenchyma. This proved to be a renal cell carcinoma, chromophobe type.

Renal cell carcinoma is the third most common tumor of the genitourinary tract after carcinoma of the prostate and bladder. CE-CT is the modality of choice for imaging renal cell carcinoma because it has proved to be effective in detection, diagnosis, characterization, and staging, with accuracy exceeding 90%.[291,292] On noncontrast CT, renal cell carcinoma appears as an ill-defined area in the kidney with HU close to that of the renal parenchyma (Fig. 25.70). After the injection of intravenous contrast material, most renal cell carcinomas show enhancement. The best phase for depiction of the mass is the nephrographic phase (see Fig. 25.70).[293–295] The corticomedullary phase is most helpful for showing the relationship of the tumor to the vascular structures because there is maximal enhancement of the arteries and veins (Fig. 25.71).[296,297] The excretory phase is most helpful for showing the relationship of the tumor to the pelvicalyceal system and in preoperative planning for nephron-sparing partial nephrectomy (see Fig. 25.70).[298,299] Clear cell renal cell carcinoma tends to have greater and more heterogenous enhancement than the papillary types (see Figs. 25.64, 25.71, 25.72, and 25.73).[300,301] Chromophobe tumors typically have a homogeneous enhancement pattern

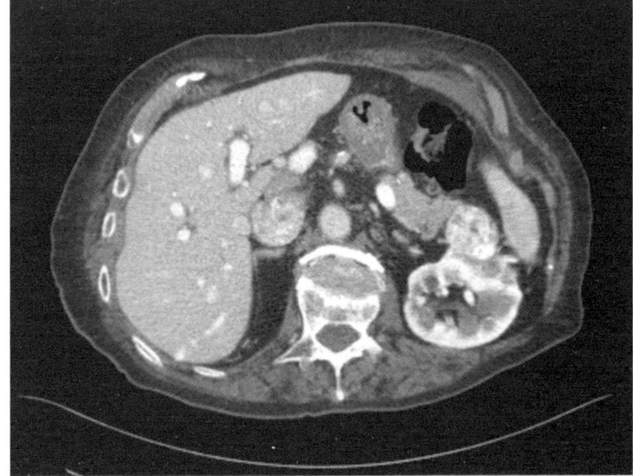

**Fig. 25.71** Renal cell carcinoma: computed tomographic scan. Contrast material-enhanced axial image in the corticomedullary phase. Note the heterogeneously enhanced mass in the anterior aspect of the left kidney. This is a stage II renal cell carcinoma, inasmuch as it has extended through the renal capsule into Gerota's fascia. This proved to be a renal cell carcinoma, clear cell type.

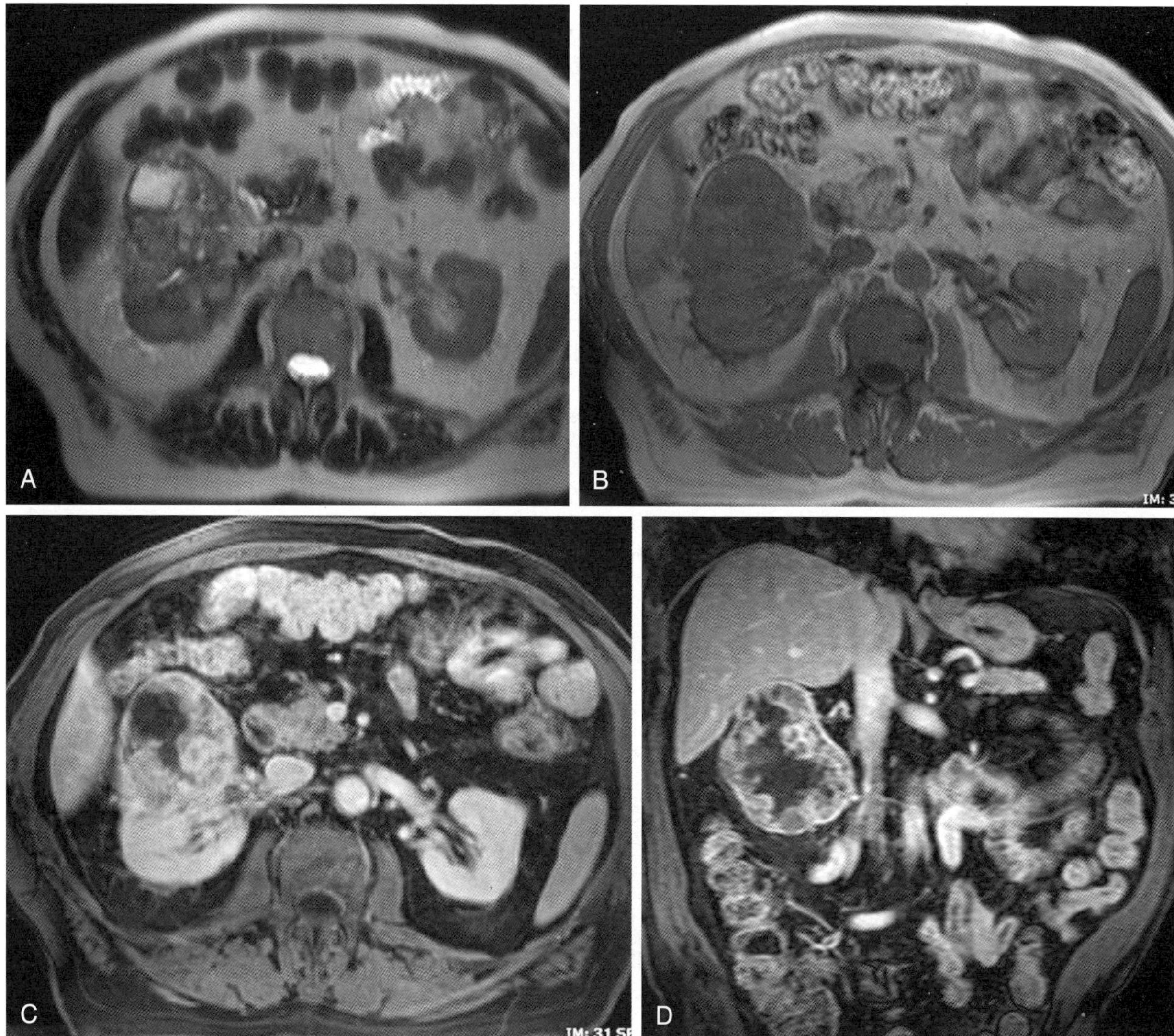

**Fig. 25.72** Clear cell renal cell carcinoma, stage IIIA. **A,** Axial T2-weighted image shows a 7.5-cm right renal mass with areas of high signal intensity, consistent with necrosis and cystic degeneration. **B,** Axial T1-weighted image shows a heterogeneous, isointense mass with increased perinephric fat stranding. Axial **(C)** and coronal **(D)** gadolinium-enhanced images confirm central areas of necrosis. No venous invasion is visible. Focal microinvasion of the perinephric fat was found at surgery.

(see Fig. 25.70).[300] Chromophobe and papillary types more often contain calcification than does the clear cell type, and they demonstrate only mild enhancement of 25 to 30 HU.[302]

The appearance of renal cell carcinoma on MRI can vary with the histologic type. For example, the clear cell type tends to be larger and is associated more frequently with hemorrhage and necrosis (Figs. 25.72 and 25.73) than is the papillary type (Fig. 25.74) and chromophobe renal cell carcinoma. The feasibility of differentiating histologic types of renal cell carcinoma by means of advanced MRI techniques such as diffusion weighting is being evaluated, but further research is required.[303] Renal cell carcinoma is most commonly heterogeneously hyperintense on T2-weighted sequences and hypointense to isointense on T1-weighted sequences (Fig. 25.75). Renal cell carcinoma enhances less than normal renal cortex tissue. The heterogeneity increases with increasing size as a result of variable amounts of necrosis and intraluminal lipid. The intraluminal lipid may make areas of the mass drop in signal intensity on opposed-phase T1-weighted sequences.

The staging of renal cell carcinoma is important in predicting survival rates and planning the proper surgical approach to the mass. Both the World Health Organization and the Robson classifications are used in the staging of renal cell carcinoma.[291] In the Robson classification of renal cell carcinoma, a stage I tumor is confined to the renal parenchyma by the renal capsule (see Figs. 25.70, 25.74, and 25.75). In stage II renal cell carcinoma, the tumor extends through the renal capsule into the perinephric fat but is still within Gerota's fascia (see Fig. 25.71 and Fig. 25.64). Stage III lesions are subdivided: IIIA tumors extend into the renal vein or IVC (Fig. 25.73 and Fig. 25.76); IIIB tumors involve regional retroperitoneal lymph nodes; and IIIC tumors involve the veins and nodes. In stage IVA renal cell carcinoma, the tumor extends outside Gerota's fascia with involvement of adjacent organs or muscles other than the ipsilateral adrenal gland

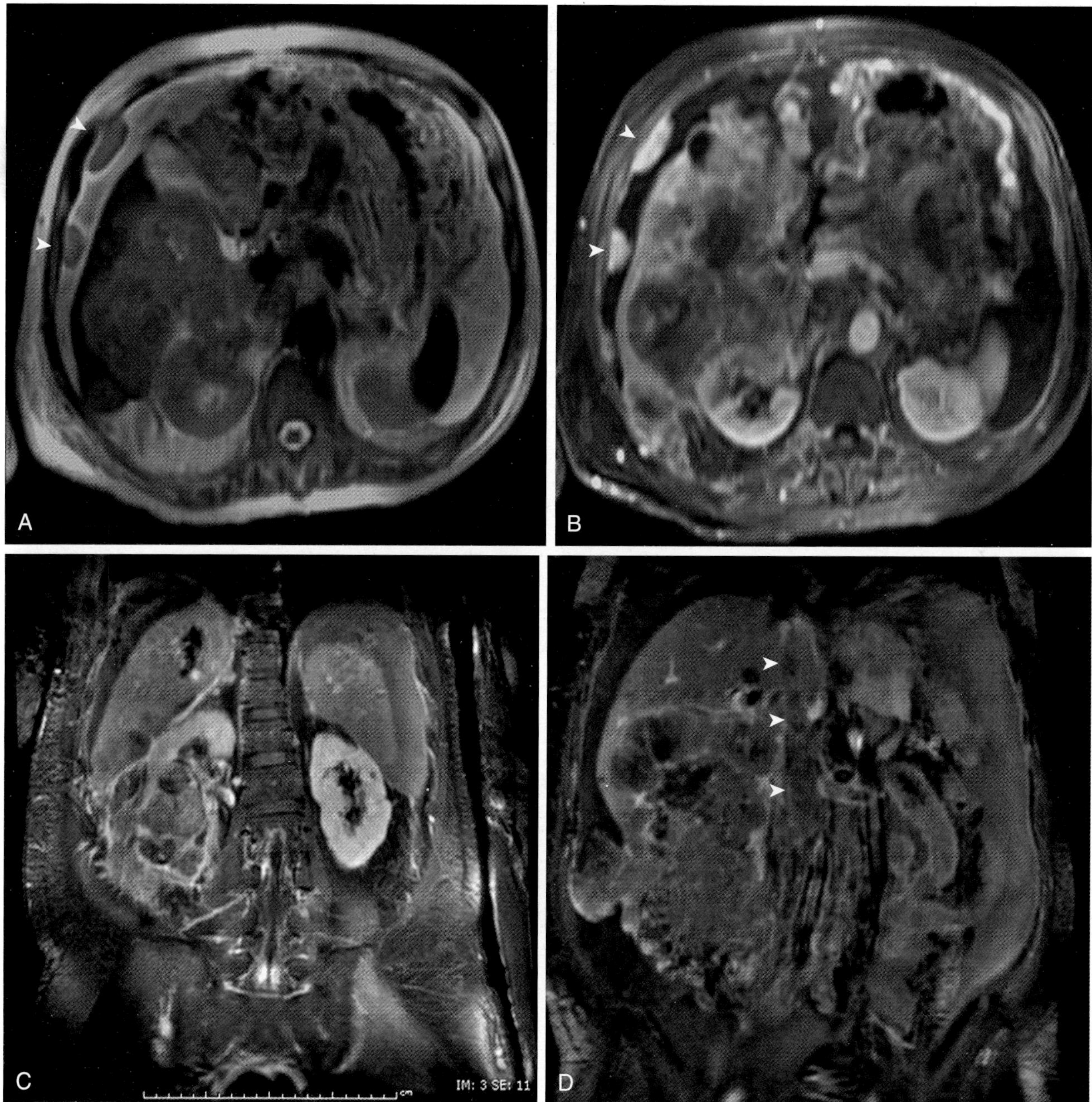


**Fig. 25.73** Metastatic clear cell renal cell carcinoma, stage IV. T2-weighted **(A)** and gadolinium-enhanced T1-weighted **(B)** axial images show a large, heterogeneous mass with invasion of the adjacent liver and peritoneal metastases *(arrowheads)*. **C** and **D,** Coronal gadolinium-enhanced T1-weighted images show the large mass extending inferiorly and medially, with invasion of the inferior vena cava to the level of the hepatic veins *(arrowheads)*.

(see Fig. 25.77). Stage IVB renal cell carcinoma represents tumor with distant metastases, the most common sites being the lungs, mediastinum, liver, and bone. Kidney cancer is further discussed in Chapter 41.

MRI has been found to be highly accurate in staging renal cell carcinoma; however, as with CT, the areas of greatest challenge remain the evaluation for local invasion of the perinephric fat and direct invasion of adjacent organs, especially with large tumors.[304] The presence of an intact pseudocapsule aids in ruling out local invasion. A pseudocapsule is a hypointense rim around the tumor, viewed best on T2-weighted images (see Fig. 25.75A) and most frequently observed in association with small or slow-growing tumors. When the tumor extends beyond the confines of the kidney, the pseudocapsule is made of fibrous tissue; otherwise it is made up of compressed normal renal tissue.[305] If the pseudocapsule is intact, the perinephric fat is unlikely to have been invaded.[305]

Detecting and assessing vascular thrombosis in patients with renal cell carcinoma is highly accurate and reliable with MRI.[304,306] Coronal imaging in the venous and delayed phases demonstrates the presence or absence of venous invasion, determines the extent of venous invasion, if present, and differentiates enhancing intravascular tumor from nonenhanced bland thrombus (Fig. 25.77). Accurate determination of renal vein, IVC, and right atrial involvement is important for deciding the surgical approach.[307]

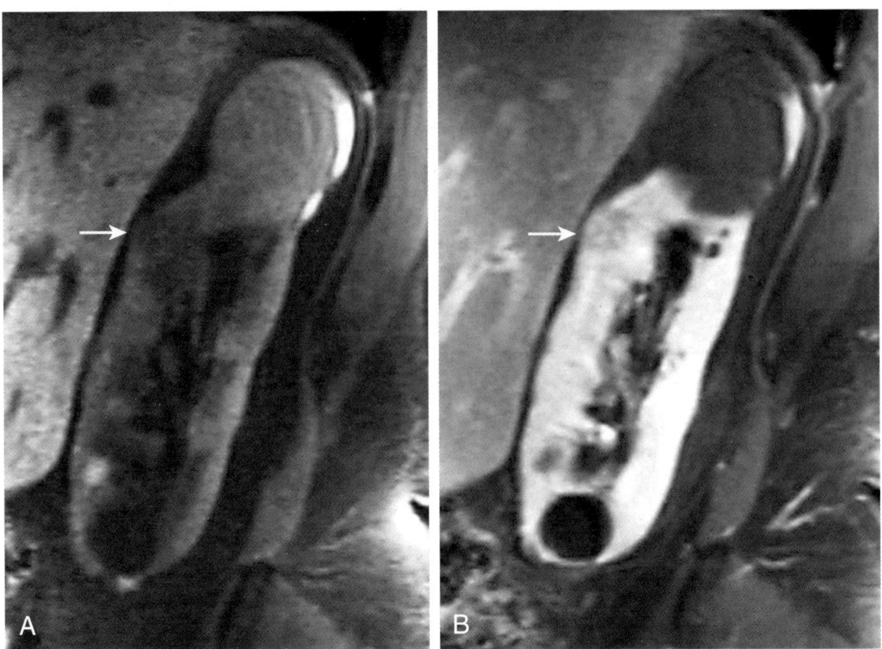


**Fig. 25.74** Papillary renal cell carcinoma, stage I. Sagittal T1-weighted images before *(arrow)* **(A)** and after **(B)** the administration of gadolinium show a subtle mass *(arrow)* in the anterior cortex and multiple nonenhanced cysts. No perinephric invasion was found at surgery.

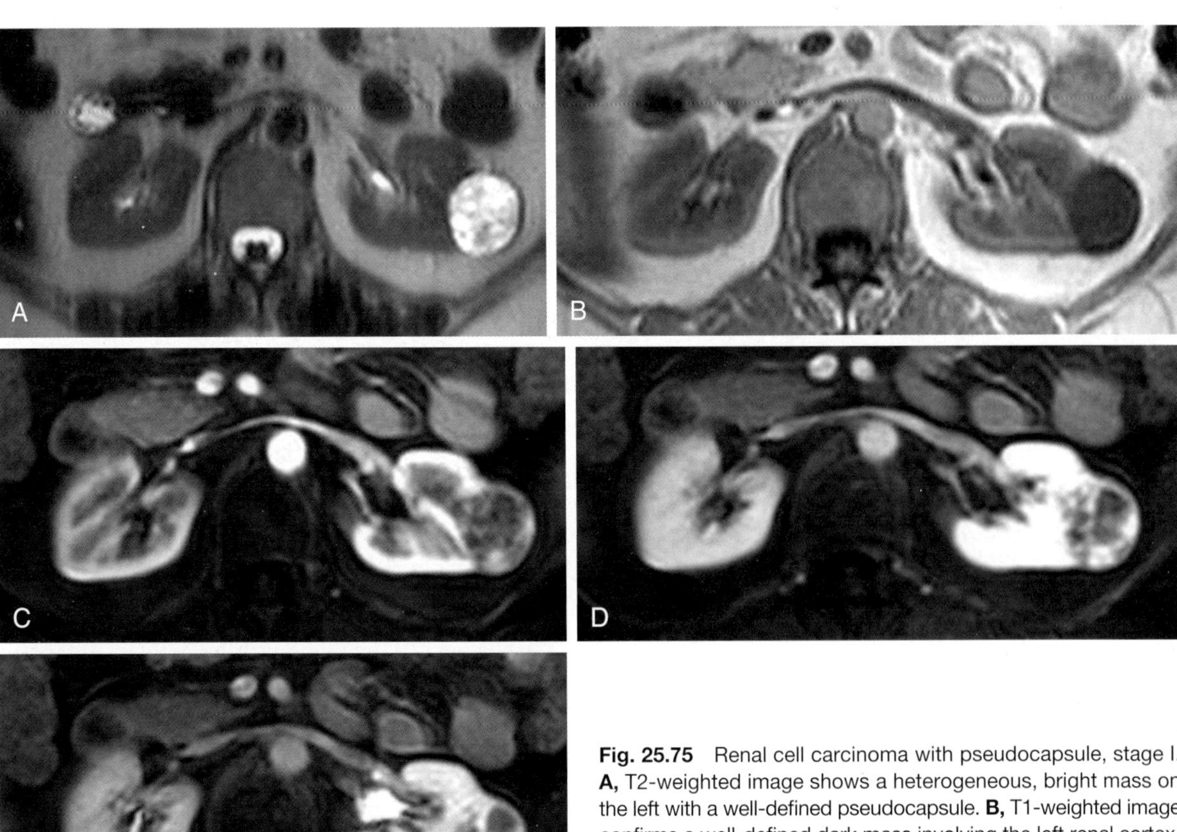


**Fig. 25.75** Renal cell carcinoma with pseudocapsule, stage I. **A,** T2-weighted image shows a heterogeneous, bright mass on the left with a well-defined pseudocapsule. **B,** T1-weighted image confirms a well-defined dark mass involving the left renal cortex. **C** to **E,** Axial gadolinium-enhanced T1-weighted images in the arterial, venous, and excretory phases demonstrate heterogeneous enhancement and no evidence of renal vein involvement. No perinephric invasion was found at surgery.

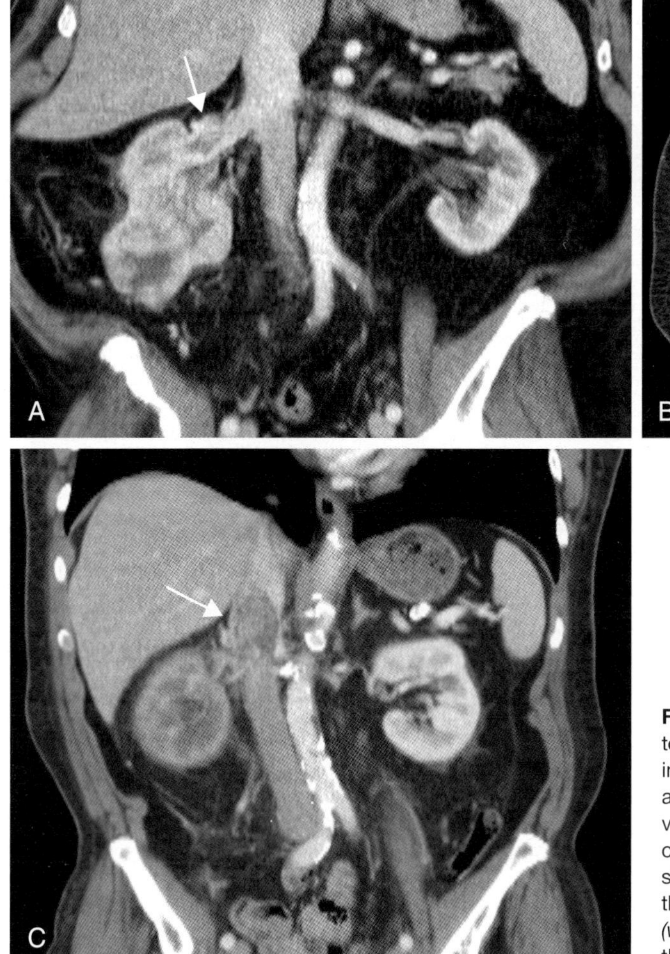


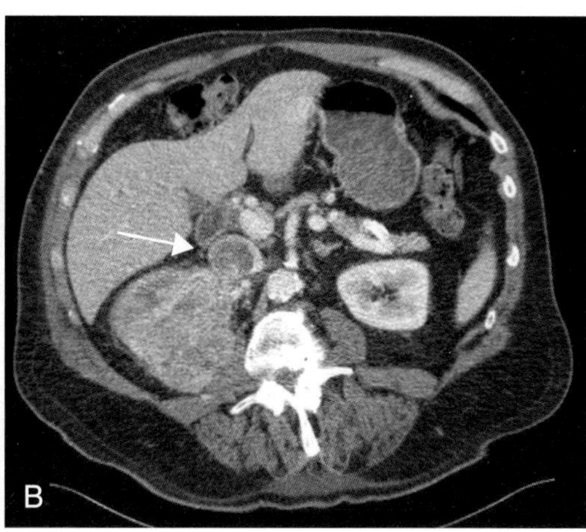


**Fig. 25.76** Renal cell carcinoma, stage IIIA: computed tomographic scan. Coronal contrast medium-enhanced image **(A)** shows a stage IIIA mass in the right kidney and a tumor thrombus extending into the right renal vein *(white arrow)*. In a different patient, axial **(B)** and coronal **(C)** contrast medium-enhanced images also show a right renal mass with a tumor thrombus, but the thrombus has extended into the inferior vena cava *(white arrows)*. Both these tumors proved to be of the clear cell type.

Although renal cell carcinoma is the most common primary malignancy in the kidney, transitional cell carcinoma also occurs within the kidneys.[308] Most transitional cell carcinomas involve the urothelium and project into the lumen of the renal pelvis or ureter. As a result, IVU images show a filling defect within the renal pelvis or ureter that can be confused with a renal stone, blood clot, or debris (Fig. 25.78). Transitional cell carcinoma of the bladder is much more common than that of the kidney or ureter.[309] The neoplasm may extend into the renal parenchyma and, on imaging, appears as a mass within the kidney. The imaging findings are similar to those of renal cell carcinoma, except the lesions tend not to enhance as much on postcontrast imaging. Renal vein involvement is rare. CTU and MRU show similar findings; transitional cell carcinoma in the upper collecting system can be either a focal or irregular mass within the collecting system (Fig. 25.79) or an ill-defined mass infiltrating the renal parenchyma. When small, they may be difficult to identify on both CT and MRI. Evaluation of the entire collecting system is required because synchronous lesions may be present. Both CTU and MRU are valuable for complete evaluation of the collecting system; however, retrograde pyelography with ureteroscopy and biopsy will make the diagnosis.

Lymphoma may involve the kidney as part of multiorgan involvement or, in rare cases, as a primary neoplasm.[310] Lymphoma may be solitary or multifocal, within one or both kidneys. Perirenal extension may be visible as well. An infiltrative picture with lymphomatous replacement of the kidney may also be observed. This form is usually accompanied by adjacent retroperitoneal adenopathy. CE-CT is the imaging method of choice in these patients. MRI findings are similar to those on CE-CT. Lymphoma typically appears hypointense on T1-weighted sequences and heterogeneous to slightly hypointense on T2-weighted sequences. Enhancement is minimal on postcontrast sequences[311] (Fig. 25.80). Vessels are usually encased, not invaded, and necrosis is usually not observed. Treated lymphoma may vary in signal intensity, as a result of the effects of therapy.[311]

Metastatic disease may also involve the kidney. Metastases are most commonly hematogenous and usually result in multiple foci of involvement, although single lesions do occur (Fig. 25.81). They are observed most frequently with CE-CT, inasmuch as CT is used in the regular follow-up of most patients with cancer. Hypodense round masses, usually in the periphery, are the typical finding. When present as a single lesion, a metastasis cannot be differentiated from a primary renal neoplasm without biopsy.

## RENAL CANCER: POSITRON EMISSION TOMOGRAPHY AND POSITRON EMISSION TOMOGRAPHY-COMPUTED TOMOGRAPHY

Preliminary studies of PET imaging of renal cell carcinoma have revealed a promising role in the evaluation of

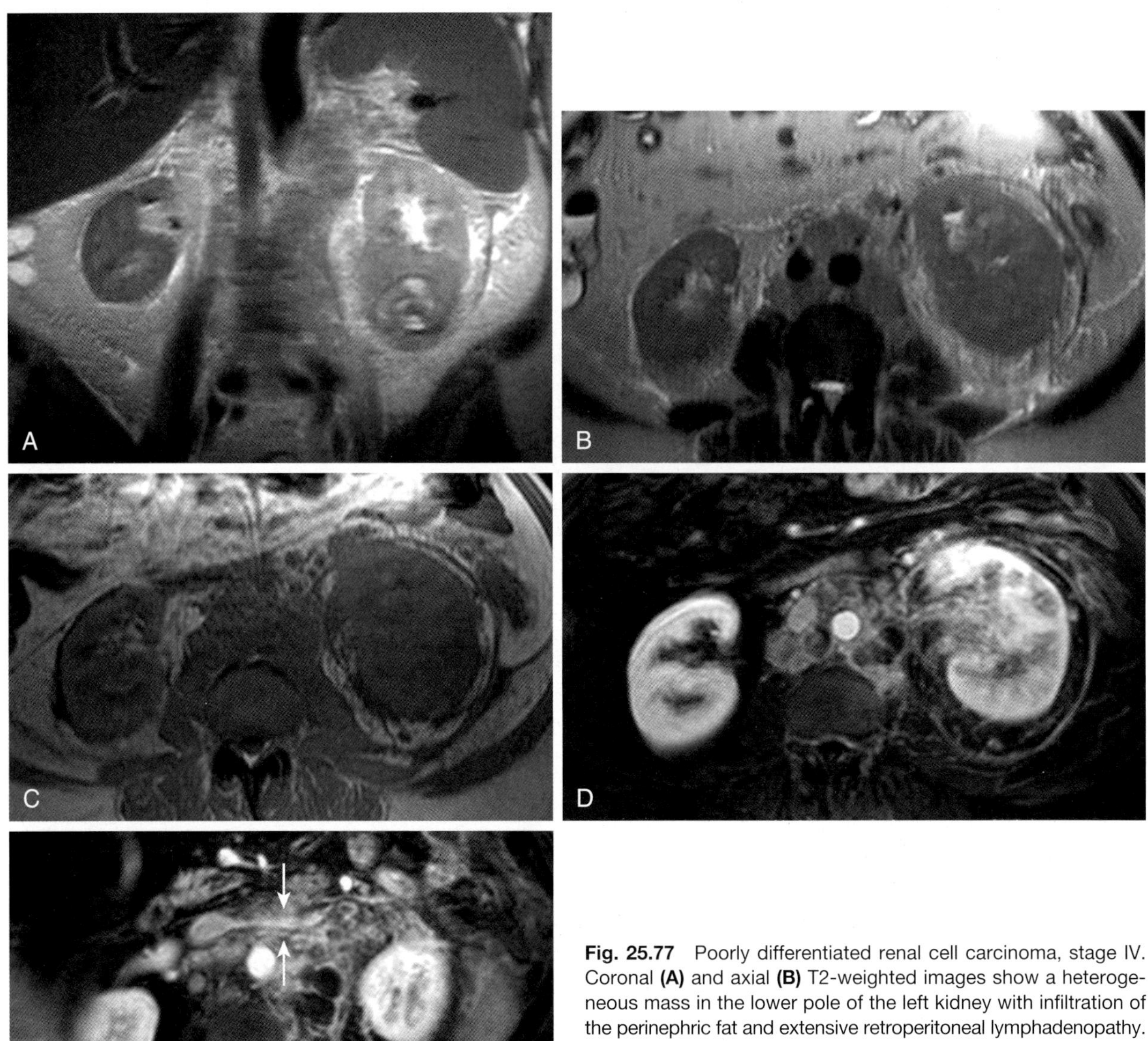


**Fig. 25.77** Poorly differentiated renal cell carcinoma, stage IV. Coronal **(A)** and axial **(B)** T2-weighted images show a heterogeneous mass in the lower pole of the left kidney with infiltration of the perinephric fat and extensive retroperitoneal lymphadenopathy. T1-weighted image **(C)** shows the masses to be intermediate in signal intensity. Gadolinium enhancement of axial T1-weighted images (**D** and **E**) make the local invasion and adenopathy more conspicuous and show that the left renal vein is encased, not invaded *(arrows)*.

indeterminate renal masses, preoperative staging and assessment of tumor burden, detection of osseous and nonosseous metastases (including vascular invasion), restaging after therapy, treatment evaluation, and the determination of effect of imaging findings on clinical management.[312–324] However, other PET studies have demonstrated less encouraging results and no advantage over standard imaging methods.[325–327]

A relatively high false-negative rate (23%) has been reported with FDG-PET in the preoperative staging of renal cell carcinoma in comparison with histologic analysis of surgical specimens.

> ***Clinical Relevance***
> Sensitivity for PET scan for detection of renal cancer and metastases is lower than CT, as the lesions may be identified on CT before they can be seen as hypermetabolic foci on PET.

In one study, PET exhibited 60% sensitivity (vs. 91.7% for CT) and 100% specificity (vs. 100% for CT) for primary renal cell carcinoma tumors. For retroperitoneal lymph node metastases or renal bed recurrence, PET had 75.0% sensitivity (vs. 92.6% for CT) and 100% specificity (vs. 98.1% for CT). For metastases to the lung parenchyma, PET had 75% sensitivity (vs. 91.1% for chest CT) and 97.1% specificity (vs. 73.1% for chest CT). For bone metastases, PET had 77.3% sensitivity and 100% specificity (in comparison with 93.8% and 87.2% for combined CT and bone scan).[328] For restaging renal cell carcinoma, 87% sensitivity and 100% specificity have been reported.[329] A comparative investigation of bone scan and FDG-PET for detecting osseous metastases in renal cell carcinoma revealed that PET had 100% sensitivity (vs. 77.5% for bone scan) and 100% specificity (vs. 59.6% for bone scan).[317] Another report revealed a negative predictive value of 33% and a positive predictive value of 94% for restaging renal cell carcinoma.[313] Other studies have

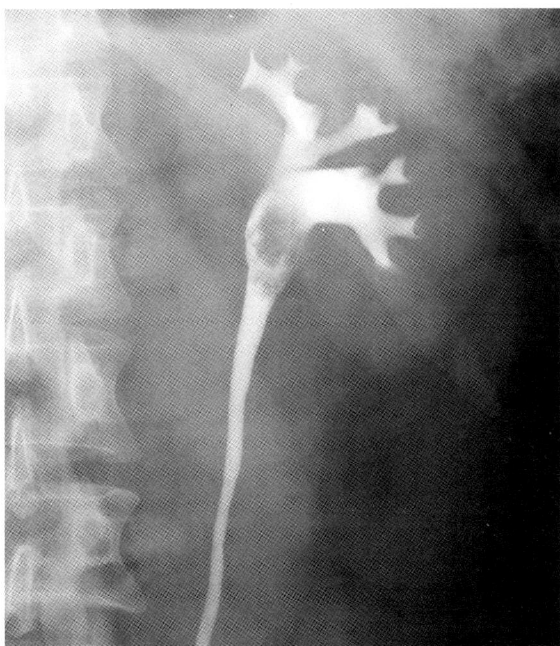

**Fig. 25.78** Transitional cell carcinoma: intravenous urogram. The irregular filling defect in the left renal pelvis represents a transitional cell carcinoma. Note that there is no significant obstruction of the left kidney, and the calyces appear normal.

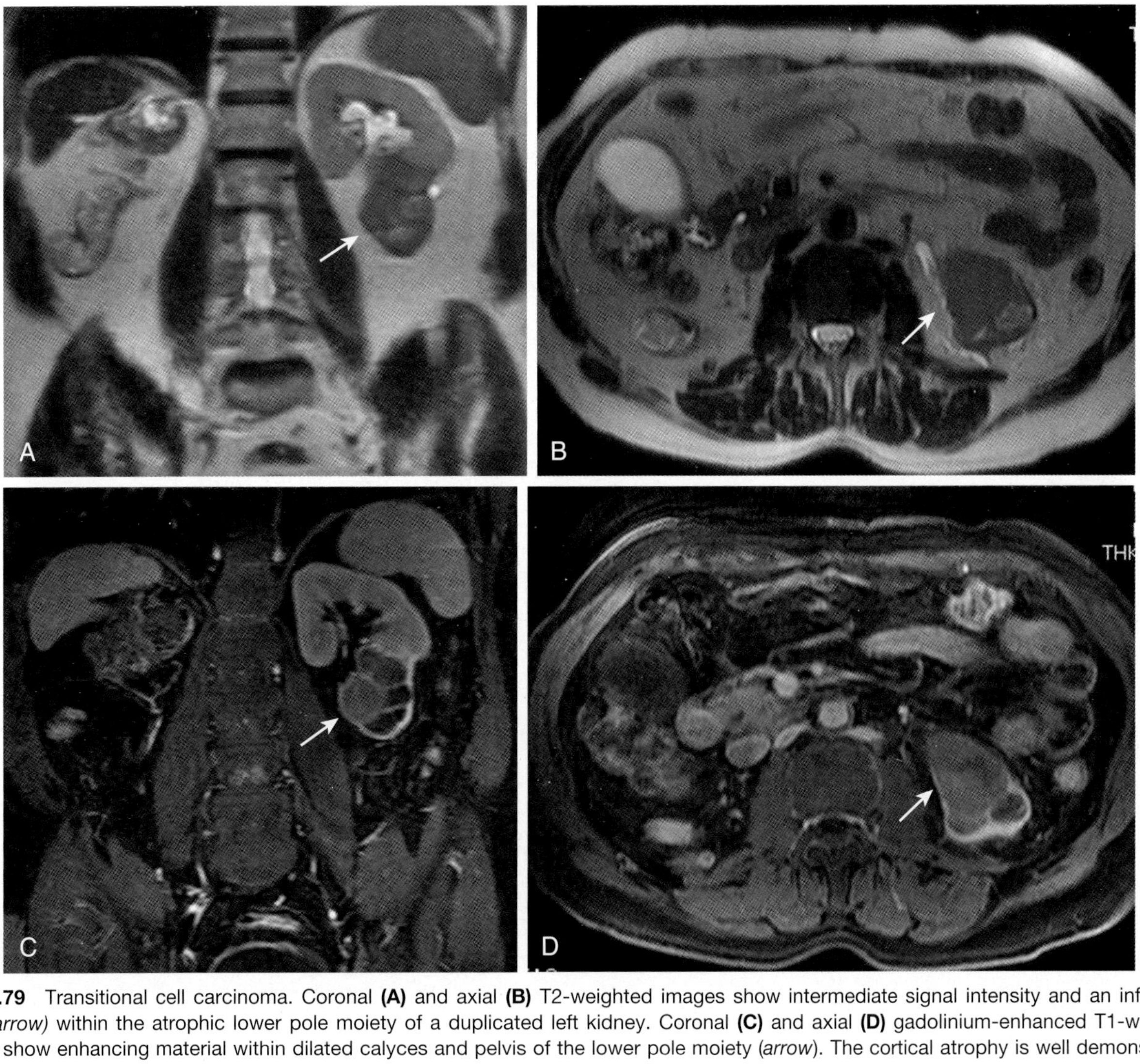

**Fig. 25.79** Transitional cell carcinoma. Coronal **(A)** and axial **(B)** T2-weighted images show intermediate signal intensity and an infiltrating mass *(arrow)* within the atrophic lower pole moiety of a duplicated left kidney. Coronal **(C)** and axial **(D)** gadolinium-enhanced T1-weighted images show enhancing material within dilated calyces and pelvis of the lower pole moiety (*arrow*). The cortical atrophy is well demonstrated.

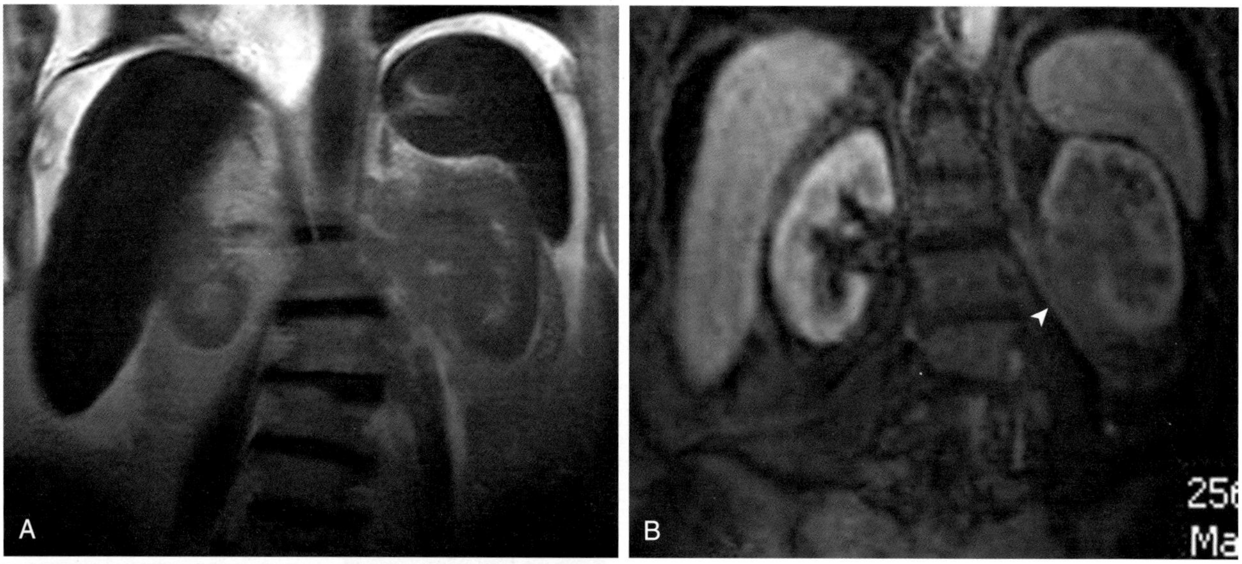

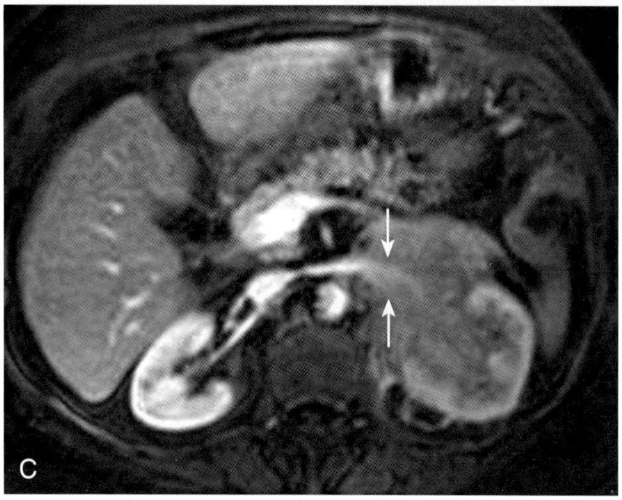

**Fig. 25.80** Lymphoma. **A,** Coronal T2-weighted image shows a large, infiltrating left renal mass extending into the perirenal fat. **B,** Coronal gadolinium-enhanced T1-weighted image better differentiates the mass *(arrowhead)* from the renal cortex. **C,** Axial gadolinium-enhanced T1-weighted image shows encasement of the left renal vein *(arrows)*.

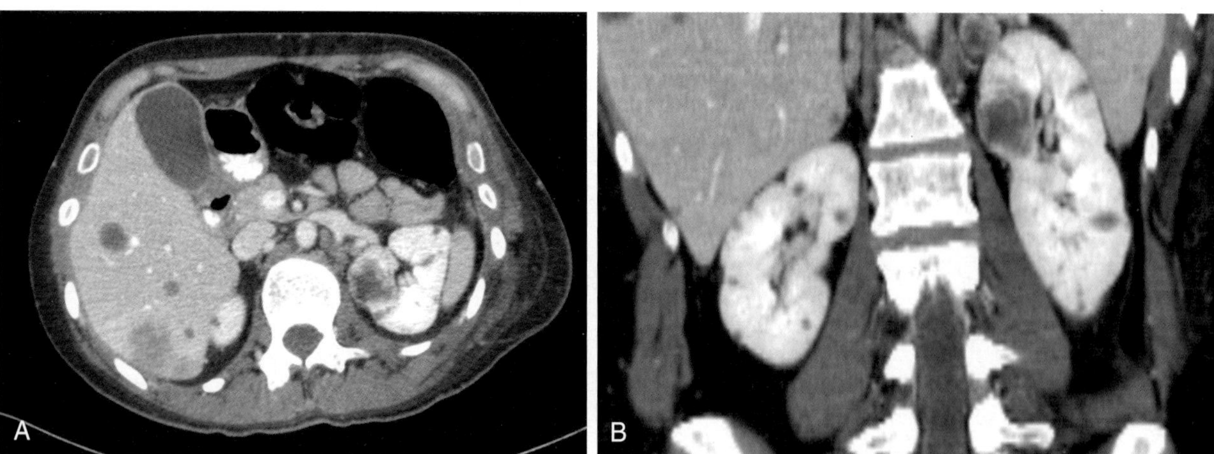


**Fig. 25.81** Metastases to the kidney: computed tomographic scan. Axial **(A)** and coronal **(B)** contrast material-enhanced images in the nephrographic phase. Multiple heterogeneous but hypodense lesions are visible in the kidneys bilaterally; the largest is in the left upper pole. These appeared in a 2-month period in a patient with metastatic lung carcinoma. Note the metastases also present in the liver.

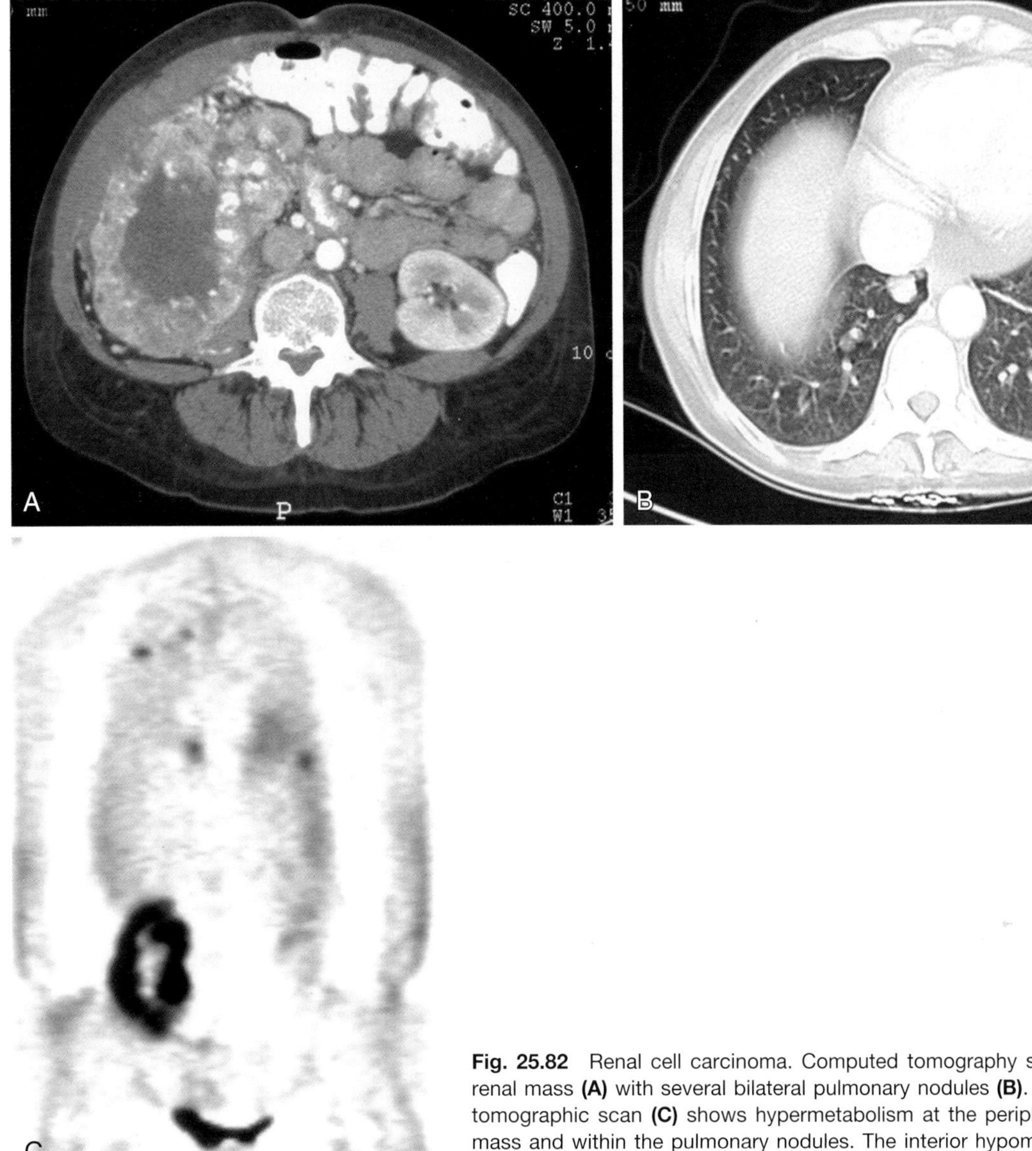

**Fig. 25.82** Renal cell carcinoma. Computed tomography shows a large necrotic renal mass **(A)** with several bilateral pulmonary nodules **(B)**. The positron emission tomographic scan **(C)** shows hypermetabolism at the periphery of the large renal mass and within the pulmonary nodules. The interior hypometabolism of the renal mass is compatible with central tumor necrosis.

revealed high accuracy in characterizing indeterminate renal masses, with a mean tumor-to-kidney uptake ratio of 3.0 for malignancy.[312]

These mixed observations are probably related to the heterogeneous expression of glucose transporter 1 in renal cell carcinoma, which may not be correlated with the tumor grade or extent.[330,331] Negative study findings may not rule out disease, whereas a positive result is highly suspect for malignancy.[332] If the tumor binds FDG avidly, then PET can be a reasonable imaging modality for follow-up after treatment and for surveillance (Fig. 25.82). In fact, it has been shown that FDG-PET can alter clinical management in up to 40% of patients with suspected locally recurrent and metastatic renal cancer.[315] A meta-analysis of 14 published studies on the diagnostic utility of FDG-PET (FDG PET-CT) in renal cell carcinoma reported a pooled sensitivity of 62% and a pooled specificity of 88% for renal lesions.[333]

Because FDG is excreted in the urine, the intense urine activity may confound lesion detection in and near the renal bed. Intravenous administration of furosemide has been proposed to improve urine clearance from the renal collecting system, although the exact benefit of such intervention in improving lesion detection remains undefined.

Many investigators since have reported on the unique diagnostic synergism of the combined PET-CT imaging systems.[334] Studies have demonstrated that FDG PET-CT has a sensitivity of 46.6% and specificity of 66.6% for primary renal cell carcinoma in the imaging evaluation of indeterminate renal masses.[335] In a study by Park et al, in South Korea, 63 patients with renal cell carcinoma underwent both FDG PET-CT and conventional imaging evaluation during follow-up after surgical treatment.[336] FDG PET-CT demonstrated 89.5% sensitivity, 83.3% specificity, a positive predictive value of 77.3%, and a negative predictive value of 92.6% in detecting recurrent and metastatic disease; these values were not significantly different from the diagnostic performance of conventional imaging studies. Park et al, concluded that FDG PET-CT can replace multiple conventional imaging studies without the need for contrast agents. The role of PET-CT in renal cancer imaging and its effect on both short- and long-term clinical management and decision making also must be investigated.

Studies have demonstrated that PET-CT might be potentially useful in treatment response evaluation and prognostication. One Japanese group of investigators reported on the use of FDG PET-CT in early assessment of therapy response to tyrosine kinase inhibitors in 35 patients with advanced renal cell carcinoma.[337] These authors found that improved progression-free survival and overall survival were both associated with favorable response to therapy (defined as decline in tumor maximum standardized uptake value by 20% or more from pretreatment scan to the scan obtained 1 month after completion of therapy). Similar findings have been reported by other investigators.[336,338–341] One study reported that although FDG PET-CT may be helpful in assessing treatment response to chemotherapy, it may not be useful in monitoring response to immunotherapy, such as with interferon alfa monotherapy or in combination with interleukin-2 and 5-fluorouracil.[342] Moreover, other studies have shown that the higher the FDG uptake in the renal cancer lesions, the higher the mortality.[343,344]

Other tracers used in PET (e.g., carbon 11–labeled acetate [$^{11}$C-acetate], $^{18}$F labeled fluoromisonidazole [$^{18}$F-FMISO], $^{18}$F–labeled sodium fluoride) have been investigated in the imaging evaluation of patients with renal cell carcinoma, but further studies are needed to establish the exact role of these and other non-FDG tracers in this clinical setting.[345–348] For example, one study revealed high accumulation of $^{11}$C-acetate in 70% of renal cell carcinomas.[349] However, an earlier similar study had demonstrated that in most kidney tumors, accumulation of $^{11}$C-acetate was not higher than in normal renal parenchyma.[350] Aside from renal cell carcinoma, $^{11}$C-acetate has also been demonstrated to be useful in the imaging-based assessment of renal oxygen consumption and tubular sodium reabsorption.[351] Another investigation using a dual-tracer ($^{11}$C-acetate and FDG) method showed that AMLs are highly avid for $^{11}$C-acetate but not at all for FDG. The uptake of $^{11}$C-acetate in renal cell cancer was lower than that in AML. In fact, this study suggested that $^{11}$C-acetate may be useful in differentiating "fat-poor angiomyolipoma" from renal cell cancer with a sensitivity of 93.8% and specificity of 98%.[352] $^{11}$C-acetate has also been found to be potentially useful in early prediction of response to the tyrosine kinase inhibitor, sunitinib, in patients with metastatic renal cell carcinoma.[353]

Murakami et al used the hypoxia imaging probe $^{18}$F-FMISO in preclinical models of renal cell carcinoma to show that $^{18}$F-FMISO hypoxia imaging can confirm "tumor starvation" as the mechanistic explanation for tumor response to anti-angiogenic therapy.[354] A pilot clinical study with $^{18}$F-FMISO also showed that patients with hypoxic metastatic tumors have shorter progression-free survival than those with non-hypoxic tumors.[355]

Other tracers that have been investigated include iodine 124 ($^{124}$I)– and zirconium 89–labeled anticarbonic anhydrase IX monoclonal antibody that is avid to clear cell renal cell carcinoma.[354] An early trial of the $^{124}$I-labeled compound for detection of clear cell renal cell carcinoma (with histopathology as reference standard) showed an average sensitivity and specificity of 86.2% and 85.9%, respectively, for PET-CT, which were statistically higher than sensitivity and specificity of 75.5% and 46.8%, respectively, for CE-CT.[356]

Schuster et al reported on their initial experience with anti-1-amino-3-$^{18}$F-fluorocyclobutane-1-carboxylic acid, which is a nonmetabolized synthetic L-leucine analog with low urinary excretion, in the imaging evaluation of renal cell carcinoma.[357] Their preliminary results in six patients showed that the uptake of this amino acid-based radiotracer may be elevated in renal papillary cell carcinoma but not in clear cell carcinoma.

Other uses of PET in the imaging evaluation of renal perfusion, function, and metabolism have also been investigated.[358] In addition, there is some effort to evaluate the role of radiolabeled antibodies as therapeutic agents in the treatment of renal cell carcinoma.[357]

## RENAL VASCULAR DISEASE

Diagnostic imaging for hypertension depends on the clinical index of suspicion for renovascular hypertension, which is found in less than 5% of the hypertensive population, but the percentage is higher in those with severe hypertension and ESKD.[359] The most common cause of renovascular hypertension is renal artery stenosis (RAS), with approximately 90% of cases due to atherosclerosis and approximately 10% due to fibromuscular dysplasia. Renovascular disease is discussed further in Chapter 47. The diagnosis of RAS at the time of screening has been problematic because the preintervention definition of significant RAS has varied. Significant RAS is best defined as a fall in blood pressure after intervention. According to the ACR, in patients with normal renal function in whom RAS is suspected, MRA or CTA is usually appropriate. Doppler US or ACE-inhibitor scintigraphy is appropriate if MRA is not desired or contraindicated, and conventional angiography is reserved for confirmation of RAS and definitive therapy. IVU has no role in the evaluation for RAS.[360]

Doppler US is a noninvasive screening test that can be used independent of the patient's renal function. In experienced hands, US has been reported to have high sensitivity and specificity; however, sensitivities have been reported as low as 0%. US screening can be technically challenging and therefore should be performed only in centers where US screening has been proven to be reliable and where there are dedicated technologists and physicians. In such centers 75% to 80% of scans are technically adequate.

Doppler US has been used with variable success to assess the main renal arteries for RAS and the intrarenal vasculature for secondary effects.[360,361] The success of Doppler US is highly operator dependent, and results may be inadequate or incomplete because of overlying bowel gas, body habitus, or aortic pulsatility.[361] A stable Doppler signal may be difficult to reproduce in some patients with renovascular hypertension. A complete examination has been possible in 50% to 90% of affected patients. Variant anatomy may also be a challenge; accessory renal arteries, which occur in 15% to 20% of affected patients, may not be imaged.[362]

The criteria used for evaluation of the main renal artery include an increase in the peak systolic velocity to more than 180 cm/sec, a renal/aortic ratio of peak systolic velocity of more than 3.0, and turbulent flow beyond the region of the stenosis.[363] Visualization of the main renal artery with no detectable Doppler signal is suggestive of renal artery occlusion. Intrarenal vascular assessment with Doppler US has depicted the shape and character of the waveform. A dampened appearance of the waveform, with a slowed systolic upstroke and delay to peak velocity (tardus-parvus), has been shown in varying degrees in RAS.[364] Using resistive indices, a difference between the kidneys of more than 5% has also been suggestive of RAS. Sensitivity and specificity for the techniques have generally been in the range of 50% to 70%. CEUS has been suggested as a means of improving the accuracy of Doppler US.[364,365]

CTA performed with MDCT has sensitivity and specificity at or near 100% (Fig. 25.83).[366–368] CTA is an effective alternative to Doppler US and MRA. When compared with MRA, CTA has higher spatial resolution and shorter examination times. CTA evaluates calcified and noncalcified atherosclerotic plaques and may be used to assess stent grafts (Fig. 25.84).[369,370] A normal result should rule out RAS.[371] The main renal artery, as well as its segmental branches, can be viewed and evaluated (Figs. 25.85 and 25.86). Accessory renal arteries as small as 1 mm in diameter can be seen.[372] CTA and MRA are of equivalent quality in the detection of hemodynamically significant RAS.[373] Both CTA and MRA can demonstrate renal cortical volume and thickness as well as secondary signs of RAS, including poststenotic dilation, renal atrophy, and decreased cortical enhancement.

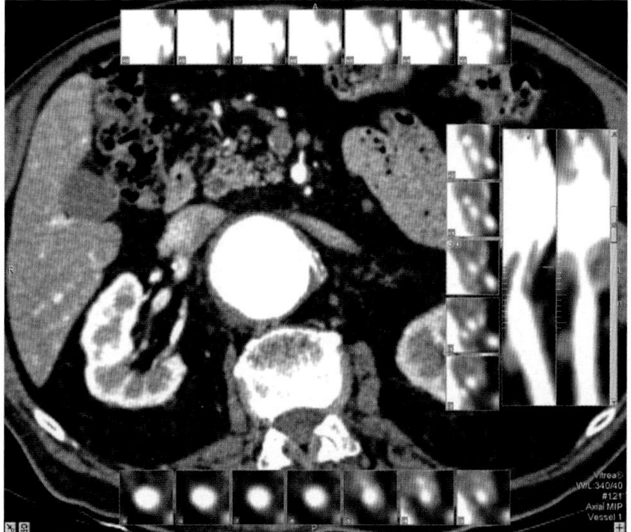

Fig. 25.83 Renal artery stenosis: computed tomographic angiogram, axial image with vessel analysis. The origin of the left renal artery is markedly narrowed by calcified and noncalcified atherosclerotic plaque. The vessel analysis demonstrates the renal artery in cross section for accurate calculation of the degree of stenosis, which in this case was greater than 70%.

Because CTA is sensitive, accurate, fast, and reproducible, MRA is reserved for patients for whom iodinated contrast material is contraindicated. Renal insufficiency is not uncommon in the population clinically at high risk for RAS. For this reason, MRA has been widely accepted as a reliable and accurate examination in the evaluation of RAS in this population.[107,118,373–375] CE-MRA is being used more selectively, given the risk for NSF in patients with CKD stage 4 and 5. Noncontrast MRA techniques are being used more frequently to reduce the amount of Gd-C needed. Like CTA, MRA is noninvasive and provides excellent visualization of the aortoiliac and renal arteries.[373]

CE-MRA is more than 95% sensitive in demonstrating the main renal arteries and has a high negative predictive value. A normal CE-MRA finding almost completely rules out a stenosis in the visualized vessels.[376] CE-MRA is a reliable examination but has been limited by incomplete visualization of segmental and small accessory vessels.[377] Whereas visualization of all accessory vessels is desired, Bude et al found isolated hemodynamically significant stenosis of an accessory artery in only 1 (1.5%) of their 68 patients.[378] Bude et al concluded that this limitation does not substantially reduce the rate of detection of renovascular hypertension by MRI. With the use of three-dimensional reconstruction, studies have demonstrated no significant difference between CE-MRA and CTA in the detection of hemodynamically significant RAS.[373] Volume rendering and multiplanar reformatting improve accuracy in depicting RAS.[117] Volume rendering increases the positive predictive value of CE-MRA by reducing the overestimation of stenosis yielded by earlier reconstruction

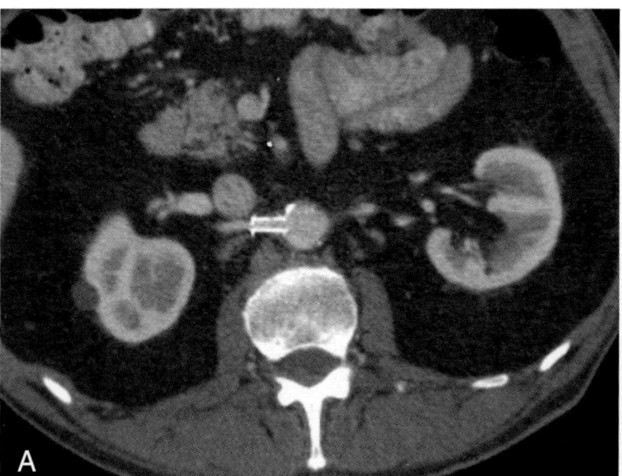


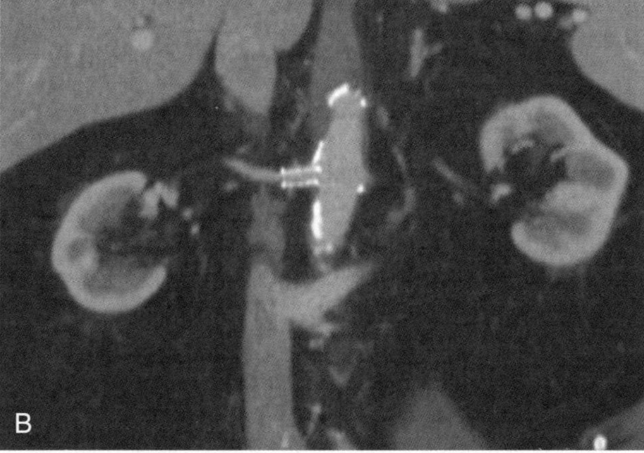


Fig. 25.84 Renal artery stent: computed tomographic scan. Axial **(A)** and coronal **(B)** images of a contrast material-enhanced scan in the corticomedullary phase. The metallic stent is visible at the origin of the right renal artery. It had been placed for treatment of renal artery stenosis that was caused by atherosclerosis. Good flow through the stent is observed as contrast material fills the lumen.

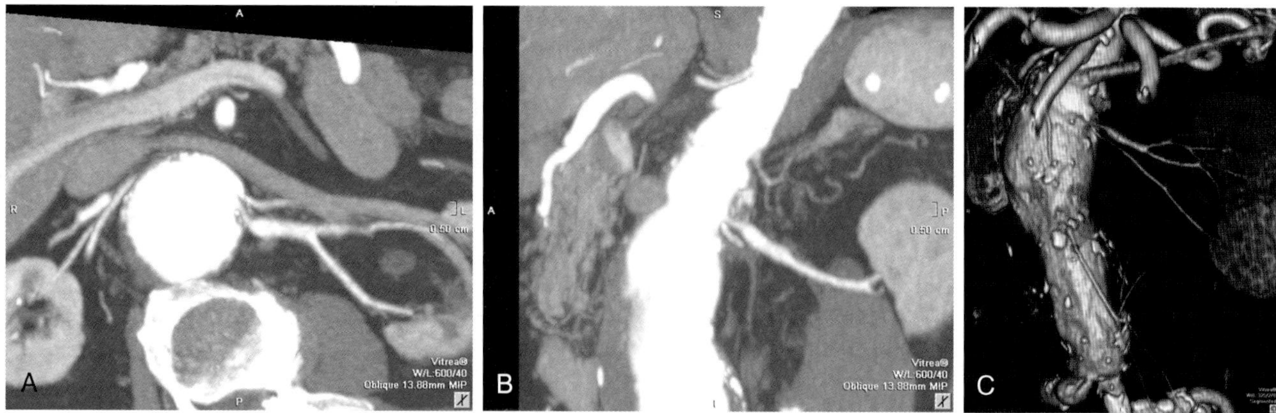

Fig. 25.85 Renal artery stenosis: computed tomographic angiography (CTA). Image processing was applied to the case depicted in Fig. 25.84. Axial **(A)** and coronal **(B)** slab maximum-intensity projection images demonstrate the atherosclerotic stenosis of the proximal renal artery. Note the accessory renal artery arising adjacent to the left main renal artery. Volume rendering of the CTA produced a three-dimensional display **(C),** which may be rotated for best viewing and analysis.

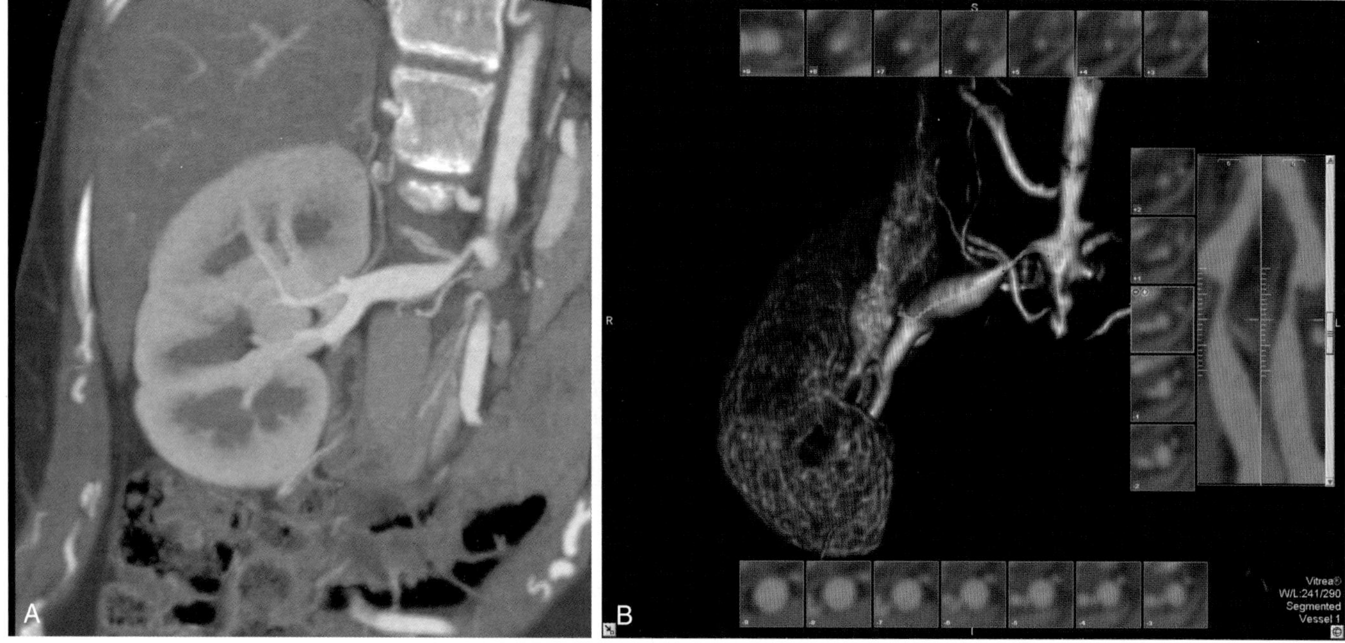

**Fig. 25.86** Renal artery stenosis: abdominal computed tomographic angiography (CTA) with image processing. **A,** Coronal slab maximum-intensity projection demonstrates the smooth narrowing of the proximal right renal artery in a patient with Takayasu's arteritis. Note the markedly abnormal aorta with occlusion distal to the origin of the renal artery. **B,** Volume rendering of the CTA with vessel analysis reveals the 80% stenosis of the right renal artery. The left renal artery had been occluded previously, and the kidney was supplied by collateral vessels.

techniques (Fig. 25.87).[118,376] Volume rendering has better correlation with digital subtraction angiography and improves delineation of the renal arteries.[118]

The usefulness of MRA is restricted in part by limitations in spatial resolution and by motion artifacts.[378,379] Advancements in magnetic resonance gradient strengths and newer MRA techniques have improved image resolution and reduced motion artifacts, while reducing imaging times.[378] Higher magnetic field strength (3 T) can result in higher spatial and temporal resolution when compared with imaging at 1.5 T. This higher resolution was found to improve the evaluation of smaller structures.[380,381] As MRI hardware and software improve, so will noncontrast MRA. Noncontrast MRA may be performed independent of renal function, and small studies have shown good results for the diagnosis of RAS.

Phase-contrast MRA can be used to calculate blood flow through the renal artery.[382] Phase-contrast flow curves can be generated, and the severity of the hemodynamic abnormalities can be graded as normal, low-grade, moderate, and high-grade stenosis. This is similar to the Doppler US method. Grading can be used to evaluate the hemodynamic significance of a detected stenosis.[383] The significance of a stenosis on parenchymal function, however, is not currently evaluated by conventional MRA. Renal MRI perfusion studies are being performed to grade the effect of RAS on parenchymal perfusion; initial results show that MRI perfusion measurements

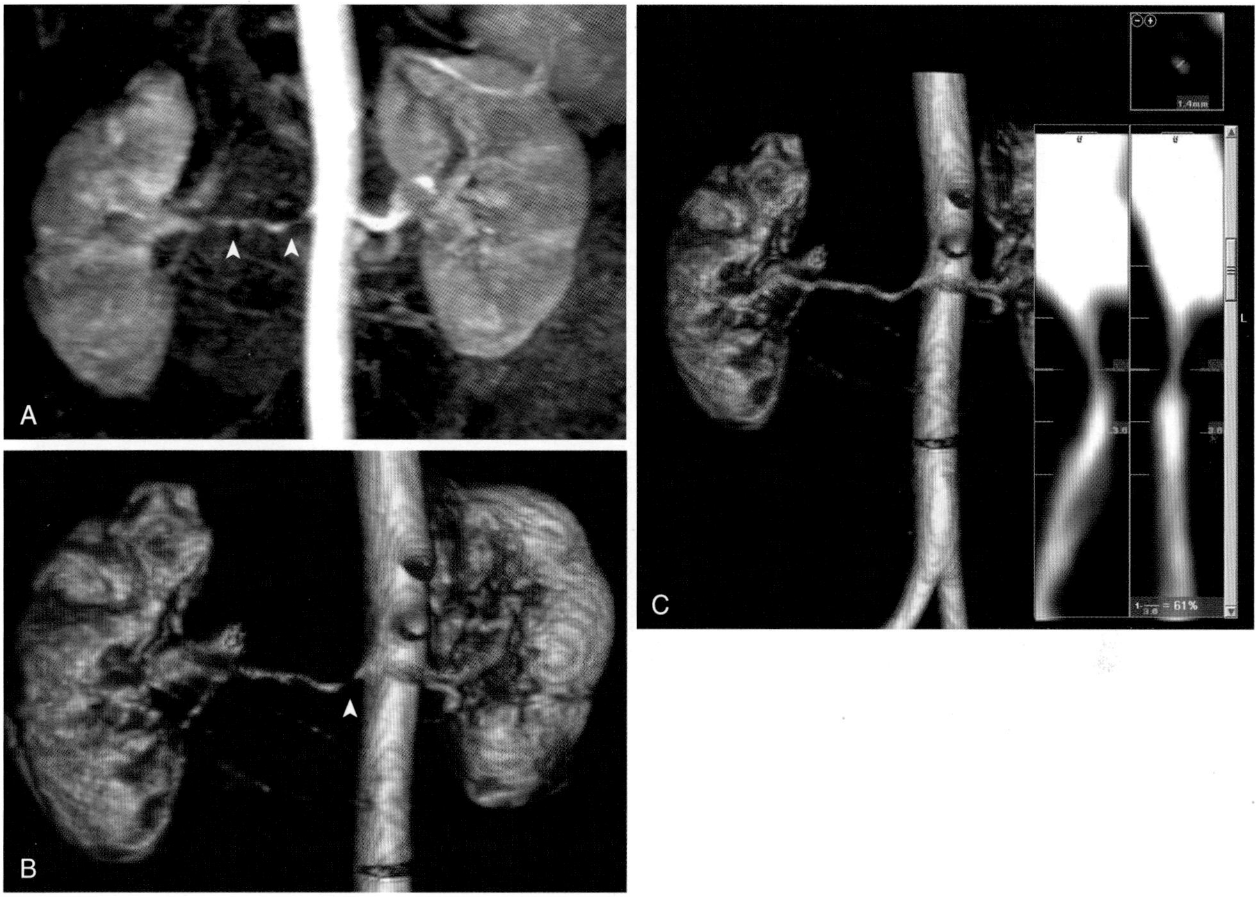

**Fig. 25.87** Renal artery stenosis. Advancements in postprocessing allow for a more accurate evaluation of stenosis with magnetic resonance angiography. **A,** Maximum-intensity projection displays a high-grade stenosis near the origin of the renal artery with areas of apparent narrowing in the midportion of the renal artery *(arrowheads),* mimicking fibromuscular dysplasia. **B,** Volume rendering shows the proximal stenosis *(arrowhead),* but the midportion of the artery is more normal in appearance. **C,** A view of the artery in two dimensions allowed measurement of the proximal stenosis and demonstrated a normal midportion of the artery. This stenosis was confirmed with angiography.

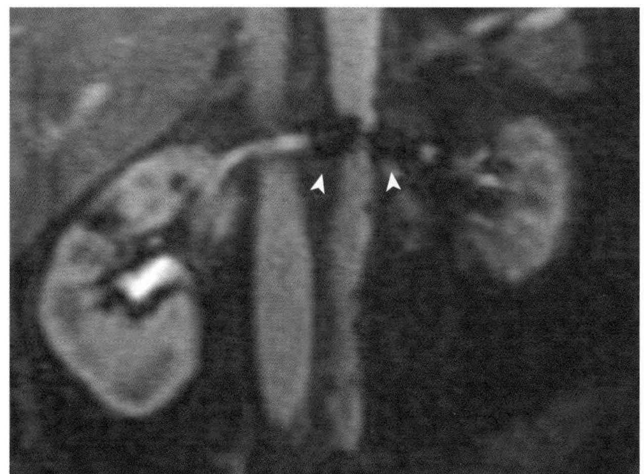

**Fig. 25.88** Magnetic resonance angiography in a patient with bilateral renal artery stents *(arrowheads).* The metal in the stent causes artifact that obscures the vessel lumen. Contrast material is visible beyond the stent, which indicates that no complete occlusion is present.

with high spatial and temporal resolution reflect renal function as measured with serum creatinine level.[384] Volumetric analysis of functional renal cortical tissue may also yield clinically useful information in patients with RAS.[385] Further research is required before this will be known, however.

MRA is currently of limited value in the evaluation of restenosis in patients with renal artery stents. Although stent technology is rapidly changing, metal artifact still obscures the stent lumen to varying degrees as a result of susceptibility artifacts (Fig. 25.88). Phase-contrast MRA may be used to measure velocities proximal and distal to the stent, but this is an indirect approach to evaluating for stenosis. Work is being done to develop a metallic renal artery stent that will allow for lumen visualization on MRI; however, this is not currently available clinically.[386]

Fibromuscular dysplasia has a characteristic appearance of focal narrowing and dilation ("string of beads"; Fig. 25.89). Because fibromuscular dysplasia frequently involves the middle to distal portions of the renal artery and segmental branches, resolution limits MRA evaluation. For this reason, MRA is not as reliable for diagnosis of fibromuscular dysplasia as it is for atherosclerotic RAS. Renal infarctions are well demonstrated on MRA as wedge-shaped areas of decreased

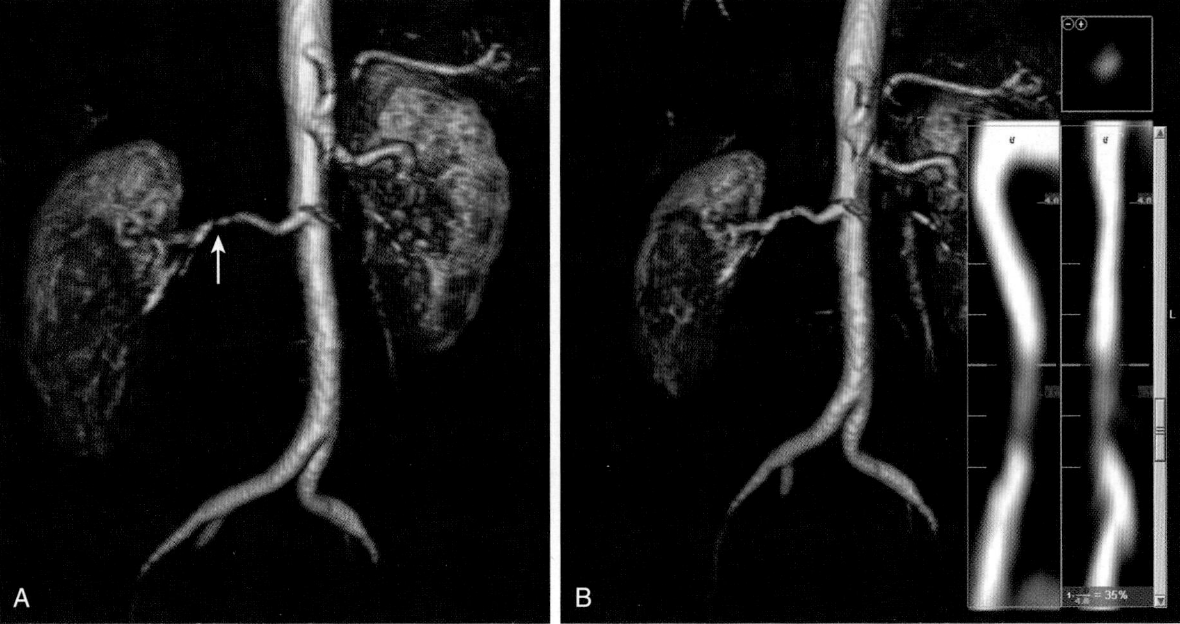


**Fig. 25.89** **A** and **B,** Magnetic resonance angiography with volume reconstruction demonstrates a subtle irregularity in the midportion of the right renal artery *(arrow)*. Fibromuscular dysplasia was confirmed with conventional angiography.

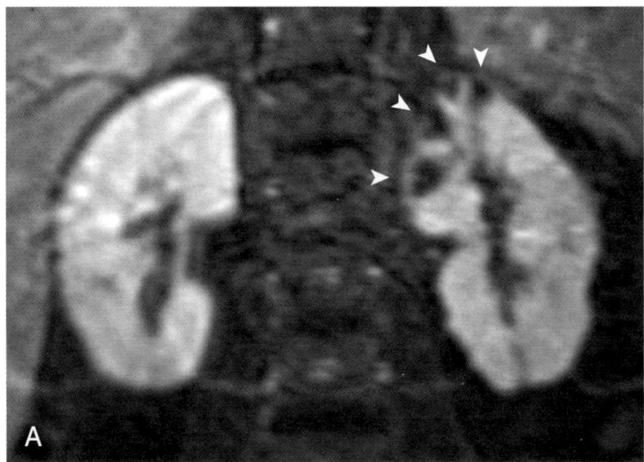


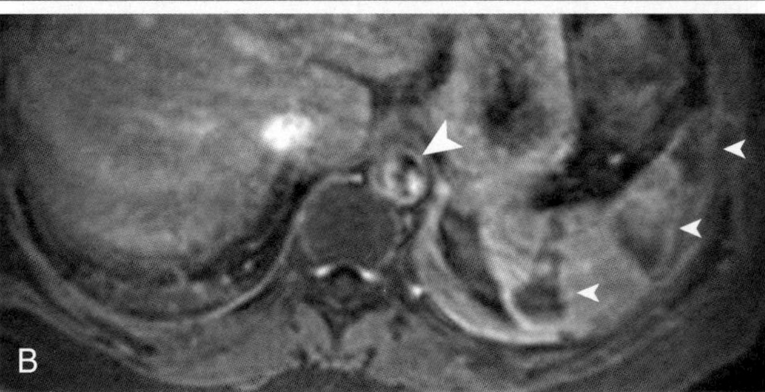


**Fig. 25.90** Renal infarcts caused by embolic disease. **A,** Coronal gadolinium-enhanced T1-weighted image shows wedge-shaped cortical areas without enhancement *(arrowheads)*. **B,** Axial gadolinium-enhanced T1-weighted image shows an irregular filling defect in the aorta *(large arrowhead)*, which is consistent with thrombus, and three focal defects in the spleen *(small arrowheads)*, which are consistent with splenic infarcts.

parenchymal enhancement. These areas are most conspicuous in the nephrographic phase. Evaluation of the arterial and venous structures may demonstrate the origin of the emboli or thrombosis (Fig. 25.90).

## NUCLEAR IMAGING AND RENOVASCULAR DISEASE

ACE inhibition prevents conversion of angiotensin I to angiotensin II. In RAS, angiotensin II constricts the efferent arterioles as a compensatory mechanism to maintain GFR despite diminished afferent renal blood flow. Therefore ACE inhibition in RAS reduces GFR by interfering with the compensatory mechanism. Captopril-enhanced renography has been successful in evaluating patients with RAS.

Before the study the patient should be well hydrated, and ACE inhibitors should be discontinued (captopril for 2 days; enalapril or lisinopril for 4–5 days) because diagnostic sensitivity may otherwise be reduced. Diuretics should also be discontinued before the study, preferably for 1 week. Dehydration resulting from diuretics may potentiate the effect of captopril and contribute to hypotension. Captopril (25–50 mg) crushed and dissolved in 250 mL water is administered orally, followed by blood pressure monitoring every 15 minutes for 1 hour. Alternatively, enalaprilat (40 μg/kg with total dose not exceeding 2.5 mg) is administered intravenously over 3 to 5 minutes. A baseline scan can be performed before captopril-enhanced renography (1-day protocol) or the next day, only if captopril-enhanced study findings are abnormal (2-day protocol).

The affected kidney in renovascular hypertension often has a renogram curve with reduced initial slope, a delayed time to peak activity, prolonged cortical retention, and a slow downward slope after the peak (Fig. 25.91). These findings are caused by the slowing of renal tracer transit as

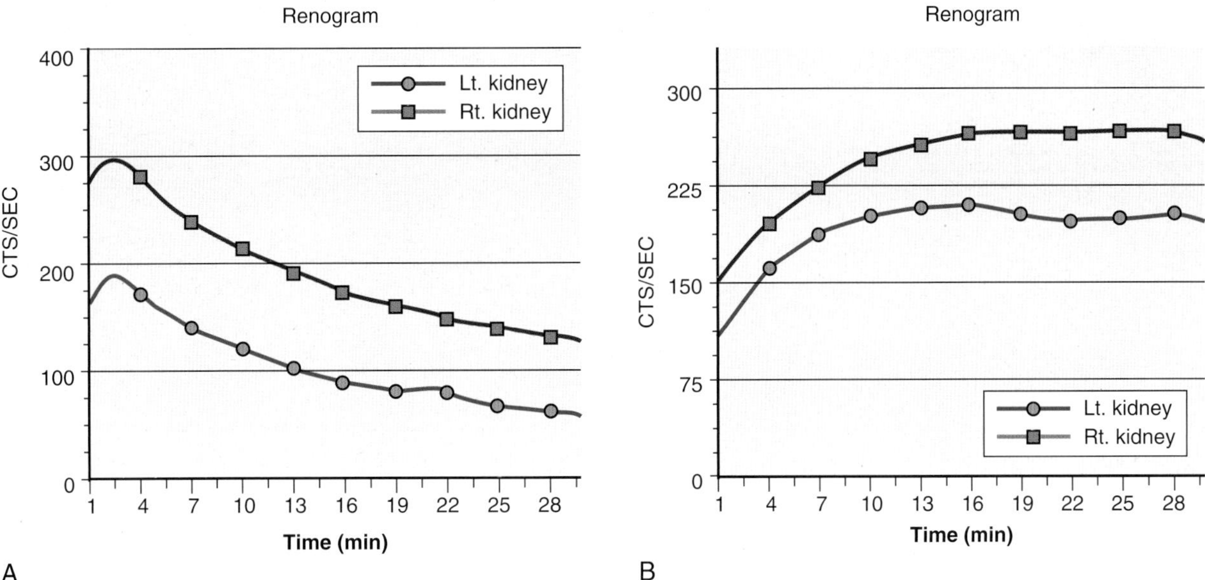


**Fig. 25.91** Technetium 99m-labeled mercaptoacetyltriglycine renograms before **(A)** and after **(B)** angiotensin-converting enzyme (ACE) inhibition with captopril. Note the relatively normal renograms **(A)** and the reduced initial slope, delayed time to peak activity, and plateau compatible with captopril-induced cortical tracer retention **(B).** These findings suggest a high probability of hemodynamically significant bilateral renal artery stenosis that is more severe on the left side *(connected circles)* than the right side *(connected squares).* Bilateral renal artery stenosis was later confirmed with angiography. (Modified from Saremi F, Jadvar H, Siegel M. Pharmacologic interventions in nuclear radiology: indications, imaging protocols, and clinical results. *Radiographics.* 2002;22:447–490.)

a result of increased retention of solute and water in response to ACE inhibition. Reduced urine flow causes delayed and decreased washout of tracer into the collecting system in $^{99m}$Tc-MAG3 and $^{131}$I-ortho-iodohippurate studies. $^{99m}$Tc-DTPA demonstrates reduced uptake on the affected side.[387]

Consensus reports regarding methods and interpretation of ACE-enhanced renograms elaborate on a scoring system of renographic curves.[388–390] It has been recommended that high (>90%), intermediate (10%–90%), and low (<10%) probability categories be applied to captopril-enhanced renography on the basis of the change of renographic curve score between baseline values and those after captopril-enhanced renograms. Among quantitative measurements, relative renal function, the time to peak activity, and the ratio of 20-minute renal activity to peak activity (20/peak) are used more commonly than other parameters. For $^{99m}$Tc-MAG3 renal scintigraphy, a 10% change in relative renal function, peak activity increase of 2 minutes or more, and a parenchymal increase by 0.15 in 20/peak after captopril-enhanced study represent a high probability of renovascular hypertension.[391]

Captopril-enhanced renography has 80% to 95% sensitivity and 50% specificity for detecting impaired GFR; the detection of stenosis by captopril-enhanced renography may be more complicated.[394] With bilateral renovascular stenosis, it is more the exception than the rule for findings to be symmetric on captopril-enhanced renography. Studies in canine models with bilateral RAS demonstrated that captopril produced striking changes in the time-activity curve of each kidney, which are even more pronounced in the more severely stenotic kidney.[387] In practice, captopril-enhanced renography has largely been replaced by CTA or MRA for the investigation of renovascular disease.

## RENAL VEIN THROMBOSIS

Renal vein thrombosis is usually clinically unsuspected. It is found in patients with a hypercoagulable state, underlying renal disease, or both.[387] The classic manifestation of acute renal vein thrombosis with gross hematuria, flank pain, and decreasing renal function is uncommon.[399] It may present clinically as nephrotic syndrome.[392] Other causes include collagen vascular diseases, diabetic nephropathy, trauma, and tumor thrombus. Renal vein thrombosis can be diagnosed by Doppler US, CT, and MRI.

IVU yields nonspecific findings in renal vein thrombosis and is no longer used for diagnosis. It may yield normal findings in more than 25% of cases. On gray-scale and Doppler US, the involved kidney appears enlarged and swollen with relative hypoechogenicity in comparison with the normal kidney.[393] The finding of a filling defect in the renal vein is both sensitive and specific for diagnosis and is the only convincing sign of renal vein thrombosis. The lack of flow on Doppler US, however, is a nonspecific finding and may be observed because of technical limitations of the study. Other findings include an absence or reversal of the diastolic waveform on Doppler US, but this may also be seen in other conditions.

CE-CT is needed to properly assess the patient with suspected renal vein thrombosis. If renal function is impaired, MRI can be used. Findings on CT include an enlarged renal vein with a low signal-attenuating filling defect that represents the clot within the renal vein.[394] Parenchymal enhancement may be abnormal, with prolonged corticomedullary differentiation and a delayed or persistent nephrogram. The kidney appears enlarged, with edema in the renal sinus leading to a striated nephrogram and attenuation of the pelvicalyceal

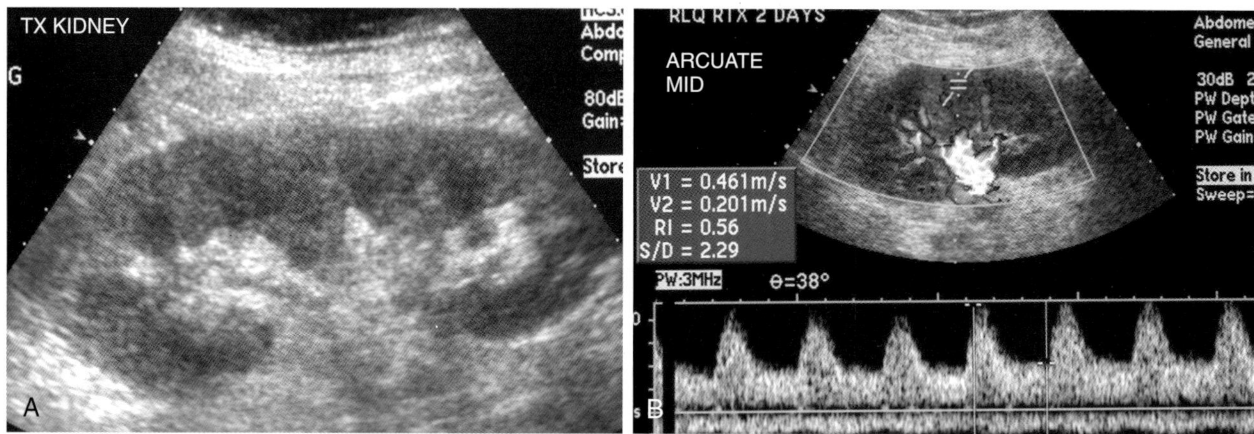


**Fig. 25.92** Normal renal transplant: ultrasonography. Coronal image **(A)** of a recently transplanted kidney in the right lower quadrant. The central echo complex, medullary pyramids, and cortex are well depicted. The duplex Doppler image **(B)** demonstrates normal flow to the transplanted kidney with a normal resistive index of 0.56.

system, and in extreme cases the pelvicalyceal system is completely compressed. Stranding and thickening of Gerota's fascia may be observed. Within chronic renal vein thrombosis, the renal vein may be narrowed because of clot retraction, and pericapsular collateral veins may be noted. Affected patients have an increased risk for pulmonary emboli as well. With renal tumors and, in rare cases, adrenal tumors, thrombus may develop in the renal vein with extension to the IVC. Imaging appearances suggesting tumor thrombus rather than bland thrombus include arterial enhancement in the thrombus, significant expansion of the vein, and continuity of the thrombus with a mass.

The appearance of renal vein thrombosis on noncontrast MRI is variable. If the thrombosis is acute, the renal vein appears distended, no normal flow void is visible, and the affected kidney appears enlarged. Renal infarction may also be present. If the thrombosis is chronic, the renal vein is small and difficult to see. A nonenhanced filling defect in the vein is visible on contrast-enhanced magnetic resonance venography, which is consistent with thrombus.

## ASSESSMENT FOR KIDNEY DONATION

The treatment of choice for patients with ESKD is renal transplantation. Although there have been significant improvements in continuous peritoneal dialysis and hemodialysis, patient survival is longer and overall quality of life is better after renal transplantation. Radiologic evaluation is performed on the potential renal transplant donor and in the postoperative assessment of the transplant recipient. Although IVU and angiography were used in the past, US, CT, MRI, and renal scintigraphy are the current methods used in evaluation of these patients (Fig. 25.92).[395–397]

A comprehensive radiologic assessment of the living renal transplant donor is crucial.[405] The anatomic information that is necessary is vascular, parenchymal, and pelvicalyceal. The renal artery must be visualized for number, length, location, and branching pattern. The parenchyma must be evaluated for scars, overall volume, renal masses, and calculi. The venous anatomy must be viewed, and the number of veins, anatomic variants, and significant systemic tributaries noted. The pelvicalyceal system must be scrutinized for anomalies such as duplication and papillary necrosis. The detailed anatomy and mapping techniques now possible have led to the increased use of laparoscopic techniques for donor kidney retrieval.[398–401]

With the development of MDCT, the complete evaluation of the living renal transplant donor is possible.[398,402,403] Noncontrast CT is performed with a low dose of radiation just to search for renal stones, locate the kidneys, and identify renal masses (see Fig. 25.9). Arterial phase scanning is generally performed at 15 to 25 seconds to demonstrate the main renal artery, branching pattern of the artery, and abnormalities such as atherosclerotic plaques or fibromuscular dysplasia (see Fig. 25.11); 25% to 40% of donors have accessory renal arteries, and 10% have early branching patterns in the main renal artery.[399,401] For transplantation the main renal artery should be free of branching for the first 15 to 20 mm. Because of the rapid transit of contrast material through the kidney, most renal veins are also well viewed in this phase (see Fig. 25.10). Venous variants occur in 15% to 28% of donors, with multiple renal veins being most common, especially on the right. On the left side, 8% to 15% have a circumaortic renal vein, and 1% to 3% have a retroaortic vein.[401,404] It is also important to visualize venous tributaries, including the gonadal, left adrenal, and lumbar veins. These are best viewed on the nephrographic phase.[399,400] Imaging in this phase is performed 80 to 120 seconds after injection of contrast material and is used to evaluate the cortex and medulla for scars and masses (see Fig. 25.12). Excretory phase imaging is performed with CT, CT digital radiography, or plain radiography to note anomalies or abnormalities in the pelvicalyceal system (see Fig. 25.13). CT has a demonstrated accuracy of 91% to 97% for arterial phase imaging, 93% to 100% for the venous phase, and 99% for the pelvicalyceal system.[403,405,406] Similar results have been noted for MRI; the biggest discrepancy is found in imaging accessory renal arteries.[407,408] Most centers today use CT in the evaluation of living renal transplant donors.

MRI, MRA, and MRU can be combined into one examination for the evaluation of the renal transplant donor.[409] MRI and CT are comparable for the evaluation of renal vasculature, structure, and function. To avoid radiation exposure and nephrotoxicity, MRI may be preferred over CT for preoperative evaluation.

In healthy renal donors it is possible to quantify functional renal volume with MRA by determining only the cortical volume. The hypothesis supported by Van den Dool et al was that glomerular filtration is an important component of renal function, and because the majority of glomeruli are in the cortex, renal function should be well correlated with cortical volume.[410] Considerations in living donors are discussed further in Chapter 71.

## ASSESSMENT OF TRANSPLANTED KIDNEYS

After surgically successful renal transplantation, radiologic evaluation is frequently necessary. Conventional US, Doppler US, CT, MRI, and renal scintigraphy are used in various settings. US assumes the primary role for assessing patients with changes in serum creatinine level, urine output, pain, or hematuria.[410] It is also used to direct kidney biopsy. Doppler US is used to evaluate renal perfusion, the patency of the renal artery and vein, and the integrity of the vascular anastomoses.[411] CT, MRI, and renal scintigraphy are adjunctive studies.

Conventional grayscale US is essential in assessing for transplant obstruction and fluid collections around the transplanted kidney.[397] Conventional US yields nonspecific findings in acute tubular necrosis and acute rejection, including obliteration of the corticomedullary junction, prominent swollen pyramids, and loss of the renal sinus echoes.[396,412] All these findings are indicative of edema of the transplanted kidney, which leads to increased peripheral vascular resistance, decreased diastolic perfusion, and elevation of the resistive index (>0.80) (Fig. 25.93).[407] Chronic rejection may lead to diffusely increased echogenicity throughout the kidney.

Doppler US adds valuable information pertaining to the integrity of the vascular elements. Despite early enthusiasm with the ability of Doppler US to differentiate acute transplant rejection from acute tubular necrosis, it is now known that the findings are nonspecific and cannot obviate the need for kidney biopsy in these cases.[413] Both acute tubular necrosis and acute rejection can cause an increase in peripheral vascular resistance.[413,414] A significant number of patients with acute rejection have a normal resistive index (<0.80).[399] It is now known that vascular rejection is no more likely to cause increases in peripheral vascular resistance than is cellular rejection.[415] Neither the timing nor clinical symptoms of the renal dysfunction can be used to differentiate acute rejection from acute tubular necrosis.[415] Doppler US is most helpful in detecting acute arterial thrombosis when signal in the artery is absent or renal vein thrombosis when the waveform is plateau-like and diastolic flow is retrograde. An abnormal Doppler waveform in the allograft indicates compromise of the transplanted kidney.[416] Sequential examinations may be used to show improvement or deterioration in the condition affecting the kidney and to note the progress of treatment.

MRI and CE-CT are useful in patients in whom the transplanted kidney is obscured by overlying bowel gas or in patients with large body habitus in whom US may be limited by the depth of the transplanted kidney. If any doubt exists after a thorough US evaluation, MRI or CT may be performed to clarify or confirm the US findings.

Fluid collections around a transplanted kidney are very common, occurring in up to 50% of cases.[418] These fluid collections may represent urinoma, hematoma, lymphocele, abscess, or seroma. The effects of the collection depend on the size and location. Urinomas and hematomas are found early, usually immediately after surgery. Lymphoceles generally are not found until 3 to 6 weeks after surgery. Abscesses are usually associated with transplant infection.

On US evaluation, extrarenal or subcapsular hematomas usually have a complex echogenic appearance, which becomes less echogenic with time (Fig. 25.94).[410] On CT they appear as high signal-attenuating fluid collections early. Such collections are usually too complex to be successfully drained percutaneously. Urine leaks and the associated urinomas are also found in the immediate postoperative period (Fig. 25.95).[410] On US these appear as anechoic fluid collection with no septations. They may rapidly increase in size. Drainage

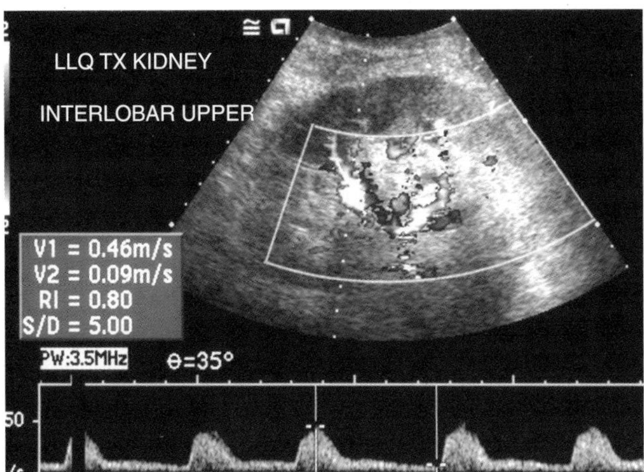


**Fig. 25.93** Renal transplant with acute tubular necrosis: ultrasonography. Duplex Doppler image of the transplanted kidney shows normal size and normal appearance with a high resistive index of 0.80 in the interlobar artery. Calculation of the resistive index (RI): *V1*, peak systolic velocity (S); *V2*, end-diastolic velocity (D). RI = (S-D)/S. The patient recovered with return of normal renal function in 5 days.

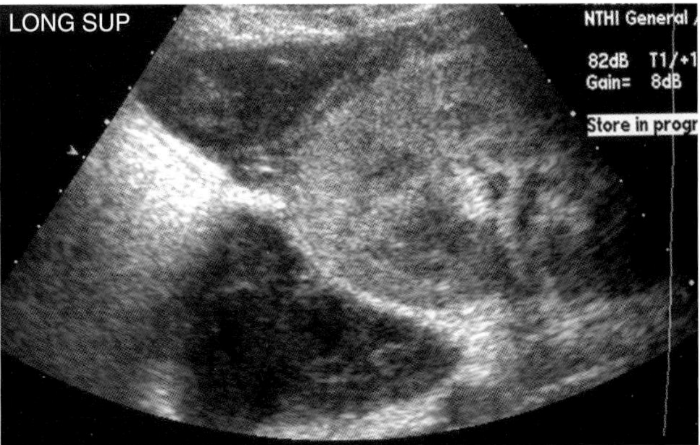


**Fig. 25.94** Renal transplant with hematoma: ultrasonography. Longitudinal image of the upper aspect of the transplanted kidney reveals two hypoechoic collections adjacent to the kidney. The heterogeneous hypoechoic nature of the collections suggests that they are hematomas, as opposed to urinomas or lymphoceles, which in general are anechoic.

may be performed under guidance by either US or CT.[417] Antegrade pyelography via a percutaneous nephrostomy is needed to detect the site of leak, usually the ureteral anastomoses. Stent placement for treatment is necessary.

Lymphoceles are recognized weeks to years after transplantation and occur in up to 20% of cases.[410] They form from the leakage of lymph fluid from the interrupted lymphatic vessels at surgery. Lymphoceles appear on US as anechoic fluid collections with septations. The size and effect on the kidney determine the need for treatment. Because lymphoceles are frequently located medial and inferior to the kidney, they are a common cause of obstruction to the kidney. US or CT guidance for drainage may be used. In a minority of cases, sclerotherapy may be needed to treat the lymphocele.[417]

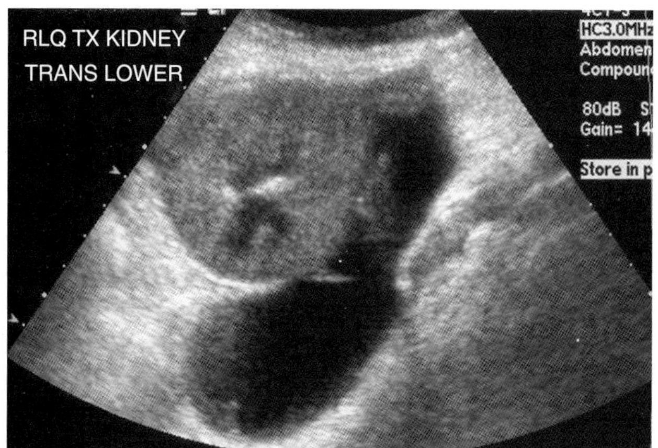


**Fig. 25.95** Renal transplant with urinoma: ultrasonography. Transverse image through the lower aspect of the transplanted kidney reveals a normal appearance with a large anechoic fluid collection adjacent to the kidney. This fluid was aspirated under US guidance, and the findings led to the diagnosis of urinoma. The patient was treated with catheter placement and drainage, also performed with US guidance.

Abscess near the transplanted kidney usually develop in association with renal infection or the infection of other fluid collections in the immunocompromised patient. On US examination, abscess appears as a complex fluid collection, possibly containing gas.[410] Fluid aspiration is usually necessary for the accurate characterization of fluid within a collection. Because blood products have characteristic signal intensities on T1- and T2-weighted sequences, MRI can provide specific diagnostic information that may help avoid an unnecessary interventional procedure in cases of hematoma.

Renal obstruction or hydronephrosis may be observed in the transplanted kidney with renal dysfunction. US is the best means for assessment.[411] In the immediate posttransplantation period, mild caliectasis is common as a result of edema at the ureteral anastomosis site. Obstruction may also be caused by fluid collections around the transplanted kidney that may be visible also with US. Blood clots within the pelvicalyceal system may also lead to hydronephrosis. Later strictures may occur, primarily at the ureteral anastomosis site. Renal stones may also cause hydronephrosis during their passage to the bladder. A functional obstruction may be visible with an overdistended bladder. With bladder emptying, US demonstrates a resolution of the hydronephrosis.

Hypertension with or without renal dysfunction may be observed in many transplant recipients.[410] Vascular and nonvascular causes must be differentiated. Doppler US is the first step of evaluation. RAS may be found in up to 23% of patients.[418] The stenosis may occur before the anastomosis in the iliac artery, at the anastomosis site, or more distally. In more than one-half the cases, the stenosis is at the anastomotic site, and it is more common in end-to-end anastomosis. CT or MRA is used to determine the site and the degree of stenosis (Fig. 25.96). Angioplasty is successful in managing most cases.[418]

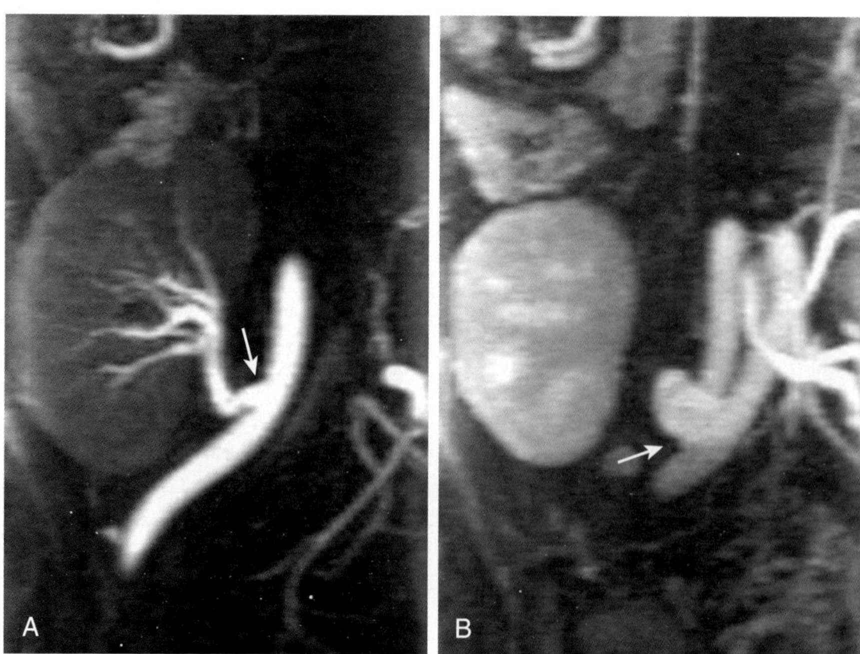


**Fig. 25.96** Renal transplant magnetic resonance angiogram, showing normal arterial (**A**) and normal venous (**B**) anastomoses *(arrows)*.

Arteriovenous fistulas may occur in transplant recipients after kidney biopsy. Most close spontaneously within 4 to 6 weeks. Grayscale images demonstrate only a simple- or complex-appearing cystic structure, whereas Doppler color-flow and duplex Doppler imaging demonstrate high-velocity and turbulent flow localized to a single segmental or interlobar artery and the adjacent vein. Arterialized flow is noted in the draining vein. If the structure is large and growing, embolization may become necessary.

Neoplasms occur in transplant recipients with increased frequency, up to 100 times more frequently than in the general population.[410] Neoplasms develop as a result of prolonged immunosuppression. The risk for renal cell carcinoma in the transplanted kidney may be increased.[419] Posttransplantation lymphoproliferative disorder may also occur in renal transplant recipients.[420] Although the transplanted kidney may be involved, the most frequent sites are the brain, liver, lungs, and gastrointestinal tract. The appearance is similar to that of conventional lymphomas with mass lesions in the organs, with or without associated adenopathy.

The MRI findings of renal transplant rejection are nonspecific (Fig. 25.97). Sadowski et al demonstrated the feasibility of using BOLD MRI to evaluate the renal transplant oxygen status and presence of acute rejection.[421] The authors concluded that MRI may differentiate acute rejection from normal function and acute tubular necrosis, but further research is required. Animal research is being performed with the hope of using noninvasive diffusion MRI techniques as a tool for monitoring early renal graft rejection after transplantation.[127]

Nuclear medicine procedures are also employed in the renal transplant recipient and play a role in the assessment of the complications associated with transplantation. These include vascular compromise (arterial or venous thrombosis), lymphocele formation, urine extravasation, acute tubular necrosis, drug toxicity, and organ rejection. Scintigraphy provides important imaging information about these potential complications, which can then guide corrective intervention.[422]

An early complication may be hyperacute rejection, which is often apparent immediately after transplantation and is caused by preformed cytotoxic antibodies. Other early complications include sudden decline in urine output and acute urinary obstruction. Scintigraphy with $^{99m}$Tc-DTPA or $^{99m}$Tc-MAG3 demonstrates absence of perfusion and function with complete thrombosis in the renal artery or renal vein. A sensitive but nonspecific sign of acute rejection is the finding of more than a 20% decline in the ratio of renal activity to the aortic activity.[423]

Renal scintigraphy performed a few days after the transplantation often reveals intact perfusion but delayed and decreased excretion of the tracer and some cortical retention of the tracer. These findings are typically caused by acute tubular necrosis and are more common with cadaveric grafts

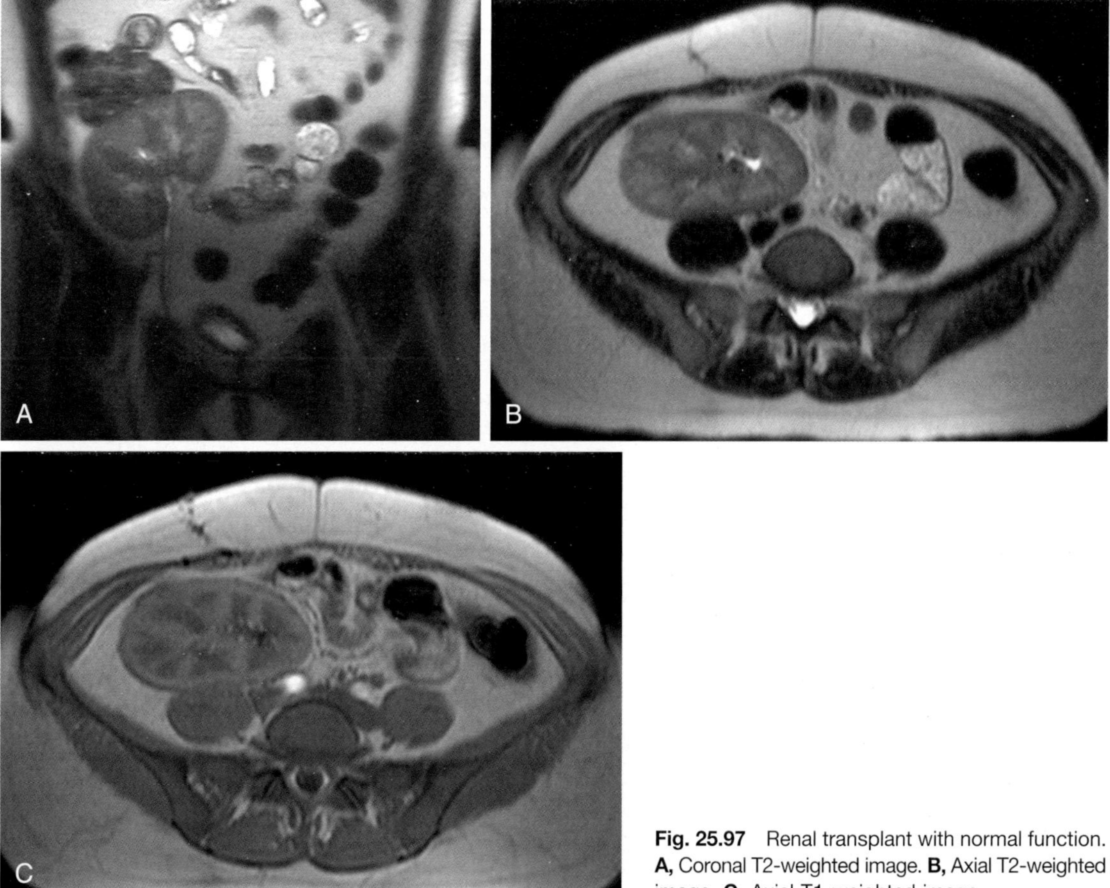


**Fig. 25.97** Renal transplant with normal function. **A,** Coronal T2-weighted image. **B,** Axial T2-weighted image. **C,** Axial T1-weighted image.

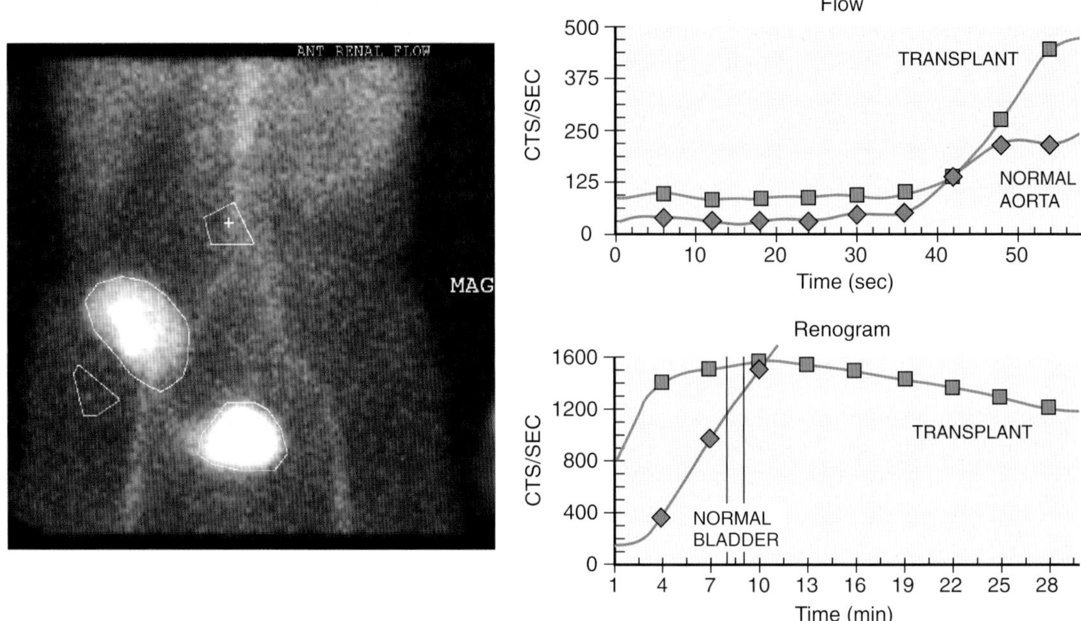


**Fig. 25.98** Abnormal technetium 99m-labeled mercaptoacetyltriglycine renogram. The pattern involving the right pelvic renal transplant from a living related donor is compatible with acute tubular necrosis.

than with grafts from living related donors (Fig. 25.98). If both perfusion and function continue to decline, then the possibility of rejection should be considered. However, acute tubular necrosis, obstruction, drug (cyclosporine) toxicity, and rejection can produce relatively similar scintigraphic appearances. The differential diagnosis should be considered in the clinical context and with regard to the interval since transplantation, although two or more of these conditions may coexist. In one report, a nonascending second phase of $^{99m}$Tc-MAG3 renogram curve was predictive of graft dysfunction. However, patients with acute tubular necrosis were not significantly more likely to have a nonascending curve than were those with acute rejection. An ascending curve was nonspecific and could be observed in both normally and poorly functioning grafts.[424]

Urine extravasation may be noted on the renal scans as collections of excreted radiotracers outside of the transplanted kidney and the urinary bladder. Because of small urine leaks and impaired renal transplant function, it may be difficult to identify a leak on scintigraphy. However, a cold-appearing defect that becomes warmer in appearance with time on the sequential images usually represents a urinoma or a urinary leak. If the activity declines with voiding, then the finding probably represents a urinoma. A chronic photopenic defect may represent a hematoma or a lymphocele (or both).[425] For assessing potential obstructive disease, scintigraphy with a diuretic may be considered, as previously discussed. Results of an animal-based study also suggested that FDG-PET may have a role in early detection of graft rejection by demonstrating significantly elevated graft tracer uptake induced by inflammatory infiltrates.[426]

## ACKNOWLEDGMENTS

The authors would like to acknowledge Sona Devedjian for manuscript preparation and William Boswell for advice.

 Complete reference list available at ExpertConsult.com.

## KEY REFERENCES

3. ACR appropriateness criteria. *Hematuria*. Available at: https://acsearch.acr.org/docs/69490/Narrative/. Accessed July 26, 2018.
4. Dyer RB, Chen MYM, Zagoria RF. Intravenous urography: technique and interpretation. *Radiographics*. 2001;21:799–824.
25. Lang EK, Macchia RJ, Thomas R, et al. Improved detection of renal pathologic features on multiphasic helical CT compared with IVU in patients presenting with microscopic hematuria. *Urology*. 2003;61:528–532.
27. Coursey CA, Nelson RC, Boll DT, et al. Dual-energy multidetector CT: how does it work, what can it tell us, and when can we use it in abdominopelvic imaging? *Radiographics*. 2010;30:1037–1055.
45. American College of Radiology Committee on Drugs and Contrast Media: *ACR manual on contrast media, V 10.3*, 2017. Available at <https://www.acr.org/Clinical-Resources/Contrast-Manual>. Accessed January 11, 2018.
48. Kidney Disease: Improving Global Outcomes: *KDIGO clinical practice guideline for acute kidney injury*. Available at: <http://www.kdigo.org/clinical_practice_guidelines/AKI.php>. Accessed June 20, 2015.
53. Davenport MS, Khalatbari S, Dillman JR, et al. Contrast material-induced nephrotoxicity and intravenous low-osmolality iodinated contrast material. *Radiology*. 2013;267:94–105.
57. Thomsen HS. European Society of Urogenital Radiology guidelines on contrast media application. *Curr Opin Urol*. 2007;17:70–76.
79. Shellock FG, ed. *Reference Manual for Magnetic Resonance Safety, Implants and Devices*. ed 2014. Los Angeles: Biomedical Research Publishing Company; 2014.
80. Rofsky NM, Weinreb JC, Bosniak MA, et al. Renal lesion characterization with gadolinium-enhanced MR imaging: efficacy and safety in patients with renal insufficiency. *Radiology*. 1991;180:85–89.
127. Zhang JL, Rusinek H, Chandarana H, et al. Functional MRI of the kidneys. *J Magn Reson Imaging*. 2013;37:282–293.
130. He W, Fischman AJ. Nuclear imaging in the genitourinary tract: recent advances and future directions. *Radiol Clin North Am*. 2008;46:25–43.
143. Esteves FP, Taylor A, Manatunga A, et al. 99mTc-MAG3 renography: normal values for MAG3 clearance and curve parameters, excretory parameters, and residual urine volume. *AJR Am J Roentgenol*. 2006;187:W610–W617.

144. *ACR appropriateness criteria: renal failure.* Available at: <http://www.acr.org/Quality-Safety/Appropriateness-Criteria/Diagnostic/~/media/ACR/Documents/AppCriteria/Diagnostic/RenalFailure.pdf>. Accessed January 11, 2018.
164. Dyer RB, Chen MYM, Zagoria RJ. Abnormal calcifications in the urinary tract. *Radiographics.* 1998;18:1405–1424.
175. *ACR appropriateness criteria: acute onset flank pain.* Available at: <http://www.acr.org/Quality-Safety/Appropriateness-Criteria/Diagnostic/Urologic-Imaging>. Accessed January 11, 2018.
182. Cheng PM, Moin P, Dunn MD, et al. What the radiologist needs to know about urolithiasis: part I: pathogenesis, types, assessment, and variant anatomy. *AJR Am J Roentgenol.* 2012;198:W540–W547.
183. Cheng PM, Moin P, Dunn MD, et al. What the radiologist needs to know about urolithiasis: part II: CT findings, reporting, and treatment. *AJR Am J Roentgenol.* 2012;198:W548–W554, 165.
198. Boll DT, Patil NA, Paulson EK, et al. Renal stone assessment with dual-energy multidetector CT and advanced postprocessing techniques: improved characterization of renal stone composition—pilot study. *Radiology.* 2009;250:813–820.
204. Takahashi N, Kawashima A, Ernst RD, et al. Ureterolithiasis: can clinical outcome be predicted with unenhanced helical CT? *Radiology.* 1998;208:97–102.
209. Kawashima A, Sandler CM, Goldman SM, et al. CT of renal inflammatory disease. *Radiographics.* 1997;17:851–866.
219. *ACR appropriateness criteria: acute pyelonephritis.* Available at: <http://www.acr.org/Quality-Safety/Appropriateness-Criteria/Diagnostic/Urologic-Imaging>. Accessed January 11, 2018.
225. Ziessman HA, Majd M. Importance of methodology on (99m) technetium dimercapto-succinic acid scintigraphic image quality: imaging pilot study for RIVUR (Randomized Intervention for Children with Vesicoureteral Reflux) multicenter investigation. *J Urol.* 2009;182:272–279.
234. Kenney PJ. Imaging of chronic renal infections. *AJR Am J Roentgenol.* 1990;155:485–494.
240. Bosniak Morton A. The use of the Bosniak classification system for renal cysts and cystic tumors. *J Urol.* 1997;157:1852–1853.
243. Israel GM, Hindman N, Bosniak MA. Evaluation of cystic renal masses: comparison of CT and MR imaging by using the Bosniak classification system. *Radiology.* 2004;231:365–371.
245. Hecht EM, Israel GM, Krinsky GA, et al. Renal masses: quantitative analysis of enhancement with signal intensity measurements versus qualitative analysis of enhancement with image subtraction for diagnosing malignancy at MR imaging. *Radiology.* 2004;232:373–378.
260. Hartman DS, Choyke PL, Hartman MS. From the RSNA refresher courses: a practical approach to the cystic renal mass. *Radiographics.* 2004;24:S101–S115.
264. Israel GM, Bosniak MA. Follow-up CT of moderately complex cystic lesions of the kidney (Bosniak category IIF). *AJR Am J Roentgenol.* 2003;181:627–633.
272. Patard JJ. Incidental renal tumours. *Curr Opin Urol.* 2009;19:454–458.
273. Berland LL, Silverman SG, Gore RM, et al. Managing incidental findings on abdominal CT: white paper of the ACR incidental findings committee. *J Am Coll Radiol.* 2010;7:754–773.
285. Bosniak M, Megibow AJ, Hulnick DH, et al. CT diagnosis of renal angiomyolipoma: the importance of detecting small amounts of fat. *AJR Am J Roentgenol.* 1988;151:497–501.
294. Davidson AJ, Hartman DS, Choyke PL, et al. Radiologic assessment of renal masses: implications for patient care. *Radiology.* 1997;202:297–305.
297. Suh M, Coakley FV, Qayyum A, et al. Distinction of renal cell carcinomas from high-attenuation renal cysts at portal venous phase contrast–enhanced CT. *Radiology.* 2003;228:330–334.
304. Kim JK, Kim TK, Ahn HJ, et al. Differentiation of subtypes of renal cell carcinoma on helical CT scans. *AJR Am J Roentgenol.* 2002;178:1499–1506.
310. Browne RFJ, Meehan CP, Colville J, et al. Transitional cell carcinoma of the upper urinary tract: spectrum of imaging findings. *Radiographics.* 2005;25:1609–1627.
325. Zukotynski K, Lewis A, O'Regan K, et al. PET/CT and renal pathology: a blind spot for radiologists? Part 1: primary pathology. *AJR Am J Roentgenol.* 2012;199:W163–W167.
335. Wang HY, Ding HJ, Chen JH, et al. Meta-analysis of the diagnostic performance of [18F] FDG PET and PET/CT in renal cell carcinoma. *Cancer Imaging.* 2012;12:464–474.
341. Kayani I, Avril N, Bomanji J, et al. Sequential FDG-PET/CT as a biomarker of response to sunitinib in metastatic clear cell renal cancer. *Clin Cancer Res.* 2011;17:6021–6028.
360. *ACR appropriateness criteria: renovascular hypertension.* Available at: <https://acsearch.acr.org/docs/69374/Narrative/>. Accessed January 11, 2018.
377. Schoenberg SO, Knopp MV, Londy F, et al. Morphologic and functional magnetic resonance imaging of renal artery stenosis: a multireader tricenter study. *J Am Soc Nephrol.* 2002;13:158–169.
379. Soulez G, Oliva VL, Turpin S, et al. Imaging of renovascular hypertension: respective values of renal scintigraphy, renal Doppler US, and MR angiography. *Radiographics.* 2000;20:1355–1368.
390. Taylor A, Nally J, Aurell M, et al. Consensus report on ACE inhibitor renography for detecting renovascular hypertension. Radionuclides in Nephrourology Group. Consensus Group on ACEI Renography. *J Nucl Med.* 1996;37:1876–1882.
420. Patel NH, Jindal RM, Wilkin T, et al. Renal arterial stenosis in renal allografts: retrospective study of predisposing factors and outcome after percutaneous transluminal angioplasty. *Radiology.* 2001;219:663–667.
427. Canadian Association of Radiologists: *Consensus guidelines for the prevention of contrast induced nephropathy.* Available at: <http://www.car.ca/uploads/standards%20guidelines/20110617_en_prevention_cin.pdf>. Accessed June 20, 2015.

# 26 The Renal Biopsy

Alan D. Salama | H. Terence Cook

CHAPTER OUTLINE



KEY POINTS

- Kidney biopsy plays an important role in the management of kidney disease.
- Percutaneous kidney biopsy is generally safe if care is taken to select and prepare the patients beforehand
- Full assessment of the biopsy requires examination by light microscopy, immunohistochemistry and (in most cases) electron microscopy
- The biopsy report should include a morphological description of the biopsy and an interpretation of the appearances in the light of the clinical presentation.
- Recommendations for the essential elements that should be present in the report have been published by the Renal Pathology Society.

## INTRODUCTION

The renal biopsy has become a fundamental component in the management of renal disease. Prior to its routine use, only autopsy material was available to investigate the pathophysiology of kidney disease, limiting antemortem diagnosis. However, its development and refinement since the late 1950s have been fundamental for the diagnosis and definition of clinical syndromes and the discovery of new pathological entities.[1] Through the critical analysis of renal biopsies taken at different disease time points, key pathophysiological features of kidney disease have been discovered, which have in turn helped to establish new paradigms in nephrology, and have led to considerable alterations in patient management, with estimates of up to 74% of patients' management changing based on the biopsy results,[2] and in two-thirds of patients, the biopsy revealed unsuspected diagnostic information. This is true for both native renal biopsies and renal transplant biopsies.[3] In addition, much is still being learnt regarding disease pathogenesis through the study of renal biopsy material, which not only remains a "gold standard" for disease diagnosis, but also has allowed the development of novel biopsy markers, which have revolutionized our concepts of pathological mechanisms.

The first percutaneous kidney biopsies were performed over 50 years ago using a liver biopsy needle and intravenous pyelograms for screening, with the patient either sitting or supine. Their success in obtaining renal tissue and in aiding management confirmed the benefit of the procedure.[1] Many innovations, including using real-time ultrasound, which allows visualization of the needle entering the kidney, spring-loaded needles,[4] or needle holders, and careful preoperative evaluation of the patient have improved the rate of obtaining renal tissue while minimizing the risks of the procedure.[5] Consequently, this has placed percutaneous renal biopsy at the very center of modern clinical nephrology. The range of diagnoses for a group of 2219 native kidney biopsies performed at the authors' institution over a 5-year period is shown in Fig. 26.1.

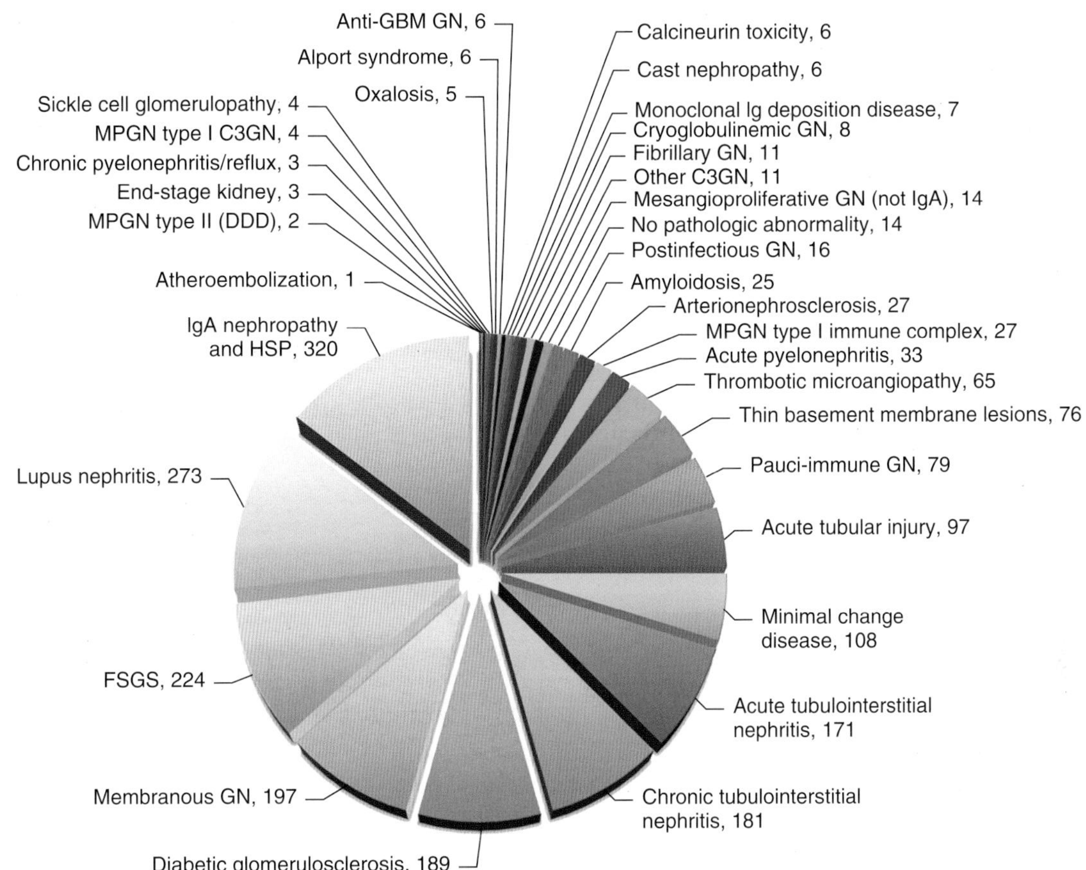


**Fig. 26.1** Proportion of diagnoses in 2219 native renal biopsies performed at Hammersmith Hospital over a 5-year period. *DDD,* Dense deposit disease; *FSGS,* focal segmental glomerulosclerosis; *GBM,* glomerular basement membrane; *GN,* glomerulonephritis; *HSP,* Henoch–Schönlein purpura; *Ig,* immunoglobulin; *MPGN,* membranoproliferative glomerulonephritis.

**Box 26.1 Indications for Renal Biopsy**

- Significant proteinuria (>1 g/day or protein-to-creatinine ratio >100 mg/mmol)
- Microscopic hematuria with any degree of proteinuria
- Unexplained renal impairment (native or transplant kidney)
- Renal manifestations of systemic disease

## SAFETY AND COMPLICATIONS OF BIOPSIES

Although generally considered safe, there is a morbidity and a small, but measurable, mortality associated with the procedure, and it is therefore imperative to subject only those patients in whom there will be a potential benefit to these risks. Indications for renal biopsy may vary from one center to another, but accepted indications are listed in Box 26.1. The significant complications related to the procedure are hemorrhage, development of arteriovenous fistulas, and to a lesser extent sepsis.[6–8] Bleeding with macroscopic hematuria and the development of perinephric hematomas may be minor and self-resolving or major and require intervention in the form of blood transfusions, embolization, or rarely surgery. Secondly, there is a risk of formation of arteriovenous fistulas, which may be asymptomatic and spontaneously resolve or lead to a significant vascular steal syndrome, compromising the rest of the kidney through ischemia. Finally, there is the risk of sepsis following the procedure, through the introduction of a septic focus or its dissemination. Overall, the risks of complication vary from center to center and between practitioners, but can be estimated between 3.5% and 13%, with the majority being minor complications (approximately 3%–9%),[6–8] although this appears to have decreased in recent years.[9,10] Mortality from the procedure is generally a result of undiagnosed bleeding with significant hematoma formation and was reported in up to 0.2% of cases from some of the larger biopsy series,[7,8] although other studies suggest that it represents an extremely rare adverse event.[5] Some degree of bleeding is common, as approximately one-half of patients have a drop in hemoglobin postbiopsy, and one-third will develop some hematoma, but only in a minority (≤7%) will bleeding be significant and require intervention.[5,8,11] Complications appear to be more common in native than transplant kidneys, and in patients with more advanced renal impairment, with prolonged bleeding times, or with lower hemoglobin (11 ± 2 vs. 12 ± 2 g/dL).[7,8] One prospective study identified the only risk factors for bleeding complications as being female, younger patients (35 ± 14.5 years vs. 40.3 ± 15.4 years), and those with a prolonged partial thromboplastin time.[12] Interestingly, needle size, number of passes, blood pressure, and renal impairment were not different between those with bleeding complications and those without. However, in this study all patients with prolonged bleeding times received DDAVP (1-deamino-8-D-arginine vasopressin) to correct the abnormality and 75% of patients had serum creatinine of less than 132 μmol/L. Conversely, others using retrospective univariate analysis have reported that blood pressure of 160/100 mm Hg or higher or a serum creatinine of greater than 2 mg/dL more than doubled the risk of bleeding.[8,13] Overall, however, no effective means has been established to identify those individuals at risk of developing "clinically" significant complications. In one small series, postbiopsy ultrasound within an hour had a 95% negative predictive value for predicting clinically significant hemorrhagic complications,[11] meaning that the absence of a hematoma on the postbiopsy scan was very suggestive of an uncomplicated clinical course. Debate continues regarding the routine use of DDAVP to counteract uremic bleeding tendencies. In part this is because its use was previously reserved for only those patients with prolonged bleeding times, and numerous studies have since demonstrated that complication rates are no different if bleeding time estimation is omitted from the preoperative assessment,[14,15] as it does not predict clinical complications.[12] However, more recent data from a randomized double blinded trial suggested a significant benefit in preventing bleeding complications with few adverse events.[16] A total of 162 low-risk adult patients undergoing biopsy were enrolled and randomized to subcutaneous DDAVP (0.3 μg/kg) or placebo. The patients were normotensive, had preserved renal function with serum creatinine of less than 1.5 mg/dL (estimated glomerular filtration rate >60 mL/min), and demonstrated a significant reduction in postbiopsy bleeds from 30.5% to 13.7% (relative risk 0.45), a significant reduction in hematoma size in those who did bleed, and a reduction in duration of hospital stay. However, hemoglobin drop after biopsy was minimal and there were no major complications, leading some to question the benefit of reduction in clinically unimportant hematomas, which can be frequently found following biopsy if looked for. No thrombotic, hyponatremic, or cardiovascular events were recorded. Whether these data, in patients with preserved renal function, could be translated to those higher-risk patients with greater renal impairment is unclear and is a question worthy of a randomized trial.

Many centers stop antiplatelet therapy prebiopsy for elective procedures, but recent data suggest that bleeding rates may be no different in those taking aspirin or stopping a week beforehand, and may avoid the increased risk of cardiovascular events following aspirin withdrawal.[9] In a center that does not routinely stop aspirin (but does stop clopidogrel), a retrospective analysis of 2563 biopsies revealed a major bleeding complication in only 2.2%, and in those in whom a complete drug record was available, no significant difference was noted on or off aspirin (357 vs. 1509, respectively, $p = .93$).[10] Very limited data are available on biopsies performed on patients taking clopidogrel.[17]

Guidelines on consenting patients and providing appropriate risk estimates have been produced by certain national renal groups and one such example is provided in Table 26.1. These estimates may err on the conservative side and should be adapted to local practice if adequate complication data are available. As well as developing procedure-related complications, there is the chance that an inadequate core of tissue is obtained for diagnosis, containing too few glomeruli or insufficient cortical material, and this is reported in between 1% and 5% of cases. The size requirements for accurate diagnosis are discussed later.

**Table 26.1 Quoted Risks of Renal Biopsy[a]**

| Complication | Quoted Risk |
|---|---|
| Macroscopic hematuria | 1:10 |
| Bleeding that requires a blood transfusion | <1:50 |
| Bleeding that may require urgent x-ray tests or even an operation to stop the bleeding | <1:1500 |
| Severe bleeding necessitating nephrectomy | <1:3000 |
| Deaths | Extremely rare |

[a]According to UK Renal Association (http://www.renal.org/information-resources/procedures-for-patients).

**Table 26.2 Contraindications to Renal Biopsy**

| Absolute Contraindications | Relative Contraindications |
|---|---|
| Uncontrolled hypertension | Single kidney |
| Bleeding diathesis | Antiplatelet/clotting agents[a] |
| Widespread cystic disease | Anatomical abnormalities |
| Hydronephrosis | Small kidneys |
| Uncooperative patient | Active urinary/skin sepsis |
| | Obesity[a] |

[a]Aspirin and body mass index >40 kg/m$^2$ were not found in recent limited cohort data to be a significant risk.

There are certain absolute contraindications, which preclude percutaneous biopsy, whereas there are a number of relative contraindications (Table 26.2) that may be circumvented depending on the importance of the biopsy, the operator's experience, and the supportive facilities available. Ideally, all efforts should be made to deal with the relative contraindications; however, in the context of acute renal failure this may not always be possible. With modern techniques evidence is emerging that previously perceived high-risk factors such as obesity, plasma cell dyscrasias such as myeloma, or amyloidosis are not actually associated with higher rates of bleeding complications.[10,18,19] The critical preoperative steps are to ensure that blood pressure is controlled, that the patient does not have a bleeding diathesis or a urinary tract infection, and that the kidneys are suitably imaged, with no evidence of obstruction, widespread cystic disease, or malignancy (although percutaneous biopsy is increasingly used to diagnose the nature of renal masses). As a result, preoperative assessment should allow those patients unsuitable for percutaneous biopsy to be referred for an alternative approach (Fig. 26.2). In these patients, there are other means of obtaining renal tissue, which include open biopsies,[20] laparoscopic biopsies, or transjugular biopsies.[21] Each is associated with certain complications and has particular merits depending on the clinical scenario (Table 26.3). Overall,

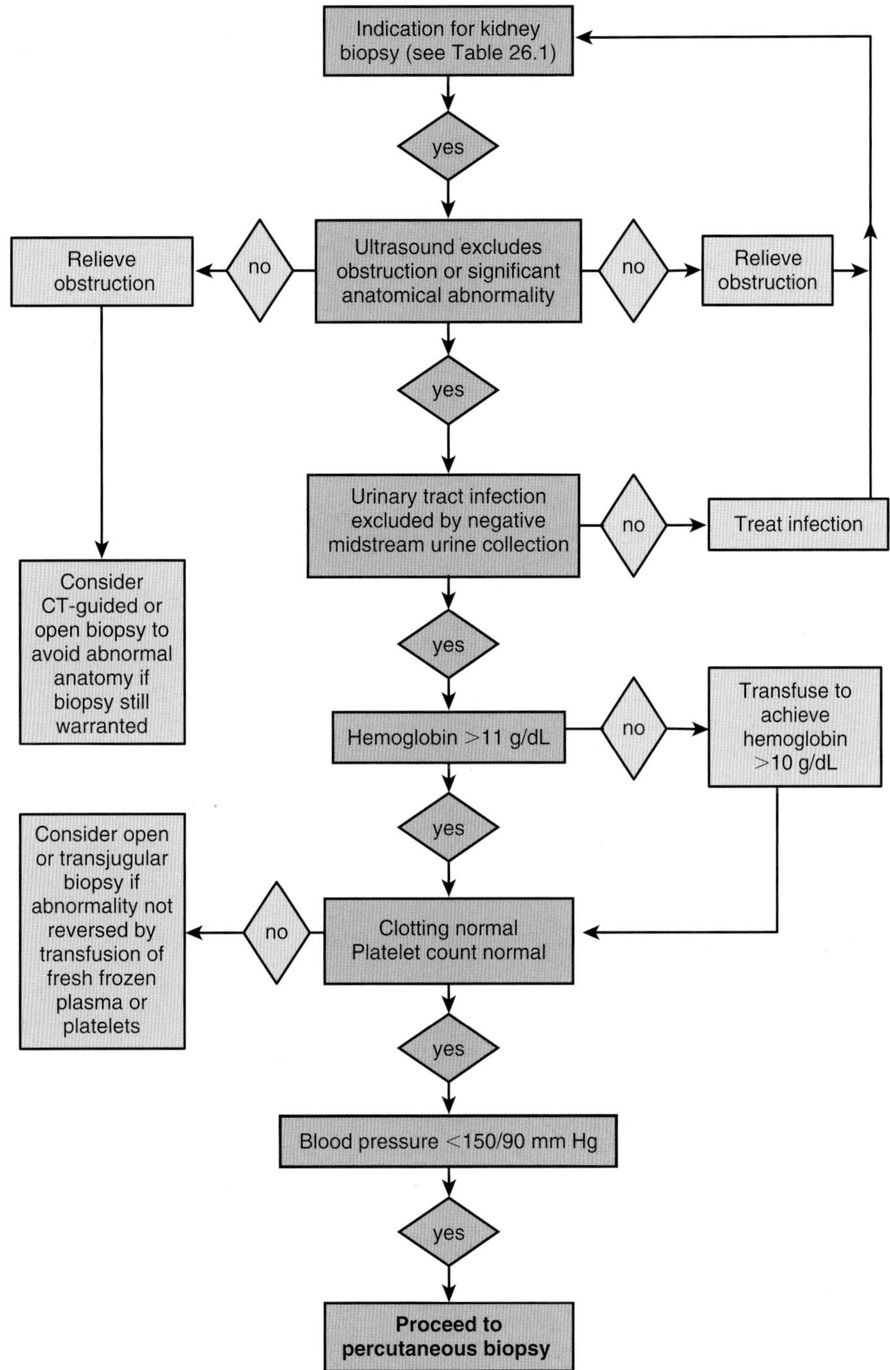


**Fig. 26.2** Renal biopsy flowchart. *CT,* Computed tomography.

these are generally only required for a minority of potential biopsy patients.

The safe duration for observation following renal biopsy has been investigated in a number of studies, which suggest that early discharge (after only 4-hour observation) will result in a number of missed complications, with many more occurring between 8 and 24 hours postprocedure. Even after 8 hours, 23% to 33% of complications will be missed. However, an overnight stay will allow an extra 20% of complications to be identified prior to discharge with between 85% and 95% of complications being identified at 12 hours and 89% and 98% following 24-hour observation.[7,22] Some units practice a policy of day biopsies with a minimum 6-hour bed rest period, which is extended only if there is evidence of bleeding, and this appears to be associated with no increased complication rates.[23] Vigilant observation of blood pressure, pulse rate, and evidence of hematuria is required in all cases.

## BIOPSY HANDLING

Detailed descriptions of methods of handling biopsies can be found in a number of publications including Churg and colleagues,[24] Furness,[25] and Walker and colleagues.[26]

**Table 26.3 Alternative Methods for Obtaining Renal Tissue and Their Risks and Benefits Compared With a Percutaneous Approach**

| Method | Advantage | Disadvantage |
|---|---|---|
| Transjugular approach | Can be of use in those with a bleeding diathesis, ventilated patients, or if combined liver and renal biopsy is required | Risk of capsular perforation<br>Inadequate material in up to 24% |
| Open approach | High yield of adequate tissue<br>Hemostasis is more secure | Requires general/spinal anesthesia; longer recovery period |
| Laparoscopic approach | High yield of adequate tissue<br>Hemostasis is more secure | Requires general/spinal anesthesia; longer recovery period |

A full assessment of the renal biopsy requires examination by light microscopy, immunohistochemistry, and electron microscopy (EM), with the use of other tests in some circumstances. Therefore it is necessary for the biopsy to be divided to provide material for each of these methods of examination. During this process it is extremely important that the biopsy is not damaged by handling, or by drying, and that the tissue is fixed in an appropriate fixative as quickly as possible, ideally within minutes. This is best achieved by dividing the biopsy at the bedside. Examination of the biopsy with a dissecting microscope allows cortex, containing glomeruli, to be distinguished from medulla and thus facilitates assessment of the adequacy of the cores and division of the biopsy so that glomeruli are present in the samples for each modality of examination. If a dissecting microscope is not available, then a standard light microscope can be used with the biopsy placed in a drop of normal saline on a microscope slide. If it is not possible to examine the biopsy in this way, then a standard approach to obtain material for EM is to take small fragments (approximately 1 mm in length) from each end of each core. In that way if there is cortex in the core, glomeruli should be sampled. The remainder of the cores can then be divided for light microscopy and for immunofluorescence (IF). The part of the biopsy for light microscopy is then placed in appropriate fixative and that for IF is either snap frozen or transported to the laboratory in a suitable transport medium such as that described by Michel et al.[27]; tissue placed in this medium can remain for several days at room temperature without loss of antigens. During division of the biopsy it is important not to introduce artifacts due to crushing or stretching. Forceps should not be used to pick up the specimen; this can be done using either a needle or a small wooden stick such as a toothpick. The biopsy should be cut using a fresh scalpel.

If the biopsy has to be taken to the histology laboratory for division, this should be done as quickly as possible with the biopsy wrapped in saline-moistened gauze or in tissue culture medium. Artifacts may be produced if the biopsy is placed on dry gauze or gauze moistened with water, or if it is placed in ice-cold saline.

If the amount of material obtained at biopsy is limited, then it may be necessary to adapt the way in which it is divided and the decision as to how this is done must depend on the clinical question. In most cases it is possible to omit frozen material for IF and instead perform immunohistochemistry on paraffin sections. However, if there is a suspicion of crescentic glomerulonephritis due to antiglomerular basement membrane (anti-GBM) disease, IF is more reliable for detecting the linear capillary wall staining. It may be possible to omit EM and perform it if necessary on material reprocessed from the paraffin block, but if this is done, it is not possible to obtain accurate measurements of glomerular capillary membrane thickness.[28]

## LIGHT MICROSCOPY

The most commonly used fixative for light microscopy is buffered 10% aqueous formaldehyde solution. This is actually a 10% solution of the 37% commercially available concentrated solution of formaldehyde, giving a final concentration of about 4%. This fixative is generally available in all histology laboratories, provides adequate fixation for light microscopy, and also allows the tissue to be used for immunohistochemistry and EM. Some more specialized fixatives such as Bouin or Zenker fixative provide better preservation of certain morphologic details, but in general the problems with handling these fixatives, and the difficulties of subsequently using the material for immunohistochemistry or EM, outweigh the advantages. For example, Bouin contains picric acid that is explosive when dry. However, we do commonly use Bouin fixative for examination of mouse kidneys where the improvement in glomerular morphology is significant. Methacarn, a modified Carnoy fixative, also provides good fixation for light microscopy and EM and may allow the immunohistochemical detection of antigens that are not detected in formalin-fixed tissue. Details of the preparation of various fixatives can be found in the appendix of Churg and colleagues.[24]

The standard method of processing tissue for light microscopy is by dehydration in graded alcohols, transfer to a clearing agent such as xylene, and embedding in paraffin wax. This is usually performed in an automated instrument but can be done by hand. Rapid processing schedules allow for same-day processing and it is possible to obtain stained slides within 3 to 4 hours of receipt of the specimen in the laboratory.

It is important to have thin uniform sections for light microscopy. These should be cut as thin as possible – no greater than 3 μm. It is often stated that renal biopsy sections should be cut at 2 μm, but this may lead to problems in cutting with damage to the tissue. Since many pathologic lesions may be focal within glomeruli, interstitium, or vessels, it is essential that the biopsy is examined at multiple levels and each laboratory will have their preferred way to achieve that. In general, serial sections should be cut with at least two placed on each slide. Multiple slides can then be stained with each stain, with some intervening unstained sections kept either for potential immunohistochemical examination or for other special stains as necessary.

## STAINING FOR LIGHT MICROSCOPY

Most renal pathologists employ a number of stains for light microscopy. The commonly used stains are hematoxylin and eosin (H&E), periodic acid–Schiff (PAS) reaction, silver methenamine, and a trichrome stain. The H&E stain is a good general histological stain for studying the overall architecture of the kidney. It is good for studying the morphology of tubular cells and the morphology of interstitial infiltrates. With experience the different staining characteristics of hyaline, fibrin, and amyloid, all of which are eosinophilic, can usually be distinguished. However, the H&E stain does not distinguish staining of glomerular matrix and basement membrane from cell cytoplasm, and therefore is less useful for the assessment of glomerular architecture. In the PAS reaction the mesangial matrix and basement membrane are stained purple and this allows a good assessment of the amount of matrix and the thickness of the GBM. PAS also stains the tubular basement membranes and hyaline deposits. The silver methenamine stain is the best stain for studying the detailed morphology of the GBM and for highlighting the membrane spikes seen in membranous glomerulonephritis and the double contours seen in membranoproliferative glomerulonephritis. Its only drawback is that a satisfactory result is more technically demanding than the other stains. A trichrome stain, such as Masson trichrome, will stain the glomerular mesangial matrix and basement membrane and may also help in highlighting fibrin and immune complex deposits. Other stains are a matter of personal preference. We always use an elastin stain to demonstrate the elastic laminae of vessels and this is counterstained with picrosirius red to stain fibrillar collagen in the interstitium. Amyloid is most specifically detected in a Congo red stain and we feel it is prudent to perform this in all native biopsies. This is the exception to the requirement for thin sections; since the Congo red stain is relatively insensitive, a section cut at 10 μm should be used. Details of staining methods are given in the appendix of Churg and colleagues.[24] Other stains that may be employed when necessary include the von Kossa stain that demonstrates calcium deposition and the Perls Prussian blue stain for iron.

## EXAMINATION OF THE BIOPSY BY LIGHT MICROSCOPY

It is important to approach the examination of the biopsy systematically. Sections should first be assessed at low power to determine what parts of the kidney (or other structures in some cases) they contain, including whether there is cortex and/or medulla. A low-power view will also allow an assessment of the amount of chronic nephron damage, as demonstrated by tubular atrophy and interstitial fibrosis, and the presence of interstitial inflammatory infiltrates. It will also allow an assessment of interstitial expansion, most commonly due to either edema or fibrosis, but occasionally due to infiltration by, for example, amyloid. Examination should then proceed by studying the glomeruli, tubules, interstitium, and vessels, including arteries, arterioles, and veins, in more detail. Features that should be looked for in glomeruli and tubules are detailed in Boxes 26.2 and 26.3. Arterioles should be examined for the presence of hyalinosis, thrombosis, and necrosis. Arteries should be assessed for intimal thickening and whether it is accompanied by reduplication of the internal elastic lamina, thrombosis, necrosis, inflammation, and cholesterol emboli.

**Box 26.2 Features to Be Assessed by Light Microscopy in Glomeruli**

- Size.
- Cellularity: if increased, then are the extra cells mesangial, in capillary lumens (endocapillary), or in Bowman's space? (NB: Normal mesangial areas contain two to three cells.)
- Capillary wall thickness (use periodic acid–Schiff or silver stain); if thickened, are there double contours or spikes on the silver stain?
- Is the mesangium expanded? If so, are there nodules?
- Is there deposition of abnormal material (e.g., amyloid)?
- Is there segmental sclerosis?
- Is there thrombosis?
- Is there necrosis?

**Box 26.3 Features to Be Assessed by Light Microscopy in Tubules**

- Percentage atrophy
- Signs of acute damage (e.g., dilatation, epithelial flattening, granular casts, mitoses)
- Tubulitis
- Casts: Granular casts suggest acute tubular injury; eosinophilic fractured casts suggest myeloma; neutrophil casts suggest acute pyelonephritis
- Crystals (e.g., oxalate)
- Viral inclusions (e.g., BK virus)

## TERMINOLOGY IN DESCRIPTION OF GLOMERULAR DISEASE

The involvement of glomeruli by a pathological process can be defined by the percentage of glomeruli involved by a lesion and by whether the lesion involves all or only part of any individual glomerulus. A lesion that involves all or nearly all glomeruli is described as "diffuse," whereas one that involves some but not all glomeruli is described as "focal." In the definitions given in the World Health Organization (WHO) atlas of glomerular diseases, it was suggested that the cutoff for focal versus diffuse should be 80% of glomerular involvement. However, in recent classifications of lupus glomerulonephritis[29] and immunoglobulin A (IgA) nephropathy,[30] the cutoff is defined as 50%. If a lesion involves only part of a glomerulus, that is, with some capillary lumens remaining uninvolved, it is called "segmental," whereas if it involves the whole glomerulus, it is called "global." In the classifications of lupus glomerulonephritis[29] and IgA nephropathy,[30] the cutoff is set at 50% glomerular tuft involvement, except for segmental sclerosis in IgA nephropathy, in which any area of sclerosis that leaves some of the glomerulus unaffected is defined as segmental.

**Box 26.4 Definitions of Terms Used in Describing Glomerular Lesions**

Sclerosis: A lesion resulting from an increase in mesangial matrix and/or collapse and condensation of the basement membranes – the sclerotic material stains with eosin, periodic acid–Schiff (PAS), and silver stains.

Hyalinosis: Lesion containing an acellular structureless material consisting of glycoproteins and sometimes lipids – stains intensely with eosin and PAS but not with silver stains.

Fibrosis: A lesion consisting of collagen fibers, which may be differentiated from sclerosis by not staining with PAS reagent or silver stains.

Necrosis: A lesion characterized by fragmentation of nuclei and/or disruption of the basement membrane, often associated with the presence of fibrin-rich material.

Extracapillary proliferation or cellular crescent: Extracapillary cell proliferation of more than two cell layers with >50% of the lesion occupied by cells.

Extracapillary fibrocellular proliferation or fibrocellular crescent: An extracapillary lesion comprising cells and extracellular matrix, with <50% cells and <90% matrix.

Extracapillary fibrosis or fibrous crescent: >10% of the circumference of Bowman's capsule covered by a lesion composed of >90% matrix.

There are a number of other terms, such as sclerosis and hyalinosis, that have specific definitions in the glomerulus and these are listed in Box 26.4.

## IMMUNOHISTOCHEMISTRY

The understanding of renal pathology was transformed in the 1960s by the use of IF microscopy. This allowed the detection and localization of immunoglobulins and complement components in glomeruli, and the identification of new entities such as IgA nephropathy. It is mandatory to perform immunohistochemistry for a full assessment of glomerular pathology in biopsies for native kidneys. The use of immunohistochemistry in transplant biopsies is discussed further later. There are a number of diagnoses that cannot be made on renal biopsy without immunohistochemistry including IgA nephropathy, C3 glomerulopathy (GN), C1q nephropathy, anti-GBM disease, and light-chain deposition disease.

In native kidneys a minimum panel of immunohistochemical stains would include antibodies for IgA, IgG, IgM, C3c, and kappa and lambda light chains. Light-chain immunohistochemistry is very important if diagnoses such as light-chain deposition disease, monoclonal immunoglobulin deposition disease, or proliferative glomerulonephritis with monoclonal immunoglobulin deposits are not to be missed. Many pathologists would also add antibodies for C1q, C4c, and fibrinogen to this routine panel. In transplant kidney biopsies staining for C4d is invaluable in assessing the activation of the classical pathway of complement by antibody and hence in the diagnosis of antibody-mediated rejection. There are a number of other antigens whose detection may be useful in particular circumstances. These include:

1. Microorganisms, including BK virus, cytomegalovirus, and Epstein–Barr virus.
2. Amyloid proteins. Antibodies are available to AA amyloid and many of the rarer inherited forms of amyloid.
3. Alpha chains of type 4 collagen. In suspected hereditary nephropathy of Alport type, it may be helpful to stain for the alpha 3 and alpha 5 chains of type IV collagen.
4. IgG subclasses in cases of suspected monoclonal immunoglobulin deposition.
5. Myoglobin in suspected myoglobinuria.
6. Lymphocyte surface antigens particularly in cases of suspected lymphoid neoplasia.
7. Type III collagen in collagenofibrotic GN.
8. Fibronectin in fibronectin GN.

Immunohistochemistry is performed either on cryostat sections of a piece of snap-frozen tissue or on paraffin sections. Antigen detection on frozen sections is usually performed using an antibody labeled with a fluorochrome and this is then viewed using a fluorescence microscope – commonly referred to as immunofluorescence or IF. The use of fluorescent-labeled antibodies on frozen sections is technically straightforward and very sensitive because the antigens have not been altered by fixation. There are some drawbacks. First, it requires a separate piece of tissue to have been obtained at the time of biopsy. Second, the morphology of frozen sections is never as good as paraffin sections and so it may be more difficult to define the site of the antigen within the glomerulus. In addition, immunofluorescent sections will fade over time but if appropriately mounted and refrigerated in the dark, they will retain staining for weeks to months.

If paraffin sections are used, then some form of antigen retrieval is essential for most antigens because they become "masked" during fixation and processing. For the detection of immunoglobulins and complement the antigen retrieval that works best is some form of protease digestion. The length of time required for protease digestion is critically dependent on a number of factors such as the length of time the biopsy has been in fixative and the particular processing schedule used; some of these may be difficult to control. This variability of the antigen retrieval process is the major drawback of immunohistochemistry on paraffin sections and means that results are highly dependent on the skills of the technician performing the staining. After the antigen retrieval step, antigens are generally detected using a primary antibody followed by a detection system that leads to the deposition of a colored reaction product that is visible by light microscopy. Commonly this product is developed by a reaction that uses the enzyme horseradish peroxidase, and hence this method is often referred to as "immunoperoxidase" staining. However, it is also possible to use fluorescent antibody staining on paraffin sections after antigen retrieval.[31]

The major advantage of immunohistochemistry on paraffin sections is that it is not necessary to take a separate piece of tissue for frozen section. In addition, it is possible to specifically localize antigens and compare this with adjacent sections examined by light microscopy. However, it is technically demanding and also it is significantly less sensitive for some antigens. Direct comparison of the two methods showed that detection of IgG, IgA, and C3c by immunoperoxidase on protease-digested deparaffinized sections of formaldehyde-fixed tissue is, with few exceptions, equal to IF on frozen sections.[32] Our experience is that it is extremely difficult to get satisfactory staining for light chains using peroxidase techniques on paraffin sections (although fluorescence on paraffin sections may be more successful) and that detection of the linear capillary wall staining of anti-GBM antibodies is more difficult in paraffin sections. It may also be more difficult to detect very early deposits of membranous glomerulonephritis in paraffin as compared with frozen tissue.

In our experience most renal pathologists find IF on frozen sections the most satisfactory way to detect immunoglobulins and complement but, regardless of preference, there will always be cases in which no material is available for frozen section, or the material is inadequate, and so laboratories should also be competent to carry out immunohistochemistry on paraffin sections.

In reporting immunohistochemical staining for immunoglobulins and complement, it is important to describe the site of staining in the glomerulus (e.g., mesangial or capillary wall), its nature (whether linear, finely or coarsely granular), and its intensity. For estimation of intensity most pathologists rely on semiquantitative subjective scale from 0 to 3+, but formal quantitation by image analysis may be useful for research. In addition to the glomerulus, staining should also be assessed in the tubules, especially the tubular basement membrane, interstitium, and vessels.

## ELECTRON MICROSCOPY

EM is invaluable for assessing structural changes in the glomerulus and for identifying immune complexes, which are seen as areas of electron density. Although the importance of EM has become much reduced in other areas of surgical pathology, because of the development of immunohistochemistry, it remains an invaluable technique for the examination of glomeruli in biopsies in native kidneys and, increasingly, for the determination of causes of dysfunction in transplant kidneys. The part of the renal biopsy on which EM is to be performed is usually placed in separate fixative, although entirely satisfactory results can be obtained using material fixed in formalin. Most laboratories prefer either ice-cold glutaraldehyde or paraformaldehyde. The material is then exposed to osmium tetroxide and processed into resin blocks. In order to select the areas to be studied, "semithin" 0.5-μm sections are first screened by light microscopy to select areas of interest that can then be examined further on the electron microscope. An ultramicrotome is then used to obtain the very thin sections required for the electron microscope. A permanent record of the electron microscopic appearances is kept either as photographs or, increasingly, as digital images. As with light microscopy, examination of the biopsy by EM should be systematic with assessment of the glomerular capillary basement membrane and its thickness; the endothelium and whether there is thickening or loss of fenestrations; the capillary lumen and particularly whether there is narrowing by cells or other material; the podocytes looking particularly at the preservation of the foot processes and whether the cell bodies show any vacuolation or microvillous change. The presence of any electron-dense deposits – most commonly due to immune complex deposition – should be noted together with their distribution – mesangial, subendothelial, or subepithelial. EM may also demonstrate a number of other structures such as fibrils in amyloidosis or fibrillary glomerulonephritis, tubules in immunotactoid GN, or the characteristic inclusion bodies of various storage diseases.

Although EM is most useful in the assessment of glomerular morphology, it may also be very helpful in demonstrating ultrastructural changes in other parts of the kidney. For example, it may help in demonstrating tubular basement membrane immune complexes, in elucidating the nature of tubular epithelial cell inclusions, and in examining the morphology of mitochondria in tubular epithelial cells, which may show abnormalities in inherited conditions or as a result of drugs.

There have been several studies that have assessed the utility of EM in the assessment of native kidney biopsies. Most studies suggest that EM provides useful information in about half of all native kidney biopsies and is essential for diagnosis in about 20%.[33] Because it is impossible to know which these are at the time of biopsy, it is prudent to always have material available for EM even if, in some cases, it is not processed further after light microscopy and immunohistochemistry. Box 26.5 lists some conditions for which EM is essential for the diagnosis and others where it is helpful. Also listed are some conditions in which the diagnosis may be reached without EM but, even in these cases, it is important to remember that EM may allow a more detailed description of the morphology of these conditions or also reveal a totally unrelated pathology.

### Box 26.5 Examples of the Use of Electron Microscopy in Diagnosis of Kidney Biopsies

**Electron Microscopy (EM) Essential for Diagnosis**

Thin basement membrane lesion
Fibrillary glomerulopathy (GN)
Immunotactoid GN
Alport syndrome
Fabry disease
Lecithin-cholesterol acetyltransferase deficiency
Nail patella syndrome

**EM Very Helpful**

Dense deposit disease
Minimal change disease
Early diabetic GN
Early membranous GN (particularly if only paraffin sections are available for immunohistochemistry)
Membranoproliferative GN
Postinfectious GN
Human immunodeficiency virus (HIV) nephropathy
Lipoprotein GN
Collagenofibrotic GN

**Diagnosis May Be Made Without EM**

IgA nephropathy
Acute tubulointerstitial nephritis
Myeloma cast nephropathy
Pauci-immune crescentic GN
Amyloid (although amyloid fibrils may be detected by EM when it has been missed on light microscopy)

Morphometric analysis of EM is mainly of importance for research. However, it is important to be able to measure the thickness of the GBM in order to quantitate the thinning that may be seen in thin basement membrane lesion or the thickening commonly seen in diabetic glomerulosclerosis. Accurate unbiased measurement of the GBM thickness requires complex morphometric techniques to avoid the bias introduced by tangential sectioning of capillary loops. However, in practice it is satisfactory to use direct measurement of GBM thickness (distance from endothelial to podocyte plasma membrane) and determination of the arithmetic mean of such measurements. Das et al.[34] found that if 16 measurements from each of two glomeruli were made using this direct method, the results were reproducible. Ideally, each laboratory should define a normal range using this method.

## OTHER STUDIES ON THE RENAL BIOPSY

In addition to examination by light microscopy, immunohistochemistry, and EM it may also be appropriate to consider other methods for studying the tissue. In cases of suspected infection, part of the biopsy may be sent for culture or for polymerase chain reaction for infective organisms. In biopsies with lymphoid infiltrates, immunoglobulin gene rearrangement studies may allow the confirmation of clonality. The chemical composition of material in the biopsy (e.g., crystalline material) may be determined by energy-dispersive x-ray spectroscopy.

There has been considerable interest in the possibilities of extracting messenger RNA (mRNA) from biopsies, in order to study differences in gene expression in different pathological conditions,[35] and in studying the range of proteins in the biopsy – the proteome.[36] These techniques have been applied to whole biopsies or to parts of the biopsy – for example, glomeruli isolated either by simple dissection under a dissecting microscope or by laser capture microdissection. Examination by mass spectrometry may allow identification of the fibril proteins of amyloid or fibrillary glomerulonephritis.[37,38] Examination of mRNA transcripts shows considerable promise for assisting in the diagnosis of kidney transplant rejection.[39]

## BIOPSIES OF TRANSPLANTED KIDNEYS

The handling of transplant biopsies differs in some respects from that of native kidneys. For biopsies taken to assess the cause of kidney dysfunction in the first few months after transplantation, it may not be necessary to carry out immunohistochemistry with a full panel of antibodies to immunoglobulins and complement, or to perform EM, unless there is a clinical suspicion of glomerular disease. However, immunohistochemistry for C4d is performed to assess antibody binding and complement activation on peritubular capillary endothelium. In later biopsies EM is very useful in the diagnosis of chronic allograft GN and its differentiation from recurrence of de novo glomerulonephritis. It is also helpful in identifying chronic rejection involving peritubular capillaries, which is associated with multilayering of the peritubular capillary basement membranes.[40] The recommendations from the Banff Conference on Allograft Pathology 2013[41] are that ultrastructural studies should be performed in all biopsies from patients who are sensitized, have documented donor-specific antibodies at any time after transplantation, and/or who have had a prior biopsy showing C4d staining, glomerulitis, and/or peritubular capillaritis. It is also advised that EM be considered in all biopsies performed more than 6 months after transplantation and in "for-cause" biopsies done more than 3 months after transplantation to determine if early changes of transplant GN are present, prompting testing for donor-specific antibodies.

## THE SIZE OF THE BIOPSY

The renal biopsy is only a small sample of the renal parenchyma and this always needs to be kept in mind when making inferences about the state of the whole kidney from changes seen in the biopsy. Some diseases may only affect the kidney focally and therefore may be missed on biopsy, for example, reflux nephropathy or arterial cholesterol emboli. Others may be segmental at the level of the glomerulus, for example, focal and segmental glomerulosclerosis or pauci-immune necrotizing glomerulonephritis, and therefore the chance of detecting them will depend on how many glomeruli are present in the biopsy and how many sections are examined. Sampling is also a problem when we make inferences from the amount of disease we see in the biopsy to the amount that affects the kidney. For example, if 20% of the glomeruli in a biopsy have crescents, we tend to assume that this is the percentage of the glomeruli in the kidney that have crescents. However, because of the small size of most biopsies, the confidence limits we can place on the true involvement of glomeruli are usually very wide. An elegant mathematical description of the problems of glomerular sampling has been published by Corwin et al.[42] This shows, for example, that to confidently exclude a segmental glomerular disease that is affecting about 5% of the glomeruli, a biopsy with 20 glomeruli is needed. The situation is worse if we consider the problem of comparing the amount of glomerular involvement in two different biopsies, a question that often arises, for example, in patients with lupus glomerulonephritis who have repeat biopsies. In that case, to confidently detect a 10% difference in glomerular involvement between two biopsies would require over 100 glomeruli in each biopsy. To detect differences of 25% to 40% glomerular involvement the minimum biopsy size is 20 to 25 glomeruli.

For some diseases, classification schemes have defined minimum sizes for biopsy adequacy. Thus, for lupus glomerulonephritis it is suggested that a biopsy should contain a minimum of 10 glomeruli.[29] In transplant biopsies the Banff group has suggested that the requirements for biopsy adequacy are 10 or more glomeruli with at least two arteries.[43] It has been shown that examining two rather than one core of tissue increases the sensitivity for the diagnosis of acute rejection from 91% to 99%.[44] In acute cellular rejection, examining slides taken at only one level, rather than at three, misses 33% of cases with intimal arteritis.[45]

## THE BIOPSY REPORT

The biopsy report should include a morphologic description of the biopsy and an interpretation of the appearances in the light of the clinical presentation. The changes seen on light microscopy, immunohistochemistry, and EM must be integrated and this is best done if a single person examines the biopsy by each modality. A Committee of the Renal Pathology Society has published recommendations for the essential elements that should be present in a renal biopsy report.[46]

The description of the light microscopy should include the number of glomeruli present and the number that show global or segmental sclerosis. It is essential to provide a quantitative estimate of the amount of irreversible nephron damage in the biopsy and, where appropriate, the severity of any active inflammatory process. The best way to estimate the irreversible damage is by specifying the number of globally sclerosed glomeruli and the amount of tubular atrophy and interstitial fibrosis. The estimate of activity will depend on the particular disease process but should include an indication of the proportion of glomeruli involved by crescents, necrosis, and endocapillary hypercellularity. For some diagnoses there are established classification schemes that should be applied to the biopsy, for example, the International Society of Nephrology (ISN)/Renal Pathology Society (RPS) classification of lupus nephritis,[29] the Oxford Classification of IgA nephropathy,[47,48] and the Banff classification of allograft pathology. International consensus groups have published recommendations for Pathologic Classification, Diagnosis, and Reporting of GN[49] and for the standardized grading of chronic changes in native kidney biopsy specimens.[50]

The interpretation of renal biopsies requires the pathologist to integrate the biopsy findings with detailed clinical information and therefore requires a thorough understanding of renal disease and the therapeutic implications of the biopsy diagnosis. Close communication between the clinician and pathologist is essential and it is generally very helpful for the biopsy to be viewed and discussed at a clinicopathologic conference so that full discussion of the implications of the biopsy specimen appearances for patient management can take place.

## CONCLUSION

Percutaneous renal biopsy is generally safe if care is taken to select and prepare the patients beforehand. It has become a cornerstone of nephrological practice and its handling and interpretation should be made by those experienced in renal pathology. The interpretation of the biopsy should be carried out with adequate clinical information for integrated clinicopathologic conclusions to be drawn.

 Complete reference list available at ExpertConsult.com.

## KEY REFERENCES


1. Cameron JS, Hicks J. The introduction of renal biopsy into nephrology from 1901 to 1961: a paradigm of the forming of nephrology by technology. *Am J Nephrol.* 1997;17:347–358.
2. Kitterer D, Gurzing K, Segerer S, et al. Diagnostic impact of percutaneous renal biopsy. *Clin Nephrol.* 2015;84:311–322.
23. Roccatello D, Sciascia S, Rossi D, et al. Outpatient percutaneous native renal biopsy: safety profile in a large monocentric cohort. *BMJ Open.* 2017;7:e015243.
24. Churg J, Bernstein J, Glassock RJ. *Renal Disease: Classification and Atlas of Glomerular Diseases.* New York: Igaku-Shoin; 1995.
25. Furness PN. Acp. Best practice no 160. Renal biopsy specimens. *J Clin Pathol.* 2000;53:433–438.
26. Walker PD, Cavallo T, Bonsib SM. Practice guidelines for the renal biopsy. *Mod Pathol.* 2004;17:1555–1563.
31. Nasr SH, Galgano SJ, Markowitz GS, et al. Immunofluorescence on pronase-digested paraffin sections: a valuable salvage technique for renal biopsies. *Kidney Int.* 2006;70:2148–2151.
46. Chang A, Gibson IW, Cohen AH, et al. A position paper on standardizing the nonneoplastic kidney biopsy report. *Clin J Am Soc Nephrol.* 2012;7:1365–1368.
50. Sethi S, D'Agati VD, Nast CC, et al. A proposal for standardized grading of chronic changes in native kidney biopsy specimens. *Kidney Int.* 2017;91:787–789.

# 27 Biomarkers in Acute and Chronic Kidney Diseases

Chirag R. Parikh | Jay L. Koyner

## CHAPTER OUTLINE



## KEY POINTS

- An ideal biomarker is easily measurable, reproducible, sensitive, organ-specific, cost-effective, easily interpretable, and present in readily available specimens (e.g., blood and urine).
- Due to the inherent variability in the serum creatinine assay, patients with advanced chronic kidney disease (CKD) may be misclassified as acute kidney injury (AKI) based on small changes in creatinine levels.
- Serum cystatin C performs on par with serum creatinine for estimates of glomerular filtration rate (GFR) in the setting of CKD and may provide additional information about a CKD patient's risk for cardiovascular morbidity and mortality.
- Urinary $\alpha_1$-microglobulin, a low-molecular-weight glycoprotein and member of the lipocalin superfamily, has been associated with the increased risk of CKD and all-cause mortality in a variety of clinical settings.
- Heart-type fatty acid binding protein, proenkephalin, and monocyte chemoattractant protein-1 are promising AKI biomarkers in the setting of cardiac surgery and intensive care unit–associated AKI
- Urinary TIMP-2 × IGFBP-7 is associated with the increased risk of development of Kidney Disease: Improving Global Outcomes stage 2 or 3 AKI in the next 12 hours in ICU patients at high risk for AKI.
- Plasma levels of *TGFR1*, *TGFR2*, EGF, and KIM-1 have been increasingly recognized as potential biomarkers for incident and progressive CKD.

Kidney disease is a global health problem. Acute kidney injury (AKI) and chronic kidney disease (CKD) are increasing in incidence.[1] In the United States, it is clear that the incidence of AKI, regardless of its severity, has been steadily increasing at a rate that is disturbingly high, and it is increasingly recognized that AKI predisposes to the progression of CKD toward end-stage renal disease (ESRD), which ultimately requires dialysis or kidney transplantation.[2–4] According to the World Health Organization, approximately 850,000 patients develop ESRD every year.[5–7] Across the globe, treatment of ESRD poses a major challenge for health care systems and the global economy. The burden of kidney disease is most significant in developing countries and is adversely influenced by inadequate socioeconomic and health care infrastructures.[5,8,9] Importantly, kidney disease progression may be curtailed if the disease is diagnosed early. Hence, detection and management of kidney diseases, whether acute or chronic, in the early, reversible, and potentially treatable stages, is of paramount importance. Biomarkers that will help diagnose kidney injury, predict progression of kidney disease, and provide information regarding the effectiveness of therapeutic intervention will be important adjuncts to our standard management strategies.

Recently, many novel, high-throughput technologies in the fields of genomics, proteomics, and metabolomics have made it easier to interrogate hundreds or even thousands of potential biomarkers at once, without prior knowledge of the underlying biology or pathophysiology of the system being studied.[10–13] As a result, there is a renewed interest in discovering novel biomarkers for use in drug development and patient care. Despite notable achievements, however, only a few biomarkers—blood urea nitrogen (BUN) level, creatinine concentration, urinalysis results and proteinuria—are routinely used to diagnose and monitor kidney injury. These commonly used gold standard biomarkers of kidney function are not optimal to detect injury or dysfunction early enough to allow prompt therapeutic intervention. Although additional candidate biomarkers have been reported, none have been adequately validated to justify their use in making patient care decisions, but a few look quite promising.

## BIOMARKER DEFINITION

In 2001, the U.S. Food and Drug Administration (FDA) standardized the definition of a biomarker as "a characteristic that is objectively measured and evaluated as an indicator of normal biologic processes, pathogenic processes, or pharmacologic responses to therapeutic intervention."[14] The National Institutes of Health further classified biomarkers based on their utility (Table 27.1).[14] Biomarkers can potentially serve a wide range of functions in drug development, clinical trials, and therapeutic management strategies. There are many different classes of biomarkers—prognostic, predictive, pharmacodynamic, and surrogate biomarkers. Of note, these categories are not mutually exclusive. Definitions of the different types of biomarkers can be found in Table 27.1. Examples of biomarkers are proteins, lipids, genomic or proteomic patterns, imaging determinations, electrical signals, and cells present in urine. Some biomarkers also serve as surrogate endpoints. A surrogate endpoint is a biomarker intended to substitute for a clinical endpoint. Furthermore, a surrogate endpoint biomarker is expected to predict clinical benefit (harm or lack of benefit) based on epidemiologic, therapeutic, pathophysiologic, or other scientific evidence.[15] An ideal biomarker is easily measurable, reproducible, sensitive, cost- effective, easily interpretable, and present in readily available specimens (blood and urine).

**Table 27.1 Biomarker Definitions**

| Term | Definition |
|---|---|
| Biomarker | A characteristic that is objectively measured and evaluated as an indicator of a normal biologic process, pathogenic process, or pharmacologic response to therapeutic intervention.<br>• A prognostic biomarker is a baseline patient or disease characteristic that categorizes patients by degree of risk for disease occurrence or progression, informing about the natural history of the disorder in the absence of a therapeutic intervention.<br>• A predictive biomarker is a baseline characteristic that characterizes patients by their likelihood for response to a particular treatment, predicting either a favorable or unfavorable response.<br>• A pharmacodynamic biomarker is a dynamic assessment that shows that a biologic response has occurred in a patient who has received a therapeutic intervention. Pharmacodynamic biomarkers may be treatment-specific or broadly informative of disease response, with the specific clinical setting determining how the biomarker is used and interpreted. |
| Clinical endpoint | A characteristic or variable that reflects how a patient fares or functions or how long a patient survives |
| Surrogate endpoint biomarker (type 2 biomarker) | A marker that is intended to substitute for the clinical endpoint. A surrogate endpoint is expected to predict clinical benefit, harm, lack of benefit, or lack of harm on the basis of epidemiologic, therapeutic, pathophysiologic, or other scientific evidence. |

## PROCESS OF BIOMARKER DISCOVERY, ASSAY VALIDATION, AND QUALIFICATION IN A CLINICAL CONTEXT

Primary challenges to the development of biomarkers for kidney injury and toxicity are discovery of candidate markers, design of an assay, validation of the assay, and qualification of the biomarker for use in specific clinical contexts. The process of biomarker identification and development is arduous and involves several phases.[16,17] For the purpose of simplicity, this process can be divided into the following five phases (adapted and modified from Pepe and colleagues[16]).

### PHASE 1: DISCOVERY OF POTENTIAL BIOMARKERS THROUGH UNBIASED OR HYPOTHESIS-GENERATING EXPLORATORY STUDIES

The primary goal of phase 1 is to identify potential leads using various technologies and to confirm and prioritize the identified leads. The search for biomarkers often begins with preclinical studies that compare either tissue or biologic fluids in diseased animals (e.g., animals with kidney injury) with those in healthy animals to identify genes or proteins that appear to be upregulated or downregulated in diseased tissue relative to control tissue. When biologic samples, such as blood and urine, are readily available from humans, it is possible to forgo the animal model stage. Innovative discovery technologies include microarray-based gene expression profiling that provides information regarding expression of genes, micro RNA (miRNA)-based expression, and proteomic technologies, as well as metabolomic, profiling of biologic fluids based on mass spectrophotometry, and other technologies. The candidate marker approach, especially when informed by the pathophysiology of the disease for which the biomarker is being evaluated, should not be ignored.

Once a promising biomarker is discovered, the validation process begins. An assay has to be developed and validated. The validation process is laborious and expensive, requiring access to patient samples with complete clinical annotation and long-term follow-up, as described in the section on phase 2. In addition, each biomarker must be qualified for specific application. This is especially true in the case of kidney diseases, for which one biomarker alone may not satisfy the requirements of an ideal biomarker. This is described in the subsequent section on phase 4. Incorporation of several of these novel biomarkers into a biomarker panel may enable simultaneous assessment of site-specific kidney injury or several mechanisms contributing to clinical syndromes.

## PHASE 2: DEVELOPMENT AND VALIDATION OF AN ASSAY FOR THE MEASUREMENT OR IDENTIFICATION OF THE BIOMARKER IN CLINICAL SAMPLES

The primary goal of phase 2 is to develop and validate a clinically useful assay that has the ability to distinguish a person with kidney disease or injury from a person with healthy kidneys in a high-throughput fashion. This phase involves development of an assay, optimization of assay performance, and evaluation of the reproducibility of the assay results within and among laboratories. Defining reference ranges of biomarker values is a crucial step before the biomarker can be used clinically.[18,19] It is important to characterize how the levels of these markers vary with patient age, gender, race, and ethnicity, and how biomarker values are related to known risk factors.[20]

## PHASE 3: DEMONSTRATION OF THE BIOMARKER'S POTENTIAL CLINICAL UTILITY IN RETROSPECTIVE STUDIES

In phase 3, the primary objectives are to as follows: (1) evaluate the biomarker potential in samples obtained from a completed clinical study; (2) test the diagnostic potential of the biomarker for early detection; and (3) determine the sensitivity and specificity of the biomarker using defined threshold values of the biomarker for utility in prospective studies. For example, if the levels of biomarker differ significantly between cases (those with acute or chronic kidney injury) and control subjects only at the time of clinical diagnosis, then the biomarker shows little promise for population screening or early detection. In contrast, if levels differ significantly at hours, days, or years before clinical symptoms appear, then the biomarker's potential for early detection is increased. This phase also involves comparing the biomarker with several other novel biomarkers or existing gold standard biomarkers and defining the biomarker's performance characteristics (i.e., sensitivity, specificity) using receiver-operating characteristic curve analysis. This latter process is particularly challenging in kidney disease, given uncertainties in the sensitivity and specificity of the gold standard used.[21]

## PHASE 4: PERFORMANCE OF PROSPECTIVE SCREENING STUDIES

The primary aim of phase 4 studies is to determine the operating characteristics of the biomarker in a relevant population by measuring detection and false referral rates. In contrast to phase 1, 2, and 3 studies, which are based primarily on stored specimens, studies in phase 4 involve screening subjects prospectively and demonstrating that clinical care is changed as a result of the information provided by the biomarker analysis.

### BIOMARKER QUALIFICATION PROCESS

The application for FDA qualification of novel biomarkers requires the intended use of the biomarker in nonclinical and clinical contexts and the collection of evidence supporting qualification. This can be a joint and collaborative effort among regulatory agencies, pharmaceutical companies, and academic scientists.[22]

Data are shared between the FDA and pharmaceutical industry or academic laboratories through voluntary exploratory data submissions (VXDSs).[23] Submission of exploratory biomarker data through VXDSs allows interaction between reviewers at the FDA and researchers in industry or academia regarding study designs, sample collection and storage protocols, technology platforms, and data analysis. This pilot process for biomarker qualification allows the Predictive Safety Testing Consortium to apply to both U.S. and European drug authorities simultaneously for qualification of new nephrotoxic biomarkers (e.g., kidney injury molecule-1, albumin, total protein, cystatin C, clusterin, trefoil factor 3, and $\alpha_2$-microglobulin) as predictors of drug-mediated nephrotoxicity.[23–25] The FDA and the corresponding European authority (European Medicines Agency [EMA]) reviewed the application separately and made decisions as to whether each would allow the new biomarkers to be "fit for purpose" in preclinical research.[24,25] Some of these markers were proposed to be qualified as biomarkers for clinical drug-induced nephrotoxicity once further supportive human data are submitted. More recently, the FDA has approved total kidney volume as a biomarker of disease progression for the purposes of clinical trial enrichment in autosomal dominant polycystic kidney disease (see also Chapter 45), thus opening to door to other novel measures as potential biomarkers of disease progression in the setting of acute kidney injury (AKI) and other forms of chronic kidney disease (CKD).[22,26]

It is notable that the process described above is specific for the FDA and United States and that the biomarker validation and approval process varies significantly around the world. In the past few years, the FDA, EMA, and other agencies have approved several biomarkers for clinical use in the United States and other countries throughout Europe and Asia.

## PHASE 5: CONTINUED ASSESSMENT OF THE VALIDITY OF THE BIOMARKER IN ROUTINE CLINICAL PRACTICE

Phase 5 addresses whether measurement of the biomarker alters physician decision making and/or reduces the mortality or morbidity associated with the given disease in the population.

# ANALYSIS OF BIOMARKER PERFORMANCE

The widely accepted measure of biomarker sensitivity and specificity is the receiver-operating characteristic (ROC) curve.[27] ROC curves display the proportion of subjects, with and without disease, correctly identified at various cutoff points. A ROC curve is a graphic display of trade-offs between the true-positive rate (sensitivity) and false-positive rate (1 − specificity, where specificity is expressed as a value from 0 to 1) when the biomarker is a continuous variable (Fig. 27.1).[28,29] Sensitivity is plotted along the ordinate, and the value of (1 – specificity) is plotted on the abscissa. Each point on the curve represents the true-positive rate and false-positive rate associated with a particular test value. The diagonal, represented by the equation true-positive rate (sensitivity) = false-positive rate (1 – specificity), corresponds to the set of points for which there is no selectivity in predicting disease. The area under this line of "unity" is 0.5, which indicates no advantage relative to the flip of a coin.

The performance of a biomarker can be quantified by calculating the area under the ROC curve (AUC). The AUC is the probability that a randomly sampled case has a larger biomarker value (or risk score) than a randomly sampled control. Although this makes the AUC easily interpretable, this interpretation is not always clinically meaningful, because cases and controls do not present to clinicians in random pairs. Thus, whereas an ideal biomarker could supply an AUC of 1.0 (a clinical rarity), in actuality the AUC lacks true direct clinical relevance.[29] Despite these flaws, the AUC is widely reported and familiar to clinicians. The shortcomings of AUC extend into the assessment of the incremental change in AUC (ΔAUC) when adding a new marker to a group of previously established predictors. The clinical impact of a ΔAUC of 0.02 is often unclear, and the statistics and *P* values behind such calculations remain problematic.[30,31]

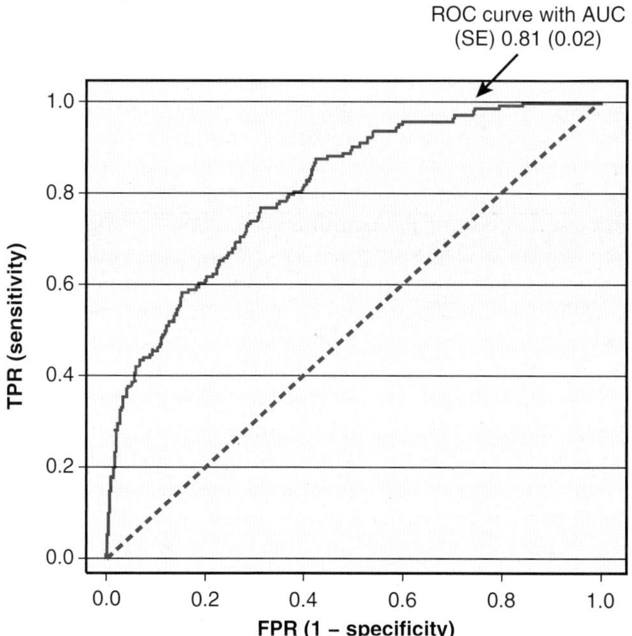


| | | True disease state | |
|---|---|---|---|
| | | Diseased | Nondiseased |
| Biomarker test | Positive (diseased) | True-positive (TP) | False-positive (FP) |
| | Negative (nondisease) | False-negative (FN) | True-negative (TN) |

**Biomarker classification by disease status**
True-positive rate (TPR) = sensitivity = TP/(TP + FN)
False-positive rate (FPR) = 1 – specifity = FP/(FP + TN)

**Fig. 27.1** Receiver operator characteristic curves.

Other important parameters related to biomarker performance, primarily with respect to the testing of larger or specific populations, are positive and negative predictive values. The positive predictive value is the proportion of persons who test positive for a disease and actually have the disease, whereas the negative predictive value represents the proportion of persons who test negative and do not have the disease. There is considerable interest in developing algorithms that use a composite of values of several biomarkers that are measured in parallel for the purpose of increasing diagnostic potential or predicting disease course and patient outcomes.

More recently, the Net Reclassification Index (NRI) and the Integrated Discrimination Improvement Indices (IDIs) have been used to evaluate the ability of new biomarkers. The NRI is simply the proportion of the population whose risk category changes with the new biomarker; a small reclassification rate means that treatment decisions will rarely be altered by the new biomarker. IDI is defined as the difference in discrimination slopes between the unadjusted and biomarker-adjusted clinic models, with large effect sizes having an IDI ≥ 0.10 and medium effect sizes having an IDI between 0.05 and 0.10.[32] Note that the NRI and IDI have not been widely accepted by all statisticians.[33]

## CHARACTERISTICS OF AN IDEAL BIOMARKER FOR KIDNEY DISEASE

Characteristics of an ideal biomarker for kidney disease are described in Table 27.2. For AKI, the biomarker should have the following characteristics: (1) be organ-specific and allow differentiation between intrarenal, prerenal, and postrenal causes of AKI, as well as acute glomerular injury; (2) be able to detect AKI early in the course and predict its course and potentially the future implications of AKI; (3) be able to identify the cause of AKI; (4) be site-specific and able to inform pathologic changes in various segments of renal tubules during AKI, as well as correlate with the histologic findings in kidney biopsy specimens; (5) be easily and reliably measured in a noninvasive or minimally invasive manner; (6) be stable in its matrix; (7) be rapidly and reliably measurable at the bedside; and (8) be inexpensive to measure.

In CKD (unlike AKI), the timing and nature of the insult are very hard to estimate, which makes the search for early biomarkers for CKD very difficult. An ideal biomarker for CKD shares many of the same requirements described earlier for AKI biomarkers, including providing insight into the following: (1) the location of the injury (e.g., glomerular, interstitial, tubular); (2) the disease mechanism; (3) the progressive course of the disease; and (4) the risk of complications from comorbid conditions such as cardiovascular disease and diabetes.

### ACUTE KIDNEY INJURY MARKERS

In the cardiac sciences, the discovery of biomarkers, such as troponins, which reflect early cardiomyocyte damage rather than decreased cardiac function, has enabled the development and implementation of novel therapeutic strategies to reduce coronary insufficiency and associated morbidity and mortality.[34,35] By contrast, the delay in diagnosis associated

**Table 27.2 Characteristics of an Ideal Kidney Biomarker**

| Functional Properties | Physiochemical Properties |
|---|---|
| • Rapid and reliable increase in response to kidney diseases<br>• Highly sensitive and specific for acute and/or chronic kidney disease<br>• Shows good correlation with degree of renal injury<br>• Provides risk stratification and prognostic information (e.g., severity of kidney disease, need for dialysis, length of hospital stay, and mortality)<br>• Site-specific to detect early injury (e.g., proximal, distal, interstitium or vasculature) and identify pathologic changes in specific segments of renal tubules<br>• Applicable across different races and age groups<br>• Allows recognition of the cause of kidney injury or disease (e.g., ischemia, toxins, sepsis, cardiovascular disease, diabetic nephropathy, lupus, or combinations)<br>• Organ-specific; allows differentiation among intrarenal, prerenal, and extrarenal causes of kidney injury<br>• Noninvasively identifies the duration of kidney failure (acute kidney injury, chronic kidney injury)<br>• Useful to monitor the response to therapeutic interventions<br>• Provides information on the risk of complications from comorbid conditions (especially in chronic kidney disease) | • Stable over time across different temperature and pH conditions, with clinically relevant storage conditions<br>• Rapidly and easily measurable<br>• Not subject to interference by drugs and endogenous substances |

**Table 27.3 Kidney Disease: Improving Global Outcomes (KDIGO) Staging of Acute Kidney Disease**

| Stage | Serum Creatinine Criteria | Urine Output Criteria |
|---|---|---|
| 1 | 1.5–1.9 times baseline<br>*or*<br>≥0.3 mg/dL (26.5 μmol/L) increase | <0.5 mL/kg for 6–12 h |
| 2 | 2.0–2.9 time baseline | <0.5 mL/kg/h for ≥12 h |
| 3 | ≥3.0 times<br>*or*<br>Increase in serum creatinine to ≥4.0 mg/dL (≥353.6 μmol/L)<br>*or*<br>Initiation of renal replacement therapy<br>*or*<br>In patients <18 years, decrease in eGFR to <35 mL/min[2] | <0.3 mL/kg/h for ≥24 h or anuria for 12 h |

with the use of kidney biomarkers, such as serum creatinine concentration, has impaired the ability of nephrologists to conduct interventional studies in which the intervention can be implemented early in the course of the disease process.[36] Although the past decade has seen a revolution in terms of diagnostic criteria for AKI with the RIFLE (*r*isk, *i*njury, *f*ailure, *l*oss, *e*nd-stage kidney disease) classification[37] and the Acute Kidney Injury Network (AKIN) definition of AKI[38] being harmonized into the Kidney Disease: Improving Global Outcomes (KDIGO) classification[39] (Table 27.3), these criteria remain limited by their reliance on the serum creatinine concentration on some level. More recently, there has been a call to expand these definitions further to potentially include biomarkers, but as of the time of this publication, these new guidelines have yet to be widely accepted.[40] These new guidelines and the concept of AKI remain reliant on the serum creatinine level and will continue to serve as a limitation, given creatinine's role as a functional biomarker. The serum creatinine level can increase in cases of prerenal azotemia when there is no tubular injury and can be unchanged under conditions of significant tubular injury, particularly when patients have good underlying kidney function and significant kidney reserve. Nonetheless, these criteria have advanced our understanding of the epidemiology of AKI, and these standardized consensus definitions have allowed for comparisons and aggregation of data from a larger number of papers.[41] Biomarkers of AKI can serve several purposes and are no longer thought of as a replacement for the serum creatinine level. Table 27.4 summarizes several of the potential uses of AKI biomarkers. Fig. 27.2 summarizes the kidney-specific location of the AKI biomarkers discussed later.

Urine and serum biomarkers each have advantages and disadvantages. Serum biomarkers are often not stable and are difficult to measure because of interference with several serum proteins. By contrast, urinary biomarkers are relatively stable and easy to assess; however, their concentrations are greatly influenced by the hydration and volume status of the patient and other conditions that affect urinary volume. To overcome this challenge, urinary biomarker concentrations have often been normalized to urinary creatinine concentrations to eliminate the influence of urinary volume on the assumption that the urinary creatinine excretion rate is constant over time, and that biomarker production or excretion has a linear relationship with the urinary creatinine excretion rate. Bonventre and colleagues have challenged this assumption, especially in AKI settings, when the urine creatinine excretion rate is not constant and changes over time, greatly influencing the normalized value of a putative urinary biomarker after normalization. They have suggested that the most accurate method to quantify biomarkers is the timed collection of urine samples to estimate the renal excretion rate[42]; however, this approach is not practical for

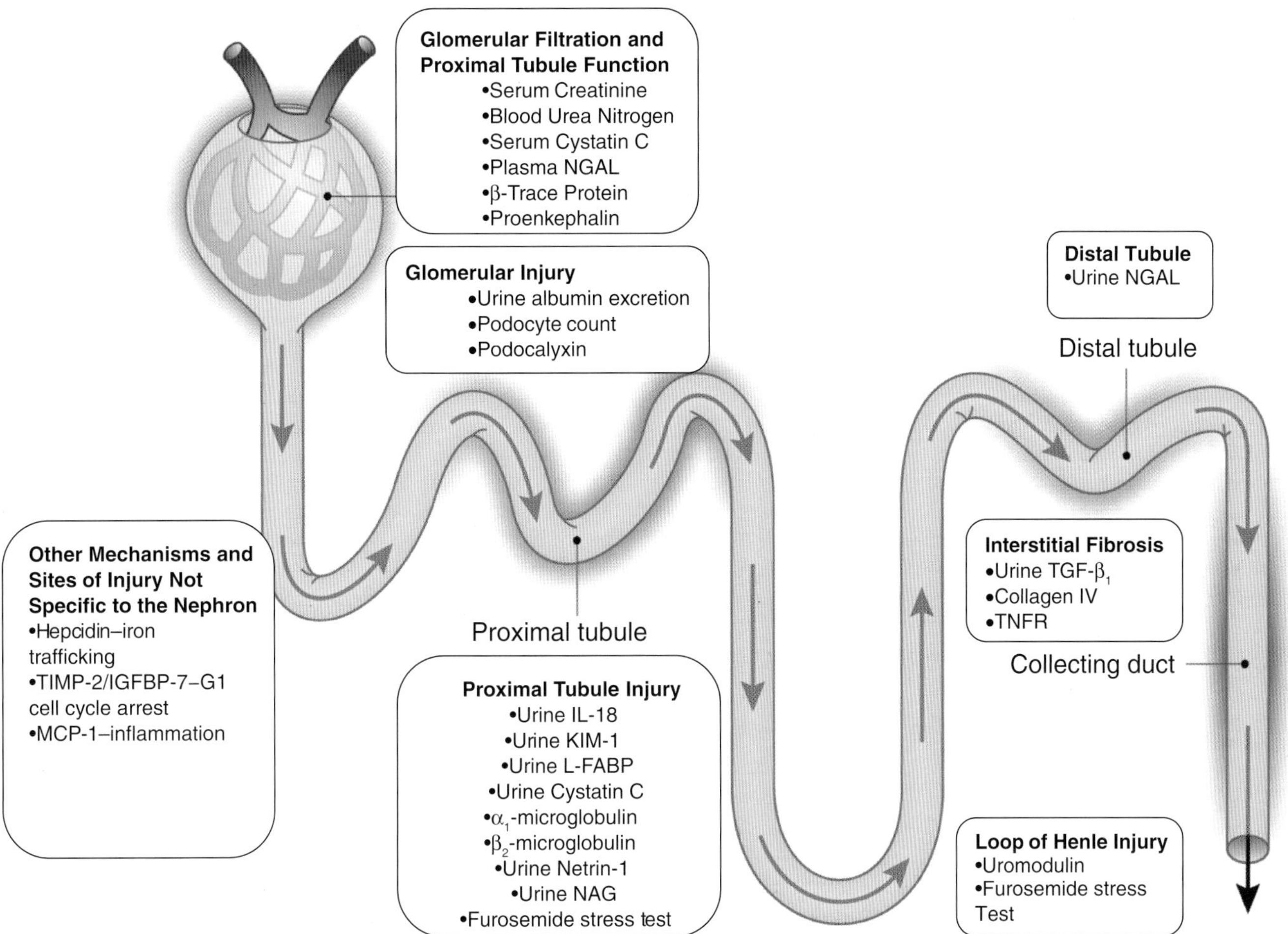


**Fig. 27.2** Biomarkers in relation to their site of injury in the nephron. *GST,* Glutathione S-transferase; *IGFBP7,* insulin-like growth factor binding protein-7; *IL-18,* interleukin-18; KIM-1, kidney injury molecule-1; *L-FABP,* liver-type fatty acid binding protein; *MCP-1,* monocyte chemotactic protein 1; *NAG,* N-acetyl-β-D-glucosaminidase; *NGAL,* neutrophil gelatinase-associated lipocalin; *TGF-β₁*, transforming growth factor-$\beta_1$; *TIMP-2,* tissue inhibitor metalloproteinase-2; *TNFR,* tumor necrosis factor receptor. (Adapted from Koyner JL, Parikh CR. Clinical utility of biomarkers of AKI in cardiac surgery and critical illness. *Clin J Am Soc Nephrol.* 2013;8:1034–1042.)

**Table 27.4 Potential Uses for Biomarkers of Acute Kidney Injury (AKI) and Chronic Kidney Disease (CKD)**

| Disorder | Potential Use |
|---|---|
| AKI | Early detection of AKI:<br>• Differential diagnosis of AKI (e.g., distinguishing between volume-mediated AKI [prerenal] and intrinsic tubular injury (e.g., acute tubular necrosis)<br>• Predicting outcomes of AKI at the time of clinical diagnosis (need for RRT, development of post-AKI CKD, short- and long-term mortality)<br>• Predicting recovery from AKI<br>• Ascertaining the nephron-specific location and cause of renal injury<br>• Monitoring the effects of an intervention |
| CKD | Early detection and diagnosis of CKD:<br>• Predicting the progression of CKD (rapid vs. slow progression)<br>• Predicting outcomes of CKD at the time of clinical diagnosis (development of ESRD, short- and long-term mortality)<br>• Predicting cardiovascular disease and outcomes in patients with CKD<br>• Monitoring the effects of an intervention |

routine clinical care. Endre and colleagues delved into this issue further by demonstrating that the ideal method for quantitating biomarkers of urinary AKI depends on the outcome of interest; absolute biomarker concentrations best diagnosed AKI at the time of intensive care unit (ICU) admission, whereas normalization to urinary creatinine improved the prediction of incipient AKI.[43] A potential explanation of the failings of normalization is that it will often amplify the signal. For example, when the glomerular filtration rate (GFR) is reduced in immediate response to a tubular injury, the amount of biomarker produced will increase, and the urinary creatinine level will decrease. The normalized value will therefore increase by a greater amount in the short term than can be explained by the increase in the absolute level of biomarker production. Currently, there is no standardized method of accounting for this issue, with some urinary biomarkers being normalized to urine creatinine and others being reported without normalization.

Because AKI and CKD share functional and structural aspects, there are overlapping as well as distinct classes of functional and structural biomarkers. Among the functional markers, the GFR is often used as the gold standard. Although the true GFR, as determined by agents that are freely filtered and undergo minimal handling by the tubule (e.g.,

**Table 27.5 Biomarker Performance in Detecting Acute Kidney Injury (AKI)[a]**

| | **Perioperative AKI** | | | | **Critically Ill** | | | **Emergency Room** | |
|---|---|---|---|---|---|---|---|---|---|
| **Parameter** | Preop AKI Risk | Early Postop AKI | AKI Progression | Long-Term Mortality | Early Diagnosis of AKI | Type of AKI (Transient vs. Intrinsic) | Need for RRT | Early Diagnosis of AKI | Type of AKI (Transient vs. Intrinsic) |
| Urine NGAL | N/A | + | – | + | + | + | + | + | + |
| Blood NGAL | – | + | + | + | – | **?** | – | **?** | **?** |
| Blood CysC | + | + | – | **?** | + | + | + | **?** | **?** |
| Urine CysC | N/A | – | – | – | + | + | + | + | + |
| Urine IL-18 | N/A | + | + | + | + | + | + | + | + |
| Urine KIM-1 | N/A | + | – | + | + | – | – | + | + |
| Urine L-FABP | N/A | – | – | + | **?** | **?** | – | + | + |
| TIMP-2 IGFBP-7 | N/A | + | + | **?** | + | **?** | + | + | **?** |
| Urine protein, albumin | + | + | + | + | **?** | **?** | **?** | **?** | **?** |

[a]From multicenter studies at a variety of clinical time points.

*CysC,* Cystatin C; *IL-18,* interleukin-18; *KIM-1,* kidney injury molecule-1; *L-FABP,* liver fatty acid binding protein; *NGAL*, neutrophil gelatinase-associated lipocalin; *Preop,* preoperative; *Postop,* postoperative; *RRT,* renal replacement therapy; *TIMP-2, IGFBP-7,* tissue inhibitor metalloprotease 2, insulin-like growth factor binding protein-7.

+, Data published display the ability to detect this aspect of AKI; –, data published do not display the ability to detect this aspect of AKI; ?, no large multicenter data published on this biomarker or aspect of AKI; *N/A,* Not applicable to the following: (1) biomarkers of tubular injury have no role in preoperative risk screening; (2) serum creatinine is intrinsic to the definitions of AKI being tested.

Adapted and expanded from Koyner JL, Parikh CR. Clinical utility of biomarkers of AKI in cardiac surgery and critical illness. *Clin J Am Soc Nephrol.* 2013;8:1034–1042.

iothalamate, iohexol, inulin), represents a sensitive measure for determining changes in kidney function, these tests are invasive and laborious to perform. Moreover, because of the renal reserve, changes in GFR may not indicate structural injury until significant injury has occurred. On the other hand, structural markers of tubular injury are expressed by tubular cells, and subtle changes in epithelial cells lead to release of these markers into the urine. It is becoming increasingly clear that many of these biomarkers serve as signals for both AKI and CKD and also may be used to monitor progression from AKI to CKD. A challenge is to define at what level of release of these markers the injury is clinically significant in either the acute or chronic setting. Failure to identify the separate impacts of CKD and AKI on these biomarker values will lead to inappropriate clinical decision and/or poor results in clinical studies.[44,45]

Table 27.5 summarizes the ability of biomarkers to detect clinical endpoints related to AKI in a variety of clinical settings.

## GLOMERULAR INJURY MARKERS

### SERUM GLOMERULAR FILTRATION MARKERS

During the course of injury, kidney function may be impaired with reduction in the GFR and accumulation of several nitrogenous compounds in the blood. Serum creatinine and BUN concentrations are routinely used as markers of kidney injury, but it is important to recognize these parameters as markers for kidney dysfunction, rather than direct markers of injury.

As discussed elsewhere in this text, the estimated GFR (eGFR), using creatinine as a biomarker, is most reliable for CKD under steady-state conditions. In the acute setting, its use is more problematic for reasons that have already been discussed. In healthy persons, the GFR is in the range of 90 to 130 mL/min/1.73 m$^2$. By definition, patients with stage 4 or 5 CKD have GFRs that are below 30 mL/min/1.73 m$^2$.[2,46] Complications of CKD are more pronounced at lower GFRs, and mild to moderate CKD may progress to end-stage renal disease (ESRD).

In AKI, the GFR is only indirectly linked to kidney injury, and changes in the GFR reflect a late consequence in a sequence of events associated with a primary insult to the kidney. Furthermore, because of renal reserve, a large amount of functioning renal tissue can be lost without significant changes in the GFR.[47,48] The functional effects of renal reserve on the GFR can be demonstrated in kidney donors, who often have only modest changes in serum creatinine levels and GFR after donating one kidney, even though 50% of the renal mass is lost.[49]

Ideally, a serum GFR marker should be freely filtered, with no reabsorption or secretion in the tubule, and should maintain a constant plasma level when kidney function is stable. GFR can be determined using exogenous and endogenous markers of filtration. Evaluation of the GFR using the exogenous markers inulin, iothalamate, or iohexol provides reliable results and represents the gold standard; however, the process is time-consuming and expensive and can be performed only in specialized settings.[46] Once the GFR level falls below 60 mL/min/1.73 m$^2$, renal functional impairment can be estimated adequately by the serum creatinine level using various equations to calculate the eGFR.[50–52] Although traditionally these equations have been less accurate for those with higher GFRs, newer formulas have been constructed using more patients with normal and near-normal GFRs.[52]

#### Creatinine

Determination of the eGFR using endogenous creatinine is cost-effective but can be problematic. Creatinine is a breakdown product of creatine and phosphocreatine, which are involved in the energy metabolism of skeletal muscle. Creatinine is freely filtered by the glomerulus, but is also to a lesser degree (10%–30%) secreted by the proximal tubule. Under normal conditions, the daily synthesis of creatinine of approximately 20 mg/kg of body weight reflects muscle mass and varies little.[53]

Accumulated data from various studies have indicated that the creatinine concentration is not an ideal marker for diagnosing AKI for a variety of reasons, including the following[54–56]:

1. Creatinine production and its release into the circulation vary greatly with age, gender, muscle mass, certain disease states and, to a lesser extent, diet. For example, in rhabdomyolysis, serum creatinine concentrations may rise more rapidly due to the release of preformed creatinine from the damaged muscle. Also, body creatinine production, as measured by 24-hour urinary excretion, decreases with older age, falling from a mean of 23.8 mg/kg of body weight in men aged 20 to 29 years to 9.8 mg/kg of body weight in men aged 90 to 99 years, largely because of the reduction in muscle mass.[57]
2. Serum creatinine concentrations are not specific for renal tubular injury. For example, intravascular volume depletion "prerenal" factors (e.g., severe dehydration, blood volume loss, altered vasomotor tone, age-related decrease in renal blood flow) and postrenal factors (e.g., obstruction or extravasation of urine into the peritoneal cavity) may falsely elevate serum concentrations in the absence of parenchymal damage. Thus, a decrease in the eGFR inferred from an increase in the serum creatinine level may not distinguish among prerenal, intrinsic renal, and postrenal causes of impaired kidney function, which may not be the case for some biomarkers of renal tubular injury.[58] Even in cases in which the serum creatinine level is elevated as a consequence of direct renal injury, it cannot be used to determine the location of the injury (glomerular vs. tubular, or proximal tubular vs. distal tubular).
3. Static measurement of the serum creatinine level does not reflect the real-time changes in the GFR resulting from acute changes in kidney function as creatinine accumulates over time. Given the large amounts of functional kidney reserve in healthy persons and the variable amounts of kidney reserve in patients with mild to moderate disease, the creatinine level is not a sensitive marker.[59]
4. Drug-induced reduction in tubular secretion of creatinine might result in underestimation of kidney function. Medications such as cimetidine and trimethoprim inhibit creatinine secretion and increase the serum creatinine concentration without affecting the true GFR.[60,61]
5. One commonly used creatinine assay—the Jaffe method—is subject to interference by intake of certain drugs or by certain pathophysiologic states, including hyperbilirubinemia and diabetic ketoacidosis.[60]
6. Small changes in serum creatinine levels are subject to high false-positive rates, and this effect is magnified in those with a higher baseline creatinine due to the inherent variability in the creatinine assay. Thus patients with CKD may be misclassified as having AKI based solely on small changes in the serum creatinine level.[62]

Similarly, the use of serum creatinine levels in CKD is limited by several patient-dependent and independent variables, including age, race, sex, and comorbid conditions. Serum creatinine concentration can significantly decrease in advanced kidney disease, unrelated to its renal clearance.[63] The sensitivity of serum creatinine levels in determining kidney function can be improved by serial measurements of timed creatinine clearance (usually, but not always, 24-hour collections). However, many individuals find this collection cumbersome, and errors (e.g., skipped voids) typically lead to underestimation of function.

The serum level creatinine is stable during long-term storage, after repeated thawing and refreezing,[64] and for up to 24 hours in clotted whole blood at room temperature.[65] The Jaffe reaction–based assay (alkaline picrate assay) is routinely used in clinical laboratories to assess creatinine levels. However, Jaffe methods overestimate serum creatinine concentration by approximately 25% due to the interference of noncreatinine chromogens, particularly proteins. Interference from glucose[66,67] and acetoacetate[68] are particularly important because diabetic patients are particularly prone to develop CKD. As a result, eGFRs are higher when Jaffe methods are used than when other approaches are used. Expert professional bodies have recommended that all methods of creatinine measurement should become traceable to a reference method based on isotope dilution mass spectrometry.[69] Several modifications of the Jaffe method have been made to increase the specificity by decreasing the influence of interfering substances.[70,71] Enzymatic methods of measuring creatinine have been widely adopted by clinical laboratories as an alternative to alkaline picrate assays. Although various substances do interfere with enzymatic assays, the assays are reported to be subject to less interference than Jaffe methods.[72–74] The high-performance liquid chromatography (HPLC)–based assay has evolved as a potential alternative approach for measurement of the serum creatinine level.[75,76] Several studies have demonstrated that HPLC methods have greater analytic specificity than conventional methods.[77–79] This approach clearly has severe limitations with respect to throughput, however.

Finally, over the past decade, there has been a dedicated national effort (within the United States) to standardize serum creatinine assays by establishing calibration traceability to an isotope dilution mass spectrometry (IDMS) reference standard. Prior to standardization, there was a large variability in serum creatinine results among clinical laboratories, with roughly a 10% to 20% bias being reported in the literature.[80] This process, which started in 2005 and has recently been completed, has led to the standardization of assays, which has led to less variation and more accurate eGFR measurements when used in conjunction with the IDMS-traceable estimating equations.[81,82]

## Blood Urea Nitrogen

Blood urea is a low-molecular-weight waste product derived from dietary protein catabolism and tissue protein turnover, and its levels are inversely correlated with decline in the GFR.[83] Urea is filtered freely, and a variable amount (≈30%–70%) is reabsorbed predominantly in the proximal tubule, with recycling between the tubule and interstitium in the kidney medulla. The normal range of urea nitrogen in blood or serum is 5 to 20 mg/dL (1.8–7.2 mmol urea/L).[83]

The wide reference range reflects the influence on BUN of nonrenal factors, including dietary protein intake, endogenous protein catabolism, fluid intake, and hepatic urea synthesis.[83,84] BUN concentrations also increase with excessive tissue catabolism, especially in cases of fever, severe burns, trauma, high corticosteroid dosage, chronic liver disease, and sepsis.[83] In addition, any factor that increases the tubular reabsorption of urea, including decreased effective arterial volume (i.e., impaired renal perfusion) and/or obstruction of urinary drainage, will increase the BUN concentration.[83,85,86] Because of these limitations, BUN is not a sensitive and specific marker for acute or chronic kidney disease. However, for those with advanced CKD (e.g., CKD 4–5), some have suggested averaging urea clearance and creatinine clearance to serve as a more accurate estimate of the true GFR. This is in part because at these lower levels of renal function, creatinine clearance will overestimate the (secretion) GFR, whereas urea clearance will underestimate the GFR.[87] BUN is measured by spectrophotometry. Because of these undesirable limitations of creatinine and BUN as markers, there has been a great deal of interest in the identification of improved biomarkers for kidney injury.

### Cystatin C

For the past 10 to 15 years, there has been a tremendous amount of research investigating serum cystatin C as a marker of GFR, and urinary cystatin C excretion has been proposed as a tubular injury marker. In 1961, Butler and Flynn studied the urine proteins of 223 individuals by starch gel electrophoresis and found a new urine protein fraction in the post–gamma globulin fraction.[88] They named this protein fraction "cystatin C." Cystatin C is a low-molecular-weight protein produced at a constant rate by all nucleated cells and eliminated exclusively by glomerular filtration. It has a small size (13 kDa) and a positive charge at physiologic pH. It is neither secreted nor reabsorbed by renal tubules but undergoes almost complete catabolism by proximal tubular cells; thus little, if any, appears in the urine under normal circumstances. Any impairment of reabsorption in proximal tubules can lead to marked increases in urinary levels of cystatin C in humans and animals. There have been a number of studies on the diagnostic potential of both serum and urinary cystatin C levels in acute and chronic kidney disease in humans.

**Chronic Kidney Disease.** Because of its short half-life (≈2 hours) and other properties described earlier, some believe that serum cystatin C levels reflect the GFR better than creatinine concentration. Initially, it was thought that the serum levels of cystatin C would be unaffected by gender, age, race, and muscle mass but, over the past several years, multiple studies have demonstrated that these factors are associated with altered levels of the biomarker.[89,90] Notably, cystatin C levels have been shown to be associated with factors similar to those associated with creatinine—namely, that these levels may be elevated in males, taller and heavier patients, and those with higher lean body mass.[89–91] However, unlike the serum creatinine level, which is usually lower in older adults, given their decreased muscle mass, a study investigating a subset of over 7500 subjects from the National Health and Nutritional Examination Survey (NHANES) III has demonstrated that cystatin C levels are elevated in more than 50% of those older than 80 years.[91]

Despite these minor limitations, cystatin C remains an excellent biomarker of CKD and performs on par, if not better than, the serum creatinine level in some cases. Equations for estimating GFR and CKD classification are discussed elsewhere in this text (Chapter 23). In a prospective cohort study of 26,643 Americans enrolled in the Reasons for Geographic and Racial Differences in Stroke (REGARDS) study, Peralta and colleagues have demonstrated that the cystatin C–based eGFR improves CKD classification and definition, as well risk stratification (for the development of ESRD and death) relative to a creatinine-based eGFR.[92] This correlation with mortality was not novel because cystatin C demonstrated a stronger risk relationship with mortality than creatinine concentration or eGFR in older adults with cardiovascular disease.[93] In the Cardiovascular Health Study cohort of 4637 community-dwelling older adults, higher serum cystatin C concentrations were associated with a significantly elevated risk of death from cardiovascular causes (hazard ratio [HR], 2.27 [1.73–2.97]), myocardial infarction (HR, 1.48 [1.08–2.02]), and stroke (HR, 1.47 [1.09–1.96]) after multivariate adjustment. In the same study, higher serum creatinine values were not independently associated with any of these three outcomes.[94] Furthermore, a study in the general population has suggested that the cystatin C level has a stronger association with cardiovascular disease outcomes than creatinine concentration or eGFR, especially among older adults.[94–96] On the other hand, a study based in primary care has reported that the use of cystatin C to estimate GFR in a predominantly older population with relatively mild CKD resulted in reclassification of a small proportion (7.7%) of participants with CKD category G3aA1, defined by creatinine to GFR (>60 mL/min/1.73 $m^2$), but a much greater proportion (59%) were reclassified to a more advanced CKD category without any improvement in risk prediction.[97] Thus, serum cystatin C levels may be a better marker of kidney function than serum creatinine concentration in some, but not all, persons.

In addition to older adults, cystatin C has proven superior to serum creatinine in those infected with HIV. Choi and colleagues have demonstrated that the cystatin C–based eGFR outperformed serum creatinine in the ability to predict 5-year all-cause mortality in a cohort of 922 HIV-infected individuals.[98] This study mirrors recent findings from a study of 908 HIV-infected women, which demonstrated that CKD risk factors are associated with an overestimation of GFR by the serum creatinine level relative to cystatin C and that cystatin C significantly improves mortality risk prediction when added to a clinical model that already includes the serum creatinine level.[99]

The concept of using cystatin C in concert, rather than in place of, serum creatinine has been gaining momentum.[100] Using a cross-sectional analyses and data from 5352 participants from 13 previously published studies, Inker and colleagues developed estimation equations using cystatin C alone and cystatin C and creatinine combined.[100] They then went on to validate these equations in a cohort of 1119 participants from 5 different studies. They demonstrated that combined equations outperformed the creatinine-alone equations and, in some cases, led to a NRI of 0.194 ($P < .001$). Although this study was performed predominantly in white subjects, thus limiting its broad applicability, it demonstrates the potential of cystatin C (and other biomarkers) to be used to augment the diagnostic scope of the serum creatinine

**Box 27.1 Cystatin C**

1. Serum cystatin C performs on par, if not, better than serum creatinine for the identification of patients with chronic kidney disease.
2. Serum cystatin C has been specifically shown to outperform serum creatinine in some older adults as well as those with HIV.
3. Additionally, serum cystatin C outperforms serum creatinine for its ability to detect those at risk for cardiovascular morbidity and mortality.
4. Serum cystatin C should be incorporated into the management and care of patients with chronic kidney disease.

level rather than replace it. Subsequently, the combined creatinine and cystatin C Chronic Kidney Disease Epidemiology Collaboration (CKD-EPI) equation has been shown to outperform each individual equation (creatinine and cystatin C) in a cohort of 805 older community-based individuals.[101] Given the mounting clinical evidence and the emergence of automated assays and cheaper reagent costs (e.g., $4), it is increasingly apparent that cystatin C should become a routine part of the nephrologist laboratory assessment of CKD and points to an increased role for cystatin C in the management of patients with CKD. However, as with any biomarker, its limitations should be considered when interpreting results (Box 27.1).[102]

**Acute Kidney Injury.** Given its success as a marker of glomerular filtration, several groups have investigated serum cystatin C as a potential biomarker of AKI. In a single-center mixed ICU population of 85 subjects (44 of whom developed RIFLE Classified AKI), Herget-Rosenthal and colleagues demonstrated that serum cystatin C had excellent diagnostic value, predicting AKI 24 and 48 hours prior to serum creatinine (AUC of 0.97 and 082, respectively).[103] These data were followed up by a study of 442 patients from 2 separate ICUs that demonstrated that plasma cystatin C increased earlier than serum creatinine and was able to significantly predict several adverse patient outcomes, including sustained AKI, death, and dialysis.[104] Similarly, in a study of 202 diverse intensive care unit (ICU) patients, of whom 49 developed AKI based on urine output and/or serum creatinine RIFLE F criteria, serum cystatin C levels showed excellent predictive value for AKI. However, the serum cystatin C concentration did not rise earlier than the serum creatinine concentration.[105]

Outside the ICU, cystatin C levels were shown to be capable of detecting a decrease in the GFR after contrast agent administration earlier than the serum creatinine value in adult patients who underwent coronary angiography.[106] In a prospective study of 87 patients who underwent elective catheterization, contrast medium–induced nephropathy occurred in 18 patients, and ROC analysis showed a higher AUC for cystatin C level than for serum creatinine concentration (0.933 vs. 0.832; $P = .012$). When a cutoff value of more than 1.2 mg/L was used, cystatin C level before catheterization exhibited 94.7% sensitivity and 84.8% specificity for predicting contrast medium–induced nephropathy.[107]

Serum cystatin C has been studied as a biomarker for both early AKI (rising earlier than serum creatinine) and AKI severity, with several smaller studies providing mixed results.[108–111] More recently, the larger multicenter Translational Research Investigating Biomarker Endpoints in AKI (TRIBE-AKI) study investigated several aspects of serum cystatin C following both adult and pediatric cardiac surgery. In 1147 adults, Shlipak and colleagues demonstrated that preoperative serum cystatin C values outperformed serum creatinine– and creatinine-based eGFRs in its ability to forecast postoperative AKI.[112] After adjustment for clinical variables known to contribute to AKI, serum cystatin C had a C-statistic of 0.70 and an NRI of 0.21 compared with serum creatinine ($P < .001$). However, when this same group investigated sensitivity and rapidity of AKI detection (defined as a 25%, 50%, and 100% increase from preoperative values) by postoperative changes in serum cystatin C, they did not demonstrate a clear advantage over changes in the serum creatinine level.[113] In a follow-up analysis, they demonstrated that postoperative elevations of cystatin C (>25%) were associated with an increased risk of death during a 3-year follow-up period. This long-term mortality risk was higher in those with changes in cystatin C alone (adjusted HR, 2.2 [1.09–4.47] compared with those with changes in just the serum creatinine level (HR, 1.50 [0.96–2.34]).[114] This mixed message of postoperative serum cystatin C in adults is in stark contrast to the results in 288 children undergoing cardiac surgery. Zappitelli and colleagues have demonstrated that serum cystatin C measured within the first 6 postoperative hours is associated with both stages 1 and 2 pediatric AKI.[115] Additionally, postoperative serum cystatin C values were also associated with adverse patient outcomes, including length of mechanical ventilation and length of ICU stay. However unlike the adult population, preoperative values were not associated postoperative AKI.

### β-Trace Protein

β-Trace protein (BTP), also referred as "prostaglandin D synthase," has emerged as another promising biomarker for the GFR. BTP is a small protein with a molecular weight of 23 to 29 kDa, depending on the size of the glycosyl moiety. BTP belongs to the lipocalin protein family, whose members are primarily involved in the binding and transport of small hydrophobic ligands. It is primarily produced in the cerebral fluid, where its concentrations are more than 40-fold higher than in the serum. BTP is primarily eliminated by glomerular filtration, and its concentrations in urine range from 600 to 1200 μg/L.[116]

The first observation of elevated BTP levels in association with impaired kidney function was reported by Hoffmann and associates in 1997.[117] Since then, several research studies have been conducted to evaluate the sensitivity and specificity of BTP as a marker of GFR and to compare it with the serum creatinine level in patients with CKD[118] and kidney transplant recipients. In two separate cohort studies, one adult and one pediatric, serum cystatin C was shown to outperform BTP for the detection of decreased renal function (as measured by inulin clearance); both markers were shown to outperform the serum creatinine level alone.[119,120]

Foster and colleagues have investigated the association of BTP, serum cystatin C, and creatinine-based eGFR with all-cause mortality in a subset of patients from the NHANES cohort.[121] They analyzed data from 6445 adults (enrolled from 1988–1994), with follow-up through December 2006. All three markers were associated with increased mortality after adjusting for demographics. However, when comparing the mortality risk of the fifth (highest) quintile with the third (middle) quintile, only BTP (HR, 95% confidence interval [CI], 2.14 (1.56–2.94) and serum cystatin C (HR, 1.94 [1.43–2.62]) remained statistically significant (creatinine eGFR, HR 1.31[0.84–2.04]). These effects remained significant when looking at either cardiovascular disease– or coronary heart disease–associated mortality. Similarly, in data from the Atherosclerosis Risk in Communities (ARIC) study. BTP was shown to outperform creatinine-based eGFR (CKD-EPI) in the prediction of mortality and development of kidney failure.[122] More recently, BTP was investigated in a pooled cross-sectional analysis of patients from three separate studies, the Modification of Diet in Renal Disease (MDRD), African American Study of Kidney Disease (AASK), and Chronic Renal Insufficiency Cohort (CRIC).[123] In 3156 patients with CKD, BTP levels were strongly associated with the serum creatinine level and urine protein excretion and demonstrated a correlation with race, where levels were lower in African Americans. Additionally, BTP was clearly associated with advanced age and male gender and inversely related to body mass index.[123]

BTP has also been investigated for its ability to predict and estimate residual kidney function in those undergoing maintenance hemodialysis.[124,125] Using interdialytic urine collections and serum BTP and $\beta_2$-microglobulin levels, Wong and colleagues derived equations to estimate GFR and residual urea clearance in 191 patients on hemodialysis.[125] Using the reciprocal of BTP and other factors, they demonstrated an $R^2$ of 0.70 with GFR and an $R^2$ of 0.625 with residual urea clearance. Similarly, Shafi and colleagues developed separate equations in 44 dialysis patients completing 24-hour urine tests and went on to validate their equations in a cohort of 826 patients from the Netherlands Cooperative Study on the Adequacy of Dialysis.[124] They demonstrated that BTP provided better accuracy than the traditional markers—creatinine and urea clearance—and that BTP had an AUC of 0.82 for detecting the gold standard–measured urinary urea clearance. Thus, BTP and other markers show promise as a method to estimate residual renal function in dialysis patients.

Concentrations of BTP are not affected by commonly used immunosuppressive medications, such as prednisone, mycophenolate mofetil, and cyclosporine.[126] This is especially useful when evaluating kidney function in kidney transplant recipients, in whom cystatin C concentrations may be falsely elevated due to steroid treatment.[127] Unlike for serum creatinine values, age and race were not associated with BTP concentrations. Several GFR estimation equations based on BTP have been developed for use in kidney transplant recipients.[126,127] However, these equations, similar to those discussed previously for dialysis patients, will require external validation in larger and more diverse patient groups. In contrast to creatinine, one limitation of using BTP is lack of widespread availability and standardization of the assay.

## URINARY GLOMERULAR CELL INJURY MARKERS

Defects in podocyte structure have been reported in many glomerular diseases, which have been classified as "podocytopathies."[128,129] Injured podocytes have been reported in immunologic and nonimmunologic forms of human glomerular disease, including hemodynamic injury, protein overload states, injury from environmental toxins, minimal change disease, focal segmental glomerulosclerosis, membranous glomerulopathy, diabetic nephropathy, and lupus nephritis.[130–135] Podocytes may be injured in many forms of human and experimental primary glomerular disease and in secondary forms of focal segmental glomerulosclerosis, including those caused by hypertension, diabetes, and tubulointerstitial disease.[136–138] Before detachment from the glomerular basement membrane, podocytes undergo structural changes, including effacement of foot processes and microvillous transformation.[128,129,139,140]

### PODOCYTE COUNT

After undergoing the aforementioned structural changes, podocytes detach from the glomerular basement membrane and are excreted into the urine. Urinary levels of viable podocytes have been extensively studied in several renal diseases.[141–144] Numerous studies have reported that the number of podocytes shed in patients with active glomerular disease is significantly higher than in healthy controls and in patients with inactive disease. Importantly, the podocyte number in urine correlates with disease activity (assessed by renal biopsy) and has been shown to decline with treatment.[145] Studies have linked podocytopenia and disease severity in immunoglobulin (IgA) nephropathy[141,142] and diabetic nephropathy.[143,144] An improved and standardized laboratory method is urgently needed to facilitate measurement of urinary podocyte number. Alternative methods that indirectly assess the number of podocytes in urine include detection of messenger RNA (mRNA) and protein levels of podocyte-specific proteins by polymerase chain reaction (PCR) assay and enzyme-linked immunosorbent assay (ELISA), respectively.

### PODOCALYXIN

Podocalyxin is the most commonly used marker protein for detecting podocytes in urine.[146] It is a highly *O*-glycosylated and sialylated type I transmembrane protein of approximately 140 kDa and is expressed in podocytes, hematopoietic progenitor cells, vascular endothelial cells, and a subset of neurons.[146] Podocalyxin participates in a number of cellular functions through its association with the actin cytoskeleton, ezrin, and $Na^+/H^+$ exchanger regulatory factor 1 and 2 (NHERF1 and NHERF2) proteins. Urinary podocalyxin has been reported as a marker of activity in a number of diseases, including IgA nephropathy, Henoch-Schönlein purpura, diabetic nephropathy, lupus nephritis, poststreptococcal glomerulonephritis, membranous nephropathy, focal segmental glomerulosclerosis, and preeclampsia.[147–155] Unfortunately, because podocalyxin is expressed on a number of cell types, the presence of podocalyxin in the urine is not always reflective of urinary podocytes.

## URINARY TUBULAR INJURY MARKERS

Microscopic examination of the urine has been used for many years to gain insight into the degree of glomerular and tubular injury. Other components of the urine have been used to quantitate tubular cell injury in a more specific and sensitive fashion. These markers have been demonstrated to be extremely valuable in detecting kidney injury in the setting of AKI. Moreover, some of these biomarkers, such as interleukin-18 (IL-18), kidney injury molecule-1 (KIM-1), neutrophil gelatinase–associated lipocalin (NGAL), and liver-type fatty acid binding protein (L-FABP), have been shown to be potentially useful in a variety of contexts in acute and chronic kidney injury. In this section, the utility of urine microscopy is described briefly. and some of the emerging biomarkers of tubular injury are discussed.

## URINE MICROSCOPY

Urine microscopy with sediment examination is a time-honored test that is routinely used to assist in the diagnosis of kidney injury.[156–158] The urine from patients with tubular injury typically contains proximal tubular epithelial cells, proximal tubule epithelial cells casts, granular casts, and mixed cellular casts. Patients with predominantly prerenal azotemia occasionally have hyaline or fine granular casts in their urine.[159–161] Several studies have shown that the increase in urinary cast excretion correlates well with AKI.[160,162,163] Marcussen and associates[162] have demonstrated that patients with tubular injury have a high number of granular casts compared with those with prerenal azotemia.

There has been a resurgence of urinalysis sediment scoring systems for the diagnosis of AKI.[161,164] Several of these systems have shown excellent specificity for AKI and correlate well with the severity of AKI.[164–166] However, their widespread acceptance has been hampered by the relatively modest sensitivity of urine microscopy for detecting AKI.[161,164,167,168] Urine microscopy remains a user-dependent tool that displays a tremendous amount of interphysician variability, which likely contributes to its suboptimal sensitivity for AKI.[169] Three of the most widely reported urine microscopy scoring systems are reviewed in Table 27.6.

Several other studies have looked at the potential of using urine microscopy in combination with other biomarkers for detecting tubular injury, with varying degrees of success.[165–167] In the near future, urine microscopy, a current mainstay in the clinical diagnosis of AKI, could be used in concert with markers of glomerular function and validated biomarkers of tubular injury to diagnose AKI.

**Table 27.6 Review of Urine Microscopy Scoring Systems**

| Study | Scoring System |
|---|---|
| Chawla et al. 2008[164] | Grade 1: No casts or RTE |
| | Grade 2: At least one cast or RTE but <10% of LPF |
| | Grade 3: Many casts or RTEs (from 10%–90% of LPF) |
| | Grade 4: Sheet of muddy brown casts and RTEs in >90% of LPF |
| Perazella et al. 2010[165] | 0 points: No casts or RTE seen |
| | 1 point each: One to five casts/LPF or one to five RTEs/HPF |
| | 2 points each: Six or more casts/LPF or ≥six RTEs/HPF |
| Bagshaw et al. 2011[167] | 0 points: No casts or RTE seen |
| | 1 point each: One cast or one RTE/HPF |
| | 2 points each: Two to four casts or RTEs/HPF |
| | 3 points each: Five casts or more or five or more RTEs/HPF |

*HPF*, High-power field; *LPF*, low-power field; *RTE*, renal tubule epithelial cells.

## $\alpha_1$-MICROGLOBULIN

$\alpha_1$-Microglobulin is a low-molecular-weight glycoprotein of approximately 27 to 30 kDa and is a member of the lipocalin superfamily. $\alpha_1$-Microglobulin is primarily synthesized by the liver and is available in free form and as a complex with IgA.[170] $\alpha_1$-Microglobulin has been detected in human serum, urine, and cerebrospinal fluid. Urine and serum levels have been found to be elevated in patients with renal tubular diseases. $\alpha_1$-Microglobulin is freely filtered at the glomerulus and completely reabsorbed and catabolized by the normal proximal tubule. Megalin mediates the uptake of this protein in the proximal tubule. Therefore, an increase in the urinary concentration of $\alpha_1$-microglobulin indicates proximal tubular injury or dysfunction.

The urinary levels of $\alpha_1$-microglobulin are influenced by age. The normal range in populations younger than 50 years of age is less than 13 mg/g of creatinine and, in those 50 years of age and older, is less than 20 mg/g of creatinine.[170] Unlike $\beta_2$-microglobulin, $\alpha_1$-microglobulin is more stable over a range of pH levels in the urine,[171] which makes it a more acceptable urinary biomarker.

### Acute Kidney Injury

$\alpha_1$-Microglobulin quantitation in the urine has been reported as a sensitive biomarker for proximal tubule dysfunction in adults and children.[170,172] In a small cohort of 73 patients, of whom 26 required renal replacement therapy, Herget-Rosenthal and colleagues compared levels of $\alpha_1$-microglobulin, $\beta_2$-microglobulin, cystatin C, retinol binding protein, $\alpha$-glutathione S-transferase, lactate dehydrogenase, and *N*-acetyl-$\beta$-D-glucosaminidase (NAG) early in the course of AKI.[173] They found that urinary cystatin C and $\alpha_1$-microglobulin had the highest ability to predict the need for renal replacement therapy. In this study, urinary $\alpha_1$-microglobulin had an AUC of 0.86 for predicting the need for renal replacement therapy. This is similar to the results of a Zheng and colleagues,[174] who measured $\alpha_1$-microglobulin levels in 58 children undergoing cardiac surgery and found that levels were higher in those who developed AKI (AKIN criteria). Four hours after cardiopulmonary bypass, $\alpha_1$-microglobulin had an AUC of 0.84 (0.72–0.95), with a value of 290 mg/g providing a sensitivity of 90% and specificity of 79%.However, follow-up studies have reported mixed results, with Martensson and colleagues[175] finding no difference in $\alpha_1$-microglobulin levels between those with and without AKI in the setting of sepsis and septic shock in a small prospective single-center study of 45 subjects.

More recently, $\alpha_1$-microglobulin levels at the time of arrival to the emergency room (ER) have demonstrated the ability to correlate with the development of AKI, with an AUC of 0.88 and a cutoff value of 35 mg/g providing reasonable sensitivity (80%) and specificity (81%). However, $\alpha_1$-microglobulin did not remain an independent predictor of AKI in the multivariable model (OR [95% CI], 1.85 [0.80–4.31]).[176] In addition, $\alpha_1$-microglobulin has also been reported as a useful marker for proximal tubular damage, and recovery in early infancy and has been shown to correlate with tubular atrophy and interstitial fibrosis on renal transplant biopsy 1 year after transplantation.[177,178]

### Chronic Kidney Disease

Increasingly, $\alpha_1$-microglobulinin has been investigated in the setting of CKD. Limited studies have demonstrated that this marker may correlate with disease activity and proximal tubule damage in the setting of diabetic nephropathy, as well as idiopathic membranous nephropathy.[179,180] In a cohort of 2948 Framingham Heart Study participants, O'Seaghdha and colleagues[181] demonstrated that although $\alpha_1$-microglobulin does not correlate with the development of CKD or albuminuria during the mean of 10.1 years follow-up, it does correlate with all-cause mortality (HR, 1.26 [1.13–1.40; $P < .001$]. In a different cohort, Jotwani and colleagues have demonstrated that $\alpha_1$-microglobulin levels in women infected with human immunodeficiency virus (HIV) are associated with both kidney function decline and mortality.[182] Compared with those with the lowest $\alpha_1$-microglobulin levels, those with the highest levels had a 2.1 (1.3–3.4)-fold increased risk of developing CKD and a 2.7-fold risk of a 10% decline of their eGFR. This correlation in CKD development and progression was separate from the 1.6-fold adjusted risk of mortality, which accounted for baseline kidney function as well as the presence of albuminuria.[182] Follow-up studies in this same cohort did not link $\alpha_1$-microglobulin levels with an *APOL1* genotype.[183]

Despite these recent data on urine concentration, the use of $\alpha_1$-microglobulin remains limited due to prior studies demonstrating variation in serum levels with age, gender,[184] and clinical conditions, including liver disease,[170] ulcerative colitis,[185] HIV infection, and mood disorders,[170] as well as the lack of international standardization. Urinary $\alpha_1$-microglobulin is measured by an immunonephelometric assay.

## $\beta_2$-MICROGLOBULIN

$\beta_2$-Microglobulin is a low-molecular-weight polypeptide with a molecular weight of 11.8 kDa. $\beta_2$-Microglobulin is present on the cell surface of all nucleated cells and in most biologic fluids, including serum, urine, and synovial fluid. $\beta_2$-Microglobulin is normally excreted by glomerular filtration, reabsorbed almost completely (≈99%), and catabolized by the normal proximal tubule in humans.[186,187] Megalin mediates the uptake of this protein in the proximal tubule.[187] In healthy individuals, approximately 150 to 200 mg of $\beta_2$-microglobulin is synthesized daily, with a normal serum concentration of 1.5 to 3 mg/L. Any pathologic state that affects kidney tubule function will result in an increase in $\beta_2$-microglobulin levels in the urine because of the impeded uptake of $\beta_2$-microglobulin by renal tubular cells. For spot urine collections, the concentration of $\beta_2$-microglobulin in healthy individuals is typically 160 μg/L or less or 300 μg/g of creatinine or less. Unlike urea, its serum levels are not influenced by food intake, which makes it an attractive marker for malnourished patients with low serum urea levels. In patients with CKD, increases in serum $\beta_2$-microglobulin levels reflect a decrease in glomerular function. In the aforementioned cross-sectional study of patients from the MDRD, AASK, and CRIC studies, serum $\beta_2$-microglobulin levels were weakly associated when male gender and non–African American race were compared; however, unlike other markers, it was strongly associated with smoking. Thus, serum $\beta_2$-microglobulin is clearly affected by nonrenal variables, demonstrating some of the limitations when implementing $\beta_2$-microglobulin as a marker of GFR.[123]

In ESRD patients, serum levels of $\beta_2$-microglobulin are usually in the range of 20 to 50 mg/L. $\beta_2$-Microglobulin accumulation is linked to toxicity because the molecule precipitates and forms fibrillary structures and amyloid deposits, particularly in bone and periarticular tissue, which leads to the development of carpal tunnel syndrome and erosive arthritis.[187,188] Elevated serum levels of $\beta_2$-microglobulin have been reported in several AKI and CKD clinical settings, including cadmium toxicity,[189] following cardiac surgery,[190,191] liver transplantation,[192] and renal transplantation.[193] In idiopathic membranous nephropathy, the $\beta_2$-microglobulin level was identified as a superior independent predictor of the development of GFR decline.[194] Other studies have reported that $\beta_2$-microglobulin performs as well as, if not better than, the serum creatinine level for the detection of AKI in critically ill children[195] or following adult cardiac surgery.[191]

Serum concentrations of $\beta_2$-microglobulin should be interpreted cautiously because they are altered significantly in various diseases, including rheumatoid disorders and several types of cancers.[196,197] Initially, it was believed that the increase in $\beta_2$-microglobulin levels in CKD is solely due to declines in kidney function, but some studies have shown that other factors, including increased synthesis of $\beta_2$-microglobulin, may contribute in patients with ESRD.[198] Another significant drawback associated with the use of urinary $\beta_2$-microglobulin as a marker of kidney injury is its instability in the urine at room temperature, particularly when the pH is less than 5.5. Because of this, the urine should be alkalinized and frozen at −80°C immediately after collection.[188,199]

## HEPCIDIN-25

Hepcidin-25 is a 2.8-kDa hormonal regulator of iron metabolism produced in the liver, heart, and kidney. Hepcidin-25 binds to and induces the internalization and degradation of the transmembrane iron exporter ferroportin.[200] Hepcidin-25 acts to downregulate iron uptake and reduce extracellular iron availability from stored iron.[201] Given its link to iron metabolism, and the fact that free iron is known to be released in the setting of the ischemia reperfusion injury and oxidative stress that occur with cardiopulmonary bypass, urinary hepcidin-25 has been investigated as a marker of kidney injury following cardiac surgery. Ho and colleagues[202] have identified urinary hepcidin-25 in a nested case-control study of 44 adults who underwent cardiac surgery. Using surface-enhanced laser desorption/ionization time-of-flight mass spectrometry (SELDI-TOF-MS), urine from 22 individuals who developed at least RIFLE risk AKI and 22 individuals whose creatinine level did not increase more than 10% from baseline during the postoperative period (no AKI), they demonstrated that hepcidin-25 is dramatically upregulated in the urine of those with no AKI. Taking this a step further, this same group quantified the concentration of hepcidin-25 in the urine (normalized to urine creatinine) and demonstrated that concentrations were higher in those who did not go on to develop postoperative AKI ($P < .0005$).

In a multivariable analysis, hepcidin-25 was significantly associated with the avoidance of AKI, with urinary concentrations on postoperative day 1 showing an AUC of 0.80.[203] The data from this small study have been corroborated by another modestly sized cohort of 100 adults undergoing cardiopulmonary bypass (CPB). Haase-Fielitz and colleagues have demonstrated that 6 hours after CPB, urinary hepcidin-25 levels are lower in the 9 subjects who developed RIFLE-based

AKI compared with those with no AKI (AUC = 0.80; $P$ = .004).[204] More recently, Prowle and colleagues measured hepcidin-25 in a 93-subject multicenter cohort of patients undergoing cardiac surgery with CPB.[205] Although this study did not have a 6-hour CPB time point, it did demonstrate that hepcidin -25 values 24 hours after surgery were different in those with and without AKI ($P$ < .001), with values being higher in those without AKI. Additionally, they demonstrated that combining hepicidin-25 with postoperative NGAL values leads to an AUC of 0.84 for the development of RIFLE- based AKI. In addition to establishing a universal commercially available assay, these results warrant further preliminary investigations in other AKI settings, as well as prompt validation in a larger cohort of cardiac surgery patients.

## INTERLEUKIN-18

IL-18 is an 18-kDa proinflammatory cytokine that is activated by caspase-1 and produced by renal tubule cells and macrophages. Animal studies have indicated that IL-18 is a mediator of acute tubular injury, including both neutrophil and monocyte infiltration of the renal parenchyma.[206,207] In studies using caspase-1 knockout mice, these mice experienced the same degree of ischemic AKI as wild-type mice injected with an IL-18 neutralizing antiserum, demonstrating that IL-18 is an important mediator of ischemic AKI.[207]

Other studies have shown that IL-18 plays a major role in macrophage activation, with mice engrafted with IL-18–deficient bone marrow experiencing a lower incidence of AKI than those with IL-18–replete marrow.[208] Similarly, in IL-18 knockout mice with AKI, tumor necrosis factor-α (TNF-α), inducible nitric oxide synthase, macrophage inflammatory protein-2, and monocyte chemoattractant protein-1 messenger RNA expression are all decreased, indicating the deleterious impact of IL-18 on AKI. In the human kidney, IL-18 is induced and cleaved mainly in the proximal tubules and released into the urine. IL-18 has been shown to participate in a variety of renal disease processes, including ischemia reperfusion injury, allograft rejection, infection, autoimmune conditions, and malignancy. IL-18 is easily and reliably measured in the urine by commercially available ELISA and microbead-based assays.

### Acute Kidney Injury

Several studies have demonstrated the usefulness of IL-18 as a biomarker for the detection of AKI. Originally, Parikh and associates studied a group of 72 patients and reported urinary IL-18 levels to be significantly higher in patients diagnosed with acute tubular necrosis than in patients with prerenal azotemia or urinary infection or in healthy control subjects with normal renal function.[209] Since then, several large multicenter studies have gone on to investigate the ability of IL-18 to detect AKI in a variety of clinical settings.

The Translational Research Investigating Biomarker Endpoints in AKI (TRIBE-AKI) consortium measured IL-18 in 1219 adults who underwent cardiac surgery. The study selected those at high risk for postoperative AKI because of the presence of one of the following: emergency surgery, preoperative serum creatinine level >2 mg/dL, left ventricular ejection fraction <35%, stage III or IV New York Heart Association cardiac failure, age >70 years, preexisting diabetes mellitus, concomitant coronary artery bypass grafting (CABG), and valve surgery or repeat cardiac surgery. Those with preoperative AKI, kidney transplants, ESRD, or a preoperative serum creatinine level >4.5 mg/dL were excluded. After dividing the cohort into quintiles, the highest quintile of IL-18 was associated with a 6.8-fold higher risk of AKI, defined as a postoperative doubling of the serum creatinine level or undergoing acute dialysis.[210] The first postoperative concentration of IL-18 (0–6 hours) had an AUC of 0.74 that increased to 0.76 after combining IL-18 with a clinical model of factors known to affect AKI risk. The TRIBE-AKI pediatric cohort (311 children) reported results in line with the TRIBE adult study, in which the highest quintile was associated with 9.4-fold increased risk of developing AKI (doubling or dialysis) compared with the first quintile. The affect was slightly attenuated after adjusting for clinical factors known to affect AKI (adjusted odds ratio [OR], 95% CI, 6.9 [1.7–28.8]).[211]

Urine IL-18 displayed a similar trend when investigating the association between biomarker concentrations and duration of AKI.[212] Stratifying the cohort of those with AKI according to the duration, 61.7% ($n$ = 251) had a duration of 1 to 2 days, 28.9% ($n$ = 118) had a duration of 3 to 6 days, and 9.3% ($n$ = 38) had a duration >7 days. The fifth quintile of IL-18 was strongly associated with the duration of AKI, providing an unadjusted OR of 3.90 (2.62–5.78). Although this effect was attenuated after adjusting for clinical factors known to affect AKI, it remained significant, at 2.90 (1.80–4.68).[212]

In another secondary analysis of the TRIBE-AKI adult cohort, Koyner and colleagues[213] have demonstrated that IL-18 at the time of AKI can forecast those with early AKI (AKIN stage 1) who go on to progress to more severe stages of AKI (AKIN stage 2 or 3). In the 380 adults who developed at least stage 1 AKI, 45 went on to progress to stage 2 or 3. In the entire cohort, the fifth quintile of IL-18 was at increased risk for developing progressive AKI (3.63 [1.64–.03]), and this effect was only slightly attenuated after adjusting for the clinical model (3.00 [1.25–7.25]).

When investigated in a separate secondary analysis of this cohort, IL-18 concentrations collected in the immediate postoperative period were associated with long-term mortality following cardiac surgery. This investigation provided a median follow-up of 3.0 years (interquartile range [IQR], 2.2–3.6) during which 139 of the 1199 subjects died (50 deaths/1000 person-years). After adjusting for clinical factors known to affect mortality, patients without AKI ($n$ = 792) in the third tertile of IL-18 were at increased risk of long-term mortality compared with the first tertile (adjusted HR, 1.23 [1.02–1.48]). This effect was magnified in subjects with perioperative AKI ($n$ = 407), with the third tertile having an adjusted HR of 3.16 (1.53–6.53) compared with the reference cohort. Thus, IL-18 provides additional prognostic information about long-term postoperative mortality in patients with and without AKI.[214]

In the setting of critical illness and ICU admission, IL-18 has not demonstrated the same robust results. In a study of 451 critically ill subjects, 86 of whom developed AKI within the first 48 hours, Siew and colleagues have demonstrated that urine IL-18 does not reliably predict AKI.[215] Although IL-18 levels at the time of ICU admission were higher in those who went on to develop AKI, the AUC was 0.62 (0.54–0.69) and only marginally improved to 0.67 after the exclusion of those with prior known CKD (eGFR < 75 mL/min). Despite the inability to detect AKI reliably, urine IL-18 levels did correlate with other adverse patient outcomes, including the need for renal replacement therapy (RRT) and 28-day mortality. This poor performance in the setting of critical illness has been corroborated by others, including data from a post hoc analysis of the EARLY ARF trial. In this prospective observational study in two large general ICUs ($n = 529$), IL-18 had an AUC of only 0.62 for the diagnosis of AKIN stage 1 AKI, but once again performed much better at forecasting the need for RRT or death (within 7 days). Unlike other biomarker studies, this IL-18 study did not demonstrate improved predictive powers, with the cohort stratified according to preadmission CKD stage.[216] In a separate post hoc analysis of this same EARLY ARF cohort, urinary IL-18 concentrations were shown to be significantly higher in those with prerenal azotemia ($n = 61$, defined as AKI that recovered within 48 hours of ICU admission, and was associated with a fractional excretion of sodium <1%), compared with those with no AKI ($n = 285$). There was a trend toward higher values in those with AKI ($n$ = 114, nonprerenal) compared with those with prerenal AKI ($P = .053$).[217]

In a single-center study of 339 mixed surgical and medical ICU patients, Doi and colleagues have demonstrated that IL-18 levels are significantly elevated in those with both established and newly diagnosed AKI at the time of ICU arrival.[218] Although biomarker concentrations and AUCs were higher in those with established AKI (AUC, 0.78) compared with newly diagnosed AKI (AUC, 0.59), both these subgroups were significantly different compared with the no-AKI cohort. In this same study, IL-18 levels were significantly higher in nonsurvivors. These results were fairly similar to those of Nickolas and colleagues,[219] who measured urinary biomarkers in 1635 ER patients at the time of admission and compared the values to adjudicated AKI outcomes, in which prerenal AKI was defined as RIFLE Risk that returned to baseline within 72 hours and in the clinical setting, suggested decreased transient effective circulating volume. They demonstrated that IL-18 values for those with more severe intrinsic AKI were significantly higher compared with those with prerenal AKI. However, there was no difference between those with prerenal AKI and no AKI.

At kidney transplantation, the IL-18 level accurately identified delayed graft function (DGF) (AUC = 0.90) and predicted the rate of increase in serum creatinine concentration.[220] To understand the utility of IL-18 and urinary NGAL in predicting graft recovery after kidney transplantation, Hall and colleagues[222] conducted a prospective, multicenter, observational cohort study of recipients of deceased donor kidney transplants. They collected serial urine samples from 91 patients for 3 days after transplantation. After adjustment for recipient and donor age, cold ischemia time, urine output, and serum creatinine concentration, NGAL and IL-18 concentrations accurately predicted the need for dialysis in transplant recipients. Furthermore, NGAL and IL-18 concentrations also predicted graft recovery up to 3 months later.[222] In further follow-up of this cohort, urine IL-18 concentrations collected at the time of surgery were correlated with 1-year posttransplantation graft outcomes. Above-median values of IL-18 on the first postoperative day had an adjusted OR of 5.5 (1.4–21.5, 95% CI) with poor graft function, defined as a GFR < 30 mL/min or return to RRT.[223]

In a study by Ling and associates involving patients who underwent coronary angiography, urinary IL-18 and NGAL concentrations were significantly increased at 24 hours postprocedure in those who developed contrast-induced nephropathy, but not in the control group. [224] ROC curve analysis demonstrated that both IL-18 and NGAL showed better performance in the early diagnosis of contrast nephropathy than the serum creatinine level ($P < .05$). Importantly, elevated urinary IL-18 concentrations 24 hours after contrast administration were also found to be an independent predictive marker for later major cardiac events (relative risk, 95% CI, 2.09 [1.15–3.77]).

### Chronic Kidney Disease

There are promising data about IL-18 in the setting of CKD. In patients with diabetic kidney disease and proteinuria, IL-18 levels in renal tubular cells are higher than in patients with nondiabetic proteinuric disease.[221] In the Women's Interagency HIV study, urine IL-18 levels were independently associated with a more rapid loss of renal function after multivariable adjustment.[225] In this cohort study of 908 HIV-infected women, urine IL-18 was the only biomarker (KIM-1 and albumin-to-creatinine ratio [ACR]) were also measured) that was associated with worsening renal function over time, as measured by eGFR–cystatin C. Urine IL-18 predicted an increased relative risk of renal function decline between 1.4 and 2.16, depending on the models used. In a follow-up study, the same group measured urine IL-18 in 908 HIV- infected and 289 noninfected women in the Women's Interagency HIV Study.[226] In this cross-sectional cohort study, they demonstrated that after multivariable adjusted linear regression analysis that IL-18 concentrations are significantly higher in those with HIV (38%; $P < .0001$). They subsequently demonstrated this same phenomenon in a cross-sectional study of 813 HIV-infected men and 331 uninfected men, with urine IL-18 being 52% higher in those with HIV.[227] Returning the female cohort, they demonstrated that urine IL-18 concentrations are significantly associated with higher HIV RNA levels and lower CD4 counts, hepatitis C infection, and high-density lipoprotein cholesterol levels, thus indicating a more extensive role for IL-18 in the setting of HIV-related kidney care.[226] This promising HIV data are in contrast to those of the Consortium for Radiologic Imaging for the Study of Polycystic Kidney Disease (CRISP), which measured IL-18 in 107 patients with autosomal dominant polycystic kidney disease and found that although there was an increased mean IL-18 over the 3-year follow-up period, there was no association between tertiles of IL-18 and change in total kidney volume or eGFR.[228]

## KIDNEY INJURY MOLECULE-1

Kidney injury molecule-1 (KIM-1 in humans, Kim-1 in rodents), which is also referred as "T-cell immunoglobulin and mucin domain–containing protein-1" (TIM-1) and "hepatitis A virus cellular receptor-1" (HAVCR-1), is a type I transmembrane glycoprotein with an ectodomain containing a six-cysteine immunoglobulin-like domains, two *N*-glycosylation sites, and a mucin domain. In an effort to identify molecules involved in kidney injury, Ichimura and colleagues originally discovered Kim-1 using representational difference analysis (a PCR-based technique) in rat models of acute ischemic kidney injury.[229,230] Importantly, KIM-1 was shown to be significantly expressed in kidneys, specifically in proximal tubular cells of humans after ischemic injury, whereas it was virtually absent or present at low levels in healthy kidneys. KIM-1 has evolved as a marker of proximal tubular injury, the hallmark of virtually all proteinuric, toxic, and ischemic renal diseases. KIM-1 has been shown to be a highly sensitive and specific marker of kidney injury in several rodent models, including models of injury due to ischemia,[229,231] cisplatin, folic acid, gentamicin, mercury, chromium,[232,233] cadmium,[234] contrast agents,[235] cyclosporine,[236] ochratoxin A, aristolochic acid, D-serine, and protein overload.[237]

In 2002, Han and associates[231] published the first clinical study linking urinary levels of KIM-1 with AKI, demonstrating that tissue expression of KIM-1 is correlated with the severity of acute tubular necrosis and corresponding levels of KIM-1 ectodomain in the urine of patients with clinically significant AKI. Since then, numerous other studies have been published on the ability of KIM-1 to detect AKI in a variety of settings, including cardiac surgery, critical illness, and general hospitalized AKI, with mixed success.[44,216,217,238–244]

KIM-1 has been investigated in several multicenter larger trials. In the TRIBE-AKI adult and pediatric cardiac surgery cohorts, the fifth quintile of urinary KIM-1 values was associated with an increased risk of AKI (those with postoperative doubling were at a 6.2-fold increased risk of AKI compared with those with the lowest KIM-1 values). This risk remained significant (4.8-fold) after adjusting for the clinical model—age, race, gender, CPB time, nonelective surgery, preoperative GFR, diabetes, hypertension, and study center. The effect was completely attenuated after including urinary IL-18 and plasma and urine NGAL into the model.[243] Urine KIM-1 concentrations were associated with duration of AKI (categories: 1 to 2 days, 3 to 6 days, and >7 days). Compared with the first quintile, the fifth quintile of early postoperative KIM-1 provided an unadjusted OR of 2.96 (2.01–4.37) for longer duration of AKI. After adjusting for clinical factors known to affect AKI (including but not limited to age, gender, race, CPB time, baseline kidney function, diabetes, and hypertension), the OR remained statistically significant 2.30 (1.51–3.53).[212]

When looking at long-term mortality in the TRIBE cohort, the third tertile of perioperative urine KIM-1 concentrations was associated with increased mortality. In those without AKI ($n$ = 792), the third tertile had an adjusted HR of 1.83 (1.44–2.33) for mortality, whereas in the 407 subjects with AKI, the adjusted HR was slightly higher 2.01 (1.31–3.1).[214] In the pediatric cohort, those in the fifth quintile of urine KIM-1 were at increased risk of AKI in the unadjusted analysis; however, this effect was attenuated and no longer significant after multivariable adjustment.[243]

The data on urine KIM-1 in the setting of critical illness–related AKI have been just as mixed as the perioperative results, with KIM-1 having an AUC of 0.66 (95% CI; 0.61–0.72) for the diagnosis of AKI in samples from the EARLY ARF study. The results were less impressive with regard to the prediction of dialysis (0.62) or death (0.56) within the first week following ICU admission.[216] On the other hand, in a cohort of 529 mixed ICU patients, urine KIM-1 outperformed other biomarkers in its ability to detect AKI at the time of ICU admission in those with a preadmission GFR < 60 mL/min (AUC = 0.70, [0.58 –0.82]). In a separate post hoc analysis of this cohort, KIM-1 levels demonstrated a significant stepwise increase when comparing those with no AKI (median, 170 μg/mmol creatinine [Cr]; interquartile range [IQR], 69 –445) to those with prerenal AKI (291 μg/mmol Cr; IQR, 121–549) and those with intrinsic AKI (lasting more than 48 hours; 376 μg/mmol Cr; IQR, 169–943).[217] In addition, urine KIM-1 was able to forecast the development of intrinsic AKI at the time of ER arrival with an AUC of 0.71 (0.65–0.76; $P < .001$). KIM-1 values again increased in a stepwise fashion, with values being lowest in those with no AKI or CKD < stable CKD < prerenal AKI < intrinsic AKI. Also, KIM-1 values were able to forecast the need for RRT, as well as inpatient mortality.[219]

The usefulness of KIM-1 has been demonstrated not only as a urinary marker but also as a tool for evaluating kidney injury in kidney biopsy specimens by immunohistochemical methods. For example, Van Timmeren and associates found that the level of KIM-1 protein expression in proximal tubule cells correlated with tubulointerstitial fibrosis and inflammation in kidney tissue specimens from 102 patients who underwent kidney biopsy for a variety of kidney diseases.[245] In a subset of patients whose urine was collected near the time of biopsy, urinary KIM-1 levels were significantly correlated with tissue KIM-1 expression in biopsy samples from patients with deterioration in kidney function and histologic changes indicative of tubular damage. In biopsy specimens from transplanted kidneys, increased KIM-1 staining was seen in 100% of patients with a deterioration of kidney function and pathologic changes indicating tubular injury, in 92% of patients with acute cellular rejection, and in 28% of patients with normal biopsy findings.[246] This is in contrast to the findings of Hall and associates, who have demonstrated that urinary KIM-1 levels do not correlate with early posttransplantation or 1-year graft function.[223,241] Similarly, Schroppel and colleagues have investigated KIM-1 RNA expression in pretransplantation biopsies collected from both living and deceased donor kidneys and found no significant correlation between KIM-1 staining and the occurrence of DGF.[247]

### Chronic Kidney Disease

KIM-1 also shows promise as a useful biomarker in CKD. In addition to serving as a marker of proximal tubule dysfunction, animal studies have demonstrated that KIM-1 is upregulated in the later phases of AKI and plays an important role in renal repair; thus, it may be a major player in the pathophysiology of repair and CKD development after AKI.[248] The ability to serve as a marker of CKD was evident in a nested case-control study from 686 participants from the Multi-Ethnic Study of Atherosclerosis (MESA). Cases were defined as those with a baseline eGFR > 60 mL/min who subsequently developed CKD stage 3 and/or had a rapid drop in kidney function over the 5-year study period. Each doubling of KIM-1 level (in pg/mL) was associated with a 1.15 (1.02–1.29) increased odds of developing CKD stage 3 or a rapid decline in GFR.

Similarly, at study entry, those in the highest decile of KIM-1 had a twofold increased risk of this same endpoint compared with the lower 90%. This ability to predict the development and progression of CKD was independent of the presence of albuminuria.[249] Similarly, when investigated in a cohort of 149 persons with chronic congestive heart failure during 5 years of follow-up, KIM-1 levels were strongly associated with the progression of CKD (defined as a >25% drop in eGFR from baseline; $P < .05$).[250] Urine KIM-1 and NAG were both independent predictors of the combined endpoint of CKD progression and all-cause mortality.[250] In a multivariable Cox proportional hazard model that included age, gender, body mass index (BMI), history of diabetes, hypertension, stroke, baseline eGFR, albuminuria, left ventricular ejection fraction, diuretic use, and brain natriuretic peptide levels, baseline eGFR, diuretic use, and KIM-1 and NAG levels were the only independent predictors of both these outcomes. More recently, in a pooled multivariable-adjusted analysis of five unique cohort studies, log-transformed urine KIM-1 levels (normalized to urine creatinine) were found to be higher in current smokers, and lower in blacks and those patients receiving angiotensin-converting enzyme inhibitors (ACE-Is) or angiotensin receptor blockers (ARBs).[251] Similarly, KIM-1 levels were higher in those with lower eGFRs and higher in those with albuminuria.

These results, which indicate the utility of KIM-1 as a biomarker for CKD, are in contrast to those of Bhavsar and colleagues, who measured KIM-1 in a case-control substudy of the ARIC study.[252] In this study of 286 subjects, 143 of whom developed new-onset CKD stage 3, KIM-1 did not display the ability to forecast or diagnose those at risk for CKD development or progression. In a follow-up case-control study by Foster and colleagues of 135 patients with ESRD and 186 controls from the same ARIC cohort (study visit 4), it was found that urinary KIM-1, normalized to urine creatinine, was associated with an increased risk of ESRD (unadjusted OR, 2.24 [1.97–4.69]; $P = .03$).[253] However, this effect was attenuated when adjusting for other factors that increase the risk for ESRD (e.g., age, baseline albuminuria, baseline eGFR).

A recent study of the 2466 participants in the Chronic Renal Insufficiency Cohort Study (CRIC) reported findings similar to those of Foster and colleagues[253] on the role of KIM-1 as a biomarker of CKD progression.[254] In this study, with 9433 person-year follow-up, there were 581 cases of CKD progression defined as incident ESRD or a 50% decrease in eGFR. All four upper quintiles of KIM-1 were associated with increased risk of progression (compared with the lowest quintile) in unadjusted analyses (e.g., fifth quintile HR of 7.68 [5.61–10.5]). However, this effect was completely attenuated after the addition of other variables known to associate with CKD progression (e.g., age, gender, race, albuminuria, diabetes, cardiovascular disease).[254]

KIM-1 has been investigated and shown promise in a variety of other clinical settings, including in children with chronic renal tubular damage from vesicoureteral reflux,[25] HIV nephropathy,[225,256] posttransplantation DGF,[257] and diabetic nephropathy.[258,259] In patients with IgA nephropathy, urinary KIM-1 levels were significantly higher than in healthy controls. Furthermore, the levels of urinary KIM-1 correlated positively with serum creatinine concentration and proteinuria and correlated inversely with creatinine clearance. Similarly, tubular KIM-1 expression, as determined by immunohistochemical analysis, correlated closely with urinary levels ($r = 0.553$; $P = .032$).[260] Sundaram and associates have evaluated the potential of KIM-1, L-FABP, NAG, NGAL, and transforming growth factor-β1 (TGF-β1), together with conventional renal biomarkers (urine albumin level, serum creatinine concentration, and serum cystatin C–GFR), to detect nephropathy early in patients with sickle cell anemia. Only KIM-1 and NAG showed a strong correlation with albuminuria; other markers did not show any association with albuminuria.[261]

More recently, plasma KIM-1 was measured in two distinct cohorts at risk for diabetic kidney disease.[262] Plasma KIM-1 was measured in subjects from the Action to Control Cardiovascular Risk in Diabetes (ACCORD) and Veterans Administration NEPHROpathy iN Diabetes (VA-NEPHRON-D) cohorts. In the ACCORD cohort, baseline KIM-1 levels were higher in those who went on to develop incident CKD. Similarly, in the NEPHRON-D study, those who went on to develop progressive CKD had higher levels at the start of the study (median IQR, 735 pg/mL [438–1172]) compared with 373 pg/mL (225–628; $P < .001$).[262] Those in the highest quartile of KIM-1 concentrations in both studies were more likely to experience adverse renal outcomes compared with those in the lowest quartiles of KIM-1 concentrations. This work expands on the limited data that link plasma KIM-1 with CKD progression.[262] Although the exact mechanism whereby KIM-1 enters the plasma circulation in the setting of renal injury remains unclear, these promising studies will undoubtedly lead to further investigation of the link between plasma KIM-1 and CKD.

## LIVER-TYPE FATTY ACID BINDING PROTEIN

Urinary fatty acid binding protein 1 (FABP1) has been proposed to be a useful biomarker for early detection of AKI and monitoring of CKD. Also known as "L-type" or "liver-type fatty acid binding protein" (L-FABP), FABP1 was first isolated in the liver as a binding protein for oleic acid and bilirubin. FABP1 binds selectively to free fatty acids and transports them to mitochondria or peroxisomes, where free fatty acids are beta-oxidized and participate in intracellular fatty acid homeostasis. There are several different types of FABP, which are ubiquitously expressed in a variety of tissues. At this time, nine different FABPs have been reported—liver (L), intestinal (I), muscle and heart (H), epidermal (E), ileal (I1), myelin (M), adipocyte (A), brain (B), and testis (T). L-FABP is expressed in proximal tubules of the human kidney and localized in the cytoplasm. Increased cytosolic L-FABP in proximal tubular epithelial cells may derive not only from endogenous expression, but also from circulating L-FABP that might be filtered at the glomeruli and reabsorbed by tubular cells.

Susantitaphong and associates[263] published a metaanalysis reporting the performance of L-FABP from 15 prospective cohorts and two case-control studies. Although the authors were only able to meta-analyze seven of the cohort studies, they demonstrated that L-FABP levels were 74.5% sensitive (60.4–84.8) and 77.6% specific (61.5–88.2) for the diagnosis of AKI. Additionally, they demonstrated that the results were more promising for the prediction of in-hospital mortality. They concluded that based on the low quality of many of the studies and the varied clinical settings, L-FABP may be a promising biomarker for the early detection of AKI.[263] In what follows we highlight some of the larger and more recent clinical investigations of L-FABP.

Portilla and colleagues have demonstrated that L-FABP predicts the development of AKI within 4 hours of surgery in children undergoing cardiac surgery.[264] Others have attempted to validate this finding in the setting of cardiac surgery, with mixed success.[242,265,266] Recently, TRIBE-AKI published the results of the largest study investigating L-FABP in the setting of adult cardiac surgery, which demonstrated that after adjusting for a clinical model that consisted of factors known to affect the development of AKI, L-FABP did not correlate with the development of AKI in either their pediatric ($n$ = 311) or adult ($n$ = 1219) cohort.[212] It was demonstrated that although L-FABP levels were statistically higher in adults with AKI compared with those with no AKI, the L-FABP concentration (in ng/mL) at the 0- to 6-hour postoperative time point had an AUC of 0.61 for subsequent AKI, and the performance was only marginally better at the 6- to 12-hour time point. Despite this suboptimal performance in detecting incident postoperative AKI, L-FABP was associated with duration of AKI, even after adjusting for factors known to affect the development of AKI. Both the fourth and fifth quintiles were associated with a longer duration of AKI, with adjusted ORs of 1.77 (1.17–2.67) and 1.92 (1.26–2.93), respectively. In the pediatric cohort, although the fifth quintile of L-FABP concentrations at the earliest postoperative time point (0–6 hours) was significantly associated with the development of an AKI odds ratio of 2.9 (1.2–7.1), this effect disappeared after adjustment to 1.8 (0.7–4.6).[243]

On a related note, heart fatty acid binding protein (H-FABP) was also measured in the TRIBE-AKI cohort.[267] H-FABP is a protein that is predominantly expressed in the cytosol of the myocardium, but can be found in the distal tubule and detects cardiac injury in less than 1 hour.[268–270] Log-transformed H-FABP concentrations in the preoperative and immediate postoperative periods were associated with an increased risk of AKI (defined by the AKIN criteria), as well as mortality. In analyses adjusted for factors known to be associated with AKI, preoperative H-FABP values were associated with all stages of AKI (adjusted OR, 2.07 [95% CI, 1.48–2.89]) and mortality 1.67 (1.17–2.37), whereas perioperative values were associated with stage 2 or higher AKI (5.39 [2.87–10.11]) in a similarly adjusted analysis.[267] In view of these promising results, we anticipate further investigation of H-FABP.

Siew and colleagues[271] have reported the performance of L-FABP in 380 critically ill subjects from medical, surgical, trauma, and cardiac ICUs, 130 of whom had AKI defined as AKIN stage 1. L-FABP levels were higher in those with AKI ($P$ = .003) and were able to discriminate incident AKI with an AUC of 0.59 (0.52–0.65). Although L-FABP was not able to predict the composite endpoint of death or RRT, L-FABP was able to predict the need for acute RRT in a multivariable analysis (HR, 2.36 [95% CI, 1.30–4.25]). These findings mirror those of Doi and colleagues, who published a prospective single-center observational cohort study examining the performance of L-FABP in 339 mixed ICU patients.[218] In their study, L-FABP outperformed NGAL, IL-18, NAG, and other biomarkers in the detection of AKI, defined by RIFLE risk. Furthermore L-FABP predicted 14-day mortality with an AUC of 0.90. This study, which followed up a smaller study ($n$ = 145) by this same group of investigators, has paved the way for L-FABP to be validated for clinical use in Japan.[272]

In a cross-sectional study of general hospitalized patients that included 92 participants with AKI and 68 control subjects (26 healthy volunteers and 42 other hospitalized patients, 29 about to undergo coronary catheterization and 13 patients in the ICU with no AKI), Ferguson and colleagues have demonstrated that urinary levels of L-FABP are significantly higher in those with AKI than in hospitalized control patients without AKI, with an AUC of 0.93 (0.88–0.97), with a sensitivity of 83% and specificity of 90% at a cutoff value of 47.1 ng/mg of creatinine.[273] Nickolas and colleagues[219] examined L-FABP at the time of ER arrival and found that it only had fair discriminatory power with regard to AKI. In their cohort of 1635 subjects, L-FABP had an AUC of 0.70 (0.65–0.76); however, there was a clear and significant stepwise increase in L-FABP concentrations across the spectrum of AKI (normal < CKD < prerenal < intrinsic AKI).

Because L-FABP is also expressed by the liver, liver injury can be a potential contributor to increased urinary levels of L-FABP during AKI. However, previous studies in patients with CKD, AKI, and sepsis have shown that serum L-FABP levels do not have an influence on urinary levels and that urinary L-FABP levels are not significantly higher in patients with liver disease than in healthy subjects.[264,274,275]

Urinary L-FABP levels have been investigated as an early diagnostic and predictive marker for contrast medium–induced nephropathy.[276,277] In a study of adult patients with normal serum creatinine concentrations who underwent percutaneous coronary intervention, serum NGAL levels rose at 2 and 4 hours, whereas urinary NGAL and urinary L-FABP levels increased significantly after 4 hours and remained elevated up to 48 hours after cardiac catheterization.[278] Nakamura and associates have demonstrated that baseline urinary L-FABP levels are significantly higher in patients who developed contrast medium–induced nephropathy after coronary angiography; however, the authors did not evaluate the diagnostic performance of urinary L-FABP in predicting AKI.[277]

Finally, L-FABP has been investigated in the setting of renal transplantation, DGF, and postoperative transplant function.[257,279,280] When measured in the deceased donor urine, prior to organ harvesting, or the early postoperative setting, urinary L-FAPB was associated with donor AKI and mildly predictive of DGF. However, although L-FABP concentrations were associated with DGF, they did not outperform postoperative urine output for this endpoint,[280] and they did not predict long-term graft function over the first posttransplantation year.[257]

### Chronic Kidney Disease

In the past, small studies investigating the excretion of L-FABP in the setting of diabetic nephropathy have been mixed. Some have reported a link between decreased urinary concentrations of L-FABP in the setting of renin-angiotensin-aldosterone blockade and preserved GFR, whereas others found no correlation.[281,282] More recently, L-FABP has been investigated in established cohorts of CKD patients (e.g., ARIC, CRIC). In a case-control study of 321 patients from the ARIC cohort, 135 with ESRD, urinary L-FABP, normalized to urine creatinine, was not associated with an increased risk of ESRD.[253] These results are slightly different from when L-FABP was investigated in the CRIC cohort. Using Cox proportional hazard models, L-FABP was assessed in 2466 members of the cohort, with an average of a 3.8-year follow-up.[254] Although several quintiles were associated with progression of CKD (50% drop in eGFR or development of ESRD; fifth quintile unadjusted HR of 10.67 [7.46–15.25]), this effect was entirely attenuated when adjusting for factors known to affect the development and progression of CKD. As such, it appears that L-FABP is not an ideal biomarker for the detection or progression of CKD.

## MONOCYTE CHEMOATTRACTANT PROTEIN-1

Monocyte chemoattractant protein-1 (MCP-1) is a chemotactic protein secreted by a variety of cells that attracts blood monocytes and tissue macrophages through interaction with the cell surface receptor CCR2 (chemokine C-C motif receptor 2).[283,284] Induction of MCP-1 at the transcript or protein level has been demonstrated in a variety of human cell types, including fibroblasts, endothelial cells, peripheral blood mononuclear cells, and epithelial cells, on proinflammatory stimuli.[284–288] Kidney cells also produce MCP-1 in response to proinflammatory cytokines, including TNF-α and IL-1β.[289]

#### Acute Kidney Injury

Plasma MCP-1 was measured in 972 participants of the TRIBE AKI cohort to determine its association with postoperative AKI and mortality.[290] In this subset of TRIBE patients, 34% of whom had AKI ($n$ = 329), MCP-1 levels were significantly higher in those who developed AKI or died (12%; $n$ = 119) in the median 2.9-year follow-up period. Preoperative MCP-1 levels in the highest tertile were associated with a 43% increased risk of AKI compared with those in the lowest preoperative tertile; however, this effect was not significant when looking only at an outcome of severe AKI. This analysis was likely limited by the low number of patients who developed severe AKI (stage 2 or 3 AKI, $n$ = 45; 5%). Those in the highest preoperative tertile were also at increased risk of death, with an adjusted HR of 1.95 (1.09–3.49).[290] Although this TRIBE study represents the largest study to date of the role of MCP-1 as a biomarker of AKI, others have investigated it in other settings, including DGF following kidney transplantation.[291] Given these limited data, as well as the strength of its role in CKD, we anticipate that MCP-1 will continue to be investigated as a biomarker of AKI over the next several years. Munshi and associates have demonstrated that urinary levels of both MCP-1 transcripts and protein were elevated in patients with AKI, as well as in experimental models of AKI; however, these data have yet to be replicated in other AKI cohorts.[292]

#### Chronic Kidney Disease

The expression of MCP-1 is induced in kidney diseases with significant inflammation, such as diabetic nephropathy and other glomerulonephropathies.[293–295] In particular, podocytes and tubular cells produce MCP-1 in response to high levels of glucose and advanced glycosylation end products.[296] Furthermore, urine levels of MCP-1 are significantly elevated in patients with diabetic nephropathy, and its levels correlate significantly with albuminuria and NAG levels in humans, as well as in experimental diabetic nephropathy.[297–300] In a prospective observational study of patients with diabetic nephropathy, urinary levels of connective tissue growth factor (CTGF) were elevated in patients with microalbuminuria and macroalbuminuria, but the urinary MCP-1 level was elevated only in those with macroalbuminuria.[301] Urinary CTGF levels correlated with progression to macroalbuminuria, whereas urinary MCP-1 levels (but not CTGF levels) correlated with the subsequent rate of eGFR decline (at a median follow-up of 6 years). The authors concluded that increased urinary CTGF concentration is associated with early progression of diabetic nephropathy, whereas MCP-1 level is associated with later-stage disease.[301] The independent association of urine MCP-1 with the risk of CKD progression has been confirmed by others.[302,303] Elevated levels of urinary MCP-1 were reported in patients with lupus nephritis, and the presence of MCP-1 in urine reflected its intrarenal expression.[304,305] Serum concentrations of MCP-1 were also shown to be elevated in patients with diabetic nephropathy and lupus nephritis, but the serum levels did not correlate with disease progression.[304–306] Moreover, the lack of correlation between urinary and serum MCP-1 levels suggests that urinary MCP-1 is the result of local production of MCP-1 by the kidney rather than simply filtration of serum MCP-1. More recently, Vianna and colleagues demonstrated that plasma and urinary levels of MCP-1 are elevated in pediatric CKD (from either glomerular disease or congenital anomalies) but were not correlated with each other. MCP-1 levels were significantly higher than in those without CKD, and there were differences in MCP-1 concentration, depending on the cause of the CKD.[295]

### NEUTROPHIL GELATINASE-ASSOCIATED LIPOCALIN

NGAL, also known as "lipocalin 2" or "lcn2," is one of the biomarkers of AKI that has been studied extensively. NGAL has many characteristics required for a good biomarker of AKI compared with serum creatinine measurement or urine output.[307] It is a 25-kDa protein with 178 amino acids belonging to the lipocalin superfamily. Lipocalins are extracellular proteins with diverse functions involving transport of hydrophilic substances through membranes, thereby maintaining cell homeostasis.[308] NGAL is a glycoprotein bound to matrix metalloproteinase-9 in human neutrophils. It is expressed in various tissues in the body, such as salivary glands, prostate, uterus, trachea, lung, stomach, and kidney,[309] and its expression is markedly induced in injured epithelial cells, including those in the kidney, colon, liver, and lung.

Transcriptome profiling studies in rodent models have identified NGAL as one of the most upregulated genes in the kidney very early after tubular injury.[310,311] Mishra and associates have demonstrated that NGAL levels are significantly elevated within 2 hours after injury in mouse models of renal ischemia–reperfusion.[312] In addition, urinary NGAL was detectable after 1 day of cisplatin administration, which suggests its sensitivity in other models of tubular injury.[312]

#### Acute Kidney Injury

Many clinical studies have followed these important observations in animals. Mishra and associates first demonstrated the value of NGAL as a clinical marker in a prospective study of 71 children undergoing CPB.[313] In this study, both serum and urinary NGAL levels were upregulated within 2 hours in patients who developed AKI. A cutoff value of 50 μg/L was 100% sensitive and 98% specific in predicting AKI. Following this seminal paper, several other papers investigating NGAL in the setting of cardiac surgery were published, with several demonstrating that both urine and serum NGAL levels were able to predict AKI earlier than serum creatinine, as well as correlate with AKI severity.*

However, no paper was able to replicate the near-perfect results published in this first study. Given the wealth of studies that have reported on NGAL over the past decade, we have chosen to highlight the larger and multicenter trials that studied NGAL.

*References 44, 45, 108, 109, 210, 211, 213, 242, 244, and 314–319.

### Urine Neutrophil Gelatinase-Associated Lipocalin

In the setting of the ER, urine NGAL was originally shown to perform well in Nickolas and colleagues'[63] first study in 635 patients, demonstrating that a cutoff of 130 μg/g of creatinine had a sensitivity of 90% and specificity of 99.5% for AKI, defined as RIFLE risk.[320] In this single-center prospective study, urine NGAL also predicted the future need for nephrology consult, admission to the ICU, and need for RRT. In a follow-up multicenter study of 1635 subjects, urine NGAL had an AUC of 0.81 (0.76–0.86) for the prediction of AKI (RIFLE risk) and had an NRI of 26.1% while demonstrating the ability to improve the classification of both AKI events and nonevents. Additionally, urine NGAL values were significantly different and increased in a stepwise fashion in those with no AKI < CKD < prerenal AKI < intrinsic AKI.

Lieske and colleagues measured urine NGAL in 363 ER patients and determined that NGAL has an AUC of 0.70 for the detection of AKIN AKI while providing only modest sensitivity (65%) and specificity (65%).[320a] In addition to demonstrating that NGAL levels increased with the severity of AKI, they demonstrated that pyuria and urinary white blood cells were associated with increased urinary NGAL levels. Urine NGAL has been studied less extensively in the pediatric ER but has demonstrated similar potential in a smaller study ($n$ = 252), with a lower AKI incidence rate ($n$ = 18; 7.1%).[240]

Urine NGAL has also been studied in the setting of critical illness by Siew and colleagues, who demonstrated that urine NGAL was able to predict AKI within the first 24 (AUC = 0.71) and 48 (AUC = 0.64) hours of ICU admission.[321] In this single-center prospective study of 451 critically ill adults, urine NGAL was independently associated with the development of AKI, even after adjusting for factors known to be correlated with the development of AKI (including severity of illness and sepsis). NGAL performed similarly when measured in a post hoc analysis of the EARLY ARF trial. Data from this prospective observational study performed in two general (mixed) ICUs in New Zealand demonstrated that urine NGAL could modestly predict the development of AKI (AKIN stage 1; AUC, 0.66) but was also able to forecast the need for RRT (AUC, 0.79) and death within the first 7 ICU days (AUC 0.66; $P < .001$ for all three). Additionally, urine NGAL performed better in predicting AKI on ICU arrival in those with higher baseline eGFRs (AUC = 0.70 for those with an eGFR from 90–120 mL/min vs. an AUC of 0.64 for those with an eGFR < 60 mL/min).[216] This improved ability to detect the future development of AKI in those with a higher eGFR has been demonstrated by others in the setting of cardiac surgery.[44,45] In a separate post hoc analysis of the EARLY ARF study, urine NGAL values again demonstrated a significant increase across the spectrum of AKI, with concentrations being lowest in those without AKI and values for those with transient AKI that lasted less than 48 hours being in between those with no AKI and those with AKI that lasted longer than 48 hours.[217] In the discovery phase of the multicenter prospective observational SAPPHIRE trial, with 522 participants, urine NGAL had an AUC of 0.66 (95% CI, 0.60–0.71) for the development of RIFLE injury or failure within the first 36 hours of study enrollment; this increased to 0.71 (0.66–0.76) when looking at RIFLE injury or failure within the first 12 hours.[322]

In the setting of cardiac surgery, urine NGAL has provided similar mixed results. In the TRIBE-AKI adult cohort, the highest quintile of urine NGAL at 0 to 6 hours following surgery was associated with an increased risk of AKI (doubling of serum creatinine or need for RRT); however, this effect was no longer significant after adjusting for factors known to contribute to AKI risk.[210] In addition to having an AUC of 0.67 for the detection of AKI in this cohort of 1219 adults, urine NGAL levels were significantly associated with the composite endpoint of inpatient mortality or receipt of RRT, as well as length of ICU stay and length of hospitalization. All quintiles of urine NGAL were associated with duration of AKI in unadjusted analyses; however, this effect was no longer significant for all but the fourth quintile after adjusting for factors known to affect the development of AKI.[212] Urine NGAL did not display the ability to detect AKI progression in the 380 adults who developed at least AKIN stage 1. Although those subjects in the fifth quintile of urine NGAL at the time of serum creatinine increase were at increased risk for more progressive AKI (e.g., going from AKIN stage 1 to AKIN stage 3), this effect was no longer significant in the adjusted analysis.[213] These results were in contrast to those of the pediatric cohort ($n$ = 311), in which those in the fifth quintile of urine NGAL remained at a significantly increased risk of developing AKI (doubling of serum creatinine or need for RRT), even after adjusting for the clinical model (OR 4.1; 95% CI, 1.0–16.3). Additionally, urine NGAL levels correlated with the length of mechanical ventilation, ICU stay, and hospitalization.[211]

In a separate secondary analysis looking at the long-term mortality of the adult TRIBE cohort in patients with AKI ($n$ = 407,) those subjects in the third tertile of urine NGAL were at increased risk of death during the median 3.0-year follow-up. The adjusted HR for this group (compared with the first tertile) was 2.52 (95% CI, 1.86–3.42). A similar effect was not seen in the third tertile of those without AKI ($n$ = 792), HR 0.90 (95% CI, 0.50–1.63).[214]

Urine NGAL has been investigated in the setting of DGF following renal transplantation, with several studies linking elevated urine NGAL levels in the posttransplantation setting with the development of DGF.[241,323] Reese and colleagues[257] shifted this paradigm slightly in measuring urine NGAL in the deceased donor urine rather than in the posttransplantation setting. They demonstrated that elevated urinary NGAL was associated the development of recipient DGF; the third tertile of NGAL had a relative risk of 1.21 (1.02–1.45) compared with the lowest tertile. Elevated deceased donor urine NGAL levels were weakly associated with slightly lower eGFR at 6 months posttransplantation in those patients who did not develop DGF. As such, although urine NGAL did correlate with donor-based AKI, it did not provide meaningful value in predicting short- and long-term outcomes posttransplantation.[257]

Urine NGAL has been investigated in several other smaller studies in more niche cohorts and has demonstrated some promise in detecting AKI and other adverse patient outcomes, including critically ill neonates,[324] individuals with cirrhosis or hepatorenal syndrome,[325,326] and 1-year graft survival following transplantation.[223] However, these trials and others require validation in larger and multicenter investigations.

**Plasma Neutrophil Gelatinase-Associated Lipocalin**

Plasma NGAL has been examined in many of the same studies with urine NGAL, including in the settings of the ER and ICU and following cardiac surgery. In the ER, Di Somma and colleagues[327] have demonstrated that the plasma NGAL drawn at the time of ER arrival had an AUC of 0.80 for the future development of AKI. In this multicenter prospective cohort study, the AUC improved to 0.90 when ER physician clinical judgment was added to plasma NGAL. This combination of physician clinical judgment and NGAL outperformed either physician judgment and serum creatinine alone, leading to a significant NRI of 32.4%.

In the setting of critical illness, plasma NGAL was measured as part of a post hoc analysis of the multicenter EARLY ARF study ($n = 528$), in which it had an AUC of 0.74 (0.69–0.79) for the development of AKIN stage 1 AKI ($n = 147$) during subsequent ICU stay. This study defined functional AKI based on the AKIN criteria but also defined structural AKI in terms of urine NGAL concentrations. Plasma NGAL performed even better (AUC = 0.79) at predicting urine NGAL–defined structural AKI ($n = 213$). In addition to strong associations with creatinine and urine NGAL–based definitions of AKI, plasma NGAL was also associated with the need for RRT ($n = 19$) but not with inpatient mortality ($n = 53$).[328] In the SAPPHIRE trial, which also examined the performance of plasma NGAL in the setting of ICU-associated AKI, NGAL had an AUC of 0.64 (0.58–0.70) for the detection of RIFLE injury or failure within the first 12 hours of study enrollment; this significant ability to forecast more severe forms of AKI did not dramatically change when assessing the ability to detect the same level of AKI over the first 36 hours (AUC, 0.64 [95% CI, 0.58–0.71]).[322]

It has been postulated that NGAL's performance in the setting of critical illness is likely attenuated in part due to the preponderance of sepsis-related AKI in the ICU, and that NGAL levels are inherently higher in those with sepsis because it is derived in part from neutrophils. De Geus and colleagues[39] published a prospective observational cohort study of 663 ICU admissions in which plasma NGAL levels were measured four times during the first 24 hours. They demonstrated that plasma NGAL levels were significantly higher in those with sepsis compared with those without sepsis, and that when the cohort was stratified according to the presence of sepsis ($n = 80$; 12% of the cohort), plasma NGAL was able to detect AKI remarkably well in both cohorts (AUC of 0.76 in those with sepsis vs. 0.78 in those without sepsis). These data corroborate the work of Katagiri and associates, which demonstrated in a prospective observational study of 139 critically ill patients that plasma NGAL levels are highest in those with sepsis associated with AKI > nonsepsis AKI > no AKI.[330] Future investigations of plasma NGAL will need to take this association with sepsis into account as we begin to construct normal ranges, as well as clinically validated cutoffs to use NGAL in interventional trials to treat those in the early stages of AKI.[331,332]

In addition to investigations in the setting of critical illness, plasma NGAL has been investigated in the setting of acute heart failure.[333] In a multicenter, prospective, observational cohort study of 927 patients with acute decompensated heart failure requiring intravenous diuretics, Maisel and colleagues evaluated plasma NGAL's ability to predict worsening of renal function, defined as a 0.5 mg/dL or ≥50% increase in serum creatinine level from baseline or the need for RRT.[333] In their study, 72 patients (7.8%) developed the primary endpoint with neither first or peak NGAL providing a significantly higher AUC compared with serum creatinine alone (0.656, 0.647, and 0.652 respectively). Similarly, plasma NGAL was predictive of in-hospital adverse events (AUC of 0.691) but did not significantly outperform serum creatinine (AUC, 0.686). This large-scale investigation does not support the use of plasma NGAL for the detection of AKI in the setting of decompensated heart failure.

Despite these disappointing findings in the setting of heart failure, plasma NGAL has been shown to predict recovery from AKI in preliminary studies. In 181 patients with community- acquired pneumonia and at least RIFLE failure AKI, plasma NGAL measures on the first day that met failure criteria were able to predict the failure of recovery of renal function. Individuals with high plasma NGAL levels were less likely to recover, with an AUC of 0.74. However, this was not significantly different from a clinical model consisting of age, serum creatinine level, and severity of illness scores.[334] This potential ability to detect nonrecovery of AKI is yet another aspect of NGAL and other biomarkers that require further investigation.

Plasma NGAL has also been extensively studied in the setting of cardiac surgery. In the TRIBE-AKI adult cohort ($n = 1219$), plasma NGAL levels were significantly higher in those who developed AKI (doubling of serum creatinine or RRT) in the early postoperative period. Those in the fifth quintile of plasma NGAL at the 0- to 6-hour time point (>293 ng/mL) were at a 7.8-fold increased risk of developing AKI compared with those in the first quintile (<105 pg/mL). This effect was attenuated after adjusting for factors known to associate with AKI but remained significant (OR, 5.0 [(95% CI, 1.6–15.3]), although it was no longer significant after adjusting for serum creatinine.[210] Additionally, plasma NGAL was significantly associated with increased length of ICU and hospital stay, as well as a composite of in-hospital death or dialysis. In this same adult cohort, plasma NGAL, measured at the time of a clinical AKI and serum creatinine increase, demonstrated a remarkable ability to detect those individuals with progressive AKI (e.g., going from AKIN stage 1 to stage 2 or 3; $n = 380$). After adjusting for the clinical model, the fifth quintile of plasma NGAL (>322 ng/mL) was nearly eight times more likely to develop progressive AKI (OR 7.72 [95% CI, 2.65–22.49]) compared with those in the first two quintiles. Plasma NGAL displayed the ability to improve the reclassification of both those with and without progressive AKI (events and nonevents), providing a category-free NRI of 0.69 ($P < .0001$).[213] The results from the TRIBE-AKI pediatric cohort were less promising, with plasma NGAL not displaying the ability to predict severe AKI (doubling of serum creatinine or need for RRT) in the early postoperative period. However, the fifth quintile of NGAL (>259 ng/mL) measured within the first 6 postoperative hours was significantly associated with the development of RIFLE risk AKI, with an adjusted OR of 2.3 (95% CI, 1.0–5.5),[211] although falling well short of the near-perfect performance published in the original Mishra paper.[335]

Outside of these large trials, there have been several smaller trials that investigated NGAL in a variety of AKI settings, so much so that Haase and colleagues conducted a pooled prospective study ($n = 2322$; 1452 with cardiac surgery and 870 with critical illness) that designated subjects as NGAL(+) or NGAL(−) and creatinine(+) or creatinine(−); creatinine (+) was defined as RIFLE-R.[41] After analyzing NGAL data from 10 separate prospective observational studies, they demonstrated that individuals who were NGAL(+) but creatinine(−) needed acute dialysis 16 times more often than those who were NGAL(−) creatinine(−) (OR, 16.4 [95% CI, 3.6–76.9]; $P < .001$). The study also demonstrated an incremental increase in ICU stay, hospital stay and mortality among the four study groups as follows: NGAL(−) creatinine(−) < NGAL(+) creatinine(−) < NGAL(−) creatinine(+) < NGAL(+) creatinine(+).

The function of NGAL as a diagnostic marker of contrast medium–induced nephropathy has also been evaluated. In a prospective study of 91 children undergoing coronary angiography, both urine and plasma NGAL levels were found to be significantly increased within 2 hours of contrast medium administration in the group that developed contrast-induced nephropathy but not in the control group. By comparison, AKI detection using increases in serum creatinine concentration was possible only 6 to 24 hours after contrast agent administration. When a cutoff value of 100 ng/mL was used, both urine and serum NGAL levels at 2 hours predicted contrast medium–induced nephropathy, with AUCs of 0.91 and 0.92, respectively.[336] In several studies of adults undergoing procedures requiring contrast, an early increase in both urine (4-hour) and plasma (2-hour) NGAL levels was documented, compared with a much later increase in plasma cystatin C levels; this provides support for the use of NGAL as an early biomarker for contrast medium–induced nephropathy.[224,337] A meta-analysis has revealed an overall AUC of 0.89 for the prediction of AKI when NGAL is measured within 6 hours after contrast agent administration when AKI is defined as a 25% or greater increase in serum creatinine concentration.[338]

The origin of plasma and urinary NGAL after AKI requires further clarification. Gene expression and transgenic animal studies have demonstrated an upregulation of NGAL in the distal nephron segments, specifically in the thick ascending limb of Henle and the collecting ducts; however, most of the injury in AKI occurs in the proximal tubules.[339,340] On the other hand, the source of plasma NGAL in AKI is not well defined. For example, in animal studies, direct ipsilateral renal vein sampling after unilateral ischemia indicates that NGAL synthesized in the kidney does not enter the circulation.[340] The increase in plasma NGAL observed in AKI may derive from the fact that NGAL is an acute-phase reactant and may be released from neutrophils, macrophages, and other immune cells. Yndestad and colleagues have reported strong immunostaining for NGAL in cardiomyocytes within the failing myocardium in studies of experimental and clinical heart failure.[341] Furthermore, any impairment in GFR resulting from AKI would be expected to decrease renal clearance of NGAL, with subsequent accumulation in the systemic circulation. However, the contribution of these mechanisms to the rise in plasma NGAL concentration after AKI has yet to be investigated.

NGAL levels are also influenced by various medical conditions, such as CKD, hypertension, anemia, systemic infections, hypoxia, inflammatory conditions, and cancer, which makes it relatively less specific for kidney injury.[342] Additionally, there is some evidence to suggest that NGAL concentrations degrade over time, with levels decreasing by nearly 50% within the first 6 months of storage at −80°C. These degradation issues also affect other biomarkers (including *N*-acetyl-β-D-glucosaminidase and KIM-1); their impact on clinical results remains unclear because this remains an area of continued investigation.[343] Nevertheless, NGAL represents a very promising candidate as a biomarker for the early diagnosis of AKI and potential prediction of outcome.

### Chronic Kidney Disease

In addition to extensive investigation in the setting of AKI, NGAL has been increasingly investigated in the setting of CKD. Some of this work was inspired by animal data that demonstrated that NGAL, like KIM-1, was highly upregulated by the persistent inflammation and late immune response following AKI and potentially contributes to the development of post-AKI CKD.[248] Moving this concept into humans, Nickolas and colleagues have reported on the correlation of NGAL with histologic changes on native kidney biopsies of subjects with CKD. They demonstrated that NGAL levels were inversely correlated with eGFR and directly correlated with both interstitial fibrosis and tubular atrophy.[320]

Over the past several years, there have been several investigations into the ability of urine NGAL to detect incident and progressive CKD, using previously collected cohorts, such as ARIC, MESA, and CRIC. In an original case-control substudy of the ARIC cohort ($n = 286$), urinary NGAL did not initially correlate with baseline eGFR. However, the fourth quartile of urine NGAL was at more than a twofold increased risk of developing incident stage 3 CKD during the follow-up period. It should be noted, however, that this effect was attenuated after adjusting for urine creatinine and urine albumin.[252] In a subsequent investigation of ARIC participants, 135 patients with ESRD and 186 matched controls (gender, race, baseline renal function, and diabetes status), there was no association of urine NGAL (normalized to urine creatinine) with the development of ESRD over time.[253]

Analysis of data from the MESA cohort was unable to find an association between urine NGAL levels and the future development of incident CKD stage 3. In a 1:1 nested case-control study, NGAL levels were not associated with the development of CKD stage 3 or a decrease in eGFR of >3 mL/min per year over a 5-year follow-up period.[249]

Finally, several analyses from CRIC have investigated the role of urine NGAL in predicting CKD and its progression. Liu and colleagues have demonstrated that there is a strong association between baseline urine NGAL and the risk of CKD progression (defined as a 50% reduction of MDRD-calculated eGFR or development of ESRD) over the mean follow-up of 3.2 years.[344] However, although this effect was significant in an unadjusted analysis, urine NGAL offered no improved prediction after adjusting for baseline age, race, eGFR, proteinuria, diabetes, and other factors known to affect CKD progression (C-statistic of 0.847 for both). Thus, in this cohort of 3386 individuals, urine NGAL offered no improvement in predicting CKD outcomes compared with more traditional markers. More recently, in a subset of 2466 CRIC enrollees with slightly longer follow-up (mean, 3.8 years) Hsu and colleagues demonstrated that the higher four quintiles of urine NGAL (normalized to urine creatinine) were associated with CKD progression. However, after adjusting for factors known to affect CKD progression, this effect was no longer significant in all quintiles.[254]

These findings from ARIC, MESA, and CRIC, which demonstrate an association with CKD progression that does not persist in adjusted models, are in direct contrast to a recent prospective observational cohort of 158 white patients with baseline CKD stage 3 or 4. This study demonstrated that urine NGAL (adjusted for urine creatinine) was associated with CKD progression; 40 patients reached the primary endpoint of all-cause mortality or need for RRT during the 2-year follow-up. The baseline urine NGAL was associated with this composite primary endpoint, with every increase of urine NGAL of 5 μg/mmol being associated with a 27% increased risk of death or RRT.[345] These findings are similar to those of Bolignano and colleagues, who performed a prospective observational study of 96 subjects with CKD, with a median follow-up of 18.5 months.[346] They demonstrated that both urine and serum NGAL were associated with a composite endpoint of either doubling of baseline serum creatinine or the development of ESRD. Conversely, in a 4-year follow-up study of 78 patients with type 1 diabetes conducted to evaluate the potential of urinary NGAL level to predict progression to diabetic nephropathy, NGAL levels were not associated with decline in GFR or development of ESRD and death after adjustment for known progression promoters.[347]

## N-ACETYL-β-D-GLUCOSAMINIDASE

NAG is a lysosomal brush border enzyme that resides in the microvilli of tubular epithelial cells. Damage to these cells results in shedding of this enzyme into the urine. NAG has a high molecular weight of 130 kDa, and hence plasma NAG is not filtered by the glomeruli. Its excretion into urine correlates with tubular lysosomal activity. Increased urinary concentrations of NAG have been found in patients with AKI, chronic glomerular disease, diabetic nephropathy, exposure to nephrotoxic drugs, delayed renal allograft function, environmental exposure, contrast medium–induced nephropathy, or sepsis and following CPB.[239,348–354] In a prospective study involving 201 hospitalized patients with AKI, patients with higher concentrations of urinary NAG and KIM-1 were more likely to die or require dialysis. This study suggests the utility of NAG in combination with KIM-1 in predicting adverse clinical outcomes in patients with AKI.[239] Urinary NAG concentrations were significantly higher in patients with contrast medium–induced nephropathy than in patients without such nephropathy within 24 hours after the administration of a contrast agent.[353]

Similarly, in a two-center Japanese study of 77 patients undergoing cardiac surgery, NAG levels were elevated in those who developed postoperative AKI.[265] In this study, biomarker performance significantly improved when NAG was combined with L-FABP (an AUC improvement from 0.75 to 0.81). This same group published a single-center study investigating the performance of NAG in predicting the development of AKI (RIFLE) in a mixed medical-surgical ICU. NAG did not perform as well in this cohort of 339 subjects, providing an AUC of 0.62 for the development of RIFLE risk.[218] In a cohort of 635 ER patients, a NAG value over 1.0 units/g had an AUC of 0.71 (95% CI, 0.62–0.81) for the development of AKI during the subsequent hospital admission. However, this effect was attenuated in a multivariable analysis that included other novel and traditional biomarkers of AKI (e.g., creatinine, BUN, NGAL).[176]

In the setting of CKD, a study of patients with type 1 diabetes and nephropathy, Vaidya and colleagues have shown that lower levels of urinary KIM-1 and NAG are associated with the regression of microalbuminuria.[259] Similarly, in a nested case-control study from the Diabetes Control and Compliance Trial, baseline NAG concentrations were shown to predict micro- and macroalbuminuria.[355]

NAG has been investigated for its ability to detect CKD progression in a few cohorts. In the CRIC cohort, NAG was associated with CKD progression in unadjusted analyses, with the fifth quintile having an HR of 15.16 (10.17–22.59).[254] However, after adjusting for age, gender, race, and albuminuria, this association was completely attenuated. Additionally, the ability of NAG to predict CKD progression was analyzed in 149 patients with chronic heart failure over 5-year follow-up.[250] Those with a urine NAG level above the median were nearly four times as likely (OR, 3.92; $P = .001$) to have their CKD progress (defined as ≥25% decrease in eGFR). NAG was also shown to be an independent predictor of all-cause mortality.[250]

There are some limitations in the use of NAG as a marker of kidney injury. Inhibition of NAG enzyme activity has been reported in the presence of metal ions and at higher urea concentrations in the urine. Moreover, increased urinary levels of NAG have been reported in several nonrenal diseases, including rheumatoid arthritis and hyperthyroidism, as well as in conditions with increased lysosomal activity without cellular damage.[356,357] Because of concerns about its specificity, the clinical utility of NAG as a biomarker has been limited.

## PROTEINURIA

In a healthy person, urinary protein excretion is less than 150 mg/day and consists mainly of filtered plasma proteins (60%) and tubular Tamm-Horsfall protein (40%).[358,359] Proteinuria can result from at least three different pathophysiologic mechanisms, including glomerular (increased permeability of glomerular filtration barrier to protein due to glomerulopathy, raised glomerular capillary hydrostatic pressure, or altered glomerular filtration coefficient), overflow (due to increased production of low-molecular-weight plasma proteins, such as immunoglobulin light chains in myeloma), and tubular processes (decreased tubular absorption of filtered proteins or increased production of tubular proteins by damaged tubules). Proteinuria mechanisms and consequences are discussed in Chapter 30. Proteinuria is diagnosed when the total urinary protein is greater than 300 mg/24 hours. Methods for detecting and monitoring proteinuria are discussed in Chapter 23.

Some reports have highlighted the diagnostic power of total protein for AKI in various drug-induced nephrotoxicities, including cisplatin and nonsteroidal antiinflammatory drugs.[360,361] A low eGFR is a known risk factor for AKI, and the utility of proteinuria in combination with the eGFR to predict the risk of this disease is now being investigated.[362] In a large cohort of nearly 1 million adult Canadians, James and colleagues demonstrated an independent association among eGFR, proteinuria, and incidence of AKI.[363] This group reported that patients with normal eGFR levels (≥60 mL/min/1.73 m$^2$) and mild proteinuria (urine dipstick, trace to 1+) have 2.5 times more risk of admission to a hospital with AKI than patients with no proteinuria. The risk was increased to 4.4-fold when they included patients with heavy proteinuria (urine dipstick ≥ 2+). Adjusted rates of admission with AKI and kidney injury requiring dialysis remained high in patients with heavy dipstick proteinuria, independent of the eGFR.[18] These findings confirm previous reports suggesting that the eGFR and proteinuria are potent risk factors for subsequent AKI.[364,365]

## ALBUMINURIA

Albuminuria is recognized as one of the most important risk factors for the progression of CKDs. Albumin is a major serum protein with a size slightly larger than the pores of the glomerular filtration membrane, so albuminuria is best known as a biomarker of glomerular dysfunction; its appearance in large amounts in urine represents compromised integrity of the glomerular basement membrane.[366] In smaller amounts, however, the presence of albumin in the urine may reflect tubular injury. Albuminuria is classified in the KDIGO classification system as A1 (UAE < 30 mg/day or urine ACR [uACR] < 30 mg/g creatinine), A2 (previously termed "microalbuminuria"; urinary albumin excretion, 30–300 mg/day, or uACR, 30–300 mg/g creatinine) and A3 (previously termed "macroalbuminuria"; urinary albumin excretion > 300 mg/day or uACR > 300 mg/g creatinine). In a number of clinical studies, albuminuria has been shown to be a sensitive biomarker of drug-induced tubular injury.[367,368] It is routinely used as a marker of kidney damage for making a CKD diagnosis at eGFR levels above 60 mL/min/1.73 $m^2$.[359] Guidelines of the National Kidney Foundation (NKF) and American Heart Association (AHA) include microalbuminuria, as well as an increase in the urinary total protein excretion, as a risk factor for renal and cardiovascular disease. Both NKF and AHA guidelines suggest measurement of the uACR in an untimed spot urine sample. Ideally, the uACR should be assessed in at least three different samples to decrease intraindividual variation.[369] Albuminuria is a continuous risk factor for ESRD and cardiovascular mortality, with no lower limit, even after adjustment for the eGFR and other established risk factors.[370–372] Urinary albumin has been used as a biomarker for monitoring CKD progression and potential therapeutic efficacy, although the FDA does not accept albuminuria as a surrogate marker. Using microalbuminuria as a marker, Levin and colleagues have demonstrated that N-acetylcysteine may attenuate contrast-induced glomerular and tubular injury.[373]

In the past several years, there have been increased investigations of albuminuria as a biomarker for AKI. In a large-scale, collaborative meta-analysis, Grams and colleagues combined data from eight general population cohorts (1,285,049 subjects) and five CKD cohorts (79,519 subjects) to investigate the association of albuminuria and other factors with AKI.[374] The primary outcome for this study was hospitalization for AKI. Using Cox proportional hazards models, they demonstrated that the incidence of AKI was higher in those with CKD (2.6%) compared with the general population (1.3%). Additionally, compared with those with an uACR < 5 mg/g, the risk of AKI with uACR > 300 mg/g was 2.73 (2.18–3.43].[374] Thus, increased uACR is a strong risk factor for the long-term risk of developing of AKI.

The TRIBE AKI measured preoperative albuminuria in 1159 adult patients, organizing the cohort into clinical risk categories based on the preoperative uACR: 10 mg/g or less (≤1.1 mg/mmol), 11 to 29 mg/g (1.2–3.3 mg/mmol), 30 to 299 mg/g (3.4–33.8 mg/mmol), and 300 mg/g or greater (≥33.9 mg/mmol). The incidence of AKI, defined as AKIN stage 1, increased across the uACR categories with those in the >300 mg/g category having a relative risk (RR) of 2.36 (95% CI,1.85–2.82) compared with the <10 mg/g group. This association was slightly attenuated after adjusting for variables known to affect proteinuria and AKI, with a RR of 2.21 (95% CI, 1.66–73).[375] Similarly, the fourth and fifth quintiles of urine albumin (in mg/L) were associated with increased duration of AKI in unadjusted analyses (fifth quintile, OR 2.83 [1.94–4.12].[212] Although this effect disappeared for the fourth quintile after adjusting for factors known to affect the development of AKI, there was only slight attenuation of the fifth quintile (2.21 [1.48–3.30].[212] These adult data are in contrast to pediatric TRIBE-AKI data ($n$ = 294), which demonstrated no association between the preoperative uACR and the development of postoperative AKI.[376] The adult uACR data represent an additional biomarker to aid in cardiac surgery AKI prediction models and supplement other recent data that point to proteinuria and albuminuria serving as biomarkers of AKI in the preoperative and postoperative setting.[377,378]

In the postoperative setting, the TRIBE-AKI cohort demonstrated that urinary albumin concentrations (mg/L) and dipstick proteinuria values within 6 hours of adult cardiac surgery correlated with the future development of AKI. Compared with the lowest quintile, the highest quintile of albuminuria (mg/L) and highest group of dipstick proteinuria were associated with the greatest risk of AKI (adjusted RR, 2.97 [95% CI, 1.20–6.91]), and adjusted RR of 2.46 (95% CI, 1.16–4.97), respectively]. However, only the postoperative urine albumin concentration (mg/L; not indexed to urine creatinine) was associated with improved risk stratification when added to the clinical model (AUC increased from 0.75 to 0.81; $P$ = .006). Urinary albumin (mg/L) in the early postoperative period was also highly predictive of long-term mortality in the TRIBE AKI adult cohort. Specifically, in those with perioperative AKI ($n$ = 407), those in the second tertile of albuminuria were at increased risk of death in the 3.0-year follow-up period (adjusted HR 2.28 [95% CI, 1.06–4.88]). Although this effect was further magnified in the third tertile of those with AKI (HR, 2.85 [95% CI, 1.36–5.99]), there was no increased mortality across any of the tertiles of urine albumin in the 792 subjects without perioperative AKI.[214] Despite its known utility in other settings, a higher early postoperative uACR (mg/g creatinine) was not statistically associated with AKI risk. The poor performance of uACR in the context of adult cardiac surgery may be explained by variations in the urine creatinine excretion within and between individuals, which could be especially prominent when renal function is not in a steady state, and may in part explain why urine albumin concentration (mg/L) outperformed uACR.

In the TRIBE AKI pediatric cohort, perioperative values of the uACR (mg/g), and not urine albumin concentration (mg/L), were found to be predictive of AKI. In children younger than 2 years, an absolute first postoperative uACR ≥ 908 mg/g (103 mg/mmol, highest tertile) predicted the development of AKIN stage 2 or 3 AKI, with an adjusted RR of 3.4 (95% CI, 1.2–9.4) when compared with the first tertile. In children 2 years of age or older, a postoperative uACR ≥ 169 mg/g (19.1 mg/mmol, highest tertile), regardless of preoperative values, predicted stage 1 AKI after adjusting for clinical factors, such as age, race, gender, and preoperative eGFR, type of cardiac surgery, and adjusted RR of 2.1 (95% CI, 1.1–4.1).[376] Although urine albumin concentration and uACR remain established and readily available laboratory tests, the diversity of results when investigating the development of postoperative AKI indicates that further studies are needed before it may be used in clinical practice.

## URINARY CYSTATIN C

Urinary cystatin C tracks the function of proximal tubular cells. In healthy individuals, the urinary levels of cystatin C are almost undetectable. Any damage to proximal tubular cells can impede the reabsorption and enhance the urinary excretion of cystatin C. Several clinical studies have sought to understand the potential of urinary cystatin C levels for the prediction of kidney injury and its prognosis. Herget-Rosenthal and associates analyzed data from 85 patients in the ICU who were at high risk of developing AKI and used the RIFLE classification to define AKI.[379,380] In their studies, the authors reported that the urine cystatin C level detected AKI 1 to 2 days before changes in serum creatinine level, with an AUC of 0.82 and 0.97 on day 2 and day 1, respectively, as well as demonstrating that urine cystatin C serves as a marker of AKI severity correlating with a future need for RRT. Urinary cystatin C-to-creatinine ratios of more than 11.3 mg/mmol were significantly associated with proteinuria. Attempts to validate urine cystatin C as a marker of ICU-associated AKI have provided mixed results. Siew and colleagues have measured urine cystatin C in 380 ICU patients (mixed surgical-medical, trauma, and cardiac) and demonstrated that there is no difference in concentrations between those with and without AKI ($P = .87$).[271] More encouraging data from the EARLY ARF trial have demonstrated that in a cohort of 529 subjects, urine cystatin C may have limited ability to detect AKI (AUC of 0.67 on ICU arrival), with no significant difference in its ability to detect AKI in those with a GFR above and below 60 mL/min.[216] Additionally, in a separate post hoc analysis of the same study, urine cystatin C values exhibited a stepwise and significant ($P < .001$) increase when comparing values from those with no AKI < prerenal AKI < intrinsic AKI (defined as AKIN stage 1 > 48 hours).

In comparison with these mixed ICU-associated AKI data, several small studies investigating urine cystatin C in the setting of cardiac surgery have demonstrated promise.[44,109,317,381] However, these results were not validated in the TRIBE-AKI cohort. In unadjusted analyses of the adult cohort, several quintiles of urine cystatin C were significantly associated with the development of both mild (AKIN stage 1) or severe (doubling of creatinine or need for RRT) AKI at both the 0- to 6-hour and 6- to 12-hour postoperative time points. However, the small associations were completely attenuated after adjusting for the clinical model. Similarly, in the TRIBE pediatric cohort, no quintile remained significantly associated with AKI (mild or severe) in the adjusted analyses.[382] Urine cystatin C demonstrated similar results when measured in a cohort of 1635 ER patients, supplying an AUC of 0.65 (95% CI, 0.58–0.72) for the future development of AKI. However, using a multivariable analysis that included traditional (creatinine) and more modern (urine NGAL, KIM-1, IL-18, and LFABP) biomarkers, urine cystatin C was not a significant contributor in predicting the composite outcome of inpatient RRT or death.[219] Finally, when investigated in a prospective multicenter observation cohort study of deceased donor kidney transplants, urine cystatin C concentration from the first postoperative day was modestly correlated with 3-month allograft function; the AUC for predicting DGF at the 6-hour postoperative time point was 0.69.[383]

A number of studies have reported increased urinary cystatin C levels in patients with proteinuria, which suggests the possibility of tubular damage as a consequence of protein overload.[384–386] Currently, urinary cystatin C level has several disadvantages as a biomarker, including lack of international standardization and expense of the assay. Although serum cystatin C has been demonstrated as a reliable biomarker of eGFR, one must remember that cystatin C synthesis is increased in smokers, patients with hyperthyroidism, those receiving glucocorticoid therapy, and those with elevated levels of inflammatory markers, such as white blood cell count and C-reactive protein level, and the impact of these factors on urine cystatin C in the setting of AKI has not been fully investigated.[387,388] Furthermore, several different commercial assays are available to measure cystatin C. Advantages are that the commercially available immunonephelometric assay provides rapid automated measurement of cystatin C, and results are available in minutes.[389] In addition, preanalytic factors, such as routine clinical storage conditions and freezing and thawing cycles, and interfering substances, such as bilirubin or triglycerides, do not affect cystatin C measurement.[389,390]

## PROENKEPHALIN

Enkephalins are small endogenous opioid peptides; because they are known to be expressed in the kidney, they have been investigated for the ability to detect both AKI and CKD.[391] Physiologically, preproenkephalin is the primary gene product of the *PENK* gene, but this propeptide is eventually cleaved, and proenkephalin (pro-ENK)is generated in this process. Given its low molecular weight, it is freely filtered at the glomerulus and, as such, is potentially ideal as a biomarker of glomerular function. Plasma pro-ENK concentrations have been shown to be stable in vitro for 48 hours, unlike other enkephalins, which have proven more difficult to measure (e.g., met-enkephalin).[392]

### Acute Kidney Injury

Pro-ENK has been investigated in a few AKI clinical settings, including a retrospective observational cohort of patients with suspected sepsis in the emergency department.[393] Given that it is freely filtered, plasma levels of pro-ENK were inversely correlated with creatinine clearance ($r = -0.72$). Additionally, pro-ENK levels were significantly higher in those who eventually developed AKI (defined by RIFLE criteria), compared with those without AKI. Pro-ENK on arrival in the ER had an AUC 0.815 ($P < .001$) for the future development of AKI. Additionally, pro-ENK was modestly associated with 7-day inpatient mortality, with an AUC of 0.69; this significantly outperformed serum creatinine for this endpoint (AUC, 0.61; $P = .045$).[393]

Pro-ENK has also been evaluated for its ability to detect AKI following adult cardiac surgery.[394] In a single-center cohort of 92 patients, 20 of whom developed postoperative AKI (AKIN definition), preoperative and early postoperative pro-ENK levels were higher in those who went on to develop AKI. Preoperative values provided a C-statistic of 0.68

($P = .013$); early postoperative values gave a C-statistic 0.72 ($P < .001$).[394]

In a separate investigation, pro-ENK levels were measured in 1908 patients with acute heart failure to investigate its relationship with renal function, as well as short- and long-term mortality.[395] Pro-ENK levels were independently associated with an increased risk of worsening of renal function ($n$ = 264), defined as 0.3 mg/dL or 50% increase in serum creatinine from the admission value within the first 5 days. In an adjusted analysis, elevated pro-ENK levels on admission were associated with increased odds of developing a subsequent rise in serum creatinine (OR, 1.58 [1.25–2.00]; $P <$ .0005). In this multicenter cohort of patients with cardiorenal syndrome and AKI, after multivariable Cox proportional hazards analyses, pro-ENK was independently associated with in-hospital and 1-year mortality. Finally, in the largest investigation of pro-ENK to date, pro-ENK was highly correlated with eGFR and plasma urea levels, with an F-statistic of 296 and 166, respectively ($P < .001$ for both).[395]

### Chronic Kidney Disease

Although pro-ENK appears to be a useful biomarker in the setting of early AKI, its relationship with eGFR requires further evaluation, because limited data have suggested that it may also serve as a biomarker of CKD.[396] In a prospective cohort of 2568 patients without CKD (defined as eGFR > 60 mL/min/1.73 $m^2$), plasma pro-ENK was found to be associated with incident CKD. Those in the highest tertile of baseline pro-ENK level had an increased incidence of CKD compared with the lowest tertile (OR 1.51 [1.18 to 1.94]; $P < .001$). Additionally, pro-ENK improved the reclassification of patients for the detection of incident CKD in over 14% of the cohort. Additionally in this same cohort, there was a signal that a minor allele in the pro-ENK gene was also associated with an increased risk of CKD. Although much like the other associations, these need to be validated in separate cohorts.[396]

## URINE TISSUE INHIBITOR METALLOPROTEINASE-2 AND INSULIN-LIKE GROWTH FACTOR–BINDING PROTEIN-7

Urine tissue inhibitor metalloproteinase-2 and insulin-like growth factor–binding protein-7 (TIMP-2 and IGFBP-7) have been shown to serve as biomarkers of AKI in the setting of critical illness. These biomarkers are unique in that they play a role in cell cycle arrest. Both IGFBP-7 (through p523 and p21) and TIMP-2 (through p27) block the effect of cyclin-dependent protein kinase complexes and cause short periods of G1 cell cycle arrest.[397–399] They were originally discovered as part of a three-center discovery cohort of 522 subjects These patients had AKI stemming from sepsis, shock, major surgery, and trauma. Over 300 potential markers were evaluated, with TIMP-2 and IGFBP-7 being the two that best predicted the development of KDIGO stage 2 or 3 AKI. This finding was then validated in a prospective international multicenter observational study of 728 subjects.[322] In this validation study, TIMP-2 and IGFBP-7 remained the top two performing biomarkers for the prediction of RIFLE injury or failure within the first 12 to 36 hours of study enrollment, with AUC values of 0.77 and 0.75, respectively (SAPPHIRE study). When these two biomarker values were multiplied together, they demonstrated an improved ability to detect this same endpoint (AUC of 0.80). The paper did not supply information about the combination of TIMP-2 and IGFBP-7 with other biomarkers of AKI (e.g., NGAL, KIM-1, L-FABP, IL-18).[322] However, these same biomarkers (TIMP-2 and IGFBP-7) were further validated in the OPAL study, where they provided a similar AUC for the detection of impending stage 2 or 3 AKI.[400] Perhaps more importantly, this study identified cut points for TIMP-2 × IGFBP-7 to help risk-stratify patients for severe AKI. Patients with a value less than 0.3 were at lowest risk for severe AKI, those with a value between 0.3 and 2.0 had a RR 4.7 (1.5–16.0) times higher, and those with a value greater than 2.0 had a RR 12.0 (4.2–40) times higher than the lowest risk group. These data cut points were further validated in a post hoc analysis of the original 728 SAPPHIRE cohort.[400]

This reproducibility of these results in distinct cohorts led the FDA to clear TIMP-2 × IGFBP-7 for clinical use in late 2014.[322,400,401] Additionally, Liu and colleagues have published data demonstrating that biomarker concentrations correlate to the clinical adjudication of a panel of three expert nephrology adjudicators who were blinded to the biomarker values.[402] Since that time, several post hoc investigations of these and other cohorts have demonstrated that these biomarkers have several strengths. In the 9-month follow-up of the SAPPHIRE cohort, TIMP-2 × IGFBP-7 levels measured at the time of study enrollment were shown to correlate with a composite endpoint of death or need for RRT.[403] There was a stepwise increase in risk of the endpoint across the biomarker cutoff strata (0.3 and 2.0) in those subjects who went on to develop AKI; those with a value greater than 2.0 had an adjusted HR of 2.16 [1.32–3.53] compared with those with values less than 0.3.[403] TIMP-2 × IGFBP-7 has also been shown to reliably forecast impending severe AKI in several subsets of critically ill patients, including those with CKD and congestive heart failure, as well as those undergoing emergent and cardiothoracic surgery.[404,405] Additionally, others have investigated these biomarkers in other clinical settings, such as pediatric AKI[406] and DGF following renal transplantation,[291] and further validation of these markers is required outside the setting of adult critical illness. Given the FDA and European clearance for clinical testing, the American Society of Nephrology's AKI Advisory group and others have published guidance documents on the potential clinical use of TIMP-2 × IGFBP-7 (Box 27.2).[407,408]

### Furosemide Stress Test

Furosemide and other diuretics have long been used in the setting of AKI to convert oliguric AKI into nonoliguric AKI, but they have seen a resurgence for the ability to ascertain

**Box 27.2 TIMP-2 × IGFBP-7**

1. Urinary TIMP-2 × IGFBP-7 has been FDA-approved for determining which high-risk critically ill patients are at increased risk of severe AKI.
2. Elevated TIMP-2 × IGFBP-7 levels (>0.3) measured early in the course of an ICU stay can forecast the development of at least stage 2 AKI and have been shown to be associated with posthospitalization outcomes, such as 9-month mortality and the need for RRT.

tubular reserve in the setting of AKI.[409–411] As a loop diuretic, furosemide (an organic anion) is not filtered by the glomerulus because it is tightly bound to serum proteins (albumin), and it therefore gains access to the tubular urinary space through active secretion in the proximal convoluted tubule via the human organic anion transporter (hOAT) system.[412,413] In the tubular lumen, furosemide inhibits the ability of the thick ascending limb of the loop of Henle to transport chloride, preventing sodium reabsorption and resulting in natriuresis and increased urine flow and potentially reducing tubular oxygen demand.[414–418] As a result of these pharmacokinetic factors, the urine output following furosemide dosing has been hypothesized to represent an approach to assess the renal tubular integrity in the setting of AKI.

In 1973, Baek and colleagues studied 15 subjects who did not yet have clinically apparent AKI (as measured by changes in serum creatinine).[410] They subjected them to a one-time furosemide challenge assessing their UOP and free water clearance ($C_{H_2O}$). Although they did not standardize the furosemide dosing, or report if any of their patients had preexisting CKD, they did report that a $C_{H_2O}$ near zero and a poor urine output response to furosemide signaled that "acute renal failure was imminent."[410]

More recently, Chawla and colleagues have modified and standardized this protocol, renaming it the "furosemide stress test" (FST).[419] They prospectively investigated the ability of the urinary response following the administration of the FST to predict adverse patient outcomes in patients with KDIGO stages 1 and 2 AKI.[39] In a cohort of 77 subjects, they reported that the 2-hour urine output response to 1.0 mg/kg FST (in the furosemide-naïve) and 1.5 mg/kg FST (in those with prior loop exposure) was able to forecast the progression to KDIGO stage 3 AKI ($n$ = 25; 32.4%), with an ROC AUC (standard error) of 0.87 (0.05). A cutoff of 200 mL at 2 hours provided a sensitivity and specificity of 87.1% and 84.1%, respectively, for progression to stage 3 AKI. This same cutoff provided an AUC (SE) of 0.86 (0.08) for the receipt of inpatient RRT ($n$ = 11; 14.2%) and 0.70 (0.09) for inpatient mortality ($n$ = 16; 20.7%).[419]

In a secondary analysis of this same cohort, FST outperformed plasma and urine NGAL, urinary IL-18, and TIMP-2 and IGFBP-7 for prediction of progression to stage 3, need for RRT, and mortality.[420] Interestingly, when the FST data were analyzed in a subset of patients with elevated biomarkers (urine NGAL > 150 ng/mL; $n$ = 44 or TIMP-2 × IGFBP-7 > 0.3; $n$ = 32), its ability to detect these same outcomes was further improved. Thus, combining AKI biomarkers with a functional assessment of tubular reserve like the FST may be an informative bedside tool to assist clinicians in the prognostication of early AKI.[420] In this study, the FST was not performed in subjects deemed to be hypovolemic, those with obstructive uropathy, or those with a baseline eGFR less than 30 mL/min/1.73 m$^2$.[419]

Conversely, Van der Voort and colleagues[421] investigated the ability of a standardized infusion of furosemide to predict renal recovery in those with advanced AKI requiring RRT. In a post hoc analysis, they reported that urine output (median IQR) was higher in patients who recovered their renal function and eventually stopped RRT (654 mL [333–1155] vs. 48 [15–207] mL; $P$ = .007). Their version of the FST for prediction of recovery had a diagnostic performance AUC ROC of 0.84. Regardless of the clinical scenario in which it is being tested, the urinary response to furosemide informs the clinician about the renal reserve present during AKI (progression or recovery). The FST provides a measure of proximal tubule secretory capacity but also assesses thick ascending limb and distal collecting duct function. Thus, the FST serves as an assessment of integrated nephron function and warrants further validation in larger and more diverse cohorts.

## GENETIC ASSOCIATIONS WITH ACUTE KIDNEY INJURY RISK

In addition to investigating novel proteins and functional aspects of the nephron, others have focused their attention on the role that genetics play in predisposing patients to an increased risk of AKI and CKD. Discussions of the genetics of chronic kidney disease can be found in Section VI of this edition and are beyond the scope of this chapter. With regard to AKI, there have been several investigations over the past few years reporting associations with several polymorphisms.

Susantitaphong and colleagues have demonstrated that a polymorphism in the promoter region of the TNF-α gene was associated with AKI severity and distant organ dysfunction.[422] Using a cohort of 262 hospitalized adults, they demonstrated that after adjustment for race, gender, age, baseline eGFR, sepsis, and the need for RRT, those with the minor allele (rs1800629) had higher peak serum creatinine and higher multiple organ failure scores, compared with the GG genotype. In a cohort of 401 patients with acute lung injury enrolled in the Fluids and Catheter Treatment Trial (FACTT), Bhatraju and colleagues have reported that two minor alleles in the nuclear factor of kappa light-chain polypeptide gene enhancer in B cells inhibitor (NFKBIA) are strongly associated with the development of AKIN criteria for AKI. For rs1050851 and rs2233417, the ORs for any AKI were 2.34 (1.58–3.46; $P = 1.06 \times 10^{-5}$; false discovery rate (FDR) = 0.003) and 2.46 (1.61–3.76; $P = 1.81 \times 10^{-5}$; FDR = 0.003) for each minor allele, respectively.[423] The associations were increased for AKIN stages 2 and 3, with respective ORs of 4.00 (2.10–7.62; $P = 1.05 \times 10^{-5}$; FDR = 0.003) and 4.03 (2.09–7.77; $P = 1.88 \times 10^{-5}$; FDR = 0.003).

In one of the larger investigations around the genetic basis for postoperative AKI, Stafford-Smith and colleagues used a discovery cohort of 873 nonemergent coronary bypass patients and then attempted to replicate their findings in a 380-subject validation cohort.[424] Using linear regression, they adjusted for a clinical AKI risk score to test single-nucleotide polymorphism (SNP) association with peak postoperative serum creatinine level. In the discovery cohort, nine SNPs that met statistical significance were detected; two of these, rs13317787 in GRM7|LMCD1-AS1 intergenic region (3p21.6) and rs10262995 in BBS9 (7p14.3), were replicated with significance in the validation cohort. Further investigation of these two regions and meta-analyses found genome-wide significance at the GRM7|LMCD1-AS1 locus and a significantly strong association at BBS9.[424] These are two new loci that had not been previously described.

More recently, the largest investigation of the genetic susceptibility to in-hospital AKI was conducted by Parikh and colleagues.[425] They performed an exploratory genome-wide association study in 760 cases of AKI and 669 controls (hospitalized patients without AKI) and attempted to validate their findings in an additional 206 cases of AKI and 1406 controls. They assessed 609,508 SNPs and, in their replication analyses, they validated four SNPs with an increased odds of association with the development of AKI. These SNPs included rs62341639 (OR, 0.64 [0.55–0.76]; $P = 2.48 \times 10^{-7}$) and rs62341657 (0.65 [0.55–0.76]; $P = 3.26 \times 10^{-7}$) on chromosome 4 near the APOL1-regulator IRF2, and rs9617814 (0.70 [0.60–0.81]; $P = 3.81 \times 10^{-6}$) and rs10854554 (0.67 [0.57–0.79] $P = 6.53 \times 10^{-7}$) on chromosome 22.[425]

Prior to these more recent larger studies, a handful of systematic reviews of the genetic predisposition to AKI were published.[426–428] They concluded that despite several gene polymorphisms with documented associations with the development, severity, and outcome of AKI, definitive conclusions would require more investigation, with replication in new cohort studies.[427] We anticipate further investigation of the role of genetics in AKI risk in the years to come.

## CHRONIC KIDNEY DISEASE BIOMARKERS

Currently, the eGFR and proteinuria are used as markers of CKD progression because of their widespread availability and ease of performing the tests. Because all forms of CKD are associated with tubulointerstitial injury, markers of tubular injury, including KIM-1, IL-18, NGAL, and L-FABP, have been investigated in CKD and shown to associate with outcomes in CKD due to a variety of causes, as discussed previously. In addition, elevated systemic levels of molecules that have impaired kidney clearance or increased production in CKD (e.g., asymmetric dimethylarginine, fibroblast growth factor 23) as well as chemokines (e.g., monocyte chemoattractant protein-1) and fibrotic markers (e.g., connective tissue growth factor, TGF-β1, and collagen IV) are discussed here. For more in-depth discussion around specific markers for glomerular diseases, cystic diseases, diabetes, and inherited forms of renal disease, please see the individual chapters covering these topics.

Table 27.7 summarizes the ability of biomarkers to detect clinical endpoints related to CKD in a variety of clinical settings.

### PLASMA ASYMMETRIC DIMETHYLARGININE

Nitric oxide is synthesized by oxidation of the terminal guanidine nitrogen of L-arginine by nitric oxide synthase (NOS). This process can be reversibly inhibited by guanidine-substituted analogs of L-arginine, such as in asymmetric dimethylarginine (ADMA).[429,430] Three types of methylated arginines have been described in vivo—ADMA, $N^G$-monomethyl-L-arginine, and symmetric dimethylarginine, an inert isomer of ADMA. Of these, ADMA is the major type of endogenously generated methylated arginine that displays inhibitor activity of NOS. However, administration of ADMA to endothelial NOS knockout mice also induces vascular lesions, which suggests that ADMA may have actions independent of nitric oxide and NOS in vivo.[431] Vallance and associates first reported that plasma levels of ADMA are elevated in patients with renal failure[432] and hypothesized that impaired renal clearance of ADMA may account for the rise in plasma levels. This assumption has been challenged by follow-up studies in animal models demonstrating that only a small portion of circulating ADMA is excreted in the urine.[433] Moreover, elevated plasma ADMA levels are also reported in patients with incipient renal disease but normal renal function.[434]

Elevated plasma levels of ADMA have been reported in patients with a variety of cardiovascular risk factors, such as hypertension, diabetes, and hyperlipidemia.[435–437] Among these groups, plasma ADMA levels are particularly high in patients with CKD, patients with ESRD undergoing hemodialysis or peritoneal dialysis, and kidney transplant recipients.[432,438,439] Plasma levels of ADMA are strongly associated with carotid intima to media thickness, left ventricular hypertrophy, cardiovascular complications, and mortality in patients with ESRD.[440–442] Plasma ADMA levels have been shown to correlate prospectively, in an inverse manner, with CKD progression in those with and without diabetes-related CKD.[443,444] Similarly, ADMA levels may also be associated with the presence of proteinuria and albuminuria.[445]

**Table 27.7 Biomarker Performance in Detecting Chronic Kidney Disease (CKD): Multicenter Studies**

| Parameter | Diagnosis of CKD | Progression of CKD to ESRD | Cardiovascular and Mortality Risk Assessment in CKD | Progression of HIV-Associated CKD |
|---|---|---|---|---|
| Urine NGAL | + | – | ? | ? |
| Blood NGAL | + | – | ? | ? |
| Blood CysC | + | + | + | + |
| Urine IL-18 | – | ? | ? | + |
| Urine KIM-1 | + | + | ? | – |
| Plasma KIM-1 | + | + | ? | ? |
| β-Trace protein | – | ? | + | ? |
| Urine protein and albumin | + | + | + | + |
| FGF23 | – | + | + | ? |
| TNFR1, R2 | + | + | ? | ? |
| suPAR | + | + | ? | ? |
| EGF | + | + | ? | ? |

*CysC*, Cystatin C; *EGF*, epidermal growth factor; *ESRD*, end-stage renal disease; *FGF23*, fibroblast growth factor 23; *IL-18*, interleukin-18; *KIM-1*, kidney injury molecule-1; *NGAL*, neutrophil gelatinase-associated lipocalin; *suPAR*, soluble urokinase-type plasminogen activator receptor; *TNFR*, tumor necrosis factor receptor; *+*, data published display the ability to detect this aspect of CKD; *–*, data published do not display the ability to detect this aspect of CKD; *?*, no large multicenter data published on this biomarker or aspect of CKD.

More recently, larger longitudinal studies have been performed linking ADMA with several forms of CKD and CKD outcomes. In a nested case-control study performed in the Genetics of Diabetes Audit and Research Tayside Study (GO-DARTS), ADMA and several other biomarkers were measured to determine their association with CKD progression in patients with type 2 diabetes.[446] In this study, progression of CKD was defined by a 40% or greater reduction in baseline eGFR over the 3.5-year study period, whereas in controls the eGFR decreased by less than 5% over this same period. ADMA levels were strongly associated with CKD progression in an analysis adjusted for clinical variables known to affect CKD progression, as well as several other biomarkers. Higher ADMA levels were associated with more rapid progression of CKD; for each standard deviation change in ADMA levels there was an increased adjusted odds of 8.36 (3.83–20.4; $P < .001$. This effect was larger than any of the other 14 biomarkers that they measured in this cohort, including KIM-1 (1.93 [1.18–3.27]; $P = .011$) and H-FABP (0.63 [0.38–1.02]; $P = .06$).[446] In a prospective observational cohort of 1157 patients (663 with diabetic kidney disease, 273 with glomerulonephritis, and 221 with cystic and/or interstitial disease), ADMA levels were measured to determine their association with mortality prior to the initiation of RRT. ADMA levels were associated with an increased risk of mortality in both the diabetic cohort (HR, 1.3 [1.1–1.6]) and the glomerulonephritis cohort (HR, 1.5 [ 1.3–1.8]).[447] Despite these emerging data, larger longitudinal studies are needed to demonstrate the ability of ADMA to identify CKD and predict its progression in cohorts with CKD due to multiple causes.

## FIBROBLAST GROWTH FACTOR 23

Fibroblast growth factor 23 (FGF23) is a 32-kDa protein consisting of 251 amino acids coded by the FGF gene located on chromosome 12 in the human genome. FGF23 serves as a endocrine hormone that is secreted by osteoblasts and osteoclasts, which binds a FGF receptor and its coreceptor Klotho and stimulates phosphaturia.[448–450] In addition to promoting phosphaturia, FGF23 also decreases levels of 1,25-dihydroxy vitamin D, as well as parathyroid hormone (PTH).[451,452] Several cross-sectional studies have demonstrated that FGF23 levels are elevated in both adult and pediatric CKD populations.[453–455] In a prospective observational study of 3879 subjects in CRIC, FGF23 levels were shown to be increased in individuals with CKD stages 2 to 4, with FGF23 elevation occurring in the absence of abnormalities in serum phosphate and PTH.[456] As such, FGF23 has emerged as a candidate biomarker to detect CKD and abnormalities of bone mineral metabolism in the absence of changes in serum phosphate and PTH.

Apart from bone, FGF23 is principally expressed in the ventrolateral thalamic nucleus in mice and is also known be secreted in minimal amounts in the liver, heart, thymus, and lymph node. Maintenance of phosphate homeostasis is carried out by the sodium-dependent phosphate cotransporters NaPi-IIa and NaPi-IIc at the brush border membrane of proximal tubule cells in kidney, and FGF23 has been shown to regulate the activity of these transporters.[457,458]

FGF23 is increased in CKD and is a prognostic indicator for cardiovascular disease in patients with CKD.[459] In a recent analysis of 3860 participants of CRIC, FGF23 levels in the highest quartiles (compared with the lowest) were independently associated with a graded risk of congestive heart failure (HR, 2.98 [95% CI 1.97–4.52]) and atherosclerotic events 1.76 (95% CI, 1.20–2.59), even after adjustment for eGFR, proteinuria, and other traditional cardiovascular risk factors.[460] Other studies have shown that elevated plasma FGF23 concentrations are associated with cardiovascular events in patients not requiring dialysis, as well as with mortality in patients receiving hemodialysis, with levels in those with ESRD reaching nearly 1000-fold above normal.[461] Interestingly, FGF23 levels have also been shown to decline rapidly in individuals with prompt allograft function in the setting of renal transplantation.[462,463] It has been reported that serum FGF23 concentrations may be a useful marker for predicting the future development of refractory hyperparathyroidism and the response to vitamin D therapy in patients receiving dialysis.[464] Similarly, FGF23 may be useful in the evaluation of calcium, phosphate, and vitamin D disorders in early-stage CKD in pediatric as well as adult patients.[465,466] Lowering FGF23 levels (e.g., with oral phosphate binders) may reduce cardiovascular morbidity in CKD patients,[467] although further studies are required to investigate this further. For further discussion of FGF23, see Chapter 53.

## SOLUBLE UROKINASE-TYPE PLASMINOGEN ACTIVATOR RECEPTOR

Although there has long been a connection between soluble urokinase-type plasminogen activator receptor (suPAR) and CKD in the setting of focal segmental glomerulosclerosis (FSGS) and other glomerular disease, this biomarker has been associated more broadly with CKD. For more on the role of suPAR in the setting of FSGS and other glomerulonephritides, see Chapter 31. suPAR is the circulating form of a glycosyl-phosphatidylinositol–anchored, three-domain membrane protein that is expressed on a variety of cells, including endothelial cells and podocytes.[468] There are circulating and bound forms of this protein, with the circulating form being produced through the cleavage of the membrane-bound form, thus making it detectable in several body fluids, including urine.[468,469] It has been proposed that soluble urokinase-type plasminogen activator receptor (suPAR) contributes to the pathogenesis of kidney disease in the setting of FGSS as well as diabetic nephropathy through the prevention of podocyte migration and apoptosis.[470,471] Although many of the specifics of these mechanisms remain an area of intense investigation, testing of human samples for suPAR has begun to yield interesting results.

Recently, Hayek and colleagues published a seminal paper measuring plasma suPAR levels in 3683 patients enrolled in the Emory Cardiovascular Biobank.[472] They then determined baseline and follow-up renal function in 2292 of these patients to determine the relationship between suPAR and baseline GFR, change in GFR, and development of CKD (defined as eGFR < 60 mL/min/1.73 m$^2$). Higher baseline suPAR levels were associated with a greater decline in eGFR/year. Patients in the highest quartile of baseline suPAR lost over four times as much eGFR/year compared with those in the lowest quartile (−4.2 mL/min compared with −0.9 mL/min). Similarly, the risk of progressing to an eGFR < 60 mL/min over the study period was 3.13 (2.11–4.65]) in those participants in the highest suPAR quartile compared with the lowest quartile ($n = 1335$ total patients who started with an eGFR > 60 mL/min). Although suPAR appears to be independently associated with the development and progression of CKD, further studies are needed to validate these findings.

## URINARY RENAL FIBROSIS MARKERS

Excessive production of extracellular matrix (collagen IV) and profibrotic growth factors including CTGF and TGF-β1 have been implicated in the progression of renal fibrosis. Several reviews on the ability of renal fibrosis markers to predict patient outcomes have been published.[473]

### CONNECTIVE TISSUE GROWTH FACTOR

CTGF (also known as "CCN2"), a member of CCN family of matricellular proteins, was first discovered by Bradham and colleagues in 1991 as a secreted protein in the conditioned media of human umbilical vascular endothelial cells.[474] CTGF has been implicated in a variety of cellular functions, including proliferation, cell adhesion, angiogenesis, and wound healing.[440,475,476] Accumulated evidence on CTFG in the past few years has indicated that CTGF is both a marker and a mediator of tissue fibrosis.[477] CTGF is an immediate early gene potently induced by TGF-β and shown to promote fibrosis primarily through TGF-β.[478] CTGF is overexpressed in several fibrotic diseases, such as scleroderma and lung and hepatic fibrosis.[479–481] In the kidney, CTGF expression has been shown to be upregulated in various forms of renal disease, including IgA nephropathy, focal and segmental glomerulosclerosis, and diabetic nephropathy.[480] CTGF has been found to be elevated in the glomeruli at early and late stages of diabetic nephropathy.[482] Riser and associates first reported that CTGF is elevated in the urine of diabetic rats and in persons with diabetes.[483] Subsequently, several groups have reported higher urinary levels of CTGF in persons with diabetes than in healthy individuals,[484,485] which indicates its potential as a marker for diabetic nephropathy. In persons with diabetes, plasma CTGF levels were shown to be higher in those with macroalbuminuria than in those with a normal urine albumin level. CTGF was an independent predictor of ESRD and correlated with the rate of decline in the GFR.[486] In another study, both blood and urine levels of intact CTGF and the N-terminal fragment were measured in 1050 patients with type 1 diabetes from the Diabetes Control and Complications Trial/Epidemiology of Diabetes Interventions and Complication (DCCT/EDIC).[487] Patients with macroalbuminuria had higher plasma levels of CTGF N-terminal fragment than those with or without microalbuminuria. Intact CTGF levels were associated with the duration of diabetes, as well as common carotid artery intima media thickness. Additionally, in regression analyses, log plasma CTGF N-terminal fragment concentrations were independently associated with the intima thickness of the common and internal carotid artery. Plasma CTGF concentration therefore serves as a risk marker for diabetic renal and vascular diseases.

More recently, urinary CTGF has been investigated for its ability to detect renal allograft fibrosis in a cohort of 315 transplant recipients.[488] Following this cohort for 2 years, Metalidis and colleagues compared CTGF concentrations with protocol biopsies at 3, 12, and 24 months posttransplantation. Urinary CTGF levels were independently associated with the degree of interstitial fibrosis.[488] In a subset of patients, CTGF levels at 3 months were associated with long-term moderate and severe fibrosis at the 24-month time point.

### TRANSFORMING GROWTH FACTOR-$\beta_1$

TGF-β is essential for the development and differentiation of various tissues.[489] Three isoforms of TGF-β have been identified in mammalian species—TGF-$\beta_1$, TGF-$\beta_2$, and TGF-$\beta_3$. TGF-$\beta_1$ is the predominant isoform in humans.[490] It is mainly secreted as a high-molecular- weight inactive complex and undergoes a cleavage process for its activation.[491] Several studies have demonstrated the association of urine levels of TGF-$\beta_1$ with the progression of CKD. Elevated urinary TGF-$\beta_1$ levels were found in patients with glomerulonephritis and diabetic nephropathy, as well as in renal allograft recipients.[491–494] In addition, some of the profibrotic molecules induced by TGF-$\beta_1$, including TGF-β–inducible gene H3 (*βig-H3*) and plasminogen activator inhibitor-1 (PAI-1), were also detected at high levels in the urine.[495,496] Because TGF-$\beta_1$ is mostly secreted as an inactive complex that requires chemical modification for its activation, βig-H3 and PAI-1 can be used as surrogate markers for TGF-$\beta_1$ activity. Urinary levels of both *βig-H3* and PAI-1 have been shown to correlate with renal injury and fibrosis in patients with diabetic nephropathy.[495,496] However, in a study of 3939 participants from the CRIC study, TGF-β levels were not shown to be significantly associated with CKD progression or the presence of macroalbuminuria.[497] This is in comparison with a much smaller case-control study looking at TGF-β in the setting of pediatric obstructive nephropathy (posterior urethral valves), in which TGF-β levels were shown to be inversely correlated with the GFR.[498]

In the Action in Diabetes and Vascular Disease: Preterax and Diamicron Modified Release Controlled Evaluation (ADVANCE) collaborative group, the addition of serum TGF-β to traditional predictors of CKD progression (e.g., diabetes, uACR, baseline eGFR) improved the prediction of doubling of serum creatinine over a 5-year follow-up period.[499] In this nested case-control study, addition of serum TGF-β significantly increased the AUC from 0.75 to 0.82 ($P < .0001$). Other more recent studies have demonstrated that urinary TGF-β can assist in determining which kidneys will recover function following unilateral obstruction.[500] In a small study of 45 subjects (11 of whom did not regain function), TGF-β levels at the time of enrollment were lower in those who went on to recover function.

### COLLAGEN IV

Collagen IV is a component of the extracellular matrix, and excess deposition of collagen IV is present in renal fibrosis. Furthermore, elevation of urinary collagen IV has been reported in patients with IgA nephropathy, as well as in those with diabetic nephropathy, and has been correlated with declining renal function.[501,502] In a prospective observational cohort study of 231 normoalbuminuric and microalbuminuric patients with type 1 diabetes, urinary collagen IV was significantly associated with a decline in the eGFR over time in both univariate and multivariate analyses, with collagen IV levels being elevated in those with the lower GFRs.[503]

### TUMOR NECROSIS FACTOR RECEPTORS

TNF is produced by immune cells and can either be membrane-bound or in a soluble circulating peptide.[504] TNF cell surface receptors have two forms (TNFR1 and TNFR2), both of which can be cleaved from the membrane with a TNF-α cleaving enzyme. TNFR1 is expressed in glomeruli and endothelial cells, and TNFR2 is variably expressed in renal cells.[505] Increasingly, both receptors have been associated with adverse outcomes in the setting of kidney disease.[262,506]

Pavkov and colleagues performed a longitudinal cohort study in Native Americans with type 2 diabetes, following them for a median duration of 9.5 years.[506] Of a total of 193 participants, 62 developed ESRD and 25 died during the follow-up period. In an age- and gender-adjusted analysis, the highest quartile of TNFR1 and TNFR2 (compared with the lowest) was associated with an increased risk of ESRD, OR of 6.6 (3.3–13.3) and 8.8 (4.3–18.0), respectively. In more complex adjusted models (including both ACR and baseline GFR) the highest quartiles of TNFR1 and TNFR2 were associated with a 60% and 70% increased risk for ESRD compared with the lowest.[506]

More recently, Coca and colleagues measured TGFR1 and TGFR2 in subjects from the Action to Control Cardiovascular Risk in Diabetes (ACCORD) and Veterans Administration NEPHROpathy iN Diabetes (VA-NEPHRON-D) cohorts.[262] They demonstrated that receptor levels were independently associated with increased decline in GFR in persons with diabetic kidney disease. In the ACCORD cohort, which enrolled subjects with early diabetic kidney disease, those who developed incident CKD had higher TNFR1 and TNFR2 levels at the time of study enrollment. Similarly, in adjusted analyses, the fourth quartiles of TNFR1 and TNFR2 (compared with lowest quartile) were both associated with increased risk of incident CKD (OR, 95 CI%, 3.0 [1.2–7.3] and 8.4 [3.0–23.4], respectively).[262] In the NEPHRON-D study, the fourth quartiles of TNFR1 and TNFR2 (compared with the lowest quartile) were again associated with the primary endpoint, CKD progression. The highest quartile of TNFR1 was associated with an adjusted odds of 3.5 (1.9–6.3) for the progression of CKD, and this effect was even larger for TNFR2 (3.8 [2.0–7.3]).[262] TNFR1 and TNFR2 were highly correlated with each other in these two cohorts (Pearson correlation coefficient > 0.75). Thus, in several cohorts with diabetic kidney disease, TNFR1 and TNFR2 levels were associated with the development and progression of CKD.

### EPIDERMAL GROWTH FACTOR

As a well-established growth factor, EGF has been shown to alter the kidney's response to tubulointerstitial injury,[507] with exogenous EGF improving outcomes in the setting of animal models of AKI.[508] However, in a recent investigation of CKD progression using a renal biopsy transcriptome-driven approach, EGF was shown to be an excellent biomarker of CKD progression, defined as the composite of a 40% reduction from baseline eGFR or the development of ESRD.[509] Intrarenal transcripts of EGF expression were correlated with baseline eGFR and patient outcomes in 164 patients from the European Renal cDNA Bank (ERCB). In this cohort, intrarenal EGF correlated with several other measures and outcomes, including urinary EGF, interstitial fibrosis and tubular atrophy, and eGFR loss. The authors were able to replicate these results in two separate CKD cohorts ($n = 55$ and $n = 48$; different samples from the ERCB cohort and Clinical Phenotyping Resource and Biobank Core [C-PROBE]).[509] Adding urine EGF to a model containing age, gender, baseline eGFR, and albuminuria significantly improved the C-statistic for the prediction of CKD progression from 0.75 to 0.87. This seminal report on EGF will be followed up with future investigations that will attempt to link this novel biomarker further with the development and incidence of progressive CKD.

## COMBINATIONS OF MULTIPLE BIOMARKERS

In the classic biomarker paradigm, one biomarker detects one disease. However, acute and chronic kidney diseases are complex, with multiple underlying causes. A single biomarker may not be optimal to make an early diagnosis and predict the longer-term outcome of the disease process. Different biomarkers provide different sets of information. As discussed above, some biomarkers excel at detecting AKI in different clinical settings (cardiac surgery vs. ICU vs. ER vs. other), whereas others detect different aspects of AKI (early diagnosis vs. AKI severity vs. prerenal). This same phenomenon is true of CKD biomarkers, with some being more likely to detect CKD in the setting of diabetes versus obstruction versus other forms of glomerulonephritis. Thus, it is important to consider the clinical utility of a panel of biomarkers for acute and chronic kidney diseases.

It is becoming increasingly clear, based in part on the evidence discussed above, that multiple biomarkers are already a viable option in the care of patients with CKD. The serum creatinine level can be used in conjunction with cystatin C for the detection and diagnosis of CKD. Proteinuria and albuminuria can be used in combination with these two markers of glomerular function to diagnose and risk-stratify individuals further. Recall that in the setting of normal serum creatinine and serum cystatin C levels, the presence of albuminuria constitutes a diagnosis of CKD.

The use of multiple biomarkers in the setting of AKI has been an area of increased investigation, with several studies attempting to combine two or more biomarkers to improve their predictive capabilities.[242,243,265,322,330] Although some studies have simply used the product of two biomarkers and then assessed the AUC, others have used logistic regression models to assess the AUC for two or more biomarkers. There has not been a consensus for the statistical methods for combining biomarkers, and this remains an area of continued investigation. More recent studies have acknowledged the aforementioned premise that individual biomarkers will have their own specific kinetics, and that combining biomarkers from different time points may improve their predictive capabilities.[243] However, the clinical implications and feasibility of collecting biomarker samples at several distinct time points following cardiac surgery or ICU admission remain untested. As more and more biomarker data are amassed, we anticipate advances in novel methods for assessing biomarker combinations. Box 27.3 summarizes a variety of rationales and approaches to combining biomarker results in the hope of achieving improved prediction of patient outcomes.

## CRITICAL PATH INITIATIVE: A NEED FOR BETTER BIOMARKERS

The Critical Path Initiative was launched in March 2004 by the FDA as a strategy for modernizing the sciences through which FDA-regulated products are developed, evaluated, manufactured, and used. In 2006, the Critical Path Initiative

**Box 27.3 Strategies for Biomarker Combination**

- Combine for different functions:
  - Combine a marker of filtration with one of tubular injury.
  - Combine a marker of proximal tubular injury with a marker of distal tubular injury.
- Combine for kinetics:
  - Combine biomarkers with different time courses to improve the duration of diagnosis.
- Combine for improved accuracy:
  - Use two or more biomarkers in statistical equations.
- Strategic combinations:
  - Combine a diagnostic biomarker with a prognostic biomarker.
  - Combine an extremely sensitive marker with an extremely specific marker.

outlined specific key areas of critical path focus identified by FDA experts and the public. Since that time, the FDA has provided guidelines stating that a biomarker can be considered "valid" only if (1) it is measured in an analytic test system, with well-established performance characteristics, and (2) there is an established scientific framework or body of evidence that elucidates the physiologic, pharmacologic, toxicologic, or clinical significance of the test result. Over the past decade there have been a few advancements in the development and approval of biomarkers of AKI and CKD.

In 2010, seven urinary proteins (KIM-1, albumin, total protein, $\beta_2$-microglobulin, cystatin C, clusterin, and trefoil factor 3) were evaluated for their utility to outperform current tests, including serum creatinine concentration and BUN concentration, in the detection of drug-induced kidney injury. The FDA and EMA qualified this panel of biomarkers for use in regulatory decision making for drug safety to detect acute drug-induced kidney injury in preclinical studies and, on a case-by-case basis, in early clinical studies in combination with standard biomarkers.[24,25,510,511] More recently, the FDA has approved total kidney volume in the setting of polycystic kidney disease as a marker of disease progression.[22] Given the aforementioned work investigating several promising biomarkers of AKI and CKD, there will undoubtedly be additionally measures approved in the next several years.

## KIDNEY HEALTH INITIATIVE

In response to the epidemic of CKD and AKI and the limited number of randomized controlled trials, the FDA, American Society of Nephrology, and their industry partners announced the founding of the Kidney Health Initiative (KHI) in 2013. This public-private partnership was designed to foster collaborations to optimize the evaluation of drugs, devices, biologics and food products in the greater kidney community. This initiative is intended to facilitate the delivery of these products to the U.S. market in a safe and expeditious manner.[512] Despite the growing evidence of their ability to predict AKI, CKD progression, and other adverse patient outcomes, no new biomarkers have been approved in the United States for clinical use; as such, it remains to be seen how this new initiative will affect the biomarker field.

## FUTURE OF BIOMARKERS

Recent advances in molecular analysis and proteomics have resulted in the identification of a wide range of potential serum and urine biomarkers for assessing renal function and injury, as well as predicting the development of kidney disease. Not only are many of these biomarkers sensitive, but some are also site-specific. A number of them have been reported to be predictive of an adverse outcome. For some, a great deal of additional work is still needed, however, to bring the biomarkers successfully to clinical practice.

Because kidney disease is complex, with multiple causes, and often presents in the setting of systemic diseases, a single biomarker may be insufficient for early diagnosis, insight into pathophysiology, and prediction of clinical course and outcome. Different biomarkers will be useful in different contexts. In some circumstances, a single biomarker may suffice, but in others, benefit will come from the use of multiple biomarkers in plasma, urine, or both to provide early evidence of risk and injury, and to distinguish between various types of kidney diseases. Many of these biomarkers can be grouped according to their association with a particular type of injury (e.g., podocyte or tubular injury) or mechanism of damage (e.g., oxidative stress, inflammation, fibrosis). Understanding the relationships between these different biomarker categories may help us better understand disease processes.

These biomarkers are not only useful for accessing kidney injury in humans in its early stages and for predicting progression of disease, but also crucial for translating novel therapeutic compounds from preclinical animal models to first human trials. Until recently, the use of newly emerged biomarkers in preclinical and clinical studies and drug development has been hindered by lack of regulatory acceptance. Hopefully, in the future, biomarker measurements obtained using biomarker test panels will not only be used to diagnose kidney injury and predict outcome, but will also be used as surrogate endpoints in clinical trials, which might speed up clinical evaluation of desperately needed therapies for kidney diseases.

### ACKNOWLEDGMENTS

Dr. Parikh was supported by NIH grant RO1HL085757 to fund the TRIBE-AKI Consortium to study novel biomarkers of acute kidney injury in cardiac surgery. Dr. Parikh is also a member of the NIH-sponsored ASsess, Serial Evaluation, and Subsequent Sequelae in Acute Kidney Injury (ASSESS-AKI) Consortium (U01DK082185).

We wish to acknowledge and thank Drs. Joseph V. Bonventre and Venkata Sabbisetti, who wrote prior versions of this chapter.

## DISCLOSURE

Dr. Koyner reports research grants from Abbott Laboratories, Abbvie, and Astute Medical for conducting observational biomarker studies. Dr. Koyner has received research funding from Argutus Medical, Satellite Medical HealthCare, and NxStage Medical and has received consulting fees from Pfizer, Astute Medical, and Sphingotec

 Complete reference list available at ExpertConsult.com.

## KEY REFERENCES


14. Biomarkers Definitions Working Group. Biomarkers and surrogate endpoints: preferred definitions and conceptual framework. *Clin Pharmacol Ther.* 2001;69(3):89–95.
16. Pepe MS, Etzioni R, Feng Z, et al. Phases of biomarker development for early detection of cancer. *J Natl Cancer Inst.* 2001;93:8.
21. Waikar SS, et al. Imperfect gold standards for kidney injury biomarker evaluation. *J Am Soc Nephrol.* 2012;23(22021710):13–21.
39. Kidney Disease: Improving Global Outcomes (KDIGO) Acute Kidney Injury Work Group. KDIGO clinical practice guideline for acute kidney injury. *Kidney Int.* 2012;Supp(2):1–138.
40. Chawla LS, et al. Acute kidney disease and renal recovery: consensus report of the Acute Disease Quality Initiative (ADQI) 16 Workgroup. *Nat Rev Nephrol.* 2017;13(4):241–257.
41. Haase M, et al. The outcome of neutrophil gelatinase-associated lipocalin-positive subclinical acute kidney injury: a multicenter pooled analysis of prospective studies. *J Am Coll Cardiol.* 2011;57(17):1752–1761.
62. Lin J, et al. False-positive rate of AKI using consensus creatinine-based criteria. *Clin J Am Soc Nephrol.* 2015;10(10):1723–1731.
94. Shlipak MG, et al. Cystatin C and the risk of death and cardiovascular events among elderly persons. *N Engl J Med.* 2005;352(15901858):2049–2060.
100. Inker LA, et al. Estimating glomerular filtration rate from serum creatinine and cystatin C. *N Engl J Med.* 2012;367(1):20–29.
115. Zappitelli M, et al. Early postoperative serum cystatin C predicts severe acute kidney injury following pediatric cardiac surgery. *Kidney Int.* 2011;80(6):655–662.
159. Perazella MA, et al. Urine microscopy is associated with severity and worsening of acute kidney injury in hospitalized patients. *Clin J Am Soc Nephrol.* 2010;5(20089493):402–408.
176. Nickolas TL, et al. Sensitivity and specificity of a single emergency department measurement of urinary neutrophil gelatinase-associated lipocalin for diagnosing acute kidney injury. *Ann Intern Med.* 2008;148(11):810–819.
209. Parikh CR, et al. Urinary interleukin-18 is a marker of human acute tubular necrosis. *Am J Kidney Dis.* 2004;43(14981598):405–414.
210. Parikh CR, et al. Postoperative biomarkers predict acute kidney injury and poor outcomes after adult cardiac surgery. *J Am Soc Nephrol.* 2011;22(9):1748–1757.
211. Parikh CR, et al. Postoperative biomarkers predict acute kidney injury and poor outcomes after pediatric cardiac surgery. *J Am Soc Nephrol.* 2011;22(9):1737–1747.
213. Koyner JL, et al. Biomarkers predict progression of acute kidney injury after cardiac surgery. *J Am Soc Nephrol.* 2012.
214. Coca SG, et al. Urinary biomarkers of AKI and mortality 3 years after cardiac surgery. *J Am Soc Nephrol.* 2014;25(5):1063–1071.
215. Siew ED, et al. Elevated urinary IL-18 levels at the time of ICU admission predict adverse clinical outcomes. *Clin J Am Soc Nephrol.* 2010;5(8):1497–1505.
216. Endre ZH, et al. Improved performance of urinary biomarkers of acute kidney injury in the critically ill by stratification for injury duration and baseline renal function. *Kidney Int.* 2011;79(10): 1119–1130.
217. Nejat M, et al. Some biomarkers of acute kidney injury are increased in pre-renal acute injury. *Kidney Int.* 2012.
219. Nickolas TL, et al. Diagnostic and prognostic stratification in the emergency department using urinary biomarkers of nephron damage: a multicenter prospective cohort study. *J Am Coll Cardiol.* 2012;59(3):246–255.
223. Hall IE, et al. Association between peritransplant kidney injury biomarkers and 1-year allograft outcomes. *Clin J Am Soc Nephrol.* 2012.
231. Han WK, et al. Kidney injury molecule-1 (KIM-1): a novel biomarker for human renal proximal tubule injury. *Kidney Int.* 2002;62:237–244.
243. Parikh CR, et al. Performance of kidney injury molecule-1 and liver fatty acid-binding protein and combined biomarkers of AKI after cardiac surgery. *Clin J Am Soc Nephrol.* 2013.
248. Ko GJ, et al. Transcriptional analysis of kidneys during repair from AKI reveals possible roles for NGAL and KIM-1 as biomarkers of AKI-to-CKD transition. *Am J Physiol Renal Physiol.* 2010;298(6):F1472–F1483.
262. Coca SG, et al. Plasma biomarkers and kidney function decline in early and established diabetic kidney disease. *J Am Soc Nephrol.* 2017.
263. Susantitaphong P, et al. Performance of urinary liver-type fatty acid-binding protein in acute kidney injury: a meta-analysis. *Am J Kidney Dis.* 2013;61(3):430–439.
267. Schaub JA, et al. Perioperative heart-type fatty acid binding protein is associated with acute kidney injury after cardiac surgery. *Kidney Int.* 2015;88(3):576–583.
290. Moledina DG, et al. Plasma monocyte chemotactic protein-1 is associated with acute kidney injury and death after cardiac operations. *Ann Thorac Surg.* 2017.
322. Kashani K, et al. Discovery and validation of cell cycle arrest biomarkers in human acute kidney injury. *Crit Care.* 2013;17(1):R25.
327. Di Somma S, et al. Additive value of blood neutrophil gelatinase-associated lipocalin to clinical judgement in acute kidney injury diagnosis and mortality prediction in patients hospitalized from the emergency department. *Crit Care.* 2013;17(1):R29.
335. Mishra J, et al. Neutrophil gelatinase-associated lipocalin (NGAL) as a biomarker for acute renal injury after cardiac surgery. *Lancet.* 2005;365(9466):1231–1238.
344. Liu KD, et al. Urine neutrophil gelatinase-associated lipocalin levels do not improve risk prediction of progressive chronic kidney disease. *Kidney Int.* 2013;83(5):909–914.
363. James M, Hemmelgarn B, Wiebe N. Glomerular filtration rate, proteinuria, and the incidence and consequences of acute kidney injury: a cohort study. *Lancet.* 2010;376:8.
364. Hsu C-P, Ordonez J, Chertow GM. The risk of acute renal failure in patients with chronic kidney disease. *Kidney Int.* 2008;74:7.
395. Ng LL, et al. Proenkephalin, renal dysfunction, and prognosis in patients with acute heart failure: a GREAT Network study. *J Am Coll Cardiol.* 2017;69(1):56–69.
400. Hoste EA, et al. Derivation and validation of cutoffs for clinical use of cell cycle arrest biomarkers. *Nephrol Dial Transplant.* 2014;29(11):2054–2061.
401. Bihorac A, et al. Validation of cell-cycle arrest biomarkers for acute kidney injury using clinical adjudication. *Am J Respir Crit Care Med.* 2014;189(8):932–939.
419. Chawla LS, et al. Development and standardization of a furosemide stress test to predict the severity of acute kidney injury. *Crit Care.* 2013;17(5):R207.
420. Koyner JL, et al. Furosemide stress test and biomarkers for the prediction of AKI severity. *J Am Soc Nephrol.* 2015;26(8):2023–2031.
423. Bhatraju P, et al. Associations between single nucleotide polymorphisms in the FAS pathway and acute kidney injury. *Crit Care.* 2015;19:368.
425. Zhao B, et al. A genome-wide association study to identify single-nucleotide polymorphisms for acute kidney injury. *Am J Respir Crit Care Med.* 2017;195(4):482–490.
460. Scialla JJ, et al. Fibroblast growth factor-23 and cardiovascular events in CKD. *J Am Soc Nephrol.* 2014;25(2):349–360.
461. Isakova T, et al. Fibroblast growth factor 23 in patients undergoing peritoneal dialysis. *Clin J Am Soc Nephrol.* 2011;6(11):2688–2695.
471. Wei C, et al. Circulating urokinase receptor as a cause of focal segmental glomerulosclerosis. *Nat Med.* 2011;17(8):952–960.
472. Hayek SS, et al. Soluble urokinase receptor and chronic kidney disease. *N Engl J Med.* 2015;373(20):1916–1925.
488. Metalidis C, et al. Urinary connective tissue growth factor is associated with human renal allograft fibrogenesis. *Transplantation.* 2013;96(5):494–500.
499. Wong MG, et al. Circulating bone morphogenetic protein-7 and transforming growth factor-beta1 are better predictors of renal end points in patients with type 2 diabetes mellitus. *Kidney Int.* 2013;83(2):278–284.
509. Ju W, et al. Tissue transcriptome-driven identification of epidermal growth factor as a chronic kidney disease biomarker. *Sci Transl Med.* 2015;7(316):316.
513. Koyner JL, Parikh CR. Clinical utility of biomarkers of AKI in cardiac surgery and critical illness. *Clin J Am Soc Nephrol.* 2013;8(6):1034–1042.

# DISORDERS OF KIDNEY STRUCTURE AND FUNCTION

SECTION V

# 28 Pathophysiology of Acute Kidney Injury

Mark Douglas Okusa | Didier Portilla

CHAPTER OUTLINE



## PATHOPHYSIOLOGY OF CLINICAL ACUTE KIDNEY INJURY

The three major pathophysiologic categories—namely, prerenal, intrinsic, and postrenal (obstructive)—provide a framework for understanding the mechanisms of acute kidney injury (AKI).

### PRERENAL ACUTE KIDNEY INJURY

Prerenal azotemia is the most common cause of AKI, accounting for approximately 40% to 55% of all cases.[1–3] It results from kidney hypoperfusion due to reductions in actual or effective arterial blood volume (EABV—the volume of blood effectively perfusing the body organs). Common conditions causing true hypovolemia include hemorrhage (traumatic, gastrointestinal, surgical), gastrointestinal (GI) losses (vomiting, diarrhea, nasogastric suction), renal losses (overdiuresis, diabetes insipidus), and third spacing (pancreatitis, hypoalbuminemia). In addition, cardiogenic shock, septic shock, cirrhosis, hypoalbuminemia, and anaphylaxis all are pathophysiologic conditions that decrease EABV, independent of total body volume status, resulting in reduced renal blood flow. Prerenal azotemia reverses rapidly if renal perfusion is restored because, by definition, the integrity of the renal parenchyma has remained intact. However, severe and prolonged hypoperfusion may result in tissue ischemia, leading to acute tubular necrosis (ATN). Therefore, prerenal azotemia and ischemic ATN are part of a spectrum of manifestations of renal hypoperfusion.

Prerenal azotemia has also been divided into volume-responsive and volume-nonresponsive forms. The former is easy to comprehend, but the latter is less straightforward. In volume-nonresponsive forms, additional intravenous volume is of no help in restoring kidney perfusion and function. Disease processes such as congestive heart failure, liver failure, and sepsis may not respond to intravenous fluids because markedly reduced cardiac output or total vascular resistance, respectively, prevent improved kidney function.

True or effective hypovolemia causes a decrease in mean arterial pressure that activates baroreceptors and initiates a cascade of neural and humoral responses, leading to activation of the sympathetic nervous system and increased production of catecholamines, especially norepinephrine. There is increased release of antidiuretic hormone, mediated primarily by hypovolemia, resulting in vasoconstriction, water retention, and urea back diffusion into the papillary interstitium. In response to volume depletion or states of decreased EABV, there is increased intrarenal angiotensin II (Ang II) activity via activation of the renin-angiotensin-aldosterone system (RAAS). Ang II is a very potent vasoconstrictor that preferentially increases efferent arteriolar resistance, preserving glomerular filtration rate (GFR) in the setting of decreased renal perfusion through the maintenance of glomerular hydrostatic pressure. In addition, Ang II increases proximal tubular sodium absorption through a combination of alterations in hydrostatic forces in the peritubular capillaries and through direct activation of sodium-hydrogen exchangers. During severe volume depletion, Ang II activity is even greater, leading to afferent arteriolar constriction, which reduces renal plasma flow, GFR, and the filtration fraction, and markedly augments proximal tubular sodium reabsorption in an effort to restore plasma volume.[4] Ang II has also been shown to have direct effects on transport in the proximal tubule through receptors located in the proximal tubule. It has also been postulated that the proximal tubule can produce Ang II locally. Hence, under conditions of volume depletion, Ang II stimulates a larger fraction of tubular transport, whereas volume expansion will blunt this response.[5–9]

Renal sympathetic nerve activity is significantly increased in prerenal azotemia. Studies have shown that in the setting of hypovolemia, adrenergic activity independently constricts the afferent arteriole and changes the efferent arteriolar resistance through Ang II. $\alpha_1$-Adrenergic activity primarily influences kidney vascular resistance, whereas renal nerve activity is linked to renin release through β-adrenergic receptors on renin-containing cells. In contrast, $\alpha_2$-adrenergic agonists primarily decrease the glomerular ultrafiltration coefficient via Ang II. Although vasodilation might be expected as a result of acute removal of adrenergic activity, a transient increase in Ang II is actually seen, maintaining GFR and renal blood flow. Even after subacute renal denervation, renal vascular sensitivity increases to Ang II as a result of major upregulation of Ang II receptors. Hence complex effects on renin-angiotensin activity occur within the kidney secondary to increased renal adrenergic activity during prerenal azotemia.[10]

All these systems work together and stimulate vasoconstriction in musculocutaneous and splanchnic circulations, inhibit salt loss through sweat, and stimulate thirst, thereby causing retention of salt and water to maintain blood pressure and preserve cardiac output and cerebral perfusion. Concomitantly, there are various compensatory mechanisms to preserve glomerular perfusion.[11] Autoregulation is achieved by stretch receptors in afferent arterioles that cause vasodilation in response to reduced perfusion pressure. Under physiologic conditions, autoregulation works only to a mean systemic arterial blood pressure of 75 to 80 mm Hg. Below this level, the glomerular ultrafiltration pressure and GFR decline abruptly. Renal production of prostaglandins, kallikrein, and kinins, as well as nitric oxide (NO), is increased, contributing to the vasodilation.[12,13] Nonsteroidal antiinflammatory drugs (NSAIDs), by inhibiting prostaglandin production, worsen kidney perfusion in patients with hypoperfusion. Selective efferent arteriolar constriction, a result of Ang II, helps preserve the intraglomerular pressure and hence the GFR. Angiotensin-converting enzyme (ACE) inhibitors inhibit synthesis of Ang II and therefore disturb this delicate balance in patients with severe reductions in EABV, such as severe congestive heart failure or bilateral renal artery stenosis and, in these settings, can worsen prerenal azotemia. On the other hand, very high levels of Ang II, as seen in circulatory shock, cause constriction of both afferent and efferent arterioles, negating its protective effect.

Although these compensatory mechanisms minimize the progression toward AKI, they too are overcome in states of severe hypoperfusion. Renovascular disease, hypertensive nephrosclerosis, diabetic nephropathy, and older age predispose patients to prerenal azotemia[14] at lesser degrees of hypotension.[14] Prerenal azotemia also predisposes patients to radiocontrast media–induced AKI and events such as anesthesia and surgery, which are known to result in further decreases in renal blood flow. Therefore it is imperative to diagnose prerenal azotemia promptly and initiate effective treatment because it is a potentially reversible condition that can lead to ischemic ATN and/or nephrotoxic AKI if therapy is delayed, or the severity of the condition increases. In patients with advanced liver disease and portal hypertension, the hepatorenal syndrome (HRS) represents an extreme form of prerenal disease, characterized by peripheral and splanchnic vasodilation, with intense intrarenal vasoconstriction unresponsive to volume resuscitation.[15–17] AKI can also result from abdominal compartment syndrome (ACS), characterized by a marked elevation in intraabdominal pressure, resulting in a clinical presentation with features similar to those of prerenal AKI.[18,19] A recent study in animal models of volume-responsive and intrinsic AKI used laser microdissection to isolate specific domains of the kidney, followed by RNA sequencing of the microdissected kidney tissue. Based on the gene expression profile, the investigators found different signal transduction pathways in the two models. Volume-responsive genes rapidly reverse with volume resuscitation, whereas intrinsic AKI genes did not change. These results suggest that volume-dependent AKI is not an attenuated form of intrinsic AKI.[20]

## INTRINSIC ACUTE KIDNEY INJURY

### DISEASES OF LARGE VESSELS AND MICROVASCULATURE

Total occlusion of the renal artery or vein is an uncommon event but can be seen in certain scenarios such as trauma, instrumentation, thromboemboli, thrombosis, and dissection of an aortic aneurysm. Stenosis of the renal artery is a slow chronic process, with or without evidence of declining GFR, and rarely presents as an acute event. Renal vein thrombosis has classically and frequently been associated with hypercoagulable states, including nephrotic syndrome, particularly when associated with membranous nephropathy. An atheroembolic source should be considered in patients who present with AKI after instrumentation with angiography, arteriography, or aortic surgery or after blunt trauma or acceleration-deceleration injury.[21] Cholesterol-laden atheroembolic plaques in the aorta or other larger arteries may become disrupted, and fragments may become trapped in smaller renal arteries, leading to hypoperfusion and an intense inflammatory reaction, akin to a vasculitis. Other organs may also be affected, leading to gastrointestinal ischemia, peripheral gangrene, livedo reticularis, and acute pancreatitis. Patients frequently develop fevers and exhibit eosinophilia, an elevated erythrocyte sedimentation rate, and hypocomplementemia, which sometimes help in differentiating this condition from other simultaneous insults (e.g., transient hypotension and/or radiocontrast media administration).

Renal artery thrombosis is usually a posttraumatic or postsurgical complication, especially in the transplantation setting, but can also occur in other hypercoagulable states, such as antiphospholipid antibody syndrome.[22–24] Diseases affecting the small vessels, generally termed *vasculitides*, include polyarteritis nodosa, necrotizing granulomatous vasculitis, hemolytic-uremic syndrome, thrombotic thrombocytopenic purpura, and malignant hypertension; they tend to occlude vessels by fibrin deposition, along with platelets. Endothelial cell damage leads to an inflammatory response in the renal microvasculature (and in other organs), leading to reduced microvascular blood flow and tissue ischemia, sometimes giving rise to superimposed ATN. One should keep in mind the intricate relationship among these inflammatory vasculitides and subsequent ischemic injury because even though the origin of these disease processes is located at a site distant from the tubules, the final result is often ATN if not treated early. Hence, virtually any disease that compromises blood flow within the renal microvasculature can induce AKI.

### DISEASES OF THE TUBULOINTERSTITIUM

Ischemic and septic ATN are the most common causes of intrinsic AKI. These are discussed extensively in later sections of the chapter on ATN. Other disorders of the tubulointerstitium causing AKI, such as acute allergic interstitial nephritis, drug-induced tubular toxicity, and endogenous toxins, are presented in the following sections.

### Interstitial Disease

Acute interstitial nephritis (AIN) results from an idiosyncratic allergic response to different pharmacologic agents, most commonly to antibiotics (e.g., methicillin and other penicillins, cephalosporins, sulfonamides, quinolones), NSAIDs (e.g., ibuprofen, naproxen),[25] chemotherapeutic agents,[26] and proton pump inhibitors..[27] Although evidence supports a role of vancomycin as a tubule toxin, most biopsy reports have described AIN.[28] The expanding list of newer targeted agents has led to more cases of acute tubulointerstitial injury. Serine-threonine protein kinase inhibitors such as vemurafenib and dabrafenib target a protein called B-Raf and have been associated with acute and chronic tubulointerstitial damage.[29] Other agents that cause acute tubulointerstitial injury include checkpoint inhibitors such as ipilimumab, nivolumab, and pembrolizumab. Programmed cell death protein 1 (PD-1), a checkpoint protein, is expressed on T cells, and PD-L1 is expressed on normal as well as cancer cells. Binding of PD-1 ligand to its receptor (PD-L1) blocks immune elimination by T cells. Cancer cells evade immune surveillance in part by this mechanism. Similarly, CTLA-4 is another checkpoint protein expressed on T cells that leads to self-tolerance and various forms of autoimmune injury, including acute interstitial injury.[30]

Other conditions such as leukemia, lymphoma, sarcoidosis, bacterial infections (e.g., *Escherichia coli*), and viral infections (e.g., cytomegalovirus) can also cause AIN, leading to AKI. Systemic allergic signs such as fever, rash, and eosinophilia are often present in antibiotic-associated AIN but are not usually present in NSAID-related AIN, in which lymphocytes tend to predominate.[31] The presence of inflammatory infiltrates within the interstitium is the key hallmark of AIN. These inflammatory infiltrates are often patchy and present most commonly in the deep cortex and outer medulla. Interstitial edema is typically seen with the infiltrates, and sometimes patchy tubular necrosis may be present in close proximity to areas with extensive inflammatory infiltrates.[25] The composition of cells in the interstitial infiltrate can suggest the cause of AIN. The presence of frequent eosinophils suggests a diagnosis of drug-induced AIN, whereas a high number of neutrophils favors bacterial infection, and a high number of plasma cells is dominant in immunoglobulin G4 (IgG4)–related tubulointerstitial nephritis and in renal allografts infected with polyomavirus.[32] Most cases of AIN are probably induced by extrarenal antigens being produced by drugs or infectious agents that may be able to induce AIN by the following: (1) binding to kidney structures; (2) modifying immunogenetics of native renal proteins; (3) mimicking renal antigens; or (4) precipitating as immune complexes and hence serving as the site of antibody- or cellular-mediated injury.[33] This reaction is triggered by many events, including activation of complement and release of inflammatory cytokines by T cells and phagocytes. In other cases, loss of tolerance from checkpoint inhibitors leads to immune-mediated inflammation and injury.[26]

### Tubular Disease—Exogenous Nephrotoxins

Nephrotoxic ATN is the second most common cause of intrinsic AKI. We shall briefly review the common drug nephrotoxicities in the context of AKI. The kidneys are vulnerable to toxicity due to the high blood flow, and they are the major elimination and metabolizing routes of many of these nephrotoxins. Furthermore, because of the medullary tonicity, the concentration of drugs within the tubular lumen increases along the nephron, exposing the tubules to toxic levels for a more prolonged exposure time. Several other well-known therapeutic agents, such as amphotericin B, vancomycin, acyclovir, indinavir, cidofovir, foscarnet, pentamidine, and ifosfamide, can all directly cause acute tubular injury and associated AKI.

**Radiocontrast Media–Induced Nephropathy.** Iodinated radiocontrast medium–induced nephropathy (CIN) is a common complication of radiologic or angiographic procedures. The incidence varies from 3% to 7% in patients without any risk factors but can be as high as 50% in patients with moderate to advanced chronic kidney disease (CKD). Other risk factors include diabetes mellitus, intravascular volume depletion, use of high-osmolality contrast media, advanced age, proteinuria, and anemia.[34,35]

Unlike many other forms of intrinsic tubular injury, radiocontrast medium–induced AKI is usually associated with urinary sodium retention and a fractional excretion of sodium ($FE_{Na}$) of less than 1%. AKI resulting from iodinated contrast media is typically nonoliguric and rarely requires dialysis. However, requirements for renal support, prolonged hospitalization, and increased mortality are associated with (although not necessarily caused by) this condition.

The pathophysiology of CIN likely consists of combined hypoxic and toxic renal tubular damage associated with renal endothelial dysfunction and altered microcirculation.[36,37] The administration of radiocontrast media causes vasoconstriction and markedly affects renal parenchymal oxygenation, especially in the outer medulla, as documented in various studies where the cortical $Po_2$ declined from 40 to 25 mm Hg and the medullary $Po_2$ fell from 26 to 30 mm Hg to 9 to 15 mm Hg.[37–39] Radiocontrast media injection leads to an abrupt but transient increase in renal plasma flow, GFR, and urinary output.[40] This effect is due to the hyperosmolar radiocontrast medium–enhancing solute delivery to the distal nephron and leads to increased oxygen consumption by enhanced tubular sodium reabsorption. Using video microscopy, it has also been documented that radiocontrast media markedly reduce inner medullary papillary blood flow, even to the extent of near-cessation of red blood cell (RBC) movement in papillary vessels, associated with RBC aggregation within the papillary vasa recta.[41] In isolated vasa recta from rats and humans, contrast medium applied to the lumen has led to constriction and enhanced vasa recta responses to Ang II.[42,43] However, it should be noted that there may be different patterns of response possibly related to the type, volume, and route of radiocontrast medium administration. Numerous neurohumoral mediators may contribute to the changes in renal microcirculation caused by radiocontrast medium injection. Intrarenal NO synthase activity, NO concentration, plasma endothelin, adenosine, prostaglandins, and vasopressin are all thought to play a role in altering the cortical and medullary microcirculation after radiocontrast medium injection. Mechanical factors may also play a role because radiocontrast media increase blood viscosity and may affect the flow in the complex, low-pressure medullary microcirculation.[39] An increased plasma viscosity after radiocontrast medium administration can interfere with blood flow, particularly under the hypertonic conditions of the (inner) renal medulla, where the plasma viscosity is already increased as a result of hemoconcentration. Indeed, there are several animal studies that have shown a correlation between experimental CIN and viscosity of the radiopaque compound.[44,45]

Evidence has also suggested direct tubular toxicity from radiocontrast media. Early studies on isolated renal tubules in vitro have shown direct toxic effects of radiocontrast media on proximal tubular cells (PTCs).[46] Radiocontrast media (e.g., diatrizoate, iopamidol) induced a decline in tubule $K^+$, adenosine triphosphate (ATP), and total adenine nucleotide contents. At the same time, there was a decrease in the respiratory rate of the tubules and an increase in $Ca^{2+}$ content. These changes were more pronounced with the very high-osmolality ionic compound diatrizoate than with the lower osmolality nonionic iopamidol. Importantly, the cytotoxic effects were aggravated by hypoxia, indicating interactions between direct cellular mechanisms and vasoconstriction-mediated hypoxia.[47] Andersen and coworkers have demonstrated the concentration-dependent radiocontrast media–mediated release of tubular marker enzymes, ultrastructural changes, and cell death in both Madin-Darby canine kidney (MDCK) and porcine kidney proximal tubule epithelial ($LLC\text{-}PK_1$) cells.[48] Radiocontrast medium–induced critical medullary hypoxia may lead to the formation of reactive oxygen species (ROS), with subsequent membrane and DNA damage. A vicious cycle of hypoxia, free radical formation, and further hypoxic injury may be activated after radiocontrast medium exposure. Clinically, CIN presents with an acute decline in the GFR within 24 to 48 hours of administration, with a peak serum creatinine concentration usually occurring in 3 to 5 days and return to baseline within 1 week, although patients with moderate to advanced CKD may take somewhat longer to return to the baseline serum creatinine concentration. Existing CKD, diabetic nephropathy, advanced age, congestive heart failure, volume depletion, and coincident use of NSAIDs also increase the risk for CIN.

Unlike the first-generation contrast media, high-osmolar contrast media (HOCM; osmolality of 1500–1800 mOsm/kg), low-osmolar contrast media (LOCM; osmolality of 600–850 mOsm/kg), and isosmolar contrast media (IOCM; osmolality of 270–320 mOsm/kg) are associated with a lower incidence of contrast-induced AKI.[49–51] However, whether the incidence of contrast-induced AKI is lower in IOCM than LOCM is still debated.[49–52] One factor that may mitigate against the theoretic value of IOCM versus LOCM is that IOCM is a dimer and has a higher viscosity than LOCM. Viscosities for HOCM, LOCM, and IOCM are 0.00275, 0.00525, and 0.0114 pascal-second (Pa·s) at 37° C, respectively.[28] According to Poiseuille's law, an increase in viscosity negatively affects flow. Following intravenous injection, contrast medium becomes diluted in the bloodstream, the viscosity and osmolality are reduced, and therefore nonkidney organs are exposed to low concentrations of contrast medium. In the kidney, however, because of the increase in medullary osmolality, the concentration of contrast medium increases in the peritubular capillary and, following filtration, the concentration of contrast rises in the tubule lumen. The consequence is that (1) the distal tubules are exposed to increasing concentration and viscosity of contrast medium, and (2) the tubule flow rate decreases, leading to prolonged exposure to contrast, potentially enhancing direct tubule nephrotoxicity.[28,53] Furthermore, when infused in animals, medullary $Po_2$ is lower in IOCM when compared with LOCM.[34]

**Aminoglycoside Nephrotoxicity.** The nephrotoxicity of aminoglycosides has best been characterized for gentamicin, a polar drug excreted by glomerular filtration. It is thought that cationic amino groups ($NH_3^+$) on the drug bind to anionic phospholipid residues on the brush border of proximal tubular cells, and the drug is then internalized by endocytosis. Although the precise cellular mechanisms responsible for renal accumulation of aminoglycosides have not been fully elucidated, binding to the endocytic complex formed by megalin and cubilin at the apical surface of proximal tubular cells appears important.[54,55] The complete elimination of aminoglycoside uptake in mice deficient in megalin has suggested that this is the major pathway responsible for renal aminoglycoside accumulation.[55] Chloride transporters, including cystic fibrosis transmembrane conductance regulator (CFTR) and the ClC-5 have been implicated because mice lacking functional CFTR ($Cftr^{\Delta F/\Delta F}$) or deficient in the $Cl^-$/$H^+$ exchanger ($Clcn5^{Y/-}$) have decreased kidney accumulation of gentamicin.[56] A three-dimensional model has described the complex between megalin and gentamicin. Gentamicin binds to megalin with low affinity and exploits the common ligand-binding motif using the indole side chain of amino acids Trp-1126 and the negatively charged residues of Asp-1129, Asp-1131, and Asp-1133.[57] Once endocytosed, aminoglycosides inhibit endosomal fusion. They are also directly trafficked to the Golgi apparatus and, through retrograde movement, to the endoplasmic reticulum (ER). From the ER, gentamicin moves into the cytosol in a size- and charge-dependent manner.[58] Once in the cytosol, either from the ER[58] or via lysosomal rupture, aminoglycosides distribute to various intracellular organelles and mediate organelle-specific toxicity, such as mitochondrial dysfunction.[58,59] Gentamicin acts on the mitochondria, activating the intrinsic pathway of apoptosis, disrupting ATP production,[60,61] and producing hydroxyl radicals and superoxide anions.[62,63] Also, delivery to the ER via retrograde transport from the Golgi apparatus allows for the binding of aminoglycosides to the 16S rRNA subunit,[64] resulting in a reduction of protein synthesis[65,66] and altering posttranslational protein folding.[67] The number of cationic groups on the molecules determines the facility with which these drugs are transported across the cell membrane and is an important determinant of toxicity.[68,69] Neomycin is associated with the most nephrotoxicity, gentamicin, tobramycin, and amikacin are intermediate, and streptomycin is the least nephrotoxic. Furthermore, blocking megalin with cilastatin is known to reduce drug-induced nephrotoxicity.[70] Risk factors for aminoglycoside nephrotoxicity include the use of high or repeated doses or prolonged therapy, CKD, volume depletion, diabetes, advanced age, and the coexistence of renal ischemia or use of other nephrotoxins.[71–73]

**Vancomycin Nephrotoxicity.** Vancomycin was discovered, developed, and approved by the US Food and Drug Administration (FDA) in 1958[74,75] and was found to be active against most gram-positive organisms, including penicillin-resistant staphylococci.[75] Initial formulations of the drug were dubbed "Mississippi mud" due to the brown color presumably due to impurities, which were thought to be responsible for nephrotoxicity and ototoxicity.[75–77] Reformulation resulted in a drug that had improved purity and was called *vancomycin* (from the word vanquish).

The incidence of vancomycin nephrotoxicity is variable, ranging from as low as 0% to over 40%, and those with vancomycin-associated nephrotoxicity were more likely to have higher trough levels and prolonged duration of treatment.[78] Durations of 7 to more than 15 days of treatment are associated with nephrotoxicity.[79–81] With modern formulations of vancomycin, the variability is due to concomitant drug use, severity of illness, and variability in the definition of AKI. Daily total dose of vancomycin of more than 4 g has been shown to be a risk factor for nephrotoxicity.[82] Vancomycin-associated nephrotoxicity is thought to be more common when combined with antipseudomonal beta-lactams. In a retrospective matched cohort study of patients receiving vancomycin and cefepime (588 patients) or vancomycin and piperacillin-tazobactam (3605 patients), the unadjusted incidence of AKI was 12.6% versus 21.4%, respectively ($P <$ .0001). Vancomycin and piperacillin-tazobactam was associated with a more than twofold increase in the risk of AKI, after matching for severity of illness.[80]

Luque and associates[83] have described a patient who received vancomycin without coadministration of an aminoglycoside. The biopsy showed obstructive tubular casts composed of noncrystal nanospheric vancomycin aggregates associated with uromodulin. In eight additional patients with AKI associated with high vancomycin levels, vancomycin-associated casts were found. These findings, which were reproduced in mice given vancomycin, demonstrate a link between vancomycin and AKI.

**Cisplatin Nephrotoxicity.** Treatment with cisplatin (cisplatinum), a platinum-based chemotherapeutic agent, is commonly associated with nephrotoxicity. The pathophysiologic mechanism of cisplatin-induced tubular damage is complex and involves a number of interconnected factors, such as accumulation of cisplatin mediated by membrane transport, conversion into nephrotoxins, DNA damage, mitochondrial dysfunction, oxidative stress, inflammatory response, activation of signal transducers and intracellular messengers, and activation of apoptotic pathways. Movement of cisplatin through the renal tubular cells occurs in a basolateral to apical direction. Two primary transporters are involved in transporting cisplatin into the tubular cells, the copper transport protein 1 (Ctrl), expressed on proximal and distal tubules, and the organic cation transporter 2 (OCT2), expressed on the basolateral side of the proximal convoluted tubule.[84] Multidrug and toxin extrusion 1 (MATE1/SLC47A1; MATE1), expressed on the apical membrane of the proximal tubule, is responsible for the efflux of cisplatin.[84,85] When cisplatin was administered to $Mate^{1-/-}$ mice, blood urea nitrogen (BUN) and creatinine levels were higher than in $Mate^{1+/+}$ mice. Furthermore cisplatin levels were higher in plasma and in kidneys of compared with $Mate1^{+/+}$ mice, suggesting that MATE1 mediates the efflux of cisplatin and could contribute to cisplatin nephrotoxicity.

The S3 segment of the proximal tubule in the corticomedullary region is the most common site of cisplatin nephrotoxicity in rats. More distal sites may be affected in humans, but glomeruli remain unaffected. A recent study in mice has examined the effects of low but frequent doses of cisplatin given once a week for 4 weeks. Mice who received multiple doses of cisplatin had increased levels of fibrotic markers in kidney tissue, including fibronectin, transforming growth factor-β, and α-smooth muscle actin, as well as interstitial fibrosis.[86] These studies in mice support observations in humans showing that adult patients with cancer who received multiple doses of experience small but permanent declines in the estimated GFR (eGFR).[87,88]

**Acute Phosphate Nephropathy.** AKI has been described as a complication following the administration of oral sodium phosphate solution as a bowel cathartic in preparation for colonoscopy and bowel surgery.[89–91] Although the mechanism linking oral sodium phosphate administration with AKI remains incompletely understood, the pathogenesis likely relates to a transient and significant rise in the serum phosphate concentration that occurs simultaneously with intravascular volume depletion.

When the urine is oversaturated and buffering factors such as pH, citrate, and pyrophosphate are overwhelmed, renal phosphorus excretion becomes compromised. This may lead to the intratubular precipitation of calcium phosphate salts when the solubility coefficient is exceeded and to obstruction of the tubular lumen, leading to direct tubular damage. ROS generated by the binding of calcium phosphate crystals further promotes tubular damage. Risk factors for acute phosphate nephropathy include preexisting volume depletion, the use of ACE inhibitors and angiotensin receptor blockers (ARBs), NSAIDs, CKD, older age, female gender, and higher dosage of oral sodium phosphate.[90,91] Patients who develop acute phosphate nephropathy typically present with elevated serum creatinine concentrations days to months following the administration of oral sodium phosphate solution and can experience progression to CKD and end-stage kidney disease. As in other conditions associated with hypercalcemia, hyperphosphatemia, or hyperphosphaturia, calcium phosphate precipitation in renal tubules is seen on renal biopsy as bluish-purple crystals that are nonpolarizable.[92]

### Tubular Disease—Endogenous Nephrotoxins

**Myoglobin and Hemoglobin.** Myoglobin and hemoglobin are the endogenous toxins most commonly associated with ATN. Myoglobin, a 17.8-kDa heme protein released during muscle injury, is freely filtered and causes red-brown urine, with a dipstick result positive for heme in the absence of RBCs in the urine. Intravascular hemolysis results in circulating free hemoglobin, which, when excessive, is filtered, resulting in hemoglobinuria, hemoglobin cast formation, and heme uptake by proximal tubular cells. The uptake in the proximal tubule may be mediated via endocytosis by megalin and cubilin. Megalin knockout mice have reduced accumulation of injected myoglobin in tubule cells and reduced nephrotoxicity.[93] The heme center of myoglobin may directly induce lipid peroxidation and, in addition, the liberation of free ferrous iron, depending on the redox potential, can promote hydroxyl radical formation by the Haber-Weiss (Fenton) reaction, resulting in the oxidation of lipids, proteins, and nucleic acids.[94,95] Iron is an intermediate accelerator in the generation of free radicals. Studies have suggested that there is increased formation of $H_2O_2$ in rat kidney models of myohemoglobinuria.[96] The subsequent hydroxyl

($OH^-$) radical plays a vital role in oxidative stress–induced AKI through mechanisms discussed in detail later in this chapter. In response, heme protein induces heme-degradative enzyme, heme oxygenase, and increased synthesis of ferritin. Ferritin, a major factor in sequestering free iron,[97] is made up of two types of 24 subunits, heavy chain and light chain. It is the ferritin heavy chain (FtH) that has ferroxidase activity necessary for iron incorporation and to limit toxicity. Zarjou and coworkers have demonstrated that proximal tubule-specific, *FtH*-knockout mice (*FtH*$^{PT-/-}$ mice) have significant mortality in myoglobin-induced AKI, indicating the protective role of proximal tubule FtH in AKI.[98] Various iron chelators such as deferoxamine and other scavengers of ROS such as glutathione provide protection against myohemoglobinuric AKI.[99] Similarly, endothelin antagonists also prevent hypofiltration and proteinuria in rats that have undergone glycerol-induced rhabdomyolysis.[100] In addition, NO supplementation may be beneficial by preventing the heme-induced renal vasoconstriction because heme proteins scavenge NO.[101,102] Finally, precipitation of myoglobin with Tamm-Horsfall protein and shed proximal tubular cells lead to cast formation and tubular obstruction, which is enhanced in acidic urine.[103] In human studies, volume expansion and perhaps alkalization of urine to limit cast formation are the preventive measures generally used because none of the experimental agents used in animal studies has been convincingly beneficial. This emphasizes the multifactorial nature of these conditions. It is unlikely that a single agent will be beneficial in this setting.[104]

**Immunoglobulin Light Chains.** *Direct tubule toxicity.* Excessive immunoglobulin light chains, produced in diseases such as multiple myeloma, are filtered, absorbed, and then catabolized in proximal tubule cells and can induce proximal tubulopathy.[105] The concentration of light chains leaving the proximal portion of the nephron depends on both the concentration of light chains in the glomerular filtrate and the capacity of the proximal tubule to reabsorb and catabolize them. Certain light chains can be directly toxic to the proximal tubules themselves.[106] In the proximal tubules, free light chains (FLCs) are reabsorbed by binding to the proximal tubule heterodimeric complex consisting of megalin and cubilin.[107–109] Accumulation of light chains in the endosomes and lysosomes of the proximal tubule leads to cellular desquamation and fragmentation, vacuolization, and focal loss of brush border.[110] Mechanisms for tubule toxicity may include blocking of transport of glucose, amino acids, or phosphate.[105] FLCs generate hydrogen peroxide,[111] which leads to the production of chemokines and cytokines,[111–114] with nuclear translocation of nuclear factor-kappa B (NF-κB), suggesting that light chain endocytosis leads to the production of inflammatory cytokines through activation of NF-κB.[115] Monoclonal FLC also promotes apoptosis through apoptosis signal-regulating kinase (ASK1), also called mitogen-activated protein kinase kinase kinase 5 (MAP3K5).[114] Subsequent inflammation leads to tubulointerstitial fibrosis.[116]

*Cast nephropathy.* Once the capacity for proximal tubule uptake is overwhelmed, a light chain load is presented to the distal tubule, where, on reaching a critical concentration, the light chains aggregate and coprecipitate with Tamm-Horsfall protein (THP) and form characteristic light chain casts.[117] FLCs bind to specific sites on Tamm-Horsfall glycoproteins through the CDR3 domain of FLC, leading to their coprecipitation in the lumen of the distal nephron and tubule flow.[118] There are critical determinants of the binding site between CDR3 and FLCs that lead to the development of a cyclized competitive peptide. This peptide inhibited binding of FLCs to THP and was effective in inhibiting intraluminal cast formation and AKI.[118] Some studies have shown that light chains, in the amount seen in plasma cell dyscrasia patients, are capable of catalyzing the formation of hydrogen peroxide in cultured HK-2 cells. Hydrogen peroxide stimulates the production of monocyte chemoattractant protein-1 (MCP-1), a key chemokine involved in monocyte or macrophage recruitment to proximal tubular cells.[111]

Any process that reduces the GFR, such as volume depletion, hypercalcemia, or NSAIDs, will accelerate and aggravate light chain cast formation. It has been proposed that acutely reducing the presented light chain load by plasmapheresis or dialysis using high-cutoff membranes might be beneficial in limiting cast formation and reducing the extent of AKI in certain select patients, allowing for the initiation of chemotherapy to decrease bone marrow– dependent light chain formation.[119,120]

**Uric Acid.** Tumor cell necrosis following chemotherapy can release large amounts of intracellular contents such as uric acid, phosphate, and xanthine into the circulation, potentially leading to AKI. Acute uric acid nephropathy with intratubular crystallization leading to obstruction and interstitial nephritis is not seen as commonly as it was in the past, mainly due to the prophylactic use of allopurinol or rasburicase before chemotherapy to lower the serum uric acid concentration acutely.

## POSTRENAL ACUTE KIDNEY INJURY

Postrenal azotemia occurs from obstruction of the ureters, bladder outlet, or urethra. AKI from ureteric obstruction requires that the blockage occur bilaterally at any level of the ureters or unilaterally in a patient with a solitary functioning kidney or CKD. Ureteric obstruction can be intraluminal or external. Bilateral ureteric calculi, blood clots, and sloughed renal papillae can obstruct the lumen, whereas external compression from a tumor or hemorrhage can block the ureters as well. Fibrosis of the ureters intrinsically or from the retroperitoneum can narrow the lumen to the point of complete luminal obstruction. The most common cause for postrenal azotemia is structural or functional obstruction of the bladder neck. Prostatic conditions, therapy with anticholinergic agents, and a neurogenic bladder can all cause postrenal AKI. Relief of the obstruction usually causes prompt return of the GFR if the duration of obstruction has not been excessive. The rate and magnitude of functional recovery are dependent on the extent and duration of the obstruction.[121]

AKI resulting from obstruction usually accounts for fewer than 5% of cases, although in certain settings (e.g., transplantation), it can be as high as 6% to 10%. Clinically, patients can present with pain and oliguria, although these are neither specific nor sensitive. Because of the availability of retroperitoneal imagining using ultrasonography or computed tomography (CT), the diagnosis is usually straightforward, although, on occasion, a volume-depleted patient or a patient with severe reduction in the GFR may not show hydronephrosis on radiologic assessment. Because the GFR is typically not affected early in the course of obstructive AKI, volume repletion can increase the sensitivity of diagnosis by increasing the GFR and urine production into the ureter, leading to dilation of the ureter proximal to the obstruction, enhancing ultrasonographic visualization. Early diagnosis and prompt relief of obstruction remain key goals in preventing long-term parenchymal damage because the shorter the period of obstruction, the better the chances for recovery and favorable long-term outcomes.

# PATHOPHYSIOLOGY OF ACUTE KIDNEY INJURY

## OVERVIEW OF THE PATHOPHYSIOLOGY OF ACUTE KIDNEY INJURY

AKI is a summation of temporally activated systems that together result in inflammation, activation of cell death pathways, tubular obstruction, backleak, altered glomerular hemodynamics and loss of the GFR. Within the kidney, mechanisms pertaining to microvascular compartments, innate immunity, and ATN result in temporary, partial, or permanent loss of the GFR. Furthermore, it is becoming widely accepted that AKI is a systemic process that affects a number of organs, leading to the high morbidity and mortality seen in patients with AKI. Systemic responses to AKI may influence the extent of injury. Hemodynamic alterations (e.g., decrease in cardiac output, low blood pressure, vasoconstriction) may initiate AKI or exacerbate intrinsic microenvironmental mechanisms of AKI. Systemic immunologic mechanisms of proinflammatory or antiinflammatory conditions may affect AKI, and neural mechanisms may attenuate AKI. Thus, the complexity of the pathogenesis of AKI requires careful understanding of its molecular mechanisms through defining important targets in humans and testing in relevant models of AKI (Fig. 28.1).[122–127]

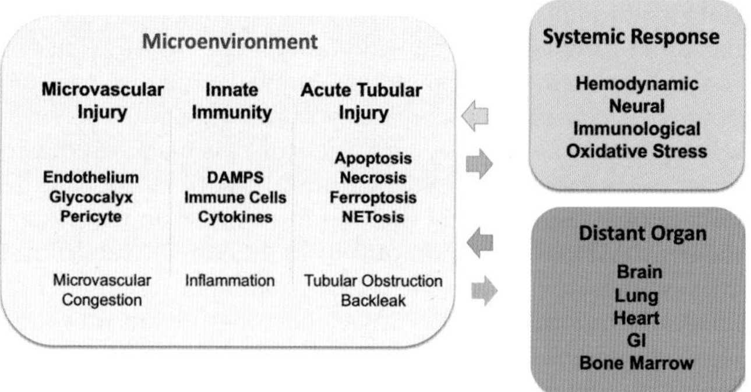


**Fig. 28.1** Overview of pathophysiology of acute kidney injury (AKI). AKI is a summation of temporally activated systems that together result in loss of the glomerular filtration rate (GFR). In the kidney, mechanisms pertaining to microvascular compartment, innate immunity, and acute tubular necrosis result in temporary, partial, or permanent loss of the GFR. Systemic responses may influence the extent of injury. Hemodynamic alterations (decrease in cardiac output, low blood pressure, and vasoconstriction) may initiate AKI or exacerbate intrinsic microenvironmental mechanisms of AKI. Systemic immunologic mechanisms of proinflammatory or antiinflammatory conditions may affect AKI, and neural mechanisms may attenuate AKI (see text for details).

## EXPERIMENTAL MODELS

The goal of preclinical AKI research is to translate basic scientific knowledge of AKI to clinical practice. Despite extensive research in AKI focusing on standardized definitions of AKI (from *R*isk, *I*njury, *F*ailure, *L*oss of kidney function, and *E*nd-stage kidney disease (RIFLE), *A*cute *K*idney *I*njury *N*etwork (AKIN), and Kidney Disease: Improving Global Outcomes [KDIGO]), biomarkers of AKI, novel drug targets, and improved clinical trial design, our knowledge remains incomplete, and effective therapies are lacking.[122,123] To advance the field, it is important that we identify relevant targets through the analysis of human tissue biopsy and necropsy specimens, develop relevant disease models of AKI, include proper pharmacokinetic, pharmacodynamic, and dose response studies and, finally, improve preclinical and human clinical trial design.[123,125,126,128] The National Institutes of Health (NIH) and National Institute of Diabetes and Digestive and Kidney Diseases (NIDDK) have initiated a bold project, the Kidney Precision Medicine Project (KPMP), whose objectives are to obtain human kidney biopsies ethically from participants with AKI and CKD with a goal to identify critical cells, pathways, and targets for therapy. The following section will focus on current animal models.

### IN VIVO MODELS OF ACUTE KIDNEY INJURY

Current investigations into the pathophysiology of AKI include a combination of animal and cell culture models of AKI designed to understand the pathophysiology of AKI better and investigate novel therapeutic agents. However, there remains a need to develop in vivo experimental models of AKI that more closely resemble clinical AKI for the development of effective therapies.[123,126,129,130] Some of the important principles in studying the pathophysiology of AKI in various models include outcome measures at multiple time points and the ability to control physiologic functions known to affect kidney function (e.g., temperature, blood pressure, anesthesia, fluid status). Current models of AKI (e.g., warm ischemia-reperfusion using a pedicle clamp) test fundamental proof of principle concepts that identify potential molecular targets. A simplified model limits confounding variables but can clearly identify potential therapeutic targets. However, additional models of AKI are necessary that should reflect human disease (e.g., aged animals, impaired kidney function, multiorgan failure, preexisting vascular changes, multiple renal insults) that often coexist in human AKI. We will briefly describe the pros and cons of using presently characterized experimental models (Table 28.1).[131–146]

The warm ischemia-reperfusion renal pedicle clamp model is one of the most widely used experimental models in rats and mice because of its simplicity and reproducibility. However, the inflammatory response differs greatly between mice and rats. It is important to realize that there is considerable variability between mice and rats, mouse strains (C57BL/6 vs. BALB/c), and the same strain from different vendors.[147] Although mice are the primary species used experimentally for examining the immune response to AKI, there are significant differences when compared with the human immune

**Table 28.1. Acute Kidney Injury–Induced Distant Organ Injury**

| Organ | Mechanism | Species | Reference |
|---|---|---|---|
| Lung | CXCL1 | Mouse | 131 |
| | TNF-α | Mouse | 132 |
| | IL-10 | Mouse | 133 |
| | Neutrophil elastase | Mouse | 134 |
| | Lung permeability | Mouse | 135 |
| | Pulmonary edema, inflammatory cytokines | Rat | 136 |
| | Oxidant stress | Rat | 137 |
| | Systemic cytokines and HMGB1 | Human (ex vivo) | 138 |
| Heart | TNF-α | Rat | 139 |
| | Mitochondrial fission protein | Mouse | 140 |
| Brain | RAAS | Mouse | 141 |
| Liver | Administration of glutathione | Rat | 142 |
| | Hepatic oxidant stress | Mouse | 143, 144 |
| Intestine | Hepatic oxidant stress | Mouse | 145 |

*AKI,* Acute kidney injury; *CXCL1,* chemokine (C-X-C motif) ligand 1; *HMGB1,* high-mobility group box protein B1; *IL,* interleukin; *RAAS,* renin-angiotensin-aldosterone system; *TNF-α,* tumor necrosis factor α.

Modified from Lee SA, Cozzi M, Bush EL, Rabb H. Distant organ dysfunction in acute kidney injury: a review. *Am J Kidney Dis.* 2018;72(6):846–856.

system.[148] Additionally, there are structural differences between rodents and humans, although pig kidneys are most similar to humans.[130]

These differences need to be taken into consideration when using mice in preclinical models to mimic human AKI. Furthermore, tubular injury and repair and medullary congestion are difficult to compare with human ischemic ATN. In human AKI, pure ischemia alone is seen in the minority of cases, and there is rarely complete cessation of blood flow to the kidneys. The parenteral delivery of prophylactic therapeutic agents is impossible in complete occlusion models. Because oxygen and metabolic substrates are unable to reach the kidney, the generation of ROS and peroxynitrite species, considered to be important mediators of injury, might have a different or delayed role as compared with low-oxygen states in hypoperfusion models. Total blood flow cessation also prevents the degradative products of the ischemic kidney from being washed out. Other factors playing a role in the pathophysiology of AKI, such as inflammatory mediators released from the spleen, ischemic gut, endothelium, and vascular smooth muscle cells, need to be taken into consideration in any experimental model. Bowel proteins released into the circulation can act as inflammatory mediators and increase the susceptibility to AKI.[149] Others have shown that short-chain fatty acids derived from gut bacteria prevent AKI[150] or germ-free conditions render mice more susceptible to AKI.[151,152] The S3 segment of the proximal tubule is characterized by severe necrosis in clamp models, a finding seen rarely in human AKI. Human biopsies, however, rarely sample the outer medulla, where most of the injury is thought to occur. In contrast to animal models, human AKI histologic biopsy data are lacking at early time points from the onset of insult.[129] Thus, the NIH/NIDDK KPMP will be vital in this regard.

The cold ischemia–warm reperfusion model resembles human kidney transplantation but is inadequately studied and experimentally difficult to perform. In the isolated perfused kidney model, the kidney is perfused ex vivo using perfusates with and without erythrocytes, and the model uses ischemic (stopping perfusate) or hypoxic (reduced oxygen tension of erythrocytes) to induce functional impairment. The morphologic patterns are different in erythrocyte-free and erythrocyte-rich perfusates. The latter system is more comparable with what is observed histologically in animal models. Additionally, limitations include exclusion of various inflammatory mediators, neuroendocrine hemodynamic regulation, and systemic cytokine and growth factor interactions known to be present and that play a pathophysiologic role in animal models and likely in human ischemia.

Cardiac arrest commonly leads to AKI. Burne-Taney and colleagues have described a whole-body ischemia-reperfusion injury (IRI) model induced by 10 minutes of cardiac arrest, followed by cardiac compression resuscitation, ventilation, epinephrine, and fluids that lead to a significant rise in serum creatinine level and renal tubular injury at 24 hours.[153] One of the unique advantages of this model is the crosstalk among vital organs such as the brain, heart, and lung and renal hemodynamics.[139] A hypoperfusion model of AKI using partial aortic clamping, first described by Zager,[154] may be more representative of human AKI, reflecting a state of reduced blood flow to the kidney, with systolic blood pressure of approximately 20 mm Hg, resulting in reproducible AKI.[154]

Toxic models of kidney failure use various known toxins, such as radiocontrast media, gentamicin, cisplatin, glycerol, and pigments, including myoglobin, folic acid, and hemoglobin. Septic models to study AKI include cecal ligation and puncture (CLP), endotoxin infusion, and bacterial infusion into the peritoneal cavity. The endotoxin model, which is simple, inexpensive, and suitable for studying new pharmacologic agents, has certain drawbacks as well. There is variability among sources of lipopolysaccharide (LPS) endotoxin, the rates and methods of administration vary, and it is usually of short duration due to the high mortality associated with the doses required to induce AKI. It also tends to be a vasoconstrictive model and does not recapitulate the early hemodynamics or inflammation of human sepsis.[155] Wichterman and colleagues were the first to describe a sepsis model in the early 1980s using the CLP laboratory model.[156] In the CLP model, there is considerable similarity to sepsis in humans, with acute lung injury, metabolic derangement, and systemic vasodilation, accompanied initially by increased cardiac output. However, there is some variability depending on the mode and size of cecal perforation. Doi and coworkers have developed a sepsis model that considers the following: (1) animals should receive the same supportive therapy that is standard for intensive care unit (ICU) patients (fluid resuscitation and antibiotics); and (2) age, chronic comorbid conditions, and genetic heterogeneity vary.[157] Another example is a hyperdynamic form of sepsis established in Merino sheep. These studies have provided important new information that cannot be derived from rodent models of sepsis.[158] Complex animal models of human sepsis that introduce these disease-modifying factors are likely more relevant and may be more pharmacologically relevant than simple animal models.[157]

This description is intended to remind the reader of the potential pitfalls in each model when evaluating experimental studies or therapeutic interventions using these models. The lack of ability to demonstrate the effectiveness of an agent in humans shown to be efficacious in animal models does not necessarily reflect a flaw with the model or the agent in question. Most often, the agent is administered late in the course of the human disease; patient heterogeneity and the difficulty in stratifying patients by severity of injury makes it even more difficult to establish efficacy.[123,159] Further studies have led to the development of zebrafish, three-dimensional (3D) microfluidic, and human kidney organoids models that are improving our understanding of AKI or facilitating pharmacologic studies for the treatment of AKI.

### Zebrafish

Given the capacity of zebrafish adult nephrons to undergo robust epithelial regeneration and to form nephrons de novo, investigations using zebrafish models of AKI have allowed a better understanding of the cellular mechanisms associated with kidney regeneration after AKI. Using chemical genetics, investigators have discovered that histone deacetylase inhibitors (HDACi) are capable of ameliorating gentamicin-induced AKI in the zebrafish embryo with an expansion of renal progenitors that express the genes *Lhx1a*, *Pax2a*, and *Pax8*.[160] Future studies using zebrafish transgenic lines in which injury can be induced in tubular cells via the nitroreductase-metronidazole system, are likely to help characterize how individual populations of cells in the nephron respond to kidney damage.[161]

### Three-Dimensional Microfluidic Models and Organoids

Side effects, and especially drug-induced nephrotoxicity, can often be an important limiting factor in the development of new pharmacotherapy. In addition to each of the current animal models of AKI having limitations in fully recapitulating human AKI, the lack of ability to predict drug-induced AKI has led to failed drug trials. Early nephrotoxicity screening studies included two-dimensional standard well plates with semipermeable filter cups. There were a number of limitations to two-dimensional standard well plates, including the following: (1) use of cell lines of nonhuman origin (MDCK; LLC-PK 1); (2) use of cell lines with limited proximal tubule characteristics (human kidney 2 [HK 2]); (3) cell lines that have features of epithelial to mesenchymal transition (HK 2); and (4) static conditions. By contrast, proximal tubule cells are subject to continuous tubule fluid flow and fluid shear stress that modulate cellular signal transduction through mechanosensing receptors, organization of the cytoskeleton, actin filaments, and adherens junctions.[162–166] More physiologically relevant models such as three-dimensional microfluidic models have been developed to bridge the step from standard two-dimensional systems to animal models or as a total replacement for costly, inefficient animal models. These three-dimensional microfluidic models, such as parallel flow-plate models and early three-dimensional perfusion models, include chip technology with cell monolayers or tubular structures that are sandwiched between two microfluidic channels. Recently, Qu and coworkers developed a multilayer microfluidic device to simulate glomerulus, Bowman's capsule, proximal tubular lumen, and peritubular endothelial cells to investigate the pathophysiology of drug-induced AKI. The authors were able to demonstrate time- and dose-dependent induction of cell death by cisplatin and doxorubicin. The use of this biomimetic device has yielded useful information about drug-induced AKI at the preclinical stage.[167]

Human kidney organoids are three-dimensional clusters of cells that are functionally and genetically similar to kidney. Human-induced pluripotent stems cells (hiPSCs) are ideally suited for human kidney organoids because of their unlimited self-renewal and ability to generate cells of all three embryonic germ layers. Major challenges to the generation of functional bioengineered kidneys are the incorporation of adequate vascularization to kidney organoids and the establishment of an effective drainage system for the removal of blood filtrate after passage and processing through the tubule system[168] Protocols that add combinations of growth factors to mimic in vivo conditions and growing cells in three-dimensional cultures have generated nephron progenitor cells and kidney organoids from human embryonic stem cells and hiPSCs.[169–172]

## ACUTE TUBULAR NECROSIS

### EPITHELIAL CELL INJURY

Although all segments of the nephron may undergo injury during an ischemic insult, the major and most commonly injured epithelial cell involved in AKI related to ischemia, sepsis, and/or nephrotoxins is the PTC. Of the three segments (S1–S3), the S3 segment of the proximal tubule in the outer stripe of the medulla is the cell most susceptible to ischemic injury for several reasons.[173] First, it has limited capacity to undergo anaerobic glycolysis due to its dependence on fatty acid oxidation as the major source of energy. Second, due to its unique primarily venous capillary regional blood flow, there is marked hypoperfusion and congestion in this medullary region after injury that persists, even though cortical blood flow may have returned to near-normal levels after ischemic injury. Endothelial cell injury and dysfunction are primarily responsible for this phenomenon, often referred to as the "extension phase" of AKI.[159] The other major epithelial cells of the nephron involved are those of the medullary

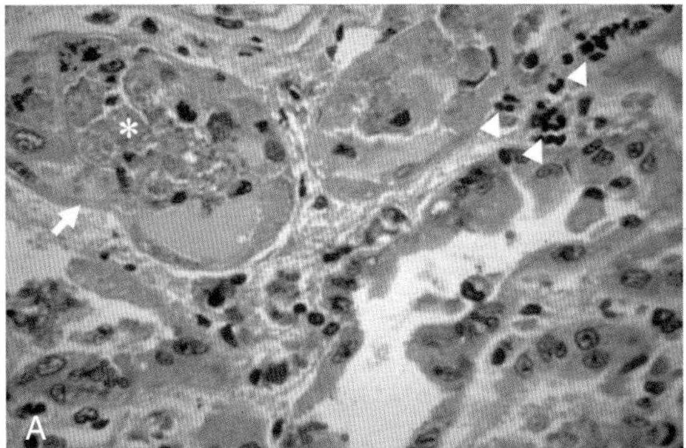

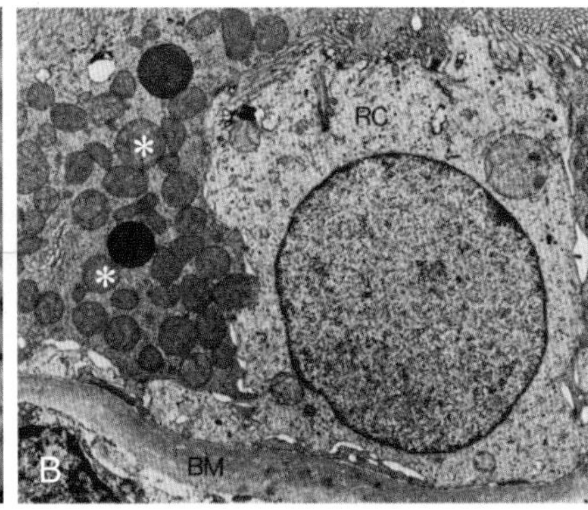

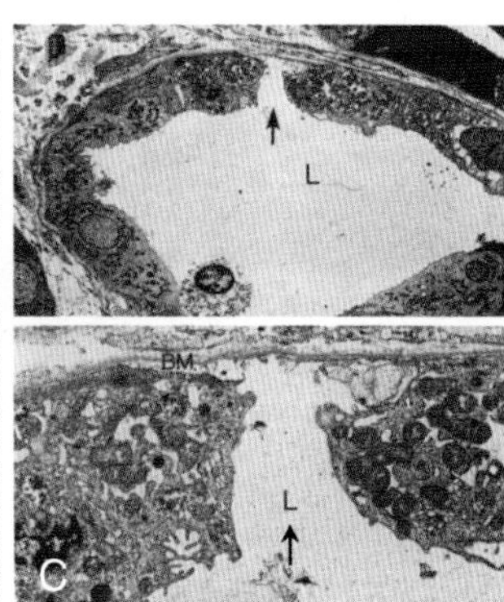


**Fig. 28.2** Morphology of human acute tubular necrosis. (A) Human biopsy specimens reveal significant proximal tubular cell damage, with intraluminal accumulation of apical membrane fragments and detached cells *(*)*, thinning of proximal tubular cells to maintain monolayer tubule integrity *(arrow)*, and dividing cells and accumulation of white cells within the microvascular space in the peritubular area *(arrowheads)*. (B) Electron micrograph of a regenerating epithelial cell. Shown are small fragmented mitochondria *(*)*. (C) Electron micrograph of renal epithelial cell showing nonreplacement site *(black arrow)* that morphologically supports the concept of backleak in the pathophysiology of AKI. (A, Courtesy M. Venkachatalam; B and C from Olsen TS, Olsen HS, Hansen HE. Tubular ultrastructure in acute renal failure in man: epithelial necrosis and regeneration. *Virchows Arch A Pathol Anat Histopathol.* 1985;406(1):75–89.)

thick ascending limb located more distally. Cells of the S1 and S2 segments are usually involved in toxic nephropathy due to their high rates of endocytosis, leading to increased cellular uptake of the toxin. PTCs and thick ascending limb of Henle (TAL) cells have been shown to be involved as sensors, effectors, and injury recipients of AKI stimuli.

Proximal tubular cell injury and dysfunction during ischemia or sepsis lead to a profound drop in the GFR through afferent arteriolar vasoconstriction, mediated by tubular glomerular feedback and proximal tubular obstruction. This phenomenon, along with tubular backleak, leads to a fall in the effective GFR[174,175] (Figs. 28.1 and 28.2).

## Morphologic Changes

The classic histologic hallmark of ATN was described in a landmark study by Oliver and coworkers, in which individual nephrons from autopsy specimens of patients dying of acute renal failure (ARF) were microdissected. Portions of glomerular ultrafiltrate had become sequestered in tubules that were obstructed (necrotic PT cells), which suggested that filtrate leaked back through damaged tubular walls and entered the interstitium, which caused it to become edematous.[176] Early on, there is the loss of the apical brush border of the PTCs. Microvilli disruption and detachment from the apical cell surface forming membrane-bound blebs occurs early, with release into the tubular lumen. Patchy detachment and subsequent loss of tubular cells exposing areas of denuded tubular basement and focal areas of proximal tubular dilation, along with the presence of distal tubular casts, are also major pathologic findings in ATN.[177] The sloughed tubular cells, brush border vesicle remnants, and cellular debris in combination with Tamm-Horsfall glycoprotein form the classic muddy brown granular casts. These distal casts have the potential to obstruct the tubular lumen. Frank necrosis itself is inconspicuous and is restricted to the highly susceptible outer medullary regions. Alternatively, features of apoptosis are more commonly seen in proximal and distal tubular cells. Glomerular epithelial cell injury in ischemic, septic, or nephrotoxic injury is not typically seen, although some studies have shown thickening and coarsening of foot processes; Wagner and associates have shown podocyte-specific molecular and cellular changes.[189] The future morphologic course of the tubular cell alterations varies according to the type and extent of injury, as discussed in the next section (see Fig. 28.2).

## Cytoskeletal and Intracellular Structural Changes

The cytoskeleton in eukaryotic cells consists of intermediate filaments, microtubules, and actin filaments.[178] The microtubule cytoskeleton is composed of α-tubulin and β-tubulin heterodimers that serve to regulate the shape, motility, and division of tubular epithelial cells. A recent study has demonstrated that IRI to the kidney causes α-tubular deacetylation in microtubules, and inhibition of microtubule dynamics induced by changes in tubulin acetylation during the recovery phase retards tubular epithelial cell regeneration.[179] Epithelial cellular structure and function are mediated in part by the actin cytoskeleton, which plays an integral role in surface membrane structure and function, cell polarity, endocytosis, signal transduction, cell motility, movement of organelles, exocytosis, cell division, cell migration, barrier function of the junctional complexes, cell-matrix adhesion, and signal transduction.[180] Based on its role in this multitude of processes, any disruption of the actin cytoskeleton results in changes and/or disruption of the functions mentioned earlier. This is especially important for PTCs, where amplification of the apical membrane by microvilli is essential for normal cell function.

Ischemic insult results in cellular ATP depletion, which in turn leads to a rapid disruption of the apical actin and disruption and redistribution of the cytoskeleton F-actin core, resulting in the formation of membrane-bound extracellular vesicles or blebs.[181] These can be exfoliated into the tubular lumen or internalized with the capability of being recycled. The core mechanism of disruption is the depolymerization mediated by actin-binding protein known as actin depolymerizing factor (ADF) or cofilin.[182] This protein family is normally maintained in the inactive phosphorylated form, which cannot bind to actin. Ischemia results in ATP depletion, which has been shown to cause Rho GTPase inactivation.[183] This can

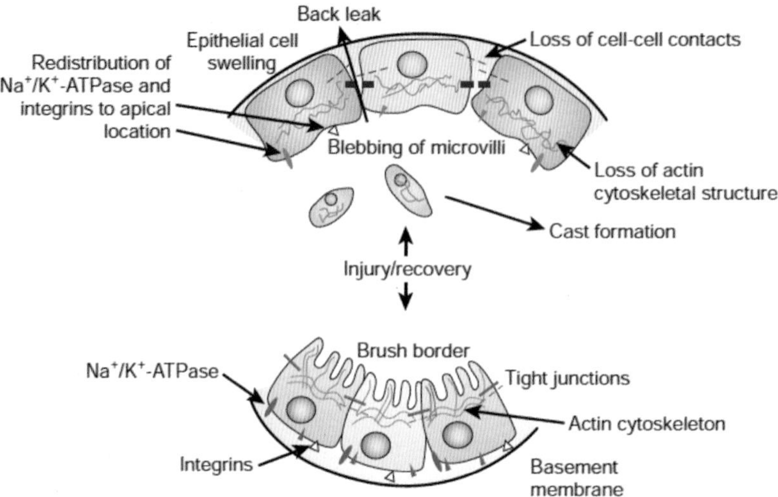


**Fig. 28.3** Overview of sublethally injured tubular cells. Sodium-potassium adenosine triphosphatase ($Na^+$-$K^+$-ATPase) pumps are normally located at the basolateral membrane. In sublethal ischemia, the pumps redistribute to the apical membrane of the proximal tubule. On reperfusion, the pumps reverse back to their basolateral location. (From Sharfuddin A, Molitoris B. Epithelial cell injury. In Vincent JL, Hall JB, eds. *Encyclopedia of Intensive Care Medicine.* New York: Springer; 2012.)

lead to activation and relocalization of ADF (cofilin) to the apical membranes, where it can mediate different effects, including depolymerization, severing, capping, and nucleation of F-actin. This destroys the actin filament core structure of microvilli and results in surface membrane instability and blebbing[184,185] (Fig. 28.3).

A recent study has used human primary tubular epithelial cells in culture to examine the role of hypoxic injury on epithelial cell cytoskeletal organization. Given previous information that stabilization of hypoxia-inducible factor (HIF) simulates hypoxic injury during AKI, the authors found that HIF stabilization in human tubular epithelial cells reduces tubular cell migration and induces the rearrangement of actin filaments and cell adhesion molecules, including paxillin and focal adhesion kinase. These data support the role of HIF stabilization during epithelial migration, which underlies a potential mechanism of renal regeneration in response to AKI.[186] Similarly, tropomyosins physiologically bind to and stabilize the F-actin microfilament core in the terminal web by preventing access to ADF. After ischemia, there is dissociation of tropomyosins from the microfilament core, resulting in access of the microfilaments in the terminal web to the binding, severing, and depolymerizing actions of ADF/cofilin.[187,188]

Another important consequence of disruption of the actin cytoskeleton is the loss of tight junctions and adherens junctions. These junctional complexes actively participate in numerous functions, including paracellular transport, cell polarity, and cellular shape. The tight junctions, also known as zonula occludens (ZO), are composed of proteins such as occludin, claudin, ZO-1, and protein kinase C with numerous barrier functions, such as adhesion, permeability, and transport. The actin present in the terminal web is linked to ZO, and hence any disruption of the terminal web results in disruption of the tight junctions. Early ischemic injury results in opening of these tight junctions, leading to increased paracellular permeability and causing further backleak of the glomerular filtrate into the interstitium.[180] In the glomerulus, ischemia also induces a rapid loss of interaction between slit diaphragm junctional proteins NEPH1 and ZO-1,[189] leading to podocyte damage, effacement, and proteinuria.

The molecular mechanisms underlying these changes have been studied as well and show that ATP depletion that results in actin polymerization is followed by a reduction in cellular adhesion ability. Pretreatment with an actin stabilizer prevented ATP depletion–induced actin polymerization and reduction of cell adhesion, indicating that the cytoskeleton reorganization decreased the cellular adhesion ability. Furthermore, the ATP depletion markedly increased the levels of p38 mitogen-activated protein (MAP) kinase and heat shock protein 27 (hsp27) phosphorylation, with enhanced translocation of phosphorylated hsp27 from cytoskeleton to cytoplasm. The inhibition of p38 MAP kinase by specific inhibitor SB203580 blocked the ATP depletion to induce hsp27 phosphorylation and actin polymerization. These findings suggest that ischemia remodels F-actin, leading to desquamation of proximal tubular epithelial cells through p38 MAP kinase–hsp27 signaling.[190]

Actin cytoskeleton alterations and dysfunction during ischemia result in changes in cell polarity and function. Normally, sodium-potassium adenosine triphosphatase ($Na^+$-$K^+$-ATPase) pumps reside in the basolateral membrane of the tubular epithelial cell, but under conditions of ischemia, they redistribute to the apical membrane as early as within 10 minutes.[191] This process occurs due to the disruption of the pumps' attachment to the membrane via the spectrin/actin cytoskeleton. Postulated mediated mechanisms include hyperphosphorylation of the protein ankyrin, with consequent loss of the binding protein spectrin, and cleavage of spectrin by the activation of proteases such as calpain. This redistribution of the $Na^+$-$K^+$-ATPase pump results in bidirectional transport of sodium and water across the epithelial cell apical membrane, as well as the basolateral membrane. This results in transport of cellular Na back into the tubular lumen, one of the major mechanisms of the high $FE_{Na}$ seen in patients with ischemic ATN,[192] and the inefficient use of cellular ATP. ATP is consumed but effective, vectorial Na transport is lost.

### Cell Death Pathways

**Necrosis and Regulated Cell Death Pathways.** Epithelial cell necrosis is a passive nonenergy dependent process that develops secondary to severe ATP depletion from toxic or ischemic insult. It is not dependent on caspase activation but results from a rise in intracellular calcium and the activation of membrane phospholipases.[193,194] Hence, morphologically, necrotic cells do not exhibit the nuclear fragmentation or chromatin condensation seen in apoptosis, and they do not form apoptotic bodies. Functionally, severe ATP depletion results first in mitochondrial injury, with subsequent arrest of oxidative phosphorylation, causing further depletion of energy stores, and robust formation of ROS, which in turn mediate further cellular injury.

In some cases, defined regulated molecular pathways may lead to necrotic cell death, a process referred to as *necroptosis*.[195] Differentiation between necrosis and necroptosis requires that necroptosis-dependent cell death involves the receptor-interacting protein kinase 3 (RIPK3).[196] Regulated cell death pathways can be grouped into a caspase-controlled cell death system (apoptosis, necroptosis, and pyroptosis) or lipid per oxidation–autoxidation-controlled necrosis system (ferroptosis; Fig. 28.4).[197]

**Apoptosis.** The fate of an epithelial cell after an injury ultimately depends on the extent of the injury. Cells undergoing sublethal or less severe injury have the capacity for functional and structural recovery if the insult is interrupted. Cells that suffer a more severe (or lethal) injury undergo apoptosis or necrosis. Apoptosis is an energy-dependent, programmed cell death after injury that results in the condensation of nuclear and cytoplasmic material, forming apoptotic bodies. These apoptotic bodies, which are plasma-membrane bound, are rapidly phagocytosed by macrophages and neighboring viable epithelial cells. In necrosis, there is cellular and organelle swelling, with loss of plasma membrane integrity and release of cytoplasmic and nuclear material into the lumen or interstitium[198] (Fig. 28.5).

The caspase family of proteases is an important initiator as well as an effector of apoptosis.[199,200] Both the intrinsic (mitochondrial) and extrinsic (death receptor) apoptotic pathways are activated in human AKI. Specifically, activation of procaspase-9 primarily depends on intrinsic mitochondrial pathways regulated by the Bcl-2 family of proteins, whereas that of procaspase-8 results from extrinsic signaling via cell surface death receptors, such as Fas and their ligand FADD (Fas-associated protein with death domain). There is also considerable crosstalk between the intrinsic and extrinsic pathways. The other group of caspases—3, 6, and 7—are effector caspases, which are more abundant and catalytically robust, cleaving many cellular proteins and resulting in the classic apoptotic phenotype. Caspase activation in

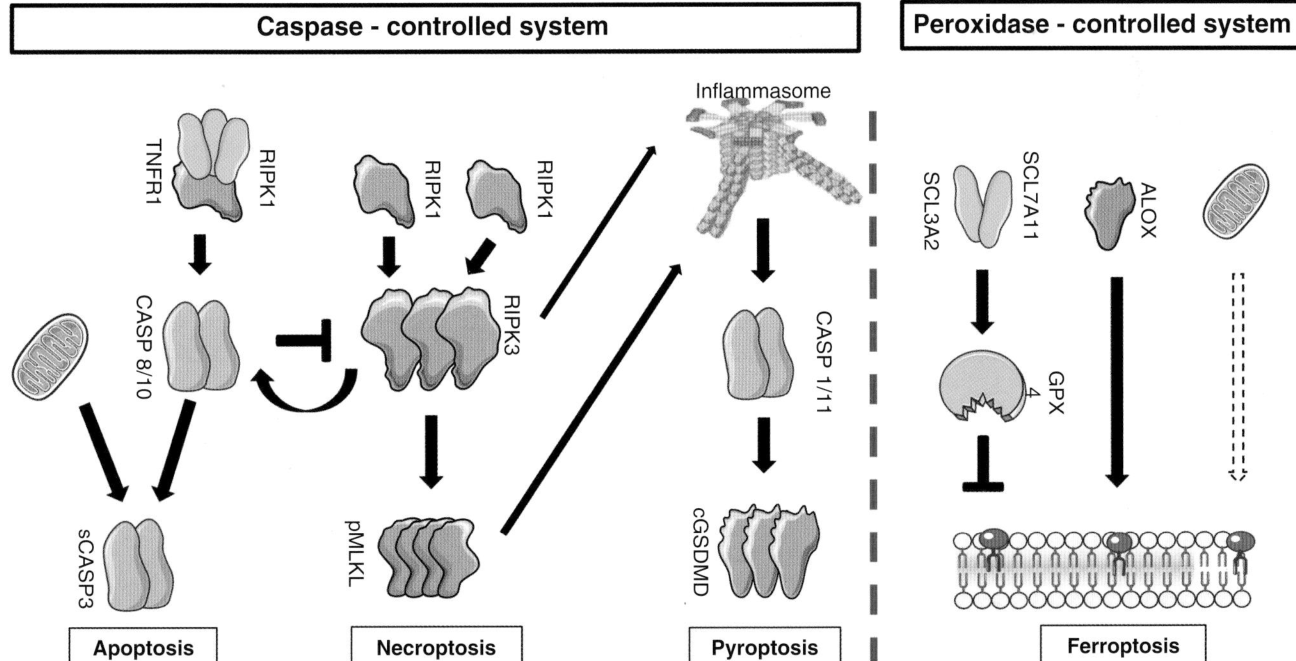


**Fig. 28.4** Overview of the pathways of regulated cell death. In general, two systems may be best differentiated when regulated cell death is considered. The caspase-controlled system includes apoptosis, necroptosis, and pyroptosis and has been studied in great detail over the last few decades. In contrast, the peroxidation-controlled system of ferroptotic cell death functions entirely independently of the caspase-controlled network. Importantly, both systems contribute to human disease. Targeting clinically relevant cell death, therefore, should at least require a combination of therapies aimed at these two systems, which may exhibit some redundant functions. Similarly, in the caspase-controlled system, inhibition of either pathway may result in alternative pathways. With the idea of necroinflammation in mind, it may be helpful to shift a deadly signal from a highly immunogenic pathway (e.g., pyroptosis) toward a pathway with less immunogenic potency (e.g., apoptosis). (From Tonnus W, Gembardt F, Latk M, et al. The clinical relevance of necroinflammation—highlighting the importance of acute kidney injury and the adrenal glands. *Cell Death Differ.* 2019;26(1):68–82.)

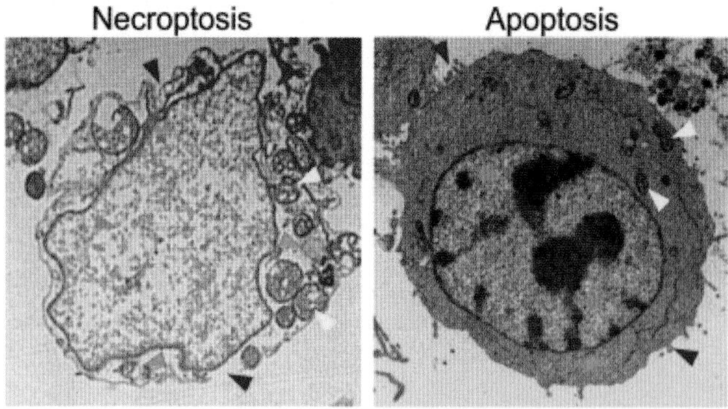


**Fig. 28.5** Morphologic features of necroptosis and apoptosis. HT29 colon cancer cells treated with an anticancer drug for 48 hours were analyzed by transmission electron microscopy. The cell undergoing necroptosis shows plasma membrane rupture and permeabilization, compared with the intact plasma membrane, with blebbing in the apoptotic cell *(red arrowheads).* The necroptotic cell exhibits cytoplasm swelling and vacuolization, which are absent in the apoptotic cell *(green arrowheads).* The necroptotic cell has swelled mitochondria, in contrast to those in the apoptotic cells *(yellow arrowheads).* The necroptotic cell also lacks the condensed and fragmented nuclei seen in the apoptotic cell *(blue arrowheads).* (From Chen D, Yu J, Zhang L. Necroptosis: an alternative cell death program defending against cancer. *Biochim Biophys Acta.* 2016;1865(2):228–236.)

epithelial cells occurs due to ischemic and other cytotoxic insults, whereas inhibition of caspase activity is protective against such injury in cultured and in vivo renal epithelial tubular AKI.[201,202]

Several pathways, including the intrinsic (Bcl-2 family, cytochrome *c*, caspase-9), extrinsic (Fas, FADD, caspase-8), and regulatory (p53 and NF-κB) pathways, appear to be activated during ischemic renal tubular cell injury. It has also been shown that the balance between cell survival and death depends on the relative concentrations of the proapoptotic (Bax, Bcl-2–associated death promoter [Bad], and Bid) and antiapoptotic (Bcl-2 and Bcl-xL) members of the Bcl-2 family of proteins. Overexpression of proapoptotic or relative deficiency of antiapoptotic proteins may lead to the formation of mitochondrial pores. Conversely, the inhibition of such pore formation may occur with the opposite imbalance.[203–205]

Other proteins that have been shown to play a significant role in the apoptotic pathways include NF-κB and p53.[206,207] The central proapoptotic transcription factor p53 can be activated by hypoxia, via HIF-1α, as well as by other noxious stimuli, such as certain drugs (e.g., cisplatin). The kinase-mediated pathways such as ERKs and c-Jun N-terminal kinases (JNKs) are responsible for mediating cellular responses involved in apoptosis, survival, and repair through their interaction with other signals from growth factors, such as hepatocyte growth factor, insulin-like growth factor-1, epidermal growth factor, and vascular endothelial growth factor (VEGF).[208,209] These independent mechanisms can inhibit proapoptotic proteins such as Bad and activate the antiapoptotic transcription of CREB (cyclic adenosine monophosphate response element binding) factors. More recent studies have indicated that there is rapid delivery of small interfering RNA (siRNA) to proximal tubular cells in AKI; targeting siRNA to minimize p53 production leads to a dose-dependent attenuation of apoptotic signaling and kidney function, suggesting potential therapeutic benefit for ischemic and nephrotoxic kidney injury.[210] In vivo, microRNA-24 (miR-24) also regulates the HO-1 and H2A histone family, member X. Overall, these results indicate that miR-24 promotes renal ischemic injury by stimulating apoptosis in endothelial and tubular epithelial cells.[211]

Considering the various pathways available for blockade or modulation, the therapeutic implications of targeting apoptosis in preventing epithelial cell injury are significant. However, it is likely that the "window" to avert lethal injury and prevent cells from progressing to necrosis is in the early initiating apoptotic phases.

Numerous studies have shown that ATP depletion leads to a rise in intracellular calcium through impairment of calcium ATPases, whereas inhibition of $Na^+$-$K^+$-ATPase activity potentiates calcium entry into the cell via the sodium-calcium exchanger. Increased cytosolic calcium causes further mitochondrial injury and cytoskeletal alterations.[212] This chain of events results in the downstream activation of proteases such as calpain and phospholipases. Phospholipases such as phospholipase A2 cause direct hydrolytic damage to membranes and also release toxic free fatty acids. They also cause release of eicosanoids that have vasoactive and hemokinetic activities, resulting in an intense surrounding inflammatory response. Calpain mediates plasma membrane permeability and hydrolysis of the cytoskeletal proteins.[213,214] Finally, there is release of lysosomal enzymes and proteases that degrade histones, resulting in accessibility of the endonucleases to the entire segment, typically seen as the smear pattern on gel electrophoresis, in contrast to the typical ladder pattern seen in apoptosis.[215]

**Necroptosis.** Necroptosis and ferroptosis are two forms of regulated, nonapoptotic cell death. Necrosis is distinguished from apoptosis by the presence of a breakdown of the integrity of the plasma membrane (see Fig. 28.5). As such, necrotic cell death is accompanied by the release of unprocessed intracellular contents, including cellular organelles, highly immunogenic proteins such as ATP, HMGB1, double-stranded DNA, and RNA components, also referred to as damage-associated molecular patterns (DAMPs), a concept known as *necroinflammation*.[216] Although tubular necrosis was thought to be accidental, work done over the last 2 decades has revealed several pathways of genetically determined and regulated necrosis in which receptor interacting serine-threonine protein kinase 1 (RIPK1),[217,218] RIPK3,[219] and its substrate, mixed-lineage kinase domain-like protein (MLKL), have been directly implicated in the regulation of this novel cell death pathway known as necroptosis.[220] The signaling pathway that triggers necroptosis includes the engagement of death receptors in the presence of caspase inhibition, stimulation of Toll-like receptors, signaling through interferons, with the activation of kinase RIPK3, and phosphorylation of pseudokinase MLKL. Phosphorylation of MLKL by RIPK3 leads to a molecular switch mechanism that induces plasma membrane rupture.[221] Demonstration of a protective effect on kidney function with the use of necrostatin-1, an inhibitor of RIPK1, suggests that necroptosis occurs in ischemic AKI.[222] Necroptosis also occurs in the model of cisplatin-induced AKI, as demonstrated by the significant protection of kidney function when using RIPK3 and MLKL-deficient mice.[223]

**Ferroptosis.** Ferroptosis is a previously unrecognized, nonapoptotic form of regulated cell death that is iron-dependent and characterized by increased lipid peroxidation resulting from lack of activity of the lipid repair enzyme glutathione peroxidase 4 (GPX4).[224–226] This leads to the accumulation of lipid-based ROS, including lipid hydroxyperoxides. This form of iron-dependent cell death is distinct from other forms of cell death such as apoptosis, unregulated necrosis, and necroptosis because it mediates cell death in a noncell autonomous and synchronized manner, providing a potential explanation for nephron loss during AKI.[227] Erastin and RSL3 are ferroptosis-inducing compounds that induce cell death in the absence of apoptotic features.[224,228,229] Erastin and RSL3 induce cell death in the absence of major components of apoptotic machinery, including caspases, BAX, and BAK.[230] In a recent study, ferroptosis was shown to play a key role in folic acid–induced AKI,[231] resulting in increased inflammation. Ferroptosis is also importantly regulated by heme oxygenase-1 (HO-1).[232] Immortalized proximal tubule cells from HO-$1^{+/+}$ mice were much more susceptible to erastin or RSL3 than cells from HO-$1^{-/-}$ mice. Iron supplementation decreased cell viability further in HO-$1^{-/-}$ compared with HO-$1^{+/+}$ cells. Finally, ferrostatin (a ferroptosis inhibitor), deferoxamine (an iron chelator), or *N*-acetyl-L-cysteine (a glutathione replenisher) attenuate erastin-induced ferroptosis[232] (see Fig. 28.4).

**Pyroptosis.** This highly inflammatory form of regulated cell death requires caspase 1,4/5 (caspase 11 in mice) for activation[197,233] (see Fig. 28.4). Intracellular damage (sterile inflammatory, such as AKI) and release of DAMPs (pathogen-associated molecular patterns [PAMPs]) activate NLRP3 inflammasome and, in turn, lead to caspase activation and cleavage of pro–interleukin-1 β (IL-1β) and pro–IL-18 to their mature forms. In addition, a newly identified pyroptosis executioner, gasdermin D (GSDMD), is activated, releasing the N-terminal fragment (GSDMD-NT).[197,234] The GDSMD-NT fragment is thought to oligomerize and form a membrane pore on the cell membrane,[235] leading to cell swelling, osmotic lysis, and release of IL-1β and IL-18 and other intracellular contents.[197,234] Thus, unlike apoptosis, pyroptosis results in plasma membrane rupture and release of DAMP molecules, leading to the activation of innate immunity and recruitment of immune cells.[236]

Understanding cell death pathways can lead to specific interventions that could involve strategies to preserve apoptosis for avoiding inflammation while blocking the more inflammatory pathways such as pyroptosis, considered the most proinflammatory of the regulated pathways.[197]

**Autophagy.** Autophagy is an essential mechanism for normal homeostasis, disease pathogenesis, and aging in kidneys.[237–240] Fig. 28.6 reviews the three forms of autophagy—macroautophagy, microautophagy, and chaperone-mediated autophagy:

- Macroautophagy starts with the de novo formation of a cup-shaped isolation double membrane that engulfs a portion of cytoplasm.

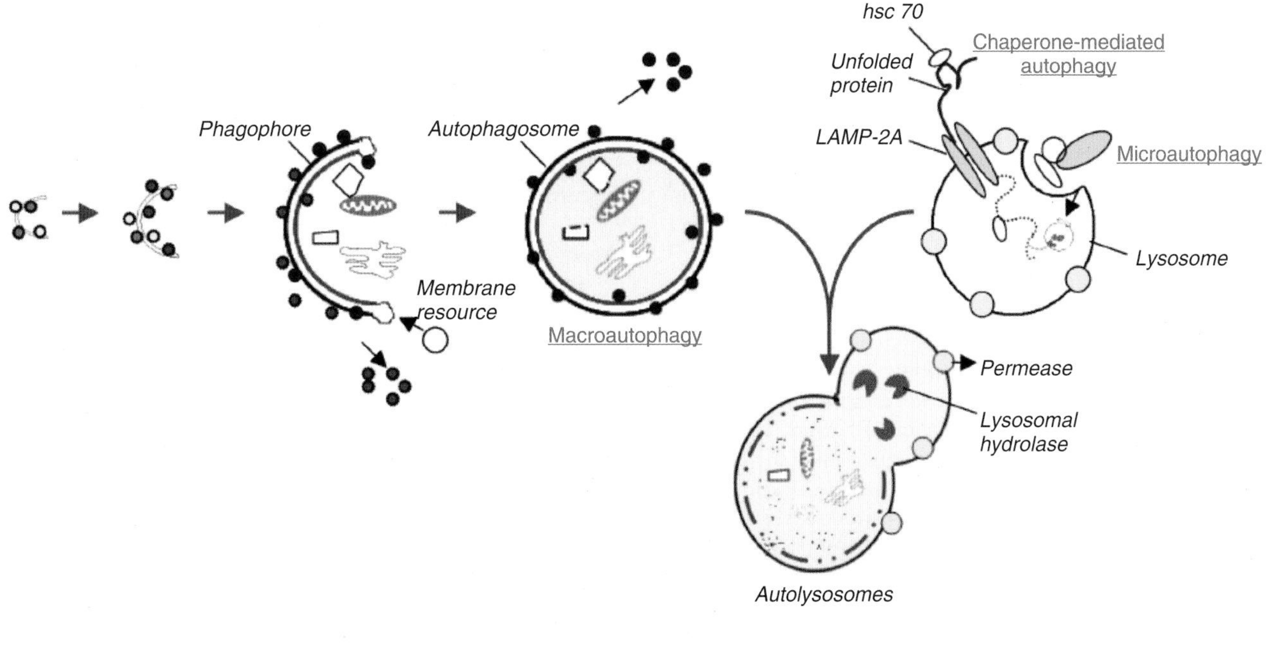


**Fig. 28.6** Autophagy. The forms of autophagy are macroautophagy, microautophagy, and chaperone-mediated autophagy. Macroautophagy starts with the de novo formation of a cup-shaped isolation double membrane that engulfs a portion of cytoplasm. Microautophagy involves the engulfment of cytoplasm instantly at the lysosomal membrane by invagination, protrusion, and separation. Chaperone-mediated autophagy is a process of direct transport of unfolded proteins via the lysosomal chaperonin hsc70 and LAMP-2A. All forms of autophagy subsequently lead to the degradation of intraautophagosomal components by lysosomal hydrolases. *PE,* Phosphatidylethanolamine. (From Periyasamy-Thandavan S, Jiang M, Schoenlein P, Dong Z. Autophagy: molecular machinery, regulation, and implications for renal pathophysiology. *Am J Physiol Renal Physiol.* 2009;297(2):F244–F256.)

- Microautophagy involves the engulfment of cytoplasm instantly at the lysosomal membrane by invagination, protrusion, and separation.
- Chaperone-mediated autophagy is a process of direct transport of unfolded proteins via the lysosomal chaperonin hsc70 and the receptor for chaperone-mediated autophagy, LAMP-2A.

Autophagy is highly conserved and is a lysosomal degradation pathway for the salvation and reuse of degraded proteins, lipids, and organelles to generate basic structural components and energy. It also removes obsolete and dysfunctional organelles and cytotoxic protein aggregates for cellular homeostasis. Under pathogenic conditions, autophagy plays a key role in ischemic, toxic, immunologic, and oxidative insults that lead to the induction of autophagy in renal epithelial cells, which plays a key role in altering the course of disease.[238] Autophagy-mediated leukocyte clearance is an important mechanism for resolving inflammation; it is a function performed by macrophages.[239] Autophagy is characterized by the formation of autophagosomes, a double-membrane vesicles wrapping cytosolic components and organelles that are destined for degradation. Autophagosomes fuse with lysosomes, the contents are degraded, and the products are salvaged and serve as building blocks for cellular function.[237] There are a number of genes and proteins associated in autophagy (autophagy-related; Atg).[237]

Autophagy serves a protective function in renal tubular cells during ischemia-reperfusion injury; it precedes the appearance of apoptotic cells, and suppression of autophagy exacerbates renal injury, in part by inhibiting apoptosis.[241,242] The importance of autophagy has been demonstrated through the generation of proximal tubule-specific ATG5 or ATG7 knockout mice.[243–245] The absence of ATG5 in proximal tubules led to the accumulation of deformed mitochondria and cytoplasmic inclusions or protein aggregates.[243] The lack of ATG5 in distal tubules did not cause significant alterations in kidney function.[244] Similar results were observed in proximal tubule-specific ATG7 knockout mice.[246] Importantly, renal ischemia-reperfusion injury was exaggerated in proximal tubule-specific ATG5 or ATG7 knockout mice.[243,244,246] Autophagy activation was also detected in cisplatin-induced AKI in mice.[247] ATG7 knockout mice demonstrated worse kidney function and injury with cisplatin treatment.[246] Chloroquine, an inhibitor of autophagy, tested in a cisplatin-induced model of AKI, blocked the lysosomal degradation of LC3 in autophagosomes and worsened kidney function.[246] Similarly, autophagy was induced in the septic AKI model of LPS treatment of mice, and inhibition by chloroquine or tubular ATG7 ablation worsened LPS-induced AKI.[248] Thus, data from pharmacologic studies and genetically deficient mice have provided strong evidence for a renoprotective role of autophagy. In addition, dysregulated autophagy can result in increased renal degeneration, leading to progressive kidney disease, as characterized by interstitial fibrosis.[249,250]

**NETosis.** NETosis is a specific form of regulated neutrophil death in which neutrophils release neutrophil extracellular traps (NETs), which are extracellular structures composed of chromatin and histones that enable immobilization and killing of bacteria.[251] On their activation by IL-8, LPS, bacteria or activated platelets, neutrophils initiate a program that leads to their death and the formation of NETs.[252] The activation pathways are known to involve Toll-like receptors (TLRs), cytokines, and Fc receptors.[251,253] This form of cell death is different from apoptosis and necrosis. Cell death is independent of caspases and is not accompanied by fragmentation.[252,254]

Infiltrating neutrophils undergoing NETosis contribute further to organ damage in ischemic AKI. Using the IRI model, Nakazawa and coworkers have demonstrated that infiltrating neutrophils undergo NETosis, leading to the release of cytotoxic DAMPs, such as histones, which exacerbate tubular epithelial cell injury and interstitial inflammation.[255] Using an inhibitor of peptidyl arginine deiminase (PAD), a key enzyme in NET formation, or depleting neutrophils with anti-Ly6G mab, reduced NET formation, tissue necrosis, and biomarkers of AKI and improved kidney function. Furthermore, the authors also demonstrated the presence of NETs in kidney biopsies of patients with ATN.

### Innate Immunity and Inflammation

**Kidney Microenvironment.** The interstitial microenvironment, between the basement membranes of epithelial cells and peritubular capillaries, is a reactive compartment containing mononuclear phagocytes, interstitial fibroblasts, and pericytes, as well as various soluble mediators.[256] The mononuclear phagocytic system consists of bone marrow-derived macrophages and dendritic cells,[257] which overlap in functional characteristics and surface biomarkers.[258] Macrophages are resident tissue phagocytic cells that function generally to clear dying cells and produce cytokines and growth factors.[259,260] Although this system is well known to be activated in response to foreign pathogens,[261] the microenvironment responds to endogenous molecules released from dying cells following tissue injury or to changes produced by conditions such as hypoxia, ischemia, or other forms of sterile inflammation. Matzinger has proposed the danger model to explain these exceptions to the classical role of immune responsiveness to foreign antigen.[262] Dendritic cells are activated by DAMPs or PAMPs[263] and are the key initiators of the innate immune system, following ischemia-reperfusion (Fig. 28.7).

**Mononuclear Phagocytes in Acute Kidney Injury.** Dendritic cells, a resident population of bone marrow–derived cells, and macrophages form a network between the basement membranes of tubular epithelia and peritubular endothelial cells.[256,264] Although dendritic cells and macrophages are often considered as distinct cell types with characteristic functions, recent studies have shown considerable overlap in cell surface markers and function between dendritic cells and macrophages[257] (Fig. 28.8). Located in the interstitial space, dendritic cells have access to endogenous and exogenous DAMPs and PAMPs released by epithelial cells, invading organisms, and infiltrating cells, and thus are key initiators, potentiators, and effectors of the innate immune system.[263,265]

Dendritic cells have enormous plasticity and can be antiinflammatory or proinflammatory.[266,267] Dendritic cells contribute early in the course of IRI-induced activation of NKT cells and the IL-17/IL-23 signaling pathway.[268,269] The importance of dendritic cells in activating the innate immune response in AKI has been determined through depletion of dendritic cells. This was accomplished using transgenic mice expressing the human diphtheria toxin receptor ([DTR]; human heparin-binding epidermal growth factor-like growth

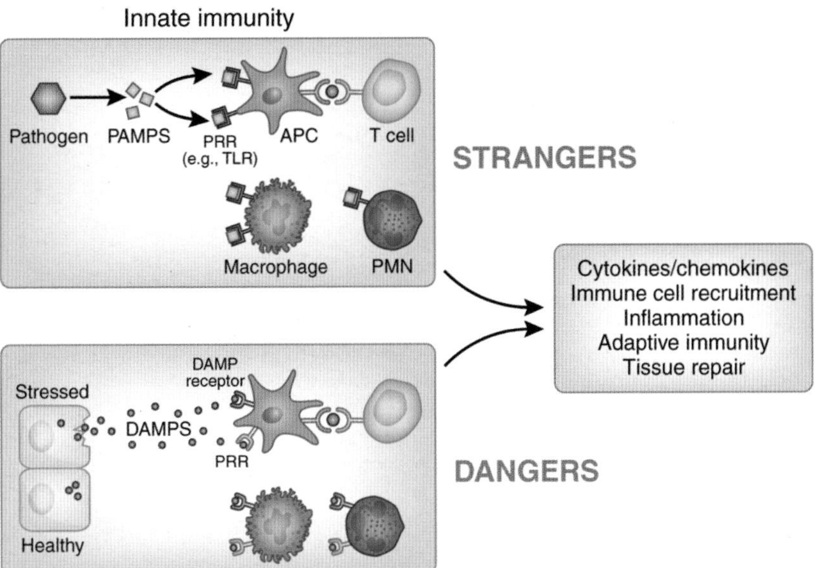


**Fig. 28.7** Danger and stranger models. Infections of pathogenic bacteria or viruses cause the release of pathogen-associated molecular patterns *(PAMPs)* that bind to pattern recognition receptors *(PRRs)*, such as Toll-like receptors *(TLRs)*, on immune cells and stimulate an innate immune response that is accompanied by inflammation and activation of adaptive immunity, and eventually processes to resolve the infection and allow for tissue repair. The danger model recognizes that similar events occur when cells are stressed or injured and that necrotic cells release molecules normally hidden within the cell. In the extracellular space, these damage-associated molecular patterns *(DAMPs)* can bind to PRRs or to specialized DAMP receptors to elicit an immune response by promoting the release of proinflammatory mediators and recruiting immune cells to infiltrate the tissue. The immune cells that participate in these processes include, for example, antigen-presenting cells *(APCs)*, such as dendritic cells and macrophages, as well as T cells and neutrophils (polymorphonuclear leukocytes *[PMNs]*). DAMPs may also stimulate adaptive immunity and participate in autoimmune responses and tissue repair. A wide variety of intracellular and extracellular molecules function as DAMPs when released from cells (see Table 28.1). The functions of such a diverse group of molecules may not yet be fully elucidated; it is unknown whether different DAMPs have specific roles, whether specific functions are elicited in different cell types or conditions, or even whether immune responses to DAMPs can be distinguished from those of PAMPs. (From Rosin DL, Okusa MD. Dangers within: DAMP responses to damage and cell death in kidney disease. *J Am Soc Nephrol.* 2011;22(3):416-425.)

factor in CD11c$^+$ cells (CD11c-DTR mouse).[270] Using diphtheria toxin (DT) and depleting kidney CD11c$^+$ dendritic cells prior to IRI, there was significantly less injury in DT-treated CD11c-DTR mice compared with CD11c DTR mice treated with a catalytically inactive mutant DT (mDT),[271] strongly supporting the concept that dendritic cells contribute to the early innate response in IRI. Depletion of dendritic cells reduced IRI, and deletion of dendritic cell sphingosine 1-phosphate receptor 3 ($S1P_3R$) or inhibition of $S1P_2R$ resulted in protection from IRI.[271–273] They are known to be the earliest producers of IL-6, tumor necrosis factor-α (TNF-α), MCP-1, and RANTES (regulated on activation, normal T cell–expressed and secreted).[274] In addition to initiating the recruitment of inflammatory cells, dendritic cells also participate in recovery via IL-10 production.[275] Dendritic cells can also induce tolerance. Tolerogenic dendritic cells are functionally immature, express inadequate positive or enhanced negative costimulatory signals and reduced proinflammatory cytokines, and can generate immune tolerance by inducing T cell anergy or deletion or by induction or expansion of regulatory T (Treg) cells.[276,277] Adenosine 2A receptor ($A_2AR$)-induced tolerized dendritic cells, suppressed NKT cell activation in vivo and attenuated kidney IRI.[278] However, mature dendritic cells also can promote tolerance.[276,279] Both immature and mature dendritic cells can prime Treg cells that prevent autoimmunity. In contrast to IRI, dendritic cell ablation in DTR mice increased injury in a cisplatin-induced model of AKI, which demonstrates the importance of dendritic cells for tissue protection in a different model of kidney injury.[280] Thus, these studies have revealed disparate roles of tissue resident dendritic cells in AKI and suggest that the differing interstitial microenvironment created by different pathogenic circumstances, such as cisplatin toxicity, IRI, or endogenous molecules (e.g., PAMPS, DAMPS, cytokines, autacoids such as adenosine) may regulate dendritic function.[266] Finally, dendritic cells migrate away from the kidney via the lymphatic system to present antigen and regulate lymphocytic responses.[281] Thus, dendritic cells serve at the crossroads of communication between the epithelium and endothelium, regulating both innate and adaptive immunity, self-tolerance, and tissue injury and repair.

Macrophages are phagocytic innate immune cells that contribute to host defense and, based on surface markers, five distinct populations have been identified.[282,283] Tissue-resident macrophages are derived from a heterogeneous population of bone marrow derived-monocytes.[260,284–286] They are characterized by low surface expression of chemokine receptor 2 (CCR2), GR-1, and Ly6C and high surface expression of the fractalkine receptor CX3CR1.[260,287] These monocytes migrate into normal tissue and differentiate into resident dendritic cells and macrophages.[286] In contrast, macrophages that infiltrate into inflamed tissue have a phenotype characterized by high surface expression of CCR2, Ly6C, and GR-1 and low surface expression of CX3CR1. It is likely that the

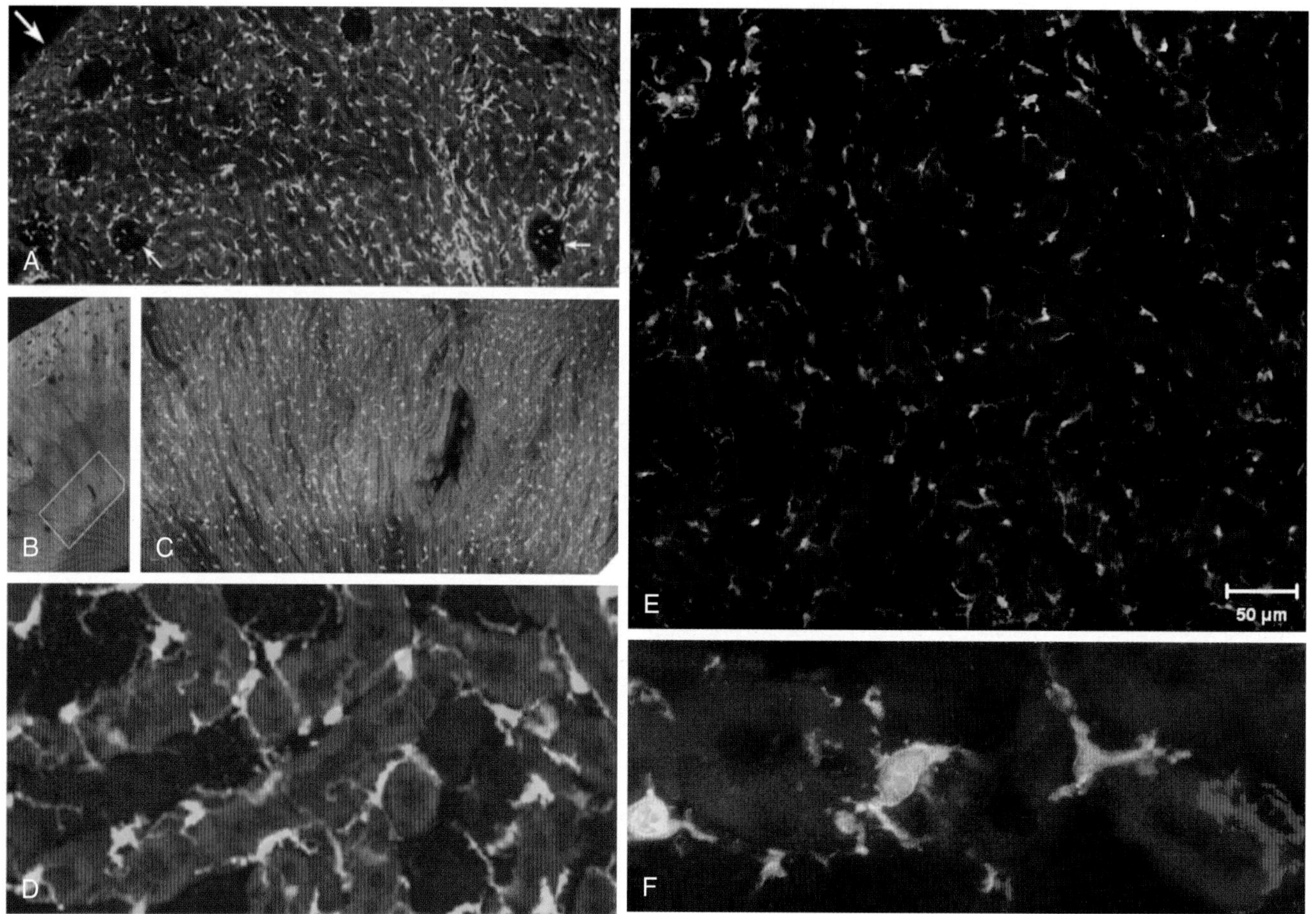


**Fig. 28.8** Heterogeneity of mononuclear phagocytes within the microenvironment. Mononuclear phagocytes within the microenvironment, identified as CX3CR1⁺/GFP⁺ cells (labelled *green*), in the kidney are shown in panels A to D, and the heterogeneity of mononuclear phagocytes is shown in panel E. (A) A heterogenous population of CX3CR1⁺/GFP⁺ mononuclear phagocytes in superficial cortex includes dendritic cells and macrophages and reside from the cortex and medulla. CX3CR1⁺ GFP⁺ cells extend to the edge of the cortex *(large arrow)* and populate the entire interstitial space abundantly. Bowman's capsule is encased by CX3CR1⁺/GFP⁺ cells *(small arrows)*. Also notable are CX3CR1⁺ GFP⁺ cells that lie within each glomeruli. (B) Rhodamine-conjugated peanut agglutinin *(red fluorescence)* highlights distal tubules and collecting ducts, capsule *(upper left)* to the papilla *(lower right)*. (C) Magnification of the boxed area in panel B showing CX3CR1⁺ GFP⁺ cells in the interstitium of the medulla, including transition into pyramidal tracks. Note the same spatial regularity as in the cortex. (D) Three-dimensional rendering of stellate-shaped CX3CR1⁺ GFP⁺ cells within the interstitium demarcated by tubular segments in the medulla *(red fluorescence)*. (E) Kidney sections from the medulla of CX3CR1⁺/GFP⁺ mice. GFP is expressed mainly on monocyte-macrophages and dendritic cells, and many CX3CR1⁺GFP⁺ green fluorescing cells are seen in the cortex; most IA⁺ cells *(red label)* are seen in the medulla. Apparent in this image is the heterogeneity of CX3CR1⁺/GFP⁺–only cells, IA⁺–only cells, and dual labeling with CX3CR1⁺/GFP⁺ and IA⁺, which in the latter case represents dendritic cells in the medulla. (F) Higher magnification, Z-stack projection image of five optical slides at 0.69-mm intervals. These results demonstrate the heterogeneity of mononuclear phagocytes within the kidney microenvironment. (A–D from Soos TJ, Sims TN, Barisoni L, et al. CX3CR1+ interstitial dendritic cells form a contiguous network throughout the entire kidney. *Kidney Int*. 2006;70(3):591–596; E, F from Li L, Huang L, Sung SS, et al. The chemokine receptors CCR2 and CX3CR1 mediate monocyte/macrophage trafficking in kidney ischemia-reperfusion injury. *Kidney Int*. 2008;74(12):1526–1537.)

microenvironment in the tissue determines their phenotype. TNF-α, IL-4, and IL-15 skew monocyte differentiation toward a dendritic cell phenotype,[288–290] whereas interferon-gamma (IFN-γ) and IL-6 direct monocyte differentiation toward a macrophage phenotype.[291,292] Following kidney IRI, through monocyte chemoattractant protein 1 (MCP-1/CCL2) signaling via monocyte CCR2 receptors,[293] monocytes migrate into inflamed kidneys within 24 hours.[269,271]

Although controversial, and challenged by recent studies, the original classification of M1 and M2 macrophages does provide an important functional framework.[294] M1 macrophages, also referred to as "classic macrophages," are activated by IFN-γ and LPS and express high levels of inducible nitric oxide synthase (iNOS). M1 macrophages have high microbicidal activity through the production of proinflammatory cytokines such as TNF-α, IL-6, and IL-12 via signal transducer and activator of transcription 1 (STAT1), NF-κB, and ROS.[283] M2 macrophages, referred to as "alternative macrophages," are activated by IL-4 or IL-13 and participate in tissue repair and resolution of inflammation through insulin-like growth factor 1 (IGF-1), mannose receptor 1 (Mrc1/CD206), and arginase-1 (Arg1) following STAT6 activation.[295]

Evidence for these disparate roles played by macrophages can be assessed in vivo through the administration of liposomal clodronate. Liposomal clodronate is engulfed by macrophages and clodronate is released from the liposome through action of lysosomal phospholipases in the macrophage, becomes toxic, and kills cells by apoptosis.[296] The functional role of macrophages was determined by liposomal clodronate depletion studies that focused on the time course for macrophage depletion (early vs. late). Depletion of kidney and spleen macrophages using liposomal clodronate before renal IRI prevented AKI, and adoptive transfer of macrophages reconstituted AKI.[297] However, depletion of macrophages 3 to 5 days after IRI slowed tubular cell proliferation and repair,[283] suggesting that M1 macrophages exhibiting a proinflammatory phenotype are important for injury, whereas M2 macrophages exhibiting an antiinflammatory phenotype are important for tissue repair.[283,298,299]

Following IRI, the proinflammatory monocyte entering into the kidney tissue is activated to a proinflammatory macrophage through the infiltration of polymorphonuclear leukocytes, T cells, and NKT cells.[268,300,301] Resident dendritic cells activate NKT cells to produce INF-γ and other inflammatory mediators such as ROS, semaphorin-3A, DAMPs, and TNF-α, which conditions the microenvironment and favors the proinflammatory macrophage phenotype.[283] These proinflammatory macrophages then produce proinflammatory cytokines, which lead to further tissue injury. Whether polarization of macrophages from M1 to M2 involves the recruitment of circulating cells or reprogramming is unclear.[283,302] Studies by Lee and colleagues have supported the concept that macrophage polarization occurs in situ.[303] In these studies, the investigators injected labeled M1 macrophages at the time of injury and examined labeled macrophages that infiltrated the injured kidneys. Most of the labeled cells maintained an M1 phenotype; however, when labeled M1 macrophages were injected 3 days after injury, most of the macrophages expressed an M2 phenotype. These studies support the concept that macrophages may be reprogrammed in situ,[283,302,304] and that the kidney microenvironment provides important conditioning cues.[266]

Early inflammation is classically characterized by the margination of leukocytes to the activated vascular endothelium via interactions between selectins and ligands that allows firm adhesion, followed by transmigration.[305,306] A number of potent mediators are generated by the injured proximal tubular epithelial cell, including proinflammatory cytokines such as TNF-α, IL-6, IL-1β, MCP-1, IL-8, transforming growth factor-β (TGF-β), and RANTES.[278,307] TLR2 is an important mediator of endothelial ischemic injury, and TLR4 has been shown to play a similar role in animal models of both ischemic and septic injury,[308] especially in PTC.[309]

**Polymorphonuclear Leukocytes in Acute Kidney Injury.** Neutrophils accumulate early in ischemic injury in animal models.[271] Both IL-17A and IFN-γ were shown to be produced by neutrophils and may positively regulate neutrophil transmigration to the injured kidney following kidney IRI[268] (Fig. 28.9). Although neutrophils are seen early in rodent models of AKI, whether they play a pathogenic role remains controversial because inhibition or depletion studies of neutrophils leads to protection[305,310,311] or lack of protection.[312] Blockade of neutrophil function or neutrophil depletion has been shown to provide only partial protection against injury.

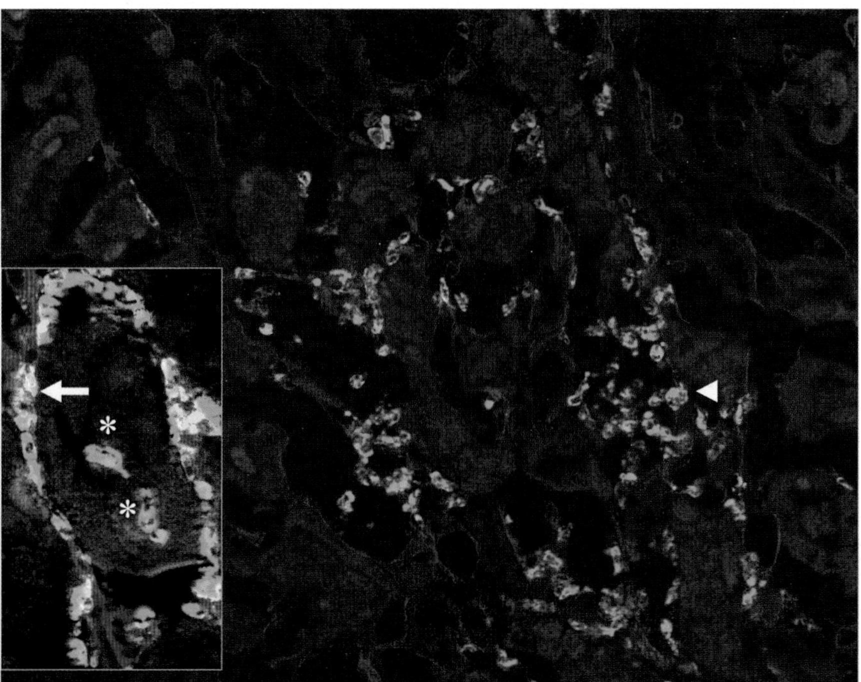


**Fig. 28.9** Localization of neutrophils to interstitial and marginated compartments in the kidney. Immunofluorescence staining of kidney outer medulla using antibodies to 7/4 (*green*, neutrophils) and CD31 (*red,* vascular endothelium). Nuclei are depicted by DAPI labeling *(blue).* Neutrophils in both sides of the vascular endothelial wall. *Inset,* Z-stack image (7.0 μm) of 12 optical slices of the kidney at 0.6-μm intervals. Shown are kidney neutrophils in the interstitium and peritubular capillaries *(arrows)*; neutrophils that have transmigrated into the lumen of the tubule *(*)* are shown in the inset. (From Awad, AS, Rouse, M, Huang, L, et al. Compartmentalization of neutrophils in the kidney and lung following acute ischemic kidney injury. *Kidney Int.* 2009;75:689–698.)

Vascular adhesion protein-1 (VAP-1) is an adhesion molecule[313,314] associated with inflammatory conditions. Tanaka and colleagues have found that VAP-1 is expressed primarily in pericytes, and a specific VAP-1 inhibitor, RTU-1096, attenuated renal IRI and decreased neutrophil infiltration. The protective effect of VAP-1 inhibition was absent in neutrophil-depleted rats, suggesting an important role of neutrophil infiltration.[315]

Other leukocytes, including but not limited to macrophages, NKT cells, B lymphocytes, and T lymphocytes contribute to kidney IRI.[297,301,316–319] Selective depletion, knockout mice models, and specific blockade have shown that all these cells do mediate tubular injury at various phases and that there are synergistic interactions between different cellular types.[297,316–319]

Whether released from the endothelium or the epithelial cell, numerous cytokines exert a concerted biochemical effort to augment the inflammatory response seen as a result of ischemic or septic injury.[317] Furthermore, mouse tubular cells when stimulated with LPS in culture, upregulate TLR2, TLR3, and TLR4 and secrete CC-chemokines such as CC motif chemokine ligand 2 (CCL2)/MCP-1 and CCL5/RANTES. These data suggest that tubular TLR expression might be involved in mediating interstitial leukocyte infiltration and tubular injury during bacterial sepsis.[320]

TLR2 and TLR4 are constitutively expressed on renal epithelium, and their expression is enhanced following renal IRI. El-Achkar and coworkers have shown that in a CLP rat model of sepsis, TLR4 expression increases markedly in all tubules (proximal and distal), glomeruli, and the renal vasculature.[321] Genetic deletion of TLR2 or TLR4 protects from renal IRI[309,322] and from cisplatin-induced AKI. In this later study, Zhang et al.,[323] using bone marrow chimeras, found that renal parenchymal TLR4, rather than hematopoietic-derived TLR4, mediated cisplatin-induced nephrotoxicity. These studies are consistent with studies by Wu and coworkers[309] and clearly demonstrate the important role TLR plays in AKI.

**T Cells in Acute Kidney Injury.** Early work by Burne-Taney and coworkers has demonstrated that T lymphocytes contribute importantly to renal IRI.[312,324,325] However, conventional CD4$^+$ T cells are thought to play an obligatory role in antigen-specific, cognate immunity that requires 2 to 4 days for T cell processing, a time course that cannot explain the rapid, innate immune response following IRI. Natural killer T (NKT) cells are a T cell sublineage[326] and, in mice, NKT cells express an invariant T cell receptor TCRα chain, Vα14-J18. In contrast to conventional T cells, the NKT cell TCR does not interact with peptide antigen presented by classic major histocompatibility complex (MHC) class I or II; rather, it recognizes glycolipids presented by the class I-like molecule, CD1d. On NKT cell activation, vigorous cytokine secretion occurs within 1 to 2 hours, including Th1-type (IFN-γ, TNF) and Th2-type (IL-4, IL-13) cytokines at the same time.[326–332] The rapid response by NKT cells following activation can amplify and regulate the function of dendritic cells, Treg cells, NK and B cells, and conventional T cells and thus link innate and adaptive immunity.[333–338] In AKI, NKT cells participate in early innate immune response to kidney IRI.[301] NKT-produced IFN-γ was found as early as 3 hours following IRI,[301] supporting previous work demonstrating that CD4$^+$ T cell IFN-γ production is responsible for kidney injury.[339,340] These data demonstrate the central role of IFN-γ from CD4$^+$ T and/or NKT cells in the pathogenesis of renal IRI.

Treg cells[318,319] have also recently been shown to play a role in ischemic AKI.[341] Liu and colleagues have shown that in a murine model of ischemic AKI, there is significant trafficking of Treg cells into the kidneys after 3 and 10 days.[342] Postischemic kidneys had increased numbers of TCR-β$^+$–CD4$^+$ and TCR-β$^+$–CD8$^+$ T cells, with enhanced proinflammatory cytokine production. These investigators also noted that Treg depletion starting 1 day after ischemic injury using anti-CD25 antibodies increases renal tubular damage, reduces tubular proliferation at both time points, and enhances infiltrating T lymphocyte cytokine production at 3 days and TNF-α generation by TCR-β$^+$–CD4$^+$ T cells at 10 days. In separate mouse studies, infusion of CD4$^+$–CD25$^+$ Treg cells 1 day after initial injury reduced IFN-γ production by TCR-β$^+$– D4$^+$ T cells at 3 days, improved repair, and reduced cytokine generation at 10 days. These studies demonstrate that Treg cells infiltrate post-IRI kidneys during the healing process and promote repair, likely through modulation of proinflammatory cytokine production of other T cell subsets.[342]

The role of Treg cells has been further extended by Kinsey and coworkers, who have shown that partial depletion of Treg cells with an anti-CD25 monoclonal antibody potentiates kidney damage induced by IRI and that reducing the number of Treg cells results in more neutrophils, macrophages, and innate cytokine transcription in the kidney after IRI.[343] Furthermore, FoxP3 (forkhead box P3)$^+$ Treg cell–deficient mice accumulated a higher number of inflammatory leukocytes after renal IRI than mice containing Treg cells, and that cotransfer of isolated Treg cells and Scurfy lymph node cells significantly attenuated IRI-induced renal injury and leukocyte accumulation.[343] Studies of adoptively transferred Treg cells have shown that IL-10 production, adenosine production through CD73, expression of the adenosine 2A receptor, and programmed cell death 1 (PD-1) on the cell surface are required by Treg cells to protect recipient mice from IRI.[319] Studies have demonstrated that PD-1, a negative costimulatory molecule expressed on T lymphocytes, monocytes, dendritic cells, and B cells,[344,345] is indispensable for Treg function. Administration of monoclonal antibodies to PD-1 or a genetic deficiency of PD-1 on Tregs exacerbated impaired kidney function and ATN after subthreshold ischemia.[346] Stremska and coworkers have synthesized a hybrid cytokine, IL233, which combines IL-2 and IL-33.[347] Tregs require IL-2 for homeostasis and upregulate IL-33, which promotes the recruitment and activation of innate lymphoid cells (ILC2s).[348] Administration of the novel hybrid cytokine, IL233, increased endogenous Tregs in blood and spleen and prevented IRI more efficiently than a mixture of IL-2 and IL-33 administered separately. IL233 also increased the proportion of ILC2s in blood and kidneys, and adoptive transfer of ILC2s protected mice from IRI.[347] Thus, the many barriers to cell-based therapy may be overcome through this hybrid cytokine, which increases endogenous Tregs. Rapid translation to human studies would be a major advancement in the field.

**B Lymphocytes.** Studies to evaluate the role of B cells and the B1 subset on ischemia-induced AKI have remained controversial, with some studies showing that B cells may be deleterious. Burne-Taney and associates have shown that μMT mice, which lack B cells and all immunoglobulins, are protected from AKI despite similar levels of infiltrating granulocytes and macrophages in the postischemic kidneys of wild type (WT) mice.[316] These investigators demonstrated that μMT mice were rendered sensitive to ischemia-induced AKI after replenishing these mice with WT serum, but not B cells, thus indicating that a serum factor enhanced the cytotoxic effect of infiltrating granulocytes and macrophages on the ischemic tubular cells. However, Renner and colleagues, using the same μMT mice, could not show that these mice were protected from ischemia-induced AKI.[349] In fact, these mice had more severe injury when compared with control WT mice. Additionally, Lobo and associates failed to show protection from ischemia-induced AKI when WT mice were acutely depleted of B cells (with anti-CD20) and not immunoglobulins.[350] More studies are needed to study the role of B cells and immunoglobulins in AKI; it may be preferable to deplete B cells or subsets of B cells acutely to study their role. μMT mice have other immune deficiencies, including low Tregs and lack of TcR diversification, which may have contributed to more severe injury in the experiments by Thurman and colleagues.[351,352]

The role of the B1 subset of B cells in murine models of ischemia has also been controversial. Ray, Zhang, and associates have clearly shown that natural IgM produced by B1 cells is deleterious in ischemia-induced injury of murine skeletal muscle, cardiac muscle, and bowel.[352–354] They demonstrated that ischemia exposed nonmuscle myosin, heavy-chain type IIA and C (NMM) neoantigen in these organs and, by immunohistochemistry, they clearly demonstrated binding of natural IgM and complement to NMM in these ischemic organs. Furthermore, they showed that natural IgM was pathogenic because these same organs were resistant to ischemic injury in immunoglobulin-deficient $Rag1^{-/-}$ mice, but become susceptible to ischemia if these mice are replenished with purified IgM. On the other hand, Lobo and colleagues have shown that natural IgM protects WT kidneys from ischemic AKI by inhibiting the innate inflammation that occurs after ischemic injury.[355] Both they and others have clearly shown that $Rag1^{-/-}$ mice are also susceptible to ischemic AKI in the absence of IgM.[350] Kidneys from IgM knockout mice, deficient in only IgM but not B cells and other immunoglobulins or Tregs, are very sensitive to minimal ischemia that is insufficient to cause AKI in WT mice.[355] Additionally, Renner and associates could not show binding of IgM to ischemic tubules or peritubular capillaries in WT mice. It is therefore possible that NMM, which is also present in the kidney, is not exposed after ischemic injury.[349] Such observations also demonstrate that the mechanisms that cause ischemic injury in the kidney may be different from those of other organs.

#### Inflammation

Altered endothelial cell function also mediates inflammation, a hallmark of ischemic injury that has been the subject of numerous studies. Ischemia induces the increased expression of a number of leukocyte adhesion molecules, such as P-selectin, E-selectin, and intercellular adhesion molecule (ICAM) and B7-1. Consequently, it has been shown that strategies to block pharmacologically or genetically ablate the expression of these molecules are protective against ischemic or septic AKI.[311] Investigators have also shown that T cells play a major role in vascular permeability during ischemic injury. Gene microarray analysis has shown that the production of TNF-α and IFN-γ protein is increased in CD3 and CD4 T cells from the blood and kidney after ischemia. Furthermore, it has also been demonstrated that in CD3, CD4, and CD8 T cell–deficient mice, there is a significantly attenuated rise in renal vascular permeability after ischemic injury. Hence, T cells directly contribute to the increased vascular permeability, potentially through T cell cytokine production.[342,356] Another feature noted during inflammation and endothelial cell injury is the phenomenon of erythrocyte trapping with rouleaux formation, prolonging the reduction in renal blood flow and exacerbating tubular injury.[357] Studies have also shown a role of the sphingosine 1-phosphate receptor (S1PR) in maintaining structural integrity after AKI. Thurman and coworkers have shown that S1PRs in the proximal tubule are necessary for stress-induced cell survival, and S1PR agonists are renoprotective via direct effects on tubular cells.[358,359]

DNA microarray analysis of ischemic kidneys from TLR4-sufficient and TLR4-deficient mice has shown that pentraxin 3 (PTX3), an endothelial induced protein, is upregulated only in TLR4-sufficient mice. Transgenic knockout of PTX3 ameliorated AKI. PTX3 was shown to be expressed predominantly on the peritubular endothelia of the outer medulla of the kidney in control mice and AKI increased PTX3 protein in the kidney and the plasma. Stimulation studies performed in primary renal endothelial cells have suggested that endothelial PTX3 is induced by pathways involving TLR4 and ROS and demonstrated that these effects could be inhibited by conditional endothelial knockout of MyD88. Compared with WT mice, PTX3 knockout mice had decreased endothelial expression of cell adhesion molecules at 4 hours of reperfusion, possibly contributing to a decreased early maladaptive inflammation in the kidneys of knockout mice, whereas later, at 24 hours of reperfusion, PTX3 knockout increased the expression of endothelial adhesion molecules when regulatory and reparative leukocytes enter the kidney. Thus, endothelial PTX3 plays a pivotal role in the pathogenesis of ischemic AKI.[360]

The role of glomerular endothelial injury in AKI is unclear. Studies in a mouse model of LPS-induced sepsis have shown decreased abundance of endothelial surface layer heparan sulfate proteoglycans and sialic acid, leading to albuminuria, likely reflecting altered glomerular filtration permselectivity and decreased expression of VEGF. LPS treatment also decreased the GFR, caused ultrastructural alterations in the glomerular endothelium, and lowered the density of glomerular endothelial cell fenestrae. These LPS-induced effects were diminished in TNF receptor 1 (TNFR1) knockout mice, suggesting the role of TNF-α activation of TNFR1, and intravenous administration of TNF also led to a decreased GFR and loss of glomerular endothelial cell fenestrae, increased fenestrae diameter, and damage to the glomerular endothelial surface layer. Thus, glomerular endothelial injury, mediated by higher TNF-α and lower VEGF levels, extends the development and progression of AKI and albuminuria in the LPS model of sepsis in the mouse.[361]

In addition to immune cells responding and sensing DAMPs and PAMPs (see later), proximal tubule cells (PTCs) function as a sensor of both self and nonself; DAMPs and PAMPs serve as recognition signals for pattern recognition receptors (PRRs) such as TLR4.[362] Proximal tubule TLR4 is upregulated and migrates to the apical domain in response to LPS in S1 PTCs, which are the earliest segments of epithelial cell postglomerular filtration.[321] Interestingly, the S1 cell internalizes and processes LPS via TLR4 receptors, which is inducible with preexposure to LPS but is protected from injury by upregulated defense mechanisms, including heme oxygenase-1 (HO-1) and sirtuin 1 (SIRT1), two cytoprotective proteins. However, S2 to S3 PTCs undergo oxidative injury with minimal uptake of LPS, implying communication, crosstalk, and coregulation between the segments following LPS exposure.[363] This injury is dependent on CD14, likely due to peroxisomal disruption, perhaps mediated by TNF-α, and the PTC injury was found to be independent of systemic cytokines.

Another role for epithelial TLR4 and MyD88 in mediating ischemic injury has been shown by Wu and colleagues.[309] In addition, in these studies, the relative contribution of epithelial versus hematopoietic TLR4 to kidney damage following IRI was assessed using bone marrow chimeras in which $TLR4^{-/-}$ mice were engrafted with WT hematopoietic cells (and vice versa). Both hematopoietic and parenchymal TLR4 contributed to kidney injury, although the effect was more pronounced when TLR4 was expressed only on parenchymal cells. These results suggest that TLR4 signaling on hematopoietic and intrinsic kidney cells contributes to mediating kidney damage but a more significant role is played by intrinsic kidney cells. Similar results with TLR2 knockout mice and chimeric mice have suggested that epithelial TLR2 plays a prominent role during ischemic injury.[364] Cytokine and chemokine production was reduced and white blood cell (WBC) infiltration was minimized in chimeric mice using antisense therapy. These studies suggest that renal-associated TLR2 is an important initiator of inflammatory responses that lead to renal injury.

Cytokines and chemokines released by PTCs in response to cell injury have direct effects on endothelial function. Using two-photon microscopy, investigators recorded cellular and physiologic responses to fluorescent cytopathologic *Escherichia coli* microinjected into early proximal tubule segments.[365–367] Attachment to the apical membrane, but without penetration into or through the PTC monolayer barrier, resulted in rapid and selective termination of blood flow to the adjacent area, and thus resulted in vascular isolation of the infected area with localized hypoxia, leukocyte migration, and necrosis. The same *E. coli* strain, missing only one virulence factor, required a far longer time to initiate this protective process. Tissue concentrations of cytokines were markedly elevated in the affected area compared with none in the injected areas.[367] Finally, prevention of this microvascular response resulted in widespread organ dissemination of the injected *E. coli* and death of the rat within 24 hours, something not seen with the intact system.[367] Therefore, communication between PTC and endothelial cells may lead to localization of the infecting agent and prevention of systemic spread.

Tamm-Horsfall protein (also known as *uromodulin*), a heavily glycosylated protein uniquely produced in the kidney by TALs,[368,369] modulates kidney innate immunity and inflammation during kidney injury.[362,368,370] Uromodulin knockout mice compared with WT controls subjected to kidney IRI showed increased S3 injury and necrosis,[370,371] neutrophil infiltration in the outer medulla, and expression of TLR4 and CXCL2 by S3 segments.[370,371] Neutralization of CXCL2 was protective, suggesting that a TLR4-CXCL2 proinflammatory pathway may be important in the pathophysiology and supporting uromodulin-dependent TAL-S3 crosstalk. Indeed, after IRI, a shift of trafficking of uromodulin was demonstrated toward the interstitium and basolateral aspects of S3 segments,[372] where a putative receptor for uromodulin is expressed.[370] This translocation of uromodulin was not the result of altered polarity of TAL. Uromodulin knockout ($THP^{-/-}$) mice, in addition to worse injury compared with WT mice, had an impaired transition of renal macrophages toward an M2 healing phenotype, suggesting that interstitial THP may not only regulate mononuclear phagocyte number, but plasticity and phagocytic activity as well.[373] A significant increase in uromodulin expression was shown in the kidney at the onset of recovery, which was concomitant with the suppression of tubular-derived cytokines and chemokines such as MCP-1, supporting the concept that the protective crosstalk mediated by uromodulin may be important in modulating recovery from AKI.[372]

## COMPLEMENT

The complement system is part of the host defense machinery that protects against microbial invasion after injury.[374] The reactivity and specificity of the complement system is accomplished via a series of circulating pattern recognition proteins (PRPs) that sense PAMPs and initiate the complement cascade. The immunomodulatory functions of complement are mediated through three canonical pathways of activation—classic pathway, alternative pathway, and lectin pathway. The classic pathway is initiated by binding of PRPs to immune complexes, whereas the lectin pathway is initiated by binding PRPs to carbohydrate structures exposed in injured cells. The alternative pathway amplifies the initial response and maintains a low level of activity via a tick-over mechanism. On recognition of foreign surfaces, PRP-associated serine proteases cleave soluble components deposited on the activating surface and form C3 convertase complexes. Subsequent convertase-mediated cleavage of C3 leads to the formation of C3 fragments that serve as ligands for a variety of complement receptors that mediate increased phagocytosis and stimulation of the adaptive immune response. In addition to C3 convertase formation, opsonization also leads to the formation of C5 convertase, which activates C5 and initiates the formation of the pore-forming membrane attack complex (MAC) that lyses susceptible microorganisms or damages cells.[375]

Previous studies have suggested that complement is only located in the intravascular space, with most components synthesized in the liver. Many reports have now documented the presence of a functionally intact intracellular complement system within lymphocytes and epithelial, endothelial, and other cell types, and several studies have identified C3- and C5-mediated activation and signaling events in the intracellular space.[376]

Complement activation causes kidney injury through direct effects on renal cells and through interactions with cells of the innate and adaptive immune systems. Small soluble peptides, named "anaphylatoxins" (C3a and C5a) are generated during complement activation. These fragments trigger a systemic inflammatory response through their receptors, including vascular changes and chemotaxis of immune cells.[377] C3a and C5a receptors are expressed on leukocytes, endothelial cells, mesangial cells, and tubular epithelial cells.[378] During ischemic injury, CR5a expression is markedly upregulated on proximal tubule epithelial cells, as well as interstitial macrophages. C5a is a powerful chemoattractant that recruits inflammatory cells. Complement cascades are activated during sepsis, and C5a, a potent complement component with procoagulant properties, is elevated in rodent models of sepsis. Blocking C5a or its receptor has shown some promise in improving survival with sepsis.[379]

To protect host cells from uncontrolled complement activation, several complement regulatory proteins are expressed in the surface of kidney cells and can directly inactivate complement convertase. Previous studies have documented complement activation in the pathogenesis of IRI-induced AKI.[380] These investigators used mice with a global deficiency to factor B or antibodies to factor B to demonstrate that the inhibition of C3 formation in kidney tissue protects mice from IRI-induced AKI. In addition to AKI, recent studies have demonstrated increased expression of complement C3 fragments and anaphylatoxin receptors C3aR and C5aR1 in PDGFRβ-positive pericytes and immune cells that were isolated from fibrotic kidneys. Inhibition of complement activation using mice with a global deletion of C3 has resulted in reduced tubulointerstitial fibrosis.[381] Given the increased awareness of the role of complement activation, not only with AKI but also in models of CKD, it is likely that emerging therapies aimed at inhibiting complement activation could be used in future studies to reduce the evolution of AKI and/or the progression of CKD.

## INTRACELLULAR MECHANISMS

### Reactive Oxygen Species

Oxidative stress plays an important role in the pathogenesis of AKI and progressive kidney disease. Low-level ROS can function as signaling molecules for cellular proliferation and vascular homeostasis under healthy conditions; however, increased ROS generation during IRI by mitochondria, nicotinamide adenine dinucleotide phosphate (NADPH) oxidases, or inflammatory cells can aggravate tissue injury. Therefore, reducing oxidative stress is considered an important therapeutic strategy to ameliorate loss of kidney function.[382]

ROS such as $OH^-$, peroxynitrite ($ONOO^-$), and hypochlorous acid (HOCl) are generated in epithelial cells during ischemic injury by catalytic conversion. These ROS can damage cells in a variety of ways (e.g., via peroxidation of lipids in plasma and intracellular membranes). They can also destabilize the cytoskeletal proteins and integrins required to maintain cell-cell adhesion, as well as extracellular matrix. These ROS can also have vasoconstrictive effects by their capacity to scavenge NO.[383]

### Heat Shock Proteins

Much of the previous discussion has been on proteins or mechanisms that promote injury. However, there are protective mechanisms that allow cells to have a defense against numerous stresses. The complex heat shock protein (HSP) system is induced to exceptionally high levels during stress conditions. The HSPs are believed to facilitate the restoration of normal function by assisting in the refolding of denatured proteins, along with aiding the appropriate folding of newly synthesized proteins. They also help in the degradation of irreparable proteins and toxins to limit their accumulation. Overexpression of HSPs before injury has protective effects.[384–386] The proteins HSP90, HSP72, and HSP25 in particular have been extensively studied (e.g., overexpression of HSP25 is protective against actin cytoskeleton disruption).[387] After renal ischemia, cytosolic HSP90 is rapidly induced in PTCs, particularly in late stages, leading to the conclusion that HSP90 may be crucial for the disposition of damaged proteins and the assembly of newly formed peptides. Intrarenal transfection with HSP90 protects against IRI with the restoration of endothelial nitric oxide synthase (eNOS)–HSP90 coupling, eNOS activating phosphorylation, and Rho kinase levels, suggesting that HSPs can regulate the NO–eNOS pathway and intrarenal vascular tone.[388] In nephrotoxic models, HSP72 has been shown to limit apoptosis through an increased Bcl-2/Bax ratio, implicating HSP72 in cell death as well.[387]

Nayak's group has described the role of myoinositol oxygenase (MIOX), a proximal tubule enzyme that participates in oxidant injury by increasing the generation of ROS in kidney tissue.[389] In a more recent study,[390] the investigators used the cisplatin model of AKI in tubule-specific MIOX-overexpressing transgenic (MIOX-TG) mice and MIOX knockout ($MIOX^{-/-}$) mice. Compared with cisplatin-treated WT mice, cisplatin-treated MIOX-TG mice had more pronounced kidney injury, evidenced by higher serum concentrations of urea, creatinine, and kidney injury molecule 1 (KIM-1), along with more prominent apoptosis, but these effects were attenuated in cisplatin-treated $MIOX^{-/-}$ mice. $MIOX^{-/-}$ mice also had reduced NADPH oxidase-4 expression and ROS generation after cisplatin treatment. Increased inflammatory cells and upregulation of cytokines were found in kidneys of cisplatin-treated MIOX-TG mice. These findings suggest that MIOX overexpression leads to worsening of AKI in cisplatin-induced injury via multiple mechanisms and that MIOX gene disruption ameliorates toxic PTC injury.

To protect cells from harmful oxidative stress, the Keap1-Nrf2 system allows the cell to sense and respond to oxidative stress. The Keap1-Nrf2 pathway is a master regulator of cytoprotective genes and a promising target for therapeutic intervention. Nrf2 (nuclear factor–like 2) is a transcription factor that can bind antioxidant response elements (AREs) in target gene regulatory regions. In kidney IRI, Nrf2 signaling is upregulated in response to injury, and Nrf2 null mice developed worse disease.[391] It was also found that bardoxolone methyl ameliorates IRI through Nrf2.[392]

Given the known adverse effects of using pharmacologic enhancers of the Keap1/Nrf2 pathway,[393] a recent study used genetically altered mice that express low levels of Keap1 protein.[394] Reduction in levels of this inhibitor of Nrf2 signaling leads to enhanced Nrf2 target transcription. The investigators demonstrated a protective effect of Nrf2 enhancement in the model of ischemia-mediated AKI, as well as in the model of unilateral ureteral obstruction. These results underscore the importance of developing drugs that selectively target increased Nrf2 transcription to ameliorate AKI.

### Iron, Ferritin, and Heme Oxygenase

Iron plays a central role in fundamental biologic functions, such as in mitochondrial respiration and DNA repair, yet at the same time plays a detrimental role in the pathophysiology of various diseases.[395] Circulating iron is mostly transferrin-bound.

A small amount bound to low-molecular-weight chelates, referred to as *labile* or *catalytic iron* is available in biologic systems and is thought to be responsible for kidney injury.[396] Although iron must undergo cyclic oxidation and reduction to perform its normal functions, this redox activity generates free radicals, leading to lipid peroxidation or generation of superoxide radicals through reaction with hydrogen peroxide (Haber-Weiss reaction).[397] The toxicity of catalytic iron to macromolecular components of the cell and its causal role in mediating disease have been demonstrated through the protection achieved by iron chelators.[62,396,398–402] Heme iron is derived primarily from erythrocyte turnover and is the major contributor to iron cycling in the body.[395]

Kidney tissue iron content increases after AKI,[403–406] suggesting that regulators of iron metabolism such as hemojuvelin and hepcidin could be used as therapeutic targets for the treatment of AKI. In a recent study, Scindia and coworkers reported that IRI caused an increase in serum iron and kidney nonheme iron levels.[404] They further demonstrated a significant reduction in IRI-induced apoptosis, oxidative stress, and inflammatory cell infiltration when hepcidin was administered 24 to 48 hours before IRI. Similar protection by the use of hepcidin was reported in the model of hemoglobin-mediated AKI.[407] Ferritin is the major regulator of intracellular iron and is composed of heavy-chain ferritin (H-ferritin) and light-chain ferritin (L-ferritin).[98] H-ferritin has ferroxidase activity converting $Fe^{2+}$ to $Fe^{3+}$, which permits the incorporation of reactive iron into ferritin to avoid iron-induced ROS generation. Mice with proximal tubules deficient of H-ferritin had higher mortality, worse tissue injury and renal function, and increased apoptosis in both cisplatin and rhabdomyolysis models of AKI. Notably, there was disrupted iron trafficking, with altered distribution of ferroportin (iron export transporter) in the proximal tubule of H-ferritin–deficient mice. These results support an important role of proximal tubule H-ferritin and iron trafficking during AKI.[98]

### Heme Oxygenase-1

The enzyme HO-1 has also emerged as a prominent player in renal tubular epithelial cell injury.[408–411] The biologic actions of HO-1 include antiinflammatory, vasodilatory, cytoprotective, and antiapoptotic effects and regulation of cellular proliferation in the setting of AKI. HO-1 is arguably one of the most readily inducible genes, responding to numerous stressors, including, but not limited to, hypoxia, hyperthermia, oxidative stress, and exposure to LPS. Induction of HO-1 has been described in various forms of AKI, including ischemic, endotoxic, and nephrotoxic models. Following ischemia-reperfusion, aged mice exhibit reduced induction of renal medullary HO-1 and worse renal injury than younger mice. A number of studies have indicated a protective effect of induction of HO-1 in AKI.[408–411] Prior induction of HO-1 by hemoglobin can reduce endotoxemia-induced renal dysfunction and mortality. Inhibition of HO-1 activity in the intact, disease-free kidney reduces medullary blood flow without exerting any effect on cortical blood flow. Overexpression of HO-1 by hemin results in a significant reduction in cisplatin-induced cytotoxicity,[412,413] and TNF-α–induced apoptosis in endothelial cells is also attenuated by the induction of HO-1.

These findings have been supported by studies of HO-1–deficient mice where glycerol-induced AKI resulted in marked exacerbation of renal insufficiency and mortality.[414] Mechanisms of HO-1–mediated protection have been extensively studied by Inguaggiato and coworkers, who showed that overexpression of HO-1 in cultured renal epithelial cells induces upregulation of the cell cycle inhibitory protein p21 and confers resistance to apoptosis.[415] Recently, HO-1 has been shown to attenuate ferroptosis in proximal tubular cells.[416] Induction of ferroptosis (erastin and RSL3) was less profound in HO-1$^{+/+}$ compared with HO-1$^{-/-}$ PTCs. Treatment with ferrostatin-1, a ferroptosis inhibitor, significantly improved viability. Macrophages in which HO-1 is upregulated by adenoviral strategies also protect against ischemic AKI. Fibroblasts from organs of transgenic pigs expressing HO-1 are resistant to proapoptotic stressors and exhibit a blunted proinflammatory response to LPS or TNF-α. Pretreatment with hemin augments glomerular HO-1 expression and renal expression of thrombomodulin and endothelial cell protein C receptor (EPCR) while reducing LPS-induced renal dysfunction, glomerular thrombotic microangiopathy, and the procoagulant state. Hemin also increases plasma levels of activated protein C in this model, suggesting its important role in the endothelial-epithelial axis in AKI.

Perhaps more importantly, HO-1 might also contribute to the repair and regeneration of tubular cells.[101,417] Following an acute insult, HO-1 is rapidly induced, but its expression subsides before renal recovery fully occurs; such abatement in HO-1 expression may allow the continued expression of proinflammatory and fibrogenic genes. In this regard, HO-1 deficiency promotes epithelial-mesenchymal transition, a process that may underlie the transition of AKI to CKD.[409] HO-1 gene expression is regulated differently in mice and humans; however, a recent study with a novel humanized transgenic mouse has confirmed the rescue of the pathologic phenotypes observed in HO$^{-/-}$ mice by the human HO-1 gene.[408] These mice offer an important tool to study the mechanisms of regulation of human HO-1 gene. In addition, the protective effects of HO-1 promoter polymorphisms in AKI could allow us to understand its significance better in clinical contexts and enable the identification of potential novel therapeutic targets.

## REPAIR AND REGENERATION

The human kidney subjected to mild injury has the ability to recover renal function, as assessed by serum creatinine levels. Experimentally, the renal tubule has the capacity to undergo regeneration within a few days after AKI.[418] Early studies that focused on progenitor-stem cells in tubular epithelial cell injury found that different types of stem cells may reside in the renal architecture. In the human kidney, CD133$^{+}$ progenitor-stem cells with regenerative potential have been identified.[419–423] Chimeric studies using enhanced GFP to label donor bone marrow have revealed the lack of significant contribution of hematopoietic cells in the repair of epithelium following injury.[424]

Currently, there are likely two major hypotheses to explain the recovery of renal function by tubule regeneration[425] (Fig. 28.10). The first hypothesis suggests that tubules regenerate from any surviving tubular epithelial cells without the contribution of a preexistent intratubular stem cell or progenitor population. Genetic fate mapping studies have demonstrated that regeneration following injury is achieved primarily by surviving epithelial cells.[426,427] Lineage-tracing studies have demonstrated that fully differentiated epithelial cells that

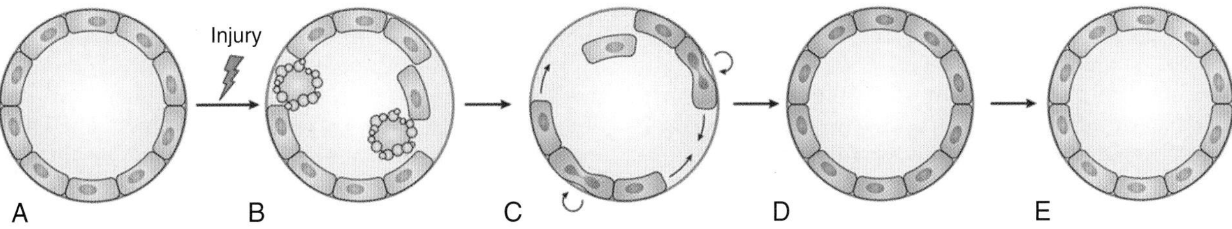


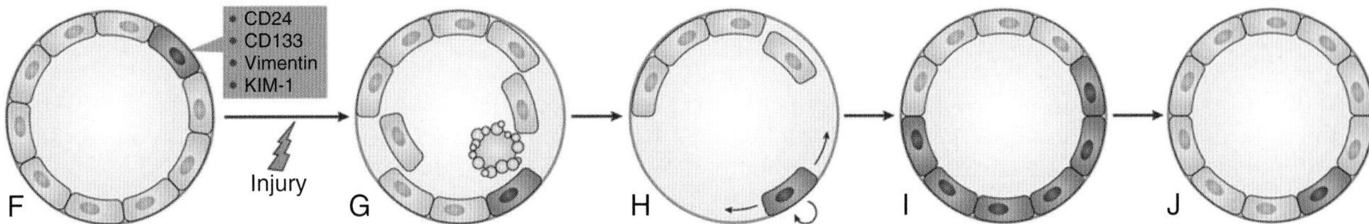


**Fig. 28.10** Tubular regeneration following acute kidney injury. *Top panel,* Tubular regeneration by dedifferentiation. (A) Healthy tubules consist of nonproliferative mature epithelial cells that express markers of differentiation. (B) After injury, the epithelium is lost through apoptosis and necrosis. (C) Surviving epithelial cells dedifferentiate, either in response to sublethal injury signals or owing to signals from other injured cells, and acquire a proliferative phenotype. (D) The surviving dedifferentiated cells reconstitute the nephron epithelium. (E) Ultimately, most dedifferentiated cells redifferentiate and downregulate the expression of dedifferentiation genes. *Lower panel,* Tubular regeneration mediated by scattered progenitor epithelial cells. (F) Scattered tubular epithelial cells express signal transducer CD24, prominin-1 (CD133), and other genes that are characteristic of proximal tubule dedifferentiation, such as vimentin and KIM-1. (G) After injury, mature tubular cells, but not scattered cells, undergo apoptosis. (H, I) Scattered tubular cells expand in response to injury and their progeny reconstitute the tubule. (J) The small subpopulation of scattered tubule cells is preserved after regeneration. (From Chang-Panesso M, Humphreys BD. Cellular plasticity in kidney injury and repair. *Nat Rev Nephrol.* 2017;13(1):39–46.)

survive an acute kidney injury episode undergo a process of reversible dedifferentiation and proliferation during repair.[428] Another independent group used the same methodology of genetic cell mapping and doxycycline-inducible parietal epithelial cell mapping (PEC)–specific transgenic mouse to label proximal tubules in the model of IRI. The authors found a significant increase in genetic labeling of proximal tubules, with increased expression of scattered tubular cell biomarkers such as CD24 and CD133, during ischemia and subsequent recovery, suggesting that scattered tubular cells arise from any surviving tubular cell.[429]

The second hypothesis suggests that tubules regenerate from a specific tubular cell subpopulation with high regenerative potential or so-called *scattered tubular cells*[428,430–432] (see Fig. 28.10). A recent study supports this hypothesis and challenges the current paradigm that functional recovery after AKI relates to a regenerative capacity of all tubular epithelial cells. These investigators applied a lineage tracing approach using conditional Pax8-Confetti mice and the models of ischemia-reperfusion and glycerol-induced AKI to demonstrate the following: (1) AKI involves a permanent loss of tubular epithelial cells (TECs), even when GFR recovery occurs; (2) Pax2-positive TECs located in the S3 segment of the proximal tubule are endowed with a higher resistance to death and are responsible for the spontaneous regeneration of necrotic tubules after AKI; (3) only Pax2-positive cells complete mitosis while other TECs go through a process of endoreplication-mediated hypertrophy that accounts for the recovery of renal function; and (4) this process of endoreplication is the dominant cell response on AKI in mice and can be detected in renal biopsy tissue of patients who developed CKD after AKI.[433] The therapeutic targeting of tubule progenitors carrying specific biomarkers of scattered tubular cell phenotype could be a promising new strategy to improve long-term outcomes after AKI.

Growth factors and signals from injured cells are crucial at this stage to promote the timely and appropriate regenerative capacity of the viable cells. In animal models, administration of exogenous growth factors accelerates renal recovery from injury. These include epidermal growth factor, IGF-1, α-melanocyte stimulating hormone, erythropoietin, hepatocyte growth factor, and bone morphogenic protein-7 (BMP-7).[434–437] These effects have not yet been validated in human clinical trials of ATN.[438,439] They all likely increase the GFR through direct hemodynamic effects and may therefore hasten tubular epithelial cell recovery.

Extracellular vesicles (EVs) derived from bone marrow mesenchymal stromal cells promote the regeneration of kidneys in models of AKI.[440] EVs represent a heterogenous group of vesicles derived from nearly all mammalian cells. Smaller vesicles or exosomes range in size from 30 to 100 nm and larger microparticles from 100 to 1000 nm.[441] Microvesicles administered to severe combined immunodeficient (SCID) mice subjected to glycerol-induced AKI induced proliferation of tubule cells and accelerated morphologic and functional recovery.[442] Tubule proliferation was mediated by

RNA-dependent effects because RNase abolished the effects of microvesicles on this process.[442] When various populations of EVs were isolated by differential centrifugation, Bruno and coworkers found that transfer of 10 K (isolation at 10,000 g) and 100 K (isolation at 100,000 g) preparations into mice had different effects on AKI. The 100 K EVs contained mRNAs regulating proliferative, antiapoptotic, and growth factors, whereas the 10-K EVs had lower expression of proproliferative molecules and were unable to induce renal regeneration.[440]

### Microvascular Function

The microvasculature consists of the endothelium and pericyte. Each of these structures contributes to barrier integrity for normal homeostatic function. During AKI, disruption may occur at each of these sites, leading to increased permeability and cell death. Normally, the microvasculature controls vascular tone, regulation of blood flow to local tissue beds, modulation of coagulation and inflammation, and permeability. Both ischemia and sepsis have profound effects on the endothelium. The renal vasculature and endothelium are particularly sensitive to these insults. When such an insult occurs, the endothelial bed becomes ineffective in performing its function, and the ensuing vascular dysregulation leads to continued ischemic conditions and further injury following the initial insult, which has been termed the "extension phase" of AKI.[443] Histopathologically, this is seen as vascular congestion, edema formation, diminished microvascular blood flow, and margination and adherence of inflammatory cells to endothelial cells.

**Vascular Tone.** Conger and associates were among the first to demonstrate that postischemic rat kidneys manifest vasoconstriction in response to decreased renal perfusion pressure and hence cannot autoregulate blood flow, even when total renal blood flow had returned to baseline values up to 1 week after injury.[444,445] Single-fiber, laser Doppler flow cytometry has revealed that blood flow is reduced to 60% and 16% of preischemic values in cortex and medulla, respectively and increased 125% in inner medulla following ischemia.[446] Selective inhibition, depletion, or deletion of iNOS has clearly shown renoprotective effects during ischemia.[447,448] NO production from the endothelium (eNOS) may be impaired at the level of enzyme activity or modified by ROS to impair normal vasodilatory activity.[449] In ischemic AKI,[450] there is an imbalance of eNOS and iNOS, and a relative decrease in eNOS, secondary to endothelial dysfunction and damage, leads to a loss of antithrombogenic properties of the endothelium and increased susceptibility to microvascular thrombosis.[450] Administration of L-arginine, the NO donor molsidomine, or the eNOS cofactor tetrahydrobiopterin can preserve medullary perfusion and attenuate AKI induced by IRI. Conversely the administration of $N^{\omega}$-nitro-L-arginine methyl ester, an NO blocker, aggravates the course of AKI following IRI.[451,452]

In a review of experimental sepsis, the pattern of renal blood flow is inconsistent. Renal blood flow was decreased in 62% of studies and unchanged or increased in 38%.[453] Langenberg and colleagues administered *E. coli* to sheep and induced hyperdynamic sepsis associated with increased cardiac output and a decrease in mean arterial pressure and AKI, as evidenced by a rise in creatinine levels.[453] Furthermore, there was marked increase in renal blood flow, decrease in urine output, and decrease in creatinine clearance. When angiotensin was dose-titrated and restored blood pressure to presepsis levels, these effects were reversed; there was a significant decrease in renal blood flow, increase in urine output, and increase in creatinine clearance.[454] These studies suggest that improvement of function may be more than simply an improvement in mean arterial pressure and that the increase in glomerular filtration pressure may be through selective constriction of efferent arterioles and/or increase in mesangial cell tone.[454] Based on these principles, in a recent clinical trial, patients with vasodilatory shock who were receiving another vasopressor were randomized to Ang II or placebo. The group that received Ang II had higher mean blood pressure[455] and, in a subgroup of patients with AKI who required renal replacement therapy, 28-day survival, mean arterial pressure, and rate of discontinuation of renal replacement were higher in the angiotensin group. These results together show the potential benefit of Ang II in hyperdynamic sepsis, which may in part be due to improved glomerular hemodynamics.

The endothelial cell structure consists of a cytoskeletal structure of actin filament bundles that form a supportive ring around the periphery, along with the adhesion complexes that provide the integrity of the endothelial layer. The assembly and disassembly of actin filaments is regulated by a large family of actin-binding proteins, including ADF-cofilin. With ischemic injury, the normal architecture of the actin cytoskeleton is markedly changed, along with endothelial cell swelling, impaired cell-cell and cell-substrate adhesion, and loss of tight junction barrier functions. ATP depletion of cultured endothelial cells has been shown to induce dephosphorylation and activation of ADF-cofilin in a direct and concentration-dependent fashion. This activity results in depolymerized and severed actin filaments, seen as F-actin aggregates at the basolateral aspects of the cell.[456]

Kidney pericytes are extensively branched cells that are scattered on the outer wall of capillaries and embedded in the capillary basement membrane; they serve a homeostatic role in angiogenesis and vessel maturation.[457] Furthermore, following kidney injury, they detach and migrate into the kidney interstitium[458] and, in some cases, transform into myofibroblasts, leading to progressive kidney fibrosis. Thus, the endothelial-pericyte crosstalk among the vascular endothelial growth factor receptors and platelet-derived growth factor receptors contribute to normal microvascular health and disease. The importance of kidney pericyte microvascular function has been demonstrated through the use of diphtheria toxin delivery to FoxD1Cre::RsDTR transgenic mice in which the diphtheria toxin receptor (heparin-binding epidermal growth factor receptor) was selectively expressed in FoxD1 cells, which are primarily pericytes.[459] The administration of diphtheria toxin selectively ablated pericytes only. Within 96 hours, there was an abrupt decline in renal function and an increase in albuminuria. These results demonstrate that pericytes are essential for normal microvascular function.

The glycocalyx is located on the blood side of the endothelium and has a depth of 1 to 3 μm. The glycocalyx is composed of cell-bound proteoglycans, glycosaminoglycan side chains, and sialoproteins.[460] Sandwiched between blood components and the endothelium, the glycocalyx is situated to play a key role in microvascular and endothelial homeostasis and endothelial physiology.[459] The specific functions served by the endothelial glycocalyx include shear stress mechanotransduction to endothelial cells, regulation of vascular permeability, inhibition of intravascular thrombosis, and protection of the endothelium from platelet and leukocyte adhesion.[460,461] The glycocalyx may be damaged by local changes in shear stress, ROS, altered oncotic pressure, altered fluid composition, and inflammatory molecules. Shedding of the glycocalyx occurs, exposing the endothelial adhesion molecules to circulating immune cells and leading to immune cell activation and inflammation and lipoprotein leakage to the subendothelial space. Coronary ischemia-reperfusion leads to shedding of the glycocalyx and an increase in neutrophil adhesion with subsequent myocardial injury.[462] Similar events are likely to occur in septic AKI and kidney IRI (Fig. 28.11).

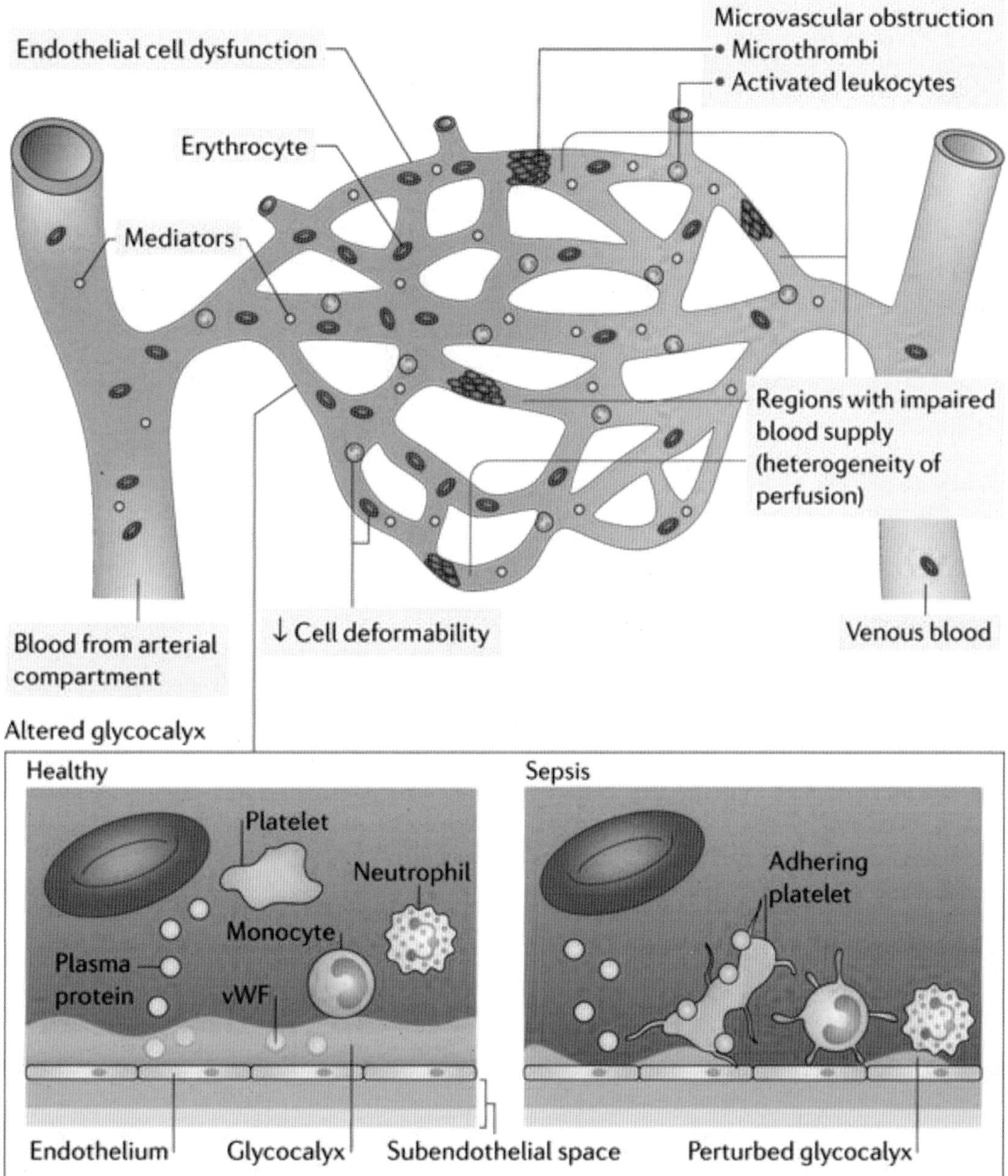


**Fig. 28.11** Microvascular dysfunction in septic acute kidney injury. Multiple mechanisms are involved in the development of sepsis-related microvascular dysfunction, among which endothelial dysfunction (related partly to circulating host-derived and pathogen-derived mediators, as well as to reactive oxygen species) and an altered glycocalyx have major roles. The glycocalyx is a thin layer of glycosaminoglycans that covers the endothelial surface, facilitating the flow of red blood cells and limiting the adhesion of leukocytes and platelets to the endothelium. The glycocalyx may be substantially altered during sepsis, so interactions between the vascular endothelium and circulating cells (e.g., leukocytes and platelets) are impaired, and leukocyte rolling and adhesion to the endothelium may occur. Activation of coagulation and the generation of microthrombi might also participate in sepsis-induced microvascular alterations, as well as alterations in erythrocyte deformability and/or their adhesion to the endothelium. All these phenomena might cause heterogeneity in microvascular blood flow, with a decrease in vascular density and nonperfused capillaries, resulting in an increased diffusion distance for oxygen and in alterations in oxygen extraction. *vWF,* von Willebrand factor. (From Lelubre, C, Vincent, JL: Mechanisms and treatment of organ failure in sepsis. *Nat Rev Nephrol.* 2018;14:417–427.)

Within 24 hours after ischemic injury, there is loss of localization in vascular endothelial cadherin immunostaining, suggesting severe alterations in the integrity of the adherens junctions of the renal microvasculature.[463] In vivo two-photon imaging has demonstrated a loss of capillary barrier function within 2 hours of reperfusion, as evidenced by leakiness of high-molecular-weight dextrans (>300,000 Da) into the interstitial space.

Critical constituents of the perivascular matrix, including collagen IV, are known to be substrates of matrix metalloproteinase-2 (MMP-2) and MMP-9, which are collectively known as gelatinases. Breakdown of barrier function may also be due to MMP-2 or MMP-9 activation, and this upregulation is temporally correlated with an increase in microvascular permeability.[443,463] MMP-9 gene deletion stabilizes microvascular density following ischemic AKI, in part by preserving tissue VEGF levels.[464] In addition, minocycline, a broad-based MMP inhibitor and the gelatinase-specific inhibitor ABT-518, both ameliorated the increase in microvascular permeability in this model. Taken together, many studies have indicated that the loss of endothelial cells following ischemic injury is not a major contributor to altered microvascular permeability, although renal microvascular endothelial cells are vulnerable to the initiation of apoptotic mechanisms following ischemic injury, which can ultimately reduce microvascular density.[465]

The endothelial cell plays a central role in coagulation via its interaction with protein C through the EPCR and thrombomoduli. The protein C pathway helps maintain normal homeostasis and limits inflammatory responses. Protein C is activated by thrombin-mediated cleavage, and the rate of this reaction is further augmented (by 1000-fold) when thrombin binds to the endothelial cell surface receptor protein thrombomodulin. The activation rate of protein C is further increased by approximately 10-fold when EPCR binds protein C and presents it to the thrombin-thrombomodulin complex. Essentially, activated protein C then has antithrombotic actions and profibrinolytic properties and participates in numerous antiinflammatory and cytoprotective pathways to restore normal homeostasis.[466] Based on these properties, the endothelial cell plays an absolutely essential and critical role in maintaining a normal and healthy vasculature and endothelial bed.

In AKI, microvascular function is ultimately compromised, resulting in disseminated intravascular coagulation and microvascular thrombosis, decreased tissue perfusion, and hypoxemia, leading to organ dysfunction and failure. It has been shown that both pretreatment and postinjury treatment with soluble thrombomodulin attenuates renal injury, with minimization of vascular permeability defects and improvement in capillary renal blood flow.[467]

The leukocyte and endothelial cell are dynamically involved in the process of adherence of leukocytes to the vascular endothelium. Leukocyte activation and cytokine release require signals through chemokines circulating in the bloodstream or through direct contact with the endothelium. Rolling leukocytes can be activated by chemoattractants such as complement C5a and platelet-activating factor. Once activated, leukocyte integrins bind to endothelial ligands to promote firm adhesion. $\beta_2$-Integrin (CD18) seems to be the most important ligand for neutrophil adherence. These interactions with the endothelium are mediated through endothelial adhesion molecules that are upregulated during ischemic conditions.[468]

The initial phase starts with slow neutrophil migration mediated by tethering interactions between adhesion molecules and their endothelial cell ligands. Within 2 to 4 hours of IRI or sepsis, endothelial P-selectin and intercellular adhesion molecule 1 (ICAM1) are expressed on endothelial cells associated with leukocyte trapping in peritubular capillaries.[306] Singbartl and Ley have found that platelet P-selectin and not endothelial P-selectin is the main determinant in neutrophil-mediated ischemic kidney injury.[468] There is also significant protection from both ischemic injury and mortality by blockade of the shared ligand to all three selectins (E-, P-, and L-selectin), which seems to be dependent on the presence of a key fucosyl sugar on the selectin ligand.[469] In a CLP model of septic azotemia, mice deficient for E-selectin, P-selectin, or both were completely protected. Furthermore, selectin-deficient mice demonstrated similar intraperitoneal leukocyte recruitment but altered cytokine levels when compared with WT mice,[470] in addition to engagement in leukocyte-endothelial cell interactions.[470] Other adhesion molecules such as VAP-1 appear to play a role in AKI.[315]

Recently, in an attempt to transition to human studies, Dehnadi and coworkers have demonstrated the critical role that leukocyte integrin CD11b–CD18 contribute to both AKI and CKD in nonhuman primates.[471] In their model, using a CD11b–CD18 inhibitor, mAb107, ischemia-reperfusion-induced a no-reflow time; plasma creatinine and ATN were markedly diminished in the mAB107 groups, indicating that the leukocyte integrin CD11b–C18 contributes to AKI. Moreover, subsequent assessment up to 9 months after AKI revealed improvement in microvascular perfusion and histology.

Recent studies have examined the role of microparticles (MPs) in sepsis-related AKI. MPs are cell membrane-derived particles of 0.2 to 2 μM in diameter that can promote coagulation and inflammation.[472] Using the cecal ligation model of sepsis, the authors found that calpastatin overexpression improved survival, organ dysfunction (including lung, kidney, and liver damage), and lymphocyte apoptosis. Increased calpastatin expression also decreased the sepsis-induced systemic proinflammatory response and disseminated intravascular coagulation by reducing the number of procoagulant circulating microparticles and therefore delaying thrombin generation.[473] The deleterious effect of microparticles in this model was confirmed by transferring microparticles from septic WT to septic transgenic mice, worsening their survival and coagulopathy. The development of therapeutics aimed to prevent the release of MPs from endothelium or other inflammatory cells may be a reasonable target in microvascular dysfunction during sepsis-induced AKI.

## ACUTE KIDNEY INJURY TO CHRONIC KIDNEY DISEASE TRANSITION

AKI is one of many initiating events that contribute to chronic, progressive kidney disease.[474,475] Some patients with AKI fully recover kidney function, whereas in others, the development of CKD is accompanied by a progressive decline in kidney function, leading ultimately to end-stage kidney disease (ESKD).[476–478] Regardless of the cause of CKD (e.g., nephrotoxic kidney injury, ischemia, infection, genetics; paraneoplastic, immunologic processes), there is a stereotypical response leading to interstitial fibrosis, tubular atrophy, and

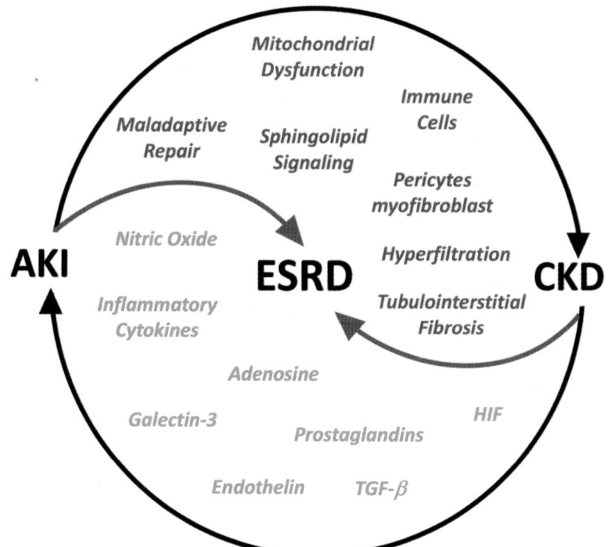


**Fig. 28.12** Conceptual framework of acute kidney injury *(AKI)* to chronic kidney disease *(CKD)* transition. AKI can lead to CKD and then to end-stage renal disease (ESRD). Conversely, CKD can lead progressively to ESKD or can predispose to AKI, which then enters a vicious circle and predisposes to CKD. A number of factors contribute to AKI to CKD transition, including traditional concepts *(green)* and emerging *(red)* concepts.

peritubular rarefaction and inflammation.[474,479,480] Incomplete repair following AKI contributes to the progression to CKD and ESKD[418,481] (Fig. 28.12).

## Role of the Endothelium

Studies have begun to elucidate the importance of the endothelium in the initiation and progression of fibrosis. Studies on human biopsies have associated microvascular rarefaction with progressive kidney failure.[482] There is also evidence in experimental AKI that acute injury to endothelial cells may have long-term implications; Basile have shown a significant reduction in blood vessel density following ischemic injury, leading to the phenomenon of vascular dropout.[483] Vascular dropout was verified by Horbelt and associates, who found a drop in the vascular density by almost 45% at 4 weeks after an ischemic insult.[465] Ehling and coworkers, using micro-CT imaging of vascular alterations, found a progressive decline of the renal relative blood volume in three models of progressive kidney disease (IRI, unilateral ureteral obstruction [UUO], and Alport) of up to 61% in late disease stages and that it preceded fibrosis.[484] Using ex vivo micro-CT imaging and three-dimensional quantification of the renal vasculature, they demonstrated macrovascular to microvascular alterations in progressive renal disease, as evidenced by a reduction in vessel diameter and in vessel branching and increased vessel tortuosity (Fig. 28.13). These findings suggest that unlike the renal epithelial tubular cells, the renal vascular system lacks comparable regenerative potential. Recent studies have suggested that renal endothelial injury can result in capillary rarefaction due to hypoxia and a lack of upregulation of VEGF in response to injury.[485–487] It is not yet clear whether apoptosis and/or necrosis play a major role in endothelial cell dropout. Ischemia has been shown to inhibit the angiogenic protein VEGF while inducing ADAMTS1, which is thought to be a VEGF inhibitor.[488] It was then postulated that the lack of vascular repair could be due to lack of VEGF, as shown by experiments where administration of VEGF-121 preserved the microvascular density.[488] Reduction of the microvasculature density increases hypoxia-mediated fibrosis and alters usual hemodynamics, which may lead to hypertension. Thus, loss of microvasculature density and its consequential effects may play a critical role in the progression of CKD following initial recovery from ischemia-reperfusion–induced AKI.[465,483,484] Using a genetic approach in the IRI mouse model of AKI, the temporal effects of endothelial sphingosine 1-phosphate receptor 1 (S1P1) during AKI were examined. Delayed deletion of S1P1 in endothelial cells after IRI, using a tamoxifen-inducible system to delete S1P1 prevented kidney recovery, resulting in chronic inflammation and progressive fibrosis. Specifically, S1P1 directly suppressed the endothelial activation of leukocyte adhesion molecule expression and inflammation. Altogether, the data indicate that activation of endothelial S1P1 is necessary to protect from IRI and permit recovery from AKI.[359]

## Epigenetic Modification

AKI is associated with histone modification[489] and DNA methylation,[490] leading to altered transcription of genes thought to contribute to renal injury.[491,492] There is evidence that epigenetic changes are closely related to renal hypoxia and CKD progression.[485,486]

## Renal Oxidative Stress in Acute Kidney Injury–Chronic Kidney Disease Transition

Renal oxidative stress has been shown to persist with resultant increased Ang II sensitivity in rats following recovery from ischemia-reperfusion–induced AKI after 5 weeks. Post-AKI rats showed significantly enhanced renal vasoconstrictor responses to Ang II, and treatment of AKI rats with apocynin normalized these responses. Expression of mRNA for common reduced NADPH oxidase subunits was not altered in kidneys following recovery from AKI; however, mRNA screening using polymerase chain reaction assays has suggested that post-AKI rats have decreased renal glutathione peroxidase 3 mRNA and an increased expression of other pro-oxidant genes such as lactoperoxidase, myeloperoxidase, and dual oxidase-1. Following infusion with Ang II, renal fibrosis was enhanced in post-AKI rats. The profibrotic response was significantly attenuated in rats treated with apocynin. These data suggest that there is sustained renal oxidant stress following recovery from AKI that alters the hemodynamic and fibrotic responses to Ang II and may contribute to the transition to CKD following AKI.[493] This also highlights the importance of managing recovering AKI very carefully to avoid further insults that might enhance ROS or sensitivity to Ang II.

## Cell Cycle Arrest

As discussed earlier, in successful repair, mature surviving cells dedifferentiate, proliferate, and repopulate proximal tubules in response to kidney injury.[426,427] Upregulation of KIM-1 is antiinflammatory through its engulfment and clearance of dead and apoptotic cells[494] but becomes maladaptive when chronically expressed.[495] Repetitive injury may result in the upregulation of cyclin-dependent kinase (CDK) inhibitors, $p16^{Ink4}$ and $P53\text{-}p21^{Cip1/Waf1}$, leading to cell cycle arrest.[496]

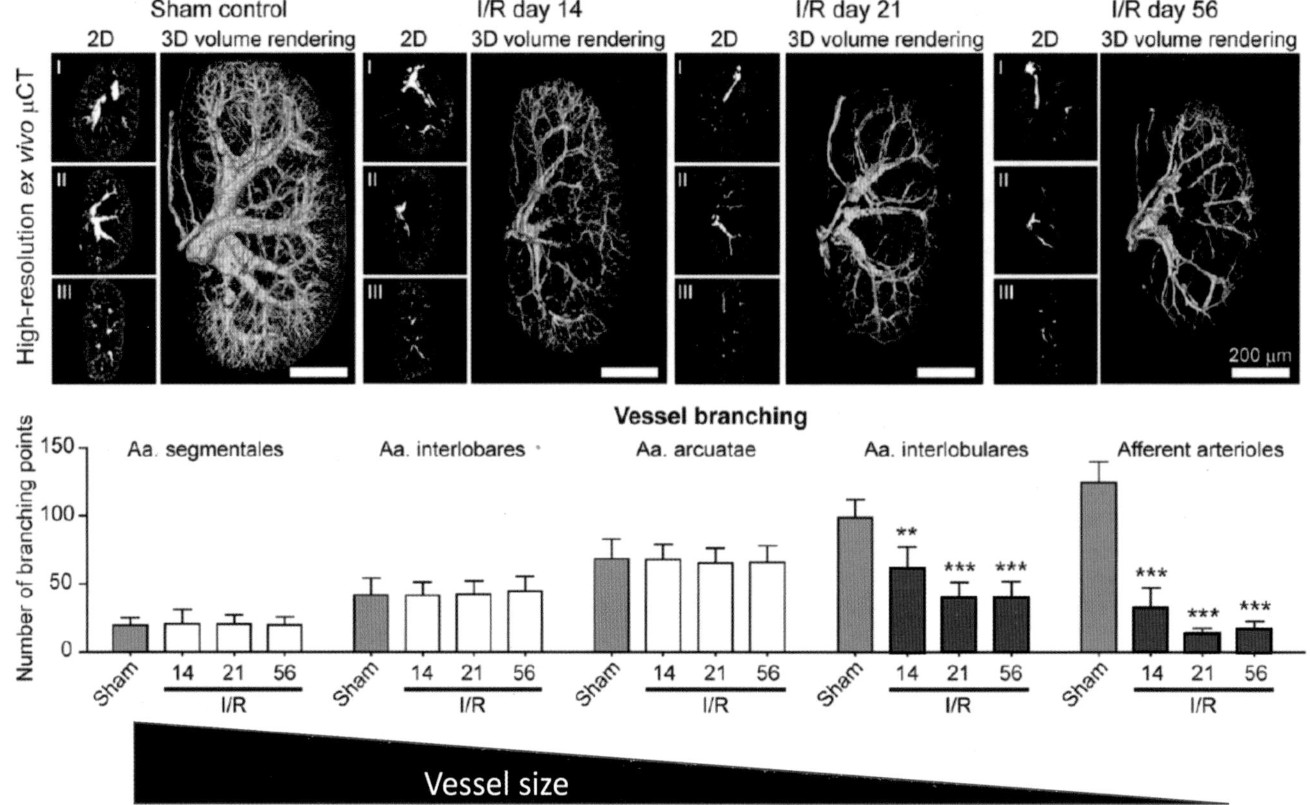


**Fig. 28.13** Ex vivo micro-computed tomography *(CT)* imaging and three-dimensional quantification of the renal vasculature reveal significant alterations of renal arteries in progressive ischemia-reperfusion (IRI) induced renal injury. *(Lower panel)* Representative high-resolution, ex vivo, micro-CT images of sham control and I/R kidneys from days 14, 21, and 56 after Microfil perfusion (two-dimensional cross-sectional images in transverse [I], coronal [II], and sagittal [III] planes, as well as three-dimensional volume renderings). Note the progressive rarefaction of functional vessels besides the continuous shrinkage of fibrotic kidneys over time. Scale bar, 200 μm. *(Upper panel)* Micro-CT–based quantification of vascular branching points per increasing vessel order (from hilus to periphery). A continuous reduction in vessel branching and vessel size was linked to an increased vessel tortuosity during fibrosis progression. **, $P < .01$; ***, $P < .001$. *AKI,* Acute kidney injury. (From Ehling J, Babickova J, Gremse F, et al. Quantitative Micro-computed tomography imaging of vascular dysfunction in progressive kidney diseases. *J Am Soc Nephrol.* 2016;27(2):520–532.)

An increase in p16$^{Ink4}$ inhibits CDK4 and CDK6 and is associated with tubulointerstitial changes leading to fibrosis; kidneys from INK4a$^{-/-}$ mice develop less fibrosis following kidney IRI.[250] Thus, cell cycle arrest and cellular senescence lead to resistance to apoptosis and persistent metabolic activity, promoting a senescence-type secretory phenotype with the secretion of TGF-β, cytokines, proteases, and other proinflammatory and profibrotic factors.[418,497] Yang, Bonventre and associates have used four models of kidney injury, including severe bilateral IRI, unilateral IRI, aristolochic acid, and UUO and demonstrated that G2/M arrest contributes to maladaptive repair and fibrosis associated with AKI-CKD transition. Similar findings have been reported and, importantly, pharmacologic inhibitors of G2/M arrest reduce fibrosis.[498,499]

### Inflammation in Acute Kidney Injury–Chronic Kidney Disease Transition

During kidney recovery, renal and extrarenal cells participate in the wound-healing response and can initiate fibrosis. Immune cells of the mononuclear phagocyte system, including macrophages and dendritic cells, not only contribute to injury but have emerged as important cells in the recovery of kidney function during adaptive repair or fibrosis during maladaptive repair. It is the balance between wound healing and progressive fibrosis that dictates the final outcome. The intrinsic plasticity of monocytes-macrophages and dendritic cells, as well as attempts to relate in vitro studies to in vivo findings, makes the functional definition and phenotype of this myeloid population in kidney pathophysiology complex.[500–503] In vitro studies have led to two well-defined mononuclear phagocytes. Classically activated macrophages—M1 mononuclear phagocytes consisting of macrophages and dendritic cells—are produced by exposure to LPS or INF-γ and are largely thought to be proinflammatory and contribute to initial kidney injury. Alternatively, activated macrophages (M2 mononuclear phagocytes) are induced by IL-4 and IL-10 and appear later, after AKI has been established, and have a genetic signature associated with wound healing and/or fibrosis.[504] These mononuclear phagocyte phenotypes depend on the complex local tissue microenvironment, which may induce phenotype switching.[303]

A key feature of fibrosis is the activation of extracellular matrix–producing myofibroblasts.[505,506] Other factors relevant in CKD progression include endothelial cell damage and vascular damage in AKI,[483] hypoxia-inducible factor (HIF),[507] innate and adaptive immunity,[508] cell cycle arrest,[509] and epigenetic mechanisms.[510,511]

Although some injured tubules undergo repair and regeneration, injury may also be accompanied by inflammation, maturation and proliferation of fibroblasts, and extracellular matrix deposition as part of the process of fibrosis. The source of fibroblasts in the injured kidney—fibrocytes, epithelial cells through epithelial mesenchymal transformation (EMT), intrinsic fibroblasts, and pericytes—remains controversial.[512,513]

Tissue fibrosis is a common component of inflammatory diseases, including various forms of CKD. Collagen deposition, characteristically formed during normal wound healing, is reversible but progressive irreversible fibrosis may occur through repeated injury due to dysregulated inflammation.[514] Some studies have focused on the role of pericytes or resident fibroblasts that contribute to normal homeostatic microvascular function but transform into myofibroblasts on activation.[513,515,516] Myofibroblasts are the primary collagen-producing cells.[512]

Although the myofibroblast is the cell type responsible for depositing collagen, investigators have been searching for its precursors. Other than interstitial fibroblasts that are known to transition, pericytes, dendritic, endothelial, and epithelial cells have been identified as potential contributors. For example, in vivo and in vitro studies have demonstrated that endothelial cells develop a myofibroblast phenotype.[517,518] Epithelial cells grown in culture can produce genes expressed in myofibroblasts, suggesting epithelial to mesenchymal transition.[519–521] Fate-mapping studies by Humphreys and associates have shown that although epithelial cells can obtain mesenchymal markers in vitro, they do not penetrate the basement membrane to enter into the interstitial space and differentiate into myofibroblasts in vivo.[513] Furthermore, lineage analysis has demonstrated that platelet-derived growth factor receptor (PDGFR)-β–positive pericytes differentiate into myofibroblasts in a UUO model. Following AKI, a potential step in the AKI-CKD transition is the dissociation of pericytes from endothelial cells.[458] Using bigenic Gli1-CreERt2; R26tdTomato reporter mice, Kramann and coworkers observed dissociation between $Gli1^+$ pericytes and endothelial cells after AKI.[458] Furthermore, following pericyte ablation, endothelial damage was observed, and pericyte loss led to a significantly reduced capillary number, a hallmark of CKD.

Two studies have shed light on this controversy. *Snail* (encodes snail family zinc finger 1, Snail1) expressed in mouse renal epithelial cells is required for kidney fibrosis.[522] Twist (encodes twist family bHLH transcription factor 1, known as Twist) genes are essential regulators of EMT.[523] Inhibition or deletion of these genes or overexpression has led to induction or inhibition of EMT, respectively.[524,525] Lineage tracing studies have demonstrated that during activation, labeled epithelial cells do not contribute to myofibroblasts or interstitial cells; however, there was downregulation of epithelial markers and loss of epithelial polarity and cell differentiation.[525] Thus, partial EMT leads to cell cycle arrest, blocks proliferation and repair, and blocks secretion of growth factors, such as TGF-β that drive proliferation of myofibroblasts[526] (Fig. 28.14).

Signaling pathways Wnt, hedgehog (Hh), and Notch pathways also play important roles during renal fibrosis. In CKD, numerous Wnt ligands are upregulated, resulting in prolonged activation of the Wnt/β-catenin pathway.[527,528] Epithelial β-catenin activation leads to epithelial dedifferentiation and interstitial fibrosis.[529] Wnt derived from tubules is necessary for myofibroblast activation and interstitial fibrosis.[530] Recently, the role of the sphingolipid pathway in progressive fibrosis. Sphingosine 1-phosphate (S1P), a pleiotropic lysophospholipid that is involved in diverse functions such as cell growth and survival, lymphocyte trafficking, and vascular stability,[531–536] is the product of sphingosine phosphorylation by two sphingosine kinase isoforms (SphK1 and SphK2). SphK2 has been localized to the nucleus and plays an important role in the production of nuclear S1P, which acts as a histone deacetylase (HDAC) inhibitor,[537] thereby allowing gene expression to be induced. Bawja demonstrated that following unilateral IRI or folic acid (FA)–induced kidney fibrosis, protection of *Sphk2*$^{-/-}$ mice from fibrosis at day 14 was thought to be due to IFN-γ. Kidneys of *Sphk2*$^{-/-}$ mice exhibited greater expression of *Ifng* and IFN-γ–responsive genes (Cxcl9 and Cxcl10) than kidneys of WT or *Sphk1*$^{-/-}$ mice. IFN-γ blocking antibody administered to *Sphk2*$^{-/-}$ mice or deletion of *Ifng* using a double-knockout mouse (*Sphk2*$^{-/-}$ *Ifng*$^{-/-}$ mice) blocked the protective effect of *Sphk2* deficiency in fibrosis. Moreover, adoptive transfer of *Sphk2*$^{-/-}$ CD4 T cells into WT mice blocked FA-induced fibrosis. Finally, a selective SphK2 inhibitor blocked FA-induced kidney fibrosis in WT mice. These studies have demonstrated that SphK2 inhibition may serve as a novel therapeutic approach for attenuating kidney fibrosis.[538,539]

Activation of myofibroblasts is also mediated through paracrine signals from immune cells (lymphocytes and antigen-presenting cells), which include cytokines, chemokines, angiogenic factors, growth factors, peroxisome proliferator-activated receptors (PPARs), and other molecules.[540] Although Th2 cytokines may induce fibrosis, Th1 cytokines such as IL-12 or IFN-γ have been shown to inhibit pulmonary[541,542] and experimental renal fibrosis.[543]

Using an unbiased approach to identify upregulated and downregulated pericyte genes in injury, Schrimpf and colleagues found increased activation and expression of ADAMTS1 (a disintegrin-like metalloprotease with thrombospondin type 1) and downregulation of its inhibitor MMP-3 (TIMP-3).[544] TIMP-3–stabilized pericytes maintained collagen capillary tube networks, whereas ADAMTS1-treated pericytes led to enhanced destabilization. TIMP-3 has many functions, including regulating VEGF signaling, pericyte migration, and MMP-2 and MMP-9 activity.[545] Furthermore, TGF-$\beta_1$ has been shown to activate the pericyte-myofibroblast transition, thus adding to the stimuli for pericyte involvement in fibrosis.[546] Injured epithelial cells reduce production of VEGF, a trophic factor for endothelial maintenance, and increase production of TGF-β and PDGFR, which enhance pericyte dedifferentiation into myofibroblasts. Finally, PDGFR blockade on pericytes or VEGF receptor 2 (VEGFR-2) on endothelial cells led to a reduction in fibrosis and stabilization of the microvasculature in the UUO model.[547] Thus, numerous factors favor microvascular maladaptation after injury, including TGF-β production and lack of VEGF production by epithelial cells, reductions in PDGF production by endothelial cells, and increased ADAMTS1 expression, with reduced TIMP-3 production by pericytes. These events also suggest several therapeutic targets that could limit microvascular dropout and loss of kidney function secondary to the fibrotic process. Normal pericyte function therefore becomes deranged following transformation to

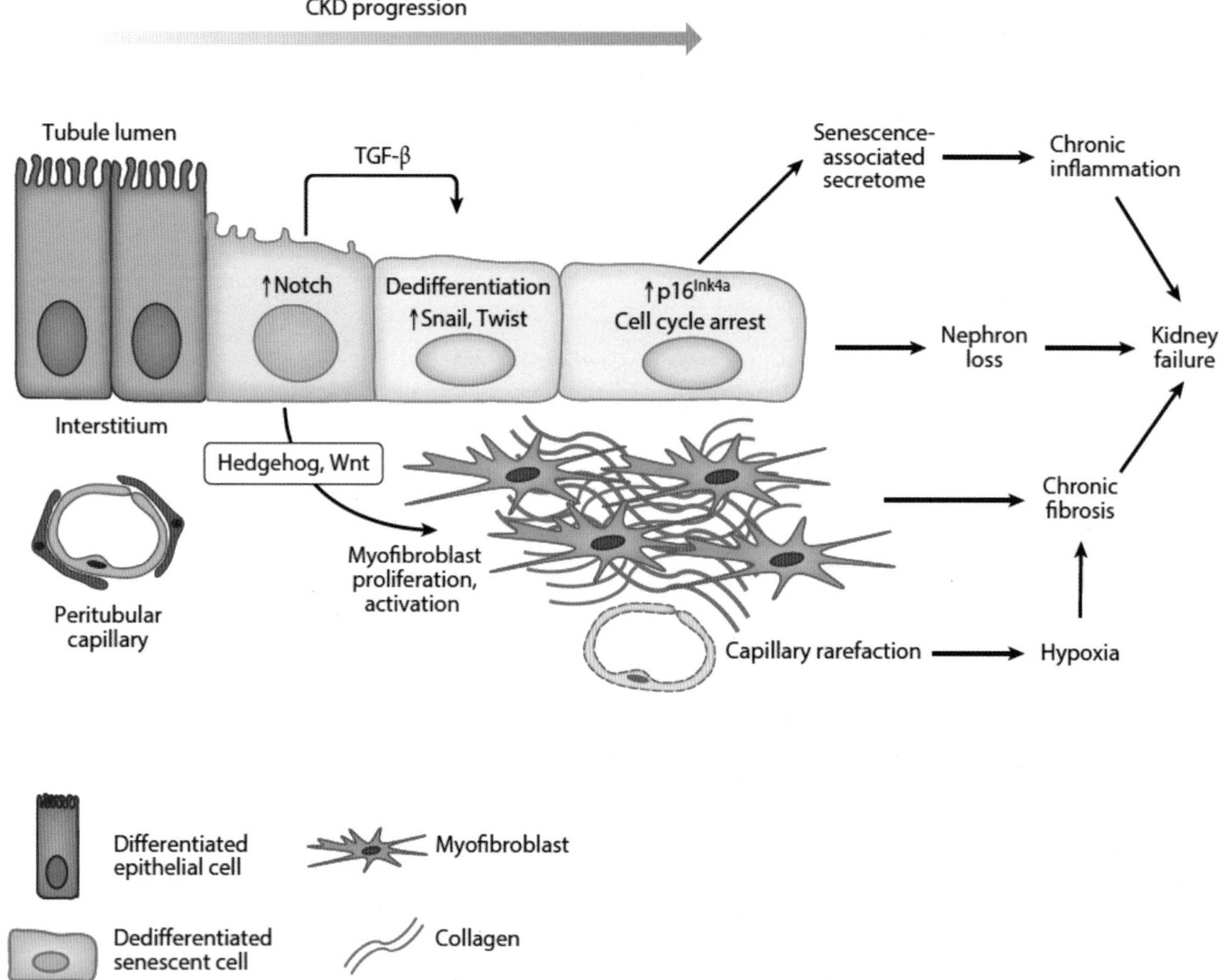


**Fig. 28.14** Critical cells and signaling pathways activated in progressive chronic kidney disease *(CKD)*. CKD is initiated by cellular injury, either to the epithelial or endothelial compartment. In the tubulointerstitium, injury leads to epithelial dedifferentiation that may be induced by transforming growth factor-β (TGF-β) and Notch pathway upregulation. Dedifferentiated epithelial cells secrete paracrine signaling factors, such as hedgehog and Wnt ligands, that act on interstitial pericytes and mesenchymal stem cell–like cells to activate myofibroblast differentiation, proliferation, and matrix secretion. This in turn causes peritubular capillary rarefaction and ongoing hypoxia. Chronic tubular injury leads to epithelial cell cycle arrest and senescence, with accompanying secretion of proinflammatory cytokines that amplify inflammation. These interrelated events ultimately drive nephron loss, ongoing interstitial fibrosis, and kidney failure. (From Humphreys BD. Mechanisms of renal fibrosis. *Annu Rev Physiol.* 2018;80:309–326.)

activated myofibroblasts, which leads to loss of microvascular stability, ineffective angiogenesis, increased permeability, and capillary rarefaction, which are all processes leading to fibrosis.[457,474]

Proximal tubules are highly metabolically active, relying on aerobic metabolism. Mitochondrial fatty acid oxidation is a major source of energy, and mitochondrial dysfunction leads to lipid accumulation, ATP depletion, and fibrosis in proximal tubule cells.[548] A number of therapeutic approaches are in development, including some agents in clinical trials for diabetic nephropathy and other kidney diseases,[549,550] but as yet there are no approved treatments to prevent the development of kidney fibrosis or accelerate repair. The development of effective treatments requires a better understanding of the inflammatory, injury, wound healing, matrix deposition, and cellular repair processes that accompany fibrosis.[497,514,526,551–553] For example, mitochondria may be an important therapeutic target in AKI to CKD progression.[554] In one approach, Birk and associates developed a novel mitoprotective drug, SS31.[555] SS peptides bind selectively to cardiolipin in the mitochondrial inner membrane to protect mitochondrial cristae. SS31 allows better function of the respiratory chain complexes, prevents peroxidase activity, and enhances electron transfer through cytochrome c to improve oxidative phosphorylation and ATP production.[555–557] SS31 administered 1 month after renal IRI attenuated glomerulosclerosis and senescence and reduced parietal epithelial cell activation and changes in podocyte and endothelial structure.[558] Perry and associates have examined the role of dynamin-related protein 1 (DRP1), a mediator of cell fission.

Proximal tubule-specific deletion of *Drp1* prevented renal IRI, inflammation, and programmed cell death and promoted epithelial recovery, which was associated with activation of the renoprotective β-hydroxybutyrate signaling pathway.[559] Importantly, delayed deletion of proximal tubule *Drp1* using a tamoxifen-inducible system after IRI attenuated kidney fibrosis. These results highlight DRP1 and mitochondrial dynamics as an important mediator of AKI and progression to fibrosis and suggest that DRP1 may serve as a therapeutic target for AKI.

### Effects of Organ Crosstalk

AKI is associated with significant morbidity and mortality. In the intensive care unit, where patients with AKI sustain multiorgan dysfunction, the mortality rate is around 60%.[560] Although AKI is associated with consequences such as accumulation of uremic toxins, metabolic acidosis, fluid and electrolyte imbalance, and fluid overload, these factors alone do not explain the mortality associated with AKI.[146,561] There is accumulating evidence that in many cases, AKI is a systemic condition in which AKI induces dysfunction in distant organs, including lung, heart, brain, liver, and intestines (Fig. 28.15). Moreover, there is evidence that distant organ function can alter kidney function. Recent studies have demonstrated that neural control of inflammation and AKI is thought to be mediated by a pathway referred to as the *cholinergic antiinflammatory pathway*, which requires an intact spleen.[562–566]

Kelly has demonstrated the effects of renal ischemia on cardiac tissues.[139] Induction of IL-1, TNF-α, and ICAM-1 mRNA was seen in cardiac tissues as early as 6 hours after renal ischemic injury and remained elevated up to 48 hours after renal ischemic injury. There was also a significant increase in myeloperoxidase activity in the heart and liver, apart from the kidneys. The increase in cardiac myeloperoxidase activity could be prevented by the administration of anti–ICAM-1 antibody at the time of renal ischemia. At 48 hours, cardiac function evaluation by echocardiography also revealed increases in left ventricular end-systolic and diastolic diameter and decreased fractional shortening. As little as 15 minutes of ischemia also resulted in significantly more apoptosis in cardiac tissue.[139] In transgenic sickle mice, bilateral renal IRI results in marked cardiac vascular congestion and increased serum amyloid P component (the murine equivalent of C-reactive protein). Kramer and colleagues have shown that renal ischemic injury leads to an increase in pulmonary vascular permeability defects that are mediated through macrophages.[135] Furthermore, they noted that in a rat model of bilateral renal ischemic injury or nephrectomy, there was downregulation of the lung epithelial Na channel, $Na^+$-$K^+$-ATPase, and aquaporin-5 expression, but not in unilateral ischemic models, suggesting the role of uremic toxins in modulating these effects in the lung.[567] Liu and colleagues have also shown effects of AKI on functional changes in the brain.[568] Mice with AKI had increased neuronal pyknosis and microgliosis in the brain; there were increased levels of the proinflammatory chemokines keratinocyte-derived chemoattractant and granulocyte colony-stimulating factor in the cerebral cortex and hippocampus and increased expression of glial fibrillary acidic protein in astrocytes in the cortex and corpus callosum. In addition, extravasation of Evans blue dye into the brain suggested that the blood-brain barrier was disrupted in mice with AKI.

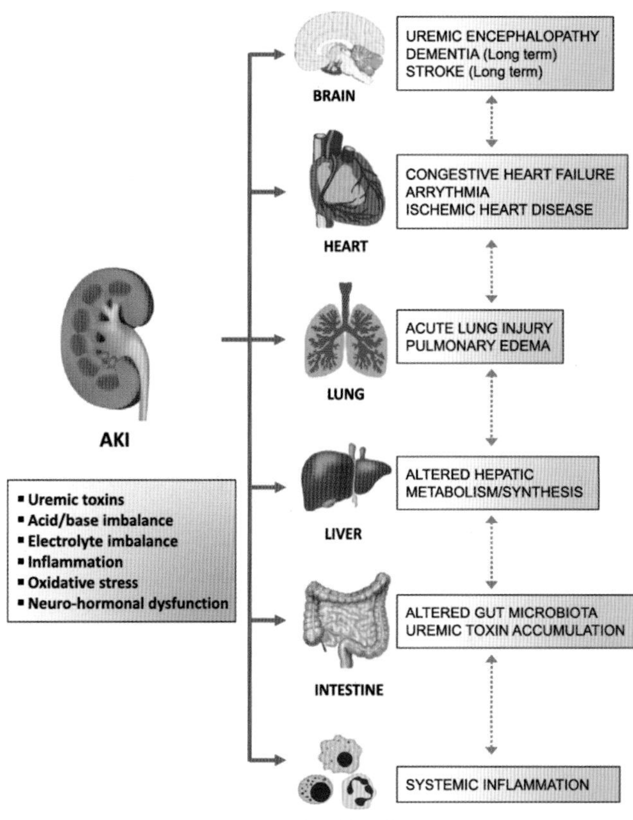


**Fig. 28.15** The impact of acute kidney injury *(AKI)* on distant organs. AKI causes hemodynamic, humoral, and immunologic changes, which lead to dysfunction of distant organs, including lung, heart, brain, liver, and intestine and the immune system. (From Lee SA, Cozzi M, Bush EL, Rabb H. Distant organ dysfunction in acute kidney injury: a review. *Am J Kidney Dis.* 2018;72(6):846–856.)

Many of the same processes involved in kidney-lung, kidney-heart, and kidney-brain interactions have been observed in the liver—increased neutrophil infiltration, vascular congestion, and vascular permeability after AKI. Following experimental AKI, levels of hepatic TNF-α, IL-6, IL-17A, ICM-1, keratinocyte-derived chemoattractant, IL-10, and MCP-1 are increased. The presence of AKI before a second-hit ischemic hepatic injury exacerbates liver injury as well, suggesting ongoing crosstalk between the kidney and liver[146] (Table 28.1).

Other organs also regulate ischemic renal injury. Patients with acute lung injury frequently have AKI, in part due to mechanical ventilation. There are three potential mechanisms whereby mechanical ventilation induces AKI—the effects of changes in arterial blood gases, barotrauma-induced systemic release of inflammatory agents, and the influence on systemic and renal blood flow.[569] Imai and coworkers have demonstrated the role of lung injury in inducing renal damage.[570] They found that in rabbits, injurious lung ventilatory strategies (high tidal volume and low peak end-expiratory pressure) alone were sufficient to induce renal epithelial cell apoptosis. This finding was further substantiated by the fact that plasma obtained from rabbits that underwent the injurious ventilation strategy induced more pronounced apoptosis in cultured LLC-$RK_1$ cells in vitro, suggesting that circulating soluble factors associated with mechanical ventilation might be involved in this process.

An example of extrarenal organs regulating ischemic AKI is evidenced by the effect of brain death on kidney transplants. Traumatic brain injury elicits a cytokine and inflammatory response. These cytokines result in renal inflammation in kidney transplants from brain-dead donors, distinct from living or cardiac-death donors.[571] Pretransplantation biopsies of brain-dead donor kidneys contain more infiltrating T lymphocytes and macrophages. Reperfusion of kidneys from brain-dead donors is associated with the instantaneous release of inflammatory cytokines, such as granulocyte colony-stimulating factor, IL-6, IL-9, IL-16, and MCP-1. In contrast, kidneys from living and cardiac death donors show a more modest cytokine response, with the release of IL-6 and small amounts of MCP-1.[572]

An important example of organ crosstalk is the one that occurs between the nervous and immune systems. Rather than two independent systems, these two systems are linked to maintain normal homeostasis and to respond to stress and pathophysiologic disorders. Studies have identified neural pathways that regulate immunity and inflammation via the inflammatory reflex pathway, thus identifying specific molecular targets that can be modulated by stimulating neurons electrically,[562,573,574] by ultrasound,[566,583] or optically.[564] The cholinergic antiinflammatory pathway (CAP) is the efferent limb of the so-called inflammatory reflex pathway mediated through the vagus nerve.[575–577] The afferent limb is activated by bacterial products (PAMPs), DAMPs, proinflammatory cytokines, immunoglobulins, and ATP.[578,579] Following detection of these inflammatory molecules at receptors, afferent signals from injured tissue and the immune cells are transmitted to the brain,[577,580] which then activates the vagus efferent nerve. Then the inflammatory reflex controls peripheral cytokine levels and inflammation through key cellular components such as macrophages and $CD4^+$ T cells. Indeed, vagus nerve stimulation shows antiinflammatory and organ-protective effects in various disorders, such as arthritis,[581] colitis,[582] ileus,[582] AKI,[563] and others. The spleen plays an integral role in linking the nervous and immune systems via the CAP. Prior splenectomy worsens AKI,[583] blocks the antiinflammatory effect of the CAP,[563,564] and worsens lung inflammation following kidney IRI.[584] Because AKI is associated with high mortality and morbidity, these studies indicate that multiorgan crosstalk that occurs in the setting of AKI is likely to be a major contributor to nonrenal organ dysfunction and may mediate clinically observable events, such as cardiac, pulmonary, and central nervous system events.

Finally, we address the issue of unilateral AKI affecting contralateral kidney function. In a model where the ischemia-reperfusion–injured kidney was removed after 5 weeks to isolate effects on the untouched kidney, challenge with higher dietary sodium yielded significant increase in blood pressure relative to sham-operated controls. Similarly, contralateral kidneys had impaired pressure natriuresis and hemodynamic responses, but reductions in vascular density were observed in the contralateral kidney. However, contralateral kidneys contained interstitial cells, some of which were identified as activated (low $CD62L/CD4^+$) T lymphocytes. Taken together, these data suggest that the salt-sensitive features of AKI on hypertension and CKD can be segregated so that effects on hemodynamics and hypertension may develop independently of direct renal damage.[585]

 Complete reference list available at ExpertConsult.com.

## KEY REFERENCES


26. Rosner MH, Perazella MA. Acute kidney injury in patients with cancer. *N Engl J Med.* 2017;376:1770–1781.
58. Sandoval RM, Molitoris BA. Gentamicin traffics retrograde through the secretory pathway and is released in the cytosol via the endoplasmic reticulum. *Am J Physiol Renal Physiol.* 2004;286: F617–F624.
83. Luque Y, Louis K, Jouanneau C, et al. Vancomycin-associated cast nephropathy. *J Am Soc Nephrol.* 2017;28:1723–1728.
97. Nath KA, Balla G, Vercellotti GM, et al. Induction of heme oxygenase is a rapid, protective response in rhabdomyolysis in the rat. *J Clin Invest.* 1992;90:267–270.
98. Zarjou A, Bolisetty S, Joseph R, et al. Proximal tubule H-ferritin mediates iron trafficking in acute kidney injury. *J Clin Invest.* 2013; 123:4423–4434.
103. Sanders PW, Booker BB, Bishop JB, et al. Mechanisms of intranephronal proteinaceous cast formation by low molecular weight proteins. *J Clin Invest.* 1990;85:570–576.
116. Zeisberg M, Neilson EG. Mechanisms of tubulointerstitial fibrosis. *J Am Soc Nephrol.* 2010;21:1819–1834.
122. Bonventre JV, Basile D, Liu KD, et al; on behalf of the Kidney Research National, D. AKI: a path forward. *Clin J Am Soc Nephrol.* 2013;8:1606–1608.
123. Okusa MD, Rosner MH, Kellum JA, et al; Acute Dialysis Quality Initiative, XW. Therapeutic targets of human AKI: harmonizing human and animal AKI. *J Am Soc Nephrol.* 2016;27:44–48.
125. Perrin S. Preclinical research: make mouse studies work. *Nature.* 2014;507:423–425.
126. de Caestecker M, Humphreys BD, Liu KD, et al. Bridging translation by improving preclinical study design in AKI. *J Am Soc Nephrol.* 2015.
139. Kelly KJ. Distant effects of experimental renal ischemia/reperfusion injury. *J Am Soc Nephrol.* 2003;14:1549–1558.
157. Doi K, Leelahavanichkul A, Yuen PS, et al. Animal models of sepsis and sepsis-induced kidney injury. *J Clin Invest.* 2009;119:2868–2878.
158. Langenberg C, Wan L, Egi M, et al. Renal blood flow in experimental septic acute renal failure. *Kidney Int.* 2006;69:1996–2002.
162. Wilmer MJ, Ng CP, Lanz HL, et al. Kidney-on-a-chip technology for drug-induced nephrotoxicity screening. *Trends Biotechnol.* 2016;34: 156–170.
169. Takasato M, Er PX, Chiu HS, et al. Kidney organoids from human iPS cells contain multiple lineages and model human nephrogenesis. *Nature.* 2015;526:564–568.
177. Solez K, Morel-Maroger L, Sraer JD. The morphology of 'acute tubular necrosis' in man: analysis of 57 renal biopsies and a comparison with the glycerol model. *Medicine (Baltimore).* 1979;58:362–376.
194. Portilla D. Role of fatty acid beta-oxidation and calcium-independent phospholipase A2 in ischemic acute renal failure. *Curr Opin Nephrol Hypertens.* 1999;8:473–477.
210. Molitoris BA, Dagher PC, Sandoval RM, et al. siRNA targeted to p53 attenuates ischemic and cisplatin-induced acute kidney injury. *J Am Soc Nephrol.* 2009;20:1754–1764.
216. Sarhan M, Land WG, Tonnus W, et al. Origin and consequences of necroinflammation. *Physiol Rev.* 2018;98:727–780.
237. Havasi A, Dong Z. Autophagy and Tubular Cell Death in the Kidney. *Semin Nephrol.* 2016;36:174–188.
240. Ravichandran KS. Beginnings of a good apoptotic meal: the find-me and eat-me signaling pathways. *Immunity.* 2011;35:445–455.
256. Kaissling B, Le Hir M. The renal cortical interstitium: morphological and functional aspects. *Histochem Cell Biol.* 2008;130:247–262.
259. Geissmann F, Manz MG, Jung S, et al. Development of monocytes, macrophages, and dendritic cells. *Science.* 2010;327:656–661.
262. Matzinger P. Tolerance, danger, and the extended family. *Annu Rev Immunol.* 1994;12:991–1045.
269. Li L, Huang L, Sung SS, et al. The chemokine receptors CCR2 and CX3CR1 mediate monocyte/macrophage trafficking in kidney ischemia-reperfusion injury. *Kidney Int.* 2008;74:1509–1511.
284. Geissmann F, Jung S, Littman DR. Blood monocytes consist of two principal subsets with distinct migratory properties. *Immunity.* 2003;19:71–82.

301. Li L, Huang L, Sung SJ, et al. NKT cell activation mediates neutrophil IFN-gamma production and renal ischemia-reperfusion injury. *J Immunol.* 2007;178:5899–5911.
303. Lee S, Huen S, Nishio H, et al. Distinct macrophage phenotypes contribute to kidney injury and repair. *J Am Soc Nephrol.* 2011;22:317–326.
324. Burne MJ, Daniels F, El Ghandour A, et al. Identification of the CD4+ T cell as a major pathogenic factor in ischemic acute renal failure. *J Clin Invest.* 2001;108:1283–1290.
347. Stremska ME, Jose S, Sabapathy V, et al. IL233, a novel IL-2 and IL-33 hybrid cytokine, ameliorates renal injury. *J Am Soc Nephrol.* 2017;28:2681–2693.
355. Lobo PI, Bajwa A, Schlegel KH, et al. Natural IgM anti-leukocyte autoantibodies attenuate excess inflammation mediated by innate and adaptive immune mechanisms involving Th-17. *J Immunol.* 2012;188:1675–1685.
377. Thurman JM, Nester CM. All things complement. *Clin J Am Soc Nephrol.* 2016;11:1856–1866.
381. Xavier S, Sahu RK, Landes SG, et al. Pericytes and immune cells contribute to complement activation in tubulointerstitial fibrosis. *Am J Physiol Renal Physiol.* 2017;312:F516–F532.
391. Liu M, Grigoryev DN, Crow MT, et al. Transcription factor Nrf2 is protective during ischemic and nephrotoxic acute kidney injury in mice. *Kidney Int.* 2009;76:277–285.
395. Swaminathan S. Iron, hormesis, and protection in acute kidney injury. *Kidney Int.* 2016;90:16–17.
417. Kapturczak MH, Wasserfall C, Brusko T, et al. Heme oxygenase-1 modulates early inflammatory responses: evidence from the heme oxygenase-1-deficient mouse. *Am J Pathol.* 2004;165:1045–1053.
418. Ferenbach DA, Bonventre JV. Mechanisms of maladaptive repair after AKI leading to accelerated kidney ageing and CKD. *Nat Rev Nephrol.* 2015;11:264–276.
426. Humphreys BD, Valerius MT, Kobayashi A, et al. Intrinsic epithelial cells repair the kidney after injury. *Cell Stem Cell.* 2008;2: 284–291.
441. Erdbrugger U, Le TH. Extracellular vesicles in renal diseases: more than novel biomarkers? *J Am Soc Nephrol.* 2016;27:12–26.
442. Bruno S, Grange C, Deregibus MC, et al. Mesenchymal stem cell-derived microvesicles protect against acute tubular injury. *J Am Soc Nephrol.* 2009;20:1053–1067.
443. Molitoris BA, Sutton TA. Endothelial injury and dysfunction: role in the extension phase of acute renal failure. *Kidney Int.* 2004;66:496–499.
474. Chawla LS, Eggers PW, Star RA, et al. Acute kidney injury and chronic kidney disease as interconnected syndromes. *N Engl J Med.* 2014;371:58–66.
475. Venkatachalam MA, Griffin KA, Lan R, et al. Acute kidney injury: a springboard for progression in chronic kidney disease. *Am J Physiol Renal Physiol.* 2010.
501. Zhang MZ, Yao B, Yang S, et al. CSF-1 signaling mediates recovery from acute kidney injury. *J Clin Invest.* 2012;122:4519–4532.
524. Lovisa S, LeBleu VS, Tampe B, et al. Epithelial-to-mesenchymal transition induces cell cycle arrest and parenchymal damage in renal fibrosis. *Nat Med.* 2015;21:998–1009.
525. Grande MT, Sanchez-Laorden B, Lopez-Blau C, et al. Snail1-induced partial epithelial-to-mesenchymal transition drives renal fibrosis in mice and can be targeted to reverse established disease. *Nat Med.* 2015;21:989–997.
562. Okusa MD, Rosin DL, Tracey KJ. Targeting neural reflex circuits in immunity to treat kidney disease. *Nat Rev Nephrol.* 2017;13:669–680.
566. Gigliotti JC, Huang L, Ye H, et al. Ultrasound prevents renal ischemia-reperfusion injury by stimulating the splenic cholinergic anti-inflammatory pathway. *J Am Soc Nephrol.* 2013;24:1451–1460.
585. Basile DP, Leonard EC, Tonade D, et al. Distinct effects on long-term function of injured and contralateral kidneys following unilateral renal ischemia-reperfusion. *Am J Physiol Renal Physiol.* 2012;302:F625–F635.

# 29 Prevention and Management of Acute Kidney Injury

Steven D. Weisbord | Paul M. Palevsky

CHAPTER OUTLINE



## DEFINITION OF ACUTE KIDNEY INJURY

Acute kidney injury (AKI) is a heterogeneous syndrome defined by rapid (hours to days) decline in the glomerular filtration rate (GFR), resulting in the retention of metabolic waste products, including urea and creatinine, and dysregulation of fluid, electrolyte, and acid-base homeostasis.[1] Although often considered a discrete syndrome, AKI represents a broad constellation of pathophysiologic processes of varied severity and cause. These include decreases in the GFR as the result of hemodynamic perturbations that disrupt normal renal perfusion without causing parenchymal injury, partial or complete obstruction to urinary flow, and a range of processes with characteristic patterns of glomerular, interstitial, tubular, or vascular parenchymal injury. AKI occurs in a heterogeneous patient population—genetics, age, kidney functional status, accompanying comorbidities—and the cause is often multifactorial.

The term *acute kidney injury* has largely supplanted the older terminology of acute renal failure (ARF). This change reflects recognition of serious shortcomings with the older terminology. Acute renal failure suggested a dichotomous relationship between normal kidney function and overt organ failure; in contrast, AKI captures the growing body of data associating small to moderate acute and transient decrements in kidney function with serious, adverse outcomes. Although the AKI terminology does emphasize the graded aspect of acute kidney disease, it should be recognized that this terminology is also imperfect. The term *injury* can be construed to imply the presence of parenchymal organ damage, which may be absent in a variety of settings associated with an acute decline in kidney function, such as early obstructive disease and prerenal azotemia associated with volume depletion. Although the term *acute kidney dysfunction* might better characterize the entire spectrum of the syndrome, AKI is the term that has been adopted by consensus and is now increasingly used in the medical literature.[2,3] In this chapter, AKI will be used to describe the entire spectrum of the syndrome. Although, in clinical practice, the term *acute tubular necrosis* (ATN) is often used synonymously with AKI, these terms should not be used interchangeably. Although ATN is the most common form of intrinsic AKI, particularly in critically ill patients, it represents only one of multiple forms of AKI. In addition, there may be a lack of concordance between the clinical syndrome and the classic histopathologic findings of ATN.[4,5]

Decreased urine output is a cardinal (although not universal) manifestation of AKI, and patients are often classified based on urine flow rates as nonoliguric (urine output >400 mL/day), oliguric (urine output <400 mL/day), or anuric (urine output <100 mL/day).[6] Transient oliguria may occur in the absence of significant decrements in kidney function, because increased tubular salt and water reabsorption is a normal physiologic response to volume depletion. In contradistinction, persistent oliguria, despite the presence of adequate intravascular volume, is virtually always a manifestation of AKI, with lower urine volume typically associated with more severe initial renal injury. The categorization of AKI based on urine volume has clinical implications for the development of volume overload, severity of electrolyte disturbances, and overall prognosis. Although oliguric AKI is associated with a higher mortality risk than nonoliguric AKI, therapeutic interventions to augment urine output (see later) have not been shown to improve patient outcomes.[7]

AKI can develop de novo in the setting of intact kidney function or can be superimposed on underlying chronic kidney disease (acute on chronic kidney injury), and the presence of underlying impaired kidney function has been shown to be one of the most important risk factors for the development of AKI.[8,9] Multiple mechanisms may contribute to this increased susceptibility, including diminished renal functional reserve, impaired salt and water conservation predisposing to intravascular volume contraction, decreased activity of detoxification mechanisms, increasing susceptibility to cytotoxic injury, impaired clearance of potential nephrotoxins, increasing the risk for and/or duration of exposure, and associated macrovascular and microvascular disease, increasing the risk of ischemic injury.

The causes of AKI are usually divided into three broad pathophysiologic categories:

1. Prerenal AKI—diseases characterized by effective hypoperfusion of the kidneys in which there is no parenchymal damage to the kidney (Box 29.1);
2. Intrinsic AKI—diseases involving the renal parenchyma (Table 29.1); and
3. Postrenal (obstructive) AKI—diseases associated with acute obstruction of the urinary tract (Box 29.2)

Although these categories are useful for didactic purposes and help inform the initial clinical assessment of patients presenting with AKI, there is often a degree of overlap between these categories. For example, renal hypoperfusion may cause a spectrum of renal injury ranging from prerenal azotemia to overt ATN, depending on its severity and duration. As a result, precise categorization of the cause of AKI in these three groups may not always be possible, and individual patients may transition between categories regarding causation.

The prior absence of a uniform operational definition of AKI impeded epidemiologic studies and hampered clinical evaluations of preventive and therapeutic interventions. Older literature was characterized by multiple definitions using varying absolute and/or relative changes in the serum creatinine concentration, with or without associated decrements in urine output, which made it difficult to compare findings

**Box 29.1 Causes of Prerenal Acute Kidney Injury**

Intravascular Volume Depletion
- Hemorrhage—trauma, surgery, postpartum, gastrointestinal
- Gastrointestinal losses—diarrhea, vomiting, nasogastric loss
- Renal losses—diuretics, osmotic diuresis, diabetes insipidus,
- Skin and mucous membrane losses—burns, hyperthermia
- Nephrotic syndrome
- Cirrhosis
- Capillary leak

Reduced Cardiac Output
- Cardiogenic shock
- Pericardial diseases—restrictive, constrictive, tamponade
- Congestive heart failure
- Valvular diseases
- Pulmonary diseases—pulmonary hypertension, pulmonary embolism
- Sepsis

Systemic Vasodilation
- Sepsis
- Cirrhosis
- Anaphylaxis
- Medications

Renal Vasoconstriction
- Early sepsis
- Hepatorenal syndrome
- Acute hypercalcemia
- Drugs—norepinephrine, vasopressin, nonsteroidal antiinflammatory drugs (NSAIDs), angiotension-converting enzyme
- Calcineurin inhibitors

Iodinated Contrast Agents

Increased Intraabdominal Pressure

Abdominal Compartment Syndrome

**Table 29.1 Major Causes of Intrinsic Acute Kidney Injury**

| Type of Injury | Examples |
|---|---|
| Tubular injury | |
| • Ischemia due to hypoperfusion | Hypovolemia, sepsis, hemorrhage, cirrhosis, CHF (see Box 29.1) |
| • Endogenous toxins | Myoglobin, hemoglobin, paraproteinemia, uric acid (see Table 29.3) |
| • Exogenous toxins | Antibiotics, chemotherapy agents, radiocontrast, phosphate preps. (see Table 29.3) |
| Tubulointerstitial injury | |
| • Acute allergic interstitial nephritis | Nonsteroidal antiinflammatory drugs (NSAIDs), antibiotics |
| • Infections | Viral, bacterial, and fungal infections |
| • Infiltration | Lymphoma, leukemia, sarcoid |
| • Allograft rejection | |
| Glomerular injury | |
| • Inflammation | Anti-GBM disease, ANCA-associated GN, postinfectious, cryoglobulinemia, membranoproliferative glomerulonephritis, IgA nephropathy, SLE, Henoch-Schonlein purpura, polyarteritis nodosa |
| • Hematologic | Hemolytic-uremic syndrome, thrombotic thrombocytopenic purpura, medications |
| Renal microvasculature | Malignant hypertension, toxemia of pregnancy, hypercalcemia, radiocontrast, scleroderma, medications |
| Large vessels | |
| • Arterial | Thrombosis, vasculitis, dissection, thromboembolism, atheroembolism, trauma |
| • Venous | Thrombosis, compression, trauma |

*ANCA,* Antineutrophil cytoplasmic antibody; *CHF,* congestive heart failure; *GBM,* glomerular basement membrane; *GN,* glomerulonephritis; *IgA,* immunoglobulin A; *SLE,* systemic lupus erythematosus.

**Box 29.2 Causes of Postrenal Acute Kidney Injury**

**Upper Urinary Tract Extrinsic Causes**

Retroperitoneal space—lymph nodes, tumors
Pelvic or intraabdominal tumors—cervix, uterus, ovary, prostate
Fibrosis—radiation, drugs, inflammatory
Ureteral ligation or surgical trauma
Granulomatous diseases
Hematoma

**Lower Urinary Tract Causes**

Prostate—benign prostatic hypertrophy, carcinoma, infection
Bladder—neck obstruction, calculi, carcinoma, infection (schistosomiasis)
Functional—neurogenic bladder secondary to spinal cord injury, diabetes, multiple sclerosis, stroke, pharmacologic side effects of drugs (anticholinergics, antidepressants)
Urethral—posterior urethral valves, strictures, trauma, infections, tuberculosis, tumors

**Upper Urinary Tract: Intrinsic Causes**

Nephrolithiasis
Strictures
Edema
Debris, blood clots, sloughed papillae, fungal ball
Malignancy

across studies. In 2002, the Acute Dialysis Quality Improvement Initiative (ADQI) proposed the first consensus definition of AKI. The ADQI work group proposed a classification scheme with three strata based on the magnitude of increases in serum creatinine levels and/or the duration of oliguria (Table 29.2).

As proposed, the first stratum provides the greatest sensitivity for diagnosing AKI, whereas higher strata provide increasing specificity of diagnosis. These three strata were combined with two outcome stages defined by the need for and duration of renal replacement therapy, resulting in the five-tiered RIFLE classification (***r***isk of renal dysfunction, ***i***njury to the kidney, ***f***ailure of kidney function, as well as the two outcome stages, ***l***oss of kidney function and ***e***nd-stage kidney disease).[10] Subsequently, the Acute Kidney Injury Network (AKIN) modified the RIFLE classification by adding an absolute increase in serum creatinine level of 0.3 mg/dL or more to the 50% relative increase in the serum creatinine level to the definition of AKI and specifying that these increments develop over no more than 48 hours[2] (see Table 29.2). This definition was further modified in the Kidney Disease: Improving Global Outcomes (KDIGO) clinical practice guideline for acute kidney injury, which clarifies that although the 0.3-mg/dL increment in the serum creatinine level needs to occur over 48 hours, from a known baseline value, the 50% increase may occur over a longer, 7-day interval.[3]

The KDIGO clinical practice guideline for AKI recognized a gap in the nosology of acute and chronic kidney disease.[3] Based on the definitions previously, AKI has an onset of less

**Table 29.2 RIFLE, Acute Kidney Injury Network (AKIN) and Kidney Disease: Improving Global Outcomes (KDIGO) Definitions and Staging of Acute Kidney Injury**

**Definitions**

| Parameter | RIFLE | AKIN | KDIGO |
|---|---|---|---|
| Serum creatinine | An increase of >50% developing over <7 days | An increase of >0.3 mg/dL or of >50% developing over <48 hours | An increase of >0.3 mg/dL developing over <48 hours or an increase of >50% developing over <7 days |
| Urine output[a] | <0.5 mL/kg/h for >6 hours | <0.5 mL/kg/h for >6 hours | <0.5 mL/kg/h for >6 hours |

**Staging Criteria**

**Increase in Serum Creatinine**

| RIFLE | | AKIN | KDIGO | Urine Output[a] |
|---|---|---|---|---|
| Risk | ≥50% | Stage 1: ≥0.3 mg/dL or ≥50% | Stage 1: ≥0.3 mg/dL or ≥50% | <0.5 mL/kg/h for >6 hours |
| Injury | ≥100% | Stage 2: ≥100% | Stage 2: ≥100% | <0.5 mL/kg/h for >12 hours |
| Failure | ≥200% | Stage 3: ≥200% | Stage 3: ≥200% | <0.3 mL/kg/h for >24 hours or anuria for >12 hours |
| Loss | Need for renal replacement therapy for >4 weeks | | | |
| End-stage | Need for renal replacement therapy for >3 months | | | |

[a]The urine output criteria for both definition and staging of AKI are the same for the RIFLE, AKIN, and KDIGO criteria.
*RIFLE,* ***R***isk of renal dysfunction, ***i***njury to the kidney, ***f***ailure of kidney function, as well as the two outcome stages, ***l***oss of kidney function and ***e***nd-stage kidney disease.

than 7 days, whereas chronic kidney disease (CKD) is defined by the presence of impaired kidney function or structural kidney damage for more than 3 months with implications for health.[11] Recognizing that some patients develop kidney disease with a more subacute onset than that of AKI, but of less than 3 months' duration, the KDIGO Acute Kidney Injury Workgroup proposed the concept of acute kidney disease (AKD), defined as AKI or a reduction in the GFR to less than 60 mL/min/1.73 m,[2] a decrease in the GFR by 35% or more, an increase in the serum creatinine level by more than 50%, or the presence of structural kidney damage of less than 3 months' duration.

Several limitations to these criteria for diagnosis and staging of AKI have been recognized.[12,13] First, although validation studies have demonstrated that the AKI stage correlates with mortality risk, it is not clear that this is the appropriate metric for assessing their validity as a definition of kidney disease. Second, there is poor correlation between AKI stage and the GFR. Because the magnitude of change in the serum creatinine level is time-dependent, a patient may demonstrate progression over time from less severe (RIFLE-R, AKIN, or KDIGO stage 1) to more severe AKI stage (RIFLE-F, AKIN, or KDIGO stage 3), despite an improving GFR. Third, the definition of AKI by serum creatinine criteria relies on a referent baseline serum creatinine level, which is often unavailable. Furthermore, variations in specifications for this referent value (e.g., admission serum creatinine level vs. most recent outpatient serum creatinine level prior to admission vs. other definitions) can alter the classification of patients.[14] Fourth, both RIFLE and AKIN definitions use relative changes in serum creatinine level to stage AKI. Analyses of creatinine kinetics have demonstrated that the time required to attain a fixed percentage change in serum creatinine level in the setting of severe AKI is dependent on the baseline level of kidney function, whereas the initial rate of change in serum creatinine level is relatively independent of kidney function.[12] Thus, early in the course of AKI, absolute changes in the serum creatinine level may be detected more readily than relative changes. Fifth, concordance between the serum creatinine level and urine output criterion is poor, even with regard to mortality risk.[15] Transient changes in urine output may reflect variation in volume status or be due to the administration of medications and do not necessarily correlate with other parameters of kidney function. Finally, it must be noted that these classification systems are independent of the various causes of AKI—prerenal, intrinsic, obstructive. Despite these shortcomings, the use of standardized classification schemes has enhanced the interpretation of epidemiologic studies and the design of clinical trials.

Conceptually, AKI comprises a spectrum of structural and functional kidney disease in which there may be an evolution from injury to organ dysfunction and, finally, overt organ failure. Reliance solely on changes in serum creatinine level and/or urine output to diagnose AKI has resulted in the inability to identify the incipient stages of intrinsic kidney damage, which may be the most opportune time for pharmacologic intervention.[16] To facilitate the early diagnosis of intrinsic injury, multiple biomarkers of tubular injury have been evaluated, including N-acetyl-β-D-glucosaminidase (NAG), kidney injury molecule 1 (KIM-1), neutrophil gelatinase-associated lipocalin (NGAL), interleukin 18 (IL-18), liver fatty acid binding protein (L-FABP), tissue inhibitor of metalloproteinase 2 (TIMP-2), and insulin-like growth factor-binding protein 7 (IGFBP7).[17–22] In addition, serum cystatin C has been proposed as more sensitive (and, in some settings, more specific) than serum creatinine for detecting changes in the GFR, and urinary cystatin C has been proposed as a marker of tubular injury.[17,23,24] Although most of these biomarkers have yet to be adequately validated for routine clinical use, they have the potential to provide an earlier diagnosis of intrinsic AKI than the serum creatinine level, differentiate volume-responsive (prerenal) AKI from intrinsic disease, diminish the confounding effect related to creatinine generation, and provide prognostic information regarding the clinical course of an episode of AKI. One or more of these biomarkers may provide a means whereby patients could be identified at the incipient stage of AKI to guide the implementation of specific therapy to ameliorate kidney damage or promote recovery of kidney function.

## INCIDENCE OF ACUTE KIDNEY INJURY

Estimates of the incidence of AKI are highly dependent on the case definition used, with rates among hospitalized patients ranging from as high as 44% when defined based on a change in serum creatinine level of at least 0.3 mg/dL to as low as 1% using an increase in serum creatinine level of at least 2.0 mg/dL.[25–29] Approximately 3% to 7% of hospitalized patients and 25% to 60% of intensive care unit (ICU) patients develop AKI, with 5% to 6% of the ICU population requiring renal replacement therapy after developing AKI.[25–29] In a single-center analysis conducted in 1996 at an urban tertiary care hospital, AKI, defined as an increase in serum creatinine level of 0.5 mg/dL for patients with a baseline serum creatinine level of 1.9 mg/dL or less, of 1.0 mg/dL for patients with a baseline serum creatinine level of 2.0 to 4.9 mg/dL, and 1.5 mg/dL for patients with a baseline serum creatinine level greater than 5 mg/dL, developed in 7.2% of 4622 consecutive patients.[25] The overall incidence of AKI is approximately 21.6% for all hospitalized adults worldwide,[30] with known associations for accelerating CKD to end-stage kidney disease (ESKD).[31–33] The more recent estimate of AKI incidence is considerably higher than the 4.9% investigators had observed in a similar study in 1979.[34] In the late 1970s, the most frequent cause for AKI was decreased renal perfusion, observed in 39% of episodes, followed by medication-associated (16%), contrast-associated (11%), postoperative (9%), and sepsis-associated (6.5%). Overall mortality was 19.4%, with higher mortality rates associated with larger maximal increments in the serum creatinine concentration.

Although definition is less of an issue with regard to rates of AKI requiring renal replacement therapy, reported rates vary considerably because of differences in the characteristics of patient populations and variability in criteria for the initiation of renal replacement therapy. In a multinational, multicenter observational study of 29,269 critically ill patients, 5.7% developed severe AKI and 4.3% received renal replacement therapy (RRT).[35] In a smaller but more recent multinational observational study, 13.5% of 1802 critically ill patients developed RRT requiring AKI.[29]

Many epidemiologic studies of AKI have relied on data from large administrative databases. Such data need to be interpreted with caution, however, because administrative coding for AKI is incomplete and may only capture 20% to 30% of all episodes of AKI.[36,37] The ascertainment of AKI requiring RRT using administrative data is substantially more complete. In an analysis of data from the National Hospital Discharge Survey in the United States, the Centers for Disease Control and Prevention have observed an increase in hospital discharges with a diagnosis of AKI from 18/100,000 population in 1980 to 365/100,000 in 2005.[38] Similar trends have been observed in analyses of the US Nationwide Inpatient Sample (NIS) and a 5% sample of US hospitalized Medicare beneficiaries. In an analysis that combined administrative and clinical data from a single integrated health care delivery system, the incidence of AKI that did not require the use of RRT increased from 322.7 to 522.4/100,000 person-years from 1996 to 2003.[39] Over the same period, AKI requiring RRT increased from 19.5 to 29.5/100,000 person-years.[39] AKI was more common among men and older adults. In a more recent analysis using data from the NIS, a nationally representative administrative database of hospitalizations, the incidence of dialysis-requiring AKI increased from 222/million person-years in 2000 to 533/million person-years in 2009, with the largest rise in incidence occurring in patients 65 to 74 years of age and 75 years of age or older.[40] Although a component of these temporal trends may be attributable to earlier initiation of dialysis and more frequent use of RRT in older patients, these changes are unlikely to account for most of the increase in incidence of severe AKI.

Preexisting kidney disease is one of the major risk factors for the development of dialysis-requiring AKI.[41] More severe baseline CKD is associated with higher levels of risk. Compared with patients with a baseline estimated GFR (eGFR) more than 60 mL/min/1.73 $m^2$, patients with eGFR values of 45 to 59 mL/min/1.73 $m^2$ have a nearly twofold increased risk of developing dialysis-requiring AKI. This risk increases to more than 40-fold among patients with baseline eGFR values less than 15 mL/min/1.73 $m^2$.[41] Underlying diabetes mellitus, hypertension, and the presence of proteinuria are also associated with the risk for hospital-acquired AKI.

## CATEGORIZATION OF ACUTE KIDNEY INJURY

Although in the clinical setting AKI is often multifactorial, the cause is commonly evaluated based on three major pathophysiologic categories—prerenal, intrinsic, and postrenal (obstructive) AKI. Prerenal azotemia is the most common cause of AKI, accounting for about 40% to 55% of all cases.[25,27,42] Prerenal AKI is caused by a reduction in blood flow to the kidneys that can result from absolute and/or effective reduction in intravascular volume. Common causes of absolute intravascular volume depletion leading to prerenal AKI include gastrointestinal losses (e.g., diarrhea, vomiting, nasogastric suction), renal losses (e.g., overdiuresis, diabetes insipidus), and sequestration of extracellular fluid (e.g., third spacing, as seen in acute pancreatitis; see Box 29.1). Common conditions that cause effective intravascular volume contraction include heart failure and liver failure. In these conditions, the absolute blood volume is increased, yet arterial blood flow to the kidneys is reduced, leading to prerenal azotemia. A more detailed narrative on prerenal AKI is presented in Chapter 28 on the pathophysiology of AKI.

Intrinsic AKI is frequently categorized based on the anatomic location of primary renal injury, including the vasculature, glomeruli, interstitium, and tubules (see Table 29.1). Diseases that affect the renal vasculature range from complete thrombosis of the renal artery or vein, which are uncommon events, atheroembolic disease typically following instrumentation of renal or extrarenal vasculature, to vasculitides that affect small renal vessels, including the glomeruli. Such vasculitides may be confined to the kidney but are commonly systemic conditions with extrarenal manifestations. Acute interstitial nephritis (AIN) most often results from an idiosyncratic allergic response to a myriad of different pharmacologic agents, most commonly to antibiotics (e.g., methicillin and other penicillins, cephalosporins, sulfonamides, quinolones) or nonsteroidal antiinflammatory drugs (NSAIDs; e.g., ibuprofen).[43] Proton pump inhibitors have more recently been associated with impaired kidney function, hypothesized to be related, at least in part, to AIN.[44–46] A multitude of other clinical conditions, including bacterial infection, can also lead to AIN. Systemic allergic signs such as fever, rash, and eosinophilia are often present in antibiotic-associated AIN, but not usually present in NSAID-related AIN.

The most common form of intrinsic AKI is acute tubular necrosis (ATN). The causes of ATN are broadly categorized as ischemic, septic, and nephrotoxic. Prolonged prerenal azotemia and hypotension, even if short-lived, can lead to necrosis of tubular epithelial cells and ATN. Nephrotoxins leading to ATN can be extrinsic, such as iodinated contrast, antibiotics, and chemotherapeutic agents, or intrinsic, such as myoglobin, hemoglobin, and intratubular crystals (Table 29.3). Sepsis-associated AKI, although previously attributed to ischemia reperfusion injury, is now believed to have a more complex pathogenesis and may develop in the absence of overt hypotension. These conditions, including their pathogenesis and pathophysiology, are discussed in detail in Chapter 28.

Postrenal (obstructive) AKI is characterized by blockage to the flow of urine. Obstruction, intrinsic or extrinsic, can occur at any point from the renal collecting system to the urethra (see Box 29.2). The development of postrenal AKI requires bilateral obstruction or unilateral obstruction in a patient with a solitary kidney or in the setting of CKD. The most common causes of postrenal AKI are functional or structural obstruction of the bladder neck due to prostatic conditions, anticholinergic agents, and neurogenic bladder. Additional causes of obstructive AKI include bilateral ureteral calculi, fibrosis, or blood clots, sloughed renal papillae (i.e., renal papillary necrosis), genitourinary malignancies, external compression from tumors or hemorrhage, and retroperitoneal fibrosis. A detailed description of renal obstruction is provided in Chapter 37.

## EVALUATION OF ACUTE KIDNEY INJURY

The assessment of the patient with AKI requires a meticulous history and physical examination, comprehensive review of medical records, evaluation of urinary findings, including the urinary sediment, review of laboratory tests, renal imaging and, when appropriate, kidney biopsy[47] (Table 29.4). Analysis

**Table 29.3 Major Causes of Endogenous and Exogenous Toxins Causing Acute Tubular Necrosis**

| Endogenous Toxins | Exogenous Toxins |
|---|---|
| Myoglobulinuria<br>• Muscle breakdown—trauma, compression, electric shock, hypothermia, hyperthermia, seizures, exercise, burns<br>• Metabolic—hypokalemia, hypophosphatemia<br>• Infections—tetanus, influenza,<br>• Toxins—isopropyl alcohol, ethanol, ethylene glycol, toluene, snake and insect bites, cocaine, heroin<br>• Drugs—HMG-CoA reductase inhibitors (statins), amphetamines, fibrates<br>• Inherited disease—deficiency of myophosphorylase, phosphofructokinase, carnitine palmityltransferase<br>• Autoimmune—polymyositis, dermatomyositis | Antibiotics<br>• Aminoglycosides<br>• Amphotericin B<br>• Antiviral agents—acyclovir, cidofovir, indinavir, foscarnet, tenofovir<br>• Pentamidine<br>• Vancomycin |
| Hemoglobinuria<br>• Mechanical—prosthetic valves, microangiopathic hemolytic anemia, extracorporeal circulation<br>• Drugs—hydralazine, methyldopa<br>• Chemicals—benzene, arsine, fava beans, glycerol, phenol<br>• Immunologic—transfusion reaction<br>• Genetic—G6PD deficiency, PNH | Chemotherapy<br>• Cisplatin<br>• Ifosfamide<br>• Plicamycin<br>• 5-Fluorouracil<br>• Cytarabine<br>• 6-Thioguanine<br>• Methotrexate |
| Intratubular obstruction from crystalluria or paraproteins<br>• Tumor lysis syndrome<br>• HGPT deficiency<br>Multiple myeloma<br>• Oxalate (ethylene glycol) | Calcineurin inhibitors<br>• Cyclosporine<br>• Tacrolimus<br>Organic solvents<br>• Toluene<br>• Ethylene glycol<br>Poisons<br>Miscellaneous<br>• Radiocontrast agents<br>• Intravenous immune globulin<br>• Nonsteroidal antiinflammatory drugs<br>• Oral phosphate bowel preparations |

*G6PD,* Glucose-6-phosphate dehydrogenase; *HGPT,* Hypoxanthine-guanine phosphoribosyltransferase; *HMG-CoA,* 5-hydroxy-3-methylglutaryl-coenzyme A; *PNH,* paroxysmal nocturnal hemoglobinuria.

of serum creatinine concentration over time is invaluable for differentiating acute from chronic kidney disease and identifying the timing of events that precipitated the acute decline in kidney function. The presence of an acute process is easily confirmed if review of laboratory records reveals a sudden rise in blood urea nitrogen (BUN) level and serum creatinine concentration from previously stable baseline values. Spurious causes of elevated BUN and serum creatinine levels must be excluded before a diagnosis of AKI is made. When prior BUN and serum creatinine measurements are not available, key findings that suggest that a chronic process is present include physical manifestations of hyperparathyroidism (e.g., resorption of distal phalangeal tufts, lateral aspect of clavicles), band keratopathy, so-called half-and-half nails, and small echogenic kidneys on radiographic imaging. Enlarged kidneys do not necessarily rule out a chronic process because diabetic nephropathy, HIV-associated nephropathy, amyloidosis, and polycystic kidney disease are characterized by enlarged kidney size, even with moderate to advanced CKD. Anemia is a less useful differentiating feature because it is often present in both AKI and CKD. Once the presence of AKI has been confirmed, attention should focus on patient, urine, laboratory, and radiographic assessments to help distinguish among prerenal, intrinsic, and postrenal processes, permit identification of the cause of AKI, and guide treatment.

## CLINICAL ASSESSMENT OF THE PATIENT

Prerenal AKI should be suspected in clinical settings associated with intravascular volume depletion, including hemorrhage, excessive gastrointestinal, urinary, or insensible fluid losses and severe burns, or with reduced effective arterial blood volume due to congestive heart failure, liver disease, or nephrotic syndrome. The risk of intravascular volume depletion is increased in comatose, sedated, or obtunded patients and in patients with restricted access to salt and water. Clinical clues to a prerenal cause of AKI on history include patient report of excessive thirst, orthostatic light-headedness or dizziness, significant diarrhea and/or vomiting, diuretic use, and recent use of medications that alter intrarenal hemodynamics, including NSAIDs, as well as inhibitors of the renin-angiotensin axis, such as direct renin inhibitors, angiotensin-converting enzyme (ACE) inhibitors, and angiotensin receptor blockers (ARBs).

Findings suggestive of volume depletion on physical examination may include orthostatic hypotension (postural

**Table 29.4 Useful Clinical Features, Urinary Findings, and Confirmatory Tests in the Differential Diagnosis of Acute Kidney Injury**

| Cause of Acute Kidney Injury | Some Suggestive Clinical Features | Typical Urinalysis | Some Confirmatory Tests |
|---|---|---|---|
| Prerenal azotemia | Evidence of true volume depletion (thirst, postural or absolute hypotension and tachycardia, low jugular venous pressure, dry mucous membranes and axillae, weight loss, fluid output >input) or decreased effective circulatory volume (e.g., heart failure, liver failure), treatment with NSAID, diuretic, or ACE inhibitor or ARB | Hyaline cases<br>$FE_{Na}$ <1%<br>$U_{Na}$ <10 mmol/L<br>SG >1.018 | Occasionally requires invasive hemodynamic monitoring; rapid resolution of AKI with restoration of renal perfusion |
| **Diseases Involving Large Renal Vessels** | | | |
| Renal artery thrombosis | History of atrial fibrillation or recent myocardial infarction, nausea, vomiting, flank or abdominal pain | Mild proteinuria<br>Occasionally RBCs | Elevated LDH with normal transaminase levels, renal arteriogram, MAG-3 renal scan, MRA[a] |
| Atheroembolism | Usually age >50 years, recent manipulation of aorta, retinal plaques, subcutaneous nodules, palpable purpura, livedo reticularis | Often normal<br>Eosinophiluria<br>Rarely casts | Eosinophilia, hypocomplementemia, skin biopsy, renal biopsy |
| Renal vein thrombosis | Evidence of nephrotic syndrome or pulmonary embolism, flank pain | Proteinuria, hematuria | Inferior venocavogram, Doppler flow studies, MRV[a] |
| **Diseases of Small Renal Vessels and Glomeruli** | | | |
| Glomerulonephritis or vasculitis | Compatible clinical history (e.g., recent infection), sinusitis, lung hemorrhage, rash or skin ulcers, arthralgias, hypertension, edema | RBC or granular casts, RBCs, white blood cells, proteinuria | Low complement levels; positive antineutrophil cytoplasmic antibodies, antiglomerular basement membrane antibodies, antistreptolysin O antibodies, anti-DNAse, cryoglobulins; renal biopsy |
| HUS, TTP | Compatible clinical history (e.g., recent gastrointestinal infection, cyclosporine, anovulants), pallor, ecchymoses, neurologic findings | May be normal, RBCs, mild proteinuria, rarely RBC or granular casts | Anemia, thrombocytopenia, schistocytes on peripheral blood smear, low haptoglobin, increased LDH, renal biopsy |
| Malignant hypertension | Severe hypertension with headaches, cardiac failure, retinopathy, neurologic dysfunction, papilledema | May be normal, RBCs, mild proteinuria, rarely RBC casts | LVH by echocardiography or EKG, resolution of AKI with BP control |
| **Ischemic or Nephrotoxic Acute Tubular Necrosis** | | | |
| Ischemia | Recent hemorrhage, hypotension, surgery, often in combination with vasoactive medication (e.g., ACE inhibitor, NSAID) | Muddy brown granular or tubular epithelial cell casts $FE_{Na}$ >1%,<br>$U_{Na}$ >20 mmol/L,<br>SG ≈ 1.010 | Clinical assessment and urinalysis usually inform diagnosis. |
| Exogenous toxin | Recent contrast-enhanced procedure; nephrotoxic medications; certain chemotherapeutic agents often with coexistent volume depletion, sepsis or chronic kidney disease | Muddy brown granular or tubular epithelial cell cases $FE_{Na}$ >1%,<br>$U_{Na}$ >20 mmol/L,<br>SG ≈ 1.010 | Clinical assessment and urinalysis usually inform diagnosis. |
| Endogenous toxin | History suggestive of:<br>Rhabdomyolysis (coma, seizures, drug abuse, trauma)<br>Hemolysis (recent blood transfusion)<br>Tumor lysis (recent chemotherapy)<br>Myeloma (bone pain) or ethylene glycol ingestion | Urine supernatant tests positive for heme in absence of red cells; urine supernatant pink and tests positive for heme in absence of red cells; urate crystals, dipstick-negative proteinuria, oxalate crystals, respectively | Hyperkalemia, hyperphosphatemia, hypocalcemia, increased CK, myoglobin; hyperkalemia, hyperphosphatemia, hypocalcemia, hyperuricemia and free circulating hemoglobin; hyperuricemia, hyperkalemia, hyperphosphatemia (for tumor lysis); circulating or urinary monoclonal protein (for myeloma); toxicology screen, acidosis, osmolal gap (for ethylene glycol) |

**Table 29.4 Useful Clinical Features, Urinary Findings, and Confirmatory Tests in the Differential Diagnosis of Acute Kidney Injury (Cont'd)**

| Cause of Acute Kidney Injury | Some Suggestive Clinical Features | Typical Urinalysis | Some Confirmatory Tests |
|---|---|---|---|
| Diseases of the tubulointerstitium—allergic interstitial nephritis | Recent ingestion of drug and fever, rash, loin pain, or arthralgias | White blood cell casts, white blood cells (frequently eosinophiluria), RBCs, rarely RBC casts, proteinuria (occasionally nephritic) | Systemic eosinophilia, renal biopsy |
| Acute bilateral pyelonephritis | Fever, flank pain and tenderness, toxic state | Leukocytes, occasionally white blood cell casts, RBCs, bacteria | Urine and blood cultures |
| Postrenal AKI | Abdominal and flank pain, palpable bladder | Frequently normal, hematuria if stones, prostatic hypertrophy | Plain abdominal x-ray, renal ultrasonography, postvoid residual bladder volume, computed tomography, retrograde or antegrade pyelography |

[a]Contrast-enhanced magnetic resonance angiography and magnetic resonance venography should be used with extreme caution in patients with AKI.

*ACE,* Angiotensin-converting enzyme; *AKI,* acute kidney injury; *ARB,* angiotensin receptor blocker; *BP,* blood pressure; *CK,* creatine kinase; *EKG,* electrocardiogram; $FE_{Na}$, fractional excretion of sodium; *HUS,* hemolytic-uremic syndrome; *LDH,* lactate dehydrogenase; *LVH,* left ventricular hypertrophy; *MRA,* magnetic resonance angiography; *MRV,* magnetic resonance venography; *NSAID,* nonsteroidal antiinflammatory drug; *RBC,* red blood cell; *SG,* specific gravity; *TTP,* thrombotic thrombocytopenic purpura; $U_{Na}$, urine sodium.

fall in diastolic blood pressure >10 mm Hg) and tachycardia (postural increase in heart rate >10 beats/min), reduced jugular venous pressure, diminished skin turgor, dry mucous membranes, and the absence of axillary sweat. However, overt signs and symptoms of hypovolemia do not usually manifest until the extracellular fluid volume has fallen by more than 10% to 20%. In addition, in patients with heart failure, liver disease, or nephrotic syndrome, renal hypoperfusion may be present, despite total body volume overload. Findings on physical examination of peripheral edema, pulmonary vascular congestion, pleural effusion, cardiomegaly, the presence of an S3 heart sound, elevated jugular venous pressure, or hepatic congestion may point to a state of reduced cardiac output and decreased effective intravascular volume. The presence of acute or chronic liver disease is suggested by evidence of icterus, ascites, splenomegaly, palmar erythema, telangiectasia, and caput medusa. In select critically ill patients, invasive hemodynamic monitoring using central venous or pulmonary artery catheters or ultrasonography of the heart and central veins may assist in assessing intravascular volume status. A definitive diagnosis of prerenal AKI is usually based on the prompt resolution of AKI after restoration of renal perfusion. In patients with underlying systolic heart failure, restoration of renal perfusion may be challenging and often requires the use of inotropic support.

There is a high likelihood of ischemic ATN if AKI follows a period of severe renal hypoperfusion, and the impairment in kidney function persists or worsens, despite restoration of renal perfusion. It should be noted, however, that significant hypotension is evident in fewer than 50% of patients with postsurgical ATN.[48] Although septic shock is a common cause of ATN, ATN may also develop in sepsis in the absence of overt hypotension.[48,49] The diagnosis of nephrotoxic ATN requires a comprehensive review of all clinical, pharmacy, nursing, radiographic, and procedural notes for evidence of the administration of nephrotoxic agents. Pigment-induced ATN may be suspected if the clinical assessment reveals risk factors for rhabdomyolysis (e.g., seizures, excessive exercise, alcohol or drug abuse, treatment with statins, prolonged immobilization, limb ischemia, crush injury) or hemolysis, as well as select signs and symptoms of the former (e.g., muscle tenderness, weakness, evidence of trauma or prolonged immobilization).[50–53]

Although most AKI is prerenal or ischemic, nephrotoxic, or septic ATN, patients should be carefully evaluated for other intrinsic renal parenchymal processes because their management and prognosis may differ substantially. Flank pain may be a prominent symptom of acute renal artery or renal vein occlusion, renal infarction (from systemic emboli), acute pyelonephritis and, rarely, necrotizing glomerulonephritis.[54–56] Interstitial edema leading to distention of the renal capsule and flank pain may be seen in up to one-third of patients with AIN.[57] Dermatologic examination can be highly informative because a maculopapular rash may accompany allergic interstitial nephritis: subcutaneous nodules, livedo reticularis, digital ischemia, and palpable purpura may suggest atheroembolism or vasculitis; a malar (butterfly) rash may be associated with systemic lupus erythematosus; and impetigo or needle tracks from intravenous (IV) drug use may underlie infection-associated glomerulonephritis. An ophthalmologic examination is useful to assess for signs of atheroembolism; hypertensive or diabetic retinopathy; the keratitis, uveitis, and iritis of autoimmune vasculitides; icterus associated with chronic liver disease; and the rare but nevertheless pathognomonic band keratopathy of hypercalcemia and flecked retina of hyperoxalemia. Uveitis may also be an indicator of coexistent allergic interstitial nephritis, sarcoidosis, and the tubulointerstitial nephritis and uveitis (TINU) syndrome.[58] Examination of the ears, nose, and throat may reveal conductive deafness and mucosal inflammation or ulceration suggestive of necrotizing granulomatous vasculitis or the neural deafness caused by aminoglycoside toxicity. Respiratory failure, particularly if associated with hemoptysis, suggests the presence of a pulmonary-renal syndrome, and ascites and other stigmata of severe chronic liver disease suggest the possibility of hepatorenal syndrome (HRS). Cardiovascular assessment may reveal marked elevation in systemic blood pressure suggesting malignant hypertension or scleroderma or may demonstrate a new arrhythmia or murmur suggesting a potential source of thromboemboli or subacute bacterial endocarditis (acute glomerulonephritis), respectively. Chest or abdominal pain and reduced pulses in the lower limbs should suggest aortic dissection or, rarely, Takayasu arteritis. Abdominal pain and nausea are frequent clinical correlates of atheroembolic disease, commonly in patients who have recently undergone angiographic evaluation, particularly in the presence of widespread atherosclerotic disease. The presence of a tensely distended abdomen may indicate the presence of abdominal compartment syndrome and should prompt transduction of bladder pressure.[59] Pallor and recent bruising are important clues to the thrombotic microangiopathies, and the combination of bleeding and fever should raise the possibility of AKI resulting from viral hemorrhagic fevers. A recent jejunoileal bypass may be a vital clue to oxalosis, a rare but reversible cause of AKI following bariatric surgery.[60] Hyperreflexia and asterixis often portend the development of uremic encephalopathy or may, in the presence of focal neurologic signs, suggest a diagnosis of thrombotic microangiopathy (i.e., hemolytic-uremic syndrome [HUS] or thrombotic thrombocytopenic purpura [TTP]; see Chapter 34).

Postrenal AKI may be asymptomatic if obstruction to the drainage of urine develops gradually. Although anuria will be seen in complete obstruction, urine volume may be normal or even increased in the setting of partial obstruction. A pattern of fluctuating urine output may also be seen in some patients with partial obstruction. Suprapubic or flank pain may be the presenting complaint if there is acute distention of the bladder or renal collecting system and capsule, respectively. Colicky flank pain radiating to the groin suggests acute ureteral obstruction, most commonly from urinary stone disease. Prostatic disease should be suspected in older men with a history of nocturia, urinary frequency, urgency or hesitancy, and an enlarged prostate on rectal examination. Urinary retention may be exacerbated acutely in such patients by medications with anticholinergic properties, such as antihistamines or antidepressants. Rectal or pelvic examination may reveal obstructing tumors in female patients. Neurogenic bladder is a likely diagnosis in patients with spinal cord injury or autonomic insufficiency and should be suspected in patients with long-standing diabetes mellitus. Bladder distention may be evident on abdominal percussion and palpation in patients with bladder neck or urethral obstruction. Definitive diagnosis of postrenal AKI usually relies on examination of the postvoid bladder volume and radiographic evaluation of the upper urinary tract and is confirmed by improvement in kidney function following relief of the obstruction.

## URINE ASSESSMENT

Urine volume is rarely helpful in distinguishing various forms and causes of AKI. Anuria can be seen with complete urinary tract obstruction but can also be seen with severe prerenal or intrinsic renal disease (e.g., renal artery occlusion, severe proliferative glomerulonephritis or vasculitis, bilateral cortical necrosis). Patients with partial urinary tract obstruction may present with polyuria caused by secondary impairment of urine-concentrating mechanisms.

Assessment of the urine is essential in patients with AKI and is an inexpensive and useful diagnostic tool.[61–63] Measured urine specific gravity above 1.015 to 1.020 often accompanies prerenal AKI, although impaired urinary concentration may be present in patients with underlying CKD or as a result of diuretic therapy. Acute glomerulonephritis may also present with concentrated urine. Isosthenuria (a urine specific gravity of 1.010, similar to that of plasma) is characteristic of ATN. Hematuria on dipstick assessment may result from urologic trauma from catheterization, urologic disease, interstitial nephritis, acute glomerulonephritis, atheroembolic disease, renal infarction, or pigment (hemoglobinuric or myoglobinuric) nephropathy. The latter are suggested when the dipstick test for blood is strongly positive but there are few or no red blood cells seen on microscopic examination of the urinary sediment.

Examination of the urinary sediment of a centrifuged urine specimen complements the dipstick analysis and is highly valuable for distinguishing among the various forms of AKI (Box 29.3). The sediment should be inspected for the presence of cells, casts, and crystals. In prerenal AKI, the urine sediment is typically bland (i.e., devoid of cells or casts) but may contain transparent hyaline casts. Hyaline casts are formed in concentrated urine from normal urinary constituents, principally Tamm-Horsfall protein secreted by epithelial cells of the loop of Henle. Postrenal AKI may also present with a bland urine sediment, although hematuria is common in patients with intraluminal obstruction (e.g., stones, sloughed papilla, blood clot) or prostatic disease. Renal tubular epithelial cells, epithelial cell casts, and pigmented, muddy brown granular casts are characteristic of ischemic or nephrotoxic ATN. These characteristic findings of ATN may be found in association with microscopic hematuria and mild tubular proteinuria (<1 g/day). Casts may be absent in approximately 20% to 30% of patients with ischemic or nephrotoxic ATN and are not a requisite for diagnosis[61,64]; however, semiquantitative scoring systems have been developed to assess the presence of epithelial cells and casts in patients with AKI to assist in the diagnosis of ATN and correlate with the clinical course.[62,65,66]

Red blood cell (RBC) casts are almost always indicative of acute glomerular disease but may be observed, albeit rarely, in AIN. Dysmorphic RBCs, best seen using phase contrast microscopy, are a more common urinary finding in patients with glomerular injury but are a less specific finding than RBC casts. Urine sediment abnormalities vary in diseases involving preglomerular blood vessels, such as HUS, TTP, atheroembolic disease, and vasculitis involving medium-sized or large vessels, and range from benign to overtly nephritic. White blood cell casts and nonpigmented granular casts suggest interstitial nephritis, whereas broad granular casts are characteristic of CKD and probably reflect interstitial fibrosis and dilation of

**Box 29.3 Urine Sediment in the Differential Diagnosis of Acute Kidney Injury**

Normal or few red blood cells or white blood cells
- Prerenal azotemia
- Arterial thrombosis or embolism
- Preglomerular vasculitis
- HUS, TTP
- Scleroderma crisis
- Postrenal AKI

Renal tubular epithelial cells and granular casts
- Acute tubular necrosis

Dysmorphic red blood cells and red blood cell casts
- Glomerulonephritis or vasculitis
- Malignant hypertension
- Rarely interstitial nephritis

White blood cell and white blood cell casts
- Acute interstitial nephritis or exudative glomerulonephritis
- Severe pyelonephritis
- Marked leukemic or lymphomatous infiltration

Eosinophiluria (>5%)
- Allergic interstitial nephritis (antibiotics >> NSAIDs)
- Atheroembolism

Crystalluria
- Acute urate nephropathy
- Calcium oxalate (ethylene glycol intoxication)
- Acyclovir
- Indinavir
- Sulfonamides
- Methotrexate

*AKI,* Acute kidney injury; *HUS,* hemolytic-uremic syndrome; *NSAIDs,* nonsteroidal antiinflammatory drugs; *TTP,* thrombotic thrombocytopenic purpura.

tubules. Eosinophiluria (from 1%–50% of urine leukocytes) is a common finding (90%) in drug-induced allergic interstitial nephritis.[67,68] However, eosinophiluria has poor sensitivity and specificity for the diagnosis of AIN, with eosinophiluria of 1% to more than 5% occurring in a variety of other diseases, including atheroembolization, ischemic and nephrotoxic AKI, proliferative glomerulonephritis, pyelonephritis, cystitis, and prostatitis. In a series of 566 patients who had urinary eosinophil testing and renal histology from kidney biopsy, eosinophiluria only had a 31% sensitivity and 68% specificity for the diagnosis of interstitial nephritis.[69] Uric acid crystals (pleomorphic) may be seen in the urine in prerenal AKI but should raise the possibility of acute urate nephropathy if seen in abundance. Oxalate crystalluria (needle- or dumbbell-shaped monohydrate crystals or envelope-shaped dihydrate crystals) may suggest a diagnosis of ethylene glycol toxicity.[70] A variety of other crystals may be seen in other medication-associated crystal nephropathies.[71–73]

Increased urinary protein excretion, characteristically less than 1 g/day, is a common finding in ischemic or nephrotoxic ATN and reflects both failure of injured proximal tubule cells to reabsorb normally filtered protein and excretion of cellular debris (tubular proteinuria). Proteinuria greater than 1 g/day suggests injury to the glomerular ultrafiltration barrier (glomerular proteinuria) or excretion of light chains.[74,75] The latter are not detected by conventional dipsticks, which detect albumin, and must be sought by other means (e.g., sulfosalicylic acid test). Heavy proteinuria is also a frequent finding (80%) in patients with allergic interstitial nephritis triggered by NSAIDs. In addition to acute interstitial inflammation, these patients have a glomerular lesion that is almost identical to that of minimal-change disease.[76] A similar syndrome has been reported in patients receiving other agents, such as ampicillin, rifampin, and interferon alfa.[77,78] Hemolysis and rhabdomyolysis may often be differentiated by inspection of plasma, which is characteristically pink in hemolysis, but clear in rhabdomyolysis.

Analysis of urine biochemical parameters may be helpful in differentiating between prerenal and intrinsic ischemic or nephrotoxic ATN (Table 29.5). Sodium is usually avidly reabsorbed from the glomerular filtrate in patients with prerenal AKI as a consequence of renal adrenergic activation, stimulation of the renin-angiotensin-aldosterone system (RAAS), suppression of atrial natriuretic peptide (ANP) secretion, and local changes in peritubular hemodynamics. In contrast, $Na^+$ reabsorption is impaired in ATN as a result of injury to the renal tubular epithelium. Renal sodium handling can be assessed based on the urinary sodium concentration ($U_{Na}$), with values of less than 10 mmol/L commonly seen in prerenal disease compared with more than 20 mmol/L in ATN. Normalizing sodium excretion to creatinine provides a more sensitive index. The fractional excretion of sodium ($FE_{Na}$) is the ratio between urine sodium excretion ($U_{Na} \times V$, where $U_{Na}$ is the urine sodium concentration and V is the urine volume) and the filtered load of sodium (calculated as $P_{Na} \times CrCl$, where $P_{Na}$ is the plasma sodium concentration and CrCl is the creatinine clearance, which can be calculated as $[(U_{Cr} \times V)/P_{Cr}]$ where V is the urine volume and $[U_{Cr}]$ and $[P_{Cr}]$ are the urine and plasma creatinine concentrations, respectively. Because urine volume is in both the numerator and denominator of this ratio, the $FE_{Na}$ can be calculated as $[(U_{Na} \div P_{Na})/(U_{Cr} \div P_{Cr})] \times 100$ using an untimed (spot) urine sample and simultaneous serum sodium and creatinine measurements; this is usually less than 1% (frequently, <0.5%) in the setting of prerenal azotemia, whereas it is typically more than 2% in patients with ischemic or nephrotoxic AKI.

The utility of the $FE_{Na}$ is limited in a variety of clinical settings. Values greater than 1% are not uncommon in the setting of prerenal AKI in patients receiving diuretics, those with metabolic alkalosis and bicarbonaturia (in whom $Na^+$ is excreted with $HCO_3^-$ to maintain electroneutrality), in the presence of adrenal insufficiency, and in the setting of underlying CKD.[79–81] Conversely, an $FE_{Na}$ less than 1% may be observed in the setting of ATN, particularly in the settings of iodinated contrast administration, rhabdomyolysis, and sepsis, although it has been reported in 15% or more of patients with ATN from a variety of other causes, including ischemia, burns, and exposure to selected nephrotoxins.[79,80,82–84]

It has been postulated that a low $FE_{Na}$ value reflects a milder degree of intrinsic renal injury in which epithelial cell damage is probably localized to the corticomedullary junction and outer medulla, with relative preservation of function in other $Na^+$-transporting segments, and may represent a transition state between prerenal azotemia and ATN. It should be recognized that an $FE_{Na}$ value of less than 1% is not abnormal and reflects normal sodium homeostasis in

**Table 29.5 Urine Indices Used in the Differential Diagnosis of Prerenal Acute Kidney Injury and Acute Tubular Necrosis**

| Diagnostic Index | Prerenal AKI | ATN |
|---|---|---|
| Fractional excretion of sodium (%) | <1[a] | >2[a] |
| Urine sodium concentration (mmol/L) | <20 | >40 |
| Urine creatinine-to-plasma creatinine ratio | >40 | <20 |
| Urine urea nitrogen-to-plasma urea nitrogen ratio | >8 | <3 |
| Urine specific gravity | >1.018 | ~1.010 |
| Urine osmolality (mOsm/kg $H_2O$) | >500 | ~300 |
| Plasma BUN-to-creatinine ratio | >20 | <10-15 |
| Renal failure index, $U_{Na}/(U_{Cr}/P_{Cr})$ | <1 | >1 |
| Urine sediment | Hyaline casts | Muddy brown granular casts |

[a]$FE_{Na}$ may be >1% in prerenal AKI associated with diuretic use and/or the setting of bicarbonaturia or chronic kidney disease; $FE_{Na}$ often <1% in acute tubular necrosis caused by radiocontrast or rhabdomyolysis.

*AKI*, Acute kidney injury; *ATN*, acute tubular necrosis; *BUN*, blood urea nitrogen; $P_{Cr}$, plasma creatinine; $U_{Cr}$, urine creatinine; $U_{Na}$, urine sodium.

patients on a moderate- to low-sodium diet. The $FE_{Na}$ is also often less than 1% in AKI caused by urinary tract obstruction, glomerulonephritis, and diseases of the renal vasculature; other parameters must be used to distinguish these conditions from prerenal AKI.

A variety of other indices has also been proposed to differentiate between causes of AKI. The renal failure index, calculated as $U_{Na}/(U_{Cr} \div P_{Cr})$ provides comparable information to the $FE_{Na}$ because clinical variations in serum $Na^+$ concentration are relatively small. The fractional excretion of urea ($FE_{urea}$) has been proposed as an alternative to the $FE_{Na}$, with particular utility in patients on diuretic therapy. Values of $FE_{urea}$ calculated as $([U_{urea} \div P_{urea}]/[U_{Cr} \div P_{Cr}] \times 100)$ less than 35% are suggestive of a prerenal state.[85–87] Similarly, indices of urinary concentrating ability, such as urine specific gravity, urine osmolality, urine-to-plasma creatinine or urea ratios, and serum urea nitrogen-to-creatinine ratio are of limited value in differentiating between prerenal and intrinsic AKI. This is particularly true for older patients, in whom urine concentrating mechanisms are frequently impaired while mechanisms for $Na^+$ reabsorption are typically preserved.

## BLOOD AND LABORATORY FINDINGS

The pattern and timing of changes of BUN and serum creatinine levels often provide clues to the cause of AKI. Enhanced tubular reabsorption of filtered urea, in parallel with sodium and water reabsorption in prerenal states, commonly leads to a disproportionate elevation in BUN relative to serum creatinine levels (ratio >20:1). Conversely, with intrinsic AKI, the increase in BUN level usually parallels the rise in serum creatinine level, maintaining a ratio of about 10:1. However, severe malnutrition and low dietary protein intake blunt the rise in BUN and creatinine levels, whereas gastrointestinal bleeding, steroid therapy, and hypercatabolic states may lead to increases in the BUN level that do not reflect prerenal physiology. In addition, aggressive volume resuscitation may rapidly expand the volume of distribution of urea and creatinine and may also obscure the acute rise in serum creatinine level. Sepsis and other forms of critical illness have also been associated with decreased creatinine generation.[88,89] The serum creatinine level typically begins to rise within 24 to 48 hours when ATN results from an ischemic insult. Although the clinical course can be highly variable, the serum creatinine level will generally peak within 7 to 10 days and, depending on the severity of the insult and underlying comorbid illnesses, AKI will resolve to varying degrees over the ensuing 1 to 2 weeks. Following iodinated contrast exposure, the peak in serum creatinine level generally occurs within 5 to 7 days. The time course of nephrotoxic ATN caused by aminoglycoside antibiotics or cisplatin is more variable, often with a delayed onset of AKI (7–10 days).

Additional clues to the diagnosis can be obtained from biochemical and hematologic tests. The presence of marked hyperkalemia, hyperuricemia, and hyperphosphatemia point to cell lysis, which, in the setting of elevated creatine kinase levels and hypocalcemia, strongly suggests rhabdomyolysis.[90,91] Biochemical signs of cell lysis with very high levels of uric acid, normal or mildly elevated creatine kinase levels, and a urine uric acid-to-creatinine ratio greater than 1.0 are suggestive of acute urate nephropathy and tumor lysis syndrome.[92,93] Severe hypercalcemia can precipitate AKI, commonly in the form of prerenal AKI from concomitant hypovolemia and renal vasoconstriction. AKI associated with a widening of both the serum anion ($Na^+ - [HCO_3^- + Cl^-]$) and osmolal (measured serum osmolality minus calculated osmolality) gaps suggests a diagnosis of ethylene glycol toxicity and should prompt a search for urine oxalate crystals. Severe anemia in the absence of hemorrhage may reflect the presence of hemolysis, multiple myeloma, or thrombotic microangiopathy (e.g., HUS, TTP, toxemia, disseminated intravascular coagulation, accelerated hypertension, systemic lupus erythematosus [SLE], scleroderma, radiation injury). Other laboratory findings suggestive of thrombotic microangiopathy include thrombocytopenia, dysmorphic RBCs on peripheral blood smear, low circulating haptoglobin concentrations, and elevated circulating concentrations of lactate dehydrogenase. Systemic eosinophilia suggests allergic interstitial nephritis but may also be a prominent feature in other diseases, such as atheroembolic disease and eosinophilic granulomatosis with polyangiitis (Churg-Strauss disease). Depressed serum complement and high titers of antiglomerular basement membrane antibodies, antineutrophil cytoplasmic antibodies, antinuclear antibodies, circulating immune complexes, or cryoglobulins are useful diagnostic tools in patients with suspected glomerulonephritis or systemic vasculitis.

## NOVEL BIOMARKERS OF KIDNEY INJURY

A number of novel biomarkers of kidney injury have been evaluated for potential roles in the early identification, differential diagnosis, and prognosis of AKI, including serum cystatin C, NGAL, KIM-1, IL-18, L-FABP, TIMP-2 and IGFBP7 among others (see earlier).[17–24] Although most of these biomarkers are not available for routine clinical use, they have the potential to provide an earlier diagnosis of intrinsic AKI, differentiate volume-responsive (prerenal) AKI from intrinsic disease, and provide prognostic information regarding the clinical course of an episode of AKI.

### Cystatin C

Cystatin C is a 13-kDa protein that is filtered by the glomerulus and completely reabsorbed and degraded by the proximal tubule. Cystatin C has been validated as an alternative marker of glomerular filtration.[94,95] As a result of its shorter serum half-life, serum cystatin C concentrations change more rapidly than serum creatinine levels in response to changes in kidney function, allowing changes in serum cystatin C to be detected sooner than changes in serum creatinine following the onset of AKI.[96] Under normal circumstances, urinary cystatin C is virtually undetectable; however, following tubular injury, tubular reabsorption of filtered cystatin is diminished, and urinary cystatin C can be detected, raising the possibility of its use as an early marker of tubular injury.[97]

### Neutrophil Gelatinase-Associated Lipocalin

NGAL is a 25-kDa protein whose expression by renal tubular epithelial cells is markedly upregulated following ischemic or nephrotoxic kidney injury.[98,99] NGAL is believed to enhance the trafficking of iron-siderophore complexes, enhancing the delivery of iron, upregulating hemeoxygenase-1, reducing apoptosis, and increasing the normal proliferation of renal tubule epithelial cells.[100] Urine and plasma NGAL have been evaluated in numerous clinical settings as an early biomarker of tubular injury.[101–111] Initial studies in children undergoing cardiac surgery have demonstrated extremely high sensitivity and specificity for the identification of AKI, with an area under the receiver operating characteristic (ROC) curve of more than 0.99; however, these early results have not been reproduced across other clinical settings.

### Kidney Injury Molecule 1

KIM-1 is a transmembrane protein whose expression is markedly upregulated in the proximal tubule following tubular injury.[112–115] The extracellular component of the KIM-1 protein is shed into the urine following tubular injury, permitting its potential use as a marker of tubular damage; however, the time course of peak KIM-1 expression in the urine is later than that seen with NGAL.[108,116–118] Moreover, more recent studies have demonstrated elevated levels of KIM-1 in non-AKI settings, including chronic kidney disease and renal cell carcinoma, which reduce its specificity for AKI.[119,120]

### Interleukin 18

IL18 is a proinflammatory cytokine whose expression is increased in the kidney following ischemic and nephrotoxic injury.[121] Urinary IL-18 levels have been shown to rise within 6 hours following tubular injury, following cardiac surgery, and in critically ill patients.[110,111,122,123]

### Liver Fatty Acid–Binding Protein

Despite its name, L-FABP is expressed in the proximal tubule.[124,125] Elevated L-FABP levels may be detected in the urine within 6 hours of ischemic or nephrotoxic injury, permitting its potential use as a marker of tubular injury.[118,126–128] In a meta-analysis of published studies, the sensitivity and specificity of urinary L-FABP for diagnosis of AKI were each approximately 75%.[129]

### Tissue Inhibitor of Metalloproteinase 2 and Insulin-Like Growth Factor–Binding Protein 7

TIMP-2 and IGFBP7 are expressed in epithelial cells and act in an autocrine and paracrine manner to arrest cell cycle in AKI.[130–132] In three discovery cohorts comprising 522 patients, these two biomarkers were identified as having the highest discriminant ability among 340 candidate biomarkers of AKI.[22] In a subsequent validation study of 728 patients, this pair of biomarkers had an area under the ROC curve of 0.80, which was significantly better than the performance of other candidate biomarkers, including NGAL, KIM-1, IL-18, and L-FABP.[22] A combination test that includes TIMP-2 and IGFBP7 is available for commercial use.

## RADIOLOGIC EVALUATION

Imaging of the abdomen is a highly useful adjunct to laboratory testing to determine the cause of AKI. In cases of suspected obstructive uropathy, postvoid residual volumes of more than 100 to 150 mL suggest a diagnosis of bladder outlet obstruction. Although plain films rarely provide definitive evidence of postrenal AKI, they may identify the presence of calcium-containing stones that can cause obstructive disease. Renal ultrasonography is the screening test of choice to assess cortical thickness, differences in cortical and medullary density, the integrity of the collecting system, and kidney size.[133] Although pelvicalyceal dilation is usual in cases of urinary tract obstruction (98% sensitivity), dilation may not be observed in the volume-depleted patient during the initial 1 to 3 days after obstruction, when the collecting system is relatively noncompliant, or in patients with obstruction caused by ureteric encasement or infiltration (e.g., retroperitoneal fibrosis, neoplasia).[134]

Alternatively, computed tomography (CT) may be used to visualize the kidneys and collecting system, although contrast administration should ideally be avoided in patients with AKI. Visualization of the collecting system may be suboptimal in the absence of contrast enhancement; however, unenhanced CT scans are useful for the identification of obstructing ureteral stones.[135,136] Ultrasonography and CT have essentially replaced the use of IV pyelography, which now has little or no role in the evaluation of AKI. Cystoscopic retrograde or percutaneous anterograde pyelography are useful tests for the precise localization of the site of obstruction and can be combined with placement of ureteral stents or percutaneous nephrostomy tubes to allow therapeutic decompression of the urinary tract. Radionuclide scans have been proposed as useful for assessing renal blood flow, glomerular filtration, tubule function, and infiltration by inflammatory cells in AKI; however, these tests lack specificity and yield conflicting or poor results in controlled studies.[137,138] Magnetic resonance angiography (MRA) of the kidneys is extremely useful for detecting renal artery stenosis and has been used in the evaluation of acute renovascular crises.[139] However, given the association of gadolinium-based contrast administration with the development of nephrogenic systemic fibrosis, contrast-enhanced MRA is contraindicated in most patients with AKI.[140,141] Doppler ultrasonography and spiral CT are also useful in patients with suspected vascular obstruction; however, contrast angiography remains the gold standard for definitive diagnosis.

### KIDNEY BIOPSY

Kidney biopsy in AKI is usually reserved for patients in whom prerenal and postrenal AKI have been excluded, and the cause of intrinsic AKI is unclear.[142,143] Kidney biopsy is particularly useful when clinical assessment, urinalysis, and laboratory investigation suggest diagnoses other than ischemic or nephrotoxic injury that may respond to specific therapy. Examples include anti–glomerular basement membrane disease and other forms of necrotizing glomerulonephritis, vasculitis, HUS and TTP, allergic interstitial nephritis, and myeloma cast nephropathy.

## CAUSES OF ACUTE KIDNEY INJURY IN SPECIFIC CLINICAL SETTINGS

The differential diagnosis of AKI in several common clinical settings warrants special mention (Box 29.4).

### ACUTE KIDNEY INJURY IN THE SETTING OF CANCER

There are several potential causes of AKI in the patient with cancer. Prerenal AKI is common in the setting of underlying malignancy and may be related to tumor- or chemotherapy-induced vomiting or diarrhea, reduced oral intake secondary to anorexia, the use of NSAIDs for pain management, and malignancy-associated hypercalcemia.[144,145]

Intrinsic AKI can be triggered by a variety of chemotherapeutic agents. Cisplatin is the classic chemotherapeutic medication associated with AKI.[146,147] The principal site of renal damage with cisplatin is the proximal tubule. The nephrotoxicity of cisplatin is dose-dependent, yet AKI can result from a single exposure. Electrolyte disturbances, including hypomagnesemia and hypokalemia, are common following cisplatin administration. Other platinum-containing chemotherapy agents, such as carboplatin and oxaliplatin, are less nephrotoxic than cisplatin but are not risk-free, particularly when high cumulative doses are administered. Ifosphamide, which has been used to treat germ cell tumors, sarcomas, other solid tumors, and occasionally lymphoma, is also associated with AKI in a dose-dependent fashion.[148–150] Methotrexate nephrotoxicity occurs following IV administration of high doses (>1 g/m$^2$), primarily as the result of precipitation of the drug and metabolites in the tubular lumen.[71,151,152] Risk factors for methotrexate nephrotoxicity include volume depletion and the presence of acidic urine. Direct tubular toxicity may also contribute to the development of AKI. Chemotherapeutic agents targeting vascular endothelial growth factor (VEGF) or the VEGF receptor, such as bevacizumab, and the tyrosine kinase inhibitor sunitinib, are associated with hypertension, proteinuria, thrombotic microangiopathy, and AKI.[153,154] Checkpoint inhibitors, such as nivolumab, may cause a variety of immune-related adverse events, including AIN.[155,156]

Renal parenchymal invasion by solid and hematologic cancers has been reported in 5% to 10% of autopsy studies but is an uncommon cause of AKI.[157,158] Infiltration of leukemic cells into the renal parenchyma can precipitate AKI and typically presents with hematuria, proteinuria, and enlarged kidneys on ultrasound imaging. Prompt diagnosis is important because the AKI may respond to chemotherapeutic intervention.

The tumor lysis syndrome, which is associated with hyperuricemia, hyperphosphatemia, and hypocalcemia, is a well-recognized cause of AKI in patients with cancer.[159,160] Tumor lysis syndrome occurs most commonly following the initiation of chemotherapy for patients with poorly differentiated, rapidly growing lymphoproliferative malignancies (e.g., Burkitt lymphoma, acute lymphoblastic or promyelocytic leukemia); however, this can occur spontaneously and in the setting of certain solid tumors that are highly sensitive to radiation and/or chemotherapy (e.g., testicular carcinoma). The Cairo-Bishop criteria, which include both laboratory and clinical criteria, have been used to provide a standard definition for the diagnosis of tumor lysis syndrome[160] (Box 29.5). AKI associated with the tumor lysis syndrome is thought to be triggered by direct tubular injury and luminal obstruction by uric acid and calcium phosphate crystals. Prophylactic therapy with aggressive volume administration and either xanthine oxidase inhibitors to inhibit uric acid synthesis or recombinant uricase to convert uric acid to allantoin has markedly reduced the incidence of this form of AKI.[161–164] Less common causes of AKI include tumor-associated glomerulonephritis and thrombotic microangiopathy induced by medications or irradiation. Chemotherapy-associated thrombotic microangiopathy is a well-recognized complication of several agents, including mitomycin C and gemcytabine.[165–167]

AKI is a common complication of multiple myeloma.[75,168] Causes of AKI in this setting include intravascular volume depletion, myeloma cast nephropathy, sepsis, hypercalcemia, ATN induced by drugs or tumor lysis during therapy, cryoglobulinemia, hyperviscosity syndrome, and plasma cell infiltration. Multiple myeloma may also result in impaired kidney function as the result of amyloidosis or light chain deposition disease; however, these usually present with proteinuria and a more subacute decline in kidney function. Myeloma cast nephropathy results from the binding of filtered immunoglobulin Bence-Jones proteins to Tamm-Horsfall glycoprotein, forming casts that obstruct the tubular lumen. Higher excretion rates of free light chains, volume depletion, and hypercalcemia are associated with higher risks for the development of myeloma cast nephropathy. Prompt treatment to lower the free light chain burden may result in recovery of kidney function. Studies of the effectiveness of plasmapheresis in the treatment of myeloma cast nephropathy have yielded conflicting results.[169–172] The use

**Box 29.4 Major Causes of Acute Kidney Injury in Specific Clinical Settings**

**AKI in the Cancer Patient**

Prerenal azotemia
- Hypovolemia (e.g., poor intake, vomiting, diarrhea)

Intrinsic AKI
- Exogenous nephrotoxins—chemotherapy, antibiotics, contrast agents
- Endogenous toxins—hyperuricemia, hypercalcemia, tumor lysis, paraproteins
- Other—radiation, HUS, TTP, glomerulonephritis, amyloid, malignant infiltration

Postrenal AKI
- Ureteric or bladder neck obstruction

**AKI After Cardiac Surgery**

Prerenal azotemia
- Hypovolemia (surgical losses, diuretics), cardiac failure, vasodilators

Intrinsic AKI
- Ischemic ATN (even in absence of hypotension)
- Atheroembolic disease after aortic manipulation, intraaortic balloon pump
- Pre- or perioperative administration of contrast agent
- Allergic interstitial nephritis induced by perioperative antibiotics

Postrenal AKI
- Obstructed urinary catheter, exacerbation of voiding dysfunction

**AKI in Pregnancy**

Prerenal azotemia—acute fatty liver of pregnancy with fulminate hepatic failure

Intrinsic AKI
- Preeclampsia or eclampsia
- Postpartum HUS, TTP
- HELLP syndrome
- Ischemia—postpartum hemorrhage, abruptio placentae, amniotic fluid embolus
- Direct toxicity of illegal abortifacients

Postrenal AKI—obstruction with pyelonephritis

**AKI After Solid Organ or Bone Marrow Transplantation (BMT)**

Prerenal azotemia
- Intravascular volume depletion (e.g., diuretic therapy)
- Vasoactive drugs (e.g., calcineurin inhibitors, amphotericin B)
- Hepatorenal syndrome, venoocclusive disease of liver (BMT)

Intrinsic AKI
- Postoperative ischemic ATN (even in absence of hypotension)
- Sepsis
- Exogenous nephrotoxins: aminoglycosides, amphotericin B, radiocontrast
- HUS, TTP (e.g., cyclosporine or myeloablative radiotherapy–related)
- Allergic tubulointerstitial nephritis

Postrenal AKI
- Obstructed urinary catheter

**AKI and Pulmonary Disease (Pulmonary-Renal Syndrome)**

Prerenal azotemia—diminished cardiac output complicating pulmonary embolism, severe pulmonary hypertension, or positive pressure mechanical ventilation

Intrinsic AKI
- Vasculitis—Goodpasture syndrome, ANCA-associated vasculitis, SLE, Churg-Strauss syndrome, polyarteritis nodosa, cryoglobulinemia, right-sided endocarditis, lyphomatoid granulomatosis, sarcoidosis, scleroderma
- Toxins—ingestion of paraquat or diquat
- Infections—Legionnaires' disease, *Mycoplasma* infection, tuberculosis, disseminated viral or fungal infection

AKI from any cause with hypervolemia and pulmonary edema

Lung cancer with hypercalcemia, tumor lysis, or glomerulonephritis

**AKI and Liver Disease**

Prerenal azotemia
- Reduced true (gastrointestinal [GI] hemorrhage, GI losses from lactulose, diuretics, large-volume paracentesis) circulatory volume or effective (hypoalbuminemia, splanchnic vasodilation)
- Hepatorenal syndrome type 1 or 2
- Tense ascites with abdominal compartment syndrome

Intrinsic AKI
- Ischemic (severe hypoperfusion; see previously) or direct nephrotoxicity and hepatotoxicity of drugs or toxins (e.g., carbon tetrachloride, acetaminophen, tetracyclines, methoxyflurane)
- Tubulointerstitial nephritis + hepatitis caused by drugs (e.g., sulfonamides, rifampin, phenytoin, allopurinol, phenindione), infections (leptospirosis, brucellosis, Epstein-Barr virus, cytomegalovirus), malignant infiltration (leukemia, lymphoma) or sarcoidosis
- Glomerulonephritis or vasculitis (e.g., polyarteritis nodosa, ANCA–associated GN, cryoglobulinemia, systemic lupus erythematosus, postinfectious hepatitis or liver abscess

**AKI and Nephrotic Syndrome**

Prerenal azotemia
- Intravascular volume depletion (diuretic therapy, hypoalbuminemia)

Intrinsic AKI
- Manifestation of primary glomerular disease
- Collapsing glomerulopathy (e.g., HIV, pamidronate)
- Associated ATN (older hypertensive men)
- Associated interstitial nephritis (NSAIDs, rifampin, interferon alfa)

Other—amyloid or light chain deposition disease, renal vein thrombosis, severe interstitial edema

*AKI,* Acute kidney injury; *ANCA,* antineutrophil cytoplasmic antibody; *ATN,* acute tubular necrosis; *GN,* glomerulonephritis; *HELLP,* ***h****emolysis,* ***e****levated* ***l****iver enzymes,* ***l****ow* ***p****latelets; *NSAIDs,* nonsteroidal antiinflammatory drugs; *SLE,* systemic lupus erythematosus.

of dialysis membranes that are permeable to light chains and other proteins with molecular weights lower than albumin (high-cutoff membranes) has also been proposed as a potential therapeutic strategy; however, data from clinical trials evaluating the efficacy of this strategy are similarly conflicting.[173–175]

## ACUTE KIDNEY INJURY IN PREGNANCY

In the industrialized world, the incidence of dialysis-requiring AKI in the setting of pregnancy is approximately 1 in 20,000 births.[176,177] The marked decline in this complication over the past 50 years is a result of improved prenatal care and

**Box 29.5 Cairo-Bishop Definition of Tumor Lysis Syndrome**

**Diagnosis of Laboratory Tumor Lysis Syndrome**

Requires at least two of the following criteria achieved in the same 24-hour interval from 3 days before to 7 days after chemotherapy initiation:

- Uric acid ≥ 8.0 mg/dL or ≥25% increase from baseline
- Potassium ≥ 6.0 mmol/L or ≥25% increase from baseline
- Phosphorus ≥ 4.6 mg/dL (≥6.5 mg/dL in children) or ≥25% increase from baseline
- Calcium ≤ 7.0 mg/dL or ≥25% decrease from baseline

**Diagnosis of Clinical Tumor Lysis Syndrome**

Laboratory tumor lysis syndrome plus at least one of the following:

- Serum creatinine ≥1.5 times the age-adjusted upper limit of normal
- Cardiac arrhythmia/sudden death
- Seizure

Modified from Cairo MS, Bishop M. Tumour lysis syndrome: new therapeutic strategies and classification. Br J Haematol. 2004;127:3–11.

advancements in obstetrics practice. In early pregnancy, ATN induced by nephrotoxic abortifacients remains a relatively common cause of AKI in developing countries, but is rare in the developed world. Ischemic ATN, severe toxemia of pregnancy, and postpartum HUS and TTP are the most common causes of AKI in later term pregnancy.[176,178,179] Ischemic ATN is usually precipitated by placental abruption or postpartum hemorrhage and, less commonly, by amniotic fluid embolism or sepsis. Glomerular filtration is usually normal in mild or moderate preeclampsia; however, AKI may complicate severe preeclampsia.[179,180] In this setting, AKI is typically transient and found in association with intrarenal vasospasm, marked hypertension, and neurologic abnormalities.

A variant of preeclampsia, the HELLP syndrome (***h**emolysis, **e**levated **l**iver enzymes, **l**ow **p**latelets*), is characterized by a benign initial course that can rapidly deteriorate with the development of thrombotic microangiopathy with hemolysis, coagulation abnormalities, derangement in hepatic function, and AKI.[180–182] Immediate delivery of the fetus is indicated in this setting. Thrombotic microangiopathy can also develop in the postpartum setting and typically occurs in patients who have had a normal pregnancy.[183] Postpartum thrombotic microangiopathy is characterized by thrombocytopenia, microangiopathic anemia, and normal prothrombin and partial thromboplastin times and frequently results in long-term impairment of renal function.

Acute fatty liver of pregnancy (AFLP) occurs in approximately 1 in 7000 pregnancies and is associated with AKI, likely as a result of intrarenal vasoconstriction, as occurs in the hepatorenal syndrome. Although the exact origin of AFLP is unknown, the incidence is increased in women who carry a fetus with a defect in fatty acid oxidation and who are themselves carriers of a genetic mutation that compromises intramitochondrial fatty acid oxidation.[182] Acute bilateral pyelonephritis may also precipitate AKI in pregnancy and should be obvious from the patient's presentation (fever, flank pain), findings on urinalysis (bacteria, leukocytes), and laboratory tests (leukocytosis, elevated serum creatinine level).[178,181,184,185] The diagnosis of postrenal AKI in the pregnant patient is particularly challenging due to the physiologic dilation of the collecting system that normally occurs in the second and third trimesters. As a result, determining the presence of abnormal findings on renal ultrasound is more difficult.

## ACUTE KIDNEY INJURY IN THE SETTING OF CARDIAC SURGERY

An acute deterioration in kidney function is a relatively common complication following cardiac surgery, with an incidence of 7.7% to 42%, depending on the criteria used to define AKI.[186–190] AKI requiring dialytic support occurs in up to 5% of patients following cardiac surgery.[186–190] AKI in the perioperative period is usually attributed to prerenal azotemia associated with decreased cardiac function or to ATN. Risk factors for cardiac surgery–associated AKI can be broadly categorized into presurgical patient-related factors, surgical factors, and postoperative events. The principal patient-related risk factors include underlying CKD, advanced age, left ventricular dysfunction, previous myocardial revascularization, diabetes mellitus, and peripheral vascular disease.[189–192] Operative factors include the need for emergent surgery, prolonged time on cardiopulmonary bypass, insertion of an intraaortic balloon pump, performance of concomitant valvular surgery, and redo coronary artery bypass grafting (CABG). Several studies have compared the incidence of AKI following on-pump versus off-pump CABG, with some data suggesting that off-pump CABG is associated with a lower incidence of AKI.[193–197] Postoperative factors associated with an increased risk for AKI include reduced cardiac output, bleeding, vasodilatory shock, and the overzealous use of diuretics and afterload reducing agents.

Additional potential causes of AKI following CABG include the administration of iodinated contrast media in the pre-, peri-, and/or postoperative period, antibiotic-associated acute interstitial nephritis, and atheroembolic disease.[198] Whereas prerenal azotemia and ATN typically occur within days of the surgical procedure, atheroembolic AKI may take longer to develop and can be distinguished by the characteristic clinical features of livedo reticularis, cyanosis, and gangrenous digital lesions, as well as the findings of eosinophilia, eosinophiluria, and hypocomplementemia.

## ACUTE KIDNEY INJURY AFTER SOLID ORGAN OR BONE MARROW TRANSPLANTATION

Nonrenal solid organ transplant recipients have a particularly high risk of AKI from cardiopulmonary and hepatic failure, sepsis, and the nephrotoxic effects of antimicrobial and immunosuppressive agents. In a large retrospective multicenter study, 25% of all nonrenal solid organ transplant recipients developed AKI, with 8% requiring RRT.[199] The development of AKI requiring dialysis was associated with a 9- to 12-fold increase in mortality. AKI developed in 35% of heart transplant recipients and in 15% of lung transplant recipients. As many as 30% of liver transplant recipients develop AKI, many of whom had CKD prior to transplantation.[200,201] There are conflicting data as to whether impaired kidney function pretransplantation predicts outcomes in patients undergoing orthotopic liver transplantation; however, patients with impaired kidney function preoperatively have longer hospital and ICU stays and are more likely to need dialysis compared with patients with intact preoperative kidney function.[202–204]

AKI is a well-recognized complication of hematopoietic cell transplantation.[144,205,206] The three types of hematopoietic cell transplantation are myeloablative autologous, myeloablative allogeneic, and nonmyeloablative allogeneic, and the incidence, severity, and outcomes of AKI following these forms of hematopoietic cell transplantation vary considerably.[205,207,208] In a study of 272 patients who underwent myeloablative hematopoietic cell transplantation (predominantly allogeneic), 53% developed AKI and 24% required dialysis.[209] Of patients with dialysis requiring AKI, the mortality rate was 84%. One study has found an incidence of severe AKI in this patient population of 73%.[210]

AKI following nonmyeloablative allogeneic hematopoietic cell transplantation is less common.[210,211] A study of 253 patients demonstrated an incidence of AKI of 40% within 3 months of hematopoietic cell transplantation, with just 4.4% of patients requiring dialysis.[211] The incidence of AKI following myeloablative autologous hematopoietic cell transplantation is considerably lower.[212,213] A study of 173 patients following autologous hematopoietic cell transplantation reported an incidence of AKI of 21%, with 5% of patients requiring dialysis.[213] The absence of graft-versus-host disease and more rapid engraftment likely account for the lower incidence of AKI in this setting. Causes of hematopoietic cell transplantation-associated AKI include hypovolemia, sepsis, tumor lysis syndrome, direct tubular toxicity from cytoreductive therapy, thrombotic microangiopathy, graft-versus-host disease, antibiotics, immunosuppressive agents, and hepatic venoocclusive disease (VOD).

VOD results from acute radiochemotherapy-induced endothelial cell injury of hepatic venules.[209,214–216] This condition usually occurs in conditioning regimens that include total body irradiation and cyclophosphamide and/or busulfan and in the setting of myeloablative allogeneic hematopoietic cell transplantation. The syndrome is characterized clinically by profound jaundice and avid salt retention, with edema and ascites within the first month after engraftment and the subsequent development of AKI. Oliguric AKI is common in moderate VOD and certain in severe cases. The mortality rate for patients with severe VOD approaches 100%.

BK virus is a human polyoma virus that is a common opportunistic infection in solid organ transplant recipients and in patients following hematopoietic cell transplantation.[217] Detectable BK viruria may be seen in as many as 50% of patients undergoing hematopoietic cell transplantation.[218] Reactivation of latent BK virus infection in immunosuppressed patients is associated with both hemorrhagic cystitis and renal involvement with tubular atrophy and fibrosis, with an inflammatory lymphocytic infiltrate with intranuclear BK virus inclusion bodies.[219] The diagnosis is suggested by rising viral titers in blood and/or urine; the mainstay of treatment is minimization of immunosuppression.

## ACUTE KIDNEY INJURY ASSOCIATED WITH PULMONARY DISEASE

The coexistence of AKI and pulmonary disease (pulmonary-renal syndrome) typically suggests the presence of Goodpasture syndrome, antineutrophil cytoplasmic antibody (ANCA)–associated vasculitis, or other vasculitides.[220–222] The detection of antiglomerular basement membrane antibodies, antineutrophil cytoplasmic antibodies, or low serum complement concentrations can be helpful in differentiating among the various causes of pulmonary-renal syndrome, although the urgent need for definitive diagnosis and treatment may mandate lung or renal biopsy. Several toxic ingestions and infections may also precipitate simultaneous pulmonary and kidney injury that mimics vasculitis-associated pulmonary-renal syndrome. Furthermore, AKI of any cause may be complicated by secondary hypervolemia and pulmonary edema. Severe lung disease and ventilator support with increased intrathoracic pressure may compromise cardiac output and induce prerenal AKI.

## ACUTE KIDNEY INJURY IN ASSOCIATION WITH LIVER DISEASE

The differential diagnosis of AKI in patients with liver disease is broad. Common causes of AKI in this setting include intravascular volume depletion, gastrointestinal bleeding, sepsis, and nephrotoxins. Most cases of AKI in advanced liver disease are due to prerenal azotemia, ATN, or HRS, and differentiating these conditions can be clinically challenging.[223–225] Although a urine sodium concentration less than 20 mmol/L and fractional excretion rate of sodium less than 1% are typical of prerenal AKI and HRS, high-dose diuretics, which are commonly prescribed in patients with advanced liver disease, may lead to higher sodium excretion rates. Differentiating ATN from other forms of AKI is further confounded by the fact that bile-stained casts, which can be seen in prerenal AKI and HRS, have a similar appearance to the classic, muddy brown, granular casts of ATN.[226] Kidney disease in patients with liver disease may also result from acute glomerular disease, including immunoglobulin A (IgA) nephropathy, hepatitis B virus–associated membranous nephropathy, and hepatitis C virus–associated membranoproliferative glomerulonephritis with cryoglobulinemia. Acetaminophen toxicity may cause nephrotoxic ATN in addition to being one of the most common causes of acute hepatotoxicity.

The term *hepatorenal syndrome* is typically reserved for a clinical syndrome marked by irreversible AKI that develops in patients with advanced cirrhosis, although it has also been described in the setting of fulminant viral and alcoholic hepatitis. HRS almost certainly represents the terminal stage of a state of hypoperfusion that begins early in the course of chronic liver disease. The precise pathophysiologic mechanisms underlying the hemodynamic alterations in HRS are incompletely understood. In the early stages of HRS, increased vascular capacitance as the result of splanchnic and systemic vasodilation is thought to trigger activation of the renin-angiotensin-aldosterone system (RAAS) and sympathetic nervous system.[223] Renal perfusion is preserved in this stage by the local release of renal vasodilatory factors; however, these compensatory mechanisms are eventually overwhelmed, and progressive renal hypoperfusion ensues.

An inadequate increase in cardiac output relative to the fall in vascular resistance is also thought to contribute to the development of HRS.

Clinically, the presentation of HRS closely resembles that of prerenal AKI. However, unlike prerenal AKI, HRS does not improve with aggressive expansion of the intravascular space. Criteria for the diagnosis of HRS have undergone revision (Box 29.6).[227] Previous criteria were based on an increase in the serum creatinine level to more than 1.5 mg/dL in the setting of cirrhosis with ascites,[228] whereas the updated criteria have been harmonized with the creatinine component of the KDIGO AKI definition.[227] Other criteria include failure of kidney function to improve after at least 2 days with diuretic withdrawal and volume expansion with albumin, the absence of shock or concurrent or recent treatment with nephrotoxic drugs, and the absence parenchymal kidney disease—defined by proteinuria more than 500 mg/day, hematuria (>50 RBC/high power field [hpf]), and/or abnormal renal ultrasonography.[227]

Two subtypes of HRS have been described. Under the prior criteria, type 1 HRS was characterized by a rapid onset of AKI defined by at least a doubling of the serum creatinine concentration to a level of at least 2.5 mg/dL or a reduction in glomerular filtration of 50% or more to a level less than 20 mL/min over a 2-week period.[229,230] In the revised criteria, the diagnosis of type 1 HRS is based on meeting KDIGO criteria for stage 2 or higher AKI (i.e., doubling of serum creatinine level from baseline).[227] Type 1 HRS typically develops in hospitalized patients and may be precipitated by variceal bleeding, overly rapid diuresis, the performance of paracentesis or, most commonly, the development of spontaneous bacterial peritonitis. Other postulated triggers include infections, minor surgery, or the use of NSAIDs or other drugs. However, caution must be exerted in these cases to exclude reversible causes of AKI. Type 1 HRS is generally characterized by a fulminant course with oliguria, encephalopathy, marked hyperbilirubinemia, and death within 1 month of the clinical presentation. However, advances in the management of HRS (discussed later) have suggested that there may be a trend toward better survival in patients who respond to therapy.[231,232] Type 2 HRS is typified by a more gradual decline in renal function that develops in the setting of diuretic resistant ascites and avid sodium retention. The prognosis of type 2 HRS is considerably better than that of type 1 HRS, with a reported median survival of 6 months and a 1-year survival rate as high as 30%.[233,234] The development of a sudden deterioration in kidney function after a prolonged stable period may occur in patients with type 2 HRS, leading to outcomes similar to those of patients with type 1 HRS.

Definitive treatment of HRS is dependent on the recovery of hepatic function or successful liver transplantation. However, the use of vasoconstrictive agents combined with volume expansion with colloid has shown promise for improving kidney function.[235–237] It is postulated that by reversing the splanchnic and peripheral vasodilation, more normal renal perfusion can be restored. Vasoconstrictive regimens that have been used include norepinephrine, combination therapy with midodrine and octreotide, and the vasopressin agonist terlipressin.[235–241] Although vasoconstrictive therapy is associated with improvement in kidney function, and patients who respond have an improved prognosis, the use of vasoconstrictive therapy has not been shown to improve overall prognosis in patients with AKI, suggesting that survival remains limited by the underlying severity of the liver disease.

**Box 29.6 Diagnostic Criteria for Hepatorenal Syndrome**

- Cirrhosis with ascites
- Acute kidney injury (AKI) defined as:
  - ≥0.3-mg/dL increase in serum creatinine over <48 hours
  - ≥50% increase in serum creatinine level known or presumed to have occurred within prior 7 days
- No improvement of serum creatinine level (decrease to a level of ≤1.5 mg/dL) after at least 2 days of diuretic withdrawal and volume expansion with albumin (1 g/kg body weight per day to a maximum of 100 g/day)
- Absence of shock
- Absence of parenchymal kidney disease as indicated by:
  - Proteinuria >500 mg/day
  - Microhematuria (>50 red blood cells/high power field); and/or
  - Abnormal renal ultrasonography

**Type 1 Hepatorenal Syndrome**

Rapid progressive AKI defined based on increase in serum creatinine level by >2× baseline

**Type 2 Hepatorenal Syndrome**

Moderate renal dysfunction with a steady or slowly progressive course

Modified from Angeli P, Gines P, Wong F, et al. Diagnosis and management of acute kidney injury in patients with cirrhosis: revised consensus recommendations of the International Club of Ascites. Gut. 2015;64:531–537.

## ACUTE KIDNEY INJURY AND THE NEPHROTIC SYNDROME

AKI in the context of the nephrotic syndrome presents a unique array of potential diagnoses. Epithelial injury, if severe, can trigger both nephrotic range proteinuria and acute or subacute kidney injury.[242,243] The epithelial injury typically occurs as a manifestation of primary glomerular disease, such as collapsing glomerulopathy or crescentic membranous nephropathy. Less dramatic visceral epithelial cell injury, in combination with proximal tubular injury (e.g., panepithelial cell injury induced by NSAIDs or possible undiagnosed viral illness) or interstitial nephritis (e.g., rifampicin- or ampicillin-induced) can also present as AKI complicating the nephrotic syndrome.[244–246] Massive excretion of light chain proteins in patients with multiple myeloma may also present in this fashion.[247,248] ATN in association with nephrotic syndrome is seen in a subpopulation of older patients with minimal change disease, and in other patients with nephrosis and severe hypoalbuminemia, particularly with overzealous diuresis. In general, patients with AKI complicating the nephrotic syndrome have higher blood pressure and urinary protein excretion than patients without AKI.[242] The higher incidence of arteriosclerosis in biopsy samples from these patients may point to preexisting hypertensive nephrosclerosis as a risk factor for the development of this complication. Renal vein thrombosis must always be considered in the differential diagnosis of the nephrotic syndrome and AKI, particularly in the pediatric population and in adults with membranous nephropathy in association with high-grade proteinuria and hypoalbuminemia.

## COMPLICATIONS OF ACUTE KIDNEY INJURY

The acute loss of kidney function in AKI results in multiple derangements in fluid, electrolyte, and acid-base homeostasis and in hematologic, gastroenterologic, and immunologic function (Table 29.6).

### POTASSIUM HOMEOSTASIS

Hyperkalemia is a common and potentially life-threatening complication of AKI.[249,250] The serum $K^+$ level typically rises by 0.5 mmol/L/day in oligoanuric patients and reflects impaired excretion of $K^+$ derived from a patient's diet, the administration of $K^+$-containing solutions and drugs administered as potassium salts, and the release of $K^+$ from the injured tubular epithelium. Hyperkalemia may be compounded by coexistent metabolic acidosis and/or hyperglycemia or other hyperosmolar states that promote $K^+$ efflux from cells. Hyperkalemia present at the time of diagnosis of AKI or the rapid development of severe hyperkalemia suggests massive tissue destruction, as might be seen with rhabdomyolysis, hemolysis, or tumor lysis.[50,90,251] Hyperuricemia and hyperphosphatemia may accompany hyperkalemia in these settings. Mild hyperkalemia (<6.0 mmol/L) is usually asymptomatic. Higher levels are frequently associated with electrocardiographic abnormalities, including, peaked T waves, prolongation of the PR interval, flattening of P waves, widening of the QRS complex, and intraventricular conduction defects.[252–254] These electrocardiographic findings may precede the onset of life-threatening cardiac arrhythmias, such as bradycardia, heart block, ventricular tachycardia, ventricular fibrillation, and asystole. In addition, hyperkalemia may induce neuromuscular abnormalities, such as paresthesias, hyporeflexia, weakness, ascending flaccid paralysis, and respiratory failure.

Hypokalemia is unusual in AKI but may complicate nonoliguric ATN caused by aminoglycosides, cisplatin, or amphotericin B, presumably because of impaired $K^+$ reabsorption resulting from epithelial cell injury in the thick ascending limb of the loop of Henle.[255,256]

### ACID-BASE HOMEOSTASIS

Normal metabolism of dietary protein yields between 50 and 100 mmol/day of fixed nonvolatile acids (principally sulfuric and phosphoric acids) that are excreted by the kidneys to maintain acid-base homeostasis. Predictably, AKI is commonly complicated by metabolic acidosis, typically with a widening of the serum anion gap due to retention of phosphates, sulfates, and organic anions.[257] Acidosis may be severe (daily fall in plasma $HCO_3^-$ >2 mmol/L) when the generation of $H^+$ is increased by additional mechanisms (e.g., diabetic or fasting ketoacidosis, lactic acidosis complicating generalized tissue hypoperfusion, liver disease, or sepsis, and metabolism of ethylene glycol).[70,225,258] In contrast, metabolic alkalosis is an infrequent finding, but may complicate overly aggressive correction of acidosis with $HCO_3^-$, overzealous use of combination loop and thiazide diuretics, or loss of gastric acid by vomiting or nasogastric aspiration.

### MINERAL AND URIC ACID HOMEOSTASIS

Mild to moderate hyperphosphatemia (5–10 mg/dL) is a common consequence of AKI, and hyperphosphatemia may be severe (10–20 mg/dL) in highly catabolic patients or when AKI is associated with rapid cell death as in rhabdomyolysis, severe burns, hemolysis, or tumor lysis.[259–262] Factors that potentially contribute to hypocalcemia include skeletal resistance to the actions of parathyroid hormone, reduced levels of 1,25-dihydroxyvitamin D, $Ca^{2+}$ sequestration in injured tissues, such as muscle in the setting of rhabdomyolysis, and metastatic deposition of calcium phosphate salts in the setting of severe hyperphosphatemia.[263–265]

**Table 29.6 Common Complications of Acute Kidney Injury**

| Metabolic | Cardiovascular | Gastrointestinal | Neurologic | Hematologic | Infectious | Other |
|---|---|---|---|---|---|---|
| Hyperkalemia | Pulmonary edema | Nausea | Neuromuscular irritability | Anemia | Pneumonia | Hiccups |
| Metabolic acidosis | Arrhythmias | Vomiting | Asterexis | Bleeding | Septicemia | Elevated parathyroid hormone level |
| Hyponatremia | Pericarditis | Malnutrition | Seizures | | Urinary tract infection | Low total triiodothyronine and thyroxine |
| Hypocalcemia | Pericardial effusion | Hemorrhage | Mental status changes | | | Normal thyroxine level |
| Hyperphosphatemia | Pulmonary embolism | | | | | |
| Hypermagnesemia | Hypertension | | | | | |
| Hyperuricemia | Myocardial infarction | | | | | |

Hypocalcemia is usually asymptomatic, possibly because of the counterbalancing effects of acidosis on neuromuscular excitability. However, symptomatic hypocalcemia can occur in patients with rhabdomyolysis or acute pancreatitis or after treatment of acidosis with $HCO_3^-$.[263] Clinical manifestations of hypocalcemia include perioral paresthesias, muscle cramps, seizures, hallucinations, and confusion, as well as prolongation of the QT interval and nonspecific T wave changes on the electrocardiogram (ECG). The Chvostek sign (contraction of facial muscles on tapping of the jaw over the facial nerve) and Trousseau sign (carpopedal spasm after occlusion of arterial blood supply to the arm for 3 minutes with a blood pressure cuff) are useful indicators of latent tetany in high-risk patients.

Mild asymptomatic hypermagnesemia is common in oliguric AKI and reflects the impaired excretion of ingested magnesium—dietary magnesium, magnesium-containing laxatives, or antacids.[266,267] More significant hypermagnesemia is usually the result of overzealous parenteral magnesium administration, as in the management of AKI associated with preeclampsia. Hypomagnesemia occasionally complicates nonoliguric ATN associated with cisplatin or amphotericin B and, as with hypokalemia, likely reflects injury to the thick ascending limb of loop of Henle, a principal site for $Mg^{2+}$ reabsorption.[256,268,269] Hypomagnesemia is usually asymptomatic but may occasionally manifest as neuromuscular instability, cramps, seizures, cardiac arrhythmias, or resistant hypokalemia or hypocalcemia.[266,270]

Uric acid is cleared from blood by glomerular filtration and secretion by proximal tubule cells, and asymptomatic hyperuricemia (12–15 mg/dL) is typical in established AKI. Higher levels suggest increased production of uric acid and may point to a diagnosis of acute urate nephropathy.[271–273] The urinary uric acid-to-creatinine ratio on a random specimen has been proposed as a means to distinguish between hyperuricemia caused by overproduction and impaired excretion. In a small series of patients, this ratio was more than 1 in 5 patients with acute uric acid nephropathy and was less than 1 in 27 patients with acute kidney injury due to other causes.[274] In a subsequent case series, elevations in the uric acid-to-creatinine ratio to values of more than 1 were described in other etiologies of AKI, most notably patients with infections who were markedly hypercatabolic.[275]

## VOLUME OVERLOAD AND CARDIAC COMPLICATIONS

Extracellular volume overload is an almost inevitable consequence of diminished salt and water excretion in AKI and may present clinically as mild hypertension, increased jugular venous pressure, pulmonary vascular congestion, pleural effusion, ascites, peripheral edema, increased body weight, and life-threatening pulmonary edema. Hypervolemia may be particularly troublesome in patients receiving multiple IV medications, high volumes of enteral or parenteral nutrition, and/or excessive volumes of maintenance IV fluids. Moderate or severe hypertension is unusual in ATN and should suggest other diagnoses, such as hypertensive nephrosclerosis, glomerulonephritis, preeclampsia, renal artery stenosis, and other diseases of the renal vasculature.[178,276–278] Excessive water ingestion or the administration of a hypotonic saline or dextrose solution can trigger hyponatremia, which, if severe, may cause cerebral edema, seizures, and other neurologic abnormalities.[279] Cardiac complications include arrhythmias and myocardial infarction. Although these events may reflect primary cardiac disease, abnormalities in myocardial contractility and excitability may be triggered or compounded by hypervolemia, acidosis, hyperkalemia, and other metabolic sequelae of AKI.[280]

## HEMATOLOGIC COMPLICATIONS

Anemia develops rapidly in AKI and is usually multifactorial in origin. Contributing factors include inhibition of erythropoiesis, hemolysis, bleeding, hemodilution, and reduced RBC survival time.[281–283] Prolongation of the bleeding time is also common, resulting from mild thrombocytopenia, platelet dysfunction, and clotting factor abnormalities (e.g., factor VIII dysfunction).

## NUTRITIONAL AND GASTROINTESTINAL COMPLICATIONS

Malnutrition remains one of the most frustrating and troublesome complications of AKI. Most patients have net protein breakdown, which may exceed 200 g/day in catabolic patients.[284–286] Malnutrition is usually multifactorial in origin and may reflect an inability to eat, loss of appetite, and/or inadequate nutritional support, the catabolic nature of the underlying medical disorder (e.g., sepsis, rhabdomyolysis, trauma), nutrient losses in drainage fluids or dialysate, and increased breakdown and reduced synthesis of muscle protein and increased hepatic gluconeogenesis, probably through the actions of toxins, hormones (e.g., glucagon, parathyroid hormone), or other substances (e.g., proteases) that accumulate in AKI.[287–291] Nutrition may also be compromised by the high incidence of acute gastrointestinal hemorrhage, which complicates up to 15% of cases of AKI. Mild gastrointestinal bleeding is common (10%–30%) and is usually due to stress ulceration of gastric or small intestinal mucosa.[292,293]

## INFECTIOUS COMPLICATIONS

Infection is the most common and serious complication of AKI, occurring in 50% to 90% of cases and accounting for up to 75% of deaths.[25,249,294–296] It is unclear whether this high incidence of infection is due to a defect in host immune responses or to repeated breaches of mucocutaneous barriers (e.g., IV cannulas, mechanical ventilation, bladder catheterization) resulting from therapeutic interventions.

## OTHER SEQUELAE OF ACUTE KIDNEY INJURY

Protracted periods of severe AKI or short intervals of catabolic anuric AKI often lead to the development of the uremic syndrome. Clinical manifestations of the uremic syndrome, in addition to those already listed, include pericarditis, pericardial effusion, and cardiac tamponade; gastrointestinal complications such as anorexia, nausea, vomiting, and ileus; and neuropsychiatric disturbances, including lethargy, confusion, stupor, coma, agitation, psychosis, asterixis, myoclonus, hyperreflexia, restless legs syndrome, focal neurologic deficit, and/or seizures. The uremic toxin(s) responsible for this syndrome has (have) yet to be defined. Candidate molecules include urea, other products of nitrogen metabolism such as guanidine compounds, products of bacterial metabolism such as aromatic amines and indoles, and other compounds that are inappropriately retained in the circulation in AKI or are underproduced, such as nitric oxide (NO).[297]

## COMPLICATIONS DURING RECOVERY FROM ACUTE KIDNEY INJURY

A vigorous diuresis may complicate the recovery phase of AKI and may precipitate intravascular volume depletion and can result in delayed recovery of kidney function. This diuretic response probably reflects the combined effects of an osmotic diuresis induced by retained urea and other byproducts of protein metabolism, excretion of retained salt and water accumulated during AKI, and delayed recovery of tubular reabsorptive function relative to glomerular filtration leading to salt wasting.[298–301] Hypernatremia may also complicate this recovery phase if free water losses are not replenished or are inappropriately replaced by relatively hypertonic saline solutions. Hypokalemia, hypomagnesemia, hypophosphatemia, and hypocalcemia are rarer metabolic complications during recovery from AKI. Mild transient hypercalcemia is relatively frequent during recovery and appears to be a consequence of delayed resolution of secondary hyperparathyroidism. In addition, hypercalcemia may complicate recovery from rhabdomyolysis because of mobilization of sequestered $Ca^{2+}$ from injured muscle.[302]

# MANAGEMENT OF ACUTE KIDNEY INJURY

The treatment of AKI varies considerably, based on its cause and clinical presentation. Evidence-based pharmacologic therapy to counteract pathophysiologic processes in the kidney and arrest renal parenchymal damage is not available for certain forms of AKI, notably ATN. In such cases, the management of AKI focuses on implementing interventions to prevent its development, when possible, providing supportive care to ameliorate derangements of fluid and electrolyte homeostasis, and instituting treatment to prevent and mitigate uremic complications (Table 29.7). In cases of severe AKI, RRT is often required. The ultimate goals of management are to prevent death, facilitate recovery of kidney function, and minimize the risk for de novo and/or progressive CKD.

## MANAGEMENT OF PRERENAL ACUTE KIDNEY INJURY

### INTRAVASCULAR VOLUME DEPLETION

Prerenal AKI is defined as hemodynamically mediated kidney dysfunction that is rapidly reversible following normalization of renal perfusion.[303] Prevention of prerenal AKI from intravascular volume depletion involves the early recognition and treatment of conditions that involve the loss of extracellular fluid, including vomiting, diarrhea, excessive diuresis, and bleeding before underperfusion

**Table 29.7 Supportive Management of Acute Kidney Injury**

| Management Issue | Treatment |
|---|---|
| Intravascular volume overload | Restriction of salt (<1–2 g/day) and water (<1 L/day) intake<br>Diuretic therapy (if nonoliguric)<br>Ultrafiltration |
| Hyponatremia | Restriction of oral and intravenous free water |
| Hyperkalemia | Calcium gluconate (10 mL of 10% solution over 5 min) if ECG changes present<br>Insulin (10–20 Units) IV push + glucose (250 mL of 20%) IV over 30–60 min<br>Albuterol (10–20 mg by nebulizer or MDI)<br>Renal replacement therapy<br>Loop diuretics (if nonoliguric)<br>$K^+$ binding resin<br>Discontinue $K^+$ supplements or $K^+$-sparing diuretics<br>Restriction of dietary potassium |
| Metabolic acidosis | Restriction of dietary protein<br>Sodium bicarbonate (if $HCO_3^-$ <15 mmol/L)<br>Renal replacement therapy |
| Hyperphosphatemia | Restriction of dietary phosphate intake<br>Phosphate binding agents (aluminum hydroxide, calcium carbonate, calcium acetate, sevelamer, lanthanum) |
| Hypocalcemia | Oral or intravenous replacement (if symptomatic or sodium bicarbonate to be administered) |
| Hypermagnesemia | Discontinue magnesium containing antacids |
| Nutrition | Caloric intake: 20–30 kcal/day<br>Protein intake:<br>Nondialysis-requiring—0.8–1.0 g/kg/day<br>Dialysis-requiring—1.0–1.5 g/kg/day<br>Continuous renal replacement therapy—up to 1.7 g/kg/day<br>Enteral route of nutrition preferred |
| Drug dosage | Adjust all doses for GFR and renal replacement modality |

*ECG*, Electrocardiographic; *GFR*, glomerular filtration rate; *MDI*, metered-dose inhaler.

of the kidneys occurs. In patients in whom intravascular volume depletion leads to prerenal AKI, treatment consists of restoration of a normal circulating blood volume. The optimal composition of administered fluids in patients with hypovolemic prerenal AKI depends on the source of fluid loss and associated electrolyte and acid-base disturbances. The initial management commonly consists of intravascular volume resuscitation with an isotonic crystalloid solution. Recent studies have demonstrated that balanced crystalloids reduce major adverse kidney events compared with isotonic saline in hospitalized patients.[304,305] Red blood cell transfusion should be used for hemorrhagic hypovolemia when there is ongoing bleeding, particularly if the patient is hemodynamically unstable, or if the blood hemoglobin concentration is dangerously low.

The relative merits of colloid and crystalloid resuscitation fluids in the management of nonhemorrhagic renal, extrarenal, and third space fluid losses are controversial, with advocates for the use of colloids positing that they are more effective at restoring circulating blood volume due to greater retention in the intravascular compartment. However, randomized controlled trials (RCTs) and meta-analyses comparing colloid with crystalloid replacement for resuscitation in critically ill patients have not confirmed this theoretic benefit and demonstrated an increased need for RRT, and other adverse outcomes were associated with colloid formulations containing hydroxyethyl starch.[306–313] In a meta-analysis of 55 trials involving 3504 patients randomly assigned to treatment with albumin or crystalloid, there was no evidence of improved outcomes, decreased mortality, or other complications associated with albumin administration.[314] These results were subsequently confirmed in a nearly 7000-patient multicenter RCT of fluid resuscitation in hypovolemic medical and surgical ICU patients, in which 28-day survival, development of single or multiple organ failure, and duration of hospitalization were similar in both groups.[315] Although specific data on the development of AKI were not described, the need for RRT was similar with saline compared with albumin resuscitation. However, in a post hoc analysis of patients with traumatic brain injury, albumin resuscitation was associated with increased mortality risk.[316]

The use of synthetic colloid solutions has been proposed as an alternative to albumin administration; however, hydroxyethyl starch preparations have been associated with an increased risk of AKI. In a multicenter RCT comparing fluid resuscitation with hydroxyethyl starch with a 3% gelatin solution in 129 patients with sepsis, hydroxyethyl starch was associated with a more than twofold increased risk of AKI.[309] A subsequent meta-analysis has confirmed the increased risk of AKI associated with hydroxyethyl starch across 34 studies that included 2604 individuals.[310] In an ensuing RCT that included 7000 critically ill patients who were assigned to receive 6% hydroxyethyl starch or isotonic saline, there was an approximately 20% increased risk of AKI treated with RRT with the use of hydroxyethyl starch.[313] Based on these data demonstrating no benefit and potential increased risk of AKI, along with the higher costs associated with colloid administration, their routine use for volume resuscitation in hypovolemia and sepsis is not advisable. In particular, hydroxyethyl starch solutions should be used very sparingly and, if used, there should be regular monitoring of kidney function. In such cases, the risk of hyperoncotic renal failure should be minimized by the concomitant use of appropriate crystalloid solutions.[3,309,310,312,313]

Experimental data have suggested that volume resuscitation with isotonic sodium chloride solutions, which contain supraphysiologic concentrations of chloride, may exacerbate renal vasoconstriction and diminish the GFR, as compared with isotonic crystalloid solutions with a lower chloride content.[317–319] In healthy patients, magnetic resonance imaging (MRI) has demonstrated that the infusion of isotonic saline is associated with reduced renal blood flow velocity and renal cortical tissue perfusion as compared with administration of a reduced chloride isotonic crystalloid solution.[320] In a subsequent open-label, sequential period study conducted in a single ICU, replacing the use of high-chloride IV solutions with fluids containing a lower chloride content was associated with a reduction in the incidence of KDIGO stage 3 AKI, from 14% to 8.4%, and in the use of RRT from 10% to 6.3%.[321] A subsequent meta-analysis that included 21 studies, 15 of which were small RCTs, found that the use of high-chloride IV fluid was associated with an increased risk of AKI, with no effect on mortality.[322] However, exclusion of heavily weighted studies in this analysis rendered the association of high-chloride fluid with AKI nonstatistically significant.

Two more recent large pragmatic, cluster-randomized clinical trials conducted in parallel at the same institution compared the administration of isotonic saline with balanced crystalloid solution (i.e., fluid with electrolyte composition that more closely resembles plasma).[304,305] In the Saline Against Lactated Ringer's of Plasma-Lyte in the Emergency Department (SALT-ED) trial of over 13,000 noncritically ill patients, balanced crystalloid was associated with a decrease in the incidence of 30-day major adverse kidney events (i.e., death, new RRT, persistent kidney impairment defined by a >200% increase in serum creatinine level at the time of hospital discharge, within 30 days) compared with saline (4.7% vs. 5.6%; $P = .01$), but not with the primary outcome of hospital-free days (days alive after discharge to day 28).[304] The Isotonic Solutions and Major Adverse Renal Events Trial (SMART), which included 15,802 critically ill patients, found that compared with isotonic saline, balanced crystalloids were associated with a decrease in 30-day major adverse kidney events (14.3% vs. 15.4%; $P = .04$).[305] In the SALT-ED trial, the benefit in the composite outcome was predominantly due to a lower rate of persistent kidney impairment, whereas in SMART, 30-day mortality predominated. Collectively, these findings support a benefit of balanced crystalloid compared with isotonic sodium chloride, yet the benefits were not homogenous. Greatest benefit was present among the critically ill patients with sepsis and among non–critically ill patients who had a baseline serum creatinine level more than 1.5 mg/dL or hyperchloremia (Cl >110 mmol/L) on initial presentation. Although the balanced fluids were more physiologic with regard to their chloride content, they were hypotonic and associated with higher rates of hyponatremia.

The volume and electrolyte content of urinary and gastrointestinal losses, as well as patients' serum electrolyte and acid-base status, should be closely monitored to guide adjustments in the composition of the replacement fluids. Although the potassium content in gastric juices tends to be low, concomitant urinary potassium losses may be quite high as the result of metabolic alkalosis.

## HEART FAILURE

The management of AKI in the setting of heart failure is dependent on the clinical setting and cause of the heart failure. In patients with heart failure in whom AKI has developed in the setting of excessive diuresis, withholding diuretics and administering cautious volume replacement may be sufficient to restore kidney function. In acute decompensated heart failure (ADHF), AKI may develop despite worsening volume overload; intensification of diuretic therapy is often required for treatment of pulmonary vascular congestion. Although diuretic therapy may exacerbate prerenal AKI, it can also result in improvement in kidney function via several postulated mechanisms:

1. Decreasing ventricular distention resulting in a shift from the descending limb to the ascending limb of the Starling curve and improvement in myocardial contractility
2. Decreasing venous congestion[318,323–326]
3. Diminishing intraabdominal pressure[327]

Additional therapies for ADHF in the setting of AKI include inotropic support, vasodilators for afterload reduction, and mechanical support, including intraaortic balloon pumps and ventricular assist devices. The use of invasive hemodynamic monitoring in ADHF has been controversial; although it is often used to guide pharmacologic management, clinical data have not demonstrated improved renal outcomes when management is guided by pulmonary artery catheters.[328] The role of isolated ultrafiltration in ADHF is also controversial. Although negative fluid balance can be achieved more readily using extracorporeal ultrafiltration than conventional diuretic therapy, studies have not demonstrated differences in kidney function or survival.[329–331] In the Ultrafiltration Versus Intravenous Diuretics for Patients Hospitalized for Acute Decompensated Heart Failure (UNLOAD) trial, hypervolemic patients with heart failure who were randomized to isolated ultrafiltration had more rapid fluid loss and decreased rehospitalizations within 90 days as compared with patients randomized to diuretic therapy, with no differences in kidney function.[330] In contrast, in the subsequent Cardiorenal Rescue Study in Acute Decompensated Heart Failure (CARRESS-HF) trial, ultrafiltration was inferior to diuretic therapy with respect to the bivariate endpoint of change in serum creatinine level and body weight 96 hours after enrollment ($P = .003$), owing primarily to worsening of kidney function in the ultrafiltration group.[331] Based on these data, extracorporeal ultrafiltration cannot be recommended for the primary management of patients with decompensated heart failure.

## LIVER FAILURE AND HEPATORENAL SYNDROME

Although volume-responsive prerenal azotemia is common in patients with advanced liver disease, differentiation from HRS and intrinsic AKI may be difficult.[223] Patients with liver failure are typically total body sodium overloaded with peripheral edema and ascites, but true hypovolemia or reduced effective systemic arterial blood volume is often an important contributory factor to the development AKI. The underlying pathophysiology of salt and water retention in cirrhosis involves multiple pathways. Portal hypertension leads directly to ascites formation, whereas splanchnic and peripheral vasodilation result in a state of relative arterial underfilling, which activates neurohumoral vasoconstrictors that produce intrarenal vasoconstriction, salt and water retention, and decreased GFR.[332] Volume-responsive AKI may develop in the setting of excessive diuresis, increased gastrointestinal losses (often as the result of therapy for hepatic encephalopathy), rapid drainage of ascites, or spontaneous bacterial peritonitis. Worsening hepatic function is often associated with diuretic resistance and progressive or precipitous worsening of kidney function. It has been postulated that an inadequate increase in cardiac output in response to the fall in peripheral vascular resistance may be central to the development of the hepatorenal syndrome.[333]

Differentiation between volume-responsive prerenal AKI and the HRS is based on the clinical response to volume loading. The optimal fluid for volume expansion in this setting has been controversial. Most recent expert opinion has advocated the use of hyperoncotic (20% or 25%) albumin at a dose of 1 g/kg per day.[228,334] However, there is an absence of rigorous data supporting this regimen as compared with volume expansion with isotonic crystalloid solutions. There are more data regarding the use of albumin infusion to prevent AKI in patients undergoing large-volume (>5 L) paracentesis[234,335,336] and in the treatment of spontaneous bacterial peritonitis.[337] In an RCT, patients undergoing paracentesis who received an infusion of approximately 10 g of albumin/L of drained ascites experienced less activation of the RAAS and a significantly lower rate of worsening kidney function than patients who did not receive albumin infusion.[335] In a subsequent study, albumin infusion was superior to the administration of dextran or gelatin solutions in preventing AKI following large-volume paracentesis.[336] Current recommendations are to infuse 6 to 8 g of albumin/L of ascites drained when the paracentesis volume exceeds 5 L. In an RCT comparing antibiotics alone with antibiotics plus albumin for the treatment of spontaneous bacterial peritonitis, infusion of 1.5 g/kg of albumin at the initiation of treatment and an additional 1 g/kg on the third day of treatment was associated with reduced rates of AKI and mortality,[337] although the benefit appears to be restricted to patients in whom the serum creatinine level is more than 1 mg/dL, the blood urea nitrogen is more than 30 mg/dL or the total bilirubin is more than 4 mg/dL.[338]

Definitive therapy of hepatorenal syndrome requires restoration of hepatic function, usually achieved through liver transplantation.[225,334] The role of peritoneovenous shunting (e.g., LeVeen and Denver shunts) in HRS has been inadequately studied. In a subset of 33 patients with HRS included in a randomized trial comparing peritoneovenous shunts to medical therapy, shunting was not associated with improved survival.[339] These data need to be interpreted with caution due to the small sample size and because data on improvement in kidney function were not reported. In addition, as a result of poor long-term patency rates and high rates of complications, particularly encephalopathy, the use of peritoneovenous shunts has largely been supplanted by the use of a transjugular portosystemic shunt (TIPS). TIPS has been demonstrated to provide better control of ascites than sequential paracentesis[340–343] and in one series, lower rates of HRS,[341] albeit with a higher risk of encephalopathy.[344] In a small case series, TIPS was reported to be effective as primary therapy for hepatorenal syndrome,[345] but has not been evaluated in a randomized trial.[334]

Pharmacologic therapy with vasoconstrictors, when combined with albumin infusion, has been associated with improvement in kidney function in patients with hepatorenal syndrome.[334,346] Agents that have shown benefit include norepinephrine,[347] the combination of octreotide and midodrine,[231,348–350] and the V1 vasopressin receptor agonist terlipressin,[235–237,351] although only terlipressin has been evaluated in RCTs. In metaanalyses of published trials, terlipressin was associated with a 3.5- to 4-fold increased odds of reversal of HRS.[352,353] Treatment of HRS with terlipressin was also associated with a modest short-term reduction in mortality; however, longer term outcomes are primarily a function of the underlying liver disease rather than treatment of HRS.[353] In addition, terlipressin was associated with a markedly increased risk of adverse cardiovascular events. More recently, the Reversal of Hepatorenal Syndrome Type 1 with Terlipressin (REVERSE) trial found similar rates of confirmed reversal of HRS with terlipressin and placebo (19.6% vs. 13.1%; $P = .22$), although the mean decrease in serum creatinine level was more pronounced with terlipressin (1.1 mg/dL vs. 0.6 mg/dL; $P = .001$).[237] At present, terlipressin is not approved for use in the United States.

### ABDOMINAL COMPARTMENT SYNDROME

Acute kidney injury can result from elevations in intraabdominal pressure, resulting in a clinical presentation with similar features to prerenal AKI. The abdominal compartment syndrome is defined by an intraabdominal pressure 20 mm Hg or higher associated with dysfunction of one or more organ systems.[354] However, intraabdominal pressures lower than 20 mm Hg may be associated with abdominal compartment syndrome, whereas values higher than this threshold do not universally lead to the abdominal compartment syndrome.[355–358] Abdominal compartment syndrome typically develops in critically ill patients, usually in the setting of trauma with abdominal hemorrhage, abdominal surgery, massive fluid resuscitation, liver transplantation, and gastrointestinal conditions, including peritonitis and pancreatitis. Mechanisms underlying the development of AKI in abdominal compartment syndrome are believed to involve renal vein compression, reduced cardiac output, and renal arterial constriction from sympathetic nervous system and RAAS activation.[359–361] Oliguria, which can lead to anuria, often develops and, as is true for other forms of AKI associated with impaired renal perfusion, urine sodium concentration is commonly reduced.

The diagnosis of abdominal compartment syndrome, which should be suspected in patients with acute abdominal distention and/or rapidly accumulating ascites or abdominal trauma, can be made by simple transduction of the bladder pressure.[59,354,355] Treatment is prompt abdominal decompression; if ascites is present, decompression may be achieved by performing large-volume paracentesis and in patients with severe ileus or colonic distention, bowel decompression may be sufficient; however, surgical laparotomy is often required for definitive therapy.

## MANAGEMENT OF POSTRENAL ACUTE KIDNEY INJURY

The principle underlying the management of postrenal AKI is the prompt relief of urinary tract obstruction. This topic is reviewed extensively in Chapter 37. Urethral or bladder neck obstruction may be relieved with the placement of a transurethral or suprapubic bladder catheter. Similarly, ureteric obstruction may be acutely relieved by placement of percutaneous nephrostomy tubes or by cystoscopically placed ureteral stents. Following the initial relief of obstruction, most patients experience a physiologic diuresis that resolves after several days as the result of the excretion of volume and solutes retained during the period of renal obstruction. However, approximately 5% of patients may have a more prolonged diuretic phase following relief of obstruction because of delayed recovery of tubule function relative to the GFR, resulting in a salt-wasting syndrome, which may require IV fluid replacement to maintain blood pressure.[300,301,362] Following initial relief of obstruction, urologic evaluation is required for definitive evaluation and management of the underlying cause of obstruction.

## PREVENTION OF INTRINSIC ACUTE KIDNEY INJURY

### GENERAL PRINCIPLES

Strategies to prevent intrinsic AKI vary based on the specific cause of the kidney injury. Optimization of cardiovascular function and restoration of intravascular volume status are key interventions to minimize the risk that prerenal AKI evolves into ischemic ATN. There is compelling evidence that aggressive intravascular volume expansion reduces the incidence of ATN after major surgery or trauma, burns, and cholera.[53,306,363,364] AKI due to sepsis is common and is associated with mortality rates as high as 80%.[35,296,365] The role of early goal-directed therapy (EGDT) using resuscitation to defined hemodynamic targets (mean arterial pressure [MAP] >65 mm Hg; central venous pressure [CVP], 10–12 mm Hg; urine output >0.5 mL/kg per hour; $ScvO_2$ >70%), using a combination of crystalloid solutions, red cell transfusion, and vasopressors guided by invasive hemodynamic monitoring in improving overall outcomes and decreasing the risk of AKI, has been controversial. In a seminal single-center RCT, EGDT resulted in a significant reduction in overall organ dysfunction and mortality in patients presenting with severe sepsis or septic shock, although specific data on the incidence of AKI were not reported.[366] However, EGDT was not associated with a reduction in dialysis-requiring AKI in the Protocolized Care for Early Septic Shock (ProCESS), Australasian Resuscitation in Sepsis Evaluation (ARISE), or Protocolised Management in Sepsis (PRoMISe) trials or in a patient-level meta-analysis that combined data from these trials (Fig. 29.1).[367–370]

Although the benefits of EGDT were not confirmed in these three later trials, early recognition of sepsis, prompt initiation of antibiotic therapy, and rapid volume resuscitation and hemodynamic stabilization were found to improve outcomes and are likely to minimize the risk of AKI.[371] The role of maintenance of normoglycemia in critically ill patients in minimizing the risk of AKI has also been controversial. Two single-center RCTs that used intensive insulin management to maintain blood glucose levels of 80 to 110 mg/dL, as compared with conventional management maintaining the glucose concentration between 180 and 220 mg/dL, each resulted in decreased rates of AKI, defined either on the basis of change in the serum

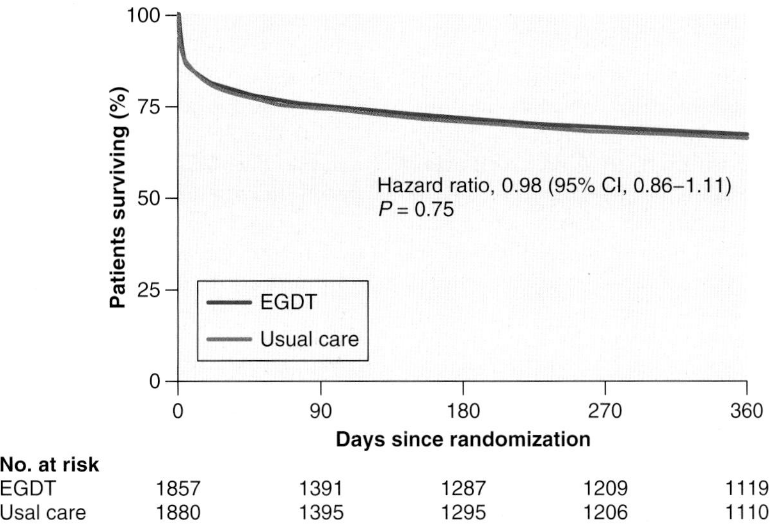


**Fig. 29.1** One-year survival comparing early goal-directed therapy (*EGDT*) with usual care in patients with sepsis. Shown are Kaplan-Meier survival curves comparing EGDT with usual care in patients with sepsis from pooled patient-level data from the ProCESS, ARISE, and ProMISe trials. Renal replacement therapy was required in 11.0% of patients who were randomized to EGDT as compared with 10.6% of patients randomized to usual care (odds ratio, 1.02; 95% confidence interval, 0.81–1.28; $P$ = .88). (From PRISM Investigators; Rowan KM, Angus DC, Bailey, et al. Goal-directed therapy for septic shock—a patient-level metaanalysis. *N Engl J Med.* 2017;376:2223–2234).

creatinine level or on the need for RRT.[372–374] However, the benefits of tight glycemic control were not confirmed in the Normoglycemia in Intensive Care Evaluation–Survival Using Glucose Algorithm Regulation (NICE-SUGAR) trial, a 6104-patient multicenter trial that compared intensive therapy to achieve a target glucose of approximately 80 to 110 mg/dL with more conventional therapy designed to maintain the blood glucose level less than 180 mg/dL.[375] In the NICE-SUGAR trial, intensive glycemic control was associated with an increased risk of hypoglycemia, an increased mortality risk (27.5% vs. 24.9%; $P$ = .02), and no reduction in the need for RRT.

In surgical patients, avoidance of hypotension has been associated with a decreased risk of AKI. In a retrospective analysis of over 33,000 patients who underwent noncardiac surgery, episodes of intraoperative hypotension with a mean arterial blood pressure less than 55 mm Hg were associated with a marked increase in the probability of AKI.[376] The adjusted odds of AKI with intraoperative hypotension increased with the duration of hypotension, from an odds ratio of 1.2 with less than 10 minutes of hypotension to 1.3 with 10 to 20 minutes of hypotension and to 1.5 with more than 20 minutes of hypotension. Volume overload is typical after surgical procedures, and small trials have suggested better patient outcomes following abdominal surgery using a restrictive fluid management strategy. However, a large RCT comparing restrictive and liberal fluid management strategies in patients undergoing major abdominal surgery at increased risk of complications found no benefit with regard to the primary outcome of 1-year disability-free survival, but found a higher rate of AKI associated with the restrictive fluid strategy (8.6% vs. 5.0%; $P < .001$).[377]

Intravascular volume depletion has been identified as a risk factor for ATN resulting from iodinated contrast, rhabdomyolysis, hemolysis, cisplatin, amphotericin B, multiple myeloma, aminoglycosides, and other nephrotoxins, crystal-associated AKI related to acyclovir and acute urate nephropathy, and AKI stemming from hypercalcemia.[74,75,160,169,251,273,364,378–380]

The restoration of adequate intravascular volume prevents the development of experimental and human ATN in many of these clinical settings. Avoidance of potentially nephrotoxic medications or insults in high-risk patients and settings is also important to reduce the risk for ATN. Specifically, among patients with advanced cardiac and/or liver disease in whom renal perfusion may be diminished, the use of selective or nonselective NSAIDs that inhibit the production of vasodilatory prostaglandins may exacerbate intrarenal vasoconstriction and precipitate AKI.[381–385] Diuretics, NSAIDs (including selective cyclooxygenase-2 [COX-2] inhibitors), ACE inhibitors, ARBs, and other inhibitors of the RAAS should be used with caution in patients with suspected absolute or effective intravascular volume depletion or in patients with renovascular disease because these agents may convert reversible prerenal AKI to ischemic ATN. The combined use of agents that block the RAAS, diuretics, and NSAIDs has been identified as a risk factor for AKI, particularly among patients with heart failure, liver failure, or other conditions with reduced baseline renal perfusion.[386,387]

Careful monitoring of circulating drug levels appears to reduce the incidence of AKI associated with aminoglycoside antibiotics and calcineurin inhibitors.[388–390] The observation that the antimicrobial efficacy of aminoglycosides persists in tissues, even after the drug has been cleared from the circulation (postantibiotic killing), has led to the use of once-daily dosing with these agents. Dosing regimens that provide higher peak drug levels but less frequent administration appear to provide comparable antimicrobial activity and less nephrotoxicity than older, conventional dosing regimens.[390–393] Nephrotoxicity of drugs may also be reduced through changes in formulation. For example, the use of lipid-encapsulated formulations of amphotericin B may decrease the risk of amphotericin-induced AKI.[394]

## CONTRAST-ASSOCIATED ACUTE KIDNEY INJURY

Contrast-associated AKI (CA-AKI) has historically been defined by and commonly manifests clinically as small absolute (>0.5 mg/dL) and/or relative (>25%) increases in serum creatinine levels that occur within 2 to 4 days following iodinated contrast administration. Although severe AKI is relatively uncommon due to iodinated contrast alone, the incidence of CA-AKI defined by relatively minor increments in the serum creatinine level has been shown in past studies to occur in up to 15% or more of high-risk patients.[395] A series of observational retrospective studies have questioned the true incidence of CA-AKI and challenged the concept that iodinated contrast is nephrotoxic.[396–399] A meta-analysis of 13 nonrandomized studies that included 25,950 patients found a similar risk of AKI in patients who received iodinated contrast IV compared with patients who underwent radiographic procedures without intravascular contrast (relative risk [RR], 0.79; 95% confidence interval [CI], 0.62–1.02).[397] Similarly, an observational study of over 29 million patient hospitalizations found that the risk for AKI among patients who received intravascular iodinated contrast during their hospitalization was comparable to the risk observed among patients who had not received contrast (RR, 0.93; 95% CI, 0.88–0.97).[400] Although the results of these retrospective analyses are adjusted for medical comorbidity and other risk factors for renal injury, such adjustment cannot fully account for all factors that influence the decision to administer contrast, rendering it likely that patients in these studies who did not receive contrast may have been at higher risk for AKI than patients who received contrast. It is therefore prudent to continue to consider intravascular iodinated contrast as potentially nephrotoxic and to implement evidence-based preventive care in patients at risk for CA-AKI (Table 29.8).

Past studies have demonstrated that the administration of IV fluids to high-risk patients prior to and following exposure to intravascular iodinated contrast diminished the risk for CA-AK, although the optimal regimen for fluid administration is unknown.[3,401,402] In a small clinical trial that was stopped early due to safety concerns, periprocedural IV isotonic saline was associated with a markedly lower rate of AKI after contrast exposure than oral fluid administration.[401] In a larger randomized trial, isotonic IV saline significantly reduced the incidence of CA-AKI following coronary angiography compared with half-normal IV saline, with a particular benefit noted in diabetic patients and those receiving large volumes of contrast.[402]

A recent study has challenged the principle that IV fluid administration reduces the risk for CA-AKI.[403] This noninferiority clinical trial randomized 660 patients with baseline CKD undergoing procedures with iodinated contrast to receive isotonic saline IV or no IV fluids and found a similar rate of CA-AKI (2.7% with saline vs. 2.6% without fluid), concluding that withholding IV fluid was not inferior to administering IV saline with regard to the prevention of small increments in the serum creatinine level. However, the patient population in this study was at relatively low overall risk for CA-AKI because more than 50% of participants received IV rather than intraarterial contrast, which is associated with lower rates of CA-AKI, and most had less advanced CKD (i.e., estimated GFR, 45–59 mL/min/1.73 m$^2$). Furthermore, this trial was powered based on the recruitment of 1300 patients, but enrolled 660 due to feasibility considerations. Thus, until additional clinical trials have demonstrated conclusively that isotonic IV fluid is ineffective, this treatment remains the standard of care for the prevention of CA-AKI.

A number of small clinical trials have compared the effects of isotonic sodium bicarbonate compared with isotonic saline for the prevention of CA-AKI.[404–413] These studies were generally underpowered and yielded conflicting results. Subsequent meta-analyses have concluded that there is an overall benefit associated with bicarbonate administration with regard to AKI defined by small changes in the serum creatinine level, although there was no demonstrable benefit with regard to the need for dialysis.[414–416] This led several clinical practice guidelines to recommend the administration of either IV isotonic sodium chloride or sodium bicarbonate to high-risk patients receiving iodinated contrast.[3,417,418] However, the Prevention of Serious Adverse Events Following Angiography (PRESERVE) trial provided more definitive findings regarding the comparative effects of sodium bicarbonate and sodium chloride for the prevention of CA-AKI.[419] PRESERVE was a multinational randomized clinical trial that used a 2 × 2 factorial design to compare IV isotonic sodium bicarbonate with IV isotonic sodium chloride and oral *N*-acetylcysteine with placebo for the prevention of serious adverse outcomes and CA-AKI following angiographic procedures in 4993 patients with CKD. IV sodium bicarbonate did not reduce the incidence of a primary outcome comprised of 90-day death, need for dialysis, or persistent decline in kidney function (odds ratio [OR], 0.93; 95% CI, 0.72–1.22). Similarly, bicarbonate did not reduce the incidence of CA-AKI assessed 3 to 5 days postangiography (OR, 1.16; 95% CI, 0.96–1.41). Although the optimal rate and duration of IV saline administration is not known, it is reasonable to administer isotonic sodium chloride at a rate of 1 mL/kg per hour for 6 to 12 hours prior to and 6 to 12 hours following a contrast-enhanced procedure in at-risk hospitalized patients. For at-risk outpatients, an alternative regimen of 3 mL/kg over 1 hour prior to the procedure, followed by 6 mL/kg administered over 2 to 6 hours following the procedure, may be more feasible.

**Table 29.8 Effectiveness of Preventive Interventions for Contrast-Associated Acute Kidney Injury**

| No Benefit | Unclear Benefit | Beneficial |
|---|---|---|
| Loop diuretics[a] | Statins | Isotonic intravenous fluids |
| Mannitol[a] | Natriuretic peptides | Low- or iso-osmolal contrast media |
| Dopamine[a] | Theophylline, aminophylline | |
| Fenoldopam[a] | Ascorbic acid | |
| Hemodialysis[a] | Hemofiltration | |
| *N*-Acetylcysteine | | |
| Sodium bicarbonate[b] | | |

[a]Potentially deleterious.
[b]As compared with isotonic saline.

*N*-acetylcysteine (NAC) is an antioxidant with vasodilatory properties that was postulated to potentially prevent CA-AKI based on its capacity to scavenge reactive oxygen species (ROS), reduce the depletion of glutathione, and stimulate the production of vasodilatory mediators, including nitric oxide.[420,421] Clinical trials of oral and IV NAC have yielded conflicting findings.[422–431] Although initially used at a dose of 600 mg bid,[422] subsequent studies suggested greater efficacy with higher doses of up to 1200 mg bid.[429,430] In the Acetylcysteine for Contrast-Induced Nephropathy (ACT) trial, 2308 patients were randomized to receive 1200 mg of NAC or placebo bid beginning prior to the procedure and continuing for three doses postprocedure.[431] No differences were observed in the incidence of CA-AKI at 48 to 96 hours postcontrast administration or in the incidence of death or need for dialysis within 30 days. However, the overall study population had relatively well-preserved kidney function, with a median serum creatinine level of 1.1 mg/dL, and fewer than 16% of patients had a baseline serum creatinine level more than 1.5 mg/dL. In the aforementioned PRESERVE trial, the administration of NAC in a dose of 1200 mg by mouth bid for 5 days beginning just prior to angiography was not associated with a reduction in 90-day death, need for dialysis, or persistent impairment in kidney function (OR, 1.02; 95% CI, 0.78–1.33) or in a reduction in CA-AKI (OR, 1.06; 95% CI, 0.87–1.28).[419] Based on these findings, NAC should not be used to reduce the risk of CA-AKI.

Trials of other pharmacologic interventions, including furosemide, dopamine, fenoldopam, calcium channel blockers, and mannitol, have failed to demonstrate significant benefit and, in some cases, have been associated with an increased risk of CA-AKI.[432–438] Studies on the benefit of natriuretic peptides, aminophylline, theophylline, and ascorbic acid have also yielded conflicting results.[439–448] Given the absence of convincing data on the efficacy of these interventions, as well as potential safety concerns with the use of natriuretic peptides, aminophylline, and theophylline in patients with cardiovascular disease, their routine use is not recommended.[447] There have been multiple trials and meta-analyses that investigated statins for the prevention of CA-AKI. Although many, albeit not all, have demonstrated a benefit of statins, particularly in a high dose, with respect to the development of CA-AKI, the effect of this class of medication on more serious outcomes, including the need for dialysis and progressive CKD, remains unclear.[449–459] Furthermore, in most patients requiring angiographic procedures, there are likely other indications for statin therapy. RRTs for the prevention of CA-AKI have been largely ineffective and, in some cases, the use of "prophylactic" hemodialysis has been associated with harm.[460–462] The interpretation of studies of hemofiltration for the prevention of CA-AKI is confounded by their use of change in the serum creatinine level as an endpoint, because hemofiltration lowers serum creatinine concentration.[463,464] Given the risks associated with IV line placement and the renal replacement procedures themselves, along with lack of definitive benefit, the use of dialysis or hemofiltration to prevent CA-AKI is not currently recommended[3,465] (Fig. 29.2).

Over the past 25 years, there has been considerable progress in developing less nephrotoxic contrast agents.[466] The use of lower osmolal contrast agents in place of the older and more nephrotoxic high-osmolal agents has resulted in a decreased incidence of CA-AKI.[467,468] Data regarding the added benefit associated with the iso-osmolal radiocontrast agent iodixanol has been less consistent[469–475] and may reflect heterogeneity in the risk of CA-AKI associated with specific lower-osmolal agents.[476]

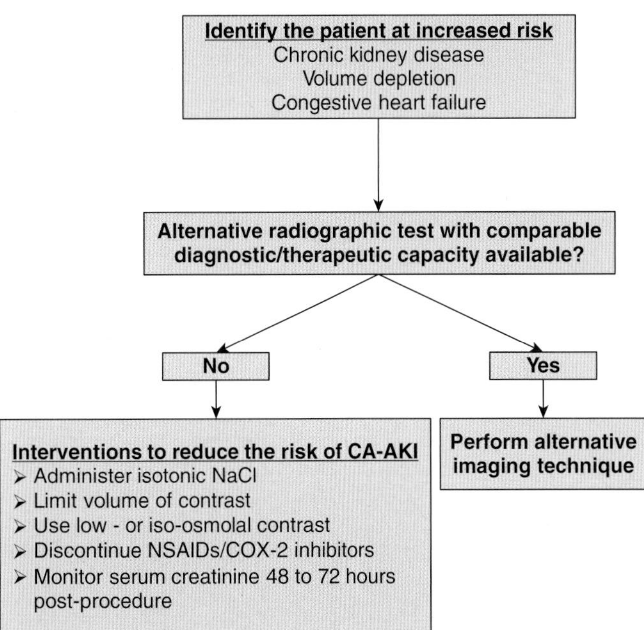


**Fig. 29.2** Algorithm for mitigation of risk of contrast-associated acute kidney injury (CA-AKI). *COX-2,* Cyclooxygenase-2; *NSAIDs,* nonsteroidal antiinflammatory drugs.

## PREVENTION OF OTHER FORMS OF INTRINSIC ACUTE KIDNEY INJURY

Allopurinol (100 mg/m$^2$ every 8 hours, maximum, 800 mg/day) is useful for limiting uric acid generation in patients at high risk for acute urate nephropathy. However, AKI can develop despite the use of allopurinol, probably through the toxic actions of hypoxanthine crystals on tubule function.*

In the setting of high rates of uric acid generation, such as tumor lysis syndrome, the use of recombinant urate oxidase (rasburicase, 0.2 mg/kg) may be more effective. Rasburicase catalyzes the degradation of uric acid to allantoin and has been shown to be effective both as prophylaxis and treatment for acute uric acid–mediated tumor lysis syndrome and to prevent the development of AKI due to tumor lysis syndrome–associated hyperuricemia.[164,251,478–481] In oligoanuric patients, prophylactic hemodialysis may be used to acutely lower uric acid levels.

Amifostine, an organic thiophosphate, has been demonstrated to ameliorate cisplatin nephrotoxicity in patients with solid organ or hematologic malignancies.[482–485] NAC limits acetaminophen-induced renal injury if given within 24 hours of ingestion, and dimercaprol, a chelating agent, may prevent heavy metal nephrotoxicity.[486,487] Ethanol inhibits ethylene glycol metabolism to oxalic acid and other toxic metabolites, but its use has been largely replaced by fomepizole, an

*References 160, 251, 271, 273, 477, and 478.

inhibitor of alcohol dehydrogenase that decreases the production of ethylene glycol metabolites and prevents the development of AKI.[488–491]

## REMOTE ISCHEMIC PRECONDITIONING

Remote ischemic preconditioning (RIPC) has been investigated as a potential intervention for the prevention of AKI. RIPC involves the implementation of brief episode(s) of ischemia and reperfusion of distant tissue—for example, with sequential brief inflation and deflation of a blood pressure tourniquet on a limb that is hypothesized to enhance the kidneys' resistance to a subsequent more prolonged period of ischemia by means of hormonal mediators, hormonal and neuronal signaling pathways, and antiinflammatory and molecular mediators (Fig. 29.3). Recent trials and meta-analyses have examined the benefits of RIPC in the setting of cardiac surgery. A trial that randomized 240 high-risk patients undergoing cardiac surgery to RIPC or sham RIPC has demonstrated a lower rate of AKI, defined by KDIGO criteria, with RIPC (37.5% vs. 52.5%; $P = .02$), with no effect on secondary endpoints, including myocardial infarction, stroke, and death.[492]

A considerably larger trial that enrolled 1612 patients undergoing cardiac surgery found no difference in the rate of AKI (a secondary endpoint) between RIPC and sham conditioning groups or in the incidence of the combined primary endpoint of death from cardiovascular causes, nonfatal myocardial infarction, coronary revascularization, or stroke within 12 months.[493] A series of meta-analyses of studies that included patients undergoing cardiac, and in some cases, vascular surgery has found lower rates of AKI with RIPC compared with control, but failed to demonstrate a benefit on the need for RRT or death.[494–496] Based on these cumulative data, the use of RIPC for the prevention of adverse outcomes following cardiac and vascular procedures is not routinely recommended.

# PHARMACOLOGIC THERAPY FOR ACUTE TUBULAR NECROSIS

During the past 2 decades, there has been extensive investigation into the pathogenesis of AKI using experimental animal models and cultured cells. These studies have resulted in substantial advances in our understanding of the pathophysiology of ATN in humans and led to the discovery of an array of potentially novel targets for the treatment of this common and serious disease. However, multiple interventions shown to ameliorate AKI in animals have failed to be effective in humans with ATN (Box 29.7). There are many possible reasons for the lack of success in translating therapeutic successes for AKI from animal models to clinical practice. Differences in the cause of ATN in animal models and human disease may contribute to differential responses to pharmacologic therapy. Another principal obstacle relates to the difficulty in identifying the incipient stage of ATN prior to elevations in the serum creatinine concentration or clinical evidence of decreased urine output. Over the past decade, several novel serum and urinary biomarkers have been investigated for their ability to identify AKI in its earliest stages and differentiate ATN from volume-responsive AKI.[17] Work in this

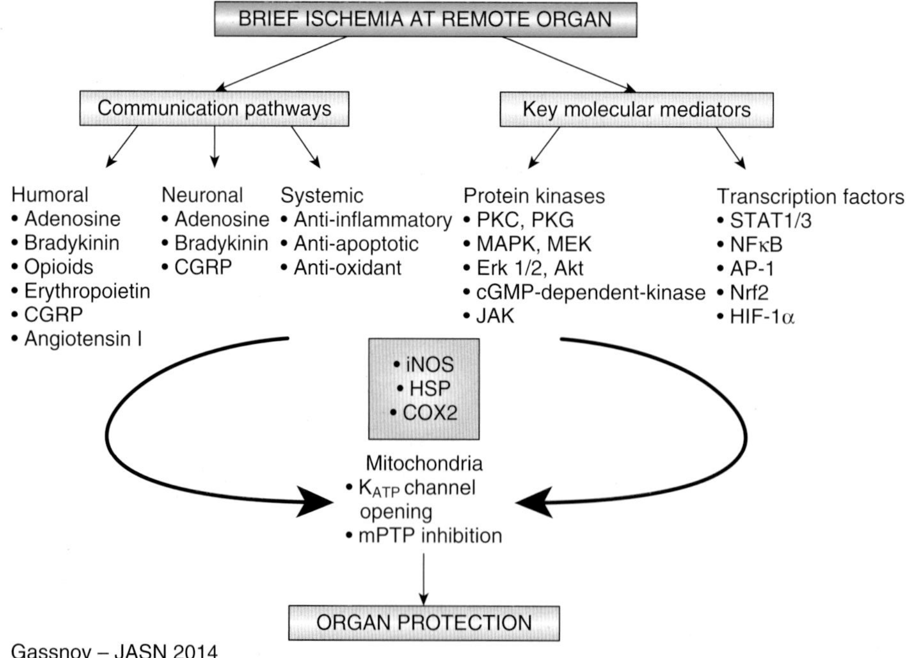


**Fig. 29.3** Postulated mechanisms for renal protective effects of remote ischemic preconditioning. *AP-1,* Activator protein-1; *cGMP,* cyclic guanosine monophosphate; *CGRP,* calcitonin gene-related peptide; *COX2,* cyclooxygenase-2; *HIF-1α,* hypoxia-inducible factor 1α; *HSP,* heat shock protein; *iNOS,* inducible nitric oxide synthase; *JAK,* Janus kinase; *MEK,* MAPK kinase; *mPTP,* mitochondrial permeability transition pore; NFkB, nuclear factor kappa B; *Nrf2,* nuclear factor (erythroid-derived 2)-like 2; *PKC,* protein kinase C; *PKG,* protein kinase G; *STAT1/3,* signal transducer and activator of transcription. (From Gassnov N, Nia AM, Caglayan E, Er F. Remote ischemic preconditioning and renoprotection: from myth to a novel therapeutic option? J Am Soc Nephrol. 2014;25(2):216–224.)

**Box 29.7 Pharmacologic Interventions Found to Be Ineffective for Acute Tubular Necrosis in Clinical Trials**

Diuretics
Dopamine
Fenoldopam
Thyroid hormone
Alpha melanocyte-stimulating hormone
Atrial natriuretic peptide
Alkaline phosphatase
Insulin growth factor
Erythropoietin
Prostaglandin A1

area may facilitate the identification of those patients most likely to respond to treatments that have been found to be effective in animal models.

## DOPAMINE

Historically, low-dose ("renal dose") dopamine (<2 mg/kg/min) was widely advocated for the management of oliguric AKI.[497–499] In experimental studies of animals and healthy human volunteers, low-dose dopamine increased renal blood flow and, to a lesser extent, the GFR. However, low-dose dopamine has not been demonstrated to prevent or alter the course of ischemic or nephrotoxic ATN in prospective clinical trials.[500–504] This absence of clinical benefit may relate to differences in the hemodynamic response to low-dose dopamine in patients with renal disease as compared with healthy individuals. In contrast to the reduction in the renal resistive index associated with low-dose dopamine in critically ill patients without kidney disease, dopamine infusion is associated with an increase in renal resistance in patients with AKI.[505] Moreover, dopamine, even at low doses, is potentially toxic in critically ill patients and can induce tachyarrhythmias, myocardial ischemia, and extravasation necrosis.[505] Thus, the routine administration of low-dose dopamine to ameliorate or reverse the course of AKI is not justified based on the balance of experimental and clinical evidence.[506,507]

## FENOLDOPAM

Fenoldopam is a selective postsynaptic dopamine agonist that acts on D1 receptors and mediates more potent renal vasodilation and natriuresis than dopamine.[508] However, fenoldopam is a potent antihypertensive agent and causes hypotension by decreasing peripheral vascular resistance. Several small studies have suggested that fenoldopam could reduce the incidence of AKI in high-risk clinical situations[509,510]; however, a subsequent larger randomized trial comparing fenoldopam with standard hydration in patients undergoing invasive angiographic procedures found no benefit in regard to decreasing the incidence of CA-AKI.[435] In another large RCT, fenoldopam administration failed to reduce mortality or the need for renal replacement therapy in ICU patients with early ATN.[511] Therefore, there is currently no clinical role for fenoldopam in the prevention or treatment of AKI.

## NATRIURETIC PEPTIDES

ANP is a 28–amino acid polypeptide synthesized in cardiac atrial muscle.[512,513] ANP augments the GFR by triggering afferent arteriolar vasodilation and constriction of the efferent arteriole.[514,515] In addition, ANP inhibits sodium transport and lowers oxygen requirements in several nephron segments.[516,517] Synthetic analogues of ANP have shown promise in the management of ATN in the laboratory setting; however, these benefits in animal models of AKI have failed to translate into clinical benefit in humans. A large multicenter, prospective, randomized, placebo-controlled trial of anaritide, a synthetic analogue of ANP, in patients with ATN failed to show clinically significant improvement in dialysis-free survival or overall mortality,[518] although there was an improvement in dialysis-free survival in oliguric patients. This benefit in oliguric patients was not confirmed in a subsequent prospective study.[519] It has been suggested that the absence of benefit may be related to both the relatively late initiation of therapy and to the effect of ANP on systemic blood pressure. In a subsequent pilot study, low-dose recombinant ANP administration in high-risk cardiac surgery patients was associated with a reduction in the requirement for postoperative RRT.[520] Until these results are confirmed in a larger, multicenter trial, the use of ANP in this setting cannot be recommended. Trials of ANP for the prevention of contrast-associated AKI have generated mixed results.[444,445] Ularitide (urodilantin) is a natriuretic pro-ANP fragment produced in the kidney. In a small randomized trial, ularitide did not reduce the need for dialysis in patients with AKI.[521] A meta-analysis of ANP for the treatment of AKI has concluded that the paucity of high-quality studies precludes a determination of the effects of this therapy.[522]

## LOOP DIURETICS

High-dose IV diuretics are commonly prescribed to increase urine output in patients with oliguric AKI. Although this strategy assists in volume management and minimizes the risk of progressive volume overload, there is no evidence that diuretic therapy alters the natural history of AKI or improves mortality or dialysis-free survival. In a retrospective analysis, diuretic therapy was associated with an increased risk of death and nonrecovery of renal function.[523] These risks were restricted, however, to patients who did not respond to diuretic administration with increased urine volume; in diuretic-responsive patients, outcomes were similar to those of untreated patients. In a prospective randomized trial, high-dose IV furosemide augmented urine output but did not alter the outcome of established AKI.[524] In a post hoc analysis of data from the Fluid and Catheter Treatment Trial, a positive fluid balance after AKI in patients with acute lung injury was strongly associated with increased mortality, whereas diuretic therapy was associated with improved 60-day patient survival.[525] Given the risks of loop diuretics in AKI, including irreversible ototoxicity and exacerbation of prerenal AKI, these agents should be used solely to facilitate the management of extracellular volume overload (see later).[526] Of note, a single administration of furosemide in a dose of 1.0 to 1.5 mg/kg has been shown to help characterize the risk for progressive AKI.[527] Specifically, a urine volume less than 200 mL in the 2 hours following furosemide administration demonstrated sensitivity and specificity for progression to AKIN stage 3 of 87.1% and 84.1%, respectively.

### MANNITOL

The osmotic diuretic mannitol, which also has renal vasodilatory and oxygen-free radical scavenging properties, has been investigated as a preventive treatment for AKI.[528,529] No adequate data exist to support the routine administration of mannitol to oliguric patients. Moreover, when administered to severely oliguric or anuric patients, mannitol may trigger an expansion of intravascular volume and pulmonary edema, as well as severe hyponatremia due to an osmotic shift of water from the intracellular to the intravascular space.[530]

## MANAGEMENT OF OTHER CAUSES OF INTRINSIC ACUTE KIDNEY INJURY

### ACUTE VASCULITIS AND ACUTE GLOMERULAR DISEASE

The management of acute vasculitis involving the kidney and acute glomerular disease is covered in detail in Chapters 31 and 32. AKI caused by acute glomerulonephritis or vasculitis may respond to corticosteroids, alkylating agents, rituximab, and plasmapheresis, depending on the primary cause of the disease. Plasma exchange is useful in the treatment of sporadic TTP and possibly sporadic HUS in adults.[531,532] The role of plasmapheresis in drug-induced thrombotic microangiopathies is less certain, and removal of the offending agent is the most important initial therapeutic maneuver.[144,533,534] Postdiarrheal HUS in children is usually managed conservatively because studies have shown that early antibiotic therapy may actually promote the development of HUS.[535] Treatment with eculizumab, a humanized monoclonal antibody that prevents cleavage of complement component C5 into C5a and C5b, inhibiting terminal complement activation, may be considered in patients with nondiarrheal (complement-mediated) HUS unresponsive to plasma exchange.[536] Hypertension and AKI associated with scleroderma may be exquisitely sensitive to treatment with ACE inhibitors.[537–539]

### ACUTE KIDNEY INJURY IN MULTIPLE MYELOMA

Early studies have suggested that plasmapheresis may be of benefit in AKI due to myeloma cast nephropathy.[169,540,541] Clearance of circulating light chains, with concomitant chemotherapy to decrease the rate of production, had been postulated to reverse renal injury in patients with circulating light chains, heavy Bence Jones proteinuria, and AKI. A subsequent RCT compared plasma exchange and standard chemotherapy with chemotherapy alone. Although the study did not demonstrate improvement with plasma exchange with regard to a composite outcome of death, dialysis dependence, or a GFR less than 30 mL/min/1.73 $m^2$ at 6 months, the study was inadequately powered to exclude a clinical benefit definitively, and there was a trend toward improved outcomes with plasmapheresis.[170–172] More recently, it has been suggested that the use of dialysis membranes that are permeable to light chains and other proteins with molecular weights lower than albumin (high-cutoff membranes) may be an effective therapeutic strategy in patients with AKI due to light chain cast nephropathy; however, data from clinical trials have yielded inconclusive results.[173–175] Thus, primary management should focus on the prompt initiation of highly effective chemotherapy. Other contributors to AKI in multiple myeloma, such as hypercalcemia, should also be promptly treated.

### ACUTE INTERSTITIAL NEPHRITIS

Most cases of acute interstitial nephritis (AIN) are due to an allergic response to a medication.[542] The initial therapeutic step in AIN is discontinuation of the offending medication or treatment of the probable inciting factor if not drug-induced. Data on the efficacy of corticosteroids have been derived from small observational studies, which have yielded highly discordant results. Although some studies have suggested that early use of corticosteroids (i.e., prior to significant renal damage and within 7–14 days of discontinuation of the offending medication)[543] may be beneficial, other studies have demonstrated no clear evidence of efficacy.[57] There have been no large, prospective RCTs investigating the role of corticosteroids in the treatment of AIN. Because corticosteroids are associated with a series of potentially serious side effects, their use should be considered on a case by case basis. If corticosteroid therapy is being considered and no patient-related contraindications exist, one potential regimen used in one study involved the IV administration of methylprednisolone (250–500 mg/day) for 3 to 4 days followed by oral prednisone at a dose of 1 mg/kg/day tapered over 8 to 12 weeks.[543] However, there are no data supporting the superiority of this specific approach over others. Mycophenolate mofetil has also been investigated as a therapeutic agent for AIN. In a study of eight patients with AIN, six experienced improvement and two experienced stabilization in kidney function with mycophenolate mofetil therapy.[544] Although this small case series suggests a possible role for mycophenolate mofetil in the treatment of AIN, additional studies are needed to confirm its safety and efficacy for this indication.

## NONDIALYTIC SUPPORTIVE MANAGEMENT OF ACUTE KIDNEY INJURY–ASSOCIATED COMPLICATIONS

Metabolic complications such as intravascular volume overload, hyperkalemia, hyperphosphatemia, and metabolic acidosis are common in oliguric AKI, and preventive measures should be implemented, beginning with the initial diagnosis (see Table 29.7). Adequate nutrition should be provided to meet caloric requirements and minimize catabolism. In addition, all medications that are normally excreted by the kidney need to be adjusted based on the severity of the renal impairment.

### EXTRACELLULAR VOLUME OVERLOAD

After correction of intravascular volume deficits, salt and water intake should be adjusted to match ongoing losses—urinary, gastrointestinal, drainage sites, insensible losses. Extracellular volume overload can usually be managed by restriction of salt and water intake and by judicious use of diuretics. High doses of loop diuretics (e.g., the equivalent of 200 mg of furosemide administered as an IV bolus infusion or 20 mg/hour as a continuous infusion) or combination therapy with both thiazide and loop diuretics may be required. If an adequate diuresis cannot be attained, further use of diuretics should be discontinued to minimize the risk of complications, such as ototoxicity. Fluid administration should be closely monitored to avoid progressive volume overload. Although there is a strong association between progressive fluid overload and mortality risk in patients with AKI,[545–547] a causal relationship has not been definitively established because volume overload may also be a surrogate for other determinants of mortality, such as hemodynamic instability and capillary leak. Fluid conservative management has, however, been demonstrated to result in improved outcomes in critically ill patients with respiratory failure.[548] Ultrafiltration or dialysis may be required for volume management when conservative measures fail.

## HYPONATREMIA AND HYPERNATREMIA

Hyponatremia associated with a fall in effective serum osmolality can usually be corrected by restriction of water intake. Conversely, hypernatremia is treated by the administration of water, hypotonic saline solutions, or hypotonic dextrose-containing solutions (the latter are effectively hypotonic because dextrose is rapidly metabolized).

## HYPERKALEMIA

Mild hyperkalemia (<5.5 mmol/L) should be managed initially by restriction of dietary potassium intake and the discontinuation of potassium supplements and potassium-sparing diuretics. More severe degrees of hyperkalemia (5.5–6.5 mmol/L) can usually be controlled by combining these measures with the administration of exchange resins to enhance gastrointestinal potassium losses. Although sodium polystyrene sulfonate has been widely used for decades, concerns have been raised regarding its safety, particularly when administered in 70% sorbitol, due to reports of bowel necrosis.[549,550] Newer exchange resins, patiromer and zirconium cyclosilicate, are also effective at decreasing the serum potassium concentration, although patiromer is not labeled for the acute management of hyperkalemia. Loop diuretics can also increase potassium excretion in diuretic-responsive patients. Emergency measures need to be used in patients with more severe hyperkalemia and in patients with electrocardiographic manifestations of hyperkalemia. In patients with severe hyperkalemia with concomitant electrocardiographic manifestations, the IV administration of calcium will antagonize the cardiac and neuromuscular effects of hyperkalemia and is a valuable emergency temporizing measure, allowing time for the additional measures described later to be implemented. IV calcium must be used with caution, however, if there is concomitant severe hyperphosphatemia or evidence of digitalis toxicity. IV insulin (10–20 U of regular insulin) promotes potassium entry into cells and lowers extracellular potassium concentration within 15 to 30 minutes, with an effect that lasts for several hours.[551,552] The concomitant administration of IV dextrose (25–50 g over 30–60 minutes) is required to prevent hypoglycemia in patients who do not have hyperglycemia. Beta-adrenergic agonists, such as inhaled albuterol (10–20 mg by nebulizer), also promote rapid potassium uptake into the intracellular compartment.[551] Although sodium bicarbonate also stimulates potassium uptake into the intracellular compartment, this effect is not sufficiently rapid to be clinically useful for the emergent management of hyperkalemia.[552] Emergent dialysis is indicated if hyperkalemia is resistant to these measures.

## METABOLIC ACIDOSIS

The treatment of metabolic acidosis is dependent on the clinical setting and cause. As a general rule, metabolic acidosis does not require emergent treatment unless the serum $HCO_3^-$ concentration falls below 15 mmol/L or the pH is lower than 7.15 to 7.20. In patients with AKI in whom metabolic acidosis is due to the underlying renal failure, more severe acidosis can be corrected by oral or IV bicarbonate administration. Initial rates of replacement should be based on estimates of the $HCO_3^-$ deficit and adjusted thereafter according to serum levels. In patients with underlying lactic acidosis, the role of bicarbonate therapy is controversial, and the primary focus of therapy should be on correction of the underlying cause.[553–556] Patients treated with IV bicarbonate need to be monitored for complications of therapy, including metabolic alkalosis, hypocalcemia, hypokalemia, hypernatremia, and volume overload.

## DISTURBANCES OF CALCIUM, PHOSPHATE, MAGNESIUM, AND URIC ACID

Hypocalcemia does not usually require treatment unless it is severe or symptomatic, as may occur in patients with rhabdomyolysis or pancreatitis or after the administration of bicarbonate. Hyperphosphatemia can often be controlled by restricting dietary phosphate intake and the use of oral phosphate binders (e.g., aluminum hydroxide, calcium salts, sevelamer carbonate, lanthanum carbonate). Caution should be used with aluminum-containing phosphate binders because prolonged use may result in aluminum intoxication, which can contribute to osteomalacia; short-term use is rarely associated with bone disease, and the feared neurologic complications of aluminum intoxication are restricted to patients with inadvertent parenteral exposure. Hypermagnesemia can be prevented through avoidance of magnesium-containing medications, such as antacids, and limiting the magnesium content of parenteral nutrition. Hyperuricemia is usually mild in AKI (<15 mg/dL) and does not require a specific intervention. Severe hyperuricemia secondary to cell lysis may be managed by blocking xanthine oxidase with allopurinol or by enhancing degradation with recombinant uricase, as previously described.

## NUTRITIONAL MANAGEMENT

Patients with AKI are clinically heterogeneous, and individualized nutritional management is required, especially in critically ill patients on RRT in whom protein catabolic rates can exceed 1.5 g/kg body weight/day.[3,285,286,288,289,557,558]

The objective of nutritional management in AKI is to provide sufficient calories to preserve lean body mass, avoid starvation ketoacidosis, and promote healing and tissue repair while minimizing production of nitrogenous waste. If the duration of impaired kidney function is likely to be short, the patient is not extremely catabolic and does not require RRT, then dietary protein should be approximately 0.8 to 1.0 g/kg body weight/day.[3] Protein intake should not be restricted in patients in whom AKI is likely to be prolonged, are hypercatabolic, or are receiving RRT. Protein intake in these patients should generally be 1.0 to 1.5 g/kg body weight per day.[285,286,557,558] There has been no evidence of improved outcomes with protein intake higher than 1.7 g/kg body weight per day, even in extremely hypercatabolic patients.[3] Total caloric intake should generally be 20 to 30 kcal/kg body weight per day and should not exceed 35 kcal/kg per day.[3,285,286,557,558] Benefits of vigorous parenteral hyperalimentation have not been consistently demonstrated;

enteral nutrition support is preferred because it avoids the morbidity associated with parenteral nutrition while providing support to intestinal function.[288] Water-soluble vitamins and trace elements should be supplemented in patients receiving RRT.[557,558]

### ANEMIA

Severe anemia is generally managed with a blood transfusion. Transfusion is usually not required for patients with a hemoglobin concentration above 7 g/dL.[559] Whether there is a role for erythropoiesis-stimulating agents in AKI has not been definitively determined.[560] Patients with AKI or another acute illness are relatively resistant to the effects of these agents, and their onset of action is delayed. In RCTs in critically ill patients, recombinant human erythropoietin decreased transfusion requirement but had no effect on other outcomes.[561,562] Uremic bleeding usually responds to desmopressin, correction of anemia, estrogens, or dialysis.

### DRUG DOSING

Doses of drugs that are excreted by the kidney must be adjusted for impaired kidney function and the use of RRT.[563–565] Whenever possible, pharmacokinetic monitoring should be used to ensure appropriate drug dosing, especially for agents with narrow therapeutic windows (see Chapter 61). In addition to careful monitoring for toxicity of agents that are normally excreted by the kidney, careful attention must be paid to dosing of antibiotics and other drugs removed by RRT to ensure that therapeutic drug levels are achieved, particularly in patients receiving augmented intensity of RRT.

## RENAL REPLACEMENT THERAPY IN ACUTE KIDNEY INJURY

### GENERAL PRINCIPLES

RRT is the generic term for the multiple modalities of dialysis and hemofiltration used in the management of kidney failure. Although kidney transplantation is also a form of RRT for ESKD, transplantation does not play a role in the management of AKI. Renal replacement therapy facilitates the management of patients with AKI, allowing correction of acid-base and electrolyte disturbances, amelioration of volume overload, and removal of byproducts of nitrogen metabolism (so-called uremic solutes). Although RRT can forestall or reverse the life-threatening complications of uremia associated with severe and prolonged AKI, it does not hasten and can potentially delay the recovery of kidney function in patients with AKI,[566] and can itself be associated with potentially life-threatening complications.[567] Despite more than 60 years of research and clinical experience,[568,569] numerous questions regarding the optimal application of RRT in AKI remain.[3,570–573]

### INDICATIONS FOR AND TIMING OF INITIATION OF RENAL REPLACEMENT THERAPY

In clinical practice, there are wide variations in the timing of initiation of RRT for patients with AKI.[574] Widely accepted indications for initiation of RRT include volume overload unresponsive to diuretic therapy, severe metabolic acidosis or hyperkalemia, despite appropriate medical therapy, and overt uremic manifestations, including encephalopathy, pericarditis, and uremic bleeding diathesis (Box 29.8). However, even these specific indications are subject to substantial clinical interpretation. In many patients, RRT is initiated in the absence of these specific indications in response to a clinical course marked by progressive azotemia or sustained oliguria. The correlation between the BUN concentration and the onset of uremic symptoms is relatively weak; although the longer the duration and the greater the severity of azotemia, the more likely it is that overt symptoms will develop. Observational series and small clinical trials dating from the 1950s through the 1980s have suggested that initiating RRT when the BUN concentration approached 90 to 100 mg/dL was associated with improved survival as compared with more delayed initiation of therapy.[575–579] Other observational studies have suggested that the initiation of RRT at an even less severe degree of azotemia may further improve survival.[580–583] These studies need to be interpreted with caution, however, because the outcomes associated with earlier initiation of RRT may reflect differences related to the reasons for initiation of therapy (e.g., volume overload or hyperkalemia vs. progressive azotemia) rather than a benefit due to the earlier therapy per se. In addition, these observational series only included patients in whom RRT was actually initiated, rather than the broader population of patients with AKI, including patients who recovered kidney function or died without receiving RRT.

**Box 29.8 Indications for Renal Replacement Therapy**

**Absolute Indications**

- Volume overload unresponsive to diuretic therapy
- Persistent hyperkalemia despite medical therapy
- Severe metabolic acidosis
- Overt uremic symptoms—encephalopathy, pericarditis, uremic bleeding diathesis

**Relative Indications**

- Progressive azotemia without uremic manifestations
- Persistent oliguria

There have been an increasing number of prospective clinical trials evaluating the timing of initiation of RRT in AKI. In a small RCT of critically ill patients randomized to early, high-volume hemofiltration, early low-volume hemofiltration, or late low-volume hemofiltration, there was no benefit associated with earlier initiation of treatment.[584] In a subsequent trial comparing earlier to later initiation of dialysis in patients with community- acquired AKI, mortality was lower in patients initiated on dialysis later than in the group of patients started earlier, with no difference in recovery of kidney function between groups.[585] This latter trial needs to be interpreted with caution, however, because almost half of the patients admitted with community-acquired AKI were excluded due to the urgent need for dialysis.

More recently, two clinical trials have compared differing strategies of early and delayed initiation of RRT in patients with AKI. The Effect of Early vs. Delayed Initiation of Renal Replacement Therapy on Mortality in Critically Ill Patients with Acute Kidney Injury (ELAIN) trial randomized 231 critically ill patients with AKI (based on KDIGO stage 2 and plasma neutrophil gelatinase-associated lipocalin level >150 ng/mL) at a single center to early or delayed initiation of RRT; it demonstrated reduced 90-day mortality (hazard ratio, 0.66; 95% CI, 0.45–0.97) with earlier initiation of RRT.[586] Patients in the early RRT group also demonstrated decreased duration of RRT (9 vs. 25 days; $P = .04$) and reduced hospital length of stay (51 vs. 82 days; $P < .001$). However, the separation in timing of the initiation of RRT between early and late groups was less than 1 day, raising questions about the therapeutic mechanisms underlying the observed marked reductions in mortality, duration of RRT, and hospital length of stay. It is possible that unrecognized differences between the two treatment groups may have contributed to the surprisingly large effect size.

The contemporaneous Artificial Kidney Initiation in Kidney Injury (AKIKI) trial was a multicenter trial that randomized 620 patients with KDIGO stage 3 AKI who required mechanical ventilation and/or catecholamine support to early or delayed initiation of RRT. It found no difference in 60-day mortality between the groups (48.5% in the early strategy group vs. 49.7% in the delayed strategy group; $P = .79$)[587] (Fig. 29.4). Notably, nearly half ($n = 151$) of patients assigned to the delayed strategy group never required initiation of RRT. Subsequently, the Initiation of Dialysis Early Versus Delayed in the Intensive Care Unit (IDEAL-ICU) trial also failed to demonstrate a benefit to the earlier initiation of RRT in 488 patients with sepsis-associated AKI.[588] In the IDEAL-ICU trial, patients were enrolled if they met the criteria for RIFLE-F AKI and had sepsis and did not have an emergent indication for RRT. In the early-treatment arm, patients initiated RRT within 12 hours of eligibility while in the delayed-treatment arm; RRT was initiated if a specific indication for RRT developed or if there was no recovery of kidney function after 48 hours. In the early treatment arm, mortality at 90 days was 58% as compared with 54% in the delayed treatment arm ($P = .38$). Of patients in the early treatment arm, 97% received RRT as compared with only 62% of patients in the delayed treatment arm. Of those in the delayed arm who did not receive RRT, 75% had spontaneous recovery of kidney function, whereas 23% died prior to specified criteria for the initiation of RRT.

Key differences between the ELAIN trial and AKIKI and IDEAL-ICU trials should be noted. In particular, the entry criterion for both the AKIKI and IDEAL-ICU trials (stage 3 or RIFLE-F AKI) was the trigger for delayed initiation of RRT in the ELAIN trial. In addition, both the AKIKI and IDEAL-ICU trials excluded individuals with an emergent indication for RRT, in whom a strategy of delayed therapy would be inappropriate. The ongoing Standard vs Accelerated Initiation of RRT in AKI (START-AKI) trial (NCT02568722) may help reconcile the divergent results between the ELAIN trial and AKIKI and IDEAL-ICU trials and clarify the benefit of early initiation of RRT in patients with AKI who do not have overt clinical or biochemical indications for this treatment.[589]

Although volume overload unresponsive to diuretic therapy is a widely accepted indication for the initiation of RRT, there are wide variations in the degree of volume overload at initiation of therapy.[546,590,591] Observational studies have demonstrated a strong association between the degree of volume overload and mortality risk, leading to the suggestion that RRT should be initiated early, prior to the development of progressive volume overload.[545,592] It should be recognized, however, that the association between volume overload and mortality risk does not establish a causal relationship; disease processes that contribute to the development of volume overload may independently contribute to mortality risk in these patients. Prospective studies will therefore be required to demonstrate that preemptive RRT, prior to the development of more severe degrees of volume overload, decreases morbidity and mortality.

Given the current level of evidence, the KDOQI clinical practice guideline for acute kidney injury does not make strong recommendations on the timing of initiation of RRT.[3] It suggests that RRT be "...initiated emergently when life-threatening changes in fluid, electrolyte, and acid-base balance exist",[3] and that "...the broader clinical context, the presence

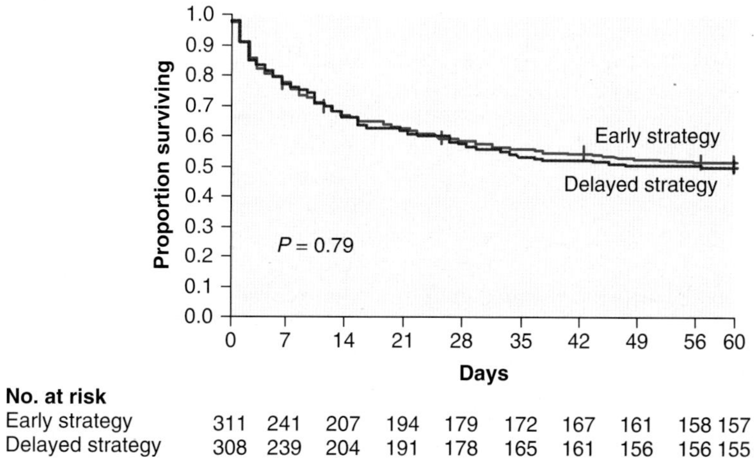


**Fig. 29.4** Probability of survival and timing of treatment with early versus delayed strategies for initiation of renal replacement therapy (RRT). Kaplan-Meier probability of survival and timing of initiation of RRT in the Acute Kidney Initiation in Kidney Injury (AKIKI) trial. In the early-treatment group, 60-day mortality was 48.5% versus 49.7% in the delayed-treatment group (hazard ratio, 1.03; 95% confidence interval, 0.81–1.29; $P = .84$). In the early-treatment group, 98% of patients imitated RRT at a median of 4.3 hours after reaching stage 3 AKI as compared with 51% of patients who initiated RRT at a median of 57 hours. (From Gaudry S, Hajage D, Schortgen F, et al. Initiation strategies for renal-replacement therapy in the intensive care unit. N Engl J Med. 2016;375:122–133.)

of conditions that can be modified by RRT, and trends of laboratory tests—rather than single BUN and creatinine thresholds alone [be considered] when making the decision to start RRT."[3]

RRT should be discontinued when kidney function recovers or because the continued provision of dialytic support is no longer consistent with the patient's overall goals of care.[3] Recovery of kidney function is usually heralded by increased urine volume. Although no specific threshold of urine output correlates with sufficient recovery of kidney function, it is unlikely that a urine output of less than roughly 1 L/day is sufficient to sustain dialysis independence. Although diuretics may increase daily urine volume, there is no evidence that diuretic therapy promotes recovery of kidney function.[593] Improved solute clearance is manifested by a spontaneous fall in blood urea and creatinine concentrations or a persistent downward trend in predialysis values. The role of creatinine clearance measurement to assess the recovery of kidney function is uncertain, with a paucity of data to define specific thresholds for recovery of kidney function. In the Acute Renal Failure Trial Network Study, RRT was continued if measured creatinine clearance on a 6-hour timed urine collection was less than 12 mL/min, RRT was stopped if the clearance was more than 20 mL/min, and the decision was left to the discretion of the clinician if the creatinine clearance was between 12 and 20 mL/min.[594,595]

## CHOICE OF MODALITY OF RENAL REPLACEMENT THERAPY

Multiple modalities of RRT are available for the management of patients with AKI, including conventional intermittent hemodialysis (IHD), peritoneal dialysis (PD), multiple forms of continuous renal replacement therapy (CRRT) and prolonged intermittent renal replacement therapies (PIRRT) such as sustained low-efficiency dialysis (SLED; also known as extended- duration dialysis, EDD). Detailed descriptions of the technical aspects of these modalities are provided in Chapters 63, 64, and 65. Objective data to guide the selection of modality for individual patients are limited, and the choice of modality is often guided by the resources of the health care institution and the technical expertise of the physicians and nursing staff. The KDIGO Clinical Practice Guideline for Acute Kidney Injury suggests that for most patients, the available modalities of RRT are complementary, with the caveats that CRRT and PIRRT be used in hemodynamically unstable patients and that CRRT be used for patients with acute brain injury or other causes of increased intracranial pressure or generalized brain edema.[3]

### Intermittent Hemodialysis

IHD has been the mainstay of RRT in AKI for more than 6 decades. Patients typically undergo dialysis treatments for 3 to 5 hours on a thrice-weekly, alternate-day, or daily schedule, depending on catabolic demands, electrolyte disturbances, and volume status. Just as with the timing of initiation of dialysis in AKI, the most appropriate dosing strategy for IHD in patients with AKI has been the subject of considerable investigation. The dose of IHD may be adjusted by altering the intensity of each individual dialysis session, usually quantified as the product of urea clearance and dialysis duration normalized to the volume of distribution of urea ($Kt/V_{urea}$) or by changing the frequency of the dialysis sessions. In an observational study, Paganini and colleagues have demonstrated a survival benefit for patients with intermediate severity of illness scores when the delivered $Kt/V_{urea}$ was more than 1.0 per treatment as compared with a delivered $Kt/V_{urea}$ less than 1.0 per treatment.[596]

However, there have been no prospective clinical trials evaluating the relationship between the delivered $Kt/V_{urea}$ and outcomes when dialysis is provided on a constant treatment schedule. Schiffl and colleagues have reported on a prospective trial of 160 patients with AKI assigned in an alternating fashion to alternate-day or daily intermittent hemodialysis.[597] The more frequent treatment schedule was associated with a reduction in mortality at 14 days after the last dialysis session, from 46% in the alternate-day dialysis arm to 28% in the daily treatment arm ($P = .01$). The duration of renal failure declined from 16 ± 6 to 9 ± 2 days ($P = .001$). This study has been criticized, however, because the delivered dose of therapy per session was low in both treatment arms ($[Kt/V_{urea}] < 0.95$), resulting in a high rate of symptoms in the alternate-day dialysis arm that may have been related to overtly inadequate dialysis.[598]

The impact of frequency of IHD was also evaluated in the Acute Renal Failure Trial Network study.[594] In this study, 1124 critically ill patients were randomized to an intensive or less intensive strategy for the management of RRT. When patients were hemodynamically stable, they received IHD and, when hemodynamically unstable, they received CRRT or sustained low-efficiency dialysis (SLED), regardless of treatment arm. Patients randomized to the less intensive treatment strategy received IHD on a thrice-weekly (alternate-day except Sunday) schedule while patients randomized to the intensive arm received IHD six times per week (daily except Sunday). All-cause mortality at 60 days was 53.6% in the intensive treatment arm compared with 51.5% in the less intensive arm ($P = .47$)[594] (Fig. 29.5). The mean delivered $Kt/V_{urea}$ was 1.3/treatment after the first IHD session. Although the study was not designed to evaluate outcomes by individual modality of RRT, there were no differences in mortality between groups when evaluated based on the percentage of time treated using IHD.[599]

Based on these results, it does not appear that there is further benefit to increasing the frequency of IHD treatments routinely beyond three times per week as long as the delivered $Kt/V_{urea}$ is at least 1.2 per treatment. More frequent treatments may be necessary if the target dose per treatment cannot be achieved—for example, in hypercatabolic patients, in patients with severe hyperkalemia or metabolic acidosis, and for issues related to volume management. The KDIGO Clinical Practice Guideline for Acute Kidney Injury recommends delivering a $Kt/V_{urea}$ of 3.9 per week when using IHD in AKI, calculating the weekly $Kt/V_{urea}$ as the arithmetic sum of the delivered dose per treatment.[3] It should be recognized, however, that this approach for calculating an equivalent weekly $Kt/V_{urea}$ is not consistent with urea kinetic principles, and that rigorous data for the appropriate dose of therapy when treatments are delivered more frequently than three times per week are not available.[13]

The selection of IHD dialyzer membrane may also affect clinical outcomes. Exposure to cellulosic membranes results in accentuated leukocyte and complement activation and delayed recovery of kidney function in experimental models of AKI as compared with exposure to more biocompatible

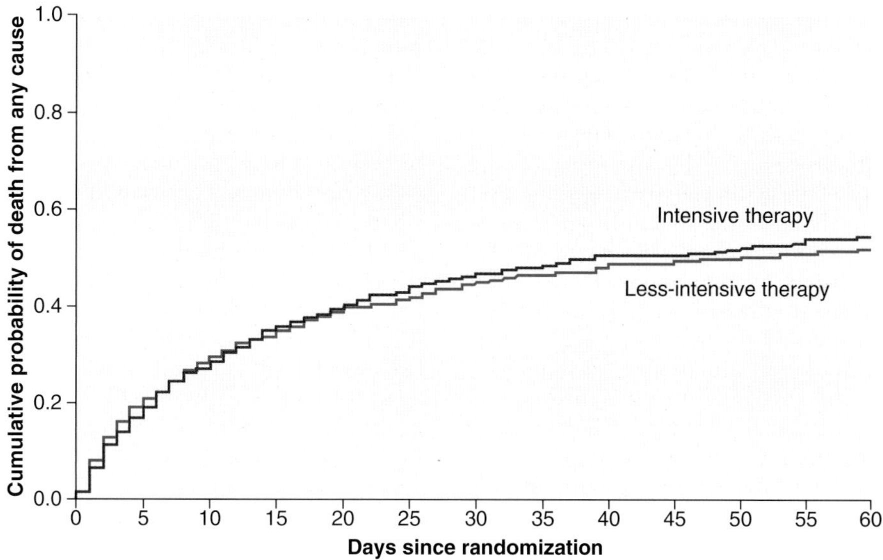


**Fig. 29.5** 60-Day mortality with intensive versus less intensive renal replacement therapy in the Acute Renal Failure Trial Network (ATN) study. Shown is the Kaplan-Meier plot of mortality in 1124 critically ill patients with acute kidney injury randomized to a strategy of more intensive renal replacement therapy (RRT; 6 times per week intermittent hemodialysis or continuous venovenous hemodiafiltration at 35 mL/kg per hour) versus less intensive RRT (3 times per week intermittent hemodialysis or continuous venovenous hemodiafiltration at 20 mL/kg per hour). At 60 days, mortality was 53.6% in the more intensive arm versus 51.5% in the less intensive arm (odds ratio, 1.09; 95% confidence interval, 0.86–1.40; *P* = .47). (From VA/NIH Acute Renal Failure Trial Network; Palevsky PM, Zhang JH, O'Connor TZ, et al. Intensity of renal support in critically ill patients with acute kidney injury. N Engl J Med. 2008;359:7–20.)

synthetic membranes.[600,601] Clinical trials comparing dialysis membranes have yielded conflicting results. Although some studies have demonstrated delayed recovery of kidney function with cellulosic membranes,[602–604] other studies have observed no difference between cellulosic and other synthetic membranes thought to be more biocompatible.[605–609] When these data have been aggregated in systematic reviews, a benefit of the synthetic membranes is not convincingly demonstrated.[610,611] Although the effect of membrane type on humoral and cellular activation may still influence recovery of kidney function in AKI, the clinical importance of this issue has diminished as the cost differential between synthetic and cellulosic membranes has narrowed, and the use of unsubstituted cellulosic membranes has decreased.

The major complications associated with IHD are related to the need to access the vasculature, the need for anticoagulation to maintain patency of the extracorporeal circuit, and intradialytic hypotension primarily resulting from shifts in solute and volume.[594,597,612] Many of these issues, particularly the need for vascular access and anticoagulation, are similar for CRRT and SLED.

Vascular access is usually obtained through the insertion of a double-lumen catheter into a large caliber central (internal jugular or subclavian) or femoral vein.[613] The major complications associated with vascular access include vascular and organ trauma during insertion, bleeding, catheter malfunction and thrombosis, and infection.[613] Although femoral catheters are generally associated with an increased risk of infection compared with catheters in the subclavian or internal jugular veins, an increased risk of infection was observed only when femoral vein catheters were used in patients with a high body mass index (BMI) in an RCT involving patients undergoing acute RRT.[614] The more prompt transition to tunneled hemodialysis catheters (or placement of tunneled hemodialysis catheters in advance of initiation) has been proposed as a means of decreasing the risk of infection in patients undergoing acute dialysis.[615,616] However, this strategy has not been rigorously evaluated in prospective clinical trials.

Anticoagulation is used to help maintain patency of the extracorporeal dialysis circuit in IHD, as well as in CRRT and SLED.[617,618] The most commonly used anticoagulant for dialysis is unfractionated heparin; with multiple protocols used to attain sufficient anticoagulation of the dialysis circuit while minimizing systemic effects.[617,618] Regional heparinization, in which heparin is infused proximally to the dialyzer, and protamine is infused into the return line to reverse heparin's effect,[619] can be used but has generally been supplanted by low-dose heparin protocols.[620] Low-molecular-weight heparin (LMWH) may be used as an alternative to unfractionated heparin; however, the benefits of this approach are unclear because LMWH is not associated with enhanced efficacy, drug half-life is variably prolonged with impaired kidney function, and monitoring of the anticoagulant effect is more difficult.[617] In patients with heparin-induced thrombocytopenia (HIT), heparin administration is contraindicated. Alternative anticoagulation strategies include regional citrate,[617,621–623] the serine protease inhibitor nafamostat,[624] the direct thrombin inhibitors hirudin, lepirudin, and argatroban[625–629] and, rarely, the prostanoids epoprostenol and iloprost.[617,618] In many patients, particularly those with underlying coagulopathy or thrombocytopenia, and in patients with active hemorrhage or recent postoperative status, acute RRT can be provided in the absence of anticoagulation.[594,630,631]

Intradialytic hypotension is common in patients undergoing acute IHD.[566,594,599,612,632] Episodes of hypotension may impair solute clearance and the efficiency of dialysis and can further compromise renal perfusion and delay recovery of kidney function.[566,633–635] Intradialytic hypotension is typically triggered by intercompartmental fluid shifts or excessive fluid removal, leading to decreased intravascular volume, and may be exacerbated by altered vascular responsiveness related to the underlying acute process.[612,636] Hypotension may be particularly problematic in critically ill patients in whom sepsis, cardiac dysfunction, hypoalbuminemia, malnutrition, or large third space losses may accompany the development of AKI. The prevention of intradialytic hypotension requires careful assessment of intravascular volume, prescription of realistic ultrafiltration targets, extension of treatment time so as to minimize the ultrafiltration rate, increasing the dialysate sodium concentration, and decreasing the dialysate temperature.[632,636–638] It is noteworthy that intradialytic hypotension can develop even among patients in whom no ultrafiltration is prescribed; the reason(s) for hypotension are not entirely clear, although many have attributed hemodynamic instability to the rapid exchange of solutes induced by high-flux, high-efficiency hemodialysis, with extra- to intracellular shifting of body water. Although there is a tendency to reduce the extracorporeal blood flow in patients prone to hypotension, there is little evidence that this provides any benefit. Reducing blood flow decreased the volume of the extracorporeal circuit in the past when parallel plate and coil dialyzers were used; however, there is little change in the volume of the extracorporeal circuit in response to changes in blood flow when hollow fiber dialyzers are used. Reducing blood flow may, however, result in reduction of the delivered dose of dialysis.

### Continuous Renal Replacement Therapy

The continuous RRTs represent a spectrum of treatment modalities. In their initial description, the continuous therapies were provided using arteriovenous extracorporeal circuits.[639–643] Although this approach provided technical simplicity, blood flow was dependent on the gradient between MAP and central venous pressure, and there was an increased risk of complications from prolonged arterial cannulation.[644] As a result, the continuous arteriovenous therapies have largely been supplanted by pump-driven, venovenous CRRT.[645–648] The modalities of venovenous CRRT vary, predominantly based on their mechanism of solute removal. With continuous venovenous hemofiltration (CVVH), solute transport occurs by convection; with continuous venovenous hemodialysis (CVVHD) by diffusion; and with continuous venovenous hemodiafiltration (CVVHDF) by a combination of the two.[648–650] Although, at the same level of urea clearance, convective therapies provide enhanced clearance of higher molecular weight solutes compared with diffusive therapies, no clear clinical benefit has been demonstrated for CVVH or CVVHDF as compared with CVVHD.[651]

The clearance of urea and other small solutes during CRRT is generally proportional to the total effluent flow rate (the sum of ultrafiltrate and dialysate flow rates),[643,648,649] and the dose of therapy is usually expressed as the effluent volume indexed to body weight. This approach to estimating solute clearance is based on the assumption of near-complete solute equilibration between blood and effluent and may overestimate the actual solute clearance.[652,653] Several single-center RCTs demonstrated an improvement in survival when doses of CVVH were increased from 20 to 25 mL/kg per hour to doses in excess of 35 to 45 mL/kg per hour[654,655]; however, other small studies did not find a similar benefit.[584,656] Two large multicenter RCTs also did not find a survival benefit associated with more intensive CRRT.[594,657] In the previously described ATN study, 1124 patients were randomized to two intensities of RRT.[594] In both treatment arms, patients received IHD when hemodynamically stable and CVVHDF or SLED when hemodynamically unstable. In the less intensive arm, CVVHDF was provided at an effluent flow rate of 20 mL/kg per hour and,in the more intensive arm at 35 mL/kg per hour. All-cause mortality at 60 days was 51.5% in the less intensive arm and 53.6% in the more-intensive arm ($P = .47$; Fig. 29.5).[594] In the Randomized Evaluation of Normal versus Augmented Level (RENAL) Replacement Therapy study, 1508 patients were randomized to CVVHDF at 25 mL/kg or 40 mL/kg per hour.[657] All-cause mortality at 90 days was 44.7% in both treatment arms ($P = .99$; Fig. 29.6).[657] Based on these data, the KDIGO Clinical Practice Guideline for Acute Kidney Injury recommends delivering an effluent volume during CRRT of 20 to 25 mL/kg per hour, recognizing that a slightly higher dose may need to be prescribed to achieve the target delivered dose to compensate for interruptions in treatment.[3]

Given the improved hemodynamic tolerance of CRRT as compared with IHD, particularly in patients with underlying hemodynamic instability, it has been postulated that CRRT would be associated with improved clinical outcomes. Five RCTs comparing outcomes with CRRT and IHD have been published. In a multicenter RCT of 166 patients with AKI, Mehta and colleagues observed ICU and hospital mortality rates of 59.5% and 65.5%, respectively, in patients randomized

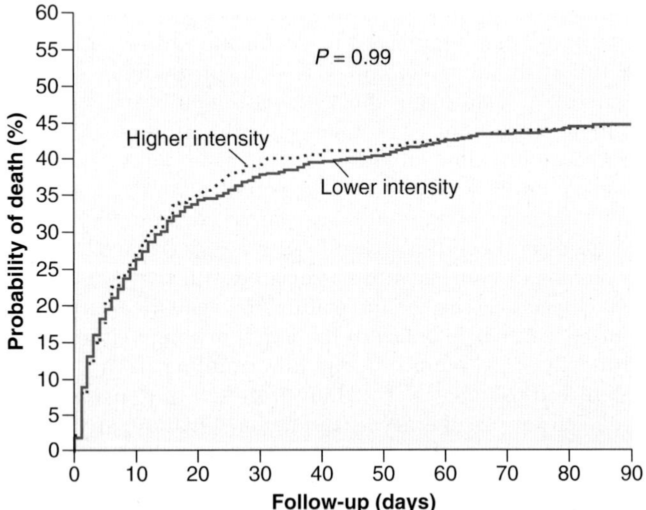


**Fig. 29.6** 90-Day mortality with intensive versus less intensive continuous venovenous hemodiafiltration (CVVHDF) in the Randomized Evaluation of Normal versus Augmented Level (RENAL) Replacement Therapy Study. Shown is the Kaplan-Meier plot of mortality in 1508 critically ill patients with acute kidney injury randomized to CVVHDF at 35 mL/kg vs. 20 mL/kg per hour. At 90 days, mortality was 44.7% in both treatment groups (odds ratio, 1.00; 95% confidence interval, 0.81–1.23; $P = .99$). (From RENAL Replacement Therapy Study Investigators; Bellomo R, Cass A, Cole L, et al. Intensity of continuous renal-replacement therapy in critically ill patients. N Engl J Med. 2009;361:1627–1638.)

to CRRT as compared with 41.5% and 47.6%, respectively, in patients randomized to IHD ($P < .02$).[658] As the result of an imbalance in randomization, patients in the CRRT arm had a higher severity of illness as measured by the APACHE III score and a higher rate of liver failure. Adjusting for the imbalanced randomization in a post hoc analysis, the investigators found no difference in mortality attributable to modality of RRT. In another single-center randomized trial ($n = 80$), Augustine and colleagues reported more effective fluid removal and greater hemodynamic stability associated with CVVHD as compared with IHD, but no difference in survival.[659] Similarly, in another single-center RCT from Switzerland, Uehlinger and colleagues observed no difference in survival in 70 patients randomized to CVVHDF as compared with 55 patients assigned to IHD.[660] In the Hemodiafe study, a multicenter RCT conducted in 21 ICUs in France, Vinsonneau and colleagues reported 60-day survival rates of 31.5% in 184 patients randomized to IHD as compared with 32.6% in 175 patients randomized to CVVHDF ($P = .98$)[632] (Fig. 29.7). Similarly, Lins and colleagues observed hospital morality rates of 62.5% in 144 patients randomized to IHD and 58.1% in 172 patients randomized to CRRT ($P = .43$).[661] Multiple meta-analyses have concluded that there is no difference in survival among patients undergoing RRT.[662–664] Although several studies have suggested that CRRT is associated with improved rates of recovery of kidney function in surviving patients as compared with IHD,[658,665–668] all these studies are confounded by higher mortality rates in the CRRT group. When analyzed across studies in which there were no differences in mortality, rates of recovery of kidney function did not appear to be affected by the modality of RRT.[566,662,664,669]

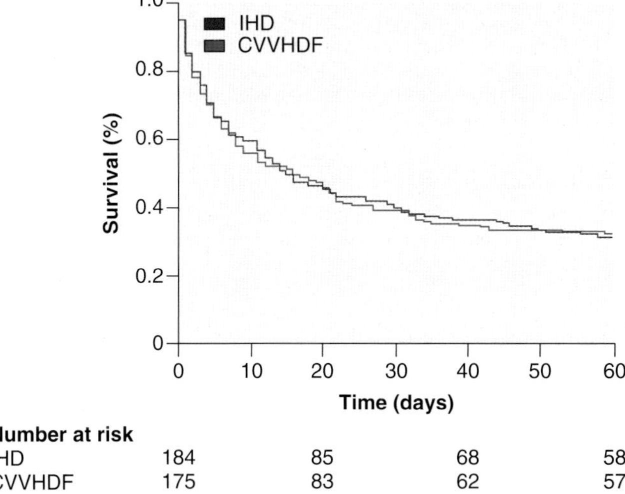


**Fig. 29.7** 60-Day survival with intermittent hemodialysis (*IHD*) versus continuous venovenous hemodiafiltration (*CVVHDF*) in the Hemodiafe Study. Shown is a Kaplan-Meier plot of survival among 359 critically ill patients with acute kidney injury randomized to intermittent hemodialysis versus continuous venovenous hemodiafiltration. At 60 days,survival was 31.5% among patients randomized to IHD versus 32.6% among patients randomized to CVVHDF ($P = .98$). (From Vinsonneau C, Camus C, Combes A, et al; Hemodiafe Study Group. Continuous venovenous haemodiafiltration versus intermittent haemodialysis for acute renal failure in patients with multiple-organ dysfunction syndrome: a multicentre randomised trial. Lancet. 2006; 368:379–385.)

### Prolonged Intermittent Renal Replacement Therapy

Prolonged intermittent renal replacement therapy (PIRRT) represents a treatment modality in which conventional hemodialysis equipment is modified to provide extended-duration hemodialysis using lower blood flow rates and dialysate flow rates.[670,671] A variety of terms have been developed to describe these therapies including SLED,[672,673] extended daily dialysis (EDD),[674] and sustained low-efficiency daily diafiltration (SLEDD-f).[675] By extending the duration of the dialysis treatment while providing slower ultrafiltration and solute clearance, these therapies are generally associated with enhanced hemodynamic tolerability compared with IHD. The degree of metabolic control attained with these treatments is comparable to that observed with CRRT.[676] In an observational study performed in three ICUs in New Zealand, Australia, and Italy that changed from using CRRT to PIRRT, there was no difference in observed outcomes following the change in modality of RRT.[671] Similarly, in a single-center prospective RCT that included 232 patients, 90-day survival rates were similar in the PIRRT and CRRT groups (PIRRT, 50.4%; CRRT, 44.4%; $P = .43$), although overall resource use was lower with PIRRT.[677] In a meta-analysis, there were no differences in mortality or recovery of kidney function comparing PIRRT with CRRT.[678]

### Peritoneal Dialysis

The use of PD in the management of AKI has diminished as the use of continuous and hybrid therapies have increased.[679–681] Peritoneal dialysis has the advantage of requiring minimal technology, facilitating its use in remote or resource-constrained areas.[682] As a result, it is still used in the treatment of AKI in regions where access to IHD or CRRT is not possible. Access for acute PD can be obtained by percutaneous placement of an uncuffed temporary peritoneal catheter or through surgical placement of a tunneled cuffed catheter. PD has the advantage of avoiding the need for vascular access or anticoagulation. Solute clearance and control of metabolic parameters may be inferior to that achieved with other modalities of RRT.[683] Although systemic hypotension is less of an issue than with other modalities of RRT, ultrafiltration cannot be as tightly controlled. Other limitations include the relative contraindication in patients with acute abdominal processes or recent abdominal surgery, the risk of visceral organ injury during catheter placement, the risk of PD-associated peritonitis, and an increased tendency toward hyperglycemia due to the high glucose concentrations in peritoneal dialysate, which in other acute settings has been associated with adverse outcomes.

Several trials have compared outcomes using PD with other modalities of RRT in AKI.[683–686] In a study of 70 patients with infection-associated AKI in Vietnam, 58 of whom had severe falciparum malaria, PD was associated with less adequate metabolic control and higher mortality than continuous hemofiltration.[683] In contrast, in a study of 120 patients in Brazil who were randomized to high-volume PD or daily hemodialysis, indices of metabolic control, recovery of kidney function, and survival were similar with both modalities.[684] In a meta-analysis that included eight observational studies and four clinical trials, Chionh and colleagues observed similar survival rates with peritoneal dialysis as compared with extracorporeal RRT in patients with AKI.[687]

## SUMMARY OF ACUTE KIDNEY INJURY MANAGEMENT

Acute kidney injury remains a common and serious disease with protean causes and variable clinical courses. The management of AKI begins with prevention in those clinical circumstances in which evidence-based preventive interventions are available. Although pharmacologic therapy is available for select causes of AKI, the treatment of established ATN is largely supportive, with pharmacology and RRTs designed to ameliorate the adverse metabolic and clinical complications of this condition. Additional research is needed to identify treatments that decrease the risk of developing AKI and, in patients with established AKI, reduce the severity of AKI and/or facilitate recovery.

 Complete reference list available at ExpertConsult.com.

## KEY REFERENCES


2. Mehta RL, Kellum JA, Shah SV, et al. Acute Kidney Injury Network (AKIN): report of an initiative to improve outcomes in acute kidney injury. *Crit Care.* 2007;11:R31.
3. Kidney Disease: Improving Global Outcomes (KDIGO) Acute Kidney Injury Work Group. KDIGO clinical practice guideline for acute kidney injury. *Kidney Int Suppl.* 2012;2:1–138.
10. Bellomo R, Ronco C, Kellum JA, et al. Acute Dialysis Quality Initiative w. Acute renal failure - definition, outcome measures, animal models, fluid therapy and information technology needs: the Second International Consensus Conference of the Acute Dialysis Quality Initiative (ADQI) Group. *Crit Care.* 2004;8:R204–R212.
13. Palevsky PM, Liu KD, Brophy PD, et al. KDOQI US commentary on the 2012 KDIGO clinical practice guideline for acute kidney injury. *Am J Kidney Dis.* 2013;61:649–672.
19. Vanmassenhove J, Vanholder R, Nagler E, et al. Urinary and serum biomarkers for the diagnosis of acute kidney injury: an in-depth review of the literature. *Nephrol Dial Transplant.* 2013;28: 254–273.
29. Hoste EA, Bagshaw SM, Bellomo R, et al. Epidemiology of acute kidney injury in critically ill patients: the multinational AKI-EPI study. *Intensive Care Med.* 2015;41:1411–1423.
59. Kirkpatrick AW, Roberts DJ, De Waele J, et al. Intra-abdominal hypertension and the abdominal compartment syndrome: updated consensus definitions and clinical practice guidelines from the World Society of the Abdominal Compartment Syndrome. *Intensive Care Med.* 2013;39:1190–1206.
101. Mishra J, Dent C, Tarabishi R, et al. Neutrophil gelatinase-associated lipocalin (NGAL) as a biomarker for acute renal injury after cardiac surgery. *Lancet.* 2005;365:1231–1238.
108. Koyner JL, Vaidya VS, Bennett MR, et al. Urinary biomarkers in the clinical prognosis and early detection of acute kidney injury. *Clin J Am Soc Nephrol.* 2010;5:2154–2165.
110. Parikh CR, Coca SG, Thiessen-Philbrook H, et al. Postoperative biomarkers predict acute kidney injury and poor outcomes after adult cardiac surgery. *J Am Soc Nephrol.* 2011;22:1748–1757.
114. Ichimura T, Hung CC, Yang SA, et al. Kidney injury molecule-1: a tissue and urinary biomarker for nephrotoxicant-induced renal injury. *Am J Physiol Renal Physiol.* 2004;286:F552–F563.
129. Susantitaphong P, Siribamrungwong M, Doi K, et al. Performance of urinary liver-type fatty acid-binding protein in acute kidney injury: a meta-analysis. *Am J Kidney Dis.* 2013;61:430–439.
133. Faubel S, Patel NU, Lockhart ME, et al. Renal relevant radiology: use of ultrasonography in patients with AKI. *Clin J Am Soc Nephrol.* 2014;9:382–394.
143. Waikar SS, McMahon GM. Expanding the role for kidney biopsies in acute kidney injury. *Semin Nephrol.* 2018;38:12–20.
144. Humphreys BD, Soiffer RJ, Magee CC. Renal failure associated with cancer and its treatment: an update. *J Am Soc Nephrol.* 2005;16:151–161.
152. Perazella MA, Moeckel GW. Nephrotoxicity from chemotherapeutic agents: clinical manifestations, pathobiology, and prevention/therapy. *Semin Nephrol.* 2010;30:570–581.
156. Cortazar FB, Marrone KA, Troxell ML, et al. Clinicopathological features of acute kidney injury associated with immune checkpoint inhibitors. *Kidney Int.* 2016;90:638–647.
164. Lopez-Olivo MA, Pratt G, Palla SL, et al. Rasburicase in tumor lysis syndrome of the adult: a systematic review and meta-analysis. *Am J Kidney Dis.* 2013;62:481–492.
175. Bridoux F, Carron PL, Pegourie B, et al. Effect of high-cutoff hemodialysis vs conventional hemodialysis on hemodialysis independence among patients with myeloma cast nephropathy: a randomized clinical trial. *JAMA.* 2017;318:2099–2110.
180. Sibai BM, Kustermann L, Velasco J. Current understanding of severe preeclampsia, pregnancy-associated hemolytic uremic syndrome, thrombotic thrombocytopenic purpura, hemolysis, elevated liver enzymes, and low platelet syndrome, and postpartum acute renal failure: different clinical syndromes or just different names? *Curr Opin Nephrol Hypertens.* 1994;3:436–445.
186. Thakar CV, Worley S, Arrigain S, et al. Influence of renal dysfunction on mortality after cardiac surgery: modifying effect of preoperative renal function. *Kidney Int.* 2005;67:1112–1119.
192. Thakar CV, Arrigain S, Worley S, et al. A clinical score to predict acute renal failure after cardiac surgery. *J Am Soc Nephrol.* 2005;16:162–168.
197. Lamy A, Devereaux PJ, Prabhakaran D, et al. Off-pump or on-pump coronary-artery bypass grafting at 30 days. *N Engl J Med.* 2012;366:1489–1497.
208. Schrier RW, Parikh CR. Comparison of renal injury in myeloablative autologous, myeloablative allogeneic and non-myeloablative allogeneic haematopoietic cell transplantation. *Nephrol Dial Transplant.* 2005;20:678–683.
227. Angeli P, Gines P, Wong F, et al. Diagnosis and management of acute kidney injury in patients with cirrhosis: revised consensus recommendations of the International Club of Ascites. *Gut.* 2015;64: 531–537.
239. Gluud LL, Kjaer MS, Christensen E. Terlipressin for hepatorenal syndrome. *Cochrane Database Syst Rev.* 2006;(4):CD005162.
249. Chertow GM, Burdick E, Honour M, et al. Acute kidney injury, mortality, length of stay, and costs in hospitalized patients. *J Am Soc Nephrol.* 2005;16:3365–3370.
304. Self WH, Semler MW, Wanderer JP, et al. Balanced crystalloids versus saline in noncritically ill adults. *N Engl J Med.* 2018;378:819–828.
305. Semler MW, Self WH, Wanderer JP, et al. Balanced crystalloids versus saline in critically ill adults. *N Engl J Med.* 2018;378:829–839.
309. Schortgen F, Lacherade JC, Bruneel F, et al. Effects of hydroxyethylstarch and gelatin on renal function in severe sepsis: a multicentre randomised study. *Lancet.* 2001;357:911–916.
354. Malbrain ML, Cheatham ML, Kirkpatrick A, et al. Results from the International Conference of Experts on Intra-abdominal Hypertension and Abdominal Compartment Syndrome. I. Definitions. *Intensive Care Med.* 2006;32:1722–1732.
366. Rivers E, Nguyen B, Havstad S, et al. Early goal-directed therapy in the treatment of severe sepsis and septic shock. *N Engl J Med.* 2001;345:1368–1377.
369. Investigators A, Group ACT, Peake SL, et al. Goal-directed resuscitation for patients with early septic shock. *N Engl J Med.* 2014;371: 1496–1506.
370. Investigators P, Rowan KM, Angus DC, et al. Early, goal-directed therapy for septic shock - a patient-level meta-analysis. *N Engl J Med.* 2017;376:2223–2234.
373. Van den Berghe G, Wilmer A, Hermans G, et al. Intensive insulin therapy in the medical ICU. *N Engl J Med.* 2006;354:449–461.
375. Finfer S, Chittock DR, Su SY, et al. Intensive versus conventional glucose control in critically ill patients. *N Engl J Med.* 2009;360: 1283–1297.
377. Myles PS, Bellomo R, Corcoran T, et al. Restrictive versus liberal fluid therapy for major abdominal surgery. *N Engl J Med.* 2018;378: 2263–2274.
395. McCullough PA, Wolyn R, Rocher LL, et al. Acute renal failure after coronary intervention: incidence, risk factors, and relationship to mortality. *Am J Med.* 1997;103:368–375.
397. McDonald JS, McDonald RJ, Comin J, et al. Frequency of acute kidney injury following intravenous contrast medium administration: a systematic review and meta-analysis. *Radiology.* 2013;267:119–128.
403. Nijssen EC, Rennenberg RJ, Nelemans PJ, et al. Prophylactic hydration to protect renal function from intravascular iodinated contrast material in patients at high risk of contrast-induced nephropathy (AMACING): a prospective, randomised, phase 3, controlled, open-label, non-inferiority trial. *Lancet.* 2017;389:1312–1322.

419. Weisbord SD, Gallagher M, Jneid H, et al. Outcomes after Angiography with Sodium Bicarbonate and Acetylcysteine. *N Engl J Med.* 2018;378:603–614.
451. Giacoppo D, Capodanno D, Capranzano P, et al. Meta-analysis of randomized controlled trials of preprocedural statin administration for reducing contrast-induced acute kidney injury in patients undergoing coronary catheterization. *Am J Cardiol.* 2014;114:541–548.
493. Hausenloy DJ, Candilio L, Evans R, et al. Remote ischemic preconditioning and outcomes of cardiac surgery. *N Engl J Med.* 2015;373:1408–1417.
523. Mehta RL, Pascual MT, Soroko S, et al. Diuretics, mortality, and nonrecovery of renal function in acute renal failure. *JAMA.* 2002; 288:2547–2553.
586. Zarbock A, Kellum JA, Schmidt C, et al. Effect of early vs delayed initiation of renal replacement therapy on mortality in critically ill patients with acute kidney injury: the ELAIN randomized clinical trial. *JAMA.* 2016;315:2190–2199.
587. Gaudry S, Hajage D, Schortgen F, et al. Initiation strategies for renal-replacement therapy in the intensive care unit. *N Engl J Med.* 2016;375:122–133.
588. Barbar SD, Clere-Jehl R, Bourredjem A, et al. Timing of renal-replacement therapy in patients with acute kidney injury and sepsis. *N Engl J Med.* 2018;379:1431–1442.
594. VA/NIH Acute Renal Failure Trial Network, Palevsky PM, Zhang JH, et al. Intensity of renal support in critically ill patients with acute kidney injury. *N Engl J Med.* 2008;359:7–20.
632. Vinsonneau C, Camus C, Combes A, et al. Continuous venovenous haemodiafiltration versus intermittent haemodialysis for acute renal failure in patients with multiple-organ dysfunction syndrome: a multicentre randomised trial. *Lancet.* 2006;368:379–385.
657. Bellomo R, Cass A, Cole L, et al. Intensity of continuous renal-replacement therapy in critically ill patients. *N Engl J Med.* 2009;361: 1627–1638.

# 30 Pathophysiology of Proteinuria

Norberto Perico | Andrea Remuzzi | Giuseppe Remuzzi

CHAPTER OUTLINE



## MECHANISMS OF PROTEINURIA

One of the most common features of glomerular diseases is an abnormal excretion of plasma proteins in the urine. Proteinuria is the cause and effect of several complications not only at a kidney but also at a systemic level. There are complex changes in the structure and function of the glomerular capillary, as well as in the entire nephron, that are responsible for the final elevation in urine protein concentration in several kidney disorders. In this chapter, before describing the consequences of proteinuria, the pathophysiology of protein excretion is reviewed.

The functional properties of the glomerular filtration barrier, tubular interaction with filtered proteins and the mechanisms of proteinuria have been reviewed in detail,[1] and the characterization of structural molecules relevant to the filtration barrier in glomerular endothelial cells and in particular on podocytes has been reported.[2,3] There are, in principle, two distinct phenomena that can result in proteinuria. The first is the elevation of glomerular filtration of circulating plasma proteins that are almost completely retained in the circulating plasma in normal physiologic conditions; the second is a defective or incomplete reabsorption of proteins by the proximal tubule. The two phenomena are interrelated, and likely are both present in so-called glomerular proteinuria, when proteins the size of albumin and larger are present in urine. Despite several experimental and clinical observations investigating the structural and molecular alterations involved in kidney diseases resulting in proteinuria,[4] the precise nature of the functional changes responsible and their quantification remain the subject of numerous ongoing investigations.[5]

### STRUCTURE AND FUNCTION OF THE GLOMERULAR CAPILLARY WALL

The function of the glomerular capillary is to allow a large amount of water and small solute filtration while efficiently restricting glomerular passage of protein macromolecules within blood circulation. This selective function is specific to the glomerular capillary membrane, which is far more permeable to water than any other capillary membrane in the body. With the development of glomerular diseases, the capillary membrane structure at molecular and/or cellular level may be altered, resulting in loss of hydraulic permeability, reduction in surface area available for filtration, and consequent loss of glomerular filtration rate (GFR). Despite the reduction in permeability to water, the capillary membrane often becomes more permeable to circulating macromolecules. Experimental research has elucidated a number of glomerular structural and molecular alterations that are responsible for these functional changes.

### GLOMERULAR CAPILLARY WALL ORGANIZATION

Morphologic studies available in the literature describe in detail the complex organization of the glomerular capillary and the capillary membrane (see Chapter 2). However, the interpretation of filtration barrier function has been largely based on major simplifications. Thus although the glomerular capillary is composed of numerous branching segments, the glomerular capillary organization has usually been considered as a simple capillary segment or as a set of several uniform segments in parallel. Similarly, the capillary membrane has been considered as a uniform three-layer structure. As described later, recent investigations allow a better understanding of the functional effects of the geometric and spatial organization of the glomerular capillary, as well as specific features of cell organization and interactions at the capillary membrane level. These aspects have revealed some new insights in the mechanisms responsible for glomerular capillary dysfunction.

#### Glomerular Capillary Network

According to classic optical microscopy observations of kidney tissue sections, the capillary network is composed of a number of capillary segments connecting afferent and efferent arterioles within a tuft that, in humans, has a mean diameter of 120–150 μm. More realistic and direct visualizations of the capillary organization are usually derived from scanning electron microscopy, but this technique allows predominantly only views from the outer surface of the capillary. Specific investigations with reconstructions from serial sections[6] or confocal microscopy[7] allow investigation of the capillary segment organization and, in particular, calculation of blood flow distribution and water filtration along the network.[8] Due to the large number of capillary segments, around 200 in the rat, and their apparent uniform size, the blood flow is expected to be uniformly distributed along the network with lower blood velocity as compared with that in the afferent arteriole. This hemodynamic arrangement allows the blood to remain in close contact with the filtration membrane. However, more detailed geometric reconstructions of the glomerular capillary show that the network has some heterogeneity. The size of some capillary segments (with diameters less than 3–4 μm)[6] would suggest that they are perfused only by plasma, excluding red blood cell transit, and may represent a sort of shunt in the network to decrease overall network pressure. This finely organized geometry is the result of cellular organization and remodeling and seems to be importantly affected by disease processes, resulting in simplification of capillary network, changes in local pressure and flow distribution, ultimately resulting in capillary obliteration in areas of segmental sclerosis.[9] These local hemodynamic changes affect the filtration function of the capillary network, as elevation of blood flow and hydraulic pressure is expected to occur in some capillary segments leading to abnormal filtration of circulating proteins.[10]

### Glomerular Capillary Wall

At a smaller scale the organization of the glomerular capillary membrane is rather heterogeneous. The arrangement that is generally described usually refers to the portion of the capillary wall that is considered the filtering surface, characterized by a three-layer composition consisting of endothelial cells, glomerular basement membrane (GBM), and epithelial cells. The structure and function of this highly differentiated arrangement of cells and matrix is presented in Chapter 2. Mechanisms whereby structural and functional changes may result in abnormal protein filtration and ultimately in proteinuria are reviewed later.

According to the classic concept, hydraulic resistance and macromolecule retention are functions of the so-called filtering surface of the glomerular capillary membrane, but recent evidence indicates that the entire structure of the epithelial cells and the relative position of the capillary membrane within the tuft may also affect water and macromolecule filtration. As reported by Neal et al.,[11] a large fraction of the filtration membrane is covered by epithelial cell bodies or by the presence of adjacent epithelial cells. The three-dimensional spaces created by these structures have been called subpodocyte (SPS) and interpodocyte spaces (IPS), respectively. Theoretical analysis of the transport of both water and macromolecules through the SPS[12] indicates that the structural organization of this compartment induces significant resistance to water flow from the filtration membrane to the urinary space. This resistance appears to not be insignificant as compared with that of the three-layer membrane structure. Macromolecule transport may also be influenced by the SPS.[13]

Specific evaluations of the structural changes that characterize SPS and IPS, and their functional consequences in experimental models of kidney disease, or in patients with renal dysfunction, are not yet available. The difficulties in obtaining such quantitative evaluations derive from the heterogeneous nature of these three-dimensional structures. In addition, they can be visualized only using electron microscopy, both transmission electron microscopy and scanning electron microscopy (SEM), but their quantification is not easy because they are in the inner portion of the glomerular capillary tuft.[14]

## ULTRASTRUCTURE OF THE GLOMERULAR CAPILLARY MEMBRANE

### Endothelial Cell Layer

Glomerular endothelial cells are the most fenestrated in the circulation, with a pore area in peripheral zone that occupies from 20% to 50% of the cell surface.[15] The surface of endothelial cells has been considered to have negative electric charge due to the presence of electrical charges of glycoproteins, glycosaminoglycans, and membrane-associated proteoglycans (glycocalyx).[16] These negative charges are expected to act as an electrostatic barrier to the transmural passage of anionic circulating proteins, such as albumin. Thus even if endothelial fenestrae are much larger than albumin (about 60 nm in diameter as compared with a radius of 3.6 nm for albumin), negatively charged circulating macromolecules stay away from the endothelial surface due to electrical repulsion and remain within the circulation. It is now evident[1] that the first restriction to albumin filtration across the glomerular membrane consists of the endothelial surface layer and its role is to substantially decrease protein concentration in the fluid that enters the GBM layer. Endothelial cell glycocalyx expression is importantly affected by fluid shear stress.[17] Increased shear stress is associated with glycocalyx formation and reorganization on the cell surface in contact with fluid flow, with lower expression in static conditions. Thus pathologic conditions in which changes in glomerular capillary flow (i.e., reduced flow) may occur are expected to decrease glycocalyx formation and consequently reduce the retention of anionic proteins within the bloodstream. It has been demonstrated[18] that disruption of the endothelial glycocalyx increases glomerular albumin filtration even in the presence of only minor changes in both the GBM and glomerular epithelial cells. The role of the glomerular polysaccharide-rich endothelial surface layer (ESL) to act as a filtration barrier for large molecules such as albumin has been recently confirmed in C57Bl/6 mice given long-term infusion of hyaluronidase, a hyaluronan degradating enzyme that disrupts the endothelial glycocalyx proteoglycans.[19,20] A new electron microscopy technique that allows visualization of the ESL and albumin transport within the entire glomerular section at nanometer resolution was used in this set of experiments.[21] It was shown that glomerular fenestrae are filled with dense negatively charged polysaccharide structures that are largely removed in the presence of circulating hyaluronidase, leaving the polysaccharide surface of other glomerular cells intact.[19] Both retention of cationic ferritin in the glomerular basement membrane and systemic blood pressure were unaltered. Hyaluronidase treatment, however, induced albumin passage across the endothelium in 90% of glomeruli, whereas this could not be observed in untreated control animals. Nevertheless, there was no net albuminuria due to binding and uptake of filtered albumin by the podocytes and parietal epithelium. The ESL structure and function completely recovered after cessation of hyaluronidase infusion. Thus the polyanionic ESL component hyaluronan is a key component of the glomerular endothelial permeability barrier whose reduction facilitates albumin passage across the endothelial layer and the GBM toward the epithelial compartment.

### Glomerular Basement Membrane Organization

The basement membrane layer that characterizes the capillary wall (see Chapter 2) has been shown to exert an important contribution to protein retention by the capillary wall. The molecular composition and organization of this basement membrane would suggest a sieving function due to both size and charge.[22] Structural proteins such as collagen type IV and laminin, as well as heparansulfate proteoglycans, represent not only a steric hindrance but also a charge effect on the filtration of circulating molecules. Both vivo and in vitro studies[23] indicate that small neutral and charged solutes are freely filtered across this extracellular matrix layer, but an important restriction is observed for macromolecules the size of albumin or larger. Thus changes in composition and/or organization of GBM molecules are expected to reduce water filtration and retention of circulating macromolecules.[24] The role of GBM in glomerular permselectivity is highlighted by the discovery of mutations affecting genes encoding GBM components in humans and mouse models.[25] Mutations in the *COL4A3*, *COL4A4*, or *COL4A5* genes that encode collagen type IV α3, α4, and α5 chains, respectively, cause Alport syndrome, a hereditary glomerular, auditory, and ocular disease.[26] Mutations in the gene encoding laminin β2 (*LAMB2*) cause Pierson syndrome, a congenital nephrotic syndrome with associated extrarenal manifestation.[27] Studies using knockout mouse models of Alport and Pierson syndromes have documented that GBM, defective of these specific components, is more permeable to ferritin or albumin than is the normal GBM, indicating it has a role in glomerular permselectivity.[28,29]

Tight adherence to the basement membrane is required to prevent podocyte detachment into the Bowman capsule. On a molecular level, a multitude of adhesion receptors including heterodimeric integrins mediate interaction of cells with the surrounding basement membrane.[30,31] One common form of integrin-mediated adhesion is focal adhesions (FAs), which have been extensively studied in cultured cells.[31] Recently, FERM-domain protein EPB41L5 has been identified as a highly enriched podocyte-specific FA component.[32] This provided the clue to document that genetic deletion of the related *Epb41l5* gene resulted in severe proteinuria, detachment of podocytes, and development of focal and segmental glomerulosclerosis.[32]

### Epithelial Filtration Slits

A large amount of experimental and clinical research has been generated in the past few decades on the molecular and structural composition of the epithelial junctional complex, known as filtration slits. The characterization of several molecular components of this structure[33] has allowed detailed definition of the proteins that compose the filtration slits (see Fig. 30.1); however, detailed information on the ultrastructure of this intracellular junction is still under investigation.[5] The original observations by Rodewald and Karnowsky[34] suggested a zipper-like structure of the epithelial filtration slit, with rectangular openings of 4 by 14 nm. These

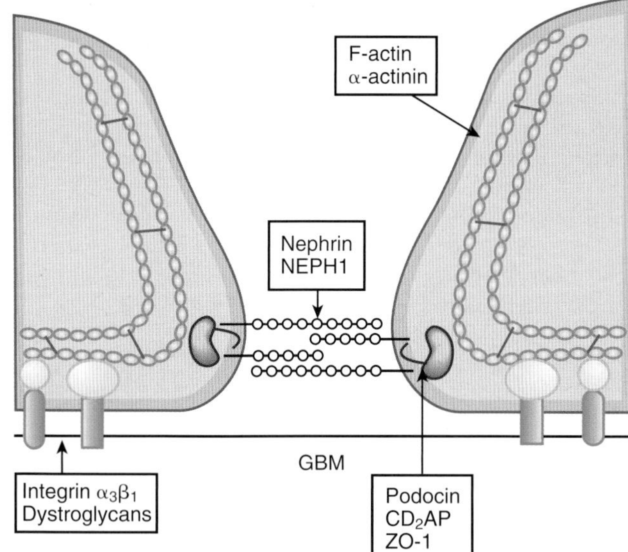


**Fig. 30.1** Hypothetical model of the podocyte slit diaphragm. See text for discussion. (From Jalanko H. Pathogenesis of proteinuria: Lessons learned from nephrin and podocin. *Pediatr Nephrol.* 2003;18:487–491, with permission.)

dimensions are in contrast with the observation that a limited amount of albumin can traverse the filtration barrier in physiologic conditions,[1] because the mean molecular radius of albumin is 3.6 nm. Observations with high-resolution SEM and three-dimensional electron microscopy reconstruction[35] suggest that the filtration slits are perforated by larger openings of the size of albumin, with more complex geometry. The morphology of the filtration slit has been further imaged with high-resolution SEM, providing evidence of a new ultrastructure composed of circular pores of different sizes with an average radius of 12 nm[36,37] (Fig. 30.2). Despite the small size of filtration slit openings, a large amount of plasma water is filtered because of the high filtration slit length per unit surface area. As mentioned earlier, under physiologic conditions about 20% of peripheral capillary filtering surface is directly in communication with the Bowman space, and the epithelial slits are the last resistance encountered by water and filtered solutes.[11] In the remaining portion of the glomerular membrane, water and solutes, after passing through the filtration slits, must traverse the SPS and the IPS before arriving in the Bowman capsule.[11]

It should also be considered that the flow of ultrafiltrate over the cell surface directly causes shear stress (SS) on the podocyte membrane associated with the filtration slit as well as to cell body. In animal models of solitary kidney where filtrate flow is increased, SS on the podocyte surface increases 1.5- to 2-fold.[38] These forces are highest within the central portion of the filtration slit diaphragm. The forces acting parallel to the GBM are balanced by the mechanical resistance produced by the slit diaphragm complex, opposing foot processes, preventing widening of the slit.[39] On the other side, SS acting perpendicular to the GBM plane, tends to detach the foot process from the GBM. However, these shear forces are balanced by the tight junctions between podocyte cell membrane and GBM proteins that allow transmission of this mechanical load into the cytoskeleton apparatus. These

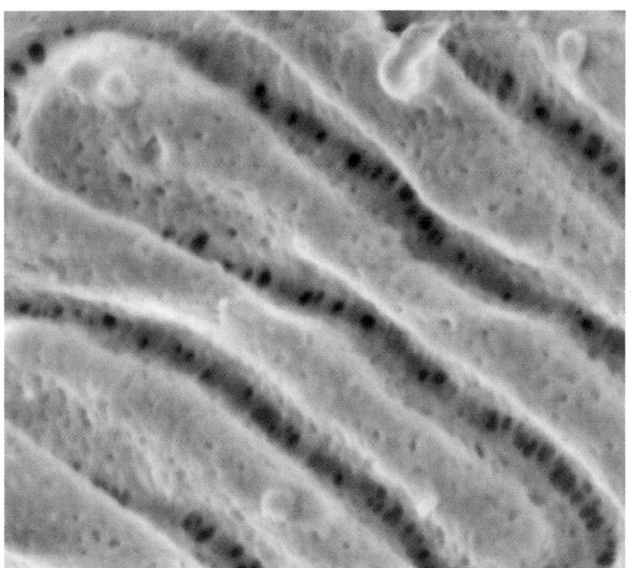

**Fig. 30.2 Visualization of epithelial filtration slits obtained using scanning electron microscopy and an in-lens detector to enhance electron detection.** Sample was obtained from a Wistar rat, dehydrated with a critical point dryer. The ultrastucture of the filtration slit appears different from the model conventionally proposed in the literature.[34] The radius of the circular pores averages 12 nm. (From Gagliardini E, Conti S, Benigni A, et al. Imaging of the porous ultrastructure of the glomerular epithelial filtration slit. *J Am Soc Nephrol.* 2010;21:2081–2089.)

complex mechanical challenges present in physiologic conditions within the podocyte, induced by glomerular ultrafiltrate flow, make mechanotransduction an important function of podocytes. In addition, SS acting on the podocyte membrane adjacent to the filtration slit, as well as to the entire cell body, seems to play a central role in the process of podocyte damage that results in foot process effacement as well as in podocyte detachment from the GBM.[39]

## THEORETICAL MODELS OF GLOMERULAR PERMSELECTIVITY

In addition to structural investigation, functional evaluations of the glomerular capillary wall permselectivity have been extensively used to characterize physiologic conditions and to quantify the effects of pathologic changes. These studies are based on the estimation of filtration of endogenous plasma molecules, such as albumin, IgG, and other proteins, or on the use of test macromolecules of different size, either neutral or electrically charged. Macromolecule filtration depends on convective and diffusive transport that is influenced by glomerular hemodynamic conditions (glomerular plasma flow and pressure) and water filtration. As described later, several investigators have developed theoretical models to derive intrinsic sieving properties of the capillary wall from estimation of macromolecule filtration in experimental and human studies.

### Heteroporous Models of Glomerular Size Selectivity

The most-used theoretical models of glomerular size-selective function are based on the assumption of water-filled pores of different sizes as functional equivalents of the glomerular membrane. The passage of water is calculated along the network taking into account the balance between hydraulic and oncotic pressure, as well as membrane hydraulic permeability.[9,40] For the calculation of solute filtration, convective and diffusive transport are taken into account, whereas pore resistance to solute filtration is based on steric and hydrodynamic hindrance.[10,40] The use of these models indicated that glomerular hypothetical pores have mean radius of 4.5–5.0 nm in humans, and a lognormal statistical distribution of pore size around the mean. However, the best simulation of experimental measurements has been obtained assuming that in parallel to restrictive pores, there is a nonselective shunt pathway.[41]

The application of these theoretical models clearly showed that in several proteinuric conditions the increased glomerular filtration of the largest neutral test macromolecules is not associated with important changes in the size of restrictive pores, but rather with changes in the nonselective shunt pathway.[42] This suggests that in normal conditions the small amount of albumin present in the urine may be the result of a small amount of protein filtration that takes place in some focal areas of the epithelial junction, while the majority of the filtration slits retain the protein.

### Fiber Models of Glomerular Size Selectivity

Fiber models of solute filtration across the glomerular membrane have also been developed and used.[1] Similar to porous models, the fiber models allow separation of the effect of glomerular hemodynamic changes from those related to intrinsic changes of glomerular membrane selective properties. The advantage of the fiber model is that other than steric hindrance, the effect of membrane and protein electrical charge can be embedded in the model, allowing the estimation of changes in membrane properties both in terms of molecular structural organization and electric charge.[43] This modeling approach indicates that filtration of albumin is importantly affected by electrical charge, whereas on the basis of size selectivity alone the molecule could easily escape the capillary membrane.

*Multilayer Membrane Models.* The structural complexity of the glomerular capillary wall suggested a need to develop more complex theoretical models to simulate more reliably the resistance to water and solute movement across the membrane. These models have been developed and tested by Deen et al.,[22] with the aim to estimate the role of individual layers on the filtration of water and solutes. In these models the resistance of endothelial cells, GBM, and epithelial cells is assumed to act in series. In normal conditions, hydraulic resistance of the endothelial layer is negligible, while GBM and epithelial resistance are comparable. The contribution of the three layers to solute hindrance has been considered and the major contribution to membrane selectivity is exerted by the filtration slit.[44] Although these models describe in detail the physical interaction of water and macromolecules with the membrane structure, their application is difficult because they require extensive measurement of utrastructural parameters.

### Models of Glomerular Charge Selectivity

As mentioned previously, the fact that negative electrical charges are present in the glomerular membrane (in the glycocalyx of endothelial cells, the negatively charged heparansulfate of the GBM and the glycoproteins of the cell membrane of podocytes) strongly suggests that circulating negatively charged proteins, like albumin, are restricted within the circulation not only for their size but also for electrical charges. The use of theoretical models for the simulation of charge-selective function of the glomerular membrane allowed estimation of the amount of electrical charge present within the membrane.[10] These studies indicated that electrical charge is an important component of glomerular permselective function, and changes in membrane electrical charge can explain abnormal albumin filtration even without changes in membrane structural parameters, such as pore size or fiber size and length per unit volume. However, the use of these models to investigate glomerular membrane charge is limited by the difficulties in measuring glomerular filtration of charged test solutes that interfere with circulating macromolecules and are not filtered simply on the basis to their molecular shape and electric charge alone.[45]

## PROTEIN REABSORPTION BY THE PROXIMAL TUBULE

### PROXIMAL TUBULE STRUCTURE AND FUNCTION

The glomerular ultrafiltrate, once flowing inside the proximal tubule, undergoes important changes in composition, due to processes of water and solute reabsorption. In addition to small solutes and electrolytes, proteins such as albumin are also reabsorbed.[46] Thus final urinary excretion of proteins depends largely on the interaction of proteins with proximal tubular epithelial cells. These cells form a compact epithelial layer with a basal side in contact with the tubular basement membrane, an intercellular junction, and a luminal surface in contact with tubular fluid. They are characterized by a large number of mitochondria, an index of important metabolic activity, and a prominent layer of microvilli (Fig. 30.3) that results in the extension of the luminal cell surface area.

The microvillar membrane is the site for receptor mediated endocytosis of low-density lipoprotein and negatively charged proteins. Albumin in the proximal tubule undergoes specific binding to the extracellular domain of a membrane receptor complex, megalin–cubilin receptor[46] (Fig. 30.4), which is followed by the internalization of the protein by membrane vesicles. These vesicles are then processed for protein degradation, amino acid transport to basal membrane of tubule cells, release into interstitial space, and ultimately into peritubular capillaries. Receptors are recycled into the luminal cell membrane by dense apical tubules.

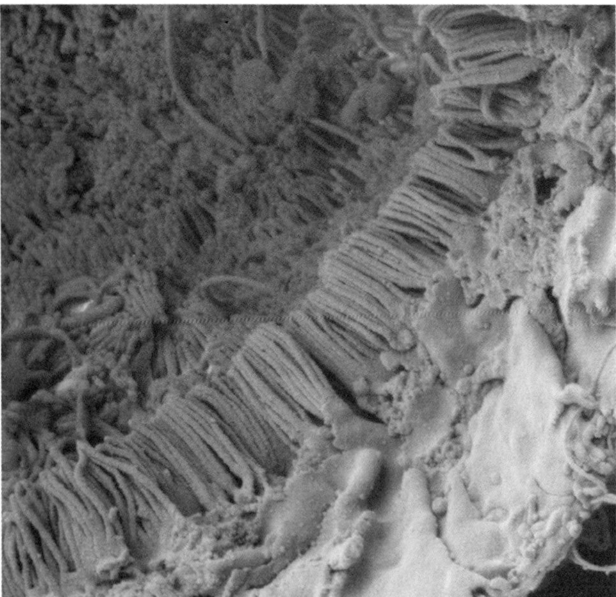

**Fig. 30.3 Scanning electron microscopy of proximal tubule cells.** Inner cell membrane is covered by microvilli of the brush border. In order to be taken up by cell receptors, albumin must diffuse through the dense layer of microvilli.

The amount of albumin filtered at glomerular level and that reabsorbed by proximal tubule cells is not easy to quantify. Ideally one would have to sample the early proximal tubule and quantify albumin concentration in these microsamples. Despite technical difficulties, micropuncture techniques have been used to avoid sample contamination with plasma present close to the puncture site (in interstitial space and peritubular capillaries). The protein concentration in the urinary space was estimated to range from 10 to 25 μg/mL.[47,48] More recently, direct in vivo imaging of fluorescent albumin by two-photon microscopy has been used to directly estimate albumin concentration in the Bowman capsule fluid.[49] It has been recently demonstrated that reliable measurements of albumin fractional clearance, the ratio between urinary space and plasma albumin concentration, allow estimation of an albumin concentration of about 60 μg/mL in the Bowman capsule in normal conditions in the rat,[50] corresponding to a fractional clearance of 0.002. Once filtered at glomerular level, albumin and smaller proteins are almost entirely reabsorbed at the proximal tubular level. In pathologic conditions, when the filtered load overwhelms the reabsorptive capacity, proteins are detected in the urine.

### THEORETICAL MODELS FOR TUBULAR REABSORPTION

The process of albumin reabsorption by proximal tubule cells has been modeled[51] to allow a quantitative assessment of the relationship between albumin ultrafiltration at the glomerular level, proximal tubular uptake, and final excretion in the urine. In this model, the process of diffusion of albumin across the microvillar space and the uptake of the protein by tubule cell receptors are taken into consideration. The amount of albumin that is reabsorbed during the proximal tubule passage is simulated assuming the presence of a high-affinity site for binding and internalization of albumin at the base of tubule cell microvilli. According to in vitro and ex vivo data, these receptors are assumed to be half-saturated at concentrations similar to those mentioned for albumin in the Bowman capsule (20–30 μg/mL). The effect of the assumption of different values for the maximum absorptive capacity ($V_{max}$) on the albumin concentration along the proximal tubule is reported in Fig. 30.5. This modeling approach showed that the transport of albumin across the microvillar space has a modest effect on the value of $V_{max}$ needed to fit micropuncture data.

The two most important parameters that determine the fraction of reabsorption of albumin are the single-nephron glomerular filtration rate (SNGFR) and the albumin concentration in the filtrate fluid (Cb). A 50% increase in SNGFR is predicted to cause a four- to fivefold increase in albumin excretion in rats and humans. For large increases in Cb, such as those measured by micropuncture,[52] there is a threshold above which the reabsorption of albumin is overwhelmed and the protein appears in the urine. According to theoretical analysis[51] this value corresponds to an albumin

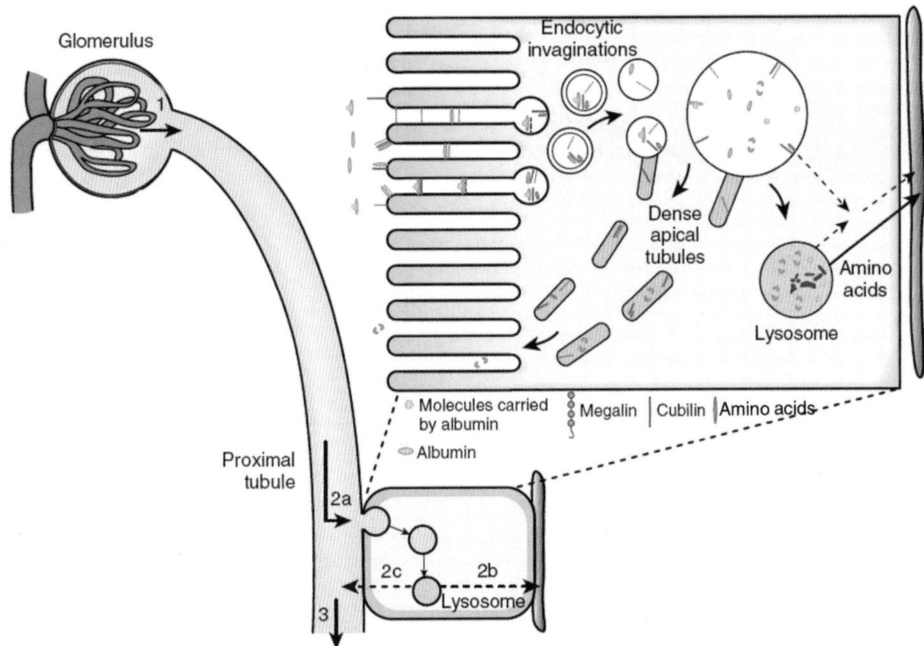


**Fig. 30.4 Pathways of albumin degradation in the proximal tubule.** Albumin is filtered in the glomeruli *(1)* and reabsorbed by the proximal tubule cells by receptor-mediated endocytosis *(2a)*. Internalization by endocytosis is followed by transport into lysosomes for degradation. Some intact albumin may escape tubular reabsorption *(3)*, the amount being greater as the glomerular filtration fraction of albumin increases or tubular function is compromised. The *upper right* shows a schematic representation of the intracellular pathways following endocytic uptake of albumin and possible associated substances. Following binding to the receptors, cubilin, or megalin, the receptor–albumin complex is directed into coated pits for endocytosis. The complex dissociates following vesicular acidification, most likely also leading to the release of any bound substances. Albumin is transferred to the lysosomal compartment for degradation. Some albumin may be degraded within a late endocytic compartment and recycled as fragments to be released at the luminal surface. Alternatively, albumin fragments may be recycled from the lysosomal compartment by a yet unknown route. Receptors recycle through dense apical tubules, whereas released substances carried by albumin may be released into the cytosol or transported across the tubular cell. (From Birn H, Christensen EI. Renal albumin absorption in physiology and pathology. *Kidney Int.* 2006;69:440–449, with permission.)

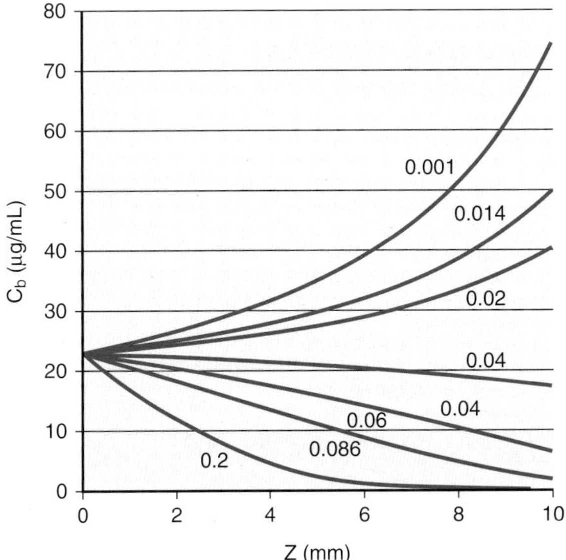


**Fig. 30.5 Theoretical calculation of albumin concentration along the proximal tubule.** Predictions of bulk albumin concentration (*Cb*) vs. axial position (*z*) in rats for $V_{max}$ ranging from 0.001 to 0.2 ng/sec per millimeter squared. The curve that most closely corresponds to normal rats is that for $V_{max}$ = 0.086 ng/sec per millimeter squared. (From Lazzara MJ, Deen WM. Model of albumin reabsorption in the proximal tubule. *Am J Physiol Renal Physiol.* 2007;292:F430–439, with permission.)

fractional clearance of approximately 0.001. The combination of increased SNGFR and elevation in filtrate albumin concentration is shown to have important additive effects.

## PROTEINURIA OF GLOMERULAR ORIGIN

Changes in glomerular protein filtration and/or defects in tubular reabsorption cause the appearance of proteins in the urine. At values exceeding 300 mg/day, or 200 mg/L the condition is termed *proteinuria.* Smaller amounts of proteins may appear in the urine in the early stages of progressive diseases, such as diabetic nephropathy. In this case an albumin excretion between 30 and 300 mg/day (20–200 mg/L) is termed *microalbuminuria.*[53] Proteinuria is considered severe or in the "nephrotic range" when protein excretion is greater than 3.5 g/day.[1] When proteins in the urine have a large molecular weight, they are considered to have glomerular origin. If the molecular weight is low, there is evidence that the defect causing proteinuria is likely related to abnormal proximal tubular reabsorption, often related to toxic damage of tubule cells.[54] Proteinuria associated with progressive kidney disease is predominantly of glomerular origin and mainly composed of plasma albumin. Mechanisms responsible for glomerular proteinuria are discussed in the next section.

## GLOMERULAR PERMSELECTIVE DYSFUNCTION

As mentioned earlier, abnormal plasma protein filtration at glomerular level may be caused by a defect in both size and charge selectivity. Glomerular size-selective dysfunction has been extensively investigated in several kidney diseases using neutral test macromolecules, usually neutral dextrans.[42,55] These studies demonstrated that in most cases there are statistically significant changes in fractional clearance of the largest test macromolecules, whereas the fractional clearance (sieving coefficient) of molecules the size of albumin is unaltered. These data consistently indicate that permselectivity defects responsible for albumin filtration must be focal and likely due to changes in glomerular cell components, most likely the podocytes. These proteinuric conditions are frequently associated with podocyte foot process effacement and simplification, and likely with defective intercellular junctions.[56]

The quantification of the contribution of charge-selectivity defects to proteinuria is more difficult. A few experimental and clinical investigations clearly indicate that proteinuria is indeed associated with abnormal filtration of charged macromolecules,[57,58] but these data have been questioned because electrically charged test or endogenous macromolecules in the circulation are expected to interfere with other circulating charged solutes and cell membranes.[1] This would result in measured fractional clearance that does not represent effective transport of probe macromolecules. However, even without direct evidence that glomerular membrane charge distribution is altered in proteinuric conditions, the evidence that glomerular albumin filtration is increased without important changes in the fractional clearance of test macromolecules of the same size strongly suggests a role for a charge-selectivity defect in proteinuria of glomerular origin.[42,58]

Experimental and clinical research has allowed the identification of molecular defects underlying some genetic disorders associated with nephrotic syndrome. In Finnish-type nephropathy a defect in the nephrin gene NPHS1 is responsible for glomerular dysfunction, proteinuria, and end-stage renal disease.[3,59] Similarly, defects in other genes (NPHS2, LMX1B and several others) have been shown to result in defective structure and function of filtration slit proteins or glomerular epithelial cells.[60]

Another condition in which proteinuria is manifest is ischemia–reperfusion injury.[61] Studies in kidney transplantation and in experimental settings suggest that abnormal elevation of protein in the urine in this condition occurs without major changes in glomerular capillary membrane structure. The evidence indicates[62] that ischemia per se is responsible for loss of glomerular endothelial glycocalyx, and the previously mentioned effect of fluid shear stress on endothelial cell glycocalyx would reinforce this evidence. Thus, abnormal elevation of glomerular protein filtration may derive from selective changes in ultrastructure and function of membrane components.

## TUBULAR HANDLING OF EXCESSIVE FILTERED PROTEINS

### EFFECTS OF PROTEIN FILTRATION ON PROXIMAL TUBULE CELLS

An excessive increase in albumin and other plasma protein filtration may result from a defective glomerular capillary membrane and/or an increase in SNGFR. Both conditions, and their combination, result in elevated protein concentration in the ultrafiltrate. These filtered proteins are expected not to be entirely reabsorbed by proximal tubule cells, because protein reabsorption is believed to operate near maximum under physiologic conditions.

The presence of high protein concentration within the renal tubule may influence the progression of disease processes. There are at least two phenomena that are expected to occur. The first is related to the fact that if albumin is still present in tubular fluid at the end of the proximal tubule, its concentration increases substantially along the remaining portion of the nephron because of water reabsorption. Thus protein concentration in the distal tubule and collecting duct can reach very high values even for a small amount of proteins filtered at glomerular level, with the possibility for these proteins to precipitate and form protein casts.[63] Tubular obstruction may then occur and the entire nephron function lost, with complete loss of glomerular water filtration.

In addition, structural changes are expected to occur with tubular atrophy, disconnection of the tubule from the Bowman capsule and glomerular capillary tuft structural changes. This condition is frequently observed in proteinuric kidney diseases at experimental and clinical level.[64]

Even before tubular obstruction, important functional changes are expected to occur in proximal tubule cells exposed to abnormal protein concentrations. The protein overload of these cells exposes them to increased workload and this can lead to loss of reabsorptive capacity due to loss of receptor activity.[65] In this condition, the elevated protein concentration along the proximal tubule further increases due to the lower level of absorption and the concomitant water reabsorption. Thus a vicious circle develops, inducing further damage in tubule cells and progressively higher protein concentration along the entire nephron. The consequences of this abnormal glomerular filtration of plasma proteins at both the organ and systemic level are discussed in the following sections.

# RENAL CONSEQUENCES OF PROTEINURIA

## GLOMERULAR DAMAGE

Data from animal models have shown that a wide variety of insults result in a common pathway of glomerular capillary hypertension, increased permeability with excess passage of proteins across the glomerular capillary wall, and progressive glomerular injury[66] (Fig. 30.6). The key glomerular lesion is sclerosis, characterized by accumulation of extracellular matrix and obliteration of the capillary tuft leading to the loss of renal function.

### PODOCYTES: CHANGES IN FUNCTION AND CELL NUMBER

Podocytes show a fairly uniform pattern of response to damage. The intercellular junction and cytoskeletal structure of the foot processes are altered, and the cell shows a simplified, effaced phenotype.[67,68] These alterations result in the disappearance of the typical slit diaphragm structures and the development of proteinuria. Although podocyte effacement is a hallmark of podocyte disease and nephrotic syndrome, damage to these cells may present as very subtle changes that are difficult to quantify.[69] Major advances in the field of live imaging have allowed the investigation of

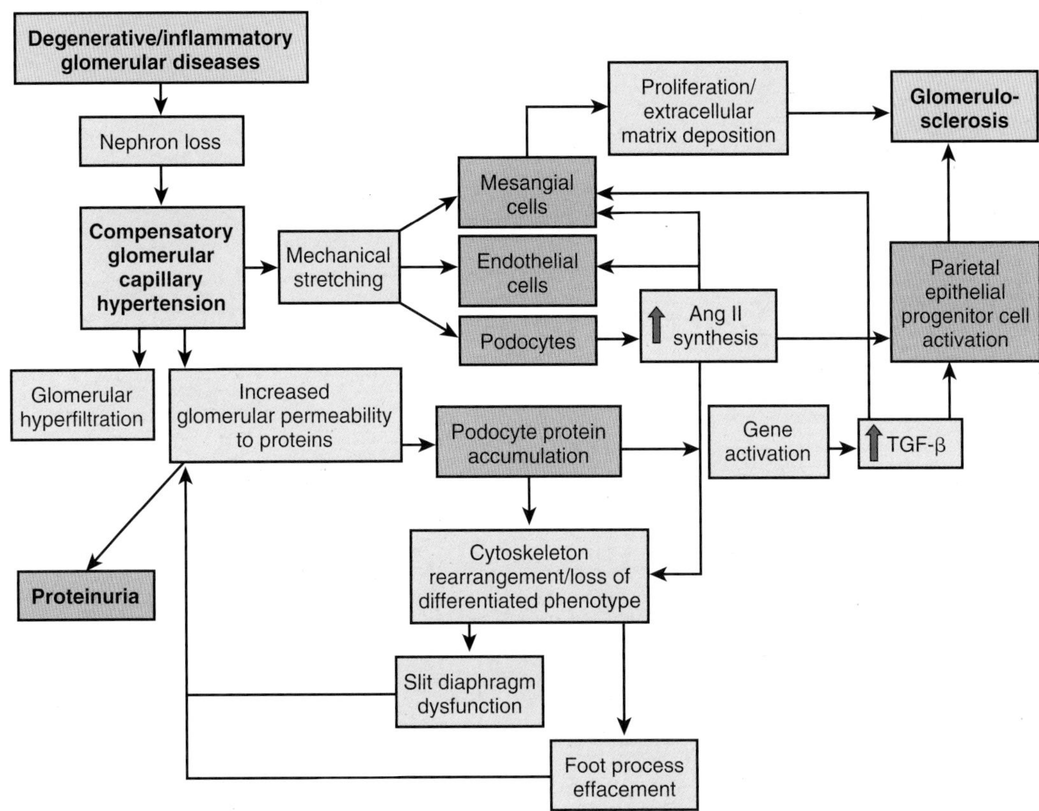


**Fig. 30.6 Mechanisms of progressive glomerular injury.** A reduction in the number of nephrons as a consequence of various glomerular diseases results in compensatory glomerular hemodynamic changes that are ultimately detrimental. In particular, by mechanical stretching, the increased glomerular capillary pressure directly injures glomerular cells. Glomerular hypertension also impairs the glomerular capillary size–selective function, which causes excessive protein ultrafiltration and eventually podocyte injury and proteinuria.

podocyte biology in unprecedented detail.[70-72] These new tools are likely to facilitate the next stage in gaining insights to podocyte responses to injury. So far there is evidence that experimental models of chronic proteinuria as well as their human counterparts (that is, minimal change glomerulopathy, focal and segmental sclerosis, diabetic nephropathy, and membranous nephropathy) have in common ultrastructural findings of severe glomerular epithelial cell damage that include vacuolization, fusion of foot processes and focal detachment of epithelial cells from the underlying basement membrane.[73] These changes appear to be the consequence mainly of persistent abnormalities in intraglomerular capillary hemodynamics. Increased capillary hydraulic pressure and flow and activation of local tissue renin–angiotensin system in podocytes[74] eventually impairs the size-selective function of the glomerular capillary wall, allowing excess plasma protein to move into the urinary space.[75]

In addition to being affected by mechanical stress, podocytes are also damaged by excessive protein load resulting from alterations of glomerular permeability to macromolecules. Protein uptake by podocytes may occur through binding to megalin, a receptor for albumin and immunoglobulin (Ig) light chains, which is endocytosed after ligand binding, as shown in cultured murine podocytes.[76] Mice with protein overload proteinuria induced by repeated injection of bovine serum albumin developed podocyte injury followed by glomerulosclerosis.[77-79] Evidence of a causal link between podocyte protein overload and podocyte damage is provided by studies showing that in rats with renal mass reduction protein accumulation in podocytes preceded cell dedifferentiation and injury, as characterized by loss of synaptopodin and an increase in desmin expression.[80]

Podocyte abnormalities were accompanied by upregulation of transforming growth factor-β (TGF-β) messenger ribonucleic acid (mRNA) and enhanced production of the related protein.[80] In vitro, albumin loading of immortalized mouse podocytes promoted actin–cytoskeleton rearrangement and upregulation of intracellular transduction signals, such as activating protein-1 (AP-1), which is a known stimulus of TGF-β1 synthesis.[81]

Podocytes possess a complex contractile structure composed of F-actin microfilaments, most abundant in the foot process, connected with adaptor molecules that anchor the slit diaphragm proteins and α3β1 integrins, transmembrane proteins that form focal adhesion complexes and mediate podocyte–GBM matrix interaction.[82,83] In vitro, actin filament disorganization, as occurs after albumin loading of mouse podocytes,[81] is closely associated with podocyte shape changes that affect cell adhesion to the extracellular matrix. Podocyte detachment from the GBM likely underlies the decrease in podocyte number in proteinuric glomerular diseases, which has been shown in many experimental and clinical studies.[84,85]

Apoptosis is considered an additional cause of podocyte loss in proteinuric glomerulopathies. Once detached from the GBM, podocytes become extremely susceptible to apoptosis.[67] Furthermore, apoptosis may be promoted by locally

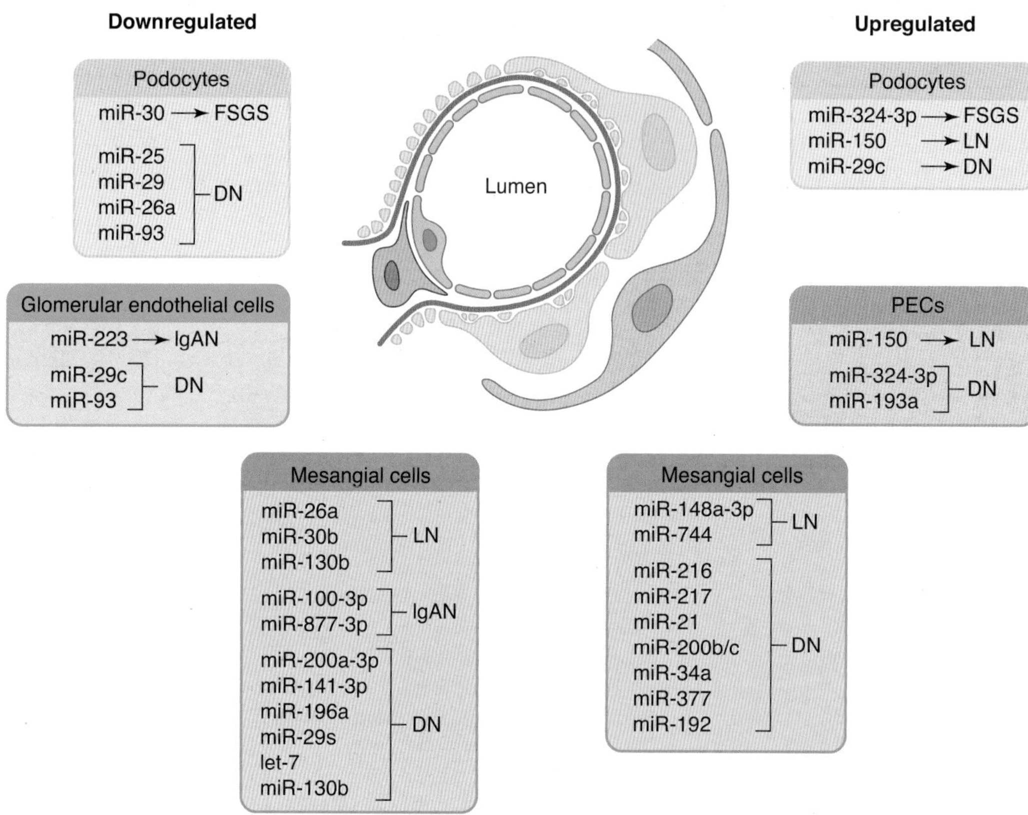


**Fig. 30.7 MicroRNA (miRNA) dysregulation in glomerular disease.** Changes in miRNAs in different populations of glomerular cells (podocytes, parietal epithelial cells, glomerular endothelial cells, and mesangial cells) occurring in focal and segmental glomerulosclerosis *(FSGS)*, lupus nephritis, IgA nephropathy, and diabetic nephropathy. *DN*, Diabetic nephropathy; *IgAN*, IgA nephropathy. (From Trionfini P, Benigni A. MicroRNAs as master regulators of glomerular function in health and disease. *J Am Soc Nephrol.* 2017;28:1686–1696.)

produced proapoptotic factors. Studies have demonstrated that exogenous TGF-β1 induced apoptosis in cultured podocytes via the p38 mitogen-activated protein kinase (MAPK) and classic caspase-3 pathways.[86] This effect occurred only in wild-type, not in p21-null cultured podocytes, indicating that the cyclin-dependent kinase (CDK) inhibitor p21 is required for TGF-β1–induced apoptosis.[87] Of note, like TGF-β1, p21 is increased in podocytes in experimental models of membranous nephropathy[88] and diabetic nephropathy.[89] In summary, protein accumulation in podocytes induces TGF-β1 production, leading to podocyte apoptosis.

Recent evidence indicates that angiotensin II (Ang II) contributes to perpetuate podocyte injury in proteinuric nephropathies eventually promoting progression to end-stage kidney disease.[90] Mechanical strain increases Ang II production and expression of Ang II type 1 ($AT_1$) receptors in podocytes[74] potentially contributing to further sustaining the glomerular hypertension-induced damage in chronic kidney disease. However, there is also evidence that, independent of its hemodynamic effect, Ang II may directly impair the glomerular barrier sieving function, possibly through inhibition of nephrin expression by podocyte, the essential protein component of the glomerular slit diaphragm.[91,92] This observation has been confirmed in studies in diabetic animals showing that blockade of Ang II synthesis/activity preserved the expression of nephrin in the glomeruli and prevented overt proteinuria.[93,94] Thus at least in diabetes, a pathogenetic relationship between Ang II and early proteinuria via functional podocyte alteration through modulation of nephrin protein level has been suggested. Moreover, in the setting of diabetes, after the initial insult of hyperglycemia and intraglomerular hypertension, Ang II plays a relevant role to sustain glomerular injury via persistent activation of Notch1 and Snail signaling in the podocyte, eventually resulting in persistent downregulation of nephrin expression.[95] The consistency of these findings in diabetic ZDF rats with overt nephropathy and in type 2 diabetic patients with established nephropathy provides robust insight to implicate an important role for the Ang II Notch1/Snail axis in perpetuating podocyte damage.

MicroRNAs (miRNAs) are a class of short (21–24 nucleotides) noncoding RNAs that regulate gene expression through posttranslational and epigenetic mechanisms, thereby affecting several cellular processes from development to disease conditions.[96] miRNAs are critical players in podocyte homeostasis (Fig. 30.7), because targeted deletion of the helicase with RNAse motif Dicer or the class II ribonuclease III enzyme Drosha in these cells leads to proteinuria and glomerulosclerosis.[97-100] Moreover, several miRNAs have been found to be dysregulated in podocyte injury, a pathologic mechanism causing glomerular injury and sclerosis. Because mature podocytes must withstand fluctuating pressures and potentially harmful molecules contained in the primary filtrate, they are unlikely to be static structures.[101] Remodeling of the actin cytoskeleton plays a primary role in the structural adaptations made by podocytes to preserve their glomerular filtration properties. The podocyte cytoskeleton is finely regulated by a set of miRNAs that are expressed mainly in the adult kidney, such as miR-30, miR-132, miR-134, and miR-29a. miR-30 family members are highly expressed in human podocytes and, in addition to protecting them against apoptosis,[102] they promote podocyte actin fiber stability by controlling calcium/calcineurin signaling through the inhibition of several components of this pathway.[103,104] Dysregulation of calcium/calcineurin signaling leads to podocyte cytoskeletal damage, which is a key feature of various glomerular diseases, such as FSGS, characterized by the early onset of podocyte injury.[103] It is notable that miR-30s are significantly downregulated in the podocytes of patients with FSGS and in the rat model of FSGS induced by the podocyte toxin puromycin aminonucleoside. Furthermore, fibrogenic factors, such as TGF-β, reduce miR-30 expression both in vivo and in cultured podocytes.[102,105] A recent study underlines the role of miRNAs in regulating podocyte cytoskeletal dynamics. The study showed that brain-derived neurotrophic factor can repair podocyte damage both in vitro and in a mouse model of FSGS by inducing miR-132 and inhibiting miR-134 expression upon binding to its receptor on podocytes. Brain-derived neurotrophic factor–induced modulation of miR-132 and miR-134 has been found to be essential for increasing actin polymerization, favoring foot process elongation that contrasts the cell flattening induced by proteinuric conditions.[106]

A crosstalk with proximal tubule cells has been recently suggested to contribute to podocyte function through the release of nicotinamide mononucleotide (NMN) that might have implications for persistent podocyte dysfunction in proteinuric diseases.[107] In a mouse model, diabetes induced downregulation of Sirtuin1 (Sirt1), a highly conserved protein deacetylase in proximal tubules.[108] The low Sirt1 expression reduces the release of nicotinamide mononucleotide by tubule cells, eventually decreasing local NMN concentrations. In vitro studies have shown that in the absence of NMN the expression of the tight junction protein claudin-1 in podocytes is no longer silenced.[107] Claudin-1 is reported to activate the intracellular β-catenin–Snail pathway[109] that eventually leads to glomerular barrier dysfunction through downregulating synaptopodin or podocin expression in podocytes.[110]

## MESANGIAL CELLS: PROLIFERATION AND DEPOSITION OF EXTRACELLULAR MATRIX

Because it is close to the capillary lumen, the mesangium may be exposed to macromolecules crossing the endothelial layer, although under normal conditions they do not accumulate.[111] However, in rats having undergone unilateral nephrectomy[112] or in puromycin-aminoglycoside–induced nephrosis,[113] intravenous infusion of colloidal carbon leads to the accumulation of the macromolecular tracer in the mesangial space. To prevent accumulation of proteins, mechanisms exist for their effective removal. These include transport along the mesangial stalk in cleft-like spaces as well as phagocytosis and degradation by mesangial cells.[114]

It has been shown that IgG and IgA can be taken up by both receptor-independent and receptor-mediated processes.[115] Another important factor for clearance of Igs from the mesangium may be complement factor D, a serine protease essential for activation of the complement system through the alternative pathway, which is constitutively expressed within the glomerulus.[116] Interestingly, mice deficient in complement factor D spontaneously develop a mesangial immune-complex deposition disease associated with albuminuria.[117] This indicates that complement factor D is necessary to prevent mesangial accumulation of immunoglobulin deposits.

Whether abnormal local accumulation of proteins promotes mesangial cell proliferation and mesangial matrix deposition remains, however, ill-defined. Nevertheless, the significance of the protein-clearing function of the mesangial cells has been illustrated by the deleterious consequences of mesangial immune complex accumulation leading to complement activation and generation of mediators of inflammation, such as reactive oxygen species, prostanoids, and cytokines, such as tumor necrosis factor-α (TNF-α) and interleukin-6 (IL-6).[118]

The mesangial cell is a critical part of the glomerular functional unit interacting closely with endothelial cells and podocytes.[116] Alterations in one cell type can produce changes in the others. As such, key survival factors for mesangial cells, including platelet-derived growth factor-B (PDGF-B) are generated by endothelial cells, and mesangiolysis has been shown in knockout mice lacking endothelial PDGF-B.[116] Whether cytokines generated by podocytes also influence mesangial cells has yet to be clearly defined, but the observation that podocyte injury frequently results in mesangial cell proliferation supports the existence of such cytokine crosstalk.[116]

Besides PDGF-B, other growth factors shown to influence mesangial cell proliferation and mesangial matrix accumulation include PDGF-C, fibroblast growth factor, hepatocyte growth factor, epidermal growth factor (EGF), connective tissue growth factor, and TGF-β.[116] Effects of vasoactive hormones such as Ang II on mesangial cell proliferation may be mediated indirectly through the generation of growth factors such as EGF.[119] In rats with renal mass ablation, glomerular TGF-β1 upregulation is associated with phenotypic transformation of mesangial cells.[80] In vitro exposure of cultured murine mesangial cells to TGF-β induced a sclerosing phenotype as shown by α-smooth muscle actin (SMA) expression, which was blocked by anti-TGF-β1 antibodies.[80] Moreover, the transfection of the TGF-β1 gene into normal kidneys in rats or the transgenic TGF-β expression in mice increased extracellular matrix accumulation in the mesangial space.[120] At least in experimental diabetes, increased matrix production in mesangial cells is induced by a fine balance between the upregulation of miR-192, miR-200b/c, miR-216a, and miR-377 and the downregulation of miR-29s and let-7. High glucose, via TGF-β, upregulates miR-377, which suppresses the expression of p21-activated kinase and superoxide dismutases, leading to enhanced susceptibility to oxidant stress and the accumulation of fibronectin.[121] In mesangial cells, TGF-β lowers the expression of miR-29s[122] and let-7,[123] antifibrotic miRNAs targeting different isoforms of collagen. Moreover, decreased miR-29a expression attenuates the Dickkopf-1/Wnt/β-catenin signaling, contributing to apoptosis and extracellular matrix deposition in streptozotocin-treated mice.[124] Notably, in mesangial cells TGF-β induces signaling loops that amplify and create a chronic state of profibrotic pathway activation, modulating the expression of miR-192, miR-200s, miR-21, and miR-130b.[125-127]

## ENDOTHELIAL CELLS: APOPTOSIS

Glomerular endothelial injury is a common feature of many human diseases, such as diabetic nephropathy, hypertension, thrombotic microangiopathy and preeclampsia. Evidence has been provided that there is close crosstalk of podocytes with glomerular endothelial cells, a key interaction for the normal function of the glomerular capillary barrier.[128] The final steps in glomerular endothelial cell differentiation involve the formation of fenestrae, plasma membrane-lined circular pores that perforate the flattened glomerular endothelium.[129] The fenestrated phenotype of glomerular endothelial cells is induced by vascular endothelial growth factor (VEGF), a molecule constitutively expressed and secreted by podocytes.[128,129] That VEGF regulates fenestrae formation was suggested by the observation that mature fenestrated endothelium is typically located adjacent to podocytes expressing high levels of VEGF mRNA.[130] There is also in vitro evidence that VEGF type A and C regulate glycosaminoglycan synthesis, charge, and shedding of glomerular microvascular endothelial cell glycocalyx.[131] Moreover, deletion of the podocyte-specific transcription factor LMX1B in mice, which results in the loss of many features of podocyte differentiation, including VEGF-A expression, is associated with failure of glomerular endothelium to differentiate and develop fenestrae.[132] Thus, loss of podocytes secondary to protein-induced cell injury may lead to reduced VEGF production influencing glomerular endothelial fenestrae formation and eventually leading to endothelial cell apoptosis.[133] However, how VEGF reaches endothelial cells against the urine flow is not yet known. Conversely, recent in vitro evidence has shown that blockade of VEGF in glomerular endothelial cells enhanced the release of endothelin-1 (ET-1), which induced nephrin shedding from podocytes,[134] leading to further glomerular protein permeability dysfunction.

Moreover, endothelin-1 activates podocytes to release heparanase.[135] In mice, podocyte-specific deletion of the endothelin receptor prevented the diabetes-induced increase in glomerular heparanase expression and consequent reduction in heparan sulfate expression, endothelial glycocalyx thickness, and development of proteinuria that was observed in wild-type mice.[135] Heparanase-deficient mice were resistant to the development of proteinuria and renal damage upon induction of type 1 diabetes mellitus.[136] In addition, proteinuria was also reduced and renal function improved by treatment with the experimental heparanase inhibitor SST0001.[136]

Taken together, these studies indicate that the toxic effects of excess ultrafiltered plasma proteins on podocytes may alter podocyte–endothelial interaction, thereby further enhancing glomerular permeability to proteins through a complex interplay of molecular signaling.

## PARIETAL EPITHELIAL CELLS: ACTIVATION

Changes in glomerular permselective function, as it occurs in proteinuric glomerulopathies, elevate the filtered load of plasma albumin and consequently its concentration in the Bowman space (Fig. 30.8). Evidence has been provided that the abnormally filtered albumin impairs the mechanism underlying regeneration of protein-induced damage to podocytes.[137] Glomerular injury caused by multiple etiologies can lead to activation and accumulation of parietal epithelial cells (PECs) within the Bowman space as a common response to damage,[138] as shown in several human proliferative glomerulonephritides. Although extracapillary proliferation is a relatively straight forward pathologic change to recognize, determining its cellular components has been more controversial. The traditional concepts, largely from immunohistochemical studies, indicate that the multilayered cellular lesions are a mixture of glomerular parietal epithelial cells, macrophages, and myofibroblasts,[139-141] the proportion of such cells in the lesion being variable. In both animal models and human tissues, PECs predominate when the Bowman capsule is intact. Recently, a heterogeneous population of renal progenitor cells, previously identified in the normal human Bowman capsule,[142] has been documented in hyperplastic lesions of human crescentic glomerulonephritis.[143] The extracapillary lesions could therefore be the result of dysregulated proliferation of renal progenitor cells in response to the injured podocytes.[143] This possibility is supported by findings in Munich Wistar Frömter (MWF) rats, which are genetically programmed to develop renal damage characterized by excessive progenitor cell migration and proliferation, leading to their accumulation into cellular lesions and glomerulosclerosis.[144] Among the factors that influence the maladaptive PEC response, ultrafiltered albumin has been regarded as a critical player that impairs podocyte regeneration.[145] Notably, albumin prevents PEC differentiation into podocytes by sequestering retinoic acid and impairing retinoic acid response element-mediated transcription of podocyte specific genes.[145]

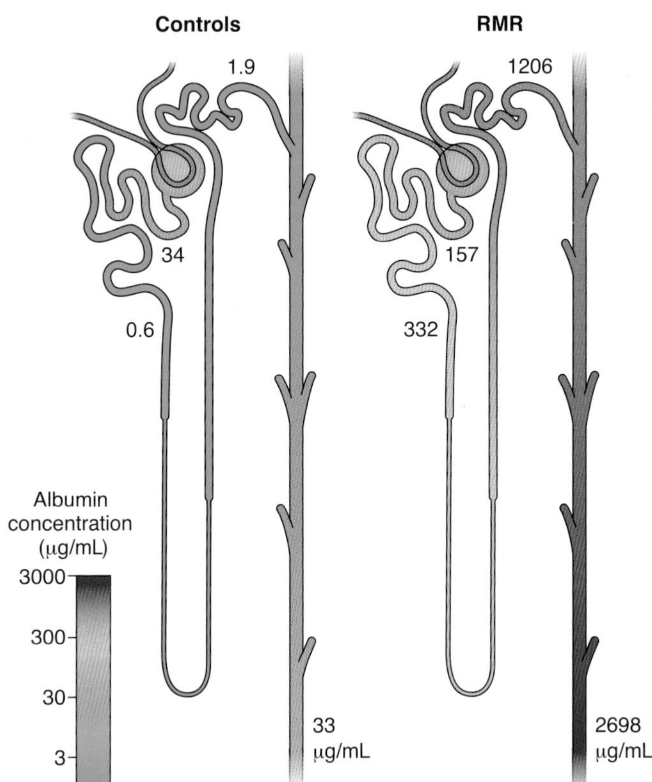


**Fig. 30.8** **Estimated albumin concentrations along the nephron.** Color-coded graphical representation of estimated albumin concentration along the entire nephron in the two animal groups (control group and renal mass reduction group). Numbers represent local group average albumin concentration in μg/mL. *RMR*, Renal mass reduction. (Modified from Sangalli F, Carrara F, Gaspari F, et al. Effect of ACE inhibition on glomerular permselectivity and tubular albumin concentration in the renal ablation model. *Am J Physiol Renal Physiol.* 2011;300: F1291–1300.)

Circulating components of the complement system are also lost in the urine in proteinuric conditions and become activated at the glomerular level, favoring progression of the lesions.[80,146-148] Thus abnormal fixation of ultrafiltered complement C3 is detected in podocytes showing signs of dedifferentiation and injury during the early stage of proteinuric disease in rats with remnant kidney,[80] and in mice with protein overload proteinuria.[148] C3-deficient mice with protein overload are protected against podocyte structural damage and sclerosis, indicating that C3 might increase susceptibility to injury. Recently, we demonstrated that complement activation via alternative pathway is a pivotal trigger for podocyte loss and PEC activation, leading to glomerulosclerosis in the model of protein-overload proteinuria.[149] Factor H ($Cfh^{-/-}$) or factor B–deficient mice were studied in comparison with wild-type littermates. Wild-type mice with protein overload induced by bovine serum albumin showed podocyte depletion accompanied by glomerular complement C3 and C3a deposits, PEC migration to capillary tuft, proliferation, and glomerulosclerosis. These changes were more prominent in $Cfh^{-/-}$ mice with protein overload induced by bovine serum albumin. The pathogenic role of the alternative pathway was documented by data that factor B deficiency preserved glomerular integrity. In protein-overload mice, PEC dysregulation was associated with upregulation of CXCR4 and GDNF/c-Ret axis. In vitro studies provided additional evidence of a direct action of C3a on proliferation and CXCR4-related migration of PECs. These effects were enhanced by podocyte-derived GDNF. In patients with proteinuric nephropathy, glomerular C3/C3a paralleled PEC activation, CXCR4, and GDNF upregulation. These results indicate that mechanistically uncontrolled alternative pathway complement activation is not dispensable for podocyte-dependent PEC activation resulting in glomerulosclerosis.[149]

Parietal epithelial cells expressing the progenitor cell marker $CD133^+CD24^+$ have also been reported to proliferate and accumulate into the multilayered cellular lesions in patients with glomerulonephritides characterized by extracapillary proliferation but not in nonproliferative nephropathies such as membranous or diabetic nephropathies.[150] Upregulation of the CXCR4 chemokine receptor on these progenitor cells was accompanied by high expression of its ligand, SDF-1, in podocytes.[150] Moreover, parietal epithelial cell proliferation was associated with increased expression of the Ang II subtype 1 receptor. Renin–angiotensin system blockade normalized CXCR4 and Ang II subtype 1 receptor expression on parietal progenitor cells concomitant with regression of crescentic lesions. Together these findings suggest that the glomerular hyperplastic lesions derive from the proliferation and migration of renal progenitors in response to injured podocytes, and that the Ang II/$AT_1$ receptor pathway may contribute, together with SDF-1/CXCR4 axis, to the dysregulated response of parietal epithelial cell precursors.

Parietal epithelial cell activation is increasingly recognized and seems to be present also in most forms of FSGS, characterized by nephrotic syndrome often leading to a progressive decline in renal function.[151] Using a lineage tagging approach in mice, it has been documented that activated parietal epithelial cells invade the affected segment of the capillary tuft and initiate glomerular and epithelial basement membrane adhesion and glomerulosclerosis.[152] The Notch signaling pathway has been proposed to play a role in orchestrating parietal epithelial cell phenotypic changes in FSGS.[153] This possibility rests on in vitro evidence that in cultured mouse parietal epithelial cells TGF-β enhanced Notch mRNA expression, which resulted in a significant upregulation of target genes associated with mesenchymal cell phenotype, such as α-smooth muscle actin, vimentin, and Snail.[153] Concurrent inhibition of Notch signaling with the γ-secretase inhibitor DBZ[154] blocked both epithelial-to-mesenchymal transition gene expression changes and cell migration in response to TGF-β, demonstrating a dependence on Notch signaling for induction of mesenchymal gene marker activation in the parietal epithelial cell line. Moreover, in LMB2 antibody-treated NEP25 transgenic mice, a model of collapsing FSGS,[155] Notch inhibition in vivo significantly decreased parietal epithelial cell lesions, pointing to the role of Notch-mediated cell activation in the formation of such lesions.[153]

miRNAs have emerged as important regulators of gene expression in parietal epithelial cells.[96] Indeed, robust miR-150 expression in PECs and podocytes of patients with lupus nephritis correlated positively with disease chronicity scores and the expression of profibrotic proteins. Increased miR-150 would foster the production of profibrotic molecules through the downregulation of its predicted target, SOCS1. The latter protein acts as a negative regulator of the JAK/STAT signaling pathway, which promotes the transcription of genes involved in cell proliferation, inflammation, and fibrosis.[156,157] Similar to miR-150, we identified miR-324-3p increased expression in PECs as well as podocytes in an FSGS rat model. Increased expression of miR-324-3p was associated with the downregulation of its target propyl endopeptidase—involved in the formation of the antifibrotic peptide Ac-SDKD—in fibrotic areas of the kidneys of diseased rats.[158] Human PECs isolated from naïve Bowman capsules express significant levels of miR-193a, which works as a suppressor of podocyte differentiation by inhibiting the expression of the transcription factor Wilms tumor protein (WT1).[159,160] WT1 is essential for the development and maintenance of podocytes and glomeruli by inducing the expression of genes governing podocyte architecture.[161] The downregulation of miR-193a is associated with PEC transdifferentiation toward a podocyte phenotype, whereas its overexpression leads to their abnormal activation, a prerequisite for the formation of crescents in proliferative glomerulonephritis.[160] In line with this, isolated glomeruli from individuals with FSGS are characterized by increased expression of miR-193a, compared with normal kidneys or kidneys affected by other glomerular diseases.[159] The involvement of miR-193a in the pathogenesis of FSGS was also supported by data from miR-193a knock in mice, which develop FSGS with extensive podocyte foot process effacement.[159] All of the previous evidence, together with findings that the number of crescents was reduced by anti-miR-193a in a mouse model of nephrotoxic nephritis,[160] concur to indicate that miR-193a is a promising therapeutic target for FSGS. The mouse model of nephrotoxic nephritis was also instrumental for identifying the key role of miRNAs in orchestrating T-cell–mediated crescentic glomerulonephritis. Mice with miRNA-deficient $CD4^+$ T cells develop less severe glomerulonephritis upon toxin injection. Moreover, the kidneys of patients with ANCA-associated crescentic glomerulonephritis and mice with nephrotoxic nephritis are characterized by the upregulation of miR-155 that drives the Th17 immune response and tissue injury.[162]

### LOSS OF GLOMERULAR CAPILLARIES: POSTGLOMERULAR HYPOXIA

Irrespective of the underlying process leading to glomerular endothelial damage, such as increased intracapillary pressure and/or podocyte loss, the net result is rarefaction of glomerular capillaries. Loss of glomerular capillary loops translates into diminished postglomerular blood flow from affected glomeruli and downstream injury of the peritubular capillary network. Microvascular dysfunction causes progressive scarring of renal tissue by creating hypoxic environment that triggers a fibrotic response in tubulointerstitial cells.[163] This, in turn, has an impact on adjacent unaffected capillaries and glomeruli, further extending the hypoxic area, and leading to a vicious cycle of progressive destruction of the kidney and decline of renal function to end-stage organ failure.

Indeed, in animal models of proteinuric chronic kidney disease, including anti-Thy1 glomerulonephritis, 5/6 remnant kidney, diabetic nephropathy, and adriamycin-induced nephrosis, the immunohistochemical detection of hypoxia-dependent pimonidazole protein adducts has revealed that renal tissue hypoxia is present early in the course of the disease.[164] Moreover, blood oxygen–dependent magnetic resonance imaging has shown hypoxia in diabetic nephropathy.[165] Although data from animal models provide a compelling argument for postglomerular hypoxia in proteinuric diseases as a primary mediator of progressive renal scarring, data in humans are scarce. Nevertheless, that hypoxia-related injury also applies to humans may be deduced by the finding that there is increased expression of hypoxia-inducible factor (HIF)—a key regulator of the adaptive response to hypoxia controlling expression of hundreds of genes[166]—in biopsies of patients with diabetic nephropathy, IgA nephropathy, and chronic allograft nephropathy.[167]

## TUBULAR DAMAGE

Glomerular ultrafiltration of excessive amounts of plasma protein-associated factors incites tubulointerstitial damage and further promotes the effects of glomerular disease on the tubular compartment. The noxious substances in the proteinuric ultrafiltrate may set off tubular epithelial injury with tubular apoptosis, secondary generation of inflammatory mediators, and peritubular inflammation.[4] The mechanisms whereby increased urinary protein concentration leads to nephrotoxic injury are multifactorial and involve complex interaction between numerous pathways of cellular damage (Fig. 30.9).

### TUBULAR CELLS: APOPTOSIS AND TUBULO GLOMERULAR DISCONNECTION

Emerging evidence suggests that proteinuria causes tubule cell apoptosis. In cultured proximal tubule cells, delipidated albumin-induced apoptosis in a dose- and time-dependent manner,[168] as characterized by internucleosomal DNA

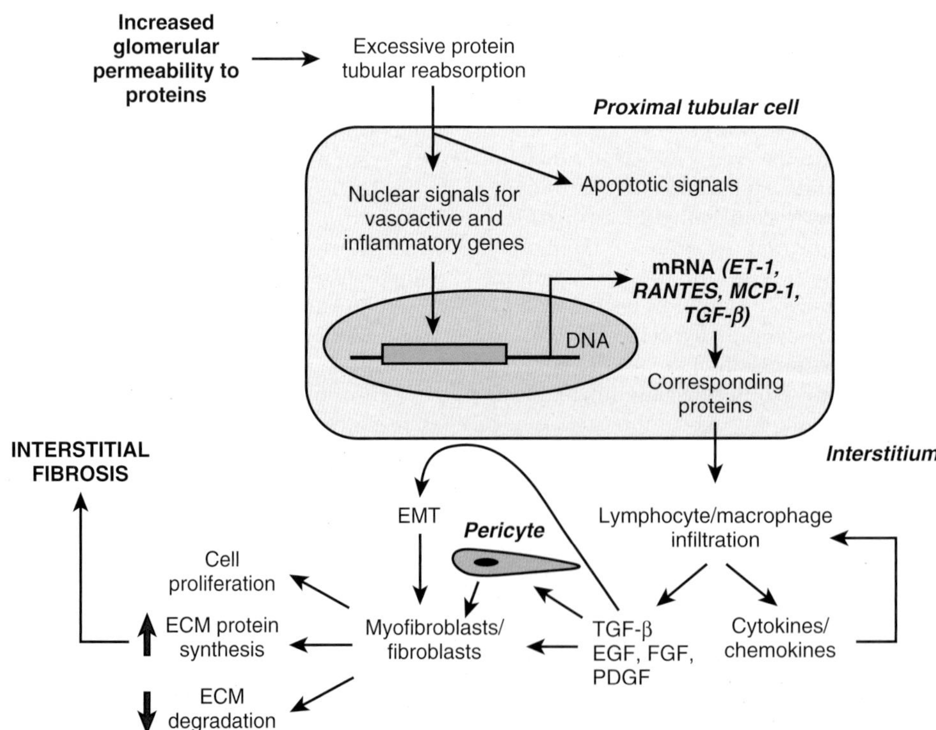


**Fig. 30.9 Mechanisms of tubulointerstitial damage induced by proteins.** Protein overload of proximal tubule cells as a consequence of increased glomerular permeability to proteins activates intracellular signals that promote cell apoptosis or cause increased production of inflammatory and vasoactive mediators and growth factors. These substances are released into the interstitium, inducing progressive inflammation and injury. *ECM*, Extracellular matrix; *EGF*, epidermal growth factor; *EMT*, epithelial-to-mesenchymal transdifferentiation; *ET-1*, endothelin-1, *FGF*, fibroblast growth factor; *MCP-1*, monocyte chemoattractant protein-1; *PDGF*, platelet-derived growth factor; *RANTES*, regulated upon activation, normal T cell expressed and secreted; *TGF-β*, transforming growth factor-β.

fragmentation, morphologic changes including cell shrinkage and nuclear condensation, and plasma membrane alterations.[168] Kidneys of rats with albumin-overload proteinuria[169] or with passive Heymann nephritis[64] showed increased numbers of terminal dUTP nick-end labeling-positive apoptotic cells in the tubulointerstitial compartment. In tubules, most of the positive cells expressed Ang II subtype 2 (AT2) receptors.[169] Findings of reduced phosphorylation of extracellular signal-regulated kinase (ERK) and Bcl-2 suggested an AT2 receptor–mediated mechanism underlying tubular cell apoptosis.[169]

Apoptotic cells expressing both proximal and distal tubular phenotypes were detected in biopsy specimens from patients with primary FSGS.[170] A strong positive correlation was found between proteinuria and incidence of tubular cell apoptosis.[170]

Renal proximal tubule cells have a remarkable ability to reabsorb large quantities of albumin through clathrin- and megalin receptor–mediated endocytosis.[65] Megalin is the sensor that determines whether cells will be protected from or injured by albumin. It has been shown that megalin binds the serine/threonine kinase PKB, crucial for the phosphorylation of Bad, the Bcl2-associated death promoter.[171] Low concentrations of albumin lead to activated PKB and phosphorylation of the Bad protein, which inhibits apoptosis.[172] On the other hand, overload of albumin leads to decreased megalin expression on the plasma membrane of proximal tubule cells that is associated with reduction of PKB activity and Bad phosphorylation.[173] The result is albumin-induced apoptosis.

In cultured proximal tubule cells, albumin repletion with fatty acids and its association with linoleic acid induced more apoptosis than the exposure to defatted albumin alone.[174] Furthermore, another study showed that nondelipidated albumin or albumin conjugated with palmitate, but not fatty acid-free albumin, altered both tubule mitochondrial variability and membrane potential and caused cytochrome *c* release.[175] In concert with the decline of mitochondrial parameters, fatty acid overload led to a redox imbalance, which deactivated the antioxidant protein peroxiredoxin 2 and caused a peroxide-mediated apoptosis through the redox-sensitive pJNK/caspase-3 pathway. These data were taken to suggest that attempts at lowering circulating fatty acid levels may be important in both preserving redox balance and limiting tubule cell damage.[175] A novel biochemical mechanism has been proposed linking lipotoxicity to tubule apoptosis in proteinuric conditions.[176] The study focused on the $Na^+/H^+$ exchanger NHE1, a regulator for proximal tubule cell survival through interaction with the membrane phosphoinositide phosphatidylinositol 4,5-bisphosphate (PI[4,5]P2), which initiates formation of a signaling complex that culminates in Akt activation and opposition to apoptotic stress. Starting from the concept that diseased glomeruli with impaired permselectivity allow filtration and proximal tubule reabsorption of nonesterified fatty acids (NEFA) bound to albumin, it was shown that an accumulation of metabolites of NEFA, long-chain acyl-CoA could stimulate lipoapoptosis by competing with the structurally similar PI(4,5)P2 for NHE1 binding, thus interrupting PI(4,5)P2 prosurvival activity.[176]

Proximal tubule cell apoptosis was found to contribute to tubulo glomerular disconnection and atrophy in response to proteinuria in animal models of proteinuric nephropathies.[64] Injured or dying cells release molecules that serve as danger signals.[177] Danger molecules trigger inflammation by engaging pattern recognition receptors such as Toll-like receptors (TLRs)[178] and nucleotide-binding domains, leucine-rich repeat-containing proteins (NLRs),[179] and are thus referred as danger-associated molecular patterns (DAMPs).[180] Through TLRs, DAMPs signal cytokine and chemokine production and upregulate the expression of cell adhesion molecules. When DAMPs interact with NLRs, they stimulate NLRs to complex with apoptosis-associated speck-like proteins to form macromolecular complexes, the inflammasomes that cleave proinflammatory cytokines to their mature forms.[181] Thus besides promoting tubulo glomerular disconnection, proximal tubular cell apoptosis contributes to create a local proinflammatory microenvironment.

## TUBULE CELLS: ACTIVATION

Receptor-mediated endocytosis of excessive proteins at the apical pole of the proximal tubule cells is also associated with phenotypic changes characteristic of an activated state.

Insights into specific mechanisms linking protein uptake to cell activation have come from in vitro studies using polarized proximal tubule cells to assess the effect of apical exposure to proteins. Collectively, they show that protein overload induces a proinflammatory phenotype.[182-185] Indeed, upregulation of inflammatory and fibrogenic genes and production of related proteins have been reported following a challenge of proximal tubule cells with plasma proteins. They include cytokines and chemokines, such as monocyte chemoattractant protein-1 (MCP-1), RANTES (regulated upon activation, normal T cell expressed and secreted), interleukin-8 (IL-8), and fractalkine.[182-185] Moreover, levels of the profibrogenic cytokine TGF-β and its type I receptor,[186] tissue inhibitors of metalloproteinase (TIMP)-1 and TIMP-2, as well as membrane surface expression of the αvβ5 integrin[187] were also highly increased in vitro upon stimulation by plasma proteins.

Investigations of the molecular mechanisms underlying chemokine and growth factor upregulation in proximal tubule cells on protein challenge have focused on the activation of transcription factor NF-κB.[182] Other studies confirmed this pathway[188,189] and revealed reactive oxygen as a second messenger.[184,190]

Extrapolation from such in vitro data to the human situation may be difficult considering the conflicting data observed with different proteins in different cell systems,[191] as well as the reported changes in the expression of several genes of unknown function.[192] However, the in vitro observations have recently been confirmed through transcription analysis by cDNA microarray of renal proximal tubule epithelial cells isolated by laser capture microdissection from patients with proteinuric nephropathies.[193] More than 160 genes—including those encoding for signal transduction, transcription, and translation, and apoptotic and inflammatory proteins—were identified as being regulated differently from those in proximal tubule cells from control subjects.

Evidence implicates megalin as a central element of the signaling pathway linking protein reabsorption and gene regulation in proximal tubule cells.[194] Megalin is subjected to regulated intramembrane proteolysis (RIP), an evolutionarily conserved process linking receptor function with transcriptional regulation.[195] Through RIP megalin is subjected to protein kinase C regulated, metalloprotease-mediated ectodomain shedding producing a membrane-associated

C-terminal fragment (MCTF).[194] The MCTF in turn forms the substrate for γ-secretase, which releases the C-terminal, cytosolic domain. The latter translocates to the nucleus where it interacts with other proteins to regulate expression of specific genes. This function may explain the phenotypic change of proximal tubules in proteinuric kidney disease.

That megalin contributes to the early activation of proximal tubule cells in nonselective proteinuria has been documented in megalin knockout/*NEP25* mice given immunotoxin LMB2, a model for nephrotic syndrome, focal segmental glomerulosclerosis, and tubulointerstitial injury.[196] Megalin-deficient proximal tubule cells reabsorbed less proteins in vivo and expressed less tubular injury markers, such as MCP-1 and heme-oxygenase 1.[196]

The proteinuric ultrafiltrate may also activate TLRs and promote an innate inflammatory immune response.[197] Besides being expressed by cells of the immune system such as macrophages, dendritic cells, neutrophils, B cells, and natural killer cells, TLRs are also expressed by nonimmune cells, including renal tubule epithelial cells.[197] The cellular effects of TLRs include the production of proinflammatory cytokines and chemokines that contribute to local inflammation and leukocyte accumulation. It has been demonstrated that proximal tubule epithelial cells were sites of robust expression of TLR-9 mRNA and protein —a receptor for CpG DNA—in NZBxNZW lupus mice with overt nephropathy.[198] Upregulation of TLR-9 expression was accompanied by the development of proteinuria and correlated with tubulointerstitial damage. Furthermore, abundant TLR-9 staining in proximal tubule cells of lupus patients correlated with tubulointerstitial damage. Thus tubular TLR activation may occur due to filtration of plasma proteins, which include immune complexes containing DNA enriched in CG motifs.[199,200]

The proximal tubule bears other receptors for ultrafiltered proteins, such as cytokines and growth factors.[4] Usually these molecules are present in high-molecular-weight precursor forms or bound to specific binding proteins that regulate their biological activity. They can be found in nephrotic tubular fluid. In experimental proteinuria in rats, there is translocation of insulin-like growth factor I (IGF-I) from plasma into tubular fluid (primarily as the 50-kDa complex).[201] Similarly, hepatocyte growth factor (HGF) is present in early proximal tubular fluid from rats with streptozotocin-induced diabetic nephropathy, and it is excreted in the urine of diabetic animals.[202] Under physiologic conditions the high molecular weight of TGF-β complexes prevents glomerular ultrafiltration of this pluripotent cytokine. However, in proteinuric glomerular diseases, TGF-β is present in early proximal tubular fluid and at least a portion is bioactive.[202] IGF-1, HGF and TGF-β are also present in the urine of patients with proteinuric diseases.[203]

Collectively the tubular response to these growth factors can be described as activation or as a moderate change toward a cell phenotype resembling cell injury, which includes a moderate increase in collagen type I and IV production in response to IGF-I[201] and upregulation of the expression of fibronectin by HGF.[204] TGF-β also increases the transcription in proximal tubule cells of the genes encoding collagen $\alpha_1$III (Col3A1) and collagen $\alpha_2$ I (Col1A2) as well as fibronectin.

With proteinuria, a putative key factor in tubule cell activation and damage is the excess glomerular filtration of serum-derived complement C3, the central molecule in the complement system that exerts proinflammatory potential.[205] Renal tubule epithelial cells appear most susceptible to luminal attack by the C5b-9 membrane attack complex because of the relative lack of membrane bound complement regulatory proteins, such as membrane cofactor protein (CD46), decay-accelerating factor, or CD55 and CD59 on the apical surface.[206] In rats with severely reduced renal mass[207,208] or with protein overload proteinuria,[148] C3 colocalized with proximal tubule cells engaged in high protein uptake. By limiting the transglomerular passage of proteins, treatment with angiotensin-converting enzyme (ACE) inhibitors was an effective maneuver to reduce C3 load of tubule cells in remnant kidneys.[207] C3 and other complement proteins are also found in proximal tubules in renal biopsy material from nephrotic patients.[205,209] Furthermore, proximal tubule cells are able to synthesize C3 and other complement factors[210] and to upregulate C3 in response to serum proteins in vitro.[211]

The injurious role of plasma-derived C3, as opposed to tubular cell–derived C3, has been documented in C3-deficient kidneys transplanted into wild-type mice.[148] Protein overload led to the development of glomerular injury, accumulation of C3 in proximal tubules, and tubulointerstitial changes. Conversely, when wild-type kidneys were transplanted into C3-deficient mice, protein overload led to a milder disease and abnormal C3 deposition was not observed. Thus ultrafiltered C3 contributes more to tubulointerstitial damage induced by protein overload than locally synthesized C3.

## INTERSTITIAL INFLAMMATION AND INJURY

In proteinuric kidney disease, progressive inflammation and injury to the renal interstitium are secondary events following glomerular or vascular injury. Tubule epithelial cells synthesize cytokines and chemokines and accumulate complement components that recruit inflammatory cells and lymphocytes into the interstitium causing progressive fibrosis.

### RESIDENT MONOCYTE/DENDRITIC CELLS

The interstitium of normal kidneys contains numerous resident monocytic myelocytes,[212] which express dendritic cell (DC) markers and can indeed present antigens.[212] DCs have recently been described to form an immune sentinel network through the entire kidney, where they probe the environment in search of antigens.[213] An inflammatory environment converts the tolerogenic status of resident DCs into an immunogenic one, favoring recruitment of T cells. It is known that cross-presentation by DCs is a major mechanism for the immune surveillance of tissue against foreign antigens.[214] In this process professional antigen-presenting cells, such as DCs, acquire proteins from other tissue cells through endocytic mechanisms, especially phagocytosis or macropinocytosis. The internalized antigen can then be processed and presented on MHC class I molecules to the extracellular environment.[215] The outcome of cross-presentation regarding immunity depends on the expression of immunostimulatory signals after the uptake of the antigen.[214]

Until recently, the role of resident DCs that accumulate in the renal parenchyma of nonimmune-mediated proteinuric nephropathies remained poorly understood. Recent studies, however, have provided new insights into the activation of DCs in the setting of proteinuria. Administration of ovalbumin—which is freely filtered by the glomerulus—to normal mice leads to concentration of the protein principally in proximal tubules and to its transfer to DCs in the kidney and renal lymph nodes.[216] Here, ovalbumin is presented to $CD8^+$ T cells, thereby inducing proliferation of these cells.

The importance of kidney DC activation to renal injury has been recently demonstrated by the fact that in transgenic NOH mice (that selectively express the model antigens ovalbumin and hen egg lysozyme in podocytes) DC depletion resolved established periglomerular mononuclear infiltrates.[217] In vitro experiments have also shown that exposure of rat proximal tubule cells to excess autologous albumin, as in the case of proteinuric nephropathies, results in the formation of the N-terminal 24-residue fragment of albumin ($ALB_{1\text{-}24}$).[218] This peptide is taken up by DCs, where it is further processed by proteasomes into antigen peptides. These peptides were shown to have the binding motif for MHC class I and to be capable of activating $CD8^+$ T cells. Moreover, in vivo, in the rat 5/6 nephrectomy model, accumulation of DCs in the renal parenchyma peaked 1 week after surgery and decreased thereafter, concomitant with their appearance in the renal draining lymph nodes. DCs from renal lymph nodes loaded with the albumin peptide $ALB_{1\text{-}24}$ activated syngeneic $CD8^+$ T cells in primary culture.[218] Thus inflammatory stimuli released from damaged tubules after protein overload may represent danger signals that, in the presence of albumin peptides, alert DCs to promote local immunity via $CD8^+$ T cells that are activated in regional lymph nodes and recruited in the renal interstitium.

## MACROPHAGES AND LYMPHOCYTES

The interstitial infiltrate of most human chronic renal diseases consists of a number of different effector cells, including macrophages, $CD4^+$ and $CD8^+$ T cells.[219] In animal models, macrophages are the dominant infiltrating cells both in the early and in later stages of chronic renal injury. More specifically, tubulointerstitial macrophage accumulation in chronic nephropathies correlates with the severity of the glomerular and interstitial lesions and the degree of renal dysfunction.[219] Direct damage to resident cells is caused through the generation by macrophages of reactive oxygen species (ROS), nitric oxide (NO), complement factors, and proinflammatory cytokines.[220] Macrophages can also affect the supporting matrix and vasculature through the expression of metalloproteinases and vasoactive peptides.

Macrophages are only one component of the cellular infiltrate that characterizes inflammation in the renal interstitium. Recent models of overload proteinuria have emphasized the importance of tubulointerstitial infiltration with mononuclear cells. Indeed, T-helper cells and cytotoxic T cells, as well as macrophages, are observed in the tubulointerstitial infiltrate 2 weeks after protein overload.[221] T-cell depletion with intraperitoneal anti-T cell monoclonal antibody administration did not modify macrophage infiltration, indicating that the influx of these cells was independent of lymphocytes,[221] and more likely resulted from local tubule cell expression of osteopontin, MCP-1 and the adhesion molecules VCAM and ICAM.

T lymphocytes are also abundantly present in the tubulointerstitial infiltrate early after renal mass ablation in rats and remain there in significant numbers for the following weeks.[222] Although the infiltration of macrophages is part of a nonspecific inflammatory reaction, the presence of lymphocytes within lesions indicates that their recruitment and activation is mediated by an antigen-specific immune response. Their role is to maintain and amplify the inflammatory response in the renal interstitium.

Because B cells are considered to be important mostly in lymph nodes, spleen, and in humoral immune responses, little attention has been paid to their potential role as intrarenal infiltrating cells.[223] However, a prominent accumulation of $CD20^+$ B cells has been described in membranous nephropathy.[224] Furthermore, $CD20^+$ B cells formed a prominent part of the infiltrating cells in renal biopsies from patients with IgA nephropathy and chronic interstitial nephritis.[225] Together with $CD3^+$ T cells, $CD20^+$ B cells formed large nodular structures, like tertiary lymphatic organs in inflamed tissues.[226]

The level of mRNA expression of the chemokine CXCL13 was increased and correlated with $CD20^+$ mRNA in the tubulointerstitial space. The localization of enhanced CXCL13 immunoreactivity to the nodular infiltrates and that of the corresponding receptor CXCR5 to B cells in the infiltrates point toward a role of CXCL13-CXCR5 for B-cell recruitment into the lymphoid follicle-like structures. In the interstitium, B cells may release proinflammatory cytokines and chemokines, present antigens, and activate T cells, as well as play a role in the development of tissue fibrosis.[226]

## BONE MARROW–DERIVED FIBROCYTES

In proteinuric renal disease, chemokines generated in the inflammatory milieu may contribute to the recruitment of bone marrow–derived fibrocytes to the renal interstitium.[227] Fibrocytes are circulating connective tissue cell progenitors with a high capacity for collagen I synthesis. In progressive kidney fibrosis induced by unilateral ureteral obstruction in mice, fibrocytes infiltrated the interstitium, and the number of these cells increased with the progression of fibrosis.[228] In addition, the number of infiltrating fibrocytes correlates well with the extent of interstitial fibrosis in several human kidney diseases.[227] Although fibrocytes isolated from mice and humans express chemokine receptors including CCR2, CCR3, CCR5, CCR7, and CXCR4,[227] the specific chemokine and receptor pair involved into the recruitment of these cells in the damaged tubulointerstitium remains uncertain.

## FIBROBLASTS: ACTIVATION AND DEPOSITION OF EXTRACELLULAR MATRIX

The process of tubulointerstitial fibrosis involves the loss of renal tubules and the accumulation of myofibroblasts and extracellular matrix (ECM) proteins.[229] Resident interstitial fibroblasts and myofibroblasts proliferate in response to macrophage-derived profibrogenic cytokines, and their number correlates with the subsequent formation of a scar.[230] These cells may be derived from transdifferentiated tubular epithelial cells or pericytes of peritubular capillaries, a process promoted by profibrogenic cytokines, including TGF-β expressed by macrophages.[231,232]

During the developmental stage embryonic epithelia of different organs, including the collecting duct epithelium of the kidney, may give rise to mesenchymal cells, a process known as epithelial to mesenchymal transition (EMT).[233] EMT has been suggested as a process that contributes to interstitial fibrosis in chronic kidney diseases by transformation of injured renal tubule cells into mesenchymal cells.[233]

However, the evidence for EMT in adult kidneys and chronic renal disease is controversial and there are no solid data supporting EMT as an in vivo process in kidney fibrosis. The most supportive data have come from a study in a model of unilateral ureteral obstruction.[234] With the use of genetically tagged proximal tubule epithelial cells, it has been demonstrated that up to 36% of all matrix-producing cells within the tubulointerstitial space may be of tubular origin.[234] However, the contribution of EMT to the formation of myofibroblasts is less in other models.[235,236] Moreover, using cell fate–tracing techniques in the unilateral ureteral obstruction model, other investigators did not find any evidence for a contribution of EMT to renal fibrosis.[237] This is in line with the finding that in the remnant kidney model in rats, after the onset of proteinuria α-smooth muscle actinin, a marker of transdifferentiation to myofibroblasts was initially expressed by nonepithelial cells in the peritubular compartment. Recently peritubular pericytes have been identified as the source of myofibroblasts in this transdifferentiation process.[237]

Activated renal fibroblasts may secrete chemokines which, in turn, may further attract macrophages and perpetuate tubulointerstitial injury.[197] Eventually activated fibroblasts produce interstitial matrix components contributing to interstitial collagen deposition and fibrosis. Increased tubulointerstitial fibrosis is a common feature of kidney injury and results from accumulation of ECM structural proteins. It is maintained by continuous remodeling through the proteolytic action of matrix metalloproteinases (MMPs) and the synthesis of new proteins.

MMPs are inhibited by tissue inhibitors of matrix metalloproteinases (TIMPs). Therefore the balance between TIMPs and MMPs determines the ECM integrity. Among the four members of the TIMP family, TIMP3 is unique in that it is ECM bound and is highly expressed in the kidney.[238] $TIMP3^{-/-}$ mice had more interstitial fibrosis, increased synthesis and deposition of type I collagen, increased activation of fibroblasts, and greater activation of MMP2 after unilateral obstruction than wild-type mice.[239] TIMP3 levels are upregulated in patients with diabetic and chronic allograft nephropathy.[239]

Recent studies link fibrosis to changes in miRNAs.[96,240,241] A number of miRNAs have been shown to be relevant to fibrotic processes in diabetic nephropathy, including miR-29 and miR-200 families, miR-192, and miR-21.[241-244] These miRNAs are regulated by TGF-β in renal cells, and normalization of their expression ameliorated fibrosis in in vitro and in vivo models of diabetes.[243]

More recently, miR-184 has been shown to be a downstream effector of albuminuria driving renal fibrosis in rats with diabetic nephropathy.[245] Indeed, in Zucker diabetic fatty (ZDF) rats, miR-184 showed the strongest differential upregulation compared with lean rats (18-fold). Tubular localization of miR-184 was associated with reduced expression of lipid phosphate phosphatase 3 (LPP3) and collagen accumulation. Transfection of NRK-52E cells with miR-184 mimic reduced LPP3, promoting a profibrotic phenotype. Albumin was a major trigger for miR-184 expression. Interestingly, anti-miR-184 counteracted albumin-induced LPP3 downregulation and overexpression of plasminogen activator inhibitor-1. In ZDF rats, ACE inhibitor treatment limited albuminuria and reduced miR-184, with tubular LPP3 preservation and tubulointerstitial fibrosis amelioration. Albumin-induced miR-184 expression in tubule cells was epigenetically regulated through DNA demethylation and histone lysine acetylation and was accompanied by binding to NF-kB p65 subunit to miR-184 promoter. These results suggest that miR-184 may act as a downstream effector of albuminuria through LPP3 to promote tubulointerstitial fibrosis and offer the rationale to investigate whether targeting miR-184 in association with albuminuria-lowering drugs may be a new strategy to achieve fully antifibrotic effects, at least in diabetic nephropathy.[245]

### CHRONIC HYPOXIA

One of the most important contributors to the development of tubulointerstitial fibrosis is chronic ischemia.[246] Production of Ang II and inhibition of production of NO underlie chronic vasoconstriction, which may contribute to tissue ischemia and hypoxia.[247] In that regard, histologic studies on biopsies from animal models and human kidneys have documented that there is often a loss of peritubular capillaries in areas of tubulointerstitial fibrosis.[233] Downregulation of VEGF may be functionally implicated in the progressive attrition of peritubular capillaries and tissue hypoxia, as shown in mouse folic acid nephropathy.[248]

Pericytes play a critical role in the stabilization and proliferation of peritubular capillaries via interaction with endothelial cells.[249-251] This process is mediated by several angioregulatory factors, including angiopoietin-1, produced by pericytes, and angiopoietin-2, produced by activated endothelial cells.[251-253] Renal ischemia, as it occurs in chronic kidney disease due to microvascular rarefaction,[254] promotes an imbalance in angiopoietins that besides leading to proliferation of pericytes may induce interstitial fibrosis in the long term.[255]

Moreover, given that the size of the interstitial compartment determines the diffusion distance between peritubular capillaries and tubule cells, interstitial fibrosis further impairs tubular oxygen supply. Focal reduction of capillary blood flow leading to starvation of tubules may underlie tubular atrophy and loss. Under these conditions, the remaining tubules are subjected to functional hypermetabolism with increased oxygen consumption, which in turn creates an even more severely hypoxic environment in the renal interstitium. In vitro, such hypoxia stimulates fibroblast proliferation and ECM production by tubular epithelial cells.[256]

## ENDOGENOUS SYSTEMS OF TISSUE REPAIR

### PROTECTIVE MACROPHAGES

Much remains to be learned about macrophages in tubulointerstitial injury. The role of interstitial macrophages was elucidated in mice with progressive adriamycin-induced nephropathy.[257] By treating mice with the monoclonal antibody ED7 directed against the CD11b/CD18 integrin, which is expressed by macrophages, renal cortical macrophages (ED1-positive cells) were reduced by almost 50%, whether ED7 was administered before or after adriamycin administration.[258] However, ED7 reduced renal structural and functional injury only when treatment was started prior to adriamycin administration.[258]

Among several possible explanations for these observations is a temporal change in the predominant macrophage phenotype. If pathogenic macrophages predominated early and protective macrophages later in the course of the disease, then only early antimacrophage treatment would be expected to protect against progression. Indeed, macrophages can exhibit distinctly different functional phenotypes and can be polarized toward proinflammatory (M1 macrophages) or tissue-reparative (M2 macrophages) phenotype.[259] In the peritubular interstitium, macrophages have been shown to mediate tissue repair in response to acute kidney injury by adopting an M2 phenotype and producing a cytokine environment that supports tubular repair and proliferation rather than inflammation.[260] Colony-stimulating factor-1 (CSF-1) signaling mediated M2 macrophage-induced recovery from renal injury, because pharmacologic blockade of CSF-1 decreased M2 polarization and eventually inhibited tissue repair.[261]

Recent observations also support the importance of macrophage phenotype. For example, in mice with unilateral ureteric obstruction reconstituted with bone marrow of Ang II subtype 1 receptor gene knockout or wild-type mice, infiltrating macrophages were shown to play a beneficial antifibrotic role.[262]

Other studies have demonstrated marked macrophage heterogeneity and context specificity, depending on the nature of the injury and location within the kidney.[263] Evidence is available that macrophages perform both injury-inducing and repair-promoting tasks in different models of inflammation. This has been shown in a reversible model of liver injury, in which the injury and recovery phase are distinct.[264] Macrophage depletion when liver fibrosis was advanced resulted in reduced scarring and fewer myofibroblasts. Macrophage depletion during recovery, by contrast, led to a failure of matrix degradation.[264] These findings provide clear evidence that a functionally distinct subpopulation of macrophages exists in the same tissue.

Further studies on possible temporal variations in the phenotype, activation status, and net effect on injury of macrophages should give a better understanding of the complex role of macrophages in tubulointerstitial injury and repair of chronic renal disease, particularly in the proteinuric setting.

## REGULATORY T CELLS

$CD4^+$ T cells constitute a critical component of the adaptive immune system and are typified by their capacity to help both humoral and cell-mediated responses. However, there is a substantial functional diversity among $CD4^+$ T cells, and certain subpopulations hinder rather than help immune response. The most well-characterized example of an inhibitory subpopulation is the $CD4^+CD25^+$, which appears to play an active role in downregulating pathogenic autoimmune responses.[265] $CD4^+CD25^+$ T cells are potent immunoregulatory cells that suppress T-cell proliferation in vitro and have the capacity to suppress immune responses to auto- and alloantigens, tumor antigens, and infectious antigens in vivo.[266]

The regulatory activity of these cells in the setting of chronic renal diseases is highlighted by studies in severe combined immunodeficient (SCID) mice reconstituted with $CD4^+CD25^+$ T cells after induction of adriamycin nephrosis.[258] Mice reconstituted with these regulatory cells had significantly reduced glomerulosclerosis, tubular injury, and interstitial expansion compared with unreconstituted mice with adriamycin-induced nephrosis.

A study using the green fluorescence protein (GFP)-*Foxp3* mouse suggests that *Foxp3* expression identifies the regulatory T-cell population.[267] In the murine model of adriamycin nephropathy, the adoptive transfer of *Foxp3*-transduced T cells protected against renal injury. Urinary protein excretion and serum creatinine were reduced, and there was significantly less glomerulosclerosis, tubular damage, and interstitial infiltrates.[268]

## KIDNEY-DERIVED PROGENITOR CELLS

In chronic proteinuric renal disease, regression of glomerular structural changes is associated with remodeling of the glomerular architecture.[269] Instrumental to this discovery were three-dimensional reconstruction studies of the glomerular capillary tuft, which allowed the quantification of sclerosis volume reduction and of capillary regeneration upon treatment.[269] The reversal of early glomerular damage in animal models and humans[270] argues for the existence of a regenerative mechanism that promotes glomerular repair. However, mature podocytes are postmitotic cells with limited capacity to divide in situ and therefore unable to regenerate.[270] A potential mechanism for podocyte replacement by bone marrow–derived stem cells has been described in the Alport mouse model as well as in kidney transplants.[271,272] Nevertheless, most studies concluded that regeneration occurs predominantly from resident renal progenitors,[56,67] although the source of these cells remains ill-defined.

Recently, a study using a triple-transgenic mouse model that allowed permanent marking of glomerular parietal cells and their progeny upon administration of doxycycline showed that parietal epithelial cells of the Bowman capsule possess the capability to migrate into the glomerular tuft via the vascular stalk, where they differentiate into podocytes.[273] Similarly, in the adult human kidney, cells localized between the urinary pole and vascular pole of the Bowman capsule—that expressed both progenitor and podocyte markers ($CD24^+CD133^+PDX^+$cells)—can differentiate into podocytes by losing stem cell markers and expressing markers indicative of a podocyte phenotype while progressing from the urinary pole to the surface of the glomerular tuft.[274]

Experimental evidence indicates that intravenous injection of human progenitor cells harvested from the Bowman capsule into SCID mice with adriamycin-induced nephropathy reduced proteinuria and mitigated chronic glomerular damage.[274] Even more intriguing from the clinical perspective is the finding that ACE inhibition induces glomerular repair in MWF rats, a model of spontaneous glomerular injury.[275] In these proteinuric animals, besides halting age-related podocyte loss, lisinopril increased the number of glomerular podocytes above baseline, which was associated with an increased number of proliferating WT1-positive cells, loss of cycling-dependent kinase inhibitor p27 expression, and increased number of parietal podocytes. This indicates that remodeling of the Bowman capsule epithelial cells contributes to the ACE inhibitor–induced restructuring of the damaged glomerular capillary, primarily by restoring the podocyte population.

Similarly, glomerular repair is augmented when glucocorticoid treatment is given to mice with experimental FSGS at a time when podocyte number was already decreased.[276] Prednisone increased podocyte number, which correlated with reduced proteinuria and decreased glomerulosclerosis. This could be the result of direct biological effects on both glomerular epithelial cells, by reducing podocyte apoptosis, and by enhancing podocyte regeneration via increasing the number of parietal epithelial cell precursors.

In addition to ACE inhibitors[144,150] and prednisone,[276] Notch inhibitors,[277] blockers of chemokine stromal-derived factor-1[278] and retinoids,[279] can be added to the list of agents that improve podocyte regeneration by augmenting the number of parietal epithelial cells progenitors. Indeed, in vitro exposure of human renal progenitor cells to human serum albumin inhibited their differentiation into podocytes by sequestering retinoic acid and preventing retinoic acid–response element (RARE)-mediated transcription of podocyte-specific genes.[145] Similarly, in mice with adriamycin-induced nephropathy in vivo, a model of human FSGS, blocking endogenous retinoic acid synthesis, increased proteinuria and exacerbated glomerulosclerosis.[145] This effect was related to a reduction in podocyte number. In RARE-lacZ transgenic mice, albuminuria reduced retinoic acid bioavailability and impaired RARE activation in renal progenitors, inhibiting their differentiation into podocytes.[145] Treatment with retinoic acid restored RARE activity and induced the expression of podocyte markers in renal progenitors, decreasing proteinuria and increasing podocyte number, as demonstrated in serial biopsy specimens.[145]

Together these experimental studies suggest that restoring the capacity of parietal epithelial progenitor cells to differentiate into podocytes could promote the regeneration of podocytes and potentially result in the regression of glomerular disease.

## SYSTEMIC CONSEQUENCES OF NEPHROTIC-RANGE PROTEINURIA

Nephrotic-range proteinuria is accompanied by a cluster of abnormalities known collectively as the nephrotic syndrome. It is characterized by systemic complications that result from profound alterations in the composition of the body protein pool, a state of sodium retention, dyslipidemia, abnormalities of coagulation factors, and a variable degree of renal insufficiency.

### HYPOALBUMINEMIA

Clinical manifestations of the nephrotic syndrome become evident in patients with levels of proteinuria in excess of 3.5 g/day. However, proteinuria in overtly nephrotic subjects usually exceeds this lower bound by a factor of 2 to 3. Immunochemical analysis shows that albumin accounts for more than 80% of the excreted proteins.[280] The second most copiously excreted protein is immunoglobulin, which, after albumin, is the next most abundant protein in plasma. One of the most common systemic abnormalities associated with nephrotic proteinuria is hypoalbuminemia, which develops in most patients.

#### PATHOGENESIS OF HYPOALBUMINEMIA

Under normal conditions, albumin production by the liver is 12–14 g/day (130–200 mg/kg). Production equals the amount catabolized, predominantly in extrarenal locations.[281] However, about 10%, is catabolized in the proximal tubule of the kidney after reabsorption of filtered albumin.[281] In patients with the nephrotic syndrome, hypoalbuminemia

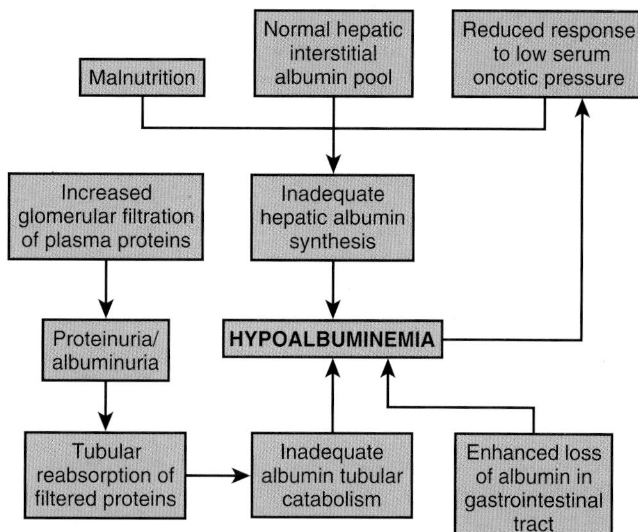


**Fig. 30.10 Schematic representation of mechanisms leading to nephrotic hypoalbuminemia.** Compensatory mechanisms, such as increase in albumin synthesis and decrease in albumin catabolism, are insufficient to correct the hypoalbuminemia.

results from excessive urinary loss, decreased hepatic synthesis, and increased rates of albumin catabolism (Fig. 30.10).

Urinary albumin loss is an important contributor to the development of hypoalbuminemia. However, it is not a sufficient cause in most patients with the nephrotic syndrome, as the rate of hepatic albumin synthesis can increase by at least threefold, thereby compensating for urinary albumin loss.[281] Enhanced loss of albumin in the gastrointestinal tract has also been proposed to contribute to hypoalbuminemia, but there is little evidence for this hypothesis.[282] Therefore for hypoalbuminemia to develop there must be either an insufficient increase in hepatic synthetic rate or an increase in albumin catabolism.

Normally the rate of hepatic albumin synthesis may increase by as much as 300%. However, studies of the nephrotic syndrome in animal models and in humans with hypoalbuminemia demonstrate that the rate of albumin synthesis is at or only slightly above the upper limit of normal as long as dietary protein is adequate.[283] This indicates an inadequate synthetic response to hypoalbuminemia by the liver.

Oncotic pressure of the plasma perfusing the liver is one major regulator of protein synthesis.[215] Experimental evidence in rats that are genetically deficient in circulating albumin showed a twofold increase in the hepatic transcription rate of the albumin gene compared with normal rats.[215] However, in these rats the increase in hepatic albumin synthesis was inadequate to compensate for the degree of hypoalbuminemia, which indicates an impaired synthetic response.[215] Similarly, in nephrotic patients, reduced oncotic pressure is unable to enhance the albumin synthetic rate of the liver to the extent required to restore plasma albumin concentration.[283] There is also evidence in normal subjects that the hepatic interstitial albumin regulates albumin synthesis.[284] Because the hepatic interstitial albumin pool is not depleted in the nephrotic syndrome, the albumin synthetic response is normal or slightly increased, but it remains inadequate relative to the level of hypoalbuminemia.[284]

Dietary protein-intake further contributes to the synthesis of albumin. Hepatic albumin mRNA and albumin synthesis was not increased in nephrotic rats when fed a low-protein diet but increased with a high-protein diet.[285] However, serum albumin levels were not altered because hyperfiltration resulting from increased protein intake led to increased albuminuria.

The contribution of renal albumin catabolism to hypoalbuminemia in the nephrotic syndrome is controversial. Some have argued that the renal tubular albumin transport capacity is already saturated at physiologic levels of filtered albumin and that any increase in filtered protein, instead of being absorbed and catabolized, is simply excreted in the urine.[286] Studies in isolated perfused proximal tubules in rabbits, however, demonstrated a dual transport system for albumin uptake.[287] In addition to a low-capacity system that became saturated when the protein load exceeded physiologic levels, a high-capacity low-affinity system was also present and allowed the tubular absorptive rate for albumin to increase as the filtered load rose. Thus an increase in the fractional catabolic rate may occur in the nephrotic syndrome.

This hypothesis is supported by the positive correlation between fractional albumin catabolism and albuminuria in rats with puromycin aminonucleoside-induced nephrosis.[288] Nevertheless, because total body albumin stores are substantially decreased in the nephrotic syndrome, absolute catabolic rates may be normal or even reduced.[282] This outcome is affected by nutritional state, as documented by the fact that in nephrotic rats nourished with a low-protein diet, absolute albumin catabolism was reduced but not in those with normal dietary protein intake.[289]

In summary, hypoalbuminemia in the nephrotic syndrome results from multiple alterations in albumin homeostasis that are not sufficiently compensated for by hepatic albumin synthesis and by decreased renal tubular albumin catabolism.

## CONSEQUENCES OF HYPOALBUMINEMIA

Impairment of kidney function is the rule in patients with nephrotic hypoalbuminemia and it usually manifests in two ways. One is the inability of the kidney to maintain sodium and fluid homeostasis. The other is loss of intrinsic ultrafiltration capacity of glomerular capillary walls, a phenomenon that leads, in turn, to fall in GFR.[290]

When viewed in physiologic terms, the GFR can be defined as the net rate of water flux across the walls of the capillaries in the glomerular tufts of the kidney. It is determined by the product of the net pressure for ultrafiltration and the ultrafiltration coefficient—$K_f$—a measure of intrinsic ultrafiltration capacity, derived from the product of the available filtering surface area(s) and the hydraulic permeability of the glomerular capillary wall (k). By estimating GFR and its determinants in humans, it has been shown that a reduced GFR in some forms of the nephrotic syndrome (minimal change and membranous nephropathy) is exclusively a consequence of profoundly lowered hydraulic permeability.[291] In the nephrotic syndrome associated with lupus nephritis, idiopathic focal and segmental glomerulosclerosis, and diabetic nephropathy, both reduction of the surface area available for filtration and impaired hydraulic permeability contribute to $K_f$ depression.[292, 293]

The principal cause of impaired hydraulic permeability in nephrotic disorders is broadening and effacement of epithelial foot processes.[291] This lowers the frequency of interpodocytic slit diaphragms through which water must pass to gain access to the Bowman space, thereby increasing the resistance to water flow. The low $K_f$ is partially offset by an increase in net ultrafiltration pressure, which is largely due to a substantial lowering of the intraglomerular capillary oncotic pressure. As a result, the fall in GFR is not proportional to the decrease in $K_f$. This compensatory elevation in net ultrafiltration pressure explains why reduced values of single-nephron GFR are not consistently observed in all experimental nephrotic models.[294]

The low ultrafiltration capacity induced by glomerular disease and protein depletion makes the nephrotic patient particularly vulnerable to acute exacerbations of hypofiltration and renal insufficiency.[295] As the prevailing level of GFR depends heavily on ultrafiltration pressure in the presence of a low $K_f$, any maneuver lowering the glomerular capillary perfusion pressure can, therefore, cause a precipitous fall in the GFR. The susceptibility of nephrotic patients to episodes of acute kidney injury should thus be borne in mind when prescribing drugs, such as diuretics, cyclooxygenase inhibitors, and cyclosporine, that can compromise the ultrafiltration pressure.

An additional consequence of hypoalbuminemia is the potential for enhanced drug toxicity.[296] Indeed, many drugs are bound to albumin. Hypoalbuminemia reduces the number of available binding sites and increases the proportion of circulating free drugs, but in a steady state this is counterbalanced by faster metabolism. Furthermore, because protein binding may enhance tubule drug secretion, diminished protein binding in the nephrotic syndrome may delay renal excretion of some drugs.[297] Although the clinical consequences of altered protein binding may be difficult to predict, higher levels of free drugs may be toxic, as shown with prednisolone.[298]

The case of diuretics is intriguing. Resistance to loop diuretics, which often occurs in patients with the nephrotic syndrome, may be due to reduced delivery of the diuretic to its site of action, secondary to hypoalbuminemia. Anecdotal reports suggest that the administration of furosemide with small amounts of albumin (6–20 g) can enhance the response to furosemide in nephrotic patients.[299] These observations are not conclusive, because others did not show a difference in the excretion of intravenous furosemide in the urine of nephrotic patients compared with normal controls.[300] On the other hand, excessive amounts of filtered albumin in the tubule may bind furosemide and make it less effective.[301]

In animals, the inhibition of fractional loop $Cl^-$ reabsorption by furosemide is blunted by the presence of albumin in the proximal tubule, and prevention of albumin–furosemide binding with warfarin and sulfisoxazole partially restored the response to the diuretic.[301] However, these findings were not confirmed in nephrotic patients given sulfisoxazole, raising doubt about the importance of excessive albumin-bound furosemide at the active tubular site in resistance to diuretics.[302] Sodium-retaining mechanisms, such as low effective arterial blood volume and activation of neurohumoral factors, may be relatively more important.

Many binding proteins are lost in the urine in the nephrotic syndrome.[303] Consequently, in patients with the nephrotic syndrome, the plasma levels of many ions (iron, copper, and zinc), vitamins (vitamin D metabolites), and hormones (thyroid and steroid hormones) are low because the level of protein-bound ligands is reduced. Urinary loss of protein-bound ligands can theoretically cause depletion, but there is little convincing clinical evidence for this, with the possible exception of vitamin D.[304] Indeed, one of the proteins lost in the urine of patients with the nephrotic syndrome is cholecalciferol binding globulin (also known as vitamin D binding protein DBP), which is a 59-kDa protein easily filtered by nephrotic glomeruli.[305] Because 25-hydroxycholecalciferol (25-[OH]$D_3$) circulates as a complex with DBP, there is also an associated urinary loss of 25-(OH)$D_3$ in the nephrotic syndrome.[306] The oral administration of $^3$H-labeled cholecalciferol indicated that the serum half-life of 25-(OH)$D_3$ was reduced and urinary excretion increased in the nephrotic syndrome.[307] Nevertheless, in general, nephrotic patients have normal to decreased plasma levels of 1,25-dihydroxycholecalciferol (1,25-[$OH_2$]$_2D_3$).[306]

Although the hypocalcemia of the nephrotic syndrome was once attributed solely to the reduction in protein-bound calcium secondary to hypoalbuminemia, a subset of patients has been noted with hypocalcemia out of proportion to the hypoalbuminemia. In these patients ionized serum calcium is decreased.[308] Secondary hyperparathyroidism is seen in some patients, even in the absence of renal failure, as are changes in bone histology consistent with mixed osteomalacia and osteitis fibrosa cystic bone disease.[309] Not all investigators, however, have observed abnormalities in calcium homeostasis in the nephrotic syndrome.[310] Why only a subset of patients is predisposed to alterations in calcium, vitamin D, and parathyroid hormone homeostasis has not been determined, but it has been suggested that factors such as age, duration of disease, renal function, degree of proteinuria, serum albumin concentration, and corticosteroid therapy might be involved.[304]

Finally, hypoalbuminemia may play a role in platelet hyperaggregability.[311] Because albumin normally binds arachidonic acid, thus limiting its conversion to thromboxane $A_2$ by platelets, hypoalbuminemia might allow increased platelet arachidonate metabolism to take place, and platelet hyperreactivity may result.[311]

## EDEMA FORMATION

The clinical manifestation that most frequently brings the nephrotic patient to medical attention is the formation of edema. This represents an increase in the size of the interstitial fluid compartment. The interstitial fluid accumulates most readily in dependent areas where tissue pressure is low. It thus manifests as periorbital edema upon awakening in the morning, and pedal edema at the end of the day. Even when edema is generalized and massive, a condition referred to as anasarca, it remains most marked in the lower extremities. Not infrequently, anasarca is also accompanied by large effusions into the peritoneal, pleural, and pericardial spaces. The mechanisms responsible for extravascular fluid accumulation in nephrotic patients are complex and only partially understood.

### REDUCED PLASMA ONCOTIC PRESSURE

Low colloid oncotic pressure as a result of hypoalbuminemia favors the movement of water from the intravascular to the interstitial space. Under normal conditions, edema formation is halted by expansion and proliferation of lymphatics that increase lymphatic flow, and by reduction of interstitial oncotic pressure due to protein-free fluid accumulation. In addition, the increased hydraulic pressure in the interstitium because of fluid accumulation lowers the transcapillary pressure gradient, further reducing the transudation of plasma fluid into the interstitial space. However, there is no clear evidence of alterations in these normal defense mechanisms against edema formation in nephrotic patients.[312] For example, comparable changes in interstitial and plasma colloid oncotic pressure have been documented during relapse and remission phases in patients with nephrotic syndrome.[312] Moreover, the capillary hydraulic conductivity is elevated in nephrotic patients,[313] possibly due to disruption of the intercellular macromolecular complex between endothelial cells, which enhances capillary filtration capacity and may lead to sustained edema formation.[314] These observations suggest that hypoalbuminemia per se may not be the primary determinant of the severity of edema formation and that intrarenal mechanisms may have a prominent contributory role.

### ALTERATIONS IN BLOOD VOLUME

According to the traditional view, lowering of the plasma albumin concentration eventually induces renal sodium and fluid retention in the nephrotic syndrome by causing hypovolemia, the so-called underfill mechanism (Fig. 30.11). Indeed, hypovolemia as a consequence of reduced plasma colloid oncotic pressure triggers a cascade of events that signal the kidney to retain the filtered sodium and water.[315] Thus hypovolemia is the afferent stimulus of a complex

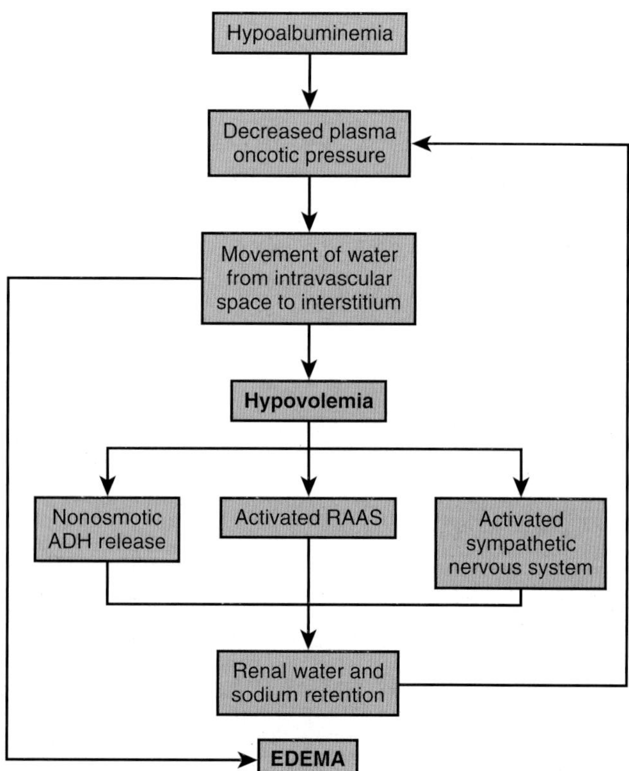


**Fig. 30.11** **The "underfill" mechanism of edema formation.** Hypovolemia, as a consequence of reduced plasma oncotic pressure, is the key event that signals the kidney to retain the filtered sodium and water. *ADH*, Vasopressin; *RAAS*, renin–angiotensin–aldosterone system.

pathway of responses mediated by low- and high-pressure baroreceptors in the cardiac atria, carotid arteries, and aorta that activate the sympathetic nervous system and the renin-angiotensin system. Moreover, hypovolemia also promotes excessive nonosmotic secretion of arginine vasopressin (AVP), which further contributes to water retention by the kidneys.[315]

The homeostatic response of renal sodium and water retention that serves to restore intravascular volume also exacerbates hypoalbuminemia, thereby sustaining transudation of plasma fluid into the interstitial space. The fact that salt retention may be the consequence of an underfilled circulation is consistent with the finding that head-out water immersion, a maneuver that increases plasma volume, is followed by a natriuretic and diuretic response in some nephrotic patients.[316]

This mechanistic scenario of edema formation in the nephrotic syndrome would also imply consistently reduced plasma volume,[317] as well as an elevated plasma renin activity (PRA),[318] and increased plasma and urinary levels of catecholamines.[319] However, only a minority of nephrotic patients have a low plasma volume[319]; in fact, approximately 70% of patients had normal or even high values in some studies.[320] In some cases, plasma volume was lower during remission than during the acute phase of the disease.[319,320] However, methodologic issues have been raised about the measurement of plasma volume in nephrotic patients that may limit the interpretation of these studies.[321]

Measurement of vasoactive hormones, which are responsive to low plasma volume and can be taken as surrogate markers of the intravascular volume, also documented that only 50% of nephrotic patients have higher than normal PRA and plasma as well as urinary aldosterone levels.[322] Moreover, pharmacologic blockade of the renin–angiotensin–aldosterone system in nephrotic patients with a high PRA does not change sodium excretion.[323] Similarly, plasma levels of norepinephrine, arginine vasopressin, and atrial natriuretic peptide (ANP) are near normal or inconsistently changed.[324] The diuretic and natriuretic response to hyperoncotic plasma or albumin infusions,[325] or to central volume expansion with head-out water immersion, also varies widely from patient to patient.[325] Evidence that PRA often increases rather than decreases after steroid-induced remission of the nephrotic syndrome is additional, albeit indirect, evidence that argues against a key role for hypovolemia in edema formation in most nephrotic patients.[322]

## INTRARENAL MECHANISMS

Alternatively, the overfill theory hypothesizes that there is a dominant mechanism by which the kidneys retain sodium independently of circulating plasma volume, leading to hypervolemia (Fig. 30.12).[315] Examination of the edema-forming, nephrotic patient during consumption of a known amount of sodium reveals a positive sodium balance. This results in increased blood volume, which by altering Starling forces across the capillary wall, leads to plasma leakage into the interstitium and overflow edema. This mechanism has been illustrated in a unilateral model of puromycin amino–nucleoside (PAN)-induced nephrosis in rats.[326] In such a model, in which albumin concentration in the systemic circulation is normal, only the proteinuric kidney (not the contralateral intact one) retained excessive amounts of sodium and water. This indicates that abnormal sodium retention by the proteinuric kidney is brought about by intrarenal rather than circulating or systemic factors.

These findings can be partly explained by a lowered filtered sodium load, a consequence of the diminished GFR that

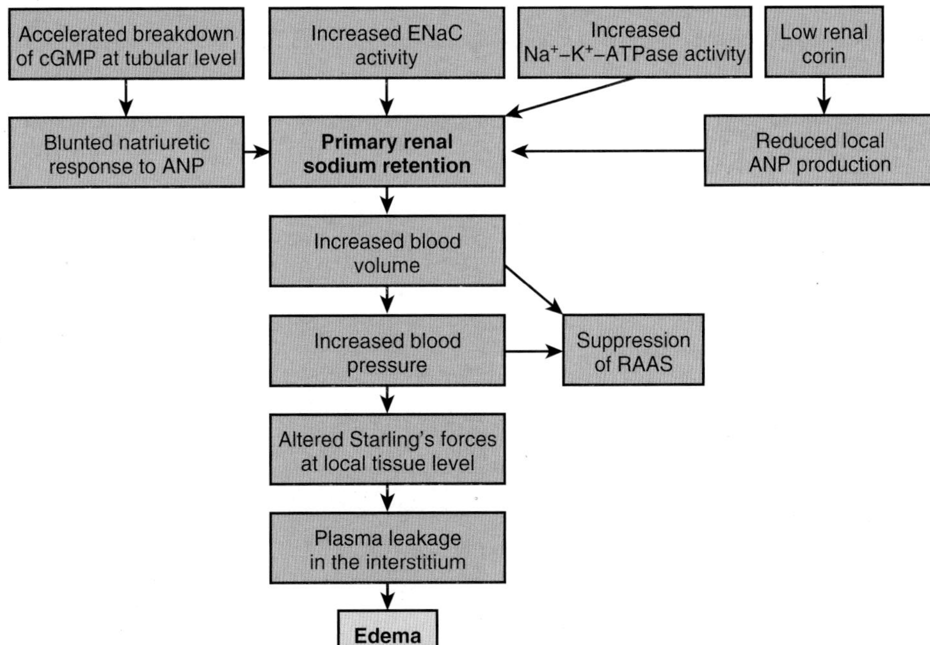


**Fig. 30.12 The "overfill" mechanism of edema formation.** The abnormal renal sodium retention is the consequence of blunted natriuretic response to atrial natriuretic peptide, increased epithelial sodium channel *(ENaC)* activity, and $Na^{+}$-$K^{+}$-ATPase activity, and is the key event of the process. The resulting hypervolemia alters Starling forces across the capillary wall at the local tissue level, leading to overflow edema. *cGMP*, Cyclic guanosine monophosphate; *RAAS*, renin-angiotensin aldosterone system.

frequently accompanies nephrotic range proteinuria. However, because the fractional sodium excretion is low, enhanced tubular sodium reabsorption appears to be the predominant cause of sodium retention in the nephrotic syndrome. Analysis of segmental sodium transport in nephrotic rats has identified the collecting duct as the major site of enhanced sodium reabsorption.[326] Refractoriness to the natriuretic action of ANP (which increases urinary sodium and water excretion) in experimental[327] and clinical[328] studies further indicates the distal segments of the nephron as the likely site of sodium retention in nephrotic syndrome. Indeed, the inner medullary segment of the collecting duct is the tubule segment most richly endowed with receptors for ANP.[329]

A crucial observation was that natriuretic and diuretic responses to intravenously infused atrial extract (from normal or nephrotic rats) or synthetic ANP were markedly reduced in nephrotic as compared with normal rats.[330] In a rat model of unilateral glomerulopathy, the blunted natriuretic and diuretic response to ANP was confined to the "nephrotic" kidney as opposed to the contralateral normal kidney, despite a comparable increase in GFR.[327] Moreover, both enhanced release of endogenous ANP during water immersion and infusion of exogenous ANP failed to promote an appropriate natriuretic response in nephrotic patients.[328]

Taken together, these findings support a role for ANP in intrarenal sodium retention in the nephrotic syndrome. In addition, it can be inferred that alterations in the intrinsic transport properties of the collecting duct render this tubule segment unresponsive to the natriuretic action of ANP.

In some studies, increased activity of efferent sympathetic nerve has been related to the blunted ANP natriuretic response.[331] More consistent evidence indicates enhanced phosphodiesterase activity in collecting duct cells from nephrotic animals, leading to accelerated breakdown of normally produced cyclic guanosine monophosphate (cGMP), which is important for intracellular signaling after ANP binding to its specific receptors.[332]

With the discovery of corin, a 1042–amino acid transmembrane serine protease that converts proANP and proBNP into the active forms ANP and BNP,[333,334] the pathogenesis of edema formation in nephrotic syndrome has been revised. In addition to being initially localized in the heart,[333] more recently, corin has been shown to also be expressed in renal tissue.[335] Using immunohistochemical analysis, colocalization of corin and ANP in renal tissue has been documented.[335] It is noteworthy that kidneys of corin$^{-/-}$ mice displayed increased amounts of renal β-epithelial $Na^+$ channel (ENaC), phosphodiesterase 5 (PDE5), and protein kinase G II, as compared with wild-type mice. Induction of nephrotic syndrome by puromycin aminonucleoside or glomerulonephritis by anti-Thy1 induced concomitant increase in proANP and decrease in ANP in the kidney in association with low renal immunoreactive levels of corin.[335,336] Upregulation of PDE5 and kinase G II resulted in reduced cGMP in the collecting duct, and subsequently in increased ENaC abundance seen in nephrotic syndrome and glomerulonephritis.[336] These findings suggest that corin deficiency by lowering locally produced ANP might be involved in primary salt retention seen in edematous glomerular diseases.[337] In this regard, reduced urinary corin levels were reported in patients with chronic kidney disease.[338]

In the kidney, the ultimate regulation of sodium reabsorption occurs in the collecting duct through the low-conductance epithelial sodium channel (ENaC),[339] located on the apical membrane of principal cells. Evidence is also available that the proteolytic removal of an inhibitory domain from the γ-subunit of ENaC by the serine protease plasmin can activate ENaC.[340] Plasmin, present in the urine of nephrotic rats and humans, has been shown to activate ENaC via this mechanism.[341] Additionally, urokinase-type plasminogen activator present in the rat and human kidney can convert inactive plasminogen (which is filtered by the nephrotic kidney) to the active form plasmin.[341] In the rat PAN nephrosis model, amiloride increased urine sodium excretion and reduced ascites volume. This effect was attributed to the ability of amiloride to inhibit both ENaC and urokinase-type plasminogen activator, and thus to reduce the amount of active plasmin present.[341]

ENaC is also regulated by aldosterone.[339] In rat models of the nephrotic syndrome, activation of ENaC together with elevated plasma aldosterone levels has been reported.[342] Nevertheless, in puromycin-induced nephrosis in rats with clamped aldosterone plasma levels, sodium retention persisted even when ENaC recruitment to the apical membrane was inhibited.[343] Conversely, the transport activity of sodium–potassium–adenosine triphosphatase ($Na^+$-$K^+$-ATPase), the ubiquitous sodium pump localized exclusively on the basolateral membrane, was increased.[343] These findings indicate that increased $Na^+$-$K^+$-ATPase activity is the driving force behind enhanced sodium reabsorption in the nephrotic syndrome, an observation confirmed by several studies in the cortical collecting ducts in nephrotic rats.[344]

Because the $Na^+$-$K^+$-ATPase pump in the basolateral membrane promotes secondary passive sodium entry from the lumen through the ENaC, Na retention in the collecting duct of nephrotic rats can result from the coordinated overactivity of these tubular sodium transporters. A role for the proximal tubule in the avid sodium retention of nephrotic syndrome has been proposed based on the observation that in PAN-nephrotic rats increased sodium reabsorption was associated with a shift of the apical $Na^+/H^+$ exchanger isoform 3 (NHE-3) from an inactive to an active pool.[345] The increase in NHE-3-specific activity may be a response to the increased albumin load presented to the proximal tubule, as indicated by the correlation between albumin exposure and enhanced NHE-3 abundance and activity in opossum kidney (OKP) cells.[346]

An additional hypothesis concerning intrarenal mechanisms of nephrotic edema proposes that interstitial inflammation of the kidney plays a major role in the pathogenesis of primary sodium retention.[347] The generation of vasoconstrictor and the reduction of vasodilator substances in the interstitium, driven by the inflammatory cell infiltrate, can lead to a reduction in Kf and single-nephron GFR. These glomerular hemodynamic changes that reduce filtered sodium load combine with the increased net tubular sodium reabsorption induced by mediators released from the inflammatory cell infiltrate leading to primary sodium retention, an overfilled intravascular volume, and increased capillary hydrostatic pressure. The decrease in plasma oncotic pressure again promotes fluid movement out of the vascular compartment, thereby buffering the changes in blood volume induced by primary sodium retention. A renal inflammatory infiltrate is, however, minimal or absent in most children with minimal-change nephrotic syndrome. Thus the nephrotic edema may derive from a combination of primary sodium retention and relative arterial underfilling. The predominance of one or the other mechanism is perhaps in accordance with the pathogenesis of nephrotic syndrome or the stage of the disease.

Deranged renal water handling is also a cardinal feature of the nephrotic syndrome. Defects in both urinary diluting ability[348] and concentrating capacity[348] have been documented in nephrotic patients. The cause of the concentrating defect has been explored in experimental models of the nephrotic syndrome. The extensive downregulation of the expression of the water channels aquaporin 1, 2, and 3 in the collecting duct,[349] and of the urea transporter,[350] as well as a marked decrease in the abundance of thick ascending limb $Na^+$ transporters represent an appropriate renal response to the extracellular volume expansion observed in the nephrotic syndrome despite increased circulating vasopressin, but may occur at the expense of decreased urinary concentrating capacity.

## HYPERLIPIDEMIA

Both quantitative and qualitative changes in lipid metabolism occur in the nephrotic syndrome, with virtually all plasma lipid and lipoprotein fractions being elevated.[351] Blood levels of cholesterol are almost always increased and continue to rise as the severity of the nephrotic syndrome increases.[351] Total cholesterol and cholesterol esters are all increased.[352] Levels of triglycerides are more variable and in many patients do not increase at all, except when the nephrotic state is very severe.[351] Plasma levels of free fatty acids are within normal limits in the nephrotic syndrome, although a smaller than normal fraction is bound to plasma albumin.[351] Levels of very low-density lipoprotein (VLDL), intermediate-density lipoprotein (IDL), and low-density lipoprotein (LDL) increased early in the nephrotic syndrome[351,353]; data on high-density lipoproteins (HDLs) are less clear. Plasma levels are usually normal but may decrease due to HDL excretion in the urine in severely proteinuric patients.[351]

The composition of the lipoprotein molecules is also abnormal. Greater than usual amounts of cholesterol and triglycerides are present in VLDL, IDL, and LDL. Moreover, an alteration in the specific type and quantity of various apoprotein moieties in the lipoprotein molecules has been described, with reduced apo C despite elevations in apo B, C-II, and E and an increased ratio of apo C-III to apo C-II.[354] These abnormalities return to normal promptly when the nephrotic syndrome remits.

### PATHOGENESIS OF NEPHROTIC HYPERLIPIDEMIA

Two mechanisms contribute to nephrotic dyslipidemia: overproduction and impaired catabolism/clearance of serum lipids and lipoproteins (Fig. 30.13). There is general agreement that hepatic lipid and apolipoprotein synthesis are both increased and that the clearance of chylomicrons (CM) and VLDL[355] is reduced in the nephrotic syndrome. Cholesterol synthesis has been shown to increase both in animals and humans in response to the hypoalbuminemia associated with the nephrotic syndrome.[356] Hepatic activity of hydroxymethylglutaryl CoA reductase, the rate-limiting step for hepatic synthesis of cholesterol, is elevated.[320] In general, serum cholesterol levels are inversely proportional to serum albumin levels,[320] and cholesterol levels generally normalize upon remission. Conversely, triglyceride synthesis does not appear to be increased.

It has been suggested that lipoprotein synthesis increases in parallel with albumin synthesis because they share a common secretory pathway.[357] This hypothesis was supported by studies showing that infusion of albumin partially corrected nephrotic hyperlipidemia. It has also been reported that apolipoprotein B (apo B) secretion by cultured hepatocytes can be reduced by increasing the oncotic pressure of the culture medium.

Most evidence still indicates that reduced extracellular albumin concentration and/or reduced extracellular oncotic

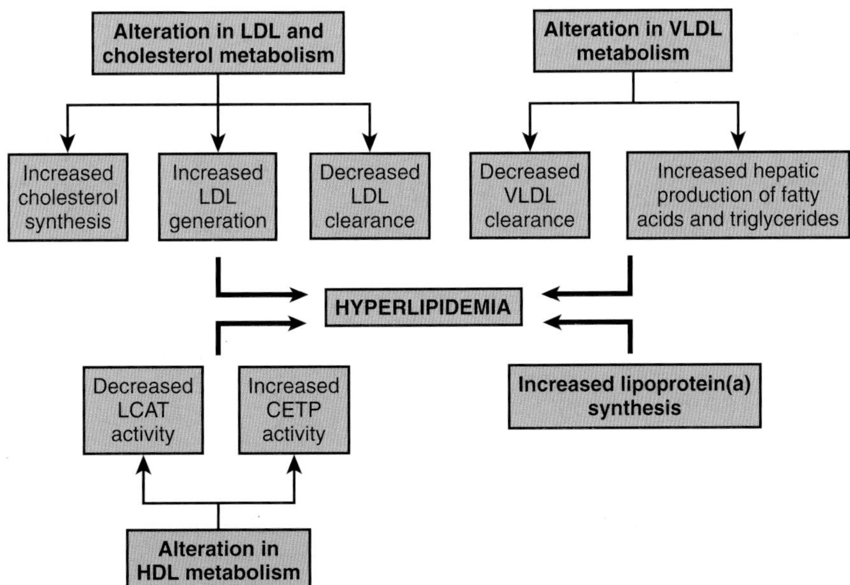


**Fig, 30.13** Pathophysiology of nephrotic hyperlipidemia. All abnormalities of lipid profile originate from alteration in low-density lipoprotein *(LDL)*, very-low-density lipoprotein *(VLDL)*, high-density lipoprotein *(HDL)*, and cholesterol metabolism and increased synthesis of lipoprotein(a).

pressure in some way regulate apolipoprotein synthesis and lipogenesis by the liver. Although hepatic apolipoprotein synthesis is increased in the nephrotic syndrome, not all apolipoproteins are affected to the same degree, and mechanisms causing increased synthesis of the various apolipoproteins are also different. Secretion of apo A is increased approximately sixfold,[357] whereas synthesis of apo B and E is only increased twofold. Synthesis of the apo C is not increased.

Apo A-I mRNA is increased transcriptionally in the livers of nephrotic and analbuminemic rats,[358] suggesting that reduced plasma oncotic pressure or albumin concentration is responsible for the change in apo A-I gene expression. Although plasma apo B and E are both increased in nephrotic and analbuminemic rats, there is little or no change in transcription rates. Thus if increased synthesis is causing increased levels of these apolipoproteins in plasma, the mechanisms involved are most likely posttranscriptional, at the level of translational or protein processing, in contrast to apo A-I.

In addition to increased synthesis, studies in animals and humans have determined alterations in the catabolism of lipids in the nephrotic syndrome. The clearance of chylomicrons and VLDL is reduced following the onset of proteinuria but is normal in rats with hereditary analbuminemia,[357,359] suggesting that urinary loss of a liporegulatory substance, and not reduced albumin concentration or oncotic pressure, may play a role in causing defective lipolysis.

One possible explanation for the defective removal of lipoproteins is a decrease in the activity of lipoprotein lipase (LPL), which hydrolyzes triglycerides in VLDL and chylomicrons, releasing free fatty acids. LPL activity is reduced in nephrotic rats, which provides a potential mechanism for delayed lipolysis.[357] Chylomicron catabolism in hearts isolated from nephrotic rats was decreased in vitro and the LPL pool bound to vascular endothelium was reduced by approximately 90%. LPL activity not bound to the vascular endothelium, and hence unable to interact with large lipoproteins, was normal.[359] Thus a specific reduction in LPL attached to the vascular endothelium may play a role in the reduced catabolism of chylomicrons and VLDL in the nephrotic syndrome.

The relationship between reduced endothelial-bound LPL activity and reduced catabolism of chylomicrons and VLDL is by no means clear. VLDL and chylomicron catabolism by analbuminemic rats is normal despite a marked reduction in heparin-releasable LPL activity.[360] Moreover, it has been reported that HDL isolated from normal animals corrects defective lipolysis of VLDL isolated from nephrotic rats, whereas HDL isolated from nephrotic animals may be dysfunctional. Indeed, HDL isolated from nephrotic animals has been found to be structurally abnormal.[361] Thus multiple separate defects in the peripheral catabolism of triglyceride-rich lipoproteins may be responsible for delayed lipolysis.

Studies in patients with the nephrotic syndrome have not been as detailed as in the rat; however, when comparable studies are evaluated both species exhibit similar disturbances in lipid metabolism. The fractional turnover rate of triglycerides is reduced in nephrotic subjects compared with controls, and the half-life of triglycerides in VLDL is prolonged from 4 to 11 hours.[362] Not only is VLDL catabolism decreased, but the concentration curve over time has an unusual shape, presumably resulting from a delay in the conversion of VLDL into LDL.[363]

It has been suggested that the delay in lipolysis in humans, as in rats, is due to a decrease in LPL activity. Evidence supporting this hypothesis is that LPL activity is reduced in children with the nephrotic syndrome and increases after remission. Furthermore, there is a strong inverse correlation between LPL activity and the concentration of triglycerides in the VLDL fraction,[364] although not all investigators report decreased LPL activity in nephrotic patients.[365]

LDL catabolism has been shown to be either normal or reduced[366] in patients with the nephrotic syndrome and only marginally reduced in nephrotic rats.[367] Reduced receptor-mediated LDL clearance has been reported in some clinical studies,[368] which may account in part for elevations in LDL. A defect in LDL receptor translation or enhanced receptor protein turnover has been hypothesized because normal LDL receptor mRNA was found in nephrotic rats despite marked reduction in LDL receptor protein expression in the liver.[369]

The nephrotic syndrome is also associated with abnormalities in the activity of enzymes required for effective function of HDL. Cholesterol ester transfer protein (CETP) catalyzes the transfer of the cholesterol ester–rich core of $HDL_2$ to VLDL remnant particles creating LDL, and thereby increasing LDL cholesterol at the expense of HDL cholesterol. CETP is increased in the plasma of nephrotic patients and correlates positively with VLDL cholesterol and negatively with HDL cholesterol.[370]

The enzyme lecithin–cholesterol acyl transferase (LCAT) catalyzes the esterification of cholesterol and its incorporation in HDL particles and promotes the conversion of $HDL_3$ to $HDL_2$. The observation that $HDL_3$ is preserved in plasma from nephrotic patients at the apparent expense of $HDL_2$ suggests that the LCAT activity is reduced in the nephrotic syndrome.[371] However, increased activity of CETP could also explain this pattern of HDL distribution by rapidly cycling the core of $HDL_2$ to VLDL remnant particles, thus increasing the flux of cholesterol from the surface of nascent HDL into the core of LDL by increased activity of this enzyme. Furthermore, mature HDL also transports a number of apolipoproteins that serve as cofactors. One of these apolipoproteins, Apo C-II, is an endogenous activator of LPL activity. Apo C-II is normally transported by $HDL_2$ to nascent VLDL and chylomicrons. Apo C-II may be lost in the urine of nephrotic patients, either as free protein or bound to HDL.[372] Additionally, an inhibitor of Apo C-II, Apo C-III, is increased in the nephrotic syndrome; with the resulting decreased Apo C-II–to–Apo C-III ratio, the activity of LPL is significantly decreased.

## CLINICAL CONSEQUENCES OF HYPERLIPIDEMIA

The most important consequence of hyperlipidemia is its potential for inducing cardiovascular disease. The changes that occur in blood lipoprotein composition in the nephrotic syndrome,[353] reduced $HDL_2$ cholesterol, a relative increase in $HDL_3$ cholesterol, and the massive increase in total cholesterol, mostly found in the LDL, IDL, and VLDL fractions, are likely to increase the risk of atherosclerotic disease. Nevertheless, the presence of additional risk factors for atherosclerosis in nephrotic patients, notably hypertension, hypercoagulability and chronic renal failure, makes it difficult to determine the individual contribution of hyperlipidemia to the increase in risk.

Given the natural history of atherosclerosis, one would predict that the patient with a protracted form of nephrotic syndrome has the highest risk of dying from premature cardiovascular disease.[373] Accelerated atherosclerosis has been reported in patients with proteinuria and hyperlipidemia and in some studies has been associated with a strongly increased incidence of cardiovascular disease and stroke.[373] One study reported an 85-fold increase in the incidence of ischemic heart disease in nephrotic patients.[374] In another retrospective analysis of 142 patients with proteinuria greater than 3.5 g/day, the relative risk of myocardial infarction was found to be 5.5 and the risk of cardiac death 2.8 compared with age- and sex-matched controls.[373]

A number of studies have indicated a potential role for hyperlipidemia in the progression of chronic kidney disease. It was proposed that filtered lipoproteins might accumulate in the mesangium and promote sclerosis.[375] In animals, lipogenic diets have been shown to induce focal sclerosis, and the extent of glomerular damage correlates with the serum cholesterol; in the obese Zucker rat, focal sclerosis correlates with hyperlipidemia and can be ameliorated by lipid-lowering drugs.[376] Similarly, free and esterified cholesterol was found in the glomeruli of nephrotic rats, and a close correlation was noted between plasma cholesterol levels and the number of sclerosing glomerular lesions.[377]

Whether hyperlipidemia also plays a role in the progression of chronic kidney disease in the human nephrotic syndrome has yet to be determined. Although there is no specific indication to treat the qualitative abnormalities that characterize the lipid disorder of the nephrotic syndrome, if it is anticipated that the duration of hyperlipidemia will be prolonged, it is wise to initiate therapy. Treatment of nephrotic patients with ACE inhibitors[378] results in a decline in both proteinuria and blood lipid levels even if plasma albumin concentration does not increase. The decline in blood lipid levels includes a decrease in total cholesterol, lipoprotein(a), a decrease in VLDL and LDL cholesterol, and a decrease in the activities of CETP and LCAT.[379]

It is prudent to restrict dietary cholesterol and saturated lipids in patients with the nephrotic syndrome. The long-term effects of dietary supplementation with fish oil (rich in omega-3-polyunsaturated fatty acids) are yet unknown and it cannot be recommended as standard treatment except within the context of a controlled investigative trial. If reduction of proteinuria and dietary fat restriction do not effectively reduce hyperlipidemia, a variety of lipid-lowering drugs, including the 3-hydroxy-3-methyl-glutaryl coenzyme A reductase inhibitors (statins), antioxidants, and fibric acid derivatives, may be useful.

## HYPERCOAGULABILITY

Urinary loss of some of the proteins involved in the coagulation cascade and the adaptive increased synthesis of others can induce a hypercoagulable state.[380] Although arterial thrombosis has been reported, it is venous thrombosis that occurs with a particularly high incidence in nephrotic subjects.[381]

### PATHOGENESIS OF HYPERCOAGULABILITY

In the nephrotic syndrome, there are widespread alterations in synthesis, turnover, and urinary losses of proteins involved both in coagulation and fibrinolysis. The numerous coagulation abnormalities that occur in the nephrotic syndrome are summarized in Fig. 30.14. Alterations in the concentrations of almost every coagulation factor, including zymogens (factors II, V, VII, IX, X, XI, and XII), cofactors (factors V and VIII), and fibrinogen, can occur.[381] Plasma proteins lost in the urine in patients with the nephrotic syndrome include factors IX, X and XII, which become deficient as there is no sufficient increase in synthetic rates.[381] In contrast, proteins of higher molecular weight, including factors V and VIII, and fibrinogen accumulate because of increased synthesis.[380] Levels of factor VIII typically increase as much as two- to three-fold.[380] However, because factor VIII is also an acute-phase reactant, high factor VIII levels may be an epiphenomenon rather than a causal factor in the development of venous thrombosis.

There is an inverse correlation between serum albumin and fibrinogen levels in the nephrotic syndrome.[382] The elevated plasma levels of fibrinogen likely result from increased hepatic synthesis, as catabolism is normal.[383] Hyperfibrinogenemia may contribute to the procoagulant state by providing more substrate for fibrin formation and by promoting platelet hyperaggregability, increased blood viscosity, and red blood cell aggregation. Increased fibrin deposition, however, may

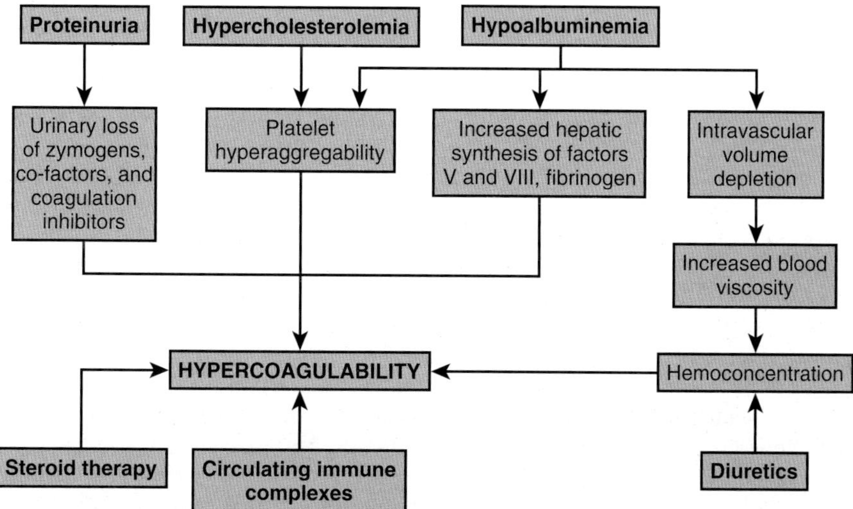


**Fig. 30.14 Mechanisms in the pathophysiology of hypercoagulability in nephrotic syndrome.** Altered levels and activity of factors in the intrinsic and extrinsic coagulation cascades, levels of antithrombotic and fibrinolytic components of plasma, platelet count and function, and other factors, such as steroids or diuretics, are the numerous abnormalities that contribute to hypercoagulability in the nephrotic syndrome.

also occur due to increased thrombin formation by the elevated levels of factors V and VIII.[384]

Nephrotic patients exhibit abnormalities in endogenous coagulation inhibitors including antithrombin III, which is deficient in 40% to 80% of patients.[385] Plasma levels of antithrombin III correlate negatively with proteinuria and positively with serum albumin levels due to urinary losses of this factor.[385] Antithrombin III deficiency has been associated with serum albumin levels of less than 2.0 g/dL[386] and correlates with deep venous thrombosis and pulmonary embolism in some studies[386] but not in others.[387]

Alterations in other endogenous anticoagulants may also occur in patients with nephrotic syndrome, but the findings are conflicting. Although plasma levels of total protein S are elevated, the active free fraction level is reduced as a consequence of urinary loss, which accounts for the reduction in the activity of this coagulation inhibitor.[388] For protein C results have been contradictory.[388] Levels of tissue factor pathway inhibitor (TFPI) were increased in patients with the nephrotic syndrome in one study despite being of relatively low molecular weight.[389] Two additional factors that may predispose to thrombosis in nephrotic patients are elevations in serum levels of thrombin activable fibrinolysis inhibitor (TAFI), as well as reductions in levels of protein Z.[390]

A number of factors may lead to a reduction in plasmin-induced fibrinolysis in the nephrotic syndrome; much of the work has focused on plasminogen, the precursor for plasmin, and two major regulators of plasmin formation, plasminogen activator inhibitor (PAI -1) and tissue plasminogen activator (t-PA). Several studies noted decreased plasminogen levels in the nephrotic syndrome correlating with the magnitude of proteinuria.[391] Furthermore, hypoalbuminemia itself has been postulated to negatively affect fibrinolysis. Albumin is a cofactor for the binding of plasminogen to fibrin and their interaction with t-PA. One study demonstrated suppressed glomerular fibrinolytic activity in nephrotic syndrome, as there was a sixfold increase in PAI-1, but not t-PA, levels in patients with membranous glomerulopathy compared with controls.[392]

Maintenance of hemostasis also involves the formation of platelet plugs through platelet activation and aggregation. Studies examining platelet abnormalities have suggested a role for enhanced, platelet–vessel wall interaction and platelet aggregation in the development of thromboembolism in nephrotic syndrome. Thrombocytosis, decreased red blood cell deformability, and increased von Willebrand factor levels all favor platelet transport toward the vessel wall and increased platelet adhesion[393] and are observed in the nephrotic syndrome.

In vitro studies have demonstrated increased platelet aggregation in nephrotic patients.[393] In addition to platelet hyperaggregability, markers of platelet activation, including plasma P-selectin levels and circulating CD62P-positive platelets, were higher in nephrotic patients than in healthy controls. Increased CD62P expression was found in pediatric patients during the nephrotic but not during remission.[394]

Platelet hyperaggregability is associated with hypoalbuminemia, hypercholesterolemia, and hyperfibrinogenemia.[394] Hypoalbuminemia results in increased availability of normally albumin-bound arachidonic acid, leading to increased formation of thromboxane $A_2$ in platelets, which promotes platelet aggregation.[395] Elevated levels of LDL cholesterol may increase platelet aggregation as suggested by the observation that lipid-lowering therapy reverses the spontaneous platelet hyperaggregability seen in such patients.[396] Such an effect, however, has not been conclusively shown in the general population.[397]

To date, observations suggest that platelet activation and aggregation may play a role in the increased risk of thromboembolism in patients with nephrotic syndrome. However, attempts at correlating in vitro functional tests with clinically overt thromboembolic events have shown conflicting results.[387] Other clinical features of the nephrotic state, such as intravascular volume depletion and exposure to steroids, also contribute to hypercoagulability. Increased blood viscosity is associated with hemoconcentration and enhanced using diuretics[398] and by hyperfibrinogenemia.[380] The nature of the underlying immunologic injury may play a role and account for the predilection of thrombosis for the renal vein and for the increased incidence of thrombotic complications in membranous glomerulopathy. The identification of circulating immune complexes in patients with membranous glomerulopathy with renal vein thrombosis, but not in those without thrombosis, supports this possibility.[381] The use of steroids has also been suggested to predispose patients to thromboembolic complications,[381] but other studies have reported a high incidence of thromboembolic complications in the absence of steroid therapy as well.[399]

Thus abnormalities in any of the steps that promote coagulation, including activation and termination of the coagulation cascade, fibrinolysis, and platelet activation and aggregation, may contribute to the hypercoagulable state seen in the nephrotic syndrome. The specific role of each of these alterations remains ill-defined.

## CLINICAL CONSEQUENCE OF HYPERCOAGULABILITY

Thromboembolic events are serious complications of the nephrotic syndrome. The most frequent site of thrombosis is the renal vein. Retrospective and prospective studies have shown an incidence of renal vein thrombosis (RVT) in the nephrotic syndrome ranging from 5% to 62%.[381] Nephrotic syndrome is associated with RVT regardless of the underlying disease. Observational studies evaluated patients who underwent renal venography.[400,401] These studies show that the prevalence of RVT is highest in patients with membranous nephropathy, on average 37%. However, the risk is still clinically important in other primary glomerular diseases, particularly in membranoproliferative glomerulonephritis and minimal change disease. Furthermore, the risk of developing RVT may have been underestimated in these largely cross-sectional studies because patients who were initially not found to have RVT may have subsequently developed it during the disease. In the largest prospective study assessing RVT in 151 patients with nephrotic syndrome, the cumulative incidence of RVT was 22%.[400]

RVT presents clinically in two ways,[400] acute and chronic. Acute RVT is usually unilateral and characterized by acute flank pain, flank tenderness, macroscopic hematuria, and some deterioration of renal function. Chronic RVT is usually asymptomatic and occurs in the elderly. Selective renal venography is the gold standard for the diagnosis of RVT, and demonstration of venous collaterals establishes chronicity. However, renal venography is invasive and associated with complications that include pulmonary embolism due to clot dislodgment, inferior vena cava perforation, and contrast-induced acute kidney injury.[402] Consequently, noninvasive diagnostic tests are preferred, including intravenous pyelography, computed tomography, and magnetic resonance imaging.[402] Nevertheless, there is need for further studies of the usefulness of these techniques in the diagnosis or exclusion of acute RVT remains unproven. Doppler ultrasonography appears to be inferior to renal venography in establishing the diagnosis of RVT and cannot be recommended based on the current data.[403]

Early data on the prognosis of nephrotic patients with RVT suggested a dismal outcome. More recently, it became clear that in the presence of anticoagulation therapy, symptomless chronic RVT is benign.[400] Deep venous thrombosis of the lower extremities is also observed in the nephrotic syndrome and can occur in isolation in up to 15% of patients,[401] or in association with RVT.[400]

Pulmonary embolism may complicate deep vein thrombosis involving the lower extremities, inferior vena cava, or RVT. In a case series of 151 patients with the nephrotic syndrome,[400] of whom 94 patients underwent ventilation–perfusion lung scanning, symptomatic pulmonary embolism was observed in 25% of patients with acute RVT and 20% of patients with chronic RVT. The incidence of asymptomatic pulmonary embolism was 12.8%. In both prospective and retrospective studies, the incidence of thromboembolic complications other than RVT ranges from 8% to 44%, with an average incidence of 20%.[381]

Many clinical studies have demonstrated an association between hypoalbuminemia and venous thromboembolism, but serum albumin levels in patients with and without thromboembolic events were not significantly different.[400] These data suggest that hypoalbuminemia is associated with, but not a prerequisite for, the development of thromboembolic complications in nephrotic patients.

The pattern of thrombosis is remarkably different between children and adults. Despite a lower incidence (1.8%–5%),[404] thromboembolic complications in children tend to be more severe, and half of the children have arterial thrombosis that may cause clinical problems, such as persistent hemiplegia, mesenteric infarction, and peripheral occlusion, leading to amputation.[404] In adults, arterial thrombosis is much less common than venous thrombosis, but it is a serious complication causing important morbidity. One case series described 43 patients with the nephrotic syndrome who had arterial thromboembolism at aortic, renal, femoral, mesenteric, cerebral, or brachial sites.[399] An increased risk of coronary events in patients with the nephrotic syndrome has been documented in a retrospective study.[373]

The treatment of venous thromboembolism in nephrotic patients is similar to that in the general population. First-line treatment consists of conventional anticoagulation with low-molecular-weight heparin and oral vitamin K antagonists.[381] When therapy is initiated early in the course of acute RVT, renal function and other symptoms of RVT have been shown to improve significantly.[400] Oral vitamin K antagonists are usually continued for the duration of nephrotic-range proteinuria,[405] as RVT can recur in the setting of ongoing nephrosis after withdrawal of anticoagulation therapy. Low-molecular-weight heparins have a reasonable safety profile but should be used cautiously in patients with renal insufficiency because of excessive anticoagulant activity and an increased risk of bleeding due to drug accumulation.[406]

Controversy exists regarding the use of prophylactic anticoagulation therapy in patients with nephrotic syndrome who do not have RVT. The potential benefit of prophylactic anticoagulant therapy for patients with membranous glomerulopathy has been documented using decision-analysis methodology.[382] Uncontrolled series show a high mortality from pulmonary embolism among patients not receiving anticoagulant therapy and very low rates of RVT and pulmonary embolism in patients given anticoagulant therapy. Prophylactic anticoagulation is warranted as long as the patient has nephrotic proteinuria, an albumin level below 2 g/dL, or both. In patients with other underlying diseases, a more cautious approach may be indicated, and prophylactic anticoagulant therapy should be initiated only if the risk of thromboembolic events is considered high.

## SUSCEPTABILITY TO INFECTION

Loss of high filtered protein load through both urinary excretion and tubular catabolism,[407] as well as a reduced rate of synthesis,[408] may result in concurrent deficiency of IgG and components of the alternate complement pathway, including factor B. Indeed, patients with nephrotic syndrome have low serum levels of various IgG subclasses. Also, IgA levels are decreased in nephrotic syndrome, whereas IgM usually is increased, particularly in patients with minimal-change disease and normal renal function.[409] Furthermore, defective cell-mediated immunity has been reported in nephrotic syndrome,[410,411] including reduced number of total circulating T lymphocytes and blunted blastogenic response by lymphocytes to the mitogens concanavalin A and phytohemagglutinin.

The defects in the humoral and cellular-mediated immunity render the nephrotic patient highly susceptible to infection.[412] The organisms most frequently encountered are *Streptococcus pneumoniae* and *Escherichia coli*. Although such susceptibility to infection is generalized, there seems to be a particular vulnerability to local infection at the sites of edema formation. Splits in the skin caused by edema and malnutrition may predispose nephrotic patients to cellulitis.[320] Peritonitis has been reported in patients who have ascitis.[412] It also occurred in approximately 6% of children with nephrotic syndrome who suffered one or more episodes of the infection.[412]

The unusual susceptibility of children to infections with encapsulated microorganisms is associated with urinary losses of the alternate pathway complement components, particularly factor B, or C3 proactivator, and D, which are essential for the destruction of encapsulated bacteria in the absence of specific antibodies.[407] The capacity to opsonize the encapsulated bacteria can be restored to normal by adding pure factor B to nephrotic serum.[407] Fungemia due to *Candida lusitaniae* has been also reported in low–birth-weight premature infants with congenital nephrotic syndrome.[413]

New potent antibiotics have contributed to considerably decreasing the incidence of fatal infections in nephrotic syndrome. However, prophylactic measures, such as pneumococcal vaccine, are recommended in adults with severely depressed immunoglobulin levels and nephrotic children over 2 years of age, especially when early remission of nephrotic syndrome is not anticipated.[414]

ACKNOWLEDGMENTS

We would like to thank Monica Cortinovis for her helpful assistance in finalizing this chapter.

 Complete reference list available at ExpertConsult.com.

## KEY REFERENCES


1. Haraldsson B, Nystrom J, Deen WM. Properties of the glomerular barrier and mechanisms of proteinuria. *Physiol Rev.* 2008;88:451–487.
3. Patrakka J, Tryggvason K. New insights into the role of podocytes in proteinuria. *Nat Rev Nephrol.* 2009;5:463–468.
6. Antiga L, Ene-Iordache B, Remuzzi G, et al. Automatic generation of glomerular capillary topological organization. *Microvasc Res.* 2001;62:346–354.
10. Deen WM, Bridges CR, Brenner BM. Biophysical basis of glomerular permselectivity. *J Membr Biol.* 1983;71:1–10.
22. Edwards A, Daniels BS, Deen WM. Ultrastructural model for size selectivity in glomerular filtration. *Am J Physiol.* 1999;276:F892–F902.
24. Hudson BG, Kalluri R, Tryggvason K. Pathology of glomerular basement membrane nephropathy. *Curr Opin Nephrol Hypertens.* 1994;3:334–339.
31. Winograd-Katz SE, Fassler R, Geiger B, et al. The integrin adhesome: from genes and proteins to human disease. *Nat Rev Mol Cell Biol.* 2014;15:273–288.
36. Gagliardini E, Conti S, Benigni A, et al. Imaging of the porous ultrastructure of the glomerular epithelial filtration slit. *J Am Soc Nephrol.* 2010;21:2081–2089.
40. Deen WM, Bridges CR, Brenner BM, et al. Heteroporous model of glomerular size selectivity: application to normal and nephrotic humans. *Am J Physiol.* 1985;249:F374–F389.
42. Remuzzi A, Remuzzi G. Assessment of glomerular size-selective function with fractional clearance of neutral dextran. *J Lab Clin Med.* 1998;132:360–362.
44. Deen WM, Lazzara MJ, Myers BD. Structural determinants of glomerular permeability. *Am J Physiol Renal Physiol.* 2001;281:F579–F596.
45. Guasch A, Deen WM, Myers BD. Charge selectivity of the glomerular filtration barrier in healthy and nephrotic humans. *J Clin Invest.* 1993;92:2274–2282.
48. Remuzzi A, Sangalli F, Fassi A, et al. Albumin concentration in the Bowman's capsule: multiphoton microscopy vs micropuncture technique. *Kidney Int.* 2007;72:1410–1411. author reply 1411.
51. Lazzara MJ, Deen WM. Model of albumin reabsorption in the proximal tubule. *Am J Physiol Renal Physiol.* 2007;292:F430–F439.
64. Benigni A, Gagliardini E, Remuzzi A, et al. Angiotensin-converting enzyme inhibition prevents glomerular-tubule disconnection and atrophy in passive Heymann nephritis, an effect not observed with a calcium antagonist. *Am J Pathol.* 2001;159:1743–1750.
66. Remuzzi G, Bertani T. Pathophysiology of progressive nephropathies. *N Engl J Med.* 1998;339:1448–1456.
69. Brinkkoetter PT, Ising C, Benzing T. The role of the podocyte in albumin filtration. *Nat Rev Nephrol.* 2013;9:328–336.
74. Durvasula RV, Petermann AT, Hiromura K, et al. Activation of a local tissue angiotensin system in podocytes by mechanical strain. *Kidney Int.* 2004;65:30–39.
80. Abbate M, Zoja C, Morigi M, et al. Transforming growth factor-beta1 is up-regulated by podocytes in response to excess intraglomerular passage of proteins: a central pathway in progressive glomerulosclerosis. *Am J Pathol.* 2002;161:2179–2193.
90. Fukuda A, Wickman LT, Venkatareddy MP, et al. Angiotensin II-dependent persistent podocyte loss from destabilized glomeruli causes progression of end stage kidney disease. *Kidney Int.* 2012;81:40–55.
96. Trionfini P, Benigni A. MicroRNAs as master regulators of glomerular function in health and disease. *J Am Soc Nephrol.* 2017;28:1686–1696.
103. Wu J, Zheng C, Wang X, et al. MicroRNA-30 family members regulate calcium/calcineurin signaling in podocytes. *J Clin Invest.* 2015;125:4091–4106.
107. Hasegawa K, Wakino S, Simic P, et al. Renal tubular Sirt1 attenuates diabetic albuminuria by epigenetically suppressing Claudin-1 overexpression in podocytes. *Nat Med.* 2013;19:1496–1504.
111. Jeansson M, Haraldsson B. Morphological and functional evidence for an important role of the endothelial cell glycocalyx in the glomerular barrier. *Am J Physiol Renal Physiol.* 2006;290:F111–F116.
122. Wang B, Komers R, Carew R, et al. Suppression of microRNA-29 expression by TGF-beta1 promotes collagen expression and renal fibrosis. *J Am Soc Nephrol.* 2012;23:252–265.
128. Eremina V, Baelde HJ, Quaggin SE. Role of the VEGF—a signaling pathway in the glomerulus: evidence for crosstalk between components of the glomerular filtration barrier. *Nephron Physiol.* 2007;106:p32–p37.
135. Garsen M, Lenoir O, Rops AL, et al. Endothelin-1 induces proteinuria by heparanase-mediated disruption of the glomerular glycocalyx. *J Am Soc Nephrol.* 2016;27:3545–3551.
143. Smeets B, Angelotti ML, Rizzo P, et al. Renal progenitor cells contribute to hyperplastic lesions of podocytopathies and crescentic glomerulonephritis. *J Am Soc Nephrol.* 2009;20:2593–2603.
149. Morigi M, Locatelli M, Rota C, et al. A previously unrecognized role of C3a in proteinuric progressive nephropathy. *Sci Rep.* 2016;6:28445.
160. Kietzmann L, Guhr SS, Meyer TN, et al. MicroRNA-193a regulates the transdifferentiation of human parietal epithelial cells toward a podocyte phenotype. *J Am Soc Nephrol.* 2015;26:1389–1401.
164. Nangaku M. Chronic hypoxia and tubulointerstitial injury: a final common pathway to end-stage renal failure. *J Am Soc Nephrol.* 2006;17:17–25.
170. Erkan E, Garcia CD, Patterson LT, et al. Induction of renal tubular cell apoptosis in focal segmental glomerulosclerosis: roles of proteinuria and Fas-dependent pathways. *J Am Soc Nephrol.* 2005;16:398–407.
173. Caruso-Neves C, Pinheiro AA, Cai H, et al. PKB and megalin determine the survival or death of renal proximal tubule cells. *Proc Natl Acad Sci U. S. A.* 2006;103:18810–18815.
176. Khan S, Abu Jawdeh BG, Goel M, et al. Lipotoxic disruption of NHE1 interaction with PI(4,5)P2 expedites proximal tubule apoptosis. *J Clin Invest.* 2014;124:1057–1068.
193. Rudnicki M, Eder S, Perco P, et al. Gene expression profiles of human proximal tubular epithelial cells in proteinuric nephropathies. *Kidney Int.* 2007;71:325–335.
194. Biemesderfer D. Regulated intramembrane proteolysis of megalin: linking urinary protein and gene regulation in proximal tubule? *Kidney Int.* 2006;69:1717–1721.
208. Nangaku M, Pippin J, Couser WG. Complement membrane attack complex (C5b-9) mediates interstitial disease in experimental nephrotic syndrome. *J Am Soc Nephrol.* 1999;10:2323–2331.
217. Heymann F, Meyer-Schwesinger C, Hamilton-Williams EE, et al. Kidney dendritic cell activation is required for progression of renal disease in a mouse model of glomerular injury. *J Clin Invest.* 2009;119:1286–1297.
237. Humphreys BD, Lin S-L, Kobayashi A, et al. Fate tracing reveals the stromal pericyte and not epithelial origin of myofibroblasts in the obstructive model of kidney fibrosis. *Am J Pathol.* 2010;176:85–95.
242. Kato M, Natarajan R. Diabetic nephropathy—emerging epigenetic mechanisms. *Nat Rev Nephrol.* 2014;10:517–530.
245. Zanchi C, Macconi D, Trionfini P, et al. MicroRNA-184 is a downstream effector of albuminuria driving renal fibrosis in rats with diabetic nephropathy. *Diabetologia.* 2017;60:1114–1125.
255. Khairoun M, van der Pol P, de Vries DK, et al. Renal ischemia-reperfusion induces a dysbalance of angiopoietins, accompanied by proliferation of pericytes and fibrosis. *Am J Physiol Renal Physiol.* 2013;305:F901–F910.
274. Ronconi E, Sagrinati C, Angelotti ML, et al. Regeneration of glomerular podocytes by human renal progenitors. *J Am Soc Nephrol.* 2009;20:322–332.
279. Zhang J, Pippin JW, Vaughan MR, et al. Retinoids augment the expression of podocyte proteins by glomerular parietal epithelial cells in experimental glomerular disease. *Nephron Exp Nephrol.* 2012;121:e23–e37.
282. Kaysen GA. Albumin metabolism in the nephrotic syndrome: the effect of dietary protein intake. *Am J Kidney Dis.* 1988;12:461–480.
321. Perico N, Remuzzi G. Edema of the nephrotic syndrome: the role of the atrial peptide system. *Am J Kidney Dis.* 1993;22:355–366.
328. Peterson C, Madsen B, Perlman A, et al. Atrial natriuretic peptide and the renal response to hypervolemia in nephrotic humans. *Kidney Int.* 1988;34:825–831.
335. Polzin D, Kaminski HJ, Kastner C, et al. Decreased renal corin expression contributes to sodium retention in proteinuric kidney diseases. *Kidney Int.* 2010;78:650–659.
351. Kaysen GA, de Sain-van der Velden MG. New insights into lipid metabolism in the nephrotic syndrome. *Kidney Int Suppl.* 1999;71:S18–S21.
380. Kanfer A. Coagulation factors in nephrotic syndrome. *Am J Nephrol.* 1990;10(suppl 1):63–68.

# 31 Primary Glomerular Disease

Manish K. Saha | William F. Pendergraft III | J. Charles Jennette | Ronald J. Falk

## CHAPTER OUTLINE



## KEY POINTS

- Primary membranous nephropathy (PMN) is an autoimmune disease characterized by circulating IgG autoantibodies against two major podocyte antigens, muscle-type phospholipase A2 receptor ($PLA_2R1$), which has been detected in 70% of cases, and thrombospondin type 1 domain-containing 7A (THSD7A) in 5% to 10% of cases.
- A new classification scheme for membranoproliferative glomerulonephritis (MPGN) has been proposed that is based on glomerular immunofluorescence. It is classified as an immune complex–mediated MPGN when both immunoglobulin and complement are deposited. Those with predominant C3 staining are classified as complement-mediated MPGN or C3 glomerulopathy.
- Fibrillary glomerulonephritis is now postulated to be an autoimmune disease based on the observation of autoantibodies targeting a putative autoantigen, DNAJB9.
- Patients with immunotactoid glomerulonephritis should be evaluated for underlying monoclonal gammopathy, malignancy, and lymphoproliferative disorders.
- In a large cohort of subjects from the European validation study of the Oxford classification of IgAN (VALIGA), no significant differences were found in respect to proteinuria or decline in renal function in patients with or without tonsillectomy.
- In anti-GBM disease, glomeruli with crescents typically have fibrinoid necrosis in adjacent glomerular segments, whereas nonnecrotic segments may look entirely normal by light microscopy or may have slight infiltration by neutrophils or mononuclear leukocytes. This differs from crescentic immune complex glomerulonephritis and C3 glomerulopathy, which typically have capillary wall thickening and endocapillary hypercellularity in the intact glomeruli.
- Autoantibodies in sporadic anti-GBM disease are directed against the NC1 domain of the $\alpha_3$ chain of type IV collagen. By contrast, the anti-GBM alloantibodies that cause posttransplantation nephritis in some patients with X-linked Alport syndrome are directed against conformational epitopes in the NC1 domain of $\alpha_5$(IV) collagen, which are normally expressed in the allograft but absent in the recipient.
- In ANCA-associated vasculitis, patients with anti–proteinase-3 (PR3) antibodies, lung involvement, or upper respiratory tract involvement are more likely to relapse than others.

Glomerular diseases may be categorized into those that primarily involve the kidney (primary glomerular diseases) and those in which kidney involvement is part of a systemic disorder (secondary glomerular diseases). This chapter focuses on primary glomerular diseases. Some forms of glomerular disease occur not only as a renal-limited (primary) disease in some patients, but also as a component of systemic disease in other patients—for example, antiglomerular basement membrane (anti-GBM) glomerulonephritis, with and without pulmonary disease, and antineutrophil cytoplasmic autoantibody (ANCA) glomerulonephritis, with and without systemic vasculitis and granulomatosis. Chapter 32 concentrates on secondary glomerular diseases and Chapter 33 focuses on therapy for glomerular disease. The separation of glomerular disease into primary versus secondary is somewhat problematic because, in some cases, what are considered primary glomerular diseases are similar, if not identical, to secondary glomerular diseases. For example, immunoglobulin A (IgA) nephropathy, pauci-immune necrotizing and crescentic glomerulonephritis, anti-GBM glomerulonephritis, membranous nephropathy (MN), and membranoproliferative glomerulonephritis (MPGN) can occur as primary kidney diseases or as components of systemic diseases such as IgA vasculitis, pauci-immune small-vessel vasculitis, Goodpasture syndrome, systemic lupus erythematosus (SLE), and cryoglobulinemic vasculitis, respectively. Of note, there has been a successful shift, as in many settings, to phase out the nosologic use of eponyms and to substitute noneponymous terms that more accurately reflect pathophysiologic specificity in the nomenclature of vasculitides. This nomenclature of vasculitides was formally revised in 2012 at the second international Chapel Hill Consensus Conference, and the following vasculitides with new names remain relevant to this edition: IgA vasculitis (formerly designated Henoch-Schönlein purpura), granulomatosis with polyangiitis (GPA, formerly designated Wegener granulomatosis) and eosinophilic granulomatosis with polyangiitis (EGPA, formerly designated Churg-Strauss syndrome).[1]

A temporal change has emerged over the past 30 years in the frequencies of glomerular disease for reasons that remain unclear but could reflect changing behavioral and/or environmental exposures. A cross-sectional observational study of 18 widely recognized glomerular diseases between 1986 and 2015, identified through diagnostic kidney biopsy specimens from the Glomerular Disease Collaborative Network spanning the southeastern United States, revealed a dramatic increase in the frequency of diabetic glomerulosclerosis.[2] The frequency of focal segmental glomerulosclerosis (FSGS) initially increased but then declined, and the frequencies of other common glomerular disease subtypes remained stable (IgA nephropathy and ANCA glomerulonephritis) or declined (minimal change glomerulopathy, MN, MPGN, and lupus nephritis).[2]

When a patient presents with glomerular disease, the clinician not only must evaluate the clinical signs and symptoms but also must be vigilant for evidence of a systemic process or disease that could be causing the kidney disease. Clinical evaluation includes assessment of proteinuria, hematuria, the presence or absence of renal insufficiency, and the presence or absence of hypertension. Some glomerular diseases cause isolated proteinuria or isolated hematuria, with no other signs or symptoms of disease. More severe glomerular disease often results in the nephrotic syndrome or nephritic (glomerulonephritic) syndrome. Glomerular disease may have an indolent course or begin abruptly, leading to acute or rapidly progressive glomerulonephritis. Although some glomerular disorders consistently cause a specific syndrome (e.g., minimal change disease [MCD] results in the nephrotic syndrome), most disorders are capable of causing features of both nephrosis and nephritis (Table 31.1). This sharing and variability of clinical manifestations among different glomerular diseases may not allow an accurate diagnosis based on clinical features alone. Therefore, kidney biopsy has an important role in the evaluation of many patients and remains the gold standard for the definitive diagnosis of many glomerular diseases.

This chapter describes the clinical syndromes caused by glomerular diseases, including isolated proteinuria, isolated hematuria, and specific forms of primary glomerular disease that cause the nephrotic or nephritic syndrome and reviews their distinctive pathologic features.

**Table 31.1 Manifestations of Nephrotic and Nephritic Features by Glomerular Diseases**

| Disease | Nephrotic Features | Nephritic Features |
|---|---|---|
| Minimal change disease | ++++ | – |
| Membranous nephropathy | ++++ | + |
| Focal segmental glomerulosclerosis | +++ | ++ |
| Fibrillary glomerulonephritis | +++ | ++ |
| Mesangioproliferative glomerulopathy[a] | ++ | ++ |
| Membranoproliferative glomerulonephritis[b] | ++ | +++ |
| Proliferative glomerulonephritis[a] | ++ | +++ |
| Acute diffuse proliferative glomerulonephritis[c] | + | ++++ |
| Crescentic glomerulonephritis[d] | + | ++++ |

[a]Mesangioproliferative and proliferative glomerulonephritis (focal or diffuse) are structural manifestations of a number of glomerulonephritides, including IgA nephropathy and lupus nephritis.

[b]Both mesangiocapillary (type I) and dense deposit disease (type II).

[c]Often a structural manifestation of acute poststreptococcal glomerulonephritis.

[d]Can be immune complex–mediated, anti–glomerular basement membrane antibody-mediated, or associated with antineutrophil cytoplasmic autoantibodies.

Modified from Jennette JC, Mandal AK: The nephrotic syndrome. In Mandal AK, Jennette JC, eds. *Diagnosis and Management of Renal Disease and Hypertension.* Durham, NC: Carolina Academic Press; 1994:235–272.

## GENERAL DESCRIPTION OF GLOMERULAR SYNDROMES

### PROTEINURIA

Proteinuria can be caused by the systemic overproduction of proteins that cross glomerular capillary walls (e.g., multiple myeloma with Bence Jones proteinuria), tubular dysfunction (e.g., Fanconi syndrome), or glomerular dysfunction. It is important to identify patients in whom proteinuria is a manifestation of substantial glomerular disease as opposed to patients who have benign functional, transient, postural (orthostatic), or intermittent proteinuria. (Proteinuria is discussed further in Chapters 23 and 30.)

Plasma proteins larger than 70 kDa cross the basement membrane in a manner normally restricted by both size-selective and charge-selective barriers.[3,4] The functional characteristics of the glomerular capillary filter have been extensively studied by the evaluation of the fractional clearance of molecules of different size and charge.[5] The size-selective barrier is most likely a consequence of functional pores within the glomerular basement membrane (GBM) that restrict the filtration of plasma proteins larger than 150 kDa. There is also a shape restriction of molecules that allows elongated molecules to cross the glomerular capillary wall more readily than other molecules of the same molecular weight, and there is a charge-selective nature of the barrier, largely a consequence of glycosaminoglycans arranged along the capillary wall. Loss of charge selectivity may be a defect in MCD, whereas a loss of size selectivity may be the cause of proteinuria in, for example, patients with MN.[4]

A number of factors have proven to be important in the disruption of the glomerular capillary wall as a consequence of tissue-degrading enzymes, complement components that assemble or deposit in it, and oxygen radicals that target both the GBM and the slit diaphragm. Heparinase and hyaluronidase alterations in the aminoglycan content of the glomerular capillary wall may play a role in increased protein excretion.[6,7] Genetic studies have provided exciting clues about the specific components of the glomerular capillary wall, including mutations in the podocyte or proteins in the slit diaphragm, that result in proteinuria (reviewed by Tryggvason and colleagues[8] and more recently by Garg and Rabelink[9]).

Another major mechanism resulting in proteinuria is impaired reabsorption of plasma proteins by proximal tubular epithelial cells. A number of low-molecular-weight proteins, including albumin and $\beta_1$-, $\beta_2$-, and $\alpha_1$- microglobulins, are filtered by the glomerulus and absorbed by tubular epithelial cells. When tubular epithelial cells are damaged, these proteins are excreted. Russo and colleagues have studied the critical importance of the tubular absorption of proteins.[10] The glomerular capillary sieving coefficient for albumin was examined in normal and nephrotic rats by two-photon (laser) intravital microscopy. The glomerular capillary sieving coefficient for albumin was $3.4 \times 10^{-2}$ rather than $6.2 \times 10^{-4}$, as found by earlier micropuncture studies in nonproteinuric rats.

Several important observations emanate from this study. First, there is a large amount of albumin filtered across the glomerular capillary bed daily in the normal rat. Second, investigators have found no evidence for a charge-based restriction to the passage of albumin through the glomerular filter. Third, in normal and nephrotic animals, the vast majority of the filtered albumin was "reclaimed" from the filtrate by a high-capacity transcytotic pathway in the proximal tubule, which returns intact (unaltered) albumin to the peritubular capillary circulation. This is an important concept, because most nephrologists view albuminuria as resulting solely from enhanced glomerular permeability (reviewed by Vallon[11]).

The term "isolated proteinuria" is used for several conditions, including mild transient proteinuria of less than 1 g protein/day that typically accompanies physiologically stressful conditions, such as fever in hospitalized patients, exercise, and congestive heart failure.[12] In other patients, transient proteinuria is a consequence of the overflow of proteins of low molecular weight due to the overproduction of light chains, heavy chains, or other fragments of immunoglobulins. Additional examples of proteinuria caused by increased circulating proteins are $\beta_2$-microglobinuria, myoglobinuria, and hemoglobinuria.

The term "orthostatic proteinuria" is defined by the absence of proteinuria while the patient is in a recumbent posture and its appearance during an upright posture, especially during ambulation or exercise.[13] The total amount of protein excretion in a 24-hour period is generally less than 1 g, but may be as much as 2 g. Orthostatic proteinuria is more common in adolescents and is uncommon in individuals older than 30 years.[13,14] About 2% to 5% of adolescents have orthostatic proteinuria. Among patients with orthostatic proteinuria who underwent kidney biopsy, 47% were found to have normal glomeruli by light microscopy, 45% to have minimal to moderate glomerular abnormalities of nonspecific nature, and the remainder to have evidence of a primary glomerular disease.[15]

Why is proteinuria increased during an upright posture in individuals with normal glomeruli by light microscopy? Although the answer to this question is not fully known, there are several likely possibilities. Orthostatic proteinuria may occur as a consequence of alterations in glomerular hemodynamics. It is possible that even in histologically "normal" glomeruli in which there are no specific lesions, subtle glomerular abnormalities exist, including abnormal basement membranes or focal changes of the mesangium.[16] Alternatively, orthostatic proteinuria has been demonstrated with anatomic entrapment and subsequent obstruction of the left renal vein between the aorta and superior mesenteric artery (commonly referred to as the "renal nutcracker").[17] In addition, the observation that surgical correction of a kink in an allograft renal vein resulted in the disappearance of orthostatic proteinuria gives credence to venous entrapment as a cause for orthostatic proteinuria.[16]

There are several approaches to the diagnosis of orthostatic proteinuria. These include comparison of protein excretion in two 12-hour urine collections, one during recumbency and one during ambulation. Another approach is to compare protein levels in a split collection of 16 hours during ambulation and 8 hours of overnight collection. It is important that patients be recumbent for at least 2 hours before their ambulatory collection is completed to avoid the possibility of contamination of the recumbent collection by urine formed during ambulation. The diagnosis of orthostatic proteinuria requires that protein excretion during recumbency be less than 50 mg during those 8 hours. Few convincing data exist on the usefulness of comparing urinary protein to creatinine ratio measurements during recumbency versus ambulation as a diagnostic test for orthostatic proteinuria.

A 20-year follow-up of orthostatic proteinuria has suggested a benign long-term course.[14] Orthostatic proteinuria resolves in most patients. It is present in 50% of patients after 10 years and in only 17% of patients after 20 years.[14] In the absence of a kidney biopsy, an underlying glomerulopathy cannot be completely excluded, and an orthostatic component of proteinuria may be found in early glomerular disease. Thus, it is important to reassess patients after an interval of about 1 year to be certain that the degree or pattern of proteinuria has not changed.

Fixed proteinuria is present whether the patient is upright or recumbent. The proteinuria disappears in some patients, whereas others will have a more ominous glomerular lesion that portends an adverse long-term outcome. The prognosis depends on the persistence and severity of the proteinuria. If proteinuria disappears, it is less likely that the patient will develop hypertension or a reduced glomerular filtration rate (GFR). These patients must be evaluated periodically for as long as proteinuria persists.

## RECURRENT OR PERSISTENT HEMATURIA

Hematuria is the presence of an excessive number of red blood cells in the urine and is categorized as microscopic (visible only with the aid of a microscope) or macroscopic (urine that is tea-colored or cola-colored, pink, or even red). Hematuria can result from injury to the kidney or to another site in the urinary tract (see Chapter 23).

Healthy individuals may excrete as many as $10^5$ red cells in the urine in a 12-hour period. An acceptable definition of hematuria is more than two red cells per high-power field (HPF) in centrifuged urine.[18] The approach to processing urine varies from laboratory to laboratory; therefore, the number of red cells/HPF that is an accurate indicator of hematuria may vary slightly among different laboratories. The urine dipstick test detects one to two red cells/HPF per and is a very sensitive test. A negative result on dipstick examination virtually excludes hematuria.[19]

Hematuria is present in about 5% to 6% of the general population[20] and 4% of schoolchildren. In most children, follow-up urinalyses are normal.[21] In most people, hematuria emanates from the lower urinary tract, especially in conditions affecting the urethra, bladder, and prostate. Less than 10% of cases of hematuria are caused by glomerular bleeding.[18] Persistent hematuria, especially in older individuals, should raise the possibility of malignancy. The incidence of malignancy, especially of the bladder, ranges from 5% in individuals with persistent microscopic hematuria to over 20% in individuals with gross hematuria.[22] Other causes of nonglomerular hematuria include neoplasms, trauma, metabolic defects such as hypercalciuria, vascular diseases, including renal infarctions and renal vein thrombosis, cystic diseases of the kidney, including polycystic kidney disease, medullary cystic disease, and medullary sponge kidney, and interstitial kidney disease, such as papillary necrosis, hydronephrosis, and drug-induced interstitial nephritis. In children with asymptomatic hematuria, hypercalciuria is the cause in 15% of cases, and 10% to 15% have IgA nephropathy. In up to 80% of children and 15% to 20% of adults with hematuria, no cause can be identified.[23]

Transient hematuria has been found in a number of settings. It is present in 13% of postmenopausal women.[24] Episodic hematuria in a cyclic pattern during a menstrual cycle is most likely a consequence of the invasion of the urinary tract by endometrial implants.[25] In 1000 men between the ages of 18 and 33 years, hematuria was present at least once in 39% and on two or more occasions in 16%. In patients with isolated asymptomatic hematuria without proteinuria or renal insufficiency, the hematuria resolves in 20% of cases; however, some of these patients will develop hypertension and proteinuria.[26] In older individuals, transient hematuria should raise a concern of malignancy.[18,27,28] In some individuals, transient hematuria may be a consequence of exercise.

Glomerular hematuria, in contrast to hematuria caused by injury elsewhere in the urinary tract, is characterized by misshapen red cells that have been distorted by osmotic and chemical stress as red blood cells pass through the nephron. Hematuria with dysmorphic cells, especially cells that have membrane blebs producing the picture of acanthocyturia, is strong evidence for glomerular bleeding.[22] The finding of protein (especially >2 g/day), hemoglobin, or red cell casts in the urine enhances the possibility that hematuria is of glomerular origin. Although brown or cola-colored urine is most commonly associated with glomerular hematuria, its absence does not exclude glomerular disease. Interestingly, blood clots do not occur in the urine with glomerular bleeding.

The differential pathologic diagnosis of glomerular hematuria without proteinuria, renal insufficiency, or red blood cell casts includes IgA nephropathy, thin basement membrane nephropathy, hereditary nephritis, and histologically normal glomeruli.[29] In a study in Europe,[30] 80 normotensive adults underwent kidney biopsy for the evaluation of recurrent macroscopic hematuria or persistent microscopic hematuria. Approximately 30% of these patients had IgA nephropathy, 20% had thin basement membrane nephropathy, and 30% had no discernible lesion. Hematuria disappeared in 13 of the latter patients. The remaining patients had mesangioproliferative glomerulonephritis, interstitial nephritis, or focal glomerulosclerosis. In contrast, in another study, 216 Chinese adults with isolated hematuria who underwent a kidney biopsy were much more likely to have IgA nephropathy than any other lesion.[31]

Table 31.2 provides data from an analysis of native kidney biopsy specimens from patients with hematuria performed by the University of North Carolina (UNC) Nephropathology Laboratory. Patients with SLE were excluded from the study. The patients selected for the study had a serum creatinine level of less than 1.5 mg/dL or more than 3 mg/dL. Patients with a serum creatinine level of less than 1.5 mg/dL were further divided into those with proteinuria less than 1 g/day and those with proteinuria of 1 to 3 g/day. The data showed that patients with a relatively normal serum creatinine level, hematuria, and proteinuria of less than 1 g protein/day were most likely to have thin basement membrane nephropathy, IgA nephropathy, or no identifiable renal lesion. When hematuria is accompanied by 1 to 3 g protein/day of proteinuria but no significant renal insufficiency, IgA nephropathy was the most likely cause. Patients with hematuria and a serum creatinine level higher than 3 mg/dL usually had aggressive glomerulonephritis with crescents.

Despite these overall tendencies, it is not possible to determine the cause of asymptomatic hematuria definitively without kidney biopsy, and even kidney biopsy specimen evaluation fails to reveal a cause in a minority of patients. Certain rules generally apply to the clinical prediction of the most likely cause. Gross hematuria is usually found in IgA nephropathy or hereditary nephritis. Patients with thin basement membrane nephropathy typically do not have substantial proteinuria.

A potential benefit of kidney biopsy in patients with isolated hematuria includes the reduction of patient and physician uncertainty by confirming a specific diagnosis. Nonetheless, the role of kidney biopsy in the evaluation of asymptomatic hematuria in patients without proteinuria, hypertension, or kidney insufficiency remains unclear. In biopsy series involving patients in whom asymptomatic hematuria was accompanied by low-grade proteinuria, specific glomerular diseases, including IgA nephropathy and membranoproliferative glomerular disease, may be discovered and, when there is no proteinuria, IgA nephropathy and thin basement membrane disease or nondiagnostic minor changes remain the most common findings.[32,33] Confirmation of a glomerular cause eliminates the need for repeated urologic studies, and a more accurate long-term prognosis can be made (e.g., thin basement membrane nephropathy is less likely to progress than is IgA nephropathy). However, isolated glomerular hematuria without proteinuria or renal insufficiency may not warrant a kidney biopsy because the findings often will not affect management. In one study of patients with isolated hematuria, the biopsy results altered patient management in only 1 of 36 patients.[34]

## GLOMERULAR DISEASES THAT CAUSE NEPHROTIC SYNDROME AND GLOMERULONEPHRITIS

### NEPHROTIC SYNDROME

The nephrotic syndrome results from proteinuria of more than 3.5 g protein/day and is characterized by edema, hyperlipidemia, hypoproteinemia, and other metabolic disorders (described in detail later). Nephrotic syndrome not only may be caused by primary (idiopathic) glomerular diseases but also may be secondary to a large number of identifiable disease states (Box 31.1). Despite the differences in these causes, the loss of substantial amounts of protein

**Table 31.2 Frequency of Kidney Disease in Patients with Hematuria Undergoing Renal Biopsy (%)[a]**

| | Hematuria | | |
|---|---|---|---|
| **Biopsy Findings** | Urinary Protein <1 g/day, Creatinine <1.5 mg/dL | Urinary protein 1–3 g/day, Creatinine <1.5 mg/dL | Creatinine >3 mg/dL |
| No abnormality | 30 | 2 | 0 |
| Thin basement nephropathy | 26 | 4 | 0 |
| Immunoglobulin A nephropathy | 28 | 24 | 8 |
| Glomerulonephritis without crescents[b] | 9 | 26 | 23 |
| Glomerulonephritis with crescents[b] | 2 | 24 | 44 |
| Other kidney disease[c] | 5 | 20 | 25 |
| Total | 100 (*n* = 43) | 100 (*n* = 123) | 100 (*n* = 255) |

[a]Based on an analysis of kidney biopsy specimens evaluated at the University of North Carolina Nephropathology Laboratory. Specimens from patients with systemic lupus erythematosus were excluded from the analysis.
[b]Proliferative or necrotizing glomerulonephritis other than immunoglobulin A nephropathy or lupus nephritis.
[c]Includes causes of nephrotic syndrome such as membranous nephropathy and focal segmental glomerulosclerosis.
Data from Caldas MLR, Jennette JC, Falk RJ, et al. Immunoelectron microscopic documentation of the translocation of proteins reactive with ANCA to neutrophil cell surfaces during neutrophil activation. [abstract]. Presented at the Third International Workshop on ANCA, November 29-30, 1990, Washington, DC.

**Box 31.1 Classification of Disease States Associated With the Development of Nephrotic Syndrome**

Idiopathic Nephrotic Syndrome Due to Primary Glomerular Disease
Nephrotic Syndrome Associated With Specific Causatives Events or in Which Glomerular Disease Arises as a Complication of Other Diseases

**1. Medications and Other Chemicals**

*Organic, inorganic, elemental mercury*[a]
*Organic gold*
*Penicillamine,* bucillamine
*Street heroin*
*Probenecid*
*Captopril*
*Nonsteroidal antiinflammatory drugs*
*Lithium*
*Interferon-α*
Chlorpropamide
Rifampin
Pamidronate
Paramethadione (Paradione), trimethadione (Tridione)
Mephenytoin (Mesantoin)
Tolbutamide[b]
Phenindione[b]
Warfarin
Clonidine[b]

Continued on following page

**Box 31.1 Classification of Disease States Associated With the Development of Nephrotic Syndrome (Cont'd)**

Perchlorate[b]
Bismuth[b]
Trichloroethylene[b]
Silver[b]
Insect repellent[b]
Contrast media
Anabolic steroids

**2. Allergens, Venoms, Immunizing Agents**

*Bee sting*
*Pollens*
Poison ivy and poison oak
Antitoxins (serum sickness)
Snake venom
Diphtheria, pertussis, tetanus toxoid
Vaccines

**3. Infections**

Bacterial: *poststreptococcal glomerulonephritis,* infective endocarditis, *shunt nephritis*, leprosy, syphilis (congenital and secondary), *Mycoplasma* infection, tuberculosis,† chronic bacterial pyelonephritis with vesicoureteral reflux
Viral: hepatitis B, hepatitis C, cytomegalovirus infection, infectious mononucleosis (Epstein-Barr virus infection), herpes zoster, vaccinia, infection with human immunodeficiency virus type 1
Protozoal: *malaria* (especially quartan malaria), toxoplasmosis
Helminthic: *schistosomiasis*, trypanosomiasis, filariasis

**4. Neoplasms**

Solid tumors (carcinoma and sarcoma): tumors of the *lung, colon, stomach, breast,* cervix, kidney, thyroid, ovary, prostate, adrenal, oropharynx, carotid body†; melanoma, pheochromocytoma, Wilms' tumor, mesothelioma, oncocytoma
Leukemia and lymphoma: *Hodgkin disease*, chronic lymphocytic leukemia, multiple myeloma (amyloidosis), Waldenström macroglobulinemia, lymphoma
*Graft-versus-host disease after bone marrow transplantation*

**5. Multisystem Disease**[c]

*Systemic lupus erythematosus*
Mixed connective tissue disease
Dermatomyositis
Rheumatoid arthritis
Goodpasture's syndrome
*IgA vasculitis (formerly Henoch-Schönlein purpura*; see also immunoglobulin A nephropathy, Berger disease)
Systemic vasculitis (including GPA, formerly Wegener)
Takayasu arteritis
Mixed cryoglobulinemia
Light- and heavy-chain disease (Randall type)
Partial lipodystrophy
Sjögren syndrome
Toxic epidermolysis
Dermatitis herpetiformis
Sarcoidosis
Ulcerative colitis
*Amyloidosis* (primary and secondary)

**6. Hereditary—Familial and Metabolic Disease**[c]

*Diabetes mellitus*
Hypothyroidism (myxedema)
Graves' disease
Amyloidosis (familial Mediterranean fever and other hereditary forms, Muckle-Wells syndrome)
Alport syndrome
Fabry disease
Nail-patella syndrome
Lipoprotein glomerulopathy
Sickle cell disease
$\alpha_1$-Antitrypsin deficiency
Asphyxiating thoracic dystrophy (Jeune syndrome)
Von Gierke disease
Podocyte slit diaphragm mutation
Nephrin mutation
*FAT2* mutation
Podocin mutation
*CD2AP mutation*
Denys-Drash syndrome (*WT1* mutation)
*ACTN4* mutation
Charcot-Marie-Tooth syndrome
Congenital nephrotic syndrome (Finnish type)
Cystinosis (adult)
Galloway-Mowat syndrome
Hurler syndrome
Familial dysautonomia

**7. Miscellaneous**

*Pregnancy-associated (preeclampsia, recurrent, transient)*
*Chronic renal allograft failure*
Accelerated or malignant nephrosclerosis
Unilateral renal arterial hypertension
Intestinal lymphangiectasia
Chronic jejunoileitis[b]
Spherocytosis†
Renal artery stenosis
Congenital heart disease (cyanotic)[b]
Severe congestive heart failure[b]
Constrictive pericarditis[b]
Tricuspid insufficiency[b]
Massive obesity
Vesicoureteric reflux nephropathy
Papillary necrosis
Gardner-Diamond syndrome
Castleman disease
Kartagener syndrome
Buckley syndrome
Kimura disease
Silica exposure

[a]Diseases and other agents in *italics* are the more commonly encountered causes of nephrotic syndrome.
[b]Based on single case reports or small series in which cause-and-effect relationship cannot be established. Other factors (e.g., use of mercurial diuretics in heart failure) may have been the true inciting event.
[c]See Chapter 33 for a detailed discussion of the secondary forms of nephrotic syndrome.
*ACTN4,* α-Actinin-4; *CD2AP,* CD2-associated protein; *FAT2*, FAT tumor suppressor homolog 2 (*Drosophila)*; *WT1,* Wilms' tumor 1.

in the urine results in a shared set of abnormalities that comprise nephrotic syndrome (Boxes 31.2 and 31.3 and Table 31.3). We are likely to witness an explosion of new insights into primary glomerular diseases responsible for nephrotic syndrome with the ongoing efforts of the Nephrotic Syndrome Study Network (NEPTUNE) and Cure Glomerulonephropathy (CureGN), both funded by the National Institutes of Health (NIH). NEPTUNE is a North American multicenter collaborative translational research consortium geared toward longitudinal clinical monitoring and blood, urine, and kidney tissue sample collection from 450 adults and children with MCD, FSGS, and MN.[35] CureGN (https://curegn.org/) is a longitudinal multicenter cohort observational study that is following 2400 children and adults with MCD, FSGS, MN, and IgA nephropathy. Both NEPTUNE and CureGN provide the infrastructure for multiple ancillary studies that will advance our understanding and management of glomerular diseases.

**Box 31.2 Alterations of Plasma Protein in the Nephrotic Syndrome**

Immunoglobulins (Ig)
- Decreased IgG
- Normal or increased IgA, IgM, or IgE
- Increased $\text{alpha}_2$ and beta globulins
- Decreased $\text{alpha}_1$ globulin

Metal-binding proteins
- Loss of metal binding proteins: iron, copper, zinc

Loss of erythropoietin
Depletion of transferrin
Transcortin deficiency
Complement deficiency
- Decreased factor B
- Decreased C3
- Decreased C1q, C2, C8, Ci
- Increased C3, C4bp

Normal C1s, C4, and C1 inhibitor
Coagulation components
- Decreased factors XI, XII, kallikrein inhibitor
- Decreased factors IX, XII
- Decreased antiplasmin, $\text{alpha}_1$ antitrypsin
- Plasminogen activator, endothelial prostacyclin stimulating factor
- Decreased antithrombin III
- Elevated beta-thromboglobulin

Procoagulant

Modified from references 504 and 1434 to 1448.

## MINIMAL CHANGE DISEASE

### EPIDEMIOLOGY

MCD was first described in 1913 by Munk, who called it "lipoid nephrosis" because of the presence of lipid in the tubular epithelial cells and urine.[36] MCD is most common in children, accounting for 70% to 90% of nephrotic syndrome in children younger than age 10 years and 50% in adults. MCD also causes 10% to 15% of primary nephrotic syndrome in adults (Fig. 31.1).

The incidence of MCD has geographic variations; MCD is more common in Asia than in North America or Europe.[37] This may be a consequence of differences in kidney biopsy practices or differences in environmental or genetic influences. The disease may also affect older adult patients in whom there is a higher propensity for the clinical syndrome of MCD

**Box 31.3 Procoagulant Factors in the Nephrotic Syndrome**

Increased blood viscosity
Hemoconcentration
Increased plasma fibrinogen
Increased intravascular fibrin formation
Increased $\alpha_2$-macroglobulins
Increased tissue type plasminogen activator
Increased factors II, V, VII, VIII, X, XIII
Decreased factors IX, XI, XII
Decreased $\alpha$-antitrypsin
Decreased fibrinolytic activity
Decreased plasma plasminogen
Decreased antithrombin III
Decreased protein S
Thrombocytosis
Increased platelet aggregability

Modified from references 507,1447, and 1449 to 1463.

**Table 31.3 Diseases that Cause the Nephrotic Syndrome[a]**

| Glomerular Lesion | No. of Patients | Male:Female Ratio | Caucasian:African American Ratio |
|---|---|---|---|
| Minimal change disease | 522 | 1.1:1.0 | 1.9:1.0 |
| Focal segmental glomerulosclerosis (FSGS; typical) | 1103 | 1.4:1.0 | 1.0:1.0 |
| Collapsing glomerulopathy FSGS | 135 | 1.2:1.0 | 1.0:7.8 |
| Glomerular tip lesion FSGS | 94 | 1.0:1.0 | 4.7:1.0 |
| Membranous Nephropathy | 1120 | 1.4:1.0 | 1.9:1.0 |
| C1q nephropathy | 114 | 1.0:1.0 | 1.0:4.8 |
| Fibrillary glomerulonephritis | 76 | 1.0:1.2 | 14.3:1.0 |

[a]Information in this table is from 9605 native kidney biopsies from the UNC Nephropathology Laboratory. This laboratory evaluates kidney biopsies from a base population of approximately 10 million throughout the southeastern United States and centered in North Carolina. The expected Caucasian-to-African American ratio in this renal biopsy population is approximately 2:1.
*FSGS,* Focal segmental glomerulosclerosis.

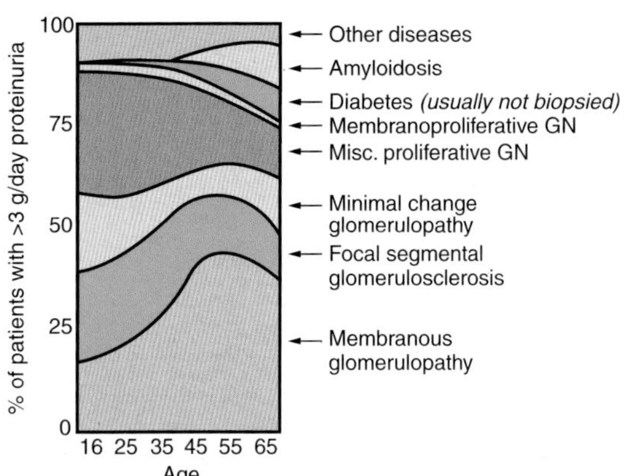


**Fig. 31.1** Graphic depiction of frequencies of different forms of glomerular disease identified in kidney biopsy specimens from patients with proteinuria of more than 3 g of protein/day evaluated at the University of North Carolina Nephropathology Laboratory. Some diseases that cause proteinuria are underrepresented because they are not always evaluated by kidney biopsy. For example, in many patients, steroid-responsive proteinuria is given a presumptive diagnosis of minimal change disease, and patients do not undergo biopsy, and most patients with diabetes and proteinuria are presumed to have diabetic glomerulosclerosis and do not undergo biopsy. *GN,* glomerulonephritis.

and acute kidney injury (AKI; discussed later). There appears to be a male preponderance of this process in some research series, especially in children, in whom the male-to-female ratio is 2:1 to 3:1[38]; however, data from our institution do not support this finding.

## PATHOLOGY

The effacement of podocyte foot processes is accompanied by increased density of the cytoskeleton, including actin filaments, in clumps near the basement membrane surface of the podocytes. However, the extent of effacement appears to correlate more with the duration of active nephrotic syndrome than with the magnitude of the proteinuria.[39]

### Light Microscopy

In MCD, no glomerular lesions are seen by light microscopy (Fig. 31.2), or only a minimal focal segmental mesangial prominence is noted.[40] This mesangial prominence should have no more than three or four cells embedded in the matrix of a segment, and the matrix should not be expanded to the extent that capillary lumens are compromised. Capillary walls should be thin and capillary lumens patent.

The most consistent tubular lesion is increased protein and lipid resorption droplets in tubular epithelial cells. These droplets stain with periodic acid–Schiff stain. Conspicuous resorbed lipid in epithelial cells prompted the designation “lipoid nephrosis” for this disease prior to the recognition of the ultrastructural glomerular lesion. Interstitial edema is rare, even in patients with severe nephrotic syndrome and anasarca. Focal proximal tubular epithelial flattening (simplification), which is histologically identical to that seen with ischemic AKI, occurs in patients who have the syndrome of MCD with AKI.[41]

Focal areas of interstitial fibrosis and tubular atrophy in a specimen that otherwise looks like MCD, especially in a young person, should raise the possibility of FSGS that was not sampled in the biopsy specimen. Examination of additional

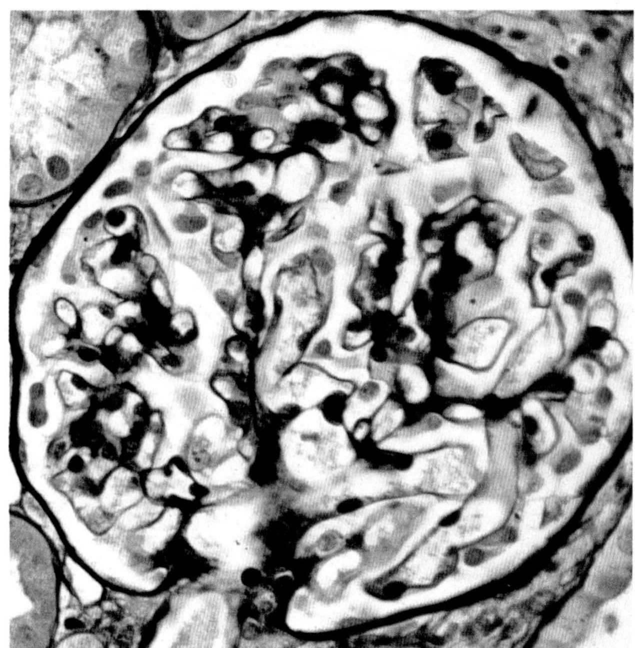

**Fig. 31.2** Unremarkable light microscopy appearance of a biopsy specimen from a patient with minimal change disease. Glomerular basement membranes are thin, and there is no glomerular hypercellularity or mesangial matrix expansion. (Jones' methenamine silver stain, ×300.)

levels of section may reveal a sclerotic glomerulus. In fact, MCD and FSGS may lie along a continuous spectrum of one unifying disease with variable manifestations.[42]

### Immunofluorescence Microscopy

Glomeruli usually show no staining with antisera specific for IgG, IgA, IgM, C3, C4, or C1q. The most frequent positive finding is low-level mesangial staining for IgM, sometimes accompanied by low-level staining for C3. If the IgM staining is not accompanied by mesangial electron-dense deposits by electron microscopy, it is consistent with a diagnosis of MCD. Patients whose specimens show mesangial IgM staining by immunofluorescence (IF) microscopy (in the absence of dense deposits by electron microscopy) do not have a worse prognosis than patients whose specimens are without IgM staining.[43,44] The presence of mesangial dense deposits identified by electron microscopy worsens the prognosis and thus justifies altering the diagnosis—for example, to IgM mesangial nephropathy.[45] Anything more than trace staining for IgG or IgA casts substantial doubt on a diagnosis of MCD. Even when no sclerotic glomerular lesions are seen by light microscopy, well-defined irregular focal segmental staining for C3 and IgM should raise the possibility of FSGS because sclerotic lesions can be enriched for C3 and IgM. Glomerular and tubular epithelial cell cytoplasmic droplets and tubular casts may stain positively for immunoglobulins and other plasma proteins when there is substantial proteinuria.

### Electron Microscopy

The pathologic sine qua non of MCD is effacement of podocyte foot processes observed by electron microscopy (Figs. 31.3 and 31.4). However, this is not a specific feature because it occurs in the glomeruli of patients with severe

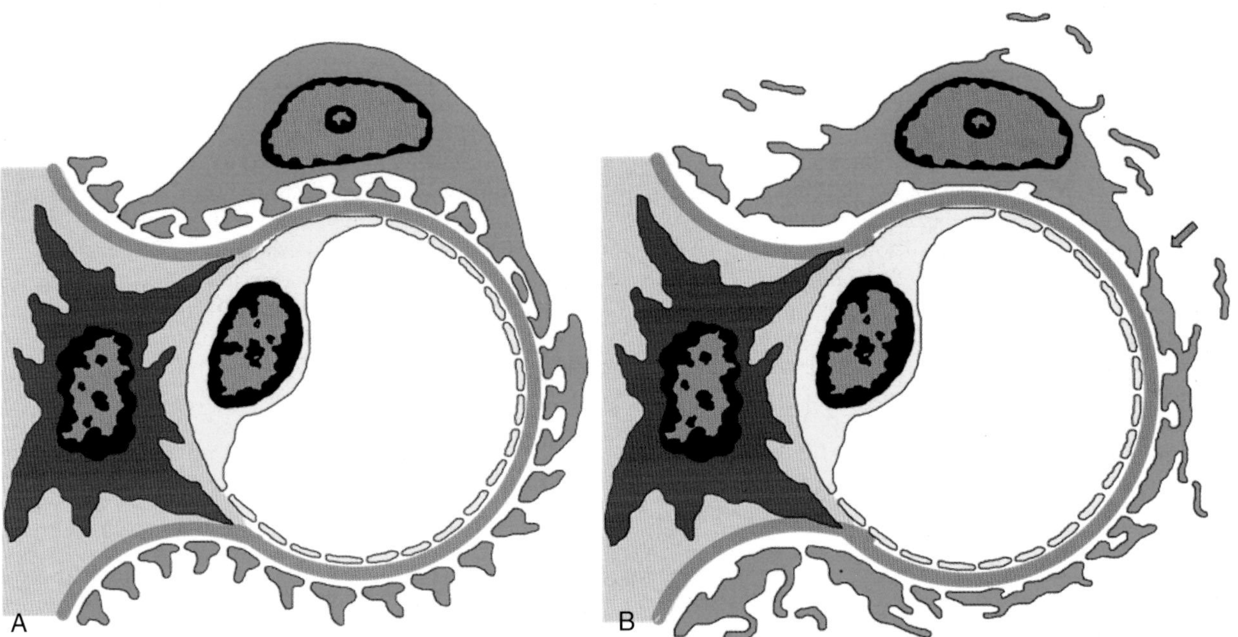


**Fig. 31.3** Diagrammatic representations of the ultrastructural features of a normal glomerular capillary loop (A) and a capillary loop with features of minimal change disease (B). The latter has effacement of podocyte foot processes and microvillous projections of podocyte cytoplasm. (Courtesy JC Jennette.)

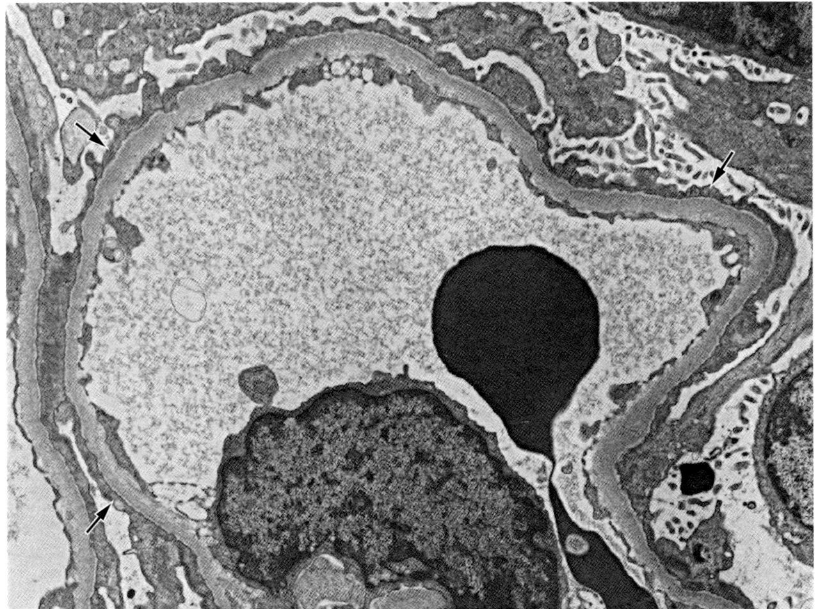

**Fig. 31.4** Electron micrograph of a glomerular capillary wall from a patient with minimal change disease showing extensive podocyte foot process effacement *(arrows)* and microvillous transformation. (×5000.)

proteinuria of any cause. During active nephrosis, the effacement often is very extensive, with only a few scattered intact foot processes. As the patient enters remission, the extent of foot process effacement diminishes. The effacement usually is accompanied by microvillous transformation, which is the development of numerous villous projections from the podocyte surface into the urinary space. These intracytoplasmic densities should not be confused with subepithelial immune complex dense deposits as a result of resorption of increased lipids and proteins in the urine. Glomerular and proximal tubular epithelial cells have increased clear and dense cytoplasmic droplets.

All these ultrastructural glomerular changes occur in other glomerular disease when there is nephrotic-range proteinuria. Therefore, MCD is a diagnosis by exclusion that is made only when there is no evidence by light, IF, and electron microscopy for any other glomerular disease.

## PATHOGENESIS

Although the pathogenesis of MCD remains unclear, this disorder is most likely a consequence of the abnormal regulation of a T cell subset[46–50] and pathologic elaboration of a circulating permeability factor. A role for the T cell is supported by the effectiveness of corticosteroids and alkylating drugs in the induction of remission of MCD, as well as by an association of MCD with Hodgkin disease,[51,52] and remissions are associated with depression of cell-mediated immunity during viral infections, such as measles. Specific evidence stems from the finding that a glomerular permeability factor is produced by human T cell hybridomas obtained from a patient with MCD. When this factor was injected into rodents, proteinuria occurred, with partial fusion of glomerular epithelial cell foot processes.[53] Although there are no recognized abnormalities in T or B cell populations in patients with relapsing or quiescent MCD,[54–57] lymphocytes have depressed reactivity when challenged with mitogens.[58–66] T cells apparently produce a product, most likely a lymphokine, which increases glomerular permeability to protein. When the glomerular permeability factor is removed from the kidney, it functions normally. This is supported by the intriguing observation that transplantation of a kidney from a patient with refractory MCD results in the rapid disappearance of proteinuria.[67]

A likely target of the pathogenic process is the podocyte, possibly a constituent of the slit pore membrane. Attention has focused on the role of plasma hemopexin in MCD.[68,69] Hemopexin is present in normal plasma, but an active isoform of the protein has been suggested to cause increased glomerular permeability due to enhanced protease activity.[68] Patients with MCD in relapse demonstrate altered isoforms of plasma hemopexin with increased protease activity compared with MCD in remission, patients with other forms of nephrotic syndrome, and normal subjects.[69] It is not understood how and why the plasma hemopexin is altered in MCD or how the enhanced protease activity results in alterations in glomerular permeability.

Differential gene expression techniques have also suggested an alteration in tumor necrosis factor–related apoptosis-inducing ligand (TRAIL) in peripheral blood mononuclear cells in MCD during relapse compared with remission.[70] Many additional genes (at least 15 of the more than 20,000 examined) were upregulated during relapse, which demonstrates the complexity of events occurring in MCD. Included among these was the IgE-dependent histamine-releasing factor gene,[71] and the well-known association of MCD with atopic allergic states could be the reason for this finding.

This factor may have specificity for podocytes that results in loss of the charge-selective barrier of the GBM. The loss of charge selectivity has been assessed by dextran studies.[72,73] In these studies, there is less evidence for a defect in the size-selective barrier and more of an alteration of the basement membrane electrostatic charge. The glomerular negative charge is reduced in relapse.[74]

Genetic aspects of MCD have been under intense investigation. Familial clustering of MCD has not generally been observed.[75] Heterozygous amino acid changes in nephrin and podocin are seen in about one-third of patients with typical MCD, but no amino acid changes were observed for *NEPH1* and *CD2AP* in a study involving 104 adults who presented with childhood-onset MCD.[75] Thus the genotype in MCD may be quite variable.

Polymorphisms in the genes encoding interleukins 4 and 13 (IL-4 and IL-13), activating transcription factor 6, and macrophage migration inhibitory factor have been described in MCD.[76–78] IL-13 polymorphisms may relate to phenotype because they have been associated with relapsing forms of MCD. IL-13 has also been suggested as a potential permeability factor in MCD. The implication of IL-13 in the pathogenesis of MCD is further suggested by the rat model of Lai and colleagues,[79] in which IL-13-transfected Wistar rats ($n = 41$) showed significant albuminuria, hypoalbuminemia, and hypercholesterolemia compared with control rats ($n = 17$). No significant histologic changes were seen in glomeruli of IL-13-transfected rats; however, electron microscopy revealed up to 80% effacement of podocyte foot process.

One observation is that podocyte-specific angiopoietin-like 4 ($ANGPTL_4$) overproduction in transgenic rats results in $ANGPTL_4$ binding to GBM with subsequent loss of GBM charge, diffuse foot process effacement, and nephrotic-range proteinuria. Furthermore, $ANGPTL_4$ expression has been observed in serum, glomeruli, and urine of patients with MCD,[80,81] and further understanding of this pathway may prove to be fruitful.

## CLINICAL FEATURES AND NATURAL HISTORY

The cardinal clinical feature of MCD in children is the relatively abrupt onset of proteinuria and the development of nephrotic syndrome with heavy proteinuria, hypoalbuminemia, and hyperlipidemia.[40] The edematous picture is typically what prompts the parents of these children to seek medical attention. Hematuria is distinctly unusual and, in children, hypertension is uncommon. The clinical features of MCD in adults tend to be somewhat different. In a group of 89 adults older than 60 years, hypertension, sometimes severe, as well as renal insufficiency, were more common.[82] Because individuals older than 60 years account for almost one-quarter of adult patients with MCD, this presentation must be considered.

MCD has been associated with several other conditions, including viral infections, use of certain pharmaceutical agents, malignancy, and allergy (Box 31.4). In some patients, there is a history of a drug reaction before the onset of MCD.

### Box 31.4 Common Associations With Minimal Change Disease

**Infections**

- Viral
- Parasitic

**Pharmaceutical Agents**

- Nonsteroidal antiinflammatory drugs
- Gold
- Lithium
- Interferon
- Ampicillin
- Rifampin
- Trimethadione
- Tiopronin

**Tumors**

- Hodgkin disease
- Lymphoma, leukemia
- Solid tumors

**Allergies**

- Food
- Dust
- Bee stings
- Pollen
- Poison ivy and poison oak
- Dermatitis herpetiformis

**Disease and Other Associations**

- Systemic lupus erythematosus
- Following allogeneic stem cell transplantation for leukemia
- Following hematopoietic cell transplantation

Modified from references 84, 101, 129 to 131, and 1464 to 1471.

The use of nonsteroidal antiinflammatory drugs (NSAIDs), and in particular fenoprofen, has been associated with and may cause MCD.[83] In this setting, most patients have not only proteinuria, but also pyuria and renal insufficiency as a consequence of the simultaneous development of acute tubulointerstitial nephritis. This same process has also been described with other compounds, including interferon,[84] penicillins, and rifampin. In most of these patients, discontinuation of the offending drug leads to resolution of the proteinuria, but it may take weeks to months for complete amelioration of pyuria and renal insufficiency.

MCD has been associated with lymphoid malignancy, usually Hodgkin disease or thymoma. In a retrospective study of adult patients,[85] MCD was associated with classic Hodgkin lymphoma of the nodular sclerosis type. MCD appeared before the diagnosis of lymphoma in 40% of patients.

MCD has also been associated with a variety of underlying exposures such as NSAIDs, as mentioned earlier,[86] and with syndromes such as SLE.[87,88] It has also occurred after allogeneic stem cell transplantation for leukemia[89] and after hematopoietic cell transplantation.

There is an association of glomerular disease with simultaneous graft-versus-host disease. Nephrotic syndrome generally follows graft-versus-host disease within 5 months in approximately 60% of hematopoietic cell–transplanted patients with either MCD or MN. Compared with MN, MCD occurred earlier after hematopoietic cell transplantation, was diagnosed soon after medication change, and exhibited a better prognosis because 90% of patients attained complete remission (vs. 27% of patients with MN).

MCD is also associated with food allergy. This is an important association because in some patients, removal of the allergen resulted in the resolution of the proteinuria. Of 42 patients with idiopathic nephrotic syndrome, 16 had positive results on skin tests for food allergy. For 13 of 42, a minimally antigenic diet was prescribed that resulted in a significant reduction in proteinuria.[90] Thus, it is important to ask patients about potential allergens, especially those found in food.

A syndrome of MCD accompanied by a reversible AKI occurs at higher incidence in adults than in children.[82,91,92] This syndrome of adult MCD with AKI was studied in 21 patients who, on presentation, had a serum creatinine level of more than 177 μmol/L and who were compared with 50 adult patients with MCD who had a serum creatinine level of less than 133 μmol/L. Patients who had AKI were older (59 vs. 40 years), had a higher systolic blood pressure (158 vs. 138 mm Hg), and had more proteinuria (13.5 vs. 7.9 g of protein/24 hours). Importantly, kidney biopsy specimens showed evidence of focal tubular epithelial simplification compatible with ischemic AKI. Of the 18 patients with renal failure for whom follow-up data were available, all showed recovery of kidney function, but only after prolonged periods of dialytic renal replacement therapy.[41]

The complications of nephrotic syndrome in MCD have been well described. The development of AKI during the course of MCD, mostly in adults older than 40 years, has been well recognized, but the underlying mechanisms are debated. Explanations for this phenomenon include a marked decrease in glomerular permeability due to extensive foot process effacement, tubular obstruction from proteinaceous casts, and intrarenal hemodynamic changes. Increased endothelin-1 expression in the kidneys of patients with MCD and AKI could indicate a hemodynamic change that underlies the pathogenesis of renal failure in these circumstances,[93] but the true cause of AKI in MCD remains uncertain and is probably multifactorial.

Another complication of MCD with nephrotic syndrome is the development of reduced bone mineral density, possibly due to the effects of glucocorticoids and/or vitamin D deficiency.[94] Statins may have a beneficial effect on bone mineral density, but the most recent study, in 2005, reported no beneficial effect of fluvastatin on the bone mineral density of children with MCD, although it did have some effect in lowering proteinuria.[95]

## LABORATORY FINDINGS

The ubiquitous laboratory feature of MCD is severe proteinuria.[40] Microscopic hematuria is seen in less than 15% of patients, with only rare episodes of macroscopic hematuria. The rapidity of the development of proteinuria in some patients is associated with evidence of volume contraction, with increased hematocrit and hemoglobin levels. The erythrocyte sedimentation rate is increased as a consequence of the hyperfibrinogenemia, as well as hypoalbuminemia. The serum albumin concentration is usually depressed, whereas the total cholesterol, low-density lipoprotein (LDL), and triglyceride levels are increased. Total serum protein concentration is usually reduced to between 4.5 and 5.5 g/dL with a serum albumin concentration generally less than 2 g/dL and, in more severe cases, less than 1 g/dL. Pseudohyponatremia has been observed in the setting of marked hyperlipidemia. The serum calcium level may be low, largely due to hypoproteinemia.

Several abnormalities that promote thrombosis are frequent in patients with severe nephrosis, including increased plasma viscosity, increased red cell aggregation, low plasminogen levels, and low levels of antithrombin III.[96] Kidney function is usually normal, although the serum creatinine level may be slightly increased at the time of presentation. A minority of patients (usually older adults) have substantial AKI, as discussed earlier.

The loss of albumin into the urine is largely a function of a loss of charge-selective permselectivity.[72,73,97,98] Consequently, the fractional excretion of albumin is proportionately greater than the fractional excretion of IgG. IgG levels may be profoundly decreased, however—a condition that occurs most notably during episodes of relapse. This low level of immunoglobulin may result in susceptibility to infections. IgM levels may be elevated after a remission.[99] Mean serum IgA levels may be substantially higher in patients with MCD than in those with another kidney disease[100] and are also elevated in association with relapse in children.[101] Among adult patients with MCD, over half have elevated levels of serum IgE, and two-thirds of patients have evidence of some allergic symptoms.[102] Elevation of IgE levels suggests a relationship between MCD and allergy. Complement levels are typically normal in patients with MCD.

## TREATMENT

The general approach to treatment of patients with MCD has been to institute corticosteroid therapy. For children, the dose of prednisone is 60 mg/m$^2$ per day. For adults, the dose of prednisone is 1 mg/kg of body weight, not to exceed 80 mg/day. In children, this form of therapy results in a complete remission, with disappearance of proteinuria in over 90% of patients within 4 to 6 weeks of therapy. A response to prednisone therapy has occurred if the patient has had no proteinuria by dipstick analysis for at least 3 days. It should be noted that the serum albumin and serum lipid levels might not return to normal for prolonged periods of time following resolution of the proteinuria.[103]

Treatment is generally continued for at least 6 weeks after complete remission of proteinuria. During those 6 weeks, the dose should be changed to alternate-day administration of prednisone or to a stepwise reduction in the daily dose of prednisone. If the dose is changed to alternate-day dosing when remission has occurred, the dosage may be decreased in children from 60 to 40 mg/m$^2$ per day.[50,104–08]

In adult patients with MCD, a response to corticosteroid treatment may take up to 15 weeks.[82] In a study of 89 adult patients with MCD, 75 of them were given prednisolone; remission occurred in 60% after 8 weeks, in 73% after 16 weeks, and in 77% over the course of the study. Of the 58 treated patients who showed a response (complete remission at 28 weeks), 24% never experienced relapse, 56% experienced relapse on a single occasion or infrequently, and only 21% had frequent relapses. Of the 89 patients, only 4 remained nephrotic, and 2 of these presented with AKI. Cyclophosphamide therapy was administered to 36 (2 of them as initial treatment, 11 with corticosteroids, and 23 with relapse) of the 89 patients and, in 66% of these patients, the disease was in remission at 5 years.

In a large retrospective analysis of 95 patients with primary adult-onset MCD, AKI complicated the nephrotic syndrome in 20% of patients.[109] The cohort was largely middle-aged, with a substantial prevalence of hypertension (45%) and microscopic hematuria (30%). Of these patients, 92 were initially treated with oral corticosteroids; two-thirds were on a daily regimen, and one-third were on an alternate-day regimen. The initial steroid dose was approximately 1 mg/kg on the daily regimen and approximately 2 mg/kg on the alternate-day regimen so that cumulative doses were similar in the two groups. There were no significant differences in demographic features between the two groups, but patients treated with alternate-day steroid regimen tended to have a lower serum albumin level at presentation than those treated with the daily regimen (1.91 ± 0.14. g/dL vs. 2.31 ± 0.1 g/dL, respectively; $P = .055$). No significant differences were seen between the daily and alternate-day treatment groups in the percentage of patients experiencing complete or partial remission (remissions in 76.8% and 73.9% of patients, respectively), or in the time to remission. It is interesting to note that the rate of relapse of nephrotic syndrome was quite elevated, at 73% of those who showed an initial response. Of the patients who were treated with at least one additional course of corticosteroids, 92% achieved a remission (complete remission in 84.4%). This nonrandomized, uncontrolled study does suggest that alternate-day and daily steroid regimens are of equivalent efficacy and safety in the treatment of MCD.

One of the most controversial issues with respect to treatment is the regimen for tapering the prednisone after the initial response. Sudden withdrawal of corticosteroids, or a rapid taper of prednisone immediately following complete remission, may prompt a relapse. Whether this is a consequence of adrenal insufficiency or depression of the hypothalamic-pituitary-adrenal axis has been a matter of debate.[108,110,111] At least in children, the likelihood of relapse is decreased with prolonged administration of corticosteroids over a 10- to 12-week period.[106,112,113] Once remission has been obtained, an alternate-day schedule should begin within at least 4 weeks of the response to decrease steroid-induced side effects.

In children who have not undergone biopsy before treatment, a kidney biopsy is usually appropriate if there is failure to respond to a 4- to 6-week course of prednisone, particularly if changes have occurred in the clinical course during this period of time suggestive of another glomerular disease. Many pediatricians advocate a biopsy at the onset of the disease if there are clinical features suggesting a diagnosis other than MCD (e.g., hypertension, red blood cell casts in the urine, or hypocomplementemia), or if the nephrotic syndrome begins in the first year of life or after 6 years of age.

After the clinical response to initial treatment, as few as 25% experience a long-term remission,[92] 25% to 30% have infrequent relapses (no more than one/year), and the remainder experience frequent relapses, steroid dependence, or steroid resistance (Box 31.5). Nephrotic patients who are steroid dependent or experience frequent relapses require additional forms of therapy. The treatment is aimed at minimizing the complications of corticosteroid therapy. In general, induction of a remission with prednisone therapy followed by the institution of cyclophosphamide treatment results in higher urine flow rates and reduced risk of hemorrhagic cystitis. When oral cyclophosphamide is given in dosages of 2 mg/kg for 8 to 12 weeks, 75% of patients remain free of proteinuria for at least 2 years.[82,114–116] The response to cyclophosphamide may be predicted from the response to corticosteroids. Patients who have experienced an immediate relapse after the cessation of corticosteroid therapy have a greater chance of experiencing relapse immediately after the cessation of cyclophosphamide treatment. Those who have had longer remissions after corticosteroid therapy have a decreased risk of relapse after cyclophosphamide therapy.[117] In one study of patients who were steroid dependent, the response to cyclophosphamide was improved by increasing

**Box 31.5 Patterns of Response of Minimal Change Disease to Corticosteroid Treatment**

- Primary responder, no relapse
- Primary responder with only one relapse in the first six months after an initial response
- Initial steroid response with two or more relapses within six months (frequent relapse)
- Initial steroid-induced remission with relapses during tapering of corticosteroid, or within 2 weeks after their withdrawal (steroid dependent)
- Steroid-induced remission, but no response to a subsequent relapse
- No response to treatment (steroid-resistant)

Modified from references 106, 107, 123, and 1472.

the duration of therapy to up to 12 weeks.[114] In at least one other investigation, however, a 12-week course of cyclophosphamide was not proven efficacious.[118]

Cyclosporine has been emerging as a reasonable alternative to cyclophosphamide.[119,120] Based on uncontrolled observations, complete remissions are common (>80%), and cyclosporine resistance is seen in only about 10% to 15% of patients. Side effects such as a rise in the serum creatinine level, hypertrichosis, and gingival hyperplasia are common. Relapses are very common after the cessation of cyclosporine treatment. The best method of monitoring cyclosporine levels has not been agreed on. Measurement of trough blood levels with twice-daily dosing, measurement of cyclosporine levels 1 to 2 hours after a once-daily dose (C1–C2) and abbreviated under the curve monitoring of cyclosporine have all been recommended.[120–122] Cyclosporine may be an acceptable alternative to cyclophosphamide therapy for relapsing or steroid-dependent MCD. The optimal duration of calcineurin inhibitor (CNI)–based therapy is not known and, because relapses are common on cessation of therapy, one may consider a prolonged course of 18 to 24 months of treatment with the lowest dose that that keeps a patient in clinical remission. Also, a thorough discussion with patient and continuing observation for adverse effects of prolonged CNI use is necessary.

### STEROID-RESISTANT MINIMAL CHANGE DISEASE

Approximately 5% of children with MCD appear to be steroid resistant. In patients who have never undergone kidney biopsy, resistance to corticosteroid therapy is an indication for kidney biopsy. Often, evaluation of the kidney biopsy specimen will demonstrate FSGS or other forms of glomerular injury other than MCD.[123]

If the diagnosis remains as MCD after kidney biopsy specimen evaluation, there may be several reasons for steroid resistance. Some patients, especially those for whom corticosteroid therapy is overly toxic, may skip doses or not fully adhere to the therapy regimen. For other patients, especially some adults, alternate-day therapy may not provide sufficient amounts of corticosteroid to induce clinical remission. In very edematous patients, oral corticosteroid therapy may not be well absorbed, and intravenous administration of a dose of methylprednisolone may provide a more reliable route. Available data suggest that pulse methylprednisolone may induce remission in some corticosteroid-resistant children. In one study, five of eight corticosteroid-resistant children had a remission with pulse methylprednisolone,[124] although this experience is not universal.[125]

Patients with MCD may have an unrecognized lesion of focal and segmental glomerulosclerosis that requires longer courses of steroid therapy (usually >4 months) to achieve a lasting remission. A regimen of CNI (cyclosporine or tacrolimus) followed by mycophenolate mofetil (MMF) and monthly intravenous pulse cyclophosphamide therapy was demonstrated in an uncontrolled study to result in a high frequency of complete remission.[126] There are anecdotal reports of the use of combinations of sirolimus and tacrolimus to treat steroid-resistant MCD,[127] but the overall safety and efficacy of this regimen are unknown. In a small nonrandomized trial, the use of cyclosporine with steroids was associated with better outcomes in those with steroid-resistant MCD.[128]

Cyclosporine can be administered at a dose of approximately 3 to 5 mg/kg per day in two divided doses. Up to 90% of patients may experience a partial or complete remission with cyclosporine.[101,106,129–131] Unfortunately, only rarely do patients experience long-term remission once cyclosporine is discontinued.[107] Two trials have examined the use of cyclosporine in steroid-resistant nephrosis. A study conducted by the French Society of Pediatric Nephrology combined cyclosporine with prednisone. Prednisone was given at a dose of 30 mg/m$^2$ per day for the first month and then changed to alternate-day dosing for 5 months. Cyclosporine was administered at a dosage of 150 to 200 mg/m$^2$ per day.[132] In this study, 48% of patients with MCD experienced complete remission, some within the first month of therapy. A minority of those who showed a response became steroid sensitive when they later experienced relapse. In a study by Ponticelli and colleagues,[133] 13 of 45 patients had MCD and were treated with cyclosporine. In those patients with MCD, partial or complete remission occurred within 2 months of the initiation of therapy. Unfortunately, in spite of the early positive results of this study, relapses occurred in all patients after cyclosporine was stopped.

In a summary of nine studies,[134] only 20% of children had complete remission with cyclosporine and many, if not most, relapsed with the cessation of therapy. Moreover, although cyclosporine and cyclophosphamide appear to have a similar degree of efficacy with respect to controlling nephrotic syndrome, one study found that cyclophosphamide-treated patients experience a more stable long-term remission.[135] In this study, the likelihood of a long-term remission was 63% in patients treated with cyclophosphamide but was only 25% in those treated with cyclosporine.

To counteract the usual relapse of nephrosis when cyclosporine has been used for 6 months, an alternative approach to cyclosporine treatment relies on a long-term course of this drug, using gradually lower doses to maintain the patient in remission. In one study,[136] patients who had been in complete remission for longer than 1 year while taking cyclosporine remained in remission if the cyclosporine was gradually tapered and then stopped. Serial biopsy specimens from patients treated for as long as 20 months showed no overt sign of nephrotoxicity.

An emerging treatment option in adults for steroid-resistant and relapsing MCD reported in numerous case reports and series to date is the B lymphocyte-depleting agent, rituximab. Most recently, the Rituximab in Nephrotic Syndrome of Steroid-Dependent or Frequently Relapsing MCD or FSGS (NEMO) Study Group conducted a multicenter trial in Italy in 10 children and 20 adults with recurrent MCD, mesangial proliferative glomerulonephritis, or FSGS who were treated with one or two doses of rituximab.[137] Interestingly, all patients were in remission at 1 year, 18 were treatment free and 15 never relapsed. There was also a significant decrease in the number of relapses and median prednisone dose across all disease groups over 1 year of follow-up, and rituximab was well tolerated. A more recent case series combined with a review of large previously published case series of patients with corticosteroid-resistant or corticosteroid-dependent MCD treated with rituximab revealed a very high likelihood of remission with this treatment strategy.[138] Although rituximab appears to be effective in some individuals, greater mechanistic understanding is needed.[139–141] Mounting evidence

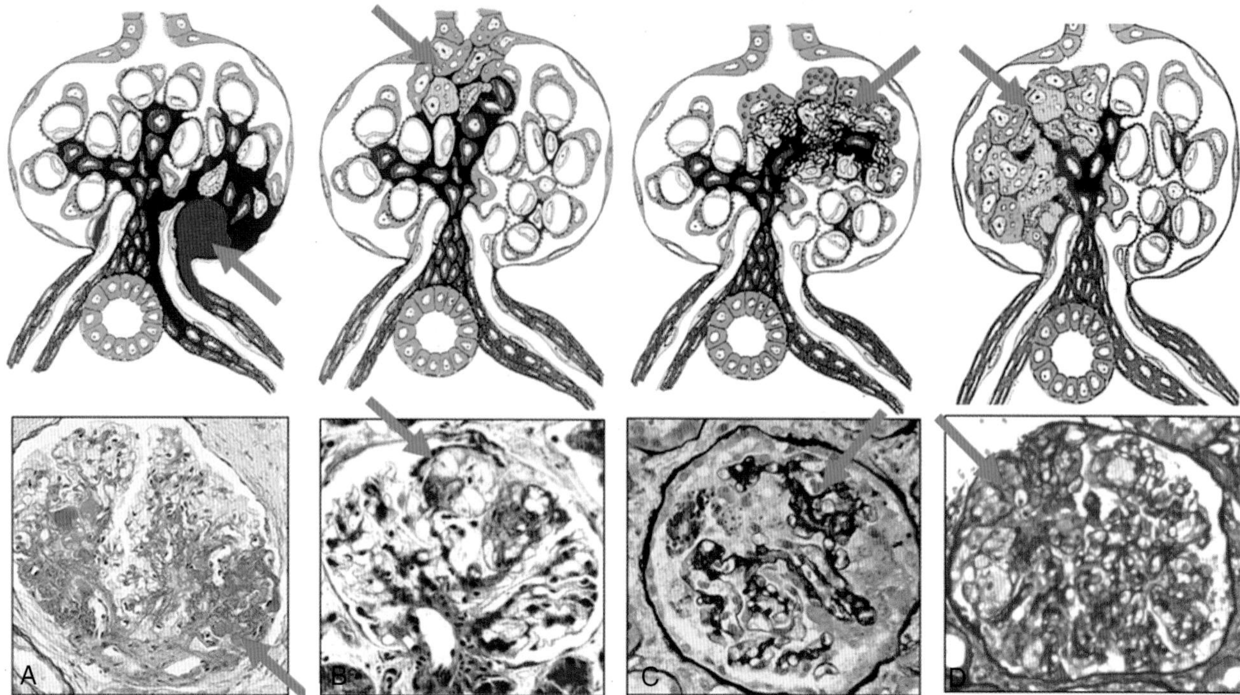


**Fig. 31.5** Light micrographs and diagrams depicting histologic variants of focal segmental glomerulosclerosis *(arrows).* (A) Perihilar variant has a predilection for sclerosis in the perihilar regions of the glomerular (periodic acid–Schiff stain). (B) Glomerular tip lesion variant has segmental consolidation confined to the segment adjacent to the origin of the proximal tubule (Masson trichrome stain). (C) Collapsing glomerulopathy variant has segmental collapse of capillaries with hypertrophy and hyperplasia of overlying podocytes (Jones' methenamine silver stain). (D) Cellular variant with endocapillary accumulation of foam cells (Jones' methenamine silver stain).

has implied that larger, prospective, randomized controlled trials are needed to assess the utility of rituximab in MCD accurately.

## FOCAL SEGMENTAL GLOMERULOSCLEROSIS

FSGS is not a single disease but rather a diagnostic term for a clinical-pathologic syndrome that has multiple causes and pathogenic mechanisms, as well as somewhat limited therapeutic options.[142–145] The ubiquitous clinical feature of the syndrome is proteinuria, which may be nephrotic or nonnephrotic. The ubiquitous pathologic feature is focal segmental glomerular consolidation or scarring, which may have several distinctive patterns (Fig. 31.5). These patterns can be classified as collapsing FSGS, tip lesion FSGS, cellular FSGS, perihilar FSGS, and FSGS not otherwise specified (NOS).[142,143] The collapsing variant of FSGS is a clinically aggressive variant that is much more common in African-Americans than in Caucasian populations and is characterized pathologically by the segmental collapse of capillaries accompanied by hypertrophy and hyperplasia of epithelial cells and accumulation of prominent protein resorption droplets in podocytes. The glomerular tip lesion variant of FSGS, which typically presents with marked nephrosis but often has a good outcome, is characterized by consolidation and sclerosis in the glomerular segment that is adjacent to the origin of the proximal tubule.[143] The term "cellular FSGS" is used when numerous cells, especially foam cells, are within consolidated segments. However, this term has been used in a number of ways in the literature, especially before the publication of the Columbia classification system. For example, the term has been used to describe the collapsing variant and tip lesion variant of FSGS. Care must be taken when reading the literature to determine if this term is being used as defined by the Columbia classification system.[142] The perihilar variant of FSGS is characterized pathologically by sclerosis at the hilum of the glomerulus that typically contains foci of hyalinosis.[142]

As shown in Box 31.6, FSGS may appear to be a primary kidney disease or may be associated with, and possibly caused by, a variety of other conditions (see Chapter 32).

### EPIDEMIOLOGY

Over the past 2 decades, the incidence of FSGS has increased, whether expressed as an absolute number of patients or as a proportion of the total incident population of patients with end-stage kidney disease (ESKD).[148] This trend appears to hold true, even when one accounts for a possible increase in the rate of diagnosis resulting from an increase in the frequency of kidney biopsies. Although this trend was previously reported to be most significant among African Americans, it has now been confirmed among Caucasians as well. A review of kidney biopsy findings performed between 1974 and 2003 in Olmstead County, Minnesota, in which 90% of the population are Caucasians of northern European extraction, FSGS was found to account for 17% of glomerulonephritides, second only to IgA nephropathy (22%), and was more frequent than MN (10%).[148] Over that period of time, the incidence of FSGS increased by 13-fold ($P < .001$), compared with a twofold increase in the incidence of all

**Box 31.6 Classification of Focal Segmental Glomerulosclerosis**

**Primary (Idiopathic) Focal Segmental Glomerulosclerosis (FSGS)**

FSGS not otherwise specified (NOS)
Glomerular tip lesion variant of FSGS
Collapsing variant of FSGS
Perihilar variant of FSGS
Cellular variant of FSGS

**Secondary FSGS**

With human immunodeficiency virus disease
With intravenous drug abuse
With other drugs (e.g., pamidronate, interferon, anabolic steroids)
With identified genetic abnormalities (e.g., in podocin, alpha-actinin-4, TRPC6)
With glomerulomegaly:
- Morbid obesity
- Sickle cell disease
- Cyanotic congenital heart disease
- Hypoxic pulmonary disease

With reduced nephron numbers:
- Unilateral renal agenesis
- Oligomeganephronia
- Reflux-interstitial nephritis
- Postfocal cortical necrosis
- Postnephrectomy

glomerular diseases ($P < .001$), and a 2.5- to threefold increase in MN and IgA nephropathy, respectively.

## PATHOLOGY

### Light Microscopy

FSGS is characterized by focal and segmental glomerular sclerosis or consolidation.[142,143,149] The sclerosis may begin as segmental consolidation caused by insudation of plasma proteins causing hyalinosis, by accumulation of foam cells, by swelling of epithelial cells, and by collapse of capillaries resulting in obliteration of capillary lumens. These events are accompanied by increased extracellular matrix material that accounts for the sclerosis component of the lesion.

FSGS is, by definition, a focal process when it begins. The limited number of glomeruli in a kidney biopsy specimen may not include any of the segmentally sclerotic glomeruli that are present in the kidney. In this case, focal tubulointerstitial injury or glomerular enlargement, which often accompanies FSGS, can be used as a surrogate marker. For example, FSGS should be considered in kidney biopsy specimens of patients with nephrotic syndrome when there is relatively well-circumscribed focal tubular atrophy and interstitial fibrosis with slight chronic inflammation, even when there are no light microscopic glomerular lesions, no immune deposits, and no ultrastructural changes other than foot process effacement. Segmental sclerosis that is adequate for diagnosis may be present only in the tissue examined by IF or electron microscopy.

Focal segmental glomerular scarring is nonspecific. Many injurious processes can cause focal glomerular scarring and must be ruled out before making a diagnosis of FSGS. For example, hereditary nephritis causes progressive glomerular scarring that can mimic FSGS, as revealed by the identification of ultrastructural changes that are characteristic of hereditary nephritis. FSGS, for example caused by IgA nephropathy, lupus nephritis, or ANCA-associated glomerulonephritis, can result in focal segmental glomerular scarring that is histologically indistinguishable from that caused by FSGS. Findings by IF, electron microscopy, and serology, can reveal a glomerulonephritic basis for focal glomerular scarring.

Based on the character and glomerular distribution of lesions, five major structural variants of FSGS can be recognized that correlate, at least in part, with outcome (prognosis) and that may be have different causes and pathogenic mechanisms.[142,143] As mentioned previously, these five pathologic variants are collapsing FSGS, tip lesion FSGS, cellular FSGS, perihilar FSGS, and FSGS NOS.[142,143]

The characteristic feature of the collapsing variant of FSGS is focal segmental or global collapse of glomerular capillaries, with obliteration of capillary lumens. Podocytes overlying collapsed segments are usually enlarged and contain conspicuous resorption droplets. Hyperplasia of podocytes raises the possibility of crescentic glomerulonephritis. The convention among most renal pathologists is not to refer to the epithelial hyperplasia of collapsing glomerulopathy as crescent formation, although the term "pseudocrescent" has been used by some. The degree of adhesion formation relative to the extent of glomerular sclerosis is much less in collapsing glomerulopathy than in typical FSGS. This may result in contracted (collapsed) tuft basement membranes and sclerotic matrix separated from Bowman's capsule by hypertrophied and hyperplastic epithelial cells. The collapsing glomerulopathy variant of FSGS is the major pathologic expression of human immunodeficiency virus (HIV) nephropathy[40,147,150,151] and also occurs with intravenous drug abuse and as an idiopathic process.[152,153] In those with a kidney transplant, this phenotype of FSGS occurs as both recurrent and de novo disease.[154,155]

Relative to the extent of glomerular sclerosis, tubulointerstitial injury is more severe in collapsing glomerulopathy than in typical FSGS. Tubular epithelial cells have larger resorption droplets, extensive proteinaceous casts, and marked focal dilation of lumens (microcystic change). There is also more extensive interstitial infiltration by mononuclear leukocytes. IF microscopy findings are similar to those observed in typical FSGS except for the usual finding of larger protein resorption droplets in glomerular podocytes and tubular epithelial cells. Electron microscopy reveals the same structural changes as seen by light microscopy. In a specimen with the collapsing glomerulopathy variant of FSGS, an important ultrastructural assessment is for the presence or absence of endothelial tubuloreticular inclusions. Endothelial tubuloreticular inclusions are identified in over 90% of patients with HIV infection and collapsing glomerulopathy, but in fewer than 10% of patients with idiopathic collapsing glomerulopathy. Other settings in which endothelial tubuloreticular inclusions are numerous are in patients with SLE and in patients treated with interferon-α.

The glomerular tip lesion variant of FSGS was first described by Howie and colleagues and is characterized by consolidation of the glomerular segment that is adjacent to the origin of the proximal tubule and thus opposite the hilum (see Fig. 31.5B).[156–160] The initial consolidation usually has obliteration of capillary lumens by foam cells, swollen endothelial cells, and an increase in collagenous matrix material (sclerosis). Podocytes adjacent to the consolidated segment are enlarged and contain clear vacuoles and hyaline droplets. These altered podocytes often are contiguous to, if not attached to, adjacent parietal epithelial cells and tubular epithelial cells at the origin of the proximal tubule, which also have irregular enlargement and vacuolation. The tip lesion may project into the lumen of the proximal tubule. Some lesions are less cellular, with a predominance of matrix and collagenous adhesions to Bowman's capsule at the origin of the proximal tubule.

The cellular variant of FSGS as defined by the Columbia classification system has lesions that resemble the cellular lesion for the tip variant, but they are distributed more widely in the glomerular tuft and are not confined to the tip.[142] Perihilar FSGS is characterized by the perihilar predilection of lesions and the presence of hyalinosis. When FSGS is secondary to obesity or reduced numbers of nephrons, it often has a perihilar pattern and is accompanied by glomerular enlargement. The FSGS NOS category is a nonspecific category, with lesions that do not have the distinctive features of any of the other four variants.

As discussed later, different pathologic variants of FSGS have distinctive demographic characteristics, clinical presentations, and outcomes.

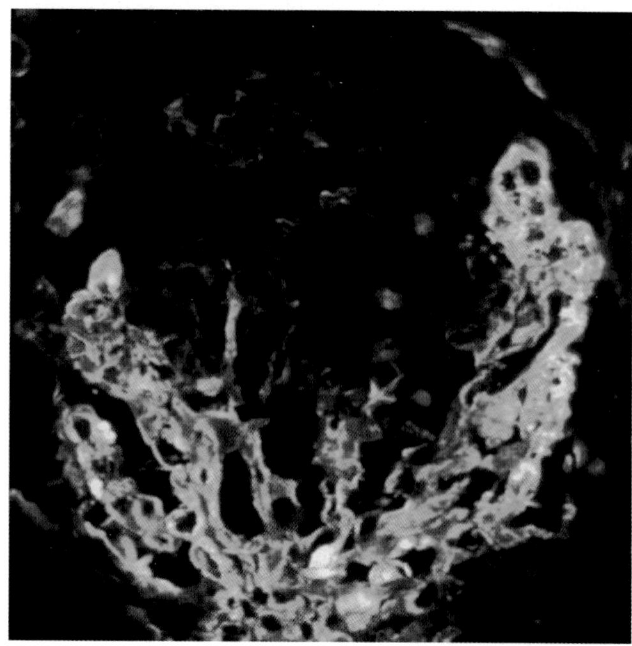

**Fig. 31.6** Immunofluorescence micrograph showing irregular segmental staining for C3 corresponding to a site of segmental sclerosis in a patient with perihilar variant focal segmental glomerulosclerosis. (Fluorescein isothiocyanate anti-C3 stain, ×3000.)

### Immunofluorescence Microscopy

In all the histologic variants, nonsclerotic glomeruli and segments usually show no staining for immunoglobulins or complement. As in patients with MCD, as well as individuals with no kidney dysfunction, a minority of patients with FSGS has low-level mesangial staining for IgM in nonsclerotic glomeruli. Low-level mesangial C3 staining is less frequent, and low-level IgG and IgA staining are uncommon. The presence of substantial staining of nonsclerotic glomeruli for immunoglobulins, especially if immune complex–type, electron-dense deposits are present, points toward the sclerotic phase of a focal immune complex glomerulonephritis rather than FSGS.

Sclerotic segments typically show irregular staining for C3, C1q, and IgM (Fig. 31.6). Other plasma constituents are less frequently identified in the sclerotic areas. Epithelial resorption droplets stain for plasma proteins.

### Electron Microscopy

The ultrastructural features of FSGS are nonspecific. Electron microscopy plays an important role in the diagnosis of FSGS by helping identify other causes for glomerular scarring that can be mistaken for FSGS by light microscopy alone.

Foot process effacement in FSGS affects sclerotic and nonsclerotic glomeruli and usually is more focal than in MCD. Foot process effacement is less extensive in some forms of secondary FSGS than in idiopathic FSGS. Occasionally, glomerular capillaries have segmental denudation of foot processes. Podocytes adjacent to collapsed segments in collapsing FSGS are cuboidal and appear dedifferentiated. Nonsclerotic glomeruli and segments should have no immune complex–type, electron-dense deposits. One must be careful not to confuse electron-dense "insudated" lesions with immune complex deposits. These lesions correspond to the hyalinosis seen by light microscopy and result from the accumulation of plasma proteins within sclerotic areas. When electron-dense material is present in sclerotic but not in nonsclerotic glomerular segments, it should not be considered as evidence for immune complex–mediated glomerular disease. Conversely, well-defined mesangial or capillary wall electron-dense deposits in nonsclerotic segments indicate immune complex-mediated glomerulonephritis with secondary scarring, which should be confirmed and further characterized by IF microscopy.

## PATHOGENESIS

The past 30 years have witnessed an explosion of interest in the role of the podocyte in FSGS, in part due to concomitant rapidly advancing genomic technology that has revealed genetic abnormalities, as well as the establishment of well-curated cohort consortia such as NEPTUNE and CureGN. Podocytes are highly differentiated postmitotic cells whose function requires a complex cellular architecture. Tremendous interest has centered on the genetics of familial FSGS, and podocyte defects have taken center stage (reviewed by D'Agati and colleagues[145] and Garg and Rabelink[9]). This has led to the identification of several proteins important to the normal function of podocytes and the development of proteinuria. Mutations in several genes have been identified and linked to familial and sporadic cases of FSGS (see also Chapter 43). These include, but are not limited to, genes coding for podocin *(NPHS2)*,[161] nephrin *(NPHS1)*,[162] α-actinin-IV *(ACTN4)*,[163,164] transient receptor potential cation channel, subfamily C, member 6 *(TRPC6)*[165–167] and phospholipase C$\varepsilon_1$ *(PLCE1)*.[168] In addition to mutations in genes encoding podocyte-specific proteins, mutations in other genes are associated with syndromes of which FSGS is often a part.[169] These include the *COQ2* gene,[170] Wilms' tumor gene *(WT1)*, and the gene for Lim homeobox transcription factor 1β

**Table 31.4 Gene Mutations With Causal Links to Focal Segmental Glomerulosclerosis**

| Gene | Protein | Mode of Inheritance |
|---|---|---|
| *NPHS1* | Nephrin | Autosomal recessive |
| *NPHS2* | Podocin | Autosomal recessive |
| *CD2AP* | CD2-associated protein | Autosomal dominant |
| *TRPC6* | Transient receptor potential cation channel 6 | Autosomal dominant |
| *PTPRO* | Protein tyrosine phosphatase receptor type O (GLEPP1) | Autosomal recessive |
| *LAMB2* | Laminin-$\beta_2$ | Autosomal recessive |
| *ITGB4* | $\beta_4$-integrin | Autosomal recessive |
| *CD151* | Tetraspanin CD151 | Autosomal recessive |
| *ACTN4* | α-actinin-4 | Autosomal dominant |
| *PLCE1* | Phospholipase C epsilon | Autosomal recessive |
| *MYH9* | Nonmuscle myosin heavy chain A (NMMHC-A) | Autosomal dominant, de novo mutation |
| *INF2* | Inverted formin 2 | Autosomal dominant |
| *MYO1E* | Myosin 1E | Autosomal recessive |
| *WT1* | Wilms' tumor suppressor protein | Autosomal dominant, de novo mutation |
| *SMARCAL1* | Smarca-like protein | Autosomal recessive |
| *mtDNA-A3243G* | tRNAleu | maternal |
| *COQ2* | Coenzyme Q2 homolog, polyprenyltransferase | Autosomal recessive |
| *COQ6* | Coenzyme Q10 biosynthesis monooxygenase 6 | Autosomal recessive |
| *SCARB2* | Lysosomal integral membrane protein (LIMP) type 2 | Autosomal recessive |
| *APOL1* | Apolipoprotein L1 | Autosomal recessive |

*(LMX1B)*, which is a transcription factor required for the expression of CD2AP and NPHS2, associated with nail-patella syndrome. The genes implicated in the pathogenesis of FSGS are summarized in Table 31.4 and have been reviewed by Rood and colleagues.[170] Whereas these genetic mutations were primarily identified based on cases of familial forms of FSGS, their implication in sporadic FSGS in children and adults, and their impact on treatment, outcome, and recurrence after transplantation, have been the focus of numerous investigations.

Mutations in *NPHS2,* the gene encoding podocin, are the most frequent genetic cause of steroid-resistant nephrotic syndrome and were initially described in early-onset disease (see recent review of all known mutations by Bouchireb and colleagues[171]). In a study of a large cohort of 430 patients from 404 different families with steroid-resistant nephrotic syndrome, recessive podocin mutations were present in 18.1%.[172] The *R138Q* mutation (a single nucleotide substitution of G to A at position 413 in the third exon of podocin gene) was found in 57% of families with two disease-causing mutations on each of the parental gene copies. Of these podocin mutations, 70% were nonsense, frameshift, or homozygous R138Q. Patients with these mutations manifested symptoms at a significantly earlier age (mean onset <1.75 years) than any other patient group, with or without podocin mutations (mean onset >4.17 years). The sequence variant R229Q was found in 9% of families in the heterozygous mutation and 0.5% as a homozygous mutation.

The significance of the R229Q sequence variant as a cause of nephrotic syndrome was addressed in a study of 546 patients (from 455 families) with familial or sporadic FSGS, only 24% of whom developed nephrotic syndrome after the age of 18 years.[173] The R229Q allele frequency was significantly higher among European and South American patients than among control individuals (0.089 for European patients vs. 0.026; for controls, $P = .00001$; and 0.17 for South American patients vs. 0.007, $P = .000002$). Compared with individuals without a p.R229Q allele, those with a p.R229Q allele had a significantly higher likelihood of having a single pathogenic *NPHS2* mutation, which strongly suggests a pathogenic role of p.R229Q in the compound heterozygous state with a *NPHS2* mutation. Patients carrying p.R229Q and one *NPHS2* mutation developed nephrotic syndrome significantly later than those carrying two pathogenic mutations (median, 19.0 vs. 1.1 years; $P < .01$). The frequency of *NPHS2* mutations in adults with treatment-resistant nephrotic syndrome was 11% in sporadic cases and 25% in familial cases. This study suggests that compound heterozygosity for p.R229Q is associated with adult-onset, steroid-resistant nephrotic syndrome. Furthermore, genetic analyses of *NPHS2* may identify individuals who are steroid-resistant before treatment initiation, as well as those who are more likely to progress to ESKD and/or have a low posttransplantation recurrence risk.[174]

The role of *NPHS2* polymorphisms in sporadic cases of late-onset idiopathic or HIV-associated FSGS was studied in 377 biopsy-confirmed FSGS cases and 919 controls without known kidney disease.[175] No homozygotes or compound heterozygotes were observed for any of five missense mutations identified on gene sequencing. R138Q carriers were five times more frequent among FSGS cases than controls ($P = .06$), but heterozygosity for the other four missense mutations (including R229Q) was equally distributed among FSGS cases and controls. Genetic variation or mutation of *NPHS2* may therefore play a role in late-onset sporadic FSGS. However, given the very low frequency of R138Q (4–8/1000) and the lack of involvement of other mutations, the attributable risk of *NPHS2* for adult sporadic or HIV-associated FSGS is extremely small. The presence of the nonsynonymous variants of *NPHS2* (p.R229Q and p.A242V) did not significantly alter the risk of albuminuria in the Nurses' Health Study participants.[176]

In summary, *NPHS2* gene mutations are associated with familial and childhood-onset, steroid-resistant nephrotic syndrome, but may not contribute significantly to adult-onset sporadic FSGS. Heterozygosity for R138Q is associated with a fivefold increased risk of FSGS in adults. When combined with other pathogenic mutations of *NPHS2*, the R229Q variant appears to be associated with disease onset at older age.

Typically, mutations in *NPHS1*, which encodes nephrin, are associated with congenital nephrotic syndrome of the Finnish type presenting within the first 3 months of life. A study of 160 patients from 142 unrelated families who presented with nephrotic syndrome at least 3 months after birth identified *NPHS1* mutations in one familial case and in nine sporadic cases.[177] Kidney biopsy at presentation revealed mesangioproliferative lesions in one patient, MCD in six patients, and FSGS in three patients. This study broadens the spectrum of kidney disease related to nephrin mutations and raises the possibility that mutations in *NPHS1* may contribute to sporadic nephrotic syndrome in combination with mutations in other genes associated with this syndrome.[177,178]

Mutations in *ACTN4*, the gene encoding the actin-binding protein α-actinin-4, are a cause of familial FSGS, with an autosomal dominant pattern of inheritance, and may be associated with a distinctive ultrastructural feature of podocyte injury consisting of cytoplasmic electron-dense aggregates that help identify patients with *ACTN4* mutations.[179] Interestingly, mechanistic investigations have revealed that *ACTN4* protein mutants lack the ability to activate protective nuclear hormone receptors in podocytes.[180]

African Americans have a disproportionate risk for several forms of kidney disease, including a fourfold increased risk for FSGS and an 18- to 50-fold increased risk for HIV-associated FSGS. The basis for that susceptibility is thought to be multifactorial, with a suspected genetic component. Two landmark studies, both of which used genome-wide mapping by admixture linkage disequilibrium, identified a chromosome 22 region that was associated with kidney disease in subjects of African ancestry.[181,182] Initial efforts focused on MYH9, which encodes a nonmuscle myosin heavy-chain type IIA expressed in kidney podocytes and possibly mesangial cells, where it binds to actin to perform intracellular motor functions. Multiple MYH9 single-nucleotide polymorphisms (SNPs) and haplotypes were recessively associated with FSGS. Nine MYH9 SNPs and the same haplotype for FSGS were associated with hypertensive ESKD (odds ratio [OR] = 2.2; 95% confidence interval [CI] = 1.5–3.4; $n = 433$), but not ESKD associated with type 2 diabetes.[181]

Unlike other mutations that are directly linked to the development of FSGS, the association of *MYH9* does not establish direct causality. In addition, more recent work has revealed coding variants within the apolipoprotein L-1 (APOL1) gene, which closely neighbors the *MYH9* gene, that are more likely responsible for the association with kidney disease.[183] Two groups have identified sequence variants in the *APOL1* gene that likely explain the genetic association of kidney disease in patients of African ancestry.[184,185] Reexamination of the interval surrounding MYH9 has led to these newer findings. Genovese and colleagues[184] and Tzur and associates[185] both used data from the 1000 Genomes Project—which conducts the sequencing of genomic DNA derived from subjects around the world, especially the Yoruba tribe of Western Africa—and identified sequence variants in the APOL1 gene that were associated with kidney disease. These variants were more strongly associated with ESKD than the previously reported MYH9 variants.

In African Americans, Genovese and colleagues[184] have found that FSGS and hypertension-attributed ESKD are associated with two independent sequence variants in the *APOL1* gene on chromosome 22 (FSGS, OR = 10.5; 95% CI = 6.0–18.4; hypertension-attributed ESKD, OR = 7.3, 95 CI = 5.6–9.5). The two *APOL1* variants were common in African chromosomes but absent from European chromosomes, and both reside within haplotypes that harbor signatures of positive selection. The *APOL1* gene product, apolipoprotein L-1, has been studied for its role in trypanosomal lysis, autophagic cell death, and lipid metabolism, as well as for its vascular effects.

APOL1 is a serum factor that lyses trypanosomes. Of interest, it was hypothesized that APOL1 variants protect patients against *Trypanosoma brucei*, the parasite that causes sleeping sickness in thousands of people in Africa. Conversely, and with great irony, these same sequences are associated with kidney disease; in vitro assays revealed that only the kidney disease-associated apolipoprotein L-1 variants lysed *T. brucei rhodesiense*, a particularly aggressive newer subspecies. Carrying two copies of the haplotype carried significantly more risk of kidney disease than carrying one copy. In some respects, therefore, kidney disease-associated APOL1 variants and protection from tsetse flies mirrors sickle cell anemia and protection from malaria.

Risk variants in MYH9 and APOL1 are in strong linkage dysequilibrium, and genetic risk that was previously attributed to MYH9 may reside in APOL1. More studies are required to test whether more complex models of risk are operative. Nonetheless, this genetic association on chromosome 22 explains, at least in part, racial disparities in nondiabetic ESKD and HIV-associated kidney disease because of the high prevalence of these haplotypes in individuals of African ancestry.[186] (For further discussion of inherited diseases of the glomerulus, see Chapter 43.)

In addition to being the site of genetic anomalies, the podocyte may be the target of injury through several mechanisms.[187] These mechanisms include infections (e.g., HIV infection), exposure to certain drugs (e.g., pamidronate, interferon), metabolic disorders (e.g., diabetes), and deposition of abnormal protein (e.g., amyloid). Podocyte injury can lead to proteinuria through abnormalities of the slit diaphragm (e.g., due to genetic mutations), podocyte loss, loss of negative charges from loss of podocyte proteins (decreased podocalyxin or glomerular epithelial protein), decreased production of these proteins (decreased heparin sulfates), or destruction of the GBM (e.g., proteases), malformation of GBM, or podocyte-related endothelial cell dysfunction (e.g., decrease in vascular endothelial growth factor).[187] In addition, the response of the podocyte to injury may be expressed differently, depending on the nature of the insult, and can result in different clinical syndromes. Thus, it has been proposed that various clinical and histologic variants of nephrotic syndromes depend on whether the podocyte injury results in apoptosis, podocyte loss, or podocyte dedifferentiation and reentry into the cell cycle and proliferation.[188] Indeed, this concept has led to proposals to change the classification of nephrotic syndromes based on the understanding of the pathogenetic mechanisms of disease, in addition to a description of histologic variants.[189]

In collapsing forms of FSGS, podocytes undergo changes in which mature podocyte markers disappear, which suggests a dysregulated podocyte phenotype in these diseases.[190–192] In fact, podocyte proliferation is seen in some examples of FSGS, which may be a consequence of the decrease in cyclin-dependent kinase inhibitors P27 and P57.[193] This has led to the concept that in collapsing FSGS, podocytes become dysregulated and proliferate.[194] However, the concept that the podocyte is a proliferating cell in collapsing FSGS has been challenged. In a mouse model of focal sclerosis, parietal epithelial and not podocytes were involved in the proliferative event.[195] This challenge is also supported from the findings of a study of two patients with HIV- and pamidronate-associated collapsing FSGS.[196]

The effacement of foot processes may be a consequence of the overproduction of oxygen radicals and accumulation of lipid peroxidase.[197] In theory, podocyte loss could result in focal areas of GBM denudation, with diminished barrier function. Podocyte dropout may be a major factor in the development of glomerulosclerosis in general and specifically in the development of collapsing FSGS.[198–201]

Some of the same pathogenic events that result in segmental scarring secondary to focal glomerular injury caused by a proliferative or necrotizing glomerulonephritis are probably operative in producing the sclerosis of FSGS. In this regard, the overproduction of transforming growth factor-β1 (TGF-β1) in glomeruli due to acute inflammatory lesions may cause glomerular sclerosis.[202] In experimental models of glomerular inflammation, the administration of antibodies to TGF-β or other inhibitors of TGF-β resulted in a decrease in matrix accumulation and a reduction in the severity of glomerular scarring.[203] Several mechanisms are associated with the fibrosis of kidney disease. Extracellular matrix and proteoglycans such as decorin and biglycan may have a pathogenic role in fibrosing diseases through the regulation of TGF-β1.[204]

FSGS also results from the loss of nephrons, which causes compensatory intraglomerular hypertension and enlargement in the remaining glomeruli. The compensatory capillary hypertension results in podocytes and endothelial cell injury, as well as mesangial alterations that lead to progressive focal and segmental sclerosis.[205–211] This process, at least in experimental animals, is made worse by increased dietary protein intake and is ameliorated by protein restriction and antihypertensive therapy.

A permeability factor has been described in some patients with FSGS. In a seminal study, 33 patients with FSGS that recurred after transplantation had a higher mean value for permeability to albumin value than normal subjects.[212] After plasmapheresis, the level of permeability factor in six patients was reduced, and proteinuria significantly decreased. The nature of the FSGS permeability factor continues to elude research efforts at identifying it. It has been hypothesized to consist of low-molecular-weight anionic proteins or proteins that alter the phosphorylation of glomerular proteins.[213] There is also a report of high affinity of the FSGS permeability factor to galactose, which appears to inhibit its activity in vitro.[214] Treatment with oral galactose has been anecdotally reported to afford remission of nephrotic syndrome.[215] Galactose treatment achieved a 50% reduction in proteinuria in three of seven patients in the FONT study,[216] but did not in another very small uncontrolled trial.[217] Another proposed permeability factor is circulating serum soluble urokinase receptor (suPAR), which has been reported to be elevated in two-thirds of patients with primary FSGS as compared to patients with other glomerular diseases.[218] Furthermore, suPAR was shown in the same study in mice to activate podocyte $\beta_3$ integrin, resulting in foot process effacement, proteinuria, and histopatholgic changes akin to human FSGS. Subsequently, serum suPAR levels were shown to be elevated in two cohorts of children and adults with FSGS and not disease controls[219]; however, some more recent studies have reported an inverse correlation between the estimated glomerular filtration rate (eGFR) and suPAR, suggesting possible confounding by the eGFR.[220–223]

Regarding the role of a circulating permeability factor in the pathogenesis of the disease, it should be noted that in a minority of patients with steroid-resistant FSGS in native kidneys, plasmapheresis may diminish proteinuria and stabilize kidney function. In most patients, however, there is no improvement in proteinuria, despite loss of the permeability factor following plasmapheresis.[224]

Glomerular enlargement accompanied by the development of FSGS occurs in the setting of hypoxemia—for example, in patients with sickle cell anemia, congenital pulmonary disease, or cyanotic congenital heart disease. Obesity predisposes to FSGS.[225,226] Weight loss and the administration of an angiotensin-converting enzyme (ACE) inhibitor decreased protein excretion by 80% to 85%.[227,228] Patients with sleep apnea may have proteinuria that is more functional in nature, but with little or no evidence of glomerular scarring or epithelial injury observed in biopsy specimens.[229,230] The association between sleep apnea and proteinuria was examined in an analysis of 148 patients referred for polysomnography who were not diabetic and had not been treated previously for obstructive sleep apnea.[231] In this patient population, clinically significant proteinuria was uncommon; it was found to be associated with older age, hypertension, coronary artery disease, and arousal index by univariate analysis, but only with age and hypertension by multiple regression analysis. Body mass index and the apnea-hypopnea index were not associated with the urine protein-to-creatinine ratio. The authors concluded that nephrotic-range proteinuria should not be ascribed to sleep apnea and deserves a more thorough nephrologic evaluation.

A number of infections cause FSGS. HIV-associated FSGS is pathologically identical to idiopathic collapsing FSGS, except that endothelial tubuloreticular inclusions are present in the former but not the latter. This close association of HIV infection with collapsing FSGS, as well as experimental evidence of focal glomerular sclerosis in mice transgenic for HIV type I genes,[146,150,232–238] raise the possibility that the HIV virus can be a causative agent of FSGS in infected patients. Whether other viral diseases, including parvovirus B19 infection, cause the idiopathic collapsing variant of FSGS remains to be elucidated.[239,240] Parvovirus B19 has been found with greater frequency in patients with idiopathic and collapsing FSGS than in patients with other diagnoses.[239] The polyomavirus SV40 may also play a role.[241]

FSGS is associated with a number of malignant conditions that have been linked to lymphoproliferative disease. In one study,[242] an association of FSGS was found with monoclonal gammopathies of undetermined significance (MGUS) and multiple myeloma. When the lymphoproliferative disease was treated, the renal lesion improved.

Finally, FSGS has been linked to exposure to a number of medications, including pamidronate[195,243] and interferon,[244] and with the use of anabolic steroids.[245] Like pamidronate and interferon therapy, the latter may also be associated with collapsing FSGS. Discontinuation of the anabolic steroids may lead to reduction of the proteinuria.

## CLINICAL FEATURES AND NATURAL HISTORY

Proteinuria is the hallmark feature of all forms of primary FSGS. The degree of proteinuria varies from nonnephrotic (1–2 g of protein/day) to over 10 g of protein/day, associated with all of the morbid features of nephrotic syndrome. Hematuria occurs in over 50% of FSGS patients, and approximately one-third of patients present with some degree of renal insufficiency. Gross hematuria is more commonly seen in FSGS than in MCD.[246] Hypertension is a presenting feature in one-third of patients. There are differences in the presentation of FSGS in adults and children.[247–250] Children tend to have more proteinuria, whereas hypertension is more common in adults.

Differences in clinical manifestations correlate with different pathologic phenotypes of FSGS.[251] Patients with perihilar FSGS accompanied by glomerular enlargement more commonly have nonnephrotic-range proteinuria than patients without glomerular hypertrophy. In addition, there are differences in the clinical presentation of the collapsing variant of FSGS and the glomerular tip lesion variant of FSGS.

Patients with collapsing FSGS have substantially more proteinuria, a lower serum albumin level, and a higher serum creatinine level than patients with perihilar FSGS.[152,153,252] The development of proteinuria, edema, or hypoalbuminemia may occur rapidly over the course of days to weeks, in contrast to the more indolent development of proteinuria in most patients with typical FSGS. Moreover, patients with collapsing FSGS more frequently have extrarenal manifestations of disease a few weeks prior to onset of the nephrosis, such as episodes of diarrhea, upper respiratory tract infections, or lower respiratory tract-like symptoms that are usually ascribed to viral or other infectious processes. However, the systemic symptoms of fever, malaise, and anorexia occur in fewer than 20% of patients at the time of onset of nephrosis. Pamidronate, a bisphosphonate that prevents bone disease in patients with myeloma and metastatic tumors, has been reported to be associated with collapsing FSGS.[195,243] After discontinuation of the drug, kidney function stabilized in all patients except those with collapsing FSGS. Treatment with interferon has also been reported to be associated with the development of collapsing FSGS.[244]

The clinical presentation of a glomerular tip lesion differs from that of both perihilar FSGS and collapsing FSGS.[215] Patients with glomerular tip lesion tend to be older Caucasian males, in contrast to the younger African-American male prevalence in collapsing FSGS. The proteinuria in these patients usually is severe, and the onset is abrupt, with the sudden development of edema and hypoalbuminemia. The rapidity of onset of the disease process is similar to the clinical presentation of MCD.[158,253,254] Patients with glomerular tip lesion may develop reversible AKI, especially at the time of initial presentation when the degree of proteinuria, edema, and hypoalbuminemia are at their peak. This also is similar to the presentation of MCD but rarely occurs with other variants of FSGS.

Several studies have addressed the clinical applicability and implications of distinguishing the variants of FSGS. An analysis of data for 197 patients followed in the Glomerular Disease Collaborative Network between 1982 and 2001 found the FSGS NOS variant in 42% of cases, the perihilar variant in 26%, the tip lesion in 17%, the collapsing lesion in 11%, and the cellular variant in 3% of patients.[143] African Americans accounted for 91% of patients with collapsing FSGS, but only 15% of patients with the tip lesion variant. Both collapsing and tip variants were associated with significantly greater amounts of proteinuria (10 ± 5.3 g protein/day and 9.7 ± 7.0 g protein/day, respectively) than perihilar or NOS variants of FSGS (4.4 ± 3.3 g protein/day and 5.5 ± 4.6 g protein/day, respectively; $P < .001$). In this retrospective uncontrolled analysis, patients with the tip lesion variant of FSGS were significantly more likely to attain a complete remission, even after adjustment for corticosteroid exposure ($P < .001$). Collapsing FSGS had the worst 1-year (74%) and 3-year renal survival rates of all other variants, regardless of differences in the histologic severity of the injury, which suggests the possibility that the nature of the injury was inherently different.

Similarly, an analysis of data for 225 patients studied at Columbia University[251] confirmed the predilection of the tip lesion variant of FSGS for Caucasians (86.2%), although the predominance of African Americans among patients with collapsing FSGS was less pronounced (53.6%). In this large cohort, 10% of patients had the cellular variant, of whom 32% were African American. The mean proteinuria (9.5 ± 1.2 g of protein/day) in these patients was comparable to that in patients with the collapsing or tip variants (8.8 ± 1.3 g of protein/day and 7.8 ± 0.6 g of protein/day, respectively). Patients with cellular FSGS showed intermediate rates of remission (44.5%) and ESKD (27.8%) compared with patients with collapsing FSGS (remission rate, 13.2%; ESKD rate, 65.3%) and tip FSGS (remission rate, 75.8%; ESKD rate, 5.7%).

A retrospective analysis of data for a cohort of 93 adult patients in the Netherlands has confirmed the improved renal survival of patients with the tip variant compared with patients with the other variants (5-year survival of 78% for tip vs. 63% for FSGS NOS and 55% for perihilar FSGS; $P = .02$).[255]

A major prospective FSGS study has evaluated the clinical impact of these histopathologic variants among participants with steroid-resistant primary FSGS in the FSGS Clinical Trial.[256,257] As in prior retrospective studies, the tip variant and collapsing variant had the strongest association with Caucasians (86%) and African Americans (63%, $P = .003$), respectively. This study also confirmed poor renal survival in participants with the collapsing variant and better renal survival in participants with the tip variant, although the sample size was small for these groups.

The degree of proteinuria is a predictor of long-term clinical outcome. Nonnephrotic-range proteinuria correlates with a more favorable renal survival of over 80% after 10 years of follow-up.[258,259] In contrast, patients who have proteinuria of more than 10 g of protein/day have very poor long-term renal survival, with most patients experiencing ESKD within 3 years.[260,261] Patients with FSGS and protein excretion that measures between nonnephrotic range and massive proteinuria have variable long-term renal outcomes. In general, these patients have a relatively poor outcome, with half experiencing ESKD by 10 years.[249,250,262]

One of the most useful prognostic indicators for patients with FSGS is whether remission of nephrotic syndrome is achieved.[248] Patients who experience remission of nephrosis have a substantially greater renal survival rate than those who do not.[248,258,259,263,264] According to Korbet and colleagues,[249,250] fewer than 15% of patients who achieve complete or partial remission progress to ESKD within 5 years of follow-up. Up to 50% of patients who do not experience remission progress to end-stage disease within 6 years of follow-up.

As in other forms of glomerular injury, the entry serum creatinine level correlates with long-term renal survival.[258,260,265,266] Patients with a serum creatinine level over 1.3 mg/dL have poorer renal survival than those with lower serum creatinine concentrations, irrespective of the level of proteinuria (10-year renal survival of 27% vs. 100%).[250] Multivariate analyses have indicated that the entry serum creatinine level may be more important than proteinuria as a predictor of progression to ESKD.*

## LABORATORY FINDINGS

Hypoproteinemia is common in patients with FSGS, with total serum protein reduced to varying extents. The serum albumin concentration may fall to below 2 g/dL, especially in patients with collapsing and glomerular tip variants of FSGS. As in other forms of nephrotic syndrome, levels of immunoglobulins are typically depressed, and levels of lipids are increased, especially the serum cholesterol level. Serum levels of complement components are generally in the normal range in FSGS. Circulating immune complexes have been detected in patients with FSGS,[267,268] although their pathogenic significance has not been determined. Serologic testing for HIV infection should be obtained for patients with FSGS, especially those with the collapsing pattern.

## TREATMENT

### Angiotensin Inhibitors

ACE inhibitors and angiotensin II receptor blockers (ARBs) have been evaluated in the treatment of FSGS. ACE inhibitors have been shown to decrease proteinuria and the rate of progression to ESKD in diabetic and nondiabetic kidney disease.[269–272] These results have been observed in the presence of diabetes, as well as in cases of nondiabetic kidney disease. A systematic review of studies has revealed that ACE inhibitors significantly reduce proteinuria in children with steroid-resistant nephrotic syndrome.[273] In a randomized controlled trial involving normotensive children with steroid-resistant nephrotic syndrome, the addition of fosinopril to prednisone resulted in a greater reduction in proteinuria than prednisone alone.[274]

In patients with glomerulomegaly and nonnephrotic-range proteinuria, an ACE inhibitor or ARB sufficiently decreases proteinuria and potentially decreases hyperlipidemia, edema, and other manifestations of persistent loss of protein in the urine, with an excellent long-term prognosis. Regardless of what other forms of antiinflammatory or immunosuppressive therapy are used, the beneficial effects of these agents indicates that they should be added, despite the well-known side effects of hyperkalemia and reduction in GFR, especially in patients with serum creatinine levels over 3 mg/dL.

Before immunomodulatory or immunosuppressive therapy is initiated in a patient with FSGS, a careful evaluation should be undertaken to exclude the possibility of an underlying cause, as described in the section on pathogenesis. Patients with secondary FSGS are unlikely to benefit from immunosuppressive therapy and may be at particularly high risk of complications. In addition, an assessment of the risks and benefits of immunosuppressive therapy should be undertaken for each patient. Patients with subnephrotic-range proteinuria have a generally good prognosis, and the initial therapy should be focused on blood pressure control, preferentially using maximal tolerated dosages of renin-angiotensin-aldosterone system (RAAS) blockers. Glucocorticoids or immunosuppressive therapy should be targeted to patients with idiopathic FSGS and nephrotic syndrome.

### Glucocorticoids

No randomized placebo-controlled trial has been conducted to assess the role of glucocorticoids in the treatment of FSGS formally. The available data are based on case series using different treatment protocols, different definitions of remission, response, relapse, and resistance and different lengths of therapy.[248,258,263,275] One review of studies has suggested that only 15% of patients with FSGS responded to treatment, in sharp contrast to those with MCD.[276] More optimistic reports have been obtained by groups in Toronto and Chicago,[248,249] which suggest that 30% to 40% of adult patients may attain some form of remission with corticosteroid treatment. A compilation of these studies by Korbet[250] has suggested that of 177 patients who received a variety of different forms of therapy, 45% experienced complete remission, 10% experienced partial remission, and 45% showed no response.[248,258,263,275,277]

In children, the initial treatment of FSGS is similar to that of MCD because treatment is typically initiated without histologic confirmation of the disease process. Thus, the International Study of Kidney Diseases in Children has recommended using an initial course of prednisone of 60 mg/day/m$^2$, up to 80 mg/day, for 4 weeks. This is followed with 40 mg/day/m$^2$, up to 60 mg/day, administered in divided doses for 3 consecutive days out of 7, for 4 weeks, and then tapered off for 4 more weeks. As in adult patients with MCD, a longer course of therapy at higher doses of prednisone may be necessary to induce remission. Thus, in those series and in retrospective analyses that showed an increased remission rate,† prednisone treatment was continued for 16 weeks to achieve remission. In adult patients, the median time for complete remission was 3 to 4 months.[136]

A portion of patients showing a positive response to corticosteroid treatment will experience relapse. Guidelines for the retreatment of relapsing patients are similar to those for treatment of patients with relapsing MCD. In patients whose remission prior to relapse was prolonged (>6 months), a repeat course of corticosteroid therapy may again induce a remission. In steroid-dependent patients who develop frequent relapses, repeated rounds of high-dose corticosteroid therapy result in unacceptable cumulative toxicity. Thus, alternative strategies, such as the addition of cyclosporine, may be useful. In patients with the glomerular tip lesion variant of FSGS, a trial of corticosteroids is appropriate because many patients experience a decline in protein excretion.[157,254,280]

Attempts at alternate-day steroid therapy have not been successful, except in older populations. The Toronto group[281]

*References 258, 259, 261, 262, 265, and 266.

†References 133, 248, 258, 263, 275, 278, and 279.

has demonstrated that a 40% remission rate could be achieved in patients older than 60 years by administering up to 100 mg of prednisone on alternate days for 3 to 5 months. This therapy was well tolerated in this population, with no obvious side effects during the study period. Alternate-day prednisone most likely works in this population because of an increased susceptibility to the immunosuppressive effects of corticosteroids and altered glucocorticoid kinetics in older adults.

The benefit of corticosteroid therapy may differ among Caucasians and African Americans. In a retrospective analysis[282] of renal survival in predominantly African American individuals with FSGS, renal survival was found to be higher when the initial serum creatinine level was lower and blood pressure was well controlled, but treatment with steroids had no effect on renal survival.

The practice of using higher dosages of corticosteroids to induce remission with the attendant risk of toxicity has resulted in the use of alternative therapeutic approaches. Administration of very high doses of corticosteroids in children, and the continuation of daily prednisone therapy for up to 6 to 9 months in adults, is not without enormous short- and long-term side effects. In studies in which long-term, high-dose corticosteroids are administered, few analyses have been undertaken to evaluate the development of osteoporosis, short- and long-term risk of infection, cataracts, diabetes, or other long-term sequelae. Thus, the available data do not allow for a careful understanding of the risk-benefit ratio. Until the use of high-dose methylprednisolone has been studied in controlled clinical trials, this potentially useful yet dangerous approach must be viewed with caution.

### Cyclophosphamide

Several studies have failed to document the effectiveness of cytotoxic drugs in the treatment of FSGS.[263,283] In one review, only 23% of 247 children with FSGS showed a response to steroid therapy, and 70 patients were treated with cytotoxic drugs. Of these, 30% showed a response. In the final analysis, the disease was in remission in fewer than 20% of the 247 children. The use of cytotoxic drugs has been evaluated in only one series of adults.[263] Although their use correlated with longer remissions and fewer relapses, no other study has corroborated these results.

The International Study of Kidney Diseases in Children carefully examined the role of cyclophosphamide in the treatment of children with FSGS.[284] Daily oral cyclophosphamide (2.5 mg/kg) was administered in addition to prednisone (40 mg/m$^2$ every other day) for 12 months, and results were compared with those for prednisone alone. The addition of cyclophosphamide had no effect on the change in proteinuria or the likelihood of achieving complete resolution of proteinuria.[284] Similarly, in a nonrandomized comparative study involving children with FSGS or steroid-resistant or frequently relapsing nephrotic syndrome, the addition of oral cyclophosphamide to prednisone for 3 months had no statistically significant effect on the rate of complete or partial remission or progression to ESKD.[285] In summary, the limited, currently available data do not support the use of cyclophosphamide in patients with FSGS.

### Cyclosporine

FSGS that is resistant to prednisone may be induced into remission by cyclosporine. The effectiveness of cyclosporine in inducing remission of proteinuria in patients with FSGS has been demonstrated in two randomized controlled trials. In the study by Ponticelli and colleagues, 45 patients with steroid-resistant nephrotic syndrome were randomly assigned to receive supportive therapy or cyclosporine (5 mg/kg/day for adults, 6 mg/kg/day for children) for 6 months, with the drug then tapered off by 25% every 2 months.[133] Remission occurred in 13 of 22 patients receiving cyclosporine, compared with 3 of 19 patients in the control group ($P < .001$). Unfortunately, relapses occurred in 69% of patients after the withdrawal of cyclosporine.

In the North America Nephrotic Syndrome Study Group trial, 49 patients were randomly assigned to treatment with low-dose prednisone alone or in combination with oral cyclosporine for 26 weeks.[286] At the end of 26 weeks of therapy, partial or complete remission of proteinuria occurred in 70% of patients in the cyclosporine-treated group compared with only 4% in the control group ($P < .001$); however, relapses occurred by 52 weeks in 40% of those experiencing remission. Treatment with cyclosporine was also associated with a 70% reduction in the risk that the GFR would decline by 50%.[286]

A randomized controlled trial compared the efficacy of cyclosporine with intravenous cyclophosphamide in the initial treatment of 22 children with steroid-resistant nephrotic syndrome related to MCD, FSGS, or mesangial hypercellularity.[287] All patients also received alternate-day prednisone therapy. Treatment with cyclosporine afforded a statistically significant higher rate of partial remission of proteinuria at 12 weeks (60% of cyclosporine-treated patients vs. 17% in the cyclophosphamide group; $P < .05$). By study's end, 12 of the 14 patients who showed no response to cyclophosphamide were patients with FSGS. Of note, all 6 patients who were heterozygous for the *NPHS2* R229Q variant or the *R6QH* mutation were assigned to the cyclophosphamide group, and only one of those showed a response to treatment. These results support the use of cyclosporine over cyclophosphamide in children with steroid-resistant nephrotic syndrome.

Results from the FSGS Clinical Trial, the largest multicenter, randomized controlled trial of its kind, compared a 12-month course of cyclosporine with a combination of oral pulse dexamethasone and MMF in 138 randomized children and young adults with biopsy-proven, steroid-resistant primary FSGS.[256] The trial was designed to determine whether treatment with MMF plus pulse steroids was superior to treatment with cyclosporine in inducing remission of proteinuria over 12 months. Partial or complete remission by the 12-month mark was achieved in only 22 MMF-treated patients and 33 cyclosporine-treated patients, with an OR of 0.59 (95% CI, 0.30–1.18) for achieving remission or better with MMF compared with cyclosporine, which was not significant. Furthermore, remission by 26 weeks after treatment cessation was not significantly different between the two groups. The investigators concluded that the lack of signal difference may have been due to insufficient sample size, and that the low rates of remission in the trial amplify the profound need for better and more targeted therapies.

Laurin and colleagues recently performed a retrospective analysis of 458 patients (173 treated with glucocorticoids alone, 90 treated with calcineurin inhibitors, with or without glucocorticoids, 12 treated with other agents, and 183 not treated with immunosuppressives) with native kidney, biopsy-proven primary FSGS diagnosed between 1980 and 2012 in the Glomerular Disease Collaborative Network.[289] Immunosuppressive therapy with glucocorticoids or calcineurin inhibitors was associated with better renal survival than no immunosuppression (hazard ratio [HR], 0.49; 95% CI, 0.28–0.86); however, calcineurin inhibitor use, with or without glucocorticoids, was not associated with a lower likelihood of ESKD compared with glucocorticoids alone (HR, 0.42; 95% CI, 0.15–1.18), thereby at least suggesting a role for immunosuppression in primary FSGS.[289] Interestingly, this same group, using a similar cohort, found that patients with collapsing or NOS FSGS had similar renal survival after controlling for exposure to immunosuppressive treatment.[288]

How long should patients be treated with cyclosporine? In a study by Meyrier and colleagues,[136] when patients remained in remission for over 12 months, cyclosporine was slowly tapered and eventually removed, without subsequent relapse. Unfortunately, long-term treatment with cyclosporine was associated with increases in tubular atrophy and interstitial fibrosis, the degree of which was positively correlated with the initial serum creatinine level, the number of segmental scars on initial biopsy specimens, and a cyclosporine dose of more than 5.5 mg/kg/day. Thus there is a clear trade-off with the use of cyclosporine over the long term, given the risk of development of interstitial fibrosis and tubular atrophy.

### Mycophenolate Mofetil

Data regarding the use of MMF in the treatment of FSGS has been largely anecdotal, with one small case series reporting transient improvement in proteinuria in 8 of 18 patients. However, two clinical trials have taken place within the past decade.

A randomized controlled trial compared the efficacy of an MMF-based regimen to treatment with corticosteroids, with or without cyclophosphamide,in adult patients with idiopathic MN ($n = 21$) or FSGS ($n = 33$).[290] MMF was given at a dosage of 2 g/day for 6 months along with prednisolone, 0.5 mg/kg/day, for 2 to 3 months. Patients with FSGS in the comparison group received prednisolone, 1 mg/kg/day, for 3 to 6 months. There was no difference between the two groups with respect to the proportion of complete or partial remissions (70% vs. 69%) or the time to remission of proteinuria at any point. Remission was achieved faster in the MMF-treated FSGS patients than in the corticosteroid-only group (5.6 vs. 10.2 months, respectively), and cumulative steroid dose was lower (1.9 ± 0.3 vs. 7.3 ± 0.9 g, respectively). Although limited to a small number of patients and relatively short follow-up, this first controlled study has suggested that the addition MMF is steroid-sparing and achieves rates of remission comparable to those for corticosteroids alone in patients with FSGS. The randomized controlled FSGS Clinical Trial, discussed in the cyclosporine section, showed no significant difference in outcomes when comparing cyclosporine with oral pulse dexamethasone and MMF.[256]

### Other Therapies

The use of sirolimus in the management of FSGS is poorly supported. Several reports have emerged of new-onset proteinuria in kidney transplant recipients who were switched from calcineurin inhibitor-based therapy to sirolimus.[291–295]

In a study of 78 solid organ transplant recipients treated with sirolimus, 18 patients (23.1%) developed proteinuria in an average of 11.2 ± 2.1 months after starting sirolimus therapy.[296] Kidney biopsy specimens obtained after the onset of proteinuria revealed various degrees of mesangial proliferation and mesangial expansion commonly seen in patients who previously had a diagnosis of chronic allograft nephropathy but showed FSGS in only 2 patients (14.3%). There was no correlation between proteinuria levels and sirolimus dose or trough blood levels. In the 6 patients in whom sirolimus was withdrawn, a complete reversal of proteinuria and edema was observed. This study certainly raises significant concern about the induction of proteinuria by sirolimus in transplant recipients.

The data pertaining to the use of sirolimus in the management of FSGS in native kidneys is rather conflicting. In a prospective open-label trial of sirolimus of 21 patients with steroid-resistant FSGS, at 6 months, 4 patients (19%) had achieved a complete remission, 8 (38%) had experienced a partial remission, and 1 patient had experienced a rapid decline in kidney function.[297] Sirolimus therapy was associated with a substantial number of adverse events, including hyperlipidemia and anemia in 43% of patients. In patients who showed no response to sirolimus, the mean serum creatinine level increased from 1.66 mg/dL at baseline to 2.2 mg/dL at 6 months and 3.24 mg/dL at 12 months (significantly different from baseline at the $P = .028$ level). In patients who did show a response to sirolimus, the mean serum creatinine level increased from 1.76 mg/dL at baseline to 1.91 mg/dL at 12 months.

In contrast, a phase II open-label clinical trial of sirolimus had to be interrupted for safety reasons after five of six patients enrolled experienced a sharp decrease in GFR, and none achieved a complete remission.[298] Three patients had a more than twofold increase in proteinuria during sirolimus therapy. Similar deleterious effects were reported in a cohort of 11 patients with a variety of glomerular diseases.[299] Although inconclusive, the bulk of the data currently available suggest that sirolimus has a deleterious effect in FSGS and should be avoided.

Future approaches to the treatment of FSGS may come from the treatment of recurrent FSGS following transplantation. One study has reported the use of CTLA-4-Ig (abatacept), an inhibitor of the T cell costimulatory molecule B7-1 (CD80), in four patients with recurrent FSGS and one with primary FSGS, given that podocytes also express B7-1 in some individuals with proteinuric kidney disease, including FSGS.[300] Surprisingly, nephrotic-range proteinuria resolved in all patients; however, much larger, more controlled studies are needed to validate this encouraging result.

Intriguing cases of recurrent FSGS after transplantation have been published, in which the proteinuria resolved after treatment with rituximab.[301] Interestingly, in one case,[302] the diagnosis of posttransplant lymphoproliferative disease (PTLD) was established 5 months after the transplantation, although recurrent nephrotic syndrome occurred within 2 weeks postoperatively. Proteinuria improved only after treatment of PTLD with rituximab. The authors suggested, however, that FSGS was probably unrelated to the viral infection due to the time gap between the two diagnoses. In addition, there have been a few reports of recurrent FSGS after transplantation that responded to rituximab (after plasmapheresis or immunoadsorption) that are not related to PTLD.[303–306] These patients may represent a specific category, and the lessons learned from their treatment may not necessarily apply to the general population of patients with FSGS.

Anecdotal reports have been emerging of treatment of primary and recurrent FSGS with rituximab, usually in combination with other immunomodulating therapies, but results have shown a mixed response to this treatment,[307,308] with several reports of failures.[309] In the largest case series, 5 of 8 adult patients with resistant FSGS failed to show a response to a course of rituximab, and 2 patients suffered a rapid deterioration of kidney function.[310] Only 2 patients had a clear and sustained improvement of kidney function and proteinuria. More recently, as discussed in the section on MCD, a small prospective trial in Italy of rituximab in 10 children and 20 adults with relapsing FSGS, MCD, and mesangial proliferative glomerulonephritis, (GN) showed significant benefit, which warrants further investigation with larger randomized clinical trials.[137] Interestingly, it has also been shown in the setting of recurrent FSGS that rituximab can bind to podocyte-derived sphingomyelin phosphodiesterase acid-like 3b (SMPDL-3b) to preserve its expression as a regulator of acid sphingomyelinase activity to prevent disruption of the actin cytoskeleton and apoptosis.[311] It is becoming clear that the use of rituximab for the treatment of FSGS requires further evaluation in the setting of a randomized controlled trial.

Another potential future approach targets renal fibrosis, which represents a common final pathway of FSGS and other chronic kidney diseases.[312] The orally available antifibrotic agent, pirfenidone, was evaluated in an open-label pilot study to determine its effect on the rate of decline in GFR in 18 patients with FSGS selected for having a monthly rate of decline in estimated GFR of more than 0.35 mL/min/1.73 $m^2$.[313] The monthly change in GFR improved from a median of -0.61 mL/min/1.73 $m^2$ during the baseline period to -0.45 mL/min/1.73 $m^2$ with pirfenidone therapy; which represented a median of 25% improvement in the rate of decline ($P < .01$). Pirfenidone had no effect on blood pressure or proteinuria and was associated with frequent dyspepsia, sedation, and photosensitive dermatitis. These enticing results provide a strong rationale for a larger placebo-controlled trial in patients with progressive chronic kidney disease.

Other forms of treatment have been used. Plasmapheresis and protein absorption strategies to remove circulating factors responsible for FSGS have led to the remission of recurrent FSGS, but do not appear to be beneficial in treating the primary disease.[224,314]

In summary, patients with primary FSGS remain frustrating patients to treat. Clearly, FSGS is a histopathologic lesion rather than a unifying disease entity, suggesting that different subtypes of FSGS require different treatment strategies. Additional investigations into the pathogenesis of this disease entity, as well as podocyte dysfunction, are warranted to identify targets that may find success in clinical trial settings.[315] Enthusiasm for the use of high-dose, prolonged corticosteroid therapy in adults and children has prompted the use of this therapy in many FSGS patients. Only a prospective randomized trial that carefully evaluates this approach will determine its effectiveness. The first step in therapy should be geared toward excellent blood pressure control using RAAS blockers. In patients who have nephrotic-range proteinuria, careful supportive care and consideration of a trial of oral corticosteroids in adult patients may be an acceptable approach after patients are carefully informed about the risks and potential benefits of 12 to 16 weeks of daily corticosteroid therapy. Alternatively, a trial of cyclosporine may be warranted for patients who have contraindications to corticosteroid therapy or in whom corticosteroid therapy fails to produce improvement.

## C1q NEPHROPATHY

Complement component 1q (C1q) nephropathy is a relatively rare cause of proteinuria and nephrotic syndrome. Unfortunately, there has been a relative dearth of new insights into C1q nephropathy compared with other primary glomerular diseases. Since the last edition of this chapter, clinical information has remained relegated to case reports and small case series. C1q nephropathy can mimic MCD or FSGS clinically and histologically, although the clinical and pathologic presentations are quite variable.[316,317] In a single-center retrospective analysis of kidney biopsy specimens from children and adolescents, C1q nephropathy was found in 6.6% of native kidney biopsy specimens.[318] In the largest case series, at the University of Ljubljana, Slovenia, which included both children and adults, C1q nephropathy was identified in 1.9% of native kidney biopsy specimens.[319] There appears to be a slight male predominance (56%–68%).[319,320] Depending on the case series, there may be an association with African American or Hispanic ethnicity.[320] Patients of all ages with C1q nephropathy have been described.

The diagnosis is based on the presence of mesangial immune complex deposits that show conspicuous staining for C1q in a patient with no clinical or laboratory evidence of SLE. The C1q staining usually is accompanied by staining for IgG, IgM, and C3. Electron microscopy demonstrates well-defined mesangial immune complex–type dense deposits. Light microscopic findings vary from no lesion (mimicking MCD), to focal glomerular hypercellularity, to proliferative glomerulonephritis with mesangial hypercellularity, and to focal segmental sclerosing lesions that may be indistinguishable histologically from those of FSGS. Anecdotal cases reports have described C1q nephropathy associated with a collapsing FSGS lesion.[321,322] The findings by immunofluorescence microscopy and electron microscopy, however, readily differentiate C1q nephropathy from MCD and FSGS. The findings by IF and electron microscopy suggest an immune complex pathogenesis, but the details of the pathogenic mechanism and the cause are unknown.

Patients with C1q nephropathy generally have proteinuria, which may or may not be associated with nephrotic syndrome. Hematuria is present in at least 50% of patients and is more common among patients with a mesangial proliferative lesion on light microscopy.[319] Likewise, hypertension affects a minority of patients with no discernible lesions on light microscopy (similar to MCD), but is much more prevalent among patients with mesangial proliferation (55%).[319] Interestingly, many patients are relatively asymptomatic, and proteinuria may first be detected at the time of a physical examination in connection with sports participation or entry into the armed forces. These patients, by definition, have no clinical or serologic evidence of SLE, despite the presence of C1q in the kidney biopsy specimen. C1q nephropathy may show spontaneous improvement.[323]

The renal outcome of patients with C1q nephropathy appears to be generally favorable,[318] especially in patients whose biopsy specimens show minimal change–like histologic features.[319,324] Studies have suggested, however, that they may experience more frequent relapses and require additional immunosuppressants more often than patients with "pure" MCD.[318,319,324] Patients whose biopsy specimens show FSGS-like or mesangial proliferative lesions on histologic analysis may show a less favorable response to immunosuppressive therapy, although the data are rather limited.

Interestingly, given the potential for C1q nephropathy to be a distinct autoimmune condition, a recent notable scientific advance in lupus nephritis is that the autoantigenicity of C1q itself may be associated with a conformational change in its globular head. This increased its hydrophobicity akin to a conformeropathy, as is seen in anti-GBM; that is, the self-antigen becomes an autoantigen through a de novo conformational change.[325]

## MEMBRANOUS NEPHROPATHY

### EPIDEMIOLOGY

Membranous glomerulopathy or nephropathy (MN) is one of the most common causes of nephrotic syndrome in adults.[326–329] MN occurs as primary form of glomerular disease usually caused by autoantibodies specific for M-type phospholipase A2 receptor (PLA2R) or secondary to multiple nonrenal diseases, including autoimmune diseases (e.g., SLE, autoimmune thyroiditis), infection (e.g., hepatitis B, hepatitis C, malaria), drugs (e.g., penicillamine, gold), and malignancies (e.g., colon or lung cancer). Secondary MN, especially that caused by hepatitis B[330–334] and lupus, is more frequent in children than in adults. In patients older than 60 years, MN is associated with a malignancy in 20% to 30% of patients.

MN is the cause of nephrotic syndrome in approximately 25% of adults with the syndrome.[326,335–343] A study of patients who had urinary excretion of more than 1 g of protein/24 hours, conducted by the Medical Research Council in the United Kingdom from 1978 to 1990, determined that 20% had MN. The peak incidence of MN is in the 4th to 5th decades of life.[326,344,345] no[346–348] A pooled analysis of studies of patients with idiopathic MN found a 2:1 predominance of males (1190 males and 598 females).[349] The adult-to-child ratio was 26:1 (1734 adults and 67 children); however, this low proportion of children among MN patients was biased by the exclusion of children from some of the studies included in the analysis. MN affects all races.

Although most patients with MN present with nephrotic syndrome, 10% to 20% of patients have proteinuria that remains at less than 2 g of protein /day.[350] It is thus likely that the frequency of MN in the general population is underestimated because asymptomatic individuals with subclinical proteinuria often do not come to diagnosis or undergo kidney biopsy.

There are geographic variations in the clinical manifestations of MN. In studies in Australia and Japan, lower percentages of patients have nephrotic syndrome at entry than in Europe or North America. The geographic differences may be related to differences in the prevalence of underlying causes of secondary MN, such as hepatitis B, malaria, and other infections.[330,332]

The association of MN with underlying malignancy is well-recognized. In a large cohort study of 240 patients in France,[351] the incidence of cancer was significantly higher in patients with MN than in the general population (standardized incidence ratio = 9.8 [5.5–16.2] for men and 12.3 [4.5–26.9] for women). In almost half the patients, the tumor was asymptomatic and was detected only because of diagnostic procedures prompted by the diagnosis of MN. The most common malignancies were cancers of the lung and prostate. The frequency of malignancy increased with age. In a separate cohort study in Norway,[352] the incidence of cancer in 161 patients with MN was significantly higher compared with the age- and gender-adjusted general Norwegian population, corresponding to a standardized incidence ratio of 2.25 (95% CI = 1.44–3.35). The median time from diagnosis of MN to diagnosis of cancer was 60 months. Patients with MN who developed cancer were older (65 vs. 52 years; $P < .001$).[352]

Risk factors for malignancy in patients with MN include older age and a history of smoking, although the clinical presentation does not differ between patients with cancer-associated MN and those with primary MN.[351] In patients with cancer-associated MN, clinical remission of the cancer is associated with a reduction of proteinuria.[351] These studies highlight the importance of thorough cancer screening among older patients with MN, not only at the time of first diagnosis, but also during subsequent long-term follow-up.

*Clinical Relevance*

**Cancer Screening in Memebanous Nephropathy**

It is important to conduct thorough cancer screening among older patients with membranous nephropathy, not only at the time of first diagnosis, but also during subsequent long-term follow-up.

### PATHOLOGY

#### Electron Microscopy

The pathologic sine qua non of MN is the presence of subepithelial immune complex deposits or their structural consequences.[353] Electron microscopy provides the most definitive diagnosis of MN, although a relatively confident diagnosis can be made based on typical light microscopic and IF microscopic findings.

Fig. 31.7 depicts the four ultrastructural stages of MN, as described by Ehrenreich and Churg.[344] The earliest ultrastructural manifestation, stage I, is characterized by the presence of scattered or more regularly distributed small immune complex–type, electron-dense deposits in the subepithelial zone between the basement membrane and the podocyte. Podocyte process effacement and microvillous transformation occur in all stages of MN when there is substantial proteinuria. Stage II is characterized by projections of basement membrane material around the subepithelial deposits. In three dimensions, these projections surround the sides of the deposits, but when observed in cross section, they appear as spikes extending between the deposits (Fig. 31.8; see Fig. 31.7). In stage III, the new basement membrane material surrounds the deposits, and thus in cross section there is basement membrane material between the deposits and

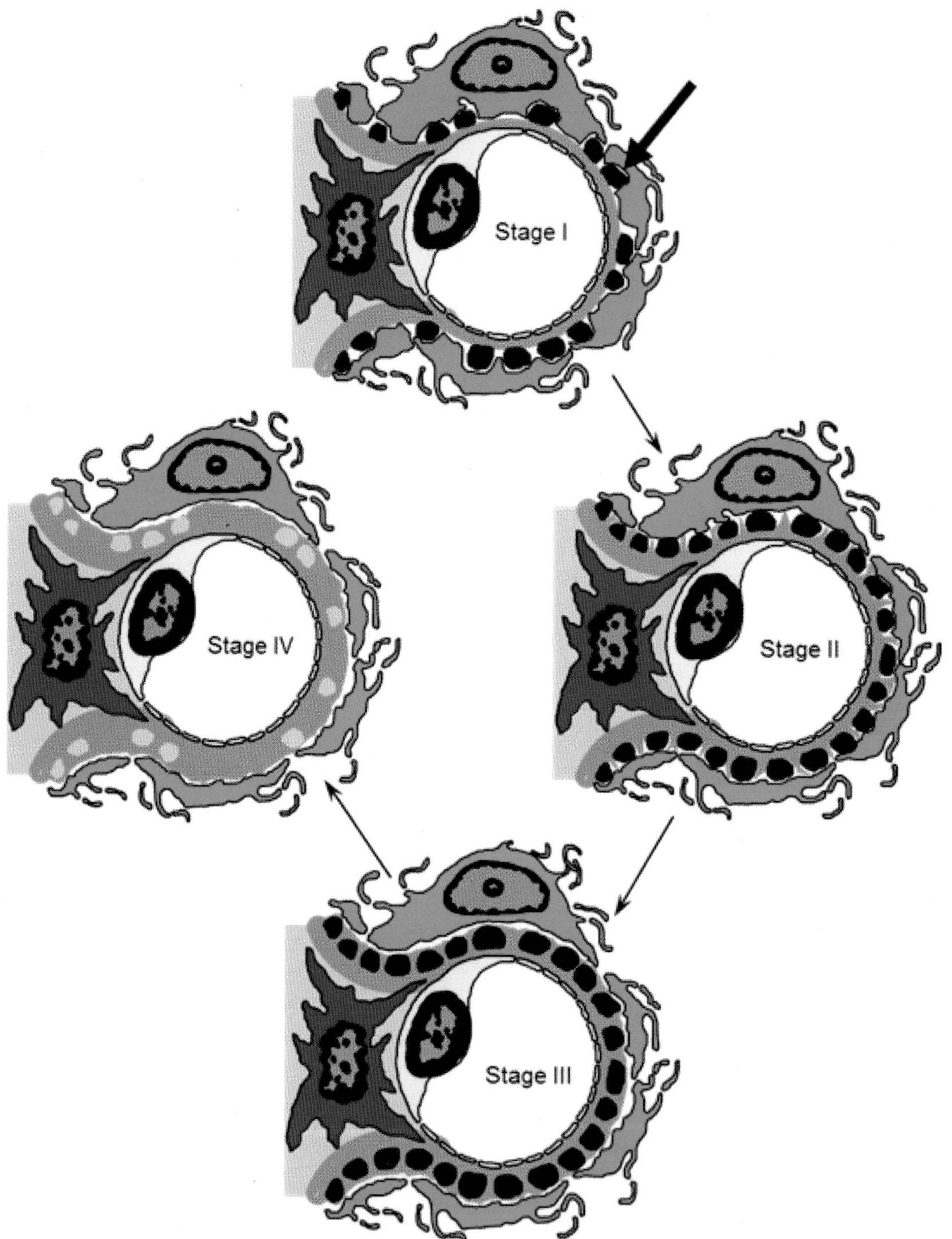


**Fig. 31.7** Diagram depicting the four ultrastructural stages of membranous nephropathy. Stage I has subepithelial dense deposits *(arrow)* without adjacent basement membrane reaction. Stage II has projections of basement membrane adjacent to deposits. Stage III has deposits surrounded by basement membrane. Stage IV has thickened basement membrane with irregular lucent zones. (Courtesy J.C. Jennette.)

the epithelial cytoplasm. At this point, the deposits are, in essence, intramembranous rather than subepithelial; however, the ultrastructural appearance allows the inference that they once were subepithelial and thus indicative of MN. Stage IV is characterized by loss of the electron density of the deposits, which often results in irregular electron-lucent zones within an irregularly thickened basement membrane. Although not described by Ehrenreich and Churg, some nephropathologists recognize stage V, which is characterized by a repaired outer basement membrane zone with the only residual basement membrane disturbance in the inner aspect of the basement membrane. At the time of kidney biopsy, most patients in the US have stage I or II disease (Table 31.5).

Mesangial dense deposits are rare in primary MN but are more frequent in secondary MN (see Table 31.5). This suggests, but does not prove, that primary MN is caused by subepithelial in situ immune complex formation with antibodies from the circulation complexing with antigens derived from the podocyte. Immune complexes formed only at this site could not go against the direction of filtration to reach

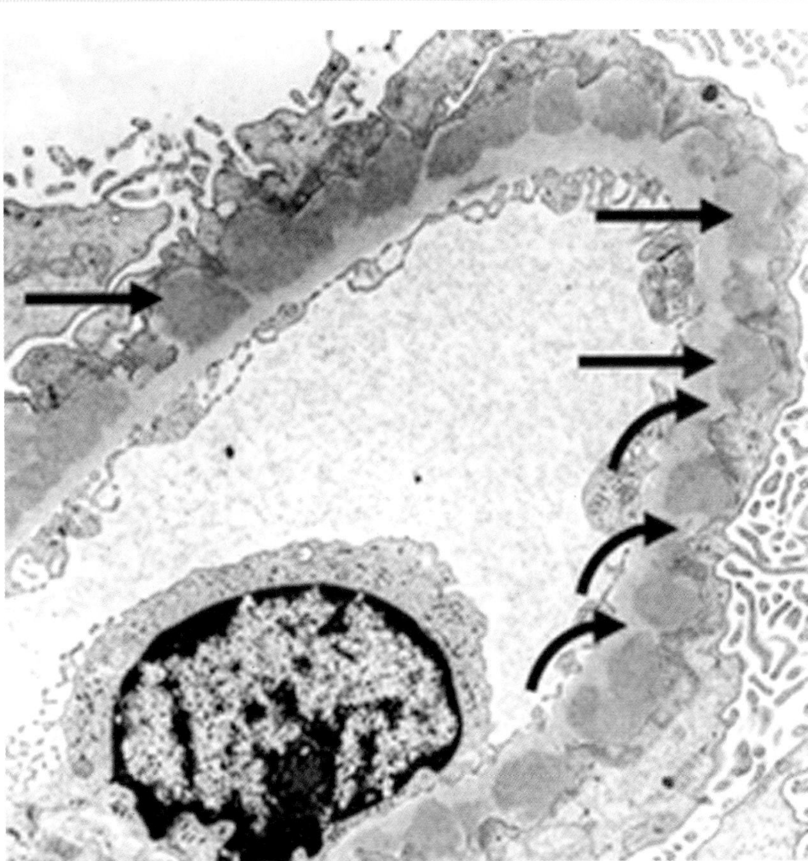

**Fig. 31.8** Electron micrograph showing features of stage II membranous nephropathy with numerous subepithelial dense deposits *(straight arrows)* and adjacent projections of basement membrane material *(curved arrows).* (×100.)

**Table 31.5 Pathologic Features of Nonlupus Membranous Nephropathy[a]**

| Procedure | Feature Present (%) |
|---|---|
| **Immunofluorescence Microscopy** | |
| IgG | 99 (3.5+)[b] |
| IgM | 95 (1.2+) |
| IgA | 84 (1.1+) |
| C3 | 97 (1.6+) |
| C1q | 34 (1.1+) |
| Kappa | 98 (3.1+) |
| Lambda | 98 (2.8+) |
| **Electron Microscopy** | |
| Subepithelial electron dense deposits | 99 |
| Mesangial electron dense deposits | 16 |
| Subendothelial electron dense deposits | 7 |
| Endothelial tubuloreticular inclusions | 3 |
| Stage I | 38 |
| Stage II | 32 |
| Stage III | 6 |
| Stage IV | 5 |
| Stage V | 1 |
| Mixed Stage | 20 |

[a]Based on an analysis of 350 consecutive kidney biopsy specimens from patients with non-lupus membranous nephropathy evaluated at the University of North Carolina Nephropathology Laboratory.
[b]Values in parentheses indicate mean intensity of positive staining on a scale of 0 to 4+.
*Ig,* Immunoglobulin.

the mesangium. Secondary forms of MN usually are caused by immune complexes containing antigens that are in the circulation, such as antigens derived from infections (e.g., hepatitis B), tumor antigens (e.g., colon cancer), or autoantigens (e.g., thyroglobulin). With both the antigens and antibodies in the systemic circulation, it is likely that some immune complexes would form, which localize not only in the subepithelial zone but also in the mesangium or subendothelial zone. This is demonstrated in the secondary form of MN that occurs in patients with SLE. In over 90% of lupus MN specimens, mesangial dense deposits are identified by electron microscopy.[354] Therefore, the presence of mesangial dense deposits should raise the index of suspicion for secondary rather than primary MN.

### Immunofluorescence Microscopy

The characteristic IF microscopy finding in MN is diffuse global granular capillary wall staining for immunoglobulin and complement that often also has capillary wall staining for PLA2R in idiopathic disease (Fig. 31.9).[353] IgG is the most frequent and usually the most intensely staining immunoglobulin, although less pronounced staining for IgA and IgM is common (see Table 31.5). IgG4 is the most prominent IgG subclass in the capillary wall deposits of primary MN.[355,356] C3 staining is present over 95% of the time but typically is of relatively low intensity. C1q staining is uncommon and of low intensity in primary MN but is frequent and of high intensity in lupus MN.[354] Although terminal complement components (i.e., components of the membrane attack complex) are not usually evaluated in routine diagnostic preparations, there is very intense staining of the capillary walls for these components. In the rare patients who have concurrent anti-GBM glomerulonephritis and MN, linear

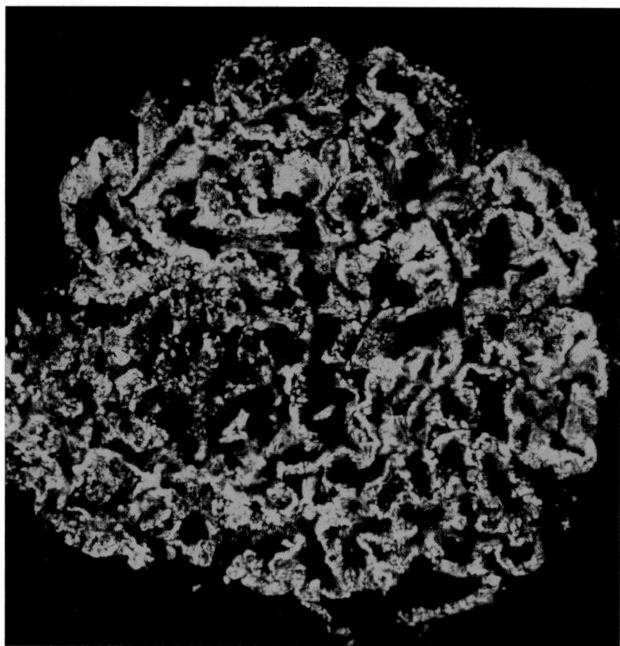

**Fig. 31.9** Immunofluorescence micrograph showing global granular capillary wall staining in a glomerulus with membranous nephropathy representative of PLA2R and also seen with immunoglobulin G in a glomerulus with membranous nephropathy (Fluorescein isothiocyanate anti-PLA2R stain, ×300).

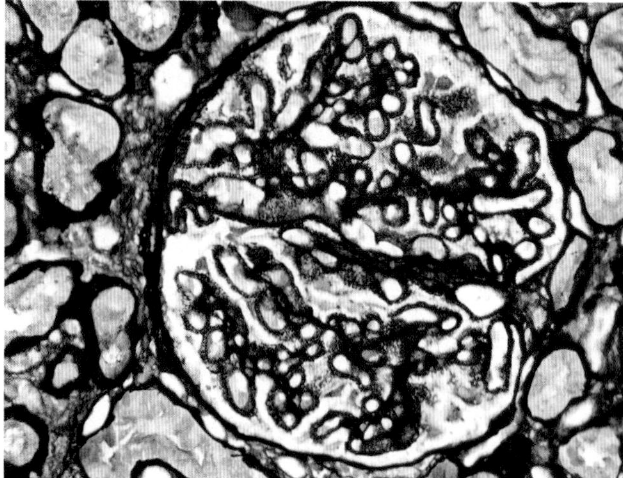

**Fig. 31.10** Light micrograph of a glomerulus with features of membranous nephropathy demonstrating spikes, craters, and other irregularities along the outer aspects of the glomerular basement membrane (see Fig. 31.2). These correspond to the projections of basement membrane material between and around the immune complex deposits. (Jones' methenamine silver stain, ×300.)

staining for IgG can be discerned just below the granular staining.[357]

Tubular basement membrane staining for immunoglobulins or complement is rare in primary MN, but is common in secondary MN, especially lupus MN.[354]

### Light Microscopy

The characteristic histologic abnormality by light microscopy is diffuse global capillary wall thickening in the absence of significant glomerular hypercellularity.[358] The light microscopic features of MN, however, vary with the stage of the disease and with the degree of secondary chronic sclerosing glomerular and tubulointerstitial injury. Mild stage I lesions may not be discernible by light microscopy, especially when only a hematoxylin and eosin stain is used. Stage II, III, and IV lesions usually have readily discernible thickening of the capillary walls.

Masson trichrome stains may demonstrate the subepithelial immune complex deposits as tiny fuchsinophilic (red) grains along the outer aspect of the GBM. However, this is not a sensitive, specific, or technically reliable method for detecting glomerular immune complex deposits. Special stains that accentuate basement membrane material, such as the Jones' silver methenamine stain, may reveal the basement membrane changes that are induced by the subepithelial immune deposits. Spikes along the outer aspect of the GBM usually are seen in stage II lesions (Fig. 31.10). Stage III and IV lesions have irregularly thickened and trabeculated basement membranes, which resemble changes that occur with membranoproliferative glomerulonephritis and chronic thrombotic microangiopathy.

Overt mesangial hypercellularity is uncommon in primary MN, although it is more frequent in secondary MN.[354] Crescent formation is rare unless there is concurrent anti-GBM disease or ANCA disease.[359–365]

With disease progression, chronic sclerosing glomerular and tubulointerstitial lesions develop. Glomeruli become segmentally and globally sclerotic, and develop adhesions to Bowman's capsule. Worsening tubular atrophy, interstitial fibrosis, and interstitial infiltration by mononuclear leukocytes parallel the progressive loss of kidney function.[358]

## PATHOGENESIS

MN is caused by immune complex localization in the subepithelial zone of glomerular capillaries. The nephritogenic antigens can be endogenous to the glomerulus itself (e.g., podocyte autoantigens) or can be exogenous (e.g., hepatitis B antigens). In the latter case, the antigen may be deposited in the subepithelial zone as part of preformed circulating immune complexes or could be produced in or planted in the subepithelial zone as free antigen to which antibodies bind to form immune complexes in situ. In rat Heymann nephritis, an animal model that closely resembles human primary MN, there is convincing evidence that the subepithelial immune deposits form in situ as a result of the binding of antibodies to glycoproteins produced by podocytes, followed by the accumulation of masses of the immune complexes in the subepithelial zone.[366–368]

The long-standing search for antigens targeted in a substantial proportion of patients with MN has witnessed significant breakthroughs over the past decade. The podocyte neutral endopeptidase was the first to be identified as the endogenous target of autoantibodies in a neonate with nephrotic syndrome. This antibody crossed the placenta and was induced in the mother, who lacked the neutral endopeptidase epitope because of a mutational deletion. Sensitization to the nascent antigen was induced during a previous pregnancy.[369–371] These findings provided the first direct support for the paradigm of in situ immune complex formation in the pathogenesis of human primary MN and constitute an example of alloimmunization leading to the generation of immune complex–mediated glomerulopathy.[371,372] It is now clear that most cases of primary MN are due to antibodies directed against the phospholipase A2 receptor ($PLA_2R1$) and the thrombospondin type 1 domain containing 7A (THSD7A; see next section).

The current understanding of these mechanisms, whereby immune complex deposition leads to proteinuria, is largely based on data emerging from studies of passive Heymann nephritis.[368,373] In this model, immune complex formation in the subepithelial zone initiates activation of the complement pathway, leading to the formation of the C5b-C9 membrane attack complex. This results in complement-mediated injury to the epithelial cells.[374–376] The proposed sequence of events includes complement activation and sublytic complement C5b-9 attack on podocytes, resulting in upregulated expression of genes for the production of oxidants, proteases, prostanoids, growth factors, connective tissue growth factor, TGF, and TGF receptors, leading to the overproduction of extracellular matrix.[370,371,377] C5b-9 also causes alterations of the cytoskeleton that lead to abnormal distribution of slit diaphragm proteins and detachment of viable podocytes. These events result in disruption of the functional integrity of the GBM and the protein filtration barrier of podocytes.

The characteristic findings of a predominance of IgG4 with less IgG3 and no IgG1 in subepithelial deposits,[355,356] and the paucity of C1q and C4 in these deposits,[378] argues against a predominant role for the classic or lectin pathways of complement activation in MN and, instead, points to a role of the alternative pathway.[379] The fact that the alternative pathway is spontaneously active in turn points to the likely importance of the complement regulatory proteins. Podocytes primarily rely on membrane complement receptor 1 (CR1; Crry in rodents) and decay-accelerating factor and have the capability to make their own factor H. The importance of complement-mediated injury (at least in passive Heymann nephritis) comes from evidence that nephritogenic serum contains antibodies to membrane complement-regulatory proteins (Crry).[380,381] In a model of active Heymann nephritis, immunization with fraction 1A (Fx1A) lacking Crry leads to the formation of anti-Fx1A antibodies and subepithelial immune complex deposits, but no complement activation or the development of proteinuria.[382] Conversely, the overexpression of Crry or treatment with exogenous Crry has a salutatory effect on immune complex–mediated glomerulonephritis.[383,384] Subsequent injury to the epithelial cell membrane and to the GBM has been hypothesized to be mediated, at least in part, by the production of reactive oxygen species and lipid peroxidation of cell membrane proteins and type IV collagen.[385]

Proteinuria may also be mediated by mechanisms independent of the formation of the C5b-9 membrane attack complex, as is suggested by the generation of proteinuria in passive Heymann nephritis in PVG rats that are deficient in complement factor 6 (PVG/C6 rats). These rats are incapable of generating the membrane attack complex. In this study, PVG/C6 and normal PVG rats developed similar levels of proteinuria after the injection of Fx1a antisera. Isolated glomeruli showed similar deposition of rat Ig and C3 staining in both groups of rats, but C9 deposition was not detected in the glomeruli of C6-deficient rats, which indicates that the C5b-9 membrane attack complex had not formed.[386] Furthermore, the alteration in the glomerular extracellular matrix seen in MN may be caused, at least in part, by a decrease in fibrinolytic activity, due to the stabilization of active plasminogen activator inhibitor I in conjunction with vitronectin in the subepithelial deposits.[387]

Complement activation also results in tubular epithelial cell injury and mediates progressive interstitial disease in MN.[388–390] Proteinuria itself may lead to tubulointerstitial damage through activation of the alternative complement pathway. Strong staining for properdin, a soluble complement regulator also known as "complement factor P," on the luminal surface of the tubules was observed in kidney biopsy specimens from patients with primary MN, but not from healthy kidney donors.[391] After spontaneous hydrolysis of C3, properdin binds to C3b and enhances complement activation by stabilizing C3 convertase. Target-bound properdin may serve as a focal point for amplification of C3 activation. Properdin was shown in vitro to bind proximal tubular epithelial cells. Exposure of proximal tubular epithelial cells with normal human serum as a source of complement, but not to properdin-depleted serum, resulted in complement activation, with the deposition of C3 and generation of C5b-9. This led to the hypothesis that in proteinuric kidney disease, filtered properdin may bind to proximal tubular epithelial cells and act as a focal point for alternative pathway activation.

The human leukocyte antigen (HLA) class II antigen DR3 has been linked with MN,[392–394] and its presence is associated with a relative risk of 12.[392] In a Japanese population, there is an increased frequency of HLA-DR2[395,396] and DQW1[397] in patients with MN. It is possible that a haplotype containing HLA-DR3 and specific HLA class I antigens may be common in these patients as well.[392] For example, HLA-B18 and HLA-DR3 haplotypes may confer an even greater risk of the development of MN.[398] Also associated with an increased susceptibility to MN are polymorphisms of the tumor necrosis factor (TNF)-α gene.[399,400] C4-null alleles are also more frequently found in patients with MN, especially in Caucasian populations.[401] A genome-wide association study (GWAS) of Caucasian patients with primary MN from the United Kingdom ($n = 335$), France ($n = 75$), and The Netherlands ($n = 146$) has identified two significant genomic loci—namely, chromosome 2q24 containing the gene encoding the culprit autoantigen PLA2R and chromosome 6p21 containing the gene encoding HLA-DQA1.[402] Despite the relative risk associated with some of these genetic markers, there are relatively few examples of familial MN.[403–408]

Other studies have also suggested a possible role for APOL1 risk alleles in increasing risk or accelerating progression of $PLA_2R$-associated MN in association with collapsing nephropathy.[409]

## $PLA_2R$, THSD7A, AND MEMBRANOUS NEPHROPATHY

Primary membranous nephropathy (PMN) is an autoimmune disease characterized by circulatory immunoglobulin G (IgG) autoantibodies against two major podocyte autoantigens. Muscle (M)-type phospholipase A2 receptor ($PLA_2R1$) has been detected in 70% of cases, and thrombospondin type 1 domain containing 7A (THSD7A) in 5% to 10% of cases. Autoantibodies to other podocyte intracytoplasmic antigens (e.g., aldose reductase, superoxide dismutase, alpha-enolase) have been detected in primary and secondary membranous nephropathy. The pathogenesis and relationship of these autoantibodies to disease activity remain to be defined.[410,411]

The team of Beck and colleagues has identified M-type $PLA_2R$ as a target autoantigen common to about 70% of patients with primary MN. In contrast, none of the sera from normal controls, patients with MN secondary to SLE or hepatitis B, patients with proteinuric conditions other than MN, or other autoimmune disorders ($n$ = 7) reacted with this antigen. $PLA_2R$ expression in podocytes was confirmed by IF microscopy and in cultured immortalized human podocytes, indicating that the target antigen is intrinsic to glomeruli rather than deposited from sera of patients with PMN.[412]

An international team has investigated a cohort of 154 patients with idiopathic membranous nephropathy and found, using mass spectrometry, that 15 patients (10%) harbor autoantibodies to the glomerular protein THSD7A and were anti–$PLA_2R$-negative.[413] A subsequent study has demonstrated that human anti-THSD7A autoantibodies administered to mice bind to murine THSD7A on murine podocytes, resulting in proteinuria and a glomerular lesion akin to MN, suggesting a causative role. Similar to $PLA_2R$ autoantibody ($PLA_2RAb$), autoantibodies against THSDA7A recognize conformation-dependent epitopes.[413,414] Patients with primary membranous nephropathy may have an autoantibody targeting $PLA_2R$ or THSD7A, but rarely against both autoantigens.

$PLA_2R$ is one of the four members of the mannose receptor family.[415] $PLA_2R$ is a 185- kDa transmembrane glycoprotein consisting of an extracellular N-terminal, cysteine-rich region (CysR), a fibronectin-like type II domain, and eight carbohydrate recognition domains (c-type lectin domain [CTLD1-8]), followed by a transmembrane and C-terminal intracellular tail.[416] The function of this human protein in podocyte remains undefined.[417] IgG4 is the predominant autoantibody against $PLA_2R$, although IgG1 and IgG3 have been reported, especially during the early phase of the disease process. This autoantibody may be present in the circulation and also colocalizes with $PLA_2R$ on the glomerular capillary wall in PMN. The genesis of this autoantibody is currently not known, but molecular mimicry between microbial or environmental antigen and $PLA_2R$ is a possibility.[418] Although the pathogenic role of this autoantibody remains to be elucidated, multiple studies have shown a correlation between the antibody titer and disease activity, suggesting its role as a useful biomarker.

When first described, Beck and colleagues[412] performed Western blot analysis after nonreducing SDS-PAGE for the detection of $PLA_2R$ antibody ($PLA_2RAb$) with recombinant $PLA_2R$ antigen. Although this method is very sensitive and specific, it is impractical for clinical use. In 2014, the U.S. Food and Drug Administration (FDA) approved recombinant cell indirect IF and enzyme-linked immunosorbent assay (ELISA). IF uses transfected cells as a substrate, whereas ELISA is based on purified recombinant human $PLA_2R$ receptors from transfected cells. Based on a metaanalysis, positive serum $PLA_2RAb$ in PMN has a summary sensitivity of 78% (95% CI, 66%–87%) and specificity of 99% (95% CI, 96%–100%). Heterogeneity in diagnostic accuracy could be related to multiple factors, including race (lower in Japanese cohort), sample size, different ELISA methodology and, most importantly, the stage and activity of the disease process.[419]

$PLA_2R$ is expressed on the cell body and foot processes of human podocytes and is absent in rodents. THSD7A is expressed at the basal surface of podocytes in humans and rodents.[420] After binding to $PLA_2RAb$, the immune complexes are shed into the lamina rara externa of the GBM. On routine immunohistochemistry (IHC) of kidney biopsy samples in healthy controls, there is a weak expression of glomerular $PLA_2R$.[421]

IHC may be performed after antigen retrieval of paraffin-embedded renal biopsy samples using polyclonal anti-$PLA_2RAb$. Patients with PMN may have enhanced expression of glomerular $PLA_2R$. Qin and colleagues have reported the presence of serum PLA2RAb in 70% of cases of PMN, of which 98% also had positive glomerular $PLA_2R$ antigen staining by IHC. In contrast, only 70% of patients who were seronegative for $PLA_2RAb$ had podocyte expression of $PLA_2R$.[422] This may be attributed to the rapid clearance of serum antibodies or immunologic remission with glomerular structural changes. Moreover, due to the high affinity of anti-$PLA_2R$ antibodies to the cysteine-rich (CysR) epitope, patients who are low producers of antibody may remain seronegative until they have fully saturated $PLA2_R$ binding sites on podocytes.[417,422] Patients may also have circulatory $PLA_2RAb$ with negative glomerular staining, suggesting that either the antibody is not pathogenic or there are inaccessible epitopes during the antigen retrieval process of kidney biopsy samples.[423]

In a number of studies, including the initial landmark study by Beck and colleagues, circulatory $PLA_2RAb$ and/or glomerular staining of $PLA_2R$ were negative in secondary membranous nephropathy.[412,424] Moreover, $PLA_2RAb$ was absent in a European cohort of SLE with membranous nephropathy and active proliferative lupus nephritis.[425] It begs the question whether positive $PLA_2R$ serology and glomerular staining obviate the need for screening of secondary causes, including malignancy. Subsequent studies have shown positive $PLA_2R$ glomerular staining in patients with many systemic disorders associated with membranous nephropathy, including sarcoidosis, chronic viral B hepatitis, hepatitis C, Sjögren syndrome, and neoplasms.[426,427] $PLA_2R$-positive glomerular staining and its colocalization with hepatitis B surface antigen (HBsAg) along capillary loops have been reported in hepatitis B virus (HBV)–associated MN.[428,429] Whether these secondary disorders induce an immunologic response against $PLA_2R$ or only a coincidental association is uncertain, but with the current body of evidence, it may be premature to obviate the need for screening of secondary causes. In contrast to $PLA_2R$-positive membranous nephropathy, THSD7A-associated membranous nephropathy has a female predominance and is associated with malignancy. Hoxha and colleagues[438] have described a case of THSD7A-MN with the concomitant presence of gallbladder carcinoma.[430] On IHC, both the tumor and lymph node metastases were positive for THSD7A. Also, messenger RNA for THSD7A was detected in the tumor but not in normal tissue. Initiation of chemotherapy led to decreased THSD7A antibody, with improvement in proteinuria. In a screening of 1000 patients with membranous nephropathy, 25 had positive THSD7A antibodies and 7 of these had a malignant tumor. It has been hypothesized that autoantibodies generated against tumor-expressed THSD7A cross-react with podocyte THSD7A in situ.[430]

Although most patients with PMN present with nephrotic range proteinuria, one-third of patients present with subnephrotic range proteinuria and usually have a favorable prognosis.[431] In a small retrospective study of biopsy-proven PMN with subnephrotic range proteinuria, the authors reported that after multivariate analysis, patients with positive $PLA_2RAb$ at entry were more likely to progress to nephrotic syndrome than $PLA_2Rab$-negative patients (HR, 3.66; 95% CI, 1.39–9.64). Moreover, $PLA_2R$-positive patients were more likely to receive immunosuppression and had a more significant rise in serum creatinine levels than $PLA_2Rab$- negative patients. Future prospective controlled studies with longer follow-up will be required to confirm these associations. If proven, patients with subnephrotic range proteinuria with positive $PLA_2R$ would require close observation and possible early initiation of immunosuppression for a favorable outcome.[432]

Based on many retrospective and observational studies, a relationship between circulatory $PLA_2RAb$, glomerular staining of $PLA_2R1$, and disease activity has been proposed. In a large study of 117 Caucasian patients with PMN and nephrotic-range proteinuria, anti-$PLA_2RAb$ was positive in about 74% of cases when measured by IF and ELISA, with a 94% agreement between the two tests. IgG4 anti-$PLA_2RAb$ titer significantly correlated with baseline proteinuria, and spontaneous remission occurred less frequently in patients with high titers (38% vs. 4% in the lowest and highest tertiles, respectively).[433] However, not all antibody titers were measured at the time of diagnosis and may have been delayed by 6 months after biopsy. In another retrospective analysis, after Cox multivariate analysis, anti-$PLA_2RAb$ titers were inversely and independently associated with the likelihood of spontaneous remission (HR, 0.37; CI, 0.17–0.84; $P = .017$).[434] In contrast to the previous study, no significant association was found between anti-$PLA_2RAb$ titers at diagnosis with baseline proteinuria, kidney function, or progression of chronic kidney disease. In primary MN, serum $PLA_2RAb$ may be detected before the development of proteinuria, and resolution of proteinuria may lag behind immunologic remission by months.[435,436] Therefore, in appropriate clinical scenarios of $PLA_2RAb$-positive PMN, monitoring of the $PLA_2RAb$ level may assist clinicians in anticipating a spontaneous remission and avoid "premature" initiation of immunosuppression. $PLA_2RAb$ values are usually high in patients with nephrotic-range proteinuria and decrease substantially with either spontaneous or treatment-induced remission. Also, antibody titers may increase again with disease relapse.[437]

In their observational study, Hoxha and colleagues reported that patients with a low antibody titer reach remission faster than patients with a high titer, although the cumulative rate of patients with remission of proteinuria was similar at the end of the study period at 24 months.[438]

The $PLA_2RAb$ recognizes only the nonreduced form of $PLA_2R$ autoantigen, suggesting the need for disulfide bonds for epitope conformation. Kao and colleagues studied sera from patients with $PLA_2RAb$-positive PMN with truncated $PLA_2R$ extracellular domains and identified the three-domain protein complex CysR, fibronectin-like type II (FnII-), and C-type lectin-like domain 1 (CTLD1) as the immunodominant humoral epitope.[439] Taking this a step further, Fresquet and colleagues have identified the CysR domain as the major humoral epitope.[440]

Epitope spreading is the diversification of epitope specificity from the initial dominant epitope-specific immune response to subdominant epitopes on that protein.[441,442] This phenomenon has been described in many autoimmune disorders, including human anti-GBM disease, rheumatoid arthritis, and Heyman nephritis. Seitz-Polski and colleagues[443] have described similar phenomena among three domains of the $PLA_2R1$ molecule in PMN. Using a series of $PLA_2R1$ deletion mutants of the extracellular domains, three reactive epitopes have been identified, with CysR being the primary dominant epitope and CTLD1 and CTLD7 being additional distinct epitopes. Patients with anti-$PLA_2R1$ reactivity against CysR had a favorable outcome, with less severe disease, younger age of onset, and a higher chance of going into spontaneous remission compared with those with antibody reactivity against other domains. The authors hypothesized that anti-$PLA_2R$ reactivity is restricted to the CysR domain in the initial stage and, after additional immune challenges, this reactivity spreads to the C-terminal region (CTLD11 or CTLD7), resulting in progressive disease that may be less responsive to therapy. Further studies are required to confirm this finding; if proven, it could guide physicians to personalize therapy based on anti-$PLA_2R$ reactivity.

In an observational study of PMN treated with cyclophosphamide or MMF, baseline anti-$PLA_2RAb$ titers did not predict initial response, but those at the end of therapy predicted long-term outcome. After a median follow-up of 5 years, 58% patients with negative antibody titers at the end of therapy maintained remission, and none of the patients with persistent seropositivity went into remission. Moreover, cyclophosphamide-based therapy was more effective in reducing antibody titers than MMF.[444] However, this observation has not been confirmed in other studies. Radice and associates could not detect statistical differences in the probability of negativization of $PAL_2RAb$ during follow-up based on different initial immunosuppressive therapies.[445] In a longitudinal observational study, the response to treatment with rituximab therapy was similar, irrespective of the presence or absence of anti-$PLA_2RAb$.[446] Among $PLA_2Rab$-seropositive patients, the probability of complete or partial remission of proteinuria progressively decreased in parallel with progressive increasing $PLA_2RAb$ titers.[446,447] The probability plateaus at a level more than 500 to 600 relative units (RU)/mL (1 RU/mL roughly equates to 2 pg/mL). Additionally, a 50% decrease in antibody titer preceded an equivalent decrease in proteinuria by 10 months.[446]

A combination of clinical parameters and $PLA_2R$ serology and glomerular staining may become very important for making appropriate and timely clinical decisions. Future randomized controlled studies with long-term follow-up are required to understand the relationship among $PLA_2RAb$ titers, glomerular staining, and clinical parameters of membranous nephropathy. With current evidence, it may not be appropriate to develop a treatment algorithm purely based on $PLA_2RAb$ titer. The process and relationship are complicated and need to be studied further and refined to put in an algorithm.

## CLINICAL FEATURES AND NATURAL HISTORY

Patients with MN usually have nephrotic syndrome with hypoalbuminemia, hyperlipidemia, peripheral edema, and lipiduria. This presentation occurs in 70% to 80% of patients.[346,448] The onset of nephrotic syndrome is usually not associated with any prodromal disease process or antecedent infections. Hypertension may be present at the outset of disease in 13% to 55% of patients.[348] Most patients present with normal or slightly decreased kidney function at presentation.

If progressive renal insufficiency develops, it is usually relatively indolent. An abrupt change to more acute renal insufficiency should prompt investigation of a superimposed condition, such as a crescentic glomerulonephritis.[449] One-third of such patients have anti-GBM antibodies, and some have ANCAs.

Other causes of sudden deterioration of kidney function include acute bilateral renal vein thrombosis and hypovolemia in the setting of massive nephrosis. The incidence of renal vein thrombosis in MN varies from 4% to 52%.[450] The diagnosis of renal vein thrombosis may be clinically apparent based on the sudden development of macroscopic hematuria, flank pain, and reduction in kidney function, but a more insidious development is also common. Although ultrasonography with Doppler studies may demonstrate the renal thrombus,[451] venography with contrast remains the gold standard. Spiral computed tomography[452] or magnetic resonance imaging with contrast have also been used.[453]

Drug-induced kidney injury is another reason for the sudden deterioration in kidney function in a patient with MN. The use of nonsteroidal antiinflammatory drugs (NSAIDs), diuretics, and antimicrobials has been linked to the occurrence of acute interstitial nephritis or acute tubular necrosis.[454,455]

An estimate of renal survival in patients with MN can be obtained from a pooled analysis of outcomes in clinical studies.[349] In this analysis of 1189 pooled patients,[326,338,347,456–468] the probability of renal survival was 86% in 5 years, 65% in 10 years, and 59% years at 15 years. Although 35% of patients may progress to ESKD by 10 years, 25% may experience a complete spontaneous remission of proteinuria within 5 years.[469]

In a retrospective study of 328 patients with MN who were not treated with immunosuppressive agents, spontaneous remission of proteinuria occurred in 32% of patients: partial remission (proteinuria ≤3.5 g/day) occurred at a mean of 14.7 ± 11.4 months, and the mean time to complete remission was 38.0 ± 25.2 months.[431] Importantly, severe proteinuria at onset of disease does not preclude the possibility of spontaneous remission because it occurred in 26% of patients with a baseline proteinuria of 8 to 12 g/day and in 21% of patients with a baseline proteinuria of more than 12 g of protein/day. Multivariate analysis has revealed that the best predictor of spontaneous remission was a decrease in proteinuria of more than 50% in the first year of follow-up (HR, 12.6;95% CI, 5.2–30.5; $P < .0001$). Other predictors were the baseline serum creatinine level, baseline proteinuria, and the use of angiotensin II inhibitors.[431]

Persistent proteinuria is more predictive of renal insufficiency than proteinuria at a single time point. Thus, persistent proteinuria of 8 g or more/day for 6 months or more was associated with a 66% probability of progression to chronic renal failure. Patients with at least 6 g of protein/day for 9 months or longer had a 55% probability of developing chronic renal insufficiency. Persistent proteinuria of 4 g or more/day for longer than 18 months was associated with an even greater risk of chronic renal insufficiency.[470] Patients with overtly declining kidney function are at higher risk for progressive renal deterioration.[469]

In addition to renal insufficiency and proteinuria, other factors may be associated with an increased risk of progressive renal failure. Male gender, advanced age (>50 years), poorly controlled hypertension, and reduced GFR at presentation have been reported as risk factors for progressive decline in kidney function.[345,463,467,469–474] In addition to the clinical prognostic features, the presence of advanced MN on kidney biopsy specimens (stage III or IV), tubular atrophy, and interstitial fibrosis can also be associated with increased risk. In fact, chronic interstitial fibrosis and tubular atrophy have been shown to be independent predictors of progressive renal failure in primary MN.[462,475–477] The presence of crescents on kidney biopsy specimens may also portend a poor long-term prognosis. The stage of glomerular lesions detected by electron microscopy has also been suggested as a risk factor for poor prognosis in some[478–480] but not all studies.[335,467,475,481] Similarly, FSGS superimposed on MN may have a worse long-term renal prognosis than MN without sclerosis.[482,483] However, the importance of these demographic and histologic risk factors was not substantiated in a retrospective analysis of a large cohort of patients from the University of Toronto that examined the rate of progression (slope).[484] Of the histologic variables, only a greater degree of complement deposition appeared to be associated with a more rapid decline in GFR.[485]

In a prospective study, urinary excretion of $\beta_2$-microglobulin level of more than 0.5 μg/min and a urinary IgG level of more than 250 mg/24 hr, assessed in a timed urine sample, were found to predict the progressive loss of GFR in a prospective cohort of 57 patients with primary MN and normal kidney function.[486] In a multivariate analysis, urine $\beta_2$-microglobulin excretion was the strongest independent predictor of the development of renal insufficiency, with a sensitivity and specificity of 88% and 91%, respectively. Unfortunately, the measurement of urine $\beta_2$-microglobulin is cumbersome because it is unstable in urine and requires alkalinization of the urine prior to collection. More recently, there have been several studies from different groups demonstrating an association between high anti-$PLA_2R$ autoantibodies and worse long-term outcomes in that there appears to be growing evidence for an inverse correlation between the level of the autoantibodies and disease.[444,487–489]

In summary, one of the strongest indicators of progressive disease appears to be the persistence of at least moderate proteinuria.[473] Impaired kidney function, severe proteinuria at presentation, the presence of substantial interstitial infiltrates on biopsy specimen, superimposed crescentic glomerulonephritis, and segmental sclerosis also portend a poorer outcome.

## LABORATORY FINDINGS

Proteinuria is the hallmark of MN. More than 80% of MN patients excrete more than 3 g of protein/day. In some patients, the amount of urinary protein may exceed 20 g/day. A Medical Research Council study has reported that 30% of patients with MN excreted more than 10 g of protein per day at the time of presentation.[350] Microscopic hematuria is present in 30% to 50% of patients at the time of presentation.[346,490,491] Macroscopic hematuria, on the other hand, is distinctly uncommon and occurs in less than 4% of adult patients,[492,493] although it may be common in children.[494] Most patients have either normal or only slightly decreased kidney function. Impaired kidney function is found in fewer than 10% of patients at the time of presentation.[490,495]

In patients with severe nephrosis, hypoalbuminemia is common, as is the loss of other serum proteins, including IgG. Serum lipoprotein levels are characteristically elevated, as they are in other forms of nephrotic syndrome. Elevated levels of low-density and very low-density lipoproteins are common in MN. In one study, elevated levels of lipoprotein(a) normalized in patients whose disease was in remission.[496]

Levels of complement components C3 and C4 are typically normal in patients with MN. The complex of terminal complement components known as C5b-9 is found in the urine of some patients with active MN. There is increased excretion of this complex in patients with active immune complex formation. The excretion may decrease during disease inactivity.[374–376,497–502]

To exclude common causes of secondary MN, one should carry out serologic tests for nephritogenic infections such as hepatitis B, hepatitis C, and syphilis, as well as tests for immunologic disorders such as lupus, mixed connective tissue disease, and cryoglobulinemia. MN has been associated with graft-versus-host disease following allogeneic stem cell transplantation, and this should be considered as well.[503]

Although hypercoagulability appears to be present in patients with nephrosis in general, this tendency may be enhanced in patients with MN.[504–506] The exact mechanisms leading to thrombophilia in this group of patients are poorly understood. Patients with MN have hyperfibrinogenemia with increased levels of circulating procoagulants and decreased levels of anticoagulant factors, such as antithrombin III.[507] The thrombotic tendency may be increased by the erythrocytosis that occurs in some patients, as well as by the effect of lipoprotein(a) to retard thrombolysis. Other possible contributors to the thrombophilic state include volume depletion, diuretic and/or steroid use, venous stasis, immobilization, and immune complex activation of the clotting cascade and anti–α-enolase antibodies.[508–510] Renal vein thrombosis has been reported more frequently in patients with MN than in those with nephrotic syndrome of other causes.[506,511–514] The prevalence of renal vein thrombosis in patients with MN ranges from approximately 5% to 63%, depending on the mode of diagnosis used and whether or not systematic screening is performed. The prevalence of all forms of deep vein thrombosis in patients with MN ranges from 9% to 44%. The combined burden of deep vein and renal vein thrombosis has been estimated to be as high as 45%.[510] Renal vein thrombosis is often silent, with pulmonary embolism being the first presenting sign. The risk of venous thromboembolic events appears to be higher when the serum albumin concentration is less than 2.5 g/dL; such events occur in as many as 40% of these patients.[510,515]

It is the concern for the morbidity and, at times, mortality associated with pulmonary embolism that has led to the use of prophylactic anticoagulation for patients with severe nephrotic syndrome and MN. A decision analysis has suggested that the risk of life-threatening complications of pulmonary embolism outweigh the risks associated with anticoagulant therapy.[516] However, this analysis may be based on an overestimate of the true incidence of thromboses among patients with MN. No direct controlled data are available to support or refute such a contention. More recently, using data from an inception cohort of 898 patients with primary MN, as well as literature review–based risk estimates of hemorrhage, a clinical tool to estimate the likelihood of benefit of anticoagulation, based primarily on bleeding risk and serum albumin concentration, was proposed as a way to begin to personalize prophylactic anticoagulation (www.gntools.com).[517] A retrospective analysis of a treatment regimen to prevent venous thromboembolism in 143 patients with nephrotic syndrome (low-molecular-weight heparin or low-dose heparin for patients with a serum albumin level <2.0 g/dL and aspirin 75, mg daily, for patients with serum albumin level of 2.0–3.0 g/dL) has appeared to be effective, with very few complications.[518] Unfortunately, there is no direct controlled support for the routine use of prophylactic anticoagulation in patients with primary MN; however, the case could be made for the judicious use of warfarin in patients with severe nephrotic syndrome who have a profoundly decreased serum albumin level (probably <2 mg/dL) if no contraindications are present. Randomized controlled trials are warranted.

## TREATMENT

### Corticosteroids

Despite numerous studies, the optimal treatment of MN remains incompletely defined. The difficulty in treating MN is a consequence of the chronic nature of the disease, the tendency for spontaneous remission and relapse, the variability of clinical severity, and the only partial efficacy of existing treatment protocols. The role of corticosteroids and alkylating agents in the treatment of this disease has been debated for decades. Common therapeutic approaches for new-onset disease include the following: (1) conservative therapy with RAAS blockade; (2) corticosteroid therapy (usually prednisone or methylprednisolone); and (3) administration of alkylating agents, such as chlorambucil or cyclophosphamide, with or without concurrent corticosteroid treatment.

Numerous studies using corticosteroid treatment have demonstrated different outcomes.*

In a pooled analysis of these studies, corticosteroid therapy was found to have no beneficial effect on renal survival.[349] Three large prospective randomized trials have examined the efficacy of oral corticosteroid therapy in adult patients with MN, with different results.[458,459,521] Findings of the US Collaborative Study[337] have suggested that 8 weeks treatment with 100 to 150 mg of prednisone, given on alternate days, resulted in a transient decrease in urinary protein excretion to less than 2 g compared with placebo. Prednisone was discontinued after 3 months unless proteinuria recurred after a partial or complete remission. Relapses were treated by reinstitution of high-dose prednisone for 1 month, followed by a taper. The results of this study have suggested that patients treated with prednisone are less likely to experience a doubling of their entry serum creatinine level and were more likely to experience a transient decrease in proteinuria to less than 2 g of protein/day, and that even a partial remission of proteinuria was associated with well-preserved, long-term kidney function. This seminal study was criticized because the control group fared substantially worse than untreated patients in several other studies.

*References 326, 337, 338, 347, 456–463,466–469, 481, 519, and 520.

A British Medical Research Council study[458] used a similar regimen except that prednisolone was discontinued after 8 weeks without tapering and without treatment of the relapse of proteinuria. Patients with lower creatinine clearance (≤30 mL/min) were included in the study. Three to 9 months after study entry, patients showed no improvement in kidney function, and the urine protein excretion and albumin level improved only transiently.

A third prospective randomized study of corticosteroid reported by Cattran and colleagues[459] included patients with relatively low levels of proteinuria (≤0.3 g of protein/day). In this study, alternate-day prednisone (45 mg/m$^2$ of body surface area) afforded no benefit with regard to proteinuria or renal function.

In a metaanalysis[349] of the U.S. Collaborative study[337] and the studies by Cameron,[458] Cattran,[459] and Kobayashi and colleagues[460] comparing glucocorticoid with supportive therapy, corticosteroid therapy was associated with a trend toward achievement of complete remission at 24 to 36 months, but this result did not reach statistical significance. A pooled analysis of randomized trials and prospective studies again demonstrated a lack of benefit of corticosteroid therapy in inducing a remission of nephrotic syndrome or preserving kidney function.[349]

An alternative to oral glucocorticoid therapy has been treatment with pulse methylprednisolone, largely in patients with deteriorating kidney function. Treatment of patients with renal insufficiency using pulse methylprednisolone at 1 g/day for 5 days followed by oral prednisone was associated with an improvement in kidney function for 6 months and a reduction in proteinuria.[522] The long-term outcomes for over 50% of these patients were discouraging; one-third experienced renal failure and 13% developed myocardial infarction with kidney dysfunction. A similar study[523] combined pulse methylprednisolone with azathioprine or cyclophosphamide. Although there may have been some improvement in proteinuria and kidney function in a minority of patients, substantial side effects were experienced by almost the entire study population. The evidence to date does not support the use of oral corticosteroids alone for the treatment of primary MN.

### Cyclophosphamide or Chlorambucil

Cytotoxic drugs, including cyclophosphamide and chlorambucil, have been used for the treatment of primary MN in conjunction with intravenous and/or oral corticosteroids. In a number of studies, Ponticelli and colleagues have demonstrated that chlorambucil has a beneficial effect in the treatment of MN.[462,479,481,524] In these studies, patients with primary MN were treated initially with intravenous pulse methylprednisolone at 1 g/day for the first 3 days of each month, with daily oral glucocorticoid therapy (methylprednisolone, 0.4 mg/kg/day, or prednisone, 0.5 mg/kg/day), given on an alternating monthly schedule with chlorambucil at a dosage of 0.2 mg/kg/day. .Both groups received a low-salt diet, diuretics, and antihypertensive agents, as needed. In patients randomly assigned to the treatment group, nephrotic syndrome lasted for a significantly shorter duration, and a complete or partial remission of proteinuria occurred in 83% of MN patients compared with 38% of control patients.[524] The slope of the mean reciprocal plasma creatinine level remained stable in the treatment group, but declined in the untreated patients beginning at 12 months. At 10-year follow-up, the probability of having a functioning kidney was 92% in the treated patients and 60% in the control patients. In only 10% of patients was therapy discontinued because of side effects. Compared with treatment with glucocorticoids alone, treatment with a combination of chlorambucil and methylprednisolone was associated with an earlier remission of nephrotic syndrome and a greater stability of complete or partial remission of proteinuria.[481] Interestingly, the overall decline in kidney function was no different in the two treatment groups. Unfortunately, although a difference in favor of the chlorambucil-treated patients persisted for the first 3 years of follow-up, it was no longer statistically significantly different by 4 years (62% without nephrotic syndrome in the group receiving combination therapy vs. 42% in the steroid-only group; $P = .102$). In a study comparing cyclophosphamide with chlorambucil, cyclophosphamide was found to be at least as effective as chlorambucil when used in a similar dosing protocol and appeared to have somewhat fewer side effects.[525]

A prospective, open-label, randomized study in India[526] involving 93 patients followed for a median of 11 years (range, 10.5–12 years) compared supportive therapy (dietary sodium restriction, diuretics, and antihypertensive agents) with a 6-month course of alternate months of steroid and cyclophosphamide treatment, similar to the Ponticelli protocol.[524,527] Unfortunately, angiotensin II blockade was withheld in all patients for at least 1 year. Study endpoints were the doubling of the serum creatinine level, development of ESKD, or patient death. Of the 47 patients who received the immunosuppressive protocol, 34 experienced remission compared with 16 of 46 in the control group ($P < .0001$). The 10-year dialysis-free survival was 89% in the immunosuppression group and 65% in the supportive treatment group ($P = .016$), and the likelihood of survival without death, dialysis, or doubling of the serum creatinine level was 79% and 44% ($P$=.0006), respectively. A significant divergence between the two groups in terms of proteinuria became apparent within the first year, and the estimated GFR was significantly lower in the control group than in the cyclophosphamide-treated group from 4 years onward. This study confirms, in a different patient population, the short- and long-term benefits associated with treatment with cyclophosphamide and corticosteroids, according to the Ponticelli protocol.[524,527]

A more recent randomized controlled trial of 108 patients with biopsy-documented primary MN in the United Kingdom compared prednisolone in combination with chlorambucil to either cyclosporine or supportive therapy alone. The primary endpoint was a further 20% decline in excretory kidney function from baseline readings, which was significantly lower in the prednisolone and chlorambucil group (HR, 0.44; 95% CI, 0.24–0.78; $P = .0042$); however, this group also had a higher frequency of serious adverse events.[528]

Despite these reported benefits, there has been a lack of corroboration in other trials regarding the salutary effects of alkylating agents combined with prednisone or other agents[461,465,468,529]; however, two metaanalyses have suggested that the use of cytotoxic agents improves the chance of a complete remission of proteinuria by four- to fivefold, but had no long-term protective effect on renal survival.[349,530] A further metaanalysis of 36 clinical trials investigating the effects of immunosuppression on adults with idiopathic MN has concluded that corticosteroids combined with alkylating agents significantly reduce all-cause mortality or ESKD (8 randomized controlled trials [RCTs], 448 participants; risk ratio, 0.44; 95% CI, 0.26–0.75; $P = .002$) and increased partial or complete remission (7 RCTs, 422 participants; risk ratio 1.46; 95% CI, 1.13–1.89; $P = .004$), but led to more adverse events (4 RCTs, 303 participants; risk ratio, 4.20; 95% CI, 1.15–15.32; $P = .03$).[531]

### Calcineurin Inhibitors

Despite the most recent trial showing the superiority of prednisolone in combination with chlorambucil over cyclosporine,[528] there has been interest in the use of cyclosporine, which has resulted in improvement in proteinuria and stability of kidney function in many patients.[532–534] In an RCT comparing 26 weeks of treatment with cyclosporine plus low-dose prednisone to treatment with placebo plus prednisone, 75% of the cyclosporine group but only 22% of the control group ($P < .001$) experienced a partial or complete remission of proteinuria by 26 weeks.[535] Relapse occurred in about 40% of patients achieving remission in both treatment groups. The fraction of patients achieving sustained remission remained significantly different between the groups until the end of the study (cyclosporine treatment, 39%; placebo, 13%; $P = .007$). Kidney function was unchanged and equal in the two groups over the test medication period.[535] This study was criticized for the rapid discontinuation of cyclosporine over 4 weeks at the end of the 26-week treatment period.

In a prospective study, treatment with cyclosporine alone (2–3 mg/kg/day) was compared with treatment with a combination of cyclosporine and oral prednisolone in 51 patients.[536] Prednisolone was started at 0.6 mg/kg/day and then gradually tapered to 10 to 15 mg/day at 6 months and continued to 12 months. Patients who experienced complete or partial remission then received long-term treatment with lower doses of cyclosporine (1–1.5 mg/kg/day) plus prednisolone (0.1 mg/kg/day) or cyclosporine alone. This study did not have a randomized design because patients with contraindications to corticosteroid use were assigned to the cyclosporine-only group. During the follow-up phase of the study, relapses were more common in patients treated with cyclosporine alone than in patients receiving cyclosporine plus oral prednisolone (47% vs. 15%, respectively; $P < .05$). However, the results suggested that the risk of relapse may be determined by the levels of cyclosporine because patients in both groups who experienced relapse had lower cyclosporine trough levels than those who did not experience relapse (72 ± 48 ng/mL vs. 194 ± 80 ng/mL, respectively; $P < .03$).

A prospective RCT was undertaken to evaluate monotherapy with tacrolimus versus supportive therapy alone in 48 patients with MN who had preserved kidney function and had persistent nephrotic syndrome for longer than 9 months, despite treatment with an ACE inhibitor or ARB.[537] Treatment with tacrolimus consisted of 0.05 mg/kg/day divided into two daily doses and adjusted to achieve a whole-blood, 12-hour trough level between 3 and 5 ng/mL. The target trough level was increased to between 5 and 8 ng/mL if a remission was not achieved after the first 2 months of treatment. Tacrolimus was continued for a total of 12 months, followed by a 6-month taper. The probability of remission in the treatment group was 58%, 82%, and 94% after 6, 12, and 18 months, but was only 10%, 24%, and 35%, respectively, in the control group. The decrease in proteinuria was significantly greater in the treatment group. Notably, 6 patients in the control group and only 1 in the treatment group reached the secondary endpoint of a 50% increase in serum creatinine level. Unfortunately, as in the previously published study of cyclosporine, almost half of the patients who had achieved remission experienced a recurrence of nephrotic syndrome by the 18th month after tacrolimus withdrawal.

An interesting pilot study from Spain[538] has studied combination therapy with corticosteroids, MMF, and tacrolimus in patients with persistent nephrotic syndrome after 6 months of treatment with full-dose RAAS blockers and a creatinine clearance of more than 60 mL/min/1.73 $m^2$. The initial dose of prednisone was 0.5 mg/kg/day for the first month, and the drug was then tapered to 7.5 mg/day at month 6. The starting dose of tacrolimus was 0.05 mg/kg/day to achieve target whole-blood trough levels of 7 to 9 ng/mL. If the level of proteinuria was less than 1 g of protein/day at the end of 3 months of this therapy, the tacrolimus dosage was reduced to maintain blood levels between 5 and 7 ng/mL and continued for a period of 9 more months. If, however, the level of proteinuria was greater than 1 g of protein/day, the dose of tacrolimus was reduced, and MMF was added at a dose of 0.5 g twice daily and adjusted to achieve target whole-blood trough levels of 2 to 4 mg/L. Triple therapy was then maintained for 9 additional months, after which immunosuppressants were tapered off over 3 months in all patients. Of the 21 adult patients enrolled, 11 had proteinuria of less than 1 g of protein/day at the end of 3 months and then received maintenance dosages of prednisolone plus tacrolimus. MMF was added after the third month in 9 patients and was associated with complete or partial remission in 5. Unfortunately, the relapse rate was very high in all groups of patients, whether treated with double or triple therapy. Clearly, additional controlled trials are required to determine the optimal duration of treatment and the benefit of adding MMF in patients who show only partial response to treatment with calcineurin-inhibitors alone.

### Adrenocorticotropic Hormone

The use of synthetic adrenocorticotropic hormone (ACTH) has been assessed in patients with nephrotic syndrome, including those with MN.[539] In one RCT,[540] 32 patients were treated with either corticosteroids and chlorambucil or cyclophosphamide administered according to the Ponticelli protocol, or with ACTH (tetracosactide) administered intramuscularly twice weekly for 1 year. Of patients in the ACTH arm, 87% experienced complete or partial remission with a dramatic reduction in proteinuria and mean serum cholesterol and remission at almost 3 years.[540] Few patients developed symptoms and signs of excess glucocorticoids.

Given lack of availability of the synthetic, long-acting ACTH analogue formulation in the United States, a retrospective case series has examined the role of a natural ACTH gel formulation for nephrotic syndrome.[541] In this study, 11 patients with primary MN out of 21 patients with nephrotic syndrome were treated with ACTH gel and 9 of 11 MN patients (82%) achieved complete (3 of 11, 27%) or partial (6 of 11, 55%) remission. A subsequent prospective, open-label study evaluated the efficacy of ACTH gel (80 units subcutaneously twice weekly for 6 months) in patients with resistant glomerular disease, defined as failure to achieve sustained remission of proteinuria off immunosuppressive therapy with at least two treatment regimens.[542] In this study, 5 patients with primary MN out of 15 patients were treated; 2 patients achieved partial remission and 3 patients achieved immunologic remission. The mechanism responsible for the beneficial effect of ACTH is unknown. Studies have pointed to the expression of the melanocortin 1 receptor on podocytes, which suggests a possible direct effect of ACTH on these cells.[543]

### Mycophenolate Mofetil

Interest has arisen in the use of mycophenolate mofetil (MMF) for the management of MN in a few small studies yielding disparate results. In an open-label study in the Netherlands, 32 patients with primary MN treated with MMF were compared with a historical matched control group treated with oral cyclophosphamide for 12 months.[544] Both groups received intermittent methylprednisolone and alternate-day prednisone. Although, on average, the degree of proteinuria decreased similarly in the MMF-treated group and in the cyclophosphamide-treated group, and although the cumulative incidence of remission of proteinuria at 12 months was comparable in the two groups, the percentage of patients who showed no response to therapy was statistically significantly higher in the MMF-treated group, as was the proportion of patients who experienced a relapse.

In a 1-year RCT of 36 patients, treatment with MMF (target dose, 2 g/day) for 12 months was compared with conservative care alone.[545] The change in the mean urine protein-to-creatinine ratio from baseline to month 12 was measured; the ratio decreased by 1834 mg/g in the control group and increased by 213 mg/g in the MMF group ($P = .3$). Complete or partial remission at month 12 was observed in 37% of patients in the MMF group and 41% in the control group.

In a separate prospective, randomized, controlled, open-label study involving 20 patients in Hong Kong and Shanghai,[546] treatment with MMF and prednisolone given for 6 months was compared with treatment that followed a modified Ponticelli regimen.[525] Over a total follow-up of 15 months, proteinuria decreased to a similar extent in both treatment groups. The rates of complete and partial remissions were 27.3% and 36.4%, respectively, in the MMF group, and 33.3% and 33.3% in the control group. These results are in marked distinction to those of the previously described study comparing MMF with conservative therapy.[545] These two studies differ in the makeup of the patient populations (Caucasians vs. Asians) and by the concomitant use of prednisolone in the Hong Kong and Shanghai study. Overall, the results of studies of MMF have been disappointing, with a notable exception of those involving Chinese patients.

### Rituximab

Given the high likelihood of antibody-mediated injury in patients with MN, there has been an explosion of interest in the use of rituximab, a humanized anti-CD20 monoclonal antibody. In an initial report of eight patients, treatment with rituximab (4 weekly doses of 375 mg/m$^2$ body surface area) was associated with prompt and sustained reduction in proteinuria.[547,548] There have been additional positive open-label studies,[447,549–552] but the effects on long-term renal outcome are unproven. The available uncontrolled data have suggested that rituximab, 375 mg/m$^2$ once weekly for 4 weeks or at 1 g on days 1 and 15, achieves a 15% to 20% rate of complete remission and 40% to 45% rate of partial remission.[553]

A cohort study has reported on the effect of rituximab in 13 patients with MN deemed to be calcineurin inhibitor-dependent (defined as the occurrence of at least four calcineurin inhibitor-responsive relapses of nephrotic proteinuria while the patient was being weaned off these drugs).[554] After rituximab therapy (375 mg/m$^2$ weekly for 4 weeks, with each dose preceded by 125 mg of methylprednisolone), proteinuria decreased significantly, and calcineurin inhibitors and other immunosuppressant drugs could be withdrawn in all patients.

Although the aggregate of these uncontrolled case series suggests a beneficial effect of rituximab in the management of MN, whether, when, and how (and how long) to use rituximab in treating MN remains to be determined. A large pharmaceutical company-funded, randomized controlled study comparing rituximab with calcineurin inhibitor therapy across 19 medical centers in the United States is now underway (www.clinicaltrials.gov, NCT01180036)[555]; however, results may be met with skepticism given prior unfavorable results seen with calcineurin inhibitors as compared with corticosteroids in combination with chlorambucil.[528]

### Other Therapies

Other forms of therapy have been tried in primary MN, with varying results. These include the use of azathioprine,[519,520] which demonstrated no positive effect either alone or in combination with prednisone. The use of pooled intravenous immunoglobulin has been evaluated only in a small case series[556] and a retrospective study.[557]

Based on the greater appreciation of the role of complement activation, and especially that of complement-regulatory proteins in the pathogenesis of MN, a great deal of interest exists in targeting this pathway for therapy. Several compounds are under development. To date, human trials have been conducted only for eculizumab, a monoclonal antibody directed against the fifth component of complement (C5). In a randomized trial of patients with de novo MN, treatment with eculizumab was not associated with a statistically significant improvement in proteinuria or preservation of kidney function. These disappointing results were likely due to insufficient dosing because consistent inhibition of complement was achieved only in a minority of patients.[558] Nevertheless, this general approach is thought to hold a great deal of promise based on early animal studies.

In the absence of a full understanding of the pathogenesis of MN, and thus an effective targeted therapy, the current approach to the treatment of MN must rely on risk stratification. The indolent disease process that results in spontaneous remissions in 25% of patients, coupled with the known adverse consequences of long-term treatment with oral glucocorticoids, alkylating agents, and calcineurin inhibitors, should prompt a careful analysis of the risk-benefit ratio in the treatment of any given patient. All patients should receive excellent supportive care, including the use of RAAS blockers[269,559–562] and lipid-lowering agents. Most patients should be observed for the development of adverse prognostic factors or the occurrence of spontaneous remissions. Adult patients with good prognostic features should be managed conservatively without the use of immunomodulatory or suppressive agents.

Patients at moderate risk (persistent proteinuria between 4 and 6 g of protein/day, despite RAAS blockade and normal kidney function) or at high risk of progression (persistent proteinuria of more than 8 g of protein/day, with or without renal insufficiency) should be considered for immunosuppressive therapy with a combination of glucocorticoids and cyclophosphamide (or chlorambucil) in alternating monthly pulses (Ponticelli protocol). This decision must be individualized to each patient with consideration of the patient's comorbidities and assessment of the risk associated with each type of therapy. The data currently available do not suggest that MMF alone is effective. Whether ACTH and/or rituximab are viable effective alternatives awaits further confirmation. Some of the difficulties associated with determining drug efficacy in clinical trials focused on MN, not to mention the other prior glomerular diseases, are related to variable endpoint definitions. Furthermore, surrogate endpoints for a treatment effect on ESKD, such as complete and/or partial remission of proteinuria used early in the disease process, could make clinical trial design more effective. A recent study has found that available data suggest that complete remission of proteinuria could potentially be used as a surrogate endpoint in primary MN in future clinical trial settings.[563]

Individuals who have advanced chronic renal failure are best managed by supportive care while awaiting dialysis and kidney transplantation. Acute renal insufficiency in this population should prompt evaluation for interstitial nephritis, crescentic nephritis, and renal vein thrombosis.

## MEMBRANOPROLIFERATIVE GLOMERULONEPHRITIS AND C3 GLOMERULOPATHY

Primary membranoproliferative glomerulonephritis (MPGN) is a collection of morphologically similar but pathogenetically distinct disorders. Overall, MPGN is identified in approximately 10% of kidney biopsy specimens.[564,565] MPGN has traditionally been classified based on electron microscopic findings into three types; MPGN type 1 is the most common form and is characterized by mesangial and subendothelial deposits. MPGN type II (dense deposit disease, DDD) has electron-dense deposits along the GBM. MPGN type III has both subepithelial and subendothelial deposits.[566,569,570] Recent advances in the understanding of the different pathogenetic mechanisms underlying the MPGN subtypes have resulted in a new classification system.[542,566–568] In the new classification, MPGN is classified based on glomerular immune deposit staining on IF, both immunoglobulin and complement (immune-complex mediated MPGN), and those with predominant C3 staining (complement- mediated MPGN, C3 glomerulopathy; Fig. 31.11). Immune complex glomerular deposits may activate the classical complement pathway, resulting in deposition of C1q, C4, and C3.[566,570] The category MPGN type 1, and probably type III, based on immunoreactant staining, involves cases of immune complex–mediated GN and cases of C3G. C3 glomerulopathy is characterized by variable light microscopic findings (with or without MPGN pattern) and defined by dominant C3 staining of glomerular deposits; the intensity of C3 staining has to be twofold greater than other immunoreactants. C3G is further subdivided based on electron microscopy into DDD and C3 glomerulonephritis.[571]

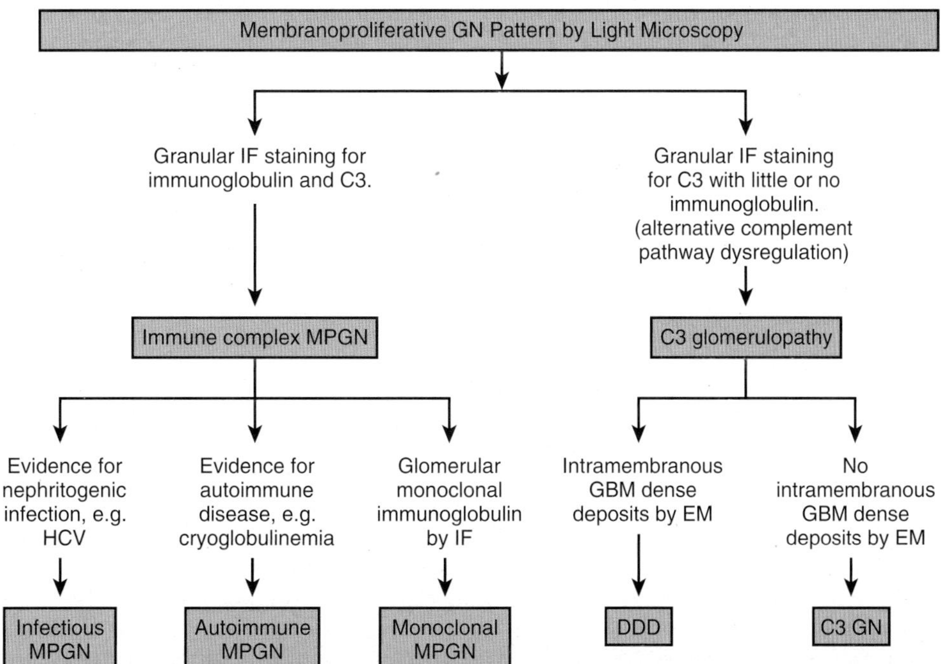


**Fig. 31.11** Algorithm for the histopathologic classification of membranoproliferative glomerulonephritis (MPGN) by immunofluorescence microscopy findings based on the presence of both immunoglobulin and C3 versus the presence of C3 with little or no immunoglobulin. This modified classification system also includes a category of diseases termed "C3 glomerulopathy," that includes dense deposit disease (DDD, formerly type II MPGN) and C3 glomerulonephritis, which comprises C3 glomerulopathy that does not have an MPGN pattern.

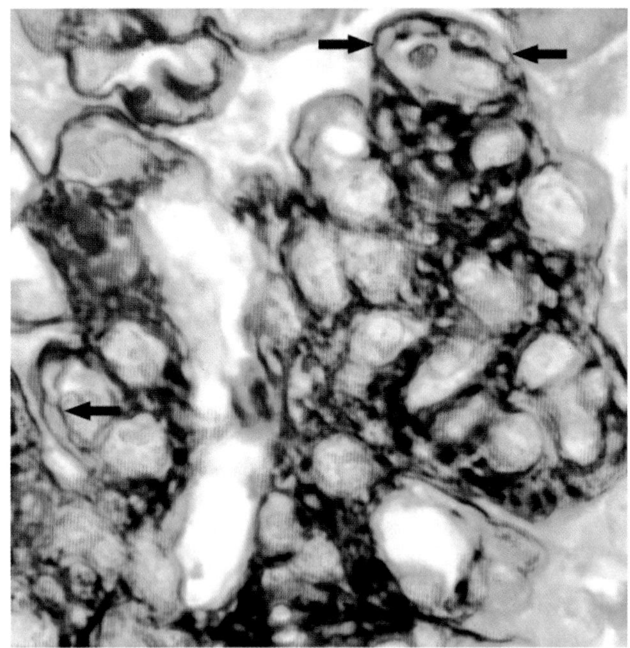

**Fig. 31.12** Light micrograph of a glomerular segment from a patient with type I membranoproliferative glomerulonephritis demonstrating doubling *(arrows)* and more complex replication of glomerular basement membranes. (Jones' methenamine silver stain, ×300.)

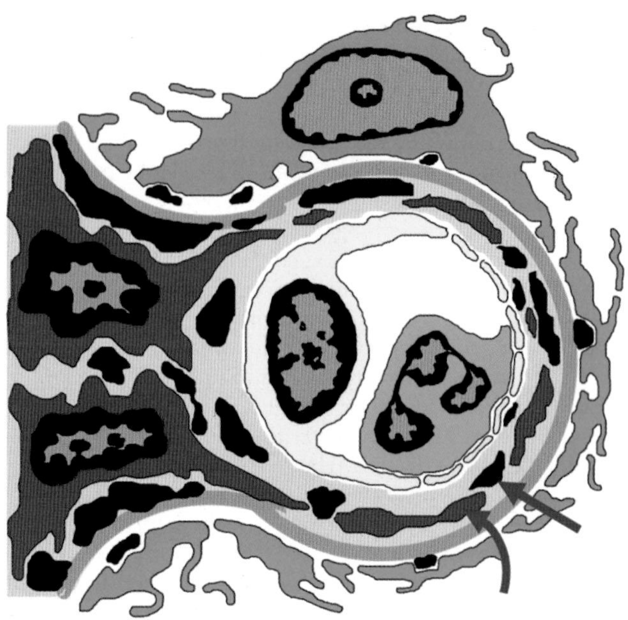

**Fig. 31.13** Diagram depicting the ultrastructural features of type I membranoproliferative glomerulonephritis. Note the subendothelial dense deposits *(straight arrow),* subendothelial mesangial cytoplasm interposition *(curved arrow),* and production of new basement material *(asterisk).* (Courtesy JC Jennette.)

A host of disorders may present as immune complex–mediated MPGN, including infections, malignancy, autoimmune disorders, and cryoglobulinemia. Rarely, immunotactoid-fibrillary GN and proliferative GN with monoclonal IgG deposits may present with a membranoproliferative pattern.[570] C3G results from a genetic or acquired dysregulation of the alternate complement pathway. C3 nephritic factor, anti-FH antibody, and monoclonal immunoglobulin are some of the acquired elements.[570–572]

## MEMBRANOPROLIFERATIVE GLOMERULONEPHRITIS TYPE I

### Pathology

**Light Microscopy.** The typical histologic features of type I MPGN are diffuse global capillary wall thickening, an increased mesangial matrix, and mesangial and endocapillary hypercellularity.[573,574] Infiltrating mononuclear leukocytes and neutrophils contribute to the glomerular hypercellularity. The consolidation of glomerular segments that results from these changes often causes an accentuation of the segmentation referred to as "hypersegmentation or lobulation." As a consequence, an earlier name for this phenotype of glomerular injury was "lobular glomerulonephritis." Markedly expanded mesangial regions may develop a nodular appearance with a central zone of sclerosis that may resemble that of diabetic glomerulosclerosis or monoclonal immunoglobulin deposition disease. However, the integration of light, IF, and electron microscopy findings differentiates type I MPGN from other diseases that can mimic it by light microscopy.

A distinctive but not completely specific feature of type I MPGN is doubling or more complex replication of GBMs that can be seen with stains that highlight basement membranes, such as Jones silver methenamine stain or periodic acid–Schiff stain (Fig. 31.12). This change is caused by the production of basement membrane material between and around projections of mesangial cytoplasm that extend into an expanded subendothelial zone, probably in response to the presence of subendothelial immune complex deposits (Fig. 31.13). The presence of so-called hyaline thrombi in capillary lumens should raise the possibility of cryoglobulinemia or lupus as the cause for the MPGN. Hyaline thrombi are not true thrombi but are aggregates of immune complexes filling capillary lumens. A minority of patients with type I MPGN have crescents, but these rarely involve more than 50% of glomeruli.[575,576] As with other types of glomerulonephritis, substantial crescent formation correlates with a more rapid progression of disease.[574]

As noted earlier, C3 glomerulopathy is divided into dense deposit disease (formerly type II MPGN) and C3 glomerulonephritis (see Fig. 31.11). C3 glomerulonephritis in turn is divided into the C3 glomerulopathy variant of type I MPGN, as well as other patterns of glomerulonephritis that do not fulfill the pathologic criteria for MPGN. Non-MPGN C3 glomerulonephritis often has focal or diffuse proliferative glomerulonephritis, with varying degrees of endocapillary and mesangial hypercellularity (Fig. 31.14).[568] Crescents may be present.

**Immunofluorescence Microscopy.** The characteristic pattern of IF staining is peripheral granular to band-like staining for complement, especially C3 (Fig. 31.15). The C3 staining is accompanied by substantial immunoglobulin staining in patients with immune complex MPGN. This positive IF corresponds to the prominent subendothelial immune deposits seen by electron microscopy. The staining pattern is less granular and less symmetric than that seen in MN. Mesangial granular staining may be conspicuous or inconspicuous. The hypersegmentation or lobulation seen by light microscopy often can be discerned by IF microscopy. A minority of patients

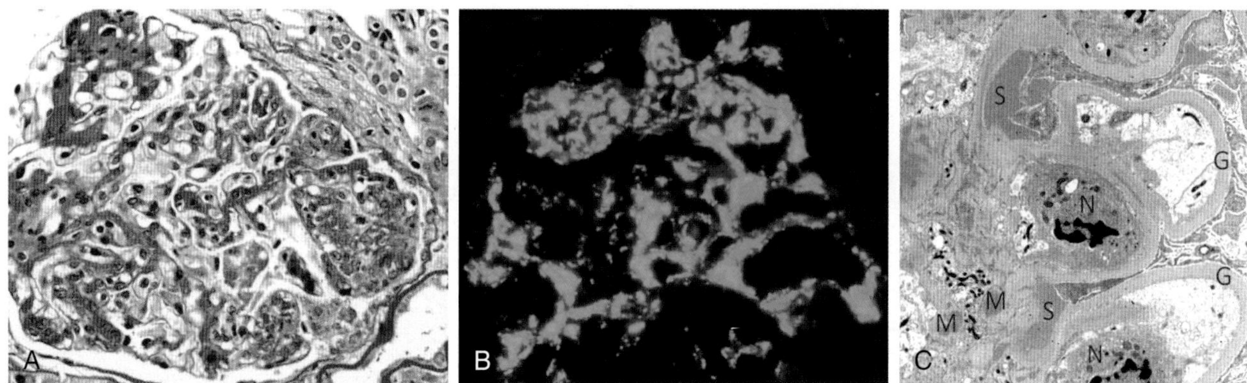


**Fig. 31.14** C3 glomerulonephritis variant of C3 glomerulopathy with light microscopy (A) showing segmental mesangial and endocapillary hypercellularity (periodic acid–Schiff stain). (B) Immunofluorescence (IF) microscopy showing granular capillary wall staining for C3 (there was no staining for immunoglobulin). (C) Electron microscopy demonstrating subepithelial electron dense deposits (S), mesangial dense deposits (M), influx of capillary neutrophils (N), and no intramembranous dense deposits in glomerular basement membranes (G).

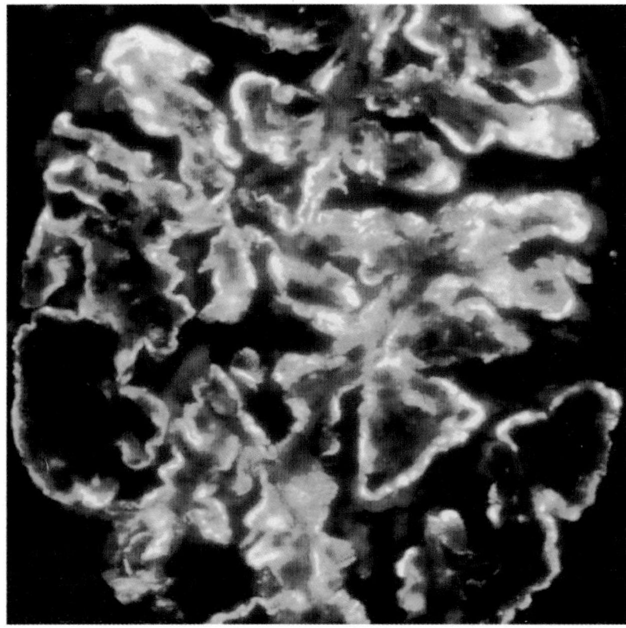

**Fig. 31.15** Immunofluorescence micrograph of a glomerulus with features of type I membranoproliferative glomerulonephritis showing global bandlike capillary wall staining for C3, as well as irregular mesangial staining. (Fluorescein isothiocyanate anti-C3 stain, ×300.)

with type I immune complex MPGN have staining along tubular basement membranes, in extraglomerular vessels, or both.

Most specimens with immune complex MPGN have more intense staining for C3 than for any immunoglobulin, but some specimens have more intense staining for IgG or IgM. Rare specimens have a predominance of IgA and can be considered an MPGN expression of IgA nephropathy. Intracapillary globular structures that stain intensely for immunoglobulin and complement correspond to the hyaline thrombi seen by light microscopy and raise the possibility of MPGN caused by lupus or cryoglobulinemia.

The C3 glomerulopathy variant of MPGN has little or no staining for immunoglobulin. However, Hou and associates[567] have noted that some specimens that seem appropriate for the C3 glomerulopathy category have minor staining for immunoglobulin rather than no staining. They have proposed a definition for C3 glomerulopathy that requires C3-dominant staining that is at least two orders of magnitude (on a scale of 0–3 or 0–4) more intense than any other immune reactant. In line with the evidence that C3 glomerulopathy is mediated by dysregulated activation of the alternative complement pathway, there is little or no staining for C4 or C1q in the C3 glomerulopathy variant of MPGN or in other histologic expressions of C3 glomerulonephritis.

**Electron Microscopy.** The ultrastructural hallmark of type I MPGN is mesangial interposition into an expanded subendothelial zone that contains electron-dense immune deposits (Fig. 31.16; see Fig. 31.13). This distinct pattern of mesangial and capillary involvement has prompted a synonym for type I MPGN, called "mesangiocapillary glomerulonephritis." New basement membrane material is formed around the subendothelial deposits and around the projections of mesangial cytoplasm, which is the basis for the basement membrane replication seen by light microscopy (see Fig. 31.12). Scattered mesangial dense deposits are usually found in association with mesangial hypercellularity and mesangial matrix expansion. Variable numbers of subepithelial electron-dense deposits occur. When they are numerous enough to resemble MN, some nephropathologists apply the diagnosis mixed membranous and proliferative glomerulonephritis or type III MPGN, as proposed by Burkholder and colleagues.[569] The term "type III MPGN" also has been applied to a very rare pattern of glomerular injury that resembles type I MPGN by light microscopy and IF microscopy, but is characterized ultrastructurally by irregularly thickened GBMs, with numerous intramembranous deposits of variable density.[577,578] Type III MPGN can be classified further as either immune complex disease or C3 glomerulopathy based on the presence or absence of staining for immunoglobulin. In the early application of the new classification system, type III MPGN as proposed by Burkholder and associates[569] tends to have an immune complex phenotype, whereas the other variant described by Strife and colleagues tends to have a C3 glomerulopathy phenotype.[577,578]

The hyaline thrombi seen by light microscopy appear as intraluminal spherical densities. When these structures, or any of the other electron-dense deposits, have a microtubular

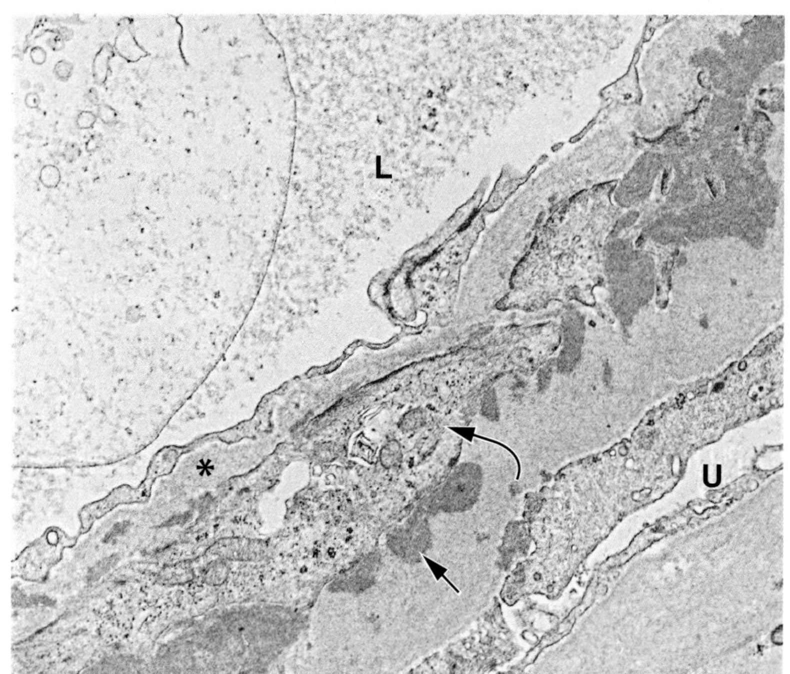


**Fig. 31.16** Electron micrograph of a capillary wall from a glomerulus with features of type I membranoproliferative glomerulonephritis. The capillary lumen (L) is in the upper left and the urinary space (U) is in the lower right. In the subendothelial zone are dense deposits *(straight arrow)*, extensions of mesangial cytoplasm *(curved arrow)*, and new basement membrane material *(asterisk)* (see Fig. 31.12). (×10,000.)

substructure, the possibility of cryoglobulinemic glomerulonephritis or immunotactoid glomerulopathy should be considered.

### Pathogenesis

As noted earlier, two major pathogenic pathways can cause the pathology pattern of glomerular injury called MPGN—immune complex localization and dysregulation of alternative pathway complement activation. A rare cause for this pattern is glomerular deposition of monoclonal immunoglobulin.

In the minority of patients with immune complex MPGN in whom the antigen has been identified, the sources have included infections, autoimmune diseases, neoplasms, and hereditary diseases (Box 31.7). The pathological finding of intense immune complex deposition with hypercellularity suggests that the inflammation caused by the immune complexes has resulted in both proliferation of mesangial and endothelial cells and the recruitment of inflammatory cells, including neutrophils and monocytes. These leukocytes are attracted to the glomerulus by activation of multiple mediator systems, including the complement system, cytokines, and chemokines.

Immune complex type I MGPN may be secondary to recognizable causes, such as cryoglobulinemia, hepatitis C, hepatitis B, osteomyelitis, subacute bacterial endocarditis, infected ventriculoatrial shunt, malignancies,[579–581] autoimmune disease (SLE or autoimmune thyroiditis[582]), light chain nephropathy,[583] and celiac sprue.[584] Serologic and clinical evidence of these processes should be sought. The precise percentage of patients with MPGN due to hepatitis C may vary according to geographic area and cultural factors. The observation that upper respiratory tract infections precede the onset of MPGN in as many as 50% of patients[585] raises the possibility that infectious agents contribute to the pathogenesis of many cases of type I MPGN.

**Box 31.7 Secondary Causes of Membranoproliferative Glomerulonephritis**

**Associated With Infection**

Hepatitis B and C
Visceral abscesses
Infective endocarditis
Shunt nephritis
Quartan malaria
*Schistosoma* nephropathy
*Mycoplasma* infection

**Associated With Rheumatologic Disease**

Systemic lupus erythematosus
Scleroderma
Sjögren syndrome
Sarcoidosis
Mixed essential cryoglobulinemia with or without hepatitis C infection
Anti–smooth muscle syndrome

**Associated With Malignancy**

Carcinoma
Lymphoma
Leukemia

**Associated With an Inherited Disorder**

$\alpha_1$-Antitrypsin deficiency
Complement deficiency (C2 or C3), with or without partial lipodystrophy

Modified from references 1106 and 1473 to 1481.

**Table 31.6 Selected Serologic Findings in Patients With Primary Glomerular Disease**

| Disease | C4 | C3 | ASO, ADNase B | Cryo Ig | aGBM | ANCA |
|---|---|---|---|---|---|---|
| Minimal change disease | N | N | — | — | — | — |
| Focal glomerulosclerosis | N | N | — | — | — | — |
| Membranous nephropathy | N | N | — | — | — | — |
| Membranoproliferative GN[a] | | | | | | |
| Type I | N or ↓↓ | ↓↓ | + | ++ | — | — |
| Type II | N | ↓↓↓ | + | — | — | — |
| Fibrillary GN | N | N | — | — | — | — |
| IgA nephropathy | N | N | — | — | — | — |
| Acute poststreptococcal GN | N or ↓ | ↓↓ | +++ | ++ | — | — |
| Crescentic GN | | | | | | |
| Anti-GBM | N | N | — | — | +++ | ± |
| Immune complex | N or ↓ | N or ↓↓ | — | N/++ | — | ± |
| ANCA-SVV | N | N | — | — | ± | +++ |

[a]Former MPGN classification schema.

*ANCA,* Antineutrophil cytoplasmic autoantibody; *aGBM,* anti-glomerular basement membrane antibody; *ASO,* antistreptolysin O; *ADNase B,* anti-deoxyribonuclease B; *cryo Ig,* cryoglobulins; *GBM,* glomerular basement membrane; *GN,* glomerulonephritis; *IgA,* immunoglobulin A; *N,* normal levels; *SVV,* small vessel vasculitis.

Modified from Jennette JC, Nickeleit V. Anti-glomerular basement membrane glomerulonephritis and Goodpasture's syndrome. In: Jennette JC, Olson JL, Schwartz MM, eds. *Heptinstall's Pathology of the Kidney.* 6th ed. Philadelphia: Lippincott Williams & Wilkins; 2006.

When immune complex type I MPGN is secondary to other disease processes such as malignancy or a rheumatic condition, the laboratory results associated with the systemic disease (e.g., SLE) are positive (e.g., antibodies to double-stranded DNA[586]; see Chapters 32 and 33). MPGN type I is also associated with underlying complement deficiency, notably of C2 and C3,[587] as well as deficiency in $\alpha_1$-antitrypsin.[586]

Even before recognition of the distinct C3 glomerulopathy variant of type I MPGN, alterations in circulating complement levels had been observed in MPGN patients (Table 31.6). The C3 level is persistently depressed in approximately 75% of MPGN patients.[564,573,588–590] This is in contrast to poststreptococcal glomerulonephritis, in which depressed C3 levels typically return to normal within 2 months.[591–593] The persistent depression of C3 levels and the presence of nephritic syndrome should suggest type I MPGN. In some patients, activation of the alternative pathway is suggested by the observation that C3 levels are depressed, whereas levels of the classical pathway activators C1q and C4 are normal. Patients with this complement profile are likely to have a C3 glomerulopathy variant of MPGN. However, when MPGN is caused by cryoglobulinemia, which is an immune complex MPGN, there may be more depression of C4 than C3.[593]

### Epidemiology

Most patients with MPGN are children between the ages of 8 and 16 years[585] accounting for 90% of cases of MPGN type I. The proportions of males and females are nearly equal.[564,565,573,577,594–600]

### Clinical Features

Type I MPGN, characterized by deposits of electron-dense material in the subendothelial zones of glomeruli, is a very heterogeneous disorder. Some combination of proteinuria (often nephrotic range), hematuria, hypertension, and renal failure are usually present.

### Treatment

The prognosis of type I MPGN has been reviewed and described in several reports.[564,573,601,602] Actuarial renal survival 10 years after renal biopsy has been calculated with life-table analysis to be 60% to 65% in type I MCGN, without significant differences between treated and untreated patients.[564] Nonnephrotic patients have an improved 10-year renal survival of 85%.[573] A minority of patients may have a spontaneous remission.[564] The features suggestive of poor prognosis in MPGN type I include hypertension,[600,603] impaired GFR,[600,603–605] and the appearance of cellular crescents in biopsy specimens.[573,605,606]

The treatment of type I MPGN is based on the underlying cause of the disease process. Thus, the therapy for MPGN associated with cryoglobulinemia and hepatitis C should be aimed at treating the hepatitis C virus infection, whereas the treatment of MPGN associated with lupus or scleroderma should be based on the principles of care for those rheumatologic conditions. Most recommendations for the treatment of type I MPGN have been derived from studies involving children.[607–613] West has touted the benefits of continuous prednisone therapy for improved renal survival.[609] Whether the benefit of low-dose prednisone therapy is seen only in children or whether similar effects can be achieved in adults has never been investigated in a prospective randomized trial. However, low-dose, alternate-day prednisone therapy may improve renal function.[611,612]

In addition to glucocorticoids, a number of other immunosuppressive and anticoagulant therapies have been used in the treatment of type I MPGN. Initial reports have indicated that treatment with aspirin and dipyridamole has a positive effect on renal survival.[565] This approach was widely accepted; however, statistical design flaws led to a reanalysis of the data, which revealed no difference in the treatment and control groups with respect to long-term outcome.[588] A subsequent study using aspirin with dipyridamole demonstrated a slight decrease in urine protein excretion by 3 years but no effect on renal function.[614] Treatment with dipyridamole, aspirin, and warfarin, with and without cyclophosphamide, was examined in both controlled and uncontrolled studies.[461,565,613–618] A regimen of warfarin, dipyridamole and cyclophosphamidekincaid[613] was suggested to improve long-term renal survival based on a retrospective analysis; however, a controlled trial in Canada has demonstrated no benefit of this approach.[286]

The use of MMF and corticosteroids has been suggested based on uncontrolled and anecdotal observations.[619] In patients with a defined underlying disease (e.g., neoplasia or hepatitis B or C), treatment should be directed at the underlying condition.[620,621] Type I MPGN is significantly ameliorated by the use of cyclosporine in the very rare condition known as "Buckley syndrome."[104,105,622]

## MEMBRANOPROLIFERATIVE GLOMERULONEPHRITIS TYPE III

Type III MPGN occurs in a very small number of children and young adults. Regardless of the pathologic distinctions of MPGN type III of Burkholder and colleagues[596] and Strife and colleagues,[578] few distinguishing clinical characteristics are noted in these patients. These patients may have clinical features of disease quite similar to those of type I MPGN, and the long-term clinical course is similar as well. Patients with MPGN described by Strife and associates[578] have low C3 levels in the absence of C3 nephritic factor. Patients with nonnephrotic proteinuria do better than patients who have nephrotic syndrome.

## C3 GLOMERULOPATHIES (DENSE DEPOSIT DISEASE AND C3 GLOMERULONEPHRITIS)

### Epidemiology

DDD (formerly MPGN II) accounts for about 25% of MPGN in children but is much less common in adults. The large majority of patients are children between the ages of 8 and 16 years[585] and account for about 70% of cases. It is estimated to affect 2 to 3 persons per million. Males and females were reported to be similarly affected in some studies,[623] whereas others reported a female predominance.[573,624,625] A retrospective of 32 cases identified through the nephropathology laboratory at Columbia University between 1977 and 2007 reported that 43% of patients were children, of whom 65% were between the ages of 5 and 10 years, and 22% of patients were adults older than 60 years. The female-to-male ratio was 1.9, and 85% of patients were Caucasian.[626] It is unclear whether the unexpectedly high representation of older adults in this cohort reflects a change in the demographics of the disease or a change in biopsy practices or selection or referral bias in this or the older studies.

C3 glomerulonephritis includes all patients with C3 glomerulopathy who do not have intramembranous dense deposits that warrant a diagnosis of DDD; this includes the C3 glomerulopathy variant of MPGN, as well as other patterns of proliferative glomerulonephritis. There is a relative paucity of epidemiologic data given that this is a rather new diagnostic category; however, one study of 19 patients with C3 glomerulonephritis revealed a median age at onset of 29.9 years (range, 7–70 years).[627] A larger and more recent study of 88 patients with C3 glomerulopathy in the United Kingdom, including 59 patients with C3 glomerulonephritis and 21 with DDD, has revealed that patients with C3 glomerulonephritis are significantly older (median age, 26 years vs.12 years; $P = .002$).[628]

### Pathology

The term *dense deposit disease* emphasizes the pathognomonic feature of discontinuous electron-dense bands in the GBM[568,574] (Figs. 31.17 and 31.18). These are accompanied by spherical to irregular mesangial dense deposits and occasional subendothelial and subepithelial deposits, some of which resemble the humps seen in postinfectious glomerulonephritis. Dense

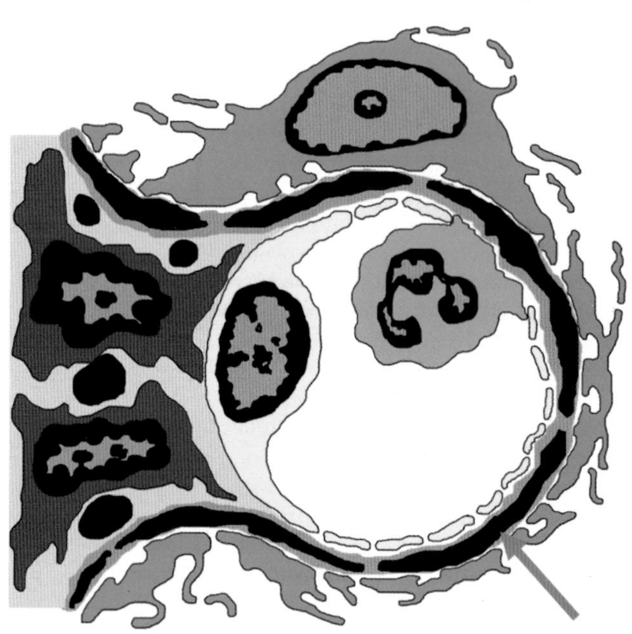

**Fig. 31.17** Diagram depicting a glomerular capillary loop with features of dense deposit disease, with bandlike intramembranous dense deposits *(arrow)* and spherical mesangial dense deposits. (Courtesy JC Jennette.)

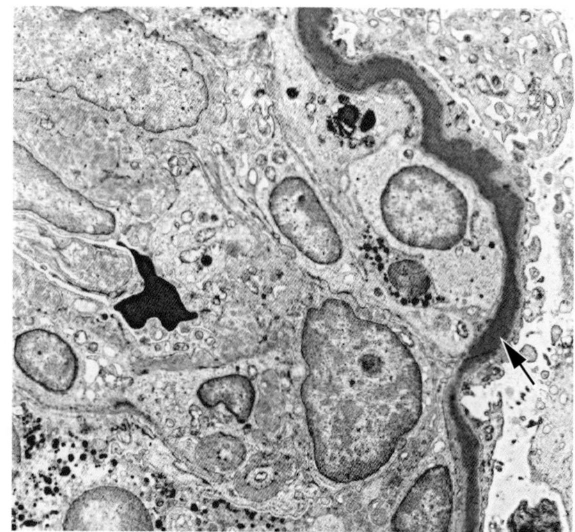

**Fig. 31.18** Electron micrograph of a glomerular capillary from a patient with dense deposit disease showing a bandlike intramembranous dense deposit that has essentially replaced the normal glomerular basement membrane. Also note the endocapillary hypercellularity. (×5000.)

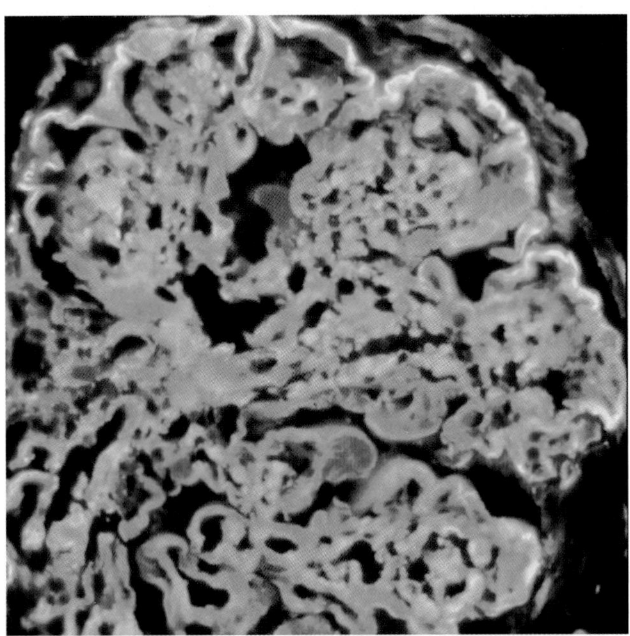

Fig. 31.19 Immunofluorescence micrograph of a glomerulus with dense deposit disease demonstrating discontinuous band-like capillary wall staining and coarsely granular mesangial staining for C3. (Fluorescein isothiocyanate anti-C3 stain, ×500.)

deposits also may be identified in Bowman's capsule and tubular basement membranes.

Immunofluorescence microscopy demonstrates intense capillary wall linear to bandlike staining for C3 (Fig. 31.19), with little or no staining for immunoglobulin.[567,568,629,630] The capillary wall staining may have a fine double contour, with outlining of the outer and inner aspects of the dense deposits. The mesangial deposits usually appear as scattered spherules or rings, with the latter resulting from staining of the outer surface but not the interior of the spherical deposits. There typically is intense staining for C3, with little or no staining for C4, C1q, or immunoglobulins.

The light microscopic appearance of DDD is much more variable than that of type I MPGN and often does not have a membranoproliferative appearance.[568] Thus the term "DDD" is preferable to the term "type II MPGN."[630,631] In a review of a large number of renal biopsy specimens obtained in North America, Europe, and Japan from patients with DDD, the light microscopy findings could be classified into five distinct patterns: (1) membranoproliferative pattern; (2) mesangioproliferative pattern; (3) crescentic pattern; (4) acute proliferative and exudative pattern; and (5) unclassified DDD. Of these, the mesangioproliferative lesion characterized by focal segmental and mesangial hypercellularity accounted for about 50% of the cases reviewed, with 28% presenting with a membranoproliferative pattern (type I) and 20% with a crescentic lesion. Although the patients' ages ranged from 3 to 67 years, nearly 75% of the patients were younger than 20 years of age, and all patients with crescentic DDD or acute proliferative DDD were between the ages of 3 and 18 years.[631] Therefore, the histologic appearance of DDD can mimic many other categories of glomerulonephritis, and the findings by IF and especially electron microscopy are required for accurate diagnosis.

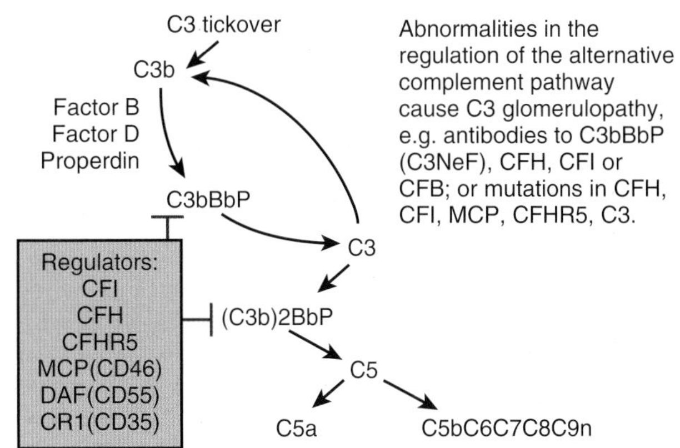


Fig. 31.20 Regulators of the alternative complement pathway and abnormalities that cause C3 glomerulopathy. *CF,* Complement factor.

As described earlier in this chapter, the pathology of the non-DDD category of C3 glomerulopathy (i.e., C3 glomerulonephritis) is extremely variable by light microscopy, but falls in the spectrum of type I MPGN, to focal or diffuse proliferative to mesangial proliferative glomerulonephritis (see Fig. 31.14).[568] As one of the variants of C3 glomerulopathy, there is C3 dominant staining by IF microscopy, with little or no staining for immunoglobulin, C4, or C1q. By definition, electron microscopy of C3 glomerulonephritis does not reveal the typical intramembranous dense deposits that are diagnostic for DDD. However, this is a somewhat subjective division, and borderline specimens are difficult to classify as DDD versus C3 glomerulonephritis. From a practical perspective, this may not be important because both are variants of C3 glomerulopathy and have similar pathogenesis and clinical features.

### Pathogenesis

As C3 glomerulopathies, DDD and C3 glomerulonephritis share a pathogenic mechanism that involves abnormal regulation of the alternative complement pathway (reviewed by Bomback and Appel).[632]

A porcine model of DDD has suggested that there is massive deposition of C3 and the terminal C5b-9 complement complex—the membrane attack complex. In the circulation, there is extensive complement activation, with very low C3 levels and high levels of circulating terminal complement components. No immunoglobulin deposits were detected in kidney tissue. In this animal model of DDD, the pathogenetic mechanism does not appear to involve immune complexes, but rather uses some other mechanism for the activation of complement and the trapping of activating complement components in the GBM.[633]

The hypocomplementemia in DDD and other forms of C3 glomerulopathy reflects dysregulated activation of the alternative complement pathway (Fig. 31.20). Under normal circumstances, the alternative complement pathway maintains low-level basal activity, termed *tickover,* which maintains C3 convertase. Any disruption in C3 convertase activity can thereby alter tickover and result in overactivation. Three distinct mechanisms result in uncontrolled activation of C3 convertase: (1) the development of an autoantibody, the C3 nephritic factor (C3NeF); (2) the absence of circulating regulators (e.g., factor H); and (3) the presence of a circulating inhibitor of factor H.[633] The most common of these is the presence of the autoantibody C3NeF. C3NeF is an antibody that protects C3 convertase (C3bBb) from dissociation by factor H and thus prolongs its half-life by 10-fold.[634] It does so in one of two ways, by binding to C3bBb or to IgG-C3b-C3bBb of the assembled convertase. The stabilization of this complex results in perpetual C3 breakdown. It is tempting to incriminate this factor as central to the pathogenesis of MPGN, especially DDD, because most affected patients harbor C3NeF in their circulation. However, C3NeF does not always correlate with disease activity and, more importantly, progressive kidney damage still occurs in patients who have normal levels of complement.[635–637] Interestingly, autoantibodies to other complement components such as factor B, factor H, factor I, or component of C3 convertase (C3b and/or CFB) can also be seen in some individuals.[632,638,639] More recently, reclassification of MPGN was strongly proposed by Sethi and colleagues,[640,641] who found higher level alternative and terminal complement pathway components, as identified by mass spectrometry, directly within the glomeruli of patients with DDD as compared with those from patients with immune complex–mediated forms of MPGN, as well as healthy individuals.

Normal protective, or regulatory, mechanisms control C3bBb levels and complement deposition, of which factor H is one of the most important. Factor H is a soluble glycoprotein that regulates complement in the fluid phase and on cell surfaces by binding to C3b.[642] Some mutations in factor H result in C3 glomerulopathy that does not have an MPGN pattern.[643,644]

The genetics of DDD are complex. Only a few families have been identified with more than one affected member, although families exist with one patient with DDD and other members affected by other autoimmune diseases. The most robust genetic association with DDD is a deficiency of factor H, associated with a mutation of the complement factor H (*CFH*) gene.[645,646] Another study has identified a family with DDD in which a C3 convertase-resistant C3 gene mutation was identified in a mother and her identical twin sons, thereby resulting in alternative complement pathway activation.[647]

C3 glomerulonephritis is a result of overactivity of the alternative complement pathway due to autoantibodies to and/or mutations in critical regulators of the pathway.[568] The underlying genetic defect in C3 glomerulonephritis has been identified in some hereditary forms of the disease such as CFHR5 nephropathy, and further insight is likely to occur rapidly given intense interest in this area.[648–650]

### Clinical Features

Patients with DDD may have hematuria, proteinuria, or both. They may have a nephrotic or acute nephritic syndrome. At least one-third of patients have all the components of the nephrotic syndrome on presentation. Microhematuria is present in the overwhelming majority of patients, whereas gross hematuria occurs only in about 15%.[626] Finally, 25% of patients have acute nephritic syndrome associated with red cells and red call casts in the urine, hypertension, and renal insufficiency.[564,573,588,589] Hypertension is typically mild, but may be severe in some cases. Kidney dysfunction occurs in at least 50% of cases and is more common among adults than in children.[626] When present at the outset of disease, kidney dysfunction portends a poor prognosis.

Hypocomplementemia of the C3 factor is present in 80% to 90% of patients with DDD. In a retrospective review from Columbia University, depressed C3 levels occurred in 100% of children, but only in 41% of adults ($P$= .001).[626] Depressed C4 levels were very uncommon in both age groups. C3 hypocomplementemia is prolonged in patients with DDD[467] and is associated with decrements in terminal complement components C5b-9. C3NeF is present in more than 80% of patients.

Respiratory tract infections precede cases of MPGN in 50% of patients, especially in children.[626] On rare occasions, the onset can be triggered by a streptococcal infection, so that the disease mimics acute poststreptococcal glomerulonephritis except for the persistence of C3 hypocomplementemia beyond 8 weeks from onset.[651] Comorbid conditions may be seen in adult patients with DDD, including plasma cell dyscrasias, which were noted in 4 of 18 patients (22%) in the Columbia University review.[626]

Patients with DDD may have deposits in the retina, along Bruch's membrane, that are similar in structure and composition to the deposits in GBM. These whitish yellow drusen develop at an early age. Initially, drusen have little impact on visual acuity, but visual loss can occur in about 10% of patients.[652] A careful retinal examination is therefore indicated in all patients with proven DDD. There is no correlation between the severity of kidney and ocular involvement; however, patients with other forms of MPGN do not typically have drusen.[653]

DDD may be associated with the syndrome of acquired partial lipodystrophy.[637] About 80% of patients with this syndrome have low C3 levels and C3NeF. About 20% of patients develop MPGN, although the lipodystrophy and glomerular disease may occur several years apart.[654] The link between acquired partial lipodystrophy and MPGN stems from the production by adipocytes of C3, factor B, and factor D (adepsine) whose function is the cleavage of factor B. In the presence of C3NeF, the alternative pathway of complement activation is dysregulated, leading to the destruction of adipocytes.[654]

Patients with C3 glomerulonephritis, as also seen with DDD, can present with hypertension, azotemia, hematuria, and proteinuria, with or without nephrotic syndrome. Interestingly, although C3 levels are usually low and C4 levels are normal, the large study of 59 patients with C3 glomerulonephritis in the United Kingdom found that C3 was more likely to be normal when compared with patients with DDD (52% vs. 11%; $P$= .003); therefore, a normal C3 level alone does not exclude C3 glomerulonephritis.[628,641] As with DDD, some patients may have C3NeF.[627,632,655]

### Treatment

The prognosis for DDD is worse than that for type I MPGN. The less favorable prognosis is in accord with a higher frequency of crescentic glomerulonephritis and chronic tubulointerstitial nephritis at the time of biopsy in DDD.[603,656,657] In DDD, clinical remissions are rare,[573,594] occurring in fewer than 5% of children. Patients generally reach ESKD in 8 to 12 years from the onset of disease. In DDD, the prognosis is worse in adults than in children.[626]

There is currently no widely agreed on treatment of DDD, and the available information that remains is based on small case series. Inhibition of angiotensin II may be helpful, but it has not been formally tested.[626] The use of corticosteroid therapy is probably not effective.[645] Immunosuppressive therapy with agents such as MMF and rituximab aimed at reducing C3NeF in DDD has been suggested.[658] It is not likely that immunosuppression, with or without plasma exchange, will be beneficial, except perhaps if an inhibitory autoantibody to complement factor H is present. There are reports of effective treatment of patients with defined deficiency of complement factor H with infusion of fresh-frozen plasma every 14 days to provide functionally intact factor H.[655,659–662] In a proof of concept study in mice genetically deficient in complement factor H, treatment with purified human complement factor H resulted in rapid normalization of plasma C3 levels and resolution of the GBM C3 deposition.[663] Based on the current understanding of the pathogenesis of DDD, inhibition of C5 activation and formation of the terminal component of complement activation (C5b-9) with the monoclonal antibody eculizumab would be theoretically beneficial. However, evidence for this approach had been lacking until a proof of concept efficacy and safety study in three patients with DDD and three patients with C3 glomerulonephritis treated in an open-label fashion with eculizumab.[661] This resulted in reduced serum creatinine levels in two subjects, reduction in proteinuria in one subject, and histopathologic improvement in one subject. It also appeared that elevated levels of the serum membrane attack complex might predict treatment response.[542]

Given that C3 glomerulonephritis represents a new diagnostic category, treatment protocols outside of supportive care are limited but will likely involve targeted therapies that correct complement dysregulation now that pathogenetic mechanisms are becoming increasingly understood. As one example, a proof of concept efficacy and safety study in three patients with DDD and three patients with C3 glomerulonephritis treated in an open-label fashion with eculizumab resulted in reduced serum creatinine levels in two subjects, reduction in proteinuria in one subject, and histopathologic improvement in one subject. It also appeared that elevated levels of the serum membrane attack complex might predict treatment response.[664]

Data are also limited with regards to prognosis; however, the study by Servais and colleagues would suggest that prognosis is poor, but possibly better than that of DDD. Of the 19 patients with C3 glomerulonephritis, 3 progressed to ESKD at the time of the study, and 6 had a creatinine clearance less than 60 mL/min.[665] It was also found in a cohort of 134 patients with C3 glomerulopathy in France, in which roughly 25% of patients with C3 glomerulonephritis progressed to ESKD over a follow-up period of 10 years.[665] Sethi and colleagues reported on 12 patients with C3 glomerulonephritis, with a mean follow-up of 26.4 months, that kidney function remained stable in every patient, except for 1 who progressed to dialysis soon after presentation.[641] With regard to kidney transplantation, one group reported their experience with 21 patients with ESKD due to C3 glomerulonephritis who underwent kidney transplantation. In this study, 14 patients (68%) developed recurrent C3 glomerulonephritis in the allograft, which was typically manifested by hematuria and proteinuria, and median time to recurrence was 28 months. Furthermore, 50% of patients with recurrent C3 glomerulonephritis experienced graft failure, with a median time to graft failure of 77 months.[666] Recurrences in those with kidney transplants for DDD are common, 80% or higher,[594,667–669] especially in the presence of C3NeF or CFH mutations.[670] Prophylactic plasma infusions or simultaneous liver transplantation can be beneficial in the latter cases.[659,660] Levels of C3 in the serum do not seem to predict recurrences.[670] Fig. 31.21 depicts a current framework for the diagnosis and management of C3 glomerulopathy, which is likely to be refined even further as additional pathogenetic insight occurs.

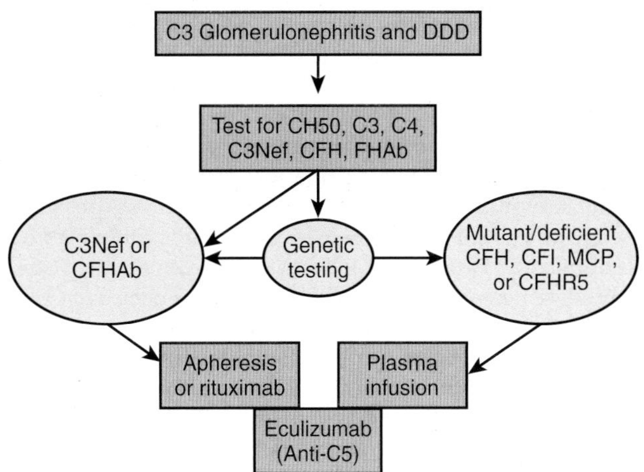


**Fig. 31.21** A framework for the diagnosis and management of C3 glomerulopathies, C3 glomerulonephritis, and dense deposit disease (DDD). *Ab,* Antibody; *CF,* complement factor; *C3Nef,* C3 nephritic factor.

## ACUTE POSTSTREPTOCOCCAL GLOMERULONEPHRITIS

### EPIDEMIOLOGY

Acute poststreptococcal glomerulonephritis (PSGN) is a disease that affects primarily children, with a peak incidence in those between the ages of 2 and 6 years. Children younger than 2 years and adults older than 40 years account for only about 15% of patients with acute PSGN. Interestingly, evidence has pointed to acute PSGN as the cause of Wolfgang Amadeus Mozart's early death at the age of 35.[671] Subclinical microscopic hematuria may be four times more common than overt acute PSGN, as documented in studies of family members of affected patients.[672–674] Only rarely do PSGN and rheumatic fever occur concomitantly.[675] Males are more likely than females to have overt nephritis. Acute PSGN may occur as part of an epidemic or sporadic disease. During epidemic infections of streptococci of proven nephrogenicity, the clinical attack rate appears to be about 12%,[676–678] but has been reported at 33%[679] or even as high as 38% in certain affected families.[674]

Differences in incidence rates among different families argue for the existence of host genetic susceptibility factors affecting the propensity for overt nephritis.[680] An association was found between PSGN and HLA-DRW4,[680] HLA-DPA*02-022, and DPB1*05-01[681] and, more recently, DRB1*03011.[682]

The rate of acute PSGN after sporadic infections with group A streptococci of potentially nephritogenic types is quite variable,[683,684] which again points to an effect of ill-defined host factors. A minority of streptococcal infections lead to nephritic syndrome, which argues for the presence of certain nephritogenic characteristics of the offending agent. In the 1950s, Rammelkamp and colleagues[683,684] identified certain strains of streptococci within Lancefield group A, in particular type XII, that are capable of leading to an acute glomerulonephritis. Other nephritogenic serotypes include M types 1, 2, 3, 4, 18, 25, 31, 49, 52, 55, 56, 57, 59, 60 and 61. There are differences among these serotypes in their propensity to be associated with nephritis, depending on the site of infection. Certain strains, such as types 2, 49, 55, 57, and 60, are usually associated with nephritis after pyoderma,[685,686] whereas M type 49 can lead to nephritis after pharyngitis or pyoderma.[686] In addition to occurring after infection with group A beta-hemolytic streptococci, acute PSGN has also been described after infection with group C streptococci and possibly group G streptococci.[687,688]

Acute PSGN has been on the decline in developed countries, but it continues to occur in developing communities.[689,690] Epidemic PSGN is frequently associated with skin infections, whereas pharyngitides are associated with sporadic PSGN in developed countries. Overt glomerulonephritis is found in about 10% of children at risk, but when one includes subclinical disease, as evidenced by microscopic hematuria, about 25% of children at risk are found to be affected.[691,692] In some developing countries, acute PSGN remains the most common form of acute nephritic syndrome among children. The incidence rate appears to follow a cyclic pattern, with outbreaks occurring about every 10 years.[693] A review of 11 published population-based studies has estimated the median incidence of PSGN in children to be 24 cases per 100,000 person-years, based on studies that examined populations in less developed countries or included substantial minority populations in more developed countries; the incidence in adults was conservatively estimated to be 2 cases per 100,000 person-years in less developed countries and 0.3 cases per 100,000 person-years in more developed countries.[694] The authors of this review have estimated that over 470,000 cases of acute PSGN occur annually, leading to approximately 5000 deaths (1% of total cases), 97% of which are in less developed countries.

Interestingly, the epidemiology of PSGN in Florida appears to have changed in the last 2 decades. Compared with the 1960s and 1970s, pharyngitis has replaced impetigo as the predominant underlying infection, a shift has occurred in racial distribution (now predominantly Caucasians are affected) and in seasonal variation, and the severity of disease has decreased.[695] These changes are thought to reflect a change in the causal agent of impetigo.[695]

## PATHOLOGY

### Light Microscopy

The pathologic appearance of acute PSGN varies during the course of the disease. The acute histologic change is the influx of neutrophils, which results in diffuse global hypercellularity (Fig. 31.22).[696–700] Endocapillary proliferation of mesangial cells and endothelial cells also contributes to the hypercellularity. The hypercellularity often is very marked and results in enlarged consolidated glomeruli. The description "acute diffuse proliferative glomerulonephritis" often is used as a pathologic designation for this stage of acute PSGN. A minority of patients has a crescent formation, which usually affects only a small proportion of glomeruli.[701] Extensive crescent formation is rare.[702,703] Special stains that have differential reactions with immune deposits may demonstrate

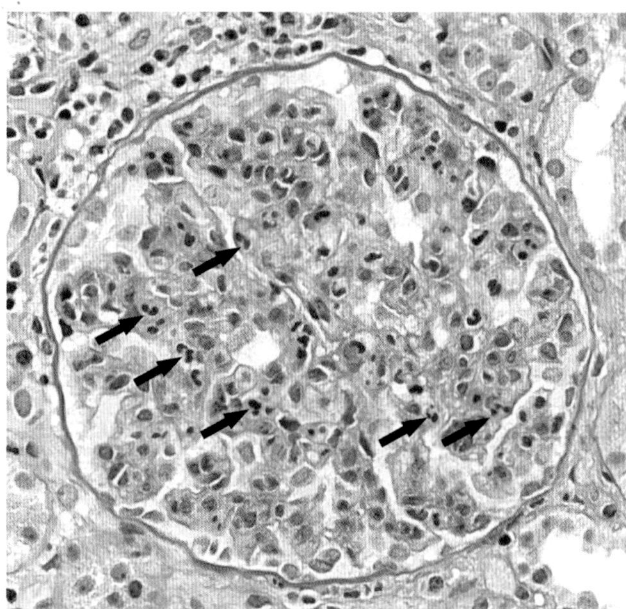

**Fig. 31.22** Light micrograph of a glomerulus with acute post-streptococcal glomerulonephritis demonstrating marked influx of neutrophils *(arrows)*. (Periodic acid–Schiff stain, ×300.)

subepithelial deposits. For example, the subepithelial deposits may stain red (fuchsinophilic) with Masson trichrome stain.

Interstitial edema and interstitial infiltration of predominantly mononuclear leukocytes usually are present and occasionally are pronounced, especially with unusually severe disease associated with crescents. Focal tubular epithelial cell simplification (flattening) also may accompany severe disease. Arteries and arterioles typically have no acute changes, although preexisting sclerotic changes may be present in older patients.

During the resolving phase of self-limited PSGN, which usually begins within several weeks of onset, the infiltrating neutrophils disappear, and endothelial hypercellularity resolves, leaving behind only mesangial hypercellularity.[696,704] This mesangioproliferative stage often is present in patients with PSGN who have had resolution of nephritis but have persistent isolated proteinuria, and it may persist for several months in patients who have complete clinical resolution. There may be focal segmental glomerular scarring as sequelae of particularly injurious inflammation, but this is seldom extensive, except in the rare patient with crescentic PSGN. Ultimately, the pathologic changes of acute PSGN can resolve completely.[704,705]

### Immunofluorescence Microscopy

IF microscopy demonstrates glomerular immune complex deposits in PSGN.[697,699,700,706] The pattern and composition of deposits change during the course of PSGN. During the acute diffuse proliferative phase of the disease, there is diffuse global coarsely granular capillary wall and mesangial staining, which usually is very intense for C3, and of varying degrees for IgG from intense to absent (Fig. 31.23). Staining for IgM and IgA is less frequent and is usually less intense. In self-limited disease, biopsy should be performed later in the disease course because it is more likely that the staining will be predominantly or exclusively for C3, with little or

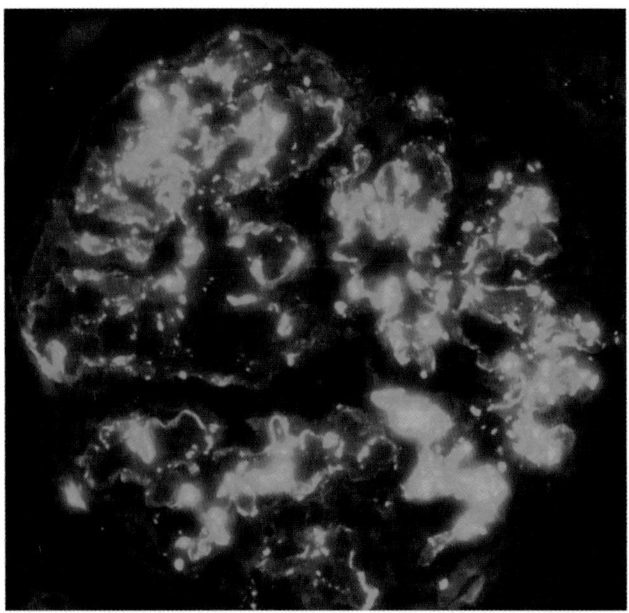

**Fig. 31.23** Immunofluorescence micrograph of a glomerular segment from a patient with acute poststreptococcal glomerulonephritis showing coarsely granular capillary wall staining for C3. Compare this to the finely granular capillary wall staining of membranous nephropathy in Fig. 31.9. (Fluorescein isothiocyanate anti-C3 stain, ×300.)

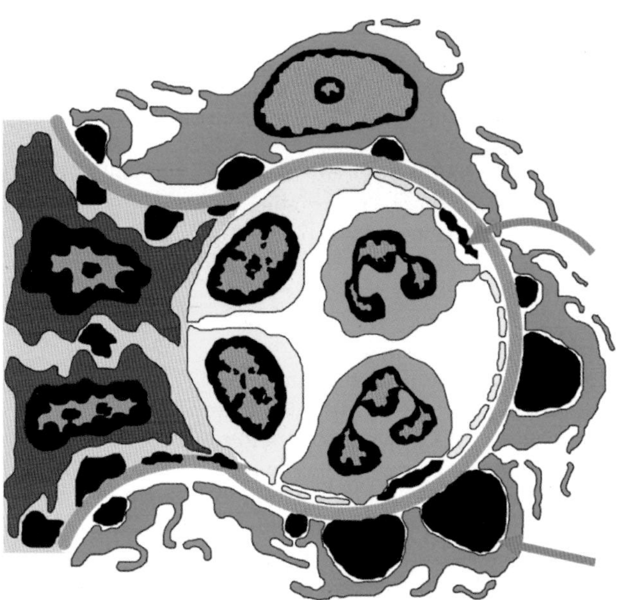

**Fig. 31.24** Diagram of the ultrastructural features of acute poststreptococcal glomerulonephritis. Note the subepithelial humplike dense deposits *(straight arrow),* subendothelial deposits *(curved arrow),* and mesangial deposits. There is endocapillary hypercellularity caused by neutrophil infiltration and endothelial and mesangial proliferation. (Courtesy JC Jennette.)

no immunoglobulin staining. Because most patients with uncomplicated new-onset acute PSGN do not undergo kidney biopsy, most biopsy specimens are obtained later in the course, when there is diagnostic uncertainty due to equivocal serologic confirmation or unusually aggressive or persistent clinical features. At this time, IF microscopy staining is usually predominantly for C3. This may reflect termination of nephritogenic immune complex localization in the kidney, with masking of residual complexes by complement. An alternative explanation for the presence of C3 in the absence of immunoglobulin is activation of complement or blockade of complement regulatory mechanisms by factors released by the infection. This could initiate a pathogenic mechanism similar to that in C3 glomerulopathy. The continued presence of intense staining for IgG 1 month or more into the course of what otherwise looks like pathologically typical PSGN is cause for concern that the process will not be self-limited.

Several patterns of immune staining have been described but are of limited prognostic value.[697,700,707] The garland pattern is characterized by numerous large, closely apposed granular deposits along the capillary walls. Patients with this pattern usually have nephrotic-range proteinuria as a component of their disease. The starry sky pattern has more scattered granular staining, which corresponds somewhat to less severe disease. The mesangial pattern, especially when it is predominantly C3 staining, corresponds to the resolving phase, with a mesangioproliferative light microscopic appearance.

### Electron Microscopy

The hallmark ultrastructural feature of PSGN is the subepithelial humplike dense deposits (Figs. 31.24 and 31.25).[699,704–706,708] However, small subendothelial and mesangial dense deposits can usually be identified with careful observation and theoretically may be more important in the pathogenesis of the

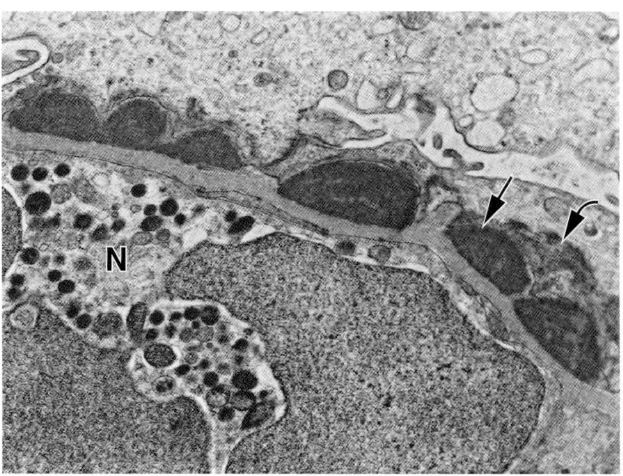


**Fig. 31.25** Electron micrograph of a portion of a glomerular capillary from a patient with acute poststreptococcal glomerulonephritis showing subepithelial dense deposits *(straight arrow),* condensation of cytoskeleton in adjacent podocyte cytoplasm *(small curved arrow),* and a neutrophil (N) marginated against the basement membrane, with no intervening endothelial cytoplasm. (×5000.)

disease, especially the neutrophilic influx and endocapillary proliferative response, than are the subepithelial humps. The subepithelial humps are covered by effaced epithelial foot processes, which usually contain condensed cytoskeletal filaments (including actin) that form a corona around the immune deposits (Fig. 31.25). Similar humps are observed in C3 glomerulopathy. During the acute phase, capillary lumens often contain marginated neutrophils, some of which are in direct contact with GBMs (see Fig. 31.25). Lesser numbers of monocytes and macrophages contribute to the leukocyte influx. Mesangial regions are expanded by increased numbers of mesangial cells and leukocytes, as well as increased matrix material and varying amounts of electron-dense material.

During the resolution phase, usually 6 to 8 weeks into the course, the subepithelial humps disappear, leaving behind only mesangial and sometimes a few scattered subendothelial and intramembranous dense deposits. The subepithelial deposits first become electron-lucent and then disappear completely. The humps in peripheral capillary loops disappear before the humps in the subepithelial zone adjacent to the perimesangial basement membrane.

## PATHOGENESIS

Acute PSGN is the prototype disease of an acute glomerulonephritis associated with an infectious cause. The first description of this link dates back to the early 19th century after scarlet fever epidemics in Florence and Vienna. Richard Bright first described the association in 1836, reporting that scarlet fever was sometimes followed by hematuria and kidney disease.[709] In 1907, Schick described an asymptomatic interval of 12 days to 7 weeks between the onset of streptococcal infection and the onset of nephritis.[710] In the early 1950s, Rammelkamp and colleagues further defined the association of PSGN with specific serotypes of streptococci.[584,711]

Despite the early recognition of an association between streptococcal infection and acute glomerulonephritis, the pathogenic mechanism of disease remains incompletely understood. Conceptually, either acute PSGN could be secondary to a direct pathogenic effect of a streptococcal protein (e.g., a protein that activates or blocks regulation of the alternative complement pathway), or the streptococcal product could induce an immune complex–mediated injury. This could occur by a number of different mechanisms: (1) by introducing an antigen into the glomerulus (planted antigen); (2) by the deposition of circulating immune complexes; (3) by alteration of a normal renal antigen that causes it to become a self-antigen; or (4) by induction of an autoimmune response to a self-antigen by way of antigenic mimicry. It is conceivable that more than one streptococcal antigen may be involved in the pathogenesis of acute PSGN, and more than one pathogenic mechanism may be at play simultaneously.

Several streptococcal proteins have been implicated in the pathogenesis of acute PSGN.[712] M protein molecules protruding from the surface of group A streptococci contain epitopes that cross-react with glomerular antigens. Shared sequences of M protein types 5, 6, and 19 have been shown to elicit antibodies that react with several myocardial and skeletal muscle proteins.[713] Conversely, monoclonal antibodies raised against human kidney cortex have been shown to cross-react with types 6 and 12 M proteins, which provides evidence that certain M proteins may share antigenic determinants between all glomeruli.[714] The glomerular cross reactivity of the amino-terminal region of type 1 M protein was further localized to a tetrapeptide sequence at position 23-26.[715] Antibodies raised against the amino-terminus of type 1 M protein was shown to cross-react with the cytoskeletal protein of glomerular mesangial cells—namely, the filament protein vimentin.[713] Two antigens have been found within the glomerular deposits in kidney biopsy specimens from patients with PSGN and have been reported to induce an antibody response characteristic for nephritogenic streptococcal infections—streptococcal proteinase exotoxin B (SPEB, zymogen)[716] and the glycolytic enzyme glyceraldehyde 3-phosphate dehydrogenase (GAPDH), which shares exact homology with the nephritis-associated plasmin receptor (NaPlr) that binds plasminogen.[717] In a study that tested antigen deposition in 17 kidney biopsy specimens and circulating antibodies in sera from 53 patients, responses to SPEB were more consistently found than deposits and antibody responses to GAPDH.[718]

Currently, the spectrum of infectious agents associated with postinfectious or periinfectious glomerulonephritis includes many more bacterial pathogens than streptococci. Other agents include staphylococci, gram-negative rods, and intracellular bacteria.[719,720] Likewise, the population at risk for periinfectious glomerulonephritis has changed to include alcoholic individuals, intravenous drug users, and patients with ventricular atrial shunts and on immunosuppressive therapy.[720] However, PSGN remains one of the most extensively studied and documented infection-associated glomerulonephritides.

## CLINICAL FEATURES AND NATURAL HISTORY

Classically, the syndrome of acute PSGN presents abruptly with hematuria, proteinuria, hypertension, and azotemia. This syndrome can show a wide spectrum of severity, from asymptomatic disease to oliguric AKI.[721] A latent period occurs from the onset of pharyngitis to the onset of nephritis. In postpharyngitic cases, the latent period averages 10 days, with a range of 7 to 21 days. The latent period may be longer after a skin infection (from 14–21 days), although this period is harder to define after impetigo.[722] The latency period can exceed 3 weeks.[723] Short latency periods less than 1 week are suggestive of a so-called synpharyngitic syndrome, typically corresponding to exacerbation of an underlying IgA nephropathy.

The hematuria is microscopic in more than two-thirds of cases but may be macroscopic on occasion. Patients commonly report gross hematuria and transient oliguria. Anuria is infrequent, however and, if persistent, may indicate the development of crescentic glomerulonephritis.

Mild to moderate hypertension occurs in more than 75% of patients. It is most evident at the onset of nephritis and typically subsides promptly after diuresis.[675] Antihypertensive treatment is necessary in only about 50% of patients. Signs and symptoms of congestive heart failure may occur and may dominate the clinical picture. These include jugular venous distention, the presence of an S3 gallop, dyspnea, and signs of pulmonary congestion.[723–726] Frank heart failure may be a complication in as many of 40% of older patients with PSGN.

Edema is the presenting symptom in two-thirds of patients and is present in as many as 90% of cases.[672] The presence of edema is based on primary renal sodium and fluid retention. The edema typically appears in the face and upper extremities. Ascites and anasarca may occur in children.

Encephalopathy presenting as confusion, headache, somnolence, or even convulsion is not common and may affect children more frequently than adults. Encephalopathy is not always attributable to severe hypertension but may be the result of central nervous system vasculitis instead.[723,725–727]

The clinical manifestations of acute PSGN typically resolve in 1 to 2 weeks as the edema and hypertension disappear after diuresis, and the patient remains typically remains asymptomatic. Both the hematuria and proteinuria may persist for several months but are usually resolved within 1 year. However, proteinuria may persist in patients who initially had nephrotic syndrome.[672] The long-term persistence of proteinuria, and especially albuminuria, may be an indication of the persistence of proliferative glomerulonephritis.[678]

The differential diagnosis of acute PSGN includes the following: (1) IgA nephropathy[728] and IgA vasculitis (formerly Henoch-Schönlein purpura), especially when the acute nephritic syndrome is associated with gross or rusty hematuria; (2) MPGN and C3 glomerulopathy; and (3) acute crescentic glomerulonephritis—rapidly progressive glomerulonephritis: immune complex–mediated, anti-GBM–mediated, or pauci-immune). The occurrence of acute nephritis in the setting of persistent fever should raise the suspicion of a periinfectious glomerulonephritis, especially with persistence of an infection such as an occult abscess or infective endocarditis.

Although rheumatic fever and PSGN rarely occur together, their concurrence has been described.[729]

## LABORATORY FINDINGS

Hematuria, microscopic or gross, is nearly always present in acute PSGN. There are, however, rare cases of documented acute PSGN with no associated hematuria.[674,730] Microscopic examination of urine typically reveals the presence of dysmorphic red blood cells[731] or red blood cell casts. Other findings on microscopy are leukocytes, renal tubule epithelial cells, and hyaline and granular casts.[675] When the hematuria is macroscopic, the urine typically has a rusty or tea color.

Proteinuria is nearly always present but is typically in the subnephrotic range. In 50% of patients, it may be less than 500 mg of protein/day.[732,733] Nephrotic-range proteinuria may occur in as many as 20% of patients and is more frequent in adults than in children.[672] The excreted proteins may include large amounts of fibrin degradation products and fibrinopeptides.[730,734]

A pronounced decline in urine GFR is common in older patients with acute PSGN, affecting nearly 60% of patients 55 years of age and older.[725] This profound decrease in GFR is uncommon in patients from childhood to middle age. Indeed, because of the accompanying fluid retention and increase in circulatory volumes, a mild decrease in GFR may not be accompanied by an increase in the serum creatinine concentration above laboratory limits of normal. Renal plasma flow, tubular reabsorptive capacity, and concentrating ability are typically not affected. On the other hand, urinary sodium excretion and calcium excretion are greatly reduced.[735]

A transient hyporeninemic hypoaldosteronism may lead to mild to moderate hyperkalemia. This may be exacerbated by a concomitant decrease in GFR and reduced distal delivery of solute. This type 4 renal tubular acidosis may resolve with the resolution of nephritis in the event of diuresis but may be persistent beyond that point in some patients.[736] The suppressed plasma renin activity may be a consequence of the volume expansion present in those patients.[737]

Cultures of throat or skin samples frequently reveal group A streptococci.[675,738] The sensitivity and specificity of these tests are likely affected by the method of obtaining a culture specimen and the test used.[739] Such cultures may be less satisfactory than serologic studies to evaluate for the presence of recent streptococcal infection in patients suspected of having PSGN.[740] The antibodies most commonly studied for the detection of a recent streptococcal infection are antistreptolysin O, antistreptokinase, antihyaluronidase, antideoxyribonuclease B, and anti–nicotinamide adenine dinucleotidase.[741] Of these, the most commonly used is the antistreptolysin O test. An elevated antistreptolysin O titer above 200 units may be found in 90% of patients with pharyngeal infection.[675] In the diagnosis of an acute PSGN, however, a rise in titer is more specific than the absolute level of the titer. The latter is likely affected by the geographic and socioeconomic prevalence of pharyngeal infections with group A streptococci. Increased antistreptolysin O titers are present in about two-thirds of patients with upper respiratory tract infection, but in only about one-third of patients following streptococcal impetigo.[672] Serial antistreptolysin O titer determinations with a twofold or greater rise in titer are highly indicative of a recent infection.[672,675]

The streptozyme test combines several antistreptococcal antibody assays and may be a useful screening test.[740] Because certain strains of type 12 group A streptococci do not produce streptolysin S or O, and in patients in whom impetigo-associated PSGN is suspected, testing for antideoxyribonuclease B and antihyaluronidase is a useful procedure.[685] Antibodies to other streptococcal cell wall glycoproteins may also increase, including those for endostreptosin.[675,742–745] On occasion, autoantibodies to collagen and laminin may be detected.[675,746] Cultures of throat or skin specimens may yield positive results in as few as 25% of patients.

The serial measurement of complement component levels is important in the diagnosis of PSGN. Early in the acute phase, the levels of hemolytic complement activity (CH-50 and C3) are reduced. These levels return to normal, usually within 8 weeks.[675,723,747–752] The reduction in serum C3 levels is especially marked in patients with C3NeF, which is capable of cleaving native C3.[591–593] The finding of low properdin and C3 levels, and concomitant normal to modestly reduced levels of C1q, C2, and C4,[747,748,753] all point to the importance of the activation of the alternate pathway of the complement cascade.[747] Immunohistochemical analysis of mannose-binding protein and mannose-binding protein–associated serine proteinase 1 suggests that the lectin pathway of complement activation is engaged in about one-third of patients.[754] There is also some evidence for activation via the classic pathway.[755] Another complement level abnormality is a mild depression of C5 levels, whereas levels of C6 and C7 are usually normal.[591,675,753] The plasma level of soluble terminal complement components (C5b-9) rises acutely and then falls to normal.[748] Because complement levels typically return to normal within 8 weeks, the persistent depression of C3 levels may be indicative of another diagnosis, such as MPGN, endocarditis, occult sepsis, SLE, atheromatous emboli, or congenital chronic complement deficiency.[747]

Circulating cryoglobulins[756,757] as well as circulating immune complexes,[758–761] may be detected in some patients with PSGN. The pathophysiologic importance of these circulating immune complexes for the development of acute nephritis is unclear.[760–762]

Abnormalities in blood coagulation systems may be detected in acute PSGN; thus, thrombocytopenia may be seen.[763] Elevated levels of fibrinogen, factor VIII, plasmin activity, and circulating high-molecular-weight fibrinogen complexes may be seen and correlate with disease activity and an unfavorable prognosis.[764–768]

Although complement studies have suggested that the alternative pathways are primarily involved in acute PSGN, there is some evidence also for activation via the classic pathway.[755]

### TREATMENT

Treatment of acute PSGN is largely supportive care. Children almost invariably recover from the initial episode.[769–771] Of concern to clinicians are patients who have AKI at presentation. An initial episode of AKI is not necessarily associated with a bad prognosis.[721] In a study of 20 adult patients with diffuse proliferative glomerulonephritis, 11 had AKI and 9 had normal or mild renal insufficiency. There were no differences between these groups in clinical, immunologic, or histological features. After 18 months of follow-up, outcomes were similar in the two groups. Thus, there is little evidence to suggest the need for any form of immunosuppressive therapy. Because of the profound salt and water retention observed in these patients—and, in some, pulmonary congestion—it is important to use loop diuretics such as furosemide to avoid volume expansion and hypertension. When volume expansion does occur, antihypertensive agents are frequently useful to ameliorate the hypertension. Interestingly, plasma renin levels are reduced; however, captopril has been shown to lower blood pressure and improve GFR in patients with PSGN.[772]

Some patients with substantial volume expansion and marked pulmonary congestion show no response to diuretic therapy. In those individuals, dialytic support is appropriate, either hemodialysis or continuous venovenous hemofiltration in adults or peritoneal dialysis in children. Some patients develop substantial hyperkalemia. In those patients, treatment with exchange resins or dialysis may be useful. Importantly, so-called potassium-sparing agents, including triamterene, spironolactone, and amiloride, should not be used in this disease state. Usually, patients undergo a spontaneous diuresis within 7 to 10 days after the onset of their illness and no longer require supportive care.[721,773] There is no evidence to date that early treatment of streptococcal disease, either pharyngitic or cellulitic, will alter the risk of PSGN. It has long been speculated that treatment with penicillin can control the spread of outbreaks of epidemic PSGN. In studies from Aboriginal communities in Australia, the use of benzathine penicillin prevented new cases of PSGN, especially in children with skin sores and household contact with affected cases.[774]

The long-term prognosis of patients with PSGN is not as benign as previously considered. Widespread crescentic glomerulonephritis results in an increased number of obsolescent glomeruli associated with tubulointerstitial disease that results in the progressive reduction of the renal mass over time.[775] A proportion of patients with streptococcal glomerulonephritis develop hypertension, proteinuria and renal insufficiency from 10 to 40 years after the illness.[775–777] Nonetheless, it is most common that the long-term disease process is marked only by mild hypertension.

In some patients, there is evidence to suggest that the original diagnosis of PSGN may have been in error. This is especially true for individuals in whom a kidney biopsy was never performed. For example, a patient who has an upper respiratory tract infection and then develops a glomerulonephritis may be considered to have PSGN when, in fact, the patient has another proliferative form of glomerulonephritis. In these patients, lack of resolution of the kidney disease should prompt a kidney biopsy to elucidate the underlying cause of the glomerular injury.

## IMMUNOGLOBULIN A NEPHROPATHY

### EPIDEMIOLOGY

IgA nephropathy remains one of, if not the, most common forms of glomerulonephritis, especially in developed countries with a low prevalence of infectious diseases.[778] Initially described in the late 1960s by Berger and Hinglais,[779,780] the disorder is characterized by deposition predominantly of IgA (and, to a lesser extent, of other immunoglobulins) in the mesangium, with mesangial proliferation and with clinical features that span the spectrum from asymptomatic hematuria to rapidly progressive glomerulonephritis. Although it was previously considered a benign disease, it is now clear that up to 40% of patients may progress to ESKD. Moreover, it has become recognized that in addition to a primary form of the disorder, IgA nephropathy is also associated with and may be secondary to a variety of disease processes (Box 31.8).

IgA nephropathy occurs in individuals of all ages, but it is still most common in the 2nd and 3rd decades of life and is much more common in males than females (Table 31.7). IgA nephropathy is uncommon in children younger than 10 years of age. In fact, 80% of patients are between the ages of 16 and 35 years at the time of kidney biopsy.[781–786] The male to female ratio has been described as anywhere from 2:1 to 6:1.[781–786]

The distribution of IgA nephropathy varies in different geographic regions throughout the world.[787] It is the most common form of primary glomerular disease in Asia,

**Box 31.8 Classification of Immunoglobulin A Nephropathy**

Primary immunoglobulin A (IgA) nephropathy
Secondary IgA nephropathy: Associated disorders
- IgA vasculitis (formerly Henoch-Schönlein purpura)
- Human immunodeficiency virus infection
- Toxoplasmosis
- Seronegative spondyloarthropathy
- Celiac disease
- Dermatitis herpetiformis
- Crohn disease
- Liver disease
- Alcoholic cirrhosis
- Ankylosing spondylitis
- Reiter syndrome
- Neoplasia
- Mycosis fungoides
- Lung CA
- Mucin-secreting CA
- Cyclic neutropenia
- Immunothrombocytopenia
- Gluten-sensitive enteropathy
- Scleritis
- Sicca syndrome
- Mastitis
- Pulmonary hemosiderosis
- Berger disease
- Leprosy

Familial IgA nephropathy

*CA*, Cytoplasmic antibody.
Modified from references 826, 850, 862, 979, 980, and 1482 to 1509.

**Table 31.7 Diseases That Cause Glomerulonephritis[a]**

| Glomerular Lesion | N | Male-Female Ratio | Caucasian:African American Ratio |
|---|---|---|---|
| IgA nephropathy | 693 | 2.0:1.0 | 14.0:1.0 |
| MPGN I | 248 | 1.2:1.0 | 3.3:1.0 |
| Anti-GBM | 82 | 1.1:1.0 | 7.9:1.0 |
| ANCA-GN | 257 | 1.0:1.0 | 6.7:1.0 |
| Fibrillary glomerulonephritis | 76 | 1.0:1.2 | 14.3:1.0 |

[a]Based on the analysis of 9605 native kidney biopsy specimens evaluated at the University of North Carolina Nephropathology Laboratory. This laboratory evaluates kidney biopsy specimens from a base population of approximately 10 million throughout the southeastern United States and centered in North Carolina. The expected Caucasian:African American ratio in this kidney biopsy population is approximately 3:2.

*ANCA-GN,* Antineutrophil cytoplasmic antibody- glomerulonephritis; *Anti-GBM*, anti- glomerular basement membrane; *MPGN I*, membranoproliferative glomerulonephritis type 1.

accounting for up to 30% to 40% of all biopsies performed for the diagnosis of glomerular disease, and it accounts for 20% of all biopsies in Europe and 10% of all biopsies in North America.[787] This wide variation in incidence is partly attributable to the differing indications for kidney biopsy in Asia compared with those in North America. In Asia, urinalyses are performed routinely in school-age children. Those with asymptomatic hematuria typically undergo biopsy, which may lead to an increased number of diagnoses of IgA nephropathy.

Genetic factors may also be important in the geographic differences. A Japanese study of biopsy specimens obtained from kidney donors immediately before transplantation showed that 16% of donors had covert mesangial deposition of IgA.[788] IgA nephropathy has been reported to be rare in African-Americans,[789,790] although population-based incidence rates of newly diagnosed IgA nephropathy have been found to be similar in African American and Caucasian populations.[791] IgA nephropathy is quite common in Native Americans of the Zuni and Navajo tribes.[792] The prevalence of IgA in the general population has been estimated to be between 25 and 50 cases/100,000[787,793] although, notably, almost 5% of all patients undergoing kidney biopsy have at least some IgA deposits in their glomeruli.[794] Population studies in Germany and in France calculated an incidence of 2 cases/10,000,[795–798] but autopsy studies performed in Singapore[799] have suggested that 2.0% to 4.8% of the population had IgA deposition in their glomeruli.

## GENETICS

IgA nephropathy is a histologically based diagnosis. It is unlikely to be related to a single genetic locus, but is probably due to the interactions of multiple susceptibility and progression genes in combination with environmental factors.[800] A number of studies have suggested that there are genes that render an individual susceptible to IgA nephropathy and genes that portend a more rapid progression of IgA nephropathy. Polymorphisms in a number of genes, including those coding for ACE, angiotensin, angiotensin II receptor, T cell receptor, IL-1 and IL-6, IL receptor antagonist, TGF, mannose-binding lectin, uteroglobin, nitric oxide synthase, and TNF, as well as major histocompatibility loci, have been evaluated as possibly affecting both the susceptibility to and progression of disease.[778,801–807] A number of studies have examined the role of ACE gene in IgA nephropathy, with or without progressive disease. The D allele of the ACE gene may be associated with susceptibility to IgA nephropathy in Asians but not in Caucasians.[808] The Polymorphism Research to Distinguish Genetic Factors Contributing to Progression of IgA Nephropathy (PREDICT-IgA nephropathy) study, which investigated associations between the progression of IgA nephropathy and 100 atherosclerotic disease-related gene polymorphisms using a retrospective candidate gene approach, has found significant associations between polymorphisms in the glycoprotein Ia and intracellular adhesion molecule- 1 genes and progression of disease.[809] In this study, the association between the ACE I/D polymorphism and progression of disease was not found to be significant after adjustment for multiple comparisons.

Familial IgA nephropathy has been reported in multiple ethnic groups worldwide, including Africa and Central America. Some studies have suggested that 4% to 14% of patients with IgA nephropathy may have a family history of kidney disease,[795,810,811] and systematic screening of asymptomatic first-degree relatives has detected hematuria in more than 25% of them.[812] Disease findings in most pedigrees are consistent with autosomal dominant transmission with incomplete penetrance.[810] However, in some families, IgA nephropathy may aggregate with other glomerular diseases.[810,813]

Linkage studies have suggested an association of IgA nephropathy with genes at several loci.[810] Based on a genomewide linkage study of 30 kindreds with IgA nephropathy, a locus on chromosome 6q22-23 was identified, with a logarithm of the odds ratio (LOD) score of 5.6.[814] This was named IGAN1 (a LOD score ≥3 signifies odds ≥1000:1 in favor of linkage).[810]

Genomewide association studies have successfully identified candidate genes and single-nucleotide polymorphisms (SNPs) that may correlate with susceptibility to or protection against IgA nephropathy. A genomewide association study (GWAS) was first performed using DNA in the UK Glomerulonephritis DNA Bank from individuals with IgA nephropathy[815] and then later in Chinese cohorts.[816,817] These studies led to the identification of seven susceptibility loci—three loci within the MHC region on chromosome 6p21, DEFA locus on chromosome 8p23, TNFSF13 locus on chromosome 17p23,

HORMAD2 locus on chromosome 22q12 and CFH/CFHR locus on chromosome 1q32—which implicate defects in innate immunity, adaptive immunity, and the alternative complement pathway.[818,819] A larger GWAS of 20,612 individuals comprising discovery and follow-up cohorts of European and East Asian decent has revealed six new associations, four in ITGAM-ITGAX, VAV3, and CARD9 and two new signals at the HLA-DQB1 and DEFA loci. The biologic nature of the risk alleles has strongly suggested a role for host–intestinal pathogen interactions, and almost all risk alleles were associated with inflammatory bowel disease risk and/or intestinal epithelial barrier maintenance and response to mucosal pathogens.[820] Notably, the major histocompatibility complex has been implicated in every GWAS to date.

The prevailing hypothesis regarding the pathogenesis of IgA nephropathy focuses on defects in protein glycosylation, particularly in B cells secreting IgA1. Studies measuring serum levels of galactose-deficient IgA1 in patients with IgA nephropathy, their relatives, and unrelated controls have found a higher level of aberrantly glycosylated IgA1 in patients with familial or sporadic IgA nephropathy and in their at-risk relatives than in unrelated individuals or control subjects.[821,822] This finding suggests that abnormal IgA1 glycosylation is an inherited rather than an acquired trait. Polymorphisms of the genes for the enzymes responsible for glycosylation of IgA1 may thus be associated with increased susceptibility to IgA nephropathy. Such genes include the core 1β-galactosyltransferase gene (*C1GALT1*),[823,824] and the molecular chaperone COSMC gene (*C1GALT1C1*), although the findings are inconsistent across studies. Interestingly, a recent GWAS for serum levels of galactose-deficient IgA1 in 2633 subjects of European and East Asian decent has identified two novel loci in *C1GALT1* and *C1GALT1C1* that encode molecular partners required for the enzymatic O-glycosylation of IgA1.[825]

## PATHOLOGY

### Immunofluorescence Microscopy

IgA nephropathy can be definitively diagnosed only by the immunohistologic demonstration of glomerular immune deposits that stain dominantly or codominantly for IgA compared with IgG and IgM (Fig. 31.26).[826–829] The staining is usually exclusively or predominantly mesangial, although a minority of specimens, especially from patients with severe disease, will have substantial capillary wall staining. By definition, 100% of IgA nephropathy specimens stain for IgA. On a scale of 0 to 4+, the mean intensity of IgA staining is approximately 3+.[828] IgM staining is observed in 84% of specimens with a mean intensity (when present) of only approximately 1+. IgG staining is observed in 62% of specimens, also with a mean intensity (when present) of approximately 1+. Early studies of IgA nephropathy described more frequent and more intense IgG staining than is seen today, but this probably was caused by the use of less specific antibodies that cross-react between IgA and IgG. Almost all IgA nephropathy specimens have substantial staining for C3. In contrast, staining for C1q is rare and weak when present. If there is intense staining in a specimen that shows substantial IgA and IgG, the possibility of lupus nephritis rather than IgA nephropathy should be considered.[828] An additional relatively distinctive feature of IgA nephropathy is that unlike

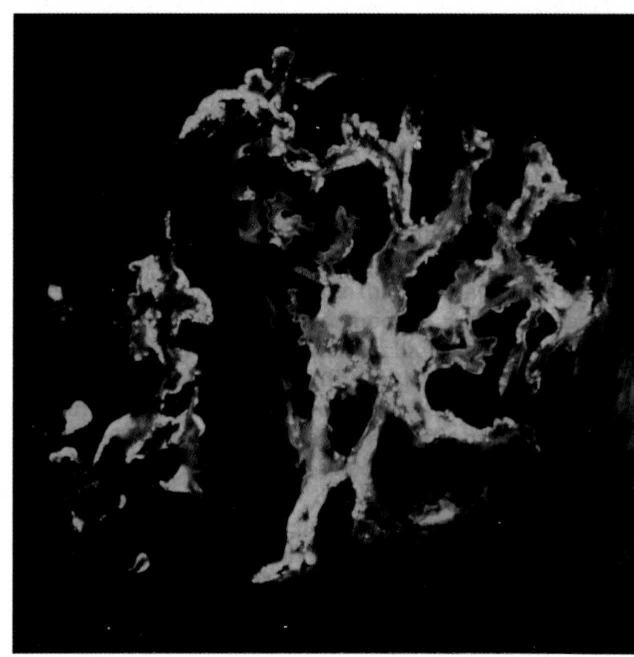

**Fig. 31.26** Immunofluorescence micrograph of a glomerulus with features of immunoglobulin A (IgA) nephropathy showing intense mesangial staining for IgA. (Fluorescein isothiocyanate anti-IgA stain, ×300.)

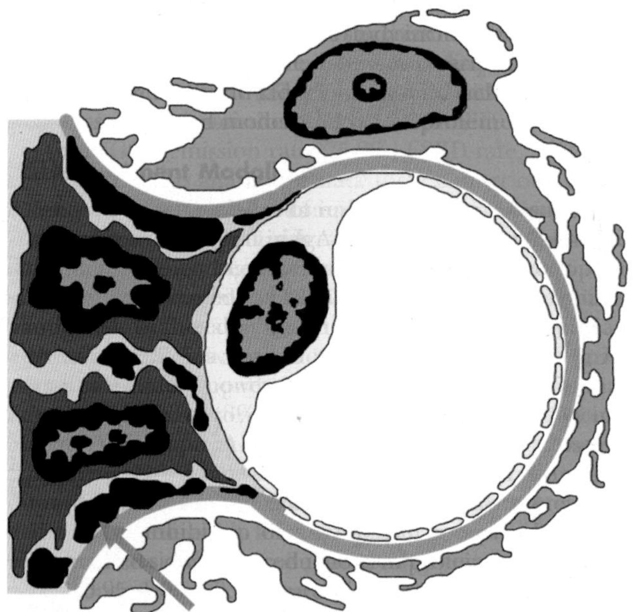

**Fig. 31.27** Diagram depicting the ultrastructural features of immunoglobulin A nephropathy. Note the mesangial dense deposits *(blue arrow)* and mesangial hypercellularity. (Courtesy JC Jennette.)

any other glomerular immune complex disease, the immune deposits usually have more intense staining for gamma (λ) light chains than kappa (κ) light chains.[826,828]

### Electron Microscopy

The ubiquitous ultrastructural finding is mesangial electron-dense deposits that correspond to the immune deposits seen by immunohistologic analysis (Figs. 31.27 and 31.28).[827] The mesangial deposits often are immediately beneath the

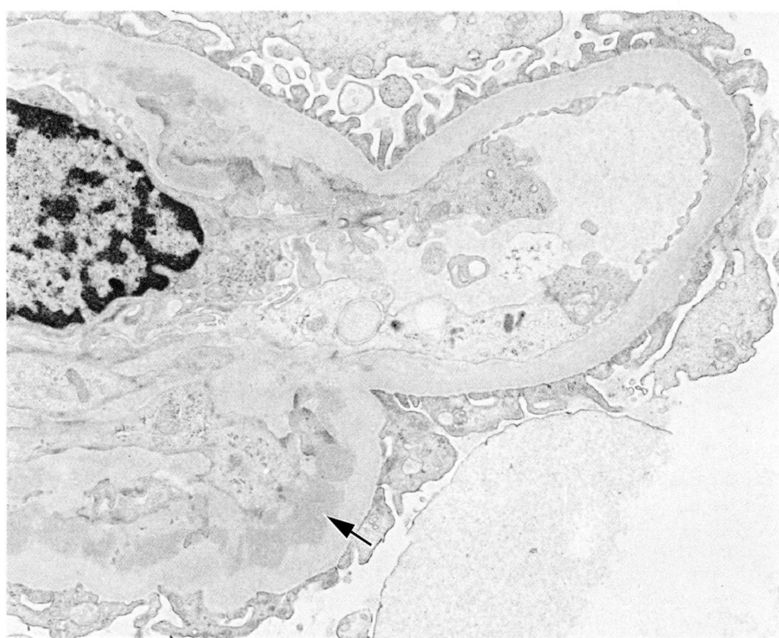

**Fig. 31.28** Electron micrograph of a capillary and adjacent mesangium from a patient with immunoglobulin A nephropathy showing mesangial dense deposits immediately beneath the perimesangial basement membrane *(arrow)*. (×7000.)

perimesangial basement membrane. They are accompanied by varying degrees of mesangial matrix expansion and hypercellularity. Most specimens do not have capillary wall deposits, but a minority, especially from patients with more severe disease, show scattered subendothelial dense deposits or subepithelial dense deposits or both. The extent of endocapillary proliferation and leukocyte infiltration parallel the pattern of injury observed by light microscopy. Epithelial foot process effacement is observed in patients with substantial proteinuria.

### Light Microscopy

IgA nephropathy can cause any of the light microscopic phenotypes of proliferative glomerulonephritis (Fig. 31.29) or may cause no discernible histologic changes.[827–834] As depicted in Fig. 31.30, this spectrum of glomerular inflammatory responses is shared by a variety of glomerulonephritides that have different causes but that induce similar or identical light microscopic alterations in glomeruli. Fig. 31.30 also depicts the most frequent clinical manifestations at the time of biopsy of the different histologic phenotypes of glomerulonephritis, all of which can be caused by IgA nephropathy. At the time of biopsy, IgA nephropathy usually manifests as a focal or diffuse mesangioproliferative or proliferative glomerulonephritis, although specimens from a few patients will have no lesion by light microscopy, those from a few will show aggressive disease with crescents, and occasional specimens will already demonstrate chronic sclerosing disease.

Different criteria for performing a kidney biopsy result in different frequencies of the various phenotypes of IgA nephropathy among distinct populations of patients. Of 668 consecutive native kidney IgA nephropathy specimens diagnosed in the UNC Nephropathology Laboratory, 4% showed no lesion by light microscopy, 13% had exclusively mesangioproliferative glomerulonephritis, 37% had focal proliferative glomerulonephritis (25% of these had <50% crescents), 28% had diffuse proliferative glomerulonephritis (45% of these had <50% crescents), 4% had crescentic glomerulonephritis (≥50% crescents), 6% had focal sclerosing glomerulonephritis without residual proliferative activity, 6% had diffuse chronic sclerosing glomerulonephritis, and 2% had lesions that did not fall into any of these categories.

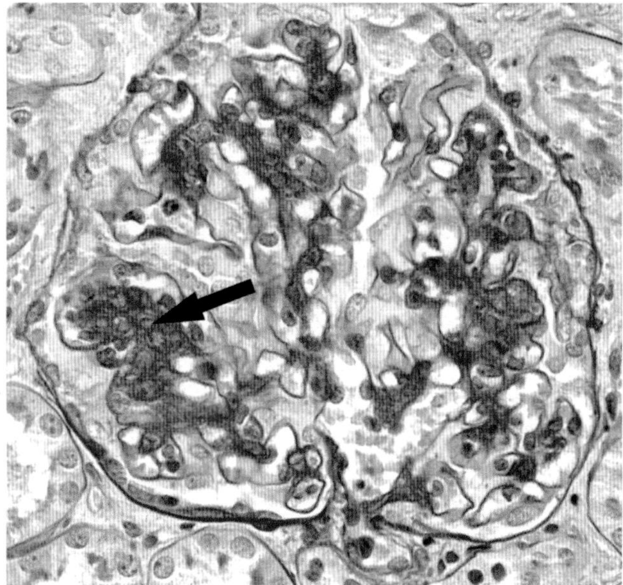

**Fig. 31.29** Light micrograph of a glomerulus with immunoglobulin A (IgA) nephropathy showing segmental mesangial matrix expansion and hypercellularity *(arrow)*. (Periodic acid–Schiff stain, ×300.)

The mildest light microscopic expression of IgA nephropathy, other than no discernible lesion, is focal or diffuse mesangial hypercellularity without more complex endocapillary hypercellularity, such as endothelial proliferation or influx of leukocytes. This is analogous to International

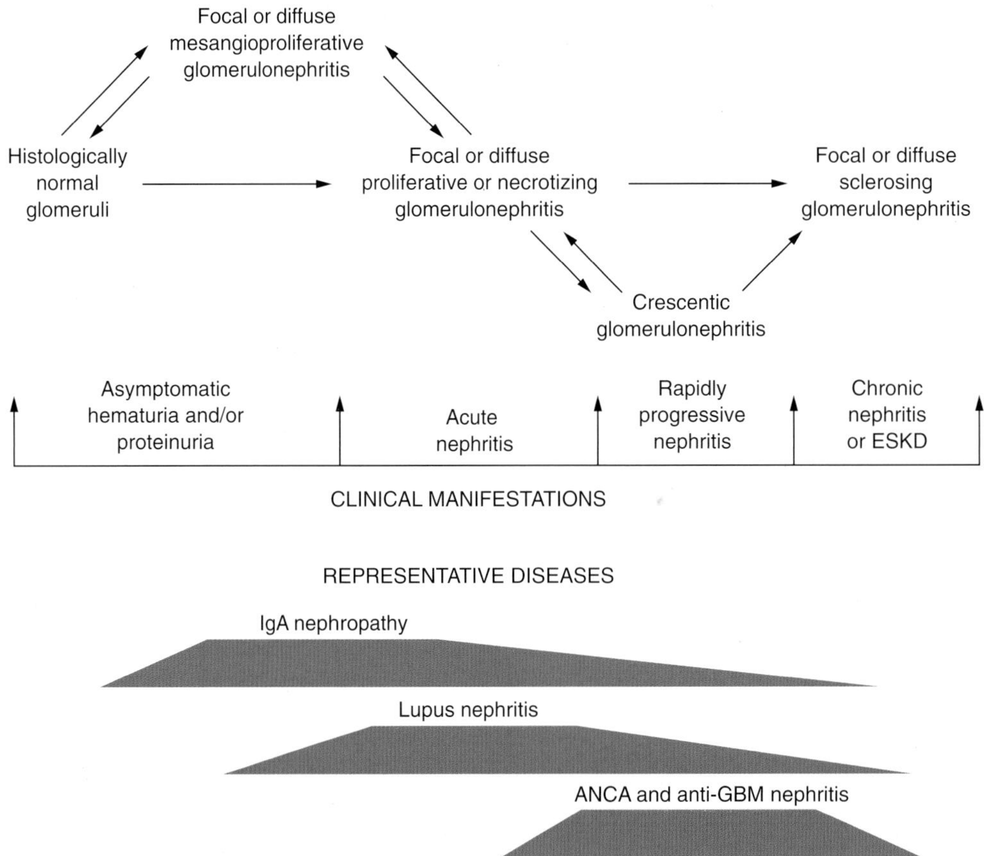


**Fig. 31.30** Diagram depicting the continuum of histological changes that can be caused by glomerular inflammation *(top),* the usual clinical syndromes caused by each expression of glomerular injury *(middle),* and the portion of the continuum that most often corresponds to several specific categories of glomerular disease *(bottom). ANCA,* Antineutrophil cytoplasmic autoantibody; *ESKD,* end-stage kidney disease; *GBM,* glomerular basement membrane; *IgA,* immunoglobulin A.

Society of Nephrology/Renal Pathology Service class II lupus nephritis.[835] More severe inflammatory injury causes focal (involving <50% of glomeruli) or diffuse proliferative glomerulonephritis as the pathologic expression of IgA nephropathy, which is pathologically analogous to classes III and IV lupus nephritis. The lesions are characterized not only by mesangial hypercellularity, but also some degree of endothelial proliferation or leukocyte infiltration that distorts or obliterates some capillary lumens. Extensive necrosis is rare in IgA nephropathy, although slight focal segmental necrosis with karyorrhexis can occur in severely inflamed glomeruli. With time, destructive glomerular inflammatory lesions progress to sclerotic lesions that may form adhesions to Bowman's capsule. Occasional patients with IgA nephropathy will have focal glomerular sclerosis by light microscopy that is indistinguishable from FSGS until the IF microscopic findings are taken into consideration. Because of the episodic nature of IgA nephropathy, many patients have combinations of focal sclerotic lesions and focal active proliferative lesions. Patients with the most severe IgA nephropathy have crescent formation because of extensive disruption of capillaries.[834] Advanced chronic disease is characterized by extensive glomerular sclerosis associated with marked tubular atrophy, interstitial fibrosis, and interstitial infiltration by mononuclear leukocytes.

Whether or not histologic features detected on kidney biopsy can be used to predict the progression of IgA nephropathy has been studied for many years. Nephropathologic findings have previously provided limited prognostic value over and above that of simple clinical parameters such as blood pressure, serum creatinine level, and degree of proteinuria. The Oxford classification of IgA nephropathy study is a seminal investigation that assessed the value of specific pathologic features in predicting the risk of progression of kidney disease in IgA nephropathy.[836,837] The study population was a multiethnic cohort of patients with IgA nephropathy that included children ($n = 59$) and adults ($n = 206$) who were followed for a mean of 69 months. By an iterative process, pathologic variables selected based on reproducibility, least susceptibility to sampling error, ease of scoring, and independent association with outcome were then correlated through multivariate analysis with three clinical outcomes—the rate of kidney function decline, survival from a 50% decline in kidney function or ESKD, and proteinuria during follow-up.[836]

Four parameters emerged as independently predictive of clinical outcomes: mesangial hypercellularity, endocapillary hypercellularity, segmental glomerulosclerosis, and tubular atrophy–interstitial fibrosis. Of these predictors, mesangial hypercellularity was significantly associated with ESKD or a 50% reduction in GFR, segmental sclerosis was associated with the rate of decline in kidney function, and tubular atrophy/interstitial fibrosis was statistically associated with both the rate of decline and ESKD or a 50% decline in kidney function. Endocapillary hypercellularity was not significantly predictive of the rate of decline of kidney function or survival from ESKD or a 50% reduction in kidney function. However, patients with endocapillary (or extracapillary) hypercellularity were more likely to receive immunosuppressive therapy, and the relationship between this pathologic variable and the rate of decline in kidney function may have been influenced by the use of immunosuppression. This latter finding indirectly suggests that patients with this type of lesion are responsive to immunosuppressive therapy.

These conclusions led to a proposal to incorporate the following scoring of the four identified parameters (known as the "Oxford-MEST score") into the pathology report for IgA nephropathy[836]:

- Mesangial hypercellularity—score ≤ 0.5 = 0 or score >0.5 = 1
- Endocapillary hypercellularity—absent = 0 or present = 1
- Segmental glomerulosclerosis: absent = 0 or present = 1
- Tubular atrophy–interstitial fibrosis—percentage of cortical area ≤ 25% = 0, 26% to 50% = 1, or >50% = 2

This scoring system was shown to be valid for both children and adults,[838] but true proof of its utility required validation in separate cohorts, especially in comparison with clinical features such as serum creatinine level and proteinuria.[839] Since the development of the Oxford classification of IgA nephropathy, a metaanalysis of 16 subsequent retrospective cohort studies between January 2009 and December 2012, assessing the utility of the scoring system, has found that M, S, T, and crescent (C) lesions (not E lesions) were strongly associated with progression to kidney failure, defined as a doubled serum creatinine level, 50% decline in eGFR, or ESKD.[840] A large validation study in Europe examined 1147 patients who had the whole spectrum of IgAN.[841] Over a median follow-up of 4.7 years, in patients with an eGFR less than 30 mL/min/1.73 m$^2$, M and T lesions independently predicted a poor survival and, in patients with proteinuria less than 0.5 g/day, both M and E lesions were associated with a rise in proteinuria to 1 or 2 g/day or more. The combination of M, S, and T lesions with clinical parameters significantly increased the ability to predict progression in the absence of substantial immunosuppressive therapy. An update from the IgA Nephropathy Classification Working Group in 2016 also found that the crescents are predictive of outcome, thereby changing the MEST score to the MEST-C score (C for crescents).[842] Additional prospective studies using the Oxford classification are warranted, and the CureGN cohort is posed to address the utility of the MEST-C score prospectively.

## PATHOGENESIS

A great deal of progress has been made in our understanding of the pathogenesis of IgA nephropathy.[778,843,844] The characteristic pathologic finding by IF microscopy of granular deposits of IgA and C3 in the glomerular mesangium, as well as the dermal capillaries in IgA vasculitis (formerly known as Henoch-Schönlein purpura), suggests that this disease is the result of the deposition of circulating immune complexes leading to the activation of the complement cascade via the alternate pathway. The deposited IgA is predominantly polymeric IgA1.[845–848] The fact that polymeric IgA1 is usually derived mainly from the mucosal immune system, as well as the association of clinical flare-ups in some cases of IgA nephropathy with syndromes that affect the respiratory tract or gastrointestinal tract, has led to the suggestion that IgA nephropathy is a consequence of defective mucosal immunity.[849] This concept was supported by the finding in some patients with IgA nephropathy of antibodies to dietary antigens or various infectious agents, both viral and bacterial,[850–863] and the clinical observation that hematuria increases acutely in some patients at the time of upper respiratory tract or gastrointestinal infections. However, it has now been determined that the elevation in polymeric IgA1 antibody synthesis does not occur in the mucosa, and polymeric IgA levels are increased after systemic immunization with tetanus toxoid.[846,864,865] In addition, an increase in IgA-secreting B cells was documented in both peripheral blood[866] and bone marrow[867] of patients.

Serum levels of IgA do not correlate with disease activity or mesangial deposits; therefore, it is unlikely that the pathogenesis of IgA nephropathy is related to a quantitative increase in serum levels of polymeric IgA1. Rather, it relates to an anomaly in the IgA molecule itself—namely, in its glycosylation, as discussed earlier.[868] This is best exemplified by patients with IgA-secreting multiple myeloma, among whom only those patients with aberrant IgA glycosylation develop glomerulonephritis.

In humans, the heavy chain of IgA1, but not that of IgA2, contains an 18-amino acid hinge region that is rich in proline, serine, and threonine residues. *O*-linked monosaccharides or oligosaccharides consisting of *N*-acetylgalactosamine can be posttranslationally added to these amino acid residues. This *N*-acetylgalactosamine is usually substituted with a terminal galactose.[869] Lectin-binding studies and carbohydrate composition analysis have demonstrated that the IgA1 in patients with IgA nephropathy contains less terminal galactose than that of healthy control subjects.[846,870] The addition of a galactose residue to the glycosyl side chain is blocked by premature sialylation of the *N*-acetylgalactosamine residues on the hinge region of IgA1. The precise cause of this has not been fully elucidated. Three mechanisms have been postulated—excessive activity of α-2,6-sialyltransferase, decreased activity of ß-1,3-galactosyltransferase, and decreased stability of ß-1,3-galactosyltransferase due to decreased activity of its chaperone (Cosmc).[871,872] Whether these abnormalities are acquired or genetically determined remains unclear.[824,873,874] IgA glycosylation may also be influenced by acquired abnormalities such as the polarity of the T cell cytokine milieu.[875]

Galactose-deficient IgA1 (Gd-IgA1) results in IgA1 hinge region exposure of *N*-acetylgalactosamine and neoepitope formation. This neoepitope is the target of IgG autoantibodies, as demonstrated in studies of immortalized B cells from patients with IgA nephropathy,[872,876] and IgG autoantibodies specific for Gd-IgA1 are found in the circulation of such patients.[877] These autoantibodies were found to be of highly restricted heterogeneity directed at the unique epitopes present on the abnormally glycosylated IgA1.[876] The autoantibodies and target Gd-IgA1 form circulating immune complexes[878,879] that escape removal by the reticuloendothelial system and deposit in glomeruli via an interaction with a mesangial IgA receptor, possibly the transferrin receptor.[880–883] Once deposited in glomerular mesangium, these immune complexes provoke mesangial proliferation.[884] The deposition of IgA in glomeruli may also occur independently of immune complex formation[885] because abnormally glycosylated IgA1 also leads to an increased binding in the kidney.[868,879,886] However, aberrantly glycosylated IgA in isolation does not cause mesangial proliferation in tissue culture.[876] Mesangial Gd-IgA1 molecules induce a variety of inflammatory mediators, including cytokines, chemokines, and growth factors, as well as complement activation through the mannose-binding lectin pathway.[887–889]

Of particular interest is the clinical relevance of Gd-IgA1 and anti-Gd-IgA1 autoantibodies. One study has demonstrated that serum levels of IgG- and IgA-based antiglycan autoantibodies from 97 patients with IgA nephropathy, compared with 30 patients with non-IgA nephropathy disease and 30 healthy controls, correlate with disease progression and poor prognosis.[890] A larger subsequent study followed 275 patients with IgA nephropathy for a median of 47 months (range, 12–96 months) and assessed renal survival. Not only was the level of Gd-IgA1 elevated compared with healthy controls, but higher levels were independently associated with a greater risk of renal failure (HR per standard deviation of natural log-transformed Gd-IgA1, 1.44; 95% CI, 1.11–1.88; $P = .006$).[891]

Another component of the pathogenesis of IgA nephropathy pertains to direct cytokine- or chemokine-induced podocyte injury, which is reflected by increased podocyturia. Podocyte damage may be the result of local complement activation and elevated levels of platelet-derived growth factor or TNF-$\alpha$ levels.[892–894]

It has been hypothesized that a subsequent autoantibody response may be triggered by an environmental cross-reacting antigen and lead to in situ immune complex formation by the interaction of circulating autoantibodies to the "planted" autoantigen. The formation of circulating immune complexes with abnormally glycosylated IgA and circulating IgA receptor molecules could also be involved.[895] Because IgA1 is normally cleared from the circulation by the liver via the asialoglycoprotein receptor,[896–898] it is also thought that the defective galactosylation of the hinge region in IgA1 may lead to decreased clearance of IgA1 molecules in patients with IgA nephropathy.[886,899]

The existence, nature, and role of other autoantibodies in IgA nephropathy has also been under investigation. A number of autoantibodies to various putative autoantigens have been described in IgA nephropathy.[900] Such autoantigens include a mesangial cell membrane antigen,[901] endothelial cells (human umbilical vein endothelial cells),[851,900] single-stranded DNA,[851] and cardiolipin,[851,902] Most of these autoantibodies were found in subsets of patients that rarely exceeded 3% of patients with IgA nephropathy and may sometimes have been the result of high circulating levels of IgA in these patients.[902] A more recent integrative "antibiomics" approach found 117 specific autoantibodies, many of which were directed to proteins in the kidney.[903] The presence of IgG ANCAs has been described to occur in a minority of patients with IgA nephropathy.[904] In addition, IgA ANCAs have been rarely associated with a systemic vasculitis, IgA vasculitis.[905–907] In the setting of IgA ANCA, the autoantigen seems to be different from the major ANCA autoantigens—namely, myeloperoxidase (MPO) and proteinase 3 (PR3). Circulating IgA-fibronectin complexes have also been described in the circulation of patients with IgA nephropathy and HIV infection.[908] These complexes may not be true immune complexes, however, and may be directly related to increased IgA levels in patients with IgA nephropathy.[909] A special form of IgA-dominant immune complex glomerulonephritis that resembles postinfectious glomerulonephritis occurs secondary to staphylococcal infection, especially but not exclusively in patients with diabetes.[910]

Given the lack of efficacy of immunosuppressive treatments focused on autoantibody production, such as plasma exchange and B cell–depleting agents, interest has greatly expanded with regard to the alternative and lectin complement pathways in IgA nephropathy.[911] As one example of many, deletion polymorphisms of complement factor H–related protein 1 (FHR-1), an endogenous antagonist of factor H, and FHR-3 are strongly associated with protection against IgA nephropathy, and plasma samples from a large cohort of patients with IgA nephropathy were found to have elevated levels of FHR-1, suggesting a role in disease progression.[912] An open-label study investigating the efficacy of an oral C5a receptor antagonist is now underway in patients with IgA nephropathy on stable RAAS blockade (www.clinicaltrials.gov, NCT02384317).

## CLINICAL FEATURES AND NATURAL HISTORY

Approximately 40% to 50% of these patients have macroscopic hematuria at the time of their initial presentation. The episodes tend to occur in close temporal relationship to upper respiratory infection, including tonsillitis and pharyngitis. This synchronous association of pharyngitis and macroscopic hematuria has been given the name *synpharyngitic nephritis*. Much less commonly, episodes of macroscopic hematuria follow infections that involve the urinary tract or gastroenteritis. Macroscopic hematuria may be entirely asymptomatic, but more often is associated with dysuria that may prompt the treating physician to consider bacterial cystitis. Systemic symptoms are frequently found, including nonspecific symptoms such as malaise, fatigue, myalgia, and fever. Some patients have abdominal or flank pain.[913,914] In a minority of patients (<5%), malignant hypertension may be an associated presenting feature.[915] In the most severe cases (fewer than 10%), acute glomerulonephritis results in acute renal insufficiency and failure.[916,917] Recovery typically occurs with the resolution of symptoms, even in patients who have been temporarily dialysis-dependent.[917]

Macroscopic hematuria due to IgA nephropathy occurs more often in children than in young adults. When it occurs in older individuals, it should raise the possibility of the more common causes of urinary tract bleeding, such as stones or malignancy.

A presentation with asymptomatic microscopic hematuria, with or without proteinuria, occurs in 30% to 40% of patients.[918] Patients with IgA nephropathy come for the evaluation of asymptomatic hematuria, with or without the presence of proteinuria. In addition to glomerulonephritis, these patients may commonly have hypertension. In fact, in Caucasian patients with hypertension and hematuria, IgA nephropathy is the most common form of hematuria.[919] Intermittent macroscopic hematuria occurs in 25% of these patients. Microscopic hematuria and proteinuria persist between episodes of macroscopic hematuria.

Patients with nephrotic syndrome at presentation may have widespread proliferative glomerulonephritis or coexisting IgA nephropathy and minimal-change glomerulopathies.[920] Finally, some patients with IgA nephropathy have reached ESKD at the time of their first presentation. These individuals typically have had asymptomatic microscopic hematuria and proteinuria that remained undetected.[916]

In addition to idiopathic IgA nephropathy, there is secondary IgA nephropathy that is the glomerular expression of a systemic disease (see Box 31.8). For example, patients with IgA vasculitis have abdominal pain, arthritis, a vasculitic rash, and a glomerulonephritis that is indistinguishable from that of primary IgA nephropathy. This condition is discussed more fully in Chapter 32.

Although IgA nephropathy was earlier thought to carry a relatively benign prognosis, it is estimated that measured from the time of diagnosis, 1% to 2% of all patients with IgA nephropathy will develop ESKD each year. In a review encompassing 1900 patients derived from 11 separate series, long-term renal survival was estimated to be 78% to 87% at 1 decade after presentation.[921] Similarly, European studies have suggested that renal insufficiency may occur in 20% to 30% of patients within 2 decades of the original presentation.[785] In a study of the natural history of IgA nephropathy and "isolated" microscopic hematuria in 135 Chinese children,[31] spontaneous clinical remission occurred in 12%, whereas 88% had persisting hematuria. Almost 30% developed new-onset proteinuria, and hypertension developed in 32%. Eventually, 20% developed renal insufficiency of varying severity. A poor outcome was associated with persistent hematuria, microalbuminuria, and tubulointerstitial changes on the kidney biopsy specimen. This study clearly demonstrates that careful follow-up is required for all patients given the diagnosis of IgA nephropathy.

Overall, about 25% of patients develop ESKD within 10 to 25 years from diagnosis, depending on the initial severity of disease. Patients with episodes of gross (macroscopic) hematuria generally have a more favorable prognosis than those with persisting microhematuria; however, after an episode of microhematuria associated with AKI, some patients (≈25%) may not recover normal kidney function.[922] The proliferative forms of IgA nephropathy seem to be associated with better outcomes in children than in adults.[923] It is unclear whether gender affects the prognosis of IgA nephropathy,[924] with some studies suggesting that the prognosis may be worse for males. Older age at disease onset may also connote a poor prognosis.[921,925–929]

Several studies have assessed features that predict a poor prognosis. Sustained hypertension, persistent proteinuria (especially proteinuria of >1 g protein/24 hours), impaired kidney function, and nephrotic syndrome are markers of a poor prognosis.[811,829,925] Controversy persists with respect to the issue of recurring bouts of macroscopic hematuria.[930] It is possible that macroscopic hematuria is an overt manifestation of disease and therefore identifies patients earlier in the course of their disease. Alternatively, macroscopic hematuria may represent an episodic process that results in self-limited inflammation, in contrast to persistent hematuria, which represents ongoing, low-grade inflammation. In general, persistent microscopic hematuria is associated with a poor prognosis.[931] In fact, remission of hematuria improves kidney survival and has a favorable effect of outcomes associated with IgA nephropathy.[932] It is important to note that AKI associated with macroscopic hematuria does not affect the long-term prognosis. The fact that AKI does occur during gross episodes of hematuria has been confirmed.[933–935] In these patients, the AKI is most likely associated with acute tubular damage and not with true crescentic disease. After the episodes of gross hematuria, kidney function typically returns to baseline, and the long-term prognosis is good.

The degree of proteinuria is more than likely an additional marker of glomerular disease. Whether this is a consequence of the relationship between proteinuria and the tubular dysfunction found in many forms of glomerular disease or is specific to IgA nephropathy is not clear. In a study by Chen and colleagues,[936] mice that had been made proteinuric by various methods had enhanced deposition of administered IgA immune complexes. This suggests that these complexes might be more easily deposited in proteinuric states. More importantly, the amount of protein excretion 1 year after diagnosis was highly predictive of the development of ESKD within 7 years of subsequent follow-up. Individuals with less than 500 mg/dL/day had no renal failure within 7 years, whereas those with over 3 g of protein excretion had approximately a 60% chance of ESKD.[937]

Many formulas have been advanced to predict the progression of IgA nephropathy in individual patients that yield different results for the same patient. The Toronto formula, based on average mean arterial pressure and proteinuria during the first 2 years of observation, is the best-validated in Caucasian U.S. and European subjects,[938] but a large fraction of the variation in progression remains unexplained by these two factors. Risk stratification for progression can be aided by algorithms using a small set of variables—age, gender, family history of chronic kidney disease, reduced estimated GFR at diagnosis, proteinuria, serum albumin and total serum protein levels, hematuria, systolic or diastolic blood pressure, and histologic variables.[939–942] An absolute renal risk score to predict dialysis or death, developed by analysis of a prospective cohort of 332 patients with biopsy-proven IgA nephropathy followed for an average of 13 years, allowed for significant risk stratification ($P < .0001$) by counting the number of risk factors present at diagnosis—hypertension, proteinuria 1 g or more/day, and severe pathologic lesions.[943] One of the most recent risk prediction scores based on a large cohort of Chinese patients with IgA nephropathy, using four baseline variables (lower eGFR, serum albumin, hemoglobin, and higher systolic blood pressure) had a significant independent effect on the risk of ESKD.[944] Treatment has also favorably influenced the long-term trends of progression in IgA nephropathy,[945] and a postdiagnosis decline in the level of protein excretion to less than 1.0 g/day is a very reliable surrogate measure of a more favorable long-term prognosis.[946]

A large number of factors other than simple clinical assessment have been examined to predict outcomes. Some have been independently correlated with outcomes, whereas others have failed to demonstrate any added value in prognostication or therapeutic decision making.[947] Some of the more recently described factors include autophagy in podocytes,[948] $CD19^+CD5^+$ B cells in kidney biopsy specimens and in blood,[949] C5b-9 glomerular deposition,[950] extensive C4d deposition in the mesangium,[951] tubular $\alpha_3\beta_1$-integrin expression,[950] granule membrane protein of 17 kDa (GMP-17)–positive T cells in renal tubules,[952] glomerular density and size,[953] urinary epidermal growth factor-to-monocyte chemotactic peptide 1 ratios,[954,955] urinary growth arrest and DNA damage-45γ (GADD45γ) expression,[956] analysis of the urinary proteome (kininogen, trypsin inhibitor chain 4, transthyretin),[957] and the fractional urinary excretion of IgG (in combination with assessment of nephron loss) in crescentic IgA nephropathy.[958] Likewise, hematuria associated with podocyturia may be associated with a poorer prognosis.[959] The clinical utility and applicability of these assays in prognostication and treatment decision making remains to be established, and individual patient-level risk prediction still remains limited until risk scoring systems are validated in multiple diverse cohorts.

In addition to these variables, obesity,[960] elevated nocturnal blood pressure,[961] increased uric acid levels,[961] and elevated levels of C4-binding protein[962] have been associated with a poorer prognosis. Moderate alcohol consumption is associated with an improved prognosis in IgA nephropathy.[963] A mildly elevated serum bilirubin level (>0.6 mg/dL) was associated with an improved long-term outcome in Korean patients with IgA nephropathy,[964] a finding that has not been confirmed in a non-Asian population. Prolonged, high-level exposure to organic solvents may also confer a worse prognosis to patients with IgA nephropathy.[965]

Women with IgA nephropathy tolerate pregnancy well.[966] Only women with uncontrolled hypertension, a GFR of less than 70 mL/min, or severe arteriolar or interstitial damage on kidney biopsy are at risk for kidney dysfunction.[967,968] Women with creatinine levels higher than 1.4 mg/dL have a greater propensity for hypertension and a progressive increase in creatinine level during the course of pregnancy, and pregnancy-related loss of maternal kidney function occurs in 43% of these patients.[969] The infant survival rate was 93% in this study; preterm delivery occurred in almost two-thirds and growth retardation in one-third of infants.[969] A more recent study of 223 women (136 and 87 in the pregnancy and nonpregnancy groups) with biopsy-proven IgA nephropathy in Italy has shown no difference in long-term outcomes of IgA nephropathy between the two groups over a minimum follow-up period of 5 years.[970]

## LABORATORY FINDINGS

To date, there are no specific serologic or laboratory tests diagnostic of IgA nephropathy or IgA vasculitis. The identification of abnormally galactosylated IgA1 has led to the development of a potential diagnostic test based on the detection of increased lectin binding in patients with IgA nephropathy.[971]

Although the serum IgA levels are elevated in up to 50% of patients, the presence of elevated IgA in the circulation is not specific for IgA nephropathy. The detection of IgA-fibronectin complexes was initially thought to be a marker in patients with IgA nephropathy but has not proven to be a useful clinical test.[972,973] As noted earlier, polymeric IgA also appears to be found in some patients with IgA nephropathy.[845,974–978] The polymeric IgA itself is of the IgA1 subclass. IgA may also be contained in circulating immune complexes that are not complement binding. Similar immune complexes have been described in IgA vasculitis.[979–996] The level of circulating immune complexes wax and wane and may sometimes correlate with episodes of macroscopic hematuria. In one interesting study, the level of circulating immune complexes was increased after patients drank cow's milk. This phenomenon occurred in 10% to 15% of patients and possibly suggests sensitivity to bovine serum albumin. Unfortunately, none of these findings is pathognomonic of IgA nephropathy.

Antibodies to the GBM,[997] the mesangium,[998,999] glomerular endothelial cells,[850,903] neutrophil cytoplasmic constituents,[852,853] IgA rheumatoid factor,[1000,1001] and a number of infectious agents, bovine serum proteins, and soy proteins[855–862,1002] have been found in patients with IgA nephropathy. Until studies demonstrate that certain patients have sensitivity to a particular pathogen or food allergen, it is difficult to know whether to perform antibody testing to identify certain foods that should be eliminated from the patient's diet. None of these antibody tests has been standardized in large patient populations. Therefore their applicability to all patients with IgA nephropathy is not known. Levels of complements, such as C3 and C4, are typically normal and, in some patients, even elevated,[1003] as are complement components C1q and C2–C9.[783,979,980,1003,1004] The fact that these complement levels are normal may belie the fact that either the alternate or classical pathway of complement may be activated. In this regard, C3 fragments are increased in 50% to 75% of patients,[1005,1006] and C4-binding protein concentrations are also increased.[1004] It has also been suggested that both a decreased C3 level and an elevated IgA/C3 ratio may have diagnostic utility for IgA nephropathy[31] and may be associated with a higher risk of progression.[1007,1008] Interestingly, a large study in Korea of 343 patients with biopsy-proven IgA nephropathy also demonstrated an independently predictive correlation between decreased C3 and mesangial C3 deposition and renal outcomes.[1009]

A typical finding is microscopic hematuria on urinalysis that may persist, even at very low levels of macroscopic hematuria. The finding of dysmorphic erythrocytes in the urine is typical.[1010] Proteinuria is found in many patients with IgA nephropathy although, in most of them, protein excretion is less than 1 g/day. Mesangial and endocapillary hypercellularity, segmental glomerulosclerosis, and extracapillary proliferation are strongly associated with proteinuria.[836]

Although older studies suggested that the detection of dermal capillary IgA deposits in the skin may be of diagnostic utility in IgA nephropathy,[1011] this test has not gained widespread acceptance, largely because of the substantial variation in sensitivity and specificity of skin biopsy findings in IgA in patients with nephropathy.[1012]

## TREATMENT

In part because of the outcome variability of patients with IgA nephropathy, the best approach to therapy remains incompletely established.[1013–1015] Treatment is indicated for patients with urinary protein excretion of more than 0.5 g of protein/day.[1016] Three major approaches have emerged and are supported by substantial direct evidence: (1) RAAS blockade; (2) oral and/or intravenous glucocorticoids; and (3) combined immunosuppressive (cytotoxic) therapy. The latter is usually reserved for patients with documented progressive disease.[1017] Combinations of these approaches have been under intense evaluation.

### Angiotensin II Inhibition

In retrospective studies, angiotensin II inhibition has been associated with a slower rate of loss of kidney function and a higher frequency of remission of proteinuria compared with either no therapy[1018] or the use of beta blockers.[1019] Several RCTs of angiotensin II inhibition in patients with IgA nephropathy have been undertaken.[1020–1025]

A metaanalysis of 11 studies (totaling 585 subjects) has revealed that the use of angiotensin II inhibition is associated with a reduction in proteinuria and preservation of GFR.[1026] The antiproteinuric effects of the ACE inhibitor appear to be more profound in patients with the ACE gene DD genotype.[1027] Observational studies of patients with IgA nephropathy have suggested that an elevated fractional excretion of IgG is a powerful predictor of the renoprotective response to angiotensin II inhibition.[1028] Higher doses of angiotensin II inhibitors may afford additional renoprotective effects. In an RCT involving 207 patients, a high-dose ARB (losartan, 200 mg/day) was compared with an ARB given at the usual dose (losartan, 100 mg/day), as well as with a usual-dose ACE inhibitor and a low-dose ACE inhibitor (equivalent to enalapril, 20 and 10 mg/day, respectively).[1029] High-dose ARB therapy was most efficacious in reducing proteinuria and slowing the rate of loss of decline of estimated GFR. The current first line of treatment consists of escalating doses of an ARB to achieve a target urinary protein excretion of less than 1 g/day, along with dietary sodium restriction, for patients of any age with IgA nephropathy and proteinuria of more than 500 mg of protein excretion/day.

### Glucocorticoids

Although prednisone was initially considered to be without effect,[921] some cohort studies have suggested that corticosteroids may afford some benefit.[1030,1031] For example, a RCT has demonstrated that a 6-month course of intravenous plus oral glucocorticoids may be useful in patients with IgA nephropathy who have well-preserved kidney function (serum creatinine level <1.5 mg/dL and proteinuria of 1–3.5 g of protein/day).[1032] After a 5-year follow-up, the risk of a doubling in plasma creatinine concentration was significantly lower in the corticosteroid-treated patients, who also showed a significant decrease in mean urinary protein excretion after 1 year that persisted throughout the follow-up.[1033] This beneficial effect was maintained after 10 years of follow-up, as reflected by a rate of renal survival (failure to double the serum creatinine level) of 97% in the treated group compared with 53% in the placebo group (log rank test, $P = .0003$).[1032] On the other hand, no benefit of corticosteroids over placebo could be demonstrated in the multicenter RCT conducted by the Southwest Pediatric Nephrology Study Group,[1034] although this negative result was mitigated by a statistically significant lower degree of proteinuria at baseline among placebo-treated patients. A metaanalysis of seven RCTs involving 366 patients suggested that glucocorticoid therapy was effective in reducing proteinuria and preventing loss of kidney function.[1035] A subsequent metaanalysis of 15 clinical trials that measured ESKD, doubling of the serum creatinine level, and urinary protein excretion as outcomes has found that corticosteroid therapy is associated with a decrease of proteinuria and with a statistically significant reduction in ESKD risk.[1036]

Another circumstance in which prednisone has demonstrated a substantial beneficial effect is in the treatment of patients with IgA nephropathy and concurrent MCD. These patients had nephrotic-range proteinuria and diffuse foot process effacement. They responded to prednisone in a manner very similar to that of patients with MCD.[129,920,1037,1038] Low doses of prednisone (20–30 mg/day, tapered to 5–10 mg/day over 2 years) may also be effective in lowering proteinuria in patients with mild inflammatory glomerular lesions.[1039] Conversely, a poor response to glucocorticoids can be predicted in patients with extensive glomerular obsolescence, tuft adhesions, severe interstitial fibrosis, low serum albumin level, low estimated GFR, and marked proteinuria.[1040] A high number of fibroblast-specific protein 1 (FSP1)–positive cells in the interstitium (>33 FSP-1$^+$ cells/high-power field) is highly predictive of a poor response to steroids.[1041]

The Therapeutic Evaluation of Steroids in IgA nephropathy (TESTING) study, assessing, as the name implies, the effects of corticosteroids in patients with IgA nephropathy and persistent proteinuria, was recently completed to assess the risk of disease progression.[1042] This multicenter, double-blind, RCT randomized 262 participants to oral methylprednisolone (0.6–0.8 mg/kg/day; maximum, 48 mg/day) or placebo for 2 months, weaned over 4 to 6 months with a primary composite outcome (ESKD, death due to kidney failure, or 40% decrease in eGFR). However, recruitment was discontinued because of excess serious adverse events, primarily in the steroid group, including serious infections and two deaths.

Of considerable recent import, the NEFIGAN trial was a phase 2b double-blind, randomized, placebo-controlled clinical trial that randomized 150 patients with native kidney biopsy–proven IgA nephropathy and persistent proteinuria despite maximal RAAS blockade to one of three arms—placebo, targeted-release formulation (TRF) budesonide, 8 mg orally daily or TRF budesonide, 16 mg daily. Primary outcome was defined as the mean change from baseline for the 9 months of treatment. Patients in the TRF budesonide arms, regardless of dose, achieved a 24.4% decrease from baseline in mean urine protein-to-creatinine ratio (UPCR; change in UPCR vs. placebo, 0.74; 95% CI, 0.59–0.94; $P = .0066$), an effect that was sustained throughout follow-up, and adverse events were similar across all groups (www.clinicaltrials.gov, NCT01728035). These results would suggest that nonsystemic corticosteroid use that more specifically targets intestinal mucosal immunity locally may prove to be an additional strategy in the treatment toolkit for IgA nephropathy.[1043]

In summary, glucocorticoid therapy is a reasonable option for the treatment of patients with adverse prognostic features with well-preserved kidney function (GFR >60 mL/min/1.73 m$^2$) who remain proteinuric despite a 3- to 6-month trial of angiotensin II inhibitors or patients with features of MCD and nephrotic syndrome.[1044]

### Combinations of Angiotensin II Inhibition and Glucocorticoid Therapy

Two RCTs in patient with IgA nephropathy have compared the combined use of glucocorticoids and angiotensin II inhibition to angiotensin II inhibition alone, but not with glucocorticoids alone.[1045,1046] In the larger of the two studies[1046] (97 subjects with IgA nephropathy, urinary protein excretion >1.0 g/day, eGFR >50 mL/min/1.73 m$^2$), 27% of the subjects receiving ramipril alone developed a doubling of the baseline serum creatinine level or ESKD, whereas only 4% of subjects in the ramipril plus steroid group developed these endpoints ($P = .003$) after a follow-up of 8 years. These studies demonstrate an added benefit of glucocorticoids over angiotensin II inhibitors alone. Whether such combined therapy should be instituted as initial therapy or only after a trial of angiotensin II inhibition alone remains to be investigated.[1047–1049]

In a retrospective analysis of the VALIGA cohort, using propensity score matching, 184 patients with IgA nephropathy treated with corticosteroids (CS) and RAAS blockade were compared with a similar number of patients on only RAAS blockade.[1047] During a median follow up of almost 5 years, the CS-treated group had a decline in renal function of −1.0 ± 7.3 mL/min/1.73 m$^2$ per year compared with 3.2 ± 8.3. mL/min/1.73 m$^2$ per year in the control group ($P = .004$). Also, among patients with more than 3 g/day of proteinuria, 64% in the CS group achieved proteinuria less than 1 g/day compared with only 4% in the RAAS blockade only group ($P < .001$). Interestingly, CS treatment in patients with an eGFR of less than 50 mL/min/1.73 m$^2$ resulted in a slower rate of renal function decline. Unfortunately, the study was limited by its retrospective nature and lack of important information, including, dosing of CS, compliance, adverse effects, and duration and timing of the CS regimen.

More aggressive treatment may be appropriate in patients with severe crescentic or progressive IgA nephropathy.[1050–1052] In an RCT, patients with a serum creatinine concentration more than 1.5 mg/dL and a GFR declining at a rate of more than 15%/year either received no immunosuppression or were treated with oral prednisolone (initially, 40 mg/day) and cyclophosphamide (1.5 mg/kg/day) for 3 months, followed by 2 years of treatment with azathioprine (1.5 mg/kg/day).[1053] Over a follow-up of 2 to 6 years, 5-year renal survival was 72% in treated patients versus only 6% in untreated patients.[1053] This approach of prednisone coupled with oral azathioprine for 2 years in patients with proteinuria of more than 2.5 g of protein/day was also observed in a retrospective survey.[1054,1055]

The use of pulse methylprednisolone, oral prednisone, and/or cyclophosphamide to treat patients who have rapidly progressive glomerulonephritis with widespread crescentic transformation has been reported.[1056–1058] It is reasonable to treat crescentic disease in IgA nephropathy in a manner similar to that for other forms of crescentic glomerulonephritis (e.g., ANCA glomerulonephritis). Of concern, however, was the finding in 12 patients of the persistence of crescents on repeat biopsy, despite the early and aggressive treatment with pulse methylprednisolone and oral prednisone, and a short-term reversal of the acute crescentic glomerulonephritis.[1058] This study suggests that there was only a diminution in the rate of progression to ESKD.

### Combinations of Angiotensin II Inhibition, Glucocorticoid Therapy, and Immunosupprression

This approach to therapy was recently the subject of a large multicenter RCT in Germany, the supportive versus immunosuppressive therapy for the treatment of progressive IgAN (STOP-IgAN) study.[1092,1093] This multicenter, open-label, randomized, controlled clinical trial enrolled 309 patients with biopsy-proven IgA nephropathy who were considered at high risk of progression (proteinuria >0.75 g/day plus hypertension, eGFR <90 mL/min/1.73 m$^2$, or both). All patients began with a 6-month run-in phase during, which they received supportive care with RAAS blockade. Over 6 months, 94 patients (30%) achieved and maintained proteinuria less than 0.75 g/day and were not included in the study, per protocol. Of the remaining patients, 162 consented and were randomized to continuing supportive therapy ($n = 80$) or immunosuppression group ($n = 82$). Patients received immunosuppression, consisting of glucocorticoids for patients with an eGFR more than 60 mL/min/1.73 m$^2$ or glucocorticoids in combination with oral cyclophosphamide, followed by azathioprine maintenance for patients with an eGFR between 30 and 59 mL/min/1.73 m$^2$. Patients with proteinuria more than 3.5 g/day, eGFR less than 30 mL/min/1.73 m$^2$, crescentic IgA, and secondary and rapidly progressive diseases were excluded. The two primary endpoints assessed at 36 months, in hierarchic order, were full clinical remission, defined by a UPCR less than 0.2 and a stable eGFR, with less than a 5-mL/min/1.73 m$^2$ decline and decrease in the eGFR of at least 15 mL/min/1.73 m$^2$ from baseline to the end of 36 months. At the final visit, 4 of 80 patients (5%) in the supportive group and 14 of 82 patients (20%) in the immunosuppression group had achieved full clinical remission. The higher rate of clinical remission was attributable solely to the reduction in proteinuria because there was no significant differences in renal function. The total number of adverse events was not significantly different between the groups, but the rate of infections were significantly higher in the immunosuppression group.

In a posthoc analysis, the same authors concluded that although corticosteroid monotherapy may reduce proteinuria, neither immunosuppressive regimen prevented GFR loss. Some of the factors noted in this study include the short-term follow-up (which may have been too early to show any beneficial effect on the kidney function), lack of histologic (MEST) scores, and modest degree of proteinuria.

### Other Treatment Modalities

Aliskiren, a direct inhibitor of renin, has been investigated as an antiproteinuric agent in IgA nephropathy. An open-label pilot study in 25 consecutive patients with IgA nephropathy in Hong Kong treated for 12 months with aliskiren resulted in a 26.3% mean reduction in the UPCR and a significant reduction in plasma renin activity (95% CI, 20.1–43.6; $P = .001$ vs. baseline); however, there were mild allergic reactions in 2 patients (8%) and transient hyperkalemia in 6 patients (24%).[1059] A subsequent randomized crossover study using aliskiren or placebo in 22 patients in China with biopsy-proven IgA nephropathy and persistent proteinuria, despite ACE inhibition or angiotensin receptor blockade, demonstrated significant reductions in proteinuria at 4 weeks (1.76 ± 0.95–1.03 ± 0.69 g protein/g creatinine; $P < .0001$) and from 4 to 16 weeks, but there was a modest but statistically significant reduction in the eGFR (57.2 ± 29.1–54.8 ± 29.3 mL/min/1.73 m$^2$; $P = .013$).[1060]

In a 3-year prospective controlled trial of cyclophosphamide, dipyridamole, and low-dose warfarin, it was reasonably clear that this treatment[1061] has very little long-term benefit in patients with IgA nephropathy. Five years after the end of a small controlled trial (total, 48 patients), there was no significant difference in the rate of ESKD between patients previously treated with cyclophosphamide, dipyridamole, and warfarin (22%) and the control group (33%). Of note, it has since been proposed that the apparent lack of benefit of cyclophosphamide therapy may have been clouded by the potential risk of a recently recognized mechanism of AKI in study subjects, termed "warfarin-related nephropathy."[1062] This observation warrants additional clinical trials using combination therapy without this potential confounder.

Whether MMF is useful in the treatment of IgA nephropathy is currently unknown. Three randomized trials of MMF have shown conflicting results.[1063–1066] The studies, based in China and Hong Kong, reported a beneficial effect of MMF on proteinuria and hyperlipidemia,[1064,1067] but no effect on kidney function in the short term.[1063] Long-term follow-up of this cohort suggested better preservation of kidney function in the MMF-treated group.[1068] On the other hand, the two placebo-controlled studies of MMF in Caucasian populations of 32 and 34 patients failed to demonstrate a benefit of MMF on proteinuria or the preservation of kidney function.[1065,1066] It is noteworthy that in one study,[1065] patients had relatively advanced renal insufficiency (mean serum creatinine level, 2.4 mg/dL). Collectively, these underpowered studies have failed to establish a role for MMF in the treatment of IgA nephropathy and raise the question as to whether certain ethnic groups (e.g., Asians) may be more responsive to this form of therapy.

With regard to azathioprine use, an RCT in Italy of 207 patients with biopsy-proven IgA nephropathy compared steroids alone or in combination with azathioprine for 6 months and found no difference in renal survival, defined as time to a 50% increase in the plasma creatinine level from baseline over a median follow-up of 4.9 years. In this study, the 5-year cumulative renal survival was not significantly different (88 vs. 89%; $P = .83$).[1069] A separate randomization list with a longer treatment course of 1 year in patients with impaired kidney function (plasma creatinine >2.0 mg/dL; proteinuria ≥1 g/day) involving 253 patients with biopsy-proven IgA nephropathy from the same group of investigators compared steroids alone or in combination with azathioprine and, similarly, found no difference in renal survival at the 6-year mark.[1070]

There has been much discussion in the literature about the use of tonsillectomy in IgA nephropathy. Results of retrospective trials have been inconsistent.[1071–1074] A single-center retrospective cohort study of 200 patients with biopsy-proven IgA nephropathy, 70 (35%) of whom received tonsillectomy, revealed by multiple regression modeling that tonsillectomy prevented GFR decline during the follow-up period (regression coefficient, 2.0; $P = .01$). This effect was also observed in non–steroid-treated patients.[1074] Based on a retrospective multivariate analysis[1072] of a large cohort of 329 patients from Japan, treatment with tonsillectomy and pulse glucocorticoid therapy (methylprednisolone, 0.5 g/day for 3 days for three courses, followed by oral prednisolone at an initial dose of 0.6 mg/kg on alternate days, with a decrease of 0.1 mg/kg every 2 months) was associated with clinical remission. Similarly, in a multivariate analysis[1075] focusing on the subgroup of 70 patients from the same cohort, with a baseline serum creatinine concentration of more than 1.5 mg/dL, treatment with the combination of tonsillectomy and pulse glucocorticoids was associated with improved long-term renal survival. Another retrospective analysis,[1071] however, showed no benefit of tonsillectomy on the clinical course of IgA nephropathy. Interestingly, a retrospective analysis of 365 patients with biopsy-proven IgA nephropathy in Japan has revealed that tonsillectomy delays disease progression to ESKD (OR, 0.09; 95% CI, 0.01–0.75; $P = .026$).[1076]

In a controlled nonrandomized trial, tonsillectomy plus pulse glucocorticoids was associated with a higher rate of remission of proteinuria and hematuria (but not kidney function) than pulse glucocorticoids alone.[1077] A multicenter RCT of patients with biopsy-proven IgA nephropathy randomly allocated patients to receive tonsillectomy with steroid pulses ($n = 33$) versus steroid pulses alone ($n = 39$).[1078] Although urinary protein excretion was significantly lower in the tonsillectomy group at the 12-month mark ($P < .05$), clinical remission (defined as the disappearance of hematuria, proteinuria, or both) was not. In contrast, in a large cohort of subjects from the European validation study of the Oxford classification of IgAN (VALIGA), no significant differences were found in respect to proteinuria or decline in renal function in patients with or without tonsillectomy.[1079] Long-term follow-up results will possibly provide further clarity.

**Omega-3 Fatty Acids.** Despite a great deal of interest in the past decade, the value of treatment with omega-3 long-chain polyunsaturated fatty acids (eicosapentaenoic and docosahexaenoic acids, found in fish oils) in IgA nephropathy remains unproven. This is based on the premise that omega-3 polyunsaturated fatty acids, eicosapentaenoic and docosahexaenoic acids, after biologic transformation into trienoic eicosanoids, may modulate the vascular reactivity and inflammatory mediators. By inhibiting cytokines, leukotriene Br, and possibly platelet-activating factor formation, fish oil may play a role in suppressing cell-mediated inflammation and limit glomerular injury.[1080,1081] In a study by the Mayo Clinic,[1081] 106 patients were randomly assigned to 12 g of omega-3 fatty acids or olive oil for 2 years. Only 6% of patients treated with fish oil experienced a doubling of their plasma creatinine concentration, compared with 33% of those treated with olive oil. In the fish oil–treated patients, only 14% excreted over 3.5 g of protein/day, in contrast to 65% of those treated with olive oil. The enthusiasm for this approach, however, was tempered by subsequent studies that showed no benefit of fish oil therapy.[1082,1083]

A metaanalysis of published trials on omega-3 fatty acids encompassing 17 trials and 626 subjects with a variety of kidney diseases, including five trials in IgA nephropathy,[1084] has revealed no beneficial effects on proteinuria or slowing in the rate of GFR decline. In an RCT involving 30 patients, the addition of omega-3 fatty acids to angiotensin II inhibition was more effective than angiotensin II inhibition alone in decreasing proteinuria and erythrocyturia over 6 months.[1085] A subsequent metaanalysis of five RCTs (totaling 233 patients) has found a significant reduction in proteinuria with omega-3 fatty acid use, but there was no significant benefit in preservation of kidney function.[1086] Unfortunately, no benefit was found in a metaanalysis published the same year.[1087] Therefore, if omega-3 fatty acids should be used at all in the treatment of IgA nephropathy, they should be used adjunctively in combination with angiotensin II inhibition and not as monotherapy.

In summary, until better long-term follow up studies are available, patients with IgA nephropathy with preserved renal function, with proteinuria more than 1 g/day, should be treated with supportive care, including RAAS blockade.[1088–1091] Should proteinuria persist despite angiotensin II inhibition, the addition of glucocorticoids (oral or intravenous plus oral) should be considered for patients with well-preserved kidney function (GFR ≥60 mL/min/1.73 m$^2$). In patients with progressive renal insufficiency, the use of prednisone and cyclophosphamide followed by azathioprine should be connsidered.[1053] In patients at high risk of progression (e.g., those fitting STOP-IgAN inclusion criteria), the use of corticosteroids or other immunosuppression requires a multifaceted approach.[1092] This challenge is best solved by assessing the risks of disease progression, MEST score, patient's clinical profile, and risks of adverse effects of immunosuppression. Also, an open discussion with patients about the study trials, risks, and benefits must be undertaken to reach a conclusion. It must be noted that the STOP-IgAN study did not address the role of immunosuppression in patients with crescentic, rapidly progressive glomerulonephritis or with nephrotic-range proteinuria because they were excluded from the study.[1093–1096]

It remains plausible that high-dose corticosteroids and/or cyclophosphamide could also be considered for patients with widespread crescentic glomerulonephritis, whereas patients with AKI associated with tubular necrosis and little glomerular damage should be treated conservatively, because these individuals have an excellent long-term response. Although there is no conclusive evidence of efficacy, the relatively benign side effect profile of omega-3 fatty acid therapy permits its use in patients who have an unfavorable prognosis. Patients with nephrotic syndrome and MCD may benefit from oral glucocorticoids.

## FIBRILLARY GLOMERULONEPHRITIS AND IMMUNOTACTOID GLOMERULOPATHY

### NOMENCLATURE

Fibrillary glomerulonephritis and immunotactoid glomerulopathy are glomerular diseases that are characterized by patterned deposits seen by electron microscopy (Figs. 31.31 and 31.32).[1097–1104] Most renal pathologists prefer to distinguish fibrillary glomerulonephritis from immunotactoid glomerulopathy based on the presence of fibrils of approximately 20 nm in diameter in fibrillary glomerulonephritis and larger, 30- to 40-nm–diameter microtubular structures in immunotactoid glomerulopathy[1097,1099–1102] (see Figs. 31.31 and 31.32). A minority of pathologists, however, have advocated grouping glomerular diseases with fibrillary deposits or microtubular deposits under the term "immunotactoid glomerulopathy."[1101,1104]

### FIBRILLARY GLOMERULONEPHRITIS PATHOLOGY

#### Electron Microscopy

The diagnosis of fibrillary glomerulonephritis (FGN) requires the identification by electron microscopy of irregular accumulations of randomly arranged. nonbranching fibrils of approximately 20-nm diameter in glomerular mesangium, capillary walls, or both[1097–1103,1105] (see Fig. 31.31A). In capillary walls, the fibrillary deposits can be subepithelial, subendothelial, or intramembranous. The fibrillary deposits often contain blotchy electron-dense material, but only rarely have associated well-defined, electron-dense deposits. The fibrils are distinctly larger than the actin filaments in adjacent cells, which is a useful observation that helps distinguish the fibrils of FGN from those of amyloidosis, which are only slightly larger than actin. The fibrils of FGN are not as large as the microtubular deposits of immunotactoid glomerulopathy or cryoglobulinemia, and they do not have the "fingerprint" configuration occasionally observed in lupus nephritis dense deposits. Most patients with FGN have substantial proteinuria, and therefore there usually is extensive effacement of visceral epithelial foot processes.

#### Light Microscopy

In FGN, extensive localization of fibrils in capillary walls causes capillary wall thickening. Mesangial localization results in an increased mesangial matrix and usually stimulates mesangial hypercellularity. Varying distributions of the

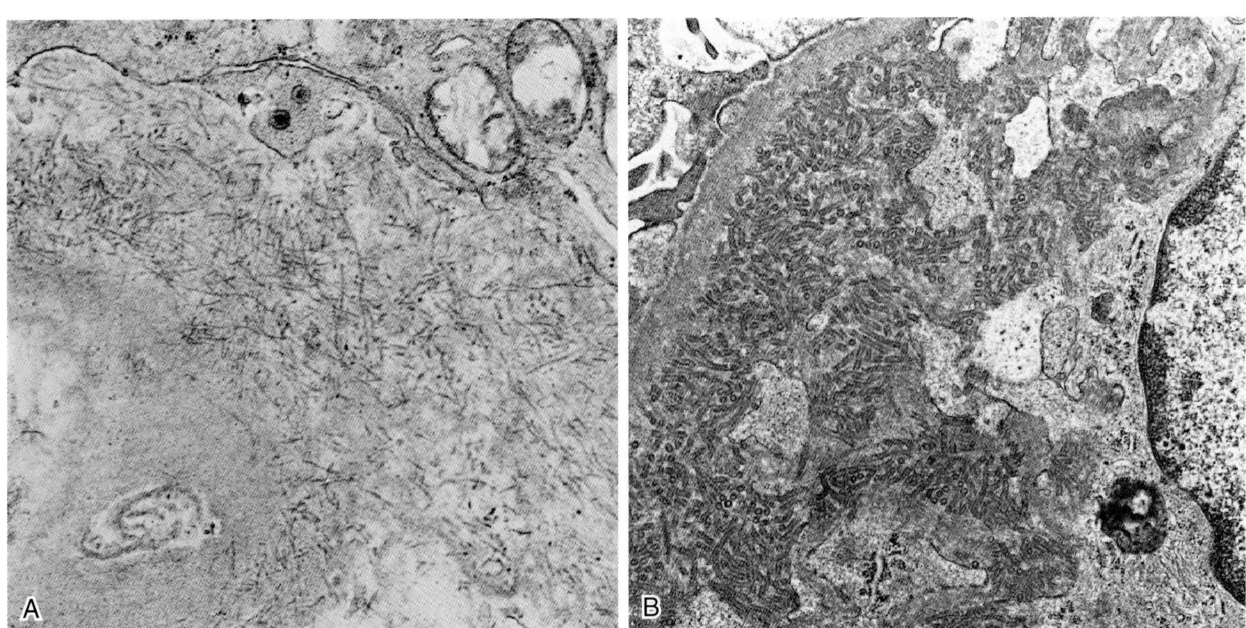


**Fig. 31.31** Electron micrographs showing the glomerular deposits of fibrillary glomerulonephritis (A) and immunotactoid glomerulopathy (B). Note the random orientation of the former and the microtubular appearance and greater organization of the latter. (×20,000.)

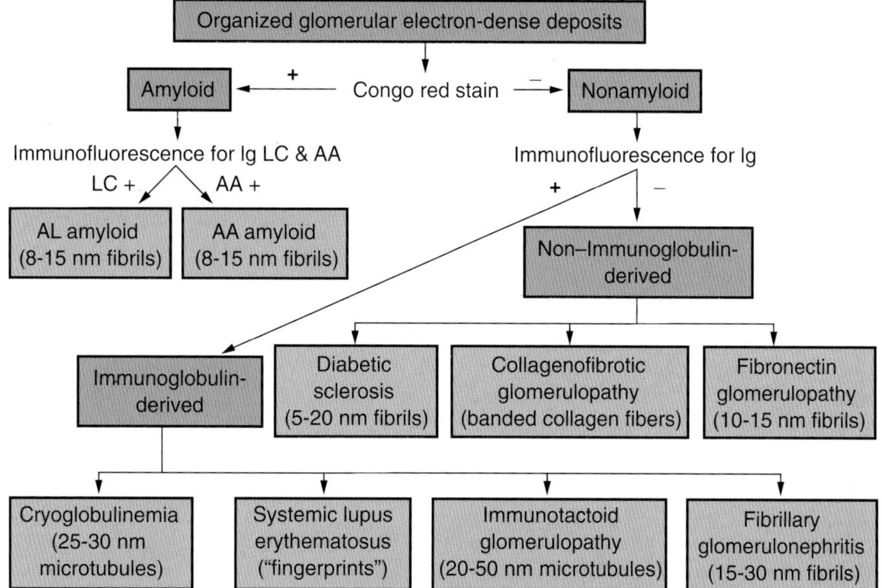


**Fig. 31.32** Algorithm for the pathologic categorization of glomerular diseases with patterned or organized deposits. The first division is into amyloid versus nonamyloid disease and the second is into diseases caused by immunoglobulin (Ig) molecule deposition and those that are not. By the approach illustrated, fibrillary glomerulonephritis is distinguished from immunotactoid glomerulopathy based on the ultrastructural characteristics of the deposits.

fibrillary deposits cause the light microscopic appearance of fibrillary glomerulonephritis to be extremely variable.[1097,1103] Therefore FGN can mimic the light microscopic appearance of MPGN, proliferative glomerulonephritis, or MN. Crescents occur in the most aggressive phenotypes. Of 74 sequential fibrillary glomerulonephritis specimens evaluated at UNC, 28% had crescents with an average involvement of 29% of glomeruli (range, 5%–80%). The fibrillary deposits typically have a moth-eaten appearance when stained with a Jones silver methenamine stain. They do not stain with Congo red, which distinguishes them from amyloid deposits.

### Immunofluorescence Microscopy

The deposits of FGN almost always stain more intensely for IgG than for IgM or IgA, and many specimens have little or no staining for IgM and IgA.[1097–1103] IgG4 is the dominant subclass. Only rare specimens have staining for only one light-chain type. C3 staining usually is intense. The IF staining pattern of fibrillary glomerulonephritis is relatively distinctive (Fig. 31.33). It is not granular or linear, but rather has an irregular bandlike appearance in capillary walls and an irregular shaggy appearance in the mesangium.

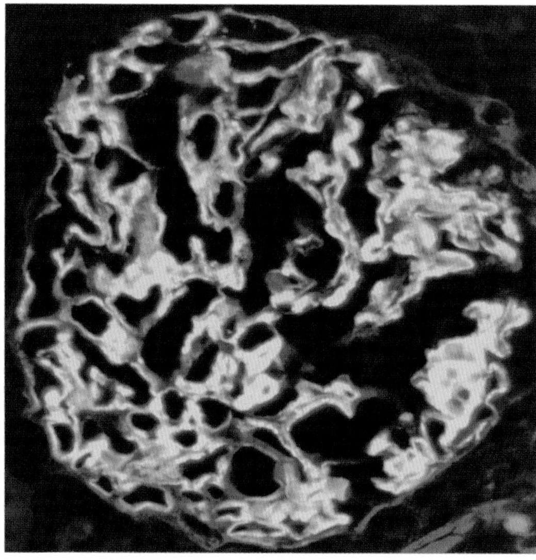

**Fig. 31.33** Immunofluorescence micrograph of a glomerulus with fibrillary glomerulonephritis showing mesangial and bandlike capillary wall staining for immunoglobulin G (IgG). (Fluorescein isothiocyanate anti-IgG stain, ×300.)

## IMMUNOTACTOID GLOMERULOPATHY PATHOLOGY

### Electron Microscopy

The tubular substructure of the deposits of immunotactoid glomerulopathy is readily discerned at 5,000 to 10,000 magnification (see Fig. 31.31B). At this magnification, the deposits of FGN have no tubular structure. The microtubules of immunotactoid glomerulopathy also have a greater tendency to align in parallel arrays, whereas the fibrils of FGN always are randomly distributed.[827] The ultrastructural deposits of immunotactoid glomerulonephritis resemble those seen in cryoglobulinemic glomerulonephritis; thus the latter must be ruled out before making a diagnosis of immunotactoid glomerulopathy. However, cryoglobulinemic microtubules typically are shorter and less well designed than immunotactoid microtubules.

### Light Microscopy

Immunotactoid glomerulopathy has a varied light microscopic appearance. Combined capillary wall thickening and mesangial expansion is most common, which often gives a membranoproliferative appearance. Immunotactoid deposits may be massive, resulting in nodular mesangial expansion in some specimens.

### Immunofluorescence Microscopy

The deposits of immunotactoid glomerulopathy usually are IgG dominant, with staining for both κ and λ light chains; however, the immunoglobulin in the deposits of immunotactoid glomerulopathy is more often monoclonal than in fibrillary glomerulonephritis.[1099] Monoclonality warrants a clinical workup for a B cell dyscrasia.

## PATHOGENESIS

The cause and pathogenesis of FGN and immunotactoid glomerulopathy are not known. Fibrillary glomerulonephritis and immunotactoid glomerulonephritis have been associated with lymphoproliferative disease (e.g., chronic lymphocytic leukemia, B cell lymphomas).[1099,1105,1106] Immunotactoid glomerulonephritis is more frequently associated with a monoclonal gammopathy.[1107] On rare occasions, FGN can also be associated with a monoclonal gammopathy.[1108,1109] The possible oligoclonal character of the deposits of FGN may facilitate self-association and fibrillar organization in a fashion analogous to that of the monoclonal light chains of immunoglobulin light-chain (AL) amyloidosis.[1102] The resemblance of immunotactoid deposits to those of cryoglobulinemia, which often contain a monoclonal component, also raises the possibility that the presence of some type of uniformity of the immunoglobulin in the deposits may be causing the patterned organization in immunotactoid glomerulopathy. Rarely, FGN may be associated with concomitant hepatitis C virus infection[1110] or an unusual IgM glomerular deposit disease.[1111]

In a recent study, FGN was postulated as an autoimmune disease caused by autoantibodies targeting putative autoantigen DNAJB9.[1112] Molecular chaperones are proteins that facilitate proper protein folding and the assembly needed for biologic functions. DNAJs are cochaperones that regulate activity of the heat shock protein (HSP), which is the major chaperone in humans. DNAJB9 (also known as "Mdg-1" or "ERdj4") is a member of the DNAJ protein located in the endoplasmic reticulum (ER). It functions as a cochaperone for Bip, which is the ER member of HSP. It is induced by many external stimuli, including heat, and also by p53 in response to DNA damage via the Ras/Raf/ERK pathway.

In two recent studies using laser capture microdissection, glomeruli were isolated from paraffin-embedded biopsy samples.[1113,1114] The proteins present in the samples were analyzed using liquid chromatography–assisted tandem mass spectrometry. DNAJB9 was a highly sampled protein found only in cases of FGN, along with IgG1and proteins of the classical complement pathway. This was specific for FGN because DNAJB9 was not detected in other glomerular diseases, including immunotactoid. Also, IF staining using DNAJB9 antibody showed specific staining in the GBM and/or mesangial regions. Dual staining was evident for the colocalization of DNAJB9 and IgG in glomerular and extraglomerular deposits. Further studies are required to understand the role of DNAJB9 and anti-DNAJB9 antibodies in the pathogenesis, of FGN.

## EPIDEMIOLOGY AND CLINICAL FEATURES

An analysis of 9085 consecutive native kidney biopsy specimens evaluated in the UNC Nephropathology Laboratory has revealed a frequency of 0.8% for fibrillary glomerulonephritis and 0.1% for immunotactoid glomerulonephritis, compared with 14.5% for MN, 7.5% for IgA nephropathy, 2.6% for type I MPGN, 1.5% for amyloidosis, and 0.8% for anti-GBM glomerulonephritis. Thus, fibrillary glomerulonephritis is about as common as anti-GBM glomerulonephritis and much more frequent than immunotactoid glomerulopathy.

Patients with fibrillary glomerulonephritis present with a mixture of nephrotic and nephritic syndrome features.[1100,1102,1105] Patients may have microscopic or macroscopic hematuria, renal insufficiency (including rapidly progressive glomerulonephritis in a few patients), hypertension, and proteinuria, which may be in the nephrotic range. In a series of 28 patients with fibrillary glomerulonephritis seen at UNC, the mean age was 49 years (range, 21–75 years), the ratio of males to females was 1 : 1.8, and the ratio of Caucasians to Afircan Americans was 8.3 : 1.[1102] After 24 months of follow-up, renal survival was only 48%.[1102] In a subsequent series of 66 patients with fibrillary glomerulonephritis seen at the Mayo Clinic in Rochester, MN, between 1993 and 2010, the mean age at diagnosis was 53 years, and the male-to-female ratio was 1 : 1.2. At presentation, 100% of patients had proteinuria, 52% had hematuria, 71% were hypertensive, and 66% had renal insufficiency. Underlying malignancy (23%), dysproteinemia (17%), or autoimmune disease (15%) was common. Of 61 patients with available data followed for an average of 52.3 months, 13% had complete or partial remission, 43% had persistent kidney dysfunction, and 44% progressed to ESKD. Not surprisingly, older age, higher creatinine level, proteinuria at biopsy, and a higher percentage of global glomerulosclerosis were independent predictors of ESKD by multivariate analysis.[1115] Overall, proteinuria is common at the time of presentation, as are hematuria, renal insufficiency, and hypertension. In patients in whom these disorders are diagnosed, malignancy, Crohn' disease, SLE, and cryoglobulinemia must be ruled out. Such patients have progressive renal failure in less than 5 years, although long-term patient survival is more than 80% at 5 years.[1107,1116]

In a group of six patients with immunotactoid glomerulopathy, the mean age was 62 years.[1100] At presentation, the clinical features in these patients looked very much like those in patients with fibrillary glomerulonephritis; they included proteinuria, hematuria, and renal insufficiency. In the largest series to date, 16 patients with immunotactoid glomerulopathy were identified from the pathology archives at the Mayo Clinic. Proteinuria was present in 100% of patients; 80% had microhematuria, 69% had nephrotic syndrome, and 50% had renal insufficiency. Interestingly, 38% of patients had a hematologic malignancy. Over an average of 48 months of follow-up of 12 patients, 50% remitted, 33% had persistent kidney dysfunction, and 17% progressed to ESKD.[1117]

Importantly, patients with immunotactoid glomerular disease are more likely to have an associated hematopoietic process and poor long-term survival.[1100] In a review study of 67 patients presenting with fibrillary glomerulopathy ($n = 61$) or immunotactoid glomerulopathy ($n = 6$), all patients had proteinuria and 50% had nephrotic syndrome, whereas hematuria occurred in approximately two-thirds of patients and hypertension in about 75% of patients.[1118] Renal insufficiency was discovered in 50% of the patient population. There were no statistically significant differences in clinical presentation between patients with fibrillary glomerulonephritis and those with immunotactoid glomerulonephritis. In regard to causative factors, patients with immunotactoid glomerulonephritis were statistically more likely to have an underlying lymphoproliferative disease, a monoclonal spike on serum protein electrophoresis, and hypocomplementemia.[1118]

Fibrillary glomerulonephritis with associated pulmonary hemorrhage has been reported anecdotally.[1119] One patient with immunotactoid glomerulopathy also had extrarenal deposits in both the liver and bone.[1120]

### TREATMENT

At this time, there is no convincingly effective form of treatment for patients with fibrillary glomerulonephritis or immunotactoid glomerulopathy.[1105] The dismal prognosis in patients with either of these diseases has prompted physicians to search for some immunosuppressive form of treatment. Fully 40% to 50% of patients with these diseases develop ESKD within 6 years of presentation.[1097,1098,1100,1102] Efforts at treatment with glucocorticoids or alkylating agents such as cyclophosphamide have typically shown no response or, at best, some amelioration of proteinuria.[1121] In our experience, prednisone therapy alone has had no benefit. One small case series (three patients) reported significant improvement in proteinuria in response to rituximab, either alone or in combination with corticosteroids, or tacrolimus.[1122] In fibrillary glomerulonephritis and other forms of glomerulonephritis associated with chronic lymphocytic leukemia or other forms of lymphocytic lymphoma, there has been a report of improvement in a minority of patients treated with chlorambucil. Thus, it is possible that the treatment of the underlying malignancy, if present, may improve the glomerulonephritis.[1106] Of note, a recent case series and review of previously published large case series have revealed a role for rituximab in patients with fibrillary glomerulonephritis if administered early in the disease process with a preserved eGFR.[1123]

The recurrence rate of fibrillary glomerulonephritis after kidney transplantation is unclear. One report has described recurrent disease in three of four patients who had received five transplants.[1124] In a larger case series, recurrent disease occurred in none of five patients with fibrillary glomerulonephritis, but in five of seven patients with monoclonal gammopathy and fibrillary deposits.[1125]

## RAPIDLY PROGRESSIVE GLOMERULONEPHRITIS AND CRESCENTIC GLOMERULONEPHRITIS

### NOMENCLATURE AND CATEGORIZATION

The term "rapidly progressive glomerulonephritis" (RPGN) refers to a clinical syndrome characterized by a rapid loss of kidney function, often accompanied by oliguria or anuria and features of glomerulonephritis, including dysmorphic erythrocyturia, erythrocyte cylindruria, and glomerular proteinuria.[1126] Aggressive glomerulonephritis that causes RPGN usually has extensive crescent formation.[1127] For this reason, the clinical term "rapidly progressive glomerulonephritis" is sometimes used interchangeably with the pathologic term "crescentic glomerulonephritis." Crescentic glomerulonephritis is the most aggressive structural phenotype in the continuum of injury that results from glomerular inflammation (see Fig. 31.30). This pathologic feature can be seen on light, IF, and electron microscopy.[1127–1129] It is the result of focal rupture of glomerular capillary walls that allows inflammatory mediators and leukocytes to enter Bowman's space, where they induce epithelial cell proliferation and macrophage influx and maturation, which together produce cellular crescents (Fig. 31.34).[1130–1132]

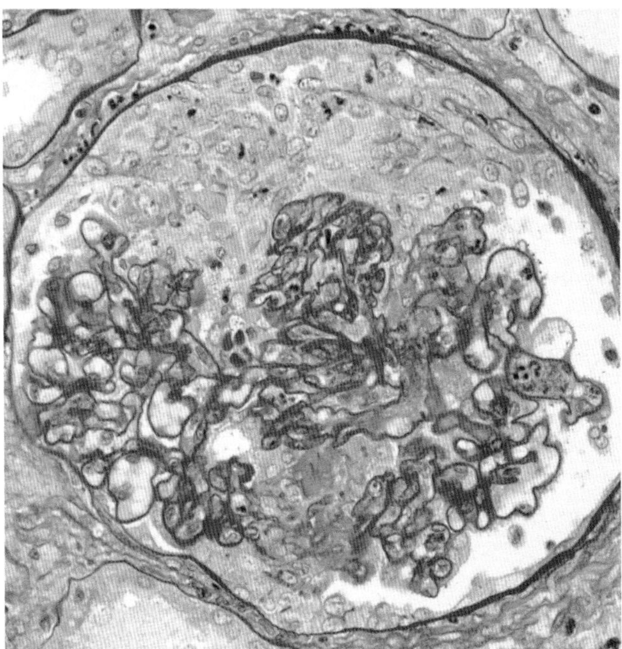

**Fig. 31.34** Light micrograph showing a cellular crescent in Bowman's space. The underlying glomerular tuft is delineated by the glomerular basement membranes. (Periodic acid–Schiff stain, ×500.)

Kidney diseases other than crescentic glomerulonephritis can cause the signs and symptoms of RPGN. Two examples are acute thrombotic microangiopathy and atheroembolic kidney disease. Although acute tubular necrosis and acute tubulointerstitial nephritis may cause rapid loss of kidney function and oliguria, these processes typically do not cause dysmorphic erythrocyturia, erythrocyte cylindruria, or substantial proteinuria.

A small minority of all patients with glomerulonephritis develops RPGN, except patients with anti-GBM disease and ANCA disease who have a high frequency of crescents. The incidence of rapidly progressive glomerulonephritis has been estimated to be as low as 7 cases/million population per year.[675,1133] The three major immunopathologic categories of crescentic glomerulonephritis have different frequencies in different age groups (Table 31.8).[1126–1128,1134] In a patient who has RPGN clinically and in whom crescentic glomerulonephritis is identified by light microscopy in a kidney biopsy specimen, the precise diagnostic categorization of the disease requires the integration of clinical, serologic, immunohistologic, and electron microscopic data (Fig. 31.35).

Immune complex crescentic glomerulonephritis is caused by immune complex localization within glomeruli. It is the most common cause of RPGN in children (see Table 31.8).[1127] The major clinical differential diagnosis in children is hemolytic uremic syndrome, which also can cause rapid loss of kidney function, hypertension, hematuria, and proteinuria.

**Table 31.8 Relative Frequency of Immunopathologic Categories of Crescentic Glomerulonephritis In Different Age Groups (%)[a]**

| | Age in Years | | | |
|---|---|---|---|---|
| **Immunopathologic Category** | All Ages (*n* = 632) | 1–20 (*n* = 73) | 21–60 (*n* = 303) | >60 (*n* = 256) |
| Antiglomerular basement membrane CGN | 15 | 12 | 15 | 15 |
| Immune complex CGN | 24 | 45 | 35 | 6 |
| Pauci-immune CGN[b] | 60 | 42 | 48 | 79 |
| Other | 1 | 0 | 30 | 0 |

[a]CGN is defined as the presence of crescents in >50% of glomeruli. Frequency is determined with respect to age in patients whose kidney biopsy specimens were evaluated at the University of North Carolina Nephropathology Laboratory. Note the very high frequency of pauci-immune disease (usually antineutrophil cytoplasmic antibody [ANCA]–associated) in older adults.
[b]Approximately 90% associated with ANCA.
*CGN*, Crescentic glomerulonephritis.
Data from Jennette JC, Nickeleit V: Anti-glomerular basement membrane glomerulonephritis and Goodpasture's syndrome. In Jennette JC, Olson JL, Silva FG, D'Agati V, eds. *Heptinstall's pathology of the kidney.* 7th ed. Wolters Klewer: Philadelphia; 2015:657–684.

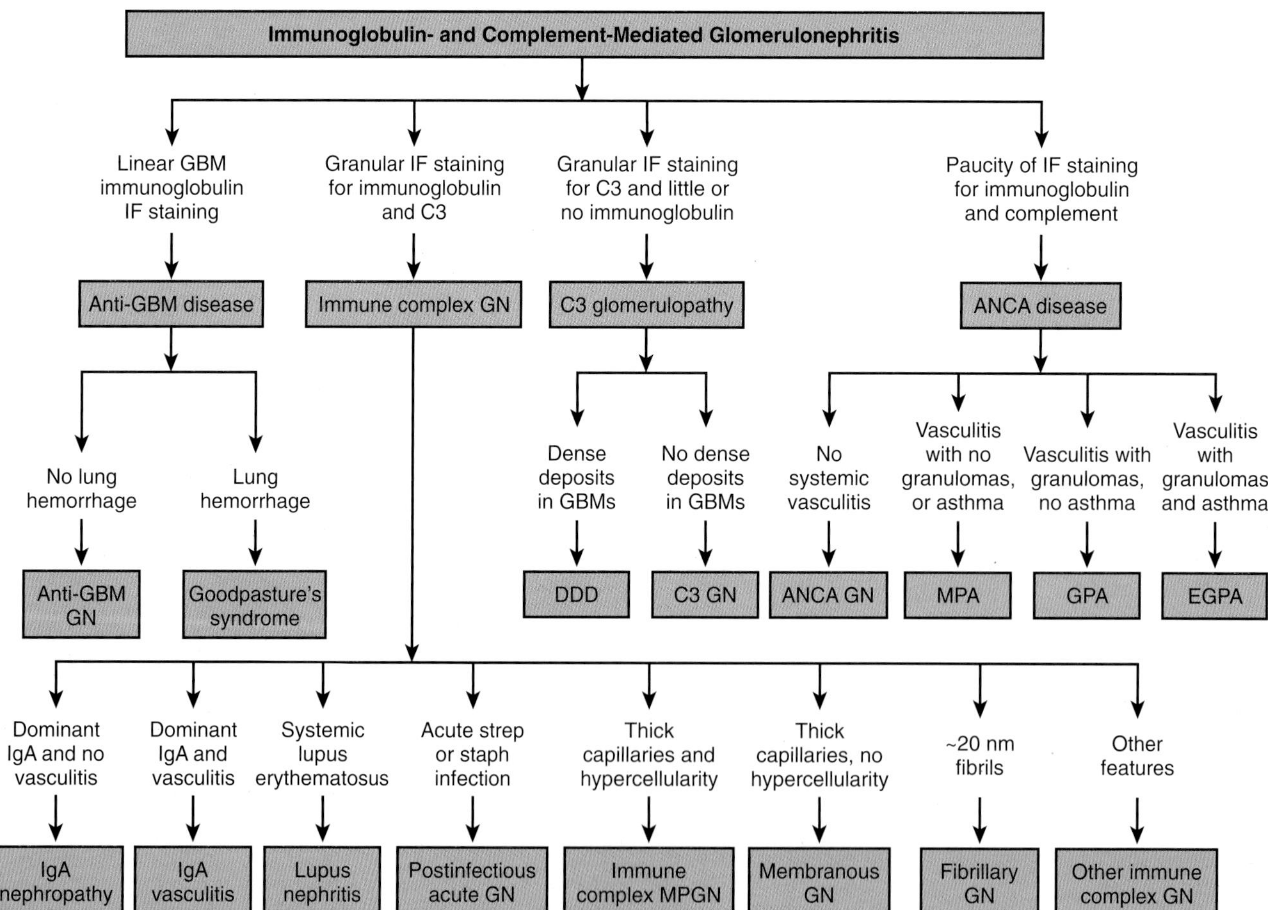


**Fig. 31.35** Algorithm for the diagnostic classification of glomerulonephritis that is known or suspected of being mediated by antibodies and complement. Note that the integration of light microscopy, immunofluorescence (IF) microscopy, electron microscopy, laboratory data, and clinical manifestations is required to diagnose glomerulonephritis (GN) precisely. *ANCA,* Antineutrophil cytoplasmic autoantibody; *DDD,* dense deposit disease; *EGPA*, eosinophilic granulomatosis with polyangiitis; *GBM,* glomerular basement membrane; *GPA*, granulomatosis with polyangiitis; *MPA,* microscopic polyangiitis.

**Table 31.9 Frequency of Immunopathologic Categories of Glomerulonephritis in Kidney Biopsy Specimens Evaluated by Immunofluorescence Microscopy[a]**

| Immunohistology | All Proliferative Glomerulonephritis (*n* = 1093) | Any Crescents (*n* = 540) | >50% Crescents (*n* = 195) | Arteritis in Biopsy (*n* = 37) |
|---|---|---|---|---|
| Pauci-immune (<2+ Ig) | 45% (496/1093) | 51% (227/540) | 61% (118/195)[b] | 84% (31/37) |
| Immune complex (≥2+ Ig) | 52% (570/1093) | 44% (238/540) | 29% (56/195) | 14% (5/37)[c] |
| Anti-GBM | 3% (27/1093) | 5% (25/540)[d] | 11% (21/195) | 3% (1/37)[e] |

[a]Based on the analysis of over 3000 consecutive nontransplant renal biopsy specimens evaluated at the University of North Carolina Nephropathology Laboratory.
[b]Of 77 patients, 70 (91%) tested positive for antineutrophil cytoplasmic antibody (ANCA), (44 for perinuclear ANCA [P-ANCA] and 26 cytoplasmic ANCA [C-ANCA]).
[c]Four patients had lupus and one had poststreptococcal glomerulonephritis.
[d]Three of 19 patients (16%) tested positive for ANCA (2 for P-ANCA and 1 for C-ANCA).
[e]This patient also tested positive for P-ANCA (myeloperoxidase ANCA).
*GBM,* Glomerular basement membrane; *IF,* immunofluorescence.
Modified from Jennette JC, Nickeleit V: Anti-glomerular basement membrane glomerulonephritis and Goodpasture's syndrome. In Jennette JC, Olson JL, Silva FG, D'Agati V, eds. *Heptinstall's pathology of the kidney.* 7th ed. Wolters Klewer: Philadelphia; 2015:657–684.

The presence of microangiopathic hemolytic anemia and thrombocytopenia are indicators that the rapid loss of kidney function is more likely caused by hemolytic uremic syndrome than crescentic glomerulonephritis. Pauci-immune crescentic glomerulonephritis, which shows little or no evidence of the localization of immune complex or anti-GBM antibodies in glomeruli, is usually associated with the presence of ANCAs and is the most common cause for RPGN and crescentic glomerulonephritis in adults, especially older adults (Table 31.9; see Table 31.8).[1126,1134–1136] In most patients, pauci-immune crescentic glomerulonephritis is a component of a systemic small-vessel vasculitis, such as GPA or MPA; however, some patients have renal-limited (primary) disease.[1127,1137] Anti-GBM disease is the least frequent cause of crescentic glomerulonephritis (see Tables 31.8 and 31.9).[1126,1127,1134,1135]

## IMMUNE COMPLEX–MEDIATED AND C3 GLOMERULOPATHY CRESCENTIC GLOMERULONEPHRITIS

### EPIDEMIOLOGY

Most patients with immune complex–mediated crescentic glomerulonephritis have clinical or pathologic evidence of a specific category of primary glomerulonephritis, such as IgA nephropathy, postinfectious glomerulonephritis, or MPGN, or they have glomerulonephritis that is a component of a systemic immune complex disease, such as SLE, cryoglobulinemia, or IgA vasculitis. A minority of patients with immune complex crescentic glomerulonephritis, however, do not have patterns of immune complex localization that readily fit into these specific categories of immune complex glomerulonephritis.[1138]

Immune complex crescentic glomerulonephritis accounts for most crescentic glomerulonephritides in children, but for only a minority of crescentic glomerulonephritis in older adults (see Table 31.8). The higher frequency in children and young adults reflects a similar trend in other types of immune complex glomerulonephritides, such as IgA nephropathy, PSGN, MPGN, DDD, and lupus nephritis.

### PATHOLOGY

#### Light Microscopy

The light microscopic appearance of crescentic immune complex glomerulonephritis depends on the underlying category of glomerulonephritis. For example, in their most aggressive expressions, MPGN, acute postinfectious glomerulonephritis, or proliferative glomerulonephritis, including IgA nephropathy, can all have crescent formation.*

This underlying phenotype of immune complex glomerulonephritis is recognized best in the intact glomeruli or glomerular segments. Immune complex–mediated glomerulonephritis and C3 glomerulopathy usually have varying combinations of capillary wall thickening and endocapillary hypercellularity in the intact glomeruli. This is in contrast to anti-GBM glomerulonephritis and ANCA glomerulonephritis, which tend to have surprisingly few alterations in intact glomeruli and segments, in spite of the severe necrotizing injury in involved glomeruli and segments. In glomerular segments adjacent to crescents in immune complex glomerulonephritis, there usually is some degree of necrosis with karyorrhexis; however, the necrosis is rarely as extensive as that typically seen with anti-GBM or ANCA glomerulonephritis. In addition, there is less destruction of Bowman's capsule associated with crescents in immune complex glomerulonephritis, as well as less pronounced periglomerular tubulointerstitial inflammation. Crescents in immune complex glomerulonephritis have a higher proportion of epithelial cells to macrophages than crescents in anti-GBM or ANCA glomerulonephritis, which may be related to the less severe disruption of Bowman's capsule and thus less opportunity for macrophages to migrate in from the interstitium.[1138]

#### Immunofluorescence Microscopy

IF microscopy, as well as electron microscopy, provides the evidence that crescentic glomerulonephritis is immune complex-mediated or complement-mediated versus anti-GBM

*References 359–363, 697, 703, 831, 1058, 1133, and 1139.

antibody-mediated or ANCA-mediated. The pattern and composition of immunoglobulin and complement staining depend on the underlying category of immune complex glomerulonephritis or C3 glomerulopathy that has induced crescent formation.[360,702,1140] For example, crescentic glomerulonephritis with predominantly mesangial IgA-dominant deposits is indicative of crescentic IgA nephropathy, C3-dominant deposits with peripheral bandlike configurations suggest crescentic MPGN, coarsely granular capillary wall deposits raise the possibility of crescentic postinfectious glomerulonephritis, and finely granular IgG-dominant capillary wall deposits suggest crescentic MN. The latter may be a result of concurrent anti-GBM disease, which also causes linear GBM staining beneath the granular staining, or concurrent ANCA disease, which can be documented serologically. About 25% of all patients with crescentic immune complex glomerulonephritis are ANCA-positive, whereas fewer than 5% of patients with noncrescentic immune complex glomerulonephritis are ANCA positive. This suggests that the presence of ANCAs in patients with immune complex glomerulonephritis may predispose to a disease that is more aggressive.

#### Electron Microscopy

As with the findings by IF microscopy, the findings by electron microscopy in patients with crescentic immune complex glomerulonephritis depend on the type of immune complex disease that has induced crescent formation. The hallmark ultrastructural finding is immune complex– type, electron-dense deposits. These can be mesangial, subendothelial, intramembranous, subepithelial, or any combination of these. The pattern and distribution of deposits may indicate a particular phenotype of primary crescentic immune complex glomerulonephritis, such as postinfectious, membranous, membranoproliferative, or DDD.[360,702,1140] Ultrastructural findings also may suggest that the disease is secondary to some unrecognized systemic process. For example, endothelial tubuloreticular inclusions suggest lupus nephritis, and microtubular configurations in immune deposits suggest cryoglobulinemia.

In all types of crescentic glomerulonephritis, breaks in GBMs usually can be identified if sought carefully, especially in glomerular segments adjacent to crescents. Dense fibrin tactoids occur in thrombosed capillaries, in sites of fibrinoid necrosis, and in the interstices between the cells in crescents. In general, the extent of fibrin tactoid formation in areas of fibrinoid necrosis is less conspicuous in crescentic immune complex glomerulonephritis than in crescentic anti-GBM or ANCA glomerulonephritis.

### PATHOGENESIS

Crescentic glomerulonephritis is the result of a final common pathway of glomerular injury that results in crescent formation. Multiple causes and pathogenic mechanisms can lead to the final common pathway, including many types of immune complex disease. The general dogma is that immune complex localization in glomerular capillary walls and mesangium, by deposition, in situ formation, or both, activates multiple inflammatory mediator systems.[211,1126,1127] This includes humoral mediator systems, such as the coagulation system, kinin system, and complement system, as well as inflammatory cells, such as neutrophils, monocytes and macrophages, lymphocytes, platelets, endothelial cells, and mesangial cells. The activated cells also release soluble mediators, such as cytokines and chemokines. If the resultant inflammation is contained internally to the GBM, a proliferative or membranoproliferative phenotype of injury ensues, with only endocapillary hypercellularity. However, if the inflammation breaks through capillary walls into Bowman's space, extracapillary hypercellularity (crescent formation) results.

Complement activation has often been considered a major mediator of injury in immune complex glomerulonephritis; however, experimental data also indicate the importance of Fc receptors in immune complex-mediated injury.[1141,1142] For example, mice deficient for the Fcγ R1 and Fcγ RIII receptors have a markedly reduced tendency to develop immune complex glomerulonephritis.[1143,1144]

### TREATMENT

The therapy for crescentic immune complex glomerulonephritis is influenced by the nature of the underlying category of immune complex glomerulonephritis. For example, acute PSGN with 50% crescents might not prompt the same therapy as IgA nephropathy with 50% crescents. However, there have been an inadequate number of controlled prospective studies to guide therapy for most forms of crescentic immune complex glomerulonephritis. Some nephrologists extrapolate from the lupus nephritis experience and choose to treat patients with crescentic immune complex disease with immunosuppressive drugs that they would not use if the glomerular lesions appeared less aggressive. For the minority of patients who have idiopathic immune complex crescentic glomerulonephritis, the most common treatment is immunosuppressive therapy with pulse methylprednisolone, followed by prednisone at a dosage of 1 mg/kg daily tapered over the second to third month to an alternate-day regimen until completely discontinued.[675,1145–1147] In patients with a rapid decline in kidney function, cytotoxic agents, with or without plasma exchange, in addition to corticosteroids, may be considered. As with anti-GBM and ANCA disease, immunotherapy should be initiated as early as possible during the course of crescentic immune complex glomerulonephritis to reduce the likelihood of reaching the irreversible stage of advanced scarring. There is evidence, however, that crescentic glomerulonephritis with an underlying immune complex proliferative glomerulonephritis is less responsive to aggressive immunosuppressive therapy than is anti-GBM or ANCA crescentic glomerulonephritis.[1058,1138]

## ANTI–GLOMERULAR BASEMENT MEMBRANE GLOMERULONEPHRITIS

### EPIDEMIOLOGY

Anti-GBM disease accounts for about 10% to 20% of crescentic glomerulonephritides.[675] This disease is characterized by circulating antibodies to the GBM (anti-GBM) and deposition of IgG or, rarely, IgA along the GBM (see also Chapter 32).[675,1138,1148–1160] Anti-GBM antibodies may be eluted from kidney tissue samples from patients with anti-GBM disease, which allows verification that the antibodies are specific to the GBM.[675,1154,1158] The antibodies eluted from kidney tissue bind to the same epitope of type IV collagen as the circulating anti-GBM antibodies from the same patient.[1161]

Anti-GBM disease occurs as a renal-limited disease (anti-GBM glomerulonephritis) and as a pulmonary-renal vasculitic syndrome (Goodpasture syndrome).[675,1138,1148–1160,1162] The incidence of anti-GBM disease has two peaks with respect to age. The first peak is in the 2nd and 3rd decades of life, and anti-GBM disease in this age group shows a higher frequency of pulmonary hemorrhage (Goodpasture syndrome). The second peak is in the 6th and 7th decades, and this later onset disease is more common in women, who more often have renal-limited disease. Interestingly, anti-GBM autoantibodies were detected in multiple serum samples from the Department of Defense Serum Repository before diagnosis in a case-control study involving 30 patients with anti-GBM disease and 30 healthy controls (50% vs. 0%; $P < .001$),[1163] which suggests the development of the autoimmune response prior to onset of disease.

Genetic susceptibility to anti-GBM disease is associated with HLA-DR2 specificity.[1164] More detailed analysis of the association with HLA-DR2 has revealed a link with the DRB1 alleles, DRB1*1501 and DQB*0602.[1165–1169] Further refinement of this association has shown that polymorphic residues in the second peptide-binding region of the HLA class II antigen segregated with disease, supporting the hypothesis that the HLA association in anti-GBM disease reflects the ability of certain class II molecules to bind and present anti-GBM peptides to helper T ($T_H$) cells.[1165]

This concept is further supported by mouse models of anti-GBM disease in which crescentic glomerulonephritis and lung hemorrhage are restricted to only certain major histocompatibility complex (MHC) haplotypes, despite the ability of mice of all haplotypes to produce antibodies to the $\alpha_3$-NC1 ("noncollagenous") domain of type IV collagen.[1170] Analyses of gene expression in the kidneys of mouse strains susceptible to anti-GBM antibody-induced nephritis, compared with those of control strains, have revealed that 20% of the underexpressed genes in these mice belonged to the kallikrein gene family, which encodes serine esterases implicated in the regulation of inflammation, apoptosis, redox balance, and fibrosis.[1171] Antagonizing the kallikrein pathway by blocking the bradykinin receptors B1 and B2 augmented disease, whereas bradykinin administration reduced the severity of anti-GBM, antibody-induced nephritis in a susceptible mouse strain. Nephritis-sensitive mouse strains had kallikrein haplotypes that were distinct from those of control strains, including several regulatory polymorphisms. These results suggest that kallikreins are protective disease-associated genes in anti-GBM antibody-induced nephritis.[1171] Whether these findings pertain to susceptibility to or severity of anti-GBM disease in humans in unknown. It should also be noted that another genetic association study of 48 Chinese patients with anti-GBM disease compared with 225 matched healthy controls revealed a genetic association of an FCγRIIB polymorphism (I232T) with disease susceptibility.[1172] This same polymorphism has been identified in patients with SLE and is thought to alter this inhibitory receptor responsible for the maintenance of B cell tolerance and activation thresholds.[1173]

## PATHOLOGY

### Immunofluorescence Microscopy

The pathologic finding of linear staining of the GBMs for immunoglobulin is indicative of anti-GBM glomerulonephritis (Fig. 31.36).[1155,1158,1159,1174–1177] The immunoglobulin is predominantly IgG; however, rare patients with IgA-dominant,

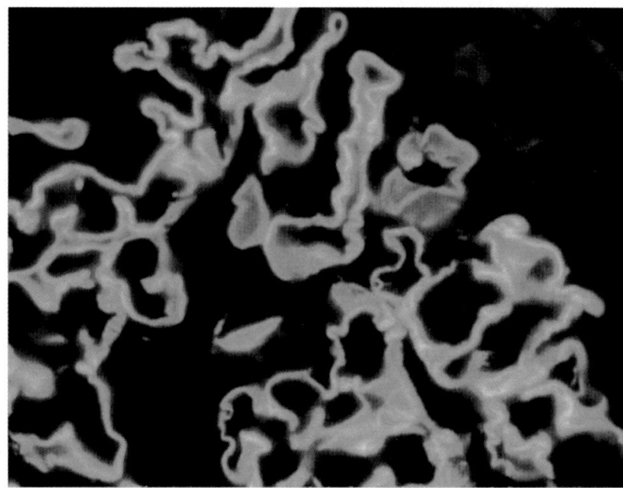

**Fig. 31.36** Immunofluorescence micrograph of a portion of a glomerulus with antiglomerular basement membrane (anti-GBM) glomerulonephritis showing linear staining of GBMs for immunoglobulin G (IgG). (Fluorescein isothiocyanate anti-IgG stain, ×500.)

anti-GBM glomerulonephritis have also been reported.[1156,1178] Linear staining for both κ and λ light chains typically accompanies the staining for γ heavy chains. Linear staining for γ heavy chains alone indicates γ heavy-chain deposition disease. Most specimens with anti-GBM glomerulonephritis have discontinuous linear to granular capillary wall staining for C3, but a minority show little or no C3 staining. Linear staining for IgG may also occur along distal tubular basement membranes.[1159]

The linear IgG staining of GBMs frequently seen in patients with diabetic glomerulosclerosis and the less intense linear staining seen in older patients with hypertensive vascular disease, must not be confused with that in anti-GBM disease. Clinical data and light microscopic findings should help make this distinction. Serologic confirmation should always be obtained to substantiate the diagnosis of anti-GBM disease.

Serologic testing for ANCAs should be ordered simultaneously because one-quarter to one-third of patients with anti-GBM disease are also ANCA-positive. This may modify the prognosis and likelihood of systemic small-vessel vasculitis.[1179,1180]

### Light Microscopy

At the time of biopsy, 97% of patients with anti-GBM disease have some degree of crescent formation, and 85% have crescents in 50% or more of glomeruli (Table 31.10).[1127,1174] On average, 77% of glomeruli have crescents. Glomeruli with crescents typically have fibrinoid necrosis in adjacent glomerular segments. Nonnecrotic segments may look entirely normal by light microscopy or may have slight infiltration by neutrophils or mononuclear leukocytes. This differs from crescentic immune complex glomerulonephritis and C3 glomerulopathy, which typically have capillary wall thickening and endocapillary hypercellularity in the intact glomeruli. Special stains that outline basement membranes, such as Jones' silver methenamine or periodic acid–Schiff stain, often demonstrate focal breaks in GBMs in areas of necrosis and also show focal breaks in Bowman's capsule. The most severely injured glomeruli have global glomerular necrosis,

**Table 31.10 Frequency of Crescent Formation in Various Glomerular Diseases[a]**

| Disease | Patients With Crescents (%) | Patients With ≥50% Crescents | Average No. of Glomeruli With Crescents (%) |
|---|---|---|---|
| Anti-GBM glomerulonephritis | 97 | 85 | 77 |
| ANCA-associated glomerulonephritis | 90 | 50 | 49 |
| Immune complex–mediated glomerulonephritis | | | |
| Lupus glomerulonephritis (classes III and IV) | 56 | 13 | 27 |
| IgA vasculitis (formerly Henoch-Schönlein purpura glomerulonephritis)[b] | 61 | 10 | 27 |
| IgA nephropathy[b] | 32 | 4 | 21 |
| Acute postinfectious glomerulonephritis[b] | 33 | 3 | 19 |
| Fibrillary glomerulonephritis | 23 | 5 | 26 |
| Type I membranoproliferative glomerulonephritis | 24 | 5 | 25 |
| Membranous lupus glomerulonephritis (class V) | 12 | 1 | 17 |
| Membranous glomerulonephritis (nonlupus) | 3 | 0 | 15 |

[a]Based on analysis of over 6000 native kidney biopsy specimens evaluated at the University of North Carolina Nephropathology Laboratory. In general, diseases in which crescents are most often seen also have the largest percentage of glomeruli involved by crescents when they are present.

[b]Because more severe cases of immunoglobulin A nephropathy and postinfectious glomerulonephritis are more often evaluated by kidney biopsy, the extent of crescent involvement is higher in the patients included in this table than in the general group of patients with these diseases.

*ANCA,* Antineutrophil cytoplasmic antibody; *GBM,* glomerular basement membrane; *GN,* glomerulonephritis; *IgA,* immunoglobulin A.

Modified from Jennette JC: Rapidly progressive and crescentic glomerulonephritis. *Kidney Int.* 2003;63:1164–1177.

circumferential cellular crescents, and extensive disruption of Bowman's capsule.

The acute necrotizing glomerular lesions and the cellular crescents evolve into glomerular sclerosis and fibrotic crescents, respectively.[1174] If the kidney biopsy specimen is obtained several weeks into the course of anti-GBM disease, the only lesions may be these chronic sclerotic lesions. There may be a mixture of acute and chronic lesions; however, the glomerular lesions of anti-GBM glomerulonephritis tend to be more in synchrony than those of ANCA glomerulonephritis, which more often show admixtures of acute and chronic injury.

Tubulointerstitial changes are commensurate with the degree of glomerular injury. Glomeruli with extensive necrosis and disruption of Bowman's capsule typically have intense periglomerular inflammation, including occasional multinucleated giant cells. There also is focal tubular epithelial acute simplification or atrophy, focal interstitial edema and fibrosis, and focal interstitial infiltration of predominantly mononuclear leukocytes. There are no specific changes in arteries or arterioles. If necrotizing inflammation is observed in arteries or arterioles, the possibility of concurrent anti-GBM and ANCA disease should be considered.

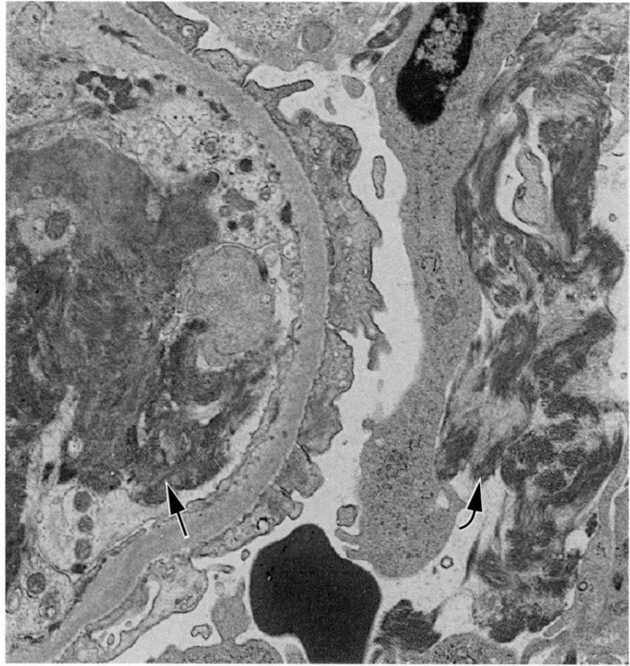

**Fig. 31.37** Electron micrograph of a portion of a glomerular capillary wall and adjacent urinary space from a patient with antiglomerular basement membrane (anti-GBM) glomerulonephritis. Note the fibrin tactoids within a capillary thrombus *(straight arrow)* and in Bowman's space *(curved arrow)* between the cells of a crescent. Also note the absence of immune complex–type, electron-dense deposits in the capillary wall. (×6000.)

### Electron Microscopy

The findings by electron microscopy reflect those seen by light microscopy.[1174,1181] In acute disease, there is focal glomerular necrosis with disruption of capillary walls. Bowman's capsule also may have focal gaps. Leukocytes, including neutrophils and monocytes, often are present at sites of necrosis, but are uncommon in intact glomerular segments. Fibrin tactoids, which are electron-dense curvilinear accumulations of polymerized fibrin, accumulate at the sites of coagulation system activation, including sites of capillary thrombosis, fibrinoid necrosis, and fibrin formation in Bowman's space (Fig. 31.37). Cellular crescents contain cells with ultrastructural features of macrophages and epithelial cells. An important negative observation is the absence of immune complex–type, electron-dense deposits. These occur only in specimens from patients with anti-GBM disease patients who have concurrent immune complex disease. Glomerular segments that do not have necrosis may appear remarkably normal, with only focal effacement of visceral epithelial foot processes. There may be slight lucent expansion of the lamina rara interna, but this is an inconstant and nonspecific feature. In chronic lesions, amorphous and banded collagen deposition distorts or replaces the normal architecture.

## PATHOGENESIS

The landmark studies opening the way to an understanding of the pathogenesis of anti-GBM disease were those of Lerner and colleagues.[1154] In these studies, antibodies eluted from kidneys of patients with Goodpasture syndrome and injected into monkeys led to the induction of glomerulonephritis, proteinuria, renal failure, and pulmonary hemorrhage, along with intense staining of the GBM for human IgG.

The antigen to which anti-GBM antibodies react was initially found to be in the collagenase-resistant part of type IV collagen, the so-called noncollagenous domain, or NC1 domain.[1182–1184] The antigenic epitopes found in the NC1 domain are in a cryptic form, as evidenced by the fact that little reactivity is found against the native hexameric structure of the NC1 domain. However, when the hexameric NC1 domain is denatured and dissociates into dimers and monomers, the reactivity of antibodies increases 15-fold.[1184] About 90% of anti–type IV collagen antibodies are directed against the $\alpha_3$ chain of type IV collagen.[1146,1185] The Goodpasture epitopes in the native autoantigen are sequestered within the NC1 hexamers of the $\alpha_3\alpha_4\alpha_5$(IV) collagen network and are a feature of the quaternary structure of two distinct subsets of $\alpha_3\alpha_4\alpha_5$(IV) NC1 hexamers. Goodpasture antibodies breach only the quaternary structure of hexamers containing only monomer subunits, whereas hexamers composed of both dimer and monomer subunits (D-hexamers) are resistant to autoantibodies under native conditions.[1186,1187] The epitopes of D-hexamers are structurally sequestered by dimer reinforcement of the quaternary complex.[1187] Extensive work over the past several decades that has focused on elucidating autoantibody-specific epitopes along the quaternary structure of the $\alpha_3\alpha_4\alpha_5$(IV) NC1 hexamer has reinforced the paradigm that this disease process is an autoimmune conformeropathy.[1188] It is presumed that environmental factors, such as exposure to hydrocarbons,[1189] tobacco smoke,[1190] and endogenous oxidants[1191] can also expose the cryptic Goodpasture epitopes. In patients with anti-GBM disease who do not have antibodies to the classic epitope on the $\alpha_3$ chain, antibodies to entactin have been detected.[1192] A small percentage of patients with anti-GBM disease may also have limited reactivity with the NC1 domains of the $\alpha_1$ or $\alpha_4$ chains of type IV collagen. These additional reactivities seem to be more frequent in patients with anti-GBM–mediated glomerulonephritis alone.[1193]

Most patients with anti-GBM disease express antibodies to two major conformational epitopes ($E_A$ and $E_B$) located within the carboxy-terminal noncollagenous (NC1) domain of the $\alpha_3$ chain of type IV collagen.[1194–1197] The immunodominant target epitope, $E_A$, is encompassed by $\alpha_3$-NC1 residues 17 to 31. A homologous region at $\alpha_3$ NC1 residues 127 to 141 encompasses the $E_B$ epitope, recognized by the autoantibodies of only a small number of patients.[1198] In a large cohort of Chinese patients,[1199] the levels of antibody against $E_A$ and $E_B$ were strongly correlated with each other. Antibody levels against $\alpha$3, $E_A$, and $E_B$ correlated with serum creatinine level and with death or ESKD at 1 year, but not with gender, age, presence of ANCAs, or hemoptysis. Interestingly, a more recent study has found that autoantibodies against $E_A$ and $E_B$ are crucial for kidney dysfunction; multivariate Cox regression analysis revealed that autoantibody reactivity to $E_B$ was an independent risk factor for renal failure (HR, 6.91;, $P$ = .02).[1200] The stimuli and mechanism(s) leading to the formation of autoantibodies remain unclear, as is the mechanism whereby the normally hidden target epitopes become accessible to circulating autoantibodies.

About one-third of patients with anti-GBM–Goodpasture syndrome also have circulating ANCAs, with most being to MPO (MPO-ANCA).[1180,1193,1196,1201,1202] In a study of a large cohort of Chinese patients with anti-GBM disease, with or without ANCAs, no differences in reactivity to the $E_A$, $E_B$, and S2 epitopes (a recombinant construct expressing the nine amino acid residues critical for the anti-GBM epitope)[1203] were detected between patients with anti-GBM plus ANCA compared with anti-GBM alone.[1204] The mechanism whereby some patients develop both anti-GBM and ANCA is unknown. It has been speculated that in such patients, ANCA may appear first and cause damage to the GBM, thus exposing the normally hidden target epitopes of anti-GBM antibodies. The coexistence of ANCA in patients with anti-GBM antibodies is associated with small-vessel vasculitis in organs in addition to the lung and kidney. In experimental models, the presence of antibodies to MPO aggravate experimental anti-GBM disease.[1180,1205,1163]

Some patients with X-linked Alport syndrome (XLAS) develop anti-GBM antibodies and glomerulonephritis post-transplantation. The main structural component of mature GBM is type IV collagen, expressed as a heterotrimer composed of three $\alpha$ chains, $\alpha_3$, $\alpha_4$, and $\alpha_5$,[1206,1207] with a central collagenous domain and noncollagenous (NC) domain at the N- and C-terminal ends. Self-reactive B cells are negatively regulated at different stages of B cell development. Deletion, anergy (functional inactivation), and receptor editing are some of the mechanisms for B cell tolerance.[1208] Patients with XLAS lack the network of $\alpha_3\alpha_4\alpha_5$ in the GBM; therefore, B cells specific for epitopes in $\alpha_3\alpha_4\alpha_5$-NC1 cannot undergo tolerance. Unlike the autoantibodies seen in anti-GBM disease that are directed to the NC1 domain of the $\alpha_3$ chain of type IV collagen, the anti-GBM alloantibodies that cause post-transplantation nephritis in some patients with XLAS are directed against conformational epitopes in the NC1 domain of $\alpha_5$(IV) collagen only, which is normally expressed in the allograft but absent in the recipient. Allograft-eluted alloantibodies mainly targeted two epitopes accessible in the $\alpha_3\alpha_4\alpha_5$-NC1 hexamers of human GBM, unlike the sequestered $\alpha$3-NC1 epitopes of anti-GBM autoantibodies.[1209]

A number of animal models of anti-GBM disease have been developed over the years, based on the immunization of animals with heterologous or homologous GBM.[1210] Alternatively, anti-GBM antibody-induced injury can be produced passively by the intravenous injection of heterologous anti-GBM antibodies.[1210] This leads to two phases of injury. The first, or so-called heterologous phase, occurs in the first 24 hours and is mediated by direct deposition of the heterologous antibodies on the GBM, with subsequent recruitment of neutrophils. This is usually followed by an autologous phase, depending on the host's immune response to the heterologous immunoglobulin bound to the GBM.[1210]

The rat model of anti-GBM disease induced by the injection of heterologous anti-GBM antibodies has permitted the study of the roles of various inflammatory mediators in the development of anti-GBM disease.[1211–1214] Thus in Wistar-Kyoto (WKY) rats injected with a rabbit antiserum to rat GBM, impairing leukocyte recruitment and monocyte-macrophage glomerular infiltrate by blocking the chemokine C-X-C motif ligand 16 (CXCL16) with a polyclonal anti-CXCL16 antiserum in the acute inflammatory or progressive phase of established glomerulonephritis, has significantly attenuated glomerular injury and improved proteinuria.[1215] Similarly, the depletion of $CD8^+$ cells has prevented the initiation and progression of anti-GBM crescentic glomerulonephritis. In the same animal model, treatment with an antibody to perforin resulted in a significant reduction in the amount of proteinuria, frequency of glomerular crescents, and number of glomerular monocytes and macrophages, although the number of glomerular $CD8^+$ cells was not changed.[1216] These results suggest that $CD8^+$ cells play a role in glomerular injury as effector cells, in part through a perforin-granzyme-mediated pathway.

The more recent development of analogous murine models of anti-GBM disease opens the way for more specific evaluations of the inflammatory processes with the use of strains of mice with specific gene knockouts.[1170] For example, the role of protease-activated receptor 2 (PAR-2) in kidney inflammation has been studied using PAR-2–deficient (PAR-$2^{-/-}$) mice.[1217] PAR-2 is a cellular receptor expressed predominantly on epithelial, mesangial, and endothelial cells in the kidney and on macrophages. PAR-2 is activated by serine proteases and coagulation factors VIIa and Xa. In the kidney, PAR-2 induces endothelium-dependent and endothelium-independent vasodilation of afferent renal arteries and renal mesangial cells proliferation in vitro. Glomerulonephritis was induced in mice by the intravenous injection of sheep antimouse GBM globulin. In this model, PAR-2–deficient mice had reduced crescent formation, proteinuria, and serum creatinine level compared with wild type mice, but this was not associated with a difference in the glomerular accumulation of $CD4^+$ T cells or macrophages or with the number of proliferating cells in glomeruli. These results demonstrate a proinflammatory role for PAR-2 in crescentic glomerulonephritis that is independent of effects on glomerular leukocyte recruitment and mesangial cell proliferation.

The theory of autoantigen complementarity states that the initiator of an autoimmune response is not necessarily the autoantigen or its mimic, but is instead an exogenous or endogenous peptide that is antisense or complementary to the autoantigen. This theory has been applied to a WKY rat model of anti-GBM disease. Rats immunized with a complementary peptide corresponding to the critical immunodominant epitope of the $\alpha_3$ chain of type IV collagen developed crescentic glomerulonephritis within 8 weeks, and sera from patients with anti-GBM disease were found to have antibodies to the complementary peptide of the $\alpha_3$ chain of type IV collagen, suggesting a role for autoantigen complementarity in anti-GBM disease. This was also previously implicated in ANCA vasculitis.[1218,1219]

Although anti-GBM disease is considered a prototypical antibody-mediated glomerulonephritis, several lines of evidence have indicated an important role for T cells in the initiation or pathogenesis of this disease. A role for T cells in the autoimmune response is suggested by the increased susceptibility to the disease associated with the presence of HLA class II antigens DRB1*1501 and DQB*0602.[1165–1169] Further evidence of the involvement of T cell activation in the development of the autoimmune response to the NC1 domain of the $\alpha_3$ chain of type IV collagen comes from studies of T cell proliferation in response to other monomeric components of the GBM[1220] and synthetic oligopeptides.[1221] The transfer of $CD4^+$ T cells specific to a recombinant GBM antigen into syngeneic rats resulted in a crescentic glomerulonephritis, without linear anti-GBM IgG deposition.[1222] Furthermore a single nephritogenic T cell epitope of type IV collagen $\alpha_3$-NC1 was demonstrated to induce glomerulonephritis in WKY rats.[1223] More recently, CD4+ T cell clones generated from HLA-DRB*1501 transgenic mice immunized with a peptide corresponding to amino acids 3136–3146 of the NC1 domain of $\alpha_3$(IV) were capable of transferring disease into HLA-DRB*1501 transgenic mice.[1224] Interestingly, cross-reactive peptides from human infection–related microbes could be identified that also induced severe proteinuria and moderate to severe glomerulonephritis in immunized rats.[1225] One peptide derived from *Clostridium botulinum* also induced pulmonary hemorrhage.[1225]

On immunization of mice with $\alpha_3$-NC1 domains of type IV collagen, the development of glomerulonephritis and lung hemorrhage depends on certain MHC haplotypes and the ability of mice to mount a $T_H1$ response.[1170] The role of T cells in this model was further documented by the fact that the passive transfer of lymphocytes or antibodies from nephritogenic strains to syngenetic recipients led to the development of nephritis, whereas the passive transfer of antibodies to T cell receptor–deficient mice failed to do so.[1170]

$CD4^+CD25^+$ regulatory T cells may play an important role in regulating the immune response in anti-GBM disease. Thus, the transfer of regulatory T cells into mice that were previously immunized with rabbit IgG, and before an injection of anti-GBM rabbit serum, significantly attenuated the development of proteinuria and dramatically decreased glomerular damage. On histologic analysis, there was reduced infiltration of $CD4^+$ T cells, $CD8^+$ T cells, and macrophages, but the deposition of immune complexes was not prevented.[1226] In humans, the action of regulatory T cells may explain, in part, the uncommon occurrence of disease relapses and the eventual disappearance of anti-GBM antibodies in patients, even without the use of immunosuppressant medications.[1227] Thus analyses of peripheral blood mononuclear cells from patients with Goodpasture syndrome have revealed the emergence of GBM-specific $CD25^+$ regulatory T cells in the convalescent period, whereas they were undetected at the time of presentation.[1228]

The role of complement in the pathogenesis of anti-GBM disease is evidenced by the deposition of C3 along the GBM. The role of complement activation has been examined largely in studies of passive injection of heterologous antibodies to GBM. Investigations using this model have suggested that the terminal components of the complement system are not involved in the pathogenesis of disease.[1229] Results of further studies in rabbits that are congenitally deficient in the sixth component of complement have also suggested that the terminal components of complement do not play a major part in the pathogenesis of the disease, except in leukocyte-depleted animals.[1230,1231] The role of complement cascade activation in a murine model of heterologous anti-GBM previously led to conflicting results in regard to the role of complement activation in this model.[1232] More recent studies involving the same model, using mice completely deficient of complement components C3 or C4, have revealed a greater protective effect of C3 deficiency, more than C4 deficiency. Both protective effects could be overcome if the dose of nephritogenic antibodies was increased.[1233]

To evaluate the role of complement activation and of Fcγ receptors further, an attenuated mouse model of anti-GBM was developed using a subnephritogenic dose of rabbit antimouse GBM antibody, followed 1 week later with an injection of mouse monoclonal antibody against rabbit IgG, which resulted in albuminuria.[1234] In this model, albuminuria was absent in Fcγ chain–deficient mice and reduced in C3-deficient mice, which indicates a role for both Fcγ receptors and complement. C1q- and C4-deficient mice did develop proteinuria, which is suggestive of involvement of the alternative complement pathway.[1234] The role of Fcγ receptors is also evidenced by the occurrence of severe lung hemorrhage in mice deficient in the inhibitory Fcγ 2b receptor that were treated with bovine type IV collagen.[1235]

Conclusions about the pathogenesis of human anti-GBM disease from animal models must be tempered because animal models may not accurately replicate human disease.

## CLINICAL FEATURES AND NATURAL HISTORY

The onset of renal anti-GBM disease is typically characterized by an abrupt, acute glomerulonephritis, with severe oliguria or anuria. There is a high risk of progression to ESKD if appropriate therapy is not instituted immediately. Prompt treatment with plasmapheresis, corticosteroids, and cyclophosphamide results in patient survival of approximately 85% and renal survival of approximately 60%.[1145,1236–1240]

Rarely, the disorder has a more insidious onset, in which patients remain essentially asymptomatic until the development of uremic symptoms and fluid retention.[675,1162,1177,1241] The onset of disease may be associated with arthralgias, fever, myalgias, and abdominal pain; however, neurologic disturbances and gastrointestinal complaints are rare.

Goodpasture syndrome is characterized by the presence of pulmonary hemorrhage concurrent with glomerulonephritis. The usual pulmonary manifestation is severe pulmonary hemorrhage, which may be life threatening; however, patients may have milder disease, which can be focal. The absence of hemoptysis does not rule out diffuse alveolar hemorrhage. For patients with early or focal disease, a high level of suspicion is necessary to establish the diagnosis, especially in the presence of unexplained anemia. The diagnosis may be aided by measurements showing an increased diffusing capacity of carbon monoxide and by findings on computed tomography of the chest. Ultimately, the diagnostic evaluation of alveolar hemorrhage usually includes bronchoscopic examination and bronchoalveolar lavage.[1242] This approach also allows exclusion of airway sources of bleeding and possible associated infections. In patients with anti-GBM disease, the occurrence of pulmonary hemorrhage is far more common in smokers in than nonsmokers[1243] and may be associated with environmental exposures to hydrocarbons[1243–1246] or upper respiratory tract infections.[1247] Occupational exposure to petroleum-based mineral oils is essentially a risk factor for the development of anti-GBM antibodies.[1248] The association of pulmonary hemorrhage with environmental exposures and infection raises the theoretic possibility that they expose the cryptic antigen in the alveolar basement membrane, thereby allowing its recognition by circulating anti-GBM antibodies.

## LABORATORY FINDINGS

Kidney involvement by anti-GBM disease typically causes an acute nephritic syndrome with hematuria that includes dysmorphic erythrocytes and red blood cells casts. Although nephrotic-range proteinuria may occur, full nephrotic syndrome is rarely seen.[1159,1172,1174,1177,1241]

The diagnostic laboratory finding in anti-GBM disease is the detection of circulating antibodies to GBM, specifically to the $\alpha_3$ chain of type IV collagen. These antibodies are detected in approximately 95% of patients by immunoassays using various forms of purified or recombinant substrates.[1249] The anti-GBM antibodies are most often of the IgG1 subclass, but may also be of the IgG4 subclass, with the latter being more often seen in females.[1250]

## TREATMENT

The standard treatment for anti-GBM disease is intensive plasmapheresis combined with corticosteroids and cyclophosphamide.[1145,1237,1251–1254] Plasmapheresis consists of removal of 2 to 4 L of plasma and its replacement with a 5% albumin solution, continued on a daily basis until circulating antibody levels become undetectable. In patients with pulmonary hemorrhage, clotting factors should be replaced by administering fresh-frozen plasma at the end of each treatment. Prednisone should be administered starting at a dose of 1 mg/kg of body weight for at least the first month and then tapered to alternate-day therapy during the second and third months of treatment. Cyclophosphamide is administered orally (2 mg/kg/day, adjusted with consideration for the degree of impairment of kidney function and white blood cell count) for 8 to 12 weeks. The role of high-dose intravenous methylprednisolone pulses remains unproven in the treatment of anti-GBM disease.[1255–1259] Nonetheless, the urgent nature of the clinical process prompts some nephrologists to administer methylprednisolone (7 mg/kg daily for 3 consecutive days) as part of induction therapy in this and other forms of crescentic glomerulonephritis.

When the regimen of aggressive plasmapheresis with corticosteroids and cyclophosphamide is used, patient survival is approximately 85%, with 40% progression to ESKD.[1145,1236–1241] These results are better than those achieved before the introduction of plasmapheresis, when patient survival was less than 50% with an almost 90% rate of ESKD. In a study at the Hammersmith Hospital in the United Kingdom, Gaskin and Pusey have demonstrated that aggressive plasmapheresis, even in patients with severe renal insufficiency, may have an ameliorative effect and provide improved long-term patient and renal survival.[1260] In that cohort, among patients who had a creatinine concentration of 500 μmol/L or more (>5.7 mg/dL) at presentation but did not require immediate dialysis, patient and renal survival were 83% and 82% at 1 year and 62% and 69% at last follow-up, respectively. The renal prognosis of patients who presented with dialysis-dependent renal failure was poor—92% of patients had ESKD at 1 year. All patients who required immediate dialysis and whose kidney biopsy specimens had crescents involving 100% of glomeruli remained dialysis dependent.[1261]

The major prognostic marker for the progression to ESKD is the serum creatinine level at the time of initiation of treatment. Patients with a serum creatinine concentration above 7 mg/dL are unlikely to recover sufficient kidney function to discontinue renal replacement therapy.[1157] At issue is whether and for how long aggressive immunosuppression should persist in dialysis-dependent patients. Aggressive immunosuppression and plasmapheresis are warranted in patients with pulmonary hemorrhage. Aggressive immunosuppression should be withheld in patients with disease limited to the kidney, whose kidney biopsy specimens show widespread glomerular and interstitial scarring and who have a serum creatinine concentration of more than 7 mg/dL at presentation. In such patients, the risks of therapy outweigh the potential benefits. In patients who have an elevated serum creatinine level, yet whose biopsy specimens show active crescentic glomerulonephritis, aggressive treatment should continue for at least 4 weeks. If there is no restoration of kidney function by 4 to 8 weeks, and in the absence of pulmonary bleeding, immunosuppression should be discontinued.

Patients who have both circulating anti-GBM antibodies and ANCA may have a better chance of recovery of kidney function than patients with anti-GBM antibodies alone. In these patients, immunosuppressive therapy should not be withheld, even with serum creatinine levels above 7 mg/dL, because the concomitant presence of ANCA was associated with a more favorable renal outcome in some studies,[1259,1262] although not in all.[1263] In a retrospective analysis comparing patients with anti-GBM autoantibodies, MPO-ANCA, and both, so-called double-positive patients and those with anti-GBM autoantibodies had significantly higher serum creatinine levels at presentation ($10.3 \pm 5.6$ and $9.6 \pm 8.1$ mg/dL, respectively) than patients with MPO-ANCA alone ($5.0 \pm 2.9$ mg/dL). One-year renal survival was better in patients with MPO-ANCA alone (63%) than in the double- positive group (10.0%; $P =$ .01) and the anti-GBM group (15.4%; $P = .17$).[1263]

Once remission of anti-GBM disease has been achieved with immunosuppressive therapy, recurrent disease occurs only rarely.[1264–1267] Similarly, the recurrence of anti-GBM disease after kidney transplantation is also rare, especially when transplantation is delayed until after the disappearance or substantial diminution of anti-GBM antibodies in the circulation.[1268]

## PAUCI-IMMUNE CRESCENTIC GLOMERULONEPHRITIS

### EPIDEMIOLOGY

In pauci-immune crescentic glomerulonephritis, the characteristic feature of the glomerular lesion is focal necrotizing and crescentic glomerulonephritis, with little or no glomerular staining for immunoglobulins by IF microscopy.[1127,1149,1174,1252,1254] Pauci-immune crescentic glomerulonephritis usually is a component of a systemic small-vessel vasculitis; however, some patients have renal-limited (primary), pauci-immune crescentic glomerulonephritis.[1127,1137,1179,1269] ANCA-associated vasculitis is also discussed in Chapter 32. Pauci-immune crescentic glomerulonephritis, including that accompanying small-vessel vasculitis, is the most common category of RPGN in adults, especially older adults (see Table 31.8). The disease has a predilection for Caucasians compared with African Americans (see Table 31.7). There are no gender differences (see Table 31.7).

### PATHOLOGY

#### Light Microscopy

The light microscopic appearance of ANCA-associated pauci-immune crescentic glomerulonephritis is indistinguishable from that of anti-GBM crescentic glomerulonephritis.[360,701,1128,1138,1269–1272] Renal-limited (primary) pauci-immune crescentic glomerulonephritis also is indistinguishable from pauci-immune crescentic glomerulonephritis that occurs as a component of a systemic small-vessel vasculitis, such as GPA (formerly Wegener granulomatosis), microscopic polyangiitis (MPA), or EGPA, formerly Churg-Strauss syndrome). As illustrated in Fig. 31.30, ANCA glomerulonephritis and anti-GBM glomerulonephritis most often manifest as crescentic glomerulonephritis.

At the time of biopsy, approximately 90% of kidney biopsy specimens with ANCA-associated pauci-immune glomerulonephritis have some degree of crescent formation, and approximately half of the specimens have crescents involving 50% or more of glomeruli (see Tables 31.9 and 31.10). Over 90% of specimens have focal segmental to global fibrinoid necrosis (Fig. 31.38). As with anti-GBM disease, the intact glomerular segments often have no light microscopic abnormalities. The most severely injured glomeruli not only have extensive necrosis of glomerular tufts but also have extensive lysis of Bowman's capsule, with resultant periglomerular inflammation. The periglomerular inflammation contains varying mixtures of neutrophils, eosinophils, lymphocytes, monocytes, and macrophages, including occasional multinucleated giant cells. This periglomerular inflammation area

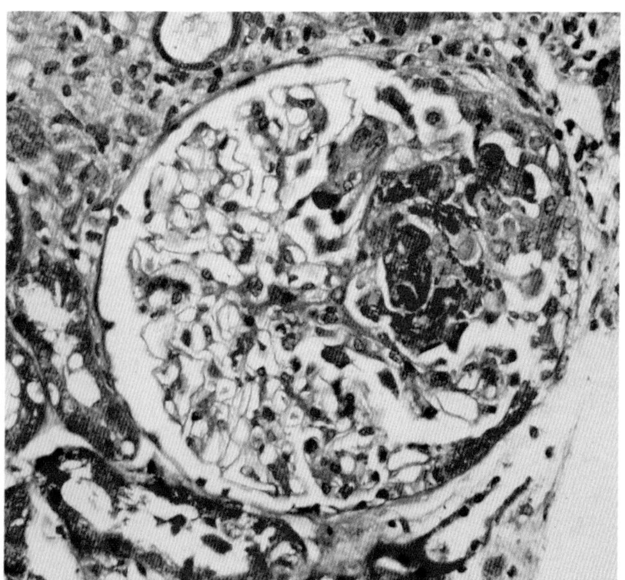

**Fig. 31.38** Light micrograph showing segmental fibrinoid necrosis (segmental bright red staining) in a glomerulus from a patient with antineutrophil cytoplasmic autoantibody–associated pauci-immune crescentic glomerulonephritis. (Masson trichrome stain, ×300.)

may have a granulomatous appearance, especially when the glomerulus that was the nidus of inflammation has been destroyed or is not in the plane of section. This granulomatous appearance is a result of the periglomerular reaction to extensive glomerular necrosis and is not specific for a particular category of necrotizing glomerulonephritis.

This pattern of injury can be seen with anti-GBM glomerulonephritis, renal-limited pauci-immune crescentic glomerulonephritis, and crescentic glomerulonephritis secondary to MPA, GPA and EGPA. Necrotizing granulomatous inflammation that is not centered on a glomerulus, but rather is in the interstitium or centered on an artery, raises the possibility of GPA or EGPA. The presence of arteritis in a biopsy specimen that has pauci-immune crescentic glomerulonephritis indicates that the glomerulonephritis is a component of a more widespread vasculitis, such as MPA, GPA, or EGPA.

The acute necrotizing glomerular lesions evolve into sclerotic lesions. During completely quiescent phases, a kidney biopsy specimen may have only focal sclerotic lesions that may mimic FSGS. ANCA-associated glomerulonephritis is also often characterized by many recurrent bouts of exacerbation. Therefore, combinations of active acute necrotizing glomerular lesions and chronic sclerotic lesions often occur in the same kidney biopsy specimen.

#### Immunofluorescence Microscopy

By definition, the distinguishing pathologic difference between pauci-immune crescentic glomerulonephritis and anti-GBM and immune complex crescentic glomerulonephritis is the absence or paucity of glomerular staining for immunoglobulins. How pauci-immune is pauci-immune crescentic glomerulonephritis? One basis for categorizing the disorder as pauci-immune crescentic glomerulonephritis is to determine whether the patient is likely to be ANCA-positive, which increases the likelihood of certain systemic small-vessel vasculitides.[365,1269,1273,1274] The likelihood of positivity for ANCA is inversely proportional to the intensity of glomerular immunoglobulin staining by IF microscopy in a specimen with crescentic glomerulonephritis.[1272] The likelihood of positive results on an ANCA serologic assay is approximately 90% if there is no staining for immunoglobulin, approximately 80% if there is trace to 1+ staining (on a scale of 0–4+), approximately 50% if there is 2+ staining, approximately 30% if there is 3+ staining, and less than 10% if there is 4+ staining. Thus, even patients with definite evidence for immune complex–mediated glomerulonephritis have a higher than expected frequency of ANCA, but the highest frequency is in patients with little or no evidence for immune complex– or anti-GBM– mediated disease.

The presence of ANCA at a higher than expected frequency in immune complex disease is intriguing and raises the possibility that ANCA contributes to the pathogenesis of not only pauci-immune crescentic glomerulonephritis, but also the most severe examples of immune complex disease.[365] Considering this issue from a different perspective, approximately 25% of patients with idiopathic immune complex crescentic glomerulonephritis (i.e., immune complex glomerulonephritis that does not fit well into one of the categories of primary or secondary immune complex disease) are ANCA-positive, compared with less than 5% of patients who have idiopathic immune complex glomerulonephritis with no crescents.[365]

Glomerular capillary wall or mesangial staining usually accompanies immunoglobulin staining and is present in occasional specimens that do not have immunoglobulin staining. There is irregular staining for fibrin at sites of intraglomerular fibrinoid necrosis and capillary thrombosis and in the interstices of crescents. Foci of glomerular necrosis and sclerosis also may have irregular staining for C3 and IgM.

#### Electron Microscopy

The findings by electron microscopy are indistinguishable from those described earlier for anti-GBM glomerulonephritis.[1181] Specimens with pure pauci-immune crescentic glomerulonephritis have no or only a few immune complex–type, electron-dense deposits. Foci of glomerular necrosis have leukocyte influx, breaks in GBMs, and fibrin tactoids in capillary thrombi and sites of fibrinoid necrosis.

### PATHOGENESIS

The pathogenesis of pauci-immune crescentic glomerulonephritis is currently not fully understood, but there is strong evidence that ANCA IgG is a major pathogenic factor.[1275–1277] In the absence or paucity of immune complex deposition in glomeruli or other vessels, classic mechanisms of immune complex–mediated damage are not implicated in the pathogenesis of pauci-immune crescentic glomerulonephritis. On the other hand, the substantial accumulation of polymorphonuclear leukocytes at sites of vascular necrosis has led to examination of the role of neutrophil activation in this disease. A large body of in vitro data has implicated a pathogenic role for ANCA based on the demonstration that these autoantibodies activate normal human polymorphonuclear leukocytes.[1272,1275,1278–1280]

For anti-MPO autoantibodies, anti-PR3 autoantibodies, or autoantibodies to other neutrophil antigens contained in the azurophilic granules to interact with their corresponding antigens, either the antibodies must penetrate the cell or those antigens must translocate to the cell surface. Indeed, small amounts of cytokine (e.g., TNF-α, IL-1) at concentrations too low to cause full neutrophil activation are capable of inducing such a translocation of ANCA antigens to the cell surface.[1281] This translocation of ANCA antigens to the cell surface has been demonstrated in vivo on the neutrophils of patients with GPA and in patients with sepsis.[1282–1284] Patients with ANCA disease aberrantly express *PR3* and *MPO* genes, and this expression correlates with disease activity.[1285] Despite the fact that these genes exist on different chromosomes, their expression appears coordinately upregulated during disease activity and downregulated during remission. Epigenetic changes occur as a result of increased unmethylated DNA at the *MPO* and *PR3* loci, and as a result of loss of recruitment of histone methylase PRC2 (polycomb recessive complex 2) by RUNX3 (Runt-related transcription factor 3) in both *MPO* and *PR3* genes with depressed gene transcription. In addition, JMJD3 (Jumonji domain-containing protein 3) appears to be expressed in these patients, which further diminishes histone H3K27me3 methylation status.[1286] In further support of epigenetic modifications contributing to autoantigen gene expression and disease state in ANCA vasculitis, measurement of gene-specific DNA methylation of the *MPO* and protein-coding proteinase 3 (*PRTN3*) genes in leukocytes of patients with ANCA vasculitis over their disease course has revealed that patients with active disease have hypomethylation of *MPO* and *PRTN3* and increased autoantigen expression, whereas DNA methylation during times of remission increased.[1287] Furthermore, patients with increased DNA methylation at the *PRTN3* promoter had a significantly greater probability of a relapse-free period ($P < .001$), regardless of ANCA serotype, suggesting the potential use of these types of measurements as bioindicators of disease activity.[1287]

Regardless of whether the antigen is expressed on the surface of the cell as a consequence of cytokine stimulation or gene expression, in the presence of circulating ANCAs, the interaction of the autoantibody with its externalized antigen results in full activation of the neutrophil, which leads to the respiratory burst and degranulation of primary and secondary granule constituents.[1288,1289] The current hypothesis stipulates that ANCAs induce a premature degranulation and activation of neutrophils at the time of their margination and diapedesis, which leads to the release of lytic enzymes and toxic oxygen metabolites at the site of the vessel wall, thereby producing a necrotizing inflammatory injury. This view has been supported by in vitro studies demonstrating that neutrophils activated by ANCAs lead to the damage and destruction of human umbilical vein endothelial cells in culture.[1290–1292]

Not only does neutrophil degranulation cause direct damage of the endothelium, but ANCA antigens released from neutrophils and monocytes enter endothelial cells and cause cell damage. PR3 can enter the endothelial cells by a receptor-mediated process[1293–1295] and result in the production of IL-8[1296] and chemoattractant protein-1. PR3 also induces an apoptotic event from both proteolytic and nonproteolytic mechanisms.[1297,1298] Interestingly, PR3-mediated apoptosis appears to be in part related to cleavage of the cell cycle inhibitor $p21^{CIP1/WAF1}$ and nuclear factor-kappa B (NF-κB).[1299,1300] Similarly, MPO enters endothelial cells by an energy-dependent process[1301] and transcytoses intact endothelium to localize within the extracellular matrix. There, in the presence of the substrates $H_2O_2$ and $NO_2^-$, MPO catalyzes the nitration of tyrosine residues on extracellular matrix proteins,[1302] which results in the fragmentation of extracellular matrix protein.[1303] It also appears that endothelial cells inhibit superoxide generation by ANCA-activated neutrophils and that serine proteases may play a more important role than reactive oxygen species as mediators of endothelial injury during ANCA-associated vasculitis.[1304]

Neutrophil activation by ANCA is likely mediated by both the antigen-binding portion of the autoantibodies ($F[ab']_2$) and by the engagement of their Fc fraction to Fc gamma receptors on the surface of neutrophils.[1137,1291,1305,1306] Human neutrophils constitutively express the IgG receptors FcγRIIa and FcγRIIIb.[1307] ANCAs have been shown to engage both types of receptors.[1291,1308] Engagement of the Fc receptors results in a number of neutrophil activation events, including respiratory burst, degranulation, phagocytosis, cytokine production, and upregulation of adhesion molecules.[1309] In particular, FcγRIIa engagement by ANCAs appears to increase neutrophil actin polymerization in neutrophils, which leads to distortion in their shape and possibly decreases their ability to pass through capillaries (the primary site of injury in ANCA vasculitis).[1310] Furthermore, polymorphisms of the FcγRIIIb receptors[1311,1312] (but not of FcγRII[1313,1314]) appear to influence the severity of ANCA vasculitis.

In addition to the Fc receptor–mediated mechanism, substantial data support a role for the $F(ab')_2$ portion of the antibody molecule in leukocyte activation. ANCA $F(ab')_2$ portions induce oxygen radical production[1306] and the transcription of cytokine genes in normal human neutrophils and monocytes. Microarray gene chip analysis has shown that ANCA IgG and ANCA-$F(ab')_2$ stimulate the transcription of a distinct subset of genes, some unique to whole IgG, some unique to $F(ab')_2$ fragments, and some common to both.[1315] It is most likely that $F(ab')_2$ portions of ANCA are capable of low-level neutrophil and monocyte activation.[1306] The Fc portion of the molecule almost certainly causes leukocyte activation once the $F(ab')_2$ portion of the immunoglobulin has interacted with the antigen, either on the cell surface or in the microenvironment.[1291] The signal transduction pathways of F(ab')2 and Fc receptor activation through a specific p21ras (Kristen-ras) pathway have also been elucidated.[1316]

Given the pathogenicity of ANCA, there has been considerable current effort directed toward identifying specific epitope(s) on MPO that are recognized by ANCAs in an effort to begin to identify therapeutic avenues to eliminate this interaction in vivo. Using a highly sensitive epitope excision and mass spectrometry approach, investigators from the United States, the Netherlands, and Australia have identified autoantibodies to specific epitopes of MPO in sera from patients with active disease that differed from those in remission. Furthermore, this same study reported what may be a seminal finding in that pathogenic MPO-ANCA were found in patients with ANCA-negative disease. These were detected after IgG purification that eliminated ceruloplasmin, the natural inhibitor of MPO, contamination from serum.[1317]

The role of T cells in the pathogenesis of pauci-immune necrotizing small-vessel vasculitis or glomerulonephritis, although suspected,[1318,1319] is somewhat less well defined. Such a role is suggested by the presence of $CD4^+$ T cells in granulomatous[1320] and active vasculitic lesions[1321–1325] and by some correlation of the levels of soluble markers of T cell activation with disease activity,[1320,1326] specifically, soluble IL-2 receptor and sCD3.[1327,1328] Much is known about T cell responsivity in ANCA disease, including the recognition of PR3 and MPO by T cells.[1329,1330] The proportion of regulatory T cells in ANCA patients increases, although these regulatory T cells seem defective in their inability to suppress proliferation of effector cells in cytokine production. In addition, the percentage of T cells secreting IL-17 increases in the periphery, and serum levels of $T_H17$-associated cytokine IL-23 correlate with the propensity for disease activity.[1331] Although yet to be replicated and validated, gene expression profiling of purified $CD8^+$ T cells from patients with ANCA-associated vasculitis has identified a signature associated with poor prognosis and that included an expanded $CD8^+$ memory T cell population.[1332] A separate study examining purified CD4+ T cells from patients with ANCA-associated vasculitis has found an increased frequency of regulatory T cells with decreased suppressive function in patients with active disease, as well as a second T cell population that was resistant to regulatory T cell suppression.[1333]

It has long been proposed that patients with ANCA-associated vasculitis and glomerulonephritis have a genetic predisposition for disease. The first ever GWAS was performed using DNA samples from 1233 patients in the United Kingdom, with ANCA-associated vasculitis and 5884 controls, and a replication cohort of 1454 Northern European case patients and 1666 controls.[1334] Interestingly, genetic associations were made most strongly with respect to ANCA serotype rather than disease phenotype in that patients with PR3-ANCA had significant associations with HLA-DP and genes encoding $\alpha_1$-antitrypsin (SERPINA1, the endogenous inhibitor of PR3) and PR3 (PRTN3) itself ($P = 6.2 \times 10^{-89}$, $P = 5.6 \times 10^{-12}$ and $P = 2.6 \times 10^{-7}$, respectively). Patients with MPO-ANCA had a significant genome-wide association with HLA-DQ ($P = 2.1 \times 10^{-8}$). Of note, ANCA-associated vasculitis is notably rare in African Americans; however, an association of the HLA-DRB1*15 alleles with PR3-ANCA-positive disease has been found, conferring a 73.3-fold higher risk in African American patients than in community-based controls.[1335] Interestingly, the DRB1*1501 allelic variant, which is of Caucasian descent, was found in 50% of African American patients, whereas the DRB1*1503, of African descent, was underrepresented in this group. A recent GWAS of 1986 patients with GPA or MPA in North America identified risk alleles associated with HLA-DPB1, SERPINA1, PTPN22, and PRTN3 loci.[1336]

Further establishment of a pathogenetic link between ANCA and the development of pauci-immune necrotizing glomerulonephritis and small-vessel vasculitis has greatly benefited from the development of animal models of this disease. Early models of disease were based on the finding of circulating anti-MPO antibodies in 20% of female MRL/lpr mice[1337] and in an inbred strain of mice, SCG/Kj, derived from the MRL/lpr mice and BXSB strains that develop a severe form of crescentic glomerulonephritis and systemic necrotizing vasculitis.[1338] Anti-MPO antibodies have been isolated from these strains of mice. Treatment of rats with mercuric chloride has led to the development of widespread inflammation, including necrotizing vasculitis in the presence of anti-MPO antibodies and anti-GBM antibodies.[1339] A more convincing model has indicated a pathogenetic role for ANCA. Aggravation of a mild, anti-GBM–mediated glomerulonephritis in rats, when the animals were previously immunized with MPO.[1205] suggests that minor proinflammatory events could be driven to severe necrotizing processes in the presence of ANCA.

More compelling models for ANCA small-vessel vasculitis now exist. MPO-deficient mice were immunized with murine MPO, and splenocytes from these mice were transferred to immunoincompetent recombination-activating gene (Rag2)–deficient mice.[1340] This resulted in the development of anti-MPO autoantibodies, severe necrotizing and crescentic glomerulonephritis and, in some animals, vasculitis in the lung and other organ systems. In a separate but similar set of experiments, anti-MPO antibodies alone were transferred into $Rag2^{-/-}$ mice and induced pauci-immune necrotizing and crescentic glomerulonephritis.[1340] These studies indicate that anti-MPO antibodies cause pauci-immune necrotizing disease. The glomerulonephritis induced by anti-MPO antibodies is aggravated by the administration of lipopolysaccharide (LPS).[1341] Conversely, the disease is abrogated when the neutrophils of anti-MPO–recipient mice are depleted by a selective antineutrophil monoclonal antibody.[1342] In experiments to assess the role of T cells using this animal model, the transfer of T cell–enriched splenocytes (>99% T cells) did not cause glomerular crescent formation or vascular necrosis. These data do not support a pathogenic role for anti-MPO T cells in the induction of acute injury.[1343] Furthermore, the role of genetic predisposition was investigated by inducing disease in 13 inbred mouse strains from the Collaborative Cross; however, a dominant quantitative trait locus was not identified, suggesting that differences in severity are likely polygenic in nature and possibly related to environmental milieu as well.[1344]

Using the same model described previously, a previously unsuspected role of complement activation was demonstrated. Glomerulonephritis and vasculitis were abolished with the administration of cobra venom factor and failed to develop in mice deficient in complement factors C5 and B, whereas C4-deficient mice developed disease comparable with that in wild-type mice.[1345] These results indicate that the alternative complement pathway is required for disease induction, but not the classic or lectin pathways. Using this same mouse model, glomerulonephritis was completely abolished or markedly ameliorated by treating the mice with a C5-inhibiting monoclonal antibody either 8 hours before or 1 day after disease induction with anti-MPO IgG and lipopolysaccharide.[1346] Thus, anti-C5 had a dramatic therapeutic effect on this mouse model of ANCA vasculitis. These results have been corroborated by in vitro experiments demonstrating that blockade of the C5a receptor on human neutrophils abrogated their stimulation.[1347]

More recent work has confirmed the immunopathogenetic importance of the alternative complement pathway in that blockade of C5a receptor (C5aR) activity protects against disease development. Mice expressing human C5aR were protected from anti-MPO autoantibody-induced disease when given an oral small-molecule antagonist of human C5aR called "CCX168."[1348] In contrast, using the same mouse model, mice deficient in complement factor 6 were not protected from disease, thereby supporting the concept that formation of the membrane attack complex is not necessary for disease development.[1348]

In aggregate, these results suggest an important role for complement activation in the pathogenesis of ANCA vasculitis and have implications for possible future therapeutic interventions using blockers of the complement cascade. Although yet to be confirmed, there is also preliminary evidence for this in humans, because abnormal levels of C3a, C5a, and soluble C5b-9 in plasma and urine have been identified in patients with active disease.[1349,1350] A randomized, placebo-controlled clinical trial, recruited adults with newly diagnosed or relapsing ANCA-associated vasculitis treated with cyclophosphamide or rituximab, as well as placebo plus corticosteroids, avacopan (oral anti-C5a receptor antagonist, 30 mg orally bid) with reduced prednisone (20 mg orally daily) or avacopan (30 mg orally bid) without steroids.[1351] The primary outcome was the proportion of patients receiving a more than 50% reduction in the Birmingham Vasculitis Activity Score (BVAS) by week 12 and no worsening in any body system; 67 patients were enrolled. Clinical response at week 12 was achieved in 14 of 20 (70%) of the placebo group, 19 of 20 (86.4%) of the avacopan plus reduced-dose steroids group, and 17 of 21 (81%) in the avacopan without prednisone group (difference from control 11.0%; two-sided 90% CI, −11.0% to 32.9%; $P$ = .01 for noninferiority). Adverse events were similar across groups.[1351] In addition, the phase 3 ADVOCATE clinical trial is underway to assess the efficacy of CCX168 (anti-C5a receptor antagonist) in a large group of patients with ANCA-associated glomerulonephritis (www.clinicaltrials.gov, NCT02994927). It is also important to note that all evidence for the role of the alternative complement pathway emanates from a model of anti-MPO autoantibody-mediated disease. and there is no direct evidence in mice or humans that this also applies to the anti-PR3 autoantibody-mediated disease.

The pathogenic role of anti-MPO antibodies has been documented in a second animal model, in which rats immunized with human MPO developed antirat-MPO antibodies and necrotizing and crescentic glomerulonephritis, as well as pulmonary capillaritis.[1352] Using intravital microscopy, elegant studies have shown that anti-MPO–activated neutrophils undergo margination and diapedesis along the vascular wall.[1352,1353] These two animal models have documented that anti-MPO antibodies are capable of causing necrotizing and crescentic glomerulonephritis and a widespread systemic vasculitis.

A model of anti-PR3–induced vascular injury was developed in PR3-neutrophil elastase-deficient mice in which the passive transfer of murine antimouse PR3 was associated with a stronger localized cutaneous inflammation, and perivascular infiltrates were observed around cutaneous vessels at the sites of intradermal injection of TNF-α.[1343,1354] In summary, these animal studies have documented that both anti-MPO and PR3 antibodies are capable of causing disease.

As is true for most autoimmune responses, the inciting events in the breakdown of tolerance and the generation of anti-MPO or anti-PR3 antibodies are not known. Although genetic predispositions[1355] and environmental exposure to foreign pathogens,[1356] notably to silica,[1357,1358] have been implicated, no direct link between these exposures and the formation of ANCAs has been established. A serendipitous finding in ANCA vasculitis has led to a theory of autoantigen complementarity.[1218,1359] This theory rests on evidence that proteins transcribed and translated from the sense strand of DNA bind to proteins that are transcribed and translated from the antisense strand of DNA.[1360] It has been demonstrated that some patients with PR3-ANCA harbor antibodies to an antigen complementary to the middle portion of PR3.[1330] These anticomplementary PR3 antibodies form an antiidiotypic pair with PR3-ANCA. Moreover, cloned complementary PR3 proteins bind to PR3 and function as a serine proteinase inhibitor. Preliminary data have suggested that the complementary PR3 antigens are found on a variety of microbes, some of which have been associated with ANCA vasculitis and have also been found in the genome of some patients with both PR3-ANCA and MPO-ANCA.[1218] Although these studies need to be confirmed and expanded to determine the source of the complementary PR3 antigen and their role (if any) in inducing vasculitis, these observations may provide a promising avenue for the detection of the proximate cause of the ANCA autoimmune response.

## CLINICAL FEATURES AND NATURAL HISTORY

Most patients with pauci-immune necrotizing crescentic glomerulonephritis and ANCA have glomerular disease as part of a systemic small-vessel vasculitis. The disease is clinically limited to the kidney in about one-third of patients.[1361] When both renal-limited and vasculitis-associated pauci-immune crescentic glomerulonephritis are considered, this category of crescentic glomerulonephritis is the most common cause of RPGN in adults.[1127,1133,1179,1361,1362] When the disorder is part of a systemic vasculitis, patients have pulmonary-renal, dermal-renal, or a multisystem disease. Frequent sites of involvement are the eyes, ears, sinuses, upper airways, lungs, gastrointestinal tract, skin, peripheral nerves, joints, and central nervous system. The three major ANCA-associated syndromes are MPA, GPA, and EGPA.[1270,1363,1364] Even when patients have no clinical evidence of extrarenal manifestations of active vasculitis, systemic symptoms consisting of fever, fatigue, myalgias, and arthralgias are common.

Most patients with ANCA-associated pauci-immune necrotizing glomerulonephritis have RPGN with rapid loss of kidney function associated with hematuria, proteinuria, and hypertension. However, some patients follow a more indolent course of slow decline in function and less active urine sediment. In the latter group of patients, episodes of focal necrosis and hematuria resolve with focal glomerular scarring. Subsequent relapses result in cumulative damage to glomeruli.

Note that patients who have only pauci-immune crescentic glomerulonephritis at presentation may later develop signs and symptoms of systemic disease, with involvement of extrarenal organ systems.[1365] An autopsy study was conducted in deceased patients with ANCA-associated vasculitis. This study revealed the widespread presence of glomerulonephritis, but also demonstrated the finding of clinically silent extrarenal vasculitis. It was found that 8% of patients died from septic infections or progressive recurrent vasculitis.[1365]

No studies currently available specifically examine the prognostic factors of pauci-immune crescentic glomerulonephritis in the absence of extrarenal manifestations of disease. In studies addressing the question of prognosis of patients with ANCA-related small-vessel vasculitis in general,[1273,1365,1366] the presence of pulmonary hemorrhage was the most important determinant of patient survival. With respect to the risk of ESKD, the most important predictor of outcome is the entry serum creatinine level at the time of initiation of treatment.[1366] This parameter remained the most important predictive factor of renal outcome in a multivariate analysis that corrected for variables such as the presence or absence of extrarenal disease. Treatment resistance and progression to ESKD is also predicted by longer disease duration and vascular sclerosis on kidney biopsy specimens—presence of glomerular sclerosis, interstitial infiltrates, tubular necrosis, and atrophy[1367]—and the presence of clinical markers of chronic disease, including cumulative organ damage (measured by the vasculitis damage index).[1368] A finding of vascular sclerosis on the biopsy was also found to be an independent predictor of treatment resistance[1369] and may be a reflection of chronic kidney damage due to hypertension or other atherosclerotic processes, with ANCA-associated nephritis providing an additional insult.

The impact of kidney damage as a predictor of resistance emphasizes the importance of early diagnosis and prompt institution of therapy. It is important to note that although the entry serum creatinine level is the most important predictor of renal outcome, there is no threshold of kidney dysfunction beyond which treatment is deemed futile, because more than 50% of patients who have a GFR less than 10 mL/min at presentation reach remission and experience a substantial improvement in kidney function.[1370] Therefore, aggressive immunosuppressive therapy is warranted in all patients with newly diagnosed disease.[1369] However, the risk of progression to ESKD is also determined by the change in GFR within the first 4 months of treatment. In the absence of other disease manifestations, the decision to continue immunosuppressive therapy in patients with a sharply declining GFR should be weighed against the diminishing chance of renal recovery.[1369]

Relapses of ANCA small-vessel vasculitis occur in up to 40% of patients. Based on a large cohort study, the risk of relapse appears to be predicted by the presence of PR3-ANCA (as opposed to MPO-ANCA) and the presence of upper respiratory tract or lung involvement.[1369] Patients with glomerulonephritis alone who have predominantly MPO-ANCA belong to the subgroup of patients with a relatively low risk of relapse, with a rate of relapse rate of about 25% at a median of 62 months.

Pauci-immune necrotizing glomerulonephritis and small-vessel vasculitis may recur after kidney transplantation.[1371,1372] The rate of recurrence for ANCA small-vessel vasculitis in general, including pauci-immune necrotizing glomerulonephritis alone, is about 20%.[1373] The rate of recurrence in the subset of patients who have pauci-immune necrotizing glomerulonephritis alone, without systemic vasculitis is unknown, but may be lower than 20%. A positive ANCA test result at the time of transplantation does not seem to be associated with an increased risk of recurrent disease.

## LABORATORY FINDINGS

Approximately 80% to 90% of patients with pauci-immune necrotizing and crescentic glomerulonephritis have circulating ANCA.[365,1273,1276,1363,1374–1376] On indirect IF microscopy of alcohol-fixed neutrophils, ANCAs cause two patterns of staining, perinuclear (P-ANCA) and cytoplasmic (C-ANCA).[1276,1376] The two major antigen specificities for ANCA are MPO and PR3.[1269,1376–1379] Both proteins are found in the primary granules of neutrophils and the lysosomes of monocytes. With rare exceptions, anti-MPO autoantibodies produce a P-ANCA pattern of staining on indirect IF microscopy, whereas anti-PR3 autoantibodies produce a C-ANCA pattern of staining. About two-thirds of patients with pauci-immune necrotizing crescentic glomerulonephritis, without clinical evidence of systemic vasculitis, will have MPO-ANCA or P-ANCA, and approximately 30% have PR3-ANCA or C-ANCA.[1270,1380] The relative frequency of MPO-ANCA to PR3-ANCA is higher in patients with renal-limited disease than in patients with MPA or GPA.[1270] A small percentage of patients will harbor both MPO- and PR3-ANCA; however, this likely represents primarily patients who have been exposed to levamisole-adulterated cocaine.[1381,1382]

As mentioned previously, about one-third of patients with anti-GBM disease and approximately 25% of patients with idiopathic immune complex crescent glomerulonephritis test positive for ANCAs; therefore, ANCA positivity is not completely specific for pauci-immune crescentic glomerulonephritis.[365] Maximal sensitivity and specificity with ANCA testing is achieved when both IF and antigen-specific assays are performed. Antigen-specific assays may be ELISA or radioimmunoassays. A variety of commercial tests are now available, and their diagnostic specificity ranges from 70% to 90% and sensitivity from 81% to 91%.[365,1383] However, tests still do not provide the necessary sensitivity, specificity, and predictive power to allow their use as the basis for initiating or altering cytotoxic therapy.

The positive predictive value (PPV) of a positive ANCA test result (i.e., the percentage of patients with a positive result who have pauci-immune crescentic glomerulonephritis) depends on the signs and symptoms of disease in the patient who is being tested. The signs and symptoms indicate the pretest likelihood of pauci-immune crescentic glomerulonephritis (predicted prevalence), which greatly influences predictive value. The PPV of a positive ANCA result in a patient with classic features of RPGN is 95%.[365] In patients with hematuria and proteinuria, the PPV of a positive ANCA result is 84% if the serum creatinine level is more than 3 mg/dL, 60% if the serum creatinine level is 1.5 to 3.0 mg/dL, and only 29% if the serum creatinine level is less than 1 mg/dL.[1384] Although the PPV is not good in this last setting, the negative predictive value is greater than 95%, and thus a negative result can allay any concerns that the patient has early or mild pauci-immune necrotizing glomerulonephritis.

Urinalysis findings in pauci-immune crescentic glomerulonephritis include hematuria with dysmorphic red blood cells, with or without red cell casts, and proteinuria. The proteinuria ranges from 1 g of protein/24 hours to as much as 16 g of protein/24 hours.[1365,1385] The serum creatinine concentration usually is elevated at the time of diagnosis and rising, although a minority of patients have relatively indolent disease. The erythrocyte sedimentation rate and C-reactive protein level are elevated during active disease. Serum complement component levels are typically within normal limits.

Whether a kidney biopsy is essential for the management of ANCA-associated pauci-immune glomerulonephritis depends on a number of factors, including the diagnostic accuracy of ANCA testing, pretest probability of finding pauci-immune glomerulonephritis, value of knowing the activity and chronicity of the renal lesions, and risk associated with immunotherapy for ANCA-associated pauci-immune necrotizing glomerulonephritis. Based on a study of 1000 patients with proliferative and/or necrotizing glomerulonephritis and a positive test for PR3-ANCA or MPO-ANCA, the PPV of ANCA testing was found to be 86%, with a false-positive rate of 14% and a false-negative rate of 16%. Considering the serious risks inherent in treatment with high-dose corticosteroids and cytotoxic agents, it is prudent to confirm the diagnosis and characterize the activity and chronicity of ANCA-associated pauci-immune crescentic glomerulonephritis by kidney biopsy, unless the patient is too ill to tolerate the procedure.[1384]

## TREATMENT

Data on the treatment of ANCA-positive pauci-immune necrotizing and crescentic glomerulonephritis have been derived from studies of ANCA-associated vasculitis, including GPA and MPA. There are scant data specifically addressing the treatment of patients with renal-limited pauci-immune necrotizing glomerulonephritis. The treatment of pauci-immune crescentic glomerulonephritis (with or without systemic vasculitis) is still based primarily on varying regimens of corticosteroids and cyclophosphamide.[1366,1386,1387]

In view of the potential explosive and fulminant nature of this disease, induction therapy should be instituted using pulse methylprednisolone at a dose of 7 mg/kg/day for 3 consecutive days in an attempt to halt the aggressive, destructive, inflammatory process. This is followed by the institution of daily oral prednisone, as well as cyclophosphamide, either orally or intravenously. Prednisone is usually started at a dosage of 1 mg/kg/day for the first month, tapered to an alternate-day regimen, and then discontinued by the end of the fourth to fifth month. When a regimen of monthly intravenous doses of cyclophosphamide is used, the starting dose should be about 0.5 g/m$^2$ and should be adjusted upward to 1 g/m$^2$ based on the 2-week leukocyte count nadir.[1387,1388] A regimen based on daily oral cyclophosphamide should begin at a dose of 2 mg/kg/day[1386] and should be adjusted downward, as needed, to keep a nadir leukocyte count above 3000 cells/mm$^3$.

The optimal form of cyclophosphamide therapy (daily oral vs. intravenous pulse) has been the subject of investigation. In general, the intravenous regimen allows for an approximately twofold lower cumulative dose of cyclophosphamide than the oral regimen and is associated with a significant decrease in the rate of clinically significant neutropenia and other complications. In a metaanalysis of three RCTs, the rate of relapse associated with pulse cyclophosphamide was not statistically higher than the rate of relapse with a daily oral regimen, but the intravenous pulse regimen was associated with a statistically higher rate of remission and lower rates of leucopenia and infections.[1389] The final outcomes (death or ESKD) were no different for the two dosing regimens.

A large RCT (CYCLOPS) of pulse versus daily oral cyclophosphamide for the induction of remission was conducted that included 149 patients with newly diagnosed generalized ANCA vasculitis with kidney involvement.[1390] Patients were randomly assigned to receive pulse cyclophosphamide, 15 mg/kg every 2 weeks times 3, then every 3 weeks, or daily oral cyclophosphamide, 2 mg/kg/day. Cyclophosphamide therapy was continued for 3 months beyond the time of remission. All patients were then switched to azathioprine (2 mg/kg/day orally) until month 18. All patients received prednisolone, starting at 1 mg/kg orally, followed by a taper. Patients with a serum creatinine level more than 500 µmol/L (5.7 mg/dL) were excluded from the study; 79% of patients achieved remission by 9 months (median time to remission was 3 months for both groups). The two treatment groups did not differ in time to remission or proportion of patients who achieved remission at 9 months (88.1% in the pulse group vs. 87.7% in the daily oral group). The GFR did not differ between the two groups at any time point. By 18 months, 13 patients in the pulse group and 6 in the daily oral group had experienced a relapse (HR, 2.01; CI, 0.77–5.30). Absolute cumulative cyclophosphamide dose in the daily oral group was almost twice that in the pulse group (15.9 vs. 8.2 g, respectively; $P < .001$). The pulse group had a lower rate of leukopenia (HR, 0.41; CI, 0.23–0.71), but the frequency of serious infections was not statistically different between the two treatment groups. The long-term results of this trial were reported with a median duration of 4.3 years follow-up and data from 90% of patients in the original trial.[1391] There was no difference in survival between the two groups; however, risk of relapse was significantly lower in the daily oral cyclophosphamide arm (HR. 0.50; CI, 0.26–0.93; $P = .029$) although kidney function was similar by the end of the study ($P = .82$), as were adverse events.

This RCT confirms that the two cyclophosphamide regimens are associated with similar remission induction rates and time to remission induction, with the pulse cyclophosphamide regimen resulting in about 50% of the cumulative medication dose of the oral regimen and a significantly lower rate of leukopenia. The long-term results would suggest that the daily oral cyclophosphamide regimen portends less relapse risk, and there was a trend toward this in the original study. At this point, clinicians must weigh the risks and benefits of either regimen to determine which is most appropriate, and this decision may likely be based more heavily now on the level of patient compliance.

The length of cyclophosphamide therapy has changed significantly, largely based on the results of a large controlled trial in which patients who attained complete remission with cyclophosphamide after 3 months of therapy were randomly assigned to switch to azathioprine or to continue taking cyclophosphamide for a total of 12 months. After 12 months, both groups received azathioprine maintenance therapy for an additional year.[1211] Changing to azathioprine after 3 months of cyclophosphamide treatment appeared to be as effective as receiving oral cyclophosphamide for 12 months followed by 12 months of azathioprine, based on kidney function and frequency of relapse. It is noteworthy that patients whose PR3-ANCA titers remained positive at the time of the switch had about a twofold increased risk of subsequent relapse compared with patients whose ANCA titers had reverted to negative.[1392]

In three relatively small RCTs addressing the role of plasmapheresis in the treatment of ANCA-associated vasculitis and glomerulonephritis,[1393–1395] plasmapheresis was not found to provide any added benefit over immunosuppressive treatment alone in patients with renal-limited disease or patients with mild to moderate kidney dysfunction. However, the use of plasmapheresis in addition to immunosuppressive therapy appears to be beneficial in the subset of patients who require dialysis at the time of presentation.[1395,1396] In a study performed by the European vasculitis study group (MEPEX trial) of 137 patients with a new diagnosis of severe biopsy-confirmed ANCA-associated glomerulonephritis, the use of plasma exchange was found to be superior to pulse methylprednisolone in producing recovery of kidney function in patients with severe kidney dysfunction at the time of entry into the study (serum creatinine level >5.8 mg/dL).[1397] Long-term follow-up of these patients did not show a significant difference in the proportion of patients free of ESKD or death; however, the small number of patients limited the power to detect differences.[1398] Because of the clinically observed increased risk of severe bone marrow suppression with the use of cyclophosphamide in patients receiving dialysis, such treatment should be pursued with extreme caution.

Patients who eventually are able to discontinue dialysis usually do so within 3 to 4 months of initiation of therapy.[1370,1388] For this reason, continuing immunosuppressive therapy beyond 4 months in patients who are still undergoing dialysis is unlikely to be of added benefit (unless they continue to have extrarenal manifestations of vasculitis). In a retrospective analysis of 523 patients with ANCA vasculitis followed over a median of 40 months, 136 patients reached ESKD.[1399]

Relapse rates of vasculitis were significantly lower in patients on long-term dialysis (0.08 episodes/person-year) than in the same patients before they reached ESKD (0.20 episodes/person-year) and in patients with preserved kidney function (0.16 episodes/person year). Infections were almost twice as frequent among patients with ESKD receiving maintenance immunosuppressants and were an important cause of death. Given the lower risk of relapse with hemodialysis and the higher risk of infection and death with long-term immunosuppression, the risk-benefit ratio does not support the routine use of maintenance immunosuppression therapy in patients with ANCA small-vessel vasculitis who are on long-term dialysis.

*Clinical Relevance*

**Immune Suppression in Dialysis Patients**

The risk-benefit ratio of maintenance immunosuppression therapy in patients with ANCA small-vessel vasculitis who are on long-term dialysis must be carefully considered because the relapse risk is lower on dialysis and infection risk is high.

Although high-dose intravenous pooled immunoglobulin has been used in the treatment of systemic vasculitis resistant to usual immunosuppressive treatment,[1400–1404] there have been no published reports of its use in patients with pauci-immune crescentic glomerulonephritis alone, without systemic involvement.

Induction therapy with methotrexate has been compared with cyclophosphamide treatment in patients with early limited GPA and mild kidney disease.[1405–1409] The rate of remission at 6 months was comparable in the two treatment groups.[1407] However, the onset of remission was delayed in methotrexate-treated patients with more extensive disease or pulmonary involvement. Methotrexate was also associated with a significantly higher rate of relapse than cyclophosphamide (69.5% vs. 46.5%, respectively), and 45% of relapses occurred while patients were receiving methotrexate. The dose of methotrexate must be reduced in patients whose creatinine clearance is less than 80 mL/min, and its use is contraindicated when creatinine clearances is less than 10 mL/min. Moreover, in the authors' experience, there are patients taking methotrexate who have progressive glomerulonephritis. Methotrexate is therefore unlikely to have any role in the treatment of pauci-immune crescentic glomerulonephritis alone.

Whether the use of cyclophosphamide can be reduced or avoided completely by the use of rituximab has been the subject of two RCTs. In the RITUXVAS trial, 44 patients with newly diagnosed ANCA vasculitis were randomly assigned in a ratio of 3:1 to receive rituximab (375 mg/m$^2$ weekly × 4) in addition to cyclophosphamide (15 mg/kg intravenously × 2; 2 weeks apart), or to cyclophosphamide (15 mg/kg intravenously every 2 weeks × 3, then every 3 weeks, for a maximum total of 10 doses) alone.[1409] Both groups received the same intravenous and oral prednisolone regimen. Patients in the rituximab group did not receive maintenance therapy, whereas those in the cyclophosphamide group were switched to azathioprine until the end of the trial. Minimum follow-up was 12 months. The rate of sustained remission was similar in the two treatment groups (76% in the rituximab group vs. 82% in the cyclophosphamide group; $P$ = .67 for risk difference). Severe adverse events were common in both groups, affecting 45% of patients in the rituximab group and 36% in the cyclophosphamide group ($P$= .60). This study has suggested that a combination of rituximab and reduced-dose cyclophosphamide may be no less effective than a traditional cyclophosphamide regimen, but it did not demonstrate a safety benefit of a rituximab-based approach. This study was not powered to establish equivalence or noninferiority.

In a large controlled trial designed to assess the noninferiority of rituximab compared with cyclophosphamide, 197 patients were randomly assigned to treatment with rituximab (375 mg/m$^2$ infusions once weekly × 4) or cyclophosphamide (2 mg/kg/day orally) for months 1 to 3, followed by azathioprine (2 mg/kg/day orally) for months 4 to 6. All patients received methylprednisolone (1 g/day intravenously for up to 3 days), followed by prednisone (1 mg/kg/day, tapered off completely by 6 months). The induction phase of this trial revealed similar rates between the two treatment groups in complete remission at 6 months (64% in the rituximab group vs. 55% in the cyclophosphamide group; $P$ = .21).[1410] No differences in relapse rates were observed between the groups. The 18-month efficacy of this single course of rituximab, as compared with cyclophosphamide followed by azathioprine, revealed persistent noninferiority; however, remission rates at the 18-month mark were 39% and 33% ($P$ = .32), respectively, signifying the critical and persistent need for more effective remission induction and maintenance strategies.[1411] Although these studies suggest that substitution of cyclophosphamide with rituximab may be effective, rituximab has not been formally evaluated in patients with severe renal failure requiring dialysis.

Studies pertaining to maintenance immunosuppression for relapse prevention are primarily geared to patients with GPA or MPA. Current data have suggested that patients with pauci-immune glomerulonephritis alone and MPO-ANCA are at a relatively low risk of relapse.[1369] The value of prolonged maintenance immunosuppression in this group of patients is unknown, and any benefit in preventing a relapse would have to be weighed against the potential toxicity of immunosuppressive agents and the risks associated with their use.

## MAINTENANCE TREATMENT

Following successful induction remission therapy, most patients with ANCA-associated vasculitis should remain on a maintenance immunosuppressive regimen to prevent relapses and limit end-organ damage. Patients with PR3-associated vasculitis or lung and upper respiratory tract involvement are more likely to relapse than others, with an HR of 1.7 for each risk factor.[1369]

Cardiovascular involvement may be associated with a higher risk of relapse, whereas poor renal function is associated with a lower risk of relapse.[1412] Patients with drug-associated ANCA vasculitis who achieve remission after initial induction therapy may be followed closely, without the need for maintenance therapy. Whether all patients with the lower risks of relapse (MPO-associated vasculitis without lung or upper respiratory tract involvement) need maintenance therapy is debatable, but patients should be assessed on a case by case basis.

Prolonged treatment (>12 months) with cyclophosphamide (CYC) and glucocorticoids (GCs) has been the standard of care for a long time. Although the mortality rate has dramatically improved, both CYC and GCs have been associated with significant morbidity and organ damage.[1368] This led to the search for a lesser toxic therapeutic regimen for maintenance therapy. Several major clinical trials have investigated different maintenance immunosuppressive regimens. These trials include CYClophosphamide versus AZAthioprine for early REMission phase of vasculitis (CYCAZAREM), WEgner Granulomatosis-ENTretein (WEGENT, comparing azathioprine versus methotrexate), MAINtenance of remission using RITuximab in Systemic ANCA-associated vasculitis (MAINRITSAN), MMF Protocol to Reduce Outbreaks of Vasculitides (IMPROVE), and prolonged REmission–MAINtenance therapy is systemic vasculitis (REMAIN).

In the CYCAZAREM study, newly diagnosed patients with ANCA-associated vasculitis (57% PR3-positive, 37% MPO-positive) underwent induction treatment with oral cyclophosphamide (2 mg/kg/day) and prednisone.[1413] Most enrolled patients had renal involvement (mean eGFR, 49 mL/min; 95% CI, 43.7–54.6). Patients with a serum creatinine level greater than 5.7 mg/dL were excluded. After induction of remission, patients were randomized to azathioprine (2 mg/kg/day) or continued CYC (1.5 mg/kg/day) with prednisone, 10 mg/day. At month 12, both groups were treated with azathioprine (1.5 mg/kg/day) and prednisone, 7.5 mg daily. At 18 months, the relapse rate was not significantly different (~15%), and neither were the rates of serious adverse effects in the two groups; there were seven deaths during the induction-remission phase. This study has suggested that a prolonged course of CYC may be avoided with the substitution of azathioprine after achieving remission. Also, there was a similar degree of improvement in renal function in both groups from study entry to 18 months (17.5 mL/min and 23.5 mL/min in both the azathioprine and CYC groups, respectively).[1413]

In the WEGENT study, a multicenter open-label randomized control study, patients with a new diagnosis of Wegener granulomatosis (55%) and microscopic polyangiitis (45%) who achieved induction remission following treatment with pulse CYC and GCs underwent randomization to azathioprine (2 mg/kg/day) or methotrexate (0.3 mg/kg/week, progressively increased to 25 mg/week) for 12 months, followed by taper over 3 months.[1414] The mean serum creatinine level at randomization was 1.46 mg/dL. The incidence of adverse events leading to discontinuation of the study drug or death was 11% in the azathioprine group and 12% in the methotrexate group, respectively. The HR was 1.65 (95% CI, 0.65–4.18) for the risk of an adverse event with methotrexate versus azathioprine. Also, grade 3 or 4 toxicity was higher with methotrexate (18%) compared with 8% with azathioprine ($P$ = .11). The relapse rate was similar at 36% and 33 % for azathioprine and methotrexate, respectively. Although, both drugs appeared similar in achieving remission, there was a trend toward more severe adverse events with methotrexate, probably due to use of higher dosing in the setting of impaired renal function. Moreover, the relapse rates were quite high in both groups.[1414]

In the IMPROVE study, patients with newly diagnosed GPA or MPA underwent induction-remission protocol of oral or intravenous CYC and GCs. Maintenance therapy constituted azathioprine (2 mg/kg/day) or MMF (2 g/day).[1415] At month 12, the dose was reduced to 1.5 mg/kg/day for azathioprine and 1.5 g/day for MMF up to month 18, and then further tapered to 1.0 mg/kg/day for azathioprine and 1 g/day for MMF until month 42. Both groups received a tapering course of prednisone for 24 months. The median follow-up was 39 months (interquartile range, 0.66–53.6 months). The median serum creatinine level was 2.7 mg/dL in the azathioprine group and 2.9 mg/dL in the MMF group. Relapses were more common in the MMF group, with an HR of 1.80 (95% CI, 1.10–2.93; $P$ = .02) after adjustment for other factors.[1415]

In the MAINRITSAN trial, the superiority of rituximab over azathioprine for relapse prevention of ANCA-associated vasculitis was reported.[1416] Among 115 patients, most patients had GPA (76%), whereas 20% of the cases had MPA. Most of the patients were newly diagnosed cases. All patients were randomized at 1:1 to rituximab or azathioprine after achieving remission following induction therapy with corticosteroids and pulse CYC. Patients received rituximab on days 0 and 14 after randomization and then at 6, 12 and 18 months thereafter. Azathioprine was dosed at 2 mg/kg/day for the first 12 months, followed by 1.5 mg/kg/day for the next 6 months and then at 1 mg/kg for 4 months. At month 28, there were 17 relapses in the azathioprine group (29%) compared with only 3 in the rituximab group (5%). In the rituximab group, 1 patient relapsed at month 8 and 1 each at months 22 and 24—that is, within 6 months of the last dose of rituximab. In contrast, 8 patients relapsed within the first 12 months, and 7 patients relapsed after azathioprine was stopped between months 24 and 28. Both groups had similar rates of adverse effects. Although the trial showed the superiority of rituximab over azathioprine for relapse prevention, it has drawn criticism. A major criticism is that most patients had GPA and only a small group of patients had MPO and renal-limited ANCA vasculitis. Thus, the superiority of rituximab may not hold true for both groups. Also, the dose of azathioprine was tapered after 1 year of standard dosing, but the dose of rituximab was kept the same. It begs the question whether the relapse rate would have been different if the dose of azathioprine had been uniform for the entire study period. All patients underwent induction therapy with CYC, so these conclusions cannot be extrapolated to patients who receive rituximab as induction therapy.[1416–1418]

The REMAIN study investigated patients with ANCA-associated vasculitis in remission after a CYC-based regimen for induction remission.[1419] In this study, patients were randomized into an azathioprine-prednisolone group for 48 months from diagnosis (continuation group) or to withdraw azathioprine/prednisolone at 24 months (withdrawal group). This prospective, randomized controlled study was designed to study the risk of relapse with prolonged duration of maintenance therapy. The study demonstrated that continuation of maintenance therapy for a longer duration (>2 years) results in a threefold reduction in relapse risk. Most relapses in the withdrawal group occurred after stopping azathioprine. Although the safety profile was not statistically different between the two groups, the study was underpowered to study the difference. Moreover, cytopenias and cardiovascular events were much more common in the continuation group. There were five deaths, with two of them due to cardiovascular events in the continuation group. There are many limitations of this study including an unknown cumulative dose of GCs and CYC, exclusion of patients with ESRKD, and prior severe relapse of disease. Although prolonged immunosuppression therapy may reduce the risk of relapse, this study did not address the risks associated with this approach.[1360,1419]

Based on the previous results, one could consider azathioprine, rituximab, or methotrexate for maintenance therapy. The patient's clinical and serologic characteristics, renal function, concomitant medications (azathioprine is best avoided with allopurinol), cost, and other factors should be considered when determining the best and most appropriate maintenance therapy. The duration of maintenance therapy remains undefined, and it must be weighed against the risks of relapse and effects of long-term immunosuppression (e.g., risks of infections, cardiovascular morbidity, malignancy). Open discussions between the clinician and patient are essential in determining the best maintenance therapy, duration, and if or when to stop therapy. Patients should be educated about the signs and symptoms of disease relapse when off therapy, and periodic urine dipstick measurement of hematuria in patients with kidney involvement should be encouraged.

Methotrexate should be avoided in patients with renal insufficiency or in those at high risk for kidney injury. Rituximab may lead to HBV reactivation, so screening for HBV infection is essential before the initiation of therapy. The optimal duration and dosing of azathioprine still needs to be determined, but because most relapses occur when the drug is stopped and/or tapered after 12 to 15 months, one could consider continuing azathioprine for a longer time. The duration of maintenance therapy also depends on the risks of relapse, tolerance of the drug, infections, adverse effects, and other factors. With rituximab, one may consider the dosing regimen used in the MAINRITSAN trial until the results of MAINRITSAN 2 (NCT01731561) and RITAZAREM (NCT01697267) trials are available. The MAINRITSAN 2 study will evaluate the dosing regimen of rituximab based on ANCA titers and CD19 lymphocytes versus infusions at a fixed interval in systemic ANCA-associated vasculitis. The RITAZAREM trial aims to compare the infusion of rituximab, 1000 mg, every 4 months for 2 years versus azathioprine at 2 mg/kg/day for patients with relapsing ANCA-associated vasculitis after an induction remission with rituximab and glucocorticoids.

Serum IgG levels should be monitored in patients receiving repeated courses of rituximab, especially if they previously received cytotoxic therapy. Because circulatory mature plasma cells, the source of most IgG, do not express CD20, a single dose of rituximab may not deplete IgG levels. Repeated dosing and depletion of B cell precursors may result in hypogammaglobulinemia. In a retrospective analysis following rituximab infusion, 34% of patients were found to have a low IgG level (<6 g/L) for at least 3 months, of whom only 4% had a severely low IgG level (<3 g/L). Although the median IgG level trended toward the hypogammaglobulinemic range in patients who received more than 6 g, this was not statistically significant.[1420] In a single-center cohort study of 29 GPA patients who received a median cumulative dose of 17 g of CYC one quarter of GPA patients developed hypogammaglobulinemia following rituximab infusion.[1421] Male gender, total cyclophosphamide exposure, and baseline serum immunoglobulin levels were independent risks factors, whereas the total cumulative rituximab dose did not influence the risk.[1421]

In another series, 4% of patients with systemic vasculitis had moderate to severe hypogammaglobulinemia with recurrent infections after rituximab infusion. Most of these patients had previously received other immunosuppressive medications. The median dose of CYC was 6 g. IgG was replaced intravenously at a dose of 0.4 g/kg monthly, titrated to achieve a goal of 8 to 10 g/L and a decrease in infection rate. This regimen resulted in a decreased incidence and severity of infections, and many patients were able to continue rituximab infusion along with IgG replacement.[1422]

Following significant response to induction therapy, GCs should be tapered over 6 months. Although data are inconsistent on the duration of therapy, a metaanalysis has suggested that low-dose GCs for longer than 12 months may result in fewer relapses. However, the authors acknowledged that the nature of relapses (major or minor) and an accurate assessment of adverse effects were lacking in their analysis.[1423] Moreover, long-term, low-dose GC use may increase the risks of infections and probably new-onset diabetes mellitus.[1424]

Sulfamethoxazole-trimethoprim (S-T) has been suggested for the maintenance treatment of ANCA-associated vasculitis.[1425,1426] It has been proposed that S-T may act as an anti-inflammatory agent by interfering with cytotoxic oxygen metabolites from activated neutrophils and prevent tissue damage.[1427] In a prospective, randomized, placebo-controlled study of 81 patients with generalized GPA, cotrimoxazole (800 mg of sulfamethoxazole plus 160 mg of trimethoprim) or placebo was given twice daily during remission following treatment with CYC and prednisolone. The mean serum creatinine clearance was more than 60 mL/min in both groups, and there was no significant difference among groups in dosing of prednisolone and CYC. At month 24, there were fewer respiratory and non–respiratory tract infections; 82% of patients in the S-T group and only 60% in the placebo group remained in remission (relative risk of relapse, 0.4; 95% CI, 0.17–0.98). In 20% of patients, the drug was stopped due to side effects, including nausea, vomiting, rash, and a single case of possible interstitial nephritis and asymptomatic hepatotoxic effects. All adverse effects resolved with cessation of drug therapy.[1425]

In a separate study of generalized GPA following induction remission with CYC and prednisone, patients were randomized to receive methotrexate or daily oral S-T (160 mg trimethoprim plus 800 mg sulfamethoxazole), with or without prednisone for maintenance therapy. In contrast to the previous study, remission (complete or partial) was maintained in 86% of patients on methotrexate but only 58% in the S-T group. Also, all patients on S-T and on low-dose prednisone relapsed after a median duration of 14 months. The discrepancy in the remission rates between the two studies could be partially explained by the use of different clinical tools for assessment of disease activity. In addition, the risk factors for relapse could have been different among different groups.[1428] Although S-T could be used in conjunction with standard maintenance immunosuppressive therapy to prevent infections and possibly reduce the risk of relapse, its use alone is not recommended to prevent relapses, especially in patients with pauci-immune glomerulonephritis.

Both PR3 ANCA-associated vasculitis (AAV) and MPO-AAV have been categorized together in most clinical trials. Multiple studies have suggested that PR3- and MPO-AAV have significant differences, including their genetic basis, histologic findings, and clinical manifestations.[1318,1334,1429] Moreover, the risk of relapse is higher with PR3-AAV than with MPO-AAV, and renal survival is worse with MPO-AAV compared with PR3-AAV and ANCA-negative vasculitis (HR, 2.1; 95% CI, 1.11–3.80; $P = .01$). Patients with PR3-AAV with pauci-immune glomerulonephritis have more active disease compared with those with MPO-AAV who may have more chronic lesions on renal histology, suggesting a smoldering disease with a delay in diagnosis and treatment.[1318,1430] Based on a post hoc clinical trial analysis, patients with PR3-AAV are more likely to achieve and maintain remission with rituximab compared with CYC ($n = 131$; 65% vs. 48%; $P = .04$).[1431]

MPO ANCA patients have been underrepresented in many clinical trials. Future clinical studies for induction and maintenance therapy should be designed by separating the MPO and PR3 ANCA serotypes.

 Complete reference list available at ExpertConsult.com.

## KEY REFERENCES


1. Jennette JC, Falk RJ, Bacon PA, et al. 2012 revised international chapel hill consensus conference nomenclature of vasculitides. *Arthritis Rheum.* 2013;65(1):1–11.
8. Tryggvason K, Patrakka J, Wartiovaara J. Hereditary proteinuria syndromes and mechanisms of proteinuria. *N Engl J Med.* 2006; 354(13):1387–1401.
14. Springberg PD, Garrett LE Jr, Thompson AL Jr, et al. Fixed and reproducible orthostatic proteinuria: results of a 20-year follow-up study. *Ann Intern Med.* 1982;97(4):516–519.
18. Mariani AJ, Mariani MC, Macchioni C, et al. The significance of adult hematuria: 1,000 hematuria evaluations including a risk-benefit and cost-effectiveness analysis. *J Urol.* 1989;141(2): 350–355.
22. Schramek P, Schuster FX, Georgopoulos M, et al. Value of urinary erythrocyte morphology in assessment of symptomless microhaematuria. *Lancet.* 1989;2(8675):1316–1319.
30. Tiebosch AT, Frederik PM, Breda Vriesman PJ, et al. Thin-basement-membrane nephropathy in adults with persistent hematuria. *N Engl J Med.* 1989;320(1):14–18.
42. Maas RJ, Deegens JK, Smeets B, et al. Minimal change disease and idiopathic FSGS: manifestations of the same disease. *Nat Rev Nephrol.* 2016;12(12):768–776.
80. Clement LC, Avila-Casado C, Mace C, et al. Podocyte-secreted angiopoietin-like-4 mediates proteinuria in glucocorticoid-sensitive nephrotic syndrome. *Nat Med.* 2011;17(1):117–122.
85. Audard V, Larousserie F, Grimbert P, et al. Minimal change nephrotic syndrome and classical Hodgkin's lymphoma: report of 21 cases and review of the literature. *Kidney Int.* 2006;69(12):2251–2260.
97. Bridges CR, Myers BD, Brenner BM, et al. Glomerular charge alterations in human minimal change nephropathy. *Kidney Int.* 1982;22(6):677–684.
113. Short versus standard prednisone therapy for initial treatment of idiopathic nephrotic syndrome in children. Arbeitsgemeinschaft f++r P+ñdiatrische Nephrologie. *Lancet.* 1988;1(8582):380–383.
153. Detwiler RK, Falk RJ, Hogan SL, et al. Collapsing glomerulopathy: a clinically and pathologically distinct variant of focal segmental glomerulosclerosis. *Kidney Int.* 1994;45(5):1416–1424.
158. Howie AJ, Brewer DB. The glomerular tip lesion: a previously undescribed type of segmental glomerular abnormality. *J Pathol.* 1984;142(3):205–220.
162. Koziell A, Grech V, Hussain S, et al. Genotype/phenotype correlations of NPHS1 and NPHS2 mutations in nephrotic syndrome advocate a functional inter-relationship in glomerular filtration. *Hum Mol Genet.* 2002;11(4):379–388.
171. Bouchireb K, Boyer O, Gribouval O, et al. NPHS2 mutations in steroid-resistant nephrotic syndrome: a mutation update and the associated phenotypic spectrum. *Hum Mutat.* 2014;35(2): 178–186.
184. Genovese G, Friedman DJ, Ross MD, et al. Association of trypanolytic ApoL1 variants with kidney disease in African Americans. *Science.* 2010;329(5993):841–845.
207. Brenner BM, Meyer TW, Hostetter TH. Dietary protein intake and the progressive nature of kidney disease: the role of hemodynamically mediated glomerular injury in the pathogenesis of progressive glomerular sclerosis in aging, renal ablation, and intrinsic renal disease. *N Engl J Med.* 1982;307(11):652–659.
209. Simons JL, Provoost AP, Anderson S, et al. Modulation of glomerular hypertension defines susceptibility to progressive glomerular injury. *Kidney Int.* 1994;46(2):396–404.
218. Wei C, El HS, Li J, et al. Circulating urokinase receptor as a cause of focal segmental glomerulosclerosis. *Nat Med.* 2011;17(8):952–960.
229. Chaudhary BA, Sklar AH, Chaudhary TK, et al. Sleep apnea, proteinuria, and nephrotic syndrome. *Sleep.* 1988;11(1):69–74.
235. Novick AC, Gephardt G, Guz B, et al. Long-term follow-up after partial removal of a solitary kidney. *N Engl J Med.* 1991;325(15): 1058–1062.
238. Border WA, Noble NA, Yamamoto T, et al. Natural inhibitor of transforming growth factor-beta protects against scarring in experimental kidney disease. *Nature.* 1992;360(6402):361–364.
272. Maschio G, Alberti D, Janin G, et al. Effect of the angiotensin-converting-enzyme inhibitor benazepril on the progression of chronic renal insufficiency. The Angiotensin-Converting-Enzyme Inhibition in Progressive Renal Insufficiency Study Group. *N Engl J Med.* 1996;334(15):939–945.
288. Laurin LP, Gasim AM, Derebail VK, et al. Renal survival in patients with collapsing compared with not otherwise specified FSGS. *Clin J Am Soc Nephrol.* 2016.
319. Vizjak A, Ferluga D, Rozic M, et al. Pathology, clinical presentations, and outcomes of C1q nephropathy. *J Am Soc Nephrol.* 2008;19(11):2237–2244.
330. Takekoshi Y, Tanaka M, Shida N, et al. Strong association between membranous nephropathy and hepatitis-B surface antigenaemia in Japanese children. *Lancet.* 1978;2(8099):1065–1068.
354. Jennette JC, Iskandar SS, Dalldorf FG. Pathologic differentiation between lupus and nonlupus membranous glomerulopathy. *Kidney Int.* 1983;24(3):377–385.
356. Haas M. IgG subclass deposits in glomeruli of lupus and nonlupus membranous nephropathies. *Am J Kidney Dis.* 1994;23(3):358–364.
363. Mathieson PW, Peat DS, Short A, et al. Coexistent membranous nephropathy and ANCA-positive crescentic glomerulonephritis in association with penicillamine. *Nephrol Dial Transplant.* 1996; 11(5):863–866.
381. Salant DJ, Belok S, Madaio MP, et al. A new role for complement in experimental membranous nephropathy in rats. *J Clin Invest.* 1980;66(6):1339–1350.
412. Beck LH Jr, Bonegio RG, Lambeau G, et al. M-type phospholipase A2 receptor as target antigen in idiopathic membranous nephropathy. *N Engl J Med.* 2009;361(1):11–21.
456. Pollak VE, Rosen S, Pirani CL, et al. Natural history of lipoid nephrosis and of membranous glomerulonephritis. *Ann Intern Med.* 1968;69(6):1171–1196.
462. Ponticelli C, Zucchelli P, Passerini P, et al. A randomized trial of methylprednisolone and chlorambucil in idiopathic membranous nephropathy. *N Engl J Med.* 1989;320(1):8–13.
492. Pruchno CJ, Burns MW, Schulze M, et al. Urinary excretion of C5b-9 reflects disease activity in passive Heymann nephritis. *Kidney Int.* 1989;36(1):65–71.
517. Lee T, Biddle AK, Lionaki S, et al. Personalized prophylactic anticoagulation decision analysis in patients with membranous nephropathy. *Kidney Int.* 2014;85(6):1412–1420.
527. Ponticelli C, Altieri P, Scolari F, et al. A randomized study comparing methylprednisolone plus chlorambucil versus methylprednisolone plus cyclophosphamide in idiopathic membranous nephropathy. *J Am Soc Nephrol.* 1998;9(3):444–450.
566. Sethi S, Fervenza FC. Membranoproliferative glomerulonephritis–a new look at an old entity. *N Engl J Med.* 2012;366(12):1119–1131.
570. Cook HT, Pickering MC. Histopathology of MPGN and C3 glomerulopathies. *Nat Rev Nephrol.* 2015;11(1):14–22.
634. Daha MR, Fearon DT, Austen KF. C3 nephritic factor (C3NeF): stabilization of fluid phase and cell-bound alternative pathway convertase. *J Immunol.* 1976;116(1):1–7.
741. Peter G, Smith AL. Group A streptococcal infections of the skin and pharynx (first of two parts). *N Engl J Med.* 1977;297(6):311–317.
771. Potter EV, Lipschultz SA, Abidh S, et al. Twelve to seventeen-year follow-up of patients with poststreptococcal acute glomerulonephritis in Trinidad. *N Engl J Med.* 1982;307(12):725–729.
780. Berger J, Hinglais N. Intercapillary deposits of IgA-IgG. *J Urol Nephrol (Paris).* 1968;74(9):694–695.
788. Suzuki K, Honda K, Tanabe K, et al. Incidence of latent mesangial IgA deposition in renal allograft donors in Japan. *Kidney Int.* 2003;63(6):2286–2294.

836. Cattran DC, Coppo R, Cook HT, et al. The Oxford classification of IgA nephropathy: rationale, clinicopathological correlations, and classification. *Kidney Int.* 2009;76(5):534–545.
878. Tomana M, Novak J, Julian BA, et al. Circulating immune complexes in IgA nephropathy consist of IgA1 with galactose-deficient hinge region and antiglycan antibodies. *J Clin Invest.* 1999;104(1):73–81.
1093. Rauen T, Eitner F, Fitzner C, et al. Intensive Supportive Care plus immunosuppression in IgA nephropathy. *N Engl J Med.* 2015;373(23):2225–2236.
1121. D'Agati V, Sacchi G, Truong L. Fibrillary glomerulopathy: defining the disease spectrum. *J Am Soc Nephrol.* 1991;2:591.
1209. Kang JS, Kashtan CE, Turner AN, et al. The alloantigenic sites of alpha3alpha4alpha5(IV) collagen: pathogenic X-linked alport alloantibodies target two accessible conformational epitopes in the alpha5NC1 domain. *J Biol Chem.* 2007;282(14):10670–10677.
1210. Wilson CB. Immunologic aspects of renal diseases. *JAMA.* 1992;268(20):2904–2909.
1218. Pendergraft WF, Preston GA, Shah RR, et al. Autoimmunity is triggered by cPR-3(105-201), a protein complementary to human autoantigen proteinase-3. *Nat Med.* 2004;10(1):72–79.
1221. Steblay RW, Rudofsky U. Autoimmune glomerulonephritis induced in sheep by injections of human lung and Freund's adjuvant. *Science.* 1968;160(824):204–206.
1243. Zimmerman SW, Groehler K, Beirne GJ. Hydrocarbon exposure and chronic glomerulonephritis. *Lancet.* 1975;2(7927):199–201.
1261. Levy JB, Turner AN, Rees AJ, et al. Long-term outcome of anti-glomerular basement membrane antibody disease treated with plasma exchange and immunosuppression. *Ann InternMed.* 2001;134(11):1033–1042.
1301. Baldus S, Eiserich JP, Mani A, et al. Endothelial transcytosis of myeloperoxidase confers specificity to vascular ECM proteins as targets of tyrosine nitration. *J Clin Invest.* 2001;108(12):1759–1770.
1340. Xiao H, Heeringa P, Hu P, et al. Antineutrophil cytoplasmic autoantibodies specific for myeloperoxidase cause glomerulonephritis and vasculitis in mice. *J Clin Invest.* 2002;110(7):955–963.
1351. Jayne DRW, Bruchfeld AN, Harper L, et al. Randomized trial of C5a receptor inhibitor avacopan in ANCA-associated vasculitis. *J Am Soc Nephrol.* 2017;28(9):2756–2767.
1364. Jennette JC, Falk RJ, Andrassy K, et al. Nomenclature of systemic vasculitides. Proposal of an international consensus conference. *Arthritis Rheum.* 1994;37(2):187–192.
1372. Rosenstein ED, Ribot S, Ventresca E, et al. Recurrence of Wegener's granulomatosis following renal transplantation. *Br J Rheumatol.* 1994;33(9):869–871.
1378. Jennette JC, Hoidal JR, Falk RJ. Specificity of anti-neutrophil cytoplasmic autoantibodies for proteinase 3. *Blood.* 1990;75(11):2263–2264.
1386. Fauci AS, Katz P, Haynes BF, et al. Cyclophosphamide therapy of severe systemic necrotizing vasculitis. *N Engl J Med.* 1979;301(5):235–238.
1414. Pagnoux C, Mahr A, Hamidou MA, et al. Azathioprine or methotrexate maintenance for ANCA-associated vasculitis. *N Engl J Med.* 2008;359(26):2790–2803.
1464. Warren GV, Korbet SM, Schwartz MM, et al. Minimal change glomerulopathy associated with nonsteroidal antiinflammatory drugs. *Am J Kidney Dis.* 1989;13(2):127–130.
1487. Kalsi J, Delacroix DL, Hodgson HJ. IgA in alcoholic cirrhosis. *Clin Exp Immunol.* 1983;52(3):499–504.
1508. Galla JH, Kohaut EC, Alexander R, et al. Racial difference in the prevalence of IgA-associated nephropathies. *Lancet.* 1984;2(8401):522.

# 32 Secondary Glomerular Disease

Jai Radhakrishnan | Gerald B. Appel | Vivette D. D'Agati

CHAPTER OUTLINE



## SYSTEMIC LUPUS ERYTHEMATOSUS

Lupus nephritis (LN) is a frequent and potentially serious complication of systemic lupus erythematosus (SLE).[1–6] Kidney disease influences morbidity and mortality both directly and indirectly through complications of therapy. Recent studies have more clearly defined the spectrum of clinical, prognostic, and renal histopathologic findings in SLE. Controlled randomized trials of induction therapy for severe LN have focused on achieving remissions of renal disease while minimizing adverse reactions to therapy. Maintenance trials have compared the efficacy of therapeutic agents in preventing renal flares and the progression of renal disease over several years. For patients who fail to respond to current treatment regimens, a number of newer immunomodulatory agents are being studied in resistant or relapsing disease.

### EPIDEMIOLOGY

The incidence and prevalence of SLE depend on the age, gender, geographic locale, and ethnicity of the population studied as well as the diagnostic criteria for defining SLE.[1,3,6–8]

Females outnumber males by about 10 to 1. However, males with SLE have the same incidence of renal disease as females. The onset of disease peaks between 15 and 45 years of age and more than 85% of patients are younger than 55 years of age. SLE is more often associated with severe nephritis in children and in males and is milder in older adults. SLE and LN are more common, and are associated with more severe renal involvement, in African-American, Asian, and Hispanic populations, although the precise roles of biologic–genetic versus socioeconomic factors have not been clearly defined. Nearly one half of all end-stage renal disease (ESKD) patients with SLE in the United States are African-Americans.[3,8–14] The overall incidence of SLE ranges from 1.8 to 7.6 cases per 100,000 with a prevalence from 40 to 200 cases per 100,000.[3,6,15] The incidence of renal involvement varies depending on the populations studied, the diagnostic criteria for kidney disease, and whether involvement is defined by renal biopsy or clinical findings. Approximately 25% to 50% of unselected lupus patients will have clinical renal disease at onset while as many as 60% of adults with SLE will develop renal disease during their course.[3,15–18]

A number of genetic, hormonal, and environmental factors influence the course and severity of SLE.[3,6,7,15,16,18] A multiplicity of genes are involved in both SLE and LN.[19] A genetic predisposition is supported by a higher concordance rate in monozygotic twins (25%) than fraternal twins (<5%), the greater risk of relatives of SLE patients developing SLE or other autoimmune disease, the association with certain human leukocyte antigen (HLA) genotypes (e.g., HLA-B8, HLA-DR2, and HLA-DR3), inherited deficiencies in complement components (e.g., homozygous C1q, C2, and C4 deficiencies), and Fc receptor polymorphisms. Some HLA alleles in SLE patients have protected against LN (HLA DR4 and DR11), whereas others increase the risk of developing renal involvement (HLA DR3 and DR13).[3,19–21] Genome-wide association studies (GWASs) have identified over 40 different genetic loci associated with an increased risk of SLE. These candidate susceptibility genes regulate diverse immune functions such as T-cell activation, B-cell signaling, Toll-like receptors (TLRs), signal transduction, neutrophil function, and interferon (IFN) production.[3,22] A meta-analysis of GWASs in SLE patients looking for risk alleles for LN have mapped these alleles to individual genes such as PDGF receptor A gene.[23] Likewise, high-risk groups for LN such as African-Americans have high frequency of genetic markers that may explain the increased risk including certain Fcgamma RIIA –R131 alleles and APOL1 risk alleles, which can almost triple the risk of ESKD in this population.[24,25] Inbred spontaneous genetic murine models of SLE and LN include the NZB B/W F1 hybrid, the BXSB, and the MRL/lpr mouse. SLE is inducible in some murine strains through injection of autoantibodies against DNA or by injection of Smith antigen peptides. Evidence for the role of hormonal factors includes the strong predominance of SLE in females of childbearing age and the increased incidence of lupus flares during or shortly after pregnancy. In the F1 NZB/NZW mice, females have more severe disease than males and disease severity is ameliorated by oophorectomy or androgen therapy. Environmental factors other than estrogens also modulate disease expression; these factors include immune responses to viral or bacterial antigens, exposure to sunlight and ultraviolet radiation, and certain medications.[3,6,7,26,27]

For study purposes, the diagnosis of SLE is established by the presence of certain clinical and laboratory criteria defined by the American College of Rheumatology (ACR).[3,17] Development of any 4 of the 11 criteria over a lifetime gives a 96% sensitivity and specificity for SLE. These criteria include malar rash, discoid rash, photosensitivity, oral ulcerations, nondeforming arthritis, serositis (including pleuritis or pericarditis), central nervous system disorder (such as seizures or psychoses), renal involvement, hematologic disorder (including hemolytic anemia, leukopenia, lymphopenia, or thrombocytopenia), immunologic disorder (including anti-DNA antibody, anti-Sm antibody, lupus anticoagulant, or antiphospholipid [APL] antibody), and positive antinuclear antibody (ANA). The criterion of renal involvement is defined by persistent proteinuria exceeding 500 mg/dL/day (or 3+ on the dipstick) or the presence of cellular urinary casts. Because some patients, especially those with mesangial or membranous LN, will present with clinical renal disease before they have fulfilled 4 of the 11 criteria, the diagnosis of SLE remains a clinical diagnosis with histopathologic findings supporting or confirming the presumed diagnosis.[3] Some centers, especially in Europe, have adopted the Systemic Lupus International Collaborating Clinics criteria for SLE, which have greater sensitivity but lower specificity than the ACR criteria for diagnosis of SLE.[28]

## PATHOGENESIS OF SYSTEMIC LUPUS ERYTHEMATOSUS AND LUPUS NEPHRITIS

In patients with SLE, abnormalities of immune regulation lead to a loss of self-tolerance, autoimmune responses, and the production of a variety of autoantibodies and immune complexes.[3,16,26,27,29–33] SLE is associated with defective regulation of T cells with decreased numbers of cytotoxic and suppressor T cells; increased helper ($CD4^+$) T cells; dysfunctional T-cell signaling; and abnormal $T_H1$, $T_H2$, and $T_H17$ cytokine production.[3,6,29–34] There is also polyclonal activation of B cells and defective B-cell tolerance. The failure of apoptotic mechanisms to delete autoreactive B-cell and T-cell clones may promote their expansion and may trigger immune responses through interactions with TLRs with subsequent autoantibody production. The result of this loss of tolerance is the production of a wide range of autoantibodies, including those directed against nucleic acids, nucleosomes (double-stranded DNA [dsDNA] in association with a core of positively charged histones), chromatin antigens, and nuclear and cytoplasmic ribonuclear proteins.[3,6,27,33,35] Viral or bacterial peptides containing sequences similar to native antigens may lead to “antigen mimicry” and stimulate autoantibody production.

In SLE, autoantibodies combine with self-antigens to produce circulating immune complexes that deposit in the glomeruli, activate complement, and incite an inflammatory response. Immune complexes are also detectable in the skin at the dermal–epidermal junction, in the choroid plexus, pericardium, and pleural spaces. Renal involvement in SLE has been considered a human prototype of classic experimental chronic immune complex–induced glomerulonephritis.[36] The chronic deposition of circulating immune complexes plays a major role in the mesangial and the endocapillary proliferative patterns of LN. Immune complex size, charge, avidity, local hemodynamic factors, and the clearing ability of the mesangium influence the localization of circulating immune complexes within the glomerulus.[6,16,30,36] In diffuse proliferative LN, the deposited complexes consist of nuclear antigens (e.g., DNA) and high-affinity complement-fixing immunoglobulin G (IgG) antibodies.[3,16,36] In some SLE patients, the initiating event may be the local binding of cationic nuclear antigens such as histones to the subepithelial region of the glomerular capillary wall, followed by in situ immune complex formation. Once glomerular immune deposits form, the complement cascade is activated, leading to complement-mediated damage, activation of procoagulant factors, leukocyte Fc receptor activation with leukocyte infiltration, release of proteolytic enzymes, and production of various cytokines regulating glomerular cellular proliferation and matrix synthesis. Transcriptome analysis of glomeruli from LN biopsies shows variable expression of B-cell genes, myelomonocytic genes, IFN-inducible genes, and fibrosis genes in both human and murine models.[37] Characterizing the immune profile of the kidney biopsy at LN flare differentiates early treatment responders from nonresponders.[38] Autoantibodies to complement components (C1q and C3b), which are found in some patients, may enhance autoantigen exposure and facilitate immune complex deposition, while autoantibodies to C-reactive protein (CRP) may also lead to further immune activation and worsening of LN.[39,40] Neutrophils undergoing cell death may release chromatin meshworks (called neutrophil extracellular traps [NETs] which are composed of chromatin, histones, and neutrophil proteins). These NETs, which are detectable in LN biopsies, are not degraded properly in patients with lupus and are a source of autoantigen presentation and induction of IFN-α by plasmacytoid dendritic cells.[41] There is also evidence for intrarenal autoantibody production in patients with LN.[42] Glomerular damage may be potentiated by mechanisms distinct from immune complex deposition, such as hypertension and coagulation abnormalities. Some lupus patients with associated antineutrophil cytoplasmic antibodies (ANCAs) have documented focal segmental necrotizing glomerular lesions without significant immune complex deposition, resembling a "pauci-immune" glomerulonephritis.[43,44] The presence of APL antibodies, with their attendant alterations in endothelial and platelet function (including reduced production of prostacyclin and other endothelial anticoagulant factors, activation of plasminogen, inhibition of protein C or S, and enhanced platelet aggregation), can also potentiate glomerular and vascular lesions. Some SLE patients develop a podocytopathy with no evidence of immune complex deposition.[44,45]

**Table 32.1 International Society of Nephrology/Renal Pathology Society (2003) Classification of Lupus Nephritis**

| | |
|---|---|
| Class I | Minimal mesangial lupus nephritis (LN) |
| Class II | Mesangial proliferative LN |
| Class III | Focal LN[a] (<50% of glomeruli) |
| III (A) | Active lesions |
| III (A/C) | Active and chronic lesions |
| III (C) | Chronic lesions |
| Class IV | Diffuse LN[b] (≥50% of glomeruli) |
| | Diffuse segmental (IV-S) or global (IV-G) LN |
| IV (A) | Active lesions |
| IV (A/C) | Active and chronic lesions |
| IV (C) | Chronic lesions |
| Class V[c] | Membranous LN |
| Class VI | Advanced sclerosing LN |
| | (≥90% globally sclerosed glomeruli without residual activity) |

[a]Indicates the proportion of glomeruli with active and with sclerotic lesions.
[b]Indicates the proportion of glomeruli with fibrinoid necrosis and with cellular crescents.
[c]Class V may occur in combination with III or IV in which case both will be diagnosed.
Indicate and grade (mild, moderate, or severe) tubular atrophy, interstitial inflammation and fibrosis, severity of arteriosclerosis or other vascular lesions.

## PATHOLOGY OF LUPUS NEPHRITIS

The histopathology of LN is pleomorphic.[3–5,16,36] This diversity is evident when comparing biopsy findings from different patients or even adjacent glomeruli in a single biopsy. Moreover, the lesions have the capacity to transform from one pattern to another spontaneously or following treatment.[16,36] The World Health Organization (WHO) classification system[46,47] classified LN by combining glomerular light microscopic (LM), immunofluorescence (IF), and electron microscopic (EM) findings. The 2003 International Society of Nephrology/Renal Pathology Society (ISN/RPS) classification of LN (Table 32.1) has proven more reproducible and provides more standardized definitions for precise clinical pathologic correlations.[48,49] Recently a minor revision of this classification has been published.[50] This provides new cutoff for mesangial hypercellularity (>3 mesangial cells per mesangial area), more precise definitions of cellular and fibrocellular crescents, and replaces the term "endocapillary proliferation" with "endocapillary hypercellularity" to acknowledge the major contribution of infiltrating leukocytes. It also eliminates the subdivisions IV-S and IV-G of class IV LN, and applies modified National Institutes of Health (NIH) activity and chronicity indices to all LN classes.

ISN/RPS class I has normal-appearing glomeruli by LM but with mesangial immune deposits detected by IF and EM. Even patients without clinical renal disease often have mesangial immune deposits when studied carefully by the more sensitive techniques of IF and EM.[51]

ISN/RPS class II has purely mesangial hypercellularity, with mesangial immune deposits on IF and EM (Figs. 32.1–32.3).[51] Mesangial hypercellularity is defined as more than three cells in mesangial regions distant from the vascular pole in 3-μm-thick sections. There may be rare minute subendothelial or subepithelial deposits visible by IF or EM but not by LM.

ISN/RPS class III, focal LN, is defined as focal segmental and/or global endocapillary and/or extracapillary glomerulonephritis affecting less than 50% of the total glomeruli sampled. Both active and chronic lesions are taken into account when determining the percentage of total glomeruli involved. There is typically focal segmental endocapillary proliferation, including mesangial cells and endothelial cells, with infiltrating mononuclear and polymorphonuclear leukocytes (Figs. 32.4–32.6).[51] Class III biopsies can have any

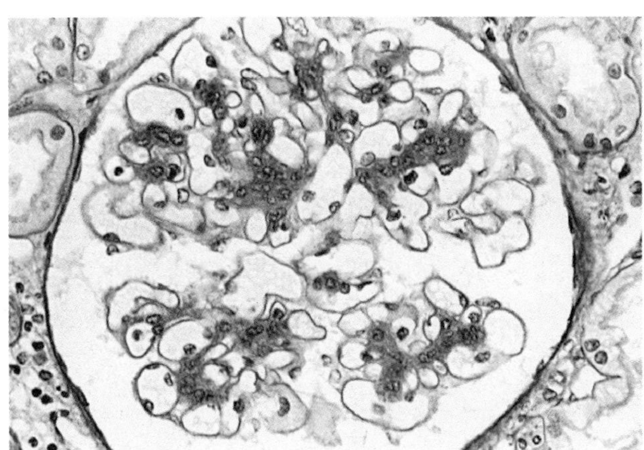

**Fig. 32.1** Lupus nephritis class II. There is mild global mesangial hypercellularity (periodic acid–Schiff, ×400).

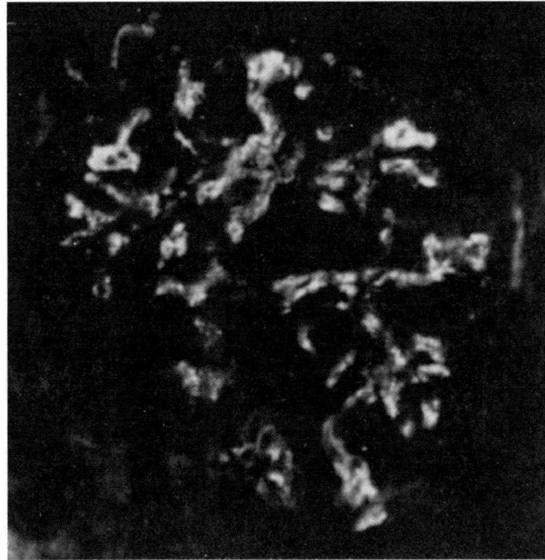

**Fig. 32.2** Lupus nephritis class II. Immunofluorescence photomicrograph showing deposits of C3 restricted to the glomerular mesangium (×400).

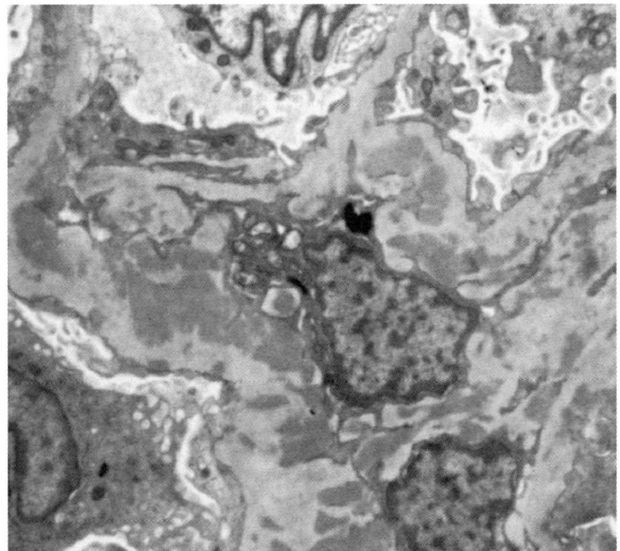

**Fig. 32.3** Lupus nephritis class II. Electron micrograph showing abundant mesangial electron-dense deposits (×12,000).

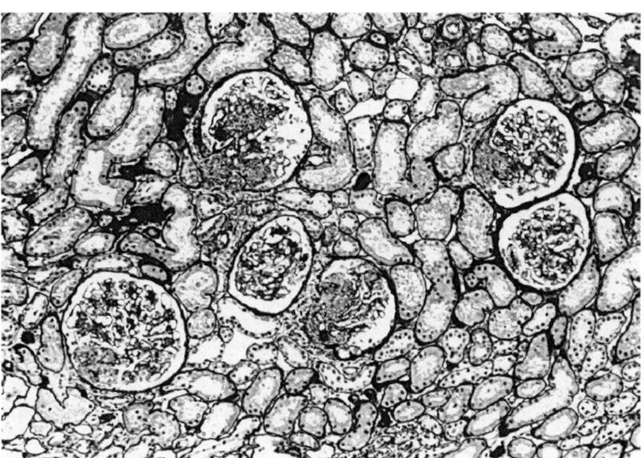

**Fig. 32.4** Lupus nephritis class III. There is focal segmental endocapillary proliferation (Jones methenamine silver, ×100).

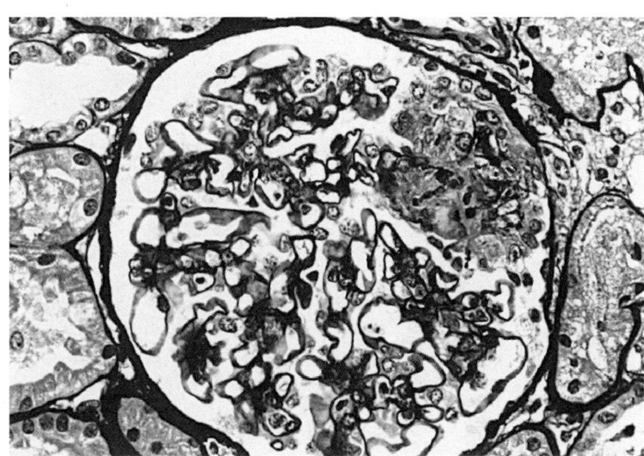

**Fig. 32.5** Lupus nephritis class III. The glomerular endocapillary proliferation is discretely segmental with necrotizing features and an early cellular crescent (Jones methenamine silver, ×400).

combination of active and chronic features. Active lesions may display cellular crescents, fibrinoid necrosis, nuclear pyknosis or karyorrhexis, and rupture of the glomerular basement membrane (GBM). Hematoxylin bodies, swollen basophilic nuclear material resulting from binding to ambient ANAs, are occasionally found within the necrotizing lesions. Subendothelial immune deposits may be visible by LM as "wire loop" thickenings of the glomerular capillary walls or large intraluminal masses known as "hyaline thrombi." Chronic glomerular lesions consist of segmental and/or global glomerular sclerosis owing to scarred glomerulonephritis with or without fibrous crescents.[51] In class III biopsies, glomeruli adjacent to those with severe histologic changes may show only mesangial abnormalities by LM. In class III, diffuse mesangial and focal and segmental subendothelial immune deposits are typically identified by IF and EM. The segmental subendothelial deposits are usually present in the distribution of the segmental endocapillary proliferative lesions.

ISN/RPS class IV, diffuse LN, has qualitatively similar glomerular endocapillary and/or extracapillary lesions as

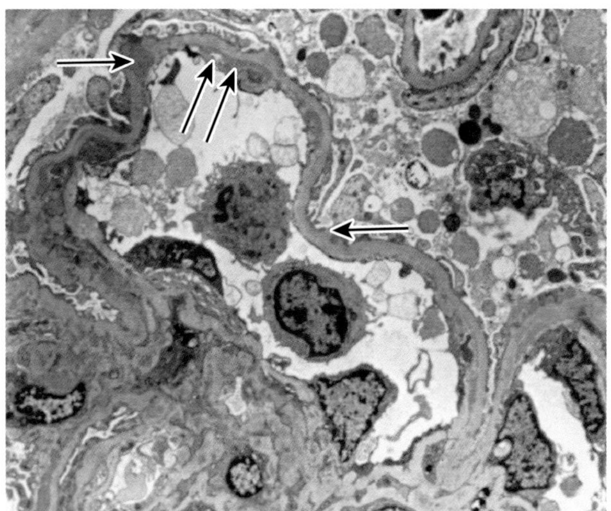

**Fig. 32.6** Lupus nephritis class III. Electron micrograph showing deposits in the mesangium as well as involving the peripheral capillary wall in subendothelial *(double arrow)* and subepithelial *(single arrows)* locations (×4900).

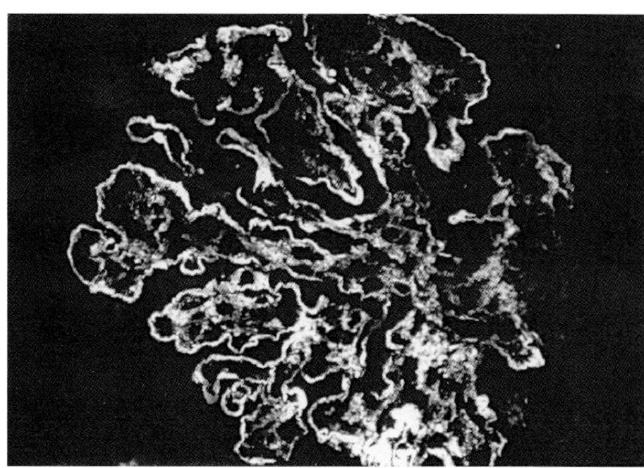

**Fig. 32.8** Lupus nephritis class IV. Immunofluorescence photomicrograph showing global deposits of immunoglobulin G in the mesangial regions and outlining the subendothelial aspect of the peripheral glomerular capillary walls (×600).

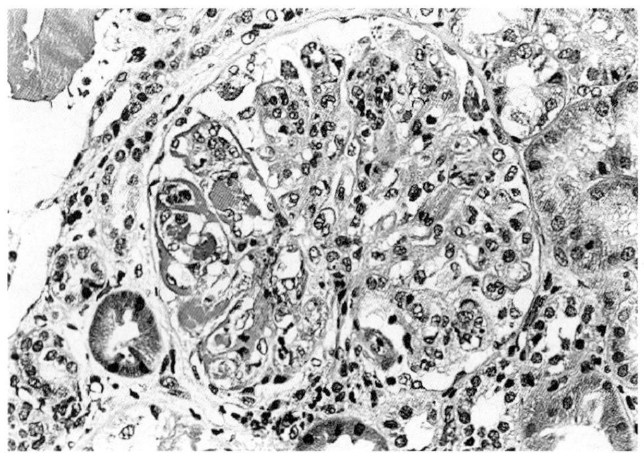

**Fig. 32.7** Lupus nephritis class IV. There is global endocapillary proliferation with infiltrating neutrophils and segmental wire loop deposits (hematoxylin–eosin, ×320).

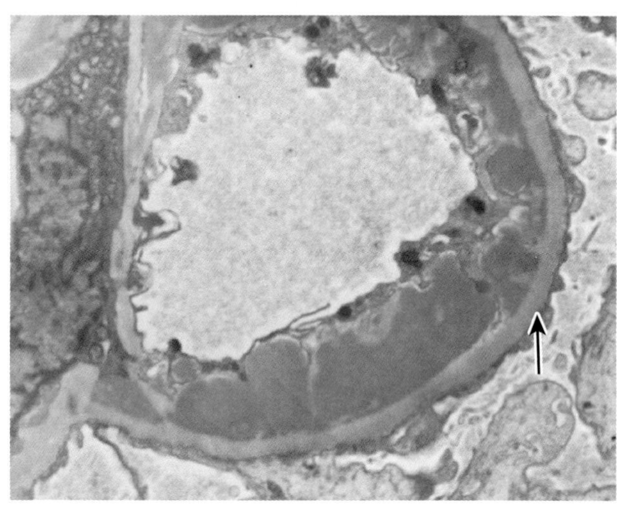

**Fig. 32.9** Lupus nephritis class IV. Electron micrograph showing a large subendothelial electron-dense deposit as well as a few small subepithelial deposits *(arrow)* (×1200).

class III but involves more than 50% of the total glomeruli sampled (Figs. 32.7–32.9).[46,51–53] Again, both active (proliferative) and chronic (sclerosing) lesions are included when determining the percentage of glomeruli affected. Class IV is subdivided into diffuse segmental proliferation, class IV-S, in which more than 50% of affected glomeruli have segmental lesions, and diffuse global proliferation, class IV-G, in which more than 50% of affected glomeruli have global lesions. All the active features described earlier for class III (including fibrinoid necrosis, leukocyte infiltration, wire loop deposits, hyaline thrombi, hematoxylin bodies, and crescents) may be encountered in class IV LN. In general, there is more extensive peripheral capillary wall subendothelial immune deposition, and extracapillary proliferation in the form of crescents is not uncommon. Class IV lesions may have features similar to those of primary membranoproliferative glomerulonephritis (MPGN; also known as mesangiocapillary glomerulonephritis) with mesangial interposition along the peripheral capillary walls and double contours of the GBMs. Some class III and IV biopsies will have focal necrotizing and crescentic lesions akin to those seen in small vessel vasculitides. Some of these patients have had circulating ANCAs.[43,54]

ISN/RPS class V is defined by regular subepithelial immune deposits producing a membranous pattern (Figs. 32.10–32.12).[51,55–57] The coexistence of mesangial immune deposits and mesangial hypercellularity in most cases helps to distinguish membranous LN from primary membranous glomerulopathy. Early membranous LN class V may have no identifiable abnormalities by LM but subepithelial deposits are detectable by IF and EM.[58] In well-developed membranous lesions, there is typically thickening of the glomerular capillary walls and "spike" formation between the subepithelial deposits. Because sparse subepithelial deposits may also be

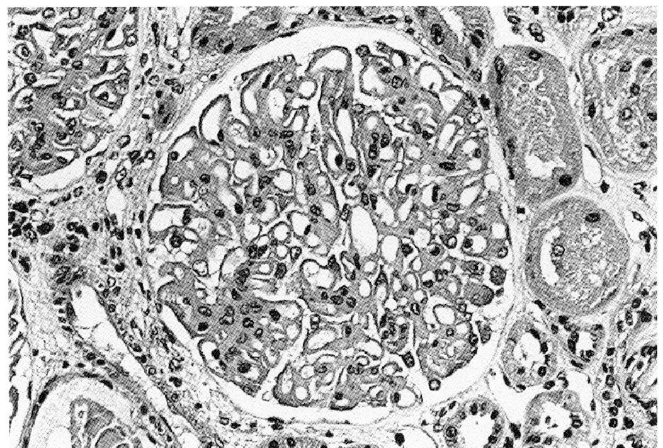

**Fig. 32.10** Lupus nephritis class V. There is diffuse uniform thickening of glomerular basement membranes accompanied by mild segmental mesangial hypercellularity (hematoxylin–eosin, ×320).

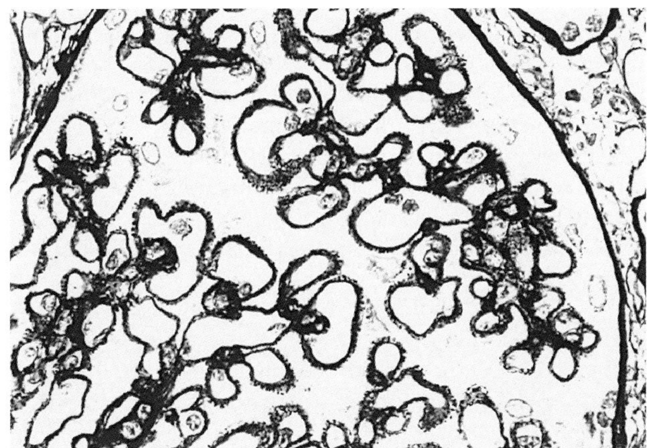

**Fig. 32.11** Lupus nephritis class V. Silver stain highlights glomerular basement membrane spikes projecting outward from the glomerular basement membranes toward the urinary space (Jones methenamine silver, ×800).

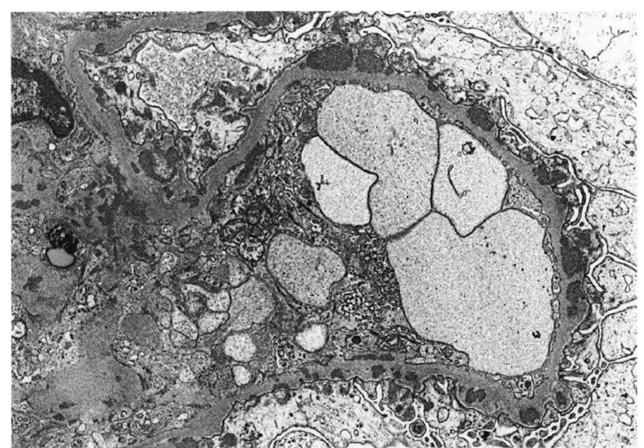

**Fig. 32.12** Lupus nephritis class V. Electron micrograph showing numerous subepithelial electron-dense deposits as well as mesangial deposits (×5000).

encountered in other classes (III or IV) of LN, a diagnosis of pure lupus membranous LN should be reserved only for those cases in which the membranous pattern predominates. When the membranous alterations involve more than 50% of the total glomerular capillaries and are accompanied by focal or diffuse endocapillary proliferative lesions and subendothelial immune complex deposition, they are classified as class V + III or class V + IV, respectively.

ISN/RPS class VI, advanced sclerosing LN, or end-stage LN is reserved for biopsies with more than 90% of the glomeruli sclerotic and no residual activity.[51] In such cases, it may be difficult even to establish the diagnosis of LN without the identification of residual glomerular immune deposits by IF and EM or a biopsy history of prior active LN.

## IMMUNOFLUORESCENCE

In LN, immune deposits can be found in the glomeruli, tubules, interstitium, and blood vessels.[4,5,16,36,58] IgG is almost universal, with codeposits of IgM, IgA, C3, and C1q common.[16,36,51] The presence of all three immunoglobulins (IgG, IgA, and IgM) along with the two complement components (C1q and C3) is known as "full house" staining and is highly suggestive of LN. Staining for fibrin–fibrinogen is common in crescents and segmental necrotizing lesions. The "tissue ANA"[58] (i.e., nuclear staining of renal epithelial cells in sections stained with fluoresceinated antisera to human IgG) is a frequent finding in any LN class. It results from the binding of patient's own ANA to nuclei exposed in the course of cryostat sectioning.

## ELECTRON MICROSCOPY

The distribution of glomerular, tubulointerstitial, and vascular deposits seen by EM correlates closely with that observed by IF.[4–6,16,17,36] Deposits are typically electron dense and granular. Some exhibit focal organization with a "fingerprint" substructure composed of curvilinear parallel arrays measuring 10 to 15 nm in diameter.[16,36] Tubuloreticular inclusions (TRIs), which are intracellular branching tubular structures measuring 24 nm in diameter located within dilated cisternae of the endoplasmic reticulum of glomerular and vascular endothelial cells, are commonly observed in SLE biopsies.[5,16,36] TRIs are inducible upon exposure to α-IFN (so-called interferon footprints) and are also present in biopsies of human immunodeficiency virus (HIV)-infected patients and those with some other viral infections.[59]

## ACTIVITY AND CHRONICITY

Current guidelines advocate that renal biopsies should be accorded an activity and chronicity score, as modified from the NIH system.[50] The purpose is to identify and quantify active (potentially reversible) lesions and chronic (irreversible) lesions. In the newly modified NIH system, activity index is calculated by grading the biopsy on a scale of 0 to 3+ for each of six histologic features; these features are endocapillary hypercellularity, glomerular neutrophil infiltration and/or karyorrhexis, wire loop deposits, fibrinoid necrosis, cellular and/or fibrocellular crescents, and interstitial inflammation. The severe lesions of crescents and fibrinoid necrosis are assigned double weight. The sum of the individual components yields a total histologic activity index score from 0 to 24. Likewise, a chronicity index of 0 to 12 is derived from the sum of global and/or segmental glomerulosclerosis, fibrous crescents, tubular atrophy, and interstitial fibrosis, each graded on a scale of 0 to 3+. Studies at the NIH correlated both a high activity index (>12) and especially a high chronicity index (>4) with a poor 10-year renal survival rate. However, in several other large studies, neither the activity index nor the chronicity index correlated well with long-term prognosis. Other NIH studies concluded that a combination of an elevated activity index (>7) and chronicity index (>3) predicts a poor long-term outcome.[60] A major value of calculating the activity and chronicity indices is in the comparison of sequential biopsies in individual patients. This provides useful information about the efficacy of therapy and the relative degree of reversible versus irreversible lesions.[4,5,16,36,61,62]

## TUBULOINTERSTITIAL DISEASE, VASCULAR LESIONS, AND LUPUS PODOCYTOPATHY

Some SLE patients have prominent changes in the tubulointerstitial compartment in association with significant glomerular activity, while much more rarely interstitial nephritis may be the major renal involvement in patients with SLE.[63–67] Active tubulointerstitial lesions include edema and inflammatory infiltrates of T lymphocytes (both $CD4^+$ and $CD8^+$ cells), B lymphocytes, monocytes, and plasma cells.[66] Tubulointerstitial immune deposits of immunoglobulin and/or complement may be present along the basement membranes of tubules and interstitial capillaries. Severe acute interstitial changes and tubulointerstitial immune deposits are most commonly found in patients with active proliferative class III and IV LN. The degree of interstitial inflammation does not correlate well with the presence or quantity of tubulointerstitial immune deposits.[63,64] Interstitial fibrosis, tubular atrophy, or both are commonly encountered in the more chronic phases of LN. One study documented a strong inverse correlation between the degree of tubular damage and renal survival.[64] In addition, the renal survival rate was higher in patients who had lower expression levels of the intercellular adhesion molecule-1 (ICAM-1) in kidney biopsy tissue.[65]

Vascular lesions are not included in either the ISN/RPS classification or in the NIH activity and chronicity indices despite their frequent occurrence and clinical significance.[44,68–70] The most frequent vascular lesion is simple vascular immune deposition, most common in patients with active class III and IV biopsies. Vessels may be normal by LM, but by IF and EM there are granular immune deposits in the media and intima of small arteries and arterioles. Noninflammatory necrotizing vasculopathy, most common in arterioles in active class IV LN, is a fibrinoid necrotizing lesion without leukocyte infiltration that severely narrows or occludes the arteriolar lumen. True inflammatory vasculitis resembling polyangiitis is extremely rare in SLE patients. It may be renal limited or part of a more generalized systemic vasculitis.[44,69,70] Thrombotic microangiopathy involving vessels and glomeruli may be associated with anticardiolipin/APL antibody or a hemolytic-uremic/thrombotic thrombocytopenic purpura (HUS/TTP)–like syndrome.[44,69,70]

A number of other renal diseases have been documented on biopsy in SLE patients, including podocytopathies with features of minimal change disease (MCD), focal segmental glomerulosclerosis (FSGS), or collapsing glomerulopathy.[45,71–73] In some, the relationship between SLE and the podocytopathy suggests that this is not a coincidence but related to SLE-induced cytokine-mediated effects on podocytes. A collapsing pattern of focal sclerosis in SLE patients of African descent has been associated with APOL1 risk alleles.[74]

## CLINICAL MANIFESTATIONS

Although SLE predominantly affects young females, the clinical manifestations are similar in both sexes and in adults and children. Organ systems commonly affected include the kidneys, joints, serosal surfaces (including pleura and pericardium), central nervous system, and skin. In addition, cardiac, hepatic, pulmonary, hematopoietic, and gastrointestinal involvement is not infrequent.

Renal involvement often develops concurrently or shortly after the onset of SLE and may follow a protracted course with periods of remissions and exacerbations. Clinical renal involvement usually correlates well with the degree of glomerular involvement. However, some patients may have disproportionately severe vascular or tubulointerstitial lesions that dominate the clinical course.[44,63,70]

Patients with ISN/RPS class I biopsies often have little evidence of clinical renal disease. Likewise, most patients with mesangial lesions (ISN/RPS class II) have mild or minimal clinical renal findings.[3–5,16,34,46] They may have active lupus serology (a high anti-DNA antibody titer and low serum complement), but the urinary sediment is inactive, hypertension is infrequent, proteinuria is usually less than 1 g/day, and the serum creatinine concentration and glomerular filtration rate (GFR) are usually normal. Nephrotic-range proteinuria is extremely rare unless there is a superimposed podocytopathy.[71,72]

Class III, focal proliferative LN, is often associated with active lupus serologies, although the degree of serologic activity does not necessarily correlate with the histologic severity.[46,52] Hypertension and active urinary sediment are common. Proteinuria is often more than 1 g/day, and one quarter to one third of patients with focal LN have nephrotic syndrome at presentation. Many patients have an elevated serum creatinine concentration at presentation. Patients with less extensive glomerular proliferation, fewer necrotizing features, and no crescents are more likely to be normotensive and have preserved renal function.

Patients with ISN/RPS class IV, diffuse proliferative LN, typically present with the most active clinical features. They often have high anti-DNA antibody titers, low serum complement levels, and very active urinary sediment, with erythrocytes, and cellular casts on urinalysis.[3–5,16,46,51,53,75] Virtually all have proteinuria and as many as 50% of the patients will have nephrotic syndrome. Hypertension and renal dysfunction are typical. Even when the serum creatinine level is in the "normal range," the GFR is usually depressed.

Patients with membranous LN, ISN/RPS class V, typically present with proteinuria, edema, and other manifestations of nephrotic syndrome.[3–5,16,46,51,55–57] However, as many as 40% will have proteinuria of less than 3 g/day, and 16% to 20% less than 1 g/day. Only about 60% of membranous LN patients have a low serum complement concentration and an elevated anti-DNA antibody titer at presentation.[46] However, hypertension and renal dysfunction may occur without superimposed proliferative lesions. Patients with membranous LN may present with nephrotic syndrome before developing other clinical and laboratory manifestations of SLE.[46,55–57] In addition, they are predisposed to thrombotic complications such as renal vein thrombosis and pulmonary emboli.[44,69] Patients with mixed membranous and proliferative biopsies have clinical features that reflect both disease components.

End-stage LN, ISN/RPS class VI, is usually the result of "burned-out" LN of long duration.[51] Some renal histologic damage may represent nonimmunologic progression of sclerosis mediated by hyperfiltration in remnant nephrons. Although the lesions are sclerosing and inactive, class VI patients may still have microhematuria and proteinuria. Virtually all have hypertension and a decreased GFR. Levels of anti-DNA antibodies and serum complement levels often normalize at this late stage of disease.

"Silent LN"[3,35,76] has been described in patients without clinical evidence of renal involvement despite biopsy evidence of active proliferative LN. Some define silent LN as active biopsy lesions without active urinary sediment, proteinuria, or a depressed GFR, whereas others require negative lupus serologies as well. Although silent LN is well described in some studies, others have been unable to find even isolated examples.[3,34] It appears to be uncommon, and it is highly likely that even patients with true "silent disease" will manifest clinical renal involvement when followed into their course.

## SEROLOGIC TESTS

The presence of antibodies directed against nuclear antigens (ANAs) and especially against DNA (anti-DNA) antibodies is included in the ACR criteria for SLE and commonly used to monitor the disease course.[3,6,27] ANAs are a highly sensitive screen for SLE, being found in more than 90% of untreated patients, but they are not specific for SLE and occur in many other rheumatologic and nonrheumatologic conditions.[3,6,27,36] Neither the particular pattern of ANA fluorescence (homogeneous, speckled, nucleolar, or rim) nor the titer correlates well with the presence or the severity of renal involvement in SLE.

Autoantibodies directed against dsDNA (anti-dsDNA) are a more specific but less sensitive marker of SLE and are found in almost three-fourths of untreated active SLE patients.[3,6,27] Anti-dsDNA IgG antibodies of high avidity that fix complement have correlated best with the presence of renal disease,[3,6,27] and such anti-dsDNA antibodies have been found in the glomerular immune deposits of murine and human LN.[3,27,77,78] High anti-dsDNA antibody titers correlate well with clinical activity.[3,6,27] Antisingle-stranded DNA antibodies (anti-ssDNA), commonly found in SLE and other collagen vascular diseases, do not correlate with clinical lupus activity.

Autoantibodies directed against ribonuclear antigens are commonly present in lupus patients and include anti-Sm and anti-nRNP against extractable nuclear antigen (ENA).[3,6,27,33] Anti-Sm antibodies, although very specific for SLE, are found in only about 25% of lupus patients and are of unclear prognostic value. Anti-nRNP antibodies, found in over one third of SLE patients, are also present in many other rheumatologic diseases, particularly mixed connective tissue disease (MCTD).[27,33,79] Anti-Ro/SSA antibodies are directed against the protein complex of a cytoplasmic RNA and are present in 25% to 30% of SLE patients. Anti-La/SSB autoantibodies, directed against a nuclear RNP antigen, are present in 5% to 15% of lupus patients. Neither of the latter two antibodies is specific for SLE and both are found in other collagen vascular diseases, especially Sjögren syndrome. Maternal anti-Ro antibodies are important in the pathogenesis of neonatal lupus and the development of cardiac conduction abnormalities in the newborn.[80] Anti-Ro antibodies are also associated with a unique dermal psoriasiform type of lupus, with SLE patients who are homozygous C2 deficient, and with a vasculitic disease associated with central nervous system involvement and cutaneous ulcers.[81] In addition, lupus patients may develop antibodies directed against histones, endothelial cells, phospholipids, the *N*-methyl-D-aspartate receptor (associated with central nervous system disease in SLE), and neutrophil cytoplasmic antigens (ANCAs).[82–84]

Levels of total hemolytic complement (CH50) and complement components are usually decreased during active SLE and especially active LN.[3–6,16] Levels of C4 and C3 often decline before a clinical flare of SLE. Serial monitoring of complement levels, with a decline in levels predicting a flare, is considered more useful clinically than an isolated depressed C3 or C4 value.[5] Likewise, normalization of depressed serum complement levels is often associated with improved renal outcome.[85] Levels of total complement and C3 may be decreased in the absence of active systemic or renal disease in patients with extensive dermatologic involvement by SLE. Several heritable complement deficiency states (including C1r, C1s, C2, C4, C5, and C8) have been associated with SLE and such patients may have depressed total complement levels despite inactive disease[86]

Other immunologic test results commonly found in lupus patients include elevated levels of circulating immune complexes, a positive lupus band test, and the presence of cryoglobulins. None correlates well with SLE or LN activity.[87–89] In both SLE and isolated discoid lupus, immune complex deposits containing IgG antibody and complement are found along the dermal–epidermal junction of involved skin lesions. The presence of granular deposits in clinically unaffected skin (the lupus band test) is usually found only in patients with systemic disease. However, the specificity and sensitivity of this test are debated, and it requires IF microscopy of the dermal biopsy. Patients with SLE commonly have a false-positive Venereal Disease Research Laboratory (VDRL) test result due to the presence of APL antibodies.[3] The surprising finding that patients with SLE often have low CRP levels was initially used to argue against the importance of using CRP levels as a biomarker for inflammation in other diseases. It is now appreciated that this reflects high titer antibodies to CRP in some SLE patients, though the clinical correlates of these unique antibodies are not clear.

## MONITORING CLINICAL DISEASE

It is important to be able to predict systemic and renal relapses and prevent their occurrence through the judicious use of immunosuppressive agents. Serial measurements of many serologic tests (including complement components, autoantibodies, erythrocyte sedimentation rate [ESR], CRP, circulating immune complexes, and, recently, levels of cytokines and interleukins [ILs]) have been used to predict lupus flares. Although there is controversy regarding the value of serum C3 and C4 levels and anti-DNA antibody titers in predicting clinical flares of SLE or LN, these have yet to be replaced by new biomarkers.[4,6,89] Serum levels of anti-dsDNA typically rise and serum complement levels typically fall as the clinical activity of SLE increases, often preceding clinical renal deterioration. In patients with active renal involvement, the urinalysis frequently reveals dysmorphic erythrocytes, red blood cell casts, and other formed elements. An increase in proteinuria from levels of less than 1 g/day to more than this amount, and certainly from low levels to nephrotic levels, is a clear indication of either increased activity or a change in renal histologic class. When there is concern about the degree of activity of the SLE and LN, a renal biopsy will often clarify whether to change therapy.[4,46]

## DRUG-INDUCED LUPUS

A variety of medications may induce a lupus-like syndrome or exacerbate an underlying predisposition to SLE. Those medications metabolized by acetylation, such as procainamide and hydralazine, have been common causes.[90,91] This occurs more commonly in patients who are slow acetylators due to a genetic decrease in hepatic *N*-acyltransferase. Diltiazem, minocycline, penicillamine, isoniazid, methyldopa, chlorpromazine, and practolol are other potential causes of drug-induced lupus.[90–93] Other drugs that have been associated less frequently with this syndrome include phenytoin, quinidine, propylthiouracil, sulfonamides, lithium, β-blockers, nitrofurantoin, Para-aminosalycilic acid (PAS), captopril, glyburide, hydrochlorothiazide, IFN-α, carbamazepine, sulfasalazine, rifampin, and tumor necrosis factor-α (TNF-α) blockers.[90,94,95] Clinical manifestations of drug-induced lupus include fever, rash, myalgias, arthralgias and arthritis, and serositis. Central nervous system and renal involvement are relatively uncommon.[90,96,97] While elevated anti-DNA antibodies and depressed serum complement levels are less common in drug-induced lupus, antihistone autoantibodies are present in more than 95% of patients.[90] These are usually formed against a complex of the core histone dimer H2A-H2B and DNA and other histone components.[90,98] Antibodies are also present in the vast majority of idiopathic, nondrug-related SLE patients, but they are directed primarily against different histone antigens (linker H1 and core H2B).[90] The presence of antihistone antibodies in the absence of anti-DNA antibodies and other serologic markers for SLE is also indicative of drug-induced disease. The diagnosis of drug-induced lupus depends on documenting the offending agent and achieving a remission following withdrawal of the drug. The primary treatment consists of discontinuing the offending drug.

## PREGNANCY AND SYSTEMIC LUPUS ERYTHEMATOSUS

Because SLE occurs so commonly in women of childbearing age, the issue of pregnancy arises often in the care of this population. Independent but related issues are the health of the mother (in terms of both flares of lupus activity and progression of renal disease) and the fate of the fetus. It is unclear whether flares of lupus activity occur more commonly during pregnancy or shortly after delivery. Some controlled studies found no increase in lupus flares in pregnant patients versus nonpregnant lupus controls.[99–102] Some controlled studies found no increase in lupus flares in pregnant patients versus nonpregnant lupus controls.[99,101,102] Patients with quiescent lupus at the time of pregnancy are less likely to experience an exacerbation of SLE. However, in two small retrospective studies, flares of lupus activity including renal involvement occurred in more than 50% of the pregnancies.[99,102] This was significantly greater than the rate of flare after delivery and in nonpregnant lupus patients.

Pregnancy in patients with preexisting LN has also been associated with worsening of renal function.[103,104] This is less likely to occur in patients who have been in remission for at least 6 months. Patients with hypertension are likely to develop higher blood pressure levels, and those with proteinuria are likely to have increased levels during pregnancy. Patients with elevated serum creatinine levels are most likely to suffer worsening of renal function and to be at highest risk for fetal loss. Although high-dose corticosteroids, cyclosporine, tacrolimus, and azathioprine have all been used in pregnant lupus patients, their safety is unclear. Cyclophosphamide is contraindicated due to its teratogenicity, and newer agents such as mycophenolate and rituximab are not recommended, thus making the treatment of severe LN difficult.

The rate of fetal loss in all SLE patients in most series is 20% to 40% and may approach 50% in some series.[99,101,103,104] While fetal mortality is increased in SLE patients with renal disease, it may be decreasing in the modern treatment era.[103–106] Patients with anticardiolipin or APL antibodies, hypertension, or heavy proteinuria are at higher risk for fetal loss. One review of 10 studies in more than 550 women with SLE found that fetal death occurred in 38% to 59% of all pregnant SLE patients with APL antibodies compared with 16% to 20% of those without these antibodies.[107]

## DIALYSIS AND TRANSPLANTATION

The percentage of patients with severe LN who progress to dialysis or transplantation varies from 5% to 50% depending on the population studied, the length of follow-up, and the response to therapy.[3,5,6,46,108–111] Many with slow progressive renal failure have a resolution of their extrarenal disease manifestations and serologic activity.[112,113] With more prolonged time on dialysis, the incidence of clinically active patients declines further, decreasing in one study from 55% at the onset of dialysis to less than 10% by the fifth year and 0% by the tenth year of dialysis.[113] Patients with end-stage kidney disease (ESKD) due to LN have increased mortality during the early months of dialysis due to infectious complications of immunosuppressive therapy.[112,113] Long-term survival of SLE patients on chronic hemodialysis or continuous ambulatory peritoneal dialysis is similar to that of nonlupus patients, with the most common cause of death being cardiovascular.[112–114]

Most renal transplant programs suggest that patients with active SLE undergo a period of dialysis from 3 to 12 months to allow clinical and serologic disease activity to become quiescent before transplantation.[113] Allograft survival rates in patients with LN are comparable with the rest of the transplant population.[3,5,114–118] The rate of recurrent SLE in the allograft has been low, less than 4% in most series,[114–118] although in several more recent reports a higher recurrence rate has been noted.[116] The prevalence of recurrent LN was only 2.4% in a 20-year study of nearly 7000 lupus transplant recipients and was more common in black, female, and younger patients.[117] When surveillance biopsies were used, however, recurrences could be detected in as many as 54% of a small cohort of lupus transplant recipients, although this was mostly subclinical mild mesangial LN.[118] The low rate of clinically important recurrence may be due, in part, to the immune suppressant action of the renal failure prior to transplantation and, in part, to the immunosuppressive regimens used following transplantation. Lupus patients with an APL antibody may benefit from anticoagulation therapy during the posttransplant period.[119,120]

## COURSE AND PROGNOSIS OF LUPUS NEPHRITIS

The course of patients with LN is extremely varied with less than 5% to over 60% of patients developing progressive renal failure.[3,5,16,46,52,61,108–111,121] This course is defined by the initial pattern and severity of renal involvement as modified by therapy, exacerbations of the disease, and complications of treatment. The prognosis has clearly improved in recent decades with wider and more judicious use of new immunosuppressive medications. Most studies have found additional prognostic value of renal biopsy versus clinical data in patients with LN.[52,122–124]

Patients with lesions limited to the renal mesangium generally have an excellent course and prognosis.[3–5,16,36] Patients with lesions that do not transform into other patterns are unlikely to develop progressive renal failure, and mortality is due to extrarenal manifestations and complications of therapy. Patients with focal proliferative disease have an extremely varied course. Those with mild proliferation involving a small percentage of glomeruli respond well to therapy and less than 5% progress to renal failure over 5 years.[3–5,16,46,124,125] Patients with more proliferation, necrotizing features, and/or crescent formation have a prognosis more akin to patients with class IV diffuse LN. Class III patients may transform into class IV over time. Some patients with very active segmental proliferative and necrotizing lesions resembling ANCA-associated small vessel vasculitis have a worse renal prognosis than other patients with focal proliferative lesions.[43,54,126]

Patients with diffuse proliferative disease have the least favorable prognosis in most older series.[3–5,16,36,46,52,53] Nevertheless, the prognosis for this group has markedly improved, with renal survival rates now exceeding 90% in some series of patients treated with modern immunosuppressive agents.[5,53,125,127] In trials from the NIH, the 5-year risk of doubling the serum creatinine concentration, a surrogate marker for progressive renal disease, in patients with diffuse proliferative lupus treated with cyclophosphamide-containing regimens ranged from 35% to less than 5%.[109,110,127] In an Italian study of diffuse proliferative LN, patient survival was 77% at 10 years and more than 90% if extrarenal deaths were excluded.[53] In a US study of 89 patients with diffuse proliferative LN, renal survival was 89% at 1 year and 71% at 5 years.[128] It is unclear whether the improved survival rates in these recent series are largely due to improved immunosuppression or better supportive care and more judicious clinical use of these medications.

In the past, some studies have found age, gender, and race to be as important prognostic variables as clinical features in patient and renal survival in SLE.[3,4,9–11,60,123,128–131] However, a consistent finding is that African-Americans have a greater frequency of LN and a worse renal and overall prognosis. This worse prognosis appears to relate to both biologic/genetic and socioeconomic factors.[3,4,10,11,60,128,130–132] In a study from the NIH of 65 patients with severe LN, clinical features at study entry associated with progressive renal failure included age, black race, hematocrit less than 26%, and serum creatinine concentration greater than 2.4 mg/dL.[60] Patients with combined activity index (>7) plus chronicity index (>3) on renal biopsy, as well as those with the combination of cellular crescents and interstitial fibrosis also had a worse prognosis. In another US study of 89 patients with diffuse proliferative LN, none of the following features affected renal survival: age, gender, SLE duration, uncontrolled hypertension, or any individual histologic variable.[128] Entry serum creatinine level higher than 3.0 mg/dL, combined activity and chronicity indices on biopsy, and black race predicted a poor outcome. Five-year renal survival rate was 95% for the Caucasian patients but only 58% for the black patients. In a study of more than 125 LN patients with WHO class III or IV from New York, both racial and socioeconomic factors were associated with the worst outcomes in African-Americans and Hispanics.[10] An evaluation of 203 patients from the Miami area confirmed worse renal outcomes in African-Americans and Hispanics related to both biologic and economic factors.[11]

More rapid and more complete renal remissions are associated with improved long-term prognosis.[133,134] Renal flares during the course of SLE also may predict a poor renal outcome.[121,135,136] Relapses of severe LN over 5 to 10 years of follow-up occur in up to 50% of patients and usually respond less well and more slowly to repeated course of therapy.[4,121,137–140] A retrospective analysis of 70 Italian patients in which over half had diffuse proliferative disease found excellent patient survival (100% at 10 years and 86% at 20 years) as well as preserved renal function with probability of not doubling the serum creatinine concentration to be 85% at 10 years and 72% at 20 years. Most patients in this study were Caucasian, which likely influenced the excellent long-term prognosis. Patients with renal flares of any type had seven times the risk of renal failure, and those with rapid rises in creatinine had 27 times the chance of doubling their serum creatinine concentration. Another Italian study of 91 patients with diffuse proliferative LN showed more than 50% having a renal flare, which correlated with a younger age at biopsy (<30 years old), higher activity index, and karyorrhexis on biopsy.[135] The number of flares, nephritic flares, and flares with increased proteinuria correlated with a doubling of the serum creatinine. The role of relapses in predicting progressive disease has been documented by others as well, although relapse does not invariably predict a bad outcome.[141]

Although an elevated anti-DNA antibody titer and low serum complement levels may correlate with active renal involvement, they do not correlate with long-term renal prognosis.[3,46,108,121,128] In several studies anemia has been a poor prognostic finding regardless of the underlying cause.[60,121] Severe hypertension has also been related to renal prognosis in some studies but not in others.[46] Renal dysfunction, as noted by an elevated serum creatinine or decreased GFR or by heavy proteinuria, and nephrotic syndrome are indicative of a poor renal prognosis in the vast majority of series.[3–6,16,52] However, not all studies have found an elevation of the initial serum creatinine to predict a poor long-term prognosis, and in some the initial serum creatinine only predicted short-term renal survival.[128] Other renal features, such as duration of nephritis and rate of decline of GFR, may also predict prognosis.[108,125]

Finally, histologic features such as the class, the degree of activity and chronicity, and the severity of tubulointerstitial damage have also predicted prognosis. In a number of studies, the pattern of renal involvement, especially when using the ISN/RPS or older WHO classification, has been a useful guide to prognosis.[3,16,46,49,75] In NIH trials, patients with severe proliferative LN with a higher activity index or chronicity index were more likely to have progressive renal failure.[125] Studies with different referral populations could not confirm this.[4,16,36,46,142] Regardless, the contribution of chronic renal scarring to a poor long-term outcome has been confirmed by many studies.[65,108,135,141,143] Some studies have found the initial renal biopsy to have little predictive value; rather, certain features on a repeat biopsy at 6 months proved to be a strong predictor of doubling the serum creatinine or progression to renal failure.[64,144] These include ongoing inflammation with cellular crescents, macrophages in the tubular lumens, persistent immune deposits (especially C3) on IF microscopy, and persistent subendothelial and mesangial deposits or an active NIH activity score.[145,146] Other studies suggest that reversal of interstitial fibrosis and glomerular segmental scarring along with remission of initial inflammation and immune deposition is an important favorable prognostic finding on the 6-month biopsy.[141] Thus chronic changes on the initial biopsy are not always cumulative or immutable, and their reversal may be crucial in preventing ultimate renal failure when new acute lesions develop.

The natural history of membranous LN is less clear. In early studies, its course appeared far better than that for active proliferative disease.[147] Subsequent studies with longer follow-up suggested a worse outcome for membranous LN with persistent nephrotic syndrome.[46] Retrospective analyses show that 5-year renal survival rates largely depend on whether patients have pure membranous lesions (class V) or superimposed proliferative lesions in a focal (class III + V) or diffuse (IV + V) distribution.[56,57] A US-based study found that the 10-year survival rate was 72% for patients with pure membranous lesions but only 20% to 48% for those with superimposed proliferative lesions.[56] Black race, elevated serum creatinine, higher degrees of proteinuria, hypertension, and transformation to another WHO pattern all portended a worse outcome.[1,3] The poor survival in blacks with membranous LN may explain the excellent results in retrospective Italian studies, which follow largely Caucasian cohorts. One such Italian study found the 10-year survival rate of membranous LN patients to be 93%.[56] Even in this Italian population, survival for pure membranous LN was far better than in patients with superimposed proliferative lesions. Thus, at least in part, the variability of prognosis in the varied, older studies can be explained by the differences in racial background, histology, and therapy.

## TREATMENT OF LUPUS NEPHRITIS

The treatment of severe LN remains controversial. Although recent controlled studies have better defined the course and therapy for this group, the most effective and least toxic regimen for any given patient is often less clear. Although cyclophosphamide has been an effective therapy for many patients with severe LN, newer regimens have been developed in the hope of attaining equal or greater efficacy with less toxicity. The concept of more vigorous initial therapy during an "induction" treatment phase followed by more prolonged lower-dose therapy during a "maintenance phase" is now widely accepted.[3,16,148,149]

Patients with ISN/RPS class I and II biopsies have an excellent renal prognosis and need no therapy directed to the kidney. Transformation to another histologic class is usually heralded by increasing proteinuria and activity of the urinary sediment. At this point, repeat renal biopsy may serve as a guide to therapy.[3] ISN/RPS class III patients with only few mild proliferative lesions and no necrotizing features or crescent formation have a good prognosis and will often respond to a short course of high-dose corticosteroid therapy or a brief course of other immunosuppressive agents. Patients with greater numbers of affected glomeruli and those with necrotizing features and crescents usually require more vigorous therapy similar to therapy for patients with diffuse proliferative LN.

Patients with diffuse proliferative disease, ISN/RPS class IV lesions, require aggressive treatment to avoid irreversible renal damage and progression to ESKD.[3,6,16,125,127,133] The ideal immunosuppressive regimen should be individualized and based on the patient's prior therapy, risk and concern over potential side effects, compliance, and tolerability. Initial regimens may include combinations of the following: oral or intravenous corticosteroids, oral or intravenous cyclophosphamide, mycophenolate mofetil (MMF), cyclosporine, tacrolimus, and/or rituximab. A number of other treatments are currently being studied for resistant or relapsing disease and for maintenance therapy.

Prednisone, despite the lack of controlled trials, is included in most treatment regimens for LN. In retrospective studies, higher initial doses of corticosteroids appeared more effective than lower dose therapy (<30 mg prednisone daily).[1–6] Initial use of high-dose corticosteroid treatment alone is still used by some clinicians for limited focal proliferative disease. However, for severe proliferative LN, either class III or class IV, corticosteroids along with other immunosuppressive agents are required.[5] Common regimens use 1 mg/kg/day of prednisone, tapering after 4 to 6 weeks of treatment so that patients are on 30 mg/day or less by the end of 3 months of therapy. Other clinicians start with daily pulses of IV methylprednisolone for 1 to 3 days followed by the oral corticosteroids.

Despite initial favorable results with pulse methylprednisolone followed by oral corticosteroids in treating severe LN, there have been few randomized trials using this regimen versus other immunosuppressive therapy.[3,109,110] Two NIH trials have found pulse corticosteroids to be less effective than intravenous cyclophosphamide in preventing progressive renal failure.[109,110] In one trial, 48% of the pulse steroid–treated patients doubled their serum creatinine at 5 years compared with only 25% of the cyclophosphamide-treated group.[110]

Controlled randomized trials at the NIH and elsewhere have helped establish the role of cyclophosphamide in the treatment of severe LN.[61,109,110,127,148–150] In one seminal trial, patients were randomly assigned to regimens of high-dose corticosteroids for 6 months or oral cyclophosphamide, oral azathioprine, combined oral azathioprine plus cyclophosphamide, or intravenous cyclophosphamide every third month, all given with low-dose corticosteroids.[127] Evaluation at 120 months showed superior renal survival in the intravenous cyclophosphamide group versus the steroid group. At longer follow-up to 200 months, the renal survival of the azathioprine group was statistically no better than that of the corticosteroid group.[127] A subsequent Dutch collaborative trial found remission rates comparable between oral azathioprine and cyclophosphamide, but more relapses and worse long-term outcome with azathioprine.[151] Thus, for a number of years, cyclophosphamide used with corticosteroids was the most widely used induction immunosuppressive agent for LN. Because side effects in the NIH trial appeared least severe when cyclophosphamide was used intravenously, subsequent NIH protocols utilized the drug in this manner given once monthly. Other trials at NIH and elsewhere have also used monthly pulses of intravenous cyclophosphamide for 6 consecutive months as opposed to the original every third-month regimen.[137,148–150]

These studies, and others, have confirmed the benefits and response rate of intravenous cyclophosphamide regimens along with corticosteroids in severe LN.[61,128,137] In most patients treated with intravenous cyclophosphamide, side effects such as hemorrhagic cystitis, alopecia, and neoplasms have been infrequent.[3,6] Exceptions are menstrual irregularities and premature menopause, which are most common in women older than 25 years of age who have received intravenous cyclophosphamide for more than 6 months.[152] The dose of intravenous cyclophosphamide must be reduced for significant renal impairment and adjusted for some removal by hemodialysis. The cytoprotective agent mesna has been used successfully by some to reduce bladder complications from cyclophosphamide.

A three-armed controlled randomized trial at the NIH of 1 year of monthly doses of intravenous methylprednisolone, versus monthly intravenous cyclophosphamide for 6 months and then every third month, versus the combination of both therapies found that the remission rate was highest with the combined treatment regimen (85%) as opposed to cyclophosphamide alone (62%) and methylprednisolone alone (29%).[109] Mortality was low and similar in all groups. Long follow-up indicated that drug toxicity was not different between the cyclophosphamide group and the combined cyclophosphamide–methylprednisolone group.[150] It is likely that through higher sustained remissions and fewer relapses, fewer patients required repeated treatments in the combined cyclophosphamide–steroid-treated group. Moreover, the long-term efficacy, especially in terms of renal outcomes, was greatest for the combination therapy group. Thus combined treatment with intravenous methylprednisolone pulses followed by oral corticosteroids along with intravenous cyclophosphamide pulses became a standard therapy for severe LN. However, it should be noted that some groups have achieved equal efficacy and few side effects using short courses of oral cyclophosphamide followed by other immunosuppressive medications.[1,2,153] Oral maintenance immunosuppressive agents other than cyclophosphamide were more effective and safer than cyclophosphamide, and have led the search for equally effective but safer regimens as induction therapy. One approach to obtain efficacy with less toxicity uses lower induction doses of the cytotoxic agent. The Euro Lupus Nephritis Trial, a multicenter prospective trial of 90 patients with severe LN, compared low-dose versus "conventional" high-dose intravenous cyclophosphamide.[154] Patients were randomized to either 6-monthly intravenous pulses of 0.5 to 1 g/m$^2$ cyclophosphamide followed by two quarterly pulses or only 500-mg intravenously every 2 weeks for a total of six doses, both followed by oral azathioprine as maintenance therapy. At 40 months' follow-up, there were no statistically significant differences in treatment failures, renal remissions, or renal flares, but twice as many infections occurred in the high-dose group. Although this trial may have included some patients with milder renal disease (mean creatinine, 1 to 1.3 mg/dL; mean proteinuria, 2.5 to 3.5 g/day for both groups) and a predominantly Caucasian patient population, it supported the use of shorter duration and lower total dose cyclophosphamide for induction therapy. Longer follow-up of this population confirms these data and suggests that early response to therapy is predictive of a good long-term outcome and that the long-term results are excellent.[133] A recent trial of this regimen as standard care in both arms of an investigational study of Abatacept in patients with severe LN confirms that this regimen is effective in black as well as Caucasian populations.[155]

MMF has proven to be an effective immunosuppressive in transplant patients and a variety of other immunologic renal diseases.[156] It is a reversible inhibitor of inosine monophosphate dehydrogenase required for de novo purine synthesis and blocks B- and T-cell proliferation, inhibits antibody formation, and decreases expression of adhesion molecules, among other effects. MMF is effective in treating murine LN.[156] MMF was shown to have good efficacy and reduced complications when compared with standard treatment regimens in a number of uncontrolled trials in LN.[156] In one 6-month Chinese trial of patients randomized to either MMF or intravenous pulse cyclophosphamide for induction therapy of severe LN,[157] proteinuria and microhematuria decreased more in the MMF-treated patients than in the cyclophosphamide-treated group, with renal impairment before and after therapy, activity index on biopsy before and after therapy, and serologic improvement equivalent. MMF was better tolerated with fewer gastrointestinal side effects and fewer infections. In another randomized controlled trial of patients given either a regimen of prednisone plus oral MMF or a regimen of prednisone plus cyclophosphamide orally for 6 months followed by oral azathioprine for another 6 months, both regimens proved similar in efficacy.[158] Of the MMF group, 81% achieved complete and 14% partial remission versus 76% complete and 14% partial remission for the cyclophosphamide–prednisone group. Treatment failures, relapses following therapy, discontinuations of therapy, mortality, and time to remission were similar. Longer follow-up at 4 years with the addition of more patients showed MMF to have comparable efficacy to cyclophosphamide with no significant difference in complete or partial remissions, doubling of baseline creatinine, or relapses. Significantly fewer MMF-treated patients developed severe infections, leukopenia, or amenorrhea, and all deaths and renal failure were in the cyclophosphamide group.[159]

A multicenter US study comparing induction therapy in 140 patients largely with severe class III and class IV LN included more than 50% blacks, most with heavy proteinuria and active urinary sediment.[160] Patients were randomized to monthly pulses of intravenous cyclophosphamide 0.5 to 1 g/m$^2$ or oral MMF 2 to 3 g/day, both with tapering corticosteroid doses for 6 months. Although designed as an equivalency study, MMF proved superior in attaining both complete remissions and complete and partial remissions. The side-effect profile also appeared better with MMF. At the 3-year follow-up, there was a trend to less renal failure and mortality with MMF. Thus in a patient population at high risk for poor renal outcomes, MMF proved superior to intravenous cyclophosphamide. A subsequent international multicenter randomized controlled trial compared similar regimens of MMF with intravenous cyclophosphamide for induction therapy in 370 LN patients with ISN/RPS classes III, IV, or V.[9] This study found virtually identical rates of complete and partial remission (>50%), improvement of renal function and proteinuria, and mortality rates between the two regimens. Diarrhea and gastrointestinal side effects were most common in the MMF group, whereas nausea, vomiting, and alopecia were more common in the cyclophosphamide group. In the small group of about 30 patients with a greatly reduced GFR (<30 mL/min), MMF proved at least as effective, if not more so, compared with intravenous cyclophosphamide.[161] In an analysis of different geographic and ethnic backgrounds, MMF proved uniformly more effective across different groups.[162] In another study of 52 patients with crescentic LN (>50% crescents on biopsy) randomized to induction therapy with MMF or intravenous cyclophosphamide, the MMF group had a higher remission rate and a lower relapse rate.[163] Thus, taken together, these two large, randomized controlled trials and a variety of other analyses support the use of MMF as a first-line treatment of severe LN. Both ACR and Kidney Disease Improving Global Outcomes (KDIGO) guidelines support either a cyclophosphamide- or a mycophenolate-based regimen as first-line therapy for severe LN. For patients who fail to achieve remission with either initial regimen at 6 months of therapy, substitution with the other regimen is recommended.[164]

A number of studies have focused on the optimal maintenance therapy for LN with the goal of avoiding relapse and flares while minimizing the long-term immunosuppressive toxicity. One randomized controlled trial examined LN patients who had successfully completed induction of remission with 4 to 7 monthly pulses of intravenous cyclophosphamide and were then randomized to either continue with intravenous cyclophosphamide every third month, oral azathioprine, or oral MMF.[3,16,165] The 54 LN patients randomized were largely composed of blacks (50%) and Hispanics and included many patients with nephrotic syndrome (64%), reduced GFR, and severe proliferative LN. Fewer patients in the azathioprine and MMF groups reached the primary endpoints of death and chronic renal failure compared with the group that continued to receive cyclophosphamide. The cumulative probability of remaining relapse free was higher with MMF (78%) and azathioprine (58%) compared with cyclophosphamide (43%), and there was increased mortality in patients given continued cyclophosphamide. Complications of therapy were also reduced in the MMF and azathioprine groups, including days of hospitalization, amenorrhea, and infections. Thus maintenance therapy with either oral MMF or azathioprine was superior to intravenous cyclophosphamide and had less toxicity.

The results of two large randomized trials further delineate the role of these oral agents in the maintenance of patients with proliferative LN.[166,167] In the European MAINTAIN trial, 105 patients were randomized to either azathioprine or MMF for at least 3 years of maintenance (mean, 53 months).[166] There was no difference between these medications in the time to renal flares or to renal remission. In the worldwide Aspreva Lupus Management Study (ALMS) maintenance trial, 227 patients who achieved remission after induction therapy with either intravenous cyclophosphamide or MMF were rerandomized in double-blind fashion to either MMF or azathioprine maintenance for 3 years.[167] MMF proved superior to azathioprine with respect to the primary endpoint of time to treatment failure (death, ESKD, doubling of serum creatinine, LN flare, or requirement for rescue therapy).[167] Differences between the two studies likely explain the differing results. The MAINTAIN trial was prerandomized from day 1, included smaller numbers of patients who were largely Caucasian, and used the endpoint of renal flare because few patients in this population progress to renal failure. Even so, there were 26% flares in the azathioprine group compared with only 19% in the MMF group, although this difference was not statistically significant. The ALMS maintenance trial included only those patients who achieved remission after induction; was international, including multiracial and diverse populations; and used harder endpoints for response (doubling creatinine, ESKD, etc.). At present, both the ACR and KDIGO recommend either agent, azathioprine or MMF, as maintenance therapy.

The calcineurin inhibitors cyclosporine and tacrolimus have been proven to increase the induction remission rate in a number of uncontrolled and controlled trials.[1,2] Tacrolimus has been successful in increasing remissions as part of a multidrug regimen for severe LN patients with combined ISN/RPS class IV and V lesions.[168] Intravenous cyclophosphamide resulted in complete remission in 5% and partial remissions in 40% at 6 months versus a "multitargeted regimen" of tacrolimus, MMF, and corticosteroids, which led to a 50% complete and a 40% partial remission rate in this period. In a large multicenter trial from China containing more than 350 patients, multitarget therapy with a CNI added to mycophenolate and corticosteroids proved superior to cyclophosphamide and corticosteroid induction therapy.[169] An extension trial of the 200 patients of this study population who responded initially to this therapy compared maintenance with the multitarget therapy to maintenance with azathioprine for the cyclophosphamide group. Both groups had similar low renal relapse rates (5% and 7%, respectively). Moreover, serum creatinine and GFR remained stable in both groups. Of note, the azathioprine group had more adverse events (44% vs. 16%) and more withdrawals due to adverse events.[170]

Rituximab, a chimeric monoclonal antibody targeting CD20 B cells, depletes them through multiple mechanisms, including complement-dependent cell lysis; FcRγ-dependent, antibody-dependent, cell-mediated cytotoxicity; and induction of apoptosis. Rituximab, which is approved by the US Food and Drug Administration (FDA) for the treatment of rheumatoid arthritis, granulomatosis with polyangiitis (GPA; formerly designated Wegener granulomatosis), and microscopic polyangiitis (MPA), has been utilized with varying success in many other immunologic and autoimmune diseases, including a variety of primary glomerular diseases.[171] It has been used in more than 300 LN patients, mostly in case reports and open-label uncontrolled trials.[1,2] However, two large randomized controlled trials have given disappointing results. In one trial of 257 SLE patients without severe renal disease, patients were randomized to receive rituximab or placebo.[172] Although subgroup analyses suggested a beneficial effect in the African-American and Hispanic subgroups, there were no significant overall differences between the placebo and the rituximab arms of therapy. In the Lupus Nephritis Assessment with Rituximab (LUNAR) trial, 140 patients with class III and IV LN were randomized to rituximab or placebo in addition to an induction regimen of MMF (goal 3 g/day) and tapering corticosteroids.[173] Although the rituximab group had a greater fall in anti-DNA antibody titers and rise in serum complement levels, there was no statistically significant difference in the primary renal response between treatment groups at 1 year.[174] At present, therefore, rituximab is not a first-line agent for induction therapy of most patients with severe LN. It continues to be used in patients resistant to other treatments and in those who do not tolerate conventional treatment.[175,176] A recent study of the use of rituximab and MMF in 50 LN patients without the use of oral corticosteroids has given excellent complete and partial remission results.[177] A large multicenter controlled randomized trial assessing the use of rituximab as a steroid-sparing agent for induction therapy is needed to define the role of this agent in LN.

Other monoclonal antibodies directed at B cells have been or are being studied. Ocrelizumab, a fully humanized anti-CD20 monoclonal antibody FDA approved for severe multiple sclerosis, had the advantages of avoiding first-dose infusion reactions and the development of human antichimeric antibodies that were potential problems with rituximab therapy.[178] A controlled randomized trial using this agent in patients with LN was terminated early due to adverse events. Obinutuzumab, another FDA-approved fully humanized anti-CD20 monoclonal therapy, is currently being evaluated in LN. Atacicept, a soluble fully humanized recombinant fusion protein that inhibits B-cell stimulating factor (BLISS) and a proliferation-inducing ligand (APRIL), failed in initial trials with patients with LN.[179] Epratuzumab, a humanized monoclonal antibody against CD22, a marker of mature B cells but not plasma cells, is currently being studied. IFN-α is an antiviral cytokine induced in SLE patients that may lead to inflammation, autoimmunity, and renal damage. Anifrolumab, a monoclonal antibody against the IFN-α type I receptor, has been shown in a trial of over 300 SLE patients to add to the efficacy of standard therapy.[180]

T-lymphocyte activation requires two signals.[171,181] The first occurs when the antigen is presented to the T-cell receptor in the context of major histocompatibility complex (MHC) class II molecules on antigen-presenting cells and the second by the interaction of costimulatory molecules on T lymphocytes and antigen-presenting cells. Disruption of costimulatory signals interrupts the (auto)immune response. Two clinical trials using different humanized anti-CD40L monoclonal antibodies in LN patients to block B- and T-cell costimulation have not been successful.[182,183] Another costimulatory pathway is mediated through the interaction of CD28 with CD80/86. CTLA4 Ig, abatacept, a fusion molecule that combines the extracellular domain of human CTLA4 with the constant region (Fc) of the human IgG1 heavy chain, interrupts the CD28CD80/86 interaction. It is FDA approved for the treatment of rheumatoid arthritis. Two major randomized controlled trials in patients with severe LN treated concurrently with intravenous cyclophosphamide and steroids have now given negative results.[3,184,185] Recently belimumab, a humanized monoclonal antibody against BLys (B-lymphocyte stimulator), has been FDA approved for the treatment of lupus based on two trials.[186,187] Although few patients in this trial had significant renal disease, a group of patients with over 1 g proteinuria daily did show improved response to belimumab.[188] There are several ongoing trials which include belimumab in one arm of therapy.

Other therapies studied in controlled trials in LN have included plasmapheresis and intravenous γ-globulin administration. Plasmapheresis was studied in a multicenter controlled trial of 86 patients with severe LN.[189] This study found no benefit in terms of clinical remission, progression to renal failure, or patient survival beyond a more rapid lowering of anti-DNA antibody titers. Likewise, plasmapheresis synchronized to intravenous cyclophosphamide pulse therapy has not proven effective.[190] At present, plasmapheresis should be reserved for only certain LN patients (e.g., those with severe pulmonary hemorrhage, those with a TTP-like syndrome, and those with APL antibodies and a clotting episode who cannot be anticoagulated due to hemorrhage).

Intravenous immune globulin has been used successfully in a number of SLE patients to treat thrombocytopenia as well as LN, leading to clinical and histologic improvement in some patients.[191,192] One controlled trial included only 14 patients but showed stabilization of the plasma creatinine, creatinine clearance, and proteinuria when intravenous immune globulin was used as maintenance therapy after successful induction of remission with intravenous cyclophosphamide.[193]

Other newer, but as yet unapproved, therapies that have been studied in LN patients include the proteasome inhibitor bortezomib, adrenocorticotropic hormone, total lymphoid irradiation, bone marrow ablation with stem cell rescue, laquinimod therapy, voclosporin (a newer calcineurin inhibitor), and use of tolerance molecules.[5,111,193–196] All are still experimental because none has yet completed multiple large successful controlled clinical trials. Immunoablative therapy with high-dose cyclophosphamide with and without stem cell transplantation has been used successfully in a limited number of SLE patients with only a short period of follow-up and relatively high risks.

For patients with class V membranous LN, there have been conflicting data regarding the course, prognosis, and response to treatment.[3,5] Class V membranous LN should be treated with antihypertensive, antiproteinuric, and lipid-lowering measures. The use of anticoagulation to prevent thromboembolic events in patients with severe nephrotic syndrome should be individualized. Experts disagree about which patients with class V membranous LN should be treated with immunosuppressive therapy. The degree of superimposed proliferative lesions greatly influences outcome in class V patients, and it is unclear if older trials included only pure membranous LN patients. Thus early trials reported low and inconsistent response rates with oral corticosteroids.[55] Excellent long-term results with intensive immunosuppressive regimens from Italian studies, and others, raise questions of whether the results are related to the therapeutic intervention, the population studied, or better supportive treatments.[57] A retrospective Italian trial found better remission with a regimen of chlorambucil and methylprednisolone than with corticosteroids alone.[197] In a small nonrandomized trial of cyclosporine in membranous LN, there was an excellent remission rate of nephrotic syndrome with mean proteinuria decreasing from 6 to 1 or 2 g/day by 6 months.[62] At long-term follow-up and rebiopsy there was no evidence of cyclosporine-induced renal damage, but two patients had developed superimposed proliferative lesions over time. An NIH trial of 42 nephrotic patients with membranous LN compared cyclosporine, prednisone, and intravenous cyclophosphamide and found superior remission rates for the cyclosporine and cyclophosphamide regimens, but a trend toward more relapses when the cyclosporine was withdrawn.[198] Tacrolimus has also been used for class V LN with good results. A study of 38 patients with pure membranous LN evaluated long-term treatment with prednisone plus azathioprine.[157] At 12 months 67% of the patients had experienced a complete remission and 22% a partial remission. At three years only 12% had relapsed, at 5 years only 16%, and at 90 months only 19% relapsed. At the end of follow-up, no patient had doubled serum creatinine. Clearly in this population a regimen of steroids plus azathioprine was highly effective. The response of patients with membranous LN to MMF has been varied.[199–201] There were 84 patients with pure ISN class V membranous LN among the 510 patients enrolled in two similarly designed randomized controlled trials comparing MMF and intravenous cyclophosphamide induction therapy.[201] Rates of remissions, relapse, and course were similar in both treatment groups. Thus MMF can also be considered a first-line therapy for certain patients with membranous LN.

Given limited data, the treatment of membranous LN should be individualized.[3,5] Patients with pure membranous LN and a good renal prognosis (subnephrotic levels of proteinuria and preserved GFR) may benefit from a short course of cyclosporine with low-dose corticosteroids along with inhibitors of the renin–angiotensin–aldosterone system and statins. For those at higher risk of progressive disease (African-Americans, those fully nephrotic), options include cyclosporine, tacrolimus, monthly intravenous pulses of cyclophosphamide, MMF, or azathioprine plus corticosteroids. Patients with mixed membranous and proliferative LN are treated in the same way as those with proliferative disease alone.

As effective and safer therapies for LN have evolved, greater attention has been directed to other causes of morbidity and mortality in the SLE population. Lupus patients have accelerated atherogenesis and a disproportionate rate of atypical coronary vascular disease leads to a high mortality rate.[202] The high cardiovascular risk rate has been attributed to concurrent hypertension, hyperlipidemia, nephrotic syndrome, prolonged corticosteroid use, APL syndrome (APS), and, in some, the added vascular risks of chronic kidney disease (CKD).[203,204] Despite limited data on therapeutic interventions in this population, aggressive management of modifiable cardiovascular risk factors may alter the morbidity and mortality of this population. Extrapolating from other proteinuric CKD populations, closely monitored blood pressure control (<130/80 mm Hg), the use of angiotensin-converting enzyme (ACE) inhibitors and/or angiotensin receptor blockers, and correction of dyslipidemia with statins are all reasonable in LN patients. In addition, use of calcium, vitamin D supplements, and bisphosphonates to prevent glucocorticoid-induced osteoporosis may be useful.

Some form of APL antibodies is present in 40% to 75% of lupus patients.[205–207] Because most do not experience thrombotic complications, they require no special treatment. However, some would recommend low-dose aspirin and hydroxychloroquine for prophylaxis of asymptomatic patients with APL antibodies. In patients with evidence of a clinical thrombotic event, most investigators use chronic anticoagulation with warfarin as long as the antibody persists. While the standard practice has been not to anticoagulate other patients, in one recent series of more than 100 SLE patients, over one-fourth had APL antibodies, of whom almost 80% had a thrombotic event. The antibody-positive patients also had a greater incidence of chronic renal failure than the antibody-negative patients.[207] (See discussion of anticardiolipin antibodies and glomerulonephritis in the following section.)

## ANTIPHOSPHOLIPID SYNDROME

APS may be associated with glomerular disease, small and large vessel renal involvement, as well as coagulation problems in dialysis and renal transplant patients.[205–208] Patients with APS have autoantibodies directed against plasma proteins bound to phospholipids. They may include IgG and/or IgM anticardiolipin antibodies, antibodies to $\beta_2$-glycoprotein I of IgG or IgM isotype, or lupus anticoagulant activity.[209–211] In some studies the presence of specific $\beta_2$-glycoprotein I antibodies has been correlated with an increased risk of thrombotic events in patients with APS.[212] APL antibodies may cause a false-positive VDRL. In addition to having one of these autoantibodies, patients with APS must have one or more episodes of venous, arterial, or small vessel thrombosis, or fetal morbidity.[213] Thrombocytopenia and prolonged partial thromboplastin time are frequent laboratory findings. The presence of APL antibodies should be documented on two or more occasions at least 12 weeks apart and within 5 years of clinical manifestations.

The pathogenesis of the APS remains unclear.[214–220] Susceptible individuals may develop APL antibodies after exposure to infectious or other noxious agents. Among SLE patients there may be a genetic predisposition associated with HLA-DRB1 loci.[221] However, despite the presence of APL antibodies, a "second hit" (such as pregnancy, contraceptive use, nephrotic syndrome, SLE, or hyperlipidemia) may be necessary for them to produce thrombotic events and the APS. The mechanism(s) of the procoagulant effect is likely to be multifactorial. APL antibodies exert procoagulant effects at multiple sites in the clotting cascade, including prothrombin, protein C, annexin V, coagulation factors VII and XII, platelets, serum proteases, and tissue factor procoagulant. They may also impair fibrinolysis through inhibition of such factors as tissue-type plasminogen activator. APL antibodies may also be procoagulant due to inhibition of the mTorc intracellular pathway.[222] The result of all these actions is endothelial damage and intravascular coagulation.

Among patients with APL antibodies, 30% to 55% have the primary APS in which there is no associated autoimmune disease.[205–207,209–211,213] APL antibodies are found in from 25% to 75% of SLE patients, although most patients never experience clinical features of the APS. A variable percentage (0%–23%) of patients in different series initially felt to have idiopathic APS have evolved into SLE-associated APS with time.[205–207,209–211,223] In an analysis of 29 published series with more than 1000 SLE patients, 34% were positive for the lupus anticoagulant and 44% for anticardiolipin antibodies.[218] Most studies have found a higher incidence of thrombotic events in SLE patients positive for APL antibodies.[219,224–226] A European study of almost 575 SLE patients found the prevalence of IgG anticardiolipin antibodies to be 23% and of IgM 14%.[227] Patients with IgG antibodies had a clear association with thrombocytopenia and thromboses. A multicenter European analysis of 1000 SLE patients found thromboses in 7% of patients over 5 years. Patients with IgG anticardiolipin antibodies again had a higher incidence of thromboses, as did those with a lupus anticoagulant.[228] APL antibodies are also found in up to 2% of normal individuals and in those with a variety of infections (commonly in patients with HIV or hepatitis C virus [HCV]) and drug reactions, but these are not usually associated with the clinical features of the APS.[229–231]

The clinical features of APS relate to thrombotic events and consequent ischemia. Among 1000 APS patients the most common features were deep vein thrombosis (32%), thrombocytopenia (22%), livedo reticularis (20%), stroke (13%), pulmonary embolism (9%), and fetal loss (9%).[228] Patients may also experience pulmonary hypertension, cardiac involvement, memory impairment and other neurologic manifestations, fever, malaise, and constitutional symptoms.[205–208,225] Patients who test positive for all three diagnostic tests (lupus anticoagulant, anticardiolipin antibodies, and $\beta_2$-glycoprotein antibodies) are at higher risk for thromboembolic events. Catastrophic APS, a rare event (occurring in 0.9% of APS patients), is associated with rapid thromboses in multiple organ systems and has a high fatality rate.[213,232,233]

Renal involvement, so-called APL nephropathy, although generally an uncommon finding in patients with APS, occurs in as many as 25% of patients with primary APS and is characterized by thrombosis of blood vessels ranging from the glomerular capillaries to the main renal artery and vein.[205,208,234,235] Lesions involving the arteries and arterioles often have both a thrombotic component and a reactive or proliferative one with intimal mucoid thickening, subendothelial fibrosis, and medial hyperplasia (Fig. 32.13).[235,236]

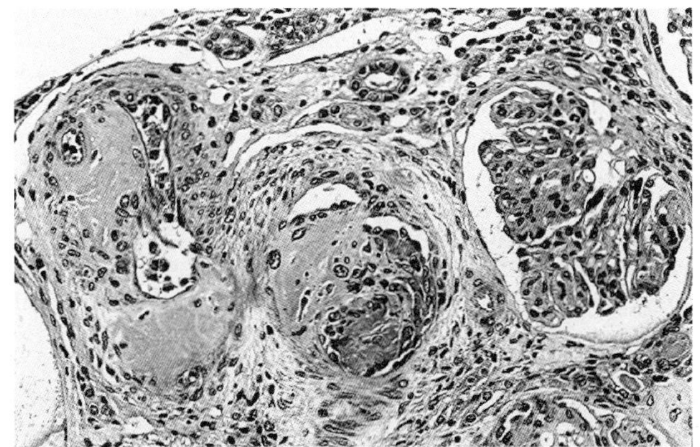

**Fig. 32.13** Antiphospholipid antibody syndrome. Organizing recanalized thrombi narrow the lumens of two interlobular arteries. The adjacent glomerulus displays ischemic-type retraction of its tuft (hematoxylin–eosin, ×200).

Interstitial fibrosis and cortical atrophy may occur due to tissue ischemia. Glomerular lesions include glomerular capillary thrombosis with associated mesangiolysis, mesangial interposition and duplication of GBMs, and subendothelial accumulation of electron-lucent, flocculent material, resembling the changes in other forms of glomerular thrombotic microangiopathy such as HUS and TTP.

A retrospective renal biopsy study found APL nephropathy in almost 40% of APL-positive patients versus only 4% of patients without APL antibody. When APL nephropathy was present, it was associated with both lupus anticoagulant and anticardiolipin antibodies.[237] Among APL-positive SLE patients, APL nephropathy was found in two-thirds of those with APS and in one-third of those without APS. Although patients with APL nephropathy had a higher frequency of hypertension and elevated serum creatinine levels at biopsy in this series, they did not have a higher frequency of progressive renal insufficiency, ESKD, or death at follow-up.[238] This is in contrast to another series of more than 100 SLE patients, which found the presence of APL antibodies to be associated with both thrombotic events and a greater progression to renal failure.[207] In patients with APL nephropathy, renal biopsies with thrombotic microangiopathy may be misclassified as FSGS, membranous nephropathy, and MPGN.[239] However, a recent study reports that some patients with APS may develop a number of other glomerular histologic patterns on LM examination, including membranous nephropathy, minimal change/focal sclerosis, mesangial proliferative glomerulonephritis, and pauci-immune rapidly progressive glomerulonephritis (RPGN).[240]

The most frequent clinical renal findings are proteinuria, at times in the nephrotic range, active urinary sediment, hypertension, and progressive renal dysfunction.[205,206,234,236,237,239,240] Some patients present with an acute deterioration in renal function.[239] With major renal arterial involvement there may be renal infarction, and renal vein thrombosis may be silent or present with sudden flank pain and a decrease in renal function. Renal artery stenosis has been reported with and without malignant hypertension. Some patients present with an acute deterioration in renal function. With major renal arterial involvement there may be renal infarction, and renal vein thrombosis may be silent or present with sudden flank pain and a decrease in renal function. Renal artery stenosis has been reported with and without malignant hypertension.[241–243]

About 10% of biopsied lupus patients have glomerular microthromboses as the major histopathologic finding. Therapy of this glomerular lesion clearly differs from that of immune complex–mediated glomerulonephritis.[69] One study of 114 biopsied SLE patients found vasoocclusive lesions in one-third of biopsies, which correlated with both hypertension and an increased serum creatinine level.[244] In SLE, features that correlate well with high titers of IgG APL antibodies are thrombocytopenia, the presence of a false-positive VDRL for syphilis (FTA [flüorescent treponemal antibody] negative), and a prolonged activated partial thromboplastin time.[205,206,244] Neither the titer of anti-DNA antibodies nor the serum complement levels correlate well with the APL antibody levels. In SLE, high titers of IgG anticardiolipin antibody usually correlate well with the risk of thrombosis. However, in one study of 114 biopsied SLE patients, renal thrombi were related to lupus anticoagulant but not anticardiolipin antibodies.[244] The clinical features of APS in SLE patients are identical to those of primary APS. An important study documents the prevalence of APL antibodies in 26% of 111 LN patients followed for a mean of 173 months.[207] Of the APL antibody–positive patients, 79% developed a thrombotic event or fetal loss, and the presence of antibodies was strongly correlated with the development of progressive CKD.

There is a high prevalence of APL antibodies (10% to 30%) in hemodialysis patients irrespective of patient age, gender, or duration of the dialysis.[245,246] By contrast, patients with renal insufficiency and those on peritoneal dialysis have a much lower incidence of APL antibodies.[205] One hemodialysis study found more patients with arteriovenous (AV) grafts than native fistulas to have a raised titer of IgG anticardiolipin antibody.[246,247] There was a significant increase in the odds of having two or more episodes of AV graft thrombosis in patients with raised anticardiolipin titer. Whether AV grafts induce anticardiolipin antibodies or whether patients with anticardiolipin antibodies require AV grafts remains unclear.[205] In another study, of 230 hemodialysis patients, titers of IgG anticardiolipin antibodies were elevated in 26% of the patients as opposed to elevated titers of IgM antibodies in only 4%.[247] The mean time to AV graft failure was significantly shorter in the group with elevated IgG antibodies, and the use of warfarin increased graft survival in these patients.

In several studies 20% to 60% of SLE patients with APL antibodies who received renal transplants had problems related to APS, such as venous thromboses, pulmonary emboli, or persistent thrombocytopenia.[119,120,248,249] In one large study of non-SLE patients, 28% of 178 transplant patients had APL antibodies which were associated with a threefold to fourfold increased risk of arterial and venous thromboses.[248] However, another study of 337 renal transplant recipients found the 18% who were IgG or IgM anticardiolipin antibody positive had no greater allograft loss or reduction in GFR than did patients who were anticardiolipin antibody negative.[250] Although most patients with APL antibodies who have tested positive for HCV do not have evidence of increased thromboses and APS, when they receive a transplant, they appear to have a higher risk of allograft thrombotic microangiopathy.[251] In many of these transplant studies, treatment with anticoagulation has proven successful in preventing recurrent thromboses and graft loss.[119,120,249]

## TREATMENT

The optimal treatment of patients with APL antibodies and the APS remains to be defined.[205,206,252] Many patients with APL antibodies do not experience thrombotic events. In asymptomatic patients with APL antibodies but no evidence of thrombotic events or the APS, low-dose aspirin may be beneficial based on limited data.[253]

Because patients with higher titers of IgG APL antibody have a greater incidence of thrombotic events, they may benefit from anticoagulation.[227,228] In patients with full APS, anticoagulation with heparin followed by warfarin has proven more effective than no therapy, aspirin, or low-dose anticoagulation in preventing recurrent thrombosis.[205,208,252] A retrospective analysis of 147 APS patients (including 62 primary disease, 66 SLE, and 19 lupus-like syndrome) reported 186 recurrent thrombotic events in 69% of the patients.[252] The median time between the initial thrombosis and the first recurrence was 12 months but with a broad range (0.5 to 144 months). Treatment with higher-dose warfarin (international normalized ratio [INR] >3) was more effective than treatment with low-dose warfarin (INR <3) or treatment with aspirin. The highest rate of thrombosis (1.3 per patient-year) occurred in patients within 6 months after discontinuing anticoagulation. Bleeding complications occurred in 29 of the 147 patients but were severe in only seven patients. There is insufficient data from comparative studies on the use of newer direct oral anticoagulants versus warfarin to recommend their use in patients with APS.[254,255] The role of immunosuppression is uncertain in APS.[205,206,229] In SLE patients the anti-DNA antibody titer and the serum complement may normalize with immunosuppression without a significant change in a high titer of IgG APL antibody.[205] In pregnant patients with APS, heparin and low-dose aspirin have been successful, whereas prednisone therapy has not.[256,257] In rare patients who cannot tolerate anticoagulation due to recent bleeding, who have thromboembolic events despite adequate anticoagulation, or who have catastrophic APS, plasmapheresis with corticosteroids and other immunosuppressives have been used with some success.[257,258] It is uncertain whether hydroxychloroquine, used mostly in SLE patients, can prevent thromboembolic events in APS.[253,259,260] There is insufficient and conflicting data on whether newer agents such as rituximab lower the levels of APLs or decrease the risk of thromboembolism.[261,262] The use of other treatments, such as eculizumab, intravenous γ-globulin, and stem cell transplant, are only reported in isolated patients.[263,264]

## MIXED CONNECTIVE TISSUE DISEASE

MCTD is defined by a combination of clinical and serologic features.[79,265,266] Patients share overlapping features of SLE, scleroderma, and polymyositis.[265–267] They also typically have distinct serologic findings with a very high ANA titer, often with a speckled pattern, and antibodies directed against a specific ribonuclease-sensitive ENA, U1RNP.[266,267] MCTD has a low incidence and prevalence, a high female-to-male sex ratio, and linkage to HLA-DR4 and DR2 genotypes.[268,269] Not all patients with clinical features of MCTD have a positive ENA, and not all ENA-positive patients have the clinical features of MCTD.[267] Because over time some patients fulfill diagnostic criteria for other connective tissue diseases, investigators have questioned whether MCTD is a distinct syndrome and have developed specific criteria to categorize patients as having MCTD.[270] The term *undifferentiated autoimmune rheumatic and connective tissue disorder or overlap syndrome* has also been used.[267,268] One study of 161 MCTD patients followed for 8 years found 60% with unclassified MCTD, 17% with systemic sclerosis, 9% with SLE, 2.5% with rheumatoid arthritis, and 11.5% with undifferentiated connective tissue disease.[270] A positive anti-DNA antibody predicted the development of SLE while hypomotility of the esophagus or sclerodactyly predicted the development of systemic sclerosis.

In early stages of MCTD, patients usually manifest nonspecific symptoms such as malaise, fatigue, myalgias, arthralgias, and low-grade fever. Over time features similar to other rheumatologic connective tissue diseases appear, including arthralgias, deforming arthritis, myalgias and myositis, Raynaud phenomenon, swollen hands and fingers, restrictive pulmonary disease and pulmonary hypertension, esophageal dysmotility, pericarditis and myocarditis, serositis, oral and nasal ulcers, digital ulcers and gangrene, discoid lupus-like lesions, malar rash, alopecia, photosensitivity, and lymphadenopathy.[266,267,271] However, patients with MCTD, especially those documented to have anti-U1RNP antibodies, infrequently have major central nervous system disease or severe proliferative glomerulonephritis.[266,267,271] Low-grade anemia, lymphocytopenia, and hypergammaglobulinemia are all common in MCTD.

The most widely used serologic test to confirm a diagnosis of MCTD is the ENA with anti-U1RNP antibodies.[267,272] The diagnosis of MCTD is even firmer in those patients with IgG antibodies against an antigenic component of U1RNP, the 68-kD protein.[272,273] Antibodies to other nuclear antigens have been found in MCTD and some correlate better with some clinical features of specific rheumatologic diseases.[266] Antibodies against dsDNA, Sm antigen, and Ro are infrequently positive in MCTD, but up to 70% of patients will have a positive rheumatoid factor.

The incidence of renal involvement has varied from 10% to 26% of adults and from 33% to 50% of children with MCTD.[267,273] Many patients have mild clinical manifestations with only microhematuria and less than 500-mg proteinuria daily. However, heavier proteinuria, severe hypertension, and acute kidney injury (AKI) reminiscent of "scleroderma renal crisis" may occur.[271,274,275] Although the titer of anti-RNP does not correlate with renal involvement, the presence of serologic markers of active SLE (e.g., high anti-dsDNA antibody titers, anti-Sm antibody) is more common with renal disease.[267] Low serum complement levels have not always correlated with the presence of renal involvement.[271] Children with MCTD more often have glomerular involvement with few clinical or urinary findings.[276]

The pathology of MCTD is diverse with the glomerular lesions resembling the spectrum found in SLE and the vascular lesions resembling those in scleroderma. Glomerular disease is most common and is usually superimposed on a background of mesangial deposits and hypercellularity as in SLE.[271,274,276–279] As many as 30% of biopsied patients have mesangial deposits of IgG and C3. Other patients have focal proliferative glomerulonephritis with both mesangial and subendothelial deposits, but fibrinoid necrosis and crescents are rare. The most common pattern of glomerular involvement is membranous nephropathy reported in up to 35% of cases,[274,276–278] with typical peripheral capillary wall granular IF staining for IgG, C3, and at times IgA and IgM. Some patients will have a mixed pattern of membranous plus mesangial proliferative GN.[276] Renal biopsy findings may transform over time from one pattern of glomerular involvement to another, similar to SLE patients. By ultrastructure analysis, LN-like findings have been reported including endothelial TRIs, deposits with "fingerprint" substructure, and tubular basement membrane deposits.[271] In a review of 100 biopsied patients with MCTD, 12% had normal biopsies, 35% mesangial lesions, 10% proliferative glomerular lesions, and 36% membranous nephropathy.[280] In addition 15% to 25% of patients had interstitial disease and vascular lesions. In autopsy series, in which two-thirds of patients had clinical renal disease, a similar distribution of glomerular lesions was found.[279] Other renal pathology findings in MCTD include secondary renal amyloidosis,[281] vascular sclerosis ranging from intimal sclerosis to medial hyperplasia, and vascular lesions resembling those in scleroderma kidney with involvement of the interlobular arteries by intimal mucoid edema and fibrous sclerosis.[271]

Therapy of MCTD with corticosteroids is effective in treating the inflammatory features of joint disease and serositis.[267,271] Steroids are less effective in treating sclerodermatous features such as cutaneous disease, esophageal involvement, and especially pulmonary hypertension. Intravenous immunoglobulin has been used to treat thrombocytopenia and hemolytic anemia.[282] Treatment of the glomerular lesions is similar to that for LN.

Originally MCTD was felt to have a good prognosis with low mortality and few patients developing other distinct connective tissue disorders. The longer patients with MCTD are followed, the greater the percentage who evolve more clearly into a specific connective tissue disorder.[267] In some series, almost half of the patients with a short duration of follow-up were still felt to have true MCTD, but in those with longer follow-up the percentage had dropped to 15% or less.[267,271] Most patients evolve toward a picture of either SLE or systemic sclerosis, but some develop features of rheumatoid arthritis[270,271] and rates have been found to range from 15% to 30% at 10 to 12 years, with patients having more clinical features of scleroderma and polymyositis faring worse.[267,271] The presence of anticardiolipin antibodies and anti-$\beta_2$-glycoprotein antibodies increases the mortality risk. In a recent study, 5-, 10-, and 15-year survival rates were 98%, 96%, and 88%, respectively.[282] The leading causes of mortality in MCTD are pulmonary hypertension and cardiovascular disease.[267,283] Other causes include vascular lesions of the coronary and other vessels, hypertensive scleroderma crisis, and chronic renal failure. Clearly MCTD is not a benign disorder but rather a disease with the potential for significant morbidity and mortality.

## ANTINEUTROPHIL CYTOPLASMIC ANTIBODY–ASSOCIATED VASCULITIS

GPA (formerly designated Wegener granulomatosis), MPA, and eosinophilic GPA (EGPA; formerly designated Churg–Strauss syndrome or Churg–Strauss vasculitis) are usually classified together as three pauci-immune small vessel vasculitides that affect the arterioles, capillaries, and venules.[284–294] There is considerable overlap in the clinical, histologic, and laboratory features of these entities. Moreover, all may be associated with a positive serologic test for ANCA. However, genetic analyses are defining differences between these entities, and differences in the course and response to therapy may be noted.[295]

### GRANULOMATOSIS WITH POLYANGIITIS

GPA has been traditionally defined by the triad of vasculitis associated with necrotizing, granulomatous inflammation of the upper and lower respiratory tracts, and by glomerulonephritis.[296] Subsequent descriptions of "limited" upper respiratory tract disease, of multiorgan system involvement, and of the nature and pathogenesis of the serologic marker, ANCA, have enhanced our understanding of this disease.[288–291] Even in the pre-ANCA era these clinical criteria yielded a sensitivity of 88% and a specificity of 92% for the diagnosis of GPA. Adding ANCA to the diagnostic criteria increases these percentages.[292–294] From 1993 to 2011, the annual hospitalization rate for GPA in the United States increased from 5.1 to 6.3 per million, a 24% increase, whereas the in-hospital mortality declined by 73%.[297]

GPA has a slight male predominance and a peak incidence in the fourth to sixth decade of life.[286,289,298,299] Pauci-immune RPGN (including GPA and MPA) is the most common form of crescentic glomerulonephritis at all ages, especially in older adults.[293,294] Most patients have been Caucasian, although with use of ANCA screening, patients of all races are being diagnosed.[298] The occurrence of GPA in more than one family member has rarely been noted.[299] Certain HLA frequencies, such as HLA-DR2, HLA-B7, and HLA-DR1 and DR1-DQW1, are reported more commonly.[299,300]

## PATHOLOGY

The classic histopathologic finding in GPA is a focal segmental necrotizing and crescentic glomerulonephritis (Fig. 32.14).[290] Although the percentage of affected glomeruli can vary widely, the necrotizing changes are usually segmental in distribution.[290,301] Unaffected glomeruli typically appear normal. Global proliferation and necrotizing glomerular tuft involvement are more common in the more severe cases. The earliest lesions are "intracapillary thrombosis" with deposition of eosinophilic "fibrinoid" material associated with endothelial cell swelling, infiltration by polymorphonuclear leukocytes, and pyknosis or karyorrhexis.[290,301] In areas of active necrotizing glomerular lesions, there are ruptures in the GBM and formation of overlying cellular crescents that range from segmental to circumferential. Crescents are frequently associated with breaks in or broad destruction of Bowman's capsule.[302] Granulomatous crescents containing epithelioid histiocytes and giant cells may involve from fewer than 15% to over 50% of cases, and the finding of large numbers of them is more typical of GPA and cytoplasmic ANCA (C-ANCA) positivity than other vasculitides. Chronic segmental or global glomerulosclerosis with fibrous crescents often occurs side by side with more active glomerular lesions. Although there is much overlap in the histologic findings between MPA and GPA, some differences have been noted. Patients with MPA and those who have antimyeloperoxidase (anti-MPO) ANCA are more likely to have a greater degree and severity of glomerulosclerosis, interstitial fibrosis, and tubular atrophy on initial biopsy.[303]

The true vasculitis in GPA may affect small- and medium-sized renal arteries, veins, and capillaries.[290,301] It is focal in nature and has been reported in 5% to 10% of GPA biopsies.[286,289,290] It is more commonly found at autopsy, with inherent tissue sampling of larger volumes of tissue, or when serial sectioning and a directed search for the lesions have been performed. The necrotizing arteritis consists of endothelial cell swelling and denudation, intimal fibrin deposition, and mononuclear and polymorphonuclear leukocyte infiltration of the vessel wall with mural necrosis (Fig. 32.15). In some cases, the arteritis displays granulomatous features. Tubules show focal degenerative and regenerative changes, and cortical infarcts may occur.[286,290] Interstitial inflammatory infiltrates of lymphocytes, monocytes, plasma cells, and polymorphonuclear leukocytes are common. Granulomas containing giant cells may form in the interstitium of the cortex and medulla in 3% to 20% of cases. Cortical granulomas may represent foci of glomerular destruction by granulomatous crescents. Papillary necrosis, often bilateral and affecting most papillae, has been reported, usually in those with necrotizing interstitial capillaritis of the vasa recta. Biopsy of extrarenal tissue may show necrotizing and granulomatous inflammation or evidence of vasculitis.[289,290]

There is no specific glomerular or vascular immune staining in most cases of GPA, hence the term pauci-immune. Low-level staining for immunoglobulins and complement likely represents nonimmunologic trapping in areas of necrosis and sclerosis. This negative or only focal low-intensity IF staining pattern is referred to as "pauci-immune."[286–290] Positivity for fibrin–fibrinogen is common in the distribution of the

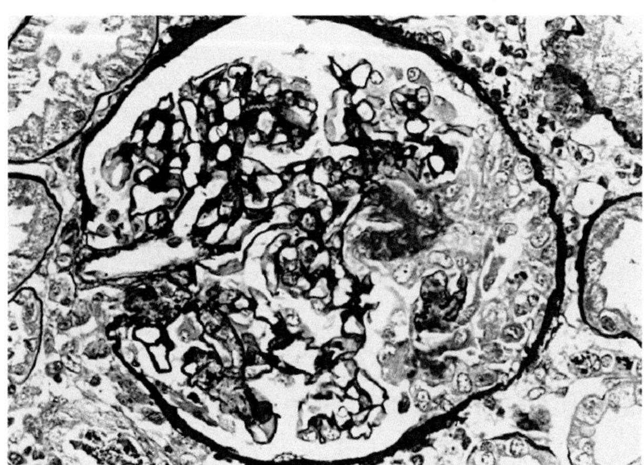

**Fig. 32.14** Granulomatosis with polyangiitis. A representative glomerulus displays segmental fibrinoid necrosis with rupture of glomerular basement membrane, fibrin extravasation into the urinary space, and an overlying segmental cellular crescent (Jones methenamine silver, ×500).

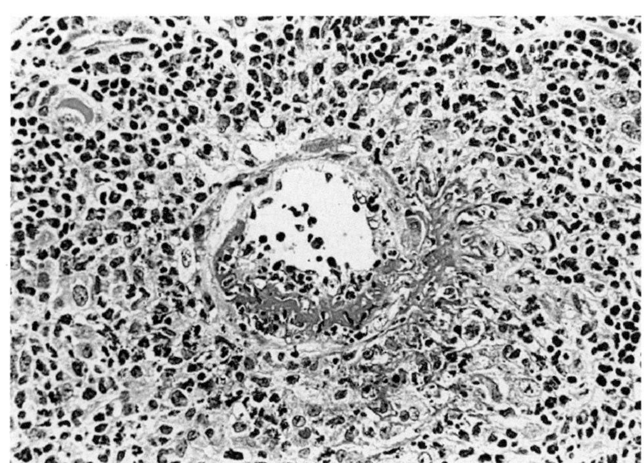

**Fig. 32.15** Granulomatosis with polyangiitis. An interlobular artery displays necrotizing vasculitis with intimal fibrin deposition and transmural inflammation by neutrophils and lymphocytes (hematoxylin–eosin, ×375).

necrotizing glomerular lesions, crescents, and vasculitic lesions. By EM, the glomeruli affected by necrotizing lesions often show areas of intraluminal and subendothelial fibrin deposition associated with endothelial necrosis and gaps in the GBM through which fibrin and leukocytes extravasate into Bowman's space.[286–290] There may be subendothelial accumulation of electron-lucent flocculent material associated with intravascular coagulation. True electron-dense immune-type deposits are not usually identified and, when present, are sparse and ill-defined.[286–290] EM of the vessels in GPA may show swelling and denudation of endothelial cells, and subendothelial accumulation of fibrin, platelets, and amorphous electron-dense material, but no typical immune-type electron-dense deposits.

## PATHOGENESIS

While the exact pathogenesis of GPA remains unknown, involvement of both humoral and cell-mediated immunity as well as the complement system has been described.[287,289,290] A GWAS found that GPA and MPA are genetically distinct diseases with informative DNA markers strongly associating with the antigenic specificity of the ANCA rather than the clinical syndrome per se.[295] A variety of initiating events, on the background of this genetic predisposition, have been proposed to incite GPA and MPA including infections, medications, exposure of the respiratory tract to toxins such as silica.[304] In vitro and animal experiments strongly support a role for ANCA in the pathogenesis of the disease.[305–309] ANCA production may relate to infectious, genetic, environmental, and other risk factors.[305] Both molecular mimicry to infectious pathogens and formation of antibody to antisense peptide have been proposed in the development of ANCA. Patients with proteinase 3 (PR3)–positive ANCA have been shown to have antibodies to complementary PR3, a protein encoded by the antisense RNA of the PR3 gene, and $CD4^+$ $T_H1$ memory cells responsive to the complementary PR3 peptide.[306] In Rag-2 mice, transfer of anti-MPO IgG causes glomerulonephritis with necrosis and crescent formation that appears identical to human ANCA-associated glomerulonephritis by LM and IF.[308] This can occur in the absence of antigen-specific T lymphocytes, strongly suggesting a pathogenetic role for the antibodies themselves. In humans, neonatal MPA with pulmonary hemorrhage and renal disease has occurred secondary to the transfer of maternal MPO-ANCA.[310] One study has found a unique subgroup of ANCA directed against lysosomal-associated membrane protein 2 (LAMP2), as opposed to MPO or PR3, to be present in more than 90% of ANCA-positive pauci-immune necrotizing glomerulonephritis.[311] Others have not been able to confirm a high incidence of anti-LAMP2 antibodies in this population. However, a recent study did find a high incidence of anti-LAMP2 antibodies in patients with pauci-immune necrotizing glomerulonephritis who were both PR3 and MPO negative.[312,313]

Cell-mediated mechanisms of tissue injury in GPA are supported by a predominance of $CD4^+$ T lymphocytes and monocytes in the inflammatory respiratory tract infiltrates, high levels of $T_H1$ cytokines, defects in delayed hypersensitivity, a rise in soluble markers of T-cell activation as soluble IL-2 receptor and CD30, impaired lymphocyte blastogenesis, and T-cell response to PR3.[291,314–316] Despite prominent respiratory tract involvement, no inhaled pathogen or environmental allergen has been identified as the initiator of the disease process. However, respiratory infections may allow the release of cytokines such as TNF from cells that can "prime" neutrophils to express PR3 and other antigens on their cell surfaces. The expression of granule proteins on the surface of neutrophils and monocytes allows for the interaction with circulating ANCA, leading to a respiratory burst in the cell, degranulation and local release of damaging proteases and reactive oxygen species, release of chemoattractant products, and neutrophil apoptosis. This results in endothelial cell injury, fibrinoid necrosis, and inflammation.[289–291,317–319] In the presence of ANCA, neutrophils exhibit exaggerated adhesion and transmigration through endothelium.[319] Recently a number of studies point to the involvement of the complement system in the pathogenesis of ANCA-associated vasculitis (AAV) and have led to therapeutic studies targeting this mechanism.[320,321]

A spectrum of glomerular and vascular disease reaction is seen depending on antigen expression, host leukocyte activation, circulating and local cytokines and chemokines, the condition of the endothelium, and the nature of T- and B-cell interactions.[289–291,317–319] The membranes of leukocytes from GPA patients may be primed to express PR3 molecules on their surfaces, making them ripe for activation of the disease process.[291,318,322,323] This priming phenomenon might explain the exacerbations of disease activity associated with respiratory infections as well as the potential benefits of prophylaxis with trimethoprim–sulfamethoxazole.[323,324]

## CLINICAL AND LABORATORY FEATURES

Patients with GPA may present with an indolent, slowly progressive involvement of the respiratory tract and mild renal findings or with fulminant acute glomerulonephritis. Despite greater awareness of the disease, more extensive use of renal biopsy, and the widespread availability of ANCA serologic testing, diagnosis is still often delayed. Most patients will have constitutional symptoms, including fever, weakness, and malaise at presentation.[286–289,325,326] From 70% to 80% of patients have upper respiratory findings at presentation and more than 90% eventually develop upper respiratory problems over time.[286–289,325,326] There may be rhinitis, purulent or bloody nasal discharge and crusting, and sinusitis, typically involving the maxillary sinus and less commonly the sphenoid, ethmoid, and frontal sinuses.[286–289,325,326] X-rays show sinus opacification, air-fluid levels, mass lesions, or rarely bony erosions. Upper respiratory tract involvement can also manifest by tinnitus and hearing loss, otic discharge, earache, perforation of the tympanic membrane, and hoarseness and throat pain.[286–289] Chronic sequelae include deafness, chronic sinusitis, and nasal septal collapse with saddle nose deformity.[288]

Lower respiratory tract disease, found at presentation in up to 75% of patients and eventually in 85%, leads to symptoms of cough (often with sputum production), dyspnea on exertion and shortness of breath, alveolar hemorrhage and hemoptysis, and pleuritic pain.[286–290,327] Chest radiographs and computed tomographic scans may reveal single or multiple nodules, some with areas of cavitation, alveolar infiltrates, and interstitial changes, and less commonly small pleural effusions and atelectatic areas.

GPA is a multisystem disease with many organs involved by the vasculitic process and its sequelae.[286–290] Cutaneous involvement, present in 15% to 50% of patients, occurs with a variety of macular lesions, papules, nodules, or purpura, usually on the lower extremities. Patients with rheumatologic involvement have arthralgias of large and small joints as well as nondeforming arthritis of the knees and ankles or, more rarely, a myopathy or myositis. Up to 65% of patients have ophthalmologic disease with conjunctivitis, episcleritis and uveitis, optic nerve vasculitis, or proptosis due to retroorbital inflammation. Nervous system involvement is most typically manifested as a mononeuritis multiplex but may involve cranial nerves or the central nervous system. Other organs involved include the liver, parotids, thyroid, gallbladder, and the heart.[286–290] Recent reports have emphasized the risks of thromboembolism, especially during active disease, perhaps related to endothelial injury and hypercoagulability induced by the vasculitis and its treatment.[328]

Abnormal laboratory tests in GPA include a normochromic, normocytic anemia, and a mild leukocytosis and thrombocytosis.[286,290] Nonspecific markers of an inflammatory disease process such as an elevated ESR, CRP levels, and rheumatoid factor tests are often positive and correlate with the general disease activity. Other serologic tests including those for ANA, serum complement levels, and cryoglobulins are normal or negative.[286]

ANCA has been detected in from 85% to over 95% of GPA patients. Patients with granulomatous lesions are more likely to be C-ANCA positive with antibody directed against PR3, a 228–amino acid serine proteinase found in the azurophilic granules of neutrophils and the lysosomes of monocytes.[285,287–289,296] However, many patients fitting the clinical and histologic definition of GPA will be perinuclear ANCA (P-ANCA) positive with antibodies directed against MPO, a highly cationic 140-kDa dimer located in a similar cellular distribution to PR3.[285,287–289,291] ANCA may also be directed to other antigens (e.g., lactoferrin, cathepsin, elastase), but these antibodies are not usually associated with vasculitis and are usually found in other immune-mediated diseases. In a study of 89 patients from China who fulfilled clinical and histopathologic criteria for GPA, 61% were MPO-ANCA positive and only 38% PR3-ANCA positive.[298] Although the specificity of C-ANCA for GPA has been as high as 98% to 99% by different assays, the sensitivity may be low in certain populations with inactive or limited disease.[329] Some patients with pauci-immune crescentic glomerulonephritis will be ANCA negative and may have a somewhat distinct disease from the more common ANCA-positive patients.[330] In a series of 141 Chinese patients with RPGN, 27% were ANCA negative and had more upper airway disease than the ANCA-positive group.[330] However, they had no difference in other clinical manifestations. Other patients with crescentic glomerulonephritis will be positive for both ANCA and anti-GBM antibodies (see the “Antiglomerular Basement Membrane Disease and Goodpasture Syndrome” section). Positive ANCA tests have been reported in patients with certain infections (e.g., HIV, tuberculosis, infective bacterial endocarditis) and neoplastic diseases.[331] A number of medications have also been associated with ANCA, usually anti-MPO, and at very high titers. The strongest association is with the antithyroid drug propylthiouracil, and hydralazine and minocycline. Methimazole, carbimazole, penicillamine, allopurinol, clozapine, rifampin, cefotaxime, isoniazid, and a number of other drugs have also been associated with ANCA-positive vasculitis.[332,333] Levamisole as an adulterant in cocaine has been associated with unique ANCA anti-MPO and anti-PR3 positivity, often with high titers of ANCA in association with positive ANAs, APL antibody titer, and other serologic tests.[334,335] While there has been debate over whether the ANCA levels parallel the clinical and histologic activity in GPA, many patients will normalize their ANCA titer during periods of quiescence.[293,329,336–340] A subsequent rise in ANCA titer from low titer has been suggested to be predictive of renal and systemic flares.[336–340] One recent study of 166 patients with AAV who were positive for PR3 or MPO and who were followed almost 50 months included 104 patients with renal involvement and 62 without kidney disease. Eighty-nine patients had a rise in ANCA titer and there were 74 relapses.[341] A rise in ANCA titer correlated with relapse in the patients with renal disease but only weakly in those without kidney disease. Another recent study also found a rise in PR3 ANCA titer to be associated with severe relapses, especially in those with renal disease and pulmonary hemorrhage.[342] Most clinicians prefer to use the ANCA level in the context of other clinical findings and often with other markers of active inflammation such as ESR and CRP. At times, renal biopsy is the only way to be certain of the clinical significance of a change in ANCA titer.

## RENAL FINDINGS

Renal findings in GPA are extremely variable and usually occur together with other systemic findings.[286–290,326] The degree of renal involvement in AAV is highly predictive of patient survival. Patients with active urinary sediment but normal GFR have a twofold increased risk of death, whereas those with impaired renal function have a fivefold greater risk of dying.[343] A number of studies confirm that severe renal disease is a negative prognostic feature. Many patients have some evidence of renal disease at presentation, and from 50% to 95% eventually develop clinical renal involvement. Proteinuria and urinary sediment abnormalities, including microscopic hematuria and red cell casts, are common. Patients with more severe glomerular involvement have a decrease in GFR and greater levels of proteinuria, but nephrotic syndrome is uncommon. The level of proteinuria may be higher in those with less severe renal insufficiency and may actually increase during therapy as the GFR improves.[326] The degree of renal failure and serum creatinine do not always correlate well with the percentage of glomerular necrotizing lesions, the percentage of glomerular crescent formation, or the presence of interstitial granulomas or vasculitis. The incidence of both acute oliguric renal failure and significant hypertension varies among reports but is higher in reports from renal centers. Intravenous pyelograms are typically normal, and vascular aneurysms are not usually present on angiography.

Other renal conditions found in GPA include pyelonephritis and hydronephrosis due to vasculitis, causing ureteral stenosis, papillary necrosis, perirenal hematoma from arterial aneurysm rupture, and lymphoid malignancies with neoplastic infiltration of the renal parenchyma in patients treated with immunosuppression.[344]

## COURSE AND TREATMENT

The course of the active glomerulonephritis in GPA is typical of RPGN with progression to renal failure over days to months.[286–290] Patients with severe necrotizing, granulomatous glomerulonephritis are more likely to develop renal failure, and patients with more global glomerulosclerosis are more likely to develop ESKD. Greater degrees of glomerulosclerosis and interstitial fibrosis predict a poor renal outcome.[345] Even with immunosuppressive therapy, a significant number of patients will eventually progress over the long term to renal failure. Patients who are dialysis dependent for more than 4 months are unlikely to recover function even with optimal immunosuppression.[346]

The introduction of effective cytotoxic immunosuppressive therapy dramatically changed the clinical course of GPA. Initial studies of untreated or corticosteroid-treated patients documented survivals of only 20% to 60% at 1 year.[286,290] Both renal and extrarenal lesions may progress during corticosteroid therapy.[286] Long-term survival with cyclophosphamide-based regimens ranges from 87% at 8 years to 64% at 10 years.[286–290,347,348] Using a regimen of combined cyclophosphamide (1.5–2 mg/kg/day) and corticosteroids, remissions were achieved in 85% to 90% of 133 GPA patients.[286] Although many patients eventually relapsed, others remained in long-term remission off immunosuppression. Other studies have confirmed these results.[288–291,347] Complete remissions of renal and extrarenal symptoms, including severe pulmonary disease and renal failure requiring dialysis, have been described. More than 50% of dialysis-dependent patients will be able to discontinue dialysis and remain stable for years. Although resistance to therapy is well documented, some patients do not benefit from treatment for reasons of nonadherence, intercurrent infection requiring decreased treatment, comorbidities, or inadequate duration of therapy.

The optimal dose, duration of treatment, route of administration, and concomitant therapy to be given with cyclophosphamide are still debated for patients with ANCA-positive small vessel vasculitis.[288–291] Many recent trials have included both GPA and MPA patients. Cyclophosphamide is usually administered with corticosteroids initially, with the dose of the steroids tapered or changed to alternate-day therapy. Some regimens include intravenous high-dose "pulse" corticosteroids initially, and others have used plasmapheresis in critically ill patients. A typical regimen for induction therapy of severe GPA or MPA RPGN might include intravenous pulse methylprednisolone (7 mg/kg, to a maximum dose of 500–1000 mg) for 3 consecutive days followed by oral prednisone 1 mg/kg/day (to a maximum of 60–80 mg/day) for the first month, with subsequent tapering of the dose along with either intravenous or oral cyclophosphamide given for approximately 6 months.[287–290] Doses are adjusted for leukopenia and other side effects as well as for treatment response. Several studies have evaluated the role of pulse intravenous cyclophosphamide versus oral cyclophosphamide in ANCA-positive small vessel vasculitis.[349–352] In one study of 50 GPA patients randomly assigned to either 2 years of intravenous or oral cyclophosphamide, remissions at 6 months occurred in 89% of the intravenous group versus 78% of the oral group.[349] At the end of the study, remissions occurred in 67% of the intravenous group and 57% of the oral group, but relapses were more common in the intravenous group (60% vs. 13%). In a meta-analysis of 11 nonrandomized studies including more than 200 AAV patients, complete remissions occurred in more than 60% of patients and partial remissions in another 15%.[350] Pulse cyclophosphamide was more likely to induce remission and less likely to cause infection than oral cyclophosphamide. However, relapses may be more frequent with intravenous use of the drug. Relapses occur in 10% to 60% of patients with AAV, depending upon the case series. This large variation in observed relapse rate depends upon initial and maintenance therapy, duration of treatment, follow-up duration, serologic type of AAV, and the criteria for diagnosing a relapse (clinical vs. laboratory based). The relapse rate was clarified by a recent large multicenter trial that randomized 149 ANCA-positive vasculitis patients to either Solu-Medrol plus pulsed intravenous cyclophosphamide (15 mg/kg every 2–3 weeks) or plus oral cyclophosphamide (2 mg/kg/day).[350] There was no difference in time to remission or percentage of patients who achieved remission by 9 months (88% of both groups) and no difference in improvement of GFR over time. Although there were more relapses in the intravenous group, this was not statistically significant. The total dose of cyclophosphamide was approximately half as much in the intravenous group versus the oral group, and infections were more common with oral cyclophosphamide. Thus both regimens are effective. However, relapses appear to be more common with intravenous therapy, but total dose and adverse effects of the cytotoxic agent are reduced by intravenous usage.[318] It is unclear how frequent the initial intravenous "pulses" of cyclophosphamide should be given; some investigators use monthly doses and others start with smaller doses every 2 to 3 weeks. It is clear that early application of an intensive immunosuppressive regimen helps prevent long-term morbidity and end-organ damage. Because the total dose of the cyclophosphamide is far less in patients receiving pulsed intravenous therapy, many prefer to use it as a less toxic regimen and try to enhance maintenance therapy to avoid relapse.

Methotrexate has been used for both induction and maintenance therapy in patients with GPA and other ANCA-associated vasculitides.[351–354] The largest trial, the NORAM trial, compared methotrexate (20–25 mg/week orally) with oral cyclophosphamide (2 mg/kg/day), both for 1 year, with corticosteroids in 95 ANCA-positive vasculitis patients (89 GPA, 6 MPA).[351] Although an equal percentage of both groups achieved remission, the time to remission was longer in the methotrexate group and the relapse rate much higher (70% vs. 47%). Given these data, methotrexate is rarely used for induction therapy in ANCA-positive vasculitis unless the disease is very mild and rapidly controllable.

The addition of plasmapheresis to therapy for GPA appears to benefit patients with severe renal failure, those with pulmonary hemorrhage, those with coexistent anti-GBM antibodies, and those failing all other therapeutic agents.[345,355] For small vessel vasculitis patients with massive pulmonary hemorrhage treated with methylprednisolone, intravenous cyclophosphamide, and plasmapheresis, all 20 patients had resolution of pulmonary hemorrhage.[355] A trial of 137 patients with ANCA-positive glomerulonephritis, the Methylprednisolone versus Plasma Exchange (MEPEX) trial, evaluated patients with a marked elevation of the serum creatinine (>500 μmol/L or 5.7 mg/dL) treated with induction therapy with either plasma exchange or intravenous pulsed methylprednisolone, both with oral corticosteroids and cyclophosphamide.[356] Although both groups had an equal and high 1-year mortality rate, the plasma exchange group had an improved short-term patient survival and a greater likelihood of not reaching renal failure at 1 year (19% vs.

43%). At longer follow-up of almost 4 years, however, this benefit in less renal failure did not translate into reduced long-term mortality, raising the question of whether adding plasma exchange therapy really provides a true benefit to patients.[357] The study design of plasma exchange versus intravenous pulsed methylprednisolone is not the same as intravenous pulsed methylprednisolone with or without plasma exchange. However, some recent guidelines recommend plasma exchange for rapidly progressive renal failure or severe diffuse pulmonary hemorrhage.[358] The addition of etanercept, a TNF-α blocker, to a standard induction regimen for GPA was evaluated in 174 patients and provided no additional benefit in terms of sustained remissions or time to achieve remission or resolution of pulmonary granulomatous disease.[359] Disease flares and adverse events were common in both treatment groups, and solid tumors developed in six of the etanercept group. The use of infliximab, another TNF-α blocker, was associated with an 80% remission rate but a high rate of infectious complications in four uncontrolled trials.[360] Likewise, a study of alemtuzumab, an anti-CD52 monoclonal antibody, gave a remission rate of 83% in 70 patients but was associated with high rates of relapse, infection, and mortality.[361] Recent studies have suggested a role for complement blockade in AAV and have led to ongoing clinical trials.[362]

Small uncontrolled trials initially found a role for rituximab in ANCA-positive vasculitis, with sustained remissions in many of the patients studied.[363,364] A retrospective analysis of 120 AAV patients found that 86% of rituximab patients achieved remission but 41% had a relapse at a median time of around 20 months.[365] This was true regardless of whether patients had two or more infusions, and suggested rituximab was beneficial even outside of a controlled trial. Two controlled randomized studies support the use of rituximab as a first-line therapy comparable in efficacy to cyclophosphamide for the treatment of AAV.[366,367] In the Rituximab versus Cyclophosphamide in ANCA-associated Renal Vasculitis (RITUXIVAS) study, 44 patients (mean age, 68 years) were randomized with two-thirds receiving four doses of intravenous rituximab and only two doses of intravenous cyclophosphamide and one dose of intravenous pulse Solu-Medrol versus the remaining one-third of patients receiving 6 to 10 pulses of intravenous cyclophosphamide.[366] Both received steroids in tapering doses. At 12 months of follow-up the number of remissions, time to remission, and side effects were similar in the two groups. Mortality and morbidity were high in both groups due to the age of the patients and their renal dysfunction. At longer follow-up (≤24 months) the composite outcome of death, ESKD, and relapse still was the same between the two treatment groups.[368] In the Rituximab in ANCA-Associated Vasculitis (RAVE) trial, 197 patients with severe AAV (75% GPA) were randomized to steroids plus either four weekly doses (375 mg/m$^2$) of rituximab or oral cyclophosphamide (2 mg/kg/day) with replacement by azathioprine maintenance only in the cyclophosphamide group.[367] Among those in the rituximab group, 64% reached remission, whereas only 53% of the cyclophosphamide group did. More patients in the rituximab arm had resolution of active vasculitis by activity scores. Adverse events were similar in both arms of the study. The subgroups with renal involvement and pulmonary hemorrhage also fared the same. Those with relapsing disease had a significantly higher remission rate with rituximab compared with cyclophosphamide therapy. Recent long-term follow-up of this population confirms the equivalency of a steroid plus rituximab regimen to that of steroids plus cyclophosphamide followed by azathioprine maintenance in leading to a complete remission in AAV.[369] There was no difference in adverse events in terms of infections or malignancies between the groups. While this does not mean rituximab will replace cyclophosphamide as standard treatment for ANCA-positive vasculitis, the evidence suggests that it offers an initial treatment option for many patients.[370] The European League Against Rheumatism (EULAR)/European Renal Association–European Dialysis and Transplant Association (ERA-EDTA) in recent guidelines recommends that for remission induction in severe organ-threatening AAV cyclophosphamide and rituximab are considered to have equal efficacy.[358] Rituximab has also been used successfully as a maintenance therapy in AAV after induction therapy.

Relapse rates from 20% to 50% have been reported often when infectious complications have led to a discontinuation of immunosuppressive therapy.[336,339,347,371] Predictors of relapse in a cohort of 350 patients with ANCA-positive vasculitis included C-ANCA or PR3 positivity, lung involvement, and upper respiratory involvement. By contrast, factors not predicting relapse include age, gender, race, and a clinical diagnosis of GPA rather than MPA or renal-limited vasculitis.[364,371] Most patients respond to another course of cyclophosphamide therapy.[347] In patients whose ANCA level has declined during remission, a major rise in titer may predict a relapse, although ANCA levels and clinical disease activity do not always correlate.[336–340]

Because of the potential for severe complications with cyclophosphamide therapy (infections, infertility, hemorrhagic cystitis, and an increased risk of long-term malignancy), once an initial remission has been achieved, patients have usually been switched to less toxic immunosuppressives such as azathioprine, low-dose methotrexate, or MMF.[371–374] A study of 155 patients with ANCA-positive vasculitis treated patients with cyclophosphamide and steroids to induce a remission and then randomized them to either oral azathioprine or continued cyclophosphamide maintenance therapy.[374] Of the 155 patients, 144 entered remission and were randomized. There was no difference in the relapse rate in the two groups or in the adverse event rate. Relapse rates were lower in patients with MPA than in the GPA group. A controlled randomized trial of MMF versus azathioprine for remission maintenance found more relapses with MMF.[375] Rituximab, timed to prevent B-cell repopulation and rise in the ANCA titer, has also been used successfully for maintenance therapy.[376,377] A retrospective analysis of 172 patients with AAV (57% MPO positive) who were treated with rituximab approximately every 4 months for a mean time of over 2 years found a major relapse rate of only 5% and no greater mortality than age- and gender-matched controls in the general population.[378] A controlled randomized trial in 115 patients compared 500 mg of intravenous rituximab given at 6 monthly intervals with daily azathioprine for preventing relapse in AAV.[379] At 28 months of follow-up, the rituximab group had a lower major relapse rate (5%) than the azathioprine group (29%) and no greater side effects (infection, cancer, serious adverse events) than the group receiving azathioprine. Because respiratory infections, perhaps through priming of neutrophils or activation of ANCA, may be associated with flares of disease activity, prophylactic use of trimethoprim–sulfamethoxazole has been advocated.[380] Although not in favor for induction, methotrexate has also been used as maintenance therapy in GPA.[353] Supportive measures for GPA patients such as sinus drainage procedures, hearing aids, and corrective surgery for nasal septal collapse may be helpful in individuals with chronic sequelae of upper respiratory involvement.[286–290] Attention to cardiovascular risks is important because patients with AAV and renal disease have more than a twofold increased risk of cardiovascular events when compared with matched controls with CKD.[381]

ESKD occurs in about 25% of patients at 3 to 4 years after presentation. Dialysis and transplantation have been performed in increasing numbers of AAV patients.[382–387] Many patients' disease activity diminishes with onset of renal failure, and relapses are significantly less frequent for patients who reach ESKD.[385] However, some patients still require intensive immunosuppression, and relapses have been reported well after the onset of ESKD. Fatality rates may be high in some ESKD populations due to slow recognition of relapses of the vasculitic process or, more often, infectious complications. Most patients receiving allografts have been maintained on prednisone and cyclosporine or tacrolimus with or without mycophenolate with very good patient and allograft survival rates.[382–387] Patients should not receive a transplant until after a prolonged period of remission.[388] Recurrent active glomerulonephritis in the allograft occurs in 15% to 37% of patients and may respond to cyclophosphamide or rituximab therapy or other more intensive therapies.[382–387] There is no evidence that regimens including MMF or tacrolimus have advantages over older immunosuppressive regimens in preventing recurrences of AAV in renal allografts.[386] There is only limited experience with sirolimus or other newer transplant immunosuppressives.[389]

## MICROSCOPIC POLYANGIITIS

The incidence of renal disease associated with this ANCA-positive small vessel vasculitis appears to be increasing.[287–290] While this may be caused by wider use of ANCA testing and renal biopsy, many investigators feel the absolute incidence has increased. In one large series, ANCA-associated crescentic glomerulonephritis made up almost 10% of all glomerular diseases diagnosed by renal biopsy in a 2-year period. In very old adults this was the most common etiologic diagnosis.[292] Vasculitis and glomerulonephritis similar to those seen in MPA have been noted in relapsing polychondritis[390] and ANCA-positive polyangiitis induced by use of a number of medications, most notably the antithyroid medication propylthiouracil.[391]

### PATHOLOGY

#### Light Microscopy

The most typical histologic finding is focal segmental necrotizing glomerulonephritis with crescents affecting from few to many glomeruli (Fig. 32.16).[287–291,392] There is segmental rupture of the GBM associated with polymorphonuclear infiltration, karyorrhexis, and fibrin deposition within the glomerular tuft and the adjacent Bowman's space. Crescents characteristically overlie areas of segmental tuft necrosis and may be segmental or circumferential. Cellular and fibrous crescents often coexist. Some crescents are voluminous with a "sunburst" appearance due to massive circumferential destruction of Bowman's capsule. Uninvolved glomeruli are typically normocellular. In the chronic or healing phase of the disease there is segmental and global glomerulosclerosis with focal fibrocellular and fibrous crescents. While there are many similarities, one study documents biopsy differences between MPA and GPA patients. Biopsies from patients with MPA and patients who are MPO-ANCA positive were more likely to show glomerulosclerosis, interstitial fibrosis, and tubular atrophy.[303] This suggests a more prolonged, less fulminant course in patients with MPA compared with GPA. An international classification differentiates glomerular lesions depending on whether they are focal, crescentic, mixed, or sclerotic and found correlates with clinical outcome.[393]

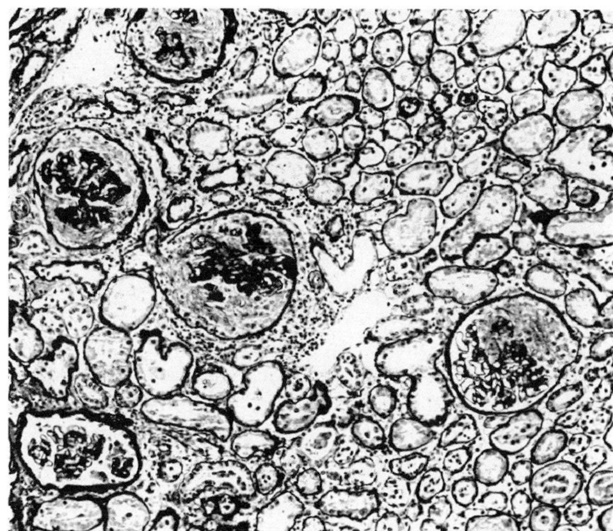

**Fig. 32.16** Microscopic polyangiitis. There are diffuse crescents with focal segmental necrosis of the glomerular tuft (Jones methenamine silver, ×125).

Patients with MPA infrequently have a true arteritis identified on renal biopsy. The frequency ranges from 11% to 22% with predominant involvement of interlobular arteries and arterioles.[392] Involvement is circumferential, lesions are generally of the same age, and aneurysm formation is rare. The acute vasculitis is usually necrotizing with fibrinoid necrosis of the vessel wall and infiltration by neutrophils and mononuclear leukocytes. Vasculitis with granulomatous features is uncommon. In later stages of the disease there may be narrowing of the lumens of small arteries due to concentric intimal fibroplasia and elastic reduplication, but medial scarring is less frequent and severe than in classic polyarteritis nodosa (PAN). In MPA there is often a diffuse interstitial inflammatory cell infiltrate with plasma cells, lymphocytes, polymorphonuclear leukocytes, and sometimes eosinophils especially around glomeruli and vessels. Interstitial inflammatory cells may penetrate the tubular basement membrane causing tubulitis.[392] In more chronic stages there is patchy tubular atrophy with interstitial fibrosis that parallels the distribution of the glomerular and vascular damage.

#### Immunofluorescence and Electron Microscopic Findings

In most cases the glomeruli show no or only weak IF staining consistent with the designation "pauci-immune" glomerulonephritis.[392,393] A review of a number of large series reported positivity for one or another immunoglobulin in 3% to 35% of cases with great heterogeneity and variability of intensity.[392] Fibrin/fibrinogen was the most common and intensely staining reactant identified in the glomeruli, followed by C3 with relatively sparse and weak IgG and Clq.[392,393] The pattern is thought to be consistent with "nonspecific trapping" rather than immune complex deposition. Vascular staining is similar.

By EM, the glomeruli in most patients with MPA have no or rarely sparse irregular, glomerular electron-dense deposits.[392,393] Glomeruli may show endothelial swelling, subendothelial accumulation of "fluffy" electron-lucent material, and subendothelial and intracapillary fibrin deposition. Through gaps in the GBM, fibrin tactoids and neutrophils exude into Bowman's space associated with epithelial crescents. Vascular changes have included swelling and focal degeneration of the endothelium; separation of the endothelium from its basement membrane with subendothelial fibrin deposition; and, with severe damage, intraluminal and intramural fibrin deposition, edema, and inflammatory infiltration of the intima and media by leukocytes.[392,393] No discrete electron-dense deposits are found in the vessels. In vessels with chronic changes, there may be expansion of the intima by concentric layers of fibrous or fibroelastic tissue, with focal scarring of the media.

### PATHOGENESIS

ANCA is felt to play a pathogenetic role in ANCA-associated MPA and glomerulonephritis in a manner similar to GPA (see the "Antiglomerular Basement Membrane Disease and Goodpasture Syndrome" section[305,307,308]; also see the section on GPA). There is initial priming of the neutrophil with cytokines and other mediators of inflammation, perhaps in response to infection, leading to expression of MPO-ANCA antigens on the surface of the neutrophil. These exposed antigens are then poised to react with circulating ANCAs. Neutrophils become activated and undergo a respiratory burst, with degranulation and release of reactive oxygen species onto endothelial surfaces. In drug-induced MPA, although ANCAs develop in relation to many different antigens (elastase, cathepsin G, lactoferrin, etc.), only patients with high titers of high avidity and complement-binding-specific anti-MPO antibodies develop the disease.[391]

### CLINICAL FEATURES

Patients with ANCA-negative pauci-immune focal segmental necrotizing glomerulonephritis and ANCA-positive RPGN have similar clinical findings and presentations regardless of whether vasculitis has been documented on renal biopsy.[287–290] Because MPA is a multisystem disease with various organs involved, many of the clinical findings are similar to those of ANCA-positive GPA, including the development of cutaneous disease, rheumatologic involvement, and neurologic disease. Pulmonary disease is common and presents with shortness of breath, dyspnea, cough, and wheezing.[287–290]

### LABORATORY TESTS

Abnormal laboratory tests may include a normochromic, normocytic anemia, thrombocytopenia, and a mild leukocytosis, at times with eosinophilia.[287–291] Nonspecific inflammatory markers such as the ESR and CRP are often elevated. ANA, serum complement levels, and cryoglobulins are normal or negative.

The widespread use of accurate enzyme-linked immunosorbent assay (ELISA)-based assays for ANCA has facilitated the clinical diagnosis of MPA.[287–291] There is considerable clinical overlap between patients with MPA, GPA, and EGPA, and all may have high rates of ANCA positivity. Although C-ANCA-positive patients are more likely to have biopsy-proven necrotizing vasculitis or granulomatous inflammation of the sinuses or lower respiratory tract, there is a large overlap in the clinical manifestations between C-ANCA-positive and P-ANCA-positive patients. For example, in a recent clinical trial of 198 patients with ANCA-positive disease, 75% of patients were clinically GPA, but only 67% were anti-PR3 positive.[367] Likewise, 25% of patients were clinically MPA, but 33% were anti-MPO positive. ANCA titers vary considerably among patients with similar clinical manifestations, and the role of the titer in predicting flares of the disease is not fully defined (see the "Granulomatosis with Polyangiitis" section under "ANCA-Associated Vasculitis"). Some patients will retain high ANCA levels despite clinical remission, and some patients are positive for anti-GBM antibodies as well as ANCA (see the "Antiglomerular Basement Membrane Disease and Goodpasture Syndrome" section).

### RENAL FINDINGS

Most MPA patients will have laboratory evidence of renal involvement at presentation with urinary sediment changes of microscopic hematuria and erythrocyte casts.[287–291] Proteinuria is common but the nephrotic syndrome is not. A decreased GFR is common in unselected series, and even more common in those selected for renal involvement. Severe renal insufficiency may be found at presentation. These renal findings are similar in patients with ANCA-positive RPGN, whether or not it is associated with systemic involvement.[287–291,303,394] In MPA the severity of the clinical renal findings generally correlates with the degree of glomerular involvement, similar to patients with GPA. Patients with normal serum creatinines or normal creatinine clearances are likely to have greater numbers of normal glomeruli on biopsy, whereas patients with reduced or deteriorating renal function are more likely to exhibit more glomeruli with severe segmental necrotizing glomerulonephritis or diffuse proliferative features.[394,395] Extensive crescent formation correlates with oliguria, severe renal failure, and a residual decrease in GFR after therapy.

### PROGNOSIS AND TREATMENT

Standard treatment for MPA has included cyclophosphamide and corticosteroids in a fashion similar to the treatment of GPA ("Granulomatosis with Polyangiitis" section under "ANCA-Associated Vasculitis"). Controlled trials of the use of intravenous versus oral cyclophosphamide, anti-TNF-α agents, methotrexate, and rituximab have all been examined in populations of ANCA-positive vasculitis patients, including those with GPA and MPA.[350,351,355,356,360,366,367,369,370,374] These regimens are discussed extensively in the section on GPA. In most studies both MPO- and PR3-ANCA-positive patients have responded equally. Likewise, the presence or absence of systemic symptoms has not dictated the response. However, even patients with a good initial response to therapy may suffer residual glomerular damage and progress to ESKD.[396]

Thus aggressive, vigorous early therapy to turn off the disease process is thought to be crucial in preventing residual organ damage. Therapeutic intervention in addition to immunosuppressive therapy includes measures to prevent nonimmunologic glomerular disease progression such as the use of renin–angiotensin–aldosterone blockade, control of dyslipidemia, antihypertensive therapy, and low-protein diets in some patients.

## EOSINOPHILIC GRANULOMATOSIS WITH POLYANGIITIS

EGPA (formerly designated Churg–Strauss syndrome or allergic granulomatosis and angiitis) is an uncommon multisystemic disease characterized by vasculitis, asthma, allergic rhinitis, organ infiltration by eosinophils, and peripheral eosinophilia.[397–400] There may be some overlap with other vasculitic and allergic processes such as GPA, MPA, PAN, Loeffler syndrome, and chronic eosinophilic pneumonitis.[397–400]

EGPA is the least frequent of the ANCA-associated small vessel vasculitides.[397–403] In a review of almost 185,000 asthmatic patients taking medications, only 21 cases of EGPA were identified.[401] The low incidence may reflect, in part, underrecognition. EGPA is part of the differential diagnosis of eosinophilic pulmonary diseases which include eosinophilic pneumonia, allergic bronchopulmonary aspergillosis, and disseminated strongyloidiasis, among other entities.[404] Diagnostic criteria from several sources which include clinical criteria (asthma, greater than 10% peripheral blood eosinophilia, neuropathy, transient pulmonary infiltrates, paranasal abnormalities, and extravascular eosinophilic infiltrates) and combined clinical and histopathologic criteria (eosinophil-rich granulomatous inflammation, necrotizing vasculitis with eosinophilia and asthma, and the presence of a positive ANCA test) are highly sensitive and specific for diagnosing the disease.[405–407] There is no gender predominance in EGPA, and the mean age at diagnosis is around 40 years.[397–403] Clinical renal involvement is clearly less prevalent than morphologic renal involvement. In autopsy series, the kidney is affected in more than 50% of patients, whereas clinical renal disease has been described in 25% to more than 90% of patients.[398–403]

A number of studies describe the rare occurrence of EGPA in steroid-dependent asthmatic patients taking leukotriene receptor antagonists (such as montelukast, zafirlukast, pranlukast), especially during reduction of the steroid therapy.[408–411] While not all investigators have been able to document this association, analysis of published reports does support it.[412,413] This may occur via unmasking of the vasculitic syndrome as the leukotriene receptor antagonist permits the steroid withdrawal. Similar cases have been reported in asthmatic patients following a change from oral to inhaled steroids. Rarely, substitution of a leukotriene receptor antagonist for inhaled steroids has also led to EGPA.[411–413]

### PATHOLOGY

Histologic findings suggestive of EGPA in any organ include a number of the following features: eosinophilic infiltrates, areas of necrosis, an eosinophilic giant cell vasculitis of small arteries and veins, and interstitial and perivascular granulomas. Renal biopsies in EGPA vary from normal kidney tissue to severe glomerulonephritis, vasculitis, and interstitial inflammation.[392,397,398,414] There may be a focal segmental necrotizing

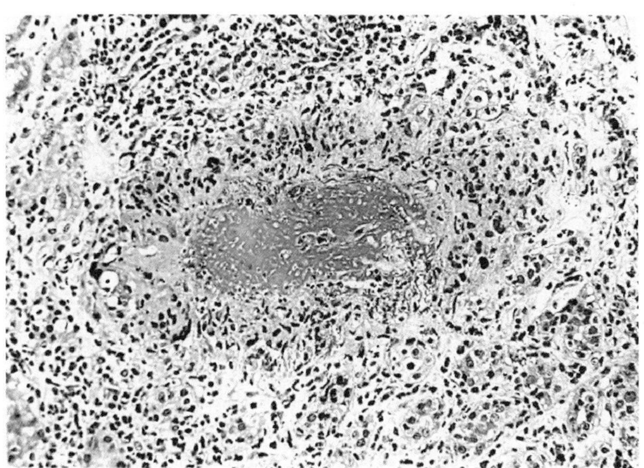

**Fig. 32.17** Eosinophilic granulomatosis with polyangiitis. Granulomatous vasculitis involves an arcuate artery. There is granulomatous transmural inflammation with focal giant cells and superimposed luminal thrombosis (hematoxylin–eosin, ×125).

glomerulonephritis, sometimes with small crescents. In most cases the glomerulonephritis is mild, affects only a minority of glomeruli, and involves the tuft segmentally. The glomerulonephritis rarely may be diffuse and global with severe necrotizing features and crescents. In some cases, there is only mesangial hypercellularity without endocapillary proliferation or necrosis.

In the original autopsy studies by Churg and Strauss, vasculitis was found in the kidney in over one half of cases, and it has been noted on renal biopsy as well.[392] It may involve any level of the renal arterial tree from arterioles to large arcuate or interlobar arteries and may vary from fibrinoid necrotizing to granulomatous. Although resembling other forms of vasculitis, the arteritis is characterized by eosinophilic granulocytes within the arterial wall and in the surrounding connective tissue (Fig. 32.17). Vascular lesions may display destruction of elastic membrane, aneurysms, and luminal thrombosis with recanalization, as well as epithelioid cells and multinucleated giant cells in the media, adventitia, and perivascular connective tissue. Active and healed lesions may coexist. Less commonly, venules and small veins of interlobular size are affected, typically with granulomatous features. The tubulointerstitial region is involved by an inflammatory infiltrate containing many eosinophils and some lymphocytes, plasma cells, and polymorphonuclear leukocytes in association with interstitial edema.[392] In some cases there are interstitial granulomas composed of a core of eosinophilic or basophilic necrotic material surrounded by a rim of radially oriented macrophages, giant cells of the Langhans type, and numerous eosinophils. Interstitial nephritis may be present without glomerular pathology.

By IF, areas of segmental necrosis in the glomeruli may contain IgM, C3, and fibrinogen.[399] The presence of IgE in renal or other tissues has not been adequately investigated. EM of the glomeruli, pulmonary granulomas, venules, and capillaries reveals no electron-dense deposits.[392,398–400]

### PATHOGENESIS

Although the pathogenesis of EGPA remains unclear, allergic or hypersensitivity mechanisms are supported by the presence of asthma, hypereosinophilia, and elevated plasma levels of IgE.[397–400,413,415] Eosinophils in patients with EGPA have prolonged survival due to inhibition of CD95-mediated apoptosis and T-cell secretion of eosinophil-activating cytokines. Human eosinophil cationic proteins (ECPs), which are capable of tissue destruction in a variety of hypereosinophilic syndromes, have been found in granulomatous tissue from patients with EGPA.[416,417] Higher serum levels of ECP, soluble IL-2 receptor, and soluble thrombomodulin levels have been associated with disease activity.[368,418] The number of peripheral T-regulatory cells producing IL-10 is reduced in EGPA and the number increases during clinical remission.[419] Hypocomplementemia and circulating immune complexes have rarely been observed, and the negative IF and EM findings do not support an immune complex mechanism. Cell-mediated immunity is likely involved, and high helper-to-suppressor T-cell ratios in the peripheral blood during active disease, as well as a preponderance of helper T cells in the granulomas of skin biopsies, have been reported.[398] In those patients with positive ANCA, the ANCA antibody likely plays a pathogenic role akin to GPA and MPA.[317,318,323]

## CLINICAL AND LABORATORY FEATURES

Patients may have initial constitutional symptoms such as weight loss, fatigue, malaise, and fever.[397–400] Characteristic extrarenal features include asthma (present in >95% of cases), an allergic diathesis, allergic rhinitis, and peripheral eosinophilia.[397–399,403] Asthmatic disease typically precedes the onset of the vasculitis by years, but it may occur simultaneously. The severity of the asthma does not necessarily parallel the severity of the vasculitis. Many patients subsequently develop eosinophilia in the blood along with eosinophilic infiltrates in multiple organs. Disease often involves the heart, with pericarditis, heart failure, and/or ischemic disease; the gastrointestinal tract, with abdominal pain, ulceration, diarrhea, or bowel perforation; and the skin, with subcutaneous nodules, petechiae, and/or purpuric lesions.[397–399,419,420] Peripheral neuropathy with mononeuritis multiplex is common, but migrating polyarthralgias and/or arthritis occur less frequently.[421] The eye, prostate, and genitourinary tract may be involved. Some patients with EGPA have overlapping features with PAN- or other ANCA-positive vasculitides.[397–400]

Laboratory evaluation may reveal anemia, leukocytosis, hypergammaglobulinemia, and elevated ESR and CRP levels.[397–400,402,403] Eosinophilia greater than 10% is universally present and may reach 50% of the total peripheral leukocyte count. The degree of eosinophilia and the ESR may correlate with disease activity as may the levels of ECP, soluble IL-2 receptor, and soluble thrombomodulin levels.[418] Rheumatoid factor is often positive, but serum complement, hepatitis markers, circulating immune complexes, ANAs, and cryoglobulins are usually negative or normal.[397–399,402,403] Elevated serum IgE levels and IgE-containing circulating immune complexes are frequently found. IgG4 levels are elevated in many EGPA patients.[404] Chest radiography may show patchy infiltrates, nodules, diffuse interstitial disease, and pleural effusion.[397–399,422] Pleural effusions may be exudative and contain large numbers of eosinophils.[422] On angiography, visceral aneurysms may be present in patients with both PAN overlap syndromes and classic EGPA. The most frequent findings on computed tomography of the chest include ground glass opacities and areas of consolidation.[404]

ANCA levels are elevated in about 40% of EGPA patients and often correlate with disease severity and, in some, the clinical course of the disease.[397–400,423–426] Most ANCA-positive patients are P-ANCA and anti-MPO positive, but some are C-ANCA and anti-PR3 positive. In one analysis of almost 100 patients 35% were ANCA positive by indirect IF with a perinuclear pattern and anti-MPO specificity in about three-quarters.[424] Patients with clinically active vasculitis and those with active glomerulonephritis are likely to be ANCA positive.[414] Many investigators have found a good correlation between ANCA positivity or ANCA titers and clinical activity, but the correlation between ANCA titer and relapse is less clear.[419,424,426,427] Clearly in some ANCA titers may remain positive despite clinical remissions. In EGPA, ANCA positivity has often correlated with active glomerulonephritis, pulmonary hemorrhage, neuropathy, and the presence of small vessel vasculitis.[397–400,423,425]

Clinical renal involvement in EGPA is quite variable. In one series of 383 patients with EGPA, renal involvement was found in 22%.[426] In another series of 116 patients, many patients had isolated urinary findings and approximately half had AKI.[414] Microscopic hematuria and mild proteinuria are common, but nephrotic-range proteinuria is infrequent. Hypertension is found in 10% to 30% of patients. In one study of patients undergoing renal biopsy, almost 70% had a necrotizing crescentic glomerulonephritis, whereas others had an interstitial eosinophilic nephritis.[414] ANCA was positive in 75% of the patients with nephropathy as opposed to 25% of patients without nephropathy.

## PROGNOSIS, COURSE, AND TREATMENT

Patients may have several phases of the syndrome over many years including an early allergic phase, then an eosinophilic phase, and finally a vasculitic phase.[397–399,402–404,426] There may be a prodromal phase of asthma or allergic rhinitis followed by a phase of peripheral blood and tissue eosinophilia that is remitting and relapsing over months to years before the development of systemic vasculitis. A shorter duration of asthma prior to the onset of vasculitis has been associated with a worse prognosis. The correlation between ANCA levels and disease activity has been variable. In general, renal disease is mild, with only 7% of patients in one large literature review having renal failure as a cause of death, even including untreated patients.[399] However, cases progressing to severe renal failure and dialysis have certainly been reported.[403] Most patients surviving the initial insult fare well with survival rates in treated patients of approximately 90% at 1 year and 70% at 5 years.[397–399,402,403,426] Patients with significant cardiac, central nervous system, and gastrointestinal involvement, and those with greater degrees of renal damage have a poorer long-term survival. A five-factor scoring system giving one point for each of five variables (age >65 years, cardiac involvement, gastrointestinal involvement, renal insufficiency, and absence of ENT involvement) at onset predicts outcome well in EGPA. For those with scores of 0, 1, or 2 and more, the 5-year mortality rate was 9%, 21%, and 40%, respectively.[428]

Corticosteroid therapy is the primary treatment for many patients with EGPA with mild disease and those with interstitial disease.[397–399,402,403,426] Patients may respond rapidly to high daily oral prednisone therapy, and even relapses respond to retreatment. Extrarenal disease often responds as well. In patients with multisystem disease, with necrotizing glomerulonephritis, and other signs of severe organ involvement, or for those with resistant or relapsing disease, other immunosuppression has been used together with corticosteroids.[429] These agents have included cyclophosphamide, azathioprine, methotrexate, leflunomide, MMF, IFN-α, intravenous immunoglobulin, TNF blocking agents, and plasma exchange.[397–399,402,403,426,430,431]

Rituximab has been shown in case reports and small series to be effective therapy for EGPA in refractory and relapsing cases.[432,433] Omalizumab (a monoclonal antibody directed against the IgE receptor has been used successfully in steroid-resistant patients)[434] and mepolizumab (a humanized monoclonal antibody to IL-5, which activates eosinophilic inflammation) has recently been associated with positive results in a phase 3 trial in EGPA.[435]

Although the prognosis for recovery is good, some patients progress to dialysis and others relapse or have chronic sequelae such as permanent peripheral neuropathy, chronic pulmonary changes, and hypertension.

## GLOMERULAR INVOLVEMENT IN OTHER VASCULITIDES

### POLYARTERITIS NODOSA (CLASSIC MACROSCOPIC POLYARTERITIS NODOSA)

Classic PAN is a systemic necrotizing vasculitis primarily affecting medium-sized, muscular arteries, often at branch points, producing lesions of varying ages with focal aneurysm formation.[296] A second "microscopic" form was originally described as manifesting necrotizing inflammation of small arteries, veins, and capillaries associated with glomerulonephritis. The microscopic form is now understood to represent ANCA-positive vasculitis and should clearly be considered as part of the spectrum of ANCA-associated small vessel vasculitides (see the sections under ANCA-Associated Vasculitis: Granulomatosis With Polyangiitis and Microscopic Polyangiitis). This section will discuss only "classic" macroscopic PAN.

PAN is more common in males than females and occurs most often in the fifth and sixth decades of life. Incidence studies and prevalence studies show that PAN is uncommon and has a major regional variation.[436] Reduced rates have been noted in parallel to the reduction of hepatitis B viral (HBV) infections.[437] Clinically, the prevalence of renal disease in patients with PAN varies from 64% to 76% in unselected series and virtually 100% in nephrology-based series.[437–440] The prevalence of pathologic renal involvement exceeds that of clinically evident disease. True idiopathic PAN is a primary vasculitis. Classic polyarteritis has also been associated with abuse of amphetamines and other illicit drugs, but it is unclear how many of these patients had associated viral infectious hepatitis.[441] The most common associated illness found in patients with classic PAN is HBV infection. The incidence ranges from 0% to 55% in different series but is probably less than 10% of all cases.[437] HBV-PAN associated with HBV has similar clinical features to idiopathic PAN and often occurs early in the course of HBV infection. It is now classified separately from the idiopathic form of the disease because its pathogenesis and treatment are different.[442] It is unclear how many of these patients have had concomitant HCV infection. In one series of 1200 patients with systemic autoimmune disorders who tested positive for HCV, 78 had PAN.[443] Hairy cell leukemia has also been reported in association with PAN. Recently, a genetic disease affecting children with features similar to PAN has been attributed to the recessive gene for loss of function of adenosine deaminase 2.[442,444,445]

#### PATHOLOGY

In classic PAN the glomeruli are usually unaffected. Some glomeruli may show ischemic retraction of the tuft and sclerosis of Bowman's capsule. Rarely, patients with large vessel vasculitis may also have a focal necrotizing glomerulonephritis akin to that seen in MPA. The vasculitis in classic PAN affects the medium-sized to large arteries (i.e., those of interlobular, arcuate, and interlobar caliber) in a segmental distribution, often producing lesions of different ages, including acute, healing, and chronic lesions.[296,440] Segments of arterial involvement are interspersed with normal areas producing "skip lesions," and even the involved portions of the vessel wall have eccentric inflammation. In areas of active vasculitis there is inflammation of the vessel wall by infiltrates of lymphocytes, polymorphonuclear leukocytes, monocytes, and occasionally eosinophils, which may involve the intima alone, the intima and media, or all three layers of the vessel wall. Lesions are often necrotizing with mural fibrin deposition and rupture of the elastic membranes. Areas of necrosis may lead to aneurysm formation particularly in larger arteries (i.e., arcuate, interlobar), which can be associated with rupture and hemorrhage into the renal parenchyma. Superimposed thrombosis with luminal occlusion is not uncommon. In the healing phase, inflammation subsides and the vessel wall is thickened by concentric cellular proliferation of myointimal cells separated by a loose ground substance. Localized destruction of elastic lamellae is demonstrable with elastic stains. Eventually the media is replaced by areas of broad fibrous scars. There may be almost total occlusion of the vessel lumen by intimal fibroplasia with areas of concentric reduplication and discontinuity of the internal elastic membrane. Wedge-shaped, macroscopic cortical infarcts are common and are usually caused by thrombotic occlusion of the vasculitic lesions.[440] In more chronic phases, tubular atrophy and interstitial fibrosis develop.

Autopsy studies in PAN describe the kidneys as being the most commonly affected organ (65%), followed by the liver (54%), adrenal tissue (41%), pancreas (39%), and, less commonly, muscle and brain.[438–440] Tissues giving high yields when biopsied for diagnostic vasculitic lesions include the testes, sural nerve, skin, rectum, and skeletal muscle.

#### PATHOGENESIS

PAN patients are typically ANCA negative; therefore this form of vasculitis is not thought to be mediated by ANCA. The vasculitis of PAN may involve diverse pathogenetic factors, including humoral vascular immune deposits, cellular immunity, and endothelial cytopathic factors. An immune complex pathogenesis of vasculitis is suggested by experiments of acute serum sickness in which an acute glomerulonephritis is produced alongside a systemic vasculitis resembling PAN.[440] The vasculitis can be largely prevented by complement or neutrophil depletion. The experimental Arthus reaction can also induce a vasculitis resulting from in situ vascular immune complex formation with vessel injury preventable by neutrophil or complement depletion.[446] MRL1 mice develop an immune complex glomerulonephritis with necrotizing vasculitis similar to PAN in association with high levels of circulating immune complexes, predominantly with autoantibodies containing anti-DNA.[447] Viral infection of the muscle cells of the vessel media by murine leukemia virus is also associated with a necrotizing vasculitis and lupus-like syndrome with vascular deposits of immunoglobulin and complement.[448] However, glomerular and vascular immune deposits are rarely found in human PAN despite significant levels of circulating immune complexes.

Two models of cell-mediated vasculitis have been produced experimentally in mice.[449] There is no evidence in these models for vascular immune deposits, and some have a granulomatous form of vasculitis similar to that of PAN in multiple organs. In Kawasaki vasculitis, IgM antiendothelial antibodies directed against endothelial surface antigens inducible by cytokines have been described.[450] Likewise, several viral infections in humans are capable of inducing direct cytopathic injury to arterial endothelium.[440]

### CLINICAL FEATURES

The clinical features of PAN are quite variable. In classic PAN, patients are ANCA negative and typically have findings related to visceral organ infarction and ischemia, including abdominal, cardiac, renal, and neurologic involvement. The most common clinical features relate to constitutional symptoms of fever, weight loss, and malaise. Gastrointestinal involvement may include nausea, vomiting, abdominal pain, gastrointestinal bleeding, bowel infarcts, and perforations.[440,451,452] Liver involvement may be associated with HBV or HCV, and vasculitis of the mesenteric vessels, hepatic arteries, and gallbladder leading to cholecystitis have all been found.[437,452] Patients may develop heart failure, coronary artery ischemia with angina or myocardial infarction, and, less commonly, pericarditis and conduction abnormalities. Disease of the nervous system may be central, with seizures and cerebrovascular accidents, or related to peripheral nerves, with mononeuritis multiplex and peripheral neuropathies.[453–455] Patients may develop muscle weakness, myalgias or myositis, and arthralgias, but frank arthritis is uncommon.[440,456] Other clinical findings relate to disease in the gonads, salivary glands, pancreas, adrenals, ureter, breast, and eyes. In general, with the exception of liver manifestations and arthralgias, there is little difference between the clinical findings of patients who are HBV positive or negative. Cutaneous disease may present with "palpable purpura" owing to leukocytoclastic angiitis, or with petechiae, nodules, papules, livedo reticularis, and skin ulcerations.

### LABORATORY TESTS

No laboratory test is diagnostic of PAN. Abnormal laboratory tests commonly include an elevated ESR, anemia, leukocytosis at times with eosinophilia, and thrombocytosis.[395,437,440] Patients with classic PAN are usually ANCA negative, and the finding of a positive ANCA should suggest the diagnosis of small vessel vasculitis such as MPA, GPA, or EGPA.[435] ANA testing is negative, and patients have normal serum complement values. Tests for rheumatoid factor are often positive. Although cryoglobulins have often been reported to be positive, it is unclear what percentage of cases have had associated viral hepatitis.[440] The incidence of hepatitis B antigenemia has ranged from 0% to 40% of PAN patients, as opposed to less than 10% of unselected patients.[435] Likewise, some patients have positive serologic tests for HCV. Screening for these two forms of hepatitis should be included in all evaluations of patients for PAN as positive results will influence therapy.

## RENAL FINDINGS

The renal manifestations in classic PAN reflect renal ischemia and infarction due to predominant involvement of the larger vessels. Hypertension, which may be mild or severe, is found initially in up to one half of patients and can develop at any time during the course of the disease.[395,437–439,451,457] Presenting renal symptoms are uncommon in PAN, but may include hemorrhage from a renal artery aneurysm, flank pain, and gross hematuria. Although mild proteinuria and microhematuria may be found, signs of glomerulonephritis such as erythrocyte casts and nephritic syndrome are absent.

Angiographic examination of the vasculature in PAN often reveals evidence of vasculitis and wedge-shaped areas of ischemia. Angiograms demonstrate multiple rounded, saccular aneurysms of medium-sized vessels in about 70% of cases, as well as thromboses, stenoses, and other luminal irregularities.[451,458] Aneurysms most commonly involve the hepatic, splanchnic, and renal vessels, are usually bilateral, multiple, and vary in size from 1 to 12 mm.[458] There is no way to clinically predict the presence of aneurysms. Vasculitic changes and even aneurysms can heal over time as documented by angiography, usually correlating with the clinical response of the patient.[457,458] Similar aneurysms have been documented in GPA, SLE, TTP, bacterial endocarditis, and EGPA.

### PROGNOSIS AND TREATMENT

In older studies, untreated patients with PAN had a dismal survival rate.[440] Many patients had a fulminant course with a high early mortality due to acute vasculitis leading to renal failure, gastrointestinal hemorrhage, or acute cardiovascular events. Late mortality has been attributed to chronic vascular changes with chronic renal failure and congestive heart failure.[438,459] In one series of more than 300 PAN patients, there were 20 deaths in the first year among the 109 HBV-positive patients and only 18 deaths among 200 non-HBV-positive PAN patients.[460] Risk factors for early mortality included older age, renal involvement, central nervous system disease, and gastrointestinal involvement. Treatment at that time had no effect on this early mortality, which was due to vasculitis and infection.

Corticosteroid use improved the survival rate of PAN patients significantly, with a 5-year survival rate of approximately 50%.[436] Nevertheless, some patients achieved only partial remissions with long-term morbidity and mortality. Even recent attempts to use corticosteroids alone only in patients with mild disease have led to high relapse rates.[461] The use of cytotoxic immunosuppression in idiopathic PAN has improved the 5-year survival rate to well over 80%.[396,437,458,462,463] While a number of immunosuppressive medications have been used, cyclophosphamide is widely accepted as the most effective agent. Initial therapy of idiopathic PAN usually consists of high doses of cyclophosphamide (e.g., 2 mg/kg/day), commonly given along with high doses of corticosteroids (e.g., prednisone, 1 mg/kg/

day), which are then tapered over time. Many use another less toxic immunosuppressive agent (e.g., azathioprine) for maintenance therapy. However, in one small trial of 19 patients with nonsevere PAN the addition of azathioprine to corticosteroids did not result in improved remission rates, lower relapse rates, or steroid sparing.[464] Successful treatment can lead to complete inactivity of the vasculitic process and even reversal of severe renal failure. For PAN associated with HBV, initial therapy should be with antiviral agents. In severe cases or those without a response to these medications several immunosuppressive regimens have been used. Thus a short 2-week course of corticosteroids with or without plasma exchange followed by antiviral agents has been used in the treatment of PAN associated with HBV and hairy cell leukemia, leading to reduced rates of relapse and mortality. Likewise, for patients with an HCV antiviral therapy would be considered first-line treatment. Hypertension control is an important part of therapy. For those patients with ESKD, immunosuppressive therapy should be continued for 6 to 12 months after the disease appears inactive. Transplantation has been performed in only a limited number of patients with PAN.

## TEMPORAL ARTERITIS (GIANT CELL ARTERITIS)

Temporal arteritis, or giant cell arteritis, is a systemic vasculitis with giant cell involvement targeting medium-sized and large arteries It is characterized by segmental transmural inflammation of medium-sized and large elastic arteries by a mixed infiltrate of lymphocytes, monocytes, polymorphonuclear leukocytes. The size and degree of the vessels involved on temporal artery biopsy correlate with clinical manifestations of the disease and morbidity.[465,466]

The disease is the most common form of arteritis in Western countries.[467–470] Temporal arteritis is primarily a disease of older adults, the average age being 72 years, with more than 95% of patients exceeding 50 years of age.[469,470] Vascular involvement occurs in 10% to 15% of patients with giant cell arteritis.[467,468,471] Temporal arteritis should be suspected in older individuals who present with persistent headaches, abrupt visual disturbances, jaw claudication, symptoms of polymyalgia rheumatica, or unexplained fevers and malaise along with anemia and elevated levels of ESR and CRP. Temporal artery biopsy is the definitive diagnostic test. However, other radiologic tests such as color Doppler ultrasonography, compression ultrasonography, and use of magnetic resonance imaging (MRI) radiologic techniques may give a high rate of sensitivity and specificity.[472–474] The ultrasound compression sign to diagnose temporal giant cell arteritis shows excellent interobserver agreement.[475] Renal manifestations are rare and generally mild, although significant renal involvement has been reported.[467,468,470,471,476]

Some patients may have positive serology for P-ANCA or less commonly C-ANCA. The renal pathology has been described as a focal segmental necrotizing glomerulonephritis with focal crescents and vasculitis, primarily affecting small arteries and arterioles. Rarely, visceral aneurysms are demonstrable angiographically. Whether these cases represent true manifestations of temporal arteritis or forms of “overlap” with small vessel vasculitis is not clear. There are also reports of LN, membranous nephropathy, and renal amyloidosis in patients with temporal arteritis.[476,477]

The most common renal manifestations of mild proteinuria and microhematuria are present in less than 10% of patients. Renal insufficiency is uncommon. Hypertension is infrequent and most often mild to moderate when present. Rare cases of renal failure have been attributed to renal arteritis affecting the main renal artery or its major intraparenchymal branches.[476] In some cases the pathology has been inadequate to diagnose the precise cause of the renal failure. Nephrotic syndrome has been reported in a patient with temporal arteritis and membranous nephropathy, with steroid therapy producing a reduction in proteinuria.[476]

The treatment of temporal arteritis with corticosteroids usually causes rapid and dramatic improvement in general well-being, specific symptomatology, and laboratory abnormalities.[467,468,470,471] Therapy is targeted to avoid the feared complication of anterior ischemic optic neuropathy. Intravenous pulse steroids and a number of corticosteroid-sparing and secondary immunosuppressives have been used successfully.[470,478–481] There are conflicting results as to whether any agent such as methotrexate is equivalent to corticosteroids in efficacy. Because relapses occur commonly, other therapies that are steroid sparing are often needed.[482,483] Some agents, such as cyclophosphamide, have led to good efficacy in steroid-dependent patients.[481,484] Some agents such as infliximab and adalimumab do not appear beneficial,[468,470,471,480] whereas others such as abatacept may reduce relapses without adding to toxicity.[485,486] Recent studies have found tocilizumab to be effective. A small single-center trial of tocilizumab along with corticosteroids showed the efficacy of this agent in induction and maintenance of remission.[487] Recently a large multicenter randomized controlled trial confirmed the efficacy of tocilizumab with regard to sustained corticosteroid-free remission.[488] With corticosteroid use, abnormalities of the urinary sediment disappear, and there is resolution of extracranial large vessel involvement. However, once established, visual loss is often permanent, despite resolution of the active disease process. Exacerbation of systemic vasculitis may occur if corticosteroids are tapered too rapidly.

## TAKAYASU ARTERITIS

Takayasu arteritis is a rare giant cell arteritis of unknown pathogenesis characterized by inflammation and stenosis of medium-sized and large arteries, with a predilection for the aortic arch and its branches.[284,489–492] The disease most commonly affects young women between the ages of 10 and 40, and Asians are much more commonly affected. Although findings are typically confined to the aortic arch (including the subclavian, carotid, and pulmonary arteries), the abdominal aorta and its branches may be affected. The histopathologic findings of the vessels include arteritis with transmural infiltration by lymphocytes, monocytes, polymorphonuclear leukocytes, and multinucleated giant cells. In the chronic phase of the disease, intimal fibroplasia and medial scarring may result in severe vascular stenoses or total luminal obliteration.

Renal disease is usually due to an obliterative arteritis of the main renal artery or narrowing of the renal ostia by abdominal aortitis leading to renovascular hypertension.[490–495] Arteriography is useful to diagnose Takayasu arteritis although computerized tomography, MRI, and positron emission tomography scan imaging also have been used.[496–498]

Laboratory abnormalities reveal mild anemia, elevated ESR, increased levels of CRP, and elevated γ-globulin levels, but other serologic tests such as ANA, VDRL, antistreptolysin O (ASLO), and serum complement levels are normal. Some patients have antiendothelial cell antibodies and others have elevated levels of pentraxin 3, a product of immune and vascular cells produced in response to inflammation.[494,499] Hypertension, which may be severe, occurs in 40% to 60% of patients and has been attributed to decreased elasticity of the aorta, increased renin secretion due to stenosis of major renal arteries, and other mechanisms.[500,501] Although mild proteinuria and hematuria are found in some patients, nephrotic-range proteinuria is uncommon.[502] The serum creatinine is usually normal but may be mildly elevated or associated with a high blood urea nitrogen-to-creatinine ratio suggestive of "prerenal" azotemia. Progressive renal failure is uncommon.[489]

A mild mesangial proliferative glomerulonephritis may occur in patients with Takayasu arteritis.[493–495] Mesangial deposits of IgG, IgM, IgA, C3, and C4 have been reported and mesangial electron-dense deposits are found. Most patients have normal renal function and only mild hematuria and proteinuria. Some patients have had glomerular involvement typical of IgA nephropathy.[489,493] Whether this is coincidental or part of the disease process is unclear. One series of patients with Takayasu arteritis had unusual glomerular histopathology with mesangial sclerosis and nodules, as well as mesangiolysis and glomerular microaneurysms resembling a chronic thrombotic microangiopathy or diabetic glomerulosclerosis.[493] IF and EM in these cases of "centrolobular mesangiopathy" did not support an immune pathogenesis. There are also reports of renal amyloidosis, MPGN, crescentic glomerulonephritis, and proliferative glomerulonephritis.[503,504]

### TREATMENT

In the majority of patients, corticosteroids are effective therapy for the vasculitis and systemic symptoms.[502,505] Other medications, including azathioprine, methotrexate, leflunomide, cyclophosphamide, and MMF, and anti-TNF therapy have also been used successfully in some individuals, as have anticoagulants, vasodilators, and acetylsalicylic acid.[506–509] Recent reports of the use of tocilizumab, a monoclonal antibody against the IL-6 receptor, have been promising.[510,511] A small controlled trial, although it did not meet its primary endpoint, did suggest that the addition of tocilizumab to corticosteroids delayed time to relapse.[512] Residual morbidity and mortality in Takayasu arteritis may result from the progressive fibrosis and stenosis of previously inflamed arteries.[513]

## HENOCH–SCHÖNLEIN PURPURA

Henoch–Schönlein purpura (HSP), also called IgA vasculitis, is a systemic vasculitic syndrome with involvement of the skin, gastrointestinal tract, and joints in association with a characteristic glomerulonephritis. In HSP, IgA-containing immune complexes deposit in association with an inflammatory reaction of the vessels. In the skin this leads to a leukocytoclastic angiitis with petechiae and purpura. In the gastrointestinal tract, there may be ulcerations, pain, and bleeding. In the kidney, an immune complex–mediated glomerulonephritis is found.[514–516]

Males are slightly more commonly affected with HSP than are females, and children are affected far more frequently than adults.[514,515,517–523] HSP is the most common vasculitis of childhood. The peak age of patients with HSP is approximately 5 to 10 years as opposed to IgA nephropathy, which has a broad age distribution.[514,515,517–520,524] HSP may account for up to 15% of all glomerulonephritis in young children. More severe renal disease occurs in older children and adults.[521,525] HSP, like IgA nephropathy, is uncommon in blacks. Familial occurrence has rarely been reported, and the frequency of HLA-Bw35 is increased in some series.[515–518] About one-fourth of patients will have a history of allergy, but exacerbations related to a specific allergen are rare. Relapses of the syndrome have occurred after exposure to allergens or the cold, and seasonal variations show peak occurrence in the winter months.

HSP may be mistaken for systemic illnesses such as SLE and MPA, with ongoing infections such as meningococcemia, gonococcemia, and *Yersinia* enterocolitis, with certain medications and vaccination-related hypersensitivity, and with some postinfectious glomerulonephritides associated with systemic manifestations. Although an upper respiratory infection precedes HSP in 30% to 50% of patients, serologic evidence of streptococcal infection is often lacking.

### CLINICAL FINDINGS

The classic tetrad of findings in HSP is dermal involvement, gastrointestinal disease, joint involvement, and glomerulonephritis, but not all patients will have clinical involvement of all organ systems.[514–516,526] Constitutional symptoms may include fever, malaise, fatigue, and weakness. Skin lesions are almost universal with HSP and are commonly found on the lower and upper extremities but may also be on the buttocks or elsewhere.[514–516,525] They are characterized by urticarial macular and papular reddish-violaceous lesions that do not blanch. Lesions may be discrete or may coalesce into palpable purpura associated with lower extremity edema. New crops of lesions may recur over weeks or months. On skin biopsy, there is a leukocytoclastic angiitis with evidence of IgA-containing immune complexes along with IgG, C3, properdin but not C4 or C1q. Gastrointestinal manifestations are present in 25% to 90% of patients and may include colicky pain, nausea and vomiting, melena, and hematochezia.[514–516,525–528] Abdominal pains may be mistaken for appendicitis, cholecystitis, or surgical emergencies, leading to exploratory laparotomy. One study of over 260 patients found that 58% had abdominal pain and 18% evidence of gastrointestinal bleeding.[528] Endoscopy may reveal purpuric lesions, and rarely patients may develop areas of intussusception or perforation. Rheumatologic disease involves the larger joints, usually the ankles and knees, and less commonly the elbows and wrists. There may be arthralgias or frank arthritis with painful, tender effusions, but patients do not develop joint deformities or erosive arthritis. Rarely, patients will have evidence of involvement of other organs (e.g., lungs, central nervous system, or ureters). Adults with HSP may present differently from children. In the largest recent study of 250 adults with HSP, manifestations at presentation included purpura (100%), arthritis/arthralgias/myalgias (61%), gastrointestinal involvement (53%), and glomerulonephritis (70%).[514–516,525,529]

Renal involvement at presentation varies from 20% to 50% of patients with HSP.[514,515,522,525] Renal disease is more frequent and of greater severity in older children and adults, and in general the severity of the clinical disease correlates with biopsy findings and outcome.[522,525,530,531] In studies routinely examining the urine, renal involvement ranges from 40% to 60% of patients. The onset of active renal disease usually follows within days to weeks after the onset of the systemic manifestations and is characterized by microscopic hematuria, active urinary sediment, and proteinuria.[514,516,525,532] In one series of more than 200 children, HSP nephritis occurred in 46% of patients at a mean of 14 days and within 1 month in the majority.[532] In a series of 250 adults with HSP, 32% had renal insufficiency, usually with proteinuria (97%) and hematuria (93%).[525] Some patients will develop nephrotic syndrome and some will have a nephritic picture. There is no relationship between the severity of extrarenal organ involvement and the severity of the renal lesions.

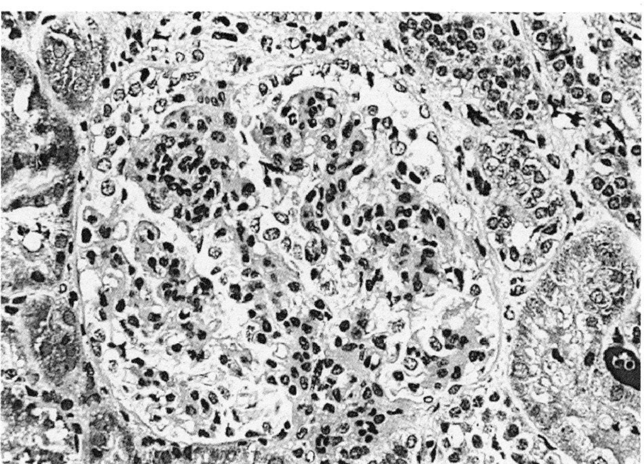

**Fig. 32.18** Henoch–Schönlein purpura nephritis. An example with global mesangial proliferation and focal infiltrating neutrophils (hematoxylin–eosin, ×500).

## LABORATORY FEATURES

In HSP, platelet counts and serum complement levels and other serologic tests are all usually normal.[514,516,526] Serum albumin may be low due to renal or gastrointestinal losses.[526] Serum IgA levels are elevated in up to one half of patients during active illness but do not correlate well with the severity of clinical manifestations or the course of the disease.[514–516,533] Patients with both IgA nephropathy and HSP have high levels of galactose-deficient IgA in their circulation.[534,535] A number of abnormal IgA antibodies have been noted, including IgA rheumatoid factor, circulating immune complexes with IgA and IgG, IgA anticardiolipin antibodies, IgA fibronectin aggregates, IgA anti–α-galactosyl antibodies, and IgA ANCA.[533,536–539] The relationship of these to active renal or systemic disease remains unclear, although concentrations of IgA and IgG immune complexes, IgA rheumatoid factor, and IgG and IgA antigalactosyl antibodies have been correlated with clinical renal disease manifestations.[533,538,540] Recent studies suggest that IgG and IgA autoantibodies against galactose-deficient IgA correlate with clinical outcome.[538]

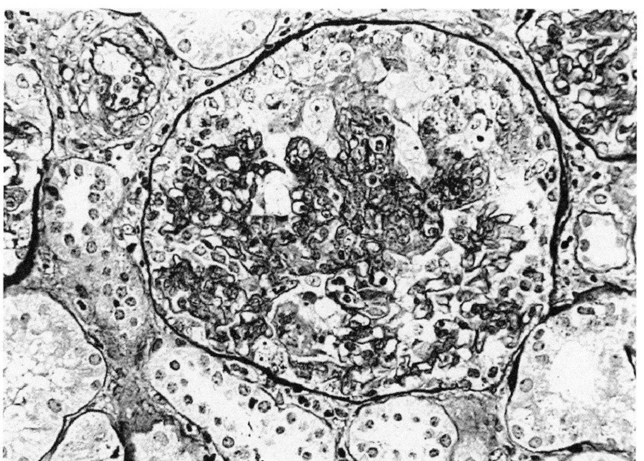

**Fig. 32.19** Henoch–Schönlein purpura nephritis. There is segmental endocapillary proliferation with an overlying segmental cellular crescent (periodic acid–Schiff, ×475).

## PATHOLOGY

The renal biopsy findings of HSP overlap with those of IgA nephropathy. The typical glomerular pathology of HSP is a mesangial and endocapillary proliferative glomerulonephritis with variable crescent formation.[514–516,541] The mesangial changes include both increased mesangial cellularity and matrix expansion that may be focal or diffuse (Fig. 32.18). In severe cases, neutrophils and mononuclear leukocytes also infiltrate the glomerular tufts in areas of endocapillary proliferation, often accompanied by fibrinoid necrosis. Increased numbers of monocyte/macrophages and CD4 and CD8 T cells are found.[542,543] Some cases have a well-developed membranoproliferative pattern with double contours of the GBM. Crescents are common and vary from segmental to circumferential, with evolution from cellular to fibrous crescents over time (Fig. 32.19). Tubulointerstitial changes of atrophy and interstitial fibrosis are consistent with the degree of glomerular damage. In general, endocapillary and extracapillary proliferation and also glomerular fibrin deposition are more frequent and severe in HSP than in IgA nephropathy. The histopathologic classification system proposed by the International Study of Kidney Disease of Childhood correlates the glomerular lesions with clinical manifestations as well as prognosis. These categories include class I, with minimal glomerular alterations; class II, with mesangial proliferation only; class III, with either focal or diffuse mesangial proliferation but less than 50% of glomeruli containing crescents or segmental lesions of thrombosis, necrosis, or sclerosis; class IV, with similar mesangial proliferation as classes IIIa and IIIb, but 50% to 75% of glomeruli with crescents; class V, with similar changes and more than 75% crescents; and class VI, a "pseudo" membranoproliferative pattern.[544] While hematuria is common to all groups, and proteinuria of some degree may be found in all, nephrotic syndrome is present in only 25% of groups I, II, and III. Likewise, groups IIIb, IV, and V tend to have a more progressive course toward renal failure. Even by LM, deposits may be seen in the mesangial regions and rarely along the capillary walls. It is unusual to find the presence of vasculitis on renal biopsy.

By IF, IgA is the dominant or codominant immunoglobulin. Co-deposits of IgG and IgM, C3, and properdin are common.

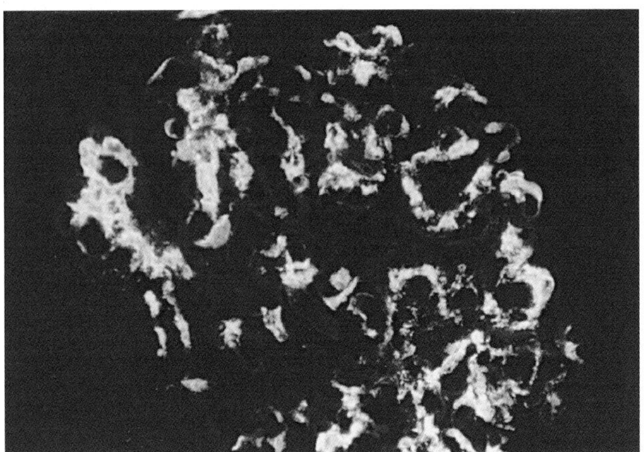

**Fig. 32.20** Henoch–Schönlein purpura nephritis. Immunofluorescence photomicrograph showing intense deposits of IgA distributed throughout the mesangium and also extending into a few peripheral glomerular capillary walls (×600).

Deposits are typically found in the mesangium, especially involving the paramesangial regions, and often extend segmentally into the subendothelial areas (Fig. 32.20).[514–516] Some cases may have more abundant peripheral capillary wall than mesangial deposits. Early classical complement components of C1q and C4 are rarely present. These findings contrast with LN in which IgG usually predominates and C1q is almost always present. The deposited IgA is usually IgA1 subclass and may have the J-chain indicating its polymeric nature, but the secretory fragment is not found.[514–516,545,546] Fibrin-related antigens are also commonly present. IgA may be deposited along with C3 and C5 in both involved and uninvolved skin in the small vessels similar to the findings in IgA nephropathy.[547,548] Similar IgA deposits may also occur in the skin in dermatitis herpetiformis and in SLE along with early and late complement components. IgA is also found in vasculitic lesions in the intestinal tract.[527,528]

By EM, characteristic immune-type electron-dense deposits are found predominantly in the mesangial regions, accompanied by increase in mesangial cellularity and matrix.[514–516,544] In some capillaries, the deposits extend subendothelially from the adjacent mesangial regions. Occasionally, scattered subepithelial deposits are also present and may resemble the humps of poststreptococcal disease. Evidence of coagulation with fibrin and platelet thrombi may be found in capillary lumens. In cases with severe crescent involvement there may be focal rupture of the GBM. Immunoelectron microscopy has confirmed the predominance of IgA in association with some C3 and IgG in the deposits.[541]

## PATHOGENESIS

The pathogenesis of HSP remains unknown. Patients with HSP and their blood relatives, like those with IgA nephropathy, have high circulating levels of galactose-deficient IgA.[534,535] HSP is clearly a systemic immune complex disease (ICD) with IgA-containing deposits that are associated with small vessel vasculitis and capillary damage. The deposits contain polymeric IgA of the IgA1 subclass and late-acting complement components. This composition suggests complement activation of the alternate or lectin pathway. Patients with IgA nephropathy have increased levels of IgG and IgA antibodies directed against galactose-deficient IgA molecules.[536] They also have evidence of oxidative stress on proteins in their circulation along with the high levels of galactose-deficient IgA.[523,549] Certain genetic polymorphisms of the inducible nitric oxide synthase gene have been found to associate with nephritis in HSP patients.[550] Evidence for preceding infections is stronger in children than adults with HSP and may be an etiologic factor in the pathogenesis in some predisposed individuals. This combination may trigger autoantibody and immune complex formation. It is unclear whether IgA immune complexes trigger complement activation and what the ultimate role of complement participation is. The presence of circulating polymeric IgA complexes, the deposition of IgA in the kidney as well as the skin, intestines, and other organs, and recurrence of disease in the allograft point to the systemic nature of the disease process. The precise mechanism(s) whereby IgA deposition causes tissue injury is unclear because IgA is deposited in some diseases such as celiac disease and chronic liver disease without causing major clinical glomerular damage.[551] Complement activation, platelet activation and coagulation, vasoactive prostanoids, cytokines, and growth factors are thought to play a role. Impaired T-cell activity has also been implicated in the pathogenesis of HSP.[552] HSP has also been reported in rare patients with IgA monoclonal gammopathy.[553]

The relationship of HSP to IgA nephropathy is not fully defined with some investigators considering the diseases separate entities and most describing them as opposite ends of a pathogenetic spectrum.[520] Similar renal histologic findings and similar immunologic abnormalities such as elevated circulating galactose-deficient IgA levels, IgA fibronectin aggregates, and antimesangial cell antibodies suggest a common mechanism of renal injury. IgG autoantibodies against mesangial cells parallel the course of the renal disease. Both IgA nephropathy and HSP have occurred in different members of the same families and in monozygotic twins after adenovirus infection.[520] Infectious agents associated with the occurrence of HSP have included varicella, measles, adenovirus, HBV and/or HCV, *Yersinia* spp., *Shigella* spp., *Mycoplasma*, HIV infection, and staphylococci including methicillin-resistant organisms, but none has been proven to be a causal agent.[515,554–556] Likewise, HSP has been reported to occur in association with vaccinations, insect bites, cold exposure, and trauma, although the causal relationship is unproven.[557]

## COURSE, PROGNOSIS, AND TREATMENT

In most patients HSP is a self-limited disease with a good long-term outcome.[513,514] Patients may have recurrences of the rash, joint symptoms, and gastrointestinal symptoms for months or years, but most patients have a benign short-term or long-term renal course. In general, there is a good correlation between the initial clinical renal presentation, renal biopsy findings, and the ultimate prognosis.[514–516,527] Patients with focal mesangial involvement and only hematuria and mild proteinuria tend to have an excellent prognosis. In one recent large pediatric study, renal survival was 100%.[532] In another series of 150 patients with 50% renal involvement, only two patients had residual hematuria and no patients had abnormal renal function at 2.5 years.[514] In most series at several years from presentation, more than 50% of the patients had no renal abnormalities, less than 25% had urinary sediment abnormalities or proteinuria, and only 10% had decreased GFR. Less than 10% of patients with severe clinical renal involvement at onset had persistent hypertension or declining GFR over the long term. A review of more than 50 patients followed over 24 years after childhood-onset HSP found seven of 20 with severe HSP at onset with residual renal impairment as adults as opposed to only two of 27 patients with mild initial renal disease.[558] In a long-term follow-up of more than 1100 children with HSP in a retrospective review of published series, no patients with a normal urinalysis developed renal impairment.[559] Renal impairment developed in less than 2% of patients with isolated urinary abnormalities and in 20% of those with full nephritic or nephrotic syndrome. Some patients have a relapsing course. In one series of over 400 patients, one-third had a relapse usually not long after initial remission of symptoms.[560] Renal relapses were found in one-fourth of patients and ultimately 8% of these relapsing patients had significant renal sequelae.

Long-term renal function is not as good in adults with HSP.[525,540,558,561,562] In a series of over 250 adults with HSP followed almost 15 years, 11% developed ESKD, 13% severe renal impairment with a clearance less than 30 mL/min, and 15% moderate renal insufficiency.[525] A poor renal prognosis is predicted by an acute nephritic presentation, older age, and especially by larger amounts of proteinuria and more severe nephrotic syndrome.[540,561–563] In one retrospective analysis of 219 patients with HSP and nephritis, no findings at initial diagnosis were predictive of ultimate functional decline, but higher proteinuria levels at follow-up did correlate with this decline.[540] On renal biopsy, a poor prognosis is predicted by IgA deposits extending from the mesangium into the peripheral capillary walls, increased interstitial fibrosis, glomerular fibrinoid necrosis, and especially a greater percentage of crescents.[525,540,562] In one study of over 150 children with HSP, those with greater than 50% of glomeruli-containing crescents had progression to ESKD in more than one-third of cases and chronic renal insufficiency developed in another 18%. Repeat biopsies in patients with HSP who have clinically improved show decreased mesangial deposits and less hypercellularity. Markers of oxidative stress on plasma proteins, circulating levels of galactose-deficient IgA, and the level of IgG and IgA antibodies directed against galactose-deficient IgA have correlated with renal prognosis.[535,538,549] While complete clinical recovery occurs in 95% of affected children, many adults with HSP have a lower recovery rate; those with nephritic syndrome, renal insufficiency, hypertension, a large percentage of glomeruli with crescents, and tubulointerstitial fibrosis are likely to have progressive disease.[540,562] More than one-third of HSP patients who become pregnant have associated hypertension or proteinuria. Mortality in HSP is less than 10% at 10 years.

The 2 weeks of corticosteroid therapy had no effect on proteinuria over time. Therapy for the majority of patients with HSP has been mostly supportive, with symptomatic pain medications and blood pressure control.[514–516] Most fare well despite the lack of any immunosuppressive intervention. The use of corticosteroids is controversial, and although they are associated with decreased abdominal and rheumatologic symptoms, they have not clearly been proven to ameliorate the renal lesions or alter the clinical course in any controlled fashion.[526,564–566] Controlled randomized trials have also shown benefit on reductions of proteinuria and preservation of renal function with longer follow-up after an approximately 6-month short course of corticosteroids in patients with IgA nephropathy.[567–569] Because the renal pathology is the same, one might extrapolate these to HSP patients. HSP patients with more severe clinical features, and especially those with nephrotic syndrome or more crescents on biopsy, have also been treated with azathioprine, cyclophosphamide, chlorambucil, other immunosuppressives, and even plasma exchange.[570–572] Although these reports have shown anecdotal success in reversing the renal progression, controlled trials and other large retrospective studies have not yet shown benefits of using cytotoxic immunosuppressive therapy.[529,563] For example, in one controlled trial of 54 adults with HSP, proliferative glomerulonephritis, and severe systemic manifestations, the addition of cyclophosphamide added no benefit over steroids alone in terms of remissions, renal outcome, or mortality.[573,574] Cyclosporine has been used successfully in a number of patients to control severe proteinuria.[575] Intravenous immune globulin has been used in several patients with nephrotic syndrome and decreased GFR in an uncontrolled nonrandomized but apparently successful fashion.[576]

ESKD occurs in 10% to 30% of adults with HSP at 15 years of follow-up.[521,525] Renal disease due to HSP may recur in the renal allograft.[577–579] As in IgA nephropathy, histologic recurrence is far more common than clinical recurrence. However, graft recurrence may lead to allograft loss in as many as 8% to 14% of patients.[578,579] This may be more common in patients who are transplanted either with living-related donors or while still active clinically within the first few years of developing ESKD. Although the severity of original disease is not correlated with recurrent disease outcome, many would suggest waiting before transplanting a patient with active disease who has reached ESKD. Patient survival after renal transplantation is excellent and reaches 95% at 15 years. Overall 5- and 10-year graft survival is similar to that of patients with IgA nephropathy and other disease leading to transplantation.[577–579]

## ANTIGLOMERULAR BASEMENT MEMBRANE DISEASE AND GOODPASTURE SYNDROME

Anti-GBM disease is caused by circulating antibodies directed against an antigenic site on type IV collagen in the GBM.[580–582] Although the original description of pulmonary hemorrhage and glomerulonephritis long antedated the discovery of the pathogenesis of anti-GBM disease, true Goodpasture syndrome should consist of the triad of (1) proliferative, usually crescentic, glomerulonephritis; (2) pulmonary hemorrhage; and (3) the presence of anti-GBM antibodies.[580–583] In anti-GBM disease the pulmonary hemorrhage may precede, occur concurrently with, or follow the glomerular involvement.[582,584] Some patients with anti-GBM antibodies and glomerulonephritis and hence anti-GBM disease never experience pulmonary involvement and thus do not have true Goodpasture syndrome. Documentation of anti-GBM antibody–induced disease may be via renal biopsy, or by establishing the presence of circulating anti-GBM antibodies.[580,582,584] Indirect IF, although highly specific for diagnosis, requires an experienced pathologist.[585,586] Radioimmunoassay, enzyme-linked immunosorbent assay, and immunoblotting for the antibodies are highly specific and sensitive and readily available.[580,586]

## PATHOGENESIS

Anti-GBM autoantibodies, produced in response to an unknown inciting stimulus, react with epitopes on the noncollagenous domain of the α3 and α5 chains of type IV collagen.[580–583] The antigenic epitope has been localized between amino acids 198 and 237 of the terminal region of the α3-chain.[580,581,584,587] The alpha 3 chain of type IV collagen is found predominantly in the GBM and alveolar capillary basement membranes, which correlates with the limited distribution of disease involvement in Goodpasture syndrome.[580,581,583] Goodpasture syndrome is now considered an autoimmune "conformeropathy" involving perturbation of the quaternary structure of the α345 NC1 hexamer of type IV collagen.[580,581,587] In Goodpasture disease, autoantibodies to both the α3 NC1 and the α5 NC1 domains bind to the kidneys and lungs. These autoantibodies bind to epitopes encompassing the Ea region in the α5 NC1 domain and the Ea and Eb region of the α3 NC1 domain, but they do not bind to nondenatured native cross-linked α345 NC1 hexamers.[587] The epitope is identical in the glomeruli and the alveolar basement membranes and may require partial denaturation for full autoantigen exposure. Eluates of antibody from the lung and kidney of patients with Goodpasture syndrome cross-react with GBM and the alveolar basement membrane and can produce disease in animal models.[580,582–584] Antibody reacting with autoantigen(s) and perhaps aided by auto-reactive T cells leads to an inflammatory response, the formation of proliferative glomerulonephritis, breaks in the GBM, and the subsequent extracapillary proliferation with exuberant crescent formation.[580,583] The pathogenetic role of ANCAs found in 10% to 50% of patients with anti-GBM disease needs to be further defined.[588,589] A large retrospective review comparing 568 contemporary patients with AAV, 41 with anti-GBM disease, and 37 "double-positive" patients, found double-positive patients to be older, more likely to recover from severe renal failure, to have a 50% relapse rate, and a mortality similar to both the single ANCA and anti-GBM-positive patients.[590] A role for T cells in Goodpasture syndrome is supported by the T-cell infiltrates on biopsy, patient T-cell proliferation in vitro in response to alpha 3 (α3) type IV NC1 domain, the correlation of autoreactive T cells with disease activity, the role of $CD4^+CD25^+$ regulatory cells controlling the autoreactive T-cell response, and a role for T-cell epitope mimicry in disease induction.[591] Data from animal models suggest that both α3 type IV collagen-specific $T_H1$ and $T_H17$ cells accumulate in the kidney and contribute to the development of anti-GBM nephritis.[592] An initial insult to the pulmonary vascular integrity may be required to produce damage to the basement membranes of the pulmonary capillaries, because alveolar capillaries are not normally permeable to passage of anti-GBM antibodies.[582,593–595] Exacerbations of disease and especially pulmonary disease with hemoptysis have been related to exposure to hydrocarbon fumes, cigarette smoking, hair dyes, metallic dust, D-penicillamine, and cocaine inhalation.[595–597] Although smokers with anti-GBM disease have a higher incidence of pulmonary hemorrhage, circulating anti-GBM antibody levels are no higher than in nonsmokers with the disease.[595,596] Goodpasture syndrome has occasionally been reported in more than one family member. Certain HLA alleles may predispose to the syndrome and perhaps more severe disease.[598] Influenza A2 infection may be associated with Goodpasture syndrome. Clustering of cases in some areas may suggest an environmental trigger for the disease.[599] Anti-GBM disease can also occur in patients with typical membranous nephropathy and in 5% to 10% of patients with Alport syndrome receiving allografts.[600] However, in Alport syndrome patients posttransplantation, the alloantibodies, in contrast to those in anti-GBM disease, bind to the Ea region of the α5 NC1 domain of the intact α345 NC1 hexamer (rather than to denatured hexamer[583]; see the "Hereditary Nephritis, Including Alport Syndrome" section).

## CLINICAL FEATURES

Anti-GBM disease is rare.[580,582–584] Although some studies suggested occurrences as high as 3% to 5% of all glomerular diseases, most reduce this to 1% to 2%. The disease has two peaks of occurrence, the first in younger males, often associated with pulmonary hemorrhage, and the second in older females, often with isolated glomerulonephritis. In the former case, the presence of clinically relevant anti-GBM antibody titers is short-lived. Despite these trends, anti-GBM disease can occur at any age and in either gender.[580,582,583,595,601] Anti-GBM disease limited to the kidney may be more common in older patients. Goodpasture syndrome is less common in blacks, perhaps due to less frequent occurrence of certain predisposing HLAs in this population. An upper respiratory infection precedes the onset of disease in 20% to 60% of cases.[5,79,582,583,595]

The most common extrarenal findings are pulmonary, including cough, dyspnea, and shortness of breath, and hemoptysis, which may vary from trivial amounts to life-threatening amounts associated with exsanguination and suffocation. In almost three-fourths of cases pulmonary hemorrhage precedes or is coincident with the glomerular disease.[580,582,595] Patients infrequently have constitutional symptoms of weakness, fatigue, weight loss, chills, and fevers. Others may have skin rash, hepatosplenomegaly, nausea and vomiting, and arthralgias at onset.[582]

The clinical renal presentation is usually an acute nephritic picture with hypertension, edema, hematuria and active urinary sediment, and reduced renal function. However, only 20% of patients are hypertensive at onset and in some series 15% to 35% have normal urinary sediment and GFR.[580,582,584,601] Renal function is usually already reduced at presentation and may deteriorate from normal to requiring dialysis in a matter of days to weeks.[580,582,601–603] There is a good correlation between the serum creatinine level and the percentage of glomeruli involved by severe crescent formation.

## LABORATORY FINDINGS

Laboratory evaluation typically shows active urinary sediment with red cells and red cell casts.[582] Proteinuria, although common, is usually not in the nephrotic range. Serologic tests such as ASLO, ANA, serum complement levels, rheumatoid factor, and cryoglobulins are all either negative or normal.[582,595,601–603] Circulating anti-GBM antibodies are present in more than 90% of patients, although the antibody titer does not always correlate well with the manifestations or course of either the pulmonary or renal disease.[583] From registry samples of plasma, anti-GBM antibodies have been found in the plasma of patients who eventually develop anti-GBM disease prior to the presentation of clinical disease.[604] Most patients have a decrease in serum antibody titer with time. From 10% to 38% of patients will have both positive anti-GBM antibodies and ANCA usually directed against MPO, but occasionally against PR3.[582,583,604,605] The anti-GBM antibodies in patients who are ANCA positive have the same antigenic specificity as in patients who are ANCA negative.[606] Some studies suggest that the course of patients double positive for anti-GBM antibodies and ANCA parallels that of patients with anti-GBM antibody disease, such that these patients are more likely to develop severe renal failure than those with purely ANCA-positive vasculitis.[605,607] Because ANCA disease is a more common cause of pulmonary renal syndrome, there is a strong possibility that patients with anti-GBM antibodies will also be ANCA positive in this setting. Some patients have a clinical systemic vasculitis with purpura and arthralgias and arthritis, findings rarely seen in isolated Goodpasture syndrome without coexistent ANCA.[605,606] In Goodpasture syndrome a microcytic, hypochromic anemia is common even without overt pulmonary hemorrhage. Other patients may have leukocytosis. Iron deposition in the lungs may be documented by Fe59 scanning, bronchopulmonary lavage, or expectorated sputum showing hemosiderin-laden macrophages.[601] In patients with pulmonary involvement the chest radiograph is abnormal in more than 75% and typically shows infiltrates corresponding to areas of pulmonary hemorrhage. It may also demonstrate atelectasis, pulmonary edema, and areas of coexistent pneumonia. Lung function discloses restrictive ventilatory defects and hypoxemia, and an increased arterial alveolar gradient is present in severe cases.[582,584,601,603]

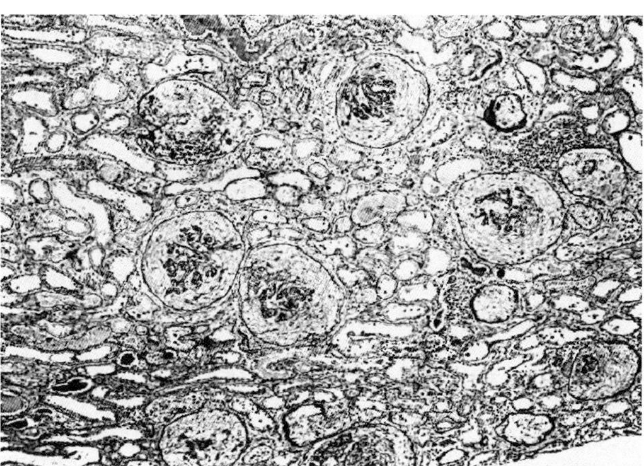

**Fig. 32.21** Antiglomerular basement membrane disease (Goodpasture syndrome). There is diffuse crescentic glomerulonephritis with large circumferential cellular crescents and severe compression of the glomerular tuft (periodic acid–Schiff, ×80).

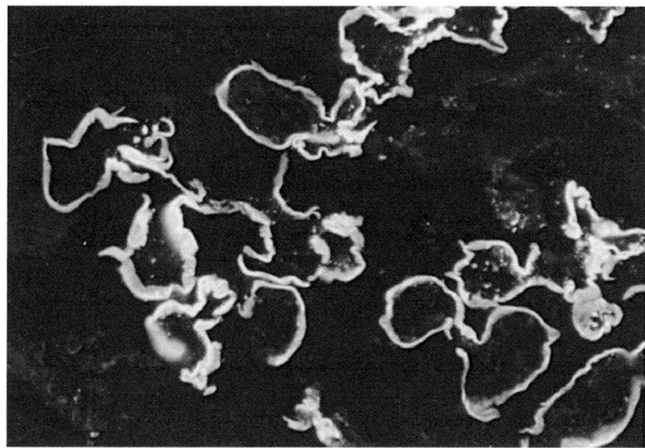

**Fig. 32.22** Antiglomerular basement membrane disease (Goodpasture syndrome). Immunofluorescence photomicrograph showing linear glomerular basement membrane deposits of immunoglobulin G. Some of the glomerular basement membranes are discontinuous, indicating sites of rupture (×800).

## PATHOLOGY

By LM, patients with mild clinical involvement often have a focal, segmental proliferative glomerulonephritis associated with areas of segmental necrosis and overlying small crescents.[582,583,603] However, the most common biopsy picture is diffuse crescentic glomerulonephritis involving more than 50% of glomeruli, with exuberant, predominantly circumferential crescents (Fig. 32.21).[302,584] The underlying tuft is compressed but displays focal necrotizing features. Disruption and destruction of large portions of the GBM and the basal lamina of Bowman's capsule may be seen on silver stain.[302] Early crescents are formed by proliferating glomerular epithelial cells and infiltrating T lymphocytes, monocytes, and polymorphonuclear leukocytes, whereas older ones are composed predominantly of spindled fibroblast-like cells, with few if any infiltrating leukocytes.[302] An associated prominent interstitial inflammatory infiltrate with interstitial edema is common. Multinucleated giant cells may be present in the crescents or tubulointerstitial regions. Some patients, especially those who are ANCA positive, have necrotizing vasculitis of small arteries and arterioles. In biopsies taken later in the disease, there is progressive global and segmental glomerulosclerosis and interstitial fibrosis. Pulmonary histology reveals intraalveolar hemorrhage with widening and disruption of the alveolar septa and accumulations of hemosiderin-laden macrophages.[582,584]

The IF findings define the disease process in Goodpasture syndrome and differentiate it from both pauci-immune– and immune complex–mediated forms of crescentic glomerulonephritis. The diagnostic finding is an intense and diffuse linear staining for IgG, especially IgG1 and IgG4, involving the GBMs (Fig. 32.22).[608,609] Rarely have IgM or IgA been identified in a linear distribution. C3 deposits are found in a more finely granular GBM distribution in many patients. C1q is typically absent. Linear IF staining for IgG may also be found along some tubular basement membranes, particularly distal tubules. Fibrin-related antigens are commonly present within the crescents and segmental necrotizing lesions. In the lungs, similar linear deposition of IgG occurs along the alveolar capillary walls. EM findings typically do not reveal immune-type electron-dense deposits. There may be widening of the subendothelial space by fibrinlike material, and gaps in the GBM and in Bowman's capsule are commonly present.[302]

## COURSE, TREATMENT, AND PROGNOSIS

The course of untreated Goodpasture syndrome is one of progressive renal dysfunction leading to uremia.[583,584,605] In early studies, almost all patients died from either pulmonary hemorrhage or progressive renal failure. Mortality is less than 10% in recent studies, probably related to improved supportive care and more rapid diagnosis and treatment.[582,610] Once the disease is quiescent, relapses are rare in anti-GBM disease as opposed to GPA-, MPA-, and other ANCA-positive vasculitides. Spontaneous remission of the renal disease is extremely rare, although with therapy many patients will have a stable course and some dramatic improvement.[582,610,611] If treatment is started early, patients may regain considerable kidney function. The plasma creatinine correlates fairly well with the degree of crescentic involvement, and if the plasma creatinine is markedly elevated and the patient requires dialysis, most such cases will develop ESKD.[581,582]

There are no large randomized studies defining the benefits of any therapy for anti-GBM disease. While pulmonary hemorrhage and even renal disease have abated in some patients with high-dose oral or intravenous corticosteroids, combination therapy with steroids, cyclophosphamide, and plasmapheresis is now standard.[582,611] A typical treatment regimen might include a combination of oral prednisone (1 mg/kg/day) or intravenous pulse methylprednisolone (30 mg/kg/day up to 1000 mg/day) for several days followed by high-dose oral corticosteroid therapy along with cyclophosphamide (2 mg/kg/day) and plasmapheresis. Plasmapheresis may have a dramatic effect in reversing pulmonary hemorrhage and renal disease when used early in the course in combination with immunosuppressive agents.[582,607] Plasmapheresis removes the circulating anti-GBM antibodies while immunosuppressive therapy prevents new antibody formation and controls the ongoing inflammatory response. One uncontrolled study found that 40% of patients had stabilized or improved renal function with plasmapheresis.[611] Patients with severe renal failure who are already on dialysis or who have serum creatinine levels greater than 5 to 8 mg/dL are less likely to respond to therapy, but some have recovered. Some studies have found that patients who were positive for both anti-GBM antibodies and ANCA behaved similar to those with anti-GBM antibodies alone, with a 1-year renal survival rate of 73% in those with a plasma creatinine concentration of less than 500 µmol/L and 0% in those on dialysis.[611] In other series, patients who are double positive have been older and had a better outcome in terms of renal recovery but a greater likelihood of relapse.[589] A large retrospective review comparing 568 contemporary patients with AAV, 41 with anti-GBM disease, and 37 double-positive patients found double-positive patients to be older, more likely to recover from severe renal failure, to have a 50% relapse rate, and a mortality similar to both the single ANCA and anti-GBM positive patients.[590,605] Although daily plasmapheresis is often maintained for weeks, its frequency can be determined by the rapidity of clinical response. Exacerbations of disease may occur with intercurrent infections. Immunosuppressive therapy is usually continued for 6 months with a tapering regimen to allow spontaneous cessation of autoantibody production. Some patients with early disappearance of circulating anti-GBM antibodies may respond to shorter therapy or tolerate change to less toxic maintenance immunosuppression such as azathioprine. There are limited data on other immunosuppressive regimens in Goodpasture syndrome.[611–615] Rituximab has been used successfully in a small and perhaps biased group of patients.[614] Immunoadsorption and double filtration plasmapheresis have also been used to remove the anti-GBM antibodies in Goodpasture syndrome.[616–618] Even in patients with initial improvement of renal function, some with severe crescentic glomerular involvement will progress to renal failure over time, perhaps related to nonimmunologic progression of disease. The incidence of ESKD in patients with significant glomerular involvement is more than 50%, and the renal outcome is usually progressively downhill unless vigorous prompt therapy is instituted.

Anti-GBM–mediated renal disease rarely recurs in the renal allograft.[589,619–621] De novo anti-GBM disease may appear in patients with hereditary nephritis (see the "Alport Syndrome" section). As with a number of other forms of glomerulonephritis, evidence of histologic recurrence (i.e., linear staining for IgG along GBMs) is far higher than clinical involvement and may be as high as 50%. The low recurrence rate recently reported in transplants probably reflects a combination of waiting sufficient time to document the absence of anti-GBM antibodies, the use of immunosuppressive medications and plasmapheresis to remove current antibody, and the "one-shot" nature of the disease.[620–622] Graft loss secondary to recurrent disease is rare. Patients should not be transplanted during the acute phase of their illness when autoantibody levels are high, and prophylactic pretransplant immunosuppression has been recommended for those receiving allografts from living-related donors. Although patients with resolving pulmonary disease may have residual diminished gas exchange, most pulmonary function tests return to normal and do not limit the renal transplant process.[622]

## SJÖGREN SYNDROME

Sjögren syndrome is characterized by a chronic inflammatory cell infiltration of the exocrine salivary and lacrimal glands and is associated with the "sicca complex" of xerostomia and xerophthalmia.[623–625] Recent classification schema using both clinical and serologic criteria give a 95% specificity and sensitivity for the diagnosis of primary Sjogren syndrome.[626] Systemic manifestations occur in approximately one-third of Sjogren patients.[627] Some patients may have involvement by a systemic inflammatory disease of the kidneys, lungs, esophagus, thyroid, stomach, and pancreas.[623–625] Others have manifestations of a connective tissue disease, most commonly rheumatoid arthritis, and less frequently SLE, scleroderma, polymyositis, or MCTD. Still other patients have different immunologic disorders such as chronic active hepatitis, primary biliary cirrhosis, Crohn disease, and fibrosing alveolitis or develop lymphoma or Waldenström macroglobulinemia. Serologic abnormalities in Sjögren syndrome include hypergammaglobulinemia, rheumatoid factor, cryoglobulins, a homogeneous or speckled pattern ANA, anti-Ro/SSA and anti-La/SSB, but serum complement levels are generally normal unless the patient has associated SLE.[623–625]

The major clinical renal manifestations of patients with Sjögren syndrome usually relate to tubulointerstitial involvement of the kidneys with tubular defects such as a distal renal tubular acidosis, impaired concentrating ability, hypercalciuria, and, less frequently, proximal tubular defects.[623–625,628,629] Most patients have no evidence of glomerular disease. In an analysis of more than 470 patients with primary Sjögren syndrome followed for a mean of 10 years, only 20 patients (4%) developed overt renal disease.[624] Ten patients had interstitial nephritis, eight patients had glomerular lesions, and two had both interstitial nephritis and lesions. In those infrequent patients with glomerular lesions, hematuria, proteinuria, nephrotic syndrome, and renal insufficiency are found. Others may develop renal vasculitis with hypertension and renal insufficiency.

In most cases the renal pathology shows a chronic active interstitial inflammation by a predominantly lymphocytic infiltrate admixed with plasma cells, with variable interstitial fibrosis and tubular atrophy.[623–625,629] A nonspecific glomerulosclerosis with mesangial sclerosis, GBM thickening and wrinkling is found in those with chronic and severe tubulointerstitial damage. Infrequent patients will have immune complex–mediated glomerular involvement.[76,624,625,628–633] In one series of biopsied patients with primary Sjogren syndrome, patients had either mesangial proliferative glomerulonephritis or MPGN.[624] Other series have had SLE features with the similar spectrum of glomerular involvement ranging from mesangial proliferative to focal proliferative, diffuse proliferative, and membranous glomerulonephritis.[76,630–633] A membranoproliferative pattern of glomerulonephritis has been reported in patients with associated cryoglobulinemia.[624,631–633] By IF and EM, immune deposits have been localized in the various patterns to the mesangial region or the subendothelial or subepithelial aspect of the GBM. Some patients with Sjögren syndrome have a necrotizing arteritis of the kidney, occasionally with extrarenal involvement.[634] Most Sjögren patients with tubulointerstitial disease respond to treatment with corticosteroids.[623–625,629] Patients with immune complex glomerulonephritis and Sjögren syndrome are generally treated in a similar fashion to those with SLE, and those with vasculitis generally receive immunosuppressive agents. In patients with systemic involvement rituximab has been used along with corticosteroids with variable long-term success, while use of rituximab for low disease activity has not been shown to be beneficial.[635–638] Small preliminary trials have also used belimumab and abatacept with promising results.[639,640]

## SARCOIDOSIS

Most manifestations of sarcoidosis are not related to the kidney.[641] The kidney can be affected by hypercalcemia. The most common renal findings are granulomatous interstitial nephritis, nephrolithiasis, and tubular functional abnormalities.[642,643] Glomerular disease is infrequent and may be coincidental. Glomerular lesions described include MCD, FSGS, membranous nephropathy, IgA nephropathy, MPGN, and proliferative and crescentic glomerulonephritis with and without a positive ANCA serology.[642–650] The IF and EM features conform to the various histologic patterns. One recent study found one-fourth of 27 patients with biopsied sarcoidosis to have IgA nephropathy. However, demographic features and biopsy selection bias may influence these findings.[651] Some patients have granulomatous renal interstitial nephritis in addition to the glomerular lesions. Glomerular disease in sarcoidosis presents with proteinuria, active urinary sediment at times, and most commonly nephrotic syndrome. Some degree of proteinuria, usually 0.5 to 1 g/day, is common in sarcoid patients with tubulointerstitial disease and no evidence of glomerular lesions. Sarcoid patients have been treated with various forms of immunosuppression, including steroids, depending on their glomerular lesions.[644–650]

## AMYLOIDOSIS

Amyloidosis comprises a diverse group of systemic and local diseases characterized by the extracellular deposition of characteristic fibrils in various organs.[652–655] Although more than 25 different proteins can produce amyloid fibrils, all share an antiparallel β-pleated sheet configuration on X-ray diffraction, leading to their amyloidogenic properties. All amyloid fibrils bind Congo red (leading to diagnostic apple green birefringence under polarized light) and thioflavin T, and have a characteristic ultrastructural appearance with randomly oriented 8- to 12-nm nonbranching fibrils. All amyloids also contain a 25-kDa glycoprotein, serum amyloid P component (SAP), a member of the pentraxin family. Amyloid deposits may also contain restricted sulfated glycosaminoglycans and proteoglycans noncovalently linked to the amyloid fibrils.[652–655] Only some amyloid proteins deposit in the kidney. Most renal amyloidoses are due to either AL amyloidosis or AA amyloidosis. In one series from a referral center for amyloidosis 1.3% of 21,500 renal biopsies over an 8.5-year period were found to have amyloidosis with 86% AL amyloid, 7% AA amyloid, and the remainder being a variety of types of hereditary amyloids.[656] In another single-center series of 474 amyloidosis patients evaluated from 2007 to 2011, 85% were AL amyloid, 7% AA amyloid, and 4% hereditary amyloid.[652] In AL amyloidosis, the deposited fibrils are derived from the variable portion of immunoglobulin light chains produced by a clonal population of plasma cells or plasmacytic B cells. AA amyloid results from the deposition of serum amyloid A (SAA) protein in chronic inflammatory states.[652,653,657] A small fraction of renal amyloidoses is due to rare hereditary forms of amyloidosis, such as those caused by inherited gene mutations encoding transthyretin (ATTR), fibrinogen A α-chain (AFib), apolipoprotein A-I (apo A-I) or A-II (apo A-II), lysozyme (ALys), gelsolin (AGel), and leukocyte chemotactic factor 2 (LECT2) peptide.[654,656,658–660] However, renal amyloidosis caused by ALECT2 defects has been noted more frequently and in some populations (e.g., Latinos from the southwest United States, Punjabis, Native Americans, and Egyptians) this is a more common cause of amyloidosis than AL amyloid.[661] Laser microdissection and mass spectrometry were necessary to determine the origin of some of these unusual amyloid subtypes.[652,656,662,663] Difficulty in IF diagnosis of AL amyloid occurs in as many as 14% to 35% of cases.[652,662,663]

It is unclear what factors confer the propensity for amyloidogenic proteins to fold into a β-pleated sheet and amyloid fibrils.[664–668] Cofactors such as amyloid P component may have an important role in the pathogenesis of tissue deposition. These may act by promoting fibrillogenesis, stabilization of the fibrils, binding to matrix proteins, or inhibiting denaturation and proteolysis. It is also possible that stabilizing cofactors are deposited after fibrillogenesis.[654,657,664–667] Amyloid fibrils generally resist biodegradation and accumulate in the tissues, resulting in organ dysfunction. However, amyloid deposits do exist in a dynamic state and have been shown to regress by radiolabeled SAP scintigraphy.[669] A critical mass of an abnormal protein is necessary to produce clinically significant amyloid of any type.[670] In SAA amyloid the SAA concentration has correlated with amyloid burden and reduction in circulating SAA with regression of amyloid deposits. Patients with AA amyloidosis, such as those with tuberculosis or bronchiectasis, have levels of circulating SAA protein no greater than those with inflammatory diseases who do not have amyloid deposition. Therefore some additional unknown stimuli are required for amyloid fibrils to form and precipitate.[668] In AL amyloid biochemical characteristics of the light chain, such as an aberrant amino acid composition at certain sites, appear important in determining amyloid formation.[671] This may account for the reproducibility of a given form of renal disease (cast nephropathy vs. amyloid) in animal models infused with monoclonal light chains from affected patients.[671] Certain light chains may also form high-molecular-weight aggregates in vitro. Patients with AL amyloid more frequently produce abnormal excessive λ- than κ-light chains, and among AL amyloid patients with renal disease λ-light chains strongly predominate over κ-light chains (by ratio of 12 : 1) as opposed to patients without renal disease (4 : 1).[652–654] Macrophage-dependent generation of preamyloid fragments with chemical properties allowing aggregation may also play a role. Mesangial cells have receptors for light chains and may modify them as well. Amyloid P component may also prevent degradation of amyloid fibrils once formed.[672]

## AL AND AA AMYLOIDOSIS

In AL amyloidosis, fibrils are composed of the N-terminal amino acid residues of the variable region of an immunoglobulin light chain. λ-Light chains predominate over κ-light chains, and there is an increased incidence of monoclonal λ subtype VI.[652–654] The diagnosis of AL amyloidosis may be suspected on clinical grounds but requires biopsy documentation. The kidneys are the most common major organ involved by AL amyloid and most patients eventually develop renal amyloid.[652–654,673] In the past, up to 10% to 20% of patients older than 60 years with presumed idiopathic nephrotic syndrome had amyloidosis on renal biopsy.[674] Multiple myeloma occurs in up to 20% of AL amyloidosis cases. Amyloidosis should be suspected in all patients with circulating serum monoclonal M proteins, and approximately 90% of primary amyloid patients will have a paraprotein spike in the serum or urine by immunofixation,[652,653,673] and a greater percentage will have an elevation and predominance of one circulating light chain. While all AL amyloid patients will have an increased production of amyloidogenic light chains, not all patients with renal disease and a monoclonal protein in the serum will have amyloid. This is especially true in older patients, because 5% of patients older than 70 years of age will have a benign monoclonal gammopathy.[675]

The incidence of AL amyloid is about 8 per million annually, but varies greatly in different locations.[653] Most patients with AL amyloidosis are older than 50 years (median age 59–63 years) and less than 1% are younger than 40 years of age. Men are affected twice as often as women.[652,653,673] Presenting symptoms include weight loss, fatigue, light-headedness, shortness of breath, peripheral edema, pain due to peripheral neuropathy (often carpal tunnel syndrome), and orthostatic hypotension. Patients may have cardiomyopathy, hepatosplenomegaly, macroglossia, or rarely enlarged lymph nodes. Multisystem organ involvement is typical, with most commonly affected organs being the kidney (50%), heart (40%), and peripheral nerves (up to 25%).[652,653,673] In one series, 25% of AL amyloid patients had one major organ system involved, 36% had two organ systems involved, and 38% had three or more involved.[676] However, a recent study comparing the presentation of over 1500 newly diagnosed AL amyloid patients at one referral center from 2000 to 2014 found that patients diagnosed in the most recent period of 2010 to 2014 were less likely to have over two involved organs.[677]

AA amyloidosis occurs in chronic inflammatory diseases and is composed of the N-terminal end of the acute phase reactant SAA protein.[652,654,666,669,678,679] SAA is produced in the liver and circulates in association with high-density lipoprotein. While in Westernized countries AA amyloid is most commonly found in association with rheumatoid arthritis and other inflammatory arthritides, it is also seen with inflammatory bowel disease, familial Mediterranean fever (FMF), quadriplegics with chronic urinary infections and decubitus ulcers, bronchiectasis, poorly treated osteomyelitis, and in chronic heroin addicts who inject drugs subcutaneously.[652,654,666,679–682] In one large multicenter study of 374 patients with AA amyloid, 60% had chronic inflammatory arthritis, 15% chronic infections, 9% periodic fever syndromes, 5% inflammatory bowel disease, 6% other etiologies, and in 6% no etiology was found.[678] In an autopsy study of 150 addicts, 14% of subcutaneous and 26% of those with chronic suppurative infections had renal amyloidosis.[681] In a more recent review from this center of 625 AA amyloid patients seen from 1990 to 2014 there were several epidemiologic changes.[683] Recent patients were older (average age 56 years), South Asians had increased in the population, and there was a reduction in patients with juvenile idiopathic arthritis but an increase in patients with chronic infections due to IV drug abuse and uncharacterized inflammatory diseases. More patients presented in ESKD. AA amyloid typically occurs in older addicts with a long history of substance abuse who have exhausted sites of intravenous access and resorted to "skin popping" or "muscling."[682,684]

The diagnosis of amyloid is usually established by tissue biopsy of an affected organ.[652–654] Liver and kidney biopsy are positive in as many as 90% of clinically affected cases. A diagnosis may be made less invasively with fat pad aspirate (60%–90%), rectal biopsy (50%–80%), bone marrow aspirate (30%–50%), gingival biopsy (60%), or dermal biopsy (50%).[685] SAP whole-body scintigraphy following injection of radiolabeled SAP allows the noninvasive diagnosis of amyloidosis as well as a quantification of the extent of organ system involvement and assessment of the response to treatment.[686] This test may be positive even when tissue biopsy has been negative and may be more accurate in AA than in AL amyloidosis. In AL amyloidosis detection of an abnormal ratio of free κ- to λ-light chains in the serum suggests plasma cell dyscrasias with a higher sensitivity than either serum or urinary protein electrophoresis and immunofixation.[687] It also allows assessment of response to therapy by following the level of abnormal free light chain in the serum.[680] Patients with hereditary amyloidosis due to deposition of abnormal transthyretin, apolipoproteins, lysozyme, or fibrinogen Aa may present in a fashion similar to AL amyloid. In one series 10% of 350 cases of hereditary amyloidosis were misdiagnosed as having AL amyloid.[659]

Although hereditary amyloidoses may present at any age, most patients are adults and present with higher serum creatinines and less proteinuria than those with AL or AA amyloidosis.[652] Targeted genetic testing of patients on dialysis and others with kidney disease in high-risk areas for hereditary amyloid, such as searching for fibrinogen A alpha chain amyloidosis in areas of Portugal, has been rewarding in diagnosing many new involved patients.[688] Some hereditary types lead to predominant amyloid deposition in the tubulointerstitial and medullary compartment (e.g., amyloid due to apo A-I, A-II, A-IV). For example, a recent clinical review of 11 patients with apolipoprotein A-IV-associated amyloidosis showed progressive renal failure with minimal proteinuria and histologically extensive medullary involvement sparing the renal cortex.[689] Other forms of hereditary amyloidosis are associated with massive glomerular obliteration (AFib),[53,652] and still others such as LECT2 deposit in all compartments of the kidney and can lead to progressive kidney failure.[656,690,691] Although the course of hereditary amyloid is often more prolonged and more benign than that of AL amyloid, presentation can be identical and in some forms the progression to CKD and ESKD is rapid. For example, a recent study of 72 patients with ALECT2 amyloid found that one-third developed ESKD in about 2 years.[691] Establishing the correct diagnosis is crucial because the treatment of hereditary amyloid may include liver transplantation rather than chemotherapy or stem cell transplantation as in AL amyloid.[656] Laser dissection of involved glomeruli and proteomic analysis by mass spectrometry, a test currently available in few specialized centers, can accurately diagnose all types of glomerular amyloid.[662]

Clinical manifestations of renal disease depend on the location and extent of amyloid deposition. Renal involvement predominates in AL amyloidosis with one-third to 70% of patients having renal manifestations at presentation.[652–654,692] Most patients have proteinuria, approximately 25% have nephrotic syndrome at diagnosis, and others present with varying degrees of azotemia.[652–654,673] Over time as many as 40% will develop nephrotic syndrome while others will have lesser degrees of proteinuria or azotemia. Urinalysis is typically bland, but microhematuria and cellular casts have been reported. Proteinuria is typically nonselective and almost 90% of patients with more than 1 g/day urinary protein will have a monoclonal protein in the urine. Hypercholesterolemia is less common than in other forms of nephrotic syndrome. The amount of glomerular amyloid deposition by LM does not correlate well with the degree of proteinuria or renal dysfunction.[652,653] Despite the literature's suggestion of enlarged kidneys in AL amyloid, by ultrasonography most patients have normal-sized kidneys.[652] Hypertension is found in 20% to 50% of patients, but many will have orthostatic hypotension due to peripheral neuropathy, autonomic neuropathy, and/or nephrotic syndrome. Patients with AA amyloid typically also have proteinuria and renal dysfunction with a progressive course. Patients with predominantly vascular involvement may have little proteinuria but rather renal insufficiency due to decreased renal blood flow. Infrequently patients will have predominantly tubulointerstitial deposition of amyloid with renal insufficiency and tubular defects such as distal renal tubular acidosis, Fanconi syndrome, and nephrogenic diabetes insipidus.[652,653,673]

## PATHOLOGY

In patients with clinical renal disease, the diagnostic sensitivity of an adequate renal biopsy approaches 100%.[653,657,693,694] Renal biopsy distinguishes AL amyloid from AA amyloid, and excludes involvement by other renal disease in patients with known amyloidosis of other organs.

By LM, there is glomerular deposition of amorphous hyaline material that usually begins in the mesangium and extends into the peripheral capillary walls (Fig. 32.23). Affected glomeruli appear hypocellular and may have a nodular aspect. This deposited material is lightly eosinophilic, weakly PAS positive, and nonargyrophilic in contrast to the findings in diabetic nodular glomerulosclerosis. In the peripheral GBM, amyloid deposits form spicular hairlike projections (Fig. 32.24). Congo red stain gives an orange staining reaction and diagnostic apple green birefringence under polarized light (Fig. 32.25). Amyloid deposits stain metachromatically with crystal or methyl violet and fluoresce under ultraviolet

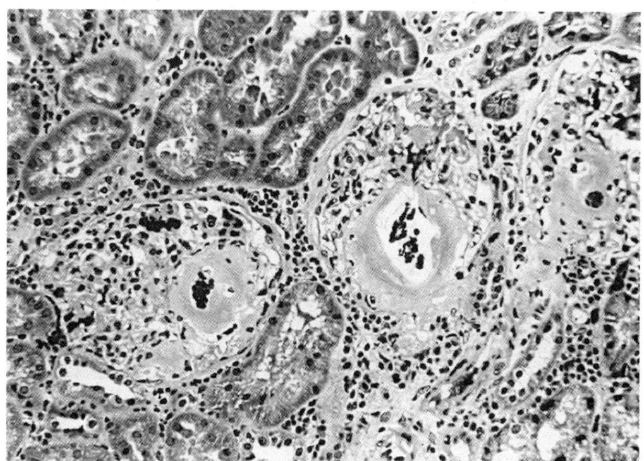

**Fig. 32.23** Amyloidosis. The glomerular tuft contains segmental deposits of amorphous eosinophilic hyaline material involving the vascular pole and some mesangial regions (hematoxylin–eosin, ×375).

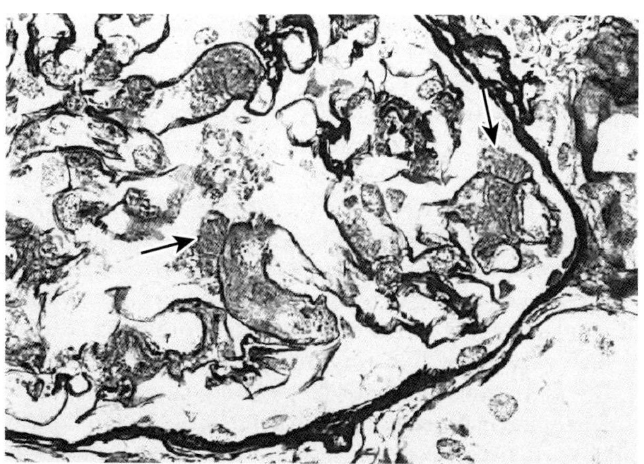

**Fig. 32.24** Amyloidosis. The amyloid deposits expand the mesangium and form focal spicular projections through the glomerular capillary walls, resembling spikes *(arrows)* (Jones methenamine silver, ×800).

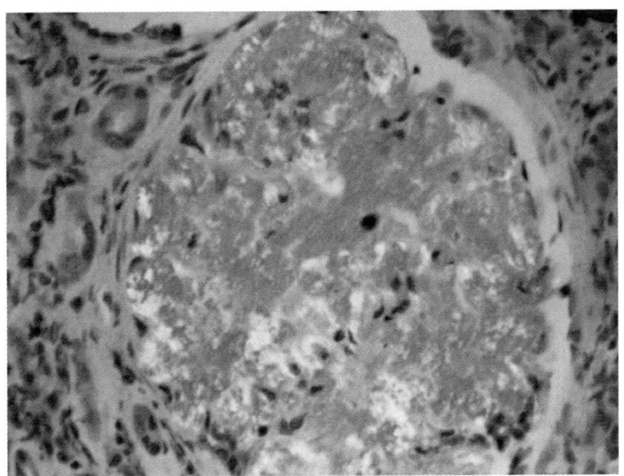

**Fig. 32.25** Amyloidosis. Congo red stain of a glomerulus that is largely replaced by amyloid demonstrates the characteristic birefringence under polarized light (×450).

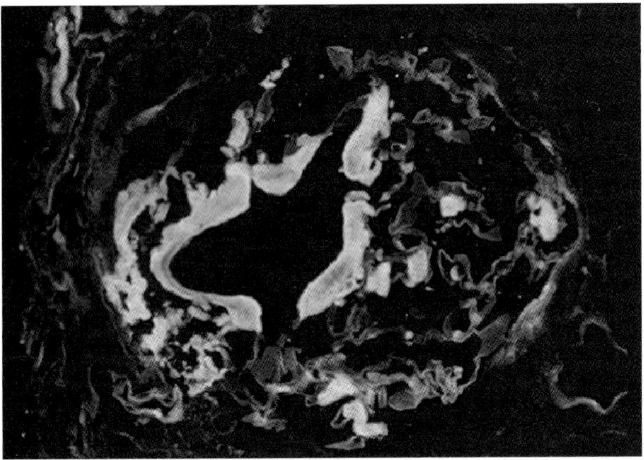

**Fig. 32.26** Amyloidosis. Immunofluorescence photomicrograph showing glomerular staining for lambda light chain in the distribution of the glomerular amyloid deposits in a patient with AL amyloidosis and plasma cell dyscrasia (×600).

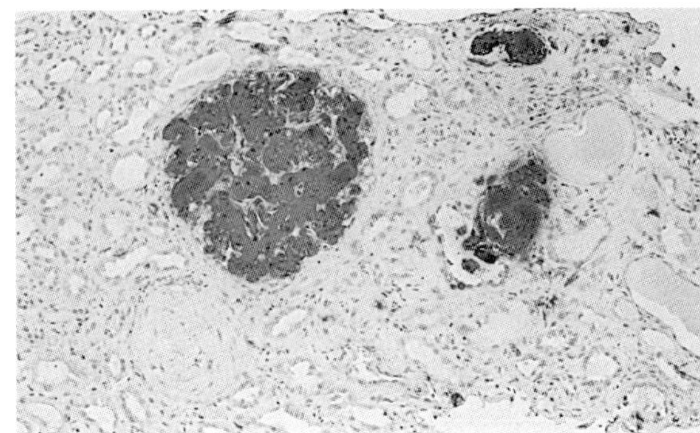

**Fig. 32.27** Amyloidosis. Immunoperoxidase staining for serum amyloid A protein stains the amyloid deposits in the glomeruli and arteries of a patient with secondary (AA) amyloidosis due to rheumatoid arthritis (×125).

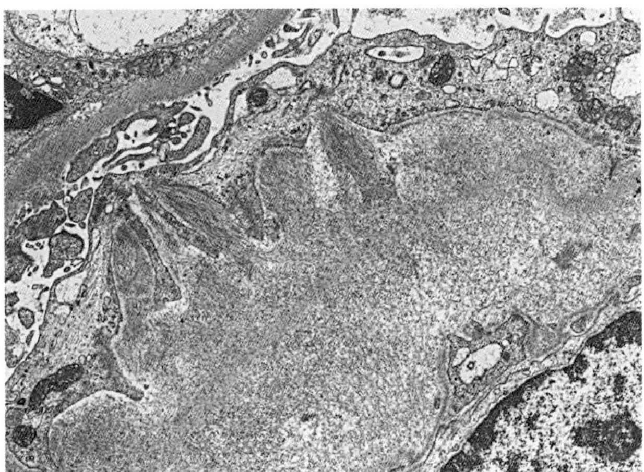

**Fig. 32.28** Amyloidosis. Electron micrograph showing extensive infiltration of the glomerular basement membrane by 10-nm fibrils that project toward the urinary space (×8000).

light following thioflavin T staining. Amyloid deposition may be confined to the glomeruli or involve tubular basement membranes, interstitium, and blood vessels as well. The IF in AL amyloidosis gives strong staining with antisera to the pathogenic light chain, usually λ (Fig. 32.26). Some less-common forms of amyloid derived from Ig precursor proteins contain only Ig heavy chain (AH amyloid) or both heavy and light chain (AHL amyloid). The heavy chain is usually γ (derived from IgG), with less frequent α (IgA) and μ (IgM) forms. In AA amyloidosis, immunostaining for immunoglobulins and complement components is usually negative or gives a generalized weak reactivity due to nonspecific trapping. Diagnosis depends on the demonstration of strong reactivity for SAA protein by IF or immunoperoxidase staining (Fig. 32.27). Hereditary amyloidoses neither stain selectively for a single light chain nor for AA protein, but stain with antisera to the particular precursor protein. Nonspecific trapping of circulating proteins, including Ig and light chains, may lead to equivocal IF results. In difficult cases, mass spectrometry–based proteomic analysis of the amyloid deposits extracted by laser capture microdissection from renal biopsy sections is required to identify the amyloid subtype.[662] By EM, in all glomerular amyloidosis, typical nonbranching 8- to 12-nm-wide fibrils are randomly distributed in the mesangium and frequently along the GBM in the subepithelial, intramembranous, and subendothelial locations (Fig. 32.28). Mild cases may have deposition limited to the mesangium. More severe cases usually have more extensive deposition in the peripheral capillary walls and obliterate the lumina. By EM, glomerular capillary wall infiltration by amyloid may form characteristic spicular, cockscomb-like projections along the subepithelial aspect of the GBMs.

## COURSE, PROGNOSIS, AND TREATMENT

The prognosis of patients with AL amyloidosis in the past was poor with some series having a median survival rate of less than 2 years.[652,653,673] The serum creatinine and the degree of proteinuria at baseline as well as hematologic response are predictive of the progression to ESKD. In older series, the median time from diagnosis to dialysis was 14 months, and from dialysis to death only 8 months.[652,653,673] Recent data suggest improved survival. Factors associated with decreased patient survival include evidence of cardiac involvement, renal dysfunction, and interstitial fibrosis on renal biopsy.[652,653,673] Cardiac involvement with associated heart failure and arrhythmias is the primary cause of death in amyloidosis, followed by renal disease.[652,653,673,695]

Recent data describe improved survival. In one recent study patients with autologous stem cell transplantation (ASCT) had a 4-year survival of 91% and the non-ASCT group had a survival of 38%. Increased survival correlated with earlier diagnosis, higher response rates to therapy, and a marked decrease in early mortality.[677]

The course of AA amyloidosis has recently been defined in a study of 374 patients followed for a median time of more than 7 years.[680] Therapy to suppress the inflammatory disease was used whenever possible. The predominant manifestation and influence on the course of the disease was renal dysfunction and the median survival was more than 10 years. The SAA concentration correlated with overall mortality, amyloid burden, and renal prognosis. Amyloid deposits regressed (as assessed by SAP scans) in patients whose SAA concentration was kept low, and patient survival was superior in this group compared with those with no amyloid regression.[680]

The optimal treatment for AL amyloid depends on the patient's age, organ system involvement, and overall health.[653,673,696] In general, healthier and younger patients have been offered ASCT (discussed later), whereas older patients with more morbid associated conditions have received chemotherapeutic regimens. For patients presenting with a very low GFR (<20 mL/min/1.73 $m^2$), renal survival depends upon the magnitude and speed of the response of the hematologic disorder to treatment.[692] Current treatment strategies focus on methods to decrease the production of monoclonal light chains. In an older review of 153 AL amyloid patients treated with melphalan and prednisone only, 18% of the patients had a regression of organ manifestations of amyloidosis with responders having a 5-year survival of 78% versus only 7% in the nonresponders.[697] Patients with renal amyloidosis fared best with 25% having a 50% resolution in nephrotic-range proteinuria and stable or improved GFR. Recent chemotherapeutic agents used successfully in conjunction with dexamethasone include a number of agents used in myeloma, including melphalan, lenalidomide, thalidomide, bortezomib, and cyclophosphamide.[697–703] In some patients, there is resolution of proteinuria, stabilization of renal function, improvement of symptoms, and occasionally evidence of decreased organ involvement such as reduced hepatosplenomegaly. Recent studies show increased use of bortezomib added to protocols based on melphalan- and corticosteroid-based regimens with higher response rates.[704] Likewise, lenalidomide has been used successfully in combination with melphalan and dexamethasone.[705] Recently, the anti-CD38-directed monoclonal antibody daratumumab has improved hematologic response rates in both multiple myeloma and amyloidosis.[706] It has been well tolerated and effective even with cardiac amyloid involvement. Some therapies used experimentally to treat AL amyloid, including dimethyl sulfoxide, colchicine, 4′-iodo-4′-deoxydoxorubicin, fludarabine, vitamin E, high-dose dexamethasone monotherapy, and IFN-α-2, have not been effective.[696,699,703] However, a recent trial using a drug that efficiently depletes SAP component followed by a monoclonal anti-SAP IgG antibody appears to safely clear AL amyloid deposits from the liver and other organs of AL amyloid patients.[707]

Reports using high-dose melphalan followed by allogeneic bone marrow transplant or stem cell transplant have given promising results.[708,709] Such regimens have led to resolution of nephrotic syndrome and biopsy-proven improvement of amyloid organ involvement in some cases. However, a renal complication of ASCT (AKI) developed in 20% of one series of 173 amyloid patients. Although there was a high mortality in early reports (20% in the first 3 months), many survivors had a complete hematologic response, and many with renal involvement survived with a major decrease in proteinuria without a worsening of GFR. One retrospective study analyzed 65 AL amyloid patients with more than 1 g/day proteinuria treated with dose-intensive ablative chemotherapy followed by autologous blood stem cell transplantation.[710] Three-fourths of the patients survived the first year, and among those, a good renal response was found in 36% at 1 year and 52% at 2 years. Patients with a complete hematologic response were more likely to have a good renal response, and patient survival was superior in younger patients with fewer than three organ systems involved and those able to tolerate higher doses of the ablative therapy. Toxicities included mucositis, edema, elevated liver function tests, pulmonary edema, gastrointestinal bleeding, and, in 23%, transient acute renal failure. Thus for younger patients with predominantly renal involvement, stem cell transplantation has been a reasonable alternative therapy.[711] Some studies have supported stem cell transplantation as a beneficial therapy for some AL amyloid patients. Even patients with ESKD due to amyloidosis may undergo this form of therapy with results no different from non-ESKD patients with AL amyloidosis.[712] However, the only large randomized trial of stem cell transplantation for amyloid found this treatment to be inferior to standard chemotherapy.[713] In this multicenter French trial, 100 patients were randomized to hematopoietic cell transplantation or melphalan plus dexamethasone. The chemotherapeutic group had a better overall survival. Although this study has been criticized for patient selection and the high subsequent mortality, it is the only large randomized trial. In recent studies the results of ASCT for amyloid have shown marked improvements in hematologic response and overall survival. One recent review showed, since 2010, an overall survival rate of 91%.[677] A review of over 1500 AL amyloid patients who underwent ASCT over a period from 1995 to 2012 showed a marked decrease in early mortality over time, improved hematologic response rates, and a 5-year overall survival rate of 77%.[714] Others have also shown marked improvements in long-term survival in AL amyloid patients treated with high-dose melphalan and ASCT with decreasing early mortality.[715]

Regardless of whether chemotherapy or marrow transplant is used, the treatment of nephrotic amyloid patients requires supportive care. This may include judicious use of diuretics and salt restriction in those with edema, and treatment of orthostatic hypotension with compression stockings, fludrocortisone, and, in some, midodrine, an oral α-adrenergic agonist.

The treatment of AA amyloid focuses on the control of the underlying inflammatory disease process.[669,678,680,716] This has included surgical débridement of inflammatory tissue, antibiotic therapy of infectious processes, and antiinflammatory and immunosuppressive agents in rheumatoid arthritis and inflammatory bowel disease. Therapy may lead to stabilization of renal function, reduction in proteinuria, and resolution of amyloid deposits.[669,678,680,716] Prognosis may be good if the underlying disease can be controlled and there is not already extensive amyloid deposition. Immunosuppressives, antiinflammatory agents, and anticytokine therapy have been used in rheumatologic diseases and Crohn disease, with evidence of increased GFR and decreased proteinuria, and in some cases with regression of renal amyloid deposits.[678,680,716,717] FMF, an autosomal recessive disease caused by mutation of the gene encoding pyrin, is primarily found in Sephardic Jews, Turks, Armenians, and Arabs. The diseases characterized by recurrent attacks of fever and serositis lead to the development of AA amyloidosis in up to 90% of untreated patients.[678] Colchicine can effectively prevent the febrile attacks and stabilize or reduce the development of proteinuria. However, renal function did deteriorate in patients with nephrotic syndrome at presentation. A retrospective analysis of FMF patients with milder renal clinical involvement and at least 5 years' follow-up concluded that high doses of colchicine were more effective in preventing renal dysfunction and that patients with lower levels of serum creatinine at presentation responded better to therapy. Once the serum creatinine level was elevated, however, increasing the dose of colchicine did not prevent progression.

Recently, newer biologics have been used to suppress inflammation in diseases like rheumatoid arthritis with improvement of AA amyloid.[718] Likewise, newer agents to block inflammation in FMF have appeared beneficial.[719] Tocilizumab, an IL-6 blocker, has also proven effective in a series of 20 patients with systemic inflammatory disorders refractory to other treatments with reductions in serum levels of AA amyloid and decrease in AA deposits when measured by SAP scans.[720] AA amyloidosis seen in drug abusers and patients with inflammatory states such as Behçet disease and inflammatory bowel disease have occasionally responded to colchicine therapy, although it is unclear if this was due to cessation of drug abuse or treatment of the underlying inflammatory disease process.[682,721]

A multicenter randomized controlled trial compared a glycosaminoglycan mimetic (used to block fibrillogenesis) with placebo in 183 patients with AA amyloid. Although the drug had no significant effect on preventing progression to ESKD or risk of death, the glycosaminoglycan mimetic did reduce the rate of progression of the renal disease.[722] This study clearly shows the need for newer therapies for amyloidosis and the value of controlled trials in studying these agents. Several promising experimental therapies for treating amyloid include the use of antiamyloid antibodies and the use of an inhibitor of the binding of amyloid P component to amyloid fibrils.

In hereditary transthyretin (ATTR) amyloidosis, the traditional treatment is to provide a liver transplant that would lead to reduced production of the mutated protein. Another approach investigated transthyretin tetramer stabilizers (tafamidis and diflunisal), which showed clinical efficacy in patients with cardiac endpoints. ATTR-specific oligonucleotides, as either small interfering RNA (patisiran) or "antisense" (inotersen) constructs, by reducing hepatocyte levels of TTR messenger RNA would lead to less synthesis of the secreted transthyretin protein and consequently less misfolded monomer to form deposits. Two randomized studies showed slower progression of neurological endpoints.[670,723,724] The novel use of RNAi therapeutics offers hope for patients with hereditary transthyretin (ATTR) amyloidosis.

### END-STAGE KIDNEY DISEASE IN AMYLOIDOSIS

In most series the median survival of amyloid patients with ESKD is less than 1 year with the primary cause of death being complications of cardiac amyloid.[725,726] However, for patients who survive the first month of ESKD replacement therapy, the survival rate is over 50% at 2 years and 30% at 5 years.[726] There is no survival difference between peritoneal dialysis and hemodialysis.[726] A report of survival data in 19 dialysis patients with AL amyloid found an 80% mortality at 35 months' follow-up, whereas 20 AA amyloid dialysis patients had a 15% mortality over this period.[727] Likewise, another series found a shorter than 1-year median survival for hemodialysis patients with AL amyloidosis.

Experience with renal transplantation in AL amyloid is limited, but transplantation may be performed either before or after ASCT.[711,712] An earlier series on transplantation in amyloid included 45 patients (42 with AA amyloid) and found an overall low patient survival, particularly in the early posttransplant period in older patients because of infectious and cardiovascular complications.[728] Graft survival, however, was not decreased despite rates of recurrence of amyloidosis in the allograft as high as 20% to 33%.[728,729] The 5- and 10-year survival rates of renal transplant patients with AA amyloid, largely FMF patients, who received living-related allografts have been as high as 80% and 66%, respectively. In hereditary amyloidosis due to fibrinogen A α-chain disease, recurrence occurred in 50% of allografts with frequent graft loss. Better results are reported with combined liver and kidney transplantation.

## FIBRILLARY GLOMERULONEPHRITIS AND IMMUNOTACTOID GLOMERULONEPHRITIS

Some uncommon glomerular diseases have fibrillar deposits differing in size from that of amyloid.[730,731] In the past, many investigators subdivided these patients into two major groups depending on fibril size, with the fibrils in fibrillary GN being approximately 16 to 24 nm (mean, 20 nm) in diameter, and in immunotactoid glomerulonephritis the deposits forming larger hollow microtubules of 30 to 50 nm in diameter.[730–733] Fibrillary GN is a distinct entity and different from immunotactoid GN with a specific immunohistochemical marker DNAJB9 found in the distribution of the fibrillary glomerular deposits.[734,735] DNAJB9 is a chaperone protein synthesized by many cell types. Because it colocalizes with IgG in the deposits of fibrillary GN, the theoretical possibility that it might represent an autoantigen has been proposed. A third, rare form of fibrillary renal disease is fibronectin glomerulopathy in which the glomeruli are infiltrated by massive deposits of fibronectin.[736,737]

Fibrillary glomerulonephritis occurs mostly in adults, in both sexes, in all age groups, and most commonly in Caucasians. Although usually considered an isolated idiopathic renal entity, it has been associated in some series with malignancies, monoclonal gammopathies, and autoimmune disorders.[730–737] Patients with immunotactoid glomerulonephritis tend to be older, may have a less rapidly progressive course, and in all series are more likely to have underlying lymphoproliferative disease (e.g., chronic lymphocytic leukemia or B-cell lymphoma), often with a circulating paraprotein and sometimes with hypocomplementemia.[730–733] Patients with both diseases usually have proteinuria, and most have hypertension and hematuria. About 70% to 75% have nephrotic syndrome at biopsy. At presentation, renal insufficiency is common and most patients progress to ESKD. Fibrillary glomerulonephritis and immunotactoid glomerulonephritis can both be associated with HCV infection.[733]

Diagnosis of these disorders requires a renal biopsy to demonstrate the defining ultrastructural features.[730–733] LM findings in fibrillary glomerulonephritis are highly variable and include mesangial proliferation; mesangial expansion by amorphous amyloidlike material; and membranous, membranoproliferative, and crescentic glomerulonephritis (Fig. 32.29).[730] In immunotactoid glomerulonephritis, glomerular lesions are often nodular and sclerosing, whereas others are proliferative or membranous (Fig. 32.30). The pathognomonic findings seen on EM consist of nonbranching fibrils of 16 to 24-nm diameter in fibrillary glomerulonephritis (as opposed to 8–12 nm for amyloid; Fig. 32.31) and hollow microtubules of diameter 30 to 50 nm in immunotactoid glomerulonephritis (Fig. 32.32). In fibrillary glomerulonephritis, fibrils are arranged randomly in the mesangial matrix and GBMs. By contrast, the microtubules of immunotactoid glomerulonephritis are often arranged in parallel stacks in the mesangium, subendothelial, and/or subepithelial regions. The fibrils and microtubules do not stain with Congo red or thioflavin T. In fibrillary glomerulonephritis, IF is almost always positive for IgG (Fig. 32.33; especially subclasses IgG1 and IgG4), C3, and both κ and λ chains, indicating polyclonal deposits.[730–733] Staining for IgM, IgA, and C1 has been reported in a minority of cases. In immunotactoid glomerulonephritis, the immunoglobulin deposits are often monoclonal, consisting of IgG with a restricted light-chain isotype (either κ or λ). IgG subtypes IgG1 and IgG3 are most common and have the capacity to fix complement, leading to glomerular codeposits of C1q and C3. In both diseases, the deposits are usually limited to the glomerulus. In fibrillary glomerulonephritis, the fibrils may be focally admixed with more granular immune-type electron-dense deposits.[730] Rare patients with fibrillary glomerulonephritis have been reported to have extrarenal deposits involving alveolar capillaries and, in the case of immunotactoid glomerulonephritis, the bone marrow.[738,739] Given the recent immunohistochemical and

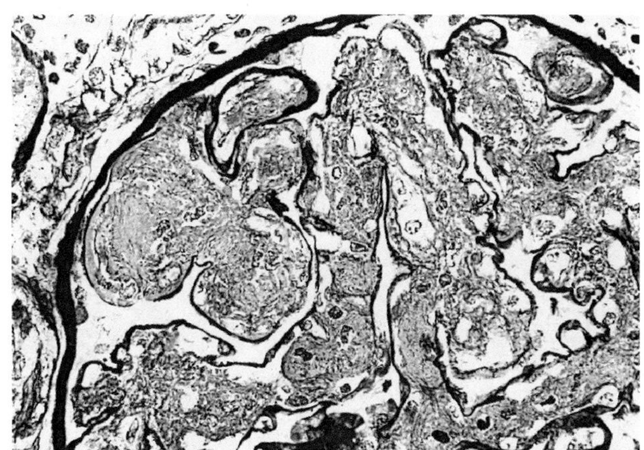

**Fig. 32.30** Immunotactoid glomerulonephritis. There is lobular expansion of the glomerular tuft by abundant mesangial deposits of silver-negative material. Segmental extension of deposits into the subendothelial aspect of some glomerular capillaries is also seen (Jones methenamine silver, ×500).

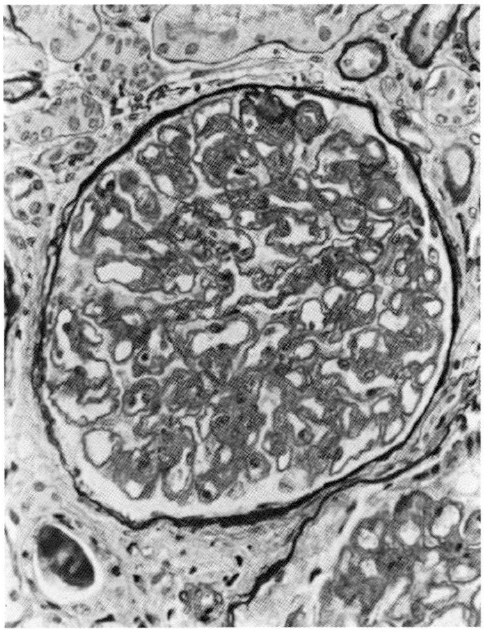

**Fig. 32.29** Fibrillary glomerulonephritis. The mesangium is mildly expanded and the glomerular capillary walls appear thickened with segmental double contours (periodic acid–Schiff, ×300).

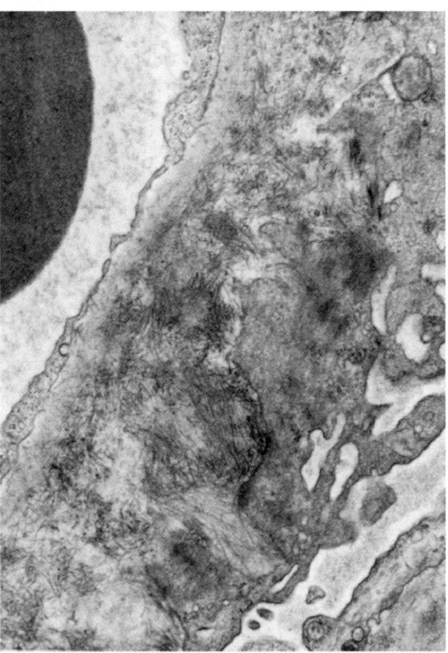

**Fig. 32.31** Fibrillary glomerulonephritis. Electron micrograph showing the characteristic randomly oriented fibrils, measuring 16 to 20 nm within the glomerular basement membrane. The foot processes are effaced (×8000).

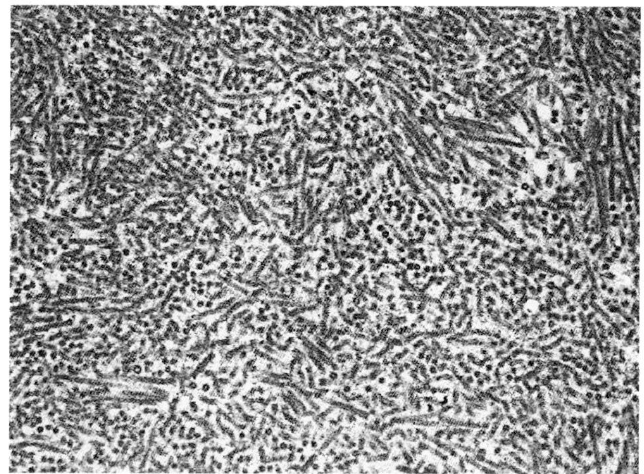

**Fig. 32.32** Immunotactoid glomerulonephritis. Electron micrograph showing abundant mesangial deposits of microtubular structures measuring approximately 35 nm in diameter (×10,000).

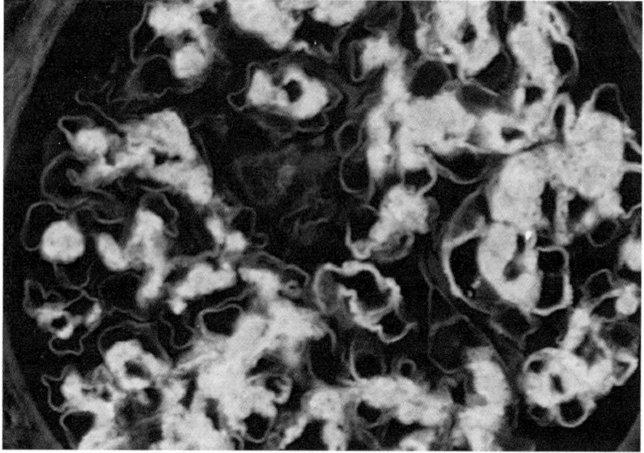

**Fig. 32.33** Fibrillary glomerulonephritis. Immunofluorescence photomicrograph showing smudgy deposits of immunoglobulin G throughout the mesangium, with segmental extension into the peripheral glomerular capillary walls (×800).

laser microdissection–mass spectrometry studies demonstrating the unique deposition of DNAJB9 in fibrillary GN, its pathogenesis and optimal therapy will hopefully be better defined in the near future.[734,735]

Almost half of patients with fibrillary glomerulonephritis or immunotactoid glomerulonephritis develop ESKD within 2 to 6 years of presentation.[730,732] Those with crescentic lesions, sclerosing glomerulonephritis, and diffuse proliferative glomerulonephritis fare worse than those with mesangioproliferative glomerulonephritis and those with a membranous pattern. Younger patients, patients with a normal GFR, and those with subnephrotic-range proteinuria have a more benign renal course.[730]

Although there is no proven therapy for fibrillary glomerulonephritis, some clinicians choose to treat the LM pattern observed on renal biopsy (e.g., membranous, membranoproliferative, crescentic).[730] Prednisone, cyclophosphamide, and colchicine have not led to consistent benefit in most patients.[730] However, in some with crescentic glomerulonephritis, cyclophosphamide and corticosteroid therapy has led to a dramatic improvement in GFR and proteinuria. Cyclosporine has also been used successfully in some patients with fibrillary glomerulonephritis and a membranous pattern on LM. Rituximab has been used in those with MPGN pattern, although recent larger series have given less promising results.[371,730,740,741] In some patients with associated chronic lymphocytic leukemia, treatment with chemotherapy has been associated with improved renal function and decreased proteinuria.[730,732] Dialysis and transplantation have been performed in both fibrillary glomerulonephritis and immunotactoid glomerulonephritis, but there is a significant recurrence rate in the allograft in both diseases.[730,742,743] Some have found a higher recurrence rate in those with an associated monoclonal gammopathy.[743]

Fibronectin glomerulopathy is a familial disease with autosomal dominant inheritance that presents with proteinuria and hematuria usually in adolescents and eventually progresses to nephrotic syndrome and slowly deteriorating renal function.[736,737] It is caused by an inherited mutation in the gene encoding fibronectin-1.[737] Patients who progress to ESKD may develop recurrent fibronectin glomerulopathy in the allograft.

## MONOCLONAL IMMUNOGLOBULIN DEPOSITION DISEASE

Monoclonal immunoglobulin deposition disease (MIDD) includes light-chain deposition disease (LCDD), combined light- and heavy-chain deposition disease (LHCDD), and heavy-chain deposition disease (HCDD). MIDD is a systemic disease caused by the overproduction and extracellular deposition of a fragment of monoclonal immunoglobulins.[744–746] LCDD is by far the most common pattern. Unlike amyloidosis, in LCDD the deposits in more than 80% of cases are composed of κ-light chains, most often of the VkIV subgroup, rather than λ-light chains.[744–747] In LCDD the deposits are granular in nature, do not have the biochemical properties necessary to form fibrils or β-pleated sheets, and thus do not bind Congo red stain or thioflavin T, and are not associated with amyloid P protein.[744–747] In amyloid, the fibrils are usually derived primarily from the variable region of the light chains, whereas in LCDD the deposits are predominantly composed of the constant region of the light chain. This may explain the far brighter IF staining for light chains found in LCDD as opposed to amyloidosis. The nature of the light chains may also explain the far more common occurrence of light-chain cast nephropathy in LCDD than in amyloidosis.[744–747] The pathogenesis of the glomerulosclerosis in LCDD involves promotion of a profibrotic mesangial cell phenotype with production of transforming growth factor-β, which acts as an autacoid to stimulate mesangial cell synthesis of extracellular matrix proteins such as type IV collagen, laminin, and fibronectin, and decreased production of collagenases.[748]

It was originally thought that patients with MIDD were generally older than 45 years.[744–747] However, in one recent series with a median age of 56 years, more than one-third of the patients were younger than 50 years of age.[745] Many such patients develop frank myeloma, and some may have a lymphoplasmacytic B-cell disease such as lymphoma or Waldenström macroglobulinemia.[744–746] As in amyloidosis, the clinical features vary with the location and extent of organ

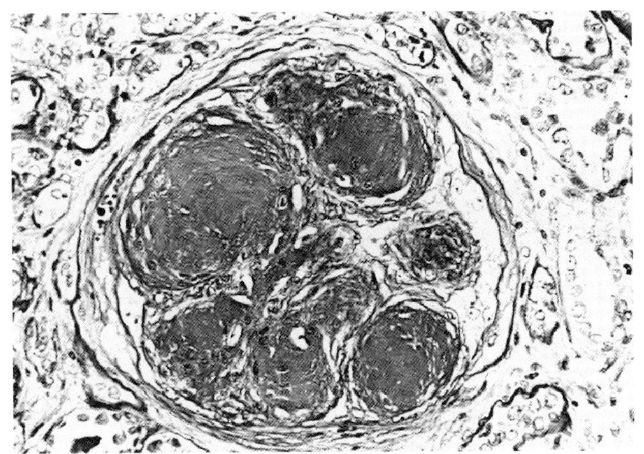

**Fig. 32.34** Light-chain deposition disease. There is nodular glomerulosclerosis with marked global expansion of the mesangium by intensely periodic acid–Schiff–positive material, but without appreciable thickening of the glomerular capillary walls (periodic acid–Schiff, ×375).

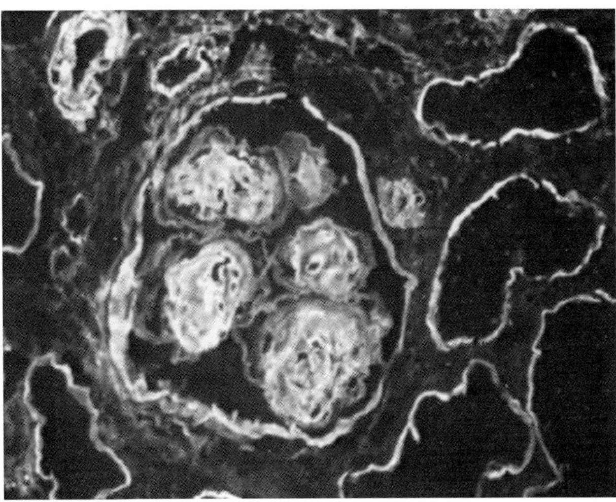

**Fig. 32.35** Light-chain deposition disease. Immunofluorescence photomicrograph showing linear staining for kappa light chain involving glomerular and tubular basement membranes, the mesangial nodules, Bowman's capsule, and vessel walls (×250).

deposition of the monoclonal protein. Patients typically have cardiac, neural, hepatic, and renal involvement, but other organs such as the skin, spleen, thyroid, adrenal glands, and gastrointestinal tract may be involved.[744–747] Patients with renal disease usually have significant glomerular involvement and present with proteinuria, nephrotic syndrome, and hypertension. Renal insufficiency is present in most, and some require dialysis. While by serum protein electrophoresis or urine protein electrophoresis 15% to 30% of patients may have no identifiable M spike, by analysis of serum-free light-chain assay, 100% have an abnormal protein and 80% have high levels of production.[745] Some patients may have greater tubulointerstitial involvement and less proteinuria along with renal insufficiency.[748]

The glomerular pattern by LM is most often nodular sclerosing with mesangial nodules of acellular eosinophilic material resembling the nodular glomerulosclerosis seen in diabetic patients (Fig. 32.34).[744–746] Glomerular capillary microaneurysms also may occur.[749] Some glomeruli have associated membranoproliferative features. In LCDD the nodules are more strongly PAS positive and less argyrophilic than in diabetes, and the GBMs in LCDD are not usually visibly thickened by LM.[744,745] Other glomeruli may be entirely normal or have only mild mesangial sclerosis. IF is usually diagnostic by demonstration of a monoclonal light-chain (κ in 80%) staining in a diffuse linear pattern along the GBMs, in the nodules, and along the tubular basement membranes and vessel walls (Fig. 32.35).[744,745] Staining for complement components is usually negative. By EM, deposition of a finely granular punctate, highly electron-dense material occurs along the lamina rara interna of the GBM, in the mesangium, and along tubular and vascular basement membranes.[744–747]

The prognosis for patients with LCDD is variable. Death is often attributed to heart failure, infectious complications, or the development of frank myeloma and renal failure.[744–747] In one series of 63 MIDD patients, 65% of patients developed myeloma and 36 patients developed uremia.[746] In another more recent series of 64 patients with MIDD, including 51 with LCDD, with a median follow-up of over 2 years, 57% had stable or improved renal function, 4% worsening of renal function, and 39% progression to ESKD.[745] Patient survival has been about 90% at 1 year and 70% at 5 years, with renal survival 67% and 37% at 1 and 5 years, respectively.[744–746,750,751] A recent series of 53 patients documented a 5.4-year renal survival and a 14-year patient survival. In that same series 62% progressed to ESKD.[752] Predictors of worse renal outcome have included increased age, associated light-chain cast nephropathy, and elevated serum creatinine at presentation.[744–746] Predictors of worse patient survival included increased age, occurrence of myeloma, higher initial serum creatinine, and extrarenal deposition of light chains.[744–746] A good hematologic response to chemotherapy has been associated with better renal and patient survivals.[752]

Treatment, akin to the treatment of myeloma or amyloidosis, has been with dexamethasone in combination with other agents, including melphalan, cyclophosphamide, bortezomib, thalidomide, and lenalidomide, and has led to stabilized or improved renal function in some MIDD patients.[744–746] However, this therapy is not usually successful in patients with significant renal dysfunction and a plasma creatinine above 4 mg/dL at initiation of treatment.[751] In one series of 32 patients treated with chemotherapy, 34% progressed to ESKD.[746] Marrow or stem cell transplantation is a therapeutic option for some patients with LCDD.[744,746] Although there are little data on dialysis and renal transplantation in LCDD, patients appear to fare as well as those with amyloidosis. Recurrences in the renal transplant have been reported[744,745,750,751,753] and recurrence rates in some series are as high as 70% to 75%.[711,745,753] Thus suppression of the abnormal paraprotein producing cell clone is crucial prior to renal transplantation. Indeed, with sustained remission of the clonal disorder in one series there were no recurrences in seven patients followed after renal transplantation for 10 years.[752]

In some patients with a plasma cell dyscrasia, monoclonal light and heavy immunoglobulin chains combined (LHCDD) or short monoclonal truncated heavy chains alone (HCDD) are deposited in the tissue (Fig. 32.36).[744,747,754,755] As in LCDD the EM deposits are granular and biopsies are Congo red

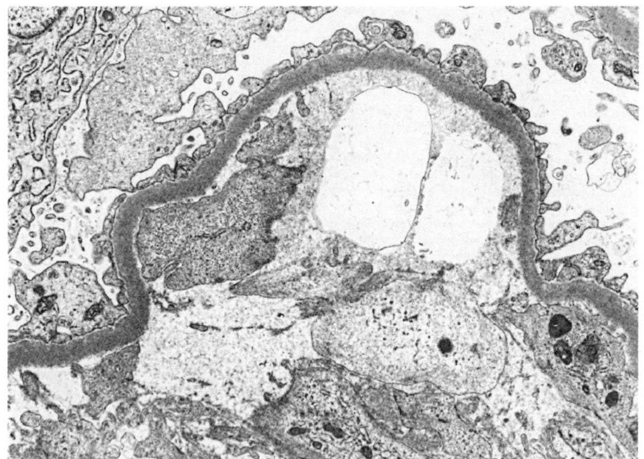

**Fig. 32.36** Heavy-chain deposition disease. Electron micrograph showing bandlike finely granular electron-dense deposits involving the glomerular basement membrane, with greatest concentration along the inner aspect (×5000).

negative. The clinical features are similar to those of LCDD and amyloidosis.[755] Most patients are middle age or older. They present with renal insufficiency, hypertension, proteinuria, and often the nephrotic syndrome. In most patients, a monoclonal protein is detected in the serum or urine. In contrast to amyloid and LCDD, HCDD may be associated with hypocomplementemia if the heavy chain avidly binds complement (especially gamma heavy-chain subtypes G1 and G3).[755] All patients with HCDD have a deletion of the CH1 domain of the heavy chain, which causes the heavy chain to be secreted prematurely by the plasma cell.[755,756] The characteristic LM finding in HCDD is a nodular sclerosing glomerulopathy at times with small crescents.[744,755–757] The diagnosis is made by IF with linear positivity for the heavy chain of immunoglobulin (usually gamma) and negativity for both kappa and lambda light chains.[755] The distribution is diffuse involving glomerular, tubular, and vascular basement membranes. Treatment has been similar to LCDD, and many patients have progressed to renal failure.[755,758] Recurrence in the renal transplant has been documented.[744]

## OTHER GLOMERULAR DISEASES AND DYSPROTEINEMIA

A proliferative glomerulonephritis resembling immune complex glomerulonephritis has also been described with increasing frequency in association with a monoclonal gammopathy.[759,760] This newly described entity is known as proliferative glomerulonephritis with monoclonal IgG deposits (PGNMIDs). These patients present with renal insufficiency and proteinuria, sometimes associated with nephrotic syndrome, but no evidence of cryoglobulinemia. LM shows an MPGN pattern in more than one-half and an endocapillary proliferative pattern with membranous features in more than one-third. PGNMID typically has ordinary-appearing granular nonorganized electron-dense deposits in the mesangial, subendothelial, and subepithelial sites, but by IF these were restricted to a single monoclonal γ heavy-chain subclass and light-chain isotype (most commonly IgG3κ). Rare cases with monoclonal IgG deposits have had a purely membranous pattern. An M spike has been identified in the serum in 20% to 30% of PGNMID cases, but most patients do not develop overt myeloma or lymphoma during the follow-up period. In one large series at 2.5 years of follow-up, 38% of patients had had a complete recovery, 38% had persistent renal dysfunction, and 22% had progressed to ESKD.[760] Higher presenting serum creatinine, higher percentage of glomerulosclerosis, and more interstitial fibrosis on biopsy predicted progression to ESKD. Despite the absence of evidence of overt hematologic malignancy on bone marrow biopsy, patients with PGNMID may benefit from treatments directed to small clonal proliferations, including therapies that include rituximab, cyclophosphamide, bortezomib, and dexamethasone.[761] PGNMID commonly recurs in the transplant and may in some cases be amenable to either rituximab, bortezomib, or cyclophosphamide therapies.[762–764]

Other rare patients with dysproteinemia have had intracellular glomerular crystals within the podocytes, sometimes in association with tubular epithelial crystalline deposits.[765] Pamidronate-induced collapsing focal sclerosis has been noted in myeloma[766] as has crescentic glomerulonephritis. MPGN has been reported rarely, particularly in patients with associated cryoglobulinemia (see the "Mixed Cryoglobulinemia" section).

## WALDENSTRÖM MACROGLOBULINEMIA

In Waldenström macroglobulinemia, patients have an abnormal circulating monoclonal IgM protein in association with a B-cell lymphoproliferative hematologic disorder.[767–770] This slowly progressive disorder occurs in older patients (median age 60 years) who present with constitutional symptoms of fatigue and weight loss, bleeding, visual disturbances, neurologic symptoms, hepatosplenomegaly, lymphadenopathy, anemia, and often hyperviscosity syndrome.[767–770] Although renal involvement occurs in less than 5% of patients, glomerular lesions can present with microscopic hematuria, proteinuria, and nephrotic syndrome.[770,771] Patients may have enlarged kidneys. The renal pathology in Waldenström macroglobulinemia is varied.[770–773] A recent review found 44 of 1391 patients with Waldenström macroglobulinemia at one institution to have had a kidney biopsy.[774] The most common findings were amyloidosis (25%), monoclonal IgM deposition disease/cryoglobulins (23%), lymphoplasmacytic lymphoma infiltration (18%), LCDD (9%), light-chain cast nephropathy (9%), and a variety of other lesions. Others have AKI with intraglomerular occlusive thrombi of the IgM paraprotein. These cases have large eosinophilic, amorphous, PAS-positive deposits occluding the glomerular capillary lumens with little or no glomerular hypercellularity (Fig. 32.37). By IF, these glomerular "thrombi" stain for IgM and a single light-chain isotype, consistent with monoclonal IgM deposits, but complement components are usually negative or only weakly positive. By EM, the deposits contain nonamyloid fibrillar or amorphous electron-dense material. Some patients develop MPGN with an associated type I or type II cryoglobulinemia (Fig. 32.38). Cases of LCDD with intratubular casts similar to those of light-chain cast nephropathy and examples of renal amyloidosis have also been reported in patients with Waldenström macroglobulinemia. Treatment

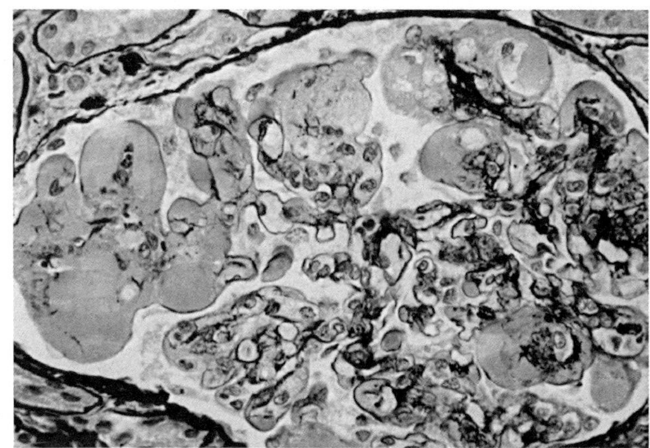

**Fig. 32.37** Waldenström macroglobulinemia. Large "protein thrombi" corresponding to the monoclonal immunoglobulin M deposits fill the glomerular capillary lumina, with minimal associated glomerular hypercellularity (Jones methenamine silver, ×600).

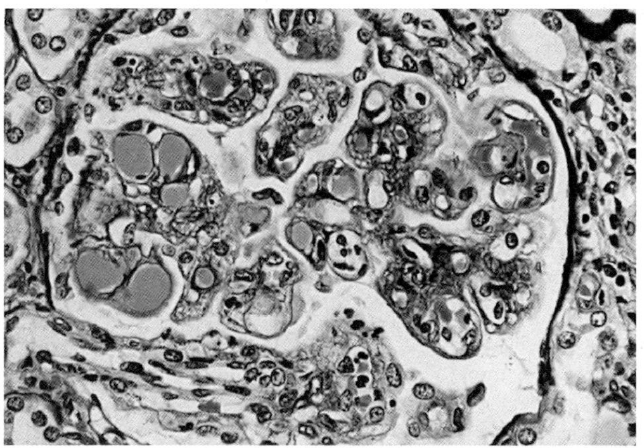

**Fig. 32.38** Waldenström macroglobulinemia. An example with cryoglobulinemic glomerulonephritis showing the characteristic intraluminal deposits, infiltrating leukocytes, and double-contoured glomerular basement membranes (Jones methenamine silver, ×600).

of Waldenström macroglobulinemia is directed against the lymphoproliferative disease with alkylating agents, melphalan, corticosteroids, rituximab, bendamustine, ibrutinib, bone marrow transplantation, and at times plasmapheresis for hyperviscosity signs and symptoms.[775–779] In one series, overall survival in Waldenström macroglobulinemia with renal involvement was 11.5 years versus 16 years for age-matched nonkidney patients.[774]

## MIXED CRYOGLOBULINEMIA

Cryoglobulinemia is caused by circulating immunoglobulins that precipitate on cooling and resolubilize on warming.[780] Cryoglobulinemia is associated with a variety of infections, especially HCV, as well as collagen vascular disease, and lymphoproliferative diseases.[443,780] Cryoglobulins have been divided into three major groups based on the nature of the circulating immunoglobulins.[780] In type I cryoglobulinemia, the cryoglobulin is a single monoclonal immunoglobulin often found associated with Waldenström macroglobulinemia or myeloma. Type II and type III cryoglobulinemia are defined as mixed cryoglobulins, containing at least two immunoglobulins. In type II, a monoclonal immunoglobulin (IgMκ in more than 90%) is directed against polyclonal IgG and has rheumatoid factor activity. In type III, the antiglobulin is polyclonal in nature with both polyclonal IgG and IgM in most cases. The majority of patients with type II and III mixed cryoglobulins have now been shown to have HCV infection.[746,781–786] To establish a diagnosis of cryoglobulinemia, the offending cryoglobulins or the characteristic renal tissue involvement must be demonstrated.

In the past, there was often no obvious cause of cryoglobulinemia and the name "essential mixed cryoglobulinemia" was appropriate.[781] It is now clear that many such patients had HCV-related disease.[783,787,788] Systemic manifestations of mixed cryoglobulinemia include weakness, malaise, Raynaud phenomenon, arthralgias–arthritis, hepatosplenomegaly with abnormal liver function tests in two-thirds to three-fourths of patients, peripheral neuropathy, and purpuric–vasculitic skin lesions.[443,780] In a recent study of 64 patients with type I cryoglobulinemia which is unrelated to hepatitis C infection, 28 patients had a monoclonal gammopathy of unknown significance and 36 had a defined hematologic malignancy.[785] The disease was characterized by severe cutaneous involvement with necrosis and ulcers and high serum levels of cryoglobulins, and a lower incidence of renal disease than in older series. Hypocomplementemia, especially of the early components (low C4 level), is a characteristic and often helpful finding in all types of cryoglobulinemia. Renal disease occurs at presentation in less than 25% of patients but develops in as many as 50% over time.[781,789,790] In one review of 279 patients with severe life-threatening HCV-associated cryoglobulinemic vasculitis, 205 had AKI.[784] In those renal patients who died, sepsis was the most common cause of death, whereas for other patients, vasculitis of the gastrointestinal tract, central nervous system, and pulmonary system led to death. These causes of death are similar to those of 242 patients in a review of noninfectious mixed cryoglobulinemic vasculitis.[785] In most, an acute nephritic picture with hematuria, hypertension, proteinuria, and progressive renal insufficiency develops, and 20% of patients have nephrotic syndrome. Few patients develop RPGN with oliguria. The majority of patients with renal disease have a slow, indolent renal course characterized by proteinuria, hypertension, hematuria, and renal insufficiency.

Many older studies of type II cryoglobulinemia have shown evidence of hepatitis B infection or other viral infections (e.g., Epstein-Barr virus [EBV]).[786] However, recent studies have clearly documented HCV as a major cause of cryoglobulin production in most patients previously felt to have essential mixed cryoglobulinemia. Antibodies to HCV antigens have been documented in the serum and HCV RNA and anti-HCV antibodies are enriched in the cryoglobulins of these patients.[783,787,789,790] This is true even for patients with normal levels of aminotransferases and no clinical evidence of hepatitis. HCV antigens have also been localized by immunohistochemistry to the glomerular deposits.[787] In cryoglobulinemia, immunoglobulin complexes deposit in the glomeruli and small- and medium-sized arteries, binding complement and inciting a proliferative response.[783,789] The serum cryoglobulin participates in the formation of the glomerular immune complex deposits. In vitro studies have shown that IgM-κ rheumatoid factor from patients with type II cryoglobulinemia is  much more likely to bind to cellular fibronectin (a component of the glomerular mesangium) than IgM from normal controls or IgM-containing rheumatoid factor from rheumatoid arthritis patients.[791] The particular physicochemical characteristics of the variable region of the immunoglobulin cryoglobulin may be important in the localization of the renal deposits.

Although by LM the glomerular lesions of cryoglobulinemia may show a variety of morphologic features (Fig. 32.39), certain findings help to distinguish cryoglobulinemic glomerulonephritis from other proliferative glomerulonephritides.[781,789,790] These features include massive glomerular exudation of monocytes/macrophages and, to a lesser degree, polymorphonuclear leukocytes; amorphous eosinophilic PAS-positive, Congo red–negative deposits along the subendothelial aspect of the glomerular capillary wall and focally filling the capillary lumens, forming "immune thrombi"; membranoproliferative features with double-contoured GBMs and interposition of deposits, mesangial cells, and monocytes; and the rarity of extracapillary proliferation (crescents) despite the intense intracapillary proliferation. The glomerular lesions may be accompanied by an acute vasculitis of small- or medium-sized vessels. By IF (Fig. 32.40), the glomeruli in type II or type III cryoglobulinemia contain deposits of both IgM and IgG, κ- and λ-light chains, and C3 and C1q in the distribution of subendothelial and mesangial deposits and the intracapillary "thrombi." Staining for both IgM and κ are often dominant, reflecting the deposition of type II cryoglobulins containing a monoclonal IgM-κ component. By EM (Fig. 32.41), deposits in the subendothelial location or filling the capillary lumens often appear as either amorphous electron-dense deposits or organized deposits of curvilinear parallel fibrils or annular–tubular curvilinear structures with a diameter of 20–35 nm.[781,789] The infiltrating macrophages are in close contact with the subendothelial deposits and contain prominent phagolysosomes, suggesting active phagocytosis of the immune deposits. In some cases, the phagocytosis is so effective that immune deposits are difficult to detect by both IF and EM.

Some patients with mixed cryoglobulinemia will have a partial or total remission of their disease while most have episodic exacerbations of their systemic and renal disease.[781,789] Before the association between mixed cryoglobulinemia and HCV was discovered, many patients were treated successfully with prednisone and cytotoxic agents such as cyclophosphamide and chlorambucil.[782] Treatments were not used in a controlled fashion. In patients with severe renal disease, in those with digital necrosis from the cryoglobulins, and in those with life-threatening organ involvement, plasmapheresis was used in combination with steroids and cytotoxics.[782,792] Most patients with cryoglobulinemia in the past did not die of renal disease but rather of cardiac or other systemic disease and infectious complications.[782] Currently, most patients with HCV-associated cryoglobulinemia are treated with antiviral agents[793] (see the "Hepatitis C" section under "Glomerular Manifestations of Liver Disease"). Aggressive immunosuppressive therapy carries the risk of promoting

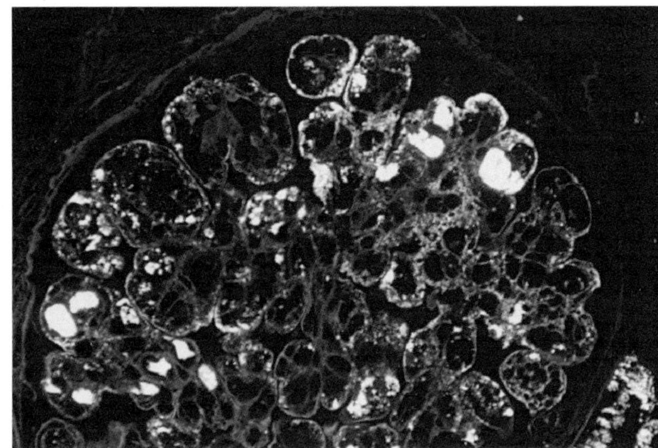

**Fig. 32.40** Cryoglobulinemic glomerulonephritis. Immunofluorescence photomicrograph showing deposits of immunoglobulin M corresponding to the large glomerular intracapillary deposits, with more finely granular subendothelial deposits outlining the glomerular capillary walls (×900).

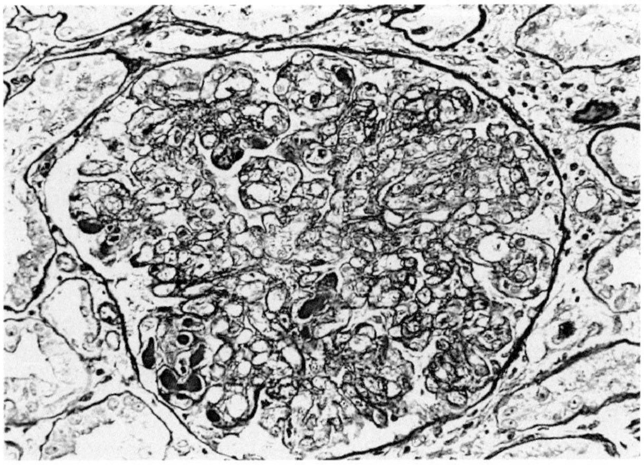

**Fig. 32.39** Cryoglobulinemic glomerulonephritis. There is global endocapillary proliferative glomerulonephritis with membranoproliferative features and focal intraluminal cryoglobulin deposits, forming "immune thrombi" (periodic acid–Schiff, ×375).

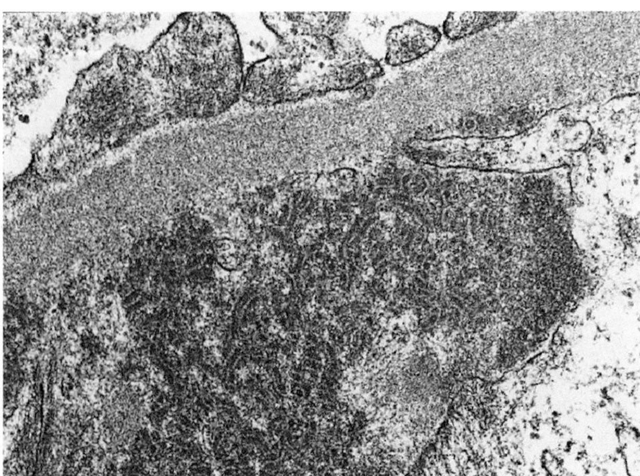

**Fig. 32.41** Cryoglobulinemic glomerulonephritis. Electron micrograph showing organized subendothelial deposits with an annular–tubular substructure. These curvilinear tubular structures measure approximately 30 nm in diameter (×30,000).

HCV replication in HCV-infected patients and of lymphoma in others. Rituximab has recently been used successfully for treatment of type II mixed cryoglobulinemia in patients with or without evidence of HCV infection and with and without prior antiviral therapy.[794–797] Rituximab has also been used successfully in small numbers of patients with HCV-related glomerulonephritis and mixed cryoglobulinemia.[798,799] In patients with type I cryoglobulins, unassociated with infections, therapy based on regimens of alkylating agents, rituximab, thalidomide–lenalidomide, and bortezomib has been effective.[781] Dialysis and transplantation in cryoglobulinemia have been used, but recurrences in the allograft have been reported.

## ALPORT SYNDROME

Alport syndrome is an inherited (usually X-linked) disorder of collagen α3α4α5(IV) with almost inevitable progression to ESKD, and is frequently associated with hearing loss and ocular abnormalities. Guthrie first reported a family with recurrent hematuria.[800] Alport reported additional observations on this family, the occurrence of deafness associated with hematuria, and the observation that affected males died of uremia whereas affected females lived to an old age.[801] Alport syndrome and other hereditary and familial disease account for 0.4% of adults with ESKD in the United States.[802] Guidelines for the diagnosis and management of disorders of collagen α3α4α5(IV) have been published.[803,804]

### CLINICAL FEATURES

The disease usually manifests in children or young adults.[805–807] Males have persistent microscopic hematuria, with episodic gross hematuria, which may be exacerbated by respiratory infections or exercise. There may be flank pain or abdominal discomfort accompanying these episodes. Proteinuria is usually mild at first and increases progressively with age. The nephrotic syndrome has also been described.[808] Hypertension is a late manifestation. Slowly progressive renal failure is common in males. ESKD usually occurs in males between the ages of 16 and 35 years. In some kindred, the course may be more delayed with renal failure occurring between 45 and 65 years of age. In most females, the disease is mild and only partially expressed; however, some females have experienced renal failure.[809] In the European Community Alport Syndrome Concerted Action (ECASCA) cohort, hematuria was observed in 95% of female carriers and consistently absent in the other 5%. Proteinuria, hearing loss, and ocular defects developed in 75%, 28%, and 15%, respectively.[810] This variability in disease severity in females can be explained by the degree of random inactivation of the mutated versus wild-type X chromosome during lyonization.

High-frequency sensorineural deafness occurs in 30% to 50% of patients. Hearing impairment is always accompanied by renal involvement. The severity of hearing loss is variable and there is no relation between the severity of hearing loss and the renal disease. Based on brain stem auditory-evoked responses, the site of the aural lesion is in the cochlea.[811,812] Families with hereditary nephritis, but without sensorineural hearing loss have been described.[812,813]

Ocular abnormalities occur in 15% to30% of patients.[814] Anterior lenticonus, which is the protrusion of the central portion of the lens into the anterior capsule, is virtually pathognomonic of Alport syndrome. Other ocular abnormalities include keratoconus, spherophakia, myopia, retinal flecks, cataracts, retinitis pigmentosa, and amaurosis.[805,806,815] Aortic disease including dissections, aneurysms, dilation, and aortic insufficiency may be an unusual feature in some patients.[816]

Other variants of the so-called *Alport syndrome*, now known to be distinct entities with different genetic bases, include the association of hereditary nephritis with thrombocytopathia (megathrombocytopenia), the so-called *Epstein syndrome*,[817,818] diffuse leiomyomatosis,[819] ichthyosis and hyperprolinuria,[820] and Fechtner syndrome (nephritis, macrothrombocytopenia, Döhle-like leukocyte inclusions, deafness, and cataract).[821]

### PATHOLOGY

The LM appearance of biopsies is nonspecific. The diagnosis rests on the EM findings. By LM, most biopsies have glomerular and tubulointerstitial lesions. In the early stages (<5 years of age), the kidney biopsy may be normal or nearly normal. The only abnormality may be the presence of superficially located fetal glomeruli involving 5% to 30% of the glomeruli or interstitial foam cells.[822,823] In the older child (5–10 years of age), mesangial and glomerular capillary wall lesions may be visible. These consist of segmental to diffuse mesangial cell proliferation, matrix increase, and irregular thickening of the glomerular capillary wall.[824] Special stains such as Jones methenamine silver or periodic acid–Schiff may reveal thickening and lamellation of the GBM. Podocytes often appear swollen. Segmentally or globally sclerosed glomeruli may be present. Tubulointerstitial changes may include interstitial fibrosis, tubular atrophy, and interstitial foam cells. The glomerular and tubular lesions progress over time. A pattern of focal segmental and global glomerulosclerosis with hyalinosis is common in advanced cases, especially those with nephrotic-range proteinuria. Of note, a significant proportion of patients with familial FSGS (without apparent GBM lamellation) may harbor mutations in COL4 genes, including COL4A5.[825] Tubulointerstitial lesions progress from focal to diffuse involvement.[822,826]

By IF, many specimens are negative,[822,827] but some may have nonspecific granular deposits of C3 and IgM within the mesangium and vascular pole and along the glomerular capillary wall in a segmental or global distribution.[805,812] The finding in rare cases of nonspecifically trapped electron-dense material with positivity for IgG and C1q within the lamellated GBMs and paramesangial regions may lead to an erroneous diagnosis of immune complex GN.[828] With segmental sclerosis, subendothelial deposits of IgM, C3, properdin, and C4 are found.[805,822] The GBM of males with Alport syndrome frequently lacks reactivity with sera from patients with anti-GBM antibody disease, or with monoclonal antibodies directed against the Goodpasture epitope.[829,830] This abnormality can help in diagnosing equivocal cases where the EM findings are not specific.[831]

In the mature kidney, collagen IV is composed of heterotrimers made up of six possible alpha chains. Collagen type IV chains composed of collagen type IV α1, α1, α2 are distributed in all renal basement membranes. Collagen IV chains composed of collagen type IV$\alpha$3, $\alpha$4, $\alpha$5 are present in mature GBM and some distal tubular basement membrane (TBM). Chains of $\alpha$5, $\alpha$5, $\alpha$6 are distributed in Bowman's capsule and collecting duct TBM, as well as in epidermal basement membrane. Commercially available antisera to the subunits of collagen IV reveal preservation of the $\alpha_1$ and $\alpha_2$ subunits but loss of immunoreactivity for the $\alpha_3$, $\alpha_4$, and $\alpha_5$ subunits from the GBM of affected males with X-linked disease. In addition, there is loss of $\alpha_5$ staining from Bowman's capsule, distal tubular basement membranes, and skin in affected males with X-linked disease. Females are chimeras with segmental loss of $\alpha_5$ in glomerular and epidermal basement membranes due to random inactivation of the mutated X chromosome in podocytes and basal keratinocytes. Patients with autosomal recessive forms of Alport disease typically lack the $\alpha_3$, $\alpha_4$, and $\alpha_5$ subunits in GBM but retain $\alpha_5$ immunoreactivity in Bowman's capsule, collecting ducts, and skin (where $\alpha$5 forms a heterotrimer with $\alpha$6). Thus absence of $\alpha_5$ staining in skin biopsies is highly specific for the diagnosis of X-linked Alport syndrome.[832]

On EM, the earliest change in young males is thinning of the GBM (which is not specific for hereditary nephritis and can occur in thin basement membrane disease). The cardinal ultrastructural abnormality is the variable thickening, thinning, basket weaving, and lamellation of the GBM (Fig. 32.42). These abnormalities may also be seen in some patients without a family history of nephritis[833]; these patients may be offspring of asymptomatic carriers, or may represent de novo mutations. The endothelial cells are intact, and foot process effacement may be seen overlying the altered capillary walls. The mesangium may be normal in early cases, but with time, matrix and cells increase and mesangial interposition into the capillary wall may be observed.[805,827] In males, the number of glomeruli showing lamellation increases from about 30% by age 10 years to over 90% by age 30 years. In females with mild disease, less than 30% of the glomeruli may be affected.[834] Some affected females have a predominantly thin basement membrane phenotype with only rare segmental areas of lamellation.

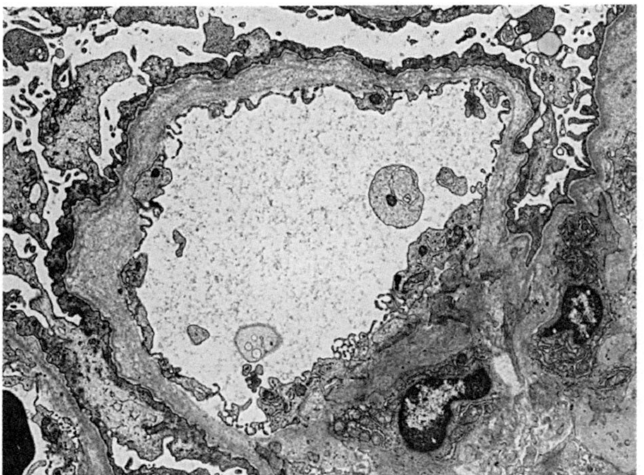

**Fig. 32.42** Alport syndrome. Electron micrograph showing a thickened, lamellated glomerular basement membrane with the characteristic "split and splintered" appearance (×4000).

The specificity of the GBM findings has been questioned.[835] Foci of lamina densa lamellation and splitting have been seen in 6% to 15% of unselected renal biopsies. These changes also may be seen focally in other glomerulopathies. Clinical correlation and IF examination are essential when the ultrastructural features suggest Alport syndrome. Although diffuse thickening and splitting of the GBM strongly suggest Alport syndrome, not all Alport kindreds show these characteristic features. Thick, thin, normal, and nonspecific changes have all been described.

## PATHOGENESIS AND GENETICS OF HEREDITARY NEPHRITIS

There are three genetic forms of hereditary nephritis (Table 32.2). In the majority of cases, the disease is transmitted via an X-linked inheritance (i.e., father to son transmission does not occur), and women are carriers, who are sometimes affected because of lyonization. Autosomal dominant and recessive inheritance have also been described, as has sporadic occurrence.[806,836,837] The frequency of the Alport gene mutations has been estimated to be 1:5000 in Utah[838] and 1:10,000 in the United States.[839]

Hereditary nephritis is caused by defects in type IV collagen. Six genes for type IV collagen have been characterized. Mutations in the COL4A5 gene (encoding the $\alpha$5 subunit of collagen type IV) on the X chromosome are responsible for the more frequent X-linked form of hereditary nephritis.[840] The six different type IV collagens exist as three distinct loci in the human gene: back-to-back orientations of $\alpha$1/$\alpha$2, $\alpha$3/$\alpha$4, and $\alpha$5/$\alpha$6, with the first pairings on autosomes and the latter pairing on the X chromosome. The identified mutations include deletions, insertions, substitutions, and duplications.[840–844] However, there are other abnormalities that are not encoded by the COL4A5 gene. Other type IV collagen peptides are abnormally distributed. The $\alpha_1$ and $\alpha_2$ peptides, which are normally confined to the mesangial and subendothelial regions of the mature glomerulus, become distributed throughout the full thickness of the GBM in hereditary nephritis. With progressive glomerular obsolescence, these peptide chains disappear, with an increase in collagen V and VI.[845] Moreover, the basement membranes of these patients do not react with anti-GBM antibodies. This implies that the NC1 domain of the $\alpha_3$ subunit of type IV collagen is not incorporated normally into the mature GBM, because the $\alpha_5$ subunit is required for normal heterotrimer assembly.[846] Cationic antigenic components are also absent.[847] The reason why these GBM abnormalities occur in not known, but may be due to alteration in the incorporation of other collagens into the GBM.[848] Autosomal recessive and autosomal dominant hereditary nephritis have been shown to involve the $\alpha_3$ or $\alpha_4$ chains, which are encoded by an autosome, specifically chromosome 2. An abnormality of any of these chains could impair the integrity of the basement membranes in the glomerulus and cochlea, leading to similar clinical findings.

Minor causes of familial hematuria, the Fechtner and Epstein syndromes, along with two other genetic conditions featuring macrothrombocytes (Sebastian syndrome and May–Hegglin anomaly), result from heterozygous mutations in the gene *MYH9*, which encodes nonmuscle myosin heavy-chain IIA (NMMHC-IIA).[849]

**Table 32.2 Unified Nomenclature for Genetic Disorders of the Collagen IV α345 Molecule**

| Inheritance | Affected Gene(s) | Generic State | Comments | Estimated Risk of ESKD |
|---|---|---|---|---|
| X-linked | *COL4A5* | Hemizygous (male subjects) | Rate of progression to ESKD and timing of extrarenal manifestations strongly influenced by genotype | 100% |
| | | Heterozygous (female subjects) | Risk factors for progression: gross hematuria, SNHL, proteinuria, GBM thickening and lamellation | Up to 25% |
| Autosomal | *COL4A3* or *COL4A4* | Recessive (homozygous or compound heterozygous) | Rate of progression to ESKD and timing of extrarenal manifestations strongly influenced by genotype | 100% |
| | | Dominant | Hematuria<br>Includes patients previously diagnosed as TBMN/BFH. Risk factors for progression: proteinuria, FSGS, GBM thickening and lamellation, SNHL, or evidence of progression in patient or family, genetic modifiers | 20% or more among those with risk factors for progression, <1% in absence of risk factors |
| Digenic | *COL4A3*, *COL4A4*, and *COL4A5* | *COL4A3* and *COL4A4* mutations in trans | Clinical findings and pedigree simulate autosomal recessive transmission | Up to 100% |
| | | *COL4A3* and *COL4A4* mutations in cis | Clinical findings and pedigree simulate autosomal dominant transmission | Up to 20% |
| | | Mutations in *COL4A5* and in *COL4A3* or *COL4A4* | Inheritance pattern does not simulate any Mendelian transmission | Up to 100% (affected male subjects) |

*BFH*, Benign familial hematuria; *ESKD*, end-stage kidney disease; *FSGS*, focal segmental glomerulosclerosis; *GBM*, glomerular basement membrane; *SNHL*, sensorineural hearing loss; *TBMN*, thin basement membrane nephropathy.

## COURSE AND TREATMENT

Recurrent hematuria and proteinuria may be present for many years followed by the insidious onset of renal failure. Virtually all affected males reach ESKD but there is considerable interkindred variability in the rate of progression. The rate of progression within male members of an affected family is usually but not always relatively constant.[805,850,851] The presence of gross hematuria in childhood, nephrotic syndrome, sensorineural deafness, anterior lenticonus, and diffuse GBM thickening portend a poor prognosis in females.[809] In the ECASCA, a 90% probability rate of progression to end-stage renal failure by age 30 years in patients with large deletions, nonsense mutations, or frameshift mutations was noted. The same risk was 50% and 70%, respectively, in patients with missense or splice site mutations. The risk of developing hearing loss before 30 years of age was approximately 60% in patients with missense mutations, compared with 90% for the other types of mutations.[852] Female carriers with the X-linked COL4A5 mutation generally have less severe disease. In the ECASCA cohort described earlier, the probability of developing ESKD before the age of 40 was 12% in females versus 90% in males. The risk of progression to ESKD appears to increase after the age of 60 in women. Risk factors for renal failure in women included the development and progressive increase in proteinuria, and the occurrence of a hearing defect.[810]

There is no proven therapy for Alport syndrome. Proteinuria-reduction strategies, such as aggressive control of hypertension and use of ACE inhibitors might slow the rate of progression in patients with hereditary nephritis.[853–855] The addition of an aldosterone antagonist may further reduce proteinuria.[856] A small number of patients showed apparent stabilization when treated long term with cyclosporine[857]; however, calcineurin inhibitor toxicity can occur with long-term use.[858] A phase II clinical trial of the antifibrotic agent targeting microRNA-21 (miR-21) has been initiated after demonstrating success in a preclinical model.[859]

Renal replacement therapy (either dialysis or transplantation) may be necessary in patients with hereditary nephritis. Allograft and patient survival were comparable to survival rates in the UNOS database.[860] In approximately 2% to 4% of male patients receiving a renal transplant, anti-GBM antibody disease may develop.[861] These antibodies are directed against the α5 noncollagenous (NC1) subunit of the intact α3,4,5 hexamer of collagen IV.[862] This antigen, which presumably does not exist in the native kidney of patients with hereditary nephritis, is present in normal donor kidneys and is thus recognized as foreign.[863,864] A profile of these patients has been compiled.[831] The patients are usually male, always deaf, and likely to have reached ESKD before the age of 30 years. There is a suggestion that certain mutations in the COL4A5 gene, such as deletions (which account for 11%–12% of Alport cases), may predispose patients to the development of allograft anti-GBM nephritis.[864] In 75% of cases, the onset of anti-GBM nephritis occurs within the first year after transplantation, and 76% of the allografts were lost. In a registry study of 296 patients with Alport syndrome, only one patient experienced anti-GBM disease. Outcomes in Alport patients were similar to matched controls in this Australia–New Zealand registry.[865]

## THIN BASEMENT MEMBRANE NEPHROPATHY

Thin basement membrane nephropathy (TBMN; also known as benign familial hematuria and thin GBM nephropathy) designates a condition that differs from Alport disease in its generally benign course and lack of progression. The typical finding on renal pathology is diffuse thinning of the GBMs. However, thin GBM may be found in other conditions as well (including early Alport disease and IgA nephropathy).[866] The true incidence of TBMN is unknown but is estimated to affect at least 1% of the population; reports evaluating patients with isolated hematuria suggest that 20% to 25% of such patients have TBMN.[867–869]

### CLINICAL FEATURES

Patients usually present in childhood with microhematuria. Hematuria is usually persistent but may be intermittent in some patients. Episodic gross hematuria may occur particularly during upper respiratory infections.[870,871] Patients do not typically have overt proteinuria, but when present, this may signal disease progression.[867,872]

### PATHOLOGY

Renal biopsies typically show no histologic abnormalities with the exception of focal erythrocyte casts. By IF, no glomerular deposits of immunoglobulins or complement are found. By EM, there is diffuse and relatively uniform thinning of the GBM (Fig. 32.43). The normal thickness of the GBM is age and gender dependent. Vogler et al.[873] have defined normal ranges for children: at birth 169 ± 30 nm, at 2 years of age 245 ± 49 nm, at 11 years 285 ± 39 nm. Steffes et al.[874] have defined normal ranges for adults as 373 ± 42 (males) or 326 ± 45 nm (females). Each laboratory should attempt to establish its own normals for GBM thickness. A cutoff value of 250 nm has been reported by some authors,[875–877] whereas other groups have used a cutoff of 330 nm.[872] There is often accentuation of the lamina rara interna and externa. Focal GBM gaps may be identified ultrastructurally. Immunostaining for the alpha subunits of collagen IV reveals a normal distribution in the GBM.

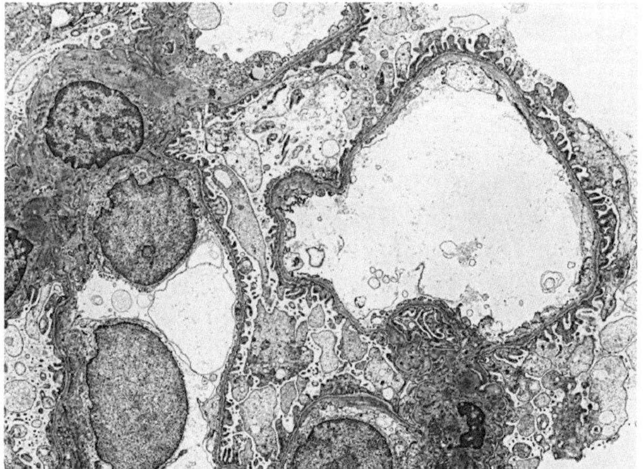

**Fig. 32.43** Thin basement membrane disease. By electron microscopy, the glomerular basement membranes are diffusely and uniformly thinned, measuring less than 200 nm in thickness (×2500).

### PATHOGENESIS

About 40% of TBMN disease has been linked to mutations of the COL4A3 and COL4A4 genes.[878] In most kindreds with TBMN, the disorder appears to be transmitted in an autosomal dominant pattern. In a few families with several affected children and apparently unaffected parents, the findings suggest a recessive mode of inheritance or that one parent was an asymptomatic carrier.[869,870,879] There appears to be a reduction or loss of the subepithelial portion of the basement membrane, which apparently contains normal relative amounts of type IV collagen.[880] The degree of GBM thinning does not appear to affect the clinical presentation or outcome.[881]

## DIFFERENTIAL DIAGNOSIS OF FAMILIAL HEMATURIAS

Type IV collagen defects can cause both TBMN and Alport syndrome. Patients with TBMN can be considered carriers of autosomal recessive Alport syndrome.[882,883] With advances in molecular biology and immunopathology, hereditary forms of hematuria have been better characterized. With the wider availability of genetic testing (which can secure the diagnosis in over 90% of Alport patients), a recommendation for a unified nomenclature for genetic disorders of the collagen IV α345 molecule has been suggested in a recent position paper and expert guidelines (Table 32.2).[803,804] The term *Alport syndrome* should be reserved for patients with the characteristic clinical features and a lamellated GBM with an abnormal collagen IV composition, and in whom a COL4A5 mutation (X-linked disease) or two COL4A3 or two COL4A4 mutations in trans (autosomal recessive disease) are identified or expected. The term thin basement membrane nephropathy (TBMN) should be reserved for individuals with persistent isolated glomerular hematuria who have a thinned GBM due to a heterozygous COL4A3 or COL4A4 (but not COL4A5) mutation. This distinction is to ensure patients who have X-linked Alport syndrome are not falsely reassured by the usually benign prognosis seen in TBMN. In those patients with renal impairment together with a heterozygous COL4A3 or COL4A4 mutation, there is likely to be a coincidental renal disease, such as IgA GN, or autosomal recessive Alport syndrome, or a second, undetected COL4 mutation. The correct diagnosis may be adjudicated after discussions among the nephrologist, pathologist, clinical geneticist, ophthalmologist, and audiologist, and interpretation of the relevant test results.[803] Genetic testing may be utilized when the diagnosis of Alport syndrome is suspected but cannot be confirmed with other techniques and when TBMN is suspected but X-linked Alport syndrome must be excluded. With current genetic techniques, the mutation detection rate is over 90% and more likely to be identified in individuals with early onset renal failure and extrarenal manifestations.[803]

Where genetic tests are not available, immunohistochemical analysis of $\alpha_3$, $\alpha_4$, and $\alpha_5$ subunits should be undertaken if

**Table 32.3 Immunostaining Patterns for $\alpha_5$ Subunit of Collagen IV in Kidney and Epidermal Basement Membranes**

| | Glomerular Basement Membrane | Bowman's Capsule | Epidermal Basement Membrane |
|---|---|---|---|
| Normal | Present/Normal | Present/Normal | Present/Normal |
| X-linked Alport males | Absent | Absent | Absent |
| X-linked Alport female carriers | Present segmentally/Mosaic | Present segmentally/Mosaic | Present focally/Mosaic |
| Autosomal recessive Alport | Absent | Present/Normal | Present/Normal |
| Thin basement membrane disease | Present/Normal | Present/Normal | Present/Normal |

From Savige J, Gregory M, Gross O, Kashtan C, Ding J, Flinter F. Expert guidelines for the management of Alport syndrome and thin basement membrane nephropathy. *J Am Soc Nephrol.* 2013;24(3):364–375.

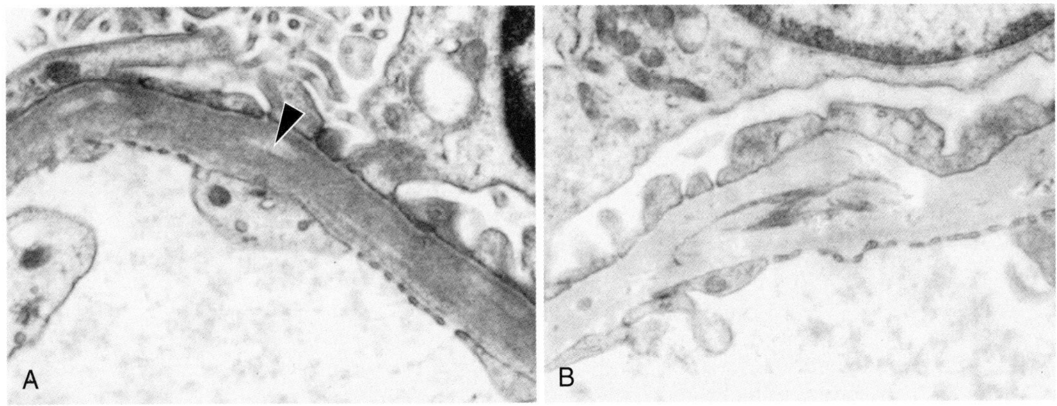


**Fig. 32.44** (A and B) Nail–patella syndrome. (A) Routine electron micrograph showing thickening of a glomerular basement membrane with focal irregular internal lucencies *(arrowhead)* (×15,000). (B) Phosphotungstic acid–stained electron micrograph demonstrating the characteristic banded collagen fibrils within the rarefied segments of glomerular basement membrane (×15,000).

available. Table 32.3 shows the typical immunostaining patterns in the kidney and skin basement membranes.

## NAIL–PATELLA SYNDROME (HEREDITARY OSTEO-ONYCHODYSPLASIA)

Nail–patella syndrome (NPS) is an autosomal dominant condition affecting tissues of both ectodermal and mesodermal origin, manifested as symmetrical nail, skeletal, ocular, and renal anomalies.

### CLINICAL FEATURES

The classical tetrad of anomalies of the nails, elbows, and knees, and iliac horns was described by Mino et al. in 1948.[884] Nail dysplasia and patellar aplasia or hypoplasia are essential features for the diagnosis of NPS. The presence of triangular nail lunulae is a pathognomonic sign for NPS. Other skeletal abnormalities include dysplasia of the elbow joints, posterior iliac horns, and foot deformities. Various ocular anomalies have sporadically been found in NPS patients, including microcornea, sclerocornea, congenital cataract, iris processes, pigmentation of the inner margin of the iris, and congenital glaucoma.[885]

Renal involvement is variable, being present in up to 38% of patients. Renal manifestations first appear in children and young adults and may include proteinuria, hematuria, hypertension, or edema. The nephrotic syndrome and progressive renal failure may occasionally occur. The course is generally benign with renal failure being a late feature.[886,887] Congenital malformations of the urinary tract and nephrolithiasis are also more frequent in these patients. Cases with renal lesions typical of NPS but without skeletal abnormalities have been reported.[888]

### PATHOLOGY

The findings on LM are nonspecific and include focal and segmental glomerular sclerosis, segmental thickening of the glomerular capillary wall and mild mesangial hypercellularity.[889] IF microscopy is nonspecific and IgM and C3 have been observed in sclerosed segments. Ultrastructural studies show a thickened basement membrane that contains irregular lucencies, imparting a "moth-eaten" appearance (Fig. 32.44A). The presence of intramembranous fibrils with the periodicity of collagen is revealed by phosphotungstic acid stains in EM sections, corresponding to the distribution of the intramembranous lucencies (Fig. 32.44B). These must be distinguished from the occasional collagen fibrils that can accumulate nonspecifically in the sclerotic mesangium in a variety of sclerosing glomerular conditions.[889]

## PATHOGENESIS

The genetic locus for this syndrome is on chromosome 9 and results from mutations in the LIM homeodomain protein *LMX1B* gene, which is transmitted in an autosomal dominant pattern and encodes a transcription factor. LMX1B plays a central role in dorsoventral patterning of the vertebrate limb.[890,891] In mice, genetic ablation of LMX1B leads to loss of Nphs2 expression as well as loss of expression of the GBM collagens Col4a3 and Col4a4, suggesting that Lmx1b potentially acts as a common upstream regulator of these genes.[892] In a study in zebrafish, expression of the podocyte gene NPHS2 is combinatorially regulated by the transcription factors Lmx1b and FoxC interacting synergistically with a common enhancer FLAT-E and forkhead.[893]

## TREATMENT

There is no specific treatment for this condition; occasional patients with renal failure have been successfully transplanted.[894]

# FABRY DISEASE (ANGIOKERATOMA CORPORIS DIFFUSUM UNIVERSALE)

Fabry disease (FD)[895] is an X-linked inborn error of glycosphingolipid metabolism involving a lysosomal enzyme, α-galactosidase A (also known as ceramide trihexosidase), and results from mutations of the *GLA* gene.[896] The enzyme deficiency leads to the accumulation of globotriaosylceramide (ceramide trihexoside) and related neutral glycosphingolipids, leading to multisystem involvement and dysfunction. Clinical guidelines for the diagnosis and treatment of FD have been published.[897,898]

## CLINICAL FEATURES

FD has been reported in all ethnic groups, and the estimated incidence in males is 1 in 40,000 to 1 in 60,000. In male hemizygotes, the initial clinical presentation usually begins in childhood with episodic pain in the extremities and acroparesthesias. Renal involvement is common in male hemizygotes and is occasional in female heterozygotes. The disease presents with hematuria and proteinuria, which often progresses to nephrotic levels. In men, progressive renal failure generally develops by the fifth decade. Data from the Fabry Registry suggest that proteinuria is a strong determinant of renal outcome.[899] In the United States, FD accounts for 0.02% of patients who began renal replacement therapy.[900]

The skin is commonly involved with reddish-purple macules (angiokeratomas) typically found "below the belt" on the abdomen, buttocks, hips, genitalia, and upper thighs. Other findings include palmar erythema, conjunctival and oral mucous membrane telangiectasia, and subungual splinter hemorrhages. The nervous system is involved with peripheral and autonomic neuropathy. Premature arterial disease of coronary vessels leads to myocardial ischemia and arrhythmias at a young age. Similarly, cerebrovascular involvement leads to early onset of strokes. In the heart, valvular disease and hypertrophic cardiomyopathy have also been reported. Corneal opacities are seen in virtually all hemizygotes and most heterozygotes. Posterior capsular cataracts, edema of retina and eyelids, and tortuous retinal and conjunctival vessels also may occur. Generalized lymphadenopathy, hepatosplenomegaly, aseptic necrosis of the femoral and humeral heads, myopathy, hypoalbuminemia, and hypogammaglobulinemia have been reported.

In carrier females, clinical manifestations may range from asymptomatic to severe disease similar to male hemizygotes. Up to one-third of female carriers have been reported to have significant disease manifestations.[901]

Atypical (later-onset) variants usually have residual alpha-Gal-A levels and may not demonstrate the classical syndrome. In the cardiac variant, patients present in their fifth to eighth decade of life with hypertrophic cardiomyopathy, conduction abnormalities, or arrhythmias.[902] The renal variant was reported in 1.2% of patients on dialysis who were previously misdiagnosed as chronic glomerulonephritis.[903]

## PATHOLOGY

Glycosphingolipid accumulation begins early in life[904] and the major renal site of accumulation is the podocyte (visceral epithelial cells). By LM, these cells are enlarged with numerous clear, uniform vacuoles in the cytoplasm causing a foamy appearance (Fig. 32.45). These vacuoles can be shown to contain lipids when fat stains (such as Oil Red-O) are used, or when viewed under the polarizing microscope where they exhibit a double refractile appearance before being processed with lipid solvents. All renal cells may accumulate the lipid. These include (in addition to podocytes) parietal epithelial cells, glomerular endothelial cells, mesangial cells, interstitial capillary endothelial cells, distal convoluted tubule cells, and to a lesser extent, cells of the loops of Henle and proximal tubular cells. Indeed, vascular endothelial cells are involved in virtually every organ and tissue.[905] In the kidney, the myocytes and endothelial cells of arteries also are commonly involved. In heterozygotes, similar changes are present but with less severity.[906] Characteristic findings are noted on EM

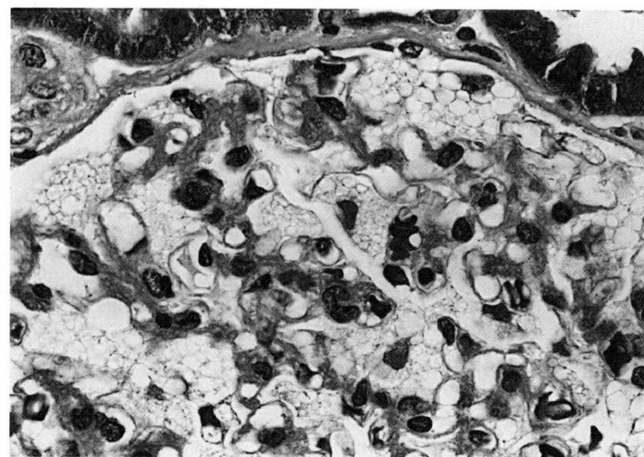

**Fig. 32.45** Fabry disease. By light microscopy, the visceral epithelial cells (podocytes) are markedly enlarged with foamy-appearing cytoplasm (trichrome, ×800).

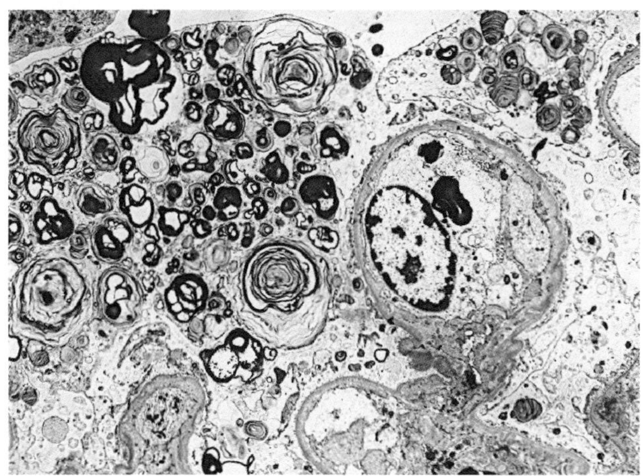

**Fig. 32.46** Fabry disease. Electron micrograph showing abundant whorled myelin figures within the cytoplasm of the podocytes. A few similar inclusions are also identified within the glomerular endothelial cells (×2000).

(Fig. 32.46). The major finding is large numbers of "myelin figures" or "zebra bodies" within the cytoplasm of the podocytes, and to a variable extent, in other renal cell types. These intracytoplasmic vacuoles consist of single membrane–bound dense bodies with a concentric whorled or multilamellar appearance. Glomerular podocytes exhibit variable foot process effacement. The GBMs are initially normal, but with progression of disease, there may be thickening and collapse of the GBM, focal and segmental glomerular sclerosis, with accompanying tubular atrophy and interstitial fibrosis.[907] Findings on IF microscopy are usually negative except in areas of segmental sclerosis, where IgM and complement may be demonstrated. Orange autofluorescence corresponding to the lipid inclusions may be found in podocytes and other renal cells.

## PATHOGENESIS

The mutations in the GLA gene generally are "private" with specific molecular defects that vary from family to family, and include rearrangements, deletions, and point mutations.[908] Deficiency of the enzyme leads to accumulation of globotriaosylceramide especially in the vascular endothelium, with subsequent ischemic organ dysfunction. Patients with blood groups B and AB have earlier and more severe symptoms, likely related to accumulation of the terminal α-galactose substance during the synthesis of the B antigen on red blood cell membranes.[909] Globotriaosylceramide accumulation in podocytes may lead to proteinuria and renal dysfunction, but functional abnormalities are not always noted, especially in female heterozygotes. A gene-knockout mouse model of FD has been produced, which shows the characteristic changes.[910]

## DIAGNOSIS

The diagnosis in affected males can be established by measuring levels of α-galactosidase-A in plasma or peripheral blood leukocytes followed by mutation analysis when positive. Hemizygotes have almost no measurable enzyme activity. Female carriers may have enzyme levels in the low to normal range; to diagnose female carriers, the specific mutation in the family must be demonstrated.[803] The measurement of urinary ceramide digalactoside and trihexoside levels may also be of use to identify the carrier state. Prenatal diagnosis can be made by measuring amniocyte enzyme levels in amniotic fluid. Screening of dialysis and renal transplant patients with undiagnosed renal failure and those with hypertrophic cardiomyopathy and strokes has yielded the diagnosis of FD in 1% to 5%.[911]

## TREATMENT

Two forms of recombinant α-Gal A are available. Agalsidase alpha (Replagal; Shire Human Genetic Therapies, Boston, MA, USA) and agalsidase beta (Fabrazyme; Genzyme, Cambridge, MA, USA). Agalsidase alpha is produced in a continuous human cell line and is administered as an intravenous infusion over 40 minutes at a dose of 0.2 mg/kg body weight every 2 weeks. Agalsidase beta is produced in Chinese hamster ovary (CHO) cells and is given as an intravenous infusion over a 4-hour period at a dose of 1.0 mg/kg body weight every 2 weeks.[897] Two pivotal randomized, controlled trials have shown that recombinant human α-galactosidase-A enzyme replacement therapy (ERT) is safe and can improve clinical parameters. In one short-term study α-galactosidase-A treatment was associated with improved neuropathic pain, decreased mesangial widening, and improved creatinine clearance.[912] In the second study, repeat renal biopsies showed decreased microvascular endothelial deposits of globotriaosylceramide.[905,913] However, a systematic review of five trials involving 187 patients did not provide robust evidence for the use of replacement therapy.[914] From a renal standpoint, open-label extension studies showed that renal function remained stable in the long-term in most patients with normal renal function at baseline.[915,916] However, patients with impaired baseline renal function may show continued decline despite ERT.[916] Clinical recommendations for the treatment of FD have been published.[897,898]

Based upon consensus criteria, treatment of FD was based on gender, and the presence of classical or nonclassical disease manifestations. The division of females into classical and nonclassical FD is based on the presence or absence of clustered angiokeratoma, cornea verticillata, or a very high (lyso)Gb3 level. For males with classical FD, treatment with ERT may be considered in patients aged over 16 years even if asymptomatic. The diagnosis of classical FD in these patients is based on the presence of a GLA mutation, absent or very low residual enzyme activity, and the presence of at least one of the following: angiokeratoma, cornea verticillata, or a very high (lyso)Gb3 level. Classically affected males and females and males with nonclassical FD should be treated as soon as there are early signs of organ involvement (kidney, heart, and/or central nervous system signs) consistent with FD and not fully explained by other pathology, whereas treatment may be considered in females with nonclassical FD and early clinical signs consistent with FD.[898] Treatment should not be withheld from patients with severe renal insufficiency (GFR <45 mL/min/1.73 $m^2$) and from those on dialysis or with cognitive decline, but carefully considered on an individual basis. Stopping ERT may be considered in patients with end-stage FD or other comorbidities, leading to a life expectancy of <1 year. In those with cognitive decline of any cause, or lack of response for 1 year when the sole indication for ERT is neuropathic pain, stopping ERT may be considered. In addition, in patients with ESKD, without an option for renal transplantation, in combination with advanced heart failure (New York Heart Association [NYHA] class IV), cessation of ERT should be considered. ERT in patients who are noncompliant or fail to attend regularly at visits is ineffective.[898]

The ERA-EDTA Registry in Europe reported that patient survival on dialysis was 41% at 5 years; cardiovascular complications (48%) and cachexia (17%) were the main causes of death. Graft survival at 3 years in 33 patients was not inferior to that of other nephropathies (72% vs. 69%), and patient survival after transplantation was comparable to that of patients under 55 years of age.[917] In the US population, survival of Fabry patients was lower than nondiabetic renal failure patients.[900] Long-term allograft function in patients with FD has been reported. Glycosphingolipid deposits do recur in allografts, but have not been reported to cause graft failure.[918]

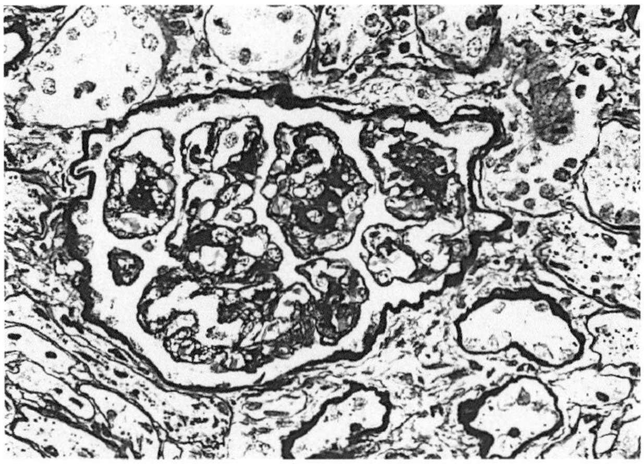

**Fig. 32.47** Sickle cell disease. An example of sickle cell glomerulopathy with membranoproliferative features. There are double contours of the glomerular basement membrane associated with segmental mesangiolysis (Jones methenamine silver, ×500).

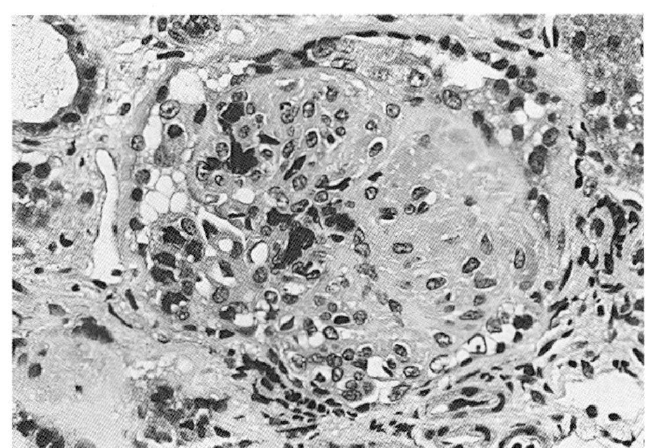

**Fig. 32.48** Sickle cell disease. An example with focal segmental glomerulosclerosis. The nonsclerotic glomerular capillaries are congested with sickled erythrocytes (hematoxylin–eosin, ×500).

## SICKLE CELL NEPHROPATHY

Renal disease associated with sickle cell disease includes gross hematuria, papillary necrosis, nephrotic syndrome, renal infarction, inability to concentrate urine, renal medullary carcinoma, and pyelonephritis.[919,920] Microscopic or gross hematuria is likely the result of microinfarcts in the renal medulla.[921] Glomerular lesions, however, are less commonly encountered and may be seen in patients with HbSS, HbSC, and sickle cell thalassemia.[922]

### CLINICAL FEATURES

In one study, the prevalence of proteinuria (>1+ on a dipstick) in HbSS disease was 26%.[918] The majority of proteinuric patients had less than 3 g/day and an elevated serum creatinine level was present in 7% of patients. In another study, 4.2% with HbSS disease and 2.4% with combined sickle C disease developed renal failure. The median age of disease onset for these patients was 23.1 and 49.9 years, respectively. Survival time for patients with HbSS anemia after the diagnosis of renal failure, despite dialysis, was 4 years, and the median age at the time of death was 27 years. The risk for renal failure was increased in patients with the Central African Republic beta s-gene cluster haplotype, hypertension, proteinuria, and severe anemia.[923] The course of HbSS renal disease is progressive; in one series, 18% of patients with HbSS disease progressed to ESKD.[924]

### PATHOLOGY

Early glomerular lesions in patients with HbSS include enlarged glomeruli and dilated and congested capillaries containing sickled erythrocytes (some of these patients may have nephrotic proteinuria).[925] Heterogeneous patterns of glomerular injury have been reported. A membranoproliferative pattern exhibits mesangial proliferation with mild to moderate capillary wall thickening due to GBM reduplication and mesangial interposition (Fig. 32.47). Some of these patients also exhibit features of chronic thrombotic microangiopathy, with narrow double contours of the GBM and mesangiolysis. A pattern of membranous glomerulonephritis has also been described. On IF microscopy, irregular granular deposits of IgG and C3 have been reported in those cases with membranous features and in a subgroup of cases with membranoproliferative pattern on LM.[925,926] Ultrastructural studies show granular dense deposits in the mesangial and subepithelial area. More commonly, those cases with membranoproliferative features have no detectable deposits, but exhibit subendothelial accumulation of electron-lucent “fluff” resembling the changes in chronic thrombotic microangiopathies. Mild mesangial proliferation and peripheral mesangial interposition are frequently seen. Sickled erythrocytes containing paracrystalline inclusions may be identified within glomerular capillaries.[926–930]

In the second form of sickle glomerulopathy, focal and segmental glomerulosclerosis occurs in association with glomerulomegaly (Fig. 32.48). Two patterns of FSGS may be observed: a “collapsing” pattern and an “expansive” pattern.[919,922,931–933] Using the modern classification of FSGS, collapsing, perihilar, tip, and not otherwise specified variants have been reported.[925] On IF, nonspecific IgM and C3 are seen in sclerosed segments. In all these forms, there may be prominent intracapillary erythrocyte sickling and congestion.

## PATHOGENESIS

The mechanism(s) for glomerular abnormalities in SS patients is not fully understood. One theory proposes that mesangial cells are activated by the presence of fragmented red blood cells in glomerular capillaries. Activated mesangial cells promote synthesis of matrix proteins and migrate into the peripheral capillary wall, leading to GBM reduplication.[934] In another study, renal tubular epithelial antigens and complement components were detected in a granular pattern along the GBM, leading the authors to hypothesize that glomerulonephritis was mediated by glomerular deposition of immune complexes containing renal tubular epithelial antigen and specific antibody to renal tubular epithelial antigen (the antigen possibly released after tubular damage secondary to decreased oxygenation and hemodynamic alterations related to SS disease).[926]

In patients with the FSGS pattern, it is proposed that there is an initial but progressive obliteration of the glomerular capillary bed by red blood cell sickling that cannot be compensated by further glomerular hypertrophy. Hemodynamic glomerular injury ensues from the sustained or increasing hyperfiltration in a diminishing capillary bed, manifesting morphologically as the expansive pattern of sclerosis.[922,931] According to one report, the hyperfiltration observed in 51% of SS patients correlated positively with lower hemoglobin levels and reticulocyte counts, implying that the hemolysis-related vasculopathy may be contributing.[935] A role for reactive oxygen species as mediator of chronic vascular endothelial injury has also been proposed.[936]

Recently, polymorphisms in the myosin, heavy-chain 9, nonmuscle (MYH9) and apolipoprotein L1 (APOL1) genes have been associated with risk for proteinuria in African-American patients with SS disease. GFR was negatively correlated with proteinuria ($P < .0001$), and was significantly predicted by an interaction between MYH9 and APOL1 in a multivariable model.[937] High-risk APOL1 genotypes were also associated with European patients of sub-Saharan African ancestry.[938]

## TREATMENT

The treatment of renal disease in sickle cell anemia has generally been unsatisfactory. Treatment of patients with sickle cell nephropathy with ACE inhibitors reduces the degree of proteinuria.[922,939] However, their effectiveness in preserving renal function remains to be established.[804] Hematopoietic stem cell transplantation in selected patients with sickle cell disease was found to be effective in preventing renal function decline compared with nontransplanted patients.[940]

SS nephropathy accounts for 0.1% of ESKD patients in the United States, with a higher mortality compared with other causes of ESKD (including diabetes).[941] Renal transplantation has been performed in SS patients. One-year graft survival in SS patients was similar to other transplanted patients; however, long-term renal outcome was worse, as was short- and long-term mortality.[942] Transplanted SS patients commonly experience sickle crises.[943,944] Recurrent sickle cell nephropathy has been reported in the transplanted kidney.[932,945] Patient survival has improved compared with previously, with survival rates comparable with diabetic recipients.[811]

# LIPODYSTROPHY

Lipodystrophies are rare diseases associated with insulin resistance in which there is loss of fat, which may be localized to the upper part of the body in partial lipodystrophy (PLD) or more diffuse in generalized lipodystrophy (GLD).[946,947]

A majority of patients with GLD (both genetic and acquired) are proteinuric and have an elevated GFR (reflecting hyperfiltration). Renal biopsy showed FSGS as the most common finding, followed by type I MPGN and only rarely diabetic nephropathy.[948]

PLD (Barraquer–Simons syndrome) is commonly associated with C3 glomerulopathy/dense deposit disease. PLD most often presents in girls between ages 5 and 15 years. In addition to the loss of fat, the lipodystrophies are associated with a wide variety of metabolic and systemic abnormalities. Hyperinsulinism, insulin resistance, and diabetes are common. Other metabolic abnormalities include hyperlipidemia, hyperproteinemia, and euthyroid hypermetabolism. Clinical findings may include tall stature, muscular hypertrophy, hirsutism, macroglossia, abdominal distension, subcutaneous nodules, acanthosis nigricans, hepatomegaly, cirrhosis, clitoral or penile enlargement, febrile adenopathy, cerebral atrophy, cerebral ventricular dilatation, hemiplegia, mental retardation, and cardiomegaly.[946,947] Renal disease occurs in 20% to 50% of patients with PLD,[946,947] and PLD occurs in 10% of patients with dense deposit disease.[949,950] Patients usually have asymptomatic proteinuria and microhematuria, but some may develop the nephrotic syndrome.[951,952] Diminished C3 levels in association with the C3 nephritic (C3NeF) is the most prominent serologic abnormality. The course of glomerular disease is fairly rapid progression to ESKD, and the prognosis of PLD is determined mainly by renal disease.[947]

In GLD, the nephrotic syndrome, nonnephrotic proteinuria, and hypertension have been reported.[946] About 88% of these patients had albumin excretion over 30 mg/24 h, 60% had macroalbuminuria (>300 mg/24 h), and 20% had nephrotic-range proteinuria over 3500 mg/24 h.[953]

The pathogenesis of PLD and GLD is poorly understood. Acquired forms of lipodystrophy are believed to be autoimmune disorders. Most patients with PLD possess an IgG autoantibody, C3 nephritic factor (C3NeF), which binds to and stabilizes the alternate pathway C3 convertase, C3bBb. In the presence of C3NeF, C3bBb becomes resistant to its regulatory proteins, factors H and I. Although the majority of patients with partial dystrophy have low serum C3, not all patients will exhibit nephritis.[954] There is no effective therapy for PLD, and although renal transplantation is the treatment of choice when ESKD ensues, recurrence in transplants has been reported.[947,955,956] In a single patient with PLD and crescentic dense deposit disease eculizumab was used successfully.[957] In GLD, leptin therapy has been associated with improvement of renal parameters.[958] A single GLD patient has undergone renal transplantation.[959]

## LECITHIN-CHOLESTEROL ACYLTRANSFERASE DEFICIENCY

Gjone and Norum reported a familial disorder characterized by proteinuria, anemia, hyperlipidemia, and corneal opacity.[960,961] Most of the initial patients were of Scandinavian origin; subsequently the disease has also been reported from other countries.[962,963] The disease arises from decreased serum LCAT activity because of mutations in the *LCAT* gene.[964,965]

### CLINICAL FEATURES

The triad of anemia, nephrotic syndrome, and corneal opacities suggests this disorder. Renal disease is a universal finding with albuminuria noted early in life. Proteinuria increases in severity during the fourth and fifth decades, often with development of the nephrotic syndrome. The latter is accompanied by hypertension and progressive renal failure. Most patients are mildly anemic with target cells and poikilocytes on the peripheral smear. There is evidence of low-grade hemolysis. During childhood, corneal opacities appear as grayish spots over the cornea accompanied by a lipoid arcus. Visual acuity is unimpaired. Fish eye disease results from a partial deficiency of LCAT and presents with corneal disease and without renal manifestations. Patients have reduced plasma high-density lipoprotein cholesterol concentrations (usually <0.3 mmol/L; 11.6 mg/dL) and plasma levels of apo A-I below 50 mg/dL. Premature atherosclerosis is unusual in complete LCAT deficiency but may occur from unknown reasons in fish eye disease.[966]

### PATHOLOGY

Abnormalities are found mainly in the glomeruli, but arteries and arterioles may also be affected.[960,961,967,968] By LM (Fig. 32.49), the glomerular capillary walls are thickened and there is mesangial expansion. Basement membranes are irregular and often appear to contain vacuoles, resembling stage 3 membranous alterations. Double contouring of capillary walls is occasionally present. Similar vacuoles in the mesangium impart a honeycomb appearance. There is no associated glomerular hypercellularity, with the exception of occasional endocapillary foam cells. By IF microscopy, there is typically negative staining for all immunoglobulin and complement components. On EM (Fig. 32.50), the vacuolated areas seen by LM correspond to extracellular irregular lucent zones (lacunae) in the mesangial matrix and GBM containing lipid inclusions. These inclusions consist of rounded, small structures, either solid or with a lamellar substructure containing electron-lucent and electron-dense zones.

### PATHOGENESIS

The disorder is inherited in an autosomal recessive pattern. Patients have little or no LCAT activity in their blood circulation because of mutations in the *LCAT* gene.[964,965] LCAT is an enzyme that circulates in the blood primarily bound to high-density lipoprotein and catalyzes the formation of cholesteryl esters via the hydrolysis and transfer of the sn-2 fatty acid from phosphatidylcholine to the 3-hydroxyl group of cholesterol. Thus patients with LCAT deficiency have high levels of phosphatidylcholine and unesterified cholesterol, with corresponding low levels of lysophosphatidylcholine and cholesteryl ester in the blood. An abnormal lipoprotein, lipoprotein-X (Lp-X), is present in patients' plasma. Lp-X is thought to arise from the surface of chylomicron remnants that remain after not being metabolized due to the absence of active LCAT. Accumulation of lipid component occurs in both intracellular and extracellular sites. Lipid accumulation in the GBM results in proteinuria. Endothelial damage and resulting vascular insufficiency may contribute to renal insufficiency. It has been proposed that Lp-X stimulates mesangial cells, leading to the production of MCP-1 (monocyte chemoattractant protein-1), promoting monocyte infiltration, foam cell formation, and progressive glomerulosclerosis in a manner similar to atherosclerosis.[969] Rarely, acquired autoimmune LCAT deficiency may occur, with renal biopsy findings similar to familial LCAT deficiency with coexisting lesion of membranous nephropathy.[970]

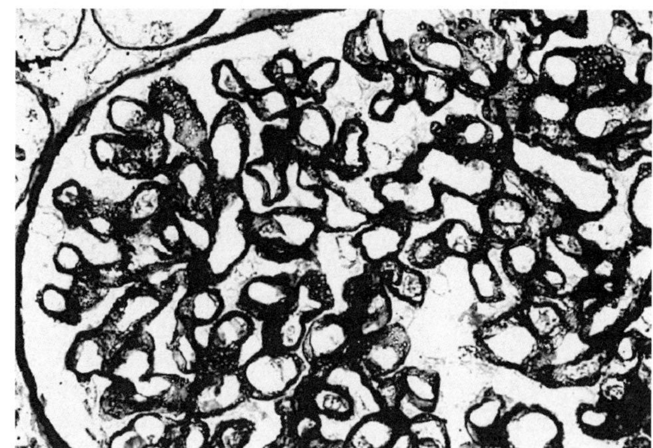

**Fig. 32.49** LCAT deficiency. The glomerular basement membranes and mesangium have a vacuolated appearance, resembling stage 3 membranous glomerulopathy (Jones methenamine silver, ×800).

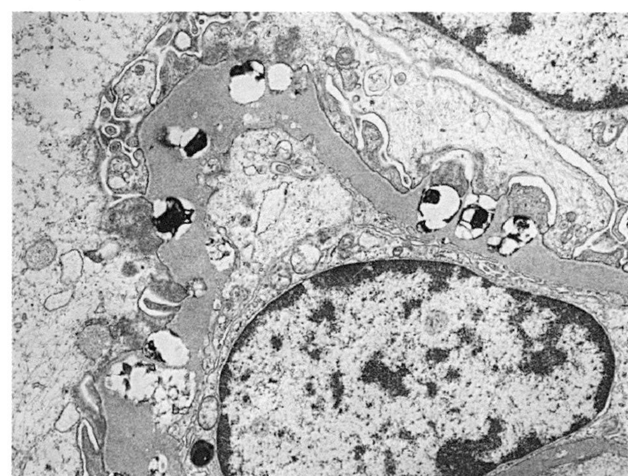

**Fig. 32.50** LCAT deficiency. Electron micrograph showing intramembranous lacunae with rounded structures containing an electron-dense membranous core and electron-lucent periphery (×5000).

### DIAGNOSIS

In patients suspected of having LCAT deficiency, measurements of plasma enzyme should be performed. The enzyme levels and activity vary amongst kindreds[971]; thus enzyme measurements should include activity as well as mass. The diagnosis can be confirmed by genetic analysis of the entire coding region, or targeted variant analysis (https://www.ncbi.nlm.nih.gov/gtr/).

### TREATMENT

A low lipid diet or lipid-lowering drugs have not shown to be of benefit.[967] Plasma infusions may provide reversal of erythrocytic abnormalities, but long-term benefits have yet to be demonstrated.[972] The lesions may recur in the allograft but renal function is adequately preserved.[973] A single-patient study of ERT rhLCAT (ACP-501) showed improved biochemical parameters.[974]

## LIPOPROTEIN GLOMERULOPATHY

Lipoprotein glomerulopathy (LPG) is a characterized by dysbetalipoproteinemia and lipid deposition in the kidney, leading to glomerulosclerosis and renal failure. The kidney is the only organ affected in this lipid disorder. The majority of reported patients have been from Japan,[975,976] but other populations can also be affected. Renal manifestations are usually detected in adulthood with rare reports of childhood onset and disease progression.

The histologic hallmark of LPG is the presence of laminated thrombi consisting of lipids within the lumina of dilated glomerular capillaries. The pathogenesis of LGP is unknown, but the presence of thrombi consisting of lipoproteins suggests a primary abnormality in lipid metabolism.[977] Indeed type III hyperlipidemia (elevated low-density lipoprotein and high apo-E levels) has been reported in Japanese patients, associated with apo-E variants (commonly apo-E2 as opposed to apo E-III).[976,978–982] Other genetic variants, such as ApoE Las Vegas, have been reported in Caucasians of European descent in the United States.[983] Furthermore, LPG-like deposits were detected in apo-E–deficient mice transfected with apo-E (Sendai), one of the apo-E variants associated with LPG.

There is no uniformly effective therapy for LPG; however, intensive lipid-lowering therapy with fibrates or double filtration plasmapheresis therapy has been reported to be effective in case reports.[984,985] Recurrence of lesions of LPG has occurred in renal allografts.[986,987]

## GLOMERULAR INVOLVEMENT WITH BACTERIAL INFECTIONS

### INFECTIOUS ENDOCARDITIS

The natural history of endocarditis-associated glomerulonephritis has changed significantly in parallel with the changing epidemiology of infectious endocarditis (IE) and the advent of effective antibiotic therapies.[988] In the preantibiotic era, *Streptococcus viridans* was the commonest organism and glomerulonephritis occurred in 50% to 80% of subacute endocarditis cases.[989] During that era, glomerulonephritis was less commonly associated with acute endocarditis.[990,991] With the use of prophylactic antibiotics in patients with valvular heart disease, and an increase in intravenous drug use, *Staphylococcus aureus* has replaced *S. viridans* as the primary pathogen. Glomerulonephritis in these patients with acute IE occurs as commonly as in subacute endocarditis.[989,992–994] The incidence of glomerulonephritis with endocarditis with *S. aureus* ranges from 22% to 78%,[992,995] being higher in those series consisting predominantly of intravenous drug users.[995,996] In a study of 49 patients with IE, the commonest organism isolated was *S. aureus* (53%), with methicillin resistance in 56%. *Streptococcus* species were the second most common pathogens found (23%). Less common causes of endocarditis were *Bartonella henselae* in four patients, *Coxiella burnetii* in two, *Cardiobacterium hominis* in one, and *Gemella* species in one. Four patients (9%) had culture-negative endocarditis.[997]

### CLINICAL FEATURES

Renal complications of IE include infarcts, abscesses, and glomerulonephritis (all of which may coexist). In focal glomerulonephritis, mild asymptomatic urinary abnormalities including hematuria, pyuria, and albuminuria may be noted. Infrequently, with severe focal glomerulonephritis, renal insufficiency or uremia may be present. Renal dysfunction, microhematuria or gross hematuria, and the nephrotic-range proteinuria may be present with diffuse glomerulonephritis.[989,992,998] Rapidly progressive renal failure with crescents has been reported.[989,999] Rarely, patients may present with vasculitic features (including purpura).[1000] Although hypocomplementemia is frequent, it is neither invariable (occurring in 60%–90% of patients with glomerulonephritis) nor specific for renal involvement.[994,995] The majority of patients demonstrate activation of the classical pathway.[995,1001] Alternate pathway activation has been described in some cases of *S. aureus* endocarditis.[995] The degree of complement activation correlates with the severity of renal impairment[995] and the complement levels normalize with successful therapy of the infection. Circulating immune complexes have been found in the serum in up to 90% of patients.[1001,1002] Mixed cryoglobulins and rheumatoid factor may also be present in the serum of patients.[994,1003] ANCA positivity has been occasionally reported in biopsy-proven immune complex glomerulonephritis associated with IE, some of which have necrotizing and crescentic features.[1004] Anti-GBM antibody in eluates from diseased glomeruli has been rarely reported.[1005]

### PATHOLOGY

On LM, focal and segmental endocapillary proliferative glomerulonephritis with focal crescents is the most typical finding. Necrotizing lesions may be present.[997] Some patients may exhibit a more diffuse endocapillary proliferative and exudative glomerulonephritis with or without crescents.[989,990,992,1006,1007] Typically IF reveals granular capillary and mesangial deposits of IgG and C3, C3 alone, or varying combinations of IgM, IgG, and C3.[989,992,1006] IgA staining may predominate in some patients, and is known as IgA-dominant infection–related GN.[997,1008,1009] The latter is particularly associated with *Staphylococcus*, especially pulmonary sources, which might make it difficult to differentiate this from IgA nephropathy/vasculitis. The finding of predominant IgM staining may be associated with *Bartonella* endocarditis.[870] EM shows electron-dense deposits in mesangial, subendothelial, and occasionally subepithelial locations, with varying degrees of mesangial and endocapillary proliferation.[989,992,1006,1010] Rarely, patients with endocarditis may be ANCA positive with renal biopsy showing concomitant necrotizing lesions and proliferative lesions with relatively scant immune complex deposition.[997,1009,1011]

## PATHOGENESIS

The diffuse deposition of immunoglobulin and the depression of complement and electron-dense deposits support an immune complex mechanism for the production of this form of glomerulonephritis. The demonstration of specific antibody in kidney eluates and the detection of bacterial antigen in the deposits further supported this view. Both *S. aureus*[1012] and hemolytic *Streptococcus*[1013] antigens have been identified.

## TREATMENT

With the initiation of antibiotic therapy, the manifestations of glomerulonephritis begin to subside. Rarely, microhematuria and proteinuria may persist for years.[989] Plasmapheresis and corticosteroids have been reported to promote renal recovery in some patients with renal failure.[999,1014] However, this approach should be taken cautiously because of the risk of promoting infectious aspects of the disease, and concomitant secondary hypogammaglobulinemia, while ameliorating the immunologic manifestations. Immunosuppression has also been used to treat patients with concomitant ANCA and immune complex–associated glomerulonephritis.[872]

## SHUNT NEPHRITIS

Ventriculovascular (ventriculoatrial, ventriculojugular) shunts (which are rarely used nowadays) for the treatment of hydrocephalus were colonized commonly with microorganisms, particularly *Staph. albus* (75%).[1015] Less often, other bacteria (e.g., *Propionibacterium acnes*) have been implicated.[1016,1017] Ventriculoperitoneal shunts are more resistant to infection. However, glomerulonephritis has been reported with these shunts as well.[1018]

Patients commonly present with fever. Anemia, hepatosplenomegaly, purpura, arthralgias, and lymphadenopathy are found on examination. Renal manifestations include hematuria (microscopic or gross), proteinuria (nephrotic syndrome in 30% of patients), azotemia, and hypertension. Laboratory abnormalities include presence of rheumatoid factor, cryoimmunoglobulins, elevated sedimentation rate and CRP levels, hypocomplementemia, and presence of circulating immune complexes.[1019,1020] Shunt nephritis usually presents within a few months of shunt placement, but delayed manifestations, as late as two decades have been reported.[1021] By LM, glomeruli exhibit mesangial proliferation or membranoproliferative pattern of glomerulonephritis. IF reveals diffuse granular deposits of IgG, IgM, and C3. IgM is often the predominant Ig deposited in shunt nephritis. Electron-dense mesangial and subendothelial deposits are found by EM.[1017,1022] Antibiotic therapy and prompt removal of the infected catheter usually lead to remission of the glomerulonephritis.[1023] However, cases progressing to chronic renal failure have been reported.[1024] Rarely, patients have elevated proteinase-3–specific ANCA titers which also improved after removal of the infected shunt, with or without corticosteroid therapy.[1025]

## VISCERAL INFECTION

Visceral infections in the form of abdominal, pulmonary, and retroperitoneal abscesses are known to be associated with glomerulonephritis.[1026] These can be clinically occult. The clinical and pathological syndrome resembles infective endocarditis. Beaufils et al. reported on 11 patients who had visceral abscesses and in whom acute renal failure developed. Circulating cryoglobulins, decreased serum complement levels, and circulating immune complexes were found in some of these patients. All renal biopsies showed a diffuse proliferative and crescentic glomerulonephritis. The evolution of the glomerulonephritis, documented by serial biopsies, closely paralleled the course of the infection. A complete recovery of renal function occurred in those cases in which a rapid and complete cure of the infection was obtained. For those patients in whom the infection was not cured or in whom therapy was delayed, chronic renal failure also developed.[1027] Outcome is worse in elderly patients and in diabetics.[988]

## OTHER BACTERIAL INFECTIONS AND FUNGAL INFECTIONS

Congenital, secondary, and latent forms of syphilis rarely may be complicated by glomerular involvement. Patients are typically nephrotic, and proteinuria usually responds to penicillin therapy.[1028–1032] Membranous nephropathy with varying degrees of proliferation and with granular IgG and C3 deposits is the most common finding on biopsies. Treponemal antigen and antibody have been eluted from deposits. Rarely, minimal change lesions[1033] and crescentic glomerulonephritis[1034] or amyloidosis may be seen.

*Bartonella henselae* is the organism responsible for bartonellosis (cat scratch disease) which typically manifests as a skin papule followed by regional lymphadenopathy. Rarely, endocarditis, central nervous system involvement (encephalopathy), generalized skin rash, and the Parinaud oculoglandular syndrome (fever, regional lymphadenopathy, and follicular conjunctivitis) may occur. Renal manifestations are rare and can include IgA nephropathy,[1035] postinfectious glomerulonephritis with IgM dominance,[1036,1037] or necrotizing glomerulonephritis.[1038] In general, spontaneous recovery may occur with control of infection; however, end-stage renal failure has been reported with aggressive renal disease.[1038]

Renal involvement including azotemia, proteinuria, nephrotic syndrome, renal tubular defects, and hematuria is not uncommon in leprosy, especially with the lepra reaction.[1039–1044] Rarely, patients present with RPGN[1045] or ESKD.[1046] Mesangial proliferation, diffuse proliferative glomerulonephritis, crescentic glomerulonephritis, membranous nephropathy, MPGN, microscopic angiitis, and amyloidosis may all be seen in kidney biopsies. Organisms consistent with *Mycobacterium leprae* have been found in glomeruli.

Aspergillosis has been associated with immune complex–mediated glomerulonephritis.[1047] Membranous nephropathy, MPGN, crescentic glomerulonephritis, and amyloidosis have been associated with *Mycobacterium tuberculosis.*[1048–1051] *Mycoplasma* has been reported to be associated with nephrotic syndrome and RPGN. Antibiotics do not seem to alter the course of the disease. Mycoplasmal antigen has been reported to be present in the glomerular lesions.[1052–1056] Acute glomerulonephritis with hypocomplementemia has been reported with pneumococcal infections. Proliferative glomerulonephritis with deposition of IgG, IgM, complements C1q, C3, and C4, and pneumococcal antigens has been observed in renal biopsies.[1057,1058] Nocardiosis has been associated with mesangiocapillary glomerulonephritis.[1059] In infections with *Brucella,* patients may present with hematuria, proteinuria (usually nephrotic), and varying degrees of renal functional impairment. There usually is improvement after antibiotics, but histologic abnormalities, proteinuria, and hypertension may persist. Glomerular mesangial proliferation, focal and segmental endocapillary proliferation, diffuse proliferation, and crescents may be found in renal biopsies. IF may show no deposits, IgG, or occasionally IgA.[1060–1064] Asymptomatic urinary abnormalities may be seen in up to 80% of patients infected with *Leptospira.* Patients usually present with acute renal failure due to tubulointerstitial nephritis. Rarely, mesangial or diffuse proliferative glomerulonephritis may be seen.[1065,1066] From 1% to 4% of patients with typhoid fever secondary to *Salmonella* experience glomerulonephritis. Asymptomatic urinary abnormalities may be more frequent. Renal manifestations are usually transient, resolving within 2 to 3 weeks. Serum C3 may be depressed. Mesangial proliferation with deposits of IgG, C3, and C4 is the commonest finding. IgA nephropathy has also been reported.[1067–1069]

## GLOMERULAR INVOLVEMENT WITH PARASITIC DISEASES

### MALARIA

Four strains of malaria parasite cause human disease: *Plasmodium vivax, Plasmodium falciparum, Plasmodium malariae* (causing quartan malaria), and *Plasmodium ovale.* Of these, renal involvement has been extensively documented and studied in *P. malariae* and *P. falciparum.* In falciparum malaria, clinically overt glomerular disease is uncommon. Asymptomatic urinary abnormalities may occur with subnephrotic proteinuria and hematuria or pyuria. Renal function is usually normal. Renal biopsies show mesangial proliferation or membranoproliferative lesions.[1070] Severe malaria may manifest with hemoglobinuric acute renal failure.[1071] In initial reports, quartan malaria was strongly associated with nephrotic syndrome in infected children. There was progression to end-stage renal failure within 3 to 5 years with no improvement following antimalarial treatment or steroids.[1072] Renal biopsies in Ugandan adults and children with quartan malaria showed some form of proliferative glomerulonephritis (diffuse, focal, lobular, or minimal). Membranous nephropathy had also been described in these patients.[1073] However, in Nigerian children, the most common lesion was a localized or diffuse thickening of glomerular capillary walls with focal or generalized double-contouring and segmental glomerular sclerosis.[1074] IF examination revealed deposits of IgG, IgM, C3, and *P. malariae* antigen in the glomeruli. By EM, electron-dense material was observed within the irregularly thickened GBM.[1075] Of note, a recent report from endemic areas in Nigeria has not found any cases of childhood nephrotic syndrome associated with quartan malaria.[1076] The propensity of malaria to cause glomerular disease may be related to impaired clearance of immune complexes owing to reduced expression of complement receptor 1 (CR1) on monocytes/macrophages by the parasite. CR1 binds complement-bound immune complexes, which is critical to their clearance from the circulation.[937]

Schistosomiasis is a visceral parasitic disease caused by the blood flukes of the genus *Schistosoma. Schistosoma mansoni* and *Schistosoma japonicum* cause cirrhosis of the liver and *Schistosoma haematobium* causes cystitis. Glomerular involvement in *S. mansoni* includes mesangial proliferation, focal sclerosis, membranoproliferative lesions, crescentic changes, membranous nephropathy, amyloidosis, and eventually end-stage kidney disease.[1077–1079] Schistosomal antigens have been demonstrated in renal biopsies is such patients.[1080] Treatment with antiparasitic agents does not appear to influence progression of renal disease.[1081] *S. haematobium* is occasionally associated with the nephrotic syndrome, which may respond to treatment of the parasite.[1077] In some patients with schistosomiasis, renal involvement may be related to concomitant *Salmonella* infection.[1082]

Leishmaniasis, also known as kala-azar, is caused by *Leishmania donovani.* Renal involvement in kala-azar appears to be mild and reverts with antileishmanial treatment. Renal biopsies show glomerular mesangial proliferation or focal endocapillary proliferation. IgG, IgM, C3 may be observed in areas of proliferation. Amyloidosis may also complicate kala-azar.[1083,1084] In trypanosomiasis, *Trypanosoma brucei, Trypanosoma gambiense,* and *Trypanosoma rhodesiense* cause African sleeping sickness and have rarely been associated with proteinuria.[1085] Filariasis is caused by organisms in the genus *Onchocerca, Brugia, Loa,* and *Wuchereria.* Hematuria and proteinuria (including nephrotic syndrome) have been described in filariasis. Renal manifestations may appear with treatment of infection. Renal biopsy findings have included mesangial proliferative glomerulonephritis with C3 deposition, diffuse proliferative glomerulonephritis, and collapsing glomerulopathy with loiasis.[1086–1091] In patients with lymphatic filariasis of the renal hilus, chyluria (the passage of milky white urine containing lymphatic fluid) may mimic nephrotic syndrome by producing nephrotic-range proteinuria, but is distinguished by the absence of hypoalbuminemia or glomerular disease on biopsy.[953] Trichinosis is caused by *Trichinella spiralis* and may be associated with proteinuria and hematuria which abated after specific treatment. Renal biopsies in patients with loiasis have shown mesangial proliferative glomerulonephritis with C3 deposition.[1092,1093] *Echinococcus granulosus* and *Echinococcus multilocularis* cause hydatid disease or echinococcosis in humans. Mesangiocapillary glomerulonephritis and membranous nephropathy have occasionally been associated with hepatic hydatid cysts.[1094,1095] Toxoplasmosis may be associated with nephrotic syndrome in infants and rarely in adults. Mesangial and endothelial proliferation may be found, with deposition of IgG, IgA, IgM, C3, and fibrinogen in areas of proliferation.[1096–1098]

## GLOMERULAR INVOLVEMENT WITH VIRAL INFECTIONS

Viruses have been postulated to cause glomerular injury by various mechanisms including direct cytopathic effects, the deposition of immune complexes, or by initiation of autoimmune mechanisms.

In a study of previously healthy people with nonstreptococcal upper respiratory infections, 4% had erythrocyte casts and glomerulonephritis on biopsy. A reduction in serum complement and serologic evidence of infection with adenovirus, influenza A, or influenza B were observed in some. Initial renal biopsy showed either focal or diffuse mesangial proliferation in all nine, with mesangial C3 deposits in six specimens. Sequential creatinine clearances were reduced in about half these patients during follow-up.[1099]

The nephrotic syndrome has been described with EBV infections.[1100] Renal biopsies in patients with urinary abnormalities have included immune complex–mediated glomerulonephritis with tubulointerstitial nephritis,[1101] minimal glomerular lesions with IgM deposition,[1102] membranous nephropathy,[1103] and widespread glomerular mesangiolysis sometimes admixed with segmental mesangial sclerosis.[1104] In addition, the presence of EBV DNA in the glomerulus is thought to worsen glomerular damage in chronic glomerulopathies.[1105] Other viruses have rarely been associated with glomerulonephritis including herpes zoster, mumps, adenovirus, echovirus, Coxsackie virus, and influenza A and B.[1106]

## HIV-RELATED GLOMERULOPATHIES

An estimated 35.3 million people are living with the HIV worldwide, with over 2 million new infections each year.[1107] A variety of glomerular lesions and in particular, a unique form of glomerular damage, HIV-associated nephropathy (HIVAN), are associated with HIV infected patients.[1108,1109] Following the introduction of combination antiretroviral therapy (cART) in 1996, patients with acquired immunodeficiency syndrome (AIDS) are living longer with a concomitant change in the epidemiology of renal diseases.[1110] The incidence of ESKD from HIVAN appears to have plateaued to 800 to 900 new cases each year, with an accompanying rise in prevalence on account of patients surviving longer because of cART and traditional comorbidities such as diabetes and hypertension.[1111] Corresponding to this observation, the histologic diagnosis of HIVAN decreased from 80% to 20% from 1997 to 2004 in HIV-infected patients. However, in resource-poor countries, HIVAN remains a common cause of ESKD.[1110]

## HIV-ASSOCIATED NEPHROPATHY

### CLINICAL FEATURES

In 1984, the first detailed account of a new pattern of sclerosing glomerulopathy in HIV-infected patients was reported.[1112] Subsequent studies largely from large urban centers confirmed the occurrence and described the features of HIVAN.[1112–1122] In these largely urban U.S. East Coast centers, the prevalence of HIVAN approached 90% in nephrotic HIV-positive patients in contrast to a prevalence of only 2% in San Francisco, where most seropositive patients were Caucasian homosexuals.[1123–1125]

There is a strong predilection for HIVAN among black HIV-infected patients. The black:white ratio among patients with HIVAN is 12 : 1.[1126] HIVAN is the third leading cause of ESKD among black Americans aged 20 to 64 years, following only diabetes and hypertension.[1119,1127] Racial factors may influence rates of mutations in HIV receptors, which may in part explain some differences in the racial predisposition to HIV infection and HIVAN.[1128–1130] Mapping by admixture linkage disequilibrium has linked HIVAN and sporadic FSGS to variants in the APOL1 gene on chromosome 22, thereby explaining most of the strong black racial predominance observed in these conditions.[1131,1132]

Although intravenous drug use has been the most common risk factor for HIVAN, the disease has been seen in all groups at risk for AIDS including homosexuals, perinatally acquired disease, heterosexual transmission, and exposure to contaminated blood products.[1108] HIVAN usually occurs in patients with a low CD4 count, but full-blown AIDS is certainly not a prerequisite for the disease. In one New York study the onset of HIVAN was most common in otherwise asymptomatic HIV-infected patients (i.e., 12/26 were asymptomatic patients).[1112,1116] There is no relationship between the development of HIVAN and patient age and duration of HIV infection, or types of opportunistic infections or malignancies.[1108] The prevalence of HIVAN in patients who test positive for HIV is reported to be 3.5% in patients screened in the clinic setting[1133]; the same group reported that HIVAN was found in 6.9% of autopsies in HIV-infected patients.[1134]

The clinical features of HIVAN include presenting features of proteinuria, typically in the nephrotic range (and often massive), and renal insufficiency. Other manifestations of the nephrotic syndrome including edema, hypoalbuminemia, and hypercholesterolemia have been common in some series but less so in others despite the heavy proteinuria.[1108,1112,1115,1116,1120,1122,1135] Likewise, the incidence of hypertension has been variable even in patients with severe renal failure. Some patients, however, present with subnephrotic-range proteinuria and urinary sediment findings of microhematuria and sterile pyuria.[1136] The renal ultrasound in HIVAN shows echogenic kidneys with preserved or enlarged size with an average of over 12 cm in spite of the severe renal insufficiency.[1116,1120] Echogenicity may correlate with the histopathologic tubulointerstitial changes better than the glomerular changes.[1120]

### PATHOLOGY

The term HIVAN is reserved for the characteristic LM pattern of FSGS of the "collapsing" type with retraction of the glomerular capillary walls and luminal occlusion either in a segmental or in a global distribution[1109,1114,1137] (Fig. 32.51). There is striking hypertrophy and hyperplasia of the visceral epithelial cells, which form a cellular crown over the collapsed glomerular lobules (Fig. 32.52). In one study analyzing the expression pattern of podocyte differentiation and proliferation markers, there was disappearance of all podocyte differentiation markers from collapsed glomeruli, associated with cell proliferation, suggesting that the podocyte phenotype is dysregulated.[1138] Subsequent studies have emphasized the proliferation of parietal epithelial cells to replace lost podocytes.[1139] Patients with HIVAN have a higher percentage of glomerular collapse, less hyalinosis, and greater visceral cell swelling than patients with classic idiopathic FSGS or heroin nephropathy even when matched for serum creatinine and degree of proteinuria.[1114] The tubulointerstitial disease is also more severe in HIVAN, including tubular degenerative and regenerative features, interstitial edema, fibrosis, and inflammation.[1109,1114] Tubules are often greatly dilated into microcysts containing proteinaceous casts (Fig. 32.53). By IF, IgM and C3 are present; however, by EM, immune deposits

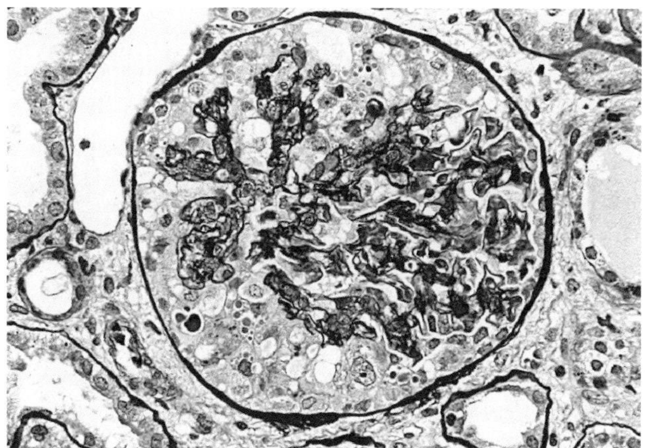

**Fig. 32.51** Human immunodeficiency virus–associated nephropathy. Electron micrograph showing wrinkling of glomerular basement membranes with marked podocyte hypertrophy, complete foot process effacement, and numerous intracytoplasmic protein resorption droplets (×2500).

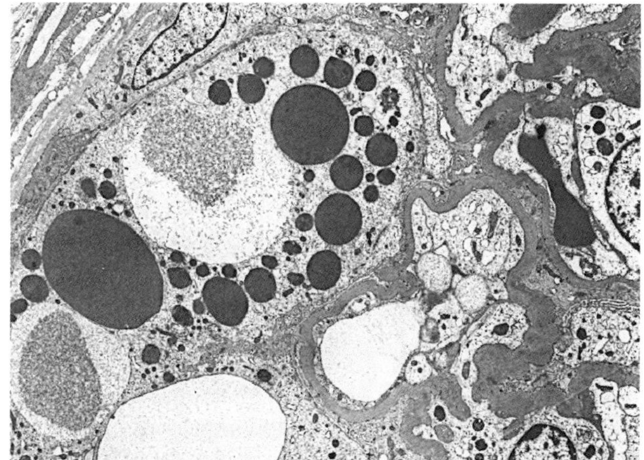

**Fig. 32.52** Human immunodeficiency virus–associated nephropathy. Glomeruli have collapsed tufts with capping of the overlying podocytes and dilatation of the urinary space. The tubules are dilated forming microcysts with abundant proteinaceous casts (periodic acid–Schiff, ×125).

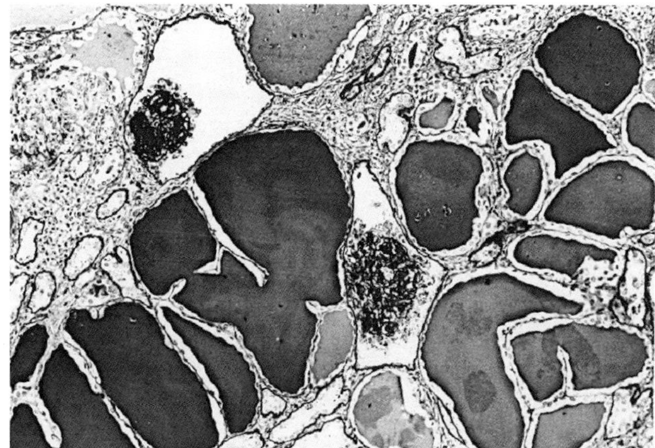

**Fig. 32.53** Human immunodeficiency virus–associated nephropathy. The characteristic pattern of collapsing glomerular sclerosis is depicted. Glomerular capillary lumina are occluded by wrinkling and retraction of the glomerular capillary walls associated with marked hypertrophy and hyperplasia of the visceral epithelial cells, forming a pseudocrescent (periodic acid–Schiff, ×325).

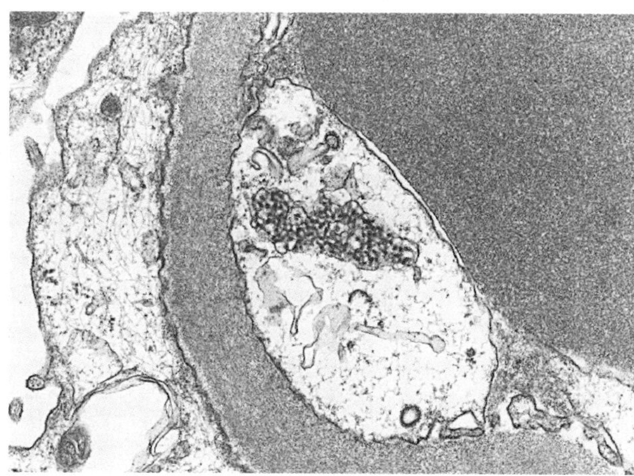

**Fig. 32.54** Human immunodeficiency virus–associated nephropathy. Electron micrograph showing a typical tubuloreticular inclusion within the endoplasmic reticulum of a glomerular endothelial cell (×6000).

are not detected (Fig. 32.51). In almost all biopsies of untreated HIVAN there are numerous TRIs within the glomerular and vascular endothelial cells (Fig. 32.54).[1108,1109,1114,1137] These 24-nm interanastomosing tubular structures are found within the dilated cisternae of the endoplasmic reticulum. Of note, patients who develop HIVAN while receiving cART usually lack collapsing features but display classic FSGS lesions on biopsy.[1111,1140]

## PATHOGENESIS

Experimental evidence strongly supports a role for direct HIV-1 infection of renal parenchymal cells. By in situ hybridization, HIV-1 RNA was detected in renal tubular epithelial cells, glomerular epithelial cells (visceral and parietal), and interstitial leukocytes.[1141] Renal epithelial cells may be an important reservoir for HIV because HIV RNA was found in the kidney of patients with undetectable viral loads in peripheral blood.[1141] Moreover, HIV-infected tubular epithelium can support viral replication, as evidenced by the detection of different HIV quasispecies in kidney epithelial cells compared with peripheral blood mononuclear cells of the same patient.[1142]

A replicative-deficient transgenic mouse model of HIVAN has been developed with lesions identical to HIV nephropathy,[1143–1145] suggesting that expression of viral gene products in renal epithelium underlies the development of nephropathy.

The lesions of collapsing glomerulopathy are associated with podocyte proliferation and dedifferentiation.[1138] The expression of two cyclin-dependent kinase inhibitors (which regulate the cell cycle), p27 and p57, was decreased in podocytes from HIVAN biopsies, whereas expression of another CDK inhibitor, p21, was increased.[1146] The specific HIV gene(s) required to produce these changes are being investigated. The nef gene (which is thought to act by activation of tyrosine kinases) was found to be essential in producing HIV-induced changes in podocyte cultures[1147] and in one murine model of HIVAN.[1148] There appears to be a synergistic role for nef and vpr in podocyte dysfunction and progressive glomerulosclerosis.[1149] Vpr has a role in G2 cell cycle arrest and possibly in the induction of apoptosis.[1150] There are several other abnormalities seen in the podocyte which are associated with an immature phenotype and subsequent loss of podocyte function. Synthesis of retinoic acid (an important differentiation factor) is impaired in association with reduced expression of the enzyme retinol dehydrogenase 9.[1151] The expression of TERT, a telomerase protein, is increased in HIVAN podocytes. TERT increases upregulation of the Wnt pathway, which also is associated with podocyte dedifferentiation. Suppressing TERT or Wnt signaling led to amelioration of podocyte lesions.[1152]

The APOL1 gene, which encodes apolipoprotein L1, in a recessive model is associated with a 29-fold higher odds for HIVAN in black patients. The lifetime risk of developing HIVAN is 50% in untreated HIV-infected black patients with two APOL1 risk alleles (G1/G1, G1/G2, or G2/G2). Further, the majority of patients with two APOL1 risk alleles had FSGS on kidney biopsies, whereas with one or zero risk alleles, immune complex glomerulonephritis was more common.[1153] The mechanism whereby APOL1-risk variants associate with HIVAN is not fully elucidated but is thought to be related to defective podocyte autophagy. IFN signaling in the podocyte has been shown in vitro to upregulate APOL1 synthesis.[1154] In mice, podocyte expression of the risk-variant APOL1 alleles was found to interfere with endosomal trafficking and blocking autophagic flux, which ultimately led to inflammatory-mediated podocyte death and glomerular scarring.[1155]

### COURSE AND TREATMENT

The natural history of HIVAN during the early part of the AIDS epidemic was characterized by rapid progression to ESKD. Case series from the United States that were published during the years that HIVAN was first described demonstrated an almost universal requirement for dialysis within 1 year of diagnosis.[1112] The role of combined antiviral therapies and the use of newer agents in the treatment of HIVAN have been associated with beneficial effects.[1140,1156–1158] The development of HIVAN is an indication for antiretroviral therapy. Corresponding to the introduction of cART, the rise in new cases of ESKD due to HIVAN slowed markedly.[1159]

There have been a few studies using corticosteroids in HIVAN. In an early study, prednisone was not associated with improvement in children with HIVAN.[1160,1161] Remissions in HIV-infected children with the minimal change pattern on biopsy treated with steroids have been noted, but not in children with sclerosing or collapsing lesions.[1108] In adults, however, several retrospective studies have shown short-term improvement in clinical parameters.[1162–1164]

Three pediatric patients with HIVAN on biopsy had sustained remissions of the nephrotic syndrome when treated with cyclosporine.[1160] They eventually developed opportunistic infections requiring the cyclosporine to be discontinued and subsequently experienced relapses of the nephrotic proteinuria and renal failure.

In isolated patients and in several small trials, use of ACE inhibitors has been shown to decrease proteinuria in HIVAN and to slow the progression to renal failure.[1165–1167] Serum ACE levels are elevated in HIV patients and ACE inhibitors may prevent proteinuria and glomerulosclerosis by either hemodynamic mechanisms or through modulation of matrix production and mesangial cell proliferation or even by affecting HIV protease activity.[1165–1167] Although some of these studies used control groups of untreated HIV patients of similar age, sex, race, and degree of renal insufficiency and proteinuria, these were not randomized, blinded trials. Nevertheless, in each study the ACE-treated group had less proteinuria, less rise in serum creatinine, and less progression to ESKD.

At present, the therapy of HIVAN should include use of multiple antiviral agents as in HIV-infected patients without nephropathy. Use of ACE inhibitors or perhaps angiotensin II receptor blockers, with careful attention to hyperkalemia and acute rises in the serum creatinine, may be beneficial. Several studies have documented favorable outcomes in HIVAN patients who received renal transplants.[1168–1171] The current opinion is that renal transplantation is no longer a contraindication in HIV-positive patients who have undetectable viral loads and CD4 over 200 cells/µL for at least 6 months.[1172,1173]

## OTHER GLOMERULAR LESIONS IN PATIENTS WITH HIV INFECTION

In the pre-cART era, HIVAN was the most common form of glomerulopathy found in HIV-infected patients, but other lesions had been reported as well. In the present era with the availability of cART, a renal biopsy in an HIV-positive patient with viral loads less than 400 copies/mL is more likely to show hypertensive nephrosclerosis[1174] or diabetic nephropathy.[1175] However, the two main entities directly associated with HIV infection, although uncommon, are HIV-associated ICD (HIV-ICD) and thrombotic microangiopathy. HIV-ICDs represent distinct glomerulopathies characterized by immune complex deposition that can lead to diverse renal histopathologies. Immune complex glomerulonephritides described in patients infected with HIV include IgA nephropathy, lupus-like glomerulonephritis, postinfectious glomerulonephritis, MPGN, and cryoglobulinemic glomerulonephritis.[1111,1176] In one series of over 100 biopsies for glomerular disease in HIV-positive patients, 73% were classic HIVAN, but other lesions included MPGN in 10%, MCD in 6%, amyloid in 3%, lupuslike nephritis in 3%, acute postinfectious glomerulonephritis in 2%, membranous nephropathy 2%, and 1% each of focal and segmental necrotizing glomerulonephritis, thrombotic microangiopathy, IgA nephropathy, and immunotactoid nephropathy.[1109,1177–1179]

IgA nephropathy has been reported in a number of series of HIV-infected patients.[1180–1184] This has occurred in both Caucasians and blacks despite the rarity of typical IgA nephropathy in black populations. The clinical features usually include hematuria, proteinuria, and some renal insufficiency. Cases with leukocytoclastic angiitis of the skin, consistent with HSP, have also been noted. The histology shows a variety of changes from mesangial proliferative glomerulonephritis to collapsing glomerulosclerosis with mesangial IgA deposits. IgA anti-HIV immune complexes have been eluted from the kidneys of several such patients, and several patients have had circulating immune complexes containing IgA idiotypic antibodies directed against viral proteins, either anti-HIV p24 or HIV gp41.[1183]

MPGN may be the most common pattern of immune complex–mediated glomerulonephritis seen in HIV-infected patients. Two series documented a high occurrence in intravenous drug abusers coinfected with HIV and hepatitis C.[1185,1186] Most patients have had microscopic hematuria, nephrotic-range proteinuria, and renal insufficiency at biopsy. Cryoglobulins are commonly positive, as is hypocomplementemia, and some have had both hepatitis B and C infection. The pathology of the glomerulopathy may be similar to idiopathic MPGN type 1 or 3, although some patients also have segmental membranous or mesangioproliferative features.[1187]

A lupuslike immune complex glomerulonephritis has been reported in a number of patients.[1119,1188–1191] Most of these patients have had positive serology for SLE with positive ANA, anti-DNA, and low complement levels. This contrasts with a low incidence of ANA positivity and almost no anti-DNA positivity in the general HIV-infected population.[1192] These patients are generally treated with corticosteroids with or without mycophenolate and concomitant highly active antiretroviral therapy. The results have been variable.[1191]

A not-infrequent association in both Caucasian and black HIV-infected patients has been thrombotic microangiopathy resembling TTP. Most have been in an advanced stage of HIV infection and had renal involvement with hematuria, proteinuria, and variable renal insufficiency. Other typical findings of TTP such as fever, neurologic symptoms, thrombocytopenia, and microangiopathic hemolytic anemia are often present. The initiation/reinitiation of cART, plasma exchange with or without adjunctive immunosuppression, can lead to remission.[1193] ADAMTS13 may be decreased (as in idiopathic TTP) and may be associated with a better prognosis.[1194] Other entities such as malignant hypertension, angioinvasive infections such as Kaposi sarcoma, and direct HIV-associated HUS need to be excluded.[1195]

## GLOMERULAR MANIFESTATIONS OF LIVER DISEASE

### HEPATITIS B

Hepatitis B antigenemia has been associated with glomerulonephritis for over 40 years. Hepatitis B has a worldwide distribution. In countries where the virus is endemic (sub-Saharan Africa, Southeast Asia, and Eastern Europe) there is vertical transmission from mother to infant and horizontal transmission between siblings. Hepatitis B–associated nephropathy occurs in these children with a 4:1 male preponderance.[1196–1198] In the United States and Western Europe, where hepatitis B is acquired by parenteral routes or sexually, the nephropathy affects mainly adults and has a different clinical course from the endemic form.[1199–1201] However, hepatitis B–associated nephropathy is rare in hepatitis B carriers.[1202] As noted earlier, PAN has also been associated with hepatitis B.[1203]

#### CLINICAL FEATURES

Most patients present with proteinuria or the nephrotic syndrome. In endemic areas, there may not be a preceding history of hepatitis. The majority of patients have normal renal function at time of presentation. There may be urinary erythrocytes but the majority have a bland sediment. Liver disease may be absent (carrier state) or chronic, and clinically mild. Serum aminotransferases may be normal or modestly elevated (between 100 and 200 IU/L). Liver biopsies in these patients often show chronic active hepatitis. Some patients ultimately develop cirrhosis. There is often spontaneous resolution of the carrier state with resolution of renal abnormalities. Spontaneous resolution of HBV-associated nephropathy is particularly common in children from endemic areas. The probability of a spontaneous remission may be as high as 80% after 10 years.[1204,1205]

#### PATHOLOGY

Most cases of hepatitis B–associated nephropathy manifest membranous nephropathy, although mesangial proliferation and sclerosis have also been reported.[1196,1197,1199–1201,1206,1207] In a cohort of Chinese patients with membranous nephropathy, HBV was found in 12%. There are fewer reports of MPGN with mesangial cell interposition, reduplication of the GBM, and subendothelial glomerular deposits.[1199,1201,1206] In a few series type III MPGN has been reported in which there are electron-dense subepithelial deposits in addition to the changes seen in type I MPGN.[1201] Crescentic glomerulonephritis in association with membranous changes and primary crescentic glomerulonephritis have also been described.[1208–1210]

The glomerular lesions appear to be immune complex mediated. HBsAg, HBcAg, and HBeAg[1211] have all been demonstrated in glomerular lesions, as has HBV DNA.[1198,1212] Rarely, staining of antiphospholipase A2 receptor (PLA2R) in the glomeruli and circulating anti-PLA2R antibody have been reported in HBV membranous nephropathy.[1210]

#### TREATMENT

In children with mild endemic form of hepatitis B–associated nephropathy, no treatment other than supportive care is advocated. In patients with progressive renal dysfunction, IFN has been used with mixed results.[1213–1216] Steroids do not significantly improve proteinuria and may potentially enhance viral replication.[1217,1218] Nucleoside analogs including lamivudine, telbivudine, adefovir, entecavir, or tenofovir suppress HBV replication by inhibiting viral DNA polymerase, and have demonstrated clinical utility in treating hepatitis B infection. Specifically, lamivudine was shown to reduce proteinuria and lead to a lesser incidence of ESKD in 10 patients with hepatitis B–associated nephropathy.[1219] The addition of corticosteroids to lamivudine did not improve renal outcome in another small randomized study in 16 patients.[1220] Preemptive lamivudine therapy in renal transplant recipients has shown improved survival compared with historical controls.[1221,1222] A meta-analysis confirmed that corticosteroids did not ameliorate proteinuria, but antiviral therapy was associated with HBeAg clearance and improvement of proteinuria.[1223] Current recommendations for hepatitis B treatment discourage the use of lamivudine in view of a high rate of drug resistance; tenofovir, entecavir, and pegylated IFN-α-2a are suggested.[1224] However, there are no data on the response of hepatitis B–related glomerulonephritis to these newer regimens.

### HEPATITIS C

Renal disease associated with HCV infection includes MPGN with or without associated mixed cryoglobulinemia and membranous glomerulopathy. The MPGN is most often of the immune complex type.[1225–1227] Rare cases of diffuse proliferative and exudative glomerulonephritis, polyarteritis, and fibrillary and immunotactoid glomerulopathy have also been described in association with HCV.[1228,1229] Most patients have evidence of liver disease as reflected by elevated plasma transaminase levels. However, transaminase levels are normal in some cases and a history of acute hepatitis is often absent.

## PATHOGENESIS

The pathogenesis of HCV-related nephropathies is immune complex mediated. A clonal expansion of B cells secreting IgM rheumatoid factors is seen in patients with chronic HCV infection. HCV drives the clonal expansion of $CD27^{+}IgM^{+}$ B cells, producing a rheumatoid factor often encoded by the $V_H$1-69 and $V_k$3-20 genes. These B cells display anergy induced by continual engagement of the B-cell receptor (BCR), such as high expression of phosphorylated extracellular signal–regulated kinase and reduced life span, and of virus-specific exhaustion, such as $CD21^{low}$ phenotype and a defective response to ligation of BCR and TLR9. After sustained virologic response, features of anergy in MC B cells rapidly revert, whereas virus-specific exhaustion imparts a durable inhibitory imprint on cell function.[1230]

HCV-specific proteins have been isolated from glomerular lesions.[1231] The disappearance of viremia in response to anti-HCV therapy (see later) is associated with a diminution of proteinuria; a relapse of viremia is accompanied by rising proteinuria.

## CLINICAL AND PATHOLOGIC FEATURES

Mixed cryoglobulinemia is associated with HCV and may cause a systemic vasculitis. Patients may exhibit constitutional systemic symptoms, palpable purpura, peripheral neuropathy, and hypocomplementemia. The renal manifestations include hematuria, proteinuria (often in the nephrotic range), and renal insufficiency. The histologic findings resemble those in idiopathic MPGN type 1 or 3 (Figs. 32.55 and 32.56) except for intraluminal protein "thrombi" on LM and the organized annular–tubular substructure of the electron-dense deposits on EM. Prior to the advent of hepatitis C serological tests, mixed cryoglobulinemia had been considered an idiopathic disease ("essential" mixed cryoglobulinemia). Up to 95% of these patients subsequently showed signs of HCV infection.[1232] Few patients with thrombotic microangiopathy associated with cryoglobulinemia have been described.[1233] MPGN without associated cryoglobulinemia may occur but is much less common.[1226]

Rarely, membranous nephropathy may be associated with HCV infection. Patients present with the nephrotic syndrome or proteinuria. Complement levels tend to be normal and neither cryoglobulins nor rheumatoid factors are present in HCV-associated membranous nephropathy.[1234] Now that staining for PLA2R, the major target antigen in primary membranous nephropathy, is being performed on renal biopsies, it has become evident that some HCV-infected patients with membranous nephropathy actually have a primary form.[1235]

Both type I MPGN (with and without cryoglobulinemia) and membranous nephropathy may recur in the allograft after renal transplantation, sometimes leading to graft loss.[1236–1239] Similar lesions have occurred in native kidneys after liver transplantation in HCV-positive patients.[1240,1241]

## TREATMENT

The treatment of HCV-associated renal disease has been revolutionized with the availability of oral direct-active antiviral (DAA) drugs. A complete virologic response can be achieved. Prior to the development of DAAs a number of early reports demonstrated a beneficial response to α-IFN therapy[1234,1242,1243] and cessation of IFN therapy; however, this was associated with recurrence of viremia and cryoglobulinemia in a majority of patients in these studies. IFN therapy may paradoxically exacerbate proteinuria and hematuria that appears to be unrelated to viral antigenic effects.[1244] The second-generation combination therapy regimens with ribavirin and pegylated IFN appeared to improve biochemical parameters of renal dysfunction in 20 HCV-GN patients and was accompanied by a virological response in 25% of patients.[1245] Another report on 18 patients showed sustained virologic responses in two-thirds of patients, which was associated with improvement in renal parameters.[1246] Combination therapy (especially ribavirin) may not be well tolerated in the presence of significant renal dysfunction.[1247] IFN-α treatment of renal transplant patients with HCV has been associated with acute renal failure[1248] and acute humoral rejection[1249] and is not recommended.

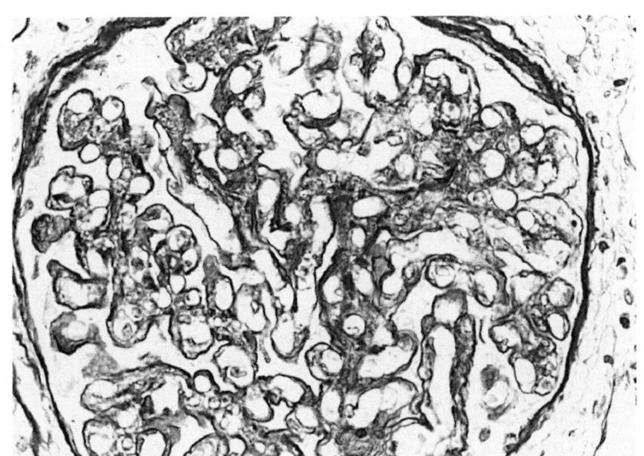

**Fig. 32.55** Hepatitis C–associated membranoproliferative glomerulonephritis type I. The mesangium is expanded by global mesangial hypercellularity associated with numerous double contours of the glomerular basement membranes (periodic acid–Schiff, ×500).

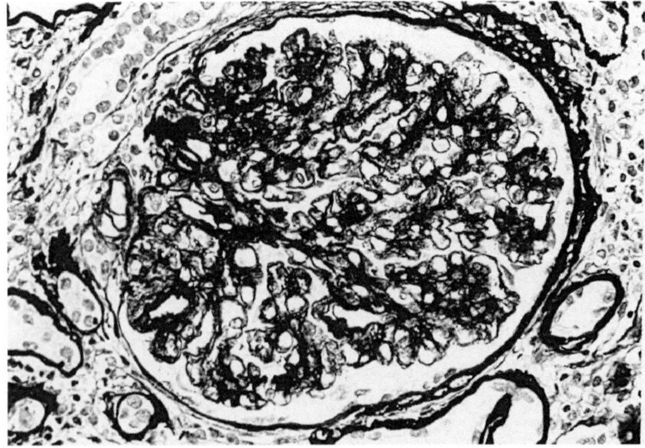

**Fig. 32.56** Hepatitis C–associated membranoproliferative glomerulonephritis type III. There are mixed features of membranoproliferative glomerulonephritis type 1 (with mesangial proliferation and duplication of glomerular basement membrane) and membranous glomerulopathy (with basement membrane spikes) (Jones methenamine silver, ×325).

Newer-generation DAAs are associated with a sustained viral response in over 90% of patients and guidelines are published by the Infectious Diseases Society of America/American Association for the Study of Liver Diseases (IDSA/AASLD).[1250] In a study of 24 consecutive patients with HCV-cryoglobulinemia vasculitis (GN in 21%), an IFN-free regimen using sofosbuvir with ribavirin was given for 24 weeks. About 74% of patients experienced sustained virological response at week 12 posttreatment; 87.5% experienced complete clinical response at week 24.

In patients with symptomatic cryoglobulinemia, immunosuppressive therapy may provide symptomatic relief. Prior to the availability of DAA, immunosuppressive regimens with or without antiviral drugs were used in symptomatic patients. Cyclophosphamide treatment has been used successfully in HCV glomerulonephritis,[1251] even if IFN resistant.[1252] Cyclophosphamide treatment may be associated with a temporary, reversible increase in viral load and a change of quasispecies.[1253] Fludarabine has been reported to decrease proteinuria in HCV-associated cryoglobulinemic MPGN.[1254] Rituximab has been associated with remissions of proteinuria in HCV-GN.[1255–1257] In renal transplant patients with HCV-GN, similar improvement in renal parameters has been reported, albeit with a higher incidence of infectious complications.[1258] Rituximab alone has been successfully used in patients with relapsing cryoglobulinemic vasculitis with a low adverse event rate.[1259]

Currently DAA alone is associated with improvement in vasculitis and many patients do not need immunosuppression. Because the sustained virological response rate is lower with IFN containing regimens,[1260] it has been suggested that with acute flare of disease with nephrotic proteinuria or rapidly progressive GN, treatment with immunosuppressive drugs (rituximab or cyclophosphamide, with corticosteroids) with or without plasmapheresis (in severe cases) can also be considered.[1261]

## AUTOIMMUNE CHRONIC ACTIVE HEPATITIS

Autoimmune chronic hepatitis is a distinctive progressive necrotic and fibrotic disorder of the liver with clinical and/or serologic evidence of a generalized autoimmune disorder.[1262] Two distinct clinical lesions have been associated with this disorder: glomerulonephritis and interstitial nephritis. Patients with the glomerular lesion present with nephrotic syndrome or renal insufficiency. On renal biopsy, they have membranous glomerulonephritis or MPGN. In two patients with membranous nephropathy, circulating immune complexes containing U1-RNP (ribonucleoprotein) and IgG have been reported. Eluates from the kidney tissue revealed higher concentrations of anti U1-RNP antibody. It is not known whether immunosuppressive therapy ameliorates the renal disorder.[1262] It is unclear if coexistent hepatitis C infection had been present in many of these patients.

## LIVER CIRRHOSIS

Glomerulonephritis is a rare manifestation of liver cirrhosis. Glomerular morphologic abnormalities with IgA deposition have been noted in more than 50% of patients with cirrhosis at both necropsy and biopsy,[1263,1264] although this has also been found in some autopsies of noncirrhotic kidneys.[1265] Clinically, there may be mild proteinuria and/or hematuria. There are two patterns on histology: a mesangial sclerosis (cirrhotic glomerular sclerosis) or MPGN. The latter may be associated with more severe renal symptoms and a depression of serum complement C3 levels.[1266] Again, it is unclear if some patients had coexistent hepatitis C infection. Rarely, HSP with RPGN has been described in association with cirrhosis.[1267]

Renal biopsies of patients with cirrhosis on LM show an increase in mesangial matrix with little or no increase in mesangial cellularity, a lesion known as "hepatic glomerulopathy." Less commonly, the distinctive pathologic findings consist of mesangial proliferative glomerulonephritis with mesangial IgA deposits usually accompanied by complement deposition and less intense IgG and/or IgM.[1263,1268,1269] By EM, the mesangium and subendothelial regions contain lucencies with dense granular and rounded membranous structures consistent with lipid inclusions (Fig. 32.57). Increased serum IgA levels are found in over 90% of cirrhotic patients with glomerular IgA deposition. Other authors have reported IgM as the dominant immunoglobulin.[1264] Cirrhotic glomerulonephritis is usually a clinically silent disease. However, the diagnosis can be suspected by finding proteinuria or abnormalities of the urine sediment. Kidney biopsies in cirrhotic patients at the time of liver transplantation may show glomerular lesions (predominantly IgA nephropathy or diabetic nephropathy) even if there is no clinical evidence of renal involvement. Diabetic lesions were associated with significantly worse renal function 5 years after transplantation compared with patients with IgA nephropathy.[1270] Rarely, cirrhotic patients may present with an acute glomerulonephritis with unusually large, exuberant glomerular immune complex deposits which are dominant or codominant for IgA. Six of nine such patients had a concurrent bacterial infection.[1271]

The pathogenesis may relate to defective hepatic clearance of IgA as well as altered processing and/or portacaval shunting of circulating immune complexes.[1270] This theory

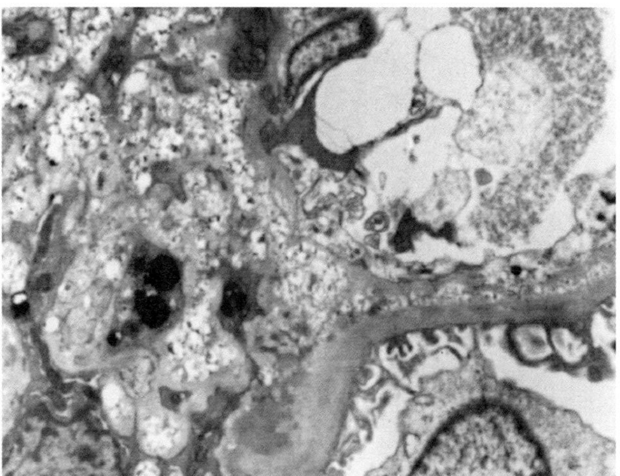

**Fig. 32.57** Hepatic glomerulopathy. A paramesangial electron-dense deposit corresponding to immune staining for immunoglobulin A is seen. In addition, there are irregular lucencies containing dense granular and rounded membranous structures within the mesangial matrix and extending into the subendothelial space (×6000).

is bolstered by the finding of increased deposits of IgA in skin and hepatic sinusoids in cirrhotic patients.[1272] Moreover, in patients with noncirrhotic portal fibrosis who underwent portal-systemic bypass procedures there was an increase in the incidence of clinically overt glomerulonephritis (from 78% to 32%) associated with deposition of IgA after the procedure. In the latter group, there was also a significant incidence of renal failure (50% after five years).[1273] Similar findings were noted in children with end-stage liver disease from α-1 antitrypsin deficiency or biliary atresia, which resolved after liver transplantation.[1274]

## GLOMERULAR LESIONS ASSOCIATED WITH NEOPLASIA

The occurrence of paraneoplastic (not related to tumor burden, metastasis. or invasion) glomerular syndromes, both nephrotic and nephritic, is rare (<1% of cancers). Glomerular disease may be seen with a wide variety of malignancies.

Some studies have shown that the risk for cancer is higher in patients with glomerular disease than in the general population. For example, the Danish Kidney Biopsy Registry, which includes all kidney biopsies performed in Denmark since 1985, reported that the risk for cancer at 1 year and 1 to 4 years after the diagnosis of glomerulopathy was increased by 2.4- and 3.5-fold, respectively, compared with the general population.[1275] Carcinomas of the lung, stomach, breast, and colon are most frequently associated with glomerular lesions.[1276] Membranous nephropathy is the commonest lesion associated with carcinoma. Patients over the age of 50 presenting with nephrotic syndrome should be reviewed for the presence of a malignancy.[1277,1278]

### CLINICAL AND PATHOLOGIC FEATURES

Clinically, the glomerulopathy of neoplasia may be manifested by proteinuria or the nephrotic syndrome, an active urine sediment, and/or diminished glomerular filtration. Significant renal impairment is uncommon, and is usually associated with the proliferative forms of glomerulonephritis. In evaluating an ESR in patients with nephrotic syndrome, it should be noted that most such patients have an ESR above 60 mm/h, with roughly 20% being above 100 mm/h. As a result, an elevated ESR alone in a patient with the nephrotic syndrome (or with ESKD) is not an indication to evaluate the patient for an occult malignancy or underlying inflammatory disease.[1279,1280]

### MEMBRANOUS NEPHROPATHY

Membranous nephropathy may be associated with malignancies in 6% to 22% of cases.[1278,1281,1282] These include carcinoma of the bronchus,[1283] breast,[1284] colon,[1285,1286] stomach, ovary,[1287] kidney,[1288] pancreas,[1289] and prostate,[1290,1291] as well as testicular seminoma,[1292] parotid adenolymphoma, carcinoid tumor,[1293,1294] Hodgkin disease (HD), and carotid body tumor.[1295] In some cases of membranous nephropathy associated with malignancy, tumor antigens have been detected within the glomeruli. It is postulated that tumor antigen deposition in the glomerulus is followed by antibody deposition, causing "in situ" immune complex formation, and subsequent complement activation.[1296,1297] Immune complexes and complement have been found in cancer patients without overt renal disease.[1296]

The kidney biopsy in cancer-associated MN may show more inflammatory cells (>8 cells/glomeruli) infiltrating the glomerulus. Indeed, increased inflammatory cells was noted in 92% of patients with cancer MN versus 25% of patients with idiopathic MN.[1281] Analysis of the IgG subclasses of the immune deposits in cancer-associated MN shows a predominance of IgG1 and IgG2, rather than IgG4 predominance that is common in idiopathic MN.[1298] Antibodies to the transmembrane glycoprotein M-type PLA2R is typical of primary MN and is now thought to distinguish this autoimmune entity from secondary MN (e.g., in lupus).[1299] However, in one study, serum anti-PLA2R antibodies were found to be present in three of 10 patients with MN in whom cancers were subsequently detected. The fact that anti-PLA2R antibodies persisted despite resection of the tumor and that IgG4 was the predominant immunoglobulin subclass may suggest that these cases were likely coincidental primary MN rather than cancer-associated MN.[1300]

In a recent study, antibodies to thrombospondin type-1 domain-containing 7A (THSD7A) were discovered in a subset of patients with MN.[1301] In a subsequent study using larger cohorts, eight of 40 patients with THSD7A MN developed a malignancy within a median time of 3 months from the time of diagnosis of MN.[1302] A previous report presented the case of a patient with THSD7A MN, in association with a mixed adenoneuroendocrine carcinoma of the gallbladder. The primary gallbladder tumor and corresponding lymph-node metastases were positive for THSD7A on immunohistochemical analysis in association with serum anti-THSD7A antibodies. After chemotherapy, anti-THSD7A antibodies in plasma became undetectable, and urinary protein-to-creatinine ratio decreased from 5.0 to 0.7.[1303]

A search for malignancy should be undertaken in older patients with newly diagnosed MN after excluding other secondary causes. The presence of anti-THSD7A antibody, absence of anti-PLA2R antibody, and/or predominant IgG1 and IgG2 deposits are other reasons to exclude malignancies thoroughly. Patients in these categories should be evaluated for cancer risk factors, prescribed gender- and age- appropriate screening (colonoscopy, prostate-specific antigen testing, and mammography), and low-dose chest computed tomography should be performed in smokers. If malignancy is not detected on initial screening, close follow-up for cancer should be undertaken.

Removal of the tumor may lead to remission of the nephrotic syndrome, which may then recur, following the development of metastasis. In the series reported by Lefaucheur et al.,[1281] in 23 patients with cancer-associated MN, a complete remission was observed in six cases. All remissions occurred in patients whose tumor was also in remission, whereas conversely, tumors were in remission in only three of 14 patients with persistent nephrotic-range proteinuria.

#### MINIMAL CHANGE DISEASE OR FOCAL GLOMERULOSCLEROSIS

MCD or focal glomerulosclerosis may occur in association with HD,[1304–1306] and, less often, non-Hodgkin lymphoma or leukemia,[1305] and rarely thymoma,[1276,1307] mycosis fungoides,[1308] renal cell carcinoma,[1309] and other solid tumors.[1310–1312]

HD is particularly associated with podocytopathies, most commonly MCD. In a series of 600 patients with HD, four patients were diagnosed with MCD.[1313] In another case series of 21 patients from France, the onset of MCD preceded the diagnosis of HD in 38% of patients, 50% of whom had steroid-resistant nephrotic syndrome. Treatment of HD was associated with remission of MCD.[1314]

Secretion of a cytokine may underlie glomerular injury in these disorders. Vascular endothelial growth factor (VEGF) may be one such cytokine; overexpression of VEGF in the podocyte is associated with podocytopathy in experimental models.[1315] Serum VEGF levels were found to be elevated in one patient with rectal carcinoma and MCD, and resection of the cancer was associated with remission of nephrotic syndrome and corresponding reduction of VEGF levels. Moreover, VEGF was highly expressed in the cancer tissue.[1316] C-Maf-inducing protein (C-Mip) was found to be expressed in podocytes and lymphoma tissue in patients with HD-associated MCD, but not in patients with HD without MCD, suggesting its potential involvement in the pathogenesis of HD-associated MCD.[1317] In another patient who presented with nephrotic syndrome from FSGS, small cell carcinoma of lung was found on testing. C-Mip was overexpressed in both podocytes and cancer cells, but was not found in control kidney and lung tissue samples. Exposure of cultured podocytes to patient's serum led to disorganization of the podocyte skeleton and expression of C-Mip that was not seen in control serum, or serum of HD patients after chemotherapy. The nephrotic syndrome resolved after remission of lung cancer.[1318]

Secondary amyloidosis (AA type) has been described with a number of malignancies, particularly renal cell carcinoma, HD, and chronic lymphocytic leukemia [1,2,4]. In HD, for example, renal amyloidosis is generally a late event resulting from a chronic inflammatory state; by comparison, MCD most often occurs at the time of initial presentation [5].

#### PROLIFERATIVE GLOMERULONEPHRITIDES AND VASCULITIDES

Both membranoproliferative and RPGN have been described in patients with solid tumors and lymphomas, although the etiologic relationship between these conditions is not proven.[1312,1319] The association is probably strongest for MPGN and chronic lymphocytic leukemia and may be associated with circulating cryoglobulins or glomerular deposition of monoclonal immunoglobulins.[1320,1321] Mesangial proliferation with IgA deposition has been associated with mucosa-associated lymphoid tissue lymphoma which resolved following treatment of the malignancy with chlorambucil.[1322] Although the association between crescentic glomerulonephritis and vasculitis with tumors may be coincidental, it has been suggested that the malignancy may act as a trigger for the vasculitis.[1323–1325] In contrast to the nephrotic states described earlier in which renal function is generally well preserved at presentation and the urine sediment is usually benign, patients with proliferative glomerulonephritis often have an acute decline in renal function and an active urine sediment.

#### THROMBOTIC MICROANGIOPATHY

Both the HUS and the related disorder TTP can occur in patients with malignancy. An underlying carcinoma of the stomach, pancreas, or prostate may be associated with HUS. More commonly, however, antitumor therapy is implicated: mitomycin, gemcitabine, the combination of bleomycin and cisplatin, and radiation plus high-dose cyclophosphamide prior to bone marrow transplantation all can lead to the HUS, which may first become apparent months after therapy has been discontinued.[1326] Anti-VEGF agents are also associated with glomerular thrombotic microangiopathy, leading to proteinuria, renal insufficiency, and hypertension.[1131,1167]

## GLOMERULAR DISEASE ASSOCIATED WITH DRUGS

### HEROIN NEPHROPATHY

In the 1970s, reports began to appear linking heroin abuse to the nephrotic syndrome and renal biopsy findings of lesions of focal and segmental glomerulosclerosis. This syndrome was referred to as heroin-associated nephropathy (HAN).[1327–1332] Similar lesions were seen in users of intravenous pentazocine (Talwin) and tripelennamine (Pyribenzamine), the so-called Ts and Blues.[1333] This syndrome occurred almost exclusively in blacks; it has been suggested that blacks may have a genetic predisposition for developing HAN.[1334,1335] The mean age was less than 30 years with 90% of the patients being males. The duration of drug abuse varied from 6 months to 30 years (mean 6 years) prior to the onset of renal disease. Most patients presented with the nephrotic syndrome. The course of HAN was relentless progression to ESKD over many years in those addicts who continued to use heroin, whereas a regression of abnormalities was seen in patients who were able to stop using the drug. Kidney biopsies of these patients showed lesions of focal segmental and global sclerosis. Nonspecific trapping leads to the deposition of IgM and C3 in areas of sclerosis. There was usually significant interstitial inflammation associated with the glomerular lesion. The pathogenesis of HAN is unknown. Abnormalities of cellular and humoral immunity have been well described in heroin addicts.[1336] It has been suggested that morphine itself could act as an antigen and that contaminants used to "cut" the heroin could contribute to the pathogenesis. Morphine (the active metabolite of heroin) has been shown to stimulate proliferation and sclerosis of mesangial cells and fibroblasts.[1337,1338] The syndrome of HAN has almost disappeared among drug addicts presenting with renal failure; for example, there has been a sharp decline in the incident case of HAN and there have been no reported cases of HAN-associated ESKD from Brooklyn, New York, during the period of 1991–1993.[1339,1340] In part this trend coincides with the rise of HIV infection and HIVAN.

### NONSTEROIDAL ANTIINFLAMMATORY DRUG–INDUCED NEPHROPATHY

Nonsteroidal antiinflammatory drugs (NSAIDs) are being used by approximately 50 million of the general public in the United States at any point in time. Approximately 1% to 3% of patients exposed to NSAIDs will manifest one of the renal abnormalities associated with its use: fluid and electrolyte disturbances, acute renal failure, and nephrotic syndrome with interstitial nephritis and papillary necrosis.[1341] The combination of acute interstitial nephritis and nephrotic syndrome is characteristic of this group of compounds. Essentially all NSAIDs can cause this type of renal disease,[1342–1344] including the cyclooxygenase-2 inhibitors.[1345,1346]

### CLINICAL AND PATHOLOGIC FEATURES

#### Minimal Change Disease With Interstitial Nephritis

The onset of NSAID-induced nephrotic syndrome is usually delayed, with a mean time of onset of 5.4 months (range 2 weeks to 18 months) after initiation of NSAID therapy. Patients may present with edema and oliguria. Systemic signs of allergic interstitial nephritis are usually absent. The urine exhibits microhematuria and pyuria. Proteinuria is usually in the nephrotic range. The extent of renal dysfunction may be mild to severe. On LM, the findings consist of MCD with interstitial nephritis. A focal or diffuse interstitial infiltrate consists predominantly of cytotoxic T lymphocytes (also other T-cell subsets, B cells, and plasma cells).[1347,1348] The syndrome usually reverses after discontinuing therapy, and the time to recovery may be between 1 month and 1 year.[1344] Complete remission is usually seen.[1349] Relapse of proteinuria has been reported.[1350] Treatment of the nephrotic syndrome is usually unnecessary, because the disorder is self-limiting. However, a short course of corticosteroids may be beneficial in patients in whom no response is seen after several weeks of discontinuation of the drug.[1351] Plasma exchange was reported as being associated with rapid recovery of renal function in two patients.[1352]

#### Other Patterns

Minimal change nephrotic syndrome without interstitial disease has been occasionally reported.[1353] Granulomatous interstitial disease without glomerular changes has also been described.[1354] Membranous nephropathy has also been reported in association with NSAID use,[1355] including the newer COX-2 inhibitors.[1346] As in minimal change nephrotic syndrome, there is rapid recovery after drug withdrawal in NSAID-induced membranous nephropathy.

**Pathogenesis.** The mechanism of NSAID-induced nephrotic syndrome has not been defined. It has been proposed that inhibition of cyclooxygenase by NSAID inhibits prostaglandin synthesis and shunts arachidonic acid pathways toward the production of leukotriene. These by-products of arachidonic acid metabolism may promote T-lymphocyte activation and enhanced vascular permeability, leading to MCD.[1342–1344]

## ANTIRHEUMATOID ARTHRITIS THERAPY–INDUCED GLOMERULOPATHY

Proteinuria and nephrotic syndrome have been reported to occur in association with both oral and parenteral gold.[1356,1357] Dermatitis may occur concurrently. Membranous nephropathy and rarely MCD have been reported.[1358] A higher incidence of nephropathy has been reported in patients with HLA B8/DR3.[1359,1360] D-Penicillamine treatment for rheumatoid arthritis can induce proteinuria. Membranous nephropathy is the commonest lesion reported. Less commonly, MCD and mesangial proliferative lesions have been reported.[1360] Goodpasture-like syndrome,[1361] minimal change nephrotic syndrome,[1362] and membranous nephropathy concurrently with vasculitis[1363] have been described rarely. HLA B8/DR3 haplotypes are also associated with penicillamine nephropathy.[1364] Tiopronin and bucillamine (a penicillamine-like compound) have also been associated with the same renal lesions described for penicillamine.[1365,1366] The onset of proteinuria with gold or penicillamine therapy is usually between 6 and 12 months after starting therapy. Proteinuria usually resolves after withdrawing the offending agent; persistent renal dysfunction is uncommon.[1360,1364,1367] Under close supervision, gold and penicillamine have been continued in patients with nephropathy with no obvious adverse effect on renal function.[1368] Anti-TNF-α agents have been reported to promote the development of lupuslike nephritis and ANCA-associated glomerulonephritis in patients with rheumatoid arthritis.[1369]

## OTHER MEDICATIONS

Organic mercurial exposure can occur with diuretics, skin lightening creams, gold refining, and industrial exposure. Proteinuria and nephrotic syndrome have been reported.[1370–1372] Renal biopsy in such patients has shown membranous nephropathy[1373,1374] or MCD.[1375] The nephrotic syndrome has been associated with the anticonvulsants ethosuccimide,[1376] trimethadione,[1377] and Paradione.[1378] Diffuse proliferative glomerulonephritis may be seen with mesantoin (mephenytoin).[1379] AAV as well as a lupuslike nephritis has been reported with propylthiouracil[1380–1383] and hydralazine.[1151] Captopril has been associated with the development of proteinuria and the nephrotic syndrome due to membranous nephropathy.[1384] Substituting enalapril for captopril has been reported to ameliorate the nephrotic syndrome.[1385] IFN-α has been associated with interstitial nephritis, MCD, focal and segmental glomerulosclerosis, and acute renal failure.[1386,1387] In patients with collapsing FSGS due to IFN therapy, discontinuation of therapy usually leads to improvement in renal function and proteinuria.[1388] Cases of thrombotic microangiopathy[1389,1390] and crescentic glomerulonephritis[1391] have also been reported. Mercaptopropionyl glycine used in the treatment of cystinuria has been associated with membranous glomerulopathy[1392]. Lithium use has been associated with MCD,[1393,1394] membranous nephropathy,[1395] and focal and segmental glomerulosclerosis.[1396,1397] The use of high-dose pamidronate in patients with malignancies has been associated with HIV-negative collapsing focal and segmental glomerulosclerosis.[1398] Cocaine may be contaminated with levamisole, a veterinary antihelminthic that is a known immunomodulator. This combination may result in an ANCA-positive systemic vasculitis, with both C- and P-ANCA positivity, with a predilection for skin necrosis and arthralgia; renal and pulmonary involvement may occur.[1399] Abuse of anabolic steroids in conjunction with a body-building regimen may produce FSGS with variable histologic subtypes. Roles for both increased glomerular filtration demand and potential direct toxic effects of anabolic steroids on glomerular cells have been proposed.[1242] Treatment of C3 glomerulopathies with eculizumab, a humanized monoclonal antibody directed to C5, may lead to binding of the drug to C5 deposits in renal tissue, producing de novo positivity for IgG-kappa that mimics an MIDD.[1243]

## MISCELLANEOUS DISEASES ASSOCIATED WITH GLOMERULAR LESIONS

Well-documented cases exist of nephrotic syndrome associated with unilateral renal artery stenosis, which improved after correction of the stenosis. The mechanism of proteinuria presumably relates to high levels of angiotensin-II.[1400–1402]

Acute silicosis has been associated with a proliferative glomerulonephritis with IgM and C3 deposits, leading to renal failure.[1403] A patient with dense lamellar inclusions in swollen glomerular epithelial cells, similar to those seen in FD, has also been described.[1404]

Membranous nephropathy and MPGN[1405] have been described in association with ulcerative colitis.[1406]

Kimura disease and angiolymphoid hyperplasia with eosinophilia (ALHE) produce skin lesions that appear as single or multiple red-brown papules or as subcutaneous nodules with a predilection for the head and neck region. Other associated features include eosinophilia and elevated IgE levels. Both Kimura disease and the similar ALHE are frequently associated with glomerular disease. Mesangial proliferative glomerulonephritis[1407] and MCD[1408] have been described.

Renal complications of Castleman disease (angiofollicular lymph node hyperplasia) are uncommon. The reported cases are very heterogeneous and their renal pathology includes MCD, mesangial proliferative glomerulonephritis,[1409] membranous nephropathy,[1410] MPGN,[1411] crescentic glomerulonephritis,[1412] fibrillary glomerulonephritis,[1413] and amyloidosis.[1414] Serum IL-6 levels appear to be elevated and decline with corticosteroid therapy.[1409] Removal of tumor mass or treatment with steroids appears to ameliorate the renal manifestations in some cases.

Angioimmunoblastic lymphadenopathy has been associated with diffuse proliferative glomerulonephritis with necrotizing arteritis and MCD.[1305,1415]

Hemophagocytic syndrome related to infections or lymphoproliferative disease has been associated with collapsing FSGS.[1416]

Complete reference list available at ExpertConsult.com.

## KEY REFERENCES


1. Almaani S, Meara A, Rovin BH. Update on lupus nephritis. *Clin J Am Soc Nephrol.* 2017;12(5):825–835.
2. Appel GB, Contreras G, Dooley MA, et al. Mycophenolate mofetil versus cyclophosphamide for induction treatment of lupus nephritis. *J Am Soc Nephrol.* 2009;20(5):1103–1112.
3. Weening JJ, D'Agati VD, Schwartz MM, et al. The classification of glomerulonephritis in systemic lupus erythematosus revisited. *Kidney Int.* 2004;65(2):521–530.
4. Bajema IM, Wilhelmus S, Alpers CE, et al. Revision of the International Society of Nephrology/Renal Pathology Society classification for lupus nephritis: clarification of definitions, and modified National Institutes of Health activity and chronicity indices. *Kidney Int.* 2018;93(4):789–796.
5. Gourley MF, Austin HA 3rd, Scott D, et al. Methylprednisolone and cyclophosphamide, alone or in combination, in patients with lupus nephritis. A randomized, controlled trial. *Ann Intern Med.* 1996;125(7):549–557.
6. Boumpas DT, Austin HA 3rd, Vaughn EM, et al. Controlled trial of pulse methylprednisolone versus two regimens of pulse cyclophosphamide in severe lupus nephritis. *Lancet.* 1992;340(8822):741–745.
7. Steinberg AD, Steinberg SC. Long-term preservation of renal function in patients with lupus nephritis receiving treatment that includes cyclophosphamide versus those treated with prednisone only. *Arthritis Rheum.* 1991;34(8):945–950.
154. Houssiau FA, Vasconcelos C, D'Cruz D, et al. Immunosuppressive therapy in lupus nephritis: the Euro-Lupus Nephritis Trial, a randomized trial of low-dose versus high-dose intravenous cyclophosphamide. *Arthritis Rheum.* 2002;46(8):2121–2131.
164. Kidney Disease: Improving Global Outcomes (KDIGO) Glomerulonephritis Work Group. KDIGO clinical practice guideline for glomerulonephritis. *Kidney Inter Suppl.* 2012;2.
165. Contreras G, Pardo V, Leclercq B, et al. Sequential therapies for proliferative lupus nephritis. *N Engl J Med.* 2004;350(10):971–980.
166. Houssiau FA, D'Cruz D, Sangle S, et al. Azathioprine versus mycophenolate mofetil for long-term immunosuppression in lupus nephritis: results from the MAINTAIN Nephritis Trial. *Ann Rheum Dis.* 2010;69(12):2083–2089.
169. Liu Z, Zhang H, Liu Z, et al. Multitarget therapy for induction treatment of lupus nephritis: a randomized trial. *Ann Intern Med.* 2015;162(1):18–26.
173. Rovin BH, Furie R, Latinis K, et al. Efficacy and safety of rituximab in patients with active proliferative lupus nephritis: the Lupus Nephritis Assessment with Rituximab study. *Arthritis Rheum.* 2012;64(4):1215–1226.
198. Austin HA 3rd, Illei GG, Braun MJ, et al. Randomized, controlled trial of prednisone, cyclophosphamide, and cyclosporine in lupus membranous nephropathy. *J Am Soc Nephrol.* 2009;20(4):901–911.
201. Radhakrishnan J, Moutzouris DA, Ginzler EM, et al. Mycophenolate mofetil and intravenous cyclophosphamide are similar as induction therapy for class V lupus nephritis. *Kidney Int.* 2010;77(2):152–160.
284. Jennette JC, Falk RJ, Bacon PA, et al. 2012 revised international chapel hill consensus Conference nomenclature of vasculitides. *Arthritis Rheum.* 2013;65(1):1–11.
309. Jennette JC, Falk RJ. Pathogenesis of antineutrophil cytoplasmic autoantibody-mediated disease. *Nat Rev Rheumatol.* 2014;10(8):463–473.
349. Guillevin L, Cordier JF, Lhote F, et al. A prospective, multicenter, randomized trial comparing steroids and pulse cyclophosphamide versus steroids and oral cyclophosphamide in the treatment of generalized Wegener's granulomatosis. *Arthritis Rheum.* 1997;40(12):2187–2198.
350. de Groot K, Harper L, Jayne DR, et al. Pulse versus daily oral cyclophosphamide for induction of remission in antineutrophil cytoplasmic antibody-associated vasculitis: a randomized trial. *Ann Intern Med.* 2009;150(10):670–680.
351. De Groot K, Rasmussen N, Bacon PA, et al. Randomized trial of cyclophosphamide versus methotrexate for induction of remission in early systemic antineutrophil cytoplasmic antibody-associated vasculitis. *Arthritis Rheum.* 2005;52(8):2461–2469.
356. Jayne DR, Gaskin G, Rasmussen N, et al. Randomized trial of plasma exchange or high-dosage methylprednisolone as adjunctive therapy for severe renal vasculitis. *J Am Soc Nephrol.* 2007;18(7):2180–2188.
358. Yates M, Watts RA, Bajema IM, et al. EULAR/ERA-EDTA recommendations for the management of ANCA-associated vasculitis. *Ann Rheum Dis.* 2016;75(9):1583–1594.
366. Jones RB, Tervaert JW, Hauser T, et al. Rituximab versus cyclophosphamide in ANCA-associated renal vasculitis. *N Engl J Med.* 2010;363(3):211–220.
367. Stone JH, Merkel PA, Spiera R, et al. Rituximab versus cyclophosphamide for ANCA-associated vasculitis. *N Engl J Med.* 2010;363(3):221–232.
374. Jayne D, Rasmussen N, Andrassy K, et al. A randomized trial of maintenance therapy for vasculitis associated with antineutrophil cytoplasmic autoantibodies. *N Engl J Med.* 2003;349(1):36–44.
379. Guillevin L, Pagnoux C, Karras A, et al. Rituximab versus azathioprine for maintenance in ANCA-associated vasculitis. *N Engl J Med.* 2014;371(19):1771–1780.
529. Audemard-Verger A, Terrier B, Dechartres A, et al. Characteristics and management of IgA vasculitis (henoch-schonlein) in adults: data from 260 patients included in a French multicenter retrospective survey. *Arthritis Rheumatol.* 2017;69(9):1862–1870.
566. Huber AM, King J, McLaine P, et al. A randomized, placebo-controlled trial of prednisone in early Henoch Schonlein Purpura [ISRCTN85109383]. *BMC Med.* 2004;2:7.
573. Pillebout E, Alberti C, Guillevin L, et al. Addition of cyclophosphamide to steroids provides no benefit compared with steroids

alone in treating adult patients with severe Henoch Schonlein Purpura. *Kidney Int.* 2010;78(5):495–502.

580. Hudson BG. The molecular basis of Goodpasture and Alport syndromes: beacons for the discovery of the collagen IV family. *J Am Soc Nephrol.* 2004;15(10):2514–2527.
662. Sethi S, Theis JD, Vrana JA, et al. Laser microdissection and proteomic analysis of amyloidosis, cryoglobulinemic GN, fibrillary GN, and immunotactoid glomerulopathy. *Clin J Am Soc Nephrol.* 2013;8(6):915–921.
714. D'Souza A, Dispenzieri A, Wirk B, et al. Improved outcomes after autologous hematopoietic cell transplantation for light chain amyloidosis: a center for international blood and marrow transplant research study. *J Clin Oncol.* 2015;33(32):3741–3749.
722. Dember LM, Hawkins PN, Hazenberg BP, et al. Eprodisate for the treatment of renal disease in AA amyloidosis. *N Engl J Med.* 2007;356(23):2349–2360.
735. Nasr SH, Vrana JA, Dasari S, et al. DNAJB9 is a specific immunohistochemical marker for fibrillary glomerulonephritis. *Kidney Int Rep.* 2018;3(1):56–64.
744. Lin J, Markowitz GS, Valeri AM, et al. Renal monoclonal immunoglobulin deposition disease: the disease spectrum. *J Am Soc Nephrol.* 2001;12(7):1482–1492.
759. Nasr SH, Markowitz GS, Stokes MB, et al. Proliferative glomerulonephritis with monoclonal IgG deposits: a distinct entity mimicking immune-complex glomerulonephritis. *Kidney Int.* 2004;65(1):85–96.
774. Vos JM, Gustine J, Rennke HG, et al. Renal disease related to Waldenstrom macroglobulinaemia: incidence, pathology and clinical outcomes. *Br J Haematol.* 2016;175(4):623–630.
803. Savige J, Gregory M, Gross O, et al. Expert guidelines for the management of Alport syndrome and thin basement membrane nephropathy. *J Am Soc Nephrol.* 2013;24(3):364–375.
804. Kashtan CE, Ding J, Garosi G, et al. Alport syndrome: a unified classification of genetic disorders of collagen IV alpha345: a position paper of the Alport Syndrome Classification Working Group. *Kidney Int.* 2018.
897. Terryn W, Cochat P, Froissart R, et al. Fabry nephropathy: indications for screening and guidance for diagnosis and treatment by the European Renal Best Practice. *Nephrol Dial Transplant.* 2013;28(3):505–517.
898. Biegstraaten M, Arngrimsson R, Barbey F, et al. Recommendations for initiation and cessation of enzyme replacement therapy in patients with Fabry disease: the European Fabry Working Group consensus document. *Orphanet J Rare Dis.* 2015;10:36.
925. Maigne G, Ferlicot S, Galacteros F, et al. Glomerular lesions in patients with sickle cell disease. *Medicine (Baltimore).* 2010;89(1):18–27.
948. Musso C, Javor E, Cochran E, et al. Spectrum of renal diseases associated with extreme forms of insulin resistance. *Clin J Am Soc Nephrol.* 2006;1(4):616–622.
960. Norum KR, Gjone E. Familial plasma lecithin-cholesterol acyltransferase defciency: biochemical study of a new inborn error of metabolism. *Scand J Clin Lab Invest.* 1967;20:231–243.
988. Nasr SH, Radhakrishnan J, D'Agati VD. Bacterial infection-related glomerulonephritis in adults. *Kidney Int.* 2013;83(5):792–803.
1111. Swanepoel CR, Atta MG, D'Agati VD, et al. Kidney disease in the setting of HIV infection: conclusions from a Kidney Disease: improving Global Outcomes (KDIGO) Controversies Conference. *Kidney Int.* 2018;93(3):545–559.
1171. Stock PG, Barin B, Murphy B, et al. Outcomes of kidney transplantation in HIV-infected recipients. *N Engl J Med.* 2010;363(21):2004–2014.
1199. Venkataseshan VS, Lieberman K, Kim DU, et al. Hepatitis-B-associated glomerulonephritis: pathology, pathogenesis, and clinical course. *Medicine (Baltimore).* 1990;69:200–216.
1281. Lefaucheur C, Stengel B, Nochy D, et al. Membranous nephropathy and cancer: epidemiologic evidence and determinants of high-risk cancer association. *Kidney Int.* 2006;70(8):1510–1517.
1314. Audard V, Larousserie F, Grimbert P, et al. Minimal change nephrotic syndrome and classical Hodgkin's lymphoma: report of 21 cases and review of the literature. *Kidney Int.* 2006;69(12):2251–2260.

# 33 Treatment of Glomerulonephritis

Heather N. Reich | Daniel C. Cattran

## CHAPTER OUTLINE



## KEY POINTS

- The incidence and prevalence of glomerulonephritis (GN) is likely underestimated.
- There is a growing body of literature guiding treatment of GN based upon randomized-controlled trials.
- Decisions regarding therapy should be tailored to the individual patient, with thoughtful balance of the risk of disease progression and the risk of treatment toxicity in the individual patient.
- The development of novel therapies and new protocols to treat GN underscore the importance of mitigation of medication toxicity.
- Age and cumulative dose modulate risk of gonadal toxicity from alkylating agents.
- Mycophenolic acid has recognized teratogenicity.
- Treatment with Eculizumab is associated with susceptibility to infections with encapsulated bacteria including *Nisseria menigitides* meningitis. Prior vaccination and prophylactic antibiotics are recommended.

## INTRODUCTION

The societal burden of glomerulonephritis (GN) on both the individual and the healthcare system is substantial. Although renal replacement therapy is an essential life-sustaining therapy for patients with kidney failure, advances in the therapeutic options available for treatment of GN offer great potential to avoid kidney failure in patients afflicted with these diseases. The field of GN treatment is also progressing quickly toward individualization of therapy—through development of more targeted and less toxic therapies and identification of patients who have the greatest potential for benefit from these medications. In this chapter we discuss strategies to individualize care of patients with GN, and opportunities to mitigate risk of currently available treatment options.

## THE GLOBAL IMPACT AND CHALLENGES

Estimating the incidence of GN and its impact on patient morbidity and mortality is challenged by several barriers. First, the incidence of GN is grossly underappreciated and

**Table 33.1. Considerations for Individualization of Therapy and Avoidance of Drug Toxicity**

| | Considerations | Example |
|---|---|---|
| Disease | Disease-specific treatment targets | A partial remission of proteinuria may portend favorable prognosis and minimize drug toxicity |
| | Disease-related risks with no treatment | Risk of thrombosis with untreated membranous nephropathy, life-threatening risks of vasculitis |
| Patient | Modifiable patient factors | Obesity, smoking |
| | Nonmodifiable patient factors | Age, comorbid conditions |
| | Exposures | Endemic and latent infections |
| Drug | Anticipation of drug-specific toxicities | Steroid avoidance in prediabetes, infection prophylaxis |

the costs underestimated because of the lack of national or international registries of GN at the level of renal pathology. Although large prospective study cohorts are now established to study the natural history and pathogenesis of these diseases (reviewed elsewhere[1]), the incidence of biopsy-proven GN cannot be calculated from these studies as the geographic region from which patients are enrolled is not as carefully delineated.

The extent of these diseases may, therefore, be better approximated by imputing incidence rates from country-wide renal pathology registries where there is prescribed reporting. Such a registry from Finland, for example, reported an incidence of GN that ranged from 8.7 to 25.4 per 100,000 population in the central hospitals and the university center, respectively, which was remarkably higher than the rates reported by the European Biopsy Registry (between 1 and 6.9).[2] The full disease impact is also substantially discounted if assessed solely from figures derived from end-stage renal disease (ESRD) registries as patients presenting with advanced chronic kidney disease (CKD) or ESRD are often not biopsied. Most recently, a study of a data set consisting of a public Medicare and two insurer databases capturing over 19 million clients also suggested that the incidence of GN may be far higher than previously estimated.[3] Based upon health claim data (International Classification of Diseases, 9th Revision [ICD-9] codes), the incidence of GN was estimated to be as high as 134 per 100,000 patient-years (95% confidence interval [CI] 132–136). Rates were lower in the privately insured but remained much higher than previously referenced registry estimates.

Understanding the incidence of GN is important. As therapy becomes more tailored, the cost of medications becomes critical from a resource perspective. Health care payers cannot estimate cost–benefit without an appreciation of the incidence and course of GN. With the emergence of more costly but targeted medications, consideration of savings from avoidance of both kidney failure and complications of therapy becomes increasingly relevant. Similarly, it is incumbent upon the nephrology community to conduct rigorously designed and high-quality therapeutic trials to expedite development and quantitate the efficacy of novel therapies.[4]

## PERSONALIZING THERAPY: BALANCING RISKS AND BENEFITS

GN is associated with significant morbidity and mortality that must be considered when making informed decisions about therapy. A recent retrospective analysis of an observational cohort derived from an insurer-based (Kaiser Permanente) integrated healthcare system highlights these risks.[5] The cohort consisted of over 2300 patients with biopsy-proven GN. At a mean follow-up of 4.5 years, 21% developed end-stage kidney failure, and 8% died before reaching this endpoint. This emphasizes the rationale for more aggressive intervention strategies on a population level. The development of the Kidney Disease Improving Global Outcomes (KDIGO) guidelines represents an important advance in harmonizing and standardizing treatment for GN and providing the evidence-based context of recommendations. However, one of the challenges of adopting clinical guidelines is individualizing treatment strategy to the patient.

A focus of our practice is developing patient-specific risk evaluation so that treatment benefits and risks can be considered at the individual patient level. This can be adopted formally through checklist-style documentation or more informally during the consultation process. Consideration of personalized treatment is critical to balance the potential risks and benefits of immunotherapy, so that both clinicians and patients can enter a treatment plan with an informed and collaborative decision making process.

Broadly, there are three primary areas for consideration when evaluating a treatment plan for an individual patient (Table 33.1). These include consideration of the specific disease-associated risks and treatment goals, the patient characteristics, and the specific medication toxicities. As one evaluates a patient, each of these categories is considered and pros and cons of various strategies are measured and reviewed with the patient—an active participant in his or her care.

## PERSONALIZING TREATMENT: DISEASE-SPECIFIC RISKS AND GOALS

Treatment cannot be personalized without understanding the specific nature of the disease and risk of disease progression. This includes the disease natural history and the therapeutic goals. To balance the risks of therapy, consideration of the individual patient's likelihood of progression and the disease natural history (including patient morbidity) should be reviewed.

Risk of disease progression is described largely in natural history studies that have yielded important information that has influenced patient management and altered how we assess treatment benefit.[6–9] These efforts have allowed a more accurate estimation of the impact of modifiable predictors

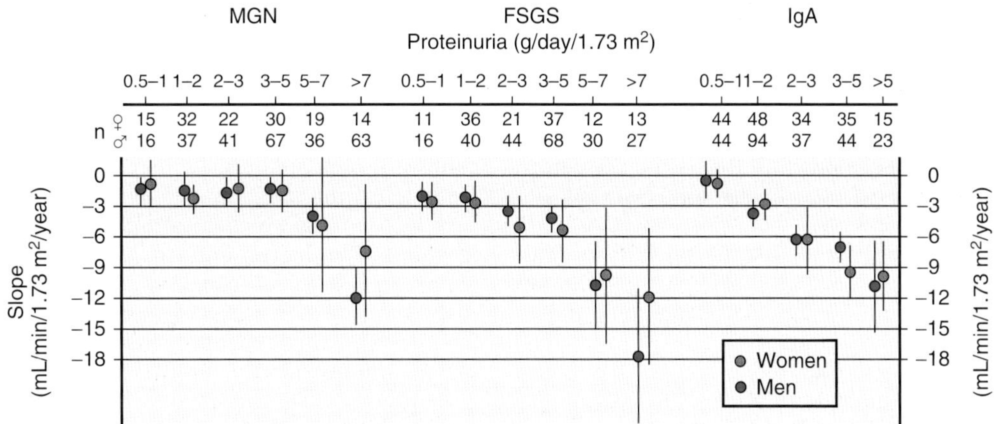


**Fig. 33.1** Differential impact of proteinuria according to sex and histologic subtype on the rate of renal function decline in membranous glomerulonephritis *(MGN)*, focal and segmental glomerulosclerosis *(FSGS)*, and immunoglobulin A *(IgA)* nephropathy. This figure illustrates the annual rate of renal function decline (*y*-axis) according to categories of time-averaged proteinuria (*x*-axis). This is described by disease subtype and gender. (From McCarthy ET, Sharma M, Savin VJ. Circulating permeability factors in idiopathic nephrotic syndrome and focal segmental glomerulosclerosis. *Clinical Journal of the American Society of Nephrology: CJASN.* 2010;5(11):2115-2121.)

**Table 33.2. Definition of Remission and Outcome by Histologic Diagnosis in Primary Glomerulonephritis**

| | Membranous Glomerulonephritis | Focal and Segmental Glomerulosclerosis | Immunoglobulin A Nephropathy |
|---|---|---|---|
| Definition of partial remission | Reduction to <3.5 g/day and 50% decrease from peak proteinuria | Reduction to <3.5 g/day and 50% decrease from peak proteinuria | Reduction to <1 g/day proteinuria |
| Rate of renal function decline | CR: −1 mL/min/year<br>PR: −2 mL/min/year<br>NR: −10 mL/min/year | CR: −0.1 mL/min/year<br>PR: −5.6 mL/min/year<br>NR: −10 mL/min/year | CR: −1.6 mL/min/year<br>PR: −2 mL/min/year<br>NR: −9 mL/min/year |

*CR,* Complete remission; *NR,* no remission; *PR,* partial remission.

on clinical outcome, thus allowing physicians to provide general and disease-specific recommendations. For example, hypertension is a risk factor for progression across all forms of primary and secondary GN, and targets may be relatively generalizable across kidney disease categories. However, the relationship between quantity of proteinuria and outcome in GN varies across diagnoses.

Traditionally, clinicians have estimated the risk of progression of GN based upon whether a patient has proteinuria in the nephrotic range or not. Comprehensive reviews of large cohorts of patients with biopsy-proven GN have highlighted that proteinuria has different implications dependent upon the underlying diagnosis. This is illustrated in Fig. 33.1. As can be seen in this figure, the rate of renal function decline according to category of sustained proteinuria does not largely differ according to patient sex, but varies greatly according to histologic diagnosis. A finding of 2 g/day of proteinuria in a patient with immunoglobulin A nephropathy (IgAN) portends a far worse prognosis than in a patient with membranous GN (MGN). Nephrotic versus nonnephrotic categorization of proteinuria is therefore too simplistic for estimating disease risk.

Natural history studies have also helped to define treatment goals and the value of proteinuria reduction in GN (Table 33.2). The quantitative value of proteinuria reduction is a crucial element in the decision making of nephrologists in terms of balancing the risks and benefits of treatment and is emerging as a surrogate endpoint for renal survival. The capacity to translate proteinuria reduction into a disease-specific estimate of improvement in long-term outcome provides an important element of the benefit in the benefit–risk equation not only in terms of whether to initiate treatment, but also more commonly today to provide help in the decision about prolonging treatment or retreating a patient to maintain or reestablish a partial remission.

## MEMBRANOUS GLOMERULONEPHRITIS

Natural history studies in MGN have demonstrated the value of complete remission of proteinuria. A prospective study of 348 nephrotic patients with MGN assessed the relative benefit of a complete, or partial, remission of proteinuria on both renal survival and rate of progression.[8] Partial remission was defined as both a reduction to less than 3.5 g/day and a 50% decrease from peak proteinuria. Over a median follow-up of 60 months, 30% had a complete remission, 40% had a partial remission, and the remaining 30% had no remission. At 10 years, renal survival in those with a complete remission was 100% with minimal loss of function over time (rate of loss of creatinine clearance −1 mL/min/year). Those achieving a partial remission had a 90% renal survival at 10 years, and a more rapid rate of progression compared with those with a complete remission, although still limited to a loss of –2 mL/min/year of creatinine clearance. In comparison, those with no remission had a renal survival of only 50% at 10 years and a significant fivefold rate of renal function loss compared with the partial remission group (–10 mL/min/year). Survival from renal failure for partial remission was significantly improved (hazard ratio for ESKD vs. the reference group of no remission of 0.08, 95% CI 0.03–0.19; $P < .001$). This study, however, did not identify the intervention required for achievement of partial remission of proteinuria; partial remission of proteinuria is also associated with favorable outcome when achieved spontaneously.[10]

A more recent analysis of the same cohort further reinforces the value of proteinuria reduction. Indeed, the quantity of time spent in either complete or partial remission imparts better preservation of renal function and a lower rate of kidney failure.[11] There is increasing support that partial remission of proteinuria is a surrogate marker of improved "hard" renal outcomes such as survival free from kidney failure.[12]

## FOCAL AND SEGMENTAL GLOMERULOSCLEROSIS

The same estimates of benefit of proteinuria reduction on long-term outcome are observed in patients with focal and segmental glomerulosclerosis (FSGS). It has been appreciated for some time that complete remission of proteinuria is the best predictor of a favorable renal survival.[13,14] Factors that have been previously associated with a poor outcome in FSGS have included the severity of initial proteinuria, renal function at presentation, and the extent of tubulointerstitial disease on histologic examinations.[10,15] Proteinuria reduction is an independent determinant of outcome.[16]

The impact of partial proteinuria reduction on disease course was addressed in a long-term cohort study of 281 nephrotic patients with biopsy-proven primary FSGS followed over an average of 65 months.[9] A partial remission is defined by both a reduction of proteinuria to the subnephrotic range (<3.5 g /day) and a 50% reduction from peak proteinuria. During the observation period 55 patients had a complete remission, 117 patients achieved a partial remission, and 109 had no remission of proteinuria. Partial remission was independently predictive of both renal survival and rate of decline in renal function, and was associated with more favorable outcome. Partial remission was associated with improved renal survival with a time-adjusted hazard ratio of 0.48 (95% CI 0.24 to 0.96; $P = .04$). Ten-year renal survival was 75% in the partial remission group compared with 35% in those with no remission. Similar to MGN, this information on the quantitative benefits of partial remission is important in the assessment of the FSGS patient because it provides equipoise for the risks of treatment.

## IGA NEPHROPATHY

Proteinuria, at far lower levels compared with MGN and FSGS, is tightly correlated with renal outcome in patients with IgAN.[17] Treatment and observational studies support the importance of proteinuria reduction in mitigating risk of progressive disease in IgAN. Donadio et al.[18] demonstrated an association between proteinuria reduction and both improved renal survival and prolonged time to doubling of serum creatinine in patients enrolled in a trial of fish oil. A cohort of more than 500 patients with primary IgAN nephropathy followed for an average of 78 months evaluated the clinical relevance of achieving a partial remission of proteinuria to <1 g/day. In the almost 200 patients that achieved and sustained partial remission of proteinuria (either spontaneously or through treatment), the mean rate of decline in renal function was only 10% of those who did not. Furthermore, regardless of the level of presenting proteinuria, those that attained a partial remission had the same long-term prognosis and slow rate of disease progression as those patients whose peak proteinuria never exceeded 1 g/d. Although there were other modifiable factors identified in the multivariate analysis associated with kidney function decline (time-averaged mean arterial pressure and exposure to renin–angiotensin system blockade), the level of sustained proteinuria was the dominant modifiable risk. The differential in progression rate and renal failure risk was dramatic and understanding the impact of even a small but sustained improvement in proteinuria is extremely valuable information for the practicing physician. Occasionally IgAN presents with the nephrotic syndrome and preserved renal function. In this subset of patients, partial or complete remission of the nephrotic syndrome is also associated with a favorable outcome.[19]

Proteinuria has strong links to cardiovascular mortality in patients without GN.[20] A longitudinal study of nearly 1400 patients with IgAN followed in Korea suggested that this disease—particularly when associated with proteinuria greater than1 g/day—may be associated with a higher standardized mortality rate.[21] The potential independent benefit of proteinuria reduction on mortality certainly merits further study.

The Supportive Versus Immunosuppressive Therapy for the Treatment of Progressive IgAN (STOP-IgAN) study suggested a disconnect between proteinuria reduction and renal survival.[22] Although more patients achieved remission of proteinuria after having received corticosteroids, this did not translate to improved long-term outcome. One possible explanation for this disconnect may be that overall the cohort had relatively low-grade proteinuria, and a very low rate of renal function decline. Therefore it would be difficult to demonstrate differences in "hard" renal endpoints. In addition, the treatment lasted only 6 months. Proteinuria reduction may not always be maintained and 6 months may be insufficient time to accrue the benefit of proteinuria reduction over the long term in this population.

## REMISSION IN LUPUS NEPHRITIS AND VASCULITIS

Estimation of the value of proteinuria remission on outcome is more complex in GN secondary to vasculitis and lupus. In secondary GN the potential morbidity associated with nonrenal manifestations may be the primary determinant for estimating patient risk and guiding decisions regarding immunotherapy. Cohorts differ greatly in terms of renal disease severity, serologic risk factors, and treatment regimens, making it challenging to distinguish the independent value of proteinuria reduction beyond these important factors. Long-term observational studies confirm the association of sustained proteinuria with long-term outcome.[23–26] However, given the relapsing and systemic nature of these diseases, even complete remission of proteinuria does not guarantee freedom from morbidity and mortality resulting from these multisystem diseases, including developing CKD.[27]

## TIMING OF RESPONSE

Expectations regarding the timing of treatment response should be well understood by patients and clinicians at the start of therapy. This helps avoid both excessive exposure to toxicities of therapy and premature escalation or interruption of a treatment protocol. For example, in the case of MGN, the earliest signs of response may only be evident at 3 months of immunotherapy. This is, in part, because of the extensive filtration barrier injury that must be remodeled to restore function. Improvement may continue for months following initiation of therapy. In the case series describing use of rituximab, the median time to remission endpoint from start of therapy was 7 months with a maximum duration extending over a year (interquartile range 3–12).[28] At 3 months, one should expect to see a trend toward improvement. However, evaluating the full response to a treatment can take 12 months.

Similarly, the time to normalization of urine sediment (i.e., resolution of hematuria) is often delayed in secondary GN. At 6 months of evaluation, less than half of patients with severe lupus nephritis enrolled in therapeutic trials will have reached a complete remission according to definitions that include renal sediment findings.[29] A recent review of long-term outcomes of patients with severe lupus nephritis treated in a prior randomized controlled study indicated that halving of proteinuria at 6 months was an important predictor of both long-term renal and patient survival.[30] Similarly, in a renal-focused trial of rituximab in vasculitis, the mean time to complete remission was 182 days (standard deviation 43 days) in the rituximab group and 202 days (standard deviation 66 days) in the cyclophosphamide/azathioprine group.[31] These findings emphasize that provided there is evidence of improvement and treatment is being well tolerated, patience is warranted before assessing for full medication response.

Disease-specific treatment goals are critical to planning individualized therapy and minimizing toxicity. However, untreated disease can also be associated with substantial morbidity and mortality. For example, a 6-month observation is commonly the first step in management of membranous nephropathy. Indeed, with prolonged observation spontaneous remission can occur beyond a year, and can occur even in patients with high-grade proteinuria.[10] However, prolonged periods of profound hypoalbuminemia will place patients at added risk of not only infections, and thrombotic events despite sparing exposure to immunosuppression, but also of progression of parenchymal damage during this waiting period. Therefore these competing risks must be weighed in each patient. Strategies to mitigate risks of postponing treatment (e.g., prophylactic anticoagulation in MGN) should also be factored into plans. Similarly, patients with advanced kidney injury with vasculitis may not have salvageable renal function and certainly toxicity of immunotherapy is higher in patients on dialysis. However, vasculitis is a systemic disease with potential for extrarenal disease–associated morbidity. Avoidance of immunosuppression may not be possible.

## INDIVIDUALIZING THERAPY: MITIGATING TOXICITIES OF THERAPY

With every one of the immunosuppressive agents used in the treatment of GN, the risks of treatment versus potential benefits must be assessed on the basis of drug exposure (a composite of dose and duration), and individual patient factors including gender, age, ethnicity, country of origin, and comorbid conditions such as obesity, diabetes mellitus, and cardiac disease. Further, there is no universal availability of many of the newer drugs and biologic agents because of the paucity of controlled data and the high costs of many of these agents. As such, careful attention must be paid to potential side effects from the therapeutic choices made by practicing clinicians with side-effect profiles often dominating the choice of therapy.

## CORTICOSTEROIDS

Glucocorticoids (GCs) are the most common antiinflammatory and immunosuppressive drugs used in the treatment of both primary and secondary GN. They have protean effects on immune responses mediated by T and B cells, including reversibly blocking T-cell and antigen-presenting cell–derived cytokine and cytokine-receptor expression. Their hydrophobic structure permits them to easily diffuse into cells and bind to specific cytoplasmic proteins, facilitating translocation of these proteins into the cell nucleus where they bind to a highly conserved GC receptor DNA-binding domain (the GC response element) and modulate gene transcription.[32] Some of the downstream effects accounting for the antiinflammatory activity of GCs include the inhibition of synthesis of proinflammatory cytokines implicated in glomerular and tubulointerstitial injury, such as interleukin-2, -6, -8 and tumor necrosis factor.[33,34] GCs also exert a host of nontranscriptional immunomodulatory effects on immune effector cells including alteration of leukocyte trafficking and chemotactic properties, and modulation of endothelial function, vasodilatation, and vascular permeability.[32] Conditions where resolution of proteinuria can be even more rapid than expected based upon immunomodulatory function (such as minimal change disease) effects on podocyte function may be more relevant. This may include alteration in podocyte function and motility.[35–37]

### MAJOR ADVERSE EFFECTS

Infection is a potential risk common to all immunosuppressant medications. Pronounced suppression of cell-mediated immunity results from the protean effects of corticosteroids on the immune system. GC exposure poses a significant short- and long-term risk of infection, particularly in older patients. A nested case–control analysis indicated a rate of serious infection as high as 46% with 6 months of continuous use of more than 5 mg/day in patients with rheumatoid arthritis.[38] In addition to the potential to cause infection, GCs have widespread systemic side effects, including but not limited to, impaired glucose tolerance, cardiovascular and gastrointestinal (GI) toxicity, potentially severe musculoskeletal damage as well as a large array of cosmetic, ophthalmological, and psychiatric side effects.

GCs affect glucose metabolism by increasing hepatic gluconeogenesis and decreasing peripheral tissue insulin sensitivity. These changes in glucose homeostasis may be ameliorated by dose reduction.[39] However, the metabolic effects of these drugs may not be completely reversible, even when the dose is reduced to physiologic range or discontinued entirely.[40] Whereas higher doses of GCs are associated with a higher risk of hyperglycemia, additional risk factors for steroid-induced hyperglycemia include African-American and Hispanic ancestry, obesity (defined as a body mass index >30 kg/m$^2$), older age, a family history of diabetes, and the presence of other components of the metabolic syndrome.[40]

GCs have important musculoskeletal effects. Muscle injury associated with chronic steroid treatment with GC produces a pattern of proximal weakness, atrophy, and myalgia. The ideal management includes discontinuation of steroid administration, although recovery can take weeks or months. Steroid myopathy is more common when the patient has been exposed to the potent fluorinated steroids (dexamethasone, betamethasone, triamcinolone), but similar patterns of muscle injury have been described with the nonfluorinated steroid such as prednisone.[41]

Corticosteroids have major effects on trabecular bone structure. Up to 10% of patients on long-term therapy will have a clinically evident fracture,[42] and risk of bone fracture is increased at doses as low as 2.5 to 7.5 mg/day,[43] rapidly declining toward baseline after stopping treatment.

Avascular necrosis is a clinically and pathophysiologically different type of bone injury than the loss of bone density. It is a devastating condition associated with destruction of the head of the femur or other long bones. The relationship between development of avascular necrosis and dose of prednisone is less clear.[44]

Vision may be affected by cataract formation, and increased intraocular pressure. Thinning of the skin, easy bruising, development of striae, and impaired wound healing may also be potentiated by GCs. Mood lability and insomnia induced by GCs also contribute to their relatively poor patient tolerance. GI effects of GCs include induction of gastritis and GI bleeding.

Given the elevated risk of cardiovascular disease in patients with kidney disease, the added cardiovascular toxicity of GCs is also an important consideration. A large cohort study of 68,781 GC users demonstrated that high-dose steroids are independently associated with cardiovascular events after adjustment for other traditional risk factors, including hypertension, glucose intolerance, and obesity.[45]

## STRATEGIES FOR REDUCING TOXICITY

There are several strategies available for minimizing steroid exposure. Alternate day steroids has been described to treat nephrotic syndrome.[46] However, cumulative dose does not differ with this approach, and efficacy and minimization of side effects is not proven in adults. An alternate strategy is shortening the course and/or a more rapid taper of the prednisone, and this approach is currently being investigated in the context of vasculitis (PEXIVAS study, www.clinicaltrials.gov). More commonly, a second non-GC immunosuppressive agent is introduced for its "steroid-sparing" potential. The introduction of these agents has allowed the total exposure to corticosteroids in many of these disorders to be limited by allowing a shorter initial total exposure to the drug. In patients at very high risk of complications, consideration may also be given to use protocols classified as "second line" to avoid toxicity. For example, a calcineurin inhibitor (CNI) may be considered as a second-line therapy for nephrotic syndrome as a result of FSGS in adults according to 2012 KDIGO guidelines.[47] However, consideration may be given to using this agent as a first-line approach in patients with significant contraindications to GCs such as preexistent significant obesity, or a history of psychosis.

Alternate strategies specifically focus on reducing or preventing the complications related to corticosteroid treatment. Such prophylactic strategies include the use of antibiotics such as trimethoprim-sulfamethoxazole to prevent *Pneumocystis jirovecii* pneumonia (previously known as pneumocystis pneumonia PCP). Retrospective studies have indicated that a corticosteroid dose equivalent to 16 mg of prednisone for a period of 8 weeks was associated with a significant risk of pneumocystis pneumonia.[48,49] Ongoing surveillance for diabetes is required along with regular eye examinations. Antihypertensive regimens may require adjustment while on high-dose therapy, and blood pressure should be evaluated regularly. Gastric protection in the form of a proton-pump inhibitor should be prescribed.

In relationship to the risk of fracture, if daily corticosteroids (0.5–1 mg/kg) are expected to be used in excess of 8 to 12 weeks in adults, consideration should be given to adding vitamin D 1000 U/day and 1 g/day of calcium, and some populations may merit more intensive therapy including addition of bisphosphonates. The American College of Rheumatology recently updated recommendations on the prevention of osteoporosis in patients on prolonged therapy.[50] These guidelines review general universal strategies to minimize risk such as optimizing calcium and vitamin D intake, and exercise. The decision to give bisphosphonates is guided by early bone density evaluation, age, and patient-specific risks that can be assessed using validated online risk calculators. Bisphosphonates may have more potent effects to prevent reduction in bone density during corticosteroid use; however, it is important to note that bisphosphonates remain in mineralized bone for months to years, posing a theoretical risk of teratogenicity when administered to women of childbearing potential.[51]

# CALCINEURIN INHIBITORS

Cyclosporine and tacrolimus are CNIs that suppress the immune response by downregulating T-cell activation. They specifically block calcium-dependent T–cell receptor signaling transduction, thereby inhibiting the transcription of interleukin-2 as well as other proinflammatory cytokines, in both T cells and antigen-presenting cells.[52] Interleukin-2 serves as the major activation factor for T cells and a key modulator of both T-and B-cell activity in numerous immunological processes.[53] Tacrolimus and cyclosporine have a common mechanism of action (i.e., inhibition of calcineurin phosphatase), although they bind different intracellular proteins. These intracellular proteins belong to the immunophilin family with cyclosporin binding cyclophilin and tacrolimus binding FKBP12.[54] The role of differential immunophilin binding in the mechanism of toxicity is not clear, but it may allow for the unique side-effect profile of each of these drugs. More recently an alternative mechanism of action of these agents has been suggested relating to their capacity to stabilize the internal cytoskeletal structure of the glomerular podocyte.[55] This is an intriguing possibility and may help explain its efficacy in some of the glomerular-based diseases at lower drug levels compared with those required in solid organ transplantation.[56]

## MAJOR ADVERSE EFFECTS

The CNI class of agents have significant adverse effects with the most concerning being its nephrotoxicity. This is particularly relevant when prolonged therapy is being contemplated. These longer treatment courses are usually given to prevent or modify the well-recognized risk of relapse of nephrotic syndrome that does occur upon treatment withdrawal. CNI-associated nephrotoxicity can be severe, and reports indicate a significant risk of CKD if the drug is given in high doses for prolonged periods, such as occurred in early recipients of nonrenal solid organ transplants.[57] However, the cyclosporine dose and duration used in these studies are no longer considered appropriate[58] and lower doses in the glomerular-based diseases versus solid organ transplant are currently advocated.[59] In addition, modifications have occurred in drug formulation of cyclosporine, which has resulted in more consistent and predictable pharmacokinetics, allowing at least potentially even lower drug exposure regimens.[59]

New onset or worsening of "hypertension" is another important and common dose-dependent adverse effect of CNI use and likely contributes to their long-term nephrotoxic potential. The reported incidence of hypertension in patients with glomerular diseases treated with CNIs varies from 10% to 30%.[60] An additional significant adverse effect is the induction of glucose intolerance and even overt diabetes.[61] This seems to be specific to CNIs and is somewhat more common with tacrolimus.[62] The transplantation literature highlights the potential contributions of CNIs to development of hyperglycemia, which is thought to be a result of both impaired insulin secretion and increased insulin resistance. The higher rate of hyperglycemia associated with tacrolimus use may reflect differential effects on pancreatic beta-cell insulin transcription and release. Even when CNIs are used as monotherapy, the risk of new-onset diabetes has been reported to be as high as 4%.[63]

As with all immunosuppressive agents, CNIs affect immune surveillance and are associated with an increased rate of infections and malignancy. The incidence of malignancy induced by CNIs alone in the glomerular diseases is very hard to determine from the literature. Very few of the GN treatment studies have been long enough to assess CNI exposure as an independent risk factor. Cyclosporine, however, has been used in the long-term management of other autoimmune diseases including rheumatoid arthritis and psoriasis. When patients with rheumatoid arthritis treated with cyclosporine were compared with control patients (who received placebo, D-penicillamine, or chloroquine) an increased cancer risk was not seen.[64] A recent review of patients with psoriasis did find an increase in the standardized incidence ratio of cancer in patients treated with cyclosporine compared with the general population. However, when examined more closely and skin malignancies, known to be more common in patients with psoriasis, were excluded, the incidence was not significantly higher in the CNI-treated patients.[65] As such, although not well-described, the incidence of drug-associated malignancy specifically in the context of GN therapy is considered to be relatively low.[66] The underlying risks of infection associated with untreated nephrotic syndrome and the potential for malignancy associated with membranous nephropathy further complicate the assessment of risk of these complications with CNI treatment.

Other common adverse effects of CNIs are cosmetic and include gum hypertrophy and hypertrichosis (less frequent with tacrolimus than cyclosporine). The excess hair growth can be severe and is likely to contribute to poor drug adherence, particularly in young female subjects. A cohort of approximately 200 pediatric nephrotic patients treated with cyclosporine for an average of 22 months[67] was recently reviewed; reported side effects of such prolonged therapy included hypertrichosis (52.3%), gum hyperplasia (25.4%), hypertension (18.8%), and renal impairment (9.1%). Close examination of the subgroup of patients with renal impairment in this study is revealing. In the small number ($N = 18$ patients) that demonstrated renal impairment, 12 recovered completely after the cyclosporine was stopped, three experienced stable but continued renal impairment, and only three (1.5% of the total number exposed) had slow progression of their renal disease. On multivariate analysis, resistance to the cyclosporine treatment was the only factor predictive of renal impairment

## STRATEGIES FOR REDUCING TOXICITY

In contrast to transplantation, long-term low-dose therapy with cyclosporine (1.0–2 mg/kg per day) with or without low-dose steroids has been shown to be both safe and effective at maintaining remission. The lower toxicity of CNIs in patients with GN is at least in part related to the lower daily maintenance dose required and the capacity to gradually increase the dose over days or weeks to achieve a therapeutic affect versus the need for a much more rapid dose escalation following solid organ transplant.[59] Although higher doses of cyclosporine may be required for the induction phase in membranous nephropathy, the initial dose can usually be reduced during the maintenance phase.[68] In renal transplant patients, CNI dose has been safely reduced after the first year with renal function remaining stable even after 20 years of exposure to this agent.[69] Nevertheless, nephrotoxicity is a risk with this therapy and careful monitoring of drug levels, a constant awareness of drug interactions (that may either increase or decrease drug levels), and frequent monitoring of renal function are mandatory.

One of the mechanisms of the nephrotoxicity that is attributable to these agents is their renal vasoconstrictive properties. This hemodynamic effect is both dose dependent and reversible,[70] but may still result in dangerous episodes of acute kidney injury, particularly when a patient is also taking concomitant renin–angiotensin system blockade. As such, patients should be cautioned as to what to do in the event of unanticipated volume contraction secondary to volume depletion. For example, patients with significant acute GI illness may be counseled to hold one dose of medication. If they are unable to safely restart the next scheduled dose, they should present for assessment and possible intravenous hydration. The more delayed chronic damage in the tubular interstitial compartment and the small arterioles is less well understood but may also be abrogated at least in part by a dose reduction or discontinuation of the agent. CNI toxicity may be more evident when used in patients with more advanced renal impairment and/or in those with significant tubular interstitial and/or vascular changes noted on histology. However, with careful monitoring and the slow escalation of dosage, even patients with significant renal dysfunction can be safely treated with CNIs.[71]

The hypertension that commonly accompanies treatment with CNIs is another adverse effect that requires attention. However, the adjustments in antihypertensive medication are usually straightforward, and its presence does not generally preclude or limit CNI usage. The vasoconstrictive effects of cyclosporine, in addition to their effects on renal potassium secretion, may limit the ability to use higher doses of inhibitors of the renin–angiotensin system to control blood pressure in patients on cyclosporine. With respect to the risk of diabetes, ongoing vigilance by the prescribing physician is required. In patients at highest risk for developing glucose intolerance including obese individuals, those with a strong family history of diabetes, older age, and metabolic syndrome,[40] strategies for preventing this adverse effect include preferential use of cyclosporine over tacrolimus and/or the use of CNI monotherapy or in combination with other steroid-sparing agents, thereby at least avoiding the additive risk of corticosteroid exposure.

## ALKYLATING AGENTS

Cyclophosphamide is the most common drug in this class used in the treatment of GN. It is a cytotoxic agent that acts largely through the alkylation of purine bases. This DNA damage induces apoptosis or altered function of both B cells and T cells.[72,73] Chlorambucil is the other drug of this class that is used, although less commonly than cyclophosphamide because of significant differences in both the short- and long-term adverse effect profile and drug tolerability.

### MAJOR ADVERSE EFFECTS

Infertility in both men and women has been reported with these agents, most commonly following cyclophosphamide and is likely the most concerning long-term side effect given the often younger age of patients with glomerular disease. This effect is closely related to total exposure but is also strongly impacted by the age of the patient.[74] One early series indicated that the rate of permanent ovarian failure was 26% in those who received between 10 and 20 g cyclophosphamide, but was greater than 70% in those whose cumulative dose was more than 30 g.[75] This effect is of particular concern in women who are increasingly delaying conception to the later part of their reproductive life because of career demands. It has been estimated that women who receive a single course of cyclophosphamide therapy (10- to 20-g exposure) before the age of 25 years are at significantly less risk of permanent sterility (0%–15% risk) compared with the same exposure after the age of 30 years (30%–40% risk).[75–77] Similar drug exposure, but an even higher risk has been estimated by Ioannidis et al. who calculated the risk of permanent ovarian failure for a standard dose of 12 g/m$^2$ to be 90% in women when treated after the age of 32.[78] This combination of age and exposure on fertility can be expressed as an odds ratio. These authors suggest an odds ratio for permanent ovarian failure of 1.48 per 100 mg/kg of cumulative dose and 1.07 per patient-year.[79] Although more difficult to estimate, there is certainly a substantial risk of infertility in men as well. However, the age effect has not been as clearly demonstrated as in women. Studies have indicated that long-term gonadal toxicity was not evident until the cumulative exposure to cyclophosphamide was greater than 300 mg/kg, but more recent information suggests a substantial risk at a cumulative dose of less than168 mg/kg (equivalent to 12 g for a 70-kg patient),[80,81] and gonadal toxicity as indicated by a reduction in sperm count has been documented with exposures as low as 100 mg/kg.[74]

The other major adverse effect is the risk of malignancy. It is suspected that this has been underestimated in the past at least in part because of the delay between exposure to the drug and the appearance of the cancer. This latent period may be many years. More recent data from an epidemiological study of 293 Danish patients with antineutrophil cytoplasmic antibody-associated vasculitis treated with cyclophosphamide suggested a much lower safety limit for exposure than previously indicated.[82] The authors of that study concluded that patients who received a cumulative dose of more than 36 g of cyclophosphamide (equivalent to 2 mg/kg for 8 months in a 70-kg patient) had a substantially increased risk for the development of a malignancy compared with the normal-age and sex-controlled population. Their standardized incidence ratio of acute myelocytic leukemia was 59.0, bladder cancer was 9.5, and nonmelanoma skin cancer was 5.2 above this cumulative cyclophosphamide exposure. They also confirmed the substantial delay between exposure and malignancies. The latent period after cyclophosphamide and malignancy diagnosis averages between 6.9 and 18.5 years, and patients therefore require lifelong screening for malignancies. This exposure of 36 g is a much lower threshold for these serious complications than previously estimated and needs to be validated in an independent data set.[83,84] In the meantime, however, the potential for toxicity at much lower exposure limit should be kept in mind when considering the more prolonged course of cyclophosphamide as a treatment option in membranous nephropathy, lupus nephritis, or vasculitis.

An additional well-recognized, short-term adverse effect of the alkylating agents is bone marrow suppression, particularly the white cell line. A recent meta-analysis reported significant leucopenia in 25% of patients with lupus nephritis who were treated with cyclophosphamide.[85] Another short-term adverse effect of cyclophosphamide is an increased susceptibility to infections. These infections can be severe and resistant to therapy and in combination with leucopenia can be overwhelming. Additional less serious but disconcerting side effects that can impact on compliance include alopecia and hemorrhagic cystitis. This long list of potentially serious complications makes monitoring, for both short- and long-term effects of these agents, a critical and necessary component of management.

Chlorambucil is an alternative alkylating agent used in the treatment of membranous nephropathy. The original regimen developed by Ponticelli et al.[86] with this agent cycled it monthly, alternating with corticosteroids over a 6-month treatment course. The adverse effects of chlorambucil are similar to cyclophosphamide, although it has not been associated with the bladder toxicity with the associated gross hematuria. Even so, chlorambucil may be less well tolerated overall than cyclophosphamide and has the added associated risk of acute myelogenous leukemia.[87]

## STRATEGIES FOR REDUCING TOXICITY

Strategies to limit exposure focus on limiting duration of therapy rather than modifying the dose. The exception to this is the use of intravenous cyclophosphamide in lupus and vasculitis wherein less frequent and smaller doses of intravenous cyclophosphamide appear to be as effective as the earlier higher-dose regimens with fewer adverse events.[73,88] A shorter-duration regimen of exposure is an established option in membranous nephropathy. The two published effective regimens vary dramatically in terms of cyclophosphamide exposure. In the original classic 6-month regimen for example, cyclophosphamide exposure is limited to 3 months[86] compared with the later published routine that employs a full year of exposure.[87] This is frequently modified to be of only 6 months' duration, but the long-term results of this reduction are still unknown.

Substitution of other agents less toxic than cyclophosphamide is another option. Mycophenolate mofetil (MPA) or azathioprine for maintenance therapy in lupus nephritis are well-established options and appear to have similar efficacy with significantly fewer adverse effects. Data from a recent randomized controlled trial in patients with diffuse proliferative lupus nephritis confirmed that MPA (3 g/day) was associated with fewer pyogenic infections than a cyclophosphamide-based regimen (relative risk 0.36).[89] Similarly, long-term therapy with azathioprine has been proven to be as efficacious as cyclophosphamide in the maintenance phase of vasculitis, with less toxicity.[90] Similar results in terms of complete and partial remissions were obtained when MPA was substituted for the year of cyclophosphamide in membranous nephropathy, but a significantly lower incidence of serious side effects was observed. This study was not a randomized controlled trial because the cyclophosphamide-treated patients were a historical control group. Although the initial response rate was equal, the relapse rate was very much higher than in the cyclophosphamide group.[91] Replacement of the cyclophosphamide with CNIs is another option. This substitution strategy could be employed when initial therapy with cyclophosphamide has failed, in the situation where the patient has relapsed, and/or when repeated exposure to alkylating agents was being considered. This strategy can be used in the management of patients with membranous nephropathy, lupus nephritis, or FSGS.

Monitoring the other potential adverse effects of cyclophosphamide by frequent blood counts, adjusting the dose relative to degree of renal impairment, age, and other comorbid conditions are additional tools to minimize cyclophosphamide toxicity. The likelihood of inducing opportunistic infections such as *pneumocystis jiroveci* pneumonia and/or cytomegalovirus can also be reduced by the use of prophylactic antibiotic/antivirals as described earlier in the "Corticosteroids" section. With respect to the potential to cause infertility in young patients, sperm banking and oocyte cryopreservation can be considered. There are limited data to suggest a gonadotropin-releasing hormone analog (GnRH-a) may provide ovarian protection, decreasing the rates of premature ovarian failure from 30% to 5% in one study.[92] However, the use of GnRH-a remains controversial. In the cancer literature, use of GnRH-a is more widely described, yet currently not universally recommended because of conflicting study data.[93] There is relatively limited experience with the use of ovarian suppression described in the renal literature. This is, in part, because of the urgency required to start therapy, without sufficient time to institute preventative strategies. Risks should be explained to patients in detail, and alternative therapies considered in patients of childbearing age. Finally, given the teratogenicity of cyclophosphamide, contraception counseling is required for sexually active men and women and the risks and benefits of various modes of contraception should be reviewed. Cryopreservation of sperm may be a realistic option for reproductive-age men requiring urgent therapy.

# AZATHIOPRINE

Azathioprine is an inhibitor of inosine monophosphate dehydrogenase, a critical enzyme involved in de novo purine synthesis, required for lymphocyte division resulting in depressed levels of both B and T lymphocytes as well as immunoglobulin synthesis. Its metabolite, 6-thio-guanosine-5′-triphosphate (trio-GTP), causes immunosuppression by blockade of guanosine-5′-triphosphatase activation in T lymphocytes specifically by blocking activation of Rac proteins.[94]

## MAJOR ADVERSE EFFECTS

GI side effects including nausea and vomiting are common, and remain the primary reason for treatment interruptions.[95] Liver toxicity with a significant increase in serum transaminase levels has also been described as has pancreatitis.[96] Dose-related bone marrow suppression primarily affects white blood cells, but can affect all cell lines, and can be severe in patients with low levels of thiopurine methyltransferase (TPMT). This genetic abnormality affects approximately 0.3% of the population wherein the enzyme is lacking, whereas 11% of individuals are heterozygous for a variant low-activity allele with intermediate activity,[97] causing diminished azathioprine metabolism. Similarly, allopurinol causes drug accumulation and can result in severe myelosuppression.[98] As with all immunosuppressive agents, bacterial and viral infections do occur, particularly in the setting of leukopenia, and increased rates of malignancies, in particular skin cancers, have been noted.[99,100]

## STRATEGIES FOR REDUCING TOXICITY

There is no consensus among physicians treating glomerular disease with respect to the assessment for TPMT deficiency. Both genetic testing and functional assays are available, but it is common practice to simply slowly dose escalate while surveying for toxicity. Myelosuppression will typically improve with dose reductions. The gout therapies, allopurinol and febuxostat, are contraindicated when using azathioprine (and other cytotoxic drugs such as cyclophosphamide) due the risk of leukopenia. Monitoring for hepatotoxicity and pancreatitis is also essential when prescribing azathioprine.

## MYCOPHENOLIC ACID

Mycophenolate acid (MPA – available as mycophenolate mofetil, or the metabolite mycophenolic acid) is a reversible inhibitor of inosine monophosphate dehydrogenase, a critical enzyme involved in de novo purine synthesis, required for lymphocyte division.[101] Several factors contribute to the lymphocyte-specific effects of MPA on purine metabolism. First, unlike other cells, lymphocytes are uniquely dependent upon de novo purine synthesis to generate RNA and DNA because they do not have a salvage pathway for purine generation. Inhibition of this pathway by MPA, therefore, predominantly affects lymphocyte metabolism. MPA also is a highly potent inhibitor of the isoform of inosine monophosphate dehydrogenase that is expressed in activated lymphocytes (the type II isoform), contributing to its specificity.[102,103] The selectivity of MPA for inhibiting lymphocyte proliferation is the concept that underlies the reduced toxicity of MPA compared with other alkylating agents that affect all dividing cells. In addition to its effects on T and B cells, MPA may affect fibroblast proliferation/activity[104] and endothelial function.[105]

### MAJOR ADVERSE EFFECTS

The principal adverse effects of MPA relate to GI symptoms including both upper GI irritation with nausea and vomiting and lower tract involvement with diarrhea. This is more common with MPA than with cyclophosphamide.[106] These symptoms tend to occur early in the course of treatment, and can improve over time.

As with all antimetabolites, MPA can cause hematologic complications including leucopenia and anemia. The myelosuppressive effects of MPA contribute to the risk of infection associated with its use, and although some data suggest a lower infection risk than with cyclophosphamide in lupus nephritis, several studies indicate similar risk of serious infection, and serious infections have been reported.[85,107–109] Furthermore, the transplantation literature suggests an increased risk of viral infections with MPA, particularly in the context of multidrug regimens.[110] Whether there is a difference with respect to risks of late-onset malignancy with MPA when used for the treatment of lupus or other variants of GN is too early to determine.

Although there is no fertility impact, MPA has now clearly emerged as a human teratogen with an identifiable pattern of malformations – craniofacial (microtia or anotia, absent auditory canal, cleft palate, hypertelorism) and limb anomalies.[111] Manufacturer data note a 33% increased miscarriage rate and at least a 22% rate of teratogenicity. As such, women may elect to terminate the pregnancy if conception occurred during exposure to MPA. The possibility of sperm-mediated MPA teratogenicity has recently been an area of controversy.[112] In the absence of clear risk of teratogenicity above population rates, risks should be weighed against the consequences of losing control of disease by altering therapy if conception is planned.[112]

### STRATEGIES FOR REDUCING TOXICITY

Unlike the transplantation context, the dose of MPA can frequently be titrated up over the course of days to weeks to minimize development of GI symptoms. Splitting the dosage into four times/day versus the standard two doses/day also reduces GI problems. Temporarily reducing the dose also may be tried, especially in the context of acute GI infections. The predominant effect on the bone marrow is leucopenia and is usually corrected by a temporary dose reduction. If the full dose is still not tolerated, the addition of MPA-sparing agents such as a low dose of steroid or a CNI may be considered. Sexually active women initiating MPA should have a negative pregnancy test before initiating the therapy, and those who desire pregnancy should be off MPA at least 6 weeks before conception. Two forms of contraception should be used by women who are taking MPA.

## RITUXIMAB AND OCRELIZUMAB

Rituximab is a genetically engineered, chimeric, murine/human monoclonal antibody directed against the CD20 antigen found on the surface of normal and malignant pre-B and mature B cells.[113] The CD20 antigen is not expressed on hematopoietic stem cells, pro-B cells, normal plasma cells, or other normal tissues. Thus it has an impressive safety record when compared with classic cytotoxic agents. The precise mechanism of action of anti-CD20 antibodies in autoimmune disease and in particular GN is unclear. It is known that B cells play an important role as immunoregulatory cells by both antigen presentation and cytokine release. Their elimination could have dampening effects on other immune cells such as T lymphocytes, dendritic cells, and macrophages. In vitro studies have demonstrated that the Fc portion of rituximab binds human complement and can lead to cell lysis of the targeted cell through complement-dependent cytotoxicity and it has been demonstrated that rituximab mediates antibody-dependent cellular cytotoxicity. Most recently, rituximab been shown to be effective in the treatment of idiopathic membranous nephropathy and may work at least in part by depletion of the autoantibody to the podocyte-located antigen phospholipase $A_2$ receptor.[114] Further, rituximab may have a direct podocyte-modulating effect via cross-reactivity with sphingomyelin phosphodiesterase acid–like 3b protein and regulation of acid sphingomyelinase essential for the lipid-raft compartmentalization of the podocyte plasma membrane as well as for the organization and signaling of podocytes in general.[115] This potential direct effect on podocytes independent of its known effect on selective depletion of the B-cell clone may make it a very effective option to consider for the treatment of idiopathic glomerular diseases.

Ocrelizumab is a genetically engineered fully humanized monoclonal antibody directed against the same CD20 antigen found on the surface of normal B cells, with the same mode of action as rituximab. Because of its fully humanized nature, this anti-CD20 antibody can be infused more rapidly and has less immediate infusion-related reactions than rituximab. In addition, because of the fully humanized construct, formation of autoantibodies directed against the drug is unlikely, thereby enhancing the potential efficacy and safety of repeated treatments.

### MAJOR ADVERSE EFFECTS

Acute infusion-related reactions can vary from minor symptoms to severe life-threatening reactions. Minor reactions occur in up to 10% of exposed individuals and include skin rash, pruritus, flushing, nausea, vomiting, fatigue, headache, flulike symptoms, dizziness, hypertension, and/or runny nose. Anaphylaxis and shock can occur but are fortunately rare (<1%). Other rare side effects that have been seen with the use of rituximab include anemia, cardiac arrhythmias, respiratory failure, and acute kidney injury (occurring in <0.1.%).[116–120] The latter severe reactions have been seen primarily—although not exclusively—with its use in the treatment of hematologic malignancies where the tumor cell burden is high and an acute tumor lysis syndrome can develop. More delayed adverse effects include serum sickness and an increased incidence of infection including reactivation of latent viral infections including hepatitis B and several cases of pneumocystis.[121] There have been several reports of the development of progressive multifocal leukoencephalopathy (PML) in patients treated with this agent. This devastating syndrome is as a result of the activation of latent JC (John Cunningham) polyomavirus, and is associated with progressive neurologic impairment and ultimately death within months of diagnosis. In the majority of reported cases, PML developed when rituximab was used in combination with additional chemotherapeutic agents.[122] Given its impact on antibody formation, vaccinations that contain live organisms should be avoided during treatment with rituximab.

Formation of human antichimeric antibodies (HACAs) does occur although their clinical significance is unclear. Despite the appearance of HACA in patients treated with rituximab and their theoretical consequences, these sequelae have not been uniformly observed in the small studies in GN.[123] The new fully humanized version of the anti-CD20 agent should either ameliorate or eliminate the issue of HACA formation.

### STRATEGIES FOR REDUCING TOXICITY

The risk of acute infusion reaction can be mitigated by careful dose infusion escalation, as well as premedication with antihistamines, and corticosteroids. Administration protocols are available[124] (see Appendix in McGeoch et al.). The precise dose and/or regimen to use in patients with autoimmune disorders is unknown. Although the relationship between peripheral CD20-positive cell depletion and response is poor, it has been suggested that a single dose, in membranous nephropathy, is adequate for B-cell depletion and provides a similar response in proteinuria as multiple doses of the agent.[125]

## ECULIZUMAB

Eculizumab is an anti-C5 (complement factor 5) monoclonal antibody designed for use in diseases characterized by functional impairment of endogenous inhibitors of the activation of the alternative complement pathway. The activation of this cascade has classically been implicated in atypical hemolytic uremic syndrome, thus providing a potential rationale for this agent in this disease and others that might involve the complement pathway.[126,127] Emerging evidence suggests that complement dysregulation may be a critical contributor to many forms of progressive glomerular injury traditionally attributed to classical or lectin-activated complement pathways. Activation of these pathways and their potential inhibition by eculizumab may have relevance in the context of C3 nephropathy and dense deposit disease, and perhaps even in the idiopathic immunoglobulin-mediated forms of membranoproliferative glomerulonephritis,[128] systemic lupus erythematosus,[129] and other variants of GN, as well as in antibody-mediated rejection in transplantation.[130]

### MAJOR ADVERSE EFFECTS

Overall, eculizumab is well tolerated, but there is the potential for an increased risk for infection by encapsulated bacteria such as *Neisseria meningitides*.

### STRATEGIES FOR REDUCING TOXICITY

As such, vaccination before instituting therapy and careful surveillance are recommended based on its use in patients with paroxysmal nocturnal hemoglobinuria and in atypical hemolytic-uremic syndrome.[131] In addition, prophylactic antibiotics are widely recommended, particularly when there is concern regarding timing and efficacy of immunization. Guidelines are available to guide choice and duration of antibiotic therapy (e.g., National Renal Complement Therapeutics Centre guidelines).[132] The precise dose and/or regimen to use in patients with glomerular diseases are presently unknown.

## ADRENOCORTICOTROPHIC HORMONE

Synthetic formulations of adrenocorticotrophic hormone (ACTH) have previously proven effective in patients with nephrotic syndrome, and the use of ACTH for the treatment of elevated cholesterol and proteinuria dates back many decades.[133,134] In Europe, the synthetic formulation of ACTH, tetracosactide (Synacthen), has proven similarly effective in both uncontrolled series and a small randomized controlled trial wherein it was compared with cytotoxic therapy.[135–137] To date, there are limited data to suggest that natural ACTH (H.P. Acthar Gel), which is currently the only available ACTH preparation in North America, may also have a beneficial effect in patients with nephrotic syndrome by lowering proteinuria, improving serum albumin, and cholesterol profiles.[138]

The active ingredients of H.P. Acthar Gel are part of the family of structurally related peptides known as melanocortin peptides. Melanocortin peptides, which include ACTH and the α-, β-, and γ-melanocyte–stimulating hormones, are derived from the natural protein proopiomelanocortin that bind to the cell surface G protein–coupled receptors known as melanocortin receptors (MCRs).[139] To date, five forms of MCRs have been cloned, each with different tissue distributions, affinities, and physiological roles. As such, its potential therapeutic mechanisms are numerous and complex.[140] Potential renoprotective mechanisms include corticosteroid-mediated systemic immunosuppression and antiinflammatory actions subsequent to ACTH-induced steroidogenesis through MCR 2 interaction as well as direct MCR-mediated immunomodulation and antiinflammatory effects (MCR 1, 3, and 5). Correction of dyslipidemia mediated by MCR 1 and 5 on hepatic cells and neurogenic antiinflammatory effects mediated by MCR 3 and 4 expressed in the central nervous system are likely also beneficial to the kidneys. Finally, a direct

MCR-mediated protective effect on kidney cells, particularly the podocytes, has been described. MCRs are expressed in glomerular podocytes and receptor stimulation has been demonstrated to reduce oxidative stress and improve glomerular morphology by diminishing podocyte apoptosis, injury, and loss in the remnant kidney animal model.[141]

## MAJOR ADVERSE EFFECTS

Although initially thought to be associated with less toxicity than GCs, studies now suggest that the frequency of adverse events associated with this regimen in membranous nephropathy has been underestimated. One open label study reported an incidence of adverse events in 95% of subjects treated with synthetic ACTH.[142] In a recent pilot study side effects were noted to be dose dependent.[138] Reported side effects associated with the use of ACTH include steroid-like effects including a cushingoid appearance, weight gain, as well as worsening of edema or bloating. Potential skin changes include acne, flushing, and bronzing. With respect to potential psychological effects of the treatment, increased irritability, depression, and improved mood have been noted along with transient insomnia, tremulousness, dizziness, muscle aches or pain, headaches, GI symptoms, blurred vision, as well as generalized weakness or fatigue. Glucose intolerance and frank diabetes are also potential rare side effects that tend to improve with the cessation of treatment.

## STRATEGIES FOR REDUCING TOXICITY

The precise dose and/or regimen to use in patients with glomerular diseases are presently unknown, limiting ability to mitigate toxicity. Given the toxicity profile described, similar strategies used in mitigating corticosteroid toxicity should be considered.

# TREATMENT ALGORITHMS AND CONSIDERATIONS

The most recent treatment recommendations are reviewed in Chapters 31 and 32. Guidelines assist in decision making, and highlight the evidence supporting different regimens. However, guidelines cannot account for all of the variations in patient and disease variability nor individual preferences in avoiding treatment toxicity (e.g., desire to preserve fertility). Therefore application of these guidelines to the individual patient requires careful consideration. In practice, we consider the following questions before making guideline-based treatment recommendations:

1. What is the risk of progression to kidney failure in this individual patient?
   - The critical question is whether the risks of the medication outweigh the risks of progression of the kidney disease. Complementary considerations are the morbidity and mortality associated with dialysis or with transplantation, where many of the same medications will be used to prevent rejection.
   - Proteinuria is one of our main considerations when we decide whether or not there is an advantage to addition of immunomodulatory treatment to conservative therapy for treatment of patients with primary idiopathic GN. Although the threshold of proteinuria associated with highest risk of disease progression varies according to disease (Fig. 33.1), this measure is a more important contributor to our treatment decisions than histologic diagnosis. For example, membranous nephropathy may be a lesion that is very amenable to immunologic therapy. However, patients with MGN with persistent subnephrotic range proteinuria have an excellent long-term prognosis.[6] The added advantage of immunotherapy versus conservative therapy alone is not established in this subpopulation. Renal insufficiency at presentation and progression of renal insufficiency during observation should also be considered. Although this may argue for a more aggressive approach to care, side effects of immunosuppressive therapy are often more frequent in patients with impaired clearance and additional susceptibility to infections. Pathologic indices of kidney injury, in particular tubulointerstitial fibrosis, are also informative to address chronicity and prognosis. Indeed, a common clinical error is to put patients with irreversible kidney injury at risk with little chance of benefit.[143] Advanced tissue injury with impaired clearance may change the risk–benefit ratio of immunotherapy.
2. What are the patient's comorbid conditions?
   - Ideally the choice of therapy should be tailored to the individual patient, considering comorbid conditions that may place patients at risk of medication toxicity. For example, guidelines suggest that a trial of a minimum of 4 weeks of corticosteroid therapy should be first considered as first-line treatment for idiopathic FSGS associated with clinical features of the nephrotic syndrome. However, in a patient with significant obesity, the weight gain and glucose intolerance induced by steroids are important potential toxicities. A CNI may be a better first choice for that individual patient.
   - Important variables to consider when selecting a patient-specific regimen include age, personal or family history of glucose intolerance, obesity, cancer history, and prior cumulative immunosuppression exposure.
3. What are plans for childbearing?
   - Important considerations in patients contemplating future pregnancy include the teratogenicity of drugs, the effects of the medications on fertility, and the optimization of renal health before pregnancy.
   - Recognizing the complexity of these patients as well as the treatment regimens recommended, treatment of patients with GN in a multidisciplinary specialized clinic, similar to predialysis and transplant clinics, may be advocated. The addition of nursing guidance and supervision, dietary counselling, pharmacy support, as well as social supports may ultimately improve both patient safety and the disease experience of this unique population. Although this setting is not feasible in all health-care centers, the benefits of the multidisciplinary specialized clinic approach merit further study.

# CONCLUSION

GN remains a leading cause of CKD and kidney failure. New data regarding clinically relevant surrogate endpoints and therapeutic goals will hopefully facilitate the development and study of novel agents to treat patients with GN and prevent loss of kidney function. The toxicity of immunotherapeutic agents requires careful consideration by clinicians; the risks of these drugs must always be weighed against the potential benefits in each individual patient, considering patient-, disease-, and drug-specific characteristics. The toxicity and complexity of current regimens also make it imperative that the nephrology community pursue development of novel targeted therapies for these important diseases, and demonstrate efficacy of these treatments in rigorous clinical trials.

 Complete reference list available at ExpertConsult.com.

## KEY REFERENCES


3. Wetmore JB, Guo H, Liu J, et al. The incidence, prevalence, and outcomes of glomerulonephritis derived from a large retrospective analysis. *Kidney Int.* 2016;90(4):853–860.
4. Ayme S, Bockenhauer D, Day S, et al. Common elements in rare kidney diseases: conclusions from a Kidney Disease: Improving Global Outcomes (KDIGO) Controversies Conference. *Kidney Int.* 2017;92(4):796–808.
7. Reich HN, Troyanov S, Scholey JW, et al. Remission of proteinuria improves prognosis in IgA nephropathy. *J Am Soc Nephrol.* 2007;18(12):3177–3183.
8. Troyanov S, Wall CA, Miller JA, et al. Idiopathic membranous nephropathy: definition and relevance of a partial remission. *Kidney Int.* 2004;66(3):1199–1205.
9. Troyanov S, Wall CA, Miller JA, et al. Focal and segmental glomerulosclerosis: definition and relevance of a partial remission. *J Am Soc Nephrol.* 2005;16(4):1061–1068.
12. Thompson A, Cattran DC, Blank M, et al. Complete and partial remission as surrogate end points in membranous nephropathy. *J Am Soc Nephrol.* 2015;26(12):2930–2937.
13. Korbet SM, Schwartz MM, Lewis EJ. Primary focal segmental glomerulosclerosis: clinical course and response to therapy. *Am J Kidney Dis.* 1994;23(6):773–783.
17. Berthoux F, Mohey H, Laurent B, et al. Predicting the risk for dialysis or death in IgA nephropathy. *J Am Soc Nephrol.* 2011;22(4):752–761.
22. Rauen T, Eitner F, Fitzner C, et al. Intensive supportive care plus immunosuppression in IgA nephropathy. *N Engl J Med.* 2015; 373(23):2225–2236.
24. Houssiau FA, Vasconcelos C, D'Cruz D, et al. The 10-year follow-up data of the Euro-Lupus Nephritis Trial comparing low-dose and high-dose intravenous cyclophosphamide. *Ann Rheum Dis.* 2010;69(1):61–64.
28. Ruggenenti P, Cravedi P, Chianca A, et al. Rituximab in idiopathic membranous nephropathy. *J Am Soc Nephrol.* 2012;23(8):1416–1425.
31. Geetha D, Specks U, Stone JH, et al. Rituximab versus cyclophosphamide for ANCA-associated vasculitis with renal involvement. *J Am Soc Nephrol.* 2015;26(4):976–985.
38. Dixon WG, Abrahamowicz M, Beauchamp ME, et al. Immediate and delayed impact of oral glucocorticoid therapy on risk of serious infection in older patients with rheumatoid arthritis: a nested case-control analysis. *Ann Rheum Dis.* 2012;71(7):1128–1133.
42. Curtis JR, Westfall AO, Allison J, et al. Population-based assessment of adverse events associated with long-term glucocorticoid use. *Arthritis Rheum.* 2006;55(3):420–426.
47. Kidney Disease: Improving Global Outcomes (KDIGO) Glomerulonephritis Work Group. KDIGO Clinical Practice guideline for glomerulonephritis. *Kidney Int Suppl.* 2012;2:139–274.
50. Buckley L, Guyatt G, Fink HA, et al. 2017 American College of Rheumatology guideline for the prevention and treatment of glucocorticoid-induced osteoporosis. *Arthritis Rheumatol.* 2017;69(8): 1521–1537.
63. Praga M, Barrio V, Juarez GF, et al. Tacrolimus monotherapy in membranous nephropathy: a randomized controlled trial. *Kidney Int.* 2007;71(9):924–930.
66. Anderka MT, Lin AE, Abuelo DN, et al. Reviewing the evidence for mycophenolate mofetil as a new teratogen: case report and review of the literature. *Am J Med Genet A.* 2009;149A(6):1241–1248.
71. Cattran DC, Greenwood C, Ritchie S, et al. A controlled trial of cyclosporine in patients with progressive membranous nephropathy. Canadian Glomerulonephritis Study Group. *Kidney Int.* 1995; 47(4):1130–1135.
73. Houssiau FA, Vasconcelos C, D'Cruz D, et al. The 10-year follow-up data of the Euro-Lupus nephritis trial comparing low-dose and high-dose intravenous cyclophosphamide. *Ann Rheum Dis.* 2010;69(1):61–64.
74. Rivkees SA, Crawford JD. The relationship of gonadal activity and chemotherapy-induced gonadal damage. *JAMA.* 1988;259(14): 2123–2125.
75. Mok CC, Lau CS, Wong RW. Risk factors for ovarian failure in patients with systemic lupus erythematosus receiving cyclophosphamide therapy. *Arthritis Rheum.* 1998;41(5):831–837.
76. Boumpas DT, Austin HA III, Vaughan EM, et al. Risk for sustained amenorrhea in patients with systemic lupus erythematosus receiving intermittent pulse cyclophosphamide therapy. *Ann Intern Med.* 1993;119(5):366–369.
77. Huong DL, Amoura Z, Duhaut P, et al. Risk of ovarian failure and fertility after intravenous cyclophosphamide. A study in 84 patients. *J Rheumatol.* 2002;29(12):2571–2576.
78. Ioannidis JP, Katsifis GE, Tzioufas AG, et al. Predictors of sustained amenorrhea from pulsed intravenous cyclophosphamide in premenopausal women with systemic lupus erythematosus. *J Rheumatol.* 2002;29(10):2129–2135.
81. Meistrich ML, Wilson G, Brown BW, et al. Impact of cyclophosphamide on long-term reduction in sperm count in men treated with combination chemotherapy for Ewing and soft tissue sarcomas. *Cancer.* 1992;70(11):2703–2712.
82. Faurschou M, Sorensen IJ, Mellemkjaer L, et al. Malignancies in Wegener's granulomatosis: incidence and relation to cyclophosphamide therapy in a cohort of 293 patients. *J Rheumatol.* 2008;35(1):100–105.
84. Westman KW, Bygren PG, Olsson H, et al. Relapse rate, renal survival, and cancer morbidity in patients with Wegener's granulomatosis or microscopic polyangiitis with renal involvement. *J Am Soc Nephrol.* 1998;9(5):842–852.
88. Houssiau FA, Vasconcelos C, D'Cruz D, et al. Immunosuppressive therapy in lupus nephritis: the Euro-Lupus Nephritis Trial, a randomized trial of low-dose versus high-dose intravenous cyclophosphamide. *Arthritis Rheum.* 2002;46(8):2121–2131.
89. Ginzler EM, Dooley MA, Aranow C, et al. Mycophenolate mofetil or intravenous cyclophosphamide for lupus nephritis. *N Engl J Med.* 2005;353(21):2219–2228.
90. Contreras G, Pardo V, Leclercq B, et al. Sequential therapies for proliferative lupus nephritis. *N Engl J Med.* 2004;350(10):971–980.
95. Singh G, Fries JF, Spitz P, et al. Toxic effects of azathioprine in rheumatoid arthritis. A national post-marketing perspective. *Arthritis Rheum.* 1989;32(7):837–843.
98. Min MX, Weinberg DI, McCabe RP. Allopurinol enhanced thiopurine treatment for inflammatory bowel disease: safety considerations and guidelines for use. *J Clin Pharm Ther.* 2014;39(2):107–111.
108. Chan TM, Li FK, Tang CS, et al. Efficacy of mycophenolate mofetil in patients with diffuse proliferative lupus nephritis. Hong Kong-Guangzhou Nephrology Study Group. *N Engl J Med.* 2000; 343(16):1156–1162.
111. Anderka MT, Lin AE, Abuelo DN, et al. Reviewing the evidence for mycophenolate mofetil as a new teratogen: case report and review of the literature. *Am J Med Genet A.* 2009;149A(6):1241–1248.
112. Canadian Transplantation Society. *Male-mediated developmental toxicity and mycophenolate exposure:Information for the transplant professional*; 2016. www.cst-transplant.ca.
114. Beck LH, Fervenza FC, Beck DM, et al. Rituximab-induced depletion of anti-PLA2R autoantibodies predicts response in membranous nephropathy. *J Am Soc Nephrol.* 2011;22(8):1543–1550.
115. Fornoni A, Sageshima J, Wei C, et al. Rituximab targets podocytes in recurrent focal segmental glomerulosclerosis. *Sci Transl Med.* 2011;3(85):85ra46.
121. Kolstad A, Holte H, Fossa A, et al. Pneumocystis jirovecii pneumonia in B-cell lymphoma patients treated with the rituximab-CHOEP-14 regimen. *Haematologica.* 2007;92(1):139–140.
122. Carson KR, Evens AM, Richey EA, et al. Progressive multifocal leukoencephalopathy after rituximab therapy in HIV-negative patients: a report of 57 cases from the Research on Adverse Drug Events and Reports project. *Blood.* 2009;113(20):4834–4840.
125. Cravedi P, Ruggenenti P, Sghirlanzoni MC, et al. Titrating rituximab to circulating B cells to optimize lymphocytolytic therapy in idiopathic membranous nephropathy. *Clin J Am Soc Nephrol.* 2007;2(5):932–937.
143. Bose B, Silverman ED, Bargman JM. Ten common mistakes in the management of lupus nephritis. *Am J Kidney Dis.* 2014;63(4):667–676.

# 34 Thrombotic Microangiopathies

David Kavanagh | Neil Sheerin

CHAPTER OUTLINE



## INTRODUCTION

Thrombotic microangiopathies (TMAs) are the consequence of severe endothelial injury with pathological features representing the tissue response to injury.[1] It can manifest in a diverse range of conditions and presentations, but acute kidney injury (AKI) is a common prominent feature because of the propensity of the glomerular circulation to endothelial damage and occlusion.

## CLASSIFICATION

Over the past 20 years the classification of TMAs has evolved to reflect our increasing understanding of the pathophysiology of disease. Historically, classifications reflected the predominant phenotype: hemolytic uremic syndrome (HUS) for renal dominant disease and thrombotic thrombocytopenic purpura (TTP) for predominant neurological involvement. More recently, severe ADAMTS13 deficiency defined TTP; the

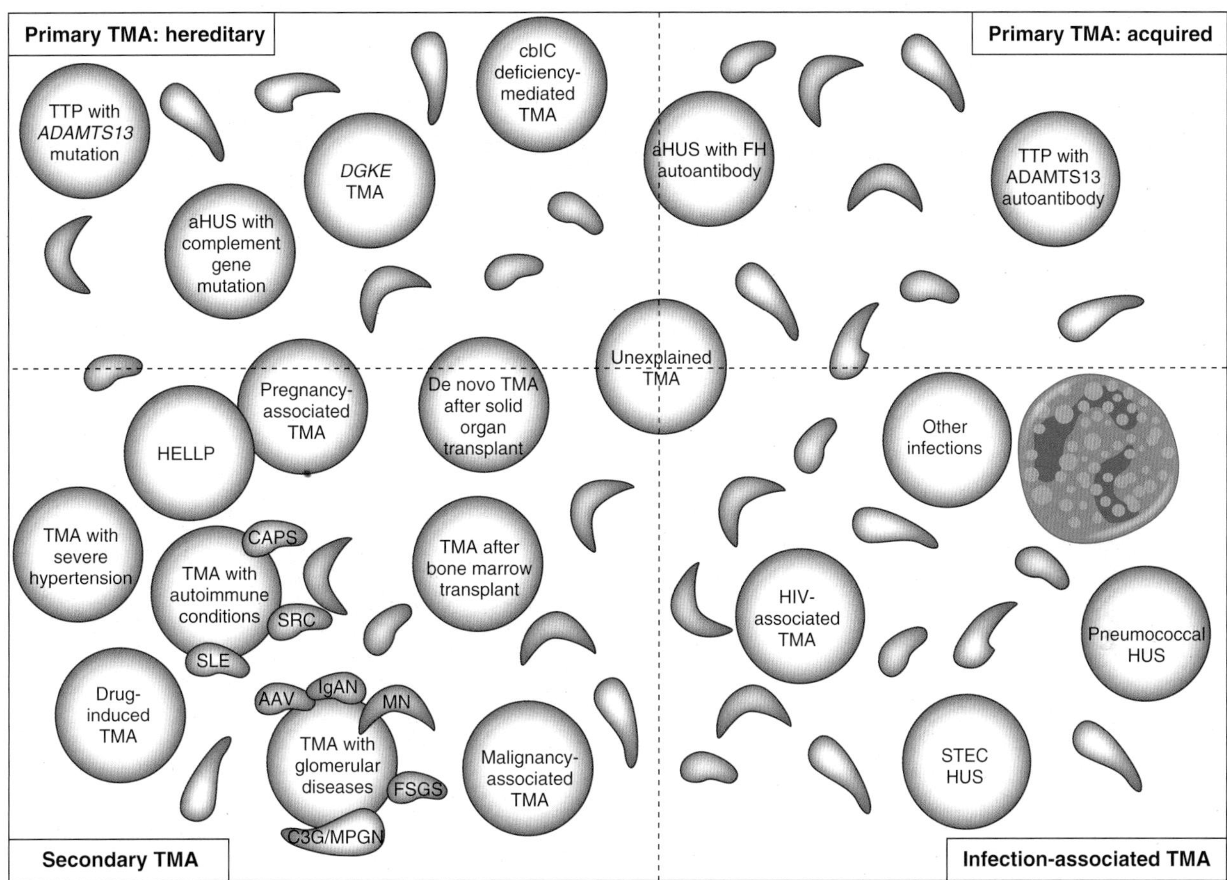


**Fig. 34.1** Classification of thrombotic microangiopathies (TMAs). TMAs are classified as primary inherited TMAs, primary acquired TMAs, infection-associated TMAs, and secondary TMAs. Primary inherited TMAs are predisposed to by mutations in *ADAMTS13, MMACHC,* or genes encoding complement proteins. Primary acquired TMAs are caused by autoantibodies to ADAMTS13 or complement FH. Infection-associated TMAs may have distinct mechanisms (e.g., Shiga toxin–producing *Escherichia coli* and pneumococcal hemolytic uremic syndrome). In other infections the processes are not defined and in some cases the infection may trigger manifestation of a primary TMA. Secondary TMAs occur in a spectrum of conditions, and in many cases the pathogenic mechanisms are multifactorial or unknown. In some secondary cases (e.g., pregnancy-associated TMA or de novo TMA after transplantation), a significant proportion of individuals will have a genetic predisposition to a primary TMA. *AAV,* ANCA (antineutrophil cytoplasmic antibody)–associated vasculitis; *ADAMTS13,* a disintegrin and metalloproteinase with a thrombospondin type 1 motif, member 13; *aHUS,* atypical hemolytic uremic syndrome; *C3G,* C3 glomerulopathy; *CAPS,* catastrophic antiphospholipid syndrome; *cblC,* cobalamin C type; *DGKE,* gene encoding diacylglycerol kinase ε; *FH,* factor H; *FSGS,* focal segmental glomerulosclerosis; *HELLP,* syndrome of *h*emolysis, *e*levated *l*iver enzymes, and *l*ow *p*latelets; *HIV,* human immunodeficiency virus; *IgAN,* IgA nephropathy; *MN,* membranous nephropathy; *MPGN,* membranoproliferative glomerulonephritis; *SLE,* systemic lupus erythematosus; *SRC,* scleroderma renal crisis; *TMA,* thrombotic microangiopathy; *TTP,* thrombotic thrombocytopenic purpura. (Modified from the National Renal Complement Therapeutics Centre 2017/2018 annual report. Available from: http://www.atypicalhus.co.uk/. Last accessed February 4, 2019.)

presence of Shiga toxin–producing bacteria categorized Shiga toxin–associated HUS (STEC-HUS) and broadly all other causes of TMA could be classified as atypical HUS (aHUS). Current classifications designate primary inherited TMAs (e.g., complement mutations, ADAMTS13 mutations), primary acquired TMAs (factor H autoantibodies, ADAMTS13 autoantibodies), infection-associated TMAs, and secondary TMAs (Fig. 34.1).[1] It is, however, necessary to remember that patients with an underlying complement genetic mutation often require a secondary trigger for aHUS to manifest.

## CLINICAL AND LABORATORY FEATURES

The clinical features of TMA reflect hemolysis and ischemic organ dysfunction and the underlying cause. Specific features of different etiologies are covered in individual sections.

Thrombocytopenia and microangiopathic hemolytic anemia (MAHA) are defining features of TMAs. Aggregation and consumption account for the low platelet count, and the MAHA is thought to be caused by mechanical fragmentation in areas of disturbed flow in small blood vessels due to partial occlusion by thrombus (Fig. 34.2A). An elevated lactate dehydrogenase is the most sensitive marker of hemolysis and is due to cell lysis and tissue ischemia. Haptoglobin levels are low in TMAs due to the binding of free hemoglobin and the uptake of haptoglobin–hemoglobin complexes in the reticuloendothelial system. A direct antiglobulin test (DAT/direct Coombs) is negative with the exception of pneumococcal HUS. AKI is a common manifestation of TMAs due to ischemia in the kidney, although rarely a severe feature of TTP. Once routine hematological and biochemical diagnostics have confirmed a TMA, investigations are aimed at determining the underlying etiology and excluding other differential

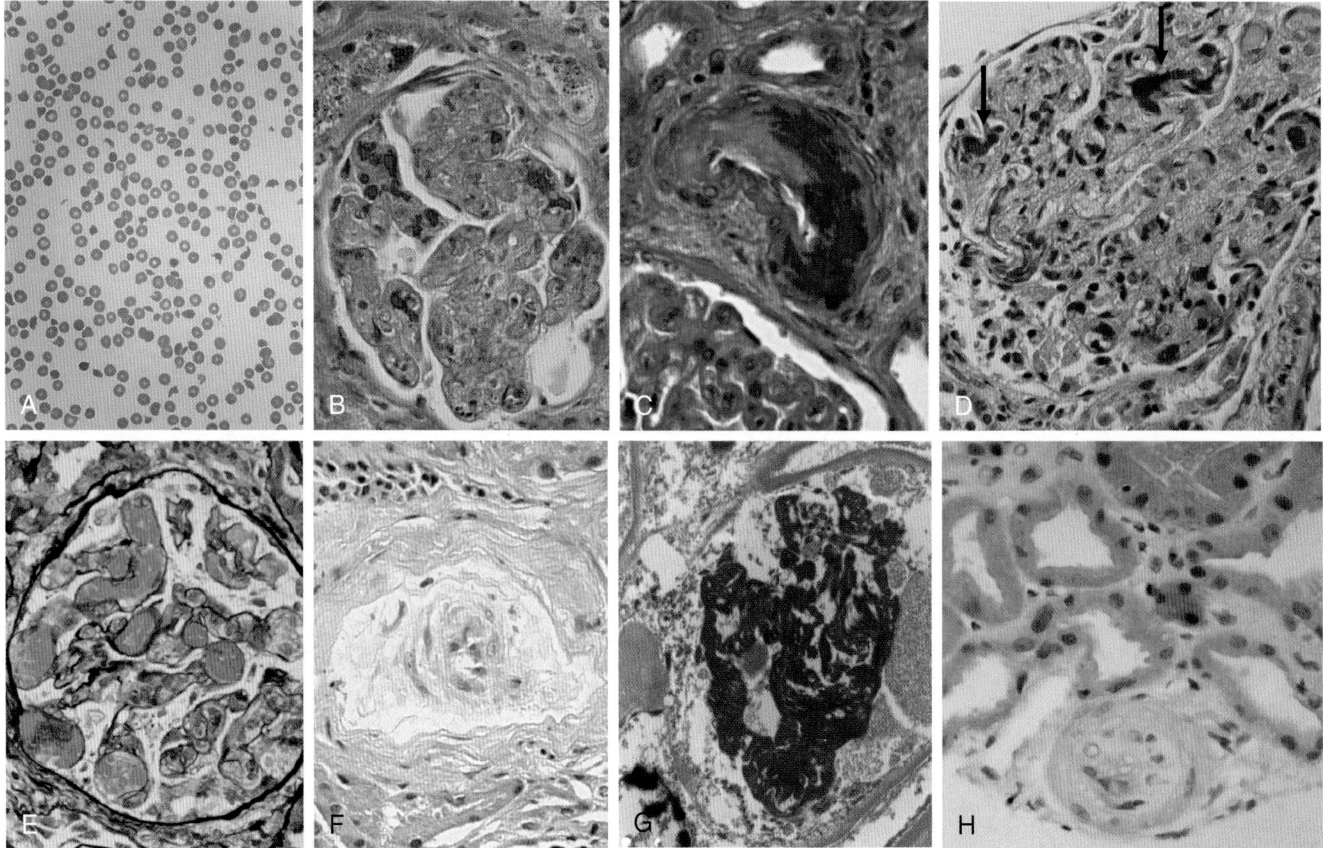

**Fig. 34.2** The pathological features of thrombotic microangiopathies. (A) Blood film of a patient with thrombotic microangiopathy demonstrating the presence of schistocytes. (B) Fibrin thrombi *(red)* and erythrocytes *(yellow)* in glomerular capillary lumina *(Martius Scarlet Blue)*. (C) Fibrinoid necrosis of arterial wall *(Martius Scarlet Blue)*. (D) Thrombi *(arrows)* in capillary loops *(Masson trichrome)*. (E) Glomerular paralysis with capillary loops containing abundant erythrocytes *(silver)*. (F) Myxoid intimal thickening of small artery *(hematoxylin and eosin)*. (G) Fibrin tactoids *(black)* in glomerular capillary (electron micrograph). (H) Mucoid thickening and obliteration of the lumen of a small artery *(hematoxylin and eosin)*.

diagnoses—the most urgent test being an ADAMTS13 assay (Fig. 34.3).[1]

## THROMBOTIC MICROANGIOPATHY PATHOLOGY

In acute HUS, glomerular capillary wall thickening is seen as a result of endothelial cell swelling and accumulation of flocculent material between the endothelial cell and the basement membrane. Fibrin and platelet thrombi may be seen, resulting in occlusion of the glomerular capillaries and glomerular paralysis. It has been noted that overt fibrin platelet thrombosis may be absent from renal biopsies of TMA, which has recently led to a suggested reclassification to microangiopathy with or without thrombosis.[2] Mesangiolysis occurs early in the disease process and subsequently is replaced by sclerotic changes. Early arterial changes are variable, ranging from only mild endothelial swelling to fibrinoid necrosis with occlusive thrombus formation. Erythrocyte fragments may be seen in the vessel wall. Subsequently, there is mucoid intimal hyperplasia with narrowing of the vessel lumen (Fig. 34.2).

Deposition of fibrin or fibrinogen in the glomeruli and in the mesangium, as well as within the vessel walls, is seen on immunofluorescence. Complement and immunoglobulin deposits along the capillary loops of glomeruli may be seen.

Evidence of TMA has also been reported in a number of glomerular diseases and autoimmune diseases; however, in published clinicopathologic studies only a small proportion of individuals with pathological evidence of TMA in these contexts had concurrent clinical and laboratory evidence. It is not possible based on current knowledge to establish TMA etiology from the histopathological morphology, though this may evolve with further research.

TTP is characterized by unusually large multimers of von Willebrand factor (vWF) and platelet-rich thrombi in capillaries and arterioles, although with current practice pathological specimens are rarely available.

## PRIMARY THROMBOTIC MICROANGIOPATHIES

### COMPLEMENT-MEDIATED ATYPICAL HEMOLYTIC UREMIC SYNDROME

A series of ground-breaking studies in the late 1990s established the role of complement overactivation in the pathogenesis of aHUS.[3]

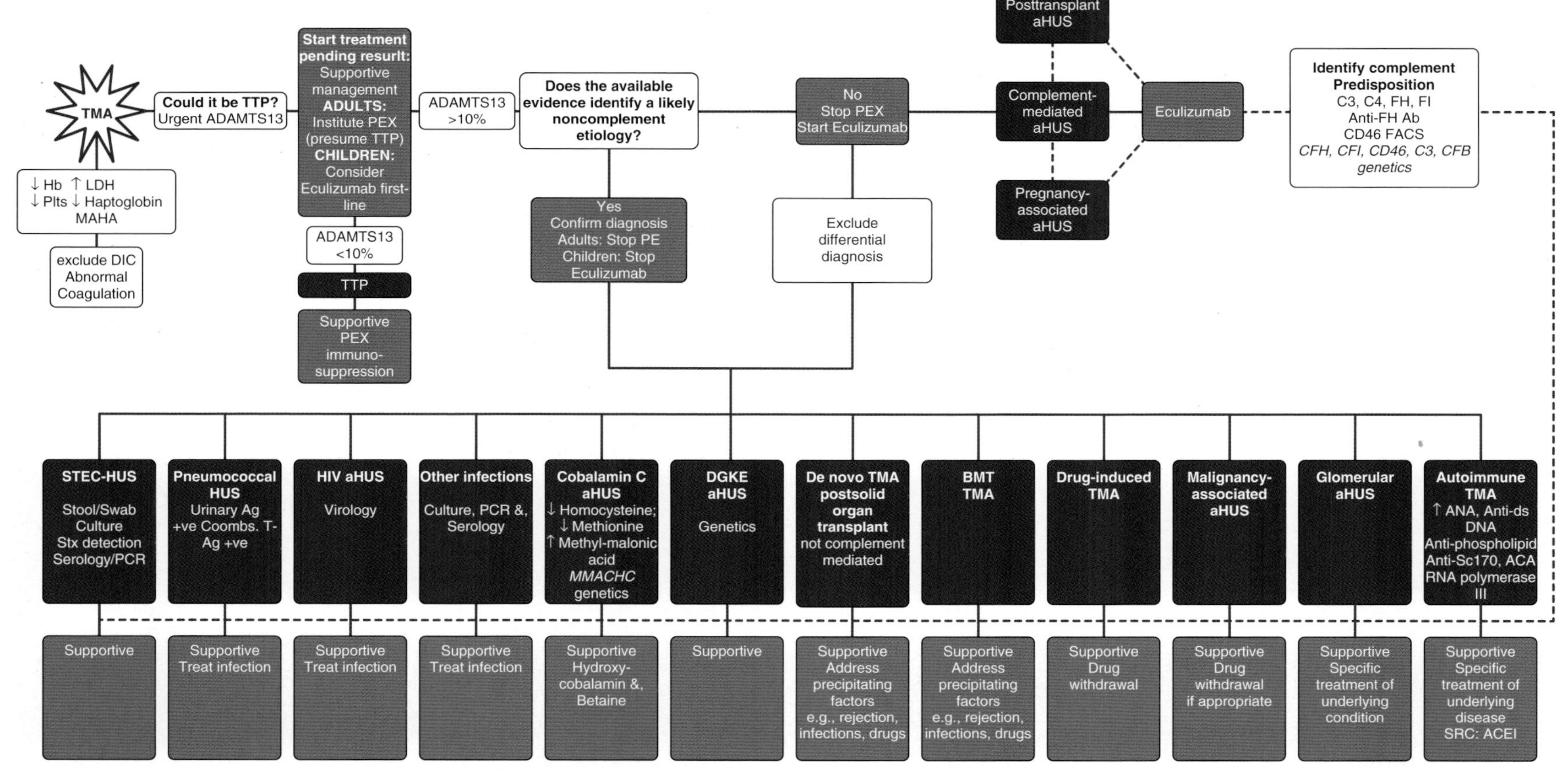


**Fig. 34.3** Algorithm for the investigation and management of a patient presenting with thrombotic microangiopathy. Urgent treatment is critical given the high mortality if untreated. In adults, plasma exchange *(PEX)* should be instituted on the presumption that it is thrombocytopenic purpura *(TTP)* unless strong evidence suggests otherwise. In children, TTP is rarer and initial treatment with eculizumab should be considered if complement-mediated atypical hemolytic uremic syndrome *(aHUS)* is suspected and should not be delayed while ADAMTS13 activity is determined. There is no rapid diagnostic test which identifies complement-mediated aHUS in the acute phase and in those with ADAMTS13 activity greater than 10% without an obvious other etiology, eculizumab should be commenced. A diagnostic screen for noncomplement etiologies should then be commenced to determine optimal long-term treatment. Where eculizumab is not available, PEX should be continued until remission is established. Complement evaluation is recommended in all cases due to secondary causes of TMA unmasking latent complement defects. *BMT,* Bone marrow transplant; *DGKE,* diacylglycerol kinase ε; *DIC,* disseminated intravascular coagulation; *FACS,* fluorescence-activated cell sorting; *FH,* factor H; *FI,* factor I; *Hb,* hemoglobin; *HIV,* human immunodeficiency virus; *LDH,* lactate dehydrogenase; *MAHA,* microangiopathic hemolytic anemia; *MMACHC,* methylmalonic aciduria and homocystinuria type C protein; *PCR,* polymerase chain reaction; *Plts,* platelets; *STEC-HUS,* Shiga-toxin–producing *Escherichia coli*-HUS; *TMA,* thrombotic microangiopathy.

The complement system comprises around 50 plasma and cell-surface proteins operating in a regulated network of signaling and amplification central to the normal physiological functioning of both innate and adaptive immune systems. Equal numbers of complement activators and inhibitors exist. In addition to opsonization and lysis of pathogens and modulation of the adaptive immune system, complement also facilitates the disposal of damaged host cells and potentially damaging immune complexes.

Complement activation can be initiated by three pathways: classical pathway (CP), lectin pathway (LP), and alternative pathway (AP; Fig. 34.4). The CP is triggered when C1q binds to one of a number of activators such as antigen–antibody complexes and other nonimmunoglobulin moieties. C1q activates the associated serine proteases, C1r and C1s, which cleave the plasma proteins C2 and C4 to form a C3 convertase complex (C4b2a) on the activating surface. The LP is activated when microbial carbohydrates are recognized by mannose-binding lectin (MBL), ficolins, or collectins and induces MBL-associated serine proteases to cleave C2/C4, once again forming C4b2a. The AP is constitutively active at a low level (tick over), but is primarily responsible for the rapid amplification of the CP and LP. The C3 convertases activate C3, resulting in the deposition of C3b and the release of C3a. Through interplay with the soluble proteases factor B and D (FB and FD, respectively), surface-bound C3b forms additional C3 convertases. Thus the alternate pathway is responsible for approximately 80% of complement activity even when initially triggered through the CP.

The terminal pathway of complement begins when continuous deposition of C3b and stabilization of convertases by properdin lead to the formation of C5 convertases, which cleave C5 to the anaphylatoxins C5a and C5b that after a conformational change bind C6, C7, C8, and C9 to form the membrane attack complexes that induce lysis or damage of targeted cells (Fig. 34.4).

## COMPLEMENT REGULATION

The amplification loop of the complement system provides a rapid response to pathogens but leaves host cells susceptible to collateral damage if the complement system is unchecked. The system is, therefore, tightly regulated by plasma proteins, including factor H and factor I and cell surface proteins such as CD46. Impaired regulation can lead to pathology and complement-mediated aHUS is the archetypal disease of excessive complement activation (Fig. 34.4).

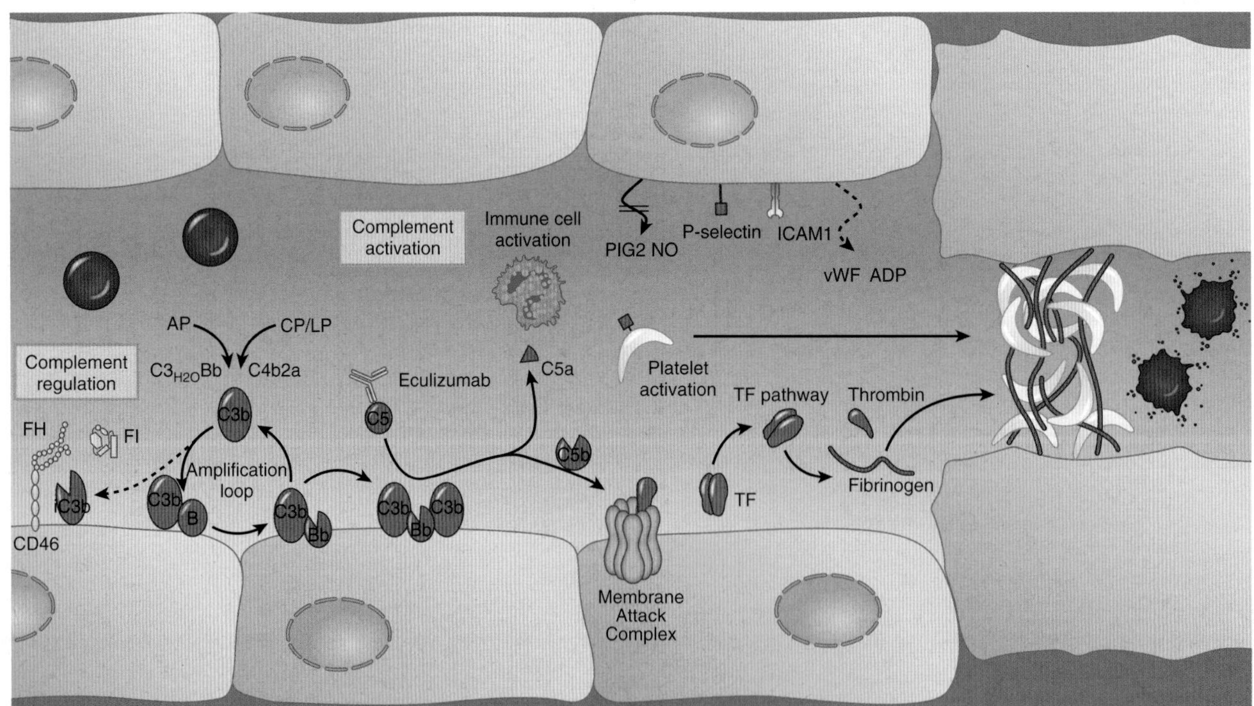


**Fig. 34.4** Complement-mediated atypical hemolytic uremic syndrome (aHUS). Complement is activated by the alternative (AP), classical (CP), and lectin (LP) pathways. The AP is a positive amplification loop. C3b interacts with factor B, which is then cleaved by factor D to form the C3 convertase C3bBb. Unfettered, this leads to activation of the terminal complement pathway with generation of the anaphylatoxin C5a and the membrane attack complex (MAC, C5b-9). The glomerular endothelium is protected from collateral damage from the AP by complement regulators including factor H (FH), factor I (FI), and CD46. In complement-mediated aHUS, loss-of-function mutations in *CFH, CFI,* and *CD46,* activating mutations in *C3* and *CFB,* and autoantibodies to FH result in overactivation of the AP. This leads to immune cell and platelet activation and endothelial cell damage and swelling, with consequent thrombus formation, platelet consumption, vascular occlusion, and mechanical hemolysis. Eculizumab binds to C5 to prevent activation of the terminal pathway inhibiting the generation of the effector molecules that cause thrombotic microangiopathy (TMA) in individuals in whom a primary defect in complement underlies the TMA pathogenesis. (Modified from the National Renal Complement Therapeutics Centre 2017/2018 annual report. Available from: http://www.atypicalhus.co.uk/. Last accessed February 4, 2019.)

## INHERITED COMPLEMENT-MEDIATED ATYPICAL HEMOLYTIC UREMIC SYNDROME

Complement-mediated aHUS is a rare disease with an incidence of about 0.4 per million population per year.

### COMPLEMENT FACTOR H

Genetic studies in 1998 first established that loss-of-function mutations in factor H (*CFH*) caused complement-mediated aHUS.[4] Since then, multiple studies have confirmed that mutations in this gene are the most common cause of disease, accounting for around 25% of cases.

The factor H protein (FH) is the most important fluid-phase regulator of the AP of complement. It consists of 20 modules called complement control proteins modules (CCPs). The four N-terminal CCPs (CCPs 1–4) mediate the complement regulatory functions of FH by (1) competing with FB for C3b binding, (2) accelerating the decay of the C3 convertase into its components, and (3) acting as a cofactor for factor I–mediated proteolytic inactivation of C3b. The C-terminal domains of FH (CCP19–20) mediate host surface protection by binding polyanions such as glycosaminoglycans. It is this C-terminal region of FH that is most commonly mutated in aHUS, resulting in impaired cell-surface complement regulation.[5]

It is the genetic architecture of the regulators of complement activation (RCA) gene cluster on chromosome 1, in which *CFH* resides, which is responsible for this mutational hotspot. The RCA cluster is thought to have arisen from several large genomic duplications and *CFH* and five factor H–related proteins thus have a very high degree of sequence identity. This homology predisposes to gene conversions and genomic rearrangements (*CFH/CFHR1* and *CFH/CFHR3* hybrid genes) through nonallelic homologous recombination and microhomology-mediated end joining.[6] These hybrid genes, as with C-terminal point mutations in *CFH*, result in loss-of-cell-surface complement regulation. From a practical perspective, this complex genomic locus is very hard to sequence when compared with other genes mutated in human disease, in part, because of large regions of repetitive genomic DNA sequences.

More recently a reverse *CFHR1/CFH* hybrid gene arising through nonallelic homologous recombination in which the C-terminal CCPs of FHR1 are replaced by the C-terminal CCPs of FH has been described. In this setting this FHR1/FH hybrid protein does not impair FH cell surface binding but instead, acts as a competitive inhibitor of FH.[7]

### CD46 MEMBRANE COFACTOR PROTEIN

Mutations in *CD46* (membrane cofactor protein) are found in approximately 10% of patients with aHUS. CD46 is a membrane inhibitor of complement activation expressed on most cell types with the exception of erythrocytes. It consists of four CCP modules containing the sites for complement interaction followed by an O-glycosylation region, enriched with serine, threonine, and proline residues (STP domain); a transmembrane anchor; and a cytoplasmic tail. Most mutations described in aHUS are found in the extracellular four CCP domains that are responsible for C3b and C4b binding. The majority of *CD46* mutations resulted in reduced cell surface expression of CD46 (75%) with the remaining producing a surface expressed but nonfunctional protein.[8]

### COMPLEMENT FACTOR I

Mutations in complement factor I (*CFI*) account for between 5% and 10% of aHUS.[9] FI is a disulfide-linked heterodimer serine protease that cleaves C3b and C4b in conjunction with a cofactor protein (FH for C3b; C4b binding protein for C4b; CD46 and complement receptor 1 for both). The *CFI* mutations described in aHUS are all heterozygous.[3]

### COMPLEMENT C3

C3 is the nexus of the complement cascade. It is cleaved to form the anaphylatoxin C3a and the highly reactive C3b which can then bind to cell surfaces via its reactive thioester. Thioesters are compounds with the functional group R–S–CO–R′. C3b can then interact with FB in the presence of FD to form the AP convertase. Mutations in C3 account for around 2% to 8% of complement-mediated aHUS.[10] They represent gain-of-function mutations. The mutations in C3 linked to complement-mediated aHUS result in complement overactivation by either binding to FB with greater affinity or preventing complement regulators binding to C3 and inactivating it. Most C3 mutations are associated with low serum C3 levels (70%–83%).

### COMPLEMENT FACTOR B

Gain-of-function mutations also have been reported in *CFB*, although these appear to be rare.[11] FB carries the catalytic site of the complement AP convertase (C3bBb). Complement overactivation occurs by impaired complement regulation or increased convertase formation.

### THROMBOMODULIN

Genetic variants in thrombomodulin *(THBD)* have been reported in some aHUS cohorts, however their causality remains to be established.[12] THBD regulates clot formation by the activation of protein C by thrombin and enhancing thrombin-mediated activation of plasma procarboxypeptidase B (CPB2), an inhibitor of fibrinolysis. THBD, however, has been suggested to have a role in the regulation of the AP by accelerating FI-mediated inactivation of C3b.[12]

### DISEASE PENETRANCE

In complement-mediated aHUS, genetic mutations are not causative per se but are instead predisposing. For a disease to manifest, additional genetic and environmental modifiers are required (Fig. 34.5). The disease penetrance is age related and has been reported to be as high as 64% by the age of 70 years in individuals with a single rare genetic variant, although this is likely to represent the upper range. Rarely aHUS patients (about 3%) will have more than one mutation with increased penetrance per additional mutation.

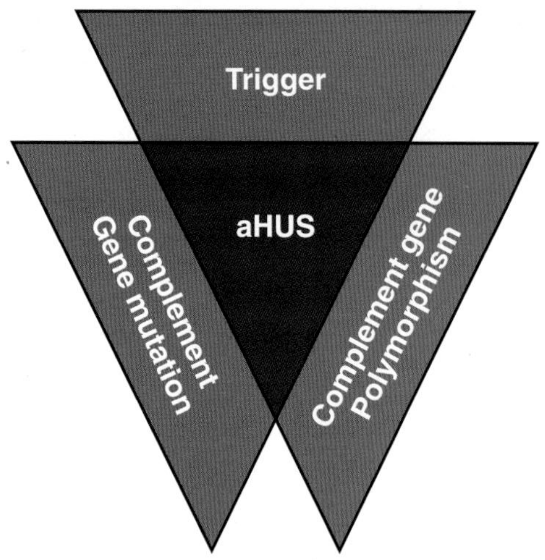


**Fig. 34.5** Multihit model of complement-mediated atypical hemolytic uremic syndrome *(aHUS)*. For complement-mediated aHUS to manifest, in addition to a rare genetic mutation in a complement gene, an individual may require common genetic variants such as an at-risk haplotype in a complement gene and the presence of a trigger (e.g., pregnancy, infection). (Modified from the National Renal Complement Therapeutics Centre 2017/2018 annual report. Available from: http://www.atypicalhus.co.uk/. Last accessed February 4, 2019.)

In addition to rare genetic variants, common genetic single-nucleotide polymorphisms (SNPs) have been associated with complement-mediated aHUS. A haplotype block in encompassing the *CFH* gene (CFH-H3; tgtgt) composed of these SNPs increases this risk of aHUS twofold to fourfold. Functional analysis has shown that the risk variant, *CFH*-Val62, has a subtle decrease in cofactor activity compared with the protective variant. Another haplotype block in the RCA cluster, $CD46_{ggaac}$, has been associated with two- to threefold increased risk of aHUS, although the functional significance has yet to be established. Even when there are multiple rare and common genetic risk factors for complement-mediated aHUS, a trigger is frequently required (e.g., pregnancy, infection) to unmask the latent complement defects and cause aHUS. These triggers usually activate complement. For instance, complement activation is the normal physiological response to infection.[3] In some cases of secondary TMA a high proportion of individuals carry a mutation (e.g., pregnancy-associated aHUS, approximately 70%, and de novo posttransplant TMA, approximately 30%) but in others the incidence of mutations is unknown or low (e.g., STEC-HUS). In other TMAs, complement activation may be seen in vivo but it is yet to be determined if in these settings complement is causative, a modifier, or simply a bystander (Fig. 34.6).

## ACQUIRED PRIMARY COMPLEMENT-MEDIATED ATYPICAL HEMOLYTIC UREMIC SYNDROME

In addition to inherited defects in the complement system, acquired defects in the form of autoantibodies to FH[13] and FI[14] have been reported in complement-mediated aHUS. FH autoantibody aHUS predominantly presents in childhood and in European cohorts accounts for 5% to 25% of cases, although in one Indian cohort this was as high as 56%.

There is a genetic predisposition to FH autoantibodies in aHUS with FHR1 deficiency either by way of whole gene deletions of *CFHR3* and *CFHR1* or *CFHR1* and *CFHR4* or by point mutations in the *CFHR1* gene strongly linked. The role of FHR1 deficiency in the generation of FH autoantibodies is obscure and several patients have been reported with factor H autoantibodies in the presence of FHR1.[15]

The FH autoantibodies predominantly bind to C-terminal epitopes on FH and perturb FH-mediated cell-surface protection. Thus these acquired defects mirror the genetic defects seen in FH-associated aHUS.

Autoantibodies against FI have also been reported but are rare and their functional relevance remains to be established.

## COMPLEMENT SCREENING IN ATYPICAL HEMOLYTIC UREMIC SYNDROME

Complement analysis in cases of aHUS should include serum levels of C3, C4, FH, FI, FB, FBb, and sC5b-9 and factor H autoantibodies prior to plasma exchange (PEX; Fig. 34.3).[2] Low C3 levels are commonly seen in patients with complement mutations and may point to a complement-mediated process; however, normal C3 levels do not exclude the presence of a mutation or autoantibodies. Flow cytometry of peripheral blood mononuclear cells to detect reduced CD46 is also advised. Mutation screening in aHUS is challenging, because most of the disease-associated mutations are individually rare. In the case of nonsense mutations, large gene rearrangements, and frame shift mutations, the functional consequences are clear. In complement-mediated aHUS, a significant proportion of variants consist of missense mutations of unknown significance which pose a challenge when reporting the genetic results. In addition to direct DNA sequencing, the high frequency of gene conversions and genomic rearrangements found in aHUS makes copy number analysis essential in aHUS screening. A polymorphism in the C5 gene (p.R885H) has been demonstrated to prevent eculizumab binding to C5 and genetic screening should be undertaken to identify those that will not respond to eculizumab therapy, allowing early reinitiation of PEX.[3]

## CLINICAL FEATURES OF COMPLEMENT-MEDIATED ATYPICAL HEMOLYTIC UREMIC SYNDROME

AKI is a predominant feature of complement-mediated aHUS.[1] Historically the prognosis for patients with aHUS was poor. Initial mortality was been reported to be higher in children (6.7% vs. 0.8% at 1 year), although adults progress to end-stage renal disease (ESRD) more frequently at initial presentation (46% vs. 16%). At 3 to 5 years after onset, 64% to 67% of adults and 36% to 48% of children had died or reached end-stage renal failure (ESRF). Prognosis varies according to genotype, with *CD46* mutations carrying the best prognosis. No patient with a *CD46* mutation from two large reported cohorts died at first episode and no children and only 25% of adults reached ESRF at first presentation. At 3

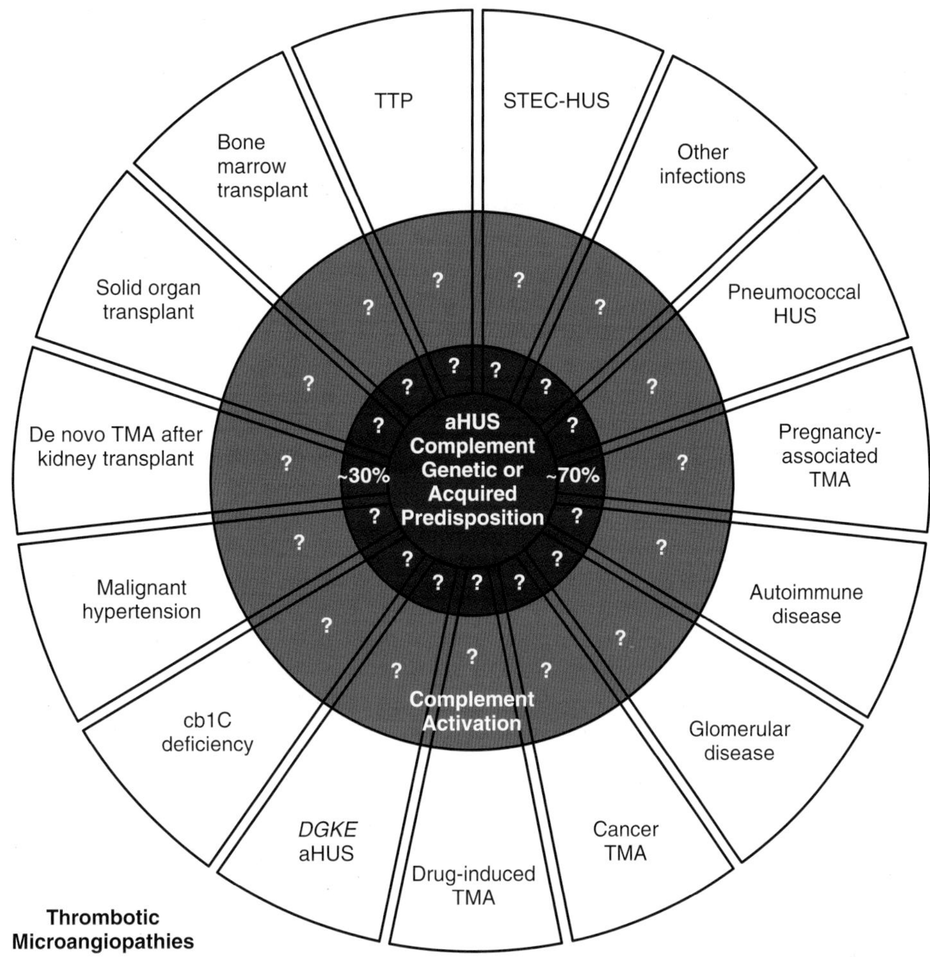


**Fig. 34.6** The role of complement in thrombotic microangiopathies *(TMAs)*. In primary inherited and acquired complement-mediated atypical hemolytic uremic syndrome *(aHUS)* a mutation or autoantibody resulting in complement dysregulation predisposes to disease. Complement-mediated aHUS frequently only manifests upon exposure to an environmental trigger, which can include other causes of TMA. In some cases of secondary TMA a high proportion of individuals carry a mutation (e.g., pregnancy-associated aHUS, about 70%, and de novo posttransplant TMA, about 30%), but in others the incidence of mutations is unknown or low (e.g., STEC-HUS). In other TMAs, complement activation may be seen in vivo but it is yet to be determined if in these settings complement is causative, a modifier, or simply a bystander. *STEC-HUS,* Shiga toxin–producing *Escherichia coli*-hemolytic uremic syndrome; *TTP,* thrombotic thrombocytopenic purpura. (Modified from the National Renal Complement Therapeutics Centre 2017/2018 annual report. Available from: http://www.atypicalhus.co.uk/. Last accessed February 4, 2019.)

years following initial presentation only 6% of both adults and children had developed ESRF. By contrast, individuals with mutations in *CFH, CFI,* or *C3* all had poor outcomes. In those with *CFH* mutations initial mortality was 30% in children and 4% in adults and evolution to ESRD at first episode in survivors was 19% to 33% in children and 48% in adults. At 5 years up to 77% of patients with *CFH* mutations had developed ESRD or had died. Only 30% to 40% of individuals with *CFI* and *C3* mutations will be alive with native kidney function at 3 to 5 years. A small proportion of patients will have multiple rare genetic variants. In those with CD46 mutations additional mutations worsened the prognosis. In those with FH autoantibody–mediated aHUS 36.5% to 63% died or reached ESRD by 5 years. Eculizumab is a recombinant humanized monoclonal antibody directed against the C5 complement protein. Eculizumab inhibits the cleavage of C5 by C5 convertase. The introduction of eculizumab has altered the natural history of disease and the outcome for those with complement abnormalities is markedly improved.

In complement-mediated aHUS extrarenal manifestations are reported in only 10% to 20% of patients with aHUS (Box 34.1). Neurological sequelae are the commonest reported symptom with symptoms ranging from irritability to coma. It is unclear whether these clinical events are a direct consequence of the TMA, a direct effect of complement activation, or complications of AKI, such as severe hypertension and uremia.[3]

## TREATMENT OF COMPLEMENT-MEDIATED ATYPICAL HEMOLYTIC UREMIC SYNDROME

### PLASMA EXCHANGE

PEX is currently recommended in TMA until an ADAMTS13 activity is available to exclude TTP. In addition to removing ADAMTS13 autoantibodies and replacing ADAMTS13, PEX will replace nonfunctioning complement proteins and remove

**Box 34.1 Extrarenal Manifestation in Complement-Mediated Atypical Hemolytic Uremic Syndrome and Shiga Toxin–Producing *Escherichia Coli*-Hemolytic Uremic Syndrome**

- Neurologic involvement, including seizures and altered consciousness
- Pancreatitis
- Diabetes mellitus
- Cardiac involvement/myocardial infarction
- Gastrointestinal involvement (including diarrhea, vomiting, abdominal pain)
- Ocular involvement
- Digital gangrene/skin
- Cerebral artery thrombosis/stenosis
- Extracerebral artery stenosis
- Pulmonary involvement
- Hepatitis
- Hemorrhagic colitis
- Bowel necrosis
- Bowel perforation
- Intussusception
- Colonic strictures

FH-autoantibodies and hyperfunctional complement components. Once TTP has been excluded eculizumab should be used, although its current high price means that PEX will remain the only option in many countries. Consensus guidelines recommend using 1–2 plasma volumes per session in adults and 50–100 mL/kg in children. PEX is initially performed daily with a reduced frequency when hemolysis is controlled. In those with complement defects plasma dependency was frequently seen and some patients required long-term plasma therapy (weekly/biweekly) to maintain remission.

## ECULIZUMAB

The discovery of the role of complement in disease provided the rationale for the use of eculizumab.[2] Eculizumab is a recombinant humanized monoclonal antibody that binds C5 and blocks its subsequent cleavage into C5a and C5b. Eculizumab appears highly effective, with approximately 85% of patients becoming disease free in both plasma-resistant and plasma-dependent aHUS.[16] No biomarker currently exists that will diagnose a primary complement-mediated aHUS in the acute setting, and the diagnosis is one of exclusion. As early initiation of eculizumab has been shown to lead to better outcomes, treatment is often commenced in patients with suspected primary complement-mediated aHUS, and discontinued if an alternative etiology is subsequently identified (Fig. 34.3).[1]

The optimal treatment duration in complement-mediated aHUS is uncertain, although currently the license is for long-term treatment. Eculizumab has been withdrawn in a large series of patients with complement-mediated aHUS with relapse reported in about 33% of patients. All individuals who relapsed had rare genetic variants in the complement system but importantly, rapid reintroduction of complement inhibition normalized the renal function. Prospective trials of disease-driven intermittent eculizumab regime are underway to define the optimal treatment duration.

## ECULIZUMAB NONRESPONSIVE ATYPICAL HEMOLYTIC UREMIC SYNDROME

With increasing use in clinical practice it has become apparent that subgroups of patients with aHUS do not respond to eculizumab.[17] In an industry study, all pediatric patients with a rare complement genetic variant or an autoantibody to FH had an improvement in estimated glomerular filtration rate, whereas 27% of individuals without an identified complement abnormality failed to show an improvement. It is not clear whether this represents late presentation of disease or true nonresponse. In addition, individuals with methylmalonic aciduria and homocystinuria type C protein (MMACHC)–,[18] diacylglycerol kinase ε (DGKE)–,[19] and inverted formin 2 (INF2)–mediated[20] aHUS have been shown to fail to respond to treatment. Individuals with the C5 polymorphism (p.R885H) will also fail to respond to treatment.[21]

## ECULIZUMAB SIDE EFFECTS

Susceptibility to infection with encapsulated gram-negative organisms, particularly *Neisseria* infections, is the most serious side effect of eculizumab treatment. Because of this, meningococcal vaccination is mandatory although its effectiveness in the context of complement blockade is uncertain. Long-term antibiotic prophylaxis is thus recommended, although meningococcal infection can occur despite these precautions and patient awareness is crucial.[2] Hepatotoxicity and deposition of eculizumab in the glomerulus have been reported.

## RENAL TRANSPLANTATION IN COMPLEMENT-MEDIATED ATYPICAL HEMOLYTIC UREMIC SYNDROME

Historically the outcome of renal transplantation in complement-mediated aHUS was poor with a 5-year death-censored graft survival of only approximately 50% with a 7% mortality.[22] Graft failure was predominantly due to aHUS recurrence, which occurred in up to 70% of patients usually early in the course of the transplant (about 70% in the first year). The outcome of renal transplantation was largely predicted by the underlying genetic abnormality.[22] In individuals with mutations in *CFH* the recurrence rate was >80%. Likewise activating mutations in *C3* and *CFB* had a high risk of renal recurrence. Unlike these fluid-phase complement proteins, *CD46* is membrane tethered and as such, a renal allograft will correct the complement defect and protect against aHUS. In keeping with this, the outcome following transplantation in those with mutations in *CD46* is much better with a very low recurrence rate. The posttransplant milieu [e.g., viral diseases, ischemia reperfusion injury, uncontrolled blood pressure, donor-specific antibodies, immunosuppressive calcineurin inhibitors (CNIs)] provides the necessary triggers to unmask the latent genetic complement defects by causing endothelial cell damage and activation of the complement cascade. The CNIs (tacrolimus and cyclosporin), although consistently linked as a trigger for aHUS, have not been demonstrated to be significantly associated in two recent studies of aHUS recurrence posttransplant. Mammalian target of rapamycin inhibitors (e.g., sirolimus), however, have been reported to increase the risk of recurrence. Plasma therapy had a low success rate in rescuing recurrent aHUS following renal transplantation, although preemptive PEX has been associated with a trend of decreased recurrence. Such regimes have now been largely replaced by preemptive eculizumab at the time of transplantation.

Living-related kidney transplantation is not recommended in aHUS given that de novo aHUS has been recorded in four donors within a year of donation with complement mutations reported subsequently. Genotyping may reveal a known mutation in a family member; however, the presence of risk haplotypes and the fact that further genetic risk factors remain to be discovered make it impossible to rule out subsequent aHUS for a donor. If live related transplantation is to be considered, the donor should be counseled about the risk of de novo TMA.

## DGKE THROMBOTIC MICROANGIOPATHY

DGKE-mediated aHUS is caused by homozygous or compound heterozygous mutations in this gene.[19] Genetic pleiotropism, where a single gene affects a number of phenotypic traits in the same organism, is also seen in DGKE-mediated renal disease with a membranoproliferative glomerulonephritis (MPGN) phenotype also reported.[23]

### PATHOGENESIS

DGKE is an intracellular lipid kinase that converts diacylglycerol (DAG) to phosphatidic acid. DAG activates protein kinase C which leads to a number of downstream effects including the release of antithrombotic factors and prothrombotic factors as well as platelet activation, changes in vascular tone, and changes in the actin cytoskeleton. The ultimate mechanisms by which DGKE abnormalities result in TMA are yet to be elucidated. The disease appears to be independent of complement activation; however, rarely concomitant mutations in complement genes have been reported.

### CLINICAL FEATURES

DGKE-mediated aHUS presents in infancy and early childhood. Heavy proteinuria is a predominant feature. The natural history of disease follows a relapsing/remitting course commonly progressing to chronic kidney disease (CKD) and ESRD.

### TREATMENT

Treatment outcome data are limited with most cases progressing regardless of treatment. The disease appears to be complement-independent with reports of poor responses to eculizumab. Relapse of DGKE-mediated aHUS posttransplantation has not been reported.

## METHYLMALONIC ACIDURIA AND HOMOCYSTINURIA, COBALAMIN C (CBLC)-TYPE HEMOLYTIC UREMIC SYNDROME

Methylmalonic aciduria and homocystinuria is a disorder of cobalamin (cbl; vitamin $B_{12}$) metabolism, which is associated with aHUS.[24] Homozygous or compound heterozygous mutations in the gene for the methylmalonic aciduria and homocystinuria type C protein, *MMACHC,* cause this disease. Cobalamin is a cofactor for both methionine synthase and methylmalonyl-coenzyme A mutase and its deficiency leads to methylmalonic acidemia with homocystinuria.

### CLINICAL FEATURES

MMACHC-mediated aHUS predominantly presents in infancy or childhood, although rare cases in early adulthood have been reported. Plasma homocysteine levels are elevated and methionine levels are low. Methylmalonic acid is elevated in the urine. This metabolic disease has many extrarenal manifestations of variable severity (comprised development, ophthalmic, neurologic, and cardiac defects). Mortality is high if untreated or if there is cardiopulmonary involvement.[24]

### TREATMENT

Metabolic therapy with hydroxocobalamin and betaine is very effective. The role of complement is not clear; there are isolated reports of concomitant complement gene mutations and polymorphisms that may modify the disease, but the small number of published reports of eculizumab use describe nonresponse.

## THROMBOTIC THROMBOCYTOPENIC PURPURA

### INCIDENCE

The incidence of acquired TTP is 0.37 per 100,000 per year. The median age for diagnosis of the acquired form is 41 with 75% of cases occurring in female patients. Acquired TTP is very rare in children.[25]

### PATHOGENESIS

TTP is mediated by ADAMTS13 (A Disintegrin And Metalloprotease with a ThromboSpondin type 1 motif, member 13) deficiency, usually acquired with anti-ADAMTS13 autoantibodies (95%) and occasionally inherited with recessive mutations in the *ADAMTS13* gene. Ultra-large von Willebrand factor (ULvWF) multimers, which are synthesized and secreted by endothelial cells, are cleaved by ADAMTS13. In areas of very high shear stress (e.g., arterioles with high flow rates) these ULvWF multimers undergo a conformational change. In the absence of functional ADAMTS13, the ULvWF multimers accumulate on the endothelium to which platelets adhere. This results in the platelet-rich thrombi in the microvasculature which mediates end organ damage.[25] There is a genetic predisposition to the development of ADAMTS13

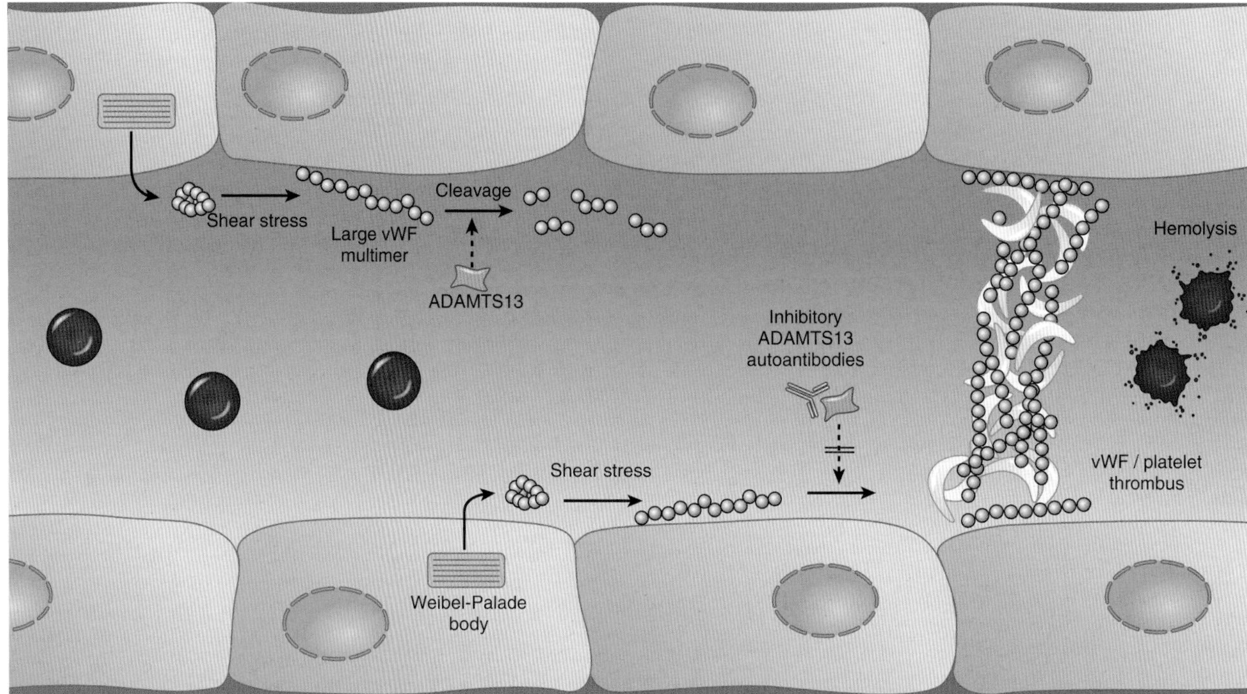


**Fig. 34.7** Thrombotic thrombocytopenic purpura. Under normal circumstances ultra-large von Willebrand factor (vWF) multimers released from Weibel–Palade bodies in endothelial cells are cleaved by ADAMTS13 to prevent and regulate platelet adherence. In thrombotic thrombocytopenic purpura (TTP), ADAMTS13 deficiency, either acquired (ADAMTS13 autoantibodies) or inherited (recessive mutations in ADAMTS13), results in reduced cleavage of secreted or anchored ultra-large vWF strings. These form vWF–platelet thrombi, which result in tissue ischemia, platelet consumption, and microangiopathic hemolytic anemia. *ADAMTS13,* A disintegrin and metalloproteinase with a thrombospondin type 1 motif, member 13. (Modified from the National Renal Complement Therapeutics Centre 2017/2018 annual report. Available from: http://www.atypicalhus.co.uk/. Last accessed February 4, 2019.)

autoantibodies with HLA-DQ7, DRB1*11, and HLA-DRB3 linked in Caucasians. ADAMTS13 deficiency by itself may be insufficient to cause TTP in isolation, often requiring a secondary inflammatory or prothrombotic trigger (Fig. 34.7).

## CLINICAL FEATURES

In comparison with complement-mediated aHUS, TTP is described to have less severe renal impairment (serum creatinine, 1.7–2.3 mg/dL) and more severe thrombocytopenia (<30 × $10^9$/L). Although a general guide to the likely cause of a TMA, these cut-offs are not absolute and cannot be relied upon in clinical practice where an ADAMTS13 activity is urgently required.[26]

Although a potentially life-threatening disease the initial presenting clinical features may be mild and not of a critically ill patient. These symptoms may include nausea, vomiting, fatigue, dyspnea, bruising, and petechiae. Neurologic involvement is very common ranging from minor (e.g., headache, confusion, weakness) to major (seizure, stroke, coma) features. Gastrointestinal features are present in around 50%. Cardiac involvement can be seen with myocardial infarction. Arrhythmias are a frequent cause of death.[25]

## TREATMENT

TTP was historically almost universally fatal, but mortality decreased to approximately 10% following the introduction of PEX. Patients with TTP should be managed in a high dependency area with monitoring. PEX should be initiated urgently.[27] Plasma infusion should only be used to temporize until the patient can be transferred to a facility able to undertake PEX. PEX is undertaken daily until recovery is seen. In refractory patients PEX may be increased to twice daily.

Immunosuppressive therapies (e.g., glucocorticoids and rituximab[28]) are now standardly used to reduce the relapse rate in acquired TTP.

Relapse of acquired TTP was seen in around 33% of cases; however, with increasing use of rituximab this rate is falling. Around 50% of relapses will occur in the first year after presentation and routine clinical monitoring is required.

# INFECTION-ASSOCIATED THROMBOTIC MICROANGIOPATHIES

## SHIGA TOXIN HEMOLYTIC UREMIC SYNDROME

Shiga toxin–induced HUS is one of the main causes of AKI in young children and occurs following infection with Shiga toxin–producing enterohemorrhagic *Escherichia coli* (STEC) or *Shigella.*[29]

## MICROBIOLOGY

Shiga toxin–producing *E. coli* is the most common cause of HUS in the developed world. *E. coli* serotypes are classified by their O and H antigens. The O antigen is a polymer of repeating oligosaccharides which forms the outermost domain of the lipopolysaccharide (LPS) in the outer membrane. The H antigen is a major component of bacterial flagella. In Europe and North America *E. coli* O157:H7 is the commonest serotype associated with STEC-HUS, although other non-O157 strains can cause disease (including O26, O80, O91, O103, O104, O111, O121, O145). In some regions non-O157:H7 strains predominate (e.g., Australia) and in May 2011 the largest recorded outbreak centered in Germany was with an *E. coli* O104:H4 strain. In Asia and Africa, *Shigella dysenteriae* serotype 1 is a major cause of HUS, again by the production of Shiga toxin.

## SOURCE OF INFECTION

Shiga toxin–producing *E. coli* colonize healthy cattle intestine and also have been isolated from deer, sheep, goats, horses, dogs, birds, and flies. Meat, contaminated at slaughter, is the most common method of human infection although other vehicles for transmission have been described (Box 34.2), including unpasteurized dairy products, contaminated water sources, and infected vegetables.[29]

*S. dysenteriae* 1 infection in the developed world is rare with contamination of food and water the usual sources. The infectious dose of *Shigella* is low and direct person-to-person spread is reported.

## INCIDENCE

STEC-HUS accounts for over 90% of cases of HUS in children and occurs more commonly in summer months. In keeping with the mode of transmission, agricultural areas have a higher incidence. The incidence of STEC-HUS is 0.7 cases per 100,000/year predominantly in children under 5 years of age. HUS arises from around 5% to 10% of STEC infections, although this figure was much higher in the German O104:H4 outbreak (about 20%).[30] Less than 10% of children infected with *S. dysenteriae* 1 will develop a TMA.

## CLINICAL FEATURES OF SHIGA TOXIN–PRODUCING ENTEROHEMORRHAGIC ESCHERICHIA COLI–HEMOLYTIC UREMIC SYNDROME

Bloody diarrhea is the classical prodromal feature of a STEC-HUS. Three days postexposure to STEC, diarrhea will develop in association with vomiting and abdominal pain. In the 5% to 10% of patients who develop HUS, this will occur around 7 days later. Although conventionally reported as bloody, this is only reported in approximately 60% of cases (Fig. 34.8). It is not clear why some patients progress and others do not.

In around 5% of cases of STEC-HUS, no diarrhea is reported and thus investigations for STEC should be carried out in all cases of TMA regardless of the absence of diarrhea.[31] Urinary tract infections with STEC have been documented to cause HUS. A high white cell count is common in STEC-HUS and correlated with a poorer outcome. Over 50% of STEC-HUS cases will require dialysis, frequently in those with concurrent decreased effective arterial volume at admission. Despite this, renal recovery is the rule in STEC-HUS with dialysis dependency for more than 2 weeks being unusual. Hypertension is also frequently observed. Mortality in STEC-HUS is low at approximately 2% and occurs predominantly in the very old and very young.[29]

**Box 34.2 Vehicles for Transmission of *Escherichia coli* O157:H7**

Meat
- Undercooked ground meat
- Undercooked steak
- Undercooked roast beef
- Salami
- Deer jerky
- Venison

Contaminated Fruit/Vegetables
- Lettuce
- Bean sprouts
- Radish sprouts
- Salad
- Melons
- Coleslaw
- Grapes
- Unpasteurized apple juice/cider

Dairy Products
- Unpasteurized milk
- Cheese curd from unpasteurized milk
- Butter from unpasteurized milk
- Ice cream bars

Water
- Lakes/ponds
- Swimming pools
- Municipal drinking water
- Other

Fecal–Oral
- Daycare centers

Airborne

## EXTRARENAL MANIFESTATIONS

Extrarenal manifestations in STEC-HUS are common. Neurological symptoms are commonly reported and these may range from headaches to coma and cortical blindness. Gut effects such as hemorrhagic colitis, bowel necrosis, perforation, and intussusception are seen with longer-term colonic strictures reported. Pancreatitis is seen in STEC-HUS and impaired glucose tolerance and diabetes mellitus may be develop (Box 34.1).

## LONG-TERM SEQUELAE

Although ESRF is unusual, impaired renal function, proteinuria, and hypertension have been reported in up to 40%. Less commonly ongoing diabetes mellitus and neurological defects and seizures may be seen.[32]

## CLINICAL FEATURES OF *SHIGELLA DYSENTERIAE* TYPE 1

*Shigella* typically presents with a similar prodrome to STEC: diarrhea (initially watery, subsequently mucoid, or bloody), abdominal pain, and vomiting. Fever is common and an

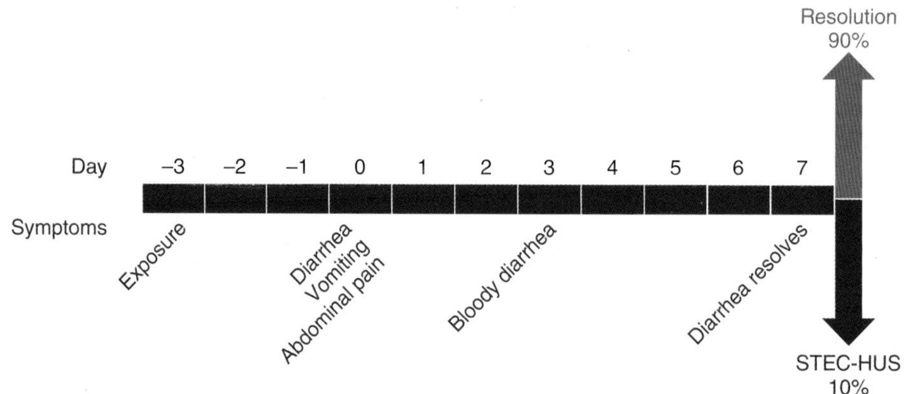


**Fig. 34.8** Clinical time line of *Escherichia coli* O157 infection. Three days postexposure to Shiga toxin–producing *Escherichia coli* (STEC), diarrhea will develop in association with vomiting and abdominal pain. Thus around day 3 bloody diarrhea may be seen. In about 10% that develop hemolytic uremic syndrome *(HUS)*, this will occur around 7 days later.

elevated white cell count may be seen. On average, symptoms develop 3 days after infection. In comparison with STEC-HUS the disease has a poorer outlook with 15% mortality and 40% of patients developing CKD. The presentation with HUS is at about day 7 when the diarrheal illness has resolved. As with STEC-HUS, gastrointestinal and neurological manifestations can arise.

## MICROBIOLOGY TESTING

Stool samples should be sent in all cases of TMA because approximately 5% of patients lack a diarrheal prodrome. Diarrhea may have stopped by the time of presentation, but STEC can still be cultured from feces or rectal swab. Culture is not a sensitive test, especially if sample collection is delayed as bacteria are usually only present for a few days and stool samples are not routinely processed after many days in hospital, especially when diarrhea has stopped. In addition, polymerase chain reaction testing for Shiga toxin 1/2 genes or enzyme-linked immunosorbent assay (ELISA) measurement to detect Shiga toxin 1/2 in the stools is now recommended. Serological detection of anti-LPS antibodies against *E. coli* (immunoglobulin M [IgM] positive/rising IgG titer) may also suggest infection.

## PATHOGENESIS

STEC reaches the gut and closely adheres to the epithelial cells of the gastrointestinal mucosa through a 97-kD outer membrane protein, intimin, resulting in the formation of effacement lesions. The intimin protein is encoded by the *eaeA* gene in the locus of enterocyte effacement. Following this attachment there is translocation of toxin (usually Shiga toxin type 2) through the epithelium into the circulation. The toxin is thought to circulate attached to leucocytes, erythrocytes, and platelets. Shiga toxins consist of an A unit and five B units. The pentameric B unit binds to globotriaosyl ceramide (Gb3) on expressing organs mediating internalization in clathrin-coated pits and retrograde transport of the toxin via the Golgi complex to the endoplasmic reticulum. The A unit inhibits ribosomal function and protein synthesis, leading to endothelial cell death and exposure of the underlying basement membrane.[29] In addition, Shiga toxin is able to enhance the release of proinflammatory cytokines (interleukin-1 [IL-1], tumor necrosis factor-α, and IL-6), amplifying the inflammatory events and contributing to the procoagulant milieu and ultimately a TMA.[33] Although Gb3 is found in other organs, the kidney is most susceptible to injury. This may be due to higher levels of Gb3 on renal cells, particularly the glomerular endothelium (but also podocytes, mesangial, and tubular epithelial cells), the high blood flow to the kidney, or a greater susceptibility of renal cells to the effects of the toxin. The expression of Gb3 at other sites (e.g., brain) may explain extrarenal manifestations of STEC-HUS. Increased expression of the Gb3 receptor in children has also been proposed as a cause for the predominant pediatric presentation, although other explanations have also been proposed (e.g., increased prevalence of anti-Shiga antibodies in adults; Fig. 34.9).

## ROLE OF COMPLEMENT IN THE PATHOGENESIS OF STEC-HUS

Complement activation, particularly the alternative complement pathway, has long been implicated in the pathogenesis of STEC-HUS with the frequent finding of low C3 levels and increased breakdown products of C3 and FB suggesting activation of the AP of complement.[34] The presence of low C3 is associated with up to 50% of cases of STEC-HUS and it has been reported that persistently low levels are associated with a poorer prognosis. In vitro studies have demonstrated that STEC induces P-selectin expression at the membrane surface, increasing complement AP activation. There is evidence from a preclinical rodent model of Shiga toxin–mediated injury that complement activation may augment the effects of the toxin on cells, although no evidence of complement activation was seen in a primate model. It remains uncertain whether this complement activation plays a role in the development of STEC-HUS and whether complement blockade may improve outcome. In rare cases functionally significant complement mutations are also present and often result in a poorer prognosis.[35]

## TREATMENT

As a self-limiting condition, supportive management with fluid resuscitation, blood pressure control, and dialysis remain

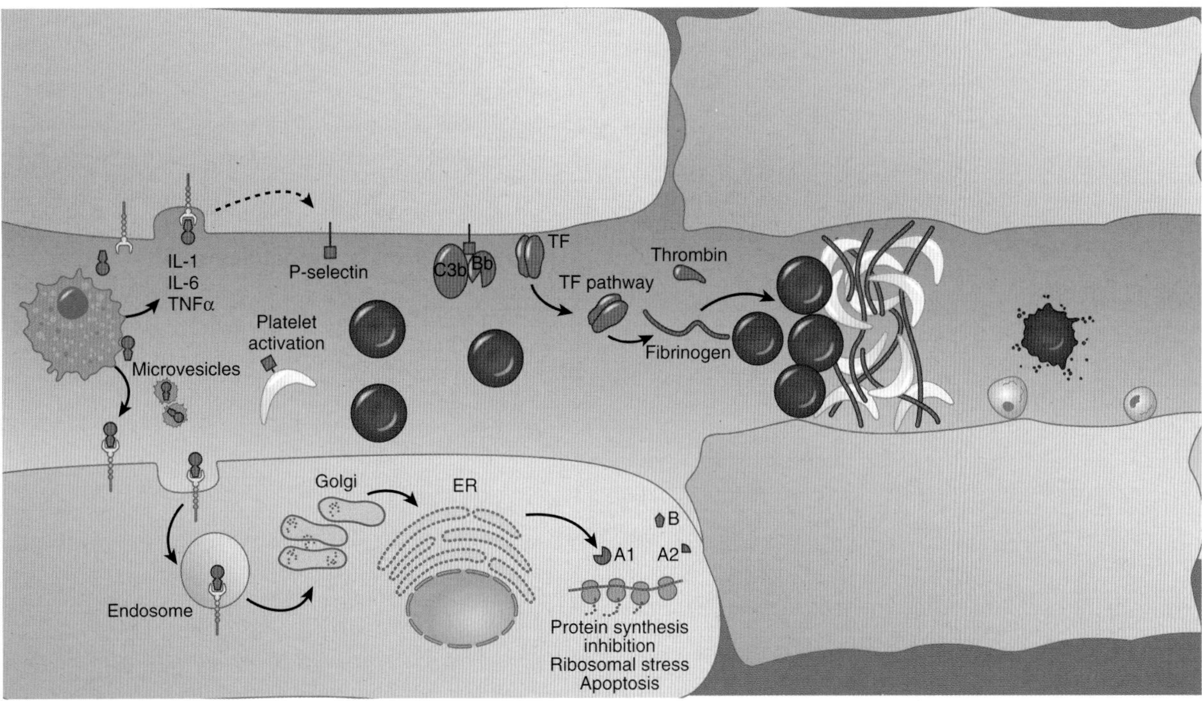


**Fig. 34.9** Shiga toxin hemolytic uremic syndrome. Shiga toxin is transported from the gut to the kidney via leucocytes, erythrocytes, and platelets. Toxin released in the circulation or within microvesicles is internalized in clathrin-coated pits and thereafter undergoes retrograde transport via the Golgi complex to the endoplasmic reticulum. The A unit of Shiga toxin inhibits ribosomal function and protein synthesis, leading to endothelial cell death and exposure of the underlying basement membrane. Shiga toxin is also able to enhance the release of proinflammatory cytokines [interleukin-1 (IL-1), tumor necrosis factor-α (TNFα), and IL-6], thus amplifying the inflammatory events. Shiga toxin can also upregulate P-selectin and cause complement activation. The consequent thrombosis results in microangiopathic hemolytic anemia and end organ damage. (Modified from the National Renal Complement Therapeutics Centre 2017/2018 annual report. Available from: http://www.atypicalhus.co.uk/. Last accessed February 4, 2019.)

the mainstay of treatment for STEC-HUS. Antimotility agents should be avoided because they increase the risk of HUS. The use of antibiotics is controversial with most centers avoiding their use in the treatment of *E. coli* O157 infection because of either no benefit or potential increase in the risk of developing HUS, although this may be dependent on the antibiotic used. Some classes of antibiotics (e.g., fluoroquinolones) dramatically increase the production and the release of Shiga toxin before bacterial lysis and worsen the outcome of STEC-HUS in animal models. Bacteriostatic agents (e.g., azithromycin) block protein synthesis and have a strong inhibitory effect on Shiga toxin production and release by STEC. A randomized controlled trial of azithromycin in STEC-HUS (NCT02336516) is underway.

By contrast, antibiotic treatment in *S. dysenteriae* type 1 has not been associated with increased HUS risk, possibly due to the differences in control of Shiga toxin production.

Although there is evidence of complement activation in STEC-HUS, the role of the complement inhibitor eculizumab remains unproven. Several case reports in 2011 described renal and neurological recovery in children treated with eculizumab for STEC-HUS.[36] Subsequently, in the 2011 O104:H4 HUS outbreak in Europe, retrospective analyses did not demonstrate a beneficial role of eculizumab or PEX over supportive care, although the patients who were treated with eculizumab had more severe disease.[30] Ultimately in a self-limiting disease a randomized clinical trial of eculizumab for STEC-HUS will be required to define the role of complement inhibition and these are underway (ECUSTEC).

Because patients usually shed STEC for a week, standard precautions to prevent person-to-person transmission and source isolation should be implemented. In children it is usual to have at least two negative stool cultures prior to returning to school.

## PNEUMOCOCCAL HEMOLYTIC UREMIC SYNDROME

TMA may occur in adults and children in the context of invasive *Streptococcus pneumoniae* infection.[37]

### INCIDENCE

Pneumococcal HUS has been reported to have a 10-year cumulative incidence rate of 1.2 per 100,000 children. It complicates 0.5% of pneumococcal disease, usually in those with pneumonia and empyema.[37]

### PATHOGENESIS

Several mechanisms have been suggested to explain the pathogenesis of pneumococcal HUS. Pneumococci produce neuraminidase, which cleaves sialic residues from glycoproteins on erythrocyte, platelet, and endothelial cell membranes, exposing the cryptic Thomsen–Friedenreich antigen (T antigen). Natural IgM antibodies can then bind and result in cell damage and a TMA.[38] The DAT (Coombs) test is thus positive. The cleavage of sialic acid has also been hypothesized to reduce FH binding, resulting in impaired endothelial complement regulation, thus contributing to disease pathogenesis.[39] The pneumococcal protein PspC has also been demonstrated to bind plasminogen and, when converted to plasmin, damage the endothelium, again contributing to the disease mechanism. Again, as with STEC-HUS, rare genetic variants in the complement system are only rarely found.

### CLINICAL FEATURES

Most pneumococcal HUS is associated with pneumonia (approximately 70%), frequently with empyema. Meningitis (around 20%), sinusitis, and otitis media have also been associated with HUS. Infected children are usually extremely unwell and frequently require prolonged hospitalization and intensive care unit admission. The majority (approximately 75%) require dialysis. The mortality is much higher than seen in STEC-HUS (around 10%) usually due to the underlying infection. Up to around 33% develop ESRD. As with all other TMAs extrarenal manifestations have been reported.[40]

### TREATMENT

Supportive management and treatment of the infection should be the focus. The role of PEX is controversial with a theoretical risk of worsening the TMA with donor plasma because it may contain anti-T IgM. The role of eculizumab in the treatment of pneumococcal HUS is unclear with only sporadic case reports documenting response.[17]

## HUMAN IMMUNODEFICIENCY VIRUS–ASSOCIATED THROMBOTIC MICROANGIOPATHIES

Human immunodeficiency virus (HIV)–associated TMA was common in the pre–highly active antiretroviral therapy era with reported incidences from 1.5% to 7%. With the currently available treatments for HIV this has fallen to approximately 0.3%. The pathogenic mechanisms are unclear but are thought to reflect glomerular endothelial damage. HIV TMAs are associated with lower $CD4^+$ cell counts, higher viral RNA levels, and opportunistic infections. Treatment consists of supportive care and antiretroviral treatment.[41]

## OTHER INFECTIONS

In addition to *E. coli*, HIV, and *S. pneumoniae*, a large number of other bacterial, viral, fungal, and parasitic infections have been described in association with TMA (Box 34.3). Unlike *E. coli* and *S. pneumoniae* it is unclear if this is a direct effect of the pathogen, a side effect of treatment, or a trigger that unmasks a latent complement defect (Fig. 34.6). In studies of complement-mediated aHUS in those with *CFH*, *CFI*, or *CD46* mutations 70% were reported to have an infectious trigger. Supportive care and treatment of the infection are recommended and complement evaluation should be undertaken. Eculizumab can be considered when the infectious agent is considered a trigger of complement-mediated aHUS.[1]

**Box 34.3 Infections Linked to Hemolytic Uremic Syndrome**

**Shiga Toxin Diarrheal Illnesses**

*Escherichia coli* O157:H7 O26, O80, O91, O103, O104, O111, O121, O145
*Shigella dysenteriae* type 1

**Non-Shiga Toxin Diarrheal Illnesses**

Norovirus
*Campylobacter upsaliensis*
*Clostridium difficile*
Respiratory infections
*Bordetella pertussis* infection
*Streptococcus pneumoniae*
*Haemophilus influenzae*

**Other Bacterial**

*Fusobacterium necrophorum*

**Viral Illnesses**

Varicella
Cytomegalovirus
Influenza H1N1
Hepatitis A
Hepatitis C
Human immunodeficiency virus
Coxsackie B virus
Epstein-Barr virus
Dengue
Human herpesvirus 6
Parvovirus B19

**Parasites**

*Plasmodium falciparum*

## SECONDARY THROMBOTIC MICROANGIOPATHIES

### PREGNANCY-ASSOCIATED THROMBOTIC MICROANGIOPATHIES

Pregnancy-associated TMAs include primary complement-mediated aHUS and TTP. Additionally, there is a broader differential diagnosis which includes preeclampsia, HELLP (*h*emolysis, *e*levated *l*iver enzymes, and *l*ow *p*latelets), fatty liver, placental abruption, and postpartum hemorrhage (Fig. 34.10). See Chapter 48 for a more detailed discussion of pregnancy-related renal disorders.

Pregnancy is a common trigger of aHUS in women, accounting for 20% of cases, usually in the postpartum.[42] It has become clear that a high proportion will have identifiable complement mutations and that pregnancy acts as a trigger in those with an underlying genetic predisposition. Historically outcomes were poor with approximately 75% developing ESRD despite PEX. The high frequency of complement mutations in pregnancy-associated aHUS provides the rationale for complement inhibition with eculizumab, although no clinical trials have been performed in this setting.[42] Many reports about the safe use of eculizumab in

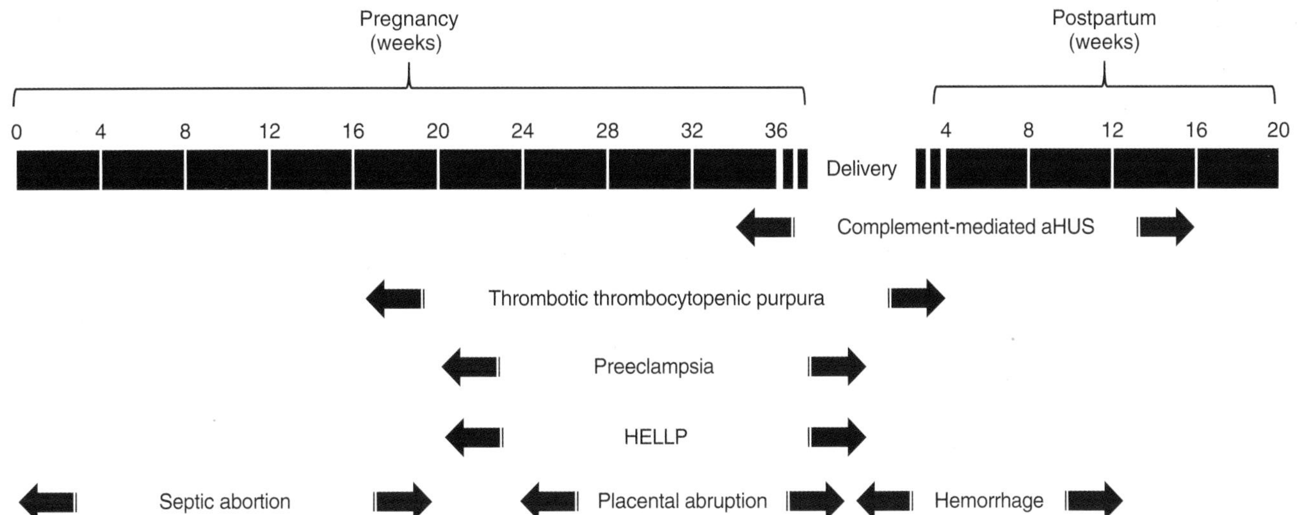


**Fig. 34.10** Presentation and differential diagnosis of thrombotic microangiopathies (TMAs) during pregnancy and postpartum. Timing of presentation can help with the differential diagnosis of TMA, with complement-mediated atypical hemolytic uremic syndrome typically presenting in the postpartum. *aHUS,* Atypical hemolytic uremic syndrome; *HELLP, h*emolysis, *e*levated *l*iver enzymes, and *l*ow *p*latelets.

pregnancy for paroxysmal nocturnal hemoglobinuria and aHUS have now been published.

A significant proportion of women present with TTP during the second and third trimesters of pregnancy.[43] The physiological increase in vWF during pregnancy, which consumes ADAMTS13, has been proposed as a predisposition and in women with a genetic predisposition its activity can fall low enough for TMA to manifest. PEX is recommended.

Preeclampsia is characterized by new-onset hypertension and proteinuria or other systemic signs (e.g., thrombocytopenia and AKI). Preeclampsia is the most common cause of AKI in pregnancy, although dialysis requirement is rarely required. Preeclampsia complicates up to 5% of all pregnancies and hypertension, diabetes mellitus, and CKD increase the risk.[43] HELLP is thought to be a severe atypical form of preeclampsia. It complicates 10% to 20% of preeclampsia cases and about 0.1% of all pregnancies. The pathogenesis of preeclampsia and HELLP is not well defined. Increased circulating levels of the syncytiotrophoblast-derived antiangiogenic factors, soluble endoglin and the soluble form of the vascular endothelial growth factor receptor (sFlt1/soluble VEGFR1), may contribute to the observed endothelial dysfunction. Although it is often difficult to differentiate clinically between HELLP and TMA, in HELLP, the predominant glomerular pathology is endotheliosis. In contrast to pregnancy-associated aHUS, only a minority (8%–10%) of patients with preeclampsia and HELLP syndrome harbor complement gene variants, mostly of unknown or nonpathogenic significance.[44] Management is supportive, with expedited delivery being the definitive treatment for HELLP. Expectant management may be considered if the woman is not at or near term. While there is some evidence of complement activation in HELLP and preeclampsia, its role in the pathogenesis of disease is uncertain. It should be noted that in women receiving eculizumab for paroxysmal nocturnal hemoglobinuria[45] or complement-mediated aHUS, preeclampsia has occurred, arguing against a role for C5 inhibition in the management of preeclampsia.

## DRUG-MEDIATED THROMBOTIC MICROANGIOPATHY

Although TMA has been linked to a large number of drugs, causality has only been established in relatively few (Box 34.4). Drug-mediated TMA occurs by two main mechanisms: direct toxicity and immune-mediated damage. For example, interferon-β[46] and bevacizumab[47] cause TMAs by a dose-dependent toxicity, whereas quinine induces the development of autoantibodies reactive with either platelet glycoprotein Ib/IX or IIb/IIIa complexes, or both.[48] Supportive care and discontinuation of the causative drug are the standard treatment options with the exception of ticlopidine which has been associated with anti-ADAMTS13 antibodies and TTP, and therefore PEX is recommended.

## MALIGNANCY-ASSOCIATED THROMBOTIC MICROANGIOPATHY

There are many reports of malignancy-associated TMAs in the literature.[3] The pathogenesis remains obscure. However, erythrocyte shearing after direct contact with microvascular embolic tumor cells has been suggested as a possible mechanism. It is frequently difficult to discriminate between a direct effect of the malignancy and chemotherapy-mediated effect in the cause of the TMA. Prognosis is poor because of malignancy-related mortality. Withdrawal of chemotherapy and supportive management are usually initiated.

## DE NOVO THROMBOTIC MICROANGIOPATHY AFTER SOLID ORGAN TRANSPLANT

De novo TMAs following solid organ transplants (liver, pancreas, lung, and heart) are reported. The pathogenesis

**Box 34.4 Drugs Associated With Thrombotic Microangiopathies**

Cisplatin
Gemcitabine
Vincristine
Mitomycin
Clopidogrel
Quinine[a]
Interferon α
Interferon β[a]
Oxaliplatin
Penicillin
Pentostatin
Quetiapine
Sulfisoxazole
Sunitinib
Ticlopidine
Muromonab-CD3
Antivascular endothelial growth factor bevacizumab[a]
Campath
Cyclosporin
Tacrolimus
Everolimus
Sirolimus
Ciprofloxacin
Oral contraceptives
Illicit drugs (e.g., cocaine, heroin, ecstasy)

[a]Although many drugs have been reported in association with thrombotic microangiopathy, compelling evidence for causality has been demonstrated in very few, including antivascular endothelial growth factors, interferon B, and quinine. (Modified from George JN. Interferon-induced thrombotic microangiopathy. *Blood.* 2016;128:2753–2754.)

is multifactorial and is likely to reflect the endothelium-damaging milieu seen posttransplant, including immunosuppressant drugs such as CNIs, ischemia reperfusion injury, antibody-mediated rejection, viral infections (e.g., cytomegalovirus), etc. In one series of de novo TMA after kidney transplantation, complement mutations were identified in about 30%.[49] Thus eculizumab therapy should be considered if the primary diagnosis is not incompatible with complement-mediated aHUS. Supportive treatment and removal of the precipitating factors (CNI discontinuation or dose reduction, treatment of antibody-mediated rejection, and viral infections) may be sufficient to stop the TMA.

## THROMBOTIC MICROANGIOPATHY AFTER BONE MARROW TRANSPLANT

TMAs are reported to complicate 10% to 40% of allogenic bone marrow transplants with mortality rates reported up to 75%. As with TMAs, following solid organ transplantation there is a multifactorial pathogenesis including CNIs, graft versus host disease, HLA mismatch, chemotherapy, radiation therapy, and infections. FH autoantibodies and rare genetic variants in aHUS-associated genes have rarely been reported in postbone marrow transplant TMA.[50]

The optimal therapeutic strategy has yet to be defined for this treatment group. The occasional reports of complement mutations and evidence of complement activation have provoked the use of eculizumab with uncontrolled retrospective analyses describing response. Prospective trials are likely needed in order to establish the optimal strategy.

## AUTOIMMUNE AND GLOMERULAR DISEASE–ASSOCIATED THROMBOTIC MICROANGIOPATHIES

TMAs have been reported in association with many glomerular diseases: MPGN/C3 glomerulopathy (C3G), focal segmental glomerulosclerosis (FSGS), IgA nephropathy, antineutrophil cytoplasmic antibody–associated vasculitis, membranous nephropathy. Frequently this is a histopathological description without hematological or biochemical features.

In MPGN/C3G, acquired and hereditary complement abnormalities are seen (Chapter 31). These are similar (mutations in *CFH* and *C3*) although subtly different to those seen in complement-mediated aHUS, and concurrent and sequential manifestation of C3G and TMA has been reported. This genetic pleiotropy is poorly understood, and may reflect the location of mutations within these genes and also genetic modifiers of disease. Genetic pleiotropy has also been reported in *DGKE*- and *INF2*-mediated disease with TMAs reported in addition to the MPGN or FSGS, respectively.

Autoimmune diseases such as systemic lupus erythematosus (SLE), catastrophic antiphospholipid syndrome (CAPS), and scleroderma renal crisis (SRC) can also present with a TMA. The exact pathogenesis has yet to be defined; however, in CAPS and SLE there is evidence of complement activation. For SLE, CAPS, and SRC with TMA, treatment should be of the underlying condition.

For SRC the use of angiotensin-converting enzyme inhibitors has been demonstrated to significantly reduce mortality.

In SLE associated with a TMA there is no evidence to suggest additional therapy other than standard lupus management. It is not clear whether a TMA in the setting of SLE worsens the outcome.

In CAPS, the incidence of TMA is about 14% with an overall mortality of 37%. Anticoagulation with glucocorticoids with or without PEX is the most common treatment. In CAPS, there is evidence of complement activation in both clinical setting and mouse models. There are case reports of successful use of eculizumab in CAPS and prospective trials are underway.

## SEVERE HYPERTENSION-ASSOCIATED THROMBOTIC MICROANGIOPATHY

Severe hypertension can present with a phenotype indistinguishable from complement-mediated aHUS in the acute setting. In practice, failure of blood pressure control and supportive management to control the TMA will often result in the pragmatic initiation of PEX or eculizumab until complement evaluation is available. In the majority of patients with TMA associated with severe hypertension, renal function and MAHA usually recover with management of blood pressure. In a retrospective case series, genetic analysis identified rare variants in complement genes in patients for whom

TMA was initially attributed to severe hypertension; eight of nine patients progressed to ESRD despite management of hypertension. This may be particularly relevant when considering kidney transplant assessment in an individual with ESRD attributed to severe hypertension with TMA, or if TMA occurs again after transplantation.

## SUMMARY

TMA can manifest in a wide range of conditions and can be associated with significant morbidity and mortality. The different pathogenesis of these TMAs mean that personalized management of patients is required to provide the targeted therapy best suited to the underlying cause.

 Complete reference list available at ExpertConsult.com.

## KEY REFERENCES

1. Brocklebank V, Wood KM, Kavanagh D. Thrombotic microangiopathy and the kidney. *Clin J Am Soc Nephrol.* 2018;13(2):300–317.
2. Goodship TH, Cook HT, Fakhouri F, et al. Atypical hemolytic uremic syndrome and C3 glomerulopathy: conclusions from a "Kidney Disease: Improving Global Outcomes" (KDIGO) Controversies Conference. *Kidney Int.* 2017;91(3):539–551.
16. Legendre CM, Licht C, Muus P, et al. Terminal complement inhibitor eculizumab in atypical hemolytic-uremic syndrome. *N Engl J Med.* 2013;368(23):2169–2181.
17. Brocklebank V, Kavanagh D. Complement C5-inhibiting therapy for the thrombotic microangiopathies: accumulating evidence, but not a panacea. *Clin Kidney J.* 2017;10(5):600–624.
19. Lemaire M, Fremeaux-Bacchi V, Schaefer F, et al. Recessive mutations in DGKE cause atypical hemolytic-uremic syndrome. *Nat Genet.* 2013;45(5):531–536.
20. Challis RC, Ring T, Xu Y, et al. Thrombotic microangiopathy in inverted formin 2-mediated renal disease. *J Am Soc Nephrol.* 2017; 28(4):1084–1091.
29. Tarr PI, Gordon CA, Chandler WL. Shiga-toxin-producing Escherichia coli and hemolytic uremic syndrome. *Lancet.* 2005;365(9464): 1073–1086.
30. Kielstein JT, Beutel G, Fleig S, et al. Best supportive care and therapeutic plasma exchange with or without eculizumab in Shiga-toxin-producing E. coli O104:H4 induced hemolytic-uremic syndrome: an analysis of the German STEC-HUS registry. *Nephrol Dial Transplant.* 2012;27(10):3807–3815.
42. Bruel A, Kavanagh D, Noris M, et al. Hemolytic uremic syndrome in pregnancy and postpartum. *Clin J Am Soc Nephrol.* 2017;12(8): 1237–1247.
46. Kavanagh D, McGlasson S, Jury A, et al. Type I interferon causes thrombotic microangiopathy by a dose-dependent toxic effect on the microvasculature. *Blood.* 2016;128(24):2824–2833.

# 35 Tubulointerstitial Diseases

Mark A. Perazella | Mitchell H. Rosner

## CHAPTER OUTLINE



## KEY POINTS

- Tubulointerstitial diseases are a relatively common cause of acute kidney injury (AKI) (10%–20% of cases) and are likely to be a significant unrecognized cause of chronic kidney disease (CKD).
- Tubulointerstitial injury can be immune mediated, driven by activation of both innate and adaptive immune responses, or nonimmune, with interstitial fibrosis as the final common pathway. Drug-induced acute tubulointerstitial nephritis (ATIN) is most commonly caused by a T-cell–mediated delayed hypersensitivity reaction.
- Autosomal dominant tubulointerstitial kidney disease (ADTKD), formerly known as familial juvenile hyperuricemic nephropathy or medullary cystic disease, is a rare group of inherited disorders that leads to slowly progressive nonproteinuric CKD. The commonest form, due to mutations in the uromodulin gene, *UMOD*, is associated with hyperuricemia and gout.
- Drugs, particularly antibiotics, proton pump inhibitors, and nonsteroidal antiinflammatory drugs (NSAIDs), are the most common cause of ATIN, with immune checkpoint inhibitors being increasingly recognized. Other causes include autoimmune and systemic disorders, such as systemic lupus erythematosus (SLE), Sjögren syndrome, and sarcoidosis, and infections such as *Legionella*, tuberculosis, polyoma virus, hantavirus, and leptospirosis.
- ATIN presents with minimal symptoms and an acute or subacute rise in serum creatinine. The classic triad of fever, rash, and eosinophilia is uncommon and seen predominantly in drug-induced ATIN due to β-lactams and sulfonamides. Urine sediment findings and urine eosinophils, and imaging tests such as gallium scanning, have limited sensitivity and specificity, so kidney biopsy is generally required to make a definitive diagnosis.
- Early use of steroids is generally recommended for the treatment of drug-induced ATIN if there is no improvement after drug discontinuation, but this is based on limited evidence from small, observational studies. Failure to diagnose and treat ATIN early may result in increased kidney fibrosis and incomplete recovery of kidney function.
- Chronic tubulointerstitial nephritis (CTIN) may develop as a late complication of ATIN, or may be the initial manifestation of exposure to toxins, such as combination analgesics, aristolochic acids, heavy metals, and lithium, or systemic and autoimmune diseases, such as sarcoidosis or Sjögren syndrome.
- CKD of uncertain etiology is a newly recognized cause of CTIN that affects predominantly young, male agricultural workers in hot climates and is a major health concern in certain countries including parts of Central America, Sri Lanka, India, and Egypt.

## INTRODUCTION

The renal interstitium consists of the intertubular, extraglomerular, and extravascular spaces of the kidney. This renal compartment can be affected by a diverse group of diseases that can elicit local inflammation, tubular cell damage, and possibly lead to fibrosis and chronic, progressive kidney disease. Tubulointerstitial diseases are traditionally referred to as interstitial nephritis and can take two broad forms: acute and chronic. Acute forms present with rapid deterioration in renal function along with marked interstitial inflammatory response characterized by mononuclear cell infiltration, interstitial edema, and varying degrees of tubular cell damage. Chronic forms are more indolent and are characterized by interstitial mononuclear cell infiltration, tubulointerstitial fibrosis, and atrophy. There is some overlap between the acute and chronic forms, especially if acute disease is not recognized and treated in a timely manner, which allows for progression to chronic kidney disease (CKD).

## PRIMARY VERSUS SECONDARY TUBULOINTERSTITIAL DISEASE

Another classification for tubulointerstitial disease is to consider whether the pathologic process in this compartment is either primary or secondary in etiology. Primary causes include those etiologies of acute and chronic tubulointerstitial injury (such as drug-induced interstitial nephritis, toxin- and heavy metal–induced chronic interstitial disease, and autoimmune-mediated diseases) that directly injure the renal tubules and surrounding interstitium. Injury typically occurs through a variety of pathologic processes, including immune cell, cytokine, and complement-mediated mechanisms, and may be acute or chronic in nature.

However, tubulointerstitial injury is also present with multiple forms of kidney disease, including those that do not primarily involve this compartment (i.e., secondary). Examples of this secondary tubulointerstitial disease are seen in patients with glomerulonephritis, diabetes mellitus, hypertension, atherosclerosis, and cystic renal diseases.[1,2] More recently, tubulointerstitial changes have been noted as a secondary process after acute kidney injury (AKI).[1–4] Furthermore, aging itself leads to significant changes and progressive fibrosis in the tubulointerstitial compartment.[1–6] As a final common pathway, these tubulointerstitial changes correlate with impaired renal function and the presence of renal fibrosis on biopsy.[1,2]

The importance of these secondary interstitial changes associated with many kidney diseases was first recognized in 1870 when it was hypothesized that interstitial changes documented in Bright disease were responsible for kidney scarring and shrinkage associated with end-stage renal disease (ESRD).[7] Subsequently, it has been found that in almost all forms of progressive experimental and human CKD, a prominent inflammatory infiltrate exists within the interstitial compartment. The extent of these infiltrates, number of fibroblasts present, and area of fibrosis all correlate with progressive decline in renal function.[8–10] Several studies have pointed out the prognostic significance of severe injury of the tubulointerstitium in lupus nephritis, membranous nephropathy, immunoglobulin A (IgA) nephropathy, and other glomerular diseases.[10–12] There is an association between the degree of renal impairment and extent of tubulointerstitial damage in patients with glomerular disease.[10] In 50 cases of persistent glomerulonephritis, the correlation between the extent of tubular lesions and alterations in renal function was far greater than the changes in glomerular structure on renal function.[10] These findings suggested, in chronic glomerulonephritis, that interstitial damage has much more effect on the glomerular filtration rate (GFR) than structural injury in the glomeruli. Subsequent work also highlighted the importance of tubulointerstitial changes on GFR in a wide variety of glomerulopathies.[13]

Several mechanisms may explain how tubulointerstitial disease affects renal function. The simplest explanation is that tubular obstruction from interstitial inflammation and fibrosis impedes urine flow, increases intratubular pressure, and eventually lowers glomerular filtration.[13,14] A second possible mechanism implicates a reduction in the volume of peritubular capillaries due to progressive fibrosis and, in this setting, the tubulointerstitial compartment becomes relatively avascular and ischemic.[15] As a result of the increase in vascular resistance in the postglomerular segment, hydrostatic pressure in glomerular capillaries also increases, impairing glomerular arteriolar outflow. A third possibility is an alteration in tubuloglomerular feedback leading to GFR reduction.[16] The presence of edema, inflammation, and fibrosis in the renal interstitium, by increasing the interstitial pressure, may lower the sensitivity of the feedback mechanism, possibly through local control of production of vasoactive substances such as angiotensin-II (Ang-II), nitric oxide, and prostaglandins.[16,17] When tubulointerstitial fibrosis develops, the autoregulation of renal blood flow is also disrupted permanently, leading to falls in GFR.[18] Fourth, glomerular–tubular disconnection, or finding atrophic tubules and glomeruli no longer connected to each other, is a well-recognized consequence of tubulointerstitial injury.[19] This may be particularly true with injury to the proximal tubule.[19–21] This is consistent with evidence from human studies showing a positive correlation between the fractional volume of the interstitium, percentage of proximal tubule without connection to a glomerulus, and decline of renal function in patients with chronic pyelonephritis.[22] Collectively, all these pathophysiologic processes are interrelated and highlight the importance of secondary fibrotic changes in the interstitium as a critical mechanism for progression of CKD.

## MECHANISMS OF TUBULOINTERSTITIAL INJURY

Tubulointerstitial injury is caused by a number of processes, many of which share various components that ultimately promote tubulointerstitial changes.[23,24] Primary innate and adaptive immune injuries in the tubulointerstitium drive inflammation and, with glomerular injury, there are secondary downstream effects from proteinuria leading to tubulointerstitial nephritis. Persistent inflammation leads to destructive progression with tubulointerstitial fibrosis. The inflammatory process may also be driven by genotypic variations among hosts.

## COMPONENTS OF THE TUBULOINTERSTITIUM

A large number of intrinsic cells and structural components, as well as infiltrating cells entering this renal compartment, make up the tubulointerstitium. A dynamic interplay exists between intrinsic and extrinsic cells and tubulointerstitial components. The renal tubules and vasculature, along with a number of endogenous and exogenous cells and the interstitium, fall within the compartment known as the tubulointerstitium.[25] In essence, the interstitium is composed of the intertubular, extraglomerular, and extravascular spaces of the kidney, which is surrounded by both tubular and vascular basement membranes.[25] Fibrillar pericytes reside at the vascular pole between the macula densa and afferent arterioles, presumably participating in renal autoregulatory responses. Vasa recta and lymphatics within the interstitium are involved in solute exchange, which is driven by a hydrostatic pressure gradient. Separation into cortical and medullary interstitia allows countercurrent medullary solute trapping and the development of the corticomedullary osmotic gradient.

Multiple cell types, extracellular matrix, and interstitial fluid are also important components of the interstitium.[25] Proximal tubules, which have antigen-presenting capability and secrete various growth factors and cytokines, directly interact with the interstitium through paracrine and juxtacrine mechanisms.[26] These cells may also participate in tubulointerstitial inflammation, which is the result of inflammatory and immunologic stimuli they are exposed to on their tubular and basolateral borders. They are influenced by a number of autocoids, which lead to both growth factor (metalloproteinases and associated inhibitors) production and cytokine (transforming growth factor-β [TGF-β]) secretion.[27] The resulting cell–matrix interactions determine extracellular matrix production, stabilization, or removal by matrix-producing fibroblast cells.[28]

Interstitial fibroblasts, which are of mesenchymal origin, are the most abundant cell within the interstitium.[29] They are different from other nonfibroblastic cells of renal mesenchymal origin (pericytes, stem cells, myofibroblasts, and vascular smooth muscle cells) and express matrix-promoting and matrix-degrading proteins that determine net matrix production and the amount of interstitial fibrosis within the tubulointerstitium.[30]

In addition to fibroblasts, macrophages, lymphocytes, lymphatic endothelial cells, mast cells, and dendritic cells inhabit the interstitium. Circulating monocytes that migrate into the kidneys transform into renal interstitial macrophages. Following recruitment of monocytes to the kidney in tubulointerstitial disorders, they subsequently differentiate into inflammatory M1 or reparative M2 phenotypes.[31] The balance between M1/M2 phenotypic expression and the interaction with T lymphocytes, fibroblasts, and dendritic cells via growth factors, and cytokines determines the extent of renal fibrogenesis and progression of chronic tubulointerstitial disease. Mast cells are sparse within the interstitium, but appear to be both profibrotic and antifibrotic.[32] Dendritic cells are antigen-presenting cells derived from bone marrow–derived precursor cells that migrate into the interstitium.[33] These cells interact with T cells within the interstitial lymphatic network to process antigens and elicit inflammatory responses.[34] They may also engage antigens presented by proximal tubular cells, which constitutively express major histocompatibility complex (MHC) class II antigens,[35] leading to inflammation and tubulointerstitial nephritis. They may also participate in tubulointerstitial injury following glomerular injury.[27]

## IMMUNE-MEDIATED TUBULOINTERSTITIAL DISEASE

When the immune system targets the renal interstitial compartment as a primary process, target antigens are derived from endogenous and exogenous sources. These include endogenous renal cells, tubular basement membrane (TBM), or other extracellular matrix components, or are exogenous antigens processed and presented by native renal cells or minor populations of dendritic cells within the interstitium.

### ANTIGENS WITHIN THE RENAL COMPARTMENT

Proximal TBM antigen is the major target of anti-TBM antibody-mediated interstitial nephritis (TIN) in humans.[36] Glycoprotein isoforms of 54 to 58 and 40 to 50 kDa are the TIN antigens recognized by anti-TBM antibodies.[36] This glycoprotein has affinity for type IV collagen and laminin and likely serves to stabilize the TBM.[37]

Drugs and/or drug–hapten complexes can also serve as nephritogenic antigens. These antigens, along with targeting antibodies, can form immune deposits in situ within the interstitium or precipitate as a circulating complex. Examples of this include members of the penicillin family, cephalosporins, and phenytoin. In some cases, antibodies directed against microorganisms may discover cross-reactive epitopes on interstitial components, as in the antibodies to nephritogenic streptococci, which cross-react with type IV collagen. Some anti-DNA antibodies also react with the extracellular matrix components, laminin and heparin sulfate.

### ANTIGEN PRESENTATION BY TUBULAR CELLS

T cells recognize foreign antigens when they are digested into small fragments and presented on the surface of antigen-presenting cells (APCs) bound to MHC antigen molecules.[38] Recognition of this complex on APCs leads to activation of T cells. $CD4^+$ T cells recognize antigens following the processing and presentation of that antigen in conjunction with class II MHC molecules. By contrast, $CD8^+$ T cells recognize antigens synthesized by the APC in conjunction with class I MHC molecules. Activation of T cells by APCs expressing processed antigen is also optimized by a number of cell–cell interactions involving cell surface costimulatory molecules and their ligands. Recognition of class II MHC molecules by $CD4^+$ T cells generally results in cell proliferation and cytokine expression, whereas $CD8^+$ T cells cause target cell death after detecting antigen–class I complex-bearing cells.

Activated tubular epithelial cells release proinflammatory cytokines and $CD4^+$ $T_H1$ chemokines, but not $T_H17$ chemokines.[39] In addition to processing multiple potentially immunogenic peptides, proximal tubular cells could also be exposed to a number of filtered low-molecular-weight proinflammatory cytokines such as interferon-γ (IFN-γ), interleukin-1 (IL-1), and tumor necrosis factor-α (TNF-α) and cytokines secreted by immune cells infiltrating the interstitium. The ability of renal epithelial cells to present antigen or serve as a target for CD8⁺ T cells depends on the cytokine milieu and whether the net effect of those mediators is proinflammatory or antiinflammatory. Proinflammatory cytokines typically augment the expression of class II MHC molecules on epithelial cells, which is markedly amplified in interstitial nephritis, as is the expression of adhesion molecules such as intercellular adhesion molecule-1 (ICAM-1).[40]

Renal tubular cells also require the augmented expression of costimulatory molecules, which are required for full activation of T cells.[41] The interaction of the costimulatory molecular pair (a T-cell receptor and an APC ligand) results in activation or inhibition of the immune response. Many of the receptors on T cells are members of the Ig superfamily, including CD28, cytotoxic T-lymphocyte–associated protein 4 (CTLA-4), inducible T-cell costimulator (ICOS), and programmed death 1 (PD-1), whereas their receptor ligands are members of the B7 family, which can be induced by proinflammatory cytokines.[42] Tubular cells can also be induced to express other accessory molecules, such as CD40, ICAM-1, vascular cell adhesion molecule 1 (VCAM-1), and ICOS-L, which are involved in T-cell activation.[43,44] In addition, renal tubular cell expression of programmed death-ligand 1 (PD-L1), the receptor for PD-1, may have inhibitory effects on T-cell proliferation and/or effector functions.[45,46] IgA nephropathy, interstitial nephritis, and systemic lupus erythematosus (SLE) nephritis demonstrate significant staining of tubules for B7-H1 (PD-L1),[47] suggesting that the expression of this costimulatory molecule is upregulated. Thus the number of receptor–ligand pairs that potentially regulate the outcome of renal tubular cell interactions with T cells is large but unpredictable.

## CELLULAR INFILTRATES

Cell-mediated immune responses are implicated in the pathogenesis of interstitial nephritis because of both in vivo (delayed-type hypersensitivity) and in vitro (lymphoblast transformation) evidence of hypersensitivity to specific inciting antigens. However, tubulointerstitial inflammation can result from either antigen-specific stimulation or may develop in the absence of antigenic stimulation.[48] In the latter case, there is growing evidence for the role of innate immune sensors (TLR2, TLR4, and MyD88 signaling) and the inflammasome complex in initiating tubulointerstitial injury.[49,50]

The interstitial infiltrate found in most human CKDs consists of a number of different effector cells, including CD4⁺ and CD8⁺ T cells and macrophages, although CD4⁺ T cells predominate.[51] Monocytes and macrophages infiltrating the renal interstitium are also important in the initiation and progression of kidney injury. Macrophages cause cellular damage by generating reactive oxygen species, nitric oxide, complement factors, and proinflammatory cytokines.[52] These cells can also affect supporting matrix and vasculature through the expression of metalloproteinases and vasoactive peptides. Macrophages may also have a beneficial role in interstitial injury, serving as markers of disease remission[53] or having an antifibrotic role.[54] Clearly, interstitial macrophages have phenotypic and functional heterogeneity in a number of interstitial injury models.

B and T lymphocytes often accompany macrophages within the interstitium. The composition of the interstitial infiltrate is similar, whether the initiating cause of injury is chronic ischemia,[55] autoimmune tubulointerstitial nephritis,[56] or protein overload.[57] It is possible that immune responses to injured interstitial cell neoantigens are a final common pathway for interstitial injury. In remnant kidney models, infiltration of the interstitium with macrophages and lymphocytes correlates with functional parameters of kidney failure, and improvement occurs with immunosuppressive treatment,[58] supporting the importance of immune-mediated injury in progressive interstitial disease observed in nonimmune forms of primary injury.

The histologic appearance of human interstitial disease can vary from granulomatous interstitial nephritis with an intense cellular infiltrate to sparse infiltrates. Although this variable appearance may reflect different stages of an immune-mediated lesion or different target antigens, it may also reflect the biologic activity of discrete populations of activated T cells.[59] Although interstitial injury can be induced by a single T-cell clone, the resultant damage to interstitial and tubular cells is most likely the end result of interactions among many cell types. The cytotoxic activity of renal antigen–reactive T-cell clones may ultimately account for tubular cell destruction and resultant tubule atrophy.

## IMMUNOLOGY AND PATHOGENESIS OF DRUG-INDUCED ACUTE TUBULOINTERSTITIAL NEPHRITIS

Drug-induced acute tubulointerstitial nephritis (ATIN) is believed to be primarily a T cell–mediated delayed hypersensitivity reaction, falling into the type IV classification.[60–65] Renal susceptibility to hypersensitivity is related to the high blood delivery as well as local drug metabolism. Hypersensitivity can be renal limited without systemic manifestations. Four phases characterize this reaction: (1) antigen recognition; (2) antigen presentation; (3) immune regulatory; and (4) effector phases.

Antigen recognition occurs after a drug induces antigenicity by an assortment of mechanisms. Drugs can act as haptens and bind to intrinsic renal proteins, rendering them antigenic.[60,61] Drugs can also act as prohaptens, which require metabolism by the kidney or liver to become haptens.[64] Another drug mechanism of antigenicity involves making a native protein immunogenic by damaging tubulointerstitial structures, thereby producing neoantigens.[66] Various medications are also structurally similar to native kidney antigens (molecular mimicry) and can incite an immune reaction.

As reviewed previously, resident dendritic cells, interstitial macrophages, and tubular cells can function as APCs in the kidneys.[66–71] Dendritic cells search for foreign material at the basolateral aspects of tubular cells and peritubular capillaries. Although phagocytosis of various native and foreign substances is a major function of macrophages, they also play a role in antigen presentation. Renal tubular cells have inducible MHC class II expression when they come into contact with foreign antigens, facilitating antigen presentation. All of these APCs present antigens to T cells located within the kidneys and regional lymph nodes.

Because immune response in the kidney is self-regulatory, drug-induced ATIN tends to be a rare phenomenon. Self-regulation involves activation of suppressor T cells and downregulation of MHC class II expression.[63] Use of checkpoint inhibitors, which activate quiescent T cells to destroy cancer cells, is an example of immune regulation disturbed by medications.

**Table 35.1 Drug-Induced Hypersensitivity Reaction Classification**

Type IVa
- $T_H1$ cell
- IFN-γ/IL-12
  - Monocyte/macrophage stimulation
  - Synthesis of complement-fixing antibody and complement-mediated injury
  - Costimulate proinflammatory responses (tumor necrosis factor, IL-12)
  - Costimulate CD8 T-cell responses

Type IVb
- $T_H2$ cell
- IL-4, IL-13, IL-5
  - B-cell production of IgE and IgG4
  - Macrophage deactivation
  - Mast cell and eosinophil responses

Type IVc
- Cytotoxic T cells
  - Injury via perforin/granzyme and FasL-dependent processes

Type IVd
- T cell (IL-8 and GM-CSF)
  - Neutrophil-mediated inflammation/sterile PMN-rich inflammation

*FasL*, Fas ligand; *GM-CSF*, granulocyte–monocyte colony stimulating factor; *IFN*, interferon; *Ig*, immunoglobulin; *IL*, interleukin; *PMN*, polymorphonuclear; $T_H$, T helper.

The effector phase of the immune system promotes interstitial inflammation and tubular injury via infiltration of lymphocytes, neutrophils, macrophages, mast cells, and eosinophils. Of these, T lymphocytes constitute 80% of the infiltrating cells.[64,65,71,72] In its most common form, drug-induced ATIN is a type IV(b) hypersensitivity reaction (Table 35.1) with production of IL-5 and presence of systemic and tissue eosinophilia.[64,71,73] However, different drugs can cause ATIN via different pathways as seen with nonsteroidal antiinflammatory drugs (NSAIDs), which lack interstitial eosinophils implicating a non–type IV(b) drug-hypersensitivity reaction.[72]

Immune-complex deposition is a rare cause of ATIN with drugs. However, anti-TBM antibody deposition occurs with medications such as methicillin, rifampin, allopurinol, and phenytoin.[51] The deposits generally consist of IgG and complement factor C3 and are deposited along the TBM in a linear or granular fashion. Finally, direct drug interaction with T cells can induce ATIN. Interaction of unprocessed drugs with T cells via T-cell receptor activates T cells, which also play a role in drug hypersensitivity.[64,74]

## NONIMMUNE-MEDIATED TUBULOINTERSTITIAL DISEASE

In addition to immune-mediated tubulointerstitial injury, a variety of nonimmune-mediated processes promote damage to this compartment.

### GLOMERULAR-RELATED EVENTS

Glomerular diseases incite tubulointerstitial injury through multiple pathways.[75] These include (1) impaired glomerular permselectivity that allows for entry of substances that are morphogenic to tubuli[75,76]; (2) intraglomerular hypertension damages the nephron,[77] and alternatively, glomerular hypoperfusion may diminish postglomerular blood flow and cause tubular ischemia; (3) immunologic mechanisms in glomeruli may incur the loss of tolerance and instigate tubulointerstitial injury[78]; and (4) inflammatory mediators enter the interstitium through the juxtaglomerular apparatus.[79] Subsequent nephron loss caused by injury to glomeruli and attached tubules may facilitate metabolic adaptations in surviving nephrons that induce tubulointerstitial injury through the renin–angiotensin system.[80]

Other possible mechanisms include (1) misdirected filtration and (2) crescentic cell proliferation. According to the misdirection mechanism, extension of a proteinaceous crescent into the outer aspect of the proximal tubule expands into the space between the tubular epithelium and TBM and may spread along the entire proximal convolution within this space. This process may cause tubulointerstitial inflammation and injury.[81,82] The other mechanism is the encroachment of a growing cellular crescent on the glomerulotubular junction, where the initial segment of the proximal tubule is incorporated into the crescent.[82,83] This results in nephron loss and subsequent fibrosis, which some consider a reparative process important for the maintenance of renal structure rather than a determinant of further injury.[84]

Ultimately, injury that spreads beyond the confines of the glomerulus allows inflammation to extend within the tubulointerstitial compartment. Chronic injury and the accompanying fibrosis, driven by glomerular processes, provide a pathway for the transmission of more inflammation into areas previously uninvolved by original disease.

### PROTEINURIA-INDUCED TUBULAR CELL INJURY

One important mechanism of glomerular–tubulointerstitial interaction is through proteinuria. Although proteinuria is considered as a surrogate marker of the severity of underlying glomerular damage, clinical and experimental data suggest that proteinuria is an independent risk factor and plays an important role in the progression of kidney disease.[85] Mechanisms underlying nephrotoxic injury induced by excessive proteinuria are multifactorial and involve numerous pathways of cellular damage.

Obstruction of tubular lumens by proteinaceous casts and obliteration of the tubular neck by glomerular tuft adhesions may contribute to tubulointerstitial damage. However, the direct effects of filtered macromolecules on tubular cells are important.[86] Proteins reaching the tubular urine are largely reabsorbed in the proximal segments of tubular epithelium, where they incite injury. Protein overload activates proximal tubular cells into acquiring a proinflammatory phenotype.[87] Upregulation of inflammatory and fibrogenic genes and production of related proteins occur with exposure of proximal tubular cells to plasma proteins. These include a number of proinflammatory and profibrogenic cytokines and chemokines.[88–90] Apoptosis and autophagy are other mechanisms that underlie protein-induced tubular cell injury.[91,92] Protein overload causes a dose- and duration-dependent induction of apoptosis in cultured proximal tubular cells.[93] It is these processes that are thought to underlie proteinuria-induced tubulointerstitial disease. See also Chapter 30 for an in-depth discussion of this topic.

### GLOMERULAR FILTERED GROWTH FACTORS AND CYTOKINES

Many growth factors and cytokines, usually in high-molecular-weight precursor forms or bound to specific binding proteins, are present in nephrotic tubular fluid.[94] Insulin-like growth factor-1 (IGF-1) and hepatocyte growth factor (HGF) both undergo glomerular ultrafiltration in proteinuric states and interact with proximal tubular cells.[95] In proteinuric glomerular diseases, TGF-β is also present in early proximal tubular fluid at concentrations that are required for biologic responses.[96] Ultrafiltered IGF-1, HGF, and TGF-β appear to act on tubular cells through their apical signaling receptors, where they induce increased expression of matrix proteins that most likely contribute to interstitial fibrosis.

### ACTIVATION OF COMPLEMENT COMPONENTS

Serum- or tubular-derived complement factors are components of urinary proteins that can be harmful to the tubulointerstitium.[97] Renal tubular epithelial cells appear most susceptible to luminal attack by C5b-9 because of the relative lack of a number of membrane-bound complement regulatory proteins.[98] Activation of C5b-9 by tubules is associated with tubular injury characterized by severe cytoskeletal alterations, bleb formation, and cytolysis. Increased production of superoxide anion and $H_2O_2$ and synthesis of proinflammatory cytokines such as IL-6 and TNF-α also contribute to injury.[99] Accumulation of complement within proximal tubular cells is followed by local recruitment of infiltrating mononuclear cells.[100] Overall, complement activation appears to play a pivotal role as a mediator of progressive tubulointerstitial damage.

## TUBULOINTERSTITIAL FIBROSIS

Fibrosis is the final common pathway leading to CKD, irrespective of initiating events. The process of tubulointerstitial fibrosis involves the loss of renal tubules and the accumulation of fibroblasts and matrix proteins, such as collagen (types I–V and VII), fibronectin, and laminin.[101] Cells infiltrating the renal interstitium have long been thought to play a role in the initiation and progression of tubulointerstitial fibrosis; however, fibroblasts have been identified as the principal effector mediating tubulointerstitial fibrosis.[102]

### EPITHELIAL–MESENCHYMAL TRANSITIONS IN FIBROSIS

Epithelial–mesenchymal transition (EMT) is a robust source of tissue fibroblasts,[103,104] which play a critical role in tubulointerstitial fibrosis.[105] Epithelial and endothelial cells that line tubules and ducts have plasticity.[106,107] Midway through development, these cells can transition into fibroblasts by EMT as part of organ growth.[106] Tubular epithelia and endothelia undergoing EMT during persistent injury in the kidney produce new renal fibroblasts, as well as resident and new fibroblasts that proliferate to expand total numbers.[103,108] Pericytes that have undergone transition are also a source of fibroblasts.[109] Persistent cytokine activity during renal inflammation and disruption of the underlying basement membrane by local proteases initiates the process of EMT.[110]

A number of proteins, including Wnt proteins, integrin-linked kinases, IGF-1 and IGF-2, epidermal growth factor (EGF), fibroblast growth factor-2 (FGF-2), and TGF-β are among the archetypal modulators of EMT.[105] However, TGF-β and EGF provide the strongest stimulus for completion of epithelial transitions. These growth factors or their intermediates enhance the transition of epithelial cells into fibroblasts. EMT also operates in human tubular cells[111,112] and pathologic renal tissues.[113,114] Importantly, mature epithelia are in a dynamic but not terminal state of differentiation.[107] As such, morphogenic forces that normally maintain epithelial phenotypes are pitted against countervailing forces trying to weaken that stability. Chronic inflammation into the interstitium destabilizes epithelial tissues by favoring fibrogenesis.

### CHRONIC HYPOXIA IN FIBROSIS

One of the most important contributors to the development of tubulointerstitial fibrosis is chronic ischemia.[115–117] Production of AngII and inhibition of nitric oxide production underlie chronic vasoconstriction, which contributes to tissue ischemia and hypoxia[118] and stimulates EMT. Loss of peritubular capillaries (rarefaction) in areas of tubulointerstitial fibrosis may develop due to downregulation of vascular endothelial growth factor, and contributes to further ischemia.[118,119] Moreover, given that the size of the interstitial compartment determines the diffusion distance between peritubular capillaries and tubular cells, interstitial fibrosis likely makes tubular oxygen supply worse. This interstitial reduction of capillary blood flow, leading to starvation of tubules, may underlie tubular atrophy and loss. Under these conditions, the remaining tubules are subject to functional hypermetabolism, with increased oxygen consumption, which further promotes the hypoxic environment and increases amounts of tubulointerstitial fibrosis.

## GENETIC CAUSES OF TUBULOINTERSTITIAL DISEASES

There are a rare group of autosomal dominant disorders where disease-causing mutations lead directly to slowly progressive ESRD that is typified by interstitial fibrosis and tubular atrophy along with thickening and lamellation of the TBM. There is no immunologic component for the pathogenesis of these conditions and there is negative immunofluorescence for complement and immunoglobulins.[120] In the past, this group of diseases has been known by a number of names, such as familial juvenile hyperuricemic nephropathy and medullary cystic disease. However, a recent consensus conference has provided standard terminology for these disorders based on their genetic mutations[120] (Table 35.2). Thus far, four genes, encoding tubular proteins, have been identified that when mutated lead to autosomal dominant tubulointerstitial kidney disease (ADTKD): uromodulin (*UMOD*), renin (*REN*), hepatocyte nuclear factor 1β (*HNF1β*), and mucin-1 (*MUC1*).[121–124] It is thought that mutations in *UMOD* and *MUC1* are more frequently encountered.[120]

The clinical manifestations as well as the age at which disease manifestations occur are highly variable in these conditions and make diagnosis a challenge. However, in most cases there is a positive family history of kidney disease and this takes the form of autosomal dominant inheritance. Furthermore, the rate of decline in kidney function is variable and the age at which ESRD occurs can range from 20 to 80 years, with most patients requiring renal replacement therapy

**Table 35.2 Autosomal Dominant Tubulointerstitial Kidney Disease**

| KDIGO Terminology | Gene Mutated | Past Terminology | Clinical Characteristics | Laboratory Characteristics | Histological Characteristics |
|---|---|---|---|---|---|
| ADTKD-UMOD | *UMOD* | – Uromodulin kidney disease<br>– Familial juvenile hyperuricemic nephropathy<br>– Medullary cystic disease type 2 | – Early onset gout and occasional renal cysts<br>– Rarely presents during childhood | – Hyperuricemia with low-fractional excretion of uric acid<br>– Low urinary excretion of uromodulin | – Intracellular deposits of uromodulin especially in the thick ascending limb of the loop of Henle |
| ADTKD-MUC1 | *MUC1* | – Mucin-1 kidney disease<br>– Medullary cystic disease type 1 | – No characteristic findings<br>– Occasional renal cysts<br>– Presents later in life | None described | Intracellular accumulation of mucin-1 frameshift protein in distal tubules |
| ADTKD-REN | *REN* | – Familial juvenile hyperuricemic nephropathy type 2 | – Mild hypotension<br>– Anemia during childhood<br>– Frequently presents during childhood | Hyperuricemia, hyperkalemia, and low urinary excretion of uromodulin | Reduced renin staining in cells of the juxtaglomerular apparatus |
| ADTKD-HNF1β | *HNF1β* | – Maturity-onset diabetes mellitus of the young type 5<br>– Renal cyst and diabetes syndrome | – Maturity-onset diabetes<br>– Few bilateral renal cysts<br>– Pancreatic atrophy<br>– Genital abnormalities<br>– Frequently presents during childhood and even prenatally | Hypomagnesemia, hypokalemia, liver function test abnormalities | Nonspecific |

*ADTKD,* Autosomal dominant tubulointerstitial kidney disease; *HNF1β,* hepatocyte nuclear factor-1β; *KDIGO,* Kidney Disease Improving Global Outcomes; *MUC1,* mucin-1; *REN,* renin; *UMOD,* uromodulin.

between ages 30 and 50. Proteinuria is typically at low levels and the urinary sediment is usually normal.[125] Although renal cysts can be seen in these conditions, they are generally found in more advanced cases and are no more frequently seen than in other noncystic renal diseases.[121–125]

There are differentiating characteristics between the various forms of ADTKD (see Table 35.2). ADTKD-UMOD is characterized in some affected individuals by a decreased fractional excretion (FE) of uric acid, hyperuricemia, and gout, which may be manifested in childhood.[126] ADTKD-REN is characterized by a transient anemia in childhood as well as an increased risk for volume depletion (due to defects in the renin–angiotensin system).[127] Patients with *HNF1β* mutations may have multiple extrarenal manifestations, including maturity-onset diabetes mellitus of the young, and some may not manifest tubulointerstitial disease.[128] ADTKD-MUC1 patients present with progressive tubulointerstitial fibrosis without unique phenotypic characteristics.[129]

ADTKD-UMOD results from mutations in the *UMOD* gene encoding the most abundant protein in the urine, uromodulin (also called Tamm–Horsfall protein).[120,121] ADTKD-UMOD is the most commonly encountered subtype of ADTKD. Mechanistically, it appears that mutant uromodulin accumulates in the endoplasmic reticulum of the tubular cells in the thick ascending limb of the loop of Henle, leading to cellular injury and defective trafficking of the $Na^+$–$K^+$–$2Cl^-$ cotransporter to the luminal surface.[130,131] These changes lead to impaired sodium conservation, decreased urinary concentrating ability, and resulting mild volume depletion. It is thought that this volume depletion may drive proximal tubular reabsorption of uric acid and lead to the characteristic finding of hyperuricemia.[130,131] Progressive CKD is likely related to tubular cell death and fibrosis. ADTKD-UMOD should be suspected in patients with a strong family history of early-onset gout, hyperuricemia, and progressive CKD with bland urinary sediment. Gout in patients with ADTKD-UMOD may occur in the teenage years and in one case series of 205 patients, 65% of patients had gout; however, some families did not display this feature and instead had asymptomatic hyperuricemia in a higher percentage.[131] CKD in these patients follows a variable course with ESRD developing at a median age of 54 years with a range of 25–70 years.[126,131] The diagnosis of ADTKD-UMOD can be confirmed with specific genetic testing, and renal biopsy does not have a diagnostic role unless specific immunofluorescence microscopy is performed with antibodies to uromodulin, which will demonstrate abnormal deposition in the tubular cell of the thick ascending limb of the loop of Henle.[132] No specific therapy is available for ADTKD-UMOD and thus therapy should focus on treatment of gout and prevention of progression of CKD. It remains controversial whether allopurinol therapy may slow the progression of kidney disease, especially when initiated early in the course of the disease.[133,134] However, given the high risk of developing gout, many clinicians recommend allopurinol therapy in patients when hyperuricemia is found. There is no evidence that angiotensin inhibitors slow the progression of CKD in patients with ADTKD-UMOD.

Mutations in the mucin-1 gene (*MUC1*), which encodes a transmembrane protein expressed in the distal tubule, lead to ADTKD-MUC1. This mutation creates a new peptide that accumulates inside renal tubular epithelial cells.[135] However, the mechanism of progressive CKD is not well understood.

Patients typically present with unexplained progressive CKD with bland urine sediment. Although a renal ultrasound is typically normal in these patients, they may show medullary cysts, which are not sensitive or specific for this condition. In some cases, a history of inherited CKD may be present. The course of CKD is highly variable with ESRD occurring over a wide range of ages (ages 20–70 years).[136] Genetic testing for ADTKD-MUC1 is not widely available. Care is supportive and follows the general principles for any CKD patient.

Mutations in *HNF1β* can lead to a variety of phenotypes because the gene is expressed in numerous tissues and regulates other downstream genes.[137] A whole spectrum of associated phenotypes has been reported, including genital malformations, autism, epilepsy, gout, hypomagnesemia, primary hyperparathyroidism, liver and intestinal abnormalities, and a rare form of kidney cancer.[138] The mechanisms involved in the development of tubulointerstitial fibrosis are not elucidated. Genetic testing is available for patients suspected of having ADTKD-HNF1β. Treatment of the renal manifestations of this syndrome is supportive.

ADTKD-REN is due to mutations of the gene encoding preprorenin. Preprorenin undergoes processing to renin, which exerts multiple effects through the prorenin receptor as well as through its protease function to control angiotensin formation.[139] Mutations in this disease disrupt the translocation of preprorenin into the endoplasmic reticulum of renin-expressing cells that are found in several segments of the renal tubule and juxtaglomerular apparatus.[122] The net effect is that preprorenin accumulates in these cells, leading to low renin levels and damage of renal tubular cells in affected individuals.[140] Low renin levels are not diagnostic in this condition. Thus some clinical manifestations of ADTKD-REN are due to the low renin state, including low-normal blood pressure, mild elevations of serum potassium, risk for developing volume depletion and prerenal azotemia, and hypoproliferative anemia with low erythropoietin levels that manifests early in life but resolves with adolescence (only to recur once advanced CKD is present).[140,141] Hyperuricemia and early-onset gout are also present. Progressive CKD begins in childhood and ESRD may be manifest between ages 30 and 60 years. Diagnosis can be confirmed with genetic testing. For some affected individuals with low blood pressure and hyperkalemia, treatment with fludrocortisone and/or a high-salt diet can be helpful. Because of the low renin state in these patients, they are prone to develop volume depletion and a low-sodium diet should be avoided. Furthermore, they are at increased risk to develop AKI when taking NSAIDs.

Kidney transplantation is an effective therapy in all forms of ADTKD because the disorder does not recur in the transplanted kidney. However, family members should be carefully screened for these mutations prior to donating a kidney.

## ACUTE TUBULOINTERSTITIAL NEPHRITIS

### GENERAL FEATURES OF ACUTE TUBULOINTERSTITIAL NEPHRITIS

ATIN is an entity that is characterized by histologic findings of interstitial inflammatory cellular infiltrate, variable degrees of tubular injury, interstitial edema, and tubulitis. Councilman defined the renal lesion of ATIN as "an acute inflammation of the kidney characterized by cellular and fluid exudation in the interstitial tissue, accompanied by, but not dependent on, degeneration of the epithelium; the exudation is not purulent in character, and the lesions may be both diffuse and focal."[142] This form of sterile interstitial nephritis was observed at postmortem in patients dying of scarlet fever and diphtheria. In addition, "allergic" interstitial nephritis was also found in association with bacterial sepsis and other systemic infectious diseases where there was no direct bacterial infection within the kidney parenchyma. As effective antimicrobial agents such as the sulfonamides and β-lactams were used to treat infections, the incidence and prevalence of infection-associated ATIN gradually decreased while pharmacologic agents became the most common etiology.[143] In subsequent years, interstitial nephritis from autoimmune processes was described and the role of various tubulointerstitial antigens, nephritogenic T cells, and the fibrogenic processes associated with ATIN was demonstrated.[144]

### INCIDENCE/PREVALENCE

The true incidence and prevalence of ATIN in the overall population are difficult to estimate and most estimates are obtained from biopsy registries.[145–148] The incidence is highly variable depending on the clinical scenario and the population studied. For example, in patients undergoing kidney biopsy for any indication, the incidence ranges from 1% to 3% (Table 35.3). In fact, most biopsy series support this incidence.[149] An incidence of 0.7% is observed in asymptomatic patients with abnormal urinary findings (hematuria or proteinuria), whereas hospitalized patients with AKI without a clear-cut cause may have an incidence ranging from 10% to 20% (Table 35.3). Of note, the proportion of biopsies showing ATIN appears to be on the rise, although another explanation is an increased rate of detection. The Spanish Registry (1994–2009) noted that the proportion of kidney biopsies with ATIN increased from 3.6% to 10.5% over the duration of the study.[146–148,150] Similar findings are reported in other studies.[151]

Medications are now the leading cause of ATIN in the United States, Europe, and other developed countries. Although ATIN can occur in all age groups, it appears to be more common in older individuals. The increase in the number of ATIN diagnoses in the Spanish Registry was driven primarily by older patients (12.3%) versus younger patients (1.6%).[146] A U.S. study reported that the proportion of biopsies showing ATIN in the elderly was 19%, which is higher than seen in the general population.[147] It may be that the increase in biopsy-proven ATIN seen in the elderly patients reflects either polypharmacy with greater drug exposure or other inciting factors in this group.

### CLINICAL HISTORY

The clinical presentation of ATIN in patients is quite varied and often challenging to clinicians trying to sort out the correct diagnosis. The presentation can be hospital-acquired AKI, a subacute decline in kidney function in hospitalized or outpatients, or only abnormal urinary findings such as hematuria, pyuria, or proteinuria.[152,153] The classically taught clinical manifestations of fever, skin rash, arthralgia, and eosinophilia are rarely seen (Table 35.4). The "triad" of ATIN (fever, rash, and eosinophilia) occurs in only approximately 5%–10% of unselected patients and should not be relied on

**Table 35.3 Kidney Biopsy Databases Reporting Acute Interstitial Nephritis From Various Countries**

| Author, Country | Study Period | Total Biopsies Performed | Overall Incidence of AIN | Incidence of AIN in AKI |
|---|---|---|---|---|
| Haas et al., USA[147] | 1991–1998 | 259 | N/R | 18.6% |
| Gesualdo et al., Italy[148] | 1996–2000 | 14,607 | 5.3% | NR |
| Davison and Jones, UK[149] | 1978–1998 | 7161 | 2.2% | 6.5% |
| Muriithi et al., USA[150] | 1993–2011 | 7575 | 1.8% | NR |
| Clarkson et al., USA[151] | 1988–2001 | 2598 | 2.6% | 10.3% |
| Valluri et al., Scotland[252] | 2000–2012 | 3604 | 4.7% | NR |
| Prendecki et al., UK[253] | 1998–2011 | 3983 | 5.9% | NR |

*AIN,* Acute interstitial nephritis; *AKI,* acute kidney injury; *NR,* not reported.

**Table 35.4 Clinical and Laboratory Manifestations of Acute Interstitial Nephritis**

| Manifestation | Comments |
|---|---|
| **Clinical Features** | |
| Manifestations of allergic reaction: fever, rash, and eosinophilia | Triad is seen in <5%–10% |
| History of exposure to a potential culprit drug | |
| Evidence of underlying systemic disease: lungs and skin in sarcoidosis, uveitis in TINU, skin/joint manifestations in SLE, dry eyes in Sjögren syndrome | |
| Age of onset | TINU and SLE more common in the young, drug-induced more common in elderly |
| **Laboratory Tests** | |
| Subacute or acute rise in glomerular filtration markers (serum creatinine and blood urea nitrogen) | |
| Elevated inflammatory markers (ESR, CRP) | Not specific for ATIN |
| Eosinophilia | Inconsistent finding, more common in drug-induced AIN |
| **Elevated IgE level** | |
| Sterile pyuria, white blood cell casts, renal tubular epithelial cells, and granular casts | Limited sensitivity: urine sediment is normal in approximately 20% of biopsy-proven ATIN |
| Hematuria, rare red blood cell cast | RBC casts are rare |
| Low-grade (tubular) proteinuria (<1 g/day) | |
| Urine eosinophils | Sensitivity 20%–30%, specificity 70%–90%, PPV 15%–30%, NPV approximately 85% |
| Fanconi syndrome (glycosuria, phosphaturia, bicarbonaturia, and aminoaciduria) | Not specific or sensitive for ATIN |
| Distal tubulopathy (distal RTA, nephrogenic diabetes insipidus, sodium wasting) | Not specific or sensitive for ATIN |
| **Imaging Tests** | |
| Gallium-67 scintigraphy shows enhanced renal uptake | Limited utility due to poor sensitivity and specificity |
| FDG-PET scanning shows enhanced renal uptake | A few positive cases reported, but studies are lacking |
| Renal ultrasound and CT scan, may show increased kidney size and echogenicity | Findings nonspecific but helpful to rule out other causes of kidney disease |
| **Kidney Biopsy** | |
| Renal histology reveals inflammatory interstitial infiltrate with tubulitis (and sometimes granuloma) | Gold standard for making the diagnosis |

*AIN,* Acute interstitial nephritis; *ATIN,* acute tubulointerstitial nephritis; *CRP,* C-reactive protein; *CT,* computed tomography; *ESR,* erythrocyte sedimentation rate; *FDG-PET,* 2-[$^{18}$F] fluoro-2-deoxy-D-glucose-positron emission tomography; *NPV,* negative predictive value; *PPV,* positive predictive value; *RBC,* red blood cell; *RTA,* renal tubular acidosis; *SLE,* systemic lupus erythematosus; *TINU,* tubulointerstitial nephritis and uveitis.

to influence the final diagnosis of ATIN.[152,153] In fact, this allergic presentation is more often seen in association with certain drugs, such as penicillin derivatives and sulfonamides (compared with NSAIDs), but is by no means a common finding. More commonly, nonspecific symptoms are noted with ATIN.[154,155] These include generalized malaise, fatigue, weakness, anorexia, and nausea. At times patients will describe myalgias and arthralgias, flank pain, and "feeling feverish." A pruritic skin rash may develop, raising suspicion for an allergic or drug-related process. However, these are not specific to ATIN and may be seen in many hospitalized patients with or without AKI.[152–155]

It is important to determine the presence and timing of suspected medication exposure in the clinical evaluation of the patient where ATIN is considered part of the differential diagnosis. As will subsequently be discussed, although any drug may cause ATIN, classic and common agents that should be sought are certain antimicrobial agents such as the β-lactams, sulfonamides, quinolones, and antiviral agents; antiulcer agents such as the proton pump inhibitors (PPIs) and $H_2$ antagonists; NSAIDs; anticonvulsants; and allopurinol.[154,155] Table 35.4 provides a list of selected medications that are more commonly associated with ATIN.

## PHYSICAL EXAMINATION

Physical examination sometimes points toward a diagnosis of ATIN. Low-grade or spiking fevers that occur in the absence of documented infection should raise suspicion for this diagnosis. In reality, however, it is often quite difficult to sort out such fevers in hospitalized patients who are receiving antibiotics for infection. This includes those with invasive devices in place, such as peripheral or central vein catheters, and indwelling bladder catheters. In addition, fever is not uniformly present, although it occurs more often with ATIN from methicillin and other penicillin derivatives.[145,146,151–163] A classic drug eruption, typically morbilliform and involving the trunk, can be very helpful in suggesting the possibility of drug-related ATIN. It is not a sensitive finding, however, and is frequently not present even in the setting of very severe biopsy-proven ATIN. In general, a drug-related rash is reported in approximately 15% to 50% of ATIN cases. This rash is more likely to develop following exposure with drugs that cause a hypersensitivity reaction such as the β-lactams, sulfonamides, and phenytoin. By contrast, rash is rarely seen or completely absent with drugs such as NSAIDs and PPIs.[145,158,164] Other physical examination findings described with ATIN include palpably enlarged, tender kidneys.[154,155] However, this is a rarity on examinations. In the absence of an underlying systemic illness, culprit drug exposure, and classic drug eruption, it is extremely difficult to diagnose ATIN in the setting of hospital-acquired AKI in the absence of other supportive data.

In patients with systemic diseases that have been associated with ATIN such as sarcoidosis, SLE, Sjögren syndrome, and other such entities, the presence of active end-organ involvement should raise suspicion of ATIN when renal abnormalities develop.[153,158,159] In patients with active systemic disease, clues for associated ATIN include various electrolyte acid–base disorders indicative of a tubulopathy (proximal/distal renal tubular acidosis [RTA], hyperkalemia, concentrating defects), an abnormal urinalysis or active urine sediment (hematuria, pyuria, proteinuria, white blood cell [WBC] casts), or the development of acute, chronic, or acute on CKD.[152,153,163,164] Table 35.4 notes some of the clinical clues to ATIN in the setting of a systemic disease.

## LABORATORY TESTING

In addition to the information provided by clinical history and physical examination in evaluating for possible ATIN, a number of diagnostic modalities are used. A definitive diagnosis of ATIN, especially when drug induced, remains a challenge as the available noninvasive tests lack the required accuracy.[152–154] As a result, kidney biopsy remains the gold-standard test for diagnosis. Laboratory and imaging tests employed to diagnose ATIN are listed in Table 35.4.

### Serum Creatinine Concentration

Increases in serum creatinine concentration, a marker of reduced GFR, can be rapid and indicative of severe AKI. However, the rate of rise in serum creatinine may be slow and not meet the Kidney Disease Improving Global Outcomes (KDIGO) diagnostic criteria of AKI. It is notable that up to 50% patients with kidney biopsy–proven ATIN do not meet currently accepted definitions of AKI.[149] In fact, only 57% of 107 patients diagnosed with ATIN met AKI criteria. Interestingly, >90% of these patients actually met the umbrella term of KDIGO Acute Kidney Disease (AKD) criteria, which is defined as the following: (1) KDIGO AKI criteria, (2) GFR < 60 mL/min/1.73 $m^2$ for <3 months, (3) decrease in GFR by ≥35% or increase in serum creatinine by >50% for <3 months, or (4) evidence of kidney damage for <3 months.[165] Thus clinicians must remember that an indolent rise in serum creatinine concentration does occur with ATIN and failure to recall this will lead to a delay in recognition of ATIN, which may ultimately be associated with the development of interstitial fibrosis and CKD.

### Serum Eosinophil Count

An elevated serum eosinophil count is one of the most helpful serum tests for raising suspicion of ATIN, in particular when due to an allergic or hypersensitivity reaction. Significant eosinophilia may tip the clinician off to an allergic drug reaction and may be very helpful diagnostically for patients with hospital-acquired AKI.[152–155] Despite the fact that eosinophilia also occurs in other settings, such as cancer, cholesterol emboli syndrome, and vasculitis, which may be associated with AKI, these disease processes are often clinically recognizable.[152–155] However, as with other tests utilized to evaluate for ATIN, serum eosinophils are not a sensitive or specific finding. Eosinophilia may be only modest and barely recognizable as abnormal or markedly elevated with severe allergic reactions and certain malignancies having eosinophils making up 50%–75% of the total WBC count.[166] An example is the DRESS (*d*rug *r*eaction with *e*osinophilia and *s*ystemic *s*ymptoms) syndrome and eosinophilic leukemias. As is observed with drug-related fever and associated morbilliform rash, a significant increase in serum eosinophils in the setting of ATIN is wide ranging (0%–50%), is more common with certain classes of drugs (β-lactams and sulfonamides), and may be absent despite the presence of eosinophil-dominant infiltrate on kidney biopsy.[145,161,164] As noted previously, the lack of diagnostic utility of the combination of fever, rash, and eosinophilia for ATIN is very disappointing as the triad is seen in only 5%–10% of patients.[151,161]

### Other Serum Tests

Markers of inflammation, such as erythrocyte sedimentation rate and C-reactive protein, are often elevated but are quite nonspecific and not helpful for diagnosis.[151–153,164] Increased IgE levels may be seen but are an inconsistent finding. Anemia is commonly seen in the setting of ATIN; however, this abnormality is nonspecific and widely prevalent in numerous hospitalized patients, especially those with isolated AKI or AKI superimposed on CKD.[151–153] Anemia likely results from a number of processes, including loss of erythropoietin production from kidney injury, as well as hyporesponsiveness or resistance to erythropoietin from concurrent inflammation and/or infection.[151–153] Liver function tests (LFTs) may also be abnormal in patients suffering from ATIN, primarily due to an associated medication-induced hepatitis. However, this finding is exceedingly rare in ATIN, and multiple other disease processes can elevate LFTs in hospitalized patients. Thus the vast majority of these tests are not otherwise useful for diagnosis.

### Serum Markers of Tubular Dysfunction

It is possible that tubular injury and abnormalities in serum markers of tubular dysfunction may precede the rise in serum creatinine concentration and development of AKI. Early serum findings of renal tubular dysfunction include hypokalemia/hyperkalemia or RTA. The alert clinician may notice the development of serum chemistry abnormalities that are suggestive of tubular injury and dysfunction. As an example, hyperkalemia with a hyperchloremic metabolic acidosis, which appears out of proportion to the severity of kidney failure, raises the specter of an associated tubulointerstitial injury.[152,153,164] In addition to these serum abnormalities, other patterns of tubulointerstitial injury such as a Fanconi syndrome, salt-wasting nephropathy, distal RTA, and urinary concentrating defects may be observed with ATIN.[152,153,164] A classic example of distal RTA associated with ATIN is Sjögren syndrome.

### Urinalysis

Urinalysis is considered an important diagnostic test for AKI and is commonly used to understand the underlying cause of AKI in hospitalized patients. This test can provide helpful clues suggestive of ATIN for the clinician.[152–155,167,168] Because of the nature of tubulointerstitial kidney injury, some urinary abnormality is often present. In general, some degree of low-grade proteinuria is almost universally (>90%) present in most forms of ATIN and generally reflects tubular proteinuria.[150,169] Trace, 1, or 2+ proteinuria may be seen on the dipstick, unless there is concomitant glomerular injury, such as minimal-change disease or membranous nephropathy associated with NSAIDs, or an underlying glomerulopathy upon which ATIN develops (diabetic nephropathy, and so on).[152,153] Quantifying the amount of proteinuria with a spot urine protein-to-creatinine ratio generally shows levels <1 g of protein/day, consistent with "tubular" proteinuria.[145,152,153]

Hematuria is seen in approximately 50% of cases, but is more common, up to 90%, with drugs such as methicillin and the β-lactam class.[152,153,164,167,168] Pyuria may be seen; sterile pyuria should always raise the specter of ATIN in the appropriate clinical setting. Urinary leukocytes are considered a fairly common urinary abnormality in the setting of ATIN. Early publications on methicillin-associated ATIN noted that leukocytes were present in up to 90% of cases.[161,166] In fact, one study noted that approximately 80% of patients with drug-induced ATIN had dipstick pyuria.[170] By contrast, in other forms of ATIN (including drug-induced forms), leukocytes are noted in ≤50% of cases.[159,162] Urinary findings described in 21 cases of biopsy-proven drug-induced ATIN noted red blood cells (RBCs) in 43% and WBCs in 57% of patients, respectively.[167] Thus these studies confirm that although hematuria and leukocyturia are relatively common, clinicians should not erroneously exclude ATIN as a cause of AKI when either hematuria or pyuria is absent.

### Urine Eosinophil Test

One of the most common diagnostic tests used for ATIN is the urine eosinophil test. In fact, most clinicians practice with the belief that eosinophiluria is part and parcel of drug-induced ATIN. This clinical approach is based on an early description of nine cases of methicillin-associated ATIN that tested positive for eosinophils, whereas none of 43 patients with AKI from another diagnosis had eosinophiluria.[171] In a subsequent small study, eosinophiluria was observed in six of nine patients with drug-induced ATIN.[172] These two small studies form the basis of the widespread use of urine eosinophils for evaluation of ATIN.

Following these two small, positive studies, variable sensitivities and specificities of this test in evaluating for ATIN were noted, raising questions as to the utility of eosinophiluria. As poor visualization of urinary eosinophils was considered a major problem, the Hansel stain rather than Wright stain was pursued to improve test sensitivity.[173] This was based on the excellent accuracy of this stain in visualizing eosinophils in nasal, bronchial, and ocular secretions of patients with allergic diseases. A small study using this stain noted an improvement in sensitivity to 91%; however, further studies of the Hansel stain[174,175] demonstrated various ranges of sensitivity and specificity.[35] The crux of the problem with this test is that many disorders other than ATIN are associated with significant eosinophiluria. These include cystitis, prostatitis, pyelonephritis, atheroembolic disease, ATN, rapidly progressive glomerulonephritis, allergic granulomatosis, bladder tumors, ileal conduits, and asthma.[175] Many of these also present with AKI.

Despite the unclear utility of the urine eosinophil test, clinicians commonly order this test to evaluate for ATIN in patients with AKI, in particular hospital-acquired AKI. Erroneous decisions based on potentially incorrect results may result—treating with steroids when ATIN is not present or allowing a patient with drug-induced ATIN to continue on the culprit medication. This approach stems from results generated by small studies with many flaws, in particular, the lack of a gold standard for ATIN diagnosis. One of the largest and best studies of the urine eosinophil test was conducted over an 18-year period at the Mayo Clinic on 566 patients who had both urinary eosinophil testing and kidney biopsies performed within the same week.[170] Approximately two-thirds of the biopsy-confirmed ATIN cases were negative for urinary eosinophils. When urinary eosinophils ≥1% was used as a positive test, this assay identified only approximately 31% of ATIN cases with a similar sensitivity for ATN (29.0%). The specificity of urinary eosinophils (>1%) for ATIN was 68.2%. A 5% urinary eosinophil cutoff improved specificity (91.2%) but with a concomitant decreased sensitivity (19.8%). Thus urinary eosinophils should no longer be considered a useful biomarker for ATIN and we recommend abandoning this diagnostic test.[170,176]

### Urine Microscopy and Sediment Examination

Thorough examination of the spun urine sediment performed by an experienced nephrologist is considered to be fairly accurate and tantamount to a "liquid biopsy" of the kidney. In the absence of pyelonephritis, urinary leukocytes and RBCs, along with WBC casts observed in the urine of AKI patients, are highly suggestive of ATIN.[145,152,153] Unfortunately, WBC casts are not necessarily specific for ATIN as they may be rarely seen with acute glomerulonephritis and acute papillary necrosis.[145,152,153,155] Other urinary sediment findings also seen with ATIN include renal tubular epithelial cells and casts and granular casts. Tubular epithelial cells and casts reflect tubular cell injury that develops from tubulitis and invading inflammatory cells. In addition, numerous hyaline and granular casts were observed in 18 of 21 patients with biopsy-proven drug-induced ATIN.[167] A surprising finding in this study was the presence of RBC casts in 26% of patients and WBC casts in only 14% of the cases. Furthermore, approximately 20% of patients with ATIN can manifest a normal urinary sediment.[145,152,153] Thus clinicians should not mistakenly exclude ATIN as a cause of AKI in the absence of pyuria or WBC casts.

### Urine Chemistries

Urine chemistries are commonly used in the evaluation of AKI. Urine concentrations of sodium (Na) and urea examined alone or as FEs of Na (FENa) or urea (FEurea) are widely used to assess AKI patients.[168] With some notable exceptions, urine chemistries' greatest utility is in distinguishing prerenal azotemia from ATN, whereas they are unhelpful for ATIN. Patients with ATIN may have FENa values that are either above or below 1%.[154,155,168] Although FEurea has not been widely examined in this setting, there is no reason to believe it offers any advantage over FENa.[168] Thus urine chemistries have no role in the evaluation of ATIN.

### Novel Urinary Biomarkers

In the field of AKI the role of novel biomarkers in the early diagnosis and prognosis of AKI has been intensely studied. Novel markers of tubular dysfunction, such as monocyte chemoattractant protein-1 (MCP-1), neutrophil gelatinase-associated lipocalin (NGAL), α1-microglobulin (α1-MG), and N-acetyl-β-D-glucosaminidase (NAG), have been shown to be elevated in ATIN.[177] However, they have only been studied in drug-induced ATIN patients in comparison with healthy controls,[177] so their value in discriminating between ATIN and other causes of AKI is unknown. Although novel and traditional tubulointerstitial biomarkers, such as urine microalbumin, α1-MG, matrix metalloproteinase (MMP)-2, MMP-9, urine NGAL, retinol-binding protein, and NAG, correlate with renal prognosis in chronic tubulointerstitial nephritis (CTIN),[178–180] they have not been adequately studied in ATIN.

### Lymphocyte Transformation Test

The lymphocyte transformation test is largely used to evaluate and detect culprit allergens (from several potential candidates) in nonrenal drug-hypersensitivity reactions.[181] The test detects in vitro activation of T cells and measures their proliferation when mixed with nonlethal doses of drug. This test is based on the hypothesis that drugs can directly interact with T-cell receptors in the absence of previous metabolism or need for protein binding. Based on this hypothesis, this test may possibly detect the exact etiology of drug-induced ATIN. Its potential advantages include high specificity (85%–100%) and the ability to simultaneously test multiple drugs. However, the lymphocyte transformation test is technically challenging and highly operator dependent, is dependent on availability of drugs in their pure form, and cannot be performed in the acute stage of hypersensitivity.[181] Furthermore, drugs such as NSAIDs that do not normally go through the usual T-cell activation pathway will give false-negative results. As a result, the test is not routinely used in the clinical evaluation of suspected drug-induced ATIN.

### Imaging Tests

**Ultrasonography and CT Scanning.** Renal ultrasound and/or computed tomography (CT) scan imaging is commonly used in the setting of AKI. Kidney imaging with either ultrasonography or CT scan provides structural information such as kidney size and number, cortical echogenicity, and presence or absence of hydronephrosis, cysts, masses, or stones.[182–184] Thus the utility of these modalities lies with their exclusion of other causes of AKI. Enlarged, swollen kidneys with increased echogenicity on ultrasound are often seen with ATIN. However, this finding is not specific and can be seen with infiltrative diseases, acute tubular necrosis, acute glomerulonephritis, and other etiologies of AKI.[154,155,183,184] Renal volume was reported to be increased by up to 100% in the setting of ATIN,[185] presumably related to inflammatory cell infiltration and interstitial edema. Similarly, CT scan may show renomegaly in the setting of ATIN, but this test has the same limitations as renal ultrasound.[182–184] Overall, these imaging tests are neither sensitive nor specific for ATIN, adding little except excluding urinary tract obstruction or another structural form of kidney injury.

**$^{67}$Gallium Scanning.** Renal imaging using $^{67}$gallium scanning has been used in the evaluation of ATIN for >30 years.[186,187] This test is based on the fact that kidneys with ATIN enhance with tracer because $^{67}$gallium binds to lactoferrin, which is produced and released by and on the surface of leukocytes (primarily lymphocytes) infiltrating the renal interstitium.[161] Tracer uptake in the kidneys, which is measured at 48 to 72 hours following $^{67}$gallium injection, is graded on a scale of 0 to 3+ and is compared with spinal intensity.[187] In general, a scan result of 2+ or greater renal intensity is considered positive. An animal model that examined the utility of gallium scanning in diagnosing ATIN supported this notion. $^{67}$Gallium scanning in rats was highly accurate in differentiating experimentally induced ATIN from both drug-induced ATN and normal rat kidneys.[186]

However, use of $^{67}$gallium scintigraphy in humans to evaluate ATIN is marked by conflicting results. Although initial studies reflected excellent sensitivity (100%) in patients with biopsy-proven ATIN,[187] subsequent studies revealed lower sensitivities ranging from 58% to 69%[188,189] with a test specificity of only 50%–60%.[152,153,161] The major limiting factor of this modality is that positive scan results are seen with other inflammatory conditions, such as pyelonephritis, renal atheroemboli, and glomerulonephritis, as well as noninflammatory condition such as ATN and normal kidney tissue.[152,153,161] Renal scanning with $^{67}$gallium scintigraphy may be useful in differentiating ATIN from ATN when kidney biopsy is high risk or is refused by the patient. However, the limitations of this imaging modality should be considered prior to using it in such patients.

**FDG-PET Scanning.** A noninvasive imaging test, the 2-[$^{18}$F] fluoro-2-deoxy-D-glucose-positron emission tomography (FDG-PET) scan is used primarily to evaluate malignant disease but has been recently used to diagnose ATIN.[165] Positive FDG-PET scans were noted in two patients with severe AKI due to biopsy-proven ATIN (one of the patients had a negative gallium scan).[190] A third patient with severe AKI from crescentic glomerulonephritis had a negative FDG-PET scan. Following treatment and resolution of ATIN in the two patients, repeat FDG-PET scans were negative. Uptake of tracer in this setting is based on the premise that FDG accumulates in the lymphocytes, macrophages, neutrophils, and fibroblasts of inflammatory lesions.[190] However, this modality cannot be considered a useful test to diagnose ATIN until its true utility is substantiated in a large group of patients.

## DIFFERENTIAL DIAGNOSIS

Evaluation of acute and subacute increases in serum creatinine concentration has become more standardized through the use of definitions such as the *r*isk-*i*njury-*f*ailure-*l*oss-*e*nd *s*tage (RIFLE), Acute Kidney Injury Network (AKIN), and KDIGO AKI criteria to diagnose and classify this entity.[156,157,191] The KDIGO criteria include a category, AKD, that includes AKI and increases in serum creatinine or other renal-focused abnormalities that do not otherwise fit into the AKI diagnostic criteria. As previously noted, ATIN often falls into both the AKI and non-AKI AKD definitions. Regardless, these criteria do not permit differentiation of the various types of AKI or AKD, including prerenal AKI, ATN, ATIN, and other entities, which ultimately require different management approaches.

As previously discussed, ATIN may present clinically as AKI or subacute increases in serum creatinine concentration often associated with other abnormal laboratory findings, in particular urinalysis and urine microscopy abnormalities. Clinicians frequently encounter these clinical presentations in patients admitted to the general hospital wards and the intensive care units, as well as in the outpatient setting.[191] Although the majority of hospital-acquired AKI cases are due to either prerenal AKI or ATN, unrecognized ATIN is likely the third most common cause and must be considered in the differential diagnosis.[147,152,153] Other potential causes of an acute/subacute serum creatinine concentration rise include various forms of immune-complex and non–immune-complex glomerulonephritis, pauci-immune vasculitis, renal-limited thrombotic microangiopathies, several non-AIN tubulointerstitial diseases (renal atheroemboli, cast nephropathy, infiltrative diseases such as lymphoma and leukemia, and so on), and obstructive nephropathy. It is notable that acute or subacute increases in serum creatinine without an obvious cause can be due to biopsy-proven ATIN in a significant percentage of cases (10% to 27%).[143,145,151–153,192,193]

Differentiating ATIN from these other causes of AKI requires a thorough clinical history, physical examination, certain laboratory data, and targeted imaging tests (Table 35.4). Ultimately, kidney biopsy to examine the underlying histology is required to accurately make a definitive diagnosis and guide therapy. The clinical and histologic features that help distinguish between different causes of ATIN are summarized in Table 35.5.

## RENAL PATHOLOGY

Diagnosis of ATIN relies on obtaining an optimal sample of kidney tissue, which includes both renal cortical and medullary tissue, via percutaneous kidney biopsy. The type of inflammatory cells, presence or absence of granuloma, interstitial edema and/or fibrosis, and other features vary based on the underlying etiology.

### Tubulointerstitial Histopathology

The characteristic findings of ATIN are found predominantly in the tubulointerstitium, with the key findings of interstitial inflammation and tubulitis present. Infiltration of the renal interstitium with inflammatory cells (Fig. 35.1) is accompanied by infiltration of inflammatory cells into renal tubules, a process called "tubulitis," and variable amounts of acute tubular injury.[194] In addition, there is some degree of interstitial edema and/or fibrosis. ATIN generally develops over days to weeks. When recognized and treated late, it can transition to a chronic form of interstitial nephritis, characterized by interstitial fibrosis and tubular atrophy developing over months to years.[194]

The interstitial infiltrate is often composed of mononuclear cells, with a predominance of lymphocytes (T cells), which are primarily $CD4^+$ and $CD8^+$ T cells. Monocytes/macrophages, intermixed with plasma cells, B cells, small numbers of eosinophils, and possibly neutrophils are also present within the interstitium.[194–196] The composition of the interstitial infiltrate may be helpful in determining the etiology of ATIN. For example, if a significant number of neutrophils are found within the infiltrate, the possibility of pyelonephritis (especially

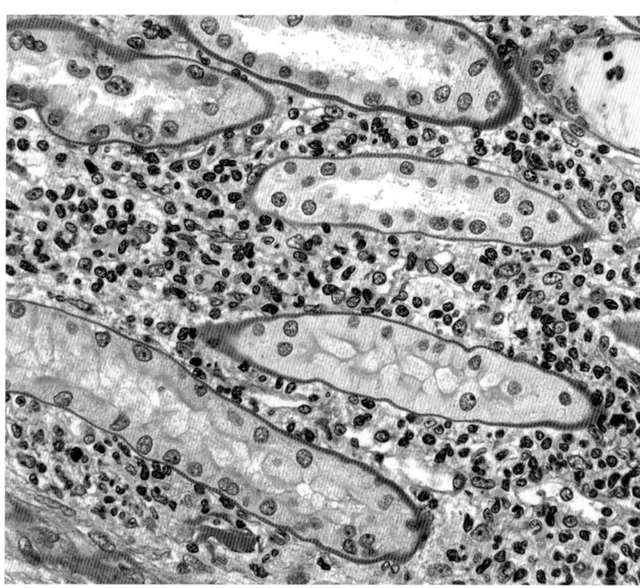

**Fig. 35.1** Renal histology observed in acute tubulointerstitial nephritis highlighting the inflammatory infiltrate. Periodic acid–Schiff stain. (From Perazella MA. Clinical approach to diagnosing acute and chronic tubulointerstitial disease. *Adv Chronic Kidney Dis*. 2017;24:57–63.)

**Table 35.5 Clinical, Laboratory, and Histologic Features to Help in Differential Diagnosis of ATIN**

| Etiology of ATIN | Clinical and Laboratory Features | Distinguishing Histopathologic Features |
|---|---|---|
| **Drug Induced** | More common in older individuals | Mixed inflammatory interstitial infiltration |
| Proton pump inhibitors and $H_2$ antagonists | Long latent period; few typical clinical features | Eosinophils may be present; rarely granulomas |
| Nonsteroidal antiinflammatory drugs | May be associated with nephrotic-range proteinuria, long latent period, allergic manifestations are rarely present | Eosinophils are often absent; glomerular lesions of minimal-change disease and membranous glomerulopathy rarely accompany the tubulointerstitial lesion |
| β-Lactams, sulfonamides, anticonvulsants | Systemic allergic manifestations of rash, eosinophilia, and fever are more common, especially with methicillin, penicillin; short latent period | Mixed inflammatory infiltrate commonly with abundant interstitial eosinophils; tubulitis and granulomas may be present |
| **Immune Mediated** | More common in younger individuals | Mononuclear cell infiltration |
| SLE | Systemic features of SLE; hematuria, proteinuria, pyuria, white cell casts; SLE serologies positive; hypocomplementemia | Usually seen in association with other renal manifestations of SLE, such as focal or diffuse proliferative glomerulonephritis and "full house" immunofluorescence staining pattern; rarely seen without glomerular disease |
| Sarcoidosis | Hypercalcemia, hypercalciuria, urinary concentrating defects, nephrocalcinosis, nephrolithiasis, and acute or chronic kidney disease | Focal lymphocytic infiltrate and interstitial noncaseating granulomas composed of giant cells, histiocytes, and lymphocytes |
| Sjögren syndrome | Dry eyes and dry mouth; positive serologies | Lymphoplasmacytic infiltrate, acute tubular injury |
| IgG4 related | Multisystem disorder with elevated serum IgG4 level involving salivary glands, pancreas, retroperitoneum, and kidneys; affects middle-aged men | Lymphoplasmacytic interstitial infiltrate with a predominance of IgG4-positive plasma cells and interstitial fibrosis in a "storiform" pattern |
| Tubulointerstitial nephritis and uveitis syndrome | Uveitis characterized by painful red eyes, photophobia; common in young women | Mixed inflammatory infiltrate (including eosinophils) with noncaseating granuloma formation |

*ATIN,* Acute tubulointerstitial nephritis; *SLE,* systemic lupus erythematosus.

with neutrophils forming microabscesses) or other infectious agents should be considered. An eosinophilic infiltrate is often present with drug-induced ATIN, which should be suspected when >10 eosinophils per ×20 field are observed. However, eosinophilic infiltration may also be present in several other etiologies of ATIN such as tubulointerstitial nephritis and uveitis (TINU) and IgG4-related kidney disease.[194–196] Importantly, the absence of interstitial eosinophils does not exclude a drug as causative, particularly in ATIN cases associated with PPIs and NSAIDs.

Tubulitis is diagnosed when lymphocytes are seen crossing the TBM in proximity to and crossing into/through the outer and inner aspects of the TBM.[194–196] Physiologically this suggests extension of the interstitial inflammatory process into the tubular epithelial cells. Tubulitis is often accompanied by tubular degenerative changes, including apoptotic figures, prominent nucleoli, luminal ectasia, irregular luminal contours, cytoplasmic simplification, and loss of brush border.[194–197] These tubular changes can be focal or diffuse and often start with denudation of the TBM as opposed to acute tubular injury, where injury often involves the villi of tubular epithelial cells with their subsequent apoptosis or necrosis.

Granulomas involving the interstitium may also be found in ATIN but is a relatively rare finding.[198,199] Granulomas may be caseating with infectious causes, such as tuberculosis, and noncaseating with a number of causes, including drugs, sarcoidosis (Fig. 35.2), and idiopathic etiologies.[198,199] Drug-induced ATIN can present pathologically as granulomatous interstitial nephritis, which is marked by the presence of "hypersensitivity granulomas" that are composed of reactive epithelioid histiocytes (macrophages) and multinucleated giant cells.[198,199] Medications more commonly associated with granuloma formation include anticonvulsants, antibiotics, NSAIDs, allopurinol, checkpoint inhibitors, and diuretics.

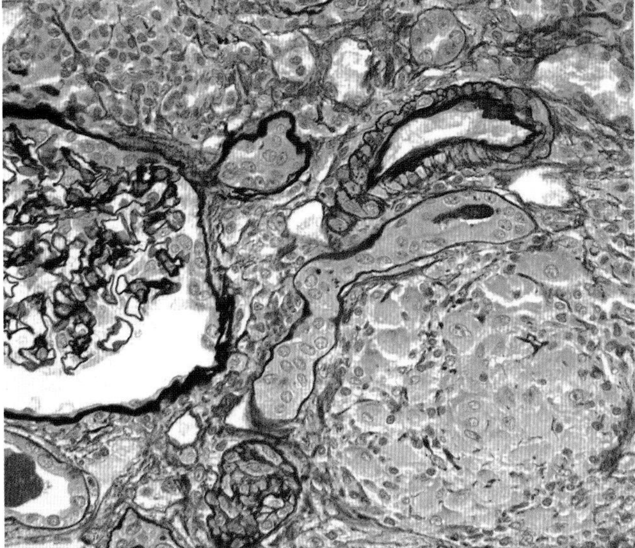

**Fig. 35.2** Renal histology in sarcoidosis highlighting the inflammatory infiltrate and nonnecrotizing granuloma. Jones silver stain. (From Perazella MA. Clinical approach to diagnosing acute and chronic tubulointerstitial disease. *Adv Chronic Kidney Dis*. 2017;24:57–63.)

Immunohistochemistry of renal tissue may rarely show findings that point to the pathomechanism of ATIN. Immune-complex deposits are relatively uncommon but may be present in SLE nephritis with tubulointerstitial disease and drugs associated with ATIN such as methicillin,[200] where linear or granular staining for IgG and C3 is present on TBMs (anti-TBM antibodies). Significant IgG4 positivity in plasma cells within the interstitial infiltrate is observed with IgG4-related kidney disease.[201–203]

#### Blood Vessels and Glomeruli

In the absence of underlying kidney disease, glomeruli and the renal vasculature are typically spared in ATIN. Changes related to underlying CKD, such as diabetic nephropathy, hypertension, and other renal lesions, might be seen with ATIN superimposed on these findings, especially when due to a drug.[194–196] Kidney biopsy performed late in the course of ATIN may reveal significant interstitial fibrosis, and tubular atrophy with dilated tubular lumens. In certain forms of drug-induced ATIN, such as following NSAID exposure, glomerular lesions such as minimal-change disease or membranous nephropathy may also be observed.[204]

### GENERAL TREATMENT PRINCIPLES

Treatment of ATIN hinges on identification of the underlying cause that is driving the interstitial disease. In rheumatologic disease, treatment of the underlying inflammatory condition improves kidney function. In the setting of infection-related ATIN, eradication of the infectious agent enhances kidney recovery. Early treatment is helpful in limiting chronic tubulointerstitial injury and fibrosis regardless of the cause. One of the best examples of this is drug-induced ATIN. The mainstay of management of drug-induced ATIN is early diagnosis, followed by rapid identification of the offending agent and its prompt discontinuation.[144] Use of immunosuppressive agents to quell the inflammatory lesion is also an attractive option (discussed in the "Drug-Induced ATIN" section). Immunosuppressant therapy is considered standard of care for many immune disorders, including sarcoidosis, Sjögren syndrome, IgG4-related kidney disease, and TINU.[201–203,205–209] However, although widely used for drug-induced ATIN, the supporting evidence for immunosuppressive agents is limited and controversial. In addition to these maneuvers, good supportive care is important. Blood pressure control, avoidance of nephrotoxin exposure, and management of any CKD issues improve overall patient outcomes. The following section on etiology of ATIN provides more details about specific treatment.

## SPECIFIC ETIOLOGIES OF ATIN AND THEIR FEATURES

Multiple causes of ATIN exist, including drugs, infections, and systemic and idiopathic diseases (Table 35.6). Prior to the widespread use of antimicrobial agents, infections were the leading cause of ATIN. In the United States, Europe, and other developed countries, medications are now the most common cause, whereas drugs and infection are equally prevalent causes of ATIN in developing countries.[210]

### DRUG-INDUCED ATIN

Medications account for >70% of AIN in developed countries and approximately 50% in developing countries.[169,210,211]

**Table 35.6 Common Causes of Acute Tubulointerstitial Nephritis**

| Class | Specific Causative Agents |
|---|---|
| **Drugs** | |
| Antimicrobials | β-Lactams (penicillin and derivatives, cephalosporins), quinolones, ethambutol, isoniazid, macrolides, rifampin, sulfonamides, tetracycline, vancomycin, antiviral agents (acyclovir, foscarnet, indinavir, and atazanavir) |
| NSAIDs and COX-2 inhibitors | Almost all agents |
| Gastrointestinal drugs | Proton pump inhibitors, $H_2$ antagonists, mesalamine, sulfasalazine |
| Diuretics | Furosemide, thiazides, triamterene |
| Anticancer agents | Ifosfamide, tyrosine kinase inhibitors, pemetrexed, immune checkpoint inhibitors |
| Miscellaneous | Allopurinol, amlodipine, azathioprine, captopril, carbamazepine, clofibrate, cocaine, creatine, diltiazem, phentermine, phenytoin, pranlukast, propylthiouracil, quinine, phenindione, synthetic cannabinoids |
| **Infectious Agents** | |
| Bacteria | *Corynebacterium diphtheriae, Escherichia coli, Legionella, Staphylococcus, Streptococcus, Yersinia, Brucella, Campylobacter, Legionella* |
| Viruses | Cytomegalovirus, Epstein-Barr virus, hantaviruses, hepatitis C, herpes simplex virus, HIV, polyoma virus, adenovirus |
| Others | *Leptospira, Mycobacterium, Mycoplasma, Chlamydia,* rickettsia, syphilis, toxoplasmosis, fungi |
| **Systemic Diseases** | |
| Immune | SLE tubulointerstitial nephritis, sarcoidosis, Sjögren syndrome, IgG4-related kidney disease, TINU, ANCA-related diseases, spontaneous tubulointerstitial nephritis |
| Neoplastic | Lymphoproliferative disorders, plasma cell dyscrasias |

*ANCA,* Antineutrophil cytoplasmic antibody; *COX-2,* cyclooxygenase; *HIV,* human immunodeficiency virus; *NSAIDs,* nonsteroidal antiinflammatory drugs; *SLE,* systemic lupus erythematosus; *TINU,* tubulointerstitial nephritis and uveitis.

Although any medication may cause ATIN, certain medications do it frequently. Importantly, the list of medications is constantly expanding. As noted in Table 35.6, common culprits include antimicrobial agents, PPIs, NSAIDs, antiepileptics, and several anticancer drugs. A retrospective case series of 133 biopsies of ATIN noted that 70% were drug induced.[169] The top three drug classes identified as causes were antibiotics (49%), PPIs (14%), and NSAIDs (11%), and the top three drugs were omeprazole (12%), amoxicillin (8%), and ciprofloxacin (8%).

### Antimicrobial Agents

The β-lactam antibiotics (penicillins and cephalosporins) are commonly associated with development of ATIN as part of a hypersensitivity syndrome.[212–214] The duration of exposure to the causative β-lactam antibiotic prior to ATIN is typically relatively short, ranging from a few days to a few weeks. Fever, rash, or eosinophilia is fairly common and seen in >75% of patients. Urinary abnormalities consisting of proteinuria, pyuria, or hematuria occur in approximately 75% of affected patients. Although most patients who develop β-lactam–induced ATIN recover kidney function, CKD may also occur.[212–214]

ATIN also occurs following exposure to non–β-lactam antibiotics such as the sulfonamide antibiotics. As with β-lactam antibiotics, these drugs may be associated with hypersensitivity reactions such as fever, rash, and eosinophilia.[210–214] Transplant recipients, human immunodeficiency virus (HIV) patients, and CKD patients tend to develop sulfonamide-induced ATIN at higher rates than other patient groups, which likely relates to their frequent use in these populations and higher drug concentrations in patients with reduced kidney function.[210,215,216]

The fluoroquinolone class of antibiotics may also cause ATIN. Ciprofloxacin is the most common offender, which likely relates to its widespread use. In contrast to the sulfonamide antibiotics, the fluoroquinolone antibiotics are rarely associated with a hypersensitivity syndrome. Although ciprofloxacin is the most common causative agent, ATIN does occur with other fluoroquinolone antibiotics, including norfloxacin, ofloxacin, and levofloxacin.[210,217,218]

ATIN complicates rifampin therapy when the drug is used intermittently to treat various mycobacterial infections.[19,23,77] In contrast to other agents, rifampin-induced ATIN is dose dependent, is associated with the production of antirifampin antibodies, and is associated with hemolytic anemia, thrombocytopenia, and hepatitis. Dialysis is required in nearly two-thirds of patients that develop rifampicin-induced ATIN.[160,164,219]

Various antiviral agents have been associated with ATIN. However, they are rare when compared with antibiotics.[220,221]

### Proton Pump Inhibitors

PPIs are the mainstay of therapy for acid-related gastrointestinal disorders. They were first recognized as a cause of ATIN in 1992,[222] with numerous case reports and case series documenting the association.[223–226] A retrospective study evaluated the records of two teaching hospitals in Australia over a 10-year period (1993–2003) and noted 28 cases of biopsy-proven ATIN, 18 (64%) of which were associated with PPI use.[227] The mean time to development of this lesion after treatment with PPIs was 11 weeks. The Therapeutic Goods Administration database in Australia revealed 34 cases of "biopsy-proven ATIN," 10 cases of "suspected interstitial nephritis," 20 cases of "unexplained renal failure," and 26 cases of "renal impairment" associated with PPIs used over a 14-year period.[227] A 2007 literature review identified 73 cases of PPI-induced ATIN, 64 of which were biopsy proven.[226] All classes of PPIs were implicated, with omeprazole being the most common cause ($n = 59$).

A population-based case–control study in New Zealand patients receiving PPIs (2005–2009) examined ATIN risk that resulted in hospitalization or death.[228] Current PPI users had fivefold higher odds of developing ATIN. There was a higher absolute risk in older patients (~0.2/1000 person-years for age >60 years) compared with younger patients (0.02/1000 person-years for age 15–49 years). A second population-based study evaluated elderly Ontario residents who were hospitalized with AKI and ATIN within 120 days of initiating PPI therapy.[229] Using a propensity score-matching algorithm, both AKI and ATIN incidence and hazard ratio (HR) were higher among patients given PPIs than among controls (AKI: 13.49 vs. 5.46/1000 person-years, HR = 2.52; ATIN: 0.32 vs. 0.11/1000 person-years, HR = 3.00). These population-based studies suggest that ATIN risk is increased in PPI users, especially the elderly population.

In contrast to ATIN induced by β-lactam antibiotics, PPI-induced ATIN is often subtle and without systemic allergic manifestations, making it challenging for clinicians to readily identify the problem. In fact, a recent study showed that only about a quarter of cases were suspected prior to a kidney biopsy.[150] Approximately 10% of affected patients have fever, rash, and eosinophilia, whereas <50% have fever only, <10% have rash only, and nearly 33% have eosinophilia only.[226] Nonspecific complaints such as weakness, fatigue, malaise, and anorexia are the most often noted symptoms. The prognosis for PPI-induced ATIN is generally favorable with early diagnosis; patients rarely required renal replacement therapy, although CKD is a complication.[227] Data suggest that clinical features and available diagnostic tests are suboptimal for diagnosing PPI-induced ATIN and kidney biopsy is required for definitive diagnosis.

A potential long-term complication of PPI exposure is CKD. Case series and several observational studies support an association between PPI use and CKD.[230,231] It is notable that the associations between PPI use and CKD have remained in analyses designed to account for confounding by indication, or that PPI users are sicker than the comparison group, making them more likely to experience adverse outcomes. PPI exposure leading to CKD also has biologic plausibility—unrecognized and untreated episodes of ATIN and AKI ultimately cause chronic interstitial disease and CKD.[232]

### Nonsteroidal Antiinflammatory Agents

NSAIDs, including both selective and nonselective cyclooxygenase (COX) inhibitors, are widely used to treat pain, fever, and inflammation. Although the main limitations to NSAID therapy are gastrointestinal adverse effects, they are also associated with a diverse range of nephrotoxic effects with hemodynamic AKI being the most common.[233–239] AKI developing in the setting of NSAID exposure may also occur due to ATIN. The selective COX-2 inhibitors (celecoxib and rofecoxib) have similar nephrotoxic manifestations as the nonselective NSAIDs.[232,236,237] The clinical and pathologic findings in NSAID-induced ATIN are slightly different from that which follows treatment with β-lactam antibiotics. Fever, rash, and eosinophilia are extremely rare, and the duration of therapy prior to the development of ATIN is long, typically in the range of 6–18 months.[204] NSAIDs may rarely cause a dual lesion of ATIN along with a glomerular lesion (minimal change disease more common than membranous nephropathy).[238,239]

Renal histology seen with these drugs demonstrates interstitial inflammation and tubulitis; however, they are less intense than in other forms of drug-induced ATIN and have few or no interstitial eosinophils.[204] The clinical and pathologic differences between NSAID-induced ATIN and other agents may be due to the antiinflammatory properties of NSAIDs and possible shunting of arachidonic acid metabolites into alternative pathways that suppress immune function.[63] Rare cases of granulomatous ATIN and ATIN with TBM immune deposits have also been reported with NSAIDs.[234,235] Despite severe AKI, most patients recover kidney function following drug withdrawal and, in some cases, treatment with prednisone.

### Anticancer Agents

Chemotherapeutic agents are increasingly recognized as causing or contributing to the development of ATIN. A retrospective review at a single center found that nearly 5% of ATIN cases were associated with cancer chemotherapy.[240] Among cancer patients undergoing kidney biopsy, approximately half were diagnosed with ATIN attributed to a chemotherapeutic agent. The four leading drug causes were ifosfamide (28%), bacillus Calmette–Guérin (BCG; 12.5%), tyrosine kinase inhibitors (14%), and pemetrexed (9%). It is important to remember that ifosfamide more commonly causes acute tubular necrosis and the tyrosine kinase inhibitors are more often associated with thrombotic microangiopathy.[241]

A unique form of drug-induced ATIN has been described with the immune checkpoint inhibitors (CPIs).[242–248] Tumors can survive and evade immune surveillance by overexpressing ligands that bind inhibitory T-cell receptors (immune checkpoint molecules), thereby decreasing activated T-cell infiltration into the tumor microenvironment and inhibiting antitumor T-cell responses. Two CPI drug classes use monoclonal antibodies to target immune checkpoints, which allow immune activation of T cells to invade the tumor environment and destroy cancer cells. However, activation of the immune system is associated with T-cell invasion of solid organs including the kidneys, leading to a form of autoimmune ATIN. An adverse drug effect initially noted with the CPIs was autoimmune involvement of the lung, gastrointestinal tract, and some endocrine organs. Ipilimumab, a monoclonal antibody against CTLA-4 approved to treat advanced malignant melanoma, has now been noted to cause ATIN, with or without granuloma.[242–244] The PD-1 inhibitors (nivolumab and pembrolizumab), which are approved to treat advanced melanoma and squamous cell lung cancer, are also associated with development of ATIN.[243–247] In a recent narrative review by the Cancer and Kidney International Network Workgroup on Immune Checkpoint Inhibitors,[249] the incidence of AKI in patients treated with CPIs was estimated to be as high as 10%–30%. Patients who received combination therapy with ipilimumab and nivolumab had an increased incidence and severity of AKI compared with monotherapy. The onset is typically 2–3 months after initiating therapy with ipilimumab but can be delayed up to 12 months with PD-1 inhibitors. Multiple case reports and case series suggest that steroids are an effective treatment for this complication. In the largest series of 12 patients with biopsy-proven CPI-induced ATIN, 10 received treatment with glucocorticoids, of whom 2 and 7 had complete or partial improvement in kidney function, respectively, and 2 patients were not given steroids and had no improvement in renal function.[244]

### Immunosuppressive Therapy of Drug-Induced AIN

As the use of corticosteroids in the setting of drug-induced ATIN is an important and controversial topic, it is briefly reviewed. The immunologic mechanism causing ATIN and extensive inflammatory infiltrate on kidney biopsy make immunosuppressive therapy a biologically plausible treatment. However, the existing evidence is limited and derived from retrospective studies rather than randomized controlled trials.

These retrospective studies reveal conflicting results about benefits of corticosteroid therapy in drug-induced ATIN (Table 35.7).[151,169,250–253] In these studies, the decision to use steroids was based on clinical judgment, which increased the risk for bias (potentially for or against steroids). Furthermore, the studies were all small and underpowered to detect any potential steroid benefit. Although these studies provide low-level evidence, they do suggest that a trial of corticosteroids in the subgroups of patients identified early (<2 weeks) without significant scarring on kidney biopsy and without significant contraindication to steroid use should be considered. Our approach is to first discontinue the offending agent. Then if kidney function does not improve within 5 days of drug discontinuation, steroid therapy should be considered. In our opinion, documentation of ATIN with kidney biopsy is preferable in all cases that are thought to be due to drugs, not only to establish the diagnosis before a potentially harmful therapy but also to evaluate the degree of scarring and possibility of response. Those responding to therapy may be continued for 4–8 weeks, whereas in the absence of response within 3–4 weeks, steroids should be promptly tapered off. A reasonable approach is to start therapy with either 3 days of intravenous pulse steroids (250–500 mg) or prednisone at 1 mg/kg. As corticosteroid therapy may not always be effective or well tolerated, other agents have rarely been used for ATIN. A 4-week trial of these agents may not be an unreasonable approach in patients where immunosuppressive therapy is deemed necessary, but glucocorticoids are not optimal.

## INFECTIONS

Prior to widespread antibiotic use, streptococcus and diphtheria infections caused inflammatory reactions within the kidney. Subsequently, infections have become an uncommon cause of ATIN in the developed world, accounting for <5% of biopsy-proven cases.[210,211] Infection may injure the tubulointerstitium either directly by renal invasion as in pyelonephritis or indirectly by an immune-mediated mechanism. Bacterial pyelonephritis should be suspected when the interstitial infiltrate consists predominantly of neutrophils and is confined to a single renal pyramid, although it becomes more diffuse when occurring in the setting of urinary obstruction. CT scanning demonstrates a wedge-shaped area of inflammation, which supports pyelonephritis rather than an allergic form of ATIN.

**Table 35.7 Selected Studies of Corticosteroid Therapy in Acute Tubulointerstitial Nephritis**

| | Sample Size | | Peak sCr (mg/dL) | | Final sCr (mg/dL) | | | |
|---|---|---|---|---|---|---|---|---|
| **Author, Year** | Steroid | Control | Steroid | Control | Steroid | Control | **Follow-Up (months)** | **Comment** |
| Clarkson et al., 2004[151] | 26 | 16 | 7.9 | 6.1 | 1.6 | 1.6 | 12 | Patients received steroids late (median delay >3 weeks) after diagnosis. |
| Gonzalez et al., 2008[250] | 52 | 9 | 5.9 | 4.9 | 2.1 | 3.7 | 19 | Patients treated with steroids with complete recovery had shorter delay in steroid onset (13 days) as compared with those without complete recovery (34 days). |
| Raza et al., 2012[251] | 37 | 12 | 6.5 | 5.2 | 2.8 | 3.4 | 19 | $P < .05$ for eGFR improvement for steroid versus control. No difference in renal outcomes based on steroid timing. |
| Muriithi et al., 2014[169] | 83 | 12 | 3.0 | 4.5 | 1.4 | 1.5 | 6 | Steroid-treated patients had superior renal outcomes with early versus late steroid therapy. |
| Valluri et al., 2015[252] | 73 | 51 | 4.03 | 3.16 | NR | NR | 12 | Steroid-treated patients had complete recovery (48%) versus control group (41%); final sCr not significantly different at 1 year. |
| Prendecki et al., 2016[253] | 158 | 29 | 20.5 mL/min (eGFR) | 25 mL/min (eGFR) | 43 mL/min (eGFR) | 24 mL/min (eGFR) | 24 | Steroid-treated patient has significantly better eGFR at 2 years and less dialysis (5.1% vs. 24.1%). Dose, duration, and time to steroid treatment initiation were variable. |

*eGFR,* Estimated glomerular filtration rate; *NR,* not reported; *sCr,* serum creatinine concentration.

ATIN has been also associated with a variety of other infectious agents. These include tuberculosis, leptospirosis, legionellosis, histoplasmosis, *Candida* infection, mycoplasmosis, rickettsial fever, babesiosis, and several viruses—cytomegalovirus, hantavirus, adenovirus, BK virus, and Epstein-Barr virus.[253–265] Tuberculosis manifests as ATIN with caseating granulomas, but noncaseating granulomas can be seen.[253,254] Histoplasmosis may present with noncaseating granulomatous interstitial nephritis.[262] Leptospirosis is a classic example of invasive ATIN where the spirochete enters the bloodstream through the mucosa and migrates into the tubulointerstitium, where the organism induces inflammation and tubulointerstitial injury.[257,258] Hantavirus is associated with an inflammatory infiltrate and edema of the interstitium. Interstitial hemorrhage accompanies renal inflammation and is associated with gross or microscopic hematuria.[255] Treatment focuses on antimicrobial treatment of underlying infection. Immunosuppressive agents are not typically used.

## SYSTEMIC DISEASES

### Immunologic Disorders

A variety of autoimmune disorders may cause ATIN. For the most part they are more common in the young as compared with older patients. A number of autoimmune diseases cross over from rheumatology to nephrology due to renal involvement; those that are associated with ATIN include SLE, sarcoidosis, Sjögren syndrome, and TINU.[211,266–272] Lupus nephritis can have ATIN alone or more commonly is associated with glomerular disease. Immune-complex deposits within the TBM drive the tubulointerstitial inflammatory lesion.

Renal sarcoidosis includes a variety of manifestations, including hypercalcemia, hypercalciuria, nephrocalcinosis, nephrolithiasis, and various glomerular lesions.[211,266,267] ATIN is the most common intrinsic kidney lesion with sarcoidosis and is characterized by a diffuse inflammatory interstitial infiltrate that is composed of lymphocytes (T cells) sometimes with noncaseating granulomas (Fig. 35.2). Steroids are an effective therapy for sarcoidosis. However, not all cases have a complete response with many patients having partial remission and sometimes no renal improvement.[211,266,267] As a result, CKD may be a long-term complication. Other immunosuppressive agents have been used for steroid-intolerant and steroid-dependent cases.

Idiopathic or secondary Sjögren syndrome is a systemic illness with multiorgan involvement characterized by lymphoplasmacytic infiltration.[268,269] Although immune-complex glomerular disease rarely occurs, kidney involvement with

ATIN is far more common and ranges from 15% to 67%.[268,269] ATIN is lymphocyte dominant and is associated with tubular atrophy, tubulitis, and variable degrees of interstitial fibrosis. Tubular involvement is clinically manifested as various tubulopathies, in particular a distal RTA. The optimal therapy for ATIN in Sjögren syndrome is unknown. Immunosuppression is generally used and may include steroids, azathioprine, cyclophosphamide, or mycophenolic acid.[268,269]

Other immune-related disorders that primarily affect the renal microvasculature and glomeruli may also have an associated ATIN lesion.[270,273–275] Examples include anti-glomerular basement membrane antibody disease (i.e., Goodpasture disease), immune-complex diseases (SLE or IgA nephropathy), or antineutrophil cytoplasmic antibody (ANCA)-related pauci-immune vasculitides.[270,273–275] The presence of a concomitant active tubulointerstitial lesion with lymphocytes, plasma cells, eosinophils, and macrophages is not uncommon.

#### Tubulointerstitial Nephritis and Uveitis Syndrome

TINU is a rare condition of unclear etiology that presents most frequently in adolescent girls, but may appear in adulthood and rarely in the elderly.[272,276,277] It consists of a clinical syndrome that primarily involves the eyes and kidneys.[272,276,277] Uveitis manifests with painful red eyes and photophobia. Weight loss, fever, anemia, and hyperglobulinemia often occur before ocular and kidney manifestations. An isolated proximal tubulopathy or Fanconi syndrome can be the initial kidney manifestation.[272,276,277] Notably, ATIN may occur before, during, or after the occurrence of uveitis. Renal histopathology reveals a mixed inflammatory infiltrate, sometimes associated with granulomas. Steroids are the mainstay of therapy for both the ocular and kidney manifestations. Therapy typically consists of 3–6 months of prednisone with a slow taper to reduce chances of relapse, which is relatively common.[272,276,277] Steroid-sparing options include mycophenolic acid, methotrexate, and cyclosporine. The mechanism and risk factors for this cause of ATIN are unknown; however, infections such as toxoplasmosis, Epstein-Barr infection, and giardiasis have been associated with TINU. No clear-cut immune or genetic cause has been described. Fortunately, treated patients have a relatively good prognosis.

#### IgG4-Related Kidney Disease

IgG4-related kidney disease is part of a relatively recently recognized group of disorders characterized by elevated serum levels of IgG4 subclass antibodies (60%), tissue deposition of IgG4, and involvement of various organ systems, including salivary glands, pancreas, retroperitoneum, and kidneys.[278–282] Middle-aged men most commonly develop this disease. IgG4-related kidney disease can be very difficult to diagnose unless the patient develops a renal lesion in the setting of known or suspected IgG4-related systemic disease. Kidney involvement from this disease is fairly wide ranging and includes acute or chronic interstitial nephritis, granulomatous ATIN, masslike kidney lesions, and obstructive nephropathy due to retroperitoneal fibrosis, which may present in the absence of hydronephrosis on imaging.[278–282] A lymphoplasmacytic interstitial infiltrate with a predominance of IgG4-positive plasma cells is observed on histology. Interstitial fibrosis with a "storiform" pattern that is typified by a cartwheel appearance of arranged fibroblasts and inflammatory cells are somewhat characteristic of this disease.[278–282] Therapy consists of long-term glucocorticoid therapy; however, steroid-sparing agents such as mycophenolic acid or rituximab have been used with some success.

### PROGNOSIS

The prognosis of ATIN is best characterized for drug-induced disease, which is generally considered reversible with early recognition and withdrawal of the offending agent. Patients with drug discontinuation within 2 weeks of disease onset are more likely to recover kidney function than those who remain on the precipitating medication for ≥3 weeks. However, renal recovery after an episode of ATIN is not complete in over half of the patients, and studies with long-term follow-up have found progression of AIN to CKD in 70%–88%.[175,283,284] In a review of three ATIN case series, it was noted that only 64.1% of patients made a full recovery, whereas 23.4% gained a partial recovery, and 12.5% developed CKD and remained on renal replacement therapy.[158] Worse prognosis is associated with increasing age, but there appears to be no correlation with severity of AKI. The severity of tubulointerstitial disease (in particular, focal vs. diffuse interstitial cellular infiltration) is not associated with outcome.[285]

## CHRONIC TUBULOINTERSTITIAL DISEASES

CTIN is characterized by progressive, often indolent, loss of kidney function along with the pathologic features of tubular atrophy, interstitial mononuclear cell infiltrates, and interstitial fibrosis. CTIN has numerous etiologies (Table 35.8) with common clinical features

### CLINICAL FEATURES

Patients with chronic tubulointerstitial disease are brought to medical attention from either the findings of abnormal laboratory testing (elevated serum creatinine or abnormal urinalysis) or symptoms due to a systemic disease (sickle cell anemia). Depending on the level of kidney disease at the time of presentation, patients may complain of nonspecific symptoms attributable to CKD, such as fatigue, weakness, decreased appetite, weight loss, and others. Because chronic tubulointerstitial diseases may lead to decreased ability to concentrate the urine, patients may complain of nocturia. Typical laboratory findings in these patients included nonnephrotic-range proteinuria that is typically low-molecular-weight (tubular) in nature (lysozyme, β2-MG, NAG, and retinol-binding protein), microscopic hematuria and pyuria (including leukocyte casts), glycosuria (due to tubular defects), and if associated with an infectious etiology, positive urine cultures. Some causes of CTIN display characteristic patterns of tubular dysfunction. Proximal tubular defects may include glycosuria, bicarbonaturia, phosphaturia, aminoaciduria, and a proximal RTA. Distal tubular defects may include hyperkalemia, sodium wasting, and a distal RTA. Medullary injury may lead to sodium wasting and urinary concentrating defects. Serum uric acid levels are usually lower than expected for the degree of renal failure, presumably because of tubular defects in the reabsorption of uric acid. Anemia occurs relatively early in the course of certain forms of chronic interstitial disease, presumably because of early

**Table 35.8 Etiologies of Chronic Tubulointerstitial Nephritis**

| Drugs and Toxins | Metabolic Disorders | Immune Mediated | Infection | Hematologic | Others |
|---|---|---|---|---|---|
| Combination analgesics | Abnormal uric acid metabolism | Sarcoidosis | Bacterial pyelonephritis | Sickle cell disease | Radiation nephritis |
| 5-Aminosalicylic acid | Hypokalemia | Behçet syndrome | Hantavirus | Light-chain nephropathy | Secondary to progressive glomerular disease |
| NSAIDs | Hypercalcemia | Sjögren syndrome | Leptospirosis | Amyloidosis | Obstruction |
| Chinese herbs | Hyperoxaluria | Inflammatory bowel disease | Xanthogranulomatous pyelonephritis | Multiple myeloma | Vesicoureteral reflux |
| Lithium | Cystinosis | TINU | Malacoplakia | | |
| Lead | | IgG4-related systemic disease | | | |
| Cadmium | | Allograft rejection | | | |
| Mercury | | Systemic lupus erythematosus | | | |
| Balkan endemic nephropathy | | | | | |
| Calcineurin inhibitors | | | | | |
| Cisplatin | | | | | |
| Herbicides (glyphosate) | | | | | |
| CKD undetermined origin | | | | | |

*CKD,* Chronic kidney disease; *Ig,* immunoglobulin; *NSAID,* nonsteroidal antiinflammatory drug; *TINU,* tubulointerstitial nephritis and uveitis.

destruction of erythropoietin-producing interstitial cells. Ultrasonography is typically normal in most patients with CTIN until late in the course when the kidneys appear echogenic and shrunken. In some cases, such as CTIN due to analgesic toxicity, the kidney may have irregular contours and calcifications.

## DIFFERENTIAL DIAGNOSIS

Patients suspected of having CTIN usually present with CKD that is progressive and often indolent in nature. The urinalysis may show nonnephrotic-range proteinuria and thus many of these patients may not undergo diagnostic renal biopsy. Therefore a high degree of suspicion for the diagnosis is required. As shown in Table 35.8, there are a myriad of etiologies for CTIN and a careful history and physical examination may uncover clues as to the cause. For instance, exposure to heavy metals, heavy NSAID use, other drug or toxin exposure, chronic infections, or other chronic systemic diseases may serve to form a narrow differential diagnosis that can be supplemented by appropriately focused laboratory testing (such as heavy-metal levels, immunologic testing, or others). Kidney biopsy can be especially useful when CTIN is secondary to immune-mediated, paraprotein-associated, or infectious etiologies.

## RENAL PATHOLOGY

Pathologic features of CTIN are largely conserved and stereotyped across a wide variety of distinct causes. These features include atrophy of tubular cells with flattened epithelial cells and tubule dilation, interstitial fibrosis, and areas of mononuclear cell infiltration within the interstitial compartment and between tubules. TBMs are frequently thickened. The cellular infiltrate in chronic tubulointerstitial disease is composed of lymphocytes, macrophages, and B cells, with only occasional neutrophils, plasma cells, and eosinophils. This infiltrate is typically less marked than in ATIN. If immunofluorescent studies are performed on biopsy specimens, they might occasionally reveal nonspecific immunoglobulin or C3 deposition along the TBMs. As described later, specific etiologies of chronic tubulointerstitial disease may show additional characteristic findings on renal biopsy.

In chronic tubulointerstitial disease, glomeruli may remain remarkably normal by light microscopy, even when marked functional impairment is present. As chronic interstitial injury progresses, glomerular abnormalities become more evident and consist of periglomerular fibrosis, segmental sclerosis and, ultimately, global sclerosis. Small arteries and arterioles show fibrointimal thickening of variable severity.

## GENERAL TREATMENT PRINCIPLES

Progressive CKD associated with CTIN is best approached by addressing any underlying systemic disease (such as appropriate immunosuppressant therapy for sarcoidosis), removing and avoiding any drug or toxin exposure, and addressing any other reversible condition that may hasten progression (such as diabetes mellitus or hypertension). Otherwise, treatment largely follows existing paradigms for the care of patients with CKD[286] (see Chapter 59: Staging and Management of Chronic Kidney Disease). An exception to this is that there are no data supporting a protective role for RAAS blockade in CTIN as there is for patients with proteinuria or glomerular-predominant diseases.

## SPECIFIC ETIOLOGIES OF CHRONIC TUBULOINTERSTITIAL NEPHRITIS

Table 35.8 lists the etiologies associated with CTIN and selected causes are discussed here.

### ANALGESIC-INDUCED CHRONIC TUBULOINTERSTITIAL NEPHRITIS (ANALGESIC NEPHROPATHY)

Long-term (years) ingestion of large quantities of combination analgesic medications has been associated in epidemiologic studies with chronic interstitial nephritis (termed analgesic nephropathy) and papillary necrosis. The incidence of analgesic nephropathy varies among different countries and among different U.S. geographic areas and is highly dependent on the period sampled. Before the removal of phenacetin (between 1960 and 1980) from analgesic mixtures, analgesic nephropathy had been reported as a common cause of CKD in Scotland, Belgium, and Australia, accounting for 10% to 20% of patients with ESRD in those countries.[287] In the United States, case–control studies support the conclusion that variations in the frequency of analgesic nephropathy track with patterns and the degree of analgesic use.[288] In the 1990s, there was a decrease in the prevalence and incidence of analgesic nephropathy among patients undergoing dialysis in several European countries and Australia. Most authors associated this decrease with the removal of phenacetin from analgesic mixtures.[289] The true prevalence of analgesic nephropathy is not known, in part because definitive diagnostic criteria do not exist. The condition is often a diagnosis of exclusion in CKD patients: a history of heavy analgesic use and no other etiologies that can explain their progressive kidney disease. No histologic features are characteristic of analgesic nephropathy.

Analgesics implicated in analgesic nephropathy are compound mixtures that contain aspirin or antipyrine in combination with phenacetin, acetaminophen (paracetamol), or salicylamide and caffeine or codeine in over-the-counter proprietary mixtures. Development of analgesic nephropathy likely requires prolonged regular ingestion of combination analgesics (at least 6 tablets daily for >3 years). Despite numerous observational studies, the relative contribution of specific drugs to the development of analgesic nephropathy is not clear and often data on individual components of analgesic combinations do not show nephrotoxicity.[290]

Data are strongest for phenacetin, an analgesic antipyretic compound that is metabolized to paracetamol and other reactive intermediates. Given the concern for renal toxicity, phenacetin has been withdrawn from the market in most countries. Supporting its association with renal toxicity, there was a marked reduction in analgesic nephropathy incidence in those countries, coinciding with this withdrawal.[289] Interestingly, phenacetin compounds remain in use in some countries, and recent Chinese data suggest that phenacetin users are more likely to have CKD than a control population of nonusers.[291] However, this study requires cautious interpretation because, after adjusting for confounders for the development of CKD, there was no statistically significant effect. It is also important to note that the risk for analgesic nephropathy with phenacetin occurs solely in compound mixtures and that experimental rat studies of long-term phenacetin monotherapy at therapeutic doses have not demonstrated nephrotoxicity, although chronic supratherapeutic administration has repeatedly been found to produce papillary necrosis.[292]

Paracetamol (acetaminophen) has also been recognized as a potential cause of analgesic nephropathy. In one prospective study, lifetime intake of >500 g of paracetamol was associated with an approximately twofold higher risk of developing a GFR decline to < 30 mL/min 1.73 $m^2$.[293] However, direct causation has not been demonstrated and several studies have not demonstrated an association between CKD and paracetamol use.[294]

There are few data to suggest that long-term aspirin monotherapy is associated with the development of analgesic nephropathy.[295,296] In a large case–control study of 11,032 men, there was no association between serum creatinine levels and aspirin consumption.[295] A more recent cohort study also failed to find an association with long-term aspirin monotherapy with CKD.[296] However, mixtures containing both paracetamol and aspirin are associated with greater renal toxicity than either agent alone.[297,298] For instance, a Swedish study demonstrated a twofold higher incidence of raised creatinine levels in users of paracetamol–aspirin as compared with users of aspirin alone.[298]

The majority of studies have failed to find an association between heavy NSAID use and CKD.[293,295] However, chronic repeated intake of NSAIDs may increase the rate of progression of CKD in those patients with preexisting renal impairment.[299]

Analgesic nephropathy is recognized far more frequently in women than in men (five to seven times). The patients typically give a history of chronic headaches, joint pain, and/or abdominal pain that prompts regular use of analgesics. An episode of flank pain with or without associated hematuria may indicate a sloughed and potentially obstructing papilla. Because these drugs are available over the counter, many patients may not come to the attention of healthcare professionals until kidney disease has reached an advanced stage. At that point, renal functional abnormalities attributable to CTIN are nonspecific, including nocturia, sterile pyuria, and azotemia. Anemia is common. Discontinuation of heavy analgesic use can slow or arrest progression of the renal disease, but reversal of the kidney dysfunction is unlikely.

Mechanistically, analgesic components such as acetaminophen can injure cells through lipid peroxidation.[300] These drugs and metabolites are present in highest concentration in the medulla and papillary tip, which is where the initial lesions of capillary sclerosis are seen.[301] In the presence of aspirin, there is competition for glutathione within the cortex and papillae of the kidney. If cellular glutathione is depleted, there is the possibility of potentiation of the renal toxicity of acetaminophen, and its reactive metabolites.[301] In addition, because aspirin and other NSAIDs can suppress the production of vasodilatory prostaglandins, renal blood flow to the medulla may be compromised, adding a hemodynamic contribution to injury.

Imaging findings may be suggestive but not diagnostic for analgesic nephropathy. Findings on noncontrast CT scans of small kidneys, with bumpy renal contours and papillary calcifications, were found to diagnose analgesic nephropathy with greater sensitivity and specificity than clinical signs and symptoms (Fig. 35.3).[302] However, these CT findings are infrequent in the U.S. ESRD population and do not occur frequently enough among those patients with heavy and sustained analgesic use to make it a sensitive tool to detect analgesic nephropathy.[303]

The late course of analgesic nephropathy may be complicated by urinary tract malignancy.[304] The major presenting symptom of this complication is microscopic or gross hematuria. It has been estimated that a urinary tract malignancy will develop in as many as 8% to 10% of patients with analgesic nephropathy, typically after 15 to 25 years of heavy analgesic use.[305] Some of these patients may not have been previously diagnosed with analgesic nephropathy.[306] Pathogenesis of these uroepithelial malignancies presumably relates to the concentration and accumulation of phenacetin metabolites with alkylating capabilities within the renal medulla and lower urinary tract.[307] Whether NSAIDs and

**Analgesic nephropathy (AN)**

Macroscopic aspect of an AN kidney

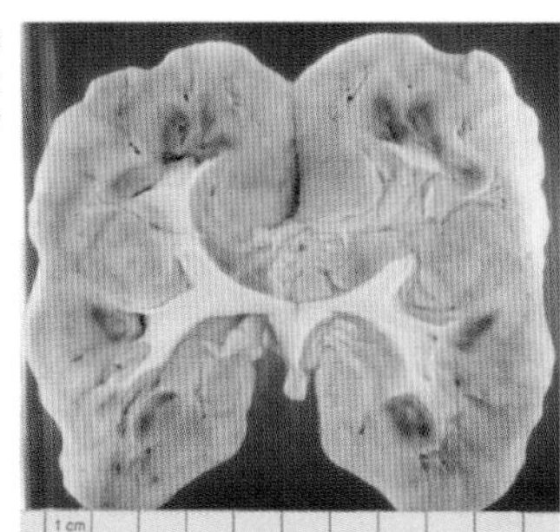


**Measurement of diagnostic criteria**

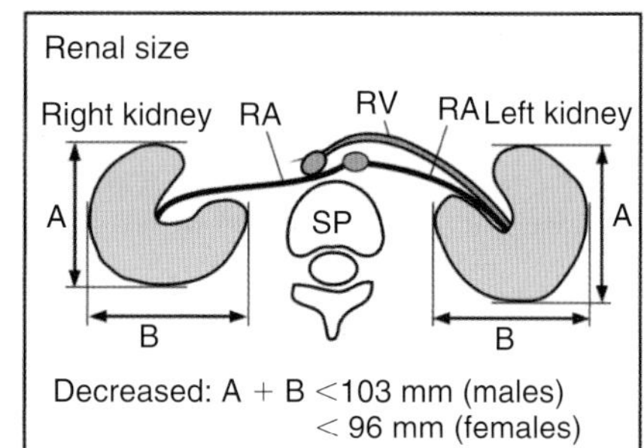


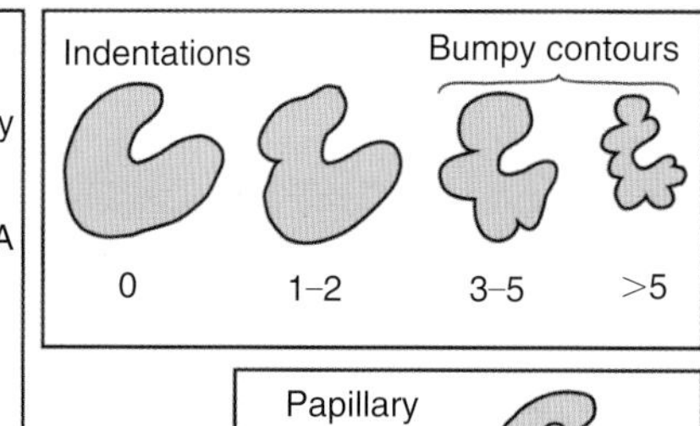


Papillary calcifications

**CT scans without contrast material**

Normal kidney

Analgesic abuse

Moderate renal failure

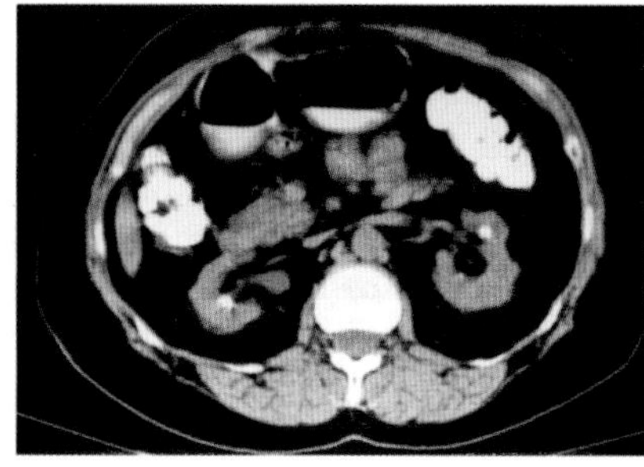

Belgian female, age 62 y, Scr 1.8 mg/dL.
*Abuse: 20 y mixture of pyrazolone derivatives*

End-stage renal failure

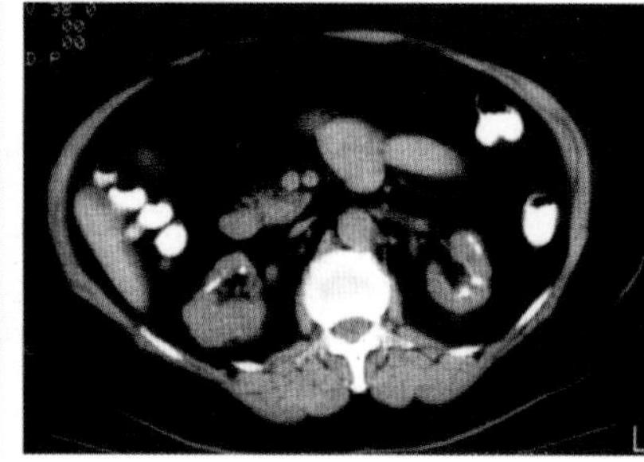

Belgian female, age 59 y, ESRF.
*Abuse: 8 y mixture of pyrazolone derivatives*
*26 y mixture of aspirin + paracetamol*

**Fig. 35.3 Renal imaging criteria of analgesic nephropathy *(AN)* as observed in a postmortem kidney and in computed tomography *(CT)* scans without contrast material.** These criteria include a decreased renal size, bumpy contours, and papillary calcifications. *RA,* Renal artery; *RV,* renal vein; *SP,* spine. (Adapted from De Broe ME, Elseviers MM. Analgesic nephropathy. *N Engl J Med.* 1998;338:446–452.)

acetaminophen are associated with these kidney tumors remains controversial. However, a recent meta-analysis of epidemiologic studies has suggested that both classes of drugs are associated with a significant increase in the risk of developing kidney cancer, regardless of the presence of analgesic nephropathy.[308]

## ARISTOLOCHIC ACID–INDUCED INTERSTITIAL NEPHRITIS (BALKAN AND CHINESE HERB NEPHROPATHY)

Aristolochic acids (AAs) are compounds derived from plants of the genus *Aristolochia* and have been used in various manners ranging from antiviral and antibacterial agents to components of weight-loss preparations.[309] Of note, two species, *Aristolochia clematitis* and *Aristolochia fangchi,* with common names of birthwort and Fang chi, have been identified as compounds responsible for kidney injury leading to progressive renal failure in a syndrome that was originally referred to as "Chinese herb nephropathy," but later became known as AA nephropathy (AAN).[310]

In the early 1990s, reports from Belgium described patients, frequently women, presenting with a rapidly progressive form of renal failure. Kidney biopsies from these patients revealed findings consistent with those of CTIN.[311] Initial reports noted that affected patients shared a history of chronic ingestion of the same preparation of Chinese slimming herbs as part of a weight-loss regimen. The number of case reports grew throughout the 1990s to over 120 cases by early 2000.[310] Cases were described throughout the world. Investigations into the cause of the initial outbreak demonstrated that an herb with no known nephrotoxicity (*Stephania tetrandra*) had been substituted with *A. fangchi,* which was toxic. Subsequent studies demonstrated several clinical subtypes, including AKI, tubular dysfunction with normal serum creatinine levels, and CTIN (the most common presentation).[310] These subtypes likely represent clinical variants that varied due to the amount and duration of exposure to AA. For example, the CTIN variant was seen more commonly in those patients with low daily intake but large cumulative doses.

Patients with AAN usually present with elevated serum creatinine values and few other symptoms. Other presenting signs and symptoms of AAN include anemia out of proportion to the degree of kidney failure (destruction of peritubular erythropoietin-producing cells), glucosuria, mild tubular proteinuria, and sterile pyuria. Renal ultrasound, especially when CKD is advanced, shows small kidneys with irregular contours.[312] Diagnostic criteria for AAN have been proposed and include an estimated GFR (eGFR) < 60 mL/min/1.73 m$^2$, and two of the three following histopathologic criteria: (1) hypocellular interstitial fibrosis decreasing from the outer to the inner cortical regions; (2) ingestion of AA-containing product, confirmed by phytochemical analysis; and (3) presence of DNA adducts in the renal tissue or urinary tract that can be identified in specialized laboratories.[313]

Evidence from clinical investigation and animal models has suggested that AA is the primary etiologic agent of these original presentations as well as having a significant contribution to the epidemiology of CKD and ESRD in Taiwan and mainland China where these herbal preparations are ingested.[314,315] AA now appears to be the common factor underlying the development of the nephropathy associated with Chinese herbs and Balkan nephropathy (see later).[316] The role of AA in producing this lesion has been supported by the creation of a similar renal lesion in rabbits and rats to which AA was administered regularly over weeks to months.[317,318] Kidneys from these animals display interstitial fibrosis, tubular atrophy, and some cellular infiltration, along with some atypical and/or malignant uroepithelial cells. Given the role of AA in causing nephropathy as well as uroepithelial malignancies, most health agencies worldwide have enacted bans on supplements containing this compound. However, due to lack of regulatory oversight over supplements, many AA-containing products can still be found for sale.[319]

Several therapies have been tried to slow the progression of AAN to ESRD.[310] Obviously, avoidance of further AA exposure is critical. However, the only therapy that has demonstrated possible benefit is glucocorticoids, which has been investigated in observational studies in very small numbers of patients and appears to delay progression of CKD.[320,321] Given the lack of other effective therapies, it is reasonable to consider a course of glucocorticoids in patients with documented AAN.

The potential for uroepithelial malignancies in patients exposed to AA is well documented. For example, in a study of 39 patients with Chinese herbal nephropathy and ESRD who underwent removal of their native kidneys and ureters, urothelial carcinoma was discovered in 18 patients and mild-to-moderate urothelial dysplasia in 19 patients.[322] The mutational footprint induced by AA has been studied and the average mutation rate induced by this compound is nearly 20-fold higher than that seen in lung cancers associated with smoking.[323] This makes AA one of the most potent carcinogens known to man. Such findings have led to recommendations that patients with a history of AA exposure should undergo regular cancer surveillance with yearly CT, cystoscopy with ureteroscopy, and biannual urine cytology.[310,312] When renal replacement therapy is started and prior to transplantation, strong consideration should be given for bilateral nephroureterectomy.

Balkan endemic nephropathy (BEN) is a chronic tubulointerstitial disease seen largely in families residing on the alluvial plains of the Danube River in Serbia, Bosnia, Herzegovina, Croatia, Romania, and Bulgaria. The prevalence is high in these areas, ranging from 0.5% to 5%.[324] Although genetic and environmental factors were suspected to play a role in its pathogenesis, current evidence suggests that AA may be the primary etiologic agent.[310] BEN may result from the ingestion of bread contaminated with seeds of *A. clematitis*, which leads to a low-grade but extended exposure to AA. This mechanism is supported by the finding of AADNA adducts in kidney and urothelial tumor specimens from BEN patients.[325]

Patients with BEN share nonspecific clinical features common to many chronic tubulointerstitial diseases. Renal and urinary abnormalities first appear after residing in an endemic area for at least 15 years. Affected individuals are not usually hypertensive. Initial renal abnormalities include tubular dysfunction characterized by tubular proteinuria, glycosuria, aminoaciduria, and impaired acid excretion. On kidney biopsy, there is a hypocellular infiltrate and tubulointerstitial fibrosis that decreases from the outer to inner cortex. This is temporally followed by impaired concentrating ability and slowly progressive azotemia, which can result in ESRD over a period of >20 years (unlike AAN, which progresses at a faster pace). A normochromic normocytic anemia is typical as well. Kidneys are of normal size early in the course of the disease, but kidney size diminishes with time. As with AAN, there is a strong association of BEN with urothelial carcinoma and thus screening for these cancers is critical in exposed individuals.[325] Diagnosis is presumptive, based on renal abnormalities consistent with chronic tubulointerstitial disease in a patient residing in an endemic area.[326] There is no specific therapy for this form of tubulointerstitial disease.

## HEAVY-METAL–ASSOCIATED CHRONIC TUBULOINTERSTITIAL NEPHRITIS

Occupational or environmental exposure to heavy metals has been implicated in the etiology of CKD. The linkage between heavy metals and nephrotoxicity is strongest for lead and cadmium. Although arsenic and uranium exposure has been hypothesized as nephrotoxins, the data in this regard are weak.[327,328]

### Lead

Epidemiologic studies have strongly implicated excessive exposure to lead as a cause of CTIN leading to renal failure.[329] Although occupational and environmental exposure to lead has significantly decreased, continued exposure to low levels of lead occurs through old water pipes, pottery, crystal, and lead-based paint in older dwellings. Most recently, lead exposures in larger amounts have occurred in contaminated water supplies such as in Flint, Michigan, in 2014. Given the prevalence of low-level lead exposure, it is critical to understand whether this exposure contributes, solely or in combination with other factors to the development of CKD. The determination of lead exposure requires a combination of careful history taking as well as the accurate measurement of body lead burden, which is accomplished through the ethylenediaminetetraacetic acid (EDTA) mobilization test. This test is required because blood lead levels only indicate recent, not chronic, lead exposure. Several studies have demonstrated correlations between elevated blood levels and/or body lead burden with the presence of kidney disease and/or accelerated rates of progression of chronic renal disease.[330,331] Using data from the Third National Health and Nutrition Examination Survey (NHANES III), Muntner and colleagues concluded that among the adult U.S. population with hypertension, even low-level exposure to lead is associated with CKD.[331] The same study also showed that in U.S. adolescents, higher blood lead levels correlated with lower GFRs.[332] Animal studies have also supported the hypothesis that ingestion of lead can accelerate CKD.[333]

The pathogenesis of chronic lead nephropathy is related to the reabsorption of filtered lead by the proximal tubule leading to defects in proximal tubule function, especially in children, including aminoaciduria, glycosuria, and phosphaturia representing Fanconi syndrome. Renal biopsies in adult patients with subclinical lead nephropathy and a mild-to-moderate decrease in GFR primarily show chronic interstitial nephritis, tubular atrophy, and interstitial fibrosis.

Adults who develop CTIN in association with lead exposure typically have hypertension and frequently gout as well. Thus the combination of progressive CKD, gout, and hypertension should prompt at least consideration of possible lead exposure. Progression to ESRD develops over years. Such slow progression has encouraged clinical investigators to examine whether chelation of lead might slow or reverse the progression of this disease. Earlier studies with small numbers of patients suggested that chronic injections of EDTA in patients with mild renal insufficiency and industrial exposure to lead could improve GFR.[334] Two larger prospective studies in patients with nondiabetic CKD, no lead exposure history, and normal or low-normal total body lead burdens demonstrated that chronic EDTA chelation can improve GFR over a 24-month period relative to the control group.[335,336] Although EDTA chelation may be exerting a benefit through processes other than lead removal, it is intriguing to consider that lead may adversely affect the progression of other forms of renal disease and that this may be positively affected by EDTA chelation. Use of EDTA chelation therapeutically for chronic lead nephropathy still requires confirmation in larger studies.

#### Cadmium

Cadmium accumulates in the body after gastrointestinal absorption or inhalation. Cadmium nephropathy can develop in those with prolonged low-level exposure to excess cadmium, such as with zinc smelter workers, or in the setting of massive environmental contamination, as occurred in Japan in the early part of the 20th century. Prominent features of this poisoning included renal failure.[337] Cadmium is bound to metallothionein, and proximal tubular cells take up the complexes. Cadmium induces a tubular proteinuria.[338] Other proximal tubule defects, including renal glycosuria, aminoaciduria, hypercalciuria, and phosphaturia, are also observed. Uncommonly, such renal damage may progress to an irreversible reduction in glomerular filtration.[339]

High levels of environmental contamination with cadmium related to mining in Japan were an unusual event. The extent to which chronic, low-level environmental exposure to cadmium affects renal function is much less clear. The Cadmibel Study recruited over 2000 adults from different areas of Belgium in an attempt to compare the relationships among hypertension, cardiovascular disease, and renal abnormalities with urinary cadmium excretion, a measure of lifetime cadmium exposure. The results demonstrated that although hypertension and cardiovascular risk were not associated with urinary cadmium excretion, there was a direct correlation of urinary cadmium excretion with serum alkaline phosphatase activity, and with urinary excretion of retinol-binding protein, NAG, β2-MG, amino acids, and calcium, suggesting that cadmium exposure is associated with renal tubular injury.[339] Interestingly, 5-year follow-up study of individuals with the highest urinary cadmium excretion did not demonstrate evidence of progressive kidney damage or loss of function.[340] Increased urinary calcium excretion seen in those exposed to cadmium has been associated with calcium phosphate kidney stones.[341]

### LITHIUM-INDUCED CHRONIC TUBULOINTERSTITIAL NEPHRITIS

Lithium has multiple nephrotoxic effects ranging from nephrogenic diabetes insipidus associated with diminished expression of the vasopressin-regulated water channel aquaporin-2 to progressive CKD from CTIN.[342–344] Animal models of chronic lithium ingestion reveal the development of focal interstitial nephritis, including tubular atrophy, interstitial fibrosis, and distal tubular dilation and microcyst formation. Glomerular sclerosis and azotemia also occurred by 12 months in these animals.[345] In a study of patients treated chronically with lithium (mean duration of therapy > 13 years), kidney biopsies from 24 patients with abnormal renal function were studied.[346] In this selected population, all the patients had findings consistent with CTIN on biopsy. Tubular dilation and cysts were also present in the cortex and medulla (Fig. 35.4). Development of these cysts is likely a direct consequence of lithium uptake by principal cells, because these cysts mainly originate from the distal tubule and collecting duct. A number of patients also had focal or global glomerulosclerosis. A serum creatinine value >2.5 mg/dL at the time of biopsy was the most powerful predictor of ultimate progression to ESRD, which occurred even if lithium was discontinued. Approximately 20% of long-term lithium patients demonstrated slowly rising serum creatinine values,

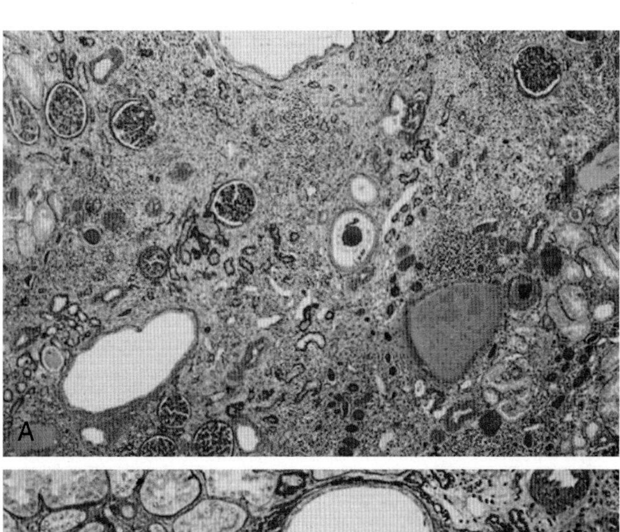


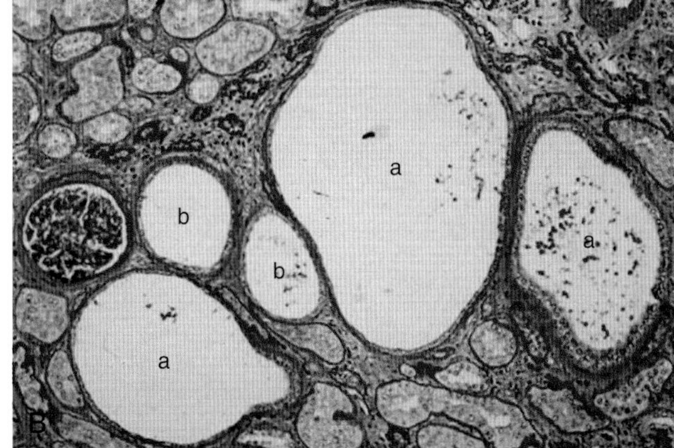


**Fig. 35.4** (A) Severe lithium-associated chronic tubulointerstitial nephropathy, with the additional finding of focal tubular cysts arising in a background of severe interstitial fibrosis and tubular atrophy. (Periodic acid–Schiff [PAS] stain, ×40.) (B) High-power view of tubular cysts lined by simple cuboidal epithelium *(a)*. Adjacent tubules show tubular dilation *(b)*. (PAS stain, ×100.) (From Markowitz GS, Radhakrishnan J, Kambham N, et al. Lithium nephrotoxicity: a progressive combined glomerular and tubulointerstitial nephropathy. *J Am Soc Nephrol.* 2000; 11:1439–1448.)

but this did not correlate with duration of therapy or cumulative dose.[347] Another study from Sweden has described a sixfold increase in prevalence for ESRD in patients taking lithium compared with the general population. Prevalence of CKD in the lithium-treated population was about 1.2%, with duration of therapy as the only identified risk factor.[348] Molecular alterations associated with lithium use are multiple and include changes in calcium signaling, inositol monophosphate, extracellular-regulated prostaglandin, sodium/solute transport, G-protein–coupled receptors, nitric oxide, vasopressin/aquaporin, and inflammation-related pathways.[349] How these may interact to lead to tubulointerstitial injury and fibrosis is not clearly elucidated, but elevated production of TGF-β1 may be a final common pathway leading to fibrosis.[350]

Clinical management of patients on chronic lithium who develop CKD requires judgment and a risk–benefit analysis in conjunction with a discussion of possible alternative medications that can be used to treat the patient. Lithium levels should be carefully monitored and maintained at the lowest level that controls symptoms. Given the more recent development of additional drugs (olanzapine, quetiapine, lamotrigine) for first-line treatment of bipolar disorder, it is reasonable to use these drugs in patients with an elevated creatinine level, preferably before irreversible interstitial damage has occurred. Although experimental and clinical evidence has demonstrated the efficacy of the epithelial sodium channel inhibitor amiloride for the treatment of lithium-induced nephrogenic insipidus, it is not known whether this drug can prevent CKD.[351]

## URIC ACID NEPHROPATHY

As the major organ responsible for the excretion of uric acid, the kidney can be affected in a number of ways by abnormal uric acid metabolism. In general, problems arise following uric acid crystallization in the tubules, collecting system, or outflow tract or the deposition of uric acid within the interstitium, with resulting inflammation. Uric acid solubility is pH and concentration dependent. Thus because uric acid in the tubular lumen is concentrated and exposed to a lower pH in the distal nephron, the likelihood of precipitation increases in these distal segments. Uric acid stones are a well-recognized entity and are discussed in Chapter 38: Urinary Stone Disease. Acute uric acid nephropathy, typically seen as an AKI phenotype following cell breakdown with tumor lysis syndrome, is also a recognized entity for which prophylactic treatment (rasburicase and allopurinol) can usually be given.

Whether sustained and chronic hyperuricemia leads to CTIN has been a controversial issue. Claims in the 1970s that up to 11% of chronic interstitial disease could be attributed to disorders of uric acid metabolism were challenged in the 1980s because of the difficulty in identifying effects of hyperuricemia independent of other risk factors, such as hypertension, vascular disease, kidney stones, or aging.[352,353] An additional controversy was related to the possibility that patients with coexisting gout and CTIN might have chronic lead intoxication as a cause of both disturbances. Recently, several studies have confirmed an association between hyperuricemia and the development and progression of CKD. In a study of >13,000 participants followed for up to 9 years, every 1-mg/dL increase in baseline uric acid level

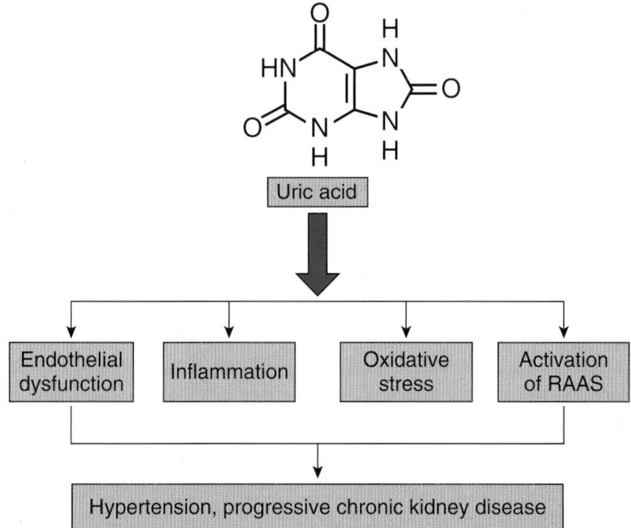


**Fig. 35.5** Pathogenesis of uric acid–associated chronic kidney disease. *RAAS,* Renin–angiotensin–aldosterone system.

was associated with a 7% increased risk for developing kidney disease after adjustment for confounders.[354] A meta-analysis of 13 observational studies also identified hyperuricemia being associated with an increased risk of new-onset CKD.[355] Other studies have documented that hyperuricemia is also associated with an increased risk of progression to ESRD.[356,357]

Given these associations, a few small trials have assessed the effect of uric acid-lowering therapies (allopurinol, febuxostat) on the progression of CKD. Although small, these studies have shown promising results with slower progression of CKD in patients treated to lower uric acid levels.[358–361] Losartan also has the ability to lower uric acid levels by decreasing uric acid absorption in the proximal tubule. In the Reduction of Endpoints in Non-insulin diabetes mellitus with Angiotensin II Antagonist Losartan (RENAAL) trial, the risk of renal events was decreased by 6% for every 0.5-mg/dL decrease in uric acid levels.[362] Larger-scale randomized trials are needed to confirm these results and to inform clinical practice. However, it seems reasonable to recommend dietary restriction of protein and purines in patients with gout and interstitial disease or patients with CKD and an elevated serum urate level.

Mechanistically, hyperuricemia may contribute to progressive CKD through several overlapping mechanisms that lead to endothelial dysfunction, inflammation, oxidative stress, and activation of the renin–angiotensin system (Fig. 35.5).[363] Furthermore, uric acid regulates critical proinflammatory pathways in vascular smooth muscle cells, potentially having a role in the vascular changes associated with hypertension and vascular disease.[364,365] Animal studies have also revealed that hyperuricemia induces hypertension and accelerates renal progression in the remnant kidney model.[366,367] Taken in aggregate, these studies provide evidence that uric acid may be a true mediator of kidney disease and progression.

## CHRONIC KIDNEY DISEASE OF UNKNOWN ETIOLOGY

In 2002, a cohort of patients with advanced CKD without a clear etiology was observed in El Salvador.[368] Subsequently, several other epidemiologic studies from the coastal regions of Nicaragua and El Salvador as well as Costa Rica and Guatemala have also documented the existence of a form of progressive CKD that, at that time, had no clear etiology[369–372] (see also discussion in Chapter 76). The CKD that has been described has the following characteristics: (1) the location is relatively restricted to a specific geographic region, the coastal Pacific area of Central America; (2) there is no association with diabetes mellitus, hypertension, or other known CKD etiologies; (3) there is both male and younger age predominance; and (4) it occurs predominantly in low-income laborers working under extreme environmental conditions of heat and recurrent dehydration, such as agricultural workers performing cotton and sugarcane harvesting.[373] The disease typically manifests as asymptomatic, progressive CKD, low-grade (<1 g/day) proteinuria, bland urine sediment, and mild hyperuricemia may be present. Kidney biopsies reveal tubulointerstitial disease and, in some cases, glomerular ischemia and glomerulosclerosis.[374] Progression to ESRD occurs at a variable pace but because renal replacement therapy is scarce in the affected regions, mortality is very high.[373]

The etiology of Mesoamerican nephropathy is not known and is likely multifactorial. However, several potential risk factors have been proposed. These include heavy metals, agrochemicals, excessive use of NSAIDs, and consumption of contaminated alcohol. Underlying these mechanisms are repeated episodes of dehydration/volume depletion and perhaps episodes of rhabdomyolysis associated with strenuous labor.[375] At this time, the best suggestion for prevention is to provide adequate hydration and limit exposure to extremes of heat. Further field studies investigating the pathogenesis of this devastating condition are ongoing.

A similar form of CKD associated with tubulointerstitial fibrosis has also been reported in Egypt, India, Tunisia, and Sri Lanka.[376] Once again, the etiology of this condition is uncertain but epidemiologic data suggest that exposure to dietary and waterborne toxins may be causative.[377] Specifically, rice and water levels of cadmium are elevated in affected regions.[378] Further data are needed to understand the role of environmental toxins in the pathogenesis of this condition.

## ACKNOWLEDGMENTS

The authors would like to thank Drs. Carolyn J. Kelly and Eric G. Neilson for their chapter in the previous edition of this book, select parts of which have been carried over for this edition.

 Complete reference list available at ExpertConsult.com.

## KEY REFERENCES


1. Zeisberg M, Neilson EG. Mechanisms of tubulointersitial fibrosis. *J Am Soc Nephrol.* 2010;21:1819–1834.
3. Basile DP, Bonventre JV, Mehta R, et al. Progression after AKI: understanding maladaptive repair processes to predict and identify therapeutic treatments. *J Am Soc Nephrol.* 2016;27:687–697.
52. Zheng G, Wang Y, Mahajan D, et al. The role of tubulointerstitial inflammation. *Kidney Int.* 2005;67(suppl):S96–S100.
64. Spanou Z, Keller M, Britschgi M, et al. Involvement of drug-specific T cells in acute drug-induced interstitial nephritis. *J Am Soc Nephrol.* 2006;17(10):2919–2927.
101. Eddy AA. Molecular insights into renal interstitial fibrosis. *J Am Soc Nephrol.* 1996;7:2495–2508.
110. Kalluri R, Neilson EG. Epithelial-mesenchymal transition and its implications for fibrosis. *J Clin Invest.* 2003;112:1776–1784.
118. Nakagawa T, Kang DH, Ohashi R, et al. Tubulointerstitial disease: role of ischemia and microvascular disease. *Curr Opin Nephrol Hypertens.* 2003;12:233–241.
120. Eckardt K-U, Alper SL, Antignac C, et al. Autosomal dominant tubulointerstititial disease: diagnosis, classification and management—a KDIGO consensus report. *Kidney Int.* 2015;88:676–683.
126. Bollee G, Dahan K, Flamant M, et al. Phenotype and outcome in hereditary tubulointerstitial nephritis secondary to UMOD mutations. *Clin J Am Soc Nephrol.* 2011;6:2429–2438.
143. Perazella MA, Markowitz GS. Drug-induced acute interstitial nephritis. *Nat Rev Nephrol.* 2010;6(8):461–470.
146. Goicoechea M, Rivera F, Lopez-Gomez JM. Increased prevalence of acute tubulointerstitial nephritis. *Nephrol Dial Transplant.* 2013; 28(1):112–115.
147. Haas M, Spargo BH, Wit E-JC, et al. Etiologies and outcome of acute renal insufficiency in older adults: a renal biopsy study of 259 cases. *Am J Kidney Dis.* 2000;35(3):433–447.
149. Davison AM, Jones CH. Acute interstitial nephritis in the elderly: a report from the UK MRC glomerulonephritis register and a review of the literature. *Nephrol Dial Transplant.* 1998;13:12–16.
151. Clarkson MR, Giblin L, O'Connell FP, et al. Acute interstitial nephritis: clinical features and response to corticosteroid therapy. *Nephrol Dial Transplant.* 2004;19(11):2778–2783.
158. Baker RJ, Pusey CD. The changing profile of acute tubulointerstitial nephritis. *Nephrol Dial Transplant.* 2004;19:8–11.
166. Buysen JG, Houtlhoff HJ, Krediet RT, et al. Acute interstitial nephritis: a clinical and morphological study in 27 patients. *Nephrol Dial Transplant.* 1990;5:94–99.
167. Fogazzi GB, Ferrari B, Garigali G, et al. Urinary sediment findings in acute interstitial nephritis. *Am J Kidney Dis.* 2012;60:330–332.
169. Muriithi AK, Leung N, Valeri AM, et al. Biopsy-proven acute interstitial nephritis, 1993-2011: a case series. *Am J Kidney Dis.* 2014; 64(4):558–566.
170. Muriithi AK, Nasr SH, Leung N. Utility of urine eosinophils in the diagnosis of acute interstitial nephritis. *Clin J Am Soc Nephrol.* 2013;8(11):1857–1862.
171. Galpin JE, Shinaberger JH, Stanley TM, et al. Acute interstitial nephritis due to methicillin. *Am J Med.* 1978;65:756–765.
172. Linton AL, Clark WF, Driedger AA, et al. Acute interstitial nephritis due to drugs: review of the literature with a report of nine cases. *Ann Intern Med.* 1980;93:735–741.
173. Nolan CR, Anger MS, Kelleher SP. Eosinophiluria—a new method of detection and definition of the clinical spectrum. *N Engl J Med.* 1986;315:1516–1519.
174. Corwin HL, Bray RA, Haber MH. The detection and interpretation of urinary eosinophils. *Arch Pathol Lab Med.* 1989;113:1256–1258.
175. Ruffing KA, Hoppes P, Blend D, et al. Eosinophils in urine revisited. *Clin Nephrol.* 1994;41:163–166.
176. Perazella MA, Bomback AS. Urinary eosinophils in AIN: farewell to an old biomarker? *Clin J Am Soc Nephrol.* 2013;8(11):1841–1843.
192. Wilson DM, Turner DR, Cameron JS, et al. Value of renal biopsy in acute intrinsic renal failure. *Br Med J.* 1976;2:459–461.
196. D'Agati VD, Theise ND, Pirani CL, et al. Interstitial nephritis related to nonsteroidal anti-inflammatory agents and beta-lactam antibiotics: a comparative study of the interstitial infiltrates using monoclonal antibodies. *Mod Pathol.* 1989;2(4):390–396.
197. Joh K, Aizawa S, Yamaguchi Y, et al. Drug-induced hypersensitivity nephritis: lymphocyte stimulation testing and renal biopsy in 10 cases. *Am J Nephrol.* 1990;10(3):222–230.
198. Joss N, Morris S, Young B, et al. Granulomatous interstitial nephritis. *Clin J Am Soc Nephrol.* 2007;2(2):222–230.
226. Brewster UC, Perazella MA. Proton pump inhibitors and the kidney: critical review. *Clin Nephrol.* 2007;68:65–72.
230. Lazarus B, Chen Y, Wilson FP, et al. Proton pump inhibitor use and the risk of chronic kidney disease. *JAMA Intern Med.* 2016; 176:238–246.
231. Xie Y, Bowe B, Li T, et al. Proton pump inhibitors and risk of incident CKD and progression to ESRD. *J Am Soc Nephrol.* 2016;27:3153–3163.
237. Esteve JB, Launay-Vacher V, Brocherious I, et al. COX-2 inhibitors and acute interstitial nephritis: case report and review of the literature. *Clin Nephrol.* 2005;63:385–389.
243. Izzedine H, Mateus C, Boutros C, et al. Renal effects of immune checkpoint inhibitors. *Nephrol Dial Transplant.* 2017;32(6):936–942.

250. Gonzalez E, Gutierrez E, Galeano C, et al. Early steroid treatment improves the recovery of renal function in patients with drug-induced acute interstitial nephritis. *Kidney Int.* 2008;73(8):940–946.
251. Raza MN, Hadid M, Keen CE, et al. Acute tubulointerstitial nephritis, treatment with steroid and impact on renal outcomes. *Nephrology.* 2012;17(8):748–753.
292. Henrich WL. Analgesic nephropathy. *Am J Med Sci.* 1988;295:561–568.
298. Fored CM, Ejerblad E, Lindblad P, et al. Acetaminophen, aspirin, and chronic renal failure. *N Engl J Med.* 2001;345:1801–1808.
299. Gooch K, Culleton BF, Manns BJ, et al. NSAID use and progression of chronic kidney disease. *Am J Med.* 2007;120:280.e1–280.e7.
308. Choueiri TK, Je Y, Cho E. Analgesic use and the risk of kidney cancer: a meta-analysis of epidemiologic studies. *Int J Cancer.* 2014; 134:384–396.
309. Krell D, Stebbing J. *Aristolochia*: the malignant truth. *Lancet Oncol.* 2013;14(1):25–26.
310. Luciano RL, Perazella MA. Aristolochic acid nephropathy: epidemiology, clinical presentation and treatment. *Drug Saf.* 2015;38:55–64.
316. De Broe ME. Chinese herbs nephropathy and Balkan endemic nephropathy: toward a single entity, aristolochic acid nephropathy. *Kidney Int.* 2012;81:513–515.
330. Yu CC, Lin JL, Lin-Tan DT. Environmental exposure to lead and progression of chronic renal diseases: a four-year prospective longitudinal study. *J Am Soc Nephrol.* 2004;15:1016–1022.
340. Hotz P, Buchet JP, Bernard A, et al. Renal effects of low-level environmental cadmium exposure: 5-year follow-up of a subcohort from the Cadmibel study. *Lancet.* 1999;354:1508–1513.
350. Alsady M, Baumgarten R, Deen PMT, et al. Lithium in the kidney: friend and foe? *J Am Soc Nephrol.* 2016;27:1587–1595.
354. Weiner DE, Tighiouart H, Elsayed EF, et al. Uric acid and incident kidney disease in the community. *J Am Soc Nephrol.* 2008;19: 1204–1211.
355. Li L, Yang C, Zhao Y, et al. Is hyperuricemia an independent risk factor for new-onset chronic kidney disease? A systematic review and meta-analysis based on observational cohort studies. *BMC Nephrol.* 2014;15:122.
373. Correa-Rotter R, Wesseling C, Johnson RJ. CKD of unknown origin in central America: the case for a mesoamerican nephropathy. *Am J Kidney Dis.* 2014;63:506–520.
374. Wijkström J, Leiva R, Elinder CG, et al. Clinical and pathological characterization of Mesoamerican nephropathy: a new kidney disease in Central America. *Am J Kidney Dis.* 2013;62:908–918.

# 36 Urinary Tract Infection in Adults

Lindsay E. Nicolle

## CHAPTER OUTLINE



## KEY POINTS

- Urinary tract infection is a common problem for all ages, affecting primarily healthy females and individuals with underlying genitourinary abnormalities.
- The optimal approach to management of urinary tract infection requires evaluation of the clinical presentation and critical interpretation of urine culture results, together with an assessment of underlying patient comorbidities and urologic abnormalities.
- The evolution of antimicrobial resistance in common uropathogens, including *Escherichia coli*, requires continuing reassessment of empiric antimicrobial treatment.
- Asymptomatic bacteriuria is common in many populations, but treatment is indicated only for pregnant women or individuals who undergo invasive urologic procedures associated with mucosal bleeding.
- Indwelling devices in the urinary tract become coated with biofilm following insertion, and the presence of the biofilm will have an impact on the urine culture and outcomes with antimicrobial therapy.
- Small renal abscesses (<5 cm) can usually be managed medically with prolonged courses of antimicrobial therapy, but larger abscesses, including most perinephric abscesses, require drainage in addition to antimicrobial therapy.
- Genitourinary tuberculosis is one of the most common forms of extrapulmonary tuberculosis, and usually presents as reactivation with involvement of only one kidney or the ureter.
- *Schistosoma mansoni*, an endemic parasite in many regions of the world, localizes to the bladder wall; acquisition of infection with this parasite is a risk for travelers to these areas.

Urinary tract infection of the bladder, the kidney, or (in men) the prostate is one of the most common human infections. Infecting organisms are usually bacteria; fungi also contribute. Much less frequently, infection is caused by viruses or parasites. Other manifestations of genitourinary tract infection are renal and perinephric abscesses, emphysematous cystitis and pyelonephritis, xanthogranulomatous pyelonephritis, and pyocystitis. Disseminated viral infections (e.g., mumps, cytomegalovirus, and other herpes viruses) and fungal infections (e.g., blastomycosis, histoplasmosis) may also involve the urinary tract but are not discussed in this chapter. Polyomavirus BK infection in kidney transplant recipients and urinary tract infection in children, including vesicoureteral reflux, are addressed in Chapters 70 and 72, respectively.

## DEFINITIONS

Urinary tract infection results from the presence of bacteria or other microorganisms in the urine or genitourinary tissues. The term "bacteriuria" describes isolation of any bacteria in the urine, although in practice it usually refers to isolation of organisms in concentrations that meet specific quantitative criteria. Infection is asymptomatic when the urine culture

**Table 36.1 Abnormalities of the Urinary Tract That May Be Associated With Complicated Urinary Tract Infection**

| Abnormality | Example(s) |
|---|---|
| Obstruction | Pelvicalyceal junction obstruction, ureteric or urethral strictures, prostate hypertrophy, urolithiasis, tumor, extrinsic compression, female genital mutilation |
| Neurologic impairment | Neurogenic bladder |
| Urologic devices | Indwelling catheter, ureteric stent, nephrostomy tube |
| Urologic abnormalities | Vesicoureteral reflux, bladder diverticuli, cystoceles, urologic procedures, ileal conduit, augmented bladder, neobladder |
| Metabolic/congenital diseases | Nephrocalcinosis, medullary sponge kidney, urethral valves, polycystic kidneys |
| Immunologic impairment | Renal transplantation |

**Table 36.2 Some Host Defenses Other Than Voiding That Contribute to Maintaining Sterility of Urine**

| Defense | Example(s) |
|---|---|
| Normal flora | Urethra, possibly bladder microbiome |
| Urine characteristics | pH, osmolality, concentrations of organic acids |
| Urine proteins | Tamm–Horsfall protein (uromodulin), secretory immunoglobulins, lactoferrin, lipocalin, cationic peptides (defensins, cathelicidins), siderophores |
| Innate immune response | Toll-like receptors, polymorphonuclear leukocytes, chemokines/cytokine production, antimicrobial peptides, myeloid dendritic cells, macrophages, mast cells |
| Uroepithelium | Mucopolysaccharide layer, glycoprotein plaque (uroplakins), epithelial barrier, shedding of superficial epithelial cell layer |
| Prostate secretions | Chemokines, immunoglobulins |

result meets quantitative criteria for bacteriuria without signs or symptoms attributable to infection. Symptomatic urinary tract infection may manifest as bladder infection (cystitis or lower tract infection), kidney infection (pyelonephritis or upper tract infection), or prostate infection (acute or chronic bacterial prostatitis). Acute uncomplicated urinary tract infection occurs in women with a normal genitourinary tract, usually manifesting as cystitis.[1–3] Pyelonephritis, also referred to as "acute nonobstructive pyelonephritis" or "acute uncomplicated pyelonephritis," also occurs in these women but much less frequently.[2] Complicated urinary tract infection occurs in individuals with functional or structural abnormalities of the genitourinary tract (Table 36.1).[4,5] In healthy postmenopausal women without genitourinary abnormalities and diabetic women without nephropathy or neurologic bladder impairment, urinary tract infection should be considered uncomplicated. Acute uncomplicated urinary tract infection rarely occurs in men. A urinary tract infection in a man should be considered complicated until underlying abnormalities have been ruled out.

Urinary tract infection commonly recurs. "Reinfection" is infection that recurs after entry of an organism into the genitourinary tract, usually from the periurethral flora. Reinfection characteristically occurs with a different organism. However, when periurethral colonization with a potential uropathogen persists, the same strain may be isolated from reinfection. "Relapse" occurs when the infecting organism persists in the urinary tract despite antimicrobial therapy; the same organism is isolated from recurrent infection after therapy.

## GENERAL CONCEPTS

### HOST DEFENSES OF THE NORMAL URINARY TRACT

Using standard microbiologic methods, the urine and genitourinary tract are normally sterile apart from the distal urethra. The normal flora of the distal urethra plays an important role in host defense by preventing colonization at this site by potential uropathogens. The flora includes aerobic bacteria that are common skin commensals, such as coagulase-negative staphylococci, viridans group streptococci, and *Corynebacterium* species.[6,7] There is also a large and complex anaerobic flora.[7] Recent studies using 16S ribosomal RNA sequence analysis of bladder urine collected by suprapubic aspiration or urethral catheterization to minimize contamination also describe a urine microbiome of predominantly nonpathogenic gram-positive organisms, with some other species present.[8,9] This microbiome shows substantial heterogenicity among women and variation with age. The role of the microbiome is not clear, but a protective role based on biofilm barrier, nutrient competition, or priming of host defenses has been suggested.

Urine is a good nutrient source for most bacterial species, and common uropathogens grow well in urine. The most important host defense that maintains sterility of the urine is normal, unobstructed voiding. A complex array of urine and uroepithelial cell components also contributes to maintenance of sterile urine in the normal genitourinary tract (Table 36.2).[10–12] Inhibitors of bacterial adherence to uroepithelial cells prevent persistence of bacteria once they have entered the urinary tract. Tamm–Horsfall protein, the most abundant protein in the urine, appears to have an important role in this regard.[11] This protein prevents attachment of *Escherichia coli* to uroepithelial cell receptors by binding to the type 1 fimbria adhesin (FimH), and removes some other uropathogens, such as *Klebsiella pneumoniae* and *Staphylococcus saprophyticus*.[13] It also may have an immunomodulatory role through activation of the innate immune response by a Toll-like receptor (TLR)-4–dependent mechanism.[11]

Adherence of bacteria to uroepithelial cells is also prevented by the surface mucopolysaccharide–glycosaminoglycan layer of the uroepithelium, by urine immunoglobulin G (IgG) and secretory immunoglobulin A (IgA), and by some low-molecular-weight oligosaccharides present in the urine. The relative in vivo importance of any of these is not yet established. Despite the many components contributing to maintaining sterility of the urine, bacteriuria is readily established once normal voiding is impaired. In the complicated urinary tract, infection occurs through increased entry of organisms into the bladder or kidney, which may be attributed to the use of urologic devices, turbulent urine flow, or ureteric reflux. Organisms may then persist despite other host defenses when infected urine is retained if voiding is incomplete, or in biofilm on urologic devices.

## IMMUNE AND INFLAMMATORY RESPONSES TO URINARY TRACT INFECTION

The innate immune system provides the major immunologic response to urinary tract infection.[12] The intensity of response is determined by the interactions of microbial pathogenicity, individual genetic regulation, and the site of infection.[14,15] Unique *E. coli* strains have a variable capacity to stimulate or evade activation of the innate immune response. Uropathogenic strains that cause symptomatic infection induce a strong innate immune response, whereas strains isolated from asymptomatic bacteriuria evoke a limited response.[16,17] Strains that successfully evade immune activation may have a pathogenetic advantage for establishing bladder colonization and persistent infection.[18,19] Host genetic polymorphisms affecting the innate immune response predispose to acute pyelonephritis or asymptomatic bacteriuria.[15,20]

Infecting organisms that gain access to the bladder adhere to uroepithelial cells, and stimulation by bacterial lipopolysaccharide leads to activation of these cells.[21] Recognition is through TLRs (TLR-4, TLR-2, TLR-5, TLR-11) and activation promotes cytokine production, particularly interleukin (IL)-1, IL-6, and IL-8 (chemokine [C–X–C motif] ligand 1 [CXCL-1]). These cytokines recruit neutrophils and other immunocompetent cells to the kidney and bladder.[11,12,15] The chemotactic cytokine IL-8 is released at the mucosal site and induces a rapid influx of neutrophils into the bladder, with subsequent phagocytosis and clearance of bacteria. Macrophages and mast cells resident in the submucosa are also recruited. Organisms may also infect superficial bladder epithelial cells, with subsequent shedding of these cells. This innate immune response rapidly clears most uropathogenic *E. coli* organisms from the bladder, but it does not produce a sterilizing immunity in murine models.[22] In humans, bacteriuria often persists despite marked pyuria.

Urine and serum IL-6 concentrations are correlated with the severity of infection. The highest levels occur in patients with pyelonephritis. Systemic elaboration of IL-1β and IL-6 produces fever and activation of the acute-phase response. The acute inflammatory infiltrate of polymorphonuclear leukocytes that develops in renal tissue during pyelonephritis limits bacterial spread and persistence within the kidney but also contributes to tissue damage and renal scarring.

IgA-producing plasma cells are found in higher numbers in the bladder submucosa of patients with bacterial cystitis than in healthy controls. However, acute cystitis is associated with a reduced or undetectable serologic response, presumably reflecting the superficial nature of the infection.[12] The local immune response is of short duration and is reactivated for each infection. This limited immunologic response to bladder infection may explain why early reinfection with the same *E. coli* strain is observed in some women with acute cystitis. However, animal studies have reported some protection against same-strain reinfection mediated by systemic and local antibodies.[22]

A vigorous local and systemic humoral immune response occurs in patients with pyelonephritis.[10,16] The antibody response is directed against surface antigens of the infecting bacteria, including O antigens, and surface proteins such as the type 1 (FimH) and P fimbriae, which are major adhesins of *E. coli*.[22,23] IgM antibodies dominate the systemic humoral response in the first episode of infection in the upper urinary tract, but subsequent episodes are characterized by an IgG response. In pyelonephritis, elevations of IgG antibodies to lipid A are correlated with severity of renal infection and parenchymal destruction. There is also a substantial urinary IgG and secretory IgA antibody response. Despite this robust response, the protective role, if any, of the antibody response in pyelonephritis is not clear. Bacteria often persist in the renal parenchyma despite very high levels of specific antibodies. In addition, the frequency of urinary tract infection is not increased in women who do not produce secretory IgA.

Cell-mediated immunity appears to have a limited role in the host defense against urinary tract infection. A small number of mucosal T lymphocytes are present throughout the urinary tract, and both $CD4^+$ and $CD8^+$ T cells can be found in the submucosa and lamina propria of the bladder and urethra. Recruitment of B and T lymphocytes to the bladder wall is observed with secondary infections. T-cell–derived proinflammatory cytokines also stimulate renal tubular epithelial cells to produce IL-6, which may increase IgA secretion of committed B cells.[22] However, women infected with human immunodeficiency virus (HIV) who have very low $CD4^+$ counts do not have an increased susceptibility to or severity of urinary tract infection[24]; this finding suggests that cell-mediated immunity is not an essential defense against such infection.

## URINE CULTURE

The definitive diagnosis and appropriate management of urinary tract infection usually require microbiologic confirmation by urine culture. Urine specimens for culture should always be obtained before antimicrobial therapy is initiated because urinary excretion of antimicrobial agents rapidly sterilizes urine. Once collected, the specimen should be forwarded promptly to the laboratory. Organisms present in small quantitative counts (i.e., contaminants) grow readily in urine at room temperature and reach high quantitative counts within a few hours. If the specimen is delayed in reaching the laboratory, it should be refrigerated at 4°C until transported.

A urine specimen for culture must be collected with a method that minimizes contamination. A clean-catch voided specimen without additional periurethral cleaning is usually appropriate. When patients cannot cooperate for the collection of a voided specimen, urine may be collected by an in-and-out catheter. For men, a specimen may be obtained in an external condom catheter after application of a clean condom catheter and collecting bag.[25] Urine samples may also be collected by suprapubic aspiration or directly from the renal pelvis when percutaneous drainage of an obstructed urinary tract is necessary. Specimens obtained from patients with short-term indwelling catheters should be collected by puncture of the catheter port. For a long-term indwelling catheter, two to five organisms are present in the catheter biofilm at any time, so urine collected through the catheter will be contaminated by organisms present in the biofilm.[26] The long-term indwelling catheter should be removed and replaced by a new catheter, and a specimen of bladder urine obtained through the newly placed catheter.[25,26]

The standard quantitative criterion for diagnosis of urinary tract infection with voided specimens is an organism count of $\geq 10^5$ colony-forming units (CFU)/mL of a potential uropathogen. Women usually have contaminating organisms from vaginal or periurethral flora isolated from voided specimens, and the quantitative criterion distinguishes bacteriuria from contamination. Application of this quantitative standard is always appropriate for the diagnosis of asymptomatic bacteriuria, but for symptomatic cases the quantitative urine culture results must be interpreted in the context of the clinical presentation and with consideration of the method of specimen collection (Table 36.3). Bacteria require several hours of incubation in bladder urine to achieve a concentration $\geq 10^5$ CFU/mL. Some patients with frequency or diuresis may not retain urine in the bladder for a sufficient time to achieve the concentration of $\geq 10^5$ CFU/mL. Quantitative counts may also be lower when infection is caused by some fastidious organisms or if the patient is receiving a urinary antiseptic. For symptomatic men, a single urine specimen in which $\geq 10^3$ CFU/mL of a uropathogen is isolated is diagnostic for bladder bacteriuria, on the basis of paired comparisons of voided specimens and suprapubic aspirates.

**Table 36.3 Quantitative Counts of Bacteria in the Urine for Microbiologic Diagnosis of Urinary Tract Infection in Patients Not Receiving Antimicrobial Therapy**

| Collection Method | Quantitative Criteria (CFU/mL) |
|---|---|
| **Voided Specimen** | |
| Asymptomatic women or men | $\geq 10^{5}$[a] |
| Women: acute uncomplicated | |
| Cystitis | $\geq 10^3$ |
| Pyelonephritis | $\geq 10^{4}$[b] |
| Men: Symptomatic | $\geq 10^3$ |
| Men: External condom collection | $\geq 10^5$ |
| **Catheter** | |
| In-and-out | $\geq 10^2$ |
| Indwelling[c] | |
| Asymptomatic | $\geq 10^5$ |
| Symptomatic | $\geq 10^2$ |
| Suprapubic or percutaneous aspiration | Any growth |

[a]Two consecutive specimens are recommended for women.
[b]In 95% of cases, values $\geq 10^5$ colony-forming units (CFU) per milliliter.
[c]A long-term catheter should be replaced and the specimen collected through a new catheter.

A urine specimen obtained by suprapubic aspiration or other percutaneous collection method such as renal pelvis drainage is assumed to be a sterile specimen, and any quantitative count of an organism represents true bacteriuria. However, in specimens collected by an in-and-out catheter, contaminating organisms are introduced from the periurethral area, and a quantitative criterion of $\geq 10^2$ CFU/mL is recommended. Other relevant considerations in interpreting a urine culture result include the number and type of organisms isolated. A single infecting organism is usual, but in patients with complicated urinary tract infection, particularly those with indwelling urinary devices, more than one organism is frequently present. Commensal bacteria of the normal skin flora, such as *Lactobacillus* spp. and coagulase-negative staphylococci, should usually be considered contaminants when they are isolated from voided urine specimens. In young healthy women, group B streptococci and *Enterococcus* species isolated in any quantitative count are also usually contaminants.[27]

## PHARMACOKINETIC AND PHARMACODYNAMIC CONSIDERATIONS FOR TREATMENT

Therapeutic success in the treatment of cystitis depends on antimicrobial levels in the urine. Antimicrobial levels in renal tissue, which are correlated with serum levels, determine outcome for pyelonephritis.[27] Treatment of urinary tract infection is unique in some respects because of the exceptionally high urine concentrations achieved by many antimicrobial agents excreted into the urine (Table 36.4). The urine concentration is determined by the interplay of glomerular filtration, active tubular secretion, and tubular reabsorption, all influenced by urine pH, protein binding, and the molecular structure of the drug. Cystitis and pyelonephritis may be successfully treated with antimicrobial agents at minimum inhibitory concentrations (MICs) to which the infecting organism would not usually be considered susceptible. The "intermediate" susceptibility designation reported by the clinical microbiology laboratory implies clinical efficacy in body sites where antimicrobial agents are physiologically concentrated, such as the urine, and is relevant to treatment of urinary tract infection. Thus when an organism isolated from the urine is reported to have intermediate susceptibility to an antimicrobial agent, the drug is usually appropriate for treatment of urinary tract infection with that organism. The urine bactericidal activity of some antimicrobial agents is modified by the urine pH. Penicillins, tetracyclines, and nitrofurantoin are more active in acidic urine, and aminoglycosides, fluoroquinolones, and erythromycin are more active in alkaline urine. This pH variability has not, however, been shown to be relevant for therapeutic outcomes, with the exception of methenamine salts, for which an acidic pH is necessary to release formaldehyde, the active component.

The prostate is a unique compartment for consideration of antimicrobial efficacy. There are no active antibiotic transport mechanisms for the gland and most antibiotics penetrate poorly into prostate tissue and fluid.[28,29] The interior of the gland is an acidic environment. Drug entry and activity are determined by concentration gradient, protein binding, lipid solubility, molecular size, local pH, and $pK_a$ of the antimicrobial agent. Alkaline drugs such as trimethoprim

**Table 36.4 Urinary Excretion of Antimicrobial Agents in Persons With Normal Renal Function**

| Antimicrobial Agent | % of Absorbed Drug Excreted Renally as Parent Metabolites (Active Metabolites)[a] | Usual Dosage for Normal Renal Function[b] |
|---|---|---|
| **Penicillins** | | |
| Penicillin G | 80 | 1–2 million U IV q4–6h |
| Amoxicillin | 90 | 500 mg PO tid |
| Amoxicillin/clavulanic acid | Clavulanate: 20–60 | 500 mg PO tid or 875 mg PO bid |
| Ampicillin | 90 (10) | 1–2 g IV q6h |
| Cloxacillin | 35–50 | 1–2 g IV q4–6h |
| Piperacillin | 50–80 | 200–300 mg/kg/day IV qid |
| Piperacillin/tazobactam | Tazobactam: 60–80 | 3.375 g IV q6h |
| Pivmecillinam | 45 | 200–400 mg bid or tid |
| **Cephalosporins** | | |
| Cephalexin | >80 (18) | 500 mg PO qid |
| Cefazolin | >80 | 1 g IV q8h |
| Cefuroxime | >80 | 250–500 mg PO bid |
| Cefotaxime | 50–60 (30) | 1 g IV q8h |
| Ceftriaxone | 50 | 1–2 g IV q24h |
| Cefepime | 85 | 1–2 g PO q12h |
| Cefixime | 15–20 | 400 mg PO qd |
| Cefpodoxime | 20–35 | 100–200 mg PO q12h |
| Cefprozil | 60 | 250–500 mg PO q12h |
| Ceftazidime | 80–90 | 1–2 g IV q8–12h |
| Ceftaroline | 50 | 600 mg IV q12h |
| Ceftolozane/tazobactam | 95/80 | 1 g/500 mg q8h |
| Ceftazidime/avibactam | 80–90/97 | 2 g/500 mg q8h |
| **Macrolides, Lincosamides** | | |
| Erythromycin | 5–15 | 500 mg PO qid or 1 g IV q6h |
| Clindamycin | ≤6 (some active metabolites) | 150–300 mg PO tid or 600–900 mg IV q6–8h |
| Clarithromycin | 20–30 (10–15) | 250–500 mg PO q12h |
| Azithromycin | 6 | 500 mg PO qd |
| **Aminoglycosides** | | |
| Gentamicin | 99 | 5 mg/kg/day IV in 1–3 divided doses |
| Tobramycin | 99 | 5 mg/kg/day IV in 1–3 divided doses |
| Amikacin | 99 | 15 mg/kg/day IV in 1–3 divided doses |
| **Carbapenems** | | |
| Imipenem/cilastatin | 70–76 | 500 mg IV q6h |
| Meropenem | 70–80 | 500 mg to 1 g IV q6–8h |
| Ertapenem | 40 | 1 g IV q24h |
| Doripenem | 70 (15) | 500 mg q8h |
| **Fluoroquinolones** | | |
| Norfloxacin | 25–40 (10–20) | 400 mg bid |
| Ciprofloxacin | 40 (10–20) | 250–750 mg PO or 400 mg IV bid |
| Levofloxacin | 70–80 | 250–750 mg PO or IV q24h |
| Moxifloxacin | 20 | 400 mg PO or IV q24h |
| **Other Antibacterials** | | |
| Vancomycin | >90 | 1 g IV q12h |
| Teicoplanin | >90 | 6–12 mg/kg IV q12h |
| Dalbavancin | 42 | 1 g IV |
| Daptomycin | 54 | 4 mg/kg IV q24h |
| Linezolid | 35 | 600 mg PO or IV q12h |
| Tigecycline | 32 | 250–500 mg IV q6h div q12h |
| Colistin | 64–70 | 1.5–2.5 mg/kg/day |
| Trimethoprim | 66–95 | 100 mg PO q12h |

*Continued on following page*

**Table 36.4 Urinary Excretion of Antimicrobial Agents in Persons With Normal Renal Function (Cont'd)**

| Antimicrobial Agent | % of Absorbed Drug Excreted Renally as Parent Metabolites (Active Metabolites)[a] | Usual Dosage for Normal Renal Function[b] |
|---|---|---|
| Sulfamethoxazole | 20–40 | |
| Trimethoprim/sulfamethoxazole | | 180/800 mg PO bid |
| Nitrofurantoin monohydrate/macrocrystals | 40–60 | 50–100 mg PO q6h |
| Fosfomycin tromethamine[a] | 30–60 | |
| Uncomplicated UTI | | 3 g, one dose; |
| Complicated UTI | | 3 g q48–72h |
| Doxycycline | 20–30 | 100 mg PO bid |
| Aztreonam | 66 | 1–2 g IV q6–8h |
| Metronidazole | 15 (30–60) | 500 mg PO or IV tid |
| Rifampin | <10/50 | 600 mg PO qd |
| **Antifungals** | | |
| Amphotericin B deoxycholate | <10 | 0.5–1 mg/kg IV qd |
| Amphotericin B lipid formulations | <1 | 1–5 mg/kg/day IV |
| 5-Flucytosine | 90 | 100–150 mg/kg/day PO in four divided doses |
| Ketoconazole | <10 | 400 mg PO qd |
| Fluconazole | 80 | 100–400 mg PO or IV q24h |
| Itraconazole | <1 | 200 mg bid PO or IV × 2 days, then 200 mg PO qd |
| Voriconazole | <1 | 6 mg/kg IV × 1 dose, then 200 mg IV bid; 200-mg PO bid × 1 day, then 100 mg bid |
| Posaconazole | <1 | 400 mg PO bid |
| Caspofungin | <1 | 70-mg loading dose, then 50 mg IV q24h |
| Micafungin | <1 | 50–100 mg IV q24h |
| Anidulafungin | <1 | 100- to 200-mg IV loading dose, then 50–100 mg IV q24h |

[a]Except where noted, values are the proportion of dose renally excreted unchanged.
[b]Not all antimicrobial agents have an indication for urinary tract infection.
*bid,* Twice a day; *IV,* intravenous; *PO,* by mouth; *qd,* once a day; *qid,* four times a day; *tid,* twice a day; *UTI,* urinary tract infection.

(TMP) diffuse into the prostate and are trapped, with high concentrations achieved, but the drug remains in an inactive, ionized form. Fluoroquinolones and macrolides, however, penetrate well and remain active.

Current pharmacodynamic models for antimicrobial treatment of infection distinguish between time-dependent and concentration-dependent bacterial killing. Bacterial killing by β-lactam antimicrobial agents is time dependent, as the therapeutic efficacy depends on how long the concentration of the antimicrobial agent remains above the MIC of the infecting organism. Bacterial killing by fluoroquinolones and aminoglycosides is concentration dependent; the therapeutic efficacy is measured by the ratio of peak antimicrobial concentration to MIC, or the ratio of the area under the curve to MIC. A pharmacodynamic model in which the urine bactericidal titer replaces the MIC has been applied to predict optimal dosing regimens for antimicrobial treatment of urinary tract infection.[27,30] The validity of these models for urinary tract infection, however, still requires confirmation in clinical trials.[31,32] In particular, the relevance to treatment of complicated urinary tract infection is uncertain because impaired renal function, voiding abnormalities, and the presence of biofilms on indwelling devices introduces variability that will affect antimicrobial efficacy.[30]

## USUAL PRESENTATIONS OF URINARY TRACT INFECTION

### ACUTE UNCOMPLICATED URINARY TRACT INFECTION: CYSTITIS

#### EPIDEMIOLOGY

Acute uncomplicated urinary tract infection manifesting as acute cystitis is a common syndrome that affects otherwise healthy women.[1,3] About 10% of young, sexually active, premenopausal women experience a urinary tract infection each year, and 60% of all women have one or more such infections in their lifetimes. From 2% to 5% of women experience frequent recurrent infection for at least some period. After a first episode of cystitis, 21% of female college students in one study reported a second infection within 6 months.[33] Among postmenopausal women aged 55 to 75 years who were enrolled in a Seattle health group, the incidence was seven infections per 100 patient-years; in 24 months, 7% of women had one infection, 1.6% had two infections, and 1% had three or more infections.[34] Acute cystitis is associated with considerable short-term morbidity.[35] Female college students reported that symptoms persisted for an average of 6.1 days,[2] and, for ambulatory women, a mean duration of symptoms was 4.9 days, with 63% of patients reporting their usual activities were compromised by the infection.[36] However, although a large number of women are affected and many have frequent recurrence of infection, there is no long-term morbidity. Acute uncomplicated urinary tract infection is uncommon in healthy young men, with an estimated incidence of <0.1% per year.

## PATHOGENESIS

### Microbiology

Acute uncomplicated urinary tract infection is primarily a disease of extraintestinal pathogenic *E. coli,* also referred to as uropathogenic *E. coli.* These organisms are isolated in 80% to 85% of episodes of acute cystitis.[1,2,34] Infection occurs via the ascending route after bacterial strains that originate in the gut flora colonize the vagina or periurethral area.[7] Although urethral colonization with a potential uropathogen appears to be a prerequisite for infection, cystitis does not subsequently develop in most women with periurethral colonization.[7] Strains of *E. coli* that colonize the periurethral area and subsequently cause urinary tract infection belong to a restricted number of phylogenetic *E. coli* groups and more frequently express diverse virulence factors than do periurethral strains that do not cause symptomatic infection.[37,38] A necessary characteristic for establishing bladder infection is production of FimH, an adhesin attaching to receptors on uroepithelial cells.[39] This surface protein, however, is common on *E. coli* strains, regardless of whether they cause infection. Other potential urovirulence characteristics include other adhesins, iron sequestration systems, toxin secretion, and motility.[38] The putative virulence factors produced by strains isolated from symptomatic infection overlap with those isolated from asymptomatic bacteriuria, and no single characteristic is uniquely correlated with symptomatic infection.[40] Uropathogenic *E. coli* strains may be acquired during travel, from ingestion of food or water, from other household members, including pets, and from sexual partners.[41,42] Clonal outbreaks may occur with transmission of a single strain within a community or larger geographic area.[43,44]

*S. saprophyticus,* a coagulase-negative staphylococcal species, is an organism virtually unique to acute cystitis. It is the second most frequently isolated species (in 5%–10% of episodes), and there is a seasonal variation of infection, with isolation more common in late summer or fall. Genetic elements described in the *S. saprophyticus* genome that may promote urovirulence include adhesins, transport systems to support growth in urine, and urease production.[45] Other Enterobacteriaceae, most commonly *K. pneumoniae,* are isolated in fewer than 5% of premenopausal women but in 10% to 15% of postmenopausal women.[34,46] Gram-positive organisms such as *Enterococcus* species and group B streptococci are uncommon pathogens in premenopausal women.[47] *Salmonella* species and bacteria associated with sexually transmitted infections, such as *Ureaplasma urealyticum, Gardnerella vaginalis,* and *Mycoplasma hominis,* are occasionally isolated.[48]

Acute uncomplicated urinary tract infection recurs in many women and is characteristically reinfection. In as many as 30% of early reinfections—those occurring within 1 month of treatment of an episode of acute cystitis—an *E. coli* strain similar to the pretherapy strain is isolated. This finding is assumed to be a consequence of failure of the antimicrobial therapy to eliminate virulent strains from the gut or vaginal flora reservoirs.[2] Intracellular persistence of *E. coli* in uroepithelial cells is an alternative mechanism proposed to explain same-strain recurrence, on the basis of observations in animal studies.[49,50] However, prospective studies in women document periurethral colonization prior to bladder infection onset for most episodes,[51] and the contribution of an intracellular reservoir to recurrent acute uncomplicated cystitis in humans remains uncertain.

### Host Factors

Acute, uncomplicated urinary tract infection is a consequence of the interaction of a virulent organism with host genetic susceptibility and behavioral variables.[10,14] The notion of genetic propensity is supported by two consistent observations: (1) an increased frequency of urinary tract infection in first-degree female relatives of women with recurrent infection[1,3,52] and (2) the fact that infection at a younger age is a major risk factor for recurrent cystitis in women of any age.[1,34,52] One well-characterized genetic association is being a nonsecretor of the ABO blood-group antigens.[52,53] Women with recurrent urinary tract infection are at least three times more likely to be nonsecretors than are those without recurrent infection. Nonsecretors express cell–surface glycosphingolipids on the vaginal epithelium, and presumably urethral mucosa, that differ from those expressed by secretors and bind uropathogenic *E. coli* more avidly.[14] Other potential genetic determinants include genetic polymorphisms of the IL-8 receptor CXCR1, TLRs, and the tumor necrosis factor promoter.[14]

The most important behavioral association of urinary tract infection in premenopausal women is sexual intercourse.[1–3,54] In young, sexually active women, 75% to 90% of episodes are attributable to intercourse, and there is a correlation between frequency of intercourse and frequency of infection.[53] Intercourse appears to promote infection by facilitating ascension of organisms from the periurethral area into the bladder. Spermicide use for birth control is another independent behavioral risk factor for acute cystitis in premenopausal women. The frequency of recurrent infection is at least twice as high among women who use spermicides as among women who do not.[53] Spermicides are bactericidal for the hydrogen peroxide–producing lactobacilli of the normal vaginal flora, which maintain the acidic pH. When these bacteria are not present, the vaginal pH increases and this facilitates colonization with potential uropathogens such as *E. coli.* Case–control studies have consistently demonstrated that behavioral variables popularly identified as risks for cystitis—such as type of underwear, bathing rather than showering, postcoital voiding, frequency of voiding, perineal hygiene practices, vaginal douching, and tampon use—are not associated with an increased risk of infection.[1,2]

A history of prior urinary tract infection at a younger age is the strongest association of recurrent acute cystitis in postmenopausal women.[55–57] Sexual intercourse is not an important contributor.[57,58] Estrogen deficiency has been proposed to promote recurrent urinary tract infection in these women through alterations in vaginal flora, including replacement of lactobacilli by potential uropathogens. However, prospective cohort studies and case–control studies uniformly demonstrate no association of oral or topical estrogen use with recurrent urinary tract infection, regardless of restoration of vaginal lactobacilli and acid pH.[59] Acute uncomplicated urinary tract infection in men is uncommon, but reported risk factors have included intercourse with a female partner with recurrent urinary tract infection, not being circumcised, and anal intercourse.[60]

## DIAGNOSIS

The classic clinical manifestation of symptomatic lower urinary tract infection is the acute onset of one or more irritative bladder symptoms, such as urgency, frequency, dysuria, stranguria, and hesitancy.[1,3] Gross hematuria is also common. The most important differential diagnoses to exclude are sexually transmitted infections[61]; vulvovaginal candidiasis and noninfectious syndromes such as interstitial cystitis should also be considered. The combination of new-onset frequency, dysuria, and urgency, together with the absence of vaginal discharge and pain, has a positive predictive value for acute cystitis of 90%.[62] Women who experience recurrent infection also have >90% accuracy in self-diagnosis on the basis of symptoms.[2]

A urine culture is not recommended routinely for women with a clinical presentation consistent with acute uncomplicated cystitis.[3,48,63] The utility of the urine culture is limited by the reliability of the clinical diagnosis, predictable microbiology, and prompt clinical response with short-course empirical antimicrobial therapy. Final culture results are often not available until therapy is completed, and quantitative bacterial counts $<10^5$ CFU/mL are isolated in as many as 30% of women with acute cystitis. Therefore interpretation of culture results may be problematic.[1,47] In fact, urine culture results are negative in as many as 10% of women with a characteristic clinical presentation, and these women have a clinical response to antimicrobial therapy similar to that of women with positive cultures.[64] These women with low quantitative counts of organisms isolated in the urine culture may have urethritis, rather than cystitis. However, both urinary frequency and increased fluid intake are characteristic of patients with acute cystitis. Thus the limited dwell time of urine in the bladder seems the likely explanation for the observation of a high frequency of urine cultures with lower quantitative counts. Culture results may be negative because organisms are present in quantitative counts below the level of detection by standard laboratory procedures (usually $<10^3$ CFU/mL) or because fastidious organisms may not be identified by routine laboratory procedures used in processing urine specimens.

A urine specimen for culture should be obtained, however, from selected women with possible acute uncomplicated urinary tract infection. When the clinical presentation is not characteristic, a urine culture may help confirm or exclude the diagnosis of urinary tract infection. Any quantitative count of an Enterobacteriaceae or *S. saprophyticus* is considered positive. *Enterococcus* spp. or group B streptococcus in any quantitative count should be interpreted as contamination.[47] Failure to respond to appropriate empirical antimicrobial therapy or an early (<1 month) symptomatic recurrence after therapy is suggestive of infection with a resistant organism. In these situations, a urine culture should be obtained to confirm whether antimicrobial resistance is present and to facilitate selection of an effective alternative regimen.

The presence of pyuria, identified by routine urinalysis or leukocyte esterase dipstick testing, is a consistent accompaniment of acute cystitis.[1,63] The absence of pyuria is suggestive of an alternative diagnosis but does not rule out urinary tract infection in women with a consistent clinical presentation.[1,64–66] Thus routine screening for pyuria is not recommended in the management of women presenting with presumed acute cystitis.[1,63] A urine nitrite dipstick test screens for the presence of bacteria, rather than leukocytes, and results are usually positive in women with infection.[66] False-negative nitrite test results may occur when there is infection with bacteria that do not reduce nitrate, such as *Enterococcus* species, or when urine has not been retained in the bladder a sufficient time to allow bacteria to convert nitrate to nitrite. Nitrite tests uncommonly have false-positive results, but these may occur when blood, urobilinogen, or some dyes are present in the urine.

## TREATMENT

For many women, the natural history of acute uncomplicated cystitis is spontaneous clinical and microbiologic resolution within a few days or weeks. In a clinical trial in which subjects were randomly assigned to receive antibiotic therapy or placebo, 28% of 277 women who received placebo were asymptomatic by 1 week, and 45% had negative culture results by 6 weeks.[67] In another study, 54% of women who received placebo were asymptomatic by 3 days and 52% at 7 days.[68] However, antimicrobial treatment is associated with a significantly shorter duration of symptoms. The rates of clinical cure were 77% with nitrofurantoin in comparison with 54% with placebo at 3 days, and 88% and 52%, respectively, at 7 days.[68] After initiation of antimicrobial therapy, 54% of women reported symptom improvement by 6 hours, 87% by 24 hours, and 91% by 48 hours. In another case series, 72% of women reported complete symptom resolution by the fourth day of effective treatment.[36] In a trial of antiinflammatory therapy with ibuprofen alone compared with empiric fosfomycin antimicrobial therapy for women with mild to moderate symptoms, antimicrobial therapy was associated with more rapid resolution of symptoms and fewer cases of pyelonephritis.[69]

Many antimicrobial agents are effective for treatment of acute cystitis (Table 36.5). The anticipated cure rate for recommended first-line empirical regimens is 80% to 95%.[3,70] TMP/sulfamethoxazole (TMP/SMX) has been a mainstay of empirical treatment of acute cystitis for decades and remains highly effective against susceptible organisms.[70,71] However, increasing rates of TMP/SMX resistance in community *E. coli* isolates compromise the use of this agent as first-line empirical therapy.[72] Some antimicrobial agents—nitrofurantoin, pivmecillinam, and fosfomycin—have indications largely restricted to acute cystitis. These drugs do not induce cross-resistance with other classes of antimicrobial agents and, to date, limited resistance has been observed in community uropathogens.[3,72] Thus they are ecologically attractive for treatment of acute cystitis.[35,70,73] Pivmecillinam, however, is not available in all countries. Fosfomycin is now also used both orally and parenterally for infections with some resistant organisms, and resistance to this agent is emerging in some settings.[74] The fluoroquinolones with urinary excretion—norfloxacin, ciprofloxacin, and levofloxacin—are not generally recommended as first-line therapy because widespread use promotes the emergence of resistance.[73] β-Lactam antimicrobial agents, including amoxicillin, amoxicillin/clavulanic acid,

**Table 36.5 Preferred Antimicrobial Regimens for Treatment or Prevention of Acute Uncomplicated Urinary Cystitis in Women With Normal Renal Function**

| First-Line Therapy | Other Therapy |
|---|---|
| **Acute Cystitis** | |
| TMP/SMX, 160/800 mg bid × 3 days<br>Nitrofurantoin, 50–100 mg qid, or monohydrate/ macrocrystals, 100 mg bid × 5 days[a]<br>Pivmecillinam, 400 mg bid × 5 days or 200 mg bid × 7 days[a]<br>Fosfomycin trometamol, 3-g single dose[a] | Norfloxacin, 400 mg bid × 3 days<br>Ciprofloxacin, 250 mg bid, or extended-release preparation, 500 mg qd × 3 days<br>Levofloxacin, 250–500 mg qd × 3 days<br>Trimethoprim, 100 mg bid × 3 days<br>Amoxicillin 500 mg tid × 7 days[a]<br>Amoxicillin/clavulanic acid, 500 mg tid or 875 mg bid × 7 days[a]<br>Cephalexin, 250–500 mg qid × 7 days[a]<br>Cefpodoxime proxetil, 100 mg bid × 3 days<br>Cefuroxime axetil, 500 mg bid × 7 days[a]<br>Cefixime, 400 mg qd × 7 days[a]<br>Doxycycline, 100 mg bid × 7 days |
| **Prophylaxis** | |
| **Long-Term Low-Dose Regimens (at Bedtime)** | |
| Nitrofurantoin, 50 mg qd, or monohydrate/ macrocrystals, 100 mg qd<br>TMP/SMX, 40/200 mg od or every other day | Cephalexin, 500 mg qd[a]<br>Norfloxacin, 200 mg every other day<br>Ciprofloxacin, 125 mg qd<br>Trimethoprim, 100 mg qd |
| **Postcoital (Single-Dose) Regimen** | |
| TMP/SMX, 40/200 mg or 80/400 mg<br>Trimethoprim, 100 mg<br>Nitrofurantoin, 50 or 100 mg[a] | Cephalexin, 250 mg[a]<br>Norfloxacin, 200 mg<br>Ciprofloxacin, 125 mg |

[a]Recommended for pregnant women.
*bid,* Twice a day; *qd,* once a day; *qid,* four times a day; *tid,* twice a day; *TMP/SMX,* trimethoprim/sulfamethoxazole.

and cephalosporins, are reported to be 10% to 15% less effective than first-line agents.[70,75] The β-lactam agents are useful, however, for treatment in pregnant women because they are safe for the fetus.[48]

To limit adverse effects, cost, and emergence of bacterial resistance, the shortest effective duration of antimicrobial therapy should be prescribed. For TMP/SMX and the fluoroquinolones, 3 days is optimum.[3,70] The minimum duration of nitrofurantoin therapy is 5 days.[76,77] For β-lactam antimicrobial agents, 7 days is recommended; shorter courses are less effective. Fosfomycin is given as a single dose. For other agents a single dose is generally 5% to 10% less effective than the recommended longer regimens.[48,70]

The antimicrobial susceptibility of uropathogenic *E. coli* strains acquired in the community evolves continually in response to antimicrobial pressure.[72,78–80] Resistance in community isolates has compromised the efficacy of ampicillin, cephalosporins, and TMP/SMX for use as empirical therapy and there is increasing resistance to fluoroquinolones.[3,72] Recent prior antimicrobial therapy is most strongly associated with isolation of a resistant organism.[80] Treatment of cystitis with an antimicrobial agent to which the infecting organism is resistant is associated with a high failure rate, despite very high urinary levels of the drug.[81,82] In fact, cure rates when the organism is resistant to the antimicrobial agent are similar to those reported with placebo: about 50%. If the local prevalence of resistance to an antimicrobial agent in community *E. coli* strains exceeds 20%, that agent should not be used for first-line empirical therapy.[70] The current increase in extended-spectrum β-lactamase (ESBL)–producing *E. coli* in community-acquired infections, attributed to global expansion of the *E. coli* clone ST131,[44] is of particular concern because these strains are usually also resistant to TMP/SMX and fluoroquinolones.[80,83] Optimal treatment of infection with ESBL-producing *E. coli* is not yet well defined. Nitrofurantoin, fosfomycin, and pivmecillinam currently remain effective for most of these strains.[80,84]

## OTHER INVESTIGATIONS

Young women with a characteristic clinical presentation and prompt response following appropriate empirical therapy do not require further diagnostic imaging or urologic investigation.[85] Fewer than 5% of these women have urologic abnormalities, and the few women in whom abnormalities are identified usually do not require further intervention. However, investigation may be appropriate to rule out alternative pathologic processes when the diagnosis is uncertain or clinical presentation is atypical.

## RECURRENT INFECTION

Episodes of acute cystitis recur frequently in many women. Effective control can be achieved with low-dose prophylactic antimicrobial therapy given either daily or every other day at bedtime or after intercourse (Table 36.5).[2,86,87] This strategy is recommended for women who experience more than two episodes in 6 months. The initial course of prophylaxis lasts 6 or 12 months. Antimicrobial prophylactic therapy decreases recurrent symptomatic episodes by about 95% while the agent is being taken, but it does not alter the frequency of recurrent infection once prophylaxis is discontinued. About 50% of women experience reinfection within 3 months of discontinuing prophylaxis. Reinstitution of prophylaxis for as long as 2 years may be considered for these women. Self-treatment is another effective strategy for managing recurrent infections; this approach is often preferred by women who are traveling or who experience less frequent recurrences.[2] A 3-day course of TMP/SMX or ciprofloxacin has been shown to be effective for empirical self-treatment in clinical trials, but other regimens are also probably effective.

The only feasible behavioral intervention to prevent recurrent urinary tract infection is to avoid spermicide use. Other proposed nonantimicrobial approaches for prevention include daily intake of cranberry products, oral or vaginal probiotics to reestablish normal vaginal flora, and estrogen replacement for postmenopausal women.[88,89] Initial studies reported that daily intake of cranberry juice or tablets decreased episodes of recurrent cystitis by 30% in comparison with placebo.[90] The proposed mechanism for this effect is inhibition of the P fimbria–mediated adherence of *E. coli* to uroepithelial cells by the proanthocyanidins present in cranberry products and excreted in the urine. However, more recent clinical trials reported no benefit of daily cranberry juice in comparison with placebo,[91] and cranberry capsules were less effective than TMP/SMX prophylaxis.[92] Trials of oral or vaginal *Lactobacillus* probiotics do not support efficacy of these products in preventing urinary tract infection.[93–95] The role of estrogen replacement to prevent urinary tract infection in postmenopausal women is controversial.[2,96] In prospective clinical trials, researchers have uniformly reported no benefit of systemic estrogen over placebo, despite restoration of an acidic vaginal pH and increased vaginal colonization with lactobacilli in subjects who received estrogen.[59] Two small clinical trials comparing vaginal estrogen with placebo in postmenopausal women with frequent, recurrent infection demonstrated a decreased frequency of symptomatic episodes in women treated with topical estrogen therapy, but in a comparative trial, an estrogen-containing pessary was substantially less effective than nitrofurantoin prophylaxis.[59,97] Currently, topical vaginal estrogen should likely only be considered for use to prevent infection in selected women with a very high frequency of recurrent infection.

Several other potential nonantimicrobial approaches for prevention of recurrent urinary tract infection are under investigation.[49,98,99] These include strategies to reinstate the glucosaminoglycan layer,[100,101] to block bacterial FimH adhesion with D-mannose,[99] using vitamin D to enhance antimicrobial peptide production,[102] vaccination using FimH or iron receptors,[99] and immune stimulation with heat-killed whole bacteria.[99] A recent trial with one of the whole bacterial immunostimulants (OM-89S), however, showed no benefit.[103] The clinical efficacy of any of these proposed interventions remains uncertain.

## ACUTE NONOBSTRUCTIVE PYELONEPHRITIS

### EPIDEMIOLOGY

Pyelonephritis is a less common manifestation of acute uncomplicated urinary tract infection than cystitis. The ratio of pyelonephritis to cystitis episodes is reported to be between 1:18 and 1:29 in women with recurrent infection.[2] The highest incidence is among women aged 20 to 30 years. Pyelonephritis is associated with substantial morbidity; hospitalization is required for as many as 20% of affected nonpregnant women.[104] Severe manifestations such as sepsis syndrome are, however, uncommon. Acute pyelonephritis complicates 1% to 2% of pregnancies. When this complication occurs at the end of the second trimester or early in the third trimester, preterm labor and delivery may occur and lead to poor fetal outcomes, as with any febrile illness in later pregnancy.[105]

Acute nonobstructive pyelonephritis is rarely a direct cause of renal failure. In the few reports of renal failure attributed to pyelonephritis, the patients were elderly[106] or had comorbid conditions such as diabetes and HIV infection.[107] Renal scarring is a complication of pyelonephritis in some women with more severe clinical presentations. An Italian study reported renal scars identified by computed tomography (CT) or magnetic resonance imaging (MRI) at a 6-month follow-up in 29% of women who required hospitalization for pyelonephritis.[108] In an Israeli study, 30% of a cohort of 203 women admitted for acute pyelonephritis were reassessed 10 to 20 years after admission; renal scars were detected in 46% of these women on technetium (Tc) 99m–labeled dimercaptosuccinic acid scanning. However, the renal scars were not associated with hypertension or renal impairment.[109] The histologic finding of "chronic pyelonephritis" in patients with renal failure was formerly attributed to infection. However, this condition is now recognized as an end stage of many chronic inflammatory conditions of the kidney, and it is attributable to infection in only a few patients in whom there is a clear history of recurrent renal infection.

### PATHOGENESIS

*E. coli* is isolated in 85% to 90% of women who present with acute uncomplicated pyelonephritis.[2,110] Infecting strains are characterized by production of the P fimbria adhesin Gal(α1–4) Galβ disaccharide galabiose. This surface protein appears to have a direct role in the pathogenesis of pyelonephritis through induction of mucosal inflammation.[38,111] A familial susceptibility to pyelonephritis has been reported and attributed to polymorphisms with decreased expression of the IL-8 receptor.[112] Other genetic and behavioral risk factors for pyelonephritis in healthy women are similar to those described for acute uncomplicated cystitis.[110] For premenopausal women, these associations are frequency of sexual intercourse, history of urinary tract infection, history of urinary tract infection in the patient's mother, a new sexual partner, and recent spermicide use. The strongest association is with recent sexual intercourse. Women who experience pyelonephritis as children remain at increased risk of pyelonephritis as adults but experience a lower frequency of episodes.[113] Diabetes is also an independent risk factor for pyelonephritis. Young diabetic women are 15 times more likely to be hospitalized for pyelonephritis than age-matched nondiabetic women. Behavioral risk factors associated with pyelonephritis in postmenopausal women have not yet been identified.

### DIAGNOSIS

The classic clinical manifestation of renal infection is costovertebral angle pain or tenderness, often accompanied by fever and variable lower urinary tract symptoms. There is a wide spectrum of severity, however, from mild irritative symptoms with minimal costovertebral angle tenderness to severe symptoms that may include high fever, nausea and vomiting, and severe pain. Acute cholecystitis, renal colic, and pelvic inflammatory disease are occasionally confused with pyelonephritis. When patients present with severe symptoms, underlying complicating factors such as obstruction and abscess must be excluded through urgent imaging. A urine specimen for culture should be obtained before initiation of antimicrobial therapy in every case of suspected pyelonephritis. The culture will confirm the diagnosis of urinary tract infection and identify the specific infecting organism and susceptibilities so that antimicrobial therapy can be optimized. In 95% of women with pyelonephritis, $\geq 10^5$ CFU/mL of organisms are isolated from the urine culture.

Bacteremia is identified in 10% to 25% of women presenting with acute pyelonephritis if blood culture specimens are collected routinely. However, the clinical utility of routine blood cultures is limited because bacteremia does not alter therapy, nor is it predictive of outcome.[114,115] Thus blood cultures should be obtained selectively, usually only if the diagnosis is uncertain or the clinical presentation is severe. Growth of the same organism from both blood and urine usually confirms a urinary source for the infection. However, bacteria isolated from the urine occasionally originate from bacteremia from a source outside the urinary tract. This finding may also reflect hematogenous seeding with development of renal microabscesses, which is well described for *Staphylococcus aureus* in particular.[116] The proportion of cases in which *S. aureus* bacteriuria has a nonurinary source, however, is controversial.[116,117]

Additional investigations recommended for most patients presenting with acute pyelonephritis are measurements of peripheral leukocyte count and serum creatinine level. The leukocyte count is usually elevated and may be useful as a parameter to monitor the response to therapy. C-reactive protein and procalcitonin values are elevated in most women with acute pyelonephritis and tend to correlate with severity of presentation.[2,118,119] The serum procalcitonin value at presentation is a marker for bacteremia[120] and septic shock,[121] but it does not reliably discriminate between patients requiring inpatient therapy and those who can undergo outpatient therapy,[122] and is not predictive of outcome.[118] An elevated C-reactive protein value at discharge has been associated with prolonged hospitalization and postdischarge recurrence.[119]

## DIAGNOSTIC IMAGING

When the clinical presentation of pyelonephritis is characteristic, symptoms are of mild or moderate severity, and the clinical response after initiation of antimicrobial therapy is prompt, routine diagnostic imaging is not indicated.[48,123] Women whose clinical presentations are severe, in whom treatment fails, or who experience early posttreatment recurrent infection should undergo prompt imaging to rule out obstruction or abscesses and to determine whether intervention is necessary. Ultrasonography is often the initial imaging modality because it is safe and widely accessible.[124] The ultrasound examination in women with uncomplicated pyelonephritis usually yields normal results, but enlargement and edema in one or both kidneys are observed in 20% of patients.[125] Ultrasonography is less sensitive or specific for pyelonephritis than is either CT or MRI.

The optimal diagnostic imaging is contrast-enhanced CT, though this may be associated with a risk of developing contrast-induced nephropathy.[125] Abnormalities observed on CT are characterized as unilateral or bilateral, focal or diffuse, focal swelling or no focal swelling, and renal enlargement or no renal enlargement.[124] In addition to renal enlargement and edema, dilation of the collecting system in the absence of obstruction, wedge-shaped areas of decreased attenuation, and rounded low-attenuation masses with delayed enhancement may be observed. Obstruction of the renal tubules by inflammatory debris or impaired function with tubular ischemia may result in a "striated nephrogram."[124] Abnormalities within the renal cortex and medulla, inflammatory changes in Gerota fascia or the renal sinuses, and thickening of the urothelium are sometimes observed. "Acute focal pyelonephritis" (also called acute lobar nephronia) is infection confined to a single lobe and may be more common in women who have diabetes or are immunocompromised. The response to treatment is similar, however, for patients with or without this imaging finding.[125] In one study the presence of a focal lesion characterized by peripheral ring enhancement without central uptake of contrast material on CT or MRI at presentation was the only imaging finding that was correlated with subsequent development of renal scars.[108]

## TREATMENT

The majority of women with uncomplicated pyelonephritis receive treatment as outpatients.[48,70] Indications for hospitalization include pregnancy, hemodynamic instability, uncertain gastrointestinal absorption or compliance with oral therapy, the need to exclude complicating factors such as obstruction and abscess, and the necessity of monitoring or treatment of associated medical illnesses. Appropriate supportive management for hypotension, nausea and vomiting, and pain should be initiated promptly. When oral tolerance is uncertain because of nausea and vomiting, a strategy frequently used in emergency department management is to provide a single parenteral dose of ceftriaxone, 1 g, or of gentamicin, 120 mg, followed by oral therapy once gastrointestinal symptoms are controlled.

Many parenteral antimicrobial regimens are effective for pyelonephritis (Table 36.6). Options for empiric parenteral therapy include aminoglycosides, extended-spectrum cephalosporins such as cefotaxime and ceftriaxone, and fluoroquinolones such as ciprofloxacin or levofloxacin.[2,70] Aminoglycosides have unique efficacy for the treatment of renal infection as they are bound in high concentrations in the renal cortex.[2] Ceftriaxone therapy is the preferred empirical regimen for pregnant women. Although it is suggested that gentamicin be avoided in pregnancy because of potential fetal ototoxicity, excess otologic impairment has not been reported in large cohorts of newborn infants stratified by gentamicin exposure in utero.[126] Thus when cephalosporins cannot be used because of antimicrobial resistance or patient intolerance, gentamicin remains an alternate antimicrobial for treatment of pregnant women. For ESBL-producing *E. coli* resistant to all first-line therapies, a carbapenem (meropenem, ertapenem, doripenem) is recommended.

Oral therapy selected on the basis of urine culture results can then be prescribed to complete the antimicrobial course. In most young, nonpregnant women, acute pyelonephritis is effectively managed with outpatient oral therapy (Table 36.6).[48,70] The recommended empirical antimicrobial choice is either ciprofloxacin or levofloxacin.[70] Oral TMP/SMX is effective, but because of the high prevalence of TMP/SMX-resistant *E. coli* in many communities, this agent is recommended only when the infecting organism is known to be susceptible. Other oral regimens are also effective and may be appropriate, depending on organism susceptibility and the patient's tolerance. The usual duration of treatment was previously 10 to 14 days, but ciprofloxacin 500 mg twice daily given for 5 or 7 days,[127,128] levofloxacin 750 mg daily for 5 days, and a course of a single dose of ceftriaxone 1 g and cefixime 400 mg daily for 6 days[129] are all effective shorter regimens.[130]

A satisfactory clinical response is usually observed by 48 to 72 hours after initiation of antimicrobial therapy. Risk factors predictive of a poor outcome are hospitalization, isolation of a resistant organism, concurrent diabetes mellitus,

**Table 36.6 Antimicrobial Regimens for Treatment of Acute Uncomplicated Pyelonephritis in Women With Normal Renal Function and Susceptible Organisms**

| First-Line Therapy | Other Therapy |
|---|---|
| **Oral** | |
| Ciprofloxacin, 500 mg bid or 1000 mg extended-release preparation, qd × 7 days | TMP/SMX, 160/800 mg bid × 7–14 days |
| Levofloxacin, 750 qd × 5 days | Amoxicillin, 500 mg PO tid × 14 days[a] |
| | Amoxicillin/clavulanic acid, 500 mg tid or 875 mg PO bid × 14 days[a] |
| | Cephalexin, 500 mg qid × 14 days[a] |
| | Cefuroxime axetil, 500 mg bid × 14 days[a] |
| | Cefixime, 400 mg qd × 14 days[a] |
| **Parenteral**[b] | |
| Ciprofloxacin, 400 mg q12h × 7 days | Ertapenem, 1 g qd |
| Levofloxacin, 750 mg qd × 5 days | Meropenem, 500 mg q6h |
| Gentamicin or tobramycin, 3–5 mg/kg qd, ± ampicillin, 1 g q4–6h | Piperacillin/tazobactam, 3.375 g q6h |
| Ceftriaxone, 1–2 g qd[a] | Doripenem, 500 mg q8h |
| Cefotaxime, 1 g q8h[a] | Ceftolozane/tazobactam, 1 g q8h |
| | Ceftazidime/avibactam, 2 g q8h |

[a]Recommended for pregnant women.
[b]Change to oral therapy to complete course once condition is clinically stable.
*bid,* Twice a day; *PO,* by mouth; *qd,* once a day; *qid,* four times a day; *tid,* twice a day; *TMP/SMX,* trimethoprim/sulfamethoxazole.

and history of renal stones.[131] All these variables are suggestive of greater severity of illness at presentation or of a complicated infection. Prophylactic antimicrobial strategies similar to those for recurrent cystitis are effective for prevention of recurrent uncomplicated pyelonephritis.

## COMPLICATED URINARY TRACT INFECTION

### EPIDEMIOLOGY

The frequency of complicated urinary tract infection is highly variable, depending on the underlying genitourinary abnormality (Table 36.1).[1,5] Some individuals with a transient abnormality, such as a ureteric stone complicated by pyelonephritis, may experience only a single infection. Other patients, including those with indwelling devices or persistent obstruction, may experience frequent recurrent infections. For instance, in men with spinal cord injury in whom voiding is managed with an indwelling catheter, the incidence is 2.72 infections/1000 days; when voiding is managed with intermittent catheterization, the infection incidence is 0.41/1000 days.[132] In residents of long-term care facilities with long-term indwelling urethral catheters, the incidence of symptomatic infection is 3.2/1000 catheter days.[133]

Complicated urinary tract infection is a frequent cause of hospitalization. The urinary tract is the most common source of community-acquired bacteremia,[134,135] and most bacteremic episodes of urinary tract infection are attributable to complicated infection.[136] Patients who have obstruction, an indwelling catheter, urologic tumors, or who have undergone recent manipulation of the urinary tract with mucosal bleeding are at increased risk of bacteremia and severe sepsis. The genitourinary tract is the source of infection in about 10% of patients admitted to critical care units with septic shock.[137]

These patients are also at risk for local suppurative complications, such as renal or perinephric abscess, or metastatic infection after bacteremia, such as septic arthritis, osteomyelitis, or endocarditis. Serious complications are more common in patients who are diabetic, are immunocompromised, or have long-term urologic devices or obstruction. Renal functional impairment in patients with complicated urinary tract infection is usually attributable to the underlying abnormality or to organ failure complicating septic shock, rather than being a direct consequence of infection. For instance, introduction of voiding strategies to maintain low bladder pressure and to prevent reflux have almost eliminated the complication of chronic renal failure in persons with spinal cord injury, despite a continued high incidence of urinary tract infection in these patients.[138]

### PATHOGENESIS

#### Microbiology

Host impairment rather than organism virulence is the major determinant of infection. *E. coli* remains the organism most frequently isolated in complicated urinary tract infection.[4,5] The *E. coli* strains are characterized by a low frequency of expression of virulence factors in comparison with strains isolated in acute uncomplicated infection.[40] Many other bacteria and yeast species are also isolated.[5,139,140] Enterobacteriaceae such as *Klebsiella* species, *Enterobacter* species, *Serratia* species, *Citrobacter* species, *Proteus mirabilis, Morganella morganii,* and *Providencia stuartii* are common. Other gram-negative organisms that may be isolated include *Pseudomonas aeruginosa, Stenotrophomonas maltophilia,* and *Acinetobacter* species. Gram-positive organisms are also frequently isolated, including group B streptococci, *Enterococcus* species, and coagulase-negative staphylococci. *S. aureus* is less commonly isolated. *Candida* species may be isolated, usually from patients who have diabetes or indwelling urologic devices or who are undergoing broad-spectrum antimicrobial therapy.[141] Organisms isolated from patients with complicated urinary tract infection often have increased antimicrobial resistance.[142] Risk factors for isolation of a resistant organism include a history of recent antimicrobial therapy or hospitalization, indwelling urethral catheter, invasive urologic procedures, nursing home residence, and some comorbidities.

Biofilm formation is universal in patients with chronic indwelling urinary devices.[143] Following insertion, a conditioning layer composed of proteins and other host components immediately coats the device. This conditioning layer provides a surface for subsequent attachment of bacteria or yeast that originate from the periurethral flora or drainage bags or are introduced after disruption of the closed drainage system. Organisms grow along the device, elaborating an extracellular polysaccharide substance, and colonies of microorganisms persist within this relatively protected environment. Urine components such as Tamm–Horsfall protein and magnesium or calcium ions are also incorporated into the biofilm. Organisms ascend in the biofilm along the interior and exterior surfaces of the device and reach the bladder within days. The initial infection is usually with a single organism, but a polymicrobial flora is invariably present on long-term indwelling devices.[26,143] Urease-producing organisms such as *P. mirabilis, K. pneumoniae, M. morganii,* and *P. stuartii* are isolated more frequently from individuals with long-term indwelling catheters and persist longer than other organisms, such as *Enterococcus* species. Complications attributed to biofilm formation with urease-producing organisms include development of renal or bladder stones and obstruction of the device.[144]

Although the most common device is the urethral catheter, the process of biofilm formation is similar with other indwelling devices, such as ureteric stents and nephrostomy tubes.[145–147] From 34% to 42% of ureteral stents are found at removal to be colonized with bacteria or yeast species, often with multiple organisms. More than 50% of organisms identified by stent biofilm analysis are not isolated from culture of urine specimens collected at the same time.

Uncommon bacteria are occasionally a cause of infection. Some of these organisms may not be identified with standard laboratory procedures for processing urine specimens. *Corynebacterium urealyticum* is a urease-producing gram-positive rod associated with the unique clinical manifestations of encrusted cystitis or pyelonephritis.[148] This infection is characterized by ulcerative inflammation and struvite encrustations on the bladder or renal pelvis wall. Pyelitis, if untreated, may lead to destruction of the kidney. *U. urealyticum* is another urease-producing bacterium that may cause cystitis or pyelonephritis, often with urolithiasis. Case reports suggest a predisposition in immunocompromised individuals, particularly those with hypogammaglobulinemia; healthy persons may also become infected. *Aerococcus sanguinicola* is a rare cause of complicated urinary tract infection; the diagnosis is usually made by isolation of the organism in the blood culture.[149] *Aerococcus urinae* was isolated in 0.3% to 0.8% of urine specimens in one clinical microbiology laboratory, usually from older persons with underlying abnormalities and bacteremia.[150] Anaerobic organisms are seldom identified in the absence of suppurative complications such as abscess.[151]

### Host Factors

Genitourinary abnormalities facilitate infection through increased entry of organisms into the bladder (e.g., by intermittent catheterization, urologic procedures) and subsequent persistence due to incomplete voiding (e.g., as a result of obstruction, urolithiasis, diverticula, reflux), or in biofilm on urologic devices.[4,5] Asymptomatic bacteriuria is common in patients with persistent abnormalities and universal in patients with long-term indwelling catheters.[152] The determinants that lead to symptomatic infection in chronically bacteriuric individuals are not well characterized. However, obstruction and mucosal trauma with bleeding are well-recognized risk factors for bacteremia and sepsis in patients with preexisting bacteriuria.

## CLINICAL PRESENTATIONS

Complicated urinary tract infection manifests across a wide clinical spectrum of signs and symptoms, from mild, irritative symptoms of lower tract infection to pyelonephritis and bacteremia, including septic shock.[4,5,153] Localizing signs and symptoms consistent with cystitis or pyelonephritis are usually present. Patients with indwelling urethral catheters or other indwelling devices usually present with fever alone, although costovertebral angle pain or tenderness, hematuria, or catheter obstruction, if present, identifies a genitourinary source. Patients with chronic neurologic impairment sometimes report symptoms that are not classic for urinary tract infection. For instance, spinal cord–injured patients experience increased bladder and leg spasms or autonomic dysreflexia,[138] whereas patients with multiple sclerosis may present with fatigue or deterioration in neurologic function.[5]

The clinical diagnosis of symptomatic infection is often problematic in older populations with cognitive impairment.[154–156] These patients frequently have chronic genitourinary symptoms and impaired communication, which limits the assessment of signs and symptoms. Because bacteriuria is very common in elderly individuals with functional impairment, nonlocalizing clinical deterioration is frequently attributed to urinary tract infection because the urine culture is positive.[157] However, nonlocalizing clinical manifestations, including fever, are unlikely to have a urinary source in elderly persons without a long-term indwelling catheter.[25,155] Changes in character of the urine, such as cloudiness and odor, are also frequently interpreted as symptoms of urinary tract infection. Cloudiness may be attributed to pyuria, which usually accompanies bacteriuria, and an unpleasant odor is suggestive of production of polyamines by bacteria in the urine. However, alterations in characteristics of the urine are neither sensitive nor specific for the diagnosis of infection. They may be attributable to other causes, such as precipitation of crystals and dehydration. Thus changes in character of the urine should not be interpreted as symptoms of urinary tract infection.

## LABORATORY DIAGNOSIS

A urine specimen for culture should be obtained before initiation of antimicrobial therapy for every patient with suspected complicated urinary tract infection. Because of the wide variety of potential infecting organisms and increased likelihood of resistant strains, definitive microbiologic characterization is necessary to optimize antimicrobial management.

The presence of biofilm on devices such as indwelling catheters and stents within the urinary tract complicates interpretation of the urine culture in some patients with complicated infection.[7,143–145] In patients with a long-term indwelling catheter, the catheter should be replaced, and the new catheter should be used to sample bladder urine and avoid contamination by organisms present in the biofilm of the old catheter.[25,26] When the intestine is interposed into the urinary tract through creation of an ileal conduit, continent cutaneous diversion, or neobladder, urine collected through the conduit or reservoir is often bacteriuric, regardless of symptoms.[158] The organisms isolated represent mixed gram-positive flora, including streptococcal species and *Staphylococcus epidermidis,* but uropathogenic strains such as *E. coli, P. mirabilis, P. aeruginosa,* and *Enterococcus faecalis* may also be present. Similar urine culture findings are reported in 30% to 60% of patients with orthoptic bladder substitution or augmentation cystoplasty[159]; individuals with these reservoirs who practice clean intermittent catheterization are more likely to have positive culture findings.[158] Thus when symptomatic urinary tract infection is suspected, results of a urine culture in such a patient must be interpreted in the context of this usual bacteriuria.

Infection with a fastidious organism should be considered when the clinical presentation suggests symptomatic urinary tract infection but urine culture results are repeatedly negative, particularly when pyuria is present. These organisms may include *C. urealyticum, U. urealyticum,* and *Haemophilus* species. A persistently alkaline pH with pyuria but a negative urine culture suggests a urease-producing organism such as *C. urealyticum* or *U. urealyticum.* The laboratory should be consulted if a fastidious organism is considered, and appropriate specimens should be collected for additional laboratory evaluation to maximize the likelihood of isolating potential infecting organisms.

Patients with genitourinary abnormalities frequently have pyuria, whether or not they have bacteriuria or symptomatic infection, and so pyuria by itself is not diagnostic for urinary tract infection.[5] The absence of pyuria, however, has a high negative predictive value for ruling out urinary tract infection in some populations, such as elderly patients.[25] The severity of clinical manifestations determines whether additional investigation, such as blood culture or a peripheral leukocyte count, is indicated. Renal function should be assessed in every patient with complicated urinary tract infection. A second urine culture after antimicrobial therapy is not recommended if the patient remains asymptomatic.

## ANTIMICROBIAL TREATMENT

The principles of management for individuals with complicated urinary tract infection include prompt specimen collection to identify the specific infecting organism, characterization of renal function and underlying abnormalities, and early institution of appropriate antimicrobial therapy. The antimicrobial regimen selected is individualized on the basis of site of infection, severity of manifestations, known or presumed infecting organism and susceptibility, and the patient's tolerance.[5] When the presenting symptoms are mild, it is preferable to delay initiation of antimicrobial therapy until results of the urine culture are available. This approach allows selection of a narrow-spectrum agent specific for the infecting organism and minimizes antimicrobial pressure, which promotes resistance.

When patients present with severe symptoms, empirical antimicrobial therapy is initiated pending urine culture results. Previous urine culture results, if available, and recent antimicrobial therapy received by the patient should be considered in the selection of the empiric regimen.[5] Parenteral therapy is indicated for patients who present with hemodynamic instability, who cannot tolerate or absorb oral medications, or who are known or suspected to have an infecting organism resistant to available oral options. Patients who present with severe sepsis, including septic shock, should receive initial empirical antimicrobial therapy that provides broad coverage for both gram-positive and gram-negative bacteria, including resistant organisms.[153] Appropriate regimens for these patients may include an aminoglycoside, with or without ampicillin; a cephalosporin with an aminoglycoside; a carbapenem (ertapenem, imipenem, meropenem); an extended-spectrum cephalosporin, or a β-lactam/β-lactamase inhibitor. The new β-lactam/β-lactamase inhibitors—ceftazidime/avibactam and ceftolozane/tazobactam—are effective for the treatment of complicated infection with resistant organisms.[160–164] Intravenous fosfomycin has also been used for some highly resistant organisms, usually in combination with another broad-spectrum antimicrobial.[165]

Fluoroquinolones with good urinary excretion and broad gram-negative coverage—norfloxacin, ciprofloxacin, and levofloxacin—are indicated for empirical oral therapy.[5] Many other oral agents are effective and may be appropriate, depending on patient tolerance and the specific infecting organism.[5] These include TMP/SMX, amoxicillin, amoxicillin/clavulanic acid, oral cephalosporins, and doxycycline. Oral fosfomycin has been used for some resistant organisms, with success rates of 50%–85% reported.[166–168] Nitrofurantoin is effective for treatment of some episodes of bladder infection, but it is not effective for renal or prostate infection. It is contraindicated for treatment of patients with renal failure because peripheral neuropathy has been reported to occur with accumulation of toxic metabolites. *K. pneumoniae, P. aeruginosa,* and *P. mirabilis* strains are uniformly resistant, but nitrofurantoin remains effective for many resistant organisms such as vancomycin-resistant *Enterococcus* and most ESBL-producing *E. coli.*

Substantial clinical improvement is expected by 48 to 72 hours after initiation of effective antimicrobial therapy. Empirical therapy is reassessed at this time, considering the clinical response and urine culture results. Therapy is usually modified to an appropriate narrow-spectrum parenteral or oral agent to complete a 7- to 10-day course. If an organism isolated in the pretherapy urine culture specimen is resistant to the empirical antimicrobial, therapy should be altered to an antimicrobial agent to which the infecting organism is susceptible, even if clinical improvement has occurred. Shorter courses of therapy with treatment durations of 5 days are effective in some patients.[169]

## OTHER INTERVENTIONS

The optimal management of complicated urinary tract infection requires characterization of the underlying genitourinary abnormality and appropriate urologic or other interventions to assist in resolution of the current infection and prevention of subsequent infections. Urgent diagnostic imaging or urologic investigation is indicated for patients who have severe systemic symptoms or whose symptoms do not respond to appropriate antimicrobial therapy despite isolation of a susceptible organism. The goal of early imaging is to identify obstruction or abscesses, for which immediate drainage may be necessary for source control.[132] When the underlying abnormality is already well characterized—as in the case of a patient with an indwelling catheter or a neurogenic bladder managed with intermittent catheterization—further investigations may still be appropriate if the patient has experienced a recent change in frequency or severity of infections. Such a patient remains at risk for development of urolithiasis, tumors, and suppurative complications.

The approach to diagnostic imaging and urologic investigation is determined by the clinical presentation and the patient's previous history. A plain radiograph of the abdomen may identify emphysematous infections and some stones. CT is the imaging modality of choice. It identifies calculi, gas, hemorrhage, calcification, obstruction, renal enlargement, and inflammatory masses. Contrast media–enhanced scans are recommended (though are associated with risk of contrast-induced nephropathy, which should be considered in clinical decision making), with helical and multislice CT to study different phases of contrast excretion.[123–125] Ultrasound examination is less sensitive and specific than other imaging modalities such as spiral CT and MRI, but it may be more accessible.[125]

Appropriate supportive care must be initiated promptly. The removal and replacement of a long-term indwelling catheter before institution of antimicrobial therapy are associated with a more rapid defervescence and a lower risk of early relapse after therapy, as well as facilitating collection of a more valid urine culture specimen.[26] The clinical benefits of catheter replacement are presumed to result from removal of the high concentration of organisms in the biofilm, which are often not eradicated by antimicrobial therapy and remain a source for relapse. Urologic investigations such as cystoscopy, retrograde pyelography, and urodynamic studies should be obtained as appropriate. If encrusted *C. urealyticum* infection is present, surgical resection of the encrustations is required together with antimicrobial therapy. *C. urealyticum* strains are generally susceptible to vancomycin, tetracyclines, and fluoroquinolones.[148]

## MANAGEMENT OF RECURRENT INFECTION

When symptoms recur early after antimicrobial treatment, the susceptibility of the pretherapy infecting organism should be reviewed to confirm that the antimicrobial agent prescribed is effective. If the organism is susceptible, underlying genitourinary abnormalities should be reviewed and further evaluation obtained, if appropriate, to identify abnormalities such as abscesses that may necessitate drainage. Even if the abnormalities cannot be fully corrected, interventions to improve urine drainage may decrease the frequency of episodes of symptomatic infection.[4,5] Indwelling devices should be removed whenever possible. Evidence-based infection control guidelines provide recommendations for prevention of catheter-acquired urinary tract infection.[170–172] and multifaceted programs are effective in decreasing catheter use and infection rates.[173,174] Specific practices include catheter use for restricted indications, limiting duration of use, safe practices for insertion and care, and appropriate catheter size. Interventions that have been shown not to be effective and that are not recommended include use of different catheter materials, antimicrobial coating of catheters, antiseptic or antimicrobial meatal care, and instillation of antiseptics into the drainage bag. Patients with long-term indwelling catheters and other indwelling devices experience infection because of biofilm formation on these devices; therefore the prevention of catheter-acquired infection will ultimately require development of biofilm-resistant biomaterials.[175,176]

Long-term prophylactic antimicrobial therapy is not recommended.[5,138,177] When patients with impaired voiding or indwelling devices are given prophylactic antimicrobial agents, there is little, if any, decrease in symptomatic infection, and rapid reinfection with resistant organisms is uniformly observed.[5] For selected patients with a persistent abnormality and who experience symptomatic relapsing infection with an organism that cannot be eradicated, suppressive therapy may be considered. The goal of suppressive therapy is not to prevent reinfection but either to control symptomatic episodes when infecting bacteria cannot be eradicated or to prevent stone enlargement when inoperable infection stones are present. The antimicrobial regimen is selected on the basis of the infecting organism and is prescribed initially at a full therapeutic dose. If the patient remains clinically stable and the urine is sterile, this dose is usually decreased to about half after 4 to 6 weeks. Suppressive therapy is not appropriate for patients with indwelling devices because biofilm formation facilitates rapid reinfection and emergence of resistant organisms. However, short-term use of such therapy (several weeks or months) for patients with complex urologic abnormalities and indwelling devices may occasionally be considered as part of a palliative care strategy.

A novel approach proposed for control of recurrent infection in patients with impaired bladder emptying is "bacterial interference."[178] This strategy establishes asymptomatic bacteriuria with a nonpathogenic *E. coli* strain in patients with impaired voiding. The avirulent strain in the bladder then prevents infection by other, potentially more virulent, strains. The proposed mechanisms for this protective effect include blocking of bacterial receptors present on uroepithelial cells, competition for nutrients in the urine, and toxin production. Preliminary clinical trials have demonstrated some efficacy of this approach in a small number of highly selected patients.[179]

# ASYMPTOMATIC BACTERIURIA

## EPIDEMIOLOGY

Asymptomatic bacteriuria is a common finding, particularly in women, older persons, and some patients with persistent genitourinary abnormalities (Table 36.7).[152] The prevalence of bacteriuria among sexually active young women ranges from 3% to 5% but is <1% among age-matched controls who are not sexually active. Bacteriuria is present in 5% to 10% of healthy postmenopausal women[152] and in 20% of women older than 80 years living in the community.[180] Asymptomatic bacteriuria is uncommon in younger men, but the prevalence increases in men older than 65 years, presumably concurrently with age-related prostate hypertrophy. Bacteriuria occurs in 10% of healthy men older than 80 years living in the community.[180] Among residents of nursing homes who do not have indwelling catheters, 20% to 50% of women and 15% to 40% of men are bacteriuric. The prevalence among persons with long-term indwelling catheters is 100%.[155] Among spinal cord–injured patients with impaired voiding and no indwelling catheter, the prevalence of bacteriuria is 50%, regardless of the method used for bladder emptying.[138]

Patients with an increased prevalence of asymptomatic bacteriuria also have a higher incidence of symptomatic urinary tract infection. However, this higher frequency of symptomatic infection is not attributable to bacteriuria. The same biologic determinants promote both asymptomatic and symptomatic infection. Bacteriuria in healthy young women is usually transient, but up to 8% have acute cystitis within 1 week of initial identification of a positive urine culture result.[181] In women with diabetes[182] and female or male residents of nursing homes,[155] persistent bacteriuria for months or years, frequently with the same strain, is often observed. No long-term negative outcomes have been attributed to asymptomatic bacteriuria.[152,182] Bacteriuric individuals are not at increased risk of hypertension or chronic renal failure, and survival is similar to that for persons without bacteriuria.

**Table 36.7 Asymptomatic Bacteriuria in Normal Populations and in Selected Patients With Underlying Genitourinary Abnormalities**

| Population/Patients | Prevalence of Bacteriuria (%) |
|---|---|
| **Healthy Women** | |
| Aged 20–50 years: | |
| Sexually active | 3–5 |
| Not sexually active | <1 |
| Aged 50–70 years | 3–9 |
| Aged ≥80 years | 14–22 |
| **Healthy Men** | |
| Aged <65 years | <1 |
| Aged ≥80 years | 6–10 |
| **Patients With Complicated Genitourinary Abnormalities** | |
| **Spinal Cord Injury** | |
| Bladder retrained | 25 |
| Intermittent catheterization | 23–89 |
| Sphincterotomy/condom | 58 |
| Ileal neobladder | 30–60 |
| **Residence in Long-Term Care Facility** | |
| Women | 25–57 |
| Men | 19–37 |
| **Indwelling Urethral Catheter** | |
| Short term | 5%–7% acquisition/day |
| Long term | 100 |
| **Urethral Stents** | |
| Temporary | 45 |
| Permanent | 100 |

Data from Nicolle LE, Bradley S, Colgan R, et al. Infectious Diseases Society of America guidelines for the diagnosis and treatment of asymptomatic bacteriuria in adults. *Clin Infect Dis.* 2005;40:643–654; and Rodhe N, Mölstad S, Englund L, et al. Asymptomatic bacteriuria in a population of elderly residents living in a community setting: prevalence, characteristics, and associated factors, *Fam Pract.* 2006;23:303–307.

Harmful short-term outcomes attributable to asymptomatic bacteriuria are recognized in only two distinct populations: pregnant women and patients who undergo traumatic genitourinary procedures.[152] The prevalence of bacteriuria during early pregnancy is 3% to 7%, similar to that among age-matched nonpregnant women. The physiologic changes that accompany the increased progesterone levels in pregnancy include smooth muscle relaxation and decreased peristalsis, which result in dilation of the renal pelvis and ureters. In later pregnancy, ureteric obstruction may result from pressure of the uterus at the pelvic brim. In 20% to 35% of pregnant women with bacteriuria that is not treated, acute pyelonephritis develops later in pregnancy, usually at the end of the second trimester or early in the third trimester. This incidence of pyelonephritis is twentyfold to thirtyfold higher among untreated women with bacteriuria than among women whose initial screening urine cultures yielded negative results or in whom bacteriuria was treated. Acute pyelonephritis in later pregnancy is associated with premature delivery and poorer fetal outcomes. The second group of bacteriuric patients at risk are those who undergo traumatic urologic procedures. If bacteriuria remains untreated, bacteremia develops in as many as 60% after the procedure, and in 5% to 10% progresses to severe sepsis or septic shock.

## PATHOGENESIS

### Microbiology

*E. coli* is isolated from 80% of healthy women with asymptomatic bacteriuria.[181] Most of the remaining bacterial strains are *K. pneumoniae, Enterococcus* species, and coagulase-negative staphylococci. For men older than 65 years of age, coagulase-negative staphylococci are isolated most frequently, followed by *E. coli* and *Enterococcus* species. In patients with underlying genitourinary abnormalities, a wider variety of organisms are isolated. *E. coli* and other organisms associated with asymptomatic bacteriuria are characterized by the relative absence of or lack of expression of recognized virulence factors.[183] Some strains that are strongly adherent but unable to stimulate an epithelial cell IL-6 cytokine response have been described. These relatively avirulent *E. coli* strains may originate from nonvirulent commensal strains or may evolve from virulent strains by attenuation of virulence genes.[184,185] Other organisms that are frequently isolated, such as coagulase-negative staphylococci and *Enterococcus* species, are relatively nonpathogenic and seldom associated with symptomatic infection. Biofilm formation results in polymicrobial bacteriuria in patients with chronic indwelling catheters.[143]

### Host Factors

The genetic and behavioral risk factors and genitourinary abnormalities associated with asymptomatic bacteriuria are similar to those described for uncomplicated and complicated symptomatic urinary tract infection. For younger women, behavioral risks are sexual activity and spermicide use.[181] Bacteriuric women older than 80 years who reside in the community are characterized by reduced mobility, urinary incontinence, and receiving estrogen treatment; and men older than 80 years with bacteriuria are characterized by prostate disease, history of stroke, and residence in supervised housing.[180] Functional impairment is the major risk factor associated with asymptomatic bacteriuria in the long-term care facility population without indwelling catheters.[155] Higher residual urine volume is not associated with increased bacteriuria in elderly populations but has been associated with bacteriuria in patients referred to an ambulatory urology clinic.[155]

## DIAGNOSIS

The criterion for identification of asymptomatic bacteriuria is an organism quantitative count of $\geq 10^5$ CFU/mL in a urine culture. For women, two consecutive urine specimens with similar culture results are recommended, but a single specimen is sufficient for men.[152] When an initial urine culture in a young woman yields positive results, a second positive result in a specimen obtained within 2 weeks confirms bacteriuria in 85% to 90% of women. If the second specimen result is negative, the initial positive culture result may have been contaminated; however, bacteriuria may also have resolved spontaneously. If a voided specimen has a low quantitative count of a single potential uropathogen, and if it is essential to rule out bacteriuria, a second urine specimen should be collected as a first morning void.

Pyuria usually accompanies bacteriuria, but there is variability in the frequency of pyuria observed in different populations. Pyuria is present in only 50% of bacteriuric pregnant women; therefore screening for pyuria is not a reliable method to rule out bacteriuria in pregnancy.[186] Pyuria is present in about 75% of diabetic women with bacteriuria, in 90% of bacteriuric patients undergoing hemodialysis, and in >90% of elderly persons with bacteriuria.[152] Pyuria also occurs in 30% to 70% of bacteriuric patients with short-term indwelling catheters and in 100% of those with long-term indwelling catheters. Some other biomarkers have been explored to be used in differentiating asymptomatic from symptomatic infection, particularly in the nursing home population. Urinary IL-6 has some association with symptomatic infection, but has not been shown, to date, to have clinical utility.[187,188]

### TREATMENT

Screening for and treatment of asymptomatic bacteriuria is recommended only for pregnant women or for patients who will undergo a traumatic genitourinary tract procedure.[152] For other patients, treatment does not improve short- or long-term clinical outcomes, whereas negative consequences such as reinfection with organisms of increased antimicrobial resistance and adverse drug effects occur.[152,189] In girls and women, an increased frequency of symptomatic infection has been reported after treatment of asymptomatic bacteriuria.[152,190] This finding may be attributable to alteration of vaginal flora by antimicrobial therapy or to replacement of a benign organism in the urine by a more virulent organism. Studies suggest no benefits of treatment of asymptomatic bacteriuria for patients with complicated infection, including renal transplant recipients.[191–193] Treatment of patients with asymptomatic bacteriuria is identified as a major contributor to inappropriate antimicrobial use, and an important target for intervention in antimicrobial stewardship programs.[194,195]

Identification and treatment of asymptomatic bacteriuria early in pregnancy reduces the risk of pyelonephritis from between 25% and 30% to between 1% and 2%.[152] A recent trial in the Netherlands enrolling only low-risk pregnant women reported a much lower rate of pyelonephritis, but a significant association of pyelonephritis and untreated asymptomatic bacteriuria was still observed.[196,197] Current recommendations are that all pregnant women should be screened for bacteriuria by urine culture at the end of the first trimester and treated if bacteriuria is found.[186] Preferred regimens include a 5- or 7-day course of nitrofurantoin[198] or a 7-day course of amoxicillin, amoxicillin/clavulanic acid, or a cephalosporin. The specific regimen is chosen on the basis of the organism isolated and the patient's tolerance. Shorter antimicrobial courses are sometimes prescribed, but these abbreviated courses are likely less effective.[199] TMP/SMX should be avoided, especially in the first trimester, and fluoroquinolones are contraindicated during pregnancy. After treatment for asymptomatic or symptomatic urinary tract infection, urine cultures should be performed at least monthly. If infection recurs, prophylactic antimicrobial therapy should be initiated and continued for the duration of the pregnancy. Nitrofurantoin and cephalexin are the preferred prophylactic regimens because these are considered safe for the fetus.

Initiation of effective antimicrobial treatment immediately before a traumatic urologic procedure prevents bacteremia and sepsis in a bacteriuric patient.[152,200] Conceptually, this approach is surgical prophylaxis rather than treatment of asymptomatic bacteriuria. A single dose of an antimicrobial agent is usually adequate, although some guidelines recommend that the antimicrobial agent be continued after transurethral resection of the prostate until the indwelling catheter is removed.[152] Antimicrobial agents are not recommended for minor urologic procedures such as cystoscopy and urodynamic studies or before replacement of a long-term urethral catheter, as the risk of bacteremia and sepsis with these interventions is low and clinical outcomes are not improved with prophylactic antimicrobial agents.[5,171,201]

## PROSTATITIS

The development of the National Institutes of Health classification of prostatitis syndromes (Table 36.8) and subsequent application of this classification in clinical trials and patient care have greatly advanced the understanding and appropriate management of this common problem.[202] Only acute or chronic bacterial prostatitis is considered attributable to infection and has indications for antimicrobial therapy.[28,203,204]

Acute bacterial prostatitis is a severe infection, which is a urologic emergency.[28] This syndrome is usually community acquired, although healthcare–associated infection may occur after prostate biopsy.[205] Affected men present with severe systemic manifestations including fever and marked urinary symptoms of dysuria and frequency. Urinary obstruction and intense suprapubic pain are often present. Bacteremia is reported in 27% of episodes. A digital rectal examination is not recommended because it may precipitate bacteremia.[28]

*E. coli* is isolated in 70% of episodes. These strains are characterized by the presence of multiple virulence factors.[206] *Proteus* species, *Klebsiella* species, *Enterococcus* species, *P.*

**Table 36.8 National Institutes of Health Classification of Prostatitis Syndromes**

| Class | Description |
|---|---|
| I | Acute bacterial prostatitis |
| II | Chronic bacterial prostatitis |
| III | Chronic pelvic pain syndrome (CPPS) |
| IIIa | Inflammatory CPPS<br>Leukocytes present in semen, in urine after prostate massage, or in expressed prostate secretions |
| IIIb | Noninflammatory CPPS<br>Absence of leukocytes in specimens |
| IV | Asymptomatic inflammatory prostatitis<br>Leukocytes in specimens similar to those in inflammatory CPPS, but no symptoms |

Data from Krieger JN, Nyberg L, Nickel JC. NIH consensus definition and classification of prostatitis. *JAMA.* 1999;281: 236–237.

*aeruginosa,* and *S. aureus* are each isolated in fewer than 10% of cases.[205] Management includes bladder drainage by insertion of a urethral or suprapubic catheter, blood and urine cultures to characterize the infecting organism, and initiation of empirical parenteral antimicrobial therapy. Most antimicrobial agents are active in the acutely inflamed prostate. A combination of a β-lactam and an aminoglycoside is considered first-line therapy, although other broad-spectrum parenteral antibiotics, such as piperacillin/tazobactam and carbapenems, are also effective.[29] Once the infecting organism and susceptibility are confirmed and there has been an adequate clinical response to parenteral therapy, the antibiotic is modified to oral therapy to complete a 6-week course. A fluoroquinolone, either ciprofloxacin or levofloxacin, is recommended as oral therapy if the infecting organism is susceptible. When there is not a prompt clinical response following bladder drainage and initiation of effective antimicrobial therapy, CT or MRI is indicated to search for the uncommon complication of prostate abscess, which occurs in about 5% of cases. When an abscess is identified, transrectal ultrasonography-guided aspiration is usually effective for drainage. A small proportion of patients, 10% to 15%, develop chronic bacterial prostatitis following acute prostatitis.[206]

Chronic bacterial prostatitis occurs in men with persistent prostate infection.[28,203,207–209] Bacteria enter the prostate from the urethra and persist because of limited antimicrobial diffusion or activity in the gland as well as the frequent presence of infected prostate stones in older men. A common clinical presentation is recurrent acute cystitis because bacteria in the prostate intermittently enter the bladder. The same organism is often repeatedly isolated, but the intervals between symptomatic episodes may last months or even years. Other symptoms are generally mild, such as irritative voiding symptoms and discomfort localized to the testicles, lower back, or perineum. Results of the prostate examination are usually normal, but tenderness may occasionally be elicited.

Chronic bacterial prostatitis is documented microbiologically in only 10% of men who present with the clinical syndrome of chronic prostatitis or chronic pelvic pain syndrome. The diagnosis requires paired cultures of midstream and post–prostatic massage urine specimens.[29] The midstream specimen confirms negative results of a urine culture, and the post–prostatic massage specimen reveals pyuria and organisms of presumed prostate origin.[28,207] Gram-negative organisms, including Enterobacteriaceae and *P. aeruginosa,* and gram-positive *Enterococcus* species, *S. aureus,* coagulase-negative staphylococci, and group B streptococci are the bacteria most commonly isolated.[206] Sexually transmitted organisms such as *Chlamydia trachomatis, U. urealyticum, Mycoplasma genitalium,* and *Trichomonas vaginalis* are uncommon and, when present, are usually identified in younger men.[29] The clinical relevance of post–prostatic massage cultures, however, remains controversial. In one study of 463 patients and 121 age-matched controls, 70% of patients were found to harbor at least one organism in a post–prostatic massage specimen, and uropathogens such as *E. coli* were isolated from 8% of patients and 8.3% of controls.[210] In another study, gram-positive organisms were isolated from 6% of 470 men after prostatic massage, but 97% of these organisms were not confirmed on second culture.[211]

Despite this uncertainty, chronic bacterial prostatitis does respond to appropriate antimicrobial treatment, although relapse after treatment is common. Ciprofloxacin and levofloxacin are the first choices for antimicrobial treatment of chronic bacterial prostatitis when susceptible organisms are isolated. These agents penetrate well into the prostate and seminal fluid, and they remain active in the acidic environment of the prostate. Cure rates at 6 months after a 4-week course are 75% to 89%,[29,203] although late relapses may still occur. Doxycycline and macrolides are considered second-line drugs but are preferred for gram-positive infections.[203] Men who present for the first time with chronic pelvic pain syndrome and with evidence of inflammation (i.e., leukocytes) in expressed prostatic secretions, but in whom cultures are negative, should be prescribed a 4-week trial of antimicrobial therapy if they have not previously received a prolonged antimicrobial course.[203,212] In reported case series, as many as 10% of men with such findings show response to antimicrobial therapy despite negative culture results; however, comparative clinical trials in treatment-naïve men with negative culture results have not been reported. If symptoms persist or recur after this 4-week antimicrobial trial, and if results of post–prostatic massage cultures remain negative, further antimicrobial therapy is not indicated.[207,213,214]

## URINARY TRACT INFECTION IN UNIQUE PATIENT POPULATIONS

### RENAL TRANSPLANT RECIPIENTS

Urinary tract infection accounts for 45% to 60% of infections that occur in patients after renal transplantation.[215–217] By 6 months after transplantation, 17% of recipients have experienced at least one urinary tract infection, and by 3 years, posttransplantation infection is reported in 60% of female recipients and 47% of male recipients.[218] The incidence is highest in the early posttransplant period, when immunosuppressive therapy is most intense and infection complicates surgical intervention and the use of urologic devices such as urinary catheters and ureteric stents.[219–221] The clinical presentation is usually asymptomatic bacteriuria, but both cystitis and pyelonephritis are also common; 3% to 14% of episodes are associated with bacteremia.[217,220,222] Early posttransplantation infections tend to be more severe and to manifest more frequently as pyelonephritis or with bacteremia.[223]

Risk factors for urinary tract infection are (1) patient specific, such as female gender, diabetes mellitus, pretransplantation urinary tract infections, prolonged prior dialysis, polycystic kidney disease, and diabetes; or (2) transplant procedure related, such as allograft trauma, microbial contamination of cadaveric kidneys, technical complications related to ureteral anastomosis, the presence of urinary catheters and ureteric stents, immunosuppression, reimplantation, and vesicoureteric reflux.[221] Independent risk factors for any symptomatic or asymptomatic infection in the first year after transplantation are reported to be older age, female gender, higher number of days of indwelling catheter after transplant, anatomic genitourinary abnormalities, and urinary infection within 1 month prior to the procedure.[224] For acute pyelonephritis at any time after transplantation, independent risk factors are female gender, experiencing acute rejection episodes, higher number of urinary infections, and receiving mycophenolate mofetil.[225] Following transplantation, the risk for development of urinary tract infection correlates with the duration of perioperative catheterization or ureteral stent.[216,226] The routine use of ureteric stents at transplantation decreases the overall transplantation complication rate, but stent implantation is associated with a small, but significant, increased risk of urinary tract infection.

Asymptomatic bacteriuria is associated with symptomatic urinary infection but is not a risk factor for graft loss or impaired graft function.[152] Transplant recipients with asymptomatic bacteriuria who progress to graft failure usually also experience symptomatic infection. Graft failure in these patients is usually attributable to urologic abnormalities that promote infection rather than a direct consequence of infection. Symptomatic urinary tract infection has also not been independently associated with graft survival.[222,227–230] However, case reports have described transplant recipients receiving stable immunosuppressive regimens who experience deterioration in graft function that is coincident with an episode of acute pyelonephritis.[231] This occurrence may be attributable to activation of the immune system by the infection.

The principles of management are similar to those for any patient with complicated urinary tract infection. They include prompt clinical diagnosis and initiation of antimicrobial therapy, obtaining appropriate specimens for culture, and urologic evaluation for underlying genitourinary abnormalities that may promote infection. Enterobacteriaceae, particularly *E. coli*, are the most common infecting organisms, but a variety of other bacteria or yeasts may be isolated. The choice of antimicrobial agent is determined by the susceptibility of the infecting organism and the patient's tolerance. A 1-week course of antimicrobial agent for cystitis and 2 weeks for pyelonephritis is recommended. The effect of type and intensity of immunosuppressive therapy on antimicrobial efficacy has not been reported. Bacteriuria does not compromise renal function[193,228] and treatment of bacteriuria does not improve clinical outcomes, including the frequency of symptomatic episodes or graft function.[191–193] Current guidelines therefore do not recommend screening for bacteriuria.[232] Treatment of asymptomatic candiduria in renal transplant recipients has also not been shown to be beneficial and is not recommended.[233]

Urinary tract infections after transplantation are limited by ensuring optimal surgical technique, which includes minimizing the perioperative duration of indwelling urinary devices. TMP/SMX prophylaxis given for the first 6 months after transplantation decreases the risk of both symptomatic and asymptomatic urinary tract infection, as well as other infections, but the effectiveness is compromised by increasing antimicrobial resistance.[234,235] When urinary tract infection is diagnosed in patients receiving TMP/SMX prophylaxis, the organisms isolated are invariably resistant to TMP/SMX. Frequent recurrent symptomatic infection after transplantation may be attributable to an inadequate duration of antimicrobial treatment, resistance of the infecting organism, the presence of urologic abnormalities such as obstruction and stones, or infection of native kidneys. When infection recurs shortly after treatment, previous urine culture results should be reviewed to establish whether reinfection or relapse is occurring and to confirm that the infecting organism is susceptible to the antimicrobial therapy given. If relapse with a susceptible organism occurs after a 2-week course of therapy, retreatment with a 4- to 6-week course is recommended, although the effectiveness of such prolonged retreatment has not been critically evaluated.[222] Repeated relapse after prolonged antimicrobial therapy in patients without identified urologic abnormalities is often caused by infection localized to the native kidneys. Such patients usually have a history of recurrent urinary tract infection before transplantation. The organisms frequently cannot be eradicated, presumably because of failure of antibiotics to achieve effective levels in the nonfunctioning kidney. Long-term suppressive therapy may be necessary to prevent further symptomatic episodes in these patients.

## PERSONS WITH RENAL FAILURE

Urinary tract infections in patients with mild-to-moderate renal failure usually respond adequately to antimicrobial therapy.[236] When renal impairment is severe, however, adequate urine or renal levels of antimicrobial agents may not be achieved because of limited kidney perfusion. If renal failure occurs with acute pyelonephritis, the response following initiation of antimicrobial therapy may be delayed or the risk of relapse after therapy may be increased. Systematic evaluation of antimicrobial efficacy for treatment of urinary tract infection in patients with renal failure has been limited.[5] Aminoglycosides have little penetration into nonfunctioning kidneys and are not recommended for treatment. Fluoroquinolones, TMP/SMX, ampicillin, and cephalosporins have all been effective for treatment in individual case reports. Ertapenem therapy for patients with cystitis or catheter-acquired urinary tract infection is effective but associated with a more prolonged time to negative cultures for patients with impaired renal function.[237] For patients with urinary infection with multiple drug-resistant organisms treated with fosfomycin, chronic kidney disease was associated with a significantly increased risk of treatment failure.[166]

Another therapeutic problem arises when infection is localized to a unilateral nonfunctioning kidney. Antimicrobial therapy sterilizes the urine and often ameliorates symptoms because high urine levels are achieved by antimicrobial excretion through the functioning kidney. However, organisms persist in the kidney with impaired function because antimicrobial penetration to the site of infection is inadequate. When antimicrobial therapy is discontinued, a prompt relapse of infection occurs. Localization of infection to one kidney can be documented by culture of urine collected directly from the ureter following bladder irrigation with normal saline to remove infected bladder urine before ureteric catheterization. For symptomatic relapsing infection when a nonfunctioning kidney is known or suspected to be infected, management options include a trial of a more prolonged course of antimicrobial therapy, continuous suppressive therapy, and surgical removal of the nonfunctioning kidney.

## PERSONS WITH URINARY STONES

Urinary tract infection complicates urolithiasis in several ways; infection may be the cause of stone formation, noninfected metabolic stones may become colonized with bacteria which persist in biofilm, and obstructing noninfected stones may precipitate infection proximal to the obstruction.[238] In any patient with urolithiasis and infection, the infection should be controlled with appropriate antimicrobial therapy before urologic manipulations.[239]

Infection stones, also called "struvite stones," are a complication of infection with urease-producing organisms such as *P. mirabilis*.[240] Urease catalyzes the hydrolysis of urea in the urine. This process produces ammonia and alkaline urine, favoring precipitation of magnesium ammonium phosphate, carbonate apatite, and monoammonium urate.[241] These crystals are incorporated into bacterial biofilm, creating the infection stone.[143] Infection stones continue to enlarge, sometimes rapidly, and ultimately cause obstruction and renal failure if not adequately treated. Patients at increased risk for development of infection stones are those with long-term indwelling catheters, urinary tract obstruction, neurogenic voiding dysfunction, distal renal tubular acidosis, and medullary sponge kidney (see also Chapter 38: Urinary Stone Disease).

Management of infection stones requires complete removal of the stone, together with sterilization of the urine.[239] Percutaneous ultrasonic lithotripsy is effective in removing 60% to 90% of these stones, whereas extracorporeal shock wave lithotripsy is 30% to 60% effective. Multiple stone fragments are passed after lithotripsy. Antimicrobial therapy, selected on the basis of urine culture results, is continued until all fragments are passed. The optimal duration of antimicrobial therapy after lithotripsy is controversial. Currently, 4 weeks is recommended, although some writers suggest a shorter duration. When percutaneous lithotripsy is not effective or is contraindicated, open surgery for stone removal or nephrectomy may be necessary. For selected elderly or debilitated patients with complex urologic or medical problems, stone removal may not be possible. In such patients, continuous suppressive antimicrobial therapy is recommended to limit stone enlargement and preserve renal function.[242] The antimicrobial agent is selected on the basis of urine culture results, and therapy is continued indefinitely if effective and tolerated.

Bacteria may adhere to the surface of a stone that is not initially infected and may subsequently persist in biofilm.[143] Culture of a voided urine specimen in such cases often does not reflect the bacteriology of the stone. In a series of 75 patients with renal stones that were not infection stones, 36 (49%) of the stones were colonized, but only 19 (53%) of these patients also had bacteriuria.[243] Organisms isolated from the colonized stones included *E. coli* (75%), *Enterococcus* species (100%), *P. aeruginosa* (19%), *Klebsiella* species (31%), *P. mirabilis* (8.3%), *Streptococcus* species (31%), *Citrobacter* species (8.3%), *S. saprophyticus* (19%), *M. morganii* (8.3%), and *Gemella* species (8.3%). Larger stones were more likely to be colonized. Patients with stones colonized with bacteria are at increased risk for postprocedure sepsis, even when the voided urine specimen culture has negative results.[244] Perioperative antimicrobial agents are recommended for all patients with stones who have indwelling catheters or stents, because they are at increased risk of stone colonization. Even with antimicrobial prophylaxis, 10% of patients undergoing percutaneous nephrolithotomy experience postoperative fever. Positive urine culture, diabetes, staghorn calculi, and preoperative nephrostomy are risk factors for postprocedure fever.[245]

A noninfected stone causing ureteric obstruction may be complicated by infection of undrained urine proximal to the stone. Complete obstruction is associated with a high risk for bacteremia and sepsis, and prompt drainage is essential for these patients.[246] When a ureter is obstructed, the microbiology of the voided urine specimen may not be consistent with that of urine sampled directly from the renal pelvis. Among patients with obstruction and a positive culture for urine sampled from the renal pelvis, the voided urine specimen culture had positive results in only 16% of cases in one report, and the organisms isolated were concordant between the two specimens in only 23% of patients.[247] Thus a urine specimen should be obtained for culture by percutaneous aspiration of the renal pelvis in patients with obstruction, whenever possible.

## OTHER INFECTIONS OF THE URINARY TRACT

### RENAL AND PERINEPHRIC ABSCESSES

Renal and perinephric abscesses are uncommon suppurative complications associated with substantial morbidity and mortality. Renal abscesses are located entirely within the renal parenchyma, whereas perinephric abscesses occupy the retroperitoneal fat and fascia surrounding the kidney. Abscesses may involve both the renal and perinephric tissues: 25% to 39% of abscesses are intranephric, 19% to 25% are both intranephric and perinephric, and 42% to 51% are perinephritic alone.[248,249] These abscesses develop following ascending urinary tract infection and pyelonephritis, or after hematogenous spread to the renal cortex or retroperitoneum following bacteremia from another site. Multiple bilateral cortical microabscesses suggest hematogenous spread. Complicating factors such as diabetes, urolithiasis, and obstruction are present in most cases. A population-based study from Taiwan reported an incidence of hospitalization for renal and perinephric abscess of 4.6/10,000 person-years for diabetic patients and 1.1/10,000 for nondiabetic patients.[250]

The organisms most commonly isolated from abscesses are *E. coli, K. pneumoniae, P. mirabilis, S. aureus,* and anaerobes. *S. aureus* abscesses are most likely to have originated with hematogenous spread from another site of infection. The clinical manifestations of both renal and perinephric abscesses mimic those of acute pyelonephritis. The characteristic findings are fever and costovertebral angle pain or tenderness. The clinical course in patients treated initially for pyelonephritis is characterized by delayed clinical response or early symptomatic relapse posttherapy. In a multivariable analysis, patients subsequently found to have renal abscess rather than pyelonephritis were more likely to have diabetes mellitus, and to present with hypotension, acute renal impairment, and a peripheral leukocyte (white blood cell [WBC]) count >20,000 WBC/mL.[251]

CT is the preferred imaging modality for diagnosing the presence of an abscess; it also characterizes the abscess size and extent and may identify the potential source.[124] Ultrasonography identifies most perinephric abscesses, but may not be able to distinguish an inflammatory lobar mass from a true renal abscess within the kidney.[125]

The management goals for renal and perinephric abscesses include prompt diagnosis, early institution of effective antimicrobial therapy, and, in selected patients, abscess drainage for both therapeutic and diagnostic purposes. Culture of the abscess fluid identifies the specific infecting organisms and directs antimicrobial choice. If abscess fluid cannot be sampled for culture, organisms isolated from blood or urine culture should be considered in the selection of antimicrobial therapy. Initial antimicrobial administration is usually intravenous. Once the patient's condition is stabilized, therapy can be continued with an appropriate oral antimicrobial agent that has good bioavailability. Small renal abscesses (up to 5 cm in diameter) may be managed medically but larger abscesses usually require drainage.[248,249,252–254] About 70% of renal abscesses resolve with medical therapy alone.[249] Perinephric or mixed abscesses are larger, and drainage is usually required. The current initial approach for these larger abscesses is to attempt percutaneous drainage and, if this is not effective, to proceed to open drainage or nephrectomy. Resolution of the abscess is monitored by repeated imaging studies. Antimicrobial therapy is continued until the abscess has completely resolved or until there is only a residual, stable scar.

## INFECTED RENAL CYSTS

The frequency of occurrence and risk factors for development of cyst infection are not well described. A French series reported that 8.4% of 389 patients with autosomal dominant polycystic kidney disease admitted to the nephrology department over a 10-year period had definite or likely cyst infection[255]; 24% of the episodes were associated with bacteremia, and two patients had more than one episode. Infected cysts complicating polycystic kidney disease may be difficult to diagnose both clinically and microbiologically.[256] Fever and abdominal pain or tenderness, often with bacteremia, are the usual clinical manifestations. However, the differential diagnosis includes pyelonephritis, infected kidney stones, perinephric abscess, cyst hemorrhage, and other intra-abdominal pathology. Most patients with infected cysts also have peripheral leukocytosis and elevated C-reactive protein values. *E. coli, K. pneumoniae, Enterococcus* species, and group B streptococci are the most common infecting organisms, but *Salmonella* spp., *P. aeruginosa, Clostridium* species, *Candida* species, and *Aspergillus* species have also been reported. In view of the wide spectrum of potential pathogens, the specific infecting organism should be confirmed by cyst aspiration whenever possible. Imaging studies are usually necessary to confirm the diagnosis and identify the implicated cyst. Ultrasonography and CT are not useful.[255] MRI and WBC-labeled scans[257,258] were successful in localizing the infected cyst in individual case reports. Positron emission tomography with fludeoxyglucose F-18 is reported to be most effective in localizing the infected cyst, but access to this technology is limited.[256,259–261]

Once the potential infected cyst is identified, a cyst aspiration, if possible, can confirm the presence of infection and provide therapeutic drainage.[262] Antimicrobial penetration into the cyst is presumed to be transepithelial. Effective concentrations of TMP/SMX, chloramphenicol, and fluoroquinolones are achieved in the cyst.[236] Cyst and serum levels of levofloxacin are similar, whereas cyst levels reported with ciprofloxacin are only 40% of serum levels.[263] Therapeutic cyst antimicrobial levels are also achieved with penicillins, cephalosporins, aminoglycosides,[236] and amphotericin B.[264] Prolonged antimicrobial therapy, for at least 4 weeks, is recommended, although clinical trials defining the optimal duration of therapy have not been reported. In the French case series described previously, the mean duration of antibiotic therapy was 5 weeks, and the initial course of therapy was successful for 71% of cases.[254] Nephrectomy is occasionally necessary when cyst drainage and appropriate antimicrobial therapy are not successful in controlling the infection (see also Chapter 45: Cystic Diseases of the Kidney).

## EMPHYSEMATOUS CYSTITIS AND PYELONEPHRITIS

Emphysematous cystitis and pyelonephritis are acute necrotizing infections characterized by gas formation. Gas within the urinary collecting system can be seen after many interventional procedures, but emphysematous infection is characterized by gas in the tissues.[125] Gas is localized to the bladder wall and lumen in cystitis[265] and in and around the kidney in pyelonephritis.[266] Emphysematous pyelitis is a gas-forming infection restricted to the collecting system; the renal parenchyma is spared. Affected patients usually have diabetes with poor glucose control. Obstruction is another common predisposing factor for emphysematous pyelonephritis. *E. coli* and *K. pneumoniae* are the organisms most commonly isolated. High levels of glucose in the urine serve as a substrate for these bacteria, and large amounts of gas are generated through natural fermentation. In affected patients who are not diabetic, protein fermentation is a proposed source of gas formation.[265] CT is considered the optimal imaging technique for confirming emphysematous infection and characterizing the extent of involvement.[124,125]

A review of 135 cases of emphysematous cystitis identified over a period of 50 years reported that the median patient age was 66 years (range, <1 to 90 years); 64% of patients were women, and 67% had diabetes.[265] Presenting symptoms ranged from pneumaturia alone through irritative lower tract voiding symptoms to severe illness suggestive of acute abdominal disease or sepsis; 7% of cases were asymptomatic. *E. coli* was isolated from 58%, *K. pneumoniae* from 21%, and *Clostridium* species and *Enterobacter aerogenes* each from 7% of cases. The diagnosis was apparent on a plain radiograph of the abdomen in 84% of cases. Medical management—including antimicrobial therapy, bladder drainage, and glycemic control—was usually effective. Surgical intervention was required for only 10% of cases and included cystectomy, partial cystectomy, and surgical debridement when concomitant emphysematous pyelonephritis was present. The overall mortality rate was only 7%.

Emphysematous pyelonephritis is a more serious infection with a substantially higher mortality rate.[267] In case series of patients with emphysematous pyelonephritis, 62% to 100% were diabetic, and the majority were women.[268–270] Serum glucose levels are often very high in the diabetic patients, and serum C-reactive protein was generally elevated. *E. coli* was isolated from 45% to 54% of episodes, and bacteremia occurred in 20% to 50% of subjects in whom blood cultures were performed. Plain abdominal radiographs identified gas in the kidney in only 50% of cases. Ultrasonography of the kidneys usually showed some abnormalities but was less accurate than CT in identifying emphysematous infection. Management includes antimicrobial therapy together with percutaneous or open drainage of abscesses and correction of obstruction.[266,267,269–271] Aggressive glucose control and supportive care are also necessary. The mortality rate ranges from 7% to 20% in patients with less severe manifestations to 70% in patients with a fulminant course characterized by necrosis, intravascular thrombosis, and microabscess formation.

Emergency nephrectomy was previously considered necessary for any patient presenting with emphysematous pyelonephritis. Currently, percutaneous drainage is the recommended initial approach. This is associated with similar or lower mortality rates than either emergency nephrectomy or medical management alone.[267,271–274] In a retrospective case series describing a relatively small number of patients, the mortality rates were 50% with medical management alone, 25% with medical management and emergency nephrectomy, and 13.5% with medical management combined with initial percutaneous drainage.[268] Delayed elective nephrectomy may subsequently be required for some patients.

### XANTHOGRANULOMATOUS PYELONEPHRITIS

Xanthogranulomatous pyelonephritis is an uncommon, severe, subacute, or chronic suppurative process characterized by destruction and replacement of the renal parenchyma by granulomatous tissue containing histocytes and foamy cells.[275,276] The inflammatory process may extend into perinephric structures such as Gerota fascia, the posterior perirenal space, the psoas muscle, the diaphragm, and the spleen. Less than 1% to 8% of kidneys removed or subjected to biopsy for inflammatory conditions are reported to show evidence of xanthogranulomatous pyelonephritis.[276] The pathogenesis of this process is unknown, but potential contributing factors include chronic urinary tract infection, abnormal lipid metabolism, lymphatic obstruction, impaired leukocyte function, and vascular occlusion. Urine culture results are positive in 62% to 89% of cases. The organisms most commonly isolated from renal tissue are *P. mirabilis* (38%), *E. coli* (33%), *Klebsiella/Enterobacter* species (8%), *P. aeruginosa* (8%), and *S. aureus* (10%).

In a single-center experience, 35 (85%) of 41 cases presenting from 1994 to 2005 were women.[277] Xanthogranulomatous pyelonephritis was responsible for 19% of 214 nephrectomies performed at this facility during the review period. The most common presenting symptoms were fever, flank or abdominal pain, weight loss, lower urinary tract symptoms, and gross hematuria. All patients had renal calculi. Of 17 cases in which urine culture was obtained, *E. coli* was isolated in 35% and *P. mirabilis* in 18%; in 35% there was no growth. A review from Greece of 39 cases occurring between 1980 and 1999 reported a female/male ratio of 2:1.[275] The presenting history included urolithiasis or renal colic, recurrent urinary tract infections, and previous urologic procedures. All patients were symptomatic at presentation; symptoms included complaints of fever, flank or abdominal pain, chills, and malaise. Anorexia, weight loss, lower tract symptoms, and gross hematuria were also reported. *E. coli* was isolated in 15 cases and *P. mirabilis* in 12. Plain radiographs or intravenous pyelography (IVP) showed a nonfunctioning kidney in 63% of cases, single or multiple calculi in 52%, staghorn calculus in 48%, calyceal deformity in 26%, and hydronephrosis in 23%. In 35 New Zealand patients presenting from 2001 to 2013,[278] 91% were female, staghorn calculi occurred in 51%, and obstructing ureteric calculi in 23%. The most common organisms isolated were *E. coli* (46%) and *P. mirabilis* (20%).

CT is considered the optimal imaging modality; it identifies the abnormality in 74% to 90% of cases.[124,125,279] Because of the current widespread access to CT, the diagnosis is now usually made preoperatively. Characteristic findings include an enlarged kidney, frequently with replacement of renal parenchyma and multiple fluid-filled cavities, together with urolithiasis. Ultrasonography identifies nonspecific abnormalities, including renal enlargement with relative preservation of renal contour and multiple hypoechoic round masses.[125] MRI shows abnormalities similar to those observed with CT.[279] The differential diagnosis includes malignancy and tuberculosis. The usual management is nephrectomy; antimicrobial therapy has only a secondary role.[276] If the diagnosis is made early, when there is only focal renal involvement, partial nephrectomy may be curative.

### PYOCYSTIS

Pyocystis, also called "vesicle empyema," is an infection characterized by a purulent fluid collection in the bladder of a patient with a nonfunctioning bladder. In effect, the bladder becomes an undrained abscess. This is a rare complication diagnosed in patients with anuric renal failure or surgically bypassed bladders. The clinical presentation includes suprapubic pain or distention, abdominal pain, foul-smelling urethral discharge, and fever or sepsis.[280,281] Organisms isolated have included *E. coli, P. mirabilis, P. aeruginosa, Serratia marcescens, Streptococcus* species, *Enterococcus* species, and *Candida* species. Mixed cultures are common. It is not known whether anaerobic organisms may also contribute.

When the condition is suspected, a specimen of bladder fluid should be obtained for diagnosis and culture. The laboratory should be requested to identify all organisms isolated, so that the specimen is processed as abscess fluid rather than urine. The treatment approach involves systemic antimicrobial agents and urethral catheterization for bladder drainage. Antimicrobial therapy is directed by the specific organisms isolated. Bladder irrigation with either saline or an antibiotic solution is sometimes recommended, but whether irrigation provides an additional therapeutic benefit is not clear.[282] Surgical intervention to achieve adequate drainage is necessary, rarely, for recalcitrant cases.

## UNCOMMON ORGANISMS

### GENITOURINARY TUBERCULOSIS

Genitourinary tuberculosis is diagnosed in 1.1% to 1.5% of all tuberculosis cases, and 5% to 6% of cases of extrapulmonary tuberculosis.[283–285] This infection is usually a consequence of local reactivation following hematogenous dissemination of *Mycobacterium tuberculosis* to the renal cortex during primary pulmonary infection. The renal cortex is also frequently involved with miliary disease, with multiple granulomas usually present. The high oxygen tension of the renal cortex is favorable for renal localization. Men are infected twice as often as women. The latent period, from the time of initial pulmonary infection to diagnosis of clinical urogenital tuberculosis, is 22 years on average with a range of 1 to 46 years.[286] Reactivation of tuberculosis usually occurs in only one kidney; thus disease is characteristically unilateral. Contiguous involvement of the collecting system leads to *M. tuberculosis* bacilluria with subsequent ureteric and bladder infection. Prostate and epididymis infection may result directly from hematogenous dissemination rather than contiguous spread. The kidneys are affected in 60% to 100% of cases, the ureters in 19% to 41%, the bladder in 15% to 20%, and the prostate or epididymis in 20% to 50% of men.[286–288]

Substantial morbidity is attributed to urogenital tuberculosis. Severe calyceal clubbing and dilation of the renal pelvis and ureters leading to total destruction of the kidney and autonephrectomy occur in 23% to 33% of cases, and renal failure occurs in 1% to 10%.[286] A summary of cases reported worldwide reported that 27% of patients had a nonfunctioning unilateral kidney at presentation, but this proportion varied from 8% to 72% in different countries, presumably reflecting the timeliness of diagnosis.[289]

Presenting genitourinary symptoms are often vague or nonspecific and may include back or flank pain, dysuria, and urinary frequency and, in women, infertility. As many as 50% of patients have no localizing genitourinary symptoms. About 25% to 33% of patients have systemic complaints, usually pulmonary symptoms, fever, and weight loss.[286,290] The subacute presentation and results of the initial evaluation can mimic those of xanthogranulomatous pyelonephritis. In men, additional features suggestive of tuberculosis include an enlarged, hard, and nontender epididymis; thickened or beaded vas deferens; indurated or nodular prostate; and nontender testicular mass.[284] Tuberculous granulomatous prostatitis may manifest as a nodular prostate with an elevation of prostate-specific antigen that is clinically indistinguishable from that in prostate carcinoma. Most patients with renal tuberculosis have evidence of concomitant extragenital disease. The most common site is the lungs, but the pulmonary disease is usually inactive. The chest radiograph is abnormal in 67% to 75% of patients, and the tuberculin skin test positive in 60% to 90%.

Urinalysis findings are abnormal in >90% of patients with genitourinary tuberculosis.[283] Sterile pyuria with hematuria is most common, but sterile pyuria alone and gross or microscopic hematuria may also occur.[283,287,288] For patients with HIV infection, an algorithm that incorporates negative results of routine urine culture and the presence of pyuria, albuminuria, or hematuria has good predictive value for detecting genitourinary tuberculosis.[291,292] As many as half of HIV-positive patients, however, have concomitant bacteriuria with other organisms at presentation, and this finding may obscure the initial assessment of the urinalysis.

IVP was traditionally the standard imaging approach, but CT is now preferred.[286] Imaging studies identify unilateral disease in 75% of cases of renal tuberculosis (Fig. 36.1). The characteristic early finding is erosions of the renal calyx; the erosions subsequently progress to papillary necrosis, hydronephrosis, renal parenchymal cavitation, and dilated calyces. Ureteric tuberculosis is characterized by a thickened ureteric wall and strictures. Lesions are most common in the distal third of the ureter. Bladder tuberculosis may manifest as reduced bladder volume with wall thickening, ulceration, and filling defects resulting from granulomatous involvement. In advanced disease, scarring results in permanent loss of volume and a residual small, irregular, calcified bladder. The

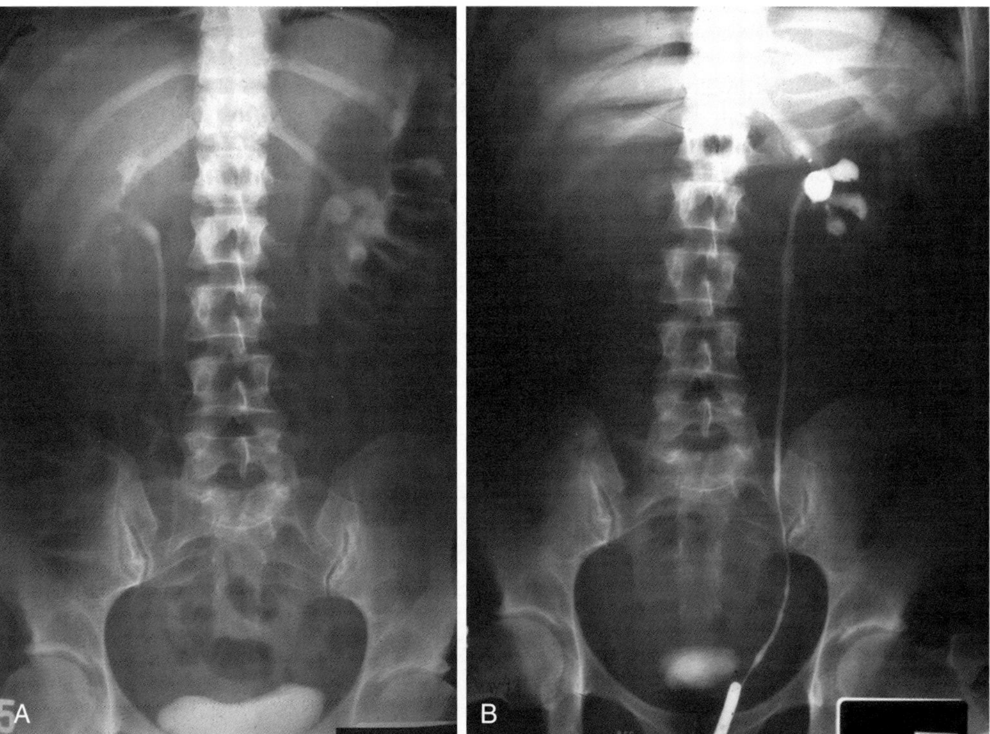


**Fig. 36.1 Renal tuberculosis.** (A) Intravenous pyelogram, showing unilateral hydronephrosis and calyceal distention. (B) Retrograde pyelogram in the same patient, showing distal ureteric narrowing.

most common finding on CT is renal calcification, present in 50% of cases.[293] Other characteristic findings are hydrocalyx secondary to infundibular stenosis and cavity formation. In advanced disease, cortical loss, uroepithelial thickening, and dystrophic calcification are present.

The diagnosis is confirmed by growth of *M. tuberculosis* in urine or tissue culture. Appropriate specimens for mycobacterial culture should be obtained whenever this diagnosis is considered. Three sequential early morning urine specimens for mycobacterial culture are recommended. Urine cultures have positive results in 75% to 90% of affected patients. A positive acid-fast bacillus smear of urine usually signifies *M. tuberculosis,* but culture confirmation is essential to rule out colonization with nonpathogenic mycobacteria and for susceptibility testing of the infecting strain.[294,295] If a suggestive renal abnormality is present but urine culture results are negative, tissue biopsy may be necessary to confirm the diagnosis. Polymerase chain reaction (PCR) nucleic acid antigen testing of urine specimens has been reported to be more sensitive than culture and, if available, provides a more rapid diagnosis.[285,292] However, culture is still necessary to isolate the organism for susceptibility testing.

Antimycobacterial treatment should be provided under the supervision of a physician with expertise in tuberculosis management. The treatment of genitourinary tuberculosis is similar to that of extrapulmonary tuberculosis at other sites. The initial regimen consists of four drugs (isoniazid, rifampin, pyrazinamide, and ethambutol) for 2 months, followed by two drugs (isoniazid and rifampin) for 4 months if the isolate is susceptible to first-line therapy. Follow-up IVP every 6 months has been recommended to identify ureteral scarring or obstruction, which may develop or progress during therapy as part of the healing process. Corticosteroid therapy does not prevent this complication.[283] Ureteral reimplantation, endoscopic balloon dilation, or implantation of ureteral stents may be necessary if progressive obstruction develops.[296] Nephrectomy is rarely required but may be indicated for intractable pain, untreatable infection proximal to a stricture, uncontrollable hematuria or hypertension, or drug resistance. Bladder augmentation surgery may be required if the bladder is scarred and contracted following treated tuberculosis infection.

## BACILLUS CALMETTE–GUÉRIN INFECTION

Intravesical vaccine instillation of bacillus Calmette–Guérin (BCG) is considered first-line treatment for superficial bladder tumors and carcinoma in situ. Treatment with this biologic therapy is complicated by systemic or local BCG infection in <5% of cases.[297–299] BCG bladder instillation is followed by local irritative symptoms such as dysuria in 80% of cases, but these symptoms do not usually persist beyond 48 hours.[300] If symptoms do persist, isoniazid for 14 days is recommended. When symptoms continue despite isoniazid therapy, a full course of antituberculous therapy is recommended.[301] Less common genitourinary infections that accompany BCG instillation include prostatitis in 1% to 3% of patients, epididymitis in 0.2%, and, in rare cases, testicular abscesses, bladder ulcers, local skin infections, or renal infection. Reflux may be a risk factor for the rare complication of BCG pyelonephritis.[302] Localized genitourinary infection tends to have a delayed onset and is usually not apparent clinically until more than 3 months after BCG treatment.[296,297] BCG may not be isolated from urine or tissue cultures.[297] Tissue biopsy usually shows necrotizing granulomatous inflammation, and this finding in the context of prior BCG therapy is sufficient for diagnosis even if subsequent culture results are negative.[299]

## FUNGAL URINARY TRACT INFECTION

Fungal urinary tract infection is usually caused by *Candida* species. These organisms have an extensive array of virulence factors that may facilitate successful colonization and invasion of the urinary tract.[303] Infection may be either antegrade, following candidemia, or retrograde via the urethra.[303] Clinical manifestations are asymptomatic candiduria, cystitis, and pyelonephritis. Bladder or renal fungus balls and systemic fungemia are rare complications.[304]

*Candida albicans* is isolated from more than 50% of episodes, followed by *Candida glabrata, Candida tropicalis,* and *Candida parapsilosis.*[305,306] Candiduria is usually identified in patients who are seriously ill with multiple comorbid conditions, and most infections are asymptomatic.[304] The most important risk factors for candiduria are the presence of an indwelling catheter or other indwelling urologic device, diabetes mellitus, and exposure to broad-spectrum antimicrobial agents.[306] Treatment of asymptomatic candiduria is not beneficial and is currently recommended only for selected patients with high-risk neutropenia (<100 WBC/mm$^3$) or before a traumatic urologic procedure.[307–309] Indwelling devices should be removed whenever possible to facilitate resolution of candiduria. Imaging studies to exclude fungus balls should be considered in patients who have recurrent symptomatic infection or urinary obstruction.[310] When fungus balls are present, surgical removal is required for cure of the infection.

Fluconazole is the treatment of choice for *Candida* urinary tract infection because it is excreted in the urine in active form and high urinary levels are achieved.[308,309] A 2-week course of fluconazole, 200 to 400 mg daily, is recommended (Table 36.9). Amphotericin B deoxycholate, 0.3 to 0.6 mg/

**Table 36.9 Treatment of Candiduria**

| | Cystitis | Pyelonephritis |
|---|---|---|
| Fluconazole (if isolate is susceptible) | 200–400 mg daily, 14 days | 200–400 mg daily, 14 days |
| Amphotericin B deoxycholate | 0.3–0.6 mg/kg daily, 1–7 days | 0.5–0.7 mg/kg daily, 14 days |
| Amphotericin B bladder irrigation | 5–50 mg/L continuous irrigation for 2–7 days | Not indicated |
| Flucytosine | 25 mg/kg qid, 7–10 days | 25 mg/kg qid, 14 days[a] |

[a]May be used in combination with amphotericin B.
*qid,* Four times a day.
From Pappas PG, Kauffman CA, Andes D, et al. Clinical practice guidelines for the management of candidiasis 2009: update by the Infectious Diseases Society of America. *Clin Infect Dis.* 2009;48:503–535.

kg daily, is the alternative treatment recommended for fluconazole-resistant strains, including most *C. glabrata* organisms, as well as in patients who are allergic to fluconazole or in whom treatment fails despite optimal fluconazole therapy and urologic management. Treatment duration with amphotericin B is 1 to 7 days for cystitis and 2 weeks for pyelonephritis. Amphotericin B may also be effective for treatment of fungal cystitis when administered as a bladder washout, but this approach is not generally recommended because it requires several days of urethral catheterization and the optimal dose, frequency, and duration are not well established.[311] With the lipid formulations of amphotericin B, concentrations of active drug achieved in renal tissue and urine are very low, so these formulations are not recommended.

The antifungal 5-flucytosine is excreted in the urine and is indicated for treatment of *Candida* urinary tract infection as a single agent or in combination with amphotericin B for renal infection.[308,309] Resistance to 5-flucytosine develops rapidly when this drug is used as a single agent, and the frequent adverse effects of bone marrow suppression and enterocolitis also limit its use, particularly in patients with renal failure. Echinocandins such as caspofungin, micafungin, and anidulafungin and other azoles such as itraconazole, voriconazole, and posaconazole, which are not excreted into the urine, are not recommended for treatment of urinary tract infection.[308,309] There are, however, case reports of successful treatment of *C. glabrata* urinary tract infection with caspofungin[312] and a case series of selected patients treated with micafungin reported a success rate of 75%.[313]

## VIRAL INFECTIONS

Viral urinary tract infections are uncommon in adults and occur largely in immunocompromised patients.[314–317] Clinical manifestations of viral infection generally follow reactivation of latent infection in immunocompromised patients, although de novo infection may occur. The usual clinical manifestation is hemorrhagic cystitis, but nephropathy has also been described.[314,318–320] The most common viruses are adenovirus, parvovirus B19, and cytomegalovirus (CMV). More than one viral infection may coexist. Most adult cases occur in recipients of hematopoietic stem cell transplants, particularly those with severe graft-versus-host disease, and in renal transplant recipients. Infection has also been reported in other immunosuppressed patients, such as HIV-infected patients with low $CD4^+$ cell counts.[316,321] HIV-associated nephropathy as a distinct clinical entity, including consideration of the role of host genetic background, glomerular cell viral entry, and replication, is considered in Chapter 32. Management of parvovirus B19 infection in the transplanted kidney is discussed in Chapter 70. Adenovirus or CMV infection is diagnosed by viral culture or PCR of the urine. Management includes minimization of immunosuppressive therapy if possible. For HIV-infected patients, antiretroviral therapy to increase the $CD4^+$ cell count should be initiated. CMV infection responds to treatment with ganciclovir or foscarnet.[314] Treatment of adenovirus infection uses cidofovir, although some efficacy has been reported with vidarabine.[314] There are also case reports of successful treatment of adenovirus with ganciclovir and ribavirin.[314,322]

## PARASITIC INFESTATIONS OF THE URINARY TRACT

The most common and important parasitic infestation of the urinary tract is with *Schistosoma haematobium*.[323–325] This parasite is acquired after exposure to contaminated water. *Schistosoma* larvae penetrate the intact skin and migrate in the blood to the liver, where they transform into young worms (schistosomulae) that mature in 4 to 6 weeks and then further migrate to the perivesical venules. The life span of the adult worm in the venule is usually 3 to 5 years but can be longer. Most eggs produced by the adult worms enter the bladder lumen and are removed in the urine. However, some eggs are retained locally in the bladder wall, where they incite an eosinophilic inflammatory and granulomatous immune response that causes progressive fibrosis. The functional abnormality early in the disease is obstruction of the bladder neck. Late complications include recurrent bacterial urinary tract infection, bladder or ureteric stone formation, renal functional abnormalities, and, ultimately, kidney failure.[324,326] *Schistosoma* infestation is also a risk factor for squamous cell carcinoma of the bladder.[327] The relative risk of cancer for persons with schistosomiasis varies from 1.8 to 23.5; the incidence is highest in the 30- to 50-year age group.[328]

The prevalence of infection in endemic areas is high. Surveys from rural Zimbabwe revealed that 60% of women younger than 20 years of age and 29% of those aged 45 to 49 years have eggs in the urine; HIV-infected women older than 35 years had a significantly higher prevalence of infestation.[329] Travelers to endemic areas may acquire infection with only minimal exposure to contaminated water[330–332] (see also Chapters 76–78 for discussion of schistosomiasis in Latin America, Africa, and the Near and Middle East).

Acute genitourinary symptoms occur in up to 50% of cases following acquisition of infection and include hematuria, which is often terminal, together with dysuria and urinary frequency. Microhematuria is reported in 41% to 100% and gross hematuria in 0% to 97% of patients with chronic schistosomal infestation. Radiologic abnormalities are present in the upper urinary tract in 2% to 62% of chronic cases.[324] Ultrasonography of the urinary tract demonstrates thickening of the bladder wall, granulomatous changes, hydronephrosis, and, on occasion, bladder or ureteric calcification. The diagnosis is established by identification of parasite eggs in the urine or biopsy specimens or by serologic findings.[325] Urine specimens collected for identification of eggs should be obtained on consecutive days between 1100 and 1300 hours because egg passage is maximal at this time. Sedimentation or filtration of the urine before examination increases the sensitivity of egg detection.[324,333]

Treatment with one dose of praziquantel, 40 mg/kg body weight, will cure 80% of cases.[325] Follow-up urine specimens for parasite examination are recommended 3 months after treatment to identify patients in whom treatment has failed and must be repeated. Bladder wall thickening and hydroureters may be reversed in the majority of affected patients if treatment is given early in the course of infestation.[334] However, when chronic disease is established and fibrotic lesions are present, changes may not be reversible, and corrective surgery or management of end-stage renal disease is required.[333]

The protozoal parasite *T. vaginalis* is commonly transmitted sexually and is occasionally identified on microscopy with routine urinalysis. In women, the parasite may originate from contamination of the urine by vaginal secretions, but the organism is a well-described cause of urethritis for both men and women. Whenever *T. vaginalis* is identified, treatment of the patient and his or her sexual partners is indicated, regardless of symptoms. The recommended treatment is a single dose of metronidazole, 2 g, or tinidazole, 2 g.[335]

*Echinococcus granulosus* infestation occasionally involves the kidneys.[320] Renal cysts are reported in 2% to 3% of cases of hydatid disease.[336,337] The diagnosis is usually made after an incidental finding of a cyst in the kidneys, ureters, bladder, or testes by imaging or in the investigation of nonspecific symptoms.[338] On occasion, flank pain or a mass is present. Hydatid cysts are not excreted in the urine. Treatment consists of surgical cyst removal or marsupialization; nephrectomy is occasionally necessary.[339] Perioperative albendazole therapy is also usually recommended for patients with hydatid disease. A less common helminthic infestation is *Wuchereria bancrofti* (filariasis), which may cause lymphatic obstruction and rupture into the urinary collecting system, producing chyluria.[323]

 Complete reference list available at ExpertConsult.com.

## KEY REFERENCES


1. Hooton TM. Uncomplicated urinary tract infection. *N Engl J Med.* 2012;366:1028–1037.
3. Grigoryan L, Trautner BW, Gupta K. Diagnosis and management of urinary tract infections in the outpatient setting. *JAMA.* 2014;312:1677–1684.
12. Abraham SN, Miao Y. The nature of immune responses to urinary tract infections. *Nat Rev Immunol.* 2015;15:655–663.
15. Ragnarsdottir B, Svanborg C. Susceptibility to acute pyelonephritis or asymptomatic bacteriuria: host-pathogen interaction in urinary tract infections. *Pediatr Nephrol.* 2012;27:2017–2029.
25. High KP, Bradley SF, Gravenstein S, et al. Clinical practice guideline for the evaluation of fever and infection in older adult residents of long term care facilities. *Clin Infect Dis.* 2009;48:149–171.
29. Lipsky BA, Byren I, Hoey CT. Treatment of bacterial prostatitis. *Clin Infect Dis.* 2010;50:1641–1652.
35. Bermingham SL, Ashe JF. Systematic review of the impact of urinary tract infections on health-related quality of life. *BJU Int.* 2012;110:e830–e836.
47. Hooton TM, Roberts PL, Cox ME, et al. Voided midstream urine culture and acute cystitis in premenopausal women. *N Engl J Med.* 1883;369:1891–2013.
59. Perrotta C, Aznar M, Mejia R, et al. Oestrogens for preventing recurrent urinary tract infection in postmenopausal women. *Cochrane Database Syst Rev.* 2008;(2):CD005131.
63. Bent S, Saint S. The optimal use of diagnostic testing in women with acute uncomplicated cystitis. *Am J Med.* 2002;113(suppl 1A): 20S–28S.
70. Gupta K, Hooton TM, Naver KG, et al. International clinical practice guidelines for the treatment of acute uncomplicated cystitis and pyelonephritis in women: a 2010 update by the Infectious Diseases Society of America and the European Society for Microbiology and Infectious Diseases. *Clin Infect Dis.* 2011;52:e103–e120.
74. Falagas ME, Rafailidis PI. Fosfomycin: the current status of the drug. *Clin Infect Dis.* 2015;61:114–1146.
77. Huttner A, Verhaegh EM, Harbarth S, et al. Nitrofurantoin revisited: a systematic reivew and analysis of controlled trials. *J Antimicrob Chemother.* 2015;70:2456–2464.
89. Beerepoot MAJ, Geerlings SE, van Haarst EP, et al. Nonantibiotic prophylaxis for recurrent urinary tract infections: a systematic review and meta-analysis of randomized controlled trials. *J Urol.* 2013;190:1981–1989.
90. Jepson RG, Craig JC. Cranberries for preventing urinary tract infections. *Cochrane Database Syst Rev.* 2008;(1):CD001321.
99. O'Brien VP, Hannan TJ, Nielsen HV, et al. Drug and vaccine development for the treatment and prevention of urinary tract infections. *Microbiol Spectr.* 2016;4:1–42.
102. Luthje P, Brauner A. Novel strategies in the prevention and treatment of urinary tract infections. *Pathogens.* 2016;5(13):1–14.
124. Demetzis J, Menias CD. State of the art: imaging of renal infections. *Emerg Radiol.* 2007;14:13–22.
128. Sandberg T, Skoog G, Hermansson AB, et al. Ciprofloxacin for 7 days versus 14 days in women with acute pyelonephritis: a randomized, open-label and double-blind, placebo controlled non-inferiority trial. *Lancet.* 2012;380:484–490.
138. D'Hondt F, Everaert K. Urinary tract infections in patients with spinal cord injuries. *Curr Infect Dis Rep.* 2011;13:544–551.
143. Marcus RJ, Post JC, Stoodley P, et al. Biofilms in nephrology. *Expert Opin Biol Ther.* 2008;8:1159–1166.
152. Nicolle LE, Bradley S, Colgan R, et al. Infectious Diseases Society of America guidelines for the diagnosis and treatment of asymptomatic bacteriuria in adults. *Clin Infect Dis.* 2005;40:643–654.
153. Nicolle LE. Urinary tract infection. *Crit Care Clin.* 2013;3:699–715.
156. Mody L, Juthani-Mehta M. Urinary tract infections in older women: a clinical review. *JAMA.* 2014;311:844–854.
158. Wullt B, Agace W, Mansson W. Bladder, bowel and bugs—bacteriuria in patients with intestinal urinary diversion. *World J Urol.* 2004;22:186–195.
171. Hooton TM, Bradley SF, Cardenas DD, et al. Diagnosis, prevention, and treatment of catheter-associated urinary tract infections in adults: 2009 international clinical practice guidelines from the Infectious Diseases Society of America. *Clin Infect Dis.* 2010;50(5): 625–663.
172. Gould CV, Umscheid CA, Agarwal RK, et al. Health Care Infection Control Practices Advisory Committee: guidelines for prevention of catheter-associated urinary tract infections 2009. *Infect Control Hosp Epidemiol.* 2010;31(4):319–326.
175. Siddiq DM, Darouiche RO. New strategies to prevent catheter-associated urinary tract infections. *Nat Rev Urol.* 2012;9:305–314.
191. Green H, Rahamimov R, Golbert E, et al. Consequences of treated versus untreated asymptomatic bacteriuria in the first year following kidney transplantation: retrospective observational study. *Eur J Clin Microbiol Infect Dis.* 2012;32:127–131.
193. Origuen J, Lopez-Medrano F, Fernandez-Ruiz M, et al. Should asymptomatic bacteriuria be systematically treated in kidney transplant recipients? Results from a randomized controlled trial. *Am J Transplant.* 2016;16(10):2943–2953.
199. Widmer M, Gulmezoglu AM, Mignini L, et al. Duration of treatment of asymptomatic bacteriuria during pregnancy. *Cochrane Database Syst Rev.* 2011;(12):CD000491.
208. Schaeffer AJ, Nicolle LE. Urinary tract infections in older men. *N Engl J Med.* 2016;374:562–571.
214. Rees J, Abrahams M, Doble A, et al. Diagnosis and treatment of chronic bacterial prostatitis and chronic prostatitis/chronic pelvic pain syndrome: a consensus guideline. *BJU Int.* 2015;116:509–525.
236. Gilbert DN. Urinary tract infections in patients with chronic renal failure. *Clin J Am Soc Nephrol.* 2006;1:327–331.
240. Flannigan R, Choy WH, Chew B, et al. Renal struvite stones—pathogenesis, microbiology, and management strategies. *Nat Rev Urol.* 2014;11:333–341.
249. Coelho RF, Schneider-Montero ED, Mesquita JLB, et al. Renal and perinephric abscess. Analysis of 65 consecutive cases. *World J Surg.* 2007;31:431–436.
253. Hung C-H, Liou J-D, Yan M-Y, et al. Immediate percutaneous drainage compared with surgical drainage of renal abscess. *Int Urol Nephrol.* 2007;39:51–55.
255. Saller M, Rafat C, Zahar J-R, et al. Cyst infections in patients with autosomal dominant polycystic kidney disease. *Clin J Am Soc Nephrol.* 2009;4:1183–1189.
256. Jouret F, Lhommel R, Devuyst O, et al. Diagnosis of cyst infection in patients with autosomal dominant polycystic kidney disease: attributes and limitations of the current modalities. *Nephrol Dial Transplant.* 2012;27:3746–3756.
265. Thomas AA, Lane BR, Thomas AZ, et al. Emphysematous cystitis: a review of 135 cases. *BJU Int.* 2007;100:17–20.
267. Pontin AR, Barnes RD. Current management of emphysematous pyelonephritis. *Nat Rev Urol.* 2009;6:272–279.
269. Bjurlin MA, Hurley SD, Kim DY, et al. Clinical outcomes of nonoperative management in emphysematous urinary tract infections. *Urol.* 2012;79:1281–1285.

286. Figuerido AA, Lucon AM. Urogenital tuberculosis: update and review of 8961 cases from the world literature. *Rev Urol.* 2008;10:207–217.
299. Perez-Jacoiste Asin MA, Fernandez-Ruiz M, Lopez-Medrano F, et al. Bacillus Calmette-Guerin (BCG) infection following intravesical BCG administration as adjunctive therapy for bladder cancer. *Medicine (Baltimore).* 2014;93:236–254.
304. Kauffman CA, Fisher JF, Sobel JD, et al. *Candida* urinary tract infections: diagnosis. *Clin Infect Dis.* 2011;52(suppl 6):S452–S456.
308. Pappas PG, Kauffman CA, Andes D, et al. Clinical practice guidelines for the management of candidiasis 2009: update by the Infectious Diseases Society of America. *Clin Infect Dis.* 2009;48: 503–535.
310. Sadegi BJ, Patel BK, Wilbur AC, et al. Primary renal candidiasis: importance of imaging and clinical history in diagnosis and management. *J Ultrasound Med.* 2009;28:507–514.
314. Paduch DA. Viral lower urinary tract infections. *Curr Urol Rep.* 2007;8:324–335.
325. Colley DG, Bustinduy AL, Secor WE, et al. Human schistosomiasis. *Lancet.* 2014;383:2253–2264.

# 37 Urinary Tract Obstruction

Jørgen Frøkiaer

## CHAPTER OUTLINE



## KEY POINTS

- Hydronephrosis and obstructive uropathy are not interchangeable terms—dilation of the renal pelvis and calices can occur without obstruction, and urinary tract obstruction may occur in the absence of hydronephrosis.
- Urinary tract obstruction may be congenital or acquired. Acquired causes can be intrinsic or extrinsic.
- There is no single diagnostic technique that can safely diagnose obstruction. Therefore obstruction must still be considered in patients with worsening renal function, chronic azotemia, or acute changes in renal function or urine output, even in the absence of hydronephrosis.
- Both intrarenal and extrarenal factors combine to decrease glomerular filtration rate and renal blood flow during and immediately after release of obstruction.
- Urinary tract obstruction disrupts the ability to concentrate and dilute urine and impairs epithelial sodium, proton, and bicarbonate transport due to downregulation of most transporter proteins in the tubules.
- Urinary tract obstruction results in development of tubulointerstitial fibrosis with irreversible kidney injury due to a complex series of mechanisms involving multiple hormonal systems as well as numerous cellular and molecular pathways.

In adults, 1.5 to 2.0 L of urine flows daily from the renal papillae through the ureter, bladder, and urethra in an uninterrupted, unidirectional flow. Any obstruction of urinary flow at any point along the urinary tract may cause retention of urine and increased retrograde hydrostatic pressure, leading to kidney damage and interference with waste and water excretion, as well as fluid and electrolyte homeostasis. Because the extent of recovery of renal function in obstructive nephropathy is related inversely to the extent and duration of obstruction, prompt diagnosis and relief of obstruction are essential for effective management. Fortunately, urinary tract obstruction in most cases is a highly treatable form of kidney disease.

Several terms describe urinary tract obstruction, and definitions may vary.[1–3] In the following discussion "hydronephrosis" is defined as a dilation of the renal pelvis and calices proximal to the point of obstruction. "Obstructive uropathy" refers to blockage of urine flow due to a functional or structural derangement anywhere from the tip of the urethra back to the renal pelvis that increases pressure proximal to the site of obstruction. Obstructive uropathy may or may not result in renal parenchymal damage. Such functional or pathologic parenchymal damage is referred to as *obstructive nephropathy*. It should be noted that hydronephrosis and obstructive uropathy are not interchangeable terms—dilation of the renal pelvis and calices can occur without obstruction, and urinary tract obstruction may occur in the absence of hydronephrosis.

## PREVALENCE AND INCIDENCE

The incidence of urinary tract obstruction varies widely among different populations and depends on concurrent medical conditions, sex, and age. Unfortunately, epidemiological reports have been based on the studies of selected "populations," such as women with high-risk pregnancies and data from autopsy series. In the United States it has been estimated that 166 patients per 100,000 population had a presumptive diagnosis of obstructive uropathy on admission to hospitals in 1985.[4] The introduction of routine prenatal ultrasound (US) scanning resulted in an increasing number of infants suspected with urinary tract obstruction,[5] and with the increasing age of the population during the past 25 years the incidence of obstructive uropathy may be expected to increase even more.

A review of 59,064 autopsies of subjects varying in age from neonate to 80 years noted hydronephrosis as a finding in 3.1% of cases (3.3% in males and 2.9% in females). In subjects under age 10 years, representing 1.5% of all autopsies, the principal causes of urinary tract obstruction were ureteral or urethral strictures, or neurologic abnormalities. It is unclear how frequently these abnormalities represented incidental findings, as opposed to being recognized clinically. Until the age of 20, there was no substantial sex difference in frequency of abnormalities (for details, please also see Chapter 72). Between the ages of 20 and 60 years, urinary tract obstruction was more frequent among women than among men, mainly due to the effects of uterine cancer and pregnancy. Above the age of 60 years, prostatic disease raised the frequency of urinary tract obstruction among men above that observed among women.

In children under age 15 years, obstruction occurred in 2% of autopsies. Hydronephrosis was found in 2.2% of the boys and 1.5% of the girls; 80% of the hydronephrosis that did occur was found in subjects aged under 1 year.[6] Consistent with this, another autopsy series of 3172 children identified urinary tract abnormalities in 2.5%. Hydroureter and hydronephrosis were the most common findings, representing 35.9% of all cases.[7] However, it was not clear what proportion of cases was diagnosed clinically before death.

Because a high proportion of these autopsy-detected cases of obstruction likely went undetected during life, the overall prevalence of urinary tract obstruction is very likely far greater than reports suggest. This conclusion is reinforced by the fact that there are several common but temporary causes of obstruction, such as pregnancy and renal calculi.

## CLASSIFICATION

Classification of urinary tract obstruction can be by duration (i.e., acute or chronic[8]), by whether it is congenital or acquired, and by its location (upper or lower urinary tract, supravesical, vesical, or subvesical, etc.). Acute obstruction may be associated with sudden onset of symptoms. Upper urinary tract [ureter or ureteropelvic junction (UPJ)] obstruction may present with renal colic. Lower tract (bladder or urethra) obstruction may present with disorders of micturition. By contrast, chronic urinary tract obstruction may develop insidiously and present with few or only minor symptoms, and with more general manifestations. For example, recurrent urinary tract infections, bladder calculi, and progressive renal insufficiency may all result from chronic obstruction. Congenital causes of obstruction arise from developmental abnormalities, whereas acquired lesions develop after birth, as a result of either disease processes or medical interventions.[9]

## ETIOLOGY

Because congenital and acquired urinary tract obstructions differ to a great degree in cause and clinical course, they will be described separately.

### CONGENITAL CAUSES OF OBSTRUCTION

Congenital anomalies may obstruct the urinary tract at any level from the UPJ to the tip of urethra, and the obstruction may damage one or both kidneys (Box 37.1). Although some lesions occur rarely, as a group they represent an important cause of urinary tract obstruction because in younger patients they often lead to severe renal impairment and may result in catastrophic end-stage renal disease.[10] Thus this condition is also presented in detail in Chapter 72.

The widespread use of fetal ultrasonography, and its increasing sensitivity, has led to early detection in an increasing number of cases. With an estimated prevalence of 2% to 5.5%, dilatation of the renal collecting system is the most common ultrasonographic abnormality found in the fetal

**Box 37.1 Congenital Causes of Urinary Tract Obstruction**

**Ureteropelvic Junction**

Ureteropelvic junction obstruction
Proximal and middle ureter
Ureteral folds
Ureteral valves
Strictures
Benign fibroepithelial polyps
Retrocaval ureter

**Distal Ureter**

Ureterovesical junction obstruction
Vesicoureteral reflux
Prune-belly syndrome
Ureteroceles

**Bladder**

Bladder diverticula
Neurologic conditions (e.g., spina bifida)

**Urethra**

Posterior urethral valves
Urethral diverticula
Anterior urethral valves
Urethral atresia
Labial fusion

urinary tract.[11] In cases of severe obstruction early detection may lead to termination of the pregnancy or attempts to ameliorate the obstruction in utero.[10,12,13] However, US may detect mild obstruction of unknown clinical significance.[10,12] In brief, UPJ obstruction is the most common cause of hydronephrosis in fetuses[14] and young children,[15] with a reported incidence of 5 cases per 100,000 population per year,[16] and it may affect adults as well.[17] There is considerable controversy as to whether all cases of obstruction early in life are clinically significant. The widespread use of fetal US has resulted in detection of many cases that remain asymptomatic and may resolve spontaneously with simple follow-up of the child.[3,18] Despite the numerous cases, there is a lack of consistency with respect to the nomenclature and grading systems used in the clinical risk assessment of infants with antenatal hydronephrosis.[5] Although most cases of congenital UPJ obstruction are diagnosed prenatally by US,[19] the most common neonatal clinical presentation is a flank or abdominal mass.[20] By contrast, adults generally present with flank pain.[17] Because intermittent obstruction may produce symptoms that mimic those of gastrointestinal disease, diagnosis may be delayed. At any age, UPJ obstruction may be associated with kidney stones, hematuria, hypertension, or recurrent urinary tract infection.[16,17] A detailed presentation of the different causes of UPJ obstruction is provided in Chapter 72, where a thorough presentation of the pathophysiology of proximal and distal congenital ureter obstruction is discussed.

Congenital bladder outlet obstruction may be caused by mechanical or functional factors and will also be discussed in Chapter 72.

Because operative complications may be high,[21] the use of fetal[13,22] or neonatal[22,23] surgery for the relief of obstruction remains controversial.[10,12,13] Although bilateral obstruction requires intervention, patients with unilateral hydronephrosis are often followed without surgery, but with aggressive observation to identify the approximately 20% of patients with congenital hydronephrosis who require pyeloplasty.[23,24] Indications for surgery in unilateral hydronephrosis include symptoms of obstruction or impaired function in a presumably salvageable hydronephrotic kidney.

## ACQUIRED CAUSES OF OBSTRUCTION

### INTRINSIC CAUSES

Acquired causes of obstruction may be intrinsic to the urinary tract (i.e., resulting from intraluminal or intramural processes) or may arise from causes extrinsic to it (Box 37.2). Intrinsic causes of obstruction may be considered according to anatomic location.

Intrinsic intraluminal causes of obstruction may be intrarenal or extrarenal. Intrarenal causes arise from formation of casts or crystals within the renal tubules. These include uric acid nephropathy[25]; deposition of crystals of drugs that precipitate in the urine, including sulfonamides,[26] acyclovir,[27] indinavir,[28] and ciprofloxacin[29]; and multiple myeloma.[30] Uric acid nephropathy usually results from the large uric acid load released when alkylating agents abruptly kill large numbers of tumor cells in the treatment of patients with malignant hematopoietic neoplasms. The risk of uric acid nephropathy relates directly to plasma uric acid concentrations.[25] Uric acid nephropathy may also occur in the setting of disseminated adenomatous carcinoma of the gastrointestinal tract.[31] Sulfonamide crystal deposition, once a common occurrence, became rare with the introduction of sulfonamides that are more soluble in acid urine than earlier drugs were. Sulfadiazine has been used as antiretroviral therapy because it is relatively lipophilic and penetrates the brain well, making it an excellent treatment for toxoplasmosis in patients with acquired immunodeficiency syndrome (AIDS). However, the same lipophilicity makes the drug prone to the formation of intrarenal crystals, which can lead to acute kidney injury when the drug is given in large doses.[26,32] Ciprofloxacin may also precipitate in the tubular fluid, resulting in crystalluria with stone formation and urinary tract obstruction.[29] A common renal complication of multiple myeloma is "myeloma kidney," a condition also known as myeloma cast nephropathy. The renal lesions (casts) are directly related to the production of monoclonal immunoglobulin free light chains (FLCs), which coprecipitate with Tamm–Horsfall glycoprotein (THP) in the lumen of the distal nephron, obstructing tubular fluid flow.[33,34] Promising experiments have identified the determinants of the molecular interaction between FLCs and THP, which permitted development of a peptide that demonstrated strong inhibitory capability in the binding of FLCs to THP in vitro.[34]

Several intrinsic intraluminal, extrarenal, or intraureteral processes may also cause obstruction. Nephrolithiasis represents the most common cause of ureteral obstruction in younger men.[35] In the US population the prevalence of symptomatic kidney stone of adults aged 20 to 74 years was estimated from self-reported incidents between 1988 and 1994 to afflict 5.2% of adults (6.3% males and 4.1% females).[36] The significance of this number is also reflected by the large number of hospital admissions due to calculus of the kidney and ureters, amounting to 166,000 hospital stays in 2006.[37] Calcium oxalate stones occur most commonly. Obstruction caused by such stones occurs sporadically and tends to be acute and unilateral, and usually without a long-term impact on renal function. Of course, when a stone obstructs a solitary kidney the result can be anuric or oliguric acute kidney injury. Less common types of stones, such as struvite (ammonium–magnesium–sulfate) and cysteine stones, more frequently cause significant renal damage because these substances accumulate over time, and often form staghorn calculi. Stones tend to lodge and to obstruct urine flow at narrowings along the ureter, including the UPJ, the pelvic brim (where the ureter arches over the iliac vessels), and the ureterovesical junction.

Other processes that cause ureteral obstruction include papillary necrosis, blood clots, and cystic inflammation. Papillary necrosis[38] may result from sickle cell disease or trait, amyloidosis,[39] analgesic abuse, acute pyelonephritis, or diabetes mellitus. Renal allografts may develop papillary necrosis as well.[40] Acute obstruction may even require surgical intervention.[41] Blood clots secondary to a benign or malignant lesion of the urinary tract or cystic inflammation of the ureter (ureteritis cystica) can also lead to obstruction and hydronephrosis.[42]

Intrinsic intramural processes that cause obstruction include failure of micturition or more rarely of ureteral peristalsis. Bladder storage of urine and micturition require complex interplay of spinal reflexes, midbrain, and cortical function.[43] Neurologic dysfunction[44] occurring in diabetes mellitus, multiple sclerosis, spinal cord injury, cerebrovascular disease,

**Box 37.2 Acquired Causes of Urinary Tract Obstruction**

**Intrinsic Processes**

***Intraluminal***

Intrarenal
- Uric acid nephropathy
- Sulfonamides
- Acyclovir
- Indinavir
- Multiple myeloma

Intraureteral
- Nephrolithiasis
- Papillary necrosis
- Blood clots
- Fungus balls

***Intramural***

Functional
- Diseases
  - Diabetes mellitus
  - Multiple sclerosis
  - Cerebrovascular disease
  - Spinal cord injury
  - Parkinson disease
- Drugs
  - Anticholinergic agents
  - Levodopa (α-adrenergic properties)

Anatomic
- Ureteral strictures
  - Schistosomiasis
  - Tuberculosis
  - Drugs (e.g., nonsteroidal antiinflammatory agents)
  - Ureteral instrumentation
  - Urethral strictures
  - Benign or malignant tumors of the renal pelvis, ureter, bladder

**Extrinsic Processes**

***Reproductive Tract***

Females
- Uterus
  - Pregnancy
  - Tumor (fibroids, endometrial or cervical cancer)
  - Endometriosis
  - Uterine prolapse
  - Ureteral ligation (surgical)
- Ovary
  - Tubo-ovarian abscess
  - Tumor
  - Cyst

Males
- Benign prostatic hyperplasia
- Prostate cancer

***Malignant Neoplasms***

Genitourinary Tract
- Tumors of kidney, ureter, bladder, urethra

Other sites
- Metastatic spread
- Direct extension

***Gastrointestinal System***

Crohn's disease
Appendicitis
Diverticulosis
Chronic pancreatitis with pseudocyst formation
Acute pancreatitis

***Vascular System***

Arterial Aneurysms
- Abdominal aortic aneurysm
- Iliac artery aneurysm

Venous
- Ovarian vein thrombophlebitis

Vasculitides
- Systemic lupus erythematosus
- Polyarteritis nodosa
- Wegener granulomatosis
- Henoch–Schönlein purpura

***Retroperitoneal Processes***

Fibrosis
- Idiopathic
- Drug induced
- Inflammatory
  - Ascending lymphangitis of the lower extremities
  - Chronic urinary tract infection
  - Tuberculosis
  - Sarcoidosis
- Iatrogenic (multiple abdominal surgical procedures)

Enlarged retroperitoneal nodes
Tumor invasion
Tumor mass
Hemorrhage
Urinoma

***Biologic Agents***

Actinomycosis

and Parkinson disease can result from upper motor neuron damage. These can produce a variety of forms of bladder dysfunction. If the bladder fails to empty properly, it can remain filled most of the time, resulting in chronic increased intravesical pressure, which is transmitted retrograde into the ureters and to the renal pelvis and kidney. In addition, failure of coordination of bladder contraction with the opening of the urethral sphincter may lead to bladder hypertrophy. In this setting, bladder filling requires increased hydrostatic pressures to stretch the hypertrophic detrusor muscle. Again the increased pressure in the bladder is transmitted up the urinary tract to the ureters and renal pelvis. Lower spinal tract injury may result in a flaccid, atonic bladder and failure of micturition, as well as recurrent urinary tract infections.

Various drugs may cause intrinsic intramural obstruction by disrupting the normal function of the smooth muscle of the urinary tract. Anticholinergic agents[45] may interfere with bladder contraction, whereas levodopa[46] may mediate an α-adrenergic increase in urethral sphincter tone, resulting in increased bladder outlet resistance. Chronic use of tiaprofenic acid (Surgam) can cause severe cystitis with subsequent ureteral obstruction.[47] In all circumstances when the bladder does not void normally, renal damage may develop as a consequence of recurrent urinary tract infections and back pressure produced by the accumulation of residual urine.

Acquired anatomic abnormalities of the wall of the urinary tract include ureteral strictures and benign as well as malignant tumors of the urethra, bladder, ureter, or renal pelvis.[48] Ureteral strictures may result from radiation therapy in children[49] and in adults[50] treated for pelvic or lower abdominal cancers, such as cervical cancer, or nowadays rarely as a result of analgesic abuse.[51] Strictures may also develop as a complication of ureteral instrumentation or surgery.

Infectious organisms may also produce intrinsic obstruction of the urinary tract. Schistosoma haematobium afflicts nearly 100 million people worldwide. Although active infection can be treated and obstructive uropathy may resolve, chronic schistosomiasis (bilharziasis) may develop in untreated cases, leading to irreversible ureteral or bladder fibrosis and obstruction.[52] Of other infections, the incidence of genitourinary tuberculosis has remained constant over the 30 years, amounting to 3% to 5% of patients with tuberculosis.[53] Mycoses caused by *Candida albicans* or *Candida tropicalis* may also result in obstruction due to intraluminal obstruction (fungus ball) or invasion of the ureteral wall.[54]

## EXTRINSIC CAUSES

Acquired extrinsic urinary tract obstruction occurs in a wide variety of settings. The relatively high frequency of obstructive uropathy from processes in the female reproductive tract such as pregnancy and pelvic neoplasms results in higher rates of urinary tract obstruction in younger women than in younger men.[2] The advent of routine abdominal and fetal ultrasonography in pregnant women has revealed that more than two-thirds of women entering their third trimester demonstrate some degree of dilation of the collecting system,[55] most often resulting from mechanical ureteral obstruction.[55] This temporary form of obstruction is usually observed above the point at which the ureter crosses the pelvic brim, and affects the right ureter more often than the left.[55] The vast majority of these cases are subclinical and appear to resolve completely soon after delivery.[56] Clinically significant obstructive uropathy in pregnancy almost always presents with flank pain.[57] In these cases, ultrasonography serves as a useful initial screening test,[20] and magnetic resonance imaging (MRI) can be used if the US is not conclusive.[57] Of course, the diagnostic evaluation must be tailored to minimize fetal radiation exposure. If the obstruction is significant, a ureteral stent can be placed cystoscopically, and its efficacy can be monitored with repeated follow-up ultrasonography.[58] The stent can be left in place for the duration of pregnancy, if needed. Clinically significant ureteral obstruction is rare in pregnancy, and bilateral obstruction leading to acute kidney injury is exceptionally rare.[57] Conditions in pregnancy that may predispose to obstructive uropathy and acute kidney injury include multiple fetuses, polyhydramnios, an incarcerated gravid uterus, or a solitary kidney.[56]

Pelvic malignancies, especially cervical adenocarcinomas, represent the second most common cause of extrinsic obstructive uropathy in women.[59] In older women, uterine prolapse and other failures of normal pelvic floor tone may cause obstruction, with hydronephrosis developing in 5% of patients.[60] In this setting prolapse may lead to compression of the ureter by uterine blood vessels. In addition, prolapse has been associated with urinary tract infection, sepsis, pyonephrosis, and renal insufficiency. Prolapse of other pelvic organs due to weakening of the pelvic floor may also result in obstruction.[60] Various benign pelvic abnormalities may cause ureter obstruction, including uterine tumors or cystic ovary and pelvic inflammatory disease, particularly a tubo-ovarian abscess. Pelvic lipomatosis, a disease with an unclear etiology seen more often in men, is another rare reason for compressive urinary tract obstruction.[61]

Although endometriosis only rarely results in ureteral obstruction,[62] it should be included in the differential diagnosis any time a premenopausal woman presents with unilateral obstruction. The onset of obstruction may be insidious, and the process is usually confined to the pelvic portion of the ureter.[62] Ureteral involvement may be intrinsic or extrinsic, with extrinsic compression arising principally from adhesions associated with the endometriosis. Because ureteral involvement may come on slowly and may be unilateral, it is important to screen for obstructive uropathy in advanced cases of endometriosis.[62] In this case using computed tomography (CT) is preferred, because US may not reveal hydronephrosis if adhesions are preventing dilatation of the ureter above the site of obstruction.[63] When surgery of any kind is contemplated in patients with endometriosis, it is all the more important to image the ureters, because they cross the anticipated surgical field and may well be near, or attached to, adhesions.[62,63] Note that 52% of inadvertent ligations of the ureter in abdominal and retroperitoneal operations occur in gynecologic procedures.[64]

Above the age of 60 years, obstructive uropathy occurs more commonly in men than in women. Benign prostatic hyperplasia, which is by far the most common cause of urinary tract obstruction in men, produces some symptoms of bladder outlet obstruction in 75% of men aged 50 years and older.[65,66] It is likely that the proportion of affected older men would be higher if physicians routinely took a detailed history for symptoms.[65,66] Presenting symptoms of bladder outlet obstruction include difficulty initiating micturition, weakened urinary stream, dribbling at the end of micturition, incomplete bladder emptying, and nocturia. The diagnosis may be established by history and urodynamic studies, as well as imaging in some cases.[65–67]

Malignant genitourinary tumors occasionally cause urinary tract obstruction. Bladder cancer is the second most common cause (after cervical cancer) of malignant obstruction of the ureter.[2] Despite stage migration to more organ-confined disease in the era of prostate-specific antigen, obstruction due to prostate cancer compressing the bladder neck and invading the ureteral orifices is still relatively common.[68] Urinary tract obstruction in advanced and metastatic prostate cancer can have a varied presentation because it may occur in multiple anatomic locations including the ureter and pelvic lymph nodes[69] Although urothelial tumors of the renal pelvis, ureter, and urethra are very rare, they also may lead to urinary obstruction.[70]

Several gastrointestinal processes may rarely cause obstructive uropathy. Inflammation in Crohn's disease may extend into the retroperitoneum, leading to obstruction of the ureters,[71] usually on the right side.[72] In addition, several gastrointestinal diseases may cause oxalosis, leading to nephrolithiasis.[73] Appendicitis may lead to retroperitoneal scarring or abscess formation in children and young adults,[74] leading to obstruction of the right ureter. Diverticulitis in older patients[75] may rarely cause obstruction of the left ureter. Fecaloma is another rare cause of bilateral ureteral obstruction.[76] Chronic pancreatitis with pseudocyst formation sometimes causes left ureteral obstruction,[77] and may very rarely cause bilateral obstruction.[78] Acute pancreatitis may result in right-sided obstruction.[79]

Vascular abnormalities or diseases may also lead to obstruction. Abdominal aortic aneurysm is the most common vascular cause of urinary obstruction,[80] which may be caused by direct pressure of the aneurysm on the ureter or associated retroperitoneal fibrosis. Aneurysms of the iliac vessels may also cause obstruction of the ureters as they cross over the vessels.[80] Rarely, the ovarian venous system may cause right ureteral obstruction.[81] In addition, and also rarely, vasculitis caused by systemic lupus erythematosus,[82] polyarteritis nodosa,[83] Wegener granulomatosis,[84] and Henoch–Schönlein purpura[85,86] has been reported to cause obstruction.

Retroperitoneal processes, such as tumor invasion leading to compression, as well as retroperitoneal fibrosis, can result in obstruction. The major extrinsic causes of retroperitoneal obstruction, accounting for 70% of all cases, are due to tumors of the colon, bladder, prostate, ovary, uterus, or cervix.[2,87,88] When idiopathic, retroperitoneal fibrosis[87,88] usually involves the middle third of the ureter and affects men and women equally, predominantly those in the 5th and 6th decades of life.[88] Retroperitoneal fibrosis may also be drug induced (e.g., methysergide), or it may occur as a consequence of scarring from multiple abdominal surgical procedures.[88] It may also be associated with conditions as varied as gonorrhea, sarcoidosis, chronic urinary tract infections, Henoch–Schönlein purpura, tuberculosis, biliary tract disease, and inflammatory processes of the lower extremities with ascending lymphangitis.[88]

Malignant neoplasms can obstruct the urinary tract by direct extension or by metastasis,[89] which may be managed by retrograde stenting as a practical but guarded treatment and should be tailored to each patient.[89] As noted earlier, cervical cancer is the most common obstructing malignant neoplasm, followed by bladder cancer.[2,90,91] Rare childhood tumors such as pelvic neurofibromas can induce upper urinary tract obstruction in up to 60% of patients.[92] Wilms tumor may obstruct via local compression of the renal pelvis.[93] Miscellaneous inflammatory processes can also result in obstruction. These include granulomatous causes such as sarcoidosis[94] and chronic granulomatous disease of childhood.[95] Amyloid deposits may produce isolated involvement of the ureter. Furthermore, a pelvic mass or inflammatory process associated with actinomycosis may cause external ureteral compression.[96,97] Retrovesical echinococcal cyst can also impede urine flow.[98] Retroperitoneal malacoplakia can also be a rare cause of urinary obstruction.[99] Polyarteritis nodosa associated with hepatitis B has also been reported to result in bilateral hydronephrosis.[100]

Hematologic abnormalities induce obstruction of the urinary tract by a variety of mechanisms. In the retroperitoneum, enlarged lymph nodes or a tumor mass may compress the ureter.[33,101] Alternatively, precipitation of cellular breakdown products such as uric acid (see discussion earlier) and paraproteins, as in multiple myeloma, may cause intrinsic obstruction. In patients with clotting abnormalities, blood clots or hematomas may obstruct the urinary tract, as can sloughing of the papillae in patients with sickle cell disease or analgesic nephropathy (see discussion earlier). Although leukemic infiltrates rarely cause obstruction in adults, in children they cause obstruction in 5% of patients.[102] Lymphomatous infiltration of the kidney occurs relatively commonly, but obstruction related to ureteral involvement in lymphoma is rarer.[103]

## CLINICAL ASPECTS

Urinary tract obstruction may cause symptoms referable to the urinary tract. However, even patients with severe obstruction may be asymptomatic, especially in settings where the obstruction develops gradually, or in patients with spinal cord injury.[104] The clinical presentation often depends on the rate of onset of the obstruction (acute or chronic), the degree of obstruction (partial or complete), whether the obstruction is unilateral or bilateral, and whether the obstruction is intrinsic or extrinsic. Pain in obstructive uropathy is usually associated with obstruction of sudden onset, as from a kidney stone, blood clot, or sloughed papilla, and appears to result from abrupt stretching of the renal capsule or the wall of the collecting system, where C-type sensory fibers are located. The severity of the pain appears to correlate with the rate, rather than the degree, of distention. The pain may present as typical renal colic (sharp pain that may radiate toward the urethral orifice), or, in patients with reflux, the pain may radiate to the flank only during micturition. With UPJ obstruction, flank pain may develop or worsen when the patient ingests large quantities of fluids or receives diuretics.[105] Early satiety and weight loss may be another symptom.[106] Ileus or other gastrointestinal symptoms may be associated with the pain, especially in cases of renal colic, so that it can be difficult to differentiate obstruction from gastrointestinal disease.

Sometimes, patients notice changes in urine output as obstruction sets in. Urinary tract obstruction is one of the few conditions that can result in anuria, usually because of bladder outlet obstruction, or obstruction of a solitary kidney at any level. Obstruction may also occur with no change in urine output. Alternatively, episodes of polyuria may alternate with periods of oliguria. Recurrent urinary tract infections may be the only sign of obstruction, particularly in children. As mentioned earlier, prostatic disease with significant bladder outlet obstruction often presents with difficulty initiating urination, decreased size or force of the urine stream, postvoiding dribbling, and incomplete emptying.[107] Spastic bladder or irritative symptoms such as frequency, urgency, and dysuria may result from urinary tract infection. The appearance of obstructive symptoms synchronous with the menstrual cycle may also be a sign of endometriosis.[108]

On physical examination, several signs may suggest urinary obstruction. A palpable abdominal mass, especially in neonates, may represent hydronephrosis, or, in all age groups, a palpable suprapubic mass may represent a distended bladder. On laboratory examination, proteinuria, if present, is generally less than 2 g/day. Microscopic hematuria is a common finding, but gross hematuria may develop occasionally, such as in rare cases with appendiceal granuloma.[109] The urine sediment is often unremarkable. Less common manifestations of urinary tract obstruction include deterioration of renal function without apparent cause, hypertension,[110] polycythemia, and abnormal urine acidification and concentration capacity.

## DIAGNOSIS

Careful history and physical examination represent the cornerstone of diagnosis, often leading to detection of urinary tract obstruction, and suggesting the reason for it. Although challenging, history and physical examination should focus on the evaluation, so that the minimum amount of time and expense are incurred in determining the cause of the obstruction.

### HISTORY AND PHYSICAL EXAMINATION

Important information in the history includes the type and duration of symptoms (voiding difficulties, flank pain, decreased urine output), presence or absence of urinary tract infections and their number and frequency (especially in children), pattern of fluid intake and urine output, as well as any symptoms of chronic renal failure (such as fatigue, sleep disturbance, loss of appetite, pruritis). In addition, relevant medical history should be reviewed in detail, looking for predisposing causes, including stone disease, malignancies, gynecologic diseases, history of recent surgery, AIDS, and drug use.

The physical examination should focus first on vital signs, which may provide evidence of infection (fever, tachycardia), or of volume overload (hypertension). Evaluation of the patient's volume status will guide fluid therapy. The abdominal examination may reveal a flank mass, which may represent hydronephrosis (especially in children), or a suprapubic mass, which may represent a distended bladder. Features of chronic renal failure, such as pallor (anemia), drowsiness (uremia), neuromuscular irritability (metabolic abnormalities), or pericardial friction rub (uremic pericarditis), may also be noted. A thorough pelvic examination in women and a rectal examination for all patients are mandatory. A careful history and a well-directed and complete physical examination often reveal the specific cause of urinary obstruction. Coexistence of obstruction and infection is a urologic emergency and appropriate studies (US, CT, MRI) must be performed immediately, so that the obstruction can be relieved promptly. Intravenous urography (IVU) is nowadays less commonly used in the diagnostic workup of these patients.

### BIOMARKERS FOR EVALUATION OF URINARY TRACT OBSTRUCTION

The effects of chronic obstruction on renal function are the result of a complex series of events that profoundly and progressively alter all components of glomerular and tubular functions. The consequence is development of tubulointerstitial injury that is characterized by dynamic changes involving tubular atrophy, inflammatory cell infiltration, and interstitial fibrosis. This leads to irreversible loss of kidney function and obstructive nephropathy, which even may continue to progress after relief of obstruction. Because the complexity of this process involves almost every cell in the kidney and many pathways, there have been many attempts to identify biomarkers, which predict the course of obstruction. These biomarkers are characterized by the current understanding of the pathophysiology of urinary tract obstruction on kidney injury and currently include biochemical assays of blood and urine as well as many imaging tools as detailed later.

### BIOCHEMICAL EVALUATION OF BLOOD AND URINE

The laboratory evaluation includes urinalysis and examination of the sediment on a fresh specimen by an experienced observer. Unexplained renal failure with benign urinary sediment should suggest urinary tract obstruction. Microscopic hematuria without proteinuria may suggest calculus or tumor. Pyuria and bacteriuria may indicate pyelonephritis; bacteriuria alone may suggest stasis. Crystals in a freshly voided specimen should lead to consideration of nephrolithiasis or intrarenal crystal deposition.

Hematologic evaluation includes the hemoglobin/hematocrit and mean corpuscular volume (to identify anemia of chronic renal disease) and white blood cell count (to identify possible hematopoietic system neoplasm or infection). Serum electrolytes ($Na^+$, $Cl^-$, $K^+$, and $HCO_3^-$), blood urea nitrogen concentration, creatinine, $Ca^{2+}$, phosphorus, $Mg^{2+}$, uric acid, and albumin levels should be measured. These will help identify disorders of distal nephron function (impaired acid excretion or osmoregulation) and uremia. Urinary chemistries may also suggest distal tubular dysfunction (high urine pH, isosthenuric urine) and inability to reabsorb sodium normally (urinary $Na^+$ >20 mEq/L, fractional excretion of $Na^+$ [$FE_{Na}$] >1%, and osmolality <350 mOsm/L). Alternatively, in acute obstruction, urinary chemistry values may be consistent with prerenal azotemia (urinary $Na^+$ < 20 mEq/L, $FE_{Na}$ <1%, and osmolality >500 mOsm/L).[8]

Novel biomarkers relevant for the functional as well as cellular and molecular changes are being developed as an index of renal injury and to predict renal reserve or recovery after reconstruction. Simple tests examining the value of risk factor proteins have suggested that elevated levels of neutrophil gelatinase-associated lipocalin and β2-microglobulin are present in the urine from obstructed kidneys.[111] Attempts to predict the clinical outcome of congenital unilateral UPJ obstruction in newborn by urine proteome analysis reveal an example of this powerful new technology. Polypeptides in the urine were identified and enabled diagnosis of the severity of obstruction, and using this technique the clinical evolution was predicted with 94% precision in neonates,[112] whereas the precision was only 20% in older children with UPJ obstruction.[113] Thus far, application of large-scale urinary proteomic analysis holds promise for better classification of individuals with hydronephrosis for early selection of surgical candidates,[114] but long-term follow-up studies are warranted to determine the true clinical value of this diagnostic approach.[115] Posterior urethral valves are diagnosed by antenatal US and by analyzing the fetal urinary peptidome; a classifier based on 12 fetal urine peptides predicted postnatal renal function with high sensitivity and specificity.[116]

In an attempt toward improved understanding of obstructive nephropathy and improved translatability of the results to clinical practice, a systems biology approach combining omics data of both human and mouse obstructive nephropathy was developed and demonstrated that novel markers can be identified only thorough a translational approach. Using the urinary miRNome of infants with UPJ obstruction and the kidney tissue miRNome and transcriptome of the corresponding neonatal partial unilateral ureteral obstruction (PUUO) mouse model revealed that let-7a and miR-29b are potentially involved in the development of fibrosis in UPJ obstruction via the control of DTX4 in both humans and mice.[117]

## EVALUATION BY MEDICAL IMAGING

The history, physical examination, and initial laboratory studies should guide the medical imaging evaluation. Pain, degree of renal dysfunction, and the presence of infection dictate the speed and nature of the evaluation. Numerous imaging techniques are available; each has its own advantages and disadvantages, including the ability to identify the site and cause of the obstruction and to separate functional obstruction from mere dilation of the urinary tract. Patient-specific factors, such as the risk of radiocontrast in the setting of renal insufficiency, or the risk of exposure to radiation in pregnant women, must also be weighed.[20]

### ULTRASONOGRAPHY

Ultrasonography (US) is the preferred screening modality when obstruction is suspected[118,119] because it is highly sensitive for hydronephrosis,[118,119] is safe and can be repeated frequently, is readily available at low cost, and avoids ionizing radiation, thus making it ideal for pregnant patients,[20] infants, and children.[118,120] Moreover, because US requires no radiographic contrast, it is well suited to rule out obstruction as a cause of renal insufficiency in patients in whom contrast is contraindicated, including those with an elevated or rising serum creatinine level,[118,119] those allergic to contrast material, and in pediatric patients.[121] In addition to detecting hydronephrosis, US can reveal dilatation of the renal pelvis and calices. It may also determine the size and shape of the kidney, and may demonstrate thinned cortex in case of severe long-standing hydronephrosis (Fig. 37.1). Finally, US may detect perinephric abscesses, which may complicate some forms of obstructive nephropathy. Importantly, in a recent multicenter comparative effectiveness trial in patients with suspected nephrolithiasis subjected to either point of care ultrasonography (emergency US), US performed by a radiologist, or abdominal CT, it was concluded that using ultrasonography as the initial test resulted in no need for CT in most patients, lower cumulative radiation exposure, and no significant differences in the risk of subsequent serious adverse events, pain scores, return emergency department visits, or hospitalizations.[122]

Ultrasonography is both highly sensitive and highly specific in detecting hydronephrosis, with the rates approaching 90%.[118,119,123,124] Importantly, US works equally well in patients with azotemia, in whom radiocontrast studies are contraindicated.[124] Hydronephrosis is detected as a dilated collecting system—an anechoic central area surrounded by echogenic parenchyma.

However, in some cases of acute urinary obstruction, US may fail to detect pathology. During the first 48 hours of obstruction,[118,119,123,124] or when hydronephrosis is absent despite obstruction evaluated by CT, the US may reveal no abnormality.[125] False-negative results also occur in cases of dehydration, staghorn calculi, nephrocalcinosis,[124] retroperitoneal fibrosis,[126] misinterpretation of caliectasis as cortical cysts,[127] and in cases of tumor encasement of the collecting system.[128] A dilated collecting system without obstruction may be observed in up to 50% of patients with urinary diversion through ileal conduits.[129] To enhance the sensitivity and specificity of US, some investigators have developed special obstructive scoring systems, which grade increased echogenicity, parenchymal rims greater than 5 mm, contralateral hypertrophy, resistive index (RI) ratio of 1.10 or higher, and other features to differentiate between obstructing and nonobstructing hydronephrosis.[120] False-positive studies may result from a large extrarenal pelvis, parapelvic cysts,[130] vesicoureteral reflux, or high urine flow rate.[124] In addition, US may only suggest, but not reveal, the presence, or cause, of the obstruction. Renal US elastography provides measurement of kidney elasticity by the shear wave technique.[131] This new imaging technique provides information about renal stiffness related to fibrosis (i.e., chronic obstruction). However, elastography is also sensitive to mechanical and functional parameters such as hydronephrosis and external pressure.[131]

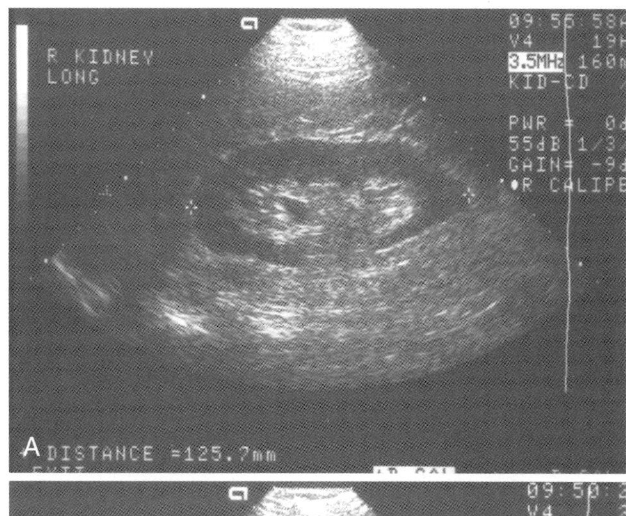


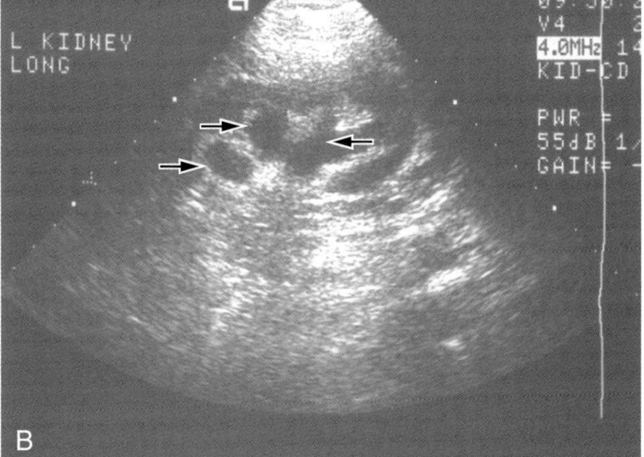


Fig. 37.1 Renal ultrasound. (A) Normal kidney. (B) Hydronephrotic kidney: dilated calices and pelvis *(arrows)*.

Importantly, although US is a useful screening test, it does not define renal function and cannot completely rule out obstruction, especially when prior clinical suspicion is high. Every experienced nephrologist has seen cases of obstruction with negative US studies. Therefore the diagnosis of obstruction must still be considered in patients with worsening renal function, chronic azotemia, or acute changes in renal function or urine output, even in the absence of hydronephrosis on the US.[132]

## ANTENATAL ULTRASONOGRAPHY

Prenatal diagnosis of renal pathology was first described in the 1970s.[133] After that, routine maternal ultrasonography devices of ever-increasing resolution resulted in a fourfold increase in antenatal detection of congenital urinary tract obstruction.[134] Prenatal hydronephrosis is diagnosed with an incidence of between 1 in 100 and 1 in 500 in maternal–fetal US studies.[10,12,102] Either obstructive or nonobstructive processes can cause dilation of the urinary tract. Overall, the etiology of urinary tract obstruction includes UPJ obstruction (44%), or the ureterovesical junction obstruction (21%), as well as multicystic dysplastic kidney, ureterocele or ureteral ectopia, duplex kidney (12%), posterior urethral valves (9%), urethral atresia, sacrococcygeal teratoma, and hydrometrocolpos (fluid distention of the uterus).[103,135–137] Nonobstructive causes include vesicoureteral reflux (14%), physiologic dilation, prune-belly syndrome, renal cystic disease, and megacalycosis (massive dilatation of the renal calyces).[103,135–137] Increased renal echogenicity and oligohydramnios (inadequate quantities of amniotic fluid) in the setting of bladder distention are highly predictive (87%) of an obstructive etiology. This finding is important in the prenatal counseling and treatment of boys with bilateral hydronephrosis and marked bladder dilation.[138]

Determining which cases require intervention and which can be treated conservatively remains a major issue in prenatal US diagnosis of urinary tract obstruction. Persistent postnatal renal abnormalities appear likely when the anteroposterior diameter of the fetal renal pelvis measures more than 6 mm at less than 20 weeks, more than 8 mm at 20 to 30 weeks, and more than 10 mm at more than 30 weeks of gestation. The long-term morbidity of mild hydronephrosis (pelviectasis without caliceal dilation) is low.[10,12] Moderate hydronephrosis (dilated pelvis and calices without parenchymal thinning) may be associated with gradual improvement in severity of dilation, without loss of anticipated relative renal function. Cases of severe hydronephrosis (pelvicalyceal dilation with parenchymal thinning) may require surgical intervention for declining renal function, infection, or symptoms. Overall, because approximately only 5% to 25% of patients with antenatal hydronephrosis will ultimately require surgical intervention,[102,139] careful long-term follow-up of these patients is required throughout childhood and into adulthood. Almost all patients with antenatal hydronephrosis will have postnatal ultrasonography performed in the first days of life, keeping in mind that most cases of the mild hydronephrosis will resolve without intervention.[140] Functional imaging is required to define residual renal function of patients with hydronephrosis and to monitor its course over postnatal life. However, in the absence of bilateral hydronephrosis, a solitary kidney, or suspected posterior urethral valve, functional imaging can be deferred until the first 4 to 6 weeks of life.[102] Otherwise, nuclear medicine examination with radioisotope renography should be performed.

In the United States most infants with prenatally detected hydronephrosis that is confirmed with postnatal studies are placed on antibiotic prophylaxis pending the outcome of further evaluation.[102] This is not the routine treatment in Europe. However, an infection in the setting of ureteral obstruction can cause significant morbidity, resulting in an infant with sepsis, and renal damage is a potential comorbidity. Oral amoxicillin (10 mg/kg/day) is the most commonly used prophylactic antibiotic.[102]

## DUPLEX DOPPLER ULTRASONOGRAPHY

As detailed earlier, US is very sensitive for the detection of collecting system dilatation (hydronephrosis); however, obstruction is not synonymous with dilatation, as either obstructive or nonobstructive dilatation may be present. To differentiate these conditions, color duplex Doppler with measurement of the RI in the intrarenal arteries may be helpful, as obstruction (except in the acute and subacute stages) leads to intrarenal vasoconstriction with a consecutive increase of the RI above the upper limit of 0.7, whereas nonobstructive dilatation does not.[103,135] Diuretic challenge to the kidney may further enhance these differences in RI between obstruction and dilatation.[136] Of clinical relevance in one study, renal colic comprised 30% to 35% of all urological emergencies, and color Doppler predicted the onset of acute dilatation with higher sensitivity, specificity, accuracy, and diagnostic efficiency than ultrasonography in patients with renal colic.[141]

## INTRAVENOUS UROGRAPHY

IVU (also known as intravenous pyelography) was for many years state-of-the-art when a patient suspected with a history of urinary tract obstruction was referred for imaging (Fig. 37.2). IVU requires administration of radiological contrast and is time-consuming to perform. It has therefore now been largely replaced by US, CT, and MRI.

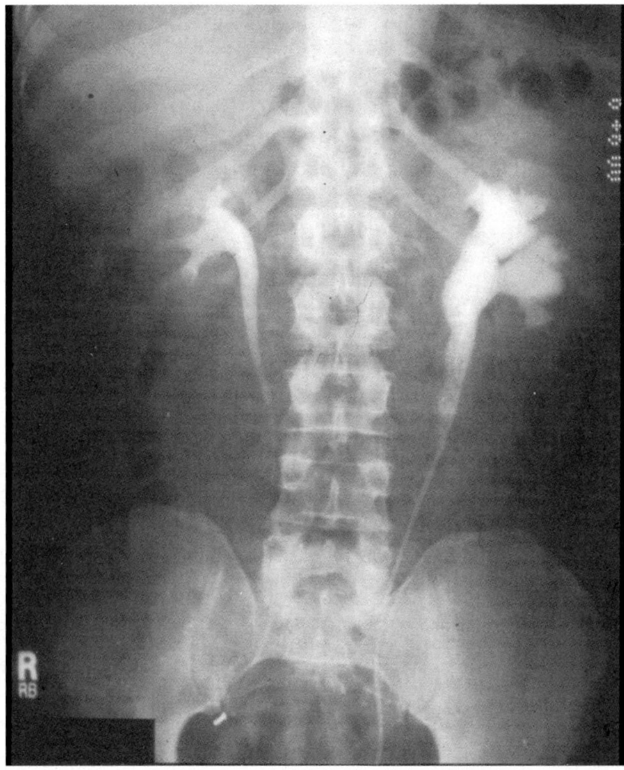


**Fig. 37.2** Intravenous pyelography. Normal right kidney and dilated collecting system on the left. The obstruction was relieved with a stent.

## COMPUTED TOMOGRAPHY

CT was initially used mainly in cases with a high index of clinical suspicion, in which US or IVU had failed to identify obstruction.[142] With the advance to higher resolution of multidetector row CT scanners, the CT scan has supplanted IVU for evaluation of the upper urinary tract.[142,143] CT has a particular advantage because it can visualize a dilated collecting system without the requirement for contrast enhancement. It can also be performed much more quickly than IVU, especially when renal impairment or obstruction would delay contrast excretion by the affected kidney in an IVU (Fig. 37.3). Noncontrast-enhanced CT identifies ureteral stones more effectively than IVU and detects the presence or absence of ureteral obstruction as effectively as IVU.[144,145] Because of its exquisite sensitivity to density, CT can identify even radiolucent stones, because even uric acid stone density is at least 100 Hounsfield units (HU), which is higher than soft tissue density on CT (usually 10–70 HU). CT is especially effective in identifying extrinsic causes of obstruction (e.g., retroperitoneal fibrosis, lymphadenopathy, hematoma). The use of CT for the diagnosis of stones has increased by a factor of 10 over the past 15 years in the United States,[146] probably because of its greater sensitivity and because it can be performed as needed in most emergency departments in the United States.[147] This was highlighted in a recent multicenter comparative effectiveness trial in patients with suspected nephrolithiasis subjected to either point of care ultrasonography (emergency US), US performed by a radiologist, or abdominal CT, which demonstrated that CT has a higher sensitivity than US, whereas US has higher specificity than CT.[122] In this regard it must be emphasized that although the cancer risk from radiation exposure to CT scans is very low, CT scans might produce a small additional cancer risk,[148] especially in those subjected to CT scans during childhood.[149]

Helical CT has also proven to be an accurate and noninvasive method of demonstrating crossing vessels in UPJ obstruction.[150] CT can detect extraurinary pathology and can establish nonurogenital causes of pain. All of these advantages establish noncontrast-enhanced helical CT as the diagnostic study of choice for the evaluation of the patient with acute flank pain.[125] CT is very useful in delineating the pelvic organs, such as the bladder and prostate, and may demonstrate abnormalities such as an obstructed and distended bladder (Fig. 37.4) secondary to an enlarged prostate. US may be the first method of diagnosis in this setting (Fig. 37.5), but CT resolution and depiction of details are usually

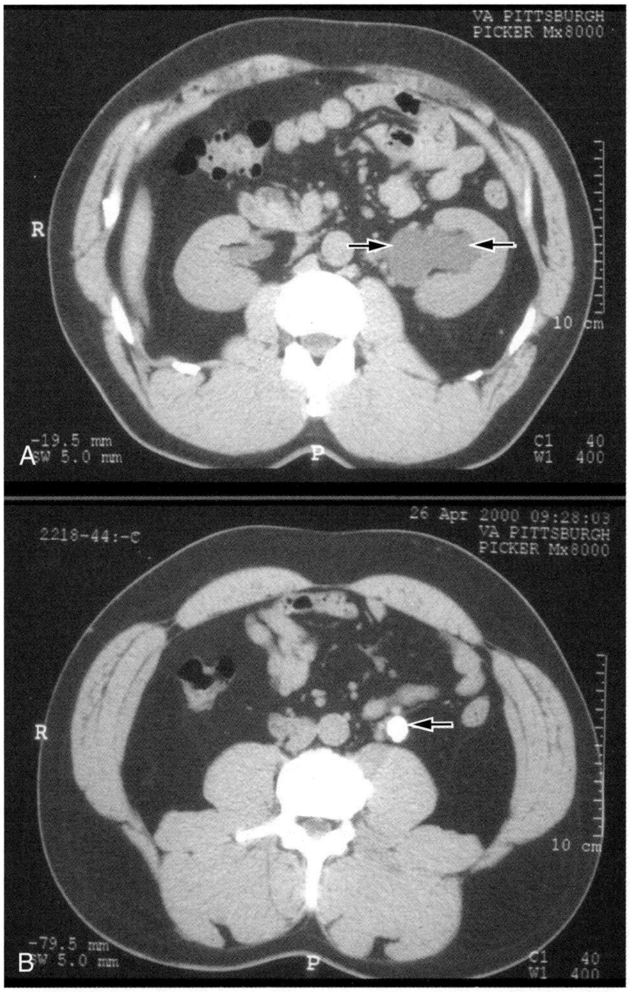

**Fig. 37.3** Computed tomography, noncontrast study. (A) Left hydronephrosis: dilated renal pelvis *(arrows)*, with normal kidney on the right. (B) Reason for obstruction: left midureteral stone *(arrow)*.

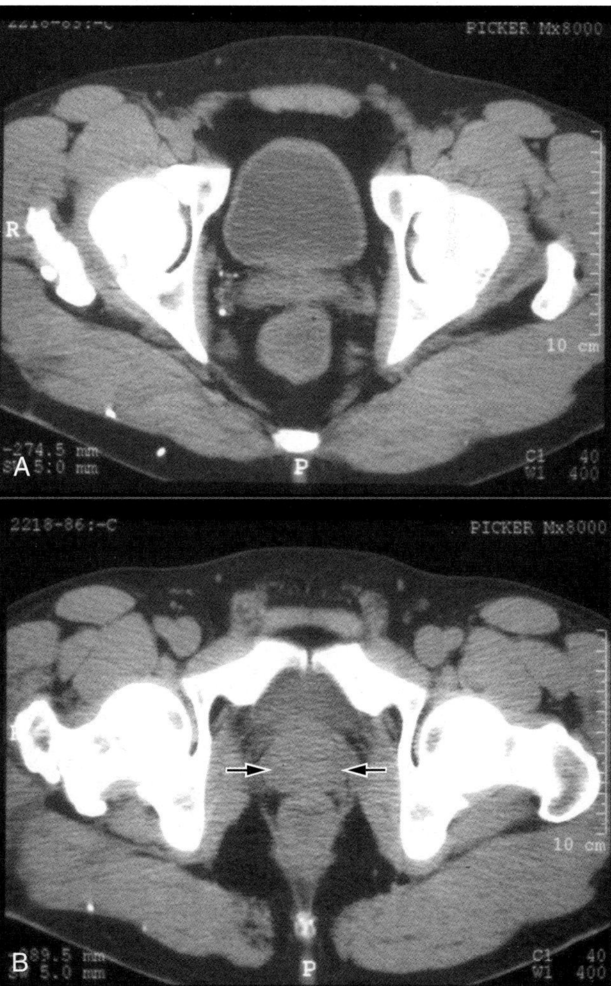


**Fig. 37.4** Computed tomography of the pelvis. (A) Large postvoiding residual urine in the bladder. (B) Enlarged prostate *(arrows)*, leading to urinary retention.

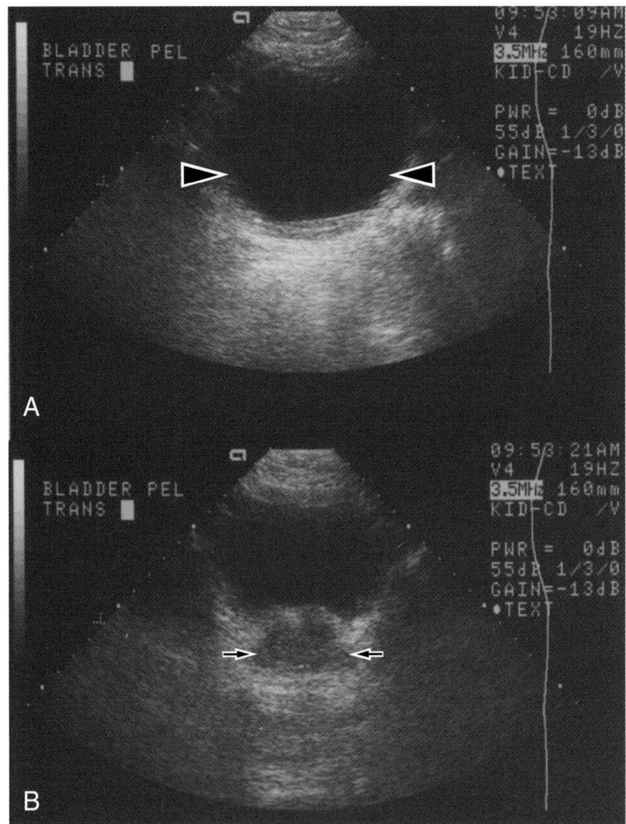


**Fig. 37.5** Pelvic ultrasound. (A) Distended bladder *(arrowheads).* (B) Enlarged prostate *(arrows),* causing infravesical urinary obstruction.

superior to those of US.[142] An exception to using a noncontrast CT is nephrolithiasis secondary to human immunodeficiency virus (HIV) protease inhibitors, primarily indinavir. These stones are not radiopaque, and signs of obstruction may be minimal or absent; thus the diagnosis may be missed with US and noncontrasted CT scan. Contrast-enhanced CT scanning may be required to establish the diagnosis in this circumstance.[151]

## ISOTOPIC RENOGRAPHY

Isotopic renography, or renal scintigraphy, is helpful in diagnosing upper urinary tract obstruction and providing information on the differential renal function (DRF) of both kidneys, while avoiding the risk of radiocontrast agents.[152,153] Radioisotope is injected intravenously, and its dynamic uptake and excretion by the kidneys are followed by using imaging with a gamma camera. Although this method gives a functional assessment of the obstructed kidney, anatomic definition is suboptimal compared with CT. Isotopic renography is typically used to estimate the fractional contribution of each kidney to overall renal function. The noninvasive character of this examination with its high reproducibility makes it excellent for monitoring patients, and it helps the urologist decide whether to perform surgical intervention or watchful waiting.[23] In addition, the test can be repeated after the relief of obstruction to gauge the extent to which relief of the obstruction has restored renal function.

Diuretic renography was introduced into clinical practice in 1978,[154] and may be used to distinguish between hydronephrosis or pelvic dilation with obstruction and dilation without obstruction. The method was developed, applied, and validated in adults.[154] In particular, this is important when applying diuretic renography in children and infants where it is not always easy to distinguish between dilation and obstruction. Following administration of radioisotope, when the isotope appears in the renal pelvis, a loop diuretic such as furosemide is given intravenously. If stasis is causing the dilation, the induced diuresis may result in prompt washout of the tracer from the renal pelvis. By contrast, when dilation is caused by obstruction, the washout does not occur.[155] Data should be interpreted visually and by quantitative measurement including the half-life ($T_{1/2}$) for the excretion of the tracer from the collecting system.[156] It is generally accepted that the clearance of the isotope from the collecting system with $T_{1/2}$ less than 15 minutes is normal, and a $T_{1/2}$ of more than 20 minutes may indicate obstruction in adults. Renal excretion of the tracer with a $T_{1/2}$ between 15 and 20 minutes is considered equivocal. An absent or blunted diuretic response resulting from decreased renal function or grossly dilated pelvis makes interpretation of the test difficult and limits its usefulness and may require support tools to increase the diagnostic performance.[157] Moreover, in children diuretic renography is a very important method for guiding the management of asymptomatic congenital hydronephrosis. The classical variables of the diuretic renogram may not allow an estimate of the best drainage. Poor pelvic emptying may be apparent because the bladder is full and because the effect of gravity on drainage is incomplete. Estimating the drainage as residual activity rather than any parameter on the slope might be more adequate, especially if the time of furosemide administration is changed. Renal function and pelvic volume can influence the quality of drainage. Misinterpretation can easily take place if the renal pelvis is very large and does not allow proper drainage within the study time and drainage may be better estimated using new tools.[158] From this examination the DRF can also be obtained, which is a robust measure, provided there is adequate background subtraction. Pitfalls are related to the drawing of regions of interest, particularly in infants, to estimating the interval during which DRF is calculated, and to an adequate signal-to-noise ratio. There is no definition of a "significant" reduction in DRF.

## POSITRON EMISSION TOMOGRAPHY

Experimentally, positron emission tomography permits quantitative imaging of the kidney at a spatial resolution appropriate for the organ. $H_2{}^{15}O$, $^{82}RbCl$, and $[^{64}Cu]$ ETS (ethylglyoxal bis[thiosemicarbazone]) are the most important radiopharmaceuticals for measuring renal blood flow.[159] Membrane organic cation and anion transporters are important for the function of the tubular epithelium and novel radiopharmaceuticals, such as copper-64-labeled mono oxo-tetraazamacrocyclic ligands and carbon-11-labeled metformin, have been used for molecular renal imaging[159,160] and potentially may play a role in detection of kidney injury in response to urinary tract obstruction.[161]

## MAGNETIC RESONANCE IMAGING

New MRI systems and specific MR contrast agents provide significant developments in the evaluation of renal function (glomerular filtration rate [GFR] measurement), assessment of potential prognostic factors (hypoxia, inflammation, cell

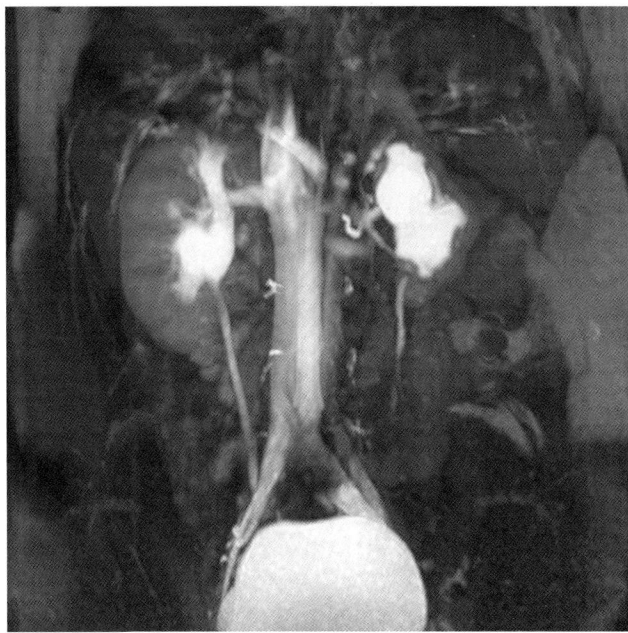

**Fig. 37.6** Magnetic resonance (MR) imaging urography of left-sided hydronephrosis with parenchymal thinning. MR urographic image shows large dilatation of the left pelvicalyceal system and narrowing of the left ureteropelvic junction segment.

viability, degree of tubular function, and interstitial fibrosis), and for monitoring new therapies.[143,162] New developments that have provided higher signal-to-noise ratio and higher spatial and/or temporal resolutions have the potential to direct new opportunities for obtaining morphologic and functional information on tissue characteristics that are relevant for various renal diseases including urinary tract obstruction with respect to diagnosis, prognosis, and treatment follow-up.[143,162] MRI can be used to explore the urinary tract when obstruction is suspected. MRI provides improved spatial resolution, and it is superior to IVU in detecting obstruction in the presence of severe renal failure.[143] MRI has very limited application for the evaluation of stone disease because it cannot directly detect calcifications or stone material.[163]

Depending on local conditions, MRI may be more expensive than other modalities. In children, MR urography (Fig. 37.6) may replace conventional uroradiological methods, and a recent study suggests that functional MR plays an important potential role in identifying those who will benefit most from pyeloplasty and those who are probably best observed.[164] Promising experimental studies have recently demonstrated that MRI may provide valuable information regarding renal function, including energy consumption from so-called BOLD (blood oxygenation level dependent) imaging; this kind of data may be helpful in the future in predicting the level of return of renal function following obstruction.[165,166] Of interest, functional MRI using BOLD demonstrated the ability to identify pathophysiological changes in patients with acute obstruction due to calculi in the ureter.[167] Using new BOLD-MRI analysis techniques, it has recently been shown that persons suffering from chronic kidney disease (CKD) have lower cortical oxygenation than normotensive controls, thus confirming the chronic hypoxia hypothesis. The acute alterations in BOLD after the administration of furosemide are smaller in CKD and represent an estimate of the oxygen-dependent tubular transport of sodium. BOLD-MRI alone or in combination with other functional MRI methods can thus be used to monitor the renal effects of drugs and may potentially be used to identify parenchymal changes in response to urinary tract obstruction. The near future will tell whether or not BOLD-MRI represents a new tool to predict renal function decline and adverse renal outcomes.[168] Recently, concerns related to the use of MRI in renal patients were highlighted by the increased risk of developing nephrogenic systemic fibrosis (NSF) induced by the toxicity of gadolinium in patients with severely impaired renal function, whereas patients with normal or moderate renal function impairment do not develop NSF. It is recommended that gadolinium contrast media should be avoided in patients with stage 4 or 5 CKD because of the risk of NSF.[169]

## WHITAKER TEST

The Whitaker test traditionally defines the functional effect of upper urinary tract dilatation by measuring the hydrostatic pressures in the renal pelvis and bladder during infusion of a saline and contrast mixture into the renal pelvis, via a catheter.[170] With a bladder catheter in place, the patient is placed in the prone position on the fluoroscopic table and a cannula is inserted percutaneously into the renal pelvis and connected to a pressure transducer. A mixture of saline and contrast material is infused through the renal cannula at a rate of 10 mL/min, and pressures are monitored. The urinary tract is considered nonobstructed if renal pelvic pressure is less than 15 cm $H_2O$, equivocal at a pressure between 15 and 22 cm $H_2O$, and obstructed if pressure exceeds 22 cm $H_2O$.[170] With the advent of noninvasive imaging techniques, this test should be reserved for assessing potential upper urinary tract obstruction only in the following circumstances: equivocal results from less invasive tests, suspected obstruction with poor kidney function, loin pain with a negative diuresis renogram, suspected intermittent obstruction, and gross dilatation with a positive diuresis renogram.[171] The test is only used rarely and interpretation relies on solid experience with the method.

## RETROGRADE AND ANTEGRADE PYELOGRAPHY

When other tests do not provide adequate anatomic detail, or when obstruction must be relieved (e.g., obstruction of a solitary kidney, bilateral obstruction, or symptomatic infection in the obstructed system), more invasive investigation, with a combination of treatments, may be necessary. When retrograde pyelography is performed, this takes place during cystoscopy, by cannulating the ureteral orifice and injecting contrast.[61,172,173] In some cases of complete obstruction, contrast may not reach the kidney, but the procedure will define the lower level of the obstruction. Retrograde pyelography can be combined with placement of a ureteral stent to relieve an obstruction, or with possible stone extraction. Because the catheter passes through the bladder to reach the upper urinary tract, the risk of introducing infection proximal to the obstruction must be kept in mind, and the obstruction should be relieved immediately after retrograde pyelography. Antegrade pyelography is performed by percutaneous cannulation of the renal pelvis, and injection of the contrast material into the kidney and ureter.[172,173] This procedure should establish the proximal level of obstruction and may

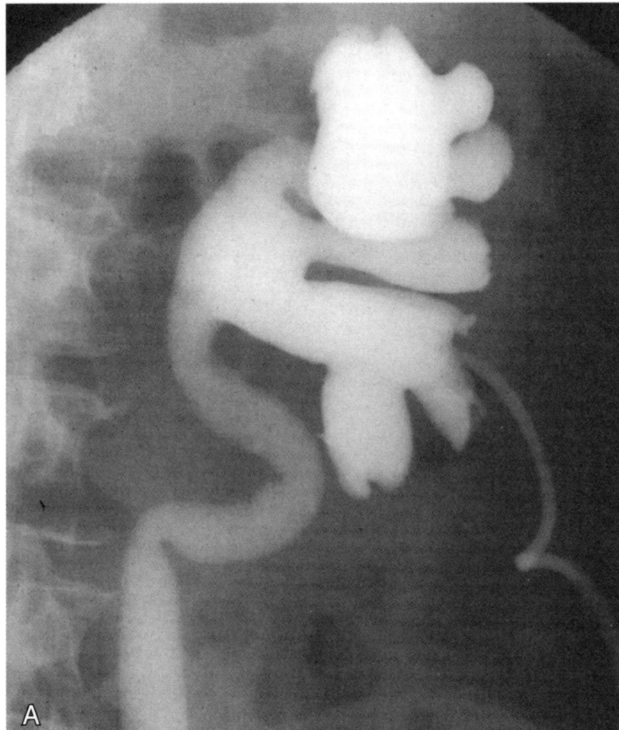


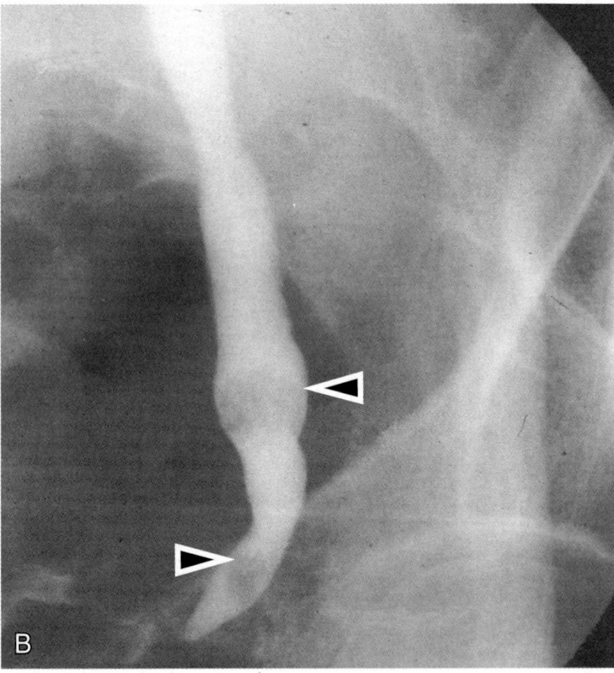


**Fig. 37.7** Antegrade pyelography. (A) Dilated renal pelvis and calices on left. (B) Stones *(arrowheads)* as filling defects in the distal ureter (not seen on plain film). Intravenous pyelography was unsuccessful owing to the obstructed and malfunctioning kidney.

also serve as a first step in relieving obstruction by means of percutaneous nephrostomy (Fig. 37.7).

## PATHOPHYSIOLOGY OF OBSTRUCTIVE NEPHROPATHY

Despite the fact that acquired obstructive nephropathy in humans usually results from partial urinary tract obstruction and is generally prolonged in its time course, most mechanistic studies of renal dysfunction in acquired obstruction use models of acute complete obstruction, usually for 24 hours. In these animal models, the extent of obstruction is clear and reproducible, and, if the kidneys are studied soon after the obstruction is performed or released, the results are not confounded by changes in renal structure brought on by inflammation or fibrosis. Complete obstruction of short duration strikingly alters renal blood flow, glomerular filtration, and tubular function, while producing minimal anatomic changes in blood vessels, glomeruli, and tubules.[2]

### EFFECTS OF OBSTRUCTION ON RENAL BLOOD FLOW AND GLOMERULAR FILTRATION

Obstruction profoundly alters all components of glomerular function. The extent of the disturbance in GFR depends on the severity and duration of the obstruction, whether it is unilateral or bilateral, and the extent to which the obstruction has been relieved or persists.[2] To describe the effects of obstruction on glomerular filtration, we must review aspects of normal GFR. Whole-kidney GFR depends on the filtration rate of all functioning glomeruli and the proportion of glomeruli actually filtering. As detailed in Chapter 3, single-nephron GFR (SNGFR) is determined by the blood flow in the glomerulus, the net ultrafiltration pressure across the glomerular capillary, and the ultrafiltration coefficient ($K_f$). Glomerular blood flow and the hydraulic pressure in the glomerular capillary ($P_{GC}$) are determined by the resistances of the afferent ($R_A$) and efferent ($R_E$) arterioles. Net ultrafiltration pressure is determined by $P_{GC}$, the hydraulic pressure of the Bowman space (which equals the proximal tubule hydraulic pressure, $P_T$), and the differences in oncotic pressure between the glomerular capillary and Bowman space. $K_f$ is determined by the permeability properties of the filtering surface and the surface area available for filtration. Obstruction can alter one or all of these determinants of GFR.

#### THE EARLY, HYPEREMIC PHASE

In the immediate 2 to 3 hours following the onset of UUO, blockade of antegrade urine flow markedly increased $P_T$. This increase in pressure in Bowman space would be expected to halt GFR immediately.[174–176] However, during this early phase of obstruction, the afferent arterioles dilate, decreasing $R_A$, increasing $P_{GC}$, and counteracting the increase in $P_T$.[174,175] Because this vasodilator or “hyperemic response” occurs in denervated kidneys in situ and in isolated perfused kidneys,[177,178] it must result from intrarenal mechanisms. In fact, glomeruli of individual nephrons exhibit the same response in in vivo micropuncture experiments when antegrade urine flow is blocked by placement of a wax block in the tubule of the nephron.[179]

Many mechanisms may mediate this afferent vasodilation, including increases in vasodilator hormones such as prostaglandins, regulation by the macula densa, and a direct myogenic reflex. This hyperemic response is not attenuated by renal nerve stimulation or infusion of catecholamines,[180] and it may be linked to changes in interstitial pressure.[178]

In the tubuloglomerular feedback response, reduced tubular flow past the macula densa induces reductions in $R_A$ and increases in $P_{GC}$, so that SNGFR rises. Similarly, because obstruction reduces urine flow past the macula densa, it would be predicted to induce afferent vasodilation.[179] However, elegant micropuncture studies separated the stoppage in flow from increases in $P_T$ by placing an additional puncture in the tubule that was proximal to the blockage of flow to the macula densa. In this setting, flow past the macula densa was halted, but $P_T$ remained normal, because accumulating tubular fluid was permitted to leak out.[175] In such nephrons the increase in $P_{GC}$ observed in obstructed tubules did not occur, indicating that the obstruction itself and not the macula densa stimulates afferent vasodilation.[175]

Renal prostaglandins and renal nerves play important roles in the hyperemic response. Indomethacin blocks the hyperemic response, indicating that vasodilator prostaglandins are critical to afferent vasodilation.[176,181] A renorenal reflex mechanism in the hemodynamic response to obstruction can be discerned from studies in bilateral obstruction, where the afferent vasodilation response is absent or markedly attenuated.[2,178] Obstruction of the left kidney augments afferent renal nerve activity from the left kidney and efferent nerve activity to the right kidney. Increased efferent nerve activity to the right kidney was accompanied by reduced blood flow to that kidney. This vasoconstrictor response was ablated by denervation of either the left or right kidney before induction of left ureteral obstruction, suggesting that increased afferent renal nerve traffic triggers vasoconstrictive renorenal reflex activity that counteracts the early intrinsic renal vasodilator effects of obstruction in bilateral ureteral obstruction.[178]

**Table 37.1 Glomerular Hemodynamics in Ureteral Obstruction**[a]

| Stage of Obstruction | $P_T$ | $R_A$ | $P_{GC}$ | SNGFR |
|---|---|---|---|---|
| 1–2 hours unilateral | ↑↑ | ↓ | ↑ | = |
| 24 hours unilateral | = | ↑↑ | ↓ | ↓↓ |
| 24 hours bilateral | ↑↑ | = | = | ↓↓ |
| After release: 24 hours unilateral | ↓ | ↑↑ | ↓↓ | ↓↓ |
| After release: 24 hours bilateral | = | ↑↑ | ↓ | ↓↓ |

[a]See text for discussion and references.

*$P_{GC}$*, Hydraulic pressure of Bowman space; *$P_T$*, proximal tubule hydraulic pressure; *$R_A$*, afferent arteriole resistance; *SNGFR*, single-nephron glomerular filtration rate; =, unchanged; ↑, increased; ↑↑, markedly increased; ↓, reduced; ↓↓, markedly reduced.

## THE LATE, VASOCONSTRICTIVE PHASE

Because obstruction results in cessation of glomerular filtration, efforts to study the regulation of SNGFR later in obstruction have measured determinants of GFR immediately after release of obstruction.[2,182] Using this approach, investigators have shown that renal blood flow declines progressively after 3 hours of unilateral obstruction, and through 12 to 24 hours of obstruction.[183,184] Interestingly, although tubular pressures rise initially after obstruction, they then decline, so that by 24 hours renal plasma flow, GFR, and intratubular pressures have all dropped below normal values.[174,176,184,185] At 24 hours into the obstruction, examination of regional blood flow in the kidney by injections of silicone rubber reveals large areas of the cortical vascular bed that are either underperfused or not perfused at all.[2,176,184] Depending on the species, the different vascular beds in the outer and juxtamedullary cortex receive differing proportions of the renal blood flow under basal conditions and following obstruction. However, it is clear that at 24 hours of obstruction, reduced whole-kidney GFR is due, in large part, to nonperfusion of many glomeruli.

Beyond 24 hours of obstruction, the SNGFR of glomeruli that remain perfused is decreased markedly, both because of reduced blood flow to the afferent arteriole and because of afferent vasoconstriction, which, in turn, reduces $P_{GC}$.[185,186] Because $P_{GC}$ responds in the same manner when the individual nephron is blocked with oil for 24 hours before micropuncture measurements are performed, it is clear that afferent arteriolar vasoconstriction plays an important role in attenuating SNGFR during the established phase of obstruction.[187] These results indicate that, like the early hyperemic response, intrarenal mechanisms play the major role in the late vasoconstrictive response to unilateral obstruction. In bilateral obstruction, renal blood flow is reduced to levels 30% to 60% below normal (Table 37.1).[185,186,188] In both unilateral and bilateral obstruction, SNGFR falls to a similar degree. However, the mechanisms involved are different in the two conditions. In unilateral obstruction, reduced $P_{GC}$ lowers the driving pressure for filtration when set against a nearly normal $P_T$. By contrast, in bilateral obstruction, $P_{GC}$ remains normal and GFR is halted by a highly elevated $P_T$.[185] These results suggest that systemic factors, such as accumulation of extracellular fluid volume and urea, increase in natriuretic substances and alterations in renal nerve activity modulate the vasoconstrictive effect of obstruction on the affected kidney.[188]

## REGULATION OF THE GLOMERULAR FILTRATION RATE IN RESPONSE TO OBSTRUCTION

The extent to which renal blood flow and GFR are reduced after release of obstruction varies with the species studied and the duration of obstruction.[2] Following release of a 24-hour complete unilateral obstruction, the GFR remains below 50% of normal in dogs and 25% of normal in rats; renal blood flow remains markedly reduced in both species.[2] After release of bilateral ureteral obstruction, renal blood flow reaches levels higher than those observed following unilateral obstruction, likely due to systemic natriuretic influences such as volume accumulation, reduced sympathetic tone, or increased circulating atrial natriuretic peptide (ANP), but the GFR remains markedly attenuated. Despite the fact that renal blood flow is increased, GFR remains low in part because of nonperfusion or underperfusion of many glomeruli as shown in silicone rubber injections.[176,184] Where glomeruli remain perfused, intense afferent vasoconstriction reduces $P_{GC}$, so that even though $P_T$ also falls with release of the obstruction, the driving force for glomerular filtration remains low.[185,186] In addition, a sharp reduction in $K_f$ augments the fall in GFR at this point following release of unilateral and bilateral obstruction.[185,186]

Several mechanisms contribute to afferent vasoconstriction and a reduced $K_f$. First, release of obstruction strikingly augments the flow of tubular fluid past the macula densa. Although the absolute rate of flow is still far below normal, the macula densa likely senses the dramatic change in the rate of flow, and this may lead to intense vasoconstriction.[2] In favor of this view, the sensitivity of the tubuloglomerular feedback mechanism is enhanced in unilateral, as compared with bilateral, obstruction, suggesting that the ability of the mechanism to regulate afferent arteriolar tone is modulated by the extrarenal hormonal milieu.[189]

There is substantial evidence that increased intrarenal secretion of angiotensin II (ANG II) participates actively in afferent vasoconstriction and reduced $K_f$ following release of ureteral obstruction. Ureteral obstruction rapidly increases renal vein renin levels at a time when renal blood flow is normal or elevated, but at later time points renal vein renin levels return to normal.[190–192] In addition, infusion of captopril attenuated the declines in renal blood flow and GFR observed in both unilateral and bilateral obstruction.[190,192] Because inhibition of angiotensin-converting enzyme can also increase kinin activity, infusions of either carboxypeptidase B, which destroys kinins, or aprotinin, which blocks kinin generation, were used to eliminate the kinin effect. Captopril remained equally effective in the presence of either agent, indicating that captopril reduced $R_A$ primarily by blocking generation of ANG II.[2] The significance of the renin–angiotensin system as an important contributor to the vasoconstriction has recently been highlighted in studies where AT1 receptor antagonist treatment attenuated the reduction in GFR in the postobstructive period in both adult rats[193] and rats with neonatally induced unilateral partial obstruction in response to long-term AT1 receptor antagonist treatment.[194]

Thromboxane $A_2$ ($TXA_2$) plays a role in the obstruction-induced vasoconstriction.[190,195] Chronically hydronephrotic kidneys exhibit increased $TXA_2$ accumulation, as measured by accumulation of its more stable metabolite $TXB_2$.[195] Furthermore, whole-kidney GFR and renal blood flow were increased in response to thromboxane synthase inhibitor treatment,[190,196] likely by reducing afferent arteriolar resistance and thereby increasing $K_f$.[197] From these results, $TXA_2$ appears to be generated in the kidney following release of obstruction and mediates afferent vasoconstriction and reductions in $K_f$.

Although the source of $TXA_2$ generation remains unclear in some cases,[198] but not all,[199] glomeruli isolated from obstructed kidneys have shown increased ability to synthesize $TXA_2$ and other studies have suggested inflammatory cells as the source of $TXA_2$. This is consistent with the observations that suppressor T cells and macrophages migrate to the renal cortex and medulla during the first 24 hours of obstruction, reaching levels fifteenfold higher than those observed in normal kidneys[200] and a parallel rise in $TXA_2$ release and the fall in GFR.[200] These changes can be attenuated by renal irradiation, indicating that obstruction stimulates migration of inflammatory leukocytes, which, in turn, generate vasoconstrictors such as $TXA_2$.[200,201] The role of ANG II for this is highlighted because glomeruli isolated from obstructed kidneys showed increased eicosanoid synthesis after ANG II stimulation and that treatment of obstructed animals with converting enzyme inhibitors enhanced GFR and reduced $TXA_2$ generation by glomeruli isolated from these animals.[202] Thus these vasoconstrictors may contribute to regulate $R_A$ and GFR following release of obstruction.

Because vasoconstriction is less severe in animals with bilateral ureteral obstruction, as noted earlier, it is likely that extrarenal factors play a major role in modulating the hemodynamic response of the kidney to obstruction and release of obstruction. In addition to renorenal reflexes already mentioned, various other factors, including accumulation of volume and solutes such as urea, ANP and its congeners, and other natriuretic substances, may ameliorate the vasoconstrictive effects of obstruction when both ureters are ligated.[203,204] Following 24 hours of obstruction, GFR is preserved to some degree if the contralateral kidney is also obstructed or removed.[203] In addition, in animals following release of 24 hours of unilateral obstruction, if the urea, salt, and water content of the urine from the contralateral kidney is reinfused into the animal, a striking increase in GFR over standard unilateral obstruction is observed,[203,205] suggesting that ANP, urea, and other excreted urine solutes have a protective effect and can ameliorate vasoconstriction following release of ureteral obstruction by direct vasodilation of afferent arterioles, constriction of efferent arterioles, and an increase in $K_f$.

Additional studies in dogs and rats have implicated endothelins as contributors to reduced GFR in obstruction and have suggested that prostaglandin $E_2$ ($PGE_2$) and nitric oxide (NO) may play an ameliorating role in glomerular vasoconstriction in the chronic obstructed kidneys.[206,207] Renal $PGE_2$ levels increase markedly in obstruction (see later) and in states of extracellular volume expansion, as occurs in bilateral ureteral obstruction. Given the vasodilator effects of $PGE_2$, it appears likely that increased levels could ameliorate falls in GFR in obstruction. Bilateral obstruction may reduce generation of NO, leading to a net vasoconstrictive effect.[202]

PUUO is associated with increased renin–angiotensin–aldosterone system activity, elevated oxidative stress, reduced NO bioavailability, and sensitized afferent arteriolar reactivity and renal autoregulation, leading to blood pressure elevation in both mice and rats.[208] Renal denervation in PUUO rats attenuated both hypertension and salt sensitivity, and normalized the renal excretion pattern, whereas the degree of renal fibrosis and inflammation was not changed. This suggests a link between renal nerves, increased blood pressure, and modulation of nicotinamide adenine dinucleotide phosphate oxidase function.

In summary, both intrarenal and extrarenal factors combine to profoundly decrease GFR during and immediately after release of obstruction. The decrease in GFR is caused by a sharp reduction in the number of perfused glomeruli and by a reduction in the SNGFR of functioning nephrons. Decreased $K_f$ and increased $R_A$ reduce SNGFR. Increases in various vasoconstrictors, such as ANG II and $TXA_2$, as well as other vasoconstrictors, some coming from inflammatory cells, augment these hemodynamic effects. In the setting of bilateral obstruction, retention of urea and other solutes, as well as volume expansion and increases in circulating levels of vasodilators such as ANP, helps offset these vasoconstrictive effects, but only partially.

## RECOVERY OF GLOMERULAR FUNCTION AFTER RELIEF OF OBSTRUCTION

The extent of recovery of glomerular filtration following release of obstruction depends on several factors, including the duration and extent of obstruction, the presence or absence of a functioning contralateral kidney, the presence or absence of associated infection, and the level of preobstruction renal blood flow.[2,209] In a classic experiment in dogs subjected to a 1-week period of complete UUO, GFR fell to 25% of normal on release of the obstruction and recovered gradually to 50% of normal levels 2 years later, indicating persisting irreversible changes.[210] In rats, release of UUO of 7- and 14-day duration left residual GFR at 17% and 9% of control levels, respectively, when the contralateral kidney was left in place, and at 31% and 14% when the animals underwent contralateral nephrectomy at the time of release of the obstruction.[211] A similar beneficial effect on the obstructed kidney of contralateral nephrectomy was observed in rats subjected to chronic partial obstruction.[211] As discussed earlier, this beneficial effect likely results from the accumulation of urea and other solutes and increased levels of ANP when the functioning contralateral kidney is absent.

The partial recovery of total GFR following release of obstruction masks a very uneven distribution of blood flow and nephron function. In micropuncture studies, some nephrons never regain filtration function, whereas others reveal striking hyperfiltration.[209] It appeared in some studies that surface nephrons exhibited normal SNGFR, whereas the whole-kidney GFR was reduced to 18% of normal.[212] These results suggest that chronic partial obstruction causes selective damage to juxtamedullary and deep cortical nephrons.[184,209,212] Similarly, studies of the long-term outcome of complete 24-hour ureteral obstruction revealed that total renal GFR recovered to normal levels by 14 and 60 days after release of obstruction. However, 15% of the glomeruli were not filtering in recovered kidneys, and other nephrons were hyperfiltering. In this model of complete obstruction, there appeared to be no selective advantage for surface glomeruli over deep cortical and juxtamedullary glomeruli.[209]

Similarly, in the developing kidney, the duration of obstruction and timing of release have a striking impact on long-term renal function. Release after 1 week of obstruction completely prevented development of hydronephrosis, and reduction in renal blood flow and GFR in rats subjected to PUUO at birth, whereas release after 4 weeks resulted in little or no renal function in the obstructed kidney, demonstrating that early release of neonatal obstruction provides dramatically better protection of renal function than release of obstruction after the maturation process is completed.[213] Consistent with this, studies in pigs subjected to neonatal unilateral partial obstruction demonstrated that impaired nephrogenesis resulted in a reduced number of glomeruli in the obstructed kidney.[214] Preserved whole-kidney function suggests some degree of glomerular hyperfiltration. In line with the hypothesis that hyperfiltration is associated with an increased risk of systemic hypertension,[215] studies in pigs and rats have demonstrated that renal expressions of neuronal nitric oxide synthase (NOS) and endothelial NOS proteins were lower in animals with hydronephrosis.[216,217] These findings suggest that the reduced NO response in the obstructed hydronephrotic kidney, and subsequent resetting of the tubuloglomerular feedback (TGF) mechanism, plays an important role in the development of hypertension in hydronephrosis.

## EFFECTS OF OBSTRUCTION ON TUBULE FUNCTION

Obstruction severely impairs the ability of renal tubules to transport $Na^+$, $K^+$, and $H^+$, and reduces their ability to concentrate and dilute the urine (Table 37.2).[2,218–224] The resulting inability to reabsorb water and solutes facilitates postobstructive diuresis and natriuresis. As is the case with glomerular filtration, the extent of disruption of tubular transport depends directly on the duration and severity of the obstruction. Pathologically, prolonged obstruction leads to profound tubular atrophy and chronic interstitial inflammation and fibrosis (see the following section), whereas at early time points following the onset of obstruction, such as at 24 hours, there are only slight structural and ultrastructural changes

**Table 37.2 Segmental Reabsorption in Superficial and Juxtamedullary Nephrons and in Collecting Ducts in Normal Rats After Release of Bilateral or Unilateral Obstruction**

| | Normal | | After Unilateral Obstruction | | After Bilateral Obstruction | |
|---|---|---|---|---|---|---|
| Site | Water Remaining (%) | $Na^+$ Remaining (%) | Water Remaining (%) | $Na^+$ Remaining (%) | Water Remaining (%) | $Na^+$ Remaining (%) |
| $S_1$ | 100 | 100 | 100 | 100 | 100 | 100 |
| $S_2$ | 44 | 44 | 26 | 26 | 45 | 45 |
| $S_3$ | 26 | 14 | 21 | 12 | 40 | 22 |
| $S_4$ | 9.4 | 5 | 3.2 | 1.9 | 25 | 7 |
| $J_1$ | 100 | 100 | 100 | 100 | 100 | 100 |
| $J_2$ | 12 | 40 | 42 | 52 | 42 | 62 |
| $CD_1$ | 3.3 | 2 | 4.2 | 3.8 | 8 | 6 |
| $CD_2$ | 0.4 | 0.6 | 2.9 | 2.5 | 16.7 | 12 |

In obstruction, increased proportions of filtered salt and water are delivered to the loop of Henle in juxtamedullary nephrons ($J_1$ and $J_2$ indicating decreased reabsorption). Delivery of sodium and water to the first accessible portion of the inner medullary collecting duct, labeled $CD_1$, was also increased, and net sodium and water reabsorption along the inner medullary collecting duct (between $CD_1$ and $CD_2$) was diminished in both bilateral and unilateral obstruction. In bilateral obstruction, there was net addition or secretion of sodium and water into the lumen of the inner medullary collecting duct, suggesting that in this setting the inner medullary collecting duct secretes sodium and water. (From Harris KP, Schreiner GF, Klahr S. Effect of leukocyte depletion on the function of the postobstructed kidney in the rat. *Kidney Int.* 1989;36:210–215.)

*$CD_1$*, Collecting duct at base of papilla, first accessible portion of inner medullary collecting duct; *$CD_2$*, end of collecting duct as it opens into renal pelvis; *$J_{1-2}$*, values found in juxtamedullary nephrons; *$J_1$*, Bowman space; *$J_2$*, tip of loop of Henle; *$S_{1-4}$*, values found in superficial nephrons: *$S_1$*, Bowman space; *$S_2$*, end of the proximal convoluted tubule; *$S_3$*, earliest portion of the distal tubule; *$S_4$*, end of the distal tubule/beginning of collecting duct.

including mitochondrial swelling, modest blunting of basolateral interdigitations in the thick ascending limb and proximal tubule epithelial cells, as well as flattening of the epithelium and some widening of the intercellular spaces in the collecting ducts.[2,225,226] The only cell death at early time points is observed at the very tip of the papilla, where focal necrosis may be observed.[225] Because there is so little cell damage, and because of the simplicity of the model, most investigators have examined the effect of 24 hours of complete ureteral obstruction on tubular function. As discussed later, regulation of tubular transport is complex and is due to both direct damage of epithelial cells and the action of extratubular mediators, arising both from the kidney and extrarenal sources.

## EFFECTS OF OBSTRUCTION ON TUBULAR SODIUM REABSORPTION

Following release of 24 hours of UUO, volume excretion from the postobstructed kidney is normal or slightly increased[2,188,203,227] (see Table 37.2). However, as discussed earlier, normal volume excretion occurs in the setting of a markedly reduced (20% of normal) GFR. Consequently, fractional excretion of sodium $FE_{Na}$ is markedly elevated in the postobstructed kidney. After release of bilateral obstruction, salt and water excretion jumps up to five to nine times normal.[2,188,218,219] Because GFR is also decreased in this setting, $FE_{Na}$ may be twentyfold higher than normal.

The micropuncture studies summarized in Table 37.2 demonstrate that the reabsorption defect following release of obstruction is localized similarly in both unilateral and bilateral ureteral obstruction. Obstruction reduced net salt and water reabsorption in the medullary thick ascending limb (MTAL), the distal convoluted tubule, and the entire length of the collecting duct, including its cortical, outer medullary, and inner medullary segments.[218]

These studies in whole animals were confirmed and extended by a series of studies from multiple laboratories using isolated perfused tubule and cell suspension preparations (Table 37.3). As shown, the segments including proximal straight tubule, MTAL, and cortical collecting duct isolated from unilaterally or bilaterally obstructed animals exhibited profound impairment of sodium reabsorptive capacity.[219,220] This finding was confirmed in studies of freshly prepared suspensions of MTAL cells from obstructed kidneys, in which transport-dependent oxygen consumption, a measure of sodium reabsorptive capacity, was markedly reduced.[221] Given the major regulatory role of mineralocorticoid in the collecting duct, it is important to note that these decreases in collecting duct sodium reabsorptive capacity occurred in tubules taken from obstructed kidneys, whether or not the animal had been pretreated with mineralocorticoid.[220,222,223] Because it is highly branched and difficult to perfuse reliably in vitro, transport in the inner medullary collecting duct has been studied in cell suspensions. In these preparations, transport-dependent oxygen consumption was markedly reduced in cells isolated from animals with bilateral obstruction.[224]

Taken together, the data derived from micropuncture, tubule perfusion, and cell suspension studies reveal a striking impairment of sodium reabsorption in the proximal straight tubule, the MTAL, and the entire collecting duct. Because these functional derangements occur in the absence of clear-cut ultrastructural damage to the epithelial cells, obstruction likely induces a selective impairment in the regulation of active cellular transport mechanisms. Unlike the situation with glomerular filtration, the functional impairment appears similar in both unilateral and bilateral obstruction.[220,223,224] Thus it appears that a major component of impaired active transport is likely due to direct tubular cell injury, rather than to the continuous action of natriuretic substances. Added onto this intrinsic injury, natriuretic substances may be responsible for the apparent secretion of sodium and water in the inner medullary collecting duct of animals following release of bilateral obstruction (see Table 37.2).

A combination of studies of cell suspensions and antibody-based targeted proteomics where long-term regulation of renal transporters and channels can be examined in intact animals to understand the integrated response to obstruction has improved the molecular understanding of mechanisms by which tubular epithelial cell sodium reabsorption is impaired in the setting of obstruction. Active tubular $Na^+$ transport requires an apical entry step (e.g., NKCC2 cotransporter in MTAL or epithelial $Na^+$ channels [ENaCs] in the

**Table 37.3 Function of Isolated Perfused Tubules in Obstructive Nephropathy**

| | $J_v$ SPCT (nL/mm/min) | $J_v$ PST (nL/mm/min) | $\Delta Cl^-$ MTAL (mEq/L) | $J_v$ CCT (ADH) (nL/mm/min) |
|---|---|---|---|---|
| Control | 0.75 ± 0.08 | 0.25 ± 0.02 | −37 ± 3 | 0.90 ± 0.08 |
| Unilateral obstruction | 0.73 ± 0.11 | 0.12 ± 0.03 | −9 ± 1 | 0.22 ± 0.04 |
| Bilateral obstruction | 0.80 ± 0.08 | 0.16 ± 0.02 | −10 ± 1 | 0.23 ± 0.04 |

The $J_V$ in the SPCT was not affected by obstruction, whereas $J_V$ in PST decreased by 52% in unilateral obstruction (0.12 ± 0.03 vs. 0.25 ± 0.02 nL/mm/min), and similarly in response to bilateral obstruction. In mTAL the ability to lower the perfusate chloride ion concentration was reduced by 76% (–9 ± 1 vs. –37 ± 3 mEq/L), and similarly in response to bilateral ureteral obstruction. Following relief of unilateral obstruction, the ability of the CCT to respond to ADH was reduced by 76% (0.22 ± 0.04 vs. 0.90 ± 0.08 nL/mm/min), and similarly following relief of bilateral obstruction.

*ADH,* antidiuretic hormone; *CCT,* cortical collecting tubule; $J_v$, net fluid reabsorption rate per length of the tubule segment; *PST,* cortical proximal straight tubule; *SPCT,* superficial proximal convoluted tubule; $\Delta Cl^-$ *MTAL,* change in $Cl^-$ concentration per length of the medullary thick ascending limb.

(Data from Reyes AA, Martin D, Settle S, Klahrs S. EDRF role in renal function and blood pressure of normal rats and rats with obstructive uropathy. *Kidney Int.* 1992;41:403–413.)

collecting duct) coupled to the basolateral $Na^+,K^+$-ATPase. In addition, the cell must generate sufficient adenosine triphosphate (ATP) to fuel active transport by the ATPase. Suspensions of MTAL cells from obstructed kidneys exhibited markedly reduced furosemide-sensitive oxygen consumption,[221] indicating striking decreases in apical NKCC2 cotransporter activity in these cells. Isotopic bumetanide binding revealed a marked reduction in the number of cotransporter protein molecules available for binding on the membrane, with no change in affinity of binding, indicating that obstruction downregulates the expression of the cotransporter protein on the membrane surface.[221] More recent studies using antibody-based targeted approaches clearly showed that obstruction diminishes expression of the cotransporter protein on the MTAL cell apical membrane.[228] Similar approaches demonstrated downregulation of $Na^+,K^+$-ATPase of both α- and β-subunits at the transcriptional and posttranscriptional levels.[228,229]

In the inner medullary collecting duct similar studies demonstrated downregulation of ENaC.[230] Consistent with this, suspensions from obstructed kidneys showed marked decreases in amiloride-sensitive oxygen consumption as well as amiloride-sensitive isotopic sodium entry into hyperpolarized cells.[224]

As occurred in MTAL cells, the rates of ouabain-sensitive oxygen consumption and of ouabain-sensitive ATPase were markedly diminished in inner medullary collecting duct cells from obstructed animals, and the levels of both pump subunits were also reduced in these preparations.[224] Patterns of messenger RNA (mRNA) expression were also similar to those in MTAL, indicating transcriptional and posttranscriptional downregulation of pump subunit expression. Using the targeted antibody-based approach demonstrated that in both unilateral and bilateral ureteral obstruction, the expressions of $Na^+/H^+$ exchanger ($NHE_3$) and the $Na^+/PO_4^{3-}$ exchanger (NaPi-2) were strikingly decreased in the proximal tubule.[228,231] These changes in sodium transporter expression occurred in both the proximal convoluted and proximal straight tubule, even though the micropuncture and tubule perfusion studies cited earlier revealed preserved proximal convoluted tubule salt reabsorption and inhibition of proximal straight tubule reabsorption.[231,232] The same studies demonstrated significant downregulation of total transporter protein and apical membrane expression of the distal convoluted tubule $Na^+/Cl^-$ cotransporter, indicating that obstruction likely reduces distal convoluted tubule $Na^+$ reabsorption by mechanisms similar to those observed in the MTAL and collecting duct.[228,231]

Taken together, these results demonstrate that obstruction downregulates membrane expression of transporter proteins responsible for apical sodium entry and of basolateral sodium exit. Interestingly, metabolic studies reveal that obstruction reduces activities as well of several enzymes of the oxidative and glycolytic pathways, consistent with a downregulation of metabolic capacity for energy generation in these cells. This may also be enhanced by the observed reductions in the extent of basolateral infolding and in the density of mitochondria in tubules of obstructed kidneys.[225] Interestingly, in MTAL and collecting duct suspensions, obstruction reduces transport-dependent but not transport-independent oxygen consumption, indicating that the rate of ATP generation (oxygen consumption) is not rate-limiting for active transport in these cells. On this basis, it appears more likely that obstruction-induced reduction of epithelial sodium transport is a regulated process as a result of reduced metabolic demands during obstruction.

The mechanisms and pathways responsible for downregulation of transport proteins in tubular epithelial cells by obstruction remain to a large extent incomplete. Possible signals include the halting of urine flow, increased hydrostatic pressure on tubular epithelial cells, changes in blood flow to the tubules or in interstitial pressure, and generation of natriuretic substances in the kidney that result in long-term inhibition of transporter function. Powerful mass spectrometry analysis of tissue from obstructed rat kidneys and mpkCCD cells has led to proteomic identification of significant changes in more than 100 proteins including those belonging to the cytoskeleton. These findings suggest that obstruction induces acute molecular changes in the renal cytoskeleton, in part, mediated by increased stretch of the renal tubular cells during obstruction.[233]

Obstruction impairs glomerular filtration and urine production is dramatically reduced (stopped in occlusion). Consequently sodium delivery to each tubular segment is reduced and apical membrane $Na^+$ entry slows dramatically because the electrochemical gradients for $Na^+$ entry between the stationary apical fluid and the cell interior become increasingly unfavorable for continued sodium transport. Reduced $Na^+$ entry might then directly stimulate downregulation of transporter activity and expression. In both MTAL and inner medullary collecting duct cells, blocking $Na^+$ entry by furosemide or amiloride, respectively, promptly reduces ouabain-sensitive oxygen consumption,[221,234] indicating acute downregulation of $Na^+,K^+$-ATPase. In addition, in mineralocorticoid-clamped animals, chronic blockade of $Na^+$ entry at the MTAL or cortical collecting duct by administration of furosemide or amiloride, respectively, reduced the levels of ouabain-sensitive ATPase in microdissected tubule segments.[235,236]

These results suggest that the halt in urine flow might represent a major signaling mechanism by which obstruction downregulates $Na^+$ transport.[234] To test this hypothesis, apical $Na^+$ entry was inhibited for 24 hours in a cell line that mimics cortical collecting duct cells, A6 cells, grown on permeable supports. When apical $Na^+$ entry was blocked either by substituting another cation for sodium in the apical solution or by adding amiloride to the apical solution, apical sodium entry was markedly reduced for some hours after the blockade was removed.[237] This downregulation is accompanied by selective reduction in the levels of expression of the β-subunit, but not the α- or γ-subunits, of ENaC in the apical membranes of the A6 cells, but not in whole cell content of these subunits.[238] At the integrated level rats with urinary tract obstruction demonstrated downregulation of α-, β-, and γ-subunits of EnaC, indicating that downregulation of all three subunits may play a role in the impaired sodium reabsorption in obstruction.[230] Interestingly, and in contrast to the results in cell suspensions or whole kidney,[221,224,228,231] inhibition of apical sodium entry had no effect on expression of either subunit of $Na^+,K^+$-ATPase.[238] These results provide direct evidence that reductions in the rate of $Na^+$ entry, which may occur when urine flow is blocked, can directly downregulate $Na^+$ transport in renal epithelial cells.

In addition to the direct effects of halting urine flow, changes in intrarenal mediators and subcellular pathways

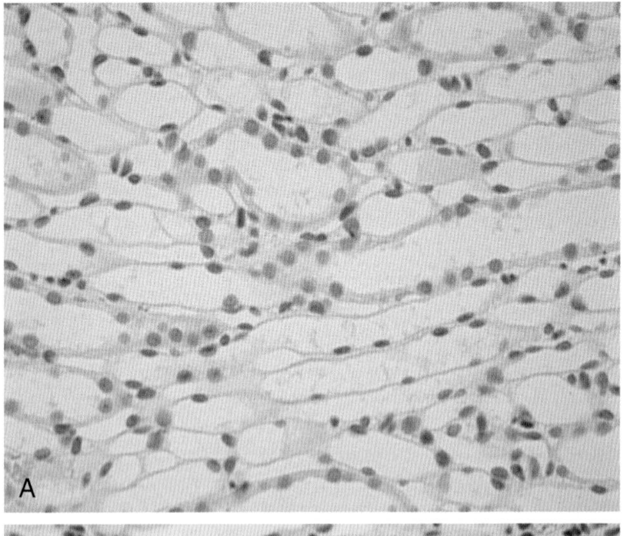


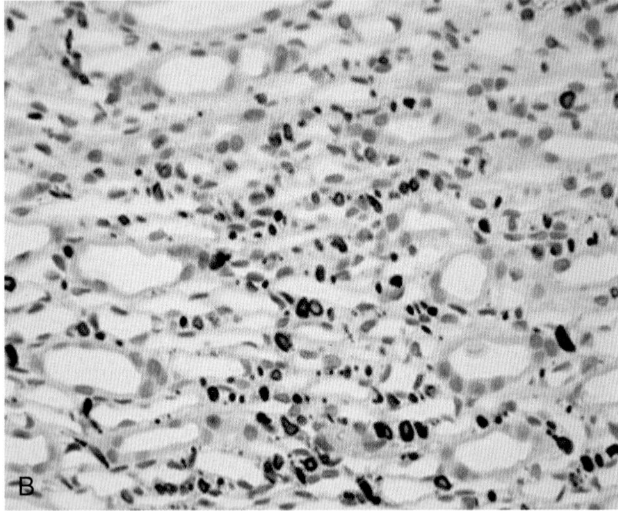


**Fig. 37.8** Immunohistochemistry for cyclooxygenase-2 in the inner medulla of the kidney of sham-operated rats (A), and rats subjected to 24 hours of bilateral ureteral obstruction (B). There is strong labeling at the base of the inner medulla in obstructed kidneys located exclusively to the interstitial cells (B), and labeling is not detectable in sham kidneys (A).

likely play a critical role in the reduction of salt transport observed with obstruction. Obstruction markedly accelerates the already rapid generation of $PGE_2$ in the renal medulla.[195,196,199,239] The molecular basis for this is a dramatic medullary cyclooxygenase-2 (COX-2) induction (Fig. 37.8).[239,240] Consistent with the known effect of $PGE_2$ to markedly inhibit $Na^+$ reabsorption in the MTAL, as well as in the cortical and inner medullary collecting ducts,[241–243] COX-2 inhibition in rats with obstruction and release of obstruction attenuated the downregulation of $NHE_2$, NKCC2, and $Na^+,K^+$-ATPase.[240,244] From these results, obstruction likely reduces apically localized sodium cotransport proteins in the tubule epithelium and sodium pump activity in tubular epithelia in part by increasing renal levels of $PGE_2$.

As discussed earlier, obstruction brings on a monocellular infiltrate in the kidney[200]; and this infiltrate tends to follow a peritubular distribution.[200] When obstructed kidneys were irradiated, the level of medullary inflammation was diminished, and there was a modest decrease in the fractional excretion of sodium.[201] In addition, it has been shown that obstruction causes an enhanced renal ANG II generation. This may have important implications for regulation of renal sodium handling. Blockade of the ANG II receptor (AT1) was associated with a marked attenuation of downregulation of $NHE_3$ and NKCC2 which was paralleled by a reduction in renal sodium loss.[57]

In summary, obstruction reduces net reabsorption of sodium in several nephron segments, including the proximal straight tubule, the MTAL, and the cortical and inner medullary collecting ducts, by downregulating the expression and activities of specific transporter proteins. Several signals mediate this downregulation, including the cessation of urine flow with its attendant reduction of the rate of $Na^+$ entry across the apical membrane, increased levels of natriuretic substances such as $PGE_2$, and infiltration of the obstructed kidney by mononuclear cells.

When both ureters are obstructed, extrarenal factors markedly enhance the sodium-wasting tendency already present in the obstructed kidney. One mechanism involves the volume expansion that occurs when bilateral obstruction ablates all renal function. Volume expansion impairs activity in the sympathetic nervous system, reduces circulating levels of aldosterone, and, along with reduced renal clearance, increases levels of ANP. Reduced sympathetic tone and aldosterone, coupled with increased ANP, markedly stimulate sodium excretion. ANP likely represents a particularly important mediator of salt wasting in bilateral obstruction. Levels of ANP are markedly elevated in bilateral, but not in unilateral obstruction.[245] ANP enhances salt wasting at several nephron segments. By blocking renin release in the macula densa and angiotensin action in the proximal tubule, ANP reduces proximal tubule sodium reabsorption.[204,245,246] ANP also reduces aldosterone release and directly inhibits sodium reabsorption in the collecting ducts.[204,245,246] In agreement with this mechanism, infusion of ANP into animals in which obstruction has just been released leads to marked increases in sodium and water excretion.[245] Moreover, efforts to reduce circulating ANP levels following bilateral obstruction attenuated sodium excretion somewhat.[245]

In addition, accumulation of urea and other solutes enhance sodium wasting by obstructed kidneys. Following release of 24 hours of unilateral obstruction, removal or obstruction of the contralateral kidney markedly enhances salt wasting by the postobstructed kidney.[203] If the contralateral kidney is left in place but amounts of urea, sodium, and water equivalent to what the contralateral kidney is excreting are infused into the animal, there is a striking increase in sodium excretion in both the obstructed and the contralateral kidney.[203,205] On this basis, bilateral obstruction induces hormonal changes and promotes accumulation of solutes and volume that together enhance natriuresis from the obstructed kidney.

## EFFECTS OF OBSTRUCTION ON URINARY CONCENTRATION AND DILUTION

Because obstruction eliminates the ability of the renal tubules to concentrate and dilute the urine, urine osmolality following release of obstruction in humans and experimental animals approaches that of plasma.[2,247,248] Dilution of the urine requires that the thick ascending limb reabsorbs sodium without water and that the collecting duct maintain the dilute urine by not reabsorbing water along its length, despite the presence of a concentrated medullary interstitium.[249] Concentration of the urine requires active sodium reabsorption in the thick limb and the action of the countercurrent multiplier to generate a concentrated medullary interstitium, as well as the ability of the collecting duct to insert the vasopressin-regulated water channel aquaporin-2 (AQP2) into the apical membrane.[250,251]

Obstructive nephropathy disrupts several of these mechanisms.[231,247,248,252] As noted earlier, obstruction also markedly reduces MTAL sodium reabsorption, limiting this segment's ability to dilute the urine and to generate a high medullary interstitial osmolality. Indeed, interstitial osmolality has been shown to be reduced in obstructed kidneys.[2] In addition, collecting ducts isolated from obstructed kidneys reveal normal basal water permeabilities, but a marked reduction in their ability to increase water permeability in response to antidiuretic hormone or other stimulants of cyclic adenosine monophosphate (cAMP) accumulation in the cells. As was the case with sodium transport, the effects were similar in unilateral and bilateral obstruction.[247,252] Detailed mechanistic studies show that obstruction markedly reduces transcription of mRNA encoding AQP2, as well as synthesis of AQP2 protein, and that collecting duct cells in obstructed kidneys do not traffic AQP2-containing vesicles effectively to the apical surface in response to vasopressin or increased cAMP.[247,251–253] Part of this failure in trafficking results from a decrease in phosphorylation of AQP2 in obstructed kidneys[231] and likely also due to the fact that V2 receptor protein expression is downregulated.[254] Redistribution of AQP2 and AQP2 phosphorylated at ser261 to more intracellular localizations after bilateral obstruction and colocalization with the early endosomal marker EEA1 and the lysosomal marker cathepsin D suggest that early downregulation of AQP2 could in part be caused by degradation of AQP2 through a lysosomal degradation pathway.[255] In addition, UUO markedly decreases synthesis and deployment to the basolateral membrane of aquaporin-3 and -4; when AQP2 is in the apical membrane, these aquaporins mediate the water flux across the basolateral membrane.[231] Enhancing the causal relationship of the changes in aquaporin activity and ability to concentrate the urine, expression of AQP2 remains suppressed for 7 days following relief of the obstruction, and the rise in urinary concentration parallels the recovery in AQP2 expression.[231,247,248,252] The fact that collecting ducts from obstructed kidneys do not respond to cAMP indicates that the lesion also involves sites beyond the receptor for antidiuretic hormone.[254]

Consistent with the hypothesis that $PGE_2$-mediated inhibition of collecting duct water permeability does not directly affect cAMP levels but may have post-cAMP effects rather than actions via cAMP regulation,[256] recent experiments have shown that COX-2 inhibition prevented dysregulation of AQP2 in obstructed kidneys where COX-2 protein expression was markedly increased (Fig. 37.8).[240,257]

On the basis of these results it can be concluded that the defect in urinary dilution in obstruction is due to reduced ability of the thick ascending limb to dilute the urine by transporting salt from the lumen of the tubule to its basolateral side. The collecting duct in obstructed kidneys maintains its low water permeability in the absence of antidiuretic hormone, so that the failure to dilute the urine is not due to collapse of osmotic gradients in the collecting duct. The inability to concentrate the urine results from the failure of the thick limb to generate a concentrated interstitium, as well as the inability of the collecting duct to synthesize and to traffic AQP2 and other water channels in response to antidiuretic hormone.

## EFFECTS OF RELIEF OF OBSTRUCTION ON URINARY ACIDIFICATION

Obstruction dramatically reduces urinary acidification in both experimental animals and humans. In humans, release of obstruction does not lead to bicarbonate wasting, indicating that proximal tubular bicarbonate reclamation is maintained. By contrast, in both experimental animals and patients following release of obstruction, the urine pH does not decrease in response to an acid load, indicating that obstruction impairs the ability of the distal nephron to acidify the urine.[258–260] This defect likely involves proton transport proteins both in the collecting duct[258,259] and in the proximal tubule and thick ascending limb of Henle.[260,261]

Reduced collecting duct acid secretion could result from defects in $H^+$ ($H^+$, ATPase or $H^+$ $K^+$-ATPase) or $HCO_3^-$ (e.g., $Cl^-/HCO_3^-$ exchange) transport pathways, backleak of protons down their electrochemical gradient from the lumen to the basolateral side of the tubule, or, in the cortical collecting duct, the failure to generate a sufficiently lumen-negative transepithelial voltage.[258,259,262] As described in detail earlier, obstruction reduces the activity of apical ENaC in the cortical collecting duct; the resulting loss of luminal negativity may attenuate acid secretion in these segments.[258,259]

In the rat inner medullary collecting duct (studied by micropuncture) and in isolated perfused rat and rabbit outer medullary collecting duct, obstruction markedly reduces luminal acidification rates.[258] Because $Na^+$ transport does not play a major role in acidification in these segments, the defect must be due to direct inhibition of acid or $HCO_3^-$ transport pathways, or backleak of protons from lumen to interstitium.[262] At low perfusion rates, outer medullary collecting ducts from obstructed animals maintain the ability to generate steep pH gradients,[258] indicating that obstruction does not block the ability of the tubule to prevent back flux of protons. By contrast, at high perfusion rates, acidification was markedly lower in tubules from obstructed, as opposed to normal, kidneys,[258] demonstrating that obstruction inhibits activity or expression of $H^+$ or $HCO_3^-$ transport pathways.

Antibody-based targeted studies examining the $Cl^-/HCO_3^-$ exchanger and subunits of the $H^+$, ATPase revealed reduced expression of these transporters in collecting ducts of unilaterally obstructed compared with contralateral, and control kidneys.[260,262] Two possible mechanisms of reduced acid secretion were explored.[262] One was that the intercalated cells in obstructed kidneys would exhibit a high proportion of "reverse" orientation, with the proton pump in the basolateral membrane, and the $Cl^-/HCO_3^-$ exchanger in the apical membrane. The other possibility was that the orientation of intercalated cells would not change, but there would be reduced expression of the $H^+$ or $HCO_3^-$ transporter. The orientation of the intercalated cells was not altered by obstruction. However, obstruction did reduce the appearance of H-ATPase along the apical membranes of intercalated cells, without altering the total content of $H^+$-ATPase in extracts of renal cortex or medulla, in unilaterally obstructed, as compared with contralateral kidneys.[262] In obstructed kidneys, fewer intercalated cells exhibited an apical labeling pattern and many that did showed discontinuities or gaps in apical membrane labeling,[262] suggesting that obstruction inhibits trafficking of $H^+$-ATPase to the apical membranes of intercalated cells. However, this disorder alone cannot account for the entire acidification defect in obstructive nephropathy, because the labeling pattern returns to control levels as the obstruction persists, while the acidification defect remains.[262] In addition, the extent of the decrease in labeling appears to be too small to account for the profound defect in acidification.

In addition to defective collecting duct, $H^+$ transport–reduced generation of the main buffer that carries acid equivalents in the urine, ammonia has also been observed in kidneys released from obstruction. Cortical slices of obstructed kidneys exhibit reduced glutamine uptake and oxidation, reduced gluconeogenesis, and reduced total oxygen consumption, all adding up to a reduced ability to generate ammonia from glutamine.[263,264]

### EFFECTS OF RELIEF OF OBSTRUCTION ON EXCRETION OF POTASSIUM

As with sodium excretion, potassium excretion increases markedly following release of bilateral obstruction.[265,266] Micropuncture and microcatheterization studies show that proximal potassium reabsorption is unchanged by obstruction while potassium is more rapidly secreted in the collecting duct, likely due to increased distal delivery and therefore more rapid distal luminal flux of sodium and volume following release of obstruction.[218,265] By contrast, following release of unilateral obstruction, potassium excretion falls roughly in proportion to the reduction in GFR,[267] an effect that may be related to reduced distal delivery of sodium. However, administration of sodium sulfate in this state does not stimulate potassium excretion in obstructed kidneys as it does in controls, suggesting that collecting ducts in unilateral obstructed kidneys have an intrinsic defect in potassium secretion.[268] This intrinsic defect may represent a response similar to the downregulation of sodium transporters in obstructed kidneys described in detail earlier. The kaliuretic effect observed in bilateral obstruction may well be due as well to the influence of elevated levels of ANP, which, at high levels, can stimulate potassium secretion in the distal nephron.

### EFFECTS OF RELIEF OF OBSTRUCTION ON EXCRETION OF PHOSPHATE AND DIVALENT CATIONS

When bilateral ureteral obstruction is released, phosphate excretion rises in proportion to sodium excretion.[228,231,269,270] Phosphate restriction before the release of the obstruction prevents phosphate accumulation during bilateral obstruction, thereby blocking the increase in phosphate excretion.[269] This can also be achieved by blockade of ANG II–mediated effects, highlighting the importance of enhanced renal ANG II levels in the obstructed kidney.[57] In addition, phosphate wasting of similar magnitude to that observed following release of bilateral obstruction can be duplicated by phosphate loading of normal animals.[269] By contrast, release of unilateral obstruction results in phosphate retention, likely due to reduced GFR and avid proximal phosphate reabsorption.[271] Calcium excretion may be increased or decreased, depending on whether the obstruction is unilateral or bilateral, and depending on the species studied.[269,271] Magnesium excretion is markedly increased following release of either bilateral or unilateral obstruction. This magnesium wasting probably occurs because both forms of obstruction markedly attenuate thick ascending limb sodium reabsorption, leading to reduced positive luminal transepithelial voltages and therefore a reduced driving force for lumen-to-basolateral magnesium flux across the paracellular pathway.[272]

## PATHOPHYSIOLOGY OF RECOVERY OF TUBULAR EPITHELIAL CELLS FROM OBSTRUCTION OR OF TUBULOINTERSTITIAL FIBROSIS

An important focus of many experimental studies in obstructive nephropathy has been devoted to the renal effects of longer-term obstruction.[273] In part these studies use UUO as a convenient model for chronic renal damage, because the timing of the injury is clear and because the extent of injury should be reproducible from animal to animal.[273] These studies, which have been conducted almost entirely in rodents, have elucidated an overall pathway for renal tubular epithelial damage, and have identified several potential targets for intervention. Obstruction inhibits oxidative metabolism and promotes anaerobic respiration, leading to decreased ATP levels and increased levels of adenosine diphosphate (ADP) and AMP.[264,274,275] In addition, obstruction alters a wide variety of metabolic enzymes, as well as the expression of many different gene products.[264,275–277] These changes are summarized in Box 37.3. Many of these changes are difficult to link mechanistically with changes in GFR or tubular transport function observed in obstruction. It is possible, however, that reduced ability to generate ATP, along with reductions in $Na^+,K^+$-ATPase expression, contributes to the natriuresis observed following release of obstruction (see earlier discussion).

It is thought that chronic obstruction damages tubular epithelial cells by increasing hydrostatic pressure, reducing blood flow (due to the renal vasoconstriction that occurs in obstruction, see earlier discussion), and increasing oxidative stress.[273] In response, tubular epithelial cells release a number of autocrine factors and cytokines, including ANG II,[273,278] transforming growth factor-beta (TGF-β),[278,279] platelet activator inhibitor,[280] and tumor necrosis factor (TNF).[281] These factors, along with the presence and increase in levels of adhesion factors, lead to the infiltration of the renal interstitium with inflammatory cells, including macrophages. These in turn release additional cytokines. All these factors accelerate the development of interstitial fibrosis by increased extracellular matrix, cell infiltration, apoptosis, and accumulation of activated myofibroblasts.[282] In addition, there is upregulation of various receptors that are targeted by autocrine factors and cytokines including both type 1 and type 2 angiotensin receptors ($AT_1R$ and $AT_2R$).[283] The complex cellular migration process may become amplified by epithelial–mesenchymal transition (EMT),[284] which is characterized by downregulation of epithelial marker proteins such as E-cadherin, zonula occludens-1, and cytokeratin; loss of cell-to-cell adhesion; upregulation of mesenchymal markers including vimentin, α-smooth muscle actin, and fibroblast-specific protein-1; basement membrane degradation; and migration to the interstitial compartment.[284] The entire cascade leads to tubulointerstitial fibrosis and permanent loss of renal function,

## Box 37.3 Effects of Urinary Tract Obstruction on Renal Enzymes and Renal Gene Expression

**Changes in Energy and Substrate Metabolism**

Decreased oxygen consumption
Decreased substrate uptake
Increased anaerobic glycolysis
Decreased ATP/(ADP + AMP)
Decreased ammoniagenesis

**Changes in Enzyme Activity**

Decreased
- Alkaline phosphatase
- $Na^+$, $K^+$-ATPase
- Glucose-6-phosphatase
- Succinate dehydrogenase
- NADH/NADHP dehydrogenase

Increased
- Glucose-6-phosphate dehydrogenase
- Phosphogluconate dehydrogenase
- Mitogen-activated protein kinases
- Matrix metalloproteinase-2/-9
- Mast cell protease 1 (chymase)

**Changes in Gene Expression**

Reduction in glomerular $G_{\alpha s}$ and $G_{\alpha q/11}$ proteins
Reduction in preproepidermal growth factor and Tamm–Horsfall protein
Transient induction of growth factors FOS and MYC
Striking induction of cellular damage (TRPM2) genes
Induction of plasminogen activator gene

*ADP,* Adenosine diphosphate; *AMP,* adenosine monophosphate; *ATP,* adenosine triphosphate; *NADH,* nicotinamide adenine dinucleotide (reduced).

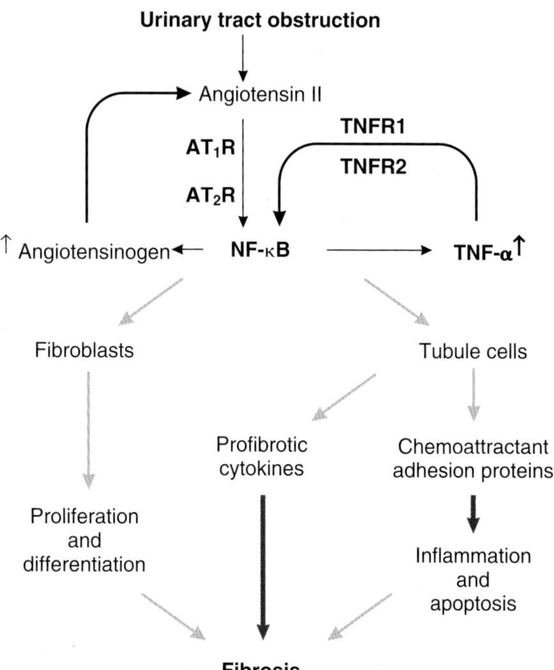


**Fig. 37.9** Urinary tract obstruction causes an enhanced expression of angiotensin II (ANG II). The regulation of gene expression by ANG II occurs through specific receptors that are ultimately linked to changes in the activity of transcription factors within the nucleus of target cells. In particular, members of the nuclear factor (NF)-κB family of transcription factors are activated, which, in turn, fuels at least two autocrine-reinforcing loops that amplify ANG II and tumor necrosis factor (TNF)-α formation. *$AT_1R$,* Type 1 angiotensin receptor; *$AT_2R$,* type 2 angiotensin receptor; *TNFR1,* TNF-α receptor 1; *TNFR2,* TNF-α receptor 2.

which may continue to progress after the obstruction has been relieved (Fig. 37.9).

It has been hypothesized that changes in the intratubular dynamic forces—so-called tubular stretch—in urinary tract obstruction also are an important determinant for development of tubulointerstitial fibrosis in the kidney.[285] Thus both in vivo[279] and in vitro models[286,287] of obstructive uropathy demonstrate that tubular stretch induces robust expression of TGF-β1, activation of tubular apoptosis, and induction of nuclear factor-κB signaling, which contribute to the inflammatory and fibrotic milieu.[285,288] Because fibrosis is absent in mast cell–deficient mice with UUO, this suggests that mast cells play an important role in induction of the inflammation and development of tubulointerstitial fibrosis in obstruction.[289] Furthermore, the importance of the renin–angiotensin system for the development fibrosis was also underscored by the observation that mast cells release renin possibly stimulated by autocrine histamine release.[289] Interaction between DNA repair and parenchymal inflammation of the kidney may also play an important role for regulating fibrosis development during ureter obstruction. Apurinic/apyrimidinic endonuclease (APE1) is a multifunctional protein with important functions in genome maintenance and the regulation of multiple transcription factors. The base excision repair pathway is the major pathway for repairing oxidative DNA base lesions. These lesions are formed when reactive oxygen species attack DNA[290] and APE1 plays a central role in base excision repair and is estimated to be responsible for more than 95% of abasic site incision activity in human cells.[291] APE1 levels were increased in almost all zones of the kidney after 7 days of unilateral ureter obstruction and the transcription regulatory activity of APE1 is involved in the regulation of the profibrotic factor connective tissue growth factor,[292] suggesting that APE1 is a protein with a potential complex role for development of tubulointerstitial fibrosis and based on dual functions: DNA repair and transcription regulation.

Thus the pathogenesis of renal fibrosis is a progressive and complicated process involving multiple molecular pathways and cellular targets including ANG II as highlighted already.[4,190] ANG II is known to stimulate production of TGF-β, which is critical for the development tubulointerstitial fibrosis.[293] This has been highlighted by the recent in vivo documentation of a relationship between ANG II and TGF-β in genetically defined mouse models of Marfan syndrome.[294] Interestingly, recent studies show that selected manifestations of Marfan syndrome reflect excessive signaling by TGF-β.[295] Moreover, systemic antagonism of TGF-β through administration of a TGF-β neutralizing antibody or treatment with losartan prevented aortic aneurysm[294] and normalized muscle architecture, repair, and function in Marfan-like fibrillin-1-deficient mice.[295] Collectively these studies propose that mast cells' release of renin and local ANG II formation in the obstructed kidney may lead to both vasoconstriction, which causes reduction in renal blood flow as well as GFR, and fibroblast and macrophage activation, which increases TGF-β levels and causes fibrosis of the kidney. Interestingly recent data suggest that mast cells also have the capacity to release chymase, a protease, which may limit development of tubulointerstitial fibrosis by decreasing infiltration of inflammatory cells and release of proinflammatory and profibrotic chemokines and cytokines.[296]

Injection of COX-2 chitosan/siRNA (small interfering RNA) nanoparticles in mice subjected to 3-day UUO diminished the obstruction-induced COX-2 expression. Likewise, macrophages in the obstructed kidney had reduced COX-2 immunoreactivity, and histological examination showed lesser tubular damage in COX-2 siRNA-treated ureter-obstructed mice.[297] Parenchymal inflammation, assessed by TNF-α and interleukin-6 (IL-6) mRNA expression, was attenuated by COX-2 siRNA. Furthermore, treatment with COX-2 siRNA reduced heme oxygenase-1 and cleaved caspase-3 in mice with ureter obstruction, indicating lesser oxidative stress and apoptosis. Thus treatment with chitosan/siRNA nanoparticles to knock down COX-2 accumulated in macrophages demonstrates a novel strategy to prevent ureter obstruction–induced kidney damage.

Several studies have shown that antagonism of ANG II, TGF-β, TNF, or factors that attract inflammatory cells may ameliorate postobstructive renal damage.[273,278–282,298–300] Similarly, augmentation of expression of factors that favor epithelial growth and differentiation, such as hepatocyte growth factor,[301] insulin-like growth factor, or BMP-7,[273] may also have a protective effect.

From multiple studies, it has been suggested that the main mechanism that is responsible for the onset of the pathophysiological cascades is the increased pressure in the renal pelvis, which leads to increased pressure in the parenchyma, and subsequently mechanical stress, which leads to activation of stretch and swelling-activated cation channels within focal adhesions of the epithelial cells causing subsequent influx of $Ca^{2+}$.[287,288] This causes oxidative stress and stimulates migration of macrophages to the obstructed kidney. However, the complexity of the process and the experience from multiple studies demonstrating that there is no single pathway responsible for the cellular changes were highlighted by the potential role of infiltrating macrophages in the pathophysiology of inflammation during UUO. It was demonstrated that activation of $AT_1R$ on macrophages in UUO is prerequisite for suppression of their release of the proinflammatory cytokine IL-1.[302] This indicates that a key role of $AT_1R$ on macrophages is to protect the kidney from fibrosis by limiting activation of IL-1 receptors in the obstructed kidney. Further, this finding may show implications for the design of novel potent therapies to overcome the shortcomings of global angiotensin receptor blockade. Thus the process leading to kidney fibrosis is complex, and numerous processes contribute to regulate the cellular responses responsible for these pathophysiological changes.

Given species differences and the fact that obstruction in humans is often partial, the animal models may not predict entirely the behavior of postobstructive kidneys in humans. However, if the studies are relevant to human obstructive nephropathy, they suggest that patients undergoing release of obstruction may benefit from therapies that block proapoptotic, proinflammatory, or profibrotic mediators, or from treatments that stimulate epithelial cell growth and differentiation.[273,278–282,298–300]

Experimentally, protection from obstruction-induced detrimental effects on renal function can also be achieved by NO supplementation. This can either be accomplished by angiotensin-converting enzyme inhibition, which increases kinin levels and subsequently increases NO formation, or by stimulation of endogenous NO synthase (NOS) with L-arginine.[303] L-Arginine is a semiessential amino acid and is also substrate and the main source for generation of NO via NOS. Importantly, chronic unilateral obstruction in mice leads to significant reduction in inducible (i)NOS activity, and the obstructed kidney of iNOS knockout mice exhibited significantly more apoptotic renal tubules than controls, underscoring the important role NO plays for protecting the cellular functions in the obstructed kidney.[304] Dietary L-arginine supplementation attenuated renal damage of a 3-day UUO in rats, indicating that L-arginine treatment may be a pharmacologically useful avenue in obstructive nephropathy.[273] It was also shown that several of the detrimental effects of obstruction can also be attenuated by treatment with α-melanocyte-stimulating hormone (α-MSH), which is a potent antiinflammatory hormone, supporting the view that inflammation is a crucial determinant for the onset of renal deterioration in urinary tract obstruction.[305] Interestingly, it was recently demonstrated that recombinant human erythropoietin (rhEPO) treatment inhibits the progression of renal fibrosis in the obstructed kidney and attenuates the TGF-β1-induced EMT, suggesting that the renoprotective effects of rhEPO could be mediated, at least partly, by inhibition of TGF-β1–induced EMT.[306]

During renal fibrosis, myofibroblasts accumulate in the interstitium of the kidney, leading to deposition of extracellular matrix and organ dysfunction, and EMT may play an important role in this. It was shown that the reactivation of *Snai1* (encoding snail family zinc finger 1, known as Snail1) in mouse renal epithelial cells is required for the development of fibrosis in the kidney. Damage-mediated Snail1 reactivation induces a partial EMT in tubular epithelial cells that, without directly contributing to the myofibroblast population, relays signals to the interstitium to promote myofibroblast differentiation and fibrogenesis and to sustain inflammation.[307] Importantly, it was shown that Snail1-induced fibrosis can be reversed in vivo and that obstructive nephropathy can be therapeutically ameliorated in mice by targeting Snail1 expression. These results reconcile conflicting data on the role of the EMT in renal fibrosis and provide avenues for the design of novel antifibrotic therapies.[307] The immune infiltrate in mouse kidneys with fibrotic obstructive nephropathy was recently characterized and demonstrated that lymphocytes and macrophages were the most abundant immune cells present in the fibrotic kidneys.[308] Interestingly, preventing tubular epithelial cells from undergoing EMT also decreased immune infiltration, suggesting that crosstalk between tubular epithelial cells and immune cells is of fundamental importance in sustaining inflammation and fibrosis.

Several other therapeutic avenues for direct targeting of specific pathways involved in the fibrotic process of obstructive nephropathy have been demonstrated. Apoptosis signal-regulating kinase 1 (ASK1) acts as an upstream regulator for the activation of p38 mitogen-activated protein kinase (MAPK) and c-Jun N-terminal kinase (JNK) in kidney disease. Mice lacking the Ask1 gene are healthy with normal homeostatic functions and are protected from renal interstitial fibrosis induced by ureteric obstruction.[309] Thus the future may show therapeutic potential for ASK1 inhibitors to treat renal interstitial fibrosis.

## FETAL URINARY TRACT OBSTRUCTION

Obstructive uropathy comprises the largest fraction of identifiable causes of renal insufficiency and renal failure in infants and children. Compared with adult obstructive nephropathy, fetal obstructive nephropathy is particularly devastating because renal growth and continued nephron development are impaired by the progression of fibrosis. Several studies have examined aspects of obstructive nephropathy in the newborn using a neonatal rat model of unilateral obstruction and the pathophysiology involved in fetal urinary tract obstruction will be discussed in Chapter 72. Briefly, fetal urinary obstruction may lead to changes in tissue differentiation. At the time of birth, the rodent kidney is not fully developed and is representative of human renal development at about the mid-trimester. Animal models reveal that fetal obstruction causes aberrations of morphogenesis, gene expression, cell turnover, and urine composition.[310,311] The earlier the kidney is obstructed in utero, the greater will be the changes in renal tissue.[310,311] After birth, obstruction may affect renal growth, especially in neonates and during the first year of life, but the obstruction will not cause tissue dedifferentiation.

Studies have demonstrated the upregulation of the renin–angiotensin system, as well as involvement of other substrates (TGF-β1, endothelin-1, and many other mediators) in obstructed kidneys.[310–313] The exact mechanisms of action of these molecules in the alteration of renal morphogenesis are not fully understood. It is not well known either if obstruction alone is enough to induce renal dysplasia[310,311] or if the latter results from secondary obstruction-induced mesenchymal disruption. To know the exact role of obstruction in the kidney malformation is very important clinically, because, as mentioned earlier, it is now possible to detect and potentially relieve obstruction in utero. The critical role of $AT_2R$ in the process of ureteric bud in kidney development has been highlighted.[314] In this regard polymorphisms in the $AT_2R$ gene have been shown to be associated with UPJ obstruction.[315] If urinary obstruction is not the cause of subsequent renal impairment, then some may argue whether it is worthwhile to relieve the obstruction in utero. However, in experimental models, obstruction in utero can cause pulmonary hyperplasia and renal impairment directly or indirectly, leading to significant morbidity and mortality.[310,311,316] In addition, shunting of urinary outflow from obstructed kidneys in animals before the end of nephrogenesis may allow reversal of the arrest of glomerulogenesis seen in this setting,[317] favoring early intervention.[316–319] The changes in renal gene expression and protein production afford many potential biomarkers of disease progression and targets for therapeutic manipulation.[320]

## TREATMENT OF URINARY TRACT OBSTRUCTION AND RECOVERY OF RENAL FUNCTION

Once the presence of obstruction is established, intervention is usually strongly indicated to relieve it. The type of intervention depends on the location of the obstruction, its degree, and its etiology, as well as the presence or absence of concomitant diseases and complications and the general condition of the patient.[321] As detailed later, treatment options for obstruction include a wide spectrum of approaches, from active surveillance or minimally invasive endourologic techniques to open, laparoscopic, or robotic pyeloplasty. The main goal of therapy is to relieve symptoms and maintain or improve renal function, but it remains difficult to define treatment success after therapy. The initial emphasis focuses on prompt relief of the obstruction, followed by the definitive treatment of its cause. Obstruction below the bladder (e.g., benign prostatic hyperplasia or urethral stricture) is easily relieved with placement of a urethral catheter. If the urethra is impassable, suprapubic cystostomy may be needed. For obstruction above the bladder, insertion of a nephrostomy tube or ureteral stent may be indicated. The urgency of the intervention depends on the degree of renal function, the presence or absence of infection, and the overall risk of the procedure.[310] The presence of the infection in an obstructed urinary tract, or urosepsis, represents a urologic emergency that requires immediate relief of the obstruction, in addition to antibiotic treatment. Acute kidney injury, associated with bilateral ureteral obstruction or with the obstruction of single functioning kidney, also calls for emergent intervention.

Calculi, the most common form of acute unilateral urinary obstruction, can usually be managed conservatively with analgesics for control of pain and intravenous fluids to increase urine flow. Approximately 90% of stones smaller than 5 mm pass spontaneously, but as they get larger, spontaneous stone passage becomes progressively less probable. Active efforts to fragment or remove the stone are indicated for persistent obstruction, uncontrollable pain, or urinary tract infection. Current possibilities for treatment include extracorporeal shock wave lithotripsy (which may require ureteral stent placement if the patient is symptomatic),[322] ureteroscopy with stone fragmentation (usually with laser lithotripsy), and, in rare cases, open excision of the stone.[172,173,323] In general, a combination of lithotripsy and endourological procedures will succeed in removing the stone. In the past, complex stones high up in the ureter or in the renal pelvis have been difficult to remove without open surgery. However, improved methods of lithotripsy, including the use of laser lithotripsy through the ureteroscope, have made more stones amenable to fragmentation, while miniaturization of flexible ureteroscopes has made the entire upper urinary tract accessible in nearly all patients, except those with severe anatomic abnormalities.[172,173] Once the stone has been removed, of course, appropriate medical therapy is needed to prevent recurrence.[173]

Intramural or extrinsic ureteral obstruction may be relieved by placement of a ureteral stent through the cystoscope.[322] If this cannot be accomplished or is ineffective (especially in cases of extrinsic ureteral compression by tumor), then nephrostomy tubes will need to be inserted to effect prompt relief of the obstruction.[322]

For infravesical obstruction due to benign prostatic hyperplasia, surgery can be safely delayed or completely avoided in patients with minimal symptoms, lack of infection, and an anatomically normal upper urinary tract.[324] If needed, transurethral resection of the prostate, laser ablation, or other techniques can be used for definitive treatment. Internal urethrotomy with direct visualization may be effective in the treatment of urethral strictures, as dilation usually has only temporary effect. Suprapubic cystostomy may be necessary in patients with impassable urethral strictures, followed by open urethroplasty to restore urinary tract continuity, when possible.

Patients with neurogenic bladder require a variety of approaches, including frequent voiding, often by external compression or Credé method, medications to stimulate bladder activity or relax the urethral sphincter, and intermittent catheterization using meticulous techniques to avoid infection.[44,325] Long-term indwelling bladder catheters should be avoided because they increase the risk of infection and renal damage. If more conservative measures such as frequent voiding or intermittent catheterization are not effective, ileovesicostomy or other forms of urinary diversion should be considered. Electrical stimulation has also been attempted with varying success.[326]

In many forms of obstruction, initial stabilization of the patient's condition is followed by a decision as to whether to continue observation or to move on to definitive surgery or nephrectomy. The actual course chosen depends on the likelihood that renal function will improve with the relief of obstruction. Factors that help decide whether to operate and what form of surgical intervention to use include the age and general condition of the patient, the appearance and function of the obstructed kidney and the contralateral one, the cause of the obstruction, and the absence or presence of infection.[327] As noted earlier, the extent of recovery of renal function depends on the extent and duration of the obstruction.

Robotic surgery has evolved from simple extirpative surgery to complex reconstructions including pyeloplasty for hydronephrosis, which is feasible and safe.[328,329] Interestingly, a recent metaanalyses comparing robotic, laparoscopic, and open pyeloplasty in children showed that robotic pyeloplasty might offer shorter hospital stays, lower analgesia requirements, and lower estimated blood loss. The postoperative success rate was comparable in the two groups, but there was a significantly higher complication rate and higher costs in the robotic group.[330] A detailed discussion of the indications and surgical techniques for intervention to treat urinary tract obstruction is beyond the scope of this chapter and may be found in other sources.[321,331]

## ESTIMATING RENAL DAMAGE AND POTENTIAL FOR RECOVERY

As noted earlier, when deciding whether to bypass or reconstruct drainage of an obstructed kidney rather than excise it, the potential for meaningful recovery of function in the affected kidney represents a critical issue. In many cases, obstruction may be partial, so that it is difficult on the basis of the history alone to predict the outcome. In addition, imaging studies that reveal both anatomy and function of the obstructed kidney predict the extent of functional recovery poorly (see earlier discussion), because the extent of anatomic distortion during obstruction correlates poorly with the extent of recovery once the obstruction is relieved.[332] Isotopic renography with a variety of isotopes can be used to examine renal function, as outlined earlier. This approach is a far more reliable indicator of potential renal function when applied well after temporary drainage of the obstructed kidney (e.g., by nephrostomy tubes) has been achieved than if it is performed while the obstruction is still present.[332] Imaging of the anatomy will provide information on the size and volume of the kidney but does not demonstrate reliable information on kidney function. All of these considerations figure into the clinical judgment as to whether attempts should be made to salvage the kidney. However, there are presently no methods available to predict reliably the functional potential recovery of an obstructed kidney.

In cases of prenatal urinary tract obstruction, clinical decision-making is complex because the risks of not intervening can be very high, as can the risks of prenatal surgery. Because fetal intervention can be associated with frequent complications and a high rate of fetal loss, subjects for intervention should be carefully chosen. Fetal renal biopsy, which demonstrated a 50% to 60% success rate, correlates well with outcome and has few maternal complications.[10,12,13,310,318] It may be used as one of the methods to determine treatment strategy. Studies demonstrate that antenatal intervention may help fetuses with the most severe forms of obstructive uropathy, otherwise usually associated with a fatal neonatal course.[10,12,13,316]

## RECOVERY OF RENAL FUNCTION AFTER PROLONGED OBSTRUCTION

In patients the potential for renal recovery depends primarily on the extent and duration of the obstruction. However, other factors, such as the presence of other illnesses and the presence or absence of urinary tract infection, play an important role as well. In dogs subjected to 40 days of ureteral ligation, release of the obstruction led to no recovery of renal function. However, recovery of renal function in humans has been documented following release of obstruction of 69 days or longer.[333,334] Because it is difficult to predict whether renal function will recover when temporary relief of obstruction has been achieved, it makes sense to measure function repeatedly with isotopic renography over time, before deciding on a definitive surgical course. Chronic bilateral obstruction, as seen in benign prostatic hyperplasia, can cause chronic renal failure, especially when the obstruction is of prolonged duration and when it is accompanied by urinary tract infections.[334,335] Progressive loss of renal function can be slowed or halted by relieving the obstruction and treating the infection.

When obstruction has been relieved and there is poor return of renal function, interstitial fibrosis and inflammation may have supervened. To ensure that there is no other process hampering recovery of renal function, renal biopsy may be indicated. As noted earlier, studies in experimental animals have implicated a variety of factors in chronic renal failure due to prolonged obstruction, including excessive production of renal vasoconstrictors such as renin and angiotensin and growth factors that may enhance fibrosis. Based on these findings, inhibitors like captopril,[322] angiotensin receptor antagonists,[312] NO supplementation,[303] α-MSH,[305] and EPO[306] have been shown experimentally to ameliorate to some degree the long-term damage to kidneys observed following prolonged obstruction.

# POSTOBSTRUCTIVE DIURESIS

Release of obstruction can lead to marked natriuresis and diuresis with the wasting of potassium, phosphate, and divalent cations. It is notable that clinically significant postobstructive diuresis usually occurs only in the setting of prior bilateral obstruction, or unilateral obstruction of a solitary functioning kidney. The mechanisms involved have been described in detail earlier and involve the combination of intrinsic damage to tubular sodium, solute, and water reabsorption, as well as the effects of volume expansion, solute (e.g., urea) accumulation, and attendant increases in natriuretic substances such as ANP. When the obstruction is unilateral and there is a functioning contralateral kidney, the volume expansion, solute accumulation, and increases in natriuretic substances do not occur, and the contralateral kidney may retain salt and water, resulting in some compensation for the natriuresis and diuresis occurring in the postobstructive kidney. Management of the patient with postobstructive diuresis focuses on avoiding severe volume depletion due to salt wasting, and other electrolyte imbalances, such as hypokalemia, hyponatremia, hypernatremia, and hypomagnesemia.

Postobstructive diuresis is usually self-limited. It usually lasts for several days to a week, but may, in rare cases, persist for months. Acute massive polyuria or prolonged postobstructive diuresis may deplete the patient of $Na^+$, $K^+$, $Cl^-$, $HCO_3^-$, and water, as well as divalent cations and phosphate. Volume or free water replacement is appropriate only when the salt and water losses result in volume depletion or a disturbance of osmolality. In many cases, excessive volume or fluid replacement prolongs the diuresis and natriuresis. Because the initial urine is isosthenuric, with an initial $Na^+$ of approximately 80 mEq/L, an appropriate starting fluid for replacement may be 0.45% saline, given at a rate somewhat slower than that of the urine output. During this period, meticulous monitoring of vital signs, volume status, urine output, serum and urine chemistry, and osmolality is imperative. This will determine the need for ongoing replacement of sodium, free water, and other electrolytes. With massive diuresis, these measurements will need to be repeated frequently, up to four times daily, with frequent adjustment of replacement fluids, as needed. With relief of uncomplicated obstruction, the kidney function usually returns to normal with adequate hormonal responses. However, some cases, especially in infants with bilateral obstructive nephropathy, have been described where the distal tubule remains refractory to aldosterone (pseudohypoaldosteronism) and the patients develop paradoxical hyperkalemia despite a returning kidney function and a falling plasma creatinine.[336] In such cases, during postobstructive diuresis, plasma potassium must be monitored carefully.

 Complete reference list available at ExpertConsult.com.

## KEY REFERENCES


2. Yarger WE. The kidney. In: Brenner BM, Rector FC, eds. *Urinary Tract Obstruction.* Philadelphia: Saunder; 1991:1768–1808.
4. Klahr S. Obstructive nephropathy. *Intern Med.* 2000;39:355–361.
9. Chevalier RL, Klahr S. Therapeutic approaches in obstructive uropathy. *Semin Nephrol.* 1998;18:652–658.
23. Ulman I, Jayanthi VR, Koff SA. The long-term followup of newborns with severe unilateral hydronephrosis initially treated nonoperatively. *J Urol.* 2000;164:1101–1105.
36. Stamatelou KK, Francis ME, Jones CA, et al. Time trends in reported prevalence of kidney stones in the United States: 1976-1994. *Kidney Int.* 2003;63:1817–1823.
43. de Groat WC, Yoshimura N. Pharmacology of the lower urinary tract. *Annu Rev Pharmacol Toxicol.* 2001;41:691–721.
44. Wein AJ. Campbell-Walsh urology. In: Wein AJ, Kavoussi LR, Novick AC, et al., eds. *Lower Urinary Tract Dysfunction in Neurologic Injury and Disease.* Philadelphia: Saunders Elsevier; 2007:2011–2045.
62. Deprest J, Marchal G, Brosens I. Obstructive uropathy secondary to endometriosis. *N Engl J Med.* 1997;337:1174–1175.
89. Chung SY, Stein RJ, Landsittel D, et al. 15-year experience with the management of extrinsic ureteral obstruction with indwelling ureteral stents. *J Urol.* 2004;172:592–595.
102. Roth JA, Diamond DA. Prenatal hydronephrosis. *Curr Opin Pediatr.* 2001;13:138–141.
108. Akcay A, Altun B, Usalan C, et al. Cyclical acute renal failure due to bilateral ureteral endometriosis. *Clin Nephrol.* 1999;52:179–182.
112. Decramer S, Wittke S, Mischak H, et al. Predicting the clinical outcome of congenital unilateral ureteropelvic junction obstruction in newborn by urinary proteome analysis. *Nat Med.* 2006;12: 398–400.
118. Shokeir AA. The diagnosis of upper urinary tract obstruction. *BJU Int.* 1999;83:893–900.
131. Grenier N, Gennisson JL, Cornelis F, et al. Renal ultrasound elastography. *Diagn Interv Imaging.* 2013;94:545–550.
140. Feldman DM, DeCambre M, Kong E, et al. Evaluation and follow-up of fetal hydronephrosis. *J Ultrasound Med.* 2001;20:1065–1069.
142. Sheth S, Fishman EK. Multi-detector row CT of the kidneys and urinary tract: techniques and applications in the diagnosis of benign diseases. *Radiographics.* 2004;24:e20.
143. Grenier N, Hauger O, Cimpean A, et al. Update of renal imaging. *Semin Nucl Med.* 2006;36:3–15.
157. Taylor A, Manatunga A, Garcia EV. Decision support systems in diuresis renography. *Semin Nucl Med.* 2008;38:67–81.
162. Grenier N, Basseau F, Ries M, et al. Functional MRI of the kidney. *Abdom Imaging.* 2003;28:164–175.
165. Prasad PV. Functional MRI of the kidney: tools for translational studies of pathophysiology of renal disease. *Am J Physiol Renal Physiol.* 2006;290:F958–F974.
179. Wright FS, Briggs JP. Feedback control of glomerular blood flow, pressure, and filtration rate. *Physiol Rev.* 1979;59:958–1006.
183. Moody TE, Vaughan ED Jr, Gillenwater JY. Relationship between renal blood flow and ureteral pressure during 18 hours of total unilateral ureteral occlusion. *Invest Urol.* 1975;13:246–251.
184. Harris RH, Yarger WE. Renal function after release of unilateral ureteral obstruction in rats. *Am J Physiol.* 1974;227:806–815.
188. Yarger WE, Aynedjian HS, Bank N. A micropuncture study of postobstructive diuresis in the rat. *J Clin Invest.* 1972;51:625–637.
190. Yarger WE, Schocken DD, Harris RH. Obstructive nephropathy in the rat: possible roles for the renin-angiotensin system, prostaglandins, and thromboxanes in postobstructive renal function. *J Clin Invest.* 1980;65:400–412.
194. Topcu SO, Pedersen M, Norregaard R, et al. Candesartan prevents long-term impairment of renal function in response to neonatal partial unilateral ureteral obstruction. *Am J Physiol Renal Physiol.* 2007;292:F736–F748.
218. Sonnenberg H, Wilson DR. The role of the medullary collecting duct in postobstructive diuresis. *J Clin Invest.* 1976;57:1564–1574.
221. Hwang SJ, Haas M, Harris HW Jr, et al. Transport defects of rabbit medullary thick ascending limb cells in obstructive nephropathy. *J Clin Invest.* 1993;91:21–28.
231. Li C, Wang W, Knepper MA, et al. Downregulation of renal aquaporins in response to unilateral ureteral obstruction. *Am J Physiol Renal Physiol.* 2003;284:F1066–F1079.
234. Zeidel ML. Hormonal regulation of inner medullary collecting duct sodium transport. *Am J Physiol.* 1993;265:F159–F173.
238. Lebowitz J, An B, Edinger RS, et al. Effect of altered Na+ entry on expression of apical and basolateral transport proteins in A6 epithelia. *Am J Physiol Renal Physiol.* 2003;285:F524–F531.
240. Norregaard R, Jensen BL, Li C, et al. COX-2 inhibition prevents downregulation of key renal water and sodium transport proteins in response to bilateral ureteral obstruction. *Am J Physiol Renal Physiol.* 2005;289:F322–F333.
247. Frokiaer J, Marples D, Knepper MA, et al. Bilateral ureteral obstruction downregulates expression of vasopressin-sensitive AQP-2 water channel in rat kidney. *Am J Physiol.* 1996;270:F657–F668.
260. Wang G, Li C, Kim SW, et al. Ureter obstruction alters expression of renal acid-base transport proteins in rat kidney. *Am J Physiol Renal Physiol.* 2008;295:F497–F506.
273. Docherty NG, O'Sullivan OE, Healy DA, et al. Evidence that inhibition of tubular cell apoptosis protects against renal damage

and development of fibrosis following ureteric obstruction. *Am J Physiol Renal Physiol.* 2006;290:F4–F13.

278. Ma LJ, Yang H, Gaspert A, et al. Transforming growth factor-beta-dependent and -independent pathways of induction of tubulointerstitial fibrosis in beta6(-/-) mice. *Am J Pathol.* 2003;163:1261–1273.
281. Misseri R, Meldrum DR, Dinarello CA, et al. TNF-alpha mediates obstruction-induced renal tubular cell apoptosis and proapoptotic signaling. *Am J Physiol Renal Physiol.* 2005;288:F406–F411.
286. Broadbelt NV, Stahl PJ, Chen J, et al. Early upregulation of iNOS mRNA expression and increase in NO metabolites in pressurized renal epithelial cells. *Am J Physiol Renal Physiol.* 2007;293:F1877–F1888.
288. Quinlan MR, Docherty NG, Watson RW, et al. Exploring mechanisms involved in renal tubular sensing of mechanical stretch following ureteric obstruction. *Am J Physiol Renal Physiol.* 2008;295:F1–F11.
289. Veerappan A, Reid AC, O'Connor N, et al. Mast cells are required for the development of renal fibrosis in the rodent unilateral ureteral obstruction model. *Am J Physiol Renal Physiol.* 2012;302:F192–F204.
295. Cohn RD, van Erp C, Habashi JP, et al. Angiotensin II type 1 receptor blockade attenuates TGF-beta induced failure of muscle regeneration in multiple myopathic states. *Nat Med.* 2007;13:204–210.
300. Anders HJ, Vielhauer V, Frink M, et al. A chemokine receptor CCR-1 antagonist reduces renal fibrosis after unilateral ureter ligation. *J Clin Invest.* 2002;109:251–259.
302. Zhang JD, Patel MB, Griffiths R, et al. Type 1 angiotensin receptors on macrophages ameliorate IL-1 receptor-mediated kidney fibrosis. *J Clin Invest.* 2014;124:2198–2203.
303. Morrissey JJ, Ishidoya S, McCracken R, et al. Nitric oxide generation ameliorates the tubulointerstitial fibrosis of obstructive nephropathy. *J Am Soc Nephrol.* 1996;7:2202–2212.
306. Park SH, Choi MJ, Song IK, et al. Erythropoietin decreases renal fibrosis in mice with ureteral obstruction: role of inhibiting TGF-beta-induced epithelial-to-mesenchymal transition. *J Am Soc Nephrol.* 2007;18:1497–1507.
307. Grande MT, Sanchez-Laorden B, Lopez-Blau C, et al. Snail1-induced partial epithelial-to-mesenchymal transition drives renal fibrosis in mice and can be targeted to reverse established disease. *Nat Med.* 2015;21:989–997.
311. Chevalier RL. Pathogenesis of renal injury in obstructive uropathy. *Curr Opin Pediatr.* 2006;18:153–160.
317. Edouga D, Hugueny B, Gasser B, et al. Recovery after relief of fetal urinary obstruction: morphological, functional and molecular aspects. *Am J Physiol Renal Physiol.* 2001;281:F26–F37.
320. Chevalier RL. Obstructive nephropathy: towards biomarker discovery and gene therapy. *Nat Clin Pract Nephrol.* 2006;2:157–168.

# Urolithiasis

# 38

Khashayar Sakhaee | Orson W. Moe

CHAPTER OUTLINE



## INTRODUCTION

Urolithiasis (nephrolithiasis, kidney stone disease) is the abnormal formation and retention of solid phase inorganic and organic concretions in the lumen of the urinary tract. Kidney stone is not a diagnosis per se but the common manifestation of a variety of underlying causative and pathophysiologic factors. Although stones are localized to the urinary tract, urolithiasis is a systemic disease. Although the surgical treatment of urolithiasis has advanced over the years, the management extends beyond the mere removal of existent stones. The need to understand how stones form is of critical importance so that they can be prevented from recurring, which is a most important objective. Overall, the metabolic evaluation of urolithiasis is still not performed with enough frequency and depth in our opinion. In addition to the potential for uncovering treatable underlying diagnoses, the pathophysiologic definition of kidney stones also guides the selection and helps the monitoring of therapy.

## EPIDEMIOLOGY

### GENERAL POINTS

#### KIDNEY STONES IN ADULTS: 1976–1994

The prevalence of kidney stones has increased steadily over 4 decades,[1,2] which is associated with a rise in both direct and indirect expenditures for this condition in the United States.[3] The estimated economic burden in the United States for kidney stone disease management is estimated to be $4.7 billion by 2030.[4] This is in part because it is estimated that more than 44% of adults are expected to be obese in the United States by 2030.[4] In 1994, data from the US National Health Examination Survey III showed a rise in the prevalence of self-reported history of kidney stones compared with the period 1976 to 1980 (from 3.8% to 5.2%). The increase was greater in females than males and higher in the aging population.[1] African-Americans had a lower risk of urolithiasis compared with whites and Mexican Americans. Age-adjusted prevalence was higher in southern parts of the United States.[1] This is consistent with cross-sectional studies showing a higher prevalence of kidney stones in Southeastern parts of the United States.[3,5]

Previous studies explored the model that environmental factors and systemic conditions, including quality of the water supply,[6] climate,[7] animal protein intake, and association with hypertension[8] may be important in increasing the risk of kidney stone disease, in addition to geographic distribution. The contribution of mineral content and the quality of the water to the prevalence of kidney stones and its geographic distribution was questioned by a study in three Midwest regions of the United States, which showed no correlation between water calcium content and the prevalence of kidney stone disease[9]; the role of other minerals were not addressed. Prevalence data from 1988 to 1994 was not able to identify dietary factors that could explain the geographic variation in the prevalence of kidney stone diseases.[1] The lack of association between diet and kidney stone prevalence may be because of the cross-sectional nature of the studies and lack of temporal association between stone disease and time of the data collection.

#### KIDNEY STONES IN ADULTS: 2007 TO 2010

A more recent National Health and Nutritional Examination Survey (NHANES) cross-sectional study from 2007 to 2010 of 12,110 subjects with a self-reported history[2] has demonstrated a marked increase in the prevalence at 8.8%, compared with the aforementioned 1994 survey with a prevalence of 5.2%. The latest estimate shows that 1 in 11 individuals in the United States has a history of kidney stones, in contrast to a previous figure of 1 in 20 U.S. citizens.[1] The overall prevalence was 10.6% in male subjects and 7.1% in females compared with the previous study,[1] which showed 6.3% in men and 4.1% in women[2] (Fig. 38.1).

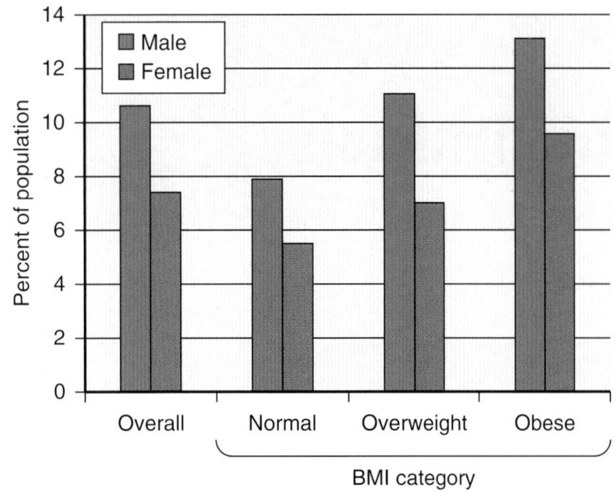


**Fig. 38.1** Prevalence of urolithiasis plotted as a function of gender and body mass index *(BMI).* (Modified from Scales CD Jr, Smith AC, Hanley JM, Saigal CS. Urologic diseases in America. Prevalence of kidney stones in the United States. *Eur Urol.* 2012;62[1]:160–165.)

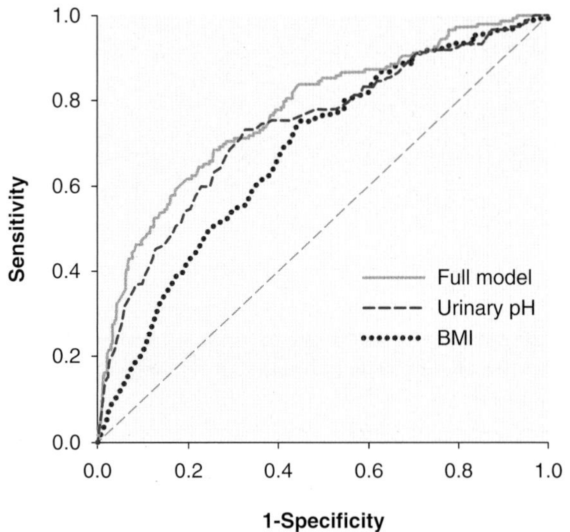


| Model | AUC | 95% Confidence interval |
|---|---|---|
| **Full model** | **0.77** | **0.73–0.82** |
| **Urinary pH** | **0.74** | **0.68–0.78** |
| **BMI** | **0.68** | **0.64–0.72** |
| Age* | 0.65 | 0.61–0.70 |
| Time periods* | 0.57 | 0.52–0.61 |
| Gender* | 0.55 | 0.51–0.58 |
| Creatinine clearance* | 0.54 | 0.49–0.59 |

**Fig. 38.2** Receiving operating characteristic curve and area under the curve *(AUC)* for clinical predictors of uric acid stone formation. The full multivariable model included urinary pH, body mass index *(BMI),* time period, gender, and creatinine clearance. Urinary pH and BMI were determined by univariable analysis; *asterisks* indicate variables that are not shown. (Modified from Xu LHR, Adams-Huet B, Poindexter JR, et al. Temporal changes in kidney stone composition and in risk factors predisposing to stone formation. *J Urol.* 2017;197[6]:1465–1471.)

Aside from gender, race, age, ethnicity, and socioeconomic class, conditions associated with the metabolic syndrome are predictive of kidney stone disease.[2] Again, the likelihood of kidney stones was lower among black and Hispanic than white populations. Furthermore, obesity, diabetes, gout, and household income of $19,999 or less were more likely to be associated with kidney stone disease. The association between features of the metabolic syndrome, such as obesity and diabetes, and prevalence of kidney stone disease is consistent with a prospective study showing that the risk of incident kidney stone disease increases with obesity and weight gain.[10,11] A multivariate Cox regression model showed that obesity is the only strong predictor of stone recurrence in first-time stone formers.[12]

Using pooled data from 1965 to 2005 from seven countries, Romero and associates have shown a continuous increase in prevalence throughout the decades, with similar gender and age distribution profiles across countries within each time period.[13] In general, the prevalence of kidney stone disease in adults is higher in the Western Hemisphere.[14] However, the highest kidney stone prevalence was in Saudi Arabia.[14] As discussed, factors such as the rise in prevalence in metabolic syndrome and dietary changes have been suggested to underlie this rise. Brikowski and coworkers[15] took a different and interesting approach using global warming trends and modeled the northward expansion of the U.S. "stone belt" in the coming decades, which predicts a dramatic increase in stone prevalence in the northern United States. In one recent cross-sectional study of 63,994 patients who had kidney stone–related procedures in California from 2010 to 2012, the authors described the association between higher precipitation and temperature and an increased rate for kidney stone intervention.[16] The authors concluded a larger trend in kidney stone prevalence with a warm wet climate than a warm arid climate.

Despite the increased global prevalence of kidney stones in recent decades, the association between changes in kidney stone composition, demographic characteristics, and biochemical profiles has not been fully explored. In one retrospective study of 1516 patients over 35 years with calcium or uric acid stones, the proportion of uric acid stones increased from 7% to 14%.[17] The proportion of females with kidney stones also increased over time, but the increase in the female gender was more significant among calcium stone formers. Both age and body mass index (BMI) increased with time in both uric acid and calcium stone formers; however, uric acid stone formers were consistently older and had a higher BMI and lower urinary pH than calcium stone formers. Urinary pH, phosphorus oxalate, and sodium increased with time in calcium stone formers, but remained unchanged in uric acid stone formers. The most significant denominators for discriminating uric acid versus calcium stone was urinary pH[17] (Fig. 38.2). This study was corroborated with another cross-sectional retrospective study performed in the United Kingdom in 2132 patients with kidney stone stratified to normal weight, overweight, and obese.[18] In this study, both obese and overweight kidney stone formers had a greater risk, principally because of an increase in urinary promoters, including calcium, sodium, uric acid and lower urinary pH, but without any change urinary inhibitors of kidney stone formation, such as citrate and magnesium.[18] Furthermore, the higher incidence of uric acid but not calcium stones was demonstrated in overweight kidney stone formers.

## CALCIUM STONES

### PREVALENCE OF CALCIUM STONES

In one study, kidney stone composition was evaluated using data from the National Veterans Administration Crystal Identification Center.[19] A comparison with a previous study showed an increased percentage occurrence of calcium oxalate and brushite stones between 1996 and 2003. Furthermore, with each recurrent stone event, there was an increased percentage occurrence of calcium phosphate stones accompanied by a decrease in occurrence of calcium oxalate stones (Fig. 38.3).[19] The underlying factors for the change in composition are not known. A retrospective evaluation of 1201 stone formers in the past 3 decades has shown that over time, an increased incidence of calcium phosphate stones coincides with increased urinary pH and the number of shockwave lithotripsy treatments.[20] Causality between stone risk and lithotripsy and urinary pH still remains to be determined. A study from France has shown an increased prevalence of calcium phosphate stone in men versus women from 1980 to 2004, from 9.4% to 26.6%,[21] and the increase was associated with a gradual rise in BMI during this period.[21]

### CALCIUM INTAKE

Several large studies have explored the association between dietary factors and the risk of kidney stone disease. The role of dietary calcium as a risk factor was assessed in a few prospective observational studies showing that low dietary calcium intake is associated with a higher risk of kidney stones in women and young men.[22–25] On the contrary, calcium supplementation was associated with a higher risk of kidney stones solely in older women.[24,26] The epidemiologic association of low dietary calcium with nephrolithiasis is consistent with the findings of a randomized controlled study in hypercalciuric men with calcium nephrolithiasis.[27] This study will be discussed later.

### VITAMIN D INTAKE

Vitamin D deficiency is endemic worldwide, influencing approximately 1 billion people.[28,29] Vitamin D deficiency is highly prevalent in kidney stone formers, of which 20% are hypercalciuric.[30,31] Thus, clinicians are reluctant to treat vitamin D deficiency in kidney stone formers because of the concern with increased kidney stone risk. The studies addressing the relationship between vitamin D supplementation and hypercalciuria are limited and contradictory.[32–37] The controversy arose in part as a result of the small sample size of the retrospective studies, nonadherence to the vitamin D supplement, and dietary indiscretion of salt and calcium intake. However, given these shortcomings, and in the absence of prospective control trials, the consensus is that among kidney stone formers with vitamin D deficiency, a short course of vitamin D repletion does not increase urinary calcium excretion, except in the subset of hypercalciuric patients.[31,35] Thus, vitamin D repletion should not be avoided in the kidney stone population, but urinary calcium excretion should be assessed during the repletion period.

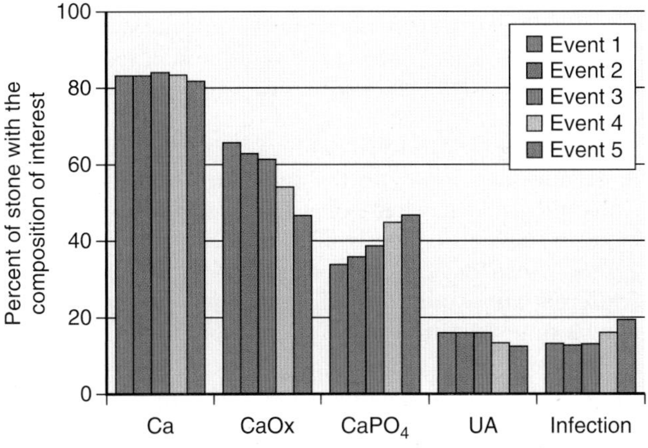


**Fig. 38.3** Percentage occurrence of stone types. Calcium *(Ca),* calcium oxalate *(CaOx),* calcium phosphate *($CaPO_4$),* uric acid *(UA),* and infection stones as function of event; that is, ranging from the first to the fifth stone. (Modified from Mandel N, Mandel I, Fryjoff K, et al. Conversion of calcium oxalate to calcium phosphate with recurrent stone episodes. *J Urol.* 2003;169[6]:2026–2029.)

### OXALATE INTAKE

One epidemiologic study using a food frequency questionnaire in men, older women, and younger women has shown that oxalate intake does not correlate with kidney stone disease.[38] One has to exercise caution in drawing conclusions about such negative studies, given the limitations of questionnaires, the heterogeneity of cause among the stone formers, and the magnitude of the effect of dietary oxalate.

### PROTEIN CONSUMPTION

Epidemiologic studies have demonstrated a positive relationship between animal protein consumption and kidney stone formation in men, but not as much in women.[22,24,26] However, in a randomized controlled trial (RCT), consumption of a low–animal protein and high-fiber diet was not shown to reduce the relative risk of recurrent kidney stones in calcium oxalate stone formers compared with those instructed to maintain a high fluid intake.[39] Nonetheless, the pathophysiologic basis and metabolic studies supporting the relationship between dietary protein and stone risk is very solid, and one interventional study, where multiple variables, including dietary protein were manipulated, showed benefits from protein restriction.[27]

## URIC ACID STONES

### PREVALENCE OF URIC ACID STONES

There are regional differences in uric acid stone prevalence. The highest prevalences are reported in the Middle East and a few European countries,[40–42] whereas uric acid stones comprise only 8% to 10% of all kidney stones in the United States.[43] In the United States, uric acid stones among Chinese and Japanese descendants have been reported to be slightly higher than in the general population at approximately 15% to 16%.[44] The highest prevalence of uric acid stones and gouty arthritis has been demonstrated in the Hmong population of East Asian and Southeast Asian heritage living in Minnesota.[44,45] The factors underlying these differences are not known. The high prevalence of uric acid stones in the Hmong population is unique, given that a low prevalence of reported uric acid stones is reported in Northeastern Thailand, which is geographically adjacent to Laos, from which the Hmong population originated.[46]

### GENETIC AND DIETARY FACTORS

The underlying causes for the global differences in uric acid stone prevalence remain unknown. However, a high prevalence of obesity, diabetes, and hypertension is commonly associated with uric acid nephrolithiasis in Western societies[47–49] and has also been shown to be present in Hmong populations born in the United States. Therefore, it is likely that an interplay between genetic factors and diet have an impact on uric acid stone formation. Among stone formers in the United States and Europe, uric acid stones occur more frequently in subjects with type 2 diabetes mellitus (T2DM) and obesity than in nonobese, nondiabetic stone formers (Fig. 38.4).[48–52]

### DATA ON STONE INCIDENCE

Compared with prevalence, precise knowledge of kidney stone incidence among adult and pediatric populations is limited. In adult populations, one small study from Minnesota has shown an incidence rate of 101.8/100,000 patients per year.[53] Two studies using a questionnaire found an overall incidence rate among adult males and females of 306 and 95/100,000 person-years, respectively.[22,26]

One study from South Carolina used data from pediatric emergency visits and deduced that the incidence of nephrolithiasis increased from 7.9 to 18.5/100,000 children (≤18 years of age) in a little over a decade.[54] It has been suggested that childhood obesity may play a key role in the rising kidney stone incidence of children in recent years. However, larger U.S. epidemiologic studies do not support this notion.[55]

Dietary factors, including increased sodium consumption[56] and decreased calcium intake[57] from milk, which has been substituted by sugar drinks,[58,59] have also been implicated to have a pathophysiologic role in the development of kidney stones in the pediatric population. Children are also consuming less water than in the past.[60] Data from Asia and Europe have also shown incidence rates consistent with those of pediatric populations in South Carolina.[61,62] Like adults, calcium-containing stones are the most predominant kidney stones in pediatric populations.[63,64] On the contrary, uric acid stones are less common, comprising only 2% to 3% of stones in this population.[65]

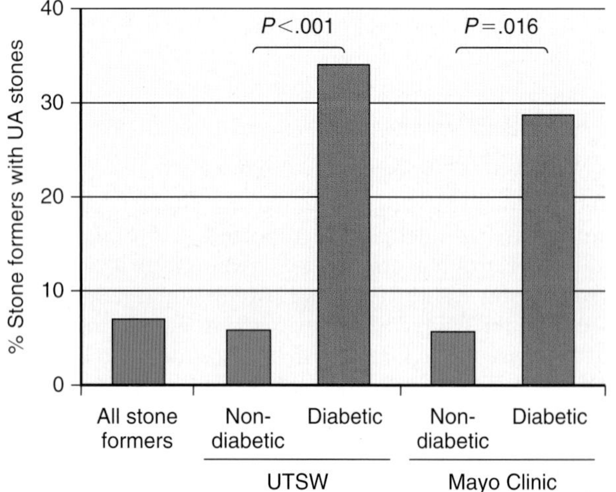


**Fig. 38.4** Prevalence of uric acid urolithiasis in the kidney stone population. *Mayo,* Mayo Clinic; *UA,* uric acid; *UTSW,* University of Texas Southwestern Medical Center. (From Lieske JC, de la Vega LS, Gettman MT, et al. Diabetes mellitus and the risk of urinary tract stones: a population-based case-control study. *Am J Kidney Dis.* 2006;48[6]: 897–904.)

## HISTOPATHOLOGY

Although urinary biochemical stone risk factors can be studied in rodents, the histopathology of urolithiasis that genuinely resembles human disease, involving both urinary and epithelial factors, is rather unusual in rodents.[66] The main source of human histopathologic data has been from clinical surgical samples. In addition to urinary factors such as solutes that comprise the chemical components of stones, known inhibitors and promoters, there are epithelial factors that initiate and promote crystal adhesion, growth, and agglomeration.[67] This field was advanced significantly by the work of Borofsky and Evan and colleagues, who used human samples from intraoperative biopsies and provided histologic descriptions that enable the formulation of pathogenic models of stone formation.[68,69]

### RANDALL'S PLAQUE

In the 1930s, Randall examined the papilla of over 1000 pairs of cadaveric kidneys and observed a cream-colored area near the papillae in one of five kidneys. These plaques are mainly interstitial rather than luminal in locale and are associated with interstitial collagen and tubular basement membranes; they are composed of calcium, nitrogen, carbon dioxide, and phosphorus.[70] More advanced lesions intrude into tubular lumens. What differentiates these plaques from more normal variants was the finding of small stones attached to some (not all) of the plaques, projecting into the renal pelvis in more than 60 kidneys. Randall concluded that the attached stones were growing from the interstitial calcium plaque, rather than directly from the normal epithelium.[70] There was no clinical information on Randall's subjects but there is a reasonable chance that they were calcium oxalate stone formers.

These observations were confirmed by many surgeons in the decades to follow, and the Indianapolis-Chicago group of investigators shed light on the importance of Randall's plaques. The pathogenesis of Randall's plaques is still an enigma, but a degenerative stress model of induction of dedifferentiation and transdifferentiation followed by pathologic biomineralization has been proposed.[71]

### IDIOPATHIC CALCIUM OXALATE STONES

Plaques form in the papillary tip in the basement membrane of the thin loop of Henle, with mineral and organic layers alternating in a concentric configuration (Fig. 38.5). Evan and coworkers have proposed that this is the final form of plaque composed of fused particles in close association with type 1 collagen, with the mineral phase covered by organic

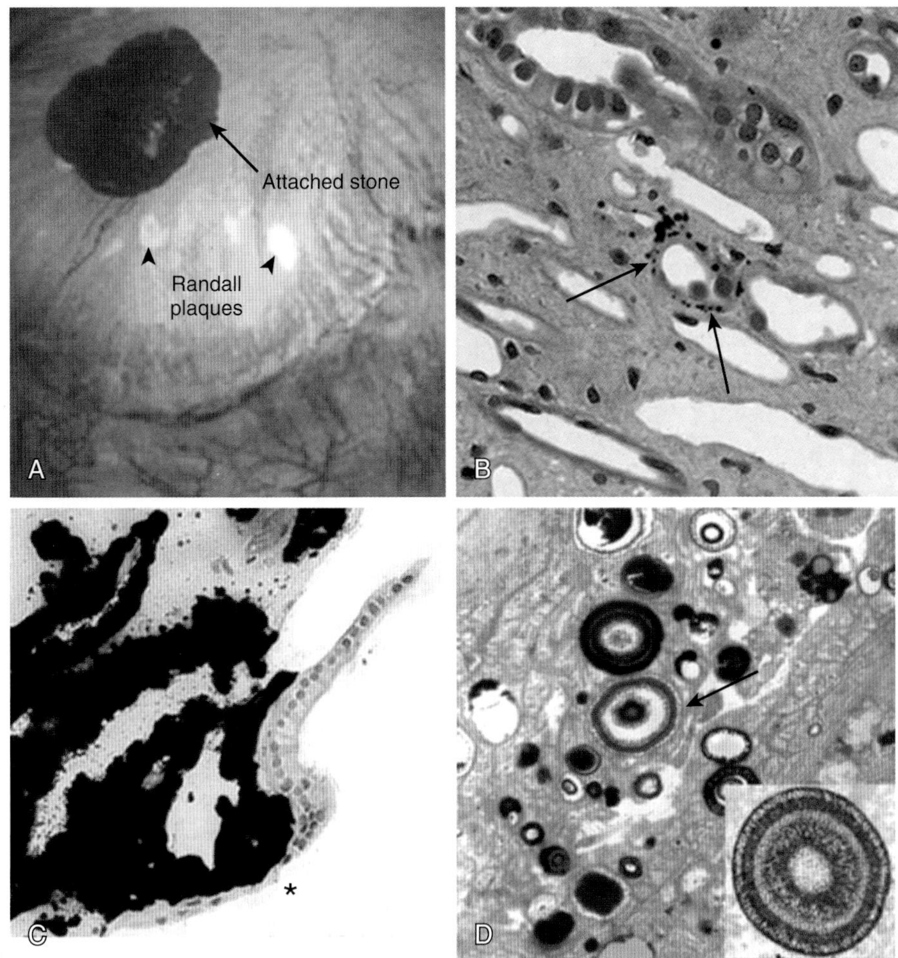


**Fig. 38.5** Histopathology of Randall's plaques in calcium oxalate stone formers. (A) View during endoscopic surgery. One plaque (not visible) has an overlying attached calcium oxalate stone *(arrow)*. Two Randall's plaques without stones are below *(arrowheads)*. (B) Light microscopic image of the locale of the initial crystal deposits in the basement membrane of the thin loops of Henle *(arrows)*. (C) Calcium phosphate (stained *black*) showing a more advanced lesion filling the interstitial space and extending *(*)*, eventually protruding into the urinary space and corresponding to the cream-colored plaques in A. (D) The individual deposits *(arrow)* assume the morphology of multilaminated spheres of alternating layers of electron-lucent inorganic crystal and electron-dense matrix *(inset)*. (From Evan AP, Lingeman JE, Coe FL, et al. Randall's plaque of patients with nephrolithiasis begins in basement membranes of thin loops of Henle. *J Clin Invest.* 2003;111[5]:607–616.)

matrix.[72] In the absence of longitudinal biopsies, extrapolation from cross-sectional data has indicated that the particles move from the tubular basement membrane into the surrounding interstitium.

En bloc examination of stones with attached tissue[73] show loss of epithelial cells at the attachment site and that the plaque is exposed to the urinary lumen. On contact with urine, the plaque is overlaid with new matrix, and new crystals and matrix form in sequential waves. Osteoprotegerin is present in the stone and plaque, and Tamm-Horsfall protein, known to be restricted to the urine and cells of the thick ascending limb, is present only on the urine space side of the interface.[73] Coe and associates have proposed that the organic material overlaying the exposed plaque comes from urine molecules adsorbed initially onto the matrix of plaque. As new crystals nucleate in this urine matrix, the crystals themselves attract molecules with affinity for them, thereby perpetuating stone formation.[74]

## CALCIUM PHOSPHATE STONES AND STONES IN RENAL TUBULAR ACIDOSIS

Although Randall's plaques are observed in calcium phosphate (CaP) stone formers, they are fewer in number compared with calcium oxalate stone formers. CaP stone formers have apatite deposits in the lumen ducts of Bellini and inner medullary collecting ducts associated with massive ductal dilation[75] (Fig. 38.6). The dilated ducts seem to have lost epithelial cells and are surrounded by interstitial fibrotic tissue. The abundance of CaP crystals is correlated with higher urinary CaP supersaturation,[20] driven mostly by a high urine pH and, to a lesser extent, by hypocitraturia and hypercalciuria. Coe and coworkers have postulated that shock wave lithotripsy may injure the epithelium and impair local luminal acidification.[76] Interestingly, a similar pattern is observed in patients with CaP stones from primary hyperparathyroidism.[77] Luminal plugging and plaque can coexist. A scenario of

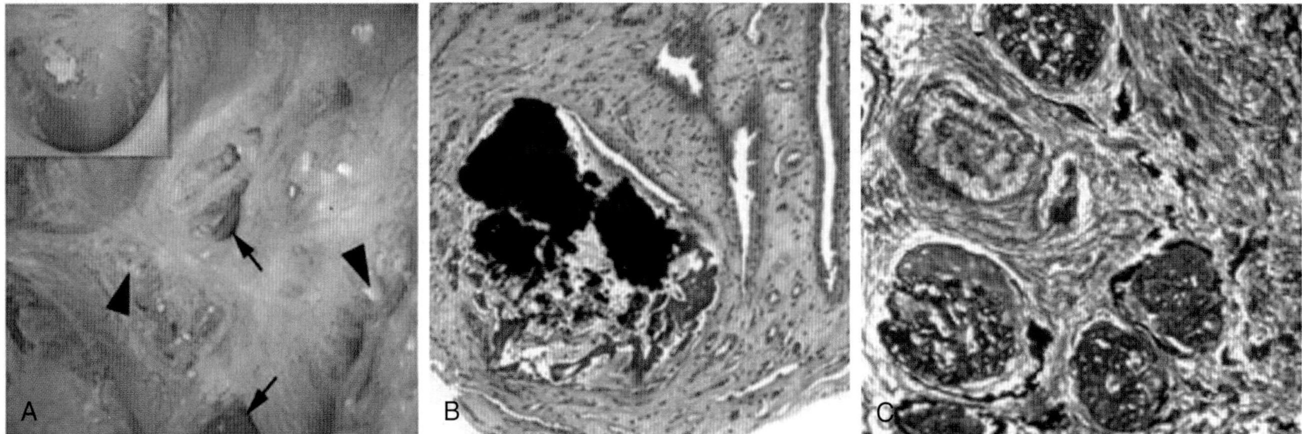


**Fig. 38.6** Histopathology of calcium phosphate stone formers. (A) View during endoscopic surgery. Depressions near the papillary tips *(arrows)* are unique to calcium phosphate stone formers, which coexist with Randall's plaques. The papillae shows yellow crystalline deposits coming out of the ducts of Bellini *(inset)*. (B) Micrograph of luminal deposits in an inner medullary collecting duct. The crystal deposits greatly expanded the lumen, and cell injury and necrosis were found. Interstitial inflammation and fibrosis surround the intraluminal crystal deposition. (C) Renal biopsy from a patient with calcium phosphate stones showing advanced glomerulosclerosis, tubular atrophy, and interstitial fibrosis. This is rarely seen in calcium oxalate stone formers. (From Evan AP, Lingeman JE, Coe FL, et al. Crystal-associated nephropathy in patients with brushite nephrolithiasis. *Kidney Int.* 2005;67[2]:576–591.)

persistently high pH is seen in CaP stone formers with distal renal tubular acidosis (dRTA) from congenital or acquired causes. Papillae show multiple dilated ducts of Bellini, with intraluminal CaP deposits. Distortion, flattening, and fibrosis are common. Atrophic remnants of nephron structures lie within the fibrotic fields of interstitium. It is plausible that the bulk bladder urine pH does not truly reflect the much higher luminal pH in damaged ducts.

## STONES IN ENTERIC HYPEROXALURIA

In patients with enteric hyperoxaluria, crystallization is mainly driven by a high urinary luminal oxalate concentration. In patients after gastric bypass surgery, the epithelium appears rather normal, but calcium oxalate crystals are lodged in the lumen.[78] In hyperoxaluric calcium oxalate stone formers from small bowel resection (e.g., as a result of Crohn disease) the inner medullary collecting ducts contain crystal deposits associated with cell injury, interstitial inflammation, and structural deformity of the papillae, tubular atrophy, and interstitial fibrosis. Interestingly, Randall's plaques are observed, similar to those seen in idiopathic calcium oxalate stone formers. The inner medullary collecting duct deposits contain apatite, with calcium oxalate in some cases.[79] The birefringent thin crystalline material scattered on the inner medullary collecting duct (IMCD) cell membranes may be the initial crystal lesion.

In summary, based mainly on histopathologic findings and aided by clinical chemistry and imaging, Coe and colleagues have postulated three morphologic pathways of stone formation.[74] First is overgrowth on interstitial apatite plaque, as seen commonly but not exclusively in idiopathic calcium oxalate stone formers; similar lesions were observed in stone formers with primary hyperparathyroidism, ileostomy, and small bowel resection and in some brushite stone formers. Second is crystal deposits in renal tubules rather than the interstitium, which was seen in all stone formers other than the idiopathic calcium oxalate stone formers. Third is free solution crystallization in the lumen, as seen in patients with cystinuria or enteric hyperoxaluria.

# PATHOPHYSIOLOGY

## PHYSICAL CHEMISTRY OF URINARY SATURATION

### GENERAL CONCEPTS

Lithogenesis involves solutes entering a solid phase in urine, among other processes. Some definitions are in order here. Using calcium oxalate as an example, equilibrium is attained when the calcium and oxalate concentrations in solution and the amount of calcium oxalate crystals bathed by that solution is constant with time. The product of the free ionized calcium and oxalate concentrations in such a solution in equilibrium is the equilibrium solubility product. However, solubility is the concentration of the calcium oxalate complex (not the individual components) in solution, which is approximately 6.2 μM. Solubility for CaP (brushite; initial phase of complex formation) is about 0.35 μM and, for uric acid, is about 520 μM. Activity refers to the portion of the ion that is chemically active (not always 100%) and is related to its chemical concentration by the activity coefficient (activity = activity coefficient × chemical concentration). States of saturation are dependent on the activities of the component ions. When free ion activity product is below the solubility product, the crystals will dissolve; this solution is undersaturated. When free ion activity product is higher than the solubility product, it is in a supersaturated state, which causes crystals to grow (Fig. 38.7).

When soluble calcium and oxalate are added to a saturated solution at equilibrium to raise the ion activity product beyond the equilibrium solubility product, there will be growth of any preformed crystals, if such were present. However, in the absence of a preexisting solid phase, no new crystals appear, despite activity products sitting above the solubility product. A solution that will cause the growth of preformed

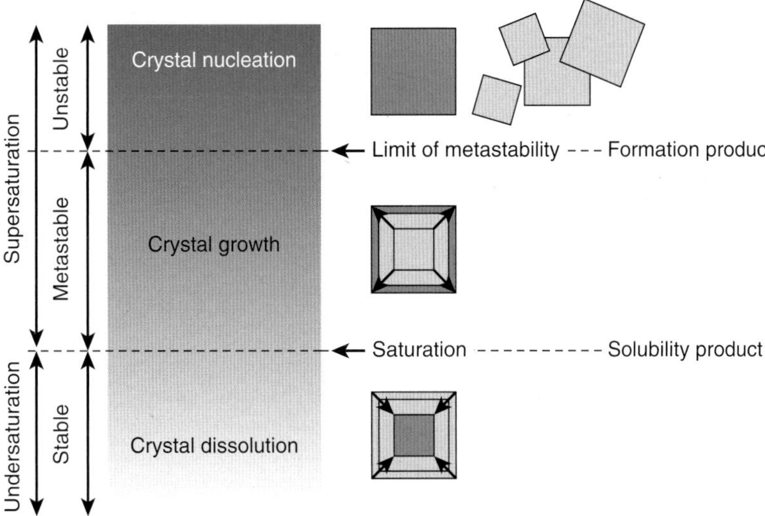


**Fig. 38.7** Physicochemical parameters used in the assessment of kidney stone risk. These are shown in relation to the three states of crystal—dissolution, growth, and nucleation.

crystals but not the appearance of a new solid phase is supersaturated and metastable. If one raises the activity product yet higher, with further calcium and oxalate addition, new crystals will appear at some point without existing crystals (see Fig. 38.7). The product of the activities of the ions has now reached the formation product, which is also called the *upper limit of metastability*. Above the formation product, a solution changes from metastable to unstable, and crystallization is inevitable. Therefore, urine may be undersaturated, metastable, or unstable with respect to calcium oxalate or CaP crystals (see Fig. 38.7).

## FACTORS INFLUENCING SATURATION

Rate of urinary excretion of the component species of the activity products (e.g., calcium, oxalate, phosphate, urate) and water (denominator) are the primary determinants of saturation. Additional factors, such as complexation and changes in urine pH, can all influence the free ion concentrations and are important in regulating saturation. Therefore,total concentration measurements may not provide full information of the actual activity product. For example, citrate readily complexes calcium, reducing the ionized calcium (activity) levels[80]; a similar relationship exists for magnesium and oxalate.[81] Changes in urine pH can drastically affect the monovalent to divalent phosphate and urate–to–uric acid ratio. For this reason, hypercalciuria, hyperoxaluria, hypocitraturia, unduly alkaline urine, and chronic dehydration all increase the risk of calcium stones, but the relationships are complex.

Thus, interpretation based solely on individual chemical concentrations can be misleading. An example is when a patient with idiopathic hypercalciuria is treated with thiazide, and the urinary calcium excretion decreases. However, a state of potassium deficiency can develop, causing secondary hypocitraturia. It is not easy for a clinician to look at the urinary calcium and citrate excretion rates and concentrations and determine whether the stone risk is reduced. Another scenario is a patient with CaP stones from distal renal tubular acidosis and profound hypocitraturia that is treated with alkali. The urinary citrate level increases but the urine pH concomitantly increases as well, so it is not easy to determine whether the risk of CaP crystallization is reduced or increased. Several methods have been designed to address these questions.

## URINE SATURATION MEASUREMENTS IN VITRO

### Upper Limits of Metastability and Formation Product

Upper limits of metastability (ULM) and formation product (FP) is an empiric entity determined in the laboratory by raising the activity product. This is done by adding ligands and noting the activity products at which solid phases begin to appear spontaneously, which is usually detected optically (see Fig. 38.7). Because this is an empiric method, it takes the concentration of the lithogenic solutes and all the inhibitors and promoters into consideration.

### Activity Product Ratio

Activity is the fraction of the total solute in free ionized form that is free to react. Crystals of interest are seeded to urine and incubated at 37°C with stirring at a constant pH until equilibrium, until the crystal mass has stabilized (neither increases nor decreases). The activity product ratio (APR) is defined as the ratio of the activity product in the original sample to that obtained after incubation and stabilization of the sample with crystals. If the crystals have grown after reaching equilibrium, the activity product will be lower than the original sample; thus the APR is less than 1, implying that the solution has high lithogenic propensity. If the crystals partially dissolved, the activity product at equilibrium is higher than the original sample and the APR is more than 1, implying that the solution is not lithogenic. Thus, the APR describes whether preexistent crystals, once formed, will grow (APR >1) or shrink (APR >1) while suspended in it.

Although the APR provides a good indication of crystal growth, it gives incomplete information about the ability of that particular urine sample to produce new crystals. In simple salt solutions, the ULM for calcium oxalate was found to occur at an APR of 8.5 by Pak and Holt[82] and at 10.0 by Robertson and associates.[83] The small difference is mainly methodologic in origin.

### Concentration Product Ratio

Activities are important chemical parameters but are difficult to ascertain definitively. Pak and colleagues have used an empiric method to measure urine saturation by comparing urine chemical concentrations (instead of activities) of the components for a given crystal to their concentrations after reaching equilibrium.[84,85] In their original assay, crystals of interest were seeded to an aliquot of urine and incubated at 37°C, with stirring at a constant pH for 2 days. At equilibrium, the crystal mass has stabilized. If the activity coefficients for calcium, oxalate, and phosphate remain stable throughout the incubation, the ratio of the concentration product at the start of incubation to the concentration product after incubation (equilibrium), must equal the APR, even though the concentration products themselves do not equal the activity products (the activity coefficients cancel out). If activity coefficients can be assumed to be stable, the empiric concentration product ratio (CPR) is a valid estimation of the APR, provided the calcium concentration is below 5.0 mM and the oxalate level is below 0.5 mM.[85] This assay has been simplified technically and was validated for the analysis of the propensity of calcium oxalate and CaP stone formation.[86–88]

## URINE SATURATION ESTIMATION IN SILICO

Physicochemical methods are informative, although empiric. An obvious drawback of physicochemical methods is the labor involved. Another option is to take clinical urine chemistry data and use a computer program to calculate urine free ion activities for calcium, oxalate, and phosphate from their measured chemical concentrations and their known tendencies to form soluble complexes with each other and with other ligands.[83,85,89]

### Relative Supersaturation Ratio

Using all the relevant association constants ($K_a$), one can calculate the free ion activity product. If one divides this by the corresponding equilibrium solubility product, one obtains the relative supersaturation ratio (RSR), which estimates the degree of saturation. An RSR above 1 connotes oversaturation and below 1, undersaturation. The validity has been confirmed by studies showing a correlation between the type of stone a patient forms and the prevailing supersaturations in two or three 24-hour urine samples, as estimated by the EQUIL2 program (a BASIC computer program for the calculation of urinary saturation).[90,91]

### Supersaturation Index

Another computer-based program, the Joint Expert Speciation System (JESS), uses the same principle as EQUIL2 but differs from it in that more thermodynamic constants are used to calculate mixed ligand speciation.[92,93] One important difference is that JESS includes the calcium phosphocitrate complex, which is soluble, and whose formation is pH-dependent. Pak and coworkers have compared the two computer-based programs to empiric physicochemical methods and found a closer approximation of JESS than EQUIL2 to physicochemical methods.[86–88] Although EQUIL2 provides relative supersaturation (RS) as a readout, JESS expresses the data as the solubility index (SI), which is calculated based on the same physicochemical principles as RS values generated by EQUIL, but the two programs use different speciation concentrations.

## URINE SATURATION IN STONE FORMERS

Pak, Robertson, Marshall, and Weber and colleagues have independently provided evidence that urine from stone formers is more supersaturated than urine from non–stone formers.[82,94–96] The results were similar, although absolute values differed for the three investigative groups, likely because of differences in methods. Stone formers have higher average values of urine saturation than normal subjects whether or not saturation is measured with respect to calcium oxalate, brushite, octocalcium phosphate, or hydroxyapatite. Weber and associates have shown that supersaturation for calcium oxalate is higher among hypercalciuric than normocalciuric patients.[96] In all studies, urine from non–stone formers is supersaturated with respect to calcium oxalate. Added crystals grow in urine from most normal persons.[82,96] Hautmann and coworkers measured calcium and oxalate concentrations in tissues from the cortex, medulla, and papilla of seven human kidneys.[97] The calcium oxalate concentration product in the papillae ($1 \times 10^{-4}$ $M^2$) exceeded that of urine ($5 \times 10^{-7}$ $M^2$) and those of the medulla and cortex ($8 \times 10^{-7}$ $M^2$ and $6 \times 10^{-7}$ $M^2$, respectively). In addition, high CaP supersaturation is common in the tip of loop of Henle because both tubule fluid pH and the $Ca^{2+}$ concentration are high because of water extraction on the descending limb.[98]

The actual ULM for calcium oxalate and brushite in human urine samples from normal subjects and from hypercalciuric, normocalciuric, and hyperparathyroid stone formers are surprisingly variable.[82] The ULM of calcium oxalate and brushite was measured in urine from calcium stone formers and gender- and age-matched control subjects[99,100]; the gap between prevailing supersaturation of the urine and the ULM was reduced in stone formers, rendering it more likely for crystallization and stone formation to occur. The reduced ULM may represent deranged crystallization inhibition. Values of APR are close enough to the ULM for calcium oxalate and CaP that new crystal formation is expected. Most urine, even from normal persons, is metastable with respect to calcium oxalate, so growth of crystal nuclei is expected.

## ASSESSMENT OF NUCLEATION

Saturation estimates the propensity to crystallize. Nucleation refers to the initial formation of a crystal nidus. Nucleation is followed by crystal growth, epitaxial growth, and aggregation. Homogeneous nucleation, the spontaneous formation of new crystal nuclei in a supersaturated metastable solution, is actually uncommon. Usually, debris particles, surface irregularities, or other existing crystals furnish a substrate on which crystal nuclei begin to form at a lower APR than what is required for true homogeneous nucleation. The metastable zone reflects the greater free energy required to create new nuclei than to simply enlarge preformed nuclei. Any surface that can serve as a substrate for ions in solution on which to organize may act as a heterogeneous nucleus, bypassing the energetically more costly process of creating a solid phase de novo. In other words, there is a lower apparent ULM for heterogeneous nucleation.

The efficiency of heterogeneous nucleation depends on the similarity between the spacing of charged sites on the preformed surface and in the lattice of the crystal that is to grow on that surface. This matching is referred to as "epitaxis," and its extent is usually referred to as a good or poor epitaxial relationship.[101] To achieve homogeneous nucleation, all potential heterogeneous nuclei must be excluded. This is an unreasonably difficult task when the urine formation product ratio (FPR) for any given crystal is conditioned by preformed heterogeneous nuclei, and the nuclei of other crystals that form as the APR is raised during the experimental determination itself.

A number of urine crystals have good epitaxial matching and behave toward one another as heterogeneous nuclei. Monosodium urate and uric acid are excellent heterogeneous nuclei for calcium oxalate,[102,103] so uric acid or urate could, by crystallizing, lower the ULM for calcium oxalate. Heterogeneous nucleation may be the mechanism linking hyperuricosuria to calcium oxalate stones.[104,105] The epitaxial overgrowth of calcium oxalate on a surface of uric acid has been experimentally documented.[106] Both brushite and hydroxyapatite can also nucleate calcium oxalate,[107,108] which is likely the basis for Randall's plaque as initiators of calcium oxalate stones.

Randall's plaque is formed in the interstitium of the papilla but can erode through the papillary epithelium to be exposed to the urinary space, thus furnishing a nucleating site for the crystallization of calcium oxalate and anchoring site. This allows retained new crystals to have sufficient time to grow to a clinically significant size. Apatite is frequently found at the core of calcium oxalate stones,[109] and there is increased prevalence and severity of Randall's plaques in stone formers as compared with non–stone formers.[110] Evan, Coe, Kuo, and colleagues have extensively studied Randall plaque formation in patients with various types of nephrolithiaisis.[72,75,111–114] Their findings are presented in the relevant sections later.

## ASSESSMENT OF CRYSTAL GROWTH AND AGGREGATION

Growth is the enlargement of a crystal, and aggregation is the coalescence of crystals. Once formed, crystals will grow if bathed in urine with an APR greater than 1. Growth and aggregation are pathogenic because microscopic nuclei are too small to cause disease. Crystals are regular lattices, composed of repeating subunits, and they grow by the incorporation of calcium and oxalate or phosphate, or uric acid, into new subunits on their surfaces. In metastable solutions at 37°C, growth rates of calcium oxalate and the stone-forming CaP crystal show appreciable changes in macroscopic dimensions over hours. The growth rate increases with supersaturation and is most rapid in urine samples with the highest APR. Small crystals aggregate into larger crystalline masses by electrostatic attraction from the charged surface of the crystals, which rapidly increase particle size, producing a crystal that can lodge in the urinary tract. Stone formers' urine contains larger crystal aggregates compared with non–stone formers.[115]

### Inhibition of Crystal Agglomeration

The inhibition of crystal agglomeration (ICA) can be measured by adding a fixed amount of solid calcium oxalate to a synthetic solution intently and metastably supersaturated with calcium oxalate (CaOx), or to a similar solution spiked with the test subject's urine. ICA is expressed as the time to reach half of the maximum decline in the [Ca] half-life ($t_{1/2}$) in synthetic solution. A higher $t_{1/2}$ indicates a higher ICA.[116]

## CELL-CRYSTAL INTERACTIONS

Finlayson and Reid have proposed that crystals cannot grow or aggregate fast enough to anchor in the urinary tract during the normal urinary transit time.[67] This is analogous to throwing a handful of sand into a sink with the faucet turned on full; the sand will simply wash into the drain. Crystals must anchor to the renal tubule epithelium to delay its passage so that they can grow large enough to be of clinical significance. Although Randall's plaques[117] may offer both an anchoring or nucleating site, it is also clear that some stones can form in the absence of Randall's plaques,[110] so alternative mechanisms are present. CaOx crystals can adhere to cultured collecting duct epithelial cells.[118] The in vitro adherence and uptake of crystals appear to be greater for CaOx than CaP.[119] The crystals bind to anionic sites on the cell membrane[120] and can be inhibited by a variety of anionic compounds normally found in urine.[121] Phosphatidylserine in the lipid bilayer appears to be a binding site, and enrichment of cell membranes with phosphatidylserine increases CaOx crystal binding by renal epithelial cells in culture, although the in vivo significance cannot be confirmed.[122]

In addition for adhesion and crystal growth, it has been proposed that cell-crystal interactions result in cell injury and death,[123,124] which constitutes an integral part of stone formation. Nano-sized crystals induce predominantly apoptotic cell death, leading to cell and nuclear shrinkage and phosphatidylserine ectropion. In contrast, micron-sized crystals primarily caused necrotic cell death, leading to cell swelling and plasma membrane and lysosomal disintegration.[125]

Thus far, the evidence on the role of cell-crystal interaction has been mostly from cell culture experiments. The importance of the cell-crystal interaction in the pathogenesis of human kidney stone disease is not clear at this time.

# INHIBITORS

## CONCEPT

Stone constituents such as CaOx, CaP, sodium urate, or uric acid are often supersaturated in normal urine, yet precipitation does not occur.[82,94–96] This suggests that there are inhibitors to stone formation present in normal urine.[126,127] The ULM is lower in patients who form stones compared with matched controls, indicating deficiency in inhibitors in stone formers.[114] Despite this phenomenologic finding, the exact role of inhibitors is far from fully understood. There has been an argument posed that the therapeutic efficacy of agents such as potassium citrate in reducing the rate of stone recurrence may be because of their effect on the supersaturation of urine with respect to CaOx and CaP, rather than to any increase in inhibitory activity[128]; this remains unresolved. One can arbitrarily classify inhibitors into four groups: (1) multivalent metallic cations such as magnesium; (2) small organic anions such as citrate; (3) small inorganic anions such as pyrophosphate; or (4) macromolecules such as osteopontin and Tamm-Horsfall protein (Table 38.1).

## MAGNESIUM

Magnesium has been touted as a kidney stone inhibitor for many years.[129] It is present in urine in millimolar

**Table 38.1 Natural Inhibitors of Stone Formation**

| Inhibitor | Examples |
|---|---|
| Inorganic | Magnesium |
| | Pyrophosphate |
| Small organic anion | Citrate |
| Macromolecules | Bikunin |
| | Calgranulin |
| | FK binding protein-12 |
| | Glycosaminoglycans |
| | Nephrocalcin |
| | Osteopontin |
| | Prothrombin F1 fragment |
| | Lithostathine |
| | Matrix Gla protein |
| | Tamm-Horsfall protein |
| | Urinary trefoil factor-1 |

concentrations, and it readily binds to oxalate. Some have expressed the notion that magnesium is efficacious in preventing stone formation by binding or complexing oxalate in both the bowel and urine,[130–132] by inhibiting CaOx crystallization,[131,133,134] and by increasing urinary citrate when given as alkali salt.[135] In vitro studies have shown that magnesium is an inhibitor of CaOx crystal growth in artificial, rodent, and human urine, but these measurements were largely made at supraphysiologic concentrations.[136–141] Magnesium inhibits both nucleation and growth of CaOx crystals.[142] In a seeded crystal growth system of constant composition, magnesium was a weak inhibitor.[143]

The clinical trial experience has not been uniform. Fifty-five stone formers were given 500 mg of Mg daily as $Mg(OH)_2$ and experienced a decrease in stone rate from 0.8 to 0.08 stones/year.[129] However, other controlled studies have suggested that magnesium does not alter the recurrence rates for CaOx stone formation, perhaps because of its poor absorption.[144] Another possibility is that the beneficial inhibitory effect of magnesium may be offset by its hypercalciuric effects because luminal Mg inhibits the calcium channel, TRPV5, in a pH-dependent manner.[145] Human metabolic studies have shown interacting effects of urinary Mg and pH on calcium excretion.[146] At any given urine pH, Mg marginally increases urine calcium levels. Provision of an alkali load significantly lowered urine calcium levels and saturation of CaOx at any given level of urinary Mg excretion. At present, magnesium supplement is not routinely recommended as antiurolithiasis therapy; Mg supplements can be used if there is evidence of Mg depletion in a stone former—potassium magnesium citrate should be used instead of Mg oxide.[147,148]

## CITRATE

Citrate is the best studied, understood, and tested stone inhibitor. It is also one that is amenable to use as therapy. In addition to chelating calcium, which reduces calcium's availability to bind oxalate and phosphate, citrate also inhibits three properties of calcium oxalate crystals: nucleation, growth, and aggregation.[149,150] Citrate therapy directly inhibits crystallization[135,151] and increases the upper limit of metastability by increasing both urine citrate and pH.[152] Potassium citrate was shown, in most clinical studies, to reduce recurrent calcium nephrolithiasis in patients with idiopathic hypercalciuria and distal renal tubular acidosis, even in stone formers considered normocitraturic.[147,153–158] Citrate is the most important base equivalent in human urine. The principal regulator of urinary citrate levels is the acid-base status of the organism, particularly proximal tubule cell pH.[159] Because urinary citrate serves dual roles as a calcium chelator and the principal urinary base, this presents a conflict when base conservation is required, thus putting the urine at risk of calcium crystallization.[160] During systemic or proximal tubule cellular acidosis, there is an increase in both proximal citrate reabsorption and metabolism, reducing the amount of citrate excreted in the urine.[161] A reduction of urinary citrate, because of an increase in the acid load generated from dietary protein ingestion or to intestinal base loss, can promote the formation of both CaOx and CaP stones.[156,162]

## PYROPHOSPHATE

The inhibitory role of pyrophosphate on calcium crystallization has been known for years,[163] and it plays important anticalcification roles outside the kidney.[164] Pyrophosphate binds to the surface of basic CaP crystals, including hydroxyapatite, and arrests or at least retards the crystal growth of both CaP and CaOx crystals.[165–167] The average pyrophosphate concentration in bulk urine is sufficient to inhibit crystal growth significantly,[167] but the concentration in the microenvironment around the stone is not known and may be inadequate. There is a reduced pyrophosphate-to-creatinine ratio in 50% of stone formers, suggesting that a lack of pyrophosphate may predispose to nephrolithiasis.[166]

## MACROMOLECULES

Macromolecules are potent inhibitors of calcium oxalate crystallization.[168] Some of the macromolecules listed in Table 38.1 will be highlighted. These molecules are generally highly anionic and contain large amounts of acidic amino acid that undergo posttranslational modification, with negatively charged side chains. Bergsland and colleagues have compared the inhibitory proteins in urine from 50 stone-forming and 50 non–stone-forming, matched, first-degree relatives of calcium stone-forming patients[169]; they found that profiles of inhibitory proteins were effective in discriminating relatives of stone formers from non–stone formers and were even more effective than conventional measurements of supersaturation. Clinical use of inhibitor profiles is hampered by the difficulty and expense of these measurements.

### Osteopontin

Osteopontin, previously termed *uropontin,* is an acidic phosphoglycoprotein that was initially isolated from bone[170–173] but is present in urine at about 4 mg/day.[171,172] In bone, osteopontin inhibits hydroxyapatite formation during oeteogenesis.[174–176] It is expressed in cells of the thick ascending limb of Henle and distal convoluted tubules and secreted into the urine. Osteopontin inhibits nucleation, growth, and aggregation of CaOx stones in vitro.[170,171,177] Osteopontin-deleted mice develop intratubular CaOx crystals when given ethylene glycol, a nephrotoxin that leads to metabolic acidosis and hyperoxaluria, at doses that do not induce crystal formation in the wild-type mice.[170,178] Osteopontin is upregulated at sites of biomineralization in genetic hypercalciuric stone-forming rats,[179] and other models have suggested that it is increased in response to crystal formation.

### Tamm-Horsfall Protein

Tamm-Horsfall protein (THP) is the most abundant protein found in human urine, with approximately 100 mg excreted/day. It is synthesized in the thick ascending limb of Henle's loop and, because of self-aggregation, is the principal component of urinary casts.[180] Also known as uromodulin (UMOD), THP is implicated and involved in a multitude of functions and pathobiologic effects, including ion transport, innate immunity, blood pressure, and acute and chronic kidney injury.[181–183] UMOD/THP protein inhibits CaOx crystal aggregation but does not alter growth or nucleation.[184,185] UMOD/THP-deleted mice spontaneously form calcium crystals in the lumen of tubules in the papilla and medulla.[186] When these mice are given ethylene glycol to induce CaOx stone formation, there is a marked induction of renal osteopontin at sites of crystal formation.[186] UMOD/THP also activates the calcium channel TRPV5[187] and can theoretically reduce calciuria. One study has described higher UMOD/THP excretion in recurrent stone formers with positive family histories but concluded that the UMOD/THP is aggregated and functionally defective in inhibiting CaOx aggregation in vitro.[188] In a urinary proteomic study, the administration of lime (calcium, oxide, hydroxide, carbonate) increased UMOD/THP, but the biologic effect on lithogenesis was unclear.[189]

### Urinary Prothrombin Fragment 1

Urinary prothrombin fragment 1 (UPTF1, crystal matrix protein) is a fragment of prothrombin made in the kidney.[190] It is a potent inhibitor of CaOx growth, aggregation, and nucleation[191] and is present in kidney stones.[192] Differences in UPTF1 levels and genetic alleles have been found between stone formers and non–stone formers.[193,194]

### Bikunin

This is the light chain of the inter-alpha-trypsin inhibitor, which inhibits both calcium oxalate growth and nucleation.[195] It is found in the proximal tubule and in the thin descending segment of the loop of Henle.[196] Bikunin, along with the heavy chains of the inter-alpha-trypsin inhibitor, have been isolated from kidney stones, suggesting that multiple fragments of this inhibitor may be active in preventing stone formation.[197] Bikunin was present only in the collecting duct apical membranes and loop cell cytoplasm of stone formers, colocalizing with osteopontin and inter-alpha-trypsin inhibitor heavy-chain 3, and extensive heavy-chain 3 was only present in stone formers and not in controls.[198] One study has shown differences in the electrophoretic mobility pattern between stone formers and non–stone formers.[199]

### Glycosaminoglycans

Glycosaminoglycans (GAGs) occurring in the urine of normal individuals typically has around 50% chondroitin sulfate, around 25% heparan sulfate, around 10% low-sulfate chondroitin sulfate, and around 5% to 10% hyaluronic acid (HA).[200] Chondroitin sulfate retards nucleation; dermatan sulfate inhibits nucleation.[201] In rodents induced to precipitate CaOx, there is increased expression of heparan sulfate in tubules.[202] HA, which is in the extracellular matrices, is thought to bind at cell surfaces.[203] Human tubular cells in primary culture bind crystals when damaged, and this is dependent on the expression of HA.[204] Canine tubular cells increase the synthesis of glycosaminoglycans to protect from toxic insults of CaOx crystals and oxalate ions in vitro.[205] Human studies have shown decreased urinary GAG levels in stone formers,[206,207] but this finding has not been universal.[208,209]

### Matrix-Gla Protein

Matrix-Gla protein (MGP) is a small (14-kDa) glycoprotein that was the first urinary protein found to have crystal inhibitory properties.[184,210,211] MGP contains five γ-carboxyglutamic acid (Gla) residues, which have a high affinity for calcium and phosphate ions and hydroxyapatite crystals[212] and inhibit crystal growth, nucleation, and aggregation. MGP protects the vasculature from calcification[213,214] and may serve a similar role in the kidney. MGP mRNA expression is increased in renal tubular epithelial cells following exposure to CaOx crystals.[215,216] Interestingly, multilaminated crystals formed in the injured tubules with lack of MGP expression.[217] In contrast, no crystal formation was seen in tubules with MGP expression. MGP genetic single-nucleotide polymorphism is associated with the individual susceptibility of nephrolithiasis.[218] MGP from some stone-forming patients lacks Gla and has diminished ability to inhibit nucleation and growth of CaOx crystals.[184,185,219]

### Urinary Trefoil Factor 1

An anionic protein was isolated with inhibitory activity against CaOx crystal growth and identified as human trefoil factor 1 (TFF1). Functional studies of urinary TFF1 have demonstrated that its inhibitory potency is similar to that of nephrocalcin. The inhibitory activity of urinary TFF1 was neutralized by anti–C-terminal antibody, consistent with a model in which the C-terminal glutamic residues of TFF1 interact with calcium. Concentrations and amounts of TFF1 in the urine of patients with idiopathic CaOx kidney stone were significantly less than those found in controls.[220]

## CALCIUM STONES

CaOx is the most prevalent kidney stone worldwide, accounting for approximately 70% to 80% of kidney stones. CaP stones contribute to a smaller percentage (15%).[221–225] However, the percentage of CaP stones appears to increase with each new stone event in individual stone formers.[19] Risk factors for CaOx stone formation include hypercalciuria, hyperuricosuria, hypocitraturia, hyperoxaluria, and altered urinary pH.[221,222] CaP stones share some common mechanisms with CaOx stones, including hypercalciuria and hypocitraturia but, in contrast to CaOx, unduly alkaline urine is characteristic among CaP stone formers but not in CaOx stone formers. An ambulatory evaluation in over 1270 patients with recurrent calcium nephrolithiasis has demonstrated hypercalciuria in 60% of the patients, whereas hyperuricosuria was found in 36%, hypocitraturia in 31%, hyperoxaluria in 8%, abnormal urinary pH in 10%, low urinary volume in 16%, and no metabolic abnormality in 4% of patients.[223] These percentages are merely approximations because all the variables in question are continuous in their distribution. A study of 82 brushite stone formers has demonstrated hypercalciuria in 80%, alkaline urinary pH in 60%, and hypocitraturia in 50% of patients; hyperuricosuria and hyperoxaluria were uncommon, comprising 18% and 10%, respectively. Low urinary volume, however, was found in nearly 60%.[224]

## HYPERCALCIURIA

Hypercalciuria is the most prevalent metabolic abnormality in patients with calcium nephrolithiasis, occurring in 60% of adults with calcium stones.[224–229] The pathophysiologic mechanisms for hypercalciuria are protean and may involve increased intestinal absorption (absorptive hypercalciuria; Fig. 38.8), diminished renal tubular calcium reabsorption (renal leak hypercalciuria), and enhanced calcium mobilization from the bone (resorptive hypercalciuria).[222,230–233] Intestinal hyperabsorption of calcium is the most common abnormality in this population,[234] but all these physiologic derangements may coexist in individual patients.

## INTESTINAL HYPERABSORPTION OF CALCIUM

Flocks first showed a link between hypercalciuria and nephrolithiasis.[235] Subsequently, Albright and Henneman have used the term "idiopathic hypercalciuria" to highlight the unknown origin of hypercalciuria in this population.[236,237] The metabolic basis of intestinal hyperabsorption of calcium was first described by Nordin and Peacock, who introduced the term "absorptive hypercalciuria" (AH).[238] Balance studies have shown a negative calcium balance in patients with hypercalciuria compared with non–stone-forming control subjects.[239,240] Compatible with the balance data was information from dietary recall, which also hinted that patients with hypercalciuria consume less calcium than they excrete.[241]

Balance studies have shown low fecal calcium content,[242] and hypercalciuria was corrected by intestinal calcium binding with sodium cellulose phosphate.[243,244] The characteristic features of absorptive hypercalciuria are hypercalciuria with normocalcemia, normal or suppressed serum parathyroid hormone (PTH), and/or urinary cyclic adenosine 3′,5′-monophosphate (cAMP; surrogate marker of PTH bioactivity in the kidney), reflective of an increased calcium load on the system. Hyperabsorption is the most prevalent feature in patients with idiopathic hypercalciuria. Furthermore, it is likely that absorptive hypercalciuria is a heterogeneous disorder, consisting of two broad subtypes, calcitriol-dependent[245–249] or calcitriol-independent.[234,242,250–252]

### 1,25-Dihydroxyvitamin D–Dependent Absorptive Hypercalciuria

Increased 1,25(OH)$_2$D concentration has been reported in four different studies in hypercalciuric nephrolithiasis patients.[245–248] The diagnosis of absorptive hypercalciuria was established by direct measurement of intestinal calcium absorption[251,253] or indirectly[247] by showing a lower serum PTH concentration. The underlying pathophysiologic mechanism responsible for an increased serum 1,25(OH)$_2$D level likely results from increased production rather than decreased metabolic clearance, This is based on studies using an infusion equilibrium technique in 9 patients with absorptive hypercalciuria (>4 mg/kg/day and/or >300 mg/day) on a defined calcium intake (Fig. 38.9).[246] The diagnosis of absorptive hypercalciuria in this study was based on a high calciuric response after oral calcium load in association with a fasting normal or decreased PTH level or nephrogenic cAMP.[246] Further support for 1,25(OH)$_2$D in enhancing urinary calcium excretion has come from a study in normal subjects who became hypercalciuric after receiving a high dose of 1,25(OH)$_2$D.[245] In a separate study, net intestinal calcium absorption significantly increased during calcitriol treatment, and urinary calcium excretion in stone formers exceeded that of controls,[254] demonstrating a negative calcium balance during calcitriol administration in stone formers. This was associated with an increase in the urinary hydroxyproline level, a marker of bone resorption, suggesting that elevated 1,25(OH)$_2$D in healthy men on a low-calcium diet enhances bone resorption. There is a direct correlation between serum 1,25(OH)$_2$D, calcium excretion, and calciuric responses, suggesting the pathogenetic role of excess 1,25(OH)$_2$D in increased intestinal absorption.[245] It is still unknown whether the calcium in 1,25(OH)$_2$D-driven hypercalciuria originates from the bone[254] or intestine.[245]

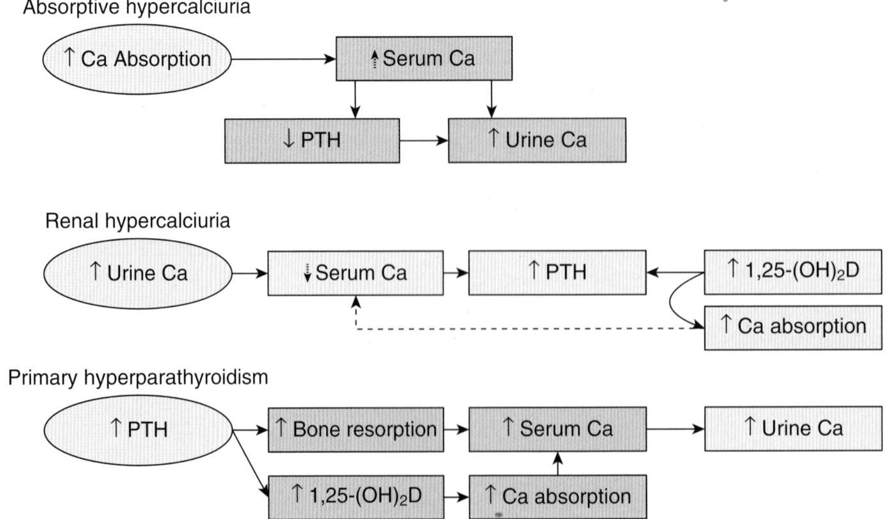


**Fig. 38.8** Pathophysiologic mechanisms of hypercalciuria. *PTH,* Parathyroid hormone. (From Pak CY. Etiology and treatment of urolithiasis. *Am J Kidney Dis.* 1991;18[6]:624–637.)[1]

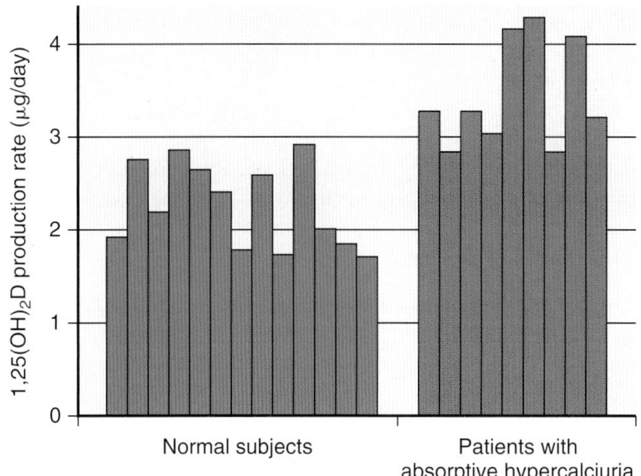


**Fig. 38.9** Individual values for 1,25(OH)$_2$D production rates in normal subjects and in those with absorptive hypercalciuria. The mean 1,25-dihydroxyvitamin D production rate was significantly higher in patients with absorptive hypercalciuria than in normal subjects (3.4 ± 0.5 vs. 2.2 ± 0.5 μg/day; $P < .001$). (From Insogna KL, Broadus AE, Dreyer BE, et al. Elevated production rate of 1,25-dihydroxyvitamin D in patients with absorptive hypercalciuria. *J Clin Endocrinol Metab.* 1985;61[3]:490–495.)

The reason for elevated 1,25(OH)$_2$D production in an absorptive hypercalciuria population is unclear. PTH, one of the main regulators of 1,25(OH)$_2$D synthesis, and urinary cAMP, a marker of PTH bioactivity, have never been found to be increased in this population.[223,225,234,247,251,252, 255–257]

There were no frank reductions in serum phosphorus concentration, the other main regulator of 1,25(OH)$_2$D production.[245–247,258]

Some studies have found that certain patients with absorptive hypercalciuria may have a primary defect in renal tubular reabsorption of phosphorus (renal phosphorus wasting), which consequently stimulates 1,25(OH)$_2$D synthesis and enhances intestinal calcium absorption.[247,259,260] However, the serum phosphorus concentration does not differ in hyperabsorptive and normal subjects under the same dietary regimen,[257,261] and hypophosphatemia and a low TmP/GFR (tubular maximum phosphate reabsorption per glomerular filtration rate) were found only in a minority of the patients with absorptive hypercalciuria.[257] Differences in urinary calcium or serum 1,25(OH)$_2$D levels between stone formers with and without a renal phosphate leak was detected in one study, but not in others.[262–265] Moreover, the underlying mechanism(s) of the renal phosphate leak in this population has not been fully investigated. An association of fibroblast growth factor 23 (FGF23) with renal phosphate leak and potential pathogenic role in patients with calcium nephrolithiasis has been reported in two studies.[265,266] It is still possible to have phosphate wasting and depletion without frank hypophosphatemia—serum phosphate is a practical but imperfect surrogate for phosphate stores.[267]

The conversion of circulating serum 25-hydroxyvitamin D (25[OH]D) occurs principally in the kidneys, and this metabolic conversion is enhanced with vitamin D deficiency.[268] However, CYP24A1 is highly expressed in the kidney and converts 1,25(OH)$_2$D and 25(OH)D to the inactive metabolites,[268] such as 1,24,25-trihydroxyvitamin D and 24,25-dihyroxyvitamin D, respectively. Thus, CYP24A1 hydroxylase acts as a potent inhibitor of vitamin D action by diminishing both 25(OH) D and 1,25(OH)$_2$D.

One study has described two patients with an elevated serum 1,25(OH)$_2$D level, nephrolithiasis, and nephrocalcinosis associated with hypercalciuria because of undetectable activity of 1,25(OH)$_2$D$_3$ 24-hydroxylase (CYP24A1), an enzyme that inactivates 1,25(OH)$_2$D.[269] This loss-of-function mendelian disease was described as being as a result of biallelic inactivating mutations of CYP24A1. The frequency of the CYP24A1 variant, based on a National Center for Biotechnology Information (NCBI) database, was estimated to be 4% to 20%. This report is proof of principle for the role of the 24-hydroxylase in D-dependent calcium stones, but it is difficult to determine whether variants in this gene predispose to urolithiasis in the general population.

An epidemiologic analysis of men in a Health Professionals Follow-Up Study over 12 years has found that the odds ratio of incident symptomatic kidney stones in the highest compared with the lowest quartile of serum 1,25(OH)$_2$D, within the normal range, was 1.73 after adjusting for body mass index, diet, plasma factors, and other covariates.[270]

### 1,25-Dihydroxyvitamin D–Independent Absorptive Hypercalciuria

In humans, two-thirds of absorptive hypercalciuria patients exhibit increased intestinal calcium absorption, with normal levels of 1,25(OH)$_2$D.[234,242,250–252,271] Moreover, a triple-lumen intestinal perfusion study has supported 1,25(OH)$_2$D-independent selective jejunal hyperabsorption of calcium in this population, which differs from the less selective gastrointestinal (GI) effects of 1,25(OH)$_2$D in normal subjects.[272]

Pharmacologic probes were used to alter serum 1,25(OH)$_2$D concentrations and assess intestinal calcium absorption in hypercalciuric subjects.[252,255–257] Ketoconazole reduces serum 1,25(OH)$_2$D in normal subjects and patients with primary hyperparathyroidism.[273–275] Nineteen patients with absorptive hypercalciuria were treated with ketoconazole (600 mg/day × 2 weeks; Fig. 38.10)[255] and, in 12 patients, ketoconazole lowered 1,25(OH)$_2$D concentration, intestinal calcium absorption, and 24-hour urinary calcium. Moreover, intestinal calcium absorption assessed directly by $^{47}$Ca absorption correlated with serum 1,25(OH)$_2$D and 24-hour urinary calcium excretion. Importantly, in 7 patients, despite the significant reduction of 1,25(OH)$_2$D, there was no change in calcium absorption or urinary calcium excretion.[255] In these patients, intestinal calcium absorption and urinary calcium excretion were not correlated with serum 1,25(OH)$_2$D levels. There have also been studies using thiazide,[252] glucocorticoids,[256] and orthophosphates[257] in hyperabsorptive patients. Results indicated that lowering 1,25(OH)$_2$D concentration is not associated with a reduction in intestinal calcium absorption, indicative of a calcitriol-independent mechanism in the development of hypercalciuria in this population.

### Increased Abundance of Vitamin D Receptor

Expression and activation of the vitamin D receptor (VDR) are necessary for vitamin D action.[276] A genetic association of intestinal hyperabsorption of calcium and calcium stone

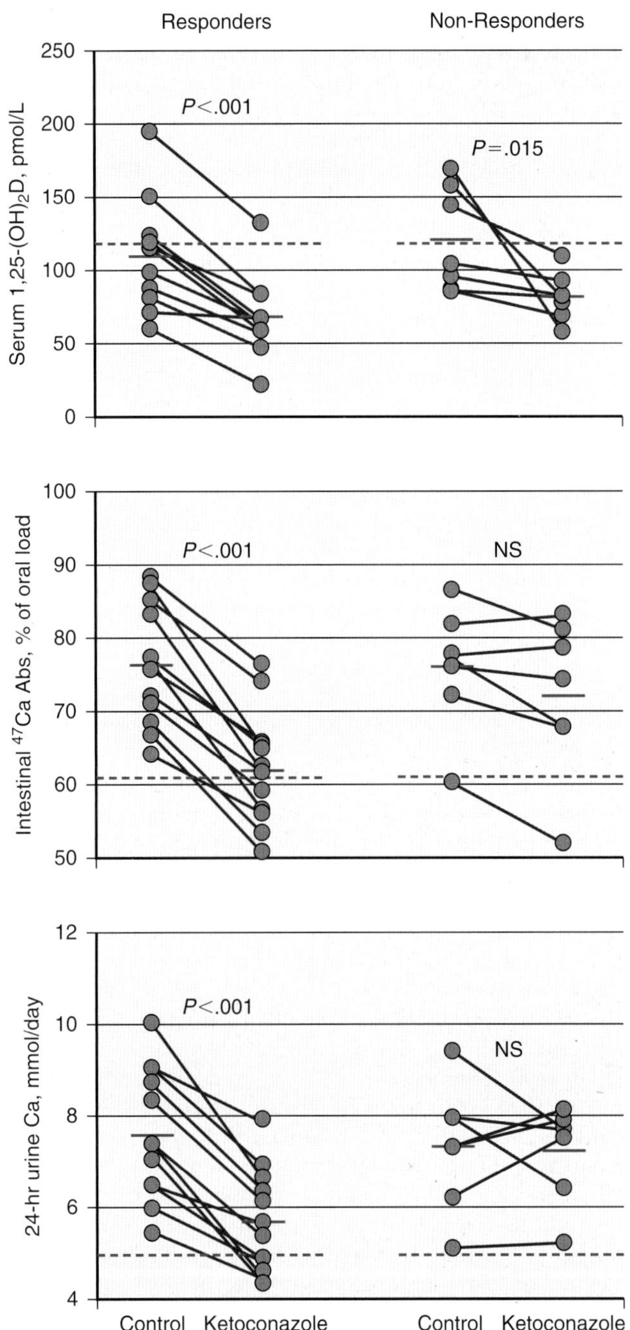


**Fig. 38.10** Heterogeneity of absorptive hypercalciuria. Shown are the responses of patients with hypercalciuria to a 2-week course of ketoconazole (600 mg/day). *Abs,* Absorption; *NS,* nonsignificant. (From Breslau NA, Preminger GM, Adams BV, et al. Use of ketoconazole to probe the pathogenetic importance of 1,25-dihydroxyvitamin D in absorptive hypercalciuria. *J Clin Endocrinol Metab.* 1992;75[6]:1446–1452.)

formation with the VDR locus has been described.[277,278] Two common single-nucleotide polymorphisms (SNPs) were linked to altered expression and/or function of VDR protein,[279–282] but these results were not confirmed by others.[283,284] Because intestinal calcium absorption in hyperabsorptive kidney stone formers mainly occurs with normal serum $1,25(OH)_2D$,[234,250–252] there might be an alteration in VDR abundance or sensitivity to $1,25(OH)_2D$. VDRs are expressed in peripheral monocytes and T and B lymphocytes.[285–289]

In 10 male hypercalciuric CaOx stone formers compared with age- and gender-matched controls without a history of stone disease, the abundance of VDR was twofold higher in peripheral blood monocytes (PBMC) in stone formers.[290] In another study of absorptive hypercalciuric patients, a Scatchard analysis has shown an increase in VDR abundance in a subset of patients with normal serum $1,25(OH)_2D$ levels. These results suggest heterogeneous patterns with respect to VDR abundance.[285]

### Genetic Hypercalciuric Stone-Forming Rat Model of Hypercalciuria

Genetic hypercalciuric stone-forming (GHS) rats are a polygenic model for hypercalciuria.[291–294] Breeding of Sprague-Dawley rats with high-end physiologic calcium excretion yielded robust constant hypercalciuria after 60 generations.[295,296] These animals have normal serum calcium and calcitriol levels, increased intestinal calcium absorption, formation of calcium stones, excessive bone resorption, and decreased renal tubular calcium reabsorption, making this a feasible model for studying the $1,25(OH)_2D$–VDR axis.[297–301] On a low-calcium diet, there was an increase in serum $1,25(OH)_2D$ levels in control and GHS rats. The increase was lower in GHS rats compared with controls, but there was greater net increase in intestinal calcium absorption in GHS rats, suggesting amplified bioactivity of $1,25(OH)_2D$.[297,302] This is analogous to patients with absorptive hypercalciuria, in whom elevated intestinal calcium absorption and urinary calcium excretion are associated with normal $1,25(OH)_2D$ levels.[234,250–252] The increased abundance of duodenal and kidney VDR[300,303,304] may account for the heightened biologic effect of $1,25(OH)_2D$ in GHS rats.[234,250–252] The high tissue VDR levels were as a result of an increase VDR gene expression, protein synthesis, and half-life of the VDR protein,[304–306] with no change in VDR DNA sequence,[305] but the transcription factor Snail, a negative regulator of VDR gene expression, seemed to be lower in GHS rats.[306]

Transcellular intestinal calcium transport involves initial calcium entry across the apical membrane, which is facilitated across the cells by the 9-kDa calbindin, followed by extrusion through the plasma basolateral membrane.[307] The biologic action of VDR in GHS rats was supported by increased expression of vitamin D–dependent genes, such as increased expression of calbindin-9 in the duodenum.[304] The 28-kDa calbindin is the principal calcium-binding protein in the renal distal convoluted tubule and plays a role in renal calcium transport.[308–310] Baseline calbindin-28k levels were higher in GHS rat kidneys and, after a single dose of $1,25(OH)_2D$, calbindin-28k increased much more in GHS rats compared with control rats.[304] One may conclude that abundance of tissue VDR in GHS rats, as well as humans with absorptive hypercalciuria, may amplify the biologic effect of normal serum $1,25(OH)_2D$ levels and consequently increase the expression of vitamin D–dependent genes and their protein products to regulate intestinal, renal, and bone calcium transport.

## RENAL LEAK HYPERCALCIURIA

Renal leak of calcium is caused by diminished renal tubular calcium reabsorption and is associated with secondary increases in serum PTH and $1,25(OH)_2D$ levels and a compensatory increase in intestinal calcium absorption.[311]

The underlying mechanisms for impaired renal tubular calcium reabsorption have not yet been fully explored. However, several potential mechanisms have been purported to affect renal tubular calcium reabsorption, including a primary proximal defect, hyperinsulinemia, calcium-sensing receptor (CaSR) gene expression and its interaction with calcitriol, and claudin-14 expression. Seminal human metabolic studies performed by Worcester and associates have demonstrated an exaggerated fractional excretion of calcium ($FE_{Ca}$) in hypercalciuric patients in a postprandial state compared with normal subjects.[312] Furthermore, increased $FE_{Ca}$ was not a consequence of differences in filtered calcium load, urinary sodium excretion, or serum PTH levels (Fig. 38.11).

It was proposed that the postprandial inhibition of renal tubular calcium reabsorption may be as a result of differences in insulin levels in hypercalciuric stone formers.[313,314] This was based on previous findings showing an exaggerated calciuric response to an oral carbohydrate load in hypercalciuric stone formers.[315–317] These studies did not segregate the effects of hyperinsulinemia from those of the serum glucose concentration. A study using euglycemic hyperinsulinemic clamp has demonstrated that the rise in insulin-induced calciuria is small and no different between hypercalciuric stone formers and non–stone-forming control subjects, suggesting that insulin is unlikely to play a significant pathogenic role in hypercalciuric stone formers.[318] Insulin resistance and hyperinsulinemia are features of obesity and are associated with hypercalciuria and the risk of kidney stone formation[10,12,319,320] but $FE_{Ca}$ was comparable in the hypercalciuric stone formers, overweight and obese non–stone formers, and lean controls, independent of peripheral insulin sensitivity measured as glucose disposal rates. This study is at variance with a previous report using semipurified insulin extracted from islets rather than recombinant insulin, which showed significant insulin-induced hypercalciuria.[321]

The CaSR is expressed in multiple tissues, including the parathyroid glands, kidney, and GI tract.[322] In the parathyroid

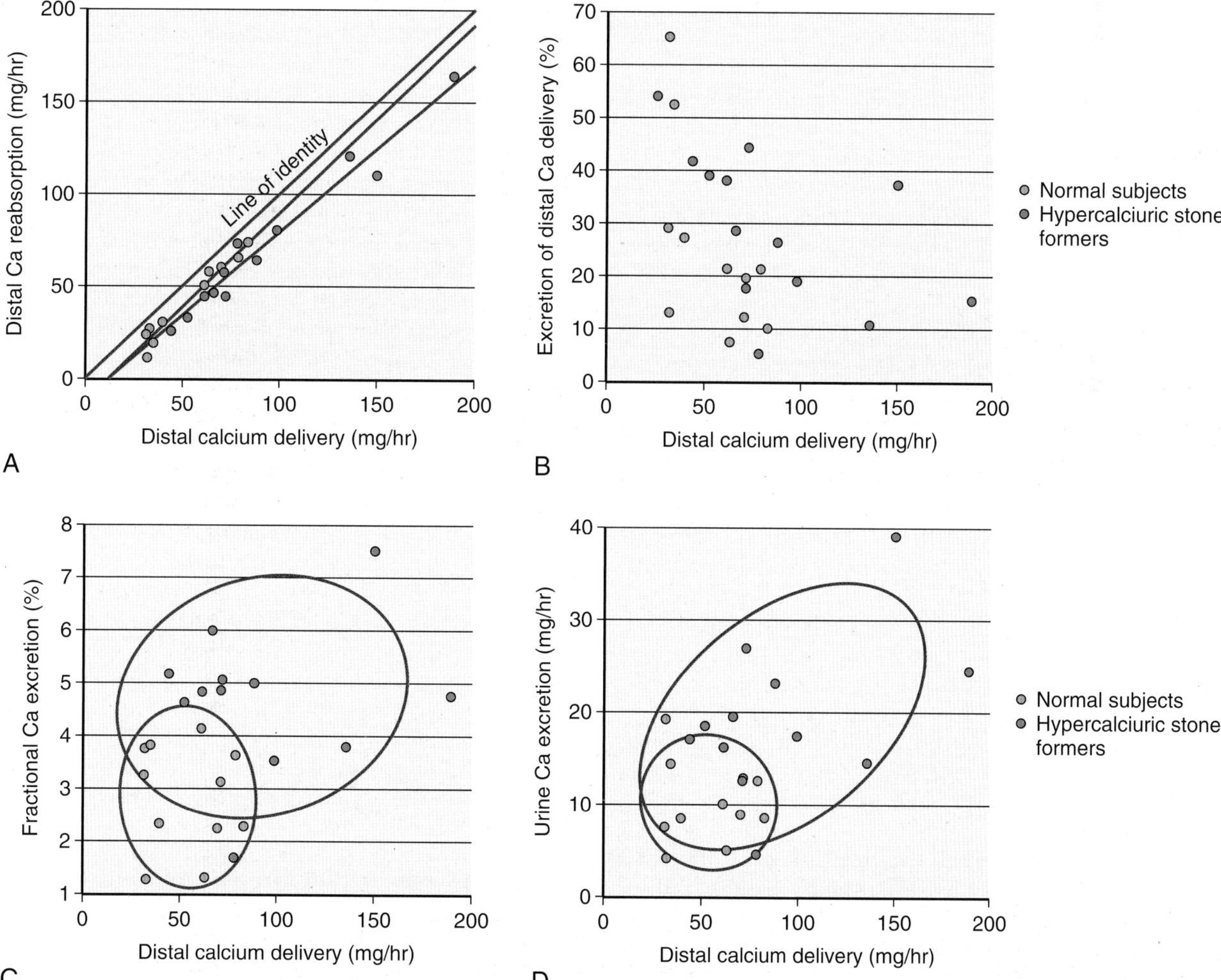


**Fig. 38.11** Relationship between distal calcium reabsorption, renal calcium excretion, and distal calcium delivery. (A) Distal calcium reabsorption increases similarly with calcium delivery in normal subjects and hypercalciuric stone formers. Both lines are positioned slightly beneath the line of identity. This suggests normal distal calcium handling but higher distal calcium delivery. (B) The actual fraction (%) of distally delivered calcium that was excreted fell with increasing distal delivery, and stone formers lie above normal at comparable distal delivery. (C) Fractional and total (D) calcium excretions were high in many stone formers versus normal subjects at comparable deliveries. (From Worcester EM, Coe FL, Evan AP, et al. Evidence for increased postprandial distal nephron calcium delivery in hypercalciuric stone-forming patients. *Am J Physiol Renal Physiol.* 2008;295[5]:F1286–F1294.)

glands, the CaSR responds to calcium and suppresses PTH release. In the kidney, the CaSR responds to increased circulating ionized calcium and reduces renal tubular calcium reabsorption in the thick ascending limb (TAL) and distal convoluted tubal (DCT).[323] An Italian cohort has linked hypercalciuria in stone formers to polymorphism in the CaSR gene. Serum calcitriol levels were not defined in these subjects. Vitamin D–responsive elements (VDREs) have been identified in the CaSR gene, which suggests that calcitriol can upregulate kidney CaSR expression and reduce renal tubular calcium reabsorption.[324] Although the physiologic function of CaSR in the GI tract has not been defined, the CaSR is highly expressed in gastric parietal G cells, which in turn increases gastric acid and gastrin release. The underlying mechanism for the intestinal hyperabsorption of calcium in kidney stone formers was suggested to be related to the increased gastrin and gastric acid secretion to oral calcium and protein load in patients with absorptive hypercalciuria.[325–328]

Tight junction proteins of the claudin family expressed in the TAL are critical for paracellular $Ca^{2+}$ reabsorption in the kidney.[329] A genome-wide association study conducted in Iceland and the Netherlands has found an association between sequence variations of the *CLDN14* gene and kidney stones and reduced bone mineral density at the hip.[330] One study has suggested that CaSR regulates claudin-14 expression via two microRNAs, miR-9 and miR-374, and that dysregulation of the renal CaSR–claudin-14 pathway might be a possible cause of hypercalciuria.[331] This model proposes that CaSR increases claudin-14, which inhibits the complex of claudin-16 and claudin-19 that regulates paracellular $Ca^{2+}$ reabsorption in the TAL.[329]

## RESORPTIVE HYPERCALCIURIA

Resorptive hypercalciuria refers to hypercalciuria caused by enhanced calcium mobilization from bone. This can be PTH-dependent or PTH-independent.

### Parathyroid Hormone-Dependent Resorptive Hypercalciuria

Primary hyperparathyroidism (PHPT) is the most common cause of resorptive hypercalciuria and is associated with calcium stones in 2% to 8% of patients.[221] Because of the much earlier diagnosis of PHPT, asymptomatic cases are common and renal complications have significantly decreased.[332] A retrospective study of 271 renal ultrasounds from asymptomatic cases with surgically proven PHPT has shown a 7% prevalence of stones compared with 1.6% in 500 age-matched subjects who underwent sonography examinations for other reasons.[333] Although hypercalciuria has been perceived as a cause of kidney stones in this population, the exact relationship between hypercalciuria and the risk of nephrolithiasis in patients with primary hyperparathyroidism is debatable.[334,335] The relative contribution from enhanced skeletal calcium mobilization versus enhanced intestinal calcium absorption is not clear.[334,336,337] The serum $1,25(OH)_2D$ level is higher, and there is increased calciuric response to oral calcium load in patients with PHPT and kidney stones.[336–339] One study has shown that kidney stones are more frequently seen in younger patients because of their higher synthetic capacity of $1,25(OH)_2D$ compared with older patients and hence higher intestinal calcium absorption.[336]

In a single-center prospective study over 5 years in 140 patients with PHPT consisting of 127 women, of whom 85% were postmenopausal women, approximately 50% had kidney stones by ultrasound, two-thirds had osteoporosis by dual-energy x-ray absorptiometry (DXA), and one-third had a history of vertebral fracture documented by x-ray. More kidney stones were detected in symptomatic than asymptomatic patients. The results of the study suggested that kidney stones and bone fractures are common in asymptomatic patients with PHPT.[340] Urinary calcium excretion was not different between kidney-stone formers and those without kidney stones, suggesting that other factors might be responsible for the development of kidney stones. The result of this study did not agree with two previous reports showing that stone-forming patients with PHPT had higher hypercalciuria than non–stone formers and higher intestinal calcium absorption.[337,341]

### Parathyroid Hormone–Independent Resorptive Hypercalciuria

Elevated serum $1,25(OH)_2D$ levels or amplified sensitivity to $1,25(OH)_2D$ at target organs may lead to enhanced bone resorption and diminished bone collagen synthesis in hypercalciuric stone-forming subjects.[290,342] In a retrospective multivariable analysis in 250 male and 182 female kidney stone formers, no significant relationship was found between urine calcium (either ad lib or restricted diet) with spine and femoral neck bone mineral density (BMD) in men and in postmenopausal women treated with estrogen. This suggests that calciuria may be a surrogate but not a causative factor in bone loss and higher fracture risk in kidney stone formers.[343] A similar phenotype has been shown in GHS rats whose bones are more sensitive to exogenous $1,25(OH)_2D$ compared with normal control rats.[303] Other mechanisms include diminished bone expression of transforming growth factor-β, which stimulates bone formation and mineralization, and/or perturbation in the RANK/RANK-L/OPG system, which increases bone resorption. The latter, in association with other cytokines and growth factors, acts synergistically with high $1,25(OH)_2D$ levels to affect bone remodeling.[230,344,345]

## HYPERURICOSURIA

Hyperuricosuria as a single abnormality is detected in much lower frequency than in combination with other metabolic abnormalities among calcium stone formers.[222,346] There is a high frequency of CaOx stones in patients with gout.[347,348] A structural similarity was described between crystals of uric acid (UA), sodium hydrogen urate, and CaOx, attributed to the growth of one crystal on another.[349] This is described in more detail later.

### Pathophysiologic Mechanism of Hyperuricosuria

UA production is from de novo synthesis, tissue catabolism, and dietary purine load. It is estimated that approximately 50% of the typical daily uric load is endogenous, with the remainder from dietary sources.[350] Increased dietary purine intake has been implicated in most hyperuricosuric calcium urolithiasis (HUCU) patients. A metabolic study comparing HUCU stone formers with age- and weight-matched normal subjects has shown that stone-forming patients ingest a higher intake of purine-rich food such as meat, fish, and poultry.[351] With kinetic studies, endogenous overproduction of UA has been suggested in approximately one-third HUCU stone formers consuming purine-free diets.[351] About one-third of synthesized UA is excreted into the intestinal tract, followed by intestinal uricolysis and the remainder by the kidney.[352] However, defective renal tubular reabsorption of UA has not been shown to be responsible for hyperuricosuria in this population.[353] In most mammals, ingested purines are converted to UA and then further to allantoin enzymatically in the peroxisomes of hepatic cells.[354] However, humans and higher primates lack functional uricase, the enzyme that converts UA to allantoin, thereby making UA the final product of purine metabolism in these species.[355,356]

### Physicochemical Mechanism of Hyperuricosuria-Induced Calcium Stones

The physicochemical basis for hyperuricosuria-induced calcium oxalate stones has been postulated but not yet been proven. There are three potential and nonmutually exclusive mechanisms.[102,357,358] In two studies, the underlying mechanisms linking UA to CaOx crystallization was attributed to heterogeneous nucleation[102,103] (Fig. 38.12). Another study showed that colloidal monosodium urate from supersaturated urine in these patients may attenuate inhibitor activity against CaOx crystallization[359,360] but, when GAGs were specifically examined, UA did not affect its inhibitor activity.[361] Monosodium urate can diminish the solubility of CaOx in solution, a process referred to as *salting out*.[357,362] Salting out is also known as *antisolvent crystallization*, which can typically be used to precipitate a nonelectrolyte multicharged macromolecule (usually protein) at a high electrolyte concentration (usually ammonium sulfate). Despite the uncertainty regarding the mechanism, clinical studies in hyperuricosuric patients have shown a drastic decline in the rate of recurrent kidney stone formation in those treated with xanthine oxidase inhibition.[363] Increasing urinary supersaturation with monosodium urate in conjunction with the decreased limit of metastability of CaOx, because of the adsorption of a macromolecular inhibitor of CaOx crystallization by monosodium urate in hyperuricosuric patients, increases the risk of CaOx stone formation.[364] Contrary to laboratory and clinical evidence, a retrospective population-based study in a large number of patients did not show a relationship between urinary UA and CaOx stone formation.[365] The urate effect is likely imperceptible in a large, unselected, calcium stone–forming population.

## HYPOCITRATURIA

Hypocitraturia as an isolated abnormality occurs in about one-third of patients with calcium nephrolithiasis.[156] The presence of citrate in human urine was described in 1917[366] and, a decade later, it was shown that acid-base homeostasis plays a key role in determining urinary citrate excretion in that a higher urinary citrate excretion rate was observed in alkalotic patients and very low excretion rate in those with metabolic acidosis or an acid load.[367] In 1954, a combination of oral sodium citrate, potassium citrate, and citric acid was used to alkalinize the urine in patients with uric acid and cystine stones.[368] Citrate is one of the most abundant organic anions (in molar quantities) in human urine and is an important inhibitor of calcium stone formation via its effects on calcium chelation, prevention of crystallization, and aggregation, in addition to its effect to reduce ionized calcium and, some have postulated, its ability to promote crystal detachment from cells (Fig. 38.13).[156,160,369,370] Tricarboxylate citrate has pKa values of 2.9, 4.3, and 5.6 and is found mostly as a trivalent anion (citrate$^{3-}$) in blood. Citrate is freely filtered, and approximately 10% to 35% of filtered citrate is excreted in urine, varying with acid-base status. The reabsorption of

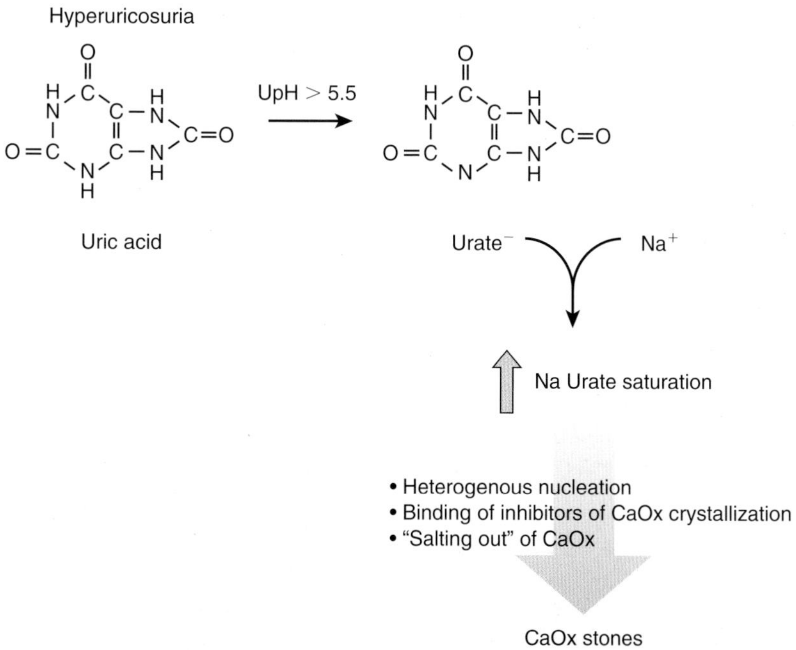

**Fig. 38.12** Physicochemical scheme for urate-induced CaOx stones. Hyperuricosuria in the absence of acidic urine renders high free urate activity levels in the urine. Sodium activity is perpetually higher than urate by two orders of magnitude. The higher sodium urate promotes calcium oxalate crystallization by three nonexclusive mechanisms. *UpH,* Urinary pH.

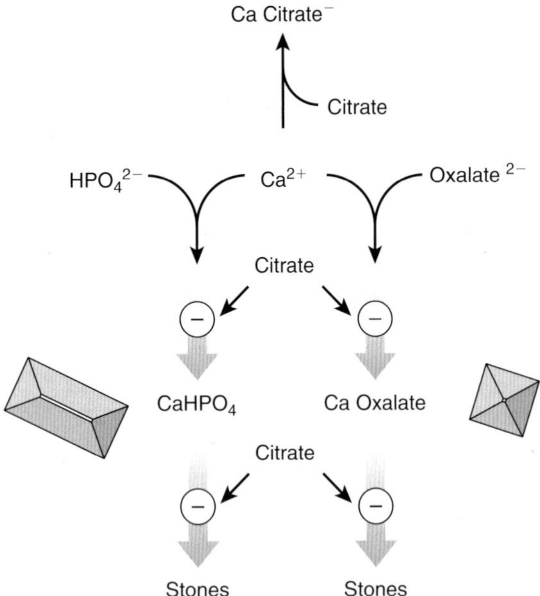


**Fig. 38.13** Protective effects of citrate against urolithiasis. Citrate binds calcium with high affinity to form soluble calcium citrate complexes and lowers the ionized calcium and calcium activity. Citrate also directly inhibits calcium oxalate and calcium phosphate crystallization and aggregation.

citrate occurs in the proximal convoluted tubule and, to a lesser extent, in the proximal straight tubule.[161,371,372] Apical membrane transport occurs through a coupled sodium-dicarboxylate cotransporter (NaDC-1).[373,374] In contrast, basolateral citrate reabsorption occurs via a tricarboxylate cotransporter (NaDC-3).[375]

### Role of Acid-Base Factors

It is well known that alterations of acid-base status plays a key role in renal tubular citrate reabsorption by multiple mechanisms (see Chapter 8). The highest $pK_a$ of citric acid is 5.6, so the concentration of $citrate^{2-}$, the transported ionic species, increases at lower luminal pH.[376] There is also a direct gating effect of pH on NaDC-1 activity, independent of the substrate concentration.[374] The abundance of NaDC-1 cotransporter increases in the apical membrane of the proximal renal tubule during acidosis. Finally, cytosolic ATP citrate lyase and mitochondrial aconitase activity increase in acidosis, which lowers the intracellular concentration of citrate and promotes its reabsorption.[377–379]

### Other Factors

The contribution of factors other than acid-base status to renal tubular citrate handling has not been extensively studied. However, it has been suggested that vitamin D, PTH, calcitonin, lithium, calcium, sodium, magnesium, and a variety of organic anions may alter urinary citrate excretion.[380,381] The effect of organic acid has been attributed to its competition with renal citrate for reabsorption via NaDC-1 transporters.[381] The effect of increasing apical calcium and magnesium has been demonstrated in cultured proximal tubular cell, showing decreased citrate uptake that may involve a transporter other than NaDC-1.[382]

**Table 38.2 Clinical Conditions Associated With Hypocitraturia**

| Low Extracellular Fluid pH | Normal or High Extracellular Fluid pH |
|---|---|
| Overproduction acidosis<br>• Chronic diarrhea<br>• Exercise-induced lactic acidosis | Potassium deficiency |
| Underexcretion acidosis<br>• Congenital or acquired distal RTA<br>• Acetazolamide, topiramate | Angiotensin II-related<br>• ACE inhibitors<br>• Salt excess<br>Excess dietary protein |

*ACE*, Angiotensin-converting enzyme; *RTA*, renal tubular acidosis.

### Clinical Conditions

Clinical conditions associated with hypocitraturia may be divided into those with systemic extracellular acidosis and those without (Table 38.2). dRTA is the most prominent cause of hypocitraturia and is frequently encountered in patients with recurrent nephrolithiasis.[383–387] Other conditions associated with systemic acidosis include carbonic anhydrase inhibition,[388,389] strenuous physical exercise,[390] and chronic diarrheal states.[391–393]

Hypocitraturia is also found in normobicarbonatemic states, including incomplete dRTA, chronic renal insufficiency, mild chronic metabolic acidosis, high protein consumption, thiazide treatment with hypokalemia, primary aldosteronism, excessive salt intake, and angiotensin-converting enzyme (ACE) inhibitor treatment.[158,380,394–398] In experimental animals and, to a certain extent, in humans, ACE inhibitors lower the intracellular pH in the proximal tubule.[398] Potassium depletion in rats upregulates renal citrate reabsorption in the proximal tubule apical membrane by altering the abundance of transporters.[399]

### Actions of Citrate

The physicochemical basis for the inhibitory role of citrate involves the formation of soluble complexes from the reduction of the ionic calcium concentration in the urine.[400] Direct inhibition of crystallization of CaOx and CaP is facilitated by the inhibition of spontaneous precipitation of CaOx and agglomeration of preformed CaOx crystals.[116,135]

## HYPEROXALURIA

Hyperoxaluria is present in isolation or in combination with other risk factors in 8% to 50% of kidney stone formers.[223,401–403] In CaOx stone formers, both urinary oxalate and calcium are responsible for driving CaOx supersaturation, although the activity of calcium is one order of magnitude higher than oxalate (Fig. 38.14).[404] Under normal circumstances, the physiologic concentration of the CaOx complex in the urine far exceeds its solubility constant.[404,405] The mechanisms underlying hyperoxaluria can stem from multiple factors and are summarized in Fig. 38.15.[406–410]

### Increased Hepatic Production

Monogenic disorders of oxalate metabolism are rare but serious causes of kidney stones. Oxalate is a dicarboxylic acid

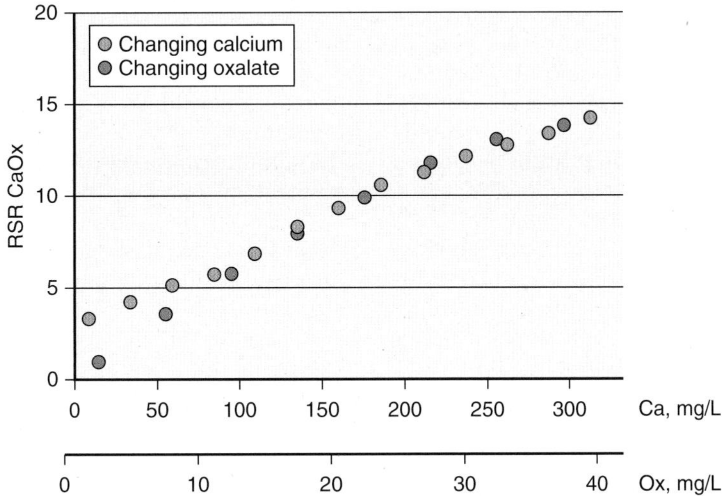


**Fig. 38.14.** Relationship between calcium oxalate relative supersaturation *(RSR)* and calcium or oxalate concentration. Calcium or oxalate was varied individually; the other was kept constant. (Modified from Pak CY, Adams-Huet B, Poindexter JR, et al. Rapid communication: relative effect of urinary calcium and oxalate on saturation of calcium oxalate. *Kidney Int.* 2004;66[5]:2032–2037.)

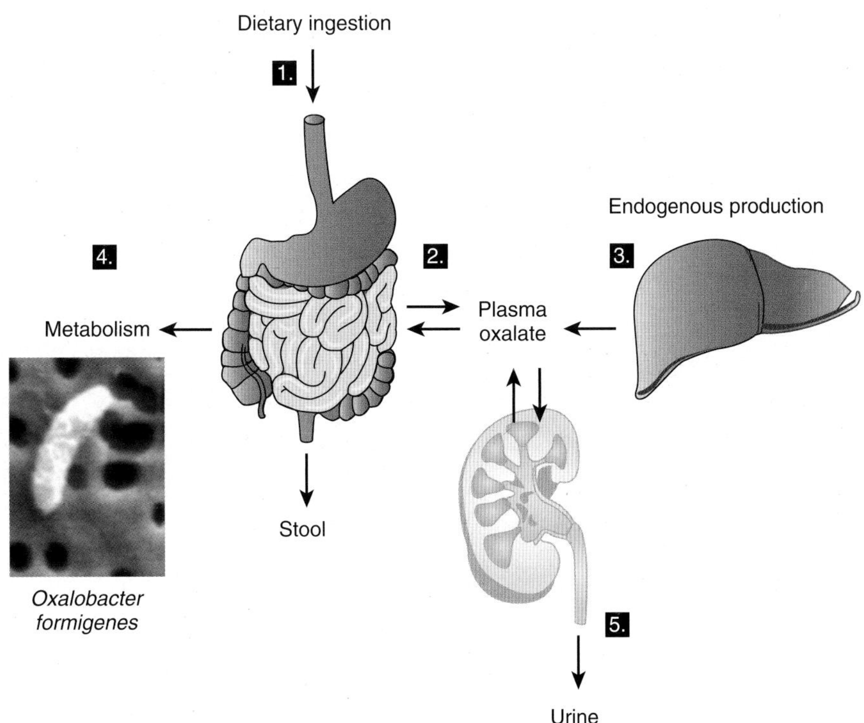


**Fig. 38.15** Pathophysiologic mechanisms of hyperoxaluria. Oxalate balance is determined by ingestion and endogenous production versus intestinal and urinary excretion. Intestinal handling can be bidirectional, and luminal degradation is facilitated by microbial degradation. Urinary excretion is the net result of filtration minus tubular reabsorption. Hyperoxaluria can be caused by the following: (1) increased dietary ingestion; (2) increased gut absorption or decreased secretion; (3) increased endogenous hepatic production; (4) decreased intestinal bacterial metabolism; or (5) renal hyperexcretion.

and in mammals is either ingested or is an end product of hepatic metabolism.[222,406,411] Primary hyperoxaluria (PH) is an autosomal recessive disorder of inborn enzymatic defects resulting in massive hepatic overproduction of oxalate. The three genetic forms converge onto the excess glyoxylate, which is the precursor of oxalate. These forms are classified into types I, II, and III. Type I PH (Online Mendelian Inheritance in Man [OMIM] 259900) is the consequence of a deficiency or mistargeting of hepatic alanine glyoxylate transferase (AGT), which is a pyridoxal 5′-phosphate–dependent enzyme that transaminates glyoxylate to glycine.[412] It accounts for about 80% of PH cases. Type II (OMIM 260000) is caused by a deficiency in the cytosolic enzyme glyoxylate reductase–hydroxypyruvate reductase (GRHPR), which reduces glyoxylate to glycolate,[413] and accounts for about 10% of cases. The least common variety, type III (OMIM 613616), is as a result of activating mutations in the mitochondrial 4-hydroxy-2-oxoglutarate aldolase enzyme (HOGA), which converts hydroxyproline to glyoxalate.[414–417] Since this is a gain-of-function mutation, type III heterozygotes can have calcium oxalate stones.[416,417] PH type 3 accounts for about 5% cases; another 5% of PH have no known genetic mutation.

Multiple other metabolic precursors of oxalate metabolism, including by-products of the breakdown of ascorbic acid—fructose, xylose and hydroxyproline—potentially contribute to oxalate production. However, their contribution under normal physiologic circumstances has not yet been fully elucidated.[418,419]

#### Dietary Intake and Bioavailability

Dietary oxalate contributes significantly to urinary oxalate excretion. There is a wide variation in estimated oral intake of oxalate, ranging from 50 to 1000 mg/day.[223,403] Dietary oxalate and its bioavailability contribute approximately 45% of the urinary oxalate excretion.[420] The main sources of most bioavailable oxalate-rich food are seeds, chocolate derived from tropical cocoa trees, leafy vegetables, including spinach and rhubarb, and tea. The relationship between oxalate absorption and dietary oxalate intake has been demonstrated to be nonlinear.[420]

#### Intestinal Absorption

Despite seminal advances in rodent intestinal physiology of oxalate handling,[421] the specific intestinal segments in the human intestine involved in oxalate absorption and secretion is not fully known. It was proposed that the main site of oxalate absorption is in the small intestine because most oxalate absorption occurs in the first 4 to 8 hours after ingestion.[401,409,422,423] Nevertheless, it has been suggested that the colon may also participate, to a lesser extent, in oxalate absorption.[423]

Oxalate is both absorbed and secreted in the GI tract through both paracellular and transcellular pathways. Paracellular oxalate absorption has not yet been confirmed in intact organisms. However, it has been proposed that at a low gastric pH, part of the dietary oxalate is converted into small hydrophobic molecules, which could possibly diffuse through the lipid bilayer[424–427] and thereby increase urinary oxalate excretion.

#### Role of Anion Exchanger Slc26a6

The anion exchanger Slc26a6 is involved in intestinal oxalate transport in rodents,[428,429] where it is expressed in the apical membrane of the duodenum, jejunum, and ileum and, to a lesser extent, the large intestine.[430] There is defective net oxalate secretion in mice with targeted inactivation of *Slc26a6*[428] (Fig. 38.16). *Slc26a6* null mice on a control oxalate diet showed increased plasma oxalate concentration, decreased fecal oxalate excretion concentration, and high urinary oxalate excretion.[428] The abnormalities were attenuated following stabilization on an oxalate-free diet, suggesting that diminished net gut oxalate secretion is responsible for the rise in plasma oxalate concentration and elevated urinary oxalate excretion. However, the influence of this putative anion exchanger on

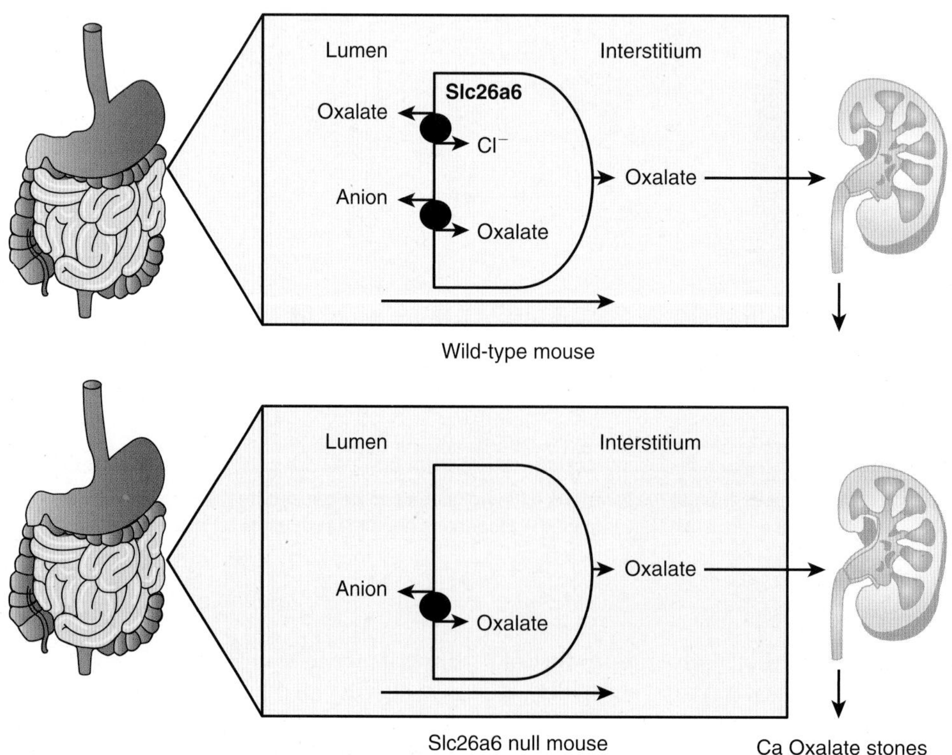


**Fig. 38.16** Comparison of the wild-type versus the Slc26a6 mouse. Slc26a6 mediates intestinal oxalate secretion in wild-type mice, so that only 10% of ingested oxalate is normally absorbed and excreted into the urine. Targeted deletion of the *Slc26a6* gene in mice unmasks a large intestinal absorptive flux of oxalate and leads to increased plasma oxalate levels, hyperoxaluria, and calcium oxalate stones.

intestinal oxalate absorption, and specifically its role in kidney stone formation in humans, has not yet been demonstrated. Studies with exogenous radiolabeled oxalate in normal humans have shown that renal excretion accounts for most of the disposal of oxalate.[431] In contrast, report of a case of enteric hyperoxaluria showed drastically diminished expression of Slc26A6 protein in the intestine.[432]

The potential underlying mechanisms of hyperoxaluria in obesity have been investigated in *ob/ob* mice.[433,434] These *ob/ob* mice had significantly higher urinary oxalate excretion than pair-fed controls, demonstrating that hyperoxaluria is not because of increased oxalate intake. When jejunal tissue was mounted on an Ussing chamber, defective oxalate secretion was shown in *ob/ob* mice. There was less *Slc26A6* mRNA and protein expression in *ob/ob* mice compared with controls. The contribution of regional and systemic inflammation in this model was supported by high plasma and jejunal tumor necrosis factor interferon and interleukin-6 levels in *ob/ob* mice.

## Role of Oxalobacter Formigenes

Many gut bacteria, including *Oxalobacter formigenes* (OF), degrade oxalate in the intestinal lumen via oxalate decarboxylse.[435] OF was initially found in ruminates, but is also present in other species, including humans.[436,437] Colonization with this bacteria begins approximately during childhood and may be found in feces of 60% to 80% of adults.[438] Dietary oxalate intake influences the colonization of in the GI tract. In animal studies, a significant decline in urinary oxalate follows administration of or increase in OF colonization.[439,440] In a cross-sectional study, patients with recurrent calcium oxalate stones had lower OF colonization than normal subjects matched for age and gender.[441] However, urinary oxalate excretion was no different between the two populations because the study was performed under an uncontrolled diet. In another study, Seiner and colleagues[442] have shown that OF- negative calcium oxalate stone formers have higher urinary oxalate excretion than OF- positive patients on a controlled diet[442] (Fig. 38.17). Intestinal oxalate absorption using $^{13}C_2$-labeled oxalate was similar in OF-positive and OF-negative patients, but plasma oxalate concentrations were significantly higher in the OF-negative population. The results supported the role of reduced oxalate secretion in OF-negative calcium oxalate kidney stone formers. An ex vivo Ussing chamber study has demonstrated that OF not only degrades intestinal luminal oxalate, but has the capacity to stimulate net intestinal oxalate secretion.[443] This pathophysiologic scheme from animal experiments was confirmed in patients with type I PH, in subjects with normal renal function, and in patients with CKD, showing a transient reduction of urinary oxalate following the oral administration of OF.[444]

## Renal Excretion

The kidney plays a major role in oxalate homeostasis. Oxalate is not significantly protein-bound and is freely filtered at the glomerulus. With impaired kidney function, plasma oxalate concentration steadily increases and exceeds its saturation in the blood, therefore enhancing the risk of systemic tissue oxalate deposition. Renal oxalate clearance studies in human subjects are more controversial. Radiolabeled oxalate studies[445,446] have demonstrated net oxalate secretion, whereas endogenous renal oxalate clearance assessments[447,448] using direct measurements of serum and urine oxalate levels have demonstrated net reabsorption. However, renal secretion of oxalate with high fractional excretion has been reported in patients with primary or enteric hyperoxaluria.[446–448]

In the renal proximal tubule, both reabsorption and secretion of oxalate have been shown.[449,450] Slc26a6 is expressed in the apical membrane of the proximal renal tubule and modulates the activity of multiple other apical anion exchangers.[451,452] However, the physiologic role of this anion exchanger in renal oxalate handling has not yet been fully demonstrated. In the *Slc26a6* null mice, the hyperoxaluria appears to be driven mostly by hyperoxalemia rather than by a renal leak of oxalate.[428]

## Clinical Hyperoxaluria

PH typically presents during early childhood with calcium oxalate stones and nephrocalcinosis. This disease is severe and is associated with frequent stone recurrence and impaired

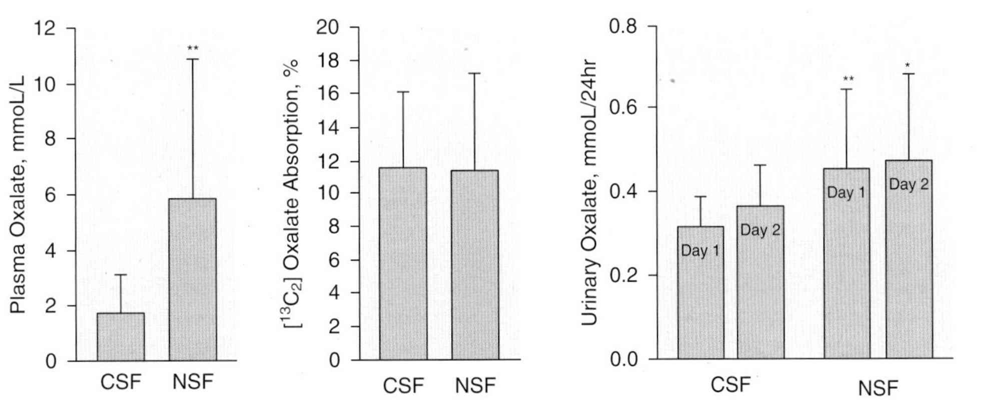


**Fig. 38.17** Impact of *Oxalobacter formigenes* on oxalate balance in stone formers. Shown is the plasma oxalate concentration, urine oxalate excretion rate, and intestinal oxalate absorption using $^{13}C_2$-labeled oxalate in *O. formigenes*-colonized stone formers *(CSF)* and noncolonized patients *(NSF)*. (From Siener R, Bangen U, Sidhu H, et al. The role of Oxalobacter formigenes colonization in calcium oxalate stone disease. *Kidney Int.* 2013;83[6]:1144–1149.)

kidney function.[453] From 1985 to 1992, the estimated prevalence of PH was reported to be 1 to 3 cases/million population, a calculated incidence rate of 1/120,000/year.[454,455] Furthermore, end-stage kidney disease (ESKD) as a result of PH has been demonstrated to occur in up to 10% of children.[456,457] Occasionally, milder forms of PH are found in adult subjects.

Enteric hyperoxaluria because of inflammatory bowel disease, jejunoileal bypass, and modern bariatric surgeries for morbid obesity are the most common cause of hyperoxaluria in the clinical practice.[458–463] Roux-en-Y gastric bypass (RYGB) is a weight reduction procedure theoretically combining restrictive and malabsorptive mechanisms for the treatment of obesity. Urolithiasis is is well-known complication of subjects who underwent RYGB. A comparison in 4690 patients following RYGB and an obese control group has shown 7.5% of kidney stones in RYGB patients compared with 4.6% in obese controls. The result of this study was confirmed by another cross-sectional study of 762 patients following bariatric surgery (mostly RYGB) matched with obese controls who did not undergo surgery.[464] Even though the prevelance of kidney stones was similar between the two populations at baseline, following RYGB, the incidence of nephrolithiasis increased to 11% compared with 4% at follow-up in obese non–stone-formers. Another retrospective cohort with 972 RYGB patients has shown an 8.8% stone prevelance before surgery, whereas 3.2% developed new stones postoperatively.[465] The pathophysiologic mechanisms for lithogenesis are complex and variable and may be because of hyperoxaluria, hypocitraturia, aciduria, and low urinary volume[392,393,466–474] (Table 38.3). A national insurance claim database from 2002 to 2006 supported the notion that gastric banding is not associated with increased kidney stone risk. After gastric banding, 1.49% of subjects formed stones compared with 5.97% in obese controls.[475]

The underlying mechanisms for hyperoxaluria following inflammatory bowel disease and bariatric procedures is not yet fully defined. Purported mechanisms have linked hyperoxaluria to intestinal fat malabsorption.[471,476] In this model, unabsorbed fatty acids sequester calcium, which would

**Table 38.3 Kidney Stone Risk Profiles Following Roux-en-Y Gastric Bypass Surgery**

| Parameter | Before RYGB | Following RYGB | Reference |
|---|---|---|---|
| Urinary oxalate (mg/day) | N/A | 79 | Nelson[466] |
| | 31 ± 16 | 65 ± 39[a] | Sinha[392] |
| | N/A | 85 ± 44[a] | Asplin[393] |
| | 31 ± 10 | 41 ± 18[a] | Duffey[468] |
| | N/A | 48 ± 4 | Penniston[472] |
| | 32 (median) | 40 (median)[a] | Park[467] |
| | N/A | 45 ± 21[a] | Maalouf[408] |
| | N/A | 61 ± 4[a] | Patel[470] |
| | 26 ± 13 | 32 ± 11 (NS) | Kumar[471] |
| | N/A | 26 (median; NS) | Froeder[473] |
| Urinary citrate (mg/day) | 660 ± 297 | 444 ± 376 (NS) | Sinha[392] |
| | N/A | 477 ± 330[a] | Asplin[393] |
| | N/A | 441 ± 71[a] | Penniston[472] |
| | 675 (median) | 456 (median)[a] | Park[467] |
| | N/A | 358 ± 357[a] | Maalouf[408] |
| | N/A | 621 ± 40[a] | Patel[470] |
| | N/A | 472 (median; NS) | Froeder[473] |
| Urinary pH | N/A | 5.72 ± 0.31[a] | Asplin[393] |
| | 5.96 ± 0.38 | 5.78 ± 0.59 (NS) | Sinha[392] |
| | 5.82 ± 0.54 | 5.66 ± 0.43 (NS) | Duffey[468] |
| | 6.03 (median) | 5.75 (median; NS) | Park[467] |
| | N/A | 5.78 (median; NS) | Froeder[473] |
| Urinary volume (mL/day) | 1380 ± 400 | 900 ± 430[a] | Duffey[468] |
| | 1800 (median) | 1440[a] | Park[467] |
| | N/A | 1900 ± 900 (NS) | Maalouf[408] |
| | 2091 ± 768 | 1316 ± 540[a] | Kumar[471] |
| | N/A | 1140[a] | Froeder[473] |
| Urinary calcium (mg/day) | 206 ± 111 | 112 ± 92[a] | Sinha[392] |
| | N/A | 141 ± 61[a] | Asplin[393] |
| | 206 ± 111 | 112 ± 92[a] | Duffey[468] |
| | 161 ± 22 | 92 ± 15[a] | Fleischer[474] |
| | N/A | 100 ± 12[a] | Penniston[472] |
| | 176 (median) | 135[a] (median) | Park[467] |
| | N/A | 115 ± 93[a] | Maalouf[408] |
| | N/A | 89[a] (median) | Froeder[473] |

[a]Significant compared with control.
*N/A*, Not available; *NS*, statistically nonsignificant; RYGB, Roux-en-Y gastric bypass.

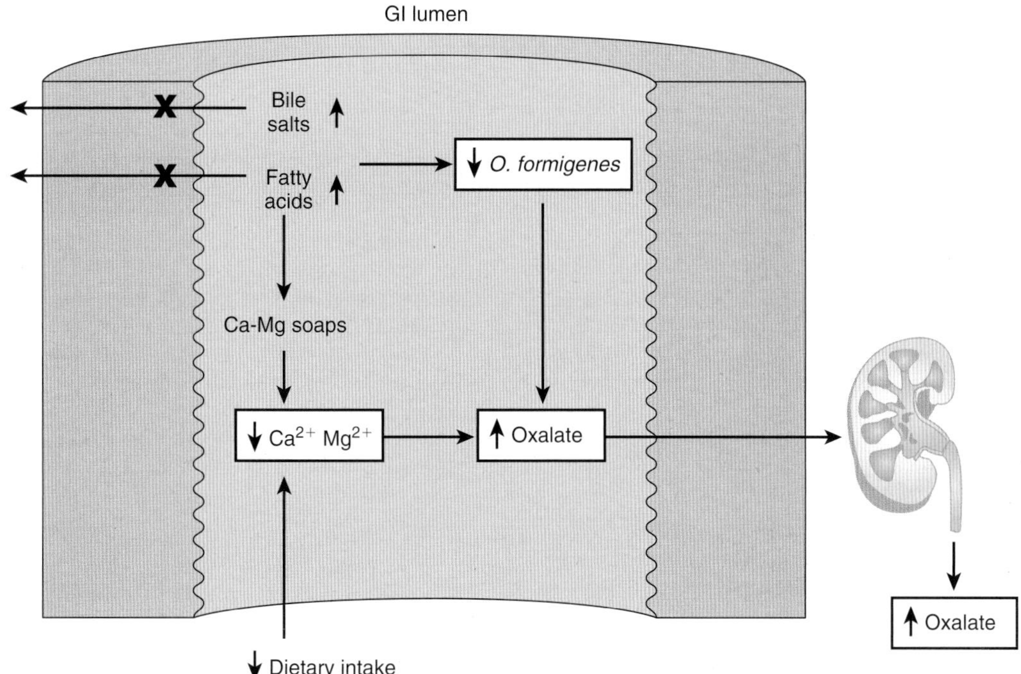


**Fig. 38.18** Pathophysiologic mechanisms of hyperoxaluria in inflammatory bowel disease or following bariatric surgery. Fatty acids and bile salts precipitate luminal calcium, which can be compounded by low dietary intake. Low luminal calcium frees up and increases unbound oxalate. Lack of *Oxalobacter formigenes* because of excess bile salts also contributes to high luminal oxalate levels. *GI,* Gastrointestinal.

otherwise bind oxalate in the intestinal lumen, and thereby increase free luminal concentrations of oxalate, enhancing its availability for absorption. An additional mechanism may involve increased permeability of the colon from exposure to unconjugated bile acids and long-chain fatty acids in both inflammatory bowel disease and bariatric procedures[410,477] (Fig. 38.18). Finally, it was proposed that changes in intestinal microbiota may occur in patients with recurrent CaOx nephrolithiasis,[439,478,479] enteric hyperoxaluria,[480,481] and cystic fibrosis,[441,482] all of which are conditions that can potentially modify the colonization of lower intestinal flora with respect to OF.[441,482]

Hyperoxaluria can develop early or late after bariatric surgery. The timing varies depending on the type of surgical procedure and nutritional and health status of the subjects.[468,469] In one study following RYGB,[464] urinary oxalate levels increased over time, with a more significant rise in those who developed kidney stones. CaOx supersaturation was found to be highest in those patients who developed kidney stones. As a result, the incidence of CaOx stones following RYGB increased but the incidence of stones with hydroxyapatite, struvite, and uric acid did not change.

### Physicochemical Effects of Hyperoxaluria

Oxalate and calcium are both important in raising calcium oxalate supersaturation in urine.[404] In human serum, the oxalate concentration is 1 to 5 μM but its concentration in the urine is 100 times higher than that of serum.[483] At physiologic pH, oxalate forms an insoluble salt with calcium. Normal urine is usually supersaturated with calcium oxalate; the solubility of CaOx in an aqueous solution is approximately 57 μM at a pH of 7. Considering that normal urine volume is between 1 and 2 L/day, normal urinary excretion is <45 μmol/day. In most cases, normal urine is supersaturated with CaOx salt but blood is undersaturated. Nevertheless, in patients with PH and renal insufficiency, when the serum oxalate concentration rises above 30 μm, the blood also becomes supersaturated with CaOx.[484]

## ALTERATIONS OF URINARY PH

Both highly acidic (≤5.5) and highly alkaline (≥6.7) urine increase the propensity for calcium kidney stone formation. With unduly acidic urinary pH, urine becomes supersaturated with undissociated uric acid that can contribute to CaOx crystallization.[102,485] Highly alkaline urine increases the abundance of monohydrogen phosphate (dissociation constant $pK_a \approx 6.7$), which, in combination with calcium, transforms to thermodynamically unstable brushite ($CaHPO_4 2H_2O$) and, finally to hydroxyapatite, $Ca_{10}(PO_4)_6(OH)_2$. Over the past 4 decades, the average CaP content of stones has progressively increased.[76]

The rise in the prevalence of CaP stones has been attributed to but not proven to be as a result of extracorporeal shock wave lithotripsy (ESWL), increasing use of medications including topiramate, and alkali therapy.[20,224,486,487] The three main risk factors for the development of brushite stone are alkaline urine, hypercalciuria, and hypocitraturia (Fig. 38.19). It has been suggested that urinary pH elevation plays the most important role in the transformation of CaOx to CaP stones. A retrospective study of 62 patients has found that high urinary pH is the primary physiologic abnormality in those who evolved from CaOx to CaP.[76] Defective renal acidification was proposed to be related to renal tissue damage from ESWL.[20] Patients with CaP stones usually carry a greater stone burden and are less likely to be stone-free after urologic

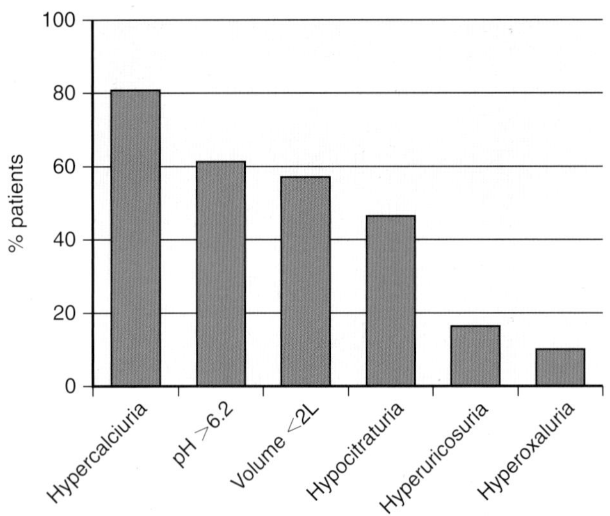


**Fig. 38.19** Urinary stone risk profiles in 82 brushite kidney stone formers. (Modified from Krambeck AE, Handa SE, Evan AP, Lingeman JE. Brushite stone disease as a consequence of lithotripsy? *Urol Res.* 2010;38[4]:293–299.)

**Table 38.4 Causes and Mechanisms for Uric Acid Nephrolithiasis**

| Causative Factors | Low Urine Volume | Low Urinary pH | Hyperuricosuria |
|---|---|---|---|
| **Acquired** | | | |
| • Diarrhea | + | + | + |
| • Myeloproliferative | | | + |
| • High animal protein | | + | + |
| • Uricosuric drugs | | | + |
| • Primary gout | | + | + |
| • Metabolic syndrome | | + | |
| **Congenital** | | | |
| • Enzyme disorders of purine metabolism | | | + |
| • Mutations in uric acid transporters | | | + |

procedures; they also experience resistance to ESWL and ultrasonic lithotripsy.[488–490]

## URIC ACID STONES

Higher primates have higher serum and urinary UA levels because of lack of the enzyme uricase, which transforms UA into more soluble allantoin.[355,356,491] Uricase deficiency is partially compensated by repression of xanthine oxidase[492] but the high serum UA level is also because of low renal fractional excretion of UA.[356] The principal sources of UA production are de novo synthesis, tissue catabolism, and dietary purine load.[350] Generally, 50% of the typical daily urate load is provided by de novo synthesis and tissue catabolism, with the remainder originating from dietary purines.[350] About 30% of synthesized UA is excreted through the intestinal tract, where it undergoes uricolysis, and the remainder by the kidney.[352]

The cause of uric acid nephrolithiasis can be genetic[355,493,494] or acquired,[390,395,495] with the metabolic syndrome being the principal cause (Table 38.4). The primary pathophysiologic mechanisms accounting for UA nephrolithiasis include hyperuricosuria, and low urinary volume; the most important contributor is an unduly low urinary pH.

### PHYSICOCHEMISTRY OF URIC ACID

Given that UA solubility in a urinary environment is limited to about 96 mg/L, and UA excretion in humans typically exceed 600 mg/day, the risk of UA precipitation is constant.[222,401] Uric acid has a $pK_a$ of 5.35 at 37°C,[496,497] so UA solubility is determined primarily by pH in that acidic urine (pH ≤5.5) titrates urate to UA, which is sparingly soluble and therefore precipitates.[401,498,499] This may also indirectly induce mixed UA-CaOx nephrolithiasis, which can be mediated through heterogeneous nucleation and epitaxial crystal growth.[104,500,501] Generally, urine is metastably supersaturated with respect to UA. This suggests that the absence of an inhibitor may influence the propensity for UA nephrolithiasis; this has been supported by experimental evidence demonstrating the presence of macromolecules that attenuate UA crystal adherence to renal tubular epithelium.[502]

### PATHOPHYSIOLOGY OF URIC ACID STONES

#### Hyperuricosuria

Hyperuricosuria may be caused by genetic, metabolic, or dietary factors.[43] Hyperuricosuria is seen in rare hereditary disorders with mutations in enzymatic pathways responsible for UA production. These conditions include X-linked phosphoribosyl synthetase overactivity, autosomal recessive glucose-6-phosphatase deficiency, and glycogenosis types III, V, and VII.[43,355,494] The clinical presentations include gout, kidney stones, and even ESKD. Biochemical abnormalities include a highly elevated serum UA concentration (≥10 mg/dL) and urinary UA excretion of 1000 mg/day or higher. The disease manifestations commonly present during childhood; however, they may remain silent until puberty.

Renal handling of UA is complex and involves secretion and reabsorption.[356] Inactivating mutation of the urate transporter, URAT1, causes renal uric acid wasting, resulting in hyperuricosuria, hypouricemia, UA kidney stones, and exercise-induced acute renal failure.[503,504] In addition, in the Sardinian population, a putative gene locus localized on chromosome 10q122 has been linked to UA nephrolithiasis. The putative culprit gene codes for a hypothetic protein with zinc finger motifs, ZNF365, of unknown function.[505]

Hyperuricosuria may also occur with excessive tissue breakdown in malignancy, especially during chemotherapy.[506,507] Certain uricosuric drugs such as high-dose salicylates, probenecid, radiocontrast agents, and losartan have been shown to increase UA excretion, which may increase the risk of UA stone formation.[497,508] In the large majority of cases of UA stones, there are no identifiable congenital or acquired causes of hyperuricosuria.

### Low Urinary Volume

Low urinary volume increases the urinary supersaturation of all stone-forming constituents.[509] Volume depletion from chronic diarrhea in inflammatory bowel disease has an impact on UA stone formation. In addition, UA stones comprise up to two-thirds of all stones in patients following ileostomy.[510] In this population, low urinary volume, in addition to the aciduria from intestinal alkali loss, is common.[511–513]

### Low Urinary pH

In the large majority of cases, hyperuricosuria or low urine volume are not the culprits. Rather, the lithogenesis is driven by a low urine pH. This is collectively called, by default, idiopathic uric acid nephrolithiasis (IUAN). The necessary requirement is unduly acidic urine, which is the single invariant feature in all patients with IUAN[47,401,514] (Fig. 38.20).

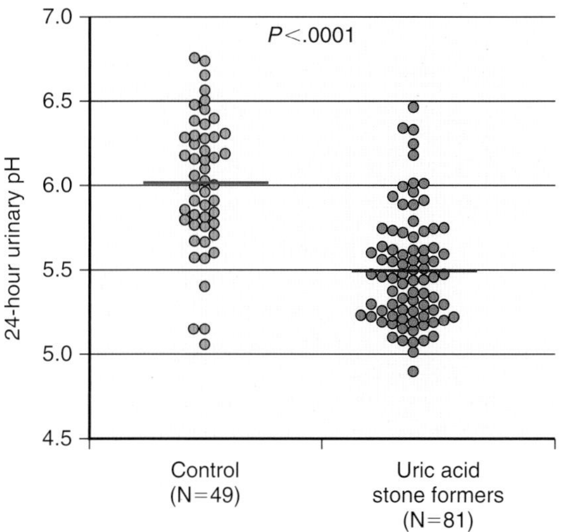


**Fig. 38.20** Shown is 24-hour urine pH in idiopathic uric acid nephrolithiasis versus control subject. Urine was collected under a fixed metabolic diet. Comparison was by an unpaired t-test.

## ORIGIN OF LOW URINARY PH

IUAN is the stone type that shares numerous common characteristics with the metabolic syndrome.[49,493,515,516] Several cross-sectional studies have supported the association between UA stones, diabetes, and obesity[48,50,51,517–520] (Fig. 38.21). Over the past 1.5 decades, two major causative factors, increased acid load to the kidneys and impaired ammonium ($NH_4^+$) excretion, have been shown to result in unduly acidic urine.[47,401]

### Increased Acid Load to Kidneys

In a steady state, net acid excretion (NAE) equals net acid production. Higher NAE can occur as a consequence of increased endogenous production, increased dietary ingestion (high dietary acid consumption or low alkali intake), or alkali loss.[521] Several metabolic studies of a constant controlled metabolic diet have shown that NAE is higher in IUAN patients and type 2 diabetics without stones compared with control subjects,[47,515,516,522–524] suggesting that endogenous acid production is elevated (Fig. 38.22). The nature and source of these putative organic acids is unknown at present but likely has an enterohepatic origin.[525] Adults with type 2 diabetes without kidney stones have similar features to those with UA stones and similar differences in gut microbiota compared with nondiabetic adults.[526]

### Impaired $NH_4^+$ Excretion

Under normal physiologic circumstances, $NH_4^+$ excretion plays a key role in the regulation of acid-base balance as a result of its high $pK_a$, of 9.3 ($NH_3/NH_4^+$ system). $NH_4^+$ can effectively buffer a major portion of secreted $H^+$ as a result of its high capacity and high $pK_a$.[527,528] The alternative source of buffering is by many $H^+$ acceptors, which are collectively referred to as titratable acid (TA).[527] In IUAN, there is defective $NH_4^+$ production and excretion (Fig. 38.23). More $H^+$ is buffered by TA (including urate) to maintain acid-base homeostasis.[47,401,516] The tradeoff is propensity for UA precipitation.[47,514] The defective $NH_4^+$ excretion in IUAN occurs at a steady state while the patient is on a fixed metabolic diet, as

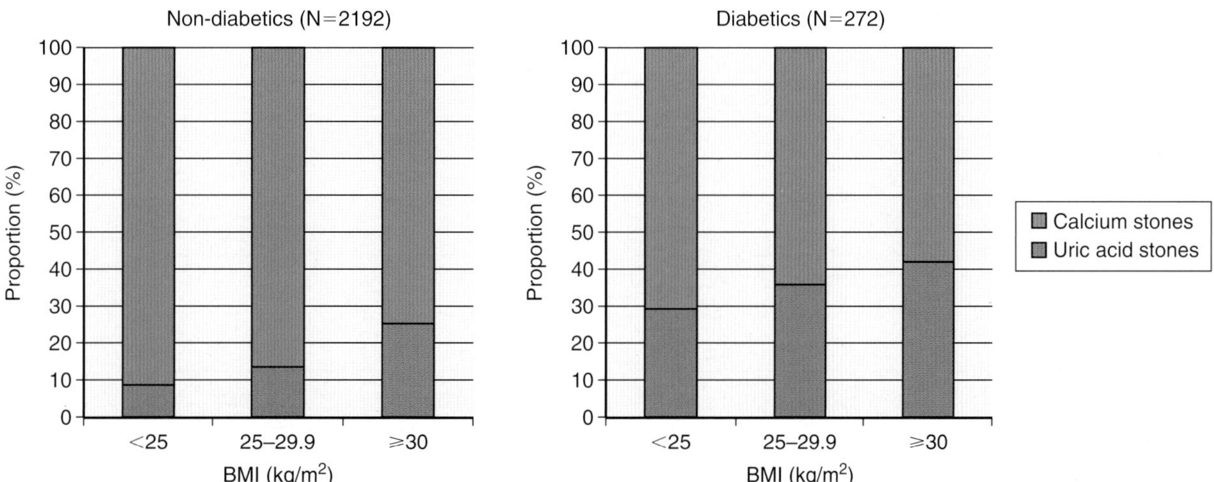


**Fig. 38.21** Distribution of stone type with respect to body mass index *(BMI)* and diabetes status. (Based on data from Daudon M, Traxer O, Conort P, et al. Type 2 diabetes increases the risk for uric acid stones. *J Am Soc Nephrol.* 2006;17[7]:2026–2033.)

well as after acute acid loads.[47] Defective $NH_4^+$ excretion is not unique to UA stone formers but remains a shared feature between metabolic syndrome and type 2 diabetic non–stone formers (Fig. 38.23).[49,493,516,520]

### Role of Renal Lipotoxicity

Most urinary $NH_4^+$ is produced and secreted by the renal proximal tubular cell.[529,530] $NH_4^+$ is directly transported by a sodium hydrogen exchanger (NHE3) as $Na^+/NH_4^+$ into the proximal tubular lumen or by nonionic diffusion of $NH_3$ into the renal proximal tubular lumen, trapped as $NH_4^+$ by luminal $H^+$ secretion by NHE3.[529–535] When energy intake exceeds utilization, as occurs in patients with IUAN, obesity, diabetes, and metabolic syndrome, fat accumulates, and this can occur in nonadipose tissues[536] (Fig. 38.24). Ectopic fat is termed *steatosis*, and the ill effect of steatosis is termed *lipotoxicity*,[536,540–544] which is the consequence of the accumulation of toxic metabolites such acyl coenzyme A, diacylglycerol, and ceramide.[545–547] In a rodent model of the metabolic syndrome, the Zucker diabetic fatty (ZDF) rat,[548] as well as in cultured proximal tubular cells, steatosis led to deranged ammoniagenesis and transport.[537] ZDF rats have higher renal cortical triglyceride content commensurate with lower urinary $NH_4^+$ and pH[537] (see Fig. 38.24). Similar findings were also seen in humans with a high BMI.[538] Kidney cell lines incubated with a mixture of long-chain fatty acids have a decrease in $NH_4^+$ production.[537] Treatment of ZDF rats with thiazolidinediones or removal of fatty acids from cultured cells reduced renal steatosis and restored acid-base parameters toward normal, demonstrating causality (see Fig. 38.24).[539] Another potential mechanism in UA stone formers and/or in ZDF rats is defective $NH_4^+$ synthesis because of substrate competition—namely, fatty acid instead of glutamine as a source of energy—thus removing the source of nitrogen for ammoniagenesis.[549]

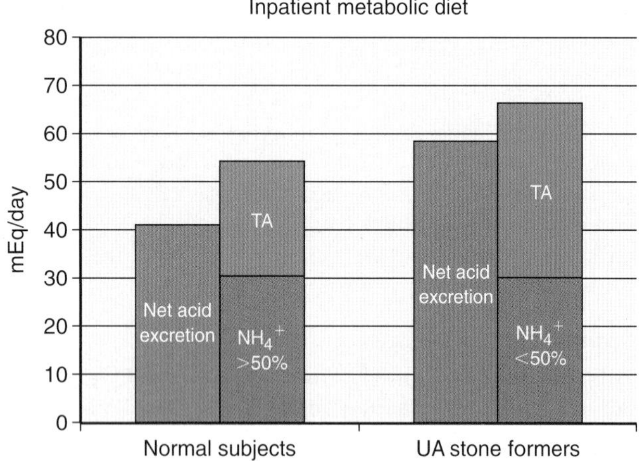


**Fig. 38.22** Comparison of net acid excretion between normal subjects and uric acid *(UA)* stone formers. Studies were performed with a controlled metabolic diet. Despite equivalent amounts of exogenous acid intake (same urinary sulfate excretion, not shown), uric acid stone formers were found to have higher net acid excretion, and a lower fraction of the net acid was carried by ammonium. *TA,* titratable acid. (Adapted from data from references 516, 523, and 524.)

## CYSTINE STONES

### OVERVIEW

Cystine stones are exclusively seen in cystinuria, which is a hereditary mendelian disorder of a heterogenous nature caused by inactivating mutations of the subunits of a dibasic amino acid transporter in the proximal tubule's rBAT or $b^{0,+}AT$ (SLC3A1 or SLC7A9—heavy and light chain, respectively); this is equivalent to the system $b^{0,+}$ of amino transport (see Chapter 8; Fig. 38.25). Cystinuria is the most common primary inherited aminoaciduria (OMIM 220100). There are no systemic symptoms of amino acid deficiency in this disorder, but it causes 1% to 2% of renal stones in adults and 6% to 8% in pediatric patients.[550] Normally, reabsorption of amino acids from the urine is almost complete. Inactivation

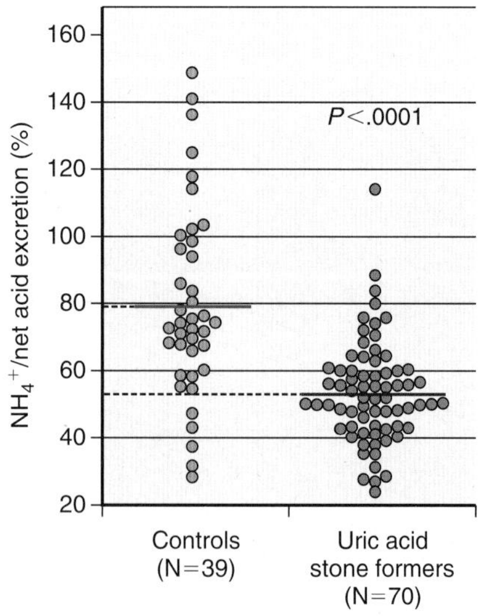


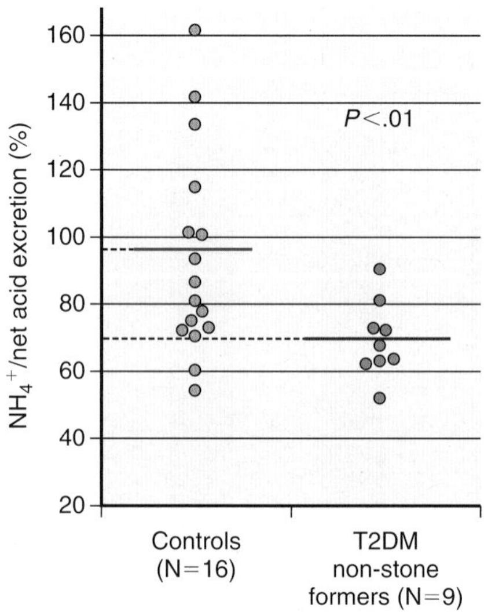


**Fig. 38.23** Decreased ammonium excretion as a fraction of net acid excretion in idiopathic uric acid stone formers and in subjects with type 2 diabetes (T2DM) without stones. Individuals were studied under controlled metabolic diet so all differences are intrinsic to the subjects. (From Maalouf NM, Cameron MA, Moe OW, Sakhaee K. Metabolic basis for low urine pH in type 2 diabetes. *Clin J Am Soc Nephrol.* 2010;5[7]:1277–1281.)

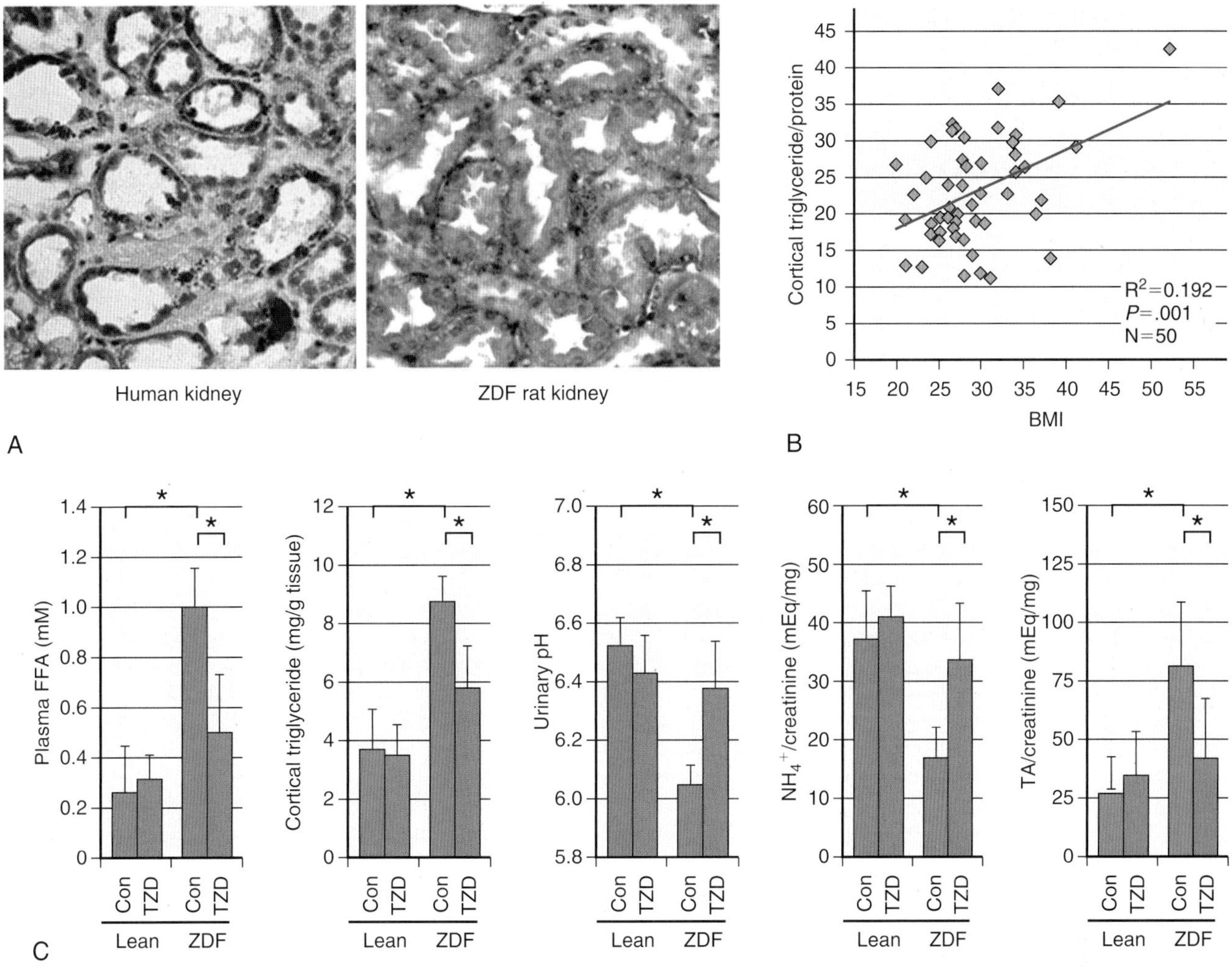

**Fig. 38.24** Renal steatosis and lipotoxicity in humans and rats. (A) Oil red O stain of triglyceride in human kidney from an obese individual and the Zucker diabetic fatty *(ZDF)* rat. (B) Cortical triglyceride content in human biopsy samples showing the relationship between triglyceride and body mass index *(BMI)*. (C) Lean rats or ZDF rats were treated with vehicle control, *(Con)*, or rosiglitazone thiazolidinedione *(TZD)*. A number of parameters were compared among the four groups. The amelioration of plasma free fatty acids *(FFAs)* and renal cortical triglycerides was accompanied by an increase in urine pH and ammonium excretion, whereas titratable acid *(TA)* excretion was decreased. (Adapted from references 537 to 539.)

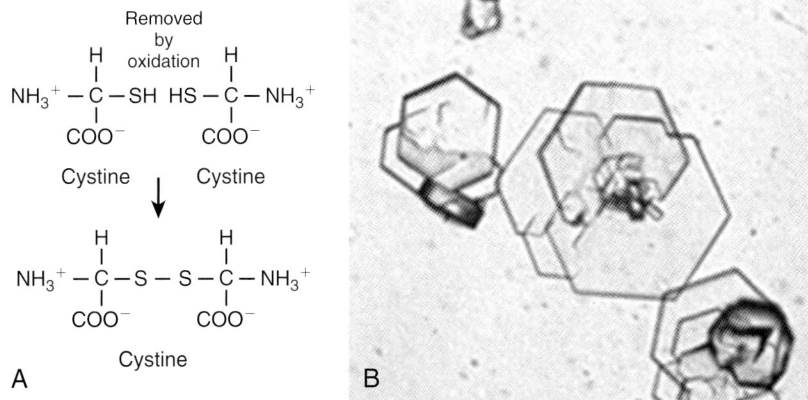


**Fig. 38.25** (A) Cystine is a dimer of cysteine formed by disulfide bonding under oxidizing conditions. (B) Appearance of cystine crystals in the urine of a patient with cystinuria.

of rBAT/$b^{0,+}$AT leads to urinary wasting of many cationic amino acids but only cystine has a low enough solubility to precipitate. Because rBAT/$b^{0,+}$AT is also present in the gut, there is some malabsorption of cationic amino acids but there is no clinically discernible intestinal phenotype.

## MOLECULAR BIOLOGY AND GENETICS

The rBAT and $b^{0,+}$AT subunits are linked by a disulfide bridge in the heterodimer, which is characteristic of the heteromeric amino acid transporters[551] and mediates obligatory exchange of cationic amino acids, (e.g., cystine = two cysteines bound by a disulfide bridge) and neutral amino acids with 1:1 stoichiometry (see Chapter 8). In addition to human disease, the causal link between rBAT/$b^{0,+}$AT and cationic aminoaciduria has been corroborated by mouse experimental models with defective rBAT (D140G mutation)[552] or $b^{0,+}$AT (knockout),[553] and by Newfoundland dogs with defective rBAT (naturally occurring nonsense mutation),[554] all of which have cystinuria similar to that in humans.

Over 130 human mutations in rBAT (*SLC3A1*; cystinuria type A) and 100 mutations in $b^{0,+}$AT (*SLC7A9*; cystinuria type B) have been identified, including missense, nonsense, splice site, frame shift, and large chromosomal rearrangements[550] in around 90% of the subjects studied. In around 3% of patients with clinical cystinuria, there are no mutations in the two candidate loci. These may be as a result of mutations in promoter, regulatory, or intronic regions. It is believed that all cases of classic and isolated cystinuria are as a result of mutations in system $b^{0+}$.

Interestingly, haplotypes with $b^{0,+}$AT polymorphisms have been reported in cystinuria and some $b^{0,+}$AT heterozygotes who are cystine stone formers.[555,556] Isolated cystinuria (cystine wasting without cationic aminoaciduria) can be caused by a heterozygous $b^{0,+}$AT mutation.[556–558] The molecular biology is in accordance with metabolic data. System $b^{0,+}$ (rBAT/$b^{0,+}$AT) is the principal transport system for cystine reabsorption in the proximal tubule. Cystine clearance approximates the GFR (glomerular filtration rate; i.e., no reabsorption) in classic cystinuria.[559] In contrast, clearance of cationic amino acids is only partly affected (GFR = 40–60 mL/min × 1.73 $m^2$) in cystinuria,[560] suggesting that other apical transport systems participate in the renal reabsorption of these amino acids.

## CLINICAL PRESENTATION

Cystine was discovered in the urine of a patient with bladder stones by Wollaston in 1810.[561] The prevalence is reported to be highest in individuals of Libyan-Jewish descent (1:2500). A history of consanguinity may or may not be present because compound heterozygotes can come from seemingly unrelated partners. Patients present with hematuria, renal colic, and urinary obstruction, although their symptoms tend to be more severe and more likely to have staghorn, surgery, and chronic kidney disease (CKD).[562] The age of onset varies widely but probably 50% of patients present to pediatricians.[563] The historical type I versus type II classification is now replaced by type A (mutations in both alleles of *SLC3A1*; genotype AA) and type B (mutations in both alleles of *SLC7A9*; genotype BB).[564] Uncommon digenic (*SLC3A1* and *ALC7A9*) inheritance (type AB) has also been described, but individuals with this pattern are less likely to suffer from kidney stones because they have a 25% chance of having a completely wild-type $b^{0+}$ system.

Urinary cystine quantification is not routinely performed in all stone formers. The features that raise suspicions are family history of cystinuria, staghorn calculi, positive non-quantitative screening test with sodium nitroprusside (>75 mg/L; 0.325 mM), and the presence of pathognomonic hexagonal cystine crystals on urinalysis (Fig. 38.25).

Quantitation of urinary cystine excretion (normal, <30 mg/day; 0.13 mmol/day) is mandatory to diagnose cystinuria. Patients with cystinuria often excrete more than 400 mg/day (1.7 mmol/day). Poor cystine solubility and precipitation can lead to misleadingly low results, so alkalinization of collected urine is often required.[565] One caveat is the inability of current assays to distinguish cystine from soluble adducted drug-cysteine complexes. Ex vivo disintegrated thiol cysteine can self-recombine to form dimeric cystine. These problems have led to the development of a solid-phase assay, which is reliable even in the presence of thiol drugs.[566] One form of physicochemical assay similar to that for calcium stones is potentially useful to empirically measure the propensity for cystine stone formation.[566]

## MANAGEMENT

Fluid, alkali, and dietary modification (salt and protein) are first-line therapies, with thiol therapy as second line. To reduce urine cystine supersaturation to less than 1.0, or concentration less than 243 mg/L (1 mmol/L) requires drinking around 4 L/day of fluids, including nocturnal intake.[567] Off-label use of a vasopressin receptor antagonist has been proposed to induce pharmacologic diabetes insipidus,[568] but the long-term effects of this drug has not been evaluated, and the cost is prohibitive. In conjunction with the safe and easily available water, it is unclear whether there is an advantage to this therapy.

Cystine excretion has been shown to be reduced by decreasing dietary sodium, although no clinical outcome studies have been performed.[569] The physiology of this effect is not known but the use of the $b^{0,+}$ system for L-DOPA (levodopa) uptake to synthesize nephrogenic dopamine is a possibility,[570] so in a high-salt diet, the $b^{0,+}$ system may be occupied with dopamine synthesis. In the absence of ill effects of salt restriction, it is reasonable to prescribe restricting salt intake to about 2 g/day. Reduction of animal protein has also been proposed because of the reduction of dietary cystine, and its precursor methionine may reduce cystine excretion,[571] and the associated increase in urinary pH (UpH).

### Pharmacologic Therapy

Cystine solubility increases with increasing pH, which is achieved with oral potassium citrate. (This is discussed in the section on alkali therapy of kidney stones.) One can start with 20 mEq bid, which may or may not be sufficient based on periodic UpH testing. In over 50% of patients, the previously mentioned measures are unlikely to suffice, and treatment with a thiol agent is indicated. The two available agents are D-penicillamine and alpha-mercaptopropionylglycine, or tiopronin. These drugs work by reducing the disulfide bond of cystine, producing mixed compounds with cysteine, which are all more soluble than cystine.[572] The incidence of adverse effects is lower with tiopronin, thus rendering it as a first-line agent. D-Penicillamine is often used for patients with adverse reactions to tiopronin. The prescription of these drugs is discussed in more detail in a subsequent section.

## INFECTION STONES

### PATHOPHYSIOLOGY

This category of stones does not form because of intrinsic host defects but because of an infected urinary environment. Struvite ($MgNH_4PO_4 \cdot 6H_2O$) stones account for a low percentage of all kidney stones and often also contain carbonate apatite, $Ca_{10}(PO_4)_6 \cdot CO_3$. These stones are rapidly growing, branch, and enlarge and fill the renal collecting system to form staghorns. The key culprits are urea-splitting bacteria. These stones are difficult to treat medically. Even with surgical removal, any remaining fragments containing the infecting bacteria furnish a nidus for further rapid stone growth. The nature of these stones to grow rapidly, recur, and cause morbidity and mortality has led to the appellation *stone cancer.*

Struvite stones occur more frequently in women than in men, largely because of the higher incidence of urinary tract infections. Chronic urinary stasis or infections predispose to struvite stones so that old age, neurogenic bladder, indwelling urinary catheters, and urinary tract anatomic abnormalities are all predisposing factors. The presence of large stones in infected alkaline urine should alert the clinician to the potential presence of struvite. Given their potential for rapid growth and substantial morbidity, early detection and eradication are essential.[573,574]

The urease of urea-splitting organisms hydrolyzes the following reactions:

$$(H_2N)_2\text{-}C = O + H_2O \rightarrow 2NH_4^+ + HCO_3^- + OH^- \quad [38.1]$$

$$(H_2N)_2\text{-}C = O + H_2O + CO_2 \rightarrow 2NH_4^+ + 2HCO_3^- \quad [38.2]$$

Urea contains two nitrogens and one carbon. On the product (right-hand) side of the equation, $2NH_4^+$ represents two acid equivalents, and either $HCO_3^-$ plus $OH^-$ or $2HCO_3^-$ represents two base equivalents. The phosphate and magnesium combines with the $NH_4^+$ to form struvite, and the calcium and phosphate combine with the carbonate to form carbonate apatite. Ammonium can bind to the sulfates on the GAGs on the urothelium,[575] impair the hydrophilic activity of the GAGs, and increase crystal adhesion. During infections with urease-producing organisms, there is a simultaneous elevation in urine $NH_4^+$, pH, and carbonate concentration. With successful antimicrobial treatment of the underlying infection, the struvite can actually dissolve because the urine is generally undersaturated with respect to struvite.[576,577] However, urine is not undersaturated with respect to carbonate apatite,[577] so successful antimicrobial therapy is not expected to dissolve this component of the stone. Whether a stone will dissolve with prolonged antibiotic is dependent on the amount of carbonate apatite.

Although many bacteria (gram-negative and gram-positive), *Mycoplasma,* and yeast species can produce urease, most urease-producing infections are caused by *Proteus mirabilis.* In addition, *Haemophilus, Corynebacterium,* and *Ureaplasma* have been identified to cause struvite stones. All these bacteria use urease to split urea and supply their need for nitrogen (in the form of $NH_3$). Colony counts may be low, so the laboratory should be instructed to identify any bacteria and determine sensitivities, no matter how low the number of colony-forming units. If routine urinary cultures are negative but a urease producer is suspected, the laboratory should be specifically instructed to culture for *Mycobacterium* and *Ureaplasma urealyticum,* which are also urease-positive.[575]

## UNCOMMON STONES

Rare kidney stone disease can be genetic or acquired. Among the genetic diseases, the most common types are xanthine stones and 2,8-dihydroxyadenine stones. Acquired causes may be iatrogenic with the use of medications or caused by toxins or other diseases.

### GENETIC CAUSES

2, 8-Dihydroxyadenine (DHA) stone is characterized by excessive production and urinary excretion of DHA as a consequence of adenine phosphoribosyl transferase deficiency (APRT), which is inherited as an autosomal recessive disorder (OMIM, 102600). In subjects with impaired APRT, adenine is converted to 8-hydroxyadenine, which is further metabolized to DHA by xanthine dehydrogenase.[578] Consequently, APRT deficiency results in high urinary levels of DHA, which is insoluble and forms crystals that aggregate, grow, and form kidney stones.[579,580] This disorder can present at any age but, in approximately 50% of subjects, symptoms do not occur until adulthood.[581] The diagnosis is made by the microscopic appearance of DHA crystals in the urine, which are pathognomonic for this disease. Typically, DHA crystals by polarized microscopy are round and reddish-brown, with a characteristic central Maltese cross pattern.[578] However, the diagnosis is established by the absence of APRT enzyme activity in red cell lysates or the identification of functionally significant mutations in *APRT.*

Xanthine stones are present in about one-third of subjects with classic xanthinuria, which is an inborn error in metabolism inherited as an autosomal recessive trait.[582,583] Hereditary xanthinuria is caused by mutations in xanthine dehydrogenase (XDH),[578] leading to the overproduction of xanthine and minimal production of uric acid. Patients have very low serum urate levels but suffer from elevated levels of xanthine in the urine, leading to xanthine stones, hematuria, and sometimes occult kidney failure.[584] Urinary excretion of xanthine and hypoxanthine are significantly increased. Xanthine stones occur more often than hypoxanthine because of the lower solubility of xanthine in urine. Xanthinuria should be suspected if a patient has significant hypouricemia and hypouricosuria in the presence of radiolucent stones.

Xanthine stones may also be acquired following allopurinol treatment in patients with significant hyperuricemia such as Lesch-Nyhan syndrome and in those undergoing chemotherapy for myeloproliferative disorders.[585,586]

### ACQUIRED CAUSES

Rare acquired kidney stones may arise from disease and also after ingesting toxins or using certain drugs with poor solubility in urinary environments.[587] Ammonium urate stones are radiolucent stones that occur in patients with chronic diarrhea, inflammatory bowel disease, ileostomy, and laxative abuse; all are associated with intestinal alkali loss and compensatory renal hyperexcretion of ammonium.[588–592] This occurs because of the relative abundance of urinary ammonium accompanied with decreased urinary sodium and potassium levels, thereby making the urine supersaturated with respect to poorly soluble ammonium urate. The catabolic state of these patients may also cause hyperuricosuria.

Consumption of over-the-counter (OTC) drugs, such as guaifenesin as an expectorant and ephedrine as a stimulant and for weight reduction, accounts for approximately one-third of the drug-induced U.S. kidney stone incidence.[593,594] After the introduction of protease inhibitors for the treatment of human immunodeficiency virus (HIV) patients, indinavir-treated patients began to show a high incidence of indinavir-associated stones.[595,596] In later years, it was shown that other antiproteases, such as nelfinavir, tenofovir, atazanavir, and antinucleosidic drugs, including efavirenz, also cause kidney stone formation.[597–600]

Other drugs such as triamterene, various antimicrobial agents, including sulfonamides, penicillin, cephalosporin, quinolones, and nitrofurantoin, as well as agents such as magnesium trisilicate, have been shown to be associated with drug-induced stones.[587]

Other environmental factors play a role in kidney stone formation. Melamine is an organic nitrogenous compound used in the industrial productions of plastics, dyes, fertilizers, and fabrics.[601] In 2008, kidney stone cases were reported in infants and children in China consuming melamine-contaminated milk.[602] A study in Taiwan screened 1129 children with potential exposure to contaminated milk formula. The results showed that those with a high exposure had an increased incidence of nephrolithiasis. The age of the group of children with kidney stones was reported to be significantly younger than those without. Metabolic workups did not disclose any evidence of hypercalciuria, and the stones were radiolucent, indicating that these stones were related to melamine ingestion.[603,604]

# GENETICS

## HUMAN GENETICS

There are a number of factors involved.

### FAMILIAL CLUSTERING

It is well accepted that a significant portion of the risk of kidney stones in humans, including its major risk factor, hypercalciuria, is hereditary in origin.[605–608] The complex polygenic trait with phenocopying, multiple loci, loci heterogeneity, and lack of intermediate phenotypes in a clinical database all render the deciphering of the genetics of hypercalciuria and kidney stones a formidable task. The familial clustering of kidney stones and of hypercalciuria has been documented for decades.[291] Despite the fact that family members share similar lifestyles, a number of studies have corrected for confounding factors and still show an increased risk of kidney stones in relatives of stone formers. This is also the anecdotal experience of most clinicians. In an epidemiologic study of more than 300,000 patient-years, adjusting for dietary factors, age, and BMI, there was a 2.6-fold higher risk of kidney stones when there was a positive family history.[609] Case-control studies with combined number of subjects in cases and controls exceeding 1000 have shown the relative risk to be two- to fourfold higher and the hereditary contribution (defined as the ratio of genetic variance to the total phenotypic variance) to be 40% to 60%.[610–613] In a segregation analysis of more than 200 stone-forming families, hypercalciuria was found to have a hereditability of 60% and to be transmitted in a polygenic fashion.[614]

### ETHNICITY

African-Americans have a lower prevalence of kidney stones than U.S. whites that cannot be accounted for by diet.[3] A longitudinal study has also shown persistently lower stone incidence in African-Americans in the 1970s through the 1990s, suggesting that the difference is intrinsic.[1] A similar difference has been noted in urinary calcium excretion, with much lower rates in blacks.[615] Values for U.S. Hispanics and Asians are intermediate between U.S. whites and blacks. In a cross-sectional, population-based study, immigrants from various ethnic backgrounds maintained the relative risk of stones of their native country, despite considerable assumption and homogenization of Western lifestyle.[616]

### HUMAN GENETIC STUDIES

#### Twin Studies

Comparison of monozygotic to dizygotic twins and/or plain siblings reared in virtually identical environments have been informative.[617,618] Goldfarb and coworkers sampled dizygotic and monozygotic twins from the Vietnam Era Twin Registry and found a concordance rate of 32% in monozygotic twins compared with 17% in dizygotic twins, an effect that cannot be explained by the documentable dietary information.[619] Other twin studies obtained urinary chemistries and found the hereditability of urinary calcium excretion rate to be around 50%.[617,618]

#### Candidate Genes

This approach is based on educated guesses of suspected loci. Studies have demonstrated an association of polymorphisms of genes along the vitamin D axis with one form of phenotypic parameter or another,[620–623] but corresponding phenotype studies have been negative.[283,284] Sib-pairs studies in French-Canadians have yielded positive results on candidate genes, including the vitamin D receptor, 1α-hydroxylase, the CaSR, and crystallization modifiers such as osteopontin, THP, and osteocalcin-related gene, but thus far no firm conclusions have been drawn.[278,624–626] Association studies in an Italian cohort have suggested that a CaSR functional polymorphism (R990G) mutation[627–629] was a possible locus. In a Swiss cohort, three nonsynonymous polymorphisms in the intestinal calcium channel, TRPPV6, were found with higher frequency in calcium stone formers. Interestingly, the contemporaneous presence of all three polymorphisms led to increased channel activity.[630]

Halbritter and associates have demonstrated the power of the candidate gene approach in a complex polygenic disease[631] by determining the percentage of cases that could be accounted for by mutations in any one of 30 known kidney stone genes. They used a high-throughput mutation analysis from multiple kidney stone clinics of 272 genetically unresolved individuals (106 children and 166 adults) from 268 families with nephrolithiasis or isolated nephrocalcinosis. In their study, 50 putative gene variants (deemed likely but not proven to be mutations) in 14 of 30 analyzed genes were detected, yielding a genetic diagnosis in 15% of all cases, with 40% previously undocumented base changes. The frequency of monogenic cases was remarkably high in both the adult (11%) and pediatric cohorts (21%). Recessive causes were more frequent among children and dominant disease more in adults. Their report showed that monogenic causes of urolithiasis are much more frequent than expected and illustrate the principle of "one who does not look will not find." One caution is that causality is still not established in these individuals.

### Genome-Wide Association Studies

To date, success using genome-wide association studies (GWAS) has been modest in regard to the identification of loci of kidney stones. A small-scale, whole-genome linkage analysis of absorptive hypercalciuria and low bone mineral density found the soluble adenylyl cyclase (sAC) as a possible locus.[632,633] Polymorphisms in this gene are also associated with BMD variation in healthy premenopausal women and men. There is a whole host of functions for the sAC protein, but one appears to be as a mediator of low bicarbonate-induced bone resorption.[634] A GWAS of >3700 cases and >42,500 controls from Iceland and the Netherlands found synonymous variants in the claudin-14 gene that were associated with kidney stones,[330] with carriers estimated to have a 1.64 times greater risk. Claudin-14 is a paracellular protein that regulates calcium transport in the renal thick ascending limb. The same variants are also associated with reduced bone mineral density.[330] From a similar Icelandic and Dutch database, another GWAS found a variant positioned next to the UMOD gene that encodes uromodulin (THP), and this variant seems to protect against kidney stones.[635] Uromodulin confers protection from kidney stones through yet unknown mechanisms.[186,636]

There is no doubt that there is a genetic component to hypercalciuria and kidney stones. However, the genes remain largely elusive after decades of study, a situation similar to that for hypertension, dyslipidemia, and diabetes mellitus. Unraveling the origins of this complex polygenic trait is a formidable challenge. Correlation of the genotype with gene product function and whole-organism physiology and pathophysiology is a critical part of this venture. The knowledge gained from monogenic diseases in humans and animals, and from polygenic animal models, is valuable in unraveling this mystery because the function and dysfunction of the gene products can be linked to physiology and pathophysiology, respectively.

## MONOGENIC CAUSES OF UROLITHIASIS

Using intermediate or endophenotypes, one can appreciate clear mendelian conditions in humans that cause hypercalciuria and a predisposition to stones. A large number of candidate loci have been identified from animal gene deletions that result in hypercalciuria. These conditions are summarized in Table 38.5. One powerful feature of mendelian diseases is that they have lesions in one gene product that allows one to connect a point of origin to a discrete phenotypic endpoint. The pathophysiologic mechanisms of hypercalciuria and/or kidney stones in these conditions are extremely diverse. This underscores the fact that defects in many organs can all converge on hypercalciuria as a phenotype. The question is whether some of these loci have alleles that contribute to the risk in the general hypercalciuric stone-forming population. It is possible that a minimal or mild form of these mutant proteins are polymorphic alleles that are more prevalent in the generation population and affect their functions only slightly but yet affect urinary stone risk. A prime example is the fact that heterozygous hypomorphic alleles of the B1 subunit of the $H^+$-ATPase can contribute to an unduly high urine pH and CaP stone risk.[652–654] Multiple loci that by themselves are each weak can then each contribute to small but yet additive effects on calciuria. This monogenic database will be most valuable in tackling the polygenic complex trait of calciuria.

## POLYGENIC ANIMAL MODEL

There are numerous animal models of monogenic stone formation.[655] However, human nephrolithiasis is clearly a polygenetic disorder, and most people with calcium-containing kidney stones are hypercalciuric.[618,656] A powerful model of polygenic hypercalciuria is the GHS rat developed by Bushinsky and coworkers and other.* After more than 90 generations of successive inbreeding of the most hypercalciuric Sprague-Dawley (SD) rats, a strain emerged with 10 times as much urinary calcium as control SD rats. GHS rats have a triple defect of increased gut absorption, renal leak, and bone resorption. The defects persisted ex vivo, with cultured bone releasing more calcium. There is an increased number of VDRs and CaSRs and an exaggerated response of VDR gene expression to $1,25(OH)_2D3$ in the intestine and kidney in GHS rats. The elevated levels of VDR are regulated by a decreased level of the transcription factor Snail.

Regions of five chromosomes—1, 4, 7, 10, 14—were linked to hypercalciuria,[660] but no specific genes have yet been identified. When normocalciuric Wistar-Kyoto rats were bred with the GHS rats to yield congenic rats with the chromosome 1 locus on the Wistar-Kyoto background, the congenic rats were also hypercalciuric but to a lesser extent than the parenteral GHS rats,[664] supporting both the importance of this locus and the polygenic nature of the hypercalciuria in the GHS rats.

# NEPHROLITHIASIS AS A SYSTEMIC DISORDER

Traditionally, kidney stone disease has been recognized as an isolated, benign, painful local condition of the urinary tract. However, the association of urolithiasis with gout and degenerative vascular disease in postmortem examinations was noted by Morgagni back in the 1760s.[665] In recent years, the prevalence of kidney stones has increased, along with the ever-expanding epidemic of obesity, T2DM, and metabolic syndrome.[10,11,666–670] Concern with metabolic syndrome and the risk for nephrolithiasis has not been limited to adults because this link was also reported in obese adolescents and the pediatric kidney stone population.[65,671] It is presently unknown whether the link between kidney stone disease and metabolic syndrome reflects the same underlying pathophysiologic mechanisms in both disorders or is simply an association.

*References 179, 298, 299, 301, 303, 305, and 657–663.

**Table 38.5 Rodent Models of Monogenic Hypercalciuria**

| Gene, Gene Product | Phenotype | Reference(s) |
|---|---|---|
| *CLC5*, chloride channel | • Hypercalciuria<br>• Hyperphosphaturia<br>• Proteinuria<br>• Increased gut calcium absorption<br>• Spinal deformities | 637–639 |
| *NPT2*, renal-I specific Na-coupled phosphate cotransporter | • Hypercalciuria<br>• Hyperphosphaturia<br>• Renal calcifications<br>• Retarded secondary ossification | 640 |
| *NHERF-1*, Na/H exchanger regulatory factor; docking protein | • Hypercalciuria<br>• Hyperphosphaturia<br>• Hypermagnesuria<br>• Female—reduced BMD and fractures | 641 |
| *TRPV5*, epithelial calcium channel | • Hypercalciuria<br>• Hyperphosphaturia<br>• Increased intestinal calcium absorption<br>• Reduced trabecular and cortical thickness of bones | 642 |
| *VDR*, vitamin D receptor | • Hypercalciuria on high-calcium and lactose diet<br>• Rickets | 643–645 |
| *CalB*, calbindin-D28k; intracellular calcium buffer | • Normocalcemia<br>• Hypercalciuria<br>• Normocalciuria | 645–648 |
| *NKCC2,* Na-K-Cl cotransporter | • Hypercalciuria<br>• Polyuria; hydronephrosis<br>• Proteinuria | 649 |
| *CAV1*, caveolin-1; scaffolding protein | • Hypercalciuria in males<br>• Bladder stone | 650 |
| *AKR1B1*, aldoketoreductase | • Hypercalciuria<br>• Hypercalcemia<br>• Hypermagnesemia | 651 |

*BMD,* Bone mineral density.

## OBESITY, WEIGHT GAIN, DIABETES MELLITUS, AND RISK FOR NEPHROLITHIASIS

A prospective epidemiologic study of over 200,000 subjects has demonstrated that obesity and weight gain increase the risk of kidney stones[10] (Fig. 38.26). The relative risk for stone formation in men with a body weight of 100 kg or more was significantly higher than men with a body weight 68 kg or less.[10]

Similarly, the relationship between T2DM and the risk of kidney stone formation was seen in three large cohorts from the Nurses' Health Study I comprising older women, the Nurses' Health Study II consisting of younger women, and the Health Professionals Follow-up Study in men. The relative risk of prevalent kidney stones in subjects with T2DM compared with those without is 1.38 in older women, 1.60 in younger women, and 1.31 in men.[11]

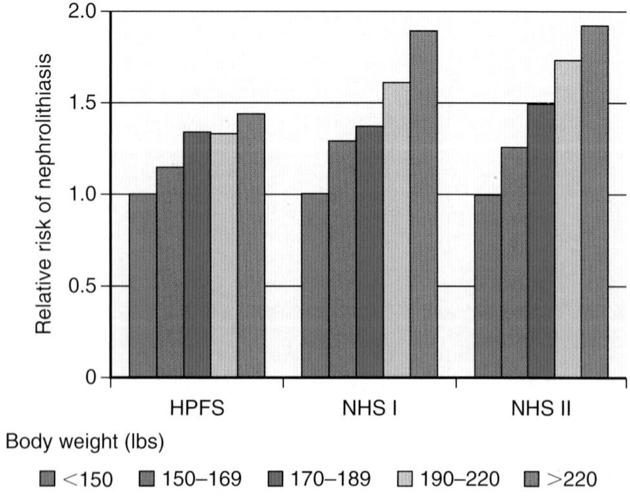


**Fig. 38.26** Obesity and the risk of nephrolithiasis. The data were pooled from three databases. *HPFS,* Health Professionals Follow-Up Study; *NHS I,* Nurses' Health Study I; *NHS II,* Nurses' Health Study II. (Modified from Sakhaee K, Maalouf NM, Sinnott B. Clinical review. Kidney stones 2012: pathogenesis, diagnosis, and management. *J Clin Endocrinol Metab.* 2012;97[6]:1847–1860.)

### ASSOCIATION BETWEEN METABOLIC SYNDROME AND NEPHROLITHIASIS

Metabolic syndrome is characterized by a cluster of features, including dyslipidemia, hyperglycemia, hypertension, obesity, and insulin resistance.[672,673] In addition to its relationship to T2DM and cardiovascular risks, metabolic syndrome is associated with nephrolithiasis and chronic renal disease.[10,11,65,666–677]

Despite this strong association between metabolic syndrome and kidney stone disease, one consistent limitation has been the lack of documentation of stone composition in most studies. The link between obesity and documented CaOx nephrolithiasis has been in part explained by dietary factors, such as higher consumption of salt and animal proteins.[319,320] The contribution of the metabolic syndrome to urinary calcium and urinary oxalate excretion in calcium stone formers has not been fully elucidated.[678] In one large Japanese cohort, hypertension and hyperlipidemia were associated with hypercalciuria, but hyperoxaluria was only associated with hyperlipidemia.[677] The result of this study was not supported by two other studies of kidney stone formers in the United States and Switzerland.[319] To this end, other investigators showed that being overweight and diabetic, but not other metabolic syndrome components, were significantly associated with increased urinary oxalate excretion in both kidney stone formers and non–kidney stone formers in the United States.[679]

Uric acid stones is more prevalent in patients with T2DM than in nondiabetic stone formers and more in obese than in nonobese stone formers.[47,48,50,51,517,519] Higher BMI and T2DM are shown to be independent risk factors for uric acid nephrolithiasis.[518] Cross-sectional studies in healthy non–stone-forming subjects and in kidney stone formers have shown an inverse relationship among urinary pH, body weight, and increasing features of metabolic syndrome.[493,520] The relationship between low urinary pH, supersaturation index of UA, and adiposity has been specifically shown to be related to fat distribution, with a significant relationship between total body fat and trunk fat associated with increased risk factors for uric acid stone formation.[680] Further evidence in ZDF rats has demonstrated the causative role of renal steatosis in the pathogenesis of urinary buffer defects in this animal model.[537] Furthermore, treatment with thiazolidinediones (TZDs) to improve insulin resistance by redistributing fat to adipocytes has been shown to restore urinary biochemical profiles in this animal model compared with control animals. These changes were associated with reduced renal triglyceride accumulation.[537]

## NEPHROLITHIASIS, CARDIOVASCULAR DISEASE, AND HYPERTENSION

Traditional Framingham risk factors for coronary artery disease such as atherosclerosis, hypertension, diabetes, and metabolic syndrome are also seen frequently in patients with kidney stones.[8,11,666,681–684] Cross-sectional studies linking coronary artery disease to kidney stones have been inconsistent,[685–687] with one study showing a positive association[685] and others demonstrating lack of such an association.[686,687] Another cross-sectional study in a large number of Portuguese subjects has shown a significant correlation between self-reported history of kidney stones and myocardial infarction solely in females, following multivariable adjustments.[688]

One longitudinal study in a U.S. population over 9 years has shown a multivariable adjusted hazard ratio (HR) for developing myocardial infarction to be higher in patients with kidney stones compared with non–stone-forming control participants[689] (Fig. 38.27). Although the study was adjusted for multiple variables, risk factors such as dietary calcium and use of thiazide diuretics were not accounted for. In a large number of patients among the two female cohorts in Nurses' Health Study I (NHS I) and Nurses' Health Study II (NHS II), a positive history of kidney stones was associated with elevated risk of coronary artery disease but such a link was not detected in a separate cohort in men in the Health Professionals Follow-Up Study (HPFS).[690] The causal relationship among kidney stones, coronary artery disease, and gender specificity has not been proven.

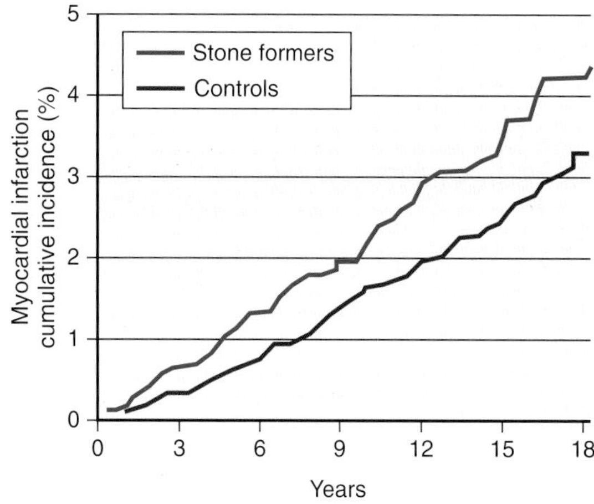


Incidence (no. at risk)

| | | | | |
|---|---|---|---|---|
| Control | 0 (10,860) | 0.8 (6,689) | 2 (3,184) | 4.2 (1,010) |
| Stone formers | 0 (4,564) | 1.3 (2,686) | 3 (1,276) | 5.2 (404) |

**Fig. 38.27** Increased risk for myocardial infarction in stone formers. Data collected from Olmsted County, Minnesota, residents. (Modified from Rule AD, Roger VL, Melton LJ 3rd, et al. Kidney stones associate with increased risk for myocardial infarction. *J Am Soc Nephrol.* 2010; 21[10]:1641–1644.)

Multiple cross-sectional studies have demonstrated an association between nephrolithiasis and blood pressure.[691–695] In 895 Swedish men whose blood pressure was measured once, the prevalence of nephrolithiasis increasing from 1% in those with the lowest blood pressure compared with 13% in those with the highest blood pressure.[691] Another study in Italian adults detected a higher prevalence of nephrolithiasis in subjects in the highest quintile of diastolic blood pressure compared with those in the lowest quintile (5.2% vs. 3.4%).[693] In study of U.S. men and women, the prevalence of nephrolithiasis was higher in hypertensive subjects compared with normotensive participants adjusted for age and race.[695] The results of these cross-sectional studies were supported by a longitudinal study conducted over an 8-year period; this study demonstrated that 17.4% of subjects with a history of nephrolithiasis versus 13.1% without a history of kidney stones received a new diagnosis of hypertension when adjusted for age, BMI, and dietary sodium, potassium, magnesium, and alcohol consumption.[696] In a Canadian study of 25,000 subjects compared with people without kidney stones, and after adjustment for potential confounders, subjects with at least one kidney stone had a higher risk of subsequent myocardial infarction, revascularization, and stroke. The magnitude of the excess risk associated with a kidney stone appeared more pronounced for younger people than for older people ($P < .001$) and for women than men ($P = .01$). The causal relationship has not yet been fully demonstrated but some have suggested that alterations in calcium metabolism may potentially link the development of kidney stone disease and hypertension.[697,698] Hypercalciuria, which is prevalent in subjects with calcium nephrolithiasis and primary hypertension, has been proposed by some as a major underlying mechanism, but the role of calcium in human hypertension has never been established.[697–701] A model of hypercalciuria and blood pressure elevation was proposed in spontaneously hypertensive rats.[702,703] The NHS showed an association among alterations in acid-base balance, hypocitraturia, and hypertension.[704] Similar associations were found in spontaneously hypertensive rats, demonstrating evidence of metabolic acidosis.[705,706]

## KIDNEY STONE DISEASE AND CHRONIC KIDNEY DISEASE

Kidney stone disease and CKD can potentially be causally related because of recurrent obstruction and infection, repeated shock wave therapy, or to the same comorbid conditions. A study conducted in Olmsted County, Minnesota, has shown that symptomatic kidney stone formers compared with matched controls followed over 9 years were at increased risk of developing ESKD, independent of diabetes, hypertension, dyslipidemia, and gout.[707] The association between kidney stones and risk of ESKD was found to be increased in those with urologic abnormalities, including a history of hydronephrosis, recurrent urinary tract infections, single kidney, neurologic bladder, and ileal conduit.[707] However, other studies have shown that the risk factors for CKD in patients with nephrolithiasis are the same as in the general population—namely, hypertension and diabetes.[11,51,708,709] Moreover, the apparent association of kidney stones to CKD has been attributed to infectious stone-causing staghorn calculi and to patients with cystinuria.[710–713] In one epidemiologic study, the prevalence of ESKD deemed to be as a result of nephrolithiasis in the general population was estimated to be approximately 3.1 cases/million per year.[714] This result is comparable to data from the US Renal Data System involving over 200,000 subjects who started dialysis between 1993 and 1997, which showed that approximately 1.2% with ESKD listed nephrolithiasis as the cause.[715] In NHANES III, the estimated glomerular filtration rate (eGFR) of 876 subjects with a history of kidney stone disease was compared with 14,000 subjects without a history of stones.[716] After adjustment for confounders, the eGFR in stone formers with a BMI of 27 kg/m$^2$ or higher was significantly lower than in non–stone formers. However, no difference in eGFR between stone formers and non–stone formers was found in subjects with a BMI of 27 kg/m$^2$ or lower. The association between kidney stones and CKD is gender-specific, with a significantly higher risk for ESKD development, doubling of serum creatinine level, and CKD (stages 3b–5) in women with a history of kidney stones than in men.[717]

## URINARY TRACT CANCERS AND KIDNEY STONES

The association of renal pelvis cancer with kidney stones has been reported in several case-control studies.[718–720] However, the association of renal parenchymal cancer has only been reported in case reports.[721] In one large population-based cohort study from a Swedish national inpatient registry and a cancer registry in 61,144 patients who were hospitalized for kidney or ureter stones from 1965 to 1983, there was an increased risk of renal pelvis, ureter, or bladder cancer beyond 10 years of follow-up. However, it was proposed that chronic infection or irritation may play a pathogenic role in the development of cancer.[722] In this large population-based cohort study, no association was found between kidney or ureteral stones and renal cell cancer. This result is contrary to the high risk reported in the case-control studies.[723–726] The possibility of selection bias may exist.

## CALCIUM STONES AND BONE DISEASE

### EPIDEMIOLOGY

Bone disease is an underemphasized condition in nephrolithiasis. Several epidemiologic studies have established an association between a history of kidney stones and a higher prevalence of fractures.[727–729] In a population-based study in Rochester, Minnesota, the incidence of first vertebral fracture in patients with symptomatic kidney stone disease followed for 19 years was fourfold higher than in the comparable general population[727] (Fig. 38.28).[230] The NHANES III study, including 14,000 men and women, demonstrated an association among a history of kidney stone, low BMD, and higher incidence of fracture.[728] This risk of fracture was found to be higher in males than females. In the most comprehensive population-based study, the Osteoporotic Fractures in Men Study ("Mr. OS"), of almost 6000 men has shown an association of kidney stones with lowered BMD at the spine and hip.[729] However, in recent studies of 9856 postmenopausal women, kidney stone formation was not shown to be associated with BMD or bone fractures after being adjusted for covariates that are linked with osteoporosis and kidney stones.[710] Major controversies have arisen from population-based cohort studies relying on self-report of kidney stone incidence, dietary composition, calcium and vitamin D supplementation, medications known to affect the risk of kidney stone and bone disease, ethnicity, and general health status of the studied

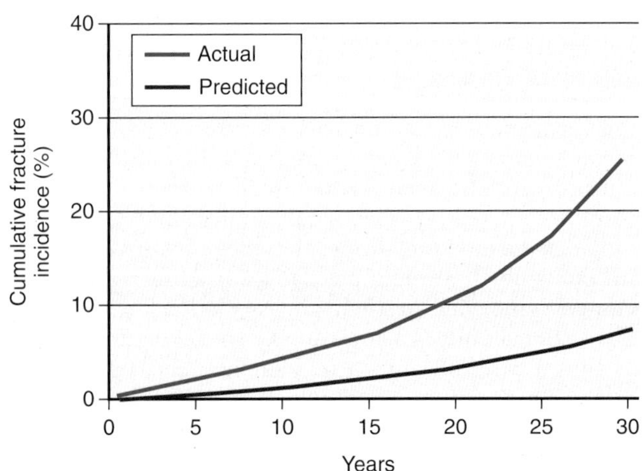


**Fig. 38.28** Cumulative incidence of vertebral fractures in stone formers; data from Rochester, Minnesota, residents following an initial episode of symptomatic nephrolithiasis. The elevated fracture risk was vertebral and was present in both genders. (Modified from Melton LJ 3rd, Crowson CS, Khosla S, et al. Fracture risk among patients with urolithiasis: a population-based cohort study. *Kidney Int.* 1998;53[2]:459–464.)

population.[27,727,730–733] A recent systematic review and comparative meta-analysis in 24 case-control studies in subjects with nephrolithiasis has shown that a lower BMD involves all skeletal sites and that the risk of osteoporosis in patients with nephrolithiasis is four times more than in healthy controls.[734]

## PATHOPHYSIOLOGIC MECHANISMS LINKING OSTEOPOROSIS AND KIDNEY STONES

Osteoporosis is a heterogeneous disorder characterized by disordered bone remodeling resulting in reduced BMD, impairment of microarchitectural integrity, reduced bone strength, and increased fracture risk.[735] Numerous studies have found reduced BMD in calcium stone-forming subjects[259,736–764] (Table 38.6).[230] The loss of BMD is generalized at all skeletal sites, with 40% of patients showing diminished BMD at the vertebral spine, 30% at the proximal hip, and 65% at the radius.[230] Although low BMD is present in hypercalciuric and normocalciuric stone formers,[738,741,745] it is most prominent in those with hypercalciuria.[738,741,745,750,756] Diminished BMD was not universally detected in normocalciuric kidney stone formers.[744,747,750,752] Given that BMD may be one of the important surrogates of bone strength, it is reasonable to suggest that hypercalciuric stone-forming subjects may carry the highest risk of bone fracture. Altered bone remodeling is a significant finding in hypercalciuric stone formers.*

Most histomorphometric studies have agreed that defective bone formation rather than excessive bone resorption plays a key role in the development of bone disease in this population[259,757–760,762,766] (Table 38.7).[230]

The pathophysiologic mechanism(s) of bone disease in stone formers is not known, although it may be related to interplay among environmental, genetic, and hormonal influences and perturbations in the formation of local cytokines.[230] A major emphasis has been placed on the link of idiopathic hypercalciuria and the development of bone disease. It has been assumed that hypercalciuria and negative calcium balance is pathogenic for bone loss in kidney stone formers in several cross-sectional studies of a small number of kidney stone formers.[241,744,767,768] However, the presence of negative calcium balance,[763] osteopenia, and osteoporosis has been demonstrated primarily in patients with dRTA, as well as medullary sponge kidney,[769] in whom there is a high prevalence of acidosis,[770,771] which can be the main cause of bone loss.

### Dietary Factors

Salt and protein intake is associated with an increased risk of kidney stones[230] and bone disease.[744,745] Multiple pathophysiologic mechanisms contribute to the high salt- and protein-induced hypercalciuria, including diminished renal tubular calcium reabsorption, hyperfiltration, reposition of acid load, and increased urinary prostaglandin excretion.[396,772–777] The presence of subclinical metabolic acidosis is common in protein-induced hypercalciuria.[775] Metabolic acidosis inhibits osteoblastic matrix protein synthesis and alkaline phosphatase activity by stimulating prostaglandin E2 production.[778–780] Increased prostaglandin E2 production may enhance the osteoblastic expression of receptor activator for nuclear factor kappa B ligand (RANKL), a major downstream cytokine, which stimulates osteoblastic production by binding to its receptor RANK.[781] Low bicarbonate in vitro alters osteoblastic extracellular matrix proteins, including type I collagen[778,780] osteopontin, matrix Gla protein,[779,782] and expression of cyclooxygenase-2[783] and RANKL.[781,784] The effect of protein is only partially mediated by its acid content[785] because, in humans, the total neutralization of the acid of dietary protein does not reverse the hypercalciuria.[786]

### Genetic Factors

The genetic link of vertebral bone loss in kidney stone patients with absorptive hypercalciuria was identified in a genome-wide linkage approach study showing polymorphism in the soluble adenylylcyclase gene *(ADCY10)* on chromosome 1q23 4-1q24.[633,787] Another genome-wide screening study associated sequence variants in the claudin-14 gene *(CLDN14)* with kidney stone and reduced BMD at the hip in a large population of kidney stone formers from Iceland and the Netherlands.[330] Although soluble *ADCY10* has been shown to regulate osteoclastic function by ambient bicarbonate concentration,[634] and claudin-14 is recognized as a paracellular protein mediating renal tubular calcium reabsorption, it is unclear in both cases how these putative genes influence bone remodeling. Others have shown an association between CaSR gene polymorphism and increased urinary calcium excretion in hypercalciuric patients[627] and reduced forearm BMD in healthy subjects and postmenopausal women.[788,789] An initial report claimed that mutation in the sodium phosphate transporter, NaPi2a, is linked to kidney stones and defective bone mineralization,[790] but additional studies did not confirm this association.[791,792]

Numerous genetically heterogeneous disorders that present in childhood or early adulthood are associated with hypercalciuria, nephrocalcinosis, nephrolithiasis, and rachitic bone disease, including Dent disease (mutation of the chloride-proton transporter, CLC-5) and Lowe syndrome (mutation of the phosphatydylinositol-4,5 bisphosphonate 5-phosphatase, OCRL1).[793–795] However, the role of these genes in bone disease in the general kidney stone-forming population has not yet been illustrated.

### Hormones and Local Cytokines

Elevated serum 1,25$(OH)_2$D levels occurs in one-third of hypercalciuric stone formers.[241,246,251,253] Peripheral blood monocyte VDR levels are increased, which may amplify the target organ action of circulating 1,25$(OH)_2$D on bone, kidney, and intestine.[290] High doses of 1,25$(OH)_2$D in vitro enhance bone resorption and decrease bone collagen synthesis.[342] Low expression of transforming growth factor-β (TGFβ), which is known to enhance bone formation and bone mineralization,[342,345] was demonstrated in bones of hypercalciuric stone formers,[344] as was increased production of bone resorptive lymphokines.[741,747,748] A study using undecalcified bone in idiopathic hypercalciuric patients has shown an elevated bone expression of RANKL.[344] Therefore it is plausible that the interplay of cytokines and RANK/RANKL/OPG (osteoprotegerin) may stimulate bone resorption, whereas lowered TGF-β, high 1,25$(OH)_2$D, and/or amplified vitamin D activity may impair osteoblastic bone formation in this population.

*References 259, 752, 757, 759, 760, 762, and 765.

**Table 38.6 Changes in Bone Mineral Density in Calcium Kidney Stone Formers**

| | | No. of Subjects | | | BMD Site | | | |
|---|---|---|---|---|---|---|---|---|
| **Reference** | **Study Subjects** | Male (M) | Female (F) | Control | Spine | Hip | Radius | **Measurement Technique** |
| Alhava[736] | Single or recurrent urolithiasis | 54 | 21 | 21 | | | ↓ | Americium-241 gamma ray attenuation |
| Lawoyin[737] | Absorptive hypercalciuria | 94 | 23 | Not reported | | | ↔ | Single-photon absorptiometry |
| | Renal hypercalciuria | 28 | 16 | | | | ↓ | |
| | Primary hyper-parathyroidism | 22 | 31 | | | | ↓ | |
| | Osteoporosis | 14 | 55 | | | | ↓ | |
| Fuss[738] | Absorptive hypercalciuria | 24 | 19 | Not reported | | | ↓ | Single-photon absorptiometry |
| | Renal or resorptive hypercalciuria | 7 | 18 | | | | ↓ | |
| | Normocalciuria | 35 | 6 | | | | ↓ | |
| Barkin[739] | Idiopathic hypercalciuria | 86 | 23 | 84 | ↓ Calcium-binding index | | | Neutron-activation analysis |
| Fuss[740] | Free diet | 63 | 0 | 16 | | | ↔ | Single-photon absorptiometry |
| | Low calcium diet | 60 | 0 | | | | ↓ | |
| Pacifici[741] | Absorptive hypercalciuria | 29 | 18 | 28 (24 M, 4 F) | ↓ | | | Quantitative computed tomography (CT) |
| | Fasting hypercalciuria | 16 | 7 | | ↓ | | | |
| Bataille[742] | Dietary hypercalciuria | 12 | 6 | 61 (41 M, 20 F) | ↔ | | | Quantitative CT |
| | Dietary independent hypercalciuria | 17 | 7 | | ↓ | | | |
| Borghi[743] | Dietary hypercalciuria | 13 | 7 | 0 | ↔ | | | Dual-photon absorptiometry |
| | Dietary independent hypercalciuria | 14 | 7 | | ↓ | | | |
| Pietschmann[744] | Absorptive hypercalciuria | 42 | 20 | 0 | ↓ | | | Dual-energy x-ray absorptiometry; dual-photon absorptiometry; single-photon absorptiometry |
| | Fasting hypercalciuria | 24 | 3 | | ↓ | | | |
| | Normocalciuric | 25 | 6 | | ↔ | | | |
| Jaeger[745] | Hypercalciuric | 49 | 0 | 234 | ↓ | ↓ | | Dual-energy x-ray absorptiometry |
| | Normocalciuric | 61 | 0 | | ↓ | ↓ | | |
| Zanchetta[746] | Fasting hypercalciuria | 15 | 23 | 50 (20 M, 30 F) | ↓ | | | Dual-photon absorptiometry |
| | Absorptive hypercalciuria | 5 | 7 | | ↓ F, ↔ M | | | |
| Weisinger[747] | Hypercalciuric | 4 | 13 | 12 (4 M, 8 F) | ↓ | | | Dual-energy x-ray absorptiometry |
| | Normocalciuric | 4 | 8 | | ↔ | | | |
| Ghazali[748] | Idiopathic hypercalciuria | 15 | 1 | 10 (8 M, 2 F) | ↓ | | | Quantitative CT |
| | Dietary hypercalciuria | 9 | 1 | | ↔ | | | |
| Giannini[749] | Fasting hypercalciuria | 8 | 23 | 13 (10 M, 3 F) | ↓ | ↓ | | Dual-energy x-ray absorptiometry |
| | Absorptive hypercalciuria | 13 | 5 | | ↓ | ↔ | | |
| Trinchieri[750] | Hypercalciuria | 10 | 0 | | ↔ | ↔ | | Dual-energy x-ray absorptiometry |
| | Normocalciuria | 34 | | | ↔ | ↔ | | |
| Tasca[751] | Fasting hypercalciuria | 27 | 12 | 15 | ↓ | | | Dual-energy x-ray absorptiometry |
| | Absorptive hypercalciuria | 20 | 11 | | Not reported | | | |
| Misael da Silva[752] | Idiopathic hypercalciuria | 11 | 11 | 10 (5 M, 5 F) | ↓ | ↓ | | Dual-energy x-ray absorptiometry |
| | Normocalciuric | 8 | 10 | | ↔ | ↔ | | |
| Asplin[753] | Stone formers | 15 | 7 | 37 (14 M, 23 F) | ↓ | ↓ | | Dual-energy x-ray absorptiometry |
| Vezzoli[754] | Hypercalciuria | 29 | 35 | 0 | ↓ | ↓ | | Dual-energy x-ray absorptiometry |
| | Normocalciuria | 15 | 27 | | ↓ | ↓ | | |
| Caudarella[755] | Stone formers (27% with hypercalciuria) | 102 | 94 | 196 (102 M, 94 F) | | | ↓ | Dual-energy x-ray absorptiometry; quantitative ultrasonography |

↓, Lower bone mineral density (BMD); ↔, no change in BMD.

Modified from Sakhaee K, Maalouf NM, Kumar R, et al. Nephrolithiasis-associated bone disease: pathogenesis and treatment options. *Kidney Int.* 2011;79(4):393–403.

Bone histomorphometric analyses performed in kidney stone formers have shown impaired bone formation as a unanimous finding.[259,762] These findings would not be expected if only hypercalciuria played a pathogenetic role in the development of bone disease in this population.[259,762] Idiopathic hypercalciuria is a heterogeneous and complex disorder that could result from increased production or sensitivity to calcitriol and affect the target organs differently. Thus, whereas there is evidence of increased intestinal calcium absorption in this population, the high levels of calcitriol attained in

**Table 38.7 Bone Histomorphometric Characteristics in Kidney Stone Formers**

| Reference | Study Subjects | No. of Subjects | Bone Histomorphometric Profiles |
|---|---|---|---|
| Bordier[259] | Dietary hypercalciuria | 20 | None |
| | Renal hypercalciuria | 19 | Increased osteoclast and osteoblast surfaces |
| | Hypophosphatemia | 21 | Increased osteoclastic and eroded surface (within normal range), decreased osteoblast surfaces, decreased osteoid parameters |
| | Controls | 12 | |
| Malluche[757] | Absorptive hypercalciuria | 15 | Low-normal osteoclastic bone resorption, low osteoblastic activity, decreased fraction of mineralizing osteoid seams, decreased mineralization apposition rate |
| | Controls | 22 | |
| de Vernejoul[758] | Idiopathic hypercalciuria | 30 (20 M, 10 F) | Decreased trabecular volume, decreased active osteoblastic surface, decreased active bone resorption surface |
| | Controls | 187 | |
| Steiniche[759] | Idiopathic hypercalciuria | 33 (22 M, 11 F) | Increased bone resorption surfaces (decreased refilling of lacunae with low bone formation), decreased bone formation rate, increased mineralization lag times |
| | Controls | 30 (19 M, 11 F) | |
| Heilberg[760] | Fasting hypercalciuria | 6 male | Increased eroded surface, decreased osteoid surface, decreased bone formation rate with a complete lack of tetracycline double labeling |
| | Controls | No information | |
| Bataille[761] | Idiopathic hypercalciuria | 24 (20 M, 4 F) | Low eroded surface, low bone volume, low osteoid surface, thickness, mineral apposition rate, adjusted apposition rate and bone formation rate |
| | Control | 18 (9 M, 9 F) | |
| Misael da Silva[752] | Idiopathic hypercalciuria | 22 | High eroded surface, increased osteoblastic bone surface, no change in trabecular thickness |
| | Control | 94 | |
| Heller[762] | Absorptive hypercalciuria | 9 (6 M, 3 F) | Relatively high bone resorption (osteoclast surface, bone surface—mean value within the normal limit), lower indices of bone formation (osteoblast surface/bone surface), decreased wall thickness |
| | Control | 9 (6 M, 3 F) | |

hypercalciuric stone formers may result in diminished osteoblastic bone formation.[255,256,290,796] The inhibitory actions of calcitriol on bone collagen synthesis, as well as in osteoblastic cell proliferation, has been shown to be exerted at $10^{-10}$ M, which is no different from the level of calcitriol attained in hypercalciuric stone formers.[253,306,342]

# EVALUATION

## CLINICAL PRESENTATION

### SYMPTOMS AND SIGNS

Kidney stones may be asymptomatic and incidentally present in patients during an imaging procedure. Renal colic, pain localized to the back and flank during passage, is a common clinical manifestation of kidney stones. The pain occurs as the kidney stone is propelled through the ureter and is a consequence of increased intraluminal pressure, causing stimulation of nerve endings in the ureteral mucosa. Pain is usually intense and intermittent, originating in the back or flank, radiating around the torso to the groin, and ending up in the testicles or labia for male or female subjects, respectively. Stones in the midportion of the ureter may imitate appendicitis on the right side or diverticulitis on the left side. Renal colic can be associated with symptoms such as nausea and vomiting because the GI tract shares common innervation with the genitourinary system. When the kidney stone approaches the urinary bladder, it frequently causes bladder symptoms such as urinary frequency, dysuria, suprapubic pain, and incontinence.[797]

The most important physical finding is costovertebral angle tenderness, although its presence and severity are not as consistent and intense as in pyelonephritis. The abdominal examination is usually negative. Hypertension and tachycardia, if present, are most likely as a result of severe relentless pain. Fever and muscle spasm are infrequent and may represent underlying diseases or complications. A toxic-appearing patient during stone passage may indicate obstruction, infection, and urosepsis.

### ENVIRONMENTAL, LIFESTYLE, AND MEDICAL HISTORY

It is important to elicit a history of any systemic disorders. These include disorders of calcium homeostasis such as primary hyperparathyroidism, conditions accompanied by extrarenal calcitriol production such as granulomatous disease, and disorders such as obesity, type 2 diabetes, gout, recurrent urinary tract infections, inflammatory bowel disease, bowel resection, pancreatic disease, bariatric surgery, distal renal tubular acidosis, and medullary sponge kidney.[222,798,799]

Patients should be asked about climate exposure, work environment, and exercise frequency and intensity because these affect the risk of development of kidney stones. Higher temperatures and prolonged summer seasons in the equatorial part of the globe increase the risk of kidney stones. Daily exposure to hot conditions, military cohorts training in a high-temperature environment, and individuals who engage in physical exercise during the summer months are also factors in stone development.[15,799,800]

Dietary history should include daily fluid intake (from water and various beverages), intake of calcium, sodium, amount and type of protein intake, food containing oxalate, and alkali-rich foods, including fruits and vegetables. The history may also detail the use of OTC medications and/or supplements, including calcium, vitamin D, multivitamins, and ascorbic acid.

A careful drug history must be taken because prescription and over-the-counter (OTC) drugs have been demonstrated to increase the risk of kidney stones.[798] In some cases, the increased risk is caused by metabolic alterations in the urinary environment—for example, calcium, vitamin D and vitamin C supplements, carbonic anhydrase inhibitors (acetazolamide, topiramate, and zonisamide), laxatives,[588,589] probenecid, ascorbic acid, lipase inhibitors,[801,802] excessive alkali treatment, and chemotherapeutic agents.[798] However, in other cases, there is a risk of crystallization of the drug in urine because of its poor solubility. This class of drugs includes triamterene, protease inhibitors (indinavir, atazinir, and nelfinavir), guaifenesin, ephedrine, antacids (magnesium trisilicate), and antimicrobials (sulfonamides and quinolones).[389,487,798,799,803]

### FAMILY HISTORY

It is very common to obtain a positive family history in a stone former. The pattern may or may not be mendelian in nature but nonetheless needs to be documented. The interpretation of whether a certain pedigree has a mendelian trait is often difficult because of phenocopy, incomplete penetrance, and loci heterogeneity. Certain monogenic diseases present with kidney stones that may have specific phenotypic characteristics. Hypercalciuric nephrolithiasis among male subjects associated with renal impairment and low-molecular- weight proteinuria that is X-linked recessive is found in patients with Dent disease.[804] The familial occurrence of kidney stones and nephrocalcinosis in male subjects with early cataracts or glaucoma is suggestive of Lowe syndrome.[805] Aggressive nephrolithiasis, nephrocalcinosis, retarded growth, and deafness can be seen in patients with dRTA, presenting with both autosomal dominance and recessive inheritance.[805,806] A presentation with nephrocalcinosis and impaired kidney function with hyperoxaluria should suggest the diagnosis of primary hyperoxaluria.[807]

## LABORATORY EVALUATION

Laboratory diagnoses include blood and urinary metabolic profiles, stone analysis, and imaging (Tables 38.8 to 38.10).[222,797] There are limited prospective studies regarding the appropriate extent of the metabolic evaluation in the kidney stone population. Therefore, the proposed evaluation varies, depending on the severity of the kidney stone disease and structure of different practices. A few studies have suggested that single stone formers share the same metabolic abnormalities with those with recurrent kidney stone disease.[808–810] Furthermore, there are no surrogate metabolic markers that identify those at high risk for recurrent nephrolithiasis, except for low urine volume.[810] However, in a recent retrospective study of a large number of first-time adult kidney stone formers followed for 15 years (Recurrence of Kidney Stones [ROKS]), a nomogram was developed to predict recurrence.[811] Among the risk factors for recurrence were younger age, male gender, white race, presence on imaging of both asymptomatic or nonobstructing stones and symptomatic renal pelvic or lower pole stones, gross hematuria, and uric acid stones. Based on this nomogram, the 10-year recurrence rate ranged from 12% to 56% in the lowest to the highest risk quintile. However, because of the lack of presentation of 24-hour urinary metabolic risk factors, no distinction was made between metabolically active and metabolically inactive stone formers.[812,813]

### SERUM CHEMISTRY

All kidney stone formers require the determination of full fasting serum chemistries (e.g., electrolytes, including calcium and phosphorus, renal function, uric acid) and PTH. Fasting glucose and a full lipid panel are also justified considering the high prevalence of diabetes and metabolic syndrome in stone formers. Increased serum total calcium concentration and low serum phosphorus levels, in association with a high PTH concentration, are indicative of primary hyperparathyroidism, although this full triad is often not present. The finding of a low serum phosphorus level with a normal serum PTH level is suggestive of a renal phosphorus leak. In the latter condition, hypercalciuria may ensue as a result of increased intestinal calcium absorption from an elevated serum calcitriol level because of hypophosphatemia. The measurement of serum $1,25(OH)_2D$ may be considered for specific situations or for research purposes. A serum 25(OH)D measurement is helpful in patients with high or high-normal PTH levels and mild hypercalcemia to exclude vitamin D deficiency as a cause of the high PTH level. The finding of a low serum potassium level and low serum total $CO_2$ content is suggestive of dRTA or a chronic diarrheal state. Hyperuricemia may suggest the diagnosis of UA nephrolithiasis.[222,656,797,799]

### URINE CHEMISTRY

#### Spot Urinalysis

A spot urine collection is of some value because of its simplicity. The UpH obtained from the colorimetric reaction of the dipstick is notoriously inaccurate, and only extreme values are informative. A very low dipstick pH (<5.5) suggests UA stones, whereas a high pH (>6.5) suggests dRTA, and a very high pH (>7.4) should raise suspicion for infection. Urine culture must be obtained in patients suspected of urinary tract infection (UTI) and in patients with established struvite stones. Crystalluria per se is not abnormal because it is found in normal urine, except that cystine crystals are never present in normal urine (see Fig. 38.22B).

To date, the available clinical studies have not shown that first-time kidney stone formers are metabolically and clinically separable from those with recurrent disease. Thus, all patients, irrespective of the severity of kidney stone disease, should have a metabolic evaluation. It has been suggested that a simplified metabolic evaluation may be considered for single

**Table 38.8 Simplified Ambulatory Metabolic Evaluation and Interpretation of Urinary Parameters[a]**

| Random 24-Hour Urinary Profile | Expected Values (per day) | Interpretation |
|---|---|---|
| Total volume | ≥2.5 L | Indicative of daily fluid intake (minus insensible losses); diminishes with low fluid intake, sweating, and diarrhea |
| pH | 5.9–6.2 | <5.5—increases risk of uric acid precipitation; commonly found in idiopathic uric acid stone patients, subjects with intestinal disease and diarrhea, and in those with intestinal bypass surgery<br>>6.7— increases risk of calcium phosphate precipitation; commonly found in patients with dRTA, primary hyperparathyroidism, alkali, and carbonic anhydrase treatment<br>>7.0–7.5— indicates urinary tract infection from urease-producing bacteria. |
| Creatinine | 15–25 mg/kg body weight (0.13–0.22 mmol/kg body weight) | Assessment of completeness of collection: 15–20 mg/kg body weight (0.13–0.15 mmol/kg body weight) in females, 20–25 mg/kg body weight (0.15–0.22 mmol/kg body weight) in males; valid only in steady state of constant serum creatinine concentration with time |
| Sodium | 100 mEq (100 mmol) | Reflects dietary sodium intake (minus extrarenal loss); much lower than dietary intake in diarrhea and with excessive sweating; high sodium intake is major cause of hypercalciuria |
| Potassium | 40–60 mEq (100 mmol) | Reflects dietary potassium intake (minus extrarenal loss); much lower than dietary intake in diarrhea states; gauge of dietary alkali intake because most dietary potassium accompanied by organic anions |
| Calcium | ≤250–300 mg (≤6.24–7.49 mmol) | A higher value expected in males; in states of zero balance, urinary calcium excretion is net gut absorption minus net bone deposition; secondary causes should be ruled out before making the diagnosis of idiopathic hypercalciuria |
| Magnesium | 30–120 mg (1.23–4.94 mmol) | Low urinary magnesium detected with low magnesium intake, intestinal malabsorption (small bowel disease), and following bariatric surgery; low magnesium may increase risk of calcium stones. |
| Oxalate | ≤45 mg (≤0.51 mmol) | Commonly encountered with intestinal disease with fat malabsorption, such as inflammatory bowel disease and following bariatric surgery; values >100 mg/day (1.14 mmol/day) suggest primary hyperoxaluria (PH); the diagnosis of PH I and PH II is further established with high urinary glycolate and L-glycerate levels. |
| Phosphorus | ≤1100 mg (35.5 mmol) | Indicative of dietary organic and inorganic phosphorus intake and absorption; a higher excretion may increase the risk of calcium phosphate stone formation. |
| Uric acid | 600–800 mg (3.57–4.76 mmol) | Hyperuricosuria is encountered with overproduction of endogenous uric acid or overindulgence of purine-rich foods such as red meat, poultry, and fish; mainly a risk factor for calcium oxalate stones when UpH is >5.5 but is a risk factor for uric acid stone when UpH < 5.5. |
| Sulfate | ≤20 mmol | Sulfate is a marker of dietary acid intake (oxidation of sulfur-containing amino acids). |
| Citrate | ≥320 mg (≥1.67 mmol) | Inhibitor of calcium stone formation; hypocitraturia is commonly encountered in metabolic acidosis, dRTA, chronic diarrhea, excessive protein ingestion, strenuous physical exercise, hypokalemia, intracellular acidosis, with carbonic anhydrase inhibitor drugs (e.g., acetazolamide, topiramate, zonisamide), but rarely with ACE inhibitors |
| Ammonium | 30–40 mEq (30–40 mmol) | Ammonium is a major carrier of $H^+$ in the urine; its excretion corresponds with urinary sulfate (acid load); a higher ammonium-to-sulfate ratio indicates GI alkali loss. |
| Chloride | 100 mEq (100 mmol) | Chloride varies with sodium intake. |
| Cystine | <30–60 mg (<0.12–0.25 mmol) | Cystine has a limited urinary solubility, at 250 mg/L. |

[a]Expected values should be cross-checked with reference laboratory recommendations because these values may differ. These limits are mean +2 standard deviations (for calcium, oxalate, uric acid, pH, sodium, sulfate, and phosphorus) or mean −2 standard deviations (for citrate, pH, and magnesium) from normal.

*ACE,* Angiotensin-converting enzyme; *dRTA,* distal renal tubular acidosis; *GI,* gastrointestinal; *UpH,* urinary pH.

stone formers, and an extensive evaluation is needed for recurrent kidney stone formers and individuals at high risk for recurrent stone formation, such as those with primary hyperparathyroidism, dRTA, chronic diarrhea, UA stones, obese subjects, patients with CKD, or bone disease and in pediatric populations with kidney stones. Kidney stone formers of a certain profession, such as pilots, and frequent travelers should also be considered for metabolic evaluation.

### Simplified Metabolic Evaluation

A simplified workup is appropriate for single stone formers with a low risk of recurrence. The evaluation should include

**Table 38.9 Simplified Ambulatory Metabolic Evaluation and Interpretation of Other Parameters**

| Other Tests | Values | Interpretation |
|---|---|---|
| Complete metabolic panel | Variable[a] | Low serum potassium, high serum chloride, and low serum total $CO_2$ content are suggestive of a diarrheal state or dRTA. |
| PTH | 10-65 pg/mL (1.06-6.90 pmol/L) | High PTH, when accompanied by high serum calcium and low serum phosphorus, is suggestive of primary hyperparathyroidism. |
| 1,25-dihydroxyvitamin D | Variable[a] | Normal serum calcium, normal PTH, and elevated 1,25 dihydroxyvitamin D is suggestive of absorptive hypercalciuria. Normal serum calcium, normal PTH, low serum phosphorus and elevated 1,25 dihydroxyvitamin D is suggestive of renal phosphorus leak. |
| Bone mineral density measurements (DXA) | Z-score >–2 T-score >–2.5 | Z-score <–2 or T-score <–2.5 indicates bone loss. This finding may be more prevalent in hypercalciuric kidney stone formers. |

[a]Expected values should be cross-checked with reference laboratory recommendations since these values may differ.
*dRTA,* distal renal tubular acidosis; *DXA,* dual-energy x-ray absorptiometry; *PTH,* parathyroid hormone.

**Table 38.10 Extensive Ambulatory Metabolic Evaluation and Interpretation[a]**

| Restricted 24-hour Urinary Profile | Expected Values (per day)[b] | Interpretation |
|---|---|---|
| Calcium | <200 mg (<4.99 mmol) | A restricted diet urinary Ca <200 mg/day (4.99 mmol/d), accompanied by a random diet urinary Ca >200–250 mg/day (6.24–7.49 mmol/day) is reflective of dietary Ca indiscretion. Persistent high urinary Ca on a restricted diet is reflective of intestinal hyperabsorption of Ca. |
| Sodium | 100 mEq (100 mmol) | Urinary Na > 100 mEq/day (100 mmol/day) may reflect high dietary salt intake. An increment of 100 mEq/day (100 mmol/day) of Na increases urinary calcium by approximately 40 mg/day (1 mmol/day). |
| Oxalate | 40 mg (<0.45 mmol) | Urinary oxalate >40 mg/day (0.45 mmol/day), in the absence of a chronic diarrheal state, is indicative of high dietary oxalate intake. |
| Sulfate | <20 mmol | Urinary sulfate >20 mmol/day indicates overindulgence of high–acid-ash diet found in animal proteins. |
| 2-hour fasting calcium-to-creatinine ratio (Ca:Cr) | <0.11 mg/100 mL GF (<2.7 μmol/100 mg GF) | Elevated fasting Ca:Cr, high serum calcium, and elevated PTH suggestive of primary hyperparathyroidism; elevated fasting Ca:Cr, normal serum calcium, and normal or suppressed PTH suggestive of resorptive hypercalciuria; Elevated fasting Ca:Cr, normal serum calcium, and elevated PTH suggestive of renal hypercalciuria. |
| 4-hour Ca:Cr following a 1-g oral calcium load | ≤ 0.20 mg/mg Cr (≤ 0.56 mmol/mmol Cr) | Elevated Ca:Cr following a 1-g oral calcium load is suggestive of absorptive hypercalciuria. |

[a]After 1 week of dietary restrictions.
[b]Expected values should be cross-checked with reference laboratory recommendations since these values may differ. These limits are mean + 2 standard deviations (for calcium, oxalate, uric acid, pH, sodium, sulfate, and phosphorus) or mean – 2 standard deviations (for citrate, pH, and magnesium) from normal.
*GF,* Glomerular filtrate; *PTH,* parathyroid hormone.

a comprehensive history and physical examination, dietary and record of fluid consumption, and review of medications.

Although it is not perfect, studies have shown a correlation between kidney stone composition and urinary biochemical profiles.[90,91] A simple evaluation includes a single, random, 24-hour urinary profile on an ad libitum diet, including total volume, pH, and creatinine, CaOx, citrate, UA, sulfate, chloride, and ammonium levels (Table 38.8). There is some controversy regarding the recommended number (one or two) of random 24-hour urine collections required to determine kidney stone risk.[814–816] Regardless of the number of samples collected, physicians should take into account the dietary intake of known risk factors such as salt and protein because these are outpatient collections from those on a random diet. Patients should be instructed to adhere to their usual daily activities and diet before and during the collection. If two collections are contemplated, restriction of dietary sodium, oxalate, and protein may be considered prior to a second collection to evaluate the contribution from dietary aberrations without embarking on a fully executed dietary control program (see later). Imaging to determine the extent of the kidney stone disease and type of stones also may be of some value. A spot urine test for the evaluation of UTI and urine culture may be useful as part of this evaluation.

### Extensive Metabolic Evaluation

An extensive evaluation is infrequently carried out in the evaluation of kidney stones.[470] One study has shown that low-risk patients with kidney stone recurrence are more interested in a complete metabolic evaluation than the practicing physician.[817] The justification for a complete metabolic evaluation is based on the economic burden of years of medical treatment in contrast to surgical intervention.[818] See Table 38.9 for a listing of other tests.

An extensive evaluation includes a 24-hour urinary sample following a 1-week instructed, fixed metabolic diet consisting of 400 mg calcium/day, 100 mEq sodium/day, and avoidance of oxalate-rich food[819] (Table 38.10). Generally, high-risk and recurrent stone formers may benefit from an extensive metabolic evaluation. These include those with a systemic illness, such as primary hyperparathyroidism, dRTA, gout, type 2 diabetes, patients with a family history of stone disease, and those with a solitary kidney. The 24-hour urine profiles may be complemented by two additional tests, which can be performed at the completion of the restricted 24-hour urine collection—2-hour urinary fasting calcium-to-creatinine ratio to assess renal leak and/or excessive skeletal calcium mobilization, urinary fractional phosphorus excretion to monitor renal phosphorus leak (TmP/GFR), and a 4-hour urinary calcium-to-creatinine ratio following a 1-g oral calcium load to determine intestinal calcium absorption. However, these tests are usually performed only as a research tool or in a specialized stone clinic.

A comprehensive metabolic workup may also include the analysis of the BMD given that both cross-sectional and epidemiologic studies have shown low BMD, abnormal bone histology, and increased fracture risks among kidney stone formers compared with the general population.[230] One major hurdle is the insurance constraints justifying BMD determination in these subjects.

In those with established cystine stones, a positive family history of cystine stone, or those suspected with the condition, urinary cystine measurement must be done. In those with urinary oxalate exceeding 100 mg/day, the diagnosis of PH may be suspected; 24-hour urine must be tested for glycolate and L-glycerate to confirm the diagnosis of PH types I and II, respectively. Increased urinary glycolate levels are detected in approximately two-thirds of PH type I subjects, so a normal urinary glycolate level does not exclude this diagnosis.[820,821] With renal impairment, there is a fall in the urinary oxalate level, so its urinary measurements may not be accurate. In these circumstances, the plasma oxalate level should be assessed to confirm the diagnosis of PH. It is typically elevated at 80 μmol/L compared with non–PH hyperoxaluric patients, in whom plasma oxalate levels vary from 30 to 80 μmol/L..[822–824] The most definitive diagnosis is by genetic analysis.[825–828] In cases in which clinical suspicion of PH is considered to be high but DNA screening is nondiagnostic, a liver biopsy can establish the diagnosis.[821]

### Spot and Fasting Urine Specimen

Some patients may be reluctant or unable to collect 24-hour urine, and one may be concerned with the accuracy of the 24-hour urine collection. Several cross-sectional studies have suggested that spot urine could be substituted for the 24-hour urine in the assessment of urinary kidney stone risk profiles.[829–835] In one study in a large population of stone and non–stone-forming subjects, fasting urinary pH correlated with a 24-hour urinary pH.[836] However, significant variability was demonstrated between these two profiles in individual subjects, suggesting that the fasting urine pH could not substitute for the 24-hour urinary pH in this population.

### Urinary Supersaturation Estimation

Urinary supersaturation measurement has not been widely used clinically (Table 38.11). However, it can be used in clinical and research settings to estimate risks and monitor response to treatment.[90,91,837] Urinary supersaturation was used in stone research using the EQUIL2 software program (now offered commercially).[83,838,839] Other programs, including JESS, have also been used in the calculation of urinary supersaturation.[92] Furthermore, urinary supersaturation ratios are reported by commercial clinical laboratories and are available to practitioners. The RSR is defined as the ratio of calculated activity product in a given urine sample and respective thermodynamic solubility product.[83] Values higher than 1 indicate supersaturation, and values less than 1 indicate undersaturation. Another method, urinary RS, is calculated as the ratio of activity product (for UA, it is the concentration of undissociated UA) in a particular urine specimen and corresponding mean activity product (for UA, it is the undissociated UA) from normal subjects. The upper limit of normal for RS of CaOx, brushite, monosodium urate, and UA is defined as 2.[509]

Despite the lack of uniform hard evidence correlating urinary biochemical abnormalities and urinary supersaturation of stone-forming salt following dietary and pharmacologic treatment with clinical stone occurrence, several observational and case-control studies have shown a correlation between

**Table 38.11 Urinary Supersaturation Estimation[a]**

| Term | Definition | Readout |
|---|---|---|
| Relative supersaturation ratio (RSR) | Ion concentration product in a given solution (activity product); ion concentration product at equilibrium (solubility product) | Values <1 represent undersaturation; values >1 represent supersaturation. |
| Relative supersaturation (RS) | Urinary activity product in urine specimen; activity product from normal subjects | Upper normal limits = 2. |

[a]The EQUIL2 software program is used for the assessment of urinary supersaturation in stone research as well as in a clinical setting. The JESS program, which is now mostly used in research programs also represents the supersaturation ratio but is defined as saturation index (SI) in that software program.

the calculated parameter and clinical outcome.[813,840,841] For example, one study at a specialized kidney stone center has shown that a reduction of CaOx supersaturation is accompanied by a reduction in the number of formed kidney stones.[842]

There is no hard rule regarding structured longitudinal monitoring of urinary parameters following the initiation of a pharmacologic and/or dietary regimen. However, it is advisable to obtain a 24-hour urine annually, depending on the activity of stone disease.[843,844]

A recent study has concluded that urinary supersaturation does not offer any diagnostic advantage in separating kidney stone formers from healthy non–kidney stone formers at presentation.[845] However, like previous studies, this study has suggested that urinary supersaturation should be analyzed in clinical and research settings during the assessment of the effectiveness of medical treatment.

### STONE ANALYSIS

Stone analysis provides valuable information that clarifies the differential diagnosis and assists in directing management.[846,847] The stone crystallographic finding also helps identify cystine- and infection-induced stones, which may completely change management. Stone analysis also assists in the diagnosis of extremely rare stones, such as 2, 8-hydroxyadenine or drug-induced stones.[798,799] Commonly, the presence of ammonium urate stones is encountered in patients with HIV-aquired immune deficiency syndrome as a consequence of laxative abuse[592] or because of protracted diarrhea.[797] In addition, the presence of CaP stones may suggest conditions such as dRTA, primary hyperparathyroidism, medullary sponge kidney, and carbonic anhydrase inhibitor treatment.[848] One may follow and reassess stone analysis in the management of recurrent stone formers who are unresponsive to specific medical treatment.

Although stone analysis plays an important role in the understanding of the underlying pathophysiology and selection of the treatment, one major limitation has been the lack of a standard method among different laboratory techniques to identify urinary stone composition.[845,849] At present, there is a general agreement that chemical analysis of urinary stone composition must be substituted with more accurate spectroscopy techniques, including Fourier-transform infrared spectroscopy (FTIR), x-ray diffraction (XRD), and possibly scanning electron microscopy. Another drawback is that all current methods involve grinding and homogenization of the specimen, thus destroying any spatial information about the distribution of different components of mixed stones.

## IMAGING STUDIES

Imaging studies could be considered in patients suspected of kidney stones and in the follow-up of treated stone formers to monitor stone activity. Various recognized imaging methods include plain abdominal radiography for the kidneys, ureters, and bladder (KUB), ultrasound examination, and noncontrast computed tomography (NCCT).

### KIDNEYS, URETERS, AND BLADDER X-RAY

KUB is a plain x-ray of the abdomen that will detect opaque calcareous or cystine stones. It has wide availability, minimal radiation exposure, and low cost. The drawback is limited sensitivity (45%–58%) and specificity (60%–77%)[850] because of body habitus, overlying bowel gas, and extragenitourinary calcifications. It does provide adequate information in following the stone load during therapy in patients with radiopaque stones. For stable patients, annual imaging is adequate; however, additional imaging must be considered according to the clinical activity of the patient.[851]

### ULTRASOUND

Although ultrasound is a reliable, noninvasive, and fast technique and does not involve ionizing radiation, its major limitation is its low sensitivity. The lack of radiation and contrast renders it safe, particularly for children and pregnant women.[852,853] It is also inexpensive and widely available. It is excellent in detecting hydronephrosis and hydroureter.[854] Renal ultrasound is suitable for most patients with radiolucent stones (e.g., UA). However, ultrasound may miss a significant fraction of ureteral stones[854] and may give a false-positive diagnosis of obstruction in patients with pyelonephritis, vesicoureteric reflux, and residual dilation following relief of obstruction. Finally, sonography tends to overestimate the size of a stone as a result of the inaccurate determination of the stone and tissue boundary.

### COMPUTED TOMOGRAPHY

NCCT, synonymous with unenhanced helical CT screening, has the highest sensitivity (94%–100%) and specificity (92%–99%)[855,856] and can be considered the current gold standard for the diagnosis of kidney stones.[857] Stones as small as 1 mm can be diagnosed by NCCT. The disadvantages of this technique include radiation exposure, limited ability to evaluate degree of obstruction, and high cost. Newer techniques have been adapted that offer lower exposure to radiation (from traditional 8 to 16 millisieverts [mSv] down to 0.5–2 mSv).[858] If NCCT imaging can be performed effectively with lower dose radiation, it will remove the only concern with this test, which is increased risk of malignancy with long-term usage in repeated stone formers.[859–861]

Another advantage of the NCCT scan is the ability to determine stone density using Hounsfield units (HU), which may have prognostic value in terms of success in shock wave therapy.[862] Similarly as a preoperative test (e.g., before percutaneous nephrolithotomy), NCCT can detect possible altered anatomy and accurately assess stone size and location, both of which have an impact on the selection of optimal surgical intervention.

### INTRAVENOUS PYELOGRAPHY

Intravenous pyelography (IVP) has been the historic gold standard imaging approach to diagnose nephrolithiasis. It provides excellent anatomic detail of the minor and major calyces, infundibula, renal pelvis, and ureters, and a calculus is visualized as a discrete filling defect. The disadvantage is the use of nephrotoxic contrast agents. The sensitivity and specificity of KUB for detecting renal calculi have been reported as 59% and 71%, respectively.[863] The use of NCCT has largely supplanted IVP.[864–866] IVP is still occasionally used following NCCT in some patients to guide in percutaneous or endoureteral surgical procedures. It is also used in diabetic patients with renal colic mimicking kidney stones caused by papillary necrosis.[850]

### MAGNETIC RESONANCE IMAGING

Magnetic resonance imaging (MRI) is a potential alternative to NCCT for the diagnosis of nephrolithiasis and urinary tract obstruction. The obvious advantage is that it does not deliver ionizing radiation. Akin to sonography, it is useful in pregnant women and in children and adolescents. A related technique, magnetic resonance urography, has been reported as a method for the diagnosis of urinary tract obstruction, specifically in pregnant women.[867] The disadvantage of MRI is its high cost.

In general, patients with a known history of previous renal colic because of stone disease may be initially evaluated by KUB or ultrasound. NCCT can be used in patients who have not been previously diagnosed and in those with atypical clinical presentation. Ultrasound is considered the method of choice in pregnant patients and children with kidney stone disease. IVP should be considered following NCCT if no stone was diagnosed or when planning an endoscopic evaluation or open intervention to assist the urologist in mapping the urinary tract. In situations in which NCCT is not available, one may start with KUB and ultrasound evaluations and only consider IVP if these two techniques fail to diagnose kidney stones. In the follow-up of patients, because of the high risk of cumulative radiation, it is advisable to select KUB and ultrasound until newer, low-radiation NCCT has been developed.

### DIGITAL TOMOSYNTHESIS

Digital tomosynthesis is a modern technique that may accurately detect radiopaque kidney stones with limited radiation (0.54 mSv).[868,869] This technique is comparable with NCCT for the detection of renal stones, but is not affected by stone size and BMI of the patient and has superb reproducibility. It has an advantage over CT scans because it offers minimal radiation with a decreased cost.

# MANAGEMENT OF STONES

## ACUTE MANAGEMENT

As an acute illness, urolithiasis is associated with significant pain, disability, and loss of productivity.[870] Approximately 50% of patients experiencing acute upper urinary tract stones require surgical intervention.[871,872] Medical treatment has been shown to facilitate spontaneous passage of ureteral stones. Stone size and location in the urinary tract are the major determinants of the likelihood of spontaneous stone passage. Spontaneous passage rates are higher for distal ureteral calculi compared with proximal and middle locations. Rates are also higher for smaller (<4 mm in diameter) compared with larger stones that are between 4 to 6 mm and those larger than 6 mm in diameter.[873,874] Overall, spontaneous passage rates are 12%, 22%, and 45% for proximal, middle, and distal ureteral calculi, respectively, and 55%, 35%, and 8% for stones smaller than 4 mm, 4 to 6 mm, and larger than 6 mm, respectively.[873] Because acute renal colic is associated with severe pain over an unpredictable time interval, adjunctive treatment to promote spontaneous stone passage and reduce symptoms is crucially important.

### MANAGEMENT OF RENAL COLIC

The management of renal colic is necessary until spontaneous passage of a stone, which usually occurs in patients with smaller (<4 mm) and more distal ureteral stones within 48 hours after the onset of acute renal colic.[875] During that period, patient will require supportive treatment, comprised of pain medications, including nonsteroidal antiinflammatory drugs (NSAIDs), opioids, hydration, and antiemetics.[876] Patients with resolving colic can be discharged from the emergency room but hospitalization is indicated in cases of persistent, relentless pain and intractable vomiting, established infection, and obstruction. Nephrostomy must be considered urgently to relieve the obstruction, which can be followed by ESWL, percutaneous lithotripsy, ureteroscopy with laser lithotripsy, retrograde basket extraction of the stone or, in rare events, open surgical removal.[877,878]

#### Medical Expulsive Therapy

Medical expulsive therapy (MET) has been used as conservative management in the treatment of ureteral stones.[879,880] It can potentially improve the patient's quality of life by reducing episodes of pain,[881,882] minimizing analgesic use,[883] and diminishing the stone transit time[883,884] and might decrease the costs and complications of ESWL and ureteroscopy.[870,885] Therapies that have been tested include glucocorticoids, hormones, NSAIDs, phosphodiesterase-5 inhibitors, calcium channel blockers, and $\alpha$-adrenergic blockers.[886–889] Most of the available studies are of $\alpha_1$-adrenergic receptor antagonists, which decrease ureteral smooth muscle tone and frequency and force of peristalsis.[4,5] There are limited data on the efficacy of calcium channel blockers, and tamsulosin has now been shown to be superior to nifedipine.[890] A recent Cochrane systematic review that included 67 studies and a total of 10,509 participants has found that alpha blockers increase stone clearance and shorten the stone expulsion time. In a subgroup analysis, alpha blockers were shown to be less effective for smaller stones (≤5 mm) than larger stones (>5 mm), perhaps because smaller stones already have a high rate of spontaneous passage.[891] In this study, only stone size, but not stone location or type of alpha blocker, was shown to affect the results.

Pradere and associates have reviewed the most recent 2016 guidelines for the management of urolithiasis.[892] Both the American Urological Association (AUA) and European Association of Urology (EAU) recommend offering alpha blockers as expulsive therapy for distal ureteral stones. The EUA recommends MET for stones larger than 5 mm, whereas the AUA recommends it for stones smaller than 10 mm. The AUA suggests 4 to 6 weeks of observation with conservative treatment from the initial clinical presentation.

## CHRONIC MANAGEMENT

### LIFESTYLE AND DIETARY MANAGEMENT

One major limitation in the field has been the scarcity of RCTs to compare the effects of specific dietary and fluid measures in recurrent kidney stone formers.

#### Fluid Intake

Fluid management should be considered in all patients with kidney stones, regardless of stone composition. Dilution of lithogenic elements in the urine should be the panacea of kidney stone therapy. The effect of fluid intake was first examined in 108 idiopathic stone formers over approximately 5 years, with significant declines in new stone formation. One limitation of this study was a lack of a control group.[893] However, in an RCT in men with recurrent CaOx stones over 5 years, high fluid intake to ensure urinary volume of approximately 2.5 L/day reduced stone recurrence by approximately 44%, compared with a control group with no dietary restrictions.[894] However, this study targeted first-time stone formers, and the results of this study are not necessarily applicable to the kidney stone–forming population with residual stones at a high-risk of kidney stone recurrence. In a 3-year RCT, 1009 kidney stone formers were randomized to a control group that continued drinking soft drinks and an intervention group that avoided consumption of soft drinks.[895] This study showed a marginal benefit in avoiding soft drinks. Another study suggested that fluid intake of fruit juices, specifically orange juice, is also effective in reducing urinary CaOx saturation.[896] The same effectiveness is not seen with apple juice, grapefruit juice, cola, or some sport drinks because of their elevated oxalate and fructose concentrations.[896–899]

Fluid therapy is also recommended for cystinuria. Cystine has a limited solubility of 243 mg/L in urine.[900] Reduction of urine cystine supersaturation to less than 1.0, or concentration to less than 243 mg/L (1 mmol/L), would require drinking around 4 L/day, including nocturnal intake.[567] Off-label use of vasopressin receptor antagonists has been proposed to induce pharmacologic diabetes insipidus,[568] but the long-term effects of this drug has not been evaluated. In conjunction with the exorbitant cost and safe and easily available water, it is unclear whether there is an advantage to this therapy.

### Dietary Adjustment

**Calcium Intake.** In general, high dietary calcium intake appears to be protective against CaOx stones. In one study of Italian men with recurrent CaOx stones, a "traditional prescription" of low calcium diet was compared against liberal calcium (1200 mg/day) but low dietary sodium (<100 mEq/day) and animal protein consumption (50–60 g/day).[27] Despite only partial adherence, the low-sodium and protein diet resulted in less recurrence of stones.

Three large epidemiologic studies using food frequency questionnaires and history of kidney stone passage have suggested that low calcium and low fluid intake,[22,24–26] sugar-containing beverages,[897] and high animal protein intake are risk factors for the development of first-time kidney stones[22,24–26] among women and younger men.

Unlike dietary calcium, supplemental calcium may increase the risk of stone formation. This association was shown in an observational study of older women treated with calcium supplements compared with those who did not take supplements.[26] However, this association was not seen in younger men and women.[24] In a large epidemiologic study (Women's Health Initiative), calcium supplementation increased the risk of CaOx stone formation; one should exercise some caution because the total calcium intake was very high in those using supplements.[32]

**Dietary Oxalate.** High urinary oxalate is associated with the risk of nephrolithiasis,[901] and dietary oxalate restriction has generally been recommended. In epidemiologic studies, however, it is difficult to demonstrate the relationship between dietary oxalate and urinary oxalate.[679] Although there is no doubt that dietary oxalate is absorbed, the huge variation in intestinal absorption, bacterial degradation, and superimposed endogenous synthesis renders it difficult to discern a clear relationship between dietary and urinary oxalate. The Dietary Approaches to Stop Hypertension (DASH) diet, which was not restricted in oxalate content, significantly reduced the risk of kidney stones.[902] However, the protective effect of the DASH diet may be caused by the ingestion of a high fruit and vegetable content (alkali) in conjunction with low animal protein intake. In general, urinary oxalate excretion is affected by calcium intake, which may determine intestinal bioavailability of oxalate and consequently its absorption. With the recommended daily dietary calcium, CaOx stone risk has been shown not to be significantly influenced, even with relatively high dietary oxalate.[38] Therefore, it is prudent to recommend patients with hyperoxaluria and CaOx stone to consume a total calcium of 1000 to 1200 mg/day ingested with meals to complex intestinal luminal oxalate. The restriction of dietary oxalate in subjects with idiopathic hyperoxaluria may not be efficacious but likely will not increase stone risk. In contrast, in patients with inflammatory bowel disease or who have undergone bariatric surgery, dietary oxalate restriction should be imposed in addition to higher total calcium intake from the diet and supplements at mealtime.[130,903,904]

**Animal Protein.** In a multicomponent dietary intervention study, it was shown that a combination of low protein (50–60 g/day) and low sodium consumption (≤100 mEq/day) associated with normal calcium intake (1200 mg/day) significantly lowered the risk of kidney stone recurrence in Italian males with hypercalciuria.[27] However, it was argued that the protective effects may not be related to low protein consumption but was because of the consumption of low-salt and normal calcium intake. The result of this study was not supported in two other studies using a low-protein and high-fiber diet[39]; another study showed no difference in stone occurrence between low animal protein intake (<three servings of fish or meat/week and dairy products <100 g/day) compared with a controlled diet.[905]

**Ascorbic Acid.** Vitamin C above the physiologic dose may increase urinary oxalate. In a metabolic study, 2 g of ascorbic acid elevated the 24-hour urinary oxalate (29–35 mg in non–stone formers; 31–41 mg in stone formers). Therefore, patients with hyperoxaluria should be cautious about OTC vitamin C supplements.[906,907] Fortunately, most preparations are less than 1 g/day.

**Dietary Intervention in Cystinuria.** Cystine excretion has been shown to be reduced by decreasing dietary sodium, although no clinical outcome studies have been performed.[567,569,908–910] The mechanism for this is not known but salt regulation of the $b^{0,+}$ system for the purpose of L-DOPA uptake and synthesis of nephrogenic dopamine is a possibility.[570] On a high-salt diet, we suggest that the $b^{0,+}$ system may be occupied with dopamine synthesis and hence unavailable for cystine reabsorption. In the absence of ill effects of salt restriction, it is reasonable therefore to recommend restricting salt intake to about 2 g/day.

Reduction of animal protein intake has also been proposed to be beneficial because it would reduce dietary intake of cystine and its precursor methionine, which might reduce cystine excretion,[571] and would also increase the solubility of urinary cystine by increasing urinary pH. One study has shown that urinary cystine excretion decreases in cystinuric patients on a low-protein diet, compared with a total of 9% of caloric intake from protein compared with higher protein intake.[571] Restriction of protein must be used cautiously in children because the restriction of essential amino acids may compromise growth in children.

**Other Dietary Interventions.** It has been suggested that lowering urinary phosphorus, magnesium, and ammonium levels via dietary manipulation will lower the risk of struvite stones. There are limited data in humans exploring the efficacy of dietary modification in this population. Low phosphorus and calcium, combined with aluminum hydroxide gel, has been proposed,[911] supposedly to lower urinary phosphorus excretion by limiting the intake and absorption of phosphorus. Treatment with estrogen over 3.5 years was proposed to diminish urinary calcium excretion mediated by decreasing bone resorption.[912] However, these interventions were also associated with side effects, including GI distress, lethargy, bone pain, and hypercalciuria.

## PHARMACOLOGIC TREATMENT

Pharmacologic treatment is essential in almost all recurrent kidney stone formers and in the management of patients with UA, cystine, recurrent calcium, and infection-induced stones, principally as a result of the lack of availability and/or consensus regarding the effectiveness of nonpharmacologic interventions.[913] One major limitation with respect to pharmacologic treatment is the paucity of randomized controlled data with stone episodes as hard evidence of treatment results.[874] This is largely because stone events are rare, and such studies must be carried out in a large number of patients over a long period of time. There is also no consensus as to whether pharmacologic treatment should be targeted at specific metabolic abnormalities or should be given empirically, irrespective of underlying biochemical abnormalities.[147,914–917] Although the benefit of directed medical treatment has not been decisively proven, some observational studies have suggested the beneficial effects of directed management of kidney stones.[918,919]

### PHARMACOLOGIC AGENTS USED

#### Thiazide Diuretics

Thiazide diuretics and their analogues are used commonly for lowering calcium excretion in hypercalciuric, recurrent, calcium stone formers.[874] To date, six RCTs have studied thiazides in recurrent calcium stone formers. One study has shown a similar decrease in stone formation among thiazide-treated versus untreated patients.[920] Another study has shown diminished hypercalciuria without any change in stone events in patients treated with hydrochlorothiazide compared with placebo.[921] The remaining four RCTs, which evaluated a total of 408 patients over durations of 26 to 36 months, have demonstrated significant reductions in recurrent kidney stones with thiazides and the thiazide analogue indapamide[916,917,922–924] (Table 38.12). The results of these RCTs are consistent with uncontrolled studies totaling over 6600 patient-years of thiazide treatment for calcium nephrolithiasis patients.[363,500,924–928,939] Two critical but often ignored facts of thiazide therapy deserve emphasis. First, the optimal effect of thiazide diuretics is attained with a low-salt diet. Although there is likely some direct effect of thiazides on the DCT, most of its effect is to induce slight extracellular volume contraction and increase proximal calcium reabsorption; thus, simultaneous ingestion of a high-salt diet will nullify the efficacy of thiazides.[940,941] Second, the successful reduction in urinary calcium can be offset by hypocitraturia because of potassium depletion and proximal tubule intracellular acidosis. One must be vigilant in detecting potassium deficiency, and potassium supplements should be prescribed to avoid hypocitraturia if dietary potassium intake is not sufficient.[397] Potassium citrate may provide an advantage over potassium chloride in these cases.[942]

Thiazide treatment, along with dietary sodium restriction to maximize the hypocalciuric effect of thiazide, is the treatment of choice in hypercalciuric calcium stone-forming subjects. The incidence of side effects on thiazide diuretic may approach 30%[924] but side effects requiring discontinuation of the drug are rare. To date, long-term side effects of thiazide treatment in the kidney stone population have not yet been documented. A meta-analysis of clinical trials in hypertensive subjects has demonstrated a relationship between changes in serum glucose and potassium concentrations.[943] This was also confirmed in a large cohort, the Antihypertensive and Lipid Lowering Treatment to Prevent Heart Attack Trial (ALLHAT), in which the incidence of diabetes mellitus was higher with chlorthalidone compared with amlodipine or lisinopril over 4 years. The exact pathophysiologic mechanism has not yet been fully uncovered.[944–946] One potential mechanism is the relationship between potassium deficiency and defective insulin secretion and action.[947,948] The list of commonly used drugs and recommended dosages in the treatment of hypercalciuric calcium nephrolithiasis with potential side effects is summarized in Table 38.13.

#### Alkali Treatment

Alkali treatment can be used alone or in combination with thiazides in recurrent calcium or uric acid stone formers. There have been four RCTs[147,153,931,949]; two of these trials targeted patients after ESWL for residual stone fragment growth or new stone formation. In three nonrandomized, non–placebo-controlled studies, one retrospective study, and one non-RCT, potassium citrate reduced the risk of clinical stone events (see Table 38.12).

One study has shown no difference in stone formation.[154] This study included a total of 50 hypocitraturic calcium nephrolithiasis patients treated with 90 mEq of potassium alkali/day over 3 years. One possibility for the lack of efficacy may have been because of the small size.

In three nonrandomized, non–placebo-controlled studies, alkali treatment showed a significant decrease in new stone events.[157,158,929] One retrospective study comparing three groups of patients with medullary sponge kidney (MSK) received potassium citrate or no treatment. The results showed that treatment with potassium citrate was effective in reducing renal stones compared with nontreated groups.[930] In one nonrandomized but placebo-controlled study, 503 subjects

**Table 38.12 Major Clinical Pharmacotherapeutic Trials of Calcium and Noncalcium Nephrolithiasis**

| Trial | Reference | Treatment | No. of Subjects | Design | Outcome |
|---|---|---|---|---|---|
| Thiazide diuretics | Laerum[917] | Hydrochlorothiazide vs. placebo | 50 | RCT | Decreased new stone formation and prolonged stone-free interval |
| | Ettinger[916] | Chlorthalidone vs. magnesium hydroxide vs. placebo | 124 | RCT | Chlorthalidone more effective than magnesium hydroxide or placebo in reducing stone events |
| | Ohkawa[922] | Trichlormethiazide vs. no treatment | 175 | RCT | Decreased calciuria and stone formation rate |
| | Borghi[923] | Diet vs. diet + indapamide vs. diet + indapamide + allopurinol | 75 | RCT | Diet + pharmacotherapy better than diet alone |
| | Yendt[924] | Hydrodiuril | 33 | NNT | Decreased number of stone events or invasive and noninvasive procedures |
| | Coe[500] | Trichlormethiazide | 37 | NNT | Decreased new stone formation |
| | Coe[363] | Trichlormethiazide vs. allopurinol vs. both | 222 | NNT | Decreased new stone formation |
| | Yendt[925] | Hydrochlorothiazide | 139 | NNT | Decreased new stone formation or stone growth |
| | Backman[926] | Bendroflumethiazide | 44 | NNT | Decreased new stone formation |
| | Maschio[927] | Hydrochlorothizide + amelioride vs. both + allopurinol | 519 | NNT | Decreased new stone formation |
| | Pak[928] | Hydrochlorthiazide | 37 | NNT | Decreased new stone formation |
| Alkali treatment | Pak[157] | Potassium citrate vs. pretreatment in calcium and uric acid stone formers | 89 | NNT | Decreased stone events |
| | Preminger[158] | Potassium citrate | 9 | NNT | Decreased new stone formation |
| | Pak[929] | Potasssium citrate | 18 | NNT | Decreased stone events |
| | Fabris[930] | Potassium citrate vs. no treatment | 65 | NNT | Decreased stone rate in those treated with potassium citrate |
| | Barcelo[153] | Potassium citrate vs. placebo | 57 | RCT | Decreased new stone formation and increased urinary citrate |
| | Hofbauer[154] | Diet + sodium potassium citrate vs. diet | 50 | RCT | No difference in stone formation |
| | Ettinger[147] | Potassium magnesium citrate vs. placebo | 64 | RCT | Decreased new stone formation |
| | Soygur[931] | Potassium citrate vs. no treatment post–shock wave lithotripsy | 110 | RCT | Decreased stone recurrence |
| | Kang[919] | Mix of potassium citrate, thiazide, allopurinol vs. no treatment after percutaneous nephrolithotomy | 226 | NCT | Decreased stone recurrence |
| Allopurinol treatment | Ettinger[932] | Allopurinol vs. placebo | 60 | RCT | Decreased stone events |
| | Coe[363] | Thiazide vs. allopurinol vs. both | 202 | RCT | Decreased stone events vs. pretreatment |
| Febuxostat | Goldfarb[567] | Febuxostat vs. allopurinol or placebo | 99 | RCT | Febuxostat decreased 24-hour urinary uric acid excretion more significantly than allopurinol; no change in stone size or number |
| Other treatment | Dahlberg[933] | D-Penicillamine | 89 | R | Decreased stone event and dissolution of stones |
| | Pak[900] | D-Penicillamine or α-mercaptoproprionylglycine vs. conservative medical therapy | 66 | R | Both drugs equally effective in reducing stone events |
| | Chow[934] | D-Penicillamine or α-mercaptopropionylglycine vs. conservative medical therapy | 16 | NNT | Decreased stone event |
| | Barbey[935] | D-Penicillamine or α-mercaptopropionylglycine vs. conservative medical therapy | 27 | R | Decreased stone events |
| | Williams[936] | Acetohydroxamic acid vs. placebo | 18 | RCT | Decreased stone size |
| | Griffith[937] | Acetohydroxamic acid vs. placebo | 210 | RCT | Decreased stone growth |
| | Griffith[938] | Acetohydroxamic acid vs. placebo | 94 | RCT | Decreased stone growth |

*N,* Number of patients; *NCT,* nonrandomized controlled trial; *NNT,* nonrandomized, non–placebo-controlled trial; *R,* retrospective; *RCT,* randomized controlled trial.

Modified from Sakhaee K, Maalouf NM, Sinnott B. Clinical review. Kidney stones: 2012: pathogenesis, diagnosis, and management. *J Clin Endocrinol Metab.* 2012;97:(6)1847–1860.

**Table 38.13 Commonly Used Drugs in the Treatment of Hypercalciuric Calcium Nephrolithiasis**

| Drug | Recommended Dosage(s) | Comments |
|---|---|---|
| Hydrochlorothiazide | 50 mg/day, 25 mg bid | A single dose is preferred because twice-daily dosage may cause nocturia, discomfort, and noncompliance. |
| Chlorthalidone | 25 mg/day, 50 mg/day | Both dosages lower urinary calcium by the same degree; long-acting; may cause hypokalemia and secondary hypocitraturia |
| Indapamide | 1.2 mg/day, 2.5 mg/day | This treatment may have fewer side effects than hydrochlorothiazide, including lower incidence of hypokalemia and hypotension. |
| Amiloride | 5 mg/day | Potassium sparing; lowers urinary calcium but to a lesser degree than hydrochlorothiazide |
| Amiloride-hydrochlorothizide | 5 mg-50 mg/day | Maintains the hypocalciuric effect of thiazide while averting the development of severe hypokalemia |
| Trichlormethiazide | 2 mg/day, 4 mg/day | Not marketed in the United States |

were treated with a mixture of potassium citrate, thiazide, and allopurinol, compared with no treatment after percutaneous nephrolithotomy, for a mean duration of 41 months; there was a decreased stone formation rate, from 1.89 to 0.46 stones/year.[919] One caveat in these studies was that alkali treatment that was given to patients with urinary citrate excretion ranged from normal to low-normal and low urinary citrate.[147,153,154]

Alkali treatment is relatively safe, with minor GI side effects, although certain susceptible individuals can have considerable gastric distress. The side effects have to be weighed against its efficacy in recurrent calcium oxalate stones[147,153,154] and uric acid stones,[499,929] as well as in patients with residual stones after shock wave lithotripsy.[931] One primary potential side effect that has been gaining attention is the risk of CaP stone formation. A rise of the urinary pH above 6.7 favors the generation of monohydrogen phosphate. Despite this concern, in two nonrandomized, non–placebo-controlled trials[158,930] in patients with dRTA and MSK with preexisting high UpH, alkali therapy was shown to be effective in reducing recurrent calcium stone formation. Larger scale prospective RCTs are still necessary to determine the effects of alkali treatment on CaP stone incidence.

Although sodium bicarbonate may offer the same degree of urinary alkalinization when used in an equivalent dose to potassium alkali, it may increase the risk of calcium stone formation because of sodium-induced hypercalciuria and promotion of monosodium urate-induced CaOx crystallization.[499,929] The initial recommended dose for alkali is 30 to 40 mEq/day. In practice, 24-hour urine will be measured to follow the increase in citraturia and titrate the alkaline dose. The goal is to maintain the UpH higher than 6.1 and less than 7 to avoid the potential complication of calcium stone formation. A 24-hour UpH, however, may not reflect diurnal variation in UpH and periods of high urinary acidity.[950] Therefore, higher doses of alkali treatment administered at night may ameliorate abnormally acidic urine in those with recurrent uric acid kidney stones.[950] Because unduly acidic urine is the predominant feature of patients with UA nephrolithiasis, alkali therapy with potassium citrate is first-line treatment in these patients.[47] Treatment with allopurinol can be considered when there is very high urinary UA levels, and alkali treatment is unsuccessful in patients with inflammatory bowel disease, bowel resection, and recurrent UA stones, despite adequate urinary alkalinization.

Alkalinization is also helpful in cystinuria because cystine solubility increases with increasing pH. Generally, it is recommended that alkalinization should be conducted conservatively, not to exceed a pH of 6.5 to 6.7, because highly alkaline urine may increase the risk of CaP stone formation. Defective acidification and high UpH was previously described in patients with mixed cystine and calcium stones.[951] It is often difficult to determine the optimal dose of alkali to be administered to each individual patient.[565,952] Therefore, it is advisable to monitor patient responses with direct measurements of urinary supersaturation with respect to cystine.[567] Both potassium citrate and sodium bicarbonate have been shown to be equally effective in alkalinizing urine in this population.[953] Sodium alkali can be used in patients with renal insufficiency to avoid hyperkalemia. The dosage of alkali is typically divided equally three or four times daily.

### Combined Pharmacologic Treatment

The effects of combined thiazide and alkali treatment were shown not be significantly different from thiazide monotherapy in reducing the risk of kidney stone recurrence in one poor-quality study.[954] Furthermore, stone recurrence was not shown to be different between thiazide combined with an allopurinol versus thiazide treatment alone.[923]

### Xanthine Oxidase Inhibitors

Allopurinol is used for the treatment of hyperuricosuric calcium stone formers rather than uric acid stone formers. One RCT in hyperuricosuric calcium stone formers, comparing allopurinol versus placebo,[932] has demonstrated significantly decreased stone events with allopurinol treatment. Another RCT in recurrent hyperuricosuric calcium stone formers, comparing thiazide versus allopurinol and combined thiazide and allopurinol, showed significantly reduced stone events with the combination treatment[363] (see Table 38.12). The efficacy of allopurinol alone in the treatment of hyperuricosuric CaOx stone-forming patients with multiple metabolic abnormalities is less evident.[955] The effective dose is 300 mg/day, which can either be administered as a single dose or divided into three equal doses throughout the day. Side effects of allopurinol are reported as uncommon, including a skin rash in 2% of treated patients and more severe but even rarer life-threatening hypersensitivity reactions, including acute interstitial nephritis and Steven-Johnson syndrome.[956] Adjustments are needed in patients with impaired kidney function because allopurinol is primarily excreted by the kidney.

A nonpurine xanthine oxidase inhibitor analogue, febuxostat, has been approved for the treatment of hyperuricemia associated with gouty arthritis. In a retrospective study, the use of febuxostat in patients with gout with allergies to allopurinol was shown to be a safe alternative.[957] In a 6-month, double-blinded RCT, hyperuricosuric calcium stone formers with one or more calcium stones detected by CT were treated with 80 mg/day of febuxostat, 300 mg/day of allopurinol, or placebo. Febuxostat reduced 24-hour urinary UA significantly more than allopurinol but there was no change in stone size or number over this period of time.[958] Therefore, no conclusion comparing the drugs can be drawn until a longer study is conducted to determine the incidence of stone events (see Table 38.12). One advantage of febuxostat is that it is principally metabolized by the liver, thereby rendering dose adjustments in those with impaired kidney function unnecessary.[959]

#### Magnesium Treatment

In only one study in calcium stone formers, treatment with magnesium lowered stone recurrence but not significantly compared with placebo.[916]

#### Cystine Chelation Therapy

The treatment of cystine stones can be challenging. Conservative management with hydration and urinary alkalinization are the first steps in the management of a cystinuric patient but, more often than not, they do not suffice. Thiol derivatives that act as chelating agents are commonly used in patients with severe cystinuria (>1000 mg/day). These drugs reduce a single cystine molecule into two cysteines and form a highly soluble disulfide compound of the drug with the cysteine molecules.[960] The effect of a disulfide compound (D-penicillamine) on stone events was first described by Dahlberg and coworkers.[933] Subsequently, α-mercaptopropionylglycine (tiopronin) was marketed for use in cystinuric patients. In two studies, pharmacologic treatment with D-penicillamine or tiopronin was shown to be superior to hydration and alkalinization alone in reducing stone events[934,935] (see Table 38.12). However, to date, no RCTs have demonstrated the superiority of pharmacologic treatment over placebo in cystinuric patients.

A few studies have suggested that captopril, which is also a thiol derivative, might also be effective in reducing urinary cystine excretion,[961,962] but its efficacy has not been confirmed by others.[935,963] The potential role of inhibitors of cystine crystal growth has been explored. The most effective inhibitors tested were L-cystine dimethyl ester (L-CDME) and L-cystine methyl ester (L-CME). However, this effectiveness has only been tested in experimental models and not yet in cystinuric populations.[964]

Tiopronin has a lower incidence of side effects compared with D-penicillamine, and it is therefore used more often.[900] The side effects include GI irritation, abnormalities in hepatic enzymes, pancytopenias, skin irritation and disorders, and proteinuria.[900] Effective therapy should be aimed at maintaining a urinary cystine concentration at 250 mg/L, although there is variability among individual patients. Therefore, assessment of urinary supersaturation with respect to cystine solubility is important. However, to date, there has been no clinical study exploring whether such measurement will avert the complications of cystine stone formation.[565,567,952] One important caveat is that urinary cystine measurement does not differentiate between a drug-cysteine complex and unbound cystine. Furthermore, urinary measurement of cystine may not change with drug treatment, which may lead to misguided attempts to increase the dose of thiol drugs to lower urinary cystine levels. Therefore, it is advisable to monitor the patient's response to treatment via urinary supersaturation, which may guide dosing of chelating agents better.

### PHARMACOTHERAPY OF INFECTION-RELATED STONES

According to the guidelines of the AUA, surgical treatment is still the best management for infectious stones (see later). However, medical treatment can be used in those with significant comorbidities who are not amenable to surgery and also to prevent stone recurrence after successful stone removal. These treatments include antibiotics, dissolution therapy, urease inhibitors, urinary acidification, dietary modification, and other supportive measures.

#### Antibiotics

Antibiotics are important during both pre- and perioperative periods to prevent urinary sepsis from surgical procedures. Antibiotics should be directed against specific microorganisms established by positive urine cultures.

#### Dissolution Therapy

Boric acid, permanganate, and other solutions have been instilled into kidneys to dissolve infectious stones.[965] However, dissolution treatment has fallen out of favor because of its cost, duration of hospitalization and, most importantly, significant associated risks. The increased mortality following internal irrigation led to a ban in the United States by the U.S. Food and Drug Association (FDA) on the use of this treatment approach.

#### Urease Inhibitors

Urease-producing microorganisms, by converting urea to ammonia, play a key role in supersaturation of urine with respect to ammonium magnesium phosphate (struvite), which usually coexists with calcium carbonate apatite stones, because both stone types are favored in an alkaline environment.[966] Although inhibition of bacterial urease has been shown to retard stone growth and prevent new stone formation, it cannot eradicate existing stones nor the underlying infection. However, when combined with antimicrobial therapy, urease inhibition provides palliation for patients who cannot undergo definitive surgical management.[575,967]

The urease inhibitor acetohydroxamic acid (AHA) is the only FDA-approved urease inhibitor that can be used orally to inhibit urease enzyme activity.[937,938] This drug is cleared by the kidney and can penetrate bacterial cell walls. It also functions synergistically with antibiotics. Three RCTs have shown significant reduction in stone growth with AHA compared with placebo.[936–938] AHA can confer serious GI, neurologic, hematologic, and dermatologic side effects in 20% of patients, but these tend to resolve on discontinuation.[936–938] The starting dose of AHA is 250 mg by mouth twice a day. AHA is also contraindicated in patients with chronic kidney disease and serum creatinine concentrations higher than

2.5 mg/dL, which increase the risk of toxicity and poor urinary concentration.[937,938]

### Urinary Acidification

Because urine alkalinity (pH >7.2) promotes the formation of struvite and carbonate apatite stones, urinary acidification has been used to control stone burden in this population. L-Methionine, which imposes an acid load ($H_2SO_4$), can lower UpH. An in vitro simulation of decreasing UpH from 6.5 to 5.7 increased the dissolution rate of struvite stones.[968] It was suggested that oral intake of L-methionine, 1500 to 3000 mg/day, can be used in humans for the dissolution of infectious stones, although there has been no trial to prove this yet.[968]

## SURGICAL MANAGEMENT OF INFECTION-RELATED STONES

Struvite staghorn calculi generally require surgical removal and, if not properly treated, may require nephrectomy.[969] The goal is eradication of stone burden and prevention of stone regrowth, renal damage, and persistent infection. A significant number of patients treated with open surgical stone removal have a recurrence following surgery because of recurrent urinary tract infections. Rather than open surgical stone removal, percutaneous nephrolithotomy can completely remove struvite stones 90% of the time,[970,971] with a recurrence rate approaching only 10% in kidneys rendered stone-free.[972] A retrospective analysis of 43 patients with pure or mixed struvite stones from Duke University Medical Center from 2005 to 2012 has found stone recurrence in 23% of patients, with stable renal function over a median follow-up of 22 months (range, 6–67 months). ESWL with ureteral stenting alone will result in stone-free rates of 50% to 75%.[973] Retrograde ureteroscopy with holmium:YAG laser stone disruption can fragment almost all minor staghorn stones, with a recurrence rate of 60% at 6 months.[974] The AUA suggests a combined approach of percutaneous nephrolithotomy and shock wave lithotripsy.

## ACKNOWLEDGMENTS

The authors are supported by the National Institutes of Health R01-DK081423, R01DK091392, R01-DK092461, U01-HL111146, O'Brien Kidney Research Center (P30 DK-079328), American Society of Nephrology, Simmons Family Foundation, and Charles and Jane Pak Foundation. We wish to acknowledge Ms. Rubyth Aguirre for her assistance in the preparation of this chapter.

 Complete reference list available at ExpertConsult.com.

## KEY REFERENCES

2. Scales CD Jr, Smith AC, Hanley JM, et al. Urologic Diseases in America P. Prevalence of kidney stones in the United States. *Eur Urol.* 2012;62(1):160–165.
13. Romero V, Akpinar H, Assimos DG. Kidney stones: a global picture of prevalence, incidence, and associated risk factors. *Rev Urol.* 2010;12(2–3):e86–e96.
17. Xu LHR, Adams-Huet B, Poindexter JR, et al. Temporal changes in kidney stone composition and in risk factors predisposing to stone formation. *J Urol.* 2017;197(6):1465–1471.
22. Curhan GC, Willett WC, Rimm EB, et al. A prospective study of dietary calcium and other nutrients and the risk of symptomatic kidney stones. *N Engl J Med.* 1993;328(12):833–838.
27. Borghi L, Schianchi T, Meschi T, et al. Comparison of two diets for the prevention of recurrent stones in idiopathic hypercalciuria. *N Engl J Med.* 2002;346(2):77–84.
47. Sakhaee K, Adams-Huet B, Moe OW, et al. Pathophysiologic basis for normouricosuric uric acid nephrolithiasis. *Kidney Int.* 2002;62(3):971–979.
49. Cameron MA, Maalouf NM, Adams-Huet B, et al. Urine composition in type 2 diabetes: predisposition to uric acid nephrolithiasis. *J Am Soc Nephrol.* 2006;17(5):1422–1428.
72. Evan AP, Lingeman JE, Coe FL, et al. Randall's plaque of patients with nephrolithiasis begins in basement membranes of thin loops of Henle. *J Clin Invest.* 2003;111(5):607–616.
153. Barcelo P, Wuhl O, Servitge E, et al. Randomized double-blind study of potassium citrate in idiopathic hypocitraturic calcium nephrolithiasis. *J Urol.* 1993;150(6):1761–1764.
161. Hamm LL. Renal handling of citrate. *Kidney Int.* 1990;38(4):728–735.
222. Sakhaee K, Maalouf NM, Sinnott B. Clinical review. Kidney stones 2012: pathogenesis, diagnosis, and management. *J Clin Endocrinol Metab.* 2012;97(6):1847–1860.
230. Sakhaee K, Maalouf NM, Kumar R, et al. Nephrolithiasis-associated bone disease: pathogenesis and treatment options. *Kidney Int.* 2011;79(4):393–403.
234. Pak CY, Oata M, Lawrence EC, et al. The hypercalciurias. Causes, parathyroid functions, and diagnostic criteria. *J Clin Invest.* 1974; 54(2):387–400.
246. Insogna KL, Broadus AE, Dreyer BE, et al. Elevated production rate of 1,25-dihydroxyvitamin D in patients with absorptive hypercalciuria. *J Clin Endocrinol Metab.* 1985;61(3):490–495.
255. Breslau NA, Preminger GM, Adams BV, et al. Use of ketoconazole to probe the pathogenetic importance of 1,25-dihydroxyvitamin D in absorptive hypercalciuria. *J Clin Endocrinol Metab.* 1992;75(6): 1446–1452.
296. Frick KK, Bushinsky DA. Molecular mechanisms of primary hypercalciuria. *J Am Soc Nephrol.* 2003;14(4):1082–1095.
318. Yoon V, Adams-Huet B, Sakhaee K, et al. Hyperinsulinemia and urinary calcium excretion in calcium stone formers with idiopathic hypercalciuria. *J Clin Endocrinol Metab.* 2013;98(6):2589–2594.
330. Thorleifsson G, Holm H, Edvardsson V, et al. Sequence variants in the CLDN14 gene associate with kidney stones and bone mineral density. *Nat Genet.* 2009;41(8):926–930.
340. Cipriani C, Biamonte F, Costa AG, et al. Prevalence of kidney stones and vertebral fractures in primary hyperparathyroidism using imaging technology. *J Clin Endocrinol Metab.* 2015;100(4):1309–1315.
342. Raisz LG, Kream BE, Smith MD, et al. Comparison of the effects of vitamin D metabolites on collagen synthesis and resportion of fetal rat bone in organ culture. *Calcif Tissue Int.* 1980;32(2):135–138.
343. Sakhaee K, Maalouf NM, Poindexter J, et al. Relationship between Urinary Calcium and Bone Mineral Density in Patients with Calcium Nephrolithiasis. *J Urol.* 2017;197(6):1472–1477.
394. Alpern RJ, Sakhaee K. The clinical spectrum of chronic metabolic acidosis: homeostatic mechanisms produce significant morbidity. *Am J Kidney Dis.* 1997;29(2):291–302.
401. Sakhaee K. Recent advances in the pathophysiology of nephrolithiasis. *Kidney Int.* 2009;75(6):585–595.
407. Holmes RP, Goodman HO, Assimos DG. Contribution of dietary oxalate to urinary oxalate excretion. *Kidney Int.* 2001;59(1):270–276.
411. Hoppe B, Beck B, Gatter N, et al. Oxalobacter formigenes: a potential tool for the treatment of primary hyperoxaluria type 1. *Kidney Int.* 2006;70(7):1305–1311.
442. Siener R, Bangen U, Sidhu H, et al. The role of Oxalobacter formigenes colonization in calcium oxalate stone disease. *Kidney Int.* 2013;83(6):1144–1149.
493. Maalouf NM, Sakhaee K, Parks JH, et al. Association of urinary pH with body weight in nephrolithiasis. *Kidney Int.* 2004;65(4):1422–1425.
515. Abate N, Chandalia M, Cabo-Chan AV Jr, et al. The metabolic syndrome and uric acid nephrolithiasis: novel features of renal manifestation of insulin resistance. *Kidney Int.* 2004;65(2):386–392.
518. Daudon M, Traxer O, Conort P, et al. Type 2 diabetes increases the risk for uric acid stones. *J Am Soc Nephrol.* 2006;17(7):2026–2033.
520. Maalouf NM, Cameron MA, Moe OW, et al. Low urine pH: a novel feature of the metabolic syndrome. *Clin J Am Soc Nephrol.* 2007;2(5):883–888.
587. Daudon M. Drug induced renal stones. In: Rao PN, Preminger GM, Kavanaugh JP, eds. *Urinary Tract Stone Disease.* London, UK: BC Decker Publishing, Springer-Verlag; 2011:225–237.

606. Moe OW, Bonny O. Genetic hypercalciuria. *J Am Soc Nephrol.* 2005;16(3):729–745.
619. Goldfarb DS, Fischer ME, Keich Y, et al. A twin study of genetic and dietary influences on nephrolithiasis: a report from the Vietnam Era Twin (VET) Registry. *Kidney Int.* 2005;67(3):1053–1061.
624. Lerolle N, Coulet F, Lantz B, et al. No evidence for point mutations of the calcium-sensing receptor in familial idiopathic hypercalciuria. *Nephrol Dial Transplant.* 2001;16(12):2317–2322.
627. Vezzoli G, Tanini A, Ferrucci L, et al. Influence of calcium-sensing receptor gene on urinary calcium excretion in stone-forming patients. *J Am Soc Nephrol.* 2002;13(10):2517–2523.
631. Halbritter J, Baum M, Hynes AM, et al. Fourteen monogenic genes account for 15% of nephrolithiasis/nephrocalcinosis. *J Am Soc Nephrol.* 2014.
642. Hoenderop JG, van Leeuwen JP, van der Eerden BC, et al. Renal Ca2+ wasting, hyperabsorption, and reduced bone thickness in mice lacking TRPV5. *J Clin Invest.* 2003;112(12):1906–1914.
652. Fuster DG, Zhang J, Xie XS, et al. The vacuolar-ATPase B1 subunit in distal tubular acidosis: novel mutations and mechanisms for dysfunction. *Kidney Int.* 2008;73(10):1151–1158.
668. Jeong IG, Kang T, Bang JK, et al. Association between metabolic syndrome and the presence of kidney stones in a screened population. *Am J Kidney Dis.* 2011;58(3):383–388.
680. Pigna F, Sakhaee K, Adams-Huet B, et al. Body fat content and distribution and urinary risk factors for nephrolithiasis. *Clin J Am Soc Nephrol.* 2014;9(1):159–165.
690. Ferraro PM, Taylor EN, Eisner BH, et al. History of kidney stones and the risk of coronary heart disease. *JAMA.* 2013;310(4):408–415.
708. Rule AD, Bergstralh EJ, Melton LJ 3rd, et al. Kidney stones and the risk for chronic kidney disease. *Clin J Am Soc Nephrol.* 2009; 4(4):804–811.
754. Vezzoli G, Rubinacci A, Bianchin C, et al. Intestinal calcium absorption is associated with bone mass in stone-forming women with idiopathic hypercalciuria. *Am J Kidney Dis.* 2003;42(6):1177–1183.
762. Heller HJ, Zerwekh JE, Gottschalk FA, et al. Reduced bone formation and relatively increased bone resorption in absorptive hypercalciuria. *Kidney Int.* 2007;71(8):808–815.
786. Maalouf NM, Moe OW, Adams-Huet B, et al. Hypercalciuria associated with high dietary protein intake is not due to acid load. *J Clin Endocrinol Metab.* 2011;96(12):3733–3740.
853. Tasian GE, Copelovitch L. Evaluation and medical management of kidney stones in children. *J Urol.* 2014;192(5):1329–1336.
878. Pearle MS. Shock-wave lithotripsy for renal calculi. *N Engl J Med.* 2012;367(1):50–57.
891. Campschroer T, Zhu X, Vernooij RWM, et al. Alpha-blockers as medical expulsive therapy for ureteric stones: a Cochrane systematic review. *BJU Int.* 2018;122(6):932–945.
892. Pradere B, Doizi S, Proietti S, et al. Evaluation of Guidelines for Surgical Management of Urolithiasis. *J Urol.* 2018;199(5):1267–1271.
929. Pak CY, Sakhaee K, Fuller C. Successful management of uric acid nephrolithiasis with potassium citrate. *Kidney Int.* 1986;30(3): 422–428.

# 39

# Epidemiology of Diabetic Kidney Disease

Alessia Fornoni | Robert G. Nelson | Behzad Najafian | Per Henrik Groop

## CHAPTER OUTLINE



## KEY POINTS

- The total number of individuals worldwide who are at risk for DKD continues to rise because of the rapidly rising prevalence of type 2 diabetes.
- The clinical course of DKD and other diabetes complications in youth-onset type 2 diabetes is more aggressive than in type 1 diabetes.
- About two-thirds of patients who develop type 2 diabetes later in life may not show classical DKD lesions despite being microalbuminuric or proteinuric. Instead they may show lesions attributable more to arterionephrosclerosis with little or mild diabetic changes in the glomeruli.
- The recommended blood pressure target for diabetic patients without albuminuria is less than 140/90, but if the patient has albuminuria, a lower target of less than130/80 might be beneficial.
- Optimal glycemic control with a hemoglobin A1C target of around 7% is crucial for the prevention of DKD.
- The main obstacle to achieving optimal glycemic control is the risk of severe hypoglycemia.
- Simultaneous pancreas-kidney transplantation has revolutionized the treatment of patients with type 1 diabetes and is generally believed to prolong patient survival beyond the survival advantage associated with renal transplantation alone.
- The presence of new-onset diabetes after transplantation (NODAT) is associated with major health outcomes such as increased risk of acute rejection, graft loss, infection, and premature mortality largely attributable to cardiovascular disease.

Diabetic kidney disease (DKD) is a chronic kidney disease attributable to diabetes, and it is increasing worldwide, largely in response to a global epidemic of diabetes. The number of people with diabetes has doubled in the last 20 years,[1] and the International Diabetes Federation estimated that in 2015, 415 million adults between 20 and 79 years of age had diabetes.[2] Approximately 91% of people with diabetes have type 2 diabetes, and three-fourths of those with diabetes (mostly type 2 diabetes) are now living in low- and middle-income countries.[2]

Several factors are responsible for the global diabetes epidemic. Improved healthcare and living standards have caused the elderly population, which is at considerable risk for type 2 diabetes, to expand. A decline in physical activity and preference for calorie-dense foods has prompted a dramatic rise in obesity, which has also contributed to an increase in type 2 diabetes in children, adolescents, and young adults[3] as well as an earlier onset of type 1 diabetes.[4–6] Adverse health effects of exposure to diabetes *in utero* are also fueling the rise in obesity and type 2 diabetes in the young, with 16% of live births now affected by hyperglycemia in pregnancy.[2] In reviewing the epidemiology of DKD, the impact of these trends will be considered.

## DEFINITION, MEASUREMENT, AND CLASSIFICATION

Although albuminuria is a continuous measurement, it is often arbitrarily divided into microalbuminuria (30–299 mg/g), which is generally characterized by a greater risk for higher levels of albuminuria than normal urine albumin excretion (<30 mg/g), and macroalbuminuria (≥300 mg/g), which is typically associated with arterial hypertension and an elevated risk of kidney failure. Microalbuminuria is also currently referred to as moderate albuminuria, and macroalbuminuria as severe albuminuria, overt nephropathy, or clinical proteinuria,[7] and this is the nomenclature favored by the Kidney Disease Improving Global Outcome (KDIGO) clinical practice guidelines.[7] The American Diabetes Association recommends simply using the term *albuminuria* for an albumin:creatinine ratio 30 or more mg/g[8].

In addition to the distinct categories of albuminuria, six categories of GFR are currently being used: G1 >90, G2 60–89, G3a 45–59, G3b 30–44, G4 15–29, G5<15 ml/min/1.73 $m^2$. Reduced kidney function is defined by a GFR of less than 60 ml/min/1.73 $m^2$, and kidney failure by a GFR of less than 15 ml/min/1.73 $m^2$.[7]

Regardless of etiology, chronic kidney disease is classified according to the combined measures of albuminuria and eGFR to indicate prognosis for acute kidney injury, progressive kidney disease, kidney failure, cardiovascular mortality, and all-cause mortality (see Chapter 59).[7] These classifications are also used to guide practitioners on the frequency of patient visits. In general, persons with diabetes have higher risks for kidney failure, cardiovascular, and all-cause mortality than those without diabetes across the range of albuminuria and eGFR, but the relative risks of these health outcomes are similar in persons with or without diabetes.[9] The likelihood that chronic kidney disease represents DKD in patients with diabetes is enhanced by knowledge of several additional clinical factors.[10] In patients with type 1 diabetes of 10 years duration or longer, chronic kidney disease is nearly always attributable to DKD.[10] An eye examination is also a useful test for determining the presence of DKD.[11,12] The presence of diabetic retinopathy in patients with albuminuria is strongly suggestive of DKD, whereas the absence of diabetic retinopathy in those with normal urine albumin excretion or microalbuminuria and GFR less than 60 ml/min/1.73 $m^2$ suggests the presence of nonDKD.[11,13] Nondiabetic causes of chronic kidney disease should also be considered in patients with diabetes in the presence of rapidly declining GFR, refractory hypertension, presence of an active urine sediment, signs or symptoms of other systemic disease, or greater than 30% reduction of GFR within 2 to 3 months after initiation of an angiotensin-converting enzyme (ACE) inhibitor or an angiotensin receptor blocker.[10] Referral to nephrology is recommended at any level of GFR for any of these atypical presentations or when the presentation is typical and the GFR is less than 30 ml/min/1.73 $m^2$.

## EPIDEMIOLOGY

Although the conceptual definition of DKD includes a characteristic pathological appearance, which is described in detail later in this chapter, the working definition used in clinical practice is based primarily on measurements of albuminuria and estimated glomerular filtration rate (eGFR). Not all patients with diabetes, elevated albuminuria, and/or reduced eGFR have DKD; however, care is required to identify clinical signs or symptoms that suggest the presence of nondiabetic kidney disease in the setting of diabetes. In such cases, kidney biopsy may be required to establish whether or not the kidney disease is attributable to diabetes.

Urinary albumin excretion is usually normal at the diagnosis of type 1 diabetes, except when ketoacidosis is present. Albuminuria in the early years of type 1 diabetes is associated with poor metabolic control, and is frequently transitory and rarely persistent,[31,73,470–472] although one study involving 3250 Europeans with type 1 diabetes reported a prevalence of microalbuminuria of 19% among patients with diabetes for 1 to 5 years.[473] With treatment, normalization of albuminuria generally occurs. Nevertheless, the annual rate of increase in urine albumin excretion in patients with type 1 diabetes and persistent microalbuminuria is about 20%,[474] although many patients with persistent albuminuria also regress to normal albuminuria,[74] as discussed in more detail later in the chapter. Once macroalbuminuria develops, albuminuria regression is less frequent.[472,475]

Because the onset of type 2 diabetes is more insidious, poor glycemic control and elevated blood pressure may be present for several years before diagnosis, and therefore albuminuria is frequently present at diabetes diagnosis. In addition, the course of urinary albumin excretion in patients with type 2 diabetes is more heterogeneous than in those with type 1 diabetes, reflecting their older age, frequent comorbidities, and greater heterogeneity of kidney lesions.[357,444]

***Clinical Relevance***

**Epidemiology**

The rapidly increasing frequency of type 2 diabetes in children, adolescents, and young adults and the more aggressive clinical course of diabetic kidney disease in these patients than in those with type 1 diabetes means that clinical care providers can expect major shifts in the demographic characteristics of their diabetic kidney disease patients in the coming years. These changes will have important management implications, as more patients will require kidney care in early and mid-adult life, and more female patients who require such care will still be of childbearing age. Given that these changes are occurring most rapidly in low- and middle-income countries, low cost means of delivering care to these complex patients will need to be developed. In all countries, more emphasis will need to be placed on preventing diabetes or delaying its development.

### PREVALENCE

About one-third of adults with diabetes in the United States have DKD, defined by a urine albumin:creatinine ratio 30 mg/g or higher, an eGFR less than 60 ml/min/1.73 $m^2$, or both.[14] Population-based data from the National Health and Nutrition Examination Survey (NHANES) indicate that the prevalence of DKD in patients with diabetes remained largely unchanged between 1988 and 2008, and did not change within any specific racial or ethnic group. The prevalence of DKD in the overall population of the United States, however, increased by 34% during the same period, indicating that the prevalence of DKD increased in direct proportion to the rising prevalence of diabetes in the population.[14] A marked increase in the use of glucose-lowering medicines and inhibitors of the renin-angiotensin-aldosterone system during this period did not change the overall prevalence of DKD, but may have modified the clinical presentation by increasing the prevalence of reduced GFR, and modestly, but not significantly, decreasing the prevalence of albuminuria.[14] A more recent study extended the analysis of the NHANES cohorts through 2014 and convincingly demonstrated declining prevalence of albuminuria and increasing prevalence of reduced GFR among people with diabetes in the United States during the last 26 years.[15] In both studies, the proportion of adults with type 1 diabetes was small, so the results are primarily relevant to adults with type 2 diabetes.

In an analysis of data from NHANES 1999–2010, the prevalence of DKD in the population of the United States was estimated by type of diabetes using a published algorithm[16] to define people with type 1 diabetes (Table 39.1). Results showed a higher prevalence of DKD in people with type 2 diabetes than in those with type 1 diabetes. In addition, a higher prevalence of DKD was found in non-Hispanic blacks than in non-Hispanic whites. DKD was also more frequent in people with hypertension or cardiovascular disease, regardless of the type of diabetes.[17]

A cross-sectional study of 24,151 patients with type 2 diabetes from 33 countries reported that about one-half of the patients had albuminuria, 22% had eGFR less than 60 ml/min/1.73 m$^2$, and 80% had high blood pressure.[18] Asian and Hispanic patients had nearly twice the risk of albuminuria than Caucasians.

**Table 39.1 Crude Prevalence of Chronic Kidney Disease Stages 1–5 in Adults Age 20 Years and Older, by Type of Diabetes, U.S., 1999–2010[17]**

| | Percent (Standard Error) | |
|---|---|---|
| Characteristics | Type 1 Diabetes (*n* = 68) | Type 2 Diabetes (*n* = 3933) |
| All | 27.6 (7.15) | 39.4 (0.88) |
| **Age (Years)** | | |
| 20–44 | 13.9 (5.68)[a] | 29.6 (2.73) |
| 45–64 | 47.0 (13.43) | 29.1 (1.38) |
| ≥65 | 65.3 (29.10)[a] | 54.8 (1.33) |
| **Sex** | | |
| Men | 27.3 (11.46)[a] | 39.1 (1.39) |
| Women | 28.1 (7.42) | 39.6 (1.35) |
| **Race/Ethnicity** | | |
| Non-Hispanic | 24.4 (8.56)[b] | 38.7 (1.09) |
| Non-Hispanic black | 47.2 (12.54) | 40.7 (1.94) |
| Mexican American[c] | | 37.7 (1.75) |
| **Cardiovascular Disease** | | |
| Yes | 57.0 (27.07)[a] | 53.3 (2.05) |
| No | 23.7 (6.07) | 34.4 (1.00) |
| **Hypertension** | | |
| Yes | 48.0 (9.87) | 44.9 (1.03) |
| No[c] | | 24.7 (1.60) |

[a]Relative standard error >40%–50%
[b]Relative standard error >30%–40%
[c]Estimate is too unreliable to present; ≤1 case or relative standard error >50%.
Type 1 diabetes includes individuals with self-reported diabetes whose age of diagnosis was younger than 30 years, who currently use insulin and who began insulin therapy within 1 year of diabetes diagnosis. Type 2 diabetes includes individuals with self-reported diabetes who are not defined as having type 1 diabetes or with undiagnosed diabetes based on A1C 6.5% (or more) or fasting plasma glucose 126 mg/dL or more. Conversions for A1C and glucose values are provided in *Diabetes in America Appendix 1 Conversions.* A1C, glycosylated hemoglobin A1C.
*Source*: National Health and Examination Surveys 1999–2010

## INCIDENCE

Microalbuminuria predicts the development of macroalbuminuria in people with either type 1[19–23] or type 2 diabetes,[24–26] and it is also associated with an increased risk of cardiovascular disease. In type 1 diabetes, the incidence rate of macroalbuminuria typically begins to increase about five years after the onset of diabetes and peaks between 10 and 20 years after diagnosis. Thereafter the incidence declines, suggesting that a subset of people with type 1 diabetes—about one-third—are susceptible to DKD.[27–30] The long-term outcomes of persistent microalbuminuria (albumin excretion rate ≥30 mg/24 h at 2 consecutive study visits) were examined in 325 participants from the Diabetes Control and Complications Trial (DCCT) and its observational extension, the Epidemiology of Diabetes Interventions and Complications (EDIC), who were followed for a median of 13 years.[31] The 10-year cumulative incidence of progression to macroalbuminuria was 28%, progression to reduced GFR (<60 ml/min/1.73 m$^2$) was 15%, and progression to end-stage kidney disease (ESKD) was 4%.

In type 2 diabetes, the incidence of albuminuria in relation to diabetes duration is less clear. No relationship between duration of type 2 diabetes and the incidence of proteinuria was found in the Mayo Clinic population in Rochester, Minnesota[32] or in Denmark,[33] whereas in Wisconsin,[34] a relationship between diabetes duration and incidence of proteinuria was stronger in people who received insulin than in those who did not. In Pima Indians, in whom the duration of type 2 diabetes is known with greater accuracy because of systematic periodic oral glucose tolerance testing in the population, the age-sex-adjusted incidence of proteinuria, defined as urine protein:creatinine ratio 0.5 g/g or higher, was strongly related to duration of diabetes and continued to increase after 20 years of diabetes, suggesting that a larger proportion of individuals with type 2 diabetes are susceptible to DKD.[35] Moreover, the cumulative incidence of ESKD in this population was 40% after 10 years of proteinuria and 61% after 15 years of proteinuria.[36]

## SECULAR TRENDS

A secular decline in the incidence of DKD has been described in type 1 diabetes.[29,37–41] In the Pittsburgh Epidemiology of Childhood-Onset Diabetes Complications Study,[38] the cumulative incidence of DKD, defined by a persistent albumin excretion rate more than 200 µg/min, was 37% lower after

20 years of diabetes in the 179 participants diagnosed with diabetes in the period between 1975 and 1980 than in the 339 participants diagnosed in between 1965 and 1974. Among those with more than 25 years of diabetes duration, the declining trend was not statistically significant, and it disappeared altogether in those with diabetes duration of greater than 35 years. Nevertheless, significant reductions in rates of ESKD and mortality for a given duration of diabetes in those diagnosed more recently suggest a slower progression to kidney failure with more recent improvements in the management of diabetes complications. Comparable data are found in people with type 1 diabetes in Sweden,[39] where the cumulative incidence of persistent albuminuria (≥1 positive test by Albustix) after 20 years of diabetes decreased from 28% in people diagnosed with type 1 diabetes in 1961 to 1965 to 6% in those diagnosed in 1980 to 1985 (Fig. 39.1B). Furthermore, none of the 51 patients in whom type 1 diabetes was diagnosed in 1976 to 1980 developed persistent albuminuria during 12 to 16 years of follow-up. The decline in the cumulative incidence of DKD coincided with improvement in glycemic control comparable with that found in the intensively treated group in the DCCT.[42] These findings were replicated in the Steno Diabetes Center cohort from Denmark.[40,41] The cumulative incidence of DKD, defined as persistent albuminuria, declined from 31% in those with onset of type 1 diabetes in 1965 to 1969 to 14% in those with onset of diabetes in 1979 to1984, with the most significant decline occurring in the most recent cohort[41] (Fig. 39.1A). In addition to improvements in glycemic control, these trends paralleled a significant trend for earlier initiation of antihypertensive treatment following the onset of diabetes, expansion of renin-angiotensin-aldosterone system inhibitor usage, and sustained improvement in mean blood pressure in these cohorts.

In contrast with type 1 diabetes, no secular decline in the incidence of proteinuria has been reported for type 2 diabetes. The 10-year cumulative incidence of persistent proteinuria in the predominantly Caucasian population age 40 years or older from Rochester, Minnesota, was 12% in those diagnosed with type 2 diabetes in 1970 to 1979 ($n$ = 483) and 12% in those diagnosed in 1980 to 1989 ($n$ = 680).[43] The 20-year cumulative incidence of proteinuria reported in this study, however, was 41%, higher than the 25% cumulative incidence reported in an earlier Rochester study of individuals diagnosed with diabetes in 1945 to 1969.[32] These secular differences may be related in part to differences in age distributions and in diabetes diagnosis criteria between the studies. In Pima Indians, the incidence of proteinuria increased between 1967 and 2002 as the proportion of people with diabetes of long duration increased. On the other hand, the incidence of ESKD attributed to diabetes declined after 1990, coinciding with improvements in blood pressure and hyperglycemia management.[44] The decline in the incidence of diabetic ESKD in the Pima Indians is consistent with a 54% decline reported in American Indians and Alaska Natives across the United States between 1996 and 2013, which followed implementation of population-based approaches to diabetes management which, in turn, led to substantial improvements in testing for albuminuria, increased usage of renin-angiotensin-aldosterone system inhibitors, and improved glycemic control.[45]

A decline in the incidence of ESKD among people with diabetes has also been reported in the United States from 1990 through 2010, with the greatest declines observed since 1995.[46] Although these data suggest that concerted efforts to improve diabetes care in recent years are effectively slowing the progression to ESKD, several factors are threatening to reverse these trends. The total number of individuals worldwide who are at risk for DKD continues to rise, and the age

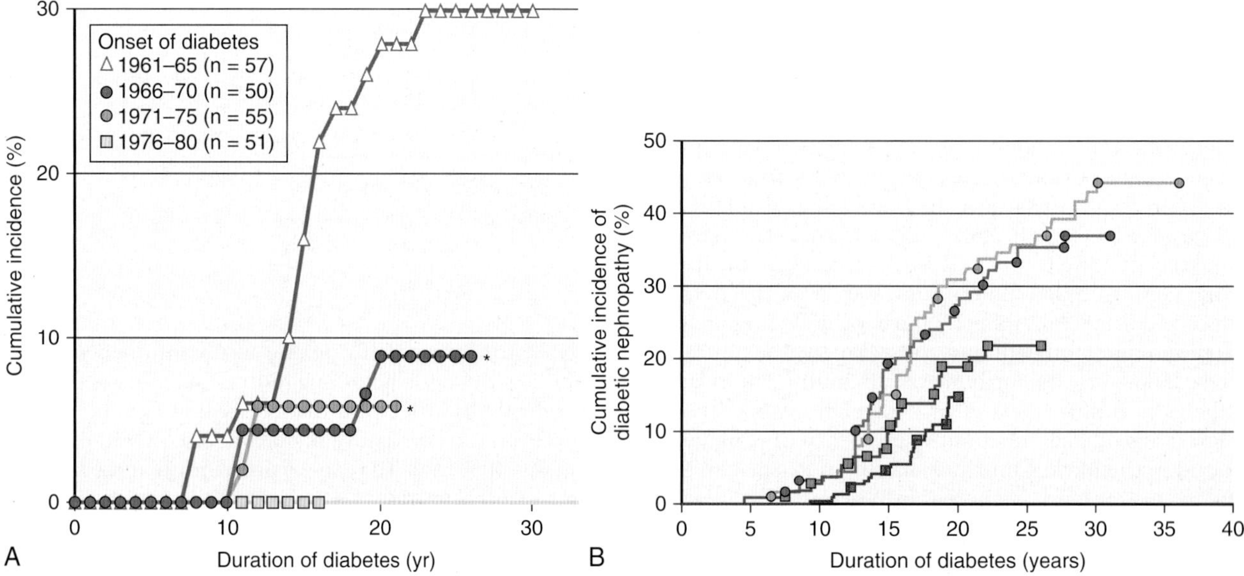


**Fig. 39.1 Cumulative incidence of diabetic kidney disease in type 1 diabetes.[41,39] A, Cumulative incidence of diabetic kidney disease in 600 type 1 diabetic patients with onset of diabetes from 1965 to 1969 ($n$ = 113, group A [○]), 1970–1974 ($n$ = 130, group B [•]), 1975–1979 ($n$ = 113, group C [□]), and 1979–1984 ($n$ = 244, group D [■]). $P$ < .001, log-rank test, pooled over strata. Not all patients in group D have yet been followed for 20 years. For pairwise log-rank test over strata after 20 years of diabetes.[41] B, Cumulative incidence of persistent albuminuria among patients in whom type 1 diabetes began before the age of 15 years, according to the year of onset.[39]**

of diabetes onset is declining,[15] supporting the observations that a greater number of persons with type 2 diabetes are developing the disease as young adults or as children.

## YOUTH-ONSET TYPE 2 DIABETES AND ITS IMPACT ON KIDNEY DISEASE

In the 1960s, reports of asymptomatic hyperglycemia in children and young adults began to appear.[47,48] These were followed by studies noting a high prevalence of glucose intolerance in obese children.[48–51] In 1979, a study in the Pima Indians reported cases of type 2 diabetes in children.[52] Subsequent studies in this population revealed a rapidly increasing prevalence of type 2 diabetes among the children that coincided with increasing childhood weight and exposure to diabetes *in utero*. The diabetes seen in these youths was unequivocally type 2 diabetes, as it did not require exogenous insulin to prevent ketosis, was not related to a single gene mutation, and was not associated with high titers of islet cell antibodies or subnormal insulin and C-peptide concentrations.[53] At the same time, reports of type 2 diabetes in children were beginning to appear in other populations.[54–59] A review of the magnitude of the problem of type 2 diabetes in North American youth confirmed the high prevalence among American Indian and First Nation youth and showed that cases were also occurring in all other racial and ethnic groups in North America.[60] A consensus statement from the American Diabetes Association in 2000 concluded that up to 45% of youth-onset diabetes in North America was type 2, with considerable variability by race and ethnicity.[61] A Cochrane review in 2005 further illustrated the global magnitude of the problem.[62] Fig. 39.2 shows the percentage of newly diagnosed diabetes identified as type 2 in children and adolescents in various regions and countries worldwide. In Japan, 80% of the new cases of diabetes are diagnosed as type 2.[62] Increasing prevalence and incidence rates of youth-onset type 2 diabetes have now been documented in large studies across the United States, particularly among racial and ethnic minorities.[63,64]

Of concern, the course of DKD in youth-onset type 2 diabetes appears to be more aggressive than in type 1 diabetes.[65–69] These findings were confirmed in a study of patients who were diagnosed with either type 1 ($n = 1746$) or type 2 ($n = 272$) diabetes before the age of 20 years and were examined for complications at equivalent durations of diabetes (mean = 7.9 years).[70] Patients with type 2 diabetes had a higher age-adjusted prevalence of hypertension, DKD, retinopathy, arterial stiffness, and peripheral neuropathy than those with type 1 diabetes. The prevalence of DKD, defined by a first-morning void urine albumin:creatinine ratio 30 or more mg/g or an eGFR 60 or less ml/min/1.73 m$^2$, was 20% in patients with type 2 diabetes and 6% in those with type 1 diabetes, for an absolute difference of 14%. After adjustment for established risk factors, the odds of DKD in patients with type 2 diabetes was nearly 3 times as high as in those with type 1 diabetes.[63]

Because youth-onset type 2 diabetes is a recent phenomenon in most populations, follow-up of individuals is generally not sufficient to assess the long-term effects of youth-onset diabetes on the kidneys. Long-term follow-up is available, however, in Pima Indians, in whom youth-onset type 2 diabetes has been present for many years.[52] In this population, the incidence of DKD, defined by a urine protein:creatinine

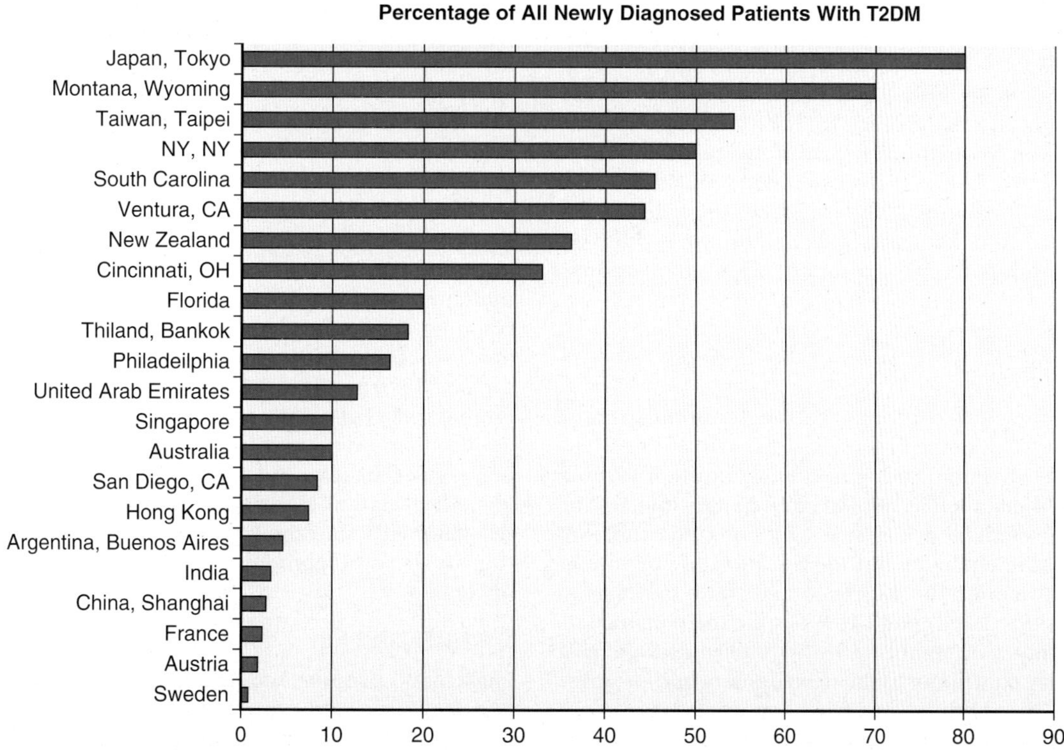


**Fig. 39.2 Reported percentage of children and adolescents in different parts of the world with newly diagnosed diabetes that have type 2 diabetes mellitus.**[62]

ratio 0.5 g/g or higher, is equivalent—as a function of diabetes duration—in those with youth-onset and older-onset type 2 diabetes,[71] and this is followed by a greatly increased incidence of ESKD by middle age in those who develop diabetes during childhood or adolescence.[72] Given the aggressive nature of the kidney complications in youth-onset type 2 diabetes in populations worldwide, we can reasonably expect to see increasing rates of ESKD in mid-life in response to the earlier onset of type 2 diabetes. Whether this expected trend will reverse the recent declines in diabetic ESKD attributed to improvements in care remains to be seen.

### REGRESSION OF ALBUMINURIA AND NONALBUMINURIC DKD

DKD was originally considered to be a progressive disease that began with the appearance of microalbuminuria, and was followed by macroalbuminuria, loss of GFR, and ultimately ESKD.[73] More recently, studies have shown that a sizeable proportion of people with diabetes do not follow this paradigm.[74]

In a study of 386 people with type 1 diabetes and microalbuminuria from the Joslin Clinic, only 19% developed macroalbuminuria and 59% regressed to normal albuminuria after 6 years of follow-up.[75] Similarly, among 325 participants from the DCCT/EDIC study who developed microalbuminuria that remained for two consecutive visits, 28% subsequently progressed to macroalbuminuria and 40% regressed to normoalbuminuria after 10 years.[31] Similar spontaneous or treatment-induced remissions are also widely observed in type 2 diabetes.[76–80]

On the other hand, many people with DKD do not develop albuminuria as their disease progresses or do so late in the disease after they have already developed reduced GFR. Of the 11% of patients with type 1 diabetes in DCCT/EDIC who developed an eGFR less than 60 ml/min/1.73 m$^2$ during a mean follow-up of 19 years, 40% did not develop macroalbuminuria before they developed reduced GFR, and 24% never exhibited albuminuria.[81] Likewise, data from the United Kingdom Prospective Diabetes Study (UKPDS),[82] the Developing Education on Microalbuminuria for Awareness of Renal and Cardiovascular Risk in Diabetes (DEMAND) study,[18] and the Australian Diabetes, Obesity, and Lifestyle Study (AusDiab)[83] indicate that as many as half of those with type 2 diabetes develop renal impairment without preceding albuminuria.

## RISK FACTORS

Numerous risk factors contribute to the development and progression of DKD. Some of these factors, such as hypertension and hyperglycemia, can be modified through various treatments. Others, such as smoking and dietary intake, can be modified through lifestyle changes. Inherited susceptibility factors cannot be changed, but modification of epigenetic factors that influence the expression of these genes may reduce the risk of developing DKD, despite the presence of the susceptibility gene. In this section, we review several risk factors that may contribute to the development and progression of DKD. In addition to widely recognized risk factors common to all people with DKD, we included others that might be relevant only in subsets of individuals experiencing uncommon exposures.

### DURATION OF DIABETES

Given the prominent role of hyperglycemia in the development of diabetic complications, including DKD, it is not surprising that the duration of diabetes is one of the most important risk factors for DKD. Its influence is far greater than that of age, sex, or type of diabetes.[88–92] Because the onset of type 2 diabetes is often insidious, duration of diabetes in type 2 diabetes is known with less certainty than it is for type 1 diabetes. For this reason, screening for DKD in type 2 diabetes is recommended from time of diabetes diagnosis, whereas screening is recommended only after 5 years of type 1 diabetes unless the patient has hypertension.[1,8]

### HYPERGLYCEMIA

Increased blood glucose concentration is the clinical hallmark of diabetes and it is the principal determinant of its complications, including DKD. Numerous studies have documented the effect of hyperglycemia on the development and progression of albuminuria in both types of diabetes.[27,30,32,34,35,84–89] Although some studies in type 2 diabetes suggest that the impact of hyperglycemia on the progression of DKD is less in more advanced diabetes,[90,91] most large observational studies indicate that hyperglycemia remains an important predictor of progression of advanced kidney disease in both type 1 and type 2 diabetes.[36,92–96]

Persistent hyperglycemia causes dysregulation of several effector molecules through various biochemical pathways in the kidney, including the generation and accumulation of advanced glycation end-products, an increased activity of the polyol pathway, and the activation of vasoactive hormones, such as angiotensin II and endothelin.[97–99] Activated prosclerotic cytokines, such as transforming growth factor beta (TGF-β) and vascular endothelial growth factor (VEGF), are important mediators between the metabolic and hemodynamic pathways affected by hyperglycemia that ultimately lead to the pathologic changes of DKD.[97]

Further evidence for the role of hyperglycemia in the development of DKD comes from biopsy studies in identical twins discordant for type 1 diabetes[100] and from morphologic studies before and after pancreas transplantation.[101] Glomerular changes, including widened glomerular and tubular basement membranes and increased mesangial fraction, are identified only in the diabetic member of twin pairs, suggesting that metabolic status, and not genetic predisposition, is responsible for the development of these diabetic kidney lesions.[100] In addition, prolonged normoglycemia following a pancreas transplant in people with type 1 diabetes and established DKD promotes virtually complete reversal of glomerular and tubular basement membrane thickness and of increases in mesangial and interstitial volumes.[101] Nevertheless, the relative contributions of hyperglycemia, insulin resistance (IR), and alterations in endogenous insulin production to the development and progression of DKD remain unclear.

### HYPERTENSION

High blood pressure is often observed in patients with DKD and may indicate both a cause and a consequence of the kidney disease. In type 1 diabetes, the elevation of blood pressure is typically coincident with the appearance of albuminuria,[102–104] illustrating that higher blood pressure is a consequence of the kidney disease. Nevertheless, other studies demonstrate the predictive value of high blood pressure in type 1 diabetes. Familial aggregation of blood pressure is widely reported and may represent a predisposition to hypertension. Higher blood pressure in the nondiabetic parents of patients with type 1 diabetes and albuminuria suggests that this predisposition to hypertension is also a risk factor for kidney disease in type 1 diabetes.[105–108] In one study, maternal blood pressure was more strongly related to albuminuria in the offspring than paternal blood pressure, suggesting a dominant effect of maternal genes or an effect of the intrauterine environment on the risk of microalbuminuria.[109] In addition, increased nocturnal blood pressure predicts the development of microalbuminuria in adolescents and young adults with type 1 diabetes.[110]

In type 2 diabetes, which typically develops later in life, the onset of hypertension generally precedes the first clinical evidence of DKD, or even the diagnosis of diabetes. Hence, to determine if high blood pressure is a risk factor for DKD, it is helpful to know the blood pressure before the onset of type 2 diabetes. In Pima Indians, blood pressure is measured at sequential research examinations that begin long before the onset of diabetes, and higher blood pressure before the onset of type 2 diabetes was strongly associated with albuminuria after the onset of diabetes.[111] In addition, the prevalence of proteinuria was significantly higher if both parents had hypertension than if only one or neither parent had hypertension.[112] Increased nocturnal blood pressure is associated with microalbuminuria in type 2 diabetes, as it is in type 1 diabetes.[113]

Sodium-lithium countertransport activity, a genetically influenced trait, is often higher in people with essential hypertension and in those whose parents have essential hypertension.[114–117] In type 1 diabetes, elevated rates of countertransport activity are reported in people with albuminuria[118–120] and elevated GFR.[121] These findings suggest that diabetic people with hypertension and with elevated sodium-lithium countertransport activity are at greater risk for DKD, although these findings have not been uniformly confirmed.[122–124] Few studies assessed this relationship in those with type 2 diabetes and some found an association between higher activity and albuminuria,[125,126] and others did not.[127–129]

## HYPERFILTRATION

Glomerular hyperfiltration is a supraphysiologic increase of GFR in all functioning nephrons, and it is caused by diabetes-induced hemodynamic and structural changes.[130] It is frequently observed in both type 1 and type 2 diabetes.[131,132] Hyperfiltration is thought to predispose to irreversible nephron damage.[133,134] Observational studies of patients with type 1 or type 2 diabetes and measured GFR demonstrated a more rapid decline of GFR in those with hyperfiltration than in those without.[135,136] Furthermore, a metaanalysis of 780 patients with type 1 diabetes from 10 cohort studies found that the odds of developing albuminuria in those with hyperfiltration at baseline was 2.7 times that of people without hyperfiltration at baseline,[137] and a study of 600 patients with type 2 diabetes found that those with persistent hyperfiltration during a 6-month period from baseline examination were more than twice as likely to develop microalbuminuria during 4 years of follow-up than those without hyperfiltration.[138] These studies suggest that hyperfiltration may indeed contribute to the development and progression of DKD, but properly controlled human studies with hard endpoints are needed to firmly establish the role of hyperfiltration as a risk factor for DKD,[139] as animal models have not well replicated the human condition.

## LIPIDS

Many of the abnormalities in plasma lipoproteins associated with kidney disease are sequelae of kidney dysfunction, yet dyslipidemia may also play a role in the pathogenesis of glomerular injury.[140–143] People with diabetes and predialysis chronic kidney disease typically have significant serum hypertriglyceridemia, elevated low-density lipoprotein (LDL), and low high-density lipoprotein (HDL) cholesterol concentrations. These abnormalities are also more pronounced in people with macroalbuminuria than in those with microalbuminuria.[31,144–146] In addition to quantitative changes, lipid particles in persons with diabetes change qualitatively, as LDL and HDL particles tend to be smaller and denser with advancing chronic kidney disease.[144]

Among 439 patients with type 1 diabetes and proteinuria who were followed at the Joslin Clinic, elevated serum cholesterol concentration was a strong predictor of a rapid loss of kidney function.[143] Specific lipids or lipid profiles may also predict progression of DKD. In 152 patients with type 1 diabetes from the United Kingdom and Finland, elevated serum LDL cholesterol concentration predicted progression of DKD during 8 to 9 years of follow-up, as defined by a doubling of albuminuria or a decline in creatinine clearance greater than 3 ml/min/year.[147] Higher triglyceride content of very low-density lipoprotein (VLDL) and intermediate-density lipoprotein (IDL) particles predicted worsening of microalbuminuria, whereas smaller LDL size was associated with declining kidney function in people with macroalbuminuria at baseline. The predictive value of these lipid profiles, however, has not been consistently observed in other studies.[84,148–150]

In type 2 diabetes, the UKPDS reported that higher serum LDL cholesterol concentration increased the risk for macroalbuminuria.[82] In a posthoc analysis of 1061 patients with type 2 diabetes in the reduction of endpoints in noninsulin dependent diabetes with the Angiotensin II Antagonist Losartan (RENAAL) trial, the risk of ESKD was 32% higher for every 50 mg/dL increase of LDL cholesterol concentration and 67% higher for every 100 mg/dL increase of total cholesterol concentration. Lowering LDL cholesterol concentrations with a statin reduced the 1-year risk of ESKD, although concurrent treatment with losartan likely contributed to this improvement.[151] Elevated plasma triglycerides are also associated with increased risk for both albuminuria[82] and ESKD in type 2 diabetes.[152] In addition, low concentrations of HDL cholesterol predict an increased risk of albuminuria progression in people with type 2 diabetes and microalbuminuria.[153] In the UKPDS, each mmol/L decline in HDL cholesterol increased the risk of doubling of serum creatinine concentration nearly threefold during a median follow-up of 15 years.[82]

Dyslipidemia may contribute to onset and progression of DKD through mechanisms like those responsible for atherogenesis.[154,155] Hypercholesterolemia may impair the kidney's hemodynamic responses and tubular function by decreasing nitric oxide production and/or increasing superoxide activity in the kidney,[156–160] with resulting antidiuretic and antinatriuretic effects.[161] Although not directly affecting GFR, these actions may play a role in the development of systemic hypertension associated with diabetes.[161] Oxidized LDL and free fatty acids can cause structural and functional damage to podocytes by inducing mitochondrial dysfunction and accumulation of reactive oxygen species,[162] suggesting a direct causal role in the development and progression of proteinuria. Nevertheless, despite much investigation and experimental evidence supporting various mechanisms, a definitive role for dyslipidemia in the development and progression of DKD in humans remains to be established.

In addition to the role of circulating lipids, the diabetic environment facilitates glomerular production of triglycerides and cholesterol, which appear to cause kidney injury both directly by accumulating in the cellular and extracellular structures and indirectly by stimulating the expression of prosclerotic, proliferative, and proinflammatory cytokines.[142,154,163] Accumulation of lipid droplets containing triglycerides and cholesterol has been described in kidney cells in experimental diabetes.[164–166] These lipid droplets are associated primarily with increased expression of sterol regulatory element-binding protein (SREBP)-1c, decreased expression of peroxisome proliferator-activated receptor (PPAR)-alpha and decreased expression of liver X receptor (LXR)-alpha, LXR-beta, and ATP-binding cassette transporter-1 *(ABCA1)*. Under normal conditions, *ABCA1* mediates the efflux of cholesterol to lipid-poor apolipoproteins (primarily Apo A1) to form HDLs. Down-regulation of glomerular expression of ABCA1 was observed in glomerular transcripts from people with DKD when compared with normal controls and was correlated with lower eGFR. The down-regulation of ABCA1 was also associated with lipid droplet accumulation in podocytes.[167,168] If and how prevention of lipid accumulation in the renal parenchyma may affect the development and progression of DKD remains to be established.

## DIETARY PROTEIN

In experimental models, excessive protein intake causes kidney vasodilation and glomerular hyperperfusion with a resulting increase in intraglomerular pressure that leads to proteinuria and glomerular damage.[133,169] Long-term high protein intake accelerates structural and functional injury in models of DKD, whereas low-protein diets offer kidney protection.[170–172] Physiologic studies in humans confirm the hyperfiltration response to a high protein diet, but only in the presence of chronic hyperglycemia.[173,174] Dietary protein of animal origin may also be a significant source of advanced glycation end-products,[175] which could accelerate kidney disease progression. Nevertheless, there are no large observational studies supporting a role for dietary protein in progressive DKD. Metaanalyses of clinical trials examining the effect of dietary protein restriction on the progression of DKD concluded that the impact of protein restriction was not associated with significant improvement in kidney function and was highly variable between individuals.[176–178]

## OBESITY

More than one-third of adults and 17% of youth in the United States are obese, and nearly 8% of adults and 6% of youth are severely obese, defined by a body mass index of 40 or more kg/m$^2$ in adults and greater than 120% of the sex-specific 95$^{th}$ percentile on the CDC BMI-for-age growth charts in youth.[179–181] Although obesity is an increasing problem in the diabetic population, it is also a major risk factor for kidney disease, independent of diabetes and hypertension. Indeed, the presence of severe obesity increases the risk of ESKD sevenfold relative to normal weight.[182,183] Obesity-associated hemodynamic changes in GFR and renal plasma flow appear to be responsible for the kidney damage.[183,184] The effects of adiposity may also impact the kidneys directly through the production of various adipokines, including leptin, adiponectin, and resistin, which activate profibrotic, proliferative, and proinflammatory mechanisms.[185–188] A retrospective clinical and histopathologic study of 6818 native kidney biopsies found diabetes-like lesions in 45% of people with obesity-related glomerulopathy.[189] The prevalence of obesity-related glomerulopathy, defined as glomerulomegaly with or without focal segmental glomerulosclerosis, increased tenfold between 1986 and 2000, attributed to the rising prevalence of obesity in the general population.[189] Although obesity-related glomerulopathy may represent a distinct entity from DKD, obesity is largely responsible for the increase in diabetes prevalence worldwide, and similarities in some underlying mechanisms of obesity-related chronic kidney disease and DKD suggest that treatments targeting obesity-related chronic kidney disease may slow the progression of kidney disease in people with diabetes.[190]

## INSULIN RESISTANCE

A cross-sectional study in 100 patients with type 2 diabetes found that albuminuric patients had lower glucose disposal rates than nonalbuminuric patients.[519] The clinical evidence that insulin resistance (IR) precedes DKD came from prospective studies in the early 1990s. A prospective analysis of 108 patients with type 2 diabetes and normoalbuminuria who underwent euglycemic clamps at enrollment demonstrated that hyperinsulinemia at baseline was strongly associated with albuminuria at the 5-year examination.[87] A larger prospective analysis of 582 nondiabetic siblings of patients with type 2 diabetes also demonstrated that IR at baseline (assessed with glucose tolerance tests and euglycemic clamps) correlated with the development of albuminuria.[520] Interestingly, in patients with type 1 diabetes or their family members, glucose disposal rates are also reduced in the presence of albuminuria,[521,522] and in a small longitudinal study of patients with type 1 diabetes and normoalbuminuria, IR predicted development of albuminuria after 3 years.[523] If and how IR affects key hemodynamic or metabolic mediators of clinical DKD, as suggested by multiple experimental studies, remains to be established.

## PREGNANCY

Among women with normal kidney function, regardless of the presence or absence of diabetes, pregnancy is associated with a rise in GFR of about 50% that persists through the 37th week of gestation[191–193] and it is accompanied by a moderate increase in urinary protein excretion.[192] Among pregnant women in Austria with type 1 diabetes, those with normoalbuminuria experience a 3.8-fold increase in albuminuria, whereas those with microalbuminuria (>15 mcg/min) have a 6.7-fold increase. Nevertheless, the albuminuria levels in both groups typically normalize within 12 weeks after delivery.[194] Much less is known about changes in albuminuria in pregnant women with type 2 diabetes, but the prevalence of albuminuria in both types of diabetes in a Danish cohort are equivalent, and pregnancy outcomes are comparable.[195]

Although neither pregnancy nor parity adversely affect the course of early kidney disease in women with diabetes,[196,197] those with poor glycemic control, hypertension, or preexisting advanced kidney disease are at increased risk of pregnancy complications and subsequent deterioration in kidney function.[193,197–200] In addition, mothers with advanced kidney disease are more likely to develop preeclampsia and have offspring with low birth weight.[201] In Finnish women with type 1 diabetes, a prior history of preeclampsia was associated with 7.7-fold higher odds of subsequent DKD than in those with normotensive pregnancies.[202] Podocyte injury due to diabetes and its impact on DKD progression will be discussed later in this chapter, but preeclampsia is also associated with podocyte injury and detachment[203–207] and could conceivably accelerate diabetic glomerular injury in a pregnant woman with diabetes who develops preeclampsia.

## INTRAUTERINE FACTORS

Fetal exposure to an abnormal intrauterine environment has lasting effects on anthropomorphic and metabolic development that lead to increased risk of disease later in life. Certain adverse intrauterine exposures, such as a shortage of maternal fuels, various drugs, vitamin A deficiency, and maternal diabetes directly affect development of the fetal kidneys and reduce nephron number in the offspring (See Chapter 21). With the resulting reduction in filtration surface area, the kidney's adaptive capacity in response to insults, such as diabetes, is reduced, thereby enhancing the risk of kidney disease.[208–210] Of concern, impaired nephrogenesis may be passed on to subsequent generations through changes in epigenetic gene regulation.[211]

Low birth weight appears to affect kidney disease risk in both type 1 and type 2 diabetes. In a case-control study of 184 Danish patients with type 1 diabetes, 75% of the women below the 10th percentile of birth weight had persistent albuminuria (≥300 mg/24 h) compared with 35% of those above the 90th percentile.[212] No relationship was found, however, between birth weight and urine albumin excretion in the men. In Pima Indians with type 2 diabetes, the prevalence of elevated urine albumin excretion (albumin:creatinine ratio ≥30 mg/g) was twice as high in both men and women of low birth weight than in those of normal birth weight, and was three times as high in those of high birth weight.[213] Two-thirds of those in the high-birth-weight category were the offspring of diabetic mothers.[222] Irrespectively of birth weight, preterm birth also appears to impose an additive risk for progression of kidney disease and such information should be collected as part of a patient's medical history.[214]

Fuel-mediated alterations in maternal metabolism in pregnancies complicated by diabetes may preferentially harm poorly replicating, terminally differentiated cells, such as those found in the nephron.[215] A proposed mechanism for this differential apoptosis during nephrogenesis is the activation of the nuclear factor NF-κB signaling pathway.[216] The adverse effect of hyperglycemia on nephrogenesis was demonstrated experimentally by exposing pregnant rats to diabetes and counting nephrons in the offspring. The number of nephrons was reduced by up to 35% in those exposed to diabetes, and even minor elevations of glucose concentration were associated with impaired metanephros development.[217] In adult offspring of women with type 1 diabetes who are exposed to maternal diabetes in utero, kidney functional reserve was significantly reduced relative to those who were not exposed, likely reflecting a reduced nephron mass because of this exposure.[218] In Pima Indians with type 2 diabetes, the odds of elevated urine albumin excretion (albumin:creatinine ratio ≥30 mg/g) was nearly fourfold higher in those exposed to diabetes in utero than in those who were not exposed.[219] Moreover, exposure to diabetes in utero among Pima Indian offspring increased nearly fourfold over a 30-year period, paralleled by a doubling in the prevalence of childhood onset diabetes attributable to this exposure,[53] suggesting that this exposure is contributing to the rising prevalence of childhood type 2 diabetes. Intrauterine exposure to diabetes was also associated with a fourfold increase in the age-sex-adjusted incidence of ESKD in young adults with type 2 diabetes, mediated largely by the younger age at onset of diabetes in those with this exposure.[220] These observations have potential relevance in the developing world and in disadvantaged groups in developed countries, where a higher proportion of type 2 diabetes develops during the childbearing years.[221] The greater frequency of diabetes during the childbearing years in these populations means that the offspring are more likely to be exposed to a diabetic intrauterine environment and to suffer the consequences of that exposure.

## SMOKING

The role of smoking in promoting DKD is controversial, but substantial evidence points to an effect on albuminuria,[88,89,222–225] although a relationship with progressive loss of GFR has not been found.[95,226] In a case-control study nested within a large population-based cohort of Swedish children with type 1 diabetes, maternal smoking during pregnancy increased the odds of having albuminuria in the offspring with type 1 diabetes by more than threefold, independent of low birth weight or blood pressure levels.[225] In 359 young people from the United States with type 1 diabetes, the risk of albuminuria was nearly threefold higher in smokers than in nonsmokers,[223] and in 509 Taiwanese men with type 2 diabetes, the odds of albuminuria were 2.8 to 3.2 times as high in those smoking more than 15 pack-years than in nonsmokers, regardless of age, blood pressure control, or diabetes duration.[224] On the other hand, no relationship was observed between smoking and GFR decline in a longitudinal study of 301 type 1 diabetic persons from Denmark who had albuminuria at baseline and serial $^{51}$Cr-EDTA GFR measurements over a median follow-up of 7 years,[226] or in 227 type 2 diabetic people from the same cohort who were also followed for 7 years.[95] Consistent with these observations, smoking increased the risk of albuminuria after 5 years of follow-up in a population-based cohort of 3,667 Swedish people with type 2 diabetes who had no kidney disease at baseline, but it was not associated with GFR decline to 60 ml/min/1.73 m$^2$ during follow-up.[222] In the Finnish Diabetic Nephropathy Study, the 12-year cumulative risk of macroalbuminuria and ESKD in 3613 patients with type 1 diabetes was 14.4% and 10.3% respectively for current smokers, 6.1% and 10.0% respectively for exsmokers, and 4.7% and 5.6% respectively for nonsmokers.[227]

There are many reasons to be concerned about a role for smoking in DKD. Nicotine induces podocyte apoptosis through increasing oxidative stress, promotes mesangial cell proliferation and extracellular matrix production, and increases TGF-β and fibronectin expression in experimental models.[228,229,230] Moreover, cigarette combustion produces over 4,000 compounds, including reactive oxygen species, carbon monoxide, nitric oxide, toxic metals, and polycyclic aromatic hydrocarbons,[231] which may enhance susceptibility to kidney disease in persons with diabetes. Tobacco smoking is also known to cause vasoconstriction, impair platelet function and coagulation, and alter blood pressure. Given that persons with diabetes already have widespread vascular damage because of their diabetes,[232] smoking may accelerate this damage. The long-term risks of electronic cigarettes are also of concern, as possible nephrotoxicity of e-cigarette refill liquid was observed in rat kidneys.[233]

## PERIDONTAL DISEASE

Periodontal disease is an inflammatory condition, which often occurs in the absence of diabetes, but is also a frequent complication of diabetes,[234] contributing to poor glycemic control, low-grade chronic systemic inflammation, and increased risk of macro- and microvascular complications.[234,235] Among patients with chronic kidney disease, periodontal disease substantially increases the risk of premature mortality.[236] In a Swedish case-control study of 78 patients with type 1 or type 2 diabetes, those with severe periodontitis, based on alveolar bone loss, had a higher frequency of dipstick positive proteinuria and cardiovascular complications after 6 years than those with mild periodontal disease.[237] Severity of periodontitis by alveolar bone loss and being edentulous predicted both albuminuria and ESKD in a dose-dependent manner among 529 Pima Indian adults with type 2 diabetes who were followed for a median of 9 years.[238] A study investigating the relationships between diabetes, periodontal disease, and chronic kidney disease in 11,211 adults from the NHANES 1988 to 1994 population suggested a bidirectional relationship between chronic kidney disease and periodontal disease, with periodontitis increasing the risk of chronic kidney disease both directly and mediated by hypertension and duration of diabetes, and chronic kidney disease having a direct effect on periodontitis.[239] Although the mechanisms linking periodontal disease to DKD remain to be established, serum lipopolysaccharide activity, which is induced by bacterial infections, is associated with the progression of DKD in Finnish patients with type 1 diabetes.[240]

Control of periodontal infection in diabetic adults improves A1c level[234] and reduces the concentration of various markers of inflammation, coagulation, and adhesion.[241] Whether such control also reduces the onset or progression of DKD is not known.

## CARDIAC AUTONOMIC NEUROPATHY

Abnormalities in heart rate control and vascular dynamics associated with diabetes is referred to as cardiac autonomic neuropathy and is the consequence of damage to and loss of the small unmyelinated nerve fibers that innervate the heart and blood vessels. Advanced cardiac autonomic neuropathy may present as resting tachycardia and orthostatic hypotension. The presence of cardiac autonomic neuropathy is a risk factor for DKD in several longitudinal studies of type 1 and type 2 diabetes. Among 35 Swedish patients with type 1 diabetes, those with cardiac autonomic neuropathy had a significant decline in GFR measured by 51Cr-EDTA clearance over a 10-year period, whereas those without cardiac autonomic neuropathy experienced almost no change.[242] More recently, cardiac autonomic neuropathy was strongly associated with both early GFR loss and progression to chronic kidney disease, defined by eGFR less than 60 ml/min/1.73 $m^2$, in a subset of the First Joslin Kidney Study, which included 204 normoalbuminuric patients with type 1 diabetes and 166 with microalbuminuria who were followed for a median of 14 years.[243] Similar associations were reported in a multiethnic cohort of 204 adults with type 2 diabetes from the United Kingdom, in whom eGFR declined more rapidly over 2.5 years in those with cardiac autonomic neuropathy (9.0% decline) than in those without (3.3% decline),[244] and in a cohort of 1,117 Korean patients with type 2 diabetes and eGFR 60 ml/min/1.73 $m^2$ or greater at baseline, in whom the presence of cardiac autonomic neuropathy increased the risk of developing chronic kidney disease by over 2.6-fold during nearly 10 years of follow-up.[245] A cross-sectional study of 63 Pima Indians who underwent research kidney biopsies demonstrated an association between cardiac autonomic neuropathy and the structural lesions of early progressive DKD.[246]

## FAMILIAL AND GENETIC FACTORS

Familial clustering of DKD and racial/ethnic differences in disease susceptibility suggest a genetic predisposition to DKD.[247–249]

Several candidate genes have been identified that may be related to DKD. One of the most intensively studied candidate genes is the insertion/deletion (I/D) polymorphism of the ACE gene (*ACE*/ID). Among 168 Japanese patients with type 2 diabetes who were followed for 10 years, analysis of the time course of the three ACE genotypes indicated that patients with the DD genotype were far more likely to progress to ESKD during follow-up than those with the other genotypes, and they had higher mortality once dialysis was initiated.[250] The deleterious effect of the D allele on kidney function was subsequently confirmed in patients from other racial groups with type 2 diabetes,[251–253] and in type 1 diabetes.[254,255] Presence of the D allele was also associated with more severe structural lesions in type 2 diabetes[256] and with greater progression of structural lesions in type 1 diabetes.[257] In the RENAAL trial, the presence of the D allele increased the likelihood of reaching the primary endpoint of doubling of baseline serum creatinine concentration, ESKD, or death in the placebo group, but treatment with losartan mitigated that risk, suggesting that losartan had its greatest effect in patients with the D allele.[258] Another candidate gene related to the renin-angiotensin system was identified by the Bergamo Nephrologic Diabetes Complications Trial (BENEDICT), which found that the Pro618Ala polymorphism of the *ADAMTS13* gene was associated with a higher risk of kidney disease progression in patients with type 2 diabetes, but patients with this polymorphism also had a better response to ACE inhibitors.[259]

ESKD is considered by some investigators to be the optimal phenotype of DKD in genetic association studies,[260,261] so the present discussion will focus on this phenotype. In a genome-wide analysis of pooled genomic data, the plasmacytoma variant 1 *(PVT1)* gene was identified as a potential susceptibility locus for ESKD in the Pima Indians,[262] and this association was subsequently confirmed in the Genetics of Kidneys in Diabetes (GoKinD) study among people of European descent with type 1 diabetes.[263] A genome-wide association study also involving the GoKinD cohort, and confirmed in the DCCT/EDIC cohort, found single nucleotide polymorphisms (SNPs) in the FERM domain-containing protein 3 *(FRMD3)* gene and near the cysteinyl-tRNA synthetase *(CARS)* gene associated with DKD, defined by overt proteinuria or ESKD.[264] A subsequent analysis in the Joslin Study of Genetics of Nephropathy in Type 2 Diabetes found that susceptibility loci near *CARS* were common to both types of diabetes.[265] The Family Investigation of Nephropathy and Diabetes (FIND) conducted a genome-wide association study in 6197 European American, African American, American Indian, and Hispanic American families in whom type 2 diabetes was the predominant cause of kidney disease.[266] Index cases all had diabetes for more than five years and/or diabetic retinopathy, with urine albumin:creatinine ratio more than 1 g/g or ESKD; unrelated controls had diabetes for at least 9 years and normal urine albumin:creatinine ratios. A replication cohort included 7539 additional European American, African American, and American Indian cases and non-nephropathy controls. The FIND investigators found and replicated a DKD associated genetic locus on chromosome 6q25.2 (rs955333) between the *SCAF8* and *CNKSR* genes across people of different ancestries. Findings were supported by significantly different gene expression patterns in this region from kidney tissue in people with DKD versus those without. Extensive work in this field over the past decade has identified several genomic areas of interest, but results thus far only support a role for multiple susceptibility genes, each with weak effects.

### EPIGENETIC FACTORS

In addition to specific genetic factors, the multifaceted cross-talk between genes and environmental factors can induce tissue-specific epigenetic changes. These changes include DNA cytosine methylation, histone posttranslational modifications in chromatin, and noncoding RNAs, all of which can modulate diabetes complications through alterations in gene expression.[267] Through epigenetic mechanisms, cells acquire metabolic memory of prior hyperglycemic exposure that appears to mediate the development and progression of DKD.[268,269] Hyperglycemia-induced epigenetic changes alter transcription factors involved in the expression of genes mediating the pathogenesis of DKD.[267] In addition, cytosine methylation changes in genes related to kidney fibrosis in human kidney tissue correlate with downstream transcript levels and provide further evidence that epigenetic dysregulation plays a role in the development of chronic kidney disease.[270] Several miRNAs and certain long noncoding RNAs also have regulatory roles in DKD, including promoting/modulating fibrotic gene expression in kidney cells by targeting transcription repressors.[268] Although the mechanisms of such cellular memory are not entirely known, its presence is supported by the regression of morphological lesions in diabetic kidneys after a prolonged period of normoglycemia following pancreas transplantation.[271] Similarly, the long-lasting effects of previous strict glycemic control observed in people with type 1 diabetes in the DCCT[272] or with type 2 diabetes in the UKPDS[273] could be attributed to cellular metabolic memory.

## BIOMARKERS OF DKD

Albuminuria is the best currently available risk marker for DKD, but it has several drawbacks, as noted earlier in the chapter. Not only does albuminuria return to normal spontaneously or in response to therapy in many people with diabetes,[31,75–80] but the absence of albuminuria does not preclude the presence of DKD.[18,81–83] Therefore investigators are searching for new biomarkers of DKD that provide additional prognostic information beyond that provided by albuminuria. Such information can be used for identifying patients at risk for progressive DKD, and may also be used to enrich clinical trials, by selectively enrolling those at highest risk of progression.[274] These markers may also reflect specific underlying molecular mechanisms relevant to the initiation and/or progression of DKD that could be targeted for therapeutic intervention.[275] In this section, we will review some of the biomarkers of greatest interest for use in assessment of DKD. We make no effort to exhaustively characterize all putative biomarkers of DKD. A more comprehensive list of potential biomarkers is shown in Table 39.2.[276] As noted in the table, biomarkers fall into several general classes that reflect underlying pathogenic mechanisms, and we will focus here on markers of tubular damage, inflammation, and oxidative stress as well as panels that combine markers from across these categories. Other emerging types of biomarkers will also be briefly considered.

Much attention has focused recently on urine concentrations of molecules predominantly expressed by renal tubular cells as biomarkers of DKD. These molecules associate strongly with acute kidney injury, and there is evidence that repeated episodes of acute kidney injury may accelerate the progression of DKD.[277–279] Tubular markers such as kidney injury molecule (KIM-1), liver fatty acid binding protein (L-FABP), N-acetyl-β-D-glucosaminidase (NAG), and neutrophil gelatinase associated lipocalin (NGAL) have been evaluated in relation to DKD, cardiovascular disease, and mortality, sometimes with conflicting results.[280–294] These inconsistencies may be due in part to differences in study design, use of surrogate or composite outcomes, or incomplete covariate adjustment in risk models. A recent study also found that the plasma concentration of KIM-1 was a stronger predictor of early progressive renal function loss in type 1 diabetes than urine concentration, suggesting that the source of this marker (plasma or urine) reflects distinct aspects of proximal tubular damage or that the plasma concentration is less susceptible to variability in the time of collection.[295] Taken together, these studies suggest that damage to the proximal tubules plays a role in DKD. In most studies, however, they do not greatly enhance risk prediction over established risk markers.

Another tubular marker that has attracted recent attention is epidermal growth factor (EGF), a growth-promoting peptide synthesized in renal tubular cells and found in the urine. Lower urine excretion of epidermal growth factor was found in persons with type 1 diabetes and elevated urine albumin excretion than in nondiabetic controls. Among persons with diabetes and GFR >90 ml/min, urine epidermal growth factor correlated directly with GFR and inversely with urine albumin excretion.[296] In addition, lower urine EGF:creatinine ratios were associated with incident impaired eGFR, greater than 5% loss of eGFR per year, or both of these outcomes in persons with type 2 diabetes who were normoalbuminuric

**Table 39.2**[276] **Biomarkers of Diabetic Kidney Disease**

| Class | Biomarkers | Method of Detection |
|---|---|---|
| Currently used | GFR | renal clearance/estimating equation |
| | Albuminuria | urine |
| | Creatinine | serum |
| | Cystatin C | serum |
| | BUN | serum |
| Oxidative stress | Pentosidine | serum/urine |
| | 8-OHdG | urine |
| | Uric acid | serum |
| | AGEs/OPs | serum |
| | IPP2K | urine |
| | Adiponectin | serum |
| Fibrosis | TGF-$\beta_1$ | serum/urine |
| | CTGF | serum/urine |
| | VEGF | serum/urine |
| Glomerular damage | Transferrin | urine |
| | Type IV collagen | urine |
| | Cystatin C | urine |
| Tubular damage | L-FABP | urine |
| | NGAL | urine |
| | KIM-1 | serum/urine |
| | ACE2 | serum/urine |
| | Angiotensinogen | urine |
| | NAG | urine |
| | $\alpha$1-microglobulin | urine |
| | FGF23 | serum |
| | EGF | urine |
| Inflammation | TNF-$\alpha$; TNFR 1/2 | serum/urine |
| | Osteoprotegerin | plasma |
| | MCP-1 | urine |
| | IL-1, IL-6, Il-8, IL-18 | serum/urine |
| | WBC counts/fractions | blood |
| | Bradykinin and related peptides | plasma |
| | hs-CRP | serum |
| | Osteopontin | serum |
| Filtration markers | Beta-trace protein | serum |
| | Beta-2 microglobulin | serum |
| Mitochondrial function | Various metabolites | urine |

*GFR*, Glomerular filtration rate; *BUN*, blood urea nitrogen; *8-OHdG*, 8-hydroxy-2'-deoxyguanosine; *AGE*, advanced glycation end-product; *OP*, oxidative product; *IPP2K*, inositol pentakisphosphate 2-kinase; *TGF-$\beta_1$*, transforming growth factor-$\beta_1$; *CTGF*, connective tissue growth factor; *VEGF*, vascular endothelial growth factor; *L-FABP*, liver fatty acid-binding protein; *NGAL*, neutrophil gelatinase-associated lipocalin; *KIM-1*, kidney injury molecule 1; *ACE2*, angiotensin-converting enzyme-2; *NAG*, *N*-acetyl-β-D-glucosaminidase; *FGF23*, fibroblast growth factor 23; *EGF*, epidermal growth factor; *TNF-α*, tumor necrosis factor-α; *TNFR ½*, tumor necrosis factor receptor 1 and 2; *MCP-1*, monocyte chemoattractant protein-1; *IL*, interleukin; *WBC*, white blood cell; hs-*CRP*, high-sensitivity C-reactive protein.

(Modified from Tables 1 and 2 from Campion CG, Sanchez-Ferras O, Batchu SN. Potential role of serum and urinary biomarkers in diagnosis and prognosis of diabetic nephropathy. *Can J Kidney Health Dis.* 2017;4:1–18. With permission.)

**Note**: This table is not intended to be an exhaustive list of potential biomarkers, but it is intended to illustrate the diversity of biomarkers and mechanisms.

and had preserved renal function at baseline.[297] Transcriptomic data obtained from kidney tissue in three chronic kidney disease cohorts, which included persons with diabetes, were used to identify potential biomarkers of chronic kidney disease. The top candidate identified by this approach was EGF, and the investigators then demonstrated that lower urine concentrations of epidermal growth factor in these patients improved prediction of progressive kidney disease beyond established risk factors.[298] What makes this study noteworthy is the transcriptomic-driven sequential strategy used for biomarker discovery and identification, an approach we can expect to see used more frequently in biomarker research in the future.

Inflammatory processes also play a key role in DKD, and several promising markers related to inflammation have been identified. Tumor necrosis factor alpha (TNF-α) was implicated in the pathogenesis of DKD in animal models in the early 1990s,[299] but its association with DKD in humans has not been convincingly established. On the other hand, circulating levels of tumor necrosis factor receptors (TNFR) 1 and 2 have recently emerged as very robust and independent predictors of the progression of DKD. In the Joslin Clinic diabetes cohorts, elevated concentrations of circulating TNFR 1 and 2 were strongly associated with impaired GFR (<60 ml/min/1.73 $m^2$) in patients with type 1 diabetes[300] and ESKD in patients with type 2 diabetes,[301] after accounting for established risk factors. Elevations of TNF receptors were subsequently found to predict macroalbuminuria in patients with type 1 diabetes in the DCCT/EDIC cohort,[302] ESKD in the FinnDiane type 1 diabetes cohort,[303] loss of renal function in the SURDIAGENE type 2 diabetes cohort,[304] and ESKD in Pima Indians with type 2 diabetes.[305] They also predicted cardiovascular events and total mortality in Swedish patients with type 2 diabetes from the CARDIPP study.[306] Research kidney biopsies performed in Pima Indians with type 2 diabetes demonstrated strong associations between higher concentrations of TNFR 1 and 2 and various morphometric lesions, including mesangial expansion, loss of endothelial cell fenestration and total filtration surface per glomerulus, increased width of the glomerular basement membrane and podocyte foot processes, and increased global glomerular sclerosis, suggesting that the TNFRs may be involved in the pathogenesis of early glomerular lesions in DKD.[307]

Monocyte chemoattractant protein-1 (MCP-1) is a cytokine secreted by mononuclear leukocytes, cortical tubular epithelial cells and podocytes that is implicated in inflammatory processes in the kidneys that ultimately lead to fibrosis.[308] Higher urine MCP-1 concentrations are associated with increased risk of renal function decline, doubling of serum creatinine concentration, and progression to dialysis or death in patients with DKD in either type 1 or type 2 diabetes.[309–311] MCP-1 is also one of several urine cytokines that predict early decline in GFR in patients with type 1 diabetes and microalbuminuria.[312] Urine MCP-1 correlates with early cortical interstitial expansion in normotensive normoalbuminuric individuals with type 1 diabetes, suggesting that it may be involved in the pathogenesis of early interstitial changes in DKD.[313]

Emerging evidence suggests that elevated serum uric acid concentrations induce oxidative stress, and promote inflammation, endothelial dysfunction, and fibrosis in the kidneys. Longitudinal studies in type 1 diabetes have found that hyperuricemia is associated with the onset and progression of albuminuria and loss of GFR,[314–317] and a double-blind randomized study of 40 patients with type 2 diabetes and DKD observed that four months of treatment with low-dose allopurinol (100 mg/day) was associated with significantly lower serum uric acid concentration and 24-hour urine protein excretion than treatment with placebo.[318] Together, these studies suggest that allopurinol may be a useful addition to established treatment of DKD. A large multicenter clinical trial is presently underway in patients with type 1 diabetes to address this hypothesis.[319] A recent study, however, questions the link between uric acid and DKD. Investigators from the FinnDiane Study examined causality between serum uric acid concentrations and progression of diabetic nephropathy in 3895 individuals with type 1 diabetes using a Mendelian randomization approach. The investigators concluded that elevated serum uric acid concentration is not causally related to DKD but is instead a downstream marker of kidney damage.[320]

Given that a spectrum of pathogenic mechanisms is operative in DKD and that there are robust markers in diverse pathways that predict progressive DKD, risk stratification may be improved by assessing markers from several different pathways simultaneously.[275,321–325] A recent study involving a subset of participants with early DKD from the Action to Control Cardiovascular Risk in Diabetes (ACCORD) trial and with advanced DKD from the Veterans Administration Nephropathy in Diabetes (VA-NEPHRON-D) study illustrated that a combination of inflammatory (plasma TNFR 1 and 2) and tubular (plasma KIM-1) biomarkers were independently associated with a higher risk of decline of eGFR in type 2 diabetes. Importantly, together these markers significantly improved risk prediction over established markers.[326] Similarly, the Genetics of Diabetes Audit and Research Tayside Study (GO-DARTS) explored a set of 207 serum proteins and metabolites in a nested case-control study of a subset of patients with type 2 diabetes and stage 3 chronic kidney disease to identify biomarkers that predicted rapid renal function decline, defined by >40% decline in eGFR within 3.5 years. Fourteen biomarkers from across several pathogenic pathways differentiated the cases with rapid renal function decline from the controls, who had no fall in eGFR, and these markers improved prediction of rapid progression over established risk factors.[327]

Other mechanisms not discussed previously are also involved in the development and progression of DKD. Evidence is accumulating that various microRNAs,[328,329] long noncoding RNAs,[262] and urine exosomes[330] may be informative biomarkers for DKD. Recent advances in imaging technology may also make it possible to improve risk stratification of early DKD using MRI-based technologies[331–333] and optical coherence tomography, which predicts 4-year incident diabetic neuropathy[334] and is being evaluated for use in DKD.

## CLINICAL COURSE

The classic course of DKD progresses through several phases in which albumin or protein excretion increases, and GFR rises and subsequently falls, eventually culminating in uremia and ESKD (Fig. 39.3).[73] As noted earlier in this chapter, much evidence has accumulated in recent years which demonstrates that progression of DKD with loss of GFR often occurs in the absence of proteinuria in both type 1 and type 2 diabetes. This phenotype is more frequently observed in women and in type 2 diabetes, particularly in the presence of obesity, dyslipidemia, hypertension, and/or early hyperfiltration; neither its causes nor its treatment are well understood.[335]

The UKPDS illustrates this new paradigm during the early course of DKD in patients with type 2 diabetes (Fig. 39.4). About 2% to 3% of enrolled patients transitioned each year from one stage of DKD to the next (i.e., normoalbuminuria → microalbuminuria → macroalbuminuria → reduced glomerular filtration rate [GFR]). At a median of 15 years after diagnosis, 38% of patients had developed albuminuria and 29% had developed reduced GFR. Half of those who developed reduced GFR did not have preceding albuminuria, and 39% never developed albuminuria during the study.[82,336]

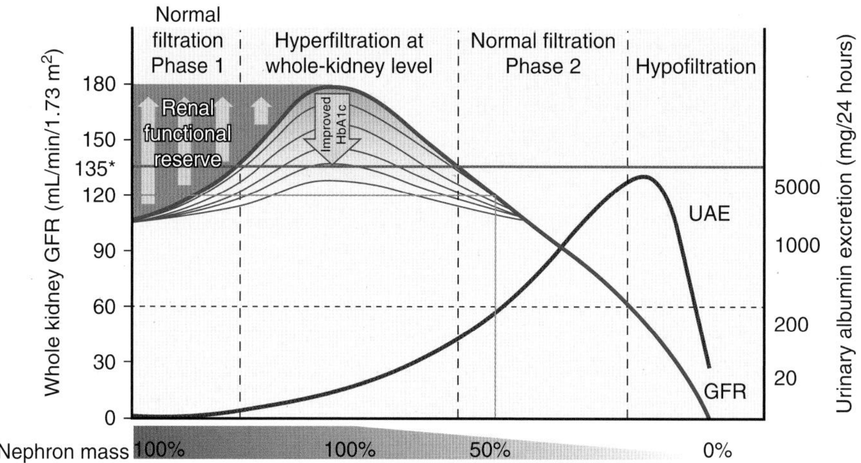


**Fig. 39.3 Classic course of whole-kidney glomerular filtration rate (GFR) and urine albumin excretion (UAE) according to the natural (proteinuric) pathway of diabetic kidney disease (DKD).[139] Peak GFR may be seen in prediabetes or shortly after diabetes diagnosis and can reach up to 180 mL/min in the case of two fully intact kidneys. Strict control of $HbA_{1c}$ and initiation of other treatments (such as RAS inhibition) mitigate this initial response. Two normal filtration phases can be encountered, in which GFR may be, for instance, 120 mL/min (indicated with the gray line): One at 100% of nephron mass and one at approximately 50% of nephron mass. Thus whole-kidney GFR may remain normal even in the presence of considerable loss of nephron mass, as evidenced by a recent autopsy study.[121] Assessing renal functional reserve and/or UAE may help identify the extent of subclinically inflicted loss of functional nephron mass. *Whole-kidney hyperfiltration is generally defined as a GFR that exceeds approximately 135 ml/min and is indicated with the red line. Heterogeneity of single-nephron filtration rate and nonproteinuric pathway[122] of DKD are not illustrated.**

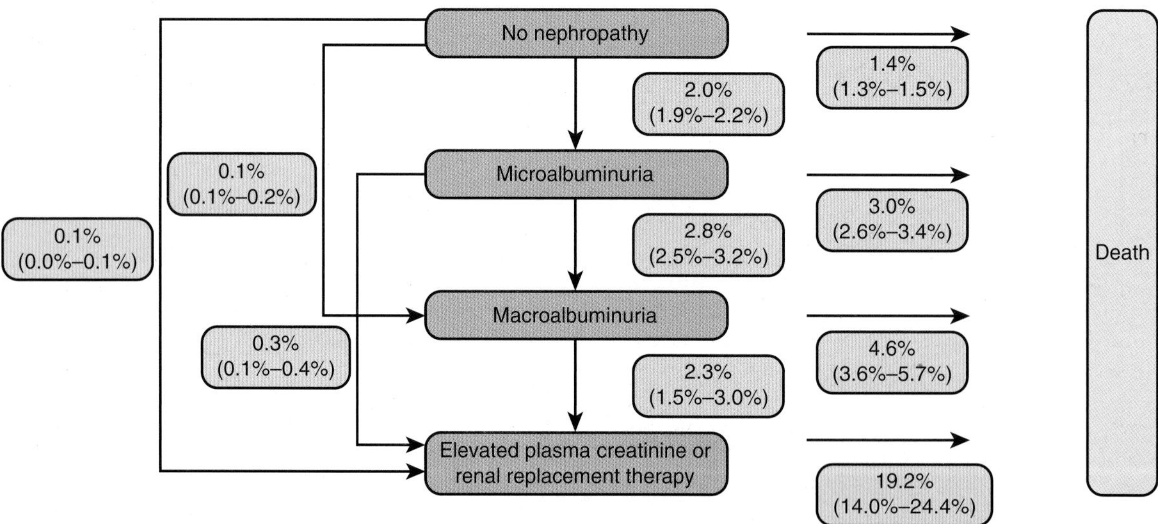


**Fig. 39.4 Annual transition rates between stages of diabetic kidney disease, and to death from any cause, in patients with type 2 diabetes in the UK Prospective Diabetes Study.[76] Confidence intervals of 95% are indicated in parentheses.**

Moreover, after developing microalbuminuria, more patients in each stage of DKD died each year than transitioned to the next stage.

## PROGNOSIS

DKD is a strong predictor of mortality, predominantly from cardiovascular and kidney disease. In the absence of proteinuria, Danish patients with type 1 diabetes have a nearly normal life expectancy.[337] The FinnDiane study and the Pittsburgh Epidemiology of Diabetes Complications Study extended these findings to show a graded association between the severity of kidney disease and mortality. In addition, they found that the excess mortality in type 1 diabetes, relative to the background population, was almost entirely observed in patients with albuminuria.[338,339] Similar findings were reported in type 2 diabetes.[340,341] Using nationally representative data from NHANES III, 10-year mortality in patients with type 2 diabetes in the United States was examined by level of kidney impairment and compared with mortality in people without diabetes and kidney disease (Fig. 39.5). Relative to this reference group, most of the excess mortality associated with type 2 diabetes was found in patients with DKD, with the greatest excess noted in those who had both albuminuria and reduced

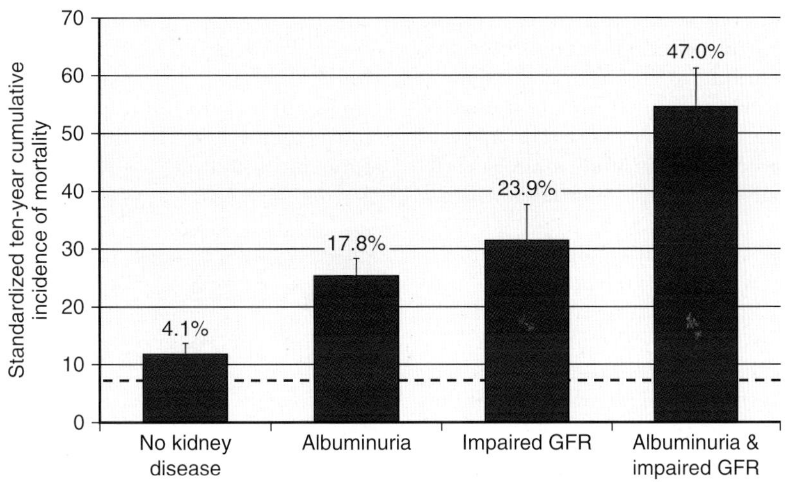


**Fig. 39.5 Ten-year mortality in type 2 diabetes by kidney disease manifestation.[341] Absolute differences in mortality risk were estimated using linear regression and were adjusted for age, sex, and race. Standardized 10-year all-cause cumulative incidences were estimated for the mean levels of the covariates in the study population. The dashed line indicates mortality in people without diabetes or kidney disease (the reference group). The numbers above bars indicate excess mortality above the reference group. Error bars indicate 95% confidence intervals.**

GFR.[341] Comparable patterns were observed for cardiovascular and noncardiovascular mortality. Widespread vascular damage associated with diabetes undoubtedly contributes to these various adverse health outcomes.[232] Importantly, the Global Burden of Disease Study noted that deaths from chronic kidney disease due to diabetes increased by nearly 107% between 1990 and 2013.[342]

Metaanalyses of large cohorts demonstrate that albuminuria, even in the microalbuminuric range, is a strong predictor of all-cause mortality, cardiovascular mortality, stroke, and ESKD in patients with diabetes and in those without.[9,343–345] More recently, the Global Burden of Disease Study, in collaboration with the Chronic Kidney Disease Prognosis Consortium, reported that cardiovascular deaths attributed to reduced GFR outnumber ESKD deaths worldwide, although the death rate from ESKD is increasing worldwide.[346] In addition, the Chronic Kidney Disease Prognosis Consortium analyzed data from 1,024,977 patients in 43 cohorts worldwide, and found that an increase in albuminuria or a decline in eGFR increased the relative risk of all-cause mortality or ESKD equivalently in patients with or without diabetes, although the absolute risk was higher in those with diabetes.[9] These findings illustrate the importance of early kidney disease as a predictor of major health outcomes, regardless of the presence or absence of diabetes. Given the comparable effects of changes in these markers across diverse types of kidney disease, predictive models have been developed to identify those at greatest risk for chronic kidney disease progression.[347] A predictive model for progression to kidney failure accurately predicted progression in two independent Canadian cohorts of patients with stage 3 to 5 chronic kidney disease.[348] In a subsequent validation study conducted by the Chronic Kidney Disease Prognosis Consortium, the accuracy of the preferred risk equations was examined in 31 multinational cohorts that included 721,357 participants from 30 countries on 4 continents. The equations provided excellent discrimination between progressors and nonprogressors in most of the North American cohorts, and the addition of a recalibration factor optimized performance in non–North American populations, which have a different level of baseline risk, suggesting that these equations can be used worldwide for prediction of kidney disease progression.[349] The 4-variable equation that includes age, sex, eGFR, and albuminuria can be implemented easily in modern health information systems and is widely available on the Internet for any practitioner interested in using it (http://kidneyfailurerisk.com).

Prediction models for development of microalbuminuria have also been developed and validated for people with type 1 diabetes.[350,351]

## EXTRARENAL COMPLICATIONS IN DKD

Diabetic retinopathy is common in type 1 diabetes, occurring in nearly all patients after 15 to 20 years of diabetes, and it is generally more severe in those with proteinuria.[352] In a population-based study in southern Wisconsin, the prevalence of proliferative diabetic retinopathy among patients with type 1 diabetes for more than 10 years was 67% in those with proteinuria and 22% in those without.[352] The severity of retinopathy also correlates strongly with the structural lesions of DKD, even in those without other clinical evidence of DKD. Among the 285 normoalbuminuric patients with normal blood pressure and type 1 diabetes in the Renin-Angiotensin System Study (RASS), mild nonproliferative diabetic retinopathy was present in 53%, moderate-to-severe nonproliferative retinopathy in 9%, and proliferative retinopathy in 2% of the cohort.[353] In the 252 patients (88%) who had both retinal photographs and a research kidney biopsy, severity of retinopathy was strongly associated with mesangial expansion, increased glomerular basement membrane width, and decreased peripheral glomerular basement membrane surface density, after adjustment for potential confounders. In a separate study of 86 patients with type 1 diabetes and advanced DKD, all the patients had diabetic retinopathy and 70% had proliferative diabetic retinopathy, reflecting their more advanced retinopathy than in the RASS cohort.[354]

The severity of retinopathy was associated with the same structural lesions, including increased mesangial fractional volume and decreased peripheral glomerular basement membrane surface density, but at a more advanced stage of these lesions. Although some discordance between DKD and diabetic retinopathy was noted in both studies, the severity of retinopathy was generally strongly concordant with the severity of the structural lesions of DKD.[353,354]

The prevalence of diabetic retinopathy in type 2 diabetes is lower than in type 1 diabetes.[352,355,356] In the population-based study in southern Wisconsin, the prevalence of diabetic retinopathy in 1370 patients with type 2 diabetes was 78% after 15 years compared with 98% in 996 patients with type 1 diabetes.[352,355] The absence of retinopathy in these patients should prompt further investigation for nondiabetic glomerulopathies. A study of 35 Danish patients with type 2 diabetes and macroalbuminuria (≥300 mg/24 hours) who underwent research kidney biopsies to ascertain the cause of their albuminuria found that diabetic retinopathy was present in 56% of those with diabetic glomerulosclerosis, and no retinopathy was observed in those with nondiabetic glomerulopathies, which accounted for a quarter of the patients with albuminuria.[357]

Blindness caused by severe proliferative diabetic retinopathy or maculopathy is approximately five times more frequent in diabetic patients with albuminuria than in those with normoalbuminuria.[356]

Macroangiopathies (e.g., stroke, carotid artery stenosis, coronary heart disease, peripheral vascular disease) are two to five times more common in patients with DKD than in those without and are the leading cause of death in patients with DKD.[356,358] Even modest elevations of albuminuria within the normal range were associated with increased numbers of cardiovascular events in 1208 hypertensive, normoalbuminuric patients with type 2 diabetes from the BENEDICT trial, who were followed for a median of 9.2 years.[359] The Multinational Study of Vascular Disease in Diabetes confirmed the importance of cardiovascular disease as the major cause of death in people with either type 1 or type 2 diabetes, but demonstrated marked ethnic variation in cardiovascular risk.[360] In populations with lower risks of cardiovascular disease, such as the Pima Indians, DKD was the leading cause of death in those with type 2 diabetes before renal replacement therapy became available. As renal replacement therapy became widely available and was accepted by the population, lives of those with DKD were prolonged, and cardiovascular disease displaced kidney failure as the leading cause of death.[361] As cardiovascular deaths decline in both types of diabetes in the developed countries, due in part to earlier detection and improved diabetes and cardiovascular care,[362-365] its impact on the frequency of DKD is uncertain. With type 2 diabetes frequently occurring at younger ages, improvements in care may be offset by the earlier onset of the disease, perhaps erasing the recent gains in longevity.

Diabetic peripheral neuropathy affects 50% of patients with diabetes in the United States,[366] and peripheral neuropathy is present in almost all patients with advanced nephropathy. Cardiac autonomic neuropathy, which may be asymptomatic or result in debilitating symptoms, increases all-cause mortality threefold in patients with diabetes.[367] Most patients with DKD have grossly abnormal results on autonomic function tests,[368] and as described above, cardiac autonomic neuropathy is a risk factor for progressive DKD, although the relationship between DKD and cardiac autonomic neuropathy may be bidirectional.[244] DKD may contribute to the progression of cardiac autonomic neuropathy by modulating leptin signaling in the hypothalamus, which, in turn, may affect sympathetic tone and function.[369]

## PATHOLOGY OF THE KIDNEY IN DIABETES

### CLASSIC LESIONS OF DIABETIC KIDNEY DISEASE

DKD was first described in 1936 by the presence of mesangial expansion and nodular glomerulosclerosis in a classic paper by Kimmelstiel and Wilson.[370] Since then much more has been learned about DKD lesions. The pathology of DKD is more homogeneous and has been more thoroughly investigated in type 1 diabetes. Therefore we will focus first on DKD in type 1 diabetes patients and then compare it with type 2 diabetes. In this section, we will describe a number of quantitative morphometric measurements that are used to describe key kidney structural parameters related to DKD. Table 39.3 provides a list of morphometric abbreviations for these parameters along with their descriptions.

The hallmark of DKD is accumulation of extracellular matrix, namely glomerular and tubular basement membranes and mesangial matrix (Fig. 39.6).[163,371] An imbalance between synthesis, controlled by transcription and translation, and degradation, regulated by the interplay between matrix metalloproteinases and their inhibitors, leads to the accumulation of extracellular matrix proteins in DKD.[372]

Characteristic features of DKD in type 1 diabetes occur in the glomeruli. These changes typically occur through a well-defined sequence. Glomerular basement membrane (GBM) thickening is the first lesion identifiable by electron microscopy morphometry. It develops within 2 years of onset of diabetes and progresses with increasing duration of diabetes, more or less in a linear fashion.[373] Thickening of GBM is associated with increased densities of $\alpha_3$ and $\alpha_4$ chains of type IV collagen, perhaps due to increased production of these molecules by podocytes in part related to hyperglycemia.[374–376]

**Table 39.3 Description of Morphometric Abbreviations Used in This Chapter**

| Morphometric Abbreviation | Description |
|---|---|
| Vv(Mes/glom) | Fraction of the volume of the glomerulus occupied by the mesangium |
| Sv(PGBM/glom) | Peripheral glomerular basement membrane filtration surface density per glomerular volume |
| Vv(Int/cortex) | Fraction of the volume of the renal cortex occupied by interstitium |
| Vv(MM/glom) | Fraction of the volume of the glomerulus occupied by mesangial matrix |
| Nv(Podo/glom) | Podocyte number density per glomerular volume |
| N(Podo/glom) | Number of podocytes per glomerulus |

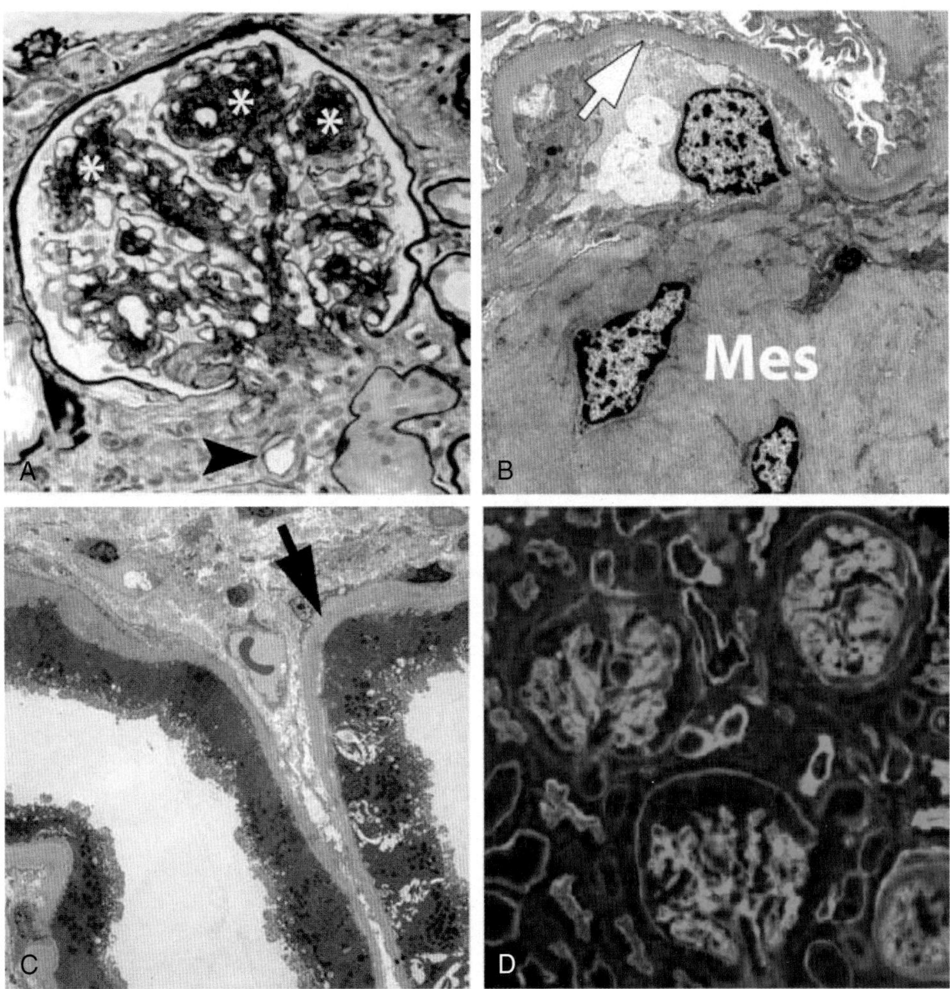


**Fig. 39.6** Classical biopsy findings in diabetic kidney disease. A, A glomerulus with nodular glomerulosclerosis or Kimmelstiel-Wilson nodules (asterisks) and mesangial expansion due predominantly to increased mesangial matrix, and arteriolar hyalinosis *(arrowhead)*; Jones methenamine silver stain. B, Thickening of glomerular basement membrane *(white arrow)* and increased mesangial matrix (Mes); transmission electron microscopy. C, Thickening of tubular basement membranes *(black arrow)*; transmission electron microscopy. D, Linear accentuation of glomerular and tubular basement membranes for immunoglobin G; immunofluorescence microscopy.

Mesangial expansion is the first lesion detected by light microscopy (best appreciated by periodic acid–Schiff stain on light microscopy). Increased fraction of the volume of the glomerulus occupied by the mesangium [Vv(Mes/glom)] can be detected as early as 4 to 5 years after the onset of type 1 diabetes.[377] The pace of increase in Vv(Mes/glom) is slower in the first few years of type 1 diabetes and becomes faster as diabetes duration increases.[378] Mesangial expansion is due primarily to increased mesangial matrix.[379] Even in those patients with Vv(Mes/glom) within the normal range, the fraction of mesangium which is matrix, as opposed to mesangial cells, is increased.[378] Mesangial expansion is associated with protrusion of mesangium into peripheral capillary walls, leading to reduced filtration surface area and an inverse relationship between Vv(Mes/glom) and peripheral GBM filtration surface density, Sv(PGBM/glom) (Fig. 39.7).[163,380] Increased glomerular volume, at least partially. compensates for reduced glomerular filtration surface density and preserves the total filtration surface area. However, increased glomerular volume, in contrast to animal models of DKD, is a relatively late finding in patients with type 1 diabetes.[381,382] Mesangial expansion can be diffuse or nodular. Nodular glomerulosclerosis (also known as *Kimmelstiel-Wilson nodules*) is characterized by prominent round expansion of hypocellular mesangial matrix, sometimes with palisading mesangial cells in the periphery of the nodule, surrounded by patent glomerular capillaries (Fig. 39.6). Mesangial matrix within the nodules may show a distinctive lamellated appearance, which is best appreciated by Jones methenamine silver stain. Nodular lesions typically occur in advanced DKD and at least 15 years after the onset of type 1 diabetes.[383,384] However, occasional nodular lesions can be seen in earlier stages of DKD when the overall mesangial expansion is mild and diffuse. It is important to note that nodular glomerulosclerosis is not pathognomonic of DKD and can be seen in other conditions, such as light chain deposition disease, immune complex processes, and idiopathic nodular glomerulosclerosis.[385] Mesangiolysis, characterized by the fraying of the mesangial matrix is considered the precursor of nodular lesions. Mesangiolysis leads to unfolding of the GBM and formation of capillary microaneurysms or nodular glomerulosclerosis (Fig. 39.8).[386,387,388]

DKD lesions associated with hyaline deposition (aside from segmental glomerulosclerosis) are termed *exudative lesions* and include arteriolar hyalinosis, fibrin caps and capsular drops (Fig. 39.9). Concomitant hyalinosis of afferent and efferent arterioles is characteristic of DKD and can be seen within 3 to 5 years after the onset of type 1 diabetes.[389] Hyalinosis starts in the subendothelial space of arterioles but can expand to totally replace the smooth muscle cells with hyaline. Aside from hyalinosis, arterioles and small interlobular arteries show increased extracellular matrix medial thickening in young patients with type 1 diabetes.[390] Efferent arterioles may proliferate at the vascular pole of glomeruli.[391] Subendothelial accumulations of hyaline in the glomerular capillary are referred to as fibrin caps, but these lesions are not composed of fibrin, and should be more appropriately be called *hyaline caps*. Capsular drops are accumulations of hyaline under the parietal epithelial cell lining of Bowman's capsule.

Podocyte injury plays a crucial role in the progression of DKD. Podocyte injury is an early phenomenon in DKD. About one-third of normoalbuminuric diabetic patients show

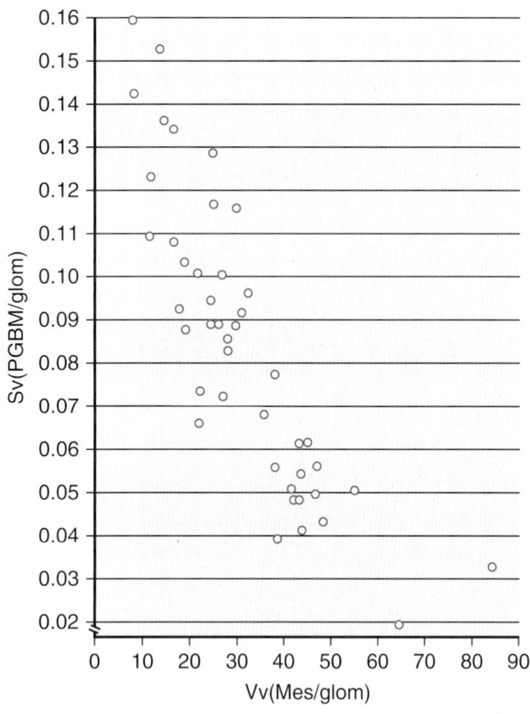


**Fig. 39.7**[163] Relationship of mesangial fractional volume per glomerulus [Vv(Mes/glom)] and filtration surface density per glomerular volume (Sv(PGBM/glom) in type 1 diabetic patients.

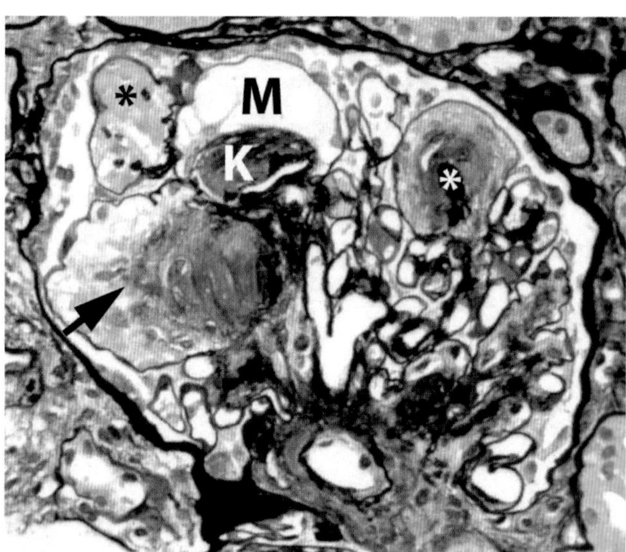


**Fig. 39.8** A glomerulus with advanced diabetic kidney disease. Mesangiolysis *(arrow)* characterized by fraying of mesangium can lead to formation of Kimmelstiel-Wilson nodules (K) and microaneurysms (M). Black asterisk shows a microaneurysm containing blood and no adjacent nodule. White asterisk shows a nodule; its associated microaneurysm is sclerotic.

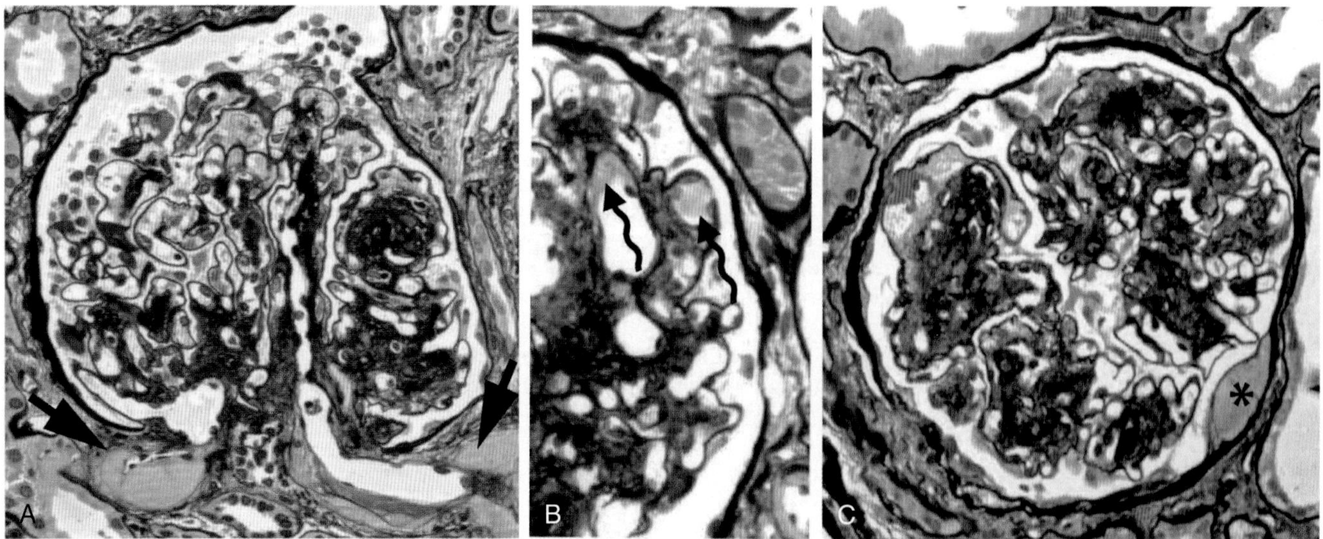


**Fig. 39.9** Exudative lesions of diabetic kidney disease. A, Concomitant hyalinosis of afferent and efferent arterioles *(arrows)*. B, Fibrin caps in glomerular capillaries *(waved arrows)*. C, Capsular drop (asterisk). Jones methenamine silver stain.

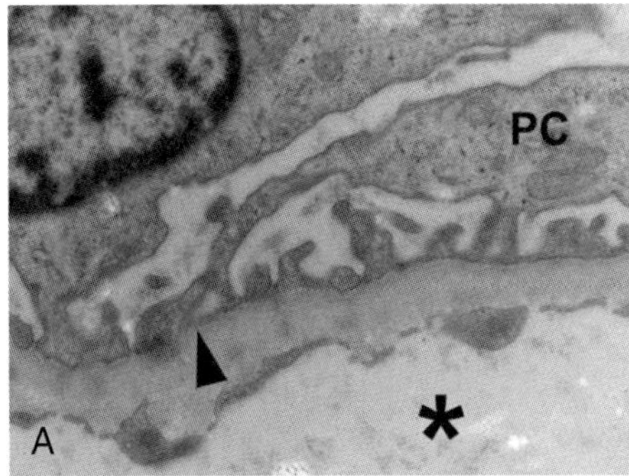

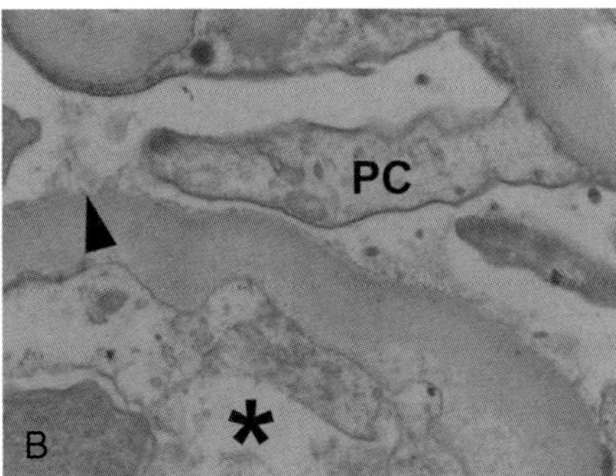

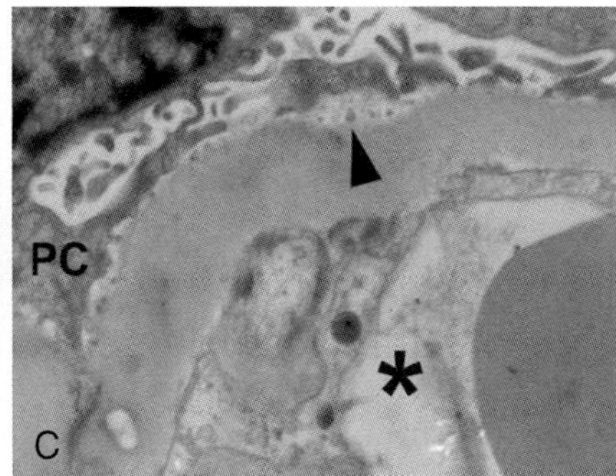


**Fig. 39.10**[394] Detachment of podocytes (PC) from the glomerular basement membrane in diabetic kidney disease (DKD) (A) glomerular basement membrane covered by intact foot processes in mild DKD. With advancement of DKD, some areas of glomerular basement membranes with complete (B), or partial (C) detachment of podocytes are observable. *Capillary lumen. Arrowhead shows the podocyte aspect of the glomerular basement membrane.

increased nephrin excretion in the urine, indicative of early podocyte injury even before the onset of microalbuminuria.[392] Similarly, widening of foot processes, a concomitant of podocyte injury, is detectable in normoalbuminuric diabetic patients[393] and becomes more severe in microalbuminuric and proteinuric patients.[394] Podocyte injury can lead to podocyte loss. Reduced expression of $\alpha_3\beta_1$ integrin,[395] apoptosis, glucose-induced oxidative stress and autophagy may be involved in this process.[396,397] Detachment of podocytes from GBM occurs early and becomes more severe as albuminuria worsens (Fig. 39.10).[394] Podocyte loss leads to secondary focal and segmental glomerulosclerosis (FSGS), which is a relatively late finding in nephropathy of type 1 diabetes and has a distinct predilection for the glomerulotubular junction area (Fig. 39.11).[398,399] This predilection may be related to a combination of enhanced shear stress to podocytes at the tubular pole of the glomerular tuft[400] and tubular epithelial cell injury secondary to the tubulotoxic effect of proteinuria.[401] FSGS directs part of the glomerular ultrafiltrate through the adhesion site into Bowman's capsule, leading to dissection of the capsular basement membrane. This dissection extends into the glomerulotubular junction, and can lead to stricture and occlusion of the glomerular tubular outlet and eventually create atubular glomeruli (Fig. 39.11).[398,399] Thus FSGS leads to nephron loss and GFR reduction, either through progression to global glomerulosclerosis or formation of atubular glomeruli.[398] Although advancement of glomerulopathy in DKD leads to global glomerulosclerosis, the sclerotic glomeruli in patients with type 1 diabetes are more often clustered in the plane vertical to the renal capsule, underscoring the importance of vascular lesions and chronic ischemia in glomerulosclerosis.[402] Severity of arteriolar hyalinosis is also associated with increased glomerulosclerosis in patients with type 1 diabetes.[403]

Tubular basement membrane (TBM) thickening is an early finding in DKD and parallels GBM thickening (Fig. 39.6).[100,371] TBM width in diabetic patients correlates strongly with GBM width and Vv(Mes/glom), but only weakly with the volume fraction of renal cortex that is interstitium [Vv(Int/cortex)],[371] indicating that TBM thickening is related to diabetes status rather than nonspecific chronic injury.

Tubulointerstitial fibrosis follows glomerulopathy in patients with type 1 diabetes. In fact, Vv(Int/cortex) initially reduces as a result of tubular hypertrophy.[404] Expansion of cortical interstitium is initially due primarily to an increase in the cellular component, while increased interstitial fibrillar collagen deposition occurs relatively late, when GFR decline is already present.[404]

GBM and TBM show modest linear staining with IgG (polytypic) and albumin in diabetic patients (Fig. 39.6), regardless of DKD. Alterations in chemical properties of extracellular matrix, immunoglobulins or both might be involved in this phenomenon, but the exact cause remains unclear. A recent study suggested that the intensity of IgG staining is directly associated with kidney outcomes, but this finding requires further validation.[405]

*Clinical Relevance*
**Pathology**

The natural history of DKD starts with an initial long clinically silent period during which albumin excretion rate remains normal and GFR is normal or high, while DKD lesions slowly progress. Therefore albuminuria is not a sensitive marker to detect early DKD. On the other hand, when patients develop micro- and, especially, macroalbuminuria DKD lesions are typically far advanced and GFR loss becomes accelerated toward ESKD. Kidney biopsy provides important insight about severity and prognosis of DKD. However, predictive value of biopsy findings in early DKD, when there is more opportunity to rescue the kidney, for later progression to ESKD remains limited. This calls for better biomarkers to identify patients at greater risk. Large studies combining clinical information with structural data as well as systems biology and biomarker discovery are needed to achieve this goal.

## STRUCTURAL-FUNCTIONAL RELATIONSHIPS OF DIABETIC KIDNEY DISEASE IN TYPE 1 DIABETES

The structural-functional relationship models of DKD mirror its clinical course and natural history, with an initial long clinically silent period characterized by normoalbuminuria and a normal or high GFR and slow progression of the disease, followed by an accelerated phase with rapid GFR decline.[406]

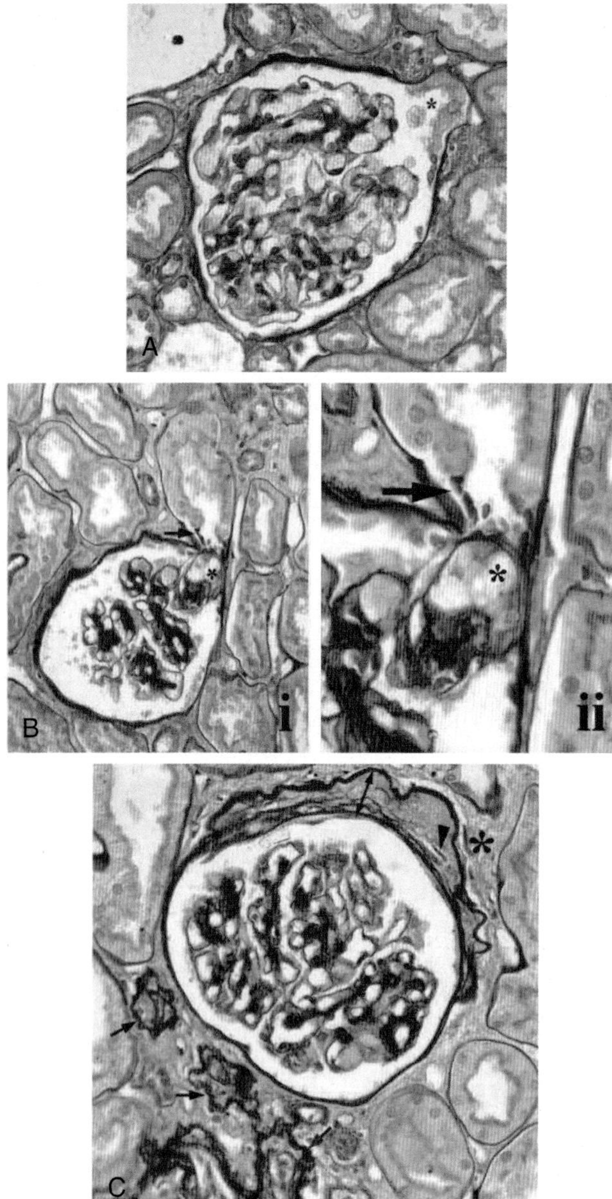


**Fig. 39.11** A, A glomerulus attached to a normal tubule (NT). *Glomerulotubular junction. B, (i) A glomerulus attached to a short atrophic tubule (SAT), with a tip lesion at glomerulotubular junction. Periodic acid–Schiff (PAS)-stained; magnification, ×630. (ii) A higher-magnification view of the tip lesion, allowing better appreciation of a dilated loop (*), with foam cells within the tip lesion and flat epithelial cells *(arrow)* covering the very beginning of the proximal tubule. C, An atubular glomerulus (AG). The glomerular tuft is indistinguishable from other glomeruli. Bowman's capsule is markedly thickened and wrinkled at a site opposite to the vascular pole, where a tubular connection is expected. ↔, reduplicated Bowman's capsule; arrowhead, a spindle-shape cell within the reduplicated Bowman's capsule; arrow, atrophic tubules adjacent to the atubular glomerulus; *periglomerular fibrosis. PAS-stained; magnification, ×630.

GBM width, Vv(Mes/glom) and Sv(PGBM/glom) in the initial normoalbuminuric phase may be within the normal range or overlap with abnormal values commonly seen in microalbuminuric, or less commonly even in proteinuric patients (Fig. 39.12A and B).[407] Persistent microalbuminuria is associated with worsening of the lesions and increased risk for progression to proteinuria.[407] Using simple linear regression analysis across a wide range of albumin excretion, from normoalbuminuria to proteinuria, Vv(Mes/glom) and GBM width correlate directly and Sv(PGBM/glom) correlate inversely with urine albumin excretion rate (Fig. 39.13A–C). Among the classical glomerular structural parameters of DKD, Vv(Mes/glom), fractional volume of mesangial matrix per glomerulus [Vv(MM/glom)] and GBM width are inversely and Sv(PGBM/glom) is directly related to GFR (Fig. 39.13).[407] Also, the total peripheral capillary filtration surface correlates directly with GFR from hyperfiltration to renal insufficiency. Increased GBM width is not only the first identifiable change in glomeruli in patients with type 1 diabetes, but it also predicts progression of DKD from normoalbuminuria to microalbuminuria or even macroalbuminuria and ESKD.[408] Importantly, in a cohort of 94 normoalbuminuric patients with long-standing type 1 diabetes, none of those with normal GBM width progressed to proteinuria or ESKD after an average follow up of 11 years.[408] On the other hand, GBM thickening is not the primary mechanism of albuminuria, as it can occur in long-standing diabetes without concomitant albuminuria.[409,410]

Structure–function relationship models derived from classical DKD glomerular structural parameters in a large cohort of patients with type 1 diabetes and a wide range of kidney functions were robust and applicable to another cohort of AER-matched patients.[411] Overall, around 70% of AER and around 20% to 30% of GFR variances are explainable by structural-functional relationship models created by multiple regression analysis based on glomerular lesions alone. On the other hand, using piecewise linear regression analysis, the predictability of the models are substantially improved, where over 80% of AER and over 65% of GFR variances can be explained. Two important conclusions can be derived from these data. First, the improved predictability of the models by piecewise linear regression analysis mirrors the natural history of DKD with an initial slow progression prior to a breakpoint and fast progression thereafter. Importantly, the breakpoints found in two separate studies were both in the microalbuminuric and normal GFR ranges,[398,411] suggesting that significant glomerular lesions are already in place, while patients are microalbuminuric and GFR is still relatively well preserved, and the shift from a slow to a fast progression phase occurs relatively early based on clinical measures. Second, these results indicate that if appropriate models are used, glomerular lesions alone explain a major proportion of AER and GFR variance in patients with type 1 diabetes. Addition of glomerulotubular junction abnormalities and Vv(Int/cortex) led to relatively minor improvements of predictability of these models.[398] These results may seem in contrast to other studies arguing that renal dysfunction in DKD is primarily driven by interstitial rather than glomerular lesions.[412,413] However, this argument was derived from studies focusing on patients with elevated serum creatinine values and in whom the interstitium was carefully measured but the glomerular structure was only subjectively estimated. Moreover, as pointed out earlier, Vv(Int/cortex) is initially decreased in the first decade of type 1 diabetes, whereas Vv(Mes/glom) and GBM width are already increased and interstitial fibrosis generally follows the glomerular lesions in type 1 diabetes. The percentage of global glomerulosclerosis

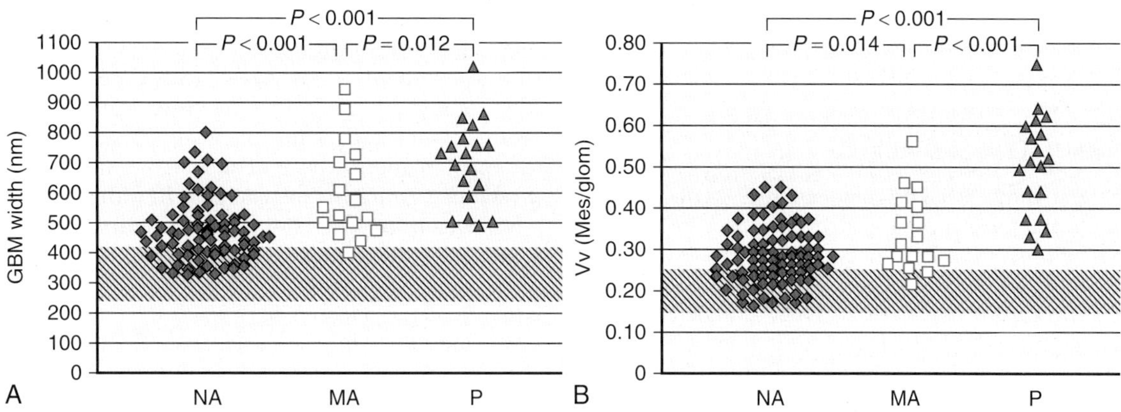


**Fig. 39.12 A, Glomerular basement membrane width in 88 normoalbuminuric (NA), 17 microalbuminuric (MA), and 19 proteinuric (P) patients with type 1 diabetes. The hatched area represents the mean ± 2 standard deviation in a group of 76 age-matched normal control subjects. All groups are different from control subjects. B, Vv (Mes/glom) in 88 normoalbuminuric (NA), 17 microalbuminuric (MA), and 19 proteinuric (P) patients with type 1 diabetes. The hatched area represents the mean ± 2 standard deviation in a group of 76 age-matched normal control subjects. All groups are different from control subjects.**

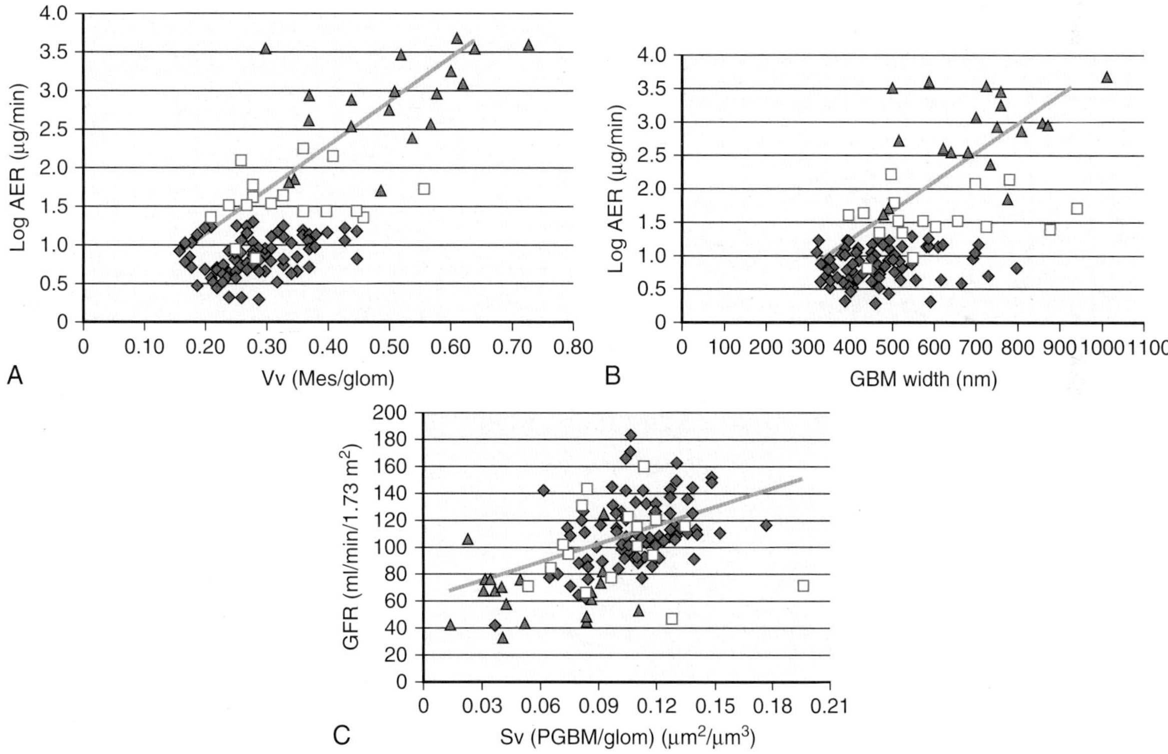


**Fig. 39.13** A, Correlation between Vv (Mes/glom) and albumin excretion rate (AER) in 124 patients with type 1 diabetes. ◆, Normoalbuminuric patients; □, microalbuminuric patients; ▲, proteinuric patients. $r = 0.75$, $P < .001$. B, Correlation between glomerular basement membrane width and AER in 124 patients with type 1 diabetes. ◆, Normoalbuminuric patients; □, microalbuminuric patients; ▲, proteinuric patients. $r = 0.63$, $P < .001$. C, Correlation between Sv (PGBM/glom) and glomerular filtration rate in 125 patients with type 1 diabetes. ◆, Normoalbuminuric patients; □, microalbuminuric patients; ▲, proteinuric patients. $r = 0.48$, $P < .001$.

is also to some extent, an independent predictor of renal dysfunction and hypertension in type 1 diabetes.

Across a wide range of albuminuria, foot process width correlates directly with AER and inversely with GFR, suggesting increasing podocyte injury as DKD progresses.[394] Podocyte number density per glomerular volume [Nv(Podo/glom)], but not number of podocytes per glomerulus [N(Podo/glom)] is inversely related to AER in normotensive proteinuric patients with type 1 diabetes.[414] These relationships were not seen in microalbuminuric patients. Moreover, podocyte structural parameters in normoalbuminuric patients with type 1 diabetes does not predict progression to proteinuria or ESKD during long-term follow-up.[415] These observations suggest that the contribution of podocyte injury to the progression of DKD in type 1 diabetes becomes more critical later in the disease process, a concept that is compatible with the notion that a glomerulus needs to lose a certain fraction of podocytes before undergoing sclerosis.[416]

## COMPARISONS OF DIABETIC KIDNEY DISEASE IN TYPE 1 VERSUS TYPE 2 DIABETES

Despite the fact that most DKD-associated ESKD cases are due to type 2 diabetes, the natural history and structural-functional relationships of DKD in type 2 diabetes is less well studied than in type 1 diabetes. There are substantial similarities between DKD lesions in type 1 and type 2 diabetes. GBM thickening, mesangial expansion, reduced glomerular filtration surface area and podocyte loss all occur in patients with type 2 diabetes as well and progress with diabetes duration.[417] However, pathologic findings are typically more heterogeneous in type 2 diabetes,[418] although this is not consistently observed in populations where type 2 diabetes occurs at earlier ages such as the Pima Indian cohort. Fioretto et al. identified three different patterns of lesions in kidney biopsies from microalbuminuric and proteinuric Northern Italian patients with type 2 diabetes: Category I with almost normal biopsies (35% of microalbuminuric and 10% of proteinuric patients) (Fig. 39.14); category II with classical lesions of DKD similar to type 1 diabetes (30% of microalbuminuric and 55% of proteinuric patients); and category III with disproportionately advanced tubulointerstitial fibrosis, arteriolar hyalinosis, arteriosclerosis or global glomerulosclerosis, despite minor diabetic glomerulopathy.[418] It is possible that this heterogeneity is due to other concomitant processes, such as aging, hypertension, obesity, and atherosclerosis, which are common in patients with type 2 diabetes, or pertain to a heterogeneous nature of mechanisms of renal injury in type 2 diabetes. Interestingly, these categories correlate with some clinical phenotypes. Category II patients with classical DKD lesions often have longer diabetes duration with poorer glycemic control, and faster GFR decline.[419,420] The great majority of

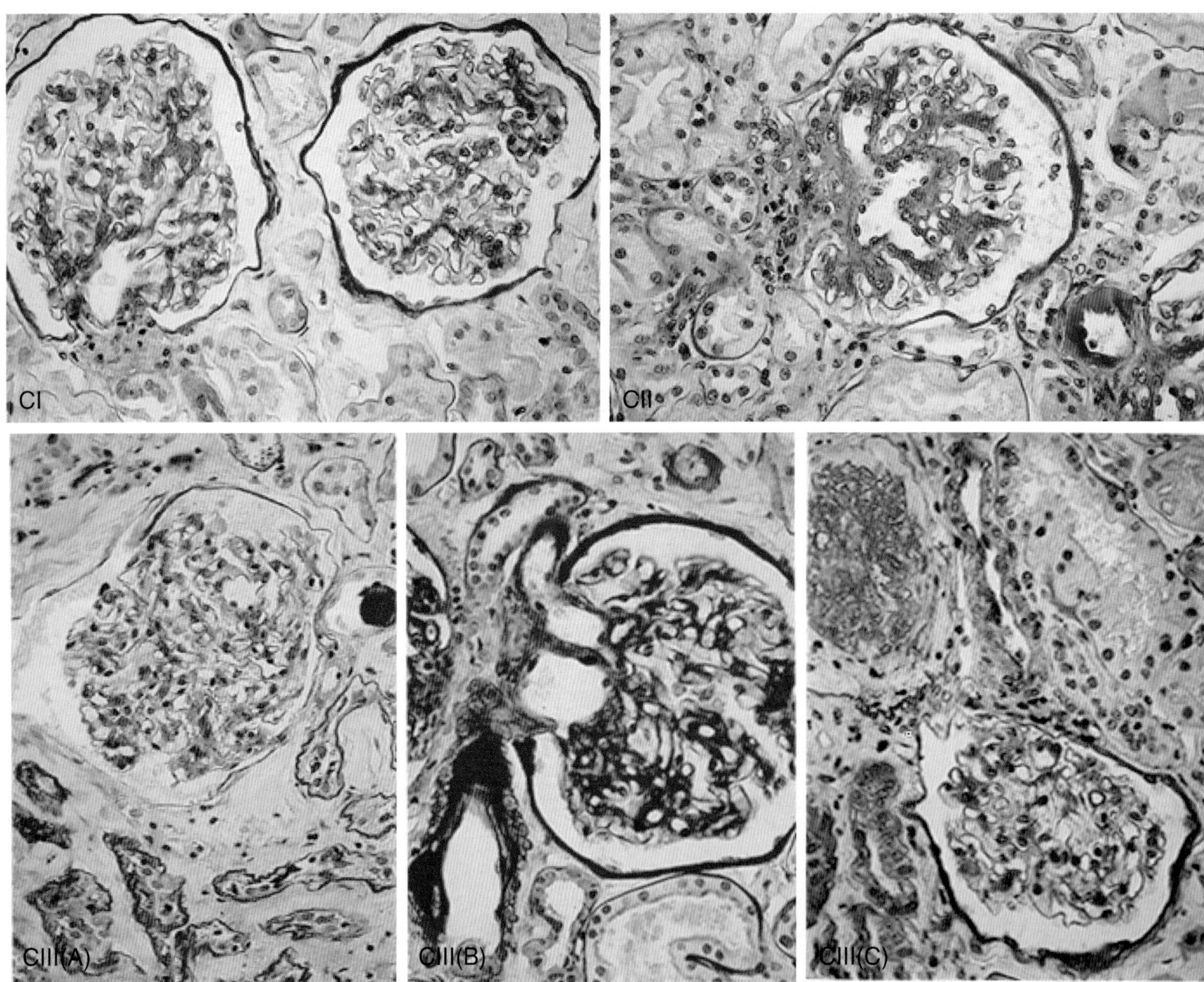


**Fig. 39.14** Glomeruli from a patient with diabetic kidney disease (DKD) in renal structural category I. Glomerular structure is near normal with minimal mesangial expansion (periodic acid–Schiff). Patterns of DKD lesions in patients with type 2 diabetes: CI, Category I with almost normal histology; CII, Category II with classical lesions of DKD; CIII, Category III includes atypical patterns with extraglomerular lesions disproportionately more severe than diabetic glomerulopathy. This category is subdivided into III(A) with advanced tubulointerstitial fibrosis, III(B) with prominent arteriolar hyalinosis, and III(C) with global glomerulosclerosis, but only minor diabetic glomerulopathy.

these patients have retinopathy, which is in contrast to category I or II patients in whom retinopathy is rare.[421] The heterogeneity of lesions in kidney biopsies from patients with type 2 diabetes and the presence of a subset of patients with micro- or macroalbuminuria, but no prominent diabetic glomerulopathy have also been confirmed by other studies.[422–424] It should be noted that this histological heterogeneity is present at an early stage of DKD in patients with type 2 diabetes, and AER is not a reliable biomarker to either distinguish among the categories of lesions or severity of DKD; therefore kidney biopsy is necessary to obtain such information. On the other hand, biopsy studies performed in Pima Indian patients with type 2 diabetes found that the relationship between albuminuria and structural changes was more similar to those seen in type 1 diabetes,[425] perhaps suggesting that DKD lesions are more homogeneous in Pima Indians with type 2 diabetes than in patients with type 2 diabetes from Europe or Japan. This observation may be related to an earlier onset of type 2 diabetes in the Pima Indians and fewer comorbidities as a consequence of their younger age.

## STRUCTURE-FUNCTION RELATIONSHIPS IN TYPE 2 DIABETES

Biopsy studies in Pima Indians have contributed substantially to our understanding of kidney structure-function relationships in type 2 diabetes. In a large cohort of Pima Indians who underwent a kidney biopsy at the end of a clinical trial testing the renoprotective effects of losartan in early DKD, greater Vv(Mes/glom), percentage of global glomerular sclerosis, nonpodocyte (mesangial and endothelial) cell number per glomerulus, GBM width, mean glomerular volume, and podocyte foot process width, lower Sv(PGBM/glom), and fewer endothelial fenestrations were each associated with GFR decline during a median follow-up of 6.6 years, after adjustment for clinical parameters, including baseline age, sex, duration of diabetes, hemoglobin A1c, measured GFR, and treatment assignment during the clinical trial.[426] The same study showed that a composite glomerulopathy index, reflecting the combined effects of the statistically significant morphometric variables, was strongly associated with renal functional loss. On the other hand, when GFR slope was modeled as a threshold, only Vv(Int/cortex) was associated with the slope. These studies underscore the significance of both glomerular and tubulointerstitial lesions in progression of DKD in type 2 diabetes. Importantly, these associations were present, even when the baseline GFR was normal or elevated. Thus the deteriorating impact of such lesions on kidney function starts at very early stages of DKD when the disease is clinically silent. A longitudinal biopsy study performed in Northern Italian patients with type 2 diabetes showed that albuminuria, GBM width and Vv(Mes/glom) predicted GFR decline over four years, even in patients who were normoalbuminuric at the baseline.[419] Likewise, in Japanese patients with type 2 diabetes, GBM width and Vv(Mes/glom) predicted progression of albuminuria after 6 years of follow-up.[427]

Podocyte injury plays an important role in progression of DKD in type 2 diabetes. Urine nephrin and/or podocin mRNA was more frequently found in urine from normoalbuminuric diabetic patients compared to nondiabetic controls, indicative that podocyte injury starts in the early stages of the disease.[428] Sustained injury leads to loss of these cells in the urine evidenced by increased podocyturia in microalbuminuric and proteinuric patients.[429] Because podocytes do not regenerate efficiently, podocyte loss leads to podocyte depletion in glomeruli, which can be assessed either in relative (i.e., podocyte number density per glomerular volume) or absolute (i.e., podocyte number per glomerulus) terms. It is likely that reduced podocyte number density starts at an early stage of DKD, leading to podocyte loss and reduced podocyte number per glomerulus, which sets the stage for glomerulosclerosis. Reduced number and number density of podocytes per glomerulus have been reported in proteinuric or microalbuminuric patients with type 2 diabetes.[425,430,431] Podocyte loss is progressive with diabetes duration and increasing albuminuria.[417] Podocyte number per glomerulus in microalbuminuric Pima Indians was the strongest predictor of increasing albuminuria and progression to overt nephropathy.[432] In a study of Caucasian patients with type 2 diabetes, podocyte number density was reduced in microalbuminuric compared with normoalbuminuric patients and was correlated with albuminuria.[430]

In summary, when compared with patients with type 1 diabetes and similar renal function, the biopsy findings in patients with type 2 diabetes are generally more heterogeneous and diabetic glomerulopathy is less severe. The heterogeneity may be less in those who develop type 2 diabetes at a younger age. Although data from kidney biopsies in young people with type 2 diabetes are not available, the finding that early onset type 2 diabetes is associated with more clinically aggressive kidney disease, as described above, suggests that the severity of diabetic glomerulopathy in young patients with type 2 diabetes may actually be greater than in patients with type 1 diabetes of similar duration, although this remains to be determined. Structure-function relationships between kidney function and glomerular structural variables are also generally similar to those in patients with type 1 diabetes, but may be less precise, perhaps at least partly related to the heterogeneity of lesions in older patients with type 2 diabetes. It is difficult to explain the phenotype of disproportionately greater albuminuria in the absence of established diabetic glomerulopathy in patients with type 2 diabetes.

## NONDIABETIC LESIONS IN DIABETIC PATIENTS

Clinically indicated kidney biopsies in diabetic patients are usually performed when the presentation raises suspicion for conditions other than DKD, such as a sudden onset of proteinuria, an onset of proteinuria less than five years from the onset of type 1 diabetes, proteinuria in the absence of retinopathy (especially in type 1 diabetes) or neuropathy, acute kidney injury, active urinary sediment, or hematuria.[433,434] Therefore it is not surprising to find a high incidence of nondiabetic kidney disease (NDKD) in clinical biopsies from diabetic patients.[357,433,435,436–438]

The reported prevalence of NDKD in the literature ranges from 10% to 85%.[439–442] However, the incidence of NDKD in research or protocol biopsies is much lower than in clinical biopsies.[443] The criteria and threshold used for indication biopsies, as well as ethnic and geographic factors, affect the likelihood of finding NDKD in biopsies from diabetic patients. Given the increasing prevalence of diabetes worldwide, it is anticipated that concomitant DKD and other renal pathologies will be seen even more frequently in the future. In a study performed at Columbia University, around 24% of all native kidney clinical biopsies were from diabetic patients, 37% of which had DKD alone, 36% had NDKD alone and 27% had DKD plus NDKD.[444] In the NDKD alone group, the most common diagnosis was FSGS (22%), followed by hypertensive nephrosclerosis, acute tubular injury, IgA nephropathy, membranous nephropathy, and pauci-immune glomerulonephritis. In the DKD plus NDKD group, however, acute tubular injury was the most common finding (43%), followed by hypertensive nephrosclerosis, FSGS, and IgA nephropathy. In multivariate analyses, longer duration of diabetes was associated with a greater likelihood of DKD and a lower likelihood of NDKD, with diabetes duration of 12 years or more being the best predictor of DKD alone. Differentiating between secondary lesions related to DKD or its common concomitants such as hypertension, and primary pathologies unrelated to DKD cannot always be readily made on examination of the kidney tissue. Focal and segmental glomerulosclerosis (FSGS), hypertensive nephrosclerosis, and acute tubular injury that are among the most commonly reported forms of NDKD in biopsies from diabetic patients are examples of such challenging conditions.[444] The challenge becomes even greater in type 2 diabetes where the biopsy may not show classical diabetic glomerulopathy. Another example would be presence of interstitial eosinophilic aggregates that are typically interpreted as evidence of a drug-induced hypersensitivity reaction. This finding, which is commonly (~40%) seen in clinical biopsies from diabetic patients, correlates with the severity of tubulointerstitial fibrosis, but does not correlate with a clinical history of drug allergy or the number of medicines used by patients, so it may not pertain to a hypersensitivity reaction.[445] Relying on clinical biopsy studies not only leads to overestimation of NDKD but may also lead to underestimation of DKD in diabetic patients. An autopsy study showed that about 20% of histologically proven DKD cases did not have DKD-associated clinical manifestations during their lifetime,[446] confirming prior results from research biopsy studies.

## CLASSIFICATION OF PATHOLOGIC LESIONS IN DIABETIC KIDNEY DISEASE

Classification of pathologic lesions facilitates uniform reporting of biopsy findings, which is of clinical importance. A proposed pathologic classification for DKD[447] (Table 39.4) includes four progressive classes based on the glomerular lesions, including glomerular basement membrane thickening (class I), mesangial expansion (class II. which divides into classes IIa if mild and IIb if severe), presence of Kimmelstiel-Wilson nodules (class III) and extensive global glomerulosclerosis (class IV). The classification also includes a separate scoring system for vascular and tubulointerstitial lesions (Table 39.5). A large-scale follow-up study of patients with type 2 diabetes showed that the severity of glomerular and interstitial lesions significantly impacts kidney prognosis and can be used as an independent risk factor for kidney outcomes.[448] Another study showed that after adjustment for clinical parameters, progression of glomerular, tubulointerstitial, and vascular lesions was associated with poor kidney outcomes.[405] However, prognostic significance of glomerular lesions according to this classification has also been challenged.[449,450] To study the net cumulative effect of various DKD lesions on renal prognosis, a D-score calculated by summing the scores of all components in the pathological classification was proposed, which led to improvement in prediction of renal outcome. Patients with a D-score or 14 or less had excellent outcomes.[451] This classification is a step towards developing a clinically useful pathology reporting system. However, all studies confirming a prognostic value for this classification basically demonstrate that more severe glomerular or tubulointerstitial lesions are associated with adverse outcomes, which is not a new finding. Whether this classification has any predictive value in early stages of DKD, when a biomarker is mostly needed to guide treatment options and outcomes, remains to be validated. Moreover, other important aspects of diabetic nephropathy, such as heterogeneity of patterns of kidney injury in type 2 diabetes,[439] and some other morphologic features with predictive value for kidney

**Table 39.4 Classification of Diabetic Kidney Disease Glomerular Lesions**

| Class | Description | Inclusion Criteria |
|---|---|---|
| I | Mild or nonspecific LM changes and EM-proven GBM thickening | Biopsy does not meet any of the criteria mentioned later for class II, III, or IV<br>GBM >395 nm in female and >430 nm in male individuals 9 years of age and older |
| IIa | Mild mesangial expansion | Biopsy does not meet criteria for class III or IV<br>Mild mesangial expansion in >25% of the observed mesangium |
| IIb | Severe mesangial expansion | Biopsy does not meet criteria for class III or IV<br>Severe mesangial expansion in >25% of the observed mesangium |
| III | Nodular sclerosis (Kimmelstiel–Wilson lesion) | Biopsy does not meet criteria for class IV<br>At least one convincing Kimmelstiel–Wilson lesion |
| IV | Advanced diabetic glomerulosclerosis | Global glomerular sclerosis in >50% of glomeruli<br>Lesions from classes I through III |

*LM*, Light microscopy. On the basis of direct measurement of GBM width by electron microscopy (EM), these individual cutoff levels may be considered indicative when other GBM measurements are used.

Adapted from Tervaert et al.[447]

**Table 39.5 Classification of DKD Interstitial and Vascular Lesions**

| Lesion | Criteria | Score |
|---|---|---|
| **Interstitial Lesions** | | |
| IFTA | No IFTA | 0 |
| | <25% | 1 |
| | 25% to 50% | 2 |
| | >50% | 3 |
| interstitial inflammation | Absent | 0 |
| | Infiltration only in relation to IFTA | 1 |
| | Infiltration in areas without IFTA | 2 |
| **Vascular Lesions** | | |
| arteriolar hyalinosis | Absent | 0 |
| | At least one area of arteriolar hyalinosis | 1 |
| | More than one area of arteriolar hyalinosis | 2 |
| presence of large vessels | – | Yes/no |
| arteriosclerosis (score worst artery) | No intimal thickening | 0 |
| | Intimal thickening less than thickness of media | 1 |
| | Intimal thickening greater than thickness of media | 2 |

Modified from Tervaert TW, Mooyaart AL, Amann K, Cohen AH, Cook HT, Drachenberg CB, et al. Pathologic classification of diabetic nephropathy. *JASN.* 2010;21(4): 556–563.

dysfunction, such as podocyte loss,[425] glomerulotubular junction abnormalities[398] or endothelial fenestration[426] are not included in this classification.

## REVERSABILITY OF DIABETIC KIDNEY DISEASE LESIONS

Normoglycemia following islet transplantation in streptozotocin (STZ)-induced diabetic rats leads to reversal of diabetic kidney lesions in two months,[452] and leptin replacement-associated normoglycemia in BTBR (black and tan, brachyuric) ob/ob diabetic mice reverses diabetic lesions in 6 weeks.[453] However, in contrast to murine models it takes a long time for human DKD lesions to fully establish. Likewise, reversibility of DKD lesions requires long-term normoglycemia. Seminal studies showed that type 1 diabetes patients with a diabetes duration of approximately 20 years showed a marked reversal of diabetic glomerulopathy lesions after 10 years, but not after 5 years[454] of normoglycemia following pancreas transplantation.[101] GBM and TBM width, Vv(Mes/glom) and Vv(MM/glom) were all reduced at 10 years compared with the baseline and 5-year values, with several patients having values at 10 years that had returned to the normal range (Fig. 39.15).[101] Perhaps most strikingly, Kimmelstiel-Wilson nodules had completely disappeared in the 10-year biopsies (Fig. 39.16). Reversal of DKD lesions in glomeruli was also associated with improvement of tubulointerstitial lesions and reduction in total cortical interstitial collagen.[455]

The effect of pharmaceutical intervention to reverse DKD or reduce its progression has also been explored. Blockade of the renin angiotensin aldosterone system (RAAS) has shown somewhat different effects in type 1 and type 2 diabetes. Thus 5 years of RAAS blockade by losartan or enalapril in normotensive normoalbuminuric patients with type 1 diabetes did not prevent progression of DKD lesions, whereas it did slow progression of retinopathy.[456] On the other hand, 6 years of treatment with losartan in microalbuminuric type 2 diabetic patients slowed progression of Vv(Mes/glom).[457]

An important question regarding reversal of DKD will be whether podocytes, which are notorious for their limited regeneration capacity, can repopulate glomeruli following reversal of lesions. Several studies have suggested the possibility that progenitor cells on Bowman's capsule could be a source for replacement of lost podocytes.[453,458–461] The study on BTBR ob/ob mice mentioned previously also showed that reversal of DKD lesions was associated with podocyte regeneration in the glomeruli[453]; however, such studies remain to be done in human DKD. Nevertheless, early DKD in clinical biopsies is associated with a remarkable increase in the number of parietal cells with a podocyte phenotype, raising the potential for podocyte replacement.[462]

## CLINICAL INDICATIONS FOR KIDNEY BIOPSY IN DIABETIC KIDNEY DISEASE

Kidney biopsy remains the gold standard for diagnosis,[463] treatment decisions, and outcome prediction in patients with kidney diseases. However, currently there are no standardized criteria or consensus about proper indications and clinical usefulness of biopsy in patients with DKD.[438] Therefore the decision to perform a kidney biopsy is usually based on personal opinion and/or single-center policies.[463] Given the prevalence of the disease, up to 25% of all clinical renal biopsies are done in patients with diabetes.[444] It may be argued that diabetic patients with macroalbuminuria and retinopathy are likely to have DKD, in which case kidney biopsy generally does not provide additional information that affects clinical management.[438] However, as discussed earlier, a significant percentage of diabetic patients may have NDKD, which may require therapeutic approaches different from DKD.[464] Moreover, biopsy remains the gold standard for the assessment of kidney damage in DKD, identifying atypical patterns of DKD in patients with type 2 diabetes, and obtaining valuable prognostic or even predictive information that can affect clinical management. It is noteworthy that the risk of complications associated with percutaneous native kidney biopsy in patients with DKD is similar to and certainly no greater than the risk in patients with most other causes of CKD.[465,466] A collective opinion of published literature on indications for kidney biopsy in diabetic patients provides the following criteria (Box 39.1):[464] (1) nephrotic range proteinuria or kidney failure in the absence of diabetic retinopathy; (2) nephrotic range proteinuria or kidney failure with diabetes duration less than 5 years; (3) nephrotic range proteinuria with normal kidney function; (4) unexplained microscopic hematuria or acute kidney injury; or (5) rapidly worsening kidney function in patients with previously stable kidney

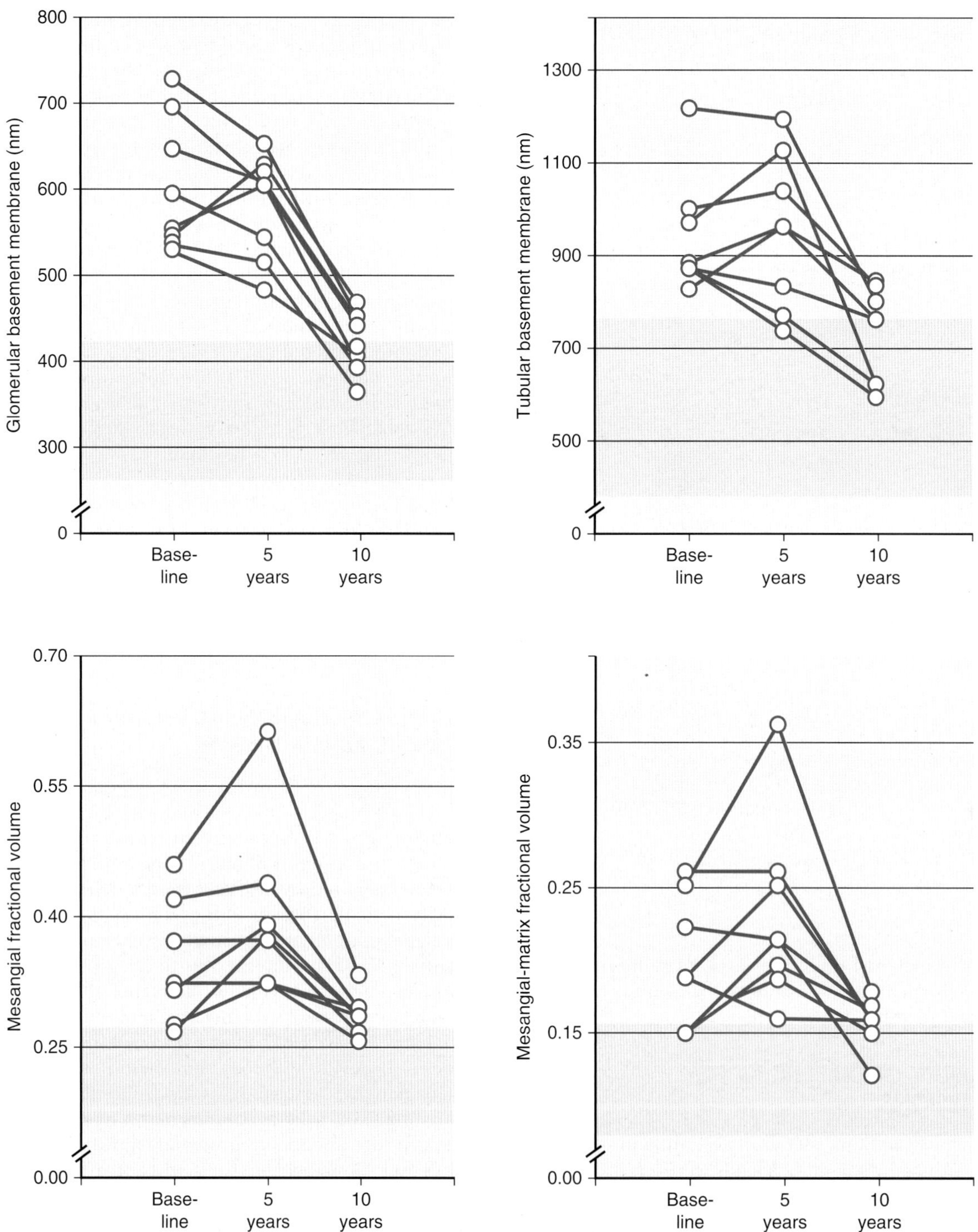


**Fig. 39.15 Thickness of the glomerular basement membrane, thickness of the tubular basement membrane, mesangial fractional volume, and mesangial-matrix fractional volume at baseline and 5 and 10 years after pancreas transplantation.** The shaded areas represent the normal ranges obtained in the 66 age- and sex-matched normal controls (means ± 2 standard deviation). Data for individual patients are connected by lines.

function. Retinopathy, which generally correlates well with the presence of DKD in type 1 diabetes, is considered a poor predictor of DKD in type 2 diabetes.[11,467]

## SYSTEMS BIOLOGY IN DIABETIC KIDNEY DISEASE

To obtain a more comprehensive understanding of the pathophysiology of DKD and to identify novel diagnostic or prognostic biomarkers and new treatment targets, one would need an understanding of molecular events involved in initiation or progression of DKD. Systems biology provides an interdisciplinary and holistic approach to deciphering the complexity of biological systems and explaining how these interactions influence systems' functions and behaviors. Correlating data obtained from systems biology with detailed morphologic information can create unique opportunities to

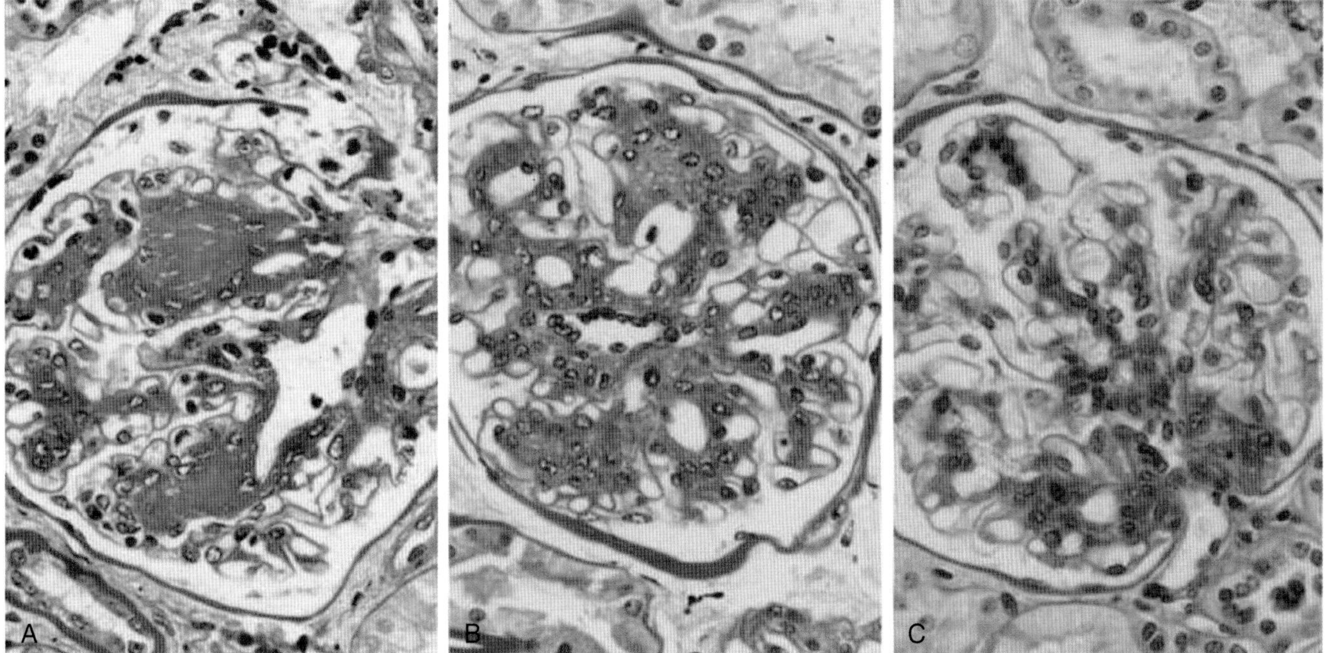

**Fig. 39.16 Photomicrographs of renal-biopsy specimens obtained before and after pancreas transplantation from a 33-year-old woman with type 1 diabetes of 17 years' duration at the time of transplantation (periodic acid–Schiff, 120).** A, A typical glomerulus from the base-line biopsy specimen, which is characterized by diffuse and nodular (Kimmelstiel–Wilson) diabetic glomerulopathy. Mesangial-matrix expansion and the palisading of mesangial nuclei around the nodular lesions are evident. B, A typical glomerulus 5 years after transplantation shows the persistence of the diffuse and nodular lesions. C, A typical glomerulus 10 years after transplantation, with marked resolution of diffuse and nodular mesangial lesions and more open glomerular capillary lumina.

**Box 39.1 List of Criteria for Kidney Biopsy in Patients With Diabetes**

1. Nephrotic range proteinuria or kidney failure in the absence of diabetic retinopathy
2. Nephrotic range proteinuria or kidney failure with diabetes duration less than 5 years
3. Nephrotic range proteinuria with normal kidney function
4. Unexplained microscopic hematuria or acute kidney injury
5. Rapidly worsening kidney function in patients with previously stable kidney function

identify pathways linked to development of specific lesions and renal dysfunction. A urine metabolomics study showed that MDM2, an E3 ubiquitin protein ligase that mediates ubiquitination of p53/TP53 had the highest significant number of protein–protein interaction connections.[468] The same study showed significant downregulation of *MDM2* gene expression in both the glomerular and tubulointerstitial compartments of kidney biopsy tissue from two independent cohorts of patients with DKD. Inhibition of this gene in mice resulted in podocyte loss and increased mortality, supporting a functional role for MDM2 in DKD. A comprehensive gene expression profiling of kidney tissue from T2D patients with early and late DKD showed a highly regulated Janus kinase-signal transducer and activator transcription (JAK-STAT) pathway in individuals with DKD compared with controls.[469] These examples demonstrate the importance of "omics" approaches in identifying key genes and pathways involved in DKD. Performing such studies requires adequate sampling and preservation of kidney tissue and biofluids. While these approaches are currently being used in research studies, it is foreseeable that they may soon become available clinically and pave the way for precision medicine in DKD.

## PATHOPHYSIOLOGY

The pathogenesis of DKD remains largely unknown and is likely to be multifactorial in origin, involving a variety of metabolic and hemodynamic factors that, combined with certain susceptibility genes, can affect different target cells in the kidney (Fig. 39.17). Nevertheless, metabolic changes that occur with the onset of diabetes substantially alter kidney physiology in ways that promote inflammation and fibrosis and may ultimately lead to kidney failure. Early perturbations in response to hyperglycemia include changes in hemodynamic function and the selective behavior of the glomerular capillary wall to macromolecules. In addition, recent experimental work is beginning to offer glimpses of the pathophysiologic mechanisms that underlie the loss of kidney function and the development of progressive fibrosis in DKD.

Glomerular endothelial cells, epithelial cells, mesangial cells and tubular cells can all be differentially affected by key elements of the diabetic milieu, and cross talk among different cell types as well as among different organs affected by diabetes is suggested by a large variety of experimental

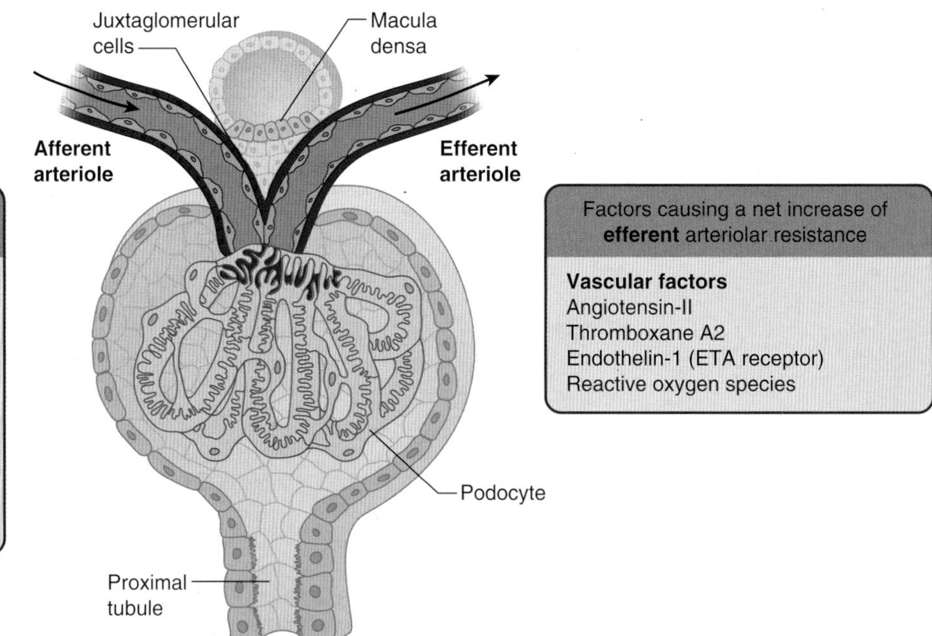


Factors causing a net reduction of **afferent** arteriolar resistance

**Vascular factors**
Nitric oxide bioavailability
COX-2 prostanoids
Kalikrein-kinins
Atrial natiuretic peptide
Angiotensin(1-7)
Hyperinsulinemia *per se*

**Tubular signals**
Inhibition of tubuloglomerular feedback (macula densa signals)

Factors causing a net increase of **efferent** arteriolar resistance

**Vascular factors**
Angiotensin-II
Thromboxane A2
Endothelin-1 (ETA receptor)
Reactive oxygen species

**Fig. 39.17 Schematic (net) effect of factors implicated in the pathogenesis of glomerular hyperfiltration in diabetes. Several vascular and tubular factors[32,48,123–126] are suggested to result in a net reduction in afferent arteriolar resistance, thereby increasing (single-nephron) glomerular filtration rate (GFR). Effects of insulin per se seem to depend on insulin sensitivity.[96,97] A net increase in efferent arteriolar resistance—leading to increased GFR—is proposed for other vascular factors.[32,42,71,124,127] Growth hormone[128] and insulin-like growth factor-1[129] likely increase filtration by augmenting total renal blood flow, without specific arteriolar preference. Glucagon and vasopressin seem to (principally) act through transforming growth factor (TGF).[48] Intrinsic defects of electromechanical coupling or alterations in signal transduction in afferent arterioles may impair vasoactive responses to renal hemodynamic (auto) regulation.[32]** Augmented filtration by increases in the ultrafiltration coefficient and net filtration pressure via reduction in intratubular volume and subsequent hydraulic pressure in Bowman's space are not depicted. Several vascular factors may be released or activated after a (high-protein) meal (e.g., nitric oxide, cyclooxygenase-2 prostanoids, angiotensin II),[48,50,130] whereas TGF becomes (further) inhibited, through increased amino acid- (and glucose) coupled sodium reabsorption in the proximal tubule[49,50] and/or increased glucagon/vasopressin-dependent sodium reabsorption in the thick ascending limb.[48] These changes may collectively play a part in postprandial hyperfiltration. *COX-2*, cyclooxygenase-2; *ETA*, endothelin A receptor.

and clinical data. Irrespective of the initiating factor and of the target cells, several key pathways modulated in DKD have been identified with systems biology approaches (Fig. 39.18). A summary of key clinical and experimental findings related to the pathophysiology of DKD are described later.

***Clinical Relevance***

**Pathogenesis**

A large body of discovery research is now available to support the need to develop new treatment strategies that go above and beyond targeting glycemia for the treatment and prevention of DKD. The ability to develop strong system biology approaches to understand the pathogenesis of clinical DKD has also helped guide discovery research towards clinically relevant targets. Elegant experiments have helped dissect autocrine, paracrine and endocrine contributors to DKD and have provided evidence of a very complex crosstalk between organs affected by diabetes and between specialized kidney cells. Finally, the biology of small noncoding RNAs and of epigenetic contributors have not only shed light on the mechanism of "glucose memory" but is now offering additional therapeutic targets.

## SELECTIVE GLOMERULAR PERMEABILITY

The excretion of albumin in the urine is determined by the amount of albumin filtered across the glomerular capillary barrier and the amount reabsorbed by the tubular cells. The glomerular capillary wall serves as a filter that discriminates among molecules based on size, electrical charge, and configuration. Studies of glomerular filtrate collected by micropuncture or narrow size fractioning of exogenous polymers, such as dextran, indicate that albuminuria is primarily the result of impairment of the electrostatic barrier within the glomerulus, consequent to a decrease in endothelial cell glycocalyx[476–478] and heparan sulfate content of the glomerular basement membrane,[479] and by changes in the size selective properties of the glomerular capillary barrier.[480–486] The size-selective defect in the glomerular capillary appears to become more prominent with higher levels of albumin excretion among patients with either type 1 or type 2 diabetes.[485,487,488] Morphometric data in kidney tissue from Pima Indians with macroalbuminuria demonstrate a significant correlation between the magnitude of this permselective defect and podocyte foot process width, which is not observed in those with microalbuminuria.[488] These findings are consistent with the view that permselective defects responsible for increased albumin excretion may be focal and are likely due to podocyte foot process effacement and simplification and to defective intercellular junctions.[489]

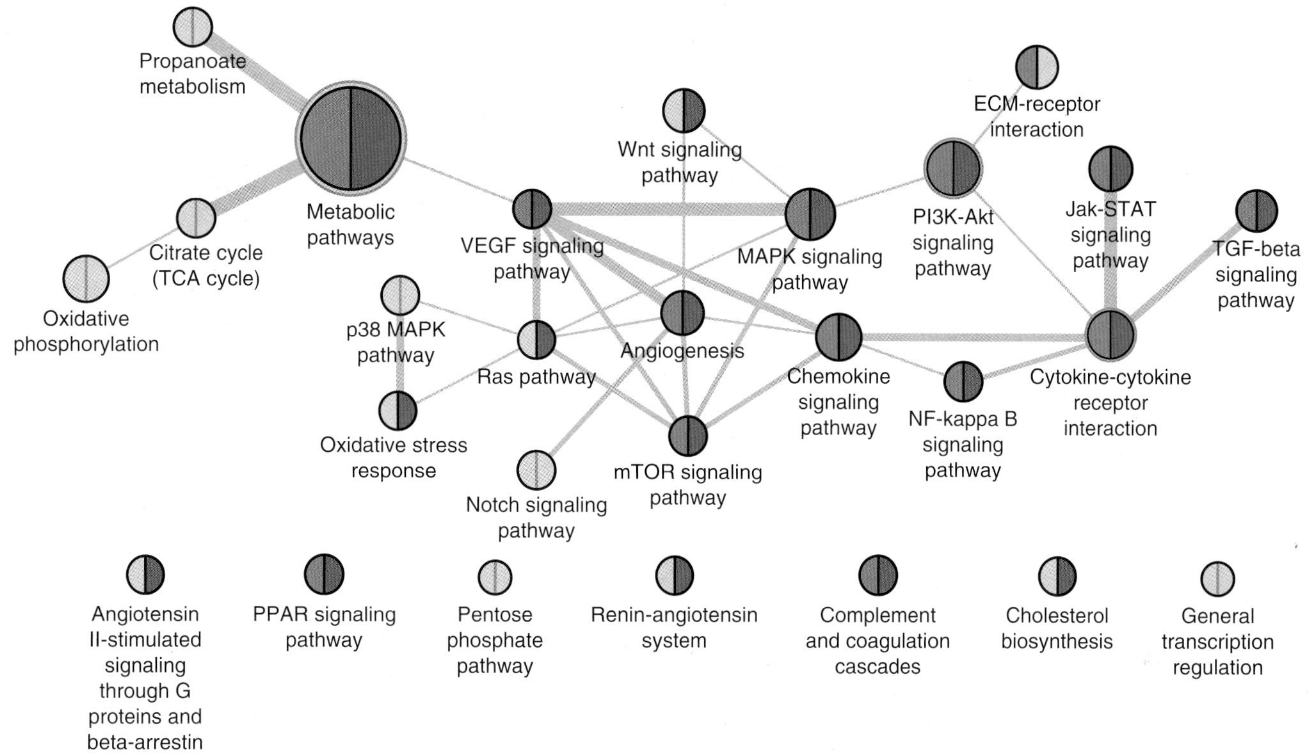


**Fig. 39.18 Pathway landscape of diabetic nephropathy. Nodes of the graph represent KEGG and Panther pathways (node diameter scales with number of protein coding genes assigned), edges between nodes scale with the number of genes overlapping, as well as interactions of genes across pathways according to the protein interaction network. Pathways are marked for holding biomarker candidates *(green)* and drug target candidates *(red)*.** (From Heinzel A, Perco P, Mayer G, Oberbauer R, Lukas A, Mayer B. From molecular signatures to predictive biomarkers: modeling disease pathophysiology and drug mechanism of action. *Front Cell Dev Biol.* 2014;2:37.)

Multiphoton fluorescence techniques permit direct imaging of the structure and function of living kidney tissue.[490] In some studies, this technique revealed what appeared to be a much higher albumin glomerular sieving coefficient than was calculated or measured by micropuncture, prompting some investigators to propose alternative explanations for the facilitated urine clearance of albumin in DKD,[490,491] including the idea that albuminuria is the result of proximal tubular cell dysfunction in retrieving and degrading albumin, and does not reflect an alteration in glomerular permselectivity.[492,493] Other studies using improved imaging techniques do not support this concept and confirm that glomerular filtration barrier permeability to macromolecules is largely restricted to areas of podocyte damage.[494–496]

## GLOMERULAR HEMODYNAMIC FUNCTION

In healthy adults, the GFR ranges from 90 to 120 ml/min/1.73 $m^2$, is stable through mid-adult life, and declines by approximately 1 ml/min per year after 50 years of age.[497–499] The onset of diabetes is associated with hemodynamic changes in the glomerular circulation that lead to increased renal plasma flow, glomerular capillary hyperperfusion, and an increased glomerular transcapillary hydraulic pressure gradient, which together contribute to an increase in GFR.[131,500–505] The prevalence of hyperfiltration, frequently defined as a GFR of at least two standard deviations above the mean GFR in persons with normal glucose tolerance, varies from 10% to 67% in persons with type 1 diabetes and from 6% to 73% in those with type 2 diabetes.[139] The large variations in these estimates are attributed to differences in age, race/ethnicity, glycemic control, duration of diabetes, absence of diet standardization, the definition of hyperfiltration, and methodologies used to measure and report GFR among different populations. Glomerular capillary hypertension and the ensuing increase in filtration pressure are partly responsible for the elevation of GFR, but various other glomerular and tubular factors also influence the magnitude of the hyperfiltration (see Fig. 39.17).[506–508]

After the initial elevation at the onset of diabetes, GFR decreases in response to metabolic control in both type 1 and type 2 diabetes[509–511] but usually not to levels found in nondiabetic persons.[503,512] In some patients, this reversal could reflect the initiation of progressive kidney disease, as suggested by the appearance of global glomerular sclerosis and the fall in the single-nephron filtration coefficient.[417] In others, it could represent a purely functional change in kidney vasomotion associated with improvement in diabetes control or simply the intrinsic variability of GFR in the absence of significant histopathologic changes.[513] Distinguishing between these two potential causes of GFR decline requires either observation of GFR over an extended period of time to determine whether it plateaus, reverses direction, or continues to decline to pathologic levels, or attention to other biomarkers, including albuminuria.[514] Nevertheless, differentiating between these possibilities is crucial, since recent studies, principally from the Joslin Clinic, suggest that progressive renal function decline indicative of underlying kidney pathology precedes the onset of albuminuria in both type 1 and type 2 diabetes.[317,515–518]

This progressive decline is predominantly linear, but the rate of decline varies widely among individuals. Importantly, half of those in the type 1 diabetes cohort at the Joslin Clinic who developed renal functional decline progressed from a normal eGFR to ESKD within 2 to 10 years.

## PRIMARY CELL TARGETS

*Glomerular Endothelial Cells.* The role of glomerular endothelial cells (GECs) and the thickness of the glycocalyx as one of the early targets in DKD has generated a lot of attention. Both a reduction in the thickness of the glycocalyx and a reduction in the fenestration of the endothelium have been described as early features of clinical DKD. GECs injury can occur via hemodynamic stimuli that cause reduced nitric oxide (NO) bioavailability via suppression of endothelial nitrix oxide synthase (eNOS), or it can result from growth factor driven altered metabolism. Triglyceride-rich lipoproteins, advanced glycation end-products and inflammatory mediators can all negatively influence the thickness of the glycocalyx.[524] Several interventions are effective in restoring the glycocalyx barrier and protecting GECs, including atrasentan,[525] C3a and C5a receptor antagonism,[526] and Vascular Endothelial Growth Factor (VEGF)A165b administration via VEGFR2 phosphorylation.[527] Among drug targets, glomerular endothelin-1 receptor type A (EdnRA) is activated in DKD and is linked to mitochondrial dysfunction.[528] The glomerular endothelium can also be the target of a "gut to kidney" connection, as the glucagon-like peptide 1 (GLP1) receptor agonist exendin-4 ameliorates lipotoxicity-induced GECs injury by improving ATP-binding cassette transporter A1 (ABCA1) dependent cholesterol efflux.[529] High glucose is sufficient to cause local upregulation of the renin angiotensin system in GECs in association with increased fenestration and decreased glycosaminoglycans content, a phenotype that can be prevented via Ang II type 1R blockade.[530]

The role of angiopoietins is potentially very important. Under physiological conditions, they regulate the integrity of the glomerular filtration barrier, but when dysregulated in diabetes they may be sufficient to drive the pathobiology of DKD.[531] These findings may lead to the development of targeted glomerular angiopoietin-1 therapies.[531,532] As GECs are also the first cells encountered by any circulating stimulus relevant to diabetes, they can be a direct target of the diabetes milieu but they can also serve as cells sending paracrine signals to adjacent mesangial cells and podocytes. Many studies suggest the presence of cross-talk between GEC and mesangial cells (primarily Platelet-derived Growth Factor (PDGF)B/PDGFRβ mediated) or GEC and podocytes (primarily mediated by angiopoietins, VEGF and Endothelin-1).[533] The possibility of an endothelial to mesenchymal transformation has also been suggested.[534]

*Podocytes.* An early and key event in the development of DKD is the loss of podocytes from the kidney glomerulus.[394,396,414,432,535] Podocytopenia correlates with disease progression,[425,432] is inversely related to the control of hypertension and diabetes,[535] but can also occur independently of blood pressure.[536] Several signaling pathways are implicated in podocyte injury in diabetes. These include loss and/or redistribution of slit diaphragm proteins such as nephrin, altered insulin receptor signaling, altered nutrient sensing via the mechanistic target of rapamycin (mTOR) pathway, and reactivation of key developmental pathways such as the Notch pathway and the Wnt/ß-Catenin pathways. Hyperglycemia is the foundation for podocyte injury in DKD through multiple pathways, including the polyol pathway, the formation of advanced glycation end-products, the modulation of protein kinase C (PKC) and the hexosamine pathway.[537] However, it is becoming more and more evident that podocyte injury in diabetes results from a multiplicity of endocrine and paracrine factors. Indeed, podocyte function is heavily modulated by a variety of circulating factors produced by other organs, suggesting a complex crosstalk between the kidney and other organs affected by diabetes. Podocytes can be the direct target of all the traditional components of the renin angiotensin system (RAS), including angiotensin II,[538–540] aldosterone[541,542] and prorenin.[543,544] The importance of the local RAS in the development of proteinuria comes from a mouse model overexpressing Ang II type 1 receptor (AT1R) in podocytes.[539] RAS blockade may also affect podocyte function through the systemic modulation of adipokines and insulin sensitivity.[545] Although the role of locally produced ACE requires further investigation, clinical and experimental evidence suggests renoprotection of selective aldosterone blockers.[546,547–549] Although both systemic and local effects may be involved, mineralocorticoid receptor (MR) activation in podocytes alters the filtration barrier and results in proteinuria.[541] Aldosterone independent MR ligands that are relevant to podocyte function, such as the small GTPase Rac1, have been identified, underlying the complexity of podocyte signaling in DKD.[542] Furthermore, insulin,[550,551] insulin-like growth factors (IGFs),[552] adiponectin,[553] sex hormones,[554] growth hormone,[555–557] adrenocorticotropic hormone (ACTH),[558] growth hormone releasing hormone (GHRH),[559] thyroid hormone[560] and vitamin D[561] are involved in the direct modulation of podocyte function. The subsequent paragraphs will describe briefly the different contribution of these factors to podocyte injury in DKD.

Podocyte-specific deletion of the insulin receptor in mice is sufficient to cause a phenotype similar to DKD in the absence of hyperglycemia, strongly supporting the importance of insulin signaling in the preservation of podocyte function.[562,563] This is supported by clinical studies, as IR correlates with the development of albuminuria in patients with either type 1 or type 2 diabetes,[519,521,523,564] their siblings[520,522] and nondiabetic individuals.[565] Furthermore, insulin sensitizing agents of the class of thiazolidinediones (TZD) offer a degree of renoprotection that is superior to other agents in patients with diabetes and DKD[566] as well as in insulinopenic experimental animal models of diabetes and DKD.[567] Experimental data support this clinical observation, as IR occurs in vitro[551] and in vivo[568] at early stages of DKD, and may occur through PKC-β-induced insulin receptor substrate-1 dysfunction. Genetic manipulation of several elements of the insulin signaling cascade other than the insulin receptor alters the course of DKD in mice and affects relevant nutrient sensing and prosurvival pathways.[569] Both glucose transporter 1(GLUT1) and glucose transporter 4 (GLUT4) expression can contribute to the pathogenesis of DKD.[570–572] In addition, several mediators of GLUT4 trafficking in podocytes are linked to podocyte function in DKD. These include septin 7,[573] CD2-associated protein (CD2AP),[574,575] nucleobindin-2,[576] Synip,[577] insulin receptor substrate 2

(IRS2), and phosphatase and tensin homolog (PTEN).[578] However, none of them has yet to translate into clinical development opportunities. Interestingly, epigenetic changes in the promoter of Src homology region 2 domain-containing phosphatase-1 (SHP-1) may also have an important role in the persistence of IR observed in podocytes in the setting of diabetes.[579]

More recently, podocyte IR has been linked to mitochondrial function, ER stress, and activation of the unfolded protein response (UPR).[580] Similar to UPR, autophagy is essential to maintain podocyte homeostasis, as haploinsufficiency of mTORC1 activates autophagy and protects from DKD while mTORC1 activation leads to acceleration of DKD.[581,582] While it was thought for many years that an increase in reactive oxygen species drives the vascular complications of diabetes, recent data suggest that increased mitochondrial superoxide production may indicate healthy mitochondria, thus opening the new theory of mitochondrial hormesis.[583] In response to excess glucose exposure or nutrient stress, the consequent reduction in mitochondrial oxidative phosphorylation may lead to the release of nonmitochondrial oxidants and to a proinflammatory and profibrotic response. Restoration of superoxide production with activation of AMPK may promote organ healing.[584]

Besides traditional hormones, additional important modulators of podocytes function include free fatty acids (FFA),[585] lipoproteins,[586,587] and angiopoietins; more studies are needed to support the specific function of these modulators in DKD before translation into new therapeutic strategies. Podocytes are also the main source of VEGFA production, with both excess and defective production of VEGFA contributing to the worsening of DKD[588] through its role as a key element in the paracrine crosstalk between podocytes and endothelial cells,[589–591] and more recently through tubulovascular crosstalk in the peritubular microvasculature of the kidney.[591] Besides the paracrine functions of VEGF-A, an autocrine function in podocytes has also been described.[592] VEGF-A is a key modulator of slit diaphragm protein interactions[593] and the actin cytoskeleton.[594,595] Nodular glomerulosclerosis resembling DKD has been described when either VEGF-A[596] or Vegf164[597] are overexpressed in podocytes in eNOS null mice or in models of type 1 diabetes. Therapeutic strategies targeting this system have failed so far, although development of soluble fms-related tyrosine kinase 1 (sFLT1) decoy peptides may stabilize podocytes through its binding to a podocyte specific GM3 ganglioside, thus increasing cell adhesion and actin remodeling.[598]

The possibility of crosstalk between the adipose tissue and the kidney is also intriguing. Podocytes express both adiponectin receptor 1 and 2 (AR1 and AR2),[553] and adiponectin null mice develop proteinuria and podocyte injury that can be reversed by the administration of recombinant adiponectin, which modulates podocyte oxidative stress through an AMPK-dependent modulation of Nox 4 in podocytes. This hallmark study establishes a cause–effect relationship between adiponectin and albuminuria.[553] Whether a similar mechanism may be at play in patients with DKD remains to be seen. The fact that several single nucleotide polymorphisms (SNPs) in the AdipoQ gene, including the promoter, are associated with increased risk of the development of type 2 diabetes and DKD strongly suggests that this is a clinically relevant pathway.[599]

Epidemiological data also suggests that estrogens may provide a protective effect against the development and progression of DKD that is lost after menopause,[600–602] and treatment with 17-β estradiol protects from experimental DKD.[603,604] Circulating 17-β estradiol affects the podocytes expression of estrogen receptor β,[554] which is involved in the modulation of extracellular matrix production via matrix metalloproteinases.[554]

Circulating vitamin D is associated with progression of CKD and mortality,[605] and vitamin D treatment reduces not only cardiovascular mortality[606–608] but also clinical proteinuria.[606–608] Vitamin D reduces podocyte loss[609] in experimental DKD and acts synergistically with AT1 receptor blockers in reducing proteinuria.[610,611,612] Among other mediators of bone and mineral metabolism, kidney expression as well as circulating concentrations of the antiaging hormone Klotho are reduced in DKD,[613–615] and Klotho replacement may ameliorate proteinuria by targeting transient receptor potential cation channel, subfamily C, member 6 (TRPC6) channels in podocytes,[616] and rescue diabetic mice from glomerular injury.[617]

Altered growth hormone (GH)/insulin-like growth factor (IGF)-1 axis has been described in diabetes and DKD.[618] Several studies suggest a direct relationship between the activity of the GH/IGF-1 axis and certain features of DKD, such as hyperfiltration and microalbuminuria,[619] and somatostatin analogues may be renoprotective in diabetes.[620] In experimental models, overexpression of GH results in severe glomerulosclerosis,[621] and inhibition of GH action through different mechanisms may improve DKD.[556,557,622] Interestingly, podocytes express GH receptor (GHR), and signaling through GHR in podocytes affects oxidative stress and actin remodeling, two important features of podocyte biology.[555] Taken together, these experimental data suggest that medicines targeting the GHR or the GH signaling cascade may represent a novel approach to prevent and/or treat DKD. High expression of GH-releasing hormone (GHRH) has been detected in the kidney,[559] but a specific function of GHRH in the kidney remains to be established.

Podocytes are also the direct target of profibrotic molecules such as transforming growth factor-ß (TGF-ß), which binds to TGF-ß receptors on podocytes and activates a SMAD7-mediated signaling pathway, leading to aberrant extracellular matrix production.[623] However, antifibrotic agents have consistently failed to protect from DKD, strongly suggesting that fibrosis is an outcome to prevent and not a disease to treat.[624] Because TGF-ß may also trigger many epigenetic changes leading to fibrosis, additional studies are required to investigate targeting the fibrotic pathways via this mechanism.

More recently, tumor necrosis factor (TNF) and nuclear factor of activated T cell (NFAT)-mediated impairment of ABCA1 dependent cholesterol efflux from podocytes was found to contribute to proteinuria and glomerulosclerosis and may open new avenues for therapeutic interventions.[625] The ability of podocytes to take up oxidized LDL[586,587] warrants further investigation, as LDL removal by apheresis in patients with proteinuric DKD improves not only the lipid profile but also decreases proteinuria and reduces the loss of podocytes in the urine.[626] The role of free fatty acid in the development of albuminuria in DKD also remains to be established, as FFA utilization by podocytes has been described[627,628] and may contribute to the development of podocyte specific IR.[585] FFA may also be responsible for the metabolic memory of diabetes via alterations in renal histones, offering a link between metabolic and epigenetic changes in DKD.[629]

*Mesangial cells.* Mesangial expansion strongly predicts the clinical manifestations of DKD.[163] The aberrant production of extracellular matrix in DKD has been reported and extensively studied, and the contribution of mesangial cells to glomerulosclerosis is well established.[630] However, discovery research specific to mesangial cells is limited by the lack of targets unique to these cells. Genetic or pharmacological blockade of the bradykinin 2 receptor, which is heavily expressed in mesangial cells in clinical DKD, results in profound mesangial sclerosis resembling human diabetic glomerulosclerosis without significantly affecting GECs or podocytes.[631] The first demonstration of a functional role of miRNA in kidney disease of any type was described in DKD, when miRNA192 was found to be a key mediator of mesangial cell function in DKD.[632] Enhanced JAK-$^{STAT}$ pathway activation in mesangial cells has been described in both clinical and experimental DKD and has led to clinical trials of JAK2 inhibitors.[633]

*Tubulointerstitial cells.* Clinicopathological correlates strongly suggest that the degree of tubule-interstitial fibrosis correlates with a decline in GFR in DKD. Several urinary biomarker-based studies on how urinary NAG, KIM-1, L-FABP and NGAL correlate with albuminuria in diabetes suggest that tubular damage starts in the early stages of DKD. In vitro and in vivo studies suggest an important role of fatty acid uptake and oxidation in the pathogenesis of CKD progression,[634] and the proximal tubule seems to be the major contributor to epithelial to mesenchymal transformation.[635] Considering the strong kidney protection observed with the use of sodium-glucose cotransporter-2 (SGLT2) inhibitors in the EMPA-REG and CANVAS trials,[636,637] it will become imperative to understand if there is a direct metabolic effect on tubular cells expressing SGLT2 that contributes to the observed effect on DKD progression. The biology of chemokines and chemokine receptors as key modulators of tubulo-interstitial damage also requires further exploration, as C-C chemokine receptor type 2 (CCR2) antagonism confers significant renoprotection in phase 2 trials and CCR2 is primarily expressed by tubular cells.[638]

*Additional common mechanisms: Epigenetic.* Irrespective of the target cell, the past few years have seen numerous reports describing the role of epigenetic changes in the pathogenesis of DKD. Epigenetic modifications include cytosine methylation of DNA (DNA methylation, DNAme), histone post-translational modifications (PTMs), and noncoding RNAs.[639–641] A critical metabolic/epigenetic switch linking the metabolic state to chromatin remodeling is miR-93, a finding that offers opportunities for therapeutic developments in this area.[642] Epigenetic modifications are reversible and are regulated in response to the changing environment. However, certain epigenetic changes can exhibit a memory of prior exposure to environmental cues and disease conditions, with consequent long-lasting effects even after the initial trigger has been removed. This is a finding validated by the clinical observation that the benefits of intensive insulin treatment in the EDIC study persisted long after treatment discontinuation, suggesting the existence of metabolic memory.[272] Both hemodynamic and metabolic factors may contribute to metabolic memory as summarized in Fig. 39.19. Epigenetic changes can occur in the intrauterine environment and be transmitted to the offspring.[643] Interestingly, different kidney cells have distinct epigenomes. While this outlines the complexity of epigenetic changes, it does offer better opportunities for cell specific therapeutic developments in this area.

*Additional common mechanisms: innate immunity.* The contribution of innate immunity by either activated local cells or infiltrating cells has also been the focus of many experimental studies during the last 10 years.[644] Pathogen-associated molecular patterns (PAMPs) and danger-associated molecular patterns (DAMPs) have been described as major activators of pattern recognition receptors (PRRs) such as membrane-bound toll-like receptors and nucleotide-binding oligomerization domain (NOD)-like receptors (NLRs), which in turn cause a local inflammatory response that may be self-perpetuating irrespective of the presence or absence of the initiating stimulus. The recent failure of bardoxolone, a drug targeting the Nrf2 antioxidant inflammatory response, in DKD,[645] challenges the possibility that intracellular inflammatory and oxidative pathways are always deleterious rather than an appropriate defense mechanism to injury. Among novel key inducers of inflammation in glomerular cells, the role of serum amyloid A (SAA) has gained a lot of attention. SAA can stimulate NF-kB as well as JAK2 and PKC leading to an autocrine amplification loop of increased endogenous production of SAA.[646] The fact that elevated baseline serum SAA can predict a composite primary outcome of death and ESKD in a cohort of patients with type 2 diabetes and a mean baseline eGFR of 56 ml/min/1.73 m$^2$ and median urine albumin:creatinine ratio of 1861 mg/g strongly suggests a potential role of causality between SSA and DKD.[647] Furthermore, in a well characterized cohort of 74 patients with type 2 diabetes and research kidney biopsies, SAA levels correlated with AER and were higher in patients with increased GBM width, although fibrinogen and IL-6 had a better correlation with GBM thickening.[648] A recent finding in a cohort of patients with type 2 diabetes and very early or no DKD (mean eGFR 128 ml/min/1.73 m$^2$ and median urine albumin:creatinine ratio of 39 mg/g) found that higher baseline serum SAA concentration was associated with a lower risk of ESKD, suggesting that early in the course of DKD, higher serum SAA concentrations may be renoprotective.[649] Identifying mechanisms that suppress early beneficial effects or promote harmful effects of SAA may enhance our understanding of progressive DKD and provide new therapeutic targets.

## TREATMENT

Annual updated guidelines for the treatment of DKD are available from the American Diabetes Association.[8] Other useful guidelines are also published by the National Kidney Foundation and the KDIGO.[650,651] These guidelines provide evidence for the control of blood pressure, hyperglycemia, dyslipidemia, protein restriction, as well as counseling about smoking cessation and lifestyle education in the management of DKD. Of note, while tight blood pressure control is superior to tight glucose control to prevent macrovascular

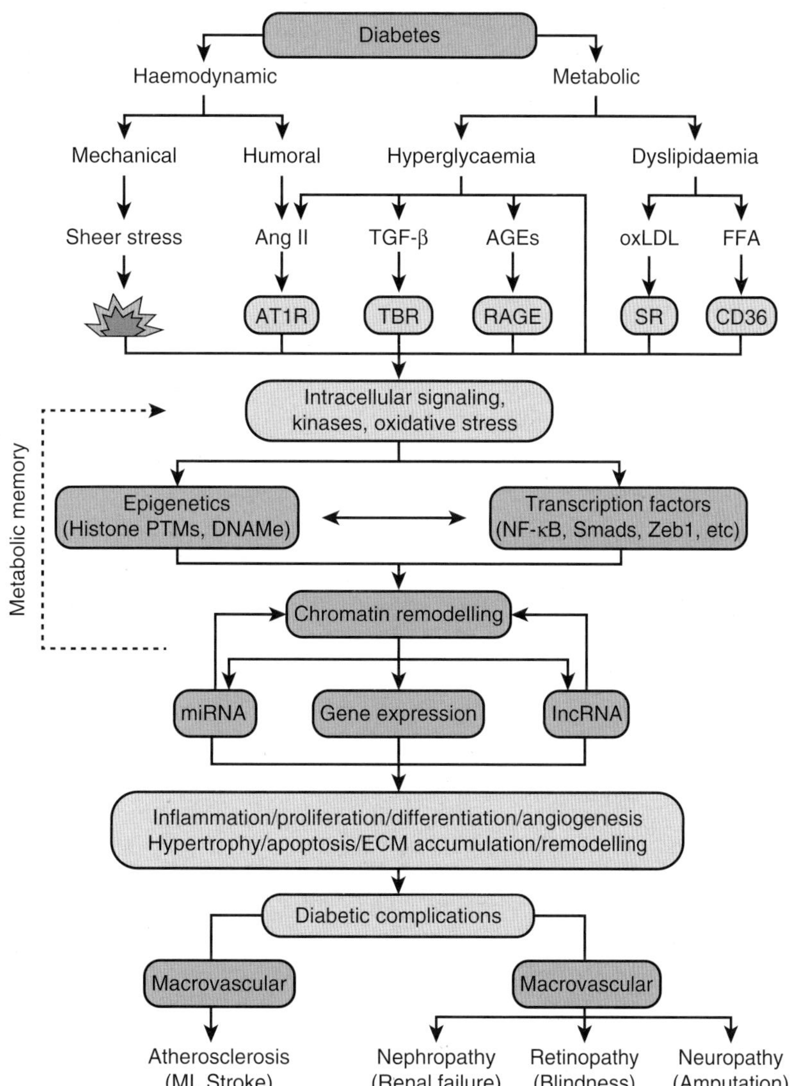


**Fig. 39.19 Signaling and epigenetic networks mediating the pathogenesis of diabetic complications and metabolic memory. Diabetes and its consequent metabolic disorders can upregulate several growth factors and lipids that can act via their receptors and other mechanisms to trigger multiple signaling pathways, transcription factors (TFs), and crosstalk with epigenetic networks. These events can lead to chromatin remodeling and changes in the transcriptional regulation of key pathological genes in cells from target tissues relevant to various complications of diabetes. Persistence of such epigenetic aberrations (including histone PTMs, DNAme, and ncRNAs) may lead to metabolic memory, which is implicated in an increased risk for developing diabetic complications even after normalization of hyperglycemia. *AT1R*, Ang II type 1 receptor; *MI*, myocardial infarction; *oxLDL*, Oxidized-LDL; *RAGE*, Receptor for AGEs; *SR*, scavenger receptors; *TBR*, TGF-β receptor.** (From Reddy MA, Zhang E, Natarajan R. Epigenetic mechanisms in diabetic complications and metabolic memory. *Diabetologia.* 2015;58(3):443–455.)

complications of diabetes, they are equally important in the prevention of microvascular complications such as DKD.[652] However, because multifactorial treatment will effectively reduce the risk of cardiovascular disease and progression of diabetic kidney disease in patients with type 2 diabetes and persistent microalbuminuria,[653] providers should consider a holistic and multifactorial approach in the management of their patients with DKD.

At more advanced stages of DKD, patients are not only at risk of progression to ESKD but also face a much higher burden of microvascular and macrovascular complications than patients at earlier stages of DKD. Physicians caring for patients with advanced DKD face a broad spectrum of therapeutic challenges.[8] They include hypertension, fluid overload, difficulties in tailoring treatment of glycaemic control due to risk of severe hypoglycaemia and reduced number of antidiabetic drugs eligible for use in patients with kidney failure, cardiovascular comorbidities, malnutrition, diabetic foot problems, autonomic neuropathy, anaemia, disturbances of the calcium and phosphorus metabolism with subsequent osteodystrophy (see Chapter 59). Nevertheless, at this stage of the disease treatment should not only address these challenges but also aim at reducing the rate of progressive decline of kidney function, avoiding any symptoms related to the disease state and at the same time preparing the patient for the future renal replacement therapy.

*Clinical Relevance*
**Treatment**

Several studies show that optimal glucose control is of utmost importance at any stage of diabetic kidney disease to reduce cardiovascular events, death and progression of kidney disease. However, the clinical obstacle to achieve favorable glycemic control has been the inherent risk of severe hypoglycemia that can counteract any positive effects of improved control. Novel medications have emerged that do not cause hypoglycemia, and that may even reduce risk of cardiovascular events, death and progression of kidney disease beyond their effect of glycemic control. However, whether these new compounds will be part of the standard care is still not known until studied in dedicated trials of patients with diabetic kidney disease. Currently, the standard care is multifactorial and focuses on lifestyle, lipid lowering, blood pressure control, and blocking of the renin-angiotensin-aldosterone system with either an ACE inhibitor or an ARB, but not in combination due to potential negative effects.

## BLOOD PRESSURE CONTROL FOR THE TREATMENT OF DIABETIC KIDNEY DISEASE

There is no doubt that blood pressure control, irrespective of the agents being used, has a strong impact on the progression of DKD,[652] and any effort should be made to resolve physician and patient-derived cultural barriers that interfere with the achievement of lower blood pressure goals (Fig. 39.20). The recommended blood pressure targets in patients with DKD are blood pressure readings below 140/90 mm Hg to reduce cardiovascular mortality and to slow down the progression of DKD.[654,655] However, in individuals with albuminuria and a blood pressure consistently above 130 mm Hg systolic and more than 80 mm Hg diastolic, physicians should consider lower blood pressure targets of less than 130/80 mm Hg.[656] Recommended blood pressure targets in patients with DKD have been extensively debated, and guidelines from different medical associations have not always found consensus. Moreover, data leading to these recommendations are based on *post hoc* analyses of studies not designed to study the effect of specific blood pressure targets in patients with DKD. Some of these studies are described later.

The Action in Diabetes and Vascular Disease: PreterAx and Diamicron-MR Controlled Evaluation (ADVANCE) trial randomized 11,140 patients with type 2 diabetes to a combination of perindopril and indapamide or placebo.[657] In the patients with lower blood pressure values (<135 mm Hg) during treatment, the risk of new-onset microalbuminuria or proteinuria, ESKD, and renal transplantation was significantly lower (−21%, $P < .0001$) than in those with higher blood pressures (~140 mm Hg). This was also the case for worsening of the kidney disease in patients with DKD at baseline, defined as an increased urine protein excretion, or a reduction in the eGFR.[658]

In a metaanalysis of trials performed in patients with chronic kidney disease, greater blood pressure reduction had greater kidney protective effects, with the slowest progression rate being exhibited by patients with a systolic blood pressure less than 120 mm Hg.[659] In studies of patients with DKD, there is a linear relationship between the magnitude of the treatment-induced blood pressure reduction and the decline in GFR (Fig. 39.21). The lowest decline in GFR is observed at an on-treatment mean arterial pressure of 89 mm Hg, which corresponds to a systolic and diastolic blood pressure of 120 mm Hg and 75 mm Hg.[660]

In the ONgoing Telmisartan Alone and in combination with Ramipril Global Endpoint Trial (ONTARGET), comprising 12,554 patients with a baseline systolic blood pressure of more than 140 mm Hg, a reduction of the blood pressure from 154 mm Hg to 125 mm Hg was accompanied by a progressive reduction in the incidence of new-onset microalbuminuria

| Outcome | No. of Studies | BP Lowering Events | BP Lowering Participants | Control Events | Control Participants | Relative Risk (95% CI) |
|---|---|---|---|---|---|---|
| Mortality | 20 | 2334 | 27,693 | 2319 | 25,864 | 0.87 (0.78–0.96) |
| Cardiovascular disease | 17 | 3230 | 25,756 | 3280 | 24,862 | 0.89 (0.83–0.95) |
| Coronary heart disease | 17 | 1390 | 26,150 | 1449 | 24,761 | 0.88 (0.80–0.98) |
| Stroke | 19 | 1350 | 27,614 | 1475 | 26,447 | 0.73 (0.64–0.83) |
| Heart failure | 13 | 1235 | 21,684 | 1348 | 20,791 | 0.86 (0.74–1.00) |
| Renal failure | 9 | 596 | 19,835 | 560 | 18,912 | 0.91 (0.74–1.12) |
| Retinopathy | 7 | 844 | 9781 | 905 | 9566 | 0.87 (0.76–0.99) |
| Albuminuria | 7 | 2799 | 13,804 | 3163 | 12,821 | 0.83 (0.79–0.87) |



**Fig. 39.20** Effect of blood pressure (BP) lowering in diabetes. Forest plot of standardized associations between 10–mm Hg lower systolic BP and all-cause mortality, macrovascular outcomes, and microvascular outcomes in a metaanalysis of clinical trials of BP lowering therapy that included patients with type 2 diabetes.[656] The area of each square is proportional to the inverse variance of the estimate. Horizontal lines indicate 95% CIs of the estimate. (From Emdin CA, Rahimi K, Neal B, Callender T, Perkovic V, Patel A. Blood pressure lowering in type 2 diabetes: a systematic review and meta-analysis. *JAMA.* 2015;313(6):603–615. With permission.)

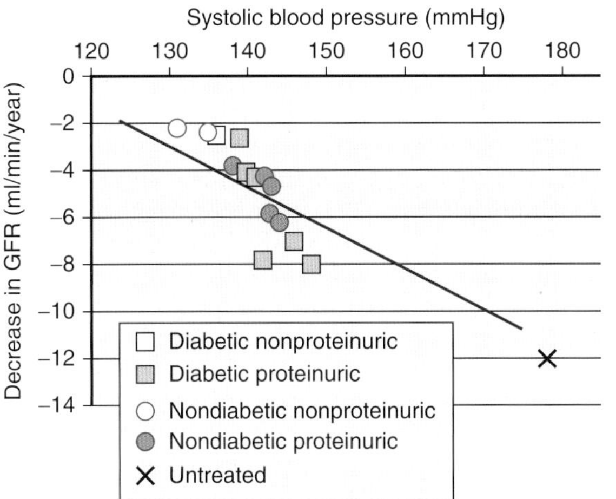


**Fig. 39.21** Data from prospective clinical trials on nephropathy progression with a follow-up duration of 2 years or more showing the relationships between the systolic blood pressure values achieved during antihypertensive drug treatment and the decrease in glomerular filtration rate (GFR).[889] (From Grassi G, Mancia G, Nilsson PM. Specific blood pressure targets for patients with diabetic nephropathy? *Diabetes Care.* 2016;39 Suppl 2:S228–S233.With permission.)

and macroalbuminuria as well as by a progressively greater return to normoalbuminuria in patients who exhibited an abnormal urine albumin excretion at baseline.[661] However, the ONTARGET trial was not a dedicated diabetes trial and the proportion of patients with diabetes in the different blood pressure responder groups varied from 47.4% in those with the smallest response (percentage of visits in which blood pressure was reduced to <140/90 mm Hg <25%) to 30.0% in those with the greatest response (percentage of visits >75%).

Finally, a pooled analysis of the 22,984 patients from the ONTARGET and Telmisartan Randomised Assessment Study in ACE intolerant participants with cardiovascular disease (TRANSCEND) trials[662,663] showed that patients who regressed from microalbuminuria to normoalbuminuria had a lower risk of loss of kidney function than those who progressed from normoalbuminuria to microalbuminuria. This finding was detected both in the overall trial cohort and in the subset of 8,454 patients with diabetes.

Thus based on the available evidence, a blood pressure target below 140/90 mm Hg is recommended for patients with diabetes and DKD, if the patient has no signs of albuminuria. However, if the patient presents with an albumin excretion rate greater than 30 mg/24 hours (or equivalent) then a lower target of less than 130/80 mm Hg might be beneficial.[654] Importantly, the guidelines also recommend the use of renin-angiotensin-aldosterone system inhibitors as standard care in patients with diabetes and albuminuria, unless there are absolute or relative contraindications. Such contraindications may be more common in patients at the later stages of DKD than in the earlier stages.

## RENIN-ANGIOTENSIN-ALDOSTERONE SYSTEM BLOCKERS

The recommendation to use ACE inhibitors or angiotensin receptor blockers (ARBs) as first-line agents in DKD is based on multiple randomized controlled clinical trials. Early evidence supporting their use was provided by the Collaborative Study Group. In their landmark study, patients with type 1 diabetes, proteinuria above 500 mg over 24 hours and serum creatinine less than 2.5 mg/dl were randomized to captopril (25 mg three times a day, $n = 207$) or to placebo ($n = 202$) on top of conventional blood pressure medication. The exposure to captopril resulted in a 51% reduction of the risk of a composite endpoint inclusive of dialysis, transplantation or death.[664] However, renoprotection with ACE inhibitors is not unique to DKD; it has been reported in other studies in chronic kidney disease of nondiabetic origin as well.[665,666] Thus in the Health Outcomes and Prevention Evaluation (HOPE) study, ACE inhibition with ramipril, in 980 patients with either mild renal insufficiency (serum creatinine between 1.4 and 2.3 mg/dl) or in 8307 patients with normal kidney function (creatinine <1.4 mg/dl), reduced the risk of cardiovascular death, stroke and myocardial infarction irrespective of the presence or absence of chronic kidney disease.[667]

Three subsequent studies established the evidence that angiotensin-receptor blockade is also an efficient method to prevent or treat DKD. In the Irbesartan in Patients with Type 2 Diabetes and Microalbuminuria (IRMA-2) study, 590 patients with type 2 diabetes and microalbuminuria were randomized to either 150 or 300 mg of irbesartan or to placebo. In the 2-year follow-up, both the low and the high dose resulted in a 39% and 70% reduction of the primary outcome, the time to onset of DKD, which was defined as persistent albuminuria in overnight specimens, with a urinary albumin excretion rate greater than 200 ug/min, and at least 30% higher than the baseline level.[668] In the Irbesartan Diabetic Nephropathy Trial (IDNT), 1715 patients with type 2 diabetes, hypertension and proteinuria were randomized to irbesartan (300 mg), amlodipine (10 mg) or placebo. In the 2.6-year follow-up, irbesartan treatment resulted in a 33% risk reduction in the proportion of patients with doubling of baseline serum creatinine, when compared with both the amlodipine and the placebo treatment arm. Although irbesartan treatment was also associated with a mean reduction in systolic blood pressure of 3.3 mm Hg, the effect on doubling of serum creatinine was independent of the effect on blood pressure.[669] In the Reduction of Endpoints in NIDDM with the Angiotensin II Antagonist Losartan (RENAAL) study, 1513 patients with type 2 diabetes and DKD were randomized to losartan or placebo. Losartan treatment over 3.4 years resulted in a 25% risk reduction of the proportion of patients with doubling of serum creatinine, 28% reduction of risk of ESKD, and 16% reduction in the composite endpoint, which was defined as doubling of serum creatinine or ESKD or death. Losartan treatment also resulted in 35% reduction of proteinuria assessed as secondary endpoint.[670]

There is no evidence of superiority of ACE inhibitors over ARBs. The prospective multicenter double-blind Diabetics Exposed to Telmisartan And enalaprIL (DETAIL) study of 250 patients with type 2 diabetes and DKD compared the effect of the ARB telmisartan (80 mg) to the ACE inhibitor enalapril (20 mg) over a 5-year period. The study clearly showed that there was no difference in the risk of reaching the primary endpoint (change in iohexol GFR) or in the secondary endpoints (serum creatinine, urinary albumin excretion or blood pressure) according to treatment assignment.[671]

Overall, the current recommendations are to treat patients with type 1 diabetes, hypertension, and albuminuria with ACE inhibitors, while in patients with type 2 diabetes, hypertension and microalbuminuria should be treated with either ACE inhibitors or ARBs, and those with overt DKD with angiotensin-receptor blockers as first-line treatment. However, when not tolerated, the recommendation is to substitute one for the other.

## COMBINATION OF ANGIOTENSIN-CONVERTING ENZYME INHIBITORS WITH ANGIOTENSIN-RECEPTOR BLOCKERS

An important clinical question is whether there is additional benefit of using a combination of an ACE inhibitor with an angiotensin-receptor blocker. The addition of candesartan, an angiotensin-receptor blocker, 16 mg once daily to the maximal recommended dose of an ACE inhibitor (either enalapril or lisinopril 40 mg daily or captopril 150 mg daily) significantly reduced albuminuria in a randomized crossover trial in 20 patients with type 2 diabetes and DKD over an 8-week period.[672] In another study with similar design, 24 patients with type 1 diabetes and DKD were randomized to either enalapril 40 mg or enalapril 40 mg plus irbesartan 300 mg daily for 8 weeks. The study showed a significant reduction in albuminuria in the combination group.[673] By contrast, the Irbesartan in the Management of PROteinuric patients at high risk for Vascular Events (IMPROVE) trial, in which 838 patients with hypertension and albuminuria were treated for 20 weeks with either ramipril or ramipril plus irbesartan, showed no significant changes in albuminuria despite a significant reduction of the blood pressure in the combination group.[674] It is of note that these studies were all short-term trials, and they were not conducted long enough to detect any potential hazards with the combination of two agents blocking the renin-angiotensin-aldosterone system.

Although the combination of an ACE inhibitor with an angiotensin-receptor blocker, as supported by some short-term clinical trials, theoretically could be more effective than either treatment alone, long-term data on safety and efficacy were missing until the ONTARGET trial investigated the renal effects of ramipril (ACE inhibitor), telmisartan (ARB), and their combination in 25,620 patients 55 years of age or older with established atherosclerotic vascular disease or diabetes with end-organ damage. The trial showed that the effects of telmisartan on major renal outcomes were similar to the effect of ramipril. Although the combination of the two agents reduced proteinuria to a greater extent than monotherapy did, overall it worsened the major renal outcomes.[675] Thus this landmark trial, instead of supporting the use of double blockade of the renin-angiotensin-aldosterone-system, discouraged it. Two other studies, the Veterans Affairs Nephropathy in Diabetes (VA NEPHRON-D) and the Aliskerin Trial in Type 2 Diabetes Using Cardiorenal Endpoints (ALTITUDE), established that double blockade in patients with type 2 diabetes and DKD might not be safe.[676,677]

The VA NEPHRON-D trial[677] prescribed the ARB losartan (100 mg daily) to patients with type 2 diabetes and DKD, defined as baseline urine albumin-to-creatinine ratio of at least 300 mg/g and an eGFR of 30 to 90 ml/min/1.73 m$^2$, and randomly assigned them to receive the ACE inhibitor lisinopril (at a dose of 10–40 mg daily) or placebo. Notably, the study was stopped early due to safety concerns, as combination therapy increased the risk of hyperkalemia (6.3 events/100 person-years vs. 2.6 events/100 person-years with monotherapy; $P < .001$) and acute kidney injury (12.2 events compared with 6.7 events/100 person-years; $P < .001$) (Fig. 39.22). There was no significant benefit regarding kidney endpoints, cardiovascular events, or mortality.[677]

The rationale for ALTITUDE was that the lack of benefit of double blockade in the ONTARGET trial could have been due to the deleterious effects of aldosterone escape and compensatory renin activation.[678,679] Therefore the ALTITUDE study was designed to determine whether the use of a direct renin-inhibitor, aliskiren, could reduce cardiovascular and renal events in patients with type 2 diabetes and DKD, cardiovascular disease, or both.[676] In the trial, a total of 8,561 patients were randomly assigned to either aliskiren (300 mg daily) or placebo on top of an ACE inhibitor or an ARB. This study was also stopped prematurely due to safety concerns. The proportion of patients with hyperkalemia was higher in the aliskiren than in the placebo group (11.2% vs. 7.2%), as was the proportion with reported hypotension (12.1% vs.8.3%) ($P < .001$ for both comparisons). It was therefore concluded that the addition of aliskiren to standard therapy with renin-angiotensin-aldosterone system blockade may be harmful.[676] Taken together these large outcome trials clearly show that double blockade of the renin-angiotensin-aldosterone system should be avoided in patients with type 2 diabetes, who are at risk for cardiovascular and renal events.

## ALDOSTERONE ANTAGONISTS IN ADDITION TO RENIN-ANGIOTENSIN-ALDOSTERONE SYSTEM BLOCKERS

Despite the discouraging results regarding double blockade, the potential use of aldosterone antagonism on top of ACE inhibition or blocking of the angiotensin II receptor, has gained interest and has also been studied in a number of small short-term trials. One example is a 1-year, placebo-controlled, double-blind, parallel-group trial in 59 patients with type 2 diabetes and albuminuria. In this study, the addition of spironolactone to an ACE inhibitor or an ARB was associated with a marked and sustained antiproteinuric effect, which was accompanied by a significant improvement in eGFR.[680] A similar effect was observed in a small study of 20 patients with type 1 diabetes with severe albuminuria and stage 2 chronic kidney disease, where 25 mg daily of spironolactone for 2 months resulted in a significant reduction of albuminuria (mg/24 hours).[681] Despite these encouraging results, caution is warranted, because of the lack of long-term safety and efficacy studies as well as the risk of hyperkalemia.

Eplerenone is a more selective aldosterone antagonist, and the effect of two different doses of this drug (50 and 100 mg daily) or placebo on top of the ACE inhibitor enalapril (20 mg daily) for 12 weeks in 268 patients with type 2 diabetes, and a baseline urine albumin-to-creatinine-ratio of 50 mg/g, resulted in significant reduction of albuminuria as early as week 4 of treatment and continued through weeks 8 and 12 ($P < .001$ for all comparisons). The effect on the albumin-to-creatinine-ratio was observed with both doses irrespective of eGFR, below 61 or above 85 ml/min/1.73 m$^2$.[547] A novel nonsteroidal mineralocorticoid receptor antagonist, finerenone, with higher selectivity for the mineralocorticoid receptor (MR) than spironolactone, was found to be safe and effective

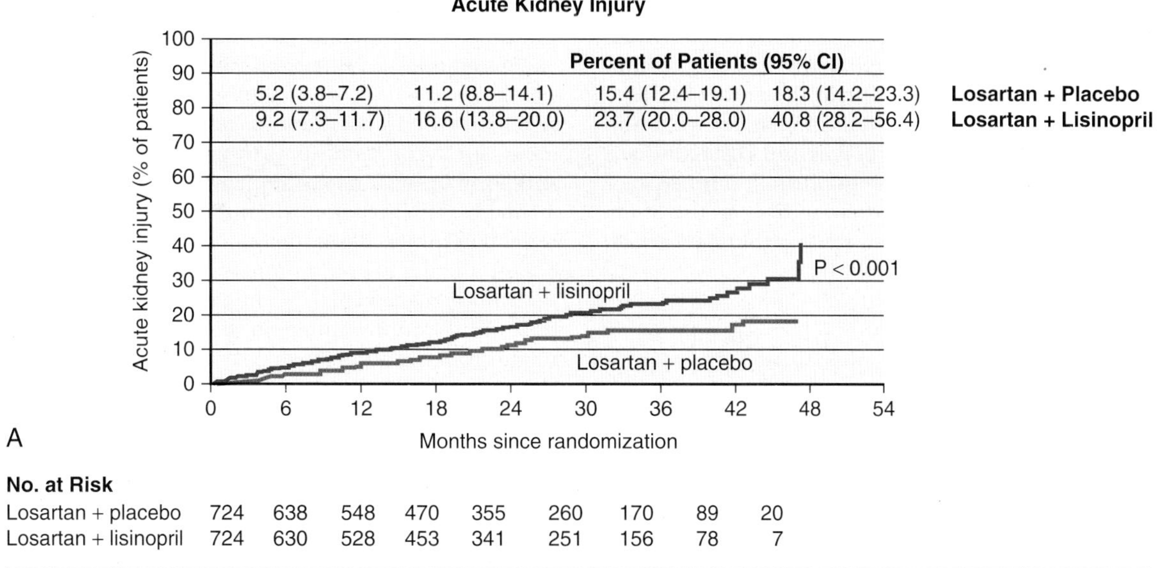


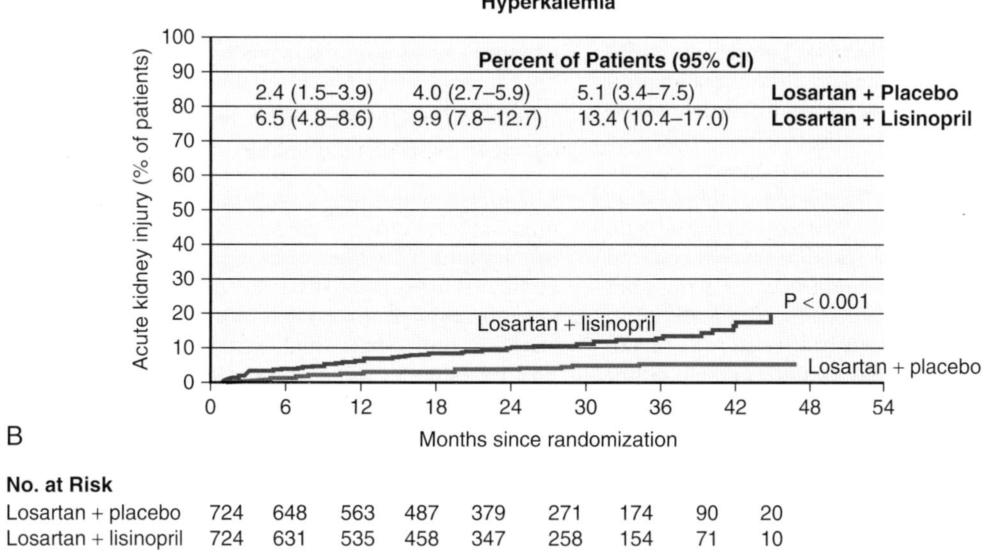


**Fig. 39.22 Kaplan–Meier plot of cumulative probabilities of acute kidney injury and hyperkalemia in patients with combined angiotensin inhibition in the VA Nephron-D trial.[677] Acute kidney injury was defined as acute kidney injury requiring hospitalization or occurring during a hospitalization. Hyperkalemia was defined as a potassium level over 6.0 mmol per liter or that required an emergency room visit, hospitalization, or dialysis. The *P* values were calculated with the use of a stratified log-rank test.**

in reducing urine albumin-to-creatinine ratio in combination with a renin-angiotensin-aldosterone inhibitor in 821 subjects with type 2 diabetes and macroalbuminuria in a 90-day phase 2 trial,[546] a study that opened the door to the design of an ongoing phase 3 trial (NCT02545049).

## ENDOTHELIN RECEPTOR ANTAGONISTS

More recently, the development of endothelin receptor antagonists has generated a lot of attention, primarily after the development of selective receptor blockers for the receptor isoform A ($ET_ARB$). Atrasentan is a selective $ET_A$ receptor blocker currently being tested in phase 3 trials after successful reduction of albuminuria in phase 2 studies.[682,683] In the first phase 2 study, 89 patients with established DKD (eGFR >20 and urine albumin-to-creatinine ratio between 100 and 3000 mg/g) were randomized to atrasentan (0.25, 0.75, or 1.75 mg) versus placebo for 8 weeks. All patients were on a stable dose of renin-angiotensin-aldosterone system blockade at enrollment. Of the atrasentan treated patients in the high-dose group, 38% experienced a 40% reduction in urine albumin-to-creatinine ratio from baseline.[682] In the subsequent study, atrasentan was evaluated as an add on to the maximum tolerated dose of renin-angiotensin-aldosterone system inhibition in 211 patients with type 2 diabetes, urine albumin-to-creatinine ratio of 300 to 500 mg/g and eGFR of 30 to 75 ml/min/1.73 $m^2$. Both 0.75 mg and 1.25 mg of atrasentan were tested against placebo for 12 weeks. Treatment resulted in a 51% and 55% reduction, respectively, in the number of participants that achieved a 30% reduction of albuminuria from baseline.[683] Discontinuation of the treatment resulted in all measured parameters returning to pretreatment levels. However, this class of agents is associated with increased fluid retention and congestive heart failure. Therefore further trials are required to prove the safety and efficacy of this class. Currently, the effects of atrasentan on kidney outcomes (time to doubling of serum creatinine or the onset of ESKD) as well as cardiovascular morbidity and mortality are being explored in patients with type 2 diabetes and DKD, who are treated with the maximum tolerated labelled daily dose of a renin-angiotensin-aldosterone system inhibitor (the Study of Diabetic Nephropathy with Atrasentan (SONAR trial), NCT01858532).

## BLOOD PRESSURE CONTROL FOR THE PRIMARY PREVENTION OF DIABETIC KIDNEY DISEASE

Although the use of ACE inhibitors and ARBs is recommended for the treatment of established DKD, their role in the primary prevention of DKD is more controversial. The BErgamo NEphrologic DIabetes Complications Trial (BENEDICT) randomized 1204 patients with type 2 diabetes, mild hypertension and normal urine albumin excretion rate (<20 ug/min), to trandolapril alone (2 mg daily), verapamil alone (240 mg daily), a combination of trandolapril (2 mg daily) and verapamil (180 mg daily) or placebo. The development of persistent albuminuria, defined as an albumin excretion of more than 20 ug/min at two consecutive visits, was assessed as the primary endpoint in a 48-month follow- up. The combination of trandolapril and verapamil as well as trandolapril alone delayed the onset of microalbuminuria by factors of 2.6 and 2.1, respectively. Notably, this trial also established the superiority of ACE inhibitors over calcium channel blockers in primary prevention because verapamil alone was no different from placebo. More importantly, the effect on albuminuria was completely independent of the effect on blood pressure, as there was no difference in either systolic or diastolic blood pressure at any time point during the study.[684]

In contrast, two other studies showed no effect at all of exposure to renin-angiotensin-aldosterone system blockade on the risk of microalbuminuria.[456,685] The Diabetic Retinopathy Candesartan Trials (DIRECT) program pooled three related randomized, double-blinded, placebo-controlled, trials to assess the effect of angiotensin-receptor blockade (candesartan) on primary prevention of DKD in normotensive patients with either type 1 ($n = 3326$) or type 2 diabetes ($n = 1905$) and normal urine albumin excretion rate (<20 ug/min). Administration of candesartan versus placebo over a 4.7-year follow-up demonstrated that candesartan (32 mg daily) had only a minor effect on the risk of microalbuminuria (hazard ratio [HR] of 0.95; $P = .60$) despite having a significant effect on blood pressure. However, these studies were powered to evaluate the effect of candesartan on diabetic retinopathy and not on DKD and therefore have to be interpreted with caution.[685] In the Renin-Angiotensin System Study (RASS), 223 normotensive patients with type 1 diabetes and normal urine albumin excretion rate (<20 ug/min) were randomized to enalapril 20 mg versus losartan 100 mg versus placebo over a 5-year period. Neither losartan nor enalapril resulted in a reduction of the cumulative incidence of microalbuminuria and/or in the change of mesangial fractional volume in research kidney biopsies. Interestingly, both treatments resulted in the protection from retinopathy progression, suggesting that the involvement of the renin-angiotensin-aldosterone system may differ in the pathogenesis of retinopathy and nephropathy.[456]

Nevertheless, a recent metaanalysis of 6 studies explored whether early blockade of the renin-angiotensin-aldosterone system in comparison with placebo can prevent the development of microalbuminuria in patients with type 2 diabetes and normal albumin excretion rate. The metaanalysis included a total of 16,921 patients, and showed a 16% relative risk reduction for the development of microalbuminuria in those exposed to renin-angiotensin-aldosterone system inhibitors as compared to placebo.[686] These findings could have implications for the future, since the side effects of these drugs are relatively few and mild in low-risk patients, such as those with normal blood pressure and well-preserved kidney function.[686] The observed hazard ratio of 0.84 corresponds to a number needed to treat (NNT) of 25, which means that for every 25 patients with normal albumin excretion rate treated with an ACE inhibitor or an angiotensin-receptor blocker, one case of new-onset microalbuminuria is prevented.[686]

Current guidelines do not yet recommend the use of an ACE inhibitor or an ARB for the prevention of DKD in patients with diabetes, who have normal blood pressure, normal albumin-to-creatinine ratio (<30 mg/g), and normal eGFR.[10,654]

## GLYCEMIC CONTROL FOR THE TREATMENT OF DIABETIC KIDNEY DISEASE

The fundamental abnormality in diabetes is abnormal glucose metabolism, and the degree of abnormality predicts the development of kidney disease.[336,687] Hence optimal glycemic control is crucial for the prevention of kidney damage and deterioration of the GFR.[419,687] Importantly, studies in both type 1[688] and type 2 diabetes[273,689] demonstrate a durable positive effect of initial intensive glucose control on kidney outcomes despite later loss of the glycemic separation in the intensive and less-intensive glucose control study arms. Today, accumulating research findings highlight that even transient glucose spikes may suffice to elicit continuous changes in the metabolic milieu perpetuating target organ damage.[690] Therefore it is not only the average blood glucose mirrored by the glycated hemoglobin that affects the kidney outcomes, but also other parameters of glucose exposure, in particular the glucose variability, that may be important in the assessment of the role of glycemic control for target organ damage.[691]

The current guidelines to control hyperglycemia for the prevention of DKD recommend a target hemoglobin A1C of about 7%. However, the target should be personalized based on patient characteristics. This is a significant change compared to prior guidelines, where A1C of less than 7% was recommended for everybody. Two hallmark studies demonstrated the importance of glycemic control in patients with type 1 diabetes (DCCT) and type 2 diabetes (UKPDS). In the DCCT trial, 1441 patients with type 1 diabetes were randomized to either intensive treatment (insulin three times a day) versus conventional treatment (1 or 2 daily insulin injections) and followed for 6.5 years. Intensive treatment resulted in a 61% reduction in albuminuria by achieving an A1C of 7.2% when compared with 9.1% in the conventional arm.[42] Most importantly, the differences in A1C were conserved throughout the trial, although after close-out of the trial the A1C levels converged.[687] Despite the convergence of the A1C levels, the beneficial effects on macrovascular,[692] and microvascular complications were sustained.[687] In the UKPDS study, 3867 patients with type 2 diabetes and a median age of 54 years were randomized to intensive treatment (sulfonylureas or insulin) versus diet and were followed for 10 years. Diet alone resulted in a median A1C of 7.9% when compared with 7.0% in the intensive treatment arm. Nevertheless, this relatively small difference in A1C resulted in a 34% reduction of albuminuria in the treatment arm. However, one of the UKPDS follow-up studies (UKPDS 33) demonstrated that a significant reduction in the proportion of patients achieving doubling of the serum creatinine in the intensive versus control arm was observed only after 12 years.[570] A clear correlation between A1C values and microvascular endpoints (retinopathy requiring photocoagulation, vitreous hemorrhage and fatal or nonfatal renal failure) was observed in the UKPDS 35 follow-up study, where the correlation with macrovascular complications was less clear.[693]

The possibility of regression of albuminuria after establishment of improved glycemic control has also been studied in patients with type 1 and type 2 diabetes. A study in 386 patients with type 1 diabetes and moderate persistent albuminuria, followed for 4 periods of two years each, demonstrated that the adjusted hazard ratio for regression of albuminuria (defined as 50% reduction in the urine albumin excretion rate from one period to another) was 1.9 when achieving a target A1C lower than 8%,[75] when compared with an A1C above 10%. Regression (50% reduction) or remission (return to normoalbuminuria) were also observed in 216 Japanese patients with type 2 diabetes that were followed for up to 6 years (3 periods of 2 years each). In this study, achieving an A1C target of less than 6.95% resulted in an adjusted odds ratio for regression of 2.2 and for remission of 3.[77]

Several studies have addressed the safety and efficacy of lowering A1C to confer additional kidney and cardiovascular protection. Both the ADVANCE and the Action to Control Cardiovascular Risk in Diabetes (ACCORD) trials were designed to test the consequences of intensive glycemic control targeting an A1C level of less than 6.5%. In the ADVANCE trial, 11,140 patients with type 2 diabetes were randomized to intensive therapy (sulphonylureas plus other agents) to achieve a A1C target of less than 6.5% versus a standard arm with target A1C of 7.0%. Although this resulted in a 21% relative reduction in nephropathy, defined by development of macroalbuminuria, doubling of the serum creatinine concentration, ESKD, or death due to renal disease, no differences were observed in macrovascular events of death of any causes.[694] In a parallel study (the ACCORD trial), 10,251 patients with type 2 diabetes were randomized to either standard versus intensive treatment (mainly insulin and thiazolidinediones). One-third of the patients had prior cardiovascular events. The trial was discontinued after 3.5 years due to a higher mortality rate in the intensive arm.[695] The outcome of these two studies provided the background to the change in guidelines from strict A1C target below 7% in all patients to a more personalized approach to glycemic control, as intensive treatment in patients with established macrovascular complication is likely to be more harmful than beneficial. A major risk of the intensive glycemic intervention, illustrated in both of these trials, is severe life-threatening hypoglycemia requiring the assistance of another person. This risk is discussed further later. Nevertheless, whereas the benefit of intensified glycemic control is typically experienced over many years, the risk of severe hypoglycemia associated with intensified glycemic control is immediate. Using data from the UKPDS, ADVANCE, ACCORD, and the Veterans Affairs Diabetes Trial (VADT), a metaanalysis of data from the Collaborators on Trials of Lowering Glucose (CONTROL) group[696] illustrated that treating 1000 patients with diabetes for 5 years with intensified glycemic control would lead to 2 fewer cases of ESKD, but to 47 additional cases of severe hypoglycemia. Accordingly, as noted above, clinicians who treat these patients must consider the benefits and risks of intensive glycemic control in each patient and adjust their treatment strategies accordingly.[697]

The clinically relevant question of whether targeting glycemia with aggressive glucose-lowering in patients with advanced DKD or ESKD will lead to cardiovascular benefit or reduced risk of premature mortality, is still open. This is mainly due to lack of trials addressing this issue in advanced kidney disease and ESKD. However, there are some data from the ADVANCE trial that randomly assigned 11,140 participants to an intensive glucose-lowering strategy targeting a HbA1c of 6.5% or less or standard glucose control.[757] Treatment effects on kidney outcomes were assessed (Fig. 39.23). After a median of 5 years, the mean HbA1c level was 6.5% in the intensive group, and 7.3% in the standard group. Notably, intensive glucose control reduced the risk of ESKD by 65% (20 vs. 7 events), macroalbuminuria by 30% (162 vs. 231 patients), and microalbuminuria by 9% (1298 compared to 1410 patients). The progression of albuminuria was reduced by 10% and regression of albuminuria increased by 15%. The study clearly showed that improved glucose control translates into major beneficial effects on renal outcomes in patients with type 2 diabetes. Nevertheless, the ADVANCE trial was not designed to focus on patients with advanced kidney disease, although a total of 2148 patients had a baseline eGFR of less than 60 ml/min/1.73 $m^2$, and 776 patients also had albuminuria.[757] During median posttrial follow-up of 5.4 years in 8494 ADVANCE participants, the in-trial reductions in the risk of ESKD (7 vs. 20 events, HR 0.35, $P = .02$) persisted after 9.9 years of overall follow-up (29 vs. 53 events, HR 0.54, $P < .01$). Importantly, the effects of glucose-lowering were not associated with an increased risk of cardiovascular events or death.[689] However, the question still remains, whether aggressive glucose-lowering in those with advanced kidney disease or ESKD will also translate into cardiovascular benefit.

## IMPACT OF TARGETING GLYCEMIA WITH DIFFERENT AGENTS IN DIABETIC KIDNEY DISEASE

Targeting $HbA_1C$ with one agent versus another may differentially affect the development and progression of DKD. Initial enthusiasm was seen a decade ago, when thiazolidinediones were thought to be superior to other agents in reducing urine albumin-to-creatinine ratio despite achieving the same A1C and fasting plasma glucose targets.[698] These data were confirmed in a metaanalysis of 15 randomized trials on 2860 patients, where thiazolidinediones were compared with either placebo or other antidiabetic agents.[699] Although these clinical findings were supported by strong experimental data discussed in the pathogenesis section of this chapter, this class of agents

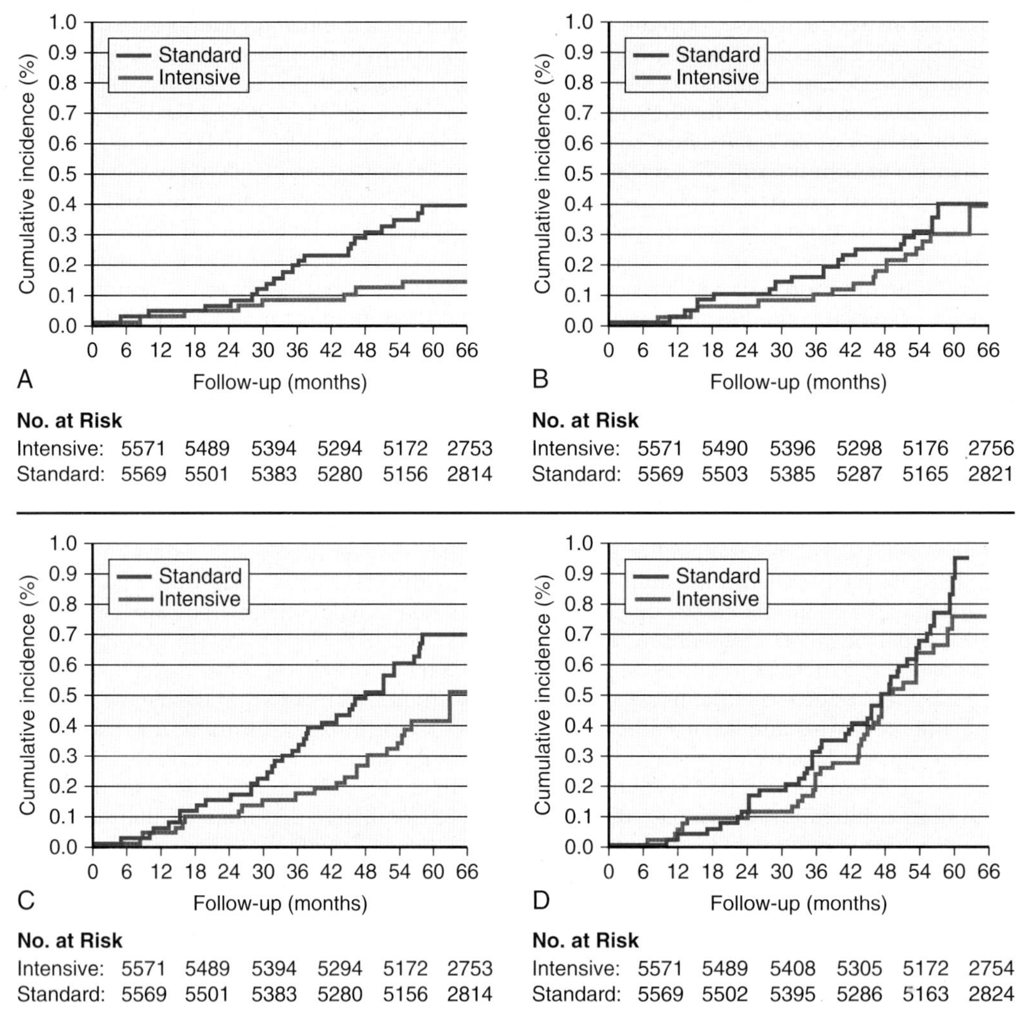


**Fig. 39.23 Effect of intensive glucose control on kidney outcomes in the ADVANCE trial.[757] Kaplan–Meier curves depicting the incidence of (A) end-stage kidney disease (ESKD), (B) renal death, (C) ESKD or renal death, and (D) doubling of creatinine to at least 200 mmol/l over time by randomized group (transient or sustained). (A) ESKD. Hazard ratio (HR) for intensive versus control: 0.35, 95% confidence interval (CI) 0.15–0.83, *P* = .01. (B) Renal death. HR for intensive versus control 0.85, 95% CI 0.45–1.63, *P* = .63. (C) Combined ESKD/renal death. HR for intensive versus control: 0.64, 95% CI 0.38–1.08, *P* = .09. (D) Sustained doubling of serum creatinine. HR for intensive versus control: 0.83, 95% CI 0.54–1.27, *P* = .38.**

was also found to cause significant side effects and there are no currently ongoing clinical trials assessing the impact of this class of agents in DKD. More recently, the Alerenal trial (NCT01893242), which was supposed to test the effect of a new dual peroxisome proliferator-activated receptor (PPAR) agonist, aleglitazar, in patients with DKD, was stopped for unreported safety reasons and this dramatically reduced the interest in this class of agents.

A new class of agents that selectively block the sodium-glucose cotransporter 2 (SGLT2) in the proximal tubule with subsequent glycosuria have generated a lot of interest.[700,701] The Empagliflozin, Cardiovascular Outcomes, and Mortality in Type 2 Diabetes (EMPA-REG OUTCOME) trial was designed to test if the SGLT2 inhibitor empagliflozin (10 mg or 25 mg) on top of standard care can reduce the risk of cardiovascular morbidity and mortality in patients with type 2 diabetes at high cardiovascular risk and with an eGFR more than 30 ml/min/1.73 m$^2$. A total of 4687 patients were treated with empagliflozin, and the study demonstrated a 38% lower rate of cardiovascular death, a 32% lower rate of death from any cause, and a 35% lower rate of hospitalization for heart failure, when compared with the 2333 patients receiving placebo.[702] In the EMPA-REG OUTCOME trial there were also prespecified kidney outcomes, and since the primary outcome was significantly reduced (HR 0.86; $P < .04$ for superiority) the prespecified testing sequence allowed assessment of the long-term kidney effects of empagliflozin as well.[636] Empagliflozin resulted in a 39% relative risk reduction in new or worsening of DKD, a 38% lower risk of progression to macroalbuminuria, a 44% lower risk of doubling of serum creatinine, and a 55% relative risk reduction in need for initiation of renal replacement therapy. Similar results were seen in the recent Canagliflozin Cardiovascular Assessment Study (CANVAS) Program in patients with type 2 diabetes and high cardiovascular risk,[637] although on the basis of their prespecified hypothesis testing sequence, the kidney outcomes were not viewed as statistically significant. However, the results showed a possible benefit of canagliflozin with respect to the progression of albuminuria (HR 0.73; 95% CI 0.67–0.79) and the composite outcome of a sustained 40% reduction

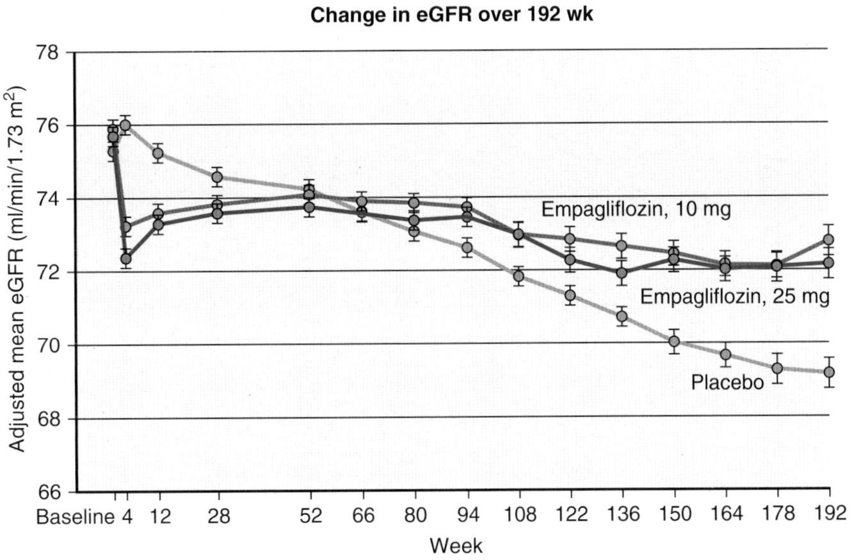

**Change in eGFR over 192 wk**

| Week | Baseline | 4 | 12 | 28 | 52 | 66 | 80 | 94 | 108 | 122 | 136 | 150 | 164 | 178 | 192 |
|---|---|---|---|---|---|---|---|---|---|---|---|---|---|---|---|
| **No. at Risk** | | | | | | | | | | | | | | | |
| Placebo | 2323 | 2295 | 2267 | 2205 | 2121 | 2064 | 1927 | 1981 | 1763 | 1479 | 1262 | 1123 | 977 | 731 | 448 |
| Empagliflozin, 10 mg | 2322 | 2290 | 2264 | 2235 | 2162 | 2114 | 2012 | 2064 | 1839 | 1540 | 1314 | 1180 | 1024 | 785 | 513 |
| Empagliflozin, 25 mg | 2322 | 2288 | 2269 | 2216 | 2156 | 2111 | 2006 | 2067 | 1871 | 1563 | 1340 | 1207 | 1063 | 838 | 524 |
| **No. in follow-up analysis** | | | | | | | | | | | | | | | |
| Total | 7020 | 7020 | 6996 | 6931 | 6864 | 6765 | 6696 | 6651 | 6068 | 5114 | 4443 | 3961 | 3488 | 2707 | 1703 |

**Fig. 39.24 Renal function over time (192 weeks) in the EMPA-REG OUTCOME Trial.**[636]

in the eGFR, the need for renal replacement therapy, or death from kidney causes (HR 0.60; 95% CI 0.47–0.77). Notably, neither the EMPA-REG OUTCOME trial nor the CANVAS Program were dedicated kidney outcome trials, and therefore the results have to be replicated in trials specifically designed to examine a kidney outcome as the primary endpoint. Such trials are ongoing or planned not only for empagliflozin but also for canagliflozin (Canagliflozin and Renal Events in Diabetes with Established Nephropathy Clinical Evaluation (CREDENCE), NCT02065791) and dapagliflozin. One of the more remarkable findings in the EMPA-REG OUTCOME trial was that empagliflozin is able to preserve kidney function by retarding the natural progression of DKD after the initial drop in eGFR[636] (Fig. 39.24) Whether the observed renoprotection is linked to restoration of the impaired tubulo-glomerular feedback observed in DKD[703] or is directly linked to changes in kidney cell metabolism remains to be established. However, although the data on SGLT2-inhibitors appear promising, these drugs are not yet indicated for the treatment of patients with an eGFR less than 45 ml/min/1.73 m$^2$. Furthermore, common side effects such as urinary tract and genital infections, and rare side effects such as euglycemic diabetic ketoacidosis in those with insulin deficiency,[704] bone fractures,[705] and amputation at the level of the toe or metatarsal,[637] have been reported.

Another class of glucose-lowering agents is the incretin analogues. In the Liraglutide Effect and Action in Diabetes: Evaluation of Cardiovascular Outcome Results (LEADER) trial[706] 9340 patients with type 2 diabetes and high cardiovascular risk were randomly assigned to liraglutide or placebo. In the 3.8 years of follow-up, the primary outcome of first occurrence of death from cardiovascular causes, nonfatal myocardial infarction, or nonfatal stroke was reduced by 13% (HR 0.87; 95% CI 0.78–0.97, $P$ = .01 for superiority). Fewer patients died from cardiovascular causes (HR 0.78; 95% CI 0.66–0.93, $P$ = .007) and the rate of death from any cause was also lower (HR 0.85; 95% CI 0.74–0.97, $P$ = .02). In subanalyses,[707] the effects of liraglutide on the primary cardiovascular outcome were only significant in the 24.7% of patients with an eGFR less than 60 ml/min/1.73 m$^2$. Importantly, because there were also prespecified kidney endpoints, the authors could also assess the effects of liraglutide on DKD. Liraglutide treatment resulted in a 22% reduction of the time to first kidney event, defined as an albumin-to-creatinine ratio of more than300 mg/g, doubling of serum creatinine, ESKD, or renal death (HR 0.78; 95% CI 0.67–0.92, $P$ = .003). This result was driven primarily by a lower incidence of new-onset persistent macroalbuminuria (HR 0.74; 95% CI 0.60–0.91, $P$ = .004), as there was no significant effect of liraglutide on the incidence of doubling of the serum creatinine concentration (HR 0.89; 95% CI 0.67–1.19, $P$ = .43), development of ESKD (HR 0.87; 95% CI 0.61–1.24), or death due to kidney disease (HR 1.59; 95% CI 0.52–4.87, $P$ = .41). Nevertheless, liraglutide was associated with a slower decline of eGFR during treatment, particularly in subgroups of patients who had evidence of kidney damage at baseline, and it highlights the need to investigate the potential role of communication between the gut and the kidney in the pathogenesis of DKD.[708]

## HYPOGLYCEMIA

The risk of hypoglycemia constitutes a major challenge in the management of DKD (Fig. 39.25).[709] Notably, in the ACCORD study, hypoglycemia in the intensively treated group was associated with an increase in mortality.[710] However, the authors could not demonstrate whether the hypoglycemia

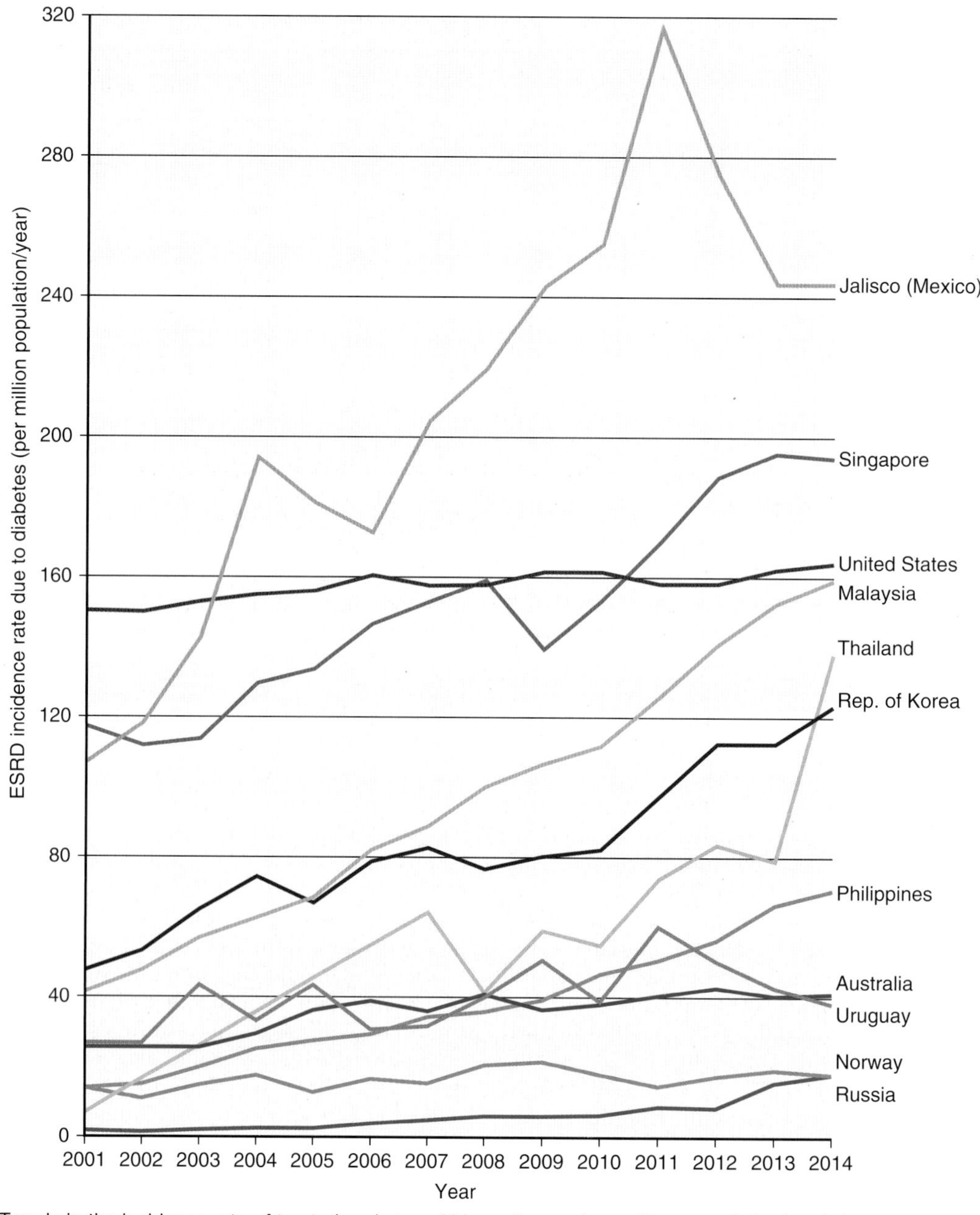


**Fig. 39.25** Trends in the incidence rate of treated end-stage kidney disease (per million population/year), by country, 2001 to 2014.[729]

itself was causative, but hypoglycemia remains a concern in the population with DKD, which constitutively carry a higher risk of hypoglycemia, cardiovascular events, and premature mortality. The reason for the increased risk of severe hypoglycemia in DKD[711] is accumulation of insulin in the circulation, inadequate compensatory gluconeogenesis, in particular during fasting, and flattening of the relationship between mean glucose control and $HbA_{1c}$. Age, an important risk factor for impaired renal function, further increases the risk of severe hypoglycemia, and given that half of the next generation type 2 diabetic patients will be above the age of 65 years, there will be a substantial proportion of patients with diabetes at risk of severe hypoglycemia. Therefore careful individualized glucose control targeting, antidiabetic medication prescription, patient education, and vigilance for hypoglycemia are all important components of the management of patients with DKD.

Data from trials[711] and epidemiological studies[712] have demonstrated the negative impact of a combination of severe hypoglycemia and DKD on the risk of premature mortality in patients with type 2 diabetes. One of the major obstacles to achieving optimal glucose control without running the risk of severe hypoglycemia is the mode of action of the majority of the currently used glucose-lowering agents; sulphonylureas, glinides and insulin all reduce the blood glucose concentration irrespective of the ambient glucose level. Consequently, there are only a limited number of glucose-lowering agents that are not associated with hypoglycemia that can be used in DKD. However, there are also other potential limitations with most of the available glucose-lowering agents, when

**Table 39.6 Potential Limitations of Glucose-Lowering Agents in Patients With Diabetic Kidney Disease**

| Drug | Limitations |
|---|---|
| Metformin | Dose modification required at reduced eGFR, discontinuation at low eGFR<br>Increased gastrointestinal side effects, hyperlactatemia, lactic acidosis |
| Sulphonylureas | Increased risk of hypoglycemia, accumulation of parent or active metabolites (with glibenclamide, glyburide, glimepiride), each require discontinuation at low eGFR |
| Thiazolidinediones | Fluid retention, increased risk of congestive heart failure |
| Dipeptidyl peptidase (DPP-4) inhibitors | Dose modification required (except linagliptin), possible heart failure |
| Glucagon-like peptide (GLP) 1 agonists | Discontinuation at low eGFR (exenatide), increased gastrointestinal side effects (nausea, vomiting, etc.) |
| Sodium glucose cotransporter (SGLT) 2 inhibitors | Reduced efficacy at low eGFR, hypovolemia, interaction with loop diuretics |
| Insulin | Increased risk of hypoglycemia, prolonged insulin half-life |

*eGFR*, Estimated glomerular filtration rate.

prescribed to patients with advanced DKD (Table 39.6).[650] The situation may change, however, with the novel glucose-lowering medications, dipeptidyl peptidase-4 (DPP-4) inhibitors, SGLT2-inhibitors and glucagon-like peptide-1 (GLP-1) agonists that may provide clinical benefits in the context of a lower risk of hypoglycemia. Whether SGLT2-inhibitors or GLP-1 agonists are efficacious and safe to use in patients with advanced kidney disease, however, remains to be demonstrated.

## LIPID-LOWERING THERAPY

The current ADA guidelines for the treatment of dyslipidaemia include an LDL-cholesterol goal of less than 70 to 100 mg/dl. All patients with DKD should be treated with a statin to prevent cardiovascular morbidity and mortality associated with DKD. Therefore the KDIGO Clinical Practice Guidelines recommend moderate-intensity therapy, with fixed dose and no additional measurements.[650,713] However, it is debatable if starting treatment may also decrease the risk of DKD in patients with diabetes and/or slow the progression of the disease. Although several studies suggest that different types of statins may reduce albuminuria and proteinuria, none of these studies have shown a significant impact on kidney function when administered alone[714] or in combination with ezetimibe.[715] The evidence that impairment of cholesterol efflux occurs in patients with DKD, and that this phenomenon may also play a key pathogenic role in the development of experimental DKD,[167,716,717] suggests the need to design new clinical trials specifically repurposing currently available agents targeting cholesterol efflux.[167] In addition, as cholesterol, triglycerides and lipid droplets all accumulate in the kidney cortex in clinical and experimental DKD, the role of niacin as well as fenofibrates in the renoprotection of DKD should be explored. Interestingly, although the Fenofibrate Intervention and Event Lowering in Diabetes (FIELD) trial was designed to test the effect of fenofibrate on retinal outcomes, the number of patients reaching ESKD was reduced in the fenofibrate group versus the placebo.[718] Finally, the response to novel agents such as the proprotein convertase subtilisin/kexin type 9 inhibitors and potentially the cholesteryl transfer protein inhibitors in patients with DKD also needs to be explored.[650]

## DIETARY PROTEIN RESTRICTION

A protein intake of 0.8 g/kg/day is currently recommended for patients affected by DKD, who have not yet reached ESKD.[8] The reduction of protein intake below this level, which was recommended previously, is no longer suggested. A 4-year prospective, randomized, controlled trial showed the beneficial effect of lowering protein intake to 0.6 g/kg/day in 82 patients with type 1 diabetes and progressive DKD (eGFR loss >7 ml/min/year), where the relative risk of ESKD or death was reduced from 27% in the control group to 10% in the low-protein diet group.[719] The authors concluded that moderate dietary protein restriction improves the prognosis of patients with type 1 diabetes and progressive kidney disease, and this was largely adopted by the guidelines. However, a review of multiple clinical trials that have examined the effects of protein restriction on DKD has not revealed consistently positive outcomes of such an intervention[720] and a too strict protein restriction may predispose to malnutrition and protein-energy-wasting, which are important risk factors for premature mortality.[10,758] Therefore the ADA guidelines state that protein intake at the level of 0.8 g/kg body weight per day slows the decline of the GFR with evidence of greater effect over time compared to higher levels of dietary protein. Notably, dietary protein intake of more than 1.3 g/kg/day or more than 20% of daily calories coming from protein, has been associated with increased albuminuria, more rapid kidney function loss, and cardiovascular mortality, and should therefore be avoided.[8] However, for patients already on dialysis, higher levels of dietary protein intake should be considered due to the imminent risk of malnutrition.

## MULTIFACTORIAL INTERVENTION

Multifactorial interventions focused on targeting hyperglycemia, blood pressure and healthy lifestyle through collaboration between interdisciplinary teams of physicians, educators, nurses, dieticians and private foundations have resulted in a significant reduction in the cumulative incidence of DKD in type 1 diabetes.[41] Similar beneficial effects are also reported in patients with type 2 diabetes and microalbuminuria at baseline.[648] Patients were either treated with an intensive multifactorial regimen (including statins, renin-angiotensin-aldosterone system blockade, aspirin and exercise) or conventional therapy. Notably, there was a clear reduction in the risk of reaching ESKD in the intensive treatment arm at both 4 and 8 years after the study started. Of note, this beneficial effect persisted 5 years after the trial was discontinued.[653]

## NEW COMPOUNDS UNDER INVESTIGATION

Novel compounds and medications that could impact the risk of DKD or reduce its progression are under investigation. A number of these compounds have failed to provide beneficial effects despite well-founded rationale and supporting experimental data. A complete review of these trials is beyond the scope of this chapter, but a number of ongoing trials are described later.

The effects of the selective $ET_A$ receptor blocker, atrasentan, on kidney outcomes are explored in patients with type 2 diabetes and DKD in the SONAR trial (NCT01858532).

The Preventing Early Renal Loss (PERL) trial (NCT02017171) is testing the potential of lowering uric acid with allopurinol as a renoprotective effect in individuals with type 1 diabetes.[319] However, as mentioned above, a recent study showed that uric acid may not be causally related to DKD, so any effects on the kidneys may arise from phenomena other than uric acid.[320]

A 90-day phase 2 trial[546] of finerenone, a novel nonsteroidal mineralocorticoid receptor antagonist with higher selectivity for the mineralocorticoid receptor than spironolactone, showed beneficial kidney effects in patients with type 2 diabetes. This trial paved the way for an ongoing phase 3 trial (NCT02545049).

Many signaling pathways are involved in the progression of chronic kidney disease. One of the major pathways that responds to and transduces inflammatory signals is the JAK-STAT pathway. Enhanced expression and augmented activity of JAK1, JAK2 and STAT3 promote DKD, and their inhibition appears to reduce disease.[721] Based on the evidence for JAK–STAT activation in DKD, baricitinib, a selective JAK1 and JAK2 inhibitor, was investigated in a 24-week phase 2, multicenter, randomized, double-blind, multidose, placebo-controlled study (NCT01683409) in patients with type 2 diabetes and reduced kidney function (eGFR 25–75 ml/min/1.73 $m^2$) and albuminuria (>300 mg/day), who were already treated with renin-angiotensin-aldosterone system inhibiting agents. Treatment with baricitinab resulted in a 40% reduction of albuminuria at both 3 and 6 months in the highest dose group. However, at 6 months there was also a decrease of hemoglobin concentration at the higher dose range, which was to be expected, since erythropoietin is dependent on JAK2 activation.[722] Therefore the question remains whether long-term administration of JAK-inhibitors is safe for the treatment of DKD[723].

Oxidative stress with increased generation of reactive oxygen species (ROS) has emerged as a critical mechanism in the pathogenesis of DKD. Interestingly, genetic targeting and pharmacologic inhibition of the NADPH oxidase Nox4 provided renoprotection in long-term DKD.[724] Deletion of Nox4, but not of Nox1, resulted in kidney protection from glomerular injury, and administration of the most specific Nox1/4 inhibitor, GKT137831, replicated these renoprotective effects of Nox4 deletion. Similar data in a mouse model resembling type 1 diabetes showed that GKT137831 significantly reduced glomerular hypertrophy, mesangial matrix expansion, urine albumin excretion, and podocyte loss.[725] Collectively, these studies identified Nox4 as a key source of ROS responsible for kidney injury in diabetes, and also provided proof of principle that GKT137831 could be a promising compound for the treatment of DKD in patients with type 1 diabetes. Indeed, GKT137831 showed considerable promise in its phase I trial in 100 patients with DKD, without major adverse effects. Consequently, a phase II trial was launched with 155 patients, but GKT137831 failed to reduce albuminuria. Whether this compound will be tested in any further trials is not known.

Chemokine (C-C motif) ligand-2 (CCL2) is the ligand of C-C motif receptor-2 (CCR2). CCL2/CCR2 signaling is suggested to play a significant role in DKD, and diabetes-induced albuminuria was improved after CCR2 antagonist treatment (RS102895). Although RS102895 did not affect blood pressure, body weight or kidney weight, it reduced mesangial expansion, and glomerular basement membrane thickening. It therefore seems that blockade of CCL2/CCR2 signaling by RS102895 may ameliorate DKD.[726] A recent study in patients with type 2 diabetes and macroalbuminuria investigated the potential albuminuria-lowering effect of the CCR2 antagonist, CCX140-B. A 12-week treatment at doses of 5 mg/day decreased albuminuria by 18% relative to placebo. The albuminuria-lowering effects persisted throughout the 52-week follow-up period, and 4 weeks after study drug discontinuation.[638] Whether CCR2 inhibitors will eventually be used for the management of patients with DKD remains to be seen.

The Pentoxifylline for Renoprotection in Diabetic Nephropathy (PREDIAN) study, an open-label, prospective, randomized trial in patients with type 2 diabetes and CKD stages 3–4, assigned pentoxifylline (1200 mg daily) to patients ($n = 82$) or to a control group ($n = 87$) for 2 years in addition to renin-angiotensin-aldosterone system inhibition. The study showed that the addition of pentoxifylline to renin-angiotensin-aldosterone inhibitors resulted in a smaller decrease in the eGFR and a greater reduction of the residual albuminuria.[727]

Overall, many clinical trials have been initiated based on encouraging efficacy and safety results from phase 2 trials. A summary of several targets being investigated in clinical trials is provided in Fig. 39.26.[728]

# END-STAGE KIDNEY DISEASE

## EPIDEMIOLOGY

People with diabetes carry the highest risk of ESKD, although hypertension, and glomerulonephritis are other common causes.[729] In recent decades, there has been a steady increase in the total number of patients with ESKD worldwide due to the increasing prevalence of diabetes. However, there are now encouraging data showing that although the prevalence of ESKD is still increasing, the incidence rates are stabilizing, and in some regions even decreasing.

## DEFINITIONS OF END-STAGE KIDNEY DISEASE IN PEOPLE WITH DIABETES

The diagnosis of ESKD is generally based on the initiation of renal replacement therapy (RRT), including dialysis or transplantation. However, many patients with diabetes and DKD will never reach the stage of ESKD because of cardiovascular comorbidities and premature death. This is due largely to the fact that the kidney and cardiac systems are inextricably linked, and an acute or chronic disorder of

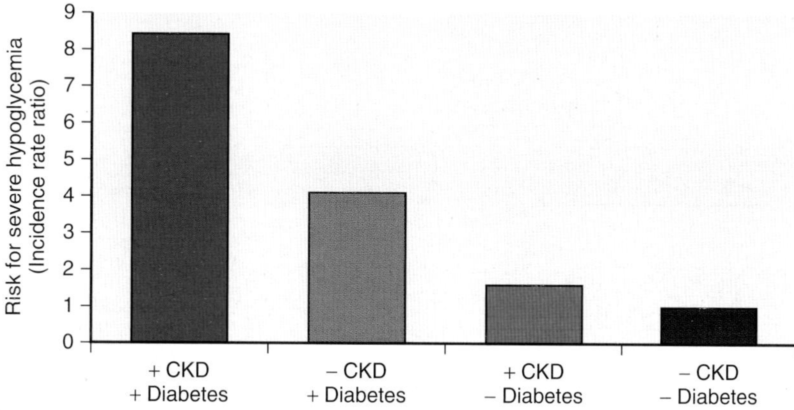


**Fig. 39.26 Impaired renal function is associated with increased risk of severe hypoglycemia in patients with type 2 diabetes.**[709] The incidence of severe hypoglycemia (blood glucose <50 mg/dL) was determined in a retrospective cohort of patients cared for at the Veterans Health Administration with (+) or without (-) chronic kidney disease (CKD), or diabetes, and expressed as an incidence rate ratio. The reference group are patients without CKD or diabetes.

one can induce dysfunction in the other.[730] Furthermore, elderly patients with diabetes and DKD are more likely to die of heart disease than advance to ESKD and dialysis.[731] Therefore the prevalence and incidence of ESKD in patients with diabetes are strongly influenced by competing causes of death. Differential mortality may also contribute to ethnicity-based disparities in diabetes-related ESKD. First Nations are the predominant aboriginal peoples of Canada, south of the Arctic. First Nations adults with ESKD are more likely than their non–First Nations counterparts to survive long enough to develop ESKD. After adjustment for sex and age at the time of diabetes diagnosis, the risk of ESKD was 2.66 times higher for First Nations than non–First Nations adults.[732] Similarly, the cumulative incidence of ESKD in Pima Indians with type 2 diabetes is 61% after 15 years of proteinuria compared with 17% after 15 years of proteinuria in Caucasians with type 2 diabetes. These differences are attributable to earlier age of onset of type 2 diabetes and lower death rates from coronary heart disease in the Pima Indians.[36]

## PREVALENCE OF END-STAGE KIDNEY DISEASE

ESKD confers a major burden on healthcare systems. According to the 2016 United States Renal Data System Annual Data Report, there were 678,383 prevalent dialysis and transplant patients (unadjusted prevalence rate of 2067 per million per year) in the United States at the end of 2014.[729] The proportion with diabetes as the primary cause of their ESKD was 37.9%. The adjusted prevalence of diabetic ESKD was 739 per million population (adjusted for age, sex, and race), and it continues to increase, although more gradually over the last 12 years. Nevertheless, DKD remains the leading contributor to the prevalence of ESKD in the United States. The prevalence varies among races and remains highest in blacks at 1986 per million, compared to 546 per million in whites.[729] The European Renal Association and the European Dialysis and Transplant Association reports that 478,990 people in Europe were receiving RRT at the end of 2013, for an overall prevalence of 738 patients per million population, 17% of whom had diabetes as the primary cause of kidney disease.[733]

## INCIDENCE OF END-STAGE KIDNEY DISEASE

Diabetes is a key contributor to the global burden of ESKD. In 2014, Singapore, Malaysia, and the Jalisco region of Mexico reported the highest proportion of patients with incident ESKD due to diabetes, at 66%, 63%, and 58% respectively.

Among the 23 countries or regions contributing data to the 2016 United States Renal Data System (USRDS) Annual Data Report,[729] incidence rates of ESKD due to diabetes more than doubled between 2001 and 2014 in Thailand, Russia, the Philippines, Malaysia, the Republic of Korea, and the Jalisco region of Mexico. Some of the countries with the largest increases are shown in Fig. 39.27.

A systematic review of 32 studies found that the incidence rates of ESKD due to any cause ranged from 132 to 167 per 100,000 person-years, whereas the incidence rates of ESKD due to diabetes varied between 38.4 and 804 per 100,000 person-years worldwide.[734] Moreover, higher incidence rates of ESKD due to diabetes were found in men as well as in blacks, Hispanics, Asians, and American Indians/First Nations people than in whites.[734] The relative risk of ESKD in diabetic populations compared to nondiabetic populations varied from 6.2 in whites to 62.0 in American Indians.[734] Notably, the incidence of ESKD due to diabetes is substantially higher in the United States than in Europe and Canada.[729] This discrepancy could be due to ethnic differences, but also to factors such as access to health care and management of ESKD risk factors.[735]

Studies from the United States have shown that after an increase during the 1980s and early 1990s,[736–738] the incidence rate of ESKD due to diabetes has decreased by approximately 3.9% per year between the mid-1990s and 2006.[736] These declines have continued through 2014 in older age groups, although they have been generally stable or increased slightly among younger individuals. Sex-adjusted incidence rates of ESKD among blacks are several-fold higher within each age category than among whites, although they are declining

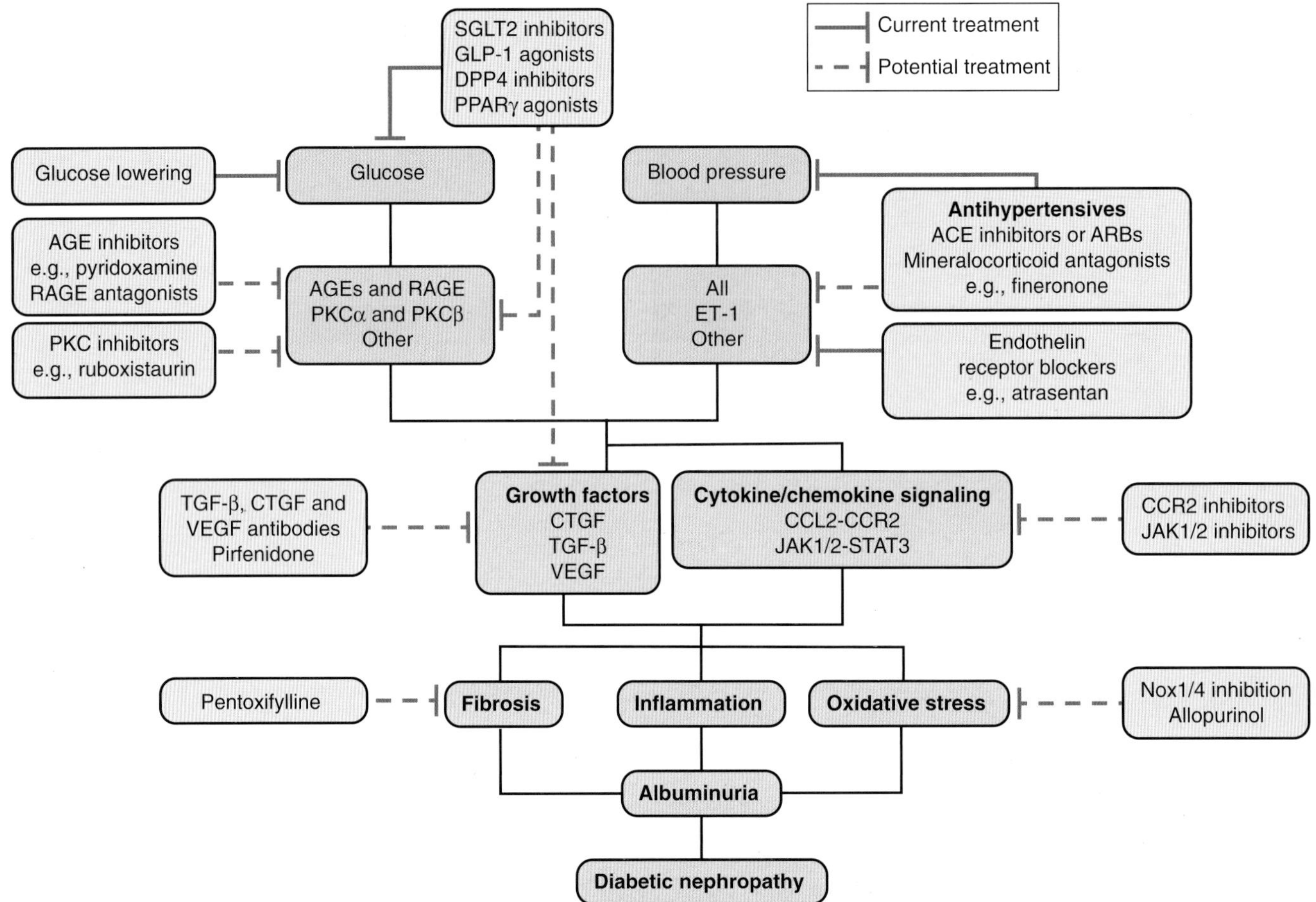


**Fig. 39.27 Putative pathways implicated in the pathogenesis of diabetic kidney disease, including established and potential new treatment strategies (*adapted*).**[728] Raised glucose and blood pressure activate various pathways that can be specifically targeted in order to reduce the classic pathological hallmarks of diabetic nephropathy, fibrosis, inflammation, and albuminuria. *ACE*, Angiotensin-converting enzyme; *AGE*, advanced glycation end product; *ARB*, angiotensin receptor blocker; *CTGF*, connective tissue growth factor; *DPP4 inhibitor*, dipeptidyl peptidase-4 inhibitor; *ET-1*, endothelin 1; *GLP-1*, glucagon-like peptide 1; *PKC*, protein kinase C; *PPARγ*, peroxisome proliferator-activated receptor γ; *RAGE*, receptor for *AGE*; *TGF-β*, transforming growth factor β; *VEGF*, vascular endothelial growth factor. Red dotted lines are added to interventions that are being tested or have recently been tested. Black arrows point to drugs targeting a specific pathway. In addition to the potential treatments shown in the original figure, finerenone is a mineralocorticoid receptor antagonist that may enhance the effect of renin-angiotensin system blockers in diabetic kidney disease (DKD) without adversely affecting serum potassium concentrations. Pyridoxamine, allopurinol, pentoxifylline, and inhibitors of Nox1-4, Janus kinase (JAK1 and JAK2), and the chemokine ligand of C-C motif receptor-2 (CCR2) may also favorably effect DKD progression through various signaling pathways involving inflammation, fibrosis, and/or oxidative stress.

more quickly in blacks than in whites. In addition, incidence rates of ESKD due to diabetes among Hispanics are similar to those for whites for ages 22 to 44 years, but are much higher than for whites for ages 44 and above. Incidence rates of ESKD due to diabetes stabilized earlier in Europe than in the United States[739–741] and have also declined in Europe since 2007, but the decline is not statistically significant.[733]

Considering the rising incidence of type 2 diabetes in Europe and the USA,[742] it is surprising that the incidence rates of ESKD due to diabetes have stabilized in Europe around 32 per million people and have actually fallen in the United States from 175 to 156 per million people. These data suggest that well-structured programs for treatment of chronic kidney disease can reduce the incidence of ESKD and perhaps ultimately the prevalence.[743] However, the prevalence will no doubt continue to increase for some time to come. There are several explanations for this. First, there is a lag time between changes in incidence and subsequent changes in prevalence. Second, some countries will continue to increase RRT acceptance rates due to social and economic progress. Third, the age of the background population will continue to increase, resulting in a greater difference between the standardized and actual incidence rates, and fourth, improved survival in patients with cardiovascular disease may increase the incidence of ESKD. Finally, the RRT survival rates may continue to increase.[743]

There are very few studies that have reported cumulative incidence rates of ESKD in people with diabetes. One exception is a report from Finland in patients with type 1 diabetes that showed a 30-year cumulative incidence ranging from 3.3% to 7.8%.[744]

## ACUTE AND ACUTE-ON-CHRONIC RENAL FAILURE

An imminent problem in patients with DKD at advanced stages of chronic kidney disease is the risk of acute kidney injury (AKI) in addition to chronic kidney disease.[767] In a retrospective analysis of the General Practice Research Database (UK) of 119,966 patients with type 2 diabetes compared with 1,794,516 nondiabetic individuals, the yearly incidence rate of AKI was 198 versus 27 per 100,000 subjects, and the difference remained statistically significant even after adjustment for other well-known AKI risk factors and comorbidities.[768] In another retrospective analysis based on the Society of Thoracic Surgeons National Database of 449,524 individuals, 33% of whom had diabetes, multivariate logistic analysis revealed diabetes as an independent risk factor for AKI after cardiac surgery.[769] Baseline GFR of less than 60 ml/min/1.73 $m^2$, the use of iodinated contrast media, hypotension, concomitant use of nephrotoxic drugs as well as diabetes (odds ratio 2.13; 95% CI, 1.01–4.49; $P = .046$) were independent AKI risk factors in a prospective study of 980 patients undergoing aminoglycoside treatment.[770] In a prospective case-control study of 318 patients with diabetes compared with 746 nondiabetic control subjects suffering from either severe septicemia or septic shock, the patients with diabetes required dialysis more often although the AKI incidence rates were similar.[771] Taken together, these data demonstrate that the risk of AKI is particularly high in patients with diabetes.

The question why patients with diabetes are especially prone to develop AKI is not fully understood, but the kidneys are in general extremely sensitive to hypoxia. Because diabetes and hyperglycemia per se cause intrarenal hypoxia, particularly in the proximal tubule cells, the diabetic milieu itself may be the culprit.[772] Experimental studies in mice have shown that as early as three days after induction of diabetes, there is pronounced and persistent intrarenal hypoxia accompanied by glomerular hyperfiltration.[773] In rats, the administration of the mitochondrial uncoupler, dinitrophenol, induced intrarenal hypoxia through increased total kidney oxygen consumption, that in turn was associated with proteinuria, increased kidney vimentin expression (cell damage) and infiltration of inflammatory cells, all hallmarks of DKD.[774] Importantly, the main driver of intrarenal oxygen consumption is sodium handling in the proximal tubule, and any increase in kidney blood flow is likely to result in a simultaneous increase in tubular electrolyte load due to increased GFR.[772,775] Therefore any increase in active tubular transport *per se* increases energy demand and results in increased kidney oxygen consumption. Altogether, increased intrarenal oxygen metabolism will inevitably result in kidney tissue hypoxia and potentially contribute to the development of AKI observed in patients with DKD. Potentially, hyperglycemia-induced intrarenal hypoxia might also contribute to the pathogenesis of DKD.

In clinical practice, it is important to recognize the most common causes of AKI, which are renal artery stenosis, inappropriate usage and dosage of RAAS-inhibitors, emergency cardiac interventions, administration of radiocontrast agents, septicemia, low cardiac output, and shock. Therefore patients should be carefully assessed before undergoing any invasive cardiologic intervention or radio-contrast examinations. Adequate preparation of the patient with saline infusion and temporary interruption of diuretics and other potentially harmful agents (e.g., metformin) may prevent kidney injury. However, not infrequently, AKI necessitates hemodialysis and might lead to irreversible kidney damage and even increased risk of premature death. AKI therefore remains a clinical and prognostic problem of fundamental importance, although the acute mortality is comparable following an AKI episode in diabetic patients compared with that in a nondiabetic cohort.[776]

## MANAGEMENT OF PATIENTS WITH END-STAGE KIDNEY DISEASE

An individual with diabetes and ESKD may be treated with hemodialysis, peritoneal dialysis and/or transplantation (kidney alone, simultaneous pancreas-kidney and pancreas after kidney). Details on general patient management with these modalities are discussed in Chapters 63, 64, and 70.

*Clinical Relevance*

**End-Stage Kidney Disease**

Physicians taking care of patients with advanced diabetic kidney disease will face a broad spectrum of therapeutic challenges such as hypertension, fluid overload, risk of severe hypoglycemia, cardiovascular comorbidities, malnutrition, diabetic foot problems, autonomic neuropathy, anemia, metabolic acidosis, disturbances of calcium and phosphorus metabolism, and osteodystrophy. Treatment should address these challenges, preserving residual renal function, implementing early transplant referral and preparing for future renal replacement therapy. Although $HbA_{1c}$ is problematic in patients with advanced kidney disease, it is still considered the gold standard. Intradialytic blood pressure phenomena have important prognostic bearing for the patient, and frequent blood pressure measurements are necessary to ensure the patient's safety during hemodialysis.

### INITIATION OF RENAL REPLACEMENT THERAPY

It was previously suggested that patients with diabetes benefited from an early dialysis start, but there is no strong evidence for this belief,[783] and the Initiating Dialysis Early and Late (IDEAL) trial provided strong evidence against it. This landmark randomized, controlled trial of early versus late initiation of dialysis in 828 adults showed that early initiation with stage 5 chronic kidney disease was not associated with an improvement in survival or clinical outcomes.[784] Of note, 33.9% in the early-start group and 34.0% in the late-start group had diabetes as the primary cause of ESKD, and 42.6% and 43.2%, respectively, had diabetes as a coexisting condition.[784]

#### Hemodialysis

Survival rates of both diabetic and nondiabetic patients with ESKD have improved over the years.[785–787] However, patient survival among patients with diabetes on maintenance dialysis is still inferior to survival of nondiabetic patients with ESKD caused by chronic glomerular disease or hypertension,[788–790] although there is no difference between patients with diabetes as primary renal disease or as a comorbid condition.[791] Both diabetic conditions are associated with increased risk of premature mortality compared to nondiabetic patients.[791] According to the 2016 USRDS, adjusted survival in 2013 based on a primary diagnosis of diabetes was 93.9% and 81.5% at 3 and 12 months.[729] Notably, survival varies with age, being the best in young patients with optimal blood pressure control and no clinically evident cardiac disease.[790,792]

Management of patients with DKD on dialysis includes a broad spectrum of therapeutic challenges. There is high risk of cardiovascular morbidity and mortality as well as challenges in managing intradialytic blood pressure, glycaemic control and accurately monitoring glycaemic control.

## CARDIOVASCULAR PROBLEMS

Patients with diabetes have a 5- to13-fold increased risk of ESKD compared with the general population,[793–795] and ESKD increases the risk of death many fold.[9,338,796] The excess mortality among the patients with diabetes appears to be largely limited to the subgroup with kidney disease and explained by their high burden of cardiovascular disease[338,339,341] (Fig. 39.28).[338] Thus it is not unexpected that the risk of premature death is the highest in those with ESKD with adjusted standardized mortality rates ranging from 18% to 38%.[338,339]

Left ventricular hypertrophy and congestive heart failure, which predominantly result from diastolic dysfunction, are highly prevalent among patients receiving RRT, including those with DKD. Left ventricular hypertrophy is estimated to affect 74% of patients with ESKD who are receiving RRT and congestive heart failure will affect about 31% of these patients.[797,798] In addition, heart failure, sudden cardiac death and ischemic and hemorrhagic stroke rates are markedly increased among all patients with ESKD.[816–819] A large study from Taiwan examined 648,851 individuals without ESKD and 71,397 with ESKD, including 53,342 and 34,754 patients with diabetes, respectively, between 1998 and 2009. This study showed a multiplicatively synergistic effect of diabetes and ESKD for cardiovascular risk, especially for acute myocardial infarction and stroke, of which the adjusted hazard ratios were 5.24 (95% CI 4.83–5.68) and 2.43 (2.32–2.55), respectively.[799] Altogether, these data indicate that diabetes and ESKD synergistically increase the risks of cardiovascular events many-fold.

Proactive screening is therefore of utmost importance and should lead to detection and treatment of not only traditional but also unique ESKD-related risk factors for atherosclerosis in the daily clinical practice. Notably, diabetes and ESKD share several risk factors for atherosclerosis such as hypertension, hyperlipidemia, endothelial dysfunction, oxidative stress and insulin resistance.[800–802] The management of these traditional risk factors are to some extent already part of standard care. However, there are also some unique risk factors in ESKD patients, such as an imbalanced calcium and phosphate metabolism, uremic toxins, hypervolemia and hemodialysis itself, which all contribute to cardiovascular disease.[803–806] These unique risk factors should also be addressed in order to minimize the risk of cardiovascular events in patients with diabetes on dialysis.

## INTRADIALYTIC BLOOD PRESSURE

*Intradialytic hypotension.* Patients with DKD are in general more hypertensive than non-diabetic patients undergoing dialysis, because blood pressure is highly volume-dependent in diabetes. However, these patients are also prone to intradialytic hypotension due to autonomic neuropathy and disturbed left ventricular compliance that may lead to an abrupt decrease in the cardiac output, when the left ventricular filling pressure is reduced by the ultrafiltration.[804,807] There are a large number of risk factors that make the patient prone to hypotension, and most of these factors are particularly detrimental and problematic in patients with diabetes. Such patient-related factors are autonomic neuropathy, antihypertensive medication, cardiovascular disease, pericardial effusion, peripheral vascular disease and meal ingestion. Hemodialysis-related factors are low dialysate sodium concentration, low dialysate calcium concentration, low plasma osmolality, warm dialysate and acetate buffer.[808] Too aggressive ultrafiltration and inaccurate target weight are also important contributors, as are anemia, hypoxia and active infection. The physiologic compensatory mechanisms in response to hypotension are increase in cardiac output, plasma refill,

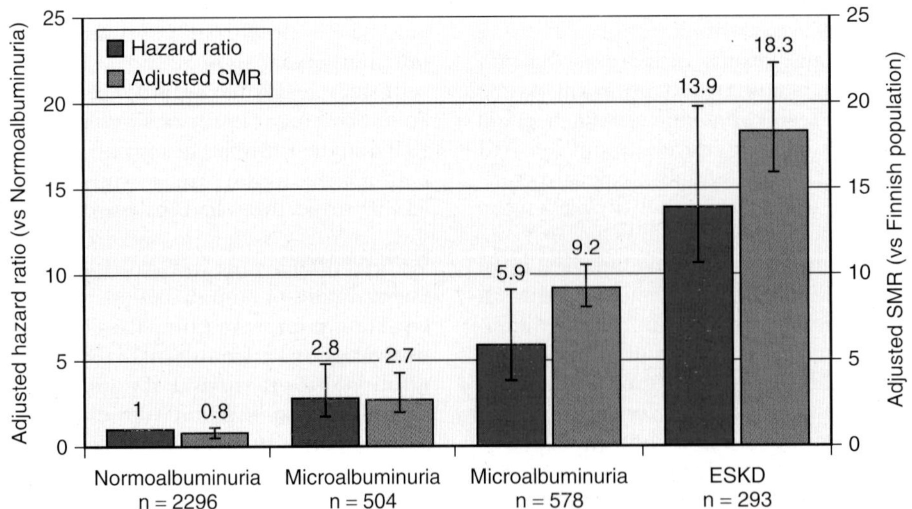


**Fig. 39.28 Risk of mortality in individuals with type 1 diabetes from the FinnDiane study associated with each level of albuminuria or end-stage kidney disease (ESKD).[338] Adjusted hazard ratios with 95% confidence intervals (CIs) are standardized against individuals with urine albumin excretion in the normoalbuminuric range (arbitrary value of 1.0). Adjusted standardized mortality ratios (with 95% CIs are provided standardized against the age- and sex-matched Finnish general population (arbitrary value of 1.0).**

passive venoconstriction and an increase in arterial tone,[807] but in patients with diabetes these compensatory mechanisms may be delayed or dysfunctional due to autonomic neuropathy. The management of intradialytic hypotension is discussed further in Chapter 63.

*Intradialytic hypertension and blood pressure variability.* Intradialytic hypertension, occurs in the range of 5% to15% in patients on maintenance hemodialysis.[809,810] In addition, blood pressure deviations from the expected course are defined as blood pressure variability, a phenomenon that has recently been shown to be another prognostic factor. Intradialytic blood pressure variability refers to such fluctuations that are independent of other blood pressure phenomena generally occurring during dialysis. In a study of 6393 prevalent hemodialysis patients, there was an association between greater intradialytic systolic blood pressure variability and increased all-cause and cardiovascular mortality.[811] The pathophysiology is not well-defined, but there are some plausible mediators such as endothelial dysfunction, chronic inflammation, increased blood vessel wall stress, baroreceptor dysfunction, enhanced sympathetic activity,[812] all factors that are associated with DKD. In clinical practice, it is therefore prudent to minimize large blood pressure fluctuations by carefully monitoring hemodynamics, volume status and medications effects.[808] This topic is discussed further in Chapter 63.

## GLYCEMIC CONTROL

The treatment of diabetes in ESKD patients is challenging, given the changes in glucose homeostasis, the unclear accuracy of glycemic control metrics, and the altered pharmacokinetics of glucose-lowering drugs by kidney dysfunction, the uremic milieu, and dialysis therapy.[813] Thus maintenance dialysis patients may experience both hyperglycemia and hypoglycemia through multifactorial mechanisms relating to the kidney dysfunction, the uremic environment, and the dialysis procedure. The role of improved glycemic control in ameliorating the exceedingly high mortality risk of diabetic patients on dialysis is unclear.[813]

Large observational studies suggest that a J-shaped relationship exists between HbA1c levels and the risk of hospitalization and all-cause mortality in patients with either type 1 or type 2 diabetes, who are receiving hemodialysis.[814–819] Among 9201 diabetic hemodialysis patients from 12 countries in the Dialysis Outcomes and Practice Patterns Study, mortality was the lowest in those with HbA1c levels of 7.0% to 7.9%, and increased progressively with either higher or lower levels, indicating that ideal HbA1c levels encompassed values that were somewhat higher than those recommended in existing guidelines.[816] Patients with indicators of poor nutritional status and lower HbA1c were particularly vulnerable to increased mortality. The ideal HbA1c range, however, varies by study and may be affected by several factors, including race and ethnicity. Among 2300 Japanese diabetic patients receiving hemodialysis, the lowest mortality was found among those with HbA1c levels of 6.0% to 7.0%.[820] A similar relationship between HbA1c and mortality was reported among 2,798 diabetic patients receiving peritoneal dialysis, in whom the glucose in dialysate fluid potentially exposes them to an additional glycemic burden.[821]

Although there are no clinical trials assessing the benefits of glycemic control in diabetic patients receiving renal replacement therapy, adjusting glucose lowering medications to achieve target HbA1c levels ascertained from observational studies may improve health outcomes. Poor glycemic control during hemodialysis is associated with higher all-cause and cardiovascular mortality post-transplantation, further emphasizing the importance of glycemic control in diabetic patients on dialysis.[822]

Interestingly, up to one-third of patients with diabetes on dialysis may experience spontaneous resolution of the hyperglycemia with HbA1c concentrations less than 6%. This phenomenon is known as *burnt-out diabetes*, but its biologic plausibility and clinical implications are undetermined.[813] Low A1c concentrations may to some extent be due to the inherent problems with glycemic control metrics in the patients with advanced DKD and ESKD as discussed earlier.

Despite the fact that the conventional methods of glycemic control assessment are confounded by laboratory abnormalities and comorbidities associated with the uremic state, the Kidney Disease Quality Outcomes Initiative (KDOQI) and the Kidney Disease Improving Global Outcomes (KDIGO) clinical practice guidelines still recommend routine measurement of long-term glycemic control using HbA1c in combination with home blood glucose monitoring.[7,823] There is, however, uncertainty regarding the optimal glycemic target in the dialysis patients. The KDOQI and KDIGO clinical practical guidelines recommend that the HbA1c target should be raised to 7% in patients with comorbidities, limited life expectancy, and in those at risk of severe hypoglycemia.[824]

*Glucose-lowering medication.* Although endogenously secreted insulin is primarily degraded by the liver and to some extent also excreted by the kidneys, the exogenous insulin is primarily excreted by the kidneys.[825] Exogenous insulin can be given to patients on dialysis, but insulin dose reductions of up to 50% are recommended.[825–827] Sulfonylureas stimulate insulin secretion irrespective of the ambient glucose concentration, and patients on dialysis may therefore run the risk of severe hypoglycemia. Most clinicians avoid the use of such agents in patients on dialysis.[825] The biguanide metformin should not be prescribed to patients with an eGFR less than 30 ml/min/1.73 m[2824] or patients on dialysis because of the risk of lactic acidosis. This risk is exaggerated by the fact that approximately 90% of the metformin is excreted by the kidneys.[828] The thiazolidinediones may promote edema, increased bone loss and fractures, and are therefore problematic in patients on dialysis despite their positive effect on glucose control.[825] Alpha-glucosidase inhibitors delay glucose absorption in the gastrointestinal tract and thereby reduce postprandial glucose peaks.[824,829] However, gastrointestinal side-effects such as abdominal pain, diarrhea and flatulence have discouraged their use, and although only less than2% of the alpha-glucosidase inhibitor acarbose and its active metabolites are excreted by the kidneys, their use in patients on dialysis is not recommended. This is mainly due to lack of data in this patient population. Miglitol is another compound that is excreted by the kidneys, and thereby not indicated for patients on dialysis.[813]

Newer glucose-lowering medications, such as DPP-4 inhibitors, SGLT2-inhibitors and GLP-1 agonists, are promising agents since they do not cause severe hypoglycemia. SGLT2-inhibitors improve glycemic control by inhibiting proximal tubular reabsorption of filtered glucose and thus promoting excretion of glucose by the kidneys,[830] but decreasing eGFR reduces the ability to inhibit glucose reabsorption.[831]

SGLT2-inhibitors are not indicated for patients on dialysis, since, on one hand, there is a lack of long-term safety and efficacy data in patients with ESKD, and, on the other hand, SGLT2-inhibitors are not anticipated to promote significant effects in patients with eGFR less than 30 ml/min/1.73 $m^2$ or in patients on dialysis.[832]

Some of the drugs affecting the incretin system can be used in patients on dialysis. DPP-4 is an enzyme expressed on the surface of various types of cells that deactivates GLP-1, a hormone that stimulates glucose-dependent insulin release. DPP-4 inhibitors promote insulin release by increasing GLP-1 availability.[833] The DPP-4 inhibitor class includes, among others, linagliptin, sitagliptin, vildagliptin, saxagliptin and alogliptin. Linagliptin is different from the other DPP-4 inhibitors in that it is only minimally (5%) excreted in the urine, whereas the other DPP-4 inhibitors are mainly excreted via the kidneys.[834–837] Therefore linagliptin does not accumulate in the circulation in patients with ESKD, and can be given to patients on dialysis without dosage adjustment.[835] However, the other DPP-4 inhibitors require dose adjustments before use in patients on dialysis. In a small retrospective study of 200 ESKD patients with type 2 diabetes on renal replacement therapy (115 on hemodialysis), who were treated with DPP-4 inhibitors sitagliptin (44 patients), vildagliptin (72 patients), and linagliptin (84 patients) were analyzed retrospectively, and there was no significant difference in the glucose-lowering effect between the different DPP-4 inhibitors tested.[838]

Exenatide and liraglutide are GLP-1 agonists that not only facilitate insulin secretion but also decrease glucagon secretion, delay gastric emptying, and promote early satiety and weight loss.[825] Exenatide is excreted by the kidneys and is thus not recommended in patients with a eGFR less than 30 ml/min 1.73 $m^2$ or in patients on dialysis. Liraglutide is neither metabolized nor eliminated by the kidneys, therefore liraglutide treatment in patients with type 2 diabetes and ESKD may be continued, although dose reduction and prolongation of the titration period is advisable.[839] A small study in 24 patients with type 2 diabetes and ESKD showed that glycemic control tended to improve after 12 weeks of exposure to liraglutide. However, the plasma liraglutide concentrations increased and the patients experienced more gastrointestinal side effects during treatment.[839]

## MONITORING OF GLYCEMIC CONTROL IN PATIENTS ON DIALYSIS

A real challenge in clinical practice is the monitoring of glycemic control in patients on dialysis. This is because the glycation rate of the hemoglobin molecule, a long-term measure of glycemic control (120 days), is influenced by a number of factors, some of which are also related to the ESKD. Thus HbA1c is influenced by: (1) the duration of glucose exposure, (2) the glucose concentration, (3) the hemoglobin concentration, (4) the pH, and (5) the temperature.[813] An elevated blood urea nitrogen concentration and metabolic acidosis are confounders that falsely increase the HbA1c concentration,[752,755,840] whereas anemia, blood transfusions, hemoglobinopathies and other disorders of shortened erythrocyte lifespan, erythropoietin-stimulating agents and protein-energy wasting are confounders that falsely decrease the HbA1c concentration.[755,815,841]

Fructosamine is a measure of intermediate-term glycemic control (approximately 7–14 days), but although fructosamine may be a more accurate measure of glycemic control in anemic patients on dialysis, it may also be confounded by a number of factors, such as altered serum protein states (i.e., peritoneal dialysate protein loss), malnutrition, hepatic disease, thyroid dysfunction, pregnancy, hyperuricemia, smoking and steroid use.[813]

Whereas fructosamine is a measure of all glycated serum proteins, glycated albumin is formed by a nonenzymatic reaction between glucose and albumin.[755,841,842] Glycated albumin is also a measure of intermediate-term glycemic control (7–14 days) and is robust in conditions of anemia and shortened erythrocyte lifespan but may be confounded by the same factors as fructosamine.[813]

Although fructosamine and glycated albumin have prompted much interest and may be more reliable measures of glycemic control than HbA1c, they have not superceded HbA1c measurements yet. Further studies are needed in order to assess their role in clinical practice.

### Peritoneal Dialysis

Many clinicians favor continuous ambulatory peritoneal dialysis (CAPD) for the treatment of diabetic ESKD for several reasons as discussed in Chapter 64. One obvious reason is that the forearm blood vessels of patients with diabetes are often affected by severe atherosclerosis, so that it is impossible to place a fistula. Another reason is that, at least as the initial mode of renal replacement therapy, survival may be better for diabetic patients treated with peritoneal dialysis than those treated with hemodialysis, with the exception of older patients.[843,844] However, although many studies have compared the clinical outcomes of diabetic patients undergoing peritoneal dialysis with those on hemodialysis, only a small number of diabetic patients have been followed up for more than 5 years on peritoneal dialysis. This is due largely to the presence of comorbid conditions at the start of dialysis and the coexistence of advanced target-organ damage, both of which are also factors that impact the choice of treatment modality and may confound any comparison between treatment modalities due to bias by selection. A recent long-term study illustrated that diabetes was a main factor shortening survival time, both in patients on peritoneal dialysis as well as on hemodialysis. When dialysis vintage over 4 years was considered, hemodialysis showed no outcome benefit over peritoneal dialysis.[845]

Problems related to the peritoneal membrane that specifically affect patients with diabetes must be considered. Apart from protein loss across the membrane, high glucose concentration in the dialysate leads to calorie gain, increased body weight and obesity with subsequent worsening of the metabolic state and further increased risk of cardiovascular comorbidities. Also important is that heat sterilization of glucose solutions creates highly reactive glucose degradation products, which are cytotoxic and contribute to the formation of advanced glycation end-products.[846] In general, advanced glycation end-products are formed by spontaneous chemical reactions between carbohydrates and tissue proteins, a reaction that is accentuated in patients with diabetes because of hyperglycemia and is speeded up by heating (browning reaction). These nonenzymatic reactions, that are known as Maillard or browning reactions, are also implicated in the development of age-related diseases such as diabetes, atherosclerosis, dialysis-related amyloidosis, and scarring of the lining of the abdominal wall and thus the peritoneal membrane with subsequent ultrafiltration failure.[847] In addition to their immediate effects on protein structure and function, advanced glycation end-products further induce oxidative stress, leading to inflammation and propagation of tissue damage.[848] In peritoneal dialysis patients using icodextrin, falsely elevated glucose concentrations are reported by glucose self-monitoring systems based on glucose dehydrogenase pyrroloquinoline quinone when compared to those based on glucose dehydrogenase nicotinamide adenine dinucleotide. The glucose dehydrogenase pyrroloquinoline quinone self-monitoring systems should not be used in peritoneal dialysis patients to avoid overinjection of insulin and hypoglycemia.[849]

### Transplantation

Whether kidney transplantation in comparison with long-term dialysis improves survival among patients with ESKD is controversial because any comparisons are subject to bias by indication; those selected for transplantation may have a lower baseline risk of premature death.[850] However, among patients with ESKD, healthier patients are generally placed on the waiting list for transplantation, and long-term survival is better for those on the waiting list, who eventually undergo kidney transplantation.[850] Thus kidney transplantation should be the ultimate goal for any patient with ESKD unless the risk associated with the operation outweighs the benefits.

One-year survival rates for kidney transplantation in patients with diabetes is now approaching 88% for deceased donors and 96% for living donors.[851] However, pancreas transplantation has become increasingly successful in recent years due to advances in surgical procedures and immunosuppression.[852,853] One-year pancreas graft survival is now nearly 95% when performed as a simultaneous pancreas-kidney transplantation, and 86% when performed as a pancreas after kidney alone transplantation.[854]

Simultaneous pancreas-kidney transplantation has revolutionized the way individuals with type 1 diabetes are managed, given that this treatment not only provides the physiological means to achieve normal glycemic control but also corrects the uremic state and renders the patients free of dialysis. Data show that the 5- and 10-year patient survival rates for simultaneous pancreas-kidney transplantation are 87% and 70%, respectively.[855] This treatment option has improved the observed lifespan compared with diabetic cadaveric and diabetic live-donor kidney transplant recipients, and has significantly reduced the annual mortality rates.[856] It is now generally accepted that simultaneous pancreas-kidney transplantation prolongs survival beyond the survival advantage associated with kidney transplantation alone in patients with type 1 diabetes.

## CARDIOVASCULAR DISEASE BEFORE KIDNEY TRANSPLANTATION

Candidates for kidney transplantation should undergo an extensive evaluation to identify risk factors that may have an adverse effect on their outcome. Thus emphasis should be put on the detection and treatment of all coexisting medical problems that may increase the risk of morbidity and mortality associated with the surgical procedure and consequently adversely impact the post-transplant course. In addition to a thorough medical examination, social issues to determine conditions that may jeopardize the outcome of the transplantation, such as a pattern of noncompliance, should be considered and addressed. A complete cardiac workup, including angiography, may not be necessary in every single transplant candidate, but patients with a significant history of cardiovascular disease, symptoms, type 1 or type 2 diabetes, or hypertensive kidney disease should undergo a thorough evaluation to rule out significant coronary artery disease.

## CARDIOVASCULAR DISEASE AFTER KIDNEY TRANSPLANTATION

By 36 months after a kidney transplantation, nearly 40% of the patients have experienced a cardiovascular event.[857] In this regard, acute myocardial infarction is particularly common in patients with diabetes and in the elderly,[858] but after infections, congestive heart failure is the most common cause of hospital admissions after renal transplantation.[857] Therefore the management of cardiovascular disease after transplantation should include modifying risk factors that contribute to congestive heart failure as well as ischemic heart disease. Such modifiable risk factors are glucose control, obesity, hypertension, hyperlipidemia, and smoking, whereas gender, age, and family history are nonmodifiable risk factors. Also, immunosuppression, anemia, proteinuria, and chronic inflammation may contribute to the development of cardiovascular disease after kidney transplantation[859] and should be both considered and addressed.

## ISLET CELL TRANSPLANTATION

Several experimental studies in rodents suggest a beneficial effect of islet cell transplantation for the reversal of early DKD.[860–863] In addition, islet cell transplantation in diabetic rodents, unlike insulin treatment, may protect the kidney from the development of thickening of the glomerular basement membrane,[864,865] although more severe diabetic glomerulopathy in rats does not improve following islet transplantation.[866] The first suggestion that islet cell transplantation may prevent albuminuria in the clinical setting came from a 10-year observational study in 10 patients with type 1 diabetes, who received cryopreserved fetal pancreatic islets, and who had a longitudinal follow-up of 10 years, and were compared with 27 patients who remained on insulin. Patients were not randomized, however, and strong selection bias may have influenced the results of this initial study,[867] because criteria for patient selection for islet transplantation are usually quite strict.[868] In a subsequent study, 36 patients with type 1 diabetes who underwent kidney-islet transplantation and had 4 years of follow-up were divided into two groups, those with successful and those with unsuccessful islet transplants. Overall, successful islet transplantation was associated with improvement in kidney function.[869] In a similar study of 42 patients with type 1 diabetes, the same authors demonstrated that successful islet and kidney transplantation was associated with improved cardiovascular function, when compared to kidney transplant alone.[870] In a longitudinal natural history study of islet transplant alone, a variable degree of proteinuria and eGFR changes were observed, with a worse outcome when tacrolimus and sirolimus were used in combination.[871] Very limited prospective studies are, however, available. In a prospective crossover study comparing islet transplantation to medical treatment, a similar rate of decline of eGFR was observed over a median of 29 months,[872] whereas protection from progressive retinopathy in the absence of a significant effect on eGFR was reported by others.[873] Patient selection and aggressive clinical management seem to be key factors for stable renal function after islet transplantation.[874] More recently, a small study in 12 recipients of allogenic islets demonstrated stable eGFR over 10.7 years of follow-up. Overall, however, islet transplantation alone has been largely abandoned and more sophisticated procedures, such as transplantation of encapsulated islets, xenotransplantation and stem cell–based approaches are being investigated.

## STEM CELL TRANSPLANTATION

The use of mesenchymal stem cell treatment to manage onset and progression of DKD is a recent development,[875] and the contribution of different circulating progenitor cell lineages to the development of microvascular complications has also gained attention.[876,877] At this stage, it is unclear if stem cell transplantation or pharmacological modulation of local kidney progenitor cell growth would be a better strategy to treat DKD.[878] The latter approach is being studied in a clinical trial, where the effect of linagliptin on endothelial progenitor cells in relation to cardiovascular protection is being investigated in patients with type 2 diabetes (ClinicalTrials.gov identifier: NCT02467478).

Although no studies have yet addressed the role of embryonic stem cells in DKD, developments around human cord blood mesenchymal stem cells (hCB-MSCs) are interesting. In experimental DKD using a murine model of streptozotocin-induced diabetes, infusion of CB-MNCs resulted in a significant improvement in serum creatinine, in blood urea nitrogen and in albumin/creatinine ratio, when compared with controls.[879]

Adult stem cells also represent an interesting development. Several studies have emphasized a critical role for bone marrow hematopoietic stem cells (HSCs), and bone marrow mesenchymal stem cells (BM-MSCs) in promoting kidney repair after injury because of their capacity for recruitment to injured areas through local release of chemokines.[880] Once recruited, these cells seem to play a major role in facilitating the development of local progenitor cells rather than in their direct differentiation into kidney cells. Infusion of BM-MSCs via the left renal artery was able to prevent kidney injury and to reduce podocyte loss in STZ-treated rats.[881] Interestingly, BM-MSCs from bone marrow of mice with glomerulosclerosis are sufficient to transmit the glomerulosclerosis phenotype to nondiabetic models,[882] as well as to diabetic mouse models.[882] Based on these promising experimental data, MSC therapy has moved into clinical trials in kidney disease, with promising initial results in lupus nephritis. With regard to DKD, there is only one ongoing recruiting clinical trial in adult patients with type 2 diabetes and DKD (ClinicalTrials.gov identifier: NCT01843387).

Interesting new data show that after administration of autologous adipose-derived MSC in STZ-induced diabetes, a reduction of mesangial expansion and of oxidative stress was observed.[883] A clinical trial is currently ongoing to determine the role of adipose-tissue-derived MSCs in moderate to severe chronic kidney disease (ClinicalTrials.gov identifier: NCT02933827).

Finally, the ability to differentiate induced-pluripotent stem cells (iPSCs) into kidney cells has also generated much interest,[884] and has markedly improved the understanding of human nephrogenesis.[885] However, although iPS derived kidney cells will be important for the dissection of clinically relevant disease mechanisms, and for new target identification, the iPSCs have not yet advanced to reliable cell replacement strategies for DKD and kidney disease in general. The evidence that iPS derived podocytes mature into vascularized glomeruli upon experimental transplantation[886] is a strong step forward in this direction.

## ACKNOWLEDGMENTS

A special thank you to the outstanding editorial support of Dr Alexis J Sloan and Ms Janessa Maidment. This work was supported in part by the Intramural Research Program of the National Institute of Diabetes and Digestive and Kidney Diseases.

 Complete reference list available at ExpertConsult.com.

## KEY REFERENCES

8. American Diabetes Association. 10. Microvascular complications and foot care. *Diabetes Care.* 2017;40(suppl 1):S88–S98. PubMed PMID: 27979897.
9. Fox CS, Matsushita K, Woodward M, et al. Associations of kidney disease measures with mortality and end-stage renal disease in individuals with and without diabetes: a meta-analysis. *Lancet.* 2012;380(9854):1662–1673. PubMed PMID: 23013602. Pubmed Central PMCID: 3771350.
10. KDOQI. KDOQI clinical practice guidelines and clinical practice recommendations for diabetes and chronic kidney disease. *Am J Kidney Dis.* 2007;49(2 suppl 2):S12–S154. PubMed PMID: 17276798.
15. Afkarian M, Zelnick LR, Hall YN, et al. Clinical manifestations of kidney disease among US adults with diabetes, 1988-2014. *JAMA.* 2016;316(6):602–610. PubMed PMID: 27532915. Pubmed Central PMCID: 5444809.
46. Gregg EW, Li Y, Wang J, et al. Changes in diabetes-related complications in the United States, 1990-2010. *N Engl J Med.* 2014;370(16):1514–1523. PubMed PMID: 24738668.
53. Dabelea D, Hanson RL, Bennett PH, et al. Increasing prevalence of type II diabetes in American Indian children. *Diabetologia.* 1998;41(8):904–910. PubMed PMID: 9726592.
100. Steffes MW, Sutherland DE, Goetz FC, et al. Studies of kidney and muscle biopsy specimens from identical twins discordant for type I diabetes mellitus. *N Engl J Med.* 1985;312(20):1282–1287. PubMed PMID: 4039409.
101. Fioretto P, Steffes MW, Sutherland DE, et al. Reversal of lesions of diabetic nephropathy after pancreas transplantation. *N Engl J Med.* 1998;339(2):69–75. PubMed PMID: 9654536.
139. Tonneijck L, Muskiet MH, Smits MM, et al. Glomerular hyperfiltration in diabetes: mechanisms, clinical significance, and treatment. *J Am Soc Nephrol.* 2017;28(4):1023–1039. PubMed PMID: 28143897. Pubmed Central PMCID: 5373460.
190. Whaley-Connell A, Sowers JR. Obesity and kidney disease: from population to basic science and the search for new therapeutic targets. *Kidney Int.* 2017;92(2):313–323. PubMed PMID: 28341271.
209. Luyckx VA, Bertram JF, Brenner BM, et al. Effect of fetal and child health on kidney development and long-term risk of hypertension and kidney disease. *Lancet.* 2013;382(9888):273–283. PubMed PMID: 23727166.
266. Iyengar SK, Sedor JR, Freedman BI, et al. Genome-wide association and trans-ethnic meta-analysis for advanced diabetic kidney disease: family investigation of nephropathy and diabetes (FIND). *PLoS Genet.* 2015;11(8):e1005352. PubMed PMID: 26305897. Pubmed Central PMCID: 4549309.
275. Van JA, Scholey JW, Konvalinka A. Insights into diabetic kidney disease using urinary proteomics and bioinformatics. *J Am Soc Nephrol.* 2017;28(4):1050–1061. PubMed PMID: 28159781. Pubmed Central PMCID: 5373465.
279. Sawhney S, Marks A, Fluck N, et al. Post-discharge kidney function is associated with subsequent ten-year renal progression risk among survivors of acute kidney injury. *Kidney Int.* 2017;92(2):440–452. PubMed PMID: 28416224. Pubmed Central PMCID: 5524434.
298. Ju W, Nair V, Smith S, et al. Tissue transcriptome-driven identification of epidermal growth factor as a chronic kidney disease biomarker.

*Sci Transl Med.* 2015;7(316):316ra193. PubMed PMID: 26631632. Epub 2015/12/04. eng.

326. Coca SG, Nadkarni GN, Huang Y, et al. Plasma biomarkers and kidney function decline in early and established diabetic kidney disease. *J Am Soc Nephrol.* 2017;PubMed PMID: 28476763.
338. Groop PH, Thomas MC, Moran JL, et al. The presence and severity of chronic kidney disease predicts all-cause mortality in type 1 diabetes. *Diabetes.* 2009;58(7):1651–1658. PubMed PMID: 19401416. Pubmed Central PMCID: 2699848.
341. Afkarian M, Sachs MC, Kestenbaum B, et al. Kidney disease and increased mortality risk in type 2 diabetes. *J Am Soc Nephrol.* 2013;24(2):302–308. PubMed PMID: 23362314. Pubmed Central PMCID: 3559486.
342. Mortality GBD, Causes of Death C. Global, regional, and national age-sex specific all-cause and cause-specific mortality for 240 causes of death, 1990-2013: a systematic analysis for the Global Burden of Disease Study 2013. *Lancet.* 2015;385(9963):117–171. PubMed PMID: 25530442. Pubmed Central PMCID: 4340604.
346. Thomas B, Matsushita K, Abate KH, et al. Global cardiovascular and renal outcomes of reduced GFR. *J Am Soc Nephrol.* 2017;28(7):2167–2179. PubMed PMID: 28408440. Pubmed Central PMCID: 5491277.
349. Tangri N, Grams ME, Levey AS, et al. Multinational assessment of accuracy of equations for predicting risk of kidney failure: a Meta-analysis. *JAMA.* 2016;315(2):164–174. PubMed PMID: 26757465. Pubmed Central PMCID: 4752167.
365. Rawshani A, Rawshani A, Franzen S, et al. Mortality and cardiovascular disease in type 1 and type 2 diabetes. *N Engl J Med.* 2017;376(15):1407–1418. PubMed PMID: 28402770.
394. Toyoda M, Najafian B, Kim Y, et al. Podocyte detachment and reduced glomerular capillary endothelial fenestration in human type 1 diabetic nephropathy. *Diabetes.* 2007;56(8):2155–2160. PubMed PMID: 17536064.
399. Najafian B, Kim Y, Crosson JT, et al. Atubular glomeruli and glomerulotubular junction abnormalities in diabetic nephropathy. *J Am Soc Nephrol.* 2003;14(4):908–917. PubMed PMID: 12660325.
411. Mauer M, Caramori ML, Fioretto P, et al. Glomerular structural-functional relationship models of diabetic nephropathy are robust in type 1 diabetic patients. *Nephrol Dial Transplant.* 2015;30(6):918–923. PubMed PMID: 25183630. Pubmed Central PMCID: 4438739.
418. Fioretto P, Stehouwer CD, Mauer M, et al. Heterogeneous nature of microalbuminuria in NIDDM: studies of endothelial function and renal structure. *Diabetologia.* 1998;41(2):233–236. PubMed PMID: 9498659.
425. Pagtalunan ME, Miller PL, Jumping-Eagle S, et al. Podocyte loss and progressive glomerular injury in type II diabetes. *J Clin Invest.* 1997;99(2):342–348. PubMed PMID: 9006003.
426. Fufaa GD, Weil EJ, Lemley KV, et al. Structural predictors of loss of renal function in American Indians with type 2 diabetes. *Clin J Am Soc Nephrol.* 2016;11(2):254–261. PubMed PMID: 26792530. Pubmed Central PMCID: 4741038. Epub 2016/01/23. eng.
439. Mazzucco G, Bertani T, Fortunato M, et al. Different patterns of renal damage in type 2 diabetes mellitus: a multicentric study on 393 biopsies. *Am J Kidney Dis.* 2002;39(4):713–720. PubMed PMID: 11920336. Epub 2002/03/29. eng.
444. Sharma SG, Bomback AS, Radhakrishnan J, et al. The modern spectrum of renal biopsy findings in patients with diabetes. *Clin J Am Soc Nephrol.* 2013;8(10):1718–1724. PubMed PMID: 23886566. Pubmed Central PMCID: 3789339.
447. Tervaert TW, Mooyaart AL, Amann K, et al. Pathologic classification of diabetic nephropathy. *J Am Soc Nephrol.* 2010;21(4):556–563. PubMed PMID: 20167701. Epub 2010/02/20. eng.
456. Mauer M, Zinman B, Gardiner R, et al. Renal and retinal effects of enalapril and losartan in type 1 diabetes. *N Engl J Med.* 2009;361(1):40–51. PubMed PMID: 19571282. Epub 2009/07/03. eng.
457. Weil EJ, Fufaa G, Jones LI, et al. Effect of losartan on prevention and progression of early diabetic nephropathy in american indians with type 2 diabetes. *Diabetes.* 2013;62(9):3224–3231. PubMed PMID: 23545707. Epub 2013/04/03. eng.
469. Harder JL, Hodgin JB, Kretzler M. Integrative biology of diabetic kidney disease. *Kidney Dis (Basel).* 2015;1(3):194–203. PubMed PMID: 26929927. Pubmed Central PMCID: 4768943. Epub 2016/03/02. eng.
515. Krolewski AS. Progressive renal decline: the new paradigm of diabetic nephropathy in type 1 diabetes. *Diabetes Care.* 2015;38(6):954–962. PubMed PMID: 25998286. Pubmed Central PMCID: 4439536.
636. Wanner C, Inzucchi SE, Lachin JM, et al. Empagliflozin and progression of kidney disease in type 2 diabetes. *N Engl J Med.* 2016;375(4):323–334. PubMed PMID: 27299675.
650. Perkovic V, Agarwal R, Fioretto P, et al. Management of patients with diabetes and CKD: conclusions from a "Kidney Disease: Improving Global Outcomes" (KDIGO) controversies conference. *Kidney Int.* 2016;90(6):1175–1183. PubMed PMID: 27884312.
677. Fried LF, Emanuele N, Zhang JH, et al. Combined angiotensin inhibition for the treatment of diabetic nephropathy. *N Engl J Med.* 2013;369(20):1892–1903. PubMed PMID: 24206457.
702. Zinman B, Wanner C, Lachin JM, et al. Empagliflozin, cardiovascular outcomes, and mortality in type 2 diabetes. *N Engl J Med.* 2015;373(22):2117–2128. PubMed PMID: 26378978.
708. Mann JFE, Orsted DD, Brown-Frandsen K, et al. Liraglutide and renal outcomes in type 2 diabetes. *N Engl J Med.* 2017;377(9):839–848. PubMed PMID: 28854085.
757. Perkovic V, Heerspink HL, Chalmers J, et al. Intensive glucose control improves kidney outcomes in patients with type 2 diabetes. *Kidney Int.* 2013;83(3):517–523. PubMed PMID: 23302714.
766. Marathias KP, Agroyannis B, Mavromoustakos T, et al. Hematocrit-lowering effect following inactivation of renin-angiotensin system with angiotensin converting enzyme inhibitors and angiotensin receptor blockers. *Curr Top Med Chem.* 2004;4(4):483–486. PubMed PMID: 14965314.
784. Cooper BA, Branley P, Bulfone L, et al. A randomized, controlled trial of early versus late initiation of dialysis. *N Engl J Med.* 2010;363(7):609–619. PubMed PMID: 20581422.
796. Tancredi M, Rosengren A, Svensson AM, et al. Excess mortality among persons with type 2 diabetes. *N Engl J Med.* 2015;373(18):1720–1732. PubMed PMID: 26510021.
799. Chang YT, Wu JL, Hsu CC, et al. Diabetes and end-stage renal disease synergistically contribute to increased incidence of cardiovascular events: a nationwide follow-up study during 1998-2009. *Diabetes Care.* 2014;37(1):277–285. PubMed PMID: 23920086.
813. Rhee CM, Leung AM, Kovesdy CP, et al. Updates on the management of diabetes in dialysis patients. *Semin Dial.* 2014;27(2):135–145. PubMed PMID: 24588802. Pubmed Central PMCID: 3960718.
829. Flynn C, Bakris GL. Noninsulin glucose-lowering agents for the treatment of patients on dialysis. *Nat Rev Nephrol.* 2013;9(3):147–153. PubMed PMID: 23358424.

# 40 Cardiorenal Syndromes

Kevin Damman | John J.V. McMurray

CHAPTER OUTLINE



KEY POINTS

- Cardiorenal syndrome represents the clinical combination of concomitant reduced heart and renal function.
- At least five subtypes of cardiorenal syndrome have been proposed.
- Worsening renal function in heart failure is not the same as acute kidney injury (AKI) in heart failure.
- Worsening renal function in the context of initiation or uptitration of renin-angiotensin-aldosterone system inhibitors in heart failure should not immediately prompt early discontinuation because the prognostic benefit is (often) maintained but requires close monitoring of kidney function.
- Pathophysiology of albuminuria in heart failure is different from that in primary kidney disease because intraglomerular pressure is presumed to be low in heart failure.

## INTRODUCTION

Heart failure (HF) is a syndrome characterized by increased cardiac filling pressures, reduced cardiac output, signs and symptoms of congestion, and evidence of structural cardiac disease.[1,2] The incidence and prevalence of HF is on the rise because of improved survival of patients with cardiovascular disease (e.g., myocardial infarction, hypertension), increased awareness, and early recognition of the syndrome, with sophisticated advanced diagnostic tests and better treatment of diagnosed HF. As such, the number of patients with HF is estimated to increase substantially in the next 10 years.[3] This dramatic increase in patient numbers will pose a challenge to health care professionals, as well as to costs in the health care system, because HF care is already responsible for 1.4% of the total medical expenditures.[4] The most important reason for these extraordinary costs are the relatively long and often repetitive admissions for HF when patients present with acute (decompensated) HF. In the syndrome of HF, the kidney plays a crucial role. It is responsible for the maladaptive and excessive salt and water retention that feeds the vicious circle of increased filling pressures, low cardiac output, and reduced organ (and renal) perfusion, which triggers even more salt and water retention.[5]

This also indicates that from a renal perspective, kidney failure itself can also induce or accelerate the progression or development of HF, as is often the case in hemodialysis patients. However, even in the early stages of chronic kidney disease (CKD), the risk of incident HF is increased, suggesting that shared cardiovascular risk factors and/or the decrease in the glomerular filtration rate (GFR) itself may predispose to HF development.

This interplay between heart and kidney is key to the pathophysiologic processes that occur in HF and end-stage renal disease (ESRD), and the synergistic failure of both organs together has been termed "cardiorenal syndrome" (CRS).[5-7] This chapter discusses the epidemiology, pathophysiology, and important clinical considerations in patients with cardiorenal failure.

## TERMINOLOGY OF CARDIORENAL SYNDROME

Followed by in-depth invasive hemodynamic research in the early 20th century,[8-10] specific interest in the importance of cardiorenal interplay was revived at the end of the 20th century. Following a number of publications around the turn of the millennium showing that a decreased creatinine clearance or GFR was associated with worse outcome in patients with chronic HF, a consensus statement on the CRS was published.[11-14] This landmark paper, by Ronco and colleagues,[14] has since led to numerous follow-up manuscripts; the current consensus is that in CRS, five subtypes exist (Table 40.1). It is important to note here that these classifications, including the term "cardiorenal syndrome," have been proposed by experts in the field. This does not mean that in daily clinical practice, distinguishing between the exact types of CRS will help guide and choose treatment. However, it does serve as a starting point to determine which organ dysfunction is the more likely initiating trigger and which one is a consequence of the other. The subclassification is based on the time relationship between the failure of both organs, one occurring before the other, and differentiating between acute and chronic situations.

CRS type 5 includes patients who do not fit the description of the other 4 and are subject to a systemic process that involves (among other organs) heart and kidney together.[15] From a biologic standpoint, one should realize that patients are not fixed within one particular type of CRS and can shift from one type to another, or even have two types at the same time. For example, a chronic HF patient who develops acute renal failure during admission with decompensated HF but who has had declining renal function over a longer period of time, preadmission, would fit both CRS types 1 and 2.[16,17] If this acute renal failure is also associated with acute worsening of HF, this means that part of the pathophysiology also fits CRS type 3.[18] This highlights that it is inherently difficult to subclassify patients within one specific subtype, let alone base treatment on this classification. For clinical practice, it would suffice to characterize a patient as having concomitant HF and renal dysfunction and to determine the initiating trigger, which also would be the target for therapy.

Since the introduction of CRS as an entity, different researchers have argued that the original definition could be broadened to include anemia also. The proposed term would then become "cardiorenal anemia syndrome" (CRAS).[19] Anemia is frequent in both HF and CKD and is associated with worse outcomes.[20] The pathophysiology is not entirely understood and is a matter of debate, but reduced erythropoietin production and responsiveness, bone marrow suppression, and fluid retention (hemodilution) are the most prominent factors.[21] It was also thought that iron deficiency might be important because it is frequently observed together with anemia in HF, but it is now clear that nonanemic HF patients are often iron-deficient as well.[22] Therefore, some argue that the terminology could even be changed to cardiorenal anemia iron deficiency syndrome (CRAIDS) or CRIDS when anemia is absent. The more subdivisions that are proposed, the more difficult it is to define a homogeneous population in which specific treatment algorithms may be proposed. It does, however, emphasize the complex pathophysiologic relationships among HF, kidney dysfunction, and other organ dysfunction and systemic abnormalities, which probably is a consequence of the heterogeneity of the cardiorenal population.

## EPIDEMIOLOGY AND PROGNOSIS

In patients with HF, renal dysfunction, mostly defined as CKD (estimated GFR [eGFR] < 60 mL/min/1.73 m$^2$) is frequently present. In the MAGGIC meta-analysis, including unselected patient cohorts with mostly chronic HF, around 50% of patients had CKD.[23] In a larger meta-analysis, including over 1,000,000 patients with HF, CKD was present in 42% of patients with chronic HF, whereas CKD was present in 53% of patients with acute HF.[24] These populations consist of different phenotypes of HF, including patients with preserved ejection fraction (HF with preserved ejection fraction [HFPEF]) and patients with HF with reduced ejection fraction (HFREF; Table 40.2). Data on the comparison between these two phenotypes are scarce, but it is thought that in general, the prevalence of CKD is similar, although patient characteristics of these patient cohorts differ substantially.[23]

In patients with chronic HF, when CKD is present, the risk of death is more than twofold greater, a risk estimate that is similar in patients with acute HF.[24] Additionally, from retrospective analyses from clinical trials, the magnitude of

**Table 40.1 Classification of Cardiorenal Syndromes**

| Type | Popular Term | Description |
|---|---|---|
| 1 | Acute cardiorenal syndrome | Acute heart failure leading to an acute renal event, including acute kidney injury (AKI), worsening renal function |
| 2 | Chronic cardiorenal syndrome | Chronic heart failure leading to renal injury or progression of renal failure |
| 3 | Acute renocardiac syndrome | AKI leading to an acute cardiac event, including acute heart failure |
| 4 | Chronic renocardiac syndrome | Chronic kidney disease (CKD) leading to cardiac injury or progression of cardiac disease, including heart failure |
| 5 | Systemic cardiorenal syndrome | A systemic event or process that results in the simultaneous development of acute heart and kidney injury, including heart failure and AKI |

**Table 40.2 Definition of Phenotypes of Heart Failure**

| Type of Heart Failure | HFREF | HFPEF |
|---|---|---|
| **Criteria** | | |
| 1 | Symptoms ± signs | Symptoms ± signs[a] |
| 2 | LVEF < 40% | LVEF ≥ 50% |
| 3 | — | Elevated levels of natriuretic peptides and either relevant structural heart disease (left ventricular hypertrophy and/or large left atrium) or diastolic dysfunction |

*HFREF,* Heart failure with reduced ejection fraction; *HPFEF,* heart failure with preserved ejection fraction; *LVEF,* left ventricular ejection fraction.

Adapted from Ponikowski P, Voors AA, Anker SD, et al. 2016 ESC guidelines for the diagnosis and treatment of acute and chronic heart failure: the Task Force for the diagnosis and treatment of acute and chronic heart failure of the European Society of Cardiology (ESC). developed with the special contribution of the Heart Failure Association (HFA) of the ESC. *Eur J Heart Fail.* 2016;18:891–975.

[a]In that guideline, a middle group, termed "heart failure with midrange ejection fraction" (HFmrEF), is specified. However, at present, there is little evidence that such a subgroup actually exists or affects treatment.

the greater risk for all-cause mortality (and HF hospitalization) was directly related to the degree of renal impairment at baseline, showing a stepwise increase in unadjusted hazard ratio—for example, 3.83 (2.92–5.01) for eGFR below 45 mL/min/1.73 $m^2$ compared with an eGFR > 90 mL/min/1.73 $m^2$.[13] In a different analysis, chronic HF patients with eGFR < 15 mL/min/1.73 $m^2$ had the highest risk for cardiovascular mortality, with the risk steeply increasing when the eGFR was lower than 60 mL/min/1.73 $m^2$.[25]

In patients with CKD, data on the prevalence of HF are scarcer. However, it is clear that with decreasing eGFR, the risk for cardiovascular disease in general increases steeply in the general population, as well as in patients. On a population level, the prevalence of HF in subjects with eGFR < 60 mL/min/1.73 $m^2$ is between 2- and 20-fold higher compared with those with preserved eGFR.[26] This higher prevalence of HF in individuals with a lower eGFR is not restricted to HF, because similar patterns are found for coronary artery disease, cerebrovascular events, and peripheral artery disease, although the association is less striking.

In the Chronic Renal Insufficiency Cohort (CRIC), which included almost 4000 patients with impaired eGFR, the risk of HF rose steeply with decreasing eGFR levels.[27] The hazard ratio (HR) for the development of HF was 1.67 (1.49–1.89) per standard deviation (15 mL/min/1.73 $m^2$) decrease in eGFR, an association that was independent of albuminuria. In the Atherosclerosis Risk in Communities (ARIC) study, including over 15,000 patients (45–64 years of age), the risk of incident HF was more than threefold higher (HR, 3.57 [1.89–6.77]) when eGFR was < 30 mL/min/1.73 $m^2$ but no albuminuria was present, whereas the HR increased to 7.98 (3.46–18.41) when macroalbuminuria was also present.[28] There are even fewer data on the risk of HF when acute kidney injury (AKI) develops. In a meta-analysis of mostly individuals with cardiovascular disease, where different definitions were pooled, the relative risk for HF associated with AKI was 58% higher than in individuals with cardiovascular disease with no AKI.[29]

## PATHOPHYSIOLOGY OF CONCOMITANT HEART FAILURE AND CHRONIC KIDNEY DISEASE

### SHARED RISK FACTORS

To understand the pathophysiology of the interplay between HF and renal dysfunction, once either one has developed, it is important to realize that the risk factors for both are remarkably similar. In particular, cardiovascular risk factors, such as hypertension, diabetes, peripheral artery disease, and obesity, predispose to failure of both organs. In many cases, these risk factors likely increase the risk of an acute event (e.g., myocardial infarction), which subsequently may lead to HF and/or CKD; on the other hand, chronic exposure to any of these risk factors may accelerate the slow progression to end-stage organ dysfunction (e.g., hypertension leading to left ventricular hypertrophy, hypertensive nephropathy, and HFPEF). Importantly, when a CRS has developed, these risk factors remain associated with worse outcomes.

### RENAL HEMODYNAMICS

#### RENAL BLOOD FLOW

In patients with chronic HF (HFREF), cardiac output is markedly reduced, leading to a decrease in organ perfusion, including perfusion of the brain, gut, liver and, most importantly, the kidney.[30] Whereas the renal perfusion normally is around 25% of cardiac output, this proportion decreases significantly when cardiac output falls.[31] Despite a fall in cardiac output, the kidney is able to preserve the GFR in a low-pressure, low-flow state because of renal autoregulation, although most patients are not severely hypotensive in the early stages of HF. In patients without renin-angiotensin-aldosterone system (RAAS) inhibition therapy, when renal blood flow (RBF) decreases and intraglomerular pressures fall, efferent autoregulation will increase the filtration fraction (FF), and the GFR will remain preserved to some extent and for some time (see Chapter 3).[31] With further deterioration in clinical status and renal perfusion (pressure), more stringent efferent and now also afferent arteriolar autoregulation will be unable to preserve GFR, and the FF will decrease. This results in loss of the GFR. Especially in these very low-flow states, where hypotension is a real issue, GFR becomes highly flow-dependent.

> ***Clinical Relevance***
>
> In patients with heart failure who are renin-angiotensin-system (RAAS) inhibitor–naïve, a reduction in cardiac output and consequently renal blood flow (RBF) does not directly translate into a reduction in glomerular filtration rate (GFR). Because of efferent arteriolar vasoconstriction, GFR is relatively preserved, resulting in increased filtration fraction. However, in patients using RAAS inhibitor therapy, this adaptive process is blocked, resulting in a reduction in GFR in parallel to the reduction in RBF, with a similar filtration fraction. This is the reason for a reduction in GFR in (some) patients with heart failure who experience an increase in the serum creatinine level. This small decrease in GFR should be distinguished from the more clinically relevant situation of an unprovoked deterioration in GFR, which requires adjustment of treatment and more elaborate assessment of the patient's clinical status.

Things are slightly different in patients who are treated with RAAS inhibitors. Angiotensin- converting enzyme (ACE) inhibitors and angiotensin II type 1 receptor blockers (ARBs) inhibit the efferent arteriolar vasoconstriction. This means that in the situation of reduced RBF, the expected efferent arteriolar vasoconstriction is prevented, resulting in loss of GFR (Fig. 40.1).[32] Only when RBF drops significantly further will the situation be similar to that without RAAS inhibitors; both efferent and afferent vasoconstriction progress (possibly due to tubuloglomerular feedback) and cause further decreases in GFR, FF, and very low intraglomerular pressures.[7] It is under these circumstances, in particular, that chronic HF patients may develop albuminuria.[32] It must be emphasized that this situation is opposite from the albuminuria that is present in hypertension, diabetes, and CKD, where high intraglomerular pressures exist; in HF, in contrast, low intraglomerular pressures are present. The actual cause of albuminuria in HF is therefore not entirely understood but could include glomerular (endothelial) damage and leakage, possibly influenced by the low-grade systemic inflammation present in HF, and abnormal tubular handling of filtered albumin or tubular dysfunction.

There have been no studies investigating renal hemodynamics in HF patients with preserved ejection fraction. It is expected that especially in the end stage of HFPEF, renal hemodynamics behave similarly to HFREF patients, because cardiac output is likely significantly reduced in these patients as well. Whether RBF is reduced in mild HFPEF is unknown. Similarly, in acute HF, where assessment of renal hemodynamics is difficult, no studies have investigated renal perfusion and GFR simultaneously. However, at least 50% of patients presenting with acute HF are actually patients with acute exacerbation of chronic HF. In such patients, RBF will already be reduced chronically. Among patients presenting with new-onset acute HF, the extent of the reduction in RBF is unknown.

In patients with CKD-AKI who develop HF (CRS types 3 and 4)[18,33] or CRS type 5,[15] no specific studies have been conducted on renal perfusion and association with GFR. CRS types 3 and 4 are discussed further in Chapter 54.

## CENTRAL AND RENAL VENOUS PRESSURE

In addition to a reduced cardiac output, patients with HF often experience not only increased left- sided filling pressure,

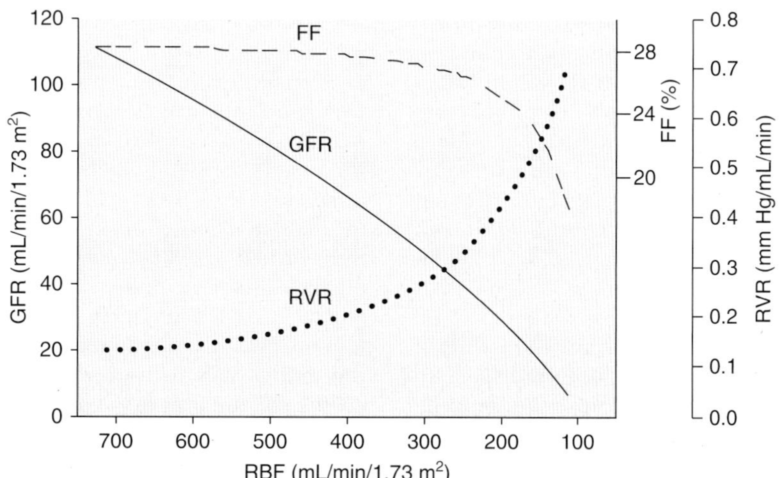


**Fig. 40.1 Renal hemodynamics in chronic HFREF in the presence of RAAS inhibition.** Shown is the relationship among RBF, RVR, FF, and GFR in the presence of RAAS inhibition. With low RBF, GFR decreases although FF is maintained when efferent arteriolar vasoconstriction is inhibited. Only when RBF decreases substantially will the FF decrease because of increased afferent arteriolar vasoconstriction. This results in increased RVR, especially in those patients who experience albuminuria. *FF,* Filtration fraction; *GFR,* glomerular filtration rate; *RAAS,* renin-angiotensin-aldosterone system; *RBF,* renal blood flow; *RVR,* renal vascular resistance. (From Smilde TD, Damman K, van der Harst P, et al. Differential associations between renal function and "modifiable" risk factors in patients with chronic heart failure. *Clin Res Cardiol.* 2009;98:121–129. Reproduced with permission from Springer.)

but also increased central venous pressure (CVP). This is the case for chronic HF patients who are relatively stable, but is even more important in patients presenting with acute or worsening HF, in whom increased CVP is one of the hallmarks of this syndrome. Because the kidney is dependent on a pressure gradient across the glomerular membrane to allow passive filtration, any change in pressure inside the glomerulus or pressure in the Bowman capsule may influence filtration. Because the renal perfusion pressure is dependent on the differences in mean arterial pressure and renal venous pressure and renal vascular resistance, a change in RBF may not only induce changes in GFR, but also change in central and renal venous pressures. This concept has long been overlooked in modern medicine. Already, in the early part of the 20th century, extensive measurements were carried out (in pateints without RAAS inhibitors), and the association between higher CVP and higher renal venous pressure was described.[8-10,34,35] Even more importantly, a higher renal venous pressure was associated with lower RBF and, subsequently, lower GFR. Therefore, because of a reduction in perfusion pressure across the kidney due to higher CVP, perfusion is decreased, and GFR deteriorates. This is the RBF-dependent effect of an increased renal venous pressure.

However, there is also an RBF-independent effect of increased renal venous pressure on the GFR. An increase in renal venous pressure leads to an increase in renal interstitial pressure.[36,37] Because the kidney is an encapsulated organ, this will lead to an increase in the pressure in the Bowman capsule, as well as lead to collapse of tubules that are compressed by the higher interstitial pressures. We now also appreciate that in patients with HF, the pressure wave caused by severe tricuspid regurgitation, together with central venous flow pattern alterations occurring in individuals with high CVP, actually reach the renal parenchyma.[38,39] These flow patterns in the large caval veins alter with a higher CVP and have been associated with worse outcomes in HF patients. Although uncertain, it is possible that this will further compromise renal function.

High central and renal venous pressures are now considered important pathophysiologic factors in patients with HF and renal dysfunction.[16,17,40] In two simultaneously published studies, higher CVP was an important predictor of worsening renal function in acute HF, whereas CVP was also the strongest independent factor associated with eGFR in a large heterogeneous cardiovascular population in another study.[41,42] There is even evidence that increased renal venous pressure, by itself, is associated with salt and water retention.[43] Although the importance of a higher CVP in relation to lower eGFR is especially important in the acute situation, where CVP is increased, it must be acknowledged that a reduction in RBF is still probably the most important determinant of GFR in any patient with HF.[44] Higher CVP does not predispose to worse renal function in every patient, because the opposite has also been found in different studies.[45] Future studies are needed to establish whether changes in CVP (reduction in the acute HF situation) are associated with changes in GFR, although some data do support this.[46,47] There have been no studies directly measuring renal venous pressure or renal interstitial pressure in HF or CRS. Fig. 40.2 summarizes the pathophysiology for CRS types 1 and 2 in patients with HF. For CRS types 3 and 4, where the first event is acute or chronic renal failure or injury, it is unknown whether compromised renal hemodynamics play a role in the pathophysiology of CRS. AKI certainly can predispose to salt and water retention, thereby increasing CVP and cardiac filling pressures. For CRS type 5, systemic processes themselves, such as shock, changes in microcirculation, redistribution of fluid to the splanchnic system resulting in hypotension, or treatment of these processes, including vasopressor therapy and fluid resuscitation, may cause higher CVP, lower renal blood flow, and induce cardiac injury.[15] However, the relative contribution and importance of these processes have not been established and therefore are speculative, at best.

## CARDIORENAL CONNECTORS

In patients with HF, it is likely that the hemodynamic variables, RBF and increased CVP, are the most important factors determining GFR. There are, however, systemic modulating factors that have been designated as "cardiorenal connectors."[5] These include endothelial dysfunction, inflammation, sympathetic nervous system (SNS) activation, RAAS activation, and reactive oxygen species (ROS) activation. These cardiorenal connectors do not only directly affect GFR, but also affect RBF, thereby also influencing GFR indirectly. In CRS types 3 and 4, levels of different inflammatory markers and markers of endothelial dysfunction are increased, and there is experimental evidence suggesting that some of these proteins (e.g., tumor necrosis factor-α, interleukin-6) have detrimental effects on cardiac function.[18,33]

Other data have suggested that uremic CKD patients experience cardiac (and renal) fibrosis, which is at least partly attributable to upregulation of the transforming growth factor-beta (TGF-β) pathway.[33,48] Inflammation by itself can also trigger more pronounced RAAS activation and the formation of ROS. RAAS activation is not only characterized by systemic effects of angiotensin II, but also by intracardiac and intrarenal effects. Angiotensin II induces cardiac remodeling, modulates the effect of renal interstitial hypertension,[37] and triggers vascular inflammation through the nuclear factor kappa B (NF-κB) pathway.[5,49]

Oxidative stress has been shown to influence cardiac function negatively and is associated with cardiac mitochondrial dysfunction.[50] Furthermore, not only is systemic ROS formation greatly increased in experimental models of CRS, but intrarenal oxidative stress also occurs, perhaps reflecting increased levels of nicotinamide adenine dinucleotide phosphate (NADPH) oxidase activity.[50] Sustained activation of the SNS is prevalent in HF and CRS and is the target of therapies such as beta-blockers. SNS activation has detrimental effects on cardiac and renal function as a consequence of recurrent cardiac and renal ischemia and mediation of fibrosis, together with RAAS activation and oxidative stress.[5,51] Furthermore, SNS activation can modify the ultrafiltration coefficient and lead to salt and water retention.[52] The detailed biologic processes and interplays between the different cardiorenal connectors are probably highly complex and are certainly poorly understood, as are their relative importance in the heart and renal impairment in CRS. It seems, however, probable that these cardiorenal connectors, together with the shared risk factors, modulate the hemodynamic relationship between heart and kidney in CRS and that activation of one system may result in activation of several others.

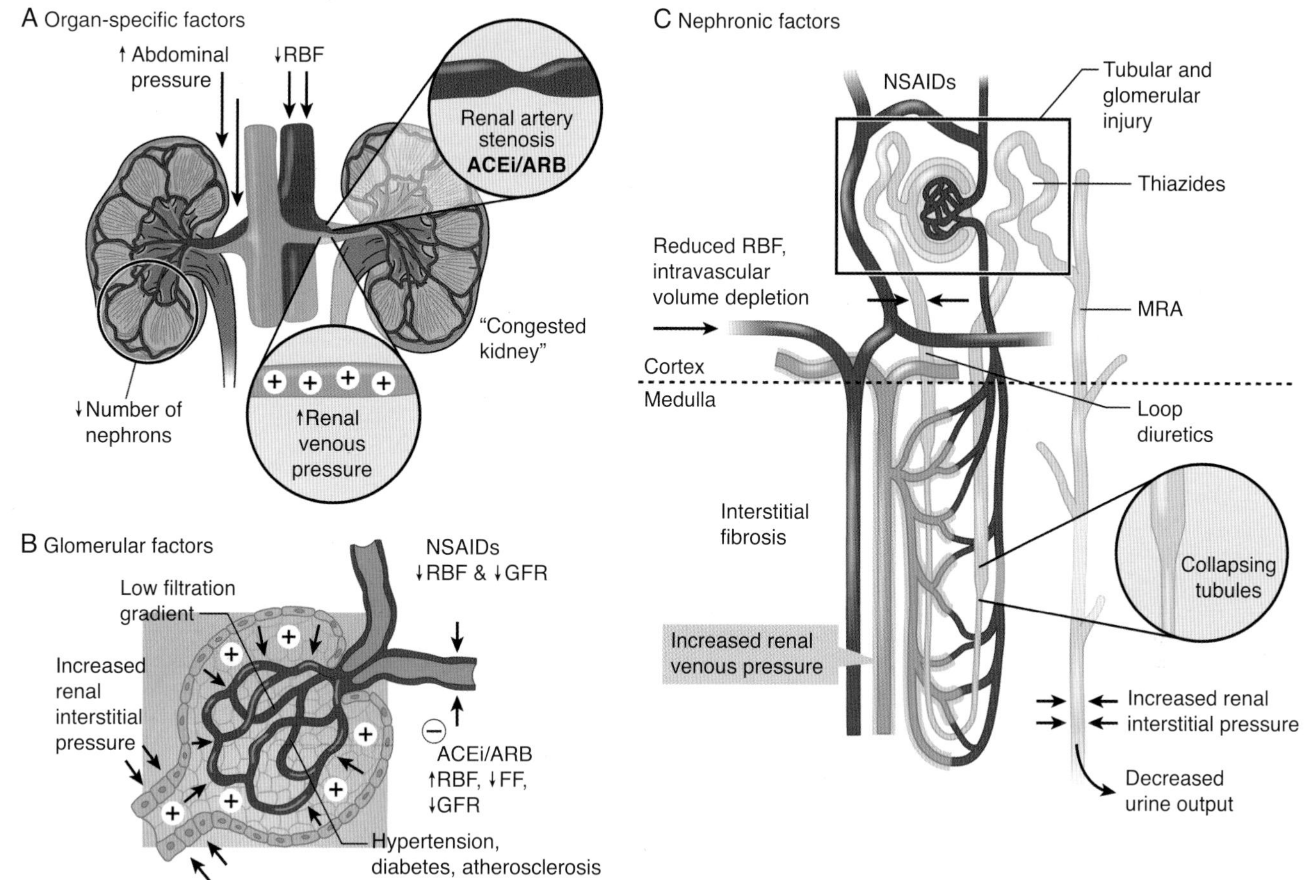


**Fig. 40.2 Factors involved in the cause of and association with outcomes of changes in renal function in heart failure.** (A) Organ-specific factors. The main determinants of decreased glomerular filtration rate are a decrease in renal blood flow and an increase in central and renal venous pressure. The latter can be caused by intravascular congestion but also by an increase in intraabdominal pressure. Owing to increased renal venous pressure, renal interstitial pressure rises, which results in a so-called congested kidney, because the kidney is encapsulated (B and C). Renal artery stenosis is present in around 25% of heart failure patients, which can further compromise renal blood flow, especially in the presence of renin-angiotensin-aldosterone system (RAAS) inhibitors. (B) Glomerular factors. Decreased renal blood flow and low blood pressure trigger renal autoregulation, preserving the glomerular filtration rate by increasing the filtration fraction by increased efferent vasoconstriction. The use of RAAS inhibitors inhibits this process, which increases renal blood flow, but leads (in some patients) to a reduction in glomerular filtration rate (pseudo–worsening renal function). Nonsteroidal antiinflammatory drugs inhibit prostaglandin synthesis, thereby impairing prostaglandin-associated increased or dependent renal blood flow. Increased interstitial pressure causes increased pressure in the Bowman capsule, which directly opposes filtration and in a glomerulus, where the filtration gradient is already low due to a decreased renal blood flow and increased renal venous pressure. Concomitant diseases have direct but differential effects on glomerular filtration, glomerular integrity, and podocyte function, as well as autoregulation. (C) Nephronic factors. Different therapies have different renal effects and exert their action at specific sites, as indicated in this diagram. Intravascular volume depletion (in the presence or absence of congestion) can lead to impaired renal perfusion and decreased glomerular filtration rate. The combination of increased interstitial pressure, reduced arterial perfusion, and concomitant disease, and therapies can cause tubular and glomerular injury. Increased renal venous pressure causes increased renal interstitial pressure, resulting in collapsing of renal tubules, which decreases the glomerular filtration rate and eventually leads to decreased urine output, sodium retention, and congestion. *ACEi,* Angiotensin-converting enzyme inhibitor; *ARB,* angiotensin II receptor blocker; *FF,* filtration fraction; *GFR,* glomerular filtration rate; *MRA,* mineralocorticoid receptor antagonist; *NSAIDs,* nonsteroidal antiinflammatory drugs; *RAAS,* renin-angiotensin-aldosterone system; *RBF,* renal blood flow. (From Damman K, Tang WH, Testani JM, et al. Terminology and definition of changes renal function in heart failure. *Eur Heart J.* 2014;35:3413–3416. Reprinted with permission from Oxford University Press.)

## WORSENING RENAL FUNCTION AND CHANGE IN RENAL FUNCTION

Not only is CKD prevalent in patients with HF, but accelerated decline in eGFR is frequently observed in these patients. There are few data from unselected patient cohorts showing overall change in eGFR across the HF population, but it has been estimated that the decrease in eGFR/year could be as high as 2 mL/min/1.73 $m^2$.[25] However, how fast eGFR may decrease depends on the clinical setting. For example, in patients admitted for acute HF, the change from admission to follow-up after 18 months in surviving patients was −7 mL/min/1.73 $m^2$, of which −2 mL/min/1.73 $m^2$ occurred in the hospital.[53] In retrospective analyses of large clinical trials, mostly with RAAS inhibitor therapy, long-term changes in eGFR have been investigated. For example, in the CHARM program, which included both HFPEF and HFREF patients, the mean change in eGFR/year was −2.8 mL/min/1.73 $m^2$, with a more significant deterioration in eGFR with the ARB candesartan compared with placebo.[54] The retrospective analysis from the GISSI-HF study in over 6000 HF patients had the benefit that the randomized treatment did not directly affect the slope of eGFR and, in this particular trial, the mean change per year in eGFR was −2.6 mL/min/1.73 $m^2$.[25] Only a few patients (15%) had a large decrease in eGFR in the first year (>15 mL/min/1.73 $m^2$ decrease), and 11% of patients actually had an increase in eGFR of the same magnitude. The greater the decrease in eGFR after 12-month follow-up, the worse the clinical outcome. Factors related to a steeper decline in eGFR in this particular analysis were the presence of obstructive lung disease, more preserved renal function at baseline, and the use of loop diuretics.

How much eGFR changes in the hospital in HF patients is difficult to establish. The serum creatinine level can fluctuate greatly in these patients during the initial phase of admission and treatment, and it is a matter of debate whether these changes in creatinine level really reflect changes in intrinsic glomerular filtration function. What we do know from large observational studies in acute HF is that the serum creatinine level may show different patterns of change, depending on patient characteristics, choice of treatment, hemodynamic alterations, and comorbid organ dysfunction.

It has, therefore, been difficult to establish the normal change in creatinine level and eGFR in patients with acute HF and how different patterns relate to differential outcomes. A significant increase in the serum creatinine level is observed in around 20% to 25% of all patients with HF.[24] Definitions vary, but mostly include an absolute increase of >0.3 mg/dL (26.5 μmol/L) and/or a relative increase in the serum creatinine level and eGFR over a certain period of time. In patients with HF, this has been termed "worsening renal function," which is distinctly different from AKI that occurs in CRS type 3 or primary kidney disease.[55] There are similarities, but the main difference seems to be that in AKI, there is evidence of actual kidney injury, with oliguria and anuria, histopathologic evidence of renal damage, and a very short time course. For worsening renal function, there is much more evidence for a transient functional change in GFR that is reversible most of the time.

The proposed definition to be used in HF differs slightly from that of AKI definitions in the nephrology literature.[55] Most important, there are additional criteria stating that a deterioration in creatinine level should be accompanied by a deterioration in clinical status to be designated as worsening renal function. Multiple studies and meta-analyses have evaluated worsening renal function in acute and chronic HF and found that overall worsening renal function is associated with worse outcomes.[24,56] However, it is now becoming clear that if the HF status of a patient improves despite the occurrence of worsening renal function, worsening renal function itself is not associated with worse outcomes. For example, in patients with acute HF, in whom the serum creatinine level can increase for various reasons, including intravascular volume depletion, loop diuretic therapy, and changes in hemodynamics, worsening renal function in these settings is not associated with increased mortality if the response to loop diuretics (decongestion) is adequate.[57,58]

Similarly, the serum creatinine level often increases after beginning and uptitration of RAAS inhibitor therapy. In contrast to patients in whom worsening renal function is unprovoked, the patients with RAAS inhibitor–induced worsening

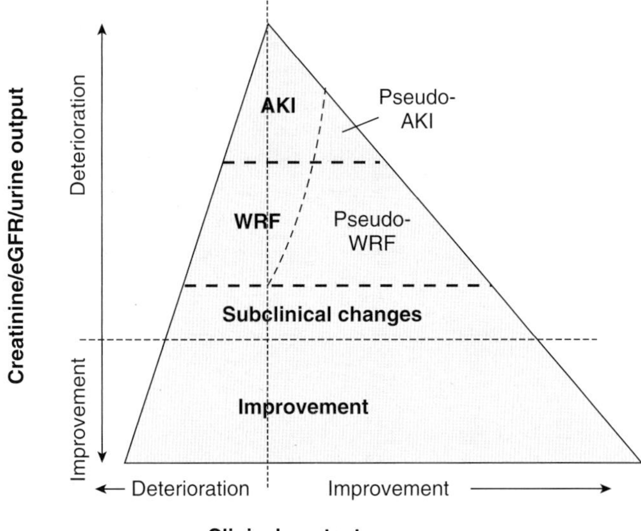


**Fig. 40.3** Visual depiction of association among changes in renal function, clinical condition, and mortality risk. Only when both deterioration in clinical status and increase in the serum creatinine level (or decrease in renal function) track together is this associated with worse clinical outcomes in heart failure. *AKI,* Acute kidney injury; *GFR,* glomerular filtration rate; *WRF,* worsening renal function. *Darker colors indicate higher mortality risk.* (From Damman K, Testani JM. The kidney in heart failure: an update. *Eur Heart J.* 2015;36:1437–1444. Reprinted with permission from Oxford University Press.)

renal function have favorable outcomes.[59] The reason for the apparently paradoxic association between deterioration in eGFR with improvement in outcomes during treatment with these agents is the attenuation of the autoregulatory response to reduced RBF, as discussed earlier. This provoked worsening of renal function without a deterioration in clinical status has now been termed "pseudo–worsening renal function" (Fig. 40.3). It highlights the importance of not relying solely on serum creatinine measurements, but also incorporating information on the patient's clinical status when evaluating the relevance of any change in renal function.[55] It must, however, be emphasized that RAAS inhibitor–induced worsening renal function can only be termed "pseudo–worsening renal function" in HFREF patients when the clinical outcome is improved with these agents; in patients with HFPEF, the worsening renal function observed with ARBs was actually associated with worse outcome.[60] Whenever the serum creatinine level does increase after initiation or uptitration of RAAS inhibitor therapy, it is important to monitor the serum creatinine and electrolyte levels (e.g., potassium) and clinical status of these patients closely.[2,61,62] An increase as much as 50% above baseline serum creatinine, or up to 3 mg/dL (266 μmol/L) and eGFR < 25 mL/min/1.73 $m^2$ is acceptable if the clinical status requires no adjustment. Changes in renal function that exceed these thresholds should be regarded as clinically significant and are a reason to lower the dose of RAAS inhibitor therapy. If the serum creatinine level increases by more than 100% or exceeds 3.5 mg/dL (310 μmol/L), and eGFR < 20 mL/min/1.73 $m^2$, RAAS inhibitor therapy needs to be stopped temporarily. Renal function and electrolytes should be checked on a regular basis thereafter and, if possible, patients should be rechallenged to evaluate whether the intolerance to RAAS inhibitors was temporary or permanent. In the situation of excessive or unexpectedly large increases in the serum creatinine level, clinicians should always consider alternative reasons, such as interactions with other medications, renal artery stenosis, dehydration, or decompensation and adherence issues. These factors should be investigated and possibly treated before rechallenge is started.

### DETERIORATION OF CARDIAC FUNCTION

In CKD, ESRD, or dialysis, there is direct evidence that maladaptive processes that normally occur during normal aging, or in hypertension, diabetes, and atherosclerosis, are markedly accelerated. Whether this is also the case in AKI is incompletely understood. In patients with ESRD or dialysis, left ventricular hypertrophy (LVH) is not only frequently observed, but there is also evidence that the progression to (more severe) LVH is often seen when eGFR decreases or (hemo)dialysis is initiated.[63] LVH is a consequence of myocyte hypertrophy, which results in myocardial stiffening and is associated with myocardial fibrosis and (subendocardial) ischemia due to myocyte–capillary mismatch. In CKD and ESRD, myocyte hypertrophy and myocardial fibrosis occur due to RAAS activation and upregulation of profibrotic pathways, which result in higher circulating levels of profibrotic molecules, such as TGF-β, galectin-3, and angiotensin II.[18] Over two-thirds of ESRD patients exhibit LVH, of which 30% have manifest LV failure. In one study of almost 600 patients, LV mass increased by over 60% 1.5 years after the initiation of dialysis, whereas almost 50% of patients exhibited evidence of HF.[64] On the other hand, among 160 patients from CRIC, there was no difference in LV mass between CKD and ESRD.[65] However, LVEF did decrease marginally from 53% to 50% in the transition to ESRD. More sophisticated echocardiographic assessments, including global longitudinal strain (GLS) measurements, have shown that with more severe renal disease, overall cardiac contractility deteriorates, even in patients with preserved LVEF.[66] Finally, as discussed above, AKI and CKD predispose to more frequent HF events (the hallmark of CRS types 3 and 4), suggesting a temporal relationship between the progression of renal disease and deterioration in cardiac function.

## ALBUMINURIA

Albuminuria and proteinuria frequently develop and are hallmarks of CKD. As such, in patients who have AKI or CKD complicated by HF (CRS type 3 or 4), albuminuria is often present and has been the focus of extensive research. In patients with HF complicated by CKD, worsening renal function, or AKI, albuminuria has been observed as well.[67,68] In patients with chronic HFREF or HFPEF, three retrospective analyses from randomized studies have shown that albuminuria is present in up to 41% of patients (20%–30% microalbuminuria, 5%–11% macroalbuminuria).[67,69] Similar prevalences were observed in one single-center study of stable HFPEF patients.[70] In acute HF, fewer data are available. Using a dipstick test to evaluate proteinuria, 55% of patients with acute HF had a positive dipstick test in a Chinese cohort.[71] In a small cohort of 100 acute HF patients from Portugal, only 26% to 40% of patients with acute HF presented with normoalbuminuria.[72] In all these analyses, including any HF phenotype, the presence of albuminuria was associated with a higher risk of cardiovascular events, independent of baseline eGFR. Furthermore, neither ARB nor statin treatment was able to reduce the urinary albumin excretion rate significantly.[67,68]

The pathophysiology of increased albumin excretion in HF, as discussed earlier, is probably different from albuminuria in hypertension, diabetes, and other cardiovascular disease, including CKD without HF. Whereas in these conditions it is thought that higher intraglomerular pressures (either primarily or as an adaptive process) induce structural glomerular changes, podocyte dysfunction, and eventually leakage of macromolecules such as albumin, in HF the intraglomerular pressures are (probably) low. The reasons for low intraglomerular pressures are a low RBF, a low efferent arteriolar tone in the presence of RAAS inhibitor therapy, and probably high afferent arteriolar tone in very low cardiac output states. Indeed, in the most severe chronic HFREF patients, RBF, GFR, and FF are low, whereas renal vascular resistance and albumin excretion are high.[32] This suggests that the pathophysiology of albumin excretion in HF must be distinctly different from that observed in hypertension, diabetes, and intrinsic renal disease. Proposed mechanisms include endothelial dysfunction and inflammation, structural glomerular damage, and changes in the glycocalyx, as well as podocyte dysfunction.

Whether higher renal venous pressure and associated higher renal interstitial pressures also contribute to albuminuria is unknown. Most interestingly, and reinforcing the notion that albuminuria must be different in HF compared with CKD, sacubitril/valsartan treatment in HFPEF and HFREF actually increases urinary albumin excretion, but leads to substantially reduced rates of adverse cardiovascular outcomes.[73,74] This essentially indicates that together with a lack of effect of both statin and ARB treatment on albumin levels, albuminuria by itself serves as a risk marker, rather than as a risk factor, in HF.[75]

## TUBULOINTERSTITIAL DAMAGE IN HEART FAILURE

Analogous to CKD, patients with HF experience not only a reduced eGFR and albuminuria, but also exhibit evidence of tubulointerstitial damage and injury.[76] However, in contrast to primary kidney disease, histologic evidence of tubulointerstitial damage is rarely obtained because biopsies are seldom performed in patients with HF. In one small study in patients with severely reduced eGFR considered for heart transplantation, renal biopsies were performed.[77] The cause of HF differed, ranging from ischemic HF to dilated cardiomyopathy and amyloid disease. The renal pathology did not correlate directly with cardiac pathology. Renal pathology ranged from ischemic nephropathy to focal global glomerulosclerosis and diabetic glomerulosclerosis. Fibrosis in the renal biopsies of the patients with severe HF ranged from 5% to 50%, but did not correlate with the amount of proteinuria or degree of eGFR decrease. These data indicate that in patients with severe HF, renal fibrosis is often present but does not correlate with a reduction in eGFR and albuminuria, unlike in primary

CKD, reflecting the superimposed physiologic component of renal dysfunction.

Most indirect evidence of tubulointerstitial damage and injury in HF patients comes from biomarker analyses. In parallel to studies in CKD, changes in urinary (and plasma) proteins that have been associated with tubular injury and damage in patients with kidney disease can also be found in a large proportion of patients with HF. In chronic HFREF patients, urinary levels of markers of tubulointerstitial damage, such as kidney injury molecule 1 (KIM-1), neutrophil gelatinase-associated lipocalin (NGAL), and N-acetyl-beta-D-glucosaminidase (NAG), were markedly elevated compared with normal values from control subjects.[76,78-81] Notably, there was only a marginal correlation between these markers of tubulointerstitial damage and albuminuria.[82] All measures of renal dysfunction, including reduced eGFR, albuminuria, and increased levels of tubulointerstitial damage, provided prognostic information in these patients. In the longer term, higher urinary KIM-1 levels were associated with more frequent occurrence of worsening renal function in the chronic outpatient setting, even outperforming baseline eGFR in predicting this.[76]

In acute HF, evidence of tubulointerstitial damage is clear as well.[78,79,83] When present either at presentation or at discharge, evidence of tubular injury predisposes to worse outcomes in these patients, especially higher mortality.[78,84] In addition to providing prognostic information, these markers of tubulointerstitial damage, especially NGAL, have been shown to predict AKI in different patient settings without HF, including patients undergoing thoracic surgery and patients with primary kidney disease.[85,86] However, the prediction of AKI and worsening renal function in acute HF has been more challenging, and these markers have not been shown to be of any help in predicting clinically relevant worsening renal function. Although small studies have suggested possible incremental information obtained with determining NGAL levels, two large studies have now shown lack of superiority of NGAL over the serum creatinine level. In the prospective AKINESIS study, plasma NGAL was not superior to the serum creatinine level in predicting AKI in those with acute HF, whereas in a retrospective analysis from the PROTECT study, serial plasma NGAL concentrations rose in parallel with the serum creatinine level in patients with worsening renal function, but did not outperform the serum creatinine level.[87,88] One small study has evaluated changes in these markers in response to loop diuretic withdrawal and re-initiation in chronic HF and showed that both NAG and KIM-1 showed significant changes in response to changes in diuretic treatment, whereas the serum creatinine level did not change.[89] Whether tubulointerstitial damage may be a target for therapy has not been established in HF.

## TREATMENT OF HEART FAILURE IN PATIENTS WITH CONCOMITANT RENAL DYSFUNCTION

In patients with acute HF who develop worsening renal function (CRS type 1), treatment is not different from that given to acute HF patients without renal dysfunction. Because no evidence-based treatments that improve outcome have been established in acute HF (rather than chronic HF), therapy is aimed at improvement of symptoms. It is, however, important to realize that patients with renal impairment at presentation (or that develops during admission) may require different doses of diuretics, vasodilators, and other therapies because their response to these treatments may be different. Most of the time these treatments will be less effective. For example, diuretic resistance and a reduced response to loop diuretic therapy in these patients is observed much more frequently. Furthermore, as alluded to in the previous sections, an increase in the serum creatinine level during decongestive therapy, without a deterioration in clinical status (or actual improvement), is often observed and acceptable. Often, these changes are transient and, when these occur in parallel, with a favorable diuretic response, are not associated with worse outcomes. It has not been established which dosage (high vs. low) or which administration type (bolus or continuous) of loop diuretics is superior, although higher dosages were associated with more frequent worsening renal function, without translating into a difference in clinical outcome.[90]

In the situation of chronic HF patients with renal dysfunction (CRS type 2), a distinction must be made for the different phenotypes of chronic HF. Treatment for HFPEF patients, with or without renal dysfunction, should focus on the underlying disease and treatment of comorbidities because there are no evidence-based treatments that improve outcomes in these patients.[1]

The cornerstone treatments in all patients with HFREF include RAAS inhibitors such as ACE inhibitors, ARBs, or preferably the combination of a neprilysin inhibitor with an ARB (i.e., sacubitril/valsartan), as well as beta-blockers and mineralocorticoid receptor antagonists (Fig. 40.4 and Table 40.3).[1,2,62] Most recent HF guidelines advocate the start of ACE inhibitor therapy (or ARB if ACE inhibitor–intolerant), together with beta-blocker therapy. These agents can safely be prescribed in HF patients with eGFR > 30 mL/min/1.73 $m^2$, and there is moderate to strong evidence of mortality benefit in HF patients with CKD stages 1 to 3. Combination therapy of ACE inhibition and ARB therapy is not recommended and is associated with a higher risk of worsening renal function and hyperkalemia, especially in CRS type 2.[61] When these treatments are at their maximum tolerable dose, and patients remain symptomatic, the next step will be addition of a mineralocorticoid receptor antagonist. This means that on top of ACE inhibition, ARB, and beta-blocker therapy, either spironolactone or eplerenone is added. In several studies in HF patients with CKD stages 1 to 3, these treatments were effective in reducing the occurrence of (cardiovascular) death or HF rehospitalization.[91] The risk of hyperkalemia with this drug combination, however, must be borne in mind, especially at lower GFRs. If despite these agents, HFREF patients remain symptomatic, the next step would be to replace ACE inhibitor or ARB therapy with sacubitril/valsartan, which is a combination of an ARB (valsartan) with a neprilysin inhibitor. This combination treatment was shown to reduce the risk of (cardiovascular) death as compared with enalapril in patients with CKD stages 1 to 3 and reduced the risk of renal adverse events.[74]

For patients who have both HFREF and reduced eGFR (CRS type 2), these treatments will generally be (and should be) prescribed without hesitation. However, none of the evidence-based treatments in HFREF have been evaluated in HF patients with eGFR below 30 mL/min/1.73 $m^2$, which

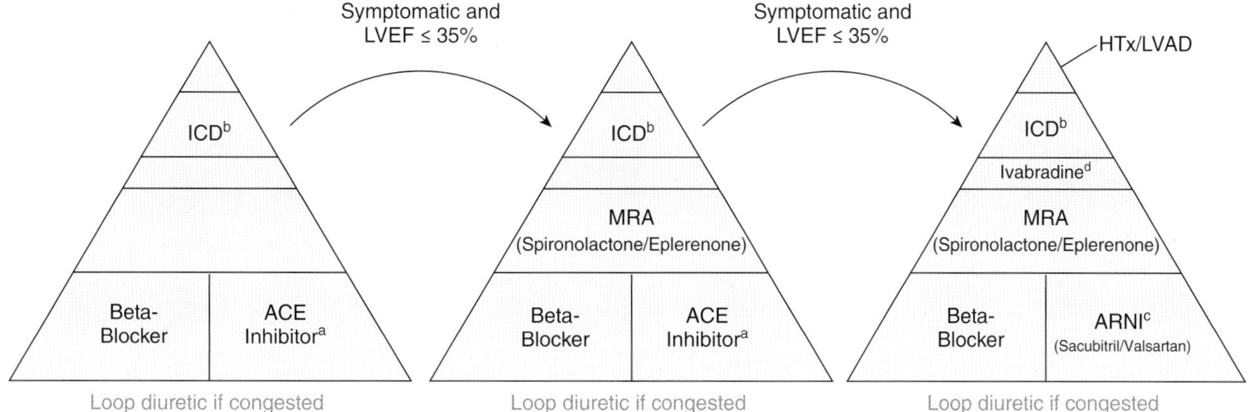


**Fig. 40.4 Treatment algorithm for HFREF patients.** This is the treatment algorithm for HFREF patients in general and for patients with CKD up to stage 3 (stages 4 and 5 not included). Initial treatment should include an ACE inhibitor and beta-blocker, uptitrated to the maximal tolerated dose. Loop diuretics are advised to relieve symptoms and signs of congestion. *ACE,* Angiotensin-converting enzyme; *CKD,* chronic kidney disease; *HFREF,* heart failure with reduced ejection fraction; *HTx,* heart transplantation. [a]Switch or start with an ARB if the ACE inhibitor is not tolerated. Do not combine an ACE inhibitor and ARB. [b]*ICD* (implantable cardioverter-defibrillator) indicated in secondary prevention or in symptomatic patients with LVEF ≤ 35%, despite optimal medical treatment (cardiac resynchronization therapy in selected patients) If patients remain symptomatic, add a mineralocorticoid receptor antagonist *(MRA)* and uptitrate to the maximum tolerated dose. [c]If, despite these therapies, the patient remains symptomatic, the ACE inhibitor can be replaced by *ARNI* (angiotensin receptor blocker neprilysin inhibitor—sacubitril/valsartan). [d]In patients with sinus rhythm and heart rate >70 beats/min, ivabradine may be added. Only select patients with advanced refractory heart failure, LVAD, and/or heart transplantation may be considered. (Adapted from Ponikowski P, Voors AA, Anker SD, Bueno H, et al. 2016 ESC guidelines for the diagnosis and treatment of acute and chronic heart failure: the Task Force for the diagnosis and treatment of acute and chronic heart failure of the European Society of Cardiology (ESC). Developed with the special contribution of the Heart Failure Association (HFA) of the ESC. *Eur J Heart Fail.* 2016;18:891–975. Also adapted from references 2, 61, and 62.)

means there is no solid scientific evidence for the use of these agents in HF patients with stage 4 or 5 CKD.[91] Furthermore, clinicians may be reluctant to maintain patients on RAAS inhibitor therapy when the serum creatinine level increases during uptitration or to start these agents when eGFR is close to 30 mL/min/1.73 m$^2$. However, the latter group represents patients who will probably benefit even more from evidence-based therapies compared with those with relatively preserved eGFR, and therefore could be initiated at low doses and uptitrated, with close follow-up.

Other therapies, such as implantable cardioverter-defibrillators (ICDs) and/or cardiac resynchronization therapy (CRT), should not be withheld in patients with concomitant cardiac and renal failure if life expectancy is sufficient to allow benefit in quality of life or life expectancy.[91] Some treatments, such as CRT and left ventricular assist devices (LVADs), have actually been shown to improve renal function in the long term.[92] LVADs are essentially extracardiac pumps that restore (part of) the circulation and thereby organ perfusion. Even though they do not provide an artificial pulse, but rather a continuous flow, renal function is often restored (to some extent), although AKI and/or worsening renal function is also often observed in the early postoperative phase of the implantation of the device. The finding that renal function improves over time with these devices suggests that for CRS type 2, impaired hemodynamics caused by worse LV function result in renal dysfunction by causing worse renal perfusion.

For patients with advanced HF who are considered possible heart transplant recipients, a greatly reduced GFR is an important relative contraindication to transplantation. Immunosuppression after transplantation is often nephrotoxic and, together with the cardiac transplant procedure itself, may initiate or exacerbate renal injury and dysfunction. A low eGFR in patients with HF is often due to hemodynamic derangement and can be restored after heart transplantation, but other comorbid organ dysfunctions, such as diabetes, atherosclerosis, and hypertension, may also have caused irreversible renal damage. The current criteria for heart transplant listing suggest thorough evaluation of renal function, and only list patients who do not have irreversible stage 4 or 5 CKD.[93] In select patients, usually young patients, a combined heart and kidney transplant may be considered, but this decision has to be made on a case-by-case basis, also taking into account donor organ availability, quality, and recipient characteristics.

For HF patients with severe CKD, treatment with evidence-based therapies should always be an individualized decision based on the balance between the risk of worsening heart and renal function and possible benefit expected with each treatment. This may mean that in the situation of palliative care in patients with very severe HF and/or renal disease, some evidence-based treatments that preserve renal and cardiac function and are associated with better outcomes in the long term may be discontinued because of worsening renal function, hypotension, and/or other discomforts to improve quality of life.

In conclusion, CRSs represent a very heterogeneous group of disorders in patients with both heart and kidney dysfunction. This chapter specifically focused on CRS types 1 and 2, where heart–kidney interactions are predominantly mediated by impaired hemodynamics. Although treatment of HF patients with renal dysfunction is in itself no different from treatment of patients without CKD, there is limited evidence of the effectiveness of these treatments in CKD stages 4 and 5. Because HF patients with concomitant renal

**Table 40.3 Characteristics of Different Treatment in HFREF Patients With Chronic Kidney Disease**

| Therapy | Incidence of Worsening Renal Function and Adverse Events | Incidence of Hyperkalemia | Effectiveness in HFREF Patients[a] | | Cautions and Remarks |
|---|---|---|---|---|---|
| | | | CKD Stage 1–3 | CKD Stage 4 or 5 | |
| ACE inhibitor | 1.5%–13.7% (35% in NYHA IV) | 1.1%–6.4% (7% in NYHA IV) | Yes | Unclear; possible | Induces early decline in eGFR; some increase in serum creatinine should be accepted. Very large increases should prompt further investigation and (temporary) stopping of drug. |
| ARB | 5.5%–17% (24% with high-dose losartan) | 1%–3% (10% with high-dose losartan) | Yes | Unclear | |
| MRA | 1.9%–17% | 2%–8% | Yes | Unclear; possible | |
| ARNI | 2.2% | 4.3% (potassium > 6 mmol/L) | Yes | Unclear; possible | Sacubitril/valsartan was superior to enalapril in reducing renal events and also slowing progression of decline in eGFR; increases urinary albumin excretion to some extent. Large increases should prompt further investigation. |
| Beta-blocker | 7%–10.1% | NA | Yes | Probable | Effect on renal function negligible compared with placebo; should be continued if possible. |
| Loop diuretics | NA | Probably low | NA | NA | Use and dose associated with worsening renal function. Long-term effects on renal function unknown. Dose should be higher in patients with CKD stage 3–5. |
| CRT | NA | NA | Yes | Unclear; possible | Improvement in renal function in parallel—improvement in clinical symptoms can be expected. |
| LVAD | NA | NA | Yes | Unclear; possible | LVAD therapy improves renal function in the long term. However, risk of AKI is peri- and postoperatively higher in patients with CKD stage 3-5 at baseline. Risk of contrast nephropathy at time of implantation. |

[a]Improvement in clinical outcome.

*ARB,* Angiotensin II receptor blocker; *ACE,* angiotensin-converting enzyme; *ARNI,* angiotensin receptor blocker neprilysin inhibitor; *CKD,* chronic kidney disease; *CRT,* cardiac resynchronization therapy; *eGFR,* estimated glomerular filtration rate; *HFREF,* heart failure with reduced ejection fraction; *LVAD,* left ventricular assist device; *NYHA,* New York Heart Association.

Adapted from Damman K, Tang WH, Felker GM, et al. Current evidence on treatment of patients with chronic systolic heart failure and renal insufficiency: practical considerations from published data. *J Am Coll Cardiol.* 2014;63:853–871.

dysfunction represent a very high-risk population, they should be monitored and evaluated closely and on a regular basis, and treatment alterations should be based on a case-by-case evaluation.

 Complete reference list available at ExpertConsult.com.

## KEY REFERENCES


1. Ponikowski P, Voors AA, Anker SD, et al. 2016 ESC guidelines for the diagnosis and treatment of acute and chronic heart failure. *Eur Heart J.* 2016;37:2129–2200.
2. Writing Committee Members, Yancy CW, Jessup M, et al. 2013 ACCF/AHA guideline for the management of heart failure: a report of the American College of Cardiology Foundation/American Heart Association Task Force on practice guidelines. *Circulation.* 2013;128:e240–e327.
6. Ronco C, Haapio M, House AA, et al. Cardiorenal syndrome. *J Am Coll Cardiol.* 2008;52:1527–1539.
7. Damman K, Voors AA, Navis G, et al. The cardiorenal syndrome in heart failure. *Prog Cardiovasc Dis.* 2011;54:144–153.
8. Maxwell MH, Breed ES, Schwartz IL. Renal venous pressure in chronic congestive heart failure. *J Clin Invest.* 1950;29:342–348.
9. Werko L, Varnauskas E, Ek J, et al. Studies on the renal circulation and renal function in mitral valvular disease. II. Effect of apresoline. *Circulation.* 1954;9:700–705.
10. Blake WD, Wegria R, Keating RP, et al. Effect of increased renal venous pressure on renal function. *Am J Physiol.* 1949;157:1–13.
16. Haase M, Muller C, Damman K, et al. Pathogenesis of cardiorenal syndrome type 1 in acute decompensated heart failure: workgroup statements from the eleventh consensus conference of the Acute Dialysis Quality Initiative (ADQI). *Contrib Nephrol.* 2013;182:99–116.
17. Cruz DN, Schmidt-Ott KM, Vescovo G, et al. Pathophysiology of cardiorenal syndrome type 2 in stable chronic heart failure: workgroup

statements from the eleventh consensus conference of the Acute Dialysis Quality Initiative (ADQI). *Contrib Nephrol.* 2013;182:117–136.
23. McAlister FA, Ezekowitz J, Tarantini L, et al. Renal dysfunction in patients with heart failure with preserved versus reduced ejection fraction: impact of the new Chronic Kidney Disease-Epidemiology Collaboration Group formula. *Circ Heart Fail.* 2012;5:309–314.
25. Damman K, Masson S, Lucci D, et al. Progression of renal impairment and chronic kidney disease in chronic heart failure: an analysis from GISSI-HF. *J Card Fail.* 2017;23:2–9.
26. Go AS, Chertow GM, Fan D, et al. Chronic kidney disease and the risks of death, cardiovascular events, and hospitalization. *N Engl J Med.* 2004;351:1296–1305.
30. Leithe ME, Margorien RD, Hermiller JB, et al. Relationship between central hemodynamics and regional blood-flow in normal subjects and in patients with congestive heart-failure. *Circulation.* 1984;69:57–64.
31. Ljungman S, Laragh JH, Cody RJ. Role of the kidney in congestive heart failure. Relationship of cardiac index to kidney function. *Drugs.* 1990;39(suppl 4):10–21.
32. Smilde TD, Damman K, van der Harst P, et al. Differential associations between renal function and "modifiable" risk factors in patients with chronic heart failure. *Clin Res Cardiol.* 2009;98:121–129.
36. Burnett JC Jr, Knox FG. Renal interstitial pressure and sodium excretion during renal vein constriction. *Am J Physiol.* 1980;238:F279–F282.
40. Damman K, Testani JM. The kidney in heart failure: an update. *Eur Heart J.* 2015;36:1437–1444.
41. Mullens W, Abrahams Z, Francis GS, et al. Importance of venous congestion for worsening of renal function in advanced decompensated heart failure. *J Am Coll Cardiol.* 2009;53:589–596.
42. Damman K, van Deursen V, Navis G, et al. Increased central venous pressure is associated with impaired renal function and mortality in a broad spectrum of patients with cardiovascular disease. *J Am Coll Cardiol.* 2009;53:582–588.
47. Mullens W, Abrahams Z, Francis GS, et al. Prompt reduction in intra-abdominal pressure following large-volume mechanical fluid removal improves renal insufficiency in refractory decompensated heart failure. *J Card Fail.* 2008;14:508–514.
51. McCullough PA, Kellum JA, Haase M, et al. Pathophysiology of the cardiorenal syndromes: executive summary from the eleventh consensus conference of the Acute Dialysis Quality Initiative (ADQI). *Contrib Nephrol.* 2013;182:82–98.
55. Damman K, Tang WH, Testani JM, et al. Terminology and definition of changes renal function in heart failure. *Eur Heart J.* 2014;35:3413–3416.
56. Damman K, Navis G, Voors AA, et al. Worsening renal function and prognosis in heart failure: systematic review and meta-analysis. *J Card Fail.* 2007;13:599–608.
61. Ponikowski P, Voors AA, Anker SD, et al. 2016 ESC guidelines for the diagnosis and treatment of acute and chronic heart failure: the Task Force for the diagnosis and treatment of acute and chronic heart failure of the European Society of Cardiology (ESC). Developed with the special contribution of the Heart Failure Association (HFA) of the ESC. *Eur J Heart Fail.* 2016;18:891–975.
67. Masson S, Latini R, Milani V, et al. Prevalence and prognostic value of elevated urinary albumin excretion in patients with chronic heart failure: data from the GISSI-heart failure trial. *Circ Heart Fail.* 2010;3:65–72.
68. Jackson CE, Solomon SD, Gerstein HC, et al. Albuminuria in chronic heart failure: prevalence and prognostic importance. *Lancet.* 2009;374:543–550.
70. Katz DH, Burns JA, Aguilar FG, et al. Albuminuria is independently associated with cardiac remodeling, abnormal right and left ventricular function, and worse outcomes in heart failure with preserved ejection fraction. *JACC Heart Fail.* 2014;2:586–596.
74. McMurray JJ, Packer M, Desai AS, et al. Angiotensin-neprilysin inhibition versus enalapril in heart failure. *N Engl J Med.* 2014;371:993–1004.
82. Damman K, Masson S, Hillege HL, et al. Clinical outcome of renal tubular damage in chronic heart failure. *Eur Heart J.* 2011;32:2705–2712.
87. Maisel AS, Wettersten N, van Veldhuisen DJ, et al. Neutrophil gelatinase-associated lipocalin for acute kidney injury during acute heart failure hospitalizations: the AKINESIS study. *J Am Coll Cardiol.* 2016;68:1420–1431.
90. Felker GM, Lee KL, Bull DA, et al. Diuretic strategies in patients with acute decompensated heart failure. *N Engl J Med.* 2011;364:797–805.
91. Damman K, Tang WH, Felker GM, et al. Current evidence on treatment of patients with chronic systolic heart failure and renal insufficiency: practical considerations from published data. *J Am Coll Cardiol.* 2014;63:853–871.

# 41 Kidney Cancer

Robert H. Weiss | Edgar A. Jaimes | Susie L. Hu

## CHAPTER OUTLINE



## KEY POINTS

- Renal cell carcinoma (RCC) is diagnosed in approximately 64,000 patients/year in the United States.
- Clear cell renal cell carcinoma (ccRCC) is the most common histologic subtype.
- ccRCC is one of the relatively few malignancies that has an increasing incidence.
- RCC is frequently asymptomatic and is commonly diagnosed incidentally in the nephrology clinic during workup of acute kidney injury, obstruction, and/or hematuria.
- ccRCC is associated with paraneoplastic syndromes, most of which are related to its reprogrammed metabolism.
- Early immunomodulating therapies have shown minimal success, but newer targeted and checkpoint inhibitor treatments have improved survival.

Kidney cancer, among the 10 most common cancers in men and women, is one of the relatively few malignancies that has been increasing in incidence. This disease has proved refractory to most systemic therapies,[1] until quite recently, with the advent of immune checkpoint inhibitor antibodies,[2] and has a dismal prognosis, with an overall 5-year survival rate of 74%. This drops to 8% of those with metastatic disease (see http://seer.cancer.gov/statfacts/html/kidrp.html). Most importantly to the readers of this chapter, kidney cancer is the most common malignancy seen in the renal clinic.

Traditionally relegated to the practice sphere of urologists and oncologists, kidney cancer has recently been the subject of a resurgence in clinical and basic research (the latter in the area of metabolic reprogramming[3]), much of it undertaken by nephrology researchers. Thus it is imperative that practitioners of this subspecialty are keenly aware of the biology, risk factors, presentation, and management of this increasingly common disease, as has been recently reviewed.[4] In this chapter, we discuss the basics of kidney cancer (also known as renal cell carcinoma, RCC), focusing on the most common type, clear cell RCC (ccRCC), so that the nephrologist will be comfortable with all aspects of a disease seen increasingly commonly in clinical practice.

## BIOLOGY OF RENAL CELL CARCINOMA

RCC is the most common malignancy that originates from the renal cortex[5] and is most often classified by histologic subtype. The most common subtype is ccRCC, comprising 75% to 85% of cases, but other histologic subtypes are also seen, many in children (Table 41.1). Each of the seven known genes that are mutated in the different types of kidney cancer are involved in a number of disparate pathways that regulate various aspects of cellular metabolism, such as oxygen and/or iron sensing, the tricarboxylic acid (TCA) cycle (also known as the Krebs cycle), glutamine metabolism, and tumor energetics.[3] For this reason, kidney cancer has been aptly labeled a "metabolic disease."[6–8] Indeed, ccRCC has also been shown to be characterized by alterations in metabolism, as evidenced by nonstandard pathways in amino acid degradation, as well as energy production and protection from oxidative stress. This phenomenon of metabolic reprogramming[9] was first described by Warburg early in the 20th century[10] and has become evident in a variety of malignancies, including RCC. Such findings have been put to use in developing new biomarkers and therapeutic paradigms.[3]

ccRCC, the most common subtype and thus the primary subject of this chapter, comprises 70% of all RCCs and is one of the most lethal subtypes. The loss of the von Hippel-Lindau tumor suppressor (pVHL) gene[11] is common in ccRCC,[12–14] which to a large degree dictates its biologic behavior. This gene loss leads to activation of hypoxia pathways, even in the absence of true hypoxia, and characterizes ccRCC as a malignancy true to the Warburg effect (i.e., aerobic glycolysis).[10] Activation of downstream events by the VHL system, including neoangiogenesis and paraneoplastic phenomena, enables ccRCC cells to thrive as their surroundings become progressively more deprived of oxygen.[15]

## RENAL CELL CARCINOMA: A METABOLIC DISEASE

ccRCC is an aggressive cancer that arises from the proximal tubular epithelium and, in its metastatic form, is associated with a high mortality. Each of the mutated genes for the various types of kidney cancer is involved in metabolic pathways, such as oxygen and iron sensing, the TCA cycle, glutamine metabolism, and tumor energetics. Studies involving different genomic platforms,[16,17] also described in proteomic[18,19] and metabolomic[20] studies, have identified a profound metabolic shift in aggressive ccRCCs involving the TCA, pentose phosphate, and phosphoinositide 3-kinase (PI3K) pathways, among others (Fig. 41.1). Furthermore, there are many reprogrammed pathways in ccRCC that have been, or can soon be, exploited for novel therapeutic approaches, with the potential to transform the treatment of a disease with currently dismal options.

The hypoxia-inducible factor (HIF)–hypoxia pathway was one of the first pathways identified as being altered in ccRCC, but subsequent research has demonstrated that RCC has a number of additional metabolic abnormalities responsible for paraneoplastic syndromes. For example, the Warburg effect (aerobic glycolysis), arginine synthetic abnormalities (due to arginosuccinate synthetase-1 [ASS1] deficiency), and glutamine pathway reprogramming are all pronounced in RCC.[18,21,22] The elucidation of these and other metabolic abnormalities turns out to be a gold mine for therapeutic exploration. Targeted therapy using pathway-specific inhibitors, which in some cases are compounds that were discarded after their discovery, would show high specificity, with fewer adverse effects.[23]

**Table 41.1 Subtypes of Renal Cell Carcinoma**

| Subtype | Incidence |
|---|---|
| Clear cell | 70%–88% of RCCs[212–214] |
| Papillary type 1 | Papillary types 1 and 2 together constitute |
| Papillary type 2 | 10%–20% of RCCs[214–216] |
| Chromophobe | 5%[7,215] |

*ccRCC*, Clear cell renal cell carcinoma; *RCC*, renal cell carcinoma.

## BIOLOGY AND RATIONALE OF CURRENT THERAPEUTICS

Prior therapeutic approaches exploited the high level of immunogenicity of RCC and used immunotherapy with interferon and interleukin-2 (IL-2), but these were associated with severe and unpleasant adverse effects and only modest success. More recently, therapies targeting newly elucidated biochemical pathways have a better response, as well as fewer adverse effects, and there are even more pipeline therapies based on metabolic reprogramming, as with tryptophan[24] and arginine[21] reprogramming. Most recently, the immune checkpoint inhibitors have shown considerable promise in treating ccRCC, and studies are currently underway to find optimal combinations using these new drugs.[2] However, the marked inter- and intratumoral heterogeneity in ccRCC[25] has made it difficult to study this disease as a single entity with respect to therapeutic response.

## RENAL CELL CARCINOMA HISTOLOGY AND GENETICS

The traditional classification of RCC is based on histomorphologic criteria that divide RCC into the three

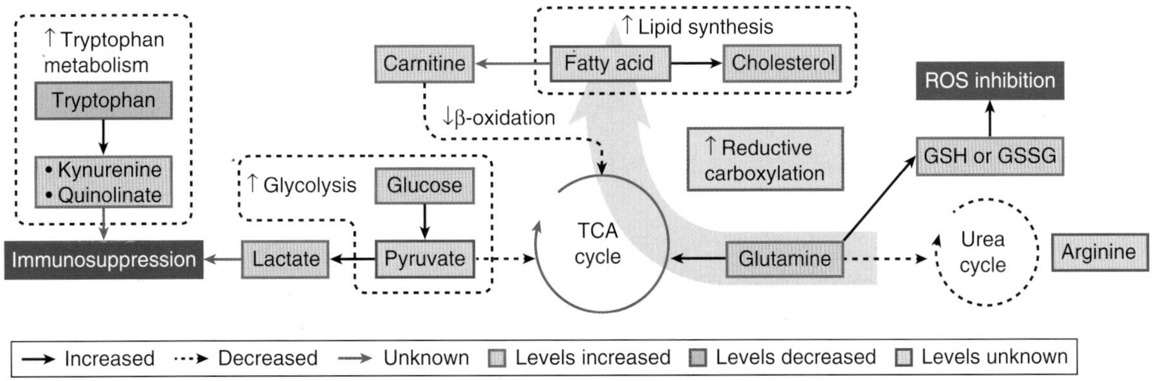


**Fig. 41.1 Metabolic reprogramming in clear cell renal cell carcinoma (ccRCC).** In ccRCC, aerobic glycolysis, carnitine and lipid synthesis, reductive carboxylation, the glutathione oxidized glutathione (GSH/GSSG) pathway, and tryptophan metabolism are upregulated, whereas the urea cycle and energy production through the tricarboxylic acid *(TCA)* cycle are downregulated. These changes are advantageous for ccRCC cells because they enable them to survive in conditions of nutrient depletion and hypoxia, provide the cellular building blocks required for proliferation, and result in the production of immunosuppressive (kynurenine and quinolinate) and antioxidant metabolites (GSH and GSSG). *GSH,* Glutathione; *GSSG,* glutathione disulfide; *ROS,* reactive oxygen species.

main types—clear cell RCC (ccRCC), papillary RCC (pRCC), and chromophobe RCC (chRCC; Table 41.1). Recent advances in the genomic profiling of RCC have resulted in further characterization of tumor types, allowing for better understanding of their biology and greater specificity of treatment targets.

### CLEAR CELL RENAL CELL CARCINOMA

ccRCC is the most common type of renal cancer and originates in proximal tubular cells. Genetic abnormalities in ccRCC are roughly divided into those affecting the VHL gene, epigenetic regulators and chromatin remodeling genes, and disruption of PI3K-AKT-mTOR signaling.[26,27]

The large majority of cases of ccRCC are sporadic, and only 2% to 3% of ccRCC cases are linked to hereditary diseases. Germline mutations in the pVHL gene on chromosome 3p25[28] lead to the formation of benign or malignant tumors and to the formation of cysts in other organs. Conversely, mutations or silencing of the same *VHL* gene are associated with more than 80% of sporadic ccRCC cases.[29,30] VHL disease is relatively common, with an estimated incidence of 1 in 36,000 live births,[31,32] and has a penetrance of more than 90% by age 65 years.[33] Most subjects affected by the disease inherit a germline mutation of the gene from the affected parent and a normal gene from the unaffected parent. All the cells of affected individuals who inherit the genetic trait will have germline mutations of *VHL*. However, tumors will develop only in those cells that undergo a deletion or mutation of the remaining wild-type allele (the so-called second hit) and, in addition, are constituents of vulnerable target organs, such as kidneys, central nervous system (CNS), adrenal glands, pancreas, and reproductive adnexal organs.

The *VHL* gene has three exons and is located on the short arm of chromosome 3 (3p25-26).[34] Since its discovery, it has been well established that this gene plays a crucial role in a variety of cellular pathways. The most important function of VHL protein (pVHL) is polyubiquitination of a variety of proteins, including HIF 1 and 2. This process marks them for degradation in the presence of normal tissue oxygenation.[35] However, under hypoxic conditions, HIF activates the transcription of hypoxia-inducible genes that results in the enhanced production of vascular endothelial growth factor (VEGF), erythropoietin, platelet-derived growth factor-β (PDGF-β), transforming growth factor-α (TGF-α), and several glycolytic enzymes.[36–38] Failure of pVHL to rein in the activity of HIF in normoxia has crucial implications for the clinical behavior and metabolic features of ccRCC. Among them are erythropoietin-dependent erythrocytosis, marked angiogenesis, and cell proliferation mediated by TGF-α and VEGF,[36,39] as well as aerobic glycolysis (Warburg effect) and the immunosuppressive effects of increased tryptophan catabolism.[40] The nature of interactions between HIF and cellular metabolism is likely bidirectional, as is evidenced by the inhibitory effects of the gluconeogenic enzyme fructose-1,6-bisphosphatase on HIF function.[41] Although some studies have shown an association between such metabolic abnormalities and tumor aggressiveness, nontargeted metabolomics analyses have not yet become a part of clinical practice.[42]

The second most common type of mutation involves several epigenetic regulators also localized on 3p25 chromosome, including polybromo 1 (PBRM1), BRCA-associated protein-1 (BAP1), and SET domain–containing 1 (SETD1) genes involved in regulation of chromatin maintenance and remodeling. Generally, hypermethylation of promoter sites is associated with the tumors carrying these mutations (with the exception of SETD1) and higher tumor grade, but their exact role in ccRCC pathogenesis is not well understood.[43–47]

Genetic aberration of mTOR pathway proteins (PTEN, AKT, PIK3CA, and mTOR) involved in cell proliferation signaling have been identified in up to 28% of RCC patients.[48] Deficiency in PTEN, in particular, is associated with more aggressive tumors.[49] Together with the abnormal expression of the focal adhesion kinase modulator of the mTOR pathway, these genetic defects are present in more than 50% of ccRCC patients.[48] As part of the Cancer Genome Atlas project, less frequent mutations of genes involved in cell metabolism and division have been described, with some of them, such as p53 overexpression, associated with a worse prognosis.[48]

### PAPILLARY RENAL CELL CARCINOMA

This second most common RCC is also of proximal tubule origin, but it has been studied less extensively than the other subtypes.[50] The type 1 papillary RCC (pRCC) is characterized by MET proto-oncogene–activating mutations taking place in germ cells in the hereditary form of the disease and 10% to 20% of cases of somatic mutations in the most common and sporadic form of the disease.[51] Additionally, trisomy 7 has been implicated in MET amplification in some cases of pRCC.[52] Type 2 pRCC is linked to activation of the NRF2 antioxidant response element pathway as the result of augmented oxidative stress. Mutations in the fumarate hydratase (FH) gene in this disorder are associated with hereditary leiomyomatosis and renal cell carcinoma (HLRCC).[29,53] Mutations in the epigenetic modifier genes *PBRM1*, *BAP1*, and *SETD1* have been described with this tumor type, but seem to be less prevalent compared with ccRCC.[52] Type 2 pRCC portends a considerably worse prognosis compared with type 1 pRCC.[54,55]

### CHROMOPHOBE RENAL CELL CARCINOMA

This rare cancer that originates from the collecting duct and that is similar to benign oncocytomas comprises less than 5% of RCC and is often linked with whole-chromosome losses and germline mutations in the folliculin gene (FLCN) found in the autosomal dominant Birt-Hogg-Dubé syndrome.[56,57] The most frequent mutation in sporadic cases of chRCC involves downregulation of p53 tumor suppressor signaling and loss of function of PTEN leading to PI3K-driven cell proliferation. ChRCC is more common in younger females and is typically the least aggressive of all RCC types, unless characterized by sarcomatous transformation.[58]

## PRESENTATION

The unusual and pleiomorphic presentation of RCC is reflective of its biologic characteristics, with clinical presentation unlike that of most other urologic tumors, and this challenge is reflected in its well-deserved appellation "the internist's tumor."[8] Thus, the diagnosis can be challenging due to its nonspecific and often systemic symptoms.[8]

The clinical presentation of RCC is variable; many patients have clinically occult disease and often present with a late and more advanced stage at the time of diagnosis. About 25% of patients have metastatic disease or advanced local disease at the time of presentation.[59–61] The classic presentation of hematuria, flank pain, and fever is seen in less than 10% of patients,[62] and more than 50% of patients are now diagnosed based on incidental findings in abdominal radiologic imaging performed for unrelated reasons.[63]

RCC patients can also present with nonspecific clinical findings, including hypertension (HTN), weight loss, malaise, night sweats, and the new onset of a varicocele. Paraneoplastic syndromes, including fever, anemia, hypercalcemia, erythrocytosis, and abnormal liver enzyme levels not due to metastatic spread (Stauffer syndrome), are seen in 7% of cases; polyneuropathy and amyloid A amyloidosis occur in 3% to 5%.[64] Fever occurs in up to 20% of patients and is often accompanied by night sweats, anorexia, weight loss, and fatigue.[64] Hypercalcemia occurs in up to 15% of cases and has been identified as a negative prognostic factor, sometimes associated with lytic bone metastases.[60] The ectopic production of parathyroid-related peptide by the tumor has been linked to hypercalcemia in the absence of bone metastases.[65–67] Erythrocytosis has been described in 1% to 5% of patients with RCC and is thought to be secondary to the unregulated production of erythropoietin by the cancer cells.[68,69]

RCC typically presents at 60 to 70 years of age. Other RCC risk factors in the general population include male gender, obesity, tobacco use, diabetes mellitus (DM), and HTN.[70] The incidence of RCC has increased more rapidly among blacks than whites, with a shift from a predominance among whites to blacks.[71] Although RCC has a higher incidence among those with obesity, this population tends to have better survival, which may be attributed to the potentially protective effect of brown fat. Furthermore, alcohol exposure paradoxically seems to lower RCC risk, unlike with other tumors, such as liver or colon cancer.[72,73] Cystic disease, which may progress to (or hide) RCC, is associated with end-stage renal disease (ESRD), and prolonged dialysis dependency also predispose ESRD patients to renal cancers, with a 100-fold increased risk.[74] A similar association has been made with chronic kidney disease (CKD), but to a lesser degree than with ESRD.[75]

## CYSTIC DISEASES AND RENAL CELL CARCINOMA

The link between cystic diseases and RCC was described in 1880 by Brigidi and Severi.[76,77] Cortical cystic disease can range from simple cysts to complex cysts, with increasing risk for malignancy, as defined by the Bosniak classification.[78–80] However, CKD-related specific cystic diseases, including acquired cystic kidney disease (ACKD) and polycystic kidney disease (PKD), have different characteristics from those of the general population and deserve further consideration, as discussed later.

### ACQUIRED CYSTIC KIDNEY DISEASE AND CHRONIC KIDNEY DISEASE

ESRD is associated with a high risk of RCC.[81] The incidence of RCC in the ESRD population ranges from 1% to 7% in various studies, which is reportedly exponentially greater than that in the general population.[82–86] Malignant transformation from ACKD that is seen primarily in the ESRD population appears to account partially for this association.[81]

The development of ACKD has been described among 7% to 22% of CKD patients, but this escalates among dialysis-dependent ESRD patients (10%–44% within 1–3 years) and increases further with prolonged duration of dialysis (>90% after 5–10 years).[84,87–89] Although the presence of ACKD leading to RCC has also been described among transplant recipients (23%), this is far less than that observed in ESRD patients on dialysis (80%).[84]

In addition to ESRD duration, risk factors for development of ACKD and likely progression to RCC include male gender, younger age at ESRD onset, and diagnosis of glomerulonephritis; however, diabetic nephropathy has been associated with a lower incidence of ACKD among Japanese dialysis patients. Furthermore, kidney volumes and the rate of volume increase appear greater in men compared with women. Other demographic factors, including race, have no association with ACKD.[84,87–89] Dialysis modality is not consistently related to ACKD risk[84,87]; however, in some reports, ACKD was less common with the peritoneal dialysis modality.[82,87,90] Much of the literature on ACKD and RCC was reported in the Japanese population, in whom transplantation is far less common, possibly because of cultural reasons. Therefore, the dialysis vintage of these ESRD cohorts is much greater than that in the United States, and these associations vary according to specific populations.

The diagnosis of ACKD is made by the presence of more than three cysts collectively in both kidneys.[87,88] ACKD cysts tend to be smaller in size (typically <0.6 cm in diameter, but can range up to 2–3 cm) compared with cysts in PKD or other cystic diseases. Symptoms related to ACKD are rare, except when related to complications. Cyst rupture with hemorrhage, cyst infections, erythrocytosis, calcium oxalate deposition, and stone formation has been described.[87,91]

It has been theorized that the acquired cysts, unlike those seen in PKD, communicate with the renal tubular system and therefore retain some normal functional properties. Cyst fluid content has been found to be higher in creatinine content, suggesting some filtering capacity, unlike simple or PCKD cysts (which have similar cyst and plasma creatinine levels). This may explain why cysts often regress with ACKD after renal transplantation when normal filtration is restored.[87,92]

The proliferation of cysts may stem from a reparative response to uremic metabolites, chronic acidosis, and ischemia.[82,87] Growth factors from cyst fluid have been proposed to induce cellular hypertrophy and hyperplasia in cell culture[82,93]; this proliferative effect was also observed in vitro with a polypeptide (15-30 kDa) isolated in plasma from dialysis patients.[94] Other potential causative factors include dialysis-related factors; however, these do not account for ACKD observed in nondialysis CKD patients. Data supporting these findings were published decades ago, without revealing a clear pathogenesis to date.[82,87]

### ACQUIRED CYSTIC KIDNEY DISEASE AND RENAL CELL CARCINOMA

The close association of ACKD with both RRC and ESRD may explain the increased risk of RCC in ESRD.[84] The annual incidence of RCC in a Japanese ACKD cohort with 20-year follow-up was 0.151%/year for those on dialysis less than 10 years and 0.340% with dialysis duration longer than 10 years,[87,89] which is higher than what has historically been observed in the general population (0.008%)[91]. Furthermore, the finding of shared risk factors between ACKD and RCC (male gender and ESRD) and related pathologic findings support the likelihood that ACKD can evolve to RCC.[87] Acquired cysts seen in dialysis patients have similar immunohistochemical profiles and histologic traits (kDaepithelial cell–lined cysts, with eosinophilic or foamy cytoplasm) compared with the RCCs associated with ACKD, suggesting that acquired cysts are precursor lesions to RCC in this population.[88,95]

Papillary RCC is the predominant pathologic subtype among ACKD and dialysis-associated tumors, in contrast to the sporadic form of RCC, ccRCC, typically seen in the general population. Distinctive immunohistochemical patterns of expression in RCC specimens appear to differentiate papillary RCC in ACKD-related cancer from ccRCC among Japanese ESRD patients. In this population, although hypoxia-inducible gene-2 (HIG2) protein expression was increased in both types of RCC, HIG2 was particularly higher with papillary RCC, whereas HIF-1α and activated nuclear factor-kappa B (NF-κB) elevation was seen primarily with ccRCC. Nontumorous but cystic regions had increased expression of all three proteins. HIG2 and HIF1-α were particularly upregulated with hyperplastic cysts. Persistent exposure to these mitogenic factors in both tubulointerstitial injury and RCC has been proposed to explain the carcinogenesis of ACKD to RCC.[96]

## POLYCYSTIC KIDNEY DISEASE AND RENAL CELL CARCINOMA

The prevalence of RCC in autosomal dominant polycystic kidney disease (ADPKD) does not appear to be greater than that in the general population, according to small case series and observational studies,[97–101] although there is some controversy in the literature on this subject. As in the general population, the histologic diagnosis of RCC in ADPKD tends to be clear cell carcinoma in the most current case series to date,[97,99,101] although in one European series, tubulopapillary pathology was prominently observed as well (42%).[100] RCC in ADPKD presents at a younger mean age (50–60 years) than spontaneous RCC, but often with advanced disease, where one-third of patients have bilateral kidney involvement or metastatic disease. Presentation with advanced disease may be caused by delayed diagnosis, given the complexity of diagnostic images in the presence of multiple benign cysts in ADPKD. Symptomatic diagnosis rather than incidental discovery of RCC is more common in this select population.[97,99,101]

## PROGNOSIS OF RENAL CELL CARCINOMA IN THE END-STAGE RENAL DISEASE POPULATION

The prognosis of RCC in the ESRD population is equivalent or better compared with that in the general population.[102–106] The 5-year survival from RCC related to ACKD was comparable between the two groups,[106] but a broader examination of RCC related to all causes in a contemporary French cohort has revealed that 5-year survival is 90.1% for the ESRD group ($n$ = 303) compared with 69.0% in the non-ESRD group ($n$ = 947). Cancer-specific mortality was much lower, at 4.3% (vs. 27.6%) for the ESRD group also. About one-third (30%) of the ESRD patients had ACKD, and RCC was incidentally diagnosed in most ESRD patients (87%). The ESRD group had more favorable characteristics, including younger age, better performance status, fewer symptoms, smaller tumor size (3.7 vs. 7.3 cm), and lower tumor grade and stage (10% vs. 42% with stage ≥3 tumor), and patients were more likely to have papillary tumor (37% vs. 7%) than observed in the general population.[105] Similar findings have been replicated in other studies.[102,104,105] Higher survival in the ESRD group is attributed to the incidental finding, presumably leading to earlier diagnosis compared with the non-ESRD group.[105] Further examination of a Japanese dialysis cohort has revealed that those with symptomatic (vs. incidental) diagnosis of RCC are more likely to have advanced tumor features, including greater size, higher stage, higher grade, and lower cancer-specific (76.9% vs. 95.3%) and overall (64.2% vs. 84.9%) 5-year survival. In addition to these features, longer dialysis duration and diabetic nephropathy were also identified as prognostic factors in a multivariable analysis for survival.[103] The less aggressive course of non-ccRCC may also explain the better outcomes associated with ERSD-related RCC.[104]

## RENAL CELL CARCINOMA RISK AND KIDNEY FUNCTION

The causal relationship between RCC and CKD is complex, with each pathology conferring risk to the other.[4] The 100-fold increased risk of RCC among ESRD patients[86] may be due to the higher prevalence of ACKD, but this does not clearly explain the association of pre-ESRD CKD with higher risk of RCC.[75] The largest cohort study to date has examined the risk of RCC due to CKD stratified by estimated glomerular filtration rate (eGFR) among 1,190,538 subjects without known RCC. With decreasing eGFR ranges, RCC risk increased as follows: stage 3a CKD, hazard ratio (HR), 1.39 (confidence interval [CI], 1.22–1.58); stage 3b, HR, 1.81 (CI, 1.51–2.17); and stages 4 and 5 CKD, HR, 2.28 (CI, 1.78–2.92).[75] The association was specifically with clear cell carcinoma and not with the other RCC subtypes. In contrast, the predominant RCC subtype seen with ESRD is pRCC, suggesting pathology that is unrelated to ACKD. Moreover, even early findings of kidney pathology, such as albuminuria, have been related to cancer, including RCC.[107] The link between kidney function and localized RCC risk was abundantly apparent among 202,195 renal transplant recipients. During periods of graft failure resulting in ESRD, the incidence of RCC rose and, during periods of graft function, RCC incidence fell (Fig. 41.2). This pattern recurred during periods of kidney function loss (repeat graft failure).[108] How loss of kidney function is related to RCC risk is largely unknown, but it has been attributed to inflammation, acidosis, or uremic factors often implicated in advanced CKD.[4,75,107]

## ACQUIRED CYSTIC KIDNEY DISEASE, RENAL CELL CARCINOMA, AND RENAL TRANSPLANTATION

Screening for RCC in renal transplant candidates who have ESRD is controversial and is not currently recommended,

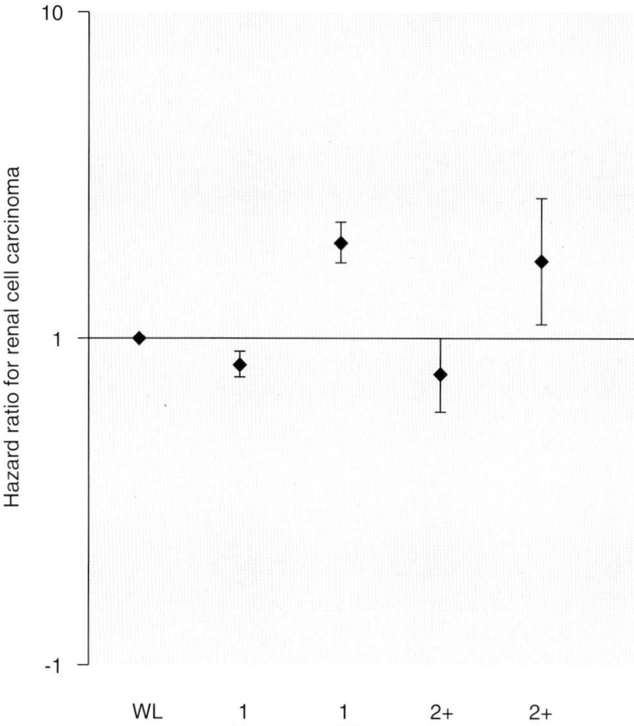


**Fig. 41.2 Risk of renal cell carcinoma (RCC) according to periods of renal function.** Shown are hazard ratios (HRs) comparing successive intervals for cancers with distinct alternating incidence patterns. Each point represents the HR comparing each interval with the immediately preceding interval. No HR estimate is given for the last interval when no cancers were observed in that interval. Vertical error bars represent end-stage renal disease–related cancers (95% confidence interval). Results are shown for cancer types that have demonstrated alternating patterns of cancer incidence across intervals—that is, based on the point estimates for the HRs, regardless of their statistical significance. *GF*, Graft failure; *Tx*, transplant; *WL*, waiting list. (Modified from Yanik EL, Clarke CA, Snyder JJ, et al. Variation in cancer incidence among patients with ESRD during kidney function and nonfunction intervals. *J Am Soc Nephrol.* 2016;27(5):1495–1504.)

despite the use of powerful immunosuppression drugs that increase cancer risk in general.[84,109,110] The question remains whether the risk of RCC is increased among transplant recipients, given the higher incidence of ACKD with ESRD. Most cohort studies have found that the prevalence of native kidney RCC for renal transplant recipients, ranging from 3% to 5%, was no different from the nontransplant ESRD population; however, this is still more than 100-fold greater than that of the general population.[86,111–113] On the other hand, donor allograft to the recipient transmission of RCC is rare (2/10,000 organs transplanted), with excellent outcomes, as reported in a meta-analysis but will not be explored further here.[114,115]

ACKD is less commonly described among transplant recipients (23%–33%) in most cohorts[86,111,116] but has been reported as high as 57%,[117] which is far less than that observed in ESRD patients on dialysis (80%).[84] The close association of ACKD and RCC is still apparent in the renal transplantation population; ACKD is higher among RCC transplant patients than among the overall, non-RCC transplant patients (60%–90% vs. 23%–33%, respectively).[86,113,117] However, there was an exception in one study, where they were found to be equivalent (33% with RCC vs. 29% without RCC).[111] Reciprocally, more transplant patients with ACKD are likely to have RCC than those without ACKD (11%–19% vs. 0.5%–0.6%). Generally, transplant recipients with RCC have favorable characteristics—younger age, smaller tumor size, less metastatic disease, more with stage T1a, and papillary subtype diagnosis—than nontransplant ESRD patients.[117] One transplant-related factor, a higher humoral rejection rate, has been observed in those diagnosed with RCC.[111]

Survival outcomes for transplant recipients with RCC have varied according to particular analyses, but generally appear to be more favorable compared with those of the general population, and possibly the dialysis population, likely due to closer surveillance of these patients. The 10-year, cancer-specific survival of 88% to 95% in transplant recipients is higher than that in the general population (75%).[116] Additionally, 97% of transplant recipients achieved a cancer-specific survival of 5 years, better than 77% in the nontransplanted ESRD group in one study.[117] The overall patient and graft survival between those with and without RCC have been comparable.[111]

Transplant recipients are a self-selected healthier cohort who, despite RCC prevalence similar to their dialysis counterparts and persistent association with ACKD, appear to have higher oncologic and overall survival than other ESRD patients and the general population. Furthermore, decision analysis did not support screening for ACKD in the entire ESRD population, given the minimal gain of life expectancy; however, the authors concluded that in younger healthier patients, screening may be considered.[109,110] Clinical judgment and risk analysis should be used to determine the benefit of screening on an individual basis.

# EVALUATION AND PROGNOSTIC ASSESSMENT OF RENAL MASSES

Renal masses are increasingly being discovered spontaneously with the frequent use of diagnostic imaging in clinical practice, in which the rate of incidental diagnosis increased from about 10% in the 1970s to 60% less than 3 decades later.[118] Incidental diagnosis has led to earlier detection of RCC at lower stages. To distinguish suspicious masses from benign tumors, clinicians rely on cyst classification systems, such as the Bosniak classification, which is based on cyst wall characteristics (thin vs. thickened), number of septae, calcification, contrast enhancement, and size (≥3 cm). Classes I and II define relatively benign lesions, starting from a simple cyst; then classes IIF and III have progressively increasing complexity, leading to class IV, composed of frankly malignant lesions (Table 41.2).[78–80] The malignancy risk of most cystic lesions can be assessed using these criteria. Prognosis is further determined with staging and grading tools, which are often incorporated into integrated staging systems for enhanced differentiation.[119,120]

## RADIOLOGIC EVALUATION OF RENAL MASSES

Along with clinical assessment, diagnostic imaging has become the mainstay of renal mass evaluation. The primary choice of imaging modality for screening and diagnosis of renal

**Table 41.2 Bosniak Classification of Renal Cystic Masses**

| Classification | Description | Likelihood of Malignancy (%) |
|---|---|---|
| Bosniak I | Simple cyst of water density with a thin wall that does not contain septa, calcifications, or other solid components | 1.7 |
| Bosniak II | Cyst may contain a few hairline septa and fine calcifications; uniform high- attenuation lesions <3 cm that do not show contrast enhancement | 18.5 |
| Bosniak IIF | Cysts may contain multiple hairline thin septa or minimal smooth wall thickening; calcifications may be thick and nodular, but no contrast enhancement | >18.5 |
| Bosniak III | More complex "indeterminate" cystic lesions, with more calcification and more prominent septation; thicker irregular or smooth walls; measurable contrast enhancement present | 33 |
| Bosniak IV | Clearly malignant cystic masses with all the criteria of category III but also contain contrast-enhancing soft tissue components adjacent to, but independent of, cyst wall or septum | 92.5 |

masses is computed tomography (CT) due to its high level of detection, particularly as higher-resolution multidetector CT scanners have come to be used more in most medical imaging centers.[118,121] Renal tumor detection by CT has high sensitivity (100%) and specificity (95%), and CT scanning can determine tumor size within 0.5 cm of the actual tumor measured histopathologically.[118] In a study examining the accuracy of tumors sizes measured by CT, 85% of renal masses identified by CT of 133 specimens were pathologically confirmed, although the tumor sizes were slightly overestimated by CT in this retrospective study.[122] Accuracy of staging by multidetector CT also excels in regard to extrarenal disease assessment, with high specificity, particularly for detection of capsular invasion (85%), perirenal fat invasion (98%), lymph node (82%), renal vein (98%), inferior vena cava (98%), and adrenal gland (98%) involvement,[118,121] and high sensitivity of 84% to 100%, except for capsular invasion (68%), perirenal fat invasion (46%), and lymph node involvement (77%).[118,121] Furthermore, RCC subtypes are identifiable on CT based on vascularity or heterogeneity of the mass, because ccRCC is more likely to be hypervascular and has heterogeneous parenchyma.[121]

Ultrasound is also commonly performed during the course of routine medical care, which has led to incidental finding of renal masses. It is particularly useful for distinguishing noncystic tumors from simple and complex cysts and equally useful for predicting T stage.[121] However, ultrasound is associated with inferior sensitivity and specificity for the detection of small tumors (1–2 cm) and is therefore a poor screening tool. Although detection rates for both ultrasound and CT for tumors are poor when evaluating masses smaller than 0.5 cm (0% and 47%, respectively), CT remains far superior to ultrasound for 1- to 2-cm lesions. Detection improves with increasing size, from 20% for 1-cm lesions to 79% for 2-cm lesions, but remains suboptimal until tumor size approaches 3 cm, where the detection rate by ultrasound (100%) finally reaches equivalence to CT.[123] Once the lesion is identified, ultrasound can be used for repeated monitoring, especially when avoidance of iodinated intravenous contrast is preferable.[121]

Novel contrast-enhanced ultrasound using microbubbles of injectable gas has been found to be even more sensitive than CT.[121] Early generations of these microbubbles were nonnephrotoxic but riddled with problems due to instability in the circulation, leading to cardiopulmonary complications and, in some cases, death. The current microbubbles, now smaller and more stable, have been approved for use by the U.S. Food and Drug Association (FDA).[124]

Magnetic resonance imaging (MRI) is traditionally considered to be the best modality for evaluating soft tissue pathology, including RCC, with optimal visualization of hemorrhage, micro- and macroscopic fat, and intracystic structures. The sensitivity and specificity for differentiating localized disease from the next stage (T3) is higher than any other modality (84% and 95%, respectively; positive predictive value of 96%) and 100% for both in detecting inferior vena cava (IVC) involvement.[125] In an advanced CKD or ESRD population, however, the use of MRI is excluded due to gadolinium-induced nephrogenic systemic fibrosis.[126] Although MRI remains highly effective in renal mass characterization and staging, the newer multidetector CT scanners have achieved an equivalent level of accuracy and detection rate as compared with MRI. Therefore, ultimately, CT has become the primary imaging modality to aid in the management of RCC.[127]

Because many ccRCCs are glutamine-avid and glutamine reprogramming has been identified in ccRCC,[3,20] this amino acid has been exploited in an experimental setting for novel positron emission tomography (PET)–based imaging techniques. A series of reports have suggested that $^{18}$F-fluorodeoxyglucose ($^{18}$F-FDG)–negative tumors might use glutaminolysis preferentially to glycolysis.[128–131] Concomitantly, we and others have found that RCC is strongly glutamine-avid and possibly even glutamine-addicted.[20,132] As a result of this work, the glutamine analog 4-$^{18}$F-(2S,4R)-fluoroglutamine was developed and shown to be taken up by cancer cells.[133] PET imaging has now been used to show glutamine uptake in animal models and in patients with glioma.[134] Moreover, glutamine uptake correlated with disease progression in these patients. In ccRCC, we have used PET scanning to show glutamine uptake in vitro and in several mouse xenograft models[134a] so that PET-based imaging based on the glutamine reprogramming of RCC could potentially be used in the future for RCC staging, patient selection, and real-time monitoring of glutaminase inhibition as a novel therapy for this disease.[3]

## DIFFERENTIATION OF BENIGN TUMORS FROM RENAL CELL CARCINOMA

The most commonly observed benign lesions are angiomyolipomas, which are composed of blood, smooth muscle, and adipose tissues. They are primarily seen among middle-aged women, 40 to 60 years of age.[135] Angiomyolipomas tend to be adipose-rich tumors that are easily distinguished from RCC, except when they are nonfatty (4.5%), which would require further assessment with MRI.[135,136] Oncocytomas are the next most frequently found benign renal mass (3%–5% of case series) generally seen among older men (aged in their 70s). These tumors are from tubular cells in the cortical collecting duct and can be difficult to differentiate from RCC due to their similar rate of growth.[135,136]

When current imaging techniques cannot adequately determine whether a tumor is benign or suspicious in a high surgical risk patient (although glutamine-based PET approaches have the potential to do this in the future; see previously), percutaneous renal biopsy can be safely performed with minimal risk of seeding (0.01% of cases), with high sensitivity (80%–100%) and specificity (83%–100%)[135,137,138] and high negative predictive value (82%) and positive predictive value (97.5%) in one series of 2474 percutaneous biopsies.[137] The rare case of seeding have been reported in transitional cell cancers, which may carry a slightly higher risk[135]; however, no case of seeding has been reported since 2001, particularly with the use of coaxial techniques, which avoid potential tumor exposure to the neighboring abdominal organs.[137,138]

## TUMOR STAGING AND GRADING

Tumor-node-metastasis (TNM) staging for RCC was first established in 1997 by the Union Internationale Contre le Cancer (UICC) and American Joint Committee on Cancer (AJCC) and was most recently updated in 2017 (Table 41.3).[139] T staging (T1–T4) is classified by the extent and size of the tumor, which differentiate cancer-specific survival. T1 tumors are limited to the kidney and are 7 cm or smaller; T2 tumors are larger, more than 7 cm, but are also in the kidney; T3 tumors extend beyond the kidney but are within Gerota fascia and may involve neighboring veins (renal vein or inferior vena cava); and T4 tumors invade Gerota fascia or extend to the ipsilateral adrenal gland. T1 and T2 are further subdivided according to renal mass size, and T3 is subdivided depending on venous involvement.[139] T staging imposes the greatest discrimination of 5-year cancer-specific survival, where T1a tumors have a survival rate as high as 98%, which declines to 10% with stage T4, as shown in Table 41.3.[120] Nodal invasion minimally alters outcomes, but distant metastases, including ipsilateral adrenal gland invasion, worsen the prognosis considerably.[120] Renal sinus fat involvement has also been found to be associated with lower survival.[140]

Composite prognostic staging (I–IV) summarizes the TNM findings. Tumors with stage I or II have kidney-limited lesions only. The prognostic stage is elevated to stage III when there is any nodal involvement, regardless of kidney size or T staging, and is escalated to stage IV when Gerota fascia invasion, adrenal gland, or distant metastasis occurs (Fig. 41.3).[139]

Grading determines prognosis based on nuclear features. Of the grading systems, the International Society of Urologic Pathology (ISUP)–defined grading system (ISUP grading system) is the currently recommend grading system; however, for some time, the Fuhrman grade has universally been used for prognostic assessment, despite some limitations. The nuclear size, irregularity, and nucleoli prominence differentiate RCC into four grades. Fuhrman grade 1 tumors have small nuclei and no nucleoli; grade 2 tumors have larger irregular nuclei and the presence of nucleoli; grade 3 tumors also

**Table 41.3 Tumor-Node-Metastasis Staging[a]**

| Stage | Category | Criteria[b] | Tumor Invasion |
|---|---|---|---|
| Tumor | T0 | No primary tumor | |
| | T1 | Tumor ≤7 cm | Confined to the kidney |
| | T1a | Tumor ≤4 cm | |
| | T1b | Tumor 4–7 cm | |
| | T2 | Tumor >7 cm | Confined to the kidney |
| | T2a | Tumor >7–10 cm | |
| | T2b | Tumor >10 cm | |
| | T3 | Major veins or perinephric tissues<br>No ipsilateral adrenal gland | Confined within Gerota fascia |
| | T3a | Renal vein and branches *or*<br>Renal pelvis and calyces *or*<br>Perirenal ± renal sinus fat | |
| | T3b | Vena cava below the diaphragm | |
| | T3c | Vena cava above the diaphragm *or*<br>vena cava wall | |
| | T4 | ± Ipsilateral adrenal gland | Extends beyond Gerota fascia |
| Node | N0 | No lymph nodes | — |
| | N1 | Any regional lymph node(s) | |
| Metastasis | M0 | No distant metastasis | — |
| | M1 | Distant metastasis | |

[a]By the American Joint Committee on Cancer (AJCC) and Union for International Cancer Control (UICC), 2017 update.
[b]Tumor size and perinephric tissue involvement.
Modified from Rini BI, McKiernan JM, Chang SS, et al., eds. *Kidney*. 8th ed. New York: Springer; 2017.

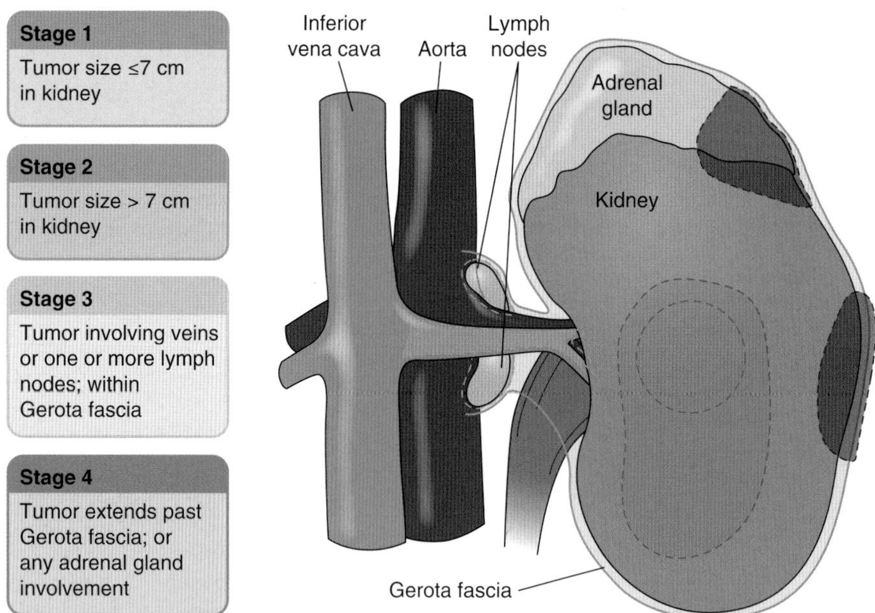


**Fig. 41.3 The tumor node metastasis (TNM) staging classification.** Shown is the general staging by the American Joint Committee on Cancer (AJCC) and Union for International Cancer Control (UICC), updated in 2017. (From Amin MB, Edge S, Greene F, et al., eds. *AJCC Cancer Staging Manual.* 8th ed. Springer International Publishing: American Joint Commission on Cancer; 2017 and Brierley JD, Gospodarowicz MK, Wittekind C, Eds. *TNM Classification of Malignant Tumours,* 8th ed. Wiley-Blackwell: 2017.)

**Table 41.4. Five-Year Cancer-Specific Survival and Prognosis of Renal Cell Carcinoma[a]**

| Prognosis | TNM Stage | Grade | Histologic Subtype | Sarcomatoid Differentiation | Rhabdoid Differentiation | Microscopic Coagulative Tumor Necrosis |
|---|---|---|---|---|---|---|
| Better | *Low stage*<br>T1a, 98%<br>T1b, 89%<br>T2a, 75%<br>T2b, 69% | *Low grade*<br>1: 51%–93%<br>2: 32%–86% | Papillary,<br>56%–92%; chromophobe,<br>78%–99% | Absence<br>79% | Absence | Absence |
| Worse | *High stage*<br>T3a, 53%<br>T3b, 31%<br>T3c, 36%<br>T4, 10% | *High grade*<br>3: 25%–50%<br>4: 10%–28% | Clear cell,<br>50%–86% | Presence,<br>15%–22% | Presence | Presence |

[a]Determined by staging, grading, and other histologic features.
*TNM,* Tumor-node-metastasis.

have large irregular nuclei, but with more visible nucleoli; and grade 4 tumors have extremely abnormal nuclei and highly prominent nucleoli apparent at low power.[141] The 5-year cancer-specific survival is highest for grade 1 and worst in grade 4, as illustrated in Table 41.4.[120] In some studies, Fuhrman grades 2 and 3 are thought to differentiate outcomes poorly.[120] Although this grading system has been reliably used for ccRCC, it has not been adequately validated for papillary or chromophobe RCC subtypes.[140,142] In 2012, the ISUP grading system further classified nuclear findings at specific magnifications and expanded criteria to include rhabdoid and sarcomatoid features (Fig. 41.4).[143]

Independent of TNM staging, higher grade and larger tumor size predict poorer survival. Histologic subtype is also a factor in survival. The most common and sporadic form of RCC, clear cell cancer (60%–90% prevalence vs. 6%–14% for papillary and 6%–14% for chromophobe), has inferior outcomes than those observed with papillary or chromophobe RCC. The 5-year survival for papillary and chromophobe RCC range is higher than that for ccRCC.[142] Other features, such as the presence of sarcomatoid or rhabdoid (eccentric large nuclei and eosinophilic cytoplasm) differentiation, now included in the ISUP grading system, and microscopic coagulative tumor necrosis add to the lower prognosis. Sarcomatoid differentiation, seen in only 4% of all RCC, reflects extreme dedifferentiation and is associated with a dismal prognosis. Each 10% increase of sarcomatoid changes is associated with a 6% increased risk of death from RCC, with less than a 1-year mean survival. Rhabdoid differentiation is even rarer, with similarly poor survival.[120,140]

Various integrated staging systems based on variables, often including TNM staging, tumor size, clinical symptoms, histologic subtype, grading, and other prognostic pathologic findings, can be used to predict outcomes preoperatively

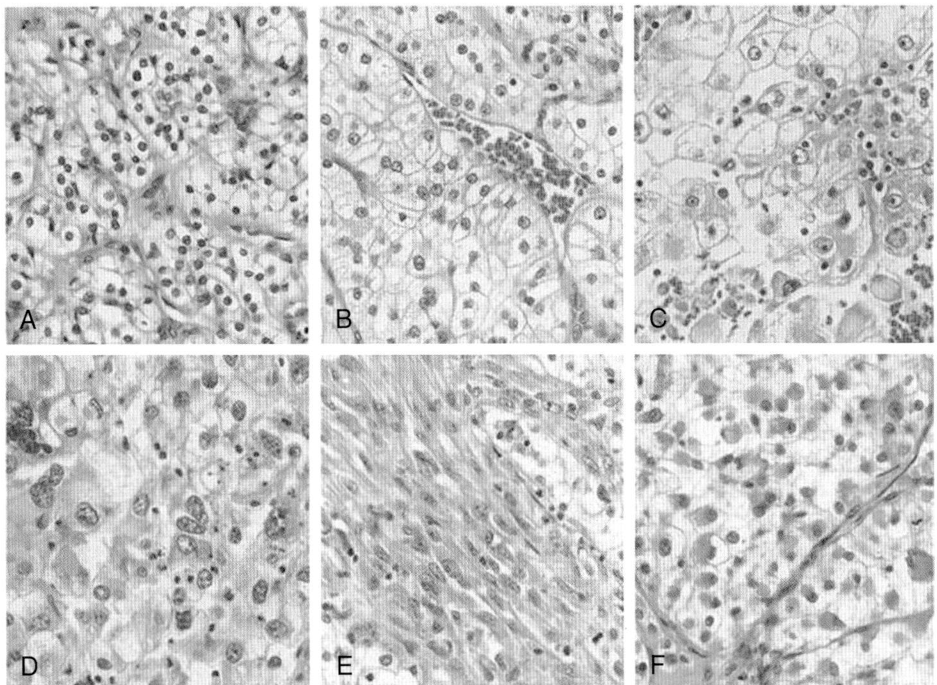


**Fig. 41.4 The International Society of Urologic Pathology (ISUP) grading system for clear cell and papillary renal cell carcinoma (RCC).** (A) Grade 1: Nucleoli are inconspicuous or absent. (B) Grade 2: Nucleoli are clearly visible at high-power magnification but are not prominent. (C) Grade 3: Nucleoli are prominent and are easily visualized at low-power magnification. (D) Grade 4: Presence of tumor giant cells and/or marked nuclear pleomorphism. (E) Grade 4: Sarcomatoid carcinoma. (F) Grade 4: Carcinoma showing rhabdoid differentiation.

and postoperatively. The accuracy of these predictions is high for RCC recurrence (66%–80%), distant metastases (78%–85%), and RCC cancer-specific survival (64%–89%).[144] Such algorithms are particularly helpful for patients with advanced disease (metastatic RCC) who are in the highest mortality range and therefore are poorly differentiated by TNM staging alone. Even the therapeutic effectiveness of antineoplastic treatments (cytokine or targeted therapy) has been examined using these staging systems to select optimal treatment regimens.[120,144]

## TREATMENT

The role of the nephrologist in the management of renal masses is evolving, because more than 50% of RCCs are being diagnosed incidentally and earlier with advanced diagnostic imaging modalities.[145,146] Although a proportion (≈20%) of these masses tends to be nonmalignant lesions, proper diagnosis often still requires surgical excision.[147,148] Fortunately, localized disease has a 5-year survival as high as 100%, particularly for those with small renal masses (T1a tumors ≤4 cm). Survival in this group is not driven entirely by cancer-related factors, but rather by complications related to their RCC treatment or comorbid diseases, which may result in CKD or cardiovascular disease.[149–151] The risk of death among those with advanced disease, however, remains high with different prognostic factors. Therefore, therapy diverges into two arms depending grossly on whether the tumor is localized or advanced. Localized disease is managed surgically, with greater emphasis on preserving kidney function, whereas advanced disease requires systemic treatment with the goal to maximize cancer-specific survival.[4]

## LOCALIZED RENAL MASSES

### PREOPERATIVE CONSIDERATIONS: CHRONIC KIDNEY DISEASE BURDEN

Shared risk factors for CKD and RCC—older age, tobacco exposure, DM, HTN, and obesity—in addition to a high prevalence of CKD in the small renal mass (≤4 cm) population, predisposes these individuals to an increased risk of new-onset CKD, CKD progression, or ESRD after surgical resection.[8,70] CKD is present in 10% to 30% of patients with RCC,[152–154] but the prevalence is even higher (10%–52%) when considering only those with small renal masses.[155–158] The higher burden of CKD risk factors in the small renal mass population (e.g., nearly 25% with DM and up to 50% with HTN) likely contributes to rising CKD incidence.[154,155,157,159,160] RCC patients were more likely than case-matched, non-RCC patients to have DM (20% vs. 8%) and HTN (31% vs. 14%) in a cohort of 26,460 patients in Taiwan.[161] Furthermore, given the increased age among those with RCC, more are likely to be saddled with preexisting CKD.[153,156]

### POSTOPERATIVE CHRONIC KIDNEY DISEASE RISK

Treatment of localized renal masses generally results in reduction of a functional nephron mass, which can lead to a decline in the eGFR. In addition to the higher burden of preexisting CKD and risk factors for CKD, as noted earlier,[162–164] the level of eGFR and poor nutrition (lower albumin), as well as surgical factors, including tumor size and acute kidney injury, has been associated with a higher incidence of CKD posttreatment[156,157,161,165–167] (Fig. 41.5). The prevalence of postnephrectomy CKD has doubled from 10% to 24% to 16% to 52% in multiple cohorts,[155–157] and

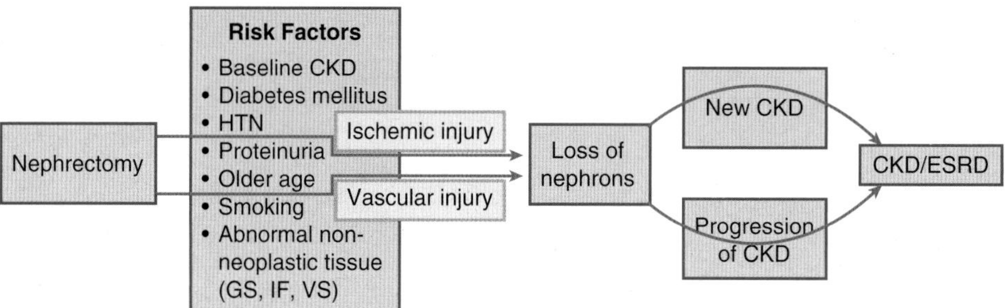


**Fig. 41.5 Risk factors for chronic kidney disease *(CKD).*** Nephrectomy performed for renal cell carcinoma is associated with nephron loss due to tissue removal, as well as ischemic and vascular injury. This loss of nephrons is associated with either new-onset CKD or progression of CKD in patients who have various risk factors, as noted. *ESRD,* End-stage renal disease; *GS,* glomerulosclerosis; *IF,* interstitial fibrosis; *HTN,* hypertension; *VS,* vascular sclerosis.

the eGFR decreased by 30% (mean, 13 mL/min/m$^2$ reduction) when followed longitudinally after nephrectomy.[167] Having DM as a comorbidity raised this risk significantly among those with small renal masses after nephrectomy, resulting in new-onset CKD, 60% in diabetics compared with 43% among all-comers with RCC. In this cohort, only 46% of diabetics were likely to remain CKD-free after 2 years compared with 76% of nondiabetics ($P$ = .006).[157] For ESRD, in a case-control study of 26,460 Taiwanese patients with 10-year follow-up, the incidence rate was 4.05% for the RCC group ($n$ = 2940) compared with 0.68% in the control group ($n$ = 23,520), with a 5.6 times more likely risk of ESRD (HR, 5.6; CI, 4.3–7.2).[161] Ultimately, RCC has been determined to be a prominent cause of ESRD in 0.5% of the population (360,000 patients), according to the US Renal Data System (USRDS).[164]

## RENAL PATHOLOGY

Although the primary purpose of pathologic evaluation is the management of RCC, proper identification of renal pathology beyond the neoplastic tissue is vital, because patients with small renal masses are outsurviving their cancer and, instead, dying from other diseases such as CKD and its complications including cardiovascular disease. The College of American Pathologists has recommended concomitant examination of nonneoplastic pathology, but compliance has been suboptimal.[168–170] As we have recently proposed,[8] a multidisciplinary team of the urologist, nephrologist, and pathologist should aim to achieve accurate diagnosis of the noncancerous renal disease (e.g., glomerular, tubulointerstitial, or vascular) to facilitate treatment of the underlying disease and promote GFR preservation.

## SURGICAL TREATMENT

### PREOPERATIVE CLINICAL EVALUATION

Before surgery or an alternative nephron-sparing procedure, risk assessment for CKD should be performed. Identification of preexisting CKD (serum creatinine level and eGFR calculation) and urinary proteinuria assessment (urine albumin-to-creatinine or urine protein-to-creatinine ratio) further allows for CKD staging using the Kidney Disease Improving Global Outcomes (KDIGO) classification criteria.[171,172] Preservation of kidney function may be achieved by addressing CKD risk factors prior to RCC intervention. Optimization of comorbid diseases encompassing glycemic control among diabetics, blood pressure adjustment for those with HTN, prevention of acute kidney injury through medication review, and avoidance of hypotension and nephrotoxicity have been recommended.[4,173,174] Further characterization of differential kidney function with renal nuclear scintigraphy prior to nephrectomy may help prognosticate the risk of CKD after treatment; however, these studies are limited because they tend to underestimate the postoperative function of the remaining kidney, which is often augmented by hyperfiltration and hypertrophy.[175] Furthermore, surgical factors, including renal mass size and duration of ischemia, correlated better with postoperative kidney function than renal functional scans.[176]

### RENAL MASS EXCISION AND NEPHRON-SPARING THERAPIES

For decades since the first nephrectomy in 1861, the primary treatment of kidney cancers had been radical nephrectomy, which involved total removal of the kidney and surrounding tissues, such as the adrenal glands or lymph nodes. Although partial nephrectomies had been performed not too long after radical nephrectomy (1867), they were generally indicated for nonmalignant lesions and did not gain acceptance until well into the 21st century[177,178]; this procedure is still not routinely performed in all centers.[179]

Nephron-sparing procedures for small renal masses have proven to be safe with comparable, if not better, outcomes than those for radical nephrectomy in numerous studies, especially with regard to CKD. A meta-analysis of 40,000 subjects in 36 studies composed of primarily retrospective cohort studies and one randomized-controlled trial (RCT) has summarized these findings. The composite all-cause mortality (19%) and cancer-specific mortality (29%) were lower in the partial nephrectomy group than in the radical nephrectomy group.[180] These findings, driven by the large number of cohort studies, differed from the one RCT, the European Organisation for Research and Treatment of Cancer (EORTC) study, which assessed 541 patients with renal masses 5 cm or smaller. The EORTC trial did not support higher overall survival with partial nephrectomy; the 10-year all-cause mortality was 81% for radical nephrectomy versus 76% for partial nephrectomy (HR; 1.5; 95% CI, 1.03–2.16). However, the difference in survival between radical nephrectomy and partial nephrectomy was no longer present when the analysis was restricted to the subgroup with a ccRCC diagnosis.[150]

Kidney function preservation in those with small renal masses is increasingly prioritized as oncologic survival approaches 100%. The CKD risk was 61% less with partial nephrectomy as compared with radical nephrectomy in the meta-analysis noted earlier.[180] Reduction of CKD risk may partially explain the lower all-cause mortality, because it has been well established that CKD is associated with cardiovascular death.[181] Likewise, eGFR decline was also lower for partial nephrectomy in the EORTC study. Compared with 86% of patients undergoing radical nephrectomy, fewer (65%) with partial nephrectomy had an eGFR decline below 60 mL/min/1.73 $m^2$. However, there was no distinction of CKD benefit between these groups when examining the risk of steeper eGFR declines (<30 or 15 mL/min/1.73 $m^2$) according to surgical modality. Despite a higher mean eGFR (67 vs. 53 mL/min/1.73 $m^2$) among those with partial nephrectomy, this did not appear to confer a survival benefit in this trial.[182] The eGFR reduction related to surgical nephron mass loss may not raise mortality like long-standing CKD.[183] Furthermore, although ESRD did not occur more frequently with radical nephrectomy than with partial nephrectomy (in a large Canadian study spanning 1995 to 2010), the risk of ESRD for those undergoing partial nephrectomy during a contemporary period (2003–2010) was lower (HR, 0.44; 95% CI 0.25–0.95) compared with radical nephrectomy. This is presumably related to the advancement of surgical practice for the former group creating disparate outcomes over time.[184]

Ablative therapies and active surveillance for the treatment of small renal masses should be considered for those who may be excluded from nephrectomy (radical or partial nephrectomy) due to the high risk of surgical complications. Radiofrequency ablation and cryoablation are well-established nephron-sparing procedures usually reserved for older adults and those with multiple comorbid conditions. These less invasive ablative therapies have the advantage of similar oncologic survival, lower procedural complication rates, fewer hospitalization days, and greater GFR preservation, but with more local and metastatic tumor recurrence compared with partial nephrectomy.[185,186] Active surveillance entails intensive and consistent monitoring of the tumor, with surgical intervention, as indicated. Compared with more aggressive measures, which start with surgical or ablative treatment, active surveillance performs well in select populations (as observed with older adults in the U.S. Surveillance Epidemiology and End Results [SEER] database)[187] and those with lower life expectancy or competing risks of death.[187,188] Surgical outcomes are similar but oncologic survival is slightly lower among those undergoing active surveillance.[18] The American Urological Association and American Society of Clinical Oncology guidelines have recommended active surveillance for those with masses 2 cm or smaller or with high operative risk, with monitoring every 3 to 6 months.[174,190] Moreover, a few prospective observational studies of those with metastatic disease (with favorable prognostic features) have found that a period of active surveillance (median, 1 year) prior to systemic therapy may possibly minimize toxicity related to treatment.[191]

### POSTTREATMENT SURVEILLANCE OF LOCALIZED TUMORS

The American Urological Association has recommended regular screening for tumor recurrence by imaging (abdominal CT, MRI, or ultrasound and chest radiography) initially after treatment. Imaging is repeated between 3 and 12 months postprocedure and thereafter yearly, up to 3 (partial nephrectomy) and 5 (ablative therapy) years, depending on the treatment modality. Among those who received ablative therapy, renal biopsy is indicated during surveillance with the discovery of concerning lesions. Anyone with preexisting or a new diagnosis of CKD (by eGFR or proteinuria criteria) should be monitored regularly for progression of kidney disease.[150,192]

## ADVANCED RENAL CELL CARCINOMA AND SYSTEMIC THERAPY

Although incidental renal mass detection has led to earlier RCC diagnosis, with favorable outcomes, nearly one-third of RCC patients continue to be diagnosed with metastatic disease or recurrent disease that is not amenable to surgical therapy. Instead, systemic therapy is the mainstay of treatment for advanced RCC, although surgical debulking may be indicated for reducing tumor burden in some cases. Advanced RCC median survival remains suboptimal; however, with the development of newer treatment options, prognoses appear to be improving.[193,194]

### INTRODUCTION TO NEW THERAPEUTIC APPROACHES

Disruption of VHL through mutation, deletion, or methylation is widely recognized as the most fundamental and critical molecular alteration in ccRCC.[11] This disruption leads to the deregulation of downstream pathways related to oxygen sensing, causing the accumulation of HIF-α and subsequent upregulation of hypoxia response genes,[195] and resulting in a clinical phenotype characterized by florid vasculature, principally modulated by VEGF signaling pathways. In the past decade, remarkable advances have been made in ccRCC drug development, primarily focusing on targeting either VEGF receptors (VEGFRs) using kinase inhibitors or the VEGF ligand using monoclonal antibodies. Such advances have led to FDA approval of several inhibitors of VEGFR (sunitinib, pazopanib, sorafenib, axitinib, cabozantinib, and lenvantinib) and VEGF (bevacizumab). These angiogenesis inhibitors were only modestly effective, however, and were often characterized by off-target effects and chronic irritative toxicities, such as fatigue and rash.[196] Furthermore, the metabolic basis of ccRCC is only partly addressed by targeting the terminal phenotype driven by VEGF. Subsequent encouraging progress in drug development efforts has attempted to exploit ccRCC metabolic reprogramming by targeting critical proteins or enzymes involved in dysregulated metabolic pathways.[3,23]

### IMMUNOTHERAPY

Interferon-alfa (IFN-α) and IL-2 were the initial immune therapies to be approved by the FDA. Cytokine therapy stimulates the immune system nonspecifically with the upregulation of T-cell and natural killer cell activity to recognize and destroy tumor cells,[197] but can also have the undesired effect of suppressing the immune system and defeating natural immunosurveillance.[24,40] Response rates have ranged roughly from 10% to 25% and median overall survival from 11 to 13 months for individual agents, without much better overall survival for combination therapy. Immunotherapy, when tolerated, is reasonably successful but is severely limited by the frequent withdrawal of treatment due to the flulike adverse effects experienced in most patients.[193]

## TARGETED MOLECULAR THERAPY

Tumor growth and angiogenesis are mediated through a number of intracellular pathways involving VEGF, HIF, and mammalian target of rapamycin (mTOR; Fig. 41.6). Treatments targeting these pathways generally inhibit the enhanced tumor cellular metabolism, cell growth, and vascular network expansion and have revolutionized the approach to cancer therapy in all solid organs, including the kidney.

### VASCULAR ENDOTHELIAL GROWTH FACTOR

The first VEGF inhibitor (bevacizumab) targets the VEGF ligand, preventing angiogenesis by the reduction of protein transcription, which promotes vascular growth and increasing oxygen delivery. VEGF inhibitors also impede tumor cell growth directly because it is present not only in endothelial cells but also in many other cell types, including tumor cells. Presently, VEGF activity is also blocked at the receptor using tyrosine kinase inhibitors (TKIs), including axitinib, pazopanib, sorafenib, sunitinib, and tivozanib.[198,199] Although highly effective, resistance can occur from the stimulation of alternative angiogenic pathways bypassing the VEGF blockage.[200]

Common adverse effects of VEGF inhibitors, which are important for the nephrologist to know and treat, are HTN (11%–43%)[201] and proteinuria (41%–63%)[202] related to the disruption of the role of VEGF in maintaining the integrity of the endothelium and slit diaphragm of the glomerular membrane. On pathology, the primary presentation is thrombotic microangiopathy, but various glomerular diseases have been reported as well.[203,204] The pathogenesis mirrors disease states of VEGF antagonism, as seen with preeclampsia.[205] The risk of HTN and proteinuria appears to increase with larger VEGF inhibitor dose.[201,202] The drug toxicity is generally treated supportively with antihypertensive agents and protein-lowering medications, such as angiotensin-converting enzyme inhibitors (ACEIs) and angiotensin receptor blockers (ARBs). Severe HTN or nephrotic syndrome resistant to medical therapy can be addressed with short-term cessation or lowering of the dose, without interruption of therapy, except for severe acute kidney injury or thrombotic microangiopathy.[206]

### PI3K/MTOR

Pathways involving mTOR and its upstream serine–threonine kinase, phosphatidylinositol-3-kinase (PI3K), also promote

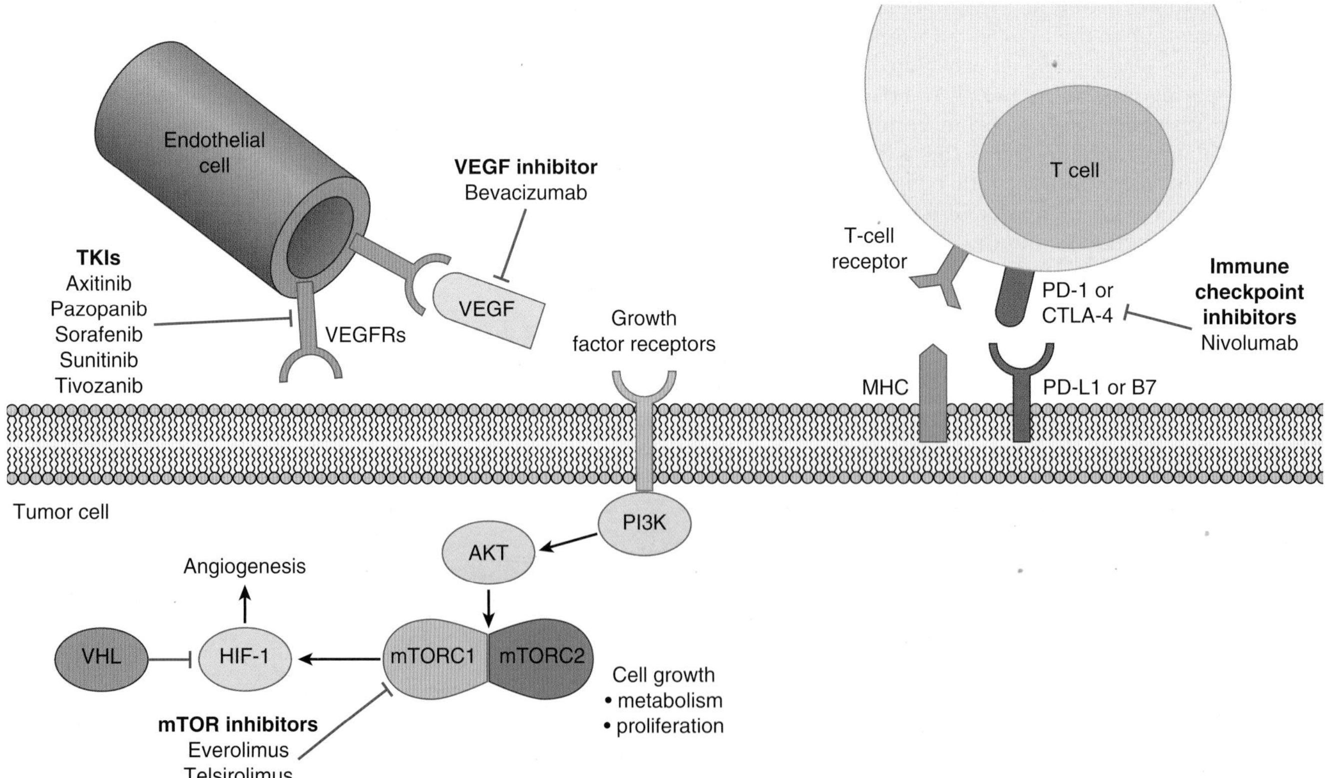


**Fig. 41.6. Tumor growth, angiogenesis, immune pathways, and associated targeted immune therapy.** Tumor cells promote growth and angiogenesis through the PI3K/mTOR and VEGF pathways and evade the T-cells and immune checkpoints. Various targeted immune therapies are listed; the site of action is indicated by the *red line*. *B7,* CD-28 ligand; *CTLA-4,* cytotoxic-T-lymphocyte–associated antigen-4; *HIF-1,* hypoxia-inducible factor-1; MHC, major histocompatibility complex; *MTOR,* mammalian target of rapamycin; *mTORC,* mammalian target of rapamycin complex; *PD-1,* programmed cell death protein-1; *PD-L1,* programmed cell death protein-1 ligand 1; *PI3K,* phosphatidylinositol-3-kinase; *TKI,* tyrosine kinase inhibitor; *VEGF,* vascular endothelial growth factor; *VEGFR,* VEGF receptor; *VHL,* von Hippel–Lindau.

tumor growth. mTOR is crucial for ribosomal activity in cell metabolism, growth, and proliferation through two separate complexes (mTORC1 and mTORC2), and the PI3K pathway controls growth factor expression and tumor cell proliferation. The reported response rate is 7% to 26%, with a higher median overall survival of 15 months compared with traditional immunotherapy, and these agents have a far more tolerable toxicity profile. The first-generation mTOR inhibitors (everolimus, temsirolimus) suppress mTORC1 activity alone; therefore, mitogenic stimulation can occur alternately through mTORC2 and PI3K. The next generation of mTOR inhibitors also block the mTORC2 and PI3K pathway, which may allow for more effective tumor suppression, and is currently undergoing investigation.[4,193,200]

## NOVEL TARGETED THERAPIES

Immune checkpoint receptors sustain normal autoregulation of our immune system by downregulating T-cell and associated immune cell (macrophage, natural killer cell) activity. Tumors cells "hijack" this function to evade circulating immune cells. Immune checkpoint inhibitors block the aberrant tumor to T-cell interaction, enabling T cells to recognize the deviant cells and stimulate the natural immune mechanisms to eradicate them. Cytotoxic T lymphocyte–associated antigen-4 (CTLA-4) and programmed cell death protein-1 (PD-1) are two receptor proteins regulating such adaptive immunity used in cancer treatment. Ipilimumab (CTLA-4–directed antibody) and nivolumab (PD-1–directed antibody) have been used successfully in the treatment of RCC.[207] The response rate for nivolumab (25%) has been respectable, although with a rare complete response; median overall survival has been reported as high as 25 months.[208] Ipilimumab appeared less effective, with a response rate of only 12.5% in one high-dose phase II trial.[209] Assessment of combination therapy is ongoing, with optimistic results so far.[207] Toxicity related to checkpoint inhibitors tends to present with cutaneous, gastrointestinal, pulmonary, and hepatic involvement. Less commonly, renal complications can occur, with acute kidney injury due to acute tubulointerstitial nephritis (lymphocytic infiltration), which typically resolves with corticosteroid administration or cessation of treatment.[210] Further investigation will help determine optimal treatment regimens for those with advanced RCC.

In most patients with metastatic renal cell cancer of the clear cell type, systemic VEGF-targeted therapy (e.g., sunitinib, pazopanib, bevacizumab/interferon) is considered a reasonable frontline standard of care. Although the mTOR inhibitor temsirolimus is also used to treat patients with a poor functional status, many of these patients are also reasonable candidates for VEGFR tyrosine kinase inhibitor (TKI) therapy. In highly selected patients with a robust functional status, high-dose IL-2 remains a treatment consideration due to its ability to induce durable responses in a small subset of patients. In the second-line setting, systemic therapy with immune checkpoint inhibitors (nivolumab) or TKIs (e.g., cabozantinib, axitinib, lenvantinib) are in the therapeutic armamentarium. The mTOR inhibitor everolimus has now been relegated to later lines of therapy.[194,211]

The use of -omics technologies to discover and validate reprogrammed metabolic pathways is starting to have an impact on RCC therapy.[18,19,40] This idea, which is especially germane to the metabolic basis of RCC, capitalizes on the availability of novel or previously discovered compounds that affect such pathways and thus are expected to affect cancer preferentially over normal tissues.[3] We foresee a bright future of newly discovered therapeutic targets using this technology, which could be rapidly and easily translated to the clinical setting.

 Complete reference list available at ExpertConsult.com.

## KEY REFERENCES


1. Choueiri TK, Motzer RJ. Systemic therapy for metastatic renal-cell carcinoma. *N Engl J Med.* 2017;376:354–366.
2. Quinn DI, Lara PN Jr. Renal-cell cancer—targeting an immune checkpoint or multiple kinases. *N Engl J Med.* 2015;373:1872–1874.
3. Wettersten HI, Aboud OA, Lara PN Jr, et al. Metabolic reprogramming in clear cell renal cell carcinoma. *Nat Rev Nephrol.* 2017;13:410–419.
4. Hu SL, Chang A, Perazella MA, et al. The nephrologist's tumor: basic biology and management of renal cell carcinoma. *J Am Soc Nephrol.* 2016;27:2227–2237.
13. Gnarra JR, Tory K, Weng Y, et al. Mutations of the VHL tumour suppressor gene in renal carcinoma. *Nat Genet.* 1994;7:85–90.
16. Cancer Genome Atlas Research Network. Comprehensive molecular characterization of clear cell renal cell carcinoma. *Nature.* 2013; 499:43–49.
37. Sufan RI, Jewett MA, Ohh M. The role of von Hippel-Lindau tumor suppressor protein and hypoxia in renal clear cell carcinoma. *Am J Physiol Renal Physiol.* 2004;287:F1–F6.
59. Ljungberg B, Campbell SC, Cho HY, et al. The epidemiology of renal cell carcinoma. *Eur Urol.* 2011;60:615–621.
62. Lowrance WT, Ordonez J, Udaltsova N, et al. CKD and the risk of incident cancer. *J Am Soc Nephrol.* 2014;25:2327–2334.
64. Bonsib SM. Renal cystic diseases and renal neoplasms: a mini-review. *Clin J Am Soc Nephrol.* 2009;4:1998–2007.
69. Truong LD, Krishnan B, Cao JTH, et al. Renal neoplasm in acquired cystic kidney disease. *Am J Kidney Dis.* 1995;26:1–12.
74. Ishikawa I. Acquired cystic disease: mechanisms and manifestations. *Semin Nephrol.* 1991;11:671–684.
84. Keith DS, Torres VE, King BF, et al. Renal cell carcinoma in autosomal dominant polycystic kidney disease. *J Am Soc Nephrol.* 1994;4:1661–1669.
89. Hashimoto Y, Takagi T, Kondo T, et al. Comparison of prognosis between patients with renal cell carcinoma on hemodialysis and those with renal cell carcinoma in the general population. *Int J Clin Oncol.* 2015;20:1035–1041.
91. Shrewsberry AB, Osunkoya AO, Jiang K, et al. Renal cell carcinoma in patients with end-stage renal disease has favorable overall prognosis. *Clin Transplant.* 2014;28:211–216.
108. Yanik EL, Clarke CA, Snyder JJ, et al. Variation in cancer incidence among patients with ESRD during kidney function and nonfunction intervals. *J Am Soc Nephrol.* 2016;27:1495–1504.
109. Sarasin FP, Wong JB, Levey AS, et al. Screening for acquired cystic kidney disease: a decision analytic perspective. *Kidney Int.* 1995;48:207–219.
119. Cohen HT, McGovern FJ. Renal-cell carcinoma. *N Engl J Med.* 2005;353:2477–2490.
127. Hallscheidt PJ, Bock M, Riedasch G, et al. Diagnostic accuracy of staging renal cell carcinomas using multidetector-row computed tomography and magnetic resonance imaging: a prospective study with histopathologic correlation. *J Comput Assist Tomogr.* 2004;28: 333–339.
134. Venneti S, Dunphy MP, Zhang H, et al. Glutamine-based PET imaging facilitates enhanced metabolic evaluation of gliomas in vivo. *Sci Transl Med.* 2015;7:274ra17.
135. Woo S, Cho JY. Imaging findings of common benign renal tumors in the era of small renal masses: differential diagnosis from small renal cell carcinoma: current status and future perspectives. *Korean J Radiol.* 2015;16:99–113.
138. Volpe A, Kachura JR, Geddie WR, et al. Techniques, safety and accuracy of sampling of renal tumors by fine needle aspiration and core biopsy. *J Urol.* 2007;178:379–386.
140. Delahunt B. Advances and controversies in grading and staging of renal cell carcinoma. *Mod Pathol.* 2009;22(suppl 2):S24–S36.

141. Fuhrman SA, Lasky LC, Limas C. Prognostic significance of morphologic parameters in renal cell carcinoma. *Am J Surg Pathol.* 1982;6:655–663.
143. Delahunt B, Cheville JC, Martignoni G, et al. The International Society of Urological Pathology (ISUP) grading system for renal cell carcinoma and other prognostic parameters. *Am J Surg Pathol.* 2013;37:1490–1504.
147. McKiernan J, Yossepowitch O, Kattan MW, et al. Partial nephrectomy for renal cortical tumors: pathologic findings and impact on outcome. *Urology.* 2002;60:1003–1009.
149. Hollingsworth JM, Miller DC, Daignault S, et al. Five-year survival after surgical treatment for kidney cancer: a population-based competing risk analysis. *Cancer.* 2007;109:1763–1768.
154. Clark MA, Shikanov S, Raman JD, et al. Chronic kidney disease before and after partial nephrectomy. *J Urol.* 2011;185:43–48.
157. Jeon HG, Jeong IG, Lee JW, et al. Prognostic factors for chronic kidney disease after curative surgery in patients with small renal tumors. *Urology.* 2009;74:1064–1068.
160. Takagi T, Kondo T, Iizuka J, et al. Postoperative renal function after partial nephrectomy for renal cell carcinoma in patients with pre-existing chronic kidney disease: a comparison with radical nephrectomy. *Int J Urol.* 2011;18:472–476.
167. Song C, Bang JK, Park HK, et al. Factors influencing renal function reduction after partial nephrectomy. *J Urol.* 2009;181:48–54.
174. Campbell S, Uzzo RG, Allaf ME, et al. Renal mass and localized renal cancer: AUA guideline. *J Urol.* 2017;198:520–529.
176. Sankin A, Sfakianos JP, Schiff J, et al. Assessing renal function after partial nephrectomy using renal nuclear scintigraphy and estimated glomerular filtration rate. *Urology.* 2012;80:343–346.
178. Pletajew S, Antoniewicz AA, Borówka A. Kidney removal: the past, presence, and perspectives: a historical review. *Urol J.* 2010;7:215–223.
179. Bjurlin MA, Walter D, Taksler GB, et al. National trends in the utilization of partial nephrectomy before and after the establishment of AUA guidelines for the management of renal masses. *Urology.* 2013;82:1283–1290.
180. Kim SP, Thompson RH, Boorjian SA, et al. Comparative effectiveness for survival and renal function of partial and radical nephrectomy for localized renal tumors: a systematic review and meta-analysis. *J Urol.* 2012;188:51–57.
182. Scosyrev E, Messing EM, Sylvester R, et al. Renal function after nephron-sparing surgery versus radical nephrectomy: results from EORTC randomized trial 30904. *Eur Urol.* 2014;65:372–377.
187. Sun M, Becker A, Tian Z, et al. Management of localized kidney cancer: calculating cancer-specific mortality and competing risks of death for surgery and nonsurgical management. *Eur Urol.* 2014;65:235–241.
193. Weiss RH, Lin PY. Kidney cancer: identification of novel targets for therapy. *Kidney Int.* 2006;69:224–232.
195. Riazalhosseini Y, Lathrop M. Precision medicine from the renal cancer genome. *Nat Rev Nephrol.* 2016;12:655–666.
196. Schmidinger M. Understanding and managing toxicities of vascular endothelial growth factor (VEGF) inhibitors. *EJC Suppl.* 2013;11:172–191.
199. Liu JY, Park SH, Morisseau C, et al. Sorafenib has soluble epoxide hydrolase inhibitory activity, which contributes to its effect profile in vivo. *Mol Cancer Ther.* 2009;8:2193–2203.
202. Zhu X, Wu S, Dahut WL, et al. Risks of proteinuria and hypertension with bevacizumab, an antibody against vascular endothelial growth factor: systematic review and meta-analysis. *Am J Kidney Dis.* 2007;49:186–193.
206. Perazella MA, Izzedine H. New drug toxicities in the onco-nephrology world. *Kidney Int.* 2015;87:909–917.
207. Carlo MI, Voss MH, Motzer RJ. Checkpoint inhibitors and other novel immunotherapies for advanced renal cell carcinoma. *Nat Rev Urol.* 2016;13:420–431.

# Onconephrology: Kidney Disease and Cancer

42

Mitchell H. Rosner | Mark A. Perazella

## CHAPTER OUTLINE



## KEY POINTS

- Acute and chronic kidney disease are common complications in cancer patients and are primarily due to the underlying malignancy or its treatment. Study of the growing connection between the two diseases is known as "onconephrology."
- Acute kidney injury (AKI) is a relatively common complication of cancer and its treatment. Both hematologic malignancies and solid cancers are associated with AKI. The causes can be classified as prerenal (e.g., volume depletion, hypercalcemia, capillary leak, renal sodium wasting), intrarenal (e.g., direct cancer invasion, paraneoplastic effects, drug toxicities), and postrenal (e.g., retroperitoneal cancer or fibrosis, bladder cancer).
- Cancer is frequently complicated by chronic kidney disease (CKD). A number of causes lead to CKD, including the underlying malignancy, drugs used to treat cancer, shared risk factors (e.g., hypertension, diabetes mellitus), nephrectomy for renal cell cancer, and therapies such as hematopoietic stem cell transplantation.
- Diseases involving the glomeruli also complicate various malignancies. Membranous nephropathy, minimal change disease, and proliferative glomerulonephritides are noted paraneoplastic effects of cancer. Paraproteinemias with monoclonal immunoglobulin or light- or heavy-chain synthesis also cause glomerular injury—for example, with AL amyloidosis and monoclonal immunoglobulin deposition disease.
- Electrolyte and acid–base disorders frequently complicate cancer and its therapy. Hyponatremia, hypernatremia, hypokalemia, and hyperkalemia, as well as imbalances in calcium, magnesium, and phosphorus, are the result of direct or paraneoplastic effects or adverse effects of drugs on the gastrointestinal tract (e.g., vomiting, diarrhea) and/or kidneys.
- Hematopoietic stem cell transplantation is a life-saving procedure for patients with certain malignancies. However, this procedure is complicated by AKI, glomerular disease, hypertension, electrolyte abnormalities, and CKD, depending on the patient's underlying risk and the conditioning regimen and type of stem cell transplant used.
- Medications used to treat cancer are associated with adverse renal effects. Conventional chemotherapeutic drugs, immunotherapies, and targeted agents are associated with AKI, glomerulopathies, and electrolyte and acid–base disturbances, and CKD.

Onconephrology refers to the intersection of the disciplines of nephrology and oncology. Kidney disease in multiple forms, ranging from glomerular diseases to electrolyte abnormalities, is common in patients with cancer. In many cases, these kidney disorders are not unique to patients with cancer but can affect the care of the patient, such as affecting the dosage of appropriate chemotherapy in patients with chronic kidney disease (CKD). In other circumstances, either the malignancy itself or its associated therapy may lead to unique kidney diseases, such as acute kidney injury (AKI), glomerulonephritis, or electrolyte disorders. It is the responsibility of the nephrologist to recognize these unique and cancer-associated kidney disorders to provide the most effective therapy.

## ACUTE KIDNEY INJURY IN PATIENTS WITH CANCER

### EPIDEMIOLOGY

Acute kidney injury (AKI) is a common occurrence in hospitalized patients with cancer and, when it occurs, it is associated with higher costs, increased hospital length of stay, and increased morbidity and mortality. In some cases, AKI may lead to changes in chemotherapy regimens that may lessen the chances of disease remission, or AKI may exclude patients from clinical trials. In the largest study on this topic, 37,267 incident cancer patients in Denmark had follow-up over a 7-year period in the early 2000s.[1] The 1-year risk of AKI, as defined by RIFLE risk (>50% increase in serum creatinine), was 17.5%. The 1-year risk for more severe AKI, the RIFLE injury (>100% increase in serum creatinine), and failure (>200% increase in serum creatinine of >4 mg/dL and requiring dialysis) risk categories was 8.8% and 4.5%, respectively. The 5-year risk for the RIFLE risk, injury, and failure AKI categories was even higher, at 27%, 14.6%, and 7.6%, respectively. Critically ill patients with cancer have a higher incidence of AKI and AKI requiring dialysis than critically ill patients without cancer.[2,3] In those patients with cancer who suffer an episode of AKI, the mortality is elevated, such that the mortality was 13.6% in those without AKI and progressively increased with higher RIFLE stage AKI (risk, 49%; injury, 62.3%; failure, 86.8%).[2] In patients with hematologic malignancies who were undergoing induction therapy, the mortality in those with RIFLE risk AKI was 13.6%, whereas the mortality in those with no AKI was 3.8% over an 8-week period.[4] Importantly, those patients who required dialysis during the period of induction therapy had a mortality of 61.7%.[4] It is important to note that more contemporary studies may demonstrate that outcomes in patients with cancer and AKI are not universally poor, with one study showing that 82% of critically ill cancer patients with AKI completely recovered kidney function, whereas partial recovery was observed in 12%, and chronic renal replacement therapy (RRT) was required in only 6% of patients.[5] The prognosis of AKI greatly depends on the underlying functional and premorbid conditions of the patient, as well as the overall state of the malignancy. Thus, individualized decisions regarding the appropriateness of RRT in these patients is warranted.

A specific group of patients with a high incidence of AKI is those undergoing hematopoietic stem cell transplantation (HSCT). Various studies have shown an incidence of AKI ranging from 23% to 73% according to the different cutoff points used to define AKI.[6–8] Furthermore, the incidence of AKI varies according to the type of HSCT, with most data supporting the finding that myeloablative allogenic transplantation is associated with a higher incidence of AKI.[8]

The risk factors for AKI in patients with cancer are multiple and depend on the specific type of cancer. These can be broadly divided into those that are modifiable and those that are not (Table 42.1). Certain cancers appear to carry a higher AKI risk than others, with renal cell carcinoma, hepatocellular carcinoma, multiple myeloma, and lymphoma having higher rates of AKI.[1] As an example, patients undergoing total (radical) nephrectomy for renal cell carcinoma have an incidence of AKI as high as 33.7%.[9] Even partial nephrectomy to spare nephron loss is associated with AKI, albeit less commonly.[10] Patients with acute lymphoma or leukemia undergoing induction chemotherapy are also at especially high risk to develop AKI, primarily due to tumor lysis syndrome and drug nephrotoxicity. In a series of 537 patients undergoing induction therapy for acute myelogenous leukemia or high-risk myelodysplastic syndrome, 36% developed AKI.[4] Whenever possible, modifiable risk factors should be addressed in an attempt to lower the incidence of AKI.

### CAUSES OF ACUTE KIDNEY INJURY IN PATIENTS WITH CANCER

The causes of AKI in patients with solid organ cancers are similar to those of the general population, with an overrepresentation of obstructive nephropathy (especially with

**Table 42.1 Risk Factors for Acute Kidney Injury in Patients With Cancer**

| Modifiable Risks | Nonmodifiable Risks |
|---|---|
| Nephrotoxic medications (nonchemotherapeutic), such as aminoglycosides, amphotericin B, calcineurin inhibitors | Age > 65 years |
| Nephrotoxic medications (chemotherapeutic), such as cisplatin, checkpoint inhibitors, ifosfamide, interferon, tyrosine kinase inhibitors, BRAF (serine–threonine protein kinase) inhibitors | Underlying chronic kidney disease, especially diabetic kidney disease |
| Hypovolemia<br>• True volume depletion—nausea, vomiting, diarrhea<br>• Effective volume depletion—cirrhosis, heart failure, nephrotic syndrome, hypoalbuminemia | Specific cancer types—multiple myeloma, hepatocellular cancer, renal cell carcinoma, pelvic malignancies |
| Intravenous radiographic contrast | Hematopoietic stem cell transplantation |
| High tumor bulk and risk for tumor lysis syndrome | Female gender |

prostate, ovarian and cervical cancer), chemotherapy-associated nephrotoxicity, sepsis-associated ischemic acute tubular necrosis in the setting of neutropenia, and AKI due to hypercalcemia.[11–13] In patients with hematologic malignancies, the causes of AKI are also similar to those of the general population, with some notable unique causes, such as AKI associated with multiple myeloma (e.g., cast nephropathy, light- or heavy-chain–associated glomerulonephritis or associated with hypercalcemia), tumor lysis syndrome, and tumor infiltration of the kidneys associated with lymphoma and leukemia.[11–13] In those patients receiving a stem cell transplant, there are other situation-specific causes of AKI, including venoocclusive disease and cytokine release syndrome.[14]

Prerenal causes of AKI are common in patients with malignancies and often result from poor oral intake, as well as chemotherapy-induced nausea, vomiting, and diarrhea. Hypercalcemia and its natriuretic effect may also lead to volume depletion and prerenal azotemia. In addition, cancer patients may be prescribed common medications, such as diuretics, angiotensin-converting enzyme inhibitors, angiotensin receptor blockers, or nonsteroidal antiinflammatory drugs (NSAIDs) that can affect renal autoregulation and exacerbate prerenal AKI. Prerenal causes are so common in this patient population that judicious trials of intravenous (IV) fluids are reasonable in most patients presenting with AKI.

Many of the causes of AKI seen in cancer patients are not unique and are covered in other chapters. However, certain intrarenal and postrenal causes are seen almost exclusively in the setting of malignancy and are covered here and shown in Table 42.2. AKI associated with glomerular disorders, chemotherapeutic agents, HSCT, and hypercalcemia and seen in the setting of renal cell carcinoma are covered in their respective sections in this chapter.

**Table 42.2 Intrarenal and Postrenal Causes of Acute Kidney Injury in the Patient With Cancer**

| Cause | Representative Example |
|---|---|
| Vascular—thrombotic microangiopathy | Gemcitabine, post–stem cell transplantation |
| Tubular injury—acute tubular necrosis | Ischemia due to sepsis, nephrotoxicity due to chemotherapeutic agents such as cisplatin |
| Tubular injury—intratubular precipitation of crystals | Methotrexate |
| Tubular injury—cast nephropathy | Multiple myeloma |
| Tubular Injury—lysozymuria | Acute promyelocytic, acute monocytic leukemia<br>Chronic myelomonocytic leukemia |
| Interstitial injury—interstitial nephritis | Checkpoint inhibitors |
| Interstitial injury—tumor infiltration of the kidneys | Lymphoma |
| Glomerular injury | Amyloidosis<br>Rapidly progressive glomerulonephritis<br>Various paraneoplastic or drug-induced glomerulonephritis<br>Paraneoplastic membranous nephropathy |
| Obstruction | Retroperitoneal lymphadenopathy (lymphoma)<br>Tumor bulk obstructing urine flow (pelvic malignancies) |

## TUMOR LYSIS SYNDROME

Tumor lysis syndrome (TLS) is encountered in patients with bulky, rapidly growing and chemosensitive malignancies, such as high-grade lymphomas (e.g., Burkitt lymphoma), leukemia, or other cancers with large cellular burdens.[15,16] Typically, TLS is seen after the administration of chemotherapy but can occur spontaneously as well. TLS has been defined by the Cairo-Bishop criteria (Table 42.3) and is biochemically typified by the findings of numerous electrolyte disorders (e.g., hyperkalemia, hyperphosphatemia, hypocalcemia, hyperuricemia) that result from the release of intracellular substances after cell lysis.[15,16] Importantly, TLS may lead to sudden death and seizures due to the electrolyte disturbances encountered in these patients. The mechanism of AKI in these patients is at least partially due to uric acid nephropathy but may also be influenced by cytokine release and nephrocalcinosis (due to high serum calcium phosphate products).[17]

Uric acid nephropathy and AKI are the result of the precipitation of insoluble uric acid in the renal tubules that occurs when purine nucleotides are released from dying cancer cells. These nucleotides are metabolized by xanthine oxidase into uric acid, which is subsequently filtered in the glomerulus and concentrated in the renal tubules. This forms an insoluble precipitate, leading to a combination of intratubular obstruction, vasoconstriction, and inflammation, culminating in a fall of the glomerular filtration rate and AKI.[18] Understanding this pathophysiology leads to rational protocols for the prevention of TLS (Fig. 42.1). The first

**Table 42.3 Cairo-Bishop Criteria for Tumor Lysis Syndrome**

| Type of Criteria | Features |
|---|---|
| Laboratory criteria for tumor lysis syndrome | Requires two or more of the following criteria within 3 days to or 7 days after initiation of chemotherapy:<br>• Uric acid level ≥ 8 mg/dL or 25% increase from baseline<br>• Potassium level ≥ 6.0 mEq/L or 25% increase from baseline<br>• Phosphorus level ≥ 6.5 mg/dL for children<br>• Phosphorus level ≥ 4.5 mg/dL for adults or 25% increase from baseline<br>• Calcium level ≤ 7 mg/dL or 25% decrease from baseline |
| Clinical criteria for tumor lysis syndrome | Laboratory tumor lysis syndrome plus one or more of the following criteria:<br>• Creatinine > 1.5 times upper limit of age-adjusted reference range<br>• Cardiac dysrhythmia or sudden death<br>• Seizure |

From Cairo MS, Bishop M. Tumor lysis syndrome: new therapeutic strategies and classification. *Br J Hematol.* 2004;127(1):3–11,2004.

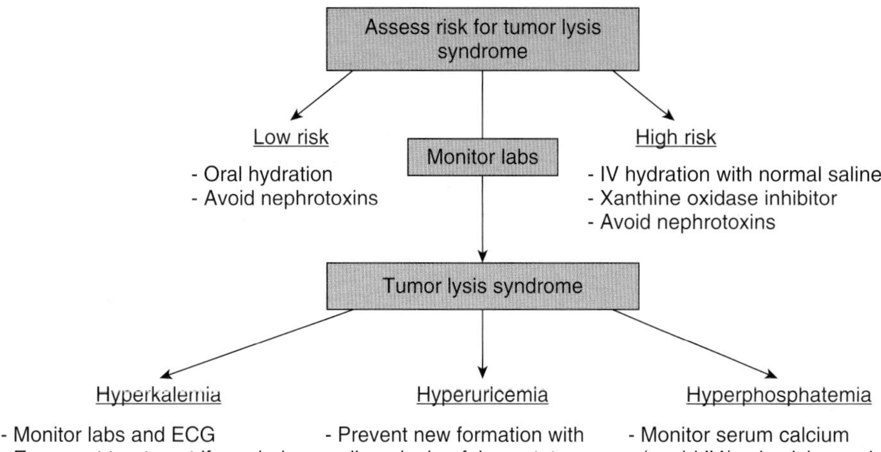


**Fig. 42.1 Approach to the management of tumor lysis syndrome.** *ECG,* Electrocardiogram; *GFR,* glomerular filtration rate; *IV,* intravenous; *SPS,* sodium polystyrene sulfonate. (From Rosner MH, Perazella MA. Acute kidney injury in patients with cancer. *N Engl J Med.* 2017; 376(18):1770–1781.)

step in a preventive strategy rests on identifying patients at risk for TLS, which should include any patient with a large, rapidly growing and chemosensitive tumor or those patients who, prior to treatment, may already be manifesting signs of tumor lysis with an associated electrolyte disturbances. Low-risk patients should be treated with oral fluids and avoidance of other nephrotoxins; high-risk patients should receive IV 0.9% saline to maintain adequate glomerular filtration and tubular flow rates that facilitate rapid clearance and dilution of uric acid, as well as the clearance of potassium and phosphate. The prophylactic use of a xanthine oxidase inhibitor (allopurinol or febuxostat) is recommended because these drugs will block de novo formation of uric acid and limit further increases in the levels of this compound. For patients who already have elevated uric acid levels, treatment with recombinant urate oxidase (rasburicase) is beneficial for rapidly lowering uric acid levels and is recommended.[19] Rasburicase converts uric acid to a soluble and readily excreted compound, allantoin.[19] It should be cautioned that rasburicase also leads to the production of hydrogen peroxide, which can cause methemoglobinemia and hemolytic anemia in patients with glucose-6-phosphate dehydrogenase (G6PD) deficiency, and at-risk patients should be tested for this condition prior to administration.[20]

For those patients manifesting signs of TLS, close monitoring of serum electrolyte levels and clinical status is required (see Fig. 42.1), and electrolyte disorders require rapid therapy. Patients should receive aggressive IV hydration, a xanthine oxidase inhibitor, and rasburicase. For patients presenting with established AKI, emergent hemodialysis to correct electrolyte disorders may be required. Urine alkalinization, which increases uric acid solubility in the renal tubules, is not recommended because it can increase the likelihood of calcium phosphate precipitation.[18]

## LYSOZYMURIA

Lysozyme can be released from certain hematologic malignancies (e.g., acute promyelocytic, monocytic, or chronic myelomonocytic leukemia) and is filtered by the glomerulus and then reabsorbed by proximal tubular cells, where it leads to tubular damage and AKI.[21] The condition is rare, and suspected cases can be confirmed by urinary protein electrophoresis, which can identify lysozyme in the urine.

## TUMOR INFILTRATION OF THE KIDNEYS

For unclear reasons, leukemia and lymphoma cells have a predilection for infiltrating the kidney and, on autopsy, up to 60% of these patients will have tumor cell infiltrates in the kidney.[22] In most cases, these infiltrates have little clinical significance but, in approximately 1% of cases, they may be so massive that they result in AKI.[22,23] AKI in these cases likely results from compression of the renal parenchyma by tumor cells, with distortion of the microvasculature and tubular architecture. Patients may present with hypertension (HTN), flank pain, and hematuria or, more often, are asymptomatic. Renal imaging with ultrasonography or computed tomography shows bilaterally enlarged kidneys with a heterogeneous texture. A kidney biopsy is diagnostic and reveals tumor cell infiltration. Appropriate chemotherapy with tumor response can lead to rapid improvement in kidney function.

## THROMBOTIC MICROANGIOPATHY

Thrombotic microangiopathy (TMA) can be a consequence from the tumor itself or, more likely, from associated chemotherapy, such as gemcitabine or vascular endothelial growth factor (VEGF) inhibitors such as bevacizumab.[24–27] TMA has been associated with mucin-producing gastric, lung, and breast cancers. TMA may also be encountered in patients undergoing HSCT, in the setting of graft-versus-host disease (GVHD, associated with cyclosporine use), and with radiation nephropathy.[27] The presentation of TMA in cancer patients may be subtle and can be acute (after a clearly defined insult) or delayed (months after starting a chemotherapy regimen, such as gemcitabine). In some patients, new-onset and relatively severe HTN and proteinuria may be a clue to the diagnosis of TMA.[26] Unfortunately, the classic laboratory signs of TMA—falling hemoglobin, falling platelet count, and

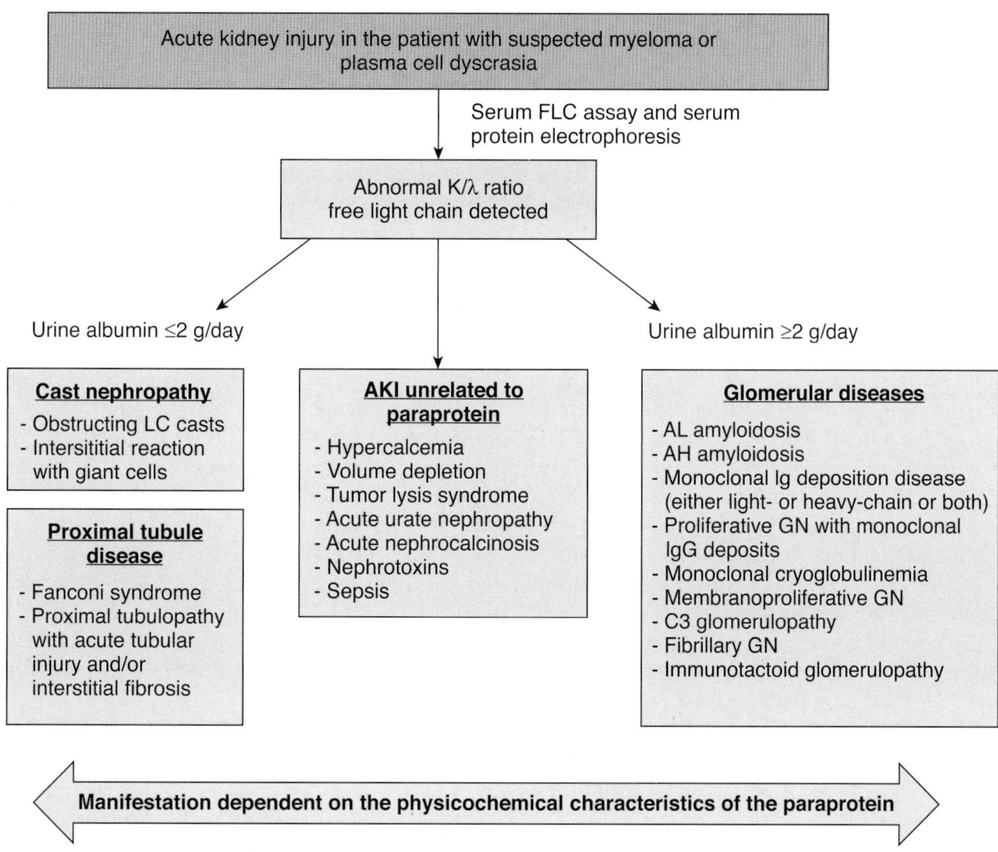


**Fig. 42.2 Approach to the patient with acute kidney injury *(AKI)* and myeloma.** *FLC,* Free light chains; *GN,* glomerular nephritis; *IgG,* immunoglobulin G; *LC,* light chain.

elevated lactate dehydrogenase level, along with falling haptoglobin and schistocytes on a peripheral blood smear—may not be present or may be mild. In some cases, renal biopsy should be considered for a definitive diagnosis, where pathologic findings of edematous intimal expansion of arteries, fibrinoid necrosis of arterioles, ischemic collapse of capillaries, and focal thrombosis of injured vessels can be seen. There are no trials that guide therapy in these cases, and treatment relies on removing any insults, such as medications, and consideration of using plasmapheresis and rituximab in more refractory cases.[26,27] Malignancy-associated TMA usually responds poorly to plasmapheresis and carries a poor prognosis overall.

## LIGHT-CHAIN CAST NEPHROPATHY AND ACUTE KIDNEY INJURY ASSOCIATED WITH MYELOMA

Patients with myeloma have an incidence of AKI that can be as high as 50%.[28] The most common cause of AKI in these patients is due to cast nephropathy, followed by light chain–related proximal tubulopathy, various glomerular diseases (including light-chain deposition disease and AL amyloidosis), hypercalcemia, hyperuricemia, and other contributing factors (Fig. 42.2).

Cast nephropathy is due to the filtration of large amounts of myeloma-produced free light chains into the renal tubules, which bind to Tamm-Horsfall protein (also known as uromodulin) to form insoluble aggregates.[29] These intratubular precipitates lead to intrarenal obstruction and local inflammation, which may be further exacerbated by the proximal tubular uptake of pathogenic light chains, which also leads to activation of inflammatory pathways.[30] Sensitive assays for serum free light chains, serum and urine protein electrophoresis, and immunofixation facilitate the diagnosis of myeloma-related AKI. Typically, patients with myeloma-related glomerular diseases will present with high levels of albuminuria (>2 g/day) indicative of the glomerular injury. Patients with cast nephropathy will demonstrate high levels of urine and serum light chains and lower levels of albuminuria.[31] Of note, 15% of patients with AKI in the setting of myeloma may have a cause of AKI completely unrelated to myeloma; thus, kidney biopsy should be performed in unclear cases.[31]

Therapy for cast nephropathy focuses on a combination of hydration and ensuring good renal tubular flow, correction of hypercalcemia, treatment of other precipitating or aggravating factors, and chemotherapy to lower the myeloma production of pathogenic light chains. Chemotherapeutic regimens for myeloma generally include a proteasome inhibitor, such as bortezomib, which does not require dosing adjustments for renal function.[32] Regimens including bortezomib (usually in combination with dexamethasone and another agent, such as thalidomide or melphalan) have led to renal response rates as high as 72% and dialysis discontinuation in 57% of patients.[33] Other effective agents include thalidomide, lenalidomide, pomalidomide, and carfilzomib.[34] A great deal of controversy remains surrounding the benefit of removing light chains by therapeutic plasma exchange or high-flux hemodialysis; currently, these methods cannot be routinely recommended.[35]

### URINARY TRACT OBSTRUCTION

Obstruction of the urinary tract is a common cause of AKI in the patient with cancer. Obstruction can be intratubular due to precipitation of uric acid, as in TLS, or from medications such as high-dose methotrexate or acyclovir.[36] In all cases, knowledge of the risk for intratubular obstruction should lead to the administration of prophylactic IV fluids to maintain urinary dilution of the drug or uric acid and maintenance of tubular fluid flow.

More commonly, urinary tract obstruction will be extrarenal and due to extrinsic compression of the ureters by a tumor mass or due to prostatic disease compressing the urethra. The clinical spectrum of patients presenting with malignant ureteral obstruction was illustrated by a case series of 102 patients.[37] Obstruction was bilateral in 68% of patients, and initial management with a percutaneous nephrostomy or ureteral stent was successful in 95% of cases. Despite successful decompression, 53% of patients developed complications, mostly urinary tract infection and obstruction of nephrostomy tubes or stents, and overall survival was poor (median, 7 months), reflecting the advanced stage of malignancy in such patients. Although renal ultrasonography will usually demonstrate hydronephrosis in patients with obstruction, patients with retroperitoneal fibrosis may not have this finding and, if clinical suspicion is high for this condition, other imaging techniques such as nuclear medicine scans should be pursued.[38]

## DECISION MAKING IN THE PATIENT WITH CANCER AND ACUTE KIDNEY INJURY

As discussed earlier, the prognosis of critically ill patients with cancer and AKI is poor, with mortality rates approaching 60% to 70% if RRT is needed. Thus, clinicians may be faced with difficult decisions when offering invasive intensive therapy for such a patient population and may appropriately opt for more conservative and palliative approaches. However, it is important to individualize these decisions because select patients (e.g., those with fewer comorbid conditions, higher functional status, and cancers that are responsive to therapy) may benefit from more aggressive therapy. Thus, decisions regarding the initiation of dialysis therapy require input from the entire care team, as well as the patient and family. These decisions should consider the reversibility of the AKI, long-term cancer prognosis, quality of life prior to critical illness, and the patient's preferences.

# CHRONIC KIDNEY DISEASE IN PATIENTS WITH CANCER

## EPIDEMIOLOGY

As has been observed with AKI, CKD is also noted to be a possible complication of numerous cancers and their associated therapy. There are a number of explanations for this observation. An important driver of this untoward complication is the fact that preexisting and often unrecognized CKD is common in patients with various types of malignancy. In addition to underlying kidney disease, incomplete renal recovery after multiple episodes of AKI, nephrectomy for kidney cancer with a reduction in nephron mass, and exposure to several courses of nephrotoxic medications can ultimately lead to the development of glomerulosclerosis and tubulointerstitial fibrosis, all of which either exacerbate underlying kidney disease or promote the development of new CKD.

In regard to preexisting CKD in cancer patients, the Renal Insufficiency and Anticancer Medications (IRMA)-1 and -2 studies clearly illustrate the extent of this problem.[39,40] In the two IRMA studies, 52.9% (IRMA-1) and 50.2% (IRMA-2) of patients with an active malignancy had an estimated glomerular filtration rate (eGFR) less than 90 mL/min/1.73 m$^2$, respectively.[39,40] In this group of patients, the prevalence of stage 3 CKD was 12% (IRMA-1) and 11.8% (IRMA-2), respectively. Stage 4 CKD was fairly rare in these two studies (0.9% and 0.7%, respectively). In an Australian cohort with various cancers ($n$ = 4077) using a prospective population cohort design, eGFR was <60 mL/min/1.73 m$^2$ in 30% of patients and <45 mL/min/1.73 m$^2$ in 8.3%.[41] In a cohort of Chinese patients with underlying cancer observed from 2000 to 2004, stage 3 CKD (defined as an eGFR < 60 mL/min/1.73 m$^2$) was noted in 12.8% (1051 of 8223).[42] The relatively common occurrence of CKD in many cancer patients has been confirmed in other studies, irrespective of the type of malignancy.

## OUTCOMES AND PROGNOSIS

Similar to cancer patients who develop AKI, CKD in patients with a malignancy may also suffer from an increased risk for death compared with those without kidney disease.[41–43] Increased cancer patient mortality is not uniformly noted in all studies; however, the effect of CKD on death occurrence appears to be specific to certain cancer types and degree of kidney dysfunction. Cancer patients with stage 3 CKD had an adjusted hazard ratio (HR) for cancer-specific mortality of 1.12 (95% confidence interval [CI], 1.01–1.26).[42] Furthermore, patients with an eGFR less than 30 mL/min/1.73 m$^2$ had an adjusted HR for cancer-specific mortality of 1.75 (95% CI, 1.32–2.32). As described in a population-based cohort study, stage 3 CKD (eGFR < 60 mL/min/1.73 m$^2$) was a significant risk factor for death from cancer.[41] In this study, the adjusted HR for cancer-specific mortality was 1.18 (95% CI, 1.08–1.29) for each 10 mL/min/1.73 m$^2$ decrease in eGFR. It is notable that mortality risk was highest for patients with breast and urinary tract cancers.[41] End-stage renal disease (ESRD) patients on hemodialysis who underwent radiofrequency ablation for hepatocellular cancer (HCC) were identified using the Japanese Diagnosis Procedure Combination database.[44] Four non-ESRD patients for each ESRD patient were matched based on age, gender, treatment hospital, and treatment year. In-hospital mortality was higher in 437 ESRD patients compared with 1345 matched controls (1.1% vs. 0.15%, respectively; odds ratio [OR] = 7.77; $P$ < .001).

In addition to CKD identified by eGFR measurement, the presence of proteinuria also appeared to increase mortality risk in cancer patients. A retrospective study of 9465 patients with newly diagnosed cancer from January to December 2010 observed an increase in all-cause mortality in patients with stage 3 CKD (eGFR < 60 mL/min/1.73 m$^2$) and proteinuria.[43] As seen in other studies, not all cancers are associated with increased mortality in the presence of CKD. To this point, an eGFR less than 60 mL/min/1.73 $m^2$ independently predicted death from hematologic (adjusted HR, 2.93; 95% CI, 1.36–6.31) and gynecologic cancers (adjusted HR, 2.82; 95% CI, 1.19–6.70), but not for other cancers. Furthermore, a study in patients with colorectal cancer ($n$ = 3379) noted that stage 3 CKD (eGFR < 60 mL/min/1.73 $m^2$) was not associated with increased mortality.[45] In addition, a prospective cohort study of cancer patients that examined the risk of death as a secondary endpoint did not show an association between CKD and mortality.[46] In fact, CKD as characterized by a reduced eGFR was not considered a risk factor for death in patients with various types of cancer.[46] Thus, it appears that underlying CKD in cancer patients is associated with increased mortality in some but not all types of malignancy. Clinicians must bear this in mind when counseling patients with cancer about the mortality risks of kidney disease.

## CANCER AND CHRONIC KIDNEY DISEASE: BIDIRECTIONAL RELATIONSHIP

As has been previously reviewed, CKD is a well-recognized complication of various malignancies and their therapies. However, in addition to the observed increase in CKD prevalence in cancer patients, both CKD and ESRD appear to be risk factors for the development of a number of malignancies.[47,48] Thus, the relationship between the kidney and cancer can be viewed as bidirectional.[47] The association between severity of kidney disease and the risk of incident cancer was examined over 6,000,420 person-years of follow-up. During this time, 76,809 incident cancers were identified in 72,875 subjects. After adjustment for time-updated confounders, a lower eGFR was associated with an increased risk of renal cancer. The adjusted HR was 2.28 (95% CI, 1.78–2.92) for an eGFR < 30 mL/min/1.73 $m^2$.[49] The authors also observed an increased risk of urothelial cancer at an eGFR < 30 mL/min/1.73 $m^2$ but no significant associations between eGFR and other types of cancer. Several observational studies have suggested an increased cancer risk in patients with ESRD on RRT[49–55] (Table 42.4). A recent study from Taiwan has demonstrated that ESRD patients have a significantly higher rate of all cancers (HR, 3.43) with higher specific risks for oral, colorectal, liver, blood, breast, renal, upper urinary tract, and bladder cancer than in the general population.[53] In one study, the observed increased risk for renal parenchymal cancer in ESRD patients was related to the development of acquired renal cystic disease, which increases with time on dialysis.[50] A U.S. study that examined data from 1996 to 2009 observed a higher incidence of cancer in ESRD patients. The cumulative 5-year incidence of any cancer was 9.48% compared with a 5-year cumulative incidence of cancer in U.S. transplant recipients of 4.4%.[54]

**Table 42.4 Standardized Incidence Rates of Cancer in Hemodialysis Patients[a]**

| Type of Cancer | Standardized Incidence Rate |
|---|---|
| All cancer types | 1.42 |
| Kidney parenchyma/pelvis | 4.03 |
| Bladder | 1.57 |
| Breast (female) | 1.42 |
| Non-Hodgkin lymphoma | 1.37 |
| Pulmonary, lung | 1.28 |
| Colonic, rectal | 1.27 |
| Pancreatic | 1.08 |
| Prostatic | 1.06 |

[a]See references 49–55.

## EFFECT OF CHRONIC KIDNEY DISEASE ON CANCER

The increased mortality observed as a complication in certain cancer patients with CKD compared with those without kidney disease has several plausible explanations. The presence of preexisting CKD may limit the use of effective agents or promote underdosing of anticancer regimens that might otherwise be curative.[47,56] In addition, underlying CKD may alter the bioavailability and/or safety profile of some anticancer drugs, which can potentially lead to different and suboptimal treatment choices. The development of AKI superimposed on CKD, which is a common complication, can lead to the cessation of effective chemotherapeutic regimens, allowing unhindered and potentially rapid tumor growth.[47,56] Furthermore, CKD and ESRD may also be associated with impaired immune surveillance, which would allow cancers to grow and metastasize, especially when combined with insufficient drug dosing. This risk is further increased when these patients receive a kidney transplant, where immunosuppressive regimens (and other factors) enhance the risk for recurrent or de novo cancers that have been associated with increased mortality.[57,58] It is also possible that the adverse renal effects of the anticancer drug used leads to acute and/or progressive kidney injury or to worsening of preexisting CKD, which leads to increased all-cause mortality unrelated to cancer.[47,56] Finally, a pessimistic view of cancer patients with CKD may lead to a nontreatment approach for potentially curable or modifiable malignancies.

## ASSESSMENT OF KIDNEY FUNCTION

Patients with cancer require frequent assessment of kidney function to ensure proper dosing of chemotherapeutic agents.[47,56,59] In addition, close monitoring during ongoing anticancer therapy is critical for timely recognition of drug-induced nephrotoxicity (either AKI or progression of underlying CKD).[56,59] The Kidney Disease: Improving Global Outcomes (KDIGO) guidelines have recommended that the glomerular filtration rate (GFR) should be the standard measure to evaluate kidney function for CKD staging and drug dosing purposes.[60] In addition, the guidelines also state that clinicians should use the most accurate method to assess kidney function in the individual cancer patient. This is of particular importance because the incidence of CKD in patients with cancer is as high as 50%.[39] Lack of appreciation for the reduced GFR in patients with CKD can lead to erroneous, harmful, and potentially life-threatening dosing of medications (and their metabolites) that are cleared predominantly by the kidneys. However, the appropriate methodology for assessing GFR in cancer patients is currently unknown. Several small studies have examined the accuracy and precision of traditional eGFR formulas in cancer patients, including the four-variable

Modification of Diet in Renal Disease (MDRD), Chronic Kidney Disease Epidemiology Collaboration (CKD-EPI), and two formulas derived specifically in cancer patients (the Wright and Martin formulas).[61,62] The previously described bedside GFR formulas all performed similarly well when compared with GFR determined by technetium-99m diethylenetriamine pentaacetic acid ($^{Tc99m}$DTPA) clearance and when used for selecting the appropriate drug dosage for carboplatin.[63] It is worth noting that all formulas significantly underdosed carboplatin, highlighting the need for continued research to determine the most accurate methodology for assessing GFR in this growing patient population. Currently, we recommend use of the CKD-EPI formula for determination of eGFR in most patients with cancer. Note that the eGFR is not reliable in the setting of AKI, and the KDIGO guidelines have therefore recommended that timed clearances of urea and creatinine may be of great value for persons with AKI.[60] See Chapter 23 for detailed discussion of methods for measuring and estimating GFR.

## DRUG DOSING IN CHRONIC KIDNEY DISEASE AND END-STAGE RENAL DISEASE

Anticancer drugs are cleared from the body predominantly by the kidneys, extrarenal pathways, or a combination of the two excretory pathways. One of the most important drug-related problems in cancer patients with impaired kidney function is inappropriate medication use and dosing errors. For example, many cytotoxic drugs and their active and potentially toxic metabolites are eliminated by the kidneys via some combination of glomerular filtration, tubular secretion, and/or tubular reabsorption. Furthermore, CKD patients receiving chemotherapeutic agents often have alterations in one or more of their pharmacokinetic parameters.[64] Alterations in medication absorption, volume of distribution and drug distribution in the body, protein binding, biotransformation, and kidney excretion may result in the accumulation of potentially toxic components and overdosage.[65,66] It is therefore critical that clinicians be wary to adjust doses of drugs that are excreted primarily by the kidneys appropriately. Drug dosing will use either the calculated or measured creatinine clearance or estimated GFR formulas (as discussed earlier), which will allow for safer use of chemotherapy in cancer patients with underlying CKD. Drug dosing and appropriate adjustments for the most commonly used chemotherapeutic agents, which may require dose modification in the setting of underlying kidney disease, are noted in Table 42.5.[63,67,68]

It is important to recognize that CKD also alters the pharmacokinetics of drugs that are cleared by nonrenal pathways. It has been demonstrated that uremia (both AKI and CKD) affects hepatic drug metabolism and coupled transport.[69] It has been shown that uremic toxins interfere with transcriptional activation, cause downregulation of gene expression mediated by proinflammatory cytokines, and directly inhibit the activity of the cytochrome P450 enzymes and drug transporters.[70] These additional nuances in pharmacokinetics will make prescribing of some drugs to CKD patients complicated, and developing a rational strategy for drug dosing in the CKD population can be quite challenging for clinicians. As a result, clinicians will need to watch closely for symptoms and signs of drug-related overdose and toxicity when the patient otherwise has had appropriate renal dosing of the anticancer drug regimen. Thus, clinicians should work closely with clinical pharmacists when these drugs are prescribed to CKD patients, and special considerations should be taken to optimize exposure to cytotoxic drugs and reduce the risk of adverse effects.[71] Precautions should include consideration of current medication pharmacokinetic and pharmacodynamic information, use of less nephrotoxic agents, and documented preventive measures, which are well integrated into oncology practice and vigilant surveillance.[72,73]

The management of cancer in the ESRD population is particularly challenging. Very little is known about anticancer drug management in ESRD patients and even less about the optimal timing and necessary dosage adjustments, depending on dialysis. In ESRD patients on RRT, kidney function no longer contributes a significant amount of drug clearance. As a result, these patients may require a reduction in drug dose to avoid excessive drug exposure and associated toxicity. This is clearly needed with drugs that are normally eliminated by the kidneys and also when extrarenal (hepatic primarily) metabolic and excretory pathways are impaired due to uremia. Because most cytotoxic drugs used are excreted predominantly in the urine as unchanged drug or active or toxic metabolite(s), any reduction in kidney clearance (as in CKD and ESRD) may result in the accumulation of potentially toxic components and overdosage.[74] The dosage of chemotherapeutic agents used in these patients will thus frequently require dosage reduction to avoid severe toxic effects. Careful dosage adjustment is mandatory to optimize exposure to cytotoxic drugs and reduce the risk of adverse effects.

The efficiency (or lack thereof) of drug clearance by the modality of dialysis must also be considered to allow for appropriate timing of chemotherapy administration. Thus, it is necessary to determine what fraction of drug(s) is removed by hemodialysis to allow chemotherapy dosing after HD sessions (medications with excellent dialytic clearance) to avoid drug removal, which may result in a loss of anticancer efficacy. Drugs that are not removed efficiently by dialysis can be administered at any time, either before or after the dialysis session. Hemodialysis influences drug pharmacokinetics primarily by the following three properties—drug clearance by dialysis, extraction coefficient, and dialysis extraction factor.[74] Hemodialysis clearance is the removal rate relative to blood concentration when entering the dialyzer. It is calculated by the amount removed (in mg/min) relative to the rate of presentation (mg/mL). Extraction coefficient, also called the "extraction ratio," is the percentage of drug removed from blood across the dialyzer. It is calculated by the rate of removal (mL/min) relative to the rate of presentation (mL/min).[75] Dialysis clearance and the extraction coefficient measure the ability of a dialysis system to remove a drug from the blood, but do not indicate how readily the drug is removed from the body. Because hemodialysis clearance and extraction ratio cannot be extrapolated to the clinical setting, the dialysis extraction factor of the drug (when available) should be used to determine the clinical impact of dialysis session on drug removal. This extraction factor, which is derived from total body clearance and the dialysis clearance of a drug, represents the actual influence of dialysis on drug pharmacokinetics. Hemodialysis is considered clinically relevant if the dialysis extraction factor exceeds 25% of the overall drug elimination.[76,77]

**Table 42.5 Dose Modifications for Commonly Used Chemotherapeutic Agents in Chronic Kidney Disease Patients**[63,67,68]

| | Creatinine Clearance (mL/min) | | | |
|---|---|---|---|---|
| **Agent** | **90–60** | **60–30** | **30–15** | **Hemodialysis** |
| Bleomycin | 100% | 75% | 75% | 50%[a] |
| Capecitabine | 100% | 75% | Avoid | Avoid |
| Carboplatin | Dosing based on AUC<br>Calvert formula—total carboplatin dose (mg) = target AUC × (eGFR + 25); AUC varies between 5 (treated pts) and 7 (untreated pts; mg/mL × min) | | | In dialysis patients, consider GFR = 0 and target dose = 125–175 mg; *E*, 84% ± 3%[b] |
| Carmustine | 100% | 80% if CrCl ≥ 45; 75% if CrCl < 45 | Consider alternative | Consider alternative |
| Cisplatin | 100% | 50% | 50% | 25%–50%[b] |
| Crizotinib | 100% | 100% | 50% | NA |
| Cyclophosphamide | 100% | 75%–100% | 75% | 75%[a]; *E*, 40%–90% |
| Cytarabine (high dose) | 100% | 60% if CrCl ≥ 45; 50% if CrCl < 45 | 30% or consider alternative | 30% consider alternative[a] |
| Dacarbazine | 100% | 80%–70% | NA | 100 mg daily for 5 days per cycle |
| Eribulin | 100% | ≥40 mL/min: 100%; <40 mL/min—NA | NA | NA |
| Etoposide | 100% | 75% | 75% | 50%[c] |
| Fludarabine | 100% | 80%, United States; 50%, United Kingdom | Avoid | Avoid |
| Hydroxyurea | 100% | 50% | 50% | 20%[b] |
| Ifosfamide | 100% | 75%–100% | 75%–100% | 75%[b]; *E*, 87% |
| Irinotecan | 100% | NA | NA | 30-40% |
| Lenalidomide | 25 mg daily | 10 mg daily | 15 mg every 2 days | 15 mg every 2 days; *E*, 31%[b] |
| Lomustine | 100% | 75% | 75% | 25%–50% |
| Melphalan | 100% | 75% | 75% | 50% |
| Methotrexate | 100% | 80% | 50% | Avoid; HD Cl, 92 ± 10 mL/min[b] |
| Mitomycin | 100% | 100% | 100% | 75%[a] |
| Oxaliplatin | 100% | 100% | Avoid if CrCl < 30 (Canada) or < 20 (United States) | Avoid |
| Pentazocine | 100% | 66% | 66% | 50% |
| Pentostatin | 100% | 50%–75% | 50% | 50% (1–2 h before dialysis) |
| Pemetrexed | 100% | 100% | Avoid | Avoid |
| Regorafenib | 100% | 100% | NA | NA |
| Sorafenib | 100% | 100% | 100% | 25% of the dose; increase to 100% according to clinical safety and efficacy[c] |
| Sunitinib | 100% | 100% | 100% | 25%; then increase to 100%, according to clinical safety and efficacy; *E*, 0[c] |
| Topotecan | 100% | 50% | 50% | 25%[b] |
| Vandetanib | 100% | 25% | NA | NA |

[a]In the absence of data on its removal during dialysis, the drug will be administered after the session.
[b]The drug is dialyzable. Therefore, it will be administered after the session, on days with HD.
[c]The drug may be administered indifferently, before or after the HD session.
*AUC*, Area under the curve; *E*, extraction coefficient (%); *NA*, not available; *pts*, patients.

Ultimately, it is very important to measure the pharmacokinetic parameters in ESRD patients on hemodialysis and to compare these data with those of patients with normal kidney function. The current lack of pharmacokinetic information of anticancer drug therapy in ESRD patients underlines the need for prospective studies in these patients.

## CANCER SCREENING IN END-STAGE RENAL DISEASE

Although cancer screening recommendations for the general population focus on early detection and treatment to improve outcomes and survival,[78] it is not clear that these same principles apply to ESRD patients. This group of patients has many unique differences from the general population that may make screening more or less relevant.[79] These include an attenuated lifespan, occurrence rates (common vs. rare) of specific cancers, unknown accuracy of screening tools, and efficacy of interventions when a cancer is identified.

The adjusted survival for incident hemodialysis and peritoneal dialysis patients in 2008 was only 55% and 66% at 3 years after ESRD onset, respectively, illustrating the marked lifespan difference as compared with the general population.[80]

ESRD patients younger than 80 years of age live less than one-third as long as their non-ESRD counterparts, whereas those aged older than 80 years are projected to live less than half as long as those without ESRD.[80] The most common cause for mortality, accounting for approximately 50% of deaths, is cardiovascular disease; malignant deaths are relatively uncommon.[80] Importantly, individual characteristics should be taken into account because groups include those with higher and lower mortality risks. For example, the 50-year-old man with uncontrolled type 2 diabetes mellitus, HTN, heart failure, and peripheral vascular disease has a much higher mortality than the 50-year-old man with polycystic kidney disease and no other significant comorbid conditions. Thus, a patient-specific understanding of the expected lifetime is required but is not routinely available for decision making. However, it is fair to conclude that ESRD patients have a shorter lifespan than the general population, and it is not clear that a uniform approach to cancer screening adds significant length or quality of life.

The goal of cancer screening is early cancer detection to enhance patient longevity. This appears to be an effective strategy for many cancers (e.g., using flexible sigmoidoscopy for colon cancer screening) in the general population when a patient's expected lifespan exceeds 10 years.[81] Thus, colon cancer screening is unlikely to be effective in many ESRD patients with multiple comorbidities whose lifespan is 3 to 5 years. In addition, screening requires patients to undergo additional procedures and tests, which have the potential for harm. Thus, in the absence of a survival benefit or if the survival benefit of screening is only realized in those with an expected lifespan of more than 10 years, cancer screening in the general ESRD population is unlikely to improve outcomes or be cost-effective. It is noteworthy, however, that certain ESRD patients enjoy life expectancies more than 10 years and may benefit from individualized cancer screening. To make this recommendation, it is important to understand the incidence of various malignancies in this population. Both CKD and ESRD are associated with an increased incidence of certain cancers,[49–55] some of which may be amenable to screening strategies.

## SCREENING TESTS FOR CANCER IN THE END-STAGE RENAL DISEASE PATIENT

Cancer screening in ESRD patients is also highly dependent on the sensitivity and specificity of screening tests used in the general population. Unfortunately, studies examining the accuracy of screening tests are generally performed on highly selected patient populations with minimal comorbidities.[82] Thus, the extrapolation of these test findings to those with ESRD is highly questionable. For most commonly used screening tests, large-scale clinical studies assessing their predictive value in detecting cancer have not been performed. In addition, there are a number of important caveats for several screening tests in the ESRD population. False-positive screening tests are observed in ESRD patients due to underlying issues such as uremic platelets (positive fecal occult blood), mammary microcalcifications, dense breast tissue (positive mammography), and elevations in several tumor markers in the absence of cancer.[83] Importantly, false-positive screening tests may lead to further inappropriate diagnostic tests and workups, unnecessary costs, and minimal benefits.

## OUTCOMES OF CANCER THERAPY IN END-STAGE RENAL DISEASE PATIENTS

In view of the increased incidence of cancer in ESRD patients, the most important question is whether a malignancy identified by screening is amenable to effective and safe therapy. Unfortunately, robust data on the outcomes of cancer therapy in patients with underlying ESRD are not available. Although cancer in this group is generally treated in the same manner as in the general population, there are important differences due to difference in pharmacokinetics and pharmacodynamics in ESRD (previously reviewed). In ESRD patients, underlying drug dosing modifications and the challenges related to the highly variable dialyzability of drugs limit the applicability of outcome data generated in the general population.[84] Cancer response rates may be very different with adjusted dosing and dialytic removal, which likely affect drug levels and overall drug exposure.

Although efficacy concerns abound for anticancer drug therapy, adverse drug effects are also higher in ESRD patients and can lead to increased morbidity and mortality. Clearly, more data are required on the efficacy of chemotherapeutic regimens in ESRD patients, and an individualized approach, which includes nephrologists, pharmacists, and oncologists, is needed to maximize outcomes and minimize the complications of drug therapy. In addition to drug toxicity, studies have observed increased adverse outcomes in patients with ESRD undergoing surgical treatment for lung and colorectal cancers.[85–87] ESRD patients with colorectal cancer undergoing tumor resection suffered a higher risk of re-intubation and a need for longer ventilator support, as well as higher rates of sepsis, deep surgical site infections, and pneumonia.[85] Most importantly, the patients also had a much higher risk of death.[85] Similar findings were found in ESRD patients undergoing surgical resection for lung cancer.[86,87] These concerns question the benefit of screening when outcomes with treatment appear to be suboptimal.

## RECOMMENDATIONS FOR CANCER SCREENING IN END-STAGE RENAL DISEASE PATIENTS

Data from routine cancer screening studies in ESRD patients have not shown this approach significantly increases life expectancy or is cost-effective.[88–91] For example, the life expectancy increase for a 60-year-old women with ESRD and type 2 diabetes mellitus who has undergone breast cancer screening would range from 1 to 16 days.[88] Furthermore, a cost analysis has demonstrated that the costs per unit of survival benefit from cancer screening range from 1.6 to 19.3 times higher in ESRD patients, with the gain in life expectancy only 5 days or less.[90] A Canadian study investigating the utility of breast and cervical cancer screening in ESRD patients has demonstrated similar results.[89] Although these points are well taken, most of these studies were performed more than 10 years ago, and mortality improvements have been seen in the ESRD population, which changes the life expectancy calculations. Also, individual patients with unique cancer risks and longer life expectancies are not usually included in these analyses. A cohort study in ESRD patients aged older than 50 years has noted that colon cancer screening is performed more often among healthier patients and those with the highest likelihood of transplantation; the overall screening rate was eight times higher than the rate in non-ESRD patients with similar limited life expectancies.[92]

Despite the fact that the general ESRD population may not benefit from universal cancer screening, an individualized approach is critical to identify patients who might benefit. The patient should be assessed for the following: (1) life expectancy; (2) risk of cancer; (3) transplantation candidacy; and (4) his or her perspective and preferences. Gauging patients prognosis and life expectancy help in the decision making process. A poor prognosis is likely when two or more of the following factors are present: (1) age older than 75 years; (2) high comorbidity score on a tool such as the Charlson score or a negative response to the surprise question (i.e., "Would I be surprised if this patient was alive in 1 year?"); and (3) poor functional status or poor nutritional state.[93] A number of prognostic scoring tools can be used to estimate life expectancy and prognosis.[93–96] In contrast, patients with an acceptable life expectancy may engender benefit from age-appropriate cancer screening, as do patients with a strong family history of cancer or another specific cancer risk (e.g., acquired cystic kidney disease). In young patients and those considered transplantation candidates, screening for acquired cystic kidney disease is appropriate. Cancer screening is reasonable for patients who are transplantation candidates determined to have an acceptable longevity. Finally, patient preferences are important, and a discussion of the risks, benefits, and costs of cancer screening is warranted.

## GLOMERULAR DISEASES ASSOCIATED WITH CANCER

Patients with cancer can present with a host of glomerular diseases either related to the primary cancer or to its therapy. Glomerular diseases associated with chemotherapy are discussed in the section on chemotherapeutic agents. Glomerular diseases associated with HSCT are discussed in the section on HSCT. Typically, patients present with hematuria, proteinuria, nephrotic syndrome, and variable degrees of renal insufficiency. For those patients with a known malignancy who develop proteinuria and/or hematuria, a malignancy-related glomerular disease should be suspected. Table 42.6 lists the commonly seen glomerular diseases associated with malignancies and their treatment. Many of these associations are based on isolated cases and case series and are likely rare associations; however, they should be considered in patients with the right presenting symptoms. Some glomerular disorders in patients with cancer represent paraneoplastic syndromes in which the clinical manifestation is not directly related to the tumor burden, invasion, or metastases but instead is caused by the action of a secreted tumor product, such as a cytokine, growth factor, or tumor cell antigen.[97] There is little information about the prevalence of paraneoplastic glomerular diseases.[98] For example, in one study of 120 patients with glomerulonephritis, 14.1% had a concomitant cancer but causality could not be determined.[99] Furthermore, it is important to realize that the treatment of certain glomerular diseases with immunosuppressive therapies (e.g., cyclophosphamide) can increase the risk for subsequent cancers.

The diagnosis of paraneoplastic glomerular diseases is difficult, and determining causation between the glomerular lesion and the cancer can be facilitated by carefully reviewing the sequence of clinical events and the timing of the cancer diagnosis in relation to the diagnosis of the glomerular lesion. In one study, most cancer diagnoses that were thought to be related to the glomerular lesion were either found at the time of renal biopsy or within the first year afterward.[99] The importance of determining the link between the cancer and glomerular disease is that if this link is present, treatment of the cancer may result in remission of the glomerular lesion.

**Table 42.6 Glomerular Diseases Associated With Cancer and Chemotherapeutic Agents**

| Glomerular Lesion | Malignancy | Drug |
|---|---|---|
| Membranoproliferative glomerulonephritis | Lung, renal cell, breast, esophageal, gastric, Wilms, melanoma, thymoma, Hodgkin and non-Hodgkin lymphoma, acute and chronic leukemia, monoclonal gammopathy, myeloma | Gemcitabine, sirolimus |
| Minimal change disease | Lung, colon, pancreas, bladder, renal cell, ovarian, mesothelioma, thymoma, Hodgkin and non-Hodgkin lymphoma, acute and chronic leukemia | Interferon-α, β, γ; pamidronate, doxorubicin, daunorubicin, sirolimus |
| Focal segmental glomerulosclerosis (FSGS) | Lung, renal cell, breast, esophageal, thymoma, Hodgkin and non-Hodgkin lymphoma, acute and chronic leukemia, T cell leukemia | Sirolimus, temsirolimus, everolimus, doxorubicin, daunorubicin, bisphosphonates |
| Collapsing FSGS | Unlikely, but causes of FSGS listed above could be considered | Interferon-α, β, γ; pamidronate, gefitinib, sirolimus, doxorubicin, daunorubicin, clofarabine, bisphosphonates |
| Membranous nephropathy | Lung, colon, gastric, pancreas, prostate, breast, head and neck, Wilms, teratoma, ovarian, cervical, endometrial, melanoma, skin, pheochromocytoma, Hodgkin and non-Hodgkin lymphoma, acute and chronic leukemia | Sirolimus |
| Lupus-like glomerulonephritis | None | Ipilimumab |
| IgA nephropathy | Lung, pancreas, renal cell, head and neck, Hodgkin and non-Hodgkin lymphoma | Sirolimus |

## MEMBRANOUS NEPHROPATHY

Membranous nephropathy is the most commonly reported glomerular disease in patients with cancer.[100–103] The database for this assertion is small and, in the largest study of 240 patients with membranous nephropathy, 10% of patients were found to have cancer that was more commonly found in the lung, prostate, and stomach.[102] In this case series, 21 cases of cancer were identified at the time of renal biopsy, and the remaining 3 cases were identified within 1 year postbiopsy. Overall, the standardized incidence ratio of cancer in patients with membranous nephropathy is 2.25, with 80% of the cancers detected before or at the time of renal biopsy.[104] From case-series data, the cancers that have been most often associated with membranous nephropathy include lung, gastric, renal cell, and prostate cancers and thymomas.[100,101] Other cancers that have been reported with membranous nephropathy include breast, colorectal, pancreatic, esophageal, and hepatic cancers.[100,101] In those patients who are aged older than 65 years or have a significant smoking history, the incidence of malignancy with membranous nephropathy may be higher.[102]

Mechanistically, malignancy-associated membranous nephropathy may be due to one of several mechanisms that lead to subepithelial deposits forming in the glomerular basement membrane.[104] Tumor cells may shed antigens that can do the following: (1) form circulating immune complexes that become trapped in the capillary wall and elicit an immune reaction in a subepithelial location; (2) form immune complexes that initially deposit in a subendothelial location but dissociate and reform in a subepithelial location; and (3) deposit in a subepithelial location (depending on the size and charge of the antigen) where they can react with a circulating antibody. A fourth mechanism may be related to an infection with an oncogenic virus or altered immune function, which can lead to both malignancy and membranous nephropathy.

Distinguishing primary versus secondary (malignancy-related) membranous nephropathy is challenging but perhaps made easier by the recognition that a high percentage of primary membranous patients have an elevated circulating level of autoantibodies to the podocyte transmembrane glycoprotein M-type phospholipase A2 receptor (anti-PLA2R) or increased expression of anti-PLA2R on kidney biopsy.[105–107] Table 42.7 lists features of malignancy- associated membranous nephropathy that can be helpful in diagnosis. There should be a high index of suspicion for an underlying malignancy in patients with a new diagnosis of membranous nephropathy, especially if there are other risk factors for cancer. However, the most efficient and cost-effective method for screening these patients has not been identified.[108] It is recommended that age- and gender-appropriate cancer screening be performed on patients with a new diagnosis of membranous nephropathy. In those patients in whom no malignancy is found on initial screening, follow-up vigilance for possible cancer should be maintained because there are case reports of cancers being detected up to 5 years after the initial diagnosis of membranous nephropathy.[109] Whether these cancers are directly related to the occurrence of glomerular disease is not known.

Malignancy-associated membranous nephropathy should resolve with surgical removal of the tumor or with effective chemotherapy.[104] In the absence of curative therapy, standard therapy for membranous nephropathy can be attempted but may have a lower likelihood of inducing remission.

**Table 42.7 Factors That Distinguish Primary From Malignancy-Associated Membranous Nephropathy**

| Parameter | Solid Tumor–Associated Membranous Nephropathy |
|---|---|
| Clinical clues | Age > 65 years, smoking > 20 pack-years, family history of malignancy, history of thromboembolism |
| Serologic | Absence of circulating anti-PLA2R autoantibodies in serum. |
| Histopathologic, kidney biopsy findings | 1. Predominance of glomerular IgG1, IgG2 deposition (idiopathic membranous nephropathy is associated with IgG4 predominance)<br>2. Normal glomerular anti-PLA2R staining<br>3. Presence of > 8 inflammatory cells/glomerulus |

## OTHER GLOMERULAR DISEASES ASSOCIATED WITH SOLID TUMORS

There are associations between solid-organ malignancies and glomerular diseases for minimal change disease (e.g., lung, colorectal, thymoma, and renal cell cancers); focal segmental glomerulosclerosis (e.g., renal cell carcinoma, thymoma); membranoproliferative glomerulonephritis (e.g., lung, renal cell, and gastric carcinomas); IgA nephropathy (e.g., renal cell carcinoma, upper respiratory tract tumors, nasopharyngeal cancers), Henoch-Schönlein purpura (e.g., lung, upper respiratory tract tumors, digestive tract tumors); crescentic glomerulonephritis (e.g., renal cell, gastric, and lung carcinomas) and AA-type amyloidosis (e.g., renal cell carcinoma).[104] These potential associations highlight the fact that in patients presenting with glomerular diseases, clinicians should remain vigilant for the possibilities of an underlying associated malignancy. Age- and gender-appropriate cancer screening should be undertaken in these patients. The association is made stronger if effective therapy for the cancer leads to concomitant remission of the glomerular disease.

## HEMATOLOGIC MALIGNANCY–ASSOCIATED GLOMERULAR DISEASES

Both lymphomas and leukemias have been associated with an increased risk of various forms of glomerular diseases.[110] The associations are strongest between Hodgkin disease and minimal change disease and chronic lymphocytic leukemia (CLL) and membranoproliferative glomerulonephritis (MPGN).

### HODGKIN DISEASE

Minimal change disease is the most frequent glomerular disease seen in association with Hodgkin disease but is uncommon, with an incidence of 0.4% in two large studies.[111] Typically, the nephrotic syndrome occurs early in the disease, with up to 40% of cases presenting at the time of or just prior to diagnosis of the cancer.[112] Minimal change disease in this setting is typically both steroid- and cyclosporine-resistant, and effective therapy of the lymphoma usually induces remission of the nephrotic syndrome.[104] Importantly, recurrence of the nephrotic syndrome in patients with previously treated Hodgkin disease can signal the recurrence of lymphoma.[111,112] The pathogenesis of minimal change disease in Hodgkin disease may be related to the induction of *c-maf*–inducing protein (c-mif), which can lead to cytoskeletal disorganization and foot process effacement of the podocyte.[113]

### CHRONIC LYMPHOCYTIC LEUKEMIA AND B-CELL LYMPHOMAS

The nephrotic syndrome is seen in approximately 1% to 2% of patients with CLL.[114] Typically, the most common glomerular lesion seen in patients with CLL is MPGN, followed by membranous nephropathy.[115] The pathogenesis of MPGN in these cases may involve cryoglobulin production by the abnormal B cell clone. In addition, B-cell lymphomas may produce a pathogenic immunoglobulin that can lead to a host of deposition diseases, including monoclonal immunoglobulin deposition disease (MIDD) and immunotactoid glomerulopathy, in which the deposits are organized in a microtubular array.[104] A clear link between the lymphoma and glomerular disease is solidified when effective chemotherapy leads to a remission of both the lymphoma or CLL and nephrotic syndrome.

### PLASMA CELL DYSCRASIA

Plasma cell dyscrasias are associated with a host of glomerular diseases and nephrotic syndrome, the most common of which is AL amyloidosis; this is found in up to 5% to 11% of patients with myeloma at autopsy.[116] Other glomerular diseases include light-chain deposition disease (up to 50% of these patients are found to have myeloma) and heavy-chain deposition disease (up to 25% of these patients have myeloma).[117] In AL amyloidosis, the predominant light-chain isotope is lambda (λ), whereas in light-chain deposition disease, it is kappa (κ).[104] The diagnosis of glomerular diseases in a patient with suspected myeloma is facilitated by finding urine albumin excretion rates > 2 g/day, and a renal biopsy is indicated in these patients (see Fig. 42.2). Several other rarer forms of glomerular disease can be found in the presence of a plasma cell dyscrasia and paraproteinemia. In all cases, effective chemotherapy or HSCT can lead to remission of the glomerular disease.[104]

## FLUID AND ELECTROLYTE ABNORMALITIES ASSOCIATED WITH MALIGNANCIES

It is not uncommon to encounter electrolyte imbalances in patients with malignancies. In general, these abnormalities may be directly linked to the malignancy as a paraneoplastic process or as a result of chemotherapeutic regimens. Conversely, they may be unrelated to the malignancy and may be similar to electrolyte disorders seen in patients without cancer (e.g., diuretic-induced hypokalemia).

### HYPONATREMIA

Disorders of water homeostasis leading to hyponatremia are among the most common electrolyte disorders encountered in patients with cancer, with a wide range of prevalence reported in the literature (4%–47%).[118,119] In patients presenting to the hospital with hyponatremia, approximately 14% had an underlying malignancy.[120] Perhaps most importantly, hyponatremia in cancer patients is associated with poor outcomes; the hospital length of stay is doubled, and mortality (within 90 days) is increased three to fivefold.[118,121–123] Whether hyponatremia has a direct link to these poor outcomes is debatable; it is more likely that hyponatremia is a marker of severity of illness, disease progression, and overall debility.

The symptoms attributable to hyponatremia are generally nonspecific (e.g., lethargy, nausea) or neurologic (e.g., headache, confusion, seizures) in origin, and the diagnosis relies on correlating laboratory studies with these symptoms. Elucidating the cause of hyponatremia requires careful history taking, physical examination, and judicious laboratory evaluation. An approach to the patient with hyponatremia and cancer is shown in Fig. 42.3. Clearly understanding the cause of a patient's hyponatremia is critical in tailoring appropriate therapy.

The syndrome of inappropriate antidiuretic hormone secretion (SIADH) is a common cause of hyponatremia in the patient with cancer and has numerous causes, ranging from paraneoplastic to medication-induced.[124] Paraneoplastic causes include small cell lung cancer (most common and seen in 10%–15% of patients) and head and neck tumors. Case reports have described SIADH with numerous other solid-organ malignancies, from brain to sarcoma.[124–126] Hyponatremia in these patients typically develops slowly and insidiously, and patients rarely have symptoms unless their serum sodium level is <125 mmol/L.[127] Serial measurements of ADH, at least for small cell lung cancer, reflect the state of the cancer, and levels fall with remission and rise with recurrence.[128] Many chemotherapeutic agents can also lead to SIADH. These include cyclophosphamide, cisplatin, vinblastine, and vincristine.[129] Many of the associations between chemotherapeutic agents and hyponatremia are derived from case reports, and the causal linkage between the drug and SIADH is not conclusive. Of note, in many cases, chemotherapeutic agents (including cyclophosphamide) are administered with aggressive IV hydration, which, depending on the levels of ADH and urine osmolality, may lower serum sodium levels further.

Therapies for hyponatremia in the patient with cancer are similar to those for other causes of hyponatremia and should be guided by three factors: (1) the presence of hyponatremia-related symptoms; (2) the duration of hyponatremia; and (3) the volume status of the patient. When possible, removal or correction of the underlying cause should always be pursued. In the vast majority of cases, hyponatremia associated with cancer is chronic in nature; thus, correction rates should be slow (no more than 6 to 8 mmol/L/day). In the presence of severe neurologic symptoms (e.g., seizures, obtundation, coma), 3% hypertonic saline can be administered as small boluses or continuous infusion to raise the serum sodium level by 4 to 6 mmol/L, which usually improves these symptoms dramatically.[130] Fluid restriction (typically defined as oral intake that is 500 mL less than urine output) is a reasonable treatment for patients with mild and transient hyponatremia due to SIADH. However, given the need for hydration protocols with several chemotherapies, as well as the need to maintain adequate nutrition, fluid restriction

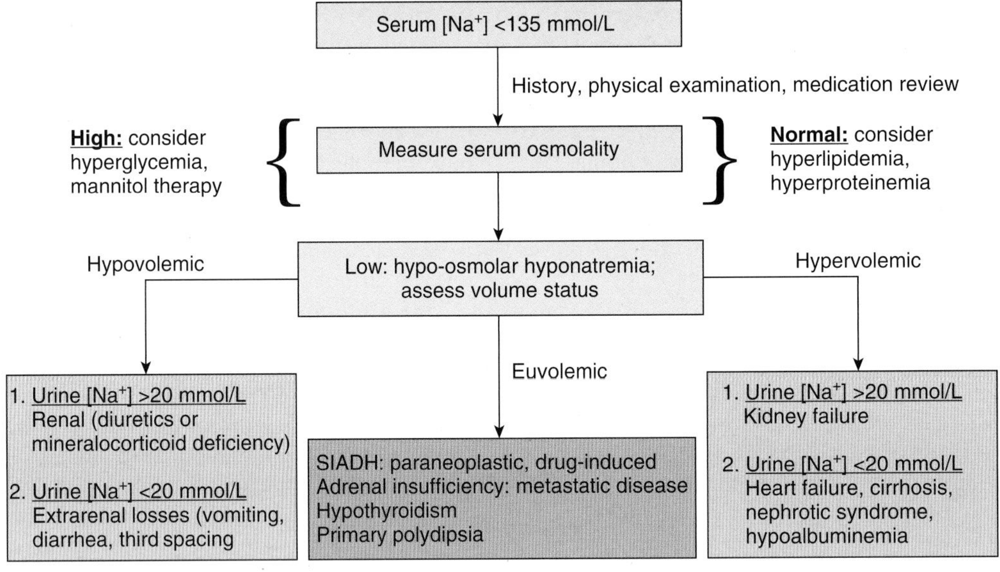


**Fig. 42.3** Diagnostic approach to hyponatremia in the patient with cancer.

can be extremely challenging. In these cases, as well as those cases of SIADH in which the urine osmolality is high (>600 mOsm/kg), the use of vasopressin type 2 receptor antagonists (e.g., conivaptan [IV only] or tolvaptan [oral only]) can be considered.[131] These drugs block the action of antidiuretic hormone (ADH) in the distal tubule and allow for the excretion of more dilute urine with increased free water excretion.[131] Tolvaptan is contraindicated in patients with hypovolemic hyponatremia, and volume depletion and in patients who cannot perceive or respond to thirst. In addition, given concerns for hepatoxicity with tolvaptan, the current recommendation is to limit its use to 1 month or less. Finally, oral urea administration can also induce a free water diuresis and can be considered as a therapy for SIADH that is not easily responsive to fluid restriction.[130]

## HYPOKALEMIA

Hypokalemia is commonly encountered in patients with cancer.[132] The causes of hypokalemia are often overlapping and multifactorial in a given patient (Table 42.8). Unique causes in the patient with cancer include the following: (1) tubular damage associated with chemotherapeutic agents and antimicrobials (e.g., cisplatin, ifosfamide, amphotericin B, aminoglycosides); (2) tubular damage associated with a light-chain–induced proximal tubulopathy, such as in multiple myeloma; (3) ectopic adrenocorticotropic hormone (ACTH) syndrome; (4) lysozymuria associated with hematologic malignancies; and (5) chemotherapy-induced gastrointestinal losses (vomiting and diarrhea).

Transcellular shifts that occur postphlebotomy, while the blood is in a sample tube, can lead to spurious hypokalemia, especially when the patient has marked leukocytosis (>100,000/μL) or when the blood is kept at room temperature for prolonged periods.[133] When this is suspected, rapid separation of the plasma and storage of blood at 4°C will usually confirm a normal serum potassium level.

**Table 42.8 Causes of Hypokalemia in the Patient With Cancer**

| Type | Cause |
|---|---|
| Tumor-related | Lysozymuria with acute leukemia<br>Mineralocorticoid excess syndromes<br>• Primary hyperaldosteronism (adrenal carcinoma)<br>• Renin-producing tumors (extremely rare)<br>• Ectopic adrenocorticotropin syndrome<br>Intracellular shifts (pseudohypokalemia) in the setting of high white blood cell counts |
| Chemotherapy-related | Chemotherapeutic agents (cisplatin, ifosfamide)<br>Antimicrobials and antifungal agents (aminoglycosides, amphotericin B)<br>Excessive gastrointestinal losses (vomiting, diarrhea) |
| Other-related | • Hypercalcemia<br>• Hypomagnesemia<br>• Postobstructive diuresis<br>• Use of growth factors |

The syndrome of paraneoplastic ACTH production can be encountered in several tumors, with the most common causes being bronchial carcinoid tumors, small cell lung carcinoma, lung adenocarcinoma, thymic cancers, and pancreatic tumors.[134] Patients typically present with signs of severe hypercortisolism—diabetes, bone loss, hyperlipidemia, HTN, and, depending on the length of symptoms, cushingoid habitus—along with severe hypokalemia.[134] The hypokalemia results from excessive cortisol production, which overwhelms the distal tubular mechanism that normally limits mineralocorticoid receptor activation by cortisol (11β-hydroxysteroid dehydrogenase). The excessive cortisol levels essentially create a syndrome similar to that of excessive aldosterone secretion, with resulting HTN and hypokalemia. Diagnosis of this syndrome is through measurement of excessive ACTH levels, hypercortisolism, and localization of the primary tumor with radiographic studies. Although optimal management is through control of the primary tumor, this may not be possible, so drugs that antagonize glucocorticoid synthesis (metyrapone and ketoconazole) are often required.[134] Rarely, adrenalectomy may be required.

A rare form of hypokalemia associated with acute myelogenous leukemia (subtypes M4 and M5) has been reported that is usually associated with other electrolyte and acid–base disorders; this includes hyponatremia, hypocalcemia, hypophosphatemia, hypomagnesemia, and a non–anion gap acidosis.[135,136] The magnitude and breadth of these electrolyte issues suggest a global tubular defect and inappropriate renal potassium losses. This defect has been postulated to be secondary to increased tumor-derived lysozyme secretion and lysozymuria-induced tubular damage.[136]

## HYPERKALEMIA

Hyperkalemia in patients with cancer is often seen in association with acute kidney injury, rhabdomyolysis, or tumor lysis syndrome. Less common causes include adrenal insufficiency (secondary to adrenal metastases) and drugs (e.g., heparin, ketoconazole, trimethoprim, and calcineurin inhibitors). An important consideration in patients with marked leukocytosis or thrombocytosis is pseudohyperkalemia, which results from a shift of potassium out of platelets or white blood cells postphlebotomy and after clotting of the sample.[137] Although patients will have hyperkalemia reported on laboratory reports, they will not display clinical or electrocardiographic signs of an elevated potassium level. In patients for whom this may be a concern, it is recommended that plasma samples be used for laboratory measurement.

## HYPERCALCEMIA

Hypercalcemia that is directly related to malignancy may occur in as many as 30% of patients with cancer at some point during their course.[138,139] When hypercalcemia occurs in these patients, it portends a very poor prognosis and a limited lifespan.[138,139] The symptoms attributable to hypercalcemia are generally nonspecific (e.g., lethargy, nausea, vomiting, confusion) and are related to both the absolute level of serum calcium and the rapidity at which the disorder develops. Patients presenting with serum calcium levels above 13 mg/dL are generally symptomatic.

There are three mechanisms that describe the pathophysiology in most cases of malignancy-associated hypercalcemia (Fig. 42.4). The most common cause is paraneoplastic production of parathyroid-related peptide (PTHrP).[140] PTHrP is very similar to parathyroid hormone (PTH) and acts to increase bone resorption (increases bone calcium release) via activation of osteoclasts and increase reabsorption of calcium in the renal tubules.[140] However, PTHrP is less likely than PTH to stimulate 1,25-dihydroxyvitamin D production. Therefore, PTHrP does not increase intestinal calcium absorption. Hypercalcemia is accompanied by hypophosphatemia, reduced tubular reabsorption of phosphorus, enhanced tubular reabsorption of calcium, and increased excretion of

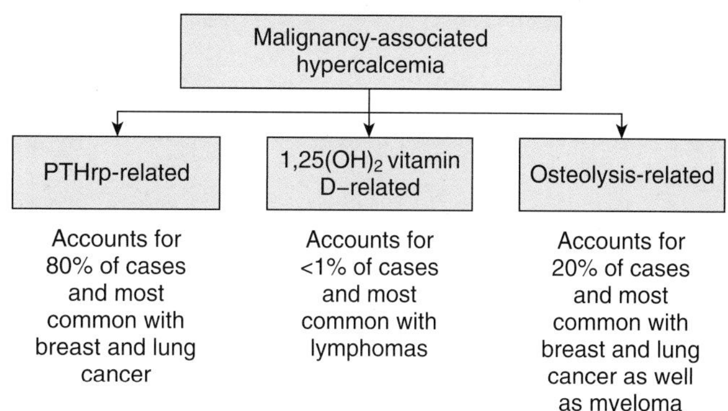


**Fig. 42.4** Causes of malignancy-associated hypercalcemia.

nephrogenous cyclic adenosine monophosphate (cAMP), reflecting the PTH-like actions of PTHrP. The second most common mechanism of malignancy-associated hypercalcemia is local osteolytic effects of the cancer and is seen in patients with myeloma, breast cancer, lymphomas, and other cancers. For example, myeloma has a predilection to grow in bone environments, and this is facilitated by the secretion of bone reabsorbing factors such as interleukin-1 (IL-1), IL-6, and tumor necrosis factor, leading to extensive bone destruction, lytic bone lesions, and the release of calcium.[141] Typically, these patients will have advanced cancers, with skeletal surveys demonstrating lytic bone lesions. The third mechanism of malignancy-associated hypercalcemia is due to activation of vitamin D by the tumor itself, which can be seen in lymphomas and, rarely, with myeloma. These patients will have elevated 1,25 dihydroxyvitamin D levels and suppressed PTH levels.[142] The elevated activated vitamin D levels facilitate increase gastrointestinal calcium absorption and increased bone calcium release leading to hypercalcemia.

The diagnostic approach to the patient with hypercalcemia is presented in Fig. 42.5. Once hypercalcemia is confirmed with measurement of an ionized calcium level, the diagnostic algorithm centers on measurement of PTH. PTH levels are suppressed in patients with malignancy-associated hypercalcemia, with the rare exceptions of tumors such as parathyroid adenocarcinomas, which produce excessive PTH. In patients with a suppressed PTH level, measurement of PTHrP and vitamin D levels is the next diagnostic step and allows for accurate diagnosis in most cases.[143]

Patients with hypercalcemia are usually severely volume-depleted due to the effects of elevated calcium levels causing nephrogenic diabetes insipidus, as well as nausea and vomiting. In addition, hypercalcemia, via activation of the calcium-sensing receptor in the thick ascending limb of the loop of Henle, leads to natriuresis and worsening of the volume depletion.[144] Thus, the cornerstone of the treatment of hypercalcemia is aggressive restoration of the extracellular volume, as well as induction of natriuresis with IV fluids (typically, 0.9% saline). This will allow excretion of excess calcium. Loop diuretics should only be added in the presence of volume overload and are not a routine part of management.[145] Data support the use of bisphosphonates as highly effective agents in the management of patients with malignancy-associated hypercalcemia, largely due to their effect to inhibit osteoclast activity.[138] Both pamidronate and zoledronic acid are U.S. Food and Drug Administration

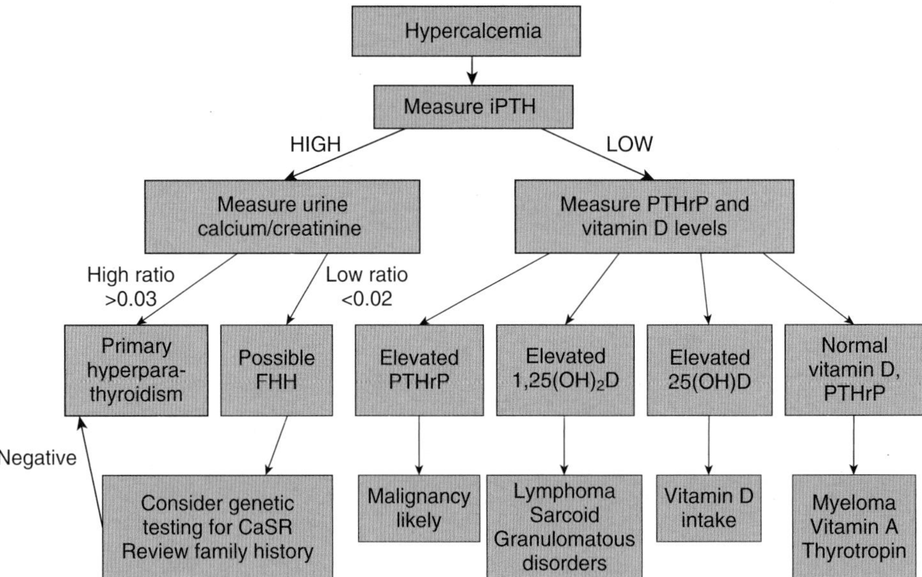


**Fig. 42.5** Diagnostic algorithm for the patient presenting with hypercalcemia. Measurement of PTH is the first step in the diagnostic approach. Patients with malignancy-associated hypercalcemia typically have low levels of PTH due to feedback inhibition of the high blood calcium levels on the parathyroid gland. In patients with low levels of PTH, measurement of PTHrP and 1,25-dihydroxyvitamin D (1,25$(OH)_2$D) levels will allow classification of patients into several diagnostic groupings. In patients with elevated PTH levels, a 24-hour urine collection for calcium and creatinine levels should be obtained. *CaSR,* Calcium-sensing receptor; *FHH,* familial hypocalciuric hypercalcemia; *iPTH,* intact parathyroid hormone; *PTH,* parathyroid hormone; *PTHrP,* parathyroid-related peptide; *25(OH)D,* 25-hydroxy vitamin D. (From Reagan P, Pani A, Rosner MH. Approach to diagnosis and treatment of hypercalcemia in a patient with malignancy. *Am J Kidney Dis.* 2013;63(1):141–147.)

**Table 42.9 Dosing Guidelines for the Use of Bisphosphonates in the Treatment of Malignancy-Associated Hypercalcemia**

| Bisphosphonate | Dosing Guidelines | Interval Between Doses |
|---|---|---|
| Pamidronate | CrCl > 60 mL/min: 90 mg IV administered over 2–3 hours<br>CrCl, 30–60 mL/min: 60 to 90 mg IV administered over 2–4 hours<br>CrCl < 30 mL/min: 60–90 mg IV administered over 4–6 hours | Every 3–4 weeks |
| Zoledronate | CrCl > 60 mL/min: 4 mg IV over 15 minutes<br>CrCl, 50–60 mL/min: 3.5 mg IV over 15 minutes<br>CrCl, 40–49 mL/min: 3.3 mg IV over 15 minutes<br>CrCl 30–49 mL/min: 3 mg IV over 15 minutes<br>CrCl < 30 mL/min: not recommended | Every 3–4 weeks |

(FDA)–approved for this indication; dosing guidelines are shown in Table 42.9. These agents are generally well tolerated, with the most common side effect being infusion-related fever, but serious nephrotoxicity of these agents has been described, including glomerular lesions and tubular toxicity.[146] Thus, the serum creatinine level should be monitored before each dose of bisphosphonate and the drug withheld in patients with worsening renal function. Urine albumin excretion should be monitored at 3- to 6-month intervals, and the drug should be held if albuminuria develops. Patients with PTHrP-mediated hypercalcemia may remain mildly hypercalcemia, even after bisphosphonate administration, due to the effects of PTHrP to decrease renal calcium excretion. An alternative antiresorptive agent is denosumab, a monoclonal antibody directed against the receptor activator of nuclear factor kappa B ligand (RANKL).[147] Denosumab does not require dose adjustment for renal insufficiency and has demonstrated benefit in reducing skeletal-related events in patients with metastatic cancer.[148] For patients with hypercalcemia secondary to tumors producing 1,25-dihydroxyvitamin D, corticosteroid therapy may be of benefit.[149] Finally, in patients with significant renal failure and hypercalcemia, hemodialysis with a low calcium dialysate can be beneficial.[138]

## HYPOPHOSPHATEMIA

Cancer can lead to disorders of phosphate homeostasis via a number of mechanisms. Hypophosphatemia can result in the setting of malnutrition and cachexia and with vitamin D deficiency; these patients typically have low normal serum calcium levels, low vitamin D levels, and elevated PTH levels. In addition, patients with hypercalcemia due to elevated PTH or PTHrP levels may have low-normal serum phosphate levels due to the effects of these hormones on renal phosphorus handling. In some cases, proximal tubular injury (either through chemotherapy such as cisplatin or ifosfamide or due to light-chain–induced tubular injury from myeloma) can lead to phosphaturia and hypophosphatemia.

A rare and unique form of hypophosphatemia is also encountered in patients with cancer, the syndrome of tumor-induced osteomalacia (TIO) or oncogenic osteomalacia.[150] In this syndrome, tumor production of phosphaturic factors such as fibroblast growth factor-23 (FGF-23) results in renal phosphate wasting, hypophosphatemia, and osteomalacia. Tumor types producing these factors include chondrosarcoma, osteoblastoma, and hemangiopericytomas. These tumors may be small and indolent and may require extensive and specialized imaging for localization. Patients with TIO typically have normal serum calcium levels, and the diagnosis is facilitated by measuring the percentage tubular reabsorption of phosphate or the tubular maximum for phosphate, corrected for the GFR.[151] Once renal phosphate wasting is confirmed, measurement of elevated levels of FGF-23 can be diagnostic of TIO. Importantly, 1,25-dihydroxyvitamin D levels are low because FGF-23 inhibits the activity of the 1α-hydroxylase. Therapy rests on surgical removal of the tumor, which is usually curative.

## HYPOMAGNESEMIA

Hypomagnesemia is a relatively common electrolyte disorder in patients with cancer; the unique causes in this patient population relate to chemotherapeutic agents such as cisplatin and cetuximab. Otherwise, patients usually develop hypomagnesemia due to gastrointestinal losses, especially with prolonged diarrhea, or renal losses due to diuretic therapy. Other drugs associated with hypomagnesemia in the patient with cancer may include proton pump inhibitors, aminoglycoside antibiotics, calcineurin inhibitors (in patients with stem cell transplants), and amphotericin B.[152]

Cisplatin causes magnesium wasting in more than 50% of treated patients, and the incidence increases with the cumulative dose.[153] Renal magnesium wasting continues after cessation of the drug for several months but can persist for years. The occurrence of magnesium wasting does not correlate with cisplatin-induced acute kidney injury. Cetuximab, a monoclonal antibody against the epithelial growth factor receptor (EGFR), has been associated with hypomagnesemia due to renal losses in as many as 30% of patients receiving this drug.[154] The mechanism of magnesium wasting during treatment with cetuximab is associated with the blockage of the EGFR-dependent transient receptor potential channel 6 (TRPM6) in the nephron, which results in insufficient activation of the TRPM6 epithelial ion channel and magnesium wasting in the distal convoluted tubule. Cessation of therapy with cetuximab leads to reversal of the magnesium wasting and return of the serum magnesium level to normal.

# KIDNEY DISEASE ASSOCIATED WITH HEMATOPOIETIC STEM CELL TRANSPLANTATION

HSCT is an important therapy for many cancer patients. However, it is complicated by acute and chronic kidney disease, which are often associated with increased morbidity and mortality. Causes of HSCT-associated kidney injury are often multifactorial, including the conditioning chemotherapy regimen, radiation exposure, nephrotoxic medications, sepsis, sinusoidal obstruction syndrome (SOS), HSCT-associated TMA and GVHD.[155,156] Short- and long-term morbidity and mortality are both increased in the setting of HSCT.[157] Other complications include fluid disturbances, electrolyte abnormalities, glomerular disease, and HTN.

HSCT involves administering lethal doses of chemotherapy and radiotherapy, followed by bone marrow rescue by engraftment of stem or progenitor cells, which are harvested from bone marrow, peripheral blood, or umbilical cord blood. Stem or progenitor cells can be autologous (patient) or allogeneic (donor). In myeloablative HSCT, high-dose chemotherapy and radiation are administered to eradicate the underlying malignancy and bone marrow, followed by marrow reconstitution with the infusion of stem or progenitor cells. However, because myeloablative HSCT is extremely toxic, older patients and those with numerous comorbidities are often excluded from transplantation candidacy. To allow this group of higher risk patients to benefit from HSCT, less toxic nonmyeloablative regimens have been created, using a so-called graft-versus-tumor effect for therapeutic efficacy.

## HEMATOPOIETIC STEM CELL TRANSPLANTATION–ASSOCIATED ACUTE KIDNEY INJURY

The incidence of AKI with HSCT is quite varied (range, 15%–73%) due to the AKI definition used, the type of HSCT performed (allogenic vs. autologous), and the chemotherapeutic conditioning regimen used (high dose vs. reduced intensity).[155] The incidence and clinical course of AKI following allogeneic HSCT are well documented. In one study, AKI developed in 53% of patients, of whom half required RRT.[158] Subsequent studies have noted that the incidence of moderate to severe AKI (defined as a doubling of the baseline serum creatinine value) ranges from 36% to 78% with allogenic HSCT.[159–161] Dialysis was required in 21% to 33% of these patients, who suffered a mortality of 78% to 90%. The incidence of AKI with autologous HSCT is less common.[159] In patients with breast cancer, autologous HSCT was associated with the development of moderate to severe AKI in 21% of patients and a mortality rate of 18%. The lower AKI incidence in this group may be due to calcineurin inhibitor avoidance.[162]

Nonmyeloablative HSCT is also associated with a lower incidence of AKI, which is attributed to the milder conditioning regimen used.[163] One study in nonmyeloablative HSCT patients demonstrated a cumulative AKI incidence of 40.4% at 4 months, and dialysis was required in 4.4% of patients. In contrast to myeloablative HSCT, AKI in these patients was usually associated with calcineurin inhibitor exposure. In addition, the development of AKI during nonmyeloablative HSCT occurs over the first 3 months, which is in contrast to myeloablative HSCT, in which AKI typically develops in the first 3 weeks.

As with AKI incidence, the risk for requiring RRT after HSCT varies widely. Overall, approximately 5% of HSCT patients with AKI require dialysis, which is associated with increased mortality risk.[163–169] However, the need for dialysis ranges from 0% to 30%,[9–15] and the risk is higher with myeloablative therapy.[170] Outcomes in patients requiring acute RRT are difficult to quantify accurately. Most

**Table 42.10 Risk Factors and Causes of Acute and Chronic Kidney Lesions With HSCT**

| Acute Kidney Injury | Chronic Kidney Disease |
|---|---|
| Prerenal—nausea, vomiting, and diarrhea associated with acute gastrointestinal GVHD, drug-induced nausea and vomiting | Thrombotic microangiopathy—calcineurin inhibitors, chronic GVHD |
| Prerenal/acute tubular injury—sepsis, sinusoidal obstruction syndrome, acute GVHD, marrow infusion syndrome | Arteriolonephrosclerosis—hypertension, radiation, TBI |
| Thrombotic microangiopathy—acute GVHD, calcineurin inhibitors, TBI | Viral nephropathy—BK virus, cytomegalovirus |
| Acute tubular injury, crystalline nephropathy—amphotericin, vancomycin, aminoglycosides, acyclovir, other nephrotoxins | Membranous nephropathy, minimal change disease—chronic GVHD, drug-induced glomerular injury |

*GVHD,* Graft-versus-host disease; *HSCT,* hematopoietic stem cell transplantation; *TBI,* total body irradiation.

studies have reported that acute dialysis in this group is associated with an extremely high mortality rate, ranging from 80% to 100%.[156,163–166,168,171,172]

Common risk factors for and causes of AKI after HSCT include volume depletion, sepsis, nephrotoxic medication exposure, SOS, and GVHD (Table 42.10).[156,169,173,174] Because of a propensity for increased gastrointestinal fluid losses and poor oral intake, HSCT patients are highly susceptible to volume depletion and prerenal AKI. GVHD is unique to HSCT and causes tissue and endothelial damage via T-cell and cytokine-mediated injury.[156] The gastrointestinal mucosa is a common site of injury by GVHD, contributing to inadequate fluid intake and increased fluid losses. SOS is also an independent risk factor for AKI and results in a picture similar to hepatorenal syndrome, with sodium avidity and edema formation. Medications commonly prescribed that cause AKI include vancomycin, aminoglycosides, acyclovir, and amphotericin. These agents cause AKI by direct tubular toxicity, acute interstitial nephritis, and crystal-related tubular injury (acyclovir). Calcineurin inhibitors can lead to renal arteriolar vasoconstriction and have been associated with the development of TMA.

## MARROW INFUSION SYNDROME

AKI associated with symptoms of nausea, vomiting, and abdominal pain may develop within 24 to 48 hours of HSCT from hemoglobin pigment nephropathy caused by the infusion of lysed red blood cells. The process of stem cell preservation is associated with exposure to various cryoprecipitants, such as dimethyl sulfoxide, which can cause red cell lysis, with hemoglobinuria in the recipient resulting in the precipitation of heme proteins in the distal tubule.[175] Renal vasoconstriction, direct cytotoxicity of hemoglobin, and intratubular hemoglobin cast formation are the mechanisms whereby AKI develops with hemoglobinuria. Management of this now rare complication includes alkalinization of the urine to increases heme solubility and mannitol-induced diuresis to prevent intratubular heme trapping.[176,177]

## HEPATIC SINUSOIDAL OBSTRUCTION SYNDROME

AKI following HSCT can also be due to acute liver injury. Hepatic SOS, formerly known as venoocclusive disease, is a commonly encountered complication after HSCT and has been implicated as an independent risk factor for the development of AKI.[175] It typically occurs within 30 days of HSCT, and the incidence varies widely, ranging from 0% to 62.3% (mean, 13.7%).[175] Although the pathophysiology of AKI in the SOS setting is poorly defined, it appears to be a variant of hepatorenal syndrome (hemodynamic AKI). Hepatic sinusoidal obstruction occurs due to iatrogenic damage to sinusoidal endothelial cells and hepatocytes, which results in fibrous narrowing of small hepatic venules and sinusoids. Injury appears to be triggered by the pretransplantation cytoreductive regimen and is more common after allogeneic than autologous HSCT. Furthermore, cytokine release and glutathione depletion in this setting cause hepatocellular necrosis and fibrosis.[178,179] The development of SOS is usually associated with pretreatment with busulfan, cyclophosphamide, and/or total body irradiation.[180]

Criteria have been established for the diagnosis of hepatic SOS. The Seattle criteria require the presence of at least two of three manifestations—jaundice, painful hepatomegaly, and fluid retention or weight gain within 20 days of HSCT.[179,180] The Baltimore criteria require a bilirubin level of >2 mg/dL, plus two or more of the following: painful hepatomegaly, weight gain >5%, or ascites, within 21 days of HSCT.[181] Hepatic SOS severity is graded as mild (the illness fulfills SOS diagnostic criteria but is self-limiting), moderate (SOS subsides with diuretic or analgesic treatment), and severe (SOS persists for more than 100 days, or death).[179]

Hepatic SOS is characterized by painful hepatomegaly, jaundice, fluid retention, and ascites. Patients have hyperdynamic vital signs along with hyponatremia, oliguria, and low fractional excretion of sodium. Urinalysis reveals minimal proteinuria and muddy brown granular casts as a result of the toxic tubular effects of bile acids and bilirubin in the urine. Hypervolemia is usually resistant to diuretics, and spontaneous recovery is rare.

Risk factors that predispose to the development of AKI include a baseline serum creatinine level > 0.7 mg/dL, weight gain, hyperbilirubinemia, and exposure to amphotericin B, vancomycin, or acyclovir. The development of AKI adversely affects survival. In patients who require RRT, the mortality rate approaches 80%.

The management of hepatic SOS has included a number of agents. Small trials using infusions of prostaglandin E, pentoxifylline, and low-dose heparin have shown promise in the prevention and treatment of SOS.[182–184] Smaller trials with defibrotide, an antithrombotic and fibrinolytic agent, have also shown benefit in patients with SOS, especially when used within the first 2 days of HSCT.[185,186] Beneficial effects are thought to be due to the prevention of platelet aggregation and antiinflammatory properties. However, bleeding risk is a concern and must be closely monitored.

## ACUTE THROMBOTIC MICROANGIOPATHY

Acute TMA is characterized by endothelial damage that leads to thickened glomerular and arteriolar vessels, fibrin thrombi in capillary loops and arterioles (Fig. 42.6), the presence of fragmented red blood cells, thrombosis, and endothelial cell swelling.[187,188] In the setting of HSCT, patients may develop subclinical kidney disease, AKI, or CKD.[189,190] Given the challenges of obtaining kidney tissue in patients with HSCT, two consensus guidelines have been published outlining clinical criteria for the diagnosis of TMA.[191,192] To meet criteria, the guidelines require the following: (1) schistocytes on a peripheral smear, and (2) an elevated lactate dehydrogenase concentration. The Blood and Marrow Transplant (BMT) Clinical Trials Network also includes AKI (doubling of serum creatinine level), unexplained central nervous system dysfunction, and a negative Coombs test result as part of diagnostic criteria.[191] The International Guidelines from the European Group for Blood and Marrow Transplantation include thrombocytopenia, anemia, and a decreased haptoglobin concentration.[192] Despite these criteria, making a diagnosis of TMA remains challenging and often requires a high index of suspicion, as supported by validation studies and autopsy studies in which clinical criteria often do not correlate with histologic findings.[193]

It is debated whether TMA is a distinct complication of HSCT or a manifestation of several other post-HSCT complications, such as GVHD, infection, and drug toxicity.[194–197] Despite histologic similarities, endothelial cell damage, primarily in the renal vasculature, underlies the pathogenesis of TMA post-HSCT, which differs from thrombotic thrombocytopenic purpura, which is characterized by low levels of von Willebrand factor–cleaving protease ADAMTS13 (genetic or acquired).[198–202] At times, HSCT may unmask a previously undiagnosed genetic mutation in the alternate complement pathway, resulting in atypical hemolytic-uremic syndrome,[203] which may respond to eculizumab.[204]

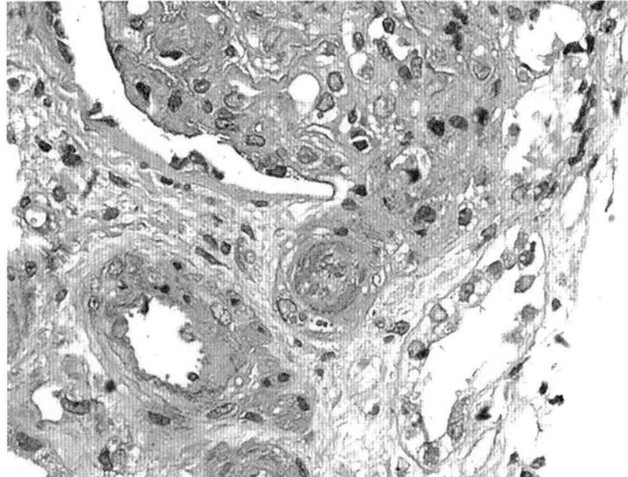

**Fig. 42.6** Kidney biopsy from a patient with thrombotic microangiopathy in the setting of HSCT exhibits a fresh fibrin thrombus in a preglomerular arteriole. (Hematoxylin & eosin, ×600.)

In addition to the conditioning regimens for and other exposures during HSCT, some studies have suggested that renal endothelial injury with subsequent TMA may also reflect direct endothelial cell injury by GVHD.[205,206] In fact, the risk of TMA diagnosed on renal pathology at autopsy was fourfold higher in patients with acute GVHD after HSCT. Renal endothelial injury may occur due to circulating inflammatory cytokines or may reflect direct injury to renal endothelial cells by GVHD. Furthermore, plasma markers of endothelial injury and coagulation activation are elevated in patients with acute GVHD after HSCT, suggesting an association among endothelial injury, acute GVHD, and the subsequent development of TMA.[205,206]

Treatment remains challenging for clinicians. Currently available studies are limited by retrospective study designs and the inclusion of heterogeneous patient populations. Options that are used include adjustment of GVHD prophylaxis (either stopping or reducing the calcineurin inhibitor dose), therapeutic plasma exchange (TPE), rituximab, and defibrotide.[191,193,207–209] In uncontrolled studies, reported response rates for TPE have ranged between 27% and 80%.[210–216] In a prospective study of 112 HSCT patients, TMA developed in 11, and 64% of these patients responded with treatment consisting of TPE and cyclosporine withdrawal.[212] Case reports have described a benefit with rituximab treatment of TMA post-HSCT.[192,217–220] More data are required to understand the true utility of rituximab for treatment of this form of TMA.

## GRAFT-VERSUS-HOST DISEASE

The use of donor stem cells requires that all allogeneic HSCT recipients receive prophylaxis against GVHD. Prophylactic regimens include cyclosporine A, mycophenolate mofetil, tacrolimus, and sometimes short-term methotrexate.[221,222] GVHD can be classified into acute and chronic categories based on the duration of onset after HSCT and the associated clinical findings. Acute GVHD has great significance because it can independently serve as a risk factor for the development of AKI in HSCT recipients.[223] GVHD may lead directly to AKI through cytokine-mediated inflammation affecting the glomeruli and/or renal tubules or indirectly from exposure to certain medications, such as cyclosporine, which itself can predispose to nephrotoxicity. Furthermore, GVHD also promotes viral reactivation, such as cytomegalovirus, which can contribute to AKI. Gastrointestinal involvement by GVHD is associated with extrarenal fluid losses from vomiting and diarrhea, which can cause prerenal AKI. Treatment options for GVHD include prednisone, antithymocyte globulin, sirolimus, and mycophenolate mofetil.[224] Supportive measures such as IV fluids and avoiding other nephrotoxins are also important in management.

CKD also develops in many patients following HSCT. In can be due to chronic TMA, various viral infections, or a sequelae of acute or chronic GVHD, particularly in patients whose pre-HSCT conditioning regimen did not include TBI.[155,225] A retrospective study of 1635 HSCT recipients has noted that neither TBI nor cyclosporine use was associated with the development of CKD (eGFR < 60 mL/min/1.73 m$^2$) at 1 year following transplantation. Subgroup analyses of patients receiving cyclosporine have supported the theory that GVHD, independent of calcineurin inhibitor therapy, increases the risk for the development of CKD.[155]

## HEMATOPOIETIC STEM CELL TRANSPLANTATION–ASSOCIATED CHRONIC KIDNEY DISEASE

HSCT also appears to be associated with the development of CKD. However, studies reporting the risk of CKD after HSCT are difficult to compare because the definitions used are not consistent, the populations studied are often heterogeneous, and follow-up times vary.[226] In general, the prevalence of CKD after HSCT ranges from 20% to 30%.[227] Microalbuminuria and macroalbuminuria, HTN, and various types of renal tubular dysfunction also complicate the course of HSCT. A meta-analysis has reviewed the published data on CKD after HSCT through 2006.[226] Kidney function was assessed with creatinine-based, radioisotope, or inulin measurements of the GFR. The overall prevalence of CKD was 16.6% (range, 3.6%–89%) and was similar in those receiving autologous and allogeneic transplants, although the allogeneic transplant recipients had a greater decrease in kidney function. Regardless of underlying cause, CKD can progress to ESRD, which increases the mortality risk post-HSCT.[228]

Causes of CKD following HSCT are quite varied (see Table 42.10). The incidence of post-HSCT TMA ranges from 2% to 21%[191] and this complication often follows an indolent course, resulting in CKD and, possibly, progression to ESRD.[229] Although several disease processes, such as TMA, radiation nephritis, nephrotic syndrome, chronic GVHD, and BK virus nephropathy, have been associated with CKD after HSCT, much of the long-term kidney injury in patients undergoing HCT remains unexplained.[230] Multiple bouts of AKI in the setting of HSCT, especially when severe and prolonged, may lead to CKD. Risk factors considered to be potentially important for the development of CKD include acute and chronic TMA post-HSCT, calcineurin inhibitor use (CNI) use, total body irradiation (TBI), and GVHD.[231] CKD occurring from GVHD-associated T-cell and cytokine-mediated damage kidney tissue is thought to be due to a chronic inflammatory state.[232] Glomerular lesions related to HSCT occur primarily in the setting of chronic GVHD. Membranous nephropathy (67%) and minimal change disease (33%) are the two most common pathologies[233,234] and occur within several months of GVHD, approximately 8 to 14 months after HSCT. Hypertension commonly complicates HSCT and likely contributes to CKD and its overall progression. BK virus–related genitourinary and renal lesions also complicate the course of HSCT and are associated with CKD.[235]

## ANTICANCER DRUGS AND KIDNEY DISEASE

The number of anticancer agents available to treat various malignancies has grown significantly in the past 10 to 20 years. Chemotherapy-related nephrotoxicity has always been an important area for the nephrologist; however, the number of agents causing kidney injury and an assortment of electrolyte and acid–base disturbances has increased dramatically.[236–242]

Furthermore, understanding renal metabolism and excretion of these drugs is critical in ensuring efficacy while also avoiding or at least reducing toxicity, especially in the setting of acute or chronic kidney disease. Nephrotoxicity associated with the more common chemotherapeutic drugs includes AKI primarily from acute tubular injury, acute interstitial nephritis, and a variety of glomerular injuries; a number of tubulopathies (alone or combined with kidney injury) may develop and result in metabolic perturbations.[236–238] In addition to conventional agents, the emergence of targeted therapies and immunotherapies has further increased the amount of drug-induced nephrotoxicity that is occurring in cancer patients[240–246] (Table 42.11).

**Table 42.11 Anticancer Drug Nephrotoxicity**

| Drug | Clinical Kidney Syndrome | Kidney Histopathology |
|---|---|---|
| **Conventional Drugs** | | |
| Platinum compounds (cisplatin, carboplatin, oxaliplatin) | • AKI<br>• Hypomagnesemia<br>• NDI<br>• Proximal tubulopathy (Fanconi syndrome)<br>• Salt wasting | • Acute tubular injury |
| Ifosfamide | • AKI<br>• NDI<br>• Proximal tubulopathy (Fanconi syndrome) | • Acute tubular injury |
| Methotrexate | • AKI | • Acute tubular injury<br>• Crystalline nephropathy |
| Gemcitabine | • AKI<br>• Hematuria<br>• Hypertension<br>• Proteinuria | • Thrombotic microangiopathy |
| Mitomycin C | • AKI<br>• Hematuria<br>• Hypertension<br>• Proteinuria | • Thrombotic microangiopathy |

**Table 42.11 Anticancer Drug Nephrotoxicity (Cont'd)**

| Drug | Clinical Kidney Syndrome | Kidney Histopathology |
|---|---|---|
| Pemetrexed | • AKI<br>• NDI<br>• Proximal tubulopathy (Fanconi syndrome) | • Acute tubular injury<br>• Interstitial fibrosis |
| Nitrosoureas | • Chronic kidney disease | • Chronic tubulointerstitial nephritis |
| **Targeted Agents** | | |
| Anti-VEGF agents (aflibercept, bevacizumab) | • AKI<br>• Hypertension<br>• Proteinuria | • Thrombotic microangiopathy |
| Tyrosine kinase inhibitors (axitinib, pazopanib, sorafenib, regorafenib, sunitinib) | • AKI<br>• Hypertension<br>• Proteinuria | • Acute tubulointerstitial nephritis<br>• Acute tubular injury<br>• Focal segmental glomerulosclerosis<br>• Thrombotic microangiopathy |
| BRAF inhibitors (dabrafenib, vemurafenib) | • AKI<br>• Electrolyte disorders | • Acute tubulointerstitial nephritis<br>• Acute tubular injury |
| ALK inhibitors (crizotinib) | • AKI<br>• Electrolyte disorders<br>• Renal microcysts | • Acute tubulointerstitial nephritis<br>• Acute tubular injury |
| EGFR inhibitors (cetuximab, erlotinib, gefitinib, panitumumab) | • Hypomagnesemia (secondary hypokalemia and hypocalcemia) | • None |
| Imatinib | • AKI<br>• Chronic kidney disease | • Acute tubular injury |
| Rituximab | • AKI (tumor lysis syndrome) | • Acute tubular injury<br>• Crystalline (uric acid) nephropathy |
| **Immunotherapy Agents** | | |
| Interferons (alfa, beta, gamma) | • AKI<br>• Nephrotic-range proteinuria | • Focal segmental glomerulosclerosis<br>• Thrombotic microangiopathy |
| Interleukin-2 | • AKI<br>• Capillary leak syndrome | • None |
| Chimeric antigen receptor (CAR) T cells | • Capillary leak syndrome with AKI, tumor lysis syndrome<br>• Electrolyte disorders | • None |
| CTLA-4 inhibitors (ipilimumab) | • AKI<br>• Proteinuria | • Acute tubulointerstitial nephritis<br>• Lupus-like glomerulonephritis<br>• Minimal change disease |
| PD-1 inhibitors (nivolumab, pembrolizumab) | • AKI | • Acute tubulointerstitial nephritis |
| **Other Drugs** | | |
| Bisphosphonates (pamidronate, zoledronate) | • AKI<br>• Nephrotic syndrome | • Acute tubular injury<br>• Focal segmental glomerulosclerosis |
| Sirolimus | • AKI<br>• Proteinuria | • Focal segmental glomerulosclerosis |

*AKI,* Acute kidney injury; *CTLA-4,* cytotoxic T lymphocyte–associated protein-4; *EGFR,* epidermal growth factor receptor; *NDI,* nephrogenic diabetes insipidus; *PD-1,* programmed death-1; *VEGF,* vascular endothelial growth factor.

## CONVENTIONAL CHEMOTHERAPEUTIC AGENTS

### GEMCITABINE

Gemcitabine is a cell cycle–specific pyrimidone antagonist used to treat a number of malignancies.[246,247] Following gemcitabine approval, TMA was described as a complication, with an incidence ranging from 0.015% to 2.4%.[11–14,246–249] The risk for TMA is associated with a higher cumulative dose and prior exposure to other chemotherapeutic agents that cause TMA.[246–249] Endothelial injury from direct drug toxicity is the most likely mechanism. Disruption of endothelial cell integrity releases von Willebrand factor (vWF) multimers and plasminogen activator inhibitor, reduces the synthesis of prostacyclin and tissue plasminogen activator, and exposes a denuded endothelial surface to fibrin and platelet, which deposit within the renal microvasculature.[246–249]

Gemcitabine-induced TMA usually develops weeks to months after initiating therapy, and AKI develops in most cases.[246–249] A case series of 29 patients with gemcitabine-associated TMA noted microangiopathic hemolytic anemia (MAHA), thrombocytopenia, and AKI in all patients, whereas new or worsening HTN, proteinuria, and hematuria were noted in 26 of 29 patients.[250] Gemcitabine discontinuation or future avoidance resulted in full ($n = 8$) or partial ($n =$

11) recovery, with CKD noted in three and ESRD in seven patients (25%). Plasma exchange and plasmapheresis had minimal or no effect on renal recovery. Reported mortality was wide-ranging (0%–90%), with TMA-specific death estimated at 15%.[246–250]

### CISPLATIN

Cisplatin is an effective and widely used chemotherapeutic agent. However, nephrotoxicity is the most common dose-limiting side effect. This relates to its renal site of elimination—, in particular, transport through the proximal tubule.[236–238] Following drug entry into the tubule cell via the organic cation transporter, direct tubular toxicity occurs in part due to a low chloride environment. In the intracellular compartment, chloride molecules are replaced with water molecules in the *cis* position of cisplatin, forming hydroxyl radicals that injure the neutrophilic binding sites on DNA.[236–238,251,252] Nonoliguric AKI, primarily from renal tubular injury (apoptosis and necrosis), typically develops after approximately 3 to 5 days of drug exposure. Furthermore, tubular injury from high-dose cisplatin is often associated with a so-called tubulopathy, which is characterized by various electrolyte (e.g., hypokalemia, hypomagnesemia, hypocalcemia) and acid–base disturbances (e.g., renal tubular acidosis).[2–4,236–238] Hypomagnesemia, which occurs with prolonged exposure, is a challenging management issue because it can be permanent and require IV supplementation[236–238,251,252]

Although kidney injury is generally reversible, repeated cisplatin doses (>100 mg/m$^2$) may cause permanent kidney injury (GFR reduction of 15%). Isotonic or hypertonic saline administration and avoidance of concomitant nephrotoxins are the most effective ways to prevent cisplatin-induced nephrotoxicity. Amifostine may reduce cisplatin nephrotoxicity through the promotion of improved DNA repair and elimination of free radicals.[2,3,18,236–238,253] Newer platinum agents (carboplatin and oxaliplatin) are less nephrotoxic than cisplatin and are available for patients with underlying kidney disease and for those who previously suffered from cisplatin nephrotoxicity.[254–256] Clinicians must recognize that these agents can still cause AKI and electrolyte disorders.

### IFOSFAMIDE

Ifosfamide is an effective alkylating agent that is associated with nephrotoxicity, predominantly injuring the renal tubules. Like cisplatin, this drug enters proximal tubular cells via the organic cation transporter.[236–238] Once inside the cell, the drug or its metabolite chloroacetaldehyde causes direct tubular epithelial cell damage.[236–238] Ifosfamide-induced tubular injury is associated clinically with AKI and a tubulopathy, which can be associated with severe hypokalemia, hypophosphatemia, hypomagnesemia, and hyperchloremia. Patients can experience Fanconi syndrome, with hypophosphatemic rickets and osteomalacia, as well as nephrogenic diabetes insipidus.[236–238,257]

Risk factors for ifosfamide nephrotoxicity include previous exposure to cisplatin, CKD, and a high cumulative dose (>84 g/m$^2$).[236–238,258,259] Amifostine may offer some protection, whereas mesna, which prevents hemorrhagic cystitis, is ineffective in the kidney. Most patients recover from ifosfamide-induced tubular injury; however, long-term complications such as CKD and tubulopathies may develop. Chronic renal fibrosis, with a progressive decline in the GFR, may rarely lead to ESRD.[236–238,260]

### METHOTREXATE

Methotrexate (MTX) is an antifolate drug that is an effective antineoplastic agent when administered in a high dose (>1 g/m$^2$).[236–238,261–265] Nephrotoxicity occurs primarily because of the precipitation of an insoluble parent drug and metabolites (7-hydroxymethotrexate) within the tubular lumens, a phenomenon known as "crystalline nephropathy."[236–238,261–265] True or effective volume depletion and acidic urine are two major risk factors for the development of AKI; direct tubular toxicity may also contribute to the development of kidney injury. The overall incidence rate of AKI is approximately 1.8% (range, 0%–12%), but can be as high as 50% with high doses in at-risk patients.[236–238,261–265] In general, kidney injury is reversible.

Preventive measures include volume repletion to achieve high urine flow rates. Isotonic saline infusion and furosemide may be necessary to maintain a high urine output. An increase in the clearance rate of MTX (and reduction in crystal precipitation) is seen when the urine pH is increased from 5.5 to 8.4, which can be accomplished with an isotonic solution containing bicarbonate. Once AKI develops, the excretion of MTX is reduced, and systemic toxicity is increased. In this case, therapy is primarily supportive. However, it may be necessary to remove the drug with hemodialysis. Hemodialysis, using high blood flow rates with a high-flux dialyzer, is an effective method of removing MTX.[266] High-dose leucovorin therapy can reduce the systemic toxicity associated with MTX and AKI. Glucarpidase (carboxypeptidase G) may be considered when severe systemic toxicity and AKI are present, and dialysis access is risky. This costly drug metabolizes MTX to benign metabolites.[267]

## IMMUNOTHERAPIES

The immune system represents a potent tool to destroy cancer cells. Enhancing the immune system as a therapy for cancer has been used for several decades. Initial therapies included interferon and IL-2. More recently, immune checkpoint inhibitors and chimeric antigen receptor T cells have been used to treat certain forms of malignancy.

### INTERFERON

Interferon is used to treat various malignancies (e.g., chronic myelogenous leukemia [CML], renal cell carcinoma) and infectious agents (e.g., hepatitis C). Treatment with interferon results in two renal lesions: (1) podocytopathy with minimal change disease (MCD) and focal segmental glomerulosclerosis (FSGS); and (2) thrombotic microangiopathy.[268,269] MCD was first described but more recent reports have described collapsing and noncollapsing FSGS. Nephrotic-range proteinuria and AKI are observed within weeks to months of commencing interferon therapy. Although proteinuria declines with interferon discontinuation, complete resolution is more common with MCD than with FSGS.[268,269] In particular, collapsing FSGS is associated with CKD. Steroids are associated with complete remission in less than one-third of patients with FSGS. Interferon-related glomerular injury may be due to the direct binding of interferon to podocyte receptors and an alteration of normal cellular proliferation. Macrophage activation and skewing of the cytokine profile toward IL-6 and IL-13, which are possible permeability factors in MCD and FSGS, are also possible mechanisms.[268,269]

### INTERLEUKIN-2

High-dose IL-2 has been used to treat renal cell carcinoma, malignant melanoma, and other cancers. High-dose IL-2 is associated with a cytokine release syndrome and capillary leak; this causes a prerenal form of AKI, which develops within 24 to 48 hours.[270] This hemodynamic disturbance is further exacerbated by concurrent NSAID therapy, which is used to reduce fever and myalgias associated with IL-2.[270] Kidney dysfunction generally reverses with drug discontinuation, although ischemic/nephrotoxic acute tubular injury can be associated with a more prolonged course of AKI.[270] This is particularly the case for patients with underlying risk factors, such as CKD, diabetes mellitus, and HTN. To reduce AKI during IL-2 therapy, antihypertensive agents should be withdrawn and fluid resuscitation initiated. Low-dose dopamine (2 μg/kg/min) may prevent some of the renal toxicity of IL-2, reversing oliguria and improving renal recovery time.[271]

### IMMUNE CHECKPOINT INHIBITORS

Another method to activate the immune system against the tumor microenvironment is the strategy of immune checkpoint inhibitor (ICI) therapy.[244,245] Activation by an immunologic event such as infection signals cytotoxic T cells to undergo damping of their response to maintain immune homeostasis by expressing several receptors, including cytotoxic T lymphocyte–associated antigen 4 (CTLA-4), programmed death-1 protein (PD-1), and programmed death ligand-1 (PD-L1) that downregulate T-cell function.[244,245,272] These checkpoints normally prevent the development of unwanted autoimmunity. Tumor survival is enhanced in malignancies that overexpress ligands that bind inhibitory T-cell receptors (PD-1), thereby decreasing activated T-cell infiltration into the tumor microenvironment and inhibiting antitumor T-cell responses. To combat this, monoclonal antibody drugs that block ligand binding to PD-1 and CTLA-4 receptors were designed to facilitate T-cell rescue and restore antitumor immunity. Ipilimumab, a fully human, immunoglobulin G1 (IgG1) monoclonal antibody blocking CTLA-4, nivolumab, a fully human IgG4 antibody blocking the PD-1 receptor, and pembrolizumab, a humanized monoclonal IgG4-kappa isotype antibody against PD-1, are the ICIs available in clinical practice. However, blocking immune checkpoints risks the development of pathologic autoimmunity and end-organ injury, such as acute tubulointerstitial nephritis (ATIN). Numerous cases of ATIN, some with granulomatous changes, have been described with the use of ICIs.[244,245] Although some patients develop rash and eosinophilia, AKI is the only consistent clinical manifestation. A small number of cases have required RRT, but most respond to drug discontinuation and steroid therapy.

## TARGETED THERAPIES

### ANTIANGIOGENESIS DRUGS

The discovery that VEGF is an important mediator of tumor growth and angiogenesis led to the development of drugs targeting this pathway for cancer therapy. However, VEGF is also an essential growth factor for maintaining glomerular and microvascular endothelial health.[240,273] In the glomerulus, VEGF is secreted by podocytes and traverses the basement membrane, where it binds to VEGF receptors on endothelial cells and maintains glomerular endothelial cell integrity and filtration barrier function.[240,273] Anti-VEGF drugs, such as the monoclonal antibody, bevacizumab, as well as drugs that inhibit tyrosine kinase, such as sunitinib, block VEGF function. This leads to glomerular endothelial cell dysfunction and filtration barrier disruption, resulting in proteinuria, thrombotic microangiopathy, HTN, and AKI. Mild and asymptomatic proteinuria is common, although heavy proteinuria occurs in <10% of subjects.[240,273] HTN or aggravation of preexisting HTN is common. The reported incidence varies between 17% and 80%. The effects of anti-VEGF therapy on the development of HTN have been reviewed in a meta-analysis of seven trials, which noted that the relative risk of HTN was three- to sevenfold higher, depending on dose.[274] Hypertension reflects the efficacy of VEGF blockade, perhaps explaining why bevacizumab-induced HTN correlates with clinical outcomes. Hypertension is managed with standard antihypertensive medications, although the use of angiotensin-converting enzyme (ACE) inhibitors or angiotensin receptor blockers (ARBs) is preferable in patients with proteinuria. Adverse kidney effects with these drugs may require dose reduction or drug discontinuation, especially with TMA.

### EPIDERMAL GROWTH FACTOR RECEPTOR INHIBITORS

The EGF pathway has multiple functions in several organs, including the kidneys.[237,238] Several novel agents that target the EGF pathway are used to treat various cancers; these include receptor antagonists, tyrosine kinase inhibitors, and antisense oligodeoxynucleotides. Cetuximab is a monoclonal antibody against the EGF receptor and was first approved for use in metastatic colon cancer. The primary abnormality observed following EGF receptor antagonism is hypomagnesemia due to renal magnesium wasting.[237,238,275] Hypocalcemia and hypokalemia may also develop as a result of the parathyroid and renal effects of hypomagnesemia.[237,238] EGF normally activates the renal magnesium channel (TRP-M6) in the apical membrane of the distal convoluted tubule to stimulate magnesium absorption. The incidence of severe hypomagnesemia is 10% to 15% but is reversible with drug discontinuation.[276] Many patients require IV magnesium repletion to continue the drug.

### B-RAF INHIBITORS

Malignant melanoma frequently has a B-RAF V600 mutation that can be effectively targeted by selective B-RAF inhibition by vemurafenib and dabrafenib. As with other effective cancer agents, these drugs have also been observed to cause nephrotoxicity. Kidney dysfunction, defined as a GFR decline at 1 and 3 months of therapy, occurred in 15 of 16 patients, which was complicated by persistent kidney injury after 8 months of follow-up.[277] In addition, eight patients developed AKI (one with ATN on biopsy) following vemurafenib therapy.[277] AKI that was clinically suggestive of AIN was observed in four patients treated with vemurafenib, with three of four patients recovering kidney function after drug discontinuation, although no biopsy data were available. Of 74 patients treated with vemurafenib, about 60% developed AKI, primarily KDIGO stage 1, within 3 months of drug exposure.[241] Biopsy in two patients revealed tubulointerstitial injury. Kidney function recovered within 3 months of B-RAF discontinuation. AKI and metabolic disturbances from B-RAF inhibitors have been described in the FDA Adverse Events Reporting System.[277] Although the mechanism of kidney injury is unknown, these drugs may interfere with the downstream MAPK pathway, increasing susceptibility to ischemic tubular injury.

### ANAPLASTIC LYMPHOMA KINASE INHIBITORS

Anaplastic lymphoma kinase 1 (ALK-1) is a member of the insulin receptor tyrosine kinase family. Small-molecule inhibitors of ALK-1 include crizotinib and ceritinib.[243,278] Crizotinib is an effective agent for the treatment of advanced ALK-positive non–small cell lung cancer; however, it is complicated by two major adverse renal effects. These include AKI and an increased risk for the development and progression of renal cysts.[243,278] In addition to these complications, crizotinib is also associated with the development of peripheral edema and electrolyte disorders (relatively rare). In regard to AKI, it appears that crizotinib is associated with both true AKI (tubulointerstitial injury) and pseudo-AKI, which is likely due to a drug-induced reduction in renal tubular creatinine secretion.

## MISCELLANEOUS AGENTS

### BISPHOSPHONATES

Bisphosphonates are administered primarily to treat patients with the hypercalcemia of malignancy and to minimize skeletal complications in the setting of bone metastases and multiple myeloma. These agents undergo renal excretion and have been associated with two major types of kidney disease—AKI from acute tubular injury and the podocytopathies, MCD and FSGS.[279] Biopsy-proven ATN has been observed in patients treated with zoledronate, which is often associated with various levels of CKD, despite drug discontinuation.[279] Pamidronate has also been shown to cause AKI, as well as the nephrotic syndrome, from a collapsing variant of FSGS.[280] The mechanism of bisphosphonate-induced kidney injury is not known, but direct toxicity to the glomerular and tubular epithelial cells is suspected. Ibandronate is a newer agent that appears to be significantly less nephrotoxic.[279] Dose modifications are recommended for pamidronate and zoledronate. Pamidronate, 90 mg, administered over 4 to 6 hours (rather than over 2 hours), is recommended for patients with stage 4 CKD, although 60 mg might be a more appropriate dose.[279] The dose of zoledronate should be reduced in patients with stage 3 CKD and avoided in those whose eGFR is <30 mL/min.[279]

 Complete reference list available at ExpertConsult.com.

## KEY REFERENCES


1. Christiansen CF, Johansen MB, Langeberg WJ, et al. Incidence of acute kidney injury in cancer patients: a Danish population-based cohort study. *Eur J Int Med.* 2011;22:399–406.
2. Libório AB, Abreu KL, Silva GB Jr, et al. Predicting hospital mortality in critically ill cancer patients according to acute kidney injury severity. *Oncology.* 2011;80(3–4):160–166.
13. Rosner MH, Perazella MA. Acute kidney injury in patients with cancer. *N Engl J Med.* 2017;376(18):1770–1781.
15. Cairo MS, Bishop M. Tumor lysis syndrome: new therapeutic strategies and classification. *Br J Hematol.* 2004;127(1):3–11.
19. Cortes J, Moore JO, Maziarz RT, et al. Control of plasma uric acid in adults at risk for tumor lysis syndrome: efficacy and safety of rasburicase alone and rasburicase followed by allopurinol compared with allopurinol alone—results of a multicenter phase III study. *J Clin Oncol.* 2010;28:4207–4213.
26. Izzedine H, Perazella MA. Thrombotic microangiopathy, cancer and cancer drugs. *Am J Kidney Dis.* 2015;66:857–868.
28. Hutchinson CA, Batumen V, Behrens J, et al. The pathogenesis and diagnosis of acute kidney injury in multiple myeloma. *Nat Rev Nephrol.* 2011;8:43–51.
29. Sanders PW, Booker BB. Pathobiology of cast nephropathy from human Bence Jones proteins. *J Clin Invest.* 1992;89:630–639.
33. Dimopoulos MA, Roussou M, Gavriatropoulou M, et al. Bortezomib-based triplets are associated with a high probability of dialysis independence and rapid renal recovery in newly diagnosed myeloma patients with severe renal failure or those requiring dialysis. *Am J Hematol.* 2016;91:499–502.
39. Launay-Vacher V, Oudard S, Janus N, et al. Prevalence of renal insufficiency in cancer patients and implications for anticancer drug management: the renal insufficiency and anticancer medications (IRMA) study. *Cancer.* 2007;110:1376–1384.
48. Lowrance WT, Ordoñez J, Udaltsova N, et al. CKD and the risk of incident cancer. *J Am Soc Nephrol.* 2014;25:2327.
52. Birkeland SA, Løkkegaard H, Storm HH. Cancer risk in patients on dialysis and after renal transplantation. *Lancet.* 2000;355(9218):1886–1887.
55. Yanik EL, Clarke CA, Snyder JJ, et al. Variation in cancer incidence among patients with ESRD during kidney function and nonfunction intervals. *J Am Soc Nephrol.* 2016;27(5):1495–1504.
57. Acuna SA, Fernandes KA, Astat CD, et al. Cancer mortality among recipients of solid-organ transplantation in Ontario, Canada. *JAMA.* 2016;2(4):463–469.
59. Aapro M, Launay-Vacher V. Importance of monitoring renal function in patients with cancer. *Cancer Treat Rev.* 2012;38:235–240.
74. Janus N, Thariat J, Boulanger H, et al. Proposal for dosage adjustment and timing of chemotherapy in hemodialyzed patients. *Ann Oncol.* 2010;21:1395–1403.
83. Rosner MH. Cancer screening in patients with end-stage renal disease: an individualized approach. *J Onco-Nephrol.* 2017;1(1):36–41.
88. LeBrun CJ, Diehl LF, Abbott KC, et al. Life expectancy benefits of cancer screening in the end-stage renal disease population. *Am J Kidney Dis.* 2000;35(2):237–243.
98. Pani A, Porta C, Cosmai L, et al. Glomerular diseases and cancer: evaluation of underlying malignancy. *J Nephrol.* 2016;29:143–152.
102. Lefaucheur C, Stengel B, Nochy D, et al. Membranous nephropathy and cancer. Epidemiologic evidence and determinants of high-risk cancer association. *Kidney Int.* 2006;70:1510–1517.
106. Beck LH Jr. Membranous nephropathy and malignancy. *Semin Nephrol.* 2010;30:635–644.
107. Qin W, Beck LH Jr, Zeng C, et al. Anti-phospholipase A2 receptor antibody in membranous nephropathy. *J Am Soc Nephrol.* 2011;22:1137–1143.
113. Audard V, Larousserie F, Grimbert P, et al. Minimal change nephrotic syndrome and classical Hodgkin's lyumphoma: report of 21 cases and review of the literature. *Kidney Int.* 2006;69:2251–2260.
124. Rosner MH, Dalkin AC. Electrolyte disorders associated with cancer. *Adv Chronic Kid Dis.* 2014;21(1):7–17.
138. Rosner MH, Dalkin AC. Onco-nephrology: the pathophysiology and treatment of malignancy-associated hypercalcemia. *Clin J Am Soc Nephrol.* 2012;7(10):1722–1729.
155. Hingorani SR, Guthrie K, Batchelder A, et al. Acute renal failure after myeloablative hematopoietic cell transplant: incidence and risk factors. *Kidney Int.* 2005;67:272–277.
174. Keating GM. Defibrotide: a review of its use in severe hepatic veno-occlusive disease following haematopoietic stem cell transplantation. *Clin Drug Investig.* 2014;34(12):895–904.
204. Zaber J, Fakhouri F, Roumenina L, et al. Use of eculizumab for atypical hemolytic uraemia syndrome and C3 glomerulopathies. *Nat Rev Nephrol.* 2012;8:643–659.
224. Kogon A, Hingorani S. Acute kidney injury in hematopoietic cell transplantation. *Semin Nephrol.* 2010;30(6):615–626.
226. Ellis MJ, Parikh CR, Inrig JK, et al. Chronic kidney disease after hematopoietic cell transplantation: a systematic review. *Am J Transplant.* 2008;8:2378–2390.

236. Porta C, Cosmai L, Gallieni M, et al. Renal effects of targeted anticancer therapies. *Nat Rev Nephrol.* 2015;11(6):354–370.
237. Perazella MA, Moeckel GW. Nephrotoxicity from chemotherapeutic agents: clinical manifestations, pathobiology, and prevention/therapy. *Semin Nephrol.* 2010;30:570–581.
242. Perazella MA. Onco-nephrology: renal toxicities of chemotherapeutic agents. *Clin J Am Soc Nephrol.* 2012;7(10):1713–1721.
245. Shirali AC, Perazella MA. Tubulointerstitial injury associated with chemotherapeutic agents. *Adv Chronic Kidney Dis.* 2014;21(1):56–63.
252. Arany I, Safirstein RL. Cisplatin nephrotoxicity. *Semin Nephrol.* 2003;23:460–464.
262. Perazella MA. Crystal-induced acute renal failure. *Am J Med.* 1999; 106:459–465.
266. Wall SM, Johansen MJ, Molony DA, et al. Effective clearance of methotrexate using high-flux hemodialysis membranes. *Am J Kidney Dis.* 1996;28:846–854.
267. Widemann BC, Schwartz S, Jayaprakash N, et al. Efficacy of glucarpidase (carboxypeptidase g2) in patients with acute kidney injury after high-dose methotrexate therapy. *Pharmacotherapy.* 2014; 34(5):427–439.
268. Markowitz GS, Bomback AS, Perazella MA. Drug-induced glomerular disease: direct cellular injury. *Clin J Am Soc Nephrol.* 2015; 10(7):1291–1299.
272. Postow MA, Callahan MK, Wolchok JD. Immune checkpoint blockade in cancer therapy. *J Clin Oncol.* 2015;33(17):1974–1982.
273. Gurevich F, Perazella MA. Renal effects of anti-angiogenesis therapy: update for the internist. *Am J Med.* 2009;122:322–328.
274. Zhu X, Wu S, Dahut WL, et al. Risks of proteinuria and hypertension with bevacizumab, an antibody against vascular endothelial growth factor: systematic review and meta-analysis. *Am J Kidney Dis.* 2007;49(2):186–193.
280. Markowitz GS, Appel GB, Fine PL, et al. Collapsing focal segmental glomerulosclerosis following treatment with high-dose pamidronate. *J Am Soc Nephrol.* 2001;12(6):1164–1172.

# Index



Note: Page numbers followed by "f" refer to illustrations; page numbers followed by "t" refer to tables; page numbers followed by "b" refer to boxes.

## C

## D

## G

## M

## O

## Q



## R

## V

ELEVENTH EDITION

# Brenner & Rector's THE KIDNEY

VOLUME TWO


**ALAN S.L. YU, MB, BChir**
Harry Statland and Solon Summerfield Professor of Medicine
Director, Division of Nephrology and Hypertension and the Jared Grantham Kidney Institute
University of Kansas Medical Center
Kansas City, Kansas

**GLENN M. CHERTOW, MD, MPH**
Norman S. Coplon/Satellite Healthcare Professor of Medicine
Department of Medicine
Division of Nephrology
Stanford University School of Medicine
Palo Alto, California

**VALÉRIE A. LUYCKX, MBBCh, MSc**
Affiliate Lecturer
Renal Division
Brigham and Women's Hospital
Harvard Medical School
Boston, Massachusetts;
Institute of Biomedical Ethics and the History of Medicine
University of Zürich
Zürich, Switzerland

**PHILIP A. MARSDEN, MD**
Professor of Medicine
Elisabeth Hofmann Chair in Translational Research
Oreopoulos-Baxter Division Director of Nephrology
University of Toronto
Toronto, Ontario, Canada

**KARL SKORECKI, MD, FRCP(C), FASN**
Dean, Azrieli Faculty of Medicine
Bar-Ilan University
Safed, Israel

**MAARTEN W. TAAL, MBChB, MMed, MD, FCP(SA), FRCP**
Department of Renal Medicine
Royal Derby Hospital
Derby, United Kingdom;
Centre for Kidney Research and Innovation
Division of Medical Sciences and Graduate Entry Medicine
School of Medicine
University of Nottingham
Nottingham, United Kingdom

*Special Assistant to the Editors*
**WALTER G. WASSER, MD**
Attending Physician, Division of Nephrology
Mayanei HaYeshua Medical Center
Bnei Brak, Israel;
Rambam Health Care Campus
Haifa, Israel


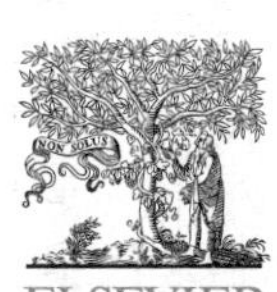

ELSEVIER

Elsevier
1600 John F. Kennedy Blvd.
Ste 1800
Philadelphia, PA 19103-2899

BRENNER & RECTOR'S THE KIDNEY, ELEVENTH EDITION

Set ISBN: 978-0-323-53265-5
Volume 1 ISBN: 978-0-323-75933-5
Volume 2 ISBN: 978-0-323-75934-2



**Notice**

Practitioners and researchers must always rely on their own experience and knowledge in evaluating and using any information, methods, compounds or experiments described herein. Because of rapid advances in the medical sciences, in particular, independent verification of diagnoses and drug dosages should be made. To the fullest extent of the law, no responsibility is assumed by Elsevier, authors, editors or contributors for any injury and/or damage to persons or property as a matter of products liability, negligence or otherwise, or from any use or operation of any methods, products, instructions, or ideas contained in the material herein.

Previous editions copyrighted 2016, 2012, 2008, 2004, 2000, 1996, 1991, 1986, 1981, and 1976.

**Library of Congress Control Number: 2019934877**

*Senior Content Strategist:* Nancy Anastasi Duffy
*Senior Content Development Specialist:* Joanie Milnes
*Publishing Services Manager:* Julie Eddy
*Senior Project Manager:* Rachel E. McMullen
*Design Direction:* Renee Duenow

Printed in India

Last digit is the print number: 9 8 7 6 5 4 3

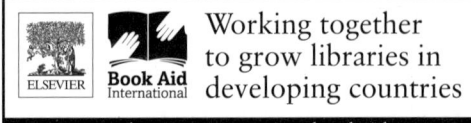

*Dedicated to*

**Barry M. Brenner, MD**
*our mentor and role model, whose vision continues to challenge and inspire us*
*and to*

**Joan Ryan**
*for her patient stewardship of The Kidney through three wonderful editions*

# Contributors

**Andrew Advani, BSc, MBChB (Hons), PhD, FRCP(UK), FASN**
Associate Professor of Medicine
University of Toronto;
St. Michael's Hospital
Toronto, Ontario, Canada

**Todd Alexander, MD, PhD**
Pediatric Nephrologist and Professor
Department of Paediatrics
University of Alberta
Edmonton, Alberta, Canada

**Michael Allon, MD**
Professor of Medicine
Division of Nephrology
University of Alabama at Birmingham
Birmingham, Alabama

**Gerald B. Appel, MD**
Professor of Clinical Medicine
Department of Medicine
Columbia University Medical Center
New York, New York

**Suheir Assady, MD, PhD**
Director, Department of Nephrology and Hypertension
Rambam Health Care Campus
Haifa, Israel

**Colin Baigent, BMBCh, MA, MSc, FRCP, FFPH**
Professor of Epidemiology
Nuffield Department of Population Health
University of Oxford
Oxford, Great Britain

**George L. Bakris, MD**
Professor and Director
American Heart Association Comprehensive Hypertension Center
Department of Medicine
University of Chicago Medicine
Chicago, Illinois

**Marisa Battistella, PharmD**
Associate Professor
University Health Network/Leslie Dan Faculty of Pharmacy
University of Toronto,
Toronto, Ontario, Canada

**Srinivasan Beddhu, MD**
Professor of Internal Medicine
Department of Internal Medicine
University of Utah School of Medicine
Salt Lake City, Utah

**Aminu K. Bello, MD, PhD**
Assistant Professor/Nephrologist
Department of Medicine
University of Alberta
Edmonton, Alberta, Canada

**Theresa J. Berndt, MD**
Assistant Professor of Medicine
Division of Nephrology and Hypertension
Mayo Clinic College of Medicine
Rochester, Minnesota

**John F. Bertram, BSc, PhD, DSc**
Biomedicine Discovery Institute
Development and Stem Cells Program
Department of Anatomy and Developmental Biology
Monash University
Clayton, Victoria, Australia

**Vivek Bhalla, MD**
Assistant Professor
Medicine/Nephrology
Stanford University School of Medicine
Stanford, California

**Daniel G. Bichet, MD**
Professor
Department of Medicine and Physiology
University of Montreal;
Nephrologist
Department of Medicine
Hôpital du Sacré-Coeur de Montréal
Montréal, Québec, Canada

**Boris Bikbov, MD, PhD**
Researcher
Department of Renal Medicine
Istituto di Ricerche Farmacologiche Mario Negri IRCCS
Ranica, Bergamo, Italy

**Detlef Bockenhauer, MD, PhD**
Professor
Department of Renal Medicine
University College London;
Doctor
Department of Nephrology
Great Ormond Street Hospital for Children
London, Great Britain

**Alain Bonnardeaux, MD, PhD**
Full Professor
Department of Medicine
Université de Montréal
Montréal, Québec, Canada

**Josée Bouchard, MD, FRCPC**
Associate Professor of Medicine
Department of Nephrology
Hôpital du Sacré-Coeur de Montréal
University of Montréal
Montréal, Québec, Canada

**Richard M. Breyer, PhD**
Professor
Division of Nephrology and Hypertension
Vanderbilt University School of Medicine
Nashville, Tennessee

**Stefan Broer, PhD**
Research School of Biology
Australian National University
Canberra, Australian Capital Territory, Australia

**Carlo Brugnara, MD**
Department of Laboratory Medicine
Boston Children's Hospital
Boston, Massachusetts

**Catherine R. Butler, MD**
Fellow
Department of Medicine, Division of Nephrology
University of Washington
Seattle, Washington

**Héloise Cardinal, MD, PhD**
Associate Professor, Division of Nephrology
Department of Medicine
Université de Montréal
Montréal, Québec, Canada

**Juan Jesús Carrero, Pharm, PhD Pharm, PhD Med, MBA**
Professor
Department of Medical Epidemiology and Biostatistics
Karolinska Institutet
Stockholm, Sweden

**Daniel C. Cattran, MD**
Professor of Medicine
Department of Medicine
University Health Network;
Senior Scientist
Toronto General Research Institute
University Health Network
Toronto, Ontario, Canada

**Tak Mao Daniel Chan, MBBS, MD**
Chief of Nephrology
Department of Medicine
University of Hong Kong, Queen Mary Hospital
Hong Kong, Hong Kong

**Tara I. Chang, MD, MS**
Associate Professor of Medicine
Division of Nephrology
Stanford University
Palo Alto, California

**Glenn M. Chertow, MD, MPH**
Norman S. Coplon/Satellite Healthcare Professor of Medicine
Department of Medicine
Division of Nephrology
Stanford University School of Medicine
Palo Alto, California

**Andrew A. Chin, MD**
Division of Nephrology
Department of Internal Medicine
University of California, Davis School of Medicine
Sacramento, California

**Yeoungjee Cho, MBBS(hons), FRACP, PhD**
Consultant Nephrologist
Nephrology
Princess Alexandra Hospital;
Clinical Trialist
Australasian Kidney Trials Network
University of Queensland
Brisbane, Queensland, Australia

**Michel Chonchol, MD**
Professor of Medicine
Division of Renal Diseases and Hypertension
University of Colorado Denver Anschutz Medical Center
Aurora, Colorado

**Marta Christov, MD, PhD**
Assistant Professor of Medicine
Westchester Medical Center and New York Medical College
Valhalla, New York

**William L. Clapp, MD**
Professor of Pathology, Director of Renal Pathology
Department of Pathology, Immunology and Laboratory Medicine
University of Florida College of Medicine
Gainesville, Florida

**Rachel Becker Cohen, MD**
Institute of Pediatric Nephrology
Shaare Zedek Medical Center;
Hadassah-Hebrew University School of Medicine
Jerusalem, Israel

**Kelsey Connelly, MD**
Faculty of Medicine
University of Manitoba
Winnipeg, Manitoba, Canada

**H. Terence Cook, MB BS, FRCPath**
Professor of Renal Pathology
Department of Medicine
Imperial College
London, Great Britain

**Josef Coresh, MD, PhD**
Professor
Epidemiology, Medicine and Biostatistics
Johns Hopkins University;
Director
G.W. Comstock Center for Public Health and Prevention
Johns Hopkins Bloomberg School of Public Health
Baltimore, Maryland

**Ricardo Correa-Rotter, MD**
Head
Department of Nephrology and Mineral Metabolism
Instituto Nacional de Ciencias Médicas y Nutrición Salvador Zubirán
Mexico City, Mexico

**Shawn E. Cowper, MD**
Associate Professor of Dermatology and Pathology
Department of Dermatology
Yale University
New Haven, Connecticut

**Vivette D. D'Agati, MD**
Professor of Pathology
Columbia University College of Physicians and Surgeons;
Director, Renal Pathology Laboratory
Columbia University Medical Center
New York, New York

**Kevin Damman, MD, PhD**
Doctor
Department of Cardiology
University Medical Center Groningen
Groningen, The Netherlands

**Mogamat Razeen Davids, MBChB, FCP(SA), MMed**
Professor
Division of Nephrology, Department of Medicine
Stellenbosch University and Tygerberg Hospital
Cape Town, South Africa

**Sara Davison, BSc, MD, MSc**
Chief of Nephrology
Department of Medicine
University of Alberta
Edmonton, Alberta, Canada

**Aleksander Denic, MD**
Division of Nephrology and Hypertension
Mayo Clinic
Rochester, Minnesota

**Bradley M. Denker, MD**
Associate Professor of Medicine
Department of Medicine
Harvard Medical School;
Clinical Chief
Renal Division
Beth Israel Deaconess Medical Center;
Chief of Nephrology
Harvard Vanguard Medical Associates
Boston, Massachusetts

**Thomas A. Depner, BS, MD**
Division of Nephrology
Department of Internal Medicine
University of California, Davis School of Medicine
Sacramento, California

**Thomas D. DuBose, Jr., MD**
Professor Emeritus of Medicine
Wake Forest School of Medicine
Winston-Salem, North Carolina

**Vinay A. Duddalwar, MD, FRCR**
Professor of Radiology and Urology
Department of Radiology
Keck School of Medicine, University of Southern California
Los Angeles, California

**Kai-Uwe Eckardt, MD**
Professor of Medicine
Director of the Medical Department,
Division of Nephrology and Internal Intensive Care Medicine
Charité–Universitätsmedizin Berlin
Berlin, Germany

**William J. Elliott, MD, PhD**
Professor of Preventive Medicine, Internal Medicine and Pharmacology
Pacific Northwest University of Health Sciences;
Head, Division of Pharmacology
Pacific Northwest University of Health Sciences
Yakima, Washington

**David H. Ellison, MD**
Professor
Department of Internal Medicine
Division of Nephrology and Hypertension
Oregon Health & Science University
Portland, Oregon

**Ronald J. Falk, MD**
Nan and Hugh Cullman Eminent Professor
Chair, Department of Medicine
Director, UNC Kidney Center
Chapel Hill, North Carolina

**Robert Andrew Fenton, BSc, MSc, PhD**
Professor of Molecular Cell Biology
Department of Biomedicine
Aarhus University
Aarhus, Denmark

**Alessia Fornoni, MD, PhD**
Professor of Medicine and Chief
Division of Nephrology and Hypertension
University of Miami Miller School of Medicine;
Director
Katz Family Drug Discovery Center
Miami, Florida

**Benjamin S. Freedman, PhD**
Assistant Professor
Department of Pathology (Adjunct) and Department of Medicine
Division of Nephrology, Kidney Research Institute, and Institute for Stem Cell and Regenerative Medicine
University of Washington School of Medicine
Seattle, Washington

**Yaacov Frishberg, MD**
Institute of Pediatric Nephrology
Shaare Zedek Medical Center;
Hebrew University Hadassah School of Medicine
Jerusalem, Israel

**Jørgen Frøkiaer, MD, DMSci**
Department of Clinical Medicine
Aarhus University
Aarhus, Denmark

**John W. Funder, MD, PhD, FRCP, FRACP**
Distinguished Scholar
Hudson Institute and Monash University
Clayton, Victoria, Australia

**Amit X. Garg, MD**
Professor
Division of Nephrology Department of Medicine
Western University
Institute for Clinical Evaluative Sciences
London, Ontario, Canada

**Marc Ghannoum, MD**
Associate Professor of Medicine
University of Montreal, Verdun Hospital
Montréal, Québec, Canada

**Mohammed Benghanem Gharbi, MD**
Nephrology Department
Faculty of Medicine and Pharmacy of Casablanca
University Hassan II of Casablanca
Casablanca, Morocco

**Richard E. Gilbert, MBBS, PhD, FRACP, FACP, FRCPC**
Professor
Department of Medicine
University of Toronto;
Head
Division of Endocrinology
St. Michael's Hospital
Toronto, Ontario, Canada

**Richard J. Glassock, MD**
Emeritus Professor
Department of Medicine
Geffen School of Medicine at UCLA
Los Angeles, California

**Nimrit Goraya, MD**
Assistant Professor
Division of Nephrology and Hypertension,
Program Director
Nephrology Fellowship Program
Baylor Scott and White Health
Temple, Texas

**Morgan E. Grams, MD, PhD**
Associate Professor
Division of Nephrology
Johns Hopkins University
Baltimore, Maryland

**Per Henrik Groop, MD, DMSc, FRCPE**
Professor
Clinicum
University of Helsinki;
Chief Physician
Abdominal Center Nephrology
Helsinki University Hospital
Helsinki, Finland

**Steven Habbous, MD**
Department of Epidemiology and Biostatistics
Western University
London, Ontario, Canada

**Yoshio N. Hall, MD, MS**
Associate Professor
Department of Medicine/Nephrology
University of Washington;
Investigator
Kidney Research Institute | Medicine
University of Washington
Seattle, Washington

**Mitchell L. Halperin, MD, FRCPC, FRS**
Emeritus Professor of Medicine
Department of Medicine/Nephrology
St. Michaels Hospital
University of Toronto
Toronto, Ontario, Canada

**L. Lee Hamm, MD**
Senior Vice President and Dean
Tulane University School of Medicine
New Orleans, Louisiana

**Peter C. Harris, PhD**
Professor of Medicine and Biochemistry and Molecular Biology
Division of Nephrology and Hypertension
Mayo Clinic
Rochester, Minnesota

**Raymond C. Harris, MD**
Ann and Roscoe R. Robinson Professor of Medicine
Department of Medicine
Vanderbilt University School of Medicine
Nashville, Tennessee

**Richard Haynes, MB, BCh, MRCP(UK)**
Clinical Research Fellow
Nuffield Department of Population Health
University of Oxford;
Honorary Consultant Nephrologist
Oxford Kidney Unit
Oxford University Hospitals NHS Trust
Oxford, Great Britain

**Marie Josée Hébert, MD**
Professor
Vice-Rector of Research
Shire Chair in Nephrology, Transplantation and Renal Regeneration
Department of Medicine
Université de Montréal
Montréal, Québec, Canada

**William G. Herrington, MA, MBBS, MD, MRCP**
Associate Professor and MRC-Kidney Research UK Professor David Kerr Clinician Scientist
MRC Population Health Research Unit
Nuffield Department of Population Health
Oxford, Great Britain

**Ewout J. Hoorn, MD, PhD**
Nephrologist and Associate Professor
Department of Internal Medicine, Division of Nephrology & Transplantation
Erasmus Medical Center
Rotterdam, The Netherlands

**Thomas H. Hostetter, MD**
Professor of Medicine and Vice Chairman for Research
Case Western Reserve University School of Medicine
Cleveland, Ohio

**Susie L. Hu, MD**
Associate Professor of Medicine
Medicine, Division of Kidney Disease and Hypertension
Warren Alpert Medical School of Brown University
Providence, Rhode Island

**Tobias B. Huber, MD**
Professor
Department of Medicine
University Medical Center Hamburg-Eppendorf
Hamburg, Germany

**Hossein Jadvar, MD**
Associate Professor of Radiology
Department of Radiology
Keck School of Medicine, University of Southern California
Los Angeles, California

**Edgar A. Jaimes, MD**
Chief, Renal Service
Department of Medicine
Memorial Sloan Kettering Cancer Center
New York, New York

**Sarbjit Vanita Jassal, MD, MB, MRCP(UK), FRCPC**
Staff Nephrologist and Director, Geriatric Dialysis Program
Division of Nephrology
University Health Network;
Professor of Medicine
University of Toronto
Toronto, Ontario, Canada

**J. Charles Jennette, MD**
Kenneth M. Brinkhous Distinguished Professor and Chair
Department of Pathology and Laboratory Medicine
School of Medicine;
Chief of Pathology and Laboratory Medicine Services, UNC Hospitals;
Executive Director, UNC Nephropathology Division
University of North Carolina at Chapel Hill
Chapel Hill, North Carolina

**David W. Johnson, MBBS (Hons), PhD, DMed(Res), FRACP, FASN**
Director of Nephrology
Department of Nephrology
Princess Alexandra Hospital;
Deputy Chair
Australasian Kidney Trials Network
Brisbane, Queensland, Australia

**Kamel S. Kamel, MD, FRCP(C)**
St. Michael's Hospital
University of Toronto
Toronto, Ontario, Canada

**S. Ananth Karumanchi, MD**
Professor of Medicine
Director, Renovascular Research
Cedars-Sinai Medical Center
Los Angeles, California

**David Kavanagh, MD, PhD**
Professor of Complement Therapeutics
National Renal Complement Therapeutics Centre
Newcastle University
Newcastle upon Tyne, Great Britain

**Frieder Keller, MD, Prof. Dr. Med.**
Internal Medicine
University Hospital
Ulm, Germany

**Christine J. Ko, MD**
Professor of Dermatology and Pathology
Yale University
New Haven, Connecticut

**Harbir Singh Kohli, MD, DM**
Professor
Department of Nephrology
Post Graduate Institute of Medical Education and Research
Chandigarh, Union Territory, India

**Jay L. Koyner, MD**
Associate Professor of Medicine
Department of Medicine
Section of Nephrology
University of Chicago
Chicago, Illinois

**Jordan Kreidberg, MD, PhD**
Division of Nephrology
Boston Children's Hospital
Harvard Medical School
Boston, Massachusetts

**Anoushka Krishnan, MBBS, FRACP**
Department of Nephrology
Sir Charles Gairdner Hospital,
Perth, Western Australia, Australia

**Rajiv Kumar, MD**
Ruth and Vernon Taylor Professor of Medicine, Biochemistry and Molecular Biology,
Distinguished Medical Investigator,
Chair Emeritus
Division of Nephrology and Hypertension
Mayo Clinic College of Medicine
Rochester, Minnesota

**Gabrielle Lafreniere, MD, FRCPC**
Assistant Professor of Medicine
Université Laval;
Geriatrician
Division of Geriatrics
Centre Hospitalier Universitaire de Québec
Québec, Quebec, Canada

**Ngan N. Lam, MD, MSc**
Doctor
Department of Medicine, Nephrology
University of Alberta
Edmonton, Alberta, Canada

**Martin J. Landray, PhD FRCP**
Professor of Medicine and Epidemiology
Clinical Trial Service Unit & Epidemiological Studies Unit
Nuffield Department of Population Health
Oxford, Great Britain

**Harold E. Layton, PhD**
Professor
Department of Mathematics
Duke University
Durham, North Carolina

**Timmy Lee, MD, MSPH**
Associate Professor of Medicine
Department of Medicine
University of Alabama at Birmingham
Birmingham, Alabama

**Colin R. Lenihan, MB BCh BAO, PhD**
Clinical Associate Professor
Department of Nephrology
Stanford University
Palo Alto, California

**Krista L. Lentine, MD, PhD**
Professor of Medicine
Center for Abdominal Transplantation
Saint Louis University
St. Louis, Missouri

**Andrew S. Levey, MD**
Chief Emeritus
William B. Schwartz Division of Nephrology
Tufts Medical Center;
Professor of Medicine
Dr. Gerald J. and Dorothy R. Friedman Professor Emeritus
Tufts University School of Medicine
Boston, Massachusetts

**Adeera Levin, BSc, MD, FRCPC**
Professor
Department of Medicine ( Nephrology)
University of British Columbia;
Director
BC Provincial Renal Agency
Vancouver, British Columbia, Canada

**Christoph Licht, MD**
Pediatric Nephrologist
Department of Paediatrics
Senior Associate Scientist
Program in Cell Biology
Research Institute
The Hospital for Sick Children
Professor
Department of Paediatrics
University of Toronto
Toronto, Ontario, Canada

**Bengt Lindholm, MD, PhD**
Adjunct Professor
Divisions of Baxter Novum and Renal Medicine
Karolinska Institutet
Stockholm, Sweden

**Kathleen Liu, MD, PhD, MAS**
Assistant Professor
Divisions of Nephrology and Critical Care Medicine,
University of California, San Francisco
San Francisco, California

**Valérie A. Luyckx, MBBCh, MSc**
Affiliate Lecturer
Renal Division
Brigham and Women's Hospital
Harvard Medical School
Boston, Massachusetts;
Institute of Biomedical Ethics and the History of Medicine
University of Zürich
Zürich, Switzerland

**David A. Maddox, PhD**
Professor
Department of Internal Medicine
University of South Dakota Sanford School of Medicine;
Senior Research Scientist (WOC)
Research & Development
Sioux Falls VA Health Care System
Sioux Falls, South Dakota

**Yoshiro Maezawa, MD, PhD**
Department of Clinical Cell Biology & Medicine
Chiba University Graduate School of Medicine
Chiba, Japan

**Gary R. Matzke, BS Pharm, PharmD**
Professor Emeritus
Pharmacotherapy and Outcomes Science
School of Pharmacy, Virginia Commonwealth University
Richmond, Virginia

**Ivan D. Maya, MD**
Associate Professor
Department of Medicine
University of Central Florida
Orlando, Florida

**Sharon E. Maynard, MD**
Associate Professor
Department of Medicine
Lehigh Valley Health Network
University of South Florida Morsani College of Medicine
Allentown, Pennsylvania

**James A. McCormick, MD**
Associate Professor
Department of Medicine
Division of Nephrology and Hypertension
Oregon Health and Science University
Portland, Oregon

**Alicia Ann McDonough, PhD**
Professor
Integrative Anatomical Sciences
Department of Cell and Neurobiology
Keck School of Medicine, University of Southern California
Los Angeles, California

**John J.V. McMurray, BSc(Hons), MB ChB(Hons), MD, FESC, FACC, FAHA**
British Heart Foundation Cardiovascular Research Centre
University of Glasgow
Glasgow, Scotland, Great Britain

**Rajnish Mehrotra, MBBS, MD, MS**
Section Head, Nephrology
Harborview Medical Center;
Division of Nephrology
University of Washington
Seattle, Washington

**Timothy W. Meyer, MD**
Professor
Department of Medicine
Stanford University
Stanford, California;
Staff Physician
Department of Medicine
VA Palo Alto HCS
Palo Alto, California

**Catherine Meyer-Schwesinger, MD**
Professor
Institute of Cellular and Integrative Physiology
University Medical Center Hamburg-Eppendorf
Hamburg, Germany

**Orson W. Moe, MD**
Professor
Department of Internal Medicine
Division of Nephrology
UT Southwestern Medical Center;
Director
Charles and Jane Pak Center for Mineral Metabolism and Clinical Research
UT Southwestern Medical Center
Dallas, Texas

**Karen M. Moritz, BSc, MSc, PhD**
Child Health Research Centre and School of Biomedical Sciences
The University of Queensland
St. Lucia, Australia

**Alvin H. Moss, MD**
Director
Center for Health Ethics and Law
West Virginia University;
Professor of Medicine
Department of Medicine
Section of Geriatrics, Palliative Medicine and Hospice
West Virginia University
Morgantown, West Virginia

**David B. Mount, MD**
Clinical Chief
Renal Division
Brigham and Women's Hospital
Boston, Massachusetts

**Karen A. Munger, PhD**
Chief, Research and Development
Sioux Falls VA Health Care System;
Associate Professor of Medicine
Department of Internal Medicine
University of South Dakota
Sioux Falls, South Dakota

**Behzad Najafian, MD**
Associate Professor
Department of Pathology
University of Washington
Seattle, Washington

**Luis Gabriel Navar, PhD**
Professor and Chairman
Department of Physiology
Tulane University
New Orleans, Louisiana

**Robert G. Nelson, MD, PhD**
Senior Investigator
Chief, Chronic Kidney Disease Section
Phoenix Epidemiology and Clinical Research Branch
National Institute of Diabetes and Digestive and Kidney Diseases
Phoenix, Arizona

**Lindsay E. Nicolle, MD**
Professor Emeritus
Department of Internal Medicine
University of Manitoba
Winnipeg, Manitoba, Canada

**Sanjay K. Nigam, MD**
Nancy Kaehr Chair in Research
Pediatrics, Medicine and Cellular Molecular Medicine
University of California, San Diego
La Jolla, California

**Mark Douglas Okusa, MD**
Professor of Medicine, Chief, Division of Nephrology
Department of Medicine
University of Virginia
Charlottesville, Virginia

**Paul M. Palevsky, MD**
Chief, Renal Section
VA Pittsburgh Healthcare System;
Professor of Medicine and Clinical & Translational Science
Renal-Electrolyte Division
Department of Medicine
University of Pittsburgh
Pittsburgh, Pennsylvania

**Suetonia C. Palmer, MB ChB, PhD, FRACP**
Doctor
Department of Medicine
University of Otago Christchurch
Christchurch, New Zealand

**Suzanne L. Palmer, MD**
Professor of Radiology
Department of Radiology
Keck School of Medicine, University of Southern California
Los Angeles, California

**Chirag R. Parikh, MD, PhD**
Director, Division of Nephrology
Ronald Peterson Professor of Medicine
Johns Hopkins School of Medicine
Baltimore, Maryland

**David Pearce, MD**
Professor
Department of Medicine
Division of Nephrology
Department of Cellular and Molecular Pharmacology
University of California San Francisco
San Francisco, California

**Aldo J. Peixoto, MD**
Professor of Medicine
Department of Internal Medicine (Nephrology)
Yale University School of Medicine;
Clinical Chief, Section of Nephrology
Department of Internal Medicine
Yale University School of Medicine
New Haven, Connecticut

**William F. Pendergraft III, MD, PhD**
Assistant Professor of Medicine
Division of Nephrology and Hypertension
Department of Medicine
University of North Carolina School of Medicine
Cambridge, Massachusetts

**Mark A. Perazella, MD, MS**
Professor of Medicine
Section of Nephrology
Yale University School of Medicine;
Director, Acute Dialysis Services
Yale-New Haven Hospital
New Haven, Connecticut

**Norberto Perico, MD**
Istituto di Ricerche Farmacologiche Mario Negri IRCCS
Bergamo, Italy

**Martin R. Pollak, MD**
Division of Nephrology
Beth Israel Deaconess Medical Center
Harvard Medical School
Boston, Massachusetts

**Didier Portilla, MD**
Professor
Department of Medicine
University of Virginia
Charlottesville, Virginia

**Susan E. Quaggin, MD**
Doctor
Feinberg Cardiovascular Research Institute
Northwestern University
Chicago, Illinois

**Jai Radhakrishnan, MD, MS**
Professor of Medicine at Columbia University Medical Center
Division of Nephrology, Department of Medicine
Columbia University Medical Center;
Clinical Chief
Division of Nephrology
New York Presbyterian Hospital
New York, New York

**Rawi Ramadan, MD**
Director, Medical Transplantation Unit
Department of Nephrology and Hypertension
Rambam Health Care Campus
Haifa, Israel

**Heather N. Reich, MD, CM, PhD, FRCPC**
Nephrologist, Clinician Scientist
Department of Nephrology
University Health Network;
Associate Professor
Gabor Zellerman Chair in Nephrology Research
Department of Medicine
University of Toronto
Toronto, Ontario, Canada

**Andrea Remuzzi, MD**
Istituto di Ricerche Farmacologicke Mario Negri IRCCS
Bergamo, Italy

**Giuseppe Remuzzi, MD, FRCP**
Istituto di Ricerche Farmacologicke Mario Negri IRCCS
Bergamo, Italy;
L. Sacco
Department of Biomedical and Clinical Sciences
University of Milan
Milan, Italy

**Leonardo V. Riella, MD, PhD**
Associate Physician
Brigham and Women's Hospital;
Assistant Professor of Medicine
Department of Medicine
Harvard Medical School
Boston, Massachusetts

**Miquel C. Riella, MD, PhD**
Professor of Medicine
Department of Medicine
Catholic University of Parana, Brazil;
Professor of Medicine
Department of Medicine
Evangelic School of Medicine
Curitiba, Brazil

**Choni Rinat III, MD**
Institute of Pediatric Nephrology
Shaare Zedek Medical Center;
Hadassah-Hebrew University School of Medicine
Jerusalem, Israel

**Darren M. Roberts, BPharm, MBBS, PhD, FRACP**
Visiting Medical Officer
NSW Poisons Information Centre
Sydney Children's Hospital Network;
Staff Specialist
Renal Medicine and Clinical Pharmacology and Toxicology
St Vincent's Hospital;
Conjoint Associate Professor
University of New South Wales
Sydney, New South Wales, Australia

**Norman D. Rosenblum, MD**
Paediatric Nephrologist
Department of Paediatrics
The Hospital for Sick Children;
Senior Scientist
Program in Developmental and Stem Cell Biology
The Hospital for Sick Children;
Professor
Department of Paediatrics
University of Toronto
Toronto, Ontario, Canada

**Mitchell H. Rosner, MD**
Professor of Medicine
Chair, Department of Medicine
University of Virginia Health System
Charlottesville, Virginia

**Andrew D. Rule, MD**
Division of Nephrology and Hypertension
Mayo Clinic
Rochester, Minnesota

**Ernesto Sabath, MD**
Department of Natural Sciences
Universidad Autonoma de Queretaro
Queretaro, Mexico

**Manish K. Saha, MD**
Assistant Professor of Medicine
Division of Nephrology and Hypertension
Department of Medicine
UNC Kidney Center
University of North Carolina, Chapel Hill
Chapel Hill, North Carolina

**Khashayar Sakhaee, MD**
Laura Kim Pak Professor in Mineral Metabolism Research
BeautiControl Cosmetics Inc.;
Professor in Mineral Metabolism and Osteoporosis
Chief, Division of Mineral Metabolism
University of Texas, Southwestern Medical Center
Dallas, Texas

**Vinay Sakhuja, MD**
Director of Nephrology and Transplant Medicine
Max Hospital
Mohali, Punjab, India

**Alan D. Salama, MBBS, PhD, FRCP**
UCL Centre for Nephrology
Royal Free Hospital
London, United Kingdom

**Jeff M. Sands, MD**
Juha P. Kokko Professor of Medicine and Physiology
Medicine—Renal Division
Emory University
Atlanta, Georgia

**Anjali Bhatt Saxena, MD**
Director of Peritoneal Dialysis
Department of Internal Medicine
Division of Nephrology
Santa Clara Valley Medical Center
San Jose, California;
Clinical Assistant Professor of Medicine
Department of Internal Medicine
Stanford University
Stanford, California

**Johannes Schlöndorff, MD**
Division of Nephrology
Beth Israel Deaconess Medical Center
Harvard Medical School
Boston, Massachusetts

**Rizaldy Paz Scott, MS, PhD**
Research Assistant Professor
Feinberg School of Medicine
Northwestern University
Chicago, Illinois

**Neil Sheerin, BSc, MBBS, PhD, FRCP**
Professor of Nephrology
Institute of Cellular Medicine
National Renal Complement Therapeutics Centre
Newcastle University
Newcastle upon Tyne, Great Britain

**Prableen Singh, MD**
Associate Professor of Medicine
Division of Nephrology and Hypertension
University of California San Diego & VA San Diego Healthcare System
San Diego, California

**Karl Skorecki, MD, FRCP(C), FASN**
Dean, Azrieli Faculty of Medicine
Bar-Ilan University
Safed, Israel

**Itzchak N. Slotki, MD**
Director
Division of Adult Nephrology
Shaare Zedek Medical Center;
Associate Professor of Medicine
Hadassah Hebrew University of Jerusalem
Jerusalem, Israel

**Miroslaw J. Smogorzewski, MD, PhD**
Associate Professor of Medicine
Division of Nephrology
Department of Medicine
University of Southern California, Keck School of Medicine
Los Angeles, California

**William E. Smoyer, MD**
Vice President and Director
Center for Clinical and Translational Research
Nationwide Children's Hospital;
Professor
Department of Pediatrics
The Ohio State University
Columbus, Ohio

**Stuart M. Sprague, DO**
Chairperson, Division of Nephrology and Hypertension
Department of Medicine
NorthShore University Health System
Evanston, Illinois;
Clinical Professor of Medicine
Department of Medicine
University of Chicago Pritzker School of Medicine
Chicago, Illinois

**Peter Stenvinkel, MD, PhD, FENA**
Professor
Department of Renal Medicine
CLINTEC
Stockholm, Sweden

**Jason R. Stubbs, MD**
Associate Professor of Medicine
Division of Nephrology and Hypertension
The Kidney Institute
University of Kansas Medical Center
Kansas City, Kansas

**Maarten W. Taal, MBChB, MMed, MD, FCP(SA), FRCP**
Department of Renal Medicine
Royal Derby Hospital
Derby, United Kingdom;
Centre for Kidney Research and Innovation
Division of Medical Sciences and Graduate Entry Medicine
School of Medicine
University of Nottingham
Nottingham, United Kingdom

**Manjula Kurella Tamura, MD, MPH**
Professor
Department of Medicine/Nephrology
Stanford University
Palo Alto, California

**Jane C. Tan, MD, PhD**
Department of Medicine
Stanford University
Stanford, California

**Navdeep Tangri, MD, FRCPC, PhD**
University of Manitoba
Department of Medicine
Chronic Disease Innovation Centre, Seven Oaks General Hospital
Winnipeg, Manitoba, Canada

**Stephen C. Textor, MD**
Professor of Medicine
Division of Nephrology and Hypertension
Mayo Clinic
Rochester, Minnesota

**Ravi I. Thadhani, MD, MPH**
Chair, Department of Biomedical Sciences
Cedars-Sinai Medical Center
Los Angeles, California

**Scott Culver Thomson, MD**
Professor
Department of Medicine
University of California;
Chief of Nephrology Section
Department of Medicine
VA San Diego Healthcare System
San Diego, California

**Kathryn Tinckam, MD, MMSc**
Associate Professor
Division of Nephrology
Departments of Medicine and Laboratory Medicine & Pathobiology
University of Toronto
Toronto, Ontario, Canada

**Vicente E. Torres, MD, PhD**
Professor of Medicine
Division of Nephrology and Hypertension
Mayo Clinic
Rochester, Minnesota

**Volker Vallon, MD**
Professor
Division of Nephrology & Hypertension
Departments of Medicine & Pharmacology
University of California San Diego & VA San Diego Healthcare System
San Diego, California

**Joseph G. Verbalis, MD**
Professor
Department of Medicine
Georgetown University
Washington, DC;
Chief
Department of Endocrinology and Metabolism
Georgetown University Hospital
Washington, Maryland

**Jill W. Verlander, DVM**
Scientist
Division of Nephrology, Hypertension, and Renal Transplantation
University of Florida College of Medicine;
Director
College of Medicine Electron Microscopy Core Facility
University of Florida
Gainesville, Florida

**Ron Wald, MDCM, MPH**
Staff Nephrologist
Division of Nephrology
Department of Medicine
Li Ka Shing Knowledge Institute of St. Michael's Hospital and the University of Toronto;
Institute for Clinical Evaluative Sciences
Toronto, Ontario, Canada

**I. David Weiner, MD**
Professor of Medicine and Physiology and Functional Genomics
Division of Nephrology, Hypertension and Transplantation
University of Florida College of Medicine;
Section Chief
Nephrology and Hypertension Section
NF/SGVHS
Gainesville, Florida

**Steven D. Weisbord, MD, MSc**
Staff Physician
Renal Section
VA Pittsburgh Healthcare System;
Associate Professor of Medicine and Clinical and Translational Science
Renal-Electrolyte Division
University of Pittsburgh School of Medicine
Pittsburgh, Pennsylvania

**Robert H. Weiss, MD**
Professor
Department of Nephrology
University of California, Davis
Davis, California

**Donald Everett Wesson, MD, MBA**
President, Baylor Scott and White Health and Wellness Center
Department of Internal Medicine
Baylor Scott and White Health;
Professor of Medicine
Department of Internal Medicine
Texas A&M College of Medicine
Dallas, Texas

**David C. Wheeler, MB ChB, MD**
Professor of Kidney Medicine
Centre for Nephrology, Division of Medicine
University College London
London, Great Britain

**Christopher S. Wilcox, MD, PhD**
Chief
Department of Nephrology and Hypertension
Georgetown University Medical Center
Washington, DC

**Jane Y. Yeun, MD**
Division of Nephrology
Department of Internal Medicine
University of California, Davis School of Medicine
Sacramento, California;
Veterans Affairs Sacramento Health Care System
Mather Field, California

**Brian Young, MD**
Health Sciences Associate Clinical Professor
Division of Nephrology
Department of Internal Medicine, Division of Nephrology
University of California, Davis Medical Center
Sacramento, California

**Alan S.L. Yu, MB, BChir**
Harry Statland and Solon Summerfield Professor of Medicine
Director, Division of Nephrology and Hypertension and the Jared Grantham Kidney Institute
University of Kansas Medical Center
Kansas City, Kansas

**Ming-Zhi Zhang, MD**
Associate Professor
Department of Medicine
Vanderbilt University
Nashville, Tennessee

# Preface

Welcome to the 11th edition of Brenner & Rector's *The Kidney*. Like the summer Olympic games, which it generally precedes by a few months, the emergence of each new edition of *The Kidney* follows a 4-year cycle, which is short enough to keep up with major advances in the field, but just long enough to complete the arduous editorial process. The purpose of this book remains unchanged from what Barry M. Brenner and Floyd C. Rector, Jr. conceived originally in 1973; namely to serve as a compendium of nephrology, from basic science to clinical diagnosis and treatment of kidney disease. The intended audience, now truly international, includes medical students, residents, nephrology fellows and practitioners, adult and pediatric renal scientists, and anyone else fascinated by the mysteries of the kidney. For those of us belonging to a certain generation, the raison d'être for *The Kidney* needs no justification. We grew up with it, considering it the definitive text of nephrology. But the modern era of medicine has been marked by a proliferation of readily accessible online digital tools that promise timely and partially digested answers to highly focused questions, catering to trainees and young physicians accustomed to the rapid pace of the modern digital age, and to established, harried clinicians with limited time for reading. While these tools are invaluable, and I confess that I, too, use them on occasion, there is clearly a place for a more considered exposition of the many complex topics in nephrology, that has both breadth and depth, combining intellectual rigor with the excitement of fresh discoveries.

The 11th edition, as with the previous two, is now edited by an international team of editors, a monumental task that remarkably was once managed singlehandedly by Barry M. Brenner. To introduce fresh perspective, we have added a new editor to the team, Valérie A. Luyckx from University of Zürich and the Brigham and Women's Hospital in Boston, a world-renowned expert in global health and management of kidney disease in underserved populations, and an advisor to the International Society of Nephrology and the World Health Organization on global health-related ethics issues. Almost one third of the chapters in this edition have been rewritten by new authors. In addition, we commissioned four entirely new chapters that address emerging areas in nephrology and are written by authoritative experts in those areas, namely "Cardiorenal Syndromes," "Supportive Care in Advanced Kidney Disease," "Considerations in Live Kidney Donation," and "Global Challenges and Initiatives in Kidney Health." To enhance the reader experience, we have introduced a listing of "Key Points" that appear at the beginning of the chapters, to summarize and highlight the important new information. In addition, some of the chapters that are focused on physiology have "Clinical Relevance" boxes to highlight points in the text that have specific relevance to clinical practice.

While some of us will look forward to the tactile experience of opening the two physical volumes of this new edition when it comes out, many of our readers will inevitably prefer the convenience of perusing our enhanced eBook online. These readers will be rewarded with additional material absent from the print version (a necessity so as to avoid occupational injury while removing from the shelf), including the full list of references for every chapter, board review-style multiple choice questions to encourage active learning and help prepare for certification or recertification, and periodic updates to the content, all of which are fully searchable.

Needless to say, an undertaking of this magnitude requires the combined effort of countless individuals. First and foremost, on behalf of the entire editorial team I would like to express deep gratitude to the 184 authors of the chapters in this edition, all of whom committed time out of their busy schedules as clinicians, scientists, and academic leaders to contribute to this project. I wish to thank my fellow editors, Glenn Chertow, Valérie Luyckx, Phil Marsden, Karl Skorecki, and Maarten Taal for their sterling work, and for entrusting me with the leadership of this edition. I also thank Walter Wasser, who has now come to our rescue twice, at short notice, to assist the editorial team finalize manuscripts, both for this edition and the previous one. All of us, in turn, are grateful to the many staff at Elsevier for shepherding this project along. Joan Ryan, a veteran of many editions of *The Kidney*, was superb as our senior content development specialist, until she had to take a leave of absence and Joanie Milnes graciously stepped in to take over. Nancy Duffy, and before her Maureen Ianuzzi, served expertly as our content strategist, and Rachel McMullen served as our senior project manager.

I would like to thank my family, as well as my trainees, colleagues, and coworkers at the University of Kansas Medical Center, for their patience during the past two years, during which this project consumed far too much of my attention and took me away from spending time with them. Finally, I would like to thank Barry M. Brenner, whose spirit of scientific rigor and exacting intellectual standards continue to guide *The Kidney*. I hope that readers will share our excitement in this new edition and savor all that it has to offer.

*Alan S.L. Yu, MB, BChir*
*Kansas City, Kansas*

# Contents

# GENETICS OF KIDNEY DISEASE

SECTION VI

# 43 Inherited Disorders of the Glomerulus

Johannes Schlöndorff | Martin R. Pollak

CHAPTER OUTLINE



## INTRODUCTION

Over the past 2 decades, there has been a rapid growth in our understanding of the influence of genetics in the development of glomerular disease. Although individual mendelian diseases make up only a small fraction of glomerular pathology,[1] it has become apparent that in aggregate they may represent a significant portion of disease in select populations such as pediatric steroid-resistant nephrotic syndrome.[2–4] The discovery that common risk variants in the *APOL1* gene are a major contributor to the increased risk of focal segmental glomerulosclerosis (FSGS), HIV-associated nephropathy (HIVAN), and nondiabetic end-stage kidney disease (ESKD) in populations of West African descent has dramatically altered our perspective of this health disparity.[5,6] Common genetic variants have been associated with increased risk of membranous nephropathy,[7,8] immunoglobulin A (IgA) nephritis,[9–12] and steroid-sensitive nephrotic syndrome.[13,14] At a basic level, genetic forms of glomerular disease have provided significant insight into the key structures necessary for the proper function and maintenance of the glomerular filtration barrier, with a particular focus on the glomerular podocyte and basement membrane. Clinically, the identification of genetic forms of glomerular disease has begun to have an impact on therapeutic considerations, risk assessment for disease recurrence posttransplantation, and counseling of potentially affected family members and kidney donors. As such, genetic factors are primed to affect the development of personalized medicine for glomerular disease.

Broadly speaking, genetic diseases are typically divided into mendelian disorders and polygenic disorders. In mendelian diseases, single-gene mutations give rise to highly penetrant pathologic phenotypes. With few exceptions, these disorders are further classified into dominant and recessive diseases, depending on whether a single mutant allele is sufficient to cause disease (dominant) or whether the lack of a normal, wild-type allele is the driver of disease (recessive). A detailed family history is often informative in suggesting the pattern of disease inheritance; dominant diseases classically affect members of multiple generations, whereas recessive disease is clustered among members of a single generation. However, it is important to realize that mendelian diseases can appear to be sporadic in the setting of small families or incompletely penetrant phenotypes and should not be ruled out by the absence of a family history. In contrast to mendelian diseases, multiple genetic variants or mutations influence the development of polygenic disorders. In these cases, individual variations are often seen in a significant proportion of the general population, but have a small effect size in regard to altering disease risk. Thus, these genetic variants are often of interest in terms of population risks and understanding the mechanism of disease, but are rarely clinically actionable.

The last 20 years have seen an explosion in the number of genes implicated in mendelian forms of glomerular disease. Mutations in over 50 genes have been reported to associate with various glomerular pathologies, including those associated with multiorgan syndromic phenotypes (Table 43.1). Studies of the gene products have identified several structural and functional components of the glomerulus that appear particularly critical for normal function or vulnerable to failure. Specifically, multiple genetic mutations target components of the glomerular basement membrane and several subcellular structures of the podocyte (Fig. 43.1).

## DISORDERS OF THE PODOCYTE

Podocytes, or visceral epithelial cells of the glomerulus, represent the outer layer of the glomerular filtration barrier. Derived from the tip of the developing nephron, these cells

**Table 43.1 Genes Involved in Inherited Human Glomerular Diseases**

| Gene | Mode of Inheritance | Protein | Site of Action | Extraglomerular Manifestations | OMIM No. |
|---|---|---|---|---|---|
| *NPHS1* | AR | Nephrin | SD | | 256300 |
| *NPHS2* | AR | Podocin | SD | | 600995 |
| *CD2AP* | AR, AD | CD2-associated protein | SD | | 607832 |
| *TRPC6* | AD | Transient receptor potential C6 | SD | | 603965 |
| *MYO1E* | AR | Nonmuscle myosin IE | SD, AC | | 614131 |
| *FAT1* | AR | FAT atypical cadherin 1 | SD | Renal tubular ectasia | *600976 |
| *MAGI2* | AR | Membrane-associated guanylate kinase, WW, and PDZ domain-containing 2 | SD, AC | Neurologic deficits | 617609 |
| *ACTN4* | AD | $\alpha$-Actinin-4 | AC | | 603278 |
| *INF2* | AD | Inverted formin 2 | AC, mito (?) | Charcot-Marie-Tooth | 613237, 614455 |
| *MYH9* | AD | Nonmuscle myosin heavy chain-9 | AC | Fechtner syndrome | 153640 |
| *ARHGAP24* | AD | Rho GTPase activating protein 24 | AC | | *610586 |
| *ARHGDIA* | AR | Rho GDP dissociation inhibitor 1 | AC | | 615244 |
| *ANLN* | AD | Anilin | AC | | 616032 |
| *AVIL* | AR | Advillin | AC | | *613397 |
| *KANK1* | AR | KN motif and ankyrin repeat domains 1 | AC | Intellectual disability | * 607704 |
| *KANK2* | AR | KN motif and ankyrin repeat domains 2 | AC | | * 614610 |
| *KANK4* | AR | KN motif and ankyrin repeat domains 4 | AC | Intellectual disability, facial dysmorphism, ASD | * 614612 |
| *TNS2* | AR | Tensin-2 | AC | | 607717 |
| *DLC1* | AR | Deleted in liver cancer 1; ARHGAP7 | AC | | 604258 |
| *ITSN1* | AR | Intersectin 1 | AC | | 602442 |
| *ITSN2* | AR | Intersectin 2; SH3D1B | AC | | 604464 |
| *CDK20* | AR | Cyclin-dependent kinase 20 | | MPGN | 610076 |
| *COL4A3,4,5* | XLR, AR, AD | Collagen 4 $\alpha_3$, $\alpha_4$, $\alpha_5$ | GBM | Alport syndrome, deafness | 104200, 203780, 301050 |
| *LAMB2* | AR | Laminin $\beta_2$ | GBM | Pierson syndrome | 609049 |
| *ITGA3* | AR | Integrin $\alpha_3$ | GBM adhesion | Interstitial lung disease, epidermolysis bullosa | 614748 |
| *CD151* | AR | CD151 (Raphe blood group) | GBM adhesion | Pretibial epidermolysis bullosa, deafness | 609057 |
| *COQ2* | AR | Coenzyme Q2 4-hydroxybenzoate polyprenyltransferase | CoQ10; mito (?) | Encephalopathy, cardiomyopathy | 607426 |
| *PDSS2* | AR | Prenyl (decaprenyl) diphosphate synthase, subunit 2 | CoQ10, mito (?) | Leigh syndrome | 614652 |
| *COQ6* | AR | Coenzyme Q6 monooxygenase | CoQ10, mito (?) | Deafness | 614650 |
| *ADCK4* | AR | aarF domain containing kinase 4 | CoQ10, mito (?) | | 615573 |
| *MT-TL1* | Maternal | Mitochondrially-encoded tRNA leucine 1 (UUA/G) | Mito | MELAS syndrome, diabetes, deafness | 590050 |
| *WT1* | AD | Wilms' tumor 1 | Gene transcription | Denys-Drash syndrome, Frasier syndrome | 194080, 136680 |
| *LMX1B* | AD | LIM homeobox transcription factor 1$\beta$ | Gene transcription | Nail-patella syndrome | 161200 |
| *SMARCAL1* | AR | SWI/SNF–related, matrix-associated, actin-dependent regulator of chromatin, subfamily A-like protein 1 | Gene transcription | Schimke immunoosseous dysplasia | 242900 |
| *PAX2* | AD | Paired box gene 2 | Gene transcription | Papillorenal syndrome | 120330 |
| *NXF5* | XLR | Nuclear RNA export factor 5 | Nuclear export | Heart block | 300319 |
| *NUP93* | AR | Nucleoporin, 93 kDa | Nuclear pore | | 616892 |
| *NUP205* | AR | Nucleoporin, 205 kDa | Nuclear pore | | 616893 |
| *XPO5* | AR | Exportin 5 | Nuclear export | | 607845 |
| *NUP107* | AR | Nucleoporin, 107 kDa | Nuclear pore | Galloway-Mowat syndrome | 616730 |
| *WDR73* | AR | WD40 repeat-containing protein 73 | Unknown | Galloway-Mowat syndrome | 251300 |
| *OSGEP* | AR | O-sialoglycoprotein endopeptidase | KEOPS complex | Galloway-Mowat syndrome | 251300 |

*Continued on following page*

**Table 43.1 Genes Involved in Inherited Human Glomerular Diseases (Cont'd)**

| Gene | Mode of Inheritance | Protein | Site of Action | Extraglomerular Manifestations | OMIM No. |
|---|---|---|---|---|---|
| *TP53RK* | AR | TP53 regulating kinase | KEOPS complex | Galloway-Mowat syndrome | 251300 |
| *TPRKB* | AR | TP53RK binding protein | KEOPS complex | Galloway-Mowat syndrome | 251300 |
| *LAGE3* | AR | L antigen family member 3 | KEOPS complex | Galloway-Mowat syndrome | 251300 |
| *SCARB2* | AR | Scavenger receptor class B, member 2 | Lysosome | Action myoclonus –renal failure syndrome | 254900 |
| *PMM2* | AR | Phosphomannomutase-2 | Protein glycosylation | Congenital disorder of glycosylation type Ia | 212065 |
| *ALG1* | AR | β-1,4-mannosyltransferase | Protein glycosylation | Congenital disorder of glycosylation type Ik | 608540 |
| *SLC35A2* | AR | UDP-galactose transporter | Protein glycosylation | Congenital disorder of glycosylation type IIm | 300896 |
| *EMP2* | AR | Epithelial membrane protein 2 | Unknown | | 615861 |
| *APOL1* | AR | Apolipoprotein L1 | Unknown | | 612551 |
| *PLCE1* | AR | Phospholipase C ε1 | Unknown, SD (?) | | 610725 |
| *DGKE* | AR | Diacylglycerol kinase ε | Unknown | Atypical HUS | 615008 |
| *SGPL1* | AR | Sphingosine-1-phosphate lyase | Sphingolipid catabolism | Ichthyosis, acanthosis, adrenal insufficiency, immunodeficiency, neuronal dysfunction | 617575 |
| *CRB2* | AR | Crumbs homolog 2 | Apical-basal cell polarity | Ventriculomegaly with cystic kidney disease | 616220, 219730 |
| *PTPRO* | AR | Glomerular epithelial protein-1 | Apical membrane | | 614196 |
| *PODXL* | AD | Podocalyxin | Apical membrane | | *602632 |
| *CUBN* | AR | Cubilin | Proximal tubule | Megaloblastic anemia | 261100 |
| *FN1* | AD | Fibronectin 1 | Fibronectin deposits | | 601894 |

*AC,* Actin cytoskeleton; *AD,* autosomal dominant; *AR,* autosomal recessive; *CoQ10,* coenzyme Q10 synthesis; *GBM,* glomerular basement membrane; *HUS,* hemolytic-uremic syndrome; *MELAS,* mitochondrial encephalomyopathy, lactic acidosis, and stroke-like episodes; *mito,* mitochondria; *OMIM,* Online mendelian Inheritance in Man; *SD,* slit diaphragm; *XLR,* X-linked recessive; *UDP,* uridine diphosphate.

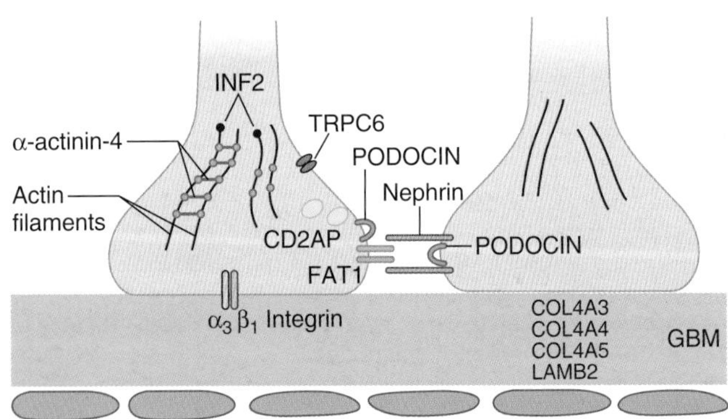


**Fig. 43.1** Schematic depiction of the glomerular filtration barrier. The three major components of the filtration barrier—the interdigitated podocyte foot processes, the glomerular basement membrane *(GBM)*, and the fenestrated capillary endothelium—are depicted. Mendelian forms of glomerular disease affect multiple proteins localized to distinct substructures of the filtration barrier, suggesting that these are potential disease nodes critical to normal function. These include components of the GBM and GBM-podocyte adhesion complexes, the slit diaphragm, a specialized cell-cell junction spanning adjacent foot processes, and the actin cytoskeleton found within foot processes, all shown here. Additional cellular structures repeatedly targeted by disease gene mutations, but not shown here, include mitochondria and the nuclear pore. In the interest of clarity, not all slit diaphragm and actin cytoskeleton components and regulators whose mutation cause human disease are depicted. A more comprehensive list of these genes and their proposed site of action, if known, can be found in Table 43.1.

form a continuous epithelial sheet lining the urinary side of the glomerular basement membrane. Podocytes are characterized by several key features:

1. A highly arborized architecture, with foot processes of adjacent podocytes forming an intricate interdigitating array dependent on the cells' actin cytoskeleton
2. The slit diaphragm, a specialized cell-cell contact spanning adjacent foot processes that has been proposed to act as the final component of the highly selective glomerular filtration barrier
3. Exposure to the large hydrodynamic pressure responsible for transglomerular filtration
4. A highly differentiated state with very limited, if any, replicative capacity

Human genetics, bolstered by in vitro and animal studies, have been instrumental in establishing several disease nodes in the podocyte.

The highly arborized architecture of podocytes is frequently disrupted, a process termed "foot process effacement," in proteinuric kidney diseases. Effacement usually also disrupts the slit diaphragm. Normally, the slit diaphragm appears as a thin, zipper-like structure by electron microscopy[15] and has been compared with a modified adherens and tight junction,[16] with unique molecular components. Passage of the primary glomerular filtrate is thought to occur through the slit diaphragm, which has been proposed to act as the final component of the highly selective glomerular filtration barrier. Human genetic studies were instrumental in establishing the importance of the slit diaphragm for proper podocyte, and hence glomerular, function when *NPHS1* and *NPHS2* genes responsible for congenital nephrotic syndrome and a form of autosomal recessive nephrotic syndrome, respectively, were found to encode components of the slit diaphragm.[17,18] Mutations in several additional slit diaphragm genes have since been identified, which, when mutated, cause nephrotic syndrome and/or FSGS. Work over the subsequent 2 decades has identified a large number of rare mendelian forms of nephrotic syndrome and FSGS, as well as common genetic variants that influence the risk of various forms of glomerular injury.

## MENDELIAN DISEASES OF THE PODOCYTE

These include congenital nephrotic syndromes and other forms of monogenic, steroid-resistant nephrotic syndrome.

### CONGENITAL NEPHROTIC SYNDROMES

#### NEPHRIN *(NPHS1)*

Mutations in the nephrin gene, *NPHS1*, cause a severe, neonatal onset form of nephrotic syndrome, referred to as "congenital nephrotic syndrome," or CNS.[18] *NPHS1* was identified through traditional positional cloning methods, in which genetic linkage analysis leads to the identification of a genomic locus containing a gene alteration segregating with disease and, ultimately, identification of the gene itself. Nephrin is a 1,241–amino acid transmembrane protein that is a member of the immunoglobulin family of cell adhesion molecules. Two founder mutations in the Finnish population—$Fin_{major}$ and $Fin_{minor}$—account for most of the disease-causing NPHS1 mutations in Finland. $Fin_{major}$ is a 2-base pair (bp) deletion early in the NPHS1 coding sequence that causes a frameshift, leading to an early stop codon. The $Fin_{minor}$ allele encodes a premature stop codon (R1109X). A founder effect explains the high rate of these two mutations and CNS in Finland. Although CNS is seen in about 1 in 8200 live births in Finland, it is much rarer outside of Finland (~1–3/100,000 births).[19]

*NPHS1* mutations occur worldwide. Over 200 distinct disease-associated mutations have been reported.[20,21] These appear to be biologically loss-of-function mutations. Most disease-associated mutations are missense but other types of mutations have also been reported (e.g., splice mutations, early termination, frameshifts).[22] Although *NPHS1* mutations are perhaps the most common cause of CNS, they are not the sole cause. *NPHS1* mutations account for virtually all cases of CNS in Finland, but from 40% to 80% of cases in other reports.[18,23,24] In addition to Finland, where CNS is more common than in other countries, founder mutations have been reported elsewhere. For example, a founder mutation in population has been described in Old Order Mennonites.[25] The large spectrum of mutations, including clear loss-of-function alleles and the knockout mouse phenotype, support the notion that this is a typical loss-of-function disorder.[26]

Nephrin localizes to the podocyte slit diaphragm.[27,28] Nephrin molecules perform structural and signaling functions.[29] Nephrin molecules on adjacent foot processes form a zipper-like structure that functions as an essential component of the glomerular filtration apparatus.[27,28] The intracellular domain of nephrin interacts with multiple intracellular signaling pathways. Nephrin interacts directly with the SH2/SH3-domain containing Nck proteins to mediate nephrin-dependent actin cytoskeleton dynamics.[30,31] Interactions between nephrin and other cytoskeletal proteins, including CD2AP, connect the nephrin signaling complex with other actin regulating proteins.[32] Nephrin and CD2AP interact with PI3-kinase (PI3K), recruit it to the plasma membrane and, with podocin, stimulate PI3K-dependent AKT signaling.[33]

Nephrin-mediated CNS is a severe disease and is lethal when untreated because of the consequences of severe nephrosis or ESKD.[18,34] Affected neonates can excrete on the order of 20 to 30 g of protein in the urine/day and demonstrate other manifestations of severe nephrosis—hypercoagulability, hypoalbuminemia, and edema.[19] Kidneys are typically somewhat enlarged. Kidney histology typically shows a normal glomerular basement membrane appearance but diffuse podocyte foot process effacement and dilation of the proximal tubules.[35] Initial supportive treatment may include the use of diuretics to control edema and albumin infusions for hypoalbuminemia. Aggressive management also includes bilateral nephrectomy to prevent nephrosis and its complications and the initiation of renal replacement therapy with peritoneal dialysis, ultimately to be followed by kidney transplantation when the affected child has reached an adequate size, typically at about 1 year of age.[36,37] Alternative treatment plans have been suggested, including a regimen including unilateral nephrectomy, renin-angiotensin system blockade, and nonsteroidal antiinflammatory drugs (NSAIDs) to reduce proteinuria and the need for albumin infusion, with later initiation of renal replacement therapy.[38] Kidney transplantation is considered standard therapy for nephrin-mediated CNS. Although nephrin-mutant CNS itself does not recur in the allograft, proteinuria secondary to the development of antinephrin antibodies is commonly observed.[39] Alpha-fetoprotein (AFP) levels in the maternal serum and amniotic fluid are elevated in CNS.[40] In a family known to be at high risk for CNS (e.g., because of Finnish parents or a previous child with CNS), prenatal genetic testing can be performed.

#### PODOCIN *(NPHS2)*

Mutations in the podocin gene *NPHS2* cause a spectrum of inherited disorders of the podocyte, ranging from neonatal nephrotic syndrome to late-onset FSGS.[17,41] In most of the reported cases, steroid-resistant nephrotic syndrome (SRNS) and FSGS associated with *NPHS2* mutations present in early childhood. *NPHS2*-associated disease is resistant to treatment with corticosteroids.[42] Causal mutations in *NPHS2* have been reported to occur in a high fraction of children with SRNS, as high as 30% in some studies[43,44]

The clinical phenotype associated with *NPHS2* mutations is highly variable. In some reports, *NPHS2* mutations are as common a cause of CNS as nephrin mutations.[24] At the other end of the clinical spectrum, *NPHS2* mutations are also associated with adult-onset FSGS, also under a recessive model of disease inheritance. In particular, a relatively common coding sequence variant in *NPHS2, R229Q*, is associated with late-onset FSGS when inherited with a second, more severe mutation.[45,46] Interestingly, the pathogenicity of the *R229Q* variant depends on the specific second allele and leads to overt disease only when inherited together with certain C-terminal *NPHS2* mutations by causing altered heterodimerization and mislocalization.[47]

Well over 100 distinct disease-associated *NPHS2* mutations have now been reported. Such mutations have been observed in all regions of the gene and include point mutations, early termination mutations (frameshift and early stop codons), and insertions and deletions.[41,48,49] An *R138Q* mutation has been reported in many apparently unrelated individuals and families and is typically associated with a severe phenotype.[50]

Podocin, a 383–amino acid integral membrane protein, localizes to the glomerular slit diaphragm.[51] Podocin traffics to the plasma membrane through the classic exocytic pathway. A direct interaction between podocin and the tyrosine-phosphorylated cytoplasmic domain of nephrin appears to facilitate nephrin-mediated signaling.[29] Podocin can also influence TRPC6 channel activity.[52,53] Most disease-causing podocin mutations lead to retention in the endoplasmic reticulum (ER).[54] Mutants that are retained in the ER appear to be associated with more severe disease than those that traffic to the cell membrane. Presumably, disease results from a consequent defect in slit diaphragm structure. Podocin may function as a dimer or oligomer via C-terminal interactions. In the presence of two *NPHS2* mutations, the specific nature of these mutations may affect the oligomerization and nature of the associated phenotype.[55] Mouse models are consistent with the human genetic findings. Mice lacking podocin demonstrate severe kidney disease and altered glomerular filtration.[56] Podocin is important in maintaining the adult filtration apparatus; mice engineered to allow podocin inactivation in adult mouse kidneys show FSGS and nephrotic syndrome.[57]

A genetic diagnosis of *NPHS2*-mediated disease can be clinically actionable. Although some immunosuppressive therapies may mediate effects on podocytes through nonimmunologic mechanisms, aggressive immunosuppressive medication is probably best avoided in individuals with *NPHS2*-associated disease.[42] Treatment of *NPHS2*-associated disease is largely supportive. Therapy with angiotensin receptor blockers (ARBs) or angiotensin-converting enzyme (ACE) inhibitors is standard. *NPHS2* mutations are not a contraindication to kidney transplantation; on the contrary, SRNS and FSGS do not tend to recur in such patients after transplantation,[4] although there are rare exceptions.[50,58] This knowledge may affect posttransplantation care.

### *ACTN4*

Mutations in the alpha-actinin 4 gene *ACTN4* cause an autosomal dominant form of kidney disease characterized by late-onset proteinuria, chronic kidney disease (CKD), and a slow progression toward kidney failure.[59] Alpha-actinin 4 is a widely expressed homodimeric actin binding and cross-linking protein. All mutations that have been convincingly shown to cause human disease are located in the actin-binding domain (ABD) of the encoded protein.[60] These mutations alter the interaction of alpha-actinin 4 with actin filaments. Despite the widespread expression of the alpha-actinin 4 protein, disease manifestations have only been observed in the glomerulus. Although *ACTN4*-associated disease is typically late in onset and usually presents with subnephrotic proteinuria, this is not always the case. Childhood-onset forms of alpha-actinin 4–associated disease have been reported.[61,62] Although clinical data are sparse, it appears that patients with *ACTN4*-mediated FSGS are resistant to immunosuppressive therapy, as might be anticipated in the setting of an altered cytoskeletal protein. Similarly, recurrence of FSGS in transplanted kidneys has not been reported in these patients.

Mice lacking *Actn4*, as well as mice with point-mutant forms of *ACTN4*, demonstrate glomerular disease.[63–65] Disease-causing ACTN4 mutations alter actin dynamics and the biophysical properties of the actin cytoskeleton.[65–67] Cells harboring disease-associated *ACTN4* mutations are stiffer and more susceptible to breakage than wild-type cells. Some studies have suggested noncytoskeletal effects of ACTN4 as well. ACTN4 has been shown to potentiate nuclear factor-kappa B (NF-κB)activity in a manner that is independent of its cytoplasmic actin-binding function.[68] Through this nuclear role, ACTN4 has been shown to regulate glucocorticoid receptor–mediated gene regulation in podocytes.[69]

### *INF2*

Mutations in the *INF2* gene cause a late-onset form of kidney disease that is clinically similar to that associated with *ACTN4* mutations.[70] INF2 is a member of the family of mammalian formin proteins. INF2, like other formins, is an actin regulatory protein. INF2 forms a homodimer that associates with the barbed end of an actin filament, promoting actin polymerization and depolymerization.[71] An FH2 domain near the C-terminus of INF2 is responsible for the actin-polymerizing activity. An interaction between a C-terminal "diaphanous autoregulatory domain" (DAD) and an N-terminal "diaphanous inhibitory domain" (DID) normally keeps INF2 in an inhibited state.[71,72] All the *INF2* mutations associated with human FSGS reported to date localize to this N-terminal region. The penetrance of *INF2*-mediated disease appears to be lower than that for *ACTN4*- and *TRPC6*-associated autosomal dominant FSGS. Mutations in *INF2* appear to be among the most common forms of podocyte-mediated autosomal dominant FSGS, with over 45 different disease-associated mutations reported to date.[70,73–76]

A subset of patients with *INF2*-associated FSGS also have Charcot-Marie-Tooth (CMT) disease.[75] CMT is a peripheral demyelinating neuropathy with several genetic causes. It is not yet clear why some *INF2* mutations cause FSGS alone and others cause FSGS plus CMT. Disease-associated *INF2* mutations appear to both inhibit the ability of the DID region to interact with the DAD, as well as the ability of the DID to interact with other formin family members.[72]

### *TRPC6*

Mutations in the *TRPC6* gene cause an autosomal dominant kidney disease characterized by proteinuria, focal and segmental glomerulosclerosis, and progressive renal failure.[77] TRPC6 is a member of the canonical (or TRPC) subfamily of transient receptor potential (TRP) channels.[78] It forms cation channels as either homotetramers or heterotetramers in conjunction with TRPC1, TRPC3, and TRPC7 and is activated by diacylglycerol; its activation leads to elevations in intracellular calcium levels.[79,80] TRPC6 is expressed in podocytes and reported to interact with nephrin and podocin, with both affecting TRPC6 function.[52,53,81,82] In rodents, TRPC6 modulates pathologic responses downstream of angiotensin

II (Ang II) signaling, Gαq activation, and several other disease models.[83–87] Numerous potential pathways downstream of TRPC6 activation have been reported,[87–93] although their relative importance in the pathogenesis of genetic forms of TRPC6-associated disease remain uncertain.

Both gain-of-function[77,81,94] and loss-of-function mutations[95] in TRPC6 have been reported to cause glomerular disease. TRPC6-mediated disease is incompletely penetrant; it predominantly becomes apparent in adults, although pediatric cases have been reported.[77,81,94,96,97] Although calcineurin inhibitors have been hypothesized as a potential treatment, this has not been reported effective in practice.[98]

## OTHER FORMS OF MONOGENIC STEROID-RESISTANT NEPHROTIC SYNDROME

A large number of other genes have been identified that when mutated, cause recessive SRNS and/or FSGS. These can be roughly categorized by the biologic pathway disrupted by mutations. The vast majority of these are early-onset recessive diseases. Some have extrarenal manifestations, and some do not.

### CYOSKELETON

#### Actin-Binding Proteins

These are in addition to *INF2, ACTN4, MYH9, MYO1E,* and *ANLN.* Mutations in the nonmuscle type II myosin gene *MYH9* cause a set of autosomal dominant disorders characterized by leukocyte inclusions, platelet abnormalities, hearing loss, and nephropathy.[99] Although different constellations of *MYH9*-associated manifestations have been given the names May-Hegglin anomaly, Sebastian syndrome, Fechtner syndrome, and Epstein syndrome, these are probably all best considered as part of a spectrum of diseases of altered *MYH9.* Approximately 30% of patients with disease-associated *MYH9* mutations have manifestations of kidney disease.[100] Kidney histology shows an FSGS-like lesion. There are correlations between mutation and phenotype. *MYH9* mutations that alter the motor domain of the encoded myosin typically show severe thrombocytopenia and deafness before 40 years of age.[101] Patients with motor domain mutations are also more likely to have severe kidney disease and progression to kidney failure.[102] Amino acid residue 702 appears to be a hot spot for mutations leading to severe disease, including a severe nephropathy.[103]

Mutations in *MYO1E* cause a rare, childhood-onset, steroid-resistant form of FSGS.[104,105] *MYO1E* encodes an atypical type 1 myosin, myosin 1E, that has been implicated in cell adhesion, migration, and endocytosis.[106] Mice deficient in myosin 1E demonstrate glomerular disease.[107]

Mutations in the gene encoding the actin-binding protein anilin *(ANLN)* have been reported as a rare cause of autosomal dominant FSGS. To date, two disease-associated point mutations have been reported. Mutations are hypothesized to disrupt normal regulation of the slit diaphragm–associated actin cytoskeleton.[108]

Mutations in the actin-associated protein advillin (*AVIL*) cause a recessive form of SRNS.[109] These mutations alter the actin-binding activity of the protein. Because disease-associated *AVIL* mutations were found to alter the association of phospholipase C epsilon with the ARP2/3 complex, *AVIL* has been hypothesized to act upstream of this enzyme to control ARP2/3-dependent actin regulation in the podocyte.

#### Cytoskeletal Regulators

Mutations in members of the kidney ankyrin repeat-containing protein family (*KANK1, KANK2, KANK4*) have been reported to cause early childhood-onset SRNS under a recessive model.[110] Individuals with *KANK4* mutations were also reported to have nonrenal features, including facial dysmorphism. These mutations are hypothesized to alter Rho GTPase signaling. Mutations in the Rho GDI-alpha gene *ARHGDIA* are a rare cause of childhood-onset recessive SRNS thought to perturb the same pathway.[111,112] The gene product is a regulator of Rho GTPase activity. Disease-associated mutations lead to altered interactions with Rho GTPase family members, as well as altered activity of some of these proteins. Mice homozygous for an inactivated *Arhgdia* gene show severe proteinuria and develop kidney failure.[113]

*ARHGAP24* encodes a RhoA-activated Rac1 GTPase-activating protein, also known as FilGAP.[114] Like other GTPase-activating proteins, ARHGAP24 regulates the activity of the Rho family members Cdc42, Rac, and RhoA. In podocytes, ARHGAP24 inactivates Rac1 activity.[115] A disease-segregating point mutation that abrogates GAP activity has been reported in a family with FSGS.[115] Mutations in *MAGI2, TNS2, DLC1, CDK20, ITSN1,* and *ITSN2* have been reported to cause rare forms of autosomal recessive, partially SRNS in children.[116] Alteration of small GTPase activity has been proposed as the unifying feature of these forms of nephrotic syndrome.

### SLIT DIAPHRAGM

In addition to *NPHS1* (nephrin) and *NPHS2* (podocin), mutations in other slit diaphragm– associated proteins have been reported as rare causes of early-onset nephrotic syndrome.

#### CD2AP

CD2-associated protein (CD2AP) is a slit diaphragm–associated scaffolding molecule involved in actin cytoskeleton regulation. CD2AP was identified on the basis of its interaction with the T cell adhesion molecule CD2.[117] Mice lacking CD2AP were found to have severe proteinuria and the development of glomerulosclerosis.[118] In the podocyte, CD2AP colocalizes with and binds to the nephrin C-terminus at lipid rafts.[119,120] CD2AP and nephrin both interact with the p85 subunit of PI3K and stimulate PI3K-dependent AKT signaling in podocytes.[33] The absence of CD2AP increases transforming growth factor beta 1 (TGF-β1)–induced activity of the proapoptotic p38 MAPK pathway.[121] Heterozygosity for loss-of-function mutations in CD2AP appears to be a rare cause of, or contributor to, human FSGS.[122] A case of apparent recessive CD2AP-associated FSGS has been reported in a 10- month-old child.[123] The small number of CD2AP-associated cases of FSGS nephrotic syndrome make it difficult to generalize as to mode of inheritance or disease mechanism.

#### *FAT1*

Mutations in the *FAT1* gene, encoding a protocadherin family member localizing to the slit diaphragm, have been reported as a cause of glomerular and tubular ectasia, as well as neurologic disease, in several families.[124]

Similarly, mice lacking FAT1 have a lethal phenotype characterized by loss of slit diaphragms and severe defects in brain development.[125]

### MAGI-2

Membrane-associated guanylate kinase inverted 2 (MAGI-2) is a large scaffolding protein present at the podocyte slit diaphragm, where it binds nephrin and regulates cytoskeletal dynamics.[126] Its transcription is regulated by Wilms' tumor 1.[127,128] MAGI-2 mutations have been reported as a rare case of autosomal recessive congenital nephrotic syndrome in children.[116,129] Mice lacking MAGI-2 similarly develop severe glomerulosclerosis, with impaired slit diaphragm formation and podocyte loss.[130–132]

## PODOCYTE-MATRIX ADHESION

Several additional gene mutations have been reported to cause FSGS or nephrotic syndrome by altering the interaction of podocytes with the glomerular basement membrane (GBM). Mutations in the integrin beta 4 gene (*ITGB4*) have been reported to cause a recessive form of epidermolysis bullosa and congenital nephrosis.[133] A recessive mutation in integrin alpha 3 (*ITGA3*) causing a gain of a glycosylation site has been reported to lead to congenital nephrosis presenting together with interstitial lung disease.[134] Mutations in the *CD151* gene (cluster of differentiation 151), encoding a tetraspanin protein that modulates integrin-laminin interactions,[135] have been reported to cause another syndrome of proteinuric kidney disease, epidermolysis bullosa and sensorineural deafness.[136] CD151-deficient mice similarly develop FSGS and kidney failure.[137] Mutations in the exostosin gene *EXT1* cause multiple exostoses type I, an autosomal dominant bone disorder.[138] EXT1 is a transmembrane glycoprotein important for the synthesis and display of cell surface heparan sulfate glycosaminoglycans.[139] A family has been reported in which steroid-sensitive nephrotic syndrome, in addition to multiple exostoses, segregated with an *EXT1* mutation.[140] The Alport syndrome–associated type 4 collagen genes and Pierson syndrome disease gene *LAMB2* are discussed later.

## MITOCHONDRIA

Alterations in mitochondria lead to a diverse set of phenotypic manifestations.[141] Inherited mitochondrial disorders are often divided into disorders of the mitochondrial genome and disorders caused by mutations in nuclear genes that encode proteins important for mitochondrial function. Mutations in the mitochondrial genome, in particular mtDNA 3243 A to G, lead to a syndrome called MELAS (*m*itochondrial myopathy, *e*ncephalopathy, *l*actic *a*cidosis and *s*trokelike episodes). Kidney disease is not a particularly common feature, but may be seen, and can present as proteinuria with FSGS histology.[141] The maternally derived inheritance and variability in phenotype make this a difficult diagnosis.

Defects in coenzyme Q10 (CoQ10) biosynthesis have been recognized as a cause of glomerulopathy, either isolated or part of a multisystem syndrome.[142] Multiple enzymatic steps are required for CoQ10 synthesis, and mutations in several of the genes encoding critical enzymes have been found to be mutated in individuals with SRNS.[143–148] Typically, affected individuals present in childhood and demonstrate proteinuria and FSGS-like histology. Although cases of isolated nephropathy have been reported, nonrenal features are common. Neurologic features, often severe, may be the predominant clinical features of disease. Mutations in *COQ2*, encoding an enzyme early in the CoQ10 synthesis pathway, were the first genetic cause of CoQ10 deficiency identified.[143] *COQ2*-related disease follows recessive inheritance, as is typical for a disease caused by an enzyme deficiency. Multiple *COQ2* mutations have since been identified in unrelated individuals.[144]

Other causes of SRNS related to defects in CoQ10 synthesis include mutations in *ADCK4*, *PDSS2*, and *COQ6*.[145–148] Importantly, disease features, including the glomerulopathy, may respond to CoQ10 supplementation.[149,150]

## NUCLEAR PORE PROTEINS

Mutations in nuclear pore genes *NUP93*, *NUP107*, *NUP205*, and *XPO5* all cause rare forms of recessive, early-onset SRNS.[151–154] Clinically, patients can also present with microcephaly, similar to Galloway-Mowat syndrome. The mechanism connecting defects in these pore proteins with nephrotic syndrome are not understood, although aberrant SMAD signaling has been proposed.[152]

## TRANSCRIPTION FACTORS

### *LMX1B*

Nail-patella syndrome is caused by mutations in the LMX1B transcription factor.[155,156] This disorder follows autosomal dominant transmission. The nonrenal phenotype is characterized by small or absent patellae and absent or dysplastic fingernails and toenails. It is estimated that a glomerular defect is present in 40% of cases of nail-patella syndrome.[157] The kidney phenotype is highly variable. Some individuals develop early-onset nephrotic syndrome, whereas others develop much milder CKD.[158] Typically, kidney histology shows FSGS and a thickened GBM.[159] Although the skeletal manifestations are present in most patients, families with apparent LMX1B-associated kidney disease but lacking skeletal manifestations have been described.[160–162]

LMX1B is a transcription factor that plays a crucial role in the transcriptional regulation of essential podocyte genes.[163,164] Studies of the activity of point mutant LMX1B have similarly supported the hypothesis that this is a loss-of-function disease.[165,166] Multiple families have been identified in which the genetic lesion appears to be a deletion of the entire *LMX1B* gene, suggesting that haploinsufficiency, rather than a gain-of-function mechanism, is responsible for this autosomal dominant disease.[167]

### *WT1*

Mutations in the Wilms' tumor gene, the tumor suppressor *WT1*, cause a spectrum of urogenital disorders that include a glomerulopathy as a prominent feature.[168] Frasier syndrome is defined by pseudohermaphroditism and a progressive glomerular disease typically showing histologic features of FSGS.[169] Affected individuals have normal external female genitalia but an XY karyotype and streak gonads and are at high risk of the development of gonadoblastoma.[170] Many Frasier syndrome mutations in *WT1* abolish an alternative splice site that leads to an alteration of the incorporation of amino acids KTS located between two zinc fingers of the WT1 protein.[169,171–173] These mutations act in a dominant manner. Denys-Drash syndrome is a related disorder defined by pseudohermaphroditism, mesangial sclerosis, Wilms' tumor, and early progression to ESKD.[174] These disorders are perhaps best viewed as part of a phenotypic spectrum caused by *WT1* mutations, rather than distinct disorders.[170,175]

Mutations in *WT1* can also cause isolated nephrotic syndrome characterized by diffuse mesangial sclerosis or FSGS on kidney biopsy.[176] WT1 regulates the transcription of multiple genes critical to podocyte development and function.[128,168,177,178] Thus, WT1-associated glomerulopathies are presumed to be a result of altered glomerular development.[179–181] Other disorders that can be caused by WT1 defects include WAGR (***W***ilms' tumor, ***a***niridia, ***g***enitourinary anomalies, and mental ***r***etardation) syndrome, seen in individuals with a deletion in a region of chromosome 11p13 that includes WT1, and Meacham syndrome, a multisystem disorder that includes urogenital abnormalities caused by point mutations in WT1.[182,183]

#### Other Transcription Factors

Mutations in the *SMARCAL1* gene cause the autosomal recessive disorder Schimke immuno-osseous dysplasia, characterized by spondyloepiphyseal dysplasia, T cell immunodeficiency, and a glomerulopathy.[184] *SMARCAL1* regulates gene transcription through its effect on chromatin structure.[185] Mutations in *SMARCAL1* have been reported to cause a nontrivial fraction of childhood SRNS.[2] The *Pax2* gene (for paired box–containing 2) is a transcription factor with important roles in the developing nervous system and kidney.[186,187] Mutations in *Pax2* cause papillorenal syndrome, also known as *renal-coloboma syndrome*, characterized by both ocular and renal anomalies.[188] Dominant-acting mutations in *Pax2* have also been reported as a rare cause of isolated, late-onset FSGS.[189] A mutation in the *NXF5* transcription factor gene has been reported to cause an X-linked phenotype characterized by FSGS and heart block in one large family.[190]

### OTHER GENES

Mutations in the phospholipase C epsilon 1 gene, *PLCE1*, cause an early-onset recessive form of nephrotic syndrome.[191] Typically, affected individuals develop early onset nephrosis and diffuse mesangial sclerosis (DMS). In nonsyndromic DMS, mutations in *PLCE1* have been reported in 10 of 35 families.[192] *PLCE1* mutations have also been reported as a cause of congenital nephrotic syndrome.[2] PLCE1 is a phospholipase protein. These proteins catalyze the formation of secondary messengers, including 1,4,5-trisphosphate and diacylglycerol. The mechanistic connection between PLCE1 mutations and DMS is not understood.

Mutations in the podocalyxin *PODXL* gene have been reported as a possible rare cause of autosomal dominant FSGS.[193] Podocalyxin is a member of the CD34 sialomucin protein family that is highly expressed in podocytes. Recently, an infant with congenital nephrotic syndrome, as well as omphalocele and microcoria, was found to harbor loss-of-function mutations on both PODXL alleles.[194] This recessive phenotype is similar to the phenotype in *PODXL*-deficient mice.[195]

Other genes that have been reported to cause rare recessive forms of nephrotic syndrome when mutated include epithelial membrane protein 2 (*EMP2*)[196] and the Crumbs cell polarity complex gene 2 (*CRB2*).[197,198]

Fibronectin glomerulopathy is an autosomal dominant disease characterized clinically by hematuria, proteinuria, frequent hypertension, and progressive renal failure, with variable penetrance and age of onset.[199] Renal histology is notable for extensive mesangial and subendothelial deposits that contain fibronectin and are largely devoid of immunoglobulin or complement. Mutations in FN1, the gene encoding for fibronectin, are detected in a significant proportion of families presenting with this disease.[200] Disease recurrence in kidney allografts suggests deposition of circulating fibronectin as the disease mechanism, although the pathophysiology is not well understood.[201]

## COMMON GENETIC FACTORS

### *APOL1* NEPHROPATHY

People of recent African ancestry have a markedly increased risk of focal segmental glomerulosclerosis, as well as other forms of nondiabetic kidney disease.[5,6] This increased risk is largely attributable to two variants in the *APOL1* gene encoding apolipoprotein L1. APOL1-associated kidney disease is inherited largely as a recessive trait. These two variants alter the APOL1 amino acid sequence and its function. The first allele, known as G1, leads to two amino acid substitutions near the C-terminus that nearly always occur together, S342G and I384M. The second allele, G2, leads to a 6-bp deletion of amino acid residues 388 and 389. G1 and G2 never occur on the same chromosome. APOL1 variants increase the risk of several subtypes of kidney disease, with inheritance of two risk alleles leading to markedly increased risk. Case-control odds ratios are approximately 7 to 10 for hypertension-attributed ESKD, 10 to 17 for FSGS, and 29 to 89 for HIVAN.[5,202,203] The G1 and G2 forms of APOL1 appear to protect individuals against the trypanosomes that cause African sleeping sickness.[5] The G1 and G2 alleles have a combined allele frequency of approximately 35% in African Americans.[5] In Africa, G1 and G2 are most frequent in western sub-Saharan Africa, with much lower frequencies in eastern Africa.[204] Although a high-risk APOL1 genotype is an extremely strong risk factor for FSGS and other forms of nondiabetic kidney disease, most people with these genotypes do not develop overt kidney disease.

The product of APOL1, apolipoprotein L1 (ApoL1), is a secreted lipoprotein that circulates as part of high-density lipoprotein 3 (HDL3) complexes, the densest HDL fraction, and is expressed in multiple tissue types.[205–209] Most but not all studies have supported a model in which the G1 and G2 forms of APOL1 have gain-of-function effects that lead to increased kidney disease risk. In cells, mice, and drosophila, expression of the G1 and G2 forms of APOL1 lead to increased death of the APOL1-expressing cells.[210–216]

### OTHER COMMON GENETIC FACTORS

Noncoding variants in the *GPC5* gene, encoding glyipcan-5, have been shown to associate with a risk of nephrotic syndrome. Glypican-5, part of a six-member family of related glypicans, is a heparin sulfate proteoglycan expressed in podocytes. The disease-associated allele is associated with higher levels of GPC5 expression.[217]

Variation near the HLA-DQ locus has been found to be associated with an increased risk of steroid-sensitive nephrotic syndrome by a genome-wide association study.[14] Subsequent work in steroid-sensitive nephrotic syndrome subjects of different ethnicities has supported the association with HLA-DQB1 and also have shown associations with HLA-BRB1 and near *BTNL2*. An increased burden of risk alleles across these three independent loci was found to be associated with a higher risk of nephrotic syndrome.[13]

## IMMUNOGLOBULIN A NEPHROPATHY

IgA is a common form of glomerular disease with a higher incidence in Asia. Multiple families segregating IgA nephropathy have been identified and studied. Early genetic studies in families from Kentucky and Italy have suggested the existence of a major IgA locus on Chr6q22-23.[218] Additional studies have suggested genetic heterogeneity of familial IgA nephropathy, implicating other genomic loci.[219] The genes and their variants underlying these familial forms have not been identified.

Several genome-wide association studies (GWAS) have been performed in an effort to identify more common genetic variations involved in susceptibility to IgA nephropathy. Several loci have been convincingly implicated as playing important roles. Loci within the MHC locus, as well as a deletion variant in CFHR1 and CFHR3 (Chr1q32), have been implicated.[9,10] Subsequent larger GWAS have identified additional loci, including signals at genes *ITGAM-ITGAX, VAV3, CARD9, DEFA, ST6GAL1,* and *ODF1-KLF10*.[12,220]

The association of IgA nephropathy with an 84 kb deletion involving *CFHR1* and *CFHR3* clearly implicates the alternative complement pathway as playing a role.[10] This deletion has been shown to associate with a reduced level of mesangial immune deposits.[221] Several of the loci implicated have also been shown to be associated with an altered risk of inflammatory bowel disease and with regulating the intestinal epithelial barrier and may reflect evolutionary pressures reflecting human interaction with intestinal pathogens.[12] For the most part, causal variants at these loci have not been clearly identified, nor their causal relationship to disease clarified. GWAS studies have also identified loci in *C1GALT1* and *C1GALT1C1*, encoding genes necessary for mucin type O–linked glycosylation as affecting levels of galactose-deficient IgA1.[222,223] Galactose-deficient IgA1 levels are higher in patients with IgA nephropathy compared with healthy controls[224] and are associated with disease progression in IgA but not membranous nephropathy.[225]

## MEMBRANOUS NEPHROPATHY

Membranous nephropathy (MN) is discussed at length in Chapter 31. Highly penetrant gene mutations causing monogenic forms of membranous nephropathy have not been reported. However, MN has significant genetic components. GWAS have identified alleles that are highly associated with the risk of idiopathic MN at two genomic loci. Variation at the M-type phospholipase A2 receptor—PLA(2)R1—gene on Chr2q24 is highly associated with MN, consistent with an alteration in the PLA(2)R antigen, which is the major target antigen in this disorder. In addition, variations at HLA-DQA1 are also highly associated with a risk of MN, in addition to risks of other forms of immune-mediated glomerulonephritis[7,8]

## DISEASES OF THE GLOMERULAR BASEMENT MEMBRANE

The GBM is one of the three major structural components that compromise the filtration barrier of the kidney. It is a fibrous extracellular matrix positioned between the glomerular podocyte on one side and the capillary endothelium and mesangium on the other. Ultrastructurally, the membrane is composed of three layers, a central lamina densa sandwiched between the lamina rara interna (on the endothelial side) and lamina rara externa (on the podocyte side). The GBM is composed of dozens of matrix proteins, the most prominent of which are type IV collagen, laminins, the heparin sulfate proteoglycan agrin, and nidogen.[226–229] During development, the immature GBM forms from the fusion of basement membrane laid down by both capillary endothelial cells and podocytes, with both cell types contributing to the formation and later maintenance of the mature GBM.[230–232] The maturation of the GBM is characterized by a significant change in its molecular composition; the laminin composition switches from laminin $\alpha_1\beta_1\gamma_1$ (LM-111) and laminin $\alpha_5\beta_1\gamma_1$ (LM-511) in the developing GBM to laminin $\alpha_5\beta_2\gamma_1$ (LM-521) in the mature glomerulus, whereas collage IV expression changes from collagen IV $\alpha_1\alpha_2\alpha_1$ (IV) to collagen IV $\alpha_3\alpha_4\alpha_5$ (IV). Additional changes in the molecular composition of the GBM take place during glomerular development and await more systematic study. Its origin as a fusion of matrix laid down by two distinct cells on opposite sides of the GBM may explain why its thickness (250–400 nm, depending on the study[233,234]) is relatively large for a basement membrane.

The GBM is thought to play several critical roles in the function of the filtration barrier. Beyond providing a structural scaffold capable of resisting transglomerular pressure, matrix components act as adhesion and signaling receptors for podocytes and endothelial and mesangial cells. In addition, the matrix is thought to act as a potential reservoir for soluble signaling molecules.[235] Morphologic and molecular changes to the GBM occur in numerous human diseases and various animal models, with diabetic nephropathy being the classic example. The role of the GBM as an actual filter in maintaining the permselectivity of the glomerulus remains an unresolved issue. Farquhar and colleagues and others have long argued that the biophysical properties of the matrix, including its electrostatic charge, play a critical role in the size and charge selectivity of the glomerular filtration barrier.[236–240] Studies by other groups have variously suggested that the endothelium and inner aspect of the GBM are the major barriers to macromolecules,[241,242] the slit diaphragm is the crucial filter,[243–245] and the GBM and slit diaphragm form a double barrier.[246–248] Detailed analysis of Lamb2-deficient mice (a model of Pierson syndrome) has demonstrated that albuminuria precedes foot process effacement in these animals,[249] supporting the notion that a properly assembled GBM functions as at least a crude prefilter. The critical importance of the GBM in maintaining glomerular structure and function is most vividly demonstrated by humans carrying mutations in the *COL4A3, -4,* or *-5* genes (and presenting with Alport syndrome or thin basement membrane nephropathy) or the *LAMB2* gene (and presenting with Pierson syndrome or congenital nephrotic syndrome).

## ALPORT SYNDROME AND COLLAGEN IV–RELATED RENAL DISEASE

The clinical syndrome of hereditary nephritis and associated hearing loss, with more severe disease in males but inheritance through females, was described by Alport in 1927.[250] Williamson, who described several pedigrees with hematuria, renal failure, and variable deafness and eye defects, proposed naming the syndrome after Alport in 1961.[251] Mutations in any one of three type IV collagen genes (*COL4A3*, *COL4A4*, and *COL4A5*) are now known to be responsible for both Alport syndrome and benign familial hematuria–thin basement nephropathy.[252] Between 30,000 and 60,000 people have been estimated to be affected by Alport syndrome in the United States,[253] accounting for 0.3% of incident ESKD patients.[254] However, more recent genetic studies have suggested that mutations in *COL4A3* and *COL4A4* may account for a significant number of cases of renal disease that have not been clinically or pathologically diagnosed as Alport syndrome or thin basement membrane disease.[255–259]

Type IV collagens are a major component of basement membranes and are composed of alpha chains encoded by six genes (*COL4A1–COL4A6*), comprising only a fraction of the different types of collagens found in vertebrates. In humans, the six collagen IV genes are arranged as three pairs of head to head genes (*COL4A1* and *COL4A2* on chromosome 13, *COL4A3* and *COL4A4* on chromosome, and *COL4A5* and *COL4A6* on the X chromosome). All six chains share a common protein structure, comprised of an amino terminal domain rich in cysteines and lysines, termed the *7S domain,* the triple helical collagenous domain, made up of several hundred Gly-X-Y repeats, and finally a carboxyl terminal noncollagenous (NC1) domain. The collagenous domains of type IV collagen alpha chains are notable for between 21 and 26 interruptions of the Gly-X-Y repeats, which provide type IV collagens with the flexibility necessary to form networks; the interruptions may also act as specific interchain cros-slinking and cell adhesion sites.[260] Type IV collagen network formation occurs through a series of distinct steps (Fig. 43.2). First, three alpha chairs form a trimeric protomer with all three chains in parallel; this assembly occurs in the secretory pathway of the cell. Once secreted, these protomers can then form higher order complexes via tetrameric head to head interactions of their 7S domain and dimeric tail to tail binding of the NC1 domains.[261] These structures are further stabilized through supramolecular twisting, lysyl oxidase–mediated cros-slinks, and disulfide and sulfilimine bonds.[262,263] Ultimately, the type IV collagens generate an irregular polygonal network in the GBM[264] with which other extracellular matrix (ECM) components can interact.

Although there are six distinct collagen IV alpha chains, only three stoichiometries of protomers—$\alpha_1\alpha_1\alpha_2$ (IV), $\alpha_3\alpha_4\alpha_5$ (IV), and $\alpha_5\alpha_5\alpha_6$ (IV)—are found. At the NC1 domain end, $\alpha_3\alpha_4\alpha_5$ (IV) protomers can only homodimerize, whereas trimerized $\alpha_1\alpha_1\alpha_2$ (IV) NC1 domains can bind either other $\alpha_1\alpha_1\alpha_2$ (IV) NC1 trimers or $\alpha_5\alpha_5\alpha_6$ (IV) NC1 trimers. This gives rise to only three potential hexamer-generated networks: $\alpha_1\alpha_1\alpha_2$ (IV)–$\alpha_1\alpha_1\alpha_2$ (IV), $\alpha_3\alpha_4\alpha_5$ (IV)–$\alpha_3\alpha_4\alpha_5$ (IV), and $\alpha_1\alpha_1\alpha_2$ (IV)–$\alpha_5\alpha_5\alpha_6$ (IV).[265–267] A defect in one component of a protomer due to a gene mutation prevents the normal expression of the other components in the network; for example, a homozygous mutation in *COL4A3* will prevent the expression of COL4A4, whereas COL4A5 will be present only when incorporated into the $\alpha_5\alpha_5\alpha_6$ (IV) network.

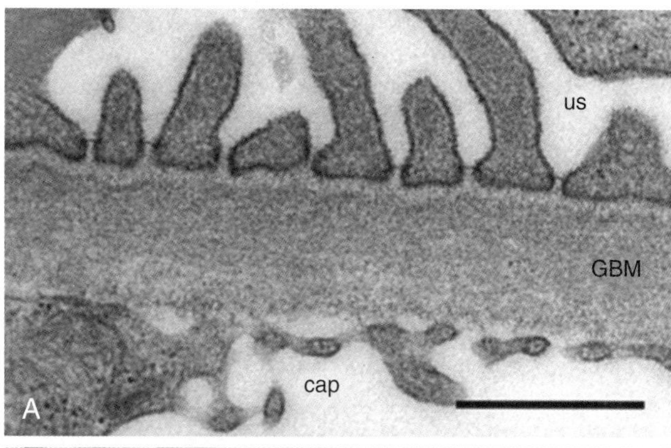


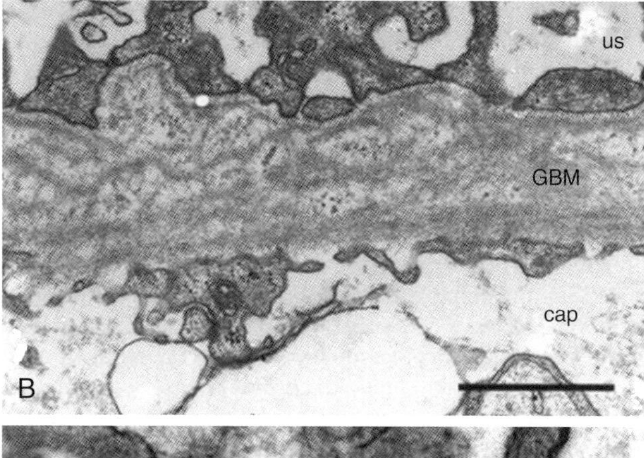


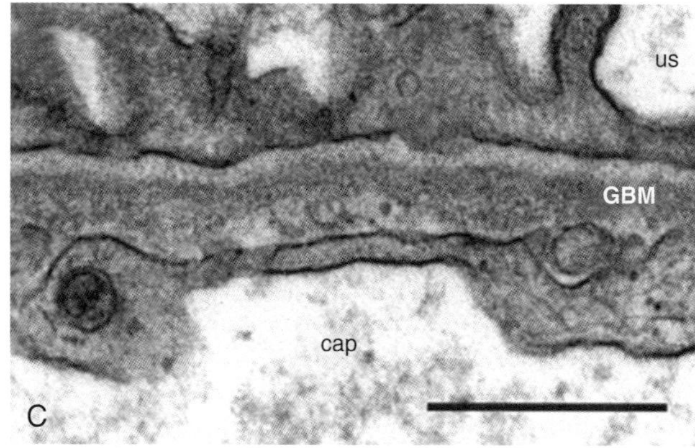


**Fig. 43.2** Transmission electron microscopy appearance of the glomerular basement membrane *(GBM)* in normal conditions, Alport syndrome, and thin basement membrane nephropathy (TBMN). (A) In the normal glomerulus, GBM width is uniform and from 250 to 400 nm in size. (B) In Alport syndrome, focal thickening and thinning of the GBM is observed with the development of a laminated GBM and a woven basket appearance. (C) In TBMN, the GBM is characteristically thinned; its thickness is only about half that of a normal kidney. *Bars* represent 500 nm. *CAP,* Capillary lumen; *US,* urinary space. (A, Courtesy Dr. Finn P. Reinholt, Karolinska University Hospital, Huddinge, Sweden; B, courtesy Dr. Kjell Hultenby, Karolinska University Hospital, Huddinge, Sweden.)

In the kidney, collagen IV $\alpha_1\alpha_1\alpha_2$ is present in the GBM, mesangium, Bowman's capsule, and tubular basement membranes. Collagen IV $\alpha_3\alpha_4\alpha_5$ expression is switched on in podocytes during glomerular maturation and largely supplants $\alpha_1\alpha_1\alpha_2$ (IV) in the GBM[230,268]; it is also found in some tubular basement membranes. Outside the kidney, $\alpha_3\alpha_4\alpha_5$ (IV) networks are also found in the cochlea, eye, lung, and testis.[269–272] The $\alpha_5\alpha_5\alpha_6$ (IV) network is present in the basement membrane of Bowman's capsule and tubules but not in the GBM,[273] a distinction that has been used to differentiate Alport syndrome driven by *COL4A5* versus *COL4A3* and *COL4A4* mutations.[274,275]

The precise mechanism whereby the absence of a functional collagen $\alpha_3\alpha_4\alpha_5$(IV) network in Alport patients leads to abnormal GBM architecture and ultimately glomerular failure remains to be established, but several pathways have been implicated. The GBM in Alport disease demonstrates persistence of the collagen $\alpha_1\alpha_1\alpha_2$ (IV) network in the GBM, as well as deposition of type V and VI collagens and laminin $\alpha_2$.[268,276] The $\alpha_1\alpha_1\alpha_2$ (IV) network is less cross-linked than the $\alpha_3\alpha_4\alpha_5$ (IV) network and therefore may be more susceptible to endoproteolysis. In addition, the $\alpha_1\alpha_1\alpha_2$ (IV) network may provide inappropriate signals to podocytes via the discoidin domain receptor 1 (DDR1), integrin $\alpha_1$, and integrin $\alpha_2$, as judged by studies in murine models.[277–280] Aberrantly expressed laminin $\alpha_2$ may also stimulate pathogenic signaling and interfere with the function of LM-521.[281,282]

Animal and human studies have also suggested a strong pathologic interplay between loss of the $\alpha_3\alpha_4\alpha_5$ (IV) network and the hemodynamic pressure across the glomerular filtration barrier. Inducing hypertension substantially aggravates disease in Alport mice,[283] whereas ACE inhibitor treatment prolongs renal survival in both mice and humans.[284–286] Accelerated detachment of podocytes from the GBM during Alport syndrome progression is likely involved,[286–288] as may be endothelin-A mediated endothelial-mesangial cross-talk,[289] a potential therapeutic target.

## GENETICS OF ALPORT SYNDROME AND COLLAGEN IV–ASSOCIATED RENAL DISEASE

Alport syndrome can be caused by mutations in *COL4A3*, *COL4A4*, and/or *COL4A5*.[290–293] *COL4A5* is located on the X chromosome and is responsible for X-linked forms of Alport syndrome, whereas mutations in *COL4A3* and *COL4A4* (both located on chromosome 2) are responsible for both autosomal recessive (AR) and autosomal dominant (AD) forms of Alport syndrome. In addition, rare digenic forms of Alport syndrome have been reported, involving either combined *COL4A3-COLA4* mutations in trans (mimicking AR disease), combined *COL4A3-COLA4* mutations in cis (mimicking AD disease), and mutations in *COL4A5* combined with *COL4A3* or *COL4A4* mutations.[294] Many dozens of distinct mutations, including deletions, frameshifts, nonsense, and missense mutations, have been described for each of these genes. Family-based studies have reported that X-linked disease accounts for about 80% of cases, with 15% showing AR inheritance and the remaining 5% demonstrating AD inheritance. However, more recent results using next-generation sequencing technology have revealed a higher incidence (20%–30%) of AD forms.[295,296]

Males carry only one X chromosome and hence will develop X-linked Alport syndrome if they carry a mutation in the *COL4A5* gene.[290] Affected males invariably experience microscopic hematuria, subnephrotic proteinuria, and progressive renal disease, usually culminating in ESKD. The rate of disease progression and extrarenal manifestations, including sensorineural deafness and ocular findings, are strongly influenced by the underlying mutation, with large deletions and nonsense, splice site, and frameshift mutations portending a worse prognosis relative to missense mutations.[297,298] The occasional association with leiomyomatosis has been attributed to coexisting mutations in the adjacent *COL4A6* gene.[299,300]

Female carriers demonstrate mosaic expression of $\alpha_3\alpha_4\alpha_5$ (IV) networks within glomeruli due to random X-linked inactivation. Although in mouse models of *COL4A5* disease, skewing of inactivation of the disease-carrying X chromosome has been correlated with disease severity in female heterozygotes,[301] data for humans are less clear, with large intrafamilial variability and no clear genotype-phenotype correlation.[302] In contrast, the development of proteinuria and hearing loss do portend a poorer renal prognosis in these carriers.[302]

AR Alport disease has been described with mutations in both *COL4A3* and *COL4A4*.[292,293] Males and females are affected equally, and the clinical presentation is similar to males with *COL4A5* mutations, with frequent sensorineural hearing loss and ocular abnormalities.[303,304] AD forms of Alport syndrome due to mutations in *COL4A3* or *COL4A4* have also been reported.[305] In general, patients with AD disease are less likely to have an ocular phenotype and tend to demonstrate slower progression of renal failure.[306–308] However, due to the broad spectrum of phenotypes associated with heterozygous mutations in these two genes,[309] differentiating between AD Alport disease and thin basement membrane nephropathy can be difficult and impractical (see later).

Thin basement membrane nephropathy is a pathologic diagnosis associated with glomerular hematuria and the finding of relatively thin GBMs on transmission electron microscopic examination. It can be seen in a variety of scenarios, including patients destined to develop Alport syndrome (e.g., young patients with AR Alport syndrome and young males with *COL4A5* mutations), female carriers of *COL4A5* mutations, persons with heterozygous *COL4A3* or *COL4A4* mutations, and patients with mutations in other genes or unknown genetics.[225,252,310–313]

Traditionally, renal disease associated with *COL4A3*, *COL4A4*, and *COL4A5* gene mutations have been divided into Alport syndrome and thin basement membrane nephropathy–benign familial hematuria based on clinical and histologic criteria. However, with the appreciation that thin basement membrane disease carries a significant risk of progression to overt CKD and even ESKD, and with the finding of heterozygous *COL4A* gene mutations in a significant proportion of patients clinically diagnosed as FSGS,[255–259] several groups, including the Alport Syndrome Classification Working Group, have suggested a new classification driven by the genetic underpinning of the disease.[309,314] The utility of such a scheme will largely depend on how widely available genetic testing becomes, but could be of particular value for patients and families with heterozygous *COL4A3* or *COL4A4* mutations. In the absence of routine genetic testing, it is important that clinicians and pathologists be cognizant of the possibility of collagen IV–associated disease as the underlying pathology, even in the absence of classic clinicopathologic findings.

### CLINICOPATHOLOGIC PRESENTATION OF ALPORT SYNDROME AND COLLAGEN IV–RELATED KIDNEY DISEASE

Clinically, Alport syndrome is characterized by glomerular hematuria, subnephrotic range proteinuria, and progressive renal failure associated with sensorineural hearing loss.[250,251] For patients with X-linked or AR Alport syndrome, microscopic hematuria is nearly universal by early childhood. Although the time to reach ESKD is variable, cohort studies have reported similar median renal survival in the mid-20s for X-linked cases[297] and AR disease.[303,304] Hearing loss is detected in more than half of these patients; it begins with loss of high tones but frequently progresses to impair conversational communication. Eye defects can include anterior lenticonus, perimacular retinal flecks, and corneal erosions and are quite frequent but only rarely impair vision.[315] Leiomyomatosis has been reported to affect a subset of patients with X-linked disease and is attributed to concomitant *COL4A6* mutations.[299,300,316]

Female carriers of *COL4A5* mutations and persons with heterozygous *COL4A3* or *COL4A4* mutations can develop a variety of findings, from isolated microscopic hematuria to gross hematuria, proteinuria, renal dysfunction, and sensorineural hearing loss. In line with this, other studies have suggested that carriers of *COL4A3* or *COL4A4* mutations and female carriers of *COL4A5* mutations, who may have initially been diagnosed with benign familial hematuria or thin basement membrane disease, have a significantly higher risk of progression to CKD and ESKD than previously suspected. Among *COL4A5* carriers, 12% progressed to ESKD by age 40 years in a large cohort study, with proteinuria and hearing loss identified as risk factors.[302] Among patients with heterozygous *COL4A3* or *COL4A4* mutations, the reported risk of progressing to ESKD is variable and probably reflects ascertainment bias of familial disease, as well as significant variability in the pathogenicity of individual mutations. One study of AD Alport syndrome reported a median renal survival of only 31 years,[308] another a median renal survival of 51 years,[306] and a third study found a lower rate and later onset of ESKD.[317] Reported risk factors for ESKD include proteinuria, hearing loss, progressive decline in GFR in the patient or family members, and biopsy findings of FSGS, GBM thickening, or GBM lamellation.[314]

Prior to the availability of genetic testing, the diagnosis of Alport syndrome was confirmed by renal pathology or skin biopsy.[275,318,319] By light microscopy, glomerular morphology can be relatively normal prior to the age of 5 years, after which mesangial cell proliferation and matrix accumulation, as well as capillary wall thickening, may be seen. This progresses to glomerular sclerosis and associated tubular and interstitial pathology over time.[320–322] Standard immunofluorescence microscopy findings are nonspecific. However, staining for collagens IV $\alpha_3$, $\alpha_4$, and $\alpha_5$ demonstrate an absence of all three chains in the GBM in the large majority of X-linked and many AR Alport cases.[271,274,275,323,324] In contrast, female *COL4A5* mutation carriers can demonstrate segmental loss of staining in skin and GBM due to random X-linked inactivation of the wild-type allele. By transmission electron microscopy, early Alport syndrome or thin basement membrane disease can demonstrate thinning of the GBM.[325,326] In more advanced disease, the classic findings of GBM lamellation and a woven basket appearance, as well as irregular thinning and thickening of the GBM, are seen (Fig. 43.3).[327] These electron microscopy findings, when paired with collagen IV immunofluorescence staining, are highly suggestive of Alport disease. Other genetic studies have demonstrated collagen IV gene mutations in a significant percentage of patients carrying diagnoses other than Alport syndrome or thin basement membrane nephropathy,[255–259] suggesting that the sensitivity of clinical and pathologic findings may be lower than previously appreciated for identifying collagen IV–associated renal disease.

### TREATMENT OF ALPORT SYNDROME

Treatment options for Alport syndrome are currently limited to the use of ACE inhibitors. Based on mouse studies,[284] ACE inhibitors and ARBs have been tested in Alport patients and have shown efficacy in reducing proteinuria.[328–330] Treatment with ACE inhibitors is associated with a significant delay in progression to ESKD and median life expectancy, with early treatment initiation providing the greatest benefit.[285] The benefit of ACE inhibitors has been extended to patients with heterozygous mutations or carriers of X-linked and AR Alport mutations.[331,332] Some experts now recommend treatment for anyone with an Alport disease gene mutation, hematuria, and either overt proteinuria or microscopic albuminuria and a severe mutation (e.g., deletion, nonsense, or splicing), hearing loss or family history of ESKD prior to the age of 30 years.[314]

Multiple treatment strategies have been explored in animal models of Alport syndrome. These include inhibition of TGF-β signaling,[277] treatment with an endothelin A antagonist,[289] and inhibition of microRNA-21 with the use of an anti-miR.[333] Clinical trials are underway to examine the potential benefit of an micro-RNA inhibitor and bardoxolone methyl in patients with Alport syndrome.

Kidney transplantation should be considered for Alport patients who progress to ESKD. Overall, patient and graft outcomes are good, although patients with severe mutations are at risk for developing de novo anti-GBM nephritis. This is due to the presence of collagen $\alpha_3\alpha_4\alpha_5$ (IV) in the allograft, which is absent in the host. Antibodies against these collagens in the serum and linear immunoglobulin deposits along the GBM are detectable in a significant proportion of allografts, but are often not associated with evidence of nephritis.[334] The reported incidence of anti-GBM nephritis in Alport patients status posttransplantation is variable, but most series have reported less than 3% of patients affected.[335–339]

## PIERSON SYNDROME

A familial form of congenital nephrotic syndrome associated with a complex eye phenotype, including microcoria (extremely narrow, nonreactive pupils) was first described by Pierson and associates in 1963.[340] Although similar cases were described in the literature in the antecedent decades, it was not until 2004 that the term *microcoria-congenital nephrotic syndrome* or *Pierson syndrome* was proposed to describe this autosomal recessive disorder.[341] Mutations in *LAMB2*, encoding for the beta-2 subunit of laminin, are responsible for the disease[342]; many aspects of the pathology are seen in *Lamb2*-deficient mice.[343,344]

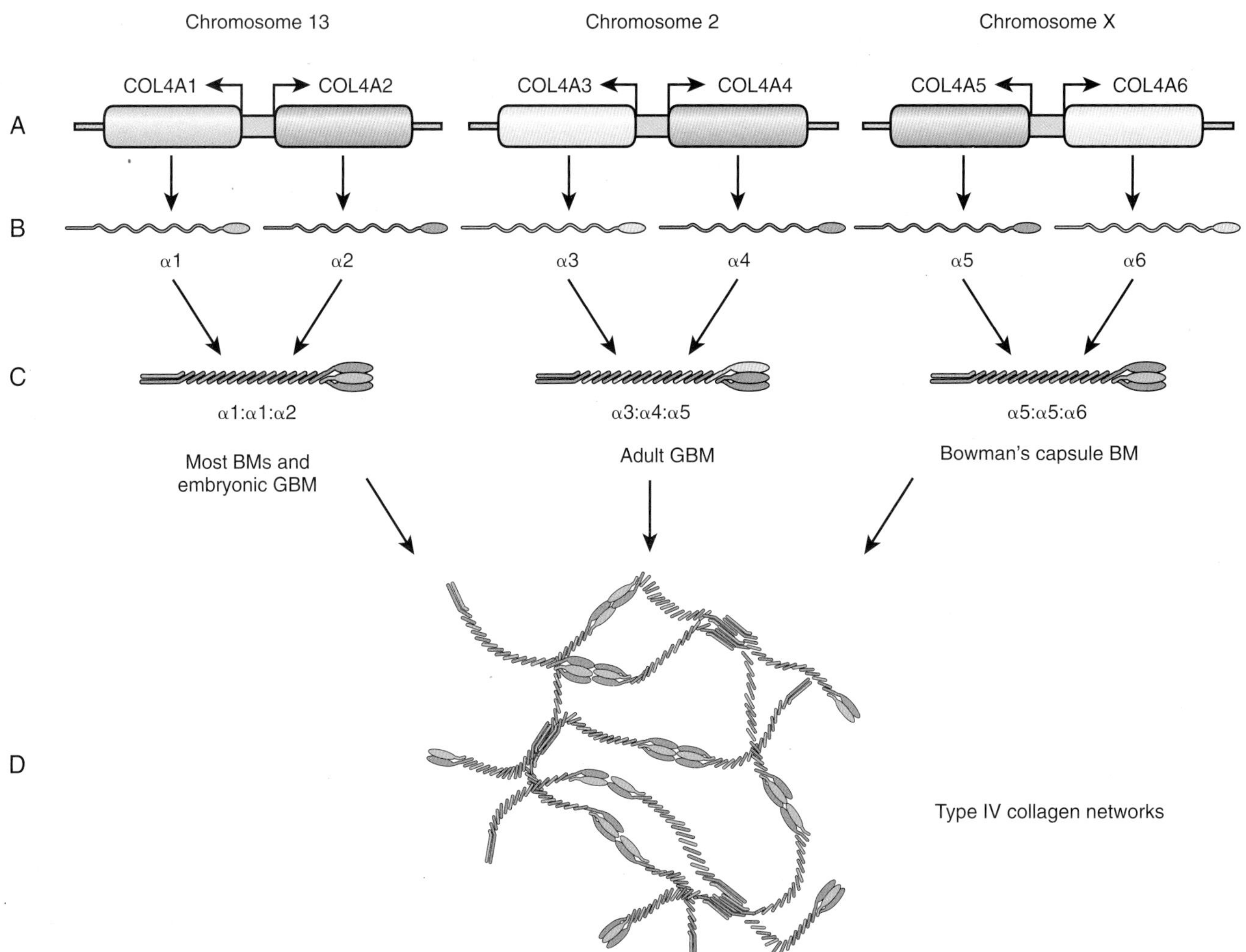


**Fig. 43.3** Type IV collagen genes, alpha chains, and glomerular isoforms. (A) The six collagen IV genes (*COL4A1* to *COL4A6*) are located pairwise in a head to head manner on three different chromosomes. (B) The *COL4A* genes generate six different alpha chains that have a globular noncollagenous domain at their C terminus. (C) Three chains form three combinations of triple-helix molecules. (D) Extracellularly, the triple-helix type IV collagen molecules form a network by associating with each other at their ends so that two molecules are cross-linked through their C-terminal globular domain (NC1), and four trimers associate with each other at the N-terminal 7S domain. The ubiquitous $\alpha_1{:}\alpha_1{:}\alpha_2$ trimer is the only isoform in the embryonic glomerular basement membrane *(GBM)*. After birth, this isoform is gradually replaced by the $\alpha_3{:}\alpha_4{:}\alpha_5$ isoform. Defects in the $\alpha_3{:}\alpha_4{:}\alpha_5$ trimers lead to a variety of glomerular pathology, ranging from thin basement membrane nephropathy to Alport syndrome (see text).

Laminins are trimeric, cross-shaped matrix proteins assembled out of one alpha, one beta, and one gamma chain. In the GBM, the major laminin isoform is laminin-521 (LM-521), consisting of the $\alpha_5$, $\beta_2$, and $\gamma_1$ subunits.[345] Trimers further polymerize to form a lattice network,[346] which can anchor additional GBM components, including agrin and nidogen. Laminins act as cell adhesion receptors, with the carboxyl terminal laminin globular (LG) domain of the alpha chain a major site for integrin and dystroglycan binding.[347] LM-521 is secreted by both endothelial cells and podocytes.[231]

Pierson syndrome is an autosomal recessive disease. Both compound heterozygous and homozygous mutations have been reported. Most mutations reported are severe truncating or frameshift mutations and appear to completely abolish laminin beta-2 protein in the GBM. Even truncation mutations smaller than 50 amino acids from the carboxyl terminus of LAMB2 appear to be functional null alleles. Missense mutations have been reported, with evidence of partial LM-521 function and milder disease, including childhood presentation of nephrotic syndrome and later development of ESKD.[348–351] Heterozygous missense and promoter variant single-nucleotide polymorphisms (SNPs) have been reported in patients with nephrotic syndrome, but their clinical significance remains uncertain.[351] Clear correlations between renal and nonrenal phenotypes and between genotype and neurologic phenotypes are lacking.

Clinically, most patients present at or shortly after birth with the symptoms of congenital nephrotic syndrome in addition to a variety of nonrenal deficits.[341,351,352] Cases of nephrotic syndrome presenting in childhood have been reported but are uncommon; most patients progress rapidly to ESKD.[351] Isolated nephrotic syndrome is rarely caused by

*LAMB2* mutations.[24,351] Ocular defects are almost universal, with microcoria, lenticonus, or cataracts and retinal detachments most common.[351,353,354] Ocular and/or neurodevelopmental defects due to *LAMB2* without renal disease has not been described, although rare cases of ocular disease preceding the development of nephrotic syndrome have been reported. Additional neurodevelopmental defects have also been reported, including muscular hypotonia and progressive neurocognitive involvement.[340,342,351] Diffuse mesangial sclerosis with associated diffuse podocyte foot process effacement is seen on renal biopsy.

Treatment for Pierson syndrome is currently limited to supportive therapy. Successful renal transplantation has been reported, with improvement in renal failure associated with growth retardation.[355] However, the presence of significant neurodevelopmental defects may limit the utility for this approach in other cases. Interestingly, recombinant LM-521 trimers infused into *Lamb2*-deficient mice appear to accumulate in the GBM and delay the development of severe proteinuria.[356] However, the LM-521 trimers appear to accumulate mainly on the endothelial half of the GBM, and a beneficial effect of the treatment on renal survival was not reported. Nonetheless, these early preclinical studies have suggested the possibility of affecting GBM composition and perhaps function through the administration of exogenous matrix components.

### *LAMA5*

*LAMA5* encodes for the laminin $\alpha_5$ subunit. *LAMA5* variants have been reported in several patients with FSGS in conjunction with additional gene mutations[256,357,358] and in homozygous form in three families with apparent recessive monogenic nephrotic syndrome.[359] In the mouse, *Lama5* deletion results in severe developmental defects, a hypomorphic allele develops a proteinuria, hematuria, and polycystic kidney disease (PKD) phenotype, and podocyte-specific *Lama5* deletion produces GBM defects and proteinuria.[360–362] However, the clinical significance of *LAMA5* variants in the development of human glomerular disease remains uncertain.

### SYSTEMIC DISEASES WITH GLOMERULAR COMPONENTS

Here we briefly review systemic monogenic diseases with glomerular components. This distinction is somewhat arbitrary because many of the forms of inherited glomerular diseases discussed previously have extrarenal components.

#### FABRY DISEASE

Fabry disease is a rare X-linked disease with both serious extrarenal and renal manifestations.[363,364] It is caused by mutations in the alpha-galactosidase gene *GLA*.[363] Dermatologic manifestations include a neuropathy characterized by reduced sensation in the palms and soles, anhidrosis, and frequent angiokeratomas. Cardiac abnormalities and neurologic symptoms are common. At a biochemical level, disease is caused by a deficiency of alpha-galactosidase activity, leading to an accumulation of globotriaosylceramide (GL3) in blood vessels and tissues, including podocytes, endothelial cells, epithelial cells, and tubular cells within the kidney. Fabry disease is treated with administration of recombinant alpha-galactosidase.[365] Treatment appears to be effective in clearing GL3 deposits from the kidney and improving the kidney prognosis.[366] Other small molecule–based therapeutic options are under investigation.[367] Because of the X-linked nature of the disease, disease manifestations are highly variable in women with GLA mutations. Kidney transplantation is a viable option for patients with Fabry disease. Kidney survival in Fabry disease is as good as those receiving transplants for other causes of ESKD.[368]

#### GALLOWAY-MOWAT SYNDROME

Galloway-Mowat syndrome is a rare, multisystem, AR disorder. Affected individuals exhibit microcephaly, severely altered central nervous system development and, often, nephrotic syndrome.[369] *WDR73* was the first Galloway-Mowat gene to be identified.[370,371] *WDR73* encodes a WD40 repeat domain–containing protein and is thought to play a role in microtubule function and microtubule-dependent cell cycle and cell proliferative functions. Mutations in the KEOPS complex genes have been recently reported also to cause Galloway-Mowat syndrome.[372] Recessive mutations in the genes *OSGEP, TP53RK, TPRKB*, and *LAGE3* encode the four subunits that comprise the KEOPS complex (for conserved kinase, endopeptidase, and other small proteins). Mutations in these genes were reported in 37 individuals from 32 families.

### NONGLOMERULAR DISEASES APPEARING AS PRIMARY GLOMERULOPATHIES

Increasingly, genetic studies are identifying variants in nonglomerular disease genes as the likely culprit in cases of apparent primary glomerular disease. There have been several reported cases of mutations in the Dent disease genes as the cause of kidney disease presenting as proteinuria or FSGS.[373–375] Similarly, mutations in nephronophthisis genes have been reported to present initially as glomerulopathies.[376–378]

## GENETIC TESTING CONSIDERATIONS

Clinical genetic testing for gene alterations underlying glomerular disease is available but is not in widespread use. A variety of academic medical centers, as well as commercial clinical laboratories, offer Clinical Laboratory Improvement Amendments (CLIA)–approved genetic testing for specific glomerular disease genes of interest, as well as panels of glomerular and/or kidney disease genes. The available test centers continue to change rapidly, and the Internet may provide the most current resource in identifying appropriate testing laboratories.

A few general considerations should be kept in mind when doing genetic testing in the evaluation and management of a patient with glomerular disease:

1. The prior probability that a gene variant is causally related to disease is related to multiple factors, including age of disease onset and clinical phenotype.
   Determination of a likely genetic cause of FSGS or nephrotic syndrome becomes less likely with increasing age. Although the likelihood of finding a genetic cause underlying congenital nephrotic syndrome in a neonate is high, it is much less likely in an adult with FSGS.[3,24,379]

2. Every gene has multiple protein sequence-altering variants. The identification of a DNA change from the most common DNA sequence seen in the human population does not mean that it has a phenotype consequence. If the prior probability of having a genetic cause of disease is high, then the meaning of the test result changes. For example, the finding of an amino acid–changing variant in a patient with FSGS and/or a strong family history of FSGS, in which this same variant is present in all the affected family members, is highly likely to be causally related to disease. However, the incidental finding of, for example, an *INF2* or *TRPC6* variant in an individual with no kidney disease, is much more difficult to interpret and, without additional information about the variant or the individual, likely has no bearing on the individual's kidney status. Such variants are often referred to as variants of uncertain significance (VUS).[380] Just like incidental findings in nongenetic testing, incidental genetic test results can create information of uncertain meaning.
3. Apparent primary glomerular disease can reflect nonglomerular gene alterations producing a phenotype that masquerades as a primary glomerular disease.
   This suggests that in the clinical setting, a clinician may want to test for a broad range of genes. These might include type 4 collagen genes or *CLCN5* in the case of familial FSGS. Finding the right balance between testing for only the most obvious candidate genes and testing for variations in a long list of possible genes requires some judgment. Interpretation of the results may benefit from the involvement of a clinical geneticist, genetic counselor, or nephrologist experienced in inherited disease.

As treatments for glomerular diseases improve, making an accurate genetic diagnosis may take on greater importance, although the clinical benefit of such testing has not been demonstrated, except for some exceptional cases.[94]

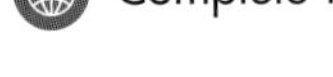 Complete reference list available at ExpertConsult.com.

## KEY REFERENCES


3. Sadowski CE, Lovric S, Ashraf S, et al. A single-gene cause in 29.5% of cases of steroid-resistant nephrotic syndrome. *J Am Soc Nephrol.* 2015;26(6):1279–1289.
5. Genovese G, Friedman DJ, Ross MD, et al. Association of trypanolytic ApoL1 variants with kidney disease in African Americans. *Science.* 2010;329(5993):841–845.
6. Tzur S, Rosset S, Shemer R, et al. Missense mutations in the APOL1 gene are highly associated with end stage kidney disease risk previously attributed to the MYH9 gene. *Hum Genet.* 2010;128(3):345–350.
7. Stanescu HC, Arcos-Burgos M, Medlar A, et al. Risk HLA-DQA1 and PLA(2)R1 alleles in idiopathic membranous nephropathy. *N Engl J Med.* 2011;364(7):616–626.
13. Debiec H, Dossier C, Letouze E, et al. Transethnic, genome-wide analysis reveals immune-related risk alleles and phenotypic correlates in pediatric steroid-sensitive nephrotic syndrome. *J Am Soc Nephrol.* 2018;29(7):2000–2013.
17. Boute N, Gribouval O, Roselli S, et al. NPHS2, encoding the glomerular protein podocin, is mutated in autosomal recessive steroid-resistant nephrotic syndrome. *Nat Genet.* 2000;24(4):349–354.
18. Kestila M, Lenkkeri U, Mannikko M, et al. Positionally cloned gene for a novel glomerular protein–nephrin–is mutated in congenital nephrotic syndrome. *Mol Cell.* 1998;1(4):575–582.
24. Hinkes BG, Mucha B, Vlangos CN, et al. Nephrotic syndrome in the first year of life: two thirds of cases are caused by mutations in 4 genes (NPHS1, NPHS2, WT1, and LAMB2). *Pediatrics.* 2007;119(4): e907–e919.
27. Ruotsalainen V, Ljungberg P, Wartiovaara J, et al. Nephrin is specifically located at the slit diaphragm of glomerular podocytes. *Proc Natl Acad Sci USA.* 1999;96(14):7962–7967.
28. Holzman LB, St John PL, Kovari IA, et al. Nephrin localizes to the slit pore of the glomerular epithelial cell. *Kidney Int.* 1999;56(4): 1481–1491.
29. Huber TB, Kottgen M, Schilling B, et al. Interaction with podocin facilitates nephrin signaling. *J Biol Chem.* 2001;276(45):41543–41546.
42. Ruf RG, Lichtenberger A, Karle SM, et al. Patients with mutations in NPHS2 (podocin) do not respond to standard steroid treatment of nephrotic syndrome. *J Am Soc Nephrol.* 2004;15(3):722–732.
52. Huber TB, Schermer B, Muller RU, et al. Podocin and MEC-2 bind cholesterol to regulate the activity of associated ion channels. *Proc Natl Acad Sci USA.* 2006;103(46):17079–17086.
59. Kaplan JM, Kim SH, North KN, et al. Mutations in ACTN4, encoding alpha-actinin-4, cause familial focal segmental glomerulosclerosis. *Nat Genet.* 2000;24(3):251–256.
70. Brown EJ, Schlondorff JS, Becker DJ, et al. Mutations in the formin gene INF2 cause focal segmental glomerulosclerosis. *Nat Genet.* 2010;42(1):72–76.
75. Boyer O, Nevo F, Plaisier E, et al. INF2 mutations in Charcot-Marie-Tooth disease with glomerulopathy. *N Engl J Med.* 2011;365(25): 2377–2388.
77. Winn MP, Conlon PJ, Lynn KL, et al. A mutation in the TRPC6 cation channel causes familial focal segmental glomerulosclerosis. *Science.* 2005;308(5729):1801–1804.
81. Reiser J, Polu KR, Moller CC, et al. TRPC6 is a glomerular slit diaphragm-associated channel required for normal renal function. *Nat Genet.* 2005;37(7):739–744.
99. Seri M, Pecci A, Di Bari F, et al. MYH9-related disease: May-Hegglin anomaly, Sebastian syndrome, Fechtner syndrome, and Epstein syndrome are not distinct entities but represent a variable expression of a single illness. *Medicine (Baltimore).* 2003;82(3):203–215.
108. Gbadegesin RA, Hall G, Adeyemo A, et al. Mutations in the gene that encodes the F-actin binding protein anillin cause FSGS. *J Am Soc Nephrol.* 2014;25(9):1991–2002.
110. Gee HY, Zhang F, Ashraf S, et al. KANK deficiency leads to podocyte dysfunction and nephrotic syndrome. *J Clin Invest.* 2015;125(6): 2375–2384.
112. Gupta IR, Baldwin C, Auguste D, et al. ARHGDIA: a novel gene implicated in nephrotic syndrome. *J Med Genet.* 2013;50(5):330–338.
115. Akilesh S, Suleiman H, Yu H, et al. Arhgap24 inactivates Rac1 in mouse podocytes, and a mutant form is associated with familial focal segmental glomerulosclerosis. *J Clin Invest.* 2011;121(10):4127–4137.
116. Ashraf S, Kudo H, Rao J, et al. Mutations in six nephrosis genes delineate a pathogenic pathway amenable to treatment. *Nat Commun.* 2018;9(1):1960.
120. Schwarz K, Simons M, Reiser J, et al. Podocin, a raft-associated component of the glomerular slit diaphragm, interacts with CD2AP and nephrin. *J Clin Invest.* 2001;108(11):1621–1629.
122. Kim JM, Wu H, Green G, et al. CD2-associated protein haploinsufficiency is linked to glomerular disease susceptibility. *Science.* 2003;300(5623):1298–1300.
129. Bierzynska A, Soderquest K, Dean P, et al. MAGI2 mutations cause congenital nephrotic syndrome. *J Am Soc Nephrol.* 2017;28(5): 1614–1621.
134. Nicolaou N, Margadant C, Kevelam SH, et al. Gain of glycosylation in integrin alpha3 causes lung disease and nephrotic syndrome. *J Clin Invest.* 2012;122(12):4375–4387.
146. Ashraf S, Gee HY, Woerner S, et al. ADCK4 mutations promote steroid-resistant nephrotic syndrome through CoQ10 biosynthesis disruption. *J Clin Invest.* 2013;123(12):5179–5189.
152. Braun DA, Sadowski CE, Kohl S, et al. Mutations in nuclear pore genes NUP93, NUP205 and XPO5 cause steroid-resistant nephrotic syndrome. *Nat Genet.* 2016;48(4):457–465.
155. Dreyer SD, Zhou G, Baldini A, et al. Mutations in LMX1B cause abnormal skeletal patterning and renal dysplasia in nail patella syndrome. *Nat Genet.* 1998;19(1):47–50.
169. Barbaux S, Niaudet P, Gubler MC, et al. Donor splice-site mutations in WT1 are responsible for Frasier syndrome. *Nat Genet.* 1997; 17(4):467–470.
191. Hinkes B, Wiggins RC, Gbadegesin R, et al. Positional cloning uncovers mutations in PLCE1 responsible for a nephrotic syndrome variant that may be reversible. *Nat Genet.* 2006;38(12):1397–1405.

196. Gee HY, Ashraf S, Wan X, et al. Mutations in EMP2 cause childhood-onset nephrotic syndrome. *Am J Hum Genet.* 2014;94(6): 884–890.
197. Ebarasi L, Ashraf S, Bierzynska A, et al. Defects of CRB2 cause steroid-resistant nephrotic syndrome. *Am J Hum Genet.* 2015;96(1): 153–161.
198. Slavotinek A, Kaylor J, Pierce H, et al. CRB2 mutations produce a phenotype resembling congenital nephrosis, Finnish type, with cerebral ventriculomegaly and raised alpha-fetoprotein. *Am J Hum Genet.* 2015;96(1):162–169.
215. Beckerman P, Bi-Karchin J, Park AS, et al. Transgenic expression of human APOL1 risk variants in podocytes induces kidney disease in mice. *Nat Med.* 2017;23(4):429–438.
226. Lennon R, Byron A, Humphries JD, et al. Global analysis reveals the complexity of the human glomerular extracellular matrix. *J Am Soc Nephrol.* 2014;25(5):939–951.
230. Abrahamson DR, Hudson BG, Stroganova L, et al. Cellular origins of type IV collagen networks in developing glomeruli. *J Am Soc Nephrol.* 2009;20(7):1471–1479.
245. Wartiovaara J, Ofverstedt LG, Khoshnoodi J, et al. Nephrin strands contribute to a porous slit diaphragm scaffold as revealed by electron tomography. *J Clin Invest.* 2004;114(10):1475–1483.
249. Jarad G, Cunningham J, Shaw AS, et al. Proteinuria precedes podocyte abnormalities in Lamb2-/- mice, implicating the glomerular basement membrane as an albumin barrier. *J Clin Invest.* 2006;116(8):2272–2279.
259. Voskarides K, Damianou L, Neocleous V, et al. COL4A3/COL4A4 mutations producing focal segmental glomerulosclerosis and renal failure in thin basement membrane nephropathy. *J Am Soc Nephrol.* 2007;18(11):3004–3016.
286. Gross O, Licht C, Anders HJ, et al. Early angiotensin-converting enzyme inhibition in Alport syndrome delays renal failure and improves life expectancy. *Kidney Int.* 2012;81(5):494–501.
290. Barker DF, Hostikka SL, Zhou J, et al. Identification of mutations in the COL4A5 collagen gene in Alport syndrome. *Science.* 1990;248(4960):1224–1227.
297. Jais JP, Knebelmann B, Giatras I, et al. X-linked Alport syndrome: natural history in 195 families and genotype- phenotype correlations in males. *J Am Soc Nephrol.* 2000;11(4):649–657.
342. Zenker M, Aigner T, Wendler O, et al. Human laminin beta2 deficiency causes congenital nephrosis with mesangial sclerosis and distinct eye abnormalities. *Hum Mol Genet.* 2004;13(21):2625–2632.
365. Eng CM, Guffon N, Wilcox WR, et al. Safety and efficacy of recombinant human alpha-galactosidase A replacement therapy in Fabry's disease. *N Engl J Med.* 2001;345(1):9–16.
372. Braun DA, Rao J, Mollet G, et al. Mutations in KEOPS-complex genes cause nephrotic syndrome with primary microcephaly. *Nat Genet.* 2017;49(10):1529–1538.
379. Santin S, Bullich G, Tazon-Vega B, et al. Clinical utility of genetic testing in children and adults with steroid-resistant nephrotic syndrome. *Clin J Am Soc Nephrol.* 2011;6(5):1139–1148.
380. Richards S, Aziz N, Bale S, et al. Standards and guidelines for the interpretation of sequence variants: a joint consensus recommendation of the American College of Medical Genetics and Genomics and the Association for Molecular Pathology. *Genet Med.* 2015;17(5):405–424.

# 44 Inherited Disorders of the Renal Tubule

Alain Bonnardeaux | Daniel G. Bichet

CHAPTER OUTLINE



Considerable progress has been made in understanding the molecular basis of inherited renal tubule disorders. These advances have allowed the identification of genes expressed in the renal tubule (Table 44.1), increasing our knowledge of basic renal physiology and pathobiology. Other benefits include potential prenatal and postnatal screening and better phenotype characterization and knowledge. Diseases described in this section are relatively rare (1:2000 or less; affecting fewer than 200,000 persons in the United States) and some were previously restricted to pediatric nephrology; however, advances in therapy have increased longevity for many patients, thus confronting the adult nephrologist with new challenges.

## INHERITED DISORDERS ASSOCIATED WITH GENERALIZED DYSFUNCTION OF THE PROXIMAL TUBULE (RENAL FANCONI SYNDROME)

Renal Fanconi syndrome is a generalized dysfunction of the proximal tubule with no primary glomerular involvement. It is characterized by variable degrees of phosphate, glucose, amino acid, and bicarbonate wasting. Isolated or partial defects are described in other sections of this chapter. The clinical presentation in children consists of rickets and impaired growth. In adults, bone disease manifests as osteomalacia and osteoporosis. Polyuria, renal sodium and potassium wasting, metabolic acidosis, hypercalciuria, and low-molecular-weight proteinuria may be part of the clinical spectrum.

There are hereditary and acquired variants of Fanconi syndrome. Acquired forms in adults are often associated with urinary excretion of protein corresponding to a paraproteinemic disorder or the nephrotic syndrome, with residual cases being secondary to tubular damage caused by toxic or immunologic factors.[1] Hereditary Fanconi syndrome occurs principally by one of two mechanisms: primary proximal tubule transport defects or accumulation of toxic metabolic products in the kidneys (Table 44.2).

### PATHOGENESIS

The proximal tubule is responsible for reclaiming most of the filtered load of bicarbonate, glucose, urate, amino acids and low-molecular-weight proteins as well as an important fraction of the filtered load of sodium, chloride, phosphate, and water. It exhibits a very extensive apical endocytic apparatus consisting of an elaborate network of coated pits and small, coated and noncoated endosomes. In addition, the cells contain a large number of late endosomes, prelysosomes, lysosomes, and so-called dense apical tubules involved in receptor recycling from the endosomes to the apical plasma membrane. This endocytic apparatus is involved in the reabsorption of molecules filtered by the glomeruli (Fig. 44.1). The process is very effective, as demonstrated by the fact that although several grams of proteins are filtered daily, the urine is virtually devoid of protein under physiologic conditions. Reabsorption of solutes by proximal tubule cells is achieved by transport systems at the brush border membrane that are directly or indirectly coupled to sodium movement, by energy production and transport from the mitochondria, and by the $Na^+$–$K^+$–adenosine triphosphatase (ATPase) at the basolateral membrane. The $Na^+$–$K^+$–ATPase lowers intracellular $Na^+$ concentration and provides the electrochemical gradient that allows $Na^+$-coupled solute to enter the cell. A second route, the paracellular pathway, is responsible for reclaiming up to half of the sodium and most of the water through tight junctions.

**Table 44.1 Impact of DNA Variation on Protein Function**

| | |
|---|---|
| Loss of function | A mutation that reduces or abolishes a normal physiologic function (likely to be recessive) |
| Gain of function | A mutation that increases the function of a protein (likely to be dominant) |
| Dominant negative | A mutation that dominantly affects the phenotype by means of a defective protein or RNA molecule that interferes with the function of the normal gene product in the same cell (likely to be dominant) |

There are several genetic forms of Fanconi syndrome, the majority of which are associated with multisystem disorders (Table 44.2). In general, the disease mechanism for these disorders can be categorized as either (i) accumulation of a toxic metabolite (e.g., cystinosis, tyrosinemia, galactosemia, Fanconi–Bickel, congenital fructose intolerance, and Wilson disease), (ii) disruption of energy provision (e.g., mitochondrial cytopathies), or (iii) disruption of endocytosis and intracellular transport (e.g., Lowe syndrome, Dent disease, and arthrogryposis-renal dysfunction-cholestasis [ARC] syndrome).[2] The field continues to evolve and a novel mechanism secondary to monoallelic mutations in the gene encoding glycine amidinotransferase (GATM), a proximal tubular enzyme in the creatine biosynthetic pathway, characterized by renal Fanconi syndrome and kidney failure has just been published.[3] All disease-related GATM mutations create an additional interaction interface within the GATM protein, promoting its linear aggregation. Aggregate-containing mitochondria in proximal tubular cells are associated with elevated production of reactive oxygen species, initiation of an inflammatory response, and increased cell death. These data establish a link between intramitochondrial GATM aggregates, renal Fanconi syndrome, and chronic kidney disease.[4]

Diseases associated with the accumulation of toxic metabolites are potentially reversible. For example, the defect is reversed after dietary restriction of tyrosine and phenylalanine in tyrosinemia,[5] fructose in hereditary fructose intolerance,[6] and galactose in galactosemia.[7] The duration of the exposure

**Table 44.2 Inherited Causes of Fanconi Syndrome**

| Gene | OMIM | Disorders/Systemic Disorders | Associated Features |
|---|---|---|---|
| **Systemic Disorders** | | | |
| *GALT* | 230400 | Galactosemia | Liver dysfunction, jaundice, encephalopathy, sepsis |
| Multiple nuclear and mitochondrial DNA variants | Multiple | Mitochondrial cytopathies | Usually multisystem dysfunction (brain, muscle, liver, heart) |
| *FAH* | 276700 | Tyrosinemia | Poor growth, hepatic enlargement and dysfunction, liver cancer |
| *ALDOB* | 229600 | Congenital fructose intolerance | Rapid onset after fructose ingestion, vomiting, hypoglycemia, hepatomegaly |
| *CTNS* | 219800 | Cystinosis | Poor growth, vomiting, rickets ± corneal cystine crystals, kidney failure |
| *GLUT2* | 227810 | Fanconi–Bickel syndrome | Failure to thrive, hepatomegaly, hypoglycemia, rickets |
| *OCRL* | 309000 | Lowe syndrome | Males (X-linked), cataracts, hypotonia, developmental delay |
| *CLCN5, OCRL* | 300009, 300555 | Dent disease I, II | Males (X-linked), hypercalciuria, nephrocalcinosis |
| *ATP7B* | 277900 | Wilson disease | Hepatic and neurological disease, Kayser–Fleischer rings |
| *VPS33B, VIPAR* | 208085, 613404 | ARC syndrome | Arthrogryposis, platelet abnormalities, cholestasis |
| *HNF4A* | 125850 | MODY1 | Neonatal hyperinsulinism, maturity-onset of diabetes in the young, mutation R76W shows RFS |
| **Isolated Renal Fanconi Syndrome** | | | |
| *GATM* | 602360 | FRTS1 | Kidney failure |
| *SLC34A1* | 613388 | FRTS2 | Phosphaturia dominating |
| *EHHADH* | 615605 | FRTS3 | No kidney failure |

*ARC,* Arthrogryposis-renal dysfunction-cholestasis; *OMIM,* Online Mendelian Inheritance in Man; *RFS,* renal Fanconi syndrome.
Modified from Klootwijk ED, Reichold M, Unwin RJ, et al. Renal Fanconi syndrome: taking a proximal look at the nephron. *Nephrol Dial Transplant.* 2015;30:1456–1460.

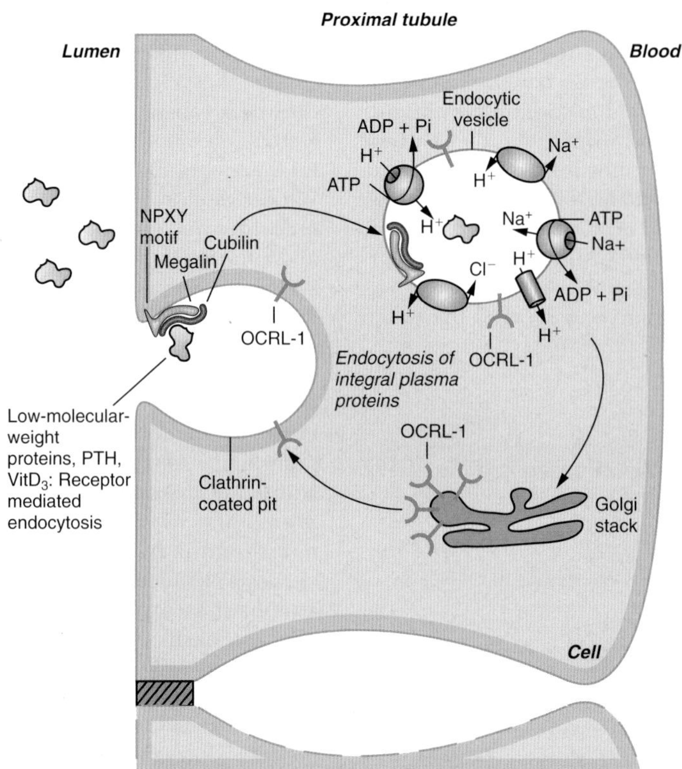


**Fig. 44.1** The glomerular filtration barrier restricts the passage of large molecules, particularly those that are negatively charged molecules. The proteins appearing in the proximal tubule are reabsorbed by endocytosis (see the luminal part of the schematic representation). Vitamins and iron that are complexed to carrier proteins bind to megalin and/or cubilin followed by endocytosis. The ligands are released from the receptors by the low pH in the endosomes, and receptors recycle through the membrane recycling compartment. The protein component is degraded, whereas the vitamin, as well as iron, is transported across the epithelial cell (not represented). 1,25-Dihydroxyvitamin $D_3$ is activated by mitochondrial 1$\alpha$-hydroxylase, implying that the vitamin is transported to the cytoplasm, possibly by diffusion, before its release to the basolateral membrane. The regulation and maintenance of an endocytic vesicle pH are represented here according to Weisz,[352] whereby protons are pumped into the organelle by vacuolar $H^+$–ATPase and can leave by the chloride proton exchanger ClC-5. The *ClC5* gene is mutated in patients with type 1 Dent disease, and the *OCRL1* gene is mutated in patients with type 2 Dent disease. OCRL1 encodes a phosphatase that is present on the trans-Golgi network and is important for regulating the traffic between the network, early endosomes, and clathrin-coated intermediate particles. *ADP,* Adenosine diphosphate; *ATP,* adenosine triphosphate; *ATPase,* adenosine triphosphatase; *NPXY,* asn-pro-any amino acid-tyrosine motif; *OCRL-1,* phosphatidylinositol 4,5-bisphosphate 5-phosphatase encoded by *OCRL1* gene; $P_i$, inorganic phosphate; *PTH,* parathyroid hormone; *Vit,* vitamin.

is also important for the disorder to be expressed and is protracted in cadmium intoxication[8] or brief in fructose intolerance following a fructose load.[9]

Considerable progress has been made in understanding the molecular basis of inherited renal tubule disorders. These advances have allowed the identification of genes expressed in the renal tubule (Table 44.1), increasing our knowledge of basic renal physiology and pathobiology. Other benefits include potential prenatal and postnatal screening and better phenotype characterization and knowledge. Diseases described in this section are relatively rare (≤1 : 2000; affecting <200,000 persons in the United States) and some were previously restricted to pediatric nephrology; however, advances in therapy have increased longevity for many patients, thus confronting the adult nephrologist with new challenges.

## CLINICAL PRESENTATION OF RENAL FANCONI SYNDROME

### AMINOACIDURIA

Amino acids are filtered by the glomerulus with more than 98% subsequently reabsorbed by multiple proximal tubule transporters. In Fanconi syndrome, all amino acids are excreted in excess. The pattern of excretion of amino acids parallels that in physiologic conditions, so those excreted at the highest levels are histidine, serine, cystine, lysine, and glycine. Aminoaciduria is usually quantified by one of several chromatographic methods in specialized centers. Clinically, losses are relatively modest and do not lead to specific deficiencies. There is no need to supplement amino acids to affected subjects.

### PHOSPHATURIA AND BONE DISEASE

Phosphate wasting is a cardinal manifestation but bone features are variable. Serum phosphate levels are usually decreased, and tubular reabsorption of phosphate (TRP) and maximal capacity—calculated by dividing maximum tubular reabsorption of phosphate ($Tm_P$) by glomerular filtration rate (GFR) or $Tm_P$/GFR—are systematically reduced. Rickets and osteomalacia, which are caused by increased urinary losses of phosphate as well as by impaired 1$\alpha$-hydroxylation of 1,25-dihydroxyvitamin $D_3$, can compose the dominant clinical picture. Rickets manifests as the bowing deformity of the lower limbs with metaphyseal widening of the proximal and distal tibia, distal femur, ulna, and radius. Bone manifestations in subjects with adult-onset renal Fanconi syndrome are severe bone pain and spontaneous fractures.

### RENAL TUBULAR ACIDOSIS

Hyperchloremic metabolic acidosis is a frequent finding and is caused by defective bicarbonate reabsorption. Hence, renal acidification by the distal tubule is normal, as demonstrated by the ability to acidify urine at a pH below 5.5 when plasma bicarbonate is below the threshold. Because the more distal segments have substantial bicarbonate reabsorptive capacity, the plasma bicarbonate concentration is usually maintained between 12 and 20 mmol/L. The diagnosis can be established by raising the plasma bicarbonate concentration with an intravenous sodium bicarbonate infusion (0.5–1 mmol/kg per hour) to 18 to 20 mmol/L. The fractional excretion of bicarbonate will usually rise to 15% to 20% in proximal renal tubular acidosis (pRTA) but will remain lower (3%) in distal RTA (dRTA). Treatment with large doses of alkali may be necessary to correct the acidosis.

### GLUCOSURIA

Glucosuria is a common manifestation although the serum glucose level is normal, and the amount of glucose lost in the urine varies from 0.5 to 10 g/day. Glucosuria (and hypoglycemia) may be massive in glycogenosis type I.[10]

### POLYURIA, SODIUM, AND POTASSIUM WASTING

Polyuria, polydipsia, and dehydration may be prominent features. Hypokalemia can contribute to decreased concentrating ability of the kidney from abnormal tubule function of the distal tubule and collecting duct. Recent studies suggest that autophagic loss of aquaporin-2 (AQP2) may contribute to the decreased urinary concentrating ability complicating hypokalemia.[11] A similar mechanism has also been proposed for the urinary concentrating defect accompanying hypercalcemia.[12] Renal sodium losses may be significant, leading to hypotension, hyponatremia, and metabolic alkalosis. Supplementation with sodium chloride is indicated and achieves clinical improvement. Potassium losses are secondary to increased delivery of sodium to the distal tubule and activation of the renin–angiotensin–aldosterone system from hypovolemia.

### PROTEINURIA

Low-molecular-weight proteinuria is almost always present in low to moderate amounts. Endosomal machinery proteins, including the vacuolar type $H^+$–ATPase (V-ATPase), ClC-5 chloride/proton exchanger channels, and the endocytotic receptors megalin and cubilin,[13] are important in protein reabsorption. The urine dipstick test result is frequently positive because of the presence of albuminuria, typically at levels of 1 g/day. Rates of $\beta_2$-microglobulin excretion are also elevated.

### HYPERCALCIURIA

Hypercalciuria is a frequent manifestation in patients with renal Fanconi syndrome. The pathogenesis is not known but could be related to abnormal recycling of proteins involved in calcium reabsorption by the proximal tubule, natriuresis, and increased vitamin D synthesis from hypophosphatemia. Hypercalciuria is only occasionally associated with nephrolithiasis, possibly because of the presence of polyuria.

## DENT DISEASE

### PATHOGENESIS

Dent disease, X-linked recessive hypophosphatemic rickets, and X-linked recessive nephrolithiasis (Online Mendelian Inheritance in Man [OMIM] entry #300009)[14] are clinical manifestations of the same disease, reviewed elsewhere.[15] Clinical features include primary Fanconi syndrome, low-molecular-weight proteinuria, hypercalciuria with calcium nephrolithiasis, nephrocalcinosis, rickets, and progressive renal failure. Dent disease 1 is caused by mutations in the *CLCN5* gene located on chromosome Xp11.22 encoding a lysosomal transport protein, ClC-5, a 2 chloride/1 proton antiporter.[16] Defects in the *OCRL1* gene (oculocerebrorenal syndrome of Lowe), encoding a phosphatidylinositol 4,5-bisphosphate ($PIP_2$) 5-phosphatase (Ocrl) and usually found mutated in patients with Lowe syndrome, can also induce a Dent-like phenotype (type 2 Dent disease [OMIM #300555]; see later)[17,18] (Fig. 44.1). Of the 32 families with the clinical diagnosis of Dent disease reported by Hoopes and colleagues,[19] 19 (60%) had mutations in *CLCN5* and 5 families (16%) had mutations in *OCRL1* (for whom the diagnosis of Lowe syndrome had been excluded because of absence of cataracts). It is possible that additional genes are involved in families not linked to *CLCN5* and *OCRL1*.[19]

*CLCN5* mutations expressed in vitro lead to a disorder manifesting as defects in receptor-mediated endocytosis and/or endosomal acidification.[20] ClC-5 colocalizes with the proton pump and internalized proteins early after uptake and is also expressed in type A intercalated cells. ClC-5 forms a dimer of two identical subunits, each of which contains a complete ion conduction pathway and is composed of 18 $\alpha$-helices. It is thought to provide an electrical shunt for the acidification of vesicles of the endocytotic pathway required for receptor–ligand interactions and cell sorting events.[21] Inhibition of the acidification interferes with cell-surface receptor recycling, reducing endocytosis of albumin and resulting in mistargeting of megalin, cubilin, $Na^+$–$H^+$-exchanger isoform 3 (NHE3), and the sodium/phosphate transporter NPT2a.

## CLINICAL PRESENTATION

The clinical presentation is explained by the predominant expression of ClC-5 in the proximal tubule. Patients have varying degrees of low-molecular-weight proteinuria, hypercalciuria with calcium nephrolithiasis, rickets, nephrocalcinosis, and renal failure.[22] There is considerable intrafamilial variability,[23] probably because of genetic and/or environmental modifiers. The disease affects male patients predominantly, and female patients have an attenuated phenotype. However, renal failure develops only in male patients.

The excretion of low-molecular-weight proteins in the urine such as albumin, $\beta_2$-microglobulin, and $\alpha_1$-microglobulin is thought to be the most reliable marker for the disease. Affected male patients usually excrete $\beta_2$-microglobulin in amounts that are more than 100-fold the upper limit of normal. Female carriers can also have low-molecular-weight proteinuria, but it is usually less pronounced than in male patients and sometimes absent. Low-molecular-weight proteinuria is not a specific finding because it can be seen in tubulointerstitial diseases as well. The degree of proteinuria is relatively constant and amounts to 0.5 to 2 g/day in adults and up to 1 g/day in children.[24–26] The nephrotic syndrome does not occur, and albumin excretion represents less than half of the proteins excreted. An attenuated form of the disease with low-molecular-weight proteinuria as the only or predominant feature appears to be prevalent in Japan.[27]

Hypercalciuria is also a common finding in this disorder and is present in most cases, beginning in childhood. It is usually overt and predominant in male patients (>7.5 mmol/day). Female patients are also frequently hypercalciuric, but their values are usually closer to the upper limit of the normal range. Nephrolithiasis is frequent, with 50% of male patients affected. Stones are composed of calcium phosphate or a mixture of calcium phosphate and oxalate.[26] Multiple episodes starting during the teenage years are common. Radiologic nephrocalcinosis of the medullary type is seen in most affected male patients and occasionally in female patients. Serum phosphate levels are usually below normal values or at the lower limit of the normal range. $Tm_P$/GFR is decreased, indicating defective reabsorption by the proximal tubule. Rickets may be present in children and is cured by the administration of pharmacologic doses of vitamin D. Osteomalacia occurs in adults and is also corrected after administration of vitamin D. Serum levels of 1,25-dihydroxyvitamin $D_3$ are normal or slightly raised, whereas 25-hydroxyvitamin D levels are normal. The cause of hypercalciuria and renal stones is not known, but one possible explanation is that renal phosphate leak and reduced degradation of luminal parathyroid hormone (PTH) results in increased 1$\alpha$-hydroxylase activity and 1,25-dihydroxycholecalciferol production. Other explanations are abnormal trafficking (recycling) of transporters or channels necessary for calcium transport to the apical membrane, and decreased reabsorption of a regulatory protein by the proximal tubule.[28]

Systemic acidosis is typically not seen before renal function deteriorates significantly. Male patients usually have urinary acidification defects detectable by an ammonium chloride load, but these are not consistent features of the phenotype. Spontaneous hypokalemia is common in male patients, and there is inability to concentrate urine maximally. Aminoaciduria and glucosuria are also frequent. Half the male patients have raised serum creatinine with progressive renal failure. End-stage kidney disease occurs at age 47 ± 13 years. Renal biopsy specimens show a pattern of a chronic interstitial nephritis with scattered calcium deposits.[24–26] The glomeruli are normal or hyalinized. There is prominent tubular atrophy with diffuse inflammatory infiltrate composed of lymphocytes, and foci of calcification around and within epithelial cells. Molecular genetic testing is available and confirms the diagnosis.

### TREATMENT

Renal stones and hypercalciuria are treated with supportive measures (and in particular, increasing fluid intake). Dietary restriction of calcium reduces calcium excretion but is not recommended because it might contribute to the bone disease.[29] Thiazide diuretics can be given in small doses and may decrease calciuria,[30] but in patients with Dent disease, who have a tendency for salt wasting, response to these agents seems to consist of excessive diuresis, kaliuresis, and blood pressure reduction.[26] Rickets are treated with small doses of vitamin D, but this treatment should be given with caution as it might increase urine calcium excretion and the risk of nephrolithiasis. Verifying urine calcium excretion before and after vitamin D therapy might be appropriate.[29] There is no specific treatment for preventing progression of renal failure, although citrate has been shown to delay progression in a *Clc-5* knockout mouse model.[31] This goal has to be balanced against the possibility of increasing calcium phosphate supersaturation and stone formation by urine alkalinization.

## OCULOCEREBRORENAL DYSTROPHY (LOWE SYNDROME)

The oculocerebrorenal syndrome (*OCRL*) of Lowe (OMIM #309000) is an X-linked recessive multisystem disorder characterized by congenital cataracts, mental retardation, and incomplete renal Fanconi syndrome with renal failure occurring later in life (reviewed elsewhere[32,33]).

### PATHOGENESIS

Mutations in the *OCRL1* gene are responsible for OCRL.[34,35] *OCRL1* encodes a 105-kDa Golgi protein with $PIP_2$ 5-phosphatase activity. Phosphorylation of phosphatidylinositol at the 3, 4, or 5 position of the inositol ring generates seven phosphoinositides (PIs) that play a central role in the regulation of diverse cellular processes, including gene expression, cytokinesis, cell motility, actin cytoskeleton remodeling, membrane trafficking, and cell signaling.[36] Therefore OCRL1 is mainly a lipid phosphatase that may control cellular levels of a critical metabolite, $PIP_2$,[37] and is involved in the inositol phosphate signaling pathway. OCRL1 is likely to regulate cellular trafficking. It is present in the trans-Golgi network, in early endosomes, and in clathrin-coated intermediates that move between these compartments[37] that play key regulatory functions in cell physiology reviewed by Pirruccello and colleagues.[38] The related soluble inositol polyphosphates and pyrophosphates, generated from inositol 1,4,5-trisphosphate ($IP_3$)—a product of phosphatidylinositol 4,5-bisphosphate [PI(4,5)$P_2$] cleavage by phospholipases—are also important signaling molecules. Phosphorylated headgroups of PIs, which are localized on the cytosolic leaflets of membranes and help define membrane identity, interact with a variety of amino acid motifs or protein domains, and regulate protein–bilayer interactions. Thus OCRL1 deficiency may result in reductions in recycling of receptors and delivery of cargo to the plasma membrane. This possibility is consistent with the apparent loss of megalin from the apical membrane and protein absorption defects seen in patients (Fig. 44.1). It is not clear why the loss of OCRL1, a ubiquitously expressed protein, should result in defects to only the eyes, brain, and kidney proximal tubule. Compensation by another enzyme with overlapping specificity in the unaffected tissues is a possible explanation.

## CLINICAL PRESENTATION

OCRL is a multisystem disorder characterized by ocular, neurologic, and renal defects. Renal dysfunction (Fanconi syndrome) is a feature that may occur in the first year of life, but with great variability in severity and age of onset. It is characterized by proteinuria (0.5–2 g of daily urinary protein per square meter of body surface area), generalized aminoaciduria (100–1000 mmol of daily urinary amino acid per kg of body weight), carnitine wasting (mean fractional excretion, 0.05–0.15), phosphaturia, and bicarbonaturia.[33] Glucosuria is variably present as well. Linear growth decreases after 1 year of age. Glomerular function decreases with age, with end-stage kidney disease predicted between the second and fourth decade of life.

Neurologic findings include infantile hypotonia, mental retardation, and areflexia. Prenatal development of cataracts is universal, and other ocular anomalies are glaucoma, microphthalmos, and corneal keloid formation. Visual acuity is frequently decreased. Mental retardation is very common. Cranial magnetic resonance imaging (MRI) shows mild ventriculomegaly and cysts in the periventricular regions. Status epilepticus is also frequent. Life span rarely exceeds 40 years.

Some patients with a phenotype indistinguishable from Dent disease (see previous discussion in the "Dent Disease" section) carry mutations in the *OCRL1* gene and have an attenuated form of OCRL.[17]

The diagnosis is established in affected individuals by the demonstration of reduced (<10% of normal) activity of inositol polyphosphate 5-phosphatase OCRL-1 in cultured skin fibroblasts. Molecular genetic testing of *OCRL* detects mutations in approximately 95% of affected males and a similar proportion of carrier females.[39] Carrier detection by slit-lamp examination has high but not absolute sensitivity. Concentrations of the muscle enzymes creatine kinase, aspartate aminotransferase, and lactate dehydrogenase, as well as of total serum protein, serum $\alpha_2$-globulin, and high-density lipoprotein cholesterol, are elevated.

## TREATMENT

Treatment of OCRL is supportive and includes taking care of ocular (cataract extraction, treatment of glaucoma), neurologic (anticonvulsants, speech therapy), and renal complications. Nasogastric tube feedings or feeding gastrostomy and antipsychotic therapy may be required. Bicarbonate therapy is usually given at a dose of 2 to 3 mmol/kg/day every 6 to 8 hours, but may vary from 1 to 8 mmol/kg/day to maintain a serum bicarbonate concentration of 20 mmol/L. Sodium or potassium phosphate can be given in amounts of 1 to 4 g/day for phosphate depletion, and vitamin D may be added if that approach is unsuccessful.

## MISTARGETING TO MITOCHONDRIA OF PEROXISOMAL EHHADH, AN ENZYME INVOLVED IN PEROXISOMAL OXIDATION OF FATTY ACIDS

Peroxisomes were first identified by Christian de Duve, and it was originally thought that the primary function of these organelles was the metabolism of hydrogen peroxide. One of their main metabolic functions is β-oxidation of very-long-chain fatty acids (for review see Lodhi and Semenkovich[40]). An EHHADH (enoyl-CoA, hydratase/3-hydroxyacyl-CoA dehydrogenase) dominant mutant has been shown to mistarget to mitochondria and not to peroxisomes, impair mitochondrial oxidative phosphorylation, and cause renal Fanconi syndrome (Fig. 44.2).[41]

## IDIOPATHIC CAUSES OF RENAL FANCONI SYNDROME

Renal Fanconi syndrome occurs in the absence of both known inborn errors of metabolism and acquired causes. Sporadic and familial cases unlinked to *CLCN5* (Dent disease), *OCRL1* (Lowe syndrome), or EHHADH[41] have been described,[19] with variable progressive renal failure.[33,42,43]

## CYSTINOSIS

### PATHOGENESIS

Cystinosis is a rare autosomal recessive disease of lysosomal transport of the disulfide amino acid cystine.[44–46] Lysosomes are intracellular organelles containing enzymes responsible for the digestion of macromolecules. Lysosomal hydrolases are optimally active at low pH. The by-products of the hydrolytic digestion exit the lysosome through specific transporters. A defect in one of the lysosomal hydrolases results in the accumulation of macromolecules or by-products that lead to lysosomal, cellular, and eventually organ dysfunction. Inactivating mutations in the *CTNS* (cystinosis) gene on chromosome 17p13, encoding an integral lysosomal membrane protein termed *cystinosin*,[47] cause cystinosis. This lysosomal cystine transporter has seven transmembrane domains and at least two lysosomal targeting signals (GYDQL in the C terminus and YFPQA in the fifth intertransmembrane loop). Cystine is poorly soluble and forms crystals in the lysosomes, but the mechanisms leading to cellular dysfunction are not clear.[48]

### CLINICAL PRESENTATION

Cystinosis, which affects 1 in 100,000 to 1 in 200,000 newborns, is the most frequent cause of the inherited forms of renal Fanconi syndrome. The clinical presentation is variable[49,50] and encompasses classic nephropathic cystinosis (OMIM #219800), a rare "adolescent" form (OMIM #219900), and also a mild adult-onset variant (OMIM #219750; Table 44.3). The most severe form manifests in the first year of life as failure to thrive, increased thirst, polyuria, and poor feeding. Affected children of Caucasian parents are frequently blond-haired and have white skin, which may be explained by the role of cystinosin in melanogenesis.[51] Additional clinical findings include phosphaturia, rickets, aminoaciduria, glucosuria, hypouricemia, and bicarbonaturia. Renal wasting of sodium, calcium (leading to nephrocalcinosis), and magnesium and tubular proteinuria are usually present. If the cystinosis is not treated, progressive renal damage culminates in end-stage kidney disease by the end of the first decade of life.

Damage in multiple organ systems, including ocular, endocrine, hepatic, muscular, and central nervous, has been reported. Cystinosis can affect most of the structures of the eye, with variable rates of progression. In the cornea, crystal deposits are absent at birth and appear by the end of the first year of life. These can be seen by slit-lamp examination as fusiform crystals involving the anterior third of the central cornea and the full thickness of the peripheral cornea. Eventually, these deposits progress to develop a characteristic haziness. They can also be found in the iridis and conjunctiva as well as in the retina, with consequent development of a characteristic peripheral retinopathy.

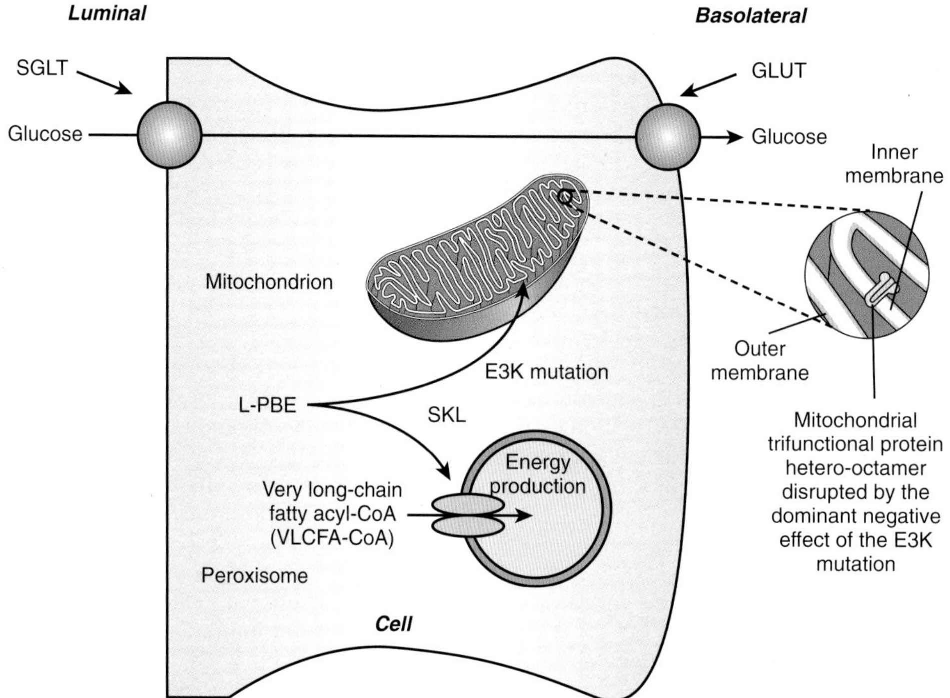


**Fig. 44.2** Proposed model of a dominant negative effect of mutant peroxisomal L-bifunctional enzyme disrupting the mitochondrial trifunctional protein heterooctamer in the renal proximal tubule. Glucose is reabsorbed from the luminal (urine-side) membranes to the basolateral (blood-side) membranes. Most of the basolateral fatty acid uptake is used for mitochondrial energy production by means of trifunctional protein. A small fraction of the fatty acid uptake is used for peroxisomal energy production by means of bifunctional protein (D-bifunctional enzyme [D-PBE]). The physiologic targeting motif, SKL (serine–lysine–leucine), normally directs L-bifunctional enzyme (L-PBE) to the peroxisome. The E3K mutation instead creates a targeting motif that directs L-PBE to the mitochondrion, where its homology causes it to interfere with the assembly and function of trifunctional protein. *GLUT,* Glucose transporter; *SGLT,* sodium-glucose linked transporter. (Modified from Klootwijk ED, Reichold M, Helip-Wooley A, et al. Mistargeting of peroxisomal EHHADH and inherited renal Fanconi's syndrome. *N Engl J Med.* 2014;370:129–138.)

**Table 44.3 Age-Related Clinical Characteristics of Untreated Nephropathic Cystinosis**

| Age (years) | Symptom or Sign | Prevalence of Affected Patients (%) |
|---|---|---|
| 6–12 months | Renal Fanconi syndrome (polyuria, polydipsia, electrolyte imbalance, dehydration, rickets, growth failure) | 95 |
| 5–10 | Hypothyroidism | 50 |
| 8–12 | Photophobia | 50 |
| 8–12 | Chronic renal failure | 95 |
| 12–40 | Myopathy, difficulty swallowing | 20 |
| 13–40 | Retinal blindness | 10–15 |
| 18–40 | Diabetes mellitus | 5 |
| 18–40 | Male hypogonadism | 70 |
| 21–40 | Pulmonary dysfunction | 100 |
| 21–40 | Central nervous system calcifications | 15 |
| 21–40 | Central nervous system symptomatic deterioration | 2 |

From Gahl WA, Thoene JG, Schneider JA. Cystinosis. *N Engl J Med.* 2002;347:111–121.

Other features include hypothyroidism from cystine crystallization in the follicular cells of the thyroid gland. It is present in more than 70% of patients older than 10 years. Insulin-dependent diabetes mellitus develops from long-standing cystine crystal accumulation in the pancreas, particularly after renal transplantation.[52] Hepatomegaly and splenomegaly with little clinical impact also occur in more than 40% of subjects older than 10 years.[49] A distal vacuolar myopathy is a late finding in 25% of cystinotic patients, with wasting in the small muscles of the hand. Facial weakness and dysphagia are often seen. In a previous study, muscle biopsies revealed marked fiber size variability, prominent acid phosphatase–positive vacuoles, and an absence of fiber-type grouping or inflammatory cells. Crystals of cystine were detected in cells of the perimysium but not within the muscle cell vacuoles. The muscle cystine content of clinically affected muscles is markedly elevated.[53] Central nervous system involvement has been described in the late stages of the disease,[45] and cystine crystal accumulation has been reported. The accumulation of intracellular cystine itself may also be a risk factor for vascular calcifications.[54]

The diagnosis is usually established by measuring the cystine content in peripheral leukocytes. Patients usually have values higher than 2 nmol of half-cystine per milligram of protein (normal <0.2 nmol). Alternatively, the diagnosis can be made through recognition of the characteristic corneal crystals on slit-lamp examination.

Approximately half of patients who have cystinosis and are of northern European descent carry at least one allele that bears a specific 57-kb deletion that encompasses the *CTNS* gene. Molecular analysis of the cystinosin gene allows early diagnosis and can be used for prenatal diagnosis as well. Prenatal diagnosis of cystinosis can also be made by measuring S-labeled cystine accumulation in cultured amniocytes or chorionic villi samples,[43] and by a direct measurement of cystine in uncultured chorionic villi samples. Over 90 mutations have been reported, with a detection ratio close to 100%.[55]

## TREATMENT

Patients with cystinosis who are treated at an early age are now expected to live a nearly normal life, but a limited access to cysteamine still exists in developing nations.[56] Before development of the cystine-depleting drug cysteamine, dialysis had to be initiated on average in patients reaching age 10. Cysteamine enters the lysosome by a specific transporter for aminothiols or aminosulfides and cleaves cystine into cysteine and a cysteine–cysteamine mixed disulfide (Fig. 44.3). Oral cysteamine is given at doses of 60 to 90 mg/kg per day every 6 hours and generally achieves approximately 90% depletion of cellular cystine, as measured in circulating leukocytes.[57] A long-acting form appears to have similar efficacy.[58] It slows the rate of progression of renal failure and increases growth in affected subjects.[59–61] Kidney function stabilizes on initiation of therapy, and even some recovery can be seen if therapy is begun in the first year or two of life.[60] The growth rate becomes normal, but there is no "catching up." Topical cysteamine eye drops[62] and a new gel formulation[63] are used to treat ocular complications of cystinosis; they cause dissolution of corneal crystals.

Symptomatic treatment also involves rehydration, particularly during episodes of gastroenteritis. Replacement of bicarbonate losses with citrate- or bicarbonate-containing salts is frequently necessary. Phosphate losses are replaced with phosphate salts and oral vitamin D therapy. Indomethacin has been used to decrease renal salt and water wasting. Recombinant human growth hormone increases growth but does not hasten the rate of progression of renal failure.[61] Kidney transplantation is routinely performed, and most recipients do well, although extrarenal late-onset complications will occur.[64] Kidneys from heterozygous family donors are widely accepted because there is no evidence of cystine accumulation in kidney transplants from such donors.

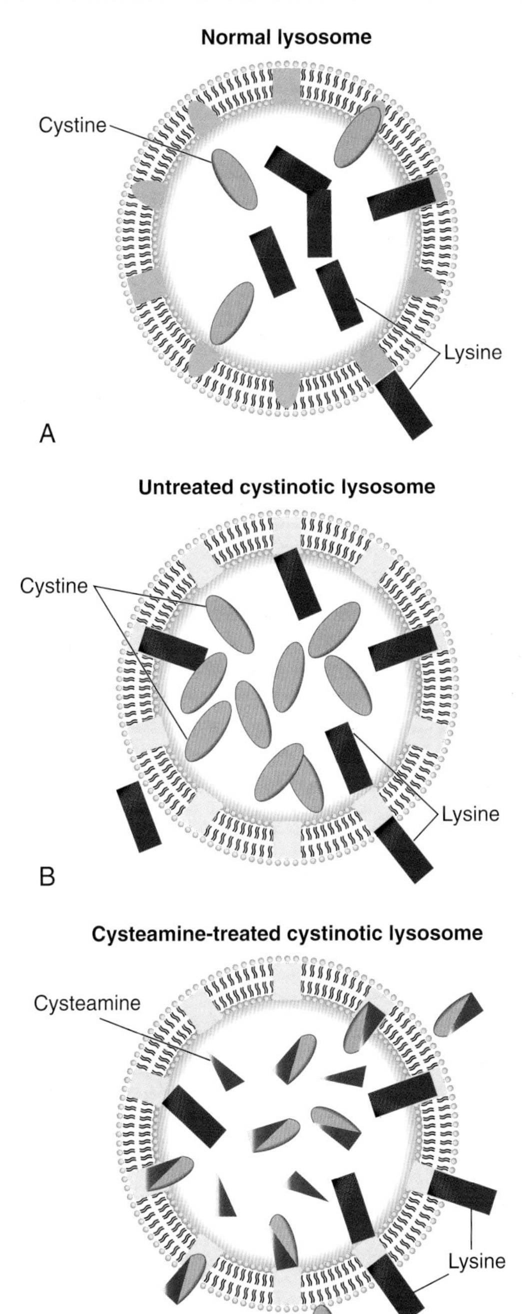


**Fig. 44.3** Mechanism of cystine depletion by cysteamine. (A) In normal lysosomes, cystine and lysine freely traverse the lysosomal membrane through specific transporters (*rectangles* for the lysine transporter; *ovals* for the cystine transporter). (B) In cystinotic lysosomes (note the absence of specific cystine transporters), lysine can freely traverse through specific transporters in the lysosomal membrane, but cystine cannot and therefore accumulates inside the lysosome. (C) In cysteamine-treated lysosomes, cysteamine combines with half-cystine (i.e., cysteine) to form the mixed disulfide cysteine–cysteamine, which uses the lysine transporter to exit the lysosome. (Modified from Gahl WA, Thoene JG, Schneider JA. Cystinosis. *N Engl J Med*. 2002;347:111–121. Copyright © 2002 Massachusetts Medical Society. All rights reserved. With permission.)

## GLYCOGENOSIS (VON GIERKE DISEASE, OMIM #232200)

Glycogen storage diseases are inherited disorders that affect glycogen metabolism (Fig. 44.4).[65] Both the liver and muscle store physiologically important quantities of glycogen. These organs are primarily affected, with the symptoms usually including hepatomegaly, hypoglycemia, muscle cramps and weakness, exercise intolerance, and fatigue. This section discusses type I glycogen storage disease because it is the only form associated with primary renal involvement. Type V glycogen storage disease (McArdle disease) as well as other rare glycogenoses associated with rhabdomyolysis, myoglobinuria, and acute tubular necrosis are not discussed further.

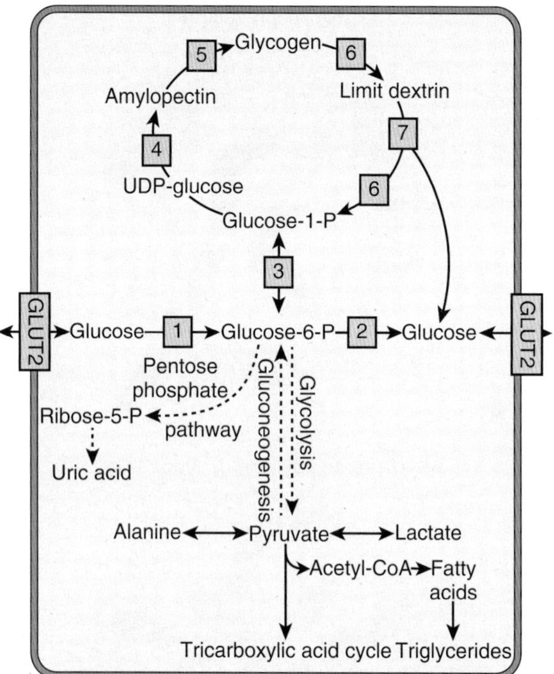


**Fig. 44.4** Simplified scheme of glycogen synthesis and breakdown. *1,* Hexokinase/glucokinase; *2,* glucose-6-phosphatase (G6Pase); *3,* phosphoglucomutase; *4,* glycogen synthase; *5,* branching enzyme; *6,* glycogen phosphorylase; *7,* debranching enzyme; *CoA,* coenzyme A; *GLUT2,* glucose transporter 2; *P,* phosphate; *UDP-glucose,* uridine diphosphoglucose. (From Wolfsdorf JI, Weinstein DA. Glycogen storage diseases. *Rev Endocr Metab Disord.* 2003;4:95–102.)

## PATHOGENESIS

Glycogen storage disease type I (GSD-I), also known as von Gierke disease, is a group of autosomal recessive metabolic disorders caused by deficiencies in the activity of the glucose-6-phosphatase (G6Pase) system that consists of at least two membrane proteins, the glucose-6-phosphate transporter (G6PT) and G6Pase.[65] G6PT and G6Pase work in concert to maintain glucose homeostasis. G6Pase catalyzes the hydrolysis of glucose-6-phosphate (G6P) to produce glucose and phosphate. GSD-Ia (G6Pase deficiency, 80% of cases)[66,67] is caused by deficiency in enzymatic activity. GSD-Ib is caused by mutations in G6PT, which translocates G6P from the cytoplasm to the lumen of the endoplasmic reticulum (ER). Other variants include GSD-Ic (defect in microsomal phosphate or pyrophosphate transport) and GSD-Id (defect in microsomal glucose transport). The molecular basis of these variants remains to be determined.

## CLINICAL PRESENTATION

GSD-I manifests as functional G6Pase deficiency, characterized by growth retardation, hypoglycemia, hepatomegaly, kidney enlargement, hyperlipidemia, hyperuricemia, and lactic acidemia. Patients with type Ib disease also suffer from chronic neutropenia and functional deficiencies of neutrophils and monocytes, resulting in recurrent bacterial infections as well as ulceration of the oral and intestinal mucosae. GSD-Ia manifests in the first year of life with hepatomegaly and/or hypoglycemic seizures with lactic acidosis. Hypoglycemia occurs because of impaired gluconeogenesis, glycogenolysis, and recycling of glucose through G6P to the glucose system. Adults usually present with hypoglycemic symptoms that are exacerbated by exercise and relieved by food. However, 48-hour fasting blood glucose levels are frequently normal.[68] The accumulation of G6P leads to an increase in glycolysis and lactic acidosis. Hyperuricemia and gout are caused by increased activity of hepatic adenosine monophosphate (AMP) deaminase and adenine nucleotide production, thus increasing uric acid production. Hyperuricemia also results from decreased renal excretion because urate competes with lactate for secretion in the proximal tubule. Gout occurs in adults but is rarely seen in children. An enlarged abdomen from hepatomegaly, short stature from impaired growth, and skin manifestations from dyslipidemia (xanthomas) are frequent findings. Dyslipidemia is a result of increased synthesis of very-low-density lipoprotein and low-density lipoprotein and decreased lipolysis. Impairment of platelet adhesion and aggregation with prolonged bleeding time lead to easy bruising and epistaxis.

A renal Fanconi syndrome occurs in GSD-I, with aminoaciduria, low-molecular-weight proteinuria, phosphaturia, and bicarbonaturia.[69,70] Renal disease is common in adult patients[71] with untreated GSD-I. It evolves slowly and is a late finding. In children, increased kidney size, hyperfiltration, and moderate proteinuria are common.[72] dRTA, hypocitraturia, hypercalciuria, and nephrocalcinosis with calcium nephrolithiasis can be variably associated,[73] but virtually all patients have impaired distal tubular acidification. The most common finding is focal and segmental glomerulosclerosis with tubulointerstitial atrophy. Glomerular changes include thickening, lamellation, and glycogen deposition in the glomerular basement membrane.[74]

The diagnosis of GSD-I is established by DNA testing of *G6PC* and *SLC37A4,* or rarely from liver biopsy.[75] A 1-mg intramuscular glucagon test can be used and the result is frequently abnormal (an increase in blood glucose level <4 mmol/L, usually at 30 minutes). Liver histology reveals prominent storage of glycogen and fat, large lipid vacuoles with hepatocyte distension, and steatosis with little fibrosis. Abnormally high glycogen levels are noted in liver biopsy samples. Electron microscopy shows moderate to large excesses of glycogen in the cytoplasm, often displacing the organelles in hepatocytes. Enzyme analysis of fresh and frozen samples can distinguish type Ia from type Ib GSD.

## TREATMENT

Life expectancy for patients with GSD-I has improved considerably. The treatment goal is to maintain normoglycemia to avoid the metabolic complications that are secondary to hypoglycemia and lactic acidosis. This can be accomplished at night with nasogastric feeding of glucose[76] or with orally administered uncooked cornstarch. A single dose of cornstarch (1.75–2.5 g/kg) at bedtime will maintain serum glucose concentrations above 3.9 mmol/L for 7 hours or longer in most young adults.[77] Because hypoglycemia and lactic acidosis occur in adults as well, treatment might also be indicated after childhood.[78] Guidelines for the management of GSD-I published by the European Study on Glycogen Storage Disease Type I[79] include a preprandial blood glucose level higher than 3.5 to 4.0 mmol/L (60–70 mg/dL), a urine lactate-to-creatinine ratio lower than 0.06 mmol/mmol, a serum uric acid concentration in the high normal range for age, a venous blood bicarbonate level above 20 mmol/L (20 mEq/L), a serum triglyceride concentration below 6.0 mmol/L (531 mg/dL), normal fecal alpha$_1$-antitrypsin concentration for GSD-Ib, and a body mass index within two standard deviations of normal. Enzyme replacement therapy is not currently available for GSD-I. Kidney transplantation has been successfully performed but does not correct the hypoglycemia.

## TYROSINEMIA

Hepatorenal tyrosinemia (tyrosinemia type I, OMIM #276700) is a rare autosomal recessive disorder caused by deficiency of fumarylacetoacetate hydrolase (FAH),[80] leading to the accumulation of fumarylacetoacetate (FAA) in body fluids and tissues, affecting principally the liver, kidneys, and peripheral nerves. The disorder is characterized by severe liver disease, which either causes liver failure in infancy or may take a more protracted course, with death often occurring during childhood or adolescence because of hepatocarcinoma.[81] Worldwide, the incidence is 1 in 100,000. The disorder is particularly prevalent in a genetic isolate in Canada (Saguenay-Lac-Saint-Jean), in which the carrier rate is 1 in 20 and the incidence is 1 in 2000.

### PATHOGENESIS

Mutations in the gene encoding FAH on chromosome 15q23-q25 are responsible for tyrosinemia type I.[82–86] The cellular toxicity is caused by accumulation of FAA, which apparently induces oxidative stress[87] and the release of cytochrome *c*, thus triggering the activation of the caspase cascade in hepatocytes as seen in affected animal models.[88] It is unlikely that tyrosine accumulation itself leads to the hepatic and renal manifestations of the disease, because hypertyrosinemia has been described in other settings without renal and liver involvement.

### CLINICAL PRESENTATION

Most patients present clinically in regions without a specific newborn screening program for tyrosinemia type 1, although a few may be identified because of affected siblings or abnormalities of plasma or urine amino acids. Renal involvement is almost always present in tyrosinemic subjects and is probably caused by succinylacetone toxicity.[89,90] It ranges from mild tubular dysfunction to renal failure. Hypophosphatemic rickets is the principal sign of tubular dysfunction, and acute decompensation can exacerbate the dysfunction. Generalized aminoaciduria is frequent. Nephrocalcinosis and nephromegaly can often be seen on renal ultrasonography.[91] Glucosuria and proteinuria are usually mild. GFR is frequently decreased. Tubular defects respond to diet but may be irreversible in chronic cases.

The liver is the main organ affected in tyrosinemia type I. Initially, liver dysfunction often affects coagulation factors, even before other signs of liver failure appear. In fact, jaundice and liver enzyme elevations are rare in the early stages of tyrosinemia. A common presentation mode is the "acute hepatic crisis," in which ascites, jaundice, and gastrointestinal bleeding are precipitated by an acute event such as an infection. Acute hepatic crises usually resolve spontaneously but on occasion progress to complete liver failure and encephalopathy. Cirrhosis eventually develops in most patients with the disease, and hepatocellular carcinoma is frequent in tyrosinemic subjects with chronic liver disease.[92] It is believed that toxic metabolites that accumulate in tyrosinemia, such as FAA, are mutagenic and contribute to the elevated rate of liver carcinoma.[93] Serial liver imaging (ultrasonography and/or MRI) is indicated. Neurologic crises are acute episodes of peripheral neuropathy with painful paresthesias and, eventually, autonomic dysfunction.[94]

The diagnosis of tyrosinemia type I is made with the detection of excess succinylacetone in urine or plasma. Succinylacetone can be detected in the biologic fluid of all untreated patients with the disorder. The increase in succinylacetone is typically detected by gas chromatography/mass spectroscopy of extracted organic acids. Confirmatory testing can be performed with the measurement of FAH in cultured skin fibroblasts or the documentation of pathogenic mutations from DNA. Enzymatic analysis of FAH is not readily available as a common clinical assay. Several laboratories perform DNA mutation analysis of the *FAH* gene. Molecular genetic studies may be needed for counseling, prenatal diagnosis, and family screening. One splice mutation is prevalent in French-Canadians, and more than 40 mutations are now known, reviewed by de Laet et al.[81]

### TREATMENT

Since 1992, nitisinone has been used in tyrosinemia.[95] It is an effective inhibitor of *p*-hydroxyphenylpyruvic acid oxidase that blocks an enzyme proximal in the catabolic pathway of tyrosine and prevents substrate from reaching the FAH enzyme. Thus the intracellular accumulation of toxic FAA and its eventual extracellular conversion to succinylacetone are prevented. A nutritionist skilled in metabolic disorders is essential to assist with the use of special formulas for infants and low-protein diet for older patients. At least 90% of patients with the acute form of tyrosinemia type I show response to nitisinone therapy. Unresponsive children require orthotopic liver transplantation, but carries a significant mortality rate (10% to 20%). The decision to perform liver transplantation depends on the patient's liver status and neurologic symptoms.[81] The renal dysfunction may persist following transplantation because the renal enzyme is still defective.[96]

## GALACTOSEMIA

Galactosemia is an autosomal recessive metabolic disorder in which the individual is unable to metabolize lactose to glucose.[97,98] Three disorders of galactose metabolism resulting in galactosemia have been described. Clinical manifestations appear after exposure to galactose and can produce failure to thrive, vomiting, inanition, liver disease, cataracts, and developmental delays.

### PATHOGENESIS

The genetic defect responsible for galactosemia may be a defect in galactose-1-phosphate uridyltransferase, galactokinase, or uridine diphosphate galactose-4-epimerase. All of these enzymes catalyze the reactions in the unique pathway converting galactose to glucose. *Classic galactosemia* (OMIM #230400), which affects approximately 1 in 30,000 to 60,000 live births, is the most frequent form. The underlying pathogenic basis of galactosemia remains poorly understood. Untreated and treated patients with galactosemia experience abnormal accumulation and/or depletion of certain metabolites. Specific abnormalities of glycosylation can also be demonstrated, suggesting that aberrant biosynthesis of glycoproteins and/or glycolipids may contribute not only to the acute but also to some of the long-term complications experienced by galactosemic patients.[98,99]

### CLINICAL PRESENTATION

The clinical manifestations of galactosemia range from cataracts caused by galactokinase deficiency to important toxicity syndromes inducing vomiting, diarrhea, jaundice, hepatomegaly, ascites, and sepsis. Tubular proteinuria, generalized aminoaciduria, and bicarbonaturia occur but may quickly disappear following withdrawal of galactose.

The diagnosis is suggested by elevation of galactose or galactose-1-phosphate in serum or of galactose in the urine. The definitive diagnosis is made by the demonstration of the enzyme deficiency in erythrocytes.[100,101] Prenatal diagnosis can be offered to parents with a family history of the disease.[102]

In the United States and many other industrialized nations, inclusion of galactosemia in the mandated panel of conditions tested during newborn screening has all but eliminated the acute presentation.

### TREATMENT

With early diagnosis and simple dietary intervention, galactosemia is no longer a lethal condition. The only therapy is a galactose-restricted diet, and initially all galactose must be removed from the diet as soon as the diagnosis is suspected.[101,103] A newborn with a positive screening result should immediately be started on a soy-based infant formula. In spite of the strict diet, long-term complications such as retarded mental development, verbal dyspraxia, motor abnormalities, and hypergonadotropic hypogonadism are frequently seen in patients with classic galactosemia.

## WILSON DISEASE

Wilson disease (OMIM #277900) is an autosomal recessive disorder in which biliary excretion of copper and its incorporation into ceruloplasmin are impaired, leading to liver, kidney, and corneal damage from accumulation of copper.[104] The frequency of the disease is approximately 1 to 3 per 100,000 live births.

### PATHOGENESIS

*ATP7B,* the gene responsible for Wilson disease, encodes a P-type ATPase, and is located on chromosome 13q14.3. More than 380 mutations in this gene have been identified in patients with Wilson disease worldwide. ATP7B protein regulates systemic copper levels by excreting excess copper into the bile[105–107] and is targeted to the ER and exocytic vesicles.[108]

### CLINICAL PRESENTATION

The primary consequence is liver disease. Most patients present with liver dysfunction, neurologic symptoms, or a combination of the two. Liver symptoms can take multiple forms, that is, chronic and acute liver failure. Copper accumulates in the liver, with progressive damage, and overflow to the brain. This causes central nervous system anomalies such as dysarthria and coordination defects of voluntary movements. Pseudobulbar palsy is frequent and is a common cause of death in undiagnosed cases. Psychiatric symptoms can encompass a spectrum of personality changes, depression, bipolar disorder, schizophrenia, and dementia.[109] Wilson disease should be suspected in all subjects with acute or chronic liver dysfunction.

Affected adults often show features of Fanconi syndrome, with aminoaciduria, bicarbonaturia, phosphaturia, glucosuria, and low-molecular-weight proteinuria,[110] probably from copper accumulation. Children do not frequently have renal manifestations. Hypercalciuria is common, and kidney stones and nephrocalcinosis have been described in several cases.[111–113] Ultrastructural findings on renal biopsies include electron-dense deposits in the tubular cytoplasm.[114]

The most useful laboratory tests for diagnostic purposes are those measuring 24-hour urinary copper excretion, and concentrations of hepatic copper, serum-free copper, and ceruloplasmin. Increased liver copper level (>300 mg/g dry weight) is a reliable finding. The Kayser–Fleischer ring is an important clinical sign for making the diagnosis; it is seen in 50% of patients with liver dysfunction and in 90% of those with neurologic disease.[115] This ring is a yellow-brown (dull copper colored) granular deposit on Descemet membrane at the limbus of the cornea, usually seen earliest at the upper and lower poles. Given the variability of the biochemical and clinical features of Wilson disease, mutation analysis is becoming more and more essential to confirm a suspicion of the disorder.[104] Molecular genetic diagnosis is available.[116] The lack of genotype–phenotype correlation remains unexplained, the causes of fulminant liver failure are not known, and the treatment of neurologic symptoms is only partially successful.[117]

### TREATMENT

Wilson disease is universally fatal if untreated. D-Penicillamine, which mobilizes copper and forms copper–penicillamine complexes that are excreted in the urine, is very effective.[118] Adults usually require 1 g/day divided in two doses, but it is best to start with small doses (125 mg/day) to avoid hypersensitivity reactions. Twenty-four-hour urinary excretion of copper should be monitored to achieve copper losses of 2 mg/day. Doses of D-penicillamine can be decreased after 1 or 2 years to achieve urinary losses of 1 mg/day. Alternative treatments include trientine, a copper chelator which can be used as a first-line treatment[119] or in case of D-penicillamine intolerance. Prevention of reaccumulation of copper can be achieved by zinc salts, which block intestinal copper absorption by inducing metallothionein synthesis in the mucosal intestinal cells. Tetrathiomolybdate, a copper chelator, appears to be an excellent form of initial treatment in patients with neurologic symptoms and signs. In contrast to penicillamine therapy, initial treatment with tetrathiomolybdate can often be effective in preventing further neurologic deterioration.[120]

Patients should be considered for liver transplantation when suitable medical therapy has failed or for the development of acute liver failure, when there is no time for other therapies to take effect. Patients with a combination of hepatic and neuropsychiatric conditions warrant careful neurologic assessment, but liver transplantation is contraindicated only in cases of severe neurologic impairment.[104]

## HEREDITARY FRUCTOSE INTOLERANCE

There are several disorders of fructose metabolism, secondary to deficiencies in aldolase B (OMIM #229600), fructose-1-phosphate aldolase, and fructokinase, respectively.[121] Aldolase B is found primarily in the liver and is involved in the metabolism of fructose so this sugar can be used as energy. Fructose-1-phosphate accumulation in liver cells results from enzyme dysfunction.

Hereditary fructose intolerance is an autosomal recessive disorder characterized by vomiting shortly after the intake of fructose. The disease can be associated with proximal tubule dysfunction and lactic acidosis. Kidney biopsies show discrete findings. Liver dysfunction, hepatomegaly, cirrhosis, and jaundice appear from prolonged exposure. Unfortunately, hypoglycemia is frequently absent. Continued ingestion of noxious sugars leads to hepatic and renal injury and growth retardation. The most common mutation has a prevalence of 1.3%, suggesting a frequency of 1 in 23,000 homozygotes.[122] Because of the difficulty in making the diagnosis, genetic analysis is useful.[123]

The pathophysiology of renal Fanconi syndrome is not clear, but could be related to vacuolar proton pump dysfunction in the proximal tubule, because a direct binding interaction between V-ATPase and aldolase was demonstrated for the regulation of the V-ATPase. This study showed that aldolase B was abundant in endocytosis zones of the proximal tubule, a subcellular domain also abundant in V-ATPase.[124] V-ATPases are essential for acidification of intracellular compartments and for proton secretion from the plasma membrane in kidney epithelial cells and osteoclasts. Perhaps the release of nonfunctional aldolase B in response to fructose ingestion impairs the coupling of the V-ATPase to glycolysis. For these reasons, mechanistic similarities in organelle dysfunction between Dent disease and hereditary fructose intolerance are apparent.

The management of hereditary fructose intolerance involves withdrawal of sucrose, fructose, and sorbitol from the diet.

## INHERITED DISORDERS OF RENAL AMINO ACID TRANSPORT

Proteins ingested in the regular diet and degraded in the intestine are absorbed by the mucosa as amino acids and small oligopeptides. Intestinal apical and basolateral transporters carry the amino acids into the blood, where they are used for metabolic needs, but are also freely filtered by the kidneys as they are not significantly bound to proteins in the plasma (except for tryptophan, which is 60%–90% bound). The proximal tubule reabsorbs 95% to 99.9% of the filtered load (reviewed elsewhere[125]). Thus the excretion of more than 5% of the filtered load of an amino acid is abnormal, except for histidine, which has a fractional excretion of 5%.[126] Renal amino acid reabsorption occurs in the proximal tubule through a variety of transporters. Most amino acids are reabsorbed by more than one transporter. Amino acids can share transporters with low affinity but high transport capacity and have a specific transporter for one amino acid that has a high affinity and low maximal transport capacity. Common carriers have been divided into five groups, which transport neutral and cyclic amino acids, glycine and imino acids, cystine and dibasic amino acids, dicarboxylic amino acids, and β-amino acids.[126] The transport of amino acids is coupled to the sodium gradient established by the basolateral $Na^+$–$K^+$–ATPase.

Aminoaciduria occurs when a renal transport defect of the proximal tubule decreases the reabsorptive capacity for one or several amino acids or when the threshold for reabsorbing an amino acid is exceeded when its plasma concentration is elevated as a result of a metabolic defect (overflow aminoaciduria).[127] This latter category is not discussed in this section. Theoretically, renal aminoacidurias can be secondary to defects in brush border or basolateral transporters and intracellular trafficking of amino acids (see also Chapter 8). They are usually detected by newborn urine screening programs, and the most frequent abnormalities identified (apart from phenylketonuria, now normally detected by blood screening) are cystinuria, histidinemia, Hartnup disease, and iminoglycinuria (Fig. 44.5).[128] Clinically, the most significant renal aminoaciduria is cystinuria (Table 44.4). In the past 10 years, all major apical neutral amino acid transporters have been identified on a molecular level.[129] This has considerably improved our understanding of inherited aminoacidurias and helped explain some of the features of Fanconi syndrome.

## CYSTINURIA

Cystinuria (OMIM #220200) is the most frequent and best known of the aminoacidurias.[130] Worldwide, the prevalence is approximately 1 in 7000 and varies according to geographic location, being 1 in 15,000 in the United States,[131] 1 in 2000 in England,[132] 1 in 4000 in Australia,[133] and 1 in 2500 in Jews of Libyan origin.[134] Newborn screening programs worldwide now help identify cases. The existence of cystinuria has been recognized since 1810,[135,136] first suspected in two patients with bladder stones, hence the name—cystic oxide and cystine to characterize their chemical composition. It is an autosomal recessive disorder associated with defective apical membrane transport of cystine and of the dibasic amino acids, ornithine, lysine, and arginine. It involves the epithelial cells of the renal tubule and gastrointestinal tract (Fig. 44.5). The formation of cystine calculi in the urinary tract is the hallmark of the disorder. Cystine is the least soluble of the naturally occurring amino acids, particularly at low pH.

### PATHOGENESIS

Cystinuria is caused by mutations in the genes that encode the two subunits that form a heterodimer—neutral and basic amino acid transport protein rBAT and $b^{(0,+)}$-type amino acid transporter 1—of the amino acid transport system $b^{(0,+)}$.[130] By itself, the subunit $b^{0,+}$AT is sufficient to catalyze transmembrane amino acid exchange (i.e., the exchange of dibasic amino acids for neutral amino acids).[137] A model for the reabsorption of cystine and dibasic amino acids is shown in Fig. 44.6. Cystinuria also manifests as defective intestinal absorption of dibasic amino acids, implying that there is a transporter defect in the gut similar to that in the renal proximal tubule cells.[130] Why defective intestinal amino acid transport does not lead to more serious metabolic problems is not known, but the reason could be either the ability of the intestine to absorb small (di- and tri-) peptides or the presence of other transporters of dibasic amino acids in the gut.

### CLINICAL PRESENTATION

Cystinuria is classified according to the gene responsible, but this classification currently has no clinical utility. Type

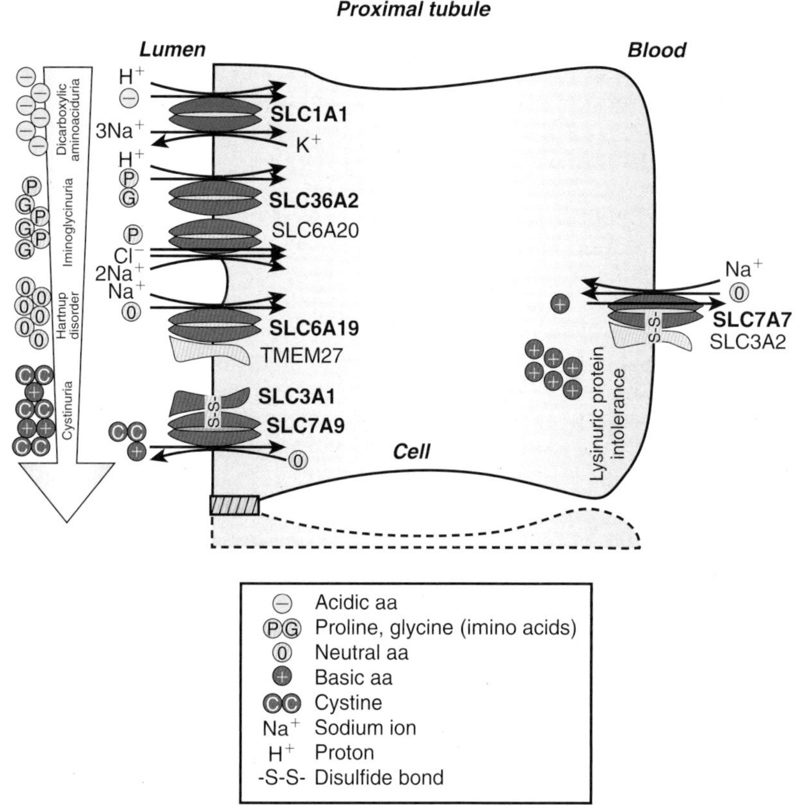


**Fig. 44.5** A model of the renal proximal tubule, illustrating the principal epithelial transporters involved in amino acid reabsorption, which are mutated in human aminoacidurias. A cross section of the proximal convoluted tubule is represented. Four of the aminoacidurias—dicarboxylic aminoaciduria (DA), iminoglycinuria, Hartnup disorder, and cystinuria—manifest at the apical surface of the renal tubule, whereas lysinuric protein intolerance manifests at the basolateral surface. Mutations in the high-affinity glutamate and aspartate transporter SLC1A1 are responsible for DA.[176] Iminoglycinuria results from complete inactivation of SLC36A2, a proline and glycine transporter, or from additional modifying mutations in the high-affinity proline transporter SLC6A20 when SLC36A2 is not completely inactivated.[175] (From Broer S, Bailey CG, Kowalczuk S, et al. Iminoglycinuria and hyperglycinuria are discrete human phenotypes resulting from complex mutations in proline and glycine transporters. *J Clin Invest.* 2008;118:3881–3892.) Mutations in the neutral amino acid transporter SLC6A19 are responsible for Hartnup disorder.[173,353] The neutral amino acid transport defect can also be exacerbated by a kidney-specific loss of heterodimerization of mutant SLC6A19 with TMEM27.[354] Cystinuria has a heterogeneous phenotype and arises from mutations in individual or both subunits of the disulfide bridge–linked heterodimer comprising the type II membrane protein SLC3A1[355] and the cystine and basic amino acid transporter SLC7A9.[356] Lysinuric protein intolerance[161,167] results from mutations in the basolaterally expressed basic amino acid transporter SLC7A7, which forms a disulfide bridge–linked heterodimer with type II membrane protein SLC3A2. *aa,* Amino acid. (Modified from Bailey CG, Ryan RM, Thoeng AD, et al. Loss-of-function mutations in the glutamate transporter SLC1A1 cause human dicarboxylic aminoaciduria. *J Clin Invest.* 2011;121:446–453.)

A cystinuria (also called type I; OMIM #220100) is caused by mutations in the *SLC3A1* gene (chromosome 2). It is a completely recessive disease because heterozygote parents excrete normal amounts of cystine (0–100 mmol/g creatinine). Jejunal uptake of cystine and dibasic amino acids is absent, and there is no plasma response to an oral cystine load. The risk of nephrolithiasis is very high. The *SLC3A1* gene encodes the renal proximal tubule S3 segment and intestinal dibasic rBAT amino acid transporter (Fig. 44.6).[138] More than 100 different mutations have been reported to date.[130] The most common point mutation, the M467T and its relative M467K, results in retention of the transporter in the ER with impaired maturation and export to the plasma membrane.[139]

Type B cystinuria (also called non–type I cystinuria; OMIM #600918) is an incompletely recessive form caused by mutations in the *SLC7A9* gene encoding BAT1 and located on chromosome 19q13. Both parents excrete intermediate amounts of cystine (100–600 mmol/g creatinine) but may also have a normal pattern. More than 90 mutations have been identified.[130] BAT1 is a subunit linked to the rBAT through a disulfide bond. It belongs to a family of light subunits of amino acid transporters, expressed in the kidney, liver, small intestine, and placenta. Cotransfection of $b^{0,+}$AT and rBAT brings the latter to the plasma membrane, and results in the uptake of L-arginine in vitro.

Type AB cystinuria is caused by one mutation in *SLC3A1* and one mutation in *SLC7A9*, but this digenic inheritance is exceptional. The observed prevalence of AB cystinuria is low because patients present with a mild phenotype and escape detection.

The only known manifestation of cystinuria is nephrolithiasis. Cystine stones account for 1% to 2% of all kidney stones (5% in children), and cystinuria should be suspected in all staghorn calculi.[140] Clinical expression of the disease frequently starts between the first and third decades of life but may occur any time from the first year up to the ninth decade. The disease occurs equally in both sexes, but male

**Table 44.4 Classification of the Aminoacidurias**

| Aminoaciduria | Gene | Gene Name | Protein | Chromosome | Hallmark (Amino Acid[s] Elevated in Urine) |
|---|---|---|---|---|---|
| Cystinuria A | *SLC3A1* | Solute carrier family 3 (cystine, dibasic, and neutral amino acid transporters, activator of cystine, dibasic, and neutral amino acid transport), member 1 | rBAT | 2p21 | Cystine, lysine, arginine, ornithine |
| Cystinuria B | *SLC7A9* | Solute carrier family 7 (cationic amino acid transporter, $y^+$ system), member 9 | $b^{0,+}AT$ | 19q13.11 | Cystine, lysine, arginine, ornithine |
| Cystinuria AB | *SLC3A1/SLC7A9* | | | | Cystine, lysine, arginine, ornithine |
| Lysinuric protein intolerance | *SLC7A7* | Solute carrier family 7 (cationic amino acid transporter, $y^+$ system), member 7 | $y^+LAT1$ | 14q11.2 | Lysine, arginine, ornithine |
| Hartnup disorder | *SLC6A19* | Solute carrier family 6 (neutral amino acid transporter), member 19 | $B^0AT1$ | 5p15.33 | Neutral amino acids |
| Iminoglycinuria | *SLC36A2* | Solute carrier family 36 (imino and glycine transporter), member 2 | PAT2 | 5q33.1 | Proline, hydroxyproline, glycine |
| Dicarboxylic aminoaciduria | *SLC1A1* | Solute carrier family 1 | $EAAT_3$ | 9p24 | Aspartate, glutamate |

Modified from Tanzi RE, Petrukhin K, Chernov I, et al. The Wilson disease gene is a copper transporting ATPase with homology to the Menkes disease gene. *Nat Genet.* 1993;5:344–350.

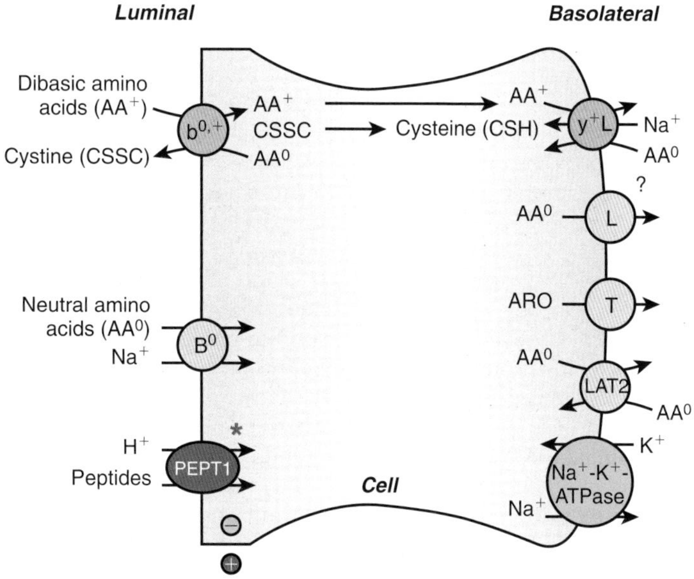


**Fig. 44.6** Trafficking of cystine and dibasic amino acids in epithelial cells of the renal proximal tubule or small intestine. The apical transport system $b^{0,+}$ mediates influx of $AA^+$ and CSSC in exchange for $AA^0$. The $Na^+$-dependent transporter $B^0$ is believed to be the major apical contributor to the high intracellular content of $AA^0$ exploited by $b^{0,+}$. In the small intestine (but not in kidney), uptake of dipeptides and tripeptides through apical $H^+$-dependent solute carrier family 15 member 1 (PEPT1) compensates the defective absorption of $AA^+$ and CSSC. $AA^+$ exits the basolateral membrane through system $y^+L$, mutations in which cause lysinuric protein intolerance. The basolateral efflux of CSH and $AA^0$ are not well understood. The general $AA^0$ exchanger LAT2 and the aromatic transporter T have been suggested to participate in the excretion of CSH and aromatic amino acids *(ARO)*. In addition, an unidentified transporter L for unidirectional efflux of $AA^0$ is believed to have a role in $AA^0$ reabsorption. *Only in intestinal cells. (Modified from Chillaron J, Font-Llitjos M, Fort J, et al. Pathophysiology and treatment of cystinuria. *Nat Rev Nephrol.* 2010;6:424–434.)

patients tend to be more severely affected. Cystine stones are made of a yellow-brown substance, are very hard, and appear radiopaque on radiographs because of their sulfur molecules. Stones are frequently multiple and staghorn, and they tend to be smoother than calcium stones. Magnesium ammonium phosphate and calcium stones can also form as a result of infection.

Diagnosis can be made through the analysis of a simple urine sample in which typical hexagonal crystals appear. Acidification of concentrated urine with acetic acid can also precipitate crystals not initially visible. Diagnosis is ultimately made from the measurement of cystine excretion in the urine usually performed in specialized centers. Molecular diagnosis is not necessary.

## TREATMENT

Cystine stone formers have significantly higher procedure rates than other stone formers, but procedure rates decline with time. The lower creatinine clearance suggests that the need for procedures is high and that close follow-up and treatment to prevent recurrences are important.[141]

Unfortunately, there have been few advances in the treatment. A regularly followed medical program based on high diuresis and alkalinization with a second-line addition of thiols slows down stone formation and precludes the need for urologic procedures in more than half of patients.[142] Patients who are poorly compliant with hyperdiuresis remain at risk for recurrence.

### Diet

Cystine production arises from the metabolism of methionine. Previous attempts at reducing methionine in the diet have been both uncomfortable and of limited usefulness.[143,144] Reducing sodium in the diet results in lower urine cystine.[145–147]

### Decreasing Urine Cystine Saturation

A combination of increasing both fluid intake and urine pH usually decreases urine cystine saturation. Fluid intake should ideally reach 4 L/day, because many cystinuric patients excrete 1 g/day or more of cysteine.[142] It is also important for patients to drink at bedtime and during sleep (using an alarm clock helps) to prevent supersaturation during periods of reduced urine output.[148] Cystine solubility can be increased by alkalinization of the urine with potassium citrate or bicarbonate, but the solubility of cystine does not increase until the pH reaches 7.0 to 7.5. Use of citrate is the preferred method because alkalinization lasts longer. The requirements for alkali often reach 3 to 4 mmol/kg/day.

### Penicillamine

Patients who are unable to comply with a regimen of high fluid intake and urine alkalinization or in whom adequate treatment fails may be given D-penicillamine in doses of 30 mg/kg per day up to a maximum of 2 g. Through a disulfide exchange reaction, D-penicillamine can form the disulfide cysteine–penicillamine, which is much more soluble than cystine. D-Penicillamine is associated with frequent side effects such as rash, fever, and, more rarely, arthralgias and medullary aplasia, leading to a significant proportion of patients discontinuing therapy.[149–152] Other reactions include proteinuria and membranous nephropathy, epidermolysis, and loss of taste. Inhibition of pyridoxine by D-penicillamine is also a potential side effect.[153]

Another drug that may be useful in cystinuria is mercaptopropionylglycine, with recommended dosing ranges of 400 to 1200 mg/day in three divided doses.[154,155] Identical in mechanism of action to D-penicillamine, mercaptopropionylglycine is as effective in reducing urine cystine excretion. Side effects are similar to D-penicillamine. Finally, captopril has been advocated as a potential treatment for cystinuria, but its efficacy is controversial.

### Surgical Management

Patients with cystinuria frequently require stone-removing procedures.[156] It is important to achieve a stone-free state because recurrent stone activity has been demonstrated to be higher in those with residual calculi.[157] The type of procedure does not impact recurrence rates. The introduction of extracorporeal shockwave lithotripsy has not been of great benefit to cystinuric patients. Cystine stones are hard and have proved difficult to pulverize. Consequently, percutaneous lithotripsy is more effective and is the preferred approach. Progress in urologic treatment of kidney stones has decreased the need for open surgery.[158] Urinary alkalinization, as well as direct irrigation of the urinary tract with D-penicillamine, *N*-acetylpenicillamine, or tromethamine to form disulfide compounds, has resulted in the dissolution of stones, but this approach requires irrigation for several weeks with a risk for potential complications of catheterization and has been largely abandoned.

Transplantation is sometimes necessary for patients with terminal renal failure from chronic obstruction or infection (or both). A kidney from an unaffected donor will not form cystine stones once transplanted.

# LYSINURIC PROTEIN INTOLERANCE

## PATHOGENESIS

Lysinuric protein intolerance (LPI; OMIM #222700) is a very rare recessively inherited dibasic amino acid transport disorder, mostly reported in Finland,[159,160] but also present in Japan and Italy. It is caused by defective basolateral membrane efflux of the cationic amino acids lysine, arginine, and ornithine in intestinal, hepatic, and renal tubular epithelia from inactivating mutations in *SLC7A7*.[161,162] *SLC7A7* encodes a 511–amino acid protein, $y^+$LAT-1, predicted to harbor 12 membrane-spanning domains, with both amino and carboxy termini located intracellularly. This protein is thought to be part of the $y^+$L multimeric unit. Cationic amino acid transport occurs through five different systems: $y^+$, $y^+$L, $b^+$, $b^{0+}$, and $B^{0+}$. Defective system $y^+$L transport explains the abnormality in cationic amino acid transport as it mediates sodium-independent high-affinity transport of cationic amino acids and the transport of zwitterionic amino acids with low affinity. It is responsible for renal reabsorption and intestinal absorption of dibasic amino acids at the basolateral membranes. $y^+$L transport is induced by a cell surface glycoprotein heavy chain (4F2hc) that represents the heavy-chain subunit of a disulfide-linked heterodimer.[159] The amino acid deficiency in LPI leads to impaired urea cycle and postprandial hyperammonemia.

## CLINICAL PRESENTATION

Infants with LPI are usually asymptomatic while breastfeeding. After weaning, they show protein aversion, a delay in bone growth, and prominent osteoporosis, hepatosplenomegaly, muscle hypotonia, and sparse hair. Jaundice, hyperammonemia, coma, and metabolic acidosis occur. Micronodular cirrhosis develops from protein malnutrition, and pulmonary alveolar proteinosis is an occasional finding.[163,164] Several immunologic abnormalities have been described[165] and are possibly secondary to low levels of arginine, the substrate for nitric oxide synthase and nitric oxide production.[166]

Various renal disorders, including immunoglobulin A (IgA) nephropathy, are associated with LPI.[167] The urinary excretion of lysine and all cationic amino acids is increased, and plasma levels are decreased. The biochemical diagnosis can be uncertain, requiring confirmation by DNA testing. So far, approximately 50 different mutations have been identified in the *SLC7A7* gene.[168]

### TREATMENT

The current treatment of LPI involves moderate protein restriction as well as supplementation with 3 to 8 g of citrulline daily during meals and lysine.[169] Citrulline is transported by a different pathway from that of dibasic amino acids and can be converted to ornithine and arginine in the liver. Lysine cannot be made from citrulline.

## HARTNUP DISORDER

### PATHOGENESIS

Described initially in 1956 in the Hartnup family, Hartnup disorder (OMIM #234500) is an autosomal recessive and usually benign condition, consisting of excessive urinary excretion of the monoamino, monocarboxylic (neutral) amino acids alanine, asparagine, glutamine, histidine, isoleucine, leucine, methionine, phenylalanine, serine, threonine, tryptophan, tyrosine, and valine. Its incidence has been estimated at 1 in 26,000 in newborn screening programs.[170] Hartnup disorder is caused by mutations in the neutral amino acid transporter $B^0AT1$ (*SLC6A19*).[171] The transporter is found in the kidney and intestine, where it is involved in the resorption of all neutral amino acids.[129] Knockout *SLC6A19* mice have improved glycemic control and pharmacological inhibitors could be a suitable target to treat type 2 diabetes.[172]

### CLINICAL PRESENTATION

Most newborns identified prospectively by genetic screening programs as having Hartnup disorder have been completely asymptomatic. In affected individuals there is also a decreased intestinal absorption of neutral amino acids, particularly tryptophan. The clinical features of this disorder, if any, are caused by deficiency of nicotinamide, which is partly derived from tryptophan. They include a photosensitive erythematous rash (pellagra-like) clinically identical with that seen in niacin deficiency, intermittent cerebellar ataxia, and, rarely, mental retardation. Emotional instability, psychosis, and depression have been rarely noted, particularly during episodes of ataxia. Although in the Hartnup family there were several cases with mental retardation, most affected subjects described subsequently have not had mental retardation. Hartnup disorder should be suspected in all subjects with pellagra and unexplained intermittent ataxia. Siblings of affected patients should be screened as well. Clinical manifestations can be triggered by periods of inadequate dietary intake or increased metabolic needs. For example, a young woman presenting with pellagra precipitated by prolonged lactation and increased activity was diagnosed with Hartnup disorder.[173]

The diagnosis is easily made with a urinary aminogram, which shows increased excretion of neutral amino acids but not of glycine, cystine, or dibasic, dicarboxylic, or imino amino acids. Thus any confusion with renal Fanconi syndrome is avoided through a complete evaluation of amino acids in the urine using one of several chromatographic methods. The pattern of amino acid excretion, rather than the total amount, is the determining factor. The reabsorption defect involves 12 amino acids, and most patients with Hartnup disorder have the same pattern of aminoaciduria. The levels of amino acids in the monoamino and dicarboxylic group (such as glutamic acid and aspartic acid), and basic group (lysine, ornithine, arginine) are normal or slightly increased. The excretion of proline, hydroxyproline, and cystine is also normal. In spite of the defect, substantial reabsorption of the involved amino acids occurs through other transporters.

### TREATMENT

Treatment of symptomatic cases involves the administration of nicotinamide in doses of 50 to 300 mg/day. The value of treating asymptomatic cases is not known, but given the harmlessness of the treatment, this might be a rational choice.

## IMINOGLYCINURIA

Familial iminoglycinuria (OMIM #242600) is a benign autosomal recessive disorder with no clinical symptoms, in which the main interest is that it suggests the presence of a common carrier for the imino acids, proline and hydroxyproline, as well as glycine.[174] Iminoglycinuria was discovered after the application of chromatographic methods to the investigation of disorders of amino acid metabolism. *SLC36A2*, the gene encoding proton amino acid transporter 2 (PAT2), has been identified as the major gene responsible for iminoglycinuria.[175] Mutations in *SLC36A2* that retain residual transport activity result in the iminoglycinuria phenotype when combined with mutations in the gene encoding the imino acid transporter *SLC6A20*. Additional mutations have been identified in the genes encoding the putative glycine transporter SLC6A18 (XT2) and the neutral amino acid transporter SLC6A19 ($B^0AT1$) in families with either iminoglycinuria or hyperglycinuria, suggesting that mutations in the genes encoding these transporters may also contribute to these phenotypes.

The diagnosis is usually suggested by increased urinary excretion of imino acids and glycine. Newborns and infants usually excrete detectable amounts of imino acids and glycine for up to 3 months. Thus the presence of increased urinary excretion of imino acids and glycine in infants older than 6 months can be considered abnormal.

## DICARBOXYLIC AMINOACIDURIA

Dicarboxylic aminoaciduria (OMIM #222730) is an autosomal recessive disorder with, in a limited number of cases, an association with mental retardation. It is secondary to loss-of-function mutations in the glutamate transporter SLC1A1, a high-affinity anionic amino acid transporter expressed in the kidney and a wide variety of epithelial tissues, the brain, and the eye.[176]

# INHERITED DISORDERS OF RENAL PHOSPHATE TRANSPORT

Inherited disorders of renal phosphate transport are hypophosphatemic conditions caused by a reduction in renal tubule reabsorption of phosphate[177] with frequent metabolic bone disease manifesting as rickets in childhood and osteomalacia in adults.

## RENAL PHOSPHATE EXCRETION

Determinants of inorganic phosphate (Pi) homeostasis are ingestion, intestinal absorption, and renal excretion. In a steady state, urine Pi excretion reflects dietary intake. Normal phosphate intake in adults varies from 800 to 1600 mg/day, and average serum phosphate levels remain normal over a wide range of intake. Unlike dietary calcium, ingested phosphate is generally efficiently absorbed (65%–90% in children) from the gastrointestinal tract, although complex plant phosphate (phytate) is almost totally excreted. Most dietary phosphate is absorbed by passive concentration-dependent processes, but the active metabolite of vitamin D increases intestinal Pi absorption marginally. Contrary to active calcium absorption, which is greatest in the duodenum with a lower rate in the jejunum, ileum, and colon, active Pi absorption is highest in the jejunum and ileum with a lower rate in the duodenum and colon.[178]

Inorganic phosphate is filtered by the glomerulus and reabsorbed in the proximal tubule. The difference between the amounts of Pi filtered and reabsorbed determines the net appearance of Pi in the urine. Phosphate reabsorption by the proximal tubule occurs by a Tm-limited active process. The fractional reabsorption of filtered phosphate is usually estimated by the tubular reabsorption of Pi (TRP). There is a simple equation to assess the renal tubular phosphate transport, as follows:

$$TRP = \frac{(1 - U_P \times P_{Cr})}{U_{Cr} \times P_P}$$

where $P_{Cr}$ and $P_P$ are plasma creatinine and phosphate concentrations, respectively; and $U_{Cr}$ and $U_P$ are urine creatinine and phosphate concentrations, respectively. Given normal renal function and normal diet, the TRP is usually above 85%. A more precise way of estimating the tubular reabsorption of Pi is to calculate the theoretical threshold, as follows:

$$\frac{Tm_P}{GFR} = P_P - \frac{(U_P \times P_{Cr})}{U_{Cr}}$$

### RENAL PHOSPHATE TRANSPORTERS

Inorganic phosphate is reabsorbed almost exclusively in the renal proximal tubule through a transcellular pathway.[179] The limiting step of this transepithelial transport system is the entry of phosphate at the apical domain of proximal tubular cells. This process requires sodium–phosphate cotransporters that use the inward sodium gradient established and maintained by the activity of $Na^+$–$K^+$–ATPase (Fig. 44.7). See Chapter 7 for more detailed discussions. There are three types of

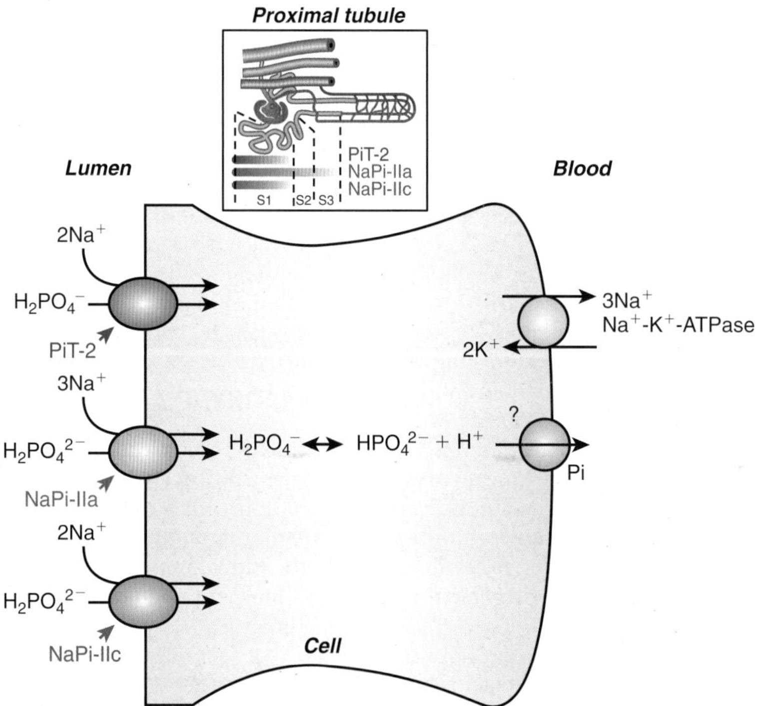


**Fig. 44.7** Cross section of mammalian kidney and schematic representation of renal tubular phosphate reabsorption in segments of the proximal tubule (S1, S2, and S3) through sodium–phosphate cotransporters. This task is accomplished by two distinct families of sodium-dependent phosphate transporters, one being NaPi-IIa/NaPi-IIc and the other PiT-2, which are expressed in the luminal membrane of proximal tubular cells. The number of sodium–phosphate cotransporter units of NPT2a/c expressed at the membrane is regulated by parathyroid hormone (PTH) and fibroblast growth factor-23 (FGF-23). NaPi-IIa and NaPi-IIc prefer transport divalent $P_i$ ($HPO_4^{2-}$), whereas PiT-2 prefers monovalent $P_i$ ($H_2PO_4^-$). The basolateral exit pathway remains unknown. The basolaterally localized $Na^+$–$K^+$–ATPase maintains an inwardly directed $Na^+$ gradient to drive cotransport. *ATPase,* Adenosine triphosphatase. (Modified from Biber J, Hernando N, Forster I. Phosphate transporters and their function. *Annu Rev Physiol.* 2013;75:535–550.)

sodium–phosphate cotransporters (members of the SLC34 and SLC20 families) at the apical (brush border) renal proximal tubular cells.[178] The putative proteins responsible for basolateral $P_i$ flux have not been identified. The transport mechanism of the two kidney-specific SLC34 proteins (NaPi-IIa and NaPi-IIc) and of the ubiquitously expressed SLC20 protein (PiT-2) has been studied by heterologous expression to reveal important differences in kinetics, stoichiometry, and substrate specificity. NaPi-IIa is central to renal phosphate reabsorption and phosphate balance. It is found almost exclusively in the apical membrane of renal proximal tubular cells. The amount of NaPi-IIa protein at the brush border membrane determines the capacity of the proximal tubule to reabsorb phosphate; this finding explains why NaPi-IIa/SLC34A1-deficient mice have increased urinary phosphate excretion and marked hypophosphatemia.[180] NaPi-IIa is the target of the two main hormones that control renal phosphate reabsorption, PTH and fibroblast growth factor-23 (FGF-23), both of which decrease the amount of NaPi-IIa at the brush border membrane (reviewed elsewhere[181]).

The contribution of NaPi-IIa to renal phosphate balance was established by Magen and coworkers when they reported autosomal recessive hypophosphatemic rickets with renal Fanconi syndrome secondary to a loss-of-function mutation in NaPi-IIa.[182]

Membrane sorting of NaPi-IIa requires sodium–hydrogen exchanger regulatory factor 1 (NHERF-1), a multifunctional intracellular protein with two structural domains, the PSD95, Discs-large, ZO-1 (PDZ1) domain and the PSD95, Discs-large, ZO-2 (PDZ2) domain. These domains can interact with specific sequences of the carboxy terminus of various membrane proteins, among them NaPi-IIa[182,183] and the PTH type 1 receptor (PTH1R).[184,185] Disruption of *NHERF1* in mice results in a phenotype that is very similar to that of *NaPi-IIa* knockout mice, including increased urinary phosphate excretion and hypophosphatemia because of decreased NPT2a in brush border membranes.[186]

Two other bone-specific proteins, PHEX [see discussion of X-linked hypophosphatemic rickets (XLH)] and dentin matrix protein 1 (DMP1), appear to be necessary for limiting the expression of FGF-23, thereby allowing sufficient renal conservation of phosphate.[187] A reduction in serum phosphate levels also leads to increased $1,25(OH)_2D_3$ levels from greater activity of the 1α-hydroxylase. The decrease in serum phosphate levels also inhibits bone deposition, and the rise in serum $1,25(OH)_2D_3$ increases bone resorption, thus favoring a net shift of phosphate from bone. Higher serum levels of $1,25(OH)_2D_3$ also increase intestinal phosphate and calcium absorption. As a consequence, serum calcium levels rise and inhibit PTH secretion. The reduction in PTH levels does not lead to a further increase in phosphate reabsorption by the kidney because the proximal tubule is insensitive to the action of PTH in states of phosphate deprivation. As a result, one should predict that a renal phosphate leak will lead to raised serum $1,25(OH)_2D_3$ levels, decreased PTH, and induction of hypercalciuria.

## X-LINKED HYPOPHOSPHATEMIC RICKETS

### PATHOGENESIS

XLH (OMIM #307800) is the most common inherited hypophosphatemic disorder, accounting for more than 50% of cases of familial phosphate wasting (Table 44.5). XLH is caused by mutations in the *PHEX* gene (phosphate-regulating gene with homologies to endopeptidases on the X chromosome). *PHEX* encodes an M13 zinc metalloprotease expressed in osteoblasts and odontoblasts but not in the kidney. Although it is not immediately apparent how loss of PHEX function leads to a decrease in renal Pi reabsorption, mutations in *PHEX* (in bone tissue) indirectly alter the degradation and production of FGF-23, causing increased circulating levels of this phosphatonin.[187,188] FGF-23 synthesis and secretion appear reduced through yet unknown mechanisms that indirectly involve PHEX.[189]

### CLINICAL PRESENTATION

XLH phenotype is characterized by hypophosphatemia secondary to renal phosphate wasting, inappropriately low concentrations of 1,25 dihydroxyvitamin D, and high circulating levels of FGF-23. Early in life, patients with XLH demonstrate short stature (growth retardation), femoral and/or tibial bowing, and histomorphometric evidence of rickets and osteomalacia. Male patients are usually more severely affected than female patients, with variable penetrance. Serum phosphate levels are lower than 0.8 mmol/L (2.5 mg/dL) and the $Tm_P$/GFR is lower than 0.56 mmol/L (1.8 mg/dL).

**Table 44.5 Inherited Hypophosphatemias – Mutated Proteins and Laboratory Findings**

| | | Laboratory Values | | | |
|---|---|---|---|---|---|
| **Disease** | Protein | Serum $Ca^{2+}$ | $1,25(OH)_2D$ | FGF-23 | PTH |
| Hypophosphatemic rickets, X-linked dominant (XLH) | PHEX | Normal | Low/Normal | High/Normal | Normal |
| Hypophosphatemic rickets, autosomal recessive (ARHR) | DMP1, ENPP1 | Normal | Normal | Normal | High/Normal |
| Hypophosphatemic rickets, autosomal dominant (ADHR) | FGF-23 | Normal | Normal | High | Normal |
| Nephrolithiasis/osteoporosis, hypophosphatemic 2 | NHERF-1 | Normal | High | Normal | Normal |
| Hypophosphatemic rickets and hyperparathyroidism | KLOTHO | High | High | High | High |
| Nephrolithiasis/osteoporosis, hypophosphatemic 1 | SLC34A1 (?) | High | n.d. | High | n.d. |
| Hypophosphatemic rickets with hypercalciuria (HHRH) | SLC34A3 | High | Low | High | High |

*DMP1,* Dentin matrix protein 1; *FGF-23,* fibroblast growth factor-23; *n.d.,* not determined; *NHERF-1,* sodium-hydrogen exchanger regulatory factor 1; *PHEX,* M13 zinc metalloprotease encoded by *PHEX*; *PTH,* parathyroid hormone; *SLC,* solute carrier.

Modified from Amatschek S, Haller M, Oberbauer R. Renal phosphate handling in human—what can we learn from hereditary hypophosphataemias? *Eur J Clin Invest.* 2010;40:552–560.

The 1,25(OH)$_2$D$_3$ levels are normal or near normal. There is apparently no correlation between the serum levels of phosphate and the severity of the disease. Affected children tend to have higher serum phosphate and Tm$_P$/GFR values than affected adults, as is the case with normal subjects. The earliest sign of the disease in children can be increased serum alkaline phosphatase levels.[189]

### TREATMENT

Early therapy with 1,25(OH)$_2$D$_3$ (1.0–3.0 mcg/day) and phosphate (1–2 g/day in divided doses) has a beneficial effect on growth, bone density, and deformations.[190] Nephrocalcinosis caused by vitamin D and phosphate therapy can lead to deterioration of renal function.

## AUTOSOMAL DOMINANT HYPOPHOSPHATEMIC RICKETS

Autosomal dominant hypophosphatemic rickets (ADHRs; OMIM #193100) is a very rare cause of rickets (Table 44.5) characterized by hypophosphatemia, phosphaturia, inappropriately low or normal 1,25(OH)$_2$D levels, and bone mineralization defects that can result in bone pain, fracture, rickets, osteomalacia, lower extremity deformities, and muscle weakness.[191] These features are similar to those of XLH. However, ADHR is far less common than XLH and has incomplete penetrance with a variable age of onset.

The gene responsible for ADHR encodes FGF-23, a 251–amino acid peptide that is secreted and processed to amino- and carboxy-terminal peptides at a consensus proprotein convertase (furin) site, RHTR (ArgHisThrArg),[192] by a subtilisin-like proprotein convertase. Missense mutations in FGF-23 are identified in all families with ADHR abrogate peptide processing.[193] The mutant FGF-23 is predicted to have a longer circulating half-life than the wild type and to be associated with higher serum concentrations. Iron deficiency may trigger late-onset ADHR (in pregnancy and adolescence, for example) by increasing FGF-23 production.[194] Treatment of ADHR involves phosphate supplementation and calcitriol.

## AUTOSOMAL RECESSIVE HYPOPHOSPHATEMIC RICKETS

Autosomal recessive hypophosphatemic rickets (ARHR1; OMIM #241520) is a very rare form of hypophosphatemic rickets caused by inactivating mutations of the DMP1 gene *(DMP1)* that result in secondary elevation of FGF-23 concentrations.[195] The *DMP1* gene is located on chromosome 4q21 and is one of a cluster of genes encoding a class of tooth and bone noncollagenous matrix proteins known as SIBLINGs (*s*mall *i*ntegrin-*b*inding *li*gand, *N*-linked *g*lycoproteins). ARHR2 (OMIM #613312) is caused by mutations in ENPP1 (ectonucleotide pyrophosphatase/phosphodiesterase family member 1), a regulator of extracellular pyrophosphate, and has previously been linked to the development of generalized arterial calcification of infancy (*GACI*; OMIM #208000).[196] The biochemical features are similar to those of XLH – hypophosphatemia, phosphaturia, and inappropriately low 1,25(OH)$_2$D$_3$. The clinical presentation is usually found not at birth but later, during childhood and even in adulthood.

## HEREDITARY HYPOPHOSPHATEMIC RICKETS WITH HYPERCALCIURIA

Hereditary hypophosphatemic rickets (OMIM #241530) associated with hypercalciuria is a rare autosomal recessive disease caused by mutations in *SLC34A3*, the gene encoding the renal sodium–phosphate cotransporter NaPi-IIc.[196,197] Affected subjects appear to have a phenotype restricted to the renal phosphate leak with an appropriate response to hypophosphatemia, because serum levels of calcitriol are increased. Consequently, intestinal calcium absorption is enhanced, resulting in hypercalciuria. Serum calcium levels are normal, and other features include variable degrees of rickets and short stature, and suppressed PTH. The condition responds to daily oral phosphate (1–2.5 g/day), which leads to an increase in serum phosphate and decreases in serum 1,25(OH)$_2$D$_3$, calcium, and alkaline phosphatase. Growth rate can be restored, and the clinical manifestations of rickets and osteomalacia disappear.

## FAMILIAL TUMORAL CALCINOSIS

Familial tumoral calcinosis (OMIM #211900) is a severe autosomal recessive metabolic disorder that manifests as hyperphosphatemia and massive calcium deposits in the skin and subcutaneous tissues.[198] It is caused by loss-of-function mutations in *FGF23*[199] as well as in *GALNT3*[200] and *KL*,[201] leading to inadequate concentrations or action of intact FGF-23. Affected individuals report recurrent painful, calcified subcutaneous masses of up to 1 kg, often resulting in secondary infection and incapacitating mutilation. The *GALNT3* gene encodes a glycosyltransferase responsible for initiating mucin-type O-glycosylation, whereas Klotho (encoded by *KL*) is a coreceptor for FGF-23.[202] Treatment involves phosphate chelators and acetazolamide.

## HEREDITARY SELECTIVE DEFICIENCY OF 1α,25(OH)$_2$D$_3$

A rare form of autosomal recessive vitamin D responsive rickets, hereditary selective deficiency of 1α,25(OH)$_2$D$_3$ (OMIM #264700) is not a disease of tubule transport per se, but a 1α-hydroxylation deficiency. It results from inactivating mutations in the *CYP27B1* gene.[202,203] Vitamin D is metabolized by sequential hydroxylations in the liver (25-hydroxylation) and the kidney (1α-hydroxylation). Hydroxylation of 25-hydroxyvitamin D$_3$ is mediated by 25(OH)D$_3$ 1α-hydroxylase in the kidney. Patients usually appear normal at birth, but muscle weakness, tetany, convulsions, and rickets start to develop at 2 months of age. Serum calcium levels are low; PTH levels are high with low to undetectable 1,25(OH)$_2$D$_3$. Serum levels of 25(OH)D$_3$ are normal or slightly increased. Once recognized, this rare disorder is easily treated with physiologic doses of calcitriol, which leads to healing of rickets and restoration of the plasma calcium, phosphate, and PTH levels.

## HEREDITARY GENERALIZED RESISTANCE TO 1α,25(OH)$_2$D$_3$

Hereditary vitamin D–resistant rickets is a rare monogenic autosomal recessive disorder caused by mutations in the vitamin D receptor and is similar to selective deficiency of $1\alpha,25(OH)_2D_3$. Its salient features are increased serum levels of $25(OH)D_3$ and $1\alpha,25(OH)_2D_3$, and the disease does not respond to doses of $1\alpha,25(OH)_2D_3$ and $1\alpha,(OH)D_3$. In addition, approximately half of the patients described with the disease have alopecia. In a subset of affected kindreds, premature stop codons in the vitamin D receptor gene lead to the absence of the ligand-binding domain.[204] Administration of very high doses of calcium (≤3 g/day) and $1,25(OH)_2D$ (≤30–60 mcg/day) may be necessary to normalize calcemia and mineralize depleted bones.

## RESISTANCE TO PARATHORMONE ACTION

Pseudohypoparathyroidism (PHP) is associated with biochemical hypoparathyroidism (i.e., hypocalcemia, hyperphosphatemia) caused by resistance to, rather than deficiency of PTH (reviewed elsewhere[204]). Patients with PHP type 1a have a generalized form of hormone resistance and a constellation of developmental defects termed *Albright hereditary osteodystrophy*. Within PHP type 1a families, some individuals show osteodystrophy but have normal hormone responsiveness, a variant phenotype termed *pseudo-PHP*. By contrast, patients with PHP type 1b manifest only PTH resistance and lack features of osteodystrophy. These various forms of PHP are caused by defects in the imprinted *GNAS1* gene that lead to decreased expression or activity of the α subunit of the stimulatory G protein ($G_{\alpha s}$). Tissue-specific genomic imprinting of *GNAS1* accounts for the variable physical and endocrine phenotypes (parathyroid, thyroid, gonads, and pituitary gland) of patients with *GNAS1* defects.[205]

# INHERITED DISORDER OF URATE TRANSPORT

## FAMILIAL RENAL HYPOURICEMIA

Renal hypouricemia is an autosomal recessive disorder characterized by impaired urate handling in the renal tubules.[206] Type 1 (>90% of cases) is caused by a loss-of-function mutation in the *SLC22A12* gene[207] (OMIM #220150) encoding the apical urate/anion exchanger URAT1 particularly prevalent in Japan and in Ashkenazi Jews, whereas type 2 is caused by defects in the *SLC2A9* gene (OMIM #612076) encoding glucose transporter 9 (GLUT9), a high-capacity urate transporter belonging to the facilitated GLUT family that is responsible for most of the basolateral urate transport.[207,208] The disorder is associated with exercise-induced acute renal failure and nephrolithiasis, particularly for carriers of *SLC2A9* mutations who show very high fractional excretion of urate (100%–150%), reflecting absent reabsorption but retained urate secretion. Carriers of *SLC22A12* mutations have a milder phenotype because of the presence of other urate anion exchangers OAT4 (SLC22A11) and OAT10 (SLC22A13).[209] Hyperuricosuria, combined with dehydration or exercise, results in acute uric acid nephropathy and causes an obstructive acute renal failure. This can be prevented by forced hydration with bicarbonate or saline solutions. Affected subjects typically have very high urate fractional excretion (≥50%) and their parents have intermediate levels.[210] Interestingly, polymorphisms in *SLC2A9* explain 1.7% to 5.3% of the variance in serum uric acid concentrations.[211]

Hereditary xanthinuria, a recessively inherited disorder, is also characterized by very low serum urate levels resulting from a deficiency of xanthine oxidase.[212] However, urine urate excretion is very low, and xanthine excretion is elevated, contrary to renal hypouricemia. Type I disease results from mutations in xanthine dehydrogenase (XDH), and type II results from a dual deficiency of XDH and aldehyde oxidase.

# INHERITED DISORDERS OF RENAL GLUCOSE TRANSPORT

Under normal conditions, glucose is almost completely reabsorbed by the proximal tubule. Thus very small amounts of glucose are present in the urine. Glucose urinary excretion (500 mg or 2.75 mmol/day in adults) is caused most often by hyperglycemia (overload glucosuria) and rarely by abnormal handling of glucose by the kidney (Box 44.1). Renal glucosuria may be part of a generalized dysfunction of the proximal tubule (Fanconi syndrome) or may manifest as an isolated defect.

## RENAL GLUCOSURIA

Familial renal glucosuria (FRG; OMIM #233100) is an inherited renal tubular disorder characterized by persistent isolated glucosuria in the absence of hyperglycemia. It is usually a benign clinical condition. Mutations in SLC5A2 encoding the sodium–glucose cotransporter SGLT2 are responsible for the disorder.[213] Some Japanese patients have mutations in GLUT2.[214]

SGLT2 and SGLT1 mediate apical glucose uptake in the S1 and S3 segments of the proximal tubule, respectively. SGLT2 inhibitors are now used in diabetic patients to control hyperglycemia by increasing urinary glucose excretion.[215] Of interest, this class of drugs also seems to show benefit in slowing the progression of diabetic nephropathy and cardiovascular complications of diabetes, with the former attributed to enhancement of tubuloglomerular feedback–mediated reduction of diabetic hyperfiltration injury[216,217] (see also Chapter 39).

**Box 44.1 Causes of Glucosuria**

**Hyperglycemia**

Diabetes mellitus
Iatrogenic:
- Glucocorticoids
- Catecholamines
- Angiotensin I–converting enzyme inhibitors
- Dextrose intravenous solutions
- Total parenteral nutrition

**Renal Glucosuria**

Idiopathic
Glucose–galactose malabsorption
Fanconi syndrome
Pregnancy

FRG is transmitted as a codominant trait with incomplete penetrance. Homozygotes can show glucosuria of more than 60 g/day, evidence of renal sodium wasting, mild volume depletion, and raised basal plasma renin and serum aldosterone levels.[218]

The definition of "glucosuria" is arbitrary, and different investigators have proposed different guidelines to distinguish abnormal from normal glucosuria. A currently accepted stringent definition of glucosuria proposes the following criteria:

- The oral glucose tolerance test result and the levels of plasma insulin and free fatty acids and of glycosylated hemoglobin should all be normal.
- The amount of glucose in the urine (10–100 g/day) should be relatively stable except during pregnancy, when it may increase.
- The degree of glucosuria should be largely independent of diet but may fluctuate according to the amount of carbohydrates ingested. All specimens of urine should contain glucose.
- The carbohydrate excreted should be glucose. Other sugars are not found (fructose, pentoses, galactose, lactose, sucrose, maltose, and heptulose).
- Subjects with renal glucosuria should be able to store and use carbohydrates normally.

## GLUCOSE–GALACTOSE MALABSORPTION

Glucose–galactose malabsorption (OMIM #606824) is a rare autosomal recessive disease resulting from a selective defect in the intestinal transport of glucose and galactose. Mutations in SLC5A1—which couples transport of sugar to sodium gradients across the intestinal brush border[218]—cause absence of the transporter in the intestine and the kidney plasma membranes, leading to glucose–galactose malabsorption. Neonatal onset of severe watery and acidic diarrhea results in death unless these sugars are removed from the patient's diet.[219] Significant weight loss from hyperosmolar dehydration and metabolic acidosis is frequent. The disease occurs occasionally in adults.[220] The acidic diarrhea results from bacterial metabolism of sugar in the stools. Normally, lactose in milk is broken down into glucose and galactose by lactase, an ectoenzyme on the brush border, and the hexoses are transported into the cell by SGLT1.

The disease is usually suspected from the clinical history and the presence of glucosuria despite normal serum glucose levels. Dramatic improvement occurs after withdrawal of glucose and galactose from the patient's diet. The acidic diarrhea can be improved with antibacterial treatment.

## INHERITED DISORDERS OF ACID–BASE TRANSPORTERS

A typical Western diet generates an acid load of approximately 1 mmol of mineral acid per kilogram of body weight, which must be excreted by the kidney. In addition, the kidney filters approximately 4000 mmol of bicarbonate daily and must reclaim most of the filtered load to maintain acid–base balance. Excretion of the ingested acid load and reabsorption of filtered bicarbonate are accomplished by complex processes requiring coordinated actions of transport and enzymatic activities in the apical and basolateral membranes (Fig. 44.8).

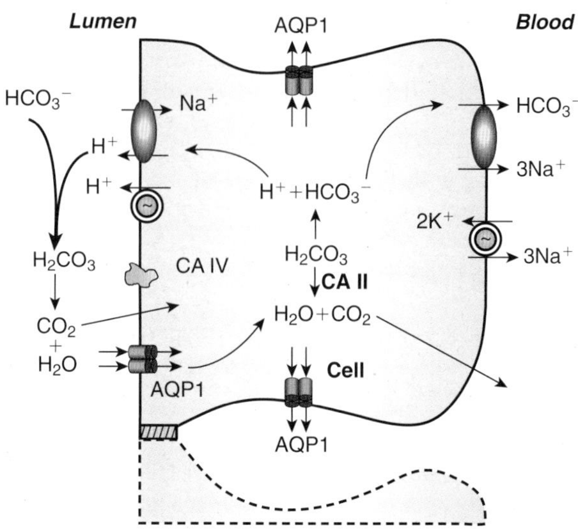


**Fig. 44.8** Mechanisms of renal acidification in the proximal tubule. *AQP1,* Aquaporin-1; *CA II/IV,* carbonic an hydrase II/IV.

In the proximal tubule, filtered bicarbonate ($HCO_3^-$) is almost completely reabsorbed by an indirect mechanism. $H^+$ and $HCO_3^-$ are generated by intracellular hydration of $CO_2$ by carbonic anhydrase II (CA II). $H^+$ secretion occurs across the apical membrane via NHE3, the $Na^+$–$H^+$ exchanger, and an $H^+$–ATPase, and $HCO_3^-$ is transferred via a basolateral $Na^+$–$HCO_3^-$ cotransporter. The secreted hydrogen ions react with filtered $HCO_3^-$ to form $H_2CO_3$, which is rapidly converted to $CO_2$ and $H_2O$ by CA IV present in the apical membrane. The $CO_2$ and $H_2O$ then diffuse into the cell. The result is the removal of a filtered $HCO_3^-$ and its replacement by another in the plasma, but the process is neutral for net urinary $H^+$ excretion because the secreted hydrogen ions are used to reabsorb filtered $HCO_3^-$. CAs are zinc metalloenzymes that catalyze the reversible hydration of $CO_2$ to form $HCO_3^-$ and protons, according to the following reaction:

$$CO_2 + H_2O \leftrightarrow H_2CO_3 \leftrightarrow H^+ + HCO_3^-$$

The first reaction is catalyzed by CA, and the second reaction occurs instantaneously. Net urinary elimination of $H^+$ depends on its buffering and excretion as titratable acid (mainly phosphate: $HPO_4^{2-} + H^+ \leftrightarrow H_2PO_4^-$), and excretion as $NH_4^+$. The production of $NH_4^+$ from glutamine by the proximal tubule and its secretion generate new plasma $HCO_3^-$. This process is stimulated in metabolic acidosis.

In the distal and collecting tubule, the connecting segment and type A intercalated cells secrete $H^+$ into the lumen via a vacuolar $Mg^{2+}$-dependent $H^+$+ATPase and an exchanger, $H^+$–$K^+$–ATPase (Fig. 44.9). The generation of $H^+$ is catalyzed by CA II and $HCO_3^-$ is transported across the basolateral membrane through the anion exchanger 1 (AE1), or $Cl^-$/$HCO_3^-$ exchanger. Luminal $H^+$ is trapped by urinary buffers, including ammonium secreted by the proximal tubule, and phosphate.

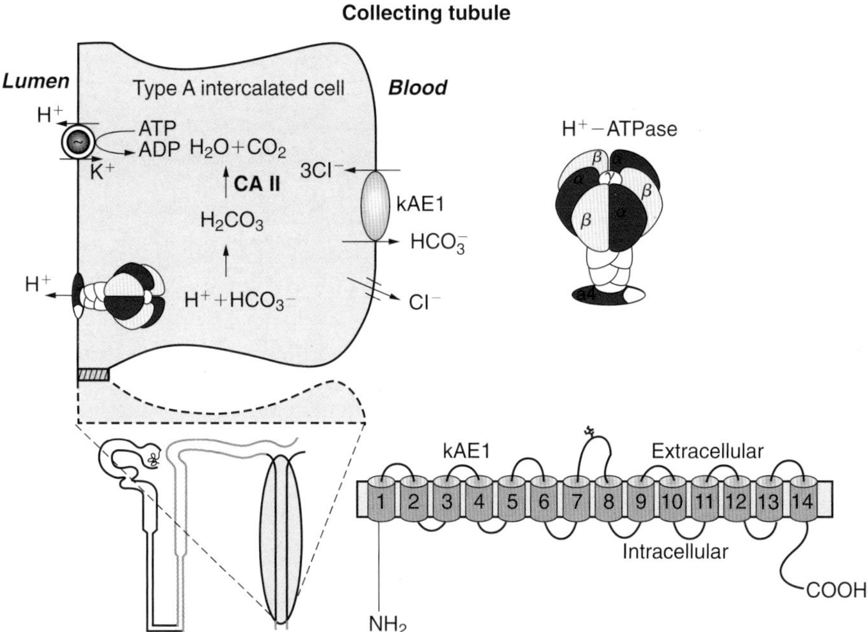


**Fig. 44.9** Mechanisms of renal acidification in the collecting tubule. Dominant distal renal tubular acidosis (RTA) is caused by mutations in the gene *SLC4A1* encoding the chloride–bicarbonate exchanger AE1.[232,357] The *AE1* gene (chromosome 17) encodes both the erythroid (eAE1) and the kidney (kAE1) isoforms of the band 3 protein.[358] Mutations in the gene encoding the $\beta_1$-subunit of $H^+$–ATPase (*ATP6V1B1;* chromosome 2p13) cause recessive distal renal tubular acidosis with sensorineural deafness.[235] Distal RTA with preserved hearing is secondary to mutations in *AIP6V0A4,* which encodes the $\alpha_4$ subunit of the proton pump.[359] Both $H^+$ and $H^+$–$K^+$–ATPases are represented. The $H^+$–ATPase is schematically represented according to the proposed structure of the F-type $F_1$-ATPase of the inner mitochondrial membrane.[360] $F_1$ is represented as a flattened sphere 80 Å high and 100 Å across. The three α- and three β-subunits are arranged alternately like the segments of an orange around a central α-helix 90 Å long. Mutations in the β-subunit cause autosomal recessive distal RTA. Autosomal recessive distal RTA has also been found, in small kindred, for the *SLC4A1* mutation G701D.[234] *ADP,* Adenosine diphosphate; *ATP,* adenosine triphosphate; *ATPase,* Adenosine triphosphatase; *RTA,* renal tubular acidosis.

RTA is a clinical syndrome characterized by hyperchloremic (normal anion gap) metabolic acidosis secondary to abnormal urine acidification.[221] It can be identified from inappropriately high urine pH, bicarbonaturia, and reduced net acid excretion. Clinical and functional studies allow classification into four types, historically numbered in the order of discovery: proximal (type 2), classical distal (type 1), hyperkalemic distal (type 4), and combined proximal and distal (type 3). Rare forms of hereditary proximal and dRTA have been identified[221–223] and are discussed here (Table 44.6).

## PROXIMAL RENAL TUBULAR ACIDOSIS

pRTA usually occurs as part of the spectrum of Fanconi syndrome, in which the excretion of glucose, amino acids, urate, and phosphate is also increased. Primary, isolated hereditary pRTA is an extremely rare disorder that may be inherited as an autosomal recessive or dominant trait.[224] The diagnosis of pRTA rests on an appropriately acid urine pH (pH <5.5) in patients with acidosis and a high fractional excretion of bicarbonate (>10%–15%) during intravenous loading with sodium bicarbonate ($NaHCO_3$). The underlying defect is a failure of proximal bicarbonate reabsorption. It results in an abnormally low threshold for renal bicarbonate reabsorption because the distal nephron is unable to compensate and reabsorb the large bicarbonate load presented to it. However, distal acidification mechanisms are intact, and acid urine can be produced. The metabolic acidosis is generally mild and associated with hypokalemia, and metabolic bone disease is common. Because of a lowering of the tubular threshold for bicarbonate reabsorption, once the plasma bicarbonate is reduced, the threshold can be reached and a steady state maintained at a serum concentration of approximately 15 mM. By contrast, levels can fall to less than 10 mM in dRTA. Administration of large amounts of alkali (10–20 mmol/kg/day) may be required to normalize serum bicarbonate in the patient with pRTA.

### SODIUM–BICARBONATE SYMPORTER MUTATIONS

Inactivating mutations in *SLC4A4,* the gene coding for the $Na^+$–$HCO_3^-$ (NBC1) symporter, cause autosomal recessive pRTA with various ocular abnormalities such as band keratopathy, glaucoma, and cataracts (OMIM #604278).[225] The $Na^+$–$HCO_3^-$ symporter is expressed in multiple ocular tissues,[226] thus explaining the abnormalities. Pancreatitis can be associated with mutations in NBC1, which is expressed in the pancreas.[227]

### CARBONIC ANHYDRASE II DEFICIENCY

Recessive mixed proximal–distal (type 3) RTA accompanied by osteopetrosis and mental retardation (OMIM #259730) is caused by inactivating mutations in the cytoplasmic CA II gene.[228] The pathogenesis of the mental subnormality and cerebral calcification is poorly understood. More than 50 cases have been described, predominantly from the Middle East and Mediterranean regions. The disorder is discovered

**Table 44.6 Classifications, Features, and Underlying Molecular Transport Defect(s) in Inherited Renal Tubular Acidoses**

| | Clinical Features | Protein | Gene |
|---|---|---|---|
| **Proximal RTA** | | | |
| Autosomal recessive PRTA with ocular abnormalities | Band keratopathy, glaucoma, cataracts, short stature, mental retardation, dental enamel defects, pancreatitis, basal ganglia calcification | NBC1 | *SLC4A4* |
| Autosomal recessive PRTA with osteopetrosis and cerebral calcification (inherited carbonic anhydrase II deficiency) | Mental retardation, osteopetrosis, cerebral calcification | CA II | *CA2* |
| Autosomal dominant PRTA | Short stature, osteomalacia | Unknown | Unknown |
| **Distal RTA** | | | |
| Autosomal dominant dRTA | Complete or incomplete dRTA, hypercalciuria, nephrocalcinosis, nephrolithiasis, hypokalemia, short stature, osteomalacia, rickets | AE1 | *SLC4A1* |
| Autosomal recessive dRTA | Complete or incomplete dRTA, other features as above | $H^+$–ATPase (A4 subunit) | *ATP6V0A4* |
| | Other features as above | (A4 subunit) | |
| | Reported in Asian populations in association with ovalocytosis | AE1 | *SLC4A1* |
| Autosomal recessive dRTA with progressive sensorineural deafness | Complete or incomplete dRTA | $H^+$–ATPase (B1 subunit) | *ATP6V1B1* |
| | As above, but with late-onset sensorineural deafness | $H^+$–ATPase (A4 subunit) | *ATP6V0A4* |

*AE1,* Ion exchanger 1; *CA II,* cytosolic carbonic anhydrase; *d,* distal; *NBC1,* $Na^+$–$HCO_3^-$ cotransporter; *P,* proximal; *RTA,* renal tubular acidosis.

Modified from Laing CM, Toye AM, Capasso G, et al. Renal tubular acidosis: developments in our understanding of the molecular basis. *Int J Biochem Cell Biol.* 2005;37:1151–1161.

late in infancy or early in childhood because of developmental delay, short stature, fracture, weakness, cranial nerve compression, dental malocclusion, and/or mental subnormality. Typical radiographic features of osteopetrosis are present, and histopathologic study of the iliac crest reveals unresorbed calcified primary spongiosa. The radiographic findings are unusual, however, in that cerebral calcification appears by early childhood and the osteosclerosis and skeletal modeling defects may gradually resolve by adulthood. Patients are usually not anemic. A hyperchloremic metabolic acidosis, sometimes with hypokalemia, is caused by RTA, which may be a proximal, distal, or combined type.[229] Bilateral recurrent renal stones, hypercalciuria, and medullary nephrocalcinosis have been described.[230] There is no established medical therapy, and the long-term outcome remains to be characterized. Treatment involves alkali supplementation for the acidosis and, potentially, bone marrow transplantation for osteopetrosis.[231]

## DISTAL RENAL TUBULAR ACIDOSIS

Hereditary dRTA is a genetically heterogeneous disorder with dominant and recessive forms caused by dysfunction of type A intercalated cells[221,222] (Fig. 44.9). Implicated transporters include the AE1 ($Cl^-/HCO_3^-$) exchanger of the basolateral membrane and at least two subunits of the apical membrane V-ATPase, the $V_1$ (head) subunit B1 (associated with deafness) and the $V_0$ (stalk) subunit A4. Clinical features include inability to acidify urine, variable hyperchloremic hypokalemic metabolic acidosis, hypercalciuria, nephrocalcinosis, and nephrolithiasis. Patients with recessive dRTA present with either acute illness or growth failure at a young age, sometimes accompanied by deafness. Dominant dRTA is usually a milder disease and involves no hearing loss.

### CHLORIDE–BICARBONATE EXCHANGER MUTATIONS

Mutations in the *SLC4A1* gene encoding AE1 can lead to dominant (OMIM #179800) or recessive dRTA.[232] AE1 is the basolateral $Cl^-/HCO_3^-$ exchanger located in alpha intercalated cells of the collecting duct.[233] The renal AE1 contributes to urinary acidification by providing the major exit route for $HCO_3^-$ across the basolateral membrane. dRTA results from aberrant targeting of AE1.

The dominant form is usually a mild disorder that can be discovered incidentally after a kidney stone episode. Serum bicarbonate concentrations are usually between 14 and 25 mmol/L, and serum potassium levels between 2.1 and 4.2 mmol/L. Minimum urine pH following an acid load varies from 5.95 to 6.8 (normal <5.30). Nephrocalcinosis and kidney stones are present in approximately 50% of subjects. Deafness is usually absent.

The recessive form of dRTA (OMIM #109270) is diagnosed at a younger age, often before 1 year. It is found in Southeast Asia (Thailand, Papua–New Guinea, and Malaysia), where it is associated with ovalocytosis.[234] Affected subjects present with vomiting, dehydration, failure to thrive, or delayed growth. Nephrocalcinosis, kidney stones, or both are frequent, and rickets can be present. Severe metabolic acidosis with serum pH less than 7.30 and serum bicarbonate less than 15 mmol/L is common. Serum potassium levels are also lower than in autosomal dominant dRTA.

### PROTON ATPASE SUBUNIT MUTATIONS

Mutations in ATP6V1B1, the $B_1$-subunit of the apical proton pump ATP6B1 that mediates distal nephron acid secretion (OMIM #267300), cause dRTA with sensorineural deafness in a significant proportion of families.[234,235] In type A intercalated cells, the $H^+$–ATPase pumps protons against an electrochemical gradient. Active proton secretion is also necessary to maintain proper endolymph pH. These findings implicate ATP6B1 in endolymph pH homeostasis and in normal auditory function, because nearly all patients with ATP6V1B1 mutations also have sensorineural hearing loss.

Mutations in the *ATP6V0A4* gene on chromosome 7 (OMIM #602722) also give rise to recessive dRTA,[236] but hearing is preserved. ATP6V0A4 encodes a kidney-specific A4 isoform of the proton pump's 116-kDs accessory a subunit. The treatment of dRTA involves the correction of dehydration, electrolyte, and bicarbonate anomalies, which will improve symptoms. In adults, administration of alkali 1 to 3 mmol kg/day usually corrects the metabolic abnormality. In children, up to 5 mmol/kg per day may be required. Potassium supplementation may be needed even after correction of the acidosis.

## BARTTER AND GITELMAN SYNDROMES

In 1962, Bartter and coworkers described two patients with hypokalemic metabolic alkalosis, hyperreninemic hyperaldosteronism, normal blood pressure, as well as hyperplasia and hypertrophy of the juxtaglomerular apparatus.[237] Since then, familial hypokalemic, hypochloremic metabolic alkalosis has been recognized as not a single entity but, rather, a set of closely related disorders.[238] Although Bartter syndrome and Bartter mutations are used commonly as diagnoses, it is likely, as explained by Jeck and colleagues, that the two patients with a mild phenotype originally described by Bartter had Gitelman syndrome, a thiazide-like salt-losing tubulopathy with a defect in the distal convoluted tubule.[237] As a consequence, salt-losing tubulopathy of the furosemide type is a more physiologically appropriate definition for Bartter syndrome. Bartter syndrome is a genetically heterogeneous disorder affecting the loop of Henle, where 30% of the filtered sodium chloride is reabsorbed, that typically manifests during the neonatal period and is associated with hypercalciuria and nephrocalcinosis (Fig. 44.10). By contrast, Gitelman syndrome is a disorder affecting the distal tubule[239] that is usually diagnosed at a later stage and is associated with hypocalciuria and hypomagnesemia, with predominant muscular signs and symptoms (Fig. 44.11).[240]

### BARTTER SYNDROME

#### PATHOGENESIS

Bartter syndrome (OMIM #601678, #241200, #607364, and #602522) is an autosomal recessive disorder affecting the function of the thick ascending limb (TAL) of the loop of Henle, giving a clinical picture of salt wasting and hypokalemic metabolic alkalosis. It is caused by inactivating mutations in one of at least four genes encoding membrane proteins (Bartter syndrome types 1 through 4)[241–245]: type 1, the $Na^+$–K–$2Cl^-$ cotransporter (*SLC12A1* encoding NKCC2); type 2, the apical inward-rectifying potassium channel (*KCNJ1* encoding ROMK); type 3, a basolateral chloride channel (*CLCNK* encoding ClC-Kb); and type 4, *BSND*, encoding Barttin, a protein that acts as an essential activator β-subunit for ClC-Ka and ClC-Kb chloride channels (Fig. 44.10). Gain-of-function mutations in the extracellular calcium-sensing receptor (CaSR) cause a variant of Bartter syndrome[241,246] with hypocalcemia. In this regard, it is of interest that a Bartter-like syndrome has been described in patients treated with aminoglycosides such as gentamicin and amikacin, characterized by transient hypokalemia, metabolic alkalosis, hypomagnesemia with urinary magnesium wasting, and hypercalciuria, which resolve weeks after drug termination. Drugs in this class are polycations acting as calcimimetics and stimulating the CaSR. This disorder can be thought of as an acquired form of type 5 Bartter syndrome. Alternatively, direct drug-induced tubular damage may be the etiologic mechanism.[247]

An additional type of Bartter syndrome has been shown to be a digenic disorder that is attributable to loss-of-function mutations in the genes that encode the chloride channels ClC-Ka and ClC-Kb.[242,245]

#### CLINICAL PRESENTATION

Most cases of Bartter syndrome present antenatally or in neonates. Polyhydramnios and premature labor are common findings. Postnatal findings include polyuria, polydipsia, failure to thrive, growth retardation, dehydration, low blood pressure, muscle weakness, seizures, tetany, paresthesias, and joint pain from chondrocalcinosis.[248] In contrast to patients with Gitelman syndrome, those with Bartter syndrome are virtually always hypercalciuric and normomagnesemic.

Nephrocalcinosis occurs in almost all patients with Bartter syndrome with NKCC2 (type 1) and ROMK (type 2) mutations but in only 20% of those with CLC-Kb mutations. This finding could be attributable to lower urine calcium excretion. Patients with ROMK mutations may show hyperkalemia at birth, which converts to hypokalemia within the first weeks of life.[249] Thus they can be misdiagnosed with pseudohypoaldosteronism type I (PHA I), vide infra. This pattern could be explained by the fact that ROMK, in addition to being required for sodium reabsorption in the TAL, is also expressed in the collecting duct. Patients do not need important $K^+$ supplementation, contrary to other patients with Bartter syndrome, but still demonstrate hypokalemia because of reduced reabsorption in the TAL and possibly to K secretion by maxi-K channels in the late distal tubule.[250] The type 3 Bartter syndrome (CLC-Kb) phenotype is highly variable and may manifest as either a typical antenatal variant or a "classic" Bartter variant characterized by an onset in early childhood and lower severity or absence of hypercalciuria and nephrocalcinosis. BSND mutations (type 4 Bartter syndrome) are usually associated with an extremely severe phenotype with intrauterine onset, profound renal salt and water wasting, renal failure, sensorineural deafness, and motor retardation.[251] Sensorineural deafness is specific for Barttin (type 4) because it is an essential subunit of chloride channels in the inner

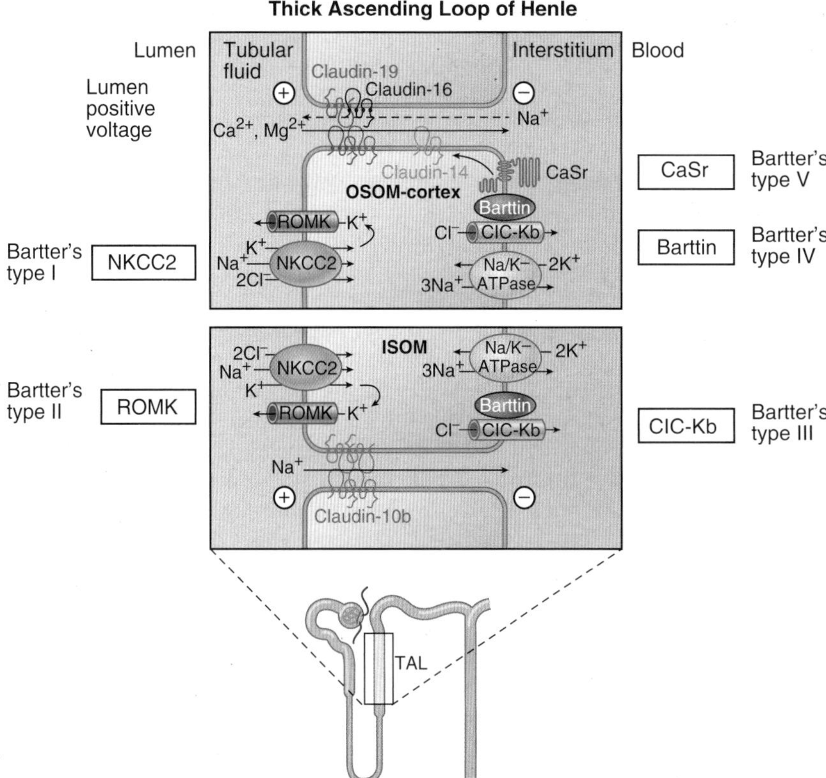


**Fig. 44.10** Schematic representation of transepithelial salt reabsorption in a cell of the thick ascending limb (TAL) of the loop of Henle. Filtered NaCl is reabsorbed through $Na^+$–$K^+$–$2Cl^-$ cotransporter type 2 (NKCC2), which uses the sodium gradient across the membrane to transport chloride and potassium into the cell. The potassium ions are recycled through the apical membrane by the potassium channel ROMK. Sodium leaves the cell actively through the basolateral $Na^+$–$K^+$–ATPase. Chloride diffuses passively through two basolateral channels, ClC-Ka and ClC-Kb. Both of these chloride channels must bind to the β-subunit of Barttin to be transported to the cell surface. The recycling of potassium maintains a lumen-positive voltage that drives calcium and magnesium reabsorption paracellularly. Claudin-16 and claudin-19 are necessary for the paracellular transport of calcium and magnesium. Four types of Bartter syndrome (types I, II, III, and IV) are attributable to recessive mutations in the genes that encode NKCC2, ROMK, ClC-Kb, and Barttin, respectively. *ClC-Kb,* Basolateral chloride channel b; *NKCC2,* $Na^+$–$K^+$–$2Cl^-$ cotransporter 2; *ROMK,* potassium channel; (Modified from Bichet DG, Fujiwara TM. Reabsorption of sodium chloride—lessons from the chloride channels. *N Engl J Med.* 2004;350:1281–1283. With permission; Olinger E, Houillier P, Devuyst O. Claudins: a tale of interactions in the thick ascending limb. *Kidney Int.* 2018;93:535–537.)

ear, necessary for generating the endocochlear potential.[252] The severity of type 4 Bartter syndrome would be consistent with contributions of both ClC-Ka and ClC-Kb to basolateral chloride exit in the TAL.

### TREATMENT

Treatment of Bartter syndrome usually involves potassium and magnesium supplements, spironolactone, and nonsteroidal antiinflammatory drugs. Indomethacin has been widely used, for which elevations of urinary prostaglandin $E_2$ have provided a rationale.[238] Angiotensin I–converting enzyme inhibitors have been used successfully in conjunction with potassium supplements.[252,253] Therapy should lead to catch-up growth in infants.[254]

## GITELMAN SYNDROME

### PATHOGENESIS

Gitelman syndrome (OMIM #263800), a milder disorder than Bartter syndrome,[255] is usually diagnosed in adolescents and adults.[255] It is an autosomal recessive trait caused by inactivating mutations in the *SLC12A3* gene encoding the thiazide-sensitive $Na^+$–$Cl^-$ cotransporter (NCC).[239] Rare cases are caused by mutations in the *CLCNKB* gene, which encodes the renal chloride channel CLC-Kb, located in basolateral membrane of cells of the TAL and the distal tubules. These patients appear to have a Gitelman and not the expected Bartter phenotype.[243] Gitelman syndrome results in a thiazide-like effect, consisting of sodium and chloride wasting with secondary hypovolemia and metabolic alkalosis. Activation of the renin–angiotensin–aldosterone system from volume depletion, plus increased sodium load to the cortical collecting duct, leads to increased sodium reabsorption by the epithelial sodium channel (ENaC), which is counterbalanced by potassium and hydrogen excretion, resulting in hypokalemia and metabolic alkalosis. Enhanced passive $Ca^{2+}$ transport in the proximal tubule rather than active $Ca^{2+}$ transport in the distal convoluted tubule explains the hypocalciuria. Downregulation of TRPM6 (epithelial $Mg^{2+}$ channel transient receptor potential channel subfamily M, member 6) explains the hypomagnesemia.[256]

### CLINICAL PRESENTATION

The carrier state of *SLC12A3* mutations occurs in 1% of the general population, suggesting a prevalence of Gitelman syndrome of 25 per million population and making it the

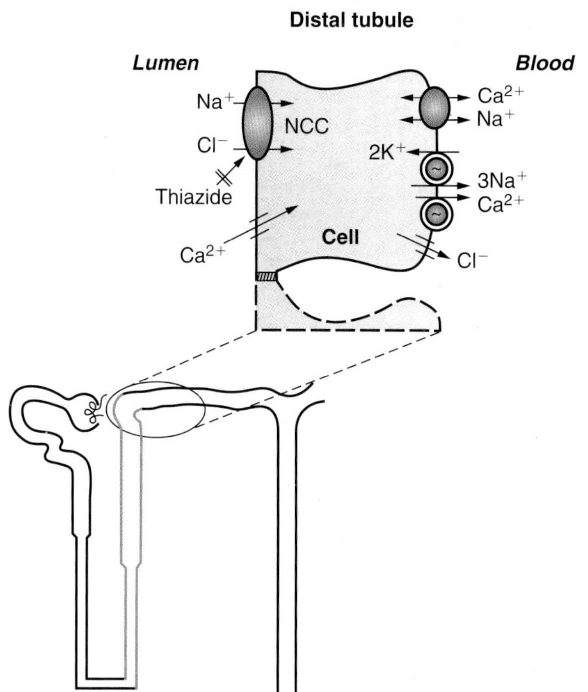


Fig. 44.11 Gitelman syndrome: loss-of-function mutations of the thiazide-sensitive Na–Cl cotransporter *(NCC)*.

most common inherited renal tubule disorder.[256,257] Contrary to patients with Bartter syndrome, those with Gitelman syndrome are usually asymptomatic in the neonatal period and often discovered incidentally (Fig. 44.12).[238] Subjects have hypokalemic metabolic alkalosis, but unlike those with Bartter syndrome, they are hypocalciuric and hypomagnesemic and do not have signs of overt volume depletion.[258] Polyuria and polydipsia are not features of Gitelman syndrome either. Patients suffer from arthritis because of chondrocalcinosis in several joints,[258] possibly secondary to hypomagnesemia. Urinary prostaglandin $E_2$ levels are normal,[259] a finding compatible with the poor response observed to prostanoid synthetase inhibition. The major conditions in the differential diagnosis of Gitelman syndrome are diuretic abuse, laxative abuse, and chronic vomiting. A careful history, as well as measurement of urinary chloride and detection of diuretics, should help differentiate among these conditions.

### TREATMENT

The treatment of Gitelman syndrome includes potassium supplementation and spironolactone.[260] Nonsteroidal anti-inflammatory drugs are usually not helpful because prostaglandin levels are normal.

## INHERITED DISORDERS WITH HYPERTENSION AND HYPOKALEMIA

Most patients with hypokalemia and hypertension have essential hypertension associated with the use of diuretics, secondary aldosteronism from renal artery stenosis, or primary hyperaldosteronism.[261] Hereditary causes of hypertension and hypokalemia include excess secretion of aldosterone or other mineralocorticoids and abnormal sensitivity to mineralocorticoids. They are primarily characterized by low or low-normal plasma renin concentration and salt-sensitive hypokalemic hypertension, suggesting enhanced mineralocorticoid activity.[262] The molecular basis for several of these traits has been elucidated.

## CONGENITAL ADRENAL HYPERPLASIA

Inherited abnormalities in steroid biosynthesis cause hypertension in some cases of congenital adrenal hyperplasia. These autosomal recessive disorders arise from deficiencies of key enzymes of the steroid biosynthesis pathway (Fig. 44.13).[263,264] The decrease in cortisol production causes an increase in adrenocorticotropic hormone (ACTH) secretion and subsequent hyperplasia of the adrenal glands. The phenotypes are determined by deficiencies as well as by overproduction of steroids unaffected by the enzymatic defect. Hypertension is observed in only two of the three major subtypes of congenital adrenal hyperplasia (11β-hydroxylase and 17α-hydroxylase deficiencies), because metabolic blockade distal to 21α-hydroxylase allows the formation of 21-hydroxyl groups necessary for mineralocorticoid precursor biosynthesis. Other clinical manifestations depend on the consequences of the enzymatic defect on androgen biosynthesis with either an increase (11β-hydroxylase) or a decrease (17α-hydroxylase) in production. In both deficiencies, overproduction of cortisol precursors that are metabolized to mineralocorticoid agonists or that have intrinsic mineralocorticoid activity induce volume and salt-dependent forms of hypertension. The elevated zona fasciculata deoxycorticosterone (DOC) produces mineralocorticoid hypertension with suppressed renin and reduced potassium concentrations. Aldosterone, the most important mineralocorticoid, regulates electrolyte excretion and intravascular volume mainly through its effects on renal distal convoluted tubules and cortical collecting ducts.

### 11β-HYDROXYLASE DEFICIENCY

Inactivating mutations in the gene encoding 11β-hydroxylase[263,265] cause the second most common form of congenital adrenal hyperplasia (OMIM #202010), representing 5% of cases (90% are caused by 21-hydroxylase deficiency). This disorder is associated with excess production of DOC, 18-deoxycortisol, and androgens. By virtue of the significant intrinsic mineralocorticoid activity of DOC, subjects with mutations in both alleles of the gene exhibit hypokalemic hypertension. Because the androgen pathway is unaffected, prenatal masculinization occurs in female patients and postnatal virilization in both sexes. The diagnosis of 11β-hydroxylase deficiency is established by means of an ACTH test showing elevation of DOC and 11-deoxycortisol and marked suppression of plasma renin activity.[263] The treatment consists of exogenous corticoids that inhibit ACTH secretion.

### 17α-HYDROXYLASE DEFICIENCY

17α-Hydroxylase deficiency (OMIM #202110) results in reduced conversion of pregnenolone to progesterone and androgens and absence of sex hormone production.[262,266] The absence of sex hormone formation in both the adrenal glands and the gonads, which causes hypogonadism and male pseudohermaphroditism, is usually detected at adolescence because of failure to undergo puberty. Patients have

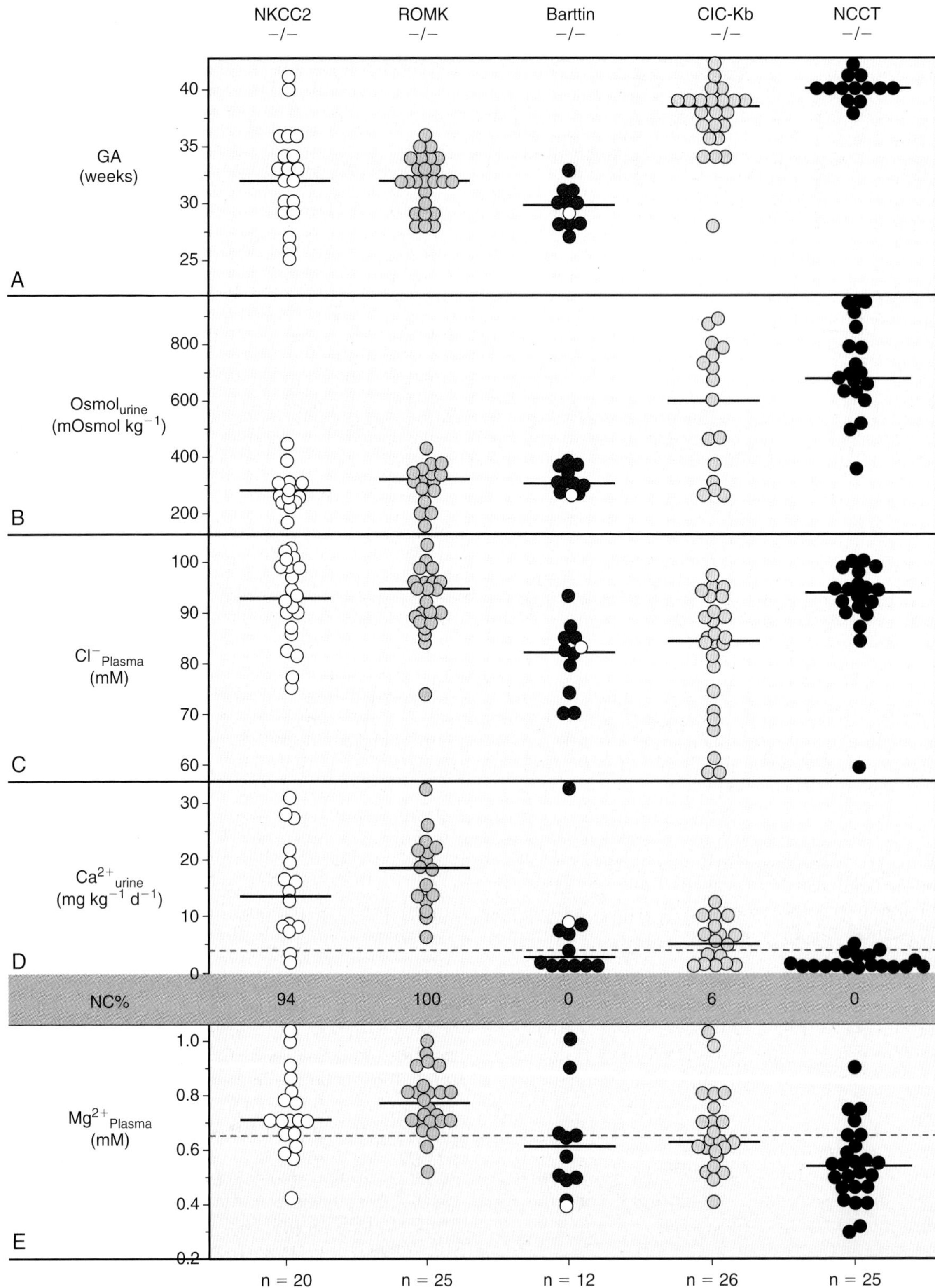


**Fig. 44.12** Genotype–phenotype correlation in untreated salt-losing tubulopathies. (A) Age of gestation at birth (GA). (B) Maximal urine osmolality in random morning urine samples. (C) Minimal plasma $Cl^-$ concentration. (D) Maximal urinary $Ca^{2+}$ excretion (*dashed line* indicates the upper normal limit, about 4 $mg{\cdot}kg^{-1}\times day^{-1}$) and percentage of medullary nephrocalcinosis (NC%). (E) Minimal plasma $Mg^{2+}$ concentration (*dashed line* indicates the lower normal limit, 0.65 mM). *Horizontal lines* indicate the median; the *open symbol* in the Barttin group indicates the digenic ClC-Ka/ClC-Kb disorder. *ClC-Kb,* Basolateral chloride channel b; *NCCT,* Na–Cl transporter; *NKCC2,* $Na^+$–$K^+$–$2Cl^-$ cotransporter 2; *ROMK,* potassium channel. (From Jeck N, Schlingmann KP, Reinalter SC, et al. Salt handling in the distal nephron: lessons learned from inherited human disorders. *Am J Physiol Regul Integr Comp Physiol.* 2005;288:R782–R795. With permission.)

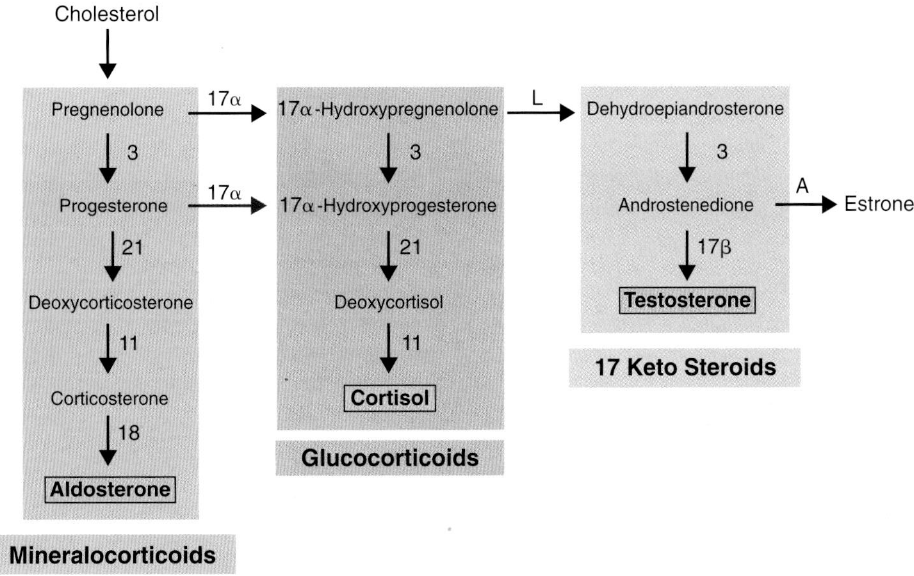


**Fig. 44.13** Key enzymes of the steroid biosynthesis pathway.

a decreased ability to synthesize cortisol, leading to elevated ACTH, which increases serum levels of DOC and, especially, corticosterone, resulting in low-renin hypertension, hypokalemia, and metabolic alkalosis. The clinical features vary depending on the enzymatic activity affected. In severe 17α-hydroxylase deficiency, both the 17α-hydroxylase and 17,20-lyase activities are reduced or absent. This deficiency results in high mineralocorticoid activity and hypertension and produces a female phenotype in all subjects because of the absence of sex steroid production in both the adrenal and gonads. Partial 17α-hydroxylase deficiency leads to sexual ambiguity in male patients without hypertension. Corticosteroid replacement corrects ACTH levels and hypertension. Women usually require hormonal therapy. Genetic male patients reared as female patients also require estrogen replacement. Genetic male patients reared as male patients require surgical correction of their external genitalia and androgen replacement therapy.

## LIDDLE SYNDROME

### PATHOGENESIS

Liddle syndrome (OMIM #177200) is an autosomal dominant form of hypertension characterized by hypokalemia and low levels of plasma renin and aldosterone, resulting from either premature termination or frameshift mutations in the carboxy-terminal tail of the ENaC β- or γ-subunits.[267] The amiloride-sensitive epithelial $Na^+$ channel is a tetramer formed by the assembly of three homologous subunits, α, β, and γ, with the α subunit being present in two copies (Fig. 44.14).[268] The $NH_2$ and carboxy-terminal terminal segments are cytoplasmic and contain potential regulatory segments that are able to modulate the activity of the channel. Mutations in the β- and γ-subunits of ENaC lead to channel hyperactivity by deleting or altering a conserved proline-rich amino acid sequence referred to as the PY motif. *SCNN1B* β-subunit or *SCNN1G* γ-subunit mutations could lead to an increase in the number of channels in the membrane or in their "openness." The identification of specific binding domains for Nedd4 (for all subunits) and α-spectrin (for the α-subunit only) within the cytosolic carboxy-terminal region of the ENaC subunits suggests that interactions with cytoskeletal elements control the expression of ENaC at the apical membrane.[269] Therefore Nedd4 (neural precursor cell expressed developmentally downregulated protein 4) and α-spectrin appear to play a role in the assembly, insertion, and/or retrieval of the ENaC subunits in the plasma membrane.[270]

### CLINICAL PRESENTATION

Liddle syndrome is characterized by inappropriate renal sodium reabsorption, blunted sodium excretion, and low-renin hypertension.[267] The features of this syndrome were described by Liddle and colleagues in 1963 in a large pedigree.[271] Affected subjects are at increased risk of cerebrovascular and cardiovascular events. Liddle syndrome can be differentiated from other rare mendelian forms of low-renin hypertension with the use of urinary/plasma hormonal profiles. Glucocorticoid-remediable aldosteronism is associated with increased production of 18-hydroxycortisol and aldosterone metabolites. Apparent mineralocorticoid excess (AME) is associated with an elevated ratio of urinary cortisol (tetrahydrocortisol) to cortisone (tetrahydrocortisone) metabolites (Table 44.7).

### TREATMENT

Hypertension is not improved by spironolactone but can be corrected by a low-salt diet and an ENaC antagonist (amiloride or triamterene).

## APPARENT MINERALOCORTICOID EXCESS

### PATHOGENESIS

The syndrome of AME (OMIM #207765) is a rare autosomal recessive disorder that results in hypokalemic hypertension with low serum levels of renin and aldosterone.[271,272] AME is

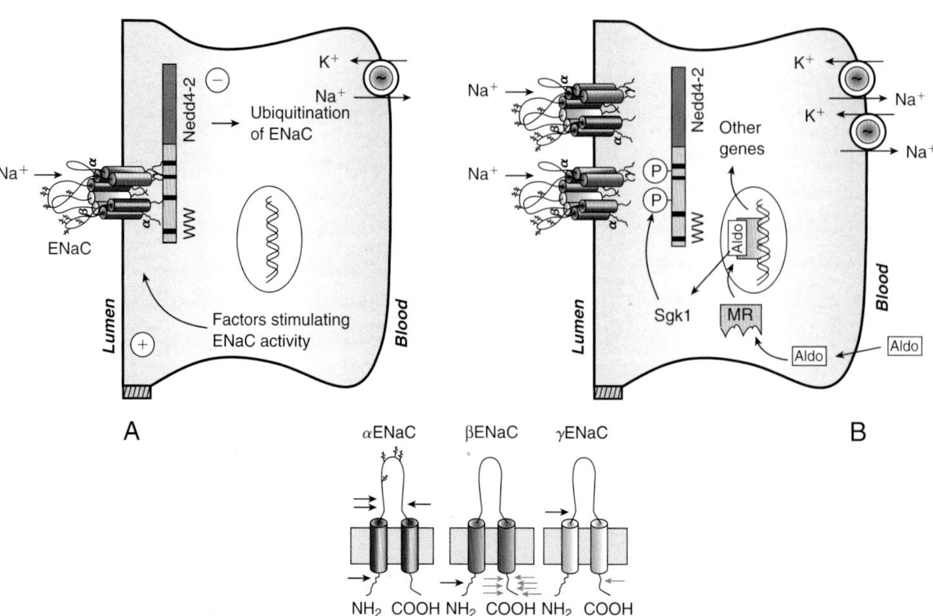


**Fig. 44.14** Disorders of the epithelial Na channel (ENaC). (*Top panel*) The mechanism of ENaC expression in an aldosterone-sensitive epithelial cell is represented. (A) In a resting state, few ENaCs, which facilitate sodium reabsorption in a rate-limiting fashion, are resident in the apical membrane. Factors known to enhance ENaC surface expression and activity are counterbalanced by retrieval of these channels from the membrane through the ubiquitin pathway mediated by ubiquitin–protein ligase Nedd4-2. (B) Shortly after aldosterone exposure and binding to the mineralocorticoid receptor (MR), transcriptional stimulation of serum and glucocorticoid-regulated kinase 1 (Sgk1) leads to phosphorylation of Nedd4-2, which subsequently disrupts ENaC/Nedd4-2 interactions. In this situation, ubiquitination of ENaCs is reduced, thus favoring both their residence in the apical membrane and enhanced sodium reabsorption. (*Bottom panel*) The ENaC is composed of two α-, one β-, and one γ-subunits surrounding the channel pore[267]. Each subunit has two transmembrane domains with short cytoplasmic amino and carboxy termini and a large ectocytoplasmic loop. Mutations in subunits of ENaC cause either Liddle syndrome (*pink arrows*; β- or γ-subunits) or the autosomal recessive form of pseudohypoaldosteronism type I [PHA I (*black arrows*)] (α-, β-, or γ-subunits).[268,284] (From Rossier BC. The epithelial sodium channel (ENaC): new insights into ENaC gating. *Pflugers Arch* 2003;446:314–316.)

**Table 44.7 Urinary Steroid Profiles in Mendelian Forms of Low-Renin Hypertension**

| | Liddle Syndrome | GRA | AME |
|---|---|---|---|
| Aldosterone | ⇓⇓ | ⇑ | ⇓ |
| TH-Aldo | ⇓⇓ | ⇑ | ⇓ |
| 18-OH-TH-Aldo | ⇓⇓ | ⇑ | ⇓ |
| 18-OH F | – | ⇑⇑ | – |
| TH-F | nl | nl | ⇑ |
| TH-E | nl | nl | ⇓ |
| TH-F/TH-E ratio | nl | nl | ⇑⇑ |

*Aldo,* Aldosterone; *AME,* apparent mineralocorticoid excess; *E,* cortisone; *F,* cortisol; *GRA,* glucocorticoid-remediable aldosteronism; *nl,* normal; *TH-,* tetrahydro-; *–,* not usually detected.

Modified from Warnock DG: Liddle syndrome: an autosomal dominant form of human hypertension. *Kidney Int.* 1998;53:18–24.

caused by a deficiency in 11β-hydroxysteroid dehydrogenase type 2 enzymatic activity (11β-HSD2), which is responsible for the conversion of cortisol to the inactive metabolite cortisone, therefore protecting the mineralocorticoid receptors from cortisol intoxication. In AME, cortisol acts as a potent mineralocorticoid and causes salt retention, hypertension, and hypokalemia with a suppression of the renin–angiotensin–aldosterone system. A milder phenotype, or type 2 variant, also results from abnormal activity of the enzyme.[273] Cushing syndrome and extremely high cortisol levels can overcome the ability of 11β-HSD2 to convert cortisol to cortisone.

## CLINICAL PRESENTATION

AME is associated with severe juvenile low-renin hypertension, hypokalemic alkalosis, low birth weight, failure to thrive, poor growth, nephrocalcinosis, and variable degrees of polyuria. The urinary metabolites of cortisol demonstrate an abnormal ratio, with predominance of cortisol metabolites (i.e., tetrahydrocortisol plus 5α-tetrahydrocortisol/tetrahydrocortisone in the range 6.7–33, the normal ratio being 1.0). The milder form of AME (type 2) lacks the typical urinary steroid profile (i.e., biochemical analysis reveals a moderately elevated ratio of cortisol to cortisone metabolites).[273] The heterozygote state is phenotypically normal but is associated with subtle defects in cortisol metabolism.

## TREATMENT

The treatment of AME is sodium restriction and triamterene, amiloride, or spironolactone. Additional antihypertensive agents may be used as needed.

## AUTOSOMAL DOMINANT EARLY ONSET HYPERTENSION WITH SEVERE EXACERBATION DURING PREGNANCY

Autosomal dominant early onset hypertension with severe exacerbation during pregnancy is a rare autosomal dominant disorder (OMIM #605115) described in a family that is associated with activating mutations in the mineralocorticoid receptor. By screening the mineralocorticoid receptor in 75 patients with early onset of severe hypertension, Geller and colleagues identified a 15-year-old boy with severe hypertension, suppressed plasma renin activity, low aldosterone, and no other underlying cause of hypertension, who had a heterozygous missense mutation (S810L) in the mineralocorticoid receptor gene.[274] Of 23 relatives evaluated, 11 had been diagnosed with severe hypertension before age 20, whereas the remaining 12 had unremarkable blood pressures. Two L810 carriers had undergone five pregnancies, all of which had been complicated by marked exacerbation of hypertension with suppressed aldosterone levels. The S810L mutation alters a conserved amino acid, resulting in a constitutively active and altered mineralocorticoid receptor. In addition, progesterone and other steroids lacking 21-hydroxyl groups, normally mineralocorticoid receptor antagonists, become potent agonists. Spironolactone is also a potent agonist of L810, so its use is contraindicated in L810 carriers.

## GLUCOCORTICOID-REMEDIABLE HYPERALDOSTERONISM

### PATHOGENESIS

Glucocorticoid-remediable hyperaldosteronism (GRA) is also known as familial hyperaldosteronism type I (OMIM #103900), aldosteronism sensitive to dexamethasone, glucocorticoid-suppressible hyperaldosteronism, and syndrome of ACTH-dependent hyperaldosteronism. It is an autosomal dominant hypertensive disorder caused by a chimeric gene duplication arising from unequal crossover between genes encoding aldosterone synthase and 11β-hydroxylase,[275] two highly similar genes with the same transcriptional orientation lying 45,000 base pairs apart on chromosome 8. Humans have two isozymes with 11β-hydroxylase activity that are required for synthesis of cortisol and aldosterone, respectively. CYP11B1 (11β-hydroxylase) is expressed at high levels and is regulated by ACTH, whereas CYP11B2 (aldosterone synthase) is normally expressed at low levels and is regulated by angiotensin II. In addition to 11β-hydroxylase activity, the latter enzyme has 18-hydroxylase and 18-oxidase activities and can synthesize aldosterone from DOC.[276] Thus with the unequal crossover between the two genes, the aldosterone synthase gene is under the control of regulatory promoter sequences of the 11β-hydroxylase. The chimeric gene product is expressed at high levels in both the zona glomerulosa and zona fasciculata and is controlled by ACTH, leading to increased production of 18-hydroxycortisol and aldosterone metabolites.

### CLINICAL PRESENTATION

The phenotype of GRA is highly variable.[277] Affected individuals may have mild hypertension and normal biochemistry and may be clinically indistinguishable from patients with essential hypertension. However, some subjects have early onset severe hypertension, hypokalemia, and metabolic alkalosis. In a study of 376 patients from 27 genetically proven GRA pedigrees, 48% of all GRA families and 18% of all patients with GRA had cerebrovascular complications, findings similar to the frequency of aneurysm in adult polycystic kidney disease.[278]

The diagnosis is usually established by measuring 18-hydroxycortisol or 18-oxocortisol metabolites in the urine or with the dexamethasone suppression test.[278] In addition, because patients with GRA secrete aldosterone in response to ACTH, glucocorticoid administration can suppress excessive aldosterone secretion.[279] The dexamethasone suppression test is a variably reliable method for establishing the diagnosis. Patients without the disease (i.e., subjects with an aldosterone-producing adenoma or with idiopathic hyperaldosteronism) can suppress aldosterone secretion.[280] The diagnosis of GRA can be definitively established by demonstration of the chimeric gene by molecular techniques.

### TREATMENT

Simple glucocorticoid replacement is the treatment for GRA. Salt restriction combined with either spironolactone or ENaC inhibition is also effective.

## FAMILIAL HYPERALDOSTERONISM TYPE II

Familial hyperaldosteronism type II (FH-II; OMIM #605635) is characterized by hypersecretion of aldosterone because of adrenocortical hyperplasia, an aldosterone-producing adenoma, or both. In contrast to familial hyperaldosteronism type I, FH-II is not suppressible by dexamethasone. Stowasser and colleagues reported five families with this phenotype with a segregation pattern supporting dominant inheritance.[281] Analysis of an extended kindred has revealed linkage between FH-II and markers on chromosome 7p22, but the gene implicated has not been clearly identified.[282]

# PSEUDOHYPOALDOSTERONISM

## PSEUDOHYPOALDOSTERONISM TYPE I

### PATHOGENESIS

PHA I is a rare disorder characterized by salt wasting, hypotension, hyperkalemia, metabolic acidosis, and failure to thrive in infants. There are two subtypes of PHA I.[283] The autosomal recessive form (OMIM #264350 and #177735) leads to severe manifestations that persist in adulthood and is caused by inactivating mutations in any of the three subunits (α, β, or γ) of ENaC. The autosomal dominant form (OMIM #177735) is associated with milder manifestations that remit with age and is caused by mutations in the mineralocorticoid receptor gene[284] that result in haploinsufficiency or in dominant negative actions. Homozygous mineralocorticoid receptor mutations are probably lethal in humans, because knockout mice show a severe salt-wasting syndrome and die a few days after birth.[285]

### CLINICAL PRESENTATION

The clinical contrast between PHA I because of ENaC and that as a result of mineralocorticoid receptor mutations is striking.[283] Autosomal recessive PHA I manifests neonatally or in childhood as renal salt wasting, hypotension, hyperkalemia, metabolic acidosis, and, on occasion, failure to thrive. Other biologic features include hyponatremia, high plasma and urinary aldosterone levels despite hyperkalemia, and elevated plasma renin activity. Autosomal dominant PHA I is associated with milder manifestations and remits with age. PHA I must be differentiated from aldosterone synthase deficiency, salt-wasting forms of congenital adrenal hyperplasia, and adrenal hypoplasia congenita, all of which cause aldosterone deficiency and are associated with hyponatremia, hyperkalemia, hypovolemia, elevated plasma renin activity, and occasionally shock and death.[286] Bartter syndrome type 2 (ROMK gene mutations) can also manifest in the neonatal period with a similar (transient) clinical picture.

### TREATMENT

Treatment of PHA I consists of salt supplementation, which can greatly improve hyponatremia, hyperkalemia, and growth. Administration of aldosterone, fludrocortisone, or DOC is not helpful. Patients with the recessive form usually need lifelong treatment for salt wasting and hyperkalemia, whereas for those with the dominant form, treatment can usually be withdrawn in adulthood.

## PSEUDOHYPOALDOSTERONISM TYPE II

### PATHOGENESIS

Pseudohypoaldosteronism type II (PHA II; OMIM #145260), also known as familial hyperkalemia and hypertension or Gordon syndrome, is a volume-dependent, low-renin hypertension characterized by persistent hyperkalemia despite a normal renal GFR. Variants within at least four genes—the with-no-lysine-(K) kinases, *WNK1* and *WNK4*, *Cullin3*, and *KLHL3* (encoding the Kelch-like 3 protein)—can cause the phenotype.[286,287] Details are still emerging for some of these genes, but it is likely that they all cause a gain of function in thiazide-sensitive NCC and, hence, salt retention. Hypertension is attributable to increased renal salt reabsorption, and hyperkalemia to reduced renal $K^+$ excretion. Reduced renal $H^+$ secretion is also commonly seen, resulting in metabolic acidosis. The features of PHA II are chloride dependent, because they are corrected when infusion of sodium sulfate or sodium bicarbonate is substituted for sodium chloride.[288]

WNK1 and WNK4 function as molecular switches, eliciting coordinated effects on diverse ion transport pathways to maintain homeostasis during physiologic perturbation. In PHA II, mutations that appear to activate WNK1 and inactivate WNK4 have been proposed to result in increased thiazide-sensitive cotransporter (NCC) activity and decreased ROMK activity (Fig. 44.15).[289] Kelch-like 3 and Cullin3 regulate electrolyte homeostasis via ubiquitination and degradation of WNK1 and WNK4.[289,290] On one hand is the overactivity of NCC and on the other is the increased paracellular reabsorption of $Cl^-$, also known as the *chloride shunt* hypothesis.

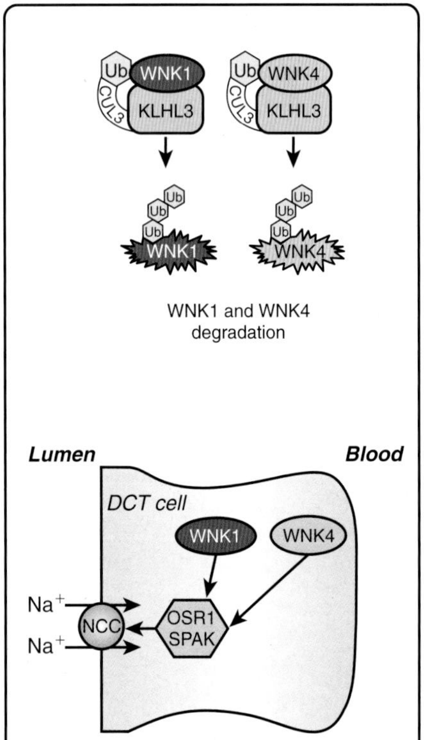


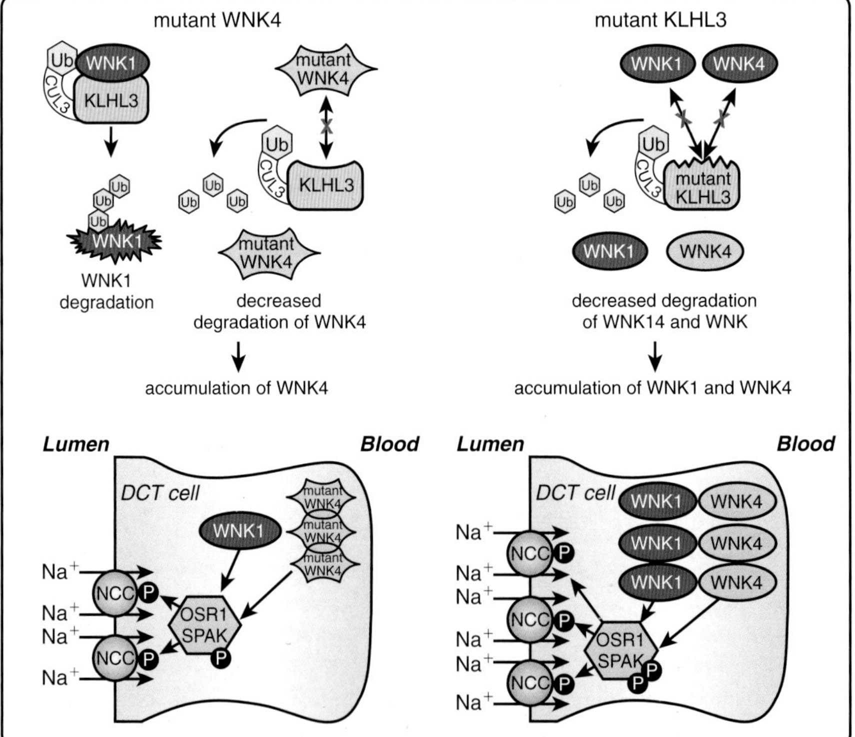


**Fig. 44.15** Molecular mechanism of pseudohypoaldosteronism type II in the distal convoluted tubule. *(Left)* Normally kinases WNK1 and WNK4 can stimulate Na–Cl cotransporter (NCC) trafficking to the plasma membrane and phosphorylation of NCC by Ste20-related proline alanine-rich kinase (SPAK) and oxidative stress–responsive kinase (OSR1). This is the WNK-OSR1/SPAK-NCC phosphorylation signaling cascade, recognized now as the major pathogenic mechanism of pseudohypoaldosteronism type II (PHA II; *shown at right*). WNK1 and WNK4 are substrates of $KLH_3$ (Kelch-like 3)–Cullin3 E3 ligase–mediated ubiquitination. *DCT,* Distal convoluted tubule; *Ub,* ubiquitin. (From Susa K, Sohara E, Rai T, et al. Impaired degradation of WNK1 and WNK4 kinases causes PHAII in mutant KLHL3 knock-in mice. *Hum Mol Genet.* 2014;23:5052–5060; Pathare G, Hoenderop JG, Bindels RJ, et al. A molecular update on pseudohypoaldosteronism type II. *Am J Physiol Renal Physiol.* 2013;305:F1513–F1520.)

The action of these kinases may serve to increase salt reabsorption and intravascular volume in volume-depleted states and decrease potassium secretion in K depletion, by enabling the distal nephron to allow either maximal NaCl reabsorption or maximal $K^+$ secretion in response to hypovolemia or hyperkalemia, respectively.

### CLINICAL PRESENTATION

PHA II is usually diagnosed in adults but can also be seen neonatally.[291] Unexplained hyperkalemia is the usual presenting feature and occurs before the onset of hypertension. The severity of hyperkalemia varies greatly and is influenced by prior intake of diuretics and salt.[292] Causes of spurious elevation of potassium should be ruled out before this diagnosis is made. In its most severe form, PHA II is associated with muscle weakness (from hyperkalemia), short stature, and intellectual impairment. Mild hyperchloremia, metabolic acidosis, and suppressed plasma renin activity are findings variably associated with the trait. Aldosterone levels vary from low to high depending on the level of hyperkalemia. Urinary concentrating ability, acid excretion, and proximal tubular function are all normal.

### TREATMENT

Thiazides reverse all biochemical abnormalities. Lower than average doses can be given if overcorrection occurs. Loop diuretics may also be used.

## INHERITED DISORDERS OF RENAL MAGNESIUM PROCESSING

Magnesium, the second most abundant intracellular cation, plays an important role as a cofactor in energy metabolism, nucleotide and protein synthesis, neuromuscular excitability, and oxidative phosphorylation and as a regulator of sodium, potassium, and calcium channels. Under normal conditions, extracellular magnesium concentration is maintained at nearly constant values (0.70–1.1 mmol/L). Hypomagnesemia results from decreased dietary intake but more commonly is caused by intestinal malabsorption, renal losses, or use of drugs including cyclosporine, omeprazole, cetuximab, and cisplatin.[293]

Primary hypomagnesemia is composed of a heterogeneous group of disorders characterized by renal and intestinal Mg wasting often associated with hypercalciuria (Table 44.8).[293–298] The genetic basis and cellular defects of a number of primary hypomagnesemias have been elucidated. These inherited conditions affect different nephron segments and different cell types, leading to variable but increasingly distinguishable phenotypic presentations.

### FAMILIAL HYPOMAGNESEMIA WITH HYPERCALCIURIA AND NEPHROCALCINOSIS

The syndrome of renal hypomagnesemia with hypercalciuria and nephrocalcinosis (OMIM #248250), or familial hypomagnesemia with hypercalciuria and nephrocalcinosis (FHHNC), is a rare autosomal recessive trait characterized by profound Mg wasting that results in severe hypomagnesemia not correctable by oral or intravenous magnesium supplementation. The disorder is caused by mutations in claudin-16 *(CLDN16)*, previously known as paracellin-1,[294] a protein located in tight junctions of the TAL and related to the claudin family of tight junction proteins (see Fig. 44.10). A study of nine additional families with severe hypomagnesemia identified mutations in *CLDN19* (OMIM #248190) that share the same renal phenotype as FHHNC. *CLDN19* encodes claudin-19, a tight junction protein expressed in renal tubules and the eye.[299]

Every patient with FHHNC has hypomagnesemia with inappropriately high urinary Mg excretion ($Mg^+$ fractional excretions >10%). Renal calcium wasting is present in every case initially and leads to parenchymal calcification (nephrocalcinosis) and renal failure, often requiring dialysis. The progression rate of renal insufficiency correlates with the severity of nephrocalcinosis. Other clinical findings are polyuria, polydipsia, ocular abnormalities, recurrent urinary tract infections, and renal colic with stone passage. Serum PTH levels are abnormally high. Serum levels of calcium, phosphorus, and potassium and urinary excretion of uric acid and oxalate are normal. In contrast to patients with a *CLDN16* defect, affected individuals with a *CLDN19* mutation have ocular symptoms that include severe visual impairment, macular colobomata, horizontal nystagmus, and marked myopia.[299] Long-term oral Mg administration does not normalize serum $Mg^{2+}$ levels. Thiazides are effective to reduce urinary Ca excretion.[300] After kidney transplantation, tubular handling of $Mg^{2+}$ and Ca is normalized.

### FAMILIAL HYPOMAGNESEMIA WITH SECONDARY HYPOCALCEMIA

Familial hypomagnesemia with secondary hypocalcemia (OMIM #602014) is an autosomal recessive disease that results in electrolyte abnormalities shortly after birth and is caused by mutations in *TRPM6* (Fig. 44.16). *TRPM6* holds 39 exons that code for a protein of 2022 amino acids. Affected individuals show extremely low serum $Mg^{2+}$ levels (0.1–0.3 mmol/L) and hypocalcemia, causing muscular and neurologic complications including seizures in early infancy that can lead to neurologic damage or cardiac arrest if left untreated. The disorder is caused by impaired intestinal uptake and renal $Mg^{2+}$ wasting.[301] Restoring the concentrations of serum magnesium to normal values with high-dose magnesium supplementation can overcome the apparent defect in magnesium absorption and in serum concentrations of calcium. Lifelong magnesium supplementation is required to overcome the defect in the seizures and magnesium handling in these individuals.

### ISOLATED DOMINANT HYPOMAGNESEMIA WITH HYPOCALCIURIA

A rare autosomal dominant disorder, isolated dominant hypomagnesemia with hypocalciuria (OMIM #154020) is caused by a dominant negative mutation of the *FXYD2* gene resulting in a trafficking defect of the γ-subunit of the $Na^+$–$K^+$–ATPase at the basolateral membrane of the distal convoluted tubule,[302] the main site of active renal $Mg^{2+}$ reabsorption. The hypomagnesemia in patients with the disorder can be as low as 0.40 mmol/L, resulting in convulsions. Mutation of *FXYD2* leads to misrouting of the $Na^+$/$K^+$-ATPase γ-subunit, so $Mg^{2+}$ reabsorption is abnormal.

**Table 44.8 Inherited Disorders of Magnesium Transport**

| Disease/OMIM[a] Entry | Gene/Inheritance | Protein | Key Clinical/Biochemical Symptoms |
|---|---|---|---|
| Gitelman syndrome/#263800 | *SLC12A3*/AR | NCC | Muscle weakness/tetany<br>Fatigue<br>Chondrocalcinosis<br>Hypomagnesemia<br>Hypocalciuria |
| Familial hypomagnesemia with hypercalciuria and nephrocalcinosis/ #248250/#248190 | *CLDN16*/AR<br>*CLDN19*/AR | Claudin-16<br>Claudin-19 | Polyuria<br>Renal stones/nephrocalcinosis<br>Ocular abnormalities<br>Severe hypomagnesemia<br>Hypercalciuria |
| Autosomal dominant isolated renal Mg loss/#154020 | *FXYD2*/AD | γ-Subunit sodium–potassium ATPase | Seizures<br>Chondrocalcinosis<br>Hypomagnesemia<br>Hypocalciuria |
| Autosomal dominant hypomagnesemia, hypermagnesuria, and hypocalciuria/#137920 | *HNF1B*/AD | Transcription factor hepatocyte nuclear factor 1 homeobox B (HNF1B) is linked to the regulation of FXYD2 | Renal malformations<br>Maturity-onset diabetes of the young (MODY) |
| Maturity-onset diabetes of the young (MODY) with hypomagnesemia and renal $Mg^{2+}$ loss/#126090 | *PCBD1*/AR | Hepatocyte nuclear factor 1 homeobox A (PCBD1) | MODY |
| Familial hypomagnesemia with secondary hypocalcemia/#602014 | *TRPM6*/AR | Epithelial magnesium channel TRPM6 | Tetany/seizures<br>Hypomagnesemia<br>Hypocalcemia |
| Autosomal recessive isolated Mg loss/#611718 | *EGF*/AR | Epidermal growth factor | Tetany/seizures<br>Hypomagnesemia<br>Normocalciuria |
| Autosomal dominant hypomagnesemia/#176260 | *KCNA1*/AD | Voltage-gated potassium channel Kv1.1 | Muscle cramps<br>Tetany<br>Tremor<br>Muscle weakness<br>Cerebral atrophy<br>Myokymia |
| Epilepsy, ataxia, sensorineural deafness and tubulopathy (EAST)/#612780 | *KCNJ10*/AR | $K^+$ channel Kir4.1 | Polyuria<br>Hypokalemic metabolic alkalosis<br>Hypomagnesemia<br>Hypocalciuria |
| Dominant and recessive hypomagnesemia with impaired brain development and seizures/#607803 | *CNNM2*/AD/AR | CNNM2<br>Mg-ATP | Mental retardation<br>Seizures |

[a]OMIM numbers. Available at http://www.ncbi.nlm.gov/omim/OMIM.
*AD,* Autosomal dominant; *AR,* autosomal recessive; *ATP,* adenosine triphosphate; *CLDN,* claudin; *CNNM2,* cyclin M2; *EGF,* epidermal growth factor; *FXYD2,* FXYD domain–containing ion transport regulator 2; *NCC,* Na–Cl cotransporter; *OMIM,* Online Mendelian Inheritance in Man; *SLC,* solute carrier; *TRPM6,* transient receptor potential channel 6.

Hypomagnesemic patients have lower urinary excretion of calcium, presumably as a consequence of increased reabsorption in the loop of Henle.[303]

The transcription factor hepatocyte nuclear factor 1 homeobox B (HNF1B) has been linked to the regulation of the *FXYD2* gene, and hypomagnesemia, hypermagnesuria, and hypocalciuria have been observed in 44% of *HNF1B* mutation carriers (OMIM #137920). Mutations have also been described in *PCBD1,* which encodes hepatocyte nuclear factor 1 homeobox A (PCBD1; see Fig. 44.16).[304]

## $CA^{2+}/MG^{2+}$-SENSING RECEPTOR–ASSOCIATED DISORDERS

An important regulator of magnesium homeostasis is the $Ca^{2+}/Mg^{2+}$(calcium)–sensing receptor (CaSR). CaSR senses ionized serum calcium and magnesium concentrations and is involved in renal calcium and magnesium reabsorption as well as in PTH secretion.[305] Activating mutations of the *CaSR* gene were first described in families affected with autosomal dominant hypocalcemia.[241,306] Affected individuals present

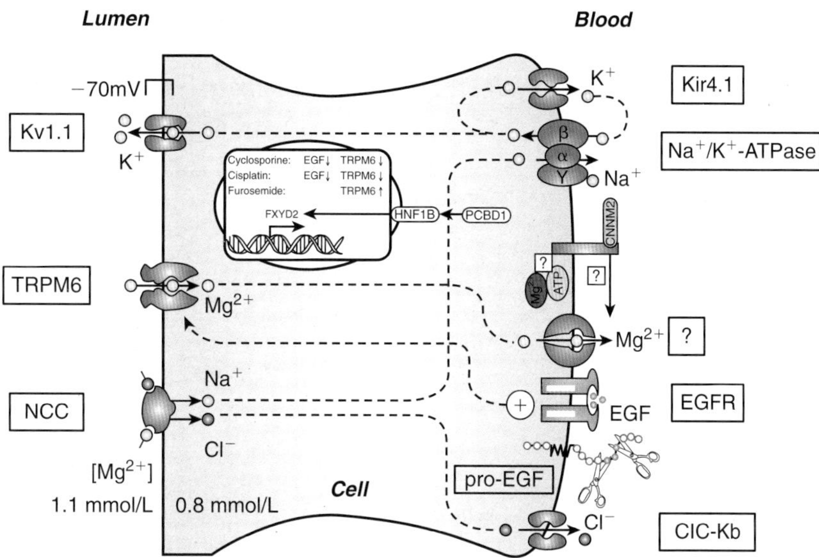


**Fig. 44.16** Magnesium reabsorption in the distal convoluted tubule. Transient receptor potential 6 (TRPM6) channels, located in the luminal membrane, facilitate transport of $Mg^{2+}$ from the prourine into the cell, which is driven primarily by the luminal membrane potential established by the voltage-gated $K^+$ channel Kv1.1. Epidermal growth factor *(EGF)* and insulin function as magnesiotropic hormones, stimulating TRPM6 activity through activation of the PI3K–Akt pathway. Insulin can also act on TRPM6 via phosphorylation of cyclin-dependent kinase 5 (CDK5). The expression of TRPM6 in the distal convoluted tubule is affected by treatment with furosemide, cyclosporine A, and cisplatin; the last two have been shown to also downregulate EGF levels. The $Mg^{2+}$ buffering and extrusion systems are not yet known. CNNM2, the gene encoding cyclin M2, is suggested as playing a role in the $Mg^{2+}$ extrusion and can bind Mg–adenosine triphosphate (ATP), which might play a role in this process. Transcription factor HNF1B, together with its regulator PCBD1, is proposed to regulate the expression of FXYD2, which encodes the γ-subunit of the $Na^+/K^+$–ATPase. The basolateral potassium channel, Kir4.1, recycles potassium to facilitate $Na^+/K^+$–ATPase activity. *ClC-Kb,* Basolateral chloride channel b; *EGFR,* EGF receptor; *NCC,* Na–Cl cotransporter; *PI3K,* phosphoinositide 3-kinase. (Modified from van der Wijst J, Bindels RJ, Hoenderop JG. $Mg^{2+}$ homeostasis: the balancing act of TRPM6. *Curr Opin Nephrol Hypertens.* 2014;23:361–369; Glaudemans B, Knoers NV, Hoenderop JG, et al. New molecular players facilitating $Mg^{2+}$ reabsorption in the distal convoluted tubule. *Kidney Int.* 2010;77:17–22.)

with hypocalcemia, hypercalciuria, and polyuria, and approximately 50% of them have hypomagnesemia.[296] Clinically, autosomal dominant hypocalcemia may be mistaken for primary hypoparathyroidism, because of the decreased PTH secretion in the setting of mild to moderate hypocalcemia. Most affected individuals have hypomagnesemia and renal magnesium wasting.

## ISOLATED RECESSIVE HYPOMAGNESEMIA WITH NORMOCALCIURIA

Isolated recessive hypomagnesemia (OMIM #131530) is a rare hereditary disease that was originally described in a consanguineous family.[307] The affected individuals presented with symptoms of hypomagnesemia during early infancy. Isolated recessive hypomagnesemia is caused by a mutation of the epidermal growth factor (EGF) precursor protein pro-EGF, which is expressed in the gastrointestinal tract, the respiratory tract, and the basolateral membrane of the distal convoluted tubule. On membrane insertion, pro-EGF is processed by unknown proteases into a functional EGF peptide hormone, which activates EGF receptors on the basolateral membrane (Fig. 44.16). As a result, EGF stimulates the trafficking of TRPM6 channels to the luminal membrane, increasing the reabsorption of $Mg^{2+}$ through TRPM6.[293]

## DOMINANT AND RECESSIVE HYPOMAGNESEMIA

Dominant and recessive hypomagnesemia with impaired brain development (recessive) and seizures secondary to *CNNM2* mutations (OMIM #607803). Mutations in the gene encoding cyclin M2 (*CNNM2*) have been found in two unrelated families with dominant isolated hypomagnesemia, mental retardation, and seizures.[308] Recessive forms have also been identified.[309]

# DIABETES INSIPIDUS

## PATHOGENESIS

The conservation of water by the human kidney is regulated by the action of the neurohypophyseal antidiuretic hormone arginine vasopressin (AVP) on cells of the collecting tubules,[310] as reviewed in detail in Chapter 10.

AVP promotes urinary concentration by allowing water to be transported passively down an osmotic gradient between the tubular fluid and the surrounding interstitium.[312]

## THE AVP–AVPR2–AQP SHUTTLE PATHWAY

Water homeostasis in the kidney is regulated by three key proteins. AVP, secreted from the posterior pituitary, activates

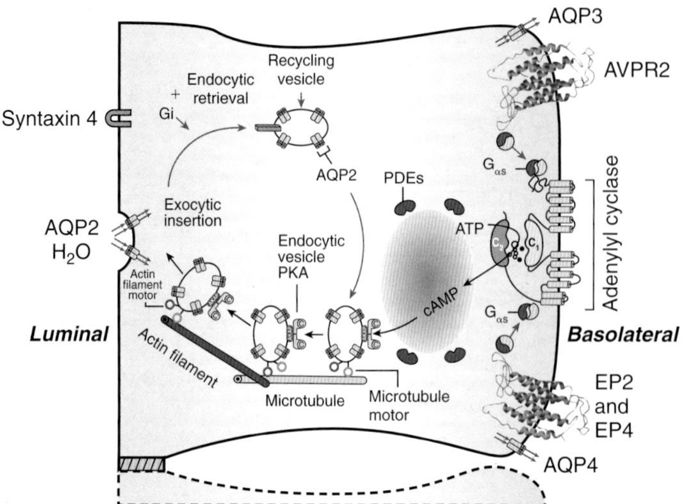


**Fig. 44.17** Effect of vasopressin to increase water permeability in the principal cells of the collecting duct. Vasopressin (AVP) binds to the $V_2$ receptor (AVPR2, a G protein–coupled receptor) on the basolateral membrane. This activates adenylyl cyclase, increasing the intracellular concentration of cyclic AMP (cAMP). Protein kinase A (PKA) is the target of the generated cAMP. The binding of cAMP to the regulatory subunits of PKA induces a conformational change, causing these subunits to dissociate from the catalytic subunits. These activated subunits as shown here are anchored to an aquaporin-2 (AQP2)–containing endocytic vesicle via an A-kinase anchoring protein. The local concentration and distribution of the cAMP gradient is limited by phosphodiesterases *(PDEs)*. Cytoplasmic vesicles carrying the water channels (represented as homotetrameric complexes) are fused to the luminal membrane in response to AVP, thereby increasing the water permeability of this membrane. The dissociation of the A-kinase anchoring protein from the endocytic vesicle is not represented. Microtubules and actin filaments are necessary for vesicle movement toward the membrane. When AVP is not available, AQP2 water channels are retrieved by an endocytic process, and water permeability returns to its original low rate. Aquaporin-3 (AQP3) and aquaporin-4 (AQP4) water channels are expressed constitutively at the basolateral membrane. Other G protein–coupled receptors, such as prostaglandin receptors EP2 and EP4, and the secretin receptor, may also contribute to an increase in intracellular cAMP. *ATP,* Adenosine triphosphate; *Gi*, inhibitory guanine nucleotide-binding protein.

the process of water excretion by binding to the vasopressin $V_2$ receptor (AVPR2; see Fig. 44.17) located on the basolateral membrane of collecting duct cells. This step activates the stimulatory G protein ($G_s$) and adenylyl cyclase, resulting in the production of cyclic AMP (cAMP) and stimulation of protein kinase A. The final step in the antidiuretic action of AVP is the exocytic insertion of a specific water channel, AQP2, into the luminal membrane, thereby increasing the water permeability of that membrane. These water channels are members of a superfamily of integral membrane proteins that facilitate water transport.[313,314]

The short-term regulation of AQP2 by AVP involves the movement of AQP2 from the intracellular vesicles to the luminal membrane; in the long-term regulation, which requires a sustained elevation of circulating AVP for 24 hours or more, AVP increases the abundance of water channels. This increase is thought to be a consequence of increased transcription of the *AQP2* gene.[317] AQP3 and AQP4 are the water channels in basolateral membranes of renal medullary collecting ducts. In addition, vasopressin increases the water reabsorptive capacity of the kidney by regulating the urea transporter UT-A1, which is expressed in the inner medullary collecting duct, predominantly in its terminal part.[318] AVP also increases the permeability of principal collecting duct cells to sodium.[319]

In summary, in the absence of AVP stimulation, collecting duct epithelia exhibit very low permeabilities to sodium, urea, and water. These specialized permeability properties permit the excretion of large volumes of hypotonic urine formed during intervals of water diuresis. By contrast, AVP stimulation of the principal cells of the collecting ducts leads to selective increases in the permeabilities of the apical membrane to water ($P_f$), urea ($P_{Urea}$), and sodium ($P_{Na}$).

In neurohypophyseal diabetes insipidus, termed "familial neurohypophyseal diabetes insipidus" (FNDI), levels of AVP are insufficient, and patients show a positive response to treatment with desmopressin (DDAVP). Growth retardation might be observed in untreated children with autosomal dominant FNDI (adFNDI).[320]

More than 85 variants in the prepro-arginine-vasopressin-neurophysin II *AVP* gene located on chromosome 20p13 have been reported in adFNDI. Autosomal dominant central diabetes insipidus is secondary to *AVP* mutations that result in misfolding and aggregation of the protein in the ER.[321] ER-associated degradation (ERAD) is a principal quality control mechanism in cells responsible for targeting misfolded ER proteins for cytosolic degradation. In mammals, the most well-characterized ERAD machinery is the highly conserved complex of suppressor-enhancer of lin-12–like and hydroxymethylglutaryl-CoA reductase degradation protein 1 (SEL1L-HRD1), which consists of the E3 ubiquitin ligase HRD1 and its adaptor protein SEL1L. WT proAVP aggregates with mutant proAVP to form complexes that are retrotranslocated and destroyed. Moreover, WT proAVP and mutant proAVP were recently shown to be substrates for Sel1L, which links these proAVPs to Hrd1 and ERAD-mediated destruction and eliminates expression of the normal allele, explaining the vasopressin deficiency before magnocellular cell death.[322,323] Recessive FNDI has also been described.[324,325]

In nephrogenic diabetes insipidus (NDI), AVP values are normal or elevated, but the kidney is unable to concentrate urine. The clinical manifestations of polyuria and polydipsia can be present at birth and must be immediately recognized to avoid severe episodes of dehydration. Most (>90%) of patients with congenital NDI have X-linked mutations in the *AVPR2* gene, the Xq28 gene coding for the vasopressin $V_2$ (antidiuretic) receptor. In less than 10% of the families studied, congenital NDI has an autosomal recessive inheritance, and more than 45 mutations have been identified in the AQP2 gene *(AQP2)*, located in chromosome region 12q13. For the *AVPR2* gene, more than 250 putative disease-causing mutations in 326 unrelated families with X-linked NDI have now been published.[326] When studied in vitro, most *AVPR2* mutations lead to receptors that are trapped intracellularly and are unable to reach the plasma membrane.[327]

A minority of the mutant receptors reach the cell surface but are unable to bind AVP or to trigger an intracellular cAMP signal. Similarly, AQP2 mutant proteins are trapped intracellularly and cannot be expressed at the luminal membrane. This AQP2 trafficking defect is correctable, at least in vitro, by chemical chaperones. Other inherited disorders with mild, moderate, or severe inability to concentrate urine include Bartter syndrome (MIM 601678),[248,328] *MAGED2* mutations with transient Bartter and severe polyhydramnios,[329] cystinosis, autosomal dominant hypocalcemia, nephronophthisis, and AME.[330]

## CLINICAL PRESENTATION AND HISTORY OF X-LINKED NEPHROGENIC DIABETES INSIPIDUS

X-linked NDI (OMIM #304800) is secondary to *AVPR2* mutations, which result in a loss of function or dysregulation of the $V_2$ receptor.[326] Male patients who have an *AVPR2* mutation have a phenotype characterized by early dehydration episodes, hypernatremia, and hyperthermia as early as the first week of life. Dehydration episodes can be so severe that they lower arterial blood pressure to a degree that is not sufficient to sustain adequate oxygenation to the brain, kidneys, and other organs. Mental and physical retardation and renal failure are the classic "historical" consequences of a late diagnosis and lack of treatment. Heterozygous female patients may exhibit variable degrees of polyuria and polydipsia because of skewed X chromosome inactivation. The "historical" clinical characteristics include hypernatremia, hyperthermia, mental retardation, and repeated episodes of dehydration in early infancy.[331] Mental retardation, a consequence of repeated episodes of dehydration, was prevalent in the Crawford and Bode study, which found that only nine of 82 patients (11%) had normal intelligence.[331]

Early recognition and treatment of X-linked NDI with an abundant intake of water allow a normal life span with normal physical and mental development.[332] Two characteristics suggestive of X-linked NDI are the familial occurrence and the confinement of mental retardation to male patients. It is then tempting to assume that the family described in 1892 by McIlraith and discussed by Reeves and Andreoli was a family with X-linked NDI.[333,334] Lacombe and Weil described a familial form of diabetes insipidus with autosomal transmission and without any associated mental retardation.[335,336] The descendants of the family originally described by Weil were later found to have neurohypophyseal adFNDI (OMIM #192340).[337] Patients with adFNDI retain some limited capacity to secrete AVP during severe dehydration, and the polyuropolydipsic symptoms usually appear after the first year of life, when the infant's demand for water is more likely to be understood by adults.

The severity in infancy of NDI was clearly described by Crawford and Bode.[331] The first manifestations of the disease can be recognized during the first week of life. The infants are irritable, cry almost constantly, and although eager to suck, will vomit milk soon after ingestion unless prefed with water. The history given by the mothers often includes persistent constipation, erratic unexplained fever, and failure to gain weight. Even though the patients characteristically show no visible evidence of perspiration, increased water loss during fever or in warm weather exaggerates the symptoms. Unless the condition is recognized early, children experience frequent bouts of hypertonic dehydration, sometimes complicated by convulsions or death. Mental retardation is a common consequence of these episodes. The intake of large quantities of water, combined with the patient's voluntary restriction of dietary salt and protein intake, lead to hypocaloric dwarfism beginning in infancy. Affected children frequently have lower urinary tract dilation and obstruction, probably secondary to the large volume of urine produced. Dilation of the lower urinary tract is also seen in patients with primary polydipsia and in patients with neurogenic diabetes insipidus.[338,339]

Chronic renal insufficiency may occur by the end of the first decade of life and could be the result of episodes of dehydration with thrombosis of the glomerular tufts. Almost 30 years ago the authors' group observed that the administration of desmopressin, a $V_2$ receptor agonist, caused an increase in plasma cAMP concentrations in normal subjects but had no effect in 14 male patients with X-linked NDI.[340]

Intermediate responses were observed in obligate carriers of the disease, possibly corresponding to half of the normal receptor response. On the basis of these results, our group predicted that the defective gene in these patients with X-linked NDI was likely to code for a defective $V_2$ receptor (Fig. 44.18).[340]

X-linked NDI is a rare disease, with an estimated prevalence of approximately 8.8 per million male live births in the province of Quebec (Canada).[341] In defined regions of North America, the prevalence is much higher. Our group estimated the incidence in Nova Scotia and New Brunswick (Canada) to be 58 per million male live births because of shared ancestry.[342]

An additional example has been identified in a Mormon pedigree whose members reside in Utah (Utah families). This pedigree was originally described by Cannon.[342] The "Utah mutation" is a nonsense mutation (L312X) predictive of a receptor that lacks transmembrane domain 7 and the intracellular COOH terminus.[342]

The largest known kindred with X-linked NDI is the Hopewell family, named after the Irish ship "Hopewell," which arrived in Halifax, Nova Scotia, in 1761. Aboard the ship were members of the Ulster Scot clan, descendants of Scottish Presbyterians who migrated to Ulster province in Ireland in the 17th century and left Ireland for the New World in the 18th century. Although families arriving with the first emigration wave settled in northern Massachusetts in 1718, the members of a second emigration wave, passengers

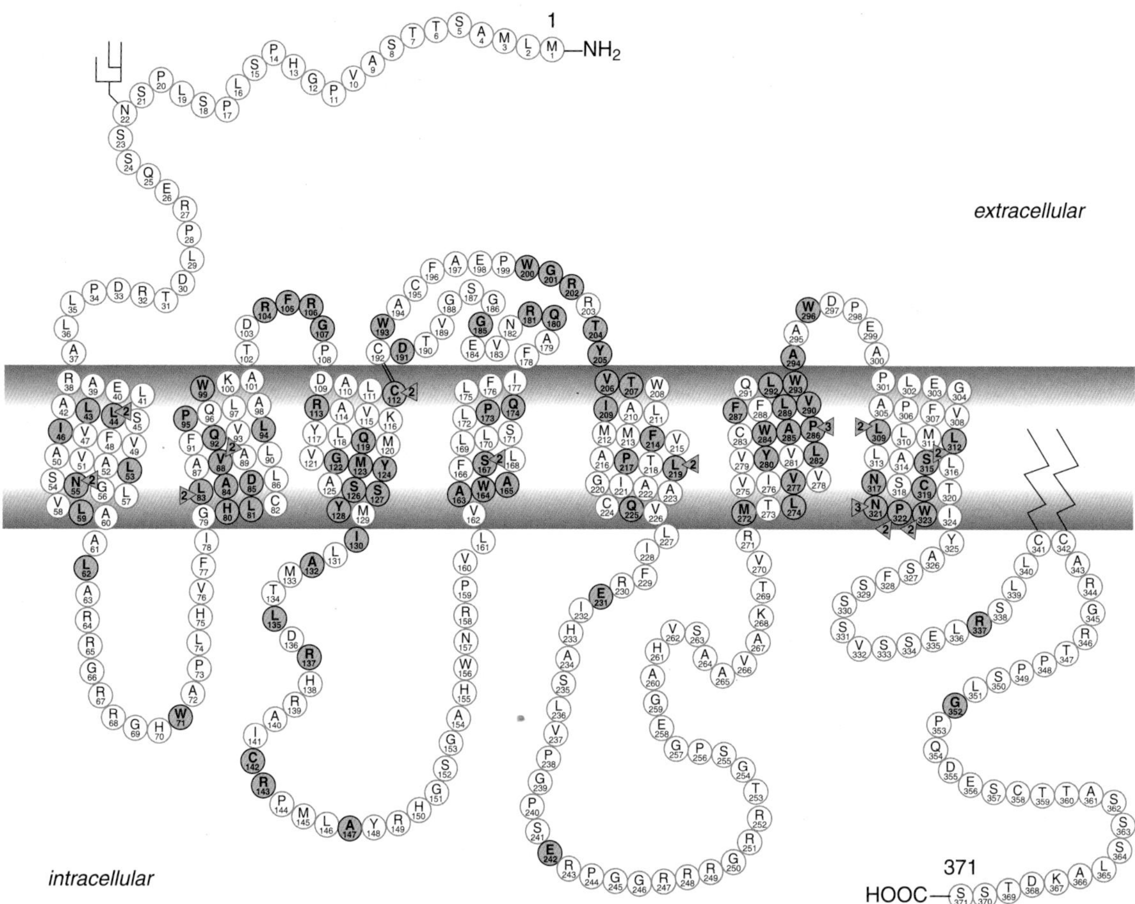


**Fig. 44.18** Schematic representation of the $V_2$ receptor (AVPR2) and identification of 193 putative disease-causing AVPR2 mutations. Predicted amino acids are shown as their one-letter amino acid codes. A *solid symbol* indicates a codon with a missense or nonsense mutation; a *number (within a triangle)* indicates more than one mutation in the same codon; other types of mutations are not indicated on the figure. There are 95 missense, 18 nonsense, 46 frameshift deletion or insertion, seven in-frame deletion or insertion, four splice-site, and 22 large deletion mutations, and one complex mutation.

of the "Hopewell," settled in Colchester County, Nova Scotia. According to the "Hopewell hypothesis,"[343] most patients with NDI in North America are progeny of female carriers of the second emigration wave. This assumption is based mainly on the high prevalence of NDI among descendants of the Ulster Scots residing in Nova Scotia. In two villages with a total of 2500 inhabitants, 30 patients have been diagnosed, and the carrier frequency has been estimated at 6%.

Given the numerous mutations found in North American X-linked NDI families, the Hopewell hypothesis cannot be upheld in its originally proposed form. However, among X-linked NDI patients in North America, the W71X mutation (the Hopewell mutation) is more common than the other *AVPR2* mutation. It is a null mutation (W71X), predictive of an extremely truncated receptor consisting of the extracellular $NH_2$ terminus, the first transmembrane domain, and the $NH_2$-terminal half of the first intracellular loop. Because the original carrier cannot be identified, it is not clear whether the Hopewell mutation was brought to North America by "Hopewell" passengers or by other Ulster Scot immigrants. The diversity of *AVPR2* mutations found in many ethnic groups (Europeans, Japanese, African Americans, and Africans) and the low frequency of the disease are consistent with an X-linked recessive disease that in the past was lethal for male patients and was balanced by recurrent mutations. In X-linked NDI, loss of mutant alleles from the population occurs because of the higher mortality of affected male patients compared with healthy male patients, whereas gain of mutant alleles occurs by mutation. If affected male patients with a rare X-linked recessive disease do not reproduce and if mutation rates are equal in mothers and fathers, then, at genetic equilibrium, one-third of new cases in affected male patients will be caused by new mutations. Our group has described ancestral mutations, de novo mutations, and potential mechanisms of mutagenesis. These data are reminiscent of those obtained from patients with late-onset autosomal dominant retinitis pigmentosa. In one-fourth of patients, the disease is caused by mutations in the light receptor rhodopsin. Here, too, many different mutations (approximately 100) spread throughout the coding region of the rhodopsin gene have been found.[344]

The basis of loss of function or dysregulation of 28 different mutant $V_2$ receptors (including nonsense, frameshift, deletion, and missense mutations) has been studied with the use of in vitro expression systems. Most of the mutant $V_2$ receptors tested were not transported to the cell membrane and were retained within the intracellular compartment. Our group also demonstrated that misfolded *AVPR2* mutants could be

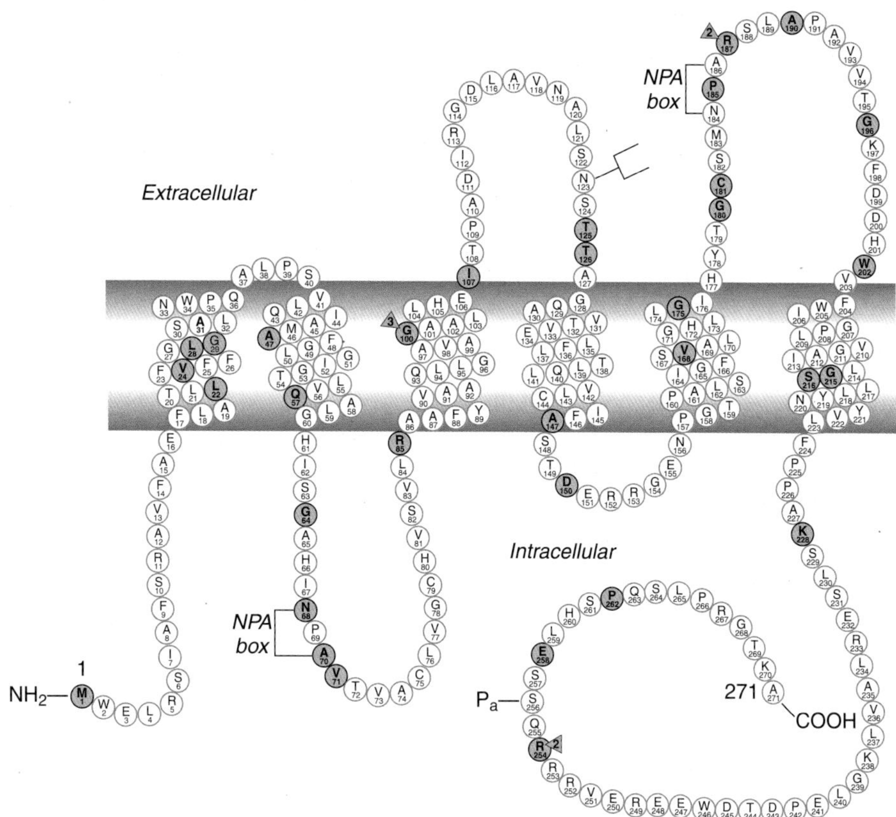


**Fig. 44.19** A representation of the aquaporin-2 (AQP2) protein and identification of 46 putative disease-causing AQP2 mutations. Predicted amino acids are shown as their one-letter amino acid codes. A monomer is represented with six transmembrane helices. The location of the protein kinase A (PKA) phosphorylation site (Pa) is indicated. The extracellular, transmembrane, and cytoplasmic domains are defined according to Deen et al. 1994.[361] *Triangles* are indicating amino acids with more than one mutation in the same codon. *Solid symbols* indicate locations of the mutations: M1I; L22V; V24A; L28P; G29S; A47V; Q57P; G64R, N68S, A70D; V71M; R85X; G100X; G100V; G100R; I107D; 369delC; T125M; T126M; A147T; D150E; V168M; G175R; G180S; C181W; P185A; R187C; R187H; A190T; G196D; W202C; G215C; S216P; S216F; K228E; R254Q; R254L; E258K; and P262L. GenBank accession numbers - AQP2: AF147092, exon 1; AF147093, exons 2 through 4. NPA (asparagine–proline–alanine) motifs and the N-glycosylation site are also indicated by the fork-like symbol on amino acid N123.

rescued in vitro but also in vivo by nonpeptide vasopressin antagonists acting as pharmacologic chaperones.[345,346] This new therapeutic approach could be applied to the treatment of several hereditary diseases resulting from errors in protein folding and kinesis.[347]

Only four *AVPR2* mutations (D85N, V88M, G201D, and P322S) have been associated with a mild phenotype.[348] In general, the male infants bearing these mutations are identified later in life and the "classic" episodes of dehydration are less severe. This mild phenotype is also found in expression studies. The mutant proteins are expressed on the plasma membranes of cells transfected with these mutants and demonstrate a stimulation of cAMP for higher concentrations of agonists.

In contrast with NDI because of inactivating mutations in *AVPR2,* mutations which result in constitutive hormone-independent activity cause nephrogenic syndrome of inappropriate antidiuresis, often manifesting as hyponatremia,[349] which is considered in greater depth in Chapter 15.

## LOSS-OF-FUNCTION MUTATIONS OF *AQP2* (OMIM #107777)

The *AQP2* gene is located on chromosome region 12q12-q13. Approximately 10% of NDI cases are caused by autosomal mutations in *AQP2.* Forty-six mutations have been reported, which are either autosomal recessive (32 mutations reported) or autosomal dominant (8 mutations reported).[350] Both male and female patients who are affected with congenital NDI have been described as homozygous for a mutation in the *AQP2* gene or carry two different mutations (Fig. 44.19). Autosomal recessive mutations give rise to misfolded proteins that are retained in the ER and are eventually degraded. Autosomal dominant mutations are believed to be restricted to the carboxy-terminal end of the AQP2 protein and to operate through a dominant negative effect whereby the mutant protein associates with functional AQP2 proteins within intracellular stores, thus preventing normal targeting and function.[351]

Oocytes of the African clawed frog (*Xenopus laevis*) have provided a useful system for studying the behavior of various AQP2 mutants on membrane water permeability. Functional expression studies showed that *Xenopus* oocytes injected with mutant complementary RNA (cRNA) had abnormal coefficient of water permeability, whereas *Xenopus* oocytes injected with both normal cRNA and mutant cRNA had coefficient of water permeability similar to that of normal constructs alone. These findings provide conclusive evidence that NDI can be caused by homozygosity for mutations in the *AQP2* gene.[350]

## POLYURIA, POLYDIPSIA, ELECTROLYTE IMBALANCE, AND DEHYDRATION IN CYSTINOSIS

Polyuria may be as mild as persistent enuresis or so severe as to contribute to death from dehydration and electrolyte abnormalities in infants with cystinosis who have acute gastroenteritis.[44]

## POLYURIA IN HEREDITARY HYPOKALEMIC SALT-LOSING TUBULOPATHIES

Patients with polyhydramnios, hypercalciuria, and hyposthenuria or isosthenuria have been found to bear *KCNJ1* (ROMK) and *SLC12A1* (NKCC2) mutations.[238,248] In a recent analysis of 115 patients bearing *CLCNKB* mutations, 29.5% had early manifestations with polyhydramnios or early manifestations in the first month of life.[328] Patients with polyhydramnios, profound polyuria, hyponatremia, hypochloremia, metabolic alkalosis, and sensorineural deafness have been found to bear *BSND* mutations.[242] The MAGED2 protein is increasing the expression of NKCC2 and NCC of the thick ascending loop of Henle and the distal convoluted tubule.[329] These studies demonstrate the critical importance of the proteins ROMK, NKCC2, and Barttin in transferring NaCl to the medullary interstitium and thereby generating, together with urea, a hypertonic milieu (see Fig. 44.10). Of clinical and diagnostic importance, polyhydramnios is never observed during the pregnancy of infants later found to have *AVPR2* or *AQP2* mutations.[326]

## CARRIER DETECTION, PERINATAL TESTING, AND TREATMENT

We encourage physicians who observe families with X-linked and autosomal recessive diabetes insipidus to recommend mutation analysis before the birth of an infant because early diagnosis and treatment can avert the physical and mental retardation associated with episodes of dehydration. Diagnosis of X-linked NDI was accomplished by mutation testing of cultured amniotic cells or chorionic villus samples ($n = 17$), or of cord blood obtained at birth ($n = 65$) in 82 of our patients from 69 families. Some 36 male patients were found to bear mutant sequences, and 26 had normal sequences. Diagnosis of AQP2 autosomal recessive mutants was made in four families for a total of six subjects, of whom three were found to be homozygous for the previously identified mutation, two were heterozygous, and one had a normal sequence on both alleles. The affected patients were immediately treated with abundant water intake, a low-sodium diet, and hydrochlorothiazide. They never experienced episodes of dehydration, and their physical and mental development was normal. Gene analysis is also important for the identification of nonobligatory female carriers in families with X-linked NDI. Most female patients heterozygous for a mutation in the $V_2$ receptor do not present with clinical symptoms, and a few are severely affected[341] (Bichet, unpublished observations). Mutational analysis of polyuric patients with cystinosis, hypokalemic salt-losing tubulopathy, nephronophthisis, and AME is also of importance for definitive molecular diagnosis.

All complications of congenital NDI can be prevented by an adequate water intake. Thus patients should be provided with unrestricted amounts of water from birth to ensure normal development. In addition to a low-sodium diet, the use of diuretics (thiazides) or indomethacin may reduce urinary output. This advantageous effect must be weighed against the side effects of these drugs (thiazides: electrolyte disturbances; indomethacin: reduction of the GFR and gastrointestinal symptoms). Many affected infants frequently vomit because of an exacerbation of physiologic gastroesophageal reflux. These young patients often improve with the absorption of a histamine $H_2$ blocker and with metoclopramide, which could induce extrapyramidal symptoms, or domperidone, which seems to be efficacious and better tolerated.

 Complete reference list available at ExpertConsult.com.

## KEY REFERENCES


2. Klootwijk ED, Reichold M, Unwin RJ, et al. Renal Fanconi syndrome: taking a proximal look at the nephron. *Nephrol Dial Transplant.* 2015;30(9):1456–1460.
3. Reichold M, Klootwijk ED, Reinders J, et al. Glycine amidinotransferase (GATM), renal fanconi syndrome, and kidney failure. *J Am Soc Nephrol.* 2018;29(7):1849–1858.
11. Khositseth S, Uawithya P, Somparn P, et al. Autophagic degradation of aquaporin-2 is an early event in hypokalemia-induced nephrogenic diabetes insipidus. *Sci Rep.* 2015;5:18311.
16. Lloyd SE, Pearce SH, Fisher SE, et al. A common molecular basis for three inherited kidney stone diseases. *Nature.* 1996;379(6564):445–449.
22. Devuyst O, Thakker RV. Dent's disease. *Orphanet J Rare Dis.* 2010;5:28.
29. Scheinman S. X-linked hypercalciuric nephrolithiasis: clinical syndromes and chloride channel mutations. *Kidney Int.* 1998;53:3–17.
32. Bokenkamp A, Ludwig M. The oculocerebrorenal syndrome of Lowe: an update. *Pediatr Nephrol.* 2016;31(12):2201–2212.
41. Klootwijk ED, Reichold M, Helip-Wooley A, et al. Mistargeting of peroxisomal EHHADH and inherited renal Fanconi's syndrome. *N Engl J Med.* 2014;370(2):129–138.
46. Wilmer MJ, Schoeber JP, van den Heuvel LP, et al. Cystinosis: practical tools for diagnosis and treatment. *Pediatr Nephrol.* 2011;26(2):205–215.
50. Gallo L, Gahl W. Nephropathic cystinosis: growing into adulthood. In: Morgan S, Grunfeld J-P, eds. *Inherited Disorders of the Kidney.* Oxford: Oxford University Press; 1998:391–405.
56. Bertholet-Thomas A, Bacchetta J, Tasic V, et al. Nephropathic cystinosis–a gap between developing and developed nations. *N Engl J Med.* 2014;370(14):1366–1367.
63. Labbe A, Baudouin C, Deschenes G, et al. A new gel formulation of topical cysteamine for the treatment of corneal cystine crystals in cystinosis: the Cystadrops OCT-1 study. *Mol Genet Metab.* 2014;111(3):314–320.
65. Wolfsdorf JI, Weinstein DA. Glycogen storage diseases. *Rev Endocr Metab Disord.* 2003;4(1):95–102.
79. Rake JP, Visser G, Labrune P, et al. Guidelines for management of glycogen storage disease type I - European Study on Glycogen Storage Disease Type I (ESGSD I). *Eur J Pediatr.* 2002;161(suppl 1):S112–S119.
81. de Laet C, Dionisi-Vici C, Leonard JV, et al. Recommendations for the management of tyrosinaemia type 1. *Orphanet J Rare Dis.* 2013;8:8.
91. Paradis K, Weber A, Seidman EG, et al. Liver transplantation for hereditary tyrosinemia: the Quebec experience. *Am J Hum Genet.* 1990;47(2):338–342.
99. Bennett MJ. Galactosemia diagnosis gets an upgrade. *Clin Chem.* 2010;56(5):690–692.
119. Weiss KH, Thurik F, Gotthardt DN, et al. Efficacy and safety of oral chelators in treatment of patients with Wilson disease. *Clin Gastroenterol Hepatol.* 2013;11(8):1028–1035, e1021–1022.
125. Makrides V, Camargo SM, Verrey F. Transport of amino acids in the kidney. *Compr Physiol.* 2014;4(1):367–403.
130. Chillaron J, Font-Llitjos M, Fort J, et al. Pathophysiology and treatment of cystinuria. *Nat Rev Nephrol.* 2010;6(7):424–434.

141. Prot-Bertoye C, Lebbah S, Daudon M, et al. CKD and Its Risk Factors among Patients with Cystinuria. *Clin J Am Soc Nephrol.* 2015;10(5):842–851.
164. Mauhin W, Habarou F, Gobin S, et al. Update on Lysinuric Protein Intolerance, a Multi-faceted Disease Retrospective cohort analysis from birth to adulthood. *Orphanet J Rare Dis.* 2017;12(1):3.
170. Broer A, Cavanaugh JA, Rasko JE, et al. The molecular basis of neutral aminoacidurias. *Pflugers Arch.* 2006;451(4):511–517.
180. Kaneko I, Tatsumi S, Segawa H, et al. Control of phosphate balance by the kidney and intestine. *Clin Exp Nephrol.* 2017;21(suppl 1): 21–26.
189. Bergwitz C, Juppner H. FGF23 and syndromes of abnormal renal phosphate handling. *Adv Exp Med Biol.* 2012;728:41–64.
206. Kaito H, Ishimori S, Nozu K, et al. Molecular background of urate transporter genes in patients with exercise-induced acute kidney injury. *Am J Nephrol.* 2013;38(4):316–320.
216. Heerspink HJL, Kosiborod M, Inzucchi SE, et al. Renoprotective effects of sodium-glucose cotransporter-2 inhibitors. *Kidney Int.* 2018;94(1):26–39.
221. Fry AC, Karet FE. Inherited renal acidoses. *Physiology (Bethesda).* 2007;22:202–211.
237. Bartter FC, Pronove P, Gill JRJ, et al. Hyperplasia of the juxtaglomerular complex with hyperaldosteronism and hypokalemic alkalosis: a new syndrome. *Am J Med.* 1962;33:811–828.
238. Jeck N, Schlingmann KP, Reinalter SC, et al. Salt handling in the distal nephron: lessons learned from inherited human disorders. *Am J Physiol Regul Integr Comp Physiol.* 2005;288(4):R782–R795.
242. Schlingmann KP, Konrad M, Jeck N, et al. Salt wasting and deafness resulting from mutations in two chloride channels. *N Engl J Med.* 2004;350(13):1314–1319.
248. Peters M, Jeck N, Reinalter S, et al. Clinical presentation of genetically defined patients with hypokalemic salt-losing tubulopathies. *Am J Med.* 2002;112(3):183–190.
262. Lifton RP, Gharavi AG, Geller DS. Molecular mechanisms of human hypertension. *Cell.* 2001;104(4):545–556.
268. Rossier BC. The epithelial sodium channel (ENaC): new insights into ENaC gating. *Pflugers Arch.* 2003;446(3):314–316.
283. Bonny O, Rossier BC. Disturbances of Na/K balance: pseudohypoaldosteronism revisited. *J Am Soc Nephrol.* 2002;13(9): 2399–2414.
290. Susa K, Sohara E, Rai T, et al. Impaired degradation of WNK1 and WNK4 kinases causes PHAII in mutant KLHL3 knock-in mice. *Hum Mol Genet.* 2014;23(19):5052–5060.
292. Hadchouel J, Delaloy C, Faure S, et al. Familial hyperkalemic hypertension. *J Am Soc Nephrol.* 2006;17(1):208–217.
293. Glaudemans B, Knoers NV, Hoenderop JG, et al. New molecular players facilitating Mg(2+) reabsorption in the distal convoluted tubule. *Kidney Int.* 2010;77(1):17–22.
296. Konrad M, Weber S. Recent advances in molecular genetics of hereditary magnesium-losing disorders. *J Am Soc Nephrol.* 2003; 14(1):249–260.
301. van der Wijst J, Bindels RJ, Hoenderop JG. Mg2+ homeostasis: the balancing act of TRPM6. *Curr Opin Nephrol Hypertens.* 2014; 23(4):361–369.
310. Zimmerman CA, Leib DE, Knight ZA. Neural circuits underlying thirst and fluid homeostasis. *Nat Rev Neurosci.* 2017;18(8):459–469.
312. Fenton RA, Knepper MA. Mouse models and the urinary concentrating mechanism in the new millennium. *Physiol Rev.* 2007; 87(4):1083–1112.
313. Noda Y, Sohara E, Ohta E, et al. Aquaporins in kidney pathophysiology. *Nat Rev Nephrol.* 2010;6(3):168–178.
314. Agre P, Preston GM, Smith BL, et al. Aquaporin CHIP: the archetypal molecular water channel. *Am J Physiol.* 1993;34:F463–F476.
318. Yang B, Bankir L. Urea and urine concentrating ability: new insights from studies in mice. *Am J Physiol Renal Physiol.* 2005;288(5): F881–F896.
322. Shi G, Somlo DRM, Kim GH, et al. ER-associated degradation is required for vasopressin prohormone processing and systemic water homeostasis. *J Clin Invest.* 2017;127(10):3897–3912.
323. Bichet DG, Lussier Y. Mice deficient for ERAD machinery component Sel1L develop central diabetes insipidus. *J Clin Invest.* 2017;127(10):3591–3593.
326. Bockenhauer D, Bichet DG. Pathophysiology, diagnosis and management of nephrogenic diabetes insipidus. *Nat Rev Nephrol.* 2015;11(10):576–588.
328. Seys E, Andrini O, Keck M, et al. Clinical and genetic spectrum of Bartter syndrome type 3. *J Am Soc Nephrol.* 2017;28(8):2540–2552.
329. Laghmani K, Beck BB, Yang SS, et al. Polyhydramnios, transient antenatal Bartter's syndrome, and MAGED2 mutations. *N Engl J Med.* 2016;374(19):1853–1863.

# 45 Cystic Diseases of the Kidney

Vicente E. Torres | Peter C. Harris

CHAPTER OUTLINE



## CLASSIFICATION OF RENAL CYSTIC DISEASES

Renal cystic diseases encompass a large number of sporadic and genetically determined congenital, developmental, and acquired conditions that have in common the presence of cysts in one or both kidneys. "Renal cysts" are cavities lined by epithelium and filled with fluid or semisolid matter. Cysts are derived primarily from tubules. Whereas cystic kidneys of different etiologies may appear morphologically similar, the same etiologic entity may cause a wide spectrum of renal abnormalities. Classifications of renal cystic diseases are based on morphologic, clinical, and genetic information (Box 45.1) and change as the understanding of the underlying etiologies and pathogeneses continues to expand.

## DEVELOPMENT OF RENAL EPITHELIAL CYSTS

Epithelial cysts develop from preexisting renal tubule segments and are composed of a layer of partially dedifferentiated epithelial cells enclosing a cavity filled with either a urinelike liquid or semisolid material. They may develop in any tubular segment between Bowman's capsule and the tip of the renal papilla, depending on the nature of the underlying disorder. After achieving a size of perhaps a few millimeters, most cysts lose their attachments to their parent tubule segment.

Pathophysiologic processes that contribute to the development of cysts include disruption of programs responsible for the establishment and maintenance of normal tubular diameter (i.e., convergent extension, or the process of cell intercalation by which cells elongate along an axis perpendicular to the proximal–distal axis of the tubule and actively crawl among one another to produce a narrower, longer tubule; and oriented cell division or alignment of the mitotic spindle axis and cell division with the proximal–distal axis of the tubule),[1,2] excessive cell proliferation, active solute and fluid transport into the expanding cysts, crosstalk between epithelial cells and interstitial macrophages, and interactions between epithelial cells and extracellular matrix (ECM)[3,4] (Fig. 45.1).

Renal cysts have been regarded as benign neoplasms that arise from individual cells or restricted segments of the renal tubule. Transgenic insertions of activated proto-oncogenes and growth factor genes into rodents result in the formation of renal cysts. Therefore processes that stimulate renal cell proliferation along with the inability to maintain planar cell polarity have the potential to generate the cystic phenotype.

Conditional knockouts of *Pkd1* or of ciliogenesis genes (*Ift88* and *Kif3a*) at various time points have shown that the timing of their inactivation determines the rate of development of cystic disease.[5–8] Inactivation in newborn mice leads to rapid cyst development. Inactivation after about 13 days leads to slowly progressive disease evident only in the adult kidneys, but progression can be hastened by maneuvers such as ischemic or reperfusion injury to stimulate cell proliferation.[9] The underlying rate of epithelial cell proliferation may account for increased susceptibility to cyst development during nephrogenesis as well as for the migration of cysts as the kidney matures in humans and in animal models of polycystic

**Box 45.1 Classification of Cystic Kidney Disorders**

Autosomal dominant polycystic kidney disease (ADPKD)
Autosomal recessive polycystic kidney disease (ARPKD)
Polycystic kidney and/or liver diseases associated with altered maturation of PKD proteins in the endoplasmic reticulum (*PRKCSH, SEC63, GANAB, ALG8, SEC61B, DNAJB11*)
Tuberous sclerosis complex
von Hippel–Lindau syndrome
Familial renal hamartomas associated with hyperparathyroidism–jaw tumor syndrome
Hepatocyte nuclear factor-1–associated nephropathy
Oro-facial-digital syndrome
Autosomal dominant tubulointerstitial kidney disease
Hereditary recessive ciliopathies with interstitial nephritis, cysts, or both:
- Nephronophthisis
- Joubert syndrome
- Meckel syndrome
- Bardet–Biedl syndrome
- Alström syndrome
- Nephronophthisis variants associated with skeletal defects (skeletal ciliopathies)

Renal cystic dysplasias:
- Multicystic kidney dysplasia

Other cystic kidney disorders:
- Simple cysts
- Localized or unilateral renal cystic disease
- Medullary sponge kidney
- Acquired cystic kidney disease

Renal cystic neoplasms:
- Cystic renal cell carcinoma
- Multilocular cystic nephroma
- Cystic partially differentiated nephroblastoma
- Mixed epithelial and stromal tumor

Cysts of nontubular origin:
- Cystic disease of the renal sinus
- Perirenal lymphangiomas
- Subcapsular and perirenal urinomas

Pyelocalyceal cysts

kidney disease (PKD) from being located predominantly proximal to appearing predominantly distal and in the collecting duct.[10] Immature early tubules (S-shaped bodies) exhibit very high rates of proliferation. Later, when the epithelium differentiates into nephron segments recognizable on light microscopy, proliferative indices become very low in proximal tubules but remain elevated in the distal nephrons and collecting ducts. In pediatric and adult kidneys, proliferative indices are very low in all tubular segments but remain higher in collecting ducts than in proximal tubules.[11,12]

The finding of fluid secretion in renal epithelial cysts led to a reinvestigation of fluid secretion mechanisms in otherwise normal renal tubules. Beyond the loop of Henle, tubule cells have the capacity to secrete solutes and fluid upon stimulation with cyclic adenosine monophosphate (cAMP).[13] This secretory flux operates in competition with the more powerful mechanism by which $Na^+$ is absorbed through apical epithelial $Na^+$ channels. Under conditions in which $Na^+$ absorption is diminished, the net secretion of NaCl and fluid can be observed at rates that could have a significant impact on the net economy of body salt and water content. Thus renal cystic disease has led to a heightened appreciation of an "ancient" solute and water secretory mechanism that has been largely overlooked in modern studies of renal physiology.[14]

Three decades ago it was noted that a germ-free environment inhibits cyst development in CFW mice and in a model of PKD induced by nordihydroguaiaretic acid; the administration of endotoxin rescued the cystic phenotype.[15,16] Chemokines and cytokines were found at high concentrations in cyst fluid and produced by epithelial cells of the cyst lining.[17] In later studies, alternatively activated (M2) macrophages aligned along cyst walls were detected in polycystic kidneys from conditional *Pkd1* knockout and the *Pkd2*$^{WS18/-}$ model.[19,20] Macrophage depletion inhibited epithelial cell proliferation and cyst growth and improved renal function. These observations led to the hypothesis that M2 macrophages contribute to cell proliferation in PKD, as has been described during development, during recovery from acute kidney injury, and in cancer.

Evidence indicates that alterations in focal adhesion complexes, basement membranes, and ECM contribute to the pathogenesis of PKD.[21] Focal adhesion complexes contain integrin αβ heterodimer receptors and multiple structural and signaling molecules, including polycystin 1 (PC1). The integrin receptors link the actin cytoskeleton, laminin αβγ heterotrimers, and collagens in the basement membrane. Integrins $\beta_4$ and $\beta_1$ may mediate the increased adhesion of cyst-lining epithelial cells to laminin-322 and collagen and are all overexpressed in cystic tissues.[22,23] Periostin, an ECM protein, and its receptor $\alpha_v$ integrin as well as $\alpha_1$ and $\alpha_2$ integrins are also overexpressed.[24,25] Laminin-322 and periostin stimulate, whereas antibodies to laminin-332 and $\alpha_v$ integrin inhibit cyst formation in three-dimensional gel culture.[18,24] Renal cystic disease develops in $\beta_1$ integrin knockout and laminin $\alpha_5$ hypomorphic mutant mice, the latter associated with overexpression of laminin-322.[26,27] Mutations to the gene *COL4A1*, which encodes procollagen type IV, have been found in patients with autosomal dominant (*h*ereditary) *a*ngiopathy with *n*ephropathy (consisting of hematuria and bilateral renal cysts), *a*neurysms, and muscle *c*ramps (HANAC syndrome).

Evidence accumulated during nearly 20 years strongly suggests that the primary cilium is essential to maintain epithelial cell differentiation and that structural and functional defects in the primary cilium of tubular epithelia have a central role in various forms of human and rodent cystic diseases. The "primary cilium" is a single hairlike organelle that projects from the surface of most mammalian cells, including epithelial and endothelial cells, neurons, fibroblasts, chondrocytes, and osteocytes. It is involved in left–right embryonic patterning as well as in mechanosensing (renal tubular and biliary epithelia), photosensing (retinal pigmented epithelia), and chemosensing (olfactory neurons).[28–32] In renal tubule epithelial cells, the cilium projects into the lumen and is thought to have a sensory role (Fig. 45.2). The cilium arises from the mother centriole in the centrosome. The centrosome comprises a mother centriole and a daughter centriole plus a "cloud" of pericentriolar material.[33] The centrosome serves as the microtubule-organizing center for interphase cells, and the mother and daughter centrioles form the poles of the spindle during cell division.

The first clue connecting PKD and cilia was that PC1 and polycystin 2 (PC2) homologs in *Caenorhabditis elegans* are

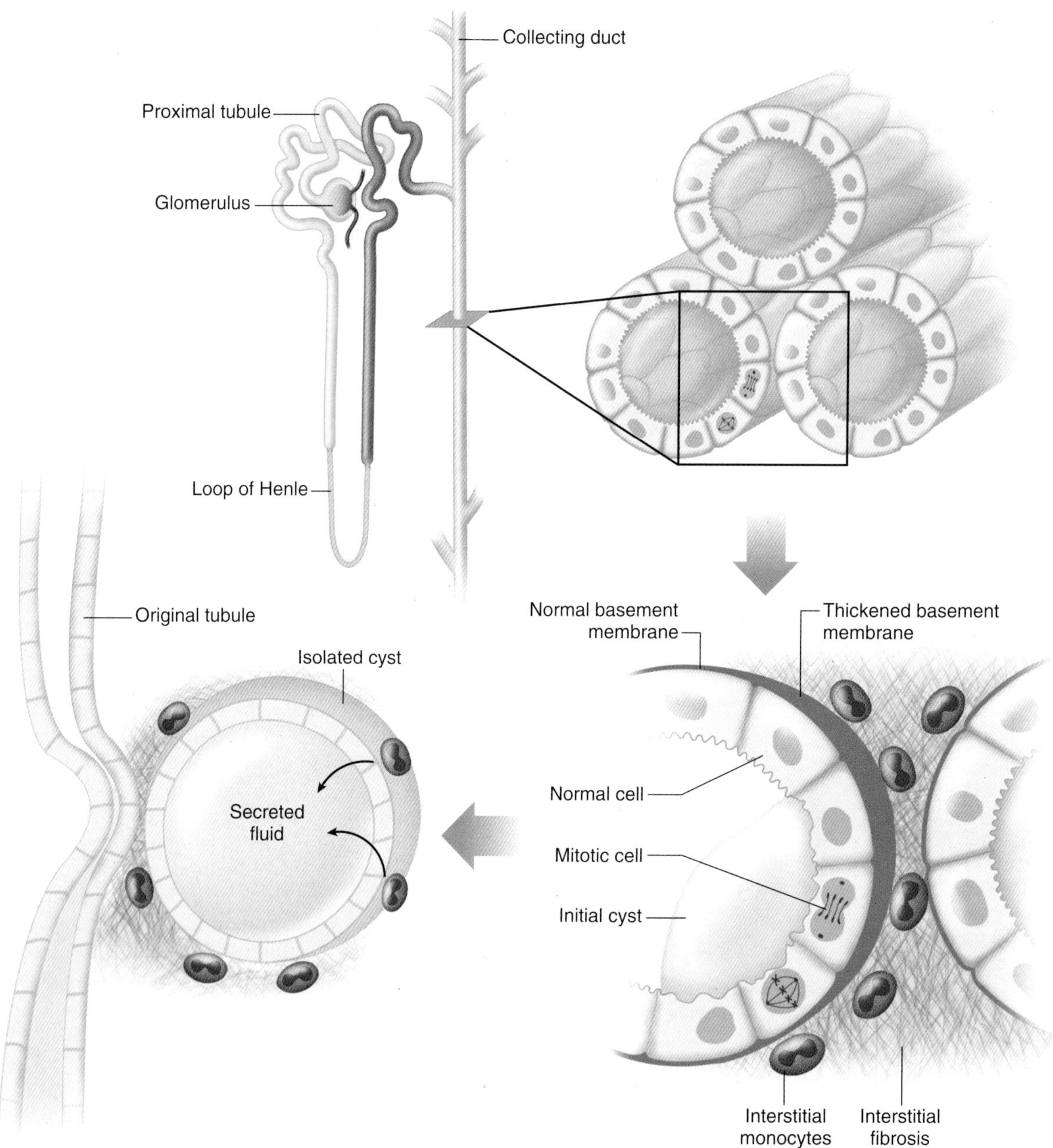


**Fig. 45.1** Evolution of cysts from renal tubules. Abnormal proliferation of tubule epithelium begins in a single cell after a "second-hit" process disables the function of the normal allele or if the level of functional polycystin falls below a specific threshold. Repeated cycles of cell proliferation lead to expansion of the tubule wall into a cyst. The cystic epithelium is associated with thickening of the adjacent tubule basement membrane and with an influx of inflammatory cells into the interstitium. The cystic segment eventually separates from the original tubule, and net epithelial fluid secretion contributes to the accumulation of liquid within the cyst cavity.

located in cilia of male sensory neurons; loss of these proteins is associated with mating behavior defects.[34] Next, a known intraflagellar transport (IFT) protein, polaris, was found to be defective in a hypomorphic mouse mutant, *orpk*, in which PKD, left–right patterning defects, and a variety of other abnormalities develop, and that has shortened cilia in the kidney.[35] Subsequently, the proteins mutated in other rodent models of PKD—such as the *cpk* (centrin) and *inv* (inversin) mice, autosomal dominant PKD (ADPKD; PC1 and PC2), autosomal recessive PKD (ARPKD; fibrocystin), autosomal recessive ciliopathies (see later in the chapter), and possibly tuberous sclerosis complex (TSC) and von Hippel–Lindau (vHL) disease—have been localized to the ciliary axoneme, the basal body, or centrosomal structures.[30,36,37] Conditional inactivation of the ciliary motor protein KIF3A (kinesin family member 3A) in collecting duct epithelial cells reproduced all of the clinical and biologic features of PKD.[38]

The polycystin complex on cilia may detect changes in flow and transduce it into a $Ca^{2+}$ influx through the PC2 channel, thus functioning as a mechanosensor,[39] although a chemosensory role or ligand receptor has not been excluded. The $Ca^{2+}$ influx may in turn induce release of $Ca^{2+}$ from

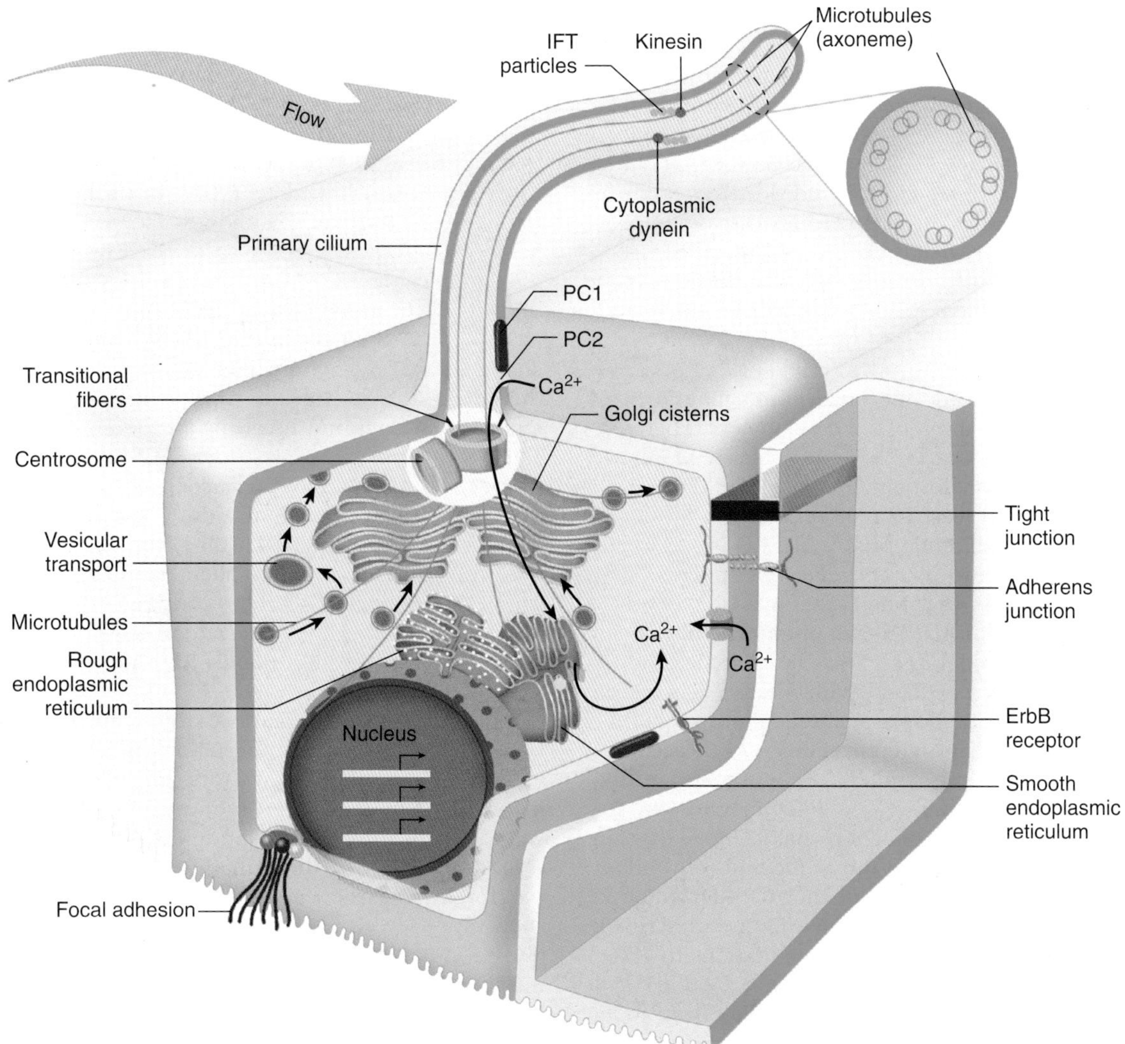


**Fig. 45.2** Diagram depicting the primary cilium and hypothetical functions of the polycystins. Polycystin 1 (PC1) and polycystin 2 (PC2) are found on the primary cilium, a single hairlike structure that projects from the apical surface of the cell into the lumen. It consists of a membrane continuous with the cell membrane and a central axoneme composed of nine peripheral microtubule doublets. It arises from the mother centriole in the centrosome, the microtubule-organizing center of the cell. The centrosome comprises a mother centriole and a daughter centriole plus a "cloud" of pericentriolar material. In response to mechanical stimulation of the primary cilium by flow, the PC1 and PC2 complex mediates $Ca^{2+}$ entry into the cell. This triggers $Ca^{2+}$-induced release of $Ca^{2+}$ from the smooth endoplasmic reticulum (ER) through ryanodine receptors. The function of the polycystins extends beyond the cilium because PC1 is also found in the plasma membrane and PC2 is predominantly expressed in the ER. PC2 is an intracellular $Ca^{2+}$ channel that is required for the normal pattern of $[Ca^{2+}]_i$ responses involving ryanodine receptors and inositol 1,4,5-trisphosphate (IP3) receptors and may also affect the activity of store-operated $Ca^{2+}$ channels. *ErbB,* Epidermal growth factor receptor; *IFT,* intraflagellar transport. (Reproduced from Torres VE, Harris PC, Pirson Y. Autosomal dominant polycystic kidney disease. *Lancet.* 2007;369:1287–1301.)

intracellular stores. The increased $Ca^{2+}$ concentration in intracellular microenvironments may then modulate specific signaling pathways that regulate cellular differentiation, proliferation, and apoptosis, such as cAMP, receptor-tyrosine kinase, extracellular signal–regulated kinase (ERK), and mammalian target of rapamycin (mTOR) signaling.[4]

The ciliocentric model of cystogenesis is attractive but may be too reductionist. Several cyst-associated proteins have other functions, including participation in cell–cell and cell–matrix interactions at adherens junctions and focal adhesions. Dysfunction of these subcellular domains most likely contributes to the aberrant epithelial growth and tubular architecture that are common to virtually all forms of renal cystic disease. Although ciliary dysfunction may be the initiating event in cystogenesis, defects in other cellular mechanisms may modulate the final cystic disease phenotype.

# HEREDITARY CYSTIC KIDNEY DISORDERS

## AUTOSOMAL DOMINANT POLYCYSTIC KIDNEY DISEASE

### EPIDEMIOLOGY

ADPKD occurs worldwide and in all races, with a prevalence estimated to be between 1 in 400 and 1 in 1000.[40] The yearly incidence rates for end-stage kidney disease (ESKD) due to ADPKD are 8.7 and 6.9 per million (1998–2001, United States),[41] 7.8 and 6.0 per million (1998–1999, Europe),[42] and 5.6 and 4.0 per million (1999–2000, Japan)[43] in men and women, respectively. Age-adjusted gender ratios greater than unity (1.2–1.3) suggest a more progressive disease in men than in women. Approximately 30,000 patients have ESKD due to ADPKD in the United States (1 : 3500 individuals aged 65–69 years).[44] The proceedings of a 2014 Kidney Disease: Improving Global Outcomes (KDIGO) Controversies Conference to assess the current state of knowledge related to the evaluation, management, and treatment of ADPKD have been published.[45]

## GENETICS AND GENETIC MECHANISMS

ADPKD is inherited as an autosomal dominant trait with complete penetrance in terms of cyst development. Therefore each child of an affected parent has a 50% chance of inheriting the abnormal gene. Most patients with ADPKD have an affected parent, but at least 10% of families can be traced to an apparent de novo mutation.[46,47] ADPKD is genetically heterogeneous with two major genes identified, *PKD1* (chromosome region 16p13.3) and *PKD2* (4q21).[48–51] Recently, two other genes with an ADPKD-like phenotype have been described, *GANAB* and *DNAJB11*[52,53] (see the "Polycystic Kidney and/or Liver Diseases Associated With Altered Maturation of PKD Proteins in the Endoplasmic Reticulum" section).

In groups identified through renal clinics, *PKD1* accounts for about 78% of pedigrees and *PKD2* about 15%, and no mutation is detected in about 7%.[54,55] *PKD2* may account for up to approximately 25% of mutation-characterized cases in population-based studies and those focused on milder patients.[56,57] In the latest version of the ADPKD Mutation Database (PKDB), 1272 *PKD1* mutations are described, accounting for 1874 families, with 202 mutations to *PKD2* causing disease in 438 pedigrees.[58] For *PKD1*, about 65% of mutations are predicted to truncate the protein, leaving about 35% nontruncating.[54,55,59,60] Corresponding levels for *PKD2* are about 87% truncating and 13% nontruncating; about 3% of ADPKD mutations are larger rearrangements involving deletion or duplication of at least one exon.[54,55,59–61] A next-generation sequencing (NGS) method for ADPKD screening based on sequencing the locus-specific long-range polymerase chain reaction products has been described.[62] Such methods can identify unusual mutations, such as gene conversions with one of the pseudogenes. Recently, exon capture and NGS approaches for screening the ADPKD have been described to efficiently screen *PKD1*, despite the segmental duplication of this locus.[63,64]

Inheritance of two *PKD1* or two *PKD2* alleles with fully inactivating mutations is lethal in utero.[65] Individuals heterozygous for both a *PKD1* and *PKD2* mutation live to adulthood but have more severe renal disease than those heterozygous for only one mutation.[66] Patients with a *PKD1* mutation have more severe disease than those with a *PKD2* mutation, the average ages at ESKD being 58.1 years and 79.7 years, respectively.[67] Viable ADPKD cases homozygous/compound heterozygous for *PKD1* pathogenic variants suggest the presence of hypomorphic alleles.[68] Some nontruncating *PKD1* changes have been suggested to be not fully penetrant alleles, resulting in ESKD at 55 years in patients with truncating *PKD1* mutations and 67 years in those with nontruncating changes.[67,69] Further bioinformatics analysis of nontruncating mutations has identified two populations, those that are fully inactivating and those that are incompletely penetrant, associated with milder kidney disease.[59]

A small number (<1%) of patients with ADPKD exhibit early-onset disease, with a diagnosis made in utero or in infancy from the presence of enlarged echogenic kidneys that may resemble those seen in ARPKD.[70,71] Most early-onset cases have been linked to *PKD1*, but a family with *PKD2* mutation and perinatal death in two severely affected infants has been described.[72] Some cases of early-onset ADPKD, or cases mimicking ARPKD, are due to an in trans combination of two *PKD1* mutations, at least one of which is hypomorphic.[68,73,74] Studies of a *Pkd1* mouse model with a missense change, p.R3277C, confirmed the hypomorphic nature of this allele and its role in causing early-onset disease.[10,68] Uniparental isodisomy involving a hypomorphic *PKD2* allele can also cause early-onset ADPKD.[75] Mutations in other cystogenes, such as *HNF1B* [associated with the autosomal dominant tubulointerstitial kidney disease (ADTKD); see later discussion] and *PKHD1* (the ARPKD gene), in combination with an ADPKD mutant allele have also been associated with early-onset PKD.[76] The contiguous deletion of the adjacent *PKD1* and *TSC2* (see later discussion of TSC) genes is characterized by childhood PKD with additional clinical signs of TSC.[77,78]

Significant intrafamilial variability in the severity of renal and extrarenal manifestations points to genetic and environmental modifying factors. Analysis of the variability in renal function between monozygotic twins and siblings supports a role for genetic modifiers.[79,80] Parental hypertension, particularly in the nonaffected parent, increases the risk for hypertension and ESKD.[81] Parents are as likely to show more severe disease as children are.[82] Mosaicism can also modulate disease presentation and result in marked intrafamilial variability.[61,83]

Cysts in ADPKD kidneys appear to be derived through clonal proliferation of single epithelial cells that occurs in fewer than 1% of the tubules. A two-hit model of cystogenesis has been proposed to explain the focal nature of the cysts. In this model, a mutated *PKD1* (or *PKD2*) gene is inherited from one parent, and a wild-type gene is inherited from the unaffected parent. During the lifetime of the individual, the wild-type gene undergoes a somatic mutation and becomes inactivated. Loss of function owing to somatic mutations of the *PKD1* and *PKD2* genes has been identified in the cells lining the cysts in both the kidney and the liver.[84,85] Support for this model of cystogenesis is provided by the embryonic lethality and severe PKD of homozygous *Pkd1* or *Pkd2* knockout mice, the late development of cysts in the kidney or liver in heterozygous mutant mice, and the increased severity of the disease in *Pkd2*$^{WS25/-}$ mice carrying a *Pkd2* allele (WS25) prone to genomic rearrangement.[86]

Evidence suggests, however, that other genetic mechanisms may also be involved. Transgenic overexpression of *PKD1* or *PKD2* can induce renal cystic disease.[87–89] The presence of somatic trans-heterozygous mutations in human polycystic kidneys (somatic mutation of the PKD gene not involved by the germline mutation) and the greater severity of cystic disease in mice with trans-heterozygous mutations of *Pkd1* and *Pkd2* than could be predicted by a simple additive effect suggest that haploinsufficiency may play a role in cyst formation.[66,90] Comparative genomic hybridization and loss of heterozygosity analysis have shown multiple molecular cytogenetic aberrations in epithelial cells from individual cysts in polycystic kidneys, suggesting the involvement of additional genes in the initiation and progression of the cystic disease.[91] Mice that are homozygous for *Pkd1* hypomorphic alleles indicate that complete inactivation of both *Pkd1* alleles is not required for cystogenesis in ADPKD.[10,92,93] *Pkd2* haploinsufficiency has been associated with a higher rate of cell proliferation in noncystic tubules of $Pkd2^{+/-}$ mice.[94] These observations suggest that diminished expression of native polycystins below a certain threshold is sufficient to induce renal cystic disease and may also be relevant for the extrarenal manifestations of the disease. Reduction of PC2 levels to 50% of normal in the vascular smooth muscle of $Pkd2^{+/-}$ mice causes significant alterations in $[Ca^{2+}]_i$ (intracellular calcium concentration) and cAMP; moreover, it results in higher rates of cell proliferation and apoptosis, contractility, and vasculature susceptibility to hemodynamic stress.[95] Reduction of PC1 levels to 50% of normal causes significant alterations in $[Ca^{2+}]_i$ homeostasis and increased vascular reactivity with compensatory changes in the transport proteins involved in calcium signaling in the aorta of $Pkd1^{+/-}$ mice.[96]

## PATHOGENESIS

PC1 (4303 aa; ≈600 kDa, uncleaved and glycosylated) is a receptorlike protein with a large ectodomain (3074 aa) that comprises a number of domains involved in protein–protein and protein–carbohydrate interactions and 16 PKD repeats with an immunoglobulin (Ig) domain–like fold (Fig. 45.3).[49,50] PC1 also has 11 transmembrane domains and a cytoplasmic tail. PC2 (968 aa; ≈110 kDa) is a six-transmembrane, $Ca^{2+}$-responsive cation channel of the transient receptor potential (TRP) family (also known as TRPP2).[51] PC1 and PC2 interact via their C-terminal tails with the resulting polycystin complex thought to play a role in intracellular $Ca^{2+}$ regulation. Data also indicate an interdependence of the proteins for maturation and localization.[90,97] The structure of a homotetrameric PC2 complex has recently been resolved by cryo-electron microscopy. It shows the presence of a large exoplasmic domain named the tetragonal opening for polycystin (TOP domain) that may regulate gating of the channel.[98,99] A 3 to 1 PC2/PC1 structure has also recently been resolved by cryo EM.[100]

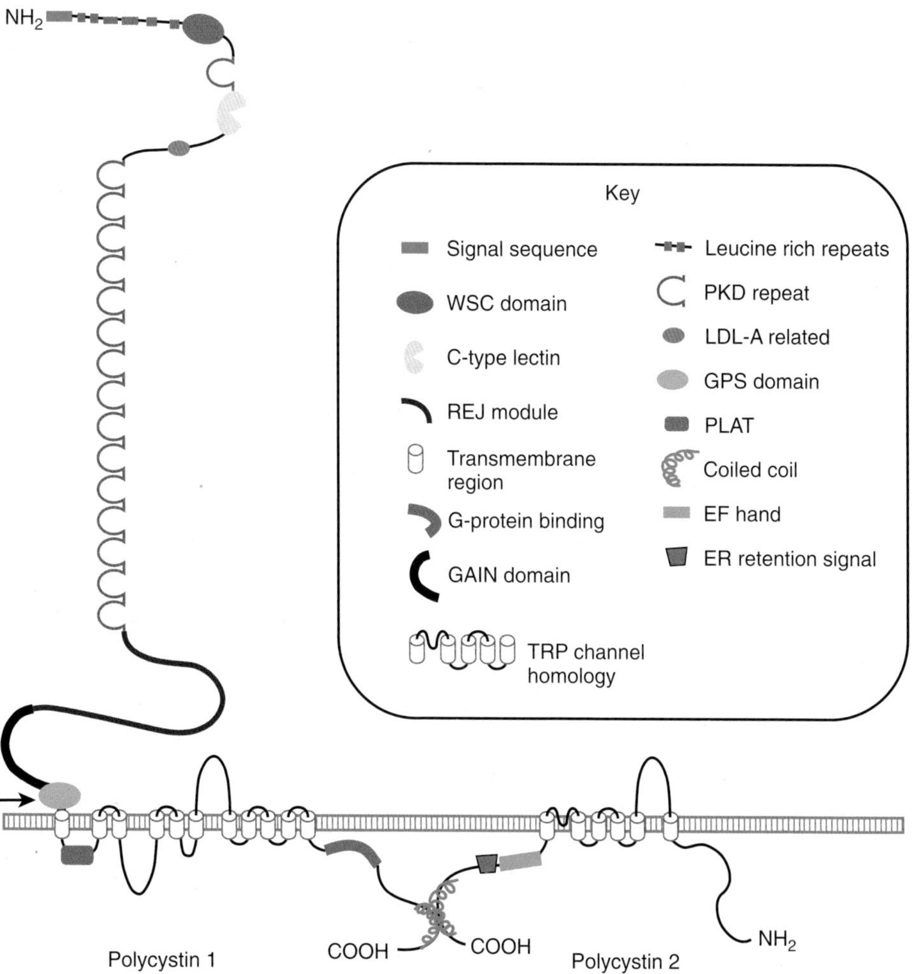


**Fig. 45.3** Structure of the polycystin proteins. Polycystin 1 (PC1) is a large protein with an extensive extracellular region, an 11-transmembrane area, and a short cytoplasmic tail. The protein contains a number of recognized domains and motifs (see Key). The protein is cleaved at the GPS (G protein–coupled receptor proteolytic site) domain *(arrow)*. Polycystin 2 (PC2) is a six-transmembrane, transient receptor potential (TRP)–like channel with cytoplasmic N and C termini. The proteins are thought to interact through coiled-coil domains. *ER,* Endoplasmic reticulum; *GAIN,* G protein–coupled receptor-autoproteolysis *in*ducing; *LDL-A,* low-density lipoprotein A module; *PKD,* polycystic kidney disease; *PLAT,* Polycystin 1, lipoxygenase, alpha-toxin; *REJ,* receptor of egg jelly protein.

Like many other proteins implicated in renal cystic diseases, the polycystins are located in the membrane overlying primary cilia.[101,102] PC2 currents have recently been recorded from patch clamping of individual cilia.[103] The polycystins may be required for the induction of calcium transients in response to ciliary bending.[39] PC1 is also found in plasma membranes at focal adhesion, desmosomes, and adherens junction sites,[104–107] whereas PC2 is found in the endoplasmic reticulum,[108–110] and both proteins are abundant in exosomes.[111,112] The PC1 protein in the plasma membrane may interact with PC2 in the adjacent endoplasmic reticulum. PC2 interacts with the inositol 1,4,5-trisphosphate receptor (IP3R), ryanodine receptor 2 (RyR2), and TRP channels TRPC1, TRPC4, and TRPV4.[113–115]

Precisely how intracellular calcium homeostasis is altered in ADPKD remains uncertain.[116] Cells overexpressing PC2 exhibit an amplified $Ca^{2+}$ release from intracellular stores after agonist stimulation.[117] A 50% reduction in PC2 lowers capacitative calcium entry, sarcoplasmic reticulum $Ca^{2+}$ stores, and $[Ca^{2+}]_i$ in vascular smooth muscle cells (VSMCs).[95] Increases in $[Ca^{2+}]_i$ levels evoked by platelet-activating factor are reduced in unciliated B-lymphoblastoid cells from patients with *PKD1* or *PKD2* mutations.[118] Loss of PC2 localization to the mitotic spindles by knockdown of the interacting cytoskeletal protein, mDia1, blunts agonist-evoked $[Ca^{2+}]_i$ increases in dividing cells that lack primary cilia.[119] The majority of studies that have measured resting intracellular calcium, endoplasmic reticulum calcium stores, and store-operated calcium entry in primary cell cultures or microdissected samples from human and rodent polycystic tissues have found them to be reduced.[95,96,113,120–126]

Tissue levels of cAMP are increased in numerous animal models of PKD, not only in the kidney[10,127–130] but also in cholangiocytes,[131] VSMCs,[132] and choroid plexus (Fig. 45.4).[133] Levels of cAMP are determined by the activities of membrane-bound (under the positive or negative control of G protein–coupled receptors and extracellular ligands) and soluble adenylyl cyclases (ACs), and of cAMP phosphodiesterases (PDEs), themselves subject to complex regulatory mechanisms. The increased levels in cystic tissues may be directly related to changes in $[Ca^{2+}]_i$ homeostasis. Reduced calcium activates calcium-inhibitable AC-6, directly inhibits calcium/calmodulin-dependent $PDE_1$ [also increasing the levels of cyclic guanosine monophosphate (cGMP)], and indirectly inhibits cGMP-inhibitable $PDE_3$[128,134] (Fig. 45.4). Additional mechanisms include the following:

1. Dysfunction of a ciliary protein complex [comprising A-kinase anchoring protein 150, AC-5/6, PC2, $PDE_{4C}$, and protein kinase A (PKA)] that normally restrains cAMP signaling via inhibition of AC-5/6 activity by PC2-mediated calcium entry and degradation of cAMP by $PDE_{4C}$ transcriptionally controlled by hepatocyte nuclear factor-1β (HNF-1β).[135]
2. Depletion of the endoplasmic reticulum calcium stores, which triggers oligomerization and translocation of stromal interaction molecule 1 (STIM1) to the plasma membrane, where it recruits and activates AC-6.[125]
3. Other contributory factors, such as disruption of PC1 binding to heterotrimeric G proteins, upregulation of the vasopressin $V_2$ receptor ($V_2R$), and increased levels of circulating vasopressin or accumulation of forskolin, lysophosphatidic acid, adenosine triphosphate (ATP), or other AC agonists in the cyst fluid.[136–139]

The marked amelioration of the cystic disease in collecting duct–specific *Pkd1* knockout mice by a concomitant *Ac6* knockout provides strong support for the central role of calcium-inhibitable AC-6.[140] PDEs are likely important in PKD because maximal rates of degradation by PDEs exceed, by an order of magnitude, those of synthesis by ACs and hence control compartmentalized pools of cAMP, which are likely more crucial than total intracellular cAMP. $PDE_1$ and $PDE_3$ may be particularly important. $PDE_1$ accounts for most PDE activity in renal tubules, it is the only PDE activated by calcium (which is reduced in PKD cells), and its activity is reduced in cystic kidneys.[134] The knockdown of *pde1a* using morpholinos induces or aggravates the cystic phenotype of wild-type or *pkd2* morphant zebrafish embryos, respectively, whereas $PDE_{1a}$ RNA partially rescues the phenotype of *pkd2* morphants.[141] $PDE_3$ controls a compartmentalized cAMP pool that stimulates mitogenesis in MDCK cells[142] as well as cystic fibrosis transmembrane conductance regulator (CFTR)–driven chloride secretion in pig trachea submucosal and shark rectal glands.[143,144] A small-molecule, nonselective PDE activator lowers cAMP and inhibits the growth of MDCK cysts.[145]

The reduction in $[Ca^{2+}]_i$ and the increase in cAMP may play a central role in the pathogenesis of PKD (Fig. 45.4). Cyclic AMP stimulates mitogen-activated protein kinase (MAPK)/ERK signaling and cell proliferation in PKD renal epithelial cells in a manner dependent on PKA, the proto-oncogene tyrosine protein kinase Src, and the protein Ras. By contrast, cAMP has an inhibitory effect in wild-type cells.[146,147] The abnormal proliferative response to cAMP is directly linked to the alterations in $[Ca^{2+}]_i$ because it can be reproduced in wild-type cells by lowering of $[Ca^{2+}]_i$.[148] Conversely, calcium ionophores or channel activators can rescue the abnormal response of cyst-derived cells.[120] Activation of mTOR signaling also occurs downstream from PKA, through ERK-mediated phosphorylation of tuberin in cystic tissues.[149,150] Activation of mTOR has in turn been linked to transcriptional activation of aerobic glycolysis and increased levels of ATP, which together with ERK-dependent inhibition of liver kinase B1 (LKB1) and inhibition of AMP kinase (AMPK)[151–153] further enhance mTOR signaling.[154] Phosphorylation and inhibition of glycogen synthase kinase type 3β[155] and direct phosphorylation and stabilization of β-catenin by PKA[156] enhance Wnt/β-catenin signaling. PKA-dependent upregulation of CREB (cAMP response element-binding transcription factor),[157] Pax-2 (paired box gene 2),[118,158] and STAT3 (signal transducer and activator of transcription 3)[159–162] also contribute to the proliferative phenotype of the cystic epithelium. Cyst-derived epithelial cells also exhibit increased expression and apical localization of the epidermal growth factor (EGF) receptors ErbB1 and ErbB2.[163,164] Activation of these receptors by EGF-related compounds, which are present in cyst fluid, is likely to contribute to the stimulation of MAPK/ERK signaling and cell proliferation.

Upregulation of PKA signaling promotes cystogenesis via phosphorylation of CFTR in the apical membrane, stimulation of chloride-driven fluid secretion,[163–170] and possibly other mechanisms such as disruption of tubulogenesis[171] and effects on cell–ECM and epithelial cell–macrophage interactions.[3]

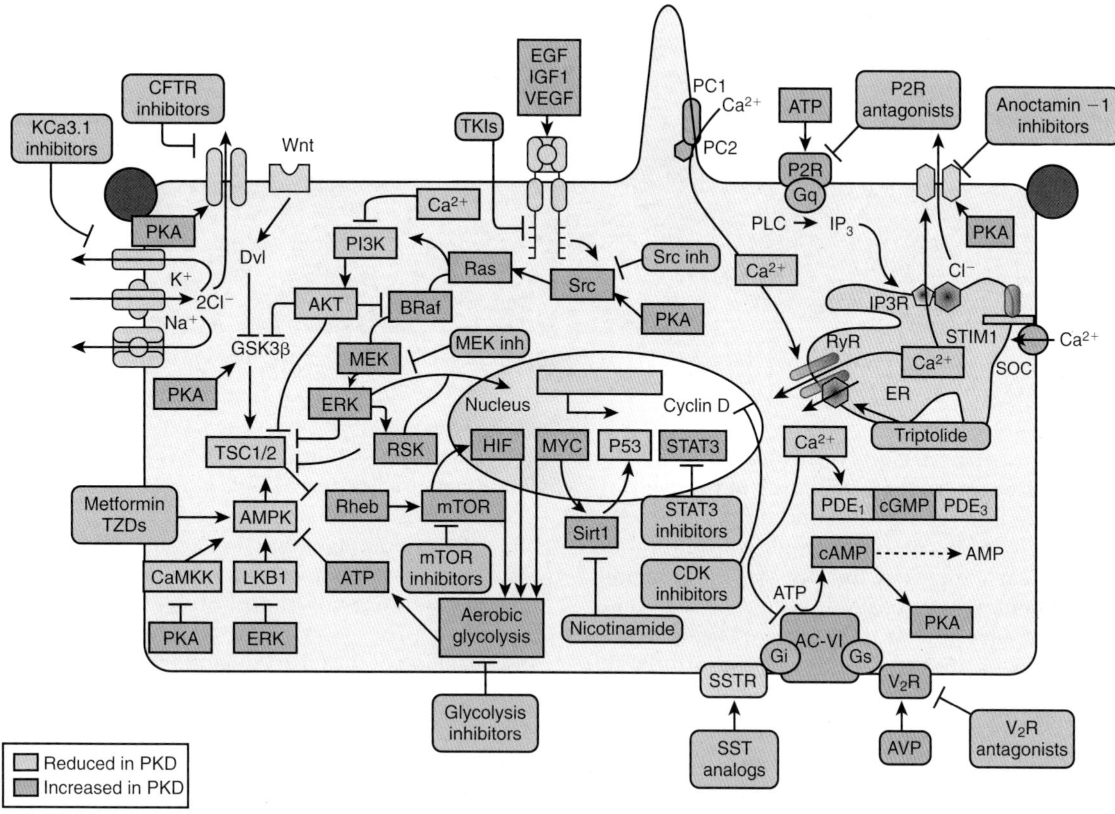


**Fig. 45.4** Diagram depicting proposed pathways upregulated or downregulated in polycystic kidney disease and rationale for treatments targeting these pathways *(green boxes)*. Aberrant crosstalk between intracellular calcium ($Ca^{2+}$) and cyclic adenosine monophosphate (cAMP) signaling may be one of the first consequences of polycystic kidney disease (PKD) mutations. Disrupted calcium may enhance cAMP and protein kinase A (PKA) signaling through activation of calcium-inhibitable adenylyl cyclases and inhibition of calcium-dependent phosphodiesterases [PDEs; $PDE_1$ and, indirectly, cyclic guanosine monophosphate (cGMP)–inhibited $PDE_3$]. Enhanced PKA activity may in turn disrupt intracellular calcium homeostasis through phosphorylation of calcium-cycling proteins in the endoplasmic reticulum. PKA-induced phosphorylation of the cystic fibrosis transmembrane conductance regulator (CFTR) allows chloride and fluid secretion into the cysts; anoctamin-1 may synergistically interact with CFTR, further enhancing fluid secretion. PKA activation inhibits cell proliferation in wild-type cells but has a stimulatory effect in PKD cells. Calcium deprivation in wild-type cells and delivery of calcium in PKD cells reverse these effects. A proposed mechanism for the proliferative response in PKD and calcium-deprived wild-type cells is inhibition of phosphoinositide 3-kinase (PI3K) and protein kinase B (AKT), which releases protein BRaf from AKT inhibition. This in turn leads to dysregulation of signaling pathways (BRaf/MEK/ERK; AMPK/mTOR) and transcription factors (HIF1, MYC, P53, STAT3) that control cell cycle progression and energy metabolism. Mislocalization of ErbB (epidermal growth factor receptor) receptors and overexpression of growth factors, cytokines, chemokines, and their receptors further contribute to disease progression. *AC-VI,* Adenylate cyclase 6; *AMPK,* AMP-activated kinase; *ATP,* adenosine triphosphate; *AVP,* vasopressin; *CaMKK,* calcium/calmodulin-dependent protein kinase kinase; *CDK,* cyclin-dependent kinase; *EGF,* epidermal growth factor; *ER,* endoplasmic reticulum; *ERK,* extracellular signal–regulated kinase; *Gi,* inhibitory G protein; *Gq,* a G-protein subunit; *Gs,* stimulatory G protein; *GSK3β,* glycogen synthase kinase 3β; *HIF,* hypoxia-inducible factor; *IGF1,* insulinlike growth factor 1; *inh,* inhibition/inhibitor; *IP3R,* inositol 1,4,5-trisphosphate (IP3) receptor; *KCa3.1,* a calcium channel; *LKB1,* liver kinase B1; *MEK,* mitogen-activated protein kinase kinase; *mTOR,* mammalian target of rapamycin; *P2R,* purinergic 2 receptor; *PC1,* polycystin 1; *PC2,* polycystin 2; *PLC,* phospholipase C; *Rheb,* Ras homolog enriched in brain; *RSK,* ribosomal s6 kinase; *RYR,* ryanodine receptor; *Sirt1,* sirtuin 1; *SOC,* store-operated channel; *SSTR,* somatostatin receptor; *STAT3,* signal transducer and activator of transcription 3; *STIM1,* stromal interaction molecule 1; *TKIs,* tyrosine kinase inhibitors; *TSC,* tuberous sclerosis proteins tuberin (TSC2) and hamartin (TSC1); *TZDs,* thiazolidinediones; *$V_2R$,* vasopressin $V_2$ receptor.

Additional ways that extracellular cues detected by the polycystin complex may be transmitted to the nucleus include canonical and noncanonical Wnt, JAK (Janus kinase)/STAT, and NFAT (nuclear factor of activated T cells) pathways.[169,170] A cleavage event in the G protein–coupled receptor proteolytic site domain, separating the extracellular region from the transmembrane part of the protein, is important for activation of PC1, as is appropriate glycosylation and trafficking.[90,172,173] It has also been proposed that PC1 may activate transcription directly by cleaving at additional sites and through the translocation of the resulting C-terminal fragments to the nucleus, a process that may be regulated by flow.[174,175]

## PATHOLOGY

Cystic kidneys usually maintain their reniform shape (Fig. 45.5). Their size ranges from minimally or moderately enlarged in early disease to >20 times normal size in advanced disease. Although unusual, striking asymmetry of cyst development may be seen. Both the outer and the cut surfaces show numerous cysts ranging in size from barely visible to several centimeters in diameter. They are distributed evenly throughout both the cortical and medullary parenchyma. The papillae and pyramids are distinguishable in early cases but are difficult or impossible to identify in advanced examples, and the calyces and pelves are often greatly distorted.

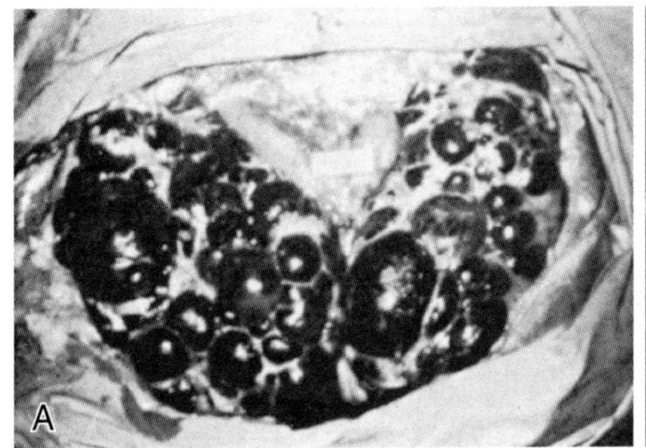

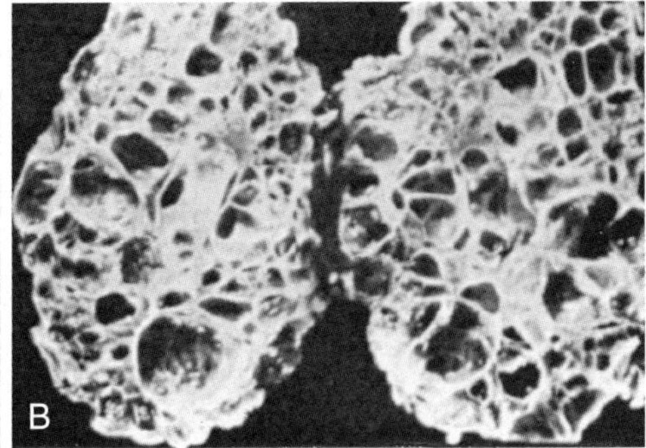


**Fig. 45.5** Autosomal dominant polycystic kidney disease (A) in situ and (B) on cut section. Note diffuse, bilateral distribution of cysts. (Courtesy FE Cuppage, Kansas City, KS.)

Nephron reconstruction and microdissection studies revealed that cysts begin as outpouchings from preexisting renal tubules. With enlargement beyond a few millimeters in diameter, most cysts become detached from the tubule of origin. In the early stages of the disease, the noncystic parenchymal elements appear relatively normal because fewer than 1% of the tubules appear to become cystic. The cells in the vast majority of the cysts are not typical of fully differentiated, mature renal tubular epithelium and are thought to be partially dedifferentiated or relatively immature. A minority of the cysts continue to function, as evidenced by their capacity to generate transepithelial electrical gradients and to secrete NaCl and fluid in vitro. The majority of cysts (75%) with $Na^+$ levels approximating the level in plasma and relatively leaky apical junctions probably represent cysts with epithelium that is less well differentiated than cysts with low Na concentrations.

Although ADPKD cysts have been thought to arise from all tubular segments, microdissection studies of ADPKD kidneys in the 1960s and 1970s suggested that collecting ducts are diffusely enlarged and that collecting duct cysts are more numerous and larger than those derived from other tubular segments. Most cysts of at least 1 mm in diameter stain positively for collecting duct markers.[176,177] Studies of *Pkd1* or *Pkd2* rodent models with postnatal development of cystic disease have shown that most cysts originate from the collecting ducts and distal nephron[86,92,93,178] but that proximal tubule cysts may be common at early stages.[10] Cultured epithelial cells from human ADPKD cysts exhibit a larger cAMP response to 1-deamino-8-D-arginine vasopressin and vasopressin than to the parathyroid hormone, a reaction consistent with a collecting duct origin.[179] These observations indicate that the majority of cysts in adults with ADPKD are derived from the distal nephron and the collecting duct (Fig. 45.6).

At the end stage of the disease, the kidneys are usually several times larger than normal and exhibit innumerable fluid-filled cysts that make up almost all of the total renal mass. In these far-advanced cases, only scant normal-appearing parenchyma may be found in isolated patches. Abundant fibrous tissue is plastered along the surface of the kidney beneath the capsule, and on the cut surfaces of transected kidneys, cysts may be found encapsulated by fibrous bands. Tubulointerstitial fibrosis and arteriolar sclerosis are cardinal features of end-stage polycystic kidney. The disappearance of noncystic parenchyma implicates apoptosis as a primary mechanism in progressive renal dysfunction in ADPKD.

Up to 90% of adults with ADPKD have cysts in the liver.[180] These cysts are lined by a single layer of epithelium resembling that of the biliary tract and contain fluid that resembles the bile salt–independent fraction of the bile. The electrolyte composition and osmolality are similar to those in the serum; the concentrations of phosphorus, cholesterol, and glucose are lower.[181] The cysts are derived by progressive proliferation and dilatation of the biliary ductules (biliary microhamartomas or von Meyenburg complexes) and peribiliary glands.[182,183] Like kidney cysts, liver cysts become detached as they grow, so macroscopic cysts usually do not communicate with the biliary system. Minimal to moderate dilation of the extrahepatic bile ducts is common. In rare kindreds, hepatic changes indistinguishable from those seen in congenital hepatic fibrosis (CHF) can be seen.

## DIAGNOSIS

The diagnosis of ADPKD in an individual with a positive family history primarily relies on imaging. Counseling should be performed before testing. Benefits of testing include certainty regarding diagnosis that may influence family planning, early detection and treatment of disease complications, selection of genetically unaffected family members for living-related donor renal transplantation, and now identification of patients for treatment. Potential discrimination in terms of insurability and employment associated with a positive diagnosis should be discussed.

Renal ultrasonography is commonly used because of its low cost and safety (Fig. 45.7). Revised criteria have been proposed to improve the diagnostic performance of ultrasonography in ADPKD (Table 45.1). For at-risk individuals with a 50% chance of having ADPKD (i.e., having a parent or sibling with ADPKD), the presence of at least three (unilateral or bilateral) renal cysts for those aged 15 to 39 years, or of two cysts in each kidney for those aged 40 to 59 years, has a positive predictive value (PPV) of 100% for the diagnosis of ADPKD.[184] For at-risk individuals aged 60 years and older, four or more cysts in each kidney are required. Although the PPVs of these criteria are very high, their sensitivity and negative predictive value (NPV) are low, particularly when applied to 15- to 59-year-old patients with PKD2, and likely hypomorphic *PKD1* alleles. This is a problem in the evaluation of potential kidney donors, in which exclusion of the diagnosis is important. Information on the age at ESKD in other affected family members may be helpful in this setting.[185] A history of at least one affected family member who had ESKD secondary to ADPKD by age 55

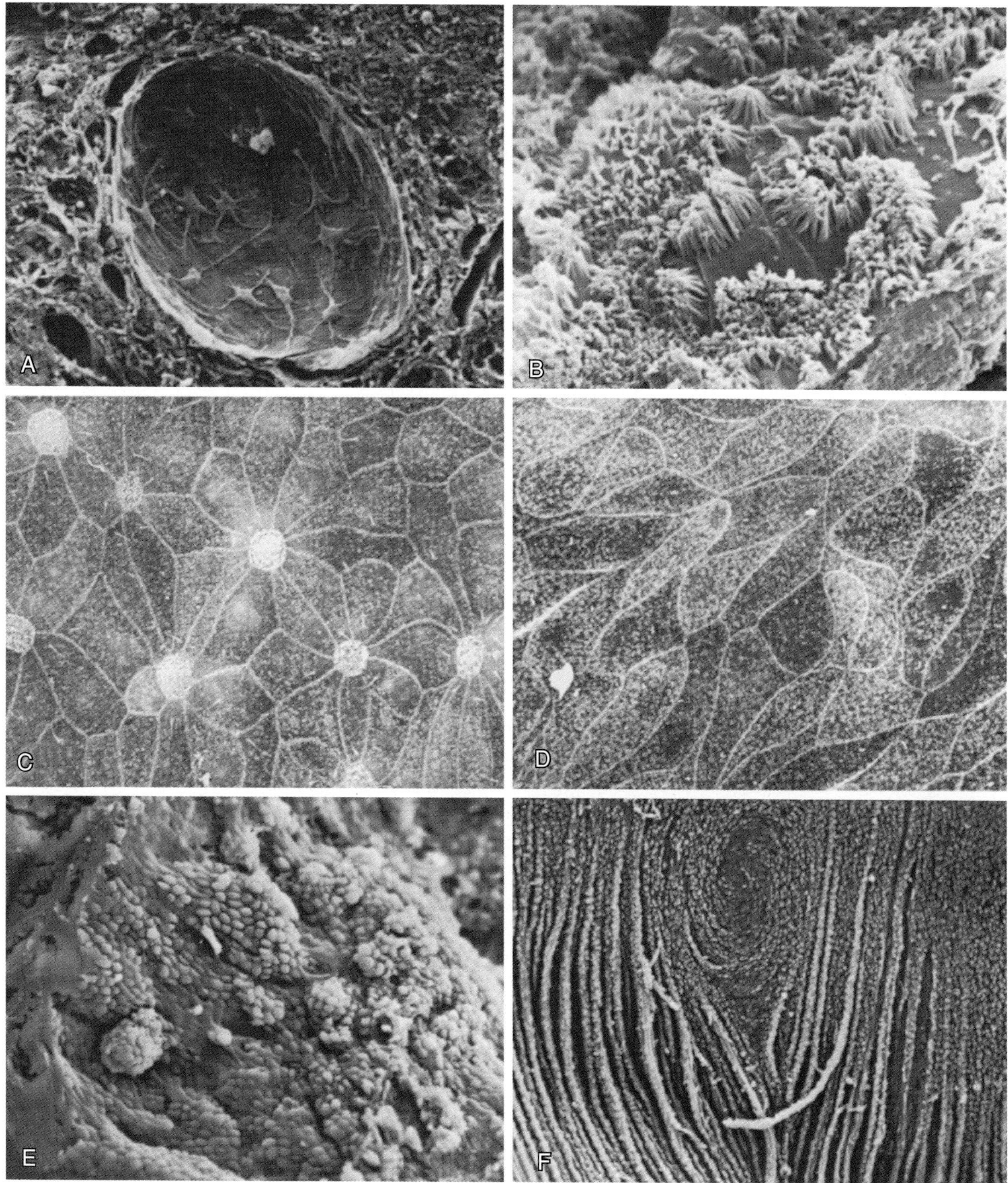


**Fig. 45.6** Scanning electron micrographs of epithelium lining a cyst in autosomal dominant polycystic kidney disease. (A) Epithelium typical of glomerular visceral layer (×250). (B) Epithelium typical of proximal tubule (×3000). (C) Epithelium typical of cortical collecting duct (×1000). (D) Epithelium not typical of any normal tubule segment (×1000). (E) Micropolyps (×250). (F) Cordlike hyperplasia (×80). (From Grantham JJ, Geiser JL, Evan AP. Cyst formation and growth in autosomal dominant polycystic kidney disease. *Kidney Int.* 1987;31:1145–1152, with permission.)

years has 100% PPV for PKD1. Conversely, a history of at least one affected family member without ESKD by age 70 or older is predictive of PKD2 or a hypomorphic *PKD1* allele. Different criteria have therefore been proposed to exclude a diagnosis of ADPKD in an individual at risk from a family with an unknown genotype (Table 45.1). An ultrasonographic finding of normal kidneys or one renal cyst in an individual 40 years or older has an NPV of 100%. The absence of any renal cyst provides near certainty that ADPKD is absent in at-risk individuals aged 30 to 39 years with an NPV of 98.3%. A negative or indeterminate ultrasonography scan result does not exclude ADPKD with certainty in an at-risk individual younger than 30 years. In this setting, the results of magnetic resonance imaging (MRI) or contrast-enhanced computed tomography (CT) provide further assurance, and one study has shown that the finding of a total of fewer than five renal cysts on MRI is sufficient for disease exclusion.[186]

In the absence of a family history of ADPKD, the finding of bilateral renal enlargement and cysts with or without hepatic cysts, as well as absence of other manifestations suggesting a different renal cystic disease, provides presumptive evidence for the diagnosis. Contrast-enhanced CT and MRI provide better anatomic definition than ultrasonography and are more helpful to ascertain the severity and prognosis of the disease (Figs. 45.8 and 45.9).

Genetic testing can be used when the imaging results are equivocal and when a definite diagnosis is required in a younger individual, such as a potential living-related kidney donor. It may also be helpful in patients with a negative family history, atypical radiologic presentations, and unusually severe or mild disease.[187] Prenatal testing is rarely considered for ADPKD.[188,189] Preimplantation genetic diagnosis, which is most commonly used in severe genetic diseases with early manifestations, such as cystic fibrosis and ARPKD, is becoming more frequently used in ADPKD, but it is available only in certain countries and the acceptance of this technique is influenced by personal values as well as the severity of the disease.[188,190]

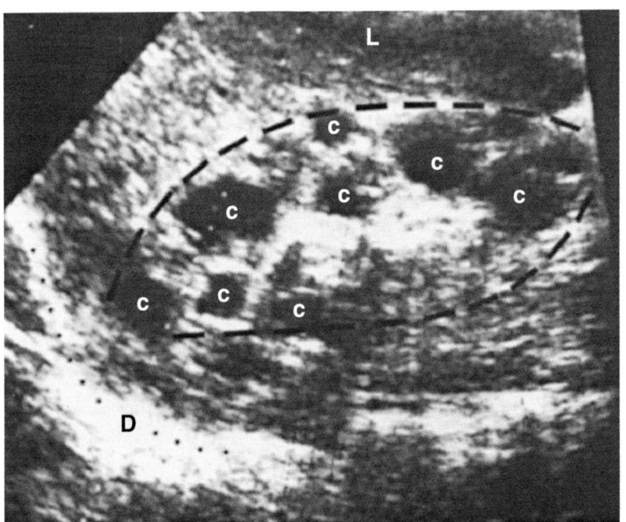


**Fig. 45.7** Autosomal dominant polycystic kidney disease seen in a parasagittal or longitudinal sonogram. This view of the right kidney was obtained with the patient in the right anterior oblique position. The approximate outline of the kidney is indicated by the *broken line*. Some of the larger renal cysts are indicated by Cs. The liver *(L)* is at the top of the figure. The right dome of the diaphragm *(D)* is at the lower left.

Genetic testing should be performed by sequence analysis. The large size and complexity of *PKD1* and marked allelic heterogeneity have been barriers to sequence-based molecular testing, but the development of multigene panels and NGS have made this more accessible. Mutation scanning by Sanger sequencing of *PKD1* and *PKD2* or employing a specifically generated NGS panel to screen PKD genes now yields detection rates >90%.[55,59,63,192] Detection of mutations in the segmentally duplicated *PKD1* gene may be lower by whole-exome sequencing. More than 50% of *PKD1* mutations are unique, with a lower level of unique pathogenic variants to *PKD2*. Approximately one-third of *PKD1* changes are in-frame; careful bioinformatic evaluation, and considering normal and ADPKD population data, can help determine pathogenic from neutral variants. The advances in NGS technologies to screen PKD genes are rendering molecular diagnostics more accessible and less costly in ADPKD and are likely to become more widely used for diagnostics and prognostics.[53]

## RENAL MANIFESTATIONS

### Cyst Development and Growth

Many manifestations of ADPKD are directly related to renal cyst development and enlargement. A longitudinal study of 241 15–46-year-old patients with creatinine clearance ≤70 mL/min followed prospectively with yearly MRI examinations by the Consortium for Radiologic Imaging Studies of Polycystic Kidney Disease (CRISP) has provided invaluable information to the understanding of how cysts develop and grow.[193,194]

**Table 45.1 Sonographic Criteria for Diagnosis or Exclusion of Autosomal Dominant Polycystic Kidney Disease in At-Risk Individuals[a]**

| | | Family Genotype | | | | | |
|---|---|---|---|---|---|---|---|
| | | Unknown | | PKD1 | | PKD2 | |
| **Age (years)** | *Criteria for Positive Diagnosis* | *PPV (%)* | *Sensitivity (%)* | *PPV (%)* | *Sensitivity (%)* | *PPV (%)* | *Sensitivity (%)* |
| 15–29 | ≥3 cysts, unilateral or bilateral | 100 | 81.7 | 100 | 94.3 | 100 | 69.5 |
| 30–39 | ≥3 cysts, unilateral or bilateral | 100 | 95.5 | 100 | 96.6 | 100 | 94.9 |
| 40–59 | ≥2 cysts in each kidney | 100 | 90.0 | 100 | 92.6 | 100 | 88.8 |
| ≥60 | ≥4 cysts in each kidney | 100 | 100 | 100 | 100 | 100 | 100 |
| | Revised Criteria For Diagnosis Exclusion | NPV (%) | Specificity (%) | NPV (%) | Specificity (%) | NPV (%) | Specificity (%) |
| 15–29 | ≥1 cyst | 90.8 | 97.1 | 99.1 | 97.6 | 83.5 | 96.6 |
| 30–39 | ≥1 cyst | 98.3 | 94.8 | 100 | 96.0 | 96.8 | 93.8 |
| 40–59 | ≥2 cysts | 100 | 98.2 | 100 | 98.4 | 100 | 97.8 |

[a]At-risk individuals are those known to have a 50% chance of having autosomal dominant polycystic kidney disease (ADPKD) by virtue of having a parent or at least one sibling with ADPKD.

*NPV,* Negative predictive value; PKD, polycystic kidney disease; *PPV,* positive predictive value.

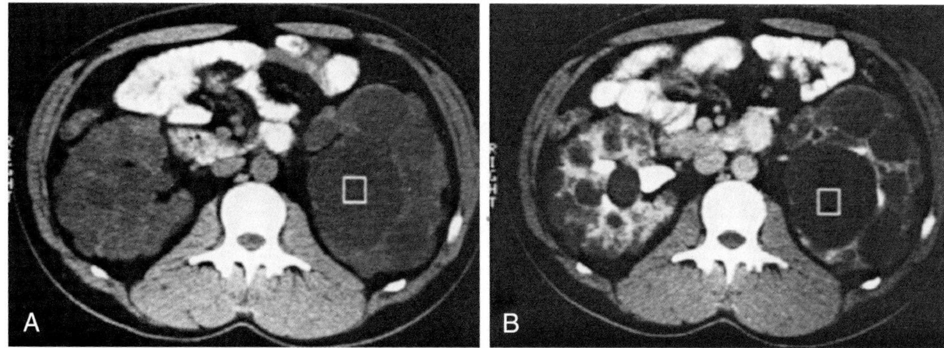


**Fig. 45.8** Computed tomography (CT) scans of polycystic kidneys. This male patient has autosomal dominant polycystic kidney disease, and his serum creatinine level is within the normal range. An oral contrast agent was given to highlight the intestine. (A) CT scan without contrast. (B) CT scan at the same level as (A) but after intravenous infusion of iodinated radiocontrast material. The cursor *(box)* is used to determine the relative density of cyst fluid, which in this case is equal to that of water. Contrast enhancement highlights functioning parenchyma, which here is concentrated primarily in the right kidney. The renal collecting system also is highlighted by contrast material in both kidneys.

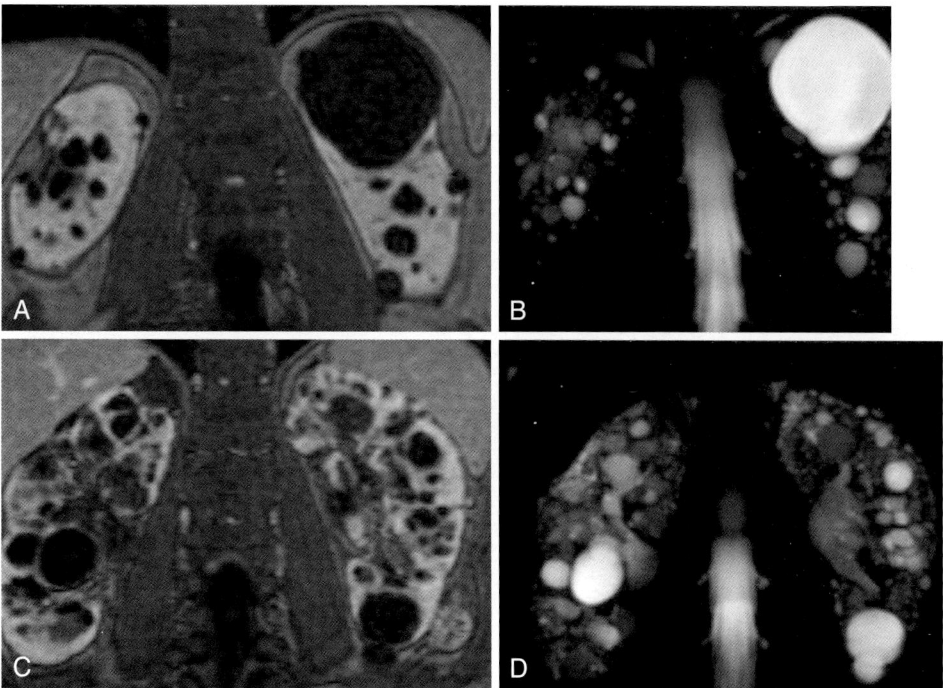


**Fig. 45.9** Magnetic resonance imaging studies of two female patients with (A and B) mild and (C and D) moderately severe disease. In neither subject was the serum creatinine value >1.1 mg/dL. For the images in (A) and (C), gadolinium was infused intravenously a few minutes previously. The residual, normal parenchyma between cysts is highlighted by gadolinium. In (B) and (D), heavy T2-weighted images are shown at the same kidney level as in (A) and (C). The cysts are emphasized, illustrating that cysts <3 mm can be detected.

MR images at baseline illustrated the large phenotypic variability in terms of total kidney volume (TKV) in ADPKD. Follow-up images showed the TKV growth to be quasi-exponential, unique to and variable among patients (Fig. 45.10). While TKV changed significantly year after year, glomerular filtration rate (GFR) started declining years later, hence TKV was a good predictor of future estimated GFR (eGFR) decline. A collaborative effort including the PKD Foundation, Food and Drug Administration (FDA), Critical Path Institute, academic centers, and the pharmaceutical industry led to FDA and European Medicines Agency qualification of TKV, together with age and eGFR, as a prognostic biomarker for risk of GFR decline.[195]

Measuring TKV, as a prognostic biomarker, does not require high precision. Measurements by the ellipsoid equation and various imaging modalities can be used to inform patients about their prognosis and determine eligibility for clinical trials and therapies as they become available. Its value is limited in atypical cases with markedly asymmetric or coexisting ischemic disease, but the Mayo imaging classification facilitates its use.[196] It is based on criteria to exclude atypical cases and stratify typical cases into five classes (A through E) based on growth rates (<1.5%, 1.5%–3%, 3%–4.5%, 4.5%–6%, or >6% per year) estimated from patient age and a theoretical starting height-adjusted TKV (150 mL/m). A model based on the classification can predict future GFR

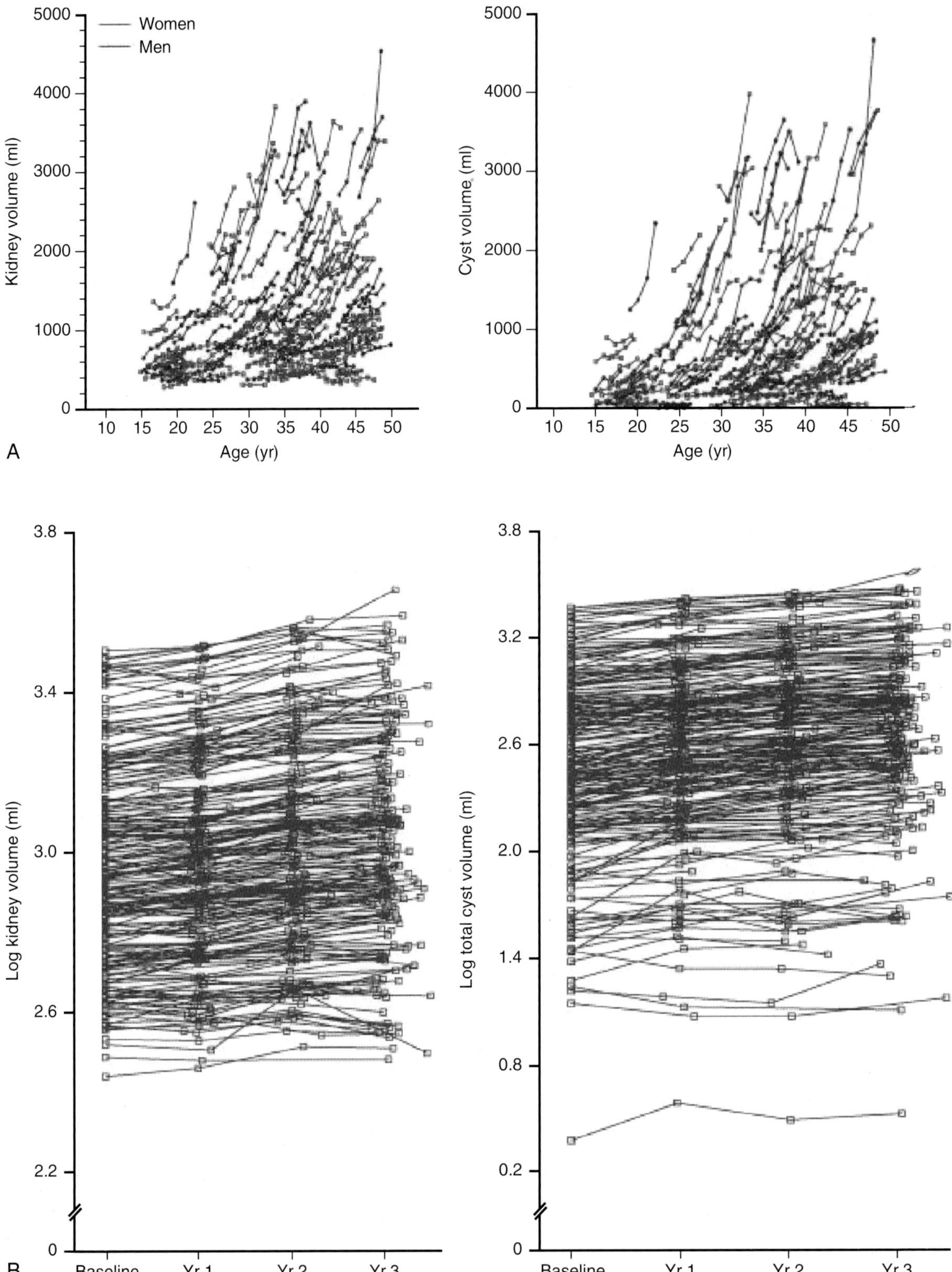


**Fig. 45.10** Progression of autosomal dominant polycystic kidney disease. (A) Combined left and right total kidney and cyst volumes in relation to age in women *(blue)* and men *(red)*. The lines connecting the four measurements for each patient in the 3 years of follow-up exhibit a concave upward sweep suggestive of an exponential growth process. (B) $Log_{10}$ combined total kidney and cyst volumes in relation to time. The linearity of the four measurements for each patient in the 3 years of follow-up is consistent with an exponential growth process. (Reproduced from Grantham JJ, Torres VE, Chapman AB, et al. Volume progression in polycystic kidney disease. *N Engl J Med.* 2006;354:2122–2130.)

decline with reasonable accuracy (http://www.mayo.edu/research/documents/pkd-center-adpkd-classification/doc-20094754). TKV has been used as an endpoint in clinical trials. Measurements for this purpose require high precision, achievable using planimetry, the gold standard, or stereology. Stereology is faster than planimetry but does not segment the kidney, a requirement for advanced image analysis. Fast, automatic segmentations, including a deep learning-based, fully automated approach, capable of replacing humans for the task of segmenting polycystic kidneys, have been developed.[197,198] Once segmented, advanced MRI processing and analysis such as texture analysis may be superior and/or complementary to TKV in predicting or measuring disease progression.[199]

## RENAL FUNCTION ABNORMALITIES

Impaired urinary concentrating capacity is common even at early stages of ADPKD. Nearly 60% of children cannot maximally concentrate their urine,[200] and plasma vasopressin levels are increased. The vasopressin-resistant concentrating defect is not explained by reduced cAMP or expression of concentration-associated genes, which are consistently increased in animal models. It has not been determined whether the defect is attributable to disruption of the medullary architecture by the cysts or to a cellular defect directly linked to disruption of polycystin function. Newer studies suggest that the urinary concentrating defect and elevated vasopressin values may contribute to cystogenesis. They may also contribute to the glomerular hyperfiltration seen in children and young adults[201] and to the development of hypertension and the progression of chronic kidney disease (CKD). Defective medullary trapping of ammonia and transfer to the urine caused by the concentrating defect may contribute to the low urine pH values, hypocitric aciduria, and predisposition to stone formation.

Reduced renal blood flow is another early functional defect.[202] It may be caused by changes in intrarenal pressures, neurohumoral or local mediators, and/or intrinsic vascular abnormalities. Mild to moderate persistent proteinuria (150–1500 mg/day) may be found in a significant number of patients in the middle to late stages of the disease and is an indicator of a more progressive disease.[203] Patients with proteinuria may also excrete doubly refractile lipid bodies (oval fat bodies).[204]

### Hypertension

Hypertension (blood pressure ≥ 140 mm Hg systolic/90 mm Hg diastolic), found in approximately 50% of 20–34-year-old patients with ADPKD and normal renal function, is present in nearly 100% of patients with ESKD.[205] Development of hypertension is accompanied by a reduction in renal blood flow, an increase in filtration fraction, abnormal renal handling of sodium, and extensive remodeling of the renal vasculature.

The association between renal size and the prevalence of hypertension supports the hypothesis that stretching and compression of the vascular tree by cyst expansion cause ischemia and activation of the renin–angiotensin–aldosterone system (RAAS).[206] The expression of PC1 and PC2 in vascular smooth muscle[207–209] and endothelium,[210] along with enhanced vascular smooth muscle contractility[211] and impaired endothelium-dependent vasorelaxation,[212] suggests that a primary disruption of polycystin function in the vasculature may also play a role in the early development of hypertension and renal vascular remodeling.

Whether circulating angiotensin is instrumental in causing hypertension is controversial.[213,214] Plasma renin activity and aldosterone values are normal in most studies, but because blood pressures are higher than those of controls, it has been argued that the renin and aldosterone levels are not appropriately suppressed. A 1990 study showed higher levels after short- or long-term administration of an angiotensin-converting enzyme (ACE) inhibitor in normotensive and hypertensive patients with ADPKD and normal renal function than in both normal subjects and patients with essential hypertension.[213] Another study found no differences in hormonal or blood pressure responses between patients with ADPKD and patients with essential hypertension matched in terms of renal function and blood pressure under conditions of high and low sodium intake and after the administration of an ACE inhibitor.[214] Sodium intake was not controlled in the former study, and differences in selection and ethnic composition of the control groups have been offered as possible explanations for the different results.

There is stronger evidence for local activation of intrarenal RAAS. It includes 1. partial reversal of the reduced renal blood flow, increased renal vascular resistance, and increased filtration fraction by short- or long-term administration of an ACE inhibitor[213,215,216]; 2. shift of immunoreactive renin from the juxtaglomerular apparatus to the walls of the arterioles and small arteries[217,218]; 3. ectopic synthesis of renin in the epithelium of dilated tubules and cysts[219,220]; and 4. ACE-independent generation of angiotensin II by a chymase-like enzyme.[220]

Nitric oxide–associated endothelium–dependent vasorelaxation has been shown to be impaired in small subcutaneous resistance vessels from patients with normal renal function before the development of hypertension.[221–223] Other factors proposed to contribute to hypertension in ADPKD include increases in sympathetic nerve activity and plasma endothelin 1 levels as well as insulin resistance.[224]

The diagnosis of hypertension in ADPKD is often made late. Twenty-four-hour ambulatory blood pressure monitoring of children or young adults without hypertension often reveals blood pressure elevations, attenuated nocturnal blood pressure dipping, and/or exaggerated blood pressure response during exercise, which may be accompanied by left ventricular hypertrophy and diastolic dysfunction. Early detection and treatment of hypertension are important because cardiovascular disease is the main cause of death in patients with ADPKD.[40,225] Uncontrolled blood pressure increases the morbidity and mortality from valvular heart disease and aneurysms as well as the risk of proteinuria, hematuria, and a faster decline of renal function. The presence of hypertension also increases the risk of fetal and maternal complications during pregnancy. Normotensive women with ADPKD usually have uncomplicated pregnancies.[226]

### Pain

Pain is the most frequent symptom (60%) reported by adult patients with ADPKD.[227,228] Acute pain may be associated with renal hemorrhage, passage of stones, and urinary tract infections. Some patients have chronic flank pain without an identifiable etiology other than the cysts.

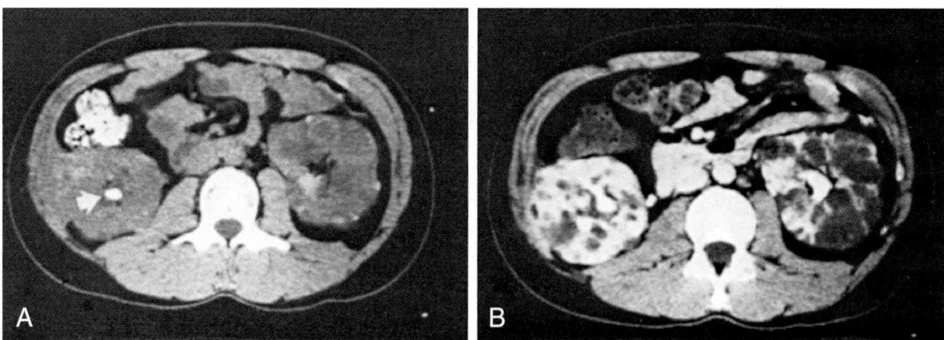


**Fig. 45.11** Computed tomography (CT) of polycystic kidneys in a male patient whose serum creatinine level is within the normal range. (A) CT scan without contrast shows a radiopaque stone in the pelvis of the right kidney *(arrow)*. (B) CT scan after intravenous administration of an iodinated radiocontrast agent. The stone now is obscured by contrast medium in the renal pelvis.

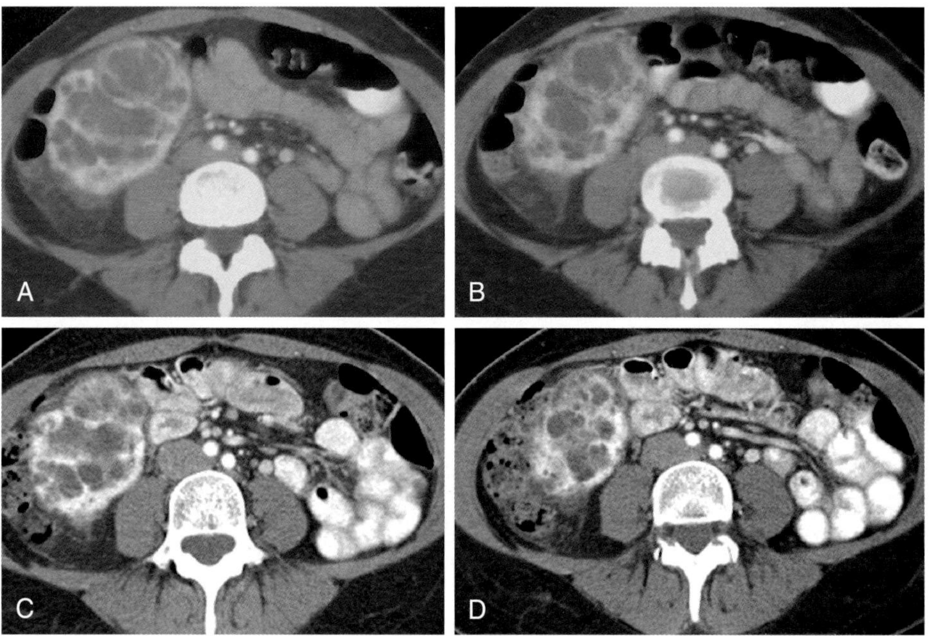


**Fig. 45.12** Cyst infection. (A and B) Contrast-enhanced computed tomography (CT) scans demonstrate a 4-cm infected cyst in the anterior portion of the lower pole of the right kidney and inflammatory stranding in the perirenal fat. (C and D) CT scans obtained after 3 weeks of antibiotic therapy show a decrease in the size of the cyst and improved enhancement of the renal parenchyma.

Vascular endothelial growth factor (VEGF) produced by the cystic epithelium[229] may promote angiogenesis, hemorrhage into cysts, and gross hematuria. Symptomatic episodes likely underestimate the frequency of cyst hemorrhage because >90% of patients with ADPKD have hyperdense (CT) or high-signal (MRI) cysts, reflecting blood or high protein content. Most hemorrhages resolve within 2 to 7 days. If symptoms last longer than 1 week or if the initial episode occurs after the age of 50 years, investigation to exclude neoplasm should be undertaken.

Approximately 20% of patients with ADPKD have kidney stones, usually composed of uric acid and calcium oxalate.[230,231] Metabolic factors include decreased ammonia excretion, low urinary pH, and low urinary citrate concentration. Urinary stasis secondary to the distorted renal anatomy may also play a role. CT of the abdomen before and after contrast enhancement is the best imaging technique to detect small uric acid stones that may be very faint on plain films with tomograms and to differentiate stones from cyst wall and parenchymal calcifications. Stones may be missed if only a contrast-enhanced CT is obtained (Fig. 45.11). Dual-energy CT can be used to distinguish between calcium and uric acid stones.[232,233]

As in the general population, urinary tract infections affect women more frequently than men. Most are caused by Enterobacteriaceae.[234] CT and MRI are useful to detect complicated cysts and provide anatomic definition, but the findings are not specific for infection (Fig. 45.12). Nuclear imaging ($^{67}$Ga- or $^{111}$In-labeled leukocyte scans) may be helpful, but false-negative and false-positive results are possible. Fluorine 18 2-fluoro-2-deoxy-D-glucose (FDG) positron emission tomography (PET) has become a promising agent for detection of infected cysts, but its use to diagnose kidney infections may be difficult because FDG is filtered by the kidneys, is not reabsorbed by the tubules, and appears in the collecting system.[235–237] Cyst aspiration should be considered when the clinical setting and imaging are suggestive and blood and urine cultures are negative.

Renal cell carcinoma (RCC) is a rare cause of pain in ADPKD. Although it does not occur more frequently than in the patients with other renal diseases,[238] it may manifest at an earlier age in patients with ADPKD, with frequent constitutional symptoms and a higher proportion of sarcomatoid, bilateral, multicentric, and metastatic tumors.[239] A solid mass on ultrasonography, speckled calcifications on CT and contrast enhancement, and tumor thrombus and regional lymphadenopathies on CT or MRI should raise the suspicion of a carcinoma.

### Chronic Kidney Disease and Renal Failure

The development of renal failure in ADPKD is highly variable. In most patients, renal function is maintained within the normal range because of compensatory adaptation, despite relentless growth of cysts, until the 4th to 6th decade of life (Fig. 45.13). By the time renal function starts declining, the kidneys usually are markedly enlarged and distorted with little recognizable parenchyma on imaging studies. At this stage, the average rate of decline in GFR is approximately 4.4 to 5.9 mL/min/year.[240] The mutated gene (*PKD1* vs. *PKD2*), type of mutation in *PKD1* (truncating versus nontruncating), and modifier genes determine to a significant extent the clinical course of ADPKD (see earlier discussion). Other risk factors are male gender, diagnosis before the age of 30 years, a first episode of hematuria before 30 years of age, onset of hypertension before 35 years of age, hyperlipidemia, low level of high-density lipoprotein cholesterol, and sickle cell trait.[59,60,241,242] As in other forms of CKD, smoking raises the risk for ESKD, at least in some patient subsets, such as male smokers with no history of ACE inhibitor treatment.[243]

While several factors contribute to renal function decline, a particularly strong relationship with renal enlargement has been noted. CRISP has confirmed this relationship and has shown that kidney and cyst volumes are the strongest predictors of renal functional decline.[244] After a mean follow-up of 7.9 years, 30.7% of CRISP enrollees reached stage 3 CKD. Correlations of htTKV at baseline with GFR at different time points increased from −0.22 (GFR at baseline) to −0.65 (GFR at year 8).[245] A htTKV of ≥600 mL/m at baseline most accurately defined the risk for development of stage 3 CKD within 8 years [area under the curve of 0.84 in a receiver operator characteristic analysis, 95% confidence interval, 0.79 to 0.90]. Kidney volume was a better predictor of GFR decline than baseline age, serum creatinine, blood urea nitrogen (BUN), urinary albumin, or monocyte chemotactic protein-1 (MCP-1) excretion. At the latest analysis, completed after a median follow-up of 13 years, 19% of patients in CRISP have now reached stage 5 CKD or end-stage renal disease (ESRD).[246] Baseline htTKV remained a strong independent predictor, with an odds ratio of 1.35 (1.18–1.55) for reaching stage 5 CKD or ESRD for each 100 mL/m increment in htTKV. While PKD genotype was also associated with CKD outcome, it was no longer independently associated with outcomes after adjusting for htTKV, suggesting that the effect of ADPKD genotype on kidney function may largely be mediated by changes in htTKV.

CRISP has also shown that reduced renal blood flow (or increased vascular resistance) is an independent predictor of GFR decline.[202] This factor points to the importance of vascular remodeling in the progression of the disease and may account for cases in which the decline of renal function seems to be out of proportion to the severity of the cystic disease. Angiotensin II, transforming growth factor-β (TGF-β), and reactive oxygen species may contribute to the vascular lesions and interstitial inflammation and fibrosis by stimulating the synthesis of chemokines, ECM, and metalloproteinase inhibitors. The expression of MCP-1 and osteopontin are increased in cyst epithelial cells. MCP-1 is found in cyst fluids in high concentrations, and the urinary excretion is increased.[247] Other factors such as heavy use of analgesics may contribute to CKD progression in some patients.

Patients with ADPKD and advanced CKD have less anemia than patients with other renal diseases because of enhanced production of erythropoietin by the polycystic kidneys.

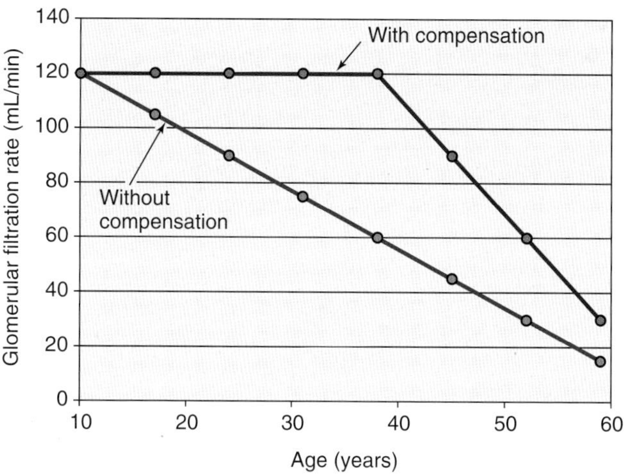


**Fig. 45.13** Effects of compensatory maintenance of glomerular filtration rate (GFR) on the pattern of progression in autosomal dominant polycystic kidney disease. It was assumed that, beginning at the age of 10 years, the patient loses an amount of parenchyma each year that normally contributes 2 mL/min of GFR. It was further assumed that each residual normal glomerulus can double the single-nephron GFR by compensatory mechanisms (as seen in normal individuals by the maintenance of total GFR after uninephrectomy for kidney donation). As seen in the model, total GFR is maintained until parenchymal loss precludes complete compensation; at that point, total GFR begins to fall at a rate that appears more "precipitous" than what had actually occurred. This model illustrates that GFR is a poor indicator of autosomal dominant polycystic kidney disease (ADPKD) progression and that more sensitive markers of parenchymal loss are needed to facilitate earlier monitoring.

## EXTRARENAL MANIFESTATIONS

### Polycystic Liver Disease

Polycystic liver disease (PLD) is the most common extrarenal manifestation of ADPKD. It is associated with both *PKD1* and non-*PKD1* genotypes.[52,248,249] Although hepatic cysts are rare in children, their frequency increases with age and may have been underestimated by ultrasonography and CT studies. Their prevalence according to MRI in the CRISP study were 58%, 85%, and 94% in 15- to 24-, 25- to 34-, and 35- to 46-year-old participants, respectively.[180] Hepatic cysts are more prevalent and hepatic cyst volume is larger in women than in men. Women who have multiple pregnancies or who have used oral contraceptive agents or estrogen replacement therapy have more severe disease, suggesting an estrogen

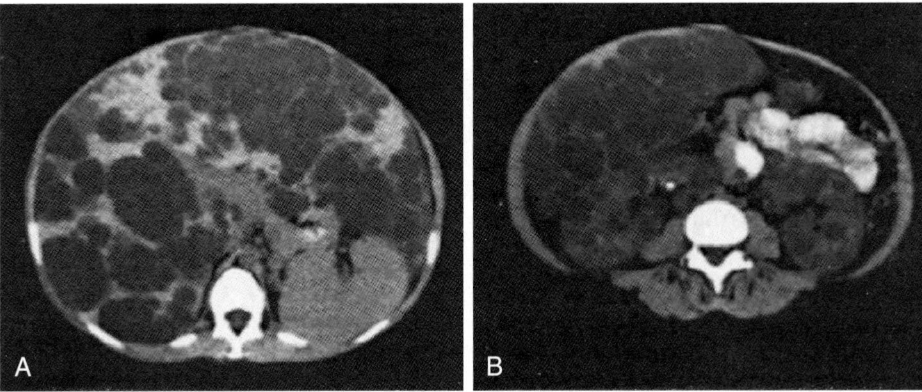


**Fig. 45.14** Computed tomography (CT) scan of polycystic liver and kidneys in a female patient with autosomal dominant polycystic kidney disease. The serum creatinine level and liver function test results were within the normal range. An oral contrast agent was given to highlight the intestine, but no intravenous contrast was used. (A) Massive enlargement of the liver caused by intraparenchymal cysts. (B) CT scan at a lower level in the abdomen shows cystic kidneys and the lower portion of the cystic liver.

effect on hepatic cyst growth.[206,250] Estrogen receptors are expressed in the epithelium lining the hepatic cysts, and estrogens stimulate proliferation of hepatic cyst–derived cells.

Typically, PLD is asymptomatic, but symptoms have become more frequent as the lifespan of patients with ADPKD has lengthened because of dialysis and transplantation. Symptoms may result from the mass effect or from complicating infection and hemorrhage (Fig. 45.14). Symptoms typically caused by massive enlargement of the liver or by mass effect from a single or a limited number of dominant cysts include dyspnea, early satiety, gastroesophageal reflux, and mechanical lower back pain. Other complications caused by mass effect include hepatic venous outflow obstruction, inferior vena cava compression, portal vein compression, and bile duct compression manifesting as obstructive jaundice.[251]

Symptomatic complications of hepatic cysts include cyst hemorrhage, infection, and, rarely, torsion or rupture. The typical manifestation of cyst infection consists of localized pain, fever, leukocytosis, elevated erythrocyte sedimentation rate, and, often, elevated alkaline phosphatase. It is usually monomicrobial and caused by Enterobacteriaceae.[252–254] MRI sensitively differentiates between complicated and uncomplicated hepatic cyst. On CT, fluid-debris levels within cysts, cyst wall thickening, intracystic gas bubbles, and heterogeneous or increased density have been associated with infection. Radionuclide imaging and FDG-PET scanning have been used for diagnosis.[255]

Mild dilation of the common bile duct has been observed in 40% of patients with PLD studied by CT and may rarely be associated with episodes of cholangitis.[256] Rare associations of PLD include CHF, adenomas of the ampulla of Vater, and cholangiocarcinoma.

Autosomal dominant PLD (ADPLD) occurs as a genetically distinct disease with no or few renal cysts. Similar to ADPKD, ADPLD is genetically heterogeneous, with initially two genes identified: *PRKCSH* (chromosome 19) and *SEC63* (chromosome 6), each accounting for approximately one-third of isolated ADPLD cases.[257–259] Subsequently, whole-exome sequencing showed that *LRP5* mutations (chromosome 11) are associated with hepatic cystogenesis,[260] and recently mutations in *GANAB, ALG8, SEC61B,* and *PKHD1* have also been associated with ADPLD.[52,249,261]

### Cysts in Other Organs

Cysts are found in the pancreas in approximately 5%, arachnoid in approximately 8%, and seminal vesicles in approximately 40% of patients with ADPKD.[262–267] Seminal vesicle cysts rarely result in infertility.[268] Defective sperm motility is another cause of male infertility in ADPKD.[269] Pancreatic cysts are almost always asymptomatic, with very rare occurrences of recurrent pancreatitis. It is uncertain whether the reported association of carcinoma of the pancreas represents more than chance. Arachnoid membrane cysts are usually asymptomatic but may increase the risk for subdural hematomas.[267,270] Spinal meningeal diverticula may occur with increased frequency and rarely manifest as intracranial hypotension due to a cerebrospinal fluid leak.[271] Ovarian cysts are not associated with ADPKD.

### Vascular Manifestations

Vascular manifestations of ADPKD include IAs and dolichoectasias, thoracic aortic and cervicocephalic artery dissections, and coronary artery aneurysms. They are caused by alterations in the vasculature directly linked to mutations in *PKD1* or *PKD2*. PC1 and PC2 are expressed in VSMCs,[207–209] $Pkd2^{+/-}$ VSMCs exhibit increased rates of proliferation and apoptosis, and $Pkd2^{+/-}$ mice have a greater susceptibility to vascular injury and premature death when hypertension is induced to develop.[95,132]

IAs occur in approximately 6% of patients with a negative family history and 16% of those with a positive family history of aneurysms[272] and are most often asymptomatic. Focal findings such as cranial nerve palsy and seizure result from compression of local structures. The risk of rupture depends on many factors (see later discussion). Rupture carries a 35% to 55% risk of combined severe morbidity or mortality.[273] The mean age at rupture is lower than in the general population (39 years vs. 51 years, respectively). Most patients have normal renal function, and up to 29% have normal blood pressure, at the time of rupture.

### Cardiac Manifestations

Mitral valve prolapse observed by echocardiography is the most common valvular abnormality, found in up to 25% of patients with ADPKD.[274,275] Aortic insufficiency may occur in association with dilation of the aortic root.[276] Although these lesions may progress with time, they rarely require valve replacement. Screening echocardiography is not indicated unless a murmur is detected on physical examination. Nonhemodynamically significant pericardial effusions are frequently observed.[277] Cardiomyopathies (dilated, hypertrophic, and left ventricular noncompaction) and atrial fibrillation may occur more frequently in ADPKD patients compared with the general population.[278]

### Diverticular Disease

Colonic diverticulosis and diverticulitis are more common in patients with ADPKD and ESKD than in those with other renal diseases. Whether this increased risk extends to patients before the onset of ESKD is uncertain.[279] There have been reports of extracolonic diverticular disease.[280] It may become clinically significant in a minority of patients. Subtle alterations in polycystin function may enhance the smooth muscle dysfunction from aging, which is thought to underlie the development of diverticula.

### Bronchiectasis

PC1 is expressed in the motile cilia of airway epithelial cells. Bronchiectasis occurs three times more frequently in patients with ADPKD than in control individuals (37% vs. 13%, respectively; $P < .002$), as detected by CT.[281]

## TREATMENT

Current therapy of ADPKD has been directed toward limiting the morbidity and mortality from the complications of the disease, but specific therapies are now becoming available.

### Hypertension

There is no proven antihypertensive agent of choice in ADPKD. ACE inhibitors or angiotensin receptor blockers (ARBs) increase renal blood flow, have a low side-effect profile, and may have renoprotective properties beyond blood pressure control. Some studies have shown better preservation of renal function or reduction in proteinuria and left ventricular hypertrophy with ACE inhibitors or ARBs than with diuretics or calcium channel blockers,[282–284] but other studies have been unable to detect the superiority of these drugs.[285] A metaanalysis of 142 patients with ADPKD in eight randomized clinical trials showed that ACE inhibitors were more effective in lowering urine protein excretion and slowing kidney disease progression in patients with higher levels of proteinuria, but the overall kidney disease progression was not significantly different (29% in the inhibitor group vs. 41% in the control group).[286] Most studies have been limited by inadequate power, short follow-ups, wide ranges of renal function, and the use of doses with inadequate pharmacologic effects.

Equally controversial has been the optimal blood pressure target. In the Modification of Diet in Renal Disease (MDRD) study, patients with ADPKD and a baseline GFR between 13 and 24 mL/min/1.73 m$^2$ assigned to a low blood pressure target (≤92 mm Hg) had faster declines in GFR than those assigned to a standard blood pressure goal (≤107 mm Hg). The reason may be the inability to autoregulate renal blood flow.[240] The rate of decline in participants with a baseline GFR between 25 and 55 mL/min/1.73 m$^2$ was not affected by the blood pressure target over a mean intervention period of 2.2 years. However, an extended follow-up of these patients showed a delayed onset of kidney failure and a reduced composite outcome of kidney failure and all-cause mortality in the low blood pressure target group (51% of them taking ACE inhibitors) in comparison with those in the standard blood pressure target group (32% of them taking ACE inhibitors).[287] The magnitude of this beneficial effect was similar to that observed in patients with other renal diseases.

In study A of the HALT Progression of Polycystic Kidney Disease (HALT-PKD) clinical trial, 558 hypertensive patients with ADPKD (15 to 49 years of age, with eGFRs > 60 mL/min/1.73 m$^2$) were randomly assigned to either a standard blood pressure target (120/70 to 130/80 mm Hg) or a low blood pressure target (95/60 to 110/75 mm Hg) and to either lisinopril plus telmisartan or lisinopril plus placebo.[288] In study B, 486 hypertensive patients with ADPKD (18 to 64 years of age, with eGFRs 25 to 60 mL/min/1.73 m$^2$) were randomly assigned to receive lisinopril plus telmisartan or lisinopril plus placebo, with the doses adjusted to achieve a blood pressure of 110/70 to 130/80 mm Hg.[289] Both studies showed that an ACE inhibitor alone adequately controlled hypertension in most patients; the addition of an ARB did not show additional benefit, justifying the use of ACE inhibitors for first-line treatment for hypertension in this disease. Study A showed that lowering blood pressure to levels below those recommended by current guidelines in young patients with good kidney function reduced the rate of increase in kidney volume by 14%, the increase in renal vascular resistance, urine albumin excretion (all identified in CRISP as predictors of renal function decline), left ventricular mass (LVM) index, and, marginally (after the first 4 months of treatment), the rate of decline in eGFR.[288] The overall effect of low blood pressure on eGFR, however, was not statistically significant, possibly because the reduction of blood pressure to low levels was associated with an acute reduction in eGFR within the first 4 months of treatment. When stratified by disease severity classification by TKV/age, class D and E patients assigned to intensive treatment had slower annual TKV increase (6.4% vs. 7.8%, $P = .033$), and eGFR decline after month 4 (−3.36 vs. −4.44, $P = .011$) and arguably overall (−3.57 vs. −4.37, $P = .051$).[290] These results underline the importance of early detection and treatment of hypertension in ADPKD.

Several studies suggest that improved blood pressure control in patients with ADPKD over the last 2 decades has been associated with reduced cardiovascular morbidity and mortality. A small prospective study from the University of Colorado showed that rigorous blood pressure control caused a greater decrease in LVM without a detectable effect on renal function.[291] A population-based study using the UK General Practice Research Database found that increased use of antihypertensive drugs over the period from 1991 to 2008 in patients with ADPKD, particularly of agents blocking the RAAS, was accompanied by reduced mortality.[292] The prevalence of left ventricular hypertrophy, assessed by MRI in 543 hypertensive HALT-PKD study A patients (mean age 36 years) with normal renal function at baseline, was 3.9% by nonindexed LVM and 0.9% by LVM index at enrollment, much lower than that observed in earlier studies.[293] This likely reflects the excellent blood pressure control (mean approximately 124/82 mm Hg) and the high utilization of RAAS blockers (61%).[294] In Danish patients with ADPKD and ESKD, cardiovascular and cerebrovascular deaths decreased from 1993 to 2008, possibly owing to a greater effectiveness of antihypertensive treatment.[295]

There is less evidence that the better control of hypertension over the last 2 decades has delayed the progression to ESKD. Two observational studies suggested that in patients with ADPKD, the average age at start of renal replacement therapy (RRT) has increased considerably during the last 2 decades.[296,297] A study of European Renal Association–European Dialysis and Transplant Association Registry data on patients starting RRT between 1991 and 2010, spanning 12 European countries with 208 million inhabitants, also showed that mean age at onset of RRT among patients with ADPKD ($n = 20{,}596$) has risen, albeit considerably less than in the two aforementioned studies, from 56.6 to 58.0 years.[298] Although the RRT incidence did not change among patients with ADPKD younger than 50 years, it increased among older patients (>70 years of age). These data suggest that the greater age of patients with ADPKD at the start of RRT may be explained by increased access of the elderly to RRT or by the lower competing risk of mortality prior to the start of RRT, rather than the consequence of effective renoprotective therapies.[299,300]

### Pain

Causes of pain in ADPKD that may require intervention, such as infections, stones, and tumors, should be excluded. Long-term administration of nephrotoxic agents such as nonsteroidal antiinflammatory drugs should be avoided, and narcotic analgesics should be reserved for acute episodes. Psychological evaluation and an understanding and supportive attitude on the part of the physician are essential to minimize the risk for narcotic and analgesic dependence in patients with chronic pain. Reassurance, lifestyle modification, avoidance of aggravating activities, tricyclic antidepressants, and pain clinic interventions such as splanchnic nerve blockade with local anesthesia or steroids may be helpful.[227,228]

When conservative measures fail, surgical interventions can be considered. Aspiration of large cysts under ultrasonographic or CT guidance is a simple procedure and may help identify the cause of the pain. Sclerosing agents may be used to prevent the reaccumulation of fluid. When multiple cysts contribute to pain, laparoscopic or surgical cyst fenestration through lumbotomy or flank incisions may be of benefit.[301] Laparoscopy is as effective as open surgical fenestration for patients with limited disease and has a shorter, less complicated recovery period.[302,303] Surgical interventions do not accelerate the decline in renal function as was once thought, but they do not preserve declining renal function either. Laparoscopic renal denervation or thoracoscopic sympatho-splanchnicectomy can be considered, particularly in polycystic kidneys without large cysts.[304,305] Percutaneous transluminal renal denervation has been proposed as a potential treatment option for PKD-related pain but has not yet been adequately tested.[306,307] Laparoscopic or retroperitoneoscopic nephrectomy is indicated for symptomatic patients with ESKD. Arterial embolization is an alternative when the surgical risk is high, but its role has not been fully defined.

### Cyst Hemorrhage

Cyst hemorrhages are usually self-limiting and respond to conservative management with bed rest, analgesics, and hydration. When a subcapsular or retroperitoneal hematoma is causing significant decrease in hematocrit and hemodynamic instability, hospitalization, transfusion, and investigation by CT or angiography become necessary. In cases of unusually severe or persistent hemorrhage, segmental arterial embolization can be successful. If not, surgery may be required to control bleeding. Segmental arterial embolization or surgery may be required in some cases. The antifibrinolytic agent tranexamic acid has been successfully used in some cases, but no controlled studies of its use have been performed,[308] and the dose needs to be reduced in the presence of renal insufficiency. Potential adverse effects of this treatment include glomerular thrombosis and ureteral obstructions due to clots.

### Cyst Infection

Cyst infections are often difficult to treat.[234] Treatment failure may occur because of poor antibiotic penetration into the cysts, but lipophilic agents such as quinolones, as well as trimethoprim–sulfamethoxazole and chloramphenicol, penetrate the cysts consistently. If fever persists after 1 to 2 weeks of appropriate antimicrobial therapy, percutaneous or surgical drainage of infected cysts or, in the case of end-stage polycystic kidneys, nephrectomy should be undertaken. If fever recurs after antibiotic therapy is stopped, a complicating feature such as obstruction, perinephric abscess, or a stone should be excluded. If none is identified, several months of antibiotic therapy may be required to eradicate the infection.

### Nephrolithiasis

Treatment is similar to that in patients without ADPKD. Potassium citrate is indicated for the three causes of stones associated with ADPKD: uric acid lithiasis, hypocitraturic calcium oxalate nephrolithiasis, and distal acidification defects. Extracorporeal shock wave lithotripsy and percutaneous nephrostolithotomy have been performed successfully without undue complications.

### End-Stage Kidney Disease

Patients with ADPKD do better on dialysis than patients with other causes of ESKD, perhaps because of higher levels of erythropoietin and hemoglobin or lower comorbidity.[309] Despite renal size and increased risk for hernias, peritoneal dialysis is usually possible.

Transplantation is the treatment of choice for ESKD in ADPKD. There is no difference in patient or graft survival between patients with ADPKD and other ESKD populations. Graft survival after living-donor transplants is also no different in patients with and without ADPKD. However, data are more limited for those with ADPKD, in whom living-related-donor transplantation was not widely practiced in the past. In 1999, for instance, 30% of kidney transplants for ADPKD patients were from living donors, compared with 12% in 1990.

Complications after transplantation are no greater in the ADPKD population than in the general population, and specific complications directly related to ADPKD are rare. Cyst infection is not increased after transplantation, and there is no significant increase in the incidence of symptomatic mitral valve prolapse or hepatic cyst infection. One study showed a higher rate of diverticulosis and bowel perforation in ADPKD. Whether ADPKD increases the risk for development of new-onset diabetes mellitus after transplantation is controversial.

Pretransplantation nephrectomy, commonly used in the past, has fallen out of favor. By 1 and 3 years following renal transplantation, kidney volumes decrease by 37.7% and 40.6%, and liver volumes increase by 8.6% and 21.4%, respectively.[310] Indications for nephrectomy include a history of infected cysts, frequent bleeding, severe hypertension, and massive renal enlargement with extension into the pelvis. There is no evidence for an increased risk for development of RCC in native ADPKD kidneys after transplantation. When nephrectomy is indicated, hand-assisted laparoscopic nephrectomy is associated with less intraoperative blood loss, less postoperative pain, and faster recovery than open nephrectomy and is increasingly being used.[303]

### Polycystic Liver Disease

PLD is usually asymptomatic and requires no treatment. When it is symptomatic, therapy is directed toward reducing cyst volume and hepatic size. Noninvasive measures include avoiding ethanol, other hepatotoxins, and possibly cAMP agonists (e.g., caffeine), which have been shown to stimulate cyst fluid secretion in vitro. Estrogens are likely to contribute to cyst growth, but the use of oral contraceptive agents and postmenopausal estrogen replacement therapy are contraindicated only if the liver is significantly enlarged and the risk for further hepatic cyst growth outweighs the benefits of estrogen therapy. Rarely, symptomatic PLD may require invasive measures to reduce cyst volume and hepatic size. Options include percutaneous cyst aspiration and sclerosis, laparoscopic fenestration, open surgical hepatic resection/cyst fenestration, selective hepatic artery embolization, and liver transplantation.[311,312] Cyst aspiration is the procedure of choice if symptoms are caused by one or a few dominant cysts or by cysts that are easily accessible to percutaneous intervention. To prevent the reaccumulation of cyst fluid, sclerosis with minocycline or 95% ethanol is often successful. Laparoscopic fenestration can be considered for large cysts that are more likely to recur after ethanol sclerosis or if several cysts are present that would require multiple percutaneous passes to be treated adequately. Partial hepatectomy with cyst fenestration is an option because PLD often spares a part of the liver with adequate preservation of hepatic parenchyma and liver function.[313] In cases in which no segments are spared, liver transplantation may be necessary.

When a hepatic cyst infection is suspected, any cyst with an unusual appearance by imaging should be aspirated for diagnostic purposes. The best management is percutaneous cyst drainage in combination with antibiotic therapy. Long-term oral antibiotic suppression or prophylaxis should be reserved for relapsing or recurrent cases. Antibiotics of choice are trimethoprim–sulfamethoxazole and the fluoroquinolones, which are effective against the typical infecting organisms and concentrate in the biliary tree and cysts.

### Intracranial Aneurysm

Widespread presymptomatic screening is not indicated because it yields mostly small aneurysms in the anterior circulation with a low risk of rupture. Indications for screening in patients with good life expectancy include a family history of aneurysm or subarachnoid hemorrhage, previous aneurysm rupture, preparation for major elective surgery, high-risk occupations (e.g., airline pilots), and patient anxiety despite adequate information.[272] MR angiography does not require intravenous contrast material. CT angiography is a satisfactory alternative when there is no contraindication to intravenous contrast agents.

When an asymptomatic aneurysm is found, the recommendation of whether to intervene depends on size, site, and morphology; prior history of subarachnoid hemorrhage from another aneurysm; patient age and general health; and whether the aneurysm is coilable or clippable. The prospective arm of the International Study of Unruptured Intracranial Aneurysms (ISUIA) provided invaluable information to assist in the decision.[314] The 5-year cumulative rupture rates for patients without a previous history of subarachnoid hemorrhage with aneurysms located in the internal carotid artery, anterior communicating or anterior cerebral artery, or middle cerebral artery were 0%, 2.6%, 14.5%, and 44.0% for aneurysms <7, 7 to 12, 13 to 24, and ≥25 mm, respectively, compared with rates of 2.5%, 14.5%, 18.4%, and 50%, respectively, for the same size categories involving the posterior circulation and posterior communicating artery. Among unruptured noncavernous segment aneurysms <7 mm in diameter, the rupture risks were higher among patients who had a previous subarachnoid hemorrhage from another aneurysm. As reported by the ISUIA, these risks also need to be balanced with those associated with surgical or endovascular surgery. The 1-year mortality and combined morbidity (Rankin score 3 to 5 or impaired cognitive status) and mortality rates were 2.7% and 12.6%, respectively, for open surgery and 3.4% and 9.8%, respectively, for endovascular repair.

The risk for development of new aneurysms or enlargement of an existing one in patients with ADPKD is very low in those with small (<7 mm) aneurysms detected by presymptomatic screening and moderate in those with a previous rupture from a different site.[315–317] On the basis of these and the ISUIA data, conservative management is usually recommended for patients with ADPKD who have small (<7 mm) aneurysms detected by presymptomatic screening, particularly in the anterior circulation. Semiannual or annual imaging studies of an aneurysm are appropriate initially, but reevaluation at less frequent intervals may be sufficient after the stability of the aneurysm has been documented. Elimination of tobacco use and aggressive treatment of hypertension and hyperlipidemia should be recommended.

The risk for development of a new aneurysm after an initial negative result is small, about 3% at 10 years in patients with a family history of IAs.[318] Therefore rescreening of patients with a family history of IAs after an interval of 5 to 10 years seems reasonable.

### Novel Therapies

A better understanding of the pathophysiology and the availability of animal models has facilitated the development of preclinical trials and identification of promising candidate drugs for clinical trials (http://www.clinicaltrials.gov).

**Vasopressin $V_2$ Receptor Antagonists.** The effect of vasopressin, via $V_2$ receptors, on cAMP levels in the collecting duct, the major site of cyst development in ADPKD, and the role of cAMP in cystogenesis provided the rationale for preclinical trials that showed effectiveness of $V_2R$ antagonists in animal models of ARPKD, ADPKD, and NPHP.[128,178,319] The initial studies with tolvaptan, conducted in small numbers of patients with ADPKD treated for 1–3 weeks, showed that split twice-daily doses were necessary for effective $V_2R$ inhibition (urine osmolality to <300 mOsm/kg continuously for 24 hours).[19] The aquaresis induced by daily split doses in patients with CKD stages 1–4 was accompanied by small reductions in GFR without significant changes in renal plasma or blood flow, likely due to activation of tubuloglomerular feedback.[320,321] These changes, which were rapidly reversible after discontinuation of tolvaptan, underlined the importance of using eGFR values either off treatment (baseline and after washout) or on treatment when comparing the effects of tolvaptan and placebo on the rate of eGFR decline.

The double-blind Tolvaptan Efficacy and Safety in Management of Autosomal Dominant Polycystic Kidney Disease and Its Outcomes (TEMPO) 3:4 trial randomly assigned 1445 patients to tolvaptan at the highest tolerated dose (45/15, 60/30, or 90/30 mg) or placebo.[322] Entry criteria were designed to enrich for patients with relatively preserved renal function and rapidly progressive disease (18–50 years, estimated creatinine clearance ≥ 60 mL/min, TKV ≥ 750 mL). TKV increased 2.8% per year in the tolvaptan group and 5.5% per year in the placebo group ($P < .001$). Tolvaptan significantly reduced the decline in eGFR from 10.1 to 6.8 mL/min/1.73 $m^2$ over 3 years, as well as the frequency of kidney pain and urine excretion of albumin and monocyte chemoattractant protein-1. The eGFR benefit at the end of TEMPO 3:4 was maintained for two additional years when all patients received tolvaptan in an open label extension (TEMPO 4:4).[323] With monitoring every 4 or 3 months in TEMPO 3:4 or TEMPO 4:4, transaminase elevations more than three times upper limit of normal (ULN) occurred in 4.4% of tolvaptan and 1% of placebo patients. A total of 3 of 1271 tolvaptan-treated patients met Hy's law criteria of hepatocellular toxicity. On the basis of the TEMPO 3:4 results, tolvaptan was approved for rapidly progressive ADPKD in Japan, Canada, the European Union, Switzerland, Norway, South Korea, and Australia. In the United States, the FDA did not approve tolvaptan and asked for additional data.

The double-blind Replicating Evidence of Preserved Renal Function: An Investigation of Tolvaptan Safety and Efficacy in later stage ADPKD (REPRISE) was designed as a randomized withdrawal trial to limit early discontinuations due to aquaretic side effects.[324] After an 8-week prerandomization, sequential placebo, and tolvaptan run-in phases, 1370 patients aged 18–55 years with eGFRs of 25–65 mL/min/1.73 m,[2] or 56–65 years with eGFRs of 25–44 mL/min/1.73 m,[2] able to tolerate 60/30-mg tolvaptan, were randomly assigned to tolvaptan or placebo for 12 months with monthly safety and serum creatinine measurements. Three additional measures of serum creatinine were obtained 7–40 days after discontinuation of tolvaptan or placebo. The eGFR change from baseline was −2.34 mL/min/1.73 $m^2$ in the tolvaptan and −3.61 mL/min/1.73 $m^2$ in the placebo group ($P< .001$). Transaminase elevations over three times ULN occurred in 5.6% of tolvaptan and 1.2% of placebo patients. No cases met Hy's law criteria, likely due to more frequent monitoring and earlier discontinuation of tolvaptan. Transaminase elevations were reversible after stopping tolvaptan. Following the results of this study, tolvaptan has now been approved for use in the US in adult ADPKD patients that are at risk of rapidly progressing disease.

**Somatostatin Analogs.** Binding of somatostatin to its receptors (somatostatin receptor 1; SSTR1 through SSTR5) inhibits AC and MAPK, cell proliferation, and secretion of several hormones (growth hormone, insulin, glucagon, gastrin, cholecystokinin, vasoactive intestinal peptide and secretin, thyroid-stimulating hormone, and adrenocorticotropic hormone) and growth factors (insulinlike growth factor 1 and VEGF).[325,326] All five SSTRs are expressed in renal tubular epithelial cells and cholangiocytes. Because somatostatin has a half-life of approximately 3 minutes, more stable synthetic peptides (octreotide, lanreotide, and pasireotide) have been developed for clinical use. They differ in stability and in affinity for the different SSTRs. Half-lives in the circulation are 2 hours for octreotide and lanreotide and 12 hours for pasireotide. Octreotide and lanreotide bind with high affinity to SSTR2 and SSTR3, with moderate affinity to SSTR5, and have no affinity to SSTR1 and SSTR4. Pasireotide binds with high affinity to SSTR1, SSTR2, SSTR3, and SSTR5. In preclinical studies, octreotide and pasireotide reduced cAMP levels and proliferation of cholangiocytes in vitro, expansion of liver cysts in three-dimensional collagen culture, and development of kidney and liver cysts and fibrosis in PCK rats and $Pkd2^{WS18/-}$ mice.[131,327] In agreement with the longer half-life and higher affinity to a broader range of SSTRs, the effects of pasireotide are more potent than those of octreotide. Pasireotide and tolvaptan have been shown to have an additive beneficial effect in the $Pkd1^{RC/RC}$ mouse model of ADPKD.[319]

Several small randomized, placebo-controlled studies of octreotide or lanreotide have been completed.[328–331] Most of these studies have been of short duration, but two of them have been extended as open-label, uncontrolled studies.[332,333] The ALADIN study randomly assigned 79 patients with ADPKD and eGFR values of ≥40 mL/min/1.73 $m^2$ to receive intramuscular injections of a long-acting form of octreotide or placebo and monitored them for 3 years.[334] The primary outcome variable, a mean increase in TKV at 3 years of follow-up, showed numerically smaller growth in the octreotide group than in the placebo group (220 vs. 454 mL). The difference, however, was not statistically significant. A favorable effect was noted on the secondary outcome of kidney function, but this endpoint also did not reach statistical significance. These findings provide support for larger randomized controlled trials to test the protective effect of somatostatin analogs, and an ongoing clinical trial involves 300 patients with ADPKD and CKD stages 3a and 3b.[335] Until the results of larger trials become available, somatostatin analogs should not be prescribed for renoprotection outside of a research study.

The somatostatin analogs have also shown a potential beneficial effect on the progression of PLD. Liver volume decreased by 4% to 6% during the first year of treatment, and this reduction was sustained during the second year. Young female patients appear to have the greatest benefit from this treatment.[336] The addition of everolimus to treatment with octreotide does not provide added benefit.

Octreotide and lanreotide are overall well tolerated. Self-resolving abdominal cramps and loose stools are common in the first few days following the injections. Other adverse effects include injection site granuloma and pain, cholelithiasis, steatorrhea, weight loss, and, rarely, hair loss. The adverse event profile of pasireotide in patients with ADPKD may include hyperglycemia because pasireotide inhibits insulin more potently than glucagon secretion, whereas the contrary is true for octreotide and pasireotide.[337]

**Rapalogs.** There is overwhelming evidence for enhanced mTOR complex 1 (mTORC1) signaling in PKD cystic tissues, and results of preclinical trials of mTOR-inhibiting rapalogs (sirolimus and everolimus) in rodent models were mostly encouraging. At doses and blood levels achievable in humans, sirolimus and everolimus were effective in a rat model of PKD affecting proximal tubules[338,339] but not in an ARPKD model affecting the distal nephron and collecting duct.[340] Mice tolerate much higher doses and blood levels than do rats and humans, and at these high levels rapalogs were consistently effective in orthologous and nonorthologous mouse models.[341,342] However, the results of clinical trials have been mostly discouraging,[343–345] likely because blood levels capable of inhibiting mTOR in peripheral blood mononuclear cells do not inhibit mTOR in the kidney.[346]

Several strategies may overcome the systemic toxicity and limited renal bioavailability of rapalogs. One is to target the drug specifically to the kidney by conjugating it to folate, and treatment of *bpk* mice was effective in reducing renal cyst growth and preserving kidney function without toxicity.[347] Another approach takes advantage of the mechanism of action of sirolimus, which forms a complex with the binding protein FKBP12 that competes with phosphatidic acid for binding to mTOR. Phosphatidic acid, a phospholipase D product generated by the hydrolysis of phosphatidylcholine, is required for the association of mTOR with component Raptor in mTORC1 and with component Rictor in mTORC2. One study showed that PKD cells have a slightly higher phospholipase D activity and that blockade of its activity by either specific inhibitors or "alcohol trap" treatment retrains mTORC1 and decreases cell viability and proliferation.[348] A third approach is the use of mTOR-catalytic inhibitors that cause a more potent and durable inhibition of mTORC1 than rapalogs, which are currently being tested in rodent PKD models.[349]

**Other Agents.** Many other drugs have been shown to be effective in preclinical trials and of potential value for the treatment of human PKD. Some act on tyrosine kinase receptors, downstream signaling pathways such as MAPK and Wnt/β-catenin signaling, effectors and inhibitors of cell cycling, or energy metabolism to inhibit cell proliferation.[163,164,350,351] Other potential therapies target fluid secretion (CFTR and KCa3.1 inhibitors) or important pathogenic interactions between epithelial cells and ECM and the interstitial inflammatory microenvironment. Of particular interest are drugs or interventions that have shown effectiveness in animal models and that can be used with relatively little toxicity, such as metformin, the thiazolidinediones, nicotinamide, and caloric restriction.[154,352–358]

#### Clinical Trials and Renal Function

In planning for clinical trials for ADPKD, the use of renal function as the primary outcome is an issue. This is because decades of normal renal function remain despite progressive enlargement and cystic transformation of the kidneys. By the time the GFR starts declining, the kidneys are markedly enlarged, distorted, and unlikely to benefit from treatment. Therefore early interventional trials would require unrealistic periods of follow-up if renal function were to be used as the primary outcome. The results of CRISP have shown that the rate of renal growth is a good predictor of functional decline and justify the use of TKV as a marker of disease progression in clinical trials for ADPKD.[194,245]

## AUTOSOMAL RECESSIVE POLYCYSTIC KIDNEY DISEASE

### EPIDEMIOLOGY

ARPKD is generally characterized by relatively rapid, symmetric, bilateral renal enlargement in infants due to collecting duct cysts in association with CHF.[359–361] Nonobstructive intrahepatic bile duct dilatation (Caroli disease) is variably seen. A minority of cases may occur in older children, teenagers, or young adults, usually with manifestations of portal hypertension or cholangitis. In rare cases, the presentation may be in older adults, mostly with complications of the liver disease but sometimes with renal manifestations such as proteinuria, nephrolithiasis, and renal insufficiency.[362,363] Prevalence and carrier frequencies are thought to be 1 in 20,000 and 1 in 70, respectively.[364] Molecular data indicate that ARPKD is likely to be found in all racial groups.[365,366]

### GENETICS

ARPKD is inherited as an autosomal recessive trait and therefore may occur in siblings but not in the parents. The disease is observed in one-fourth of the offspring of carrier parents. All cases of typical ARPKD are caused by mutations in a gene on chromosome 6p21.1-p12 (*PKHD1*).[367–369] Studies have shown that *PKHD1* mutations are also responsible for nonsyndromic CHF and Caroli disease.[362] Biallelic mutations to the ciliopathy gene *DZIP1L* have recently been associated with an ARPKD-like phenotype in humans.[370] Likewise, specific mutations to *PMM2* can result in an ARPKD-like phenotype (see the "Polycystic Kidney and/or Liver Diseases Associated With Altered Maturation of PKD Proteins in the Endoplasmic Reticulum" section).[371]

*PKHD1* is among the largest genes in the human genome, extending approximately 470 kb and including 67 exons.[372,373] Mutations are scattered throughout the gene without "hot spots."[365,366] Most have been described in just a single family, but some are more frequent in particular populations (e.g., p.R496X in Finland and c.9689delA in Spain).[374,375] One missense substitution, p.T36M, has been found on approximately 16% of mutant alleles and seems to be an ancestral mutation that arose in Europe more than a 1000 years ago.[376] There is evidence of genotype–phenotype correlations. The presence of two truncating mutations results in a lethal phenotype by the neonatal period. Surviving patients with severe or milder renal disease have at least one nontruncation mutation, indicating that many nontruncating mutations are hypomorphic.[374,375,377] Despite the importance of the germline mutations, affected sibling pairs may exhibit phenotypes of markedly discordant severity, most likely because of the effect of modifier genes.

### PATHOGENESIS

The ARPKD protein, fibrocystin (460 kDa), has a single-transmembrane pass, a large extracellular region containing IPT/TIG (immunoglobulin-like fold shared by plexins and transcription factors) and PbH1 (parallel beta-helix 1) repeats,

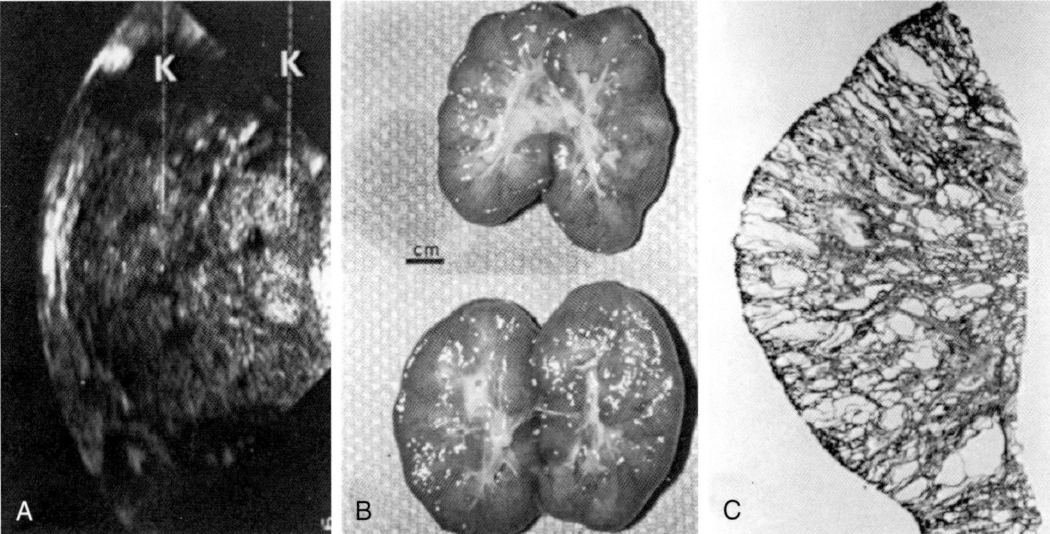


**Fig. 45.15** Autosomal recessive polycystic kidney disease in a 32-week-old fetus. (A) A sonogram showing cystic kidneys (K) of a fetus in utero. (B) Gross and (C) microscopic sections show radially oriented cysts of collecting ducts.

and an intracellular carboxyl tail.[372,373] Cleavage of the protein in the extracellular region at the proprotein convertase site is likely important to form a functional protein.[112,378] This possibility suggests that fibrocystin may be a cell surface receptor implicated in protein–protein interactions. Like the polycystins, fibrocystin is localized in primary cilia. Fibrocystin, PC2, and the kinesin-2 motor subunit KIF3B (kinesin family member 3B) have been suggested to form a protein complex in which KIF3B acts as a linker between fibrocystin and PC2.[379] However, more recent data do not place fibrocystin and PC2 in the same complex.[380] Normal kidney and liver in an animal model with the C-tail of the protein deleted also question whether signaling occurs through this part of the protein,[380] and highlights the secreted extracellular region that is found in urine alone and on exosomes. *PKHD1* has limited expression to the kidney, pancreas, and liver and the expression of fibrocystin in ureteric bud branches, intrahepatic and extrahepatic biliary ducts, and pancreatic ducts during embryogenesis is consistent with the histologic features of ARPKD.[381]

## PATHOLOGY

ARPKD affects both the kidneys and the liver in approximately inverse proportions. That is, the disease may be viewed as a spectrum ranging from severe renal damage and mild liver damage at one end to mild renal damage and severe liver damage at the other. The form with severe renal damage is the more common and is the form that manifests at or near the time of birth. The form with less severe renal damage and more severe liver damage is less common and usually manifests in infancy, childhood, or later.

Kidneys in the perinatal and neonatal forms of ARPKD are symmetrically and bilaterally enlarged up to more than 20 times normal (Fig. 45.15) and may be the cause of dystocia because of their size. Average combined weight of the kidneys in one series was about 300 g (range, 240 to 563 g), a normal combined weight being about 25 g. The renal enlargement is caused by fusiform dilation of collecting ducts to 1 to 2 mm in the cortex and medulla. Almost 100% of collecting ducts are affected in the most severe cases. Dilation of the collecting ducts occurs in the fetal period, and the glomeruli and more proximal tubular elements of the nephron appear normal. However, there is evidence in early human fetuses (14–24 weeks) that proximal tubule cysts occur, as in some rodent models of recessive PKD,[382–384] but these are no longer evident after 34 weeks of gestation.[385] The dilated collecting ducts are lined by typical cuboidal cells.[386,387] In many cases of neonatal ARPKD, an overall reduction in size may occur as the children age, and macroscopic cysts may develop. Renal calcifications are common in children with the disease.

In later presentations of ARPKD, mainly with complications of portal hypertension caused by CHF or episodes of cholangitis caused by Caroli disease, the renal involvement may be much less prominent, consisting of medullary ductal ectasia with minimal or no renal enlargement. The picture resembles and may be confused with medullary sponge kidney (MSK), a distinct disease with a far different prognosis (see later discussion).

The hepatic lesion is diffuse but limited to the portal areas. CHF is characterized by enlarged and fibrotic portal areas with apparent proliferation of bile ducts, absence of central bile ducts, hypoplasia of the portal vein branches, and sometimes prominent fibrosis around the central veins. Bulbar protrusions from the walls of dilated ducts also occur, and bridges sometimes form. This malformation has been found to occur occasionally as an isolated event (Caroli disease), but most often it is associated with ARPKD.

## DIAGNOSIS

The diagnosis is often made by sonography in utero or shortly after birth. The typical sonogram (Fig. 45.15) shows enlarged kidneys with increased echogenicity in the cortex and medulla, with poor definition of the collecting system and fuzzy delineation of the kidneys from surrounding tissues. Although the appearance of the kidneys on sonography, CT, and MRI may be very suggestive of ARPKD, a definite diagnosis based on renal imaging alone is not possible, particularly in utero and in the neonatal period, when the appearance of the

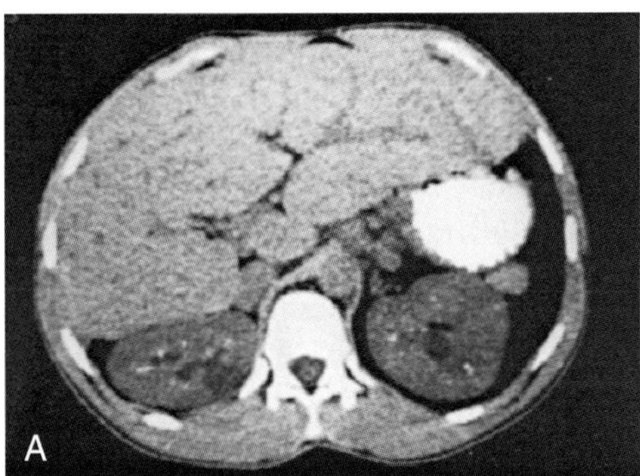


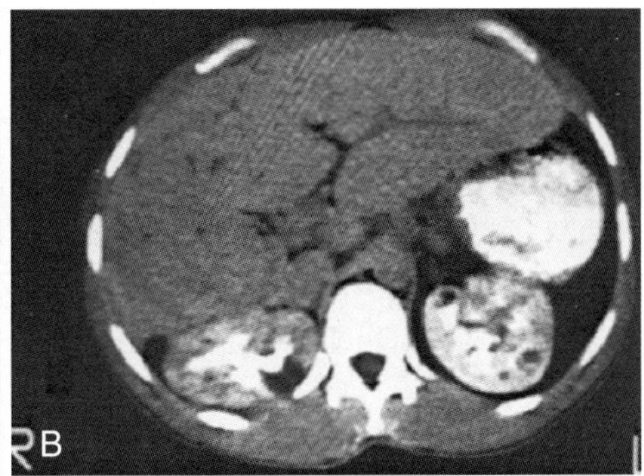


**Fig. 45.16** Computed tomography (CT) scan of autosomal recessive polycystic kidney disease in an 18-year-old man whose serum creatinine and liver function test results were within normal ranges. The patient had clinical evidence of portal hypertension (gastric varices and enlarged spleen). An oral contrast agent was given to highlight the intestines. (A) CT scan without contrast enhancement. The liver is enlarged but not cystic. The kidneys are slightly enlarged and contain focal radiodense areas (nephrolithiasis). (B) CT scan after intravenous administration of iodinated radiocontrast agent showing cystic areas in both kidneys. The renal calcifications are now obscured by contrast medium in the collecting systems.

kidney may be indistinguishable from ADPKD and other recessive renal cystic diseases. The family history, ultrasonographic or histologic evaluation of the liver for the presence of hepatic fibrosis, absence of extrarenal malformations associated with multiple malformation syndromes and renal dysplasia, and molecular analysis help in the diagnosis. Family history evaluation is complicated by the finding of increased kidney echogenicity and/or multiple small liver cysts in approximately 10% of *PKHD1* mutation carriers.[261,388]

Older children and adolescents may present with symptoms and signs related to the hepatic fibrosis and portal hypertension, including gastrointestinal bleeding from varices, hepatosplenomegaly, and hypersplenism, with or without associated renal manifestations such as a urinary concentrating defect, nephrolithiasis, hypertension, and renal insufficiency. Collecting duct ectasia and macrocystic changes may be observed in the kidneys of these patients (Fig. 45.16). Combined use of conventional and high-resolution ultrasonography with MR cholangiography in patients with ARPKD and CHF allows detailed definition of the extent of kidney and hepatobiliary manifestations without requiring ionizing radiation and contrast agents.[389]

Owing to the severity of disease in ARPKD, there is significant demand for prenatal and preimplantation diagnostics. This interest largely comes from couples with a previously affected pregnancy, detected either in utero (which may have resulted in termination) or with the birth of an affected child (who may have died in the neonatal period).[390] Preimplantation genetic diagnosis, which avoids the trauma of a termination of pregnancy in the case of an affected fetus, has been performed in only a few cases.[391] There is also demand for molecular diagnostics in older patients with less severe disease to differentiate ARPKD from other causes of childhood PKD. Molecular diagnostics is offered using mutation-based diagnostics by Sanger sequencing of the single gene, or now more commonly as a panel of PKD genes including also ciliopathy genes using an NGS approach.[249,392] Molecular diagnostics have the advantage that DNA from a previously affected family member is not required and that patients with an uncertain diagnosis can be tested. However, it is complicated by the marked allelic heterogeneity of *PKHD1* and prevalence of novel missense variants of uncertain significance (VUS). If two clearly pathogenic mutations are identified, the diagnosis is highly reliable. However, if only novel VUS are identified, careful bioinformatic and population evaluation is required, although simultaneous evaluation of other PKD/ciliopathy genes can improve the reliability of the molecular results.[249] In one study, a definitive prenatal diagnosis (presence or absence of two identified mutations) was feasible in 72% of the cases, and an improved risk assignment (presence or absence of one identified mutation) was possible in an additional 25% of the studied families.[365]

The phenotype of greatly enlarged and echogenic kidneys in neonates is not pathognomonic for ARPKD, and other cystic disorders should be considered. Rarely (<1% cases), ADPKD manifests in utero or in the neonatal period as clinical symptoms very similar to those of ARPKD.[70,249,393] In approximately 50% of these cases, an affected parent is recognized only after the diagnosis of a severely affected child.[394] In addition, rare de novo, early-onset ADPKD may occur. Most early-onset cases have been linked to *PKD1*, although two *PKD2* families with early-onset disease have been described.[72,395] CHF is not normally part of the ADPKD phenotype, but rare reports of an association have been described.

The high risk of recurrence of early-onset ADPKD in affected families suggested a common familial modifying background for early and severe disease expression (e.g., mutations or variants in genes encoding other cystoproteins).[70] Emerging family data suggested that in trans inheritance of a null and an incompletely penetrant *PKD1* allele could result in early-onset ADPKD with an ARPKD-like phenotype.[68,73,75,249,396] This hypothesis has been confirmed by a knockin mouse model mimicking the naturally occurring *PKD1* variant p.R3277C highlighted by later family studies.[68,73] Mirroring observation in the human studies, gradual cystic disease developed in $Pkd1^{RC/RC}$ animals over 1 year, whereas early-onset, rapidly progressive disease occurred in $Pkd1^{RC/null}$ mice.[10] Early-onset severe ADPKD has also been linked to contiguous deletion of *PKD1* and *TSC2*[397,398] as well as coinheritance of an ADPKD and an *HNF1B* or *PKHD1* allele.[76]

Glomerulocystic kidney disease can rarely manifest in the neonatal period with an ARPKD-like phenotype.[399] Rare families with ARPKD-like disease and skeletal and facial anomalies,[400,401] or recessively inherited renal and hepatic cystic diseases with hypoglycemia,[376,402] now identified as hyperinsulinemic hypoglycemia with PKD (HIPKD) due a specific *PMM2* promoter mutation, have been described.[371] Infantile NPHP and related disorders may also be confused with ARPKD. A number of syndromic congenital hepatorenal disorders (ciliopathies) including ones lethal in infancy can be associated with renal abnormalities resembling those in ARPKD and with CHF. These include Joubert syndrome (JBTS), Meckel syndrome (MKS), Elejalde (acrocephalopolysyndactyly), and Ivemark (renal–hepatic–pancreatic dysplasia) syndromes and glutaric aciduria type II. Mutations to *ANKS6* have also been shown to sometimes result in an ARPKD-like phenotype but usually also with cardiovascular abnormalities.[403] Biallelic mutations to *DZIP1L* result in an ARPKD-like phenotype.[370]

## MANIFESTATIONS

Children with ARPKD are typically identified in utero from the finding of enlarged, echogenic kidneys. In the most severe cases, poor urine output may result in oligohydramnios and the Potter sequence, characterized by typical facies, wrinkled skin, compression deformities of the limbs, and pulmonary hypoplasia. The presentation of ARPKD at birth may be dominated by respiratory difficulties from pulmonary hypoplasia or from restrictive disease caused by massive kidney enlargement. The need for neonatal ventilation predicts the development of CKD and death. Approximately 30% of affected neonates die shortly after birth.[404–407]

Most patients who survive the neonatal period live to adulthood. Hypertension, electrolyte abnormalities, and renal insufficiency are the major disease complications in surviving infants, with liver disease becoming more important in older patients. Hypertension developed in between 55% and 86% of patients reported in two studies, with blood pressure elevations often seen at birth or at diagnosis.[404,405] The ectopic expression of components of the RAAS in cystic-dilated tubules suggests that increased intrarenal angiotensin II production contributes to hypertension development.[408] However, the circulating plasma renin level is usually low,[406] and the intravascular volume expanded, particularly in patients with concomitant hyponatremia.[405] Increased sodium reabsorption in the ectatic collecting ducts may contribute to the hypertension,[409,410] but conflicting data have been reported.[411] The inability to concentrate and dilute urine can cause major electrolyte abnormalities. During the first year or two of life, renal function can improve, and renal size relative to body mass often decreases.[386,412,413] Renal function may remain stable for many years or may slowly progress to renal failure. The consequences of chronic renal insufficiency, growth failure, anemia, and osteodystrophy can become apparent during childhood. Because complications of liver disease become more important as ARPKD children age, careful examination for splenomegaly and blood counts for cytopenias should be regularly performed.

Adolescents and adults present most often with complications of portal hypertension (variceal esophageal bleeding, splenomegaly and hypersplenism with leukopenia, thrombocytopenia, or anemia).[362] Up to 50% of patients with CHF may exhibit segmental dilation of intrahepatic bile ducts (Caroli disease), sometimes with episodes of cholangitis or sepsis and complications of biliary sludge or lithiasis. Hepatocellular function is rarely deranged, and enzyme values are only occasionally mildly elevated. Increased bilirubin or enzyme values suggest the possibility of cholangitis. The kidneys in these patients may be normal or may exhibit various degrees of medullary collecting duct ectasia or macrocystic disease without marked renal enlargement.

Three reports have described cases of ARPKD with IAs.[414–416] It is not clear whether the prevalence of IAs is increased in ARPKD or whether these cases are coincidental findings.

Heterozygote carriers of *PKHD1* mutations have usually been considered to be entirely normal. However, an ultrasonographic study of 110 obligate carriers of ARPKD showed increased medullary echogenicity in 6 (5.5%), multiple small liver cysts in 10 (9.1%), a moderately increased liver echo pattern suggestive of CHF in 4 (3.6%), and mild splenomegaly in 9 (8.2%) patients.[417] A second study recently identified liver cysts in approximately 10% of *PKHD1* mutation carriers.[261]

## TREATMENT

Later studies suggest that the prognosis of ARPKD for children who survive the first month of life is far less bleak than was initially thought.[359,404–406] In patients with respiratory insufficiency, the cause (pulmonary hypoplasia, abdominal mass, pneumothorax, pneumomediastinum, atelectasis, pneumonia, heart failure) should be assessed fully, and artificial ventilation and aggressive resuscitative measures are indicated. Severely affected neonates may require unilateral or bilateral nephrectomies because of respiratory and nutritional compromise. An aggressive nutritional program and correction of acidosis and other electrolyte disorders are needed to optimize linear growth. The hypertension generally responds to salt restriction and antihypertensive drugs. Like patients with other renal cystic disorders, patients with ARPKD are susceptible to urinary tract infections, so urinary tract instrumentation is best avoided.

For infants with ESKD, peritoneal dialysis is preferable, but hemodialysis is also an option for children with renal failure. Kidney transplantation is limited by body size, but in experienced centers, it can be performed even in small children with a minimal weight of 7 kg.[418] Pretransplantation splenectomy may be indicated for patients with marked leukopenia or thrombocytopenia due to hypersplenism. These patients should receive pneumococcal vaccinations. Rejection rates and survival beyond 3 years for such patients are not different from those in patients with other renal diseases who undergo transplant surgery. Biliary sepsis is a frequent contributor to the mortality in patients with ARPKD who undergo transplant surgery.[419]

Surviving patients and those whose disease manifests during adolescence are likely to require portosystemic shunting to prevent life-threatening hemorrhages from esophageal varices. The renal disease may progress to renal failure years later even after successful shunting. Patients with associated nonobstructive intrahepatic biliary dilation (Caroli disease) may have recurrent episodes of cholangitis and may require antimicrobial therapy or segmental hepatic resection. Combined kidney and liver transplantation has been advocated for selected patients with ESKD who have significant bile duct dilation and episodes of cholangitis.[420–422]

## POLYCYSTIC KIDNEY AND/OR LIVER DISEASES ASSOCIATED WITH ALTERED MATURATION OF PKD PROTEINS IN THE ENDOPLASMIC RETICULUM

In the last few years, mutations in genes encoding proteins responsible for the glycosylation, quality control, or translocation across the endoplasmic reticulum membrane of membrane/secreted proteins have been associated with development of cysts in the kidneys and or liver, likely due to inefficient maturation and trafficking of the polycystins (Fig. 45.17). The disease associated with *PRKCSH* (encoding glucosidase II beta) and *SEC63* (a translocon complex protein) mutations majorly consist of PLD without renal cysts (ADPLD), although a few kidney cysts have been described in 28%–35% of cases, and renal involvement may have been underestimated.[423–425] Renal inactivation of *Prkcsh* or *Sec63* in mice induces a cystic phenotype that can be rescued by *Pkd1* overexpression.[426] More recently, mutations in *GANAB* (glucosidase II alpha), *ALG8* (alpha 1,3-glucosyltransferase), and *SEC61B* (a translocon complex protein) have been identified in patients with phenotypes compatible with ADPKD or ADPLD (Fig. 45.18).[52,261] Biallelic mutations, including at

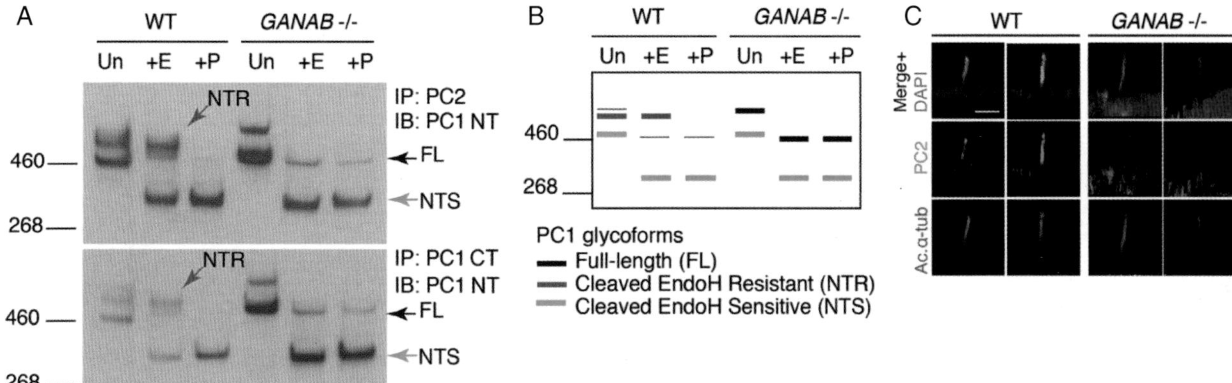


**Fig. 45.17** Mutation of the glucosidase II alpha gene, *GANAB*, leads to inefficient maturation and trafficking of polycystins. (A) Deglycosylation analysis of wild-type (WT) and *GANAB*$^{-/-}$ renal cortical tubular epithelial cell membrane protein treated with endoglycosidase H (endoH, +E), PNGase F (+P), or untreated (Un). Immunoprecipitation was used to enrich for the PC1 complex, using C-terminal PC1 (PC1 CT) or PC2 (YCE2) antibodies and immunodetected with the N-terminal PC1 (PC1 NT) antibody (7e12). Complete loss of the mature, N-terminal endoH-resistant PC1 glycoform (NTR; *red arrow*) was observed in *GANAB*$^{-/-}$ cells, with full-length PC1 (FL) and the immature, N-terminal endoH-sensitive PC1 glycoform (NTS; *green arrow*) becoming more abundant. (B) Schematic representation of the observed PC1 banding pattern in WT and *GANAB*$^{-/-}$ cells (A). (C) Confocal Z-stack rendering of primary cilia in confluent WT and *GANAB*$^{-/-}$ cells immunostained for acetylated α–tubulin (Ac. α–tub) and PC2, showing no cilia PC2 signal in *GANAB*$^{-/-}$ cells. *PC1,* Polycystin 1; *PC2,* polycystin 2. (Modified with permission from Porath B, Gainullin VG, Cornec-Le Gall E, et al. Mutations in GANAB, encoding the glucosidase iiα subunit, cause autosomal-dominant polycystic kidney and liver disease. *Am J Hum Genet.* 2016;98:1193–1207.)

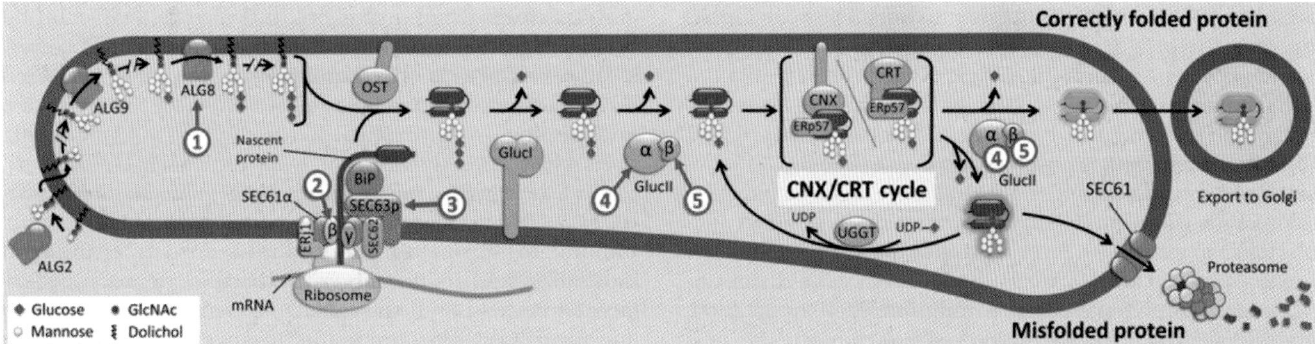


**Fig. 45.18** Schematic of the function of autosomal dominant polycystic kidney disease (ADPKD) and ADPLD genes in the endoplasmic reticulum (ER) protein biogenesis pathway. The genes are numbered 1–5. Lipid-linked oligosaccharide precursors of N-linked glycans are initially assembled on dolichol on the cytoplasmic aspect of the ER membrane. These are flipped into the ER lumen, where ALG8 (1) catalyzes the addition of the second glucose residue. Nascent polypeptides undergo cotranslational translocation via the SEC61 translocation pore that is composed of α-, β- (2), and γ-subunits and is associated with SEC62. SEC63 (3) and ERJ1 act in concert with the major ER HSP70 chaperone BiP to facilitate this translocation process. Oligosaccharyltransferase (OST) catalyzes the attachment of the glycan moiety to asparagine residues. Glucosidase I removes the outermost glucose before glucosidase II, composed of GIIα (4) and GIIβ (5) subunits, removes the second glucose. This step is necessary for the nascent peptide to enter the calnexin (CNX)/calreticulin (CRT) protein folding and quality control cycle. Glucosidase II (4, 5) subsequently removes the innermost glucose from the N-linked glycan, allowing for exit from the CNX/CRT cycle. If the protein has attained its properly folded conformation, it proceeds along the secretory pathway. Misfolded proteins are recognized and reglucosylated by UGGT, allowing for more time in the folding environment of the CNX/CRT cycle. Eventually, proteins that fail to fold properly undergo ER-associated degradation by retrotranslocation through the SEC61 translocon complex into the cytoplasmic compartment, where they are degraded by the proteasome. (Modified with permission from Besse W, Dong K, Choi J, et al. Isolated polycystic liver disease genes define effectors of polycystin-1 function. *J Clin Invest.* 2017;127(9):3558.)

least one specific in the promoter region of *PMM2* (encoding phosphomannomutase 2, a key enzyme in N-linked glycosylation), have been associated with polycystic kidneys, occasional liver cysts, and hyperinsulinic hypoglycemia[371] and HIPKD. Mutations in *DNAJB11* (a BiP cofactor, a key chaperone in the endoplasmic reticulum) have been identified in patients with nonenlarged polycystic kidneys with small renal cysts plus liver cysts in some cases leading to ESKD at advanced age.[53] Mutations in *SEC61A1* (a translocon complex protein) have been described in two families with ADTKD with anemia.[427]

## TUBEROUS SCLEROSIS COMPLEX

### EPIDEMIOLOGY

TSC is an autosomal dominant disease that affects up to 1 in 6000 individuals.

### GENETICS

It is caused by mutations in either *TSC1* or *TSC2*. *TSC1* is located on chromosome 9q34 and encodes for hamartin. *TSC2* is located on chromosome 16p13 and encodes for tuberin. The disease tends to be less severe in patients with *TSC1* mutations than in those with *TSC2* mutations.[428–430]

### PATHOGENESIS

Hamartin and tuberin physically interact, and this interaction is important for their function. The hamartin–tuberin complex antagonizes an insulin-signaling pathway that plays an important role in the regulation of cell size, cell number, and organ size.[431,432] In the absence of growth factor stimulation, tuberin–hamartin complexes maintain Rheb (Ras homolog enriched in the brain) in an inactive guanosine diphosphate–bound state by stimulating its intrinsic guanosine triphosphatase activity and inhibit downstream signaling from Rheb via mTOR. Growth factor stimulation of phosphoinositide 3-kinase signaling leads to Akt-dependent phosphorylation of tuberin, dissociation of the tuberin–hamartin complex, and activation of Rheb and mTOR. Tuberin or hamartin mutations prevent the formation of tuberin–hamartin complexes and lead to constitutive activation of mTOR.

### DIAGNOSIS

A definite clinical diagnosis of TSC requires one of the following conditions:

- Two major features from the following list: renal angiomyolipoma (AML), facial angiofibromas or forehead plaques, nontraumatic ungual or periungual fibroma, three or more hypomelanotic macules, shagreen patch, multiple retinal nodular hamartomas, cortical tuber, subependymal nodule, subependymal giant cell astrocytoma, cardiac rhabdomyoma, lymphangioleiomyomatosis
- One major feature from the previous list plus two minor features from the following list: multiple renal cysts, nonrenal hamartoma, hamartomatous rectal polyps, retinal achromic patch, cerebral white matter radial migration tracts, bone cysts, gingival fibromas, “confetti” skin lesions, multiple enamel pits

A diagnosis can also be made by the detection of a pathogenic variant in the *TSC1* or *TSC2* gene.

### MANIFESTATIONS

Renal involvement is second only to the involvement of the central nervous system (CNS) as a cause of death in patients with TSC. The main renal manifestations are AMLs (including rare epithelioid AMLs), cysts, oncocytomas, clear cell RCC, lymphangiomatous cysts, and (rarely) focal segmental glomerulosclerosis.[433–436]

AMLs are benign tumors consisting of abnormal blood vessels, smooth muscle, and fat cells. They are derived from perivascular epithelioid cells (PEComas) and exhibit immunoreactivity for both melanocytic markers (as detected by the antibodies HMB-45 and melan-A) and smooth muscle markers (actin and desmin). The diagnosis of renal AML relies on the demonstration of fat in the tumor by imaging studies. The fat appears hyperechogenic on ultrasonography, has a low attenuation value on CT, and on MRI appears bright on T1-weighted images, dark on T2-weighted images with fat saturation, and intermediate on T2-weighted images.[7,38,42,437] Approximately 5% of renal AMLs contain minimal amounts of fat and are called minimal-fat or fat-poor lesions. The differential diagnosis can be challenging and includes classic AMLs (predominantly composed of smooth muscle cells), epithelioid AMLs, RCC, and oncocytoma. When the distinction between minimal-fat renal AMLs and RCC cannot be reliably established by imaging techniques, imaging-guided percutaneous needle biopsy and staining for melanocyte markers should be considered as an alternative to surgical exploration.[438] The risk of bleeding after needle biopsy of a minimal-fat AML does not appear to be higher than that of a biopsy for other renal tumors, particularly when fine needles are used.

In patients with TSC, AMLs are extremely common, are usually multiple and bilateral, and affect both genders, in contrast to the general population, in which they are uncommon, usually single, and mainly found in middle-aged women. They develop after the first year of age, and by the third decade, 60% of patients with TSC have renal AMLs. The lesions express receptors for estrogen and progesterone, and women have more and larger AMLs than men. The early small lesions have a characteristic radial, striated, or wedge-shaped pattern with the base of the wedge facing the surface of the kidney. As the lesions increase in size, they penetrate deeper into the renal parenchyma or become exophytic, extending into the perirenal fat. The main manifestations relate to their potential for hemorrhage (hematuria, intratumoral, or retroperitoneal) and mass effect (abdominal or flank mass and tenderness, hypertension, or renal insufficiency). Because of the potential for renal AML development and growth, it is recommended that renal surveillance in patients with TSC be performed with ultrasonography at diagnosis and thereafter every 1 to 2 years (3 years in those in whom no AMLs are identified and at least yearly in patients with known AMLs).[439] In patients with known renal lesions, the serum creatinine concentration should be measured at least once a year.

The epithelioid AML variant is differentiated from the classic variant by the presence of an epithelioid cell component with abundant eosinophilic and granular cytoplasm.[440] There is no consensus on the percentage of epithelioid cells that is required to make a diagnosis of the epithelioid variant, with values ranging from 10% to 100% in published studies.[441,442]

In contrast to the uniformly benign prognosis of classic renal AMLs, as described in the preceding section, epithelioid variants infrequently undergo malignant transformation that manifests as local recurrence and/or distal metastases.

Unlike AMLs, renal cysts may be present in the first year of life, and cystic disease may be the presenting manifestation of TSC. *TSC2* and *PKD1* lie adjacent to each other in a tail-to-tail orientation at chromosome 16p13.3. Deletions inactivating both genes are associated with polycystic kidneys diagnosed during the first year of life or early childhood (*TSC2/PKD1* contiguous gene syndrome).[397,398] Therefore a contiguous gene syndrome should be considered in children with renal cysts and no family history of PKD. Rarely, *TSC2/PKD1* contiguous gene syndrome can be diagnosed in adults.[443] Patients with the contiguous gene syndrome usually reach ESKD at an earlier age than patients with ADPKD alone, but the disease severity in patients who have mosaicism is more variable.[398] Patients with *TSC1* or *TSC2* mutations without the contiguous gene syndrome also can have renal cysts. The renal cysts in TSC are often lined by a very distinct, perhaps unique, epithelium of markedly hypertrophic and hyperplastic cells with prominent eosinophilic cytoplasm. The combination of cystic kidneys and AMLs has been said to be virtually pathognomonic for TSC.

Oncocytomas—benign tumors derived from intercalated cells in the collecting ducts—and clear cell RCCs occur with increased frequency in TSC. RCCs in TSC have a female predominance and an earlier age of presentation as well as increased bilaterality. Early detection is essential. They should be suspected in cases of enlarging lesions without demonstrable fat and in the presence of intratumoral calcifications.

### TREATMENT

AMLs are benign lesions and often require no treatment. Because of their increased frequency and size in women and reports of hemorrhagic complications during pregnancy, patients with multiple AMLs should be cautioned about the potential risks of pregnancy and estrogen administration. Annual reevaluations with ultrasonography or CT are necessary to assess for growth and development of complications. Renal-sparing surgery is indicated for symptoms such as pain and hemorrhage, growth with compromise of functioning renal parenchyma, and inability to exclude an associated RCC. Because AMLs >4 cm are more likely to grow, develop microaneurysms and macroaneurysms, and cause symptoms, some writers suggest that prophylactic intervention should be considered in these cases. Some lesions, because of their size or central location, may be more amenable to selective arterial embolization. Radiofrequency ablation and cryoablation have also been successful in the treatment of renal AMLs <4 cm in diameter without bleeding complications.[444–446]

Elucidation of the TSC protein function at a molecular level and preclinical studies have identified mTOR as a target for intervention in TSC.[447,448] The efficacy of mTOR inhibitors has also been demonstrated in patients with TSC who have subependymal giant cell astrocytomas or pulmonary lymphangioleiomyomatosis. Multiple open-label, nonrandomized studies have shown that sirolimus produces a reduction in the volume of renal AMLs, mostly achieved in the first few months of treatment,[449–452] but the effect is not maintained after discontinuation of treatment. The best data on the efficacy of mTOR inhibitors come from the double-blind EXIST-2 study (Efficacy and safety of everolimus for subependymal giant cell astrocytomas associated with tuberous sclerosis complex or sporadic lymphangioleiomyomatosis), which included 118 patients, 18 years or older, who had a definite diagnosis of TSC ($n = 113$) or sporadic lymphangioleiomyomatosis ($n = 5$) and at least one renal AML ≥3 cm in its largest diameter. The patients were randomly assigned in a 2/1 ratio to everolimus 10 mg/day or placebo, and treated for a median duration of 38 or 34 weeks, respectively.[453] At the data cutoff, therapy had been discontinued in 20 patients, because of disease progression in 9 receiving placebo and because of adverse effects in 1 receiving everolimus and 4 receiving placebo. The primary endpoint, at least a 50% reduction in the total volume of all target AMLs identified at baseline, was achieved in 42% of the patients treated with everolimus and in none of the patients treated with placebo ($P < .001$). The median time to response to everolimus was 2.9 months. Progression of AMLs was significantly more common in the placebo group (21% vs. 4%). The response rate of skin lesions was significantly more common with everolimus (26% vs. 0%). The patients treated with everolimus had significantly higher rates of stomatitis (48% vs. 8%) and acnelike skin lesions (22% vs. 5%). On the basis of these findings, the FDA approved everolimus tablets for the treatment of adults with renal AMLs and TSC who do not require immediate surgery. At present, the place of everolimus or other mTOR inhibitors for the treatment of renal AMLs needs to be further defined. Benefits and risks need to be balanced, because the administration of mTOR inhibitors can be associated with significant adverse events, the reduction in renal AML volume is reversible after discontinuation of treatment, and long-term outcome results are not available.

Case reports have suggested efficacy of mTOR inhibitors in patients with unresectable or metastatic malignant epithelioid AMLs.

The main clinical problems associated with cystic disease in TSC are hypertension and renal failure. The treatment consists of strict control of hypertension. Bilateral nephrectomy should be considered before transplantation surgery because of the risk of life-threatening hemorrhage and the development of RCC.

## VON HIPPEL–LINDAU SYNDROME

### EPIDEMIOLOGY

VHL syndrome is a rare autosomal dominant disease with a prevalence of 1 in 36,000. It is characterized by retinal hemangiomas, clear cell RCCs, cerebellar and spinal hemangioblastomas, pheochromocytomas, and, less frequently, pancreatic cysts and neuroendocrine tumors, endolymphatic sac tumors of the inner ear, and epididymal cystadenomas.[454,455] Approximately 20% of patients with VHL syndrome have a de novo mutation: they do not have a family history of VHL syndrome.

### GENETICS

The VHL protein (pVHL) is encoded by a highly conserved tumor suppressor gene in chromosome 3p25-p26. Genotype–phenotype correlations in VHL syndrome have classified four VHL subtypes.[307] Patients with VHL type 1 have no pheochromocytomas. Mutations in patients with VHL type 1 are mostly loss-of-function type, leading to a truncated pVHL or no pVHL at all. Patients with complete germline deletions have a lower rate of RCC than patients with partial deletions (22.6% vs. 49%, respectively).[456] Mutations in patients with VHL type 2 are mostly missense mutations with some residual function. Whereas type 2 families have pheochromocytomas and are divided into subtypes with a low (type 2A) or high (type 2B) risk of RCC, type 2C families present with pheochromocytoma only. Dysregulation of VHL-dependent degradation of the α-subunit of hypoxia-inducible factor (HIF-α) is observed in subtypes 1, 2A, and 2B. By contrast, VHL-dependent HIF-α degradation is not observed in type 2C VHL mutants.

## PATHOGENESIS

*VHL* encodes two protein isoforms with relative molecular masses of approximately 30 and 19 kDa. Although these isoforms may have different functions, both are capable of suppressing RCC growth in vivo. However, the best-characterized function of pVHL is to act as an essential component in the degradation of HIF-α subunits. pVHL is the substrate-binding subunit of an E3 ubiquitin ligase that ubiquitinates HIF-α.[457] The HIF transcription factors consist of an oxygen-sensitive α-subunit and a constitutively expressed β-subunit, also known as the aryl hydrocarbon receptor nuclear translocator. There are three isoforms of the α-subunit (HIF-1α, HIF-2α, and HIF-3α) and one β-subunit (HIF-1β). In normoxic conditions, HIF-1α and HIF-2α are hydroxylated by prolyl hydroxylases, recognized by pVHL, and targeted for proteasomal degradation. In conditions of low oxygen tension, HIF-1α and HIF-2α are stable and bind to HIF-1β. HIF-α/HIF-β dimers are translocated to the nucleus, bind to R-C-G-T-G DNA sequences called "hypoxia response elements," and induce expression of numerous proteins, including proteins controlling angiogenesis (e.g., VEGF), erythropoiesis (e.g., erythropoietin), glucose uptake and metabolism (e.g., the Glut1 glucose transporter and various glycolytic enzymes), extracellular pH (e.g., carbonic anhydrases IX and XII), and mitogenesis [e.g., TGF-α and platelet-derived growth factor (PDGF)].[458]

Upregulation of HIF is not sufficient but is necessary to induce the RCC and CNS tumors associated with *VHL* mutations. A homozygous *VHL* missense mutation (p.R200W) causes Chuvash polycythemia. This condition is endemic to the Chuvash population of Russia, but it occurs worldwide.[459] VHL p.R200W homozygosity causes elevations of HIF, VEGF, erythropoietin, and hemoglobin; vertebral hemangiomas; varicose veins; low blood pressure; and premature mortality (42 years; range, 26 to 70 years) related to cerebral vascular events and peripheral thrombosis. The absence of RCCs, spinocerebellar hemangioblastomas, and pheochromocytomas typical of classic VHL syndrome, however, suggest that overexpression of HIF and VEGF is not sufficient for tumorigenesis. By contrast, HIF upregulation is required for the development of VHL-associated RCC, and short hairpin HIF RNAs suppress tumor formation by VHL-defective renal carcinoma cells.

The demonstration that HIF upregulation is not sufficient to induce RCC suggests that pVHL has other cellular functions in addition to controlling HIF levels.[460,461] These include its ability to regulate apoptosis and senescence as well as its role in the maintenance of primary cilia and orchestration of the deposition of ECM.

Loss of heterozygosity at the *VHL* locus in microscopic renal cysts from patients with inherited VHL syndrome established cyst formation as an early step in the pathogenesis of RCC.[462] Renal cysts and RCCs from patients with VHL syndrome show increased concentrations of both HIF-1α and HIF-2α. Renal cysts in patients with VHL syndrome and in renal clear cell carcinoma cell lines lacking pVHL have either no cilia or sparse, rudimentary cilia.[36,37,463] Importantly, ectopic expression of the VHL gene in renal clear cell carcinoma cell lines restores cilia formation, suggesting that pVHL directly supports ciliogenesis.

## DIAGNOSIS

The diagnosis of VHL syndrome should be made in a person with multiple CNS or retinal hemangioblastomas or a single hemangioblastoma plus one of the other characteristic physical abnormalities, or in families with a history of VHL syndrome. In some cases, the diagnosis may be warranted in a patient with a positive family history but without CNS or retinal lesions who has one or more of the less specific findings, with the exception of epididymal cysts, which are too nonspecific.

The molecular genetic diagnosis of VHL syndrome has greatly facilitated the evaluation and management of families whose members have the disease. Using a variety of techniques, the current detection rate of mutations is nearly 100%. Candidates for mutation analysis are patients with classic VHL syndrome (meeting clinical diagnostic criteria) and their first-degree family members and members of a family in which a germline *VHL* gene mutation has been identified (presymptomatic test). Genetic testing should also be considered for patients with findings suggestive but not diagnostic for VHL syndrome (i.e., multicentric tumors in one organ, bilateral tumors, two organ systems affected, one hemangioblastoma or pheochromocytoma in a patient younger than 50 years, or one RCC in a patient younger than 30 years) and for family members who have hemangioblastomas, RCCs, or pheochromocytomas only.

## MANIFESTATIONS

Renal cysts usually, but not always, precede the development of renal tumors. VHL syndrome–associated RCC manifests early in life, with a mean age at diagnosis of 35 years. The histology is uniformly clear cell. The cumulative probability of development of RCCs rises progressively beginning at age 20 years, reaching 70% by age 60 years. In contrast to RCCs in the general population, RCCs in individuals with VHL syndrome are more often multicentric and bilateral. Metastatic RCC is the leading cause of death from the syndrome.

## TREATMENT

Patients with VHL syndrome need annual physical and ophthalmologic examinations; annual measurements of blood or urinary catecholamines and metanephrines; yearly ultrasonography, MRI, or CT of the abdomen; and yearly or biannual MRI or CT of the head and upper spine.[464] PET or iodine 131 ($^{131}$I)-metaiodobenzylguanidine scanning may be indicated for further evaluation of biochemical or imaging abnormalities. Early detection of complications, especially RCC and CNS lesions, followed by appropriate treatment is essential to reduce mortality from VHL syndrome. Because it tends to be recurrent, bilateral, and multifocal, strategies have been developed to preserve renal parenchyma and minimize the number of invasive procedures. The National Cancer Institute developed the 3-cm rule for surgical intervention on the basis of absence of documented metastasis from tumors <3 cm. Renal-sparing surgery provides effective initial treatment, with 5- and 10-year cancer-specific survival rates similar to those obtained with radical nephrectomy. Minimally invasive techniques that include percutaneous or laparoscopically guided cryotherapy or radiofrequency ablation represent suitable treatment options for selected patients with VHL syndrome that have high technical success rates and cause minor changes in renal function.[465,466]

The demonstration that HIF is required for VHL-associated carcinogenesis provides a rationale for therapies targeting this transcription factor.[467,468] HIF can be downregulated by mTOR inhibitors, heat shock protein 90 inhibitors such as geldenamycin and 17-(allylamino)-17-demethoxygeldanamycin, histone deacetylase inhibitors, topoisomerase I inhibitors, thioredoxin-1 inhibitors, and microtubule disrupters. Two mTOR inhibitors, temsirolimus and everolimus, have shown efficacy in the treatment of sporadic RCC.[469] Treatments can be directed against HIF-responsive gene products, such as VEGF, or against receptors for VEGF, PDGF, or TGF-β. Sunitinib, a VEGF and PDGF tyrosine kinase inhibitor, is currently used in patients with VHL-associated advanced RCC, pancreatic neuroendocrine tumors, and malignant pheochromocytomas.[470]

## AUTOSOMAL DOMINANT TUBULOINTERSTITIAL KIDNEY DISEASE

ADTKD, previously called medullary cystic kidney disease (MCKD), is characterized by the pathologic appearance of the kidneys (small to normal size with cysts at the corticomedullary junction, irregular thickening of the tubular basement membrane, and marked tubular atrophy and interstitial fibrosis; see Fig. 45.19) and clinical manifestations (polydipsia and polyuria followed by development of renal insufficiency with low-grade proteinuria and a benign urine sediment) similar to those seen in NPHP (see later). The distinguishing features are the pattern of inheritance, distinct pathogenesis, later age at diagnosis and ESKD, and absence of extrarenal organ involvement except for gout.[471–473]

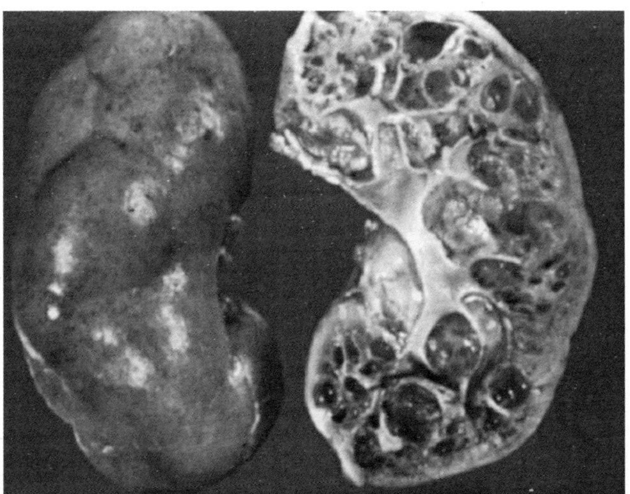

**Fig. 45.19** Outer and cut surface of kidney with severe medullary cystic disease.

ADTKD is caused by mutations in at least five genes[474,475]: *MUC1* encoding the mucoprotein mucin-1 (MUC-1; chromosomal location 1q22)[476]; *UMOD* encoding uromodulin, also known as Tamm–Horsfall protein (chromosome 16p12.3)[477,478]; *HNF1B* encoding HNF-1β (chromosome 17q12; see earlier); and *REN* encoding renin (chromosome 1q32.1). Recently mutations in two additional genes, *SEC61A* and *DNAJB11*, have been associated with a renal phenotype overlapping with other forms of ADTKD.[53,427] Intracellular accumulation of renin or uromodulin in renal tubules of renal biopsies of patients with *SEC61A* or *DNABJ11* mutations, respectively, suggests a role in the folding and trafficking of these proteins.

ADTKD-*MUC1* (or MCKD type 1) is caused by a heterozygous mutation in the variable-number tandem repeat (VNTR) region of *MUC1*.[476] The common mutation adds one cytosine to a tract of seven cytosine nucleotides, resulting in a frameshift mutation causing truncation of the VNTR and the creation of a new amino acid sequence on the terminal end of the MUC-1 protein. Other rare ADTKD-*MUC1*-associated frame-shifting mutations also result in the same novel amino acid region.[479] This new protein appears to be improperly processed in the cytoplasm, leading to apoptosis of tubular cells and slowly progressive tubular cell death and nephron dropout, resulting in CKD.[476] ADTKD-*MUC1* mutations are not readily detected by sequencing methods, including NGS panel analysis, with mass spectrometry of the abnormal VNTR most reliable for diagnostics.[480]

ADTKD-*UMOD* (or MCKD type 2) is caused by a heterozygous mutation, usually a missense mutation in exon 3, 4, 5, 6, 7, or 8, that adds or removes a cysteine residue.[481,482] The correct protein folding is disrupted, leading to intracellular accumulation of mutant uromodulin, retention in the endoplasmic reticulum, and increased apoptosis.[483,484] This gain-of-function process explains the fact that $Umod^{-/-}$ mice do not have an MCKD phenotype, although they are more susceptible to urinary tract infections and stone formation.[485–487] A consanguineous family with multiple heterozygous cases and three more severely affected but viable homozygous cases for the same mutation has been described.[488] The association of a *UMOD* mutation and glomerulocystic kidney disease has been described in one family.[489] Furthermore, single-nucleotide polymorphisms in *UMOD* have been associated with an increased risk of CKD.[490] Polydipsia, polyuria, and a tendency to waste sodium are common manifestations of the disease. ADTKD-*UMOD* is frequently but not always associated with hyperuricemia and gout at an early age. It is thought that the accumulation of abnormal uromodulin in the epithelial cells of the thick ascending limb of the loop of Henle prevents the proper function of ion channels, results in mild natriuresis, and increases proximal tubular reabsorption of urate. Hyperuricemia and gout also occur in ADTKD-*MUC1*, but usually at advanced stages of the disease. Patients with ADTKD-*MUC1* and ADTKD-*UMOD* reach ESKD at median ages of 62 and 32 years, respectively, with large patient-to-patient variability.

A diagnosis of ADTKD should be considered in patients with a family history of CKD, bland urinary sediment, and segregation suggesting autosomal dominant inheritance.[491] A history of gout at an early age or a strong family history of gout suggests *UMOD* mutations,[471] whereas a history of anemia in childhood and mildly elevated serum potassium concentrations implicates *REN* mutations.[492] NGS panel analysis including all the ADTKD genes is recommended for molecular diagnostic testing, with specific analysis for *MUC1* VNTR variants employed in genetically unresolved cases.[472,480]

The treatment of choice for ESKD secondary to ADTKD is kidney transplantation.[493] If a kidney from a living related donor is considered for transplantation, precautions should be taken to obtain it only from an older relative, who should be subjected to meticulous diagnostic evaluation.

## AUTOSOMAL DOMINANT TUBULOINTERSTITIAL KIDNEY DISEASE-HEPATOCYTE NUCLEAR FACTOR-1B–(ADTKD-*HNF1B*)

HNF-1β is a transcription factor encoded by the gene *HNF1B* (*TCF2*), which is expressed in polarized epithelia of the pancreas, liver, renal, and genital tracts. HNF-1β is expressed in the Wolffian duct, the developing mesonephros and metanephros, and the müllerian ducts from the earliest stages of differentiation. In adults, it is expressed in kidney tubules and collecting ducts, oviducts, uterus, epididymis, vas deferens, seminal vesicles, prostate, and testes. HNF-1β regulates the transcription of a number of genes involved in tubulogenesis, nephron maturation, and tubular transport, including genes mutated in PKD (*PKHD1* and *PKD2*) and another ADTKD gene (*UMOD*) and in autosomal dominant renal hypomagnesemia with hypocalciuria (*FXYD2*).[494]

Heterozygous mutations of *HNF1B* are responsible for a dominantly inherited disease with renal and extrarenal phenotypes, ADTKD-*HNF1B*.[495–497] As much as 30% to 50% of patients have de novo mutations, and whole-gene deletions occur in approximately 40% of the patients diagnosed in adulthood and in a higher percentage of the patients diagnosed in utero or infancy.[498–500] The disease is characterized by high phenotypic heterogeneity even within the same family.

The renal manifestations include structural and tubular transport abnormalities.[495,496,498] The structural abnormalities, often detected in utero, include bilateral hyperechogenic kidneys,[501] unilateral or bilateral agenesis or hypoplasia, multicystic dysplasia, abnormal calyces and papillae, and renal cysts. Histologic evaluation may reveal glomerular cysts and oligomeganephronia. Approximately 80% of congenital solitary kidneys are due to *HNF1B* mutations.

During childhood, the disease is characterized by defective kidney growth and impairment of renal function in approximately 50% of cases with evolution to ESKD in approximately 5% to 10%.[502]

The renal phenotype in adults is that of a chronic tubulointerstitial nephropathy with bland urinalysis, absence of hematuria, absence of or low-grade proteinuria, low prevalence of hypertension, and slowly progressive kidney failure (yearly eGFR decline of 2 to 2.5 mL/min/1.73 $m^2$). Renal cysts are present in 60% to 80% of the patients but usually are few in number, and unlike in ADPKD, the course of the cystic disease is not characterized by a progressive increase in the number of cysts or in kidney size.

Hypomagnesemia is present in approximately 50% of patients, likely because of the control of the expression of *FXYD2* by HNF-1β.[503] Hypokalemia is also present in 40% of adult patients but has not been observed in children; the underlying mechanism is uncertain. Hyperuricemia and gout have also been associated with the disease with variable frequency. Rarely a generalized dysfunction of proximal tubular function results in renal Fanconi syndrome. Chromophobe RCCs have been described in a few patients.

The extrarenal manifestations include maturity-onset diabetes of the young type 5 (MODY5), exocrine pancreatic failure, fluctuating liver test abnormalities, and genital tract abnormalities.[495,496,498] Pancreatic atrophy is found in approximately one-third and diabetes mellitus in approximately half of the patients. For reasons not understood, diabetic nephropathy is extremely rare in these patients. Liver function abnormalities, mainly fluctuating levels of serum alkaline phosphatase and γ-glutamyl transpeptidase, may occur in 40% to 80% of the patients, but liver biopsy findings are usually normal. The genital tract malformations may include absence of fallopian tubes or uterus, vaginal atresia, fusion abnormality such as bicornuate uterus or biseptate vagina, and male genital tract abnormalities. *HNF1B* mutations are found in approximately 18% of women with both renal and uterine malformations but not in patients with isolated uterine malformations. Cognitive defects, autistic features, and epilepsy have also been associated with *HNF1B* mutations.

Patients with ADTKD-*HNF1B* are good candidates for kidney transplantation, but they are at risk for early development of new-onset diabetes after transplantation. The immunosuppressive regimen should avoid tacrolimus and reduce corticosteroid dosage to minimize the risk of development of diabetes mellitus in nondiabetic transplant recipients.[504] In diabetic patients with ADTKD-*HNF1B* and ESKD, simultaneous pancreatic and kidney transplantation should be considered.

## FAMILIAL RENAL HAMARTOMAS ASSOCIATED WITH HYPERPARATHYROIDISM–JAW TUMOR SYNDROME

The autosomal dominant disease familial renal hamartomas associated with hyperparathyroidism–jaw tumor syndrome is characterized by primary hyperparathyroidism (parathyroid adenoma or carcinoma) and ossifying fibroma of the jaw. Kidney lesions may also occur as bilateral cysts, renal hamartomas, or Wilms tumors.[505] Renal cysts are a common finding, and in some cases they have been clinically diagnosed as PKD. The gene mutated in this disease (*HRPT2*) is ubiquitously expressed and evolutionarily conserved and encodes a protein of 531 amino acids (parafibromin) with moderate identity and similarity to a protein of *Saccharomyces cerevisiae* (cdc73p) that is important in transcriptional initiation and elongation.[506]

# AUTOSOMAL RECESSIVE CILIOPATHIES WITH INTERSTITIAL NEPHRITIS AND RENAL CYSTIC DISEASE

Autosomal recessive ciliopathies with interstitial nephritis and renal cystic disease are a large group of diseases caused by mutations in genes encoding ciliary or basal body proteins.[507,508] The primary cilium is a single hairlike organelle that projects from the surface of most mammalian cells, including epithelial and endothelial cells, neurons, fibroblasts, chondrocytes, and osteocytes.[509] It arises from the mother centriole, or basal body, in the centrosome. In addition to the basal body, the cilium comprises a transition zone, which regulates protein traffic in and out of the cilium, and the axoneme, which contains a ring of microtubule bundles

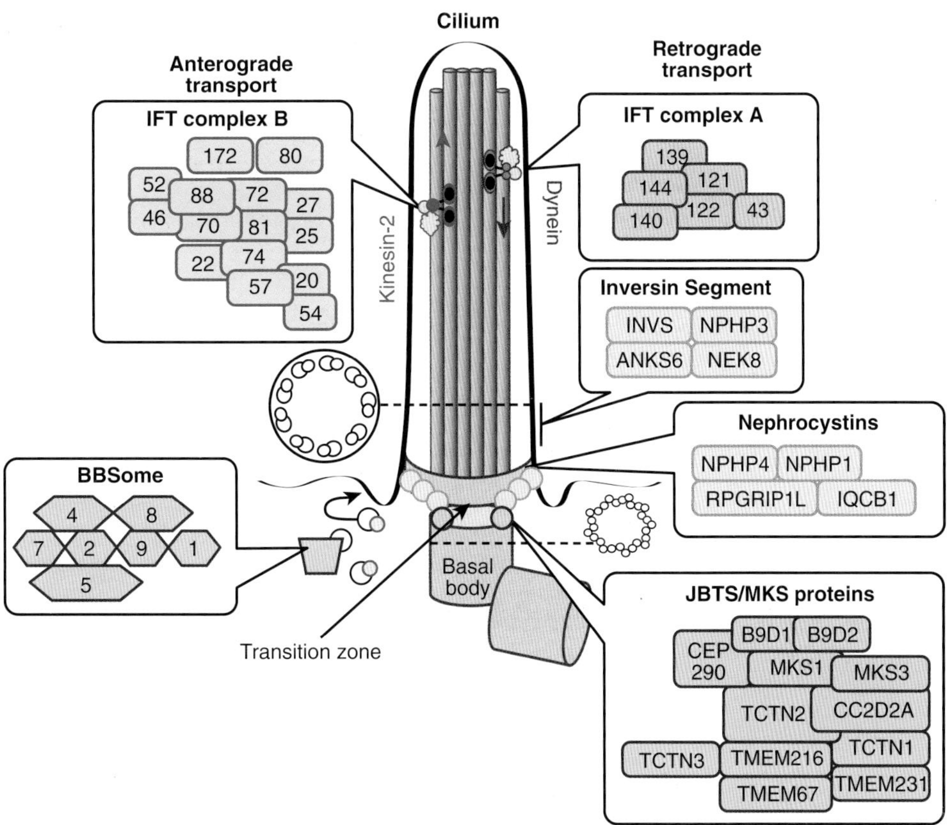


**Fig. 45.20** Structure of the primary cilium showing localization of groups of cilioproteins. Primary cilia are sensory organelles that have been implicated in the pathogenesis of polycystic kidney disease, and a large group of the proteins that cause ciliopathies have now been identified. Intraflagellar transport (IFT) moves proteins along the cilium and is involved in cilia formation. Two specific complexes of IFT proteins are involved in anterograde (IFT complex B; kinesin 2 motor) and retrograde (IFT complex A, dynein motor) movements within the cilium. (Numbers inside each complex signify specific IFT proteins). Many of the proteins involved in Meckel syndrome (MKS) and Joubert syndrome (JBTS), and some of the nephronophthisis (NPHP) proteins form a complex at the transition zone and are thought to regulate the protein composition of the cilium. Another group of proteins, including inversin (INVS), are localized to the proximal region of the ciliary axoneme (inversin segment), but their function is less clear. Many of the Bardet–Biedl syndrome (BBS) proteins form the BBSome and regulate trafficking of membrane proteins to the cilium. (Numbers inside BBSome signify various BBS proteins.) Mutations in these ciliopathy proteins alter the normal composition, sensory functions, and signaling of the cilium and are associated with the pleiotropic phenotypes typical of these diseases. *ANKS6,* Ankyrin repeat and SAM (sterile alpha motif) domain–containing protein 6; *B9D1/2,* B9 domain containing proteins 1/2; *CC2D2A,* coiled-coil and C2-domain containing 2A protein; *CEP290,* centrosomal protein of 290 kDa; *IQCB$_1$,* IQ motif containing B$_1$; *NEK8,* serine/threonine-protein kinase 8; *RPGRIP1L,* RPGR (retinitis pigmentosa guanosine triphosphatase regulator)–interacting protein 1–like protein; *TCTN,* tectonic family member; *TMEM,* transmembrane protein.

connecting the ciliary base to the tip (Fig. 45.20). There is a distinctive proximal segment of the ciliary axoneme known as the inversin compartment, but its function is uncertain. A specific process of IFT involving anterograde transport of cargo toward the tip of the cilium [using the kinesin II motor in association with the IFT complex B (IFT-B) proteins] and retrograde movement [employing the cytoplasmic dynein motor 2 in association with the IFT complex A (IFT-A) proteins] is required for ciliary formation and function.

Primary cilia are important for cell migration or fate determination and tissue patterning during development and for maintenance of cell differentiation thereafter.[509] The ciliopathies exhibit marked genetic heterogeneity and multiple organ involvement (pleiotropy). NPHP, JBTS, and MKS are autosomal recessive ciliopathies manifesting with cystic kidneys/interstitial nephritis, retinal degeneration, cerebellar/neural tube malformation, and hepatic fibrosis. The impact of the gene involved, the combination of mutations, and likely other genetic and nongenetic factors determine whether the resulting phenotype is mainly of a developmental (e.g., vermis aplasia, encephalocele, severe renal cystic disease) or degenerative (e.g., retinitis pigmentosa, interstitial nephritis, hepatic fibrosis) nature.[508] Mutations in the same gene can result in different phenotypes. For example, two *TMEM67* truncating mutations can cause MKS, but also JBTS and NPHP with liver fibrosis [COACH (*c*erebellar vermis hypoplasia/aplasia, *o*ligophrenia, *a*taxia, *c*oloboma, and *h*epatic fibrosis) syndrome]. In the case of the latter disorders, although there is a higher frequency of missense changes, a complete genotype–phenotype correlation has not been defined. Therefore NPHP, JBTS, and MKS can be considered to be allelic disorders.[510] There is also substantial phenotypic and some genetic overlap between these diseases and other disorders such as Bardet–Biedl syndrome (BBS) and Alström syndrome (ALMS). A remarkable feature of these ciliopathies is their large and overlapping genetic heterogeneity, with a total of 68 genes now implicated: NPHP (20), JBTS (34), MKS (13), BBS (21), and ALMS (1; see Table 45.2 for details).[511]

**Table 45.2 Genes Mutated in Autosomal Recessive Ciliopathies With Interstitial Nephritis, Cysts, or Both**

| Offical Gene Name | | Disease Designations | | | | | | |
|---|---|---|---|---|---|---|---|---|
| | **NPHP** | LCA | SLS | JBTS[a] | MKS | BBS | ALMS | OFDS |
| *NPHP1* | NPHP1 | | SLS1 | JBTS4 | | | | |
| *INVS* | NPHP2 | | | | | | | |
| *NPHP3* | NPHP3 | | | | MKS7 | | | |
| *NPHP4* | NPHP4 | | SLS4 | | | | | |
| *IQCB1* | NPHP5 | | SLS5 | | | | | |
| *CEP290* | NPHP6 | LCA10[b] | SLS6 | JBTS5 | MKS4 | BBS14 | | |
| *GLIS2* | NPHP7 | | | | | | | |
| *RPGRIP1L* | NPHP8 | | | JBTS7 | MKS5 | | | |
| *NEK8* | NPHP9 | | | | | | | |
| *SDCCAG8* | NPHP10 | | SLS7 | | | BBS16 | | |
| *TMEM67* | NPHP11 | | | JBTS6 | MKS3 | | | |
| *TTC21B* | NPHP12 | | | | | | | |
| *WDR19* | NPHP13 | | SLS8 | | | | | |
| *ZNF423* | NPHP14 | | | JBTS19 | | | | |
| *CEP164* | NEPH15 | | | | | | | |
| *ANKS6* | NPHP16 | | | | | | | |
| *IFT172* | NPHP17 | | | | | | | |
| *CEP83* | NPHP18 | | | | | | | |
| *DCDC2* | NPHP19 | | | | | | | |
| *MAPKBP1* | NPHP20 | | | | | | | |
| *INPP5E* | | | | JBTS1 | | | | |
| *TMEM216* | | | | JBTS2 | MKS2 | | | |
| *AHI1* | | | | JBTS3 | | | | |
| *ARL13B* | | | | JBTS8 | | | | |
| *CC2D2A* | | | | JBTS9 | MKS6 | | | |
| *OFD1* | | | | JBTS10 | | | | OFDSI |
| *KIF7* | | | | JBTS12 | | | | |
| *TCTN1* | | | | JBTS13 | | | | |
| *TMEM237* | | | | JBTS14 | | | | |
| *CEP41* | | | | JBTS15 | | | | |
| *TMEM138* | | | | JBTS16 | | | | |
| *CPLANE1* | | | | JBTS17 | | | | OFDSVI |
| *TCTN3* | | | | JBTS18 | | | | OFDSIV |
| *TMEM231* | | | | JBTS20 | MKS11 | | | |
| *CSPP1* | | | | JBTS21 | | | | |
| *PDE6D* | | | | JBTS22 | | | | |
| *KIAA0586* | | | | JBTS23 | | | | |
| *TCTN2* | | | | JBTS24 | MKS8 | | | |
| *CEP104* | | | | JBTS25 | | | | |
| *KIAA0556* | | | | JBTS26 | | | | |
| *B9D1* | | | | JBTS27 | MKS9 | | | |
| *MKS1* | | | | JBTS28 | MKS1 | BBS13 | | |
| *TMEM107* | | | | JBTS29 | MKS13 | | | OFDSXVI |
| *ARMC9* | | | | JBTS30 | | | | |
| *CEP120* | | | | JBTS31 | | | | |
| *SUFU* | | | | JBTS32 | | | | |
| *PIBF1* | | | | JBTS33 | | | | |
| *B9D2* | | | | JBTS34 | MKS10 | | | |
| *KIF14* | | | | | MKS12 | | | |
| *BBS1* | | | | | | BBS1 | | |
| *BBS2* | | | | | | BBS2 | | |
| *ARL6* | | | | | | BBS3 | | |
| *BBS4* | | | | | | BBS4 | | |
| *BBS5* | | | | | | BBS5 | | |
| *MKKS* | | | | | | BBS6 | | |
| *BBS7* | | | | | | BBS7 | | |
| *TTC8* | | | | | | BBS8 | | |
| *PTHB1* | | | | | | BBS9 | | |

**Table 45.2 Genes Mutated in Autosomal Recessive Ciliopathies With Interstitial Nephritis, Cysts, or Both (Cont'd)**

| Offical Gene Name | NPHP | Disease Designations LCA | SLS | JBTS[a] | MKS | BBS | ALMS | OFDS |
|---|---|---|---|---|---|---|---|---|
| *BBS10* | | | | | | BBS10 | | |
| *TRIM32* | | | | | | BBS11 | | |
| *BBS12* | | | | | | BBS12 | | |
| *WDPCP* | | | | | | BBS15 | | |
| *LZTFL1* | | | | | | BBS17 | | |
| *BBIP1* | | | | | | BBS18 | | |
| *IFT27* | | | | | | BBS19 | | |
| *IFT74* | | | | | | BBS20 | | |
| *C8ORF37* | | | | | | BBS21 | | |
| *ALMS1* | | | | | | | ALMS1 | |

[a]Includes CORS (cerebellooculorenal syndrome) and COACH (cerebellar vermis hypoplasia/aplasia, oligophrenia, ataxia, coloboma, and hepatic fibrosis) syndrome.
[b]Hypomorphic mutations.
*ALMS,* Alström syndrome; *BBS,* Bardet–Biedl syndrome; *JBTS,* Joubert syndrome; *LCA,* Leber congenital amaurosis; *MKS,* Meckel syndrome; *NPHP,* nephronophthisis; *OFDS,* oral-facial-digital syndrome; *SLS,* Senior-Løken syndrome.

Proteomics and assays of ciliogenesis and epithelial morphogenesis have suggested that the NPHP/JBTS/MKS proteins are organized into a network of functionally connected modules.[512,513] The role of these complexes seems to be to regulate protein trafficking into the cilium. In most cases, mutation leads not to ciliary loss but to an impaired functionality of the cilium. The NPHP1, NPHP4, and RPGRIP1L module localizes to the ciliary transition zone and to cell–cell contacts. It is not essential for ciliogenesis, but it is important for the organization of specialized structures at the apical surface of polarized cells and for epithelial morphogenesis. The IQCB1 and CEP290 module is localized to centrosomes and transition fibers and is indispensable for ciliogenesis in terminal inner medullary collecting duct (IMCD3) cells and for tissue organization. The module consisting of MKS proteins is localized to the transition zone and functionally connected to hedgehog signal transduction. Inversin (INVS), NPHP3, and NEK8 interact in the inversin compartment but their function is unknown. The NPHP–JBTS–MKS network does not overlap with the module integrated by the proteins mutated in BBS (BBSome),[514] despite significant phenotypic overlap, nor with the components of the IFT-A or IFT-B complex proteins despite the fact that defects in IFT may lead to cystic kidney disease and retinal degeneration.

The convergence of proteins mutated in these related ciliopathies at cilia and centrosomes is starting to reveal the pathogenesis of these diseases, which are likely associated with abnormal regulation of protein entry into cilia.[515] Multiple signaling pathways require cilia for proper functioning and have been implicated in ciliopathies, including Wnt and sonic hedgehog signaling.[508] The pleiotropic features seen in ciliopathies are likely a combination of defects of cilia sensor/mechanosensory functions and cilia-associated signaling that are disrupted by an abnormal cilia-gating process. The observation that proteins that cause NPHP and related ciliopathies when mutated exhibit dual localization at centrosomes and at nuclear foci and play a role in DNA damage response has led to the hypothesis that defects in DNA damage response participate in the pathogenesis of these diseases.[516]

## NEPHRONOPHTHISIS

NPHP is an autosomal recessive disorder with an estimated prevalence of 1 in 50,000 live births. It accounts for approximately 5% of ESKD in North American children.[517] It is genetically heterogeneous, with 20 genes identified (see Table 45.2).[518–524] Homozygous deletions in *NPHP1* account for approximately 21% of all cases of NPHP; the other genes contribute <3% each. No mutations in any of the known genes are found in approximately 60% of patients, indicating that many other genes remain to be discovered.[525] Recently, homozygous entire deletion of *NPHP1* has been found in 0.5% of adults with ESKD.[526]

Mutations in *INVS* and less frequently *NPHP3* lead to renal failure between birth and age 3 years (infantile NPHP). Mutations in the other genes, including *NPHP3,* cause renal failure in the first 3 decades of life (juvenile NPHP).[520] Severe retinitis pigmentosa (Senior-Løken syndrome) is frequently associated with *IQCB1, CEP290,* and *RPGRIP1L* mutations, but it is less severe and more rarely associated with mutations in other *NPHP* genes. Oculomotor apraxia (Cogan syndrome) is occasionally observed with *NPHP1* and *NPHP4* mutations. *CEP290* and *RPGRIPL1* mutations are frequently associated with cerebellar aplasia or hypoplasia and mental retardation (overlap with JBTS; see later). *INVS* and, more rarely, *NPHP3* mutations can be associated with situs inversus, cardiac ventricular septal defect, hepatic fibrosis, and retinitis pigmentosa. Hypomorphic mutations of *TMEM67* cause NPHP associated with hepatic fibrosis.

The nephrocystins form a multifunctional complex localized in primary cilia, centrosomes, and actin- and microtubule-based structures involved in cell–cell and cell–matrix adhesion signaling as well as in cell division.[519,521,522,524,527–529] In the kidney, these functional roles could be particularly important for establishing and maintaining the differentiated state of tubular epithelial cells. Localization of nephrocystins to the cilia explains the association with renal cystic disease and hepatic fibrosis (primary cilia in tubular epithelial cells and cholangiocytes; see earlier discussions of ADPKD and ARPKD), retinitis pigmentosa (rods and cones are modified cilia), and situs inversus and ventricular septal defect (primary cilia in the embryonic node are essential for left–right axis determination).

In the juvenile form, the kidneys are small with a granular capsular surface. On cut sections, the cortex and medulla are thinned, and the corticomedullary margin is indistinct with a variable number of small, thin-walled cysts of distal convoluted and collecting tubule origin. Similar cysts may also be present in the medulla. Grossly visible cysts are often absent. The tubular basement membranes are thickened, even fairly early in the course of the disease, and tubule segments of a single nephron may be encompassed by very dense sclerotic interstitium with sparse chronic inflammatory cell infiltrates. In the infantile form, the kidneys are often enlarged and cystic, and thickening of the tubular basement membranes is less prominent.

Excretory urography and ultrasonography frequently fail to detect cysts because they are small.[530] Excretory urography may show inhomogeneous streaking in the medulla caused by accumulation of contrast material in the collecting ducts. Contrast-enhanced CT and MRI are more sensitive to detect small corticomedullary and medullary cysts, but failure to detect cysts does not exclude the diagnosis.

The onset of the disease is insidious. Polyuria and polydipsia are the presenting symptoms. Hypertension is common in the infantile form, but whether absent or present, it is not a prominent feature in the juvenile form. Sodium wasting is common. The urine sediment is characteristically benign. Proteinuria is absent or low grade and there is no microhematuria. Progression to ESKD occurs within the first 3 years in the infantile form and within the first 2 to 3 decades in the juvenile form.

The treatment of NPHP is supportive. Because of the tendency for sodium wasting, volume contraction, and renal azotemia, unnecessary sodium restriction or use of diuretics should be avoided. If kidneys from siblings are considered for transplant surgery, precautions should be taken to obtain them only from unaffected, older relatives, who should be subjected to meticulous diagnostic evaluation.[531]

## JOUBERT SYNDROME

JBTS is an autosomal recessive neurologic disease characterized by cerebellar vermis aplasia or hypoplasia with abnormal superior cerebellar peduncles (the "molar tooth sign"), mental retardation, hypotonia, an irregular breathing pattern, and eye movement abnormalities.[532] In addition to these core features, patients may exhibit retinal defects (ranging in severity from Leber congenital amaurosis to slowly progressive retinopathies with partially preserved vision), renal defects (NPHP or cystic dysplastic kidneys), and CHF. Rarer features include chorioretinal or optic nerve colobomas, congenital heart malformations, situs inversus, severe scoliosis, skeletal dysplasia, Hirschsprung disease, and midline oral and facial defects, such as cleft lip, cleft palate, or both, notched upper lip, lobulated tongue with multiple frenula, and lingual or oral soft tumors. The association of JBTS with polydactyly and midline orofacial defects defines the so-called oro-facial-digital type VI syndrome. A distinct subgroup of JBTS defined by *c*erebellar vermis hypoplasia/aplasia, *o*ligophrenia, congenital *a*taxia, *c*oloboma, and *h*epatic fibrosis is known by the acronym COACH, which is usually associated with *TMEM67, CC2D2A,* or *RPGRIP1L* mutations. Gentile syndrome applies to patients who present with JBTS and CHF in the absence of other clinical features.

Like NPHP and MKS, JBTS exhibits marked genetic heterogeneity. The genetic bases of JBTS are extremely complex and only partly understood, despite the tremendous acceleration in gene discovery enabled by NGS techniques. So far, 34 causative genes have been identified, with autosomal or X-linked recessive inheritance (see Table 45.2).[532]

## MECKEL SYNDROME

MKS is characterized by bilateral renal cystic dysplasia or PKD, CNS defects (typically occipital encephalocele, but can include the Dandy–Walker malformation or hydrocephalus), postaxial polydactyly, and biliary dysgenesis/CHF. It is a lethal disorder, and most affected infants are stillborn or die within few hours or days after birth.

MKS is genetically heterogeneous with 13 genes so far identified (see Table 45.2).[533–537] The MKS proteins have been localized to the centrosome, the pericentriolar region, or the cilium itself, and their function is likely involved in forming the barrier between the cell and the cilium at the transition zone.[515]

## BARDET–BIEDL SYNDROME

BBS is characterized by retinitis pigmentosa, obesity, postaxial polydactyly, learning disabilities, hypogenitalism, and renal abnormalities. Four of these six cardinal features are required for the diagnosis. Other manifestations are diabetes, hypertension, congenital heart disease, ataxia, spasticity, deafness, hepatic fibrosis, and Hirschsprung disease. The manifestations may appear after several years of development.[538] Although rare (1 in 120,000 live births), its prevalence in certain geographically isolated communities, such as the Canadian province of Newfoundland and in Kuwait, is more common (1 in 13,500 to 1 in 17,500).[390]

BBS is genetically heterogeneous, with 21 known BBS genes accounting for approximately 80% of patients clinically diagnosed with the syndrome.[538–541] The majority of pathogenic mutations are found in *BBS1* and *BBS10,* accounting for 23.2% and 20%, respectively. The disease is primarily inherited in an autosomal recessive manner but with some evidence of a more complex, oligogenic form of inheritance (triallelism and digenic).[542,543] The localization of the BBS proteins at a subcellular level points to a role in the function of the cilium–centrosome axis. BBS4, BBS6, and BBS8 interact with the pericentriolar material protein 1, a protein important for centriolar duplication. BBS6, BBS10, and BBS12 are chaperonelike proteins. BBS proteins 1, 2, 4, 5, 7, 8, and 9 constitute the BBSome, implicated in vesicular transport toward the cilium. BBS7 and BBS8 play a role in IFT and BBS11 is an ubiquitin ligase.[514,544]

The diagnosis of BBS is often missed in childhood and made only later in life. Targeted fetal sonography in the second trimester of pregnancy to detect digital and renal abnormalities has been proposed for the prenatal diagnosis of the disease. The prenatal appearance of enlarged hyperechoic kidneys without corticomedullary differentiation should prompt the diagnosis in a family with BBS, especially when polydactyly is present.[545,546] In nonaffected families, BBS should be included in the differential diagnosis whenever such an appearance is discovered in utero. The postnatal evolution of the renal ultrasonographic findings is variable, and normalization generally occurs by the age of 2 years.

Renal abnormalities are very common in BBS.[547] Calyceal clubbing, diverticula, or cysts can be detected in up to 96% of cases. The most common and earliest functional abnormality is a reduced ability to concentrate the urine, resulting in polyuria and polydipsia. Hypertension develops in approximately 50% of patients, and chronic renal insufficiency in 25% to 50%. Despite mental retardation, obesity, and severe visual problems, patients tolerate hemodialysis well. Renal transplantation can be performed, but special attention must be given to controlling hyperphagia and obesity.

## ALSTRÖM SYNDROME

ALMS is an autosomal recessive disease that has some phenotypic overlap with BBS. It is characterized by obesity, type 2 diabetes mellitus, retinitis pigmentosa, nerve deafness, CHF, cardiomyopathy, chronic respiratory tract infections, and, frequently, slowly progressive chronic tubulointerstitial nephropathy.[548,549] The ALMS protein (ALMS1) is of unknown function, is widely expressed in human and mouse tissues, and localizes to centrosomes and the base of cilia.

## NEPHRONOPHTHISIS VARIANTS ASSOCIATED WITH SKELETAL DEFECTS (SKELETAL CILIOPATHIES)

Short-rib thoracic dysplasia (SRTD) with or without polydactyly refers to a group of autosomal recessive skeletal ciliopathies that are characterized by a constricted thoracic cage, short ribs, shortened tubular bones, and a "trident" appearance of the acetabular roof. SRTD encompasses Ellis–van Creveld syndrome (EVC) and the disorders previously designated as Jeune syndrome or asphyxiating thoracic dystrophy, short-rib-polydactyly syndrome, and Mainzer–Saldino syndrome. The disease is genetically heterogeneous, with 20 causative genes identified.[550,551] Some patients have an NPHP-like renal disease, and there is genic overlap between SRTD and JBTS and NPHP (such as *WDR19, CEP120,* and *KIAA0586*). Cranioectodermal dysplasia, also known as Sensenbrenner syndrome, is characterized by skeletal abnormalities (e.g., craniosynostosis, narrow rib cage, short limbs, brachydactyly), ectodermal defects, NPHP leading to progressive renal failure, hepatic fibrosis, heart defects, and retinitis pigmentosa. Four genes have been identified with overlap with SRTD and NPHP. Other syndromic forms of NPHP with skeletal disorders include EVC (short stature, short ribs, postaxial polydactyly, nail dystrophy, oral and cardiac defects), with *EVC* and *EVC2* as causative genes, and RHYNS syndrome (*r*etinitis pigmentosa, *h*ypopituitarism, *n*ephronophthisis, and *s*keletal dysplasia).

Whereas proteins associated with NPHP, JBTS, and MKS mainly function at the ciliary transition zone, most proteins associated with skeletal ciliopathies have been shown to participate in IFT. Ciliary proteins found to be defective in skeletal disorders currently encompass the following four main subgroups: 1. IFT-A subunits and its motor protein, DYNC2H1, whose defects disrupt retrograde transport and cause IFT protein accumulation at the ciliary tip; 2. IFT80 and IFT172, 2 of 14 subunits of IFT-B; 3. NEK1, a serine–threonine kinase involved in cell-cycle control and ciliogenesis; and 4. EVC- and EVC2-positive regulators of sonic hedgehog signaling located at the basal body.[552–562]

## ORO-FACIAL-DIGITAL SYNDROME TYPE 1

Oro-facial-digital syndrome type 1 is a rare X-linked dominant disorder with prenatal lethality in boys.[563] Affected girls may have kidneys indistinguishable from those in ADPKD. The diagnosis is suggested by the extrarenal manifestations, which may include oral (hyperplastic frenula, cleft tongue, cleft palate or lip, malposed teeth), facial (broad nasal root with hypoplasia of nasal alae and malar bone), and digital (brachydactyly, syndactyly, clinodactyly, camptodactyly, polydactyly) anomalies. Some patients have structural CNS anomalies such as agenesis of the corpus callosum, cerebellar agenesis, or the Dandy–Walker malformation. Renal cystic disease is present in 60% of cases after 18 years of age.[564] These individuals may also have liver and pancreatic cysts.[565] Mental retardation and tremor can be present in up to 50% of patients. The *OFD1* gene is located in chromosome Xp22.[566] A combination of Sanger sequencing and gene dosage methods, to detect deletions, yield an 85% mutation detection rate, although inclusion in an NGS panel of ciliopathy genes is now generally used for diagnostics.[567] Most mutations are private. The 120-kDa OFD1 protein contains an N-terminal LisH motif, which is important in microtubule dynamics. This protein is a core component of the human centrosome throughout the cell cycle.[568] Most reported *OFD1* mutations are predicted to cause protein truncation with loss of coiled-coil domains necessary for centrosomal localization. A novel X-linked mental retardation syndrome associated with recurrent respiratory tract infections and macrocephaly caused by ciliary dyskinesia, but no renal phenotype, has been associated with an *OFD1* mutation.[569]

# RENAL CYSTIC DYSPLASIA

Renal cystic dysplasia results from an interference with a normal ampullary activity that leads to abnormal metanephric differentiation. When the inhibition of the ampullary activity occurs very early, few collecting ducts are formed and few nephrons develop. The kidney becomes a cluster of cysts with little or no residual parenchyma, and the ureter is absent or atretic. These kidneys may be normal sized, larger than normal [multicystic dysplastic kidney (MCDK)], or markedly shrunken (hypodysplastic kidney). These variations probably represent different stages of the same pathologic process because renal cysts can involute and disappear completely during intrauterine life. When the interference with the ampullary activity occurs later (e.g., as the result of urethral or ureteral obstruction), there may be mild irregularities in branching with a mild generalized dilation of the collecting tubules in the medulla. Most nephrons, however, except the

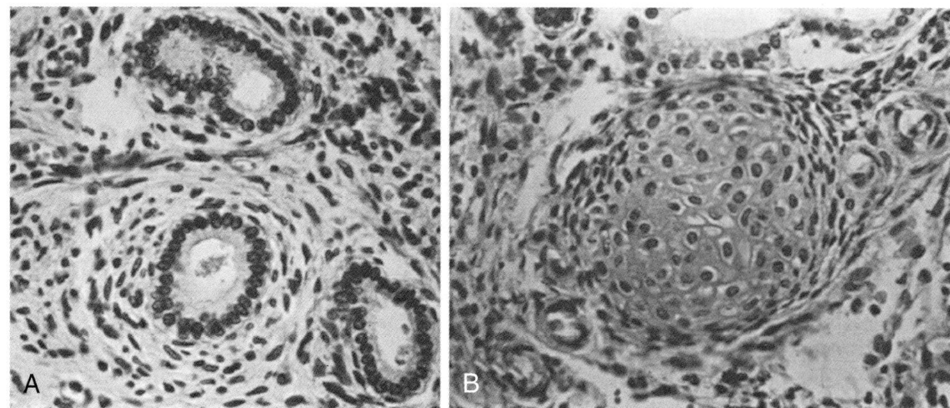


**Fig. 45.21** Renal dysplasia. The diagnostic microscopic features include (A) primitive ducts and (B) metaplastic cartilage.

last to be formed, are normal. The cysts are found under the capsule and generally derive from Bowman's spaces (glomerular cysts), the loop of Henle, or terminal ends of collecting tubules. A variety of renal abnormalities in the contralateral kidney can be found in association with cystic dysplastic kidneys. These include renal agenesis, ectopy or fusion, and ureteral duplication or obstruction that may result from injury to the ureteric bud during various stages of development. When the injury to the ureteric bud occurs before a communication with the metanephric blastema has been established, secondary atrophy of the metanephric blastema and renal agenesis ensue. By contrast, if the injury of the bud or ureteral obstruction occurs after renal development is completed, dysplasia does not occur. Thus a spectrum of renal abnormalities ranging from agenesis and severe dysplasia to mild cystic dysplasia with glomerular cysts and a variety of related renal and ureteral abnormalities may result from interferences with normal ampullary activity and metanephric differentiation.

Renal cystic dysplasia may be the consequence of an intrinsic (malformation) or extrinsic (disruption) defect in organogenesis. An intrinsic defect may be caused by a single gene mutation, a chromosomal aberration, or a combination of genetic and environmental factors (multifactorial determination). Extrinsic causes include teratogenic chemicals, metabolic abnormalities, and infections. Evidence for intrinsic or extrinsic defects should be sought by careful review of the pregnancy, family history, and physical examination (pattern of associated abnormalities) as well as by the study of the karyotype. Renal cystic dysplasia frequently occurs as a sporadic event, but they can also occur in the context of many multiorgan malformation syndromes, several of which have defined genetic bases, with these disorders now grouped under the category of congenital anomalies of the kidneys and urinary tract.[570,571]

Although most dysplastic kidneys are grossly deformed in a fairly characteristic way, most writers accept only two absolute criteria for dysplasia, both of which require histologic confirmation (Fig. 45.21). Of greater importance is the finding of primitive ducts encompassed by mantles of variably differentiated mesenchyma and lined by cuboidal to columnar, sometimes ciliated, epithelium unlike that in any normally developing or mature ducts. Somewhat less important, because of its variable presence, is the finding of metaplastic cartilage (see Fig. 45.21). Cysts of glomerular,

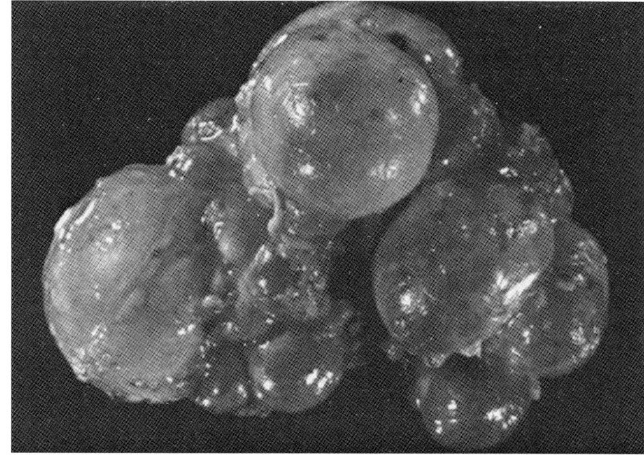

**Fig. 45.22** Severe renal cystic dysplasia (multicystic kidney). The renal architecture is markedly distorted.

tubule, and ductal origin may also be present, but because they might represent either a maldevelopment or a histologically similar degenerative change in previously normal but immature structures, they do not provide absolute evidence of parenchymal maldevelopment.

## MULTICYSTIC DYSPLASTIC KIDNEY

MCDK is the most common cause of an abdominal mass in infancy and the most common type of bilateral cystic disease in newborns (Fig. 45.22). With the widespread use of fetal sonography, MCDK is now most often diagnosed in utero, usually during the third trimester. MCDK is more often unilateral than bilateral, and boys are more frequently affected than girls. Because affected kidneys tend to involute over weeks or months prenatally and postnatally, the prevalence of unilateral MCDK is higher on fetal screening (1 in 2000) than on neonatal screening (1 in 4000).

Differentiation of MCDK from hydronephrosis in fetuses and newborns is essential because the therapeutic approaches to these conditions differ. The most useful sonographic criteria for identifying an MCDK include the presence of interphases between cysts, a nonmedial location of the larger cysts, absence of an identifiable renal sinus in 100% of the cases, and the absence of parenchymal tissue. The diagnosis can be confirmed by retrograde pyelography, which shows an absence or atresia of proximal ureter, and by angiography, which demonstrates absence or hypoplasia of the renal artery. Cyst walls often calcify in older patients and may appear as ringlike densities in the region of the kidney.

The manifestations of MCDK depend on whether it is bilateral or unilateral. Bilateral MCDK results in oligohydramnios and the Potter sequence and is incompatible with life. Unilateral MCDK may be diagnosed in a newborn during an evaluation of a renal mass or may go unnoticed until later in life, during evaluation for abdominal or flank discomfort caused by the mass effect of the lesion.[572] Serial ultrasonography shows that 33% of the MCDKs have completely involuted at 2 years of age, 47% at 5 years, and 59% at 10 years. The development of hypertension or malignant degeneration is very rare.[573] Because of its low risk and tendency to involute, MCDK in children is usually managed conservatively.[574] When indicated, laparoscopic nephrectomy is preferable to open nephrectomy. Attention should be paid to an increased risk for associated urinary tract malformations of the contralateral kidney (e.g., pelviureteric junction obstruction and vesicoureteric reflux), but voiding cystography is indicated only when the ultrasonographic findings in the contralateral kidney or ureter are abnormal.[575]

# OTHER CYSTIC KIDNEY DISORDERS

## SIMPLE CYSTS

### PREVALENCE

Simple cysts are the most common cystic abnormality encountered in human kidneys.[576] They may be solitary or multiple and are filled with a fluid that is chemically similar to an ultrafiltrate of plasma. The cysts are very rare in children, but the frequency increases with age.[577] In autopsy studies and as incidental CT findings, they are found in approximately 25% and 50% in patients 40 and 50 years of age, respectively. A more sensitive CT angiographic study of 1948 potential kidney donors (42% men; mean age, 43 years) showed that 39%, 22%, 7.9%, and 1.6% of 19- to 49-year-old individuals and 63%, 43%, 22%, and 7.8% of 50- to 75-year-old individuals had at least one cortical or medullary cyst at least 2, 5, 10, and 20 mm in diameter, respectively. The 97.5th percentile for the number of cortical and medullary cysts ≥5 mm increased with age (1 cyst in men and 1 in women 18–29 years old, 2 in men and 2 in women 30–39 years old, 3 in men and 2 in women 40–49 years old, 5 in men and 3 in women 50–59 years old, and 10 in men and 4 in women 60–69 years old).[578]

### PATHOGENESIS

Simple renal cysts are acquired, although there is now evidence that genic and allelic forms of ADPKD associated with mild disease can be mistaken for simple cysts.[249,579] Several hypotheses have been proposed to explain their pathogenesis. Tubular obstruction and ischemia might play a role. Microdissection studies revealed that diverticula of distal convoluted and collecting tubules are common after age 20 years and increase in number with age. Cysts are thought to derive from progressive dilation and detachment of these diverticula. The cyst walls also appear to be relatively impermeable to low-molecular-weight solutes and to antibiotics. Nonetheless, the turnover of cyst fluid may be as great as 20 times per day, as measured by tritiated water diffusion. Another study has shown a positive association between the plasma levels of copeptin, a surrogate for vasopressin, and the presence of renal cysts, suggesting the possibility that vasopressin may favor the development of simple renal cysts.[580]

### PATHOLOGY

Simple renal cysts are usually lined by a single layer of epithelial cells and filled with a clear, serous fluid. They grow slowly, but huge cysts, up to 30 cm in diameter, have been described. The inner surface of these cysts is glistening and usually smooth, but some cysts may be trabeculated by partial septa that divide the cavity into broadly interconnecting locules. These septated simple cysts should not be confused with multilocular cysts. The cysts are often cortical and distort the renal contour, but they may be deep cortical or apparently medullary in origin. They do not communicate with the renal pelvis. The walls typically are thin and transparent but may become thickened, fibrotic, and even calcified, possibly from earlier hemorrhage or infection.

### DIAGNOSIS

Most simple cysts are found on routine imaging studies (Fig. 45.23). Differentiation of simple cysts from RCC is a common problem. Because the appearance of a renal mass on the excretory urogram alone never excludes a malignancy, ultrasonography, CT, or MRI is commonly required to characterize the lesion. Acceptance of definite criteria for the diagnosis of a simple cyst by these imaging techniques has eliminated the use of renal angiography and percutaneous cyst aspiration to characterize renal masses. Calcium deposits are found in 2% of simple cysts and 10% of RCCs. Whereas calcifications appear to be peripheral in simple cysts, they are more central in tumors. Improvements in imaging techniques have also reduced the indications for surgery in the management of patients with benign simple cysts. When the cysts are numerous and bilateral, differentiation from ADPKD may be difficult if liver cysts are not also found. Because of the obvious implications, it is important to avoid a diagnosis of ADPKD in questionable cases unless a familial history consistent with autosomal dominant transmission can be documented or the diagnosis can be confirmed by genetic testing.

### MANIFESTATIONS

The cysts are usually asymptomatic, being discovered at the time of a nephro-urologic evaluation for some unrelated problem. They should not distract from the diagnosis of more important intrarenal or extrarenal lesions. Large renal cysts may cause abdominal or flank discomfort, often described as a sensation of weight or a dull ache. Frequently, however, this pain can be explained by a coexisting abnormality such as nephrolithiasis. Rare cases of gross hematuria due to vascular erosion by an enlarging cyst have been documented. However, hematuria is usually attributable to another cause. When the simple cysts lie at or near the hilus, a urographic pattern of calyceal obstruction or hydronephrosis is frequently found. In most but not all cases, these apparent obstructive changes are of no functional significance. A dynamic hippuran/diethylenetriaminepentaacetic acid radioactive renal scan before and after administration of

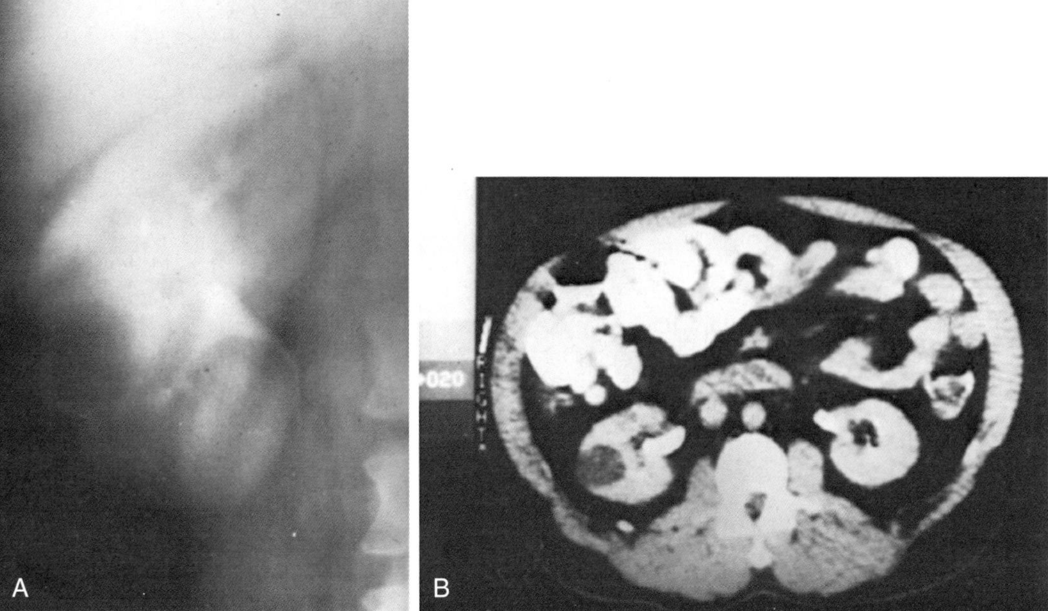


**Fig. 45.23** Simple renal cysts. (A) Solitary cortical cyst of the right kidney seen on intravenous urography. (B) Solitary cyst of right renal cortex seen on computed tomography with intravenous contrast enhancement. Oral contrast material was given to highlight the intestine.

furosemide can help assess the degree of obstruction. Rare cases of renin-dependent hypertension caused by solitary intrarenal simple cysts have been described. The proposed mechanism is arterial compression by the cyst that causes segmental renal ischemia. Infection is a rare but dramatic complication of a renal cyst. Simple cysts are not thought to impair renal function, but the presence of simple cysts has been associated with reduced renal function in hospitalized patients younger than 60 years of age.[581] A CT angiographic study of 1948 potential kidney donors showed an association of cortical and medullary cysts 5 mm or larger with higher 24-hour urine albumin excretion as well as with increased body surface area, hypertension, and higher GFR in some analyses, after adjustment for patient age and sex.[578] Renal cysts are common, particularly in older men, and may be a marker of early kidney injury because they associate with albuminuria, hypertension, and hyperfiltration. Simple cysts infrequently become infected; affected patients present with high fever, flank pain and tenderness, and, frequently, a sympathetic pleural effusion. Most patients are women, and the most common pathogen is *Escherichia coli*. Urine culture results can be negative. Carcinomas do not arise from benign simple cysts. For asymptomatic patients with unequivocal simple cysts, periodic follow-up with ultrasonography is reasonable.

### TREATMENT

Treatment of simple renal cyst is indicated only if it is symptomatic or causing obstruction. Intermediate-sized cysts can be aspirated percutaneously, and a sclerosing agent can be instilled into the cavity in an attempt to prevent recurrence. Cysts more than 500 mL in volume are usually drained surgically. Laparoscopic methods are now used routinely. Hypertension has sometimes disappeared after successful aspiration of the cyst fluid or surgical removal of the cyst. Renal vein plasma renin activity is usually elevated in such cases, and the mechanism is thought to be compression of adjacent vessels by cysts with selective renal ischemia and increased renin production. A surgical approach is usually taken to infected renal cysts, but percutaneous aspiration and drainage of infected cysts have also been used.

## LOCALIZED OR UNILATERAL RENAL CYSTIC DISEASE

Localized or unilateral renal cystic disease is a rare condition that involves part or, more rarely, the whole of one kidney with cysts that are indistinguishable from those in ADPKD.[582] The absence of a family history and the fact that the remaining renal tissue and the liver appear intact help differentiate this condition from asymmetric forms of ADPKD, although mosaicism of an ADPKD mutation is a possible cause. Its etiology and pathogenesis are not understood. The clinical presentation includes a palpable mass, flank pain, gross or microscopic hematuria, and hypertension with well-preserved renal function.

## MEDULLARY SPONGE KIDNEY

### EPIDEMIOLOGY

MSK, or precalyceal canalicular ectasia, is a common disorder characterized by tubular dilation of the collecting ducts and cyst formation strictly confined to the medullary pyramids, especially to their inner, papillary portions.[583] In studies using strict criteria for the quality of acceptable intravenous urograms, the incidence of MSK has been about 13% in patients with calcium urolithiasis but only about 2% in otherwise normal patients. In particular, MSK is associated with a 60% lifetime risk for renal stones, and the prevalence of MSK in patients with renal stones is significantly higher (8.5%; $P <$ .01) than in the control population[584] (1.5%). Among all patients with calcium stones, women have a greater incidence of MSK than men.

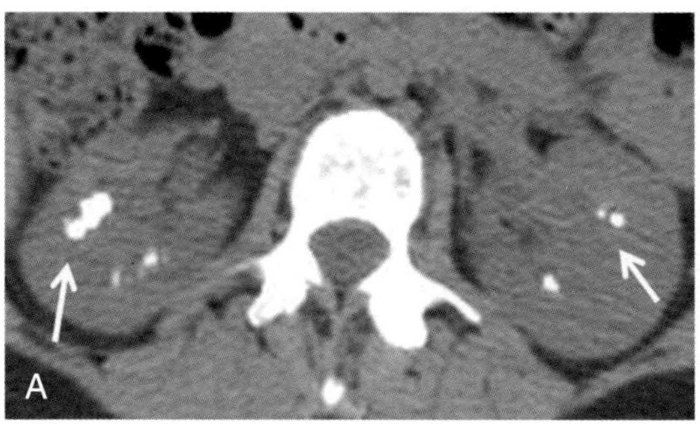


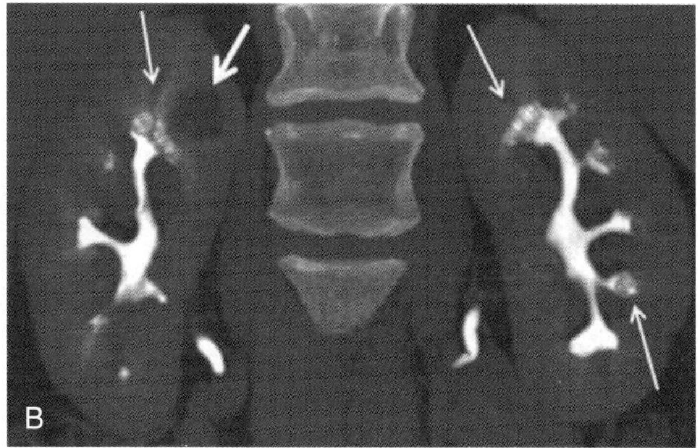


**Fig. 45.24** Medullary sponge kidney diagnosed by computed tomography (CT) scan. (A) Noncontrast axial image at the level of the kidneys demonstrates medullary calcinosis *(arrows)*. (B) Coronal maximum intensity projection during the excretory phase of contrast-enhanced CT urography shows a medullary cyst *(thick arrow)* and dilated collecting tubules showing a papillary brush pattern in both kidneys *(thin arrows)*. (Reprinted with permission from Koraishy FM, Ngo TT, Israel GM, Dahl NK. CT urography for the diagnosis of medullary sponge kidney. *Am J Nephrol.* 2014;39:165–170.)

## PATHOGENESIS

MSK has been usually regarded as a nonhereditary disease, but autosomal dominant inheritance has been suggested in several families. In five MSK families, *GDNF* (glial cell–derived neurotrophic factor) gene variants were found to cosegregate with the disease.[585] A study of family members of 50 patients with MSK identified 59 first- and second-degree relatives of 27 probands in all generations who also had MSK.[586] There were progressively lower values for urine volume, pH, and excretion of sodium and calcium, and progressively higher levels of serum phosphate noted in probands compared with relatives with bilateral MSK, those with unilateral MSK, and those unaffected by MSK. The investigators interpreted these observations as indicative of a milder form of MSK in the affected relatives. These findings suggest that familial clustering of MSK is common and that the disease has an autosomal dominant inheritance, reduced penetrance, and variable expressivity.

There have been several reports of MSK in patients with Ehlers–Danlos syndrome and in patients with hemihypertrophy. Precalyceal canalicular ectasia can be observed frequently in patients with ADPKD. MSK has been associated with primary hyperparathyroidism. The rarity of reported cases of this disorder among children favors the interpretation that this is an acquired rather than a congenital disease. Progression of the tubular ectasia and development of tubule dilation and medullary cysts have been documented in some patients.

## PATHOLOGY

Despite the name of this disorder, the affected kidney does not closely resemble a sponge. It is usually normal in size or slightly enlarged. The precalyceal canalicular ectasia may involve one or more renal papillae in one or both kidneys, and the lesions are bilateral in 70% of cases. The dilated ducts communicate proximally with collecting tubules of normal size and often show a relative constriction to approximately normal diameter at the point of their communication with the calyx. Their diameter is often 1 to 3 mm, occasionally 5 mm, and rarely up to 7.5 mm. They often contain small calculi and may be surrounded by normal-looking medullary interstitium or, in cases of more prominent cystic disease, inflammatory cell infiltration or interstitial fibrosis.

## DIAGNOSIS

A definitive diagnosis of MSK can be made by excretory urography when the dilated collecting ducts are visualized on early and later radiographs without the use of compression and in the absence of ureteral obstruction (Fig. 45.24). Deposition of calcium salts within these dilated tubules occurs as renal calculi or nephrocalcinosis. The distribution of the renal calculi in MSK patients is characteristically found in clusters fanning away from the calyx. Because conventional CT has almost completely replaced excretory urography, the diagnosis of MSK may now be made less often. The finding of medullary nephrocalcinosis on CT or medullary hyperechogenicity on ultrasonography may be suggestive, but is not diagnostic, of MSK. Diagnosis of MSK by CT requires multidetector-row CT using high-resolution three-dimensional displays and late urographic images.

## MANIFESTATIONS

MSK is usually a benign disorder that may remain asymptomatic and undetected for life. The disease is associated with gross and microscopic hematuria that may be recurrent and with urinary tract infections that often are the first signs of an underlying abnormality. Renal stones consisting of calcium oxalate, calcium phosphate, and other types of calcium salts commonly form in the ectatic collecting ducts and are the most common presentation of this disease.

Impairment of tubular functions, such as a mild concentration defect, a reduced capacity to lower the urine pH after administration of ammonium chloride in comparison with controls, and, possibly, a low maximal excretion of potassium after short-term intravenous potassium chloride loading, may be documented in patients with MSK. Incomplete distal renal tubular acidosis may be found in as many as 30% to 40% of patients.

Whether patients with MSK exhibit specific metabolic abnormalities that predispose them to stone formation different from abnormalities in other patients with stone-forming disorders has been a controversial issue.[587] Hypercalciuria and hypocitraturia, a marker of renal tubular acidosis, have been the metabolic risk factors for stone formation more frequently identified in patients with ADPKD. Many, but not all, studies find hypocitraturia to be more common in patients with MSK with stones than in patients with other stone-forming disorders, and the same can be said for hypercalciuria. Some small studies have shown that the hypercalciuria is due to increased intestinal absorption but others have demonstrated a calcium leak. The calcium leak hypothesis could explain reported associations with parathyroid hyperplasia or adenomas and with osteopenia and osteoporosis. An alternative hypothesis is that hypercalciuria in patients with MSK reflects an abnormally high bone turnover as a result of the incomplete renal tubular acidosis seen in many patients with the disease.

Several studies have emphasized the association of hypocitraturia, distal renal tubular acidosis,[588,589] and hypercalciuria[587] with MSK. However, other studies have not found hypocitraturia to occur more frequently in patients with MSK than in other patients with renal stones. It has also been suggested that hypercalciuria from a calcium leak may lead to the development of parathyroid adenomas.[590] However, a critical examination of calcium excretion in patients with MSK and other stone-forming disorders showed that absorptive hypercalciuria was the most common abnormality in MSK, occurring in 59% of patients, whereas only 18% had hypercalciuria resulting from a renal calcium leak.[591] MSK seldom progresses to ESKD, although reduced GFRs have been observed, and a few patients have a relatively poor prognosis because of recurring urolithiasis, bacteriuria, and pyelonephritis.

### TREATMENT

There is no specific treatment for MSK. Most patients discovered incidentally can be advised that the disorder is benign and that they can anticipate no serious morbidity and that it is not life-threatening. The treatment of nephrolithiasis and urinary tract infection, when present, is the same as it would be for any patient with these problems. As a general rule, patients with nephrolithiasis should excrete about 2.5 L of urine each day to reduce the risk of stone formation. Potassium citrate and thiazides have been found to be effective in preventing stones in these patients. Fabris and colleagues recommend using potassium citrate as the first step in patients with MSK and a metabolic risk factor regardless of whether this is hypercalciuria, hypocitraturia, hyperuricosuria, or hyperoxaluria.[592] They recommend starting with 20 mEq of citrate per day in two divided doses, increasing the administration gradually by 10 mEq at a time, if tolerated, for patients in whom a citraturia level >450 mg/24 hours is not achieved initially, until the desired citrate level is reached, provided that the urine pH in a 24-hour collection is less than 7.5. Careful monitoring of the urine pH is necessary to ensure that pH stays below 7.5 in a 24-hour urine collection so as to prevent further formation of calcium phosphate stones in the ectatic tubules. With this regimen, these investigators have achieved not only an increase in urine citrate but also a significant reduction in urine calcium excretion (presumably as a result of the activation of the epithelial calcium channel TRPV5 in the distal nephron by the higher luminal pH) and, most importantly, a marked reduction in the stone event rate, from 0.58 to 0.10 stones per year per patient. They also observed an improvement in bone densitometry, with a total vertebral T-score increasing from −2.82 to −1.98 and a total hip T-score increasing from −2.03 to −1.86 after an average follow-up of 6.5 years.[593] These investigators reserve the use of thiazides for patients who continue to pass stones or have hypercalciuria despite receiving an optimal dose of citrate.

Patients with MSK appear to be more susceptible to urinary tract infections, and routine preventive measures seem warranted, especially in female patients. Repeated unnecessary investigations for hematuria should be avoided. Relapsing urinary tract infections may be due to infected renal stones and may require long-term antimicrobial suppression when the source of the infections cannot be eliminated.

## ACQUIRED CYSTIC KIDNEY DISEASE

### EPIDEMIOLOGY

Acquired cystic kidney disease (ACKD) is characterized by small cysts distributed throughout the renal cortex and medulla of patients with ESKD and is unrelated to inherited renal cystic disease. There is no agreement on the extent of cystic change required for the diagnosis, ranging from one to five cysts per kidney in radiologic studies to cystic changes in 25% to 40% of renal volume for tissue-based studies. Its prevalence and severity are higher in men than in women and increase with the duration of azotemia. Acquired cysts are found in 7% to 22% of patients with renal failure and serum creatinine values exceeding 3 mg/dL before dialysis, in 35% who have undergone dialysis for <2 years, in 58% for 2 to 4 years, in 75% for 4 to 8 years, and in 92% for longer than 8 years.[594] ACKD is unrelated to age, dialysis methods, race, and the cause of renal failure. In one study, no reduction in the frequency or severity of this disease was observed in 43 patients treated with hemodiafiltration in comparison with 43 patients treated with conventional hemodialysis after a mean follow-up of 63 months despite significantly lower levels of serum parathyroid hormone and alkaline phosphatase with hemodiafiltration. Multiple logistic regression analysis indicated that the duration of RRT was the only risk factor for the presence of ACKD.[595] Cysts can regress after successful renal transplant surgery but conversely can develop in transplanted kidneys affected by long-term rejection. Cyclosporine has been incriminated as predisposing native kidneys to cyst formation.

A very important feature in ACKD is the occurrence of renal tumors. The overall prevalence of RCC in patients undergoing hemodialysis evaluated radiologically or at autopsy is approximately 1% to 4%.[596] Carcinoma in dialysis recipients is three times more common in the presence than in the absence of acquired renal cysts, and six times more common in large than in small cystic kidneys. Overall, the incidence of renal malignancy in patients undergoing dialysis has been estimated to be 50 to 100 times greater than in the general population. The RCCs associated with ACKD have a lower risk for metastasis and a better prognosis than RCCs not associated with ACKD.

The risk for RCC remains high after renal transplantation in patients with ACKD. A study of 961 patients who received a kidney transplant between 1970 and 1998 included 561 patients who underwent prospective ultrasound screening of the native kidneys between 1997 and 2003.[597] Approximately 23% of them were found to have ACKD. Including 19 patients with formerly diagnosed RCC, the study found that the prevalence of RCC was 4.8% among all patients, 19.4% among the patients with ACKD, and 0.5% in those without ACKD. RCC was bilateral in 26% of cases. Tumor histology was clear cell RCC in 58% and papillary RCC in 42% of cases. Only one patient had a lung metastasis, and no patient died. Another study conducted ultrasound examination of the native kidneys every 6 months after renal transplantation between 1991 and 2007.[598] RCCs were diagnosed in 10 patients after a mean follow-up of 61.8 months. Two lesions were solid and eight were cystic, with the average size 2.1 cm. Four were clear cell type, and six papillary carcinomas. None of the patients had metastatic disease.

## PATHOGENESIS

The development of the cysts and tumors seems to be tied to the pronounced epithelial hyperplasia observed microscopically. The hyperplasia, in turn, seems to be a result of the uremic state even though there appears to be no relation between the occurrence of acquired cysts and the efficacy of dialysis. If ACKD is present at the time of successful transplantation, that process seems to regress or at least not to increase in severity. Conceivably, the loss of renal mass causes the production of renotropic factors that stimulate hyperplasia.

## PATHOLOGY

ACKD is usually bilateral and equal, with even severely affected kidneys weighing <100 g (30% <50 g), although about 25% weigh >150 g, including a few exceptional specimens of >1000 g (Fig. 45.25). In nephrectomy and autopsy specimens, the cysts vary in number and type from a few subcapsular cysts up to 2 to 3 cm in diameter to numerous smaller cysts that are diffusely distributed. The cysts are generally smaller than those in ADPKD. Microdissection studies have demonstrated the continuity of the cysts with both proximal and distal tubules and have suggested their origin both in the fusiform dilation of tubule segments and in multiple small tubule diverticula. Some, but not all, immunohistochemical studies have shown that the cysts in ACKD are mostly derived from proximal tubules.[599]

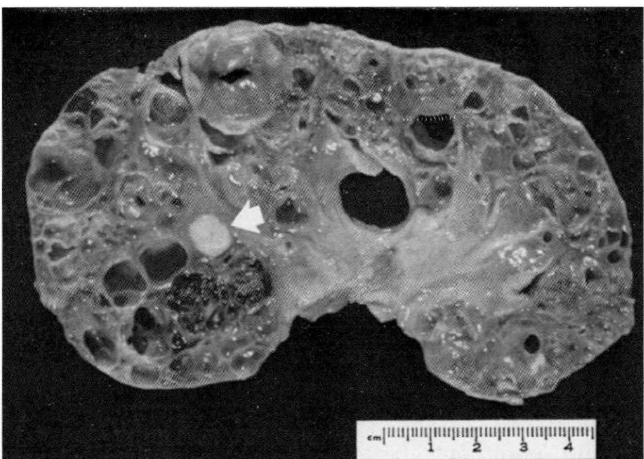

**Fig. 45.25** Acquired cystic disease in a 320-g kidney from a patient with a 10-year history of hemodialysis. There were bilateral, multifocal renal cell carcinomas *(arrow)* with multiple systemic metastases.

In a significant fraction of reported cases, the cysts contain single or, more often, multiple papillary, tubular, or solid neoplasms arising from the cyst lining and consistent with renal cell "adenomas" or adenocarcinomas. The genetic changes underlying the development of most of these tumors are different from those occurring in sporadic clear cell RCCs. Compared with sporadic RCC, ACKD-associated RCC tends to display lower Fuhrman nuclear grade, less proliferative activity, and diploidy in most cases, reflecting less aggressive behavior. The predominant type is clear cell, but papillary RCCs are overrepresented in comparison with the sporadic RCC in the general population.[596,597] In addition, RCC with distinctive histologic features has been associated with ACKD. These tumors are characterized by abundant eosinophilic cytoplasm; a variably solid, cribriform, tubulocystic, and papillary architecture; and deposits of calcium oxalate crystals.[600–602] For more discussion of ACKD-associated RCC, please see Chapter 41.

## DIAGNOSIS

Ultrasonography is a sensitive method to detect renal cysts and ACKD. However, complex cysts with intracystic septations, intracystic hemorrhage, mural nodules, and peripheral calcifications are sometimes difficult to distinguish from RCC with this method. CT with contrast enhancement is superior to ultrasonography in the evaluation of complex cysts (Fig. 45.25), but contrast enhancement is required to differentiate between benign and potentially malignant cystic lesions, and the intravenous administration of iodinated contrast media carries a risk of worsening the renal function in patients who are not yet undergoing dialysis or who have impaired renal function after transplantation. MRI, by contrast, provides high-resolution images with excellent tissue contrast even without the administration of gadolinium, which is contraindicated in patients with impaired renal function.[603] T1- and T2-weighted turbo spin-echo MRI sequences provide very good contrast among different tissues, and modern techniques such as diffusion-weighted sequences help improve diagnostic accuracy.

Because RCC is an important complication of ACKD, screening with ultrasonography has been recommended after 3 years of dialysis, followed by screening for neoplasm at 1- or 2-year intervals thereafter. However, because RCC is a relatively rare cause of death among dialysis recipients, a more aggressive renal imaging program, including annual screening, would be unlikely to significantly reduce mortality and therefore would not be cost-effective.[604] In the end, the clinical decision must be based on the individual patient, with consideration given to both the known risk factors for carcinoma—including prolonged dialysis, the presence of ACKD, large kidneys, and male sex—and the patient's age and general fitness. Screening with ultrasonography or MRI at 1- to 2-year intervals may be beneficial in selected populations such as young dialysis recipients or in transplant recipients with ACKD.

## MANIFESTATIONS

ACKD develops insidiously. Most patients have no symptoms. When symptoms occur, gross hematuria, flank pain, renal colic, fever, palpable renal mass, and rising hematocrit are most common. Retroperitoneal hemorrhage may manifest as acute pain, hypotension, and shock. Rarely, the presentation

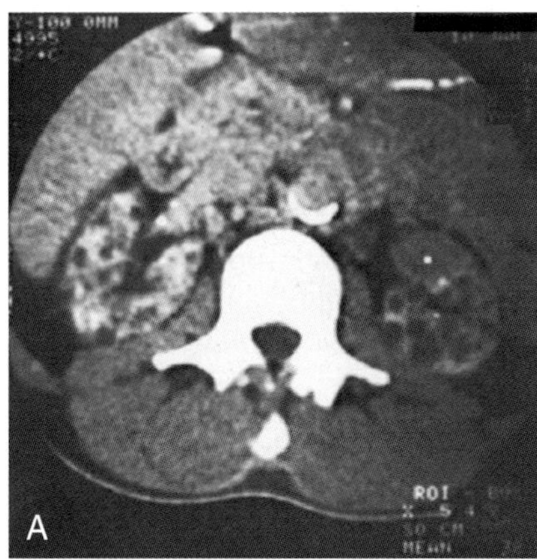


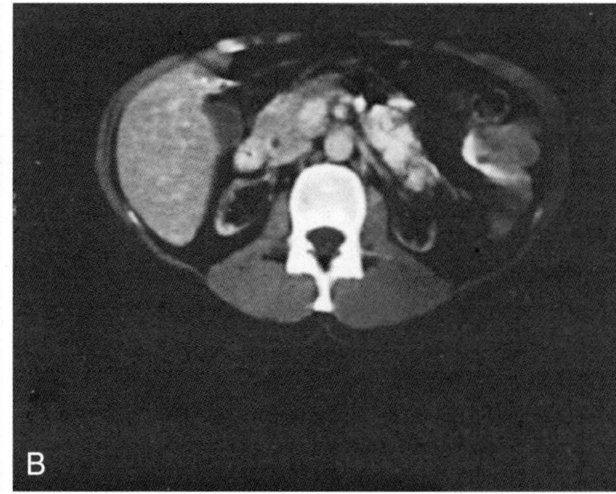


**Fig. 45.26** Acquired renal cystic disease. (A) Computed tomography (CT) scan with intravenous contrast. This man had renal failure caused by diabetic nephropathy and had received hemodialysis for 6 years before this examination. There is bilateral renal enlargement with diffuse cysts in the cortex and medulla. A solid tissue tumor *(white dot)* is seen in the anterior part of the left kidney. (B) CT scan of the original kidneys in a patient with a functioning renal allograft. Note the marked atrophy of the renal parenchyma in contrast to the cystic changes seen in (A).

consists of symptoms from metastatic RCC. Approximately 20% of ACKD-associated RCCs metastasize (vs. 50% for sporadic RCCs).

### TREATMENT

Bleeding episodes in ACKD, either intrarenal or perirenal, are often treated conservatively with bed rest and analgesics. Persistent hemorrhage, however, may require nephrectomy or therapeutic renal embolization and infarction. Because the risk of undetected RCC is high in patients with retroperitoneal hemorrhage, nephrectomy is recommended in those in whom carcinoma cannot be ruled out. If a few larger cysts are associated with flank pain, percutaneous aspiration (with cytologic examination) is a reasonable temporizing measure. ACKD may regress after successful renal transplantation (Fig. 45.26).

Renal masses larger than 3 cm detected in patients with ACKD are treated by excision. For tumors smaller than 3 cm, the options are nephrectomy for those who can undergo surgery or annual CT follow-up with resection if the lesions enlarge. Although metastases are less likely to occur from small than from large tumors, small tumor size is not a guarantee against metastasis. Resection even of small neoplasms seems prudent in preparation for transplantation. Because carcinoma in the setting of ACKD is often multicentric and bilateral, some writers recommend bilateral nephrectomy in these cases. If this procedure is not performed, frequent monitoring of the contralateral kidney is advised. Laparoscopic bilateral radical nephrectomy in patients with ESKD, ACKD, and suspicious tumors has been proposed as a more desirable alternative to traditional open surgery.[605]

## RENAL CYSTIC NEOPLASMS

Renal cystic neoplasms encompass a number of entities that cannot be reliably distinguished from one another on preoperative imaging studies. These entities include cystic RCC, multilocular cystic nephromas, cystic partially differentiated nephroblastomas, and mixed epithelial and stromal tumors.[606]

### CYSTIC RENAL CELL CARCINOMA

Multilocular and unilocular RCCs account for about 5% of RCCs and are characterized by their cystic nature—<25% of solid component—and by the absence of necrosis. They are usually clear cell type and of low grade and virtually never metastasize or cause death.[607] They should be distinguished from RCCs with a large cystic component due to extensive necrosis (pseudocystic necrotic carcinoma), which have an aggressive behavior, often leading to metastasis and death. Surgical excision is usually needed for diagnosis because fine-needle aspiration is not sufficiently accurate.

### MULTILOCULAR CYSTIC NEPHROMA

Cystic nephroma is a rare benign cystic neoplasm encountered in children and adults, with a bimodal distribution of age and gender (65% in patients younger than 4 years of age with a male:female ratio of 2:1 and the remainder in patients older than 30 years of age with a male:female ratio of 1:8). Cystic nephroma appears as an encapsulated multilocular mass, the locules of which are not connected to each other or to the pyelocalyceal system. They are lined by a single layer of nondescript, flattened, or cuboidal cells and "hobnail" cells with abundant eosinophilic cytoplasm and large apical nuclei. The septa are composed of connective tissue and may contain scattered atrophic renal tubules. Multilocular cystic nephroma is a benign lesion, but malignant transformation can occur in rare cases.

### CYSTIC PARTIALLY DIFFERENTIATED NEPHROBLASTOMA

Cystic partially differentiated nephroblastoma is a rare benign cystic renal neoplasm that is histologically identical to cystic nephroma except for Wilms tumor elements within the septa. It mostly occurs in children younger than 2 years of age, with rare adult occurrences. It is cured by complete excision.

## MIXED EPITHELIAL AND STROMAL TUMOR

Mixed epithelial and stromal tumor is a rare type of cystic renal neoplasm, with about 50 cases reported. Contrary to cystic nephroma and cystic partially differentiated nephroblastoma, which are purely cystic and have thin septa, the mixed epithelial and stromal tumor is partly cystic and has thicker wall-forming solid areas. All affected patients but one have been female, with a mean age of 46 years. The role of female hormones in the pathogenesis of this tumor is supported by a female predominance, a history of long-term estrogen treatment in many patients, and the expression of estrogen and progesterone receptors by tumor stromal cells. Mixed epithelial and stromal tumors are benign, and resection is curative.

# RENAL CYSTS OF NONTUBULAR ORIGIN

## CYSTIC DISEASE OF THE RENAL SINUS

The cystic disorders of the renal sinus are benign conditions that with modern imaging techniques can be clearly distinguished from more serious mass-occupying lesions of the renal pelvis or renal parenchyma. Two types of cystic lesions have been described in this area: hilus cysts and parapelvic cysts.

Hilus cysts, which have been identified only at autopsy, are thought to be caused by regressive changes in the fat tissue of the renal sinus, especially in kidneys with abundant fat in the renal sinus associated with renal atrophy. The cysts result from fluid replacement of adipose tissue that undergoes regressive changes owing to localized vascular disease and atrophy because of recent wasting. A single layer of flattened mesenchymal cells lines the wall of such a cyst, and the cystic fluid is clear and contains abundant lipid droplets.

Parapelvic cysts are of lymphatic origin and are much more common. The walls of the cysts are very thin and are lined by flat endothelial cells. The composition of the cystic fluid resembles that of lymph. The mechanism responsible for the dilation of the lymphatics is not known. Parapelvic cysts may be multiple and bilateral. They are in direct contact with the extrarenal pelvic surface and extend into the renal sinus, distorting the infundibula and calyces. The kidneys may appear slightly enlarged, but the enlargement is exclusively caused by the expansion of the renal sinus, and the area of the renal parenchyma remains normal. Bilateral parapelvic cysts (cystic disease of the renal sinus) can be confused with ADPKD on excretory urography, but the distinction between the two entities is straightforward on CT or MRI.

Parapelvic cysts are most frequently diagnosed after the fourth decade of life. They are usually discovered in the course of evaluations for conditions such as urinary tract infections, nephrolithiasis, hypertension, and prostatism. Despite considerable calyceal distortion, the pressure in these lymphatic cysts is low and not likely to result in significant functional obstruction. Indeed, renal function in patients with bilateral multiple parapelvic cysts is usually normal. Occasionally, parapelvic cysts are the only finding in the course of evaluation for otherwise unexplained lumbar or flank pain. The therapeutic approach to parapelvic cysts should be conservative.

## PERIRENAL LYMPHANGIOMAS

Perirenal lymphangiomas are characterized by dilation of the lymphatic channels around the kidneys that leads to the development of unilocular or multilocular cystic masses.[608] Lymphatic obstruction may play a role in its pathogenesis, and rare familial cases suggest a genetic component. Perirenal lymphangiomas have also been observed in patients with TSC.[609] Pregnancy is reported to exacerbate the condition, possibly because the renal lymphatics play a role in handling an enhanced interstitial fluid flow during this condition.[610] Mild renal functional impairment and hypertension can occur transiently and revert to normal in the postpartum period.

## SUBCAPSULAR AND PERIRENAL URINOMAS (URINIFEROUS PSEUDOCYSTS)

Subcapsular and perirenal urinomas are encapsulated collections of extravasated urine in the subcapsular and perirenal spaces. They are usually secondary to obstructive uropathies, such as posterior urethral valve, pelviureteric junction, or vesicoureteric junction obstruction, ureteric calculus, or trauma. They are caused by pyelosinus backflow, which can occur when the intrapelvic pressure rises to ≥35 cm $H_2O$, leading to rupture of calyceal fornices. Whereas subcapsular urinomas are situated between the renal parenchyma and renal capsule, perirenal urinomas are located between the renal capsule and Gerota fascia. Treatment includes temporary decompression by placement of a pigtail catheter in the most dependent point of the urinoma and correction of the underlying disorder.

## PYELOCALYCEAL CYSTS

Also termed "pyelocalyceal diverticula" or "calyceal or pyelorenal cysts" or "diverticula," pyelocalyceal cysts represent congenital, probably developmental, saccular diverticula from a minor calyx (type I) or from the pelvis or adjacent major calyx (type II). Type I is more common, is usually located in the poles (especially the upper), and tends to be smaller and less often symptomatic than the centrally located type II. Both types are usually <1 cm in diameter but occasionally may be quite large. The cysts are encompassed by a muscularis, are lined by a usually chronically inflamed transitional epithelium, and usually contain urine or cloudy fluid.

Pyelocalyceal cysts occur sporadically, affect all age groups, and usually are unilateral. They may be detected in as many as 0.5% of excretory urograms but normally are asymptomatic unless they are complicated by nephrolithiasis or infection. The frequency of stone formation in calyceal diverticula has been reported to be between 10% and 40%. Transitional cell carcinoma arising in a pyelocalyceal cyst has been seldom reported. Surgical intervention is indicated only when conservative management of this complication fails.

 Complete reference list available at ExpertConsult.com.

## KEY REFERENCES

3. Torres VE, Harris PC. Strategies targeting cAMP signaling in the treatment of polycystic kidney disease. *J Am Soc Nephrol.* 2014;25:18–32.
10. Hopp K, Ward CJ, Hommerding CJ, et al. Functional polycystin-1 dosage governs autosomal dominant polycystic kidney disease severity. *J Clin Invest.* 2012;122:4257–4273.

67. Cornec-Le Gall E, Audrezet MP, Chen JM, et al. Type of PKD1 mutation influences renal outcome in ADPKD. *J Am Soc Nephrol.* 2013;24:1006–1013.
69. Harris PC, Hopp K. The mutation, a key determinant of phenotype in ADPKD. *J Am Soc Nephrol.* 2013;24:868–870.
76. Bergmann C, von Bothmer J, Ortiz Bruchle N, et al. Mutations in multiple PKD genes may explain early and severe polycystic kidney disease. *J Am Soc Nephrol.* 2011;22:2047–2056.
116. Chebib FT, Sussman CR, Wang X, et al. Vasopressin and disruption of calcium signaling in polycystic kidney disease. *Nat Clin Nephrol.* 2015;[Epub April 14].
120. Yamaguchi T, Hempson SJ, Reif GA, et al. Calcium restores a normal proliferation phenotype in human polycystic kidney disease epithelial cells. *J Am Soc Nephrol.* 2006;17:178–187.
184. Pei Y, Obaji J, Dupuis A, et al. Unified criteria for ultrasonographic diagnosis of ADPKD. *J Am Soc Nephrol.* 2009;20:205–212.
185. Barua M, Cil O, Paterson AD, et al. Family history of renal disease severity predicts the mutated gene in ADPKD. *J Am Soc Nephrol.* 2009;20:1833–1838.
186. Pei Y, Hwang YH, Conklin J, et al. Imaging-based diagnosis of autosomal dominant polycystic kidney disease. *J Am Soc Nephrol.* 2014;26: 746–753.
191. Harris PC, Bae KT, Rossetti S, et al. Cyst number but not the rate of cystic growth is associated with the mutated gene in autosomal dominant polycystic kidney disease. *J Am Soc Nephrol.* 2006;17:3013–3019.
196. Irazabal MV, Rangel LJ, Bergstralh EJ, et al. Imaging classification of autosomal dominant polycystic kidney disease: a simple model for selecting patients for clinical trials. *J Am Soc Nephrol.* 2015;26:160–172.
237. Jouret F, Lhommel R, Beguin C, et al. Positron-emission computed tomography in cyst infection diagnosis in patients with autosomal dominant polycystic kidney disease. *Clin J Am Soc Nephrol.* 2011;6:1644–1650.
238. Wetmore JB, Calvet JP, Yu AS, et al. Polycystic kidney disease and cancer after renal transplantation. *J Am Soc Nephrol.* 2014;25: 2335–2341.
245. Chapman AB, Bost JE, Torres VE, et al. Kidney volume and functional outcomes in autosomal dominant polycystic kidney disease. *Clin J Am Soc Nephrol.* 2012;7(3):479–486.
252. Lantinga MA, Drenth JP, Gevers TJ. Diagnostic criteria in renal and hepatic cyst infection. *Nephrol Dial Transplant.* 2014;[Epub June 20].
253. Suwabe T, Ubara Y, Sumida K, et al. Clinical features of cyst infection and hemorrhage in ADPKD: new diagnostic criteria. *Clin Exp Nephrol.* 2012;16:892–902.
288. Schrier RS, Abebe KZ, Perrone RD, et al. Angiotensin blockade, blood pressure and autosomal dominant polycystic kidney disease. *N Engl J Med.* 2014;371:2255–2266.
289. Torres VE, Abebe KZ, Chapman AB, et al. Angiotensin blockade in late autosomal dominant polycystic kidney disease. *N Engl J Med.* 2014;371:2267–2276.
292. Patch C, Charlton J, Roderick PJ, et al. Use of antihypertensive medications and mortality of patients with autosomal dominant polycystic kidney disease: a population-based study. *Am J Kidney Dis.* 2011;57:856–862.
295. Orskov B, Sorensen VR, Feldt-Rasmussen B, et al. Changes in causes of death and risk of cancer in Danish patients with autosomal dominant polycystic kidney disease and end-stage renal disease. *Nephrol Dial Transplant.* 2012;27:1607–1613.
298. Spithoven E, Kramer A, Meijer E, et al. Renal replacement therapy for autosomal dominant polycystic kidney disease (ADPKD) in Europe: prevalence and survival—an analysis of data from the ERA-EDTA Registry. *Nephrol Dial Transplant.* 2014;29(suppl 4): iv15–iv25.
310. Yamamoto T, Watarai Y, Kobayashi T, et al. Kidney volume changes in patients with autosomal dominant polycystic kidney disease after renal transplantation. *Transplantation.* 2012;93:794–798.
311. Abu-Wasel B, Walsh C, Keough V, et al. Pathophysiology, epidemiology, classification and treatment options for polycystic liver diseases. *World J Gastroenterol.* 2013;19:5775–5786.
312. Drenth JP, Chrispijn M, Nagorney DM, et al. Medical and surgical treatment options for polycystic liver disease. *Hepatology.* 2010;52: 2223–2230.
317. Irazabal MV, Huston J 3rd, Kubly V, et al. Extended follow-up of unruptured intracranial aneurysms detected by presymptomatic screening in patients with autosomal dominant polycystic kidney disease. *Clin J Am Soc Nephrol.* 2011;6:1274–1285.
319. Hopp K, Hommerding CJ, Wang X. Tolvaptan plus pasireotide shows enhanced efficacy in a PKD1 model. *J Am Soc Nephrol.* 2015; 26(1):39–47.
322. Torres VE, Chapman AB, Devuyst O, et al. Tolvaptan in patients with autosomal dominant polycystic kidney disease. *N Engl J Med.* 2012;367:2407–2418.
333. Hogan MC, Masyuk TV, Page L, et al. Somatostatin analog therapy for severe polycystic liver disease: results after 2 years. *Nephrol Dial Transplant.* 2012;27:3532–3539.
334. Caroli A, Perico N, Perna A, et al. Effect of long acting somatostatin analogue on kidney and cyst growth in autosomal dominant polycystic kidney disease (ALADIN): a randomised, placebo-controlled, multicentre trial. *Lancet.* 2013;382:1485–1495.
336. Gevers TJ, Inthout J, Caroli A, et al. Young women with polycystic liver disease respond best to somatostatin analogues: a pooled analysis of individual patient data. *Gastroenterology.* 2013;145:357–365, e1–2.
343. Serra AL, Poster D, Kistler AD, et al. Sirolimus and kidney growth in autosomal dominant polycystic kidney disease. *N Engl J Med.* 2010;363:820–829.
345. Walz G, Budde K, Mannaa M, et al. Everolimus in patients with autosomal dominant polycystic kidney disease. *N Engl J Med.* 2010;363: 830–840.
417. Gunay-Aygun M, Turkbey BI, Bryant J, et al. Hepatorenal findings in obligate heterozygotes for autosomal recessive polycystic kidney disease. *Mol Genet Metab.* 2011;104:677–681.
421. Telega G, Cronin D, Avner ED. New approaches to the autosomal recessive polycystic kidney disease patient with dual kidney-liver complications. *Pediatr Transplant.* 2013;17:328–335.
453. Bissler JJ, Kingswood JC, Radzikowska E, et al. Everolimus for angiomyolipoma associated with tuberous sclerosis complex or sporadic lymphangioleiomyomatosis (EXIST-2): a multicentre, randomised, double-blind, placebo-controlled trial. *Lancet.* 2013;381:817–824.
455. Maher ER, Neumann HP, Richard S. Von Hippel-Lindau disease: a clinical and scientific review. *Eur J Hum Genet.* 2011;19:617–623.
474. Ekici AB, Hackenbeck T, Morinière V, et al. Renal fibrosis is the common feature of autosomal dominant tubulointerstitial kidney diseases caused by mutations in mucin 1 or uromodulin. *Kidney Int.* 2014;86:589–599.
481. Moskowitz JL, Piret SE, Lhotta K, et al. Association between genotype and phenotype in uromodulin-associated kidney disease. *Clin J Am Soc Nephrol.* 2013;8:1349–1357.
490. Trudu M, Janas S, Lanzani C, et al. Common noncoding UMOD gene variants induce salt-sensitive hypertension and kidney damage by increasing uromodulin expression. *Nat Med.* 2013;19:1655–1660.
491. Bleyer AJ, Kmoch S, Antignac C, et al. Variable clinical presentation of an MUC1 mutation causing medullary cystic kidney disease type 1. *Clin J Am Soc Nephrol.* 2014;9:527–535.
495. Faguer S, Decramer S, Chassaing N, et al. Diagnosis, management, and prognosis of HNF1B nephropathy in adulthood. *Kidney Int.* 2011;80:768–776.
508. Hildebrandt F, Benzing T, Katsanis N. Ciliopathies. *N Engl J Med.* 2011;364:1533–1543.
538. Forsythe E, Beales PL. Bardet-Biedl syndrome. *Eur J Hum Genet.* 2013;21:8–13.
547. Putoux A, Attie-Bitach T, Martinovic J, et al. Phenotypic variability of Bardet-Biedl syndrome: focusing on the kidney. *Pediatr Nephrol.* 2012;27:7–15.
578. Rule AD, Sasiwimonphan K, Lieske JC, et al. Characteristics of renal cystic and solid lesions based on contrast-enhanced computed tomography of potential kidney donors. *Am J Kidney Dis.* 2012;59:611–618.
580. Ponte B, Pruijm M, Ackermann D, et al. Copeptin is associated with kidney length, renal function, and prevalence of simple cysts in a population-based study. *J Am Soc Nephrol.* 2014;[Epub September 30].
587. Fabris A, Anglani F, Lupo A, et al. Medullary sponge kidney: state of the art. *Nephrol Dial Transplant.* 2013;28:1111–1119.

# SECTION VII

# HYPERTENSION AND THE KIDNEY

# 46 Primary and Secondary Hypertension

William J. Elliott | Aldo J. Peixoto | George L. Bakris

CHAPTER OUTLINE



Hypertension has consistently been one of the major contributors to premature morbidity and mortality in the United States.[1] Hypertension was ranked first worldwide in an analysis of all risk factors for global disease burden in 2010[2] (Fig. 46.1) and again in 2015. By the year 2025, hypertension is expected to increase in prevalence worldwide by 60% and will affect 1.56 billion people.[3] Developing nations will experience an 80% increase (from 639 million to 1.15 billion afflicted persons). As emerging countries have improved sanitation and other basic public health measures, cardiovascular (CV) disease has or soon will become the most common cause of death, and hypertension will be its most common reversible risk factor, as it is already in the United States.

The major public health importance of hypertension can be amply demonstrated using data from the United States, but similar conclusions have been emerging as other industrialized countries analyze national health care databases.[4] Hypertension was listed as the principal or a contributing cause of death in 16.4% of Americans older than 45 years who died in 2013, a 48% increase since 2000.[1]

Hypertension is the most important modifiable risk factor for stroke,[1] which fell from the second most common cause of death in the United States in 1958, to third between 1959 and 2007, to fourth between 2008 and 2012, and to fifth in 2013 and 2014.[5] Current estimates are that 77% of those who have a first stroke have had a blood pressure (BP) above 140/90 mm Hg.

High BP is the leading antecedent condition for heart failure—regardless of whether left ventricular function is diminished or preserved—which is the most common reason for acute care hospitalization among Medicare beneficiaries (~1.023 million in 2010); approximately 74% of people experiencing an initial hospitalization for heart failure either had or have BP of 140/90 mm Hg or higher.[1]

Currently, end-stage kidney disease (ESKD) has the highest per-patient annualized cost to Medicare, amounting to about 20% of Medicare expenditures for Americans older than 65 years,[6] and hypertension is the second most common cause of ESKD. After tobacco use and diabetes, hypertension is the most important risk factor for peripheral vascular disease, the second leading cause of loss of limbs in the United States.[1] Hypertension is likely the most important treatable cause of (vascular) dementia, which ranked sixth among causes of death in the United States in 2014 and is the third leading cause of admission to nursing homes. Hypertension ranks first among the chronic conditions for which Americans visit a health care provider. This may be secondary to its high age-adjusted prevalence (33.5% of adults >18 years in the US National Health and Nutrition Examination Survey [NHANES], 2013–2014) and the fact that treatment clearly improves prognosis.

All health care providers routinely encounter people who are likely to benefit from lowered BP levels. In the future, more people will likely become candidates for antihypertensive therapy because the prevalence of hypertension is increasing secondary to the increasing prevalence of obesity and increased longevity of the general population.[7]

## HYPERTENSION DEFINITIONS

Traditionally, high blood pressure has been defined as a persistent BP elevation in the office at or above 140/90 mm Hg.[8–11] Blood pressure is the phenotypic expression of the genetically predisposed disease hypertension. Blood pressure is a continuous variable. The threshold BP value to secure a diagnosis of hypertension has come from large epidemiologic studies demonstrating a higher mortality at levels above

**1990**

| Mean rank (95% UI) | Risk factor |
|---|---|
| 1.1 (1–2) | 1 Childhood underweight |
| 2.1 (1–4) | 2 Household air pollution |
| 2.9 (2–4) | 3 Smoking (excluding SHS) |
| 4.0 (3–5) | 4 High blood pressure |
| 5.4 (3–8) | 5 Suboptimal breastfeeding |
| 5.6 (5–6) | 6 Alcohol use |
| 7.4 (6–8) | 7 Ambient PM pollution |
| 7.4 (6–8) | 8 Low fruit |
| 9.7 (9–12) | 9 High fasting plasma glucose |
| 10.9 (9–14) | 10 High body mass index |
| 11.1 (9–15) | 11 Iron deficiency |
| 12.3 (9–17) | 12 High sodium |
| 13.9 (10–19) | 13 Low nuts and seeds |
| 14.1 (11–17) | 14 High total cholesterol |
| 16.2 (9–38) | 15 Sanitation |
| 16.7 (13–21) | 16 Low vegetables |
| 17.1 (10–23) | 17 Vitamin A deficiency |
| 17.3 (15–20) | 18 Low whole grains |
| 20.0 (13–29) | 19 Zinc deficiency |
| 20.6 (17–25) | 20 Low omega-3 |
| 20.8 (18–24) | 21 Occupational injury |
| 21.7 (14–34) | 22 Unimproved water |
| 22.6 (19–26) | 23 Occupational low back pain |
| 23.2 (19–29) | 24 High processed meat |
| 24.2 (21–26) | 25 Drug use |
| | 26 Low fiber |
| | 30 Lead |

**2010**

| Risk factor | Mean rank (95% UI) | % change (95% UI) |
|---|---|---|
| 1 High blood pressure | 1.1 (1–2) | 27% (19 to 34) |
| 2 Smoking (excluding SHS) | 1.9 (1–2) | 3% (−5 to 11) |
| 3 Alcohol use | 3.0 (2–4) | 28% (17 to 39) |
| 4 Household air pollution | 4.7 (3–7) | −37% (−44 to −29) |
| 5 Low fruit | 5.0 (4–8) | 29% (25 to 34) |
| 6 High body mass index | 6.1 (4–8) | 82% (71 to 95) |
| 7 High fasting plasma glucose | 6.6 (5–8) | 58% (43 to 73) |
| 8 Childhood underweight | 8.5 (6–11) | −61% (−66 to −55) |
| 9 Ambient PM pollution | 8.9 (7–11) | −7% (−13 to −1) |
| 10 Physical inactivity | 9.9 (8–12) | 0% (0 to 0) |
| 11 High sodium | 11.2 (8–15) | 33% (27 to 39) |
| 12 Low nuts and seeds | 12.9 (11–17) | 27% (18 to 32) |
| 13 Iron deficiency | 13.5 (11–17) | −7% (−11 to −4) |
| 14 Suboptimal breastfeeding | 13.8 (10–18) | −57% (−63 to −51) |
| 15 High total cholesterol | 15.2 (12–17) | 3% (−13 to 19) |
| 16 Low whole grains | 15.3 (13–17) | 39% (32 to 45) |
| 17 Low vegetables | 15.8 (12–19) | 22% (16 to 28) |
| 18 Low omega-3 | 18.7 (17–23) | 30% (21 to 35) |
| 19 Drug use | 20.2 (18–23) | 57% (42 to 72) |
| 20 Occupational injury | 20.4 (18–23) | 12% (−22 to 58) |
| 21 Occupational low back pain | 21.2(18–25) | 22% (11 to 35) |
| 22 High processed meat | 22.0 (17–31) | 22% (2 to 44) |
| 23 Intimate partner violence | 23.8 (20–28) | 0% (0 to 0) |
| 24 Low fiber | 24.4 (19–32) | 23% (13 to 33) |
| 25 Lead | 25.5 (25–29) | 160% (143 to 176) |
| 26 Sanitation | | |
| 29 Vitamin A deficiency | | |
| 31 Zinc deficiency | | |
| 33 Unimproved water | | |

——— Ascending order in rank
- - - - Descending order in rank

**Fig. 46.1** Global risk factor ranks with 95% uncertainty interval for all ages and genders combined in 1990 and 2010 and percentage change. *PM,* Particulate matter; *SHS,* secondhand smoke. (From Lim SS, Vos T, Flaxman AD, et al: A comparative risk assessment of burden of disease and injury attributable to 67 risk factors and risk factor clusters in 21 regions, 1990-2010: a systematic analysis for the Global Burden of Disease Study 2010. *Lancet*. 2012;380:2224–2260.)

**Table 46.1 Categorization of Blood Pressure for Hypertension and Its Related Diagnoses in the United States[a]**

| BP Category[b] | SBP | | DBP |
|---|---|---|---|
| **Normal** | <120 mm Hg | and | <80 mm Hg |
| **Elevated** | 120–129 mm Hg | and | <80 mm Hg |
| **Hypertension** | | | |
| • Stage 1 | 130–139 mm Hg | or | 80–89 mm Hg |
| • Stage 2 | 140–159 mm Hg | or | 90–99 mm Hg |

[a]If the systolic and diastolic blood pressure levels fall into two different diagnostic categories, the higher category is used (e.g., 162/92 mm Hg is stage 3 hypertension; 134/72 mm Hg is stage 1).

[b]Definitions are from Whelton PK, Carey RM, Aronow WS, et al. 2017 ACC/AHA/AAPA/ABC/ACPM/AGS/APhA/ASH/ASPC/NMA/PCNA Guideline for the Prevention, Detection, Evaluation, and Management of High Blood Pressure in Adults: Executive Summary: A Report of the American College of Cardiology/American Heart Association Task Force on Clinical Practice Guidelines. *Hypertension*. 2018;71:1269–1324. Different classification schemes are used outside the United States.

*BP*, Blood pressure; *DBP*, diastolic blood pressure; *SBP*, systolic blood pressure.

**Box 46.1 Essential Elements of Proper Blood Pressure Measurement in the Office**

Allow patient to rest in the seated position for at least 3 to 5 minutes prior to measuring blood pressure (BP).

Neither patient nor examiner should talk during measurements.

The patient should have his or her legs uncrossed and should be seated comfortably on a chair with arm and back support.

Use the arm as the preferred site of measurement.

Make sure the measuring device is adequately maintained and calibrated.

Use a cuff that fits the arm circumference properly. The bladder length should cover at least 80% of the arm circumference. Recommended cuff sizes for adults are as follows:

- Small adult (12 × 22 cm): for arm circumferences between 22 and 26 cm
- Adult (16 × 30 cm): for arm circumferences between 27 and 34 cm
- Large adult (16 × 36 cm): for arm circumferences between 35 and 44 cm
- Adult thigh (16 × 42 cm): for arm circumferences between 45 and 52 cm

Place the lower end of the cuff approximately 2 to 3 cm above the antecubital fossa.

Have the arm positioned at the level of the heart.

Take at least two BP measurements and average them. Obtain more measurements if there is disparity between the first two values.

Measure BP in both arms to identify interarm differences (~20% of individuals may have a difference >10 mm Hg). If different, report the values obtained on the arm with higher BP.

If using the auscultatory method with a stethoscope, use Korotkoff phase I (appearance) and V (disappearance) to define systolic and diastolic BP, respectively.

If using an aneroid or mercury manometer, use a deflation rate of 2–3 mm Hg/sec. (Deflation rates with automated oscillometric devices vary substantially and are defined based on proprietary algorithms.)

Data from Whelton PK, Carey RM, Aronow WS, et al. ACC/AHA/AAPA/ABC/ACPM/ AGS/APhA/ASH/ASPC/NMA/PCNA Guideline for the Prevention, Detection, Evaluation and Management of High Blood Pressure in Adults: A Report of the American College of Cardiology/American Heart Association and Task Force on Clinical Practice Guidelines. *Hypertension.* 2018;71(6):e13–e115.

140/90 mm Hg.[12] In the United States, national guidelines promulgated by the Seventh Report of the Joint National Committee on Prevention, Detection, Evaluation, and Treatment of High Blood Pressure (JNC 7) in 2003 simplified the classification of hypertension and related conditions.[8] This classification has been endorsed and expanded by more recent guidelines (Table 46.1).[13] The five categories of BP—normal, elevated, stages 1, 2, and 3 hypertension—are associated with progressively increasing CV risk and are independent of any other risk factor (including age; see Table 46.1).[13] The most recent guidelines have defined the level of raised blood pressure that should be considered for beginning treatment based not only on BP level, but also on a more than 10% cardiovascular risk over the ensuing 10 years. Thus, in people with chronic kidney disease (CKD), all people with a BP more than 130/80 mm Hg not only need lifestyle intervention but treatment with at least one antihypertensive medication.[13]

Office BP readings often display less accuracy and reproducibility than is desired, particularly if great care is not taken during the procedure (Box 46.1)[8,10] As a result, there is growing interest in other methods of measuring BP that either remove human error from the process or involve more expensive equipment (see later).

## EVOLUTION OF BLOOD PRESSURE GOALS

As more data became available, the guideline-based definition of hypertension has evolved over the last 40 years (Fig. 46.2). The change of the diastolic threshold from 95 to 90 mm Hg occurred concomitantly with the recommendation to use Korotkoff phase V (disappearance of sound), rather than phase IV (muffling of sounds) in diagnosis. The inclusion of systolic BP in the definition of hypertension has been much more gradual (see Fig. 46.2).

In JNC 1 and 2 (1977–1982), the diagnosis of hypertension was made solely on diastolic BP values. In JNC 3 and 4, "isolated systolic hypertension" (systolic BP ≥160 mm Hg, but diastolic BP <90 mm Hg) was defined, but no recommendations about therapy were made (see Fig. 46.2).

Since 1993, many guidelines have recognized isolated systolic hypertension as worthy of treatment.[7,11] BP-lowering therapy in this subgroup of older adults has morbidity and mortality benefits.[14,15] A pooling of data from nearly 1 million people from 61 long-term epidemiologic studies has concluded that systolic BP predicts approximately 89% of age-stratified stroke deaths and 93% of coronary heart disease deaths, whereas diastolic BP is much less predictive (83% and 73%, respectively).[9]

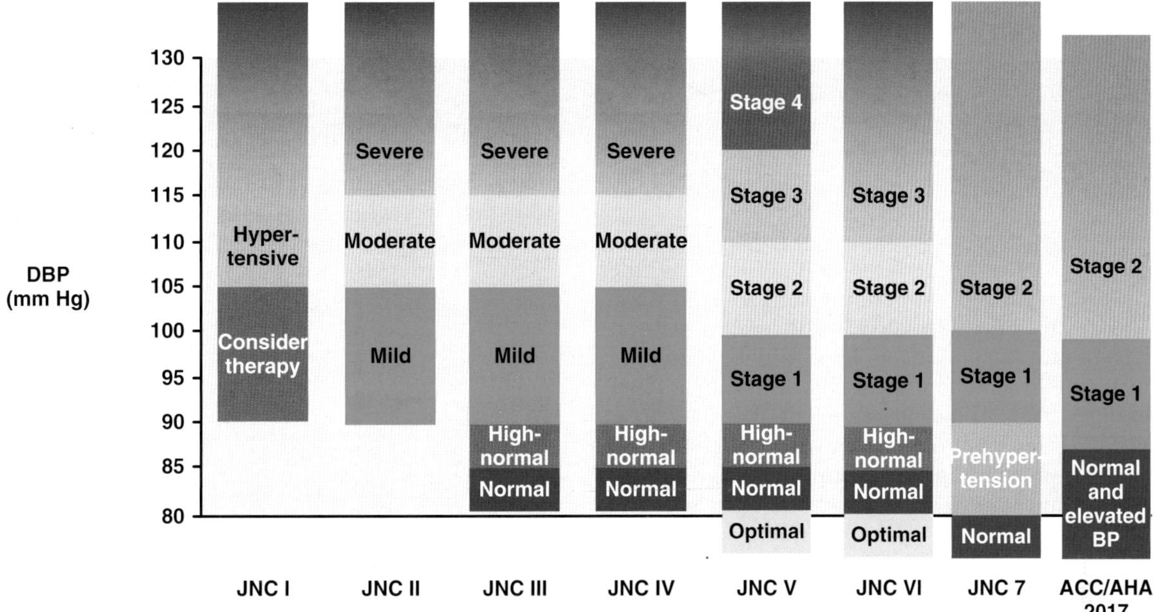


A

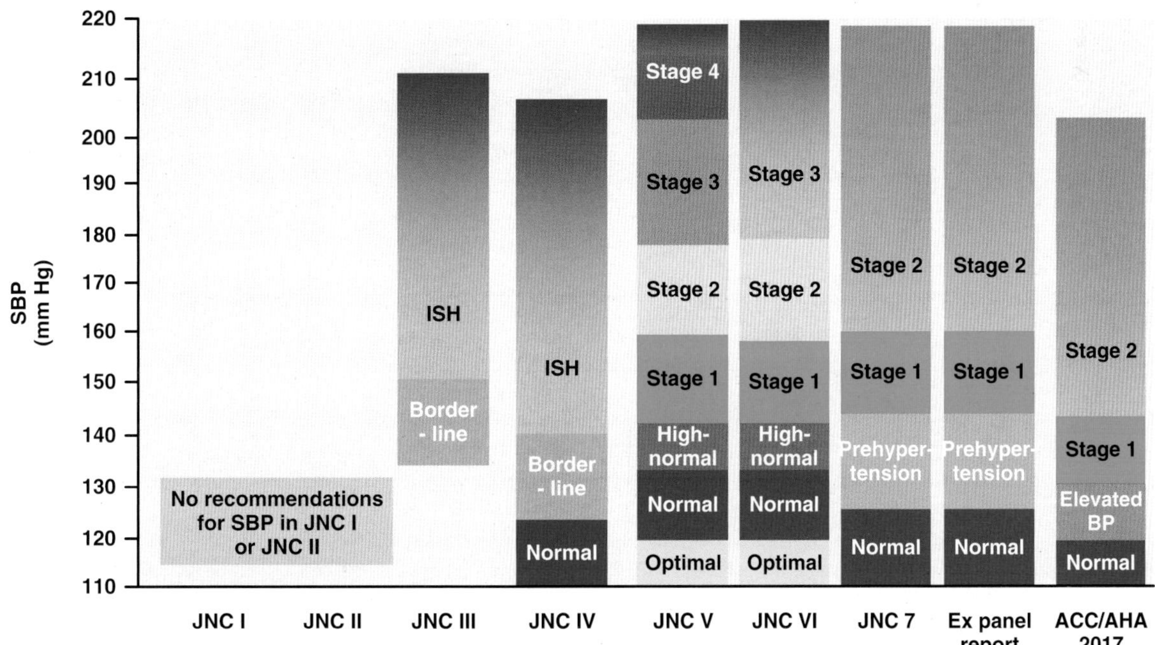


B

**Fig. 46.2** (A) Joint National Committee on Prevention, Detection, Evaluation, and Treatment of High Blood Pressure (JNC)/American Heart Association (AHA)/American College of Cardiology (ACC) DBP classifications. (B) JNC/AHA/ACC SBP classifications. *DBP,* Diastolic blood pressure; *ISH,* isolated systolic hypertension; *SBP,* systolic blood pressure.

In addition to a large body of epidemiologic data linking elevated systolic BP with cardiovascular events,[2–4,9,16] 11 clinical trials have compared active antihypertensive drugs to either placebo or no treatment in 28,436 patients. These trials demonstrated morbidity and mortality benefits of treatment tied to reductions in systolic but not diastolic BP.[14]

## EPIDEMIOLOGY

Hypertension is widely treated because of its increased risk for long-term CV and renal morbidity and mortality and the fact that antihypertensive treatment prevents some of these events. The risks attributable to elevated BP levels have been documented in numerous epidemiologic studies, beginning in 1948 with the Framingham Heart Study and extending to the present.[2–4,9,15,16] Meta-analyses of pooled data have confirmed the robust continuous relationship between BP level and cerebrovascular disease and coronary heart disease in both Western and Eastern populations.[2–4,9,15–17] In addition, BP has been linked directly in epidemiologic studies to incident left ventricular hypertrophy (LVH), heart failure, peripheral vascular disease, carotid atherosclerosis, ESKD, and subclinical CV disease. A natural history study that involved almost 12,000 veterans, followed over 15 years, has noted that the level of BP correlates with the risk for ESKD (Fig. 46.3).[18] Note that in this study, the highest risk for ESKD was found at levels above the renal autoregulatory range (i.e., a systolic BP >180 mm Hg).

CV risk factors tend to cluster; thus, hypertensive individuals are much more likely than normotensive people to have type 2 diabetes mellitus or dyslipidemia, especially elevated triglyceride levels and low high-density lipoprotein cholesterol levels. The common denominator may be insulin resistance, perhaps because of the frequent coexistence of hypertension and obesity.

## AGE AND HYPERTENSION

Increasing age is a major risk factor for developing hypertension (Fig. 46.4), as well as a very strong confounder of its independent influence on CV and renal events. In the analysis

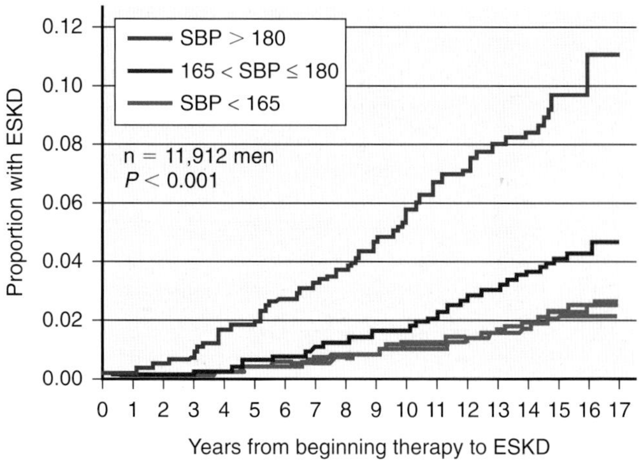


**Fig. 46.3** A 17-year follow-up from Veterans Affairs hypertension clinics on end-stage kidney disease *(ESKD)*. *SBP,* Systolic blood pressure (in mm Hg).

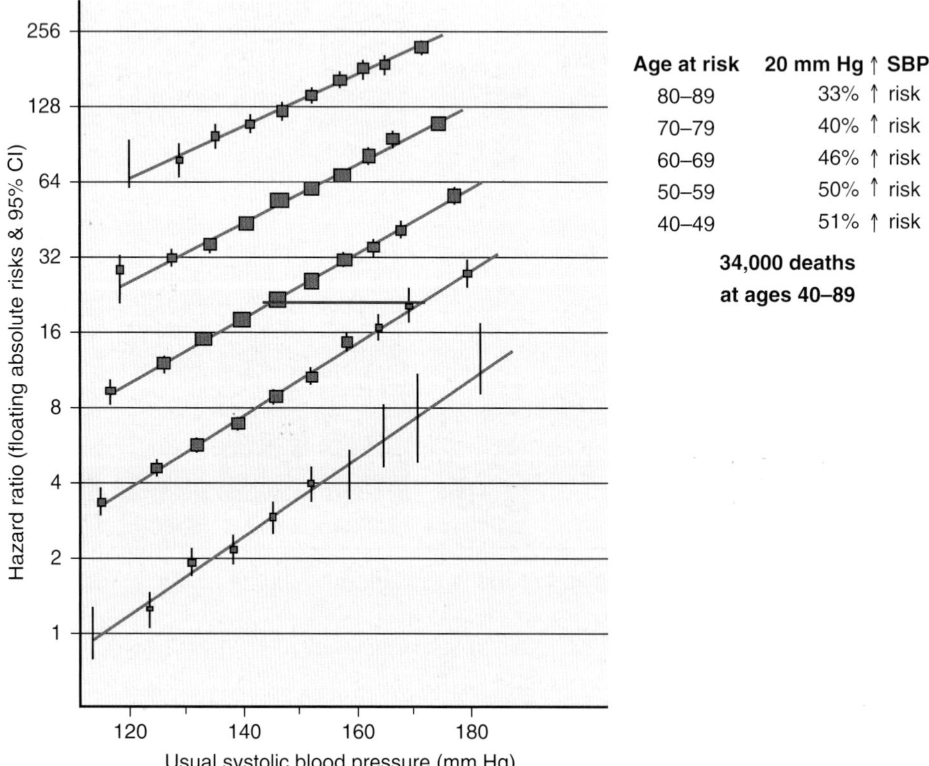


**Fig. 46.4** Coronary heart disease mortality in each decade of age versus systolic blood pressure (SBP) at the start of that decade. *CI,* Confidence interval.

of nearly 1 million individuals in 61 epidemiologic studies followed for an average of 13.3 years, those with BP levels in the highest decile had roughly the same risk for death from ischemic heart disease or stroke as people who were 20 years older but had BP levels in the lowest decile.[9] In the Framingham study, the lifetime risk of 55- to 65-year-old men or women for developing hypertension was above 90%.[19] In this study, of those who survived to age 65 to 89 years, systolic BP elevations were found in 87% of the hypertensive men and 93% of the hypertensive women. In an analysis of the Framingham data set, classification of people with hypertension who were older than 60 years into the appropriate BP stages was done correctly in 99% of the cases using systolic rather than diastolic BP.[12]

These data highlight the great public health importance of systolic BP, particularly among people older than 50 years. In such individuals, systolic BP is a much better predictor of hypertensive target organ damage and future CV and renal events than diastolic BP.[9,20,21] Overall, each 20-mm Hg increase in systolic BP doubled the risk for CV death.[9] Systolic BP was less likely to be controlled to less than 140 mm Hg than diastolic to less than 90 mm Hg in the general US population, according to every NHANES data set from 1974 to 2014. Nearly 54% of people with uncontrolled hypertension in the United States in 2013 to 2014 were 60 years of age and older.[22] Yet, antihypertensive drug therapy reduces the risk for CV events across the full age spectrum and has its greatest absolute benefit in older people, including individuals older than 80 years.[23–25]

The diagnosis of hypertension in children and adolescents is becoming more important due to the epidemic of obesity in young Americans.[26] Current US guidelines recommend BP measurement in children at least annually, but normative values depend on gender, age, and height of the child.[27] As a result, interpretation of BP levels in children and adolescents usually involves comparison of a child's average BP (from three visits) to a comprehensive table that provides threshold values for elevated (traditionally, BP between the 90th and 95th percentiles), hypertension (BP between the 95th and 99th percentiles), and severe hypertension (99th percentile or higher).

## GENDER AND HYPERTENSION

Hypertension is a major problem for both men and women, but men tend to develop it at an earlier age (Fig. 46.5), which is also true of the adverse clinical consequences of hypertension. Among individuals older than 70 years, women are more likely to have hypertension[1,22] and to have a CV event compared with men. Age and body mass index have been much stronger predictors of incident hypertension than gender in epidemiologic studies. Drug treatment of hypertension has roughly the same benefits for women and men.[28,29]

## RACE AND ETHNICITY AND HYPERTENSION

Similar to previous surveys, NHANES 2011–2014 concluded that non-Hispanic blacks had approximately a 50% higher prevalence of hypertension than non-Hispanic whites, even after age adjustment (41.2% vs. 28.0%).[22] The prevalence of hypertension in either non-Hispanic Asians or Hispanics was slightly but not significantly lower (at 24.9% and 25.9%, respectively) than in non-Hispanic whites. The prevalence of hypertension is geographically heterogeneous, with the highest prevalence in both blacks and whites in the southeastern United States (the so-called stroke belt). Perhaps because of persistent public health initiatives, non-Hispanic blacks had the highest awareness (at 85.7%) and treatment (at 77.4%) of hypertension in NHANES 2011–2012, but their BP control rate in 2011–2014 lagged behind that of non-Hispanic whites (48.5% to 55.7%, age-adjusted). This pattern has been consistent over the last decade.

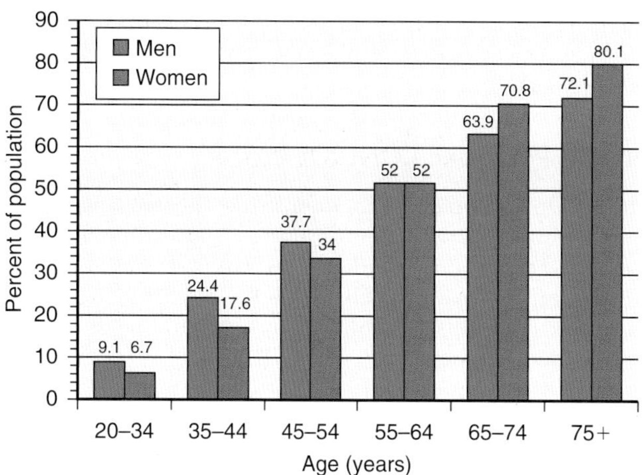


**Fig. 46.5** Prevalence of high blood pressure in US adults (≥20 years of age) by age and gender, according to the National Health and Nutrition Examination Surveys 2007–2010.

Although the prevalence of hypertension has increased between NHANES 1988–1991 and 2011–2014, the increase was greatest for non-Hispanic blacks compared with Mexican Americans or non-Hispanic whites. In contrast to non-Hispanic whites and Mexican Americans, a slightly higher prevalence of hypertension was observed in NHANES 2011–2014 for non-Hispanic black women, compared with men (41.5% vs. 40.8%). In all three racial and ethnic groups, women had higher rates of awareness, treatment, and control of BP than men in NHANES 2011–2014.

Perhaps because of the persistent historical difference in BP control rates, the adverse long-term consequences of hypertension are still more common in blacks than whites, but disparities have decreased in the last decade.[1] In 2014, the age-adjusted death rate from heart disease was 24% higher in blacks, as was stroke (by 41%) and hypertension or hypertensive renal disease (by 111%).[5] Incident ESKD was 3.1 or 1.2 times more common in 2014 in blacks or Native Americans, compared with whites.[30] Although diuretics or calcium channel blockers (CCBs) may have an advantage as initial therapy for reducing CV events in blacks, an angiotensin-converting enzyme (ACE) inhibitor was better than either a CCB or a beta-blocker in preventing the decline of renal function in African-Americans with hypertensive nephrosclerosis.[1,29,31] Most current hypertension guidelines therefore recommend controlling BP with multidrug regimens in all racial and ethnic groups.[11,13,32,33]

Although the prevalence of hypertension in Hispanics is lower than in non-Hispanic blacks and whites, hypertension is a concern. Mexican Americans continue to have the lowest age-adjusted prevalence of controlled hypertension in both men and women (25.6% and 31.9%, respectively, in NHANES 1999–2006, compared with 37.0% and 49.2% in NHANES 2007–2014).[1]

## BLOOD PRESSURE CONTROL RATES

Despite major progress in identifying the risks associated with elevated BP and demonstration that reducing BP to within a certain range reduces the risk for death from CV disease and stroke, as well as kidney disease progression, improved methods of achieving and sustaining BP control are needed. We have more than 125 different medications, most of which are generically available, from 8 different antihypertensive drug classes, to help lower BP, as well as more than 20 fixed-dose combination single-pill agents. In spite of this, BP control remains suboptimal in many parts of the world.[2,3,16,22,34,35]

BP control rates (to <140/90 mm Hg) have improved substantially in the United States since 1974 (Fig. 46.6) and have stabilized at just over 50% in the last four biennial NHANES reports.[1] Successful national efforts to increase hypertension treatment and control rates have been associated with significant reductions in CV hospitalizations or death in both Canada[35] and the United Kingdom.[36]

The prevalence of uncontrolled hypertension is greater for undiagnosed, untreated, or older individuals and for systolic (rather than diastolic) BP. Some health care delivery organizations have reported BP control rates in excess of 60% to 80%.[37] These improvements in BP control have been attributed to system improvements that routinely call the health care provider's attention to the uncontrolled BP at every clinical encounter, development of a registry of hypertensive patients, increasing convenience for BP measurements, and more widespread use of fixed-dose combination single-pill therapy.[37]

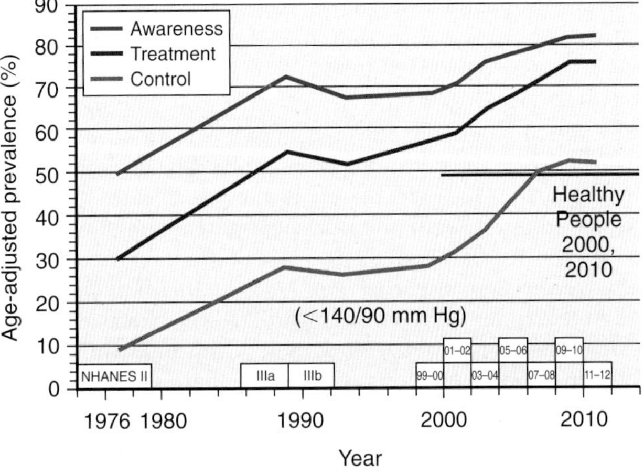


**Fig. 46.6** Awareness, treatment, and control of hypertension to less than 140/90 mm Hg in US National Health and Nutrition Examination Surveys (NHANES), from 1973 to 2012. The *horizontal line* at 50%, starting at the year 2000, corresponds to the national target for hypertension control promulgated by Healthy People 2000 and 2010, which has been increased to 61.2% by Healthy People 2020. The *small numbers* (e.g., IIIa, IIIb, 99-00) in boxes just above the *x*-axis of the figure reflect the nomenclature of the NHANES data collection period.

The wisdom of controlling BP over a relatively short time course after its discovery, rather than taking months to do so, has been most clearly demonstrated in the Valsartan Antihypertensive Long-term Use Evaluation (VALUE) trial.[38] Although the randomized comparison was between high-risk patients with hypertension who received valsartan or amlodipine initially, prevention of CV events was clearly better among individuals who achieved their goal BP during the first 6 months of treatment, regardless of initial randomized therapy. Similar long-term benefits of early control of BP have been seen for stroke or CV events in the Systolic Hypertension in Europe trial[39] and for death in the Systolic Hypertension in the Elderly Program (SHEP).[40]

## ECONOMICS OF HYPERTENSION

Although greater availability of generic antihypertensive medications (including every class except renin inhibitors) has greatly reduced the cost of treatment in the United States, limited financial resources and drug shortages have always been a major concern in the rest of the world. Even in the United States, restricted formularies, prior authorization processes, "step-edits" (which start with the most cost-effective drug therapy and progress to more costly therapies as necessary), and other barriers to prescribing and dispensing limit overall BP control rates. Currently, many of the single-pill combinations are priced generically, and the cost is often less than what would be paid for the individual components, purchased separately. Many single-pill combinations that include a thiazide diuretic cost no more than the nondiuretic component alone.

A proper analysis of the economics of hypertension and its treatment should include more than what is spent on drugs, patient visits, and/or laboratory tests.[41] For many high-risk patients, the expensive complications of untreated hypertension far outweigh the inconvenience and costs associated with effective treatment. For the United States in 2012–2013, hypertension was expected to cost approximately $51.2 billion (related to CV disease)[1] and roughly another $58 billion related to CKD in 2014,[30] although there is an undefined overlap (e.g., a hypertensive patient with CKD who is hospitalized for heart failure). Antihypertensive drugs cost approximately $19.7 billion or 18% of the total expenditures for hypertension. This proportion of expenditures has decreased steadily over the last decade due to wider use of generics, which recently constituted about 90% of the dispensed antihypertensive medications in the United States.

## PATHOPHYSIOLOGY

The physiology that generates BP involves the integration of cardiac output (CO) and systemic vascular resistance (SVR):

$$BP = CO \times SVR$$

Each of these parameters has its own determinants:

$$CO = \text{heart rate} \times \text{stroke volume}$$
$$SVR = 80 \times (\text{mean arterial pressure} - \text{central venous pressure})/CO$$

This view is simplified, but it provides a framework to define the relevant factors in BP regulation. Changes in CO typically produce short-lived BP changes (hours to days) as adaptive mechanisms adjust SVR to normalize BP. However, changes in SVR are able to produce sustained increases in BP. The following sections summarize relevant mechanisms leading to BP regulation.

## PRESSURE NATRIURESIS AND SALT SENSITIVITY

A key factor in the regulation of BP as a factor of CO and SVR is the phenomenon of pressure natriuresis. Pressure natriuresis is defined as the increase in renal sodium excretion because of mild increases in BP, typically due to extracellular fluid volume expansion, allowing BP to remain in the normal range.[42–44] This concept is essential to the understanding of the sustainability of hypertension. If one understands the set point BP as the BP at the point when extracellular volume and pressure natriuresis are in equilibrium, it necessarily follows that a change in BP can only be sustained if pressure natriureis is abnormal. Pressure natriuresis occurs over hours to days and is modulated by biophysical and humoral factors.

In the normal state, increased sodium intake causes an increase in extracellular volume and BP. Because of the steep relationship between volume and pressure, small increases in BP produce natriuresis that restores sodium balance and returns BP to normal (Fig. 46.7). Expansion of extracellular fluid volume and increased BP result in a rise in blood flow through the vasa recta, which stimulates the production of paracrine factors such as nitric oxide (NO) and adenosine triphosphate (ATP), which can inhibit tubular sodium reabsorption at multiple sites of the nephron.[45] Nitric oxide also blunts the myogenic response of arteriolar autoregulation, thus allowing increased blood flow, which is necessary to increase renal blood flow and interstitial pressure (see later).[44,45]

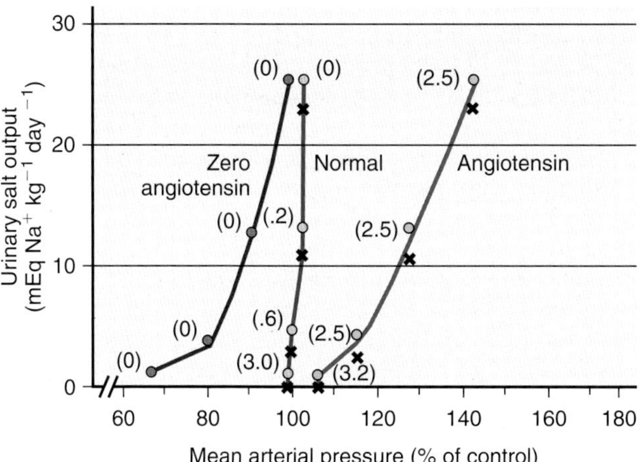


**Fig. 46.7** Pressure natriuresis curves in dogs at different levels of sodium intake (reflected in urinary salt output, *y*-axis). In the normal state, massive fluctuations in sodium intake produce minimal changes in blood pressure (BP). In states of high angiotensin II (Ang II) levels (Ang II infusion in this model), BP increases significantly, even with modest increases in sodium intake. Conversely, in states where Ang II is absent or low (administration of captopril in this model), the increased sodium results in increased BP only at low BP levels; once BP becomes normal, the relationship is similar to that of normal kidneys. Values in *parentheses* are the relative estimated concentrations of Ang II (1 being the reference). (From Elliott W. Economic considerations in hypertension management. In: Izzo JL J, Black HR, eds. Hypertension Primer. Dallas: American Heart Association; 2008; 331–334.)

The ability of the kidneys to adjust to sodium loading is remarkable, adapting to fluctuations in sodium intake as high as 50-fold,[43] but this response is markedly blunted in the setting of chronic hypertension, resulting in a need for much higher BP levels to promote natriuresis. These states of abnormal sodium handling lead to sodium-sensitive hypertension, such as in conditions of a reduced glomerular filtration rate (GFR) or high levels of Ang II (see Fig. 46.7). In such situations, the change in extracellular fluid volume is relatively small (3%–5%), but a state of chronic high BP develops, resulting from increased SVR. The mechanisms responsible for this vascular effect are not completely understood but likely involve increased activity of the renin-angiotensin-aldosterone system (RAAS; high Ang II level) and several other vasoconstricting substances,[44] as will be discussed later in this section.

The pressure natriuresis process is also mediated by biophysical factors. Increased renal interstitial hydrostatic pressure is an important factor. Sodium loading results in increased pressure in the vasa recta, which have noticeably poor autoregulation, whereas pressure in cortical peritubular capillaries remains normal.[46,47] Vasa recta blood flow approximates 10% of total renal blood flow. This increase in interstitial pressure inhibits sodium transport largely by increasing 20-hydroxyeicosatetraenoic acid, a lipoxygenase product of arachidonic acid and an inhibitor of the sodium-potassium adenosine triphosphatase ($Na^+$-$K^+$-ATPase), whose inhibition causes decreased activity of the $Na^+$-$H^+$-exchanger isoform 3 (NHE3).[46] In addition, increased interstitial pressure limits proximal tubular paracellular pathways, thus maximizing natriuresis.

Because abnormalities in pressure-sodium relationships are essential to maintaining chronic elevations in BP, they represent a fundamental step in the pathogenesis of any type of hypertension—not only primary, but also in the maintenance phase of most secondary causes, such as renal and renovascular hypertension, hyperaldosteronism, glucocorticoid excess, coarctation of the aorta, and pheochromocytoma.

The interplay between renal sodium retention and hypertension involves changes in sodium handling throughout the nephron. A theory with substantial experimental support has proposed that increased renal vasoconstriction due to a variety of possible mechanisms (e.g., increased levels of angiotensin II, catecholamines, or uric acid, progressive aging) induces a preglomerular (afferent) arteriolopathy that results in impaired sodium filtration.[48,49] In addition, renal vasoconstriction results in tubular ischemia, another mediator of increased sodium avidity.

## GENETICS OF HYPERTENSION

Hypertension clusters in families; an individual with a family history of hypertension has a fourfold greater chance of developing hypertension,[50] and it has been estimated that the heritability of hypertension ranges from 31% to 68%. Genome-wide association studies (GWAS) in several multinational cohorts have identified a large number of single-nucleotide polymorphisms (SNPs) associated with hypertension.[51] However, these individual SNPs are responsible for only minor BP effects (0.5–1 mm Hg), and the overall impact of these identified SNPs on the overall BP variance is only approximately 1% to 2%.[50] Among these genes, *FOS* (fos protooncogene) and *PTGS2* (cyclooxygenase-2 [COX-2]) have been replicated in a number of studies. There are many shortcomings of the use of GWAS and other large population approaches.[52] For example, the SNP platforms used for testing are not hypothesis-driven; they simply include common genetic variants for exploratory analyses that might provide clues for molecular pathways leading to better understanding of disease or new targets for therapy.

To advance this use in the progress toward personalized medicine in hypertension, a recent GWAS based on the large United Kingdom Biobank Study cohort also performed functional and transcript expression analyses of candidate genes in target tissues in vitro (vascular smooth muscle cells, aortic fibroblasts, and endothelial cells), with the goal of identifying potential therapeutic targets.[51] The study also developed and validated an unbiased genetic risk score that included clinical and genotype information, including data on 107 independent risk loci to generate estimates of the risk of hypertension and the risk of specific hypertension-related outcomes (e.g., stroke, coronary disease, any cardiovascular outcome). These analyses showed a gender-adjusted systolic BP difference of 9.3 mm Hg between the lowest and highest risk quintile (higher in the high-risk group, which also had 2.3-fold greater odds of hypertension and a 1.35-fold increase in the odds of any cardiovascular outcome).[51] These results indicate the potential value for genetic risk-based clinical scoring.

BP measurement is another important concern, as it is not uniform in these very large, population-based GWAS. In addition, large numbers of patients are receiving treatment at the time of testing, thus limiting the strength of any associations. Finally, hypertensive phenotypes are not well defined, so patients with very different phenotypes (e.g., isolated diastolic hypertension, isolated systolic hypertension of the young, isolated systolic hypertension of older adults) are all lumped together.[53] We now understand that each of these phenotypes likely has different underlying pathophysiologic mechanisms, and that even within each group there is substantial variability in a hemodynamic profile.[54,55]

With the improvement in techniques that allow expeditious and cheaper whole-exome or whole-genome analyses and the expansion of precision medicine, it is possible that greater mechanistic insights on the genetics of hypertension will become available. Unfortunately, compared with other clinical phenotypes, the heavy influence of lifestyle and environmental factors in hypertension makes it unlikely that the simple analysis of genome sequence will have a great impact on hypertension.[56] Instead, the systematic evaluation of epigenetic modifications associated with detailed functional phenotyping is more likely to allow us to move forward in the understanding of this complex interplay in patients with primary hypertension.[56,57]

Whereas the attempts at using current genetic approaches to understand essential hypertension in general have not been very fruitful, the study of monogenic hypertension has. Monogenic causes of hypertension, although rare, have provided substantial insight into the pathogenesis of hypertension. Of the monogenic forms of hypertension with well-described molecular mechanisms, all have one thing in common—a defect in renal sodium handling. This commonality points to the primacy of the kidney in regulating BP by way of sodium balance.

In Liddle syndrome, mutations in the epithelial sodium channel (ENaC) lead to increased ENaC expression and decreased channel removal from the luminal membrane, both of which contribute to persistent channel activation. This leads to sodium avidity, volume expansion, hypertension, hypokalemia, and metabolic alkalosis with suppressed aldosterone levels.[58]

In Gordon syndrome (pseudohypoaldosteronism type 2), a variety of mutations have been described leading to changes in the function of the thiazide-sensitive sodium-chloride cotransporter (NCC).[58] These mutations were initially mapped to the with-no-lysine (WNK) kinases 1 and 4, which regulate NCC phosphorylation and activity. Mutations in two E3 ubiquitin ligase complex proteins (kelchlike 3 and cullin 3) were discovered later.[59] These mutations are responsible for most cases of the syndrome. The presumed mechanism is related to decreased channel ubiquitination—and therefore persistent presence in the luminal membrane and augmented sodium removal from the tubular fluid—leading to the clinical phenotype of hypertension, hyperkalemia, and metabolic acidosis.

Mutations in the mineralocorticoid receptor can also produce hypertensive syndromes, such as hypertension exacerbated by pregnancy (Geller syndrome), in which there is constitutive activity of the receptor in addition to marked sensitivity to progesterone, leading to hypertension during pregnancy in addition to chronic severe hypertension with hypokalemia.[60] Likewise, increases in the aldosterone level due to a chimeric gene duplication involving the 11β-hydroxylase and the aldosterone synthase genes result in control of aldosterone synthase by adrenocorticotropic hormone (ACTH), independently of sodium balance or angiotensin II (Ang II) or serum potassium levels. Such patients have hyperaldosteronism that is only blunted by ACTH suppression—thus, the term "glucocorticoid-remediable hyperaldosteronism."[61]

Other patients may have apparent mineralocorticoid excess due to mutations in the 11β-hydroxysteroid dehydrogenase type 2 gene. This enzyme is responsible for the conversion of cortisol to the inactive cortisone in target epithelia, including the kidneys. As a result, excess cortisol, which is 1000-fold more abundant in blood than aldosterone, is available to activate the mineralocorticoid receptor, leading to a state of apparent mineralocorticoid excess (salt-sensitive hypertension, hypokalemia, metabolic alkalosis) in the absence of aldosterone.

Similarly, patients with congenital adrenal hyperplasia due to 11β-hydroxylase or 17α-hydroxylase deficiency have an excess production of 21-hydroxylated steroids such as deoxycorticosterone and corticosterone, which are potent activators of the mineralocorticoid receptor. Thus, also the syndrome of apparent mineralocorticoid excess is also produced, in addition to the well-known sexual developmental abnormalities of the syndromes.[62] Taken together, this is strong evidence of the importance of renal sodium handling in the genesis of hypertension.

It must be noted, however, that the recent elucidation of the molecular genetics of the rare syndrome of autosomal hypertension with brachydactyly points to a vascular cause that does not involve the kidney.[63] This is a monogenic form of salt-independent and age-related hypertension transmitted via gain-of-function mutations in the phosphodiasterase 3A gene (*PDE3A*), which results in increased protein kinase A–mediated PDE3A phosphorylation and increased cyclic adenosine monophosphate (cAMP) hydrolytic activity. These cellular actions result in enhanced cell proliferation in fibroblasts and vascular smooth muscle and dysregulated parathyroid hormone–related peptide physiology, accounting for the hypertensive and skeletal phenotypes.[63]

## NONOSMOTIC SODIUM STORAGE

The paradigm of sodium balance described earlier assumes that sodium and its accompanying anion are osmotically active and therefore retained isosmotically with water. However, this paradigm cannot explain the observation that acute sodium loading in humans and animals results in positive sodium balance, without the expected water (weight) gain. Consequently, sodium may accumulate without water, most prominently in the skin,[64] where negatively charged glycosaminoglycans bind sodium.[65] This system of interstitial sodium buffering adds to the classical Guytonian approach, wherein nonosmotic accumulation occurs acutely and is presumably followed by increased removal from skin (via an enhanced lymphatic network) for ultimate renal excretion.

The mechanisms explaining isosmotic sodium storage have been under intense investigation.[66] Mice and rats receiving a high-salt diet develop hypertonicity of the skin interstitium, which triggers a series of mechanisms to keep interstitial volume constant.[67] The hypertonic sodium content activates the tonicity-responsive enhancer-binding protein (TonEBP) present in mononuclear cells infiltrating the skin. Consequently, these skin macrophages act as local osmosensors and secrete vascular endothelial growth factor type C, resulting in increased density and hyperplasia of the skin lymphocapillary network and increased endothelial nitric oxide synthase (eNOS). If these responses are blocked, salt-sensitive hypertension develops.[67,68] These findings link the mononuclear phagocyte system to extracellular fluid volume control.

The translation of these findings into clinical implications was addressed in a study evaluating sodium balance in cosmonauts undergoing prolonged training (up to 205 days) in a facility simulating life in space.[69] By carefully monitoring water and electrolyte intake and excretion, as well as factors regulating sodium balance, these individuals exhibited a large variability in sodium excretion on a daily basis, despite relatively stable diets. In the long term, approximately 95% (70%–103%) of ingested sodium was recovered, but daily sodium excretion during stable sodium intake varied considerably and was independent of BP and sodium intake. Instead, urine sodium excretion varied as a function of circaseptan fluctuations (6–9 days in this case) in levels of aldosterone, cortisol, and cortisone. Moreover, total body sodium stores had even longer infradian variations (averaging several weeks).

The factors regulating these intriguing changes are still unknown. These observations have clinical implications for the use of urine sodium excretion to assess sodium intake because they suggest wide daily variations that cannot be captured in a single 24-hour urine collection.[69]

## RENIN-ANGIOTENSIN-ALDOSTERONE SYSTEM

The RAAS has wide-ranging effects on BP regulation. Fig. 46.8 summarizes the most relevant elements of the RAAS and its role in the pathogenesis of hypertension and its complications (see Chapter 11 for greater detail). The different elements of the RAAS have key roles in mediating sodium retention, pressure natriuresis, salt sensitivity, vasoconstriction, endothelium dysfunction, and vascular injury, and the use of RAAS blockers is an effective means of treating hypertension. Taken together, the RAAS has an important role in the pathogenesis of hypertension. However, there are some still unanswered issues about this relationship. For example, in a very large GWAS of 2.5 million genotyped or imputed SNPs in 69,395 individuals of European ancestry from 29 studies,[70] the meta-analysis showed that most SNPs involved issues with natriuretic peptide abnormalities. Thus, these hormones play a prominent role in the pathogenesis of hypertension and may be more important than the RAAS system, which did not have prominent SNPs associated with this analysis. Another meta-analysis evaluating the relationship between polymorphisms in key RAAS genes (ACE, AGT, and CYP11B2) and salt sensitivity also found no significant role for these polymorphisms.[71]

Despite these genetic inconsistencies, there is a wealth of experimental evidence linking the RAAS to hypertension, which we review concisely later. In addition, a classic paradigm has been to highlight the role of the circulating (systemic) RAAS. However, it is known that tissue expression of different elements of the RAAS is also important, including the protection of animals from the development of hypertension after targeted elimination of renal ACE activity.[72] Interestingly, these very same experiements have also indicated that the absence of ACE in other tissues may also be protective from hypertension caused by triggers that do not involve the RAAS (e.g., nitric oxide inhibition), therefore raising the possibility that other (extrarenal) sites may also be relevant.[73]

Renin and prorenin are synthesized and stored in the juxtaglomerular cell apparatus and released in response to decreased renal afferent perfusion pressure, decreased sodium delivery to the macula densa, activation of renal nerves (via $\beta_1$-adrenergic receptor stimulation), and a variety of metabolic products, including prostaglandin E2 and several others. The main function of renin is to cleave angiotensinogen into angiotensin I. Prorenin, previously regarded as an inactive substrate for renin production, is known to also stimulate the (pro)renin receptor (PRR). This receptor leads to more efficient cleavage of angiotensinogen and activates downstream intracellular signaling through the mitogen-activated protein (MAP) kinases extracellular signal–regulated kinases 1 and 2 (ERK1/2) pathways that have been associated with profibrotic effects in some, but not all, experimental models.[74–76] It is still uncertain if the PRR is involved in the genesis or complications of hypertension in a manner that is independent of the effects of Ang II .[74]

Angiotensin II, formed by the cleavage of angiotensin I by ACE, is at the center of the pathogenetic role of the RAAS in hypertension. Primarily through its actions mediated by the Ang II type 1 receptor (AT1R), Ang II is a potent vasoconstrictor of vascular smooth muscle, causing systemic vasoconstriction and increased renovascular resistance and decreased medullary flow, which is a mediator of salt sensitivity.

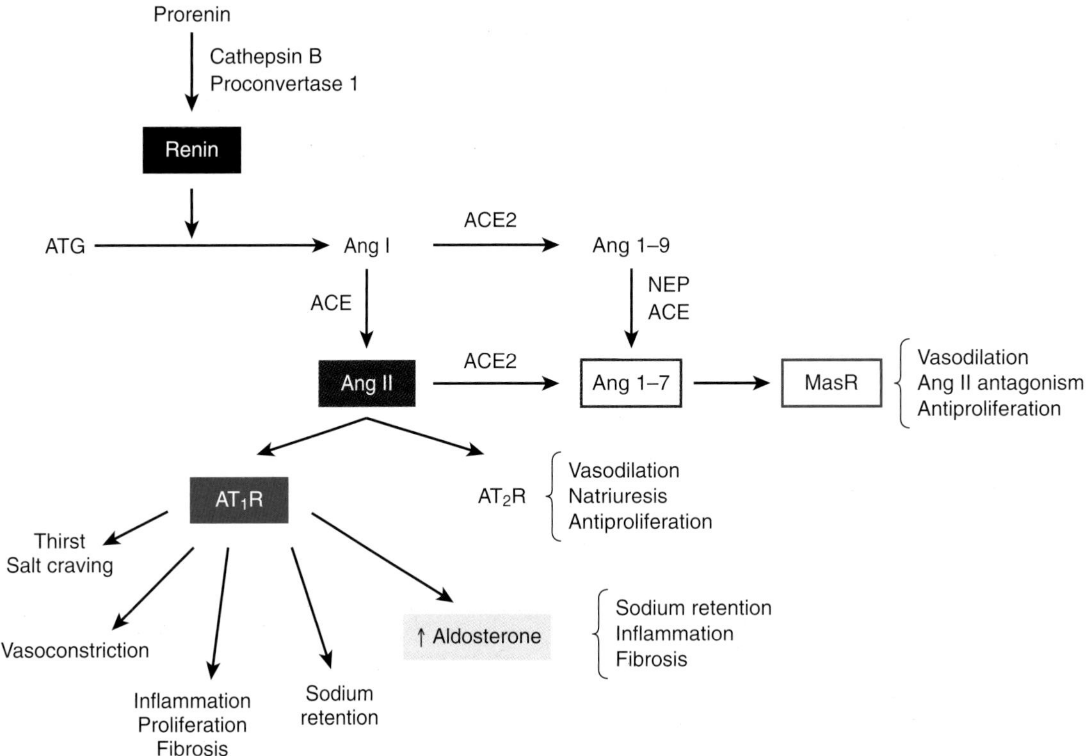


**Fig. 46.8** Key elements of the renin-angiotensin-aldosterone system. *ACE,* Angiotensin-converting enzyme; *ACE2,* Angiotensin-converting enzyme type 2; *Ang,* angiotensin; *ATG,* angiotensinogen; *$AT_1R$,* Ang II type 1 receptor; *$AT_2R$,* Ang II type 2 receptor; *MasR,* Mas receptor; *NEP,* neutral endopeptidase.

It produces increased sodium reabsorption in the proximal tubule by increasing the activity of NHE3, the sodium-bicarbonate exchanger, and $Na^+$-$K^+$-ATPase and by inducing aldosterone synthesis and release from the adrenal zona glomerulosa. In addition, it is associated with endothelial cell dysfunction and produces extensive profibrotic and proinflammatory changes, largely mediated by increased oxidative stress, resulting in renal, cardiac, and vascular injury, thus giving Ang II a tight link to target organ injury in hypertension. Conversely, stimulation of the Ang II type 2 receptor (AT2R) is associated with opposite effects, resulting in vasodilation, natriuresis, and antiproliferative effects.

The relative importance of the renal and vascular effects of Ang II has been evaluated in classic cross-transplantation studies using both wild-type mice and mice lacking the AT1R.[77,78] By cross-transplanting the kidneys of wild-type mice into AT1R knockout mice and vice versa, investigators were able to generate animals that were selective renal AT1R knockouts or selective systemic (nonrenal) AT1R knockouts. In physiologic conditions, renal, systemic, and total knockout animals had lower BP than wild-type animals, indicating a role of both renal and extrarenal AT1R in BP regulation.[78] The systemic AT1R absence was associated with approximately 50% lower aldosterone levels, but the lower BP observed in this group was independent of this lower aldosterone production. This was because BP remained low, despite aldosterone infusions to supraphysiologic levels following adrenalectomy in the systemic knockout animals. In addition, the BP reduction in kidney knockout animals occurred despite normal aldosterone excretion, again confirming the importance of aldosterone-independent renal Ang II effects.

In the hypertensive environment, it is the presence of renal AT1R that mediates hypertension and organ injury[78] (Fig. 46.9). When animals were infused with Ang II for 4 weeks, animals lacking renal AT1R did not develop sustained hypertension, whereas wild-type and systemic knockout mice had a significant increase in BP. Additionally, only animals with elevated BP developed cardiac hypertrophy and fibrosis. This indicates that cardiac injury is largely dependent on hypertension and not on the presence of AT1R in the heart, because the (hypertensive) systemic knockout animals developed significant cardiac abnormalities, despite the absence of AT1R in the heart.[77] In summary, these experiments have indicated that both systemic and renal actions of Ang II are relevant to physiologic BP regulation but, in hypertension, the detrimental effects of Ang II are mediated via its renal effects.

It must be understood that there may be a role for extrarenal RAAS activation in hypertension, albeit likely less important than its renal role.[72,73] Because Ang II is necessary for normal renal development, experimental manipulation of the intrarenal RAAS demands the presence of some level of activity of the system. In experiments where the ACE gene was knocked out systemically then reintroduced in myelomonocytic cells, there was no demonstrable renal ACE activity, but the systemic levels generated from the myelomonocytic cells were enough to allow normal renal development.[72] These animals, with absent renal ACE activity, have markedly blunted hypertensive responses to the infusion of Ang II or N(ω)-nitro-L-arginine methyl ester (L-NAME, a low-renin, Ang II–independent model of hypertension). At face value, this indicates that the absence of renal ACE protects against

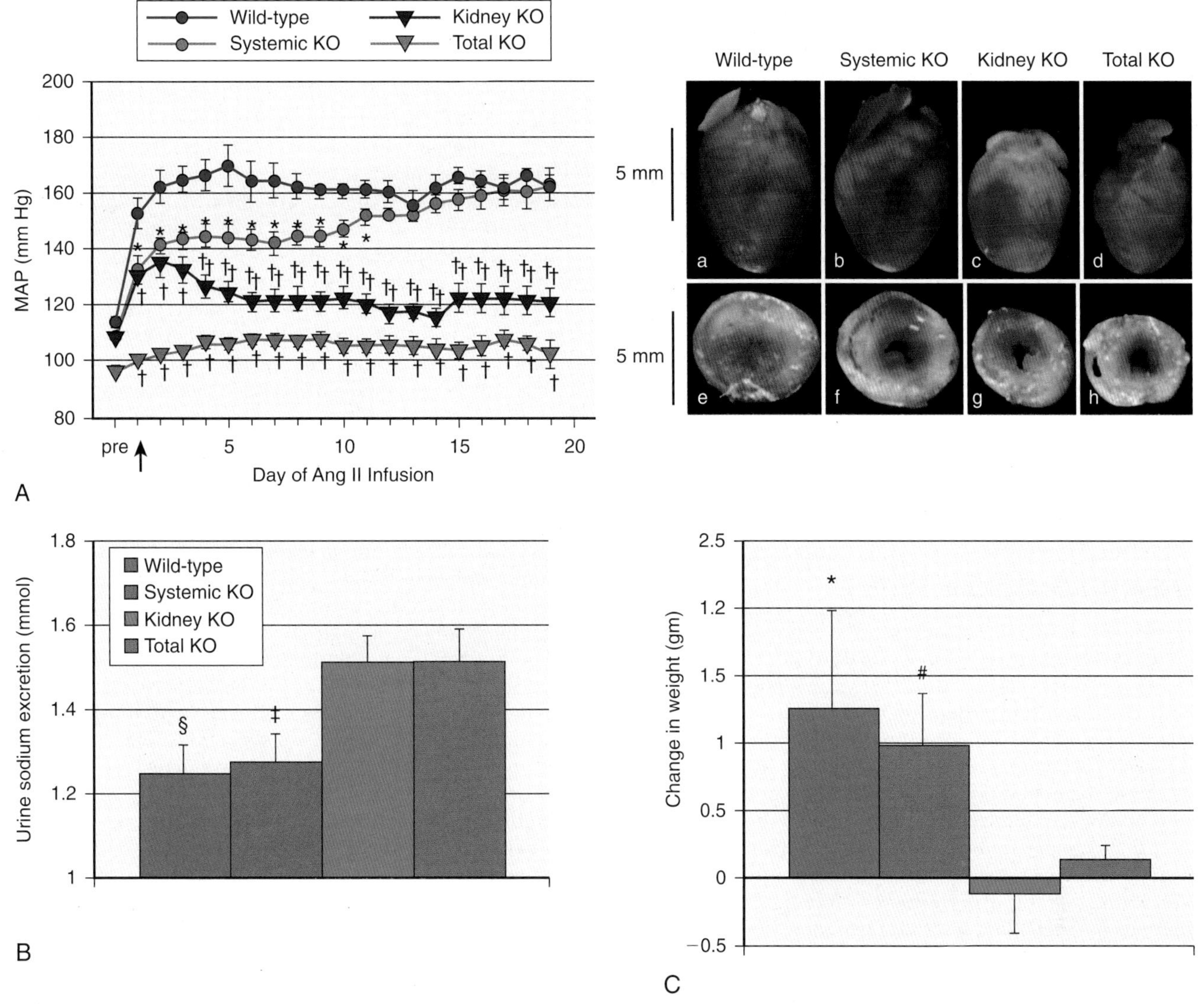


**Fig. 46.9** Effects of angiotensin II *(Ang II)* infusion on blood pressure (A), urinary sodium excretion (B), body weight (C), and cardiac hypertrophy (photos) according to renal and extrarenal presence of Ang II type 1 receptor. See text for details. *KO,* Knockout; *MAP,* mean arterial pressure. (From Crowley SD, Gurley SB, Herrera MJ, et al. Ang II causes hypertension and cardiac hypertrophy through its receptors in the kidney. *Proc Natl Acad Sci U S A.* 2006;103:17985–17990.)

hypertension, regardless of the plasma Ang II levels. This is an unexpected finding given the traditional view of the RAAS, in which an infusion of Ang II bypasses ACE and produces sustained hypertension, regardless of ACE activity,[79] but well in line with the growing evidence for the importance of ACE-induced intrarenal tubular generation of Ang II in the mediation of hypertension. However, because ACE was not expressed in other organs, it is also possible that the hypotensive effects of the absence of ACE activity was the result of the absence of an effect in other locations, such as the vasculature.[73,80] This question remains unanswered while developments continue to occur in the understanding of the function of tissue RAAS (especially intrarenal). This system has different regulators from the systemic RAAS and, differently from the endocrine RAAS, has feed-forward mechanisms that generate further augmentation of local responses on activation by the circulating RAAS.[80]

Aldosterone, the adrenocortical hormone synthesized in the zona glomerulosa, plays a critical role in hypertension through its well-known effects on sodium reabsorption that are largely mediated by transcriptional effects via activation of the mineralocorticoid receptor, leading to increased expression of ENaC. An extensive body of literature has identified other genomic and nongenomic effects of aldosterone with relevance to hypertension. Extensive nonepithelial effects include vascular smooth muscle cell proliferation, vascular extracellular matrix deposition, vascular remodeling and fibrosis, and increased oxidative stress, leading to endothelial dysfunction and vasoconstriction.[81]

Several other elements of the RAAS have been identified as having potentially important roles in hypertension. The importance of ACE2 and Ang–1-7 to BP regulation and Ang II–associated target organ injury has become apparent. ACE2 is expressed largely in heart, kidney, and endothelium; it has partial homology to ACE and is unaffected directly by ACE inhibitors.[82] It has a variety of substrates, but its most important action is the conversion of Ang II to Ang–1-7. Ang–1-7 is formed primarily though the hydrolysis of Ang

II by ACE2. Its actions are opposite to those of Ang II, including vasodilatory and antiproliferative properties mediated by the Mas receptor, a G protein–coupled receptor that on activation, forms complexes with the AT1R, thus antagonizing the effects of Ang II. The vasodilatory effects are mediated by increased cyclic guanosine monophosphate (cGMP), decreased norepinephrine release, and amplification of bradykinin effects. Studies have identified ACE2 and Ang–1-7 as protective factors in the development of atherosclerosis and cardiac and renal injury.[82,83] The administration of recombinant ACE2 or its activator, xanthenone, has resulted in improved endothelial function, decreased BP, and improved renal, cardiac, and perivascular fibrosis in hypertensive animals.[84–86] However, a phase 1 study of recombinant ACE2 in healthy humans did not show any BP-lowering effects, despite appropriate modulation of the RAAS, including a sustained increase in Ang–1-7 levels.[87] Therefore, the clinical value of the manipulation of any of the elements of this vasodepressor component of the RAAS remains to be determined.[88]

## SYMPATHETIC NERVOUS SYSTEM

The sympathetic nervous system (SNS) is activated consistently in patients with hypertension compared with normotensive individuals, particularly in those who are obese (Fig. 46.10). Many patients with hypertension are in a state of autonomic imbalance that encompasses increased sympathetic and decreased parasympathetic activity.[89,90] SNS hyperactivity is relevant to the generation and maintenance of hypertension and is observed in human hypertensives from the very earliest stages. For example, studies in humans have identified markers of sympathetic overactivity in normotensive individuals with a family history of hypertension.[89] Among patients with hypertension, increasing severity of hypertension is associated with increasing levels of sympathetic activity as measured by microneurography.[91,92] In human hypertension, plasma catecholamine levels, microneurographic recordings, and systemic catecholamine spillover studies have consistently found elevation of these markers in obesity, the metabolic syndrome, and hypertension complicated by heart failure or kidney disease.[89] In addition, SNS hyperactivity is observed in most hypertensive subgroups, although it appears more pronounced in men than in women and in younger than in older patients.

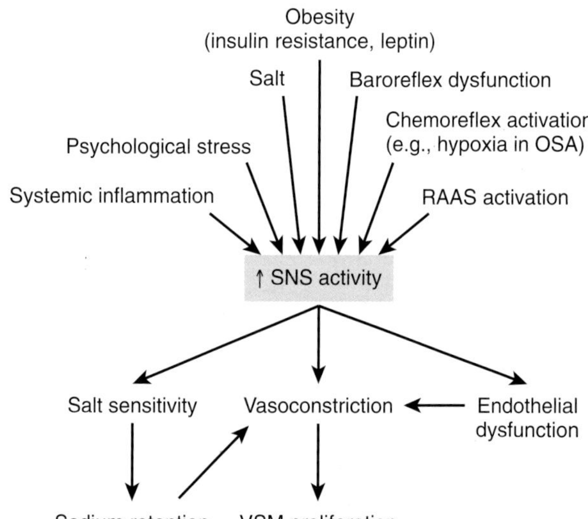


**Fig. 46.10** Causes and consequences of sympathetic nervous system activation in the pathogenesis of hypertension. *OSA,* Obstructive sleep apnea; *RAAS,* renin-angiotensin- aldosterone system; *SNS,* sympathetic nervous system; *VSM,* vascular smooth muscle.

Several experimental models have outlined the importance of the SNS in generating hypertension. Different models of obesity-related hypertension have indicated that the SNS is activated early in the development of increased adiposity,[90] and the key factor in the maintenance of sustained hypertension is increased renal sympathetic nerve activity and its attendant sodium avidity.[90]

SNS-mediated induction of salt sensitivity is a key element for sustaining high BP in other models of hypertension as well. For example, rats receiving daily infusions of phenylephrine for 8 weeks developed hypertension during the infusions, but BP normalized under a low-salt diet after discontinuation of phenylephrine.[93] However, once exposed to a high-salt diet, the animals again became hypertensive. The degree of BP elevation on a high-salt diet was directly related to the degree of renal tubulointerstitial fibrosis and decrement of GFR. These findings can be interpreted within the paradigm that catecholamine-induced hypertension causes renal interstitial injury that is associated with a salt-sensitive phenotype, even after sympathetic overactivity is no longer present.[93] In addition, enhanced SNS activity results in $\alpha_1$ receptor–mediated endothelial dysfunction, vasoconstriction, vascular smooth muscle proliferation, and arterial stiffness, all of which contribute to the development of hypertension. Finally, studies have shown that sympathetic overactivity results in salt sensitivity due to a reduction in the activity of WNK4, which causes increased sodium avidity through the thiazide-sensitive NCC.[94] Fig. 46.10 summarizes the causes and consequences of SNS activation in the genesis of hypertension.

Renalase is a flavoprotein highly expressed in kidney and heart that metabolizes catecholamines and catecholamine-like substances to aminochrome.[95] Tissue and plasma renalase is decreased in experimental models with renal mass reduction, and renalase knockout mice have increased BP and elevated circulating catecholamine levels. A normal phenotype is restored by the administration of recombinant renalase. Also of relevance to catecholamine metabolism is catestatin, a product of the proteolysis of the neuroendocrine peptide chromogranin A.[96] Catestatin acts at nicotinic cholinergic receptors in adrenal chromaffin cells as an inhibitor of catecholamine release. Chromogranin A knockout mice are hypertensive and have elevated catecholamine levels, both of which are normalized by the administration of catestatin. Moreover, serum catestatin levels are decreased in patients with hypertension and their normotensive offspring, raising the possibility of a regulatory role in the development of hypertension. The role of renalase and catestatin in the modulation of SNS-mediated hypertension, as well as their possible value in the treatment of hypertension in humans, remains uncertain.

Because increased SNS activity is associated with vascular smooth muscle proliferation, LVH, large artery stiffness, myocardial ischemia, and arrhythmogenesis, there is also a mechanistic role for the SNS in the complications of hypertension. In support of this concept, several cohort studies have reported an association between physiologic or biochemical markers of SNS activation and adverse outcomes in heart failure, stroke, and ESKD.[89,97] However, there are no such studies among patients with hypertension, and the indirect evaluation of the impact of treatment-induced heart rate reduction in hypertension has yielded paradoxic results.

In a meta-analysis of hypertension trials, heart rate reduction during treatment with beta-blockers was associated with increased risk for death and CV events in patients with hypertension.[98] In contrast, in a very large ($n$ = 10,000) patient outcome trial, a post hoc analysis of heart rate at baseline has demonstrated that those with a resting heart rate above 80 beats/min, even with a BP below 140/90 mm Hg, had a higher mortality rate.[99] Therefore, although it is apparent that SNS activation is deleterious to patients with CV disease, and presumably with hypertension, a cause for the overactivity should be sought and an attempt made to affect that mechanism.

## OBESITY

Obesity-related hypertension is characterized primarily by impaired sodium excretion and endothelial dysfunction, both of which are dependent on SNS overactivity, activation of the RAAS, and increased oxidative stress.[89,100] Fat tissue in obesity is hypertrophied, meaning larger cells versus more cells, and marked by increased macrophage infiltration in the adipose tissue.[101] It is now well described; adipose tissue is not inert and secretes a wide range of cytokines and chemokines whose profile is abnormal in obesity, marked by increased levels of leptin, resistin, interleukin-6, and tumor necrosis factor-α secretion; elevated free fatty acid release; and reduced adiponectin levels. Decreased adiponectin level results in insulin resistance, decreased induction of eNOS, and possibly increased sympathetic activity.

Resistin impairs nitric oxide (NO) synthesis (eNOS inhibition) and enhances endothelin-1 (ET-1) production, shifting the vasodilation-vasoconstriction balance toward vasoconstriction. Hyperleptinemia directly stimulates the SNS through complex mechanisms that involve central leptin receptors, as well as activation of the pro-opiomelanocortin system (via the melanocortin 4 receptor).[100]

Finally, visceral adipocyte mass is directly correlated with aldosterone secretion by the zona glomerulosa, a process mediated by angiotensinogen production by adipocytes, as well as increased secretion of Wnt-signaling molecules that modulate steroidogenesis.[102–104] In addition, despite yet unclear mechanisms, there is consistent evidence that obese individuals tend to have lower natriuretic peptide levels than lean individuals,[100] and this relative deficiency is amplified in obese hypertensives.[105] All these factors compound the tendency toward sodium retention and shifting the pressure-natriuresis curve to the right. Activation of these same systems leads to a proinflammatory state related to increased reactive oxygen species, factors directly associated with endothelial dysfunction and vascular proliferation. Therefore, multiple mechanisms contribute to the development and maintenance of hypertension in obese individuals.

## NATRIURETIC PEPTIDES

Natriuretic peptides—atrial natriuretic peptide (ANP), brain natriuretic peptide (BNP), and urodilatin—play an important role in salt sensitivity, heart failure, and hypertension.[106] These peptides have important natriuretic and vasodilatory properties that allow maintenance of sodium balance and BP during sodium loading. On administration of a sodium load, atrial and ventricular stretch lead to the release of ANP and BNP, respectively, which result in immediate BP lowering due to systemic vasodilation and decreased plasma volume. The latter is caused by fluid shifts from the intravascular to the interstitial compartment.[107] All natriuretic peptides directly increase GFR, which in volume-expanded states is mediated by an increase in efferent arteriolar tone and increased $K_f$. They also inhibit renal sodium reabsorption through direct and indirect effects. Direct effects include decreased activity of $Na^+$-ATPase and the sodium-glucose cotransporter in the proximal tubule and inhibition of the ENaC in the distal nephron.[106] The inhibitory effects of natriuretic peptides on renin and aldosterone release mediate indirect effects. Unfortunately, understanding the contribution of natriuretic peptides to the development of hypertension in humans is complicated by the elevation of their levels in association with increased BP (due to increased afterload) and hypertensive heart disease.

Some studies have tested whether polymorphisms in ANP or BNP genes resulting in higher levels of these peptides would associate with lower BP; results of these studies have been inconsistent, and effects have been small.[108–110] There have been no published studies evaluating sequential changes in natriuretic peptides and risk for incident hypertension.

Attention has been given to corin, the serine protease that is largely expressed in the heart and converts pro-ANP and pro-BNP to their active forms. Corin activates ANP. Genetic variants and defects of the enzyme that activates corin have been found in people with hypertension, heart failure, and preeclampsia. Corin intereacts with natriuretic peptides and hence impaired corin intracellular trafficking, cell surface expression, and zymogen activation will result in fluid retention.[111,112] Experiments have suggested that states of corin deficiency are associated with sodium overload, heart failure, and salt-sensitive hypertension,[111,112] and recent clinical studies have observed an association between low corin levels and increased risk of adverse cardiovascular outcomes in patients with coronary disease, heart failure, and stroke.[111]

## THE ENDOTHELIUM

The endothelium is a major regulator of vascular tone and thus plays a key role in BP regulation. Endothelial cells produce a host of vasoactive substances, of which NO is the most important to BP regulation. NO is continuously released by endothelial cells, especially in response to flow-induced shear stress in arteries and arterioles, leading to vascular smooth muscle relaxation through the activation of guanylate cyclase and generation of intracellular cGMP.[113] Interruption of NO production via inhibition of the constitutively expressed eNOS causes BP elevation and development of hypertension in animals and humans. Using brachial artery flow-mediated vasodilation and measurement of urinary excretion of NO metabolites as methods to evaluate NO activity in humans, several studies have demonstrated decreased whole-body production of NO in patients with hypertension compared with normotensive controls.

Several elements are responsible for endothelial dysfunction in hypertension. Normotensive offspring of patients with hypertension have impaired endothelium-dependent vasodilation, despite normal endothelium-independent responses, thus suggesting a genetic component to the development of endothelial dysfunction.[114] Besides direct pressure-induced injury in the setting of chronically elevated BP, a mechanism of major importance is increased oxidative stress. Reactive oxygen species are generated from enhanced activity of several enzyme systems—reduced nicotinamide adenine dinucleotide phosphate oxidase (NADPH oxidase), xanthine oxidase, and cyclooxygenase in particular—and decreased activity of the oxygen free radical detoxifying enzyme superoxide dismutase.[113,115] Excess availability of superoxide anions leads to their binding to NO, resulting in decreased NO bioavailability, in addition to generating the oxidant, proinflammatory peroxynitrite. It is the decreased NO bioavailability that links oxidative stress to endothelial dysfunction and hypertension.[114] Ang II is a major enhancer of vascular NADPH-oxidase activity and plays a central role in the generation of oxidative stress in hypertension, although several other factors are also involved, including cyclic vascular stretch, ET-1, uric acid, systemic inflammation, norepinephrine, free fatty acids, and tobacco smoking.[116]

ET-1 is the endothelial cell product that counteracts NO to maintain the balance between vasodilation and vasoconstriction. ET-1 expression is increased by shear stress, catecholamines, Ang II, hypoxia, and several proinflammatory cytokines, such as tumor necrosis factor-α, interleukins 1 and 2, and transforming growth factor-β.[113] ET-1 is a potent vasoconstrictor through stimulation of ET-A receptors in vascular smooth muscle.[117] In hypertension, increased ET-1 levels are not consistently found. However, there is a trend of increased sensitivity to the vasoconstrictor effects of ET-1. ET-1, therefore, is considered a relevant mediator of BP elevation—ET-A and ET-B receptor antagonists attenuate or abolish hypertension in several experimental models of hypertension (e.g., Ang II–mediated models, deoxycorticosterone acetate–salt hypertension, and Dahl salt-sensitive rats) and are effective in lowering BP in humans.[118]

Endothelial cells also secrete a variety of other vasoregulatory substances. These include the vasodilating prostaglandin prostacyclin (PGI2), CNP, and several vasodilating endothelium-derived hyperpolarizing factors, the identity of which remains uncertain. There are also endothelium-derived contracting factors in addition to ET-1, such as locally generated Ang II and vasoconstricting prostanoids such as thromboxane A2 and prostaglandin A2. The balance of these factors, along with NO and ET-1, determine the final impact of the endothelium on vascular tone.

Other non–endothelium-derived factors may be of relevance to the genesis of hypertension via endothelium dysfunction. Much attention has been given to uric acid, which can induce endothelial dysfunction and produce salt-sensitive hypertension through mechanisms that involve renal microvascular injury.[119,120] These changes can be abrogated by therapies that lower uric acid in animals and may be of value in lowering BP and limiting renal injury in humans with hyperuricemia. Current evidence from randomized trials, however, have only supported a modest BP-lowering effect of allopurinol in hyperuricemic hypertensive adolescents,[121] with no observable effect of allopurinol or probenecid on flow-mediated vasodilation in obese nonhypertensive adults with mild hyperuricemia.[122] This implies an age-dependent effect or an effect of duration of exposure to the hyperuricemia, even if mild. Also of relevance is the possible role of high dietary fructose consumption in intracellular adenosine triphosphate (ATP) depletion, increased oxidative stress, increased uric acid production, and endothelial dysfunction.[123,124]

Nitric oxide is not the only gasotransmitter relevant to vascular biology. Hydrogen sulfide ($H_2S$) is another compound that has received recent attention due to potential treatment relevance.[125] $H_2S$ is a vasodilating gas produced from sulfated amino acids by the action of one of two key enzymes, cystathione gamma-lyase (CSE) and cystathione beta-synthase. CSE homozygous knockout mice have around 80% decreased $H_2S$ expression in the heart and aorta and around 60% reduction in serum, and both homozygous and heterozygous animals demonstrate impaired endothelial function and develop age-dependent hypertension.[126] The mechanisms underlying the BP effects of $H_2S$ are multiple, including enhanced NO-mediated vasodilation, activation of potassium ATP channels, activation of protein kinase G1α, inhibition of phosphodiesterase type 5, and inhibition of SNS activity.[125] Modulation of $H_2S$ levels with the administration of gaseous $H_2S$ or $H_2S$ donors (sodium hydrosulfide or sodium thiosulfate) has resulted in lower BP and decreased cardiovascular and renal injury in several experiemental models.[125] If delivery systems permit, and successful oral use of these agents is developed, it is possible that $H_2S$ may become a therapeutic target in hypertension and vascular disease.

Taken together, the net result observed in patients with hypertension is one of endothelial dysfunction. In cross-sectional analyses, the lower the degree of forearm flow-mediated vasodilation, the greater the prevalence of hypertension.[115,127] Prospective cohort studies have used flow-mediated vasodilation as a measure of endothelial dysfunction, regardless of a specific mechanism, to evaluate its relationship with hypertension and test whether endothelial dysfunction is a cause or consequence of hypertension, or both.[128] These studies have shown conflicting results, but the larger of them was unable to demonstrate an association between endothelial dysfunction and incident hypertension among 3500 patients followed for 4.8 years.[128]

Furthermore, endothelial dysfunction carries a genetic predisposition that is independent of BP and may be improved by agents that have little or no impact on BP (e.g., some antioxidants).[129] Therefore, as it stands, the evidence is stronger for endothelial dysfunction as a consequence, not a cause, of hypertension.[127,129]

## ARTERIAL STIFFNESS IN HYPERTENSION

Arterial stiffness is an important factor in the pathogenesis of hypertension, particularly the syndrome of isolated systolic hypertension, because it is a common accompaniment of elevated systolic BP and pulse pressure. Arterial stiffness develops as a result of structural changes in large arteries, particularly elastic arteries.[130] These include loss of elastic fibers and substitution with less distensible collagen fibers.

Factors strongly associated with arterial stiffening include aging, hypertension, diabetes mellitus, CKD, smoking, and high-sodium intake.[131]

The most commonly used measure to assess arterial stiffness in humans is carotid-femoral pulse wave velocity (cf-PWV). The traditional view linking arterial stiffness (measured as increased cf-PWV) to hypertension noted that faster PWV produced faster reflection of the incident pulse wave, which resulted in an earlier reflected wave that returned to the central circulation before the end of systole, resulting in increased systolic BP.[132] Although these mechanisms still hold true, later data have indicated the importance of two other factors, increased amplitude of the forward wave and increased characteristic impedance of the proximal aorta.[132] When these specific factors are taken into account, the relative contribution of wave reflection to the observed age-dependent change in pulse pressure is only 4% to 11%.

Arterial stiffness was previously thought to be a consequence of hypertension. Cyclic pulsatile load is associated with fracture of elastin fibers and wall stiffening, and increased distending pressure demands recruitment of the less distensible collagen fibers, thus making vessels stiffer.[130] Evidence from several studies, however, have indicated that arterial stiffness may precede and predispose to hypertension.[132] For example, in the Framingham Heart Study, markers of arterial stiffness (cf-PWV and amplitude of the forward pressure wave) were associated with a 30% to 60% increased risk for incident hypertension (per standard deviation of each variable) during 7 years of follow-up in a cohort with a baseline mean age of 60 years.[133] Conversely, baseline BP levels were not associated with future changes in arterial stiffness. Some studies have corroborated these findings, but other studies have also suggested a bidirectional relationship, so that arterial stiffness is also a consequence of chronic hypertension.[132] In contraposition, a recent cohort study of younger adults (baseline age, 36 years) has indicated that higher BP is associated with higher large artery stiffness, not the opposite.[134] These differences in results between younger and older adult populations may indicate that earlier in life, hypertension is mediated by factors that are largely independent of large vessel stiffness, whereas later in life, arterial stiffness has a more important causal role in the development of hypertension.

Arterial stiffening is relevant to target organ damage in hypertension. Increased PWV is associated with increased mortality and CV events,[135] as well as with a variety of subclinical CV injury markers, such as coronary calcification, cerebral white matter lesions, ankle-brachial index, and albuminuria. A relationship with cardiac complications has been suggested—increased impedance to left ventricular ejection results in LVH, diastolic dysfunction, and subendocardial myocardial ischemia.

The relationship to brain and renal complications is more complex. It is apparent that the mechanism of damage of these organs, which are characterized by vasculatures with high flow and low impedance, is mediated by the increased transmission of increased pulsatile pressure to the brain and renal parenchyma. The reason for this is related to the abnormal process of impedance matching. For individuals with normal vessels, the elastic arteries are much less stiff than muscular arteries, thus creating an impedance mismatch. This mismatch provokes wave reflection, thereby protecting the tissue located distally to this reflection point from injury from the traveling pulse wave. In states of increased arterial stiffness, the stiffening of elastic arteries approximates the stiffness of muscular arteries, thus eliminating the protective impedance mismatch. Once impedances become matched, there is less reflection and greater tissue injury, as supported by a growing body of clinical and experimental literature.[132] Therefore, it is clear that the relationship between hemodynamic forces and blood vessel pathology warrants greater attention in the study of hypertension.

## ROLE OF THE IMMUNE SYSTEM IN HYPERTENSION

Immune responses, both innate and adaptive, participate in several of the mechanisms discussed earlier, including the generation of reactive oxygen species, mediation of the afferent arteriolopathy thought to be important to maintain salt sensitivity, and participation in the inflammatory changes noted in the kidneys, vessels, and brain in hypertension.[136,137] Innate responses, especially those mediated by macrophages, have been linked to hypertension induced by Ang II, aldosterone, and NO antagonism. Reductions in macrophage infiltration of the kidney or periadventitial space of the aorta and medium-sized vessels have led to improvements in BP and salt sensitivity in several experimental models.[137,138] Adaptive responses via T cells have been linked to the genesis and complications of hypertension. T cells express AT1R and mediate Ang II–dependent hypertension, as demonstrated by the observations that adoptive transfer of T cells restores the hypertensive phenotype in response to Ang II infusion that was absent in mice without lymphocytes.[138] Abnormalities in both proinflammatory T cells and regulatory T cells are implicated in complications of hypertension because they appear to regulate vascular and renal inflammation that underlies target organ injury.

Suppression of these inflammatory responses can improve BP control.[136,137,139] B lymphocytes may also play a causative role in hypertension. This has been suggested by reports of the effects of several autoantibodies, including agonistic antibodies against adrenergic receptors, vascular calcium channels, and AT1R, and antibodies against endothelial cells causing endothelial dysfunction, or heat shock proteins (hsp70) causing salt-sensitive hypertension. Further research will determine if manipulation of immune targets is of value in the prevention and treatment of hypertension.

## OTHER METABOLIC PEPTIDES AND HYPERTENSION

Several vasodilating substances act as compensatory vasodilators to balance the heavily provasoconstrictive milieu in hypertension. Some of these vasodilators act primarily through an increase in NO release from endothelial cells, such as calcitonin gene–related peptide, adrenomedullin, and substance P. The glucose-regulating, gut hormone glucagon-like peptide-1 (GLP-1) has vasodilating properties, and its administration to Dahl salt-sensitive rats improves endothelial function, induces natriuresis, and lowers BP.[140] Additionally, the use of recombinant GLP-1 to treat diabetes in humans (exenatide) results in significant BP reduction, especially in those with high BP at baseline.[141]

## GUT MICROBIOME

The gut microbiome may have a relationship with several humoral and hemodynamic aspects of hypertension, including neuroimmunologic aspects of BP regulation, such as activation of the SNS and regulation of the RAAS.[142] Bacteria that produce short-chain fatty acids (especially acetate, propionate, and butyrate) are seen as favorable to producing an environment of lower BP.[142] A proof of concept study has demonstrated an unfavorable gut microbiome profile (i.e., one that leads to less available short-chain fatty acids) in spontaneous hypertensive rats as compared with normotensive Wistar Kyoto rats and has been observed in animals exposed to Ang II infusions.[143] In addition, analyses of stool samples of 10 normotensive and seven hypertensive patients have shown a similar pattern.[143] The use of probiotics, typically as yogurt or other dairy products, is the most commonly used approach to alter the gut microbiome. A meta-analysis of nine randomized clinical trials investigating the use of probiotics to lower BP has shown an average BP reduction of 3.6/2.4 mm Hg.[144] Only one study included hypertensive patients (average BP reduction, 9.7/4.4 mm Hg), but an analysis of BP lowering according to baseline BP above or below 130/85 mm Hg has shown no differences in systolic BP and a small difference in diastolic BP reduction (2.7 vs. 0.9 mm Hg). These early results indicate that modification of the gut microbiome may alter hemodynamics and that the use of probiotics, presumably through such microbiome changes, may have salutary effects on BP, although the magnitude and clinical relevance of this effect remain to be determined.

## CLINICAL EVALUATION

The evaluation of patients with hypertension focuses on six key components:

1. The confirmation that the patient is indeed hypertensive through careful measurements of BP
2. An assessment of clinical features that might suggest specific remediable causes of hypertension
3. The identification of comorbid conditions that confer additional CV risk or that may affect treatment decisions
4. The discussion of patient-related lifestyle factors and preferences that will affect management
5. The systematic evaluation of hypertensive target organ damage
6. Shared decision making about the treatment plan

To accomplish this, the clinician often needs multiple visits, a targeted clinical examination, and selected laboratory and imaging tests.

### HISTORY AND PHYSICAL EXAMINATION

The medical history and physical examination are essential to uncovering possible secondary causes of hypertension, identifying symptoms suggestive of hypertensive target organ damage, and diagnosing comorbid conditions that may affect treatment decisions. Although the focus is traditionally on the CV, neurologic, and renal systems, a complete review of systems is indicated when the patient is first evaluated. This is because some patients will present with hypertension because of sleep apnea (snoring, witnessed apneas or gasping), hyperthyroidism or hypothyroidism (each with their litany of possible symptoms), hyperparathyroidism (symptoms of hypercalcemia), Cushing syndrome (symptoms of cortisol excess), pheochromocytoma or paraganglioma (symptoms of catecholamine excess), or acromegaly with its distinctive physical findings. These conditions are discussed in detail later in this chapter.

High BP is typically asymptomatic, but some symptoms are common among patients with very high BP levels, such as headaches, epistaxis, dyspnea, chest pain, and faintness, all of which were present in more than 10% of patients presenting with diastolic BP levels above 120 mm Hg.[145] Other common symptoms are nocturia and unsteady gait; treated patients often complain of fatigue in addition to symptoms of overtreatment and those related to specific side effects of medications. In patients with lower BP levels, the occurrence of symptoms is often difficult to tie to observed BP, as demonstrated in a study evaluating the relationship between headaches and BP levels, where the frequently observed headaches in patients with hypertension did not correlate well with office or ambulatory BP levels.[146]

When searching for target organ damage, one looks for symptoms to suggest a previous stroke or transient ischemic attack, previous or ongoing coronary ischemia, heart failure, peripheral arterial disease, or a past history of kidney disease or current symptoms, such as hematuria or flank pain.

Obtaining a detailed family history as it pertains to hypertension is essential. Focus should be on the development of hypertension at a young age or clustering of endocrine problems (e.g., pheochromocytoma, multiple endocrine neoplasia, primary aldosteronism) or renal problems (e.g., polycystic kidney disease or any inherited form of kidney disease). The young patient with hypertension and a family history of hypertension poses a particular challenge and should be evaluated in detail. Table 46.2 provides a guide to possible causes to be considered.[147]

Knowledge of conditions with potential relevance to treatment is important. For example, issues related to CV risk management, such as diabetes mellitus, hypercholesterolemia, inflammation (C-reactive protein [CRP]), obesity, and tobacco smoking need to be evaluated. Patients with established CV disease will need some treatment for their hypertension and underlying disorder (e.g., beta-blockers for angina pectoris), so knowledge of specific CV diagnoses is essential. Finally, some non-CV conditions may have an impact on treatment options. For example, patients with reactive airways disease (asthma) probably should not receive beta-blockers, patients with prostatic hyperplasia may benefit from a regimen that includes an alpha-blocker, and patients with attention-deficit/hyperactivity disorder or anxiety may benefit from a central sympatholytic (e.g., guanfacine), but those with major depression should probably not be treated with this drug class.

It is also important to recognize that it is while obtaining the history that the clinician has the opportunity to explore issues related to lifestyle, cultural beliefs, and patient preferences that will be essential in designing an effective treatment plan. It is important to define dietary and physical activity patterns and, when problems are identified, to determine if the patient is willing and/or able to modify them. Cultural

**Table 46.2 Clinical Clues to Guide the Investigation in Young Patients with Hypertension with a Potential Hereditary Cause**

| Specific Conditions | Possible Causes of Familial Hypertension | Clinical Clues |
|---|---|---|
| **Catecholamine-Producing Tumors** | | |
| Pheochromocytoma, paraganglioma | Familial cases are responsible for ~30% of cases, including MEN2A and MEN2B, von Hippel–Lindau disease, neurofibromatosis, and familial paraganglioma syndromes (SDH complex mutations) | Paroxysmal palpitations, headaches, diaphoresis, pale flushing; syndromic features of any of the associated disorders |
| Neuroblastomas (adrenal); aortic or renovascular lesions | 1%–2% of neuroblastomas are familial | |
| Coarctation of the aorta | Overrepresented in families but no familial distribution | Asymmetry between upper- and lower-extremity BP, radial-formal pulse delay; associated with Turner syndrome, Williams' syndrome, and bicuspid aortic valve |
| Renal artery stenosis caused by fibromuscular dysplasia or inherited arterial wall lesions | <10% familial with AD pattern | Abnormal renal vascular imaging results; vascular disease in the carotid territory at an early age; common in neurofibromatosis and Williams' syndrome; also present in tuberous sclerosis, Ehlers-Danlos syndrome, and Marfan syndrome |
| Parenchymal kidney disease GN | Alport disease (X-linked, AR, or AD), familial IgA nephropathy (AD with incomplete penetrance) | Proteinuria, hematuria, low eGFR |
| PKD | ADPKD type 1 or 2, ARPKD | Multiple renal cysts (as few as three in patients <30 years) |
| Adrenocortical disease; glucocorticoid-remediable aldosteronism (familial hyperaldosteronism type I) | AD chimeric fusion of the 11β-hydroxylase and aldosterone synthase genes | Cerebral hemorrhages at young age, cerebral aneurysms; mild hypokalemia; high plasma aldosterone, low renin |
| Familial hyperaldosteronism | AD; unknown defect | Severe type 2 hypertension in early adulthood; high plasma aldosterone, low renin; no response to glucocorticoid treatment |
| Familial hyperaldosteronism type III | AD; unknown defect | Severe hypertension in childhood with extensive target organ damage; high plasma aldosterone, low renin; marked bilateral adrenal enlargement |
| Congenital adrenal hyperplasia | AR mutations in 11β-hydroxylase or 21-hydroxylase | Hirsutism, virilization; hypokalemia and metabolic alkalosis; low plasma aldosterone and renin |
| **Monogenic Primary Renal Tubular Defects** | | |
| Gordon syndrome | AD mutations of *KLHL3*, *CUL3*, *WNK1*, and *WNK4*; AR mutations of *KLHL3* | Hyperkalemia and metabolic acidosis with normal renal function |
| Liddle syndrome | AD mutations of the epithelial sodium channel | Hypokalemia and metabolic alkalosis; low plasma aldosterone and renin |
| Apparent mineralocorticoid excess | AD mutation in 11β-hydroxysteroid dehydrogenase type 2 | Hypokalemia and metabolic alkalosis; low plasma aldosterone and renin |
| Geller syndrome; hypertension-brachydactyly syndrome | AD mutation in the mineralocorticoid receptor<br>AD mutations in the phosphodiesterase E3A enzyme | Hypokalemia and metabolic alkalosis; low plasma aldosterone and renin; increased BP during pregnancy or exposure to spironolactone; short fingers (small phalanges) and short stature; brain stem compression from vascular tortuosity in the posterior fossa |
| Essential hypertension | Polygenic | When obesity or metabolic syndrome is present, likelihood of essential hypertension is higher |

*AD,* Autosomal dominant; *ADPKD,* autosomal dominant polycystic kidney disease; *AR,* autosomal recessive; *ARPKD,* autosomal recessive polycystic kidney disease; *BP,* blood pressure; *eGFR,* estimated glomerular filtration rate; *GN,* glomerulonephritis; *IgA,* immunoglobulin A; *MEN,* multiple endocrine neoplasia; *PKD,* polycystic kidney disease; *SDH,* succinate dehydrogenase.

beliefs related to the treatment of hypertension, health illiteracy, and mistrust in physicians and the pharmaceutical industry are several of the factors that can affect the relationship with the patient and should be discussed openly. It is only then that patients will be able to participate in shared decision making about their treatment, an essential tenet of patient-centered care.

The physical examination is designed to complement the items discussed in the history. One should pay attention to syndromic features of cortisol excess (e.g., moon face, central obesity, frontal balding, cervical and supraclavicular fat deposits, skin thinning, abdominal striae), hyperthyroidism (e.g., tachycardia, anxiety, lid lag or proptosis, hypertelorism, pretibial myxedema), hypothyroidism (e.g., bradycardia, coarse facial features, macroglossia, myxedema, hyporeflexia), acromegaly (e.g., frontal bossing, widened nose, enlarged jaw, dental separation, acral enlargement, carpal tunnel syndrome), neurofibromatosis (e.g., neurofibromas, café au lait spots, because neurofibromatosis is associated with pheochromocytoma and renal artery stenosis), or tuberous sclerosis (e.g., hypopigmented ash leaf patches, facial angiofibromas, because tuberous sclerosis is associated with renal hypertension, usually related to angiomyolipomas). Many other even rarer associations exist but are beyond the scope of this chapter.

In younger patients or patients with unexplained, difficult to treat hypertension, it is worth exploring the possibility of coarctation of the aorta by measuring BP in both arms and in one thigh. If present, there will be a significantly lower BP in the thigh (typically by >30 mm Hg). Sometimes, in case of a lesion proximal to the left subclavian, there may be a significant interarm difference, lower on the left. In addition, there is a significant decrease in intensity of the femoral pulses and a palpable radial-femoral pulse delay.

All patients should have a funduscopic examination to evaluate vascular changes associated with hypertension. The retinal changes are associated with severity of acute and chronic BP elevation. Acute changes can happen quite abruptly (hours to days); these range from arteriolar spasm in most patients with uncontrolled BP to retinal infarcts (exudates) and microvascular rupture (flame hemorrhages) to papilledema once the protection afforded by vasoconstriction is overcome. Chronic changes take much longer to develop and include vascular tortuosity (arteriovenous nicking) due to perivascular fibrosis, followed by progressive arteriolar wall thickening that prevents visualization of the blood column, thus leading to the appearance of copper wiring and then silver wiring. Several studies have demonstrated a relationship between severity of hypertensive retinopathy and risk for LVH and stroke.

An important recent development is the availability of smartphone-based technology that allows the use of a condensing lens coupled with the smartphone's own camera for video and photography of the retina in place of a conventional ophthalmoscope.[148,149] In a study of hypertensive patients seen in the emergency room, use of this technology has resulted in improved identification of abnormal retinal findings (e.g., exudates, hemorrhages, papilledema) by an observer with very little clinical experience compared with conventional bedside opththalmoscopy, while requiring about half the time to complete the examination (74 vs. 130 seconds).[148] The price for these devices (~$450 for the D-EYE camera, D-EYE, Truckee, CA) is higher than conventional ophthalmoscopes (~US$150–US$300) but competitive with that of panoptic hand-held scopes (~US$500).

The CV examination focuses on the identification of volume overload (e.g., jugular venous distention, lung crackles, edema), cardiac enlargement (e.g., deviated cardiac impulse), and the presence of a third or fourth heart sound as markers of impaired left ventricular compliance. We also routinely look for bruits over the carotid arteries because the prevalence of carotid atherosclerosis is increased in patients with hypertension, as well in the abdomen, primarily looking for renal arterial bruits heard over the epigastrium and/or flanks. These bruits are of greater significance if they occur on both systole and diastole. Finally, detailed palpation of the peripheral pulses of the arms and legs is important to look for signs of peripheral arterial disease.

To finish the examination, a focused neurologic examination looks for obvious cranial nerve abnormalities, motor deficits, or speech or gait abnormalities. Any further testing is based on specific symptoms or on focal findings on the screening examination.

## BLOOD PRESSURE MEASUREMENT

Because treatment decisions are based largely on BP levels, accurate BP measurement is essential. Cuff-based brachial BP is the method most used to measure BP, typically in the office setting. However, a rapidly growing body of evidence has indicated the value of out-of-office BP methods, such as 24-hour ambulatory BP monitoring (ABPM) and home BP monitoring, as superior methods to evaluate BP burden and evaluate BP-related risk in patients with hypertension.[32,150] Additionally, the most recent guidelines point to much more careful assessment of blood pressure in the office setting.[13]

### OFFICE BLOOD PRESSURE MEASUREMENT

Office BP measurement is the time-honored method for the diagnosis and management of hypertension. It is strongly associated with hypertension-related outcomes based on more than 50 years of observational and clinical trial data. Accordingly, guidance provided to clinicians for the diagnosis and treatment of hypertension by most major guidelines is based on office BP values (see Box 46.1).[11] The British National Institute for Health and Care Excellence (NICE)[151] and US Preventive Services Taskforce (https://www.uspreventiveservicestaskforce.org/ Page/Document/UpdateSummaryFinal/high-blood-pressure-in-adults-screening) guidelines recommend ABPM or home BP monitoring as preferred methods for the initial diagnosis of hypertension but still recommend office BP for monitoring treatment. Additionally, the most recent American Heart Association (AHA)– American College of Cardiology (ACC) guidelines on hypertension assessment strongly recommend the following approach for blood pressure assessment in the office setting, as shown in Box 46.1. Attention to measurement technique is essential; Box 46.1 summarizes essential elements of the proper BP measurement technique. Most patients should have their BP measured in the arm in the seated position. In some situations, such as malformations, injuries, or extensive vascular disease of the upper extremities, or when comparing BP levels in the upper and lower extremities, it may be necessary to use thigh measurements with an appropriately sized thigh cuff, which should be obtained with the patient in the prone position to allow the cuff to be at the level of the heart. Mercury sphygmomanometers are now seldom available in clinical practice because of environmental concerns. Aneroid and electronic oscillometric manometers are accurate but should have periodic maintenance (every 12 months) to ensure that they are properly calibrated, as well as whenever poor function is suspected.

A recent development in office BP measurement is the use of an electronic oscillometric device for multiple

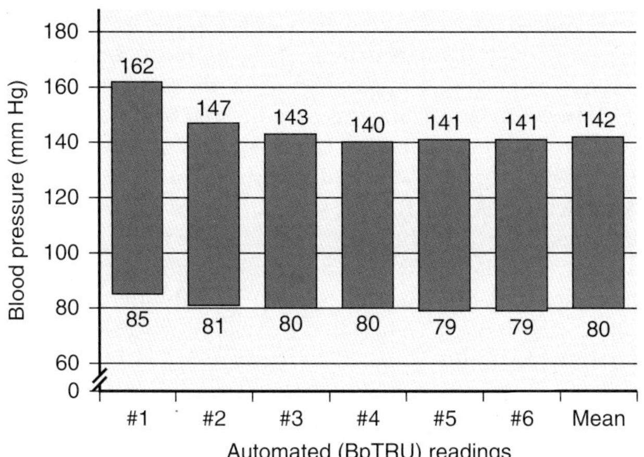


**Fig. 46.11** Blood pressure *(BP)* behavior with multiple measurements in the office in 50 patients with hypertension. The first BP reading was taken by the physician. The following five readings were taken by the patient, with only the patient in the examination room. *BpTRU,* Automated blood pressure monitor. (From Myers MG. The great myth of office blood pressure measurement. *J Hypertens.* 2012;30:1894–1898.)

measurements, but with the patient alone in the room for five automated readings. Using this method, the "white coat effect" can be largely eliminated (Fig. 46.11).[152] In addition, this automated approach results in better correlations with ambulatory BP averages and with left ventricular mass than routine office BP,[153,154] but there is a risk of underestimating masked hypertension, which is potentially problematic given the increased risk associated with this condition. The phenomenon of masked hypertension is defined as a clinical condition in which a patient's office BP level is normal but ambulatory or home BP readings are in the hypertensive range. This phenomenon, the opposite of white coat hypertension (WCH), would suggest the necessity for measuring out-of-office BP in those with apparently normal or well-controlled office BP.

## ORTHOSTATIC BLOOD PRESSURE MEASUREMENT

Orthostatic hypotension commonly accompanies uncontrolled hypertension, especially among older patients, where it occurs in 8% to 34% of patients.[155] Some guidelines now provide specific recommendations for the measurement of standing BP to screen for orthostatic hypotension in older patients with hypertension, as well as in patients at increased risk for autonomic dysfunction, such as those with diabetes and kidney disease.[156,157]

The frequency of orthostatic hypotension increases with increasing age, the presence of hypertension, and the number of antihypertensive drugs, but whether the type of antihypertensive drug has any specific impact is unclear. The development of orthostatic hypotension is important because it is a risk factor for syncope and falls. Therefore, evaluation for the presence of orthostatic hypotension should be part of the assessment of risks and benefits of drug treatment.

Orthostatic vital signs (heart rate and BP) are best obtained after at least 5 minutes in the supine position followed by immediate assumption of the patient in the standing position, when sequential measurements are taken for up to 3 minutes. The difficulties of following this protocol in a busy clinical practice are recognized, so it is acceptable to compare values in the seated position with those after standing for 1 minute; this approach results in decreased sensitivity for the detection of orthostatic hypotension but is better than no measurement at all.[158] To account for this, it has been proposed that a fall of 15/7 mm Hg be used for the definition of orthostatic hypotension when the test is performed using the seated BP as baseline, as compared with the the generally accepted definition of orthostatic hypotension as a drop in BP of more than 20/10 mm Hg that occurs after 3 minutes of standing.[159] Among patients with supine hypertension, it is recommended that the definition of systolic fall in BP for the diagnosis is a decrease of more than 30 mm Hg because the level of baseline BP is directly proportional to the orthostatic BP fall.

Integration of the heart rate response to changes in BP during orthostasis is important to guide the differential diagnosis and further evaluation of orthostatic hypotension. In the absence of medications with a negative chronotropic effect, the lack of a tachycardic response to orthostatic hypotension is indicative of baroreflex or sympathetic autonomic dysfunction. Patients with a robust tachycardic response, on the other hand, likely have effective arterial volume depletion or excessive vasodilation.

Management of orthostasis is dependent on the pathophysiology of the cause. If a baroreceptor abnormality or autonomic dysfunction is a cause, a general approach using nocturnal clonidine or nitrates to mitigate the hypertension—while requiring compression garments and increased morning sodium intake—has been shown to be beneficial to reduce the symptoms and close the pressure gap.[160]

## OFFICE VERSUS OUT-OF-OFFICE BLOOD PRESSURE

Office BP measurement is the time-honored method to evaluate hypertension. It is easy to perform and is widely available at low cost. Home BP is also widely available, although accessibility to low-income patients is still a problem, despite the availability of low-cost devices. ABPM, on the other hand, is less widely available due to costs and limited reimbursement by third-party payers in the United States. Both home BP monitoring protocols and ABPM include larger numbers of readings, thus decreasing variability and improving reproducibility.[161]

In the last 30 years, ABPM and home BP have become accepted as better markers of hypertensive target organ damage and adverse clinical outcomes. ABPM has stronger associations with several measures of LVH, albuminuria, kidney dysfunction, retinal damage, carotid atherosclerosis, and aortic stiffness than office BP, although this is not consistent among studies.[162] Likewise, home BP is a better marker than office BP for LVH and proteinuria, although it is not consistently superior for other measures of target organ damage.

In the assessment of hard CV endpoints, out-of-office BP has consistently outperformed office BP in studies that account for the values observed in the office. In other words, no matter what the office BP, it is the out-of-office BP that decisively drives outcomes. In a systematic review by the NICE clinical guidelines group in the United Kingdom of nine cohort studies comparing ABPM with office BP, ABPM was superior in eight and equal to office BP in one.[163] For home BP, they identified three studies compared with office BP; home BP was superior in two and equal in one. Finally, two studies compared ABPM, home BP, and office BP; of these, one showed superiority of both ABPM and home BP, whereas the other study did not show differences among any of the three methods.

In meta-analyses of studies that evaluated both office and ABPM on outcomes, only ABPM values retained significance.[164,165] Likewise, in the largest home BP cohort study that included simultaneous use of office and home BP to predict CV events and mortality, only home BP remained significantly associated with these adverse outcomes.[166] Similar observations of the superior prognostic performance of out-of-office methods have been made for patients with resistant hypertension, CKD, hemodialysis, and the general population.

In summary, evidence from prospective cohort studies has convincingly demonstrated the superiority of out-of-office BP measurements as predictors of hypertension outcomes. There are several possible explanations for the superiority of out-of-office measurements in outcomes assessment:

1. There is lower variability and better reproducibility afforded by the larger number of readings across a longer period of observation, thus making ABPM/home BP better reflections of so-called BP burden.
2. Home BP and ABPM can detect white coat and masked hypertension (see Fig. 46.12).

White coat hypertension, or isolated office hypertension, is the occurrence of high BP in the office and normal BP values in the out-of-office environment. It occurs in 20% to 30% of patients with a diagnosis of office hypertension.[167] It has generally been noted that patients with WCH have similar CV outcomes as normotensive individuals.[168] However, data from the large International Database of Home Blood Pressure in Relation to Cardiovascular Outcome have shown a significant increase in fatal and nonfatal CV events among untreated WCH patients diagnosed based on home BP compared with untreated normotensive persons (hazard ratio [HR], 1.42; $P = .02$).[169] Interestingly, treated patients with hypertension who retained a white coat effect had the same overall risk as treated patients whose BP was controlled both in the office and at home (HR, 1.16; $P = .45$). Moreover, an updated meta-analysis of 14 observational ABPM studies revealed an increase in risk of CV events (HR, 1.7) and CV mortality (HR, 2.8) among WCH patients compared with normotensive controls, but no statistically significant increase in stroke or all-cause death. As in previous analyses, sustained normotension was associated with a much larger risk.[170]

In addition, WCH has been associated with an intermediate phenotype between normotension and hypertension as it pertains to left ventricular mass, carotid intima-media thickness, aortic pulse wave velocity, and albuminuria.[169] However, there are no data available to demonstrate that patients with WCH benefit from drug therapy. Therefore, it appears that WCH may not be as benign as previously considered, and patients should be advised on general lifestyle changes to improve BP levels and overall vascular risk, especially as their risk for progressing to sustained hypertension is approximately 40% to 50% after 10 to 11 years of follow-up.[171,172] Masked hypertension, conversely, consists of normal BP in the office but high BP in the ambulatory setting, with an estimated prevalence of 10% to 15% in population studies. It has been

White coat hypertension vs. normotension

| Study name | Hazard ratio | Lower limit | Upper limit | *Z* value | *P* value |
|---|---|---|---|---|---|
| Verdecchia 1994 | 1.170 | 0.253 | 5.402 | 0.201 | 0.841 |
| Kario 2001 | 0.760 | 0.164 | 3.529 | −0.350 | 0.726 |
| Fagard 2005 | 1.000 | 0.372 | 2.686 | 0.000 | 1.000 |
| Ohkubo 2005 | 0.950 | 0.389 | 2.322 | −0.112 | 0.910 |
| Hansen 2006 | 0.960 | 0.500 | 1.842 | −0.123 | 0.902 |
| Pierdomenico 2008 | 0.970 | 0.381 | 2.468 | −0.064 | 0.949 |
| **Summary** | 0.964 | 0.654 | 1.421 | −0.186 | 0.852 |

Statistics for each study; Hazard ratio and 95% CI (0.1 0.2 0.5 1 2 5 10)

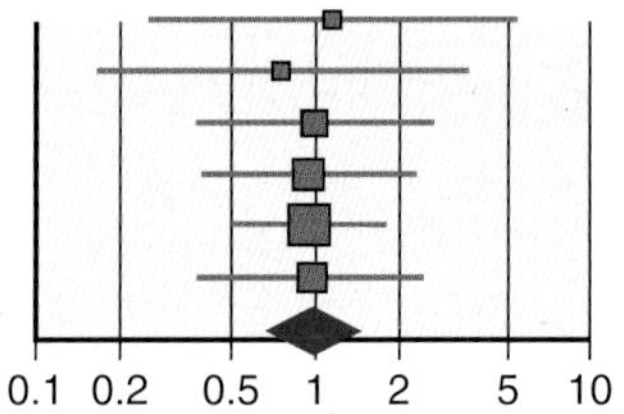

Masked hypertension vs. normotension

| Study name | Hazard ratio | Lower limit | Upper limit | *Z* value | *P* value |
|---|---|---|---|---|---|
| Bjorklund 2003 | 2.770 | 1.149 | 6.676 | 2.270 | 0.023 |
| Fagard 2005 | 1.650 | 0.526 | 5.172 | 0.859 | 0.390 |
| Ohkubo 2005 | 2.560 | 1.410 | 4.649 | 3.088 | 0.002 |
| Hansen 2006 | 1.660 | 1.056 | 2.610 | 2.195 | 0.028 |
| Pierdomenico 2008 | 2.650 | 1.177 | 5.966 | 2.354 | 0.019 |
| **Summary** | 2.088 | 1.550 | 2.812 | 4.844 | 0.000 |

Statistics for each study; Hazard ratio and 95% CI (0.1 0.2 0.5 1 2 5 10)

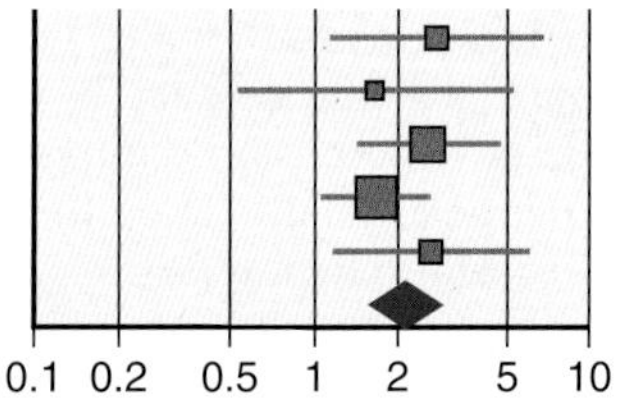

**Fig. 46.12** Results of a meta-analysis of the effects of white coat hypertension *(top)* and masked hypertension *(bottom)* on the occurrence of fatal and nonfatal cardiovascular events. There is no statistical difference between white coat hypertension and normotension (hazard ratio, 0.96; $P = .85$), whereas masked hypertension is associated with a 2.09-fold increase in risk ($P < .0001$). *CI*, Confidence interval. (From Pierdomenico SD, Cuccurullo F. Prognostic value of white-coat and masked hypertension diagnosed by ambulatory monitoring in initially untreated subjects: an updated meta-analysis. *Am J Hypertens.* 2011;24:52–58.)

consistently and strongly associated with increased risk for adverse CV endpoints and mortality to a level indistinguishable from that associated with sustained hypertension.[168] The very existence of masked hypertension is troublesome because its identification is only possible with BP measurement in the out-of-office environment. This finding has important public policy implications related to screening, which remain unresolved at this time. However, in a first step to address this issue, the ACC/AHA guidelines have indicated that it may be reasonable to use out-of-office BP to screen for masked hypertension in adults with office BP readings consistently between 120 to 129/80 to 84 mm Hg.

Because WCH and masked hypertension afflict such a substantial number of patients and have a diametrically different impact on outcomes, their identification improves outcome prediction in patients with hypertension.

3. The ability to evaluate BP during sleep was a feature until now restricted to ABPM, although newer home BP monitors can be programmed for activation during sleep. In some, but not all, studies, nighttime BP is a better marker of CV disease than daytime or 24-hour average BP.[173–175] The importance of nighttime BP (compared with daytime levels) appears greater among treated patients, perhaps because antihypertensive treatment, often taken in the morning, might result in better BP control during the day than during the night.[176]

The pattern of BP fluctuation between day and night is also associated with prognosis. The normal circadian BP pattern includes a decrease in BP of approximately 15% to 20% during sleep. Patients who lack this normal BP dip during sleep are called *nondippers* (arbitrarily defined as a sleep BP that falls by less than 10% compared with awake levels); they have increased target organ damage and overall CV risk. In large observational studies, patients whose systolic BP falls by 20% or more during the night have lower fatal and nonfatal CV event rates than those whose BP decreases by less than 20%, and those whose BP does not decrease at all during the night have significantly worse CV outcomes than all other patients.[177]

4. ABPM also provides information on BP variability throughout the day, which may add further prognostic information. Increased BP variability (measured as the standard deviation of BP) has been associated with increased event rates, although these findings are of small magnitude when taken independently from BP values.[178]

Despite these observations, objective evidence demonstrating that outcomes are better when patients are managed using an out-of-office method is lacking. Three randomized clinical trials have compared management of hypertension with office or out-of-office BP, one using 24-hour ABPM[179] and two using home BP.[39,180,181] All these studies have shown that more patients managed with out-of-office methods could have treatment stopped or deescalated, thus resulting in marginal cost savings. However, none of them could demonstrate the superiority of ABPM or home BP in achieving better BP control (the primary outcome of all three trials) or less LVH (evaluated in all studies as a secondary outcome).

## CLINICAL USE OF AMBULATORY AND HOME BLOOD PRESSURE MONITORING

ABPM has been in clinical use for almost 50 years. In the United States, problems related to limited reimbursement have significantly limited its expansion compared with other parts of the world. Despite this limitation, there is general agreement on its value in several clinical circumstances, as outlined in Table 46.3.

ABPM is performed, typically, over a period of 24 hours, although it can be extended for longer periods (e.g., 48 hours) to provide information covering more than one wake-sleep cycle or to cover a specific period in detail, such as a 2-day interdialytic period for a patient undergoing hemodialysis. Clinicians should use an independently validated monitor (for a list, refer to www.dableducational.org). A typical measurement interval is every 20 minutes during the daytime (7 AM to 11 PM) and every 30 minutes at night (11 PM to 7 AM), although the frequency and time windows can be adjusted based on clinical needs, such as the need to identify factors such as frequent BP swings and atypical sleep patterns. Patients should keep a log of activities during

**Table 46.3 Indications for 24-Hour Ambulatory and Home Blood Pressure Monitoring**

| Indication | Home BP Monitoring | ABPM | Comment |
|---|---|---|---|
| Identify white coat hypertension. | ++ | +++ | ABPM still the gold standard when patients have home BP values that are borderline (125–135/80–85 mm Hg) |
| Identify masked hypertension. | ++ | +++ | |
| Identify true resistant hypertension. | ++ | +++ | |
| Evaluate borderline office BP values without target organ damage. | ++ | +++ | |
| Evaluate nocturnal hypertension. | — | +++ | |
| Evaluate labile hypertension. | ++ | ++ | Home BP better for infrequent symptoms or paroxysms; ABPM better if frequent within a 24-hr period |
| Evaluate hypotensive symptoms. | +++ | ++ | |
| Evaluate autonomic dysfunction. | + | ++ | Home BP useful to monitor orthostatic hypotension; ABPM useful to quantify supine hypertension and determine overall (average) BP levels |
| Clinical research (treatment, prognosis) | ++ | +++ | |

*ABPM,* Ambulatory blood pressure monitoring; *BP,* blood pressure.

the day, the time of retiring to bed and waking up, and the time of taking vasoactive medications (if applicable). It is preferred that the periods designated as "night" and "day" reflect the actual periods of sleep and wakefulness obtained from the patient's diary. Most patients tolerate the procedure well, although sometimes sleep is compromised (<10% of cases) and, rarely, patients have excessive bruising or discomfort from the frequent cuff inflations. Up-to-date instructions on how to perform and interpret ABPM studies are available in guideline format from the European Society of Hypertension.

Home BP is performed by the patient in the home (or sometimes work) environment. It is used commonly in clinical practice and is associated with improved adherence to therapy. It has also been used successfully for the treatment self-titration of BP medications and is amenable to telemedicine approaches, in which the patient can upload BP values via telephone or direct entry to an Internet server so that clinicians can inspect the BP logs and make treatment decisions remotely.

Just as with office BP, it is important that the equipment fits the patient well and that measurements are obtained using the same technique as outlined earlier for office BP. Independently validated devices are listed at www.dableducational.org; unfortunately, many of the marketed devices have not been independently validated. The preferred devices use arm cuffs.[182] Finger cuffs are inaccurate and should not be used. Wrist cuffs often provide incorrect readings because of inappropriate technique but, if used correctly, can be convenient and accurate and particularly useful in obese patients.

Smartphone applications are often marketed to obtain biologic information from users, including BP, and it is likely that in the near future their use will become important in the care of hypertensive patients. However, at the present time, none of the available technologies has been adequately validated, and a clinical validation study of the best-sold BP application (Instant Blood Pressure [IBP]) has shown wildly unreliable performance, leading to immediate removal of the application from the market on publication of the article.[183]

To allow management decisions, home BP monitoring is best performed using specific periods of monitoring. For most patients, a BP log obtained over 7 days before each office visit suffices because it has excellent reproducibility.[182] We recommended that the patient obtain readings in duplicate (~1 minute apart), twice daily (in the morning before taking medications and in the evening before dinner). In some situations, more frequent or more prolonged monitoring may be needed. For example, patients with hypotensive symptoms may benefit from BP measurements during the peak action of medications, such as in the mid to late morning or late evening, depending on when medications are taken. Likewise, patients with a labile BP can be monitored more often to capture the overall BP variability better, although we prefer to use ABPM in such patients. As for ABPM, detailed home BP guidelines are available from the European Society of Hypertension[150] and the ACC/AHA.[10]

Normative values for the interpretation of ABPM and home BP results are available based on observed outcomes in longitudinal studies[184] (Table 46.4). For ease of use, these thresholds were matched to specific office BP levels at which the observed rate of CV events was the same, thus allowing clinicians to relate to office values that have historically driven clinical decisions. For ABPM, other measures, such as the nocturnal dip, early morning surge (magnitude of BP rise during the first hours postawakening), BP load (percentage of time BP remains above a certain threshold, such as 140/90 mm Hg during the day and 120/80 mm Hg during the night), and overall BP variability (standard deviation of the 24-hour BP or awake BP), were not studied in relationship to hard outcomes for precise normative results. Table 46.5 also presents general home and ambulatory BP values that mirror office BP values; these represent consensus-based values and are provided to allow the clinician to relate values seen out of the office with the heretofore more commonly used office readings.

**Table 46.4 Normative Values for Ambulatory Blood Pressure Monitoring and Home Blood Pressure Monitoring[a]**

| Parameter | Blood Pressure Equivalent to Office Blood Pressure of: 120/80 mm Hg | 140/90 mm Hg |
|---|---|---|
| **24-Hour Ambulatory BP Monitoring** | | |
| 24-hour BP | 117/74 mm Hg | 131/79 mm Hg |
| Awake BP | 122/79 mm Hg | 138/86 mm Hg |
| Sleep BP | 101/65 mm Hg | 120/71 mm Hg |
| **Home BP Monitoring** | | |
| Average BP[b] | 121/78 mm Hg | 133/82 mm Hg |

[a]Based on clinical outcomes.
[b]Average of all values during the monitoring period, usually 7 days.
Normative data based on equivalent of cardiovascular event rates observed at each level of office BP.
*ABPM,* Ambulatory blood pressure monitoring; *BP,* blood pressure.
Data from Richards EM, Pepine CJ, Raizada MK, Kim S. The gut, its microbiome, and hypertension. *Curr Hypertens Rep.* 2017;19(4):36; and Kikuya M, Hansen TW, Thijs L, et al. Diagnostic thresholds for ambulatory blood pressure monitoring based on 10-year cardiovascular risk. *Circulation.* 2007;115;2145–2152.

## INTEGRATING OUT-OF-OFFICE BLOOD PRESSURE INTO CLINICAL PRACTICE

All current hypertension guidelines recognize the value of out-of-office BP in the diagnosis of hypertension; the UK NICE guidelines, the US Preventive Services Taskforce, and the ACC/AHA guidelines formally recommend its use to confirm the diagnosis of hypertension in patients with elevated office BP prior to initiating treatment. The ACC/AHA guidelines also recommend the use of out-of-office BP to evaluate patients who are receiving treatment for hypertension but remain above goal in the office, with the explicit caveat that the recommendation is on the basis of expert opinion. A finding to support this recommendation is the high prevalence (~40%–51%) of a white coat effect in patients with

**Table 46.5 Consensus-Based Home and Ambulatory Blood Pressure Values[a]**

| Clinic | Home BP | Daytime BP | Nighttime | 24-hour BP |
|---|---|---|---|---|
| 120/80 | 120/80 | 120/80 | 100/65 | 115/75 |
| 130/80 | 130/80 | 130/80 | 110/65 | 125/75 |
| 140/90 | 135/85 | 135/85 | 120/70 | 130/80 |
| 160/100 | 145/90 | 145/90 | 140/85 | 145/90 |

[a]And their equivalent office values.

*BP*, Blood pressure.

Data from Whelton PK, Carey RM, Aronow WS, et al. 2017 ACC/AHA/AAPA/ABC/ACPM/AGS/APhA/ASH/ASPC/NMA/PCNA Guideline for the Prevention, Detection, Evaluation, and Management of High Blood Pressure in Adults: Executive Summary: A Report of the American College of Cardiology/American Heart Association Task Force on Clinical Practice Guidelines. *Hypertension*. 2018;71:1269–1324.

**Box 46.2 Proper Method of Measurement and Integration of Out-of-Office Blood Pressure**

**Method**

1. Make sure BP device is validated by medical personnel (nurse)-annually
2. Measure BP in morning before breakfast (maximal risk for CV events between 4-10 AM)
3. Method of measurement: (1) sit in chair with back firmly supported; (2) place appropriate sized BP cuff on arm and rest arm on comfortable surface at heart level; (3) rest for 5 minutes with no distractions (e.g., TV, radio, computer, phone; (4) obtain three readings 1 minute apart and average the last two readings.
4. Once BP is controlled and stabilized, do this on average four or five times a month.

**Integration**

1. Use the average range of BPs at home and compare with office readings. If home BPs are at least 10 or more mm Hg higher than office BPs, then a white coat effect is present.
2. Tailoring therapy to home BPs rather than office BPs has resulted in fewer medication side effects, especially hypotension.

*BP*, Blood pressure.

resistant hypertension. Another caveat is that patients with an office BP above 160/100 mm Hg do not need confirmation and should be treated.

We are also in agreement with the recommendation to use out-of-office BP to guide treatment, which reflects our clinical practice of systematically using this approach. Box 46.2 summarizes the steps involved in the integration of out-of-office BP in the diagnosis and management of hypertension using the proposed ACC/AHA BP thresholds for diagnosis and treatment.

## LABORATORY AND OTHER COMPLEMENTARY TESTS

Similar to the history and physical examination, laboratory tests, imaging, and other complementary tests also focus on the evaluation of comorbid conditions, established target organ damage, and possible secondary causes. In the absence of worrisome signs or symptoms during the initial evaluation, the clinician should obtain a basic set of tests, including renal function, levels of electrolytes, calcium, glucose, and hemoglobin, lipid profile, urinalysis, and electrocardiogram (Table 46.6).

Further testing may be required in case any of these initial test results are abnormal or there are specific symptoms or physical findings suggesting a diagnosis (see "Secondary Hypertension"). Likewise, patients who are resistant to treatment during follow-up have higher rates of secondary causes of hypertension—in particular, sleep apnea, hyperaldosteronism, and renovascular disease—thus deserving a more dedicated search for secondary causes in their evaluation.

### ECHOCARDIOGRAPHY

LVH is the most common target organ damage in hypertension and is independently associated with a worse prognosis, marked by increased risk for CV events (coronary, cerebrovascular), heart failure, and death.[185] The electrocardiogram is very specific but insensitive for the detection of LVH. Not surprisingly, the prevalence of LVH among patients with hypertension is only approximately 18% based on electrocardiographic criteria, whereas this number increases to approximately 40% when more sensitive echocardiographic criteria are used. The echocardiogram also provides information on left ventricular diastolic function, which is often impaired early in the course of hypertensive heart disease and does not require the presence of LVH. Finally, it allows the assessment of left ventricular systolic dysfunction, which is uncommonly present in hypertension (~4%) but is associated with a worse prognosis. Even though echocardiography is not recommended as a routine test in patients with hypertension, it often provides important information to help guide treatment, such as defining the need to initiate or escalate treatment in patients with borderline office or ambulatory BP levels.

### EVALUATION OF SODIUM AND POTASSIUM INTAKE

Because of the importance of sodium and potassium as dietary interventions in hypertension, it is often useful to quantify intake objectively. Dietary recall is the method used most often in clinical practice; however, it is often problematic because many patients have difficulty defining portions. In situations where detailed knowledge of sodium and potassium intake is important to management, our practice is to obtain a 24-hour urine collection to evaluate sodium and potassium on a stable diet. These ions are measured in milliequivalents per day and then converted to dietary target in milligrams per day (1 mEq of sodium = 23 mg of sodium or 58 mg of salt as NaCl; 1 mEq of potassium = 39 mg of potassium). A diuretic can be maintained as long as the dose has been stable over time. One must recognize that sodium excretion may follow a circaseptan rhythm[60] and may therefore be imprecise on a single 24-hour collection, but it is still

**Table 46.6 Initial Laboratory Evaluation of the Hypertensive Patient[a]**

| Test | Clinical Usefulness |
|---|---|
| Serum creatinine (and estimated glomerular filtration rate) | Assessment of renal function. Identifies parenchymal kidney disease as a possible secondary cause, as well as established TOD. |
| Serum potassium | Low potassium (of renal origin) suggests mineralocorticoid excess (primary or secondary), glucocorticoid excess, Liddle syndrome; high potassium with normal renal function suggests Gordon syndrome; low levels raise caution about the use of thiazides and loop diuretics; high levels preclude the use of ACE inhibitors, ARBs, renin inhibitors, and potassium-sparing diuretics. |
| Serum sodium | If high, suggests primary aldosteronism; if low, alerts to the need to avoid thiazide diuretics. |
| Serum bicarbonate | If high, suggests aldosterone excess (primary or secondary); if low with normal renal function, suggests Gordon syndrome (with high potassium) or primary hyperparathyroidism (with high calcium). |
| Serum calcium | If high, suggests primary hyperparathyroidism. |
| Serum glucose | Identifies prediabetes or diabetes; in the appropriate setting, suggests glucocorticoid excess, pheochromocytoma, or acromegaly. |
| Lipid profile | Identifies hyperlipidemia. |
| Hemoglobin, hematocrit | If high, in the absence of other hematologic abnormalities or underlying lung disease, suggests sleep apnea. |
| Urinalysis[b] | Proteinuria and hematuria identify a possible secondary cause (glomerulonephritis); proteinuria can also be a marker of TOD. |
| Electrocardiography | Identifies left ventricular hypertrophy, old myocardial infarction, or other ischemic changes; identifies conduction abnormalities that may preclude the use of beta-blockers or nondihydropyridine CCBs. |

[a]To investigate the presence of comorbid conditions, secondary causes, or established target organ damage.

[b]Some organizations recommend screening microalbuminuria as a more sensitive tool to identify early renal injury. The most recent guidelines do not recommend BUN measurement alone, whereas some recommend the measurement of uric acid (as a marker of cardiovascular risk) and thyroid-stimulating hormone (to more specifically screen for hypo- and hyperthyroidism).

*ACE,* Angiotensin-converting enzyme; *ARB,* angiotensin receptor blocker; *BUN,* blood urea nitrogen; *CCB,* calcium channel blocker; *TOD,* target organ damage.

valuable as a general guide to allow more precise dietary advice to patients.

### RENIN PROFILING

The evaluation of plasma renin activity has been proposed by Laragh as an empiric method for the evaluation and treatment of hypertension.[186] The premise for this approach is mechanistic; patients with high plasma renin activity levels (>0.65 ng/mL/h, and particularly >6.5 ng/mL/h) have vasoconstriction mediated by the RAAS as the primary operative mechanism of hypertension, whereas those with suppressed plasma renin activity levels (<0.65 ng/mL/h) are volume-overloaded. Accordingly, patients with high levels of plasma renin activity are treated with blockers of the RAAS (ACE inhibitors, angiotensin receptor antagonists, renin inhibitors, beta-blockers), and those with low levels of renin are treated with diuretics (including aldosterone antagonists), CCBs, or alpha-blockers. The approach not only includes using drugs that address the underlying pathophysiology directly but also proposes removal of drugs from the opposite group because there have been reports of paradoxic BP elevations in such cases.[187] A case series has reported streamlined drug regimens and improved BP control in patients with resistant hypertension, and a small randomized trial of renin-guided therapy versus conventional therapy has yielded greater systolic BP lowering with the renin-guided system (−29 vs. −19 mm Hg; $P = .03$).[188] It is reasonable to entertain renin profiling, especially in patients who do not respond to initial therapy. In such cases, renin measurement, along with plasma aldosterone measurement, will also be useful to rule out primary hyperaldosteronism.

### SYSTEMIC HEMODYNAMICS AND EXTRACELLULAR FLUID VOLUME

An alternative to the renin-profiling approach is to measure systemic hemodynamics and extracellular fluid volume noninvasively. Such measurements can be achieved with several methodologies, but impedance cardiography has the advantage of simultaneously obtaining both volume (thoracic fluid content) and hemodynamic (CO, SVR) data. This approach has been used in patients with resistant hypertension, with some success in two randomized trials.[189,190] In one study, patients managed using the hemodynamic approach achieved better BP control while receiving more diuretics, whereas in the other, control was also better but was not associated with the specific extra use of any particular drug class. Direct measurement of volume excess and hemodynamics and availability of the information at the point of care make this methodology more attractive than renin profiling. However, relatively high costs associated with the technology and lack of reimbursement in the current health care environment make the wide use of this method out of reach for most physicians and their patients.

## SECONDARY HYPERTENSION

Secondary (or remediable) hypertension is elevated BP due to a specific cause.[8,32] For several reasons, it should always be considered in every newly diagnosed or referred patient with hypertension, especially those with a history of hypokalemia. First, the proportion of patients with secondary hypertension who can eventually be cured is far greater than those with primary hypertension. This is particularly important in young hypertensive people, especially in children and adolescents,[27] who are more likely to harbor nearly all types of secondary hypertension,with the important exception of atherosclerotic renovascular hypertension. For such people, and those with an otherwise long life expectancy, the cost of diagnosis and treatment (and even cure) of secondary hypertension may be less than the cost of chronic medical therapy, including drugs, office visits, and laboratory monitoring. Finally, it is intellectually appealing to consider the possibility of cure for patients with hypertension, which not only keeps the health care provider mentally awake, but also may help avoid failure to diagnose disease in patients who actually harbor a secondary cause, but its presence is never contemplated or formally evaluated. The most common cause of secondary hypertension is primary hyperaldosteronism.[191,192]

## RISK FACTORS AND EPIDEMIOLOGY

In general clinical practice, there is a higher probability of secondary hypertension in patients: (1) with higher levels of untreated blood pressure (except in some cases of primary hyperaldosteronism); (2) with characteristic physical signs (for details, see later); (3) with refractory hypertension (now more commonly called "resistant hypertension," defined as a patient who has had all secondary causes of hypertension excluded, as well as white coat and masked hypertension, and is confirmed to be adherent with their medications (despite proper doses of three appropriately chosen antihypertensive drugs, one of which is a diuretic, and has a persistent office blood pressure ≥140/90 mm Hg); or (4) seen in tertiary referral centers (largely caused by referral bias). Because of these factors, the prevalence of secondary hypertension varies widely.

The largest prospective study reported from a primary care setting evaluated 1020 consecutive patients with hypertension in Yokohama, Japan. The authors found that 9.1% of patients had a secondary cause, which was primary hyperaldosteronism in 6%, Cushing syndrome (full-blown in 1% and preclinical in 1%), pheochromocytoma (0.6%), and renovascular hypertension (0.5%).[193]

The largest series of consecutive patients evaluated by a whole-day protocol from 1976 to 1994 in a tertiary referral center was from Syracuse, New York. In this study, 10.1% of 4429 patients with hypertension had secondary hypertension—3.1% with renovascular hypertension, 1.4% with primary hyperaldosteronism, 0.5% with Cushing syndrome, 0.3% with pheochromocytoma, 3% with primary hypothyroidism, and 1.8% with hypertension attributed to CKD.[194] Later series from worldwide studies have suggested that primary hyperaldosteronism (especially due to sleep-disordered breathing and obstructive sleep apnea) is far more common than before the year 2000, with an average prevalence of approximately 10% to 11.2% in population-based studies; its prevalence is about doubled in resistant hypertension.[149] This change in the most common cause of secondary hypertension represents a marked reduction in smoking and much higher use of cholesterol-lowering medications—hence, a major reduction in the incidence of atherosclerotic arterial disease.

### EVALUATION OF SECONDARY HYPERTENSION

Hypertension guidelines and a great deal of clinical experience have suggested a more detailed evaluation for secondary causes in patients with hypertension younger than 30 years who have no family history of hypertension. Additionally, those older than 55 years, with new-onset hypertension, sudden worsening of BP control (despite years of previously controlled BP levels), recurrent flash pulmonary edema, an abdominal bruit (especially with a louder diastolic component), and sudden increases of the serum creatinine level by 30% or more after an RAAS blocker, should prompt evaluation for secondary causes of hypertension. Such patients have a higher pretest probability of renovascular hypertension.

The initial set of laboratory tests recommended for newly diagnosed patients with hypertension includes serum levels of urea and creatinine and a urinalysis, which is generally sufficient for identifying patients with underlying intrinsic renal disease, even if the 3-month criterion for CKD is not yet met (see Table 46.6). Hyperthyroidism or hypothyroidism can be a cause of hypertension, but the presence of either is commonly detected by a serum ultrasensitive thyroid-stimulating hormone (thyrotropin) level.

Sometimes the demographic and clinical features of the patient help direct the search for a secondary cause. Fibromuscular dysplasia is much more common in young white women, whereas atherosclerotic renovascular disease is more common in older smokers (both current and former). Some symptoms, when elicited by a careful history, are also quite suggestive, although incompletely sensitive and not very specific.

Typically, paroxysmal spells occur in approximately 25% to 30% of patients with pheochromocytoma; the associated symptoms are variable across patients but are commonly experienced repetitively in a given patient. Sadly, the specificity of these paroxysms, even when they include headache, sweating, and elevated BP levels, is less than 5% in most large series. Similarly, the classic symptoms of large muscle weakness (particularly when rising from a chair or climbing stairs) reported with Cushing syndrome, or lower extremity weakness and leg cramps reported in primary hyperaldosteronism and attributed to hypokalemia, are uncommon in today's literature and patients. Given the relatively low prevalence of secondary hypertension, the decision to undertake a formal evaluation for specific causes can (and should) be individualized.

### EXACERBATION OF PREEXISTING HYPERTENSION ATTRIBUTED TO LIFESTYLE FACTORS

Although generally not considered in most discussions of secondary (or remediable) hypertension, BP can be influenced by prescription or nonprescription medications or both,[195] excessive dietary sodium intake,[196] body weight and obesity, and excessive alcohol intake.[8] The health care provider or patient may not immediately appreciate some of these factors. Appropriate attention to these issues can result in improved BP profiles and a better prognosis.[197]

Modification of these factors is the cornerstone of therapy for primary hypertension and can mimic secondary hypertension. Of these factors, the most common issues relate to excessive sodium intake, poor sleep hygiene (i.e., getting <6 hours of uninterrupted sleep a night),[198] excessive caffeine or other stimulants, and use of nonsteroidal antiinflammatory drugs (NSAIDs).

## INTRINSIC KIDNEY DISEASE

Hypertension can be both a cause and consequence of CKD—that is, estimated GFR (eGFR) is less than 60 mL/min/1.73 $m^2$. It is often difficult to discern which occurred first when a patient presents initially with both, but the screening and diagnostic processes are identical to those used for each individually. CKD is currently diagnosed using the 2012 Kidney Disease: Improving Global Outcomes (KDIGO) criteria from the National Kidney Foundation: persistent (≥3 months) evidence of kidney damage (e.g., proteinuria, abnormal urinary sediment, abnormal blood or urine chemistry levels, imaging studies, or biopsy), but primarily based on the eGFR.[199] Although it is possible to have CKD with eGFR greater than 60 mL/min/1.73 $m^2$, most authorities recommend this threshold for common use. Management strategies for hypertension due to CKD are also identical to those used in primary hypertension, except that doses and frequency of antihypertensive (and other) medications normally cleared by the kidney are decreased inversely to the eGFR. Although most antihypertensive drugs do not need dose adjustments in stage 3b or higher CKD, some agents that affect the RAAS mechanistically should theoretically be reduced. Renally excreted beta-blockers (e.g., atenolol, metoprolol, bisoprolol, nadolol, acebutolol) and all ACE inhibitors, except fosinopril and trandolapril, are reduced in dose or dosing frequency, but no serious adverse effects (other than possibly hyperkalemia) have been reported, even if no adjustment of dosing is performed. Also note that losartan and valsartan, normally twice-daily agents from the angiotensin receptor blocker (ARB) class when kidney function is normal, should be dosed once daily in those with an eGFR less than 60 mL/min/1.73 $m^2$.

Restriction of dietary protein intake had been recommended in the distant past, based on several small trials (primarily in Australia), but had marginal success in the Modification of Diet in Renal Disease trial.[200] It is usually challenging to carry out effectively, even in tertiary centers with a dedicated renal nutritionist. Dietary sodium restriction, although a somewhat lesser challenge, has benefits in patients with CKD and hypertension, not only to lower BP, but also to reduce urinary protein (and albumin) excretion.[201]

## PRIMARY HYPERALDOSTERONISM

This form of secondary hypertension has been increasing in prevalence worldwide over the last 25 years[195,202] and is generally due to one of six subtypes: (1) an aldosterone-producing (Conn) adenoma, nearly always in one adrenal gland (~35% of cases); (2) bilateral adrenal hyperplasia (also known as *idiopathic primary hyperaldosteronism*, ~60% of cases); (3) primary (or unilateral) adrenal hyperplasia (~2% of cases); (4) aldosterone-producing adrenal carcinoma (~35 cases in the world literature); (5) familial hyperaldosteronism, which takes one of two forms—glucocorticoid-suppressible hyperaldosteronism, due to a chimeric chromosome 8, in which the 5′-regulatory sequence for corticotropin responsiveness of 11β-hydroxylase is fused to the enzyme coding sequence for aldosterone synthase (<1% of cases), or familial occurrences of either an aldosterone-producing adenoma or bilateral adrenal hyperplasia (<2% of cases); or (6) ectopic production of aldosterone by an adenoma or carcinoma outside the adrenal gland (<0.1% of cases). In addition, obstructive sleep apnea and sleep-disordered breathing also cause hyperaldosteronism. This is classically described as secondary hyperaldosteronism, but its evaluation and medical treatment are often quite similar to that of bilateral adrenal hyperplasia.

The prevalence of primary hyperaldosteronism depends on where and how one looks and is controversial. Some referral centers have reported a prevalence of hyperaldosteronism related to sleep apnea at approximately 20%, similar to the original prevalence of aldosterone-secreting adenomas estimated by Conn in the 1950s. In large population-based studies, the prevalence of primary hyperaldosteronism has been estimated at approximately 10% to 11.2% of hypertensives. The condition appears to be more common in people with higher levels of BP (2% for BP levels of 140–159/90–99 mm Hg, 8% for BP levels of 160–179/100–109 mm Hg, and 13% for BP levels > 180/110 mm Hg), treatment-resistant hypertension (17%–23% in several series), patients with hypertension with spontaneous or diuretic-associated hypokalemia, and hypertension and a serendipitously discovered adrenal mass (1%–10%).

In the last millennium, hypokalemia was thought to be very common—if not nearly universal—among patients with primary hyperaldosteronism, particularly if provoked by diuretic therapy. Today, however, more afflicted patients have eukalemia than hypokalemia, although sometimes more severe cases have weakness, muscle cramps, and even periodic paralysis. Patients with primary hyperaldosteronism experience higher CV morbidity and mortality than age-, gender-, and BP-matched patients with primary hypertension.[203]

Screening for primary hyperaldosteronism is most efficiently performed in potassium-repleted patients using the ratio of plasma aldosterone concentration to plasma renin activity (ARR; Table 46.7). The ARR can be affected by many factors, including antihypertensive drug therapy, dietary sodium restriction, posture, time of day, and sample handling (see Table 46.7). Most authorities recommend sustained-release verapamil, hydralazine, and peripheral $\alpha_1$-adrenoceptor antagonists as medications that have little, if any, effect on the ARR. The likelihood of a false-positive ARR is increased by a low plasma renin activity (e.g., <0.5 ng of Ang II/mL per hour), so some investigators require the plasma aldosterone concentration to be above a given threshold (e.g., >15 ng/dL), for the screening to be considered positive, but levels between 12 and 15 ng/dL need to be considered individually, because some patients with proven aldosteronism have values in this range. Confirmation of primary aldosteronism in patients with aldosterone levels below 10 ng/dL, on the other hand, are rare. The most common cutoff value for an ARR that usually leads to further investigation is 30 (when the aldosterone level is measured in nanograms per deciliter and plasma renin activity in nanograms of Ang II per milliliter per hour), but higher thresholds lead to more falsely negative tests.

Clinical practice guidelines from the Endocrine Society have recommended one of four confirmatory tests before proceeding to an imaging study because of the expense and radiation involved in the latter. There have been only a few comparative studies of these four tests; they seem to have similar performance characteristics (75%–90% sensitivity,

**Table 46.7 Factors That May Cause False-Positive or False-Negative Results of the Aldosterone/Renin Ratio**

| Factor | False-Positives | False-Negatives |
|---|---|---|
| Aldosterone relatively high | Potassium loading | |
| Renin relatively low | Beta-blockers; central alpha-adrenoceptor agonists; direct renin inhibitors; nonsteroidal antiinflammatory drugs; chronic kidney disease; sodium loading | |
| Aldosterone relatively low | | Hypokalemia |
| Renin relatively high | | Diuretics; ACE inhibitors, angiotensin receptor blockers; calcium channel blockers (dihydropyridines); acute sodium depletion |

*ACE,* Angiotensin-converting enzyme.

80%–100% specificity). Cost, patient preference, local experience, local laboratory methods, and insurance reimbursement all factor into which confirmatory test is chosen.

The traditional saline-loading test (2 L infused over 4 hours) is confirmatory if the postinfusion plasma aldosterone concentration is greater than 10 ng/mL. Patients with aldoserone concentrations from 5 to 10 ng/mL are considered indeterminate and should be restested. Needless to say, intravenous saline is not often recommended for patients with heart failure, CKD, or uncontrolled hypertension.

Many centers have reported success with an oral sodium-loading protocol, which involves liberalizing sodium intake to approximately 6 g/day for 3 to 5 days and then assaying 24-hour urine collections for sodium (to ensure loading) and aldosterone content. The test is considered positive if the urinary aldosterone excretion is greater than 12 to 14 µg/day, but oral sodium loading can be as problematic in some patients as intravenous saline.

The fludrocortisone suppression test involves giving 0.1 mg of fludrocortisone every 6 hours for 4 days and then assaying the plasma aldosterone concentration when the patient is standing upright. It is considered confirmatory if the concentration is greater than 6 ng/dL, and plasma renin activity and serum cortisol levels are low. Execution of the test may be difficult for patients who have a long journey to the office or who are nonadherent.

Finally, the captopril challenge test is performed by assaying the plasma aldosterone concentration before and 1 and 2 hours after administration of 25 to 50 mg of oral captopril. It is considered confirmatory if the plasma aldosterone concentration remains elevated (and unchanged from baseline); many false-negative and equivocal captopril challenge test results have been reported, although several Japanese series have shown excellent results with this method.

After the diagnosis of primary aldosteronism is confirmed, a computed tomography (CT) scan of the adrenals is undertaken, which is useful in detecting large masses that might be adrenal carcinomas. Adrenal carcinomas typically are larger (>4 cm in diameter), an inhomogeneous character (often with internal hemorrhage), internal calcifications (in ~40%), and irregular borders (often because of micrometastases) and show enhancement after intravenous contrast medium is administered. Aldosterone-producing adenomas are usually small (<2 cm in diameter), hypodense, unilateral nodules. Idiopathic hyperaldosteronism usually has normal-appearing adrenal glands, but sometimes nodular changes and/or general enlargement are visible in one or both adrenals. Magnetic resonance imaging (MRI) is no better at detecting these abnormalities than CT, which is usually less expensive. Both techniques often detect nonfunctioning nodules, especially in older patients. At some centers, patients with hypertension with proven primary hyperaldosteronism who are younger than 40 years with a single typical hypodense nodule in one adrenal gland are offered an adrenalectomy directly.

Because CT scans identify unilateral adrenal disease with a sensitivity of only 78% and specificity of only 75%, the Endocrine Society has recommended adrenal venous sampling for most surgical candidates.[204] Despite being invasive, expensive, technically challenging, and potentially dangerous, and requiring an experienced and well-coordinated team, it has sensitivity and specificity of 95% and 100%, respectively, for detecting unilateral aldosterone production. It is commonly performed at 8 AM, with continuous cosyntropin administration, and simultaneous adrenal vein cortisol level measurement. Most centers use a 4:1 cutoff value of the cortisol-corrected aldosterone ratio (i.e., the ratio between the aldosterone/cortisol ratios on each side) to define a positive lateralization.

Several older (some prefer classic) tests remain available for the presumably rare circumstance in which adrenal venous sampling was technically unsuccessful or nondiagnostic. These are usually much less expensive and therefore can sometimes be preauthorized when financial and other roadblocks can affect adrenal venous sampling. The postural stimulation test, developed in the 1970s, depends on the propensity of patients with an aldosterone-producing adenoma to retain diurnal variation in the plasma aldosterone concentration, whereas those with idiopathic hyperaldosteronism often show an increased sensitivity to small increases in Ang II levels (e.g., after standing). In some centers, this test is performed by drawing two additional blood samples (before and after standing) at the conclusion of the intravenous saline infusion test. In a review of the Mayo Clinic experience from the last millennium in 246 patients with surgically proven adenomas, the test was only 85% accurate. There are also other tests. For example, iodocholesterol scintigraphy was developed at the University of Michigan in the 1970s; its sensitivity correlates directly with tumor size, so it is not very helpful in discerning microadenomas from bilateral hyperplasia. Also, serum 18-hydroxycorticosterone levels, typically measured with the patient in the recumbent position at 8 AM, are often higher than 100 ng/dL in patients with an adenoma, but the opposite is true in patients with bilateral hyperplasia, so blood was traditionally taken for this analyte before the 2-L saline infusion test. However, the accuracy of this test has been found to be even lower than the postural stimulation test.

Genetic testing for familial forms of primary hyperaldosteronism is recommended for those who are younger than 20 years at diagnosis and in those with a family history of primary aldosteronism or stroke at an early age (typically, <30 years). This strategy was successful in approximately half of large, qualifying, unrelated cohorts. Genetic testing by a Southern blot or long polymerase chain reaction assay is both sensitive and specific for glucocorticoid-remediable hyperaldosteronism (familial hyperaldosteronism, type I, the most common monogenetic cause of hypertension). Such testing is expensive, so many managed care organizations will not pay for the test unless an appropriate response (in both BP and plasma aldosterone concentration) is seen after weeks of empiric glucocorticoid administration. Familial hyperaldosteronism type II is genetically heterogeneous, despite being autosomal dominant in most affected cases. Genetic testing is not yet available for this more common type of familial hyperaldosteronism, so the diagnosis is primarily clinical, based on the biochemical findings and the pedigree.

Laparoscopic procedures for unilateral adrenalectomy have improved to the point that most patients with adrenal venous sampling–proven hyperaldosteronism have shorter hospital stays, fewer complications, and lower costs than those who have undergone an open procedure. Although nearly all return to eukalemia, hypertension is cured (i.e., follow-up BP levels of <140/90 mm Hg without antihypertensive drug therapy) in only approximately 50%. Cure is more likely in younger people, those with a short duration of hypertension, prior BP control with only one or two agents, and a pedigree that includes fewer than two first-degree relatives with hypertension. Typically, plasma aldosterone concentration and plasma renin activity are measured shortly after successful surgery, and potassium supplementation and aldosterone antagonists are discontinued. Intravenous saline is often required because the remaining adrenal gland needs to recover its normal function, which may take a few weeks. The nonsurgical option for patients with idiopathic hyperaldosteronism is spironolactone, which has had significantly better efficacy than its successor, eplerenone, in an international randomized clinical trial in hypertensive subjects with primary aldosteronism. Most physicians use dexamethasone or prednisone at bedtime (over twice-daily hydrocortisone) for glucocorticoid-remediable hyperaldosteronism, but the doses are kept low to avoid iatrogenic Cushing syndrome (see later).

## HYPERALDOSTERONISM ASSOCIATED WITH SLEEP-DISORDERED BREATHING

Several reports have highlighted this association, which is thought to account for approximately 20% of resistant hypertension and typically responds very nicely to selective aldosterone antagonists. Polysomnography is the gold standard test for obstructive sleep apnea diagnosis, but requires overnight evaluation and is expensive. The Berlin questionnaire, which includes questions about snoring, daytime somnolence, body mass index, and hypertension, is a brief and validated screening tool that identifies persons in the community who are at high risk for obstructive sleep apnea. The ratio of serum aldosterone to plasma renin activity is used most often to diagnose the condition. A therapeutic trial of spironolactone may be warranted, especially if the Berlin questionnaire or the sleep study is sufficiently suggestive.

## APPARENT MINERALOCORTICOID EXCESS STATES

Several unusual diagnoses manifest with a similar set of signs and symptoms (especially hypokalemia and often other Cushingoid features) that result from an apparent mineralocorticoid excess. These are most easily distinguished from the several types of hyperaldosteronism by the suppressed plasma aldosterone level.

The most common type, classic congenital adrenal hyperplasia, is due to one of several autosomal recessive genetic deficiencies in enzymes involved in adrenal steroidogenesis, usually resulting in mineralocorticoid and androgen excess. Although most common in infants and children, some patients (especially those with milder loss-of-function mutations) go undiagnosed until adulthood. The most common deficiency, 21-hydroxylase, accounts for approximately 95% of cases and is often discovered by universal screening programs, particularly for female newborns with ambiguous genitalia. If left untreated, approximately 75% of such babies suffer salt wasting, failure to thrive, hyponatremia, hypovolemia, shock, and death.

Hypertension occurs in approximately two-thirds of patients with congenital adrenal hyperplasia due to either 11β-hydroxylase deficiency (~5% of cases of congenital adrenal hyperplasia and a prevalence of approximately 1:100,000 in whites) or 17α-hydroxylase deficiency, which is rare. More than 40 mutations have been identified that lead to 11β-hydroxylase deficiency, which results in high circulating levels of deoxycorticosterone and 11-deoxycortisol, with increased production of adrenal androgens. Thus girls present in infancy or childhood with hypertension, hypokalemia, acne, hirsutism, and virilization, whereas boys present with pseudoprecocious puberty. Because 17α-hydroxylase is required for the production of both cortisol and sex steroids, its deficiency can delay puberty and present as pseudohermaphroditism or phenotypic female features (in genetic 45,XY boys), or as primary amenorrhea in girls. After appropriate diagnosis, typically by determination of levels of steroid precursors in serum, patients with congenital adrenal hyperplasia receive supplementation with glucocorticoids, which suppress corticotropin secretion and reduce the signs and symptoms of mineralocorticoid excess. Long-term care of adults with congenital adrenal hyperplasia is challenging.

Very rare causes of apparent mineralocorticoid excess include deoxycorticosterone-producing tumors, which are usually quite large and often malignant, primary cortisol resistance, or 11β-hydroxysteroid dehydrogenase deficiency, of which approximately 50 cases worldwide are congenital. Most are acquired and associated with imported licorice or licorice-flavored chewing tobacco. Some would also include Liddle syndrome—hypertension, hypokalemia, and inappropriate kaliuresis, associated with low plasma aldosterone and renin activity—due to an autosomal dominant condition that results in mutations in the beta or gamma subunits of the renal amiloride-sensitive ENaC.

## RENOVASCULAR HYPERTENSION

Hypertension due to renal artery stenosis (fibromuscular dysplasia or atherosclerotic disease) has been studied extensively since the pioneering work of Harry Goldblatt (see Chapter 47).

The probability of renovascular hypertension can be calculated based on clinical characteristics in a given patient, which eliminates the need for a screening test in most cases. The choice among the several screening tests for renovascular hypertension is usually based on patient and physician preference, local expertise, and a favorable decision about prior authorization for the test from insurance companies. This has become less common since the publication of several outcome studies that showed no significant benefit to renal angioplasty (usually with stenting) over medical management in atherosclerotic renal artery disease.[160]

## PHEOCHROMOCYTOMA

Although chromaffin tumors (pheochromocytomas and paragangliomas) that secrete catecholamines are rare (estimated incidence, two to eight cases/million per year), their diagnosis and management are important because of the following: (1) they might cause fatal hypertensive crises, despite otherwise appropriate treatment; (2) probably more than 10% are metastatic at diagnosis; (3) specific therapy can be curative; and (4) a much higher proportion of cases are more familial than once thought.[205]

Catecholamine-secreting tumors are found in 0.2% to 0.6% of patients with hypertension, may be more common in hypertensive children (1.7%), and are too often found incidentally, or worse, only at autopsy. The clinical presentation of patients with these tumors is variable because symptoms may occur constantly or in paroxysms. The classic triad of headache, sweating attacks, and hypertension was said to be present in 95% of patients in one large French series, but most centers reported having to see more than 100 such patients on referral before one is positively diagnosed.

The differential diagnosis includes many disorders, some of which are functional or factitious, so a high index of suspicion is required, even when faced with common admitting conditions (e.g., heart failure, which can be precipitated, if not exacerbated, by a functioning tumor). Some familial conditions that include pheochromocytoma have characteristic physical signs (e.g., café au lait spots and neurofibromas, retinal hemangiomas, port wine stains, subungual fibromas, ash leaf or shagreen patches, adenoma sebaceum, marfanoid body habitus) that provide clues to the underlying syndromes.[205]

There seem to be more exceptions to pheochromocytoma than with many other conditions: approximately 10% of such tumors are extraadrenal, multiple or bilateral, recurrent (after surgical extirpation), discovered as incidentalomas, or in children. More than 10% are likely familial or metastatic at presentation, and both of these have increased in the last 30 years. Although approximately 90% of pheochromocytomas are found in or in close proximity to the adrenal gland, paragangliomas can occur anywhere along the sympathetic ganglia, but most commonly in or near the organ of Zuckerkandl (at the aortic bifurcation) or near the bladder, which gives rise to rather unusual symptoms of so-called micturition headache, syncope, or similar problems.

Pheochromocytomas play important parts in the multiple endocrine neoplasia (MEN) syndromes, especially MEN2A (pheochromocytoma in ~50%, usually bilateral, medullary carcinoma of the thyroid, parathyroid adenomas, and cutaneous lichen amyloidosis, associated with the *RET* proto-oncogene) and MEN2B (usually bilateral pheochromocytomas, medullary carcinoma of the thyroid, submucosal neuromas, hyperplastic corneal nerves, joint laxity, Hirschsprung disease, and sometimes marfanoid body habitus). Pheochromocytomas are also found in patients with phakomatoses.

Approximately 20% of patients with von Hippel-Lindau disease type 2 (retinal and/or cerebellar hemangioblastomas, occasionally with clear cell renal carcinoma, pancreatic neuroendocrine tumors, retinal angiomas or hemangioblastomas, mediated by the *VHL* tumor suppressor gene, located on chromosome 3p25-26) will have pheochromocytomas or paragangliomas. Approximately 2% of patients with neurofibromatosis type 1 (autosomal dominant von Recklinghausen disease; neurofibromas, with café au lait spots, axillary and/or inguinal freckling, hamartomas of the iris—Lisch nodules, bony abnormalities, central nervous system gliomas, and sometimes macrocephaly, or cognitive deficits, mediated by the *NF1* tumor suppressor gene on chromosome 17q11.2) will develop a catecholamine-secreting tumor, usually an adrenal pheochromocytoma. Both these conditions can be diagnosed using genetic screening, although this is often more fruitful for screening family members after an index case has been identified.

Neither the prevalence nor genetics of pheochromocytoma in Sturge-Weber syndrome (choroidal and leptomeningeal angiomas, port wine stain in the trigeminal distribution) or tuberous sclerosis (sometimes called Bourneville or Pringle disease—adenoma sebaceum, subungual fibromas, and occasionally mental retardation) are as well understood. Familial paraganglioma is an autosomal dominant syndrome with paragangliomas in the skull base and neck, thorax, abdomen, pelvis, or urinary bladder wall. A number of studies in the last 2 decades have characterized mutations in one of several genes that code for components of the mitochondrial succinate dehydrogenase complex—*SDHD,* located on chromosome 11q23, or *SDHB,* located on chromosome 1p35-36. Availability of genetic testing for these mutations has made disease surveillance for those who carry these genes (typically relatives of index cases) much simpler.

The process of case finding for catecholamine-secreting tumors typically begins with biochemical testing for catecholamine metabolites. Measurements of plasma-free or urinary fractionated metanephrines are usually recommended, but a wide variety of factors are known to produce both false-positive and false-negative results. In some centers, plasma-free metanephrines (which provide a very brief picture of catecholamine production and metabolism) can be assayed quickly and accurately; in others, integration of catecholamine production and metabolism over a longer time period is less expensively performed using urinary collections. False-negative urinary collections are common in patients with pheochromocytomas that are familial, normotensive, dopamine β-hydroxylase deficient, or intermittently secreting. Pharmacologic testing for pheochromocytoma is occasionally used in equivocal cases; clonidine suppression testing is usually preferred over glucagon stimulation testing, although most managed care organizations recommend a repeat plasma or urinary collection 6 months or more after the initial evaluation.

To improve cost-effectiveness and reduce radiation exposure, imaging studies for pheochromocytoma and related tumors are generally not ordered until after biochemical evidence of catecholamine overproduction has been obtained. In this setting, the higher resolution available from CT scans, with thin cuts of the adrenals, outweighs the more specific finding of a T2-weighted bright spot via MRI. For some patients (e.g., those with metastatic disease, intraabdominal surgical clips, allergies to radiocontrast media, pregnant), MRI may be a more suitable option. Positron emission tomography scans using fluorine 18-labeled fludeoxyglucose or nuclear medicine scans using Iodine[123]-labeled *m*-iodobenzylguanidine ($^{123}$I-MIBG) can localize and define the extent of metastatic disease, especially if delivery of a $^{131}$I-MIBG scan is a viable therapeutic option. Prior to obtaining this scan, certain antihypertensive medications should be discontinued, if possible, for at least 7 to 10 days before the test. These classes include calcium antagonists (e.g., amlodipine), alpha- and beta-blockers (e.g., labetolol), and many other non–BP-lowering agents.[206]

The role of genetic testing in the routine care of patients with pheochromocytoma is evolving; current guidelines recommend a shared decision-making process, often involving more family members than just the index patient.[207] Eight studies have shown a high prevalence of germline mutations in patients with presumed sporadic pheochromocytoma or ganglioma, so some authorities recommend genetic screening for all afflicted patients; others base the decision on the pedigree, syndromic features, and/or extent of disease (e.g., multifocal, bilateral, or metastatic tumors at diagnosis).

Proper pharmacologic preparation of the patient with pheochromocytoma is critical for successful extirpation of the tumor; alpha-blockers (e.g., phentolamine intravenously or phenoxybenzamine orally) are given first, followed by beta-blockers if needed to control tachycardia. Most experts use a calcium antagonist before adding a beta-blocker and recommend delaying the operation for 7 to 14 days after localization of the tumor to normalize BP, heart rate, and intravascular volume, which helps minimize hypotension after removal of the tumor. Metyrosine is also used occasionally in people with very large tumors or nonsurgical candidates.

Most surgeons favor laparoscopic procedures for small adrenal pheochromocytomas or paragangliomas in accessible locations. Postoperatively, vigilant monitoring may reduce the risk for severe hypotension, hypoglycemia, or adrenal insufficiency. The diagnostic technique that originally demonstrated the overproduction of catecholamines in a given patient is usually repeated 4 to 6 weeks postoperatively to document successful tumor removal and occasionally (often annually) during long-term follow-up. The specific frequency is best individualized, based on the pedigree, results of genetic testing, and risk factors that predict recurrence.

## HYPERCORTISOLISM

Most cases of Cushing syndrome today are iatrogenic due to prescribed oral corticosteroids, but occasional sporadic cases are still seen and were found in 0.5% to 1.0% of hypertensive subjects in two large series. The pathophysiology of hypertension in Cushing syndrome overlaps somewhat with mineralocorticoid excess states. This is because excess cortisol often overwhelms the capacity of 11β-hydroxysteroid dehydrogenase type 2 to degrade cortisol to cortisone selectively in the aldosterone-producing cells of the adrenal cortex and can increase circulating levels of deoxycorticosterone, which has only mineralocorticoid activity.

The full-blown syndrome of hypertension, truncal obesity with striae, diabetes, hirsutism, acne, hyperglycemia, hypokalemia, and muscular weakness is less common today than in Cushing's era, and the recommended diagnostic sequence is also much shorter. After an appropriate screening test (urinary-free cortisol, late night salivary cortisol, or overnight dexamethasone suppression test) has positive results, an endocrine referral for a second test is recommended before imaging studies are ordered. In some centers, plasma corticotropin levels are used to discriminate between corticotropin-dependent Cushing syndrome (>15 pg/mL, probably 85%–90% of cases) and corticotropin-independent Cushing syndrome (<5 pg/mL). In most cases, dynamic testing of the hypothalamic-pituitary-adrenal axis is performed next, with a corticotropin-releasing hormone test, which assays plasma cortisol and corticotropin levels before and after intravenous releasing hormone, or a high-dose dexamethasone (2 mg every 6 hours) suppression test, which assays the serum cortisol level.

Most expert centers have reported that this localizes the tumor to the pituitary in 60% to 75% of cases, a single adrenal gland in approximately 20% (split ~60 : 40 between adenomas and carcinomas), or ectopic production of corticotropin (10%–12%, usually by small cell lung cancers), with less than 1% due to ectopic production of corticotropin-releasing hormone, typically by bronchial carcinoid tumors. Petrosal venous sinus sampling is not needed very often today. The anatomic site of hormonal overproduction is then usually approached surgically, although other modalities (e.g., radiation of the sella turcica) can be used in special circumstances. Medical therapy is also possible in some cases, especially those patients for whom surgery is not feasible.

## THYROID DYSFUNCTION

The literature about thyroid dysfunction being associated with hypertension is inconsistent. Many patients with hyperthyroidism have wide pulse pressures (and therefore elevated systolic BP levels) and high pulse rates, but this is seldom missed, especially in younger patients. The ultrasensitive serum thyroid-stimulating hormone (TSH) level is widely available and is most commonly used for screening. After diagnosis, a nonselective beta-blocker such as propranolol may be specifically useful because it treats the tachycardia and hypertension and allegedly inhibits peripheral conversion of thyroxine to triiodothyronine. However, some now question these "classic" clinical pharmacologic reports.

The role of hypothyroidism as a potential cause of hypertension, especially isolated diastolic, is less clear, despite the experience in upstate New York, in which 3% of patients with hypertension reverted to normotension after treatment of hypothyroidism.[151] The hypertension in hypothyroidism is predominantly diastolic and usually in the range of stage 1 (i.e., diastolic BP < 99 mm Hg). In children and adolescents, especially in areas of iodide deficiency, a positive association between serum TSH and BP has been noted. A pooling of seven population-based European data sets has shown similar findings in adults, but there was no consistent relationship with either a 5-year change in BP or incident hypertension. It is likely that targeted screening of patients with hypertension for hypothyroidism with determination of the serum TSH level may be useful, but routine screening for all newly diagnosed patients with hypertension is not currently recommended by any set of national or international guidelines.

### HYPERPARATHYROIDISM, CALCIUM INTAKE, VITAMIN D, AND HYPERTENSION

Although hypercalcemia and hypertension associated with hyperparathyroidism often improve after appropriate treatment, causal relationships between calcium and vitamin D intake, serum parathyroid hormone levels, and BP have not been seen consistently in large populations.[208] As a result, most current guidelines recommend a serum calcium level (and not parathyroid hormone) determination during blood testing for patients with an initial diagnosis of hypertension.

### COARCTATION OF THE AORTA

Although most discrete isthmic constrictions of the aorta occur in or near the ductus arteriosus, there has been growing awareness that this fifth most common form of congenital cardiovascular disorders constitutes a spectrum of aortic and vasculopathic disorders and is not always cured by surgical procedures that relieve the obstruction. Most patients with the condition are hypertensive[209,210] and are diagnosed in infancy or childhood, but some escape detection until adulthood. Many cases are identified by suggestive physical findings (e.g., murmur, BP lower in the legs than the arms, radial-femoral pulse delay), some after imaging studies done for other reasons (e.g., rib notching or a "3" sign on chest radiograph; the latter results from indentation of the aorta, with prestenotic and poststenotic dilation), and others during investigation of associated abnormalities (e.g., bicuspid aortic valve).

Echocardiography is highly recommended for diagnosis and localization of the coarctation, although some patients (especially adults and those with associated anomalies) may require cardiac catheterization. Most pediatric patients undergo percutaneous catheter balloon dilation with stent placement; this can be followed by definitive surgical correction later, if needed. In a systematic review, 25% to 68% of patients with a coarctation had persistent hypertension despite satisfactory procedure results, with age at the time of surgery, age at follow-up, and the type of intervention being strong predictors of persistent hypertension.[211] A beta-blocker can lower BP and is often used in patients with coarctation, but this is not an indication approved by the US Food and Drug Administration (FDA).

### ACROMEGALY

Hypertension occurs in more than 40% of patients with excessive growth hormone release causing acromegaly, and it can be exacerbated by concomitant sleep apnea.[212] Most such patients are easily identified by symptoms or signs of acral bony overgrowth, particularly in children or adolescents before epiphyseal closure, although some patients ignore or tolerate these changes for a decade or more. The vast majority (98%) of cases are caused by a pituitary adenoma; serum insulin-like growth factor-1 is the most useful initial laboratory screening test, although other tests, including the response of plasma growth hormone levels to an oral 75-g glucose load and prolactin levels, are often performed.

As with coarctation, successful treatment of acromegaly usually lowers BP, but hypertension often persists, especially in older and overweight patients.[213] No specific antihypertensive drug therapy seems to be more effective than others but, because acromegaly is a very unusual cause of resistant hypertension, antihypertensive drug therapy is usually effective.

## SLEEP DEPRIVATION AND SLEEP-DISORDERED BREATHING

Poor sleep quality, if chronic, yields the same symptomology of paroxysmal hypertension and elevated BP, especially during the afternoon and evening hours. Poor sleep quality is not just the result of obstructive sleep apnea (OSA) but a host of sleep disorders, including restless legs syndrome and insomnia of a various causes.[214] Often, these different sleep disorders coexist and prevent the patient from achieving proper restful sleep.

The mechanism of poor sleep quality contributing to elevated BP and paroxysmal bouts of very high BP relates to activation of both the sympathetic and RAAS.[215,216] Sympathetic activity is also increased in sleep deprivation, restless legs syndrome, and OSA.[215,216]

Patients without OSA who suffer from sleep deprivation, defined as less than a minimum of 6 hours of uninterrupted sleep, also have increased sympathetic activity. In this case, it is a consequence of reduced time in non–rapid eye movement (NREM) or slow wave sleep that also affects the nocturnal dip in BP.[216] This supports the hypothesis that disturbed NREM sleep quantity or quality is a mechanism whereby sleep deprivation or restless legs syndrome leads to an increase in sympathetic tone.

OSA should be suspected in patients (men more so than women) who report severe snoring, daytime somnolence, witnessed nocturnal choking or gasping, and have a "crowded oropharynx" (limited or no visualization of the soft palate) on physical examination. Formal diagnosis is based on an ambulatory sleep study or in-center polysomnography.[217]

In contrast to reduced sleep time and quality, the increase in sympathetic activity associated with OSA is a function of intermittent hypoxia because the acute rise in BP parallels the severity of oxygen desaturation at night.[218] Indeed, increased sympathetic activity is seen in animal models subjected exclusively to intermittent hypoxia.[219] It is also important to note that OSA associated hypertension is only slightly reduced by continuous positive airway pressure (CPAP) treatment.[220] Nevertheless, addressing sleep disorders or sleep habits is relevant when considering the risk of developing or controlling preexistent hypertension.

Treatment of OSA with CPAP has a modest BP lowering effect (~1-mm Hg/hour use). However, patients who have more severe hypertension, more severe OSA, higher daytime sleepiness scores, and greater adherence to CPAP (average use >4 hours/night) tend to have greater responses.[221]

## DRUG-INDUCED HYPERTENSIOM

Patients presenting with hypertension should be questioned about exposure to substances that can raise BP (Box 46.3).

**Box 46.3 Drugs Commonly Associated With Hypertension**

Oral contraceptives
Nonsteroidal antiinflammatory drugs (NSAIDs; selective and nonselective)
Sympathomimetics: pseudoephedrine, phenylpropanolamine, phentermine, cocaine, amphetamines (prescription or illegal); yohimbine (alpha-2 antagonist)
Selective serotonin reuptake inhibitors (SSRIs) and serotonin-norepinephrine reuptake inhibitors (SNRIs)
Monoamine oxidase inhibitors (MAOIs)
Cyclosporine and tacrolimus
Erythropoietin and darbepoetin
Corticosteroids, mineralocorticoids (fludrocortisone)
Anti-VEGF antibodies (e.g., bevacizumab, ramucirumab) and certain tyrosine kinase inhibitors with anti-VEGF activity (e.g., sorafenib, sunitinib)
Licorice
Ethanol

*VEGF,* Vascular endothelial growth factor.
From Peixoto AJ. Secondary hypertension. In: Gilbert S, Weiner D, eds. *Primer in kidney diseases.* Philadelphia: Elsevier, 2018.

These include drugs of abuse and over-the-counter and prescription medications. Oral contraceptive pills (OCPS) can cause hypertension, although modern low-estrogen pills do so at rates much lower than with older preparations. Stopping the OCP cures the hypertension after several weeks to months in most but not all women. NSAIDs result in a modest average hypertensive effect (up to ~5 mm Hg), but some patients can have larger, clinically significant BP elevation. NSAID-induced hypertension may also present as loss of BP control in patients taking a diuretic or a blocker of the RAAS, whereas CCBs tend to be less affected in NSAID users.

Sympathomimetic amines (legal or illegal) usually cause hypertension acutely following their ingestion. Alcohol has an acute hypotensive effect, but chronic use in large amounts (more than four or five drink equivalents/day) is associated with increased BP. Glucocorticoids and mineralocorticoids can produce a dose-dependent rise in BP. Glucocorticoids with low mineralocorticoid activity (e.g., dexamethasone, budesonide) induce lesser pressor responses.

Selective serotonin reuptake inhibitors (SSRIs) and serotonin-norepinephrine reuptake inhibitors (SNRIs) can increase BP modestly, but some patients receiving SNRIs can have a severe hypertensive response. Interestingly, when used for hypertensive patients with depression, BP often improves as depressive symptoms improve. Angiogenesis inhibitors, such as anti–vascular endothelial growth factor (VEGF) antibodies (e.g., bevacizumab, ramucirumab) and tyrosine kinase inhibitors (e.g., sorafenib, sunitinib) can produce hypertension that often persists, despite discontinuation. Because hypertension during the use of these drugs correlates with better oncologic outcomes (likely a reflection of a successful antiangiogenic effect), treatment is usually continued unless reasonable BP control is not achievable, or if severe kidney injury develops.[222]

## HYPERTENSIVE URGENCY AND EMERGENCY

A hypertensive emergency is the combination of elevated BP levels (with no specific diagnostic BP level) and signs or symptoms of acute, ongoing, target organ damage. Such patients are traditionally admitted to an intensive care unit and given parenteral infusions of short-acting antihypertensive agents to restore autoregulation in vascular beds. This is done because historical data from the 1920 to 1940 era (antedating effective antihypertensive drug therapy) showed a very poor prognosis, similar to that of many cancers. Traditionally, patients who presented with very elevated BP levels, but no acute, ongoing, target organ damage, were diagnosed with a "hypertensive urgency," observed for a few hours after treatment with one or more oral antihypertensive agents, and then discharged to a site of ongoing care for their hypertension. This practice is now undertaken primarily for medicolegal reasons. Two retrospective studies, one involving 1016 patients seen in an emergency department[223] and another involving 58,535 outpatients,[224] demonstrated very low rates of morbidity and mortality and no significant differences in prognosis for those treated acutely, compared with those who were discharged with rapid follow-up.

The initial evaluation of a severely hypertensive patient includes a thorough inspection of the optic fundi (looking for acute hemorrhages, exudates, or papilledema), a mental status assessment, a careful cardiac, pulmonary, and neurologic examination, a quick search for clues that might indicate secondary hypertension (e.g., abdominal bruit, striae, radial-femoral delay), and laboratory studies to assess renal function—dipstick and microscopic urinalysis, determination of serum creatinine level.

Several options for intravenous drug treatment exist, but nitroprusside is the least expensive and most widely available. It must be kept in the dark and is metabolized to cyanide and/or thiocyanate, particularly during long-term infusions. Fenoldopam mesylate, a dopamine-1 agonist, is very effective and acutely improves several parameters of renal function. Clevidipine is a dihydropyridine (DHP) calcium antagonist that is hydrolyzed within minutes by ubiquitous serum esterases; it is administered in an emulsion containing soy and egg proteins, either of which can cause immunologic reactions in allergic patients. Its elimination is not importantly affected by hepatic or renal functional impairment. Clevidipine and its older, longer acting cousin, nicardipine, are often used for patients with coronary disease because the reflex tachycardia is usually offset by coronary vasodilation. Nimodipine is typically used only for subarachnoid hemorrhage.

The quickest therapeutic response to a hypertensive emergency is recommended for an acute aortic dissection. In this condition, the BP should be lowered within 20 minutes to a systolic BP below 120 mm Hg (neither of which is supported by a strong evidence base), typically with a beta-blocker to reduce shear stress on the dissection and a vasodilator. Controversy exists about if and when BP lowering should be attempted in the setting of an acute ischemic stroke. If the patient is a candidate for acute thrombolytic therapy and the BP is higher than 180/110 mm Hg, acute BP lowering is recommended. Most US authorities suggest attempting slow and gradual BP lowering only if the BP is very high (e.g., ≥180/110 mm Hg) with a short-acting, rapidly titratable drug. However, two large, randomized trials done outside the United States have suggested that BP lowering in this setting is safe, but does not produce significant outcome benefits in ischemic[225] or hemorrhagic stroke.[226]

All other types of hypertensive emergencies can be handled with a gradual lowering of BP, typically 10% to 15% during the first hour and a further 10% to 20% during the next hour, for a total of approximately 25%. (See Table 46.8.)

Frequent monitoring of the patient's clinical status is important because not all patients can reestablish the normal autoregulatory capacity of the circulation in important vascular beds during the same short time period. Because hypertensive encephalopathy is a diagnosis of exclusion, it is often very rewarding to monitor these patients closely because their mental status improves markedly (and usually rather quickly) as the BP is carefully lowered.

Patients who present with hypertensive crises involving cardiac ischemia or infarction or pulmonary edema can be managed with nitroglycerin, clevidipine, nicardipine, or nitroprusside, although typically a combination of drugs (including an ACE inhibitor for heart failure or left ventricular dysfunction) is used in these settings. Efforts to preserve myocardium and open the obstructed coronary artery by thrombolysis, angioplasty, or surgery also are indicated.

Hypertensive emergency involving the kidney is commonly followed by a further deterioration in renal function, even when the BP is lowered properly. The most important predictor of the need for acute dialysis is not the BP level, but the degree of renal dysfunction (both eGFR and degree of albuminuria). Some physicians prefer fenoldopam to nicardipine or nitroprusside in this setting because of its lack of toxic metabolites and specific renal vasodilating effects. The need for acute dialysis often is precipitated by BP reduction in patients with preexisting stage 3 to 5 CKD, but many patients can avoid dialysis (and a remarkable few can even discontinue it) in the long term if BP is carefully well controlled during follow-up.

Hypertensive crises resulting from catecholamine excess states (e.g., pheochromocytoma, monoamine oxidase inhibitor crisis, cocaine intoxication) are most appropriately managed with an intravenous alpha-blocker (e.g., phentolamine), with a beta-blocker added later, if needed. Many patients with severe hypertension caused by sudden withdrawal of antihypertensive agents (e.g., clonidine) are easily managed by giving one acute dose of the missed drug.

Hypertensive crises during pregnancy must be managed in a more careful and conservative manner because of the

**Table 46.8 Hypertensive Emergencies, Therapies, and Target Blood Pressures**

| Type of Emergency | Drug of Choice | Blood Pressure Target |
|---|---|---|
| Aortic dissection | Beta-blocker plus nitroprusside[a] | 120 mm Hg systolic in 20 min (if possible) |
| **Cardiac** | | |
| Ischemia, infarction | Nitroglycerin, nitroprusside,[a] nicardipine, or clevidipine | Cessation of ischemia |
| Heart failure (or pulmonary edema) | Nitroprusside[a] and/or nitroglycerin | Improvement in failure (typically only a 10%–15% decrease is required) |
| **Hemorrhagic** | | |
| Epistaxis, gross hematuria, or threatened suture lines | Any (perhaps with anxiolytic agent) | To decrease bleeding rate (typically only 10%–15% reduction over 1–2 hours is required) |
| **Obstetric** | | |
| Eclampsia or preeclampsia | $MgSO_4$, hydralazine, methyldopa | Typically <90 mm Hg diastolic, but often lower |
| **Catecholamine Excess States** | | |
| Pheochromocytoma | Phentolamine | To control paroxysms |
| Drug withdrawal | Drug withdrawn | Typically only one dose necessary |
| Cocaine (and similar drugs) | Phentolamine | Typically only 10%–15% reduction over 1–2 hours |
| **Renal** | | |
| Major hematuria or acute kidney injury | Nitroprusside,[a] fenoldopam | 0%–25% reduction in mean arterial pressure over 1–12 hours |
| **Neurologic** | | |
| Hypertensive encephalopathy | Nitroprusside[a] | 25% reduction over 2–3 hours |
| Acute head injury, trauma | Nitroprusside[a] | 0%–25% reduction over 2–3 hours (controversial) |

[a]Many physicians prefer an intravenous infusion of clevidipine, fenoldopam, or nicardipine, none of which has potentially toxic metabolites, over nitroprusside, especially if a long duration of treatment is planned. Acute improvements in renal function occur during therapy with fenoldopam, but not with nitroprusside.

presence of the fetus. Magnesium sulfate, methyldopa, and hydralazine are the drugs of choice, with oral labetalol and nifedipine being drugs of second choice in the United States; nitroprusside, ACE inhibitors, and ARBs are contraindicated.[227] Delivery of the infant is often hastened by the obstetrician to assist in managing the hypertension in pregnancy.

Whether hypertensive urgencies (e.g., elevated BP, but without acute ongoing target organ damage) ought to be treated acutely is controversial because there is no evidence that such treatment improves prognosis. The BP in many such patients spontaneously falls during a 30-minute period of quiet rest. Conversely, immediate-release nifedipine capsules can cause precipitous hypotension, stroke, myocardial infarction, and death. According to the FDA, they "should be used with great caution, if at all." In such cases, true "hypotension" (e.g., systolic BP <90 mm Hg) may not be observed, yet the BP may fall below the autoregulatory threshold. This is likely different for every patient and may be unknown to the treating physician until it is surpassed, precipitating ischemia.

Clonidine, captopril, labetalol, several other short-acting antihypertensive drugs, and even amlodipine, have been used in this setting, but none has a clear advantage over the others, and each is usually effective in most patients. The most important aspect of managing a hypertensive urgency is to refer the patient to a good source of ongoing care for hypertension, where adherence to antihypertensive therapy during long-term follow-up will be more likely.

In short, patients presenting with a hypertensive emergency should be diagnosed quickly and started promptly on effective parenteral therapy (often, nitroprusside 0.5 µg/kg per minute) in an intensive care unit. BP should be gradually reduced by approximately 25% over 2 to 3 hours. Oral antihypertensive therapy should be instituted, usually after approximately 8 to 24 hours of parenteral therapy; evaluation for secondary causes of hypertension may be considered after transfer from the intensive care unit. Because of advances in antihypertensive therapy and management, the term *malignant hypertension* should be relegated to the dustbin of history (and used only by billers and coders) because the prognosis of patients with this condition has improved greatly since the term was introduced in 1927.

## GOALS OF ANTIHYPERTENSIVE THERAPY

There are hundreds of clinical studies that have evaluated the efficacy and safety of the eight different classes of antihypertensive medications. All BP-lowering agents need to have at least two appropriately powered, placebo-controlled studies to meet specific FDA criteria for approval as antihypertensive agents. This section will not focus on the details of these studies but rather on data supporting BP reductions with certain BP-lowering classes and the impact on CKD progression, as well as trials evaluating CV outcomes in patients with kidney disease.

Meta-analyses of all commonly used antihypertensive drug classes have demonstrated that regardless of the agent used, reduction in BP corresponds to reduction in CV events if BP reduction is achieved.[228–230] This reduction in CV risk, however, is predominantly seen in people with stage 2 hypertension (systolic, 140–159 mm Hg, or diastolic, 90–99 mm Hg) with much less outcome data to support risk reduction in stage 1 hypertension (systolic, 130–139 mm Hg, or diastolic, 80–89 mm Hg).

Events that drive the risk reduction are derived predominantly from a reduced incidence of stroke, myocardial infarction, and heart failure. In all trials to date it is the group with the best overall BP control that has the best outcomes. An exception to this generalization is Avoiding Cardiovascular Events Through Combination Therapy in Patients Living with Systolic Hypertension (ACCOMPLISH), a CV outcome trial that included over 11,000 people.[231] In this trial, both groups had similar BP control, and both were randomized to the same ACE inhibitor (benazepril), yet the group initially randomized to a single-pill combination of benazepril with a calcium antagonist had a 20% CV risk reduction compared with the ACE inhibitor plus diuretic group (Fig. 46.13). The observed benefit for the benazepril-amlodipine combination also extended to slowing CKD progression.[232]

Almost all people with an eGFR of less than 60 mL/min/1.73 m$^2$ and hypertension will require two or more medications to achieve a BP goal of less than 140/90 mm Hg. Single-pill combinations, including the combination of an RAAS blocker with a calcium antagonist or diuretic, are preferred agents.[7,233] These combinations, when given generally in an additive fashion, reduce CV events and CKD progression. Other combinations that are efficacious for reducing BP but have not been tested in clinical trials include beta-blockers with a dihydropyridine (DHP) calcium antagonist and DHP calcium antagonists with diuretics.[233]

There have been a number of trials assessing both CV outcome and changes in CKD progression. All these trials have assumed adherence with antihypertensive medications. However, according to one report, only 71% of subjects with hypertension in the United States were on treatment, and only 48% had their BP under adequate control (<140/90 mm Hg). Moreover, two separate studies, one in the United Kingdom and the other in Germany, evaluating medication adherence, have shown that only approximately 45% of patients who claimed to be taking BP-lowering medication actually were, as assessed by urinalysis of drug metabolites.[234,235] Although there has been significant reduction in the age-adjusted death rate for stroke and coronary artery disease since the early 1980s as a result of better BP control (and better treatment of other risk factors, such as hyperlipidemia), heart disease and stroke remain the first and third leading causes of death in Western countries, which emphasizes the importance of identifying and treating patients with hypertension. This section will discuss outcome trials focused on BP reduction that evaluated CKD progression as well as CV outcomes in people with CKD.

### BLOOD PRESSURE CONTROL AND CHRONIC KIDNEY DISEASE PROGRESSION

#### NONDIABETIC CHRONIC KIDNEY DISEASE

The rationale for antihypertensive therapy in nondiabetic CKD is discussed in detail in Chapter 59. There is clear evidence that partial blockade of the RAAS slows nephropathy progression in those with stage 3 or higher proteinuric kidney disease.[236–238] Although there is no evidence as to whether an ACE inhibitor versus ARB yields a better CKD

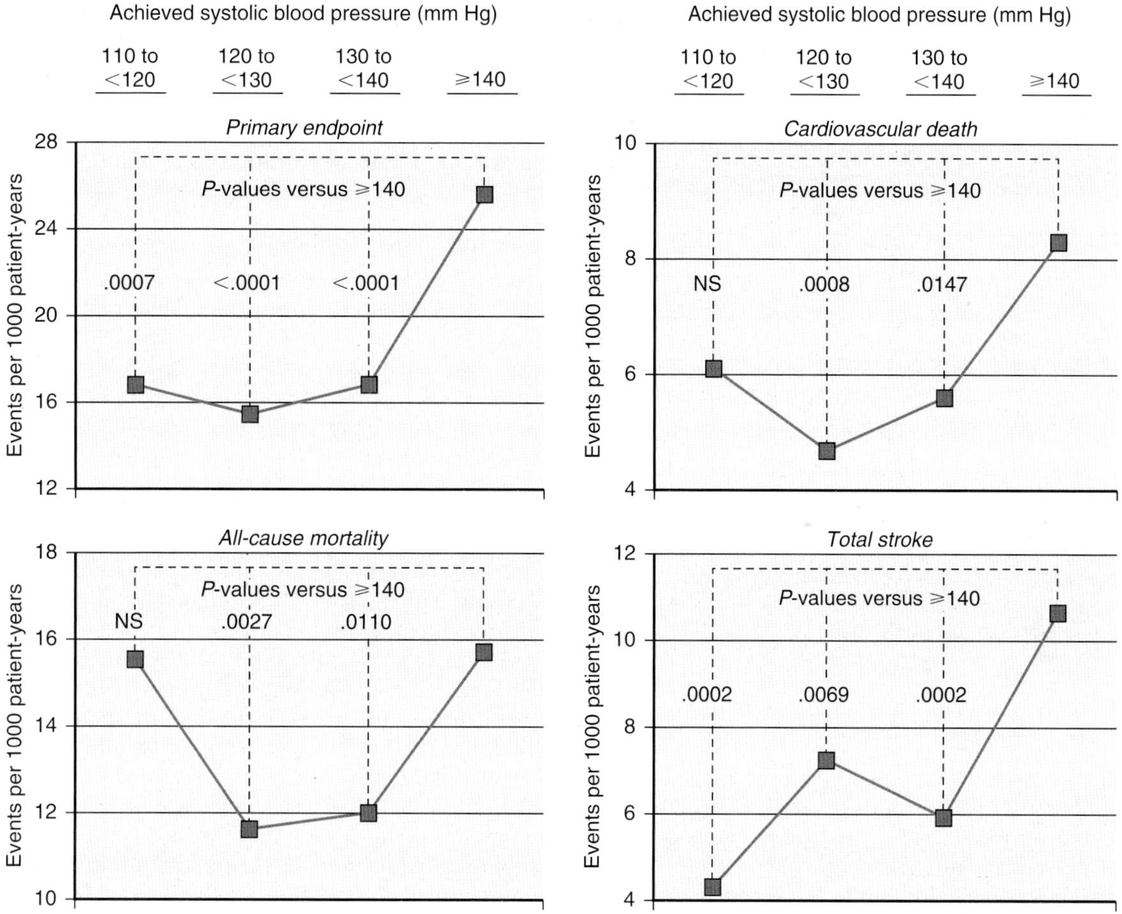


**Fig. 46.13** Event rates (per 1000 patient-years) for major clinical outcomes in the Avoiding Cardiovascular Events Through Combination Therapy in Patients Living with Systolic Hypertension (ACCOMPLISH) trial categorized by systolic pressure. *NS,* Not significant. (From Weber MA, Bloch M, Bakris GL, et al. Cardiovascular outcomes according to systolic blood pressure in patients with and without diabetes: an ACCOMPLISH substudy. *J Clin Hypertens*. 2016;18:299–307.)

outcome, it is clear that both classes have similar benefits between trials.

In contrast to the protection afforded by RAAS blockade, it is also clear that a lower level of BP does not slow nephropathy progression in hypertensive patients per se. Four prospective, randomized, long-term CKD outcome trials in nondiabetic kidney disease (discussed in the following section) have failed to show a benefit on slowing nephropathy progression among the groups with the lower BP.[200,239–241] Hence, the updated KDIGO BP guidelines recommend a BP goal of less than 140/90 mm Hg in those with CKD and is backed by the highest level of evidence. The previous goal of less than 130/80 mm Hg has a much lower level of evidence and is endorsed in the presence of a very high urine albumin level (>300 mg/day). A lower level of blood pressure further reduces cardiovascular events in people with CKD, even though it does not slow CKD progression, and should be sought for that reason.[241]

## Modification of Diet in Renal Disease Study

This was the first appropriately powered study to test whether a lower BP goal was associated with a slower progression of CKD. A low BP goal (target mean arterial pressure ≤92 mm Hg for patients ≤60 years old or 98 mm Hg for patients ≥61 years old) was associated with a significant reduction in proteinuria and to a slower subsequent decline in GFR. However, this was not significant compared with the higher pressure group with a mean arterial pressure of 102 to 107 mm Hg.

## African American Study of Kidney Disease and Hypertension

The effect of antihypertensive therapy on the progression of CKD secondary to hypertension is more controversial. In the Multiple Risk Factor Intervention Trial (MRFIT), in which thiazide diuretics and beta-blockers were primarily used to control BP, slowing or stabilization of kidney function was not seen in black men but was seen in all other racial groups studied.[33]

In the African American Study of Kidney Disease and Hypertension (AASK), the use of an ACE inhibitor (ramipril) was found to be more effective at slowing CKD progression compared with either amlodipine (a dihydropyridine CCB) or metoprolol[31] (Fig. 46.14). This trial, in over 1000 blacks, failed to show superior protection with BP reduced to levels below 130/80 mm Hg compared with conventional BP targets of 140/90 mm Hg in subjects with hypertensive nephrosclerosis, even with a total of a 10-year follow-up.[240] Masked hypertension may be a confounder to these outcomes. A subanalysis of over 50% of the AASK participants who had

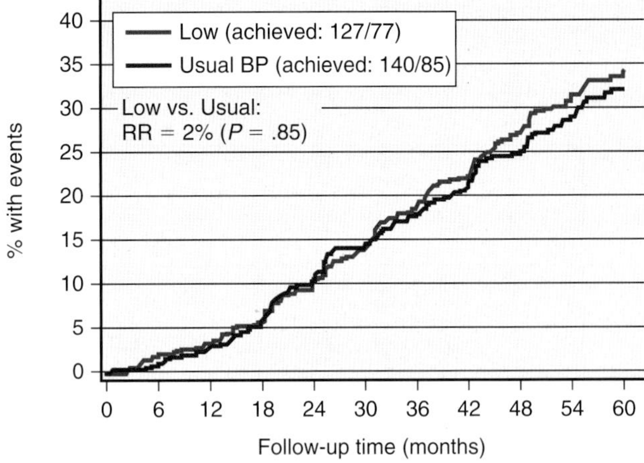


**Fig. 46.14** Composite primary clinical endpoint decline in glomerular filtration rate, end-stage kidney disease, or death in the African American Study of Kidney Disease. *BP,* Blood pressure; *RR,* relative risk. (From Bakris GL, Sarafidis PA, Weir MR, et al. Renal outcomes with different fixed-dose combination therapies in patients with hypertension at high risk for cardiovascular events (ACCOMPLISH): a prespecified secondary analysis of a randomised controlled trial. *Lancet.* 2010;375(9721): 1173–1181.)

24-hour ABPM showed inadequate 24-hour BP control in approximately 36% of the cohort.[242] Masked hypertension and failure of nocturnal dipping were the two most common reasons for poor out-of-office BP control.

Further studies were performed to assess whether changes in antihypertensive dose timing corrected the failure of nocturnal dipping, but the results were negative.[243] In contrast, studies performed in Spain in white patients with CKD stages 2 to 3b have demonstrated an improvement in dipping status when dosing BP medications at night.[243]

### Ramipril Efficacy in Nephropathy Trial (REIN-2)

This multicenter, randomized controlled trial was conducted in Italy in patients with proteinuria associated with nondiabetic kidney disease who were receiving background treatment with the ACE inhibitor ramipril (2.5–5 mg/day).[239] The aim was to assess the effect of intensified versus conventional BP control on progression to ESKD. Subjects were randomly assigned to conventional (diastolic <90 mm Hg; $n = 169$) or intensified (systolic/diastolic <130/80 mm Hg; $n = 169$) BP control. To achieve the intensified BP level, patients received add-on therapy with the dihydropyridine calcium channel blocker (DCCB) felodipine (5–10 mg/day). The primary outcome measure was time to ESKD over 36 months' follow-up. The authors found that over a median follow-up of 19 months, 38 of 167 patients (23%) assigned to intensified BP control and 34 of 168 patients (20%) who were allocated to conventional control progressed to ESKD (HR, 1.00; 95% confidence interval [CI], 0.61–1.64; $P = .99$). Hence, there was no benefit of aggressive BP lowering in slowing this nondiabetic nephropathy.

### Systolic Blood Pressure Intervention Trial

The Systolic Blood Pressure Intervention Trial (SPRINT) randomized participants to intensive BP lowering (systolic BP [SBP] <120 mm Hg) versus standard BP control (SBP <140 mm Hg) on clinical outcomes. In 2646 patients who had CKD at baseline, the composite kidney outcome of a 50% decrease or more in eGFR from baseline or ESKD, was no different between the groups (HR, 0.90 for the intensive group; 95% CI, 0.44–1.83).[241] However, the intensive group had a lower rate of cardiovascular outcomes and all-cause death.

## DIABETIC KIDNEY DISEASE

There have been no randomized trials of BP level and CKD outcome among patients with diabetes mellitus. The recommendation for a lower BP goal in diabetes has resulted from post hoc analyses of trials that evaluated CV outcomes in subjects with diabetic kidney disease. All these studies showed a benefit on CV risk reduction and some benefit in slowing CKD progression in the group randomized to the lower pressures.

The Hypertension Optimal Treatment (HOT) trial was not powered for a blood pressure diabetes outcome but was the first CV outcome trial that evaluated different levels of diastolic BP (80 mm Hg, 85 mm Hg, and 90 mm Hg) in 18,790 patients with hypertension, from 26 countries, mean age 61.5 years. In the subgroup of patients with diabetes mellitus, a post hoc analysis showed a 51% reduction in major CV events in the target group of 80 mm Hg or less compared with the target group of 90 mm Hg or less (*P* for trend = .005).[244] Nevertheless, because the primary endpoint of the trial failed to reach statistical significance on the CV outcome at the lowest randomized BP level, the diabetes subgroup could not be considered positive, even if it was statistically significant; the hypothesis tested was not specifically predefined for this subgroup.

The Ongoing Telmisartan Alone and in combination with Ramipril Global Endpoint Trial (ONTARGET) and the International Verapamil-Trandolapril Study (INVEST), like the Action to Control Cardiovascular Risk in Diabetes (ACCORD) trial, have failed to show a benefit on CV outcomes.[245–247] Taken together, these three studies demonstrated no additional benefit of BP lowering below 130/80 mm Hg on CV risk reduction compared with 130 to 139/80 to 85 mm Hg (Table 46.9).

It should be noted that there have been four recent systematic reviews of these trials and many others in diabetes that were summarized in the American Diabetes Association (ADA) Position Paper of Blood Pressure Goals in Diabetes. The committee supported a BP goal of less than 140/90 mm Hg, but acknowledged that most patients will achieve a greater CV risk reduction at blood pressure levels of less than 130/80 mm Hg. Thus, this suggests that most patients with diabetes strive for this goal.[157] Moreover, there is general agreement between the AHA/ACC BP guidelines and the ADA guidelines with regard to a BP approach in diabetes.[248]

Although there is no evidence of additional slowing of nephropathy progression at BP levels below 130/80 mm Hg, CV risk reduction did occur among those with CKD, as seen in the ACCORD trial.[249] The only prospective outcome trials that randomized groups to different BP levels and were powered statistically for CV outcomes were the United Kingdom Prospective Diabetes Study (UKPDS) and ACCORD. However, only the intensive treatment group in the ACCORD study attained a BP of less than 130/80 mm Hg.[246,250]

**Table 46.9 Achieved Blood Pressure Levels in Cardiovascular Outcome Trials Involving Patients with Diabetes**

| Clinical Outcome Trial | Achieved Level of Systolic Blood Pressure (mm Hg) |
|---|---|
| ACCORD (primary) | 119 (intensive); 133 (conventional) |
| UKPDS (primary) | 144 (intensive); 154 (conventional) |
| ACCOMPLISH (secondary) | Overall mean, 133 |
| INVEST (secondary) | 144 (tight control); 149 (conventional) |
| ONTARGET (secondary) | Averaging approximately 140 |
| VADT (secondary) | 127 (intensive); 125 (conventional) |
| ADVANCE (secondary) | 145 (in both intensive and conventional glucose control) |

*ACCOMPLISH,* Avoiding Cardiovascular Events Through Combination Therapy in Patients Living with Systolic Hypertension; *ACCORD,* Action to Control Cardiovascular Risk in Diabetes; *VADT,* Veterans Affairs Diabetes Trial; *ADVANCE,* Action in Diabetes and Vascular Disease: Preterax and Diamicron Modified Release Controlled Evaluation; *INVEST,* International Verapamil-Trandolapril Study; *ONTARGET,* Ongoing Telmisartan Alone and in combination with Ramipril Global EndpoinT trial; *UKPDS,* United Kingdom Prospective Diabetes Study.

In ACCORD, there was no significant difference in the primary endpoint, all-cause and CV mortality, between the standard and intensive BP groups. However, the long-term follow-up ACCORDION study demonstrated a major interaction between the intensive glycemic control group and intensive blood pressure goal, such that the outcomes were confounded. When reevaluating the ACCORD data in the context of these statistical limitations, a benefit was seen trending for further CV risk reduction in a lower blood pressure group, albeit not significant.[251] Two important studies using ACCORD data are important. One study used SPRINT criteria applied to the ACCORD database and compared CV outcomes; there was a significant reduction in the intensive BP group in the primary endpoint.[251a] A second equally important study evaluated change in serum creatinine levels and CV outcome in ACCORD and demonstrated that up to a 30% increase in the serum creatinine level during the trial was associated with a reduced CV outcome.[251b] This was not seen among those with a greater than 30% increase in their serum creatinine level.

The UKPDS did not show a benefit from the lower BP group, which averaged above 140/90 mm Hg. Additional findings from post hoc analyses of diabetes subgroups of other trials have also failed to show benefit of BP levels below 130/80 mm Hg, demonstrating an additional CV outcome benefit.

A number of studies have demonstrated that some classes of antihypertensive drugs should be used preferentially in patients with diabetes who have nephropathy. The effect of blockers of the RAAS system in diabetic nephropathy to retard hard kidney endpoints, such as ESKD, has now been well documented in multiple studies.[252–254] However, this class of agents does not possess any specific advantages over other antihypertensive classes in diabetics who do not have nephropathy. Moreover, there is no evidence that blockers of the RAAS benefit people with normotension, with or without microalbuminuria, from developing declines in kidney function.[157,255,256] See Chapter 39 for an in-depth discussion of therapy in diabetic kidney disease.

## ANTIHYPERTENSIVE THERAPY IN OLDER ADULTS

### Clinical Trials in Older Adults

All major clinical trials involving persons older than 65 years are summarized in Table 46.10. Most patients recruited in these trials prior to the Hypertension in the Very Elderly Trial (HYVET) were younger than 80 years, limiting information about octogenarians.[24] Results in these trials have shown a reduction in the incidence of stroke and CV morbidity. Previous clinical trials have shown that lowering BP in older adults has no effect on overall mortality or on the incidence of fatal or nonfatal myocardial infarction.[210,257] The recent results of the older subgroup of the SPRINT, with a mean age of 79 years, however, has shown a clear benefit on all CV outcomes, especially heart failure risk, among those treated to a lower blood pressure.[25] Thus, clinical practice guidelines prior to HYVET, and subsequently the ACC/AHA, have recommended that in subjects aged 80 years and older, evidence for benefits of antihypertensive treatment is as yet inconclusive.[8]

The release of the HYVET,[23] and the subsequent publication of the "ACCF/AHA 2011 Expert Consensus Document on Hypertension in the Elderly" study,[211] changed the management of hypertension, particularly in patients older than 80 years. Before SPRINT, there were five trials performed in older people, only two of which randomized to different BP levels that were below a systolic BP of 140 mm Hg. The trials were SHEP—Systolic Hypertension in Europe (Syst-Eur)—HYVET, Japanese Trial to Assess Optimal Systolic Blood Pressure in Elderly Hypertensive Patients (JATOS), and Valsartan in Elderly Isolated Systolic Hypertension (VALISH; see Table 46.10).[212] Both randomized BP trials with the lower BP levels were carried out in Japan. The results from these two studies have shown no additional benefit of achieving a BP of less than 140/90 mm Hg compared with less than 150/90 mm Hg.

A concern in patients with isolated systolic hypertension is the reduction of diastolic BP after the initiation of antihypertensive therapy. A diastolic BP that is too low may interfere with coronary perfusion and possibly increase CV risk. The relationship between diastolic BP and CV death, particularly myocardial infarction, is like a J-shaped curve; thus, excessive reduction in diastolic pressures should be avoided in patients with coronary artery disease who are being treated for hypertension.[258,259] A BP of 119/84 mm Hg was identified as a nadir when treating patients with coronary artery disease[260]; however, among patients with CKD, a nadir of 131/71 mm Hg was identified as a level below which higher CV mortality was present[260] (Fig. 46.15).

When treating patients with isolated systolic hypertension, the JNC 7 has suggested a minimum posttreatment diastolic BP of 60 mm Hg overall, or perhaps 65 mm Hg in patients with known coronary artery disease, unless symptoms that could be attributed to hypoperfusion occur at higher pressures. This was seen in the findings of the SHEP trial,[261]

**Table 46.10 Clinical Trials in Older Adults**

| Clinical Trials | Mean Age | No. of Subjects | Drugs Used | Achieved BP (Control) | Achieved BP (Rx) | Outcome |
|---|---|---|---|---|---|---|
| EWHPE, 1985 | 72 | 840 | HCTZ + triamterene, ± methyldopa | 159/85 | 155/84 | + CV risk reduction |
| Coope and Warrender, 1986 | 68 | 884 | Atenolol ± bendroflumethiazide | 180/89 | 178/87 | Stroke reduction |
| SHEP, 1991 | 72 | 4736 | Chlorthalidone ± atenolol or reserpine | 155/72 | 143/68 | Stroke reduction |
| STOP, 1991 | 72 | 1627 | Atenolol ± HCTZ or amiloride | 161/97 | 159/81 | Stroke and MI reduction |
| MRC, 1992 | 70 | 3496 | HCTZ ± amiloride vs. atenolol | ≈169/79 | ≈150/80 | Stroke, MI, and CHD reduction |
| CASTEL, 1994 | 83 | 665 | Clonidine, nifedipine and atenolol + chlorthalidone | 181/97 | 165.2/85.6 | Reduced mortality |
| STONE, 1996 | 67 | 1632 | Nifedipine | 155/87 | 147/85 | Stroke and CV event reduction |
| Syst-Eur, 1997 | 70 | 4695 | Nitrendipine + enalapril or HCTZ | 161/94 | 151/79 | Stroke and CVD reduction |
| Syst-China, 2000 | 67 | 2394 | Nitrendipine + captopril or HCTZ | 178/93 | 151/76 | Stroke, CVD, and HF reduction |
| HYVET, 2008 | 84 | 3845 | Indapamide + perindopril | 158.5/84 | 143/78 | Stroke and HF reduction |
| JATOS, 2008 | 75 | 4418 | Efonidipine hydrochloride | 145.6/78.1 | 136/74 | No difference between aggressive BP on renal and CV events |

*BP,* Blood pressure; *CASTEL,* Cardiovascular Study in the Elderly; *CHD,* coronary heart disease; *CV,* cardiovascular; *CVD,* cardiovascular disease; *EWHPE,* European Working Party on High Blood Pressure in the Elderly; *HCTZ,* hydrochlorothiazide; *HF,* heart failure; *HYVET,* Hypertension in the Very Elderly Trial; *JATOS,* Japanese Trial to Assess Optimal Systolic Blood Pressure in Elderly Hypertensive Patients; *MI,* myocardial infarction; *MRC,* Medical Research Council; *Rx,* medication; *SHEP,* Systolic Hypertension in the Elderly Program; *STONE,* Shanghai Trial of Nifedipine in the Elderly; *STOP,* Hypertension, Swedish Trial in Old Patients with Hypertension; *Syst-China,* Systolic Hypertension in China; *Syst-Eur,* Systolic Hypertension in Europe.

where older patients with lower diastolic BP had higher CV event rates.

Additionally, in some trials involving older individuals, there is concern about thiazide diuretic use, hyponatremia, and worsening of kidney function in subjects with hypertension. In the European Working Party on High Blood Pressure in the Elderly trial, a significantly higher incidence of impaired kidney function was found in those receiving diuretics compared with placebo.[262] In the SHEP trial, the serum creatinine level increased significantly in subjects treated with thiazide diuretics compared with placebo. In ALLHAT, the chlorthalidone-treated group showed worse kidney function than the amlodipine- or lisinopril-treated group at both the 2- and 4-year endpoints.[263] Although this could likely be accounted for by volume depletion in many cases, diuretics have been shown to induce mild renal injury in various animal models, possibly because of hypokalemia, hyperuricemia, and stimulation of the RAAS related to the reduction in renal perfusion pressure.

The HYVET trial, in 2008, changed how hypertension in older adults is managed. It randomly assigned almost 4000 patients who were 80 years of age and older and had systolic BP above 160 mm Hg to indapamide or placebo. Results of HYVET have provided clear evidence that BP lowering with treatment using antihypertensive medications is associated with definite CV benefits. The use of indapamide supplemented by perindopril showed reductions in the incidence of stroke, congestive heart failure, and CV fatal events.

Stricter BP goals have shown no benefit in CV morbidity and mortality in older populations. The JATOS study has shown that systolic BP goals of less than 140 mm Hg had no statistical significance in the CV mortality of patients older than 65 years.[264] The results of the Japanese trials can be contrasted with the results of SPRINT, which demonstrated significantly lower CV event rates in the group randomized to a lower BP well below 130 mm Hg.[25]

There have been no specific trials powered to assess CKD progression in older people. There are prespecified and post hoc analyses of trials where the mean age is above 65 years that examined changes in CKD progression. A notable example is the prespecified analysis of the ACCOMPLISH trial, where more than 40% of the people with CKD were 70 years of age or older. This trial showed a benefit of the RAAS blocker–CCB combination over the RAAS blocker–diuretic for slowing progression and time to dialysis.[232] A post hoc analysis of the ALLHAT study in people older than 65 years also has shown that BP control slows progression.[263] However, in this trial, we had no information about albuminuria.

### Nonpharmacologic Intervention in Older Adults

In the Trial of Nonpharmacologic Interventions in the Elderly (TONE),[265] the combination of weight loss and sodium restriction showed a drop of 5.3 ± 1.2 mm Hg in the systolic BP and 3.4 ± 0.8 mm Hg diastolic BP in obese older patients with hypertension. The goal of sodium restriction was 1.8 g/24

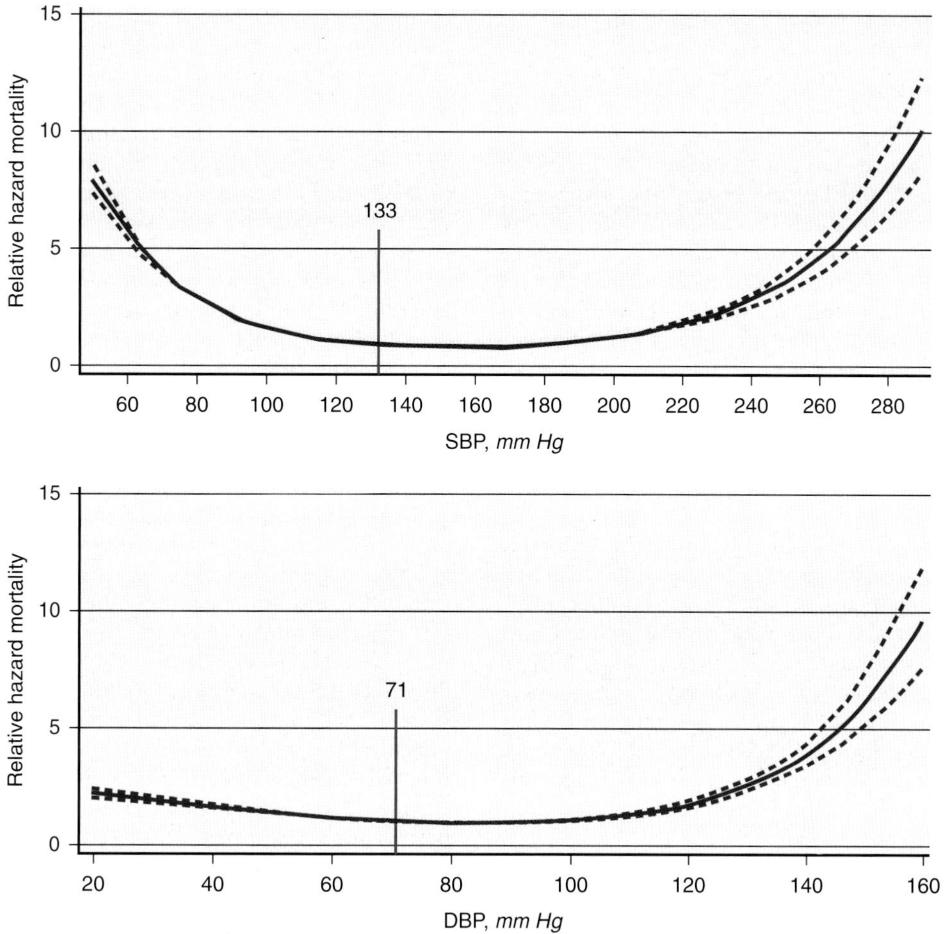


**Fig. 46.15** Blood pressure and mortality in US veterans with chronic kidney disease. Shown are multivariable-adjusted relative hazards (hazard ratios [95% confidence intervals]) of all-cause mortality associated with systolic blood pressure *(SBP)* and diastolic blood pressure *(DBP)* relative to a hypothetical patient with the mean time-varying SBP (133 mm Hg) and DBP (71 mm Hg).

hours, and the goal for weight reduction was 10 lb. Other lifestyle changes recommended in the older patient include watching the potassium intake to keep the level of serum potassium in a safe range. Patient education about high-potassium foods is important. Intake of NSAIDs should also be decreased to a minimum because these patients are more likely to take NSAIDs for arthritis and pain. These drugs are known to cause elevations in BP by inhibiting the production of vasodilatory prostaglandins and may increase BP by as much as 6 mm Hg.[266,267] Their BP-raising effects can be blunted by calcium antagonists and, to a lesser extent, diuretics.[268]

## Pharmacologic Intervention in Older Adults

The following is a brief summary of the approach to antihypertensive drug therapy in older adults. A more detailed discussion of the pharmacology and use of antihypertensive medications may be found in Chapter 49. The primary agents used in the treatment of hypertension include thiazide-type diuretics, ACE inhibitors, ARBs, and CCBs. Although many other drugs and drug classes are available, confirmation that these agents decrease clinical outcomes to a similar extent as the primary agents is lacking, or safety and tolerability may relegate their role to use as secondary agents.[13] In particular, there is inadequate evidence to support the initial use of beta-blockers for hypertension in the absence of specific cardiovascular comorbidities.

In considering the initial drug treatment of someone with a high BP, several different strategies may be contemplated. Many patients can be started on a single agent, but consideration should be given to starting with two drugs for those with BP higher than 20/10 mm Hg above the goal of 130/80 mm Hg. Many patients started on a single agent will subsequently require two or more drugs from different pharmacologic classes to reach their BP goals.

Knowledge of the pharmacologic mechanisms of action of each agent is important. Drug regimens with complementary activity, where a second antihypertensive is used to block compensatory responses to the initial agent or effect a different pressor mechanism, can result in additive lowering of BP. The use of combination therapy may also allow for treatment with lower doses of individual agents, which serves to minimize adverse effects and improve adherence. Several two and three fixed-dose drug combinations of antihypertensive drug therapy are available in generic form, with complementary mechanisms of action among the components.

The full dose of the drug is the highest pharmacologic dose of drug available; the maximum dose is the highest dose that the person can tolerate without side effects. If the person is having no therapeutic response or has had significant side effects, a drug from another class should be substituted. In fact, most older patients require two or more drugs to achieve the recommended goals in clinical trials.

Either a diuretic or calcium antagonist may be an initial drug, or a diuretic should be one of the first two agents when starting combination drugs (Box 46.4).[13] When the BP is more than 20/10 mm Hg above the goal, the recommendation is to initiate with two antihypertensive medications, with one of the choices being a diuretic. Single-pill combinations that incorporate logical doses of two agents may enhance convenience and compliance in older patients.[211] However, there is still a need for individualization of treatment; thus, treatment options should be carefully considered for older adults. The benefits of lowering BP must be weighed against the risks of side effects and the concomitant morbidity of the patient.

Thiazide diuretics such as hydrochlorothiazide, chlorthalidone, indapamide, and bendrofluazide, as well as calcium antagonists, are recommended for initiating therapy.[8,13] Diuretics cause an initial reduction of intravascular volume, peripheral vascular resistance, and BP in more than 50% of patients and are well tolerated and inexpensive.[269,270] However, they can cause hypokalemia, hypomagnesemia, and hyponatremia and are therefore not recommended for patients with baseline electrolyte abnormalities or those with a history of hyponatremia. The serum potassium level should be monitored, and supplementation should be given if needed.

Calcium antagonists are well suited for older patients whose hypertensive profile is based on increasing arterial dysfunction secondary to decreased atrial and ventricular compliance. This class of drugs dilates coronary and peripheral arteries in doses that do not severely affect myocardial contractility.[271,272] Most adverse effects relate to vasodilation, such as ankle edema, headache, and postural hypotension. Ankle edema is not secondary to sodium retention because calcium antagonists are natriuretic when given initially, but the profound vasodilation with poor venous return in older people is the major contributor.

First-generation drugs, such as nifedipine, verapamil, and diltiazem, should be avoided in patients with left ventricular dysfunction. Nondihydropyridines can precipitate heart block in older adults with underlying conduction defects.

RAAS blockers, such as ACE inhibitors, ARBs, and direct renin inhibitors, may be used in older adults.[273] Theoretically, as aging occurs, there is a reduction in angiotensin levels; thus, ACE inhibitors may not be an effective medication for hypertension in older adults. However, several clinical trials have shown otherwise. The use of ACE inhibitors is beneficial in the reduction of morbidity and mortality in patients with myocardial infarction, reduced systolic function, heart failure, and reduction in the progression of diabetic renal disease and hypertensive nephrosclerosis.[274,275] Finally, it appears that use of an RAAS blocker may provide greater benefit for CV and renal risk reduction than the use of a diuretic, based on data from ACCOMPLISH, a large outcome trial of 11,506 persons with a mean age of 68 years. Although there are very few data on kidney disease in older adults, ACCOMPLISH did provide some evidence worthy of being tested in a prospective trial—that is, a calcium antagonist–ACE inhibitor combination led to fewer people going on dialysis than a diuretic–ACE inhibitor combination.[232,276] Note that this outcome could not be explained by differences in BP of 1.2 mm Hg systolic. It must be noted that those older than 70 years tend to drink small amounts of fluid, and hence this makes them more vulnerable to decline in kidney function by RAAS blockade, as already discussed. Thus it is recommended that they increase their fluid intake to prevent volume depletion.

The clinical benefits of beta-blockers as monotherapy in uncomplicated older patients are poorly documented. They may have a role in combination therapy, especially with diuretics. Beta-blockers have established roles in patients with hypertension complicated by certain arrhythmias, migraine headaches, senile tremors, coronary artery disease, or heart failure.[277,278] Nebivolol, a selective beta-1 blocker with NO properties, does not show any associated symptoms of depression, sexual dysfunction, dyslipidemia, and hyperglycemia in older adults, unlike earlier generations of beta-blockers.[279]

Potassium-sparing diuretics are useful when combined with other agents. Aldosterone-blocking agents such as spironolactone and eplerenone reduce vascular stiffness and systolic BP.[280,281] They are also useful for hypertensive patients with heart failure or primary hyperaldosteronism. Gynecomastia and sexual dysfunction are the limiting adverse events, reactions that occur in men using spironolactone but are less frequent with eplerenone. The epithelial sodium transport

### Box 46.4 American Society of Hypertension Evidence-Based, Fixed Dose Antihypertensive Combinations

**Preferred**

- ACE inhibitor, diuretic[a]
- ARB, diuretic[a]
- ACE inhibitor, CCB[a]
- ARB, CCB[a]

**Acceptable**

- Beta-blocker, diuretic[a]
- CCB (dihydropyridine), beta-blocker
- CCB, diuretic
- Renin inhibitor, diuretic[a]
- Renin inhibitor, ARB[a]
- Thiazide diuretics, $K^+$-sparing diuretics[a]

**Less Effective**

- ACE inhibitor, ARB
- ACE inhibitor, beta-blocker
- ARB, beta blocker
- CCB (nondihydropyridine), beta-blocker
- Centrally acting agent, beta-blocker

[a]Single-pill combination available in the United States.

*ACE*, Angiotensin-converting enzyme; *ARB*, angiotensin receptor blocker; *CCB*, calcium channel blocker.

From Gradman AH, Basile JN, Carter BL, Bakris GL; American Society of Hypertension Writing Group. Combination therapy in hypertension. *J Clin Hypertens (Greenwich)*. 2011;13(3):146–154.

antagonists (e.g., amiloride, triamterene) are most useful when combined with another diuretic.

Other agents, such as alpha-blockers, centrally acting drugs (e.g., clonidine), and nonspecific vasodilators (e.g., minoxidil) should not be used as first- or second-line agents in an older adult with hypertension. Instead, they are reserved as part of a combination regimen to maximize BP control after other agents have been deployed.

## BLOOD PRESSURE MANAGEMENT IN PATIENTS UNDERGOING DIALYSIS

Elevations in BP in dialysis patients are almost exclusively due to excessive volume. Hence, hypertension control related directly to volume management is a more common problem in hemodialysis than in peritoneal dialysis. There have been no large, multicenter, randomized trials in patients undergoing dialysis to evaluate different levels of BP on CV outcomes. However, there is a prospective randomized trial that has evaluated the effects of an ACE inhibitor versus a beta-blocker on LVH and as a secondary endpoint of CV mortality in patients undergoing dialysis.[282]

The purpose of the study was to determine, in 200 hypertensive patients undergoing hemodialysis with echocardiographic LVH, whether a beta-blocker or an ACE inhibitor used for BP lowering results in a greater regression of LVH. Subjects were randomly assigned to open-label lisinopril ($n = 100$) or atenolol ($n = 100$), each administered three times/week after dialysis. Monthly monitored home BP was controlled to less than 140/90 mm Hg with medications, dry weight adjustment, and sodium restriction. The primary outcome was the change in left ventricular mass index from baseline to 12 months. The results demonstrated that there was no between-group difference in 44-hour ambulatory BP. However, the monthly measured home BP was consistently higher in the lisinopril group, despite the need for a greater number of antihypertensive agents and a greater reduction in dry weight. An independent data safety monitoring board recommended termination because of CV safety. Serious CV events were more prominent in the lisinopril group (20 events; atenolol vs. 43 events, lisinopril; $P = .001$). Combined serious adverse events of myocardial infarction, stroke, and hospitalization for heart failure or CV death were much lower in the atenolol group ($P = .021$). Thus, it appears that beta-blocker therapy is superior to RAAS blockade in patients undergoing hemodialysis to reduce CV morbidity and all-cause hospitalizations.

Retrospective analyses of patients on hemodialysis have also supported other beta-blockers such as carvedilol for lowering CV events in hypertensive patients who were undergoing hemodialysis and Japanese investigators have further corroborated the results supporting beta-blocker use in patients undergoing dialysis. The effect of beta-blocker use on mortality in a cohort of patients undergoing hemodialysis was evaluated in a database analysis from the Dialysis Outcomes and Practice Patterns Study phase II of 2286 randomly selected patients on hemodialysis in Japan.[283] The main outcome measure was all-cause mortality. The authors found beta-blocker use was low (i.e., only 247 patients [10.8%] were administered beta-blockers, and 1828 patients [80%] were not). A Kaplan-Meier analysis revealed that all-cause mortality rates were significantly decreased in patients treated with beta-blockers ($P < .007$) compared with the group not on beta-blockers. In multivariable, fully adjusted models, treatment with beta-blockers was also independently associated with reduced all-cause mortality (HR, 0.48; $P = .02$).[236]

Data from the US Renal Data System have demonstrated a U-shaped relationship between systolic BP goals in patients undergoing dialysis and CV outcomes, suggesting that BP should be consistently above 120 mm Hg and below 150 mm Hg.[284] A meta-analysis by Agarwal and Sinha of antihypertensive medications in patients undergoing dialysis has demonstrated that regardless of class, reducing BP reduces CV events.[285] Data from epidemiologic studies have consistently shown that in patients undergoing maintenance dialysis, low BP values are associated with higher death rates when compared with normal to moderately high values.

Although there is no generalizable approach to manage BP in those undergoing dialysis, the following points are vital to have an accurate assessment of BP: (1) the most representive BP is the one taken the morning after dialysis; and (2) there should be a minimum of two and ideally three readings obtained 1 or 2 minutes apart during those morning readings and then averaged.[285,286] Given that heart failure and sudden death are the most common causes of death in dialysis patients, beta-blockers have an important role in the BP-lowering armamentarium, unlike in the general population. Ensuring euvolemia is the key, however. The clinical examination is important, but newer techniques of bioimpedance, blood volume monitoring, and inferior vena cava ultrasound are effective in improving the definition of dry weight and could be considered, particularly in patients with uncontrolled BP, despite conventional dry weight probing using the clinical examination.[190,287]

## MANAGEMENT OF HYPERTENSION IN CHRONIC KIDNEY DISEASE

There are many guidelines written on the management of hypertension in the general population, and those have been summarized at the beginning of this chapter. Both the Kidney Disease Outcomes Quality Initiative (KDOQI) and KDIGO guidelines focus on the evidence for certain BP levels and classes of medication in patients with CKD. These guidelines have also been discussed in this chapter.

To summarize the key findings, the strongest level of evidence supports a BP goal below 140/90 mm Hg and the use of RAAS-blocking agents in people with stage 3 or higher CKD who have very high albuminuria. Nevertheless, there is weaker evidence to support RAAS blocker use in people with CKD in general, as well as very weak evidence supporting a BP of less than 130/80 mm Hg for those who have a urine albumin level of 1 g or more and an eGFR less than 60 mL/min/1.73 $m^2$.[288,289] These BP levels and recommendations for RAAS blockers are focused on the primary outcome of slowing CKD progression. A summary of all trials and effects on eGFR decline are shown in Fig. 46.16.

The most recent AHA/ACC BP guidelines have modified the approach slightly, with a focus on CV risk reduction rather than a focus on renal preservation. This is because the BP range of 125 to 130 mm Hg has not been shown to harm the kidneys yet reduce further CV events.[241] An algorithm proposed for BP management in CKD is shown in Fig. 46.17.

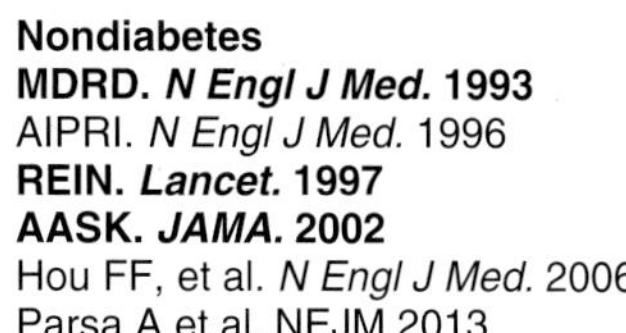


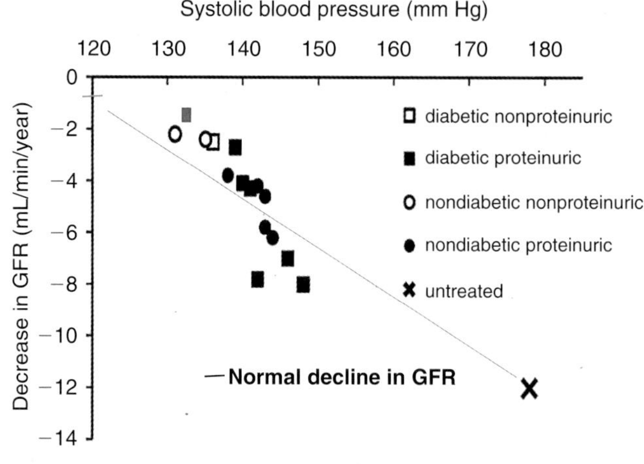


**Fig. 46.16** Relationship between achieved blood pressure and decline in kidney function from primary renal endpoint trials. *GFR,* Glomerular filtration rate. (From Kalaitzidis R, Bakris GL. Update on reducing the development of diabetic kidney disease and cardiovascular death in diabetes. In Daugirdas JT, editor. *Handbook of chronic kidney disease management*. Philadelphia: Elsevier, 2018.)

Nuances in the management of BP in the patient with CKD are necessary because these patients have problems that are not seen in the general population. First, hyperkalemia is a risk in certain subgroups of patients. A review of clinical trials where hyperkalemia developed when managing hypertension in CKD has found three risk predictors. If a patient was already receiving an appropriate diuretic for her or his level of kidney function, then these were reliable risk predictors for hyperkalemia (i.e., $[K^+]_s > 5.5$ mEq/L): (1) eGFR of less than 45 mL/min/1.73 $m^2$; (2) serum potassium level above 4.5 mEq/L; and (3) body mass index less than 25.[290] Hyperkalemia has limited our ability to assess whether RAAS blockers are effective in slowing CKD progression in stage 3b and higher CKD. Newer agents to manage hyperkalemia will open the door to safer management and expanded research.[291,292]

Another nuance in BP management in the CKD patient is the critical importance of sodium restriction to less than 2400 mg/day and reduced alcohol consumption, as well as aerobic, not isometric, exercise.[293,294] To demonstrate the importance of exercise, a recent study has randomized 296 dialysis patients to normal physical activity (control, $n = 145$) or walking exercise ($n = 151$) over a 6-month period. Those who were in the active group using a simple, personalized, home-based, low-intensity exercise program managed by dialysis staff improved physical performance and quality of life.[294]

Studies evaluating the effect of sodium intake on BP control in people with stage 4 CKD have shown that approximately every 400 mg above a sodium intake base of 3000 mg/day requires an additional BP medication to maintain BP control.[293] Moreover, failure to reduce sodium intake suppresses the RAAS system and hence reduces the efficacy of RAAS blockers. Thus, failure to reduce sodium intake is a cause of resistant hypertension, as noted earlier in the chapter. Additionally, BP targets need to be clearly defined. Finally, the appropriate antihypertensive agents indicated as initial therapy by evidence-based guidelines should be used.

The role for initial combination therapy in patients with CKD with a BP that is 20/10 mm Hg above the goal has been championed for almost 2 decades to enhance adherence and efficacy.[8,233] Studies evaluating initial monotherapy versus single-pill combination among those with an eGFR greater than 60 mL/min/1.73 $m^2$ have uniformly shown an advantage of achieving the BP goal more quickly and with better tolerability.[295,296]

These new guidelines and concepts have been integrated into an algorithm that was in the original National Kidney Foundation consensus report.[297] It is meant to provide an approach to pharmacologically meaningful agents that when combined, actually further reduce BP. Box 46.4 provides an approved list of combination agents, noting which are meaningful for optimal BP reduction and which are not. Fig. 46.17 presents an evidence-based algorithm to help achieve BP control in the patient with advanced CKD.

## RESISTANT HYPERTENSION

Resistant hypertension is currently defined as the failure to achieve a goal BP of less than 140/90 mm Hg in patients who are adherent with maximal tolerated doses of a minimum of three antihypertensive drugs, one of which must be a diuretic appropriate for kidney function.[152] The increasing prevalence of obesity and hypertension in the general population has resulted in this disorder gaining attention in the past decade. Large-scale population-based studies such as NHANES have specifically examined the prevalence and incidence of resistant hypertension and associated risk factors. These findings have suggested that the prevalence of resistant hypertension is approximately 8% to 12% of adult patients with hypertension (6–9 million people).[298] The increasing prevalence of resistant hypertension has contrasted with the improvement in BP control rates during the same period. Studies have also shown that patients with resistant hypertension who are older than 55 years, who are black, with a high

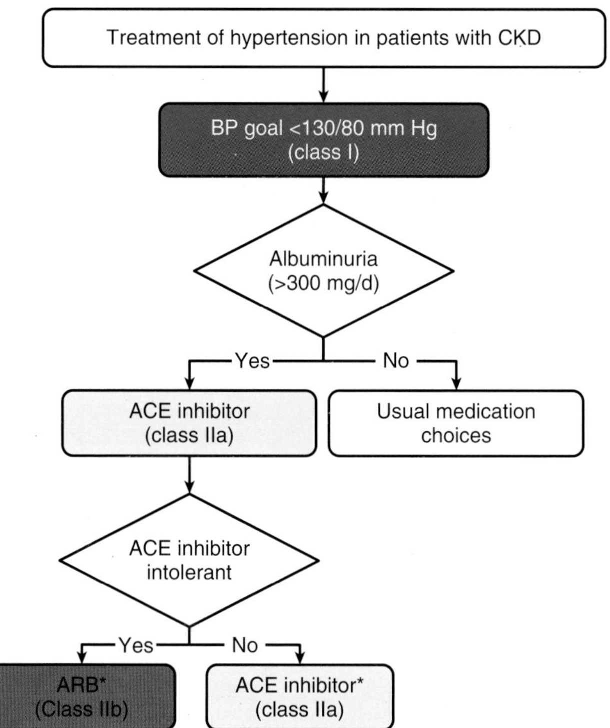


**Fig. 46.17** Management of hypertension in patients with chronic kidney disease *(CKD)* according to American Heart Association (ACC)/ American Heart Association (AHA) guidelines. Colors correspond to class of recommendation: *green,* class I (strong); *yellow,* class IIa (moderate); *orange,* class IIIb (weak). *CKD stage 3 or higher or stage 1 or 2 with albuminuria ≥300 mg/day or ≥300 mg/g creatinine. It should be noted that treating blood pressure *(BP)* in CKD patients to <140/90 mm Hg with an angiotensin receptor blocker or ACE inhibitor as first-line therapy is recommended for slowing progression of CKD by KDIGO guidelines. To further reduce CV risk, levels of <130/80 mm Hg need to be achieved. The use of combination therapy with diltiazem in the subgroup with very high albuminuria has an additive reduction, in addition, to lower BP further compared with other calcium channel blockers. *ACE,* Angiotensin-converting enzyme; *ARB,* angiotensin receptor blocker. (From Whelton PK, Carey RM, Aronow WS, et al. ACC/AHA/AAPA/ABC/ACPM/AGS/APhA/ASH/ASPC/NMA/PCNA Guideline for the Prevention, Detection, Evaluation and Management of High Blood Pressure in Adults: A Report of the American College of Cardiology/American Heart Association and Task Force on Clinical Practice Guidelines. *Hypertension.* 2018;71(6):e13–e115.)

body mass index, diabetes, or CKD have an increased risk for CV events compared with patients with nonresistant hypertension. However, the effects of white coat hypertension and pseudoresistant hypertension have not been factored into many of the prevalence studies, and hence the true prevalence is not known. The white coat effect contributes greatly to the high perceived incidence of resistant hypertension, as was evidenced by the over 60% screen failure in the Renal Denervation in Patients with Uncontrolled Hypertension (SYMPLICITY HTN-3) trial of renal denervation due to WCH.[299,300]

Thus this is a diagnosis frequently seen by nephrologists and is usually the result of nonadherence with medication, as well as volume overload secondary to poor kidney function and nonadherence to a low-sodium diet. Once a diagnosis of resistant hypertension has been made using a 24-hour ABPM, and a fourth drug is needed after the use of a calcium antagonist, diuretic, and RAAS blocker, a mineralocorticoid inhibitor has demonstrated significant benefit in controlling BP in more recent studies.[301–304] A detailed discussion of this topic is beyond the scope of this chapter, but the reader is referred to the most recent consensus report by the AHA/ACC.

 Complete reference list available at ExpertConsult.com.

# 47 Renovascular Hypertension and Ischemic Nephropathy

Stephen C. Textor

CHAPTER OUTLINE



## INTRODUCTION

Few areas within nephrology have undergone more dramatic paradigm shifts with competing treatment options than occlusive renovascular disease (RVD). Aging population demographics, coupled with advances in imaging technology, effective medical therapy, and negative clinical trials, must be reconciled with an established record of clinical success and improving techniques of renal revascularization. Although prospective trial data have failed to provide compelling evidence in favor of stenting for many patients with atherosclerotic disease, experienced clinicians recognize that renal revascularization in these disorders sometimes should be undertaken to improve hypertension and protect renal function. Selecting patients and determining optimal timing for vascular intervention at reasonable risk are rarely straightforward.

The evaluation and treatment of RVD overlaps numerous medical disciplines and subspecialties, including nephrology, internal medicine, cardiovascular diseases, interventional radiology, and vascular surgery. These subspecialty groups often deal with different patient subgroups and clinical issues that shape different points of view. Cardiologists, for example, usually manage more patients with refractory congestive heart failure (CHF) at risk for flash pulmonary edema than internists, who may deal with hypertensive patients with progressive hypertension or a rise in serum creatinine levels (Fig. 47.1). Nephrologists regularly encounter declining kidney function with high-grade stenosis to a solitary functioning kidney. All these conditions can represent clinical manifestations of RVD but present different comorbid risk and management issues. Not surprisingly, perceptions related to renovascular hypertension and ischemic nephropathy differ, even among informed clinicians. Initial results from prospective randomized trials, such as the Angioplasty and Stenting for Renal Artery Lesions (ASTRAL) in the United Kingdom and Cardiovascular Outcomes in Renal Artery Lesions (CORAL) in the United States comparing optimal medical therapy, with or without endovascular stent procedures, continue to provoke controversy. Some individual authors of these negative trials have separately reported high-risk subsets not enrolled in those studies that have major clinical and mortality benefits from restoring renal blood flow.[1–3]

These diverse observational studies underscore the ambiguity that clinicians encounter in practice. Ultimately, RVD and impaired blood flow not only affect blood pressure and cardiovascular risk but also threaten the viability of the kidney. These can lead to irreversible loss of kidney function, sometimes designated as "ischemic nephropathy" or "azotemic RVD."[4] Restoring blood flow and perfusion by relieving vascular occlusion intuitively offers a means to halt or reverse this process. It must be recognized, however, that renal revascularization is a double-edged sword. The benefits include the potential to improve systemic arterial blood pressures and preserve or salvage renal function. The potential risks of renal intervention are all too familiar to nephrologists. Endovascular procedures themselves may threaten the affected kidney through vascular thrombosis, dissection, restenosis, or atheroemboli. These events sometimes precipitate the need for renal replacement therapy, including dialysis or transplantation. It is therefore important that nephrologists

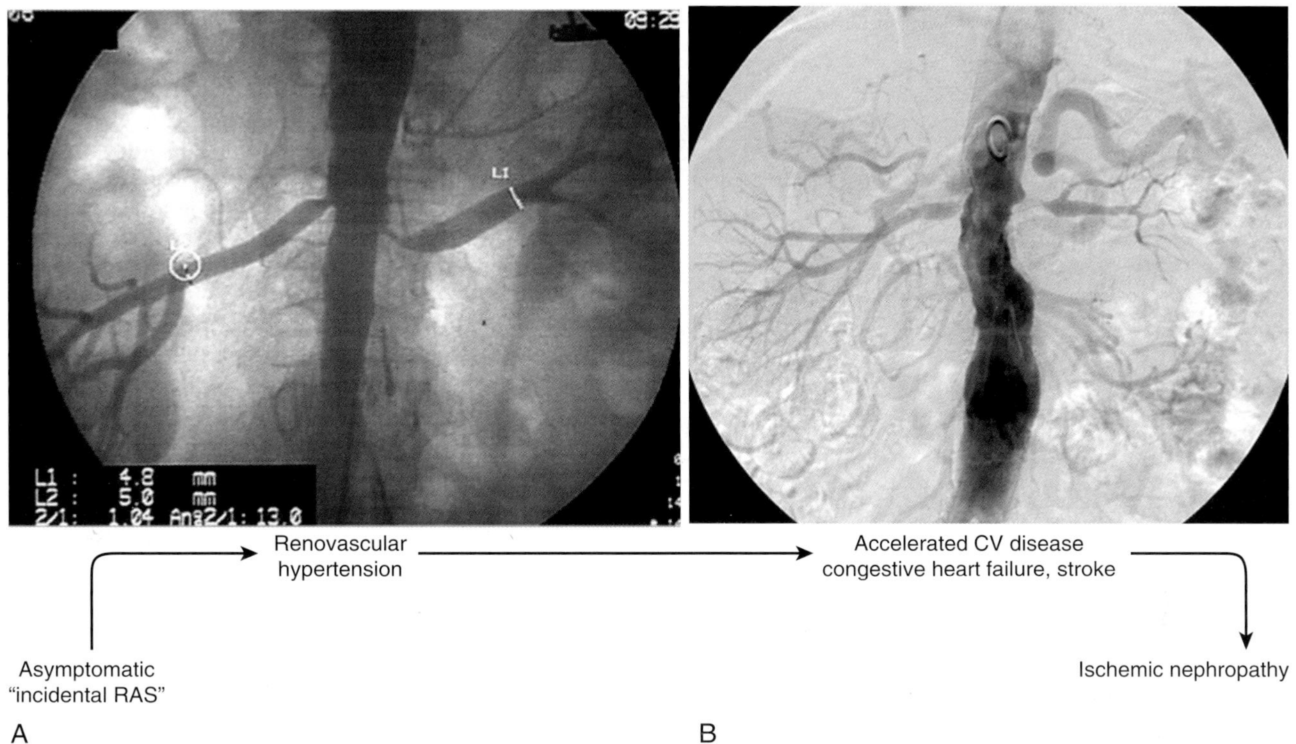


**Fig. 47.1** (A and B) Spectrum of atherosclerotic renovascular disease (ARVD) manifestations. *Left panel,* Aortogram obtained during coronary angiography demonstrating moderate incidental stenosis of both renal arteries in a 67-year-old man with symptomatic coronary disease. *Right panel,* More severe occlusive disease observed in a 68-year-old woman presenting with severe hypertension and episodes of flash pulmonary edema. RVD commonly develops in the setting of atherosclerotic disease elsewhere and may be associated with any of many clinical syndromes, ranging from renovascular hypertension to accelerated cardiovascular decompensation and ischemic nephropathy. Recent trends favor initial management with effective medical therapy, often including agents that block the renin-angiotensin system. Clinicians face the challenge of recognizing the role of RVD in more advanced disease and balancing the risks and benefits of renal revascularization in high-risk subsets. *RAS,* renal artery stenosis. (Modified from Herrmann SM, Saad A, Textor SC. Management of atherosclerotic renovascular disease after Cardiovascular Outcomes in Renal Atherosclerotic Lesions (CORAL). *Nephrol Dial Transplant.* 2015;30(3):366–375.)

have a solid foundation related to the implications of reduced renal perfusion and the risks and benefits of medical management and restoration of renal artery patency.

## HISTORICAL PERSPECTIVE

RVD is among the most extensively studied forms of secondary hypertension. Early observations regarding blood pressure regulation have revealed important connections among fluid volume, renal arterial pressures, and vascular resistance. The sequence of these observations related to identification of the renin-angiotensin-aldosterone system has been reviewed by Basso and Terragno[5] and is summarized here. In 1898, Tigerstedt and Bergman established that extracts of the kidney had pressor effects in the whole animal and are credited with the identification of "renin." Identification of each component of the renin-angiotensin system represents a remarkable series of research ventures, spanning more than a half-century and investigators in many countries.

Goldblatt and others carried out seminal experiments with the development of an animal model in which reduced renal perfusion regularly produced hypertension, published between 1932 and 1934. Numerous investigators thereafter identified the peptide nature of angiotensin, the role of renin substrate or angiotensinogen, the role of nephrectomy in sensitizing the animal to the pressor effects of angiotensin, and the sequential phases of renovascular hypertension. Hence, the renin-angiotensin-aldosterone system owes its initial discovery and nomenclature primarily to early studies related to the regulation of blood pressure by the kidney. Only recently have many additional actions of angiotensin become evident regarding vascular remodeling, modulation of inflammatory pathways, and interaction with fibrogenic mechanisms. Understanding that reduced renal blood flow produces sustained elevations in arterial pressure has led to broad study of the mechanisms underlying many forms of hypertension. Experimental models of two-kidney and one-kidney "Goldblatt" hypertension—animals undergo clipping of one renal artery to reduce blood flow, with or without nephrectomy of the contralateral kidney (i.e., two-kidney, one-clip and one-kidney, one-clip models)—represent some of the most widely applied models of blood pressure and cardiovascular regulation. Extension of these studies into clinical medicine followed soon thereafter. Some forms of hypertension were designated as "malignant" in character during the late 1930s and 1940s based on poor survival if patients were untreated.

Few antihypertensive agents were known until the 1950s; intervention consisted mainly of lumbar sympathectomy and/or extremely low sodium intake diets. Some of the major

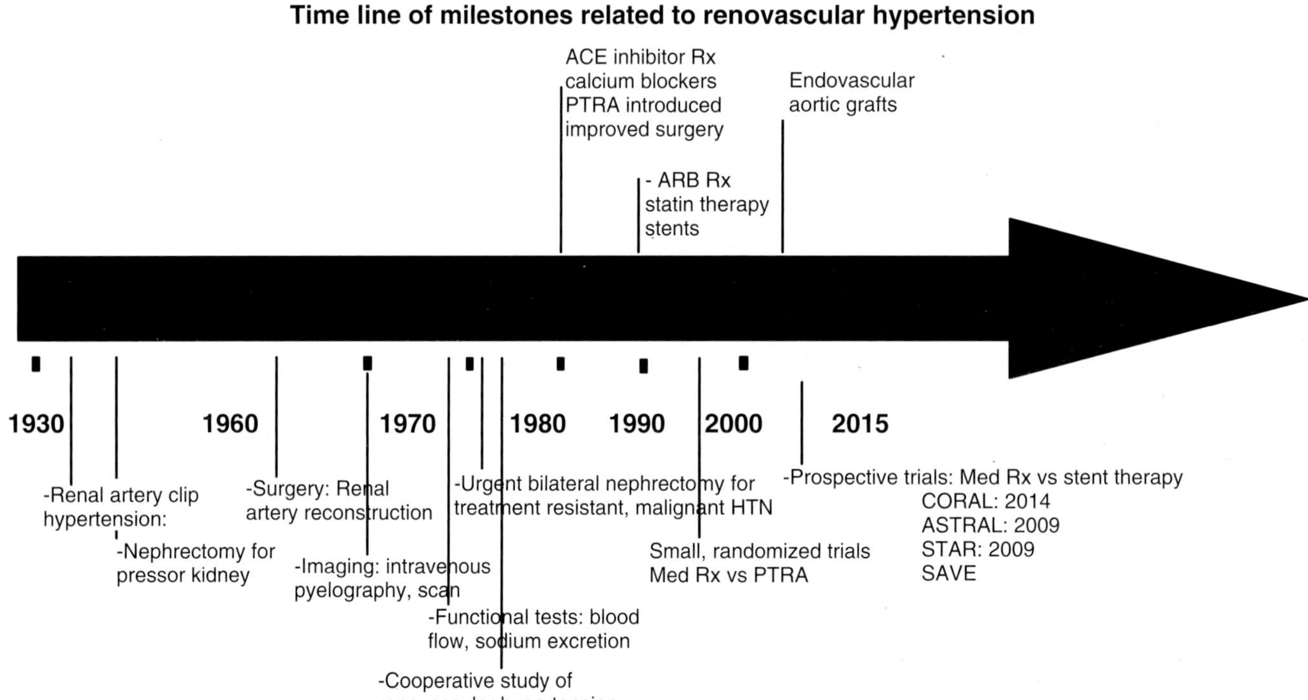


**Fig. 47.2** Historical time line of major milestones in renovascular disease (RVD). Although pressor substances derived from the kidney were identified more than a century ago, recognition that renal perfusion regulates arterial blood pressure occurred only in the 1930s. Technical advances allowing surgical reconstruction, more effective arterial imaging, and endovascular revascularization gradually evolved from 1960 to the present era. Important advances in antihypertensive drug therapy, particularly with agents that block the renin-angiotensin system, and other advances in managing atherosclerotic disease such as statins, continue to define optimal medical management of patients with RVD. The introduction of endovascular aortic stent grafts represents an iatrogenic form of RVD that benefits from protection of the renal artery patency. Results from several prospective, randomized clinical trials indicate that renal revascularization often fails to add substantial benefits to effective medical therapy in the near term for patients with moderate atherosclerotic RVD, although high-risk subsets are an exception. *ACE,* Angiotensin-converting enzyme; *ARB,* angiotensin receptor blocker; *PTRA,* percutaneous transluminal renal angioplasty.

events in the identification and treatment of renovascular hypertension are summarized in Fig. 47.2.[6] Recognition that some forms of severe hypertension were secondary to occlusive vascular disease in the kidney led surgeons to undertake unilateral nephrectomy for small kidneys in 1937.[6] The fact that some of these were indeed pressor kidneys, and blood pressure fell to normal levels, provided proof of concept and led to more widespread use of nephrectomy. Unfortunately, achieving cure of hypertension after nephrectomy was rare, and Smith reviewed the poor results overall in a 1956 paper discouraging this practice.[7]

The 1960s marked the introduction of methods of vascular surgery to restore renal blood flow. These carried substantial morbidity but offered an opportunity to improve the renal circulation and potentially to reverse renovascular hypertension. One result of this development was a series of studies that characterized the functional role of each vascular lesion in producing hypertension, thereby allowing prediction of the outcomes of vascular surgery.[6] A large cooperative study of renovascular hypertension included major vascular centers and reported on the results of more than 500 surgical procedures.[8] These results provided limited support for vascular repair but identified relatively high associated morbidity and mortality, particularly for patients with atherosclerotic disease.

In the 1980s and 1990s, further developments led to improved medications and the introduction of endovascular procedures, including percutaneous angioplasty and stents.[9] These both broadened the options for treating patients with vascular disease and raised new issues regarding timing and overall goals of intervention. Recent developments have highlighted the need for intensive cardiovascular risk factor reduction and more stringent standards of blood pressure control. Antihypertensive medications have improved dramatically, both in regard to efficacy and tolerability. As emphasized later, broad application of angiotensin-converting enzyme (ACE) inhibitors and angiotensin receptor antagonists for reasons other than hypertension alone changed the clinical presentation of disorders associated with renal artery stenosis (RAS). Recent prospective randomized trials have emphasized the limited additional benefits from restoring renal blood flow for many patients with moderate vascular disease.[1]

Uncontrolled hypertension is now less commonly the reason to intervene in RVD than in the past. Often, the main objective is long-term preservation of renal function. In recent years, endovascular techniques have made renal revascularization possible with relatively low morbidity in many patients previously considered unacceptable surgical candidates. The challenge for clinicians is how and when to apply these tools most effectively in the management of individual patients.[10]

# PATHOPHYSIOLOGY OF RENOVASCULAR HYPERTENSION AND ISCHEMIC NEPHROPATHY

## RENAL ARTERY STENOSIS VERSUS RENOVASCULAR HYPERTENSION

As with most vascular lesions, the presence of a renovascular abnormality alone does not translate directly into functional importance. Some degree of RAS can be identified in as many as 20% to 45% of patients undergoing vascular imaging for other reasons, such as coronary angiography or lower extremity peripheral vascular disease.[11,12] Most of these incidentally detected stenoses are of minor hemodynamic and/or clinical significance. Failure to limit treatment trials to patients with clinically important lesions has been a serious barrier to understanding the role for renal revascularization (see later). The term *renovascular hypertension* refers to a rise in arterial pressure definitely induced by reduced renal perfusion. A variety of lesions can lead to the syndrome of renovascular hypertension, some of which are listed in Box 47.1. Studies of vascular obstruction using latex rubber casts have indicated that from 70% to 80% of lumen obstruction must occur before measurable changes in blood flow or pressure across the lesion can be detected.[13] Measurements of pressure gradients during renal angiography confirm that a pressure gradient of at least 10 to 20 mm Hg between the aorta and poststenotic renal artery is required before measurable renin release occurs.[14,15] When advanced stenosis is present, the pressure and flow drop steeply as illustrated in Fig. 47.3. When lesions have reached this degree of hemodynamic significance, they are deemed "critical" stenoses.

When renal artery lesions reach critical dimensions, a series of events leads to a rise in systemic arterial pressure and restoration of renal perfusion pressure, as illustrated in Fig. 47.4. Hence, one can view the development of rising pressures in this context as an integrated renal response to maintain renal perfusion of the stenotic kidney. It is important to distinguish between experimental models of clip stenosis, at which time a sudden change in renal perfusion is induced, and the more common clinical situation of

**Box 47.1 Some Vascular Lesions Producing Renal Hypoperfusion and Renovascular Hypertension Syndrome**

Unilateral disease (analogous to one-clip, two-kidney hypertension)
Unilateral atherosclerotic renal artery stenosis
Unilateral fibromuscular dysplasia (FMD)
Medial fibroplasia
Perimedial fibroplasia
Intimal fibroplasia

**Medial Hyperplasia**

Renal artery aneurysm
Arterial embolus
Arteriovenous fistula (congenital, traumatic)
Segmental arterial occlusion, dissection (posttraumatic)
Extrinsic compression of renal artery (e.g., pheochromocytoma)
Renal compression (e.g., metastatic tumor)
Bilateral disease or solitary functioning kidney (analogous to one-clip, one-kidney model)
Stenosis to a solitary functioning kidney
Bilateral renal arterial stenosis
Aortic coarctation
Systemic vasculitis (e.g., Takayasu arteritis, polyarteritis)
Atheroembolic disease
Vascular occlusion due to endovascular aortic stent graft

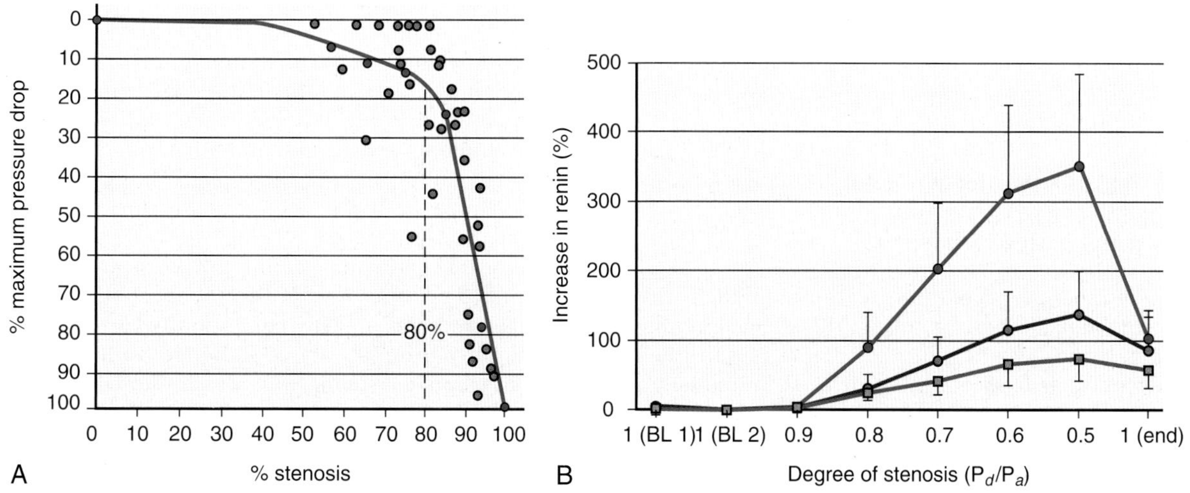


**Fig. 47.3** (A) Measured fall in arterial pressure and blood flow across stenotic lesions induced in experimental animals. The degree of stenosis was determined using latex casts after completion of the experiment. These data indicate that "critical" lesions require 70% to 80% luminal obstruction before hemodynamic effects can be detected. (B) Studies from human subjects with translesional pressure gradients indicate that an aortic-renal pressure gradient of 10% to 20% is necessary to detect renin release. $P_a$, aortic pressure; $P_d$, distal pressure. (A from May AG, Van de Berg L, DeWeese JA, et al. Critical arterial stenosis. *Surgery.* 1963;54:250–259; B from De Bruyne B, Manoharan G, Pijls NHJ, et al. Assessment of renal artery stenosis severity by pressure gradient measurements. *J Am Coll Cardiol.* 2006;48:1851–1855.)

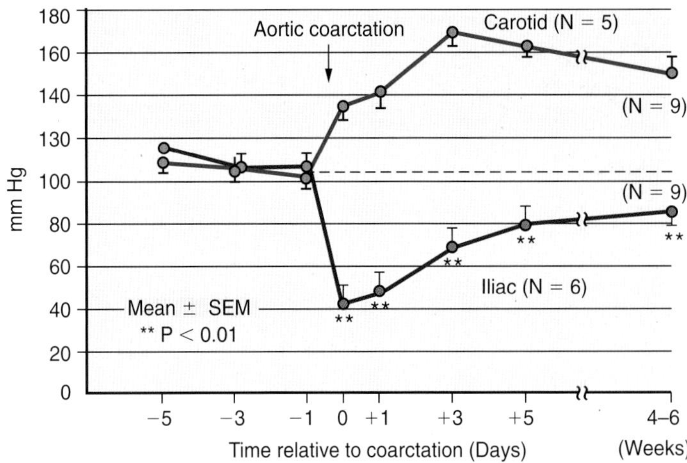


**Fig. 47.4** Systemic arterial pressure (carotid) and poststenotic renal perfusion pressures (iliac) in an aortic coarctation model with a clip placed between the right and left renal arteries. Measurements were obtained in conscious animals during the development of renovascular hypertension. They illustrate the fact that despite a persistent gradient across the stenosis, renal perfusion pressure (inferred from Iliac pressure) returns to near-normal levels as a result of systemic hypertension. A corollary of this pressure gradient is that reduction of systemic pressures would reduce poststenotic perfusion pressures, sometimes below the range of autoregulation. *SEM,* Standard error of the mean. From Textor SC, Smith-Powell L. Post-stenotic arterial pressures, renal haemodynamics and sodium excretion during graded pressure reduction in conscious rats with one- and two-kidney coarctation hypertension. *J Hypertens.* 1988;6(4):311–319.)

gradually progressive lumen obstruction. In the latter case, hemodynamic characteristics change slowly and are likely to produce hypertension over a prolonged time interval. The rise in systemic pressure restores normal renal perfusion, often with normal-sized kidneys and no discernible hemodynamic compromise. If the renal artery lesion progresses further (or is experimentally advanced), the cycle of reduced perfusion and rising arterial pressures repeats until malignant-phase hypertension develops. Experimental models in swine have used gradually progressing vascular lesions to mimic human RVD.[16]

A corollary to critical arterial stenosis is that treatment aimed at the normalization of elevated systemic pressures in renovascular hypertension reduces renal perfusion pressure beyond the stenotic lesion. Poststenotic pressures may fall below the levels of autoregulation that maintain blood flow. This underperfusion of the kidney activates counterregulatory pathways and leads to a sequence of events, again directed toward restoring kidney perfusion.

## ROLE OF THE RENIN-ANGIOTENSIN SYSTEM IN ONE-KIDNEY AND TWO-KIDNEY RENOVASCULAR HYPERTENSION

Reduction in renal perfusion pressures activates the release of renin from juxtaglomerular cells in the affected kidneys. Experimental studies have indicated that hypertension in two-kidney, one-clip models can be delayed indefinitely as long as agents that block this system are administered. Animals genetically modified to lack the angiotensin 1 (AT1) receptor fail to develop two-kidney, one-clip hypertension, as illustrated in Fig. 47.5.[17] Experiments using kidney transplantation from AT1 receptor knockout mice have indicated that both systemic and renal angiotensin receptors participate in blood pressure regulation in additive fashion.[18]

Demonstration of the role of the renin-angiotensin axis in renovascular hypertension depends in part on whether or not a contralateral nonstenotic kidney is present. Most human renovascular hypertension is considered analogous to two-kidney, one-clip experimental (Goldblatt) hypertension. The contralateral nonstenotic kidney is subjected to elevated systemic perfusion pressures. Effects of rising perfusion pressure force natriuresis from the nonstenotic kidney and suppress renin release. Hence, the nonstenotic kidney tends to prevent the rise in systemic pressures, thereby perpetuating reduced perfusion to the stenotic side and promoting continued renin release from the stenotic kidney. Blood pressure in these models is demonstrably angiotensin-dependent and is associated with elevated circulating levels of plasma renin activity, as illustrated in Fig. 47.6. The two-kidney, one-clip model of renovascular hypertension provided the basis for many of the early functional studies of surgically curable hypertension in which side-to-side function was compared regarding factors such as glomerular filtration and odium excretion. This paradigm forms the basis for comparing kidneys side to side using radionuclide studies, such as captopril renography and renal vein renin determinations. Unilateral renal ischemia is a classic model for the study of angiotensin-dependent hypertension and target organ injury.

When no such contralateral kidney is present or able to respond to pressure natriuresis, the mechanisms sustaining hypertension differ. This corresponds to the one-kidney, one-clip hypertensive model. Although renin release occurs initially, elevated systemic pressures develop with sodium and volume retention because there is limited sodium excretion by the contralateral kidney. Rising pressures eventually restore renin levels to normal. Hypertension in this model is not demonstrably dependent on angiotensin II (Ang II) unless prior sodium depletion is achieved. Clinical examples of this situation include bilateral RAS or stenosis in a solitary functioning kidney, in which the entire renal mass is affected. In such cases, diagnostic comparison of side-to-side renin release is not possible or has little meaning.

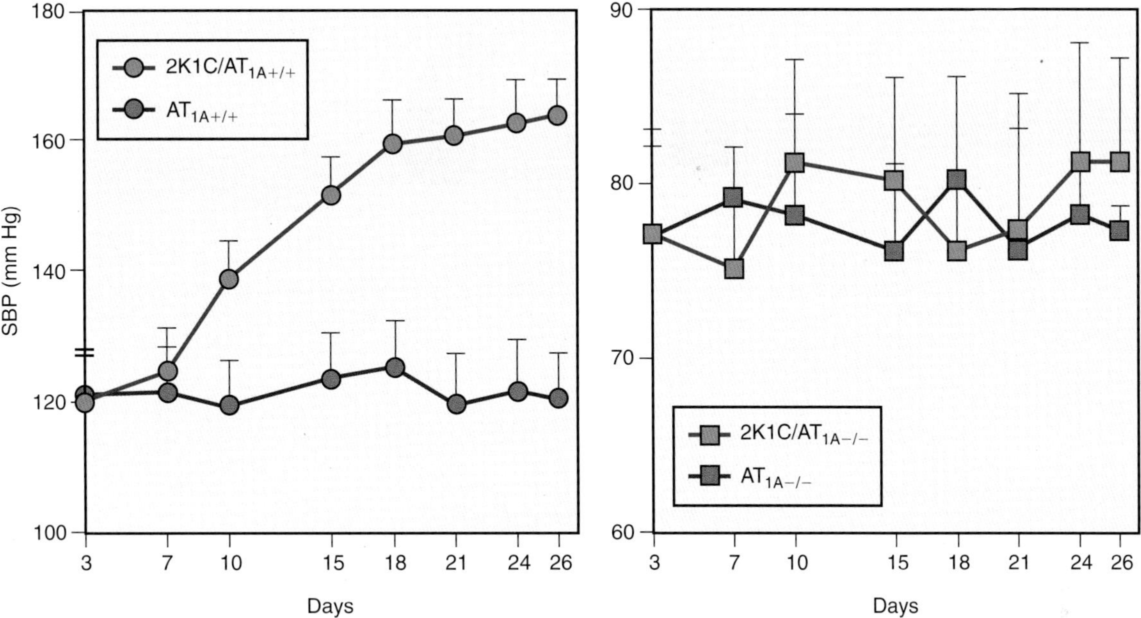


**Fig. 47.5** Systolic blood pressures in mice before and after placement of a renal artery clip in experimental two-kidney, one-clip renovascular hypertension (2K1C). The rise in systolic blood pressure *(SBP)* after clip placement develops rapidly only in mice with an intact angiotensin 1A receptor ($AT_{1A+/+}$; *solid circles, left panel*). This rise is blocked by administration of an angiotensin receptor blocker (*open circles, left panel*). A genetic knockout mouse strain with no AT1A receptor ($AT_{1A-/-}$) has a lower SBP and no change after renal artery clipping *(solid circles, right panel).* No additional effect is noted with an angiotensin receptor blocker *(open squares, right panel).* These data reinforce the essential role of the renin-angiotensin system and an intact angiotensin 1 receptor for the development of renovascular hypertension. (Modified from Cervenka L, Horacek V, Vaneckova I, et al. Essential role of AT1-A receptor in the development of 2K1C hypertension. *Hypertension.* 2002;40:735–741.)

## MECHANISMS SUSTAINING RENOVASCULAR HYPERTENSION

For more than a century, the kidney has been recognized has a source of multiple pressor substances. Recruitment of numerous pathways that raise arterial pressure increases the complexity of managing hypertension in this setting. Identification of components of the renin-angiotensin system provided a crucial link to understanding several of these systems. Circulating renin is derived primarily from the kidney in response to a reduction in renal perfusion pressure, detected by loss of afferent arteriolar stretch.[19] Renin itself has biologic activity directed mainly at the enzymatic release of angiotensin I (Ang I) from its circulating substrate, angiotensinogen, in plasma and possibly other sites.[5] Two more peptides are cleaved through the action of ACE to produce Ang II. Generation of Ang II in plasma occurs mainly during passage through the lung. Hence, the signal of reduced kidney pressures is amplified and transmitted through a major systemic vasopressor system and is one mechanism whereby renovascular hypertension develops.

### RENIN-ANGIOTENSIN SYSTEM

Following its discovery, the renin-angiotensin system has been found to have widespread effects beyond its vasoconstrictor action in renovascular hypertension.[20,21] Some actions of Ang II are illustrated in Fig. 47.7. Activation of this system increases vascular resistance, sodium retention, and aldosterone stimulation. Further studies have indicated that complex interactions between Ang II and tissue and cellular systems occur, leading to vascular remodeling, left ventricular hypertrophy, and activation of inflammatory and fibrogenic mechanisms.

Hypertension and peripheral vasoconstriction reflect further complex interactions between angiotensin and other vasoactive systems. RVD leads to disturbances in sympathetic nerve signaling, which may differ between one-kidney and two-kidney models. Muscle sympathetic nerve activity is increased in humans with renovascular hypertension, and blood pressure responses to adrenergic inhibition are amplified.[22]

A major transition occurs with recruitment of altered oxidative stress within the systemic vasculature, leading to increased oxygen free radicals.[23] Experimental animals with two-kidney, one-clip hypertension develop an increase in oxidative stress (reflected by F2 isoprostanes) that can be reversed in part with angiotensin blockade and/or antioxidants.[24] Vascular injury itself produces disturbances in endothelium-derived mechanisms, such as endothelin (ET) production and vasodilator systems, including prostacyclin.[25]

The roles of endothelial dysfunction and increased oxidative stress in human RVD have been supported by clinical studies in patients with both atherosclerotic and fibromuscular RAS showing reversal after revascularization.[22,26] Studies in a swine model of RVD have demonstrated an important interaction between atherosclerosis induced by cholesterol feeding and RVD.[27,28] Endothelial dysfunction in the kidney and tissue fibrosis are augmented by the atherosclerotic process. Some of these changes can be abrogated experimentally by intensive therapy with statins and antioxidants. These data are supported by observations of a rise in nitric oxide (NO) levels and reduction in malondialdehyde within 24 hours of endovascular revascularization in atherosclerotic RVD.[29]

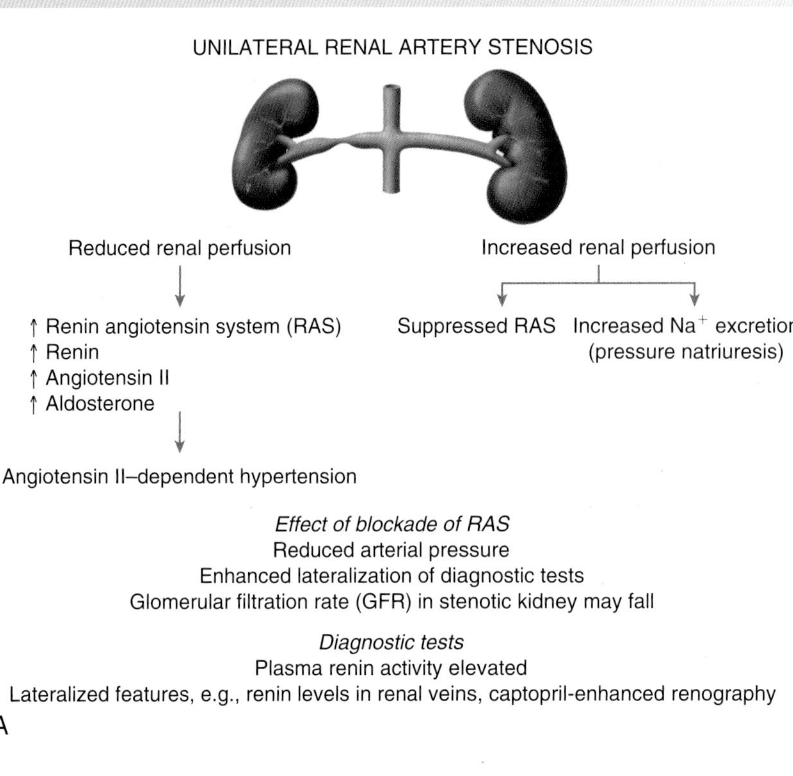


*Effect of blockade of RAS*
Reduced arterial pressure
Enhanced lateralization of diagnostic tests
Glomerular filtration rate (GFR) in stenotic kidney may fall

*Diagnostic tests*
Plasma renin activity elevated
Lateralized features, e.g., renin levels in renal veins, captopril-enhanced renography

A

BILATERAL RENAL ARTERY STENOSIS

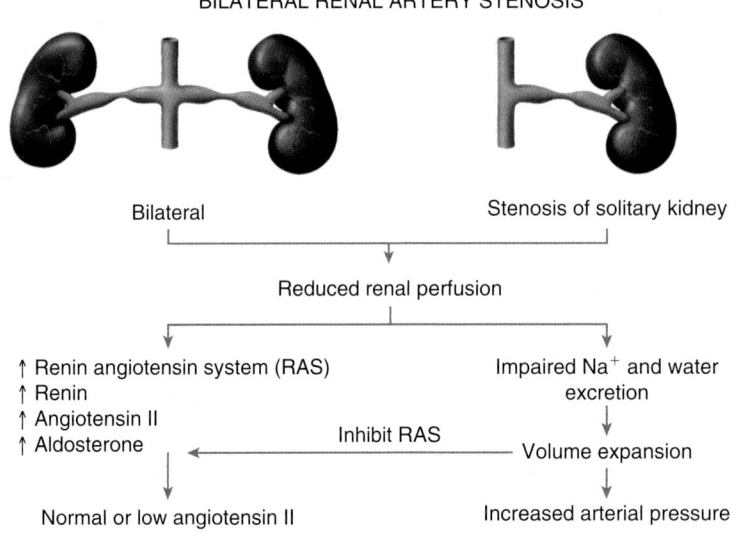

Bilateral | Stenosis of solitary kidney

Reduced renal perfusion

↑ Renin angiotensin system (RAS)
↑ Renin
↑ Angiotensin II
↑ Aldosterone

Impaired Na$^+$ and water excretion

Volume expansion

Inhibit RAS

Normal or low angiotensin II

Increased arterial pressure

*Effect of blockade of RAS*
Reduced arterial pressure only after volume depletion
May lower GFR

*Diagnostic tests*
Plasma renin activity normal or low
Lateralized features: none

B

**Fig. 47.6** Schematic view of two-kidney (A) and one-kidney (B) renovascular hypertension. These models differ by the presence of a contralateral kidney exposed to elevated perfusion pressures in two-kidney hypertension. The nonstenotic kidney tends to allow pressure natriuresis to ensue and produces ongoing stimulation of renin release from the stenotic kidney. The one-kidney model eventually produces sodium retention and a fall in renin, with minimal evidence of angiotensin dependence unless sodium depletion is achieved. *GFR,* Glomerular filtration rate; *RAS*, renin angiotensin system.

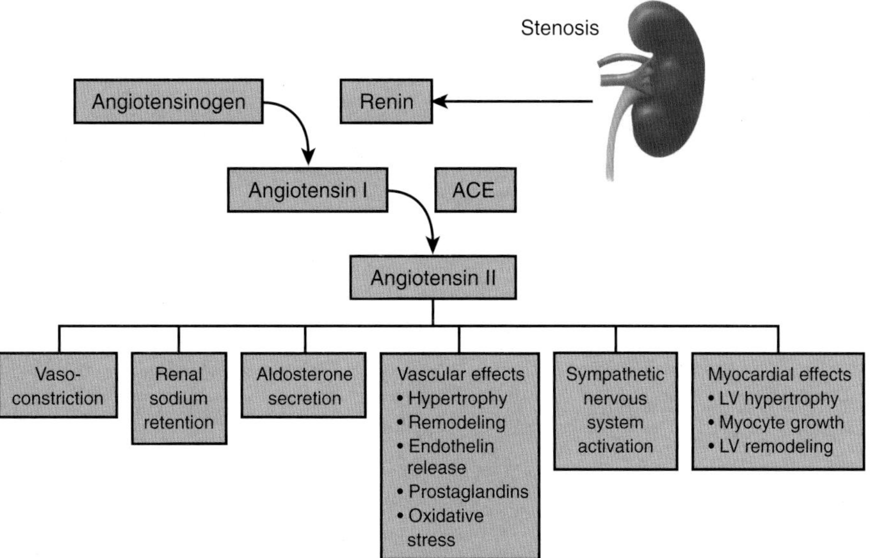


**Fig. 47.7** Schematic view of activation of the renin-angiotensin system beyond a renal artery stenotic lesion. The generation of circulating and local angiotensin II leads to widespread effects, including sodium retention, efferent arteriolar vasoconstriction, and elevated systemic vascular resistance. Additional studies implicate angiotensin II in many other pathways of vascular and cardiac smooth muscle remodeling, activation of inflammatory and fibrogenic cytokines, coagulation factors, and induction of other vasoactive systems. *ACE,* Angiotensin-converting enzyme; *LV,* left ventricular.

Studies have suggested that oxidative stress can be reversed by infusion of antioxidants and successful revascularization.[20] Experimental infusion of agents that protect mitochondria from reactive oxygen species by inhibiting opening of mitochondrial transition pores has been associated with improved recovery of microvascular structures and renal function after revascularization.[30]

## PHASES OF DEVELOPMENT OF RENOVASCULAR HYPERTENSION

Experimental models of renovascular hypertension have indicated that mechanisms sustaining hypertension change over time (Fig. 47.8).[31] Even before occlusive lesions are evident, accumulation of inflammatory monocytes in the renal vascular wall and elevation of circulating cytokines are evident.[32] An early pressor phase is characterized by elevated circulating renin activity and hypertension, both of which return to normal after removing the vascular lesion (e.g., the clip). A second phase is described with a return of circulating renin activity to normal or low levels, during which hypertension persists and blood pressure can still respond to clip removal. A third phase occurs, during which removal of the clip no longer leads to a reduction in arterial pressure. These observations highlight the transition between differing mechanisms of vascular resistance, some of which become independent of renal perfusion. Some authors have suggested that microvascular injury in the contralateral kidney sustains hypertension in the third phase.[31] Studies in a swine model have indicated that the fall in renin activity follows the transition to mechanisms related to oxidative stress, with persistent elevation of oxidative metabolites such as isoprostanes.[23] Whether these phases translate directly to human RVD is not well known.

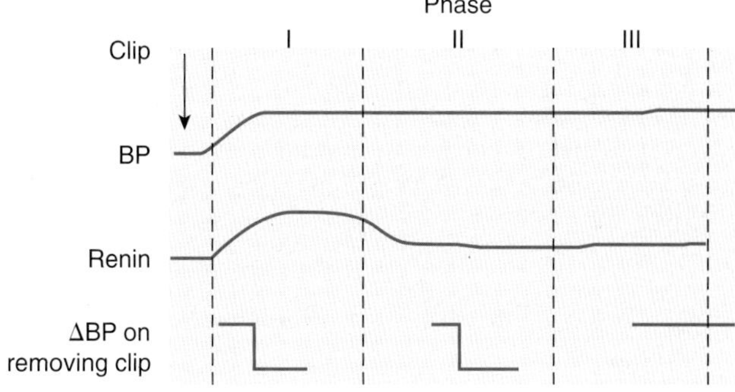


**Fig. 47.8** Schematic depiction of phases observed in experimental renovascular hypertension. Initially, high levels of renin activity fall in the chronic phase, although removal of the renal artery clip corrects hypertension. These observations support the concept of renal artery stenosis leading to the recruitment of additional structural and pressor mechanisms after initial activation of the renin-angiotensin system. The degree to which human renovascular hypertension follows these patterns is not well known. *BP,* blood pressure. (From Textor SC. Renovascular hypertension and ischemic nephropathy. In: Skorecki K, Chertow GM, Marsden PA, et al., eds. *Brenner and Rector's: The kidney.* 10th ed. Philadelphia: Elsevier; 2016:1567–1609.)

## MECHANISMS OF ISCHEMIC NEPHROPATHY

Reduced renal perfusion beyond critical stenosis ultimately leads to a loss of viable kidney function, as illustrated in Fig. 47.9.[33] Patients with stenosis affecting the entire renal mass develop reduced blood flow and glomerular filtration when poststenotic pressures fall below the range of autoregulation. This process can be reversible if pressure is restored and/or the vascular lesion is removed. The mechanisms whereby this occurs differ from those that govern the development

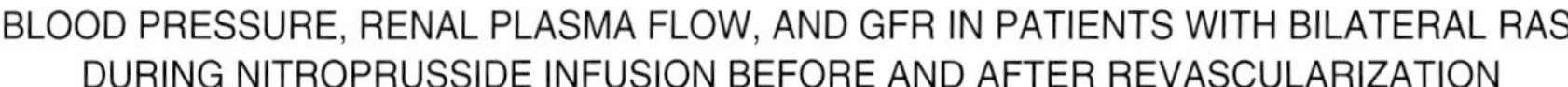


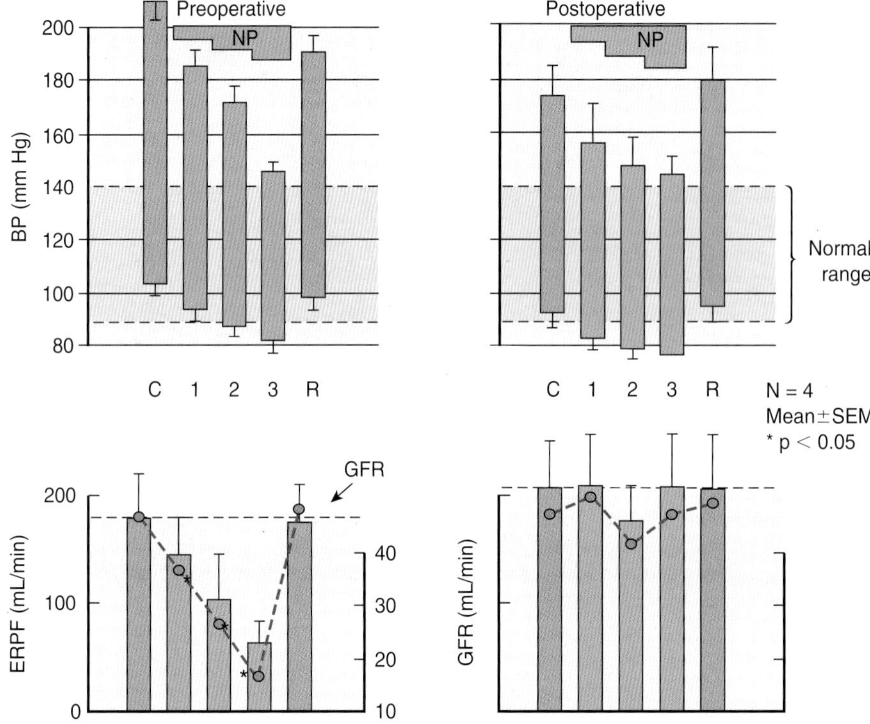


**Fig. 47.9** Effective renal plasma flow *(ERPF)* and glomerular filtration rate *(GFR)* in patients with critical bilateral renal artery stenosis during pressure reduction with sodium nitroprusside (NP). Reducing systemic blood pressure to normal levels produced a reversible fall in both plasma flow and GFR. Repeat studies in the same patients *(right-hand panel)* after unilateral surgical revascularization demonstrates that the sensitivity of blood flow and GFR to pressure reduction can be reversed. *SEM,* Standard error of the mean. (From Textor SC. Renovascular hypertension and ischemic nephropathy. In: Skorecki K, Chertow GM, Marsden PA, et al., eds. *Brenner and Rector's: The kidney.* 10th ed. Philadelphia: Elsevier; 2016:1567–1609.)

of hypertension. The term *ischemic nephropathy* may itself be a misnomer.[15,34]

## ADAPTIVE MECHANISMS TO REDUCED RENAL PERFUSION

Unlike brain or cardiac tissue, the kidney is highly perfused with oxygenated blood, consistent with its function as a filtering organ. Measurements of renal vein oxygen saturation and erythropoietin in patients with high-grade renovascular lesions indicate that whole-organ ischemia is rarely present.[35] It has long been postulated that local areas of reduced oxygen delivery in the kidney predispose to injury. The kidney maintains autoregulation of blood flow in the face of reduced arterial diameters of up to 75%. Under basal conditions, renal blood flow is among the highest of all organs reflecting its filtration function. Less than 10% of delivered oxygen is sufficient to maintain overall renal metabolic needs. Imaging using blood oxygen level–dependent (BOLD) magnetic resonance imaging (MRI) has demonstrated markedly reduced oxygenation in deeper medullary regions, despite preserved cortical oxygenation in normal kidneys and in patients with RAS.[34]

Much of the oxygen consumption in the kidney occurs during solute transport. Studies of patients with RAS sufficient to reduce blood flow, kidney volume, and glomerular filtration rate (GFR) have indicated remarkable preservation of tissue oxygenation using BOLD MRI[36] (Fig. 47.10). This stability of oxygen gradients is due partly to the surplus of oxygenated blood perfusing the cortex and to reduced oxygen consumption as a result of reduced solute filtration leading to reduced reabsorptive work of the affected kidney.[37,38] When severe, reduced blood flow leads to the accumulation of deoxygenated molecular hemoglobin (Fig. 47.11).[39,40] Under conditions of impaired renal perfusion, oxygen delivery may be maintained by the development of collateral vessels associated with intrarenal redistribution of blood flow. The renal medulla normally functions at levels close to hypoxia and is therefore sensitive to acute changes in perfusion.[37] During chronic reduction of blood flow, the medulla is partially protected by adaptive maintenance of tissue perfusion at the expense of cortical blood flow, which parallels whole-kidney renal blood flow.[41] Hence, gradual reduction of renal perfusion pressures allows recruitment of protective mechanisms that remain incompletely understood and that lead to different functional and morphologic changes from those observed after acute ischemic injury.

More severe vascular occlusion produces cortical hypoxia as these adaptive measures are overwhelmed, and tissue injury ensues.[38] Eventually, structural atrophy of the renal tubules occurs, partly due to necrosis and apoptosis.[42] The latter is an active, programmed form of cellular death, which appears to be closely regulated and differs from tissue necrosis. Tubular

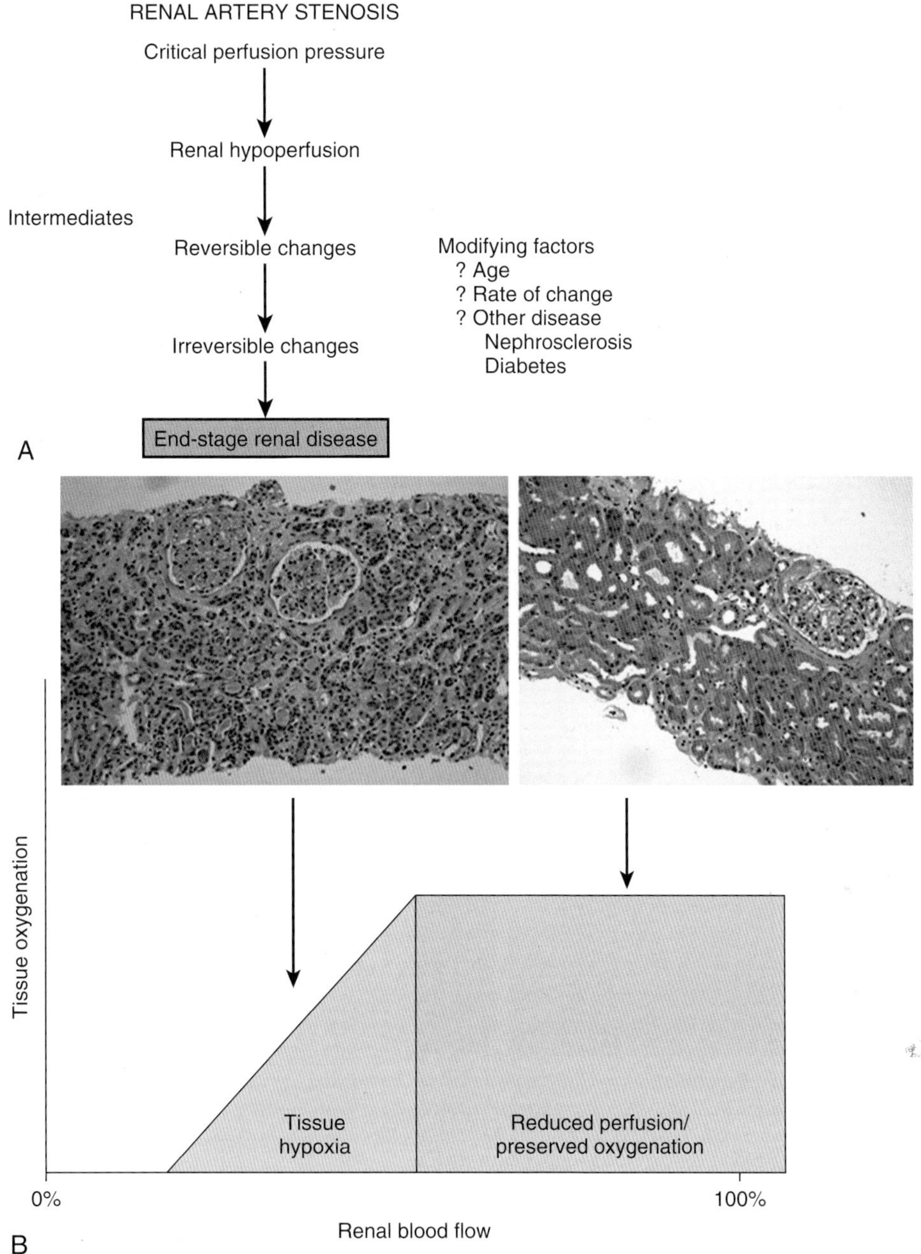


**Fig. 47.10** (A) General clinical paradigm that a reduction in the glomerular filtration rate (GFR) related to hypoperfusion of the kidney can be reversible, but can undergo a transition to irreversible injury eventually that no longer responds to restoration of blood flow alone. (B) Schematic depiction of the adaptation of tissue oxygenation in the kidney to moderate reductions in blood flow. Lowering renal blood flow up to 30% to 40% in human subjects *(right side)* is associated with preservation of both oxygen gradients *(lower graph)* and tissue histology *(upper images).* The fact that such adaptation occurs partly explains the stability of kidney function during antihypertensive drug therapy that lowers systemic pressure and renal blood flow in patients with atherosclerotic renal artery stenosis. Eventually, more severe reductions of blood flow overwhelm "adaptation," leading to overt tissue hypoxia *(left side).* Transjugular biopsy samples from patients with cortical hypoxia demonstrate loss of tubular structures and accumulation of inflammatory mmmT cells and macrophages with diffuse activation of transforming growth factor beta (TGF-β). (Magnification: low power: ×40.) (Modified from Gloviczki ML, Keddis MT, Garovic VD, et al. TGF expression and macrophage accumulation in atherosclerotic renal artery stenosis. *Clin J Am Soc Nephrol.* 2013;8(4):546–553; and Textor SC, Lerman LO. Paradigm shifts in atherosclerotic renovascular disease: where are we now? *J Am Soc Nephrol.* 2015;26:2074–2080.)

atrophy is potentially reversible, and the kidney maintains the capacity for tubular cell regeneration under many conditions. These features support the concept that underperfused kidney tissue sometimes can achieve a "hibernating" state capable of restoring function if blood flow is restored.[43] In late stages, histologic examination demonstrates reduced glomerular volume, loss of tubular structures near underperfused glomeruli, and areas of local inflammatory reaction, as illustrated in Fig. 47.10B.[44]

## MECHANISMS OF TISSUE INJURY IN AZOTEMIC RENOVASCULAR DISEASE

Reduction of blood flow to the kidney activates numerous pathways of vascular and tissue injury, including increased

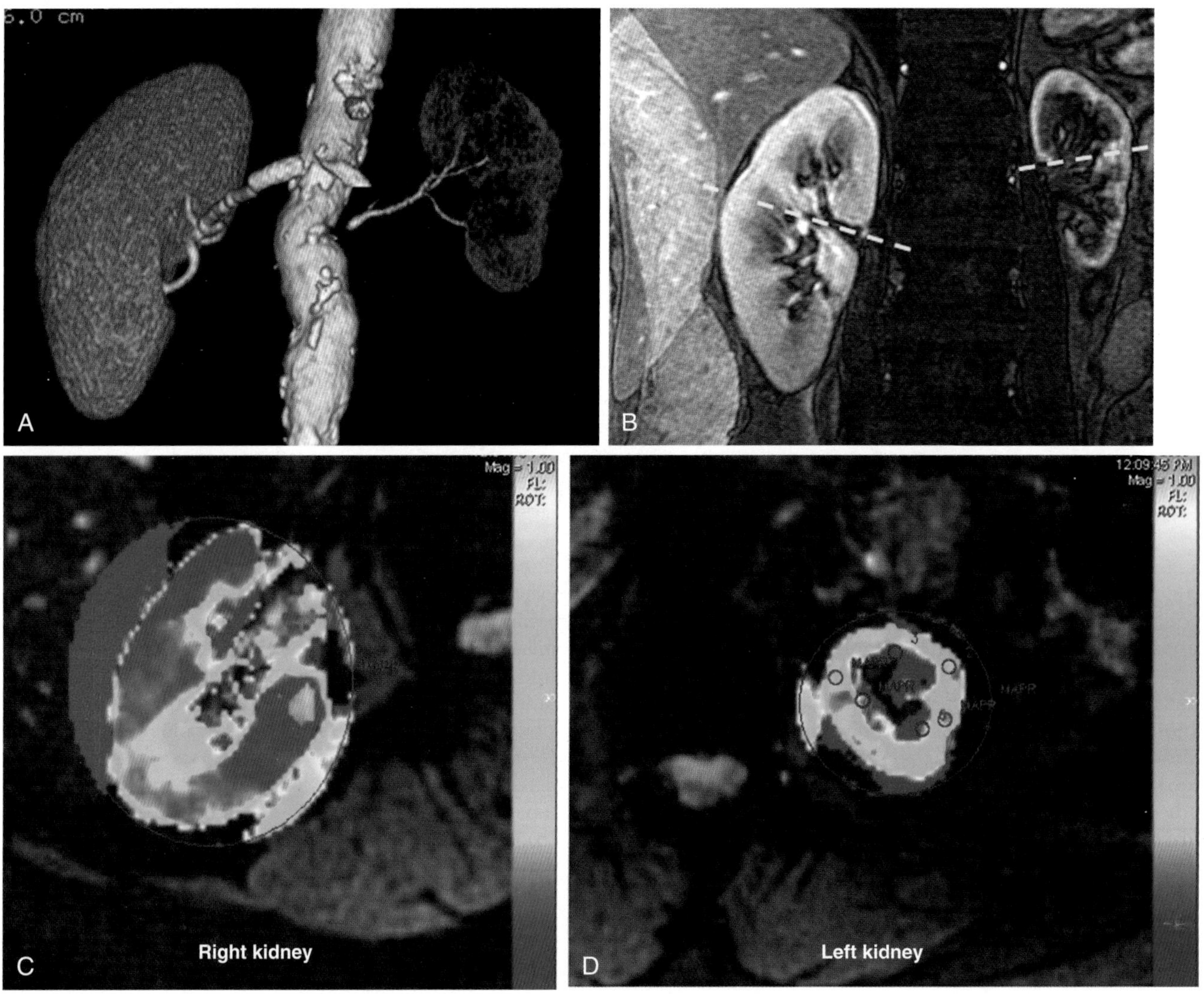


**Fig. 47.11** (A) Computed tomography angiogram of high-grade vascular occlusion leading to left kidney atrophy while the right kidney is well perfused beyond an endovascular stent. (B) T2 signals from magnetic resonance imaging (MRI) illustrate a gradient of perfusion from the cortex to lower levels in the deeper medullary sections, especially in the left kidney (*dashed line* depicts the level of axial sections shown in panels [C] and [D]). (C and D) Mapping of the blood oxygen level–dependent (BOLD) magnetic resonance R2* levels (a function of deoxyhemoglobin) illustrates the normal gradient in the right kidney from the cortex (low R2*, *blue*) to deeper medullary segments that have progressively higher levels of R2* *(green to red).* The R2* map of the left kidney (D) illustrates overt cortical hypoxia evident beyond critical vascular occlusion associated, with a larger fraction of the slice having high R2* values *(red)* and fractional medullary hypoxia.

Ang II, ET release, and oxidative stress, as noted previously. Experimental studies have demonstrated complex interactions with renal microvessels, leading to vascular rarefication (Fig. 47.12), stimulation of inflammatory signaling, and cellular infiltration in injured renal tubules.[44] Under the right conditions, these factors trigger the ongoing release of inflammatory cytokines, which eventually activates fibrogenic mechanisms and tissue fibrosis.

The role of Ang II during renal hypoperfusion is complex. The generation of Ang II acts to raise perfusion pressure and protect glomerular filtration through efferent arteriolar constriction.[45] Ang II induces hypertrophy and hyperplasia in several cell types, in addition to direct stimulation of local hormone production and ion transport.[46] Experimental infusion of Ang II leads to parenchymal renal injury, with focal and segmental glomerulosclerosis.[47] ACE inhibition and Ang II receptor blockade in several experimental models diminish renal cell proliferation and suppress infiltration of mononuclear cells, which triggers expression of extracellular matrix proteins and progressive nephrosclerosis.[43] Ang II may also participate in vascular smooth muscle cell growth, platelet aggregation, generation of superoxide radicals, activation of adhesion molecules and macrophages, induction of gene transcription for protooncogenes, and oxidation of low-density lipoproteins (LDLs).[48] These observations demonstrate the multiple roles of Ang II in the adaptation and maintenance of kidney function and the modulation of many steps along the cascade toward progressive renal injury.

Experimental studies have suggested an independent effect of hypercholesterolemia in modifying parenchymal renal injury in ischemic nephropathy. Cholesterol feeding is used as a model of early atherosclerosis and itself alters renal

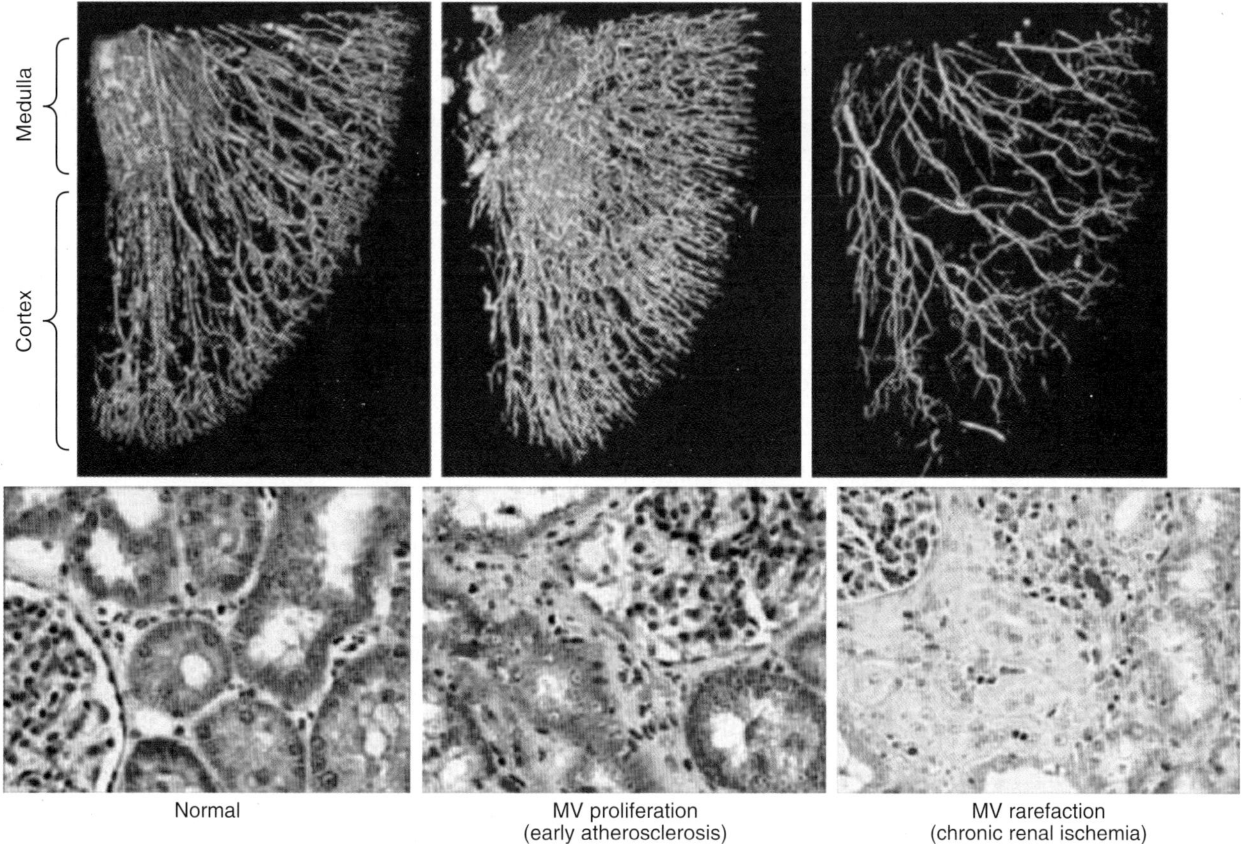


**Fig. 47.12** *Upper panels,* Micro-computed tomography reconstructions of vessels in experimental atherosclerosis and superimposed large-vessel renovascular disease at an early stage *(middle)* and after chronic ischemia *(right),* compared with normal *(left). Lower panels,* Corresponding renal histology (trichrome stain ×400). Complex microvascular dysfunction and rarefaction develop in poststenotic kidneys. These are accelerated and/or modified by angiogenic stimuli, oxidative stress pathways, and a variety of cytokines, leading eventually to interstitial fibrosis. Studies in experimental animals suggest that angiogenic stimuli such as intrarenal infusion of endothelial progenitor cells or mesenchymal stem cells may offer the potential to repair microvascular injury. *MV,* microvascular. (From Lerman LO, Chade AR. Angiogenesis in the kidney: a new therapeutic target? *Curr Opin Nephrol Hyper.* 2009;18:160–165.)

vascular reactivity to acetylcholine and changes renal tubular functional characteristics.[49] Levels of oxidized LDLs rise in this model, associated with markers of oxidative stress and activation of tissue nuclear factor kappa B (NF-κB), transforming growth factor beta (TGF-β), and inducible nitric oxide synthase. The effect of these changes in producing kidney fibrosis is magnified in the presence of RAS. Many of these effects can be reduced experimentally by ET blockade, antioxidants, statins,[50] or mitochondrial protection.[51]

The vascular endothelium is a source of multiple vasoactive factors, the most widely recognized of which are NO and ET. Endothelial NO is synthesized from L-arginine by a family of NO synthases and participates in the regulation of kidney function by counteracting the vasoconstrictor effects of Ang II.[52] In addition to its effects on blood flow and tubular reabsorption of sodium, NO inhibits the growth of vascular smooth muscle cells, mesangial cell hypertrophy and hyperplasia, and synthesis of extracellular matrix.[52]

A reduction in renal perfusion leads to diminished shear stress distal to the stenosis.[53] This condition reduces the production of NO and accelerates the release of renin and generation of AII in the stenotic kidney. Hence, the effects of NO are diminished in the poststenotic kidney, allowing predominance of intrarenal vasoconstrictors, including Ang II and vasoconstrictor prostaglandins, such as thromboxane.[54] The antithrombotic effects and the inhibition of responses to tissue injury of NO are also lost. A direct consequence of reduced perfusion in the poststenotic kidney is progressive rarefaction of small vessels in both the cortex and medulla, eventually producing tubular collapse[55] (see Fig. 47.12).

Glomerulosclerosis is a late event and usually reflects severe loss of the GFR. Experimental studies infusing autologous endothelial progenitor cells and/or vascular endothelial growth factors (VEGF) into the renal artery have demonstrated that functional recovery of GFR and restoration of vascular function can sometimes be achieved, suggesting that angiogenesis may be an achievable goal in this vascular bed.[56,57]

The ET peptides are potent and long-lasting vasoconstrictor peptides produced and released from endothelial cells. ET itself is released from renal epithelial cells after simulation with a variety of substances, such as thrombin and local cytokines, including TGF-β, interleukin-1, and tumor necrosis factor (TNF).[58] Renal ischemia is a potent stimulus for expression of ET-1 in the kidney. Sustained vascular effects of ET may contribute to hypoperfusion that lasts well beyond the vascular insult in postischemic kidneys.

The kidney is a rich site for the production of prostaglandins, which are cyclooxygenase derivatives of arachidonic acid. These mediators are produced in arteries, arterioles, and glomeruli in the cortex, where they have important actions to maintain renal blood flow and filtration, particularly under conditions of elevated levels of Ang II.[59] Enhanced synthesis of prostacyclin (prostaglandin I2 [PGI2]) and prostaglandin E2 (PGE2) occurs during tissue hypoperfusion and ischemia, which may protect against some forms of hypoxic injury.[60] Conversely, thromboxane A2 (TXA2) is a vasoconstrictor prostaglandin that lowers the GFR by reducing renal plasma flow and can accelerate structural renal damage.[61] It is stimulated by the production of Ang II and reactive oxygen species and may in turn modify the hemodynamic properties of Ang II. TXA2 modulates ET in its actions on vascular permeability, which may contribute to interstitial matrix composition and target organ damage. Blockade of TXA2 receptors in some models can reduce the severity of experimental tissue damage, including acute ischemic injury.

The term *oxidative stress* refers to an imbalance between tissue oxygen radical–generating systems and radical scavenging systems toward prooxidant species.[62] This process increases the presence and toxicity of reactive oxygen species, which in turn can promote the formation of vasoactive mediators including ET-1, leukotrienes, and prostaglandin F2 alpha and isoprostanes, which are products of lipid peroxidation. As noted previously, these mediators affect renal function and hemodynamics, both by inducing renal vasoconstriction and by changing glomerular capillary ultrafiltration characteristics.[63] Reactive oxygen species themselves can magnify ischemic renal injury by causing lipid peroxidation of cell and organelle membranes. These disrupt structural integrity and the capacity for cell transport and energy production, particularly in the proximal tubule. Other cytokine pathways, including activation of NF-κB and growth factors, may play a role.[64]

The role of TGF-β merits emphasis. It belongs to a family of polypeptides that regulate normal cell growth, development, and tissue remodeling after injury.[65] TGF-β is an important and ubiquitous fibrogenic factor, which modifies extracellular matrix synthesis by glomerular and extraglomerular mesenchymal cells.[65] These actions modify tissue healing and progression to advanced renal failure. TGF-β is essential for tissue repair after many forms of injury, including ischemic conditions during which it participates in restoring extracellular matrix in proximal tubular basement membranes. Activation of the AT1 receptor stimulates the generation of TGF-β, which plays a major role in tissue fibrosis through increases in type IV collagen deposition. TGF-β acts synergistically with ET and has interactions with platelet-derived growth factor (PDGF), interleukin-1, and basic fibroblast growth factor in progressive interstitial fibrosis.[66] Investigators have proposed that some forms of renal scarring represent an overabundance of TGF-β activity due to failure to suppress its activity after repair of an original injury.[67] Activation of TGF-β develops in experimental models of RAS and is magnified by hypercholesterolemia. Biopsies from patients with atherosclerotic RAS demonstrate diffuse TGF-β staining and macrophage infiltration.[68] Conversely, animals lacking downstream effector pathways for TGF-β (e.g., Smad3 knockout mice) are protected from parenchymal injury in RVD models.[69]

Although whole-kidney oxygen saturation and delivery remain preserved in the poststenotic kidney, it is inescapable that local areas in the kidney are exposed to at least intermittent recurrent ischemia. The potential for repetitive acute renal injury to induce long-term irreversible fibrosis is evident from studies of acute heme protein exposure.[70] The hallmark of acute ischemia is a rapid decline in cellular adenosine triphosphate (ATP), which in turn allows the accumulation of intracellular calcium, activation of phospholipases, and generation of oxygen free radicals.[71]

Tissue ischemia appears to be a common denominator in many forms of progressive tubulointerstitial injury.[72] Such injury is associated commonly with interstitial inflammatory reactions and activation of fibroblasts and heat shock proteins. Disruption of the tubular epithelium alters the antigenic profile of these cells, initiating a cell-mediated immune response, sometimes associated with B lymphocyte, T lymphocytes, and macrophage infiltrates.[73] As noted, sustained tubulointerstitial injury leads to increased TGF-β production, enhanced expression of plasminogen activator inhibitor 1 (PAI-1), tissue inhibitor of metalloprotease-1 (TIMP-1), alpha 1 (IV) collagen, and fibronectin-EIIA and thus to increased synthesis of extracellular matrix.[74]

Many of the mechanisms mentioned interact with each other. Taken together, the kidney is subject to a wide variety of vasoactive and inflammatory mediators, which can be disturbed by loss of blood flow and perfusion pressure. These disturbances appear to activate a variety of fibrogenic and local destructive mechanisms, which can lead to irreversible parenchymal damage in the kidney. For further discussion of vasoactive molecules in the kidney, see Chapter 11.

## CONSEQUENCES OF RESTORING RENAL BLOOD FLOW

As illustrated in Fig. 47.9A, restoring renal perfusion can allow recovery of renal function if accomplished when these changes remain reversible. At some point, both inflammatory and fibrogenic mechanisms no longer to respond appear with recovery of renal function.

### RENAL REPERFUSION INJURY

The course of recovery after restoration of blood flow in an underperfused kidney depends on the extent and duration of the reperfusion injury, in addition to the adequacy of reperfusion.[75] Paradoxically, some tissues subjected to ischemia undergo morphologic and functional changes, which worsen during the reperfusion phase.[76] This is thought to reflect vascular endothelial damage and activation of leukocytes, which may be primed to obstruct distal capillaries after restoration of perfusion pressure contributing to a so-called no-reflow phenomenon. Under experimental conditions, reperfusion injury appears to require major degrees of prooxidant stress with excess PGF2 alpha isoprostanes and free oxygen radicals, particularly with a deficit of NO.[77] Hence, antioxidants and reactive oxygen metabolite scavengers improve outcomes following experimental reperfusion. In the kidney, ischemia-reperfusion injury is most pronounced in the proximal tubules, with local necrosis and tubular obstruction, as observed in acute tubular necrosis (ATN). Studies in experimental RVD in swine have suggested that pretreatment with a mitochondrial transition pore-inhibiting agent allows improved recovery of blood flow, preservation of microvascular integrity, and improved function, consistent with prevention of ischemia and reperfusion injury.[51]

Ang II may participate in some of these changes because the activation of AT1 receptors impairs glomerular filtration in the postischemic kidney.[78] Local imbalance of NO production in the kidney and the dual actions of NO have the potential drawback of accelerating reoxygenation injury and initiating lipid peroxidation.[76] However, systemic treatment with NO donors improves renal function and blunts local inflammation before reperfusion in some conditions.[79]

## EPIDEMIOLOGY OF RENAL ARTERY STENOSIS AND RENOVASCULAR HYPERTENSION

The syndrome of renovascular hypertension can be produced by a wide variety of lesions affecting renal blood flow. In unselected mild to moderate hypertensive populations, the frequency appears to be between 0.6% to 3%, whereas in a referral clinic of treatment-resistant hypertensive patients, the prevalence may exceed 20%.[80] Some specific example lesions producing renal ischemia are listed in Box 47.1. A rapidly developing form of this disorder can be seen after spontaneous or traumatic renal artery dissection or iatrogenic occlusion, sometimes caused by endovascular aortic stent grafts.[9] Most stenotic lesions are fibromuscular diseases or atherosclerotic RAS. The reported prevalence depends heavily on differences between patient groups studied. As noted later, the prevalence of anatomic RAS far exceeds that of renovascular hypertension.

***Clinical Relevance***

Renal artery stenosis is much more common than renovascular hypertension. Not all stenoses are associated with hypertension.

Fibromuscular disease (FMD) commonly refers to one of several noninflammatory conditions affecting the intima or fibrous layers of the vessel wall. In some cases, multiple layers of the vessel wall may be affected. Reports from arteriograms obtained in "normal" renal organ donors have indicated that 3% to 5% of individuals may have one of these lesions, many of which are present at an early age and do not affect renal blood flow or arterial pressure.[81] Such lesions can lead to renovascular hypertension, sometimes associated with dissection or progression. Smoking is a risk factor for disease progression. Medial fibroplasia is the most common subtype, often associated with a string-of-beads appearance, as illustrated in Fig. 47.13A.[82] These lesions consist primarily of intravascular webs, each of which may have only moderate hemodynamic effect. The combination of multiple webs in series, however, can impede blood flow characteristics and activate responses in the kidney to reduce perfusion. FMD appears in the renal arteries in 65% to 70% of cases and in cerebral arteries in 25%.[81] Both renal and cerebral vessels may be abnormal in 10% to 25% of patients. The preponderance of hypertensive cases requiring vascular intervention occur in women, with a bias toward the right renal artery.[83]

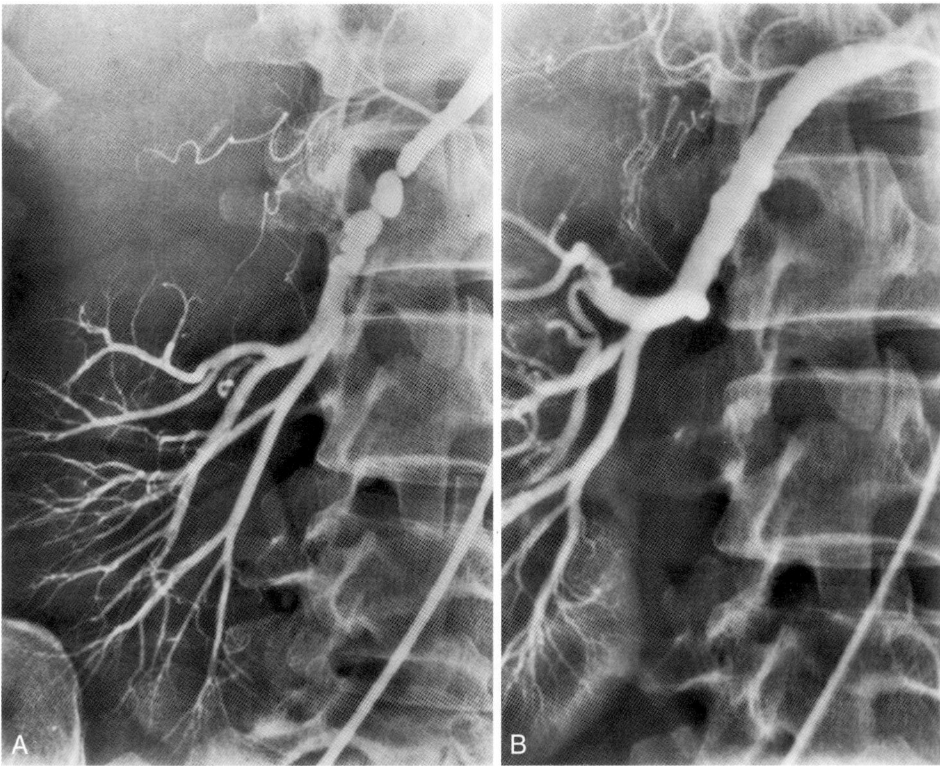


**Fig. 47.13** (A and B) Angiographic appearance of medial fibroplasia with serial intravascular webs and small aneurysmal dilations between them. These lesions appear in the midportion of the vessel, have a predilection for the right renal artery, and are most commonly found in women. As shown in B, these lesions can often be improved substantially by balloon angioplasty.

FMD lesions are typically located away from the origin of the renal artery, often in the midportion of the vessel or at the first arterial bifurcation.[81] Some of these expand to develop small vascular aneurysms. Although less common, other dysplastic lesions, particularly intimal hyperplasia, can progress and lead to renal ischemia and atrophy. Although loss of renal function is unusual with FMD, quantitative imaging of cortical and medullary kidney volumes indicate that parenchymal thinning occurs both in the stenotic and contralateral kidneys beyond FMD.[84] Interventional studies have suggested that among patients referred for renal revascularization for hypertension, FMD accounts for 16% or less.[85]

Atherosclerosis affecting the renal arteries is the most common renovascular lesion in the United States. Atherosclerotic renal artery stenosis (ARAS) can be identified commonly in patients with disease affecting other vascular beds and may be magnified by inflammatory vascular injury.[32] Population-based surveys have identified incidental RAS (>60% occlusion by Doppler criteria) in 6.8% of individuals older than 65 years in the United States.[86] A systematic review of imaging studies for other vascular conditions has confirmed that the prevalence of lesions with more than 50% luminal occlusion rises progressively with the extent of overall atherosclerotic burden.[12] Hence, patients undergoing coronary angiography have identifiable ARAS in 14% to 20% of cases.[11,87,88] Studies of patients with peripheral vascular disease have indicated that 30% to 50% of such patients have renal artery lesions of some degree.[12] Table 47.1 summarizes multiple reports related to the coexistence of atherosclerotic lesions in various vascular territories. The prevalence of ARAS increases with age and with the presence of atherosclerotic risk factors such as elevated cholesterol levels, smoking, and hypertension. The probability of identifying high-grade renal arterial stenosis in hypertensive patients with azotemia rises from 3.2% in the sixth decade to above 25% in the eighth decade.[89] Additional population-based studies in the United States have confirmed that more than 70% of older patients with RAS above 60% occlusion have clinical manifestations of cardiovascular disease.[90] The prevalence of ARAS may be rising as a result of more people surviving to older ages. These figures confirm previous postmortem observations indicating that many patients dying of cardiovascular disease have renal artery lesions at autopsy. They underscore the fact that some renal artery lesions remain undetected on clinical grounds for many years (see later).

The location of atherosclerotic disease is usually near the origin of the artery (Fig. 47.14A), although it can be observed anywhere. Many such lesions represent a direct extension of an

**Table 47.1 Prevalence Rates of Atherosclerotic Renal Artery Stenosis[a]**

| Vascular Disease | Prevalence Rate (%) |
|---|---|
| Suspected renovascular hypertension | 14.1 |
| Coronary angiography | 10.5 |
| With hypertension | 17.8 |
| Peripheral vascular disease | 25.3 |
| AAA | 33.1 |
| ESKD | 40.8 (?)[b] |
| Congestive heart failure | 54.1 (?)[b] |

[a]40 studies, 15,879 patients. Shown are prevalence rates of patients with vascular disease affecting other regional beds identified by angiography.

[b](?) marks refer to limited data suggesting high prevalence in unexplained advanced chronic kidney disease (CKD) in older subjects and patients with congestive heart failure.

*AAA,* Abdominal aortic aneurysm; *ESKD,* end-stage kidney disease.

Modified from de Mast Q, Beutler JJ. The prevalence of atherosclerotic renal artery stenosis in risk groups: a systematic literature review. *J. Hypertens.* 2009;27: 1333–1240.

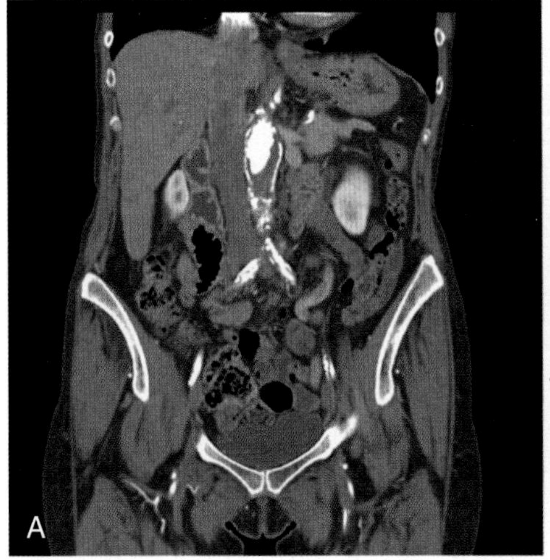


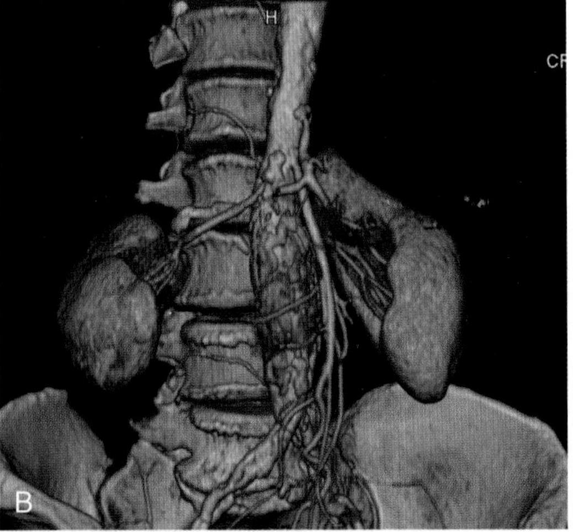


**Fig. 47.14** (A and B) Atherosclerotic disease commonly affects the renal arteries and abdominal aorta. Shown is a computed tomography angiogram with high-grade stenosis to a small right kidney arising from diffuse aortic disease. (A) The coronal section demonstrates extensive thrombotic debris along the calcified aortic wall. (B) A reconstructed view of the aorta demonstrates diffuse calcification and early aortic aneurysm formation. The mean age of series presenting for renal revascularization for atherosclerotic disease has risen to more than 70 years. The decision about endovascular or surgical intervention in such cases must balance the hazards of aortic manipulation against the potential benefits regarding blood pressure control and/or renal function.

aortic plaque into the renal arterial segment. ARAS is strongly associated with preexisting hypertension, cardiovascular lipid risk, diabetes, smoking, and abnormal renal function.[11,87]

## CLINICAL FEATURES

### RENOVASCULAR HYPERTENSION: FIBROMUSCULAR DISEASE VERSUS ATHEROSCLEROSIS

As noted earlier, renovascular hypertension may develop as a result of many lesions (see Box 47.1). The two most common are FMD and atherosclerosis. FMD represents several types of noninflammatory intimal or medial disorders of the vessel wall, commonly affecting midportions of the renal artery detected in individuals between 15 and 55 years of age.[82] These lesions rarely lead to major renal functional loss, although some progression may be seen, particularly in smokers. FMD lesions most often appear clinically as hypertension of early onset (in those between 30 and 50 years of age) and unusual severity. Occasionally, it presents as hypertension during pregnancy. Many lesions respond well to percutaneous angioplasty (see Fig. 47.13B).[91]

By contrast, atherosclerotic lesions usually arise near the origin of the renal artery and amplify the risks of systemic atherosclerosis elsewhere. ARAS is commonly associated with a reduced glomerular filtration rates.[92] Clinical manifestations fall across a wide spectrum (see Fig. 47.1) and are not related simply to the anatomic severity of the lesion.[93] Ambulatory blood pressure recordings indicate exaggerated systolic pressure variability and frequent loss of the circadian pressure rhythm,[94] commonly associated with left ventricular hypertrophy.[95] Sympathetic nerve traffic recordings indicate heightened adrenergic outflow.[96] A population-based study of 870 subjects older than 65 years has indicated that those with RAS had a two- to threefold increased risk for adverse cardiovascular events during the subsequent 2 years.[90] These data are supported by a review of Medicare claims data between 1999 and 2001 for a random sample of Medicare recipients older than 67 years.[97] The authors indicated that the incidence of newly identified atherosclerotic RVD was 3.7/1000 patient-years and was associated with preexisting peripheral and coronary disease. After detection, subsequent development of claims for heart disease, transient ischemic attack, renal replacement therapy, and CHF are 3- to 20-fold higher in such patients as compared with contemporaries without RVD.[97] Adverse cardiovascular events developed more than tenfold more commonly than the need for renal replacement therapy. As a result, a persistent controversy in cardiovascular disease has been how to manage clinically significant RAS as a modifying factor for cardiovascular outcomes. The major US trial of renal revascularization (CORAL) specifically targeted overall combined cardiovascular outcomes in treating this disorder (see later).[98] This controversy is compounded by changes produced by evolving medical therapy and changing population characteristics.

### RENAL ARTERY STENOSIS

Manifestations of renal artery disease vary widely across a spectrum, as illustrated in Fig. 47.1, Box 47.2, and Table 47.2.

**Box 47.2 Syndromes Associated With Renovascular Hypertension[a]**

1. Early- or late-onset hypertension (<30 years or >50 years)
2. Acceleration of treated essential hypertension
3. Deterioration of renal function in treated essential hypertension
4. Acute renal failure during treatment of hypertension
5. Flash pulmonary edema
6. Progressive renal failure
7. Refractory congestive cardiac failure

[a]These "syndromes" should alert the clinician to the possible contribution of renovascular disease in a given patient. Syndromes 5 to 7 are most common in patients with bilateral disease, many of whom are treated as "essential hypertension" until these characteristics appear.

**Table 47.2 Clinical Features of Patients With Renovascular Hypertension[a]**

| Clinical Feature | Essential HTN (%) | Renovascular HTN (%) |
|---|---|---|
| Duration <1 year | 12 | 24 |
| Age of onset >50 years | 9 | 15 |
| Family history of HTN | 71 | 46 |
| Grade 3 or 4 fundi | 7 | 15 |
| Abdominal bruit | 9 | 46 |
| Blood urea nitrogen > 20 mg/dL | 8 | 16 |
| Potassium <3.4 mEq/L | 8 | 16 |
| Urinary casts | 9 | 20 |
| Proteinuria | 32 | 46 |

[a]Clinical features that differed ($P < .05$) between closely matched groups of 131 patients with essential versus renovascular hypertension taken from the Cooperative Study of Renovascular Hypertension in the 1960s. (From Simon N, Franklin SS, Bleifer KH, Maxwell MH. Clinical characteristics of renovascular hypertension. *JAMA.* 1972;220:1209–1218.) These observations underscore the potential severity of hypertension in candidates for surgery, but none of these features allows clinical discrimination with confidence.
*HTN,* Hypertension.

This spectrum ranges from an incidental finding noted during imaging for other indications to advancing renal failure leading to the need for dialysis support. As lesions progress to more severe levels of occlusion, hypertension develops, and multiple manifestations may appear. As described previously, a number of mechanisms raise systemic arterial pressure and tend to restore renal perfusion pressures to levels close to baseline. Clinical features of patients with essential hypertension have been compared with those in patients subjected to revascularization for renovascular hypertension in the Cooperative Study in the 1960s are summarized in Table 47.2.[99] Many features, including short duration of hypertension, early age of onset, funduscopic findings, and hypokalemia, were more common in those with renovascular hypertension, but they have limited discriminating or predictive value.[99]

As renal artery lesions progress to critical stenosis, they can produce a rapidly developing form of hypertension, which may be severe and associated with polydipsia, hyponatremia, and central nervous system findings.[100] Such cases are usually seen with acute renovascular events, such as the sudden occlusion of a renal artery or branch vessel.

More commonly, RAS presents as a progressive worsening of preexisting hypertension, often with a modest rise in serum creatinine level. Because the prevalence of hypertension and atherosclerosis increases with age, this disorder must be considered particularly in older subjects with progressive hypertension. Some of the most striking examples of renovascular hypertension are older individuals whose previously well-controlled hypertension has deteriorated, with an accelerated rise in systolic blood pressure and target injury, such as stroke. Studies from hypertension referral centers in the Netherlands are typical in this regard. Of 477 patients undergoing detailed evaluation for RAS because of treatment resistance, 107 (22.4%) were identified with RVD (>50% stenosis by angiography).[85] Clinical features predictive of RAS included older age, recent progression, other vascular disease (e.g., claudication), an abdominal bruit, and elevated serum creatinine levels. The authors derived a multivariate regression equation of predictive features for the presence of angiographic RAS. They presented a clinical scoring system to determine the pretest probability of identifying renal artery disease (Fig. 47.15).[85] The strongest predictors include age and serum creatinine level. Clinical features alone could provide pretest predictive value nearly as accurate as radionuclide scans.[85]

Declining renal function during antihypertensive therapy is a common manifestation of progressive renal arterial disease. Not surprisingly, blood flow and perfusion pressures to the kidney fall distally to a critical RAS. This can be worsened by reduction in systemic arterial pressure by any antihypertensive regimen. A reduced GFR during antihypertensive therapy has become particularly common since the introduction of ACE inhibitors and angiotensin receptor blockers (ARBs). A precipitous rise in serum creatinine levels soon after starting these agents may occur due to a loss of transcapillary filtration pressure produced by removing the efferent arteriolar vasoconstriction from Ang II. This particular "functional" loss of GFR is reversible if detected promptly and should lead the clinician to consider large-vessel RVD when it occurs.[101,102] Clinically important changes in serum creatinine levels become apparent mainly when the entire renal mass is affected, such as with bilateral RAS or stenosis to a solitary functioning kidney. Most such patients tolerate the reintroduction of renin-angiotensin blockade when challenged after successful revascularization.[103]

Other syndromes heralding occult RAS have become more commonly recognized. Among the most important are rapidly developing episodes of circulatory congestion (so-called "flash" pulmonary edema).[104] These usually arise in patients with hypertension and with left ventricular systolic function, which may be well preserved. Underlying arterial compromise may favor volume retention and resistance to diuretics in such cases. A sudden rise in arterial pressure impairs cardiac

| Predictor | Score | |
|---|---|---|
| | Persons who never smoked | Former or current smokers |
| Age (yr) | | |
| 20 | 0 | 3 |
| 30 | 1 | 4 |
| 40 | 2 | 4 |
| 50 | 3 | 5 |
| 60 | 4 | 5 |
| 70 | 5 | 6 |
| Female | 2 | 2 |
| Signs and symptoms of atherosclerosis | 1 | 1 |
| Onset of HTN within 2 yr | 1 | 1 |
| BMI <25 kg/m$^2$ | 2 | 2 |
| Abdominal bruit | 3 | 3 |
| Serum creatinine concentration ($\mu$mol/L) | | |
| 40 | 0 | 0 |
| 60 | 1 | 1 |
| 80 | 2 | 2 |
| 100 | 3 | 3 |
| 150 | 6 | 6 |
| 200 | 9 | 9 |
| Serum cholesterol level >6.5 mmol/L or cholesterol-lowering therapy | 1 | 1 |

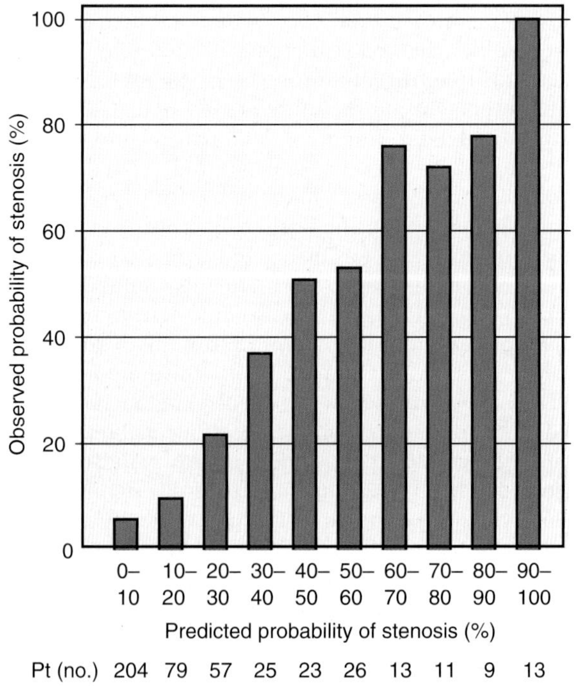

Observed probability of stenosis (%)
100
80
60
40
20
0
0–10 10–20 20–30 30–40 40–50 50–60 60–70 70–80 80–90 90–100
Predicted probability of stenosis (%)
Pt (no.) 204 79 57 25 23 26 13 11 9 13

**Fig. 47.15** Probability of identifying renal artery stenosis based on clinical features. These data were derived from 477 patients in referral centers for treatment-resistant hypertension *(HTN)* in the Netherlands. Overall prevalence was 22.4%, illustrating that even in "enriched" patient populations, renovascular disease is not present in the majority. Clinical features allowed selection of patients for testing with a relatively high pretest probability of disease, which affects the validity of testing schemes. (From Krijnen P, van Jaarsveld BC, Steyerberg EW, et al. A clinical prediction rule for renal artery stenosis. *Ann Intern Med.* 1998;129:705–711.)

function due to rapidly developing diastolic dysfunction. These episodes tend to be rapid both in onset and in resolution. Patients with treatment-resistant CHF, often with reduced arterial pressures, may also harbor unsuspected RVD. Restoration of renal blood flow in such patients can improve volume control and sensitivity to diuretics, with a lower risk of azotemia during therapy.[105] A similar sequence of events may produce symptoms of "crescendo angina" from otherwise stable coronary disease.[106] Registry data have indicated that patients with episodic pulmonary edema with RAS have substantially increased hospitalization and mortality rates, which can be reduced with successful revascularization.[107,108]

Another clinical presentation of RAS is advanced renal failure, occasionally at end stage, requiring renal replacement therapy. This manifestation has been controversial partly because it raises the possibility of an undetected, potentially reversible form of chronic kidney disease. As discussed earlier, this is designated by some as ischemic nephropathy or azotemic RVD[109] and is defined as a loss of renal function distal to an arterial stenosis due to impaired renal blood flow. Studies in patients with bilateral RAS have indicated that reduction of systemic pressures to normal levels using sodium nitroprusside can abruptly reduce renal plasma flow and the GFR, indicating that poststenotic pressures are at critical levels beyond autoregulation (see Fig. 47.9).[110] Some estimates have suggested that as many as 12% to 14% of patients reaching end-stage kidney disease (ESKD), with no other identifiable primary renal disease, may have occult, bilateral RAS.[111,112] A survey using spiral CT angiography has examined 49 of 80 patients starting dialysis therapy identified as having ARAS (estimated as >50% lumen occlusion); in 20 of them (41%) and in 8 (16%) it was bilateral. Assuming that these lesions somehow were the primary cause of ESKD, the authors have proposed that up to 27% of new ESKD patients may have lost kidney function on this basis.[113] A more conservative review of US Renal Data System (USRDS) data for patients older than 67 years in the United States starting dialysis has suggested that identified RVD may be present in between 7.1% and 11.1% of patients, although clinicians caring for such patients attributed their renal failure to RAS in only 5.0%.[114] Multivariate analysis has indicated that male gender and advancing age correlated positively with this disorder, whereas a African-American, Asian, or Native American background correlated negatively.[111] Importantly, patients with rapidly progressive dysfunction and accelerated hypertension have the potential to recover kidney function and a mortality benefit from revascularization.[2,108,115] However, such individuals have rarely been included in prospective, randomized trials (see later).

The causal role of vascular impairment in producing renal dysfunction is established most firmly when renal revascularization leads to recovery of renal function. Unfortunately, this does not occur commonly.[1,4] Studies over the last decade have produced several paradigm shifts related to hemodynamically induced renal dysfunction. As noted, the overall high perfusion of the kidneys protects against significant tissue hypoxia to some extent.[36] Hence, many subjects can be treated with antihypertensive drug therapy without evident further loss of GFR, sometimes for many years as demonstrated by prospective randomized controlled trials (RCTs) such as ASTRAL and CORAL.[116] A subset of patients with more severe or long-standing vascular occlusion (usually defined as a peak systolic velocity >385 cm/s on duplex ultrasound) manifests overt cortical hypoxia using BOLD MRI.[117] Such patients demonstrate more advanced tissue histologic injury with loss of tubular structures on biopsy and interstitial cellular infiltrates, consistent with inflammatory injury[44,117] (see Figs. 47.10B and 47.11). These observations support the gradual transition from a primarily hemodynamic reduction in kidney function (potentially improved by restoring blood flow) to inflammatory-mediated injury that no longer recovers predictably after the restoration of vessel patency. Patients with advanced renal dysfunction have high comorbidity associated with cardiovascular disease and commonly have interstitial renal injury on biopsy.[118,119] Prospective treatment trials specifically directed at slowing the loss of kidney function by renal revascularization have failed to identify much benefit in the intermediate term.[98,120,121] Those with declining renal function have a poor survival rate regardless of intervention, the strongest predictor of which is a low baseline GFR.[122]

The potential benefit of revascularization regarding salvage, or at least stabilization, of renal function is greatest when the serum creatinine level is less than 3 mg/dL, so the diagnosis of ischemic nephropathy is best considered early in its course.[122] Remarkably, RAS can be associated with proteinuria, occasionally to nephrotic levels.[123–125] Proteinuria can diminish or resolve entirely following renal revascularization,[126] suggesting that intrarenal hemodynamic changes and/or stimulation of local hormonal or cytokine activity alter glomerular membrane permeability in a reversible fashion. Although other glomerular diseases can develop in patients with renal artery disease, including diabetic nephropathy and focal sclerosing glomerulonephritis (FSGS), the presence of proteinuria alone does not establish a second disorder.

Clinical manifestations and prognosis differ when RVD affects one of two kidneys or affects the entire functioning renal mass. Although poststenotic kidneys may lose GFR and tissue volume, the contralateral kidney without stenosis undergoes compensatory hypertrophy. These changes mask the damage to the affected kidney, making the overall GFR an unreliable marker of the severity and progression of atherosclerotic RAS.[127,128] Although blood pressure levels may be similar, the fall in blood pressure after renal revascularization is greater in bilateral disease.[129] Most patients with episodic pulmonary edema have bilateral disease or a solitary kidney. Long-term mortality during follow-up is higher when bilateral disease is present, regardless of whether renal revascularization is undertaken.[93,130,131] These data have suggested that the extent and severity of RVD reflect the overall atherosclerotic burden of the individual. Patients with incidental RAS (>70%) managed without revascularization have reduced survival with bilateral disease, despite reasonable blood pressure control, as illustrated in Fig. 47.16.[9] The causes of death are mainly related to cardiovascular disease, including stroke and CHF.

## PROGRESSIVE VASCULAR OCCLUSION

Atherosclerosis is a progressive disorder, although individual rates of progression vary widely. The clinical manifestations from RAS depend partly on the severity and extent of vascular occlusion. The most ominous of these manifestations, such as renal failure or pulmonary edema, are related to bilateral disease or stenosis to a solitary functioning kidney and pose

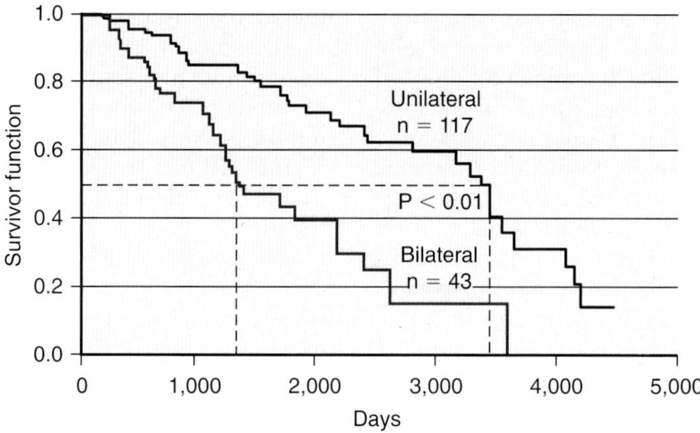


**Fig. 47.16** Kaplan-Meier survival curve of 160 patients with more than 70% renal artery stenosis managed without revascularization. Those with bilateral disease had lower survival, primarily due to associated cardiovascular disease. The mean age of death was 79 years. These data underscore the close relationship between the extent of vascular disease and mortality. Less than 10% of these subjects developed advanced kidney disease during follow-up, although long-term survival, even in treated patients, is related to levels of kidney function at the time of intervention. Recent prospective randomized clinical trials indicate that between 16% and 22% of medically treated patients with atherosclerotic renal artery stenosis progress more advanced renal dysfunction over 3 to 5 years. (From Foster JH, Maxwell MH, Franklin SS, et al. Renovascular occlusive disease: results of operative treatment. *JAMA.* 975;2231:1043–1198; Textor SC. Renovascular hypertension and ischemic nephropathy. In: Skorecki K, Chertow GM, Marsden PA, et al, eds. *Brenner and Rector's: The kidney.* 10th ed. Philadelphia: Elsevier; 2016:1567–1609.)

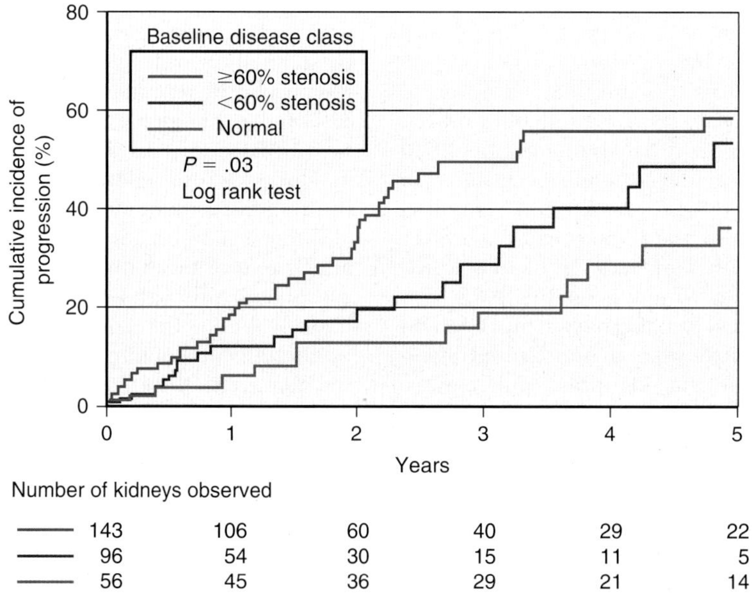


**Fig. 47.17** Cumulative rates of anatomic disease progression in atherosclerotic renal artery stenosis, as measured by renal artery Doppler ultrasound. During a follow-up period of 5 years, overall progression was 31%, but those with the most severe baseline lesion progressed in 60% of cases. The progression of vascular disease was not closely related to changes in serum creatinine levels or renal atrophy. (Modified from Caps MT, Perissinotto C, Zierler RE, et al. Prospective study of atherosclerotic disease progression in the renal artery. *Circulation.* 1998;98:2866–2872.)

the greatest hazard when total arterial occlusion develops. Hence, the impetus to intervene in RAS depends heavily on predicting or establishing the natural history of vascular stenosis in an individual. Retrospective studies of serial angiograms obtained in the 1970s and early 1980s have indicated that atherosclerotic lesions progress to more severe levels in 44% to 63% of patients followed from 2 to 5 years.[132] Up to 16% of renal arteries developed total occlusion. Subsequent prospective studies in patients undergoing cardiac catheterization or serial Doppler ultrasound measurements have suggested that current rates of progression may be lower.[133] Zierler and colleagues have reported a 20% rate of disease progression overall, with 7% advancing to total occlusion over 3 years.[133] A later report from the same group using different Doppler velocity criteria has suggested higher rates of progressive stenosis.[134] Overall progression was detectable in 31%, but primarily those with the most severe baseline stenosis (>60%) and severe hypertension were more likely to progress (51%; Fig. 47.17). The occurrence of total occlusion was uncommon (9 of 295 [3%]). Data from medical treatment trials have suggested that progressive occlusion can develop silently in up to 16% of treated subjects.[135] These observations are supported by the development of renal endpoints (defined as progressive renal deterioration) ranging from 16% to 22% in recent prospective RCTs (ASTRAL and CORAL).[1]

Importantly, clinical events such as detectable changes in renal function or accelerating hypertension bear only a limited relationship to anatomic vascular progression. The occurrence of renal "atrophy" (loss in renal size by 1 cm or more by ultrasound) developed in 20.8% of the most severe lesions in the prospective series.[106] Most series of medically treated patients have indicated that despite evident progression of vascular disease, changes in kidney function are modest and uncommon.[136] Results reported during medical follow-up of 41 patients managed medically before the introduction of ACE inhibitors for an average of 36 months have identified a loss of renal length in 35%, whereas a significant rise in serum creatinine levels developed in 8 of 41 (19.5%).[136] Blood pressure control improved during the intervals followed in the 1980s, associated with the introduction of ACE inhibitors and angiotensin-blocking agents. Medical management was associated with increased requirements for antihypertensive agents. The percentage developing clinical progression with refractory hypertension or progressive renal insufficiency fell from 21% in the earliest period to less than 10% in the later cohort after the introduction of ACE inhibitors.[130] This conclusion is consistent with long-term studies from Europe, in which incidental renal artery lesions were rarely associated with progressive renal failure over more than 9 years of follow-up.[137] These data support the observation that renal artery lesions remain stable in some patients over many years, without adverse clinical effects or evident progression[138] as observed in treatment trials, including ASTRAL and CORAL.[139] It is likely that overall rates of atherosclerotic disease progression have been falling due to the more widespread use of statins, aspirin, diminishing tobacco use, and more intense antihypertensive therapy. Hence, worsening vascular occlusion is an important clinical risk but does not occur in all patients.

## DEVELOPMENTS IN MEDICAL AND ANTIHYPERTENSIVE DRUG THERAPY

Before the 1980s, the literature of RVD was concerned primarily with the identification of functionally important lesions in patients with severe hypertension. Drug therapy was limited in scope and often produced intolerable side effects. Most importantly, the available drugs did not yet include agents capable of interrupting the renin-angiotensin system (see Fig. 47.2). As a result, patients commonly appeared with accelerated or malignant hypertension, a large fraction of which was related to RAS. Among 123 patients whose average age was 44 years presenting with accelerated hypertension, more than 30% of whites were identified as having renovascular hypertension.[140] Some patients could not be effectively controlled with available medications and were subjected to urgent bilateral nephrectomy as a lifesaving measure. Evaluation for RAS has centered on identifying patients whose blood pressures could be improved, perhaps cured, by renal revascularization. Since the 1980s, antihypertensive agents have expanded to include calcium channel blockers and, most importantly, drugs that functionally block the renin-angiotensin system, such as ACE inhibitors, ARBs, and direct renin inhibitors (i.e., aliskiren). The impact of these agents has been significant.

Reviews of medical therapy for renovascular hypertension older than indicated that regimens using these agents increase the likelihood of achieving good blood pressure control from 46% to more than 90%.[92] The concept of emergency bilateral nephrectomy for control of hypertension has effectively disappeared. It is likely that many patients with RVD and hypertension now go undetected because blood pressure and renal function are well controlled and stable.[88] Importantly, systematic efforts to reach goal blood pressure levels, optimize statin and aspirin use, and withdraw tobacco exposure have been part of treatment trials, including CORAL.[98] Reduction of cardiovascular risk may be even more effective with the expanded use of ACE inhibitors for CHF, proteinuric renal disease, and other constellations of cardiovascular risk factors, particularly since the publication of the HOPE trial[141] and others. Whether the use of ACE inhibitors and/or ARBs actually delays the onset of renovascular hypertension in humans, as it does in experimental animals, cannot be established with the present data.

## CHANGING POPULATION DEMOGRAPHICS

The last several decades have been characterized by longer lifespans in many western countries. These likely result from several factors, including major declines in mortality related to stroke and cardiovascular disease. Population groups older than 65 years are now among the most rapidly growing segments in the United States.[90] One consequence of lower mortality from coronary and cerebrovascular events has been the emergence of vascular disease affecting other areas, such as the aorta and kidneys. As a result, clinical manifestations of RAS are appearing in older individuals, often combined with other comorbid conditions.[89,142]

These features change the clinical presentation and affect the risk-benefit considerations inherent in undertaking renal revascularization. Series with renal artery intervention now routinely include average age values between 68 and 75 years, whereas 2 decades ago the mean age was between 61 and 63 years.[143,144] These mean values are more than 15 years higher than those from the 1960s and 1970s. As might be expected, the prevalence of advanced coronary disease, CHF, previous stroke or transient ischemic attack (TIA), and aortic disease, as well as impaired renal function, has been rising in patients with atherosclerotic renal artery disease.[90]

## ROLE OF CONCURRENT DISEASES

Atherosclerotic RAS rarely occurs in isolation. It is a manifestation of atherosclerotic disease, which often affects multiple other sites. Follow-up studies related to the survival of incidentally identified renal artery disease have suggested that the presence of RAS independently predicts mortality, particularly in the presence of elevated serum creatinine levels,[145] although the mortality risk of a patient with a serum creatinine level above 1.4 mg/dL (but <2.3 mg/dL), for any reason, is higher than that of those with normal serum creatinine levels.[141] The major causes of death are cardiovascular events, including CHF, stroke, and myocardial infarction.[97] It is essential to consider these competing risks in planning the management of patients with all forms of vascular disease, especially older adults.[146]

> *Clinical Relevance*
> **Competing Risks**
> Competing risks of death from cardiovascular disease must be considered when weighing the risks and benefits of revascularization.

These disorders often dominate the clinical outcomes of patients with renal arterial disease, independently of the level of renal function. It has been difficult to establish improved survival in prospective trials of patients treated with medical therapy or renal revascularization.

Although many patients experience better blood pressure control, and some recover renal function, current methods of revascularization are not free of risks.[147] Even after successful renovascular procedures, other comorbid events may obscure any long-term benefit, challenging the cost-effectiveness of renal revascularization. Reviews of Medicare claims in the United States for 2 years after identification of atherosclerotic RAS have indicated that the risk of cardiovascular events, many of which are fatal, are more than tenfold more likely than progression to advanced renal failure.[97] Conversely, others have argued that RAS accelerates these cardiovascular risks by increasing arterial pressures and activating adverse neurohumoral pathways, predisposing both to CHF and renal dysfunction.[148] These divergent views have formed the basis for several prospective RCTs related to renal revascularization over the past decade (see later) that partly address these issues.

**Box 47.3 Renovascular Disease and Ischemic Nephropathy**

**Goals of Diagnostic Evaluation**

Establish presence of renal artery stenosis, location and type of lesion.
Establish whether unilateral or bilateral stenosis (or stenosis to a solitary kidney) is present.
Establish presence and function of stenotic and nonstenotic kidneys.
Establish hemodynamic severity of renal arterial disease.
Evaluate progression of vascular occlusion, renal atrophy.
Plan vascular intervention—degree and location of atherosclerotic disease.

**Goals of Therapy**

1. Improved blood pressure control
   - Prevent morbidity and mortality of high blood pressure.
   - Improve blood pressure control and reduce medication requirements.
2. Preservation of renal function
   - Reduce risk of renal adverse perfusion from use of antihypertensive agents.
   - Reduce episodes of circulatory congestion (flash pulmonary edema).
   - Reduce risk of progressive vascular occlusion causing loss of renal function—preservation of renal function.
   - Salvage renal function—that is, recover glomerular filtration rate.
3. Recovery of volume regulation and fluid excretion
   - Reduce circulatory overload and diuretic resistance.
   - Reduce episodes of flash pulmonary edema.

# DIAGNOSTIC TESTING FOR RENOVASCULAR HYPERTENSION AND ISCHEMIC NEPHROPATHY

## GOALS OF EVALUATION

The literature related to the diagnosis and evaluation of renovascular hypertension is complex and inconsistent (Box 47.3). Some of the confusion likely reflects the widely different patient groups being considered for evaluation and divergent goals for intervention. The clinician must identify the objectives of initiating expensive and sometimes ambiguous investigations beforehand. As with all tests, the reliability and value of diagnostic studies depend heavily on the pretest probability of disease[149] (Table 47.3) Furthermore, it is essential to consider from the outset exactly what is to be achieved:

- Is the major goal to exclude high-grade renal artery disease?
- Is it to exclude bilateral (as opposed to unilateral) disease?
- Is it to identify stenosis and estimate the potential for clinical benefit from renal revascularization?
- Is it to evaluate the role of RVD in explaining deteriorating renal function?

The specific approach to diagnosis will differ, depending on which of these is the predominant clinical objective.

## DIAGNOSTIC TESTS

Noninvasive diagnostic tests for renovascular hypertension and ischemic nephropathy remain imperfect. For the purposes of this discussion, diagnostic tests fall into general categories as follows (Table 47.3): (1) perfusion and imaging studies to identify the presence and degree of vascular stenosis; (2) physiologic and functional studies to evaluate the role of stenotic lesions particularly related to activation of the renin-angiotensin system; and (3) studies to predict the likelihood of benefit from invasive maneuvers, including renal revascularization.

### IMAGING OF THE RENAL VASCULATURE

The diagnosis of RVD fundamentally requires identification of vascular abnormalities. Therefore imaging of the renal vasculature is essential for these disorders. Advances in Doppler ultrasound, radionuclide imaging, magnetic resonance arteriography (MRA), and computed tomography angiography (CTA) continue to introduce major changes in the field of renovascular imaging. The details of these methods are discussed further in Chapter 25. The following is a discussion of some of the specific merits and limitations of each modality as they apply to renovascular hypertension and ischemic nephropathy.[149]

Current practice favors limiting invasive arteriography to carrying out endovascular intervention (e.g., stenting and/or angioplasty). Although angiography remains the gold standard for evaluation of the renal vasculature, its invasive

**Table 47.3 Noninvasive Assessment of Renal Artery Stenosis**

| Study | Rationale | Strengths | Limitations |
|---|---|---|---|
| **Vascular Studies to Evaluate the Renal Arteries** | | | |
| Duplex ultrasonography | Shows the renal arteries and measures flow velocity as a means of assessing the severity of stenosis | Inexpensive, widely available; suitable for sequential measurement to follow disease progression and/or restenosis | Heavily dependent on operator's experience; less useful than invasive angiography for diagnosis of fibromuscular dysplasia and abnormalities in accessory renal arteries |
| Magnetic resonance angiography | Shows the renal arteries and perirenal aorta | Not nephrotoxic, but concerns for gadolinium toxicity exclude use in GFR <30 mL/min/1.73 $m^2$; provides excellent images | Expensive; gadolinium excluded in renal failure, unable to visualize stented vessels |
| Computed tomography angiography | Shows the renal arteries and perirenal aorta | Provides excellent images; stents do not cause artifacts | Expensive, moderate volume of contrast required, potentially nephrotoxic |
| **Perfusion Studies to Assess Differential Renal Blood Flow** | | | |
| Captopril renography with technetium $^{99m}$Tc-mertiatide ($^{99m}$Tc-MAG3) | Captopril-mediated fall in filtration pressure amplifies differences in renal perfusion | Normal study excludes renovascular hypertension | Multiple limitations in patients with advanced atherosclerosis or creatinine >2.0 mg/dL (177 µmol/L) |
| Nuclear imaging with technetium mertiatide or technetium-labeled pentetic acid (DTPA) to estimate fractional flow to each kidney | Estimates fractional flow to each kidney | Allows calculation of single-kidney GFR | Results may be influenced by other conditions (e.g., obstructive uropathy) |
| **Physiologic Studies to Assess the Renin-Angiotensin System** | | | |
| Measurement of peripheral plasma renin activity | Reflects the level of sodium excretion | Measures the level of activation of the renin-angiotensin system | Low predictive accuracy for renovascular hypertension; results influenced by medications and many other conditions |
| Measurement of captopril-stimulated renin activity | Produces a fall in pressure distal to the stenosis | Enhances the release of renin from the stenotic kidney | Low predictive accuracy for renovascular hypertension; results influenced by many other conditions |
| Measurement of renal vein renin activity | Compares renin release from the two kidneys | Lateralization predictive of improvement in blood pressure with revascularization | Nonlateralization has limited predictive power of the failure of blood pressure to improve after revascularization; resultsinfluenced by medications and many other conditions |

*DTPA,* Diethylenetriamine pentaacetic acid; *GFR,* glomerular filtration rate; *MAG3,* $^{99m}$Tc-mercaptoacetyltriglycine.
Modified from Safian RD, Textor SC. Medical progress: renal artery stenosis. *N Engl J Med.* 2001;344:431–442.

nature, potential hazards, and cost make it most suitable for those in whom intervention is planned, often during the same procedure. As a result, most clinicians favor preliminary noninvasive studies. When noninvasive studies are equivocal, arterial angiography may be warranted to establish the presence of transstenotic pressure gradients, as recommended in treatment trials.[150,151]

## Noninvasive Imaging

**Doppler Ultrasound of the Renal Arteries.** Duplex interrogation of the renal arteries provides measurements of localized velocities of blood flow and characteristics of renal tissue. In many institutions, this provides an inexpensive means for measuring vascular occlusive disease at sequential time points, both to establish the diagnosis of RAS and monitor its progression. After renal revascularization, Doppler studies are commonly used to monitor restenosis and target vessel patency[152,153] (Fig. 47.18). The main drawbacks relate to the difficulties of performing adequate studies in obese patients, operator dependency, and time required. These factors vary considerably among institutions.

The primary criteria for renal artery studies are a peak systolic velocity above 180 cm/sec and/or a relative velocity above 3.5, as compared with the adjacent aortic flow.[154,155] Using these criteria, sensitivity and specificity with angiographic estimates of lesions exceeding 60% can surpass 90% and 96%, respectively,[154] although not universally.[156] Increasing the threshold for peak systolic velocities reduces the rate of false-positive estimates of stenosis. When main vessel velocities cannot be determined reliably, segmental waveforms in the

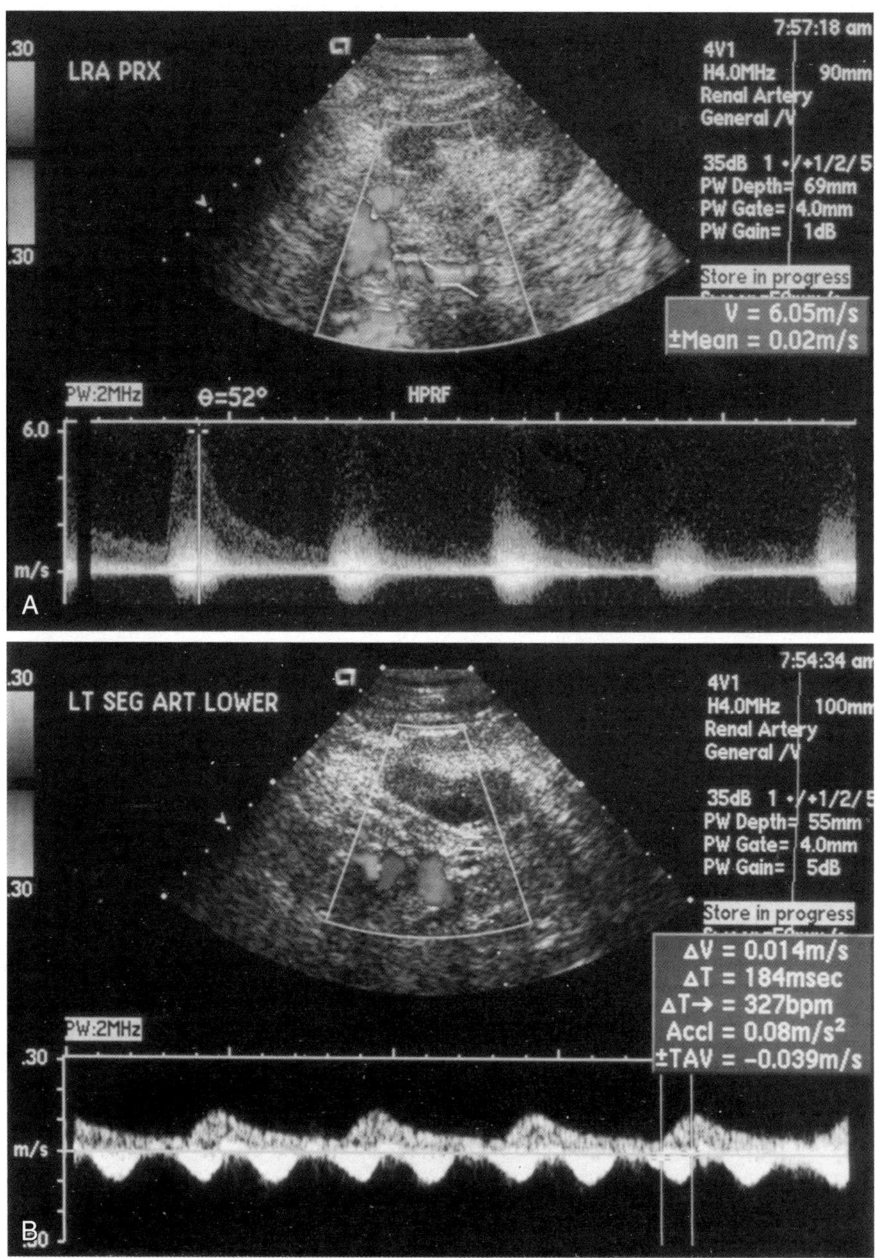


**Fig. 47.18** (A) Duplex ultrasound velocity measurement in a patient with high-grade renal artery stenosis affecting the proximal left renal artery *(LRA PRX)*. Peak systolic velocities reach 605 cm/s (6.05 m/s), well above the normal upper limit of 180 cm/s. (B) Segmental arterial branch ultrasound in the distal segmental renal arteries demonstrates "parvus" and "tardus" dampening of the signal characteristic of poststenotic waveforms. The utility of these measurements depends on the ability to obtain reliable identification of vessel segments and the skills of the operator. Once the location of a vascular lesion is known, subsequent studies can be performed more easily to track progression of vascular occlusion, restenosis, and/or the results of endovascular intervention.

arcuate vessels in the renal hilum can provide additional information. Damping of these waveforms, labeled as "parvus" and "tardus," have been proposed as indirect signs of upstream vascular occlusive phenomena.[157] Some authors have challenged the use of angiographic estimates of stenosis as representing a gold standard altogether.[158] These authors argue that Doppler velocities correlate highly ($R = .97$) with a truer estimate of vascular occlusion, specifically luminal stenosis determined by intravascular ultrasound.

Doppler study of the renal arteries is highly reliable when adequate images of the renal arteries can be obtained. Positive Doppler velocities in an artery clearly identified as the renal artery are rarely proven to be negative later. False-negative studies are more common. In subjects with accessible vessels, Doppler ultrasound provides the most practical means of following vessel characteristics sequentially over time. A drawback of renal artery Doppler studies includes a frequent failure to identify accessory vessels. Because the correlation between velocity and degree of stenosis is only approximate, clinical trials such as CORAL have raised the peak systolic velocity threshold to 300 cm/s.[154] This seems warranted, particularly when the risk of overdiagnosis of renal arterial

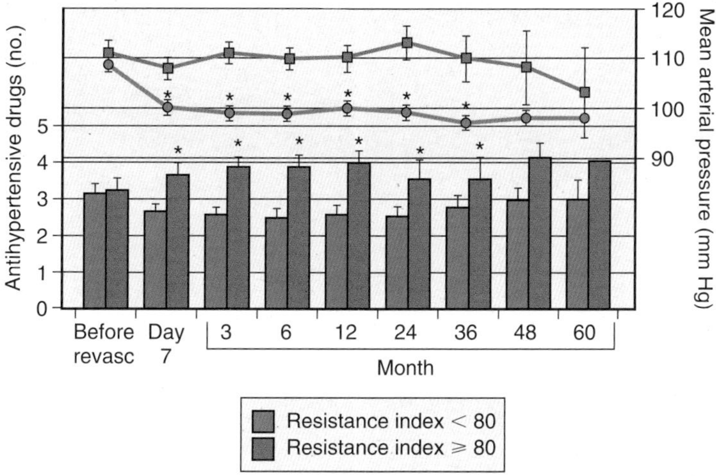


**Fig. 47.19** Outcome of revascularization as measured by mean arterial blood pressure and number of antihypertensive agents in 138 patients with renal artery stenosis. These patients were divided into groups with ultrasound-determined resistive index above 80 and those lower than 80 in the most severely affected kidney. The authors indicate that a high resistive index reflects intrinsic parenchymal and small vessel disease in the kidney that does not improve after revascularization. Those with lower indices had both lower blood pressures during follow-up and lower antihypertensive medication requirements. (From Radermacher J, Chavan A, Bleck J, et al. Use of Doppler ultrasonography to predict the outcome of therapy for renal-artery stenosis. *N Engl J Med.* 2001;344:410–417.)

lesions is high, as in the STAR trial, in which 18 of 64 patients assigned to stenting were found not to have significant RVD at the time of angiography, despite noninvasive estimates to the contrary.[120]

Additional studies have emphasized the potential for Doppler ultrasound to characterize small-vessel flow characteristics in the kidney.[159] The resistive index provides an estimate of the relative flow velocities in diastole and systole. In a study of 138 patients with RAS, a resistive index above 80 provided a predictive tool for the identification of parenchymal renal disease that did not respond to renal revascularization (Fig. 47.19). A sizeable portion of this group eventually progressed to renal failure. A resistive index less than 80 was associated with a more than 90% favorable blood pressure response and stable or improved renal function. The authors emphasized that accurate predictive power depend on using the highest resistive index observed, even when present in the nonstenotic kidney. A subsequent study of 215 subjects with mean preintervention serum creatinine levels of 1.51 mg/dL failed to confirm the predictive value of resistive index measurements.[160] Of 99 subjects with improved renal function after 1 year, 18% had a resistive index above 0.8 before intervention, whereas 15% of 92 subjects with no improvement had a resistive index above 0.8 (not significantly different [NS]). In this series, a preintervention level of serum creatinine itself was the strongest predictor of improved renal function. Most clinicians agree that detecting a low resistive index indicates a well-preserved vasculature in the kidney, with improved likelihood of recovering or stabilizing after vascular intervention.[161,162]

**Computed Tomography Angiography.** CTA using helical and/or multiple detector scanners and intravenous contrast can provide excellent images of both kidneys and the vascular tree. Resolution and reconstruction techniques render this modality capable of identifying smaller vessels, vascular lesions, and parenchymal characteristics, including malignancy and stones[163] (Fig. 47.20). When used for the detection of RAS, CTA agrees well with conventional arteriography (correlation, 95%), and sensitivity may reach 98% and specificity 94%.[164] Studies have indicated that CTA also provides excellent accuracy regarding the evaluation of in-stent restenosis,[165] and evolving quantitative, three-dimensional image analysis may improve on intraarterial methods.[164] Although this technique offers excellent noninvasive examination of the vascular tree, it does require iodinated contrast. As a result, it raises concerns for the evaluation of renovascular hypertension and/or ischemic nephropathy for older patients with impaired renal function and/or diabetes. Remarkably, patients with atherosclerotic RAS tolerate contrast from CTA imaging without evident toxicity, despite advanced age and a low GFR.[166] Some studies have suggested that release of cell cycle arrest markers tends to protect from acute injury in this setting.

Concerns regarding systemic toxicity associated with MRA contrast nonetheless have encouraged wider use of multidetector CT imaging for patients suspected of having RVD. Limitations include reduced visibility of vessel lumens in the presence of substantial calcium deposition. A single study comparing both CTA and MRA with intraarterial studies in 402 subjects has indicated lower CT performance for the detection of lesions with more than 50% stenosis.[167] In this particular study, CTA had a sensitivity of 64% and specificity of 92%, respectively, whereas MRA had a sensitivity of 62% and specificity of 84%, respectively. This was an unusual population, with only 20% of the screened population having stenotic lesions, nearly half of which were FMD. The results of such studies have reinforced the importance of careful patient selection for study and establishing exactly the purpose for which imaging is being undertaken in advance.[168]

**Magnetic Resonance Angiography.** Gadolinium-enhanced images of the abdominal and renal vasculature had been a mainstay of evaluating RVD in many institutions.[163,169]

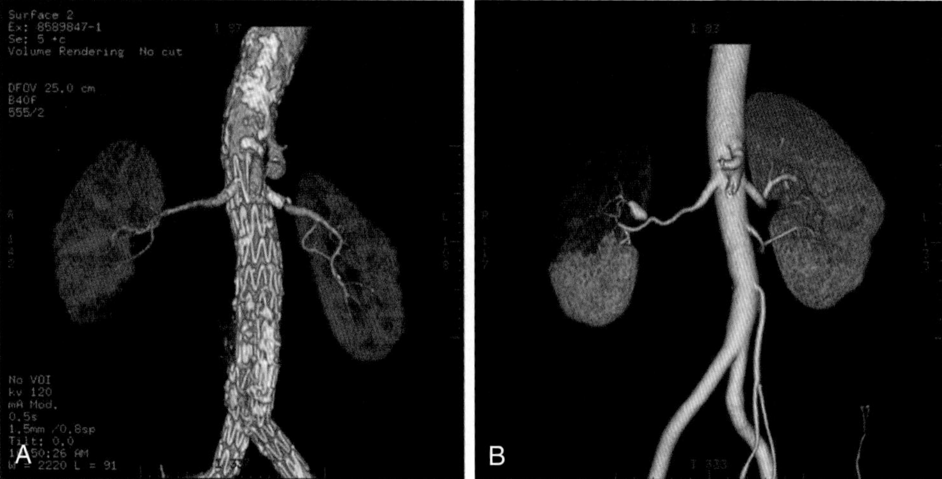


**Fig. 47.20** Computed tomography (CT) angiograms illustrating reconstructed views of complex vascular disease. (A) Aortic endovascular stent extending beyond the origins of the renal arteries. Renal artery stents have been placed through the aortic graft to restore blood flow, although the nephrograms demonstrate patchy defects consistent with small-vessel occlusion and/or atheroembolic events. (B) CT angiogram with a small aneurysm of the right renal artery that has produced segmental infarction, leading to accelerated hypertension. Although CT angiography requires contrast, current multidetector CT studies allow excellent image resolution at rapid acquisition times and less contrast exposure than before.

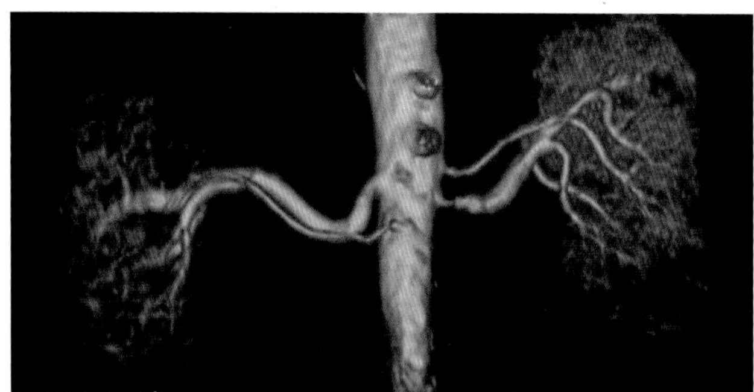

**Fig. 47.21** Magnetic resonance (MR) angiogram reconstructed without gadolinium contrast. After warnings about the association of gadolinium with nephrogenic systemic fibrosis, contrast MR is less commonly used for atherosclerotic renovascular imaging than it was used previously. Newer techniques can allow excellent vascular imaging without contrast, as shown here.

Comparative studies have indicated that sensitivity ranges from 83% to 100% and specificity from 92% to 97% in RAS.[170,171] Meta-analyses of published literature including 998 subjects have found more than 97% sensitivity using gadolinium-enhanced imaging.[172] The nephrogram obtained from gadolinium filtration provides an estimate of relative function and filtration, as well as parenchymal volume. The quantitative measurement of parenchymal volume determined by MRI appears to correlate closely with isotopically determined single-kidney GFR in some institutions.[173] Since 2006, however, concerns about the potential for gadolinium-based contrast to produce nephrogenic systemic fibrosis have effectively eliminated the use of contrast-enhanced MRI for patients with impaired kidney function in the United States.[174] This topic is further discussed in Chapter 25 because gadolinium may be used at lower renal function in other regions.

Technologic advances allow the use of high-resolution vascular MRI without contrast in many patients. An example of MRA without contrast is shown in Fig. 47.21. Drawbacks include expense and the tendency to overestimate the severity of lesions, which appear as a signal void.[163,175] The limits of resolution with current instrumentation, however, make the detection of small accessory vessels and quantitating fibromuscular lesions difficult. Both of these have been improving with use of the newer generations of scanners. High spatial resolution, three-dimensional, contrast-enhanced MR scanners provide up to 97% sensitivity and 92% specificity for renal artery stenotic lesions.[176] Signal degradation in the presence of metallic stents renders MRA unsuitable for follow-up studies after endovascular procedures in which stents are used.

**Captopril Renography.** Imaging the kidneys before and after the administration of an ACE inhibitor (e.g., captopril) can provide a functional assessment of the change in blood flow and GFR to the kidney, related both to changes in arterial pressure and removal of the efferent arteriolar effects of Ang II. Because hypertension often is not the primary motivation for evaluating RVD, these tests are less frequently carried out currently. The most commonly used radiopharmaceuticals are technetium-99 ($^{99m}$Tc) diethylenetriamine pentaacetic acid (DTPA) and $^{99m}$Tc-mercaptoacetyltriglycine (MAG3). The latter agent has clearance characteristics similar to those of Hippuran and is often taken as reflecting renal plasma flow. Both can be used, although specific interpretive criteria differ.[177,178] Both provide information regarding the size and filtration of both kidneys; the change in these characteristics after ACE inhibition allows inferences regarding the dependence of glomerular filtration on Ang II. Studies of patient groups with prevalence rates of RVD from 35% to 64% have indicated that sensitivity and specificity range from 65% to 96% and 62% to 100%, respectively.[178] Because of its high specificity, captopril renography can be used in populations with low pretest probability, with an expectation that a normal study will exclude significant renovascular hypertension in more than 96% of cases.[179] Some series have reported 100% accurate negative predictive values.[180]

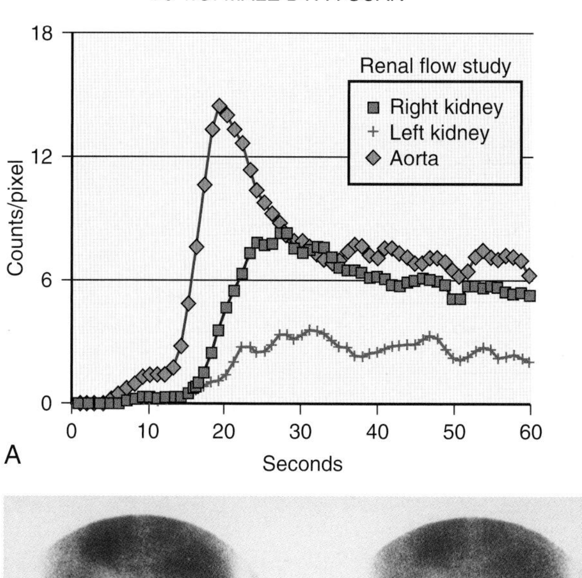


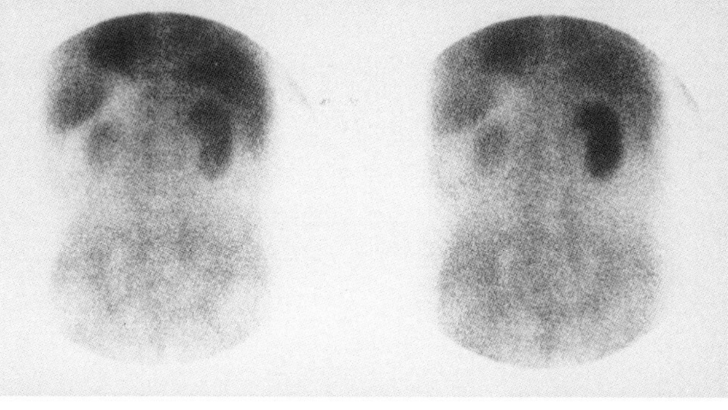


**Fig. 47.22** (A and B) Isotope renography in a patient with unilateral renal artery stenosis. (A) A $^{99m}$Tc-DTPA scan demonstrates delayed circulation and excretion of isotope on the *left.* (B) A hippuran scan (now replaced with $^{99m}$Tc-mercaptoacetyltriglycine) provides a renogram demonstrating a small kidney with impaired renal function on the affected side. Radionuclide scans provide a comparative estimate of function from each kidney that may facilitate selection of intervention, including the potential effect of nephrectomy. *DTPA,* Diethylenetriamine pentaacetic acid.

Renographic imaging studies are less sensitive and specific for RVD in the presence of renal insufficiency (usually defined as creatinine level >2.0 mg/dL). These performance characteristics also deteriorate for patients who cannot be prepared carefully (i.e., withdrawal of diuretics and ACE inhibitors for 4–14 days before the study).[178] Renography, however, only provides functional information and no direct anatomic information—the location of renal artery disease, the number of renal arteries or associated aortic, and/or ostial disease (Fig. 47.22). Prospective studies of RVD from the Netherlands did observe changes in the renogram during follow-up but did not find captopril renography predictive of angiographic findings or outcomes of revascularization.[135] A prospective study of 74 patients undergoing both renography and Doppler ultrasound evaluation before renal revascularization has reported a limited predictive value of scintigraphy (sensitivity, 58%; specificity, 57%) regarding blood pressure outcomes.[181]

Under carefully controlled conditions, some authors have argued that changes in renographic appearance correlate with changes in blood pressure to be expected after revascularization. Changes in split renal function indicate that stenotic kidneys regain GFR after revascularization, sometimes with a decrement in contralateral GFR, thereby maintaining overall kidney function unchanged.[127,182] Currently, radionuclide studies have a role in identifying the relative contributions of each kidney to overall GFR—often as part of the evaluation for residual renal function after nephrectomy.[183]

## Invasive Imaging

Intraarterial angiography currently remains the gold standard for the definition of vascular anatomy and stenotic lesions in the kidney, often performed at the time of a planned intervention, such as endovascular angioplasty and/or stenting. The role of including angiography of the renal arteries during imaging of other vascular beds, such as so-called drive-by angiography during coronary artery imaging, is unclear. Studies have confirmed that the prevalence of renal artery lesions exceeding 50% lumen occlusion in patients with hypertension and coronary artery disease is high, usually from 18% to 24%.[148] Some individuals (7% to 10%) will have high-grade stenoses above 70% occlusion, and some will be bilateral. Noting that an arterial puncture and catheterization of the aorta and coronary vessels produce some risk, the added risk from including aortography of the renal vessels may be small. Follow-up studies of individuals with incidental renal artery lesions have suggested that the presence of these lesions does provide additive predictive risk for mortality.[90,184] Screening angiography has been less commonly performed since the publication of prospective RCTs suggesting limited benefit of revascularization in stable patients with atherosclerotic RVD (see later).[148,185] Hence, endovascular procedures for such lesions should be confined to those with strong indications for renal revascularization, as even ardent advocates of catheter-based intervention have suggested.

Contrast toxicity remains an issue with conventional iodinated agents given intraarterially.[186] Intravascular ultrasound procedures have been undertaken using papaverine to evaluate flow reserve beyond stenotic lesions.[187] Various reports have indicated that either a reduction in or preserved flow reserve may identify a poststenotic kidney that may benefit from successful revascularization.[187,188] Previous studies of pressure gradients measured across stenotic lesions failed to predict the clinical response to renal revascularization. Measurements using currently available low-profile wire probes do, however, indicate a relationship between pressure gradients and activation of the renin-angiotensin system.[14] Outcomes of patients with translesional pressure gradients measured after vasodilation have suggested that measurement of the hyperemic systolic gradient above 21 mm Hg (defined after vasodilation with papaverine) most accurately predicts high-grade stenosis (average, 78% by intravascular ultrasound) and a beneficial response of blood pressure after stenting.[189] The latter observation, and increasing reliability of technical measurements, underscore the value of measuring gradients to establish a hemodynamic role for vascular lesions of marginal severity.

## Physiologic and Functional Studies of the Renin-Angiotensin System

Efforts have long been made to use activation of the RAS as a marker of underlying renovascular hypertension.[161,190]

Although these studies are promising when performed in patients with known renovascular hypertension, they are less reliable when applied to wider populations. Plasma renin activity is sensitive to changes of sodium intake, volume status, renal function, and many medications. The sensitivity and specificity of such maneuvers are heavily dependent on the a priori probability of renovascular hypertension. In practice, the major utility of these studies depends on their negative predictive value, specifically the certainty with which one can exclude significant RVD if the test is negative. Because the negative predictive value rarely exceeds 60% to 70%, these tests offer limited value in clinical decision making.[191]

Measurement of renal vein renin levels previously had been widely used in planning surgical revascularization for hypertension. These measurements are obtained by sampling renal vein and inferior vena cava blood individually. The level obtained from the vena cava is taken as comparable to the arterial levels in each kidney and allows estimation of the contribution of each kidney to total circulating levels of plasma renin activity. Lateralization is defined usually as a ratio exceeding 1.5 between the renin activity of the stenotic kidney and nonstenotic kidney.[192] Some authors have proposed a detailed examination, not only of the relative ratio between kidneys, but also the degree of suppression of renin release from the nonstenotic or contralateral kidney.[192] In general, the greater the degree of lateralization, the more probable that blood pressure will benefit from surgical or other revascularization.

Results from many studies have supported the observation that large differences between kidneys identify high-grade RAS.[193] These findings have been supported by studies of renal vein measurements before consideration of nephrectomy for refractory hypertension and advanced RVD.[183] As with many tests of hormonal activation, study conditions are crucial. A number of measures to enhance renin release and magnify differences between kidneys have been proposed, including sodium depletion with diuretic administration, hydralazine, tilt table stimulation, or captopril.[194] Strong and colleagues have demonstrated that nonlateralization can be changed to strongly lateralizing measurements by the administration of diuretics between sequential studies.[195] A review of more than 50 studies of renal vein renin measurements has indicated that when lateralization could be demonstrated, clinical benefit regarding blood pressure control could be expected in more than 90% of cases.[194] Failure to demonstrate lateralization, however, was still associated with significant benefit in more than 50% of cases.[130]

More recent series have reached similar conclusions, indicating that overall sensitivity of renal vein renin measurements is no better than 65% and that the positive predictive value is 18.5%.[196] For these and other reasons, renal vein assays are now performed less commonly. A major additional factor is that the goals of renal revascularization have shifted substantially and are often directed toward preservation of renal function, rather than for blood pressure control alone. In cases for which it is important to establish the degree of pressor effect of a specific kidney or site, such prenephrectomy measurement of renal vein renin levels can provide strong supportive evidence.[183]

**Studies of Individual Renal Function.** Serum creatinine levels, iothalamate clearance, and other estimates of the total GFR are measures of total combined renal excretory function and do not address changes within each kidney. A large body of literature has addressed the potential for individual split renal function studies to establish the functional importance of each kidney in RVD.[197]

Split renal function studies classically used separate ureteral catheters to allow individual urine collection for the measurement of separate GFRs, renal blood flow, sodium excretion, concentrating ability, and the response to blockade of Ang II. These studies have demonstrated that hemodynamic effects of renal artery lesions can produce functional changes, such as avid sodium retention, even before major changes in blood flow occur.[198] They emphasize that autoregulation of blood flow and GFR can occur over a wide range of pressures in humans and may be affected in both stenotic and contralateral kidneys by the effects of Ang II.[199,200] These studies require urinary tract instrumentation and provide only indirect information regarding the probability of benefit from revascularization. They are now rarely performed.

Separate renal functional measurements can be obtained less invasively with radionuclide techniques. These methods use a variety of radioisotopes (e.g., $^{99}$Tc-MAG3 or DTPA) to estimate fractional blood flow and filtration to each kidney. Prior administration of captopril magnifies differences between kidneys, primarily by delaying excretion of the filtered isotope due to removal of the efferent arteriolar effects of Ang II.[201] Some authors have advocated such measurements to follow progressive renal artery disease and its effect on unilateral kidney function as a guide to consider revascularization. Serial measurements of individual renal function allow more precise identification of progressive ischemic injury to the affected kidney in unilateral renal artery disease than can be determined from the overall GFR.[202] The poststenotic kidney is susceptible to gradual loss of filtration that is accompanied by a rise in blood flow and filtration in the contralateral kidney, both of which can partially reverse after restoring blood flow.[127] Single-kidney GFR measurements using radionuclide scans accurately reflect changes in three-dimensional volume parameters measured by MRI.[173] These authors argued that demonstrating preserved parenchymal volume with a disproportionate reduction in single-kidney GFR supports the concept of so-called hibernating kidney parenchyma and might provide a predictive parameter for the recovery of kidney function after revascularization.[173]

## MANAGEMENT OF RENAL ARTERY STENOSIS AND ISCHEMIC NEPHROPATHY

### OVERVIEW

The last decade has fostered a major shift from promoting renal revascularization for a cure of renovascular hypertension to primary reliance on medical antihypertensive therapy for atherosclerotic RVD. This pendulum swing may be excessive in some cases, however, eventually requiring nephrologists to confront advanced renal failure that might have been prevented. Considering the array of potential interventions and the complexity of these patients, clinicians need to formulate a clear set of therapeutic goals for each patient. Because all therapeutic measures—ranging from medical therapy alone to endovascular or surgical revascularization

**Table 47.4 Summary of Observational Series in Renal Revascularization**

**T1 Outcomes of Renal Artery Angioplasty, ±Stent Placement; Hypertension**

| | Cured[a] | Improved | No Change |
|---|---|---|---|
| 14 series, 678 patients, 98% technical success | Weighted mean, 17%; range, 3%–68% | Weighted mean, 47%; range, 5%–61% | Weighted mean, 36% range, 0%–61% |
| Renovascular hypertension, 472 patients, | 12% | 73% | 15% |

**T1 Renal Artery Stents: Effect on Renal Function[b] in Azotemic Patients**

| | "Improved" | "Stabilized" | Worse |
|---|---|---|---|
| 14 series; reporting "impaired renal function"; 496 patients | Weighted mean, 30%; range, 10%–41% | Weighted mean, 42%; range, 32%–71% | Weighted mean, 29%; range, 19%–34% |
| Ischemic nephropathy; 469 patients | 41% | 37%; no change | 22% |

[a]Cured, blood pressures at normal levels, no medication; improved, blood pressure lower by at least 10 mm Hg, fewer medications; no change, same blood pressure and/or same medications

[b]Renal function—variably defined as improved, persistent fall in creatinine, variable from 0.3–1.0 mg/dL or more; worse, variable, but persistent increase in creatinine 0.3–1.0 mg/dL or more.

Modified from Textor SC. Renovascular hypertension and ischemic nephropathy. In: Skorecki K, Chertow GM, Marsden PA, et al, eds. *Brenner and Rector's: The kidney.* 10th ed. Philadelphia: Elsevier; 2016:1567–1609.

with adjunctive therapy—carry both benefits and risks, the clinician's task is to weigh the role of each of these within the context of the individual's comorbidity.

In most cases, long-term management of the RVD patient requires integrated pharmacologic management of blood pressure and cardiovascular risk combined with optimal timing of renal revascularization for those with high-risk manifestations and/or disease progression. The objective of this section is to provide a framework in which to plan a balanced approach to the patient with unilateral or bilateral RAS. It should be emphasized that consideration of renal artery disease takes place in the context of managing other cardiovascular risk factors, cessation of tobacco use, reduction of cholesterol levels, and treatment of diabetes and obesity.

## MEDICAL THERAPY OF RENOVASCULAR DISEASE

The overall goals of therapy are summarized in Box 47.3. Foremost among these is the objective identified from multiple reports from the Joint National Committee of the National High Blood Pressure Education Program (NHBPEP): "The goal of treating patients with hypertension is to prevent morbidity and mortality associated with high blood pressure."[203] This may include the effort to simplify or potentially eliminate long-term antihypertensive drug therapy, particularly in younger individuals with FMD. A further goal is to preserve kidney function and prevent loss of kidney function related to impaired renal blood flow. In some cases, renal revascularization is undertaken to allow improved management of salt and water balance in the process of managing patients with CHF. This may allow safer use of diuretic agents, ACE inhibitor, and ARB classes of medication in patients with critical renal artery lesions affecting the entire renal mass. Because prospective clinical trial data have been limited to relatively low-risk patients included for randomization, each patient must be considered individually.

Several prospective RCTs have been undertaken since 2005. Although each has limitations, results of medical therapy over periods ranging from 2 to 5 years have been equivalent to those observed with medical therapy plus renal revascularization, with relatively few treatment crossovers (Tables 47.4–47.6).[139] Taken together, these studies underscore the importance of optimizing medical antihypertensive therapy as part of the decision-making process. If blood pressure can be well controlled with a tolerable regimen, and kidney function remains stable, it is difficult to justify moving forward with costly and potentially hazardous imaging and/or vascular intervention procedures. As a practical matter, these measures must be considered within the entire context of patient management over time.

## RENAL ARTERY STENOSIS

### UNILATERAL VERSUS BILATERAL RENAL ARTERY STENOSIS

"Bilateral" in this context refers to the circumstances when the entire functional renal mass is affected by vascular occlusion. This may be caused by bilateral stenoses or stenosis to a solitary functioning kidney. Not only are the putative mechanisms related to blood pressure and volume control different in the presence of a nonstenosed, functioning contralateral kidney with unilateral disease (as described earlier), but the potential hazards of intervention and/or medical therapy differ. Patient survival is reduced in patients with bilateral disease or stenosis to a solitary functioning kidney. Progressive arterial disease in this group also poses the most immediate hazard of declining renal function. Patient survival depends on the extent of vascular involvement,[131] regardless of whether renal revascularization is undertaken.

### UNILATERAL RENAL ARTERY STENOSIS

Most patients with atherosclerotic renal artery disease have preexisting hypertension.[204] As a result, many are exposed to antihypertensive drug therapy before identification of the lesion and may be well controlled with only moderate

**Table 47.5 Prospective Randomized Trials of Medical Therapy Versus Angioplasty for Hypertension[a]**

| Source | Inclusion, Blood Pressure Measurement | Blood Pressure Outcome (mm Hg) | Renal Outcome (mm Hg) | Comments |
|---|---|---|---|---|
| SNRAS, Webster et al, 1998[129]; *n* = 55 (unilateral = 27); *n* = 135 eligible; RAS > 50% | DBP ≥95 mm Hg, two drugs; exclusion: CVA, MI within 3 mo; creatinine >500 µmol/L; BP, random-zero device; no ACE inhibitors allowed | Unilateral—PTRA, 173/95 Med Rx, 161/88 Bilateral—PTRA, 152/83; Med Rx, 171/91; *P* < .01 | Creatinine (µmol/L), bilateral PTRA,188 Med Rx, 157 Unilateral PTRA, 144 Med Rx, 168 | "…unable to demonstrate any benefit in respect of renal function or event free survival" (F/U 40 mos). |
| EMMA: Plouin et al, 1998[243]; *n* = 49 (unilateral RAS only); RAS >75% or >60%, lateralizing study | Age <75 years; normal contralateral kidney; exclusion: malignant HTN CVA, CHF, MI within 6 mo; BP, automated sphygmomanometer, ABPM at 6 mo | PTRA, 140/81 Med Rx, 141/84 No. drugs (DDD)— PTRA, 1.0 Med Rx, 1.78, *P* <.01 Crossover to PTRA: 7/26 (27%) | Creatinine Clearance mL/min: (6 mos) PTRA: 77 Med Rx: 74 Renal artery occlusion: PTRA: 0 Med Rx: 0 | "BP levels and the proportion of patients given antihypertensive treatment were similar one year after randomization in the control and angioplasty groups, confirming that the BP-lowering effect of angioplasty in the short and medium terms is limited in atherosclerotic RAS." |
| DRASTIC: Van Jaarsveld, et al. 2000[135]; *n* = 106 ASO RAS >50% | Resistant: two drugs; DBP >95 mm Hg or creatinine rise with ACEI; exclusion: creatinine ≥2.3 mg/dL; solitary kidney, total occlusion—kidney <8 cm; BP, automated oscillometric | BP outcomes at 3 mo— PTRA, 169/89 Med Rx, 163/88 At 12 mo—PTRA,152/84 Med Rx,: 162/88 No. of drugs, 1.9 vs. 2.4, *P* < .01 | Creatinine Cl (3 mos) mL/min: PTRA: 70 Med Rx: 59 (*P* = .03) Abnormal renograms PTRA: 36% Med Rx: 70% (*P* = .002) Renal artery occlusion PTRA 0 Med Rx 8 | "In the treatment of patients with hypertension and renal artery stenosis, angioplasty has little advantage over antihypertensive drug therapy." |

[a]In patients with atherosclerotic renal artery stenosis.

*ABPM*, Overnight ambulatory reading; *ACEI*, angiotensin-converting enzyme inhibitor; *ASO*, atherosclerotic occlusive disease; *BP*, blood pressure; *CHF*, congestive heart failure; *CVA*, cerebrovascular accident; *DBP*, diastolic blood pressure; *DDD*, defined daily doses; *DRASTIC*, Dutch Renal Artery Stenosis Intervention Cooperative; *EMMA*, Essai Multicentrique Medicaments vs Angioplastie; *F/U*, follow-up; *HTN*, hypertension; *Med Rx*, medical therapy; *MI*, myocardial infarction; *n*, number of patients; *PTRA*, percutaneous renal artery angioplasty; *RAS*, renal artery stenosis; *SNRAS*, Scottish and Newcastle Renal Artery Stenosis Collaborative Group; *Tx*, therapy.

medication use.[88] As noted, such patients commonly come to clinical attention when recognizable clinical progression occurs. Occasionally, clinical decision making is strongly influenced by concerns about the hazards of medical therapy and failing to achieve restored blood flow soon enough. Examination of the results of medical therapy alone is important before evaluating the role of vascular reconstruction or dilation.

Since the introduction of agents blocking the renin-angiotensin system have been introduced, most patients (86%–92%) with unilateral renal artery disease can achieve blood pressure levels lower than 140/90 mm Hg with medical regimens based on these medications. Treatment trials have confirmed that target blood pressure levels can regularly be achieved.[98,121] Given the widespread use of these agents for patients with many forms of cardiovascular disease, it is likely that subcritical cases of RVD are treated without being identified.

The crux of clinical debates centers around whether the treatment of RAS with antihypertensive drug therapy poses a long-term hazard to kidney function. Early studies with experimental "clip" hypertension have described renal fibrosis and scarring in the stenotic kidney in animals treated with ACE inhibitors. It is well recognized that removal of the efferent arteriolar effects of Ang II leads to loss of glomerular filtration in a kidney with reduced renal perfusion (Fig. 47.23). Experimental studies in two-kidney, one-clip rats have indicated that the loss of kidney function is sometimes irreversible, although survival is improved with the use of ACE inhibitors compared with minoxidil-treated animals.[205] The unique role of ACE inhibitors and ARBs must be understood in this regard. Any drug capable of reducing systemic arterial pressure has the potential to lower renal pressures beyond a critical stenosis. As a result, successful antihypertensive therapy in RVD has the theoretic result of reducing blood flow to the poststenotic kidney sufficient to induce vascular thrombosis.

The unique feature of renin-angiotensin system blockade is the specific reduction of angiotensin-dependent efferent arteriolar resistance sufficient to lower transcapillary filtration pressures. This can occur despite preserved blood flow to the glomerulus (see Fig. 47.23 B).[206,207] This property is central

**Table 47.6 Prospective Randomized Clinical Trials for Renal Function and/or Cardiovascular Outcomes Comparing Medical Therapy With Renal Artery Stenting**

| Trial | N | Population | Inclusion Criteria | Exclusion Criteria | Outcomes |
|---|---|---|---|---|---|
| STAR (2009)[120]: 10 centers, f/up 2 years | Med Tx, 76; PTRA, 64 | Patients with impaired renal function, ostial ARVD detected by various imaging studies and stable blood pressure (BP) on statin and aspirin | ARVD >50%; creatinine clearance <80 mL/min/1.73 m²; Controlled blood pressure 1 month before inclusion | Kidney <8 cm, renal artery diameter < 4 mm<br>eCrCl < 15 mL/min/1.73 m²<br>DM with proteinuria (>3 g/day), malignant hypertension | No difference in GFR decline (primary endpoint ≥20% change in clearance), but many did not undergo PTRA<br>ARVD <50% on angiography<br>Serious complication in the PTRA group<br>Study was underpowered |
| ASTRAL (2009)[121]: 57 centers, f/up 5 years | Med Tx, 403; PTRA, 403 | Patients with uncontrolled or refractory hypertension or unexplained renal dysfunction with unilateral or bilateral ARVD on statin and aspirin | ARVD—substantial disease suitable for endovascular Rx and patient's physician uncertainty of clinical benefit from revascularization | High likelihood of PTRA in <6 months<br>Without ARVD, previous ARVD, PTRA, FMD | No difference in BP, renal function, mortality, CV events (primary endpoint: 20% reduction of in the mean slope of the reciprocal of serum creatinine level)<br>Substantial risk in PTRA group |
| CORAL (2013)[98]: 109 centers, f/up 5 years | Med Tx, 480; PTRA, 467 | Hypertension, two or more antihypertensives or CKD stage ≥3 with ARVD, with unilateral or bilateral disease on statin | SBP >155 mm Hg, at least two drugs; ARVD > 60%; subsequent changes included no longer requiring systolic hypertension if eGFR was <60 mL/min | FMD Creatinine >4.0 mg/dL Kidney length <7 cm and use of more than one stent | No difference of death from CV or renal causes modest improvement of SBP in stented group<br>Total, 26 complications (5.5%) |

*ARVD,* Atherosclerotic renovascular disease; *CKD,* chronic kidney disease; *CV,* cardiovascular; *DM,* diabetes mellitus; *eClCr,* estimated creatinine clearance; *FMD,* fibromuscular dysplasia; *f/up,* follow-up; *GFR,* glomerular filtration rate; *Med Tx,* medical therapy; *N,* number of patients; *PTRA,* percutaneous renal artery angioplasty; *RVD,* renovascular disease; *SBP,* systolic blood pressure; *Tx,* therapy.

Modified from Herrmann SM, Saad A, Textor SC. Management of atherosclerotic renovascular disease after Cardiovascular Outcomes in Renal Atherosclerotic Lesions (CORAL). *Nephrol Dial Transplant.* 2015;30(3):366–375.

to the benefits of this class of agent in hyperfiltration states thought to accelerate renal damage in other settings, such as diabetes. In the presence of RVD, the fall in glomerular filtration beyond a stenotic lesion can be observed despite relatively preserved plasma flows.[207] The fall in the GFR heralds an approaching degree of critical vascular compromise before blood flow itself is reduced.[206] Studies in a porcine renovascular model suggested that angiotensin receptor blockade may have microvascular protective effects in the kidney as compared with drug therapy without renin-angiotensin system blockade.[208] Earlier studies in renovascular hypertensive animals confirmed that despite a reduction in filtration, renal structural integrity can be preserved and recovered after removal of the clip and/or removal of the ACE inhibitor.[209] Hence, it is unlikely that ACE inhibitors or ARBs themselves pose a unique hazard beyond that attributable to reduction in renal blood flow.

It is important to recognize that the contralateral kidney usually supports total glomerular filtration, despite reduced filtration in the stenotic kidney. Changes in overall GFR may be undetectable, in part due to increased filtration in the contralateral kidney.[127] This fact may be used in several ways. Some authors have argued in favor of using "split" renal function measurements, such as radionuclide renal scans, to detect loss of individual kidney function as a means of timing revascularization.[202] Depending on the circumstances, loss of one kidney might be acceptable if one can ensure the patient that the remaining kidney has adequate function and blood supply. The fall in the GFR from a loss of one kidney may represent a loss of the GFR analogous to that of nephrectomy for malignancy or donating a kidney for renal transplantation. In such cases, the long-term hazard to the remaining kidney is small, although not negligible.[210–212] As the age and comorbidity of the population at risk rise, the loss of one kidney may pose an acceptable additional hazard if the overall glomerular filtration is adequate. Subsequent follow-up to monitor the condition of the remaining kidney is essential.

The experience with ACE inhibition in trials of CHF is reassuring in this regard. Thousands of patients with marginal arterial pressures and clinical heart failure have been treated with a variety of ACE inhibitors and ARBs.[206] These patients are at high risk for undetected renal artery lesions as part of the atherosclerotic burden associated with coronary disease. Although a minor change in the creatinine level is observed in 8% to 10% of these individuals, a rise sufficient to lead

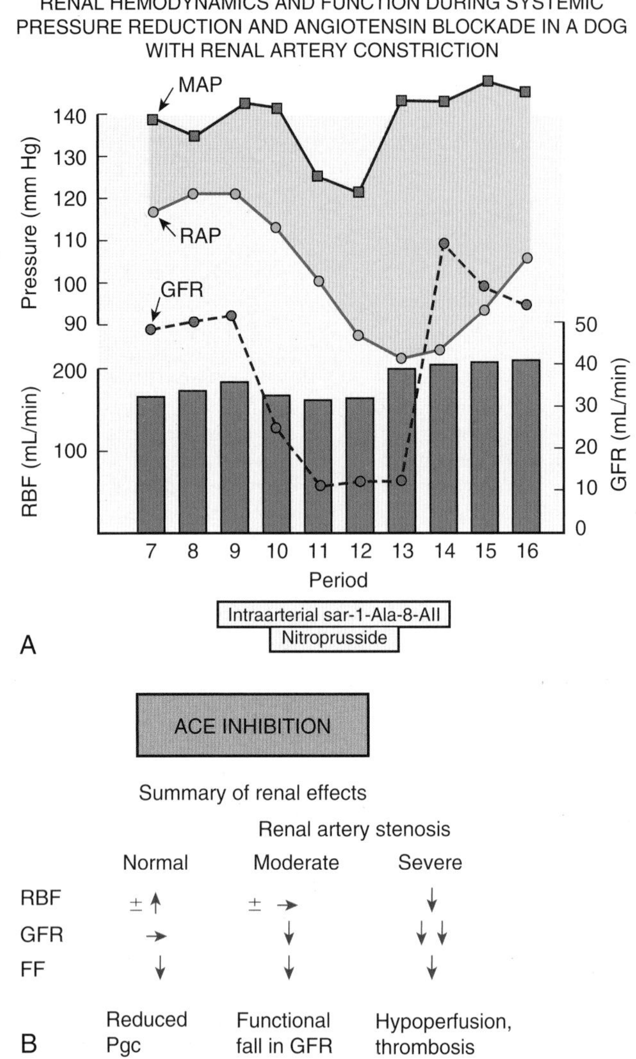


**Fig. 47.23** (A) The glomerular filtration rate *(GFR)* falls beyond a renal artery stenotic lesion during blockade of angiotensin II (produced by intrarenal infusion of sar-1-ala-8-angiotensin II) and pressure reduction induced by sodium nitroprusside. The fall in GFR occurs despite preserved renal blood flow *(RBF)*, measured by electromagnetic flow probe. These observations illustrate the specific role of angiotensin II in maintaining GFR in the poststenotic kidney at reduced perfusion pressures. (B) Summary of the effects of angiotensin-converting enzyme *(ACE)* inhibition and/or angiotensin receptor blockade on RBF, GFR, and filtration fraction *(FF)* in normal, moderate, and severe levels of renal artery stenosis. As compared with other antihypertensive agents, ACE inhibitors and angiotensin receptor blockers (ARBs) lead to a fall in GFR and filtration fraction due to removal of the efferent arteriolar effects of angiotensin II. When stenosis is sufficiently severe that pressure reduction compromises renal blood flow, the potential for complete occlusion is present, as with other effective antihypertensive agents as well. *MAP,* Mean arterial pressure; *RAP,* renal artery pressure. (From Textor SC. Renal failure related to ACE inhibitors. *Semin Nephrol.* 1997;17:67–76.)

to withdrawal of these agents under trial monitoring conditions occurs in only 1% to 2%. Data from patients with high cardiovascular disease risk treated with ramipril included patients with creatinine levels up to 2.3 mg/dL. Those with creatinine between 1.4 and 2.3 mg/dL were at higher risk for cardiovascular mortality and had a major survival benefit from ACE inhibition.[141] Close follow-up of kidney function has indicated that withdrawal of ACE inhibition due to deterioration of renal function is less than 5% and no greater than placebo.[141] All participants in the CORAL trial were treated with an ARB, with rare discontinuation.[98] Registry data from the United Kingdom have further supported the tolerability of renin-angiotensin system blockade in more than 90% of cases of atherosclerotic RVD, including more than 75% of patients with bilateral disease.[103] Importantly, there appeared to be a mortality benefit in patients treated with these agents.[213]

## PROGRESSIVE RENAL ARTERY STENOSIS IN MEDICALLY TREATED PATIENTS

The potential for vascular occlusive disease to progress further is central to long-term management of patients with RVD. It may be argued that failure to revascularize the kidneys exposes the individual to the hazard of undetected progressive occlusion, potentially leading to irreversible loss of renal function. Because the treatment trials have been relatively short (2–4 years), this issue remains an important consideration for the long-term treatment of atherosclerotic RVD. A firm understanding of the evidence regarding progressive atherosclerotic disease of the kidney is important for planning endovascular and surgical revascularization.

Atherosclerosis is a variably progressive disorder. Those involved in the management of disorders of the carotid, coronary, aortic, and peripheral vasculatures all recognize the potential for progression, which occurs at widely different individual rates. Medical therapy of all of these should incorporate measures aimed at intensive risk factor reduction. Treatment of these risk factors reduces mortality rates from cardiovascular disease.[214]

An important clinical question is whether progressive renal artery occlusive disease affects the progression of renovascular hypertension. Moderate anatomic progression alone does not reliably predict functional changes in terms of deteriorating blood pressure control or renal function. Results from prospective Doppler ultrasound studies have indicated that a decrement in measured renal size by 1 cm (renal atrophy) developed in 5.5% of those with normal initial vessels and 20.8% of those with baseline stenosis greater than 60% during a follow-up interval of 33 months.[215] Changes in the serum creatinine level were infrequent but did occur in a subset of patients, particularly those with bilateral RAS. These findings are in general agreement with early studies during medical therapy of renovascular hypertension, in which 35% had a detectable fall in measured renal length, but only 8 of 41 (19%) had a significant rise in the creatinine level during a follow-up of 33 months.[136] Follow-up of the medical treatment arms during short-term studies have failed to show major changes in kidney function, although occasional loss of renal perfusion was observed by radionuclide scanning.[135]

Another important question is whether the management of RAS without revascularization leads to clinical progression, either in terms of refractory hypertension or advancing renal insufficiency. Follow-up of patients with incidentally identified RAS is helpful in this regard. A review of peripheral aortograms has identified 69 patients with high-grade renal arterial stenoses (>70%) followed without revascularization for more than 6 months.[216] Their long-term follow-up identified generally satisfactory blood pressure control, although some required more intensive antihypertensive therapy during an average of 36 months of follow-up. Of these, 4 eventually underwent renal revascularization for refractory hypertension and/or renal dysfunction, and 5 developed ESKD, of which only one case was thought to be related to RAS directly. Overall, the serum creatinine level rose from 1.4 to 2.0 mg/dL. These data indicate that many of these patients can be managed without revascularization for years, and that clinical progression leading to urgent revascularization develops in 10% to 14% of them. Expansion of this data set to 160 individuals has allowed comparison of different antihypertensive regimens.[130] The rates of progression were not specifically related to the introduction of ACE inhibitors, although the level of blood pressure control improved in later years with all medications.[130]

These observations have been supported by a report of 126 patients with incidental RAS compared with 397 patients matched for age.[137] The measured serum creatinine level was higher, and the calculated GFR (estimated using the Cockcroft-Gault equation) was lower in patients with RAS followed for 8 to 10 years. However, no patient progressed to ESKD. These observations are consistent with the results of prospective trials of medical versus surgical intervention, which started in the 1980s and extended into the 1990s.[217] Remarkably similar data are evident from other RCTs, in which both the medical therapy and revascularization arms progressed to a renal endpoint in 16% to 22% of cases in the CORAL and ASTRAL trials (see Table 47.6).[98,121] No differences in patient survival or renal function were identified. Taken together, these studies suggest that the rates of progression of RVD are moderate and occur at widely varying rates. Many of these patients can be managed without revascularization for years, although some will inevitably progress. These observations underscore the importance of close follow-up for those identified with RVD.

Although these reports are informative, they leave many questions unanswered:

- How often does suboptimal blood pressure control of renovascular hypertension accelerate cardiovascular morbidity and mortality?
- Does one lose the opportunity to reverse hypertension effectively by delaying renal revascularization?

These issues require further prospective studies. It is clear that progressive disease develops in a subset of high-risk patients who present with pulmonary edema, accelerating hypertension, and rapidly falling GFR. In such patients, optimal stability of kidney function and blood pressure control over the long term can be achieved by successful surgical or endovascular restoration of the renal blood supply.[108,218]

## ENDOVASCULAR RENAL ANGIOPLASTY AND STENTING

The ability to restore renal perfusion in high-risk patients with renovascular hypertension and ischemic nephropathy using endovascular methods represents a major advance in regard to treatment of this disorder. Restoration of blood flow to the kidney beyond a stenotic lesion intuitively should provide a means to improve renovascular hypertension and halt progressive vascular occlusive injury. In the 1990s, a major shift from surgical reconstruction ensued, toward preferential application of endovascular procedures.[9] The total volume of renal revascularization procedures registered for the US Medicare population older than 65 years rose 62%, from 13,380 to 21,600 between 1996 and 2000.[219] This change reflected an increase in endovascular procedures by 2.4-fold, whereas surgical renovascular procedures fell by 45%. The trend continued, with an estimate of 35,000 endovascular procedures in 2005.[219,220] Since the publication of the ASTRAL trial, this trend has reversed dramatically, leading to few revascularization procedures in the United Kingdom.

Revascularizing the kidney has benefits and risks. With older patients developing RAS in the context of preexisting hypertension, the likelihood of a total cure for hypertension is low, particularly in atherosclerotic disease. Although complications are not common, they can be catastrophic, including atheroembolic disease and aortic dissection. Knowing when to pursue renal revascularization is central to the dilemma of managing RVD.

### ANGIOPLASTY FOR FIBROMUSCULAR DISEASE

Most lesions of medial fibroplasia are located at a distance away from the renal artery ostium. Many of these have multiple webs within the vessel, which can be successfully traversed and opened by balloon angioplasty. Stenting is rarely required unless vessel dissection occurs. Experience in the 1980s indicated more than 94% technical success rates.[221] Some of these lesions (≈10%) develop restenosis, for which repeat procedures have been used.[91] Clinical benefit regarding blood pressure control has been reported in observational outcome studies in 65% to 75% of patients, although the rates of cure are less secure.[83] Cure of hypertension, defined as sustained blood pressure levels less than 140/90 mm Hg with no antihypertensive medications, may be obtained in 35% to 50% of patients.[222] Predictors of cure—normal arterial pressures without medication at 6 months and beyond after angioplasty—include lower systolic blood pressures, younger age, and shorter duration of hypertension.[222,223]

A large majority of patients with FMD are female, at younger ages than those with atherosclerotic disease.[83] In general, such patients have less aortic disease and are at a lower risk for major complications of angioplasty. Because the risk for major procedural complications is low, most clinicians favor early intervention for hypertensive patients with FMD with the hope of reduced antihypertensive medication requirements after successful angioplasty.

### ANGIOPLASTY AND STENTING FOR ATHEROSCLEROTIC RENAL ARTERY STENOSIS

After the introduction of percutaneous transluminal renal angioplasty (PTRA), it was soon evident that ostial lesions commonly failed to respond, in part because of extensive recoil of the plaque, which extended into the main portion of the aorta.[224] These lesions develop restenosis rapidly, even after early technical success. Endovascular stents were introduced for ostial lesions in the late 1980s and early 1990s.[225]

The technical advantage of stents is indisputable. An example of successful renal artery stenting is shown in Fig. 47.24. Prospective comparisons between angioplasty alone versus angioplasty with stents has shown that intermediate

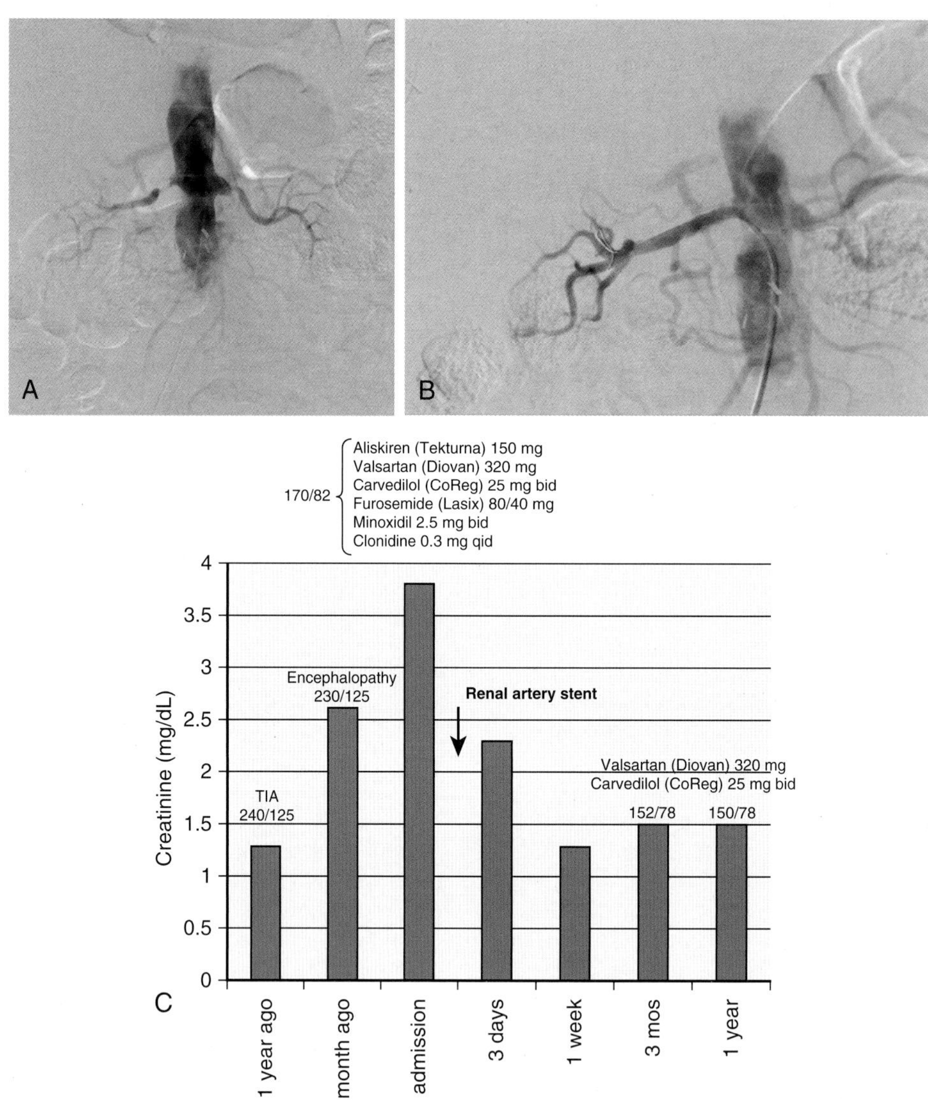


**Fig. 47.24** (A) Renal aortogram illustrating high-grade, bilateral renal arterial lesions in a 73-year-old male who developed accelerated hypertension a few months before. (B) Aortogram after placement of endovascular stents, illustrating excellent vessel patency and early technical success. This was followed by resolution of his hypertension. (C) Serum creatinine levels, blood pressure levels, and antihypertensive drug regimen in an individual with high-grade bilateral renal artery stenosis. Rapidly developing hypertension and loss of glomerular filtration rate were associated with transient neurologic deficits. Successful renal artery stenting led to sustained reduction in serum creatinine, improved blood pressure levels, and reduced medication requirements. Such cases reflect high-risk subsets that were not well represented in the prospective randomized controlled trials. (Modified from Textor SC. Attending rounds: a patient with accelerated hypertension and an atrophic kidney. *Clin J Am Soc Nephrol.* 2014;9(6):1117–1123.)

(6–12 months) vessel patency is 29% and 75%, respectively.[224] Restenosis fell from 48% to 14% in stented patients. As technical success continues to improve, many reports have suggested nearly 100% technical success in early vessel patency, although rates of restenosis continue to reach 14% to 25%.[9,148,226] The introduction of endovascular stents has expanded renal revascularization, in part because of improved technical patency possible with ostial atherosclerotic lesions and applicability in older patients with substantial comorbidity.

Regarding outcomes of renal stenting, a systematic analysis under the direction of the Agency for Health Care Research and Quality has found that the "strength of evidence" through 2016 regarding the benefits and risks of stent revascularization is low, in part because of major differences between subjects included in prospective RCTs and those reported in observational series.[227] These outcomes are commonly considered in terms of the following: (1) blood pressure control; and (2) preservation or salvage of renal function in ischemic nephropathy. Observational cohort blood pressure studies after stenting face the same limitations as those observed with angioplasty alone. Results over 1- to 4-year follow-ups are summarized from representative series in Tables 47.4 to 47.6 and reviewed in detail elsewhere.[228,229] Typically reported falls in blood pressure in observational cohorts are in the range of 25 to 30 mm Hg systolic, the best predictor of the initial systolic blood pressure.[230] Some authors have reported 42% improvement in blood pressure with fewer medications needed, although cures were rare, and renal function was unchanged.[231] Careful attention to the degree of residual patency in 210 patients with stents reported more than 91% patency at 1 year and 79% patency at 5 years.[153] Blood pressures were cured or improved in more than 80%. In some cases, episodes of angina and recurrent CHF subside.[104,232] As noted in the trials summarized later, prospective RCTs have been less impressive regarding the benefits of stenting[98,120,121] (Fig. 47.25).

Outcomes regarding the recovery of renal function after endovascular revascularization are summarized in Tables 47.4 to 47.6. In general, average changes in renal function for atherosclerotic RAS, as reflected by serum creatinine levels, have been small.[109] Remarkably, the changes in renal function in azotemic patients after surgical reconstruction are similar.[233,234] The average group changes in kidney function can be misleading. Careful evaluation of the literature indicates that three distinctly different clinical outcomes are routinely observed. In some cases (≈27%), revascularization produces clinical improvements in kidney function.[109] For this group, in one reported series, the mean serum creatinine level fell from a mean value of 4.5 mg/dL to an average of 2.2 mg/dL. There can be no doubt that such patients benefit from the procedure and avoid the major morbidity (and probably mortality) associated with advanced renal failure. The bulk of patients (≈52%) have little measurable change in renal function, however.[109] Whether such patients benefit clinically depends on the actual likelihood of progressive renal injury if the stenotic lesion were managed without revascularization, as discussed previously. Those without much risk of progression gain little, other than potential reversal of hypertrophy in the unaffected kidney.

The most significant concern, however, is the group of patients whose renal function deteriorates further after a revascularization procedure. In most reports, this ranges from 19% to 25%.[109,235] In some cases, this represents atheroembolic disease or a variety of complications, including vessel dissection with thrombosis.[236] Hence, nearly 20% of azotemic patients face progression of renal insufficiency and the potential of requiring renal replacement therapy.[234,237,238] Predictors of both mortality and ESKD include the level of renal function before intervention and the levels of proteinuria.[122] Importantly, patients with minimal proteinuria enrolled in CORAL had improved mortality outcomes.[3] Deterioration of renal function after stenting sometimes develops rapidly and may reflect atheroembolic injury, which may be nearly universal after any vascular intervention,[239] and acceleration of oxidative stress, producing interstitial inflammation and fibrosis.[240,241] Whether improved techniques, including the application of distal protection devices for endovascular catheters, will reduce these complications is not yet certain.

Several studies have suggested that the progression of renal failure attributed to ischemic nephropathy can be reduced by endovascular procedures.[108,235,242] Harden and coworkers presented reciprocal creatinine plots in 23 (of 32 patients), suggesting that the slope of loss of the GFR could be favorably changed after renal artery stenting.[235] Renal function improved or stabilized in 69%, indicating that in 31% it worsened, consistent with results from other series. These reports and a guideline document from the American Heart Association

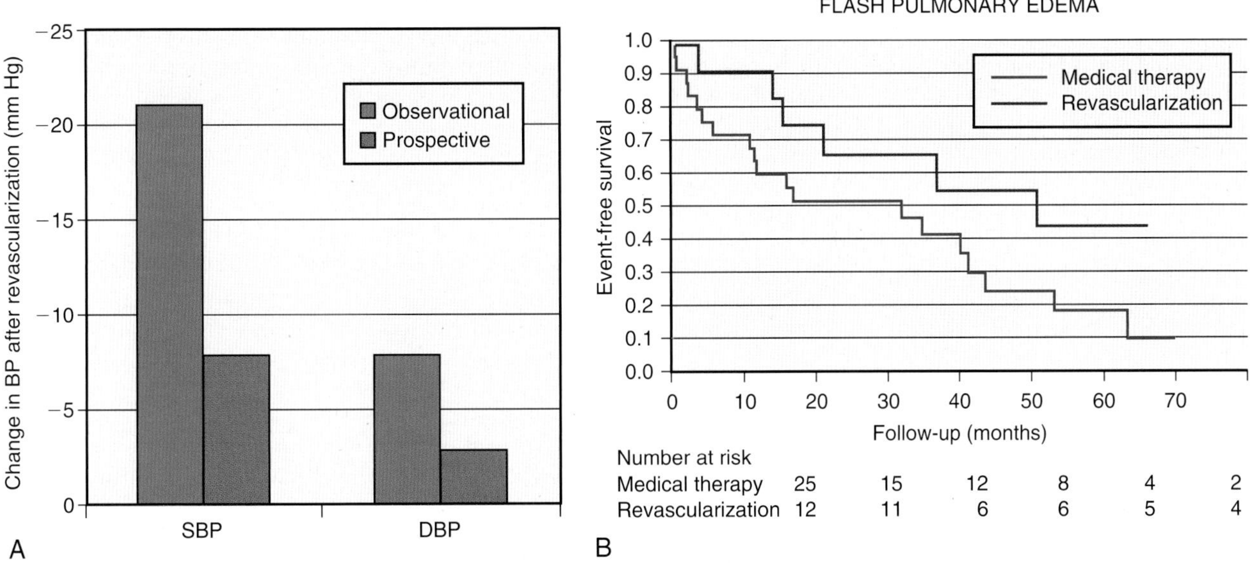


**Fig. 47.25.** (A) Comparison of blood pressure *(BP)* changes reported after renal revascularization from a large observational registry (>1000 patients) and from a meta-analysis of three prospective randomized trials (210 patients). The large difference between these BP effects is reflected in variable enthusiasm for intervention between clinicians. Initial results from prospective trials (ASTRAL and CORAL; see text) identified only minor differences in achieved BP levels. Although results from observational series may overstate treatment benefits, results from prospective trials likely underestimate changes, in part due to limitations in patient recruitment and crossover between treatment arms, ranging from 27% to 44% in early series (see text). (B) Follow-up data from a registry in the United Kingdom, most of whom were not considered candidates for ASTRAL. This report identified a major mortality risk for patients with renal artery stenosis and episodes of pulmonary edema that was reduced for patients submitted for renal revascularization. A similar mortality benefit was identified for patients with rapidly progressive renal failure (see text). *DBP*, Diastolic BP; *SBP*, systolic BP. (From Ritchie J, Green D, Chrysochou C, et al. High-risk clinical presentations in atherosclerotic renovascular disease: prognosis and response to renal artery revascularization. *Am J Kidney Dis.* 2014;63(2):186–197.)

have promoted the use of breakpoint analysis to analyze and report the results of renovascular procedures.[151] Caution must be applied regarding the application of breakpoints using reciprocal creatinine plots in this disorder, however. Vascular disease does not affect both kidneys symmetrically, nor is it likely to follow a constant course of progression, in contrast to diabetic nephropathy, for example. As a result, a gradual loss of renal function with subsequent stabilization can be observed equally with unilateral disease leading to total occlusion, as well as successful revascularization.

Perhaps the most convincing group data in this regard derives from serial renal functional measurement in 33 patients with high-grade (>70%) stenosis affecting the entire renal mass (bilateral disease or stenosis in a solitary functioning kidney), with creatinine levels between 1.5 and 4.0 mg/dL.[242] Follow-up over a mean of 20 months has shown that the slope of GFR loss converted from negative (–0.0079 dL/mg/month) to positive (0.0043 dL/mg/month). These studies agree with other observations that long-term survival is reduced in bilateral disease and that the potential for renal dysfunction and accelerated cardiovascular disease risk is highest in such patients.

## PROSPECTIVE TREATMENT TRIALS

### MEDICAL THERAPY COMPARED WITH ANGIOPLASTY PLUS STENTS

In regard to renovascular hypertension, as noted previously, many patients with unilateral RAS are managed without restoration of blood flow for a long period, sometimes indefinitely. The judgment about endovascular intervention in a specific case is based on the anticipated outcome, as summarized later. There are now several prospective randomized trials comparing medical therapy with revascularization using PTRA plus stents on which to base conclusions. Familiarity with the available trials and their limitations is important. The major features of these trials are summarized in Tables 47.5 and 47.6.

Three small trials in renovascular hypertension from the 1990s have addressed the relative value of endovascular repair, specifically PTRA as compared with medical therapy for atherosclerotic RAS.[129,135,243] To the credit of these investigators, care was taken to standardize blood pressure measurement before and after endovascular repair and to select antihypertensive regimens carefully. All these trials have limitations, but they are instructive.

Webster and colleagues randomized 55 patients with atherosclerotic RAS to medical therapy or PTRA.[129] Follow-up blood pressures were obtained using a random-zero sphygmomanometer after a run-in period. The run-in period produced considerable reduction in blood pressures in all patients. Those with unilateral disease showed no difference between medical therapy and PTRA[129] after 6 months. There was greater blood pressure benefit after PTRA in those with bilateral RAS. The authors concluded that they were "unable to demonstrate any benefit with respect to renal function or event free survival" during follow-up, up to 40 months.

Plouin and colleagues randomized 49 patients with unilateral atherosclerotic RAS more than 75% or more than 60% with lateralizing functional studies.[243] Blood pressure measurements were based on overnight ambulatory readings (ABPM), which are thought to yield more reproducible data and to be relatively free from placebo or office effects. Seven of 26 subjects assigned to medical therapy eventually crossed over to the PTRA group (27%) for refractory hypertension. There were six procedural complications in the PTRA group, including branch dissection and segmental infarction. Final blood pressures were not different between groups, but fewer medications were required in the PTRA group. Taken together, this trial suggested that PTRA produced more complications in the short term, was useful in some medical treatment failures, and required slightly fewer medications after 6 months. Medical therapy for this study specifically excluded renin-angiotensin system blockers.

A third prospective trial included 106 patients enrolled in the DRASTIC study.[135] These patients were selected for resistance to therapy, including two drugs, and were required to have serum creatinine values below 2.3 mg/dL. Blood pressures were evaluated using automated oscillometric devices at 3 and 12 months after entry. Patients were evaluated on an intention to treat basis. Blood pressures did not differ between groups overall at 3 or 12 months, although the PTRA group was taking fewer medications (2.1 + 1.3 vs. 3.2 + 1.5 defined daily doses; $P < .001$). The authors concluded that in the treatment of hypertension and RAS, "angioplasty has little advantage over antihypertensive drug therapy."[135] Many critics emphasize, however, that 22 of 50 patients (44%) assigned to medical therapy were considered treatment failures and referred for PTRA after 3 months. There were eight cases of total arterial occlusion in the medical group, as compared with none in the angioplasty group.

Many clinicians interpret these data to support an important role for PTRA in the management of patients with refractory hypertension and RAS. Regardless, the results of these trials indicate that benefits of endovascular procedures, even in the short term, are moderate compared with effective antihypertensive therapy. Patients failing to respond to medical therapy often improve after revascularization. Some authors have combined these prospective studies into meta-analyses, indicating that taken together, renal revascularization produces modest but definite reductions in blood pressures, averaging –7/–3 mm Hg.[227,244,245]

### STENTS FOR PROGRESSION OF RENAL INSUFFICIENCY AND CARDIOVASCULAR OUTCOMES

Several prospective RCTs have sought to compare medical therapy with endovascular stenting targeted primarily to the progression of chronic kidney disease (CKD) and/or adverse cardiovascular (CV) outcomes, such as stroke and coronary disease events. Among these, the largest are the US-based CORAL trial and the UK-based ASTRAL trial (see Table 47.6).[98,246] Although these have been published and add important information, they have substantial limitations.

CORAL was designed to test whether renal artery stenting, when added to optimal (standardized) medical therapy, including blockade of the renin-angiotensin system, improves CV outcomes for individuals with atherosclerotic RAS.[98] The authors listed more than 110 participating centers, with a total of 947 participants enrolled over a 5-year period to stenting plus medical therapy (467 patients) or to medical therapy alone (480 patients). Average entry estimated GFR (eGFR) values were 58 mL/min/1.73 $m^2$. This trial attempted to standardize the evaluation of stenosis by requiring translesional gradient measurement and review by an angiographic core laboratory. After a mean follow-up of 43 months, no differences were apparent for any or all of the composite endpoints—death from CV or renal causes, myocardial infarction, stroke, hospitalization for CHF, progressive renal insufficiency, or the need for renal replacement therapy—between the stent and medical therapy alone groups (35.1% and 35.8%, respectively; hazard ratio, 0.94; 95% confidence interval, 0.76–1.17; $P = .58$).[98] Systolic blood pressure was slightly lower in the revascularization arm (−2.3 mm Hg). Post hoc analysis of 413 participants in CORAL, with a urine albumin-to-creatinine ratio below the median (22.5 mg/g), showed reduced cardiovascular event rates and improved mortality compared with those with higher entry levels of proteinuria.[3] Importantly, procedural complications per vessel treated were only 5.2% in the stent group (Box 47.4). CORAL has several important limitations, which are discussed elsewhere and listed later.[1,115]

The authors acknowledged that recruitment for CORAL was difficult and took longer than anticipated. Most centers enrolled fewer than 10 subjects over the 4- to 5-year period. Several criteria for enrollment and intervention changed during the trial. The original intention had been to include patients with severe RAS and systolic blood pressure above 155 mm Hg while receiving two or more antihypertensive medications. "Severe RAS" was defined as more than 80% stenosis in isolation or 60% to 80% with a gradient of at least 20 mm Hg. As the protocols evolved, patients could be enrolled with or without hypertension if their eGFR was less than 60 mL/min/1.73 m$^2$. Requirements for translesional gradients were dropped, and patients could be enrolled using duplex ultrasound, MRA, or CTA criteria. Ultimately, the average level of stenosis (67%) measured in the core laboratory was lower than estimates by the investigators on site (73%).

As with other RCTs, it is likely that many of these lesions were below the threshold of 75% to 80% usually required to produce a reduction in blood flow in experimental studies. Of these patients, 25% had reached goal blood pressures before entry. Specific high-risk groups, including those with CHF within 30 days, were excluded. Based on Medicare claims data indicating more than 20,000 renal artery stent procedures annually (estimates from 2000), it is clear that screening and enrollment for CORAL included only a small fraction of treatment candidates, for whom no contemporaneous US registry comparison is available. Based on difficult enrollment and relaxed criteria, it appears that the CORAL cohort represented a relatively low-risk atherosclerotic population. This is supported by well-preserved levels of eGFR at baseline, easily controlled blood pressures, and exclusion of recent CHF and low 5-year CV mortality. Remarkably, fewer than 5% of enrolled patients died of cardiovascular causes during CORAL, substantially less than the registry population reported by Ritchie and associates,[108] and less even than the ASTRAL cohort,[121] which specifically excluded patients that clinicians thought would definitely benefit from revascularization.

Results from the Angioplasty and Stenting for Renal Atherosclerotic Lesions (ASTRAL) trial from the United Kingdom were published for 806 subjects followed for several years.[246] The mean serum creatinine level was above 2.0 mg/dL, and the severity of vascular occlusion estimated by a variety of imaging methods was above 70%. Patients were considered eligible for the trial if clinicians were uncertain about optimal management. No differences were apparent regarding changes in kidney function, blood pressure, hospitalizations, mortality, or episodes of circulatory congestion.[121] Rates of progression to a renal endpoint were 16% to 22% in both medically treated and revascularized groups. A smaller trial, Stent Placement in patients with Atherosclerotic Renal Artery Stenosis (STAR), enrolled 140 subjects and aimed to evaluate progression of CKD based on initial creatinine clearance of less than 80 mL/min and atherosclerotic stenosis of over 50%. No differences in change in creatinine clearance were detected at 2 years, although some substantial complications occurred in the stent-treated group.[120] This study highlights the drawbacks of including trivial vascular lesions in a treatment trial. Only 46 of 64 patients assigned to stent therapy underwent stenting, predominantly because lesions were often not hemodynamically significant.

These modest benefits present a striking contrast between the current era and a few decades ago. Reports from the 1970s underscore the fact that some patients experienced recurrent episodes of malignant phase hypertension, with encephalopathy, fluid retention, and progressive renal insufficiency. Since then, malignant hypertension has become

**Box 47.4 Complications After Percutaneous Transluminal Renal Angioplasty and Stenting of the Renal Arteries**

Minor—most frequently reported)
- Groin hematoma
- Puncture site trauma

Major—reported in 71/799 treated arteries (9%)[249]
- Hemorrhage requiring transfusion
- Femoral artery pseudoaneurysm needing repair
- Brachial artery traumatic injury needing repair
- Renal artery perforation leading to surgical intervention
- Stent thrombosis, surgical or antithrombotic intervention
- Distal renal artery embolus
- Iliac artery dissection
- Segmental renal infarction
- Cholesterol embolism: renal
- Peripheral atheroemboli
- Aortic dissection[167]
- Restenosis, 16% (range, 0%–39%)
- Deterioration of renal function: 26% (range, 0%–45%)

Combined complication rate over 24 months—stenting after failed PTRA, 24%[222]

Mortality attributed to procedure, 0.5%

Procedure-related complications—51/379 patients in 10 series, 13.5%

Procedural complications reported from CORAL angiographic core laboratoryt (2014)[159]
- Dissection 11/495 (2.2%)
- Branch occlusion 6/495 (1.2%)
- Distal embolization 6/495 (1.2%)

Single events—wire perforation, vessel rupture, pseudoaneurysm

Total events: 26/495 (5.2%)

*PTRA, Percutaneous transluminal renal angioplasty.*

**Table 47.7 Clinical Scenarios in Which Treatment of Significant Renal Artery Stenosis May Be Considered[a]**

| Type of Care | Examples |
|---|---|
| Appropriate care | • Cardiac disturbance syndromes (flash pulmonary edema or acute coronary syndrome [ACS]) with severe hypertension<br>• Resistant hypertension (HTN; uncontrolled with failure of maximally tolerated doses of at least three antihypertensive agents, one of which is a diuretic, or intolerance to medications)<br>• Ischemic nephropathy with chronic kidney disease (CKD), with eGFR <45 mL/min/1.73 $m^2$ and global renal ischemia (unilateral significant RAS with a solitary kidney or bilateral significant RAS) without other explanation |
| May be appropriate care | • Unilateral RAS with CKD (eGFR <45 mL/min/1.73 $m^2$)<br>• Unilateral RAS with prior episodes of congestive heart failure (stage C)<br>• Anatomically challenging or high-risk lesion (early bifurcation, small vessel, severe concentric calcification, severe aortic atheroma or mural thrombus) |
| Rarely appropriate care | • Unilateral, solitary, or bilateral RAS with controlled BP and normal renal function.<br>• Unilateral, solitary, or bilateral RAS with kidney size <7 cm in pole to pole length<br>• Unilateral, solitary, or bilateral RAS with chronic end-stage kidney disease on hemodialysis >3 months<br>• Unilateral, solitary, or bilateral renal artery chronic total occlusion |

[a]Significant RAS is an angiographically moderate lesion (50%–70%) with physiologic confirmation of severity or >70% stenosis.
*BP*, Blood pressure; *eGFR*, estimated glomerular filtration rate.
Modified from Parikh SA, Shishehbor MH, Gray BH, et al. SCAI expert consensus statement for renal artery stenting appropriate use. *Catheter Cardiovasc Intervent.* 2014;84:1163–1171.

less prevalent in most Western countries. The introduction of ACE inhibitors and calcium channel blockers in the 1980s led to reductions in the number of people with severe hypertension and improved the medical management of patients with high-renin states, including renovascular hypertension. Results from the prospective trials of angioplasty are less favorable now than those from retrospective series. A registry report from 2002 of over 1000 successfully stented patients has suggested that average blood pressure levels fall during follow-up, −21/−10 mm Hg[143] (see Fig. 47.23). The differences between prospective trials and registry data may reflect outcome reporting bias. Alternatively, enrollment in prospective trials itself may reflect recruitment bias in favor of more stable patients in less urgent clinical need of restoring renal circulation. Hence, the randomized trials almost certainly underestimate the benefits of renal revascularization for patients at the greatest risk of accelerated hypertension and/or renal failure.[185,227] Taken together, however, results of recent trials underscore the efficacy of medical therapy for many patients and weaken the argument for revascularization for moderate atherosclerotic RAS. Recent consensus recommendations regarding appropriate use of renal revascularization from the Society for Cardiovascular Angiography and Interventions are summarized in Table 47.7.[185]

## COMPLICATIONS OF RENAL ARTERY ANGIOPLASTY AND STENTING

Atherosclerotic plaque is commonly composed of multiple layers, with calcified, fibrotic, and inflammatory components. The physical expansion of such lesions applies considerable force on the wall and may lead to cracking and release of particulate debris into the bloodstream. Effective balloon angioplasty and stenting require techniques to limit damage to blood vessels during the procedure. A review of 10 published series with 416 stented vessels has indicated that significant complications arise in 13% of cases, not counting those that lead to the need for dialysis.[9] Complications are listed in Box 47.4; these include hematomas and retroperitoneal bleeding requiring transfusion. On average, renal function deteriorated in 26% of subjects in these series, and 50% (7 of 14) of those with preprocedure creatinine levels above 400 μmol (4.5 mg/dL) progressed to ESKD requiring dialysis.[237] Follow-up data regarding both mortality and ESKD for recent stented cohorts tend to support these observations.[122] Most complications are minor, including local hematomas and false aneurysms at the insertion site. Occasional severe complications develop, including aortic dissection,[236] stent migration, and vessel occlusion with thrombosis.[9] Local renal dissections can be managed by the judicious application of additional stents. Mortality related directly to this procedure is low, but has been reported in 0.5% to 1.5% of patients.[237,247]

Restenosis remains a significant clinical limitation. Rates vary widely, from 13% to 30%, usually developing within the first 6 to 12 months.[226,248,249] Most more recent series have reported 13% to 16% restenosis, sometimes leading to repeat procedures.[226]

## RENAL DENERVATION

Activation of sympathoadrenergic pathways has long been recognized as a major regulatory pathway for blood pressure. Studies of the renal nerves identify afferent and efferent signaling between the kidney and brain.[250,251] These pathways affect numerous mechanisms, including renin release, sodium transport, and peripheral sympathetic nerve activity. Clinical studies in patients with resistant hypertension have indicated that systemic blood pressures fall after bilateral renal denervation using radiofrequency or ultrasonic energy.[252,253] Initial studies suggested that reductions in blood pressure may exceed 34/14 mm Hg after 36 months.[254] Follow-up studies in wider ranges of patients using sham controls had smaller decrements in pressure, in the range of 14 mm Hg systolic as compared with 11 mm Hg in controls.[255] Additional studies in less resistant subjects have observed decreases of 6 to 8 mm Hg (systolic) as compared with controls.[253,256] The durability of these changes is not yet known, and most patients continue to require antihypertensive drug therapy. Experimental studies in RVD rats have indicated that denervation may reduce blood pressure and vascular remodeling. Importantly, human studies using endovascular denervation have excluded patients with RVD to this point, specifically to minimize safety concerns regarding renal arterial injury.

## SURGICAL TREATMENT OF RENOVASCULAR HYPERTENSION AND ISCHEMIC NEPHROPATHY

Early experience with vascular disease of the kidney was based entirely on surgical intervention, either nephrectomy or vascular reconstruction, with the objective of "surgical curability."[6] For that reason, much of the original data regarding split renal function measurement was geared toward identifying functionally significant lesions as a guide for patient selection for a major surgical procedure. Surgical intervention is less commonly performed today and is usually reserved for complex vascular reconstruction and/or failed endovascular procedures. Generally, age and comorbidities in patients with atherosclerotic disease favor endovascular procedures, when feasible.

Methods of surgical intervention have changed over the decades. A review in 1982 emphasized the role for ablative techniques, including partial nephrectomy.[257] The use of ablative operative means was guided by the difficulty of controlling blood pressure during this period. Such interventions have become less common since the introduction of effective medication regimens. In some cases, nephrectomy of a totally infarcted kidney provides major improvement in blood pressure control at low operative risk. The introduction of laparoscopic surgical techniques makes nephrectomy technically easier in some patients for whom vascular reconstruction is not an option. These series reflect widely variable methods of determining blood pressure benefit, as discussed later.[183,257]

Surgical series from the 1960s and early 1970s indicated that cure of hypertension occurred in only 30% to 40% of subjects, despite attempts at preselection.[6,258] Survival of groups chosen for surgery appeared to be better than those chosen for medical management. This likely reflected the high preoperative risks identified in those for whom surgery was excluded. The cooperative study of RVD in the 1960s and 1970s examined many of the clinical characteristics of renovascular hypertension.[33] These studies identified some of the limitations and hazards of surgical intervention and reported mortality rates of 6.8%, even in excellent institutions. The mean age in this series was 50.5 years. Definitions of operative mortality included events as late as 375 days after the procedure and may have overestimated the hazard. Had the authors considered only deaths within the first week, for example, the immediate perioperative mortality would be 1.7%.

The subsequent development of improved techniques for patient selection, including screening for coronary and carotid disease, for renal artery bypass and endarterectomy, and for combined aortic and renal artery repair have altered the practice of vascular surgery.[6,259] Some options developed for renal artery reconstruction are listed in Box 47.5. Most methods focus on reconstruction of the vascular supply for preservation of the nephron mass. Transaortic endarterectomy can effectively restore circulation to both kidneys. It requires aortic cross-clamping and may be undertaken as part of a combined procedure with aortic replacement. Identification and treatment of carotid and coronary disease have led to reductions in surgical morbidity and mortality. By addressing associated CV risk before surgery, early surgical mortality falls below 2% for patients without other major diseases.[260]

Surgical reconstruction of the renal blood supply usually requires access to the aorta. A variety of alternative surgical procedures have been designed to avoid manipulation of the badly diseased aorta or when previous surgical procedures make access difficult. These include extraanatomic repair of the renal artery using hepatorenal or splenorenal conduits that avoid manipulation of a badly diseased aorta.[261] An example of contemporary surgical reconstruction to protect renal function is illustrated in Fig. 47.26. Success with extrarenal conduits depends on the integrity of the alternative blood supply. Hence, careful preoperative assessment of stenotic orifices of the celiac axis is undertaken before using the hepatic or splenic arteries. Results of these procedures have been good, both in short- and long-term follow-up studies.[262] Analysis of 222 patients treated over 10 years earlier has shown that these procedures were performed with 2.2% mortality, low rates of restenosis (7.3%), and good long-term survival.[262] The predictors of late mortality were age older than 60 years, coronary disease, and previous vascular surgery.

The durability of surgical vascular reconstruction is well established. Follow-up studies after 5 and 10 years for all forms of renal artery bypass procedures indicate excellent

**Box 47.5 Surgical Procedures Applied to Reconstruction of the Renal Artery and/or Reversal of Renovascular Hypertension**

Ablative surgery: removal of a "pressor" kidney
- Nephrectomy: direct or laparoscopic
- Partial nephrectomy

Renal artery reconstruction (requires aortic approach)
- Renal endarterectomy
- Transaortic endarterectomy
- Resection and reanastomosis: suitable for focal lesions
- Aortorenal bypass graft

Extraanatomic procedures (may avoid direct manipulation of the aorta)—require adequate alternate circulation without stenosis at celiac origin
- Splenorenal bypass graft
- Hepatorenal bypass graft
- Gastroduodenal, superior mesenteric, iliac to renal bypass grafts
- Autotransplantation with exvivo reconstruction

Modified from Bower TC, Oderich GS. *Surgical Revascularization.* London: Springer; 2014; and Libertino JA, Zinman L. Surgery for renovascular hypertension. In: Breslin DL, Swinton NW, Libertino JA, Zinman L, eds. *Renovascular hypertension.* Baltimore: Williams and Wilkins; 1982:166–212.

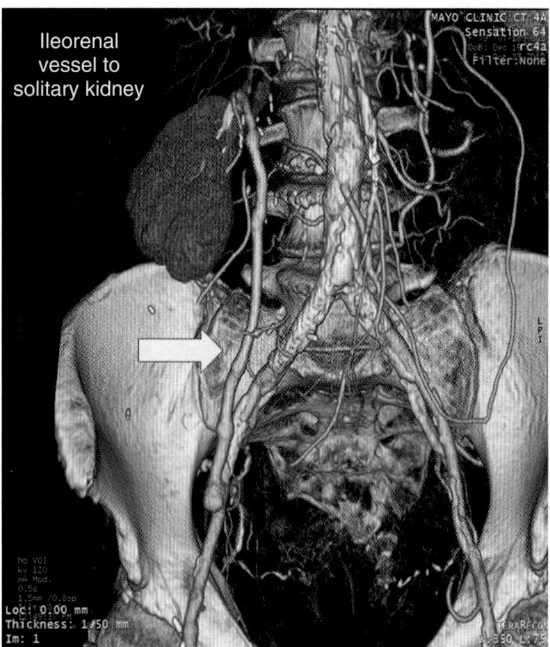


Fig. 47.26 Computed tomography angiogram illustrating complex surgical repair of aortic and vascular perfusion to a solitary functioning kidney. There is a vascular graft from the right common iliac artery to the right renal artery *(arrow)*. Although surgical reconstruction of the renal vessels is less commonly performed since the introduction of endovascular techniques, it provides an essential alternative for complex occlusive disease and failed endovascular stenting in selected patients.

long-term patency (>90%), both for renal artery procedures alone and when combined with aortic reconstruction.[263] Results of surgery have been good, despite increasing age of subjects in the reported series. Patient selection has been important in all these series. Although long-term outcome data are established for surgery, limited information is available for endovascular stent procedures, which are more prone to restenosis and technical failure. Some studies have compared endovascular intervention (PTRA without stents) and surgical repair. A single study of nonostial, unilateral atherosclerotic disease, in which patients were randomly assigned to surgery or PTRA, has shown that although surgical success rates were higher and PTRA was needed on a repeat basis in several cases, the 2-year patency rates were 90% for PTRA and 97% for surgery.[264] A prospective comparison of endovascular stents compared with open surgical renal revascularization has suggested that patency over 4 years is better with open surgical repair, but that overall the outcome of the two procedures does not differ.[265]

In many institutions, surgical reconstruction of the renal arteries is now most often undertaken as part of aortic surgery.[266] In one series, patients with impaired renal function (creatinine >2.0 mg/dL) underwent simultaneous aortic and renal procedures in 75% of cases.[233] Studies have indicated that combining renal revascularization with aortic repair does not increase the risk of the aortic operation. As with endovascular techniques, the results regarding changes in renal function include improvement in 22% to 26%, no change in 46% to 52% (some consider this as stabilization), and progressive deterioration in 18% to 22% (Fig. 47.27).

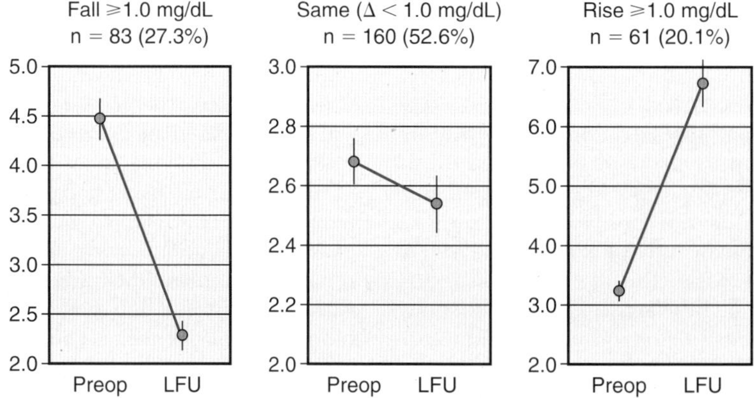


Fig. 47.27 Renal functional outcomes after surgical renal revascularization in 304 azotemic patients (creatinine >2.0 mg/dL) with atherosclerotic renal artery stenosis. On average, the mean serum creatinine level does not change during a follow-up period exceeding 36 months, as observed with most reported series. Group mean values obscure major differences in clinical outcomes, as shown here. Some patients experience major clinical benefit (defined as a fall in serum creatinine of >1.0 mg/dL; *left panel*). The largest group has minor changes (<1.0 mg/dL), which might be considered "stabilization" of renal function. The degree of benefit in these patients depends on whether renal function has been deteriorating before intervention. The data for the group in the *right panel* emphasize the failure to observe consistent overall improvement in function because 18% to 22% of patients developed worsening renal function. The exact causes of this deterioration are not clear, although atherosclerotic disease is responsible for a portion. This potential hazard of revascularization must be considered when offering these procedures. *LFU,* Latest follow-up: *RAS*, renin angiotensin system (Modified from Textor SC, Wilcox CS: Renal artery stenosis: a common, treatable cause of renal failure? *Annu Rev Med.* 2001;52:421–442.)

**Table 47.8 Selected Series of Surgical Renal Artery Revascularization, 2000–2005**

| | | No. of Patients (%) | | Renal Function Response (%) | | Hypertension Response (%) | | Perioperative Outcome (%) | |
|---|---|---|---|---|---|---|---|---|---|
| **Source** | **No. of Patients** | Bilateral Repair | Preoperative RI | Improved | Unchanged | Cured | Improved or stable | Death | Morbidity |
| Hansen | 232 | 64 | 100 | 58 | 35 | 11 | 76 | 7.3 | 30 |
| Paty[a] | 414 | NR | 4 | 26 | 68 | NR | | 5.5 | 11.4 |
| Cherr | 500 | 59 | 49 | 43 | 47 | 73 | 12 | 4.6 | 16 |
| Marone | 96 | 27 | 100 | 42 | 41 | NR | | 4.1 | NR |
| Mozes | 198 | 65 | 57 | 28 | 67 | 2 | 59 | 2.5 | 19 |

[a]Patients operated for hypertension or renal salvage. Improvement was noted in 26%, 68% remained stable, and 6% worsened. Specific renal function decline occurred in 3%.

*NR,* No response; *RI,* resistive index.

Modified from Bower TC, Oderich GS. *Surgical revascularization.* London: Springer; 2014.

Using intraoperative color flow Doppler ultrasound allows for the immediate correction of suboptimal results and improves long-term patency.[267] Results from several surgical series are summarized in Table 47.8. Despite good results, the number of open operations for renal artery revascularization continues to decline. A review of the national inpatient sample indicates relatively high mortality rates (≈10%) overall, leading the authors to support lower-risk endovascular methods, where possible, or referral to high-volume surgical centers.[268] For experienced centers using current techniques, operative risk is below 4% in good risk candidates.[269,270] Risk factors for higher risk include advanced age, elevated creatinine level (>2.7–3.0 mg/dL), and associated aortic or other vascular disease.

Studies in patients with bilateral renal artery lesions or vascular occlusion to the entire renal mass have indicated that restoration of blood flow can lead to the preservation of renal function in some cases.[271] Usually this has been undertaken when evidence for preserved blood supply, sometimes from capsular vessels, is evident by renography. Occasionally, revascularization can lead to functional recovery sufficient to eliminate the need for dialysis.

## PREDICTORS OF LIKELY BENEFIT REGARDING RENAL REVASCULARIZATION

Identification of patients most likely to improve blood pressure and/or renal function after renal revascularization remains elusive. As noted previously, functional tests of renin release, such as measurement of renal vein renin levels, have not performed universally well. Many of these studies are most useful when positive, for example, the likelihood of benefit improves with more evident lateralization, but have relatively poor negative predictive value—that is when such studies are negative, outcomes of vessel repair may still be beneficial. Clinically, recent progression of hypertension, deterioration of renal function, and/or pulmonary edema remain among the most consistent predictors of improved blood pressure after intervention.

*Clinical Relevance*

**Predictors**

Progressive hypertension, worsening renal function, and pulmonary edema are the most consistent predictors of improved blood pressure after revascularization.

Predicting favorable renal functional outcomes is also difficult. Surgical and endovascular procedures are least likely to benefit those with advanced renal insufficiency, usually characterized by a serum creatinine level above 3.0 mg/dL. Nonetheless, occasional patients with recent progression to advanced renal dysfunction can recover their GFR, with durable improvement over many years (see Fig. 47.27). Small kidneys, as identified by length less than 8 cm, are less likely to recover function, particularly when little function can be identified on radionuclide renography.[272] Reports of the renal resistance index measured by Doppler ultrasound in 5950 patients have indicated that identification of lower resistance was a favorable marker for improvement in GFR and blood pressure, whereas an elevated resistance index was an independent marker of poor outcomes[159] (see Fig. 47.20). None of these associations are absolute, and recent studies have identified favorable outcomes in some patients with adverse predictors.[247] As noted, outcomes for patients with a low urinary albumin-to-creatinine ratio are distinctly better than for those with higher levels.[3,122] Some authors have suggested that detecting abnormalities in fractional flow reserve measured by translesional flows and gradients after dilation with papaverine may predict benefits of revascularization.[189,273] Recent deterioration of kidney function or hypertension portends a more likely improvement with revascularization.

## FUTURE RESEARCH IN RENOVASCULAR DISEASE

How best to identify and recover filtration in poststenotic kidneys remains a challenging area of investigation. Measurement of renal vein cytokines have indicated that poststenotic kidneys exhibit abundant proinflammatory signaling, even

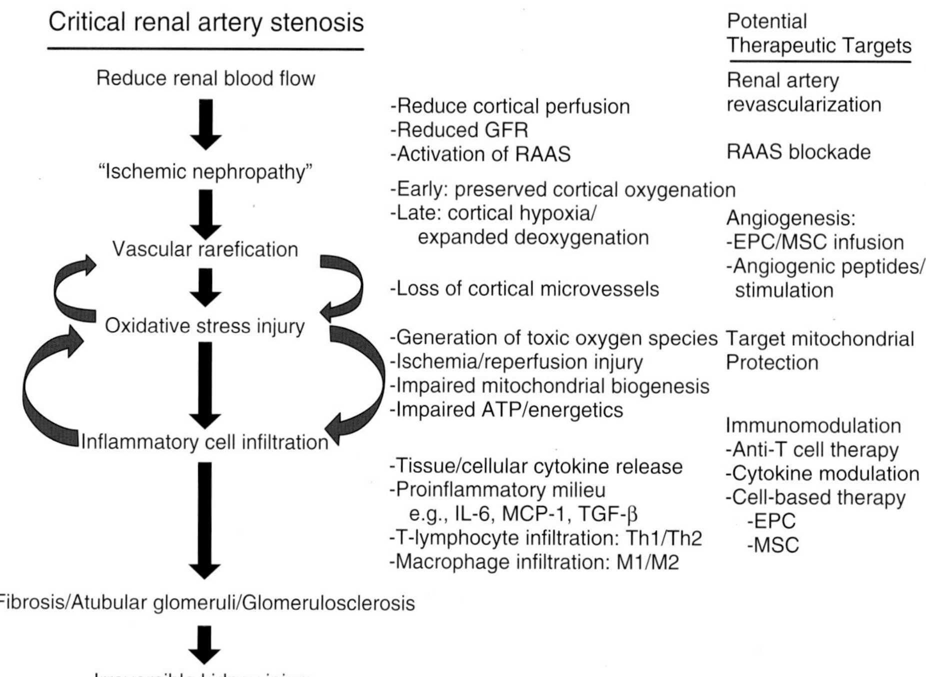


**Fig. 47.28** Injury pathways and targets in renovascular disease. The working diagram highlights recent experimental studies delineating specific pathways of oxidative stress injury and inflammatory injury pathways in the poststenotic kidney. *Right panel,* Specific therapeutic targets are identified that may alleviate these injury pathways, over and above simply restoring blood flow. Many of these pathways likely overlap in many forms of kidney injury. *EPC,* Endothelial progenitor cells; *GFR,* glomerular filtration rate; *IL-6,* interleukin 6; *MCP,* monocyte chemoattractant protein; *RAAS,* renin-angiotensin-aldosterone system; *TGF-β,* transforming growth factor beta. (From Textor SC, Lerman LO. Paradigm shifts in atherosclerotic renovascular disease: where are we now? *J Am Soc Nephrol.* 2015;26:2074–2080.)

with relatively preserved oxygenation.[241] Studies of human kidneys undergoing temporary arterial occlusion have indicated that mitochondrial swelling and disruption develop rapidly.[274] These data support experimental models showing increased oxidative stress and mitochondrial dysfunction under conditions of chronically reduced renal blood flow.[275,276] Protection of mitochondrial structure and function using infused agents that stabilize cardiolipin and inhibit opening of the mitochondrial transition pore appears to facilitate microvascular recovery and kidney regeneration after renal revascularization.[51] Preliminary studies in human subjects have supported this approach.[277]

Some studies have emphasized the role of inflammatory pathways and accumulation of activated T cells and macrophages with vessels and tissue of the atherosclerotic kidney.[32] Experimental models using infused endothelial progenitor cells[56] and mesenchymal stem cells[278] respond to revascularization with improved microvascular regeneration. Initial studies in human atherosclerotic RAS using autologous mesenchymal stem cells delivered into the renal artery have suggested that cortical blood flow and tissue oxygenation increase over a 3-month period.[279]

Recognition of the role and interactions among these pathways offers the possibility for targeted therapy in patients with occlusive RVD. Some of these are highlighted in Fig. 47.28.

## SUMMARY

RVD is common, particularly in older subjects with other atherosclerotic disease. It can have multiple clinical consequences, ranging from asymptomatic incidentally discovered disease to accelerated hypertension and progressive renal failure. With improved imaging and increasing patient age, significant renal artery disease is being detected more frequently. The clinician must evaluate the impact of the renal artery disease in the individual patient and the potential risk-benefit ratio for renal revascularization. Many patients with fibromuscular dysplasia and other disorders benefit from restoring renal artery patency in terms of blood pressure control. An algorithm to guide the treatment and reevaluation of patients with atherosclerotic RAS is presented in Fig. 47.29. Application of this strategy relies heavily on considering comorbid risks and the evolution of blood pressure control and kidney function over time. The management of cardiovascular risk and hypertension are the primary objectives of medical therapy.

For most patients, the realistic goals of renal revascularization are to reduce blood pressure medication requirements and stabilize renal function over time. Patients with bilateral disease or stenosis in a solitary functioning kidney may have a lower risk of circulatory congestion (flash pulmonary edema or its equivalent) and lower risk for advancing renal failure after revascularization of the kidney. It is essential to appreciate the risks inherent in surgical or endovascular manipulation of the diseased aorta. These include atheroembolic complications and potential deterioration of renal function related to the procedure itself (estimated at 20% for patients with preexisting kidney dysfunction). Hence, the decision to undertake these procedures should include consideration of whether the potential gain warrants such risks. In many cases, improved blood pressure and recovery of renal function

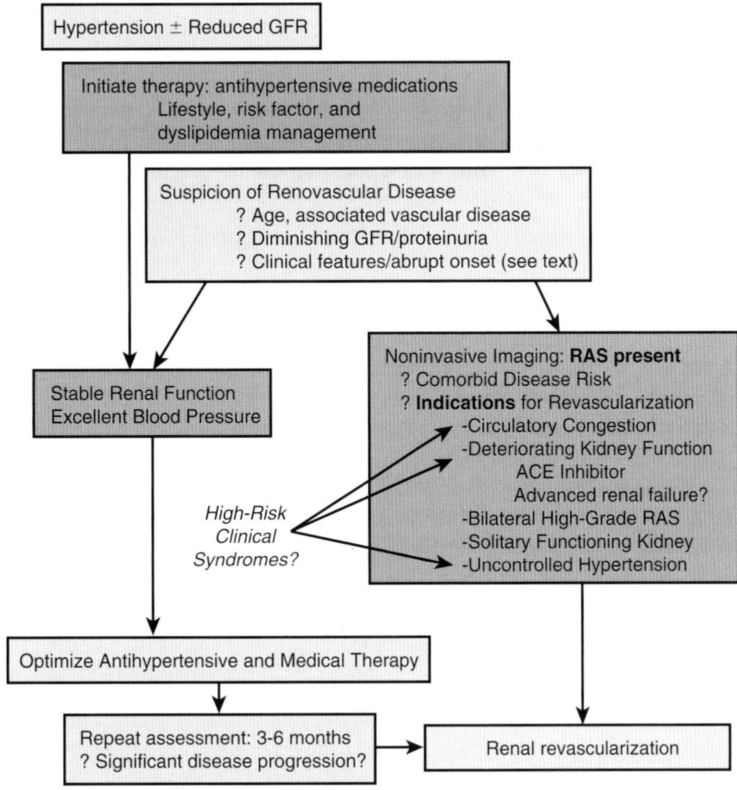


**Fig. 47.29** Algorithm summarizing a management scheme for patients with renovascular hypertension and/or ischemic nephropathy. Optimizing antihypertensive and medical therapy for comorbid conditions, including dyslipidemia and smoking, is paramount to reducing cardiovascular morbidity and mortality in atherosclerotic disease. Decisions regarding the timing of renal revascularization procedures depend on the clinical manifestations (see text) and whether blood pressures and kidney function remain stable. *ACE,* Angiotensin-converting enzyme; *GFR,* glomerular filtration rate; *PTRA,* percutaneous renal angioplasty; *RAS,* renal artery stenosis.

justify the costs and hazards. Long-term follow-up of blood pressure and renal function is important in all cases, whether revascularization is performed or not, particularly because of the potential for disease progression, restenosis, and/or recurrent disease. Optimal selection and timing for medical management and revascularization depend largely on the comorbid conditions for each patient.

 Complete reference list available at ExpertConsult.com.

## KEY REFERENCES

9. Textor SC, Misra S, Oderich G. Percutaneous revascularization for ischemic nephropathy: the past, present and future. *Kidney Int.* 2013;83(1):28–40.
36. Gloviczki ML, Glockner JF, Lerman LO, et al. Preserved oxygenation despite reduced blood flow in poststenotic kidneys in human atherosclerotic renal artery stenosis. *Hypertension.* 2010;55(4):961–966.
81. Olin JW, Gornik HL, Bacharach JM, et al. Fibromuscular dysplasia: state of the science and critical unanswered questions: a scientific statement from the American Heart Association. *Circulation.* 2014;129(9):1048–1078.
92. Garovic VD, Textor SC. Renovascular hypertension and ischemic nephropathy. *Circulation.* 2005;112(9):1362–1374.
97. Kalra PA, Guo H, Kausz AT, et al. Atherosclerotic renovascular disease in United States patients aged 67 years or older: risk factors, revascularization and prognosis. *Kidney Int.* 2005;68:293–301.
98. Cooper CJ, Murphy TP, Cutlip DE, et al. Stenting and medical therapy for atherosclerotic renal-artery stenosis. *N Engl J Med.* 2014;370(1):13–22.
104. Messerli FH, Bangalore S, Makani H, et al. Flash pulmonary oedema and bilateral renal artery stenosis: the Pickering Syndrome. *Eur Heart J.* 2011;32(18):2231–2237.
108. Ritchie J, Green D, Chrysochou C, et al. High-risk clinical presentations in atherosclerotic renovascular disease: prognosis and response to renal artery revascularization. *Am J Kidney Dis.* 2014;63(2):186–197.
122. Misra S, Khosla A, Allred J, et al. Mortality and renal replacement therapy after renal artery stent placement for atherosclerotic renovascular disease. *J Vasc Interv Radiol.* 2016.
134. Caps MT, Perissinotto C, Zierler RE, et al. Prospective study of atherosclerotic disease progression in the renal artery. *Circulation.* 1998;98:2866–2872.

# 48 Pregnancy and Kidney Disease

Sharon E. Maynard | S. Ananth Karumanchi | Ravi I. Thadhani

CHAPTER OUTLINE



KEY POINTS

- Preeclampsia is now considered a major risk factor for long-term cardiovascular disease, including stroke, end-stage kidney disease, and cardiovascular death. Women with a history of preeclampsia should be screened and treated for modifiable risk factors, such as diabetes, hypertension, tobacco use, and obesity.
- The 2013 American College of Obstetrics and Gynecology diagnostic criteria for preeclampsia include hypertension and EITHER proteinuria OR another feature of severe preeclampsia (Table 48.3).
- Intensive dialysis (≥36 hours/week) is associated with improved fertility and pregnancy outcomes in women with end-stage renal disease.
- Medications that are safe in pregnant transplant recipients include calcineurin inhibitors (tacrolimus and cyclosporine), azathioprine, and prednisone. Rapamycin and mycophenolate are teratogenic and contraindicated in pregnancy.

## INTRODUCTION

Pregnancy is characterized by a myriad of physiologic changes, of which the emergence of a placenta and growing fetus are the most dramatic. Hypertension and renal disease occurring in the setting of pregnancy present a unique set of clinical challenges. This chapter will include a detailed discussion of preeclampsia, a syndrome specific to pregnancy that remains one of the most enigmatic human disorders and continues to claim the lives of thousands of mothers and neonates yearly. The approach to acute renal failure in pregnancy will also be discussed. Current data on epidemiology and management of chronic hypertension, chronic renal disease, glomerular disease, and kidney transplantation in pregnancy will be reviewed. This chapter will offer the reader insights into the emerging understanding of the pathogenesis of preeclampsia, and provide a sound basis for the management of pregnancy from a nephrologist's perspective.

## PHYSIOLOGIC CHANGES OF PREGNANCY

### HEMODYNAMIC AND VASCULAR CHANGES OF NORMAL PREGNANCY

Normal pregnancy is characterized by profound vascular and hemodynamic changes that reach far beyond the fetus and placenta (Table 48.1). Early in pregnancy, systemic vascular resistance (SVR) decreases and arterial compliance increases.[1] These changes are evident by 6 weeks' gestation, prior to the establishment of the uteroplacental circulation.[2] This decrease in SVR leads directly to several other cardiovascular changes. Mean arterial blood pressure (BP) falls by an average of 10 mm Hg, reaching its lowest point at 18–24 weeks' gestation (Fig. 48.1). Sympathetic activity is increased, reflected in a 15% to 20% increase in heart rate.[3] The combination of increased heart rate and decreased afterload leads to a large increase in cardiac output in the early first trimester, which peaks at 50% above prepregnancy levels by the middle of the third trimester (Fig. 48.2).

**Table 48.1 Physiologic Changes in Pregnancy**

| Physiologic Variable | Change in Pregnancy |
|---|---|
| **Hemodynamic Parameters** | |
| Plasma volume | Increases 30%–50% above baseline |
| Blood pressure | Decreases by approximately 10 mm Hg below prepregnancy level, with nadir in second trimester; gradual increase toward prepregnancy levels by term |
| Cardiac output | Increases 30%–50% |
| Heart rate | Increases by 15–20 beats/min |
| Renal blood flow | Increases to 80% above baseline |
| Glomerular filtration rate | 150–200 mL/min (increases to 40%–50% above baseline) |
| **Serum Chemistry and Hematologic Changes** | |
| Hemoglobin | Decreases by an average of 2 g/L (from 13 to 11 g/L) owing to plasma volume expansion out of proportion to the increase in red blood cell mass |
| Creatinine | Decreases to 0.4–0.5 mg/dL |
| Uric acid | Decreases to a nadir of 2.0–3.0 mg/dL by 22–24 weeks, then increases back to nonpregnant levels toward term |
| pH | Increases slightly to 7.44 |
| Partial pressure of carbon dioxide ($pCO_2$) | Decreases by approximately 10 mm Hg to an average of 27–32 mm Hg |
| Calcium | Increased calcitriol stimulates increases in both intestinal calcium reabsorption and urinary calcium excretion |
| Sodium | Decreases by 4–5 mEq/L below nonpregnancy levels |
| Osmolality | Decreases to a new osmotic set point of approximately 270 mOsm/kg |

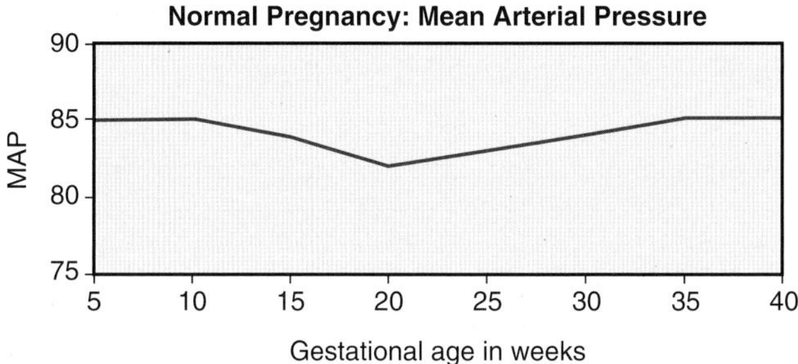


**Fig. 48.1** Changes in mean arterial pressure in normal pregnancy. Mean arterial blood pressure (MAP) according to gestational age in weeks in a large representative cohort of pregnant women followed longitudinally. (Adapted from Thadhani R, Ecker JL, Kettyle E, et al. Pulse pressure and risk of preeclampsia: a prospective study. *Obstet Gynecol.* 2001;97:515–520.)

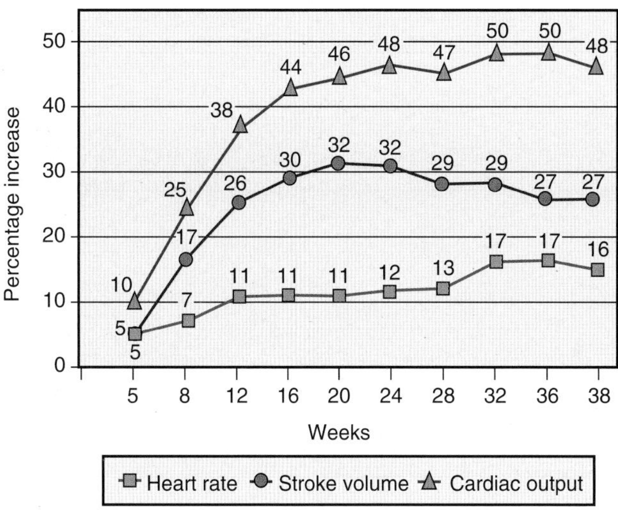


**Fig. 48.2** Hemodynamic changes in pregnancy. Shown are the percentage changes from prepregnancy values in heart rate, stroke volume, and cardiac output measured throughout pregnancy. (Modified from Robson SC, Hunter S, Boys RJ, et al. Serial study of factors influencing changes in cardiac output during human pregnancy. *Am J Physiol.* 1989;256:H1060–H1065.)

The renin–aldosterone–angiotensin system is activated in pregnancy,[4] leading to renal salt and water retention. Renal interstitial compliance is increased, whereby the renal interstitial pressure remains low despite increased renal interstitial volume. This may contribute to volume retention via an attenuation of the renal pressure natriuretic response.[5] Total body water increases by 6 to 8 liters, leading to both plasma volume and interstitial volume expansion. Thus most women have clinical edema at some point during pregnancy. There is also cumulative retention of about 950 mmol of sodium distributed between the maternal extracellular compartments and the fetus.[6] The plasma volume increases out of proportion to the red blood cell mass, leading to mild physiologic anemia.[7] Plasma volume expansion is followed by increased atrial natriuretic peptide secretion by the late first trimester.[2]

## RENAL ADAPTATION TO PREGNANCY

In pregnancy, the kidney length increases by 1–1.5 cm and kidney volume increases by up to 30%.[8] There is physiologic dilatation of the urinary collecting system in approximately 50% of pregnant women, more frequently on the right than the left (Fig. 48.3).[9] These changes may be due to mechanical compression of the ureters between the gravid uterus and the linea terminalis,[10] and the effects of estrogen, progesterone, and prostaglandins on ureteral structure and peristalsis. Hydronephrosis of pregnancy is usually asymptomatic, but abdominal pain, and rarely obstruction, can occur (see the "Obstructive Uropathy and Nephrolithiasis" section).

Glomerular filtration increases by about 40% within weeks of conception, and is maintained at this level until delivery. In early pregnancy, this is mediated primarily by an increase in renal plasma flow (Fig. 48.4). In the second half of pregnancy, renal plasma flow declines toward prepregnancy levels, yet glomerular filtration rate (GFR) remains high, reflecting relatively increased filtration fraction.[11] The maintenance of high GFR despite a fall in renal plasma flow is possible due to decreased capillary oncotic pressure and increased $K_f$ (the product of hydraulic permeability and total surface area available for filtration).[12]

The increase in GFR results in a physiologic decrease in serum creatinine, urea, and uric acid. Normal creatinine clearance in pregnancy rises to 150–200 mL/min, and average

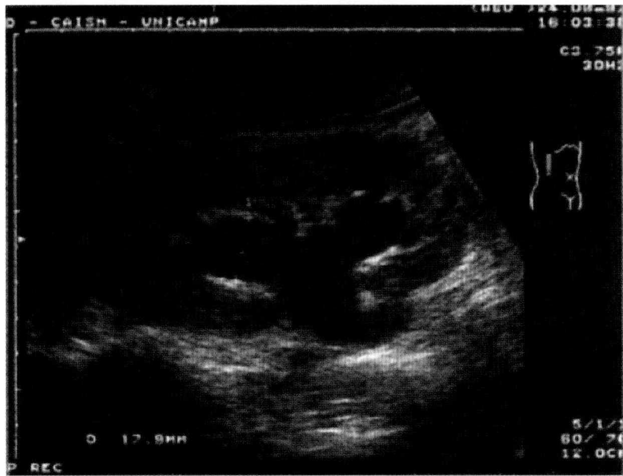

Fig. 48.3 Physiologic hydronephrosis. Renal ultrasound of the right kidney at 37 weeks' gestation, showing grade 3 (>15 mm) physiologic hydronephrosis of pregnancy. (From Faúndes A, Brícola-Filho M, Pinto e Silva JL. Dilatation of the urinary tract during pregnancy: proposal of a curve of maximal caliceal diameter by gestational age. *Am J Obstet Gynecol,* 1998;178:1082–1086.)

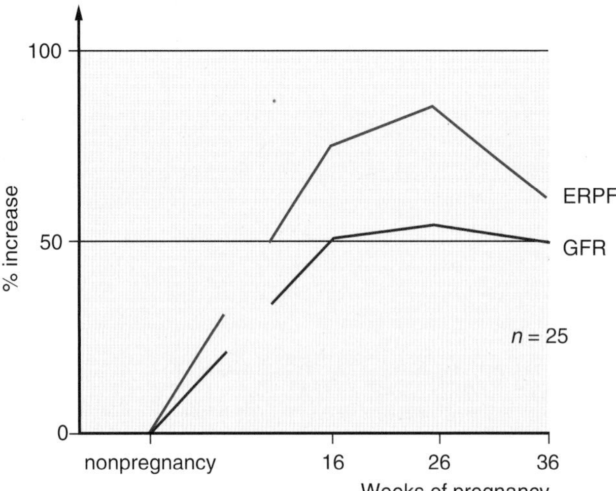


Fig. 48.4 Effect of pregnancy on glomerular filtration rate (GFR) and effective renal plasma flow (ERPF). Renal plasma flow rises out of proportion to the GFR, leading to a decrease in filtration fraction. Both GFR and ERPF peak at midgestation, at approximately 50% and 80% above prepregnancy levels, respectively, and decrease slightly toward term. (From Davison JM. Overview: kidney function in pregnant women. *Am J Kidney Dis.* 1987;9:248.)

serum creatinine falls from 0.8 to 0.5–0.6 mg/dL. Hence a serum creatinine of 1.0 mg/dL, which would be considered normal in a nonpregnant individual, reflects renal impairment in a pregnant woman. Similarly, urea (measured as blood urea nitrogen) falls from an average of 13 mg/dL in the nonpregnant state to approximately 8–10 mg/dL.

Urinary protein excretion rises in normal pregnancy from the nonpregnant level of about 100 to about 180–200 mg/day in the third trimester and occasionally up to 300 mg/day prior to delivery. In women carrying a multiple gestation, physiological proteinuria is even greater, with almost half of women excreting >300 mg/day.[13] This may result in positive urine dipstick testing for protein, particularly on a concentrated urine sample. The increased proteinuria in pregnancy results from a combination of increased GFR, increased permeability of the glomerular basement membrane, and reduced tubular reabsorption of filtered protein.[12] Likewise, women with preexisting proteinuric renal disease appear to have an exacerbation of proteinuria in the second and third trimesters, which is more exaggerated than that which would be expected from the increased GFR alone.[14] (see the "Chronic Kidney Disease in Pregnancy" section).

Serum uric acid declines in early pregnancy because of the rise in GFR, reaching a nadir of 2.0 to 3.0 mg/dL by 22–24 weeks.[15] Thereafter, the uric acid level begins to rise, reaching nonpregnant levels by term. The late gestational rise in uric acid levels is attributed to increased renal tubular absorption of urate.

Pregnancy is characterized by several changes in renal tubular function. Due to the large increase in GFR, glomerular tubular balance requires a concomitant increase in tubular solute reabsorption in order to avoid excessive renal losses. The kidney achieves this balance flawlessly, and sodium balance is maintained normally: pregnant women have normal excretion of an exogenous solute load, and appropriately conserve sodium when intake is restricted.[16]

The ability to excrete a water load is also normally maintained, albeit at a lower osmotic set point. The osmotic threshold for stimulation of both antidiuretic hormone release and thirst is decreased, by a mechanism that appears to be mediated by human chorionic gonadotropin (hCG)[17] and relaxin.[18] This results in mild hyponatremia: The serum sodium typically falls by 4–5 mM/L below nonpregnancy levels. Animal studies suggest that increased aquaporin 2 expression in the collecting tubule may contribute to this effect.[19]

Mild glycosuria and aminoaciduria can occur in normal pregnancy. This occurs in the absence of hyperglycemia or renal disease. These are thought to be due to a combination of the increased filtered load of glucose and amino acids and less efficient tubular reabsorption.

## RESPIRATORY ALKALOSIS OF PREGNANCY

Minute ventilation begins to rise by the end of the first trimester, and continues to increase until term. Progesterone mediates this response by direct stimulation of respiratory drive and by increasing sensitivity of the respiratory center to $CO_2$.[20] This results in a mild respiratory alkalosis—partial pressure of carbon dioxide ($pCO_2$) falls to approximately 27–32 mm Hg—and a compensatory increase in renal excretion of bicarbonate. This large increase in minute ventilation allows maintenance of high-normal partial pressure of oxygen ($pO_2$) despite the 20%–33% increase in oxygen consumption in pregnancy.

## DIABETES INSIPIDUS OF PREGNANCY

For reasons that are obscure, circulating levels of vasopressinase, an enzyme that hydrolyzes arginine vasopressin, are increased during normal pregnancy. The gene product mediating placental vasopressinase activity was recently characterized as a novel placental leucine aminopeptidase.[21] Occasionally, this increase is so pronounced that circulating antidiuretic hormone (arginine vasopressin) disappears, resulting in the polyuria and polydipsia of diabetes insipidus. This syndrome of transient diabetes insipidus presents during the second trimester and disappears after delivery.[22] It is important to recognize this entity because affected women may become dangerously hypernatremic, especially with cesarean section using general anesthesia and/or water restriction in the delivery room. The polyuria can be controlled by the administration of deamino-8-D-arginine vasopressin, which is not destroyed by vasopressinase.[23]

## MECHANISM OF VASODILATION IN PREGNANCY

The mechanisms mediating the widespread pregnancy-induced decrease in vascular tone are not fully understood. The fall in SVR is only partially attributable to the presence of the low-resistance circulation in the pregnant uterus, as BP and SVR are noted to fall before this system is well developed. Reduced vascular responsiveness to vasopressors such as angiotensin-2 ($AT_2$), norepinephrine, and vasopressin in pregnancy is well-documented (Fig. 48.5).[24] Altered vascular receptor expression may contribute to vascular relaxation in pregnancy. For example, animal studies suggest that gestational upregulation of the $AT_2$ receptor, which produces vasodilation rather than vasoconstriction when stimulated by $AT_2$, contributes to the fall in BP with pregnancy.[25,26] Multiple hormones and signaling pathways, including estrogen, progesterone, relaxin, and prostaglandins, also contribute to the systemic vasodilatory response.

Pregnancy differs fundamentally from other conditions of peripheral vasodilation, such as sepsis, cirrhosis, and high-output congestive heart failure, all of which are characterized by increased, rather than decreased, renal vascular resistance. This suggests that in pregnancy there is a specific renal vasodilating effect that overrides vasoconstricting factors such as renin–angiotensin–aldosterone activation. Recent advances—mostly from studies of pregnant rats—have suggested that the hormone relaxin is central to this global vasodilatory response, and specifically to the increase in glomerular filtration and renal blood flow.[27] Relaxin is a 6-kDa peptide hormone first isolated from pregnant serum in the 1920s and noted to produce relaxation of the pelvic ligaments.[28] Relaxin is released predominantly from the corpus luteum and rises early in gestation in response to hCG. Gestational renal hyperfiltration and vasodilation were completely abolished in pregnant rats administered relaxin neutralizing antibodies or lacking a functional corpus luteum, suggesting a critical role for relaxin in mediating the renal circulatory changes during pregnancy.[29] Relaxin acts by upregulating endothelin and nitric oxide production in the renal circulation, leading to generalized renal vasodilation, decreased renal afferent and efferent arteriolar resistance, and a subsequent increase in renal blood flow and GFR.[27]

The low-resistance, high-flow circulation of the fetoplacental unit also contributes to the low SVR characteristic of the second and third trimesters of pregnancy. During placental development, the high-resistance uterine arteries are transformed into larger-caliber capacitance vessels (Fig. 48.6). This transformation appears to be driven by invasion of the maternal spiral arteries by fetal-derived cytotrophoblasts, which transform from an epithelial to an endothelial phenotype as they replace the endothelium of the maternal spiral arteries.[30] The mechanisms governing this process, termed "pseudovasculogenesis," are still being elucidated. Angiogenic factors, such as vascular endothelial growth factor (VEGF) and angiopoietins, have a complex spatial and temporal expression in developing placenta, and these factors may be involved in placental vascular development.[31–33]

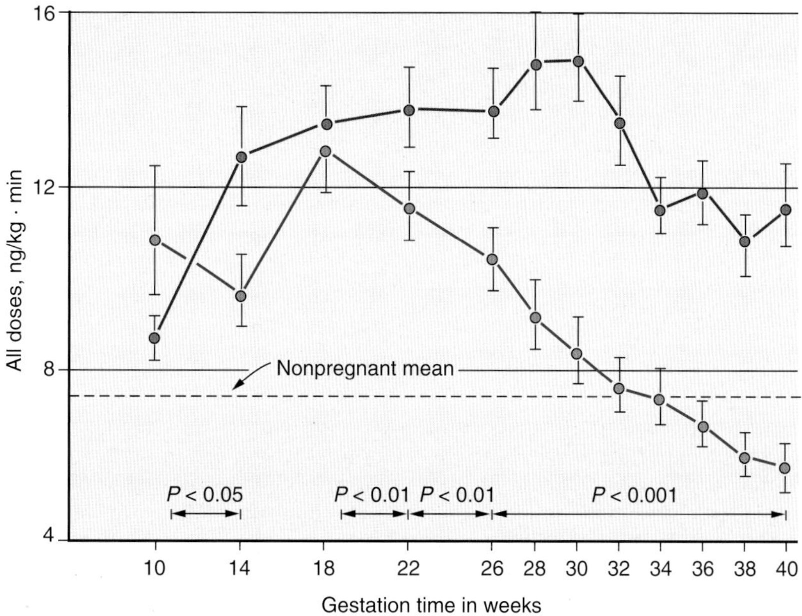


**Fig. 48.5** Effect of pregnancy on sensitivity to the pressor effects of angiotensin II. The ordinate displays the dose of angiotensin II needed to raise diastolic blood pressure by 20 mm Hg. In normal pregnancy (*red circles; N* = 120), a higher dose was required than for nonpregnant women *(dashed line).* In women in whom preeclampsia ultimately developed (*blue circles; N* = 72), insensitivity to angiotensin II was lost beginning in mid–second trimester. (From Gant NF, Daley GL, Chand S, et al. A study of angiotensin II pressor response throughout primigravid pregnancy. *J Clin Invest.* 1973;52:2682–2689, by copyright permission of the American Society for Clinical Investigation.)

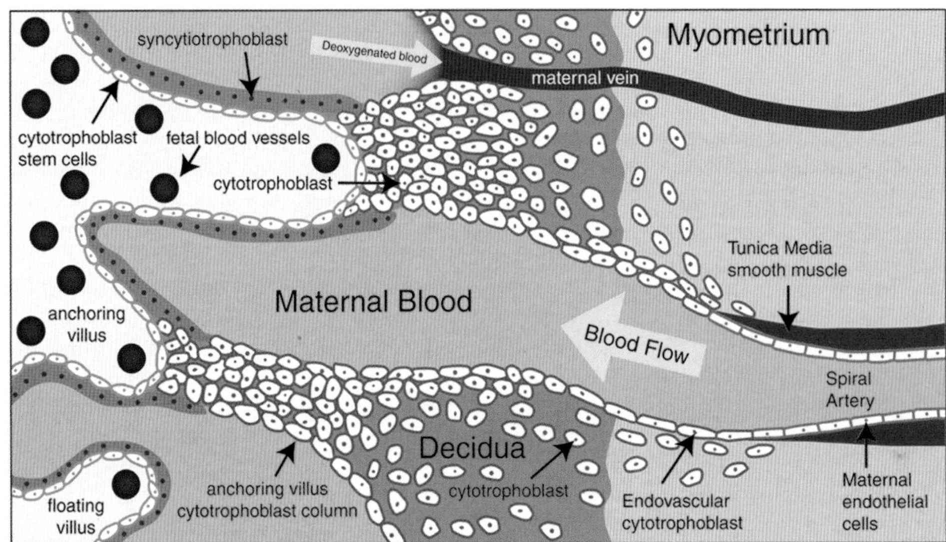


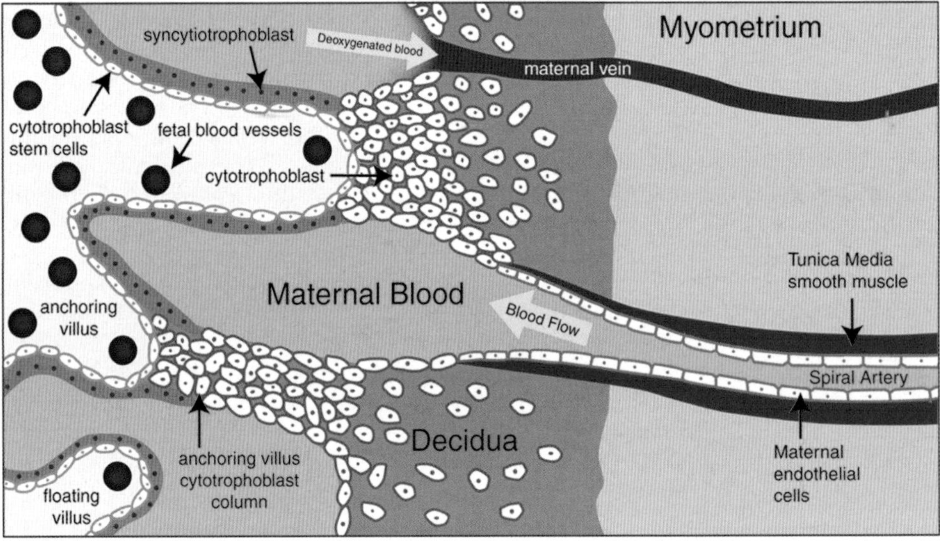


**Fig. 48.6** Placentation in normal and preeclamptic pregnancies. In normal placental development *(upper panel)*, invasive cytotrophoblasts of fetal origin invade the maternal spiral arteries, transforming them from small-caliber resistance vessels to high-caliber capacitance vessels capable of providing placental perfusion adequate to sustain the growing fetus. During the process of vascular invasion, the cytotrophoblasts differentiate from an epithelial phenotype to an endothelial phenotype, a process referred to as "pseudovasculogenesis" or "vascular mimicry." In preeclampsia *(lower panel)*, cytotrophoblasts fail to adopt an invasive endothelial phenotype. Instead, invasion of the spiral arteries is shallow, and they remain small-caliber resistance vessels. (From Lam C, Kim KH, Karumanchi SA. Circulating angiogenic factors in the pathogenesis and prediction of preeclampsia. *Hypertension* 2005;46:1077–1085.)

Increased skin capillary density in pregnancy[34] suggests that angiogenic factors may be acting systemically, as well as locally in the placenta. Dysregulation of these angiogenic factors may contribute to disorders of placental vascular development, such as preeclampsia. This is more fully discussed in the next section, "Pathogenesis of Preeclampsia."

## PREECLAMPSIA AND HELLP SYNDROME

Preeclampsia is a systemic syndrome that is specific to pregnancy, characterized by the new onset of hypertension and proteinuria after 20 weeks' gestation. Preeclampsia affects approximately 5% of pregnancies worldwide.[35] Despite many advances in our understanding of the pathophysiology of preeclampsia, delivery of the neonate remains the only definitive treatment. Hence preeclampsia is still a leading cause of preterm birth and consequent neonatal morbidity and mortality in the developed world. Maternal mortality from preeclampsia is avoidable with appropriate prenatal and peripartum care, and is now uncommon in developed countries.[36] Globally, where access to safe, emergent delivery is less readily available, preeclampsia continues to claim the lives of over 60,000 mothers every year.[37]

## EPIDEMIOLOGY AND RISK FACTORS

The incidence of preeclampsia varies among populations. Most cases of preeclampsia occur in healthy nulliparous women in whom the incidence of preeclampsia has been reported as high as 7.5%.[38] While classically a disorder of first pregnancies, multiparous women who are pregnant with a new partner appear to have an elevated preeclampsia risk similar to that of nulliparous women.[39] This effect may be due to increased interpregnancy interval rather than the change in partner per se.[40]

Although most cases of preeclampsia occur in the absence of a family history, the presence of preeclampsia in a first-degree relative increases a woman's risk of severe preeclampsia twofold to fourfold,[41] suggesting a genetic contribution to the disease. Several large genome-wide scans seeking a specific linkage to preeclampsia have been fairly discordant and disappointing, with significant logarithm of odds (LOD) scores in isolated Finnish (2p25, 9p13)[42] and Icelandic (2p12)[43] populations. Specific genetic mutations consistent with these loci have remained elusive.

Several medical conditions are associated with increased preeclampsia risk, including chronic hypertension, diabetes mellitus, renal disease, obesity, and antiphospholipid antibody syndrome (Table 48.2).[44] Women with preeclampsia in a prior pregnancy have a high risk of preeclampsia in subsequent pregnancies. Women with early preterm preeclampsia have the highest rate of recurrence.[45]

Adults who were born with low birth weights are at increased risk of pregnancy complications including preeclampsia and gestational hypertension.[46] Conditions associated with increased placental mass, such as multifetal gestations and hydatidiform mole, also are associated with increased preeclampsia risk. Trisomy 13 is associated with a high risk of preeclampsia.[47,48] Use of assisted reproductive technologies has also emerged as an important risk factor for preeclampsia,[49] particularly those methods that involve oocyte donation, such as in vitro fertilization.[50] Although none of these risk factors is fully understood, they have provided insights into pathogenesis.

Several putative risk factors remain controversial. Teen pregnancy has been identified as a risk factor in some studies,[51,52] but this has not been confirmed in a meta-analysis and systematic review.[53] Congenital or acquired thrombophilia is associated with preeclampsia in some[54,55] but not all[56,57] studies. Racial differences in the incidence and severity of preeclampsia have been difficult to assess due to confounding by socioeconomic and cultural factors. Although population-based studies have reported a higher rate of preeclampsia among black women,[58,59] these findings have not been confirmed in studies confined to healthy, nulliparous women.[60,61] This suggests that the increased preeclampsia incidence noted in some studies may be attributable to the higher rate of chronic hypertension in African Americans, as chronic hypertension is itself a strong risk factor for preeclampsia.[62] Black women with preeclampsia also have a higher case-mortality rate,[63] which may be due to more severe disease or to deficiencies in prenatal care. In Hispanics, the incidence of preeclampsia appears to be increased with a concomitant decrease in risk of gestational hypertension (for a discussion on new onset of hypertension without proteinuria, after 20 weeks' gestation, see Chronic Hypertension and Gestational Hypertension).[64]

The possibility that infection may contribute to preeclampsia risk has continued to have sporadic support. A systematic review and meta-analysis of 49 studies reported a small but significant association between preeclampsia and urinary tract infections [odds ratio (OR) 1.57] and periodontal disease (OR 1.76), but no association with other infections, including human immunodeficiency virus (HIV), cytomegalovirus, *Chlamydia*, and malaria.[65] Subsequent studies have supported the association between preeclampsia and urinary tract infection[66] and periodontal disease.[67] It is hypothesized that maternal inflammation predisposes to preeclampsia by causing endothelial stress.

**Table 48.2 Risk Factors for Preeclampsia**

| Risk Factor | Pooled Relative Risk (95% CI) |
|---|---|
| Antiphospholipid antibody syndrome | 2.8 (1.8–4.3)[44] |
| Chronic kidney disease | 1.8 (1.5–2.1)[44] |
| Prior preeclampsia | 8.4 (7.1–9.9)[44] |
| Nulliparity | 2.1 (1.9–2.4)[44] |
| Chronic hypertension | 5.1 (4.0–6.5)[44] |
| Pregestational diabetes mellitus | 3.7 (3.1–4.3)[44] |
| Multiple gestations | 2.9 (2.6–3.1)[44] |
| Strong family history of cardiovascular disease (heart disease/stroke in two or more first-degree relatives) | 3.2 (1.4–7.7)[474] |
| Systemic lupus erythematosus | 2.5 (1.0–6.3)[44] |
| Obesity (prepregnancy BMI > 30 kg/m²) | 2.8 (2.6–3.1)[44] |
| Family history of preeclampsia | 2.4 (1.8–3.6)[41] |
| Advanced maternal age (>40 years) | 1.5 (1.2–2.0)[44] |
| Excessive gestational weight gain (>35 lbs) | 1.9 (1.7–2.0)[273] |
| Assisted reproductive technology | 1.8 (1.6–2.1)[44] |
| Previous episode of acute kidney injury | 5.9 (3.6–9.7)[475] |

*BMI*, Body mass index; *CI*, confidence interval.

## PREECLAMPSIA: DIAGNOSIS AND CLINICAL FEATURES

For many years, the diagnosis of preeclampsia required the new onset of both hypertension and proteinuria after 20 weeks' gestation. In 2013, the Task Force of the American College of Obstetrics and Gynecology published updated criteria for the diagnosis of preeclampsia (Table 48.3) that allow preeclampsia to be diagnosed in the absence of proteinuria if one or more features of severe preeclampsia are present.[68] These guidelines help to distinguish preeclampsia from other hypertensive disorders of pregnancy such as chronic or gestational hypertension. The diagnosis of preeclampsia in women with chronic hypertension and/or underlying proteinuric renal disease on clinical criteria alone remains challenging.

### HYPERTENSION

For the diagnosis of preeclampsia, hypertension is defined as a systolic blood pressure (SBP) of ≥140 mm Hg or a diastolic

**Table 48.3 Diagnostic Criteria for Preeclampsia**

| **Diagnostic Criteria for Preeclampsia** | |
|---|---|
| Hypertension | ≥140 mm Hg systolic or ≥90 mm Hg diastolic after 20 weeks of gestation on two occasions at least 4 hours apart in a woman with a previously normal blood pressure<br>*OR*<br>With blood pressures ≥160 mm Hg systolic or ≥105 mm Hg diastolic, hypertension can be confirmed within a short interval (minutes) to facilitate timely antihypertensive therapy |
| *AND* | |
| Proteinuria | ≥300 mg/24 h (or this amount extrapolated from a timed collection)<br>*OR*<br>Protein-to-creatinine ratio ≥ 0.3 mg protein/mg creatinine<br>*OR*<br>Dipstick 2+ (used only if other quantitative methods not available) |
| *OR in the absence of proteinuria, new-onset hypertension with the new onset of any of the following:* | |
| Thrombocytopenia | ≤100,000 platelets/mL |
| Renal insufficiency | Serum creatinine concentrations >1.1 mg/dL or a doubling of the serum creatinine concentration in the absence of other renal disease |
| Impaired liver function | Elevated blood concentrations of liver transaminases to twice normal |
| Pulmonary edema | |
| Cerebral or visual symptoms | |
| **Diagnostic Criteria for Superimposed Preeclampsia** | |
| Hypertension | A sudden increase in blood pressure in a woman with chronic hypertension that was previously well controlled or escalation of antihypertensive medications to control blood pressure |
| *OR* | |
| Proteinuria | New onset of proteinuria in a woman with chronic hypertension or a sudden increase in proteinuria in a woman with known proteinuria before or in early pregnancy |

Adapted from American College of Obstetricians and Gynecologists, Task Force on Hypertension in Pregnancy. Hypertension in pregnancy. Report of the American College of Obstetricians and Gynecologists' Task Force on Hypertension in Pregnancy. *Obstet Gynecol.* 2013;122:1122–1131 and ACOG Practice Bulletin No 202: Gestational Hypertension and Preeclampsia. *Obstet Gynecol.* 2019;133(1):e1–e25.

blood pressure (DBP) of ≥90 mm Hg after 20 weeks' gestation in a woman with previously normal BP.[68] Hypertension should be confirmed by two separate measurements at least 4 hours apart. The severity of hypertension in preeclampsia can vary widely, from mild BP elevations easily managed with antihypertensive medication to severe hypertension associated with headache and visual changes resistant to multiple medications. The latter situation can often herald seizures (eclampsia) and is an indication for urgent delivery. Medical management of hypertension in preeclampsia is discussed in the next section.

## PROTEINURIA

Proteinuria is a hallmark of preeclampsia. For the diagnosis of preeclampsia, proteinuria is defined as >300 mg protein in a 24-hour urine collection or a urine protein-to-creatinine (P:C) ratio >0.3 mg/mg, or urine dipstick of ≥2+ (if quantitative methods are unavailable). However, preeclampsia can be diagnosed even in the absence of proteinuria, if other severe features are present (Table 48.3).

Routine obstetric care includes dipstick protein testing of a random voided urine sample at each prenatal visit – a screening method that has been shown to have a high rate of false-positive and false-negative results when compared with 24-hour urine protein measurement.[69] However, the 24-hour urine collection for proteinuria is cumbersome for the patient, often inaccurate due to undercollection,[70] and the availability of results is delayed for at least 24 hours, while the collection is being completed. The urinary P:C ratio has become the preferred method for quantification of proteinuria in the nonpregnant population. A meta-analysis showed a pooled sensitivity of 84% and specificity of 76% using P:C ratio cutoff of >0.3, as compared with the gold standard of 24-hour urine protein excretion >300 mg/day.[71] Hence it is reasonable to use the urine P:C ratio for the diagnosis of preeclampsia, with 24-hour collection undertaken when the result is equivocal. A 12-hour urine collection showing >150 mg protein may also be used as a surrogate for 24-hour urine collection, according to a meta-analysis of several studies.[72]

The degree of proteinuria in preeclampsia can range widely, from minimal to nephrotic range. However, the degree of proteinuria is a poor predictor of adverse maternal and fetal outcomes,[73] thus heavy proteinuria alone is not an indication for urgent delivery. New-onset proteinuria is particularly useful among women with chronic hypertension to diagnose superimposed preeclampsia (Table 48.3). However, among women with underlying proteinuria, other signs of preeclampsia such as elevated transaminases, thrombocytopenia, or cerebral signs/symptoms are more useful to diagnose superimposed preeclampsia.[68]

## EDEMA

Although edema was historically part of the diagnostic triad for preeclampsia, it is also recognized to be a feature of normal pregnancy, diminishing its usefulness as a specific pathologic sign. Still, the sudden onset of severe edema—especially edema of the hands and face—can be an important presenting symptom in this otherwise insidious disease and should prompt evaluation.

## URIC ACID

Serum uric acid is elevated in most women with preeclampsia primarily as a result of enhanced tubular urate reabsorption. It has been suggested that hyperuricemia may contribute to the pathogenesis of preeclampsia by inducing endothelial dysfunction[74] or by impairing trophoblast invasiveness, a key element in placental vascular remodeling.[75] Serum uric acid levels are correlated with the presence and severity of preeclampsia and with adverse pregnancy outcomes,[76] even in gestational hypertension without proteinuria.[77] Unfortunately, uric acid is of limited clinical utility in either distinguishing preeclampsia from other hypertensive disorders of pregnancy or as a clinical predictor of adverse outcomes.[78–80] One clinical scenario where serum uric acid may be useful is in the diagnosis of preeclampsia in women with chronic kidney disease (CKD), in whom the usual diagnostic criteria of new-onset hypertension and proteinuria are often impossible to apply. In such patients, a serum uric acid level >5.5 mg/dL in the presence of stable renal function might suggest superimposed preeclampsia.

## CLINICAL FEATURES OF SEVERE PREECLAMPSIA

Several clinical and laboratory findings suggest severe or progressive disease, and should prompt consideration of immediate delivery.[68] Oliguria (<500 mL urine in 24 hours) is usually transient; acute kidney injury (AKI), though uncommon, can occur. Persistent headache or visual disturbances can be a prodrome to seizures. Pulmonary edema complicates 2%–3% of severe preeclampsia,[39] and can lead to respiratory failure. Epigastric or right upper quadrant pain may be associated with liver injury. Elevated liver enzymes and thrombocytopenia can occur alone or as part of the HELLP (*h*emolytic anemia, *e*levated *l*iver enzymes, and *l*ow *p*latelets) syndrome (see later).

## ECLAMPSIA

Seizures complicate approximately 2% of preeclampsia cases in the United States.[81] Although eclampsia most often occurs in the setting of hypertension and proteinuria, it can occur without these warning signs. Up to one-third of eclampsia occurs postpartum, sometimes days to weeks after delivery.[82] Late postpartum preeclampsia in particular is often a difficult and potentially missed diagnosis, often seen by nonobstetricians in the emergency room. Radiologic imaging by head computed tomography (CT) or magnetic resonance imaging (MRI) is usually not indicated when the diagnosis is apparent, but typically shows vasogenic edema, predominantly in the subcortical white matter of the parietooccipital lobes (see "Etiology of Pathogenesis of Preeclampsia: Cerebral Changes"). Women who have had eclampsia may have subtle long-term impairment in cognitive function.[83]

## HELLP SYNDROME

"HELLP" is an acronym for the syndrome of *h*emolytic anemia, *e*levated *l*iver enzymes, and *l*ow *p*latelets. There remains considerable variability regarding diagnostic criteria for the HELLP syndrome in the medical literature. The HELLP syndrome is a severe form of preeclampsia, which can occur in the absence of proteinuria. As its name suggests, a diagnosis of HELLP syndrome is suggested by evidence of hemolytic anemia, thrombocytopenia (platelet count < 100,000/μL), and impaired liver function (liver enzyme levels more than twice the upper limit of normal). This syndrome is sometimes challenging to distinguish from thrombotic thrombocytopenic purpura (TTP), hemolytic uremic syndrome (HUS), and acute fatty liver of pregnancy (AFLP), which can present similarly (Table 48.4). The HELLP syndrome is associated with particularly high rates of adverse maternal and neonatal adverse outcomes, including eclampsia (affecting 6% of cases), placental abruption (10%), acute renal failure (5%), disseminated intravascular coagulation (8%), pulmonary edema (10%),[84] and (rarely) hepatic hemorrhage and rupture.[85]

**Table 48.4 Comparison of Clinical and Laboratory Characteristics, Effect on Delivery, and Management of HELLP, HUS/TTP, and AFLP**

| | HUS/TTP | HELLP | AFLP |
|---|---|---|---|
| **Clinical Characteristic:** | | | |
| Hemolytic anemia | +++ | ++ | ± |
| Thrombocytopenia | +++ | ++ | ± |
| Coagulopathy | – | ± | + |
| CNS symptoms | ++ | ± | ± |
| Renal failure | +++ | + | ++ |
| Hypertension | ± | +++ | ± |
| Proteinuria | ± | ++ | ± |
| Elevated AST | ± | ++ | +++ |
| Elevated bilirubin | ++ | + | +++ |
| Anemia | ++ | + | ± |
| Ammonia | Normal | Normal | High |
| Effect of delivery on disease | None | Recovery | Recovery |
| Management | Plasma exchange | Supportive care, delivery | Supportive care, delivery |

*AFLP,* Acute fatty liver of pregnancy; *AST,* aspartate aminotransferase; *CNS,* central nervous system; *HELLP, h*emolytic anemia, *e*levated *l*iver enzymes, and *l*ow *p*latelets; *HUS/TTP,* hemolytic uremic syndrome/thrombotic thrombocytopenic purpura; –, absent; ±, present or absent; +, mild; ++, moderate; +++, severe.

Data derived from Allford SL, Hunt BJ, Rose P, et al. Guidelines on the diagnosis and management of the thrombotic microangiopathic haemolytic anaemias. *Br J Haematol*. 2003;120:556–573; Egerman RS, Sibai BM. Imitators of preeclampsia and eclampsia. *Clin Obstet Gynecol*. 1999; 42:551–562; Stella CL, Dacus J, Guzman E, et al. The diagnostic dilemma of thrombotic thrombocytopenic purpura/hemolytic uremic syndrome in the obstetric triage and emergency department: lessons from 4 tertiary hospitals. *Am J Obstet Gynecol.* 2009;200:381–386.

## MATERNAL AND NEONATAL MORTALITY

Approximately 300,000 women die in childbirth each year worldwide, and hypertensive disorders of pregnancy are estimated to account for 10% to 20% of these deaths.[37,86] In the United States, the rate of severe preeclampsia has been increasing since the 1980s,[51] and preeclampsia and eclampsia account for 16%–20% of all pregnancy-related maternal mortality.[63,87] Maternal death is most often due to eclampsia, cerebral hemorrhage, renal failure, hepatic failure, pulmonary edema, and the HELLP syndrome. Most preventable errors in preeclampsia management leading to maternal death involve inattention to BP control and signs of pulmonary edema.[87] Risk of death in preeclampsia is increased for women with little or no prenatal care, women of black race, those over 35 years of age, and those with early-onset preeclampsia.[63] Adverse maternal outcomes can often be avoided with timely delivery; hence in the developed world the burden of morbidity and mortality falls on the neonate.

Worldwide, preeclampsia is associated with a perinatal and neonatal mortality rate of 10%[88]; as with maternal mortality, the risk of neonatal mortality increases substantially for preeclampsia presenting earlier in gestation. Neonatal death is most commonly due to iatrogenic prematurity undertaken to preserve the health of the mother. In addition, fetal growth restriction can occur, likely as a result of impaired uteroplacental blood flow or placental infarction. Oligohydramnios and placental abruption are less common complications.

## POSTPARTUM RECOVERY

Generally, preeclampsia begins to remit soon after delivery of the fetus and placenta and complete recovery is the rule. However, normalization of BP and proteinuria often takes days to weeks.[89] Postpartum monitoring is important because, as discussed, eclampsia can occur after delivery.

## LONG-TERM CARDIOVASCULAR AND RENAL OUTCOMES

Previously, women with preeclampsia were reassured that the syndrome remits completely after delivery, with no long-term consequences aside from increased preeclampsia risk in future pregnancies. Epidemiologic studies have refuted this claim.[90,91] Fifty percent of women with preeclampsia develop hypertension later in life. As early as 1 year after the affected pregnancy, women with preeclampsia have an increased risk of hypertension, obesity, hypercholesterolemia, microalbuminuria, and new-onset diabetes mellitus, when compared with control women who have not had preeclampsia.[92–94] Relative risk (RR) of ischemic heart disease, stroke, cardiomyopathy, and cardiovascular mortality are more than doubled in women who have had preeclampsia.[90,91,95] (Fig. 48.7) Severe preeclampsia, recurrent preeclampsia, preeclampsia with preterm birth, and preeclampsia with intrauterine growth restriction (IUGR) are most strongly associated with adverse cardiovascular outcomes. The American Heart Association Guidelines include a history of preeclampsia as a risk factor for cardiovascular disease in women.[96]

Preeclampsia, especially in association with low neonatal birth weight, also carries an increased risk of later maternal kidney disease requiring a kidney biopsy.[97] A large Norwegian study by the same authors, using birth and renal registry data on >570,000 women, showed that preeclampsia increases the

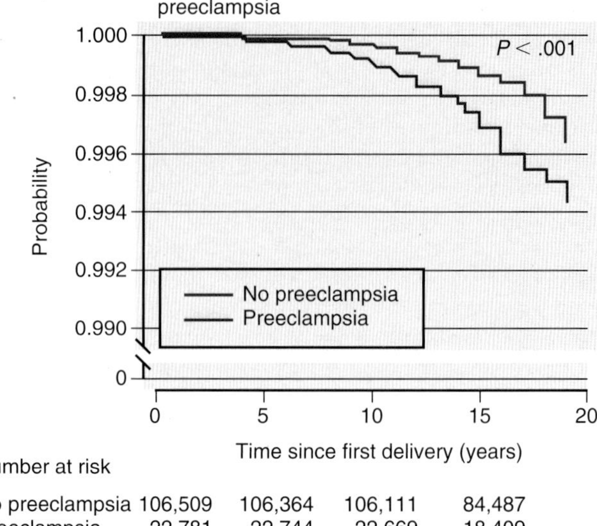


**Fig. 48.7** Preeclampsia increases the risk for cardiovascular disease later in life. Kaplan–Meier plot of the cumulative probability of survival without admission to the hospital for ischemic heart disease or death from ischemic heart disease in women with and without a history of preeclampsia. (From Smith GC, Pell JP, Walsh D. Pregnancy complications and maternal risk of ischaemic heart disease: a retrospective cohort study of 129,290 births. *Lancet* 2001;357:2002–2006.)

risk of subsequent end-stage renal disease (ESRD) by almost fivefold.[98] This finding has subsequently been confirmed in other populations.[99] Familial aggregation of risk factors does not seem to explain increased ESRD risk after preeclampsia.[100] Although it appears that preeclampsia is associated with increased risk of subsequent ESRD, the absolute risk is low (e.g., 4.72 per 10,000 person-years in the Taiwanese study).[99]

Preeclampsia and cardiovascular disease share many common risk factors, such as chronic hypertension, diabetes, obesity, renal disease, and the metabolic syndrome. Still, the increase in long-term cardiovascular mortality holds even for women who develop preeclampsia in the absence of any overt vascular risk factors. Whether these observations result from vascular damage or persistent endothelial dysfunction caused by preeclampsia, or simply reflect the common risk factors shared by preeclampsia and cardiovascular disease, remains speculative. Regardless of etiology, it is recommended that women who experience preeclampsia, especially with preterm birth or IUGR, receive screening for potentially modifiable cardiovascular and renal disease risk factors (hypertension, diabetes mellitus, hyperlipidemia, obesity) at their postpartum obstetrician visit and yearly thereafter.[68,101,102]

Epidemiologic evidence suggests that low birth weight (with or without preeclampsia) is associated with the development of hypertension, diabetes, cardiovascular disease, and CKD in the offspring of affected pregnancies.[103–106] It has been hypothesized that this may be in part due to low nephron number as is further discussed in Chapter 21.

# PATHOGENESIS OF PREECLAMPSIA

## THE ROLE OF THE PLACENTA

Observational evidence suggests that the placenta has a central role in preeclampsia. Preeclampsia only occurs in the presence of a placenta—though not necessarily a fetus, as in the case of hydatidiform mole—and almost always remits after its delivery. In a case of preeclampsia with extrauterine pregnancy, removal of the fetus alone was not sufficient; symptoms persisted until the placenta was delivered.[107] Severe preeclampsia is associated with pathologic evidence of placental hypoperfusion and ischemia. Findings include acute atherosis, a lesion of diffuse vascular obstruction that includes fibrin deposition, intimal thickening, necrosis, atherosclerosis, and endothelial damage.[108] Infarcts, likely due to occlusion of maternal spiral arteries, are also common. Although these findings are not universal, they appear to be correlated with severity of clinical disease.[109]

Several clinical and laboratory observations strongly support the role of placental ischemia in the pathophysiology of preeclampsia. Abnormal uterine artery Doppler ultrasound, consistent with decreased uteroplacental perfusion, is observed before the clinical onset of preeclampsia.[110] The incidence of preeclampsia is increased twofold to fourfold in women residing at high altitude, implying hypoxia may be a contributing factor.[111] Indeed, global gene expression profiles are similar when comparing hypoxia-treated placental explants, high-altitude placentae, or placentae from preeclamptic pregnancies.[112] Pregnant subjects with sickle cell disease, who often have pathologic evidence of placental ischemia and infarction, have an increased risk for preeclampsia.[113–115] Hypertension and proteinuria can be induced by constriction of uterine blood flow in pregnant primates and other mammals.[116] These observations suggest that placental ischemia may be an important trigger for the maternal syndrome.

However, evidence for a causative role for placental ischemia alone remains circumstantial, and several observations call the hypothesis into question. For example, the animal models based on uterine hypoperfusion fail to induce several of the multiorgan features of preeclampsia, including seizures, elevated liver enzymes, and thrombocytopenia. In most cases of preeclampsia, there is no evidence of growth restriction or fetal intolerance of labor, which are expected consequences of placental ischemia. It may be that the placental ischemic damage that accompanies late-stage preeclampsia may be a secondary event.

## PLACENTAL VASCULAR REMODELING

Early in normal placental development, extravillous cytotrophoblasts invade the uterine spiral arteries of the decidua and myometrium (see Fig. 48.6). These invasive fetal cells replace the endothelial layer of the uterine vessels, transforming them from small resistance vessels to flaccid, high-caliber capacitance vessels.[117] This vascular transformation is most dramatic in the myometrial vessels and allows the increase in uterine blood flow needed to sustain the fetus through the pregnancy.[118] In preeclampsia, this transformation is incomplete.[119] Cytotrophoblast invasion of the arteries is limited to the superficial decidua, and the myometrial segments remain narrow and undilated.[120] Fisher et al[121] have shown that in normal placental development, invasive cytotrophoblasts downregulate the expression of adhesion molecules characteristic of their epithelial cell origin and adopt an endothelial cell-surface adhesion phenotype, a process dubbed pseudovasculogenesis. In preeclampsia, cytotrophoblasts do not undergo this switching of cell-surface integrins and adhesion molecules, and fail to adequately invade the myometrial spiral arteries.

The factors that regulate this process are just beginning to be elucidated. Hypoxia-inducible factor-1 (HIF-1) activity is increased in preeclampsia and HIF-1 target genes such as encoding transforming growth factor β-3 *TGFB3,* may block cytotrophoblast invasion.[122] Invasive cytotrophoblasts express several angiogenic factors and receptors, also regulated by HIF, including VEGF, placental growth factor (PlGF), and VEGF receptor 1 (VEGFR-1 orFlt1); expression of these proteins by immunolocalization is altered in preeclampsia.[123] A genetic study identified polymorphisms in *STOX1,* a paternally imprinted gene and member of the winged helix gene family, in a Dutch preeclampsia cohort.[124] The authors hypothesized that loss-of-function mutations in this gene could result in defective polyploidization of extravillous trophoblast, leading to loss of cytotrophoblast invasion. However, a subsequent cohort failed to confirm an association between preeclampsia and STOX polymorphisms.[125] More work is needed to uncover the molecular signals governing cytotrophoblast invasion early in placentation, defects in which may underlie the early stages of preeclampsia.

***Clinical Relevance***

Inadequate early placental vascular development leads to development of placental ischemia later in pregnancy, culminating in preeclampsia. Dysregulation of angiogenic factors, such as vascular endothelial growth factor (VEGF), placental growth factor, and soluble fms-like tyrosine kinase-1 (sFlt1), may play a role in both early placental development and later stages of clinical preeclampsia.

## MATERNAL ENDOTHELIAL DYSFUNCTION

Although the origins of the preeclampsia syndrome appear to be placental, the target organ is the maternal endothelium. The clinical manifestations of preeclampsia reflect widespread endothelial dysfunction, resulting in vasoconstriction and end-organ ischemia.[126,127] Incubation of endothelial cells with serum from women with preeclampsia results in endothelial dysfunction; hence it has been hypothesized that factors present in maternal serum, likely originating in the placenta, are responsible for the manifestations of the disease (Fig. 48.8).

Dozens of serum markers of endothelial activation are deranged in women with preeclampsia, including von Willebrand antigen, cellular fibronectin, soluble tissue factor, soluble E-selectin, platelet-derived growth factor, and endothelin.[127] C-reactive protein[128] and leptin[129] are increased early in gestation. There is evidence for oxidative stress and platelet activation.[130] Decreased production of prostaglandin $I_2$, an endothelial-derived prostaglandin, occurs well before the onset of clinical symptoms.[131] Inflammation is often present; for example, there is neutrophil infiltration in the vascular smooth muscle of subcutaneous fat, with increased vascular smooth muscle expression of interleukin-8 (IL-8) and intercellular adhesion molecule 1 (ICAM-1).[132] Several of these aberrations occur well before the onset of symptoms, sup-

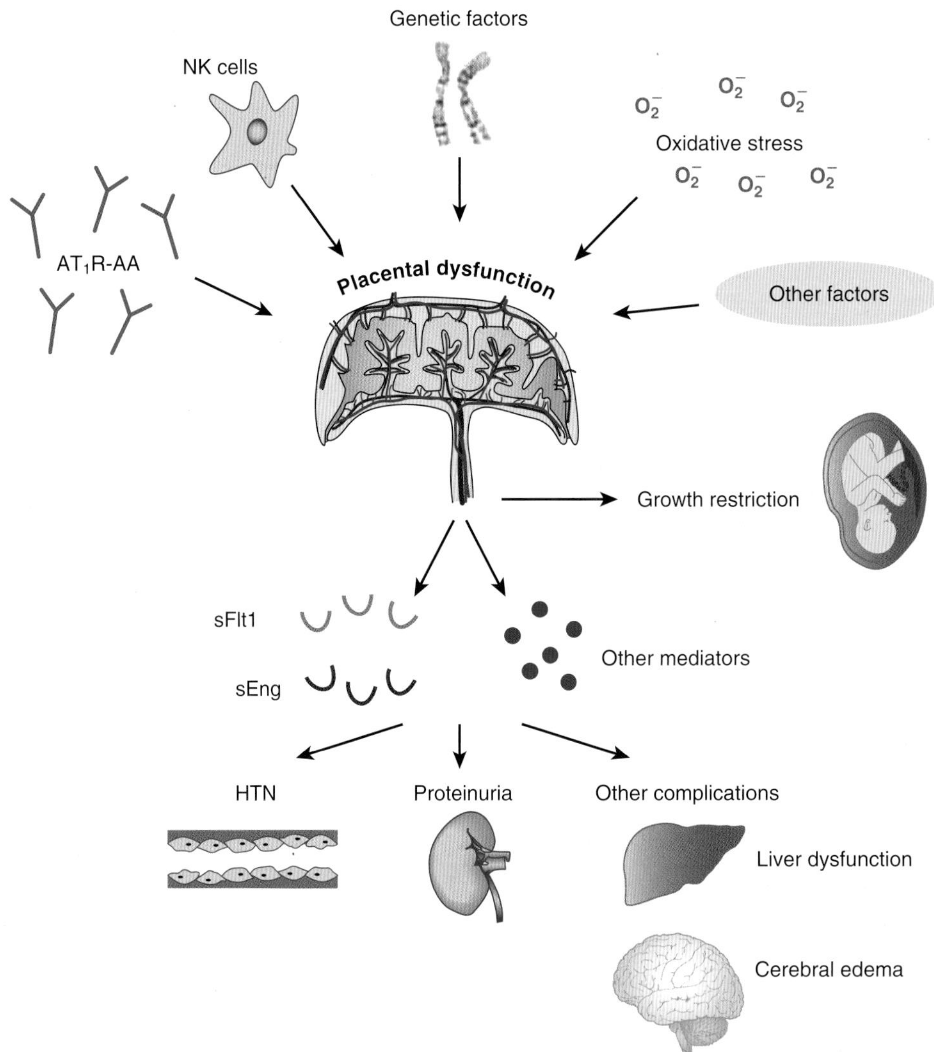


**Fig. 48.8** Placental dysfunction and endothelial dysfunction in the pathogenesis of preeclampsia. Placental dysfunction triggered by genetic, immunologic [natural killer (NK) cells and angiotensin receptor autoantibodies ($AT_1R$-AAs)], and other factors (altered heme oxygenase expression, oxidative stress) plays an early and primary role in the pathogenesis of preeclampsia. The diseased placenta in turn secretes antiangiogenic factors [soluble fms-like tyrosine kinase-1 (sFlt1), soluble endoglin (sEng)] and other toxic mediators into the systemic circulation, causing maternal endothelial dysfunction. Nearly all the manifestations of preeclampsia, including hypertension, proteinuria (glomerular endotheliosis), seizures (cerebral edema), and HELLP (*h*emolytic anemia, *e*levated *l*iver enzymes, and *l*ow *p*latelets) syndrome, can be attributable to vascular endothelial damage secondary to excess circulating antiangiogenic factors. (Adapted from Powe CE, Levine RJ, Karumanchi SA. Preeclampsia, a disease of the maternal endothelium: the role of antiangiogenic factors and implications for later cardiovascular disease. *Circulation* 2011;123: 2856–2869.)

porting the central role of endothelial dysfunction in the pathogenesis of preeclampsia.

## HEMODYNAMIC CHANGES

The decreases in peripheral vascular resistance and arterial BP that occur during normal pregnancy are absent or reversed in preeclampsia. SVR is high and cardiac output is low when compared with normal pregnancies.[133] These changes are due to widespread vasoconstriction resulting from endothelial dysfunction. This hypothesis is supported by both in vivo and in vitro evidence. Women with preeclampsia have impaired endothelium-dependent vasorelaxation, which has been noted prospectively prior to onset of hypertension and proteinuria[134] and persists for years after the preeclampsia episode.[135] There is exaggerated sensitivity to vasopressors such as angiotensin II and norepinephrine (see Fig. 48.5).[127] Subtle increases in BP and in pulse pressure are present prior to the onset of overt hypertension and proteinuria, suggesting that arterial compliance is decreased early in the course of the disease.[53,136] Mechanisms underlying endothelial dysfunction are discussed in the next section.

## RENAL CHANGES

The pathologic swelling of glomerular endothelial cells in preeclampsia was first described in 1924.[137] Thirty years later, Spargo et al[138] coined the term "glomerular endotheliosis" and characterized ultrastructural changes, including generalized swelling and vacuolization of the endothelial cells and loss of the capillary space (Fig. 48.9). There are deposits of fibrinogen and fibrin within and under the endothelial cells,

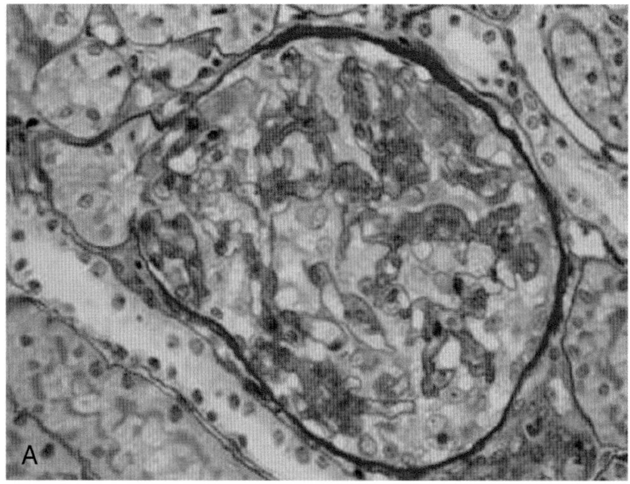


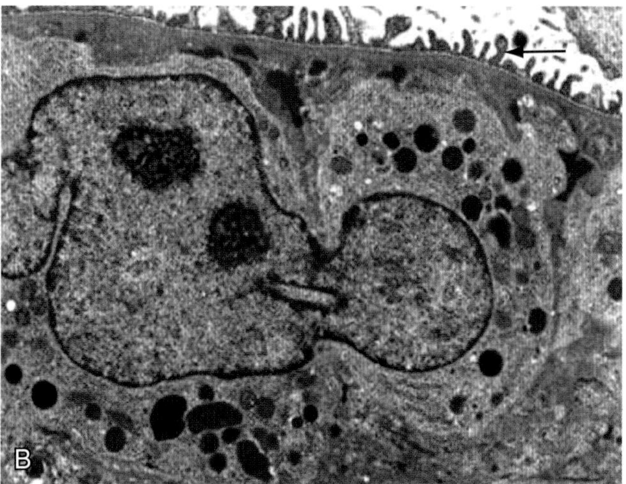


**Fig. 48.9** Glomerular endotheliosis. (A) Human preeclamptic glomerulus on light microscopy (periodic acid–Schiff stain). Renal biopsy findings from a 29-year-old woman with twin gestation and severe preeclampsia are shown. Patient's blood pressure was 170/112 mm Hg, and random urine protein-to-creatinine ratio was 9.8. Note the "bloodless" appearance of the glomeruli and absence of the capillary lumen. (Original magnification, ×40.) (B) Electron microscopy of biopsy specimen of the glomerulus from the same patient. Note occlusion of capillary lumen cytoplasm and expansion of the subendothelial space with some electron-dense material. Podocyte cytoplasm shows protein resorption droplets and relatively intact foot processes. (Original magnification, ×1500.) (Courtesy IE Stillman.)

and electron microscopy shows loss of glomerular endothelial fenestrae.[139] The primary injury is specific to endothelial cells: the podocyte foot processes are intact early in disease, a finding atypical of other nephrotic diseases. However, podocyte injury as evidenced by podocyturia has been observed in preeclampsia.[140] Changes in the afferent arteriole, including atrophy of the macula densa and hyperplasia of the juxtaglomerular apparatus, have also been described.[141] Although once considered pathognomonic for preeclampsia, recent studies have shown that mild glomerular endotheliosis also occurs in pregnancy without preeclampsia, especially in gestational hypertension.[142] This suggests that the endothelial dysfunction of preeclampsia may in fact be an exaggeration of a process present toward term in all pregnancies.

Both renal blood flow and GFR are low in preeclampsia as compared with normal pregnancy. Renal blood flow falls as a result of high renal vascular resistance, primarily due to increased afferent arteriolar resistance. GFR falls as a result of both the fall in renal blood flow and a decrease in the ultrafiltration coefficient ($K_f$), attributed to endotheliosis in the glomerular capillary.[143] Although AKI can occur in preeclampsia, typically proteinuria (with a bland urinary sediment) and renal sodium and water retention are the only renal manifestations of disease.

## CEREBRAL CHANGES

Cerebral edema and intracerebral parenchymal hemorrhage are common autopsy findings in women who died from eclampsia. The presence of cerebral edema in eclampsia correlates with markers of endothelial damage but not the severity of hypertension,[144] suggesting that the edema is secondary to endothelial dysfunction rather than a direct result of BP elevation. Findings on head CT and MRI are similar to those seen in hypertensive encephalopathy, with vasogenic cerebral edema and infarctions in the subcortical white matter and adjacent gray matter, predominantly in the parietooccipital lobes.[82] A syndrome that includes these characteristic MRI changes, together with headache, seizures, altered mental status, and hypertension, has been described in patients with acute hypertensive encephalopathy in the setting of renal disease, eclampsia, or immunosuppression.[145] This syndrome, termed reversible posterior leukoencephalopathy, has subsequently been associated with the use of calcineurin inhibitors (CNIs) or antiangiogenic agents for cancer therapy.[146] This latter observation supports the role of innate antiangiogenic factors in the pathophysiology of preeclampsia/eclampsia, as detailed later in this section.

## OXIDATIVE STRESS AND INFLAMMATION

Oxidative stress, the presence of reactive oxygen species in excess of antioxidant buffering capacity, is a prominent feature of preeclampsia. Oxidative stress is known to damage proteins, cell membranes, and DNA and is a potential mediator of endothelial dysfunction. It has been hypothesized that in preeclampsia, placental oxidative stress is transferred to the systemic circulation, resulting in oxidative damage to the maternal vascular endothelium.[130] However, the absence of any clinical benefit of antioxidant supplementation in the prevention of preeclampsia suggests that oxidative stress is likely to be a secondary phenomenon in preeclampsia, and not a promising therapeutic target.[147] Circulating placental cytotrophoblast debris and the accompanying inflammation have also been proposed as pathogenic mechanisms to explain the maternal endothelial dysfunction; however, causal evidence for this hypothesis is still lacking.[148]

## IMMUNOLOGIC INTOLERANCE

The possibility of immune maladaptation remains an intriguing but unproven theory of the pathogenesis of preeclampsia. Normal placentation requires the development of immune tolerance between the fetus and the mother. The fact that preeclampsia occurs more often in first pregnancies or after a change in partners suggests an etiologic role for abnormal maternal immune response to paternally derived fetal antigens. This could result in failure of fetal cells to successfully invade the maternal vessels during placental vascular development.

Observational studies suggest that preeclampsia risk increases in cases of exposure to novel paternal antigens – not only in first pregnancies, but also in pregnancies with a new partner[149] and with long interpregnancy interval.[40] Women using contraceptive methods that reduce exposure to sperm have increased preeclampsia incidence.[150] Women impregnated by intracytoplasmic sperm injection in which sperm were surgically obtained (i.e., the woman was never exposed to partner's sperm in intercourse) had a threefold increased risk of preeclampsia compared with intracytoplasmic sperm injection cases where sperm were obtained by ejaculation.[151] Conversely, prior exposure to paternal antigens appears to be protective. The risk of preeclampsia is inversely proportional to the length of cohabitation,[152] and oral tolerance to paternal antigens by oral sex and swallowing is associated with decreased risk.[153] None of these clinical observations have yet provided insights into immunologic triggers or pathogenic links to the paternal syndrome.

On a molecular level, HLA-G expression appears to be abnormal in preeclampsia. HLA-G is normally expressed by invasive extravillous cytotrophoblasts and may play a role in inducing immune tolerance at the maternal–fetal interface. In preeclampsia, HLA-G expression by cytotrophoblasts is reduced or absent,[154] and HLA-G protein concentrations are reduced in maternal serum[155] and in placental tissue.[156] These alterations in HLA-G expression could contribute to the ineffective trophoblast invasion seen in preeclampsia. Decidual natural killer (NK) cells, which promote angiogenesis and are involved in trophoblast invasion, have also been hypothesized to contribute to abnormal placental development seen in the disease.[157,158] Genetic studies have noted that the susceptibility to preeclampsia may be influenced by polymorphisms in killer immunoglobulin receptors (KIRs, present on NK cells) and HLA-C (KIR ligands present on trophoblasts).[159]

## ANGIOGENIC IMBALANCE

Overwhelming evidence from epidemiological studies and experimental studies in animals suggests that excess placental production of soluble VEGFR-1, referred to as soluble fms-like tyrosine kinase-1 (sFlt1, or sVEGFR-1), plays a causal role in mediating the signs and symptoms of preeclampsia.[160] sFlt1, a truncated splice variant of the VEGFR Flt1, antagonizes VEGF and PlGF by binding them in the circulation and preventing interaction with their endogenous receptors in the vasculature (Fig. 48.10). sFlt1 inhibits VEGF- and PlGF-mediated angiogenesis and is upregulated in the placenta of women with preeclampsia, resulting in elevated circulating levels.[161] The increase in maternal circulating sFlt1 precedes the onset of clinical disease (Fig. 48.11)[162–164] and is correlated with disease severity.[164,165] Increased circulating sFlt1 is accompanied by decreased circulating free PlGF in serum (Fig. 48.12). In vitro effects of sFlt1 include vasoconstriction and endothelial dysfunction. Exogenous sFlt1 administered to pregnant rats produces a syndrome resembling preeclampsia, including hypertension, proteinuria, and glomerular endotheliosis.[161] The preeclampsia-like syndrome induced by sFlt1 in animals can be rescued by exogenous VEGF or PlGF administration.[166–168] In summary, this work has suggested that sFlt1 is a key pathogenic circulating toxin that mediates the signs and symptoms of preeclampsia (see Fig. 48.8). Recently, several novel isoforms of sFlt1 have been identified

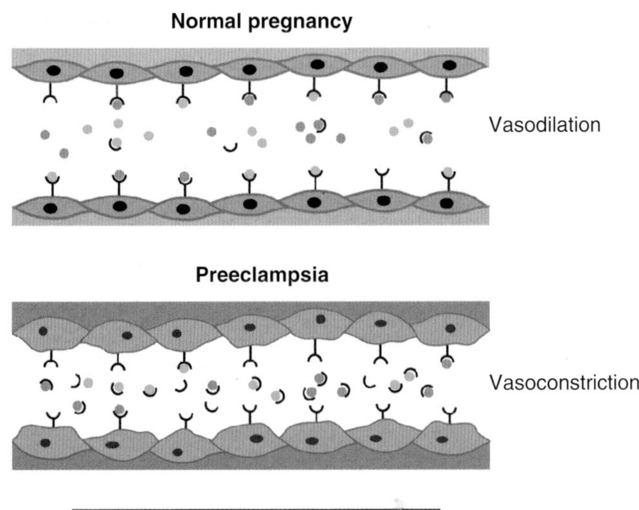


**Fig. 48.10** Proposed mechanism of soluble fms-like tyrosine kinase-1 (sFlt1)–induced endothelial dysfunction. sFlt1 protein, derived from alternative splicing of Flt1, lacks the transmembrane and cytoplasmic domains but still has the intact vascular endothelial growth factor (VEGF) and placental growth factor (PlGF) binding extracellular domain. During normal pregnancy, VEGF and PlGF signal through the VEGF receptors (Flt1) and maintain endothelial health. In preeclampsia, excess sFlt1 binds to circulating VEGF and PlGF, thus impairing normal signaling of both VEGF and PlGF through their cell surface receptors. Thus excess sFlt1 leads to maternal endothelial dysfunction. (From Bdolah Y, Sukhatme VP, Karumanchi SA. Angiogenic imbalance in the pathophysiology of preeclampsia: newer insights. *Semin Nephrol.* 2004;24:548–556.)

in the human placenta; however, the exact role of the various forms in human disease is still being investigated.[169,170]

Derangements in other angiogenic molecules have also been observed. Levels of endostatin, another antiangiogenic factor, are elevated in preeclampsia.[171] Expression of $VEGF_{165b}$, an antiangiogenic isoform of VEGF, are reduced in the first trimester in women who later develop preeclampsia.[172] Circulating levels of soluble endoglin (sEng), a truncated form of the transforming growth factor-β (TGF-β) receptor, are elevated in preeclampsia. sEng amplifies the vascular damage mediated by sFlt1 in pregnant rats, inducing a severe preeclampsia-like syndrome with features of the HELLP syndrome.[173] Maternal serum levels of sEng rise prior to preeclampsia onset,[174–176] in a pattern similar to sFlt1.[177] As TGF-β regulates podocyte VEGF-A expression,[178] sEng may result in impaired local VEGF signaling in the glomerulus. Notably, individuals who were born preterm have elevations in sEng, as well as sFlt1, as compared with individuals who were born term to uncomplicated pregnancies (intergenerational programming of preeclampsia risk is further discussed in Chapter 21).[179] It was recently reported that semaphorin 3B, a novel trophoblastic-secreted antiangiogenic protein, was also upregulated in preeclamptic placentas and that semaphorin 3B inhibits trophoblast migration and invasion by downregulating VEGF signaling.[180] The precise role of these novel antiangiogenic proteins and their relationship with sFlt1 in the systemic vasculature continues to be explored.

There is circumstantial evidence suggesting that interference with VEGF signaling may lead to preeclampsia.[160] VEGF appears to be important in the stabilization of endothelial

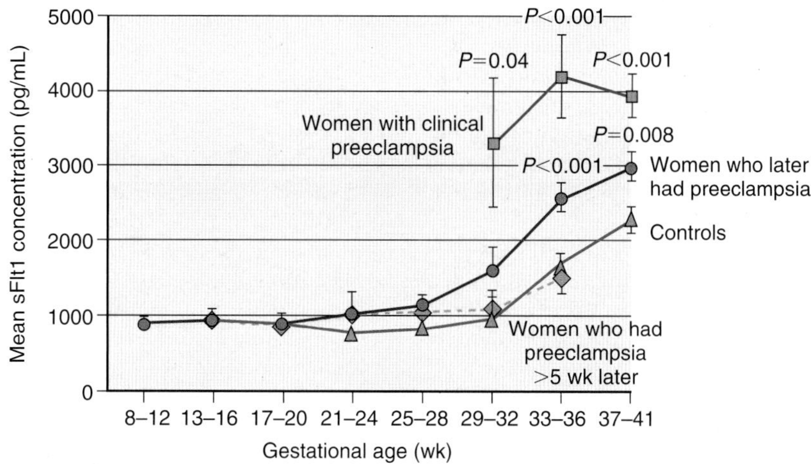


**Fig. 48.11** Concentrations of soluble fms-like tyrosine kinase-1 (sFlt1) in preeclampsia and normal pregnancy. Shown are the mean serum sFlt1 concentrations (± standard error of mean) before and after onset of clinical preeclampsia according to the gestational age of the fetus. The *P* values given are for comparisons, after logarithmic transformation, with specimens from controls obtained during the same gestational-age interval. All specimens were obtained before labor and delivery. (From Levine RJ, Maynard SE, Qian C, et al. Circulating angiogenic factors and the risk of preeclampsia. *N Engl J Med.* 2004;350:672–683.)

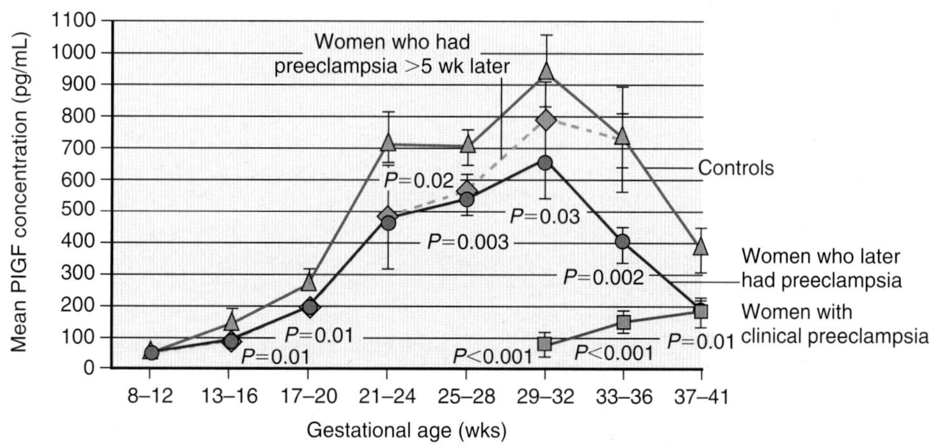


**Fig. 48.12** Concentrations of placental growth factor (PlGF) in preeclampsia and normal pregnancy. Shown are the mean serum PlGF concentrations (± standard error of the mean) before and after onset of clinical preeclampsia according to the gestational age of the fetus. The *P* values given are for comparisons, after logarithmic transformation, with specimens from controls obtained during the same gestational-age interval. All specimens were obtained before labor and delivery. (From Levine RJ, Maynard SE, Qian C, et al. Circulating angiogenic factors and the risk of preeclampsia. *N Engl J Med.* 2004;350:672–683.)

cells in mature blood vessels. VEGF is particularly important in the health of the fenestrated and sinusoidal endothelium found in the renal glomerulus, brain, and liver[181,182] – organs disproportionately affected in preeclampsia. VEGF is highly expressed by glomerular podocytes, and VEGF receptors are present on glomerular endothelial cells.[183] In experimental glomerulonephritis, VEGF is necessary for glomerular capillary repair.[184] In a podocyte-specific VEGF knockout mouse, heterozygosity for VEGF-A resulted in renal disease characterized by proteinuria and glomerular endotheliosis.[185] In antiangiogenesis cancer trials, VEGF antagonists produce proteinuria and hypertension in human subjects.[186–189] This evidence suggests that VEGF deficiency induced by excess sFlt1 has the capacity to produce the characteristic renal lesion of preeclampsia.

Although the glomerular capillary endothelial cell appears to be the primary glomerular target in preeclampsia, the podocyte is clearly affected in severe disease as evidenced by podocyturia during clinical disease and even before overt proteinuria.[140,190] However, podocyturia is also noted in other proteinuric disorders and is not specific for preeclampsia. Renal autopsy examination from women who died with preeclampsia demonstrates markedly reduced podocyte expression of nephrin,[191] and serum from preeclamptic women reduces nephrin expression by cultured podocytes.[192] Using a mouse model of preeclampsia induced by administration of anti-VEGF antibodies, it was noted that nephrin expression is reduced in podocytes.[193] The effect of sFlt1 on podocyte nephrin expression appears to be via increased endothelin-1 release by endothelial cells,[192] again implicating the glomerular endothelial cell as the primary site of injury in preeclampsia.

Alterations in circulating sFlt1 have been noted in certain preeclampsia risk groups. Higher sFlt1 levels have been noted in first versus second pregnancies,[194] in twin versus singleton pregnancies,[195,196] in women with prior preeclampsia,[197] and in women carrying fetuses affected by trisomy 13,[198,199] potentially accounting for the increased preeclampsia risk in these groups. In the case of twin pregnancies, the increased sFlt1 production appears to be due to increased placental mass, rather than placental ischemia.[196] Conversely, lower levels of sFlt1 in pregnant smokers[177,200] may explain the protective effect of smoking in preeclampsia.[201,202]

Angiogenic factors are likely to be important in the regulation of placental vasculogenesis. VEGF ligands and receptors are highly expressed by placental tissue in the first trimester.[203] sFlt1 decreases cytotrophoblast invasiveness in vitro.[123] Circulating sFlt1 levels are relatively low early in pregnancy, and begin to rise in the third trimester. This may reflect a physiologic antiangiogenic shift in the placental milieu toward the end of pregnancy, corresponding to completion of the vasculogenic phase of placental growth. It is intuitive to hypothesize that placental vascular development might be regulated by a local balance between proangiogenic and antiangiogenic factors, and that excess antiangiogenic sFlt1 in early gestation could contribute to inadequate cytotrophoblast invasion in preeclampsia. By the third trimester, excess placental sFlt1 is detectable in the maternal circulation, producing end-organ effects. In this case, placental ischemia may not be causative, but rather the earliest organ affected by this derangement of angiogenic balance.

The pathways regulating placental angiogenic factor expression, and the reasons for their dysregulation in preeclampsia, are yet unknown (see Fig. 48.8). Pieces of the puzzle may be starting to emerge, however. Animal models of preeclampsia based on induction of uteroplacental ischemia are characterized by increased endogenous sFlt1[116,204] and sEng.[205] Agonistic $AT_1$ autoantibodies produce a preeclampsia-like syndrome in mice (see later), in association with increased circulating sFlt1 levels.[206] Elaboration of the upstream pathways involved in placental angiogenic factor expression remains an area of intense research. Heme oxygenase 1 and its downstream metabolite carbon monoxide acts as a vascular protective factor by inhibiting the production of sFlt1.[207] Animal studies suggest that cystathionine γ-lyase (that regulates hydrogen sulfide) may also contribute to preeclampsia by disrupting placental angiogenesis.[208] However, human studies demonstrating alterations in heme oxygenase or cystathionine γ-lyase expression prior to alterations in antiangiogenic factor are still lacking.

In addition to angiogenic alterations, women who develop preeclampsia also have evidence of insulin resistance.[209] Moreover, women with pregestational or gestational diabetes mellitus have an increased risk for developing preeclampsia.[53] In accordance with this finding, in vitro models suggest that insulin signaling and angiogenesis are intimately related at a molecular level,[210] and recent epidemiological data find that evidence of altered angiogenesis and excess insulin resistance may be additive insults that lead to preeclampsia.[211] Furthermore, altered levels of biomarkers linked with angiogenesis and insulin resistance persist in the postpartum state,[212] possibly explaining the long-term cardiovascular risk in these women.

### ANGIOTENSIN-1 RECEPTOR AUTOANTIBODIES

In preeclampsia, plasma renin levels are suppressed relative to normal pregnancy as a secondary response to systemic vasoconstriction and hypertension. As noted in the prior section, preeclampsia is characterized by increased vascular responsiveness to angiotensin II and other vasoconstrictive agents. Wallukat et al[213] identified agonistic angiotensin-1 ($AT_1$) receptor autoantibodies in women with preeclampsia. They hypothesized that these antibodies, which activate the $AT_1$ receptor, may account for the increased angiotensin II sensitivity of preeclampsia. The same investigators later showed that these $AT_1$ autoantibodies, like angiotensin II itself, stimulate endothelial cells to produce tissue factor, an early marker of endothelial dysfunction. Xia et al[214] found that $AT_1$ autoantibodies decreased invasiveness of immortalized human trophoblasts in an in vitro invasion assay, suggesting that these autoantibodies might contribute to defective placental pseudovasculogenesis as well. The same group showed that $AT_1$ autoantibodies isolated from the serum of women with preeclampsia produce a preeclampsia-like syndrome in pregnant rats, with increased endogenous sFlt1 production,[206] suggesting that $AT_1$ autoantibodies and sFlt1 may be part of the same pathophysiologic pathway leading to preeclampsia. Increased endogenous sFlt1 and the phenotype of proteinuria and glomerular endotheliosis were seen in the pregnant dams but not in nonpregnant animals, providing further evidence that placental sFlt1 specifically mediates the proteinuria secondary to $AT_1$ autoantibodies.

$AT_1$ autoantibodies are not limited to pregnancy; they also appear to be increased in malignant renovascular hypertension in nonpregnancy.[215] In addition, these antibodies have been identified in women with abnormal second-trimester uterine artery Doppler studies who did not develop preeclampsia, suggesting that this antibody may be a nonspecific response to placental hypoperfusion.[216]

The angiotensinogen T235 polymorphism, a common molecular variant associated with essential hypertension and microvascular disease, has been associated with preeclampsia in several studies across different populations, though with significant ethnic heterogeneity.[217] Functional implications of this polymorphism remain unclear. Work by Abdalla and colleagues[218] have suggested that heterodimerization of $AT_1$ receptors with bradykinin 2 receptors may contribute to angiotensin II hypersensitivity in preeclampsia. This work remains to be validated in other studies.

## SCREENING

Although there is not yet any definitive therapeutic or preventive strategy for preeclampsia, clinical experience suggests that early detection, monitoring, and supportive care is beneficial to the patient and the fetus. For example, lack of adequate antenatal care is strongly associated with poor outcomes, including eclampsia and fetal death.[219] Risk assessment early in pregnancy is important to identify those who require close monitoring after 20 weeks. Women with first pregnancies or other preeclampsia risk factors (Table 48.2) should be assessed frequently after 20 weeks' gestation for the development of hypertension, proteinuria, headache, visual disturbances, or epigastric pain.

Higher BP in the first or second trimesters, even in the absence of overt hypertension, is associated with elevated risk for preeclampsia in healthy nulliparous women.[220] Unfortunately, these small elevations in midtrimester BP are subtle and the positive predictive value as a screening test is low (especially given the relatively low prevalence), limiting routine clinical utility.

Presumably as a result of failed placental vascular remodeling, preeclampsia is associated with increased placental vascular resistance and uterine artery waveform abnormalities in the second trimester, as measured by uterine artery Doppler ultrasound.[221] Dozens of studies have investigated the use of uterine artery Doppler for prediction of preeclampsia. Test performance varies widely among studies based on differences in populations studied, the gestational age at the time of measurement, the definition of an abnormal result, and the severity and timing of preeclampsia detected: sensitivities and specificities range from 65% to 85%. Even meta-analyses have differed in their conclusions, with some reporting limited diagnostic accuracy in predicting preeclampsia,[221,222] while others suggest that it is accurate enough to be recommended for preeclampsia screening in routine clinical practice.[223] Thus there is wide regional variability in the use of uterine artery Doppler for routine screening, and it remains uncommon in the United States. Recent data suggest that there may be promise in combining uterine artery Doppler with serum biomarkers for preeclampsia.[224,225]

Of dozens of putative serum markers for preeclampsia, only a handful have been shown to be elevated prior to the onset of clinical disease, and none have yet proven to be an effective and useful screening test for preeclampsia. Placental protein 13 (PP-13) and angiogenic biomarkers (sFlt1, PlGF, and sEng) hold promise for screening and/or early diagnosis of preeclampsia.

PP-13 is thought to be involved in normal placentation and maternal vascular remodeling. Low levels of PP-13 could identify women at high risk for preeclampsia as early as the first trimester,[226,227] although it appears to be a robust biomarker only for early onset disease and may be less useful for preeclampsia close to term.[228] Polymorphisms in *LGALS13*, the gene encoding PP-13, have been detected in cases of preeclampsia.[229] This polymorphism may result in production of a shorter splice variant of PP-13, which is not detected by conventional assays, contributing to low circulating levels and decreased local activity of PP-13.

Alterations in circulating levels of the angiogenic factors sFlt1 and sEng occur weeks prior to the onset of preeclampsia and may be useful for screening and/or diagnosis.[230,231] Significant elevations in maternal sFlt1 and sEng are observed from midgestation onward,[162,174–177,232,233] and appear to rise 5–8 weeks prior to preeclampsia onset (see Fig. 48.11).[164] Maternal sFlt1 levels are particularly elevated in severe preeclampsia, early onset preeclampsia, and preeclampsia complicated by a small-for-gestation infant.[164,234] Serum levels of PlGF are lower in women who go on to develop preeclampsia from the first[235] or early second[164,236–238] trimester (see Fig. 48.12). Since PlGF passes into the urine, low urinary PlGF has been identified as a potential marker for preeclampsia. Urinary levels of PlGF are significantly lower in women who develop preeclampsia from the late second trimester,[239] and may prove to be useful in screening and diagnosis of preeclampsia, especially in early onset and severe preeclampsia. Prospective studies are ongoing to evaluate the clinical utility of these biomarkers for preeclampsia screening and risk assessment.

***Clinical Relevance***

Preeclampsia is characterized by marked alterations in angiogenic factors. Measurement of maternal serum sFlt1, placental growth factor (PlGF), and the sFlt1-to-PlGF ratio may inform diagnosis and risk stratification in women with suspected preeclampsia.

Recent studies have suggested that circulating angiogenic factors in plasma or serum can be used to differentiate preeclampsia from other diseases that mimic preeclampsia such as chronic hypertension, gestational hypertension, lupus nephritis, and CKD.[240–244] Zeisler et al[245] demonstrated in a prospective multicenter clinical trial that serum sFlt/PlGF can be used to rule out preeclampsia among patients with suspected disease with negative predictive value >99%. Several groups have also demonstrated a role for angiogenic biomarkers in the prediction of preeclampsia-related adverse outcomes among women evaluated for suspected preeclampsia.[246–250] Measurements of circulating angiogenic factors (sFlt1, PlGF, and sEng) robustly predicted adverse maternal and perinatal outcomes in women presenting with signs or symptoms of preeclampsia and these biomarkers outperformed the standard battery of clinical diagnostic measures including BP, proteinuria, uric acid, and other laboratory assays. Importantly, sFlt1 and/or PlGF levels at presentation were strongly associated with the remaining duration of pregnancy.[246,249] By providing more accurate identification of women at high risk for adverse pregnancy outcomes, use of angiogenic biomarkers may reduce costs and unnecessary resource use in women with possible preeclampsia.[251] For example, women with mild-to-moderate preeclampsia, in whom biomarker testing indicates low risk of imminent delivery or severe complications, may be able to be safely discharged and observed in an outpatient setting, rather than remain under indefinite inpatient observation until delivery.

## PREVENTION OF PREECLAMPSIA

### ANTIPLATELET AGENTS

Aspirin for the prevention of preeclampsia has been evaluated in dozens of trials, both in high-risk and in healthy nulliparous women. The most recent meta-analyses suggest that aspirin reduces the risk of preeclampsia by at least 10%.[252] Some analyses suggest a risk reduction closer to 24% when aspirin is initiated prior to 16 weeks' gestation, and using a dosage of at least 100 mg daily (Fig. 48.13).[253] The absolute risk reduction is greatest among women at high baseline preeclampsia risk; thus current guidelines recommend treatment with acetylsalicylic acid (aspirin) in women with at least one major, or two moderate, preeclampsia risk factors.[254] Based on consistent safety and efficacy in both high- and low-risk populations, some experts recommend universal aspirin for all pregnant women, regardless of baseline preeclampsia risk.[255] Recent data on long-term follow-up of children exposed to low-dose aspirin in utero demonstrate a modest risk of childhood asthma.[256] This potential risk should be considered before widespread use of aspirin for those at low risk of preeclampsia is universally advocated. Rolnik et al[257] recently published results with an impressive 62% reduction in the risk of preterm

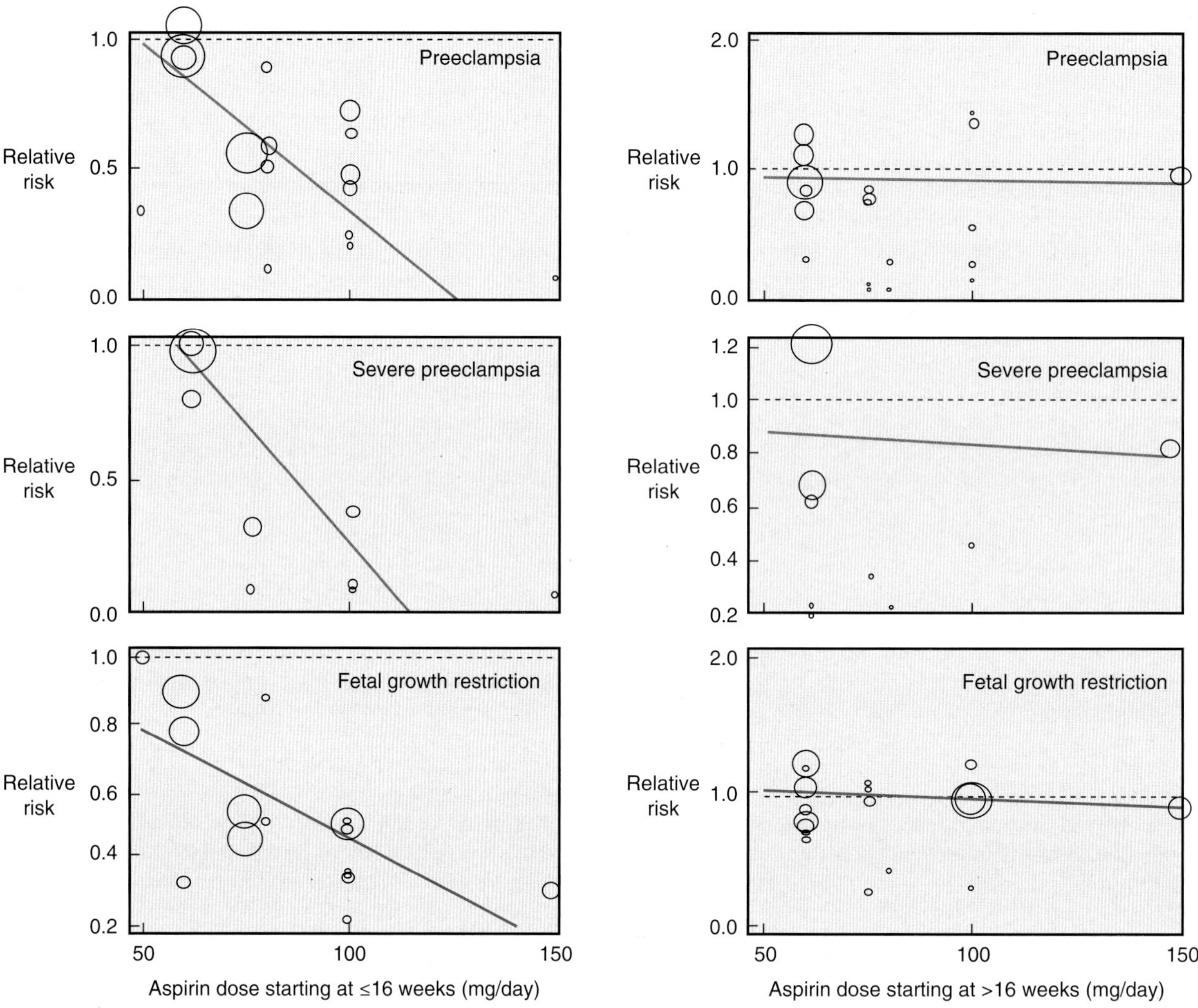


**Fig. 48.13** The effect of aspirin on preeclampsia, severe preeclampsia, and fetal growth restriction. Bubble plots with fitted metaregression line showing the relationship between aspirin dosage and relative risks for each adverse pregnancy outcome, according to gestational age at initiation of aspirin therapy. Data are based on meta-analysis of 45 randomized controlled trials, including 20,909 pregnant women. *RR,* Relative risk. (From Roberge S, Nicolaides K, Demers S, et al. The role of aspirin dose on the prevention of preeclampsia and fetal growth restriction: systematic review and meta-analysis. *Am J Obstet Gynecol.* 2017;216:110–120.e6.)

preeclampsia with utilization of aspirin (150 mg) in high-risk women identified by a previously studied algorithmic score combining mean arterial pressure, uterine-artery pulsatility index, biochemical markers – PIGF and pregnancy-associated plasma protein-A. This new trial provides early evidence that a select group of women with a higher predicted risk of preterm preeclampsia using biophysical algorithms may greatly benefit from receiving aspirin prophylaxis.

## CALCIUM FOR THE PREVENTION OF PREECLAMPSIA

Low baseline dietary calcium intake is associated with increased preeclampsia risk.[258] Several studies have examined the effectiveness of calcium supplementation to prevent preeclampsia. Among low-risk primiparous North American women, calcium supplementation did not reduce incidence of preeclampsia.[61] However, a metaanalysis of 13 trials, including 15,730 women from various parts of the world, reported a significant reduction in preeclampsia risk with high-dose (>1 g/day) calcium supplementation [RR 0.45, 95% confidence interval (CI) 0.31–0.65], with the greatest effect among women with low baseline calcium intake and at high preeclampsia risk.[259] This was tested directly in a large randomized, placebo-controlled trial of calcium supplementation in >8000 women with low baseline calcium intake (<600 mg/day).[260] Although there was no difference in the incidence of preeclampsia, the calcium group had a lower rate of eclampsia, gestational hypertension, preeclampsia complications, and neonatal mortality. Thus calcium supplementation may be useful, especially in women with low baseline calcium intake.

## ANTIOXIDANTS AND NUTRITIONAL INTERVENTIONS

Based on the hypothesis that oxidative stress may contribute to pathogenesis, it has been suggested that antioxidants may prevent preeclampsia.[261] However, four large randomized, controlled trials have failed to show a benefit of vitamin C and vitamin E supplementation for the prevention of preeclampsia in various populations,[262–266] even in women at high preeclampsia risk recruited from communities at risk for poor nutritional status.[262] Vitamin D deficiency has been associated with preeclampsia in some studies.[267–269] However, a randomized, controlled trial failed to demonstrate a reduction in preeclampsia with vitamin D supplementation.[270] More work is needed to evaluate whether treatment of vitamin D insufficiency reduces preeclampsia risk.

Nutritional interventions have generally not been effective in decreasing preeclampsia risk. Protein and calorie restriction for obese pregnant women shows no reduction in the risk of preeclampsia or gestational hypertension, and may increase risk for IUGR, so should be avoided.[271] However, obese women with lower gestational weight gain (<15 kg) have a reduced incidence of preeclampsia.[272,273] Women who have had bariatric surgery for severe obesity have a reduced incidence of preeclampsia compared with obese controls in some,[274] but not in all,[275] studies.

### LOW-MOLECULAR-WEIGHT HEPARIN

Low-molecular-weight heparin (LMWH) is commonly used to prevent recurrent pregnancy loss in women with antiphospholipid syndrome and inherited thrombophilias, such as factor V Leiden mutation. Several studies have evaluated the potential benefit of LMWH for the prevention of preeclampsia and other placental-mediated pregnancy complications in women with a history of these complications in prior pregnancies. A meta-analysis summarized six of these randomized, controlled trials.[276] The analysis suggested a significant reduction in the composite outcome of preeclampsia, birth of a small-for-gestational-age newborn (<10th percentile), placental abruption, or pregnancy loss >20 weeks in women treated with prophylactic LMWH (18.7% of treated women vs. 42.9% of controls). However, a subsequent multicenter open-label randomized controlled trial failed to show a reduction in the incidence of preeclampsia or IUGR among high-risk women treated with LMWH.[277] More studies are needed before LMWH can be recommended for preeclampsia prevention in high-risk women.

## MANAGEMENT AND TREATMENT OF PREECLAMPSIA

### TIMING OF DELIVERY

The timing of delivery in severe preeclampsia is controversial. In women presenting prior to 24 weeks' gestation, perinatal and neonatal mortality are extremely high (>80%) even with attempts to postpone delivery, and maternal complications are common.[278] For this reason, termination is usually recommended in women with severe preeclampsia presenting prior to 24 weeks. By contrast, in women presenting after 37 weeks' gestation, the neonatal benefit of prolonging pregnancy is minimal, and immediate delivery is almost always indicated to avoid potential maternal and fetal complications. For women presenting between 24 and 37 weeks' gestation, the potential neonatal benefit of continuing pregnancy must be balanced against the possibility of maternal morbidity and mortality with delaying delivery. In general, the presence of nonreassuring fetal testing; suspected abruptio placentae; thrombocytopenia; worsening liver and/or kidney function; and symptoms such as unremitting headache, visual changes, nausea, vomiting, or epigastric pain are generally considered indications for expedient delivery.

Two small, randomized controlled trials demonstrated that in women presenting with severe preeclampsia between 28 and 32 weeks' gestation, expectant management (with delivery postponed 1–2 weeks after presentation) resulted in decreased neonatal complications and decreased neonatal intensive care unit stay, with no significant increase in maternal complications.[279,280] Subsequent observational studies have confirmed that delivery can be safely and effectively postponed in women with severe preeclampsia with careful and intensive fetal and maternal monitoring.[278] Similarly, in women with nonsevere preeclampsia presenting between 34 and 37 weeks' gestation, a strategy of expectant monitoring (aimed at prolonging pregnancy until 37 weeks' gestation) led to a reduction in neonatal respiratory distress syndrome, without apparent adverse maternal effects.[281] Expectant management also appears to decrease subsequent respiratory disorders in childhood.[282]

There are no randomized controlled trials to evaluate optimal mode of delivery in severe preeclampsia. Retrospective studies suggest that maternal and neonatal outcomes are similar among women undergoing induction of labor and those undergoing cesarean section.[283]

### BLOOD PRESSURE MANAGEMENT

Management of BP in preeclampsia is substantially different from that in the nonpregnant population. Rather than seeking to minimize long-term cerebrovascular and cardiovascular complications, the goal of care is to maximize the likelihood of successful delivery of a healthy infant, while minimizing the chance of acute complications in the mother. Acute aggressive lowering of BP can lead to fetal distress or demise, especially if placental perfusion is already compromised. Because of this, antihypertensive therapy for preeclampsia is usually withheld unless the BP rises above 150–160 mm Hg systolic or 100–110 mm Hg diastolic, above which the risk of cerebral hemorrhage becomes significant.[68] In the next section we review details regarding the use of specific antihypertensive agents for BP management in pregnancy.

### MAGNESIUM AND SEIZURE PROPHYLAXIS

Magnesium has been widely used for the management and prevention of eclampsia for decades. Prior to the mid-1990s, evidence for its use was largely derived from clinical experience and from small uncontrolled studies. Over the last 10 years, magnesium has been proven to be superior to other agents in the prevention and treatment of seizures in preeclampsia, although not for the prevention of preeclampsia per se. In 1995, two randomized controlled trials in an international and a US population showed that magnesium sulfate was superior to diazepam and phenytoin in reducing risk of seizures in women with preeclampsia/eclampsia.[284,285] Subsequently, the Magpie study confirmed this benefit with a randomized, controlled trial of magnesium versus placebo for seizure prevention in >10,000 women with preeclampsia from 33 countries, finding that magnesium decreased the incidence of eclamptic seizure by 50% (0.8% vs. 1.9%).[88] A global public health effort over the past 10–15 years has led to improved access to magnesium in developing countries, where use of magnesium in preeclampsia/eclampsia has now reached 75% to 90%.[286]

Magnesium is now categorized by the US Food and Drug Administration with a warning label, due to adverse fetal bone effects with long-term (>5–7 days) use as a tocolytic in preterm labor (http://www.fda.gov/Drugs/DrugSafety/ucm353333.htm). Despite this labeling change, short-term (<48 hours) intravenous magnesium is still recommended by the American College of Obstetrics and Gynecology for the prevention and treatment of seizures in women with preeclampsia and eclampsia.[287] Magnesium is generally given intravenously as a bolus, followed by a continuous infusion. In the therapeutic range (5 to 9 mg/dL), magnesium sulfate slows neuromuscular conduction and depresses central nervous system irritability. Women receiving continuous infusions of magnesium should be monitored carefully for signs of toxicity, including loss of deep tendon reflexes, flushing, somnolence, muscle weakness, and decreased respiratory rate. Such monitoring is especially important in women with impaired renal function who have impaired urinary magnesium excretion.

### MANAGEMENT OF THE HELLP SYNDROME

The clinical course of the HELLP syndrome usually involves inexorable and often sudden and unpredictable deterioration. Given the high incidence of maternal complications, some authors recommend immediate delivery in all cases of confirmed HELLP. Among women in the 24–34 weeks' gestational window whose clinical status appears relatively stable and with reassuring fetal status, expectant management is often a viable alternative. For many years intravenous steroids have been suggested as an adjunct to usual management, based on retrospective and uncontrolled studies. A recent randomized controlled trial showed no benefit to high-dose dexamethasone treatment in HELLP syndrome.[288] Post hoc analysis suggested that the subgroup with severe preeclampsia (platelet count < 50,000) may have a shorter average platelet count recovery and shorter hospitalization with steroids, so further studies are required to evaluate the benefit in this population.

Based on pathophysiologic similarities to TTP, there are reports of using plasmapheresis in the management of the HELLP syndrome. Data for the antepartum period are limited to a few cases series with mixed results and no clear benefit.[289] Potential drawbacks include fetal compromise due to diminishment of already compromised placental blood flow.

### NOVEL THERAPIES FOR PREECLAMPSIA

Recent advances in our understanding of the pathophysiology of preeclampsia have revealed new potential therapeutic targets. Interfering with the production or signaling of sFlt1 may ameliorate the endothelial dysfunction of preeclampsia, allowing delivery to be more safely postponed. In a pilot study limited to three severe early preeclamptics (24–32 weeks' gestation), Thadhani et al[290] depleted sFlt1 levels using dextran sulfate apheresis and prolonged pregnancy by 2–4 weeks. Importantly, this therapy promoted fetal growth with no adverse effects to the fetus or the mother. More recently, Thadhani et al[291] demonstrated that therapeutic apheresis using a plasma-specific dextran sulfate column produced a 18% reduction in sFlt1, a 44% reduction in P:C ratio, and a prolongation of pregnancy as compared with untreated contemporaneous preeclampsia subjects. If confirmed, this approach could lead to targeted therapy for patients with preterm preeclampsia that present with an abnormal angiogenic profile.[290] Other modalities for targeting the angiogenic imbalance are administration of agents that neutralize sFlt1 such as PlGF and VEGF, or small molecules that block sFlt1 production, which are currently being evaluated in preclinical settings.[160,292–295]

Hydroxymethylglutaryl-coenzyme A reductase inhibitors, or statins, have been proposed as potential therapeutic agents for preeclampsia through their effects on promoting heme oxygenase activity and improving angiogenic imbalance in animal models of preeclampsia.[207,296] These agents were once considered contraindicated in pregnancy due to potential teratogenic effects, but recent data suggest that they are probably safe.[297] Early pilot data suggest that statins may be effective clinically both for the treatment[298] and for the prevention[299] of preeclampsia. Randomized, controlled trials to assess the safety and efficacy of pravastatin for the prevention and treatment of preeclampsia are ongoing.[300]

## CHRONIC HYPERTENSION AND GESTATIONAL HYPERTENSION

The diagnosis of chronic hypertension in pregnancy is usually based on a documented history of hypertension prior to pregnancy or a BP >140/90 prior to 20 weeks' gestation. Gestational hypertension, by contrast, is usually first noted after 20 weeks' gestation and, by definition, resolves after delivery. These diagnoses, based on the timing of the first recorded BP elevation, can be subject to pitfalls, however. The physiologic dip in BP in the second trimester, which nadirs at about 20 weeks' gestation (see Fig. 48.1), occurs in women with chronic hypertension and can mask the presence of underlying chronic hypertension early in pregnancy. In such cases, a woman with chronic hypertension may be inappropriately labeled as having gestational hypertension when the BP rises in the third trimester. The diagnosis of chronic hypertension is established when hypertension fails to resolve postpartum. By contrast, preeclampsia can occasionally present prior to 20 weeks' gestation; hence preeclampsia should always be considered in women presenting with new hypertension and proteinuria close to midgestation.

The incidence of chronic hypertension in pregnancy is increasing in the United States, from 1.01% in 1995–1996 to 1.76% in 2007–2008.[301] Chronic hypertension is more common with advanced maternal age, obesity, and black race.[302] Pregnant women with chronic hypertension have an increased risk of preeclampsia (21%–25%), premature delivery (33%–35%), IUGR (10%–15%), placental abruption (1%–3%), and perinatal mortality (4.5%).[303–305] However, most adverse outcomes occur in women with severe hypertension (DBP > 110 mm Hg) and those with preexisting cardiovascular or renal disease. Women with mild, uncomplicated chronic hypertension usually have obstetric outcomes comparable with the general obstetric population.[302] Both the duration and the severity of hypertension are correlated with perinatal morbidity and preeclampsia risk.[306,307] The presence of baseline proteinuria increases the risk of preterm delivery and IUGR, but not preeclampsia per se.[304]

The diagnosis of preeclampsia superimposed on chronic hypertension can be difficult. In the absence of underlying kidney disease, the new onset of proteinuria (>300 mg/day), usually with worsening hypertension, is the most reliable sign of superimposed preeclampsia.[68] When proteinuria is present at baseline, preeclampsia is likely when a sudden increase in BP is observed in a woman whose BP was previously well-controlled. The presence of other signs and symptoms of preeclampsia such as headache, visual changes, epigastric pain, pulmonary edema, and laboratory derangements (e.g., thrombocytopenia, new or worsening renal insufficiency, and elevated liver enzymes) also should prompt consideration of preeclampsia, and when present, are an indication of preeclampsia severity.[68]

## SECONDARY HYPERTENSION IN PREGNANCY

Secondary causes of hypertension are present in at least 10% of women with chronic hypertension in pregnancy.[301] Women with secondary forms of hypertension have pregnancy complication rates even higher than women with primary chronic hypertension, and failing to recognize these diagnoses can lead to significant maternal morbidity and mortality. Hence prepregnancy evaluation of women with chronic hypertension should include consideration of secondary causes of hypertension, including renal artery stenosis, primary hyperaldosteronism, obstructive sleep apnea (OSA), and pheochromocytoma. Unfortunately, diagnosis of these conditions during pregnancy is hampered by the fact that screening tests (e.g., the plasma aldosterone-to-renin ratio) have not been validated in pregnancy, and imaging involving radiation exposure (e.g., CT scanning, angiography, and fluoroscopy) is relatively contraindicated.

Renal artery stenosis due to fibromuscular dysplasia or atherosclerotic vascular disease occasionally presents in pregnancy, and should be suspected when hypertension is severe and resistant to medical therapy. Diagnosis with MR angiography followed by successful angioplasty and stent placement in the second and third trimesters of pregnancy has been described.[308]

Although rare, pheochromocytoma can be devastating if it first presents during pregnancy. This syndrome occasionally is unmasked during labor and delivery, when fatal hypertensive crisis can be triggered by vaginal delivery, uterine contractions, and anesthesia.[309] Maternal and neonatal outcomes are much better when the diagnosis is made antepartum, with attentive and aggressive medical management.[310] Surgical intervention is typically postponed until after delivery whenever possible.

Hypertension and hypokalemia from primary hyperaldosteronism might be expected to improve during pregnancy, as progesterone antagonizes the effect of aldosterone on the renal tubule. However, such remission is not universal and many women with primary hyperaldosteronism have a pregnancy-induced exacerbation of hypertension.[311] In the case of a functional adrenal adenoma, there are little data to favor either immediate surgical adrenalectomy or medical management until after delivery, though case reports have suggested success with both approaches. Although the use of spironolactone has been reported during pregnancy, there is a theoretical risk of inadequate virilization of male fetuses due to its antiandrogenic effects. Eplerenone appears to be a safe alternative in cases where conventional antihypertensive agents and potassium supplementation are inadequate.[312]

OSA has emerged as an important secondary cause of hypertension in pregnancy. In one study, 40% of women with hypertension in pregnancy had evidence of OSA by polysomnography.[313] Risk factors for OSA include snoring and obesity.[314] Screening for OSA should be considered in high-risk women.

A rare cause of early onset hypertension is due to a mutation in the mineralocorticoid receptor. This results in inappropriate receptor activation by progesterone, and affected women develop a marked exacerbation of hypertension and hypokalemia in pregnancy, but without proteinuria or other features of preeclampsia.[315]

## APPROACH TO MANAGEMENT OF CHRONIC HYPERTENSION IN PREGNANCY

In women with chronic hypertension who are planning pregnancy, BP should be controlled prior to conception using agents that are safe in pregnancy. When pregnancy is unplanned, inappropriate antihypertensive medications should be stopped as soon as possible after conception. Women should be counseled regarding the risks of adverse pregnancy outcomes, including preeclampsia, preterm birth, and IUGR. Women with chronic hypertension in pregnancy should be followed closely during pregnancy, with appropriate adjustments in antihypertensive therapy, and monitoring for superimposed preeclampsia.

### GOALS OF THERAPY

When hypertension is severe (SBP ≥ 160 or DBP ≥ 105 mm Hg), antihypertensive therapy is clearly indicated for the prevention of stroke and cardiovascular complications.[68] However, there is little evidence to guide management of mild-to-moderate hypertension in pregnancy. Dozens of small ($n < 300$) clinical trials have evaluated the impact of antihypertensive therapy versus no treatment in such women, and these have been evaluated in meta-analyses.[316–319] Although antihypertensive therapy lowered the risk of developing severe hypertension, there was no beneficial effect on the development of preeclampsia, neonatal death, preterm birth, small for gestational age babies, or other adverse outcomes. Some studies suggested that aggressive treatment of mild-to-moderate hypertension in pregnancy may impair fetal growth, presumably as a result of decreased uteroplacental perfusion.[320] For this reason, the 2013 American College of Obstetrics and Gynecology Task Force on Hypertension in Pregnancy recommends against antihypertensive medication use in pregnant women with chronic hypertension and BP < 160/105 mm Hg in the absence of evidence of end-organ damage.[68]

***Clinical Relevance***

The CHIPS (Control of Hypertension in Pregnancy Study) trial showed that treatment of hypertension in pregnancy to a "tight" blood pressure target [diastolic blood pressure (DBP) 85 mm Hg], as compared with a "less-tight" target (DBP 100 mm Hg), was safe, with no significant differences in the rate of pregnancy loss or need for high-level neonatal care. Women treated to the tight blood pressure target had a significantly lower rate of maternal complications, including severe hypertension, thrombocytopenia, and transaminitis with symptoms.

**Table 48.5 Outcomes in Women With Hypertension in Pregnancies Randomized to Tight Versus Less-Tight Blood Pressure Control**

| Outcome | Less-Tight Control (DBP 100 mm Hg) | Tight Control (DBP 85 mm Hg) | Adjusted Odds Ratio (95% CI) |
|---|---|---|---|
| **Neonatal and Pregnancy Complications** | | | |
| Pregnancy loss, *n* (%) | 15 (3.0) | 13 (2.7) | 1.14 (0.53–2.45) |
| High-level neonatal care for >48 h *n* (%) | 141 (29.4) | 139 (29.0) | 1.00 (0.75–1.33) |
| Gestational age at delivery (wk) | 36.8 ± 3.4 | 37.2 ± 3.1 | |
| Small-for-gestational-age newborns (birth weight < 10th percentile), *n* (%) | 79 (16.1) | 96 (19.7) | 0.78 (0.56–1.08) |
| Placental abruption | 11 (2.2) | 11 (2.3) | 0.94 (0.40–2.21) |
| **Maternal Complications** | | | |
| Serious maternal complications, *n* (%) | 18 (3.7) | 10 (2.0) | 1.74 (0.79–3.84) |
| Severe hypertension | 200 (40.6) | 134 (27.5) | 1.80 (1.34–2.38) |
| Preeclampsia | 241 (48.9) | 223 (45.7) | 1.14 (0.88–1.47) |
| Platelet count < 100 × $10^9$/L | 21 (4.3) | 8 (1.6) | 2.63 (1.15–6.05) |
| Elevated AST or ALT with symptoms | 21 (4.2) | 9 (1.8) | 2.33 (1.05–5.16) |
| HELLP syndrome | 9 (1.8) | 2 (0.4) | 4.35 (0.93–20.35) |

*ALT,* Alanine aminotransferase; *AST,* aspartate aminotransferase; *CI,* confidence interval; *DBP,* diastolic blood pressure; *HELLP,* hemolytic anemia, elevated *l*iver enzymes, and *l*ow *p*latelets.

Adapted from Magee LA, von Dadelszen P, Rey E, et al. Less-tight versus tight control of hypertension in pregnancy. *N Engl J Med.* 2015;372:407–417.

In 2015, CHIPS (Control of Hypertension in Pregnancy Study) added to the evidence base on this topic.[321] CHIPS was an open, international, randomized, controlled clinical trial of tight (target DBP 85 mm Hg) versus less-tight (target DBP 100 mm Hg) BP control in 987 women with mild-to-moderate hypertension in pregnancy. They found no difference in the primary outcome of pregnancy loss or need for high-level neonatal care (Table 48.5). There was no significant difference in the incidence of small-for-gestational-age newborns between the two groups. However, women in the less-tight control group had a higher incidence of severe hypertension, thrombocytopenia, and symptomatic transaminitis. There was a trend toward an increase in HELLP syndrome in the less-tight control group. This study, by far the largest of its kind, provides reassurance that treatment of mild-to-moderate hypertension in pregnancy to a DBP target of 85 mm Hg is safe for the fetus, and lowers risk of short-term maternal pregnancy complications. The study did not report long-term maternal cardiovascular outcomes with tight antihypertensive treatment, but a benefit seems likely given the strong evidence of benefit in nonpregnant persons with chronic hypertension.[322]

## GESTATIONAL HYPERTENSION

Gestational hypertension is defined as the new onset of hypertension without proteinuria after 20 weeks' gestation that resolves postpartum. Gestational hypertension likely represents a mix of several underlying etiologies. A subset of women with gestational hypertension have previously existing essential hypertension that is undiagnosed. In such cases, if the woman presents for medical care during the second-trimester nadir in BP, she may be inappropriately presumed to be previously normotensive. In such a circumstance the diagnosis of chronic hypertension is established postpartum, when BP fails to return to normal.

Gestational hypertension progresses to overt preeclampsia in ~10%–25% of cases.[323] When gestational hypertension is severe, it carries similar risks for adverse outcomes as preeclampsia, even in the absence of proteinuria.[324] A renal biopsy study suggests that a significant proportion of women with gestational hypertension have renal glomerular endothelial damage.[142] Hence gestational hypertension may share the same pathophysiologic underpinnings as preeclampsia, and should be monitored and treated as such. In recognition of the syndromic nature of preeclampsia, new American College of Obstetricians and Gynecologists (ACOG) guidelines have eliminated the dependence of proteinuria for the diagnosis of preeclampsia (Table 48.3). In a subset of women with gestational hypertension, it may represent a temporary unmasking of an underlying predisposition toward chronic hypertension. Such women often present with a strong family history of chronic hypertension and develop hypertension in the third trimester with a low uric acid and no proteinuria. Although the hypertension often resolves after delivery, these women are at risk for the development of hypertension and cardiovascular disease later in life.[325,326]

## MANAGEMENT OF HYPERTENSION IN PREGNANCY

### CHOICE OF AGENTS

Recommendations for the use of antihypertensive agents in pregnancy are summarized in Table 48.6. Methyldopa continues to be the first-line oral agent for the management of hypertension in pregnancy. Methyldopa is a centrally acting alpha-2 adrenergic agonist now seldom used outside of pregnancy. Of all antihypertensive agents, it has the most

**Table 48.6 Safety of Antihypertensive Medications in Pregnancy**

| Drug | Advantage(s) | Disadvantage(s) |
|---|---|---|
| **First-Line Agents** | | |
| Oral | | |
| Methyldopa | First line; extensive safety data | Short duration of action/multiple daily dosing |
| Labetalol | Preferred over other β-blockers owing to theoretical beneficial effect of α-blockade on uteroplacental blood flow | Short duration of action/multiple daily dosing. May exacerbate reactive airway disease |
| Long-acting nifedipine | Once-daily dosing (slow-release preparation) | Edema |
| Intravenous | | |
| Labetalol | Good safety data | |
| Nicardipine | Extensive safety data on use as a tocolytic during labor; effective | |
| **Second-Line Agents** | | |
| Hydralazine | Extensive clinical experience | Increased risk of maternal hypotension and placental abruption when used acutely |
| Metoprolol | Potential for once-daily dosing using long-acting formulation | Safety data less extensive than for labetalol |
| Verapamil, diltiazem | No evidence of adverse fetal effects | Limited data |
| **Generally Avoided** | | |
| Diuretics | No evidence of adverse fetal effects | Theoretically may impair pregnancy-associated expansion in plasma volume |
| Atenolol | | May impair fetal growth |
| Nitroprusside | | Risk of fetal cyanide poisoning if used for >4 hours |
| **Contraindicated** | | |
| Angiotensin-converting enzyme (ACE) inhibitors | | Multiple fetal anomalies; see text |
| Angiotensin receptor antagonists | | Similar risks as ACE inhibitors |

extensive safety data and appears to have no adverse fetal effects. Drawbacks include a short half-life, sedation, and rare adverse effects include elevated liver enzymes and hemolytic anemia. Clonidine appears to be comparable with methyldopa in terms of mechanism and safety, but data are fewer.

β-Adrenergic antagonists have been used extensively in pregnancy and are effective without known teratogenicity or known adverse fetal effects. One possible exception is atenolol, which has been associated with fetal growth restriction.[327] Labetalol, which may result in better preservation of uteroplacental blood flow due to its alpha-blocking action, has found widespread use and acceptance, both as an oral and as an intravenous agent.[328]

Calcium channel blockers appear to be safe in pregnancy, and clinical experience with them is growing. Long-acting nifedipine is the most well-studied, and it appears to be safe and effective.[328,329] Nondihydropyridine calcium channel blockers such as verapamil have also been used without apparent adverse effects. However, experience with these agents is more limited than some other classes.

Although diuretics are often avoided in preeclampsia, with the reasoning that circulating volume is already low, there is no evidence that diuretics are associated with adverse fetal or maternal outcomes. Similarly, diuretics are not considered first line in the management of chronic hypertension in pregnancy due to their theoretical impact on the normal plasma volume expansion of pregnancy. When hypertension in pregnancy is complicated by pulmonary edema, diuretics are appropriate and effective.

Angiotensin-converting enzyme inhibitors (ACEIs) and angiotensin receptor antagonists (angiotensin II–receptor blockers or ARBs) are contraindicated in the second and third trimesters of pregnancy. Exposure during this time leads to major fetal malformations including renal dysgenesis, perinatal renal failure, oligohydramnios, pulmonary hypoplasia, hypocalvaria, and IUGR.[330] Evidence for teratogenicity with first-trimester exposure is less compelling. In a large population-based study, Cooper et al[331] reported that congenital malformations of the central nervous and cardiovascular systems were higher among women with first-trimester exposure to ACE inhibitors. However, this study has been criticized for the presence of potential confounders and ascertainment bias. Women with a compelling indication for ACE-I/ARBs (such as diabetic nephropathy) can probably be continued on these agents while attempting conception, with discontinuation as soon as pregnancy is diagnosed. However, risks and benefits of this strategy should be discussed with the patient, with shared and individualized decision making. Women inadvertently exposed in early pregnancy can be reassured by a normal midtrimester ultrasound examination. Fewer data are available on the effects of ARBs, but a case series strongly suggests that fetal effects are similar to ACE-I,[332] as would be expected on a theoretical basis.

### INTRAVENOUS AGENTS FOR URGENT BLOOD PRESSURE CONTROL

Severe hypertension in pregnancy occasionally requires inpatient management with intravenous agents. There is a lack of controlled studies in humans for the use of all intravenous medications commonly used for urgent control of severe hypertension during pregnancy. Nevertheless, there is extensive clinical experience with several agents, which are widely used with no evidence of adverse effects. Options for intravenous use include labetalol, calcium channel blockers such as nicardipine, and hydralazine.

Intravenous labetalol, like oral labetalol, is safe and effective, with the major drawback being its short duration of action. Intravenous nicardipine has been used safely for tocolysis during premature labor, and recent reports suggest that it is safe in treatment of hypertension as well.[333] The use of short-acting nifedipine is controversial due to well-documented adverse effects in the nonpregnant population. However, a recent meta-analysis suggests that oral short-acting nifedipine can be safely used for severe hypertension during pregnancy,[334] and it may be a good option in areas where intravenous agents are unavailable.

Hydralazine has been widely used as a first-line agent for severe hypertension in pregnancy. However, a meta-analysis of 21 trials comparing intravenous hydralazine with either labetalol or nifedipine for acute management of hypertension in pregnancy suggested an increased risk of maternal hypotension, maternal oliguria, placental abruption, and low Apgar scores with hydralazine.[335] Hence hydralazine should probably be considered second line and its use limited when possible. Nitroprusside carries risk of fetal cyanide poisoning if used for >4 hours and is generally avoided.

### ANTIHYPERTENSIVE DRUGS IN BREASTFEEDING

There are few well-designed studies of the safety of antihypertensive medications in breastfeeding women. In general, the agents that are considered safe during pregnancy remain so in breastfeeding. Methyldopa, if effective and well tolerated, should be considered first-line. β-Blockers with high protein binding, such as labetalol and propranolol, are preferred over atenolol and metoprolol, which are concentrated in breast milk.[328] Diuretics may decrease milk production and should be avoided.[328] ACE inhibitors are poorly excreted in breast milk and generally considered safe in lactating women.[336] Enalapril and captopril have been best studied and are preferred in lactating women. Hence in women with proteinuric renal disease, reinitiation of ACE inhibitors should be considered immediately after delivery. Finally, specific data on the pharmacokinetics of each medication should be used to guide mothers to timing breastfeeding intervals before or well after peak breast milk excretion to avoid significant exposure to the baby.

## ACUTE KIDNEY INJURY IN PREGNANCY

The incidence of AKI in pregnancy in the developed world has fallen dramatically during the second half of the 20th century.[337] This decline was attributed to improved availability of safe and legal abortion, more widespread and aggressive antibiotic use (both of which decreased the incidence of septic abortion), and improvement in overall prenatal care. However, more recently the incidence of AKI complicating pregnancy has increased in the United States and Canada.[338,339] This trend is likely attributable to the increasing incidence of hypertensive disorders of pregnancy and preeclampsia.[339] Indeed, most cases of AKI in pregnancy in the modern era occur in the setting of hypertensive disorders: gestational hypertension, chronic hypertension, or preeclampsia.[340] Most cases of AKI in pregnancy are mild and self-limited; AKI requiring dialysis is rare, affecting approximately 1:10,000 pregnancies.[341]

Prerenal azotemia—for example, with hyperemesis gravidarum or severe pyelonephritis—is a common cause of AKI in pregnancy. Pregnancy-specific conditions such as preeclampsia, the HELLP syndrome, and AFLP are also common causes of AKI. Obstetric complications such as septic abortion, peripartum sepsis, and placental abruption are associated with severe acute tubular necrosis and rarely bilateral cortical necrosis. Obstructive uropathy is an unusual cause of renal failure in pregnancy.

### ACUTE TUBULAR INJURY AND RENAL CORTICAL NECROSIS

Volume depletion complicating hyperemesis gravidarum or uterine hemorrhage (due to placental abruption, placenta previa, failure of the postpartum uterus to contract, or uterine lacerations and perforations) can lead to renal ischemia and subsequent acute tubular injury. AKI may also occur following intraamniotic saline administration, amniotic fluid embolism, and diseases or accidents unrelated to pregnancy.

Renal cortical necrosis is a severe and often irreversible form of acute tubular necrosis that is associated with septic abortion and placental abruption. Septic abortion is an infection of the uterus and the surrounding tissues, most commonly following nonsterile illicit abortions. Septic abortion is now rare where safe therapeutic abortion is available, but remains a serious clinical problem in countries where induced abortion is illegal and/or inaccessible. Women with septic abortion usually present with vaginal bleeding, lower abdominal pain, and fever hours to days after the attempted abortion. Renal failure, which complicates up to 73% of cases,[342] is often characterized by gross hematuria, flank pain, and oligoanuria.

The bacteria associated with septic abortion are usually polymicrobial and derived from the normal flora of the vagina and endocervix, in addition to sexually transmitted pathogens. *Clostridium welchii, Clostridium perfringens, Streptococcus pyogenes,* and gram-negative organisms such as *Escherichia coli* and *Pseudomonas aeruginosa* are all known pathogens. Fatal toxic shock syndrome with *Clostridium sordellii* has been reported following medical termination of pregnancy using mifepristone (RU-486) and intravaginal misoprostol.[343] Pregnancy has long been known to confer a peculiar susceptibility to the vascular effects of gram-negative endotoxin (Shwartzman phenomenon).

AKI with cortical necrosis can also be precipitated by placental abruption. Cortical necrosis can involve the entire renal cortex, often leading to irreversible renal failure, but more commonly is incomplete or patchy. In such cases, a protracted period of oligoanuria is followed by a variable return of renal function. The diagnosis of renal cortical necrosis can usually be established by CT scan, which characteristically demonstrates hypodense areas in the renal cortex.

The treatment of AKI in pregnancy is supportive with prompt restoration of fluid volume deficits, and in later pregnancy, expedient delivery. No specific therapy is effective in acute cortical necrosis except for dialysis when needed. Both peritoneal and hemodialysis have been used during pregnancy; however, peritoneal dialysis carries the risk of impairing uteroplacental blood flow.[344] Maternal mortality with pregnancy-associated AKI requiring dialysis remains high, in both developed (4.3%)[341] and developing countries (18.3%).[345]

## ACUTE KIDNEY INJURY AND THROMBOTIC MICROANGIOPATHY

The presence of thrombotic microangiopathy (TMA) and acute renal failure in pregnancy is one of the most challenging differential diagnoses to face the nephrologist caring for pregnant patients. Five pregnancy syndromes share many clinical, laboratory, and pathologic features: preeclampsia/HELLP syndrome, TTP/HUS, AFLP, systemic lupus erythematosus (SLE) with the antiphospholipid antibody syndrome, and disseminated intravascular coagulation (usually complicating sepsis). Although it is difficult to establish clinical distinctions between these entities with certainty, the confluence of clinical clues can often establish a likely diagnosis (see Table 48.4).

### SEVERE PREECLAMPSIA

AKI affects approximately 1% of women with preeclampsia.[346] However, in patients with severe preeclampsia and HELLP syndrome, the incidence of AKI is much higher, ranging from 10% to 25% in various studies.[347,348] When acute renal failure occurs in the setting of preeclampsia, urgent delivery is indicated.

### ACUTE FATTY LIVER OF PREGNANCY

AFLP is a rare but potentially fatal complication of pregnancy, affecting about 1 in 10,000 pregnancies, with a 10% case fatality rate.[349] The clinical picture is dominated by liver failure, with elevated serum aminotransferase levels and hyperbilirubinemia. Severely affected patients have elevations in blood ammonia levels and hypoglycemia. Preeclampsia can also be present in up to half of cases. Hemolysis and thrombocytopenia are not prominent features, and the presence of these findings should suggest the diagnosis of HELLP syndrome or TTP (Table 48.4). Acute renal failure in association with acute fatty liver is seen mainly near term but can occur any time after midgestation.[350] The kidney lesion is mild and nonspecific, and the cause of renal failure is obscure. It may be due to hemodynamic changes akin to those seen in the hepatorenal syndrome or to a TMA.

Although liver biopsy is rarely undertaken clinically, AFLP is a pathologic diagnosis: histologic changes include swollen hepatocytes filled with microvesicular fat and minimal hepatocellular necrosis. This histological picture resembles that seen in Reye syndrome and Jamaican vomiting sickness. A defect in mitochondrial fatty acid oxidation due to mutations in the long-chain 3-hydroxyacyl-coenzyme A dehydrogenase gene has been hypothesized as a risk factor for the development of AFLP.[351] Women with AFLP and their offspring should be tested for this and other genetic defects of fatty acid oxidation, as early diagnosis and treatment of affected neonates may be lifesaving.[352]

Management of AFLP includes supportive care, including aggressive management of the coagulopathy, and prompt termination of the pregnancy. The use of plasmapheresis has been reported both antepartum[353] and postpartum,[354] but there are no controlled trials evaluating its use. The syndrome typically remits postpartum with no residual hepatic or renal impairment, though it can recur in subsequent pregnancies.

### THROMBOTIC THROMBOCYTOPENIC PURPURA

TTP is a primary TMA caused by severe ADAMTS13 deficiency. TTP is characterized by thrombocytopenia, hemolysis, and variable organ dysfunction. Acute renal failure may occur, though is not universal.[355] Pregnancy is associated with an increased risk of TTP, usually presenting prior to 24 weeks' gestation,[356] and pregnancy can precipitate relapse in women with a history of TTP.[357] Deficiency in the von Willebrand factor cleaving protease (ADAMTS13) has been linked to the pathogenesis of TTP in nonpregnant states, but this has not been well-studied in pregnancy. ADAMTS13 levels fall during the second and third trimester, potentially contributing to the increased incidence of TTP in pregnancy.[358]

The often challenging clinical distinction between TTP and preeclampsia/HELLP is important for patient management, because plasma exchange is beneficial in TTP but not in the HELLP syndrome. A history of preceding proteinuria, hypertension, and severe liver injury is more suggestive of the HELLP syndrome, whereas the presence of renal failure and severe nonimmune hemolytic anemia is more typical of TTP (Table 48.4). Although plasmapheresis for HUS/TTP in pregnancy and postpartum has not been evaluated in controlled studies, case series suggest that it is safe and effective.[357] Termination of pregnancy does not appear to alter the course of HUS/TTP, thus it is not generally recommended unless the fetus is compromised.

## HEMOLYTIC UREMIC SYNDROME

Atypical HUS, can cause the abrupt onset of acute renal failure, often in the peripartum or early postpartum period.[359] This disorder is due to a hereditary or acquired deficiency of complement regulatory proteins, leading to activation of the alternative complement pathway. Most of the reports of "HUS" in pregnancy predated the discovery of the role of complement pathway dysregulation in the pathogenesis of this disorder. In one series of 21 patients with pregnancy-associated HUS, 57% had low C3, and 86% of women had a detectable complement gene mutation; the most common abnormalities were CFH mutation (45%), CFI mutation (9%), and C3 mutation (9%).[360] No patients in this series had antibody-mediated disease. Long-term renal outcomes in the pre-eculizumab era were poor, with the majority of women progressing to ESRD.[360] Although data are limited, there are reports of the successful use of eculizumab for the treatment of complement-mediated TMA in pregnancy, without overt adverse fetal effects.[361] Unlike preeclampsia, delivery does not alter the course of TTP or complement-mediated TMA.

## OBSTRUCTIVE UROPATHY AND NEPHROLITHIASIS

AKI due to bilateral ureteral obstruction is a rare complication of pregnancy. Because of the physiologic hydronephrosis of pregnancy (see the "Physiologic Changes of Pregnancy" section), the diagnosis of urinary obstruction can be challenging. If clinical suspicion is high (e.g., marked hydronephrosis, abdominal pain, elevated serum creatinine), a percutaneous nephrostomy may be needed as a diagnostic and therapeutic trial to confirm the diagnosis of obstructive uropathy. If present, obstruction can be managed with ureteral stenting[362] or delivery.[363]

Circulating levels of 1,25-dihydroxyvitamin $D_3$ are increased during normal pregnancy, resulting in increased intestinal calcium absorption. Urinary excretion of calcium is also increased, leading to a tendency in some women to form kidney stones. Excessive intake of calcium supplements can lead to hypercalcemia and hypercalciuria. Although intestinal absorption and urinary excretion of calcium are increased, there is no evidence that the risk of nephrolithiasis is increased, possibly due to a concomitant increase in urine flow and physiological dilation of the urinary tract.

Calcium oxalate and calcium phosphate constitute the majority of the stones produced during pregnancy. As in nonpregnant patients, ureteral calculi in pregnancy produce flank pain and lower abdominal pain with hematuria. Premature labor is sometimes induced by the intense pain, and the risk of infection is increased. Ultrasonography and MRI are the preferred methods to exclude obstruction and visualize stones.[364] The management of renal calculi is conservative with adequate hydration, analgesics, and antiemetics. Thiazide diuretics and allopurinol are avoided during pregnancy. Twenty-four-hour urine collection to quantify urinary calcium and uric acid excretion is recommended after delivery. Nephrolithiasis complicated by urinary tract infection should be treated with antibiotics for 3–5 weeks, followed by suppressive treatment after delivery, because the calculus may serve as a nidus of infection. Most stones pass spontaneously, but placement of a ureteral stent may be required if ureteral obstruction occurs.[365] Lithotripsy is relatively contraindicated during pregnancy due to its adverse effects on the fetus. However, extracorporeal shock wave lithotripsy has been used during the first 4–8 weeks of pregnancy without known adverse consequences to the fetus.[366]

## URINARY TRACT INFECTION AND ACUTE PYELONEPHRITIS

Infections of the urinary tract represent the most frequent renal problem encountered during gestation.[367] Although the prevalence of asymptomatic bacteriuria—which ranges between 2% and 10%—is similar to that in nonpregnant populations, it needs to be managed more aggressively for several reasons. Urinary stasis predisposes pregnant women to ascending pyelonephritis in the setting of cystitis. Hence while asymptomatic bacteriuria in the nonpregnant state is usually benign, untreated asymptomatic bacteriuria in pregnancy can progress to overt cystitis or acute pyelonephritis in up to 40% of patients.[368] Acute pyelonephritis is a serious complication during pregnancy, usually presenting between 20 and 28 weeks of gestation with fevers, loin pain, and dysuria. Sepsis resulting from pyelonephritis can progress to endotoxic shock, disseminated intravascular coagulation, acute renal failure, and respiratory failure.[368] Asymptomatic bacteriuria has also been associated with an increased risk of premature delivery and low birth weight.[369] Treatment of asymptomatic bacteriuria during pregnancy has been shown to reduce these complications and improve perinatal morbidity and mortality.[370] Thus early detection and treatment of asymptomatic bacteriuria are warranted.

The usual signs and symptoms of urinary tract infection can be unreliable in pregnancy. Dysuria and urinary frequency are common during the latter half of pregnancy in the absence of infection, due to pressure on the bladder from the gravid uterus. Low-grade pyuria is often present because of contamination by vaginal secretions. The use of the urinary dipstick to screen for bacteriuria is associated with a high false-negative rate and quantitative urine culture is preferred for screening. More than $10^5$ bacteria/mL of a single species indicates significant bacteriuria. Screening for asymptomatic bacteriuria is recommended during the first prenatal visit and is only repeated in high-risk women such as those with a history of recurrent urinary infections or urinary tract anomalies.

If asymptomatic bacteriuria is found, prompt treatment is warranted (usually with a cephalosporin) for at least 3–7 days.[371] Treatment with a single dose of fosfomycin has also been used successfully. Trimethoprim-sulfa and tetracycline are contraindicated in early pregnancy because of their association with birth defects. A follow-up culture 2 weeks after treatment is necessary to ensure eradication of bacteriuria. Suppressive therapy with nitrofurantoin or cephalexin is recommended for those patients with bacteriuria that persists after two courses of therapy.[372] Prolonged suppressive treatment of bacteriuria has been shown to reduce the incidence of pyelonephritis.[373] Because of the high maternal morbidity and mortality associated with pyelonephritis, it is usually treated aggressively with hospitalization, intravenous antibiotics, and hydration. Infections of the urinary tract are further discussed in Chapter 36.

## CHRONIC KIDNEY DISEASE IN PREGNANCY

Women who enter pregnancy with CKD are at increased risk for adverse maternal and fetal outcomes, including rapid decline of renal function and perinatal mortality. Although the frequency of live births now exceeds 90% in these women, the risks for preterm delivery, IUGR, perinatal mortality, and preeclampsia are significantly elevated.[374,375] Preterm delivery results in both immediate and long-term morbidity for the offspring, with an increased risk of cardiovascular and renal disease later in life.[376] The goals for pregnancy in women with CKD are to preserve maternal renal function during and after pregnancy, and to maximize the likelihood of successful term or near-term delivery for the fetus.

The physiologic increase in renal blood flow and GFR characteristic of normal pregnancy is attenuated in chronic renal insufficiency.[375] The stress of greater renal blood flow during pregnancy may exacerbate renal damage in the setting of preexisting renal disease, similar to nonpregnant states in which the impaired kidney is more sensitive to such insults.

Indeed, worsening of hypertension and proteinuria are common during pregnancy if these conditions exist prior to pregnancy,[377] and in concert with these observations, overall maternal and fetal prognosis correlates with the degree of hypertension, proteinuria, and renal insufficiency prior to conception.

Fortunately, there is good evidence to suggest that women with underlying kidney disease but only mild renal impairment, normal BP, and no proteinuria have good maternal and fetal outcomes, with little risk for accelerated progression toward ESRD.[375,378] However, even women with stage 1 CKD are at increased risk of cesarean section, preterm delivery, and the need for neonatal intensive care as compared with low-risk control pregnancies.[379] Although debate exists whether specific renal diseases are more commonly associated with an accelerated decline in renal function, data suggest that the degree of renal insufficiency, presence and severity of hypertension, and severity of proteinuria, rather than the underlying renal diagnosis, are the primary determinants of outcome.[379] Women who become pregnant with a serum creatinine >1.4–1.5 mg/dL are more likely to experience a decline in renal function than women with a comparable degree of renal dysfunction who do not become pregnant.[375] Initiating pregnancy with a serum creatinine >2.0 mg/dL carries a high risk (>30%) for accelerated decline in renal function both during and after pregnancy.[374] Furthermore, among women with a serum creatinine >2.5 mg/dL, over 70% experience preterm delivery, and over 40% experience preeclampsia.[374,377] Measures to predict which women will experience rapid decline postpartum do not exist, and terminating pregnancy does not reliably reverse the decline in renal function. Recent data in women with autosomal dominant polycystic kidney disease and normal renal function suggest that there is a high rate of successful uncomplicated pregnancies.[380] Other specific conditions including diabetic nephropathy and lupus nephritis are discussed later. Regardless of cause of renal disease, the tenet that an elevated serum creatinine >1.4–1.5 mg/dL puts women at increased risk for renal decline holds true. An overall approach to preconception counseling and prenatal care of women with CKD is shown in Fig. 48.14.

## DIABETIC NEPHROPATHY

The incidence and prevalence of diabetes throughout the world is increasing,[381] and the number of women entering pregnancy with diabetes is rising.[382] However, the incidence of diabetic nephropathy among pregnant women with diabetes has been declining in recent years,[383,384] likely due to improvements in glycemic control, hypertension management, and more widespread use of inhibitors of the renin–angiotensin–aldosterone system among young women with diabetes.

Women with pregestational diabetes, with or without nephropathy, have a higher risk of adverse fetal and maternal outcomes, including congenital malformation, preterm birth, macrosomia, preeclampsia, and perinatal mortality.[44,385] The presence of albuminuria confers a particularly high risk for preeclampsia and preterm delivery.[386] Poor glycemic control before and during pregnancy is strongly linked to adverse pregnancy outcomes, including preeclampsia and serious adverse fetal outcomes; hence, endocrine consultation before pregnancy is strongly advised.[387,388]

Pregnancy itself does not appear to accelerate the progression of kidney disease if kidney function is normal or near normal prior to pregnancy.[389] The prognosis changes, however, if renal function is impaired at pregnancy onset. Compared with preconception measures, creatinine clearance is notably lower even within the first few months postpartum in women initiating pregnancy with impaired renal function.[390] In a study of 11 patients with diabetic nephropathy and serum creatinine >1.4 mg/dL at pregnancy onset, >40% progressed to end-stage renal failure within 5–6 years after pregnancy.[391] Aggressive BP control before and after pregnancy may attenuate the postpartum decline in renal function.[389] Nevertheless, inexorable decline in renal function following pregnancy is common in women initiating pregnancy with diabetic nephropathy and impaired renal function. For this reason, women with diabetic nephropathy are usually advised to postpone pregnancy until after renal transplantation, which improves fertility status and fetal outcomes.

ACEIs and ARBs are contraindicated in the second and third trimesters of pregnancy, leading to birth defects including hypocalvaria (hypoplasia of the membrane bones of the skull), renal tubular dysplasia, and IUGR.[328] The inability to use these medications may contribute to progression of renal failure in pregnant women with diabetic nephropathy and impaired renal function. However, population-based studies find no adverse fetal effects with first-trimester ACEI and ARB exposure.[328,392,393] Unfortunately, it is difficult to exclude first-trimester teratogenicity completely: for example, a case of exencephaly and unilateral renal agenesis was reported in a fetus of a mother who was taking an ARB at conception.[394] Some experts suggest an approach whereby women with a strong indication for ACEI or ARB, such as those with diabetic nephropathy, be continued on these medications while attempting conception, with instructions to discontinue them as soon as pregnancy is recognized. This approach minimizes both fetal risk and the amount of time that women must be off these agents which have clear maternal benefit.

The diabetic milieu during pregnancy may also subsequently affect metabolism and renal function in the offspring.[395,396] For example, in a cross-sectional study of 503 Pima Indians with type 2 diabetes, the prevalence of albuminuria was significantly higher in the offspring of mothers with diabetes during pregnancy (58%) compared with offspring of mothers without evidence of diabetes during pregnancy (40%).[396] It is speculated that abnormal in utero exposure in the offspring of diabetic mothers leads to impaired nephrogenesis and reduced nephron mass, and this puts the offspring at higher risk for developing renal disease and hypertension in later life (see also Chapter 21).

## LUPUS NEPHRITIS AND PREGNANCY

SLE is common in women of childbearing age. During pregnancy, women with SLE are at increased risk for preterm birth, IUGR, spontaneous abortions, and preeclampsia.[397,398] The presence of superimposed renal disease increases the risk of these complications even further.[399,400] Over the past few decades, improvements in disease management and perinatal monitoring have led to a decrease in pregnancy loss and preterm deliveries.[401] Outcomes, however, still appear to be poor in developing countries.[402] With careful planning, monitoring, and management, the majority of patients with

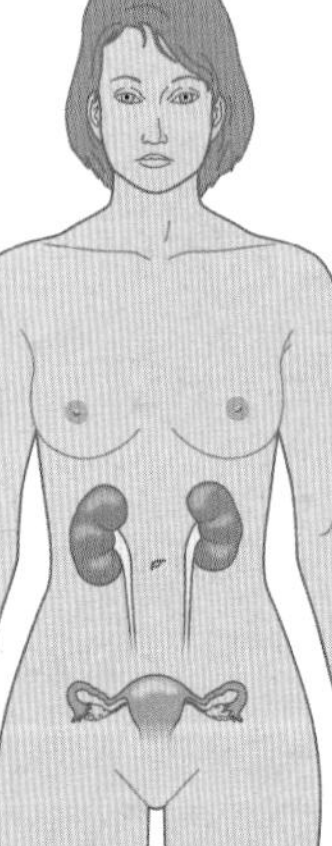

Medications when planning a pregnancy
• Initiate prenatal vitamins
• Stop medications not compatible with pregnancy (e.g., statins)
Contraception when avoiding pregnancy
• Avoid, if possible, estrogen-containing preparations in women with hypertension, vascular disease, or significant proteinuria or who are smokers
• IUDs are not contraindicated in women on immunosuppression
Immunosuppression
• Optimization of preexisting disease (e.g., lupus inactivity for 6 months)
• Ensure disease stability for 3 months on pregnancy-safe immunosuppression
• Switch mycophenolate mofetil to alternative agent (e.g., azathioprine or a calcineurin inhibitor where appropriate)
• Consider repeat kidney biopsy if remission status is unclear
BP management
• Intensive hypertension control with pregnancy-safe antihypertensive agents
• Target <140/90 130/80 mm Hg
Proteinuria
• Suppression of proteinuria with maximal ACEI/ARB until attempting conception or until conception in women where benefits outweigh potential risks
Weight reduction if necessary
• Nutritional consultation
• Encourage active lifestyle
A
Medications
• Folic acid 5 mg od
• Aspirin 150 mg od to be started <16 weeks' gestation and continued until 34–36 weeks' gestation
• Vitamin D and iron replacement as required
Monitoring of renal disease
• Renal function tests including serum creatinine, urea and creatinine clearance, and proteinuria should be repeated every few weeks based on the severity and rate of progression of kidney disease
• Levels of uric acid, liver enzymes, platelet count, and urine protein should be documented to use as a baseline in the case that superimposed preeclampsia is suspected later in pregnancy
BP management
• Intensive hypertension control with pregnancy-safe antihypertensive medications
• Target <140/90 mm Hg
• Blood pressure should be monitored and logged using a home device validated in early pregnancy
• Measure blood pressure at each office visit
Fetal surveillance
• Biophysical profiles
• Fetal growth assessments
• Placental function studies Monthly (first trimester) then alternate week (second trimester) then weekly (third trimester)
B


**Fig. 48.14** (A) Prepregnancy optimization in women with chronic kidney disease. (B) Antenatal care in women with chronic kidney disease. *ACEI,* Angiotensin-converting enzyme inhibitor; *ARB,* angiotensin receptor blocker; *BP,* blood pressure; *IUD,* intrauterine device; *od,* once daily. (Figure adapted from Hladunewich MA, Melamad N, Bramham K. Pregnancy across the spectrum of chronic kidney disease. *Kidney Int.* 2016;89:995–1007.)

SLE—especially those with normal baseline renal function—can complete pregnancy without serious maternal or fetal complications.[403]

Among pregnant women with SLE, risk factors for adverse pregnancy outcomes include lupus disease activity, history of lupus nephritis, antihypertensive use, the presence of antiphospholipid antibodies, thrombocytopenia, and nonwhite or Hispanic race.[398,404,405] Proliferative [World Health Organization (WHO) class III or IV] lupus nephritis is associated with a higher risk of preeclampsia and lower birth weight than mesangial (WHO class II) or membranous (WHO class V) lupus nephritis.[406] Alterations in circulating angiogenic factors (high sFlt1 and low PlGF) measured in the first half of pregnancy are strongly associated with adverse pregnancy outcomes, including preterm preeclampsia, fetal/neonatal death, and indicated preterm delivery < 30 weeks.[407] In the future, these may prove to be useful biomarkers for risk stratification in women with lupus in pregnancy.

Active nephritis at conception (defined in most studies as proteinuria > 500 mg/day and/or an active urinary sediment) is also a risk factor for preterm birth.[404,405] Hence, women should postpone pregnancy until lupus activity is quiescent for ~6 months and immunosuppressives are minimized.[408,409] Mycophenolate mofetil (MMF) is teratogenic and should be switched to azathioprine at least 3 months prior to conception; this approach is associated with a low risk of renal flares.[410]

Approximately 10%–15% of women with a history of lupus nephritis experience a nephritis flare during pregnancy.[411,412] De novo lupus nephritis in pregnancy is less common, affecting only 2% of women with SLE but without renal disease prior to pregnancy. Low C4, but not low C3 or anti-double-stranded DNA antibody positivity, is predictive of pregnancy-associated lupus nephritis flare.[411] Prophylactic therapy with steroids does not appear to prevent a lupus flare during pregnancy.[413] Discontinuation of hydroxychloroquine in pregnancy is associated with an increased risk of lupus flare, so this agent should generally be continued.[414] Steroids, azathioprine, and hydroxychloroquine may be used to manage lupus nephritis flares, and treat extrarenal lupus symptoms, during pregnancy.[415]

Pregnant women with SLE are at risk for both lupus nephritis flare and preeclampsia. Unfortunately, both syndromes share the common presenting symptoms of hypertension and proteinuria, hence distinguishing the two can be a clinical challenge. The distinction between preeclampsia and lupus flare is critical, however, especially in women presenting prior to 37 weeks' gestation because the treatments differ. For a lupus nephritis flare, steroids, azathioprine, and CNIs may quell the disease, allowing pregnancy to continue, whereas for preeclampsia, induction of delivery is the definitive treatment. Even in the medical literature, reports of preeclampsia in the setting of lupus renal disease are prone to misclassification, because the diagnosis of preeclampsia is usually based on hypertension and proteinuria, and not on renal biopsy or specific serologic testing. Alterations in components of the complement cascade (e.g., reductions in C3, C4, CH50) may be useful to help identify pregnant women with a lupus flare, and to distinguish lupus flare from preeclampsia.[416] An active urinary sediment suggests lupus nephritis, as the sediment in preeclampsia is typically bland. However, none of these clinical findings are definitive and kidney biopsy during pregnancy is sometimes indicated (see the "Kidney Biopsy in Pregnancy" section). On the horizon, measurement of circulating angiogenic factors may aid clinical decision making, especially during the critical period before term.[76,417,418]

Treatment of severe proliferative lupus nephritis in pregnancy is challenging, as conventional induction therapies are contraindicated due to risk for congenital malformations (mycophenolate[419]) and fetal loss (cyclophosphamide[420]). Prednisone is safe, though the risk of gestational diabetes is increased.[408] CNIs are nonteratogenic and can be used to treat lupus nephritis in pregnancy, with some data to support their efficacy in the nonpregnant population.[408] Rituximab lacks safety data in pregnancy, and it is not recommended.[421] Azathioprine is considered relatively safe in pregnancy, and is commonly used as adjunctive or maintenance therapy in pregnant patients with lupus nephritis.[415]

## KIDNEY BIOPSY IN PREGNANCY

Indications for kidney biopsy during pregnancy are similar to those in the nonpregnant population; specifically, clinical suspicion of glomerular disease where pathologic diagnosis is likely to change management. The best data on the safety of kidney biopsy during pregnancy are from a 2013 systematic review of 243 kidney biopsies performed during pregnancy, and 1236 kidney biopsies performed during the postpartum period.[422] Kidney biopsies performed during pregnancy had a higher complication rate than biopsies performed after pregnancy (7% vs. 1%). However, most complications were minor: Only four cases of major bleeding occurred, all in women who were biopsied between 23 and 26 weeks of gestation. For this reason, and because this is a period of uncertain fetal viability should complications require preterm delivery, kidney biopsy should be avoided between 23 and 26 weeks' gestation. Later in gestation, kidney biopsy becomes technically difficult, and often can be postponed until after delivery.

## PREGNANCY IN END-STAGE KIDNEY DISEASE

End-stage kidney disease is characterized by severe hypothalamic–pituitary–gonadal dysfunction, which is reversed by transplantation but not by conventional dialysis. Women of childbearing age on dialysis frequently have menstrual disturbances, anovulation, and infertility.[423] Animal studies suggest that uremia impairs fertility via aberrant neuroendocrine regulation of hypothalamic gonadotropin-releasing hormone secretion.[424] Gonadal function is impaired in men as well, who can experience testicular atrophy, hypospermatogenesis, infertility, and impotence. However, in recent decades the Toronto experience has suggested that fertility in women with ESRD may be improved by intensive hemodialysis (≥36 hours/week or more).[425]

Conception on dialysis is unusual, but not impossible. Hence contraception remains important in women of childbearing age who do not wish to become pregnant. In fact, pregnancy and live birth rates have been increasing in young women receiving dialysis.[426] Survey data from Japan, Belgium, and the United States from the 1990s reported pregnancy rates among women of childbearing age with ESRD of 0.3% to 2%.[375,427–430] In these studies, approximately half of pregnancies resulted in successful delivery of a live infant, though the majority (84% in the 1994 study) were premature.

More recent reports of pregnancies in the setting of chronic hemodialysis have reported somewhat higher neonatal survival (70%–75%).[431–433] Live birth rates of up to 86% have been reported with intensive dialysis (see later).[434] Adverse fetal outcomes are most often due to preterm labor, premature rupture of membranes, polyhydramnios, and IUGR. The likelihood of successful pregnancy is higher in women who conceive prior to initiation of dialysis, as compared with women who conceive after initiation of dialysis.[433]

When pregnancy does occur in a woman on chronic hemodialysis, a large increase in dialysis time appears to improve pregnancy outcomes.[435] Initial reports suggested that women who received ≥20 hours/week of hemodialysis had improved neonatal outcomes and longer gestations.[428,429,436] In 2014, Hladunewich and colleagues[434] pushed the envelope even further, reporting an impressively high live birth rate of 86.4% and mean gestational age at delivery of 36 weeks among women who received 43 ± 6 dialysis hours/week, compared with a live birth rate of 61.4% and mean gestational age at delivery of 27 weeks among historical control women who received 17 ± 5 dialysis hours/week. They observed a dose–response relationship between dialysis dose and pregnancy outcomes, with the highest live birth rate and longest gestation among women who received ≥37 hours/week of hemodialysis. This extremely high dialysis intensity requires a major commitment on the part of the patient and the dialysis provider, and is most realistically attained by daily nocturnal dialysis.

Volume management is challenging, as the dry weight increases up to 0.5 kg/week throughout pregnancy, and hypovolemia needs to be vigilantly avoided. Medications must be carefully reviewed so as to avoid drugs toxic to the fetus, such as ACE inhibitors. Erythropoietin and iron requirements increase in pregnancy, and dosing should be adjusted to approximate the physiologic anemia of pregnancy (10–11 g/L), as low hematocrit has been associated with adverse fetal outcomes.[437] Exacerbation of hypertension is common, though the incidence of preeclampsia is difficult to ascertain due to the inability to apply standard diagnostic criteria. If preeclampsia occurs, intravenous magnesium for seizure prophylaxis should be dosed cautiously, as magnesium excretion is impaired in ESRD. Magnesium levels should be measured frequently, and patients should be monitored for signs of toxicity such as hyporeflexia, weakness, and sedation. Close monitoring of fetal growth and well-being, in collaboration with an obstetrician, is essential after 24 weeks' gestation as IUGR and fetal distress are common.

Data on pregnancy outcomes in women on peritoneal dialysis are limited to case reports and small case series. Reports suggest a relatively high rate of complications such as peritonitis, catheter malfunction, and exit site infection.[429,438,439] Peritoneal dialysis may be associated with a higher rate of small-for-gestational-age infants, as compared with hemodialysis.[435] Supplementation of peritoneal dialysis with intermittent hemodialysis has been reported as a strategy to increase dialysis dose in pregnancy.[440]

## PREGNANCY IN THE KIDNEY TRANSPLANT RECIPIENT

While women with ESRD on dialysis are often infertile, kidney transplantation results in a return to normal hormonal function and fertility within 6 months in approximately 90% of women of childbearing age.[441] Because pregnancy in advanced CKD is associated with a high risk of pregnancy complications and accelerated loss of kidney function, women with advanced CKD are often counseled to delay pregnancy until after kidney transplantation, when pregnancy outcomes are more favorable. Over 14,000 pregnancies in renal allograft recipients have been documented since 1958 (Fig. 48.15).[442] However, the pregnancy rate among female kidney transplant recipients aged 20–45 has declined since 1990 in both the United States and Australia/New Zealand.[443,444] Reasons for this decline are speculative, but may include avoidance of pregnancy in patients receiving mycophenolate immunosuppression (introduced in 1995), and more advanced maternal age and comorbidities among more recent transplant recipients.

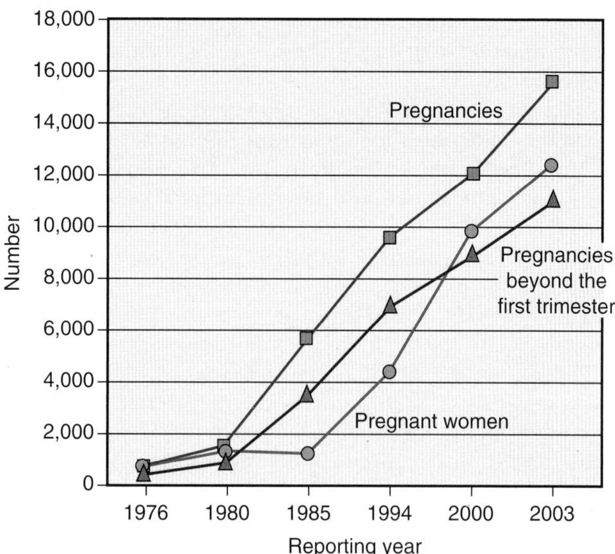


**Fig. 48.15** Pregnancies in kidney transplant recipients worldwide. The *circles* represent the numbers of pregnancies reported worldwide in kidney transplant recipients during the indicated year. The *numbers* include therapeutic terminations, spontaneous abortions, ectopic pregnancies, and stillbirths. The *squares* represent the numbers of transplant recipients reported to have been pregnant during that year, again including all outcomes. The *triangles* represent the numbers of pregnancies beyond the first trimester reported in the literature during the indicated year. The data are from the US National Transplantation Pregnancy Registry, the European Dialysis and Transplant Association Registry, and the UK Transplant Pregnancy Registry. (From McKay DB, Josephson MA. Pregnancy in recipients of solid organs—effects on mother and child. *N Engl J Med.* 2006;354:1281–1293.)

Although the majority of pregnancies following kidney transplantation lead to excellent outcomes for both mother and fetus, such pregnancies are not without risk and require close monitoring and collaboration between the nephrologist and the obstetrician. The goals of care in these patients are to optimize maternal health, including graft function and hypertensive disorders of pregnancy, and to maximize the likelihood of a healthy newborn.

### FETAL AND NEONATAL OUTCOMES

Four major registries, the US National Pregnancy Transplantation Registry,[445] the European Dialysis and Transplant Association Registry,[446] the UK Transplant Pregnancy

Registry,[447] and the Australia and New Zealand Dialysis and Transplant Registry,[448] have documented pregnancy outcomes on >2600 pregnancies in women with solid organ transplants. In addition, a 2011 meta-analysis summarized 50 studies on pregnancy outcomes from >4700 pregnancies in transplant recipients.[449] Statistics on the major complications of pregnancy from these studies are remarkably consistent. Approximately 20% of pregnancies among renal transplant recipients end in the first trimester, half due to miscarriage and the remainder due to elective termination. The live birth rate is 73%–79%; however, there is a substantial risk of low birth weight (40%–54%) and preterm delivery (45%–52%). Ectopic pregnancy appears to be slightly increased, especially in pregnancies that occur soon after transplant, but the rate remains below 1%.[449] The rate of structural birth defects is no higher than the general population. Vaginal delivery is safe, and cesarean section should be performed only for obstetrical indications.

## TIMING OF PREGNANCY AFTER TRANSPLANTATION

Pregnancy within the first 6–12 months following transplantation is undesirable for several reasons. The risk of acute rejection is relatively high, immunosuppressant medications are at higher dosages, and risk of infection is greatest.[442] Traditionally it has been recommended that women wait ~2 years after transplant prior to attempting conception.[450] However, many kidney transplant recipients are of advanced maternal age, hence delaying pregnancy may lead to age-related decrease in fertility. The American Society of Transplantation suggests that conception could be safely considered as early as 1 year posttransplant for women on stable doses of nonteratogenic immunosuppressive agents, with normal renal function (Cr < 1.5 mg/dL and urine protein excretion of <500 mg/day), no concurrent fetotoxic infections (such as cytomegalovirus), and with no rejection episodes within the past year.[442]

## EFFECT OF PREGNANCY ON RENAL ALLOGRAFT FUNCTION

Pregnancy itself does not appear to adversely affect graft function in transplant recipients, provided baseline graft function is normal and significant hypertension is not present.[450] In general, when pregnancy occurs 1–2 years after transplant, the rejection rate is similar to that seen in non-pregnant controls (3%–4%).[449,451] When moderate renal insufficiency is present (serum creatinine >1.5–1.7 mg/dL), pregnancy does carry a risk of progressive renal dysfunction,[452] as well as an increased risk of a small-for-gestational-age infant and of preeclampsia.[453]

Only two small case–control studies have reported long-term (>10 years) graft function after pregnancy. One study suggested that 10-year graft survival may be diminished in transplant recipients who become pregnant compared with controls who did not become pregnant.[454] A second study reported no significant difference.[455] Further studies reporting long-term outcomes in the era of CNIs are needed.

Due to ongoing immunosuppression, transplant recipients are at risk for infections that have implications for the fetus, including cytomegalovirus, herpes simplex, and toxoplasmosis. The rate of bacterial urinary tract infections is increased (~13%–40%),[452] but these are usually treatable and uncomplicated.

The most common complication of pregnancy in transplant recipients is hypertension, which affects between 30% and 75% of pregnancies among transplant recipients.[449,451,456] Hypertension is likely due to a combination of underlying medical conditions and the use of CNIs. Preeclampsia complicates 25%–30% of pregnancies in kidney transplant patients,[449,451,452,457] and diagnosis is often challenging due to the frequent presence of hypertension and/or proteinuria at baseline. The American Society of Transplantation recommends that hypertension in pregnant renal transplant recipients should be managed aggressively, with target BP close to normal – a goal which differs from somewhat higher BP goals in women with hypertension in pregnancy in the absence of a transplant.[328,442] Agents of choice (Table 48.6) include methyldopa, nonselective β-adrenergic antagonists (e.g., labetalol), and calcium channel blockers. ACE inhibitors and angiotensin receptor blockers should be avoided in pregnancy, particularly in the second and third trimesters. Details about the use of these agents in pregnancy are discussed in greater detail in the section Chronic Hypertension and Gestational Hypertension.

## MANAGEMENT OF IMMUNOSUPPRESSIVE THERAPY IN PREGNANCY

The US Food and Drug Administration replaced the former pregnancy risk letter categories on prescription and biological drug labeling with new information to make them more meaningful to both patients and health-care providers.[458] The benefit-to-risk ratio for most immunosuppressive agents used in the treatment of transplant recipients favors medication continuation during pregnancy. Certain immunomodulators, however, can cause extreme fetal harm and should be used with caution. There is a significant amount of published data that can inform decisions to use these agents safely in pregnancy (Table 48.7).

CNIs (either cyclosporine or tacrolimus) and steroids, with or without azathioprine, form the basis of immunosuppression during pregnancy. Corticosteroids at low to moderate doses (5–10 mg/day) are safe and prednisone is therefore the agent of choice during pregnancy.[459] Stress-dose steroids are indicated in the peripartum period. Azathioprine is generally considered safe at dosages <2 mg/kg per day. Higher doses of azathioprine are associated with congenital anomalies, immunosuppression, and IUGR, and should be avoided if possible.[450]

CNIs are widely used in pregnancy, and generally considered safe.[459–461] Clinical data have not demonstrated an increased incidence of congenital malformations, with the possible exception of low birth weight.[459] Owing to decreased gastrointestinal (GI) absorption, increased volume of distribution, and increased renal clearance, dosages of CNIs generally need to be increased in pregnancy to maintain therapeutic levels, and close monitoring of drug levels is essential.[462,463]

Sirolimus causes fetal toxicity in animal studies, and is generally contraindicated in pregnancy.[459] Whenever possible, sirolimus should be discontinued at least 12 weeks prior to conception. The risk of fetal malformations is highest at 30–71 days' gestation, so there is a window to stop sirolimus if pregnancy is detected early. Nevertheless, sirolimus should be discontinued preemptively in women of childbearing age who are not using contraception.

**Table 48.7 Immunosuppressive Medications in Pregnancy**

| Drug | Recommendations |
|---|---|
| Prednisone | Safe when used long term at low to moderate doses (5–10 mg/day)<br>Safe when given acutely at high doses for treatment of acute rejection |
| Cyclosporine | Extensive clinical data suggest safe at low-to-moderate clinical doses<br>Changes in absorption and metabolism require close monitoring of levels and frequent dose adjustments in pregnancy |
| Tacrolimus | Similar to those for cyclosporine, although somewhat less data available |
| Sirolimus | Embryo/fetal toxicity in rodents was manifested as mortality and reduced fetal weights (with associated delays in skeletal ossification); human studies are lacking |
| Azathioprine | Considered safe at dosages < 2 mg/kg per day, but at higher doses associated with fetal growth restriction |
| Mycophenolate mofetil | Contraindicated in pregnancy (teratogenic in animal and human studies) |
| Muromonab-CD3 (OKT-3) | Case reports of successful use for induction in unsuspected pregnancy and for acute rejection, but data are limited |
| Antithymocyte globulin (C) | Animal studies have not been reported, and there are no controlled data from use in human pregnancy |
| Belatacept, basiliximab, alemtuzumab | Avoid in pregnancy; inadequate safety data in humans |

Adapted from McKay DB, Josephson MA. Pregnancy after kidney transplantation. *Clin J Am Soc Nephrol.* 2008;3:S117–S125.

MMF is associated with developmental toxicity, malformations, and intrauterine death in animal studies at therapeutic dosages. Human data are limited to isolated case reports, but suggest that MMF may be associated with spontaneous abortions and with major fetal malformations,[464] especially in combination with cyclosporine.[459] Hence MMF, like sirolimus, should be avoided in pregnancy. For a more detailed discussion of data on effects of these agents on neonatal immunologic function and long-term outcomes, the reader is referred to reviews by Josephson and McKay.[465,466]

## MANAGEMENT OF ACUTE REJECTION IN PREGNANCY

The incidence of acute rejection during pregnancy is approximately 4%, similar to the nonpregnant population.[449] However, the diagnosis of acute rejection during pregnancy can be difficult. Acute rejection should be suspected if fever, oliguria, graft tenderness, or deterioration in renal function are noted. Biopsy of the renal graft should be performed to confirm the diagnosis prior to initiation of treatment. High-dose steroids are the mainstay of treatment of acute rejection during pregnancy.[450,467] Little data are available on the safety of agents such as OKT-3, antithymocyte globulin, belatacept, alemtuzumab, daclizumab, and basiliximab in pregnancy, and they are generally avoided (Table 48.7).[459] The National Transplantation Pregnancy Registry reported five cases of OKT-3 use during pregnancy, with four surviving infants.[451] Polyclonal and monoclonal antibodies would be expected to cross the placenta, but fetal effects are largely unknown.

## BREASTFEEDING AND IMMUNOSUPPRESSIVE AGENTS

Studies on transfer of CNIs to the babies of breastfeeding mothers are inconsistent, with some studies reporting undetectable levels,[459,468] and others reporting high neonatal blood concentrations.[469] There are no reports on adverse neonatal effects with cyclosporine or tacrolimus use in breastfeeding. Limited data suggest that tacrolimus levels are very low in breast milk. Investigators from the National Transplantation Pregnancy Registry suggest that breastfeeding should not be discouraged in women taking tacrolimus.[470] When cyclosporine or tacrolimus is used in a lactating mother, consideration should be given to monitoring neonatal blood concentrations for potential toxicity. Theoretically, MMF should be safe in breastfeeding because the active metabolite secreted in breast milk, MMA, is not GI bioavailable; however, human evidence of safety is lacking. Nevertheless, breastfeeding among transplant recipients remains controversial.[466]

## PREGNANCY OUTCOME FOLLOWING KIDNEY DONATION

Gestational hypertension and preeclampsia are more common among living kidney donors as compared with matched nondonors.[471] There are conflicting data on whether adverse pregnancy outcomes, such as preterm delivery and fetal loss, are also increased among kidney donors.[472,473] Women of reproductive age who are considering kidney donation should be counseled regarding these potential risks.

# CONCLUSION

Recent decades have brought significant advances in our understanding of the pathogenesis of preeclampsia. We have more data than ever before to guide management of hypertension, CKD, and glomerular disease in pregnancy. Nevertheless, large evidence gaps remain with regard to BP targets and use of novel immunosuppressive and biologic agents in women with hypertension and kidney disease in pregnancy. Preeclampsia continues to cause major maternal and neonatal morbidity and mortality worldwide, as delivery remains the only effective treatment. In the future, we look toward better and larger trials to assess the impact of interventions for hypertension, preeclampsia, and primary kidney disease in pregnant women.

Complete reference list available at ExpertConsult.com.

## KEY REFERENCES

2. Chapman AB, Abraham WT, Zamudio S, et al. Temporal relationships between hormonal and hemodynamic changes in early human pregnancy. *Kidney Int.* 1998;54:2056–2063.
11. Odutayo A, Hladunewich M. Obstetric nephrology: renal hemodynamic and metabolic physiology in normal pregnancy. *Clin J Am Soc Nephrol.* 2012;7:2073–2080.
27. McGuane JT, Debrah JE, Debrah DO, et al. Role of relaxin in maternal systemic and renal vascular adaptations during gestation. *Ann N Y Acad Sci.* 2009;1160:304–312.

29. Novak J, Danielson LA, Kerchner LJ, et al. Relaxin is essential for renal vasodilation during pregnancy in conscious rats. *J Clin Invest.* 2001;107:1469–1475.
40. Skjaerven R, Wilcox AJ, Lie RT. The interval between pregnancies and the risk of preeclampsia. *N Engl J Med.* 2002;346:33–38.
67. Ruma M, Boggess K, Moss K, et al. Maternal periodontal disease, systemic inflammation, and risk for preeclampsia. *Am J Obstet Gynecol.* 2008;198:389 e1–e5.
71. Cote AM, Brown MA, Lam E, et al. Diagnostic accuracy of urinary spot protein:creatinine ratio for proteinuria in hypertensive pregnant women: systematic review. *BMJ.* 2008;336:1003–1006.
91. Bellamy L, Casas JP, Hingorani AD, et al. Pre-eclampsia and risk of cardiovascular disease and cancer in later life: systematic review and meta-analysis. *BMJ.* 2007;335:974.
98. Vikse BE, Irgens LM, Leivestad T, et al. Preeclampsia and the risk of end-stage renal disease. *N Engl J Med.* 2008;359:800–809.
102. Bokslag A, Teunissen PW, Franssen C, et al. Effect of early-onset preeclampsia on cardiovascular risk in the fifth decade of life. *Am J Obstet Gynecol.* 2017;216:523 e1–e7.
121. Zhou Y, Fisher SJ, Janatpour M, et al. Human cytotrophoblasts adopt a vascular phenotype as they differentiate. A strategy for successful endovascular invasion? *J Clin Invest.* 1997;99:2139–2151.
123. Zhou Y, McMaster M, Woo K, et al. Vascular endothelial growth factor ligands and receptors that regulate human cytotrophoblast survival are dysregulated in severe preeclampsia and hemolysis, elevated liver enzymes, and low platelets syndrome. *Am J Pathol.* 2002;160:1405–1423.
136. Thadhani R, Ecker JL, Kettyle E, et al. Pulse pressure and risk of preeclampsia: a prospective study. *Obstet Gynecol.* 2001;97:515–520.
148. Redman CW, Sargent IL. Latest advances in understanding preeclampsia. *Science.* 2005;308:1592–1594.
160. Powe CE, Levine RJ, Karumanchi SA. Preeclampsia, a disease of the maternal endothelium: the role of antiangiogenic factors and implications for later cardiovascular disease. *Circulation.* 2011;123: 2856–2869.
161. Maynard SE, Min JY, Merchan J, et al. Excess placental soluble fms-like tyrosine kinase 1 (sFlt1) may contribute to endothelial dysfunction, hypertension, and proteinuria in preeclampsia. *J Clin Invest.* 2003;111:649–658.
164. Levine RJ, Maynard SE, Qian C, et al. Circulating angiogenic factors and the risk of preeclampsia. *N Engl J Med.* 2004;350:672–683.
170. Sela S, Itin A, Natanson-Yaron S, et al. A novel human-specific soluble vascular endothelial growth factor receptor 1: cell type-specific splicing and implications to vascular endothelial growth factor homeostasis and preeclampsia. *Circ Res.* 2008;102:1566–1574.
173. Venkatesha S, Toporsian M, Lam C, et al. Soluble endoglin contributes to the pathogenesis of preeclampsia. *Nat Med.* 2006;12: 642–649.
177. Levine RJ, Lam C, Qian C, et al. Soluble endoglin and other circulating antiangiogenic factors in preeclampsia. *N Engl J Med.* 2006;355:992–1005.
185. Eremina V, Sood M, Haigh J, et al. Glomerular-specific alterations of VEGF-A expression lead to distinct congenital and acquired renal diseases. *J Clin Invest.* 2003;111:707–716.
188. Eremina V, Jefferson JA, Kowalewska J, et al. VEGF inhibition and renal thrombotic microangiopathy. *N Engl J Med.* 2008;358:1129–1136.
190. Garovic VD, Wagner SJ, Turner ST, et al. Urinary podocyte excretion as a marker for preeclampsia. *Am J Obstet Gynecol.* 2007;196:320 e1–e7.
209. Wolf M, Sandler L, Munoz K, et al. First trimester insulin resistance and subsequent preeclampsia: a prospective study. *J Clin Endocrinol Metab.* 2002;87:1563–1568.
225. Poon LC, Kametas NA, Maiz N, et al. First-trimester prediction of hypertensive disorders in pregnancy. *Hypertension.* 2009;53:812–818.
231. Noori M, Donald AE, Angelakopoulou A, et al. Prospective study of placental angiogenic factors and maternal vascular function before and after preeclampsia and gestational hypertension. *Circulation.* 2010;122:478–487.
239. Levine RJ, Thadhani R, Qian C, et al. Urinary placental growth factor and risk of preeclampsia. *JAMA.* 2005;293:77–85.
240. Verlohren S, Herraiz I, Lapaire O, et al. The sFlt-1/PlGF ratio in different types of hypertensive pregnancy disorders and its prognostic potential in preeclamptic patients. *Am J Obstet Gynecol.* 2012;206:58 e1–e8.
243. Rolfo A, Attini R, Nuzzo AM, et al. Chronic kidney disease may be differentially diagnosed from preeclampsia by serum biomarkers. *Kidney Int.* 2013;83:177–181.
244. Perni U, Sison C, Sharma V, et al. Angiogenic factors in superimposed preeclampsia: a longitudinal study of women with chronic hypertension during pregnancy. *Hypertension.* 2012;59:740–746.
245. Zeisler H, Llurba E, Chantraine F, et al. Predictive value of the sFlt-1:PlGF Ratio in women with suspected preeclampsia. *N Engl J Med.* 2016;374:13–22.
246. Rana S, Powe CE, Salahuddin S, et al. Angiogenic factors and the risk of adverse outcomes in women with suspected preeclampsia. *Circulation.* 2012;125:911–919.
257. Rolnik DL, Wright D, Poon LC, et al. Aspirin versus placebo in pregnancies at high risk for preterm preeclampsia. *N Engl J Med.* 2017;377:613–622.
260. Villar J, Abdel-Aleem H, Merialdi M, et al. World Health Organization randomized trial of calcium supplementation among low calcium intake pregnant women. *Am J Obstet Gynecol.* 2006;194:639–649.
280. Sibai BM, Mercer BM, Schiff E, et al. Aggressive versus expectant management of severe preeclampsia at 28 to 32 weeks' gestation: a randomized controlled trial. *Am J Obstet Gynecol.* 1994;171:818–822.
281. Broekhuijsen K, van Baaren GJ, van Pampus MG, et al. Immediate delivery versus expectant monitoring for hypertensive disorders of pregnancy between 34 and 37 weeks of gestation (HYPITAT-II): an open-label, randomised controlled trial. *Lancet.* 2015;385:2492–2501.
285. Lucas MJ, Leveno KJ, Cunningham FG. A comparison of magnesium sulfate with phenytoin for the prevention of eclampsia. *N Engl J Med.* 1995;333:201–206.
290. Thadhani R, Kisner T, Hagmann H, et al. Pilot study of extracorporeal removal of soluble fms-like tyrosine kinase 1 in preeclampsia. *Circulation.* 2011;124:940–950.
291. Thadhani R, Hagmann H, Schaarschmidt W, et al. Removal of soluble Fms-Like Tyrosine Kinase-1 by Dextran sulfate apheresis in preeclampsia. *J Am Soc Nephrol.* 2016;27:903–913.
305. Bramham K, Parnell B, Nelson-Piercy C, et al. Chronic hypertension and pregnancy outcomes: systematic review and meta-analysis. *BMJ.* 2014;348:g2301.
321. Magee LA, von Dadelszen P, Rey E, et al. Less-tight versus tight control of hypertension in pregnancy. *N Engl J Med.* 2015;372:407–417.
331. Cooper WO, Hernandez-Diaz S, Arbogast PG, et al. Major congenital malformations after first-trimester exposure to ACE inhibitors. *N Engl J Med.* 2006;354:2443–2451.
351. Ibdah JA, Bennett MJ, Rinaldo P, et al. A fetal fatty-acid oxidation disorder as a cause of liver disease in pregnant women. *N Engl J Med.* 1999;340:1723–1731.
360. Fakhouri F, Roumenina L, Provot F, et al. Pregnancy-associated hemolytic uremic syndrome revisited in the era of complement gene mutations. *J Am Soc Nephrol.* 2010;21:859–867.
379. Piccoli GB, Attini R, Vasario E, et al. Pregnancy and chronic kidney disease: a challenge in all CKD stages. *Clin J Am Soc Nephrol.* 2010;5:844–855.
411. Buyon JP, Kim MY, Guerra MM, et al. Kidney outcomes and risk factors for nephritis (Flare/De Novo) in a multiethnic cohort of pregnant patients with lupus. *Clin J Am Soc Nephrol.* 2017;12:940–946.
434. Hladunewich MA, Hou S, Odutayo A, et al. Intensive hemodialysis associates with improved pregnancy outcomes: a Canadian and United States cohort comparison. *J Am Soc Nephrol.* 2014;25:1103–1109.
471. Garg AX, Nevis IF, McArthur E, et al. Gestational hypertension and preeclampsia in living kidney donors. *N Engl J Med.* 2015;372: 124–133.
475. Tangren JS, Powe CE, Ankers E, et al. Pregnancy outcomes after clinical recovery from AKI. *J Am Soc Nephrol.* 2017;28:1566–1574.

# 49 Antihypertensive Therapy

Tara I. Chang | Srinivasan Beddhu | Glenn M. Chertow

CHAPTER OUTLINE



This chapter is divided into three major sections. The first section reviews the pharmacology of nondiuretic antihypertensive drugs to provide clinicians with a complete overview of how to use these therapies safely in practice (Table 49.1; see Chapter 50 for a review of diuretic drugs). The first section also discusses individual drug classes and highlights the class mechanisms of action, renal effects, and efficacy and safety. Individual similarities and differences within and between classes are then addressed. The second section reviews clinical decision making with regard to blood pressure (BP) goals, selection of antihypertensive therapy, and methods of treating resistant hypertension. The third section reviews the pharmacology of the parenteral and oral drugs available for the management of hypertensive urgencies and emergencies and discusses clinical considerations in seeking to achieve rapid reduction of BP. The history of the development of modern antihypertensive drug therapy is shown in Fig. 49.1.

## PHARMACOLOGY OF THE NONDIURETIC ANTIHYPERTENSIVE DRUGS

### ANGIOTENSIN-CONVERTING ENZYME INHIBITORS

#### CLASS MECHANISMS OF ACTION

Angiotensin-converting enzyme (ACE) inhibitors inhibit the activity of ACE, which converts the inactive decapeptide angiotensin I (Ang I) into the potent hormone angiotensin II (Ang II) (Fig. 49.2). Because Ang II plays a crucial role in maintaining and regulating BP levels by promoting vasoconstriction and renal sodium and water retention, ACE inhibitors are powerful tools for targeting multiple pathways that contribute to hypertension. ACE inhibitors directly reduce the circulating and tissue levels of Ang II, thus blocking the potent vasoconstriction induced by the hormone (Table 49.2).[1] The resulting decrease in peripheral vascular resistance is not accompanied by changes in cardiac output or glomerular filtration rate (GFR) changes; the heart rate is unchanged or may be reduced in patients with baseline heart rates higher than 85 beats per minute.[2]

A reduction in systemic and local levels of Ang II leads to effects beyond vasodilation that contribute to the antihypertensive efficacy of ACE inhibitors (Table 49.2).[3] Additional mechanisms include the following: (1) inhibition of the breakdown of vasodilatory bradykinins catalyzed by ACE or kininase II (the hypotensive action of ACE inhibitors is blocked, in part, by bradykinin antagonists)[4]; (2) enhancement of vasodilatory prostaglandin synthesis; (3) improvement of nitric oxide–mediated endothelial function[5,6] and upregulation of endothelial progenitor cells[7]; (4) reversal of vascular hypertrophy[8]; (5) decrease in aldosterone secretion; (6) augmentation of renal blood flow to induce natriuresis[9]; (7) blunting of sympathetic nervous system (SNS) activity[10–12] through presynaptic modulation of norepinephrine release; (8) inhibition of postjunctional pressor responses to norepinephrine or Ang II[11,13]; (9) inhibition of central Ang II-mediated sympathoexcitation, norepinephrine synthesis, and arginine vasopressin release; (10) inhibition of centrally controlled baroreceptor reflexes, which results in increased baroreceptor sensitivity[13]; (11) decrease in vasoconstrictor endothelin-1 levels[14]; (12) inhibition of thirst; (13) inhibition of cholesterol oxidation[15]; and (14) inhibition of collagen deposition in target organs.[16]

#### CLASS MEMBERS

Currently, there are more than 15 ACE inhibitors in clinical use. Each drug has a unique structure that determines its potency, tissue receptor binding affinity, metabolism, and prodrug compound, but they have remarkably similar clinical effects (Tables 49.3 and 49.4).[3] The drugs are classified into sulfhydryl, carboxyl, or phosphinyl categories on the basis of the ligand that binds to the ACE–zinc moiety.

##### Sulfhydryl Angiotensin-Converting Enzyme Inhibitors

Captopril is a sulfhydryl-containing ACE inhibitor that is available in tablets of 12.5, 25, and 50 mg (see Tables 49.3

**Table 49.1 Pharmacologic Classification of Nondiuretic Antihypertensive Drugs**

Angiotensin-converting enzyme inhibitors
- Sulfhydryl
- Carboxyl
- Phosphinyl

Angiotensin II type 1 receptor antagonists
- Biphenyl tetrazoles
- Nonbiphenyl tetrazoles
- Nonheterocyclics

β-Adrenergic antagonists and α1- and β-adrenergic antagonists
- Nonselective β-adrenergic antagonists
- Nonselective β-adrenergic antagonists with partial agonist activity
- β1-Selective adrenergic antagonists
- β1-Selective adrenergic antagonists with partial agonist activity
- Nonselective β-adrenergic and α1-adrenergic antagonists

Calcium antagonists
- Benzothiazepines
- Dihydropyridines
- Diphenylalkylamines
- Tetralines

Central $\alpha_2$-adrenergic agonists
Central and peripheral adrenergic-neuronal blocking agents
Direct-acting vasodilators
Moderately selective peripheral $\alpha_1$-adrenergic antagonists
Peripheral $\alpha_1$-adrenergic antagonists
Peripheral adrenergic-neuronal blocking agents
Renin inhibitors
Selective aldosterone receptor antagonists
Tyrosine hydroxylase inhibitors
Vasopeptidase inhibitors[a]

[a]Not approved for the treatment of hypertension.

**Table 49.2 Antihypertensive Mechanisms of Action of Angiotensin-Converting Enzyme Inhibitors**

Lower peripheral vascular resistance.
Inhibit the breakdown of vasodilatory bradykinins.
Enhance vasodilatory prostaglandin synthesis.
Improve nitric oxide–mediated endothelial function.
Reverse vascular hypertrophy.
Decrease aldosterone secretion.
Induce natriuresis.
Augment renal blood flow.
Blunt sympathetic nervous system activity and pressor responses.
Inhibit norepinephrine and arginine vasopressin release.
Inhibit baroreceptor reflexes.
Reduce endothelin-1 levels.
Inhibit thirst.
Inhibit oxidation of cholesterol.
Inhibit collagen deposition in target organs.

and 49.4).[12,17,18] The usual starting dosage for hypertension treatment is 25 mg two or three times daily (Table 49.3), and the dosage can be titrated at 1- to 2-week intervals.[12] Captopril has 75% bioavailability, with peak onset within 1 hour. The half-life is 2 hours; with long-term administration, the hemodynamic effects are maintained for 3 to 8 hours.[12] Food may decrease captopril absorption by up to 54%, but this decrease is clinically insignificant.[19] Captopril is partially metabolized in the liver into an inactive compound; 95% of the parent compound and metabolites are eliminated in the urine within 24 hours. The elimination half-life increases markedly in patients with creatinine clearances of less than 20 mL/min/1.73 m$^2$. In such patients, the initial dosages should be reduced, and smaller increments should be used for titration. Hemodialysis removes approximately 35% of the dose.[12,20]

### Carboxyl Angiotensin-Converting Enzyme Inhibitors

Benazepril hydrochloride is a long-acting, nonsulfhydryl-containing, carboxyl ACE inhibitor that is available as 10- or 20-mg tablets alone or in combination with amlodipine.[18] The usual initial dosage is 10 mg daily, with maintenance dosages of 20 to 40 mg daily. Some patients respond better to twice-daily dosing (Tables 49.3 and 49.4).[21] The onset of action occurs in 2 to 6 hours; maximal antihypertensive responsiveness occurs in 2 weeks. Benazepril is a prodrug that is rapidly bioactivated in the liver into the active benazeprilat compound, which is 200 times more potent than benazepril. The elimination half-life of benazeprilat is 22 hours. Benazeprilat is excreted primarily in the urine. Dialysis does not remove benazepril, but the initial dose should be no more than 10 mg in patients with a creatinine clearance of less than 60 mL/min/1.73 m$^2$, and the dose should be reduced to 5 mg in patients with a creatinine clearance of less than 30 mL/min/1.73 m$^2$.[22]

Cilazapril is a nonsulfhydryl prodrug of the long-acting ACE inhibitor cilazaprilat.[12,18] The usual dosage is 2.5 to 10 mg daily or in divided doses. After absorption, cilazapril is rapidly deesterified in the liver to its active metabolite, cilazaprilat. The initial antihypertensive response occurs in 1 to 2 hours, peaks at 6 hours, and lasts for 8 to 12 hours.[23] Dosages should be reduced by 25% in patients with end-stage kidney disease (ESKD).[22,24]

Enalapril maleate is a nonsulfhydryl prodrug of the long-acting ACE inhibitor enalaprilat.[18,25] The oral preparations are available in tablets of 2.5, 5, 10, and 20 mg. The initial dosage of enalapril is 5 mg once daily (Table 49.3). The usual daily dose is 10 to 40 mg, singly or in divided doses. Initial responses occur in 1 hour, and peak serum levels of enalaprilat are achieved in 3 to 4 hours. Enalapril undergoes biotransformation in the liver into the active compound enalaprilat (Table 49.4). Enalapril is excreted primarily in the urine. Dosages should be reduced by 25% to 50% in patients with ESKD.[22]

Imidapril is the nonsulfhydryl prodrug of the long-acting ACE inhibitor imidaprilat.[18,26] The usual daily dose is 10 to 40 mg (Table 49.3). The peak response occurs in 5 to 6 hours and lasts for 24 hours. Imidapril is metabolized in the liver (Table 49.4). The elimination half-life of the metabolites is 10 to 19 hours. No dosage adjustments are necessary in patients with impaired kidney function. Imidapril has a unique

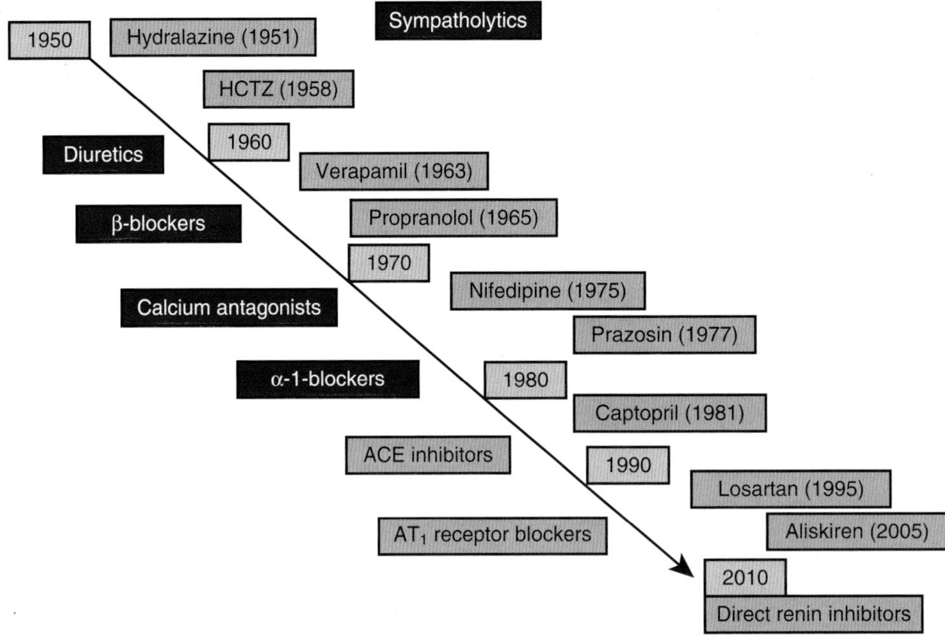


**Fig. 49.1** History of modern antihypertensive drug therapy. The first antihypertensive drug, hydralazine, was a nonspecific vasodilator discovered in the 1950s. This was followed by blockade of calcium channels on vascular smooth muscle cells, the calcium channel blockers in the 1960s, and blockade of postsynaptic α-adrenoceptors on peripheral sympathetic neurons, the α-blockers in the late 1970s. Blockade by the renin–angiotensin–aldosterone system by angiotensin-converting enzyme inhibitors was discovered in the 1980s, angiotensin receptor blockers in the 1990s, and direct renin inhibitors just 10 years ago. *ACE,* Angiotensin-converting enzyme; *$AT_1$,* angiotensin II type 1; *HCTZ,* hydrochlorothiazide. (From Sever PS, Messerli FH. Hypertension management 2011: optimal combination therapy. *Eur Heart J.* 2011;32:2499–2506.)

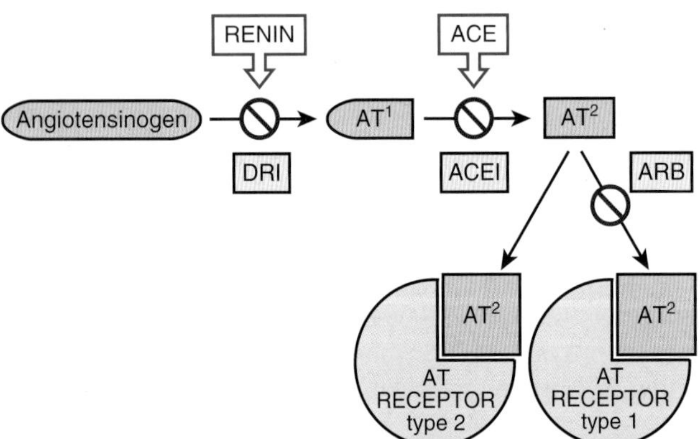


**Fig. 49.2** Renin–angiotensin–aldosterone system (RAAS)–effect site for each type of RAAS blocking drugs. The two major classes of drugs that target the RAAS are the angiotensin-converting enzyme *(ACE)* inhibitors and the selective $AT_1$ receptor blockers *(ARBs).* Both these drug classes target angiotensin II, but the differences in their mechanisms of action have implications for their effects on other pathways and receptors. Both ACE inhibitors and ARBs are effective antihypertensive agents that have been shown to reduce the risk of cardiovascular and renal events. Direct inhibition of renin—the most proximal aspect of the RAAS—became clinically feasible in 2007 with the introduction of aliskiren. *AT,* Angiotensin; *DRI,* direct renin inhibitor. (From Robles NR, Cerezo I, Hernandez-Gallego R. Renin-angiotensin system blocking drugs. *J Cardiovasc Pharmacol Ther.* 2014;19:14–33.)

advantage over other ACE inhibitors in that it is less likely to cause cough.[27]

Lisinopril is a nonsulfhydryl analog of enalaprilat.[18,28] The initial dosage is 10 mg/day, and the usual daily dose is 20 to 40 mg (Table 49.3). The initial antihypertensive response occurs in 1 hour, peaks at 6 hours, and lasts for 24 hours (Table 49.4). The maximal effect may not be observed for 24 hours. The elimination half-life is 12 hours. Lisinopril is not metabolized, and it is exclusively eliminated in the urine unchanged. Lisinopril is dialyzable, and patients undergoing dialysis may require supplemental doses. The initial dosage should be reduced to 2.5 to 7.5 mg/day in patients with moderate to advanced chronic kidney disease (CKD).[22]

Moexipril hydrochloride is the nonsulfhydryl prodrug of the ACE inhibitor moexiprilat.[18,29] The usual daily dose is 7.5 to 30 mg in single or divided doses (Table 49.3).[12] The oral bioavailability of moexipril is approximately 20%, and its absorption is impaired by high-fat meals. The peak response occurs at 3 to 6 hours and lasts for 24 hours (Table 49.4). Moexipril is rapidly converted in the liver to moexiprilat, which is 1000 times more potent than the parent compound. The dosage should be reduced by 50% in patients with ESKD.[22,30]

Perindopril is a nonsulfhydryl prodrug of the long-acting ACE inhibitor perindoprilat.[12,30] The usual daily dose is 4 to 8 mg (Table 49.3). The response peaks at 3 to 7 hours. A single dose has a duration of action of 24 hours. Perindopril undergoes extensive first-pass hepatic metabolism into the

**Table 49.3 Pharmacodynamic Properties of Angiotensin-Converting Enzyme Inhibitors**

| Generic Name (Trade Name) | Initial Dose (mg) | Usual Dose (mg) | Maximum Dose (mg) | Interval | Peak Response (h) | Duration of Response (h) |
|---|---|---|---|---|---|---|
| Alacepril (Cetapril) | 12.5 | 12.5–100 | 100 | qd | 3 | 24 |
| Captopril (Capoten) | 25 | 12.5–50 | 150 | tid | 1–2 | 3–8 |
| Benazepril (Lotensin) | 10 | 20–40 | 40 | qd | 2–6 | 24 |
| Enalapril (Vasotec) | 5 | 10–40 | 40 | qd, bid | 3–4 | 12–24 |
| Moexipril (Univasc) | 7.5 | 7.5–30 | 30 | qd, bid | 3–6 | 24 |
| Quinapril (Accupril) | 10 | 20–80 | 80 | qd | 2 | 24 |
| Ramipril (Altace) | 2.5 | 2.5–20 | 40 | qd, bid | 2 | 24 |
| Trandolapril (Mavik) | 1 | 2–4 | 8 | qd | 2–12 | 24 |
| Fosinopril (Monopril) | 5 | 5–40 | 40 | qd, bid | 2–7 | 24 |
| Cilazapril (Dynorm) | 2.5 | 2.5–10 | 10 | qd, bid | 6 | 8–12 |
| Perindopril (Aceon) | 4 | 4–8 | 8 | qd | 3–7 | 24 |
| Spirapril (SCH 33844) | 6 | 6 | 6 | qd | 3–6 | 24 |
| Zofenopril (SQ 26991) | 15 | 30–60 | 60 | qd | — | — |
| Lisinopril (Zestril, Prinivil) | 10 | 20–40 | 40 | qd | 6 | 24 |
| Imidapril (TA 6366) | 5 | 10–40 | 40 | qd | 5–6 | 24 |

**Table 49.4 Pharmacokinetic Properties of Angiotensin-Converting Enzyme Inhibitors**

| Drug | Absorption (%) | Bioavailability (%) | Affected by Food | Peak Blood Level (h) | Elimination Half-Life (h) | Metabolism | Excretion | Active Metabolites |
|---|---|---|---|---|---|---|---|---|
| Alacepril | — | 70 | — | 1 | 1.9 | L | U (70%) | Captopril |
| Captopril | 60–75 | 75 | Yes | 1 | 2 | L | U | Inactive |
| Benazepril | 35 | >37 | No | 2–6 | 22 | L, K | F, U | Benazeprilat |
| Enalapril | 55–75 | 73 | — | 3–4 | 11–35 | L | F, U | Enalaprilat |
| Lisinopril | 25 | 6–60 | — | 1 | 12 | K | U | Enalaprilat |
| Moexipril | >20 | 13–22 | Yes | 1.5 | 2–10 | L | F (50%), U | Moexiprilat |
| Quinapril | 60 | 50 | Yes | 1 | 25 | L | U (50%) | Quinaprilat |
| Ramipril | 50–60 | 60 | — | 1–2 | 13–17 | L | F, U | Ramiprilat |
| Trandolapril | 70 | 10 | No | 2–12 | 16–24 | L | F (66%), U | Trandolaprilat |
| Fosinopril | 36 | 36 | — | 1 | 12 | L, K, I | F, U | Fosinoprilat |
| Cilazapril | — | 57–76 | No | 1–2 | 30–50 | L | U (52%) | Cilazaprilat |
| Spirapril | — | 50 | Yes | 1 | 33–41 | L | F (60%), U (40%) | Spiraprilat |
| Perindopril | — | 75 | Yes | 1.5 | 3–10 | L | F, U (75%) | Perindoprilat |
| Imidapril | — | 40 | — | 3–10 | 10–19 | L | U | Imidaprilat |
| Zofenopril | >80 | 96 | Yes | 5 | 5 | K | F (26%), U (69%) | Zofenoprilat |

*F*, Feces; *I*, intestine; *K*, kidney; *L*, liver; *U*, urine.

active metabolite perindoprilat (Table 49.4). Renal excretion accounts for 75% of the clearance. The dosage should be reduced by 75% and 50% in patients with creatinine clearances of less than 50 and less than 10 mL/min/1.73 $m^2$, respectively.[22,30]

Quinapril hydrochloride is a nonsulfhydryl prodrug of the ACE inhibitor quinaprilat.[18,30,31] The initial dose is 10 mg, and the usual daily dose is 20 to 80 mg, which should be adjusted at 2-week intervals (Table 49.3). Twice-daily therapy may provide a more sustained BP reduction. The onset of action occurs in 1 hour, and the peak response occurs in 2 hours and lasts for 24 hours. Quinapril is extensively metabolized in the liver into the active metabolite, quinaprilat (Table 49.4). Renal excretion by way of filtration and active tubular secretion accounts for 50% of the clearance. Quinapril is not dialyzable. The dosage should be reduced by 25% to 50% in patients with ESKD.[22]

Ramipril is a potent, nonsulfhydryl prodrug of the ACE inhibitor ramiprilat.[12,18] Ramipril capsules are available in 1.25, 2.5, or 5 mg. The initial daily dose is 2.5 mg (Table 49.3). The usual daily dose is 2.5 to 20 mg, and it can be titrated by doubling the current dose at 2- to 4-week intervals. Ramipril is well absorbed from the gastrointestinal tract; peak concentrations are achieved in 1 to 2 hours (Table 49.4). The peak response occurs in 2 hours and lasts for 24 hours. Ramipril is extensively metabolized in the liver into the active metabolite ramiprilat. The elimination half-life of the active compound is 13 to 17 hours, and it is prolonged in renal failure patients to approximately 50 hours. The dosage should be reduced by 50% to 75% in patients with a creatinine clearance of less than 50 mL/min/1.73 $m^2$.[18,22]

Trandolapril is a nonsulfhydryl ethyl ester prodrug of the ACE inhibitor trandolaprilat.[12,18] It is available in tablets of 1, 2, and 4 mg or in combination with verapamil. The usual starting dosage is 1 mg/day (Table 49.3). Trandolapril is only 10% bioavailable, and its absorption is not affected by food (Table 49.4).[32] Trandolapril undergoes extensive first-pass hepatic metabolism into trandolaprilat. The peak serum concentrations of trandolaprilat occur within 2 to 12 hours; the duration of action is 24 hours, but it may be as long as 6 weeks. The recommended starting dose in patients with a creatinine clearance of less than 30 mL/min/1.73 $m^2$ is 0.5 mg.

### Phosphinyl Angiotensin-Converting Enzyme Inhibitor

Fosinopril sodium is a nonsulfhydryl prodrug of fosinoprilat, a long-acting ACE inhibitor.[18,33] The usual daily dose is 5 to 40 mg (Table 49.3). Its maximal effects may not occur until 4 weeks. The initial response occurs in 1 hour, the peak response occurs in 2 to 7 hours, and the duration of response is 24 hours, which is prolonged in patients with ESKD (Tables 49.3 and 49.4). The elimination half-life of fosinoprilat is 12 hours. All metabolites are excreted in the urine and feces. Hepatic biliary clearance increases significantly as kidney function declines. Thus the dosage must be reduced by 25% in patients with ESKD.[22]

## CLASS RENAL EFFECTS

There has been considerable interest in the ability of ACE inhibitors to protect the kidney from the unrelenting deterioration that occurs with hypertension and many etiologies of CKD. ACE inhibitors have extensive hemodynamic and nonhemodynamic effects that afford such protection (Table 49.5). In hypertensive patients, ACE inhibitors can restore the pressure-natriuresis relationship to normal, thereby maintaining sodium balance at a lower arterial BP.[34] The response is exaggerated in the setting of dietary sodium restriction. The mechanism responsible for this effect is the direct inhibition of proximal, and possibly distal, tubule sodium reabsorption.[35] The increased renal excretory capacity plays a major role in the long-term antihypertensive activity of the drugs. Clinically, the increase in sodium excretion is transitory because the reduced arterial pressure allows the sodium excretion to return to normal. However, the maintenance of normal sodium excretion at lower arterial pressures correlates with increased excretion in the setting of hypertension.[34] After several days, inhibition of Ang II and aldosterone contributes to the natriuresis.[36] The long-term effects on water excretion are less certain. ACE inhibitors initially induce an increase in free water clearance, but there are no long-term changes in total body weight, plasma, or extracellular fluid volume. The decrease in aldosterone caused by ACE inhibition also correlates with decreased potassium excretion,[36] particularly in patients with impaired kidney function. The antikaliuretic effect appears to be transient, but it can be exacerbated by concomitant administration of potassium-sparing diuretics, oral potassium supplements, and nonsteroidal antiinflammatory drugs (NSAIDs); it should be monitored rigorously.

**Table 49.5 Renal Protective Mechanisms of Angiotensin-Converting Enzyme Inhibitors**

| |
|---|
| Restore pressure-natriuresis relationship to normal. |
| Inhibit tubule sodium resorption. |
| Decrease arterial pressure. |
| Decrease aldosterone production. |
| Decrease proteinuria. |
| Improve altered lipid profiles. |
| Decrease renal blood flow. |
| Decrease filtration fraction. |
| Decrease renal vascular resistance. |
| Reduce scarring and fibrosis. |
| Attenuate oxidative stress and reduce free radicals. |

The effects of ACE inhibitors on angiotensin peptide levels depend on the responsiveness of renin secretion.[37,38] All ACE inhibitors decrease circulating concentrations of Ang II and increase circulating concentrations of angiotensin-(1–7) (a potential vasodilator) and plasma renin. When renin levels show little increase in response to ACE inhibition, the levels of Ang II and its metabolites decrease markedly, with little change in the levels of Ang I. Large increases in renin levels in response to ACE inhibition increase the levels of Ang I and its metabolites. The increased levels of Ang I can produce higher levels of Ang II through uninhibited ACE and other pathways, thereby blunting the effect of reduced Ang II. This phenomenon is termed "ACE escape" and may contribute to reduced ACE inhibitor efficacy when used over a long term.[39]

Recent experimental reports have highlighted the potential importance of the tissue specificity of ACE inhibitors,[40] as well as disagreement about the role played by systemic generation of Ang II versus the local generation of Ang II within the kidneys and its relative importance in terms of hypertension. An important role for intrarenal ACE has been demonstrated in murine hypertension models, as mice lacking only renal ACE are protected against hypertension.[40] The intrarenal Ang II production and local regulation of renal sodium transport represents a new mechanistic understanding of the underlying inappropriate regulation of salt and water balance. However, what remains unclear is the role that intrarenal renin–angiotensin–aldosterone system (RAAS) plays in human disease. It is clear that local inhibition of ACE in the vascular wall and renal vessels contributes to the antihypertensive activity of hypertension drugs. ACE inhibitor–induced changes in BP correlate with the degree of inhibition of RAAS in plasma and tissues.[41] The ACE inhibitors with the greatest tissue specificity, however, are associated with prolonged activity at the tissue level, even after serum ACE levels have returned to normal.[41] Consequently, they are more efficacious with once-daily dosing.[41] Other potential renoprotective effects that have been noted in experimental models include attenuation of oxidative stress,[42] scavenging of free radicals, and attenuation of lipid peroxidation.[43] The clinical importance of these effects is under investigation.

Because the degree of proteinuria correlates (inversely) with the rate of decline in kidney function, and a decrease in proteinuria correlates better with renal protection than with decreased BP, the reduction of proteinuria can have a substantial impact.[44] All ACE inhibitors decrease urinary protein excretion[45–47] in normotensive and hypertensive patients with kidney disease of various etiologies. Individual response rates vary from an increase of 31% to a decrease of 100%, and they are strongly influenced by drug dosage and dietary sodium intake.[46,48] There is a clear dose–response relation between increased doses and reduced proteinuria, and this relationship is not dependent on changes in BP, renal plasma flow, or GFR. Furthermore, the effect of ACE inhibitors on the reduction of proteinuria is eliminated with high salt intake.

Studies have demonstrated that in normotensive patients with diabetes mellitus, ACE inhibitors can normalize GFR, markedly reduce the progression of kidney disease, and normalize microalbuminuria.[49,50] These findings are discussed in depth in Chapter 39. The effect is noted in the first month of therapy and is maximal at 14 months. Several mechanisms account for the reduction in urinary protein excretion, including the following: a decrease in glomerular capillary hydrostatic pressure; a decrease in mesangial uptake and clearance of macromolecules; and improved glomerular basement membrane perm-selectivity.[3,51] ACE inhibitors have better antiproteinuric efficacy than other classes of antihypertensive agents, with the exception of angiotensin receptor blockers (ARBs). In the treatment of proteinuria, the noninferiority of ARBs to ACE inhibition was confirmed in a meta-analysis of 24 studies.[47] Furthermore, the antiproteinuric effect is additive with the ARBs, but because of the risk of hyperkalemia and higher risk of acute kidney injury (AKI), combination therapy is not recommended. The beneficial effects of ACE inhibition may not be enhanced by combined nondihydropyridine calcium channel antagonist therapy beyond BP lowering.[52,53] A suggested goal of ACE inhibition or ARB therapy is to reduce proteinuria to less than 1000 mg/day or reduce proteinuria to more than 50% from baseline, in addition to protein excretion at less than 3.5 g/day.[54] BP should be reduced to less than 130/80 mm Hg as recommended by the recent American College of Cardiology/American Heart Association Task Force (ACC/AHA) guidelines.[55]

Most of the vasoconstrictive action of Ang II is confined to the efferent arteriole. ACE inhibitors preferentially dilate the efferent arteriole by reducing the systemic and intrarenal levels of Ang II. The effect is a reduction in intraglomerular capillary pressure. In patients with hypertension, ACE inhibitors uniformly increase renal blood flow, decrease filtration fraction, decrease renal vascular resistance, reduce urinary protein excretion, impair microvascular autoregulation, and restore normal circadian BP patterns,[56–58] with variable to no effect on GFR. In patients with nondiabetic glomerular disease, short-term ACE inhibitor administration causes a decrease in renal perfusion, glomerular filtration and pressure, and an increase in afferent resistances.[59] Long-term administration is associated with a decrease in renal perfusion, as well as a tendency toward a higher filtration fraction and lower afferent resistances. Marked improvement in GFR occurs and is sustained for up to 3 years.[60,61] However, many patients with impaired renal function exhibit a reversible fall in GFR with ACE inhibitor therapy that is not detrimental. The GFR declines initially because of hemodynamic changes, but the long-term reduction in perfusion pressure is renoprotective. Even in patients receiving hemodialysis, ACE inhibitor therapy significantly preserves residual kidney function and helps maintain urine output.[62] Patients with type 1 diabetes who have the largest initial decline in GFR have the slowest rate of loss of kidney function over time.[63] It should be emphasized that ACE inhibitors need not be withdrawn immediately in response to an increase in serum creatinine; a 20% to 30% decline in GFR can be expected, and close monitoring is warranted.

An inherited trait of disordered regulation of the RAAS contributes to the pathogenesis of hypertension in approximately 45% of patients.[64] Such patients have sodium-sensitive hypertension, abnormalities in renal vascular responses to changes in sodium intake and Ang II, blunted decrements of renin release in response to saline or Ang II, and accentuated vasodilator responses to ACE inhibition; they have been termed "nonmodulators."[64] In these patients, ACE inhibition not only increases renal blood flow substantially more than it does in normal patients, but also restores the renal vascular and adrenal responses to Ang II, renin release, renal sodium handling, and BP.[64,65]

Treatment with ACE inhibitors is frequently associated with an initial decrease in kidney function, as reflected by an increase in the serum creatinine concentration.[66] The significance of an increase in serum creatinine after the initiation of RAAS inhibitor therapy is uncertain because it is due in part to a reduction in intraglomerular pressure, which might be expected to contribute to the slowing of disease progression in the long term. An initial elevation in the serum creatinine level of up to 30% above baseline, which stabilizes within the first 2 months of therapy, has been considered acceptable, and it is no reason to discontinue therapy in the absence of hypotension or hyperkalemia.[67,68] Suggesting otherwise, a review of 12 randomized trials has shown that in patients receiving ACE inhibitors, a stable rise in the serum creatinine of less than 30% was associated with long-term preservation of kidney function.[67,68]

In patients with an activated RAAS, however, ACE inhibitors can decrease GFR and may precipitate AKI. Patients with severe bilateral renal artery stenosis,[69] unilateral renal artery stenosis of a solitary kidney, severe hypertensive nephrosclerosis, volume depletion, congestive heart failure, cirrhosis, or a transplanted kidney[70] are at higher risk for deterioration in kidney function with ACE inhibitor therapy.[71,72] These patients typically have a precipitous drop in BP and deterioration of kidney function when treated with ACE inhibitors. In these states of reduced renal perfusion related to low effective arterial circulating volume or reduced perfusion because of narrowing of arterial inflow, the maintenance of renal blood flow and GFR is highly dependent on increased efferent arteriolar vasoconstriction mediated by Ang II. Interruption of the increased tone causes a critical reduction in perfusion pressure and can lead to dramatic reductions in GFR and urinary flow, worsening of renal ischemia and, in rare cases, anuria. The hemodynamic effect described here is typically reversible with cessation of therapy.[73] Even paradoxic severe hypertension has been described in rare patients with renal artery stenosis treated with ACE inhibitors.[74] Among 26 older patients with hemodynamically significant renal artery stenosis who received renin–angiotensin blockers and experienced a decline in kidney function of 25% or more, 19% (5 of 26) developed ESKD, and 73% (19 of 26) showed improvement in estimated GFR (eGFR).[75]

Although instances of reversible azotemia have provoked disproportionate fear among prescribers, multiple randomized controlled trials (RCTs) have shown that RAAS blockade effectively decreases the progression of kidney disease,[76–78] and observational studies have demonstrated the benefit of RAAS blockade on BP control, adverse cardiovascular outcomes, and all-cause mortality. Recent studies of atherosclerotic renovascular disease demonstrating the efficacy of medical therapy, including use of ACE inhibitors and ARBs over renal artery stenting, have indicated that the risks of RAAS blockade (e.g., azotemia, hyperkalemia, angioedema) can be balanced by their benefits when patients are carefully monitored.[79–81]

It should be noted that in the studies of renoprotection by ACE inhibitors, those with advanced stage 4 or nondialysis-dependent stage 5 CKD were excluded. Some have raised the possibility that withdrawal of ACE inhibitors/ARB therapy in advanced CKD may preserve kidney function. In an observational study, withdrawal of ACE inhibitor/ARB therapy in 52 older patients with advanced CKD led to a mean increase in eGFR of 10 mL/min/1.73 m$^2$ over 12 months and an increase or stabilization in eGFR in all but four patients.[82] However, RCTs are needed to establish the safety and efficacy of this approach.

## CLASS EFFICACY AND SAFETY

ACE inhibitors are recommended for initial monotherapy in patients with mild, moderate, and severe hypertension, regardless of age, sex, or ancestry.[83] They are effective in patients with diabetes, obesity, and/or following kidney transplantation,[84] and are safe to use in patients with mild, moderate, and severe CKD. In general, patients with high-renin hypertension and chronic renal parenchymal disease respond particularly well, presumably because they have inappropriately high intrarenal renin and Ang II levels. African Americans with hypertension have been found to respond less well (vis-à-vis BP reduction) to lower dosages than whites, but higher dosages are equally effective.[85–87] In most studies, ACE inhibitors elicit an adequate response in 40% to 60% of patients.[88] An immediate fall in BP occurs in 70% of patients. The enhanced efficacy of ACE inhibitors in the presence of salt restriction is paralleled by the additive effects of diuretic therapy.[89] The addition of low-dose hydrochlorothiazide (HCTZ) enhances the efficacy more than 80%, normalizing BP in another 20% to 25% of patients.[90] Adding a diuretic is more effective than increasing the dosage of the ACE inhibitor.[90,91] Recent clinical trials have examined the use of the combination of an ACE inhibitor and ARB to prevent target-organ damage.[92] The Renal Outcomes with Telmisartan, Ramipril, or Both, in People at High Vascular Risk (ONTARGET) trial compared the ACE inhibitor ramipril with the ARB telmisartan, alone and in combination, in patients at high risk for vascular disease.[93,94] Although the achieved mean BP was lower in the patients who received telmisartan or both agents than in those who received ramipril alone, there was no difference in the primary outcomes between any of the groups, and more adverse outcomes were noted in the combination group. Importantly, this trial did not evaluate ARB and ACE inhibitor therapy in patients with advanced proteinuric renal disease. The VA NEPHRON-D study, a trial using combination therapy (ACE inhibitor and ARB therapy vs. ARB monotherapy) in patients with proteinuric diabetic nephropathy, was stopped because of increased adverse events of hyperkalemia and AKI.[95] The Aliskiren Trial in Type 2 Diabetes Using Cardiorenal Endpoints (ALTITUDE) randomly assigned 8561 patients to aliskiren (300 mg daily), a direct renin inhibitor, or placebo as an adjunct to ACE or ARB monotherapy. The trial was stopped prematurely because of adverse events (hyperkalemia and hypotension).[96] Therefore, among patients with type 2 diabetes and kidney disease, ACE inhibitors should not be used concomitantly with ARBs and renin inhibitors because of an increased risk of hypotension, hyperkalemia, and aggravated renal dysfunction.[97]

Many studies have attempted to achieve further benefit from ACE inhibitors and other RAAS blocking agents by increasing the doses of these drugs. This reasoning is based on the original observation that the optimal antiproteinuric dose does not necessarily equal the optimal antihypertensive dose. Many of these study results have shown further proteinuria reduction,[98–102] whereas others have not.[103–105] However, similar to the initial studies of the combination therapy with RAAS blocking agents, many of these high-dosage studies were also short-term studies that used BP and albuminuria as outcome variables. These studies have not been sufficiently powered, or they lacked duration to detect safety signals and side effect rates that may emerge with endpoint trials.[97] Therefore before ultrahigh-RAAS blocking agent dosing as renoprotective therapy can be recommended, more studies with hard kidney and cardiovascular event points are warranted.[97]

Neither the duration nor the degree of BP lowering is predicted by the effect on blood ACE or Ang II levels, and all ACE inhibitors appear to have comparable efficacy. The response may be due in part to interindividual variability of the ACE genotype.[87,106] The activity of ACE is partially dependent on the presence or absence of a 287–base pair element in intron 16, and this insertion–deletion (I/D) polymorphism of a human Al repetitive DNA element accounts for 47% of the total phenotypic variation in plasma ACE. Deletion–deletion cases have the highest ACE concentrations, I/D cases have intermediate ACE concentrations, and insertion–insertion cases have the lowest. Genotype also influences tissue ACE activity, but the clinical implications remain incompletely understood.

ACE inhibitors are indicated as first-line therapy in hypertensive patients with heart failure and systolic dysfunction,[107] type 1 diabetes and proteinuria,[63] reduced systolic function after myocardial infarction (MI),[108] coronary artery disease or new atrial fibrillation,[109,110] and left ventricular dysfunction,[83,110,111] as well as patients undergoing dialysis.[112] ACE inhibitors reduce ventricular hypertrophy independent of the BP decrease.[113] All patients with diabetes, even those without evidence of nephropathy, should be given ACE inhibitors for cardiovascular risk reduction.[114–118] Primary and secondary prevention trials[114,119,120] have shown that ACE inhibitors improve endothelial dysfunction and cardiac and vascular remodeling, retard the progression of atherosclerosis, improve arterial distensibility, and reduce the risk of myocardial ischemia and infarction, stroke, and cardiovascular death. Some but not all studies have shown a small decrease in the risk of new and recurrent atrial fibrillation because of the beneficial structural and electrical effects on the atria.[121,122] The use of ACE inhibitors is also associated with improved exercise performance in patients with hypertension and intermittent claudication,[123] reduced pain perception,[124] and reduced perioperative myocardial ischemia,[108] as well as the retardation of the progression of aortic stenosis,[125] protection against cognitive decline and dementia,[126,127] promotion of atrial structural remodeling,[128] prolongation of the survival of arteriovenous polytetrafluoroethylene grafts,[129] and possible reduced risk of pneumonia[130] and prevention of osteoporosis.[131] Long-term use of these agents has been associated with a lower risk for breast cancer, but the importance of this finding has yet to be substantiated.[132]

ACE inhibitors may cause fetal or neonatal injury or death when used during the second and third trimesters of pregnancy[133] because angiotensin appears to be required for normal fetal growth and development.[134] Concern has been expressed regarding first-trimester use of ACE inhibitors because their use during this period might be associated with congenital malformations, but these malformations may also be related to maternal factors.[135] A recent study has found that maternal use of ACE inhibitors in the first trimester shows a risk profile similar to that of other antihypertensive agents.[136] Recognizing that the benefits of ACE inhibitors are largely long term, we advise women attempting conception to transition to an alternative antihypertensive agent with a proven safety profile in pregnancy (e.g., labetalol).

A systemic review of published case reports and case series dealing with intrauterine exposure to ACE inhibitors or ARBs has shown 118 cases of ACE inhibitor exposure and 68 cases of ARB exposure. Among 118 cases of ACE inhibitor exposure, 27% were taken only in the first trimester; in 68 cases of ARB exposure, 38% were taken throughout the entire pregnancy. Neonatal complications were more frequent following exposure to ARBs; 52% of the newborns exposed to ACE inhibitors did not exhibit any complications, whereas only 13% of the newborns exposed to ARBs did not ($P < .0001$); however, many of the patients exposed to ARBs received therapy throughout the pregnancy.[137] In 26 children, 23% developed kidney failure, 8% required dialysis, 15% demonstrated hypertension, 8% developed acidosis, 12% developed polyuria, 15% showed small or echogenic kidneys on ultrasound, 8% had polycythemia, 15% had growth retardation, and 12% experienced neurodevelopmental delay. The outcome was normal in 50% of cases, mild in 42%, and bad in 8%. Complications were similar whether the children were exposed to ACE inhibitors or ARBs. The authors commented that the congenital malformations that occurred following in utero RAAS exposure might have resulted from the drug as well as the underlying maternal illness, usually hypertension or diabetes.

A prospective, observational, controlled cohort study of ACE inhibitors and ARB exposure during the first trimester was reported in 2012.[138] Participants were enrolled from an unselected sample of women contacting a teratogen information service. There were two comparison groups, women with hypertension treated with other antihypertensives (including methyldopa or calcium channel blockers [CCBs]) and healthy controls. In the ACE–ARB and disease-matched groups, the offspring exhibited significantly lower birth weights and gestational ages than those of the healthy controls ($P < .001$ for both variables). A significantly higher rate of miscarriage was noted in the ACE–ARB group ($P < .001$). These results suggest that ACE inhibitors and ARBs are not major human teratogens during the first trimester. There was, however, a higher rate of spontaneous abortions in the ACE–ARB group.

When a patient becomes pregnant during treatment with an ACE inhibitor or ARB, the drug should be discontinued immediately, and alternative antihypertensive therapy should be started. Pregnancy termination is at the discretion of the patient and treatment team, but physicians and patients can derive some reassurance from the small studies quoted earlier if the drug is discontinued during the first trimester. Recognizing that the benefits of ACE inhibitors are largely long term, we advise women attempting conception to transition to an alternative antihypertensive agent with a proven safety profile in pregnancy (e.g., labetalol) (Table 49.6; see also Chapter 48).

ACE inhibitors are transferred into breast milk, but the drug levels in milk are low. Captopril and enalapril have been reviewed by the American Academy of Pediatrics[139] and the National Institute for Health and Care Excellence (NICE) guidelines for the management of hypertension in pregnancy from the United Kingdom,[140] and they are compatible with lactation. However, newborns may be more susceptible to the hemodynamic effects of these drugs (e.g., hypotension) and sequelae (e.g., oliguria, seizures).

Overall, ACE inhibitors are well tolerated and have relatively neutral or beneficial metabolic effects. ACE inhibitors are associated with 8% to 11% reductions in levels of low-density lipoprotein (LDL) cholesterol and triglycerides and 5% increases in levels of high-density lipoprotein (HDL) cholesterol.[141] They do not cause perturbations of serum sodium or uric acid levels. ACE inhibitors reduce the levels of plasminogen activator inhibitor-1 and may improve fibrinolysis.[142]

The effects of ACE inhibitors on glucose metabolism are favorable.[143] They may improve glucose tolerance by augmenting the insulin secretory response to glucose[143] and may also help ameliorate obesity and hyperinsulinemia.[144] The use of ACE inhibitors has been clinically associated with a 25% to 30% reduction in the risk of developing diabetes.[145] Several large clinical trials have evaluated the clinical relevance of this finding.[146] Many of the ACE inhibitors require dosage adjustment in the presence of impaired kidney function, as described earlier[22] (Table 49.7).

There are relatively few adverse effects (AEs) of this class of drugs, and AEs may occur with all ACE inhibitors. The newer agents appear to have a lower incidence of AEs, possibly because of lack of the sulfhydryl moiety found in captopril. The most common AE of ACE inhibitors is a dry, hacking, nonproductive cough, which has been reported in up to 20% of patients.[147] In the ONTARGET trial, cough sufficiently severe to permanently discontinue the drug was described in 4.2% of patients treated with ramipril[148]; cough is much less common with ARBs. The ACE inhibitor-induced cough is thought to be secondary to hypersensitivity to bradykinins, which are increased by ACE,[149] increased levels of prostaglandins,[150] accumulation of substance P,[147] a potent bronchoconstrictor,[151] or polymorphisms in the neurokinin-2 receptor gene.[152] The cough can begin initially or many months after the start of therapy.[153] It is more common in women, African Americans,[154] and Asians in Hong Kong[155] and Korea,[156] and it may spontaneously disappear.[153] It may be more common in patients with bronchial hyperreactivity, but ACE inhibitors are safe to use in asthmatic patients.[157] NSAIDs, oral iron supplements, and sodium cromoglycate have been reported to improve the cough,[158] but cessation of ACE therapy is the only absolute cure. In a dosage of 600 mg twice daily, picotamide (a thromboxane antagonist) was effective in treating ACE inhibitor–induced cough.[159] Patients may be effectively switched to ARBs if an antihypertensive effect is observed with ACE inhibitors.

**Table 49.6 Antihypertensive Therapies Commonly Used in Pregnancy**

| Agent | Indication | Dose Range | FDA Classification | Potential Side Effects | Comments |
|---|---|---|---|---|---|
| α2-Methyldopa | Often used as first line | 250 mg to 1.5 g orally twice a day | B | Lethargy | Data on offspring up to 7.5 years of age demonstrating long-term safety |
| Labetalol | Often used as first line | 100–1200 mg | C | Exacerbation of asthma | Widely used in pregnancy |
| Calcium channel blockers | Second line of alternative first line (nifedipine) | Varies according to drug used | C | Concern for synergy with magnesium sulfate for neuromuscular depression | |
| β-Blockers | Second line | Varies according to drug used | C | Exacerbation of asthma | Some recommend avoiding atenolol during pregnancy and lactation |
| Thiazide diuretics | Second line | 12.5–50 mg orally once a day | C | Volume depletion and hypokalemia | |

Angiotensin-converting enzyme inhibitors and angiotensin receptor blockers are contraindicated in the second and third trimesters of pregnancy and are class D. Safety in the first trimester is controversial: in this trimester, they are class C.
*FDA,* U.S. Food and Drug Administration.

FDA Classification of Drugs in Pregnancy
Category A: Controlled studies in pregnant women have demonstrated no risk of fetal abnormalities
Category B: Reproduction studies in animals indicate no fetal risk, but there are no adequate and well-controlled studies in pregnant women; or animal reproduction studies have shown an adverse effect of the drug but not in well-controlled studies in pregnant women.
Category C: Animal reproduction studies have shown an adverse effect on the fetus but no adequate human or animal studies; or animal reproduction studies have been conducted and it is not known whether the drug can cause fetal harm when administered to a pregnant woman.
Category D: Evidence of human fetal risk, but benefits outweigh risks. Women taking this drug during pregnancy should be informed of potential fetal risk.
Category X: Evidence of human fetal risk. Drug is contraindicated in women who are pregnant or who may become pregnant. If this drug is used during pregnancy or if the patient becomes pregnant while taking this drug, the patient should be apprised of the potential hazard to a fetus.

**Table 49.7 Dose Modifications of Antihypertensive Drugs Required for Renal Insufficiency**

| | Estimated Glomerular Filtration Rate (Creatinine Clearance; mL/min/1.73 m²) | | | |
|---|---|---|---|---|
| **Drug** | >50 | 10–15 | <10 | **Dialysis**[a] |
| **Angiotensin-Converting Enzyme Inhibitors** | | | | |
| Benazepril | No change | 50% | 25% | Negligible |
| Captopril | No change | 50% | 25% | H: 50% |
| Cilazapril | No change | 50% | 25% | H: 50% |
| Enalapril | No change | 50% | 25% | H: 50% |
| Fosinopril | No change | No change | 75% | — |
| Imidapril | No change | No change | — | — |
| Lisinopril | No change | 50% | 25% | H: 50% |
| Moexipril | No change | 50% | 25% | — |
| Perindopril | No change | 75% | 50% | — |
| Quinapril | No change | 50% | 25% | — |
| Ramipril | No change | 50% | 25% | — |
| Trandolapril | No change | 50% | 25% | — |
| Zofenopril | No change | — | — | — |
| **Angiotensin Receptor Blockers** | | | | |
| Candesartan | No change | No change | No change | Negligible |
| Eprosartan | No change | No change | 50% | Negligible |
| Irbesartan | No change | No change | — | Negligible |

**Table 49.7 Dose Modifications of Antihypertensive Drugs Required for Renal Insufficiency (Cont'd)**

| | Estimated Glomerular Filtration Rate (Creatinine Clearance; mL/min/1.73 m²) | | | |
|---|---|---|---|---|
| **Drug** | >50 | 10–15 | <10 | **Dialysis**[a] |
| Losartan | No change | No change | No change | Negligible |
| Olmesartan | No change | — | — | — |
| Telmisartan | No change | No change | No change | Negligible |
| Valsartan | No change | No change | No change | — |
| **Adrenergic Antagonists** | | | | |
| Nadolol | No change | 50% | 25% | H: 50% |
| Carteolol | No change | 50% | 25% | — |
| Penbutolol | No change | No change | 50% | Negligible |
| Pindolol | No change | No change | 50% | Negligible |
| Atenolol | No change | 50% | 25% | H: 50% |
| Betaxolol | No change | No change | 50% | H: 50% |
| Bisoprolol | No change | 50% | 25% | Negligible |
| Acebutolol | No change | 50% | 30%–50% | H: 50% |
| Celiprolol | No change | 50% | Avoid | — |
| Nebivolol | No change | 50% | — | — |
| **Calcium Channel Blockers** | | | | |
| Diltiazem | No change | No change | No change | Negligible |
| Verapamil | No change | No change | No change | Negligible |
| Nifedipine | No change | No change | No change | Negligible |
| Amlodipine | No change | No change | No change | Negligible |
| Felodipine | No change | No change | No change | Negligible |
| Isradipine | No change | No change | No change | Negligible |
| Manidipine | No change | No change | No change | Negligible |
| Nicardipine | No change | No change | No change | Negligible |
| Nisoldipine | No change | No change | No change | Negligible |
| Lacidipine | No change | No change | No change | Negligible |
| Lercanidipine | Dosage adjustment in renal failure unknown | | | |
| **Central $\alpha_2$-Adrenergic or $I_1$ Imidazole Receptor Agonists** | | | | |
| Methyldopa | No change | No change | 50% | H: 50% |
| Clonidine | No change | 50% | 25% | Negligible |
| Moxonidine | No change | 50% | — | — |
| Rilmenidine | No change | 50% | 25% | — |
| **Direct-Acting Vasodilators** | | | | |
| Hydralazine | No change | No change | 75%[b] | Negligible |
| Minoxidil | No change | 50% | 50% | H and P: 50% |
| **Peripheral Adrenergic Neuronal Blocking Agents** | | | | |
| Guanethidine | No change | No change | — | — |
| Guanadrel | No change | 50% | 25% (avoid) | — |
| **Renin Inhibitor** | | | | |
| Aliskiren | No change | No change | Not studied | Not studied |
| **Tyrosine Hydroxylase Inhibitor** | | | | |
| Metyrosine | No change | 50% | 25% | — |
| **Selective Aldosterone Receptor Antagonist** | | | | |
| Eplerenone | Dosage adjustment in renal failure unknown<br>Caution in regard to hyperkalemia | | | |

Percentage of usual dose given.
[a]Replacement dose at end of dialysis as percentage of dose prescribed for patient with glomerular filtration rate <10 mL/min.
[b]Slow acetylators.
*H,* Hemodialysis; *P,* peritoneal dialysis; —, not applicable.

Angioedema is a rare but potentially life-threatening complication of ACE inhibitor therapy. It occurs in 0.1% to 0.7% of patients within hours of the first dose of ACE inhibitor or after prolonged use.[160–162] In the ONTARGET Trial, the occurrence of angioedema, although potentially life-threatening, was reported and was listed as a reason to discontinue from the study permanently in just 0.3% of more than 8500 individuals given ramipril.[148]

This absolute risk of ACE inhibitor–induced angioedema is low, but with large numbers of prescriptions written annually, many patients are at risk for this disorder.[163] ACE inhibitor–induced angioedema accounts for one-third of all cases of angioedema seen in emergency departments.

Our understanding of the mechanism of ACE inhibitor–induced angioedema is evolving. The side effect occurs five times more frequently in individuals of African ancestry. ACE inhibitors act by inhibiting bradykinin breakdown in addition to blocking the conversion of Ang I to Ang II. ACE inhibitor–induced angioedema involves several components, including tissue accumulation of bradykinin and inhibition of C1 esterase activity.[160,164] Susceptible individuals typically have defects in non-ACE, nonkininase I vasoactive pathways of bradykinin degradation, possess the XPNPEP2 gene variant,[165–172] have elevated des-Arg9-BK,[167] or are taking dipeptidyl peptidase inhibitors (e.g., sitagliptin, saxagliptin, linagliptin) to treat diabetes.[160,168–170] Some patients also have defective degradation of substance P, thereby increasing vascular permeability.[171]

Clinical features, including asymmetric swelling confined to the face, subcutaneous or submucous membranes, and lips, usually resolve with discontinuation of the therapy, but obstructive sleep apnea may be exacerbated.[172] If the ACE inhibitor is not discontinued, the episode usually resolves, but the frequency and severity of future episodes will escalate.[173,174] Angioedema of the small intestine and acute appendicitis have also been reported.[175–178]

Involvement of the glottis and larynx requiring airway management occurs in 10% of all cases and may result in laryngeal obstruction and death.[179] Administration of epinephrine, histamine-2 blockers, glucocorticoids, and/or fresh-frozen plasma is indicated.[180] Recently, icatibant, a selective bradykinin B2 receptor antagonist approved for the treatment of hereditary angioedema, has also been shown to be effective for the treatment of ACE inhibitor–induced angioedema in a multicenter, double-blind, phase 2 study. In 27 patients, the median time to resolution was 8 hours with icatibant (interquartile range, 3.0 to 16.0 hours) compared with 27.1 hours with standard therapy (interquartile range, 20.3 to 48.0 hours) with a glucocorticoid and an antihistamine. Patients experiencing an episode of angioedema associated with ACE inhibitor usage should be switched to ARBs or other agents.[181] ACE inhibitors are contraindicated in patients with a known hypersensitivity to ACE inhibitors.

First-dose hypotension, with a reduction in BP of up to 30%, has been reported with all ACE inhibitors in up to 2.5% of patients. In the Studies of Left Ventricular Dysfunction (SOLVD trial), hypotension was observed in 14.8% of patients versus 7.1% of individuals who received a placebo ($P < .0001$).[182] In the ONTARGET Trial, of the 8579 patients who received ramipril, only 1.7% and 0.2% permanently stopped therapy because of hypotension and syncope, respectively.[160]

Hypotension occurs more commonly in patients with effective arterial volume depletion, patients with high-renin hypertension, and those with systolic heart failure.[182,183] Hypotension is usually well tolerated, although occasionally it is associated with syncope. In older patients, ACE inhibitor therapy more frequently causes nocturnal hypotension.[184] The accompanying increase in the plasma norepinephrine concentration may explain the low incidence of orthostatic symptoms.[184] In patients at high risk of orthostatic symptoms, therapy should be initiated at lower dosages, preferably after discontinuing diuretics. Rebound hypertension has not been reported with discontinuation of ACE inhibitors.

AEs related to the chemical structure are more frequently seen with the sulfhydryl-containing captopril than with the other agents. Dysgeusia appears to be related to the binding of zinc by the ACE inhibitors.[185] Approximately 2% to 4% of patients experience a diminution or loss of taste sensation that is associated with a metallic taste. It is usually self-limited and resolves in 2 to 3 months, even with continued therapy. However, it may be severe enough to interfere with nutrition and cause weight loss.[186]

Cutaneous reactions manifest as a nonallergic, pruritic, maculopapular eruption that appears during the first few weeks of therapy. These reactions may be associated with a fever or arthralgias and may disappear, even with continuation of the ACE inhibitor.[187]

Leukopenia and anemia have been reported with ACE inhibitor therapy. Among patients with normal kidney function, ACE inhibitors may reduce hemoglobin concentrations in a dose-dependent manner.[188] ACE inhibitors have been demonstrated to interfere with the response to erythropoietin. Patients receiving hemodialysis and kidney transplant recipients receiving erythropoietin frequently require higher dosages to maintain hemoglobin concentrations.[189] Consequently, ACE inhibitors can be used effectively to reduce posttransplantation erythrocytosis,[190] but appear to have little effect on erythropoiesis in patients receiving hemodialysis.[191] Neutropenia (<1000 neutrophils/mm$^3$) with myeloid hypoplasia occurs almost exclusively in patients with impaired kidney function, immunosuppression, collagen vascular disease, or autoimmune disease.[12] Neutropenia occurs within 3 months of initiation of therapy and generally resolves 2 weeks after therapy is discontinued.[12,187]

Anaphylactoid reactions ranging from mild pruritus to bronchospasm and cardiopulmonary collapse have been reported in patients treated with ACE inhibitors who undergo dialysis with equipment that uses high-flux polyacrylonitrile, cellulose acetate, or cuprophane membranes or who undergo apheresis with equipment that uses dextran sulfate membranes.[192] The frequency of reactions is unknown, but they occur within the first few minutes of treatment. Such membranes should be avoided when patients are receiving ACE inhibitors. The use of ACE inhibitors in patients on plasmapheresis or an exchange protocol is safe as long as effective arterial volume is managed appropriately.

Few significant drug interactions occur with ACE inhibitors. Studies have shown that aspirin dosages of 100 mg/day or less do not negate the effects of ACE inhibitors.[193] Ang II stimulates the production of vasodilatory prostaglandins. Aspirin inhibits the production of vasodilator and antithrombotic prostaglandins. Theoretically, either agent may antagonize the effectiveness of the other. Concomitant use of ACE inhibitors and cyclosporine may exacerbate renal hypoperfusion.[12] Use of the mammalian target of rapamycin inhibitors sirolimus or everolimus in transplant recipients decreases the metabolism of bradykinins and predisposes them to angioedema with ACE inhibitors.[194]

Hyperkalemia of more than 5.5 mmol/L was observed in 3.3% of patients taking ramipril in the ONTARGET study.[148] Production of Ang II systemically and locally in the zona glomerulosa of the adrenal gland, which is blocked by ACE inhibitors, will reduce subsequent aldosterone synthesis and urinary potassium excretion. In a Veterans Administration Medical Center case–control study of 1818 patients using ACE inhibitors, 194 (11%) developed hyperkalemia.[195] The results of laboratory studies indicated that a serum urea nitrogen concentration higher than 6.4 mmol/L and a serum creatinine concentration higher than 136 μmol/L, as well as congestive heart failure and long-acting ACE inhibitors, were independently associated with hyperkalemia; concurrent use of a loop or thiazide diuretic agent was associated with reduced risk. After 1 year of follow-up, 15 (10%) of 146 patients who remained on a regimen of an ACE inhibitor developed severe hyperkalemia (serum potassium >6.0 mmol/L). A serum urea nitrogen level higher than 8.9 mmol/L and age older than 70 years were independently associated with subsequent severe hyperkalemia.

Hyperkalemia has been effectively and safely treated with patiromer and sodium zirconium cyclosilicate recently in an outpatient setting.[196,197] These two new drugs add to the outpatient pharmacopoeia that until now has been limited to sodium and calcium polystyrene sulfonate. Correction of metabolic acidosis, if present, may also reduce the incidence and severity of hyperkalemia.

## ANGIOTENSIN II TYPE 1 RECEPTOR ANTAGONISTS

### CLASS MECHANISMS OF ACTION

The Ang II receptor blockers (ARBs) allow more specific and complete blockade of the RAAS than the ACE inhibitors because they circumvent all pathways that lead to the formation of Ang II (Fig. 49.2). For example, Ang I is metabolized not only by ACE to form Ang II but also by chymase, cathepsin G, tissue plasminogen activator, and other enzymes.[198] Ang II can be formed at sites other than those in the systemic circulation, such as the brain, kidney, and heart. Furthermore, long-term ACE inhibitor therapy is associated with a return of Ang II levels to baseline, which possibly contributes to reduced efficacy. The ARBs selectively antagonize Ang II directly at the Ang II type 1 ($AT_1$) receptor, regardless of the source of production. Because Ang II plays a crucial multifactorial role in maintaining and regulating BP, blockade of the $AT_1$ receptor with ARBs is a powerful tool for targeting multiple pathways that contribute to hypertension.

Like ACE inhibitors, ARBs directly block the vasoconstrictive action of Ang II and cause a decrease in peripheral vascular resistance.[199] Interruption of the binding of Ang II at the tissue level also leads to other effects (beyond vasodilation) that contribute to the antihypertensive effect. Additional mechanisms include the following: (1) augmentation of renal blood flow and reduction of aldosterone release to induce natriuresis and attenuate the compensatory increase in sodium retention that accompanies a fall in BP; (2) direct depression of tubular sodium reabsorption[200,201]; (3) improvement of nitric oxide–mediated endothelial function[202]; (4) reversal of vascular hypertrophy[202]; (5) blunting of SNS activity and presynaptic norepinephrine release; (6) inhibition of postjunctional pressor responses to norepinephrine or Ang II; (7) inhibition of central Ang II–mediated sympathoexcitation and vasopressin release[203–205]; (8) inhibition of centrally controlled baroreceptor reflexes[206]; (9) inhibition of central nervous system (CNS) norepinephrine synthesis; (10) inhibition of thirst[207]; and (11) possible inhibition of RAAS-mediated action on endothelin-1.[208] The antihypertensive action of ARBs is dependent on activation of the RAAS and is associated with clinically insignificant increases in circulating levels of Ang II.[199] ARBs also increase bradykinin levels by antagonizing Ang II at its type 1 receptor and diverting Ang II to its counterregulatory type 2 receptor, which potentiates vasodilation.[209] ARBs also increase the level of other angiotensin peptides, including angiotensin-(1-7), Ang II, and angiotensin IV, which can act on their respective receptors to modulate vasoconstriction, renal blood flow, and vascular hypertrophy.[210–215]

### CLASS MEMBERS

The ARB class is composed of peptide and nonpeptide analogs that vary in structure, mechanism of receptor inhibition, metabolism, and potency. There are currently eight drugs in clinical use. Many of the newer drugs were developed by modifying losartan, the first biologically active ARB oral agent. These drugs are categorized according to the substitution of carboxylic and other moieties into several groups—the biphenyl tetrazoles (derivatives of losartan), nonbiphenyl tetrazoles, and nonheterocyclic compounds. They are also classified according to their ability to antagonize Ang II.[216] The competitive (surmountable) antagonists shift the dose–response curve for Ang II–mediated contraction to the right without depressing the maximal response to Ang II. The noncompetitive (insurmountable) antagonists also depress the maximal response to Ang II. The variable effects of ARBs are mediated by differences in the interaction with allosteric binding sites on the receptor, dissociation of the drug–receptor complex, removal of the agonists from tissues, or by the ability to modulate the amount of internalized receptors[216] (Tables 49.8–49.10).

**Table 49.8 Pharmacokinetic Interactions Between Angiotensin II Type 1 ($AT_1$) Receptor Blockers and Receptor**

| Agent | $AT_1$ Receptor–Receptor Antagonist Dissociation Rate | Affinity ($K_d$) | Type of $AT_1$ Antagonism |
|---|---|---|---|
| Candesartan cilexetil (candesartan) | Slow | 280 | Noncompetitive |
| Irbesartan | Slow | 5 | Noncompetitive |
| Valsartan | Slow | 10 | Noncompetitive |
| Telmisartan | Slow | 10 | Noncompetitive |
| Losartan | Fast | 50 | Competitive |
| Eprosartan | Fast | 100 | Competitive |

**Table 49.9 Pharmacodynamic Properties of Angiotensin Receptor Blockers**

| Generic Name (Trade Name) | Initial Dose (mg) | Usual Dose (mg) | Maximum Dose (mg) | Interval | Peak Response (h) | Duration of Response (h) |
|---|---|---|---|---|---|---|
| Eprosartan (Teveten) | 200 | 400–800 | 800 | qd, bid | 4 | 24 |
| Irbesartan (Avapro) | 150 | 150–300 | 300 | qd | 4–6, 14 | 24 |
| Losartan (Cozaar) | 50 | 50–100 | 100 | qd/bid | 6 | 12–24 |
| Valsartan (Diovan) | 80 | 80–160 | 320 | qd | 4–6 | 24 |
| Candesartan (Atacand) | 16 | 8–32 | 32 | qd | 6–8 | 24 |
| Telmisartan (Micardis) | 40 | 40–80 | 80 | qd | 3 | 24 |
| Azilsartan (Edarbi) | 40 | 40–80 | 80 | qd | 1.5–3 peak response | ≥24 |
| Olmesartan (Benicar) | 20 | 20–40 | 40 | qd | 1–2 | 24 |

*bid,* Two times a day; *qd,* once a day.

**Table 49.10 Pharmacokinetic Properties of Angiotensin Receptor Blockers**

| Drug | Absorption (%) | Bioavailability (%) | Affected by Food | Peak Blood Level (h) | Elimination Half-Life (h) | Metabolism | Excretion | Active Metabolites |
|---|---|---|---|---|---|---|---|---|
| Eprosartan | >80 | 13 | Yes | 4 | 6 | L | F (70%), U (7%) | Inactive |
| Irbesartan | >80 | 60–80 | No | 1.5–2 | 10–14 | L, K | F (65%), U (20%) | Inactive |
| Losartan | >80 | 25 | No | 1 | 4–9 | L, K | F (60%), U (40%) | Active |
| Valsartan | >80 | 25 | Yes | 2–4 | 6–9 | L, K | F (83%), U (13%) | Inactive |
| Candesartan | — | 15 | No | 2–4 | 9 | I, L, K | F (67%), U (33%) | None |
| Telmisartan | — | 42 | Yes | 0.5–1 | 24 | L | F | Inactive |
| Olmesartan | — | 26 | No | 1 | 13 | I | F (50%), U (50%) | Active |

*F,* Feces; *I,* intestine; *K,* kidney; *L,* liver; *U,* urine.

### Biphenyl Tetrazole and Oxadiazole Derivatives

Azilsartan medoxomil is a selective $AT_1$ receptor blocker that has demonstrated a potent 24-hour sustained antihypertensive effect. At the approved dosage, it reduces systolic BP (SBP) by 12 to 15 mm Hg and diastolic BP (DBP) by 7 to 8 mm Hg.[217–219] Azilsartan medoxomil is a prodrug that is hydrolyzed to azilsartan in the gastrointestinal tract during absorption. It possesses a unique moiety (5-oxo-1,2,4-oxadiazole) in place of the tetrazole ring that offers a very strong inverse antagonism at the $AT_1$ receptor.[220,221] This bond is chemically stronger than that of its predecessors, which may explain its added potency when compared with other members of its class or ACE inhibitors.[220] The estimated oral bioavailability is about 60%; peak plasma concentration is reached after 1.5 to 3 hours following ingestion.[222] Food does not affect the bioavailability of the drug. More than 99% of azilsartan is bound to albumin. The initial starting dose is 20 mg once daily, and it is available in 20-, 40-, and 80-mg tablets. The terminal half-life is 9 hours, and approximately 55% of the parent compound is excreted by the kidney.[222] In a recent study to assess the pharmacokinetics of kidney disease of azilsartan, no dosage adjustment was advised for kidney disease or hemodialysis.[223] In a report, 17 patients receiving hemodialysis who switched to azilsartan showed a decrease in SBP from 150.9 ± 16.2 to 131.3 ± 21.7 mm Hg ($P$ < .008) and a decrease in DBP from 84.1 ± 6.3 to 74.9 ± 8.3 mm Hg.[224]

Candesartan cilexetil is an esterified prodrug imidazole that is rapidly and completely converted into the active 7–carboxylic acid candesartan (CV-11974) in the intestinal wall.[12] Candesartan is a selective, nonpeptide, noncompetitive (insurmountable) ARB with the second highest receptor binding affinity and a slow detachment rate from the receptor (Table 49.8). Consequently, the effects are long-lasting and unlikely to be overcome by the upregulation of Ang II that commonly accompanies $AT_1$ receptor blockade. The initial dose is 16 mg daily, and the usual daily dose is 8 to 32 mg in one or two divided doses. The antihypertensive response occurs initially in 2 to 4 hours, peaks at 6 to 8 hours, and lasts for 24 hours (Tables 49.9 and 49.10).[216,225] Radioreceptor assays demonstrate the presence of candesartan at the receptor site for longer than predicted periods (from plasma half-life analysis), which correlates with the clinical observation of a sustained effect beyond 24 hours.[225,226] Maximal response is achieved in 4 weeks. The terminal half-life of candesartan is approximately 9 hours, and it is not affected by kidney failure. No unchanged parent compound is detected in the serum or urine. Candesartan is not dialyzable.

Eprosartan is a nonpeptide selective ARB that was modified to more closely resemble Ang II.[227] It is a noncompetitive antagonist, with a high affinity for the $AT_1$ receptor (Table 49.8).[12] The initial daily dose is 200 mg (Table 49.9), and the usual daily dose is 200 to 400 mg. Eprosartan is rapidly absorbed, but its absorption is delayed by food (Table 49.10). The initial response occurs in 4 hours and lasts for 24 hours. The elimination half-life is 6 hours. Dosages should be reduced by 50% in patients with kidney failure.

Irbesartan is a nonpeptide-specific imidazolinone derivative of losartan that acts as a noncompetitive $AT_1$ receptor blocker with a very high receptor binding affinity[228] (Table 49.8).[12] The initial dose is 150 mg daily, and the usual daily dose is 150 to 300 mg. The initial response occurs in 2 hours. The peak response is bimodal; in hypertensive patients, peak responses occur in 4 to 6 hours and 14 hours, corresponding to the peak increases in plasma renin activity and Ang II levels, respectively.[228] With continuous dosing, the maximal effect may not be seen for up to 6 weeks. The duration of action is 24 hours. Irbesartan is not dialyzable.

Losartan potassium is the prototype ARB. The tetrazole moiety on the biphenyl ring accounts for its activity in oral form and its duration of action. It was the first oral active agent, and it is a nonpeptide competitive, selective $AT_1$ receptor inhibitor, with moderate receptor binding affinity (Table 49.8).[12,229] The usual starting dosage is 50 mg once daily (Table 49.9). Dosage adjustments should be made at weekly intervals. The antihypertensive efficacy may be improved with divided doses. The usual daily dose is 50 to 100 mg. The potassium content of the 25-, 50-, and 100-mg tablets is 0.054, 0.108, and 0.216 mEq, respectively. The oral bioavailability of losartan is 25%, and it is unaffected by food (Table 49.10). The initial response occurs in 1 hour, and the response peaks at 6 hours and lasts for 24 hours. Only 5% of losartan is recovered unchanged in the urine, which supports extensive metabolism and biliary secretion. Neither the parent drug nor metabolites are removed by dialysis.[22]

Olmesartan medoxomil is a nonpeptide selective ARB prodrug that is rapidly and completely bioactivated by hydrolysis to olmesartan during absorption from the gastrointestinal tract.[230] The initial dosage is 20 mg daily, and the usual dosage is 20 to 40 mg daily (Table 49.9). The peak plasma concentration is reached in 1 hour (Table 49.10). The BP-lowering effect lasts for 24 hours and peaks at 2 weeks. Olmesartan is eliminated in a biphasic manner, with a terminal half-life of 13 hours. Dosing and pharmacokinetics have not been studied in dialysis patients.

#### Nonbiphenyl Tetrazole Derivatives

Telmisartan incorporates a carboxylic acid as the biphenyl acidic group. Telmisartan is a nonpeptide, noncompetitive ARB, with high specificity and receptor affinity.[12,231] The usual starting dosage is 40 mg daily, and the usual daily dose is 40 to 80 mg. The initial response occurs in 3 hours, and it is dose dependent (Table 49.10). The duration of action is 24 hours but may last up to 7 days after discontinuing the drug. Women typically achieve plasma levels two to three times higher than those of men, but this result is not associated with differences in BP response. Less than 3% of the drug is metabolized in the liver into inactive compounds. The elimination half-life is 24 hours. Telmisartan is not dialyzable, and dosage adjustment is not necessary in patients with kidney disease.

#### Nonheterocyclic Derivatives

Valsartan is a nonheterocyclic ARB in which the imidazole of losartan is replaced by an acetylated amino acid.[12] Valsartan is a noncompetitive antagonist with high specificity and receptor binding affinity (Table 49.8). The initial starting dosage is 80 mg once daily (Table 49.9), and the usual dosage is 80 to 160 mg daily. The maximal BP response is achieved after 4 weeks of therapy. The initial response occurs in 2 hours, peaks at 4 to 6 hours, and lasts 24 hours. Valsartan does not undergo significant metabolism. The elimination half-life is 6 to 9 hours, and it is not affected by kidney failure (Table 49.10).

### CLASS RENAL EFFECTS

Intrarenal Ang II receptors are widely distributed in the afferent and efferent arterioles, glomerular mesangial cells, inner stripe of the outer medulla, and medullary interstitial cells,[232] as well as on the luminal and basolateral membranes of the proximal and distal tubule cells, collecting ducts, podocytes, and macula densa cells.[233] Most receptors are of the $AT_1$ subclass. Circulating and predominantly locally produced Ang II interacts with the receptors; the complex is internalized and Ang II is released into the intracellular compartment, where it exerts its effects. Studies have suggested that most renal interstitial Ang II is formed at sites not readily accessible to ACE inhibition or is formed by non-ACE pathways.

ARBs antagonize the binding of Ang II and cause a number of intrarenal changes. The overall renal hemodynamic responses of $AT_1$ receptor blockade are variable, depending on the counteracting influences of the decrease in arterial pressure.[200,234] Decreases in systemic arterial pressure by ARBs may be associated with compensatory activation of the intrarenal SNS, resulting in decreased renal function. This effect is more pronounced in sodium-depleted states because activation of the renin–angiotensin system helps maintain arterial and renal pressure. By contrast, direct intrarenal infusions of ARBs cause an increase in sodium excretion.[235] The enhanced sodium excretion has been shown to be caused by direct inhibition of sodium reabsorption by the proximal tubules, but it may also be caused by hemodynamic changes in medullary blood flow and tubule absorption in distal nephron segments. Because Ang II blockade enhances the ability of the kidneys to excrete sodium, sodium balance can be maintained at lower arterial pressures. Ang II blockade also reduces tubuloglomerular feedback sensitivity by decreasing macula densa transport of sodium chloride to the afferent arteriole.[236] This leads to increased delivery of sodium chloride to the distal segments for excretion, without compensatory changes in GFR.

In addition to the natriuretic and diuretic actions, short-term administration of some ARBs has been observed to induce reversible kaliuresis in salt-depleted normotensive patients in the absence of changes in GFR.[237] However, long-term Ang II receptor blockade does not cause appreciable changes in urinary electrolyte excretion or volume. The kaliuretic effect may be caused by specific intrinsic pharmacologic effects of the losartan molecule.

Another property unique to the losartan molecule is induction of uricosuria.[238] This effect is not observed with ACE inhibitors or other ARBs, including the active metabolite of losartan, and does not appear to be related to inhibition of the RAAS.[238] Losartan has a greater affinity for the urate-anion exchanger than other antagonists, and it inhibits urate reabsorption in the proximal tubule.[239] The uricosuria is associated with a concomitant decrease in serum urate concentrations in normal individuals, hypertensive individuals, and patients with kidney disease including kidney transplant recipients.[239] The effect occurs within 4 hours of drug administration and is dose dependent. Long-term administration reduces serum urate concentrations by approximately 0.4 mmol/L.[240] The clinical implications of this effect are unknown. Concerns that increased uric acid supersaturation might perpetuate renal uric acid deposition have not been borne out clinically, perhaps because losartan simultaneously increases urinary pH, which protects against crystal nucleation.[241] However, the decrease in the serum urate might be beneficial because it has been suggested that hyperuricemia is a risk factor for kidney disease progression[242] and coronary artery disease.[243]

Hypertensive patients treated with ARBs—including those with normal and those with impaired kidney function—exhibit renal responses similar to or slightly greater than the responses of patients treated with ACE inhibitors.[244] In addition to decreases in SBPs and DBPs, patients demonstrate increases in renal blood flow and decreases in filtration fraction and renal vascular resistance, with no substantial changes in GFR.[245] These effects are probably a result of combined decreases in preglomerular and postglomerular resistances. It has been suggested that elevated intrarenal Ang II levels in the presence of $AT_1$ receptor blockade stimulates $AT_2$ receptors, which can increase the preglomerular vasodilator actions of bradykinin, cyclic guanosine monophosphate, and nitric oxide.[246] ACE inhibitors can potentiate this effect, but the clinical importance of this finding has not been established. Ang II blockade may significantly reduce GFR in underperfused kidneys. Patients with low perfusion pressures, volume depletion, or renovascular disease may experience severe decreases in GFR but less severe decreases than with ACE inhibitors.[247] Under conditions of overperfusion, such as in hypertension associated with glomerulosclerosis and nephron loss or diabetes, Ang II blockade is protective. Such patients often have a suboptimal suppression of the RAAS. The lowering of efferent arteriole resistance reduces intraglomerular hydrostatic pressure, which attenuates the progression of kidney injury, and increases renal sodium excretory capacity. In concert with the reduction in systemic arterial pressure, these actions provide more renal protection than other classes of antihypertensive agents, despite equivalent reductions in BP.[76,248,249]

In healthy and hypertensive patients, ARBs produce dose-dependent increases in circulating Ang II levels and plasma renin activity.[250] The increases occur at the peak plasma drug levels and persist for up to 24 hours; they remain elevated with long-term administration. Decreases in plasma concentrations of aldosterone have been reported, but they are variable.[251] In normal individuals, decreases in aldosterone coincide with the peak interval of ARB activity; in hypertensive patients consuming a fixed-sodium diet, there are no significant changes in plasma aldosterone concentrations relative to baseline.[237] ARBs suppress the Ang II–mediated adrenal cortical release of aldosterone, but these effects appear to be quantitatively less important than the intrarenal suppression of Ang II action. Long-term $AT_1$ receptor blockade does not appear to induce aldosterone escape.[252]

Urinary protein excretion is significantly decreased with administration of ARBs and parallels findings with ACE inhibitor therapy.[47] Antiproteinuric effects have been described in diabetic and nondiabetic patients, as well as renal transplantation patients.[47,253] The antiproteinuric effect has a slow onset, and the dose–response curves differ from those of the antihypertensive effects, in which the maximal effect occurs at 3 to 4 weeks. Whether the antiproteinuric effects are equivalent to or better than those of ACE inhibitors remains to be determined, but it is evident that the suppression of albuminuria is equivalent at all stages of CKD.[254] Combining ACE inhibitors and ARBs for renoprotection and proteinuria reduction is no longer recommended owing to the significant development of hyperkalemia, hypotension, and renal hypoperfusion, particularly in patients with underlying CKD.[97,148,255,256] Like ACE inhibitors, ARBs have nonhemodynamic effects that may contribute to renoprotection, including antiproliferative actions on the vasculature and mesangium, inhibition of transforming growth factor-β (TGF-β),[30,257] inhibition of atherogenesis[258] and vascular deterioration,[259] improved superoxide production and nitric oxide bioavailability,[260] reduction of collagen formation, reduction of mesangial matrix production, improved vascular wall remodeling, decreased vasoconstrictor effects of endothelin-1, improved endothelial function,[259] reduction of oxidative stress and inflammation,[261] modulation of peroxisome proliferator–activated receptor γ activity, and protection from calcineurin inhibitor injury. ARBs also reduce salt sensitivity by restoring renal nitric oxide synthesis.[262] The clinical importance of these effects remains under investigation.

## CLASS EFFICACY AND SAFETY

All $AT_1$ receptor blockers have been demonstrated to lower BP effectively and safely in patients with mild, moderate, and severe hypertension, regardless of age, sex, or ancestry.[263–265] ARBs are indicated as first-line monotherapy or add-on therapy for hypertension and are comparable in efficacy to other agents.[266–268] They are safe and effective in patients with CKD (even when used at high dosages), diabetes, heart failure, coronary artery disease, arrhythmias, and left ventricular hypertrophy (LVH)[269–272] and kidney transplant recipients, and have been shown to protect against hypertensive end-organ damage,[148,273,274] such as LVH, stroke, ESKD,[47,275] retinopathy,[276] exercise-induced inflammatory and prothrombotic stress, and possibly diabetes and dementia.[272,277–281] Some but not all studies have shown a weak lowering of the risk for new and recurrent atrial fibrillation because of the beneficial structural and electrical effects on the atria.[121,122] ARBs have been shown to diminish the rate of persistent atrial fibrillation in patients with preexisting recurrent atrial fibrillation.[282] The Prevention Regimen for Effectively Avoiding Second Strokes (PRoFESS) study did not show any significant benefit of ARBs for the prevention of recurrent stroke but may have been underpowered to show an effect in its well-treated patient population.[283]

Although ARBs may not be the most efficacious agents in terms of BP reduction in African Americans, they are equally or more efficacious in providing target-organ protection and arresting disease progression compared with other antihypertensive agents that do not inhibit the RAAS.[284] Moreover, their antihypertensive activity is not attenuated by high-salt diets in African Americans.[267,284,285] In most patients, ARBs offer BP lowering comparable to that of all other antihypertensive drug classes, with an improved tolerability profile.[286]

ARBs provide effective control over a 24-hour period and are generally suitable for once-daily dosing.[287,288] Response rates vary from 40% to 60%. ARBs do not affect the normal circadian BP variation.[289] The long onset of action (4–6 weeks) avoids the first-dose hypotension and rebound hypertension that are commonly observed with other drugs. There is a dose-dependent response with newer agents, but losartan and valsartan have a relatively flat dose–response curve.[290] Azilsartan, candesartan, irbesartan, and olmesartan may have the greatest efficacy, with a longer duration of action because of their noncompetitive binding, and telmisartan may have an added advantage by the inhibition of SNS activation through an antioxidant effect in experimental models.[291,292]

The addition of thiazide or thiazide-type diuretics to ARBs potentiates the therapeutic effect, increases response rates to 70% to 80%, and is more effective than increasing the ARB dosage. ARBs may also abrogate the adverse metabolic effects of thiazides.[293]

An enhanced BP-lowering efficacy after 16 weeks of olmesartan-based treatment ($P = .0005$) may be observed in hypertensive patients with CKD-associated sympathetic hyperactivity, as evidenced by a baseline morning home SBP of 165 mm Hg or higher and patients with a morning home pulse rate of 70 beats/min or more in the Home BP Measurement With Olmesartan-Naive Patients to Establish Standard Target Blood Pressure (HONEST) study.[294] Similarly, the addition of mineralocorticoid receptor antagonists (MRAs) to ARBs provides added benefits for BP control and reduction of proteinuria in diabetic patients over the long term but has not been found to be protective from the decline in eGFR.[295] As with ACE inhibitor ARB combination therapy, the combination of ARBs with MRAs should be used with caution, with attention to the risks of hyperkalemia and impaired kidney function. Combination therapy with ARBs plus dihydropyridines has additive effects in reducing BP and is well tolerated.[296]

ARBs may decrease kidney function and elevate serum potassium concentrations; serum chemistries should be checked after initiation or increase in dosage of these drugs. The overall incidence of hyperkalemia from ARBs is 3.3%, similar to that of ACE inhibitors.[148] Participants in the CHARM (Candesartan in Heart Failure-Assessment of Reduction in Mortality and Morbidity; $n = 7599$) program were randomized to standard heart failure therapy plus candesartan or placebo, with recommended monitoring of serum potassium and creatinine levels.[297] The authors assessed the incidence and predictors of hyperkalemia over the median 3.2 years of follow-up. Candesartan increased the risk of incident hyperkalemia compared with placebo from 5.2% from 1.8% (difference, 3.4%; $P < .0001$). Risk factors for hyperkalemia in treated patients with symptomatic heart failure include advanced age, male sex, baseline hyperkalemia, impaired kidney function, diabetes, or combined RAAS blockade. As with ACE inhibitors, hyperkalemia associated with ARB use has been treated with patiromer and sodium zirconium cyclosilicate in addition to sodium and calcium polystyrene sulfonate.[196,197]

ARBs should be stopped immediately at the onset of pregnancy with the first missed menstrual period in the first trimester, as discussed previously in the context of ACE inhibitor use, because ARBs may cause fetal or neonatal death and congenital abnormalities when used during the second and third trimesters of pregnancy.[138] Breastfeeding is not contraindicated, according to Kidney Disease Improving Global Outcomes (KDIGO) and NICE guidelines; however, low drug levels are detected in breast milk.[139,140]

Overall, ARBs have neutral metabolic effects and are superior to other hypertensive classes with respect to tolerability. ARBs do not cause hypernatremia or hyponatremia, and hyperkalemia is relatively uncommon. In the ONTARGET study, a serum potassium concentration higher than 5.5 mmol/L was observed in 3.3% of patients who resigned from the study and is comparable to that observed with ACE inhibitor therapy.[148] ARBs have no effect on serum lipids in hypertensive patients but may improve the abnormal lipoprotein profile of patients with proteinuric renal disease and reduce obesity-related morbidity.[298,299] ARBs have favorable effects on serum glucose concentrations and insulin sensitivity.[300–302] Clinical trials comparing ARB-based therapy with treatment with other antihypertensive agents in patients with hypertension with and without LVH demonstrated a 25% reduced risk of the development of diabetes in the ARB-treated group.[303,304] The mechanism for this effect has not been defined.[277,305] Increased levels of liver transaminases are occasionally reported, but the effects are usually transient, even with continued therapy.[12]

Clinically relevant AEs are not observed more frequently than in placebo-treated patients. Because ARBs do not interfere with kinin metabolism, cough is rare, which is a major clinical advantage.[148] The incidence of cough in patients with a history of ACE inhibitor–induced cough is no greater than in those receiving placebo.[306] Similarly, the incidence of angioedema and facial swelling is no greater than that with placebo, but such swelling can occur.[307] ARBs are typically associated with a more potent antiinflammatory response than ACE inhibitors.[308] The most frequent AEs are headache (14%), dizziness (2.4%), and fatigue (2%), which occur at rates lower than those with placebo.[309] ARB therapy not only does not worsen sexual activity, but may also improve it.[310] Like ACE inhibitors, ARBs may cause minor decreases in the hemoglobin concentration; they may also lower the hemoglobin effectively in posttransplantation erythrocytosis.[311] There have been rare associated cutaneous eruptions.

A spruelike enteropathy associated with olmesartan therapy has been reported.[312,313] In a recent systematic review of 54 patients,[313] the clinical presentation was diarrhea (95%) and weight loss (89%). Less common symptoms were fatigue, nausea, vomiting, and abdominal pain. The patients had been taking olmesartan for 6 months to 7 years. A laboratory examination showed a normochromic, normocytic anemia (45%) and hypoalbuminemia (39%). HLA-DQ2 or HLA-DQ8 was observed in more than 70%. Antibody testing for celiac disease was negative. Duodenal villous atrophy in varying degrees was described in all the reported patients, and they all showed resolution of diarrhea. The US Food and Drug Administration (FDA) issued a drug safety communication on July 13, 2013 (http://www.fda.gov/Drugs/DrugSafety/ucm359477.htm).

ARBs have not been shown to increase the risk of cancer. A meta-analysis showed a slightly increased risk of cancer (relative risk [RR], 1.08; 95% confidence interval [CI], 1.01 to 1.15) relative to other antihypertensive agents.[314] The study's methodology was criticized because some RCTs were not included; had they been, the cancer signal would have disappeared. Subsequent meta-analyses[315–318] and cohort studies[319–322] were performed. The conclusion was that there was no evidence that ARBs are associated with cancers of any type in large populations, and one study suggested that

ARBs may actually lower the incidence.[319] A subsequent systematic review of observational and interventional studies suggested that the use of ACE inhibitors and ARBs may improve cancer outcomes.[323]

Drug interactions with ARBs are uncommon but, as with ACE inhibitors, NSAIDs may blunt the natriuretic effect of ARBs.[324] ARBs have an increased incidence of hypotension and impaired kidney function compared with ACE inhibitors.[148] Acute reversible renal failure has been reported with Ang II receptor blockade therapy in salt-depleted patients.[325] Thus therapy should not be instituted in hypovolemic patients or in the setting of active diuresis. Concomitant use with ACE inhibitors and direct renin inhibitors should be discouraged, especially in patients with a GFR lower than 60 mL/min and is contraindicated in patients with type 2 diabetes mellitus because of an increased risk of hypotension, hyperkalemia, and renal dysfunction.[97,256,326]

## β-ADRENERGIC RECEPTOR ANTAGONISTS

### CLASS MECHANISMS OF ACTION

β-Adrenergic receptor antagonists (β-blockers) exert their antihypertensive effects by attenuating sympathetic stimulation through the competitive antagonism of catecholamines at the β-adrenergic receptor.[327] However, the precise mechanism of the antihypertensive effect of β-blockers remains incompletely understood. $\beta_1$-Adrenergic receptor blockade has generally been considered responsible for the BP-lowering effect; however, $\beta_2$-receptor blockade has an independent antihypertensive effect.[328] Inhibition of $\beta_1$-adrenergic receptors in the juxtaglomerular cells in the kidney may inhibit renin release. A direct action on the CNS, with a reduction in CNS sympathetic outflow, may also be involved. Attenuation of cardiac pressor stimuli related to β-blockade may result in baroreceptor resetting. In addition, adrenergic neuron output may be blocked because of the inhibition of $\beta_2$-adrenergic receptors at the vascular wall.

$\beta_1$-Selective blockers may have a slightly more potent antihypertensive effect than nonselective agents. This effect may be in the range of 2 to 3 mm Hg. It may be that $\beta_2$-blockade in some fashion blunts the antihypertensive effects of $\beta_1$-blockade.[329] The $\beta_2$ partial agonist activity may mediate peripheral vasodilator effects that could contribute to the antihypertensive action. A $\beta_1$-selective antagonist with partial agonist activity at the $\beta_1$ receptor may result in less hypotensive effect. The magnitude and clinical significance of these differences are unclear.

In addition to β-adrenergic antagonist properties, certain drugs have antihypertensive effects that are mediated through different mechanisms (Table 49.11), including $\alpha_1$-adrenergic antagonist activity and effects on nitric oxide–dependent vasodilator action. Partial agonist activity is a property of certain β-blockers that results from a small degree of direct stimulation of the β-adrenergic receptor by the drug, while simultaneously blocking the same receptor to access by stimulating catecholamines.[329–331] Whether the presence of partial agonist activity is advantageous or disadvantageous remains unclear. Drugs with partial agonist activity slow the resting heart rate less than drugs that lack this pharmacologic effect.[332] The exercise-induced increase in heart rate is similarly blocked by both groups of drugs.[332] However, β-blockers with nonselective partial agonist activity may reduce peripheral vascular resistance and cause less atrioventricular (AV) conduction depression than drugs without partial agonist activity. The specificity of partial agonist activity for $\beta_1$ or $\beta_2$ receptors may also have a role in the antihypertensive response to a given drug.

β-Blockers may be nonspecific and block $\beta_1$- and $\beta_2$-adrenergic receptors, or they may be relatively specific for $\beta_1$-adrenergic receptors. $\beta_1$-adrenergic receptors are found predominantly in heart, adipose, and brain tissue, whereas $\beta_2$ receptors predominate in the lung, liver, smooth muscle, and skeletal muscle. Many tissues, however, have both $\beta_1$ and $\beta_2$ receptors, including the heart, and it is important to realize that the concept of a cardioselective drug is only relative.

β-Blockers differ significantly in gastrointestinal absorption, first-pass hepatic metabolism, protein binding, lipid solubility, penetration into the CNS, and hepatic or renal clearance. β-Blockers that are eliminated primarily by hepatic metabolism have a relatively short plasma half-life; however, the duration of the clinical pharmacologic effect does not correlate well with the plasma half-life in many of these drugs. Water-soluble

**Table 49.11 Pharmacologic Properties of β-Adrenergic Antagonists**

| Generic Name (Trade Name) | $\beta_1$ Selectivity | Partial Agonist Activity | Membrane-Stabilizing Activity | α-Adrenergic Antagonist Activity |
|---|---|---|---|---|
| Nadolol (Corgard) | | | | |
| Propranolol (Inderal) | | | + | |
| Carteolol (multiple) | | + | | |
| Penbutolol (Levatol) | | + | | |
| Pindolol (Visken) | | + | + | |
| Labetalol (Trandate) | | + | | + |
| Carvedilol (Coreg) | | | + | + |
| Atenolol (Tenormin) | + | | | |
| Metoprolol (Lopressor) | + | | | |
| Betaxolol (Kerlone) | + | | + | |
| Acebutolol (Sectral) | + | + | + | |
| Celiprolol (none in the United States) | + | | | + |
| Bisoprolol (Zebeta) | + | | | |
| Nebivolol (Bystolic) | + | | | |

drugs that are eliminated by the kidney may have longer half-lives. Bioavailability varies greatly across the class, as does the degree to which individual agents are dialyzed.[333]

### Nonselective β-Adrenergic Antagonists

Nadolol is a nonselective β-blocker without partial agonist activity (Table 49.11). The average adult dosage is 40 to 80 mg given once daily, with a maximum daily dose of 320 mg (Tables 49.12 and 49.13). Nadolol is not appreciably metabolized, and elimination occurs predominantly in the urine and feces. Dosage adjustment is indicated in patients with CKD. Dosage intervals should be increased to 24 to 36 hours, 24 to 48 hours, and 40 to 60 hours in patients with creatinine clearances of 30 to 50, 10 to 30, and less than 10 mL/min/1.73 m$^2$, respectively.[22] Dosage adjustment is not necessary in patients with hepatic insufficiency. Hemodialysis reduces the serum concentration of nadolol, but specific recommendations for dosage during dialysis are not available.

Propranolol is a noncardioselective β-blocker that has no partial adrenergic activity. The usual daily dosage range is 80 to 320 mg. The drug may be administered in a single daily dose if a long-acting preparation is used. The drug is metabolized by the liver. The major metabolite, 4-hydroxypropranolol, has β-blocking activity. Renal excretion is less than 1%. Dosage adjustment in patients with CKD is not necessary.[22] Patients with liver disease may require variable dosage adjustments and more frequent monitoring.

Timolol is a nonselective β-blocker agent without partial adrenergic activity. The recommended initial dosage of timolol in the management of hypertension is 10 mg twice daily. The maintenance dosage generally ranges from 20 to 40 mg daily. No dosage adjustment is necessary in patients with CKD.[22] Because timolol undergoes extensive hepatic metabolism, patients with liver disease may require a dosage adjustment and frequent monitoring. Timolol is not removed by dialysis.

Penbutolol is a nonselective β-blocker[334] with low partial agonist activity. Usually, dosages are 20 to 40 mg given as a single dose or divided twice daily. Hepatic metabolism to inactive metabolites occurs with subsequent renal elimination. The optimal antihypertensive effect is observed at an average of 14 days after initiation of therapy. Dosage adjustments for patients with CKD are not recommended, but adjustment may be required for patients with hepatic insufficiency.[22]

Pindolol is a nonselective β-blocker with high partial agonist activity. The usual adult oral dosage is 5 mg twice

**Table 49.12 Pharmacokinetic Properties of β-Adrenergic Antagonists**

| Drug | Bioavailability (%) | Affected by Food | Peak Blood Level (h) | Elimination Half-Life (h) | Metabolism | Excretion | Active Metabolites |
|---|---|---|---|---|---|---|---|
| Nadolol | 20–40 | No | 2–4 | 20–24 | — | U, F | — |
| Propranolol | 16–60 | Yes | — | 3–4 | L | — | — |
| Timolol | 50–90 | — | — | 2–4 | L | U (20%) | — |
| Penbutolol | 100 | No | — | 17–24 | L | U | — |
| Pindolol | 95 | No | 2 | 3–11 | L | U (40%) | — |
| Atenolol | 40–60 | Yes | — | 14–16 | — | U, F | — |
| Metoprolol | 50 | — | 1.5–2 | 3–7 | L | U | — |
| Betaxolol | 78–90 | No | 2–6 | 12–22 | L | U | — |
| Bisoprolol | 90 | — | 2.3 | 9.6 | L | U | — |
| Acebutolol | 90 | No | 2–3 | 3–8 | L | U | — |

*F*, Feces; *L*, liver; *U*, urine.

**Table 49.13 Pharmacodynamic Properties of β-Adrenergic Antagonists**

| Drug | Initial Dose (mg) | Usual Dose (mg) | Maximum Dose (mg) | Interval | Peak Response (h) | Duration of Response (h) |
|---|---|---|---|---|---|---|
| Nadolol | 40 | 40–80 | 320 | qd | — | — |
| Propranolol | 40 | 80–320 | 640 | bid | — | — |
| Timolol | 10 | 20–40 | 60 | bid | — | — |
| Penbutolol | 10 | 20–40 | 80 | qd, bid | 2 | 20–24 |
| Pindolol | 5 | 10–40 | 60 | qd, bid | — | 24 |
| Atenolol | 25 | 50–100 | 200 | qd | 3 | 24 |
| Metoprolol | 12.5–50 | 100–200 | 400 | qd, bid | 1 | 3–6 |
| Betaxolol | 10 | 10–40 | 40 | qd | 3 | 23–25 |
| Bisoprolol | 5 | 2.5–20 | 20 | qd | 2–4 | 24 |
| Acebutolol | 400 | 400–800 | 1200 | qd | 3 | 24 |

*bid*, Two times a day; *qd*, once a day.

daily, with incremental doses of 10 mg every 3 to 4 weeks. The maximum daily recommended dose is 60 mg. Approximately 40% of a dose of pindolol is excreted unchanged in the urine; 60% is metabolized in the liver. The drug half-life increases modestly in patients with impaired kidney function. Dose adjustments do not appear be necessary.[22] Dose adjustments may be necessary in patients with cirrhosis and advanced CKD.

### $\beta_1$-Selective Adrenergic Antagonists

Atenolol is a long-acting $\beta_1$-selective blocker with no partial agonist activity. The usual dosage is 50 to 100 mg once daily. Approximately 50% of the drug is eliminated by the kidneys, and 50% is excreted in the feces. Dosages of more than 100 mg/day are unlikely to produce additional benefits. The time required to achieve the optimal antihypertensive effect is 1 to 2 weeks. In patients with moderate CKD, the dosing interval should be increased to 48 hours, and in patients with advanced CKD, dosing intervals should be increased to 96 hours.[22] Atenolol is not significantly metabolized by the liver, and no dosage adjustment is necessary in patients with liver disease. Atenolol is removed by dialysis, and a maintenance dose should be given after a dialysis treatment.

Metoprolol is a $\beta_1$-selective blocker with no partial agonist activity. Extensive hepatic metabolism occurs primarily by the cytochrome P450 (CYP) 2D6 system (CYP2D6), and 3% to 10% of the drug is excreted unchanged in the urine. Metoprolol pharmacokinetics is heavily influenced by the CYP2D6 genotype and metabolizer phenotype, with up to a 15-fold difference in clearance between ultrarapid and poor metabolizers.[335] The initial oral dosage is 12.5 to 50 mg once or twice daily, increasing to 100 to 200 mg twice daily. Sustained-release (SR) preparations may be substituted as a once-daily dose. Metoprolol is extensively removed by hemodialysis.[333]

Betaxolol is a long-acting $\beta_1$-selective blocker[336] with no partial agonist activity. The usual oral dosage for hypertension is 10 to 40 mg once daily. Therapy is typically started at a dosage of 10 mg once daily. Most patients respond to 20 mg once daily. The time to achieve the optimal antihypertensive effect is approximately 1 to 2 weeks. Betaxolol is metabolized predominantly in the liver, with metabolites excreted by the kidney. Approximately 15% of the dose is recovered unchanged in the urine. CKD results in a decrease in betaxolol clearance and titration should begin at 5 mg once daily in these patients.

Bisoprolol is a long-acting $\beta_1$-selective blocker[337] with no partial agonist activity. The usual oral dosage is 2.5 to 20 mg given once daily. Hepatic metabolism occurs with the renal excretion of metabolites; however, 50% of the drug is excreted by the kidney unchanged. In patients with CKD, the initial oral dosage should be 2.5 mg once daily, with careful monitoring of dose titration. The maximum recommended dosage of bisoprolol in patients with CKD is 10 mg/day. Similar dosage reduction is also required for patients with hepatic insufficiency. It is modestly removed during hemodialysis.[333]

Acebutolol is a $\beta_1$-selective blocker with low partial agonist activity. Dosages of 400 to 1200 mg/day are effective in treating hypertension. The drug is metabolized to diacetolol, an active metabolite, with the parent compound being excreted renally and in bile. Diacetolol is excreted mainly by the kidneys. Dosage reduction of 50% to 75% is recommended for patients with advanced CKD.[22]

### Nonselective $\beta$-Adrenergic Antagonists With $\alpha$-Adrenergic Antagonism or Other Mechanisms of Antihypertensive Action

Labetalol is a nonselective $\beta$-blocker[338] with weak partial agonist activity and $\alpha_1$-receptor blocking activity (Tables 49.14

**Table 49.14 Pharmacokinetic Properties of $\beta$-Adrenergic Antagonists With Vasodilatory Properties**

| Drug | Bioavailability (%) | Affected by Food | Peak Blood Level (h) | Elimination Half-Life (h) | Metabolism | Excretion | Active Metabolites |
|---|---|---|---|---|---|---|---|
| Labetalol | 25–40 | Yes | 1–2 | 5–8 | L | U (50%–60%) | — |
| Carvedilol | 25–35 | No | 1–1.5 | 6–8 | L | F | — |
| Celiprolol | 30–70 | Yes | — | 5–6 | — | F, U | — |
| Nebivolol | 12–96 | No | 2.4–3.1 | 8–27 | L | — | — |

*F,* Feces; *L,* liver; *U,* urine.

**Table 49.15 Pharmacodynamic Properties of $\beta$-Adrenergic Antagonists With Vasodilatory Properties**

| Drug | Initial Dose (mg) | Usual Dose (mg) | Maximum Dose (mg) | Interval | Peak Response (h) | Duration of Response (h) |
|---|---|---|---|---|---|---|
| Labetalol | 100 | 200–800 | 1200–2400 | bid | 3 | 8–12 |
| Carvedilol | 6.25 | 12.5–25 | 50 | bid | 4–7 | 24 |
| Celiprolol | 200 | 200–400 | 400 | qd | — | — |
| Nebivolol | 5 | 5 | 40 | qd | 6 | 24 |

*bid,* Two times a day; *qd,* once a day.

and 49.15). The drug is approximately equipotent in blocking $\beta_1$- and $\beta_2$-adrenergic receptors. With oral administration, the ratio of $\alpha_1$- to β-blocking potency is approximately 1:3. With intravenous administration, the β-blocking potency is more prominent. The usual initial dosages for treatment of hypertension are 100 mg orally twice daily, increasing gradually to a maintenance dosage of 200 to 400 mg twice or thrice daily. The drug is metabolized in the liver, with 50% to 60% of a dose excreted in the urine and the remainder in the bile. Dose adjustment is not required in CKD.[22] Chronic liver disease has been demonstrated to decrease the first-pass metabolism of labetalol, and dosage reduction is required in these patients.

Carvedilol is a nonselective β-blocker with peripheral $\alpha_1$-blocker activity (Tables 49.14 and 49.15)[339,340] and no partial agonist activity. The drug is approximately equipotent in blocking $\beta_1$- and $\beta_2$-adrenergic receptors. The ratio of $\alpha_1$- to $\beta_1$-blocking activity is estimated to be 1:7.6. There is evidence that the therapeutic actions of carvedilol may depend in part on the endogenous production of nitric oxide, which may improve endothelial dysfunction in hypertensive patients. For the management of hypertension, an initial oral dosage of 6.25 mg twice daily is recommended and may be increased to 12.5 to 25 mg twice daily, if needed. Dose adjustments are not required for patients with CKD. Carvedilol is extensively metabolized in the liver, and dose reductions are suggested for patients with hepatic insufficiency. Carvedilol is not removed by hemodialysis.[333]

Celiprolol is a β-blocker with several unique properties.[341,342] It is a $\beta_1$-selective blocker with $\alpha_2$-receptor blocking activity (Tables 49.14 and 49.15). Celiprolol also causes vasodilation through $\beta_2$-receptor stimulation and possibly nitric oxide, with a subsequent decrease in systemic vascular resistance. In contrast to other β-blockers, celiprolol does not appear to induce bronchospasm or have negative inotropic effects. It does have moderate partial agonist activity. The initial dosage of celiprolol is 200 mg once daily and can be increased to 400 mg once daily. Renal excretion is 35% to 42%. A 50% dosage reduction is suggested in patients with a creatinine clearance of 15 to 40 mL/min/1.73 m$^2$. Celiprolol is not recommended for patients with a creatinine clearance less than 15 mL/min/1.73 m$^2$. It is not currently available in the United States.

Nebivolol is a long-acting, $\beta_1$-selective blocker (Tables 49.14 and 49.15).[343–347] The compound is a 1:1 racemic mixture of two enantiomers: D-nebivolol and L-nebivolol. The actions of nebivolol, which are unique and unlike those of other β-blocking agents, are attributable to the individual effects of the isomers. When administered alone, the L-isomer does not produce significant effects on BP, but its presence enhances the antihypertensive effects of the D-isomer. The L-isomer may potentiate the effects of endothelium-derived nitric oxide to induce decreases in BP and peripheral vascular resistance. These effects may improve endothelial dysfunction and potentially influence cardiovascular risks.[348,349] The L-isomer may also inhibit norepinephrine actions at the presynaptic β receptors. The initial oral dosage is 5 mg once daily. The drug is metabolized in the liver; rapid and slow metabolizers have been identified. The half-life of nebivolol is 8 hours in rapid metabolizers and 27 hours in slow metabolizers. Reduced initial dosages are recommended for patients with CKD.

## CLASS RENAL EFFECTS

α- and β-Adrenergic receptors in the kidney mediate vasoconstriction and vasodilation as well as renin secretion. β-Blockers may influence renal blood flow and GFR through their effects on cardiac output and BP in addition to direct effects on intrarenal adrenergic receptors. β-Adrenergic receptors have been localized to the juxtaglomerular apparatus in autoradiographic studies.[350] $\beta_2$ Receptors predominate in the kidney. The degree of specificity of β-adrenergic blockers for $\beta_1$ and $\beta_2$ receptors might be expected to influence the effect on kidney function, as might the degree of intrinsic partial agonist activity. In general, the short-term administration of a β-adrenergic blocker usually results in a reduction of GFR and effective renal plasma flow.[351] This effect is independent of whether the drug has $\beta_1$ selectivity or intrinsic partial agonist activity. Nebivolol, carvedilol, and celiprolol, however, have vasodilatory properties and have been shown to increase GFR and renal plasma flow.[352] Nebivolol dilates glomerular afferent and efferent arterioles by a nitric oxide–dependent mechanism, in contrast to metoprolol, which had no similar effect.[353] This effect may be mediated by the increased synthesis of vasodilatory nitric oxide. Nadolol, when administered intravenously, has been shown in some studies to increase renal plasma flow and glomerular filtration, whereas oral administration may result in decreased blood flow and GFR. $\beta_1$-Selective drugs, when administered orally, tend to produce smaller reductions in GFR and renal plasma flow. The long-term use of propranolol has been characterized by a 10% to 20% decrease in renal plasma flow and GFR. The degree of reduction in GFR and renal plasma flow is modest and probably not of clinical significance in most cases. Labetalol, with its combined α and β blockade with labetalol, has shown little effect on renal hemodynamics. The fractional excretion of sodium has been observed to decrease by up to 20% to 40% in some studies of the acute renal effects of β blockade.[354]

## CLASS EFFICACY AND SAFETY

β-Blockers provide effective therapy for the management of mild-to-moderate hypertension but their use as first-line therapy was not recommended[355–357] in the 2017 ACC/AHA guidelines based on results from a contemporaneous systematic review and network meta-analysis. In that review, β-blockers were found to be less effective than CCBs or thiazide diuretics for reducing stroke and cardiovascular risk.[358] No significant differences in outcomes were observed in these class-to-class comparisons by age, sex, race, and diabetes mellitus status.

β-Blockers are recommended for patients with specific comorbid conditions.[327,359–361] For example, the use of β-blockers after an acute MI has been shown to reduce morbidity and mortality,[362] regardless of SBP, age, or ejection fraction. Other studies have shown a 20% reduction in total mortality and a 32% to 50% reduction in sudden death with β-blocker therapy in patients who have experienced an MI.[363] Therefore for treatment of hypertension in patients with a history of MI (at least in the last year), β-blockers may be the drugs of choice.[83,364,365]

Patients with coexisting heart failure and hypertension are another group that benefit from treatment with β-blockers.[366–368] The Cardiac Insufficiency Bisoprolol Study II demonstrated a 20% reduction in mortality in patients with moderate heart failure randomly assigned to therapy with a β-blocker.[369] Hospitalizations for heart failure and sudden cardiac death were also significantly lower in the β-blocker group. Similar benefits were observed in randomized trial of metoprolol succinate and carvedilol.[370] Over the long term, treatment with β-adrenergic blockers improves exercise tolerance, left ventricular geometry, and left ventricular structure and reduces myocardial oxygen demand. The magnitude of heart rate reduction with β-blockers, but not the dose, is significantly associated with the survival benefit in heart failure.[371] β-Blockers may differ in effects on cardiovascular outcomes. A meta-analysis has suggested that the vasodilatory β-blocker carvedilol has a greater benefit on all-cause mortality in heart failure with reduced ejection fraction (HFrEF) compared with $\beta_1$-selective β-blockers, although this distinction has not been observed in all studies.[371–373] Genetic polymorphisms affecting the $\beta_1$-adrenergic receptor, the $\alpha_{2C}$-adrenergic receptor, and the G protein–coupled receptor kinase have been suggested to modify heart failure risk and the response to β-blocker therapy.[374]

Agents with $\beta_1$-selectivity or intrinsic sympathetic activity have a therapeutic advantage over nonselective β-adrenergic antagonists in the treatment of patients with bronchospastic airway disease, chronic obstructive pulmonary disease, peripheral vascular disease, and diabetes mellitus.[330,375,376] Bronchoconstriction is mediated in part by $\beta_2$-adrenergic receptors in the airways. β-Blockade with nonselective agents can lead to increased airway resistance. This increase is less likely to occur with $\beta_1$-selective agents. $\beta_1$-Selectivity is relative, however, and may be less apparent at higher dosages. In general, patients with severe bronchospastic airway disease should not receive β-blockers. In patients with mild-to-moderate disease, $\beta_1$-selective agents may be used cautiously; it has been proposed that they have beneficial effects on airway hyperresponsiveness.[377]

Symptoms of peripheral artery disease may be exacerbated by β-blocker therapy.[378] Cold extremities and absent pulses have been described in patients with severe disease. Raynaud phenomenon has been reported with nonselective β-blockade.[379] Blockade of $\beta_2$-receptor–mediated skeletal muscle vasodilation as well as decreased cardiac output may contribute to vascular insufficiency.[380] However, a meta-analysis showed that treatment with β-blockers does not worsen intermittent claudication or walking capacity in patients with mild-to-moderate peripheral artery disease,[381] and current treatment guidelines do not recommend against the use of β-blockers in patients with peripheral artery disease, although the evidence is relatively limited.[55]

The CNS symptoms of sedation, sleep disturbance, depression, and visual hallucinations have been reported with β-blockers. In a review of 15 randomized trials involving more than 35,000 patients, β-blockers were not associated with a significant increase in the risk of reported depressive symptoms (6/1000 patient-years; 95% CI, −7 to 19). β-Blockers were associated with a small but significant annual increase of reported fatigue (18/1000 patient-years; 95% CI, 5–30). These symptoms may be more common with lipid-soluble β-blockers and less common with nebivolol.[382]

β-Blockers are associated with weight gain and an increased risk of new-onset diabetes mellitus,[383,384] perhaps by mediating increases in glycogenolysis and gluconeogenesis from amino acids and glycerol and inhibiting glucose uptake in the periphery. β-Blockers differ in terms of their effects on glucose metabolism. Nonvasodilating β-blockers such as metoprolol decrease insulin sensitivity and are associated with a worsening of glycemic control, whereas nebivolol does not.[385,386] In patients with established diabetes mellitus, β-blockers can blunt the effects of epinephrine secretion resulting from hypoglycemia and lead to hypoglycemia unawareness.[387,388]

Nonselective β-blockers and, to a lesser degree, $\beta_1$-selective agents have been associated with a rise in the serum potassium level.[389] Suppression of aldosterone and inhibition of $\beta_2$-linked, sodium–potassium membrane transport in skeletal muscle have been proposed as possible mechanisms.[390,391] This effect is of limited clinical importance in patients who have normal kidney function and are not taking other medications that might affect serum potassium concentrations.

β-Blockers can affect plasma lipids.[392] Long-term use of β-blockers has been associated with an increase in triglyceride levels and a decrease in the level of HDL cholesterol. β-Blockers with increased $\beta_1$ selectivity or with partial agonist activity appear to have less effect on the lipid profile. Nonselective β-blockers without partial agonist activity may decrease the HDL cholesterol level by up to 20%; an increase in triglyceride levels of up to 50% has been reported. The effects of β-blockade on lipid metabolism are due primarily to the modulation of lipoprotein lipase activity. Very-low-density lipoprotein (VLDL) cholesterol and triglyceride metabolism is reduced in the setting of unopposed β-adrenergic stimulation of lipoprotein lipase activity. Decreased VLDL metabolism results in decreases in HDL cholesterol levels.

β-Blockers were associated with a small but significant annual increase in reported sexual dysfunction (5/1000 patients; 95% CI, 2–8). None of the AEs differed by lipid solubility.[393]

Abrupt withdrawal of β-blockers may be associated with rebound hypertension and worsening angina in patients with coronary artery disease.[394] MI has been reported. These withdrawal symptoms may be caused by increased sympathetic activity, which could reflect adrenergic receptor upregulation during long-term sympathetic blockade. Gradual tapering of β-blockers decreases the risk of withdrawal. Withdrawal symptoms have been reported more commonly with abrupt discontinuation of relatively short-acting drugs.[395]

## CALCIUM CHANNEL BLOCKERS

### CLASS MECHANISMS OF ACTION

CCBs remain an important therapeutic class of medications for a variety of cardiovascular disorders.[396–399] Initially introduced in the 1960s as antianginal agents, CCBs are now advocated as first-line therapy for hypertension.[83,401] The pharmacologic effects of these drugs are related to their ability to attenuate cellular calcium uptake.[400–404] CCBs do not directly antagonize the effects of calcium; rather, they inhibit the entry of calcium or its mobilization from intracellular stores.

Calcium channels have binding sites for activators and antagonists. The voltage-dependent, L-type calcium channel is a multimeric complex composed of $\alpha_1$-, $\alpha_2$-, ω-, β-, and γ-subunits.[396] These channels have different binding sites for the various CCBs and are regulated by voltage-dependent and receptor-dependent events involving protein phosphorylation and G-protein coupling resulting from, for example, β-adrenergic stimulation.[405] Each class of CCB is quantitatively and qualitatively unique; the CCB classes possess different sensitivities and selectivities for binding pharmacologic receptors and the slow calcium channel in various vascular tissues. Even within the dihydropyridine class, there is considerable pharmacologic variability.[406] This differential selectivity of action has important clinical implications for the use of these drugs and explains why the CCBs vary considerably in their effects on regional circulatory beds, sinus and AV nodal function, and myocardial contractility. The selectivity further explains the diversity of indications for clinical use, ancillary effects, and side effects.[407]

CCBs uniformly lower peripheral vascular resistance in patients, regardless of age, sex, ancestry, salt sensitivity, or comorbid conditions. There are at least three mechanisms through which CCBs lower BP. First, CCBs reduce peripheral vascular resistance by attenuating the calcium-dependent contractions of vascular smooth muscle. Contraction of vascular smooth muscle depends on the total cytosolic calcium concentration, which in turn is regulated by two distinct mechanisms. Depolarization of vascular smooth muscle tissue depends on the inward flux of calcium through voltage-sensitive L-type and T-type calcium channels. Hypertensive patients have an abnormal influx of calcium, which promotes increased peripheral vascular resistance.[400] Calcium is released from the sarcoplasmic reticulum in response to extracellular calcium influx via a nonvoltage-dependent pathway. Cytosolic calcium binds to calmodulin, initiating a sequence of cellular events that promotes the interaction between actin and myosin and results in smooth muscle contraction. Therefore the importance of the calcium channels lies in their pivotal role in linking cell membrane electrical activity to biologic responses. Calcium influxes through L-type channels from extracellular sources and intracellular sources are both attenuated by CCBs.[398,401]

Second, CCBs decrease vascular responsiveness to Ang II and the synthesis and secretion of aldosterone.[403] CCBs also interfere with $\alpha_2$-adrenergic receptor–mediated vasoconstriction and possibly $\alpha_1$-adrenergic receptor–mediated vasoconstriction.[402,408] The maximal vasodilatory response, as measured by forearm blood flow, appears to be inversely related to the patient's plasma renin activity and Ang II concentration. Thus it is possible that there is a greater influence of the calcium influx–dependent vasoconstriction in patients with low-renin hypertension, such as African Americans, which explains the clinical observation that CCBs are often more potent than other agents in these patients.

Finally, CCBs may induce a mild diuresis. It is well-known that the dihydropyridines, in particular, reduce preglomerular resistance and maintain or increase the GFR because of their preferential vasodilatory action on the renal afferent arteriole.[404] Subsequently, decreased tubular sodium reabsorption and improved renal blood flow and natriuresis are observed. The sodium excretion rate tends to correlate with the reduction in BP.

Antihypertensive activity has not uniformly been demonstrated to be secondary to changes in nitric oxide release. The vasorelaxant properties of nifedipine and verapamil appear to be nitric oxide independent, whereas those of amlodipine are partly nitric oxide dependent.[409,410] This effect of amlodipine is thought to be mediated by the inhibition of local ACEs and increases in vasodilatory bradykinins.

## CLASS MEMBERS

Despite their shared mechanism of action, the CCBs are a very heterogeneous group of compounds. They differ with respect to pharmacologic profile, chemical structure, pharmacokinetic profile, tissue specificity, receptor binding, clinical indications, and side-effect profile (Tables 49.16 and 49.17). Two primary subtypes are distinguished on the basis of their behavior: dihydropyridines and nondihydropyridines. The nondihydropyridines are further divided into two classes – benzothiazepines (diltiazem) and diphenylalkylamines (verapamil). Their distinctly different pharmacologic effects are summarized in Tables 49.16 and 49.17.

Although all CCBs vasodilate coronary and peripheral arteries, the dihydropyridines are the most potent. Because medications in this subclass of CCBs are membrane-active drugs, they exert a greater effect on the peripheral vessels than on myocardial cells, which depend less heavily on the external calcium influx.[401] Their potent vasodilatory action prompts a rapid compensatory increase in sympathetic nervous activity, as mediated by baroreceptor reflexes creating a neutral or positive inotropic stimulus.[411] Longer-acting dihydropyridines, however, do not appear to activate the SNS.[412] By contrast, the nondihydropyridines are moderately potent arterial vasodilators but directly decrease AV nodal conduction and have negative inotropic and chronotropic effects, which are not abrogated by the reflex increase in sympathetic tone. Because of their negative inotropic action, their use is contraindicated in patients with HFrEF. As expected, these drugs are more effective at reducing stress-induced cardiovascular responses than dihydropyridines.[413]

A clinically useful classification system for CCBs categorizes them by their duration of action into short-acting and long-acting agents (Tables 49.16 and 49.17). This schema is helpful because the short-acting agents are no longer recommended for the management of hypertension because of their stimulation of the SNS, which may predispose patients to angina, MI, and stroke.[414] The long-acting drugs are commonly divided into three generations. First-generation agents, such as nifedipine, have shorter half-lives and require multiple daily doses. Second-generation agents have been modified into extended-release (ER) formulations, requiring once-daily dosing. The third-generation agents have intrinsically longer plasma or receptor half-lives, possibly related to their greater lipophilicity.[415]

### Benzothiazepines

Diltiazem hydrochloride is the prototype of the benzothiazepine CCBs. Diltiazem is 98% absorbed from the gastrointestinal tract, but because of extensive first-pass hepatic metabolism, its bioavailability is only 40% compared with intravenous dosing[12] (Tables 49.16 and 49.17). In vivo, the competitively inhibited liver CYP2D6 isoenzyme is the most important metabolic pathway and probably accounts for the substantial proportion of drug interactions that occur with diltiazem.[416] The rates of elimination are lower in older persons and those with chronic liver disease but unchanged in patients with CKD.

Oral forms of diltiazem have been modified to improve delivery and currently include tablets, SR capsules, controlled-diffusion capsules, Geomatrix ER capsules, ER capsules, and buccoadhesive formulations.[417–419] The usual starting dosage

**Table 49.16 Pharmacodynamic Properties of Calcium Channel Blockers**

| Generic Name (Trade Name) | First Dose (mg) | Usual Daily Dosage (mg) | Maximum Daily Dose (mg) | Peak Response (h) | Duration of Response (h) |
|---|---|---|---|---|---|
| Diltiazem (Cardizem) | 60 | 60–120 tid, qid | 480 | 2.5–4 | 8 |
| Diltiazem SR (Cardizem SR) | 180 | 120–240 bid | 480 | 6 | 12 |
| Diltiazem CD (Cardizem CD) | 180 | 240–280 qd | 480 | — | 24 |
| Diltiazem XR (Dilacor XR) | 180 | 180–480 qd | 480 | 3–6 | 24 |
| Diltiazem ER (Tiazac) | 180 | 180–480 qd | 480 | 4–6 | 24 |
| Amlodipine (Norvasc) | 5 | 5–10 qd | 10 | 30–50 | 24 |
| Felodipine (Plendil ER) | 2.5 | 2.5 qd | 10 | 2–5 | 24 |
| Isradipine (DynaCirc) | 2.5 | 2.5–5 bid | 20 | 2–3 | 12 |
| Isradipine CR (DynaCirc CR) | 5 | 5–20 qd | 20 | 2 | 7–18 |
| Nicardipine (Cardene) | 20 | 20–40 tid | 120 | 0.5–2 | 8 |
| Nicardipine SR (Cardene SR) | 30 | 30–60 bid | 120 | 1.4 | 12 |
| Nifedipine (Procardia, Adalat) | 10 | 10–30 tid, qid | 120 | 0.1 | 4–6 |
| Nifedipine GITS (Procardia XL) | 30 | 30–90 qd | 120 | 4–6 | 24 |
| Nifedipine ER (Adalat CC) | 30 | 30–90 qd | 120 | 2–6 | 24 |
| Nisoldipine (Sular) | 20 | 20–40 qd | 60 | — | 24 |
| Verapamil (Calan, Isoptin) | 80 | 80–120 tid | 480 | 6–8 | 8 |
| Verapamil SR (Calan SR, Isoptin SR) | 120 | 120–240 bid | 480 | — | 12–24 |
| Verapamil SR Pellet (Verelan) | 120 | 240–480 qd | 480 | — | 24 |
| Verapamil COER-24 (Covera-HS) | 180 | 180–480 qhs | 480 | >4–5 | 24 |
| Mibefradil (Posicor) | 50 | 50–100 qd | 100 | 2–4 | 17–25 |

*bid,* Two times a day; *CD,* Controlled-diffusion; *COER,* controlled-onset extended-release; *CR,* controlled release; *ER,* extended release; *GITS,* gastrointestinal therapeutic system; *qd,* once a day; *qhs,* every bedtime; *qid,* four times a day; *SR,* sustained release; *tid,* three times a day; *XR,* extended release.

**Table 49.17 Pharmacokinetic Properties of Calcium Channel Blockers**

| Drug | Oral Absorption (%) | First-Pass Effect | Bioavailability (%) | Peak Blood Level | Elimination Half-Life (h) | Metabolism and Excretion | Protein Binding (%) | Active Metabolites |
|---|---|---|---|---|---|---|---|---|
| Diltiazem | 98 | 50% | 40 | 2–3 h | 4–6 | L, F, U | 77–93 | Yes |
| Diltiazem SR | >80 | 50% | 35 | 6–11 h | 5–7 | L, F, U | 77–93 | Yes |
| Diltiazem CD | 95 | E | 35 | 12 h | 5–8 | L, F, U | 77–93 | Yes |
| Diltiazem XR | 95 | E | 41 | 4–6 h | 5–10 | L, F, U | 95 | Yes |
| Diltiazem ER | 93 | E | 40–60 | 4–6 h | 10 | L, F, U | 95 | Yes |
| Amlodipine | >90 | M | 88 | 6–12 h | 30–50 | L/U | >95 | Yes |
| Felodipine | >90 | E | 13–18 | 2.5–5 h | 11–16 | L/U | >95 | No |
| Isradipine | >90 | E | 15–25 | 2–3 h | 8 | L, F, U | >95 | No |
| Isradipine CR | >90 | E | 15–25 | 7–18 h | — | L, F, U | >95 | No |
| Nicardipine | >90 | E | 35 | 0.5–2 h | 8.6 | L, F, U | >95 | No |
| Nicardipine SR | >90 | E | 35 | 1–4 h | — | L, F, U | >95 | No |
| Nifedipine | >90 | 20%–30% | 60 | <30 min | 2 | L, U | 98 | Yes |
| Nifedipine GITS | >90 | 25%–35% | 86 | 6 h | — | L, U | 98 | Yes |
| Nifedipine ER | >90 | 25%–35% | 86 | 2.5–5 h | 7 | L, U | 98 | Yes |
| Nisoldipine | >85 | E | 4–8 | 6–12 h | 10–22 | L, F, U | 99 | No |
| Verapamil | >90 | 70%–80% | 20–35 | 1–2 h | 2.8–7.4 | L, F, U | 85–95 | Yes |
| Verapamil SR | >90 | 70%–80% | 20–35 | 5–6 h | 4–12 | L, F, U | 85–95 | Yes |
| Verapamil SR pellet | >90 | 70%–80% | 20–35 | 7–9 h | 12 | L, F, U | 85–95 | Yes |
| CODAS Verapamil | >90 | 70%–80% | 20–35 | 11 h | — | L, F, U | 85–95 | Yes |

*CD,* Controlled-diffusion; *CODAS,* chronotherapeutic oral drug absorption system; *CR,* controlled release; *E,* extensive; *ER,* extensive release; *F,* feces; *GITS,* gastrointestinal therapeutic system; *L,* liver; *M,* minimal; *SR,* sustained release; *U,* urine; *XR,* extended release.

for the drug in tablet form is 180 mg/day in three divided doses, and the drug may be titrated to a total dosage of 480 mg/day (Table 49.16).

### Diphenylalkylamine

Verapamil hydrochloride, the oldest CCB, is the prototype diphenylalkylamine derivative. Verapamil inhibits membrane transport of calcium in myocardial cells, particularly the AV node, and smooth muscle cells, which renders it antiarrhythmic, antihypertensive, and a negative inotrope. The drug is available for oral administration as film-coated tablets containing 40, 80, or 120 mg of racemic verapamil hydrochloride.[12] The usual daily dose is 80 to 120 mg three times (Table 49.16). The elimination half-life increases with long-term administration and in older patients with CKD (Table 49.17).

The SR caplets are available in scored 120-, 180-, and 240-mg forms. The usual antihypertensive dose is equivalent to the total daily dose of immediate-release tablets and can be given as 240 to 480 mg/day. An adequate antihypertensive response may be improved by divided twice-daily dosing.

The SR pellet–filled verapamil capsules are gel-coated capsules with an onset of action of 7 to 9 hours that is not affected by food. The peak concentrations are approximately 65% of those of immediate-release tablets, but the trough concentrations are 30% higher. The usual daily dose is 240 to 480 mg.

The controlled-onset, ER and chronotherapeutic oral drug absorption system (CODAS) tablets have unique pharmacologic properties and deliver verapamil 4 to 5 hours after ingestion. A delay coating is inserted between the outer semipermeable membrane and active inner drug core. As the delay coating expands in the gastrointestinal tract, the pressure causes drug from the inner core to be released through laser-drilled holes in the outer membrane, making this formulation ideal for nighttime dosing by providing maximal plasma levels in the early morning hours, from 6 AM to noon, and minimizing nighttime diurnal BP variations.[420] A buccal gel formulation of verapamil that provides SR of the drug up to 6 hours has been reported.[421]

Of the 13 known metabolites of verapamil, norverapamil is the only one with cardiovascular activity; it has 20% of the potency of the parent compound. Renal excretion accounts for 70% of clearance and occurs within 5 days. The remainder is excreted in the feces. Clearance decreases with increasing age and decreasing weight.[422] With long-term administration, there is a significant increase in bioavailability, possibly as a result of saturation of hepatic enzymes. Dose adjustment is necessary in patients with liver disease but not CKD. However, verapamil should be used with caution in patients who ingest large amounts of grapefruit juice or patients taking concurrent AV nodal blocking agents.[423]

### Dihydropyridines

Nifedipine is a dihydropyridine CCB that causes decreased peripheral resistance, with no clinically significant depression of myocardial function. Because of the reflex sympathetic stimulation triggered by vasodilation, nifedipine has no tendency to prolong AV conduction or sinus node recovery or slow the sinus rate. Clinically, there is usually a small increase in heart rate and cardiac index. The labeling for immediate-release nifedipine capsules has been revised to recommend against using this dosage form for the management of hypertension.[12,424] In older persons, use of the immediate-release form has been associated with a more than threefold increase in mortality compared with the use of other antihypertensive agents, including other CCBs.[425] In most patients, immediate-release nifedipine causes a modest hypotensive effect that is well tolerated. However, in occasional patients, the hypotensive effect is profound and has resulted in MI, stroke, and death.[424] This effect appears to be more pronounced in patients also taking β-blockers.[426] Consequently, its use should be reserved for short periods, but not in the setting of acute syndromes. The usual adult dosage is 10 to 30 mg three times daily, and the dose can be titrated weekly (Table 49.16). Nifedipine is rapidly and fully absorbed, and drug levels are detectable within 10 minutes of ingestion. Peak levels are achieved within 30 minutes, and the half-life is 2 hours. There is no clinical advantage to ingestion using the technique of bite and swallow or bite and hold sublingually.

Nifedipine is extensively metabolized in the liver and then excreted in the urine. Most of the population is reported to metabolize the drug rapidly. Because nifedipine is 98% protein bound, the dosage should be adjusted in patients with hepatic insufficiency or severe malnutrition.

The ER tablets of nifedipine are available in 30-, 60-, and 90-mg doses. These tablets consist of an outer semipermeable membrane surrounding an active drug core.[427] The core is composed of an inner active drug layer surrounded by an osmotically active, inert layer that forces the dissolution of the drug core as it swells from gastrointestinal juice absorption. The drug is then slowly and steadily released over 16 to 18 hours. This method of delivery is termed the “gastrointestinal therapeutic system” formulation. The ER form should not be bitten or divided. The time to peak concentration is 6 hours, and plasma levels remain steady for 24 hours. The bioavailability of the ER tablet is 86% compared with that of immediate-release forms, and tolerance does not develop.[427] Of the metabolites, 80% are excreted in the urine. The remainder is excreted in the feces, along with the outer semipermeable membrane shell. The usual adult maintenance dosage is 30 to 90 mg/day. Conversion from the immediate-release form to ER tablets can be done on an equal-milligram basis.

A similar ER formulation is composed of a coat and core.[428] The outer layer contains a slow-release form of nifedipine; the inner core is a fast-release preparation. Peak concentrations are reached within 2.5 to 5 hours, and there is a second peak after 6 to 12 hours as the inner core is released. When the drug is administered in this way, the half-life is extended from 2 to 7 hours. The usual daily dose is 30 to 90 mg, and the dose should be titrated by 30-mg increments in 7 to 14 days for maximal effect. Because of the unique delivery system, which provides a rapid-release core, peak plasma concentrations are not always reliable. Ingestion of three 30-mg tablets simultaneously, but not two, results in a 29% higher peak plasma concentration than the ingestion of a single 90-mg tablet. Consequently, two tablets may be substituted for 60 mg, but the substitution of three 30-mg tablets to make 90 mg is not recommended.[12]

Amlodipine besylate is unique among the dihydropyridine CCBs. It appears to bind to dihydropyridine and nondihydropyridine sites to produce peripheral arterial vasodilation without significant activation of the SNS.[22] The parent compound has substantially slower but more complete absorption than others in the class (Table 49.17). After ingestion, amlodipine is almost completely absorbed, peak plasma concentrations are achieved in 6 to 12 hours, and the clinical response can be detected at 24 hours. The mean peak serum levels are linear, age independent, and achieved after 7 to 8 days of continuous dosing.[429] The elimination half-life is long, ranging from 30 to 50 hours, and is prolonged in older adults. The long half-life permits once-daily dosing; the hypotensive response may last up to 5 days,[430] 90% of amlodipine is metabolized in the liver, and 10% is excreted unchanged. The metabolites are excreted primarily in the urine, but no dosage adjustment is necessary with renal impairment. The minimum effective dose is 2.5 mg, particularly in older patients. Most patients require a dosage of 5 to 10 mg/day.

Benidipine is a long-acting dihydropyridine CCB that is available currently in Asia for the management of mild-to-moderate hypertension. It has several unique mechanisms of action[431]: It has a high vascular selectivity and inhibits L-, N-, and T-type calcium channels. The usual dosage is 2 to 4 mg once daily, but the dosage can be increased to 4 mg twice daily for those with angina pectoris.

Felodipine is a dihydropyridine CCB that is administered in ER tablets of 2.5, 5, and 10 mg (Table 49.16).[12] Felodipine is almost completely absorbed from the gastrointestinal tract, with a time to peak concentration of 2 to 5 hours (Table 49.17). There is extensive first-pass hepatic metabolism. Bioavailability is influenced by food. Large meals and the flavonoids in grapefruit juice increase the bioavailability by approximately 50%.[433] The overall half-life is 11 to 16 hours. Felodipine is metabolized in the liver to inactive metabolites, most of which are excreted in the urine. The usual daily dose is 2.5 to 10 mg, and titration can be instituted at 2-week intervals. The dosage should be adjusted for liver disease but not for CKD.

Isradipine is a dihydropyridine CCB that is effective alone or in combination with other antihypertensive agents for the management of mild-to-moderate hypertension[12] (Tables 49.16 and 49.17). Isradipine is rapidly and almost completely absorbed after oral administration. Extensive first-pass hepatic metabolism reduces bioavailability to less than 25%. The hypotensive effect peaks at 2 to 3 hours for the regular release form. The drug is active for 12 hours; however, the full antihypertensive response does not occur until 14 days. The usual dosage is 2.5 to 5 mg two to three times daily. The onset of action of the SR formulation is achieved in 2 hours and lasts for 7 to 18 hours. The usual daily dose of the controlled-release tablet is 5 to 20 mg. Isradipine is extensively protein bound. The elimination half-life is biphasic, with a terminal half-life of 8 hours. Dosage adjustment is unnecessary in liver disease or CKD.

Manidipine is a third-generation dihydropyridine CCB that is structurally related to nifedipine.[434,435] The usual adult dosage is 10 to 20 mg once daily. Dosage should be adjusted at 2-week intervals. Manidipine is highly protein bound and extensively metabolized in the liver. Metabolism is impaired by grapefruit juice[436]; 63% of the drug is excreted in the feces. The peak plasma concentration occurs after 2 to 3.5 hours, with an elimination half-life of 5 to 8 hours. Dose adjustment is not necessary in CKD. Manidipine may be less likely to cause significant ankle edema than amlodipine.[437]

Nicardipine hydrochloride is a dihydropyridine CCB available as 20- and 40-mg immediate-release gelatin capsules or 30-, 45-, and 60-mg SR capsules.[12] The usual dosage is 20 to 40 mg three times daily for the immediate-release form and 30 to 60 mg twice daily for the SR preparation. When conversion is made to the SR form, the previous daily total of immediate-release drug should be administered on a twice-daily regimen. Titration should be instituted at least 3 days after administration. Nicardipine is well absorbed orally but has only 35% systemic bioavailability because of its extensive first-pass hepatic metabolism. The time to peak concentration is 30 minutes to 2 hours for immediate-release capsules and 1 to 4 hours for SR forms. The elimination half-life is 8.6 hours. Nicardipine is 100% oxidized in the liver to inactive pyridine metabolites. There is no evidence of microsomal enzyme induction. Metabolites are excreted primarily in the urine and feces. The parent compound is not dialyzable. Dosage adjustments are necessary with liver disease but not CKD.

Nisoldipine is a dihydropyridine CCB that is formulated as ER tablets of 10, 20, 30, and 40 mg (Tables 49.16 and 49.17).[12] The initial starting dose is 20 mg, and the usual maintenance dose is 20 to 40 mg given once daily, which can be titrated at weekly intervals. The bioavailability of nisoldipine is low and variable (4%–8%). The coat core design affords a full 24-hour effect after oral administration. The drug reaches therapeutic concentrations in 6 to 12 hours, and absorption is slowed by high-fat meals. The elimination half-life ranges from 10 to 22 hours. Nisoldipine is metabolized in the liver and intestine. Variable hepatic blood flow induced by the drug probably contributes to its pharmacokinetic variability. Most of the metabolites are excreted in the urine and the remainder in the feces. Dose adjustments are necessary with liver disease but not CKD.

Lacidipine is a second-generation dihydropyridine CCB that is available in tablet form. It is reported to be unusually potent and long acting, possibly because it diffuses deeper into lipid bilayer membranes. A unique attribute of this drug is its apparently greater vascular selectivity, but the clinical relevance of this remains unclear.[438] The usual dosage is 4 to 6 mg once daily, and the dose should be titrated at 2- to 4-week intervals.[439] The duration of action is 12 to 24 hours. The elimination half-life is 12 to 19 hours. The parent compound is converted 100% by the liver into inactive fragments that are excreted primarily in the feces (70%) and kidney. Dosage adjustment is necessary in older persons and in patients with liver disease but not CKD.

Lercanidipine is a dihydropyridine CCB whose molecular design imparts greater solubility within the arterial cellular membrane bilayer, conferring a tenfold higher vascular selectivity than that of amlodipine.[439] In contrast to amlodipine, lercanidipine has a relatively short half-life but a long-lasting effect at the receptor and membrane levels and is associated with significantly less peripheral edema.[439] The drug is administered at a starting dose of 10 mg and increased to 20 mg daily as needed. It has a gradual onset of action, and its effects last for 24 hours.[440] Lercanidipine also appears to dilate the efferent renal arteriole.[441]

## CLASS RENAL EFFECTS

All CCBs exert natriuretic and diuretic effects.[442,443] Experimental studies and studies in humans with hypertension have indicated that the increase in sodium excretion is, in part, independent of vasodilatory action or changes in GFR, renal blood flow, or filtration fraction. This effect is probably the result of changes in renal sodium handling that can potentiate the antihypertensive vascular effect. In normal persons, CCBs acutely increase sodium excretion, frequently in the absence of changes in BP. In hypertensive persons, the short-term administration of CCBs uniformly increases sodium excretion 1.1- to 3.4-fold; the magnitude of the increase is not related to the decrease in BP.[442]

The natriuretic effect appears to persist in the long term. Long-term administration of CCBs to hypertensive patients results in a cumulative sodium deficit that is abruptly reversed with the discontinuation of the drug. Natriuresis frequently occurs 3 to 6 hours after the morning dose.[443] The net negative sodium balance levels off after the first 2 to 3 days of administration but persists for the duration of therapy.[444] There are no significant changes in long-term body weight, serum concentrations of potassium, urea nitrogen, catecholamines, or GFR. Moreover, stimulation of renin release and aldosterone does not occur to an appreciable degree. It has been postulated that the natriuresis induced by CCBs increases distal sodium delivery to the macula densa, suppressing renin release. Because Ang II mediates aldosterone synthesis by way of cytosolic calcium messengers, CCBs blunt this response as well.[445]

The mechanism whereby CCBs induce natriuresis appears to be direct inhibition of renal tubular sodium and water absorption. Dihydropyridines increase urinary flow rate and sodium excretion without changing the filtered water and sodium load. Studies have suggested that CCBs may diminish sodium uptake at the amiloride-sensitive sodium channels.[446] Inhibition of water reabsorption occurs distally to the late distal tubule. Proximal tubular sodium reabsorption may be inhibited by higher dosages. One possible mediator of this effect is atrial natriuretic peptide. In human studies, CCBs augment atrial natriuretic peptide release and potentiate its action at the level of the kidney. Other potential mediators are under investigation. How much the natriuretic effects contribute to the antihypertensive response is unknown, but unlike effects of other vasodilators, the changes attenuate the expected adaptive changes in sodium handling.

The renal hemodynamic effects of CCBs are variable and depend primarily on which vasoconstrictors modulate the renal vascular tone.[447] Experimentally, CCBs improve GFR in the presence of the vasoconstrictors norepinephrine and Ang II, as well as others, by preferentially attenuating afferent arteriolar resistance.[448] The efferent arteriole appears to be refractory to these vasodilatory effects. Patients with primary hypertension appear to be more sensitive to the renal hemodynamic effects of CCBs than normotensive patients, and this effect is more pronounced with more advanced CKD.[449] Short-term administration of CCBs results in little change in, or augmentation of, GFR and renal plasma flow, no change in the filtration fraction, and reduction of renal vascular resistance. Long-term administration is not associated with significant changes in renal hemodynamics. The response is maximal in the presence of Ang II, which selectively causes postglomerular vasoconstriction. Clinically significant changes are counteracted by the reduction in renal perfusion pressure coincident with a reduction of BP.

The long-term effects of CCBs on kidney function are variable.[450,451] In hypertensive patients, the effects on renal hemodynamics vary. Some patients exhibit no change in GFR, whereas others have an exaggerated increase in GFR and renal plasma flow.[447] Even normotensive patients with a family history of hypertension have an exaggerated hemodynamic response.[452]

The effects of CCBs on proteinuria also vary with respect to the specific drug and the degree of BP reduction achieved.[453] Some dihydropyridines increase protein excretion by up to 40%. It is not clear whether this increase is a result of hemodynamic vasodilation at the afferent arteriole, resulting in increased glomerular capillary pressure (because CCBs directly impair renal autoregulation), changes in glomerular basement membrane permeability, or increased intrarenal Ang II. By contrast, felodipine, diltiazem, verapamil, and others do not appear to have this effect and may lower protein excretion, possibly by also decreasing the efferent arteriolar tone and glomerular pressure.[454] Clinical implications of these differential effects remain to be determined.

Large clinical trials underscore this controversy. In African Americans with hypertension and mild-to-moderate CKD, treatment with an ACE inhibitor demonstrated superior renoprotective effects compared with amlodipine.[455] This effect was independent of BP reduction and was more evident in proteinuric patients; it was also suggestive in patients with less than 300 mg of protein/day at baseline. Hypertensive patients with diabetic nephropathy also fared worse with amlodipine than with ARB therapy.[248] Patients experienced higher rates of progression of CKD and all-cause mortality in the amlodipine- and placebo-treated groups. This effect was also independent of the achieved BP. However, it should be emphasized that coadministration of a dihydropyridine and an ARB does not abrogate the ARB's protective effect on kidney function.[76] It has been postulated that the selective dilation of the afferent arteriole favors an increase in glomerular capillary pressure that perpetuates progression.

## CLASS EFFICACY AND SAFETY

All CCBs are considered among first-line antihypertensive agents and appear to be equally efficacious and safe.[397,456] In contrast to other vasodilators, CCBs attenuate the reflex increase of neurohormonal activity that accompanies a reduction in BP and in the long term, they inhibit or do not change the sympathetic activity.[457,458] The longer-acting agents produce sustained BP reductions of 16 to 28 mm Hg systolic and 14 to 17 mm Hg diastolic, with no appreciable development of tolerance. The CCBs are effective in young, middle-aged, and older patients with white coat hypertension and mild, moderate, or severe hypertension.[459–462] Their efficacy may be determined by genetic polymorphisms.[463] CCBs are equally efficacious in men and women, in patients with a high or low plasma renin activity regardless of dietary salt intake, and in African American, white, and Hispanic patients.[464] Effects of CCBs are diminished in smokers.[465] CCBs are effective and safe in patients with hypertension and coronary artery disease,[466] as well as in patients with ESKD.[467] CCBs also reduce adverse cardiovascular events and slow the progression of atherosclerosis in normotensive patients with coronary artery disease.[468]

The use of CCBs is contraindicated in patients with HFrEF (except, perhaps, amlodipine or felodipine). These drugs should not be used as first-line antihypertensive agents in patients with heart failure, a history of MI, or unstable angina.[455]

Among the different categories, dihydropyridines appear to be the most powerful for reducing BP but may also be associated with more pronounced activation of baroreceptor reflexes.[469] Dihydropyridines induce a more prominent shift in the sympathovagal balance that favors sympathetic predominance compared with nondihydropyridines.[413] In general, however, compared with other vasodilators, CCBs attenuate the reflex increase in sympathetic activity – increased heart rate, cardiac index, and plasma norepinephrine levels and renin activity.

Verapamil and, to a lesser extent, diltiazem exert greater effects on the heart and have less vasoselectivity. These drugs typically reduce the heart rate, slow AV conduction, and depress contractility (Table 49.18). Generally, they should not be used together with β-blockers because of increased risk for heart block. The second- and third-generation CCBs consist of pharmacologically manipulated formulations, whose half-lives are progressively longer.[415]

CCBs are not associated with significant impairments in glycemic control or sexual dysfunction.[397] The rapid antihypertensive action of CCBs may encourage patient adherence. Orthostatic changes do not occur because venoconstriction remains intact. AEs are usually transient and are the direct result of vasodilation. Hypotension is most common with intravenous administration. The most common AE of the dihydropyridines is peripheral edema[470]; it is dose related and thought to be the result of uncompensated precapillary vasodilation, which causes increased intracapillary hydrostatic pressure. The edema is not responsive to diuretics but improves or resolves with the addition of an ACE inhibitor or ARB, which preferentially vasodilates postcapillary beds and reduces intracapillary hydrostatic pressure.[471] Other AEs related to vasodilation include headache, nausea, dizziness, and flushing, and occur more commonly in women. The nondihydropyridines verapamil and isradipine more commonly cause constipation and nausea. The gastrointestinal effects are directly related to the inhibition of calcium-dependent smooth muscle contraction–reduced peristalsis and relaxation of the lower esophageal sphincter. Another common AE of the dihydropyridines is gingival hyperplasia, which is exacerbated in patients who are also taking cyclosporine. Dihydropyridines lead to the accumulation of gingival inflammatory B-cell infiltrates as stimulated by bacterial plaque, immunoglobulins, and folic acid, which causes the growth of the gingiva.[472] This growth can be controlled with regular periodontal treatment and reversed with discontinuation of the drug.[473]

CCBs are notable among antihypertensive agents because of their metabolic neutrality. Because the calcium influx across β-cell membranes helps regulate insulin release,[474] CCBs might predispose to low insulin levels. At typical therapeutic levels, CCBs have no effect on serum glucose concentrations, insulin secretion, or insulin sensitivity in persons with and without diabetes mellitus. The use of CCBs was not significantly associated with incident diabetes compared with other antihypertensive agents in a meta-analysis of RCTs.[475] The association with diabetes was lowest for ACE inhibitors and ARBs, followed by CCBs, β-blockers, and diuretics.[475] Furthermore, it was recently demonstrated that CCBs can even prevent diabetes and increase β-cell survival in vitro. The mechanism behind the β-cell mass destruction is the human islet cell protein TXNIP (thioredoxin-interacting protein), which is upregulated by hyperglycemia. Orally administered verapamil resulted in a reduction of TXNIP expression and β-cell apoptosis, enhanced endogenous insulin levels, and rescued mice from streptozotocin-induced diabetes. Verapamil also promoted β-cell survival and improved glucose homeostasis and insulin sensitivity in ob/ob mice.[476] CCBs do not increase triglyceride or LDL cholesterol and do not reduce HDL cholesterol. CCBs do not precipitate hyponatremia, hyperkalemia, hypokalemia, or hyperuricemia. Therefore they are suitable agents for patients with dysmetabolic syndromes or diabetes.

Properties beyond their antihypertensive actions make the CCBs particularly useful in certain clinical situations. CCBs not only lower arterial pressure but also have variable effects on cardiac function. All CCBs are vasodilators and increase coronary blood flow. With the exception of the short-acting dihydropyridines, most CCBs reduce heart rate, improve myocardial oxygen demand, improve ventricular filling, diminish ventricular arrhythmias, reduce myocardial ischemia, and conserve contractility,[477,478] making them suitable for patients with angina or diastolic dysfunction.[466] In short-term use, CCBs improve diastolic relaxation; when administered over a long term, they reduce left ventricular wall thickness,[479] may prevent the development of hypertrophy, and may improve arterial compliance.[480–482] These effects may be crucial in hypertensive patients because LVH is one of the strongest risk predictors for cardiovascular morbidity and mortality.[483] Verapamil may also be used for secondary cardioprotection to reduce reinfarction rates in patients who are intolerant of β-blockers (unless they have concomitant heart failure)[484] and in patients with chronic headaches.[485] The BP-independent

**Table 49.18 Hemodynamic Effects of Calcium Channel Blockers**

| Class | Arteriolar Dilation | Coronary Dilation | Cardiac Afterload | Cardiac Contractility | Myocardial $O_2$ Demand | Cardiac Output | AV Conduction | SA Automaticity | Heart Rate: Short Term/ Long Term | Activation of Baroreceptor Reflexes |
|---|---|---|---|---|---|---|---|---|---|---|
| Dihydropyridines | ↑↑↑ | ↑↑↑ | ↓↓ | ↔ | ↓ | ↓ or ↔ | ↔ | ↔ | ↑/↑ | ↑ or ↔ |
| Diltiazem | ↑↑ | ↑↑↑ | ↓ | ↓ | ↓ | ↔ | ↓ | ↓↓ | ↓/↓ or ↔ | ↔ |
| Verapamil | ↑↑ | ↑↑ | ↓ | ↓↓ | ↓ | ↔ | ↓↓ | ↓ | ↓/↓ or ↔ | ↔ |

*AV*, Atrioventricular; *SA*, sinoatrial.

inhibition of atherogenesis by CCBs may be another indication to use a CCB, particularly in high-risk patients, such as those with diabetes and ESKD.[486,487]

The use of CCBs may prevent or slow the decline of dementia. In the Systolic Hypertension in Europe (SYST-EUR) trial,[488] nitrendipine use was associated with a lower risk of incident dementia. The potential benefit of CCBs on dementia has also been suggested in observational studies.[489,490]

In general, the antihypertensive effects of CCBs are enhanced more in combination with β-blockers or ACE inhibitors than in combination with diuretics.[491–494] Perhaps this reflects the fact that CCBs themselves have intrinsic diuretic activity. It has been theorized that this particular combination (a dihydropyridine and ACE inhibitor) maximizes precapillary and postcapillary vasodilation to lower peripheral vascular resistance.

The combination of dihydropyridine CCBs with β-blockers is efficacious and even desirable in selected patients. CCBs have the potential to blunt the AEs associated with β-blockade, such as vasoconstriction, and β-blockers have the ability to attenuate the increased sympathetic stimulation induced by dihydropyridine CCBs. By contrast, concomitant therapy with β-blockers and nondihydropyridine CCBs is ill advised because they may have additive effects in suppressing heart rate, AV node conduction, and cardiac contractility (Table 49.19). This combination may be particularly dangerous in patients with ESKD because of the effects of hyperkalemia on cardiac conduction.

Drug interactions are not uncommon (Table 49.19). Concurrent use of a CCB and amiodarone exacerbates sick sinus syndrome and AV block. Diltiazem, verapamil, and nicardipine have been shown to increase the levels of cyclosporine (including the microemulsion formulation), tacrolimus, and sirolimus by 25% to 100%.[495] This interaction may be clinically useful for reducing the dosage and cost associated with immunosuppressive therapy. Frequent monitoring of serum concentrations of calcineurin inhibitor is recommended. By contrast, nifedipine and isradipine exert no effect on serum concentrations of calcineurin inhibitors and can be used safely. Diltiazem is a potent inhibitor of CYP3A4, which is responsible for the metabolism of methylprednisolone. Coadministration of diltiazem and methylprednisolone resulted in a more than a 2.5-fold increase in the steroid blood level and enhanced adrenal suppressive responses.[496] Coadministration of diltiazem also increased nifedipine levels by 100% to 200%.[497] This combination has additive antihypertensive efficacy and appears to be safe.[498] Concomitant administration of CCBs with the digitalis glycosides resulted in up to a 50% increase in serum digoxin concentrations because of reduced renal clearance of digoxin, an effect that appears to be dose dependent.[499] Insofar as dihydropyridine CCBs partially suppress aldosterone synthesis, they provide an attractive alternative for patients who cannot tolerate blockade of the RAAS.[500]

Several issues regarding the inherent safety of CCBs have come under scrutiny. CCBs may be associated with an increased risk of gastrointestinal hemorrhage, particularly in older persons.[501] Diltiazem inhibits platelet aggregation in vitro,[502] but the clinical relevance of this finding has not been substantiated. Nonetheless, it is prudent to use caution when coadministering CCBs with NSAIDs because NSAIDs may exacerbate the risk of bleeding and may antagonize the antihypertensive effects of CCBs.[503,504]

There have been concerns regarding a possible relation between the long-term use of CCBs and breast cancer.[132,505] A population case–control study of breast cancer showed that the use of CCBs for more than 10 years was associated with ductal breast cancer (odds ratio [OR], 2.4; 95% CI, 1.2 to 4/9; *P* = .04) and lobular breast cancer (OR, 2.6; 95% CI, 1.3 to 5.3; *P* = .01), respectively. However, two recent large population-based observational studies demonstrated no association between CCB use and breast cancer.[506,507]

Short-acting CCBs have been associated with a small increased risk of MI in meta-analyses[424,508] when compared with other agents. It has been speculated that the disadvantageous activation of the RAAS and SNS induced by the

**Table 49.19 Drug–Drug Interactions With Calcium Channel Blockers**

| Calcium Channel Blocker | Interacting Drug | Result |
|---|---|---|
| Verapamil | Digoxin | Digoxin level ↑ by 50%–90% |
| Diltiazem | Digoxin | Digoxin level ↑ by 40% |
| Verapamil | β-Blockers | AV nodal blockade, hypotension, bradycardia, asystole |
| Verapamil, diltiazem | Cyclosporine-tacrolimus and sirolimus | Cyclosporine level ↑ by 25%–100% |
| Verapamil, diltiazem | Cimetidine | Verapamil and diltiazem levels ↑ by decreased metabolism |
| Verapamil | Rifampin–phenytoin | Verapamil level ↓ by enzyme induction |
| Dihydropyridines | Amiodarone | Exacerbation of sick sinus syndrome and AV nodal blockade |
| Dihydropyridines | α-Blockers | Excessive hypotension |
| Dihydropyridines | Propranolol | Increases propranolol level |
| Dihydropyridines | Cimetidine | Increased area under the curve and plasma level of calcium channel blocker |
| Nicardipine | Cyclosporine | Cyclosporine level ↑ by 40%–50% |
| Amlodipine | Cyclosporine | Cyclosporine level ↑ by 10% |
| Felodipine | Flavonoids | Bioavailability ↑ by 50% |
| Diltiazem | Methylprednisolone | Methylprednisone ↑ 2.5-fold |
| Nifedipine | Diltiazem | Nifedipine level ↑ 100%–200% |

*AV*, Atrioventricular.

short-acting agents may predispose to myocardial ischemia. Currently, there is no evidence to prove the existence of additional beneficial or detrimental effects of CCBs on coronary disease events, including fatal or nonfatal MIs and other deaths from coronary heart disease. Because of a potential risk, however, as well as for simplicity and improved patient adherence, longer-acting agents should be considered over short-acting CCBs for the management of hypertension.

## CENTRAL ADRENERGIC AGONISTS

### CLASS MECHANISMS OF ACTION

Central adrenergic agonists act by crossing the blood–brain barrier and have a direct agonist effect on $\alpha_2$-adrenergic receptors located in the midbrain and brain stem.[494,509,510] Binding to the $I_1$ imidazoline receptors in the brain may also play a role in the inhibition of central sympathetic output.[5,511–516] Drugs in this class bind to the α-adrenergic or $I_1$ imidazoline receptors with some degree of specificity (Table 49.20). Moxonidine and rilmenidine have a 30-fold greater specificity for the $I_1$ imidazoline receptor than the $\alpha_2$ receptor. Clonidine, by contrast, exhibits a fourfold greater specificity for the $I_1$ imidazoline receptor than for the $\alpha_2$ receptor. The central AEs are thought to be largely related to $\alpha_2$-receptor binding. Moxonidine and rilmenidine have reduced central side effects because of the lower activity at the $\alpha_2$ receptor relative to other agents.[516,517] In addition to decreasing the total sympathetic outflow, binding to these receptors results in increased vagal activity. A reduction in catecholamine release and turnover, as evidenced by decreased biochemical markers of noradrenergic activity, such as plasma concentrations of norepinephrine, correlated with the magnitude of BP lowering.

Stimulation of both receptor types is probably mediated through the same neuronal pathways.[517] The classic $\alpha_2$-receptor agonists, such as clonidine and α-methyldopa (acting through its active metabolite, α-methylnorepinephrine), result in vasodilation in the resistance vessels and thus a reduction in peripheral vascular resistance. Despite vasodilator action, reflex tachycardia generally does not occur, probably as a result of peripheral sympathetic inhibition.

The selective $I_1$ receptor agonists moxonidine and rilmenidine are predominantly arterial vasodilators that lead to a reduction in peripheral vascular resistance.[512] Moxonidine is associated with a reduction in plasma renin activity. The central $\alpha_2$-adrenergic agonists may also stimulate peripheral $\alpha_2$-adrenergic receptors. This effect predominates at high drug concentrations. These receptors mediate vasoconstriction, which may result in a paradoxic increase in BP.[509] Overall, these drugs generally result in a decrease in peripheral vascular resistance, slowing of the heart rate, and either no change or a mild decrease in cardiac output.[517,518] Orthostatic hypotension is generally not a feature of these drugs. The pharmacokinetic and pharmacodynamic properties of these drugs are shown in Tables 49.21 and 49.22.

**Table 49.20 Receptor Binding of Centrally Acting Antihypertensives**

| Drug | Receptor |
|---|---|
| Clonidine | α2, $I_1$ |
| α-Methyldopa | α2 |
| Guanabenz | α2 |
| Guanfacine | α2 |
| Rilmenidine | $I_1$ > α2 |
| Moxonidine | $I_1$ > α2 |

*$I_1$*, Imidazole receptor; *α2*, α2-adrenergic receptor.

### CLASS MEMBERS

Methyldopa is a methyl-substituted amino acid that is active after conversion to an active metabolite. This active metabolite, α-methylnorepinephrine, accumulates in the CNS and is selective for $\alpha_2$-adrenergic receptors. The initial dosage of methyldopa in hypertension is 250 mg two to three times daily. This dose may be increased at intervals of not less than 2 days until a therapeutic response is achieved. The usual maintenance dosage is 500 mg to 2 g daily in two to four doses. The maximum recommended daily dose is 3 g. An initial response occurs within 3 to 6 hours after dosing. The peak response occurs at 6 to 9 hours. The drug is approximately 50% metabolized by the liver. The drug half-life is increased in patients with CKD. Excretion in the urine is largely in the form of an inactive metabolite. The dosing interval should be increased to every 12 to 24 hours in patients with advanced CKD. Approximately 60% of methyldopa is removed with hemodialysis. A supplemental dose is recommended after dialysis treatment.

**Table 49.21 Pharmacokinetic Properties of Central Adrenergic Agonists**

| Drug | Bioavailability (%) | Affected by Food | Peak Blood Level (h) | Elimination Half-Life (h) | Metabolism | Excretion | Active Metabolites |
|---|---|---|---|---|---|---|---|
| Clonidine (Catapres) | 50 | — | — | 6–23 | L | F (30%–50%)<br>U (24%) | Methyldopa-o-sulfite |
| α-Methyldopa (ALDOMET) | 65–96 | — | 1.5–5 | 6–23 | L | F (22%)<br>U (65%) | — |
| Guanabenz (Wytensin) | 75 | — | 2–5 | 7–10 | L | F (16%) | — |
| Guanfacine (Tonex) | 80 | — | 1–4 | 17 | L | U (40%–75%) | — |
| Rilmenidine (Hyperium) | 80–90 | No | 2 | 2–3 | L | U (90%) | — |
| Moxonidine (Physiotens) | 100 | No | 0.5–3 | 2 | L | U (90%) | — |

*F*, Feces; *L*, liver; *U*, urine.

**Table 49.22 Pharmacodynamic Properties of Central Adrenergic Agonists**

| Drug | Initial Dose (mg) | Usual Dose (mg) | Maximum Dose (mg) | Interval | Peak Response (h) | Duration of Response (h) |
|---|---|---|---|---|---|---|
| Clonidine | 0.1 | 0.3–0.9 | 2.4 | bid, tid | 2–4 | 6–10 |
| α-Methyldopa | 250 | 250–500 | 3000 | bid, tid, qid | 6–9 | 24–48 |
| Guanabenz | 4 | 16–32 | 64 | bid | 2–4 | 10–12 |
| Guanfacine | 1 | 1–3 | 3 | qd | 6 | 24 |
| Moxonidine | 0.1–0.2 | 0.2–0.3 | 0.6 | bid | 1.5–4 | 48–72 |
| Rilmenidine | 1 | 1–2 | 2 | qd, bid | 1–2 | 10–12 |

*bid,* Two times a day; *qd,* once a day; *qid,* four times a day.

Clonidine is a central-acting α-adrenergic agonist.[151,513,519] The usual oral dosage is 0.1 mg two to three times daily, adjusted as necessary in 0.1- to 0.2-mg increments. The usual maintenance dosage is 0.3 to 0.9 mg daily in two to three divided doses. Total doses more than 1.2 mg daily are usually not associated with a greater effect. The onset of activity is 30 to 60 minutes after an oral dose. The peak antihypertensive activity occurs within 2 to 4 hours. The duration of the antihypertensive effect is 6 to 10 hours. The half-life of the absorbed drug is 6 to 23 hours. Hepatic metabolism to inactive metabolites is followed by renal excretion. Transdermal patches are available and may be applied on a once-weekly basis. The drug half-life with the transdermal patch is approximately 20 hours after removal of the patch. With a transdermal patch, steady-state drug levels are reached within approximately 3 days. Dose adjustment is not needed for patients with any degree of CKD including ESKD. Approximately 5% of clonidine body stores are removed after a 5-hour hemodialysis session.

Guanabenz is an orally active, central $\alpha_2$-adrenergic agonist.[509] The usual starting dosage for the management of hypertension is 4 mg twice daily. Doses may be increased by 4 to 8 mg/day at 1- to 2-week intervals. The onset of antihypertensive activity usually occurs within 60 minutes, and the activity lasts approximately 10 to 12 hours. The drug is highly protein bound and extensively metabolized. Less than 1% of the unchanged drug is excreted in the urine. The half-life of the drug is 7 to 10 hours. Dose adjustment in patients with CKD is not necessary but may be necessary in patients with severe hepatic insufficiency. Because of extensive protein binding, drug removal by dialysis is minimal.

Guanfacine is a centrally acting antihypertensive drug with actions similar to those of clonidine.[520] Effective dosages are 1 to 3 mg daily. Peak levels are noted between 1 and 4 hours. The drug half-life is approximately 17 hours. The drug is 70% protein bound. It is metabolized in the liver, with renal excretion of 40% to 75% as an unchanged drug. Limited data are available on dosing in CKD, but dosage adjustments do not appear warranted.

Moxonidine is a central $I_1$ imidazole and $\alpha_2$-receptor agonist.[151,521,522] Serum concentration peaks are reached within 30 to 180 minutes; 90% of the dose is excreted through the urine within 24 hours, and 50% of this is as unchanged drug. The average half-life is 2 hours. For the management of hypertension, the starting dosage is 0.2 to 0.4 mg/day. The dose may be increased after several weeks to 0.2 to 0.3 mg twice daily. The maximum daily dose is 0.6 mg. Selectivity for the $I_1$ imidazoline receptor results in fewer central AEs, such as dry mouth and sedation, compared with those of clonidine. Drug clearance is delayed in patients with impaired kidney function. Single doses of 0.2 mg and a maximum daily dosage of 0.4 mg should not be exceeded in patients with CKD.

Rilmenidine is a centrally acting imidazole receptor and $\alpha_2$-adrenergic receptor agonist.[151,515,523–527] Rilmenidine binds preferentially to central $I_1$ imidazoline receptors in the brain stem. At higher doses, rilmenidine can bind and activate central $\alpha_2$-adrenergic receptors. Antihypertensive effects occur within 1 hour after a single 1-mg dose. The duration of action is 10 to 12 hours. The concentration after oral dosing peaks at approximately 2 hours. Steady-state plasma levels are reached by day 3. Rilmenidine is eliminated primarily unchanged in the urine. The usual oral dosage is 1 mg once or twice daily. Dose reductions are required for patients with impaired kidney function. In patients with advanced CKD, the dose should be decreased to 1 mg every other day.

## CLASS RENAL EFFECTS

Central $\alpha_2$- and $I_1$ imidazoline receptor agonists have little if any clinically important effect on renal plasma flow, GFR, or the RAAS. The fractional excretion of sodium is unchanged. Body fluid composition and weight are not altered. A water diuresis may be associated with the use of guanabenz through inhibition of the central release of vasopressin or altered renal responsiveness to vasopressin. These agents may result in decreased renal vascular resistance, as mediated by a decrease in preglomerular capillary resistance related to decreased levels of circulating catecholamines.

## CLASS EFFICACY AND SAFETY

The antihypertensive efficacy of this class of drugs has been confirmed in large numbers of patients. These agents provide effective monotherapy for hypertension.[509] Combination with a diuretic is associated with additive effects. Drugs in this class are effective for young and old patients, and the effects do not differ in different racial or ethnic groups. Moxonidine and rilmenidine have been associated with decreased plasma glucose concentrations and may improve insulin sensitivity. These drugs may also decrease total cholesterol, LDL, and triglyceride levels[511,528,529] and may play a role in the management of metabolic syndrome. They may also be of benefit in patients with congestive heart failure. Treatment with rilmenidine and moxonidine reverses LVH and improves arterial compliance. This effect was associated with a reduction in plasma levels of atrial natriuretic peptide.

Stimulation of $\alpha_2$-adrenergic receptors in the CNS induces several AEs of these drugs, including sedation and drowsiness. The most common AE related to $\alpha_2$-adrenergic activation is dry mouth caused by a decrease in salivary flow. This decrease is attributed to centrally mediated inhibition of cholinergic transmission. Clonidine in high doses may precipitate a paradoxic hypertensive response related to the stimulation of postsynaptic vascular $\alpha_2$-adrenergic receptors.[509] Methyldopa use has been associated with a positive result on the direct Coombs test in patients with and without hemolytic anemia.[509] Because of a long history of safe use during pregnancy, methyldopa remains a common therapeutic agent for hypertensive disorders of pregnancy and for essential hypertension during pregnancy.[494,510] The $\alpha_2$-adrenergic agonists are associated with sexual dysfunction and may produce gynecomastia in men and galactorrhea in men and women.

Abrupt cessation of $\alpha_2$-adrenergic blockers may result in rebound hypertension, which occurs 18 to 36 hours after the cessation of short-acting agents.[530] Patients may experience tachycardia, tremor, anxiety, headache, nausea, and vomiting. This syndrome may be related to downregulation of the $\alpha_2$-adrenergic receptors in the CNS in the setting of long-term use of these agents. These agents have a higher specificity for the $I_1$ receptor and appear to produce significantly fewer CNS effects, such as dry mouth and drowsiness. Rebound hypertension secondary to abrupt withdrawal has not been associated with moxonidine or rilmenidine.

## CENTRAL AND PERIPHERAL ADRENERGIC NEURONAL BLOCKING AGENT

### MECHANISMS OF ACTION AND CLASS MEMBER

Reserpine, a *Rauwolfia* alkaloid, reduces BP by decreasing the activity of central and peripheral noradrenergic neurons. Reserpine blocks norepinephrine and dopamine uptake into the storage granules of noradrenergic neurons. The result is norepinephrine depletion. A similar effect is seen in central dopaminergic and serotoninergic neurons. At the dosages currently used to treat hypertension, the major effect of the use of reserpine is in the CNS. Reserpine results in a rapid reduction in cardiac output, heart rate, and peripheral vascular resistance. Enhanced vagal activity may also be involved. Tolerance to the antihypertensive effects of reserpine does not occur.

Reserpine is used at initial dosages of 0.1 to 0.25 mg daily.[531] Approximately 40% of an oral dose is absorbed. The half-life is 50 to 100 hours. Extensive hepatic metabolism occurs; 1% is recovered as unchanged compound in the urine. The maximal clinical effect is observed 2 to 3 weeks after initiation of therapy. No dosage adjustment is necessary for patients with renal insufficiency. Dosage supplementation is not required after hemodialysis.

### RENAL EFFECTS

The GFR and renal plasma flow are not affected by reserpine therapy. Renal vascular resistance may be reduced, perhaps mediated by decreased sympathetic stimulation of vascular $\alpha$-adrenergic receptors. Significant effects on the RAAS have not been observed. Renal handling of sodium and potassium is unchanged.

### EFFICACY AND SAFETY

Reserpine provides effective therapy as a single agent or in combination with HCTZ or HCTZ and hydralazine.[531,532] This has been observed in numerous large and small trials, including the Veterans Administration Cooperative Study on Antihypertensive Agents, Hypertension Detection and Follow-up Program, and the Multiple Risk Factor Intervention Trial. Reserpine used in combination with a diuretic has shown comparable efficacy to combinations of β-blockers and diuretics. In these studies, the dose of reserpine was between 0.1 and 0.3 mg daily, which is many times lower than the doses used in the 1960s that led to reserpine's reputation as having a poor side-effect profile. The most common AE of reserpine is nasal congestion, which is reported in 6% to 20% of patients. Unlike other AEs, nasal congestion does not appear to decrease at lower drug dosages and is thought to be related to the cholinergic effects of the drug. Increased gastric motility and gastric acid secretion can occur; however, the incidence of dyspepsia or peptic ulcer disease with reserpine therapy is not greater than that with other antihypertensive drug treatments. Inability to concentrate, sedation, sleep disturbance, and depression have been reported. Other AEs include weight gain, increased appetite, and sexual dysfunction.

## DIRECT-ACTING VASODILATORS

### CLASS MECHANISMS OF ACTION

The direct-acting vasodilators reduce SBPs and DBPs by decreasing peripheral vascular resistance. These drugs act directly on vascular smooth muscle with the selective vasodilation of the arteriolar resistance vessels and have little or no effect on the venous capacitance vessels.[533] There is no effect on the functioning of carotid or aortic baroreceptors. The vasodilating effects are thought to involve inhibition of calcium uptake into the cells. Decreases in arterial pressure are associated with a decrease in peripheral resistance and a reflex increase in cardiac output. Sodium and water retention are promoted secondary to the stimulation of renin release and possibly by direct effects on renal tubules. The arteriolar dilation produced by these drugs causes a decrease in cardiac afterload,[533] and the absence of venodilation leads to an increase in venous return to the heart, which produces an elevated preload. These combined effects result in increased cardiac output.[533] The pharmacokinetic and pharmacodynamic properties of these drugs are shown in Tables 49.23 and 49.24.

### CLASS MEMBERS

The initial oral dose of hydralazine for hypertension should be 10 mg four times daily, increasing to 50 mg four times daily over several weeks. Patients may require doses of up to 300 mg/day. Dosing can be changed to twice daily for maintenance. The drug may also be used as an intravenous bolus injection or as a continuous infusion. The elimination half-life is 1.5 to 8 hours and varies with the acetylation rate in the liver. Slow and fast acetylators have been described. The onset of action is approximately 1 hour. In patients with mild-to-moderate CKD, the dosing interval should be increased to every 8 hours. In patients with advanced CKD, the dosing interval should be increased to every 8 to 24 hours. No dose

**Table 49.23 Pharmacokinetic Properties of Direct-Acting Vasodilators**

| Drug | Bioavailability (%) | Affected by Food | Peak Blood Level (h) | Elimination Half-Life (h) | Metabolism | Excretion | Active Metabolites |
|---|---|---|---|---|---|---|---|
| Hydralazine (Apresoline) | 20–50 | No | 1–2 | 1.5–8 | L | U (3%–14%)<br>F (3%–12%) | — |
| Minoxidil (Loniten) | 90–100 | — | 1 | 4.2 | L | U (90%)<br>F (3%) | Glucuronide |

*F,* Feces; *L,* liver; *U,* urine.

**Table 49.24 Pharmacodynamic Properties of Direct-Acting Vasodilators**

| Drug | Initial Dose (mg) | Usual Dose (mg) | Maximum Dose (mg) | Interval | Peak Response (h) | Duration of Response (h) |
|---|---|---|---|---|---|---|
| Hydralazine | 10 | 200–400 | 400 | bid, qid | 1 | 3–8 |
| Minoxidil | 2.5 | 10–20 | 40 | qd, qid | 4–8 | 10–12 |

*bid,* Two times a day; *qd,* once a day; *qid,* four times a day.

supplement is required after hemodialysis or peritoneal dialysis (Table 49.7).

Minoxidil is more potent than hydralazine. For severe hypertension, the initial recommended starting dose is 2.5 mg as a single daily dose, increasing to 10 to 20 or 40 mg in single or divided doses. Minoxidil is usually used in conjunction with salt restriction and diuretics to prevent fluid retention. Concomitant therapy with a β-adrenergic blocking agent is often required to control tachycardia related to minoxidil use. The onset of the antihypertensive effect is within 30 to 60 minutes. The peak response occurs at 4 to 8 hours. The drug is 90% metabolized by the liver. The glucuronide metabolite has reduced pharmacologic effects but accumulates in patients with ESKD. Renal excretion is 90%. Dose adjustments may be required for patients with advanced CKD, although the mean daily doses required to control BP are similar in patients with normal and impaired kidney function (Table 49.7).

The effectiveness of minoxidil in patients with resistant hypertension has been well established.[534,535] Minoxidil is frequently a therapy of last resort in patients with CKD unresponsive to other therapies. It must nearly always be used in combination with a β-blocker and a loop diuretic to prevent tachycardia and fluid retention.

### CLASS RENAL EFFECTS

Hydralazine and minoxidil both increase the juxtaglomerular cell secretion of renin, which is associated with increased Ang II and aldosterone levels. Long-term use is associated with the return of plasma aldosterone levels to baseline. Retention of salt and water may be attributed to direct drug effects on the proximal convoluted tubule. Renal vascular resistance is decreased in association with a relaxation of resistance vessels.[533] GFR and renal plasma flow are preserved.

Hydralazine may reduce BP compared with placebo in patients with essential hypertension; however, these results are based on before and after studies, not on RCTs. It is more commonly used in practice to reduce afterload in heart failure among patients with reduced left ventricular function.

### CLASS EFFICACY AND SAFETY

Minoxidil is commonly reserved for severe or intractable hypertension. Because of its propensity to cause salt and water retention, administration with a loop diuretic is usually required. Hypertrichosis is a common AE. Pericarditis and pericardial effusions have been described.[536] An increase in left ventricular mass has been reported, which may be related to adrenergic hyperactivity.

In addition to adrenergic activation and fluid retention, long-term treatment with hydralazine has been associated with the development of systemic lupus erythematosus. Generally, this syndrome occurs early in therapy, but can develop after many years of treatment. It has been estimated that between 6% and 10% of patients receiving high doses of hydralazine for longer than 6 months develop hydralazine-induced lupus.[537] It is seen most frequently in women and rarely in African Americans. This syndrome occurs primarily in slow acetylators and is reversible when hydralazine is discontinued, but months may be required for complete clearing of symptoms. Hydralazine has been frequently used to treat pregnancy-associated hypertension in view of its relatively low teratogenicity.

## ENDOTHELIN RECEPTOR ANTAGONISTS

Endothelin is among the most potent endogenous vasoconstrictors known.[538] It also enhances mitogenesis and induces extracellular matrix formation. Endothelin is also thought to be involved in vascular remodeling and end-organ damage under several different cardiovascular conditions.[539] As a result, endothelin receptor antagonists have been studied as targets for treatment of hypertension. However, concerns about their safety and tolerability have limited their use largely to treatment of pulmonary hypertension.

### CLASS MECHANISM OF ACTION AND CLASS MEMBERS

The two primary receptor sites, endothelin type A (ET-A) and endothelin type B (ET-B), can be selectively blocked with different chemicals, or both sites can be blocked simultaneously. Bosentan, a mixed ET-A/ET-B receptor antagonist, was studied in a large placebo-controlled trial lasting 4 weeks and demonstrated a dose-dependent reduction in BP compared with placebo when bosentan was dosed from 100 mg once daily up to 1000 mg twice daily.[540] The mean reduction in DBP of 5.8 mm Hg across all dosages at or above 5 mg/day was almost identical to that seen with 20 mg of enalapril. The most common AEs were peripheral edema, flushing, headache, and some alterations in liver enzyme levels.

### CLASS RENAL EFFECTS

Endothelin receptor antagonists have been used to study the role of endothelin in the development of acute CKD in different experimental models.[541] Clinical studies using endothelin receptor blockers have shown improvement in proteinuria. This effect is independent of the antiproteinuric effects of inhibition of the RAAS and may help relieve renal injury.[542] What is unknown is whether the selective blockage of the ET-A receptor over the ET-B receptor will not only control BP but also mitigate renal ischemia and reduce proteinuria.

## MODERATELY SELECTIVE PERIPHERAL $\alpha_1$-ADRENERGIC ANTAGONISTS

### CLASS MECHANISMS OF ACTION

The nonselective agents phentolamine and phenoxybenzamine have an occasional role in hypertension management. Phentolamine is administered parenterally, and the longer-acting agent phenoxybenzamine has been used orally for the management of hypertension associated with pheochromocytoma.[543] Phenoxybenzamine is a moderately selective, peripheral $\alpha_1$-adrenergic antagonist. Its specificity for the $\alpha_1$-adrenergic receptor is 100 times greater than that for the $\alpha_2$-adrenergic receptor.

### CLASS MEMBERS

Phenoxybenzamine is a long-acting α-adrenergic blocking agent. This agent irreversibly and covalently binds to α receptors only. β Receptors and the parasympathetic system are not affected by phenoxybenzamine. The total peripheral resistance is decreased, and cardiac output increases with phenoxybenzamine. Phenoxybenzamine is also believed to inhibit the uptake of catecholamines into adrenergic nerve terminals and extraneural tissues. The usual oral dose of phenoxybenzamine for the treatment of pheochromocytoma is initially 10 mg twice daily, with the dose gradually increased every other day to dosages ranging between 20 and 40 mg two or three times daily. The final dosage should be determined by the BP response. Phenoxybenzamine may be administered with a β-blocking agent if tachycardia becomes excessive during therapy. The pressor effects of a pheochromocytoma must be controlled by α-blockade before β-blockers are initiated. With oral use, the pheochromocytoma symptoms decrease after several days. The oral bioavailability is 20% to 30%. The drug is extensively metabolized by the liver. Phenoxybenzamine should be administered cautiously to patients with renal impairment. Specific dosage recommendations are not available.

Phentolamine is an α-adrenergic blocking agent that produces peripheral vasodilation and cardiac stimulation, with a resulting decrease in BP in most patients. The drug is used parenterally. The usual dose is 5 mg, repeated as needed. The onset of activity with intravenous dosing is immediate. The drug is not absorbed well orally; its half-life is 19 minutes. Phentolamine is metabolized by the liver, with 10% excreted in the urine as unchanged drug.

### CLASS RENAL EFFECTS

Phenoxybenzamine has no clear effect on the RAAS. Blood volume and body weight are not altered. Salt and water retention do not occur. GFR and effective renal plasma flow would be expected to increase. Renal vascular resistance probably decreases in proportion to the degree of blockade of α-adrenergic receptors.

### CLASS EFFICACY AND SAFETY

Phenoxybenzamine is used primarily as an agent to counteract the excessive α-adrenergic tone associated with pheochromocytoma. Tachycardia may result from an α-adrenergic blockade, which unmasks β-adrenergic effects with epinephrine-secreting tumors. This may be controlled with concurrent use of a β-adrenergic antagonist. α-Adrenergic blockade must be initiated before β-adrenergic blockade to avoid paradoxic hypertension. AEs of phenoxybenzamine are sedation, weakness, nasal congestion, hypertension, and tachycardia.

## PERIPHERAL $A_1$-ADRENERGIC ANTAGONISTS

### CLASS MECHANISMS OF ACTION

Drugs of the peripheral $\alpha_1$-adrenergic antagonist class, including doxazosin, prazosin, and terazosin, are selective antagonists of the postsynaptic $\alpha_1$-adrenergic receptor. These drugs, which blunt the increases in arteriolar and venous tone mediated by norepinephrine released from sympathetic nerve terminals, act at the $\alpha_1$-adrenergic receptor located postjunctionally in the blood vessel wall. The affinity of these drugs for the $\alpha_2$ receptor is very low. Because of the selective $\alpha_1$ action, there is no interference with the negative feedback control mechanisms that are mediated by the prejunctional $\alpha_2$ receptors. As a result, the reflex tachycardia associated with the blockade of the presynaptic $\alpha_2$ receptor decreases substantially. The pharmacokinetic and pharmacodynamic properties of these drugs are shown in Tables 49.25 and 49.26.

### CLASS MEMBERS

Doxazosin is a selective long-acting $\alpha_1$-adrenergic antagonist. The initial antihypertensive dosage is 1 mg daily. This dose can be titrated up to a maximum of 16 mg daily. The maximal antihypertensive effect is seen 4 to 8 hours after a single dose. The drug is highly plasma protein bound and extensively metabolized. Most of the administered dose is excreted in the feces. The estimated half-life ranges from 9 to 22 hours. Doxazosin pharmacokinetics are not altered in patients with impaired kidney function. The drug should be used with caution in patients with advanced liver dysfunction.

Prazosin is a selective $\alpha_1$-adrenergic antagonist that is structurally related to doxazosin. Oral dosing is 3 to 20 mg/

**Table 49.25 Pharmacokinetic Properties of Peripheral $\alpha_1$-Adrenergic Antagonists**

| Drug | Bioavailability (%) | Affected by Food | Peak Blood Level (h) | Elimination Half-Life (h) | Metabolism | Excretion | Active Metabolites |
|---|---|---|---|---|---|---|---|
| Doxazosin (Cardura) | 62–69 | No | 2–5 | 9–22 | L | F (63%–65%)<br>U (1%–9%) | — |
| Prazosin (Minipress) | — | No | 1–3 | 2–4 | L | F | — |
| Terazosin (Hytrin) | 90 | Yes | 1 | 12 | L | F (45%–60%)<br>U (10%) | — |

*F,* Feces; *L,* liver; *U,* urine.

**Table 49.26 Pharmacodynamic Properties of Peripheral $\alpha_1$-Adrenergic Antagonists**

| Drug | Initial Dose (mg) | Usual Dose (mg) | Maximum Dose (mg) | Interval | Peak Response (h) | Duration of Response (h) |
|---|---|---|---|---|---|---|
| Doxazosin | 1 | 8 | 16 | qd, qid | 4–8 | 24 |
| Prazosin | 1 | 3–20 | 20 | bid, qid | 0.5–1.5 | 10 |
| Terazosin | 1 | 5 | 20 | qd, bid | 3 | 24 |

*bid,* Two times a day; *qd,* once a day; *qid,* four times a day.

day. Full therapeutic effects are seen within 4 to 8 weeks after initiation of therapy. Peak serum levels are reached 1 to 3 hours after an oral dose. The drug is highly protein bound with an elimination half-life of 2 to 4 hours. There is extensive hepatic metabolism followed by renal excretion of a very small amount of unchanged drug. Dose adjustment is not required for patients with CKD. Patients with significant liver disease may require dose adjustment and more frequent monitoring.

Terazosin is a selective, long-acting $\alpha_1$-adrenergic antagonist that has structural similarities to prazosin and doxazosin. The initial dosage is 1 mg orally at bedtime, with titration to 5 mg daily. Doses of 10 to 20 mg orally have been given. Peak serum levels after oral administration occur within 1 hour. The half-life is approximately 12 hours. Terazosin is extensively metabolized in the liver and eliminated primarily through the biliary tract. Pharmacokinetics are not affected by CKD, and dose adjustment is not required. Patients with severe hepatic insufficiency may require dose adjustments.

## CLASS RENAL EFFECTS

GFR and renal blood flow are maintained during long-term treatment. In some studies, there was a slight increase in renal blood flow. Renal vascular resistance may be reduced, perhaps mediated by a reduction in preglomerular capillary resistance related to inhibition of $\alpha_1$-mediated vasoconstriction. Urinary protein excretion has been reported to be reduced. The RAAS is not significantly affected by specific $\alpha_1$-adrenergic antagonists. Extracellular fluid volume has been reported to be increased, and fractional excretion may be decreased.

## CLASS EFFICACY AND SAFETY

Comparative clinical studies of the efficacy of $\alpha_1$-adrenergic blockers have shown that the antihypertensive responses are similar to those elicited by other antihypertensive drugs.[88] The availability of ER formulations of these drugs has improved tolerability. These drugs have been shown to increase insulin sensitivity[544] to exert potentially beneficial effects on lipid metabolism.[92,545–548] They can cause a modest reduction in total and LDL cholesterol and a small increase in HDL cholesterol levels. This metabolic benefit may be linked to the beneficial effect on insulin responsiveness, leading to increased peripheral glucose uptake.

There are also potential AEs of $\alpha_1$-adrenergic receptor blockers. In the Antihypertensive and Lipid-Lowering Treatment To Prevent Heart Attack Trial (ALLHAT), patients randomized to receive doxazosin as their initial antihypertensive drug were found to have poorer BP control than those receiving a chlorthalidone-based treatment.[549] No difference was seen in the primary outcomes of fatal coronary heart disease or nonfatal MI in patients, but patients randomized to doxazosin had higher rates of stroke and congestive heart failure.[550] Data from ALLHAT have largely relegated doxazosin and other peripheral $\alpha_1$-adrenergic antagonists to second-line agents in the management of hypertension.

$\alpha_1$-Adrenergic receptor blockers can also cause a first-dose orthostatic hypotension effect, resulting in ligh-theadedness, palpitations, and occasionally syncope. This is related to the drug effect on the venous capacitance vessels, which results in venous dilation and inadequate venous return. It may occur when peak drug levels are reached 30 to 90 minutes after the first dose; it can be minimized by initiating therapy with a small dose taken at bedtime.[551] This effect can be exacerbated in patients with underlying autonomic insufficiency.

$\alpha_1$-Adrenergic antagonists are also used for the symptomatic management of prostatic hypertrophy. Prostatic smooth muscle has significant $\alpha_1$-adrenal receptor expression. Blockade of these receptors results in smooth muscle relaxation within the prostate.[552,553] Terazosin has been marketed in combination with amlodipine for male patients with hypertension and lower urinary tract symptoms.[554]

### Renin Inhibitors

The earliest renin-inhibiting compounds in development included aliskiren, zankiren, and remikiren. However, because of problems with oral bioavailability, only aliskiren has been approved for the treatment of hypertension.

#### CLASS MECHANISM OF ACTION AND CLASS MEMBER

Aliskiren is an oral nonpeptide, low-molecular-weight renin inhibitor used for the management of hypertension (Fig. 49.2).[555,556] Renin inhibition interferes with the first and rate-limiting step in the renin enzyme cascade, the interaction of renin with its substrate angiotensinogen. The renin blockade step is an attractive target for hypertension therapeutics, in large part because of the remarkable specificity of renin for its substrate.[557] This specificity reduces the likelihood of unwanted interactions and possible AEs. In addition, unlike ACE inhibitors or ARBs, which lead to a reactive increase in renin and associated angiotensin peptides, direct renin inhibition renders the RAAS quiescent. Although aliskiren has low inherent bioavailability (2.6%), it is potent in reducing BP and has an effective half-life of 40 hours.[558] The drug is not actively metabolized by the liver and is primarily excreted in the urine, with most of it as unchanged drug. CYP enzymes are not involved in the metabolism of aliskiren. Thus clinically significant CYP inhibition by aliskiren is unlikely.[559]

#### CLASS RENAL EFFECTS

Experimental animal studies suggested that aliskiren may provide renal protection by reducing BP and urinary albumin excretion.[560–563] Clinical trial data in humans indicated that aliskiren reduces proteinuria in conjunction with decreasing BP.[557] In a study involving 600 patients with hypertension, diabetes, and nephropathy, the administration of aliskiren, 300 mg/day, facilitated a 20% incremental reduction in proteinuria compared with placebo in patients being treated concurrently with losartan, 100 mg/day. The baseline BP was 135 mm Hg with losartan treatment before random assignment to aliskiren therapy and did not change with the addition of aliskiren.[326] Renal vascular response curves for ACE inhibition or renin inhibition at the top of the dose–response curve indicated greater increase in renal blood flow with the renin inhibitor, despite similar changes in BP.[557] However, despite these encouraging clinical observations, a subsequent clinical trial, ALTITUDE, did not demonstrate an incremental benefit of aliskiren when used with an ACE inhibitor or ARB in patients with diabetic kidney disease when examining cardiovascular and renal endpoints.[256] From a safety standpoint, there were more adverse events in the patients receiving both classes of RAAS-blocking drugs.

#### CLASS EFFICACY AND SAFETY

Clinical trials of aliskiren have demonstrated a dose-dependent efficacy in reducing SBP and DBP. In an 8-week, double-blind, placebo-controlled trial, aliskiren was studied in dosages from 150 to 600 mg/day.[563] The placebo-corrected reduction in sitting SBP was approximately 10 to 11 mm Hg for both the 300- and 600-mg doses. Also evaluated in the same study was irbesartan, an ARB, at a dosage of 150 mg/day, which effectuated BP reduction comparable to that of aliskiren at a dosage of 150 mg/day. Other clinical studies have confirmed the antihypertensive efficacy of aliskiren compared with placebo or with other active therapies, such as the ARB losartan. As expected, BP reduction was comparable with that produced by the active agents. The only observed difference was suppression of plasma renin activity and Ang I and Ang II levels with aliskiren but increased levels of Ang I and Ang II with ARB therapy.

The tolerability of aliskiren is comparable to that of placebo, with a relatively low incidence of adverse events at all dosages tested in the 150- to 600-mg range.[563] Aliskiren treatment was comparable in tolerability to treatment with an ARB or placebo, with a low discontinuation rate and no statistical difference in the incidence of different types of adverse events, except for some diarrhea at the 600-mg dose.

Aliskiren has also been studied in combination with HCTZ, CCBs, ARBs, and ACE inhibitors in the management of hypertension.[564–567] In one small clinical trial, all patients received aliskiren 150 mg once daily for 3 weeks. Patients who had a daytime BP above 130/80 mm Hg, as measured by ambulatory BP monitoring, were given HCTZ, 25 mg daily, for an additional 3 weeks. Adding 25 mg of HCTZ resulted in an additional 10 mm Hg of SBP reduction. Not surprisingly, there was no difference in plasma renin activity between the patients receiving aliskiren with HCTZ and those receiving aliskiren alone. Adding aliskiren to amlodipine, valsartan, or ramipril provides incremental and statistically significant improvements in BP reduction. However, the ALTITUDE study did raise safety concerns about using aliskiren with other RAAS blocking drugs due specifically to declining kidney function and hyperkalemia.[255] The additional BP reduction may or may not be related to the neutralization of plasma renin activity that occurs with the addition of the renin inhibitor.

## SELECTIVE ALDOSTERONE RECEPTOR ANTAGONISTS

#### CLASS MECHANISM AND CLASS MEMBERS

Spironolactone and eplerenone are members of the class of MRAs. The mineralocorticoid receptor forms part of the steroid–thyroid–retinoid–orphan receptor family of nuclear transactivating factors.[568] When unbound, these receptors are in an inactive multiprotein complex of chaperones. On binding of aldosterone, the chaperones are released, and the receptor hormone complex is translocated into the nucleus, where it binds to hormone response elements on DNA and interacts with transcription initiation complexes, which ultimately modulate gene expression.[569] In the kidney, mineralocorticoid receptors are located primarily in the epithelial cells of the distal nephron. These receptors bind physiologic glucocorticoids and mineralocorticoids with a similar affinity. Activation of mineralocorticoid receptors by aldosterone results in the activation of epithelial sodium channels, which leads to a rapid increase in sodium and water reabsorption and promotes the tubular secretion of potassium.[570,571] A persistent increase in sodium balance does not occur, even with continued stimulation of mineralocorticoid receptors by aldosterone. The mechanism of the aldosterone escape phenomenon has not been fully elucidated.

There is evidence indicating the presence of biologic activity of mineralocorticoid receptors in nonepithelial tissues.[572] These receptors have been identified in blood vessels of the heart and brain and may be involved in vascular injury and repair responses.[520,573] Aldosterone mediates fibrosis and collagen formation through the upregulation of Ang II receptor responsiveness.[519,572] Aldosterone increases sodium influx in vascular smooth muscle and inhibits norepinephrine uptake in vascular smooth muscle and myocardial cells.[574] Aldosterone also directly participates in vascular smooth muscle cell hypertrophy.

Spironolactone and eplerenone are both inhibitors of the mineralocorticoid receptor. Spironolactone is a prodrug that is metabolized in the liver and excreted in the urine. The half-life of the prodrug is 1.3 to 2 hours whereas the half-life of the active metabolites ranges from 14 to 17 hours.

Eplerenone is approximately 24 times less potent than spironolactone but is more specific for blocking mineralocorticoid receptors with little agonist activity at estrogen and progesterone receptors.[575] Therefore eplerenone is associated with a lower incidence of gynecomastia, breast pain, and impotence in men and diminished libido and menstrual irregularities in women. The time to peak concentration is 1 to 2 hours. No significant accumulation occurs with multiple-dose administration, but up to 4 weeks may be required for the full antihypertensive effects to be evident. It appears to be well absorbed, but absolute (oral vs. intravenous) data are unavailable; specific data on protein binding and metabolism are also unavailable. The elimination half-life of eplerenone is 4 to 6 hours. Bioavailability is 69%, with approximately 50% protein binding. It is metabolized primarily by the hepatic CYP3A4 system to inactive metabolites excreted two-thirds in the urine and one-third in the feces.

### CLASS RENAL EFFECTS

Selective aldosterone receptor antagonism may have benefits for the kidney, independently of its effects on BP. Experimental and clinical studies have demonstrated that Ang II may be the primary mediator of the RAAS associated with the progression of renal disease.[576,577] The relative importance of aldosterone in this cascade has been the subject of experimental and clinical studies. Hyperaldosteronism and adrenal hypertrophy are common observations in remnant kidney models and correlate with progressive loss of renal function.[576] Hypertension, proteinuria, and structural injury are less prevalent in subtotally nephrectomized rats that have undergone adrenalectomy, even when administered large doses of replacement glucocorticoids.[578] Other investigators have demonstrated that aldosterone infusion can reverse the renal protective effects of an ACE inhibitor in stroke-prone, spontaneously hypertensive rats.[579] Interestingly, in this model, the kidney injury induced by aldosterone was independent of increases in BP, suggesting a toxic tissue effect of aldosterone. Other experimental studies have indicated that aldosterone receptor antagonism can prevent the development of proteinuria.[579]

Even though selective aldosterone receptor antagonists have no observable effects on glomerular hemodynamics, therapy with these drugs may provide an incremental effect in protecting the kidney when added to ACE inhibitors or ARBs by inhibiting the effects of aldosterone that persist, despite treatment with the latter drugs. Studies in patients with diabetic nephropathy or other glomerular diseases have demonstrated that the addition of spironolactone to ACE inhibition markedly reduces albuminuria.[580,581]

### CLASS EFFICACY AND SAFETY

These medications can be very effective for BP control, particularly in patients with resistant hypertension. In the PATHWAY-2 trial, a double-blind, placebo-controlled, crossover trial, 285 patients with resistant hypertension received spironolactone, doxazosin, bisoprolol or placebo as the fourth agent.[581a] During spironolactone therapy versus placebo, the participants' average home systolic BP decreased by 8.7 mm Hg (95% CI, 7.7 to 9.7 $P < .001$). Spironolactone was also superior to doxazosin and bisoprolol. The drug was generally well tolerated; the rates of discontinuations due to renal impairment, hyperkalemia, and gynecomastia were not increased with spironolactone relative to other treatments and placebo. Collectively, these data suggest that spironolactone at 25 to 50 mg/day is an effective treatment option for individuals with resistant hypertension (uncontrolled on three or more medicines including a diuretic).

Eplerenone is less potent than spironolactone and has a shorter half-life (3–4 hours), leading to reduced antihypertensive efficacy and a requirement for twice-daily dosing.[582] A study of 52 patients has demonstrated the efficacy of the selective aldosterone blocker eplerenone at a dose of 50 to 100 mg daily in patients with resistant hypertension. After eplerenone treatment, the clinical BP was reduced by 18/8 mm Hg compared with baseline ($P < .0001$ for SBPs and DBPs).[583] Individuals treated with aldosterone antagonists require careful monitoring for hyperkalemia.

A meta-analysis of RCTs has shown a positive effect of these agents on changes in the cardiac structure and left ventricular function in patients with heart failure.[584] The role of aldosterone antagonists in treating hypertensive obese patients with sleep apnea has been reported, representing approximately 20% of all individuals with sleep apnea. The aldosterone production relates directly to the adipocyte.[585–588] In the PATHWAY-2 trial, patients with resistant hypertension (defined as uncontrolled BP despite three antihypertensive agents) were randomized to receive add-on treatment with spironolactone, doxazosin, bisoprolol, or placebo. Spironolactone was the most effective, reducing SBP by approximately 4 mm compared with the other active antihypertensive agents.

When using MRAs, patients must be monitored for hyperkalemia, particularly among those with CKD, and those without CKD using ACE inhibitor or ARBs. MRAs are not recommended for use among patients with eGFR lower than 30 mL/min/1.73 m$^2$.

## TYROSINE HYDROXYLASE INHIBITOR

### MECHANISMS OF ACTION

Metyrosine, the only drug in the tyrosine hydroxylase inhibitor class, blocks the rate-limiting step in the biosynthetic pathway of catecholamines. Metyrosine inhibits tyrosine hydroxylase, the enzyme responsible for the conversion of tyrosine to dihydroxyphenylalanine. This inhibition results in decreased levels of endogenous catecholamines. In patients with pheochromocytomas, metyrosine reduces catecholamine biosynthesis by up to 80%, resulting in a decrease in total peripheral vascular resistance. Heart rate and cardiac output increase because of the vasodilation. It is used primarily for the management of pheochromocytoma.

#### CLASS MEMBER

The recommended initial dosage of metyrosine is 250 mg four times a day orally. The dose may be increased by 250 to 500 mg every day until a maximum of 4 g/day is given. Following oral absorption, metyrosine is eliminated primarily unchanged in the urine. The half-life is 7.2 hours. Dose reduction is appropriate in patients with CKD.

#### RENAL EFFECTS

Little information is available on the renal effects of metyrosine. On the basis of its mechanism of action, which would counteract the renal effects of excessive circulating catecholamines, renal plasma flow and glomerular filtration would be expected to increase and renal vascular resistance would be expected to decrease.

#### EFFICACY AND SAFETY

Metyrosine is used in the preoperative or intraoperative management of pheochromocytoma. Hypertension and reflex tachycardia may result from vasodilation. These effects can be minimized by volume expansion. AEs include sedation, changes in sleep patterns, and extrapyramidal signs. Metyrosine crystals have been noted in the urine in patients receiving high dosages. Patients taking metyrosine should maintain a generous fluid intake; some patients have occasionally experienced diarrhea.

**Table 49.27 Categories of Blood Pressure in Adults**

| BP Category | SBP | | DBP |
|---|---|---|---|
| Normal | <120 mm Hg | And | <80 mm Hg |
| Elevated | 120–129 mm Hg | And | <80 mm Hg |
| Hypertension | | | |
| Stage 1 | 130–139 mm Hg | Or | 80–89 mm Hg |
| Stage 2 | >140 Hg | Or | >90 mm Hg |

Individuals with SBP and DBP in 2 categories should be designated to the higher BP category.

*BP,* Blood pressure (based on an average of ≥2 readings obtained on ≥2 occasions); *DBP,* diastolic blood pressure; *SBP,* systolic blood pressure.

From Whelton PK, Carey RM, Aronow WS, et al. ACC/AHA/AAPA/ABC/ACPM/AGS/APhA/ASH/ASPC/NMA/PCNA guideline for the prevention, detection, evaluation, and management of high blood pressure in adults: executive summary: a report of the American College of Cardiology/American Heart Association Task Force on clinical practice guidelines. *Circulation*. 2018;138:e426–e483.

## SELECTION OF ANTIHYPERTENSIVE DRUG THERAPY

### DETERMINATION OF BLOOD PRESSURE GOAL

Numerous factors confound the management of hypertension, which is often a lifelong, progressive, asymptomatic disease process.

The purpose of treating BP elevation is to primarily decrease the risk of cardiovascular events and improve survival and quality of life.

Clinicians must ask themselves three major questions:

- How low should the BP go?
- What drugs should be used?
- What are the best strategies for facilitating the attainment of the target BP?

The recent ACC/AHA guidelines defined normal BP as less than 120/80 mm Hg, stage 1 hypertension as SBP of 130 to 139 mm Hg or DBP of 80 to 89 whereas stage 2 hypertension was defined by SBP of 140 mm Hg (or higher) or DBP of 90 mm Hg (or higher) (Table 49.27).[55] These BP thresholds significantly revised the previous BP cut-offs recommended by the Seventh Report of the Joint National Committee on Prevention, Detection, Evaluation, and Treatment of High Blood pressure (JNC7).[83] Apart from metaanalyses of observational studies that suggested an excess risk of stroke, MI, heart failure, and cardiovascular death with SBP greater than 120 mm Hg, the landmark SPRINT trial demonstrated that compared with the standard SBP goal of less than 140 mm Hg, the intensive SBP goal of less than 120 mm Hg resulted in 25% lower risk of a cardiovascular composite (nonfatal MI, acute coronary syndrome, nonfatal stroke, or cardiovascular death or hospitalized heart failure) and a 27% lower risk of all-cause mortality.[18,20,589]

However, the American College of Physicians/American Academy of Family Physicians (ACP/AAFP) guidelines still recommended an SBP goal of less than 150 mm Hg in persons aged 60 years or older and less than 140 mm Hg in persons with cardiovascular risk.[590] The concerns for the widespread adoption into routine clinical practice of SPRINT findings include questions on generalizability to the elderly, in persons with diabetes or advanced CKD, potential AEs including on the kidneys, and the effects of lowering SBP on DBP. These issues are discussed sequentially later.

The SPRINT trial included a subgroup of 2636 adults aged 75 years or older (mean baseline age 79.9 years). In a prespecified analysis of this subgroup, treatment to the intensive SBP goal was associated with a 34% (95% CI, 15%–49%) lower risk of the primary composite outcome relative to a standard SBP target.[591] By contrast, the incidence of serious adverse events (hazard ratio [HR], 0.99; 95% CI, 0.89–1.11) and injurious falls (HR, 0.91; 95% CI, 0.65–1.29) in the intensive and standard SBP groups were similar in the older SPRINT subgroup. Furthermore, in the older patient subgroup, the benefits of intensive SBP lowering did not differ substantially by baseline frailty status, and indeed, participants who were the frailest at baseline had the most pronounced reduction in risk of the primary composite cardiovascular outcome with the intensive SBP target. Similarly, in the Hypertension in the Very Elderly Trial (HYVET), frailty also did not modify the benefits of BP lowering.[592]

The current ACC/AHA guideline recommends a BP target less than 130/80 mm Hg for persons with diabetes. The issue of BP targets in adults with diabetes has been controversial because the primary results of the ACCORD BP trial did not show evidence of beneficial effects of intensive SBP lowering

(SBP goal <120 mm Hg) compared with standard SBP goal (<140 mm Hg) in 4733 adults with type 2 diabetes mellitus. Differences in BP measurement techniques, differences in the achieved SBP separation,[593,594] and differences in selection criteria have been proposed as potential explanations for the discrepant findings between SPRINT and ACCORD BP. Perhaps, the most widely cited reason is a lack of statistical power in ACCORD BP.[594,595] However, this reason is unlikely because the number of events and event rates were actually higher in the ACCORD BP compared with SPRINT.

Of note, in addition to randomization to the intensive or standard SBP goals, ACCORD BP participants were randomized in a 2 × 2 factorial design to either standard glucose lowering (target hemoglobin A1c 7.0%–7.9%) or intensive glucose lowering (glycosylated hemoglobin A1c <6.0%).[596] The intensive glucose lowering arm was discontinued after 3.5 years because of an increased risk of all-cause death (HR, 1.35; 95% CI, 1.04–1.76)[596] but the two BP arms were completed over 5 years and were not terminated prematurely. An alternative explanation for the discrepant findings of ACCORD BP and SPRINT is that an interaction between the intensive glycemia intervention and the intensive SBP-lowering intervention in ACCORD BP may have masked the potential beneficial effects of the SBP intervention. This hypothesis is supported by a recent reanalysis of ACCORD BP and SPRINT data.[597] Intensive SBP lowering decreased the hazard of the composite CVD endpoint similarly in SPRINT (HR, 0.75; 95% CI, 0.64–0.89) and the ACCORD BP standard glycemia arm (HR, 0.77; 95% CI, 0.63–0.95, interaction $P$ = .87). However, the effect of intensive SBP lowering on the composite CVD endpoint in the ACCORD BP intensive glycemia arm (HR, 1.04; 95% CI, 0.83–1.29) was significantly different from SPRINT (interaction $P$ = .02).

Intensive SBP lowering in SPRINT resulted in a 3.5-fold higher hazard of incident CKD among participants without CKD at baseline[597] and a 65% higher risk of AKI.[597,598] Although the cardiovascular and survival benefits of intensive SBP lowering appear to outweigh the risk of these kidney events during the trial, the long-term effects on kidney outcomes and kidney function remain to be determined.

Despite the success of SPRINT, lowering of DBP as a consequence of the SPRINT intensive therapy intervention has been cited as a cause for concern in adopting SPRINT findings in routine clinical practice.[599,600] There are a number of reports of J-shaped curves indicating associations of both low and high DBPs with worse CVD outcomes. The concept was first reported by Stewart in 1979[601] and subsequently championed by Cruickshank in the 1980s.[602] An appraisal of studies conducted in the 1980s concluded that low on-treatment DBP levels (i.e., <85 mm Hg) were associated with increased risk of cardiac events.[603] These findings were supported by subsequent cohort (observational) studies.[604,605] Secondary analyses of achieved BPs in RCTs of BP-lowering treatments[606–608] or non–BP-lowering interventions[609] also suggested that a low achieved DBP was associated with worse CVD outcomes.

Biological plausibility for the J-curve phenomenon has been proposed.[602,603] As most of the ventricular myocardial perfusion occurs during diastole, particularly in persons with LVH (increased oxygen demand) and coronary artery disease (decreased oxygen supply), lower DBP could potentially lead to myocardial hypoperfusion and associated damage. Indeed, in the Atherosclerosis Risk In Communities (ARIC) cohort, lower DBP was associated with increased serum concentrations of cardiac troponin T, a marker of myocardial injury.[600]

Based on the aforementioned observational studies of cohort or postrandomization achieved BP data sets, strong causal inferences on lowering DBP have been drawn.[600,603–607,609] For instance, depending upon the observed threshold in the given study, various lower bounds of DBP have been proposed below which DBP lowering is considered deleterious.

Although the existence of the J-curve phenomenon has been disputed by some,[610–612] the central question is whether the J-curve phenomenon observed in some of the aforementioned studies reflects a causal effect of lower DBP on CVD outcomes. It is conceivable that underlying processes (such as increased arterial stiffness) that lead to a decline in DBP rather than the level of DBP per se might be the reason for the observed associations of worse outcomes with lower DBP. Statistical modeling and multivariable regression are typically employed in observational data analyses, but residual confounding could still explain observed results. The most direct and valid method of testing the J-curve hypothesis is to actively intervene to lower DBP, particularly in those with DBP lower than 70 mm Hg; if lowering DBP is deleterious below a certain DBP level, one would expect that the effects of lowering SBP on CVD outcomes and death would be modified by baseline level of DBP.

In SPRINT, irrespective of the randomized treatment, baseline DBP had a U-shaped association with the hazard of the primary CVD outcome.[613] However, in randomized comparisons between the intensive and standard treatment groups, the effect of the intensive SBP intervention on the primary outcome was not modified by baseline DBP. Results were similar for all-cause death and kidney events; in other words, the beneficial effect of intensive SBP lowering on survival and the deleterious effect on incident CKD were present and similar in magnitude irrespective of the baseline DBP. Therefore there was no evidence that lowering SBP in those with low DBP worsened CVD outcomes. A recent causal mediation analysis of achieved low DBP in SPRINT also supports this observation.[614]

Thus the ACC/AHA guidelines of SBP goal of less than 130 mm Hg is supported by evidence.

The promptness of achieving BP control has long been thought to be an important strategy for the clinical care for patients with hypertension. Clinical trials and observational studies have indicated that initiating treatment with a two-drug combination of medications results in a more rapid achievement of target BP goals compared with monotherapy. A retrospective analysis of the Valsartan Antihypertensive Long-term Use Evaluation (VALUE) trial has indicated that earlier BP control results in a significant reduction in the 5-year risk of cardiovascular events, regardless of the type of medication used.[615] A matched cohort study has demonstrated that initial combination therapy reduces the risk of cardiovascular events in hypertensive patients.[365] This reduction was thought to be related to an earlier achievement of target BP as the main contributor of risk reduction.

Decisions about which drug(s) should be used for a given patient require careful consideration and individualization. As addressed later, the appropriate pharmacotherapy may depend on age, sex, race, obesity, and associated cardiovascular or renal disease. Clinical trials in patients with vascular disease, heart disease, or kidney disease have demonstrated the important therapeutic advantage of drugs that block the RAAS—ACE inhibitors or ARBs[76,248,249,616–621] to prevent progression of cardiovascular or kidney disease as part of a multidrug regimen to lower BP. In the aggregate, RAAS inhibitors provide an approximately 20% RR reduction benefit compared with other therapies. These drugs should be part of every antihypertensive regimen in patients with heart disease or kidney disease unless there are specific contraindications.[618] RAAS-blocking drugs are also some of the best-tolerated therapies available for treating hypertension. Although these drugs provide important risk reduction opportunities, they are not a substitute for achieving BP control.

## SINGLE-PILL COMBINATION THERAPY

Most available antihypertensive drugs, when appropriately dosed, reduce SBP by approximately 8 to 10 mm Hg (Fig. 49.3). For many patients, three or four drugs may be required. Ideally, medications that are long-acting, can be taken once daily, are well tolerated, and preferably work well with other medications to facilitate BP control should be used. In addition, there has been a marked increase in the number of single-pill, fixed-dose combination antihypertensive drugs that are available in the marketplace, developed in large part to facilitate adherence by reducing the complexity of the antihypertensive regimen (Table 49.28).[622]

The recommended first-line agents include thiazide diuretics, CCBs, and ACE inhibitors or ARBs. Chlorthalidone is a more potent antihypertensive than HCTZ. The advantage of a low-dose thiazide or thiazide-like drug is that it nearly doubles the antihypertensive effects of the parent drug without adding toxicity to the regimen (Fig. 49.4).[623] Drugs that block the RAAS system, such as ACE inhibitors or ARBs in combination with chlorthalidone or HCTZ, are a very effective combination to control BP. Single-pill combinations of an ACE inhibitor or ARB with CCB are also available. Clinical studies have demonstrated that these drugs are also additive in their ability to lower DBPs and SBPs.[624–628] Moreover, use of an ACE inhibitor or ARB in combination with a CCB abrogates the development of pedal edema, a common AE of CCBs.[629] Two triple single-pill combinations (ARB, CCB, and HCTZ) have been approved for the treatment of hypertension.[630] An ARB has also been formulated with the thiazide-like diuretic chlorthalidone. Some single-pill combinations are now approved by the U.S. FDA for initial treatment in patients with moderate-to-severe hypertension.

Considerations for physicians about how to consolidate and simplify pharmacotherapy to control BP are of great interest, given the complexity of the current multidrug regimens that many patients require. Administering four drugs

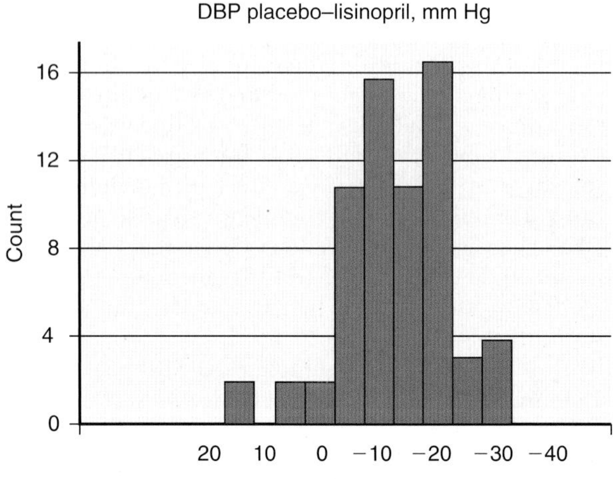


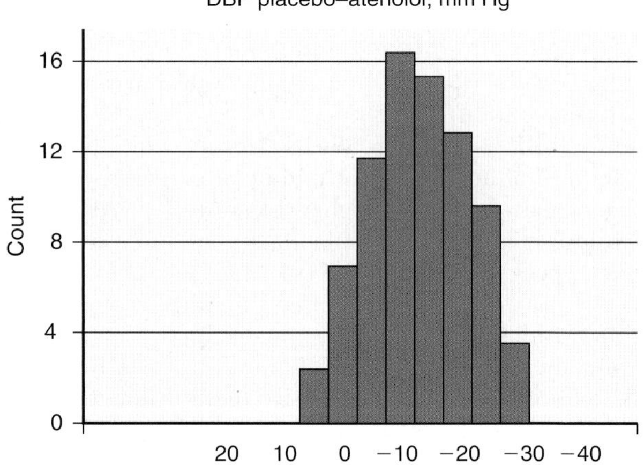


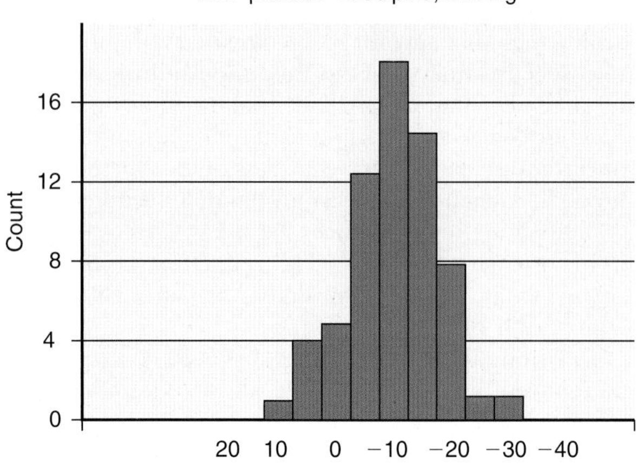


**Fig. 49.3** Frequency distribution of changes in diastolic blood pressure *(DBP)* produced by three different antihypertensive drugs. Negative values represent placebo-corrected reductions in diastolic pressure. A meta-analysis of placebo-controlled trials of monotherapy in unselected hypertensives reports averaged placebo-corrected blood pressure responses to single agents of 9.1 mm Hg systolic and 5.5 mm Hg diastolic pressures. These average values disguise the extremely wide-ranging responses in individuals across a fall of 20 to 30 mm Hg systolic pressure at one extreme, to no effect at all, or even a small rise in blood pressure at the other. (Modified from Attwood S, Bird R, Burch K, et al. Within-patient correlation between the antihypertensive effects of atenolol, lisinopril and nifedepin. *J Hypertens.* 1994;12:1053–1060.)

**Table 49.28 Single-Pill Combinations Available for the Treatment of Hypertension[622]**

| Type of Combination | First Drug (Doses) | Second Drug (Doses) | Third Drug (Doses) |
|---|---|---|---|
| **Dual Combinations** | | | |
| Thiazide/K sparing diuretic | HCTZ (25/50) | Triamterene (37.5/75) | |
| | HCTZ (25/50) | Spironolactone (25/50) | |
| | HCTZ (25/50) | Amiloride (2.5/5) | |
| | Furosemide (20) | Spironolactone (50) | |
| ACE inhibitor/diuretic | Captopril (25/50) | HCTZ (15/25) | |
| | Enalapril (10/20) | HCTZ (12.5/25) | |
| | Lisinopril (10/20) | HCTZ (12.5/25) | |
| | Cilazapril (5) | HCTZ (12.5) | |
| | Fosinopril (10/20) | HCTZ (12.5) | |
| | Quinapril (10/20) | HCTZ (12.5) | |
| | Benazepril (5/10/20) | HCTZ (6.25/12.5/25) | |
| | Moexipril (7.5/15) | HCTZ (12.5/25) | |
| | Ramipril (2/5) | HCTZ (12.5/25) | |
| | Ramipril (5) | Piretanide (6) | |
| | Zofenopril (30) | HCTZ (12.5) | |
| | Perindopril (2.5/5/10) | Indapamide (0.625/1.25, 2.5) | |
| ACE inhibitor/CCB | Perindopril (5/10) | Amlodipine (5/10) | |
| | Benazepril (10/20/40) | Amlodipine (2.5/5/10) | |
| | Enalapril (5) | Diltiazem (180) | |
| | Enalapril (10) | Nitrendipine (20) | |
| | Enalapril (10/20) | Lercanidipine (10) | |
| | Ramipril (2.5/5) | Felodipine ER (2.5/5) | |
| | Trandolapril (1/2/4) | Verapamil (180, 240) | |
| | Delapril (10) | Manidipine (30) | |
| ARB/diuretic | Losartan (50/100) | HCTZ (12.5/25) | |
| | Valsartan (80/160) | HCTZ (12.5/25) | |
| | Irbesartan (150/300) | HCTZ (12.5/25) | |
| | Candesartan (8/16/32) | HCTZ (12.5/25) | |
| | Telmisartan (40/80) | HCTZ (12.5) | |
| | Eprosartan (600) | HCTZ (12.5/25) | |
| | Olmesartan (20/40) | HCTZ (12.5/25) | |
| | Azilsartan (40) | Chlorthalidone (12.5/25) | |
| ARB/CCB | Valsartan (80/160) | Amlodipine (5/10) | |
| | Telmisartan (40/80) | Amlodipine (5/10) | |
| | Olmesartan (20/40) | Amlodipine (5/10) | |
| | Candesartan (8) | Amlodipine (5)[a] | |
| | Irbesartan (100/150) | Amlodipine (5/10)[a] | |
| Renin inhibitor/diuretic | Aliskiren (150/300) | HCTZ (12.5/25) | |
| Renin inhibitor/CCB | Aliskiren (150/300) | Amlodipine (5/10) | |
| β-Blocker/diuretic | Atenolol (50/100) | Chlorthalidone (25) | |
| | Atenolol (50) | HCTZ (25) | |
| | Metoprolol (50/100) | HCTZ (25/50) | |
| | Bisoprolol (2.5/5/10) | HCTZ (6.25) | |
| | Bisoprolol (1) | Chlorthalidone (25) | |
| | Nadolol (40/80) | Bendroflumethiazide (5) | |
| | Oxprenolol (120) | Chlorthalidone (20) | |
| | Pindolol (10) | Clopamide (5) | |
| | Propranolol (40/80) | HCTZ (25) | |
| | Propranolol LA (80/160) | HCTZ (50) | |
| | Timolol (10) | HCTZ (25) | |
| β-Blocker/CCB | Atenolol (25/50) | Nifedipine (10/20) | |
| | Metoprolol (50/100) | Felodipine (5/10) | |
| α-Blocker/diuretic | Methyldopa (250) | HCTZ (15) | |
| | Clonidine (0.1/0.2/0.3) | Chlorthalidone (15) | |
| | Reserpine (0.1) | HCTZ (10) | |
| **Triple Combinations** | | | |
| ARB/CCB/diuretic | Valsartan (160/320) | Amlodipine (5/10) | HCTZ (12.5/25) |
| | Olmesartan (20/40) | Amlodipine (5/10) | HCTZ (12.5/25) |
| | Telmisartan (40/80) | Amlodipine (5/10) | HCTZ (12.5/25) |
| ACE inhibitor/CCB/diuretic | Perindopril (5/10) | Amlodipine (5/10) | Indapamide (1.25/2.5) |
| Renin inhibitor/CCB/diuretic | Aliskiren (150/300) | Amlodipine (5/10) | HCTZ (12.5/25) |

[a]Some dosages may be available only in certain countries. The list is not exhaustive.

*ACE,* Angiotensin-converting enzyme; *ARB,* angiotensin receptor blocker; *CCB,* calcium channel blocker; *ER,* extended release; *HCTZ,* hydrochlorothiazide; *K,* potassium; *LA,* long acting.

From Burnier M. Antihypertensive combination treatment: state of the art. *Curr Hyperten Rep*. 2015;17:51.

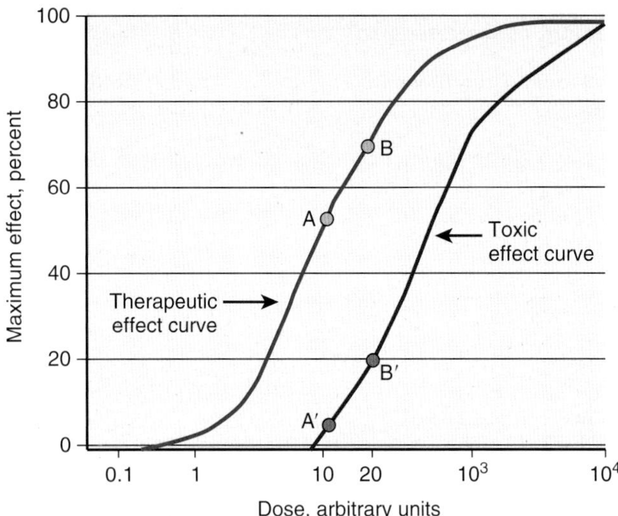


**Fig. 49.4** Dose relationship between therapeutic effect and toxicity with antihypertensive drugs. For the initial therapy of hypertension, a strategy to reduce side effects and enhance the tolerability of multiple antihypertensive drugs in combination has been identified using low doses of more than one antihypertensive agent with different combined modes of action to minimize side effects. With a low dose of drug A, a partial therapeutic effect is obtained, and adverse effects (A′) are minimal. If the dose is raised to B, a greater therapeutic effect will be accompanied by more adverse effects (B′). If a low dose of a second drug is added with its own minimal side effects, an extra effect will be obtained without more adverse effects, which will remain at A′. (Modified from Epstein M, Bakris G. Newer approaches to antihypertensive therapy. Use of fixed-dose combination therapy. *Arch Intern Med.* 1996;156:1969–1978.)

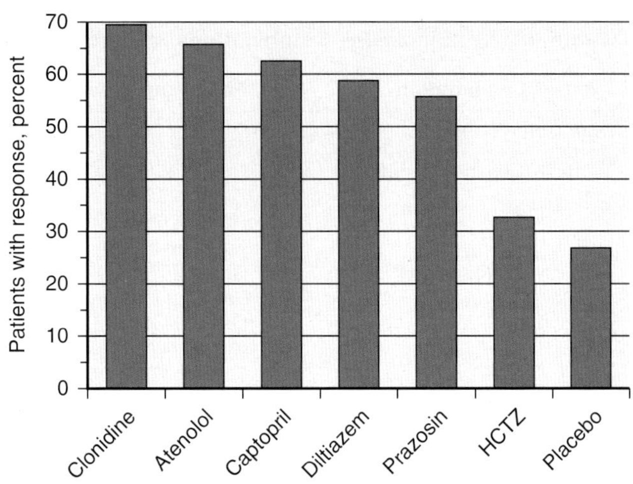


**Fig. 49.5** Antihypertensive response to different drugs for white individuals younger than 60 years of age. Hydrochlorothiazide *(HCTZ)* appears to be the least effective as a single agent. (From Materson BJ, Reda DJ, Cushman WC, et al. Single-drug therapy for hypertension in men. A comparison of six antihypertensive agents with placebo. The Department of Veterans Affairs Cooperative Study Group on Antihypertensive Agents. *N Engl J Med.* 1993;328:914–921.)

in two pills or three drugs in a single pill is possible with available fixed-dose combinations. This goal is important because many patients require eight to ten or more medications to control their various medical problems, including diabetes, dyslipidemia, and angina. Hypertension is a disease that is largely asymptomatic and, consequently, to optimize adherence, the therapeutic approach should be simple, effective, and well tolerated.

## CHOICE OF APPROPRIATE AGENTS

This section considers the initial therapy for various types of patients depending on factors such as age, sex, race/ethnicity, obesity, and coexistent cardiovascular or renal disease. These suggestions are primarily generalizations based on clinical experience and should not be viewed as rigorous guidelines. Because each patient is different, variation in the approach is frequently necessary (Fig. 49.5).

### TREATMENT OF OLDER PATIENTS

Older patients frequently have vascular stiffening, leading to an increase in SBP, decrease in diastolic pressure, and wider pulse pressure.[631] Management of isolated systolic hypertension in older patients frequently requires multiple drugs. A careful assessment of the metabolic and excretory routes of the drugs, as well as possible drug–drug interactions, is recommended because older patients frequently have impaired metabolic function. As shown by the SPRINT experience, BP control can be safely achieved in elderly individuals, even in those who are frail.[591]

Older patients have a higher likelihood of orthostasis than younger patients, due in part to a reduction in cardiovascular baroreceptor reflex function. As many as 18% of untreated older patients with hypertension have a decrease in SBP of more than 20 mm Hg after standing for 1 to 3 minutes.[632] Older patients may also have pseudohypertension, which may interfere with a true determination of BP.[633] Consequently, three-position BP measurements should always be used during the initiation and titration of medications. Older patients are also more likely to have hypertrophic cardiomyopathy with impaired diastolic function than are younger patients, which may impair cardiac output.[634]

Older patients may benefit from the use of a vasodilators such as CCBs, α-blockers, or ACE inhibitors and ARBs (Table 49.29). They are much better tolerated in the lower half of their dosing range and are quite effective even in the presence of a high-salt diet, perhaps owing to their natriuretic effects[635] or intrinsic vasodilatory effects.[636,637] α-Blockers may be useful in older men with benign prostatic hyperplasia because they facilitate prostatic urethral relaxation and improve urinary stream. ACE inhibitors and ARBs are well tolerated, and their efficacy is enhanced when they are combined with thiazide and thiazide-type diuretics.

Thiazide and thiazide-type diuretics may also have a vasodilating effect.[55] The ACC/AHA guidelines recommend chlorthalidone as the preferred thiazide as it is more potent than HCTZ. An ongoing pragmatic point-of-care clinical trial will randomize veterans aged 65 years and older to receive chlorthalidone or HCTZ to assess whether there is a difference in cardiovascular events.[638] The initial dose of chlorthalidone is 12.5 mg/day and if needed, can be increased to 25 mg/day. At doses more than 25 mg/day, the risk of side effects is higher with a lower incremental BP benefit. Hence, instead of increasing chlorthalidone to more than 25 mg another

**Table 49.29 Considerations for Initial Therapy in Older Patients**

| Clinical Observation | Pharmacologic Considerations |
|---|---|
| Decreased vascular compliance and peripheral vascular resistance | Use vasodilator (e.g., HCTZ, ACE inhibitor, ARB, CCB, α-blocker). |
| Isolated systolic hypertension and wide pulse pressure | Use vasodilator (e.g., HCTZ, CCB). |
| Reduction of cardiovascular baroreflex function with blood pressure lability | Avoid sympatholytics and volume depletion. Use β-blockers cautiously. |
| Orthostatic hypertension during recumbency | Consider using short-acting medications (<8-h duration) at bedtime. |
| Reduced metabolic capability | Adjust all medications for renal and hepatic function; start at half-dose. |
| Prostatic hypertrophy | Use α-blocker. |
| >20 mm Hg from systolic goal | Use fixed-dose combination therapy (ACE inhibitor/CCB, ARB/CCB, ACE inhibitor/HCTZ, ARB/HCTZ, β-blocker/HCTZ). |

*ACE,* Angiotensin-converting enzyme; *ARB,* angiotensin II receptor blocker; *CCB,* calcium channel blocker; *HCTZ,* thiazide diuretic.

agent should be added if BP control is not achieved with 25 mg/day of chlorthalidone.

## TREATMENT BASED ON SEX

Sex differences may help to guide the selection of antihypertensive therapy (Table 49.30).[639] Men and women benefit equally from a more intensive control of BP, which results in a reduction in the risk of cardiovascular events.[640] In general, men have a lower resting heart rate, longer left ventricular ejection fraction time, and higher pulse pressure when stressed than women.[639] Women tend to have lower peripheral vascular resistance and a relatively higher blood volume for overall size than men[639]; they also have a lower likelihood of coronary disease before menopause. However, when menopause occurs, or in the presence of diabetes, women have the same risk of coronary disease as men.[639] Vasodilation is always a good choice for treatment because elevated peripheral vascular resistance is almost always involved in BP elevation, regardless of sex. Thiazide diuretics, ACE inhibitors, ARBs, and CCBs are all effective treatments. Many patients require two or more of these drugs, and fixed-dose combinations can be used.

Women should avoid the use of ACE inhibitors and ARBs in pregnancy because of their possible teratogenic effects. CCBs may delay labor. Optimal therapy in a pregnant woman remains α-methyldopa, hydralazine, or β-blockers because they have a safety record with a minimal risk of teratogenic effects on the fetus (Table 49.6).

Women experience higher rates of osteoporosis and osteopenia than do men. In women (and men) with osteoporosis, thiazide and thiazide-like diuretics may antagonize calciuria and facilitate bone mineralization.[641]

**Table 49.30 Considerations for Initial Therapy Based on Gender**

| Clinical Observation | Pharmacologic Considerations |
|---|---|
| Men have lower resting heart rate, longer left ventricular ejection time, and higher stressed pulse pressure compared with women. | Use vasodilator (e.g., HCTZ, ACE inhibitor, ARB, CCB). |
| Women have lower total peripheral resistance and greater blood volume compared with men. | Use drugs that provide vasodilation, heart rate reduction; may need diuresis (e.g., HCTZ, ACE inhibitor, ARB, β-blocker, CCB). |
| Postmenopausal women more frequently have coronary artery disease with atypical chest pain. | Use drugs that counter angina and reduce heart rate (β-blocker, CCB). |
| Osteoporosis | Antagonize calciuria (HCTZ). |
| Pregnancy | Avoid teratogenic drugs (ACE inhibitor, ARB). Avoid drugs that may cause ureteroplacental insufficiency (loop diuretics). Optimal choices are α-methyldopa, hydralazine, and β-blockers. |
| Women report more pedal edema with CCBs and cough with ACE inhibitors than men. | Adjust dosage or discontinue drug. |
| More than 20 mm Hg from systolic goal | Use fixed-dose combination therapy (ACE inhibitor/CCB, ARB/CCB, ACE inhibitor/HCTZ, β-blocker/HCTZ, ARB/HCTZ). |

*ACE,* Angiotensin-converting enzyme; *ARB,* angiotensin II receptor blocker; *CCB,* calcium channel blocker; *HCTZ,* thiazide diuretic.

Women experience more cough with ACE inhibitors and more pedal edema with CCBs than men.[642] These differences in AEs may require adjustment in the dose or switching of medications. Interestingly, despite sex differences in the underlying pathophysiologic mechanisms of high BP, there does not appear to be a substantial difference in the response rate to similar doses of commonly used antihypertensive drugs.

## RACE AND ETHNICITY

African Americans frequently present with hypertension at an earlier age, have more substantial elevations in BP, and earlier development of target-organ damage, than matched persons of white race.[643–645] Racial differences in the response to antihypertensive medications have been demonstrated in numerous clinical trials.[636,643] The mechanisms for these differences are not yet elucidated but appear to be independent of dietary salt or potassium intake. Some investigators have suggested possible genetic differences in renal sodium handling, but clinical trials have not been conclusive. Irrespective of the mechanism, African Americans frequently display BP salt sensitivity.[646,647] A careful assessment of the dose–response for different medication classes, with adjustment for differences in dietary sodium consumption and body mass index among races and ethnic groups, has not been performed.

In general, thiazide diuretics and CCBs have more robust antihypertensive effects at lower dosages in African Americans than other commonly used therapeutic classes.[636,637,648] Drugs that block the RAAS are effective in African Americans, but higher dosages are frequently required to achieve the same degree of BP reduction as observed in non–African Americans.[284] As in most population groups, elevated peripheral vascular resistance contributes to BP elevation. Some investigators have suggested that African Americans have a modest volume component contributing to BP elevation that may also contribute to antihypertensive drug resistance.[646] It is not uncommon for multiple drugs to be required to reach the target BP. Consequently, fixed-dose combinations may be most useful in this population group as part of a strategy to simplify the approach.

Hispanics and Asians do not appear to have different hypertensive responses to commonly used drugs compared with whites.[643] However, Caribbean Hispanics who have a higher proportion of African ancestry may respond to commonly prescribed antihypertensive agents in a way that is characteristic of non-Hispanic blacks.[647]

## OBESE PATIENTS

Obese patients with hypertension frequently have other medical problems that complicate the management of hypertension (Table 49.31).[86] These patients tend to have a hyperdynamic circulation, increased peripheral vascular resistance, expanded plasma volume, and a greater sensitivity to the influence of dietary salt in increasing BP.

**Table 49.31 Considerations for Initial Therapy in Obese Patients With Hypertension**

| Clinical Observation | Pharmacologic Considerations |
|---|---|
| Hyperdynamic circulation | Reduce heart rate and sympathoadrenal outflow (β-blocker). |
| Increased peripheral vascular resistance | Use vasodilator (e.g., HCTZ, ACE inhibitor, ARB, CCB). |
| Salt sensitivity | Use natriuretic (HCTZ, ACE inhibitor, ARB, CCB). Have patient reduce salt intake. |
| Expanded plasma volume | Use diuretic (HCTZ). Have patient reduce salt intake. |
| Hypoventilation | Order sleep study to evaluate need for positive pressure ventilation at night. |
| >20 mm Hg from systolic goal | Use fixed-dose combination therapy (ACE inhibitor/CCB, ARB/CCB, ACE inhibitor/HCTZ, β-blocker/HCTZ, ARB/HCTZ). |

*ACE,* Angiotensin-converting enzyme; *ARB,* angiotensin II receptor blocker; *CCB,* calcium channel blocker; *HCTZ,* thiazide diuretic.

β-Blockers may be helpful in diminishing sympathoadrenal drive. Vasodilators such as ACE inhibitors, ARBs, and CCBs are useful for reducing peripheral vascular resistance. Combinations of these drugs may also be helpful. Because of the tendency toward expanded plasma volume, thiazide or thiazide-like diuretics can be helpful because they provide an opportunity to produce vasodilation and mild volume reduction. Frequently, obese patients require multiple drugs to achieve BP goals. β-Blockers may increase the likelihood of weight gain and may compromise glucose tolerance.[636,649] Aldosterone receptor blockers may be preferred in obese, hypertensive individuals requiring treatment with multiple medications because of adipocyte production of aldosterone.[585–588]

## TREATMENT OF PATIENTS WITH CARDIOVASCULAR OR KIDNEY DISEASE

### Cardiovascular Disease

Patients with hypertension and cardiac diseases such as stable ischemic heart disease, HFrEF, and heart failure with preserved ejection fraction (HFpEF) frequently require multiple agents for the joint control of hypertension and heart disease. The choice of specific antihypertensive medications will generally be guided by first-line therapies. For example, for patients with a history of stable ischemic heart disease, the first choice of agents should include a β-blocker and an ACE inhibitor or ARB, given evidence from randomized trials indicating a benefit in terms of cardiovascular morbidity and mortality. Other agents such as CCBs and diuretics can be added as needed to achieve the BP goal. Patients with HFrEF should also be treated with β-blockers, ACE inhibitors or ARBs, and MRA, whereas nondihydropyridine calcium channels should generally be avoided, based on data from randomized clinical trials. Less is known about optimal treatment choices in HFpEF, but the current guidelines[55] recommend management of volume overload with diuretics, followed by the addition of ACE inhibitors or ARBs and β-blockers as needed to achieve a target SBP of less than 130 mm Hg.

### Kidney Disease

In patients with kidney disease (Table 49.32), BP control is more difficult to achieve because these patients not only have increased vascular resistance but also frequently have elevated blood volume.[650] The understanding of renal autoregulation provides some insight into the appropriate levels of BP control and the relative importance of different types of antihypertensive drugs in preserving kidney function.

Glomerular circulation operates optimally at one-half to two-thirds of the systemic BP.[651] Preglomerular vasoconstriction is necessary to decrease the systemic pressure to glomerular capillary pressure levels that are optimal for filtration yet low enough to avoid mechanical injury to the filtering apparatus.[651,652] The efferent glomerular arteriole also serves an important purpose—it vasoconstricts during situations of diminished effective arterial blood volume to maintain adequate pressure for glomerular filtration. With the development of vascular disease, the afferent glomerular arteriole does not vasoconstrict properly, which permits the transmission of systemic BP into the glomerulus. A clinical clue that could indicate the failure of autoregulation is the presence of microalbuminuria or protein in the urine. Under these

**Table 49.32 Considerations for Initial Therapy in Patients With Renal Disease**

| Clinical Observation | Pharmacologic Considerations |
|---|---|
| Increased blood volume (common in glomerular diseases) | Reduce blood volume |
| Decreased blood volume (common in tubular diseases) | Salt supplementation may be needed. |
| Increased peripheral vascular resistance | Use vasodilator (ACE inhibitor, CCB, ARB). |
| Proteinuria | Reduce proteinuria (ACE inhibitor, ARB, NDCCB; recommended target systolic blood pressure ≤130 mm Hg). |
| Diabetes with proteinuria | Control blood pressure and glycemia (ACE inhibitor if type 1 diabetes, ARB if type 2; recommended target systolic blood pressure <130 mm Hg). |
| >20 mm Hg from systolic goal | Use fixed-dose combination therapy (ACE inhibitor/CCB, ARB/CCB, ACE inhibitor/HCTZ, β-blocker/HCTZ, ACE inhibitor/CCB). Use of HCTZ depends on renal function. |

All medications adjusted according to renal function.
*ACE,* Angiotensin-converting enzyme; *ARB,* angiotensin II receptor blocker; *CCB,* calcium channel blocker; *HCTZ,* thiazide diuretic; *NDCCB,* nondihydropyridine calcium channel blocker.

circumstances, systemic BP should be reduced more substantially to minimize the risk of mechanical injury to the glomerulus.

Drugs that block the RAAS, such as ACE inhibitors[616,617] and ARBs,[620,624] provide a more consistent opportunity to reduce the progression of kidney disease as part of an intensive BP–lowering strategy than other commonly used antihypertensive drugs. The benefit of these drugs resides, in part, on their ability to facilitate efferent glomerular arteriolar dilation by antagonizing the effects of Ang II as they lower BP.[653] Renin inhibitors have similar clinical effects on reducing both BP and proteinuria to those of ACE inhibitors and ARBs, but have not been studied alone in renal protection trials.[654] Overall, there is a more consistent reduction in systemic and glomerular capillary pressures with RAAS-blocking drugs. Additional medications can be added to these drugs to achieve better BP control and help reduce glomerular capillary pressure and proteinuria. Sufficient doses of diuretics to control the blood volume should also be used. When kidney function declines to a range of eGFR of 30 mL/min/1.73 $m^2$ or below, volume reduction is more amenable to the provision of loop diuretics as opposed to thiazide or thiazide-type diuretics, although chlorthalidone and metolazone retain antihypertensive efficacy.

Some investigators have questioned the safety of using CCBs in patients with kidney disease, given their preferential effects on dilating the afferent glomerular arteriole.[52] Some studies have demonstrated that CCBs can increase proteinuria, despite lowering BP.[655] However, there is no clinical evidence that these drugs are detrimental and worsen the progression of kidney disease if they are given with ACE inhibitors or ARBs, which dilate the efferent glomerular arteriole. If anything, the lower BP achieved using these drugs in combination may provide better protection against the loss of kidney function, as was observed in the ACE inhibitors and CCBs for hypertension (ACCOMPLISH) study.[656]

Antiproteinuric strategies should be considered in patients with kidney disease because a reduction in proteinuria by specific antihypertensive drugs, such as ACE inhibitors or ARBs, correlates with slowing the progression of kidney disease.[657,658] However, dual RAAS blockade, despite reducing proteinuria, has not provided incremental benefit on kidney disease progression and is associated with a higher risk for declining kidney function and hyperkalemia.[95,255] For further discussion of drugs for the treatment of hypertension associated with kidney disease, see Chapter 59.

## STRATEGIES FOR SELECTING THE OPTIMAL COMBINATION ANTIHYPERTENSIVE THERAPY

A meta-analysis involving 40,000 treated patients evaluated the usefulness of low-dose combination treatments separately and in combination.[659] The average BP reduction achieved with low-dose therapy was only 20% in 354 randomized, double-blind, placebo-controlled trials of thiazides, β-blockers, ACE inhibitors, ARBs, and CCBs. Thiazides and CCBs cause side effects infrequently at a half-standard dose (2% and 1.6%, respectively), whereas side effects occur commonly at standard doses (9.9% and 8.3%, respectively). β-Blockers, however, cause an equivalently high number of side effects at both dosage levels (5.5% vs. 7.5%; $P = .04$). The only side effect observed with ACE inhibitors was cough (3.9%), which did not vary with dosage. ARBs were not associated with an excess of side effects at a standard dose. The reduction in BP was additive; however, the prevalence of AEs was not additive. Therefore combinations of two or three drugs at low doses may be preferable to one or two drugs at standard doses. In the absence of cough, ACE inhibitors and ARBs can be used at higher doses because of the lack of AEs associated with these drugs. In a subsequent meta-analysis, the authors quantified the effect of a combination of drugs from the four drug classes on BP reduction. The extra BP reduction achieved by combining two drugs from different classes is approximately five times greater than that achieved when the dosage of one drug is doubled.[660] This confirms what might be expected based on knowledge of the dose–effect relationship between the therapeutic effects of antihypertensive drugs and their toxicity (Fig. 49.4).

The rationale for fixed-dose combination therapy is as follows[661]:

- To combine drugs acting on different systems, thus initiating a pharmacologic attack on two systems with greatly enhanced impact compared with monotherapy.
- To combat counterregulatory responses that interfere with BP reduction.

For example, CCBs activate the SNS and RAAS, which can attenuate BP-lowering effects.[662,663] This action can be buffered by RAAS blockers. The antihypertensive effect of an RAAS blocker can be enhanced by the negative sodium balance created by the diuretic and natriuretic properties of diuretics or CCBs.[664]

- To decrease the pill burden and enhance adherence to prescribed therapy.

Many individuals with BPs that are 20 mm Hg (systolic) and 10 mm Hg (diastolic) above the target pressure will require more than one drug. Clinical trials have documented that achieving BP targets necessitates the use of multiple drugs. In the ALLHAT study, for example, only one-third of patients achieved their target BP with monotherapy after 5 years.[665]

- To decrease BP variability.

BP has been shown to be less variable with combination therapy versus monotherapy.[666] Variability in visit-to-visit SBPs was shown to be a strong predictor of stoke and MI.[667] CCBs and diuretics were found to be the most useful agents for reducing this variability, whereas β-blockers increased the variability.[667]

- To decrease AEs.

Combining two antihypertensive drugs at lower doses may actually reduce AEs compared with higher doses of both drugs. Studies have shown that the combination of an ACE inhibitor and ARB with a CCB reduces the incidence of CCB-related peripheral edema by as much as 38%.[668] Combining an RAAS blocker with a thiazide reduces the occurrence of diuretic-induced hypokalemia.

In the TRIple Pill vs. Usual care Management for Patients with mild-to-moderate Hypertension (TRIUMPH) trial,[669] 700 patients with hypertension from 11 urban hospitals in Sri Lanka were randomly assigned to receive a once-daily fixed dose triple combination pill containing 20 mg of telmisartan, 2.5 mg of amlodipine, and 12.5 mg of chlorthalidone versus usual care. A higher proportion of patients in the triple combination pill arm achieved target BP at 6 months (70% vs. 55%; $P < .001$). There were no significant differences in the proportion of patient withdrawal from BP-lowering therapy because of adverse events (6.6% vs. 6.8%). Limitations have been identified with the single-pill combination approach, however, and are listed in Table 49.33.

**Table 49.33 Advantages and Limits of the Use of Single-Pill Combinations in Hypertension**

| |
|---|
| **Advantages** |
| • Reduction of the pill burden |
| • Simplification of the treatment schedule |
| • Increased adherence to therapy (better long-term persistence) |
| • Improved efficacy with reduced incidence of side effects |
| • Better prevention of cardiovascular events (to be demonstrated prospectively) |
| **Limits** |
| • Reduction of the prescription flexibility |
| • Difficulty to identify the precise cause of an unexpected side effect |
| • Difficulty to memorize the exact content of the single-pill combinations |
| • Risk of a more pronounced rebound hypertension in case of repeated omissions |
| • Risk of acute hypotension when restarting a triple combination after interruptions |
| • Increased cost versus free combinations of generics |

From Burnier M. Antihypertensive combination treatment: state of the art. *Curr Hyperten Rep*. 2015;17:51.

## PREFERRED COMBINATIONS

### Renin–Angiotensin–Aldosterone System Inhibitors and Calcium Channel Blockers

The ACCOMPLISH trial demonstrated the superiority of an ACE inhibitor and CCB in single-pill form versus an ACE inhibitor plus HCTZ. The ACCOMPLISH trial compared BP reduction and cardiovascular outcomes achieved with two combination therapies, benazepril–amlodipine and benazepril–HCTZ in a single tablet. The trial included more than 11,000 participants, and the mean BP was nearly equivalent between the benazepril–amlodipine and benazepril–HCTZ groups (131.6 and 73.3 vs. 132.5 and 74.3, respectively). The outcome in this study was time to reach a primary endpoint—a composite of cardiovascular events or death. The trial was terminated early (after a mean of 36 months) because the benazepril–amlodipine group had reached a lower event rate (9.6%) than the benazepril–HCTZ group (11.8%; RR, 19.6%; HR, 0.80; $P < .001$).

### Renin–Angiotensin–Aldosterone System Inhibitors and Thiazide-Type Diuretics

By depleting intravascular volume, diuretics activate the RAAS system, which causes vasoconstriction as well as salt and water retention. The RAAS blockade attenuates the counterregulatory response and causes additional BP reduction. This combination has several advantages—the RAAS mitigates diuretic-induced hypokalemia and glucose intolerance. In the HYVET trial, indapamide, a thiazide-type diuretic, combined with the ACE inhibitor perindopril reduced the incidence of stroke (by 30%) and heart failure (by 64%).

## ACCEPTABLE COMBINATIONS

### β-Blockers and Thiazide-Like Diuretics

There are multiple commercially available β-blocker-diuretic formulations (e.g., bisoprolol, metoprolol, propranolol, timolol with HCTZ, and atenolol with chlorthalidone). β-Blockers and diuretics have both been shown to reduce cardiovascular endpoints in RCTs; however, meta-analyses have suggested that they are less effective than other agents.[355,670] The addition of diuretics increases the effectiveness of β-blockers in individuals of African ancestry and in other persons with low-renin hypertension. These drug classes have several overlapping AEs, including the development of glucose intolerance, new-onset diabetes, fatigue, and sexual dysfunction. In 2007, the European Society of Hypertension warned against the use of this combination for patients with metabolic syndrome or for those at high risk of diabetes.[671]

A meta-analysis has demonstrated a 35% risk of new-onset diabetes with diuretics compared with non–β-blocker antihypertensives and a 31% risk of new-onset diabetes with diuretics compared with nondiuretic antihypertensives.[672] Given the possibility of adverse metabolic consequences, it seems reasonable to avoid the use of this combination for initial therapy without other compelling indications.[673]

#### Calcium Channel Blockers and Thiazide-Like Diuretics

The combination of a CCB and diuretic provides a partially additive antihypertensive effect.[674] CCBs increase kidney sodium excretion, albeit not to the same extent as diuretics. This combination performed well in the VALUE trial, in which HCTZ was administered to participants randomized to amlodipine as a second step compared with the valsartan arm.[675] AEs included peripheral edema and hypokalemia as well as a slight increase in the incidence of new-onset diabetes.

#### Calcium Channel Blockers and β-Blockers

Additive BP reduction can be achieved with the combination of a β-blocker and a dihydropyridine CCB. In one study, the antihypertensive effects of combination ER metoprolol succinate and ER felodipine produced dose-related BP-lowering effects over a wide dose range; moreover, the incidence of edema and AEs was low. Nondihydropyridine CCBs such as verapamil and diltiazem should not be given together with β-blockers because of dual negative chronotropic effects, which may result in heart block or severe bradycardia.

#### Dual Calcium Channel Blockade

In a meta-analysis of six studies consisting of 153 patients, dual CCB therapy (dihydropyridine CCB with verapamil or diltiazem) was shown to have additive antihypertensive effects without an increase in adverse events.[676] Long-term prospective clinical trials are required to assess the long-term safety of this combination and to obtain cardiovascular outcome data. Dual CCB therapy should not be used as an alternative treatment for resistant hypertension until outcome data are available.

### UNACCEPTABLE OR INEFFECTIVE COMBINATIONS

#### Dual Renin–Angiotensin Blockade

In the ALTITUDE trial, aliskiren or placebo was added to ACE inhibitors or ARBs, which inhibit RAAS, in persons with CKD and type 2 diabetes.[96] The trial was halted early because of an increased incidence of hypotension, AKI, hyperkalemia, and stroke. In the ONTARGET trial, there were more adverse events, including declining kidney function, with a combination of telmisartan and ramipril than with the individual drugs, and the combination did not improve cardiovascular outcomes.[148] The 2013 Veterans Affairs Nephropathy in Diabetes (VA NEPHRON-D)[95] study enrolled 1448 patients with type 2 diabetes and diabetic nephropathy to receive losartan 100 mg daily plus either lisinopril or placebo. That trial was terminated early because of safety concerns, as patients in the dual ACE inhibitor/ARB arm had higher rates of hyperkalemia and AKI, and no benefits were observed in the primary endpoint of reduction in eGFR, ESKD, or death.

#### β-Blockers and Central Adrenergic Agonists

β-Blockers and central adrenergic agents (e.g., clonidine, α-methyldopa) both interfere with the SNS. No studies have explored the potential additive antihypertensive effects of these agents. However, combination therapy can result in bradycardia and heart block, particularly in elderly patients. Moreover, rebound hypertension with abrupt discontinuation would be another concern.

## BEDTIME ANTIHYPERTENSIVE DOSING VERSUS MORNING DOSING

Shifting one nondiuretic antihypertensive medicine from morning to evening can reduce the total 24-hour mean BP and restore the normal nocturnal BP decrease. This failure of the BP to decrease at night, termed "nondipping," is a cardiovascular disease risk factor.[677] After a median follow-up of 5.4 years, patients who took at least one BP-lowering medication at bedtime had an adjusted risk for total cardiovascular events (a composite of death, MI, angina pectoris, revascularization, heart failure, arterial occlusion of lower extremities, occlusion of the retinal artery, and stroke) that was approximately one-third that of patients who took all medications on awakening (adjusted HR, 0.31; 95% CI, 0.21 to 0.46; $P \leq .001$).[678] Similar results were demonstrated in patients with CKD.[679]

### RESISTANT HYPERTENSION

"Resistant hypertension" is a term used to characterize high BP that fails to respond to what the clinician thinks is an adequate antihypertensive regimen (Table 49.34).[680,681] Resistant hypertension has also been defined as the inability to reach SBP goal of less than 130 mm Hg, despite the use of three optimally dosed drugs, one of which is a diuretic, or the need for four or more medications to reach the desired SBP goal of less than 130 mm Hg.[682] Before a diagnosis of resistant hypertension, it is important to exclude "pseudoresistance" by verifying adherence to the medication regimen, ensuring that BPs are measured accurately, and excluding white coat hypertension.

A variety of factors can interfere with the ability of what is deemed to be appropriate antihypertensive therapy to normalize BP. Perhaps most important is nonadherence to the therapy regimen. Nonadherence is common and is one of the most serious problems that interfere with attaining the BP goal. This problem has many sources, including inadequate education, poor clinician–patient relationship, lack of understanding of side effects, and complexity of multidrug regimens. The health care provider should make every effort to determine whether adherence to therapy is part of the problem before pursuing other potential explanations for resistant hypertension. If nonadherence is eliminated, a methodologic approach can be used to help diagnose the cause of resistant hypertension and then correct it.

A checklist for accurate measurement of office BP has been proposed by the ACC/AHA guidelines on hypertension (Table 49.35).[55] Common reasons for falsely elevated office BP readings is not following the 5-minute rest, improper positioning of the patient, and improper positioning or size of BP cuff. If office BP is elevated despite proper technique, white coat hypertension where the out-of-office BP readings are acceptable but in-office BP readings are high needs to

**Table 49.34 Causes of Resistant Hypertension**

Pseudoresistance
- White coat hypertension or office elevations
- Pseudohypertension in older patients
- Use of small cuff on very obese arm

Nonadherence to therapeutic regimen

Volume overload

Drug-related causes
- Antihypertensive drug dosage too low
- Wrong type of diuretic
- Inappropriate combinations of antihypertensive drugs
- Drug actions and interactions
  - Sympathomimetics
  - Nasal decongestants
  - Appetite suppressants
  - Cocaine
  - Caffeine
  - Oral contraceptives
  - Adrenal steroids
  - Licorice (may be found in chewing tobacco)
  - Cyclosporine, tacrolimus
  - Erythropoiesis-stimulating agents and erythropoietin
  - Antidepressants
  - Nonsteroidal antiinflammatory drugs

Concomitant conditions
- Obesity

Sleep apnea
- Ethanol intake >1 oz (30 mL)/day
- Anxiety, hyperventilation

Secondary causes of hypertension
- Renovascular hypertension
- Primary aldosteronism
- Pheochromocytoma
- Hypothyroidism
- Hyperthyroidism
- Hyperparathyroidism
- Aortic coarctation
- Renal disease

be excluded with home BP monitoring or 24-hour ambulatory BP measurements. Again, proper technique of home BP measurements is critical as proposed by the ACC/AHA guidelines. Although 24-hour ambulatory measurements are very useful to exclude white coat hypertension and to get accurate measurements outside the office, the need to wear the device for 24 hours, the need to bring back the device to the clinic, costs, and insurance coverage are issues that might limit the practical use of these devices in all patients.

Corresponding values of SBP/DBP for clinic, home BP monitoring, daytime, nighttime, and 24-hour ambulatory blood pressure monitoring (ABPM) measurements are presented in Table 49.36.[55] Underlying lifestyle factors that contribute to resistant hypertension need to be addressed. These include obesity, physical inactivity, excessive alcohol consumption, smoking, and high salt intake.

Volume overload is an important and common cause of resistant hypertension. It may be related to excessive salt intake or to the inability of the kidney to excrete an appropriate salt and water load because of endocrine abnormalities or intrinsic kidney disease.

High dietary salt intake offsets the antihypertensive activities of all antihypertensive medications.[636] Some patients are more salt sensitive than others. Salt sensitivity is common in patients of African ancestry.[647] This sensitivity is also a more common problem in patients with CKD and heart failure. A careful clinical examination coupled with the judicious use of a thiazide-type or loop diuretic (depending on the level of kidney function) is critical in achieving an ideal blood volume to restore the antihypertensive efficacy of most classes of drugs. It is also appropriate to consider educating the patient about avoiding foods that are high in salt content, such as processed foods.

Drug-related causes of resistant hypertension are common and need to be carefully assessed in each patient. Oral contraceptives, immunosuppressants (e.g., cyclosporine, tacrolimus), erythropoiesis-stimulating agents, and some antidepressants can increase BP. Perhaps the most common drugs that cause resistant hypertension are over-the-counter (OTC) preparations of sympathomimetics, such as nasal decongestants, appetite suppressants, and NSAIDs.[683] Caffeine and licorice may also increase BP. Unfortunately, patients may not always recognize OTC preparations as medications. Therefore careful questioning specifically focusing on these types of medications should be routine during the evaluation for refractory hypertension. In addition, alcohol use, smoking, and cocaine use can be complicating factors that interfere with the ability of medications to lower BP.

Some medications may interfere with the antihypertensive activity of other drugs. For example, NSAIDs interfere with the antihypertensive activity of diuretics and ACE inhibitors.[680] Interestingly, only the antihypertensive activity of CCBs appears to be unaffected by the effects of NSAIDs.[684] Drug–drug interactions that can interfere with drug absorption, drug metabolism, or the pharmacodynamics of the concomitantly administered drugs can also interfere with antihypertensive activity.

Secondary causes of hypertension should also be considered in the evaluation of resistant hypertension. These causes can be divided into renal, endocrine, and other (principally sleep apnea). Kidney disease is the most common cause of secondary hypertension. A chemistry profile and urinalysis facilitate the diagnosis. Renal artery stenosis is often considered a common cause of secondary hypertension. Although renal artery disease caused by fibromuscular dysplasia in young women often responds to interventional procedures, revascularization of atheromatous renovascular diseases often seen in elderly persons with widespread atherosclerosis has not been shown to improve BP control, progression of CKD (because of ischemic nephropathy),[685] or cardiovascular outcomes compared with conservative treatments in three large RCTs.[55] According to the ACC/AHA guidelines, in the setting of significant atherosclerotic renal artery stenosis (>60%) with inability to control BP with medical management, stenting of the atherosclerotic renal artery could be considered but evidence is weak, as shown by a class IIb recommendation (weak) and C level evidence (observational studies). Therefore whether renal vascular assessment with Doppler ultrasonography or a direct imaging technique should be part of the workup for resistant hypertension is debatable.

Associated endocrine abnormalities include primary hyperaldosteronism, Cushing disease, pheochromocytoma, hypothyroidism or hyperthyroidism, and hyperparathyroidism. Rarely, aortic coarctation can be a cause of resistant hypertension. With the realization that hyperaldosteronism explains

**Table 49.35 Checklist for Accurate Measurement of Blood Pressure**

| Key Steps for Proper BP Measurements | Specific Instructions |
|---|---|
| Step 1: Properly prepare the patient | 1. Have the patient relax, sitting in a chair (feet on floor, back supported) for >5 min.<br>2. The patient should avoid caffeine, exercise, and smoking for at least 30 minutes before measurement.<br>3. Ensure patient has emptied his/her bladder.<br>4. Neither the patient nor the observer should talk during the rest period or during the measurement.<br>5. Remove all clothing covering the location of cuff placement.<br>6. Measurement made while the patient is sitting or lying on an examining table do not fulfill these criteria. |
| Step 2: Use proper technique for BP Measurements | 1. Use BP measurement device that has been validated, and ensure that the device is calibrated periodically.<br>2. Support the patient's arm (e.g., resting on a desk).<br>3. Position the middle of the cuff on the patient's upper arm at the level of the right atrium (the midpoint of the sternum).<br>4. Use the correct cuff size, such that the bladder encircles 80% of the arm, and note if a larger-or-smaller-than-normal cuff size is used.<br>5. Either the stethoscope diaphragm or bell may be used for auscultatory readings. |
| Step 3: Take the proper measurements needed for diagnosis and treatment of elevated BP/hypertension | 1. At the first visit, record BP in both arms. Use the arm that gives the higher reading for subsequent readings.<br>2. Separate repeated measurements by 1–2 min.<br>3. For auscultatory determination, use a palpated estimate of radial pulse obliteration pressure to estimate SBP. Inflate the cuff 20–30 mm Hg above this level for an auscultatory determination of the BP level.<br>4. For auscultatory readings, deflate the cuff pressure 2 mm Hg per second, and listen for Korotkoff sounds. |
| Step 4: Properly document accurate BP readings | 1. Record SBP and DBP. If using the auscultatory technique, record SBP and DBP as onset of the first Korotkoff sound and disappearance of all Korotkoff sounds, respectively, using the nearest even number.<br>2. Note the time of most recent BP medication taken before measurements. |
| Step 5: Average the readings | Use an average of ≥2 readings obtained on ≥2 occasions to estimate the individual's level of BP. |
| Step 6: Provide BP readings to patient | Provide patients with the SBP/DBP readings both verbally and in writing. |

*BP*, Blood pressure; *DBP*, diastolic blood pressure; *SBP*, systolic blood pressure.
From Whelton PK, Carey RM, Aronow WS, et al. 2017 ACC/AHA/AAPA/ABC/ACPM/AGS/APhA/ASH/ASPC/NMA/PCNA guideline for the prevention, detection, evaluation, and management of high blood pressure in adults: executive summary: a report of the American College of Cardiology/American Heart Association Task Force on clinical practice guidelines. *Circulation*. 2018;138:e426–e483. With permission.

at least 15% to 20% of resistant hypertension, all patients with resistant hypertension should be screened for occult hyperaldosteronism by measuring the ratio of plasma aldosterone level to plasma renin activity. In a retrospective study, more widespread use of the plasma aldosterone concentration-to-plasma renin activity ratio in hypertensive patients resulted in a 1.3- to 6.3-fold increase in the annual detection rate for primary aldosteronism (1%–2% before screening and 5%–10% after screening). Although these results are complicated by selection bias, they suggest that screening for primary hyperaldosteronism should be considered for patients with resistant hypertension, despite the fact that it is unusual to find an adenoma.[686] Often, patients with subtle hyperaldosteronism respond to the addition of a selective aldosterone receptor blocker to their antihypertensive regimen.

Observational data suggest an association of sleep apnea with hypertension. However, the effects of continuous positive airway pressure (CPAP) on BP is only modest; for instance, in a meta-analysis of 16 RCTs,[687] compared with controls, CPAP resulted in a mean net change in SBP of −2.46 mm Hg (95% CI, −4.31 to −0.62) and a mean net change in DBP of −1.83 mm Hg (95% CI, −3.05 to −0.61). In a more recent RCT including 2717 patients with obstructive sleep apnea, CPAP treatment did not improve cardiovascular outcomes. However, other studies demonstrated that CPAP treatment improves quality of life and daytime somnolence.[688] Therefore CPAP treatment in sleep apnea might be indicated for quality of life rather than improving BP or cardiovascular outcomes.

Strategies to control BP in patients with refractory hypertension should first address issues related to adherence, simplification of the medical regimen, and determination of whether side effects play a role. Subsequently, one can evaluate the medications and try to choose those that work well with one another to facilitate an almost additive antihypertensive response. As previously noted, most drugs reduce SBP by approximately 8 to 10 mm Hg. Consequently, it is not unusual for patients who are 40 or 50 mm Hg from their target SBP to require multiple medications. Lifestyle issues should also be emphasized. Weight loss, dietary salt restriction, and mindfulness-based stress reduction and other relaxation

**Table 49.36 Corresponding Values of Systolic Blood Pressure/Diastolic Blood Pressure for Clinic, Home Blood Pressure Monitoring, Daytime, Nighttime, and 24-Hour Ambulatory Blood Pressure Monitoring Measurements**

| Clinic | HBPM | Daytime ABPM | Nighttime ABPM | 24-Hour ABPM |
|---|---|---|---|---|
| 120/80 | 120/80 | 120/80 | 100/65 | 115/75 |
| 130/80 | 130/80 | 130/80 | 110/65 | 125/75 |
| 140/90 | 135/85 | 135/85 | 120/70 | 130/80 |
| 160/100 | 145/90 | 145/90 | 140/85 | 145/90 |

*ABPM,* Ambulatory blood pressure monitoring; *HBPM,* home blood pressure monitoring.

From Whelton PK, Carey RM, Aronow WS, et al. 2017 ACC/AHA/AAPA/ABC/ACPM/AGS/APhA/ASH/ASPC/NMA/PCNA guideline for the prevention, detection, evaluation, and management of high blood pressure in adults: executive summary: a report of the American College of Cardiology/American Heart Association Task Force on clinical practice guidelines. *Circulation*. 2018;138:e426–e483. With permission.

techniques should be considered, as for patients with milder forms of hypertension.

One should also be careful to ensure that volume excess is controlled and that there are no drug–drug interactions or clinical situations that would promote diuretic resistance, such as excessive salt intake, impaired drug bioavailability, impaired diuretic secretion by the proximal tubule, increased protein binding in the tubule lumen, or reduced GFR. True resistant hypertension is unusual, and a methodologic approach should be taken to help facilitate BP control in these patients because a lack of control puts these patients at a greater risk of cardiovascular complications.

"Refractory hypertension" refers to patients whose BP cannot be controlled with maximal medical therapy (more than four drugs with complementary mechanisms, given at maximal tolerable doses) under the care of a specialist.[689] It is an important clinical phenotype that is commonly associated with those of African heritage, patients with diabetes, and/or those with albuminuria.[689] Recent large observational studies have noted that 0.5% of patients receiving antihypertensive treatment and 3.6% of individuals with resistant hypertension have refractory hypertension, and that these individuals have much higher 10-year Framingham Coronary Heart Disease and Stroke risk scores. Strategies for improving treatment in these types of patients are unknown but may require higher doses of MRAs.

Many hypertensive patients are not controlled because of nonadherence or lack of tolerance to available antihypertensive therapy. In one study, in as many as 35% of these individuals, who may be prescribed as many as three to five antihypertensive medications, blood and urine samples revealed no trace of medication.[690,691] Thus there is a need for novel drug therapies and devices to lower BP in individuals with refractory hypertension. Fortunately, there are many new drugs in preclinical and clinical trials.[692] A recent large, blinded clinical trial evaluating catheter-based renal denervation did not show a significant reduction of SBP 6 months after the procedure compared with that of sham controls.[693] However, it has become clear that results are difficult to interpret because of the procedural and technical shortcomings of the renal denervation procedure itself as only a few participants (9 of 253) received a complete four-quadrant ablation (covering 360 degrees of the renal artery), and SBP was significantly higher in participants who underwent incomplete renal denervation compared with those with complete renal denervation.[692,694]

Hopefully, one may be optimistic that these shortcomings will be resolved in the near-future to allow renal denervation procedures to reach clinical applicability.[692] Drugs in development and innovative novel interventional approaches should provide physicians with the tools to provide better care for their patients with hypertension that is not yet controlled. Novel antihypertensive drug and device treatments are the subject of a recent review[692] (Table 49.37).

## DRUG TREATMENT OF HYPERTENSIVE URGENCIES AND EMERGENCIES

It is important to distinguish between hypertensive urgency and hypertensive emergency. These terms are used loosely in clinical practice, with a great deal of overlap. The distinction between the two is important because the management approach is substantially different.

A hypertensive emergency is a clinical syndrome in which marked elevation in BP results in ongoing target-organ damage in the body (Table 49.38). The syndrome can be manifested by encephalopathy, retinal hemorrhage, papilledema, acute MI, stroke, or AKI. Any delay in the control of BP may lead to irreversible sequelae, including death. This syndrome is unusual but requires immediate hospitalization in an intensive care unit (ICU), with judicious use of intravenous vasodilators to lower SBPs and DBPs to approximately 140/90 mm Hg.

Hypertensive urgency is a clinical situation in which a patient may have a marked elevation in BP (e.g., >200/130 mm Hg) but no evidence of ongoing target-organ damage. Such a patient can be treated with rapid-onset drugs, such as captopril or clonidine, and be observed cautiously, with the administration of long-acting medications on an outpatient basis as progressive restoration of a more appropriate BP level is attained.

Thus the history and physical examination findings are the critical factors in delineating the difference between these two syndromes. The decision about whether to hospitalize the patient in an ICU and use intravenous medication or to observe the patient carefully and use oral medications to facilitate better BP control depends in large part on the presence or absence of ongoing target-organ injury.

### PARENTERAL DIRECT-ACTING VASODILATORS

Hydralazine is a direct-acting vasodilator and may be given intramuscularly or as a rapid intravenous bolus injection (Table 49.39). It acts rapidly, and the BP effect persists for up to 6 hours.[695,696] Hydralazine is less potent than diazoxide, and the BP response is less predictable. It may also

**Table 49.37 New Drugs for Hypertension**

| Drug | Mechanism of Action | Status |
|---|---|---|
| BAY-94-8862 (Finerenone) | Mineralocorticoid receptor antagonist | Phase IIb |
| LCI699 | Aldosterone synthase inhibitor | Phase II trials[a] |
| C21 | $AT_2$ receptor agonist | Preclinical |
| XNT | ACE2 activator | Preclinical[a] |
| DIZE | ACE2 activator | Phase 1 |
| rhACE2 | ACE2 activator | Phase 1 |
| HP-β-CD/Ang 1-7 | Ang 1-7 analogue | Preclinical |
| AVE0991 | Nonpeptide agonist of Mas receptor | Preclinical |
| CGEN-856S | Peptide agonist of Mas receptor | Preclinical |
| Alamandine/HPβCD | Mas-related-G-protein coupled receptor, member D agonist | Preclinical |
| PC18 | Aminopeptidase N inhibitor | Preclinical |
| RB150 (OGC001) | Aminopeptidase N inhibitor | Phase 1 |
| LCZ696 | Dual-acting angiotensin receptor-neprilysin inhibitor | Phase III |
| SLV-306 (Daglutril) | Dual-acting endothelin-converting enzymes-neprilysin inhibitor | Phase II |
| PL-3994 | Natriuretic peptide A agonist | Phase II |
| C-$ANP_{4-23}$ | ANP analog, selective for natruiuretic peptide clearance receptor (NPR-C) | Preclinical |
| AR9281 | Soluble epoxide hydrolase inhibitors | Phase II[a] |
| Vasomera (PB1046) | Vasoactive intestinal peptide receptor 2 (VPAC2) agonist | Phase II |
| AZD1722 (Tenapanor) | Intestinal $Na^+/H^+$ exchanger 3 inhibitor | Phase 1 |
| Etamicastat | Dopamine β-hydroxylase inhibitor | Phase 1 |
| Vaccines | | |
| CYT006-Ang0β | Vaccine against angiotensin II | Phase II |
| Angil-KLH | Vaccine against angiotensin II | Preclinical |
| pHAV-4Anglis | Vaccine against angiotensin II | Preclinical |
| ATROβ-001 | Vaccine against angiotensin II | Preclinical |
| ATR12181 | Vaccine against angiotensin II type 1 receptor | Preclinical |
| Preeclampsia Drugs | | |
| DIF | Antidigoxin antibody fragment | Phase II expedited |
| ATryn | Recombinant antithrombin | Phase III |

[a]Stopped.

*ANP*, Atrial natriuretic peptide; *ATR*, angiotensin II type 1 receptors; *DIF*, digoxin-immune Fab; *KLH*, keyhole limpet hemocyanin; *rhACE2*, recombinant human ACE2.

From Oparil S, Schmieder RE. New approaches in the treatment of hypertension. *Circ Res.* 2015;116:1074–1095.

cause a reflex increase in heart rate and sodium and water retention.

Sodium nitroprusside is the most potent of the parenteral vasodilators.[695,696] Nitroprusside acts on the excitation–contraction coupling of vascular smooth muscle by interfering with the intracellular activation of calcium. Unlike diazoxide and hydralazine, nitroprusside dilates arteriolar resistance and venous capacitance vessels. It has the advantages of being immediately effective when given as an infusion and of having an extremely short duration of action, which permits minute-to-minute adjustments in BP control (Table 49.39). Disadvantages of nitroprusside therapy include the following: (1) need for intraarterial BP monitoring; (2) need for the drug to be prepared fresh every 4 hours; (3) need to protect the solution from light during infusion; and (4) potential for toxic effects from metabolic side products. Nitroprusside is not excreted intact; it is rapidly metabolized to cyanide and thiocyanate through a reaction with hemoglobin, which yields methemoglobin and an unstable intermediate that dissociates to release cyanide. The major elimination pathway of cyanide is conversion in the liver and kidney to thiocyanate. Back conversion of thiocyanate to cyanide may occur. Thiocyanate is largely excreted in the urine; it has a plasma half-life of 1 week in normal individuals and accumulates in patients with CKD.

Toxic concentrations of cyanide or thiocyanate may occur if nitroprusside infusions are given for longer than 48 hours or at infusion rates higher than 2 mg/kg/min; the drug should not be administered at the maximal dose of 10 mg/kg/min for longer than 10 minutes.[697] Toxic manifestations include air hunger, hyperreflexia, confusion, and seizures. Lactic acidosis and venous hyperoxemia are laboratory indicators of cyanide intoxication. The appearance of drug unresponsiveness may reflect an increase in the concentration of free cyanide. In such cases, the drug should be promptly discontinued and the levels of cyanide measured. Nitroprusside is hemodialyzable.

Intravenous nitroglycerin produces dilation of arterial and venous beds in a dose-related manner. At lower dosages, the primary effect is on preload; at higher infusion rates, afterload is reduced. Nitroglycerin may also dilate epicardial coronary vessels and their collaterals, increasing the blood supply to ischemic regions. Effective coronary perfusion is maintained, provided that the BP does not fall excessively or that the heart rate does not increase significantly. Nitroglycerin has an immediate onset of action but is rapidly metabolized to dinitrates and mononitrates (Table 49.39). Because nitroglycerin is absorbed by many plastics, dilution should be performed only in glass parenteral solution bottles. Nitroglycerin is also absorbed by polyvinyl chloride (PVC) tubing; non-PVC intravenous administration sets should be used.

Patients with normal or low left ventricular filling pressure or pulmonary wedge pressure may be hypersensitive to the effects of nitroglycerin. Therefore continuous monitoring of BP, heart rate, and pulmonary capillary wedge pressure must be performed to assess the correct dose. Intravenous nitroglycerin may be the drug of choice in the treatment of patients with moderate hypertension associated with coronary ischemia because it provides collateral coronary vasodilation, a property that is not seen with the other direct-acting arteriolar vasodilators. The principal AEs are headache, nausea, and vomiting. Tolerance may develop with prolonged use.

**Table 49.38 Hypertensive Emergencies**

Hypertensive encephalopathy[a]
Acute aortic dissection[a]
- Central nervous system bleeding[a]
- Intracranial hemorrhage
- Thrombotic cerebrovascular accident
- Subarachnoid hemorrhage

Acute left ventricular failure refractory to conventional medical therapy[a]
Myocardial ischemia or infarction associated with persistent chest pain[a]
Accelerated or malignant hypertension[b]
Toxemia of pregnancy – eclampsia[a]
Renal failure or insufficiency[b]
Hypertension associated with hyperadrenergic states[a]
- Pheochromocytoma
- Interaction between monoamine oxidase inhibitors and tyramine-containing foods
- Interaction between an $\alpha$-adrenergic agonist and nonselective $\beta$-adrenergic antagonist
- After abrupt withdrawal of clonidine or guanabenz
- After severe body burns
- Neurogenic hypertension

Hypertension in the surgical patient[b]
- Associated with postoperative bleeding
- After open heart or vascular surgery
- Preceding emergency surgery
- After kidney transplantation
- Hypertension in a diabetic patient with retinal hemorrhage[a]

[a]Considered by some authors to be a true hypertensive emergency.
[b]Considered by some authors to be a hypertensive urgency.

## $\beta_1$-SELECTIVE ADRENERGIC ANTAGONIST

Esmolol hydrochloride is a short-acting, $\beta_1$-selective adrenergic antagonist. Esmolol hydrochloride concentrate for injection must be diluted to a final concentration of 10 mg/mL.[695,696] Extravasation of esmolol hydrochloride may cause serious local irritation and skin necrosis. Esmolol shares all the toxic potential of the $\beta_1$-adrenergic antagonists, as previously discussed.

After intravenous injection of a loading dose of 250 to 500 mg/kg and then infusion of a maintenance dose ranging from 50 to 100 mg/kg/min, steady-state blood concentrations are achieved within 5 minutes (Table 49.39). Efficacy should be assessed after the 1-minute loading dose and 4 minutes of maintenance infusion. If an adequate therapeutic effect is observed, as assessed by BP and heart rate response, then the maintenance infusion should be maintained. If an adequate therapeutic effect is not observed, the same loading dose can be repeated for 1 minute, followed by maintenance infusion at an increased rate.

Esmolol has pharmacologic actions similar to those of other $\beta_1$-selective adrenergic antagonists; it produces negative chronotropic and inotropic activity. It has been used to prevent or treat hemodynamic changes induced by surgical events, including increases in SBPs and DBPs and doubling of the product of heart rate multiplied by SBP. Esmolol may be particularly useful for the treatment of postoperative hypertension and hypertension associated with coronary insufficiency.[695,696] Esmolol is hydrolyzed rapidly in the blood, and negligible concentrations are present 30 minutes after discontinuance. Because the kidneys eliminate the de-esterified metabolite of esmolol, the drug should be used cautiously

**Table 49.39 Parenteral Drugs Used in the Treatment of Hypertensive Emergencies**

| Drug | Dosage | Onset of Action | Peak Effect | Duration of Action |
|---|---|---|---|---|
| Hydralazine | 0.5–1.0-mg/min infusion or 10–50 mg intramuscularly | 1–5 min | 10–80 min | 3–6 h |
| Nitroglycerine | 5–100-μg/min infusion | 1–2 min | 2–5 min | 3–5 min |
| Nitroprusside | 0.25–10-μg/kg/min infusion | Immediate | 1–2 min | 2–5 min |
| Esmolol | 250–500 μg/kg/min × 1 (loading dose), then 50–100 μg/kg/min × 4 (maintenance); maintenance dosage may be increased to maximum of 300 μg/kg/min | 1–2 min | 5 min | 0–30 min |
| Labetalol | 20 mg bolus then 0.5 to 2 mg/minute infusion | 5 min | 10 min | 3–6 h |
| Methyldopa | 250–500-mg bolus every 6 h (2 g maximum) | 2–3 h | 3–5 h | 6–12 h |
| Trimethaphan | 0.5–10-mg/min infusion bolus over 2 min (300 mg maximum) | Immediate | 1–2 min | 5–10 min |
| Enalaprilat | 0.625–5.0-mg bolus over 5 min q6h | 5–15 min | 1–4 h | 6 h |
| Phentolamine | 0.5–1.0-mg/min infusion or 2.5–5.0-mg bolus q5–15 minutes | Immediate | 3–5 min | 10–15 min |
| Nicardipine | 5–15 mg/h | 5–10 min | 45 min | 50 h |
| Clevidipine | 1–2 mg/hour (16 mg/hour maximum) | 2–4 min | 5–6 min | 15 min |
| Fenoldopam | 0.01–1.6-μg/min constant infusion | 5–15 min | 30 min | 5–10 min |

in patients with CKD. Esmolol is the preferred agent for treatment of acute aortic dissection.

### $\alpha_1$- AND β-ADRENERGIC ANTAGONISTS

The $\alpha_1$- and β-adrenergic antagonist labetalol may be given by repeated intravenous injection or slow continuous infusion[695,696] (Table 49.39). The maximal BP-lowering effect occurs within 5 minutes of the first injection. The drug should be administered to patients in the supine position to avoid symptomatic postural hypotension. The AEs of labetalol have been previously discussed. This drug has been proven safe and useful in hypertensive urgencies and emergencies in pregnant women.

### CENTRAL $\alpha_2$-ADRENERGIC AGONIST

Methyldopate hydrochloride is a central $\alpha_2$-adrenergic agonist that may be administered intravenously as a bolus infusion[695,696] (Table 49.39). It has a delayed onset of action and peak effect, and its effect on BP is unpredictable. The AEs of methyldopa are addressed earlier.

### ANGIOTENSIN-CONVERTING ENZYME INHIBITOR

Enalaprilat, the active metabolite of the oral ACE inhibitor enalapril, can be administered as a slow intravenous infusion for 5 minutes (Table 49.39) in an intravenous dose that is approximately 25% of the oral dose. The onset of action occurs within 15 minutes, and the maximal effect is observed within 1 to 4 hours.[698] The duration of action is approximately 6 hours. In patients with CKD, the initial dose should be no more than 0.625 mg.

### α-ADRENERGIC ANTAGONIST

Phentolamine mesylate is a nonselective, α-adrenergic antagonist used primarily in the treatment of hypertension associated with pheochromocytoma.[695,696] It has a rapid onset of action when administered intravenously as a bolus or continuous infusion (Table 49.39). The duration of action is 10 to 15 minutes. The drug has a plasma half-life of 19 minutes. Approximately 13% of a single dose appears in the urine as unchanged drug. AEs include those associated with nonselective α-adrenergic blockade, as previously discussed.

### CALCIUM CHANNEL BLOCKERS

Nicardipine hydrochloride, a dihydropyridine CCB, is administered by slow continuous infusion at a concentration of 0.1 mg/mL; each 1-mL ampule (25 mg) should be diluted with 240 mL of a compatible intravenous fluid (not including sodium bicarbonate or lactated Ringer's solution) to produce 250 mL of solution at a concentration of 0.1 mg/mL.[699] There is a dose-dependent decrease in BP. The onset of action is within minutes; 50% of the ultimate decrease in BP occurs within 45 minutes, but a final steady state is not reached for approximately 50 hours (Table 49.39). The discontinuation of infusion is followed by a 50% offset of action within 30 minutes, but gradually decreasing antihypertensive effects exist for approximately 50 hours. This drug has been shown to be safe and effective in the treatment of pediatric hypertensive emergencies.[699,700]

Clevidipine is a dihydropyridine CCB that is available in a lipid emulsion for intravenous infusion for the treatment of hypertensive emergencies.[701] Steady-state concentrations of clevidipine in arterial or venous blood are attained within 2 and 10 minutes in healthy volunteers receiving 0.91 and 3.2 μg/kg/min, respectively. The relationship between the intravenous infusion dose and steady-state blood concentrations is linear in patients with mild-to-moderate hypertension and in healthy volunteers. Clevidipine is highly protein bound and rapidly distributed. This drug is rapidly hydrolyzed by esterases in the blood and extravascular tissues. Blood concentrations decrease rapidly after termination of the infusion. The initial phase is rapid (half-life of ≈1 minute) and accounts for 85% to 90% of elimination. The terminal elimination half-life is 15 minutes. Clevidipine treatment results in a prompt reduction in BP (≥15% from baseline) in less than 6 minutes.[702] Clevidipine has a safety profile comparable to that of nitroglycerin, sodium nitroprusside, and nicardipine. The most common adverse events are sinus tachycardia, headache, nausea, and chest discomfort.[703]

### DOPAMINE $D_1$–LIKE RECEPTOR AGONIST

Fenoldopam mesylate, a dopamine $D_1$–like receptor agonist, is formulated as a solution to be diluted for intravenous infusion for the treatment of acute hypertension.[701,704] It is a rapid-acting agent that produces vasodilation by functioning as an agonist for dopamine $D_1$–like receptors and has moderate affinity for $\alpha_2$-adrenoreceptors.

Fenoldopam is a racemic mixture in which the R isomers are responsible for its biologic activity. It has vasodilatory effects on coronary, renal, mesenteric, and peripheral arteries in experimental studies; however, not all vascular beds respond uniformly. In humans, the drug increases renal blood flow in hypertensive and normotensive patients.

Fenoldopam comes in 1-mL ampules that contain 10 mg of fenoldopam and is diluted for administration as a constant infusion at a rate of 0.01 to 1.6 mg/kg/min (Table 49.39). It produces steady-state plasma concentrations in proportion to its infusion rate, its elimination half-life is 5 minutes, and steady-state concentrations are reached within 20 minutes.

Clearance of the active compound is not altered by ESKD or hepatic disease. Approximately 90% of infused fenoldopam is eliminated in urine and 10% in feces. Elimination occurs largely by conjugation that does not involve CYP enzymes. There are no data on drug–drug interactions.

AEs include reflex increase in heart rate, increase in intraocular pressure, headache, flushing, nausea, and hypotension.

## RAPID-ACTING ORAL DRUGS

A more gradual, progressive reduction in systemic BP may be achieved after the oral administration of drugs with rapid absorption.[622] These drugs include the following: (1) $\alpha_1$- and β-adrenergic antagonist labetalol; (2) central $\alpha_2$-adrenergic agonist clonidine; (3) CCBs diltiazem and verapamil; (4) ACE inhibitors captopril and enalapril; (5) postsynaptic $\alpha_1$-adrenergic antagonist prazosin; and (6) a combination of oral therapies. The dosages and pharmacodynamic effects of rapid-acting oral drugs that are commonly used in the treatment of hypertensive emergencies are given in Table 49.40. Note that rapid-acting oral dihydropyridine CCBs, such as sublingual nifedipine, are no longer recommended because they may cause large and unpredictable reductions in BP, with resultant ischemic events.[705]

**Table 49.40 Rapid-Acting Oral Drugs Used in the Treatment of Hypertensive Emergencies**

| Drug | Dosage | Onset of Action | Peak Effect | Duration of Action |
|---|---|---|---|---|
| **$\alpha_1$- and β-Adrenergic Antagonist** | | | | |
| Labetalol | 100–400 mg q12h (2400 mg maximum) | 1–2 h | 2–4 h | 8–12 h |
| **$\alpha_1$-Adrenergic Antagonist** | | | | |
| Prazosin | 1–5 mg q2h (20 mg maximum) | <60 min | 2–4 h | 6–12 h |
| **Central $\alpha_2$-Agonist** | | | | |
| Clonidine | 0.2 mg initially, then 0.1 mg/h (0.8 mg maximum) | 30–60 min | 2–4 h | 6–8 h |
| **Calcium Channel Blockers** | | | | |
| Diltiazem | 30–120 mg q8h (480 mg maximum) | <15 min | 2–3 h | 8 h |
| Verapamil | 80–120 mg q8h (480 mg maximum) | < 60 min | 2–3 h | 8 h |
| **Angiotensin-Converting Enzyme Inhibitors** | | | | |
| Captopril | 12.5–25 mg q6h (150 mg maximum) | <15 min | 1 h | 6–12 h |
| Enalapril | 2.5–10 mg q6h (40 mg maximum) | <60 min | 4–8 h | 12–24 h |

## CLINICAL CONSIDERATIONS IN THE RAPID REDUCTION OF BLOOD PRESSURE

The rapid reduction of BP carries the risk of impairing blood supply to vital structures, such as the brain and heart. The 2017 ACC/AHA guidelines[55] recommend an initial reduction in SBP by no more than 25%, except in certain clinical scenarios such as acute aortic dissection or preeclampsia/eclampsia, when a larger and more rapid reduction in BP may be preferred. The risk of overreduction of BP in a rapid fashion is linked to the use of sublingual nifedipine capsules with stroke and heart attack in hypertensive patients.[705] Because this approach is variable and rapid, clinicians are unable to set a lower limit of BP that is achieved with therapy.

Cerebral blood flow is normally carefully autoregulated so that perfusion is maintained at a sufficient level when BP is low but is diminished during states of chronic hypertension to avoid cerebral edema. With chronic hypertension, the short-term, rapid reduction of BP may decrease cerebral blood flow sufficiently to precipitate ischemia and infarction. This decrease may be particularly important in patients with atherosclerotic disease of the cerebral blood vessels in whom there may be areas of uneven cerebral perfusion. Although drugs that do penetrate the blood–brain barrier, such as hydralazine, sodium nitroprusside, and nicardipine, dilate cerebral vessels, which may lessen the likelihood of ischemia, intrinsic vascular disease may render some areas more ischemic than others with BP reduction. In addition, potent cerebral vasodilators can conceivably cause an increase in intracranial pressure, creating the potential for cerebral edema and possible herniation.

Sudden drops in BP can also interfere with coronary perfusion during diastole and result in myocardial ischemia, infarction, or arrhythmia. In addition, rapid reduction of BP may result in a reflex increase in heart rate, which would also interfere with coronary perfusion during diastole. For these reasons, a cautious and controlled reduction in BP is necessary for these patients. For most hypertensive emergencies, a parenteral drug, such as sodium nitroprusside, is ideal. However, if the patient has coronary disease, the use of intravenous nitroglycerin, esmolol, or both is a useful approach because these drugs can induce coronary dilation and slow heart rate, respectively. Intravenous nicardipine can also be used because it facilitates coronary vasodilation. Patients with acute aortic dissection are best treated with a β-adrenergic antagonist first, followed by a vasodilating agent. Patients with hypertensive encephalopathy or CNS hemorrhage are best treated with drugs that do not cause cerebral vasodilation, such as hydralazine, nitroprusside, nicardipine, or fenoldopam.

## ACKNOWLEDGMENTS

We acknowledge the contributions of Drs Matthew R. Weir, Donna S. Hanes, David K. Klassen, and Walter G. Wasser to this chapter in the 10th edition, substantial parts of which are carried forward here.

 Complete reference list available at ExpertConsult.com.

## KEY REFERENCES

40. Gonzalez-Villalobos RA, Janjoulia T, Fletcher NK, et al. The absence of intrarenal ACE protects against hypertension. *J Clin Invest.* 2013;123:2011–2023.

47. Kunz R, Friedrich C, Wolbers M, et al. Meta-analysis: effect of monotherapy and combination therapy with inhibitors of the renin angiotensin system on proteinuria in renal disease. *Ann Intern Med.* 2008;148:30–48.

53. Remuzzi G, Macia M, Ruggenenti P. Prevention and treatment of diabetic renal disease in type 2 diabetes: the BENEDICT study. *J Am Soc Nephrol.* 2006;17:S90–S97.

55. Whelton PK, Carey RM, Aronow WS, et al. 2017 ACC/AHA/AAPA/ABC/ACPM/AGS/APhA/ASH/ASPC/NMA/PCNA guideline for the prevention, detection, evaluation, and management of high blood pressure in adults: a report of the American College of Cardiology/American Heart Association task force on clinical practice guidelines. *Circulation.* 2018;138(17):e484–e594. doi:10.1161/CIR.0000000000000596. PMID: 30354654. No abstract available.

69. Hricik DE, Browning PJ, Kopelman R, et al. Captopril-induced functional renal insufficiency in patients with bilateral renal-artery stenoses or renal-artery stenosis in a solitary kidney. *N Engl J Med.* 1983;308:373–376.
79. Cohen JB, Townsend RR. Use of renin-angiotensin system blockade in patients with renal artery stenosis. *Clin J Am Soc Nephrol.* 2014;9:1149–1152.
82. Ahmed AK, Kamath NS, El Kossi M, et al. The impact of stopping inhibitors of the renin-angiotensin system in patients with advanced chronic kidney disease. *Nephrol Dial Transplant.* 2010;25(12): 3977–3982. doi:10.1093/ndt/gfp511. [Epub 2009 Oct 10]; PMID: 19820248.
94. Investigators O, Yusuf S, Teo KK, et al. Telmisartan, ramipril, or both in patients at high risk for vascular events. *N Engl J Med.* 2008;358:1547–1559.
95. Fried LF, Emanuele N, Zhang JH, et al. Combined angiotensin inhibition for the treatment of diabetic nephropathy. *N Engl J Med.* 2013;369:1892–1903.
96. Parving HH, Brenner BM, McMurray JJ, et al. Cardiorenal end points in a trial of aliskiren for type 2 diabetes. *N Engl J Med.* 2012;367:2204–2213.
132. Li CI, Daling JR, Tang M-TC, et al. Use of antihypertensive medications and breast cancer risk among women aged 55 to 74 years. *JAMA Intern Med.* 2013;173:1629–1637.
254. Ogawa S, Matsushima M, Mori T, et al. Identification of the stages of diabetic nephropathy at which angiotensin II receptor blockers most effectively suppress albuminuria. *Am J Hypertens.* 2013;26: 1064–1069.
256. Parving H-H, Brenner BM, McMurray JJV, et al. Cardiorenal end points in a trial of aliskiren for type 2 diabetes. *N Engl J Med.* 2012;367:2204–2213.
293. Sowers JR, Raij L, Jialal I, et al. Angiotensin receptor blocker/diuretic combination preserves insulin responses in obese hypertensives. *J Hypertens.* 2010;28:1761–1769.
333. Tieu A, Velenosi TJ, Kucey AS, et al. β-blocker dialyzability in maintenance hemodialysis patients: a randomized clinical trial. *Clin J Am Soc Nephrol.* 2018.
356. Poirier L, Lacourcière Y. The evolving role of β-adrenergic receptor blockers in managing hypertension. *Can J Cardiol.* 2012;28:334–340.
359. Ellison KE, Gandhi G. Optimising the use of beta-adrenoceptor antagonists in coronary artery disease. *Drugs.* 2005;65:787–797.
365. Gradman AH, Parisé H, Lefebvre P, et al. Initial combination therapy reduces the risk of cardiovascular events in hypertensive patients: a matched cohort study. *Hypertension.* 2013;61:309–318.
506. Grimaldi-Bensouda L, Klungel O, Kurz X, et al. Calcium channel blockers and cancer: a risk analysis using the UK Clinical Practice Research Datalink (CPRD). *BMJ Open.* 2016;6(1):e009147.
507. Raebel MA, et al. Risk of breast cancer with long-term use of calcium channel blockers or angiotensin-converting enzyme inhibitors among older women. *Am J Epidemiol.* 2017;185(4):264–273. doi:10.1093/aje/kww217.
542. Barton M. Endothelin antagonism and reversal of proteinuric renal disease in humans. *Contrib Nephrol.* 2011;172:210–222.
589. SPRINT Research Group, Wright JT Jr, Williamson JD, et al. A randomized trial of intensive versus standard blood-pressure control. *N Engl J Med.* 2015;373(22):2103–2116. doi:10.1056/NEJMoa1511939. [Epub 2015 Nov 9]; PMID: 26551272.
591. Williamson JD, Supiano MA, Applegate WB, et al. Intensive vs standard blood pressure control and cardiovascular disease outcomes in adults aged ≥75 years: a randomized clinical trial. *JAMA.* 2016.
592. Beckett NS, Peters R, Fletcher AE, et al. Treatment of hypertension in patients 80 years of age or older. *N Engl J Med.* 2008;358:1887–1898.
593. Huang C, Dhruva SS, Coppi AC, et al. Systolic blood pressure response in SPRINT (systolic blood pressure intervention trial) and ACCORD (action to control cardiovascular risk in diabetes): a possible explanation for discordant trial results. *J Am Heart Assoc.* 2017;6(11).
598. Rocco MV, Sink KM, Lovato LC, et al. Effects of intensive blood pressure treatment on acute kidney injury events in the systolic blood pressure intervention trial (SPRINT). *Am J Kidney Dis.* 2017.
630. Calhoun DA, Lacourcière Y, Chiang YT, et al. Triple antihypertensive therapy with amlodipine, valsartan, and hydrochlorothiazide: a randomized clinical trial. *Hypertension.* 2009;54:32–39.
633. Agarwal R, Andersen MJ. Blood pressure recordings within and outside the clinic and cardiovascular events in chronic kidney disease. *Am J Nephrol.* 2006;26:503–510.
656. Jamerson K, Weber MA, Bakris GL, et al. Benazepril plus amlodipine or hydrochlorothiazide for hypertension in high-risk patients. *N Engl J Med.* 2008;359:2417–2428.
669. Webster R, Salam A, de Silva HA, et al. Fixed low-dose triple combination antihypertensive medication vs usual care for blood pressure control in patients with mild to moderate hypertension in Sri Lanka: a randomized clinical trial. *JAMA.* 2018;320(6):566–579. doi:10.1001/jama.2018.10359. PMID: 30120478. Erratum in: *JAMA.* 320(18):1940, 2018.
682. Calhoun DA, Jones D, Textor S, et al. Resistant hypertension: diagnosis, evaluation, and treatment. A scientific statement from the American Heart Association Professional Education Committee of the Council for High Blood Pressure Research. *Hypertension.* 2008;51:1403–1419.
687. Bazzano LA, Khan Z, Reynolds K, et al. Effect of nocturnal nasal continuous positive airway pressure on blood pressure in obstructive sleep apnea. *Hypertension.* 2007;50(2):417–423. PMID: 17548722.

# 50 Diuretics

Ewout J. Hoorn | Christopher S. Wilcox | David H. Ellison

## CHAPTER OUTLINE



## KEY POINTS

- Dietary sodium restriction, selection of a diuretic with a prolonged action, or more frequent administration of the diuretic will enhance NaCl loss by limiting postdiuretic salt retention.
- During prolonged diuretic administration, and in the case of diuretic resistance, subjects may be particularly responsive to another class of diuretic.
- Torsemide is the preferred loop diuretic in heart failure because of better bioavailability, absence of hypokalemia, and superior outcomes compared with other loop diuretics.
- In heart failure, diuretic responsiveness is impaired, as shown by a shift to the right in the natriuresis-excretion relationship of diuretics.
- Compensatory distal reabsorption rather than reduced delivery drives diuretic resistance in heart failure.
- In chronic kidney disease, the maximal increase in fractional excretion of $Na^+$ produced by loop diuretics is maintained, but the absolute response is limited.
- The addition of an SGLT2 inhibitor may help relieve loop diuretic resistance in patients with diabetes mellitus while providing protection from progressive loss of the GFR.
- The risk of thiazide-induced hyponatremia increases in subjects with a variant in *SLCO2A1*, which inactivates a prostaglandin transporter and allows prostaglandin E2 to stimulate $EP_4$ receptors and insert aquaporin-2 water channels.

This chapter reviews the mechanisms of actions, physiologic adaptations, clinical uses, and adverse effects of diuretics. The term *diuretics* refers to several groups of drugs that share the effect of increasing urinary output. Most diuretics target sodium transport proteins in the kidney (natriuretics). Novel targets for which drugs are in preclinical development also include potassium and urea channels (urearetics; see "Novel Diuretics in Preclinical Development"). Other targets of diuretics include enzymes (e.g., carbonic anhydrase, neprilysin) or receptors (e.g., mineralocorticoid receptors) that indirectly control renal sodium reabsorption. Vasopressin receptor antagonists (vaptans) increase diuresis by selectively inhibiting water reabsorption (aquaretics). Osmotic diuretics are filtered but not reabsorbed and create a reverse osmotic gradient that inhibits the reabsorption of water and, indirectly, NaCl (solvent drag). Other diuretics also rely on osmotic diuresis, including the novel sodium-glucose transporter type 2 (SGLT2) inhibitors and the urea channel inhibitors.

The major sodium transport targets for diuretic drugs have been defined and their genes cloned. The effects of disease on diuretic kinetics are discussed in this chapter because they predict the required dosage modifications. Loop diuretics and thiazides are the most widely used diuretics, and the physiologic adaptations to their prolonged use are described. Diuretic resistance, its management, and major adverse effects of therapy are discussed. This discussion provides a framework for the design of strategies to maximize the desired actions while minimizing the unwanted effects. The chapter also includes a discussion of the practical use of diuretics in the treatment of specific clinical conditions.

Other chapters discuss the treatment of hypertension by diuretic drugs (Chapter 49), diuretic-induced changes in potassium excretion (Chapter 17), acid-base disturbances (Chapter 16), divalent cation excretion and nephrolithiasis (Chapters 18 and 38), the syndrome of inappropriate antidiuretic hormone (SIADH) secretion (Chapter 15), and

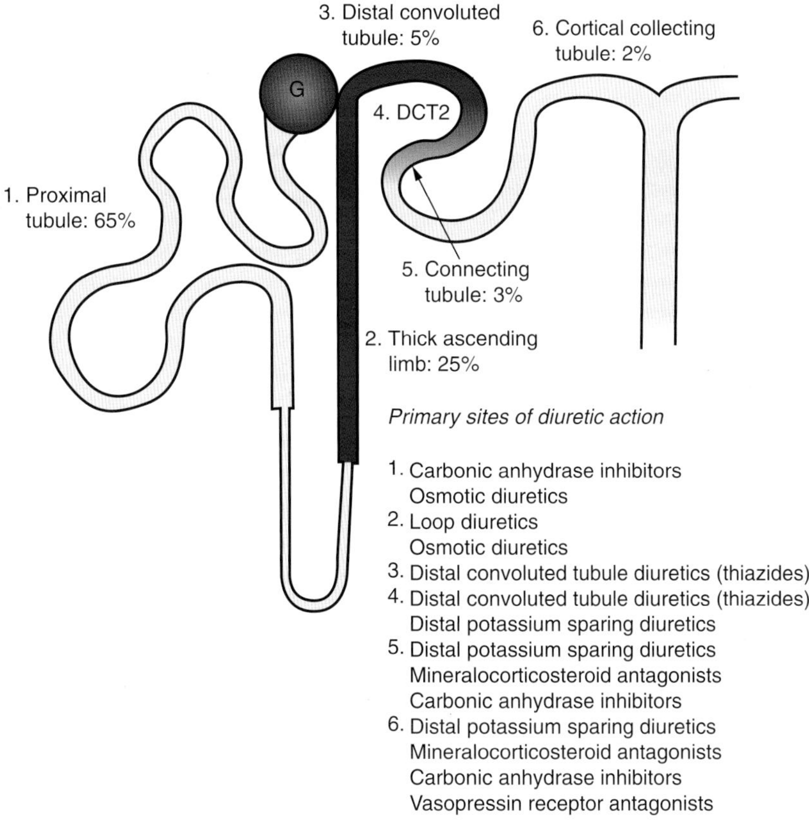


**Fig. 50.1** Nephron diagram showing the primary sites of diuretic action and the approximate percentage of filtered sodium reabsorbed at each. *DCT2,* Late segment of distal convoluted tubule; *G,* glomerulus.

acute kidney injury ([AKI]; Chapter 28). Diuretics have been reviewed extensively.[1–4] More extensive and historical references appeared in previous editions of this chapter; the interested reader is referred to editions 7 to 10 of *Brenner & Rector's The Kidney* for more detailed references.

## INDIVIDUAL CLASSES OF DIURETICS

The major sites of action of diuretics and fractions of filtered $Na^+$ reabsorbed at the corresponding nephron segments are summarized in Fig. 50.1.

### CARBONIC ANHYDRASE INHIBITORS

#### SITES AND MECHANISMS OF ACTION

In the kidney, carbonic anhydrase inhibitors (CAIs) act primarily on proximal tubule cells to inhibit bicarbonate absorption (Fig. 50.2). An additional, more modest, effect along the distal nephron, however, is also observed.[5] Carbonic anhydrase (CA), a metalloenzyme containing one zinc atom per molecule, is important in sodium bicarbonate reabsorption and hydrogen ion secretion by renal epithelial cells. The biochemical, morphologic, and functional properties of carbonic anhydrase have been reviewed.[6,7]

CA is expressed by many tissues, including erythrocytes, kidney, gut, ciliary body, choroid plexus, and glial cells. Although at least 14 isoforms of CA have been identified, two play predominant roles in renal acid-base homeostasis, CA II and CA IV. CA II is widely expressed, comprising the

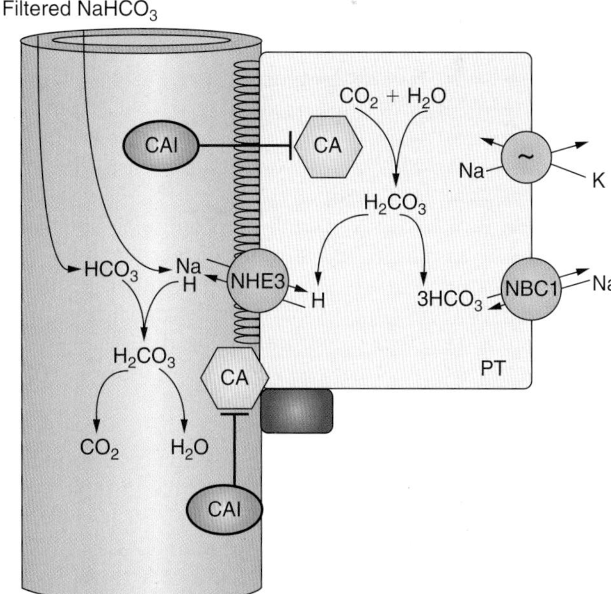


**Fig. 50.2** Mechanisms of diuretic action in the proximal tubule. The figure shows a functional model of proximal tubule cells; many transport proteins are omitted from the model for clarity. Inside the cell, carbonic anhydrase *(CA)* catalyzes the formation of $HCO_3^-$ from $OH^-$ and $CO_2$. Bicarbonate leaves the cell via the sodium-bicarbonate transporter (NBC1). A second pool of carbonic anhydrase is located in the brush border. This participates in disposing of the carbonic acid formed from filtered bicarbonate and secreted $H^+$. Both pools of carbonic anhydrase are inhibited by acetazolamide and other carbonic anhydrase inhibitors (*CAIs*; see text for details). *NBC1,* Sodium-bicarbonate cotransporter 1.

enzyme expressed by red blood cells and a variety of secretory and absorptive epithelia. In the kidney, CA II is expressed in the cytoplasm and accounts for 95% of renal CA.[7] It is present in proximal tubule cells and intercalated cells of the aldosterone-sensitive distal nephron (ASDN).[7] CA IV is expressed at the luminal border of the cells of the proximal thick ascending limb (TAL) of the loop of Henle and α-intercalated cells of the ASDN.[8]

The prototypic CAI is acetazolamide. However, many diuretics have some CAI action.[9] This characteristic contributes to the weak inhibition of proximal reabsorption by furosemide and chlorothiazide and to the relaxation of vascular smooth muscle cells by high-dose furosemide.[9]

CAIs block the catalytic dehydration of luminal carbonic acid at the brush border of the proximal tubule, decrease the intracellular generation of $H^+$ required for countertransport with $Na^+$, and decrease the peritubular capillary fluid uptake.[10] CAIs also are also weak inhibitors of reabsorption in the TAL,[11] but the natriuretic efficacy of CAIs and loop diuretics (see later) is additive, confirming their independent mechanisms of action.[12] CAIs also inhibit bicarbonate reabsorption along the distal tubule, presumably by interfering with the action of α-intercalated cells.[7] The first administration of a CAI causes a brisk alkaline diuresis. The excretion of $Na^+$, $K^+$, $HCO_3^-$, and $PO_4^{2-}$ increases, whereas the excretion of titratable acid and $NH_4^+$ decrease sharply. Excretion of $Ca^{2+}$ remains essentially unchanged. There is substantial kaliuresis owing to the presence of nonreabsorbable $HCO_3^-$ and high flow rates in the distal nephron. However, hypokalemia is uncommon, because acidosis partitions $K^+$ out of cells.

Long-term CAI administration causes only a modest natriuresis, despite the magnitude of CA-dependent proximal $Na^+$ reabsorption. Several factors account for this:

1. CA is required for the reabsorption of $HCO_3^-$, whereas about two thirds of the proximal $Na^+$ reabsorption is accompanied by $Cl^-$.
2. Some proximal $HCO_3^-$ reabsorption persists, even after apparently full inhibition of CA.[13]
3. Some of the $HCO_3^-$ that is delivered out of the proximal tubule can be reabsorbed at more distal sites.[13]
4. The metabolic acidosis that develops limits the filtered load of $HCO_3^-$ and thereby curtails the natriuresis.
5. The increased delivery of filtered $Na^+$ to the macula densa elicits a tubuloglomerular feedback (TGF)–induced reduction in the glomerular filtration rate (GFR).[14]

Micropuncture studies of mice with deletion of the proximal $Na^+$-$H^+$ exchanger, NHE3, have shown that inhibition of proximal Na reabsorption is largely balanced by reduced GFR,[15] supporting this mechanism. Although CAIs only cause a modest natriuresis, the combined use of a thiazide and acetazolamide results in a brisk natriuresis.[16] This observation may be explained by the fact that acetazolamide inhibits the $HCO_3^-/Cl^-$ exchanger pendrin, which is upregulated secondary to upstream sodium chloride cotransporter (NCC) inhibition by thiazide diuretics.[16,17]

## PHARMACOKINETICS

Acetazolamide (Diamox) is readily absorbed. It is eliminated with a half-life ($t_{1/2}$) of 13 hours by tubular secretion, which is diminished during hypoalbuminemia.[18] Methazolamide (Neptazane) has less plasma protein binding, a longer $t_{1/2}$, and greater lipid solubility, all of which favor penetration into aqueous humor and cerebrospinal fluid. This agent has less renal effect and therefore was used to treat glaucoma.

## CLINICAL INDICATIONS

The use of CAIs as diuretics is limited by their transient action, the development of metabolic acidosis, and a spectrum of adverse effects. They can be used with $NaHCO_3$ infusion to initiate an alkaline diuresis that increases the excretion of weakly acidic drugs (e.g., salicylates, phenobarbital) or acidic metabolites (e.g., urate). Chloride depletion metabolic alkalosis is best treated by the administration of $Cl^-$ with $K^+$ or $Na^+$. However, if this produces unacceptable extracellular volume (ECV) expansion, acetazolamide (250–500 mg/day) and KCl can be used to increase $HCO_3^-$ excretion.

Metabolic alkalosis due to loop diuretics or thiazides can depress respiration in patients with chronic respiratory acidosis—for example, due to chronic obstructive pulmonary disease. This effect provides the rationale for use of a CAI. Indeed, the administration of acetazolamide to such subjects can reduce the arterial partial pressure of arterial carbon dioxide ($Pa_{CO_2}$) and improve the partial pressure of oxygen ($Pa_{O_2}$). Because both $Pa_{CO_2}$ and the plasma bicarbonate concentration ($P_{HCO_3}$) decrease, there is little change in blood pH.[19] However, a reduction in $P_{HCO_3}$ limits the buffering capacity of blood. CAIs can increase the $Pa_{CO_2}$ during metabolic acidosis or exercise, perhaps by depressing hypoxic ventilatory drive[20] and hypoxic pulmonary vasoconstriction,[21] and can cause ventilation-perfusion imbalance.[22] Nevertheless, acetazolamide (250 mg bid) can improve blood gas parameters in patients with chronic obstructive pulmonary disease.[23] Careful surveillance is required when CAIs are administered to such patients.

When used to treat glaucoma, CAIs diminish the transport of $HCO_3^-$ and $Na^+$ by the ciliary process, thereby reducing the intraocular pressure.[24] CAIs also limit the formation of cerebrospinal fluid[25] and endolymph.[26] Currently, their use to treat glaucoma is typically limited to topical preparations, most commonly as combination agents. On the other hand, oral acetazolamide is still widely used as one of the therapeutic interventions in the management of idiopathic intracranial hypertension (IIH; also sometimes referred to as *pseudotumor cerebri*).[27]

Acute mountain sickness is characterized by headache, nausea, drowsiness, insomnia, shortness of breath, dizziness, and malaise after an abrupt ascent. Acetazolamide is useful in dosages of 250 to 750 mg daily as prophylaxis against mountain sickness, probably through stimulating respiration and diminishing cerebral blood flow and cerebrospinal fluid formation.[28–30] Used in established mountain sickness, acetazolamide improves oxygenation and pulmonary gas exchange.[31] It can stimulate ventilation in patients with central sleep apnea.[32] In patients with IIH, acetazolamide administration, along with a low-sodium weight reduction diet, modestly improves visual field function.[33]

CAIs are effective in the prophylaxis of hypokalemic periodic paralysis because they diminish the influx of $K^+$ into cells.[34] Paradoxically, they are also useful in the treatment of hyperkalemic periodic paralysis.[35]

It was recently shown, in mice, that acetazolamide attenuates lithium-induced nephrogenic diabetes insipidus, with fewer adverse effects than thiazides and amiloride.[36] This effect was ascribed to a reduction in the GFR and activation of TGF, but may also indicate a specific effect in the collecting duct. Clinical data are needed to assess the corresponding effect in humans.

Other indications for CAIs are experimental. They include possible applications in diseases as diverse as obesity, cancer, and infection.[37]

### ADVERSE EFFECTS

Patients taking CAIs may complain of weakness, lethargy, abnormal taste, paresthesia, gastrointestinal distress, malaise, and decreased libido. These symptoms can be diminished by $NaHCO_3$ but this agent increases the risk of nephrocalcinosis and nephrolithiasis.[38] Overall, symptomatic metabolic acidosis develops in 50% of patients with glaucoma treated with CAIs.[39]

Older patients or those with diabetes mellitus or chronic kidney disease (CKD) can experience a serious metabolic acidosis if given a CAI.[39] An alkaline urine favors partitioning of renal ammonia into blood rather than its elimination in urine. An increase in blood ammonia may precipitate encephalopathy in patients with liver failure.[39]

Acetazolamide increases the risk of nephrolithiasis by more than tenfold.[40] CAIs occasionally cause allergic reactions, hepatitis, and blood dyscrasias.[41] They can cause osteomalacia when used with phenytoin or phenobarbital.[42]

## OSMOTIC DIURETICS

### SITES AND MECHANISMS OF ACTION

Osmotic diuretics are substances that are freely filtered but poorly reabsorbed.[43] Mannitol is the prototypic osmotic diuretic, although sorbitol and glycerol have similar actions. In the water-permeable nephron segments of the proximal nephron and thin limbs of the loop of Henle, fluid reabsorption concentrates filtered mannitol sufficiently to diminish tubular fluid reabsorption. Ongoing $Na^+$ reabsorption lowers the tubular fluid [$Na^+$] and creates a gradient for backflux of reabsorbed $Na^+$ into the tubule. Increased distal flow stimulates $K^+$ secretion.

Mannitol is a hypertonic solute that abstracts water from cells. The increase in total renal blood flow (RBF) relates in part to hemodilution and a decrease in hematocrit and viscosity. Mannitol increases the medullary blood flow and decreases the medullary solute gradient, thereby preventing urinary concentration. The rise in renal plasma flow and drop in plasma colloid osmotic pressure can increase the GFR.[44]

### PHARMACOKINETICS AND DOSAGE

Mannitol is distributed exclusively to the extracellular fluid. It is filtered freely at the glomerulus. Consequently, the $t_{1/2}$ for plasma clearance of mannitol depends on the GFR and is prolonged from 1 to 36 hours in those with advanced CKD.[45] It can be infused intravenously in daily doses of 50 to 200 g as a 15% or 20% solution or 1.5 to 2.0 g/kg of 20% mannitol over 30 to 60 minutes to treat elevated intraocular or intracranial pressure.[43]

### CLINICAL INDICATIONS

Mannitol has been evaluated for the prophylaxis of AKI, but controlled trials of its use in patients at risk for AKI have not had positive results.[46,47] The rationale for such trials includes mannitol's ability to expand the ECV, block TGF, maintain the GFR, increase RBF and tubule fluid flow, prevent tubule obstruction from shed cell constituents or crystals, reduce renal edema, redistribute blood flow from the outer cortex to the relatively hypoxic inner cortex and outer medulla, and scavenge oxygen radicals.[43,44] It can protect against AKI in cadaveric kidney transplant recipients.[43] The use of diuretics to convert oliguric to nonoliguric AKI is discussed later (see "Clinical Uses of Diuretics").

A trial of mannitol therapy for cerebral edema complicating hepatic failure has demonstrated a markedly better survival of 47%, compared with only 6% in the control group.[48] Mannitol is recommended for the management of severe head injury.[49,50] It is more effective than loop diuretics or hypertonic saline in reducing brain water content.[51] Mannitol can reverse the dialysis disequilibrium syndrome.[52]

### ADVERSE EFFECTS

The effects of mannitol on plasma electrolyte concentrations are complex. The osmotic abstraction of cell water initially causes hypertonic hyponatremia and hypochloremia. Later, when the excess extracellular fluid (ECF) is excreted, the decrease in cell water concentrates $K^+$ and $H^+$ within cells, thereby increasing the gradient for their diffusion into the ECF and leading to hyperkalemic acidosis. Normally, these electrolyte changes are rapidly corrected by the kidney, provided that renal function is adequate. Later, hypernatremic dehydration may develop if free water is not provided because urinary concentrating ability is inhibited.[53]

Expansion of ECV, hemodilution, and hyperkalemic metabolic acidosis occur in patients with renal failure who cannot eliminate the drug. Circulatory overload, pulmonary edema, central nervous system depression, and severe hyponatremia require urgent hemodialysis.[54] Doses of more than 200 g/day can cause renal vasoconstriction and AKI.[43]

## LOOP DIURETICS

### SITES AND MECHANISMS OF ACTION

The primary action of loop diuretics occurs from the luminal aspect of the TAL (Fig. 50.3). An electroneutral Na-K-2Cl cotransporter, termed "NKCC2," is located at the luminal membrane.[55,56] This cotransporter, a member of the solute carrier family 12 (gene symbol *SLC12A1*), mediates $Na^+$ and $Cl^-$ movement across the cell. A high luminal $K^+$ conductance, via the renal outer medullary $K^+$ (ROMK) channel, allows most of the $K^+$ to recycle across the luminal membrane.[57] Coupled with the electrogenic exit of $Cl^-$ across the basolateral membrane, the activity of the NKCC2 generates a transepithelial voltage, oriented positively with the lumen relative to interstitial fluid. The primary energy for transport across TAL cells is provided via the basolateral sodium pump, $Na^+$-$K^+$–adenosine triphosphatase (ATPase), which maintains a low intracellular [$Na^+$]. Additional details concerning mechanisms of solute reabsorption by TAL cells can be found in Chapter 6. Loop diuretics are organic anions that bind to the NKCC2 from the luminal surface. Early studies have shown that [$^3$H] bumetanide binds to membranes that express the NKCC proteins and that $Cl^-$ competes for the same binding site on the transport protein.[58] Studies using chimeric NKCC molecules have investigated sites of bumetanide binding and

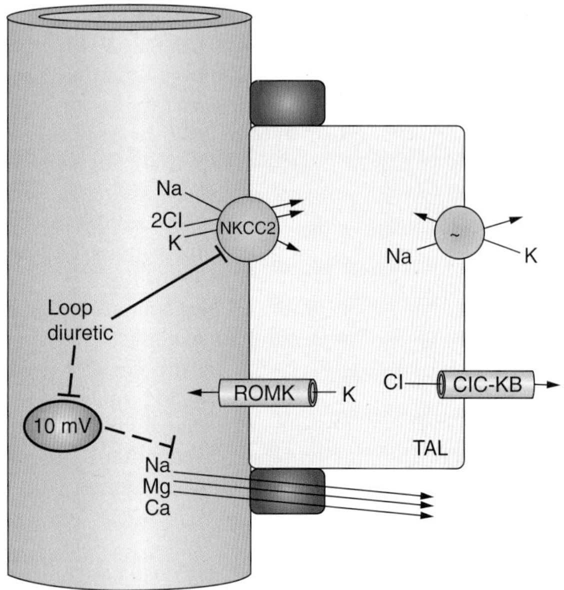


**Fig. 50.3** Mechanisms of diuretic action along the loop of Henle. The figure shows a model of thick ascending limb cells. $Na^+$ and $Cl^-$ are reabsorbed across the apical membrane via the loop diuretic–sensitive Na-K-2Cl cotransporter 2 *(NKCC2)*. Loop diuretics bind to and block this pathway directly. Note that the transepithelial voltage along the thick ascending limb is oriented with the lumen positive relative to blood (*circled* value, given in millivolts [mV]). This transepithelial voltage drives a component of $Na^+$ (and calcium and magnesium; see Fig. 50.4) reabsorption via the paracellular pathway. This component of $Na^+$ absorption is also reduced by loop diuretics because they reduce the transepithelial voltage. *ClC-KB,* Chloride channel protein; *ROMK,* renal outer medullary $K^+$ channel; *TAL,* thick ascending limb.

interactions with ions by determining effects on the ion transport of heterologously expressed NKCC proteins; it was found that changes in amino acids that affect bumetanide binding are not the same as patterns of changes affecting the kinetics of ion translocation.[59,60] Nevertheless, the second membrane-spanning segment of NKCC2 does appear to participate in both anion affinity and bumetanide affinity.[59,60] A clearer picture of the details of diuretic and ion interaction with the NKCC protein must await structural biology advances for atomic level resolution.

NKCC2 is expressed on the apical membranes of medullary and cortical TALs and macula densa segments.[61,62] Its abundance is increased by prolonged infusion of saline or furosemide.[61] A closely related gene, *NKCCl,* encodes a protein that is widely expressed in transporting epithelia.[55] In contrast to NKCC2, *NKCCl* is implicated in the uptake and secretion of $Cl^-$ and $NH_4^+$ at the basolateral membrane of the medullary CDs.[63]

Hormones that stimulate cyclic adenosine monophosphate (cAMP), such as arginine vasopressin (AVP), enhance TAL reabsorption and should enhance the response to loop diuretics.[64] In contrast, those that stimulate cyclic guanosine monophosphate (cGMP), such as nitric oxide and atrial natriuretic peptide (ANP), those that increase intracellular [$Ca^{2+}$], such as 20-hydroxyeicosatetraenoic acid (20-HETE), or those that activate the $Ca^{2+}$ (polyvalent cation)–sensing protein[65] inhibit TAL reabsorption and reduce the response to loop diuretics.[66]

The rat TAL also transports $NH_4^+$,[67] which can substitute for $K^+$ on NKCC2. In the rat, there is a luminal $Na^+$-$H^+$ countertransporter that contributes to tubular fluid acidification. Loop diuretics block the luminal entry of $Na^+$ via NKCC2, but not the peritubular exit via the $Na^+$-$K^+$-ATPase, and thereby reduce the intracellular [$Na^+$] sufficiently to promote luminal $Na^+$ uptake via the $Na^+$-$H^+$ countertransport process. This is one reason that furosemide stimulates acid excretion in the rat.[68,69] In some studies, furosemide has not affected net acid excretion or urine pH in normal human subjects.[70]

Loop diuretics reduce proximal fluid reabsorption modestly. This effect has been ascribed to a weak CAI action. However, furosemide depresses proximal reabsorption in tubules perfused with $HCO_3^-$-free solutions.[71] Moreover, bumetanide, which is a much less potent inhibitor of CA, also impairs proximal fluid reabsorption.[72]

Furosemide exerts two contrasting effects on reabsorption in the superficial distal tubule. Increased delivery to the unsaturated distal tubule reabsorption process increases $Na^+$ reabsorption.[68] However, Velazquez and Wright perfused rat distal tubules in vivo to obviate the confounding effects of altered delivery.[73] They concluded that furosemide, but not bumetanide, was a weak inhibitor of the thiazide-sensitive NCC, although the cloned NCC from flounder was not sensitive to furosemide when expressed in *Xenopus laevis* oocytes.[74] Loop diuretics also inhibit NaCl transport in short descending limbs of the loop of Henle[75] and collecting ducts (CDs).[76] Although the TAL is clearly the major site of action of loop diuretics, actions at other nephron segments contribute to the natriuresis by blunting the expected increase in reabsorption in the proximal tubule (in response to volume depletion) and the distal nephron (in response to increased load). Reabsorption of solute from the water-impermeable TAL segments dilutes the tubular fluid and concentrates the interstitium. Its inhibition by loop diuretics impairs free water excretion during water loading and free water reabsorption during dehydration.[77]

Loop diuretics increase the fractional excretion of $Ca^{2+}$ by up to 30%.[78] The predominant mechanism is a decrease in the magnitude of the lumen-positive transepithelial potential (Fig. 50.4; see Fig. 50.3). A large fraction of transepithelial $Ca^{2+}$ transport along the TAL traverses a paracellular pathway involving claudins 16 and 19 and is driven by the lumen-positive transepithelial potential.[79] By reducing the magnitude of this potential, loop diuretics lower passive calcium absorption along this segment. A second mechanism has been observed in some experiments, involving active $Ca^{2+}$ transport, but this pathway is not affected by loop diuretics.[80]

The loop of Henle is also a major nephron segment for the reabsorption of $Mg^{2+}$.[78] $Mg^{2+}$ transport along the TAL, like $Ca^{2+}$ transport, traverses a paracellular pathway that involves claudins and is driven by the transepithelial potential difference. Loop diuretics can increase fractional $Mg^{2+}$ excretion by more than 60%[74] by diminishing voltage-dependent paracellular transport[78] (see Figs. 50.3 and 50.4 and see later discussion of adverse effects). Loop diuretics initially increase urate excretion by inhibiting proximal urate transport.[81] However, there is a succeeding reduction in urate clearance that is largely secondary to volume depletion.[82] The total RBF is maintained or increased and the GFR is little changed during the administration of loop diuretics to

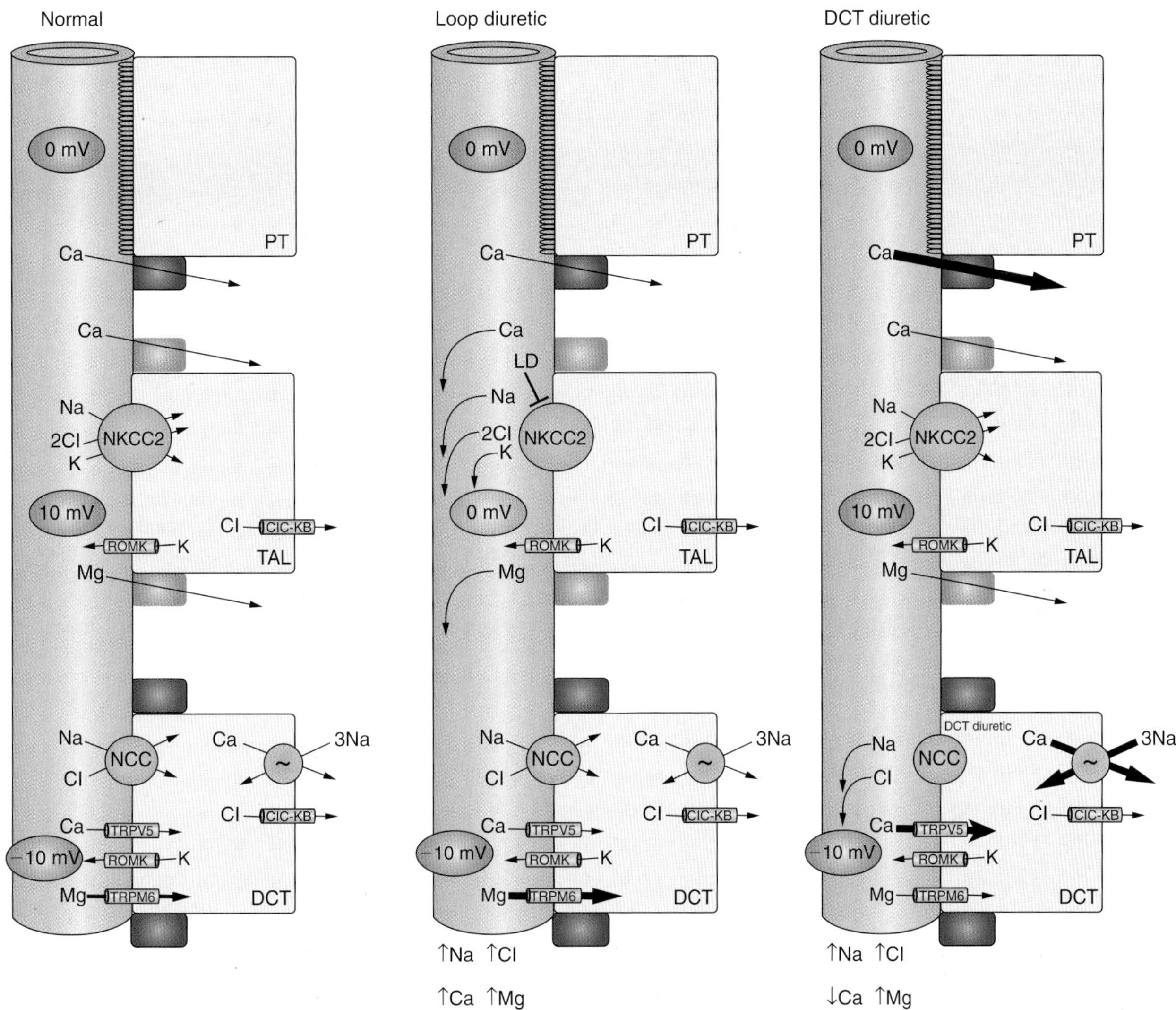


**Fig. 50.4** Possible mechanisms of diuretic effects on calcium and magnesium excretion. Typical cells from the proximal tubule *(PT)*, thick ascending limb *(TAL)*, and distal convoluted tubule *(DCT)* are shown. Calcium reabsorption occurs along the distal convoluted tubule largely via a transient receptor potential channel *(TRPV5)*. Magnesium reabsorption occurs along the distal convoluted tubule largely via a transient receptor potential channel *(TRPM6)*. Transepithelial voltages (representative but arbitrary values, given in millivolts [mV]) are shown. Net effects on electrolyte excretion are shown at the *bottom*. Normal conditions are at the *left*. Treatment with loop diuretics (LDs) is shown in the *middle*; treatment with DCT diuretics is shown on the *right*. Loop diuretics reduce the magnitude of the lumen-positive transepithelial voltage, thereby retarding passive calcium and magnesium reabsorption. Passive calcium and magnesium reabsorption appears to traverse the paracellular pathway. Long-term treatment, especially with DCT diuretics, increases proximal $Na^+$ and $Ca^{2+}$ reabsorption; thus, less calcium is delivered distally. Enhanced distal calcium absorption, driven by DCT diuretics, also occurs. Effects of DCT diuretics to increase magnesium excretion remain incompletely understood. *ClC-KB,* Chloride channel protein; *NCC,* Na-Cl transporter; *NKCC2,* Na-K-2Cl cotransporter 2; *ROMK,* renal outer medullary $K^+$ channel; ↑, increase(d); ↓, decrease(d).

normal subjects.[83] However, there is a marked redistribution of blood flow from the inner to the outer cortex.[84] The fall in papillary plasma flow depends on angiotensin II.[85] Furosemide increases the renal generation of prostaglandins.[86] Blockade of cyclooxygenase prevents furosemide-induced renal vasodilation.[87]

The macula densa participates importantly both in renin secretion and in TGF-mediated control of GFR. NaCl entry into macula densa cells regulates both processes; thus, loop diuretics affect both TGF and renin secretion. When the luminal NaCl concentration at the macula densa rises, as during ECV expansion, NaCl entry into macula densa cells leads to the production of adenosine, which interacts with adenosine 1 receptors on vascular smooth muscle and/or extraglomerular mesangial cells, activating phospholipase C. This activation leads to the depolarization and activation of voltage-dependent $Ca^{2+}$ channels, which contract afferent arterioles and reduce the GFR (the TGF response).[88] NaCl transport across the luminal membrane of macula densa cells traverses the NKCC2.[62] Loop diuretics, by blocking NaCl entry into macula densa cells, block TGF completely.[89] This is one reason that loop diuretics tend to preserve GFR despite ECV depletion.

Loop diuretics also stimulate renin secretion, both in the short term and long term. Although this effect results, in part, from ECV depletion, a major component is from direct effects of loop diuretics on the macula densa. NaCl uptake into macula densa cells inhibits renin secretion acutely and inhibits renin synthesis chronically.[90] Macula densa cells were shown to express cyclooxygenase-2 (COX-2). Schnermann has shown that lowering NaCl concentration bathing a macula densa cell line acutely increases the release of prostaglandin E2 (PGE2), followed by a delayed induction of COX-2 expression.[90] A similar stimulation of COX-2 expression was also caused by furosemide and bumetanide. A lowering of the medium chloride concentration was followed by rapid phosphorylation of p44/42 and p38 MAP kinases, and the presence of p44/42 and p38 inhibitors prevented the stimulation of COX-2 expression by low chloride. In summary, a decrease in luminal NaCl concentration activates and transcriptionally induces COX-2, causing PGE2 release, and PGE2 receptor type 4 (EP4)–mediated stimulation of renin secretion and renin synthesis. Nitric oxide synthase inhibition with L-NAME ($N^G$-nitro-L-arginine methyl ester) has been found to completely block the increase in renin messenger RNA (mRNA) after the administration of furosemide for 4 days by minipump infusion.[91] Similarly, the increase in renin content in renal microvessels caused by a 5-day furosemide treatment was completely prevented by L-NAME.[92] However, mice made deficient in both the neuronal and endothelial forms of nitric oxide synthase display relatively normal renin responses to loop diuretics.[93] These data have been interpreted to suggest that nitric oxide synthesis plays a permissive role in macula densa–mediated renin secretion.

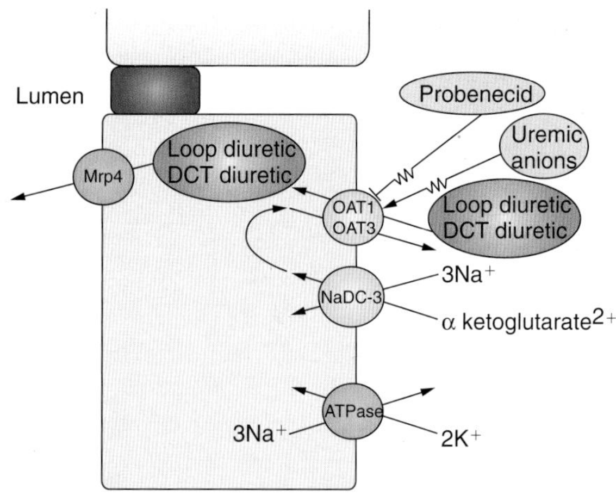


**Fig. 50.5** Mechanisms of diuretic secretion by proximal tubule cells. Cell diagram of the S2 segment of the proximal tubule shows secretion of anionic diuretics, including loop diuretics and distal convoluted tubule *(DCT)* diuretics. Peritubular uptake by an organic anion transporter (primarily OAT1, although OAT3 may play a smaller role) occurs in exchange for α-ketoglutarate, which is brought into the cell by the $Na^+$-dependent cation transporter NaDC-3. Luminal secretion can occur via a voltage-dependent pathway or in exchange for luminal hydroxyl or urate. A portion of the luminal transport traverses multidrug resistance–associated protein 4 *(Mrp4)*. *ATPase,* Adenosine triphosphatase.

## PHARMACOKINETICS AND DIFFERENCES BETWEEN DRUGS

Loop diuretics are absorbed promptly after ingestion, but their bioavailabilities vary. Because bumetanide and torsemide are more completely absorbed than furosemide, changing from intravenous to oral dosing may require a doubling of the furosemide dose but does not require changing the bumetanide or torsemide dose. Moreover, there is considerable variation in furosemide absorption, both between patients and over time,[94] that is accentuated by food intake.[95,96]

The highly variable bioavailability of furosemide compared with torsemide and the absence of hypokalemia with usual doses,[97] combined with the superior outcomes of torsemide in two clinical trials of patients with heart failure[98,99] have prompted consideration that torsemide become the loop diuretic of choice, at least for heart failure.[100–102] However, a class problem shared with all available loop diuretics is their short duration of action, 2 to 4 hours.[97] The resulting torrential diuresis (termed the *Niagara effect*) can be troubling, especially for patients with prostatism or stress incontinence. Moreover, the limited time of action of a daily dose of diuretic on the tubules provides some 20 hours for the kidneys to regain salt and water losses (see Fig. 50.10). An investigational extended-release formulation of torsemide that delivers torsemide to the circulation over 8 to 12 hours doubled salt and water losses in normal volunteers in the day after a single dose, without increasing potassium excretion.[103] Remarkably, one dose of the extended-release torsemide given to subjects ingesting 300 mmol of $Na^+$ daily, caused a negative daily $Na^+$ balance, whereas prior studies with furosemide at this level of salt intake reported no net loss of $Na^+$ because of postdiuretic salt retention.[104]

Once absorbed, loop diuretics circulate largely bound to albumin (91%–99%), greatly limiting their clearance by glomerular filtration. The diuretic volume of distribution varies inversely with the serum albumin concentration,[105] but this is not usually a major determinant of diuretic responsiveness (see later).[106] The metabolism of loop diuretics is comprised of both hepatic and renal mechanisms; the relative fractions that are cleared by each mechanism differ among agents. Loop diuretics, thiazides, and CAIs are all secreted avidly by a probenecid-sensitive organic anion transporter in proximal tubule cells (Fig. 50.5).[107,108] Diuretics gain access to tubular fluid almost exclusively by proximal secretion. Studies have characterized this weak organic anion ($OA^-$) transport process. Four isoforms of an OA transporter (OAT) have been cloned and are expressed in the kidney.[108,109] Peritubular uptake by an OAT is a tertiary active process (see Fig. 50.5). Energy derives from the basolateral $Na^+$-$K^+$-ATPase providing a low intracellular [$Na^+$] that drives an uptake of $Na^+$ coupled to α-ketoglutarate (α-KG) to maintain a high intracellular level of α-KG. This in turn drives a basolateral OA–α-KG countertransporter. OAT1 is expressed on the basolateral membrane of the S2 segment of the proximal tubule.[110] A mouse colony deficient in OAT1 was generated and shown to exhibit dramatically impaired renal OA secretion and furosemide resistance.[111] A similar effect was observed in OAT3-deficient mice, suggesting that both OAT1 and OAT3 mediate the secretion of loop diuretic by proximal cells, and that a lack of either is not fully compensated by the other.[112]

OATs translocate diuretics into the proximal tubule cell, where they can be sequestered in intracellular vesicles. They are secreted across the luminal membrane by a voltage-driven OA transporter[113] and by a countertransporter in exchange for urate or $OH^-$.[109] The orphan transporter hNPT4 (human sodium phosphate transporter 4; SLC17A3) has been identified as an organic anion efflux transporter that likely also secretes furosemide and bumetanide.[114] In addition, the multidrug resistance–associated protein 4 (MRP4) has been identified as the third type of transporter involved in the urinary excretion of diuretics. Mice lacking MRP4 exhibited an almost twofold lower excretion of furosemide and hydrochlorothiazide.[115] Approximately 50% of furosemide is eliminated by metabolism to the inactive glucuronide. Only the unmetabolized and secreted fraction is available to inhibit NaCl reabsorption. In contrast, bumetanide and torsemide are metabolized in the liver.[116,117] Slow-release furosemide is more effective in reducing blood pressure and treating edema, highlighting the importance of pharmacokinetics in diuretic responsiveness.[118] Torsemide's action is approximately twice as long as furosemide's,[119] and bumetanide's action is shorter than that of furosemide. These differences may be clinically relevant.[98,120] Unlike the elimination of bumetanide or torsemide,[119] the elimination of furosemide in patients with CKD is greatly reduced because its metabolism to the inactive glucuronide occurs in the kidney; in contrast, metabolic inactivation of bumetanide and torsemide occurs mainly in the liver and therefore they are unaffected by uremia.[4] This difference prolongs the $t_{1/2}$ of furosemide in CKD, leading to drug accumulation. However, the fraction of a dose excreted unchanged in patients with CKD is greater for furosemide, leading to an enhanced natriuretic response (Fig. 50.6). There is therefore a tradeoff in the selection of a loop diuretic in CKD: Furosemide can accumulate and cause ototoxicity at high doses, whereas bumetanide retains its metabolic inactivation but is therefore somewhat less potent.

Renal clearance of the active form of loop diuretics is reduced in CKD in proportion to the creatinine clearance.[121] There is competition both for peritubular uptake[108] and for luminal secretion[113] with other OAs, including urate, which accumulate in uremia. Metabolic acidosis depolarizes the membrane potential of proximal tubule cells,[122] which decreases OA secretion,[113] an effect that may explain why diuretic secretion is enhanced by alkalosis.[123] Therefore, the increased plasma levels of OAs and urate and the metabolic acidosis of CKD impair proximal tubule secretion of diuretics and, hence, impair their delivery to their active sites in the nephron.

Proximal secretion of active furosemide is potentiated by albumin.[124] In the rabbit, an equal fraction of administered furosemide is taken up by probenecid-sensitive mechanisms in the S2 (secretory) or S1 segment of the proximal tubule, where it is conjugated and excreted as the inactive glucuronide (Fig. 50.7).[125] Unlike the uptake and secretion of active furosemide by the S2 segment, uptake and metabolism by the S1 segment is enhanced by a drop in albumin concentration. Therefore, a low serum albumin concentration enhances furosemide metabolism[126] yet decreases tubular secretion of active diuretic.[124] The consequences of this process are described later (see "Nephrotic Syndrome").

There is a similar sigmoidal relation between fractional sodium excretion and the log of the urinary diuretic concentration (Fig. 50.8). Inhibition of proximal secretion with probenecid shifts the curve of the plasma dose-response to the right but does not perturb the relationship between natriuresis and diuretic excretion.[127] Thus, natriuresis is related to the urinary concentration, but not the plasma concentration, of diuretic. The administration of indomethacin or other nonsteroidal antiinflammatory drugs (NSAIDs) reduces the responsiveness of the tubule to furosemide.[128] This reduction is due predominantly to reduced generation of PGE2, because a natriuretic response to furosemide can be restored in indomethacin-treated rats by the infusion of PGE2.[129] Both a reduced dietary salt intake and repeated administration of furosemide during salt restriction[104] diminish the renal tubular response to furosemide (see Fig. 50.8).

Although knowledge of the pharmacogenetics of diuretics is still rudimentary, a number of studies have demonstrated that certain polymorphisms contribute to individual differences in the response to loop diuretics. For example, in 97 healthy whites, one study reported that the acute effects of loop diuretics were greater in subjects with polymorphisms

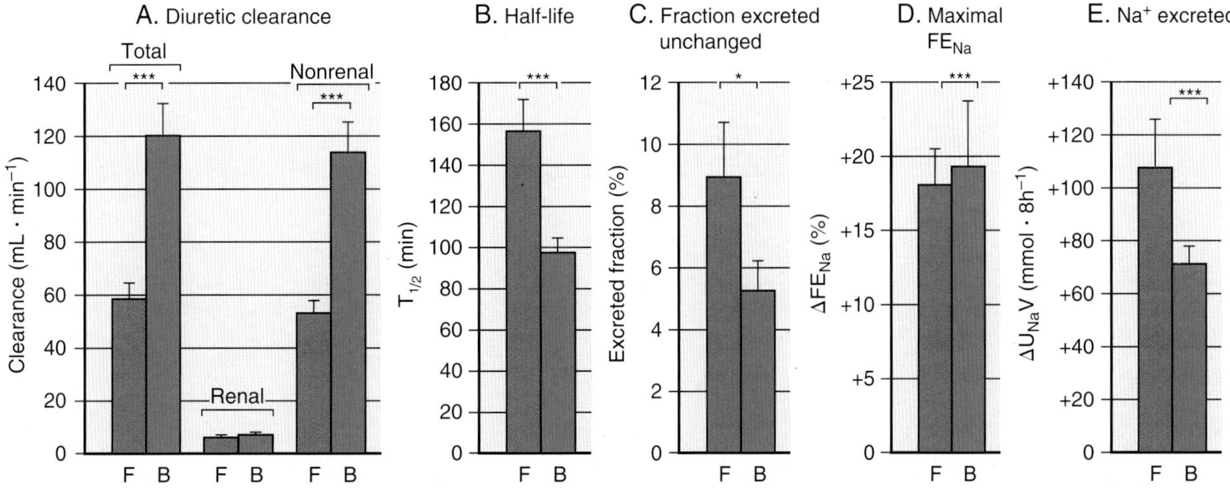


**Fig. 50.6** (A–E) Comparison of the pharmacokinetics and dynamics of furosemide (F, 160 mg; metabolically inactivated in the kidney) and bumetanide (B, 4 mg; metabolically inactivated in the liver) in 10 subjects with chronic kidney disease (mean creatinine clearance, 12 ± 2 mL/min). Significance of difference: *, $P < .05$; ***, $P < .005$. $FE_{Na}$, Fractional excretion of sodium; $T_{1/2}$, half-life; $U_{Na}$, urinary sodium. (Redrawn from data in Voelker JR, Cartwright-Brown D, Anderson S, et al. Comparison of loop diuretics in patients with chronic renal insufficiency. *Kidney Int.* 1987;32:572–578.)

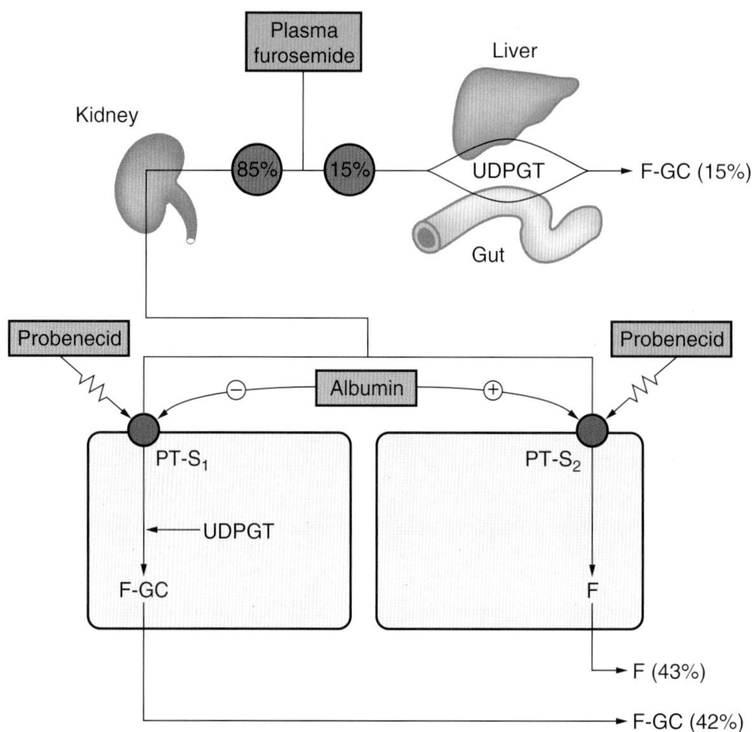


**Fig. 50.7** Diagrammatic representation of the disposition of intravenous furosemide and the effects of hypoalbuminemia or probenecid in normal or hypoalbuminemic rabbits. After intravenous administration of furosemide, 15% is metabolized by uridine diphosphate glucuronyl transferase *(UDPGT)* in the liver and gut to the inactive furosemide glucuronide *(F-GC)*. Of the remainder, 85% is transported by the kidney. Some 42% is taken up in the S1 segment of the proximal tubule *($PT-S_1$)* and metabolized to the inactive glucuronide, and the remainder is taken up by the S2 segment *($PT-S_2$)* and secreted in active form into the lumen. Both uptake processes are inhibited by probenecid. The plasma albumin concentration facilitates uptake and secretion by $PT-S_2$ but inhibits uptake and metabolism by $PT-S_1$. (Modified from Pichette V, Geadah D, du Souich P. The influence of moderate hypoalbuminemia on the renal metabolism and dynamics of furosemide in the rabbit. *Br J Pharmacol.* 1996;119:885–890.)

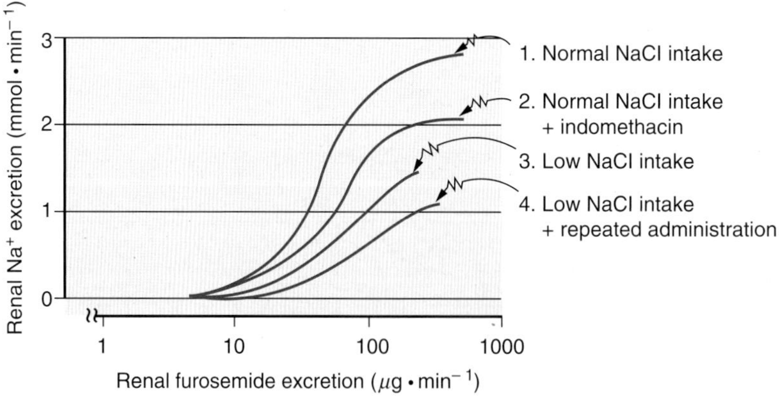


**Fig. 50.8** Relationship between the excretion of $Na^+$ and furosemide (log scale) following a bolus intravenous injection of 40 mg furosemide in normal subjects with a normal NaCl intake (1), with a normal NaCl intake after indomethacin (2), with a low $Na^+$ intake (20 mmol/24 hours) (3), and for the third day of furosemide administration with a low $Na^+$ intake (4). (Modified from Wilcox CS, Mitch WE, Kelly RA, et al. Response of the kidney to furosemide. *J Lab Clin Med.* 1983;102:450–458; and Chennavasin P, Seiwell R, Brater DC. Pharmacokinetic-dynamic analysis of the indomethacin-furosemide interaction in man. *J Pharmacol Exp Ther.* 1980;215:77–81.)

in the genes encoding NCC and the beta subunit of the epithelial $Na^+$ channel (ENaC), but smaller in those with a polymorphism in the gene encoding the gamma subunit of ENaC.[130] This finding suggests that individual variations in loop diuretic response may, in part, be attributed to lower or higher activities of transporters located distal to NKCC2. Another pharmacokinetic study has identified female gender and polymorphisms in the gene encoding the organic anion transporter OATP1B1 as predictors for the slower elimination of torsemide.[131]

## CLINICAL INDICATIONS

Clinical indications for the use of loop diuretics are discussed later (see "Clinical Uses of Diuretics").

## ADVERSE EFFECTS

Adverse effects of loop diuretics are discussed later (see "Adverse Effects of Diuretics").

# THIAZIDES AND THIAZIDE-LIKE DIURETICS (DISTAL CONVOLUTED TUBULE DIURETICS)

## SITES AND MECHANISMS OF ACTION

Thiazides and thiazide-like diuretics are moderately active drugs that increase the excretion of sodium, chloride, and potassium while reducing the excretion of calcium. The major site of action of thiazide and thiazide-like diuretics is the distal convoluted tubule (DCT), where they block coupled reabsorption of $Na^+$ and $Cl^-$ (Fig. 50.9).[73,96,132] The true thiazides (benzothiadiazines) are chlorothiazide, hydrochlorothiazide, bendroflumethiazide, and others. Subsequent to their development, nonthiazide drugs with similar activities were developed. Substitution of the ring sulfone in the thiazides with a carbonyl group provides a group of quinazolinones with diuretic activity similar to that of the thiazides (e.g., metolazone). Chlorthalidone, a substituted benzophenone that does not contain the benzothiadiazine molecular structure, exhibits strong CA activity and a prolonged half-life and has seen widespread use as an antihypertensive.

The predominant effect of the thiazide diuretics is to inhibit the thiazide-sensitive NCC (gene symbol *SLC12A3*). This protein is expressed in the DCT[133,134] and is inhibited directly by thiazides (see later). Several thiazides and thiazide-like drugs (e.g., chlorothiazide, hydrochlorothiazide, chlorthalidone) also inhibit CA, contributing to their natriuretic efficacy.[135] However, patients with Gitelman syndrome, who have a loss-of-function mutation in the NCC, and mice lacking NCC demonstrate a dramatically impaired natriuretic response to thiazides,[136] confirming that the principal effect of these drugs is to inhibit NCC. A small component of thiazide-sensitive

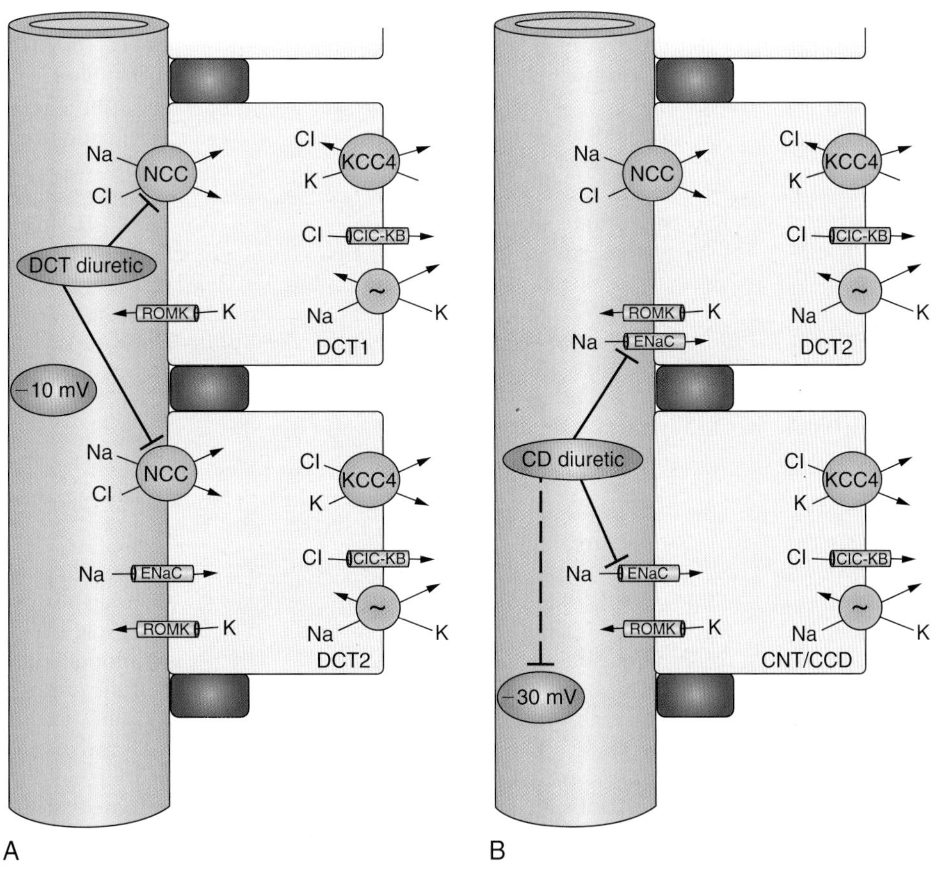


**Fig. 50.9** Mechanisms of distal convoluted tubule *(DCT)* and collecting duct *(CD)* diuretics. (A) Mechanism of action of DCT diuretics. In rat, mouse, and human, two types of DCT cells have been identified, referred to here as DCT1 and DCT2. $Na^+$ and $Cl^-$ are reabsorbed across the apical membrane of DCT1 cells only via the thiazide-sensitive $Na^+$-$Cl^-$ cotransporter *(NCC)*. This transport protein is also expressed by DCT2 cells where $Na^+$ can also cross through the epithelial $Na^+$ channel (ENaC; see text for details). Thus, the transepithelial voltage along the DCT1 is near to 0 mV, whereas it is finite and lumen-negative along the DCT2. (B) Mechanism of action of CD diuretics. The late distal convoluted tubule cells (DCT2 cells) and connecting tubule *(CNT)* or cortical collecting duct *(CCD)* cells are shown. $Na^+$ is reabsorbed via ENaC, which lies in parallel with a renal outer medullary $K^+$ channel (ROMK). The transepithelial voltage is oriented with the lumen negative, relative to the interstitium (shown in the *circled value*), generating a favorable gradient for transepithelial $K^+$ secretion. Drugs that block the epithelial $Na^+$ value reduce the voltage toward 0 mV (effect indicated by *dashed line*), thereby inhibiting $K^+$ secretion. *ClC-KB,* Chloride channel protein; *KCC4,* Potassium-chloride cotransporter 4.

Na+ excretion was observed in mice lacking NCC, which has been attributed to the inhibition of a sodium-dependent chloride-bicarbonate exchange process.[137] Furthermore, $Na^+$ reabsorption by the proximal tubule is enhanced during long-term treatment with thiazides, even when the drug has significant CA-inhibiting capacity.[138]

Like loop diuretics, diuretics that are active in the DCT, including the thiazides, are organic anions that bind to the transport protein from the luminal surface. The mechanism(s) of NCC inhibition have been studied using two approaches. First, Beaumont and Tran and colleagues have shown that [$^3$H]-metolazone binds avidly to kidney membrane proteins; its binding is inhibited competitively by $Cl^-$, suggesting that $Cl^-$ and diuretics compete for the same binding site.[139,140] These results are reminiscent of studies that used [$^3$H]-bumetanide to study properties of the NKCC proteins and were used to develop a kinetic model for the NCC.[141] Moreno and colleagues have expressed chimeras of the NCC in *Xenopus* oocytes and defined thiazide affinity on the basis of transport inhibition. The results suggest a more complicated picture. They concluded that thiazide diuretic affinity is conferred by transmembrane segments 8 through 12, whereas transmembrane segments 1 through 7 affect chloride affinity. Both domains are involved in determining $Na^+$ affinity.[142] These data suggest that the affinity of thiazide diuretics for binding to the transport protein is in a region distinct from the region that participates in $Cl^-$ transport.

Thiazides increase potassium excretion, but do not augment DCT secretion of $K^+$ directly.[96,143] Instead, their effects result from their tendency to stimulate aldosterone secretion, increase distal flow, and increase calcium reabsorption.[144] Mineralocorticoids, glucocorticoids,[145] and estrogens[146] enhance thiazide binding and tubular actions. Thiazides reduce $Ca^{2+}$ excretion. Three potential and nonredundant mechanisms have been postulated (see Fig. 50.4).[147,148] First, blockade of luminal NaCl entry reduces the tubule cell intracellular [$Na^+$] sufficiently to enhance basolateral $Na^+$-$Ca^{2+}$ exchange.[149] Second, thiazide-induced blockade of luminal NaCl entry reduces cell $Cl^-$ concentration, thereby hyperpolarizing the membrane voltage (making the interior of the cell more negative, electrically). Hyperpolarization increases calcium entry via the transient receptor potential channel subfamily V, member 5 (TRPV5) channel, which is expressed at the apical membrane of DCT and connecting tubule cells.[150,151] Third, thiazides stimulate proximal reabsorption of $Ca^{2+}$ owing to ECV depletion.[152] The importance of this proximal effect has been highlighted because thiazides reduce $Ca^{2+}$ excretion, even when TRPV5, the major distal calcium reabsorptive pathway, has been knocked out and is absent.[153]

However, other mechanisms in the DCT must also play a role because a study in mice deficient for the DCT-specific protein parvalbumin has shown that hydrochlorothiazide does not increase natriuresis but does induce hypocalciuria.[154] Similarly, a study in humans has shown that hypovolemia is not the sole cause of hypocalciuria in patients with Gitelman syndrome who have a genetic inactivation of NCC.[155] Thiazides produce a sustained reduction in renal $Ca^{2+}$ excretion that is accompanied by a small rise in serum $Ca^{2+}$ concentration. $Mg^{2+}$ excretion is enhanced by thiazide diuretics, at least during prolonged therapy[156] (see Fig. 50.4). It has also been shown that transient receptor potential channel melastatin 6 (TRPM6) is a magnesium channel of the distal nephron.[157,158] Long-term thiazide treatment of mice diminishes TRPM6 mRNA expression modestly and reduces TRPM6 protein abundance by approximately 80%. Such changes would be expected to reduce magnesium reabsorption along the distal nephron, leading to $Mg^{2+}$ wasting. $Mg^{2+}$ depletion that can occur during chronic thiazide administration may be augmented by $K^+$ depletion.[156] Thiazides reduce urate clearance secondary to ECV depletion[82] and competition for tubular uptake.[107]

Expression of the water channel aquaporin-2 (AQP2) begins at the junction between the DCT and connecting tubule. Thus, the NCC-expressing DCT comprises the terminal diluting segment of the kidney. Thiazides impair maximal urinary dilution but not maximal urinary concentration.[159] Thiazides also enhance water absorption from inner medullary collecting ducts in an AVP-independent manner.[160] This effect is correlated with an increase in AQP2 expression during long-term thiazide treatment.[161] These effects may contribute to the tendency of thiazide diuretics to produce hyponatremia. Central effects on thirst, however, may also contribute (see later discussion of adverse effects).

*Clinical Relevance*

**Implications of Differential Effect of Diuretics on Electrolyte and Acid-Base Handling**

The classes of diuretics have different effects on acid-base and electrolyte balance. Hyponatremia is a specific adverse effect of thiazide diuretics. Loop and thiazide diuretics increase urinary magnesium and potassium excretion, whereas distal $K^+$-sparing diuretics reduce this. Urinary calcium excretion is increased by loop diuretics and decreased by thiazide diuretics. All diuretics tend to cause metabolic alkalosis, except for carbonic anhydrase inhibitors, which cause metabolic acidosis. Diuretic combinations may be used to prevent clinically significant acid-base and electrolyte disturbances.

## PHARMACOKINETICS OF AND DIFFERENCES AMONG THIAZIDES

Thiazides are readily absorbed and are extensively bound to plasma proteins. They are eliminated largely through secretion by the S2 segment of the proximal tubule, mostly via OAT1 and OAT3.[108,112] The $t_{1/2}$ is prolonged in renal failure and in older adults, reducing natriuretic efficacy.[162] The more lipid-soluble drugs (e.g., bendroflumethiazide, polythiazide) are more potent, have a more prolonged action, and are more extensively metabolized.[163] Chlorthalidone has a particularly prolonged action.[163] Indapamide is sufficiently metabolized to limit accumulation in renal failure.[163] Extrarenal effects of thiazide diuretics, including effects on platelet aggregation and vascular permeability, vary among the types of thiazide diuretics. This may explain why thiazide-like diuretics (e.g., chlorthalidone, indapamide) appear to have superior cardioprotective effects compared with thiazide-type diuretics (e.g., chlorothiazide, hydrochlorothiazide).[164–166]

As stated above, little is known about the pharmacogenetics of diuretics, but available studies have suggested that differences in individual responses are important. In one study, diuretic therapy in carriers of a variant of α-adducin, a cytoskeleton protein important for the function of renal $Na^+$-$K^+$-ATPase, was found to be associated with a lower risk of combined myocardial infarction and stroke than other antihypertensive therapies.[167] In another study, polymorphisms in with-no-lysine kinase 1 (WNK1), a kinase involved in the regulation of NCC, also affected the response to a thiazide diuretic.[168] Finally, polymorphisms in Nedd4-2, a ubiquitin ligase that regulates the sodium chloride cotransporter,[169] predicts the blood pressure response to hydrochlorothiazide in white subjects and cardiovascular outcome with hydrochlorothiazide in black subjects.[170]

### CLINICAL INDICATIONS AND ADVERSE EFFECTS

The clinical indications for the use of thiazides and thiazide-like drugs are discussed below (see "Clinical Uses of Diuretics"). Adverse effects of thiazides and thiazide-like drugs are discussed below (see "Adverse Effects of Diuretics").

## DISTAL POTASSIUM-SPARING DIURETIC AGENTS

Distal $K^+$-sparing diuretics comprise those that directly block the ENaC (amiloride and triamterene) and antagonists of the mineralocorticoid receptor (spironolactone and eplerenone). Finerenone is the first of a class of dihydropyridine derivatives with antimineralocorticoid actions currently under development.[171]

### SITES AND MECHANISMS OF ACTION

Distal $K^+$-sparing diuretics act on the cells in the late DCT, connecting tubule, and cortical CD (the ASDN), where they inhibit luminal $Na^+$ entry via ENaC (see Fig. 50.9).[132,172] They depolarize the lumen-negative transepithelial voltage, diminishing the electrochemical gradient for $K^+$ and $H^+$ secretion.[132,173]

Both amiloride and triamterene are organic cations that block ENaC directly from the luminal surface. Amiloride also inhibits NHE3, but the affinity of amiloride for NHE3 is low enough that the distal effects predominate in clinical use. In experimental work, congeners of amiloride that are more selective for ENaC or NHE3 have been developed, although they have not been used clinically. Amiloride appears to bind ENaC in its conducting pore and is thus a pore blocker.[174] Amiloride binding is sensitive to the electric field, and the agent appears to compete with $Na^+$ for binding to the pore of the channel.[175] Amiloride may interact with several regions on the ENaC protein, but one amiloride-binding region comprises a short amino acid stretch within the extracellular loop.[176] In addition to their natriuretic effects, amiloride and triamterene also reduce the excretion of $Ca^{2+}$ and $Mg^{2+}$.[156,177]

Spironolactone and eplerenone are competitive antagonists of the mineralocorticoid receptor. Mineralocorticoid receptor antagonists (MRAs; also called "aldosterone receptor antagonists") were developed when it was discovered that aldosterone is an 18-aldehyde derivative of corticosterone and that progesterone increases $Na^+$ excretion by blocking exogenously administered mineralocorticoid. Eventually, spironolactone was developed. It was found not to have any effect on urinary $Na^+$ or $K^+$ directly, but instead competitively blocks the mineralocorticoid receptor. Structurally, spirolactone strongly resembles aldosterone. Eplerenone was developed as an attempt to find an MRA with fewer estrogenic side effects.

These drugs were used for many years primarily to reduce the excretion of $K^+$ and net acid, especially when used in combination with other diuretics, because these drugs cause a very modest natriuresis. Under certain circumstances, however, their natriuretic efficacy can be significant. For example, spironolactone is more effective than furosemide in reducing cirrhotic ascites.[179] Furthermore, spironolactone is often an effective adjunct in the treatment of resistant hypertension.[180] This agent has achieved an important role in the treatment of heart failure with a reduced ejection fraction,[181] although the mechanisms whereby it achieves protection continue to be debated.

### PHARMACOKINETICS

Triamterene is well absorbed. It is rapidly hydroxylated to active metabolites.[182] The drug and its metabolites are secreted by the organic cation pathway in the proximal tubule,[3] with half-lives of 3 to 5 hours. Triamterene and its active metabolites accumulate in patients with cirrhosis because of decreased biliary secretion,[183] and in older adults[184,185] and patients with CKD[162] because of decreased renal excretion.

Amiloride is incompletely absorbed. Its duration of action is approximately 18 hours. It is secreted into the tubular fluid by the organic cation transport pathway.[186] Other organic cations, such as cimetidine, inhibit its secretion and prolong its half-life.[186] It accumulates in renal failure[187] and may worsen renal function.[188] Spironolactone is readily absorbed and circulates bound to plasma proteins. Its intrinsic half-life is short, but it is metabolized to active compounds with considerably prolonged actions. Spironolactone is metabolized to canrenones ($t_{1/2}$ = 16 hours) and to sulfur-containing metabolites, predominantly 7-alpha-thiomethylspirolactone ($t_{1/2}$ = 13 hours).[189] Canrenones are metabolized by the cytochrome P-4503A system.[190] Clinically, spironolactone has a $t_{1/2}$ of approximately 20 hours. It takes 10 to 48 hours to become maximally effective.[191] It is lipid-soluble and enters distal renal tubules from the plasma.[192] Eplerenone has fewer antiandrogenic and proestrogenic effects.[193,194] However, it is metabolized with a half-life of 3 hours and therefore should be given twice daily.[195]

### CLINICAL INDICATIONS

Distal $K^+$-sparing agents are used to prevent or treat hypokalemic alkalosis, especially in combination with a thiazide diuretic.[196] Amiloride can prevent amphotericin-induced hypokalemia and hypomagnesemia.[197] Spironolactone is indicated as a first-line agent for ECV expansion in the setting of cirrhotic ascites, in which it is more effective than daily furosemide,[198–200] although current guidelines suggest that it should be used in combination with furosemide at a dose ratio of spironolactone 100 mg/furosemide 40 mg.[201] It is also indicated for heart failure with a reduced ejection fraction, in which its effects may include renal and extrarenal mineralocorticoid receptor blockade,[202] and recommended doses are limited to 25 and 50 mg/day, respectively. Spironolactone is also commonly used to treat hypertension associated with hyperaldosteronism and for resistant hypertension,[180,203,204] and it may reduce proteinuria and progressive loss of kidney function in CKD.[205,206] However, see the following discussion of adverse effects. Eplerenone is indicated to prevent cardiac remodeling and systolic dysfunction in the setting of recent myocardial infarction.[207,208] Preliminary experimental data have suggested that spironolactone may help prevent the development of CKD after ischemic AKI (AKI-induced CKD).[209]

### ADVERSE EFFECTS AND DRUG INTERACTIONS

Hyperkalemia is the most common complication of the distal $K^+$-sparing diuretics. The risk is dose-dependent and increases considerably in patients with CKD or in those receiving $K^+$ supplements, angiotensin-converting enzyme (ACE) inhibitors, angiotensin receptor blockers (ARBs), NSAIDs, beta-blockers, heparin, or ketoconazole. The incidence of hyperkalemia-associated morbidity and mortality in Canada rose sharply after the publication of the Randomized Aldactone Evaluation Study (RALES). This study demonstrated the efficacy of spironolactone in improving outcomes in heart failure and may relate to the consequent widespread use of this agent in patients with congestive heart failure and impaired renal function.[211] It is important to note that the original RALES study specifically excluded patients with several of these comorbidities. Renal failure appears to be another complication in this group.[212]

Gynecomastia may occur in men, especially as the dose is increased[213] but, even at low doses,[214] decreased libido and impotence have also been reported. Women may experience menstrual irregularities, hirsutism, or swelling and tenderness of the breast. Impaired net acid excretion can cause metabolic acidosis,[215] which worsens hyperkalemia.

Amiloride and triamterene accumulate in renal failure,[185,216] and triamterene accumulates in cirrhosis.[183] Therefore, these drugs should be avoided in patients with these conditions. Triamterene occasionally precipitates in the urinary collecting system and causes obstruction.[217] It can cause acute kidney injury when given with indomethacin.[218]

## MISCELLANEOUS AGENTS

### DOPAMINERGIC AGENTS

When given to normal subjects in low doses (1–3 μg/kg per minute), dopamine causes a modest increase in the GFR, reduces proximal reabsorption via a cAMP-induced inhibition of the $Na^+$-$H^+$ antiporter, and increases $Na^+$ excretion.[219] Fenoldopam is a selective dopamine type 1 receptor agonist, with little cardiac stimulation.[219] Unfortunately, these beneficial effects are reduced in patients who are critically ill and/or receiving vasopressors.[220] A comprehensive review of the literature has concluded that in controlled trials, low-dose dopamine universally fails to improve renal outcomes in patients at high risk for AKI and that in the largest trials, it had no effect on renal function, need for dialysis, or mortality in critically ill patients with early renal dysfunction.[220] Thus, there is currently no justification for the use of low-dose dopamine for renal protection.[221] Dopamine infusion at higher rates has a role as a pressor agent in septic shock or refractory heart failure, but the benefits can be offset by arrhythmias.[220]

### VASOPRESSIN RECEPTOR ANTAGONISTS

Vasopressin receptor antagonists are nonpeptide molecules that competitively inhibit one or more of the human vasopressin receptors, V1aR, V1bR, and V2R.[222] Conivaptan is a combined V1aR/V2R antagonist for intravenous use, whereas tolvaptan, mozavaptan, and lixivaptan are orally active V2R-selective antagonists. All these agents cause a free water diuresis without appreciable natriuresis or kaliuresis and they are therefore sometimes referred to as "aquaretics."[223] This effect is mainly attributed to the inhibition of V2R in the collecting duct, which prevents vasopressin from recruiting AQP2 water channels to increase water reabsorption. Therefore, vasopressin receptor antagonists can be used to treat hypervolemic or euvolemic hyponatremia, in which increased vasopressin is considered inappropriate. Co-inhibition of V1aR, which is located in vascular smooth muscle, could be beneficial to reduce coronary vasoconstriction, myocyte hypertrophy, and vascular resistance in patients with heart failure,[224] but definitive studies on this effect are lacking. At present, some 20 clinical trials have tested these agents against placebo or conventional therapy in patients with liver cirrhosis, heart failure, or hyponatremia secondary to SIADH.[225] In all trials, vasopressin receptor antagonists effectively raised serum sodium levels and helped correct hyponatremia. In addition, a positive effect on some secondary end points was observed in patients with heart failure, including improved mental condition and reductions in body weight, dyspnea, and ascites.[226–228] However, the Efficacy of Vasopressin Antagonist in Heart Failure Outcome Study with Tolvaptan (EVEREST), which involved 4133 patients hospitalized for heart failure (with or without hyponatremia), did not show a beneficial effect of tolvaptan on the primary outcome of death and rehospitalization for heart failure.[227] Thus, vasopressin receptor antagonists appear effective in the correction of hyponatremia but have not yet shown an effect on primary outcomes.

### ADENOSINE TYPE I RECEPTOR ANTAGONISTS

Aminophylline is an adenosine receptor antagonist that inhibits NaCl reabsorption in the proximal tubule and diluting segments and causes a modest increase in GFR.[229] Highly selective adenosine 1 (A1) receptor antagonists are natriuretic[230] and antihypertensive, and they potentiate furosemide-induced natriuresis in normal humans[231] and in patients with diuretic-resistant heart failure. A1 antagonists disrupt glomerulotubular balance and TGF, thereby decreasing proximal reabsorption and increasing the GFR.[230] Several A1 receptor antagonists have been tested in patients with acute heart failure, but a large trial with the drug rolofylline did not show improvement in survival, heart failure status, or kidney function.[232]

### NESIRITIDE

Nesiritide is the recombinant form of B-type natriuretic peptide, which can be administered intravenously in acute decompensated congestive heart failure (see later discussion of clinical uses of diuretics in congestive heart failure). By stimulating cGMP, this agent causes both a natriuresis and relaxation of smooth muscle.

### NEPRILYSIN INHIBITORS

Neprilysin inhibitors prevent the breakdown of natriuretic peptides, and therefore contribute to natriuresis. The combined use of an ARB and neprilysin inhibitor (LCZ696) has been shown to reduce rates of cardiovascular death and hospitalization for heart failure in patients with class II, III, or IV heart failure.[233]

### SODIUM GLUCOSE-LINKED TRANSPORTER 2 (SGLT2) INHIBITORS

Sodium glucose-linked transporter 2 (SGLT2) inhibitors block glucose reabsorption in the proximal tubule, thereby delivering much of the filtered glucose to the urine and inducing an osmotic diuresis. Empagliflozin, canagliflozin, and dapagliflozin are three SGLT2 inhibitors that are licensed for the treatment of type 2 diabetes mellitus. Because SGLT2 cotransports $Na^+$ with glucose, and the filtered load of glucose is increased in uncontrolled diabetes mellitus, a significant fraction of proximal tubular $Na^+$ reabsorption is blocked by these drugs, thereby delivering more $Na^+$ to the loop of Henle and macula densa segments.[234] The result is increased renal $Na^+$ excretion and activation of TGF that increases preglomerular vascular tone and reduces the GFR. The resulting reduction in glomerular capillary pressure and glomerular blood flow reduces hyperfiltration and, in combination with a fall in blood pressure, may account for the slowing or prevention of the progressive loss of the GFR in patients with diabetic nephropathy treated with empagliflozin.[235] Moreover, the prolonged increase in $Na^+$ delivery from the proximal tubule leads to an adaptive increase in NaCl reabsorption in the loop of Henle[234] that could account for the observation of an adaptive synergistic natriuresis when a loop diuretic is given to subjects adapted to an SGLT2 inhibitor.[236] Thus, the addition of an SGLT2 inhibitor may help relieve loop diuretic resistance in patients with diabetes mellitus while providing some protection from progressive loss of the GFR.[237,238]

#### NOVEL DIURETICS IN PRECLINICAL DEVELOPMENT

Several novel diuretics are being developed targeting urea channels, ROMK, or pendrin in the kidney. Urea channel inhibitors induce an osmotic diuresis by inhibiting urea reabsorption in the renal medulla.[239] An inhibitor of the urea channel UT-B (SLC14A1) increased urine output in rats without commensurate urinary sodium and potassium loss.[240] Recently, a small- molecule screen also identified selective inhibitors of UT-A1 (SLC14A2).[241]

Dimethylthiourea was found to inhibit both UT-B and UT-A1 and produced a greater diuresis in rats than furosemide while preserving sodium levels better. This compound was also effective in preventing hyponatremia in a model of SIADH.[242] ROMK inhibitors induce a robust natriuresis in rats but, unlike loop and thiazide diuretics, do so without kaliuresis.[243] A ROMK inhibitor caused greater diuresis and natriuresis when combined with hydrochlorothiazide or amiloride, but not bumetanide, suggesting that the diuretic target site of ROMK inhibitors is the TAL.[243] Pendrin is a $Cl^-/HCO_3^-$ exchanger in intercalated cells involved in $Na^+$ reabsorption and acid-base balance.[244] Small-molecule pendrin inhibitors have been identified from a high-throughput screen.[245] Pendrin inhibitors alone are not effective diuretics.[246] In contrast, the addition of a pendrin inhibitor to mice treated with furosemide further increased urine output by 30% to 60%.[246] This confirms the importance of pendrin upregulation in chronic treatment with diuretics that target $Na^+$ transport upstream.[247] Accordingly, pendrin inhibitors may prove useful compounds for combined diuretic treatment or in diuretic resistance (see below).

## ADAPTATION TO DIURETIC THERAPY

Diuretics entrain a set of homeostatic mechanisms that limit their fluid-depleting actions and contribute to resistance to these agents and their adverse effects.

### DIURETIC BRAKING PHENOMENON

The first dose of a diuretic normally produces a reassuring diuresis. However, in normal subjects, a new equilibrium is rapidly attained when body weight stabilizes and daily fluid and electrolyte excretion no longer exceeds intake.[104] This reaction is called the "diuretic braking phenomenon." The effects of dietary salt intake on the diuretic braking phenomenon during 3 days of loop diuretic administration to normal human subjects are shown in Fig. 50.10.[104,248–250] During high $Na^+$ intake (270 mmol/24 hours), the first dose of furosemide ($F_1$) causes a large negative $Na^+$ balance over the ensuing 6 hours (*blue bars* in Fig. 50.10A), followed by 18 hours during which $Na^+$ excretion is reduced well below intake (postdiuresis salt retention), which results in a positive $Na^+$ balance (*light green areas* in Fig. 50.10A) that offsets the preceding negative $Na^+$ balance. The natriuresis caused by the third daily dose of furosemide ($F_3$) is comparable to that caused by the first dose and also is followed by a restoration of $Na^+$ balance. Consequently, at high levels of $Na^+$ intake, subjects regain neutral $Na^+$ balance within 24 hours of each dose of furosemide and maintain their original body weight. A similar diuretic braking phenomenon occurs during established furosemide therapy.[83] During severe dietary $Na^+$ restriction (20 mmol/24 hours; Fig. 50.10C), the first dose of furosemide produces a blunted natriuresis. However, $Na^+$ balance cannot be restored because of the low level of dietary $Na^+$ intake. Consequently, virtually all the $Na^+$ lost during the diuretic phase is represented as a negative $Na^+$ balance for the day. Unlike in the high-salt protocol, tolerance manifests as a 40% reduction in the natriuretic response to the drug over 3 days. However, despite a blunted initial response and the development of tolerance, all subjects lose $Na^+$ and body weight. A loop diuretic given during an $Na^+$ intake of 120 mmol/24 hours (equivalent to a salt-restricted diet) causes $Na^+$ loss, but the loss is curtailed by a combination of postdiuretic renal salt retention and diuretic tolerance (see Fig. 50.10B).[250]

> ***Clinical Relevance***
> **Diuretic Braking Phenomenon**
>
> The diuretic braking phenomenon refers to the observation that diuretics no longer produce a negative sodium balance. It is explained by postdiuretic renal salt retention and compensatory distal reabsorption. Dietary sodium restriction or the addition of a second diuretic are effective strategies to overcome the diuretic braking phenomenon.

Furosemide kinetics and the GFR are unchanged over 3 days of furosemide administration. During a low NaCl intake, the curve representing the relationship between natriuresis and furosemide excretion on a graph is shifted to the right

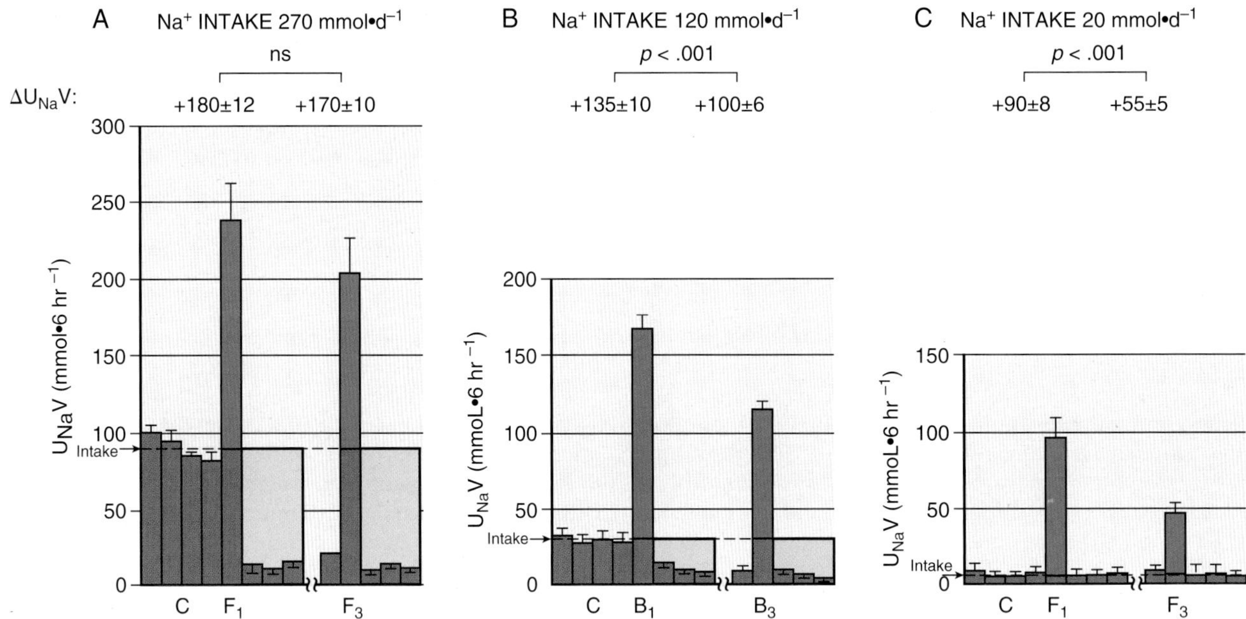


**Fig. 50.10** Effects of dietary salt intake on the diuretic braking phenomenon. Renal $Na^+$ excretion (mmol/6 hours) for 24 hours before and after the first ($F_1$) and third ($F_3$) daily doses of furosemide (A and C; 40 mg intravenously) and (B) bumetanide ($B_1$, $B_3$, 1 mg intravenously) in groups of 8 to 10 normal subjects equilibrated to fixed daily $Na^+$ intakes. The average level of $Na^+$ intake (mmol/6 hours) is shown by *broken horizontal lines*. Negative $Na^+$ balance is indicated by *blue bars* and positive $Na^+$ balance by *light green areas*. The mean ± standard error of the mean (SEM) values for diuretic-induced increases in $Na^+$ excretion above baseline values ($\Delta U_{Na}V$) for 6 hours after the administration of the diuretic are shown at the *top*. (Modified from Wilcox CS, Mitch WE, Kelly RA, et al. Response of the kidney to furosemide. *J Lab Clin Med.* 1983;102:450–458.)

by the third day of diuretic administration (see Fig. 50.8), indicating a blunting of diuretic responsiveness.

One month of furosemide therapy for hypertension reduces the natriuretic response to a test dose of furosemide by 18%.[83] This tolerance cannot be ascribed to aldosterone nor to a fall in plasma or ECV, because tolerance to furosemide is not prevented by spironolactone and does not develop during thiazide therapy, which causes similar reductions in body fluids. In fact, the natriuretic response to a test dose of a thiazide is augmented during furosemide therapy. Thus, tolerance to furosemide is class-specific and depends on increased NaCl reabsorption at a downstream, thiazide-sensitive nephron site.

Furosemide activates the renin-angiotensin-aldosterone system (RAAS) and the sympathetic nervous system (SNS). However, postdiuretic $Na^+$ retention is not blunted by doses of an ACE inhibitor, which prevents any changes in plasma angiotensin II or aldosterone concentrations,[248,251,252] or by prazosin, which blocks adrenergic receptors, even when an ACE inhibitor and prazosin are given in combination.[249]

Micropuncture studies have shown that the blunted natriuretic response to furosemide during repeated administration can be attributed to three factors: (1) reduced NaCl delivery to the site of furosemide action; (2) limited inhibition of NaCl reabsorption by furosemide in the loop of Henle; and (3) enhanced ability of the distal tubule to reabsorb the extra NaCl load delivered during furosemide's upstream action.[253] A recent clinical study has suggested that the third factor is the primary driver for loop diuretic resistance in acute heart failure.[254]

Rats receiving prolonged infusions of loop diuretics have considerable structural hypertrophy of the DCT, connecting tubule, and intercalated cells of the CD[255] that is partially dependent on angiotensin II.[256] The DCT and CD have a large increase in mRNA for insulin-like growth factor–binding protein-1[257] and increases in both $Na^+$-$K^+$-ATPase[258] and $H^+$-ATPase.[259] The $Na^+$-$K^+$-ATPase activity of rat cortical CD segments increases abruptly following an increase in cellular $[Na^+]$, owing to the mobilization of a latent pool of enzyme.[260] There is doubling of NCC expression in the distal tubules of rats adapted to diuretics.[261] Microperfusion studies of rats adapted to prolonged diuretic infusion have shown enhanced, aldosterone-independent distal $Na^+$ and $Cl^-$ absorption and $K^+$ secretion.[262] Therefore, diuretics induce structural and functional adaptations of downstream nephron segments, apparently in response to increased rates of NaCl delivery and. to some extent, to RAAS activation. Nephronal adaptation could underlie the inappropriate renal $Na^+$ retention that can persist for up to 2 weeks after abrupt cessation of diuretic therapy.[263]

Normal subjects fully eliminate a modest NaCl load (100 mmol) over 2 days.[264] However, when these subjects are challenged with the same NaCl load delivered after the administration of bumetanide during simultaneous infusion of sufficient fluid, $Na^+$, $K^+$, and $Cl^-$ to prevent any losses, elimination of the load is prevented.[264] Thus, diuretics can entrain an ECV-independent NaCl retention; this is apparent when distal delivery is enhanced, as during high NaCl intake. Even a single dose of loop diuretic can cause a $Cl^-$ depletion "contraction" alkalosis, which may contribute to diuretic

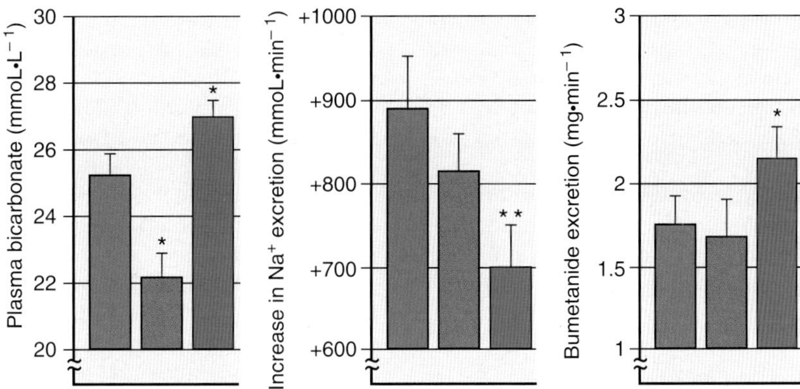


**Fig. 50.11** Mean ± standard error of the mean values for plasma bicarbonate concentration, increase in $Na^+$ excretion with bumetanide (1 mg intravenously), and rate of bumetanide excretion in normal subjects ($n$ = 8) after equilibration to equivalent diets containing 100 mmol/24 hours of NaCl (control, *blue bars*), $NH_4Cl$ (mild metabolic acidosis, *pink bars*), or $NaHCO_3$ (mild metabolic alkalosis, *green bars*). Compared with control: *$P < .05$; **$P < .01$. (Modified from Loon NR, Wilcox CS. Mild metabolic alkalosis impairs the natriuretic response to bumetanide in normal human subjects. *Clin Sci [Colch].* 1998;94:287–292.)

**Box 50.1 Strategies to Overcome Diuretic Braking**

1. Restrict dietary salt to prevent postdiuretic salt retention.
2. Consider adding another class of diuretic.
3. Consider multiple daily dosing or a diuretic with prolonged action.
4. Do not stop diuretic therapy abruptly.
5. Prevent or reverse diuretic-induced metabolic alkalosis.

tolerance and the braking phenomenon.[70] In a study of normal subjects in whom mild metabolic alkalosis was produced by the equimolar substitution of $NaHCO_3$ for NaCl, bumetanide-induced natriuresis was reduced during alkalosis. despite enhanced delivery of bumetanide to the urine (Fig. 50.11).[123] This finding implies a profound defect in tubular responsiveness to the diuretic. Several mechanisms may contribute:

1. The Na-K-2Cl cotransporter has affinities for $Na^+$, $K^+$, and $Cl^-$ of 7.0, 1.3, and 67 mM, respectively. Thus, the $[Cl^-]$ of tubular fluid may be low enough during $Cl^-$ depletion alkalosis to limit reabsorption by this transporter and thereby limit the responsiveness to loop diuretics.
2. Alkalosis causes glycosylation of the NKCC2, which could alter its transport function.[61]
3. The thiazide-sensitive NCC in the rat DCT is increased by 40% during $NaHCO_3$ administration.[265]

Findings from these studies have several clinical implications (Box 50.1):

1. Dietary salt intake must be restricted, even in subjects receiving powerful loop diuretics, to obviate postdiuretic salt retention and ensure the development of a negative NaCl balance.
2. During prolonged diuretic administration, subjects may be particularly responsive to another class of diuretic.
3. Diuretic therapy should not be stopped abruptly unless dietary salt intake is curtailed because the adaptive mechanisms limiting salt excretion persist for days after diuretic use.
4. Selection of a diuretic with a prolonged action, or more frequent administration of the diuretic, will enhance NaCl loss by limiting the time available for postdiuretic salt retention. Indeed, a continuous infusion of a loop diuretic is somewhat more effective than the same dose given as a bolus injection in volunteers[266] and in patients with CKD,[267] despite a similar delivery of diuretic to the urine. Although a previous study has shown that a continuous infusion is also more effective in cardiac disease,[268] a later study showed similar efficacy.[269]
5. Prevention or reversal of diuretic-induced metabolic alkalosis may enhance diuretic efficacy.

There are similar patterns of furosemide-induced $K^+$ loss followed by renal $K^+$ retention[270] associated with an increase in the transtubular $K^+$ gradient.[271] In contrast, loop diuretics induce ongoing renal $K^+$ losses during severe salt restriction due to hyperaldosteronism,[270] which can be countered by distal, $K^+$-sparing diuretics.[271]

## HUMORAL AND NEURONAL MODULATORS OF THE RESPONSE TO DIURETICS

### RENIN-ANGIOTENSIN-ALDOSTERONE SYSTEM

Diuretic therapy increases plasma renin activity and serum aldosterone concentrations, as described previously. The initial rise in plasma renin activity with loop diuretics is independent of volume depletion or the SNS and is related to the inhibition of NaCl reabsorption at the macula densa.[272] Loop diuretics also stimulate renal prostacyclin release, which promotes renin secretion.[273] In longer term use of loop diuretics, renin secretion depends on ECV depletion and the SNS.

Activation of the RAAS in patients treated with diuretics and salt restriction for edema limits the natriuresis.[274] In a study of patients with heart failure (HF), ACE inhibition potentiated the diuretic and natriuretic responses to furosemide, despite a drop in blood pressure.[275] However, severe volume depletion and azotemia can complicate overzealous therapy with ACE inhibitors, particularly in patients with HF who are receiving high doses of diuretics or in those with stenosis of both renal arteries or the artery to a single or dominant kidney.[276] Thus, the combination of diuretics and ACE inhibitors can be highly effective but requires careful surveillance.

During stimulation of the RAAS by severe dietary salt restriction, further diuretic-induced increases in serum aldosterone concentration promote renal $K^+$ losses.[277] ACE inhibitors counter diuretic-induced increases in serum aldosterone concentration and blunt diuretic-induced hypokalemia.[270]

## EICOSANOIDS

PGE2 acting on $EP_4$ inhibits NaCl reabsorption via the NKCC2[278] and inhibits free water and $Na^+$ reabsorption in the CDs via changes in cAMP (Fig. 50.12).[279] Loop diuretics, thiazides, triamterene, and spironolactone increase prostaglandins substantially.[280] Inhibition of PG synthesis by NSAIDs can diminish the natriuresis and diuresis induced by furosemide,[281] hydrochlorothiazide,[282] spironolactone,[280] or triamterene (see Fig. 50.12).[283] Microperfusion of the loop segment with PGE2[129] restores the response to furosemide in indomethacin-treated rats. Indomethacin also blunts furosemide-induced renal[284] and capacitance vessel vasodilation[285] and stimulation of renin.[286] The blunting of furosemide-induced natriuresis by NSAIDs is potentiated by salt depletion[287] and is prominent in edematous patients.[281] The NSAIDs ibuprofen, naproxen, and sulindac similarly blunt furosemide-induced natriuresis. A COX-2 inhibitor blocks furosemide-induced renin secretion but not natriuresis, although other studies have shown an effect of COX-2 inhibition on $Na^+$ reabsorption.[288] It is COX-1 that facilitates natriuresis in the distal nephron.[289] Salt-sensitive hypertensive subjects have a blunted natriuretic response to furosemide that may be related to a paradoxic reduction in the renal excretion of 20-HETE. Thus, COX-1 products mediate a part of furosemide-induced natriuresis, whereas COX-2 products mediate renin secretion. 20-HETE may be an important positive modulator of salt excretion.

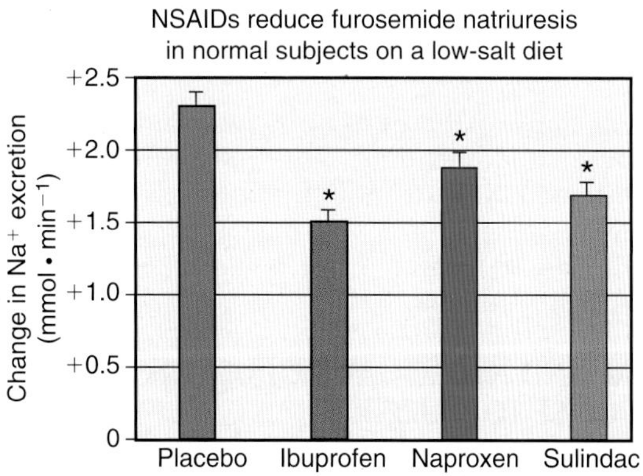


Mean ± SEM (n=11) studied in crossover design after equilibration to 10 mmol 24h$^{-1}$ $Na^+$ diet

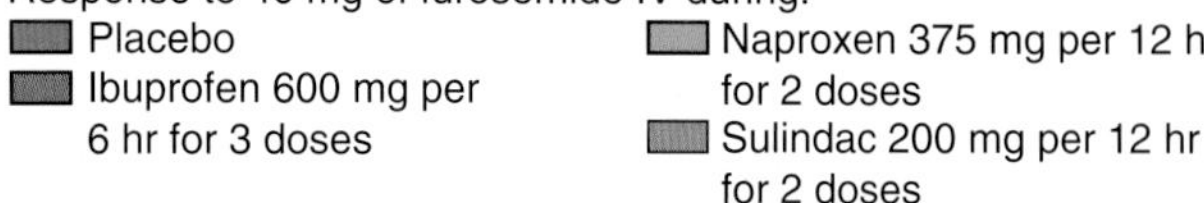


Compared to placebo: *, $P<0.05$ vs placebo

**Fig. 50.12** Mean ± standard error of the mean *(SEM)* values for change in $Na^+$ excretion for 11 normal subjects given 40 mg of furosemide intravenously after placebo or after each of three nonsteroidal antiinflammatory drugs: ibuprofen, 600 mg/6 hr for three doses; naproxen, 375 mg/12 hr for two doses; or sulindac, 200 mg/12 hr for two doses. *NSAIDs,* Nonsteroidal antiinflammatory drugs. (Modified from Brater DC, Anderson S, Baird B, et al. Effects of ibuprofen, naproxen, and sulindac on prostaglandins in men. *Kidney Int.* 1985;27:66–73.)

Loop diuretics also increase the excretion of the thromboxane A2 (TXA2) metabolite TxB2. Inhibition of TXA2 synthesis or receptors in the rat increases furosemide diuresis[290] and diminishes the renal vasodilation.[291] Thus, TxA2 may antagonize the actions of loop diuretics.

## ARGININE VASOPRESSIN

AVP levels increase after the administration of furosemide.[292] This may be a response to a reduced blood volume. Plasma AVP levels are increased in many edematous states, such as HF and liver cirrhosis,[293] especially in those who demonstrate hyponatremia during thiazide treatment.[294] AVP stimulates $K^+$ secretion in the rat distal tubule.[295] Diuretic-induced AVP release contributes to hypokalemia because the kaliuretic response to furosemide is reduced by 40% in subjects whose AVP release is suppressed by a water load.[277] In addition, despite its classic role as a water balance hormone, AVP has been shown to increase the activity of both the NCC and ENaC, possibly aggravating sodium retention in edematous states.[296,297]

## CATECHOLAMINES AND SYMPATHETIC NERVOUS SYSTEM

The first dose of furosemide raises the heart rate and plasma catecholamine concentrations.[123,249] Blockade of $\alpha_2$-adrenergic receptors with prazosin does not modify the ensuing renal salt retention[249] but blockade of these receptors blunts the renin release.[272] Short-term, furosemide-induced ECV depletion in the conscious rat activates sympathetic nerve activity that stabilizes the blood pressure.[298]

## ATRIAL NATRIURETIC PEPTIDE

Diuretics are often used to treat patients who have an expanded blood volume and elevated levels of ANP. Administration of furosemide to dogs with heart failure reduces ANP levels.[299] Infusion of ANP in this dog model promotes furosemide-induced natriuresis and blunts activation of the RAAS and the fall in the GFR. Thus, a drop in ANP levels contributes to postdiuretic renal NaCl retention.[299]

# DIURETIC RESISTANCE

Diuretic resistance implies an inadequate clearance of edema, despite a full dose of diuretic.[300] The principal causes are summarized in Box 50.2. The first step in addressing inadequate diuretic response is to select the appropriate target response (e.g., a specific body weight) and to ensure that the edema is due to inappropriate renal NaCl and fluid retention, rather than to lymphatic or venous obstruction or redistribution (Fig. 50.13). Diuretics do not prevent edema caused by dihydropyridine calcium channel blockers.[301]

The next step is to exclude poor adherence, severe blood volume depletion, and concurrent NSAID use. Thereafter,

**Box 50.2 Common Causes of Diuretic Resistance**

Incorrect diagnosis (e.g., venous or lymphatic edema)
Inappropriate NaCl or fluid intake
Inadequate drug reaching tubule lumen in active form because of:
- Noncompliance
- Dose inadequate or too infrequent
- Poor absorption (e.g., due to uncompensated HF)
- Decreased renal blood flow (e.g., due to HF or cirrhosis of liver, or in older patient)
- Decreased functional renal mass (e.g., due to AKI or CKD, or in older patient)
- Proteinuria (e.g., due to nephrotic syndrome)

Inadequate renal response because of:
- Low glomerular filtration rate (e.g., due to AKI, CKD)
- Decreased effective extracellular fluid volume (e.g., due to edematous conditions)
- Activation of renin angiotensin aldosterone system (e.g., due to edematous conditions)
- Nephron adaptation (e.g., due to prolonged diuretic therapy)
- Nonsteroidal antiinflammatory drugs (e.g., indomethacin, aspirin)

*AKI,* Acute renal failure; *HF,* heart failure; *CKD,* chronic kidney disease.

dietary NaCl intake should be quantitated. In the steady state, this can be assessed from measurements of 24-hour $Na^+$ excretion. For patients with mild edema or hypertension, a daily $Na^+$ intake of 100 to 120 mmol may be sufficient. For patients with diuretic resistance, the help of a dietitian is usually necessary to reduce daily $Na^+$ intake to 80 to 100 mmol. In patients who are not in a steady state (e.g., patients with worsening heart failure), urine sodium levels will be low, and this observation may be used as an indication to intensify diuretic therapy.[302] The diuretic dose must be above the natriuretic threshold (the steep part of the dose-response curve in Fig. 50.8). Outpatients should be able to detect an increase in urinary volume within 4 hours of an administered dose; urine volume or body weight can be measured directly in patients who are hospitalized. If a diuresis does not occur, the next step is to double the dose until an effective dose or the maximum safe dose is reached.

The next step is to give two daily doses of the diuretic. Furosemide and bumetanide act for only 3 to 6 hours. Two daily half-doses, by interrupting postdiuretic salt retention, produce a greater response than the same total dose given once daily, as long as both are above the diuretic threshold. Concurrent disease may impair absorption of the diuretic. Thus, a more bioavailable diuretic, such as torsemide, may be preferable to furosemide.[98] Diuretic resistance is often accompanied by a pronounced metabolic alkalosis,[123] which may be reversed by the administration of KCl or addition of a distal $K^+$-sparing diuretic.

A progressive increase in diuretic dosage may produce an inadequate reduction in body fluids because of activation of NaCl-retaining mechanisms. ACE inhibitors can sometimes restore a diuresis in resistant patients with HF,[274] but a fall in blood pressure often limits the response. Adaptive changes in downstream nephron segments during prolonged diuretic therapy[83,255] provide a rational basis for combining diuretics (see the following section). Highly resistant patients can be admitted for a trial of intravenous infusion of a loop diuretic or ultrafiltration.[303]

## DIURETIC COMBINATIONS

Full doses of more than one diuretic acting on the same transport mechanism are less than additive, whereas use of several diuretics acting on a separate mechanism may be synergistic.[5,304]

### LOOP DIURETICS AND THIAZIDES

A loop diuretic and a thiazide or thiazide-like drug (e.g., hydrochlorothiazide, metolazone) are synergistic in normal subjects and in subjects with edema or renal insufficiency.[304–308] Metolazone is equivalent to bendrofluazide in enhancing NaCl and fluid losses in furosemide-resistant subjects with HF or the nephrotic syndrome.[309] During prolonged furosemide therapy, the responsiveness to a thiazide is augmented.[83] Patients with advanced CKD (eGFR <30 mL/min/1.73 $m^2$) that is unresponsive to a thiazide alone show a marked natriuresis when a thiazide is added to loop diuretic therapy,[307] probably by blockade of enhanced distal tubular $Na^+$ reabsorption.[310] However, such combination therapy should be initiated under close surveillance because of a high associated incidence of hypokalemia, excessive ECV depletion, and azotemia.[311]

### LOOP DIURETICS OR THIAZIDES AND DISTAL POTASSIUM-SPARING DIURETICS

Amiloride or triamterene increases furosemide natriuresis only modestly but curtails the excretion of $K^+$ and net acid[68] and preserves total body $K^+$.[312] Distal $K^+$-sparing agents are generally contraindicated in renal failure because they may cause severe hyperkalemia and acidosis.

# CLINICAL USES OF DIURETICS

A general algorithm for diuretic therapy in the treatment of CKD, nephrotic syndrome, liver cirrhosis, and HF is shown in Fig. 50.14.[313]

## EDEMATOUS CONDITIONS

The first aim in the treatment of edema is to reverse the primary cause by restoring hemodynamics and cardiac output in patients with heart failure (e.g., use of vasodilators or elimination of cardiac depressant drugs), by improving hepatic function in patients with cirrhosis and ascites (e.g., stopping alcohol intake), or by diminishing proteinuria in patients with the nephrotic syndrome (e.g., administration of ACE inhibitors or ARBs). Although the GFR is not reduced by low-dose diuretic therapy in normal subjects, it can be reduced in those with CKD or if there is an abrupt fall in blood pressure (BP), especially if this is complicated by orthostatic hypotension. Moreover, overzealous diuresis decreases the cardiac output, BP, and renal function, and stimulates the RAAS, SNS, prostaglandins, and AVP, all of which may compromise the desired hemodynamic and renal responses.[314] Therefore, diuretic therapy for edema should be initiated

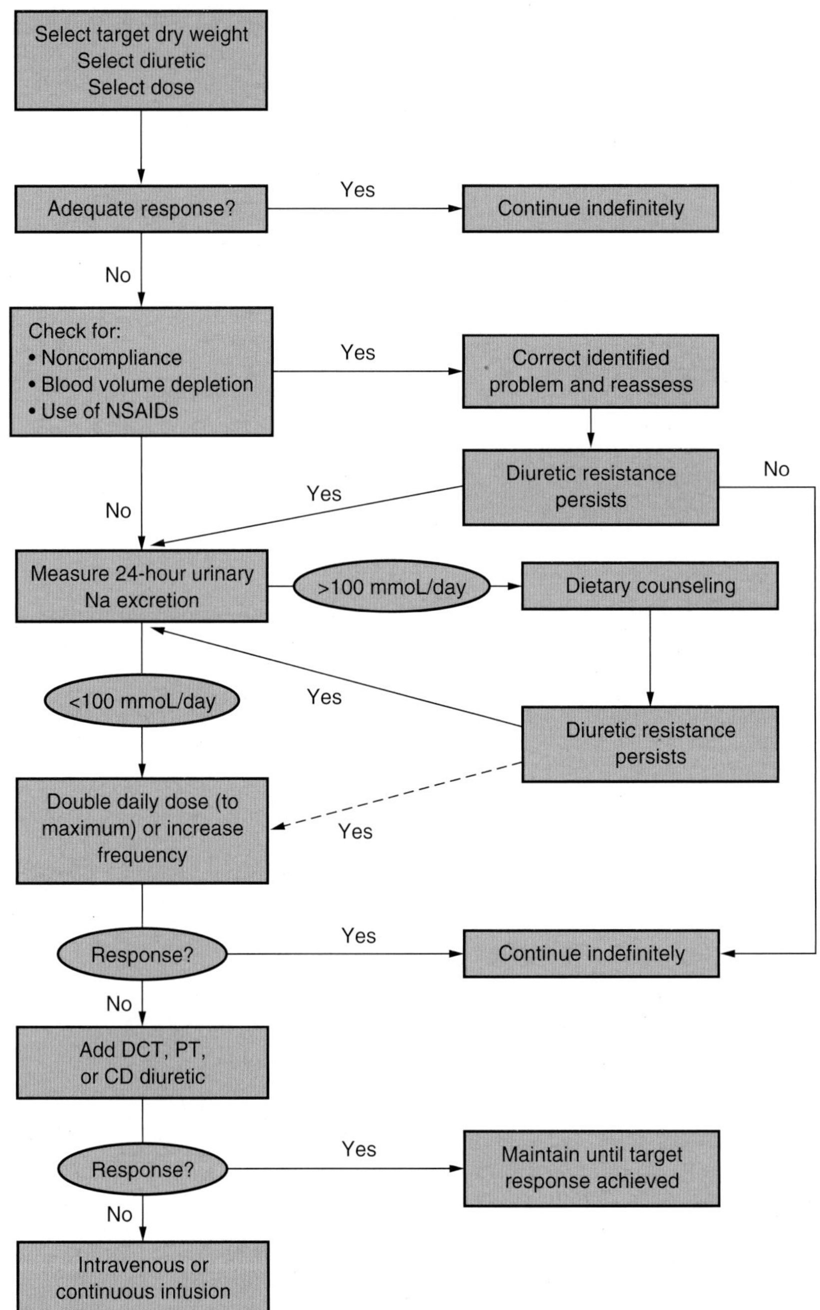


**Fig. 50.13** Diagrammatic representation of an approach to the management of a patient with resistance to a loop diuretic. *CD,* Collecting duct diuretic (e.g., amiloride, triamterene, or spironolactone); *DCT,* distal convoluted tubule diuretic (e.g., thiazide); *NSAIDs,* nonsteroidal antiinflammatory drugs; *PT,* proximal tubule diuretic (e.g., acetazolamide). (From Ellison DH, Wilcox CS. Diuretics: use in edema and the problem of resistance. In Brady HR, Wilcox CS, eds. *Therapy in Nephrology and Hypertension.* ed 2. London: Elsevier Science; 2003.)

with the lowest effective dose.[315] Additional drugs can be used to counteract unwanted actions. For example, ACE inhibitors, ARBs, or MRAs can prevent RAAS activation and enhance fluid losses, yet diminish $K^+$ depletion (see Fig. 50.20). The use of a second diuretic can have a synergistic action, whereas the use of a distal $K^+$-sparing agent may counteract unwanted hypokalemia, alkalosis, or $Mg^{2+}$ depletion (see "Adaptation to Diuretic Therapy").

Dietary $Na^+$ intake should be restricted to 2.5 to 3 g daily (corresponding to 107–129 mmol/24 hours) in patients with mild edema. Increasingly severe $Na^+$ restrictions to 2 g daily (86 mmol/24 hours) are required for patients with refractory edema.

Some resistance to diuretic therapy should be anticipated in all patients with CKD and those with more than mild edema (Fig. 50.15).

## HEART FAILURE

HF is classified as occurring with reduced or preserved ejection fraction, yet both forms of HF require diuretics as cornerstones

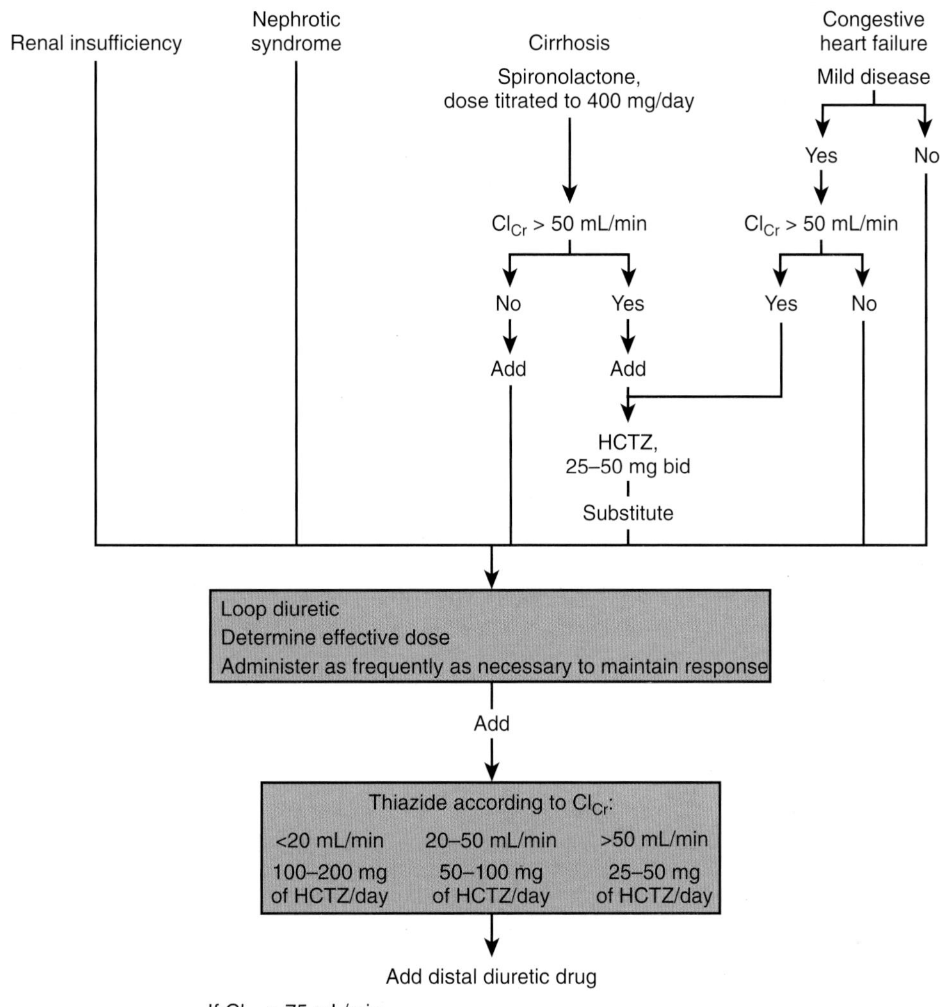


**Fig. 50.14** Algorithm for diuretic therapy in patients with edema due to renal, hepatic, or cardiac disease. *bid,* Twice a day; *$Cl_{Cr}$,* creatinine clearance; *HCTZ,* hydrochlorothiazide. (From Brater DC. Diuretic therapy. *N Engl J Med.* 1989;339:387–395.)

of therapy. The approach to cardiac failure depends on the cause and whether there is acute decompensation or a compensated chronic state.[316,317] This section first reviews the role of diuretics in acute decompensated HF in general and as secondary to acute coronary syndrome and then discusses the role of diuretics as maintenance therapy in systolic and diastolic HF. The reader is also referred to a recent review[318] and to the joint guidelines published by the American College of Cardiology and American Heart Association for more detailed recommendations and an overview of the level of evidence for each treatment.[319]

## Acute Decompensated Heart Failure

In the absence of obvious causes such as acute coronary syndrome and valve abnormalities, acute decompensated HF (ADHF) often results from an imbalance in the neurohumoral systems that regulate cardiac and renal function.[320] Therefore, it is rational to target these mechanisms with selective therapy. After initial stabilization, the mainstay of treatment is vasodilator and diuretic therapy. Intravenous vasodilators such as nitroglycerine, nitroprusside, and nesiritide counteract the effects of baroreceptor-dependent increases in sympathetic tone, angiotensin II and aldosterone, endothelin, and AVP. Vasodilators are usually combined with intravenous loop diuretics (e.g., furosemide, 40 mg; bumetanide, 1 mg; torsemide, 10–20 mg). For example, a study in patients with severe HF has shown that therapy with vasodilators and diuretics aimed at improving overall hemodynamic status leads to rapid neurohumoral improvement when central filling pressure declined.[321] Another study has found that although "aggressive decongestion" during ADHF is associated with worsening renal function, survival is actually improved.[322] In a carefully performed randomized trial, no differences between continuous dosing and bolus dosing of furosemide were observed; furthermore, no differences in global symptom improvement were observed between a low dose (equivalent of an oral dose) and a high dose (2.5 times the oral dose).[269] It should be noted, however, that this trial did not study

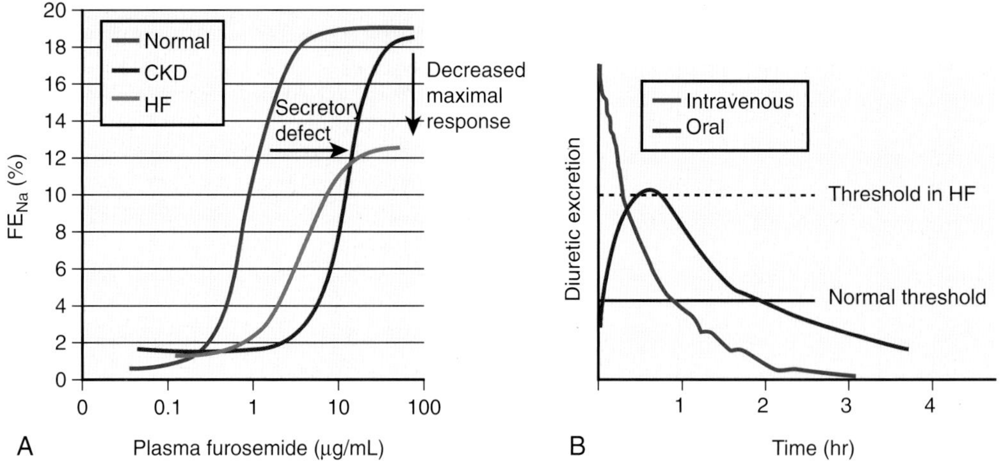


**Fig. 50.15** Dose-response curves for loop diuretics. (A) The fractional $Na^+$ excretion ($FE_{Na}$) as a function of plasma loop diuretic concentration. Compared with normal subjects, patients with chronic kidney disease *(CKD)* show a rightward shift in the curve owing to impaired diuretic secretion. The maximal response is preserved when expressed as $FE_{Na}$, but not when expressed as absolute $Na^+$ excretion. Patients with congestive heart failure *(HF)* demonstrate a rightward and downward shift, even when expressed as $FE_{Na}$, and thus are relatively diuretic-resistant. (B) Comparison of the response to intravenous and oral doses of loop diuretics. In a normal individual, an oral dose may be as effective as an intravenous dose because the time during which this individual is above the natriuretic threshold (indicated by the *Normal threshold* line) are approximately equal. If the natriuretic threshold increases (as indicated by the *Threshold in HF* line), then the oral dose may not provide a high enough plasma level to elicit natriuresis.

patients shown to be diuretic-resistant. Longer acting loop diuretics, such as torsemide[323] and azosemide,[324] produce less neurohumoral activation and may be preferable.

Diuretic kinetics are impaired in decompensated HF.[325,326] The bioavailability of furosemide, unlike that of bumetanide or torsemide, is erratic in HF.[327] This feature, and a longer duration of action, may account for the finding of a 50% reduction in the requirement for readmission to hospital in patients with HF randomly assigned to receive torsemide rather than furosemide.[98] There is decreased plasma clearance in decompensated HF because of a decreased RBF.[325] Together, these effects can limit the peak diuretic concentration in the tubular fluid to the foot of the dose-response curve and thereby diminish the response (see Fig. 50.15).

Nesiritide is a recombinant human B-type natriuretic peptide (BNP) that was approved by the US Food and Drug Administration (FDA) for the treatment of ADHF.[328] Studies of mice deficient in natriuretic peptide receptor A have implicated this system in the natriuretic response to blood volume expansion[329] and provide a rationale for BNP in the treatment of ADHF. Nesiritide given short term to patients with decompensated HF can reduce pulmonary capillary wedge pressure.[330] However, some subsequent studies have shown that nesiritide is not a diuretic in patients with HF and, in comparison with placebo, may be associated with higher risks of death and worsening renal function.[331–333] Conversely, other studies have indicated a potential role for nesiritide in the perioperative treatment of patients with left ventricular dysfunction who are undergoing cardiac surgery. In this context, these agents may improve renal function and possibly even survival.[334,335] Current guidelines recommend nesiritide for alternative vasodilator therapy in patients with ADHF without hypotension and with volume overload who remain dyspneic, despite receiving intravenous loop diuretics.[319,336]

In the past few years, there has been substantial interest in venovenous ultrafiltration as treatment for ADHF.[337] Nevertheless, a randomized trial conducted by the Heart Failure Clinical Research Network, comparing diuretic therapy with ultrafiltration, found that creatinine levels rose more in the ultrafiltration group than in the diuretic group, despite similar volume losses.[338] It should be emphasized, however, that this trial specifically excluded individuals in whom dialysis, in addition to volume removal, was indicated. The supplementary material in this publication[338] also provides protocols that have been widely promulgated by the Heart Failure Clinical Research Network for volume reduction in decompensated CHF. A recent meta-analysis has shown that ultrafiltration results in better clinical decongestion than intravenous loop diuretics, but does not improve rehospitalization or mortality rates.[339] Furthermore, ultrafiltration may cause serious product-related adverse events.[340]

Finally, the intravenous inotropes dobutamine and milrinone are reserved for situations in which ADHF is complicated by unresponsiveness to standard therapies, diminished peripheral perfusion, end-organ dysfunction, and/or hypotension (low-output syndrome). One trial has shown no added benefit of low-dose dopamine or nesiritide in decongestion or kidney function.[341]

## ACUTE DECOMPENSATED HEART FAILURE IN ACUTE CORONARY SYNDROME

Patients with acute myocardial infarction (AMI) require the rapid establishment of coronary reperfusion (e.g., by thrombolysis and percutaneous coronary intervention) and treatment of arrhythmias. The aim of concomitant treatment is to counter the increase in left ventricular end-diastolic pressure, which enhances wall tension and $O_2$ usage, and the accumulation of pulmonary edema without further curtailing the cardiac output. Judicious use of diuretics may meet these requirements. In one study, intravenous furosemide for left ventricular failure (LVF) complicating acute AMI reduced the left ventricular filling pressure from 20 to 15 mm Hg within 5 to 15 minutes and increased the venous capacitance by 50%.[342] This rapid venodilation is blocked by NSAIDs[285] and ACE inhibitors.[343] The ensuing diuresis reduces left ventricular end-diastolic pressure further.

A study of first-line therapy for 48 patients with acute LVF following AMI compared the responses to intravenous furosemide, a venodilator (isosorbide dinitrate), an arteriolar dilator (hydralazine), and a positive inotrope (prenalterol).[344] The venodilator and furosemide both reduced left ventricular filling pressure while maintaining the cardiac index and heart rate. The investigators concluded that these were the best first-line agents but that they should be combined with an arteriolar vasodilator. In contrast, a study randomly assigned 110 patients with acute LVF to receive either high-dose isosorbide dinitrate (3 mg intravenously every 5 minutes) or high-dose furosemide (80 mg intravenously every 15 minutes).[345] An adverse end point occurred more frequently in those receiving furosemide (46%) than in those receiving nitrate (25%). The investigators cautioned against the use of high-dose furosemide in acute LVF. Although intravenous furosemide decreases left ventricular filling pressure in patients with LVF, the shape of the Frank-Starling ventricular function curve predicts little change in cardiac output at elevated filling pressures. Nevertheless, most investigators recommend a trial of loop diuretics after ECV depletion and preload-dependent right HF have been ruled out by targeted volume boluses.[346]

Furosemide can be given as an IV bolus of up to 100 mg or as a short-term infusion to limit the risk of ototoxicity. Although controversial, an intermittent infusion produces a slightly greater natriuresis in most comparative studies.[347] Ideally, lower doses are used initially and titrated up to a good effect—for example, a pulmonary capillary wedge pressure of 16 mm Hg.[347] Hemodynamic and biochemical parameters should be monitored frequently during loop diuretic therapy, especially because patients with AMI are usually also treated with beta-blockers, ACE inhibitors, or vasodilators.

### Chronic Heart Failure

Diuretics are extremely useful in the long-term management of chronic HF with reduced ejection fraction. Avid renal NaCl and fluid retention leads to pulmonary edema that limits ventilation. Cardiac dilation limits cardiac function and increases wall tension and $O_2$ usage. This combination can create a spiral of decreasing oxygenation and cardiac output. In a study of 13 patients with severe edema due to HF, furosemide therapy increased stroke volume by 15% and decreased peripheral vascular resistance, despite reducing body weight by an average of 10 kg.[348] In another study, combined therapy using a diuretic and vasodilator reduced left and right atrial volumes, corrected atrioventricular valvular regurgitation, and improved stroke volume by 64%.[344] A meta-analysis of trials for HF has concluded that odds ratios were reduced to 0.25 for mortality and 0.31 for hospitalization for subjects randomly selected to receive diuretics.[349] These remarkable data strongly support the use of diuretics in HF.

On the other hand, the failing heart has a decreased capacity to regulate its contractility in response to changes in venous return, so if diuretic therapy is too abrupt or severe, the patient suffers from a decreased effective blood volume—orthostatic hypotension, weakness, fatigue, decreased exercise ability, and prerenal azotemia. This is especially true for patients with diastolic dysfunction, an increasingly recognized form of symptomatic HF with preserved ejection fraction.[350] Therefore, salt-depleting therapy requires continual reassessment and judicious use of other measures (e.g., vasodilators, ACE inhibitors, ARBs, or MRAs). Mild HF often responds to dietary $Na^+$ restriction (100–120 mmol/day) and low doses of a thiazide diuretic. As cardiac failure progresses, larger, more frequent doses of loop diuretics and tighter control of dietary salt (80–100 mmol/day) are required. It is important to emphasize that diuretic responsiveness is impaired in patients with advanced HF, as shown by a shift to the right in the natriuresis-excretion relationship of diuretics (see Fig. 50.15).[326] For the refractory patient, the addition of a second diuretic acting at the proximal tubule (e.g., acetazolamide) or a downstream site (e.g., a thiazide) can produce a dramatic diuresis, even in individuals with impaired renal function.[351,352] For example, additional therapy with metolazone[353] or hydrochlorothiazide[354] can increase fluid losses by an average of 7 to 8 kg. By comparing the fractional lithium and sodium excretion after intravenous loop diuretics, a recent study has confirmed that distal tubular compensatory sodium reabsorption is the primary driver of diuretic resistance in heart failure.[355]

Although drug therapy for chronic HF should be individualized, a suggested step-up algorithm consists of diuretics and ACE inhibitors or ARBs as the first agents, beta-blockers second, and MRAs or hydralazine-isosorbide dinitrate (in blacks) third, with digoxin, cardioverter-defibrillator, and resynchronization devices being saved as a final resort.[356] The lesson from the excess morbidity from hyperkalemia observed during trials of spironolactone therapy is to use MRAs within guidelines.[211] The guidelines exclude men with serum creatinine concentrations greater than 2.5 mg/dL (221 μmol/L) and women with serum creatinine concentrations greater than 2.0 mg/dL (177 μmol/L).[357] However, within guidelines, both MRAs and loop diuretics are important because they can improve ventricular remodeling.[358,359] In patients with preserved ejection fraction, spironolactone may improve left ventricular diastolic dysfunction, but it has been found not to improve symptoms and outcome.[360,361]

Despite these options, HF often progresses and introduces a vicious cycle. Decompensated HF stimulates the RAAS and AVP,[362] predisposing to hypokalemia, hypomagnesemia, hyponatremia, and arrhythmias. Hypokalemia potentiates the binding of digitalis to cardiac myocytes,[363] decreases its renal elimination,[364] and enhances its cardiac toxicity.[365] Although this cycle can be curtailed by higher doses of diuretics or continuous intravenous infusion of a loop diuretic,[366] the risks of volume depletion, azotemia, and electrolyte abnormalities increase sharply.[367] Continuous infusion should be tried in patients known to show a response to maximum bolus doses of diuretics because bolus therapy results in higher initial serum concentrations and therefore higher initial rates of urinary diuretic excretion than continuous infusion. If the patient has received one or more intravenous boluses within the previous few hours, then an infusion can be started without a loading dose.

Furosemide infusion rates of up to 240 mg/hour have been reported in the literature. The risk of ototoxicity and other side effects associated with these infusion rates must be weighed against alternative strategies, such as the addition of a thiazide-type diuretic or fluid removal via ultrafiltration.

Therefore, new therapies are required because a decrement in renal function predicts a bad outcome in patients treated for HF.[368] Renal dysfunction can be ameliorated by an ARB, provided that BP is maintained. The combination of an ARB with a neprilysin inhibitor, which prevents the breakdown of natriuretic peptides, may be especially advantageous in terms of cardiovascular and renal outcomes.[233,369] In the scenario in which deteriorating HF worsens kidney function, often referred to as the *cardiorenal syndrome*, therapy must be aimed at improving cardiac function (if possible) and treating congestion with diuretics, beta-blockers, ACE inhibitors, or ARBs and MRAs.[370]

### Right Ventricular Failure

The requirement for diuretic therapy in patients with pure right HF or cor pulmonale is not compelling. A decrease in venous return induced by vigorous diuresis may worsen right heart function. Furosemide administration increases angiotensin II–induced hypoxic pulmonary vascular resistance.[365] Therefore, the emphasis should be on the reversal of chronic hypoxemia.

## CIRRHOSIS OF THE LIVER

Most patients with cirrhotic ascites and peripheral edema have expansion of the ECV owing to arteriolar underfilling, which is caused by peripheral vasodilation and impaired cardiac function.[371–373] Studies in patients with cirrhosis have also demonstrated increases in proximal reabsorption in response to a diminished effective arterial blood volume.[374] Finally, patients with liver cirrhosis have increases in both the natriuretic response to a thiazide and serum aldosterone concentrations.[375] Thus the use of diuretics acting on the distal nephron and MRAs are rational for cirrhosis and are usually well tolerated.[179] The American Association for the Study of Liver Disease practice guidelines have suggested that first-line treatment of patients with cirrhosis and ascites should consist of sodium restriction (2000 mg, or 88 mmol daily) and diuretics (oral spironolactone, with or without oral furosemide).[376] The guideline suggests an initial regimen of 40 mg furosemide and 100 mg spironolactone, with titration upward maintaining the same diuretic ratio.[376] Maximally recommended doses are 400 mg of spironolactone and 160 mg of furosemide.

Patients with cirrhosis and ascites cannot usually tolerate ACE inhibitors or ARBs because of a fall in BP.[377] Mild edema without ascites can be treated with dietary restriction of $Na^+$ (100 mmol/day). Dietary fluid restriction is not necessary in most patients with cirrhotic ascites. The guideline does not recommend fluid restriction in patients with cirrhosis and ascites, unless the serum sodium level falls below 125 mmol/L.[376] Although it has never been shown that treating hyponatremia in liver disease improves prognosis, hyponatremia by itself has been a consistent predictor of poor prognosis.[378] Ascitic fluid is largely cleared by the lymphatics. Diuretics increase thoracic duct lymph flow.[379] Thus, diuretics decrease ascites formation by decreasing venous and portal hydraulic pressures, concentrating the plasma proteins,[380] and increasing ascites absorption.[379,381]

The maximal daily ascites drainage into the systemic circulation is limited to 300 to 900 mL.[382] Therefore, the maximum daily weight loss in nonedematous patients should not exceed 0.3 to 0.5 kg. In patients with ascites and edema, daily diuretic-induced weight losses of 1 to 3 kg do not perturb the plasma volume or renal function.[383] The same diuretic regimen maintained after the peripheral edema has cleared, however, or given to nonedematous patients, reduces plasma volume by as much as 24% and raises the risks of hyponatremia, alkalosis, and azotemia. Furthermore, the reduced serum albumin level and an increased portal venous pressure, coupled with preexisting diuretic use, can lead to true "underfill edema." Diuretic therapy for patients with these findings is complicated by hypotension, azotemia, and electrolyte dysfunction. Thus, a diuretic prescription that is initially safe must be reviewed continuously. In addition, patients with ascites but without peripheral edema seem more prone to the development of the side effects of diuretics.[383]

The most common problems with furosemide in cirrhosis are electrolyte disturbances and volume depletion. Hypokalemia, which is related to preexisting $K^+$ depletion and hyperaldosteronism, can be countered with the use of spironolactone, eplerenone, or a distal $K^+$-sparing agent, as noted previously. However, hyperkalemic metabolic acidosis can develop in patients with cirrhosis who are given spironolactone.[384] More severe diuretic resistance requires paracentesis. It is important, however, to differentiate diuretic resistance from poor adherence to NaCl restriction. This can be done by determining 24-hour NaCl excretion or by using a spot urine Na/K ratio; higher ratios suggest poor adherence and lower ratios diuretic resistance; the optimal cutoff varies among studies, between 1 and 2.5.[385] Controlled trials in patients with refractory ascites have shown that large-volume paracentesis is more effective than diuretic therapy in reducing hospital stay and electrolyte complications but does not influence mortality.[386] Even repeated, large-volume paracenteses (4-6 L/day) are safe if intravenous albumin (40 g with each procedure) is administered.[386] Most investigators, however, recommend paracentesis only for cases that are relatively resistant to diuretics and dietary $Na^+$ restriction (Fig. 50.16).[387]

Patients with mild cirrhosis of the liver have a normal or reduced natriuretic response to furosemide, with little change in diuretic kinetics.[2] However, in those with advanced disease, furosemide absorption is slowed,[388] its volume of distribution is increased because of hypoalbuminemia and an expanded ECV, and its elimination is delayed because of hypoalbuminemia, which limits proximal tubule diuretic secretion, and a low RBF, which limits renal clearance.[2] Resistance to loop diuretics in early cirrhosis is largely due to decreased responsiveness to the drug, which correlates with elevated serum aldosterone levels.[179] With the development of ascites, a further decrease in natriuretic response correlates with decreased delivery of furosemide to the urine[389] and with further stimulation of the RAAS.[179]

Diuretic resistance is common in advanced cirrhosis. In addition to the usual causes (see Box 50.2), it may herald the development of infection, bleeding, or a critical drop in cardiac output. Patients whose disease is refractory and who

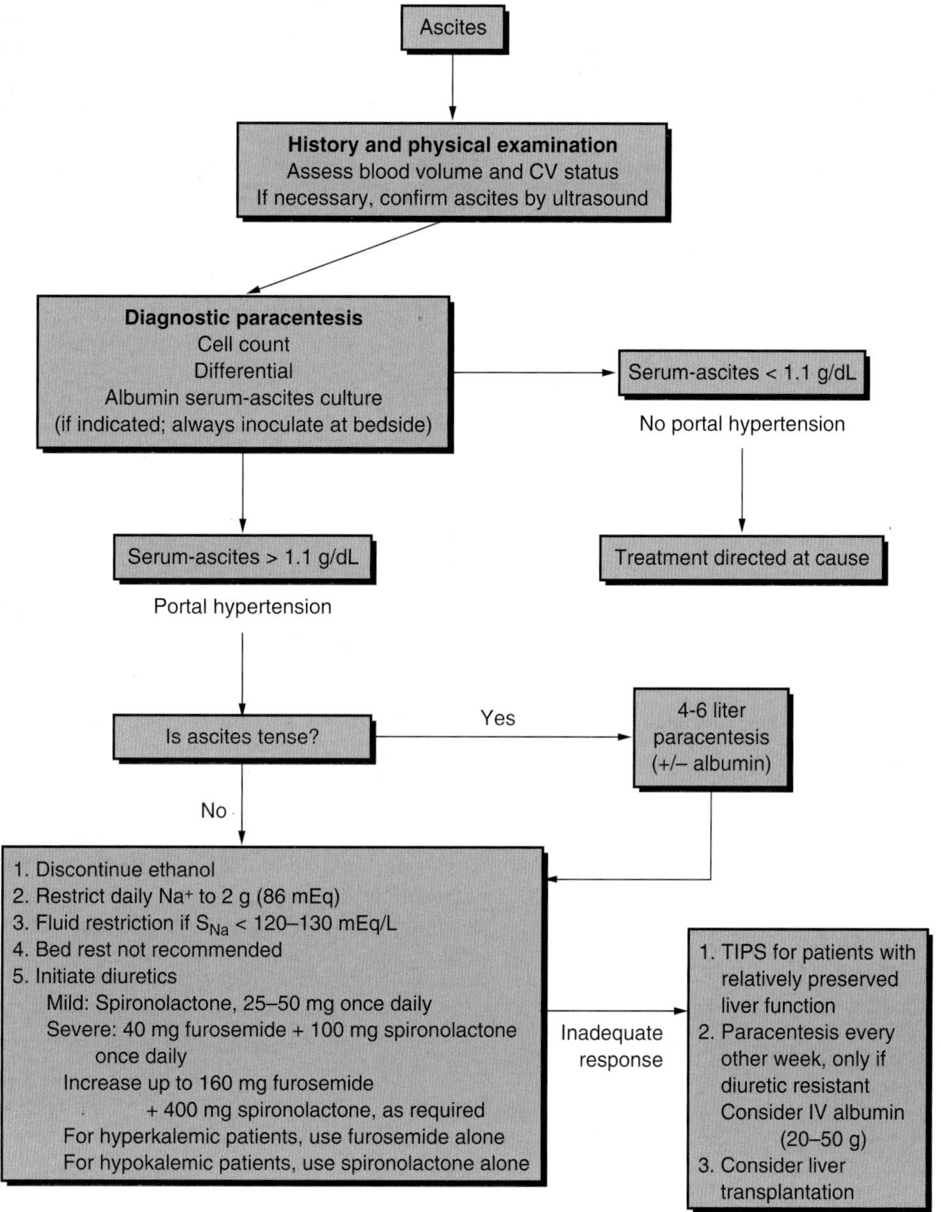


**Fig. 50.16** Treatment algorithm for the management of fluid retention in patients with hepatic cirrhosis and ascites. *CV,* Cardiovascular; *IV,* intravenous; $S_{Na}$, serum $Na^+$ concentration; *TIPS,* transjugular intrahepatic portosystemic shunt. (From Ellison DH, Wilcox CS. Diuretics: use in edema and the problem of resistance. In Brady HR, Wilcox CS, eds. *Therapy in Nephrology and Hypertension.* ed 2. London: Elsevier Science; 2003.)

are disabled by recurrent paracentesis may show response to body compression[390] or a transjugular intrahepatic portosystemic shunt.[391] Intravenous loop diuretics are generally discouraged because they may precipitate the hepatorenal syndrome.

## NEPHROTIC SYNDROME

Urinary albumin losses and reduced hepatic synthesis in the nephrotic syndrome eventually lead to hypoalbuminemia. The ensuing fall in plasma oncotic pressure increases the flux of fluid into the interstitial spaces, leading to underfill edema.[392,393] Additionally, a primary renal salt retention can lead to overfill edema (Fig. 50.17). Patients with minimal change disease often have contracted plasma volume and stimulated RAAS, whereas those with other causes of nephrotic syndrome usually have an expanded plasma volume and suppressed RAAS.[394] Micropuncture studies of sodium-retaining animal models of the nephrotic syndrome have demonstrated pronounced NaCl reabsorption in the distal nephron and TAL.[395,396] The proteinuric kidney of a rat model of unilateral nephrotic syndrome has an enhanced $Na^+$ reabsorption in the CDs[397] and a diminished response to ANP.[398] Hyperaldosteronism reinforces NaCl reabsorption at these sites. Renin and aldosterone levels are highly variable in patients with the nephrotic syndrome.[399] Hypoalbuminemia reduces the binding of furosemide to plasma proteins and thereby enlarges its volume of distribution.[400] Whereas one study has reported that premixing furosemide with albumin in the syringe prior to intravenous injection enhances the diuresis of patients with the nephrotic syndrome,[105] this finding

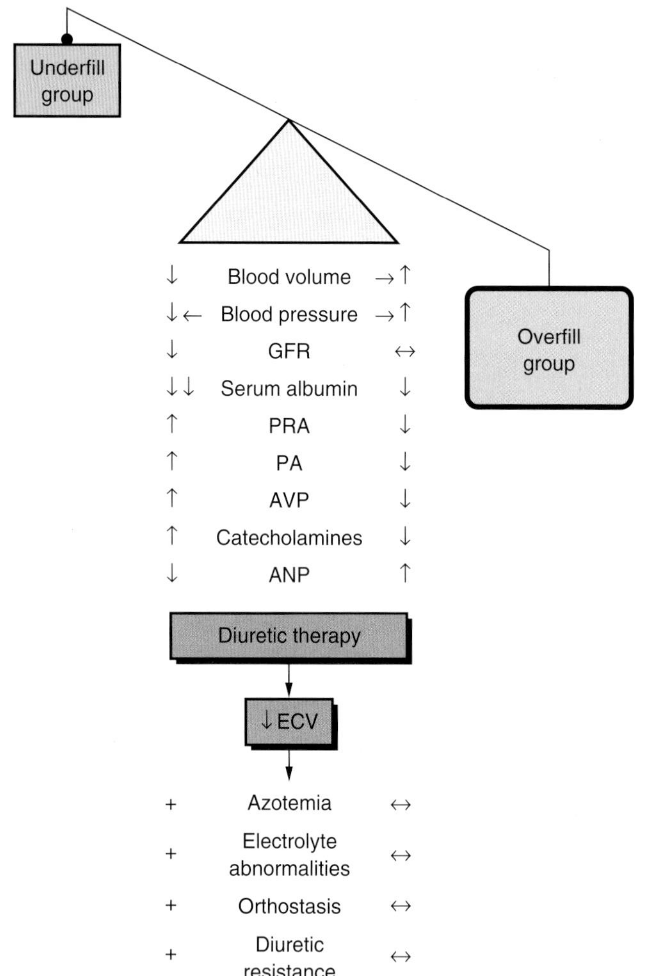


**Fig. 50.17** Comparison of clinical and biochemical characteristics and responses in patients with nephrotic syndrome and underfill edema versus overfill edema. *ANP,* Atrial natriuretic peptide; *AVP,* arginine vasopressin; *↓ECV,* decrease in extracellular fluid volume; *GFR,* glomerular filtration rate; *PA,* plasma aldosterone; *PRA,* plasma renin activity; *↑,* increase; *↓,* decrease; *↔,* no effect; *+,* potential side effect. (Modified from Schrier RW, Fassett RG. A critique of the overfill hypothesis of sodium and water retention in the nephrotic syndrome. *Kidney Int.* 1998;53:1111–1117.)

has not been confirmed.[106,401,402] Indeed, two studies have shown that patients with a serum albumin level of 2 g/dL can deliver normal quantities of furosemide into the urine.[400,403] Iso-oncotic plasma volume expansion with albumin in patients with the nephrotic syndrome fails to induce negative NaCl balance[404] or enhance the response to furosemide[401] and so is not generally recommended for the treatment of resistant nephrotic syndrome.[401,405] One study has found that a fractional sodium excretion of 0.2% differentiates volume-contracted from volume-expanded nephrotic syndrome in children; treatment with diuretics alone has proven effective and safe for the volume-expanded group.[406]

A more logical approach to diuretic resistance is to limit albuminuria with an ACE inhibitor, ARB, or both, which also may combat the associated coagulopathy, dyslipidemia, edema, and progressive loss of renal function. The addition of a loop diuretic to an ACE inhibitor or an ARB reduces proteinuria further but increases the serum creatinine concentration.[407]

The tubular secretion of CAIs[18] and loop diuretics[125] by the S2 segment of the proximal tubule depends on albumin. However, in the rabbit, the uptake of loop diuretics into the S1 portion of the proximal tubule, where furosemide is inactivated by glucuronidation, is inhibited by albumin (see Fig. 50.7).[126,408] Albumin infusion into nephrotic patients does indeed increase renal furosemide excretion, whereas hypoalbuminemia enhances its metabolic clearance.[409]

The interaction of furosemide with its target in the lumen of the TAL is restricted by binding to filtered albumin.[410] Addition of albumin to the tubular perfusate of the loop of Henle attenuates the response to perfused furosemide because of binding to albumin and is reversed by coperfusion with warfarin, which displaces it from its albumin-binding site.[411] However, Agarwal and colleagues have found that displacing furosemide from albumin via the coadministration of sulfisoxazole did not affect natriuresis in patients with the nephrotic syndrome.[412] This study's results are not definitive, however, because subjects did not have diuretic resistance.

Animal studies have demonstrated five mechanisms that could impair the responsiveness to loop diuretics in patients with the nephrotic syndrome: (1, 2) decreased delivery and/or decreased tubular secretion of the diuretic; (3) increased renal metabolism; (4) decreased blockade by the diuretic; and (5) increased NaCl reabsorption by other nephron segments. Clinical studies have confirmed that nephrotic patients have an impaired tubular response to loop diuretics.

Nephrotic edema is best managed with dietary salt and fluid restriction. Most patients show an initial response to a loop diuretic when it is required. Spironolactone or eplerenone is effective in some patients.[393] Decreasing renal function[292] or the administration of indomethacin[281] causes marked resistance to loop diuretics in these patients. The combination of a thiazide diuretic with furosemide dissipates edema but at the expense of marked kaliuresis.[413] Studies have suggested that primary sodium retention in nephrotic syndrome is related to the presence of plasma proteinases in nephrotic urine, such as plasmin, which can activate ENaC.[414,415] A recent study has shown that this mechanism is also present in patients with proteinuric CKD.[416] This would provide a rationale for the ENaC blockers amiloride or triamterene, but requires clinical study.

### IDIOPATHIC EDEMA

Idiopathic edema predominantly affects women. It causes fluctuating salt retention and edema, exacerbated by orthostasis.[417] The effects of diuretic withdrawal during controlled salt intake were studied in 10 such patients.[418] Although their body weight increased by 0.5 to 5.0 kg within 2 to 8 days, 7 returned to their original weight by 3 weeks, without the reinstitution of diuretic therapy. The investigators concluded that diuretic abuse could cause idiopathic edema. However, this conclusion has been challenged.[419] Remarkably, 83% of habitual furosemide abusers who consume high doses over prolonged periods demonstrate medullary nephrocalcinosis and tubulointerstitial fibrosis.[420] Patients with idiopathic edema are best treated with salt restriction.

## NONEDEMATOUS CONDITIONS

### HYPERTENSION

Hypertension is discussed in Chapters 46 to 49.

## ACUTE KIDNEY INJURY

A review of 11 randomized trials of loop diuretics or mannitol for prophylaxis or treatment of established AKI found no benefit.[421] Diuretics can be used to convert oliguric to nonoliguric AKI. One study involving 58 patients has found that sustained diuresis can be provoked in most patients given 1 g furosemide orally three times daily, but this very large dose produced deafness in two patients, which was permanent in one,[422] and therefore cannot be recommended. Older observational and randomized studies have indicated that furosemide does not improve the prognosis of AKI,[423–425] and some have suggested that diuretics worsen the prognosis.[426] Evidence of adverse effects of ECV overload in critically ill patients has been growing. The Fluid and Catheter Treatment Trial was a randomized trial comparing treatment strategies in patients with respiratory distress syndrome. A posthoc analysis of patients in this trial in whom AKI developed has suggested that patients randomly assigned to lower central venous pressure (CVP) targets exhibited lower mortality. These patients received substantially higher diuretic doses than those randomly assigned to higher CVP targets. Because this approach eliminated the confounding by indication that has complicated other studies, it provides substantial evidence that loop diuretics can be used safely in this population.[427] Furosemide can reduce the need for dialysis by diminishing hyperkalemia, acidosis, or fluid overload.[421] One protocol is to give 40 mg of furosemide, 1 mg of bumetanide, or 25 mg of torsemide intravenously and to double the dose every 60 minutes if there is no response, up to a total daily dose of 1 g of furosemide or the equivalent.[421] Bumetanide and torsemide are metabolized by the liver and so may be preferred to furosemide, which is metabolized by the kidney and therefore accumulates to a greater degree in patients with renal insufficiency (see Fig. 50.6).

## CHRONIC KIDNEY DISEASE

In subjects who are in balance, the fractional reabsorption of NaCl and fluid by the renal tubules is reduced in proportion to the fall in the GFR. The renal clearance of loop diuretics falls in parallel with the GFR because of a decreased renal mass and the accumulation of organic acids that compete for proximal secretion.[428] Thus, although the maximal increase in fractional excretion of $Na^+$ produced by furosemide is maintained quite well in CKD,[5,429,430] the absolute response to diuretics is limited by reductions in the absolute rate of NaCl reabsorption and in delivery of the diuretic to its target (see Fig. 50.15). Although CKD decreases proximal reabsorption, there is enhanced fractional reabsorption in the loop segment, distal tubule, and CDs,[431] with a relative increase of threefold to fourfold per residual nephron in the expression of the NKCC2 in the TAL and the NCC in the DCT.[432]

Torsemide has the greatest oral bioavailability in CKD.[117] For refractory cases, a loop diuretic infusion (e.g., bumetanide, 1 mg/hour for 12 hours) produces a greater natriuresis and less myalgia than two bolus injections.[268] Thiazides when used alone are considered relatively ineffective in patients with creatinine clearance below 35 mL/min/1.73 m$^2$, although this notion has been challenged.[433] When used in combination with a loop diuretic that increases NaCl delivery and reabsorption at the distal tubule, larger doses of thiazides are effective in patients with moderate azotemia, although at the cost of a sharp further rise in the serum creatinine and blood urea concentrations and a high incidence of hypokalemia and electrolyte disorders.[311] Moreover, high plasma levels of furosemide can cause ototoxicity.[434] Therefore, care should be taken not to exceed the ceiling dose (Table 50.1).[429,430] Epidemiologic studies have correlated diuretic use with end-stage CKD,[435] but this is likely an epiphenomenon.[436] In fact, continuing diuretics in patients undergoing dialysis who have residual renal function was associated with lower interdialytic weight gain, less hyperkalemia, and lower cardiac-specific mortality.[437] In CKD patients using diuretics, the presence of hyponatremia indicated volume overload or depletion and was associated with the earlier initiation of renal replacement therapy.[438] (See Wilcox[4] and Sica and Gehr[584] for further reading on diuretics in CKD.)

## RENAL TUBULAR ACIDOSIS

Furosemide increases the distal delivery of NaCl and fluid and stimulates aldosterone secretion and phosphate elimination, which enhance acid elimination.[439] In addition, a direct

**Table 50.1 Ceiling Doses of Loop Diuretics (in mL)**[a]

| Condition | Furosemide IV | Furosemide PO | Bumetanide, IV or PO | Torsemide, IV or PO |
|---|---|---|---|---|
| Chronic renal insufficiency: | | | | |
| • Moderate (GFR = 20–50 mL/min/1.73 m$^2$) | 80–160 | 160 | 6 | 50 |
| • Severe (GFR <20 mL/min/1.73 m$^2$) | 200 | 240 | 10 | 100 |
| Nephrotic syndrome with normal GFR | 120 | 240 | 3 | 50 |
| Cirrhosis with normal GFR | 40–80 | 80–160 | 1 | 20 |
| Heart failure with normal GFR | 40–80 | 80–160 | 1 | 20 |

[a]From Skott P, Hommel E, Bruun NE, et al: The acute effect of acetazolamide on glomerular filtration rate and proximal tubular reabsorption of sodium and water in normal man. *Scand J Clin Lab Invest.* 1989;49:583–587; Schwartz GJ: Physiology and molecular biology of renal carbonic anhydrase. *J Nephrol.* 2002;15(Suppl 5):S61–S74; Kaunisto K, Parkkila S, Rajaniemi H, et al: Carbonic anhydrase XIV: luminal expression suggests key role in renal acidification. *Kidney Int.* 2002;61:2111–2118.

*GFR,* Glomerular filtration rate; *IV,* intravenous; *PO,* oral.

effect of both furosemide and thiazide on distal acidification with increased abundance of the $H^+$-ATPase B1 subunit has been demonstrated.[440] Hence, furosemide can be used in patients with hyperkalemic (type IV) renal tubular acidosis to increase renal acid excretion.[441,442] Because hyperkalemic renal tubular acidosis is usually due to hypoaldosteronism, mineralocorticoid therapy is also often indicated.[443]

### HYPERCALCEMIA

$Ca^{2+}$ excretion is increased by osmotic or loop diuretics but decreased by thiazides and distal agents. Hypercalcemia activates the $Ca^{2+}$-sensing receptor[444,445] that inhibits fluid and NaCl reabsorption in the TAL and impairs renal concentration. The ensuing ECV depletion further limits $Ca^{2+}$ excretion by reducing the GFR and enhancing proximal fluid and $Ca^{2+}$ reabsorption. Therefore, the initial therapy for hypercalcemia is volume expansion with saline, with or without bisphosphonates or steroids, depending on the cause. Loop diuretics may help prevent or treat fluid overload, but there is little evidence to support a role in the treatment of hypercalcemia.[446]

### NEPHROLITHIASIS

Thiazides reduce stone formation in hypercalciuric and even normocalciuric patients by reducing the excretion of $Ca^{2+}$ and oxalate.[447] Some patients continue to form stones and require additional citrate therapy.[448] $Ca^{2+}$ reabsorption can be enhanced further by the addition of amiloride[449] or a low-salt diet. $KHCO_3$ produces a greater reduction in $Ca^{2+}$ excretion than KCl when given with hydrochlorothiazide.[450]

### OSTEOPOROSIS

Bone cells express an $Na^+$-$Cl^-$ cotransporter[451] that when blocked by a thiazide, enhances bone $Ca^{2+}$ uptake.[452] Thiazides inhibit osteocalcin, an osteoblast-specific protein that retards bone formation,[453] and directly stimulate the production of the osteoblast differentiation markers.[454,455] They inhibit bone reabsorption[456] and augment bone mineralization, independently of parathyroid hormone.[457] Thus, thiazides may promote bone mineralization both by reducing renal $Ca^{2+}$ excretion and through direct effects on bone. These biologic effects are supported by epidemiologic studies and clinical trial data. Thiazide therapy is associated with an increase in bone mineral density and a reduction in hip and pelvic fractures in older persons.[458–460] In a placebo-controlled trial in postmenopausal women,[461] hydrochlorothiazide (50 mg/day) slowed cortical bone loss significantly. Surprisingly, despite having opposite effects on $Ca^{2+}$ excretion, a thiazide and a loop diuretic both enhance bone formation in postmenopausal women, at least in the short term.[462] However, loop diuretics alone have been associated with hip bone loss in older men, increased risk of fractures in postmenopausal women, and increased risk of revision following primary total hip arthroplasty in men and women.[463–465]

### GITELMAN SYNDROME

In addition to potassium supplementation, potassium-sparing diuretics may be used in Gitelman syndrome to treat hypokalemia. Spironolactone (200–300 mg/day) was shown to be more effective than amiloride (10–30 mg/day).[466] In a later study, the efficacies of indomethacin (75 mg/day), amiloride (30 mg/day), and eplerenone (150 mg/day) in correcting hypokalemia were compared in a crossover trial.[467] Although all three drugs significantly increased plasma potassium levels, indomethacin was most effective but also was associated with the most adverse effects.

### DIABETES INSIPIDUS

Thiazides can reduce urine flow by up to 50% in patients with central or nephrogenic diabetes insipidus.[468,469] This paradoxic effect is related to decreased GFR, enhanced water reabsorption in the proximal and distal nephron,[470,471] and an increase in papillary osmolarity leading to distal water reabsorption. A small placebo-controlled crossover trial and an animal study have shown that amiloride prevents lithium-induced polyuria.[472,473] This effect is attributed to blockage by amiloride of the entry of lithium via ENaC in the principal cell, where it can downregulate the water channel AQP2 via glycogen synthase kinase 3.[474]

# ADVERSE EFFECTS OF DIURETICS

## FLUID AND ELECTROLYTE ABNORMALITIES

### EXTRACELLULAR VOLUME DEPLETION AND AZOTEMIA

Diuretics normally do not decrease the GFR.[83,475] However, a GFR decrease can be precipitated by vigorous diuresis in patients with CKD, severe edema, or cirrhosis and ascites. A rise in the ratio of blood urea nitrogen to creatinine suggests ECV depletion. This change can be ascribed to decreased renal urea clearance because of greater urea reabsorption in the distal nephron[476] and to increased urea generation. The latter is is due to greater uptake by the liver of arginine, which is metabolized by arginase.[477–479] In addition, combining diuretics with ACE inhibitors and NSAIDs raises the risk of AKI.[480,481]

### HYPONATREMIA

This effect is relatively specific for thiazides, which inhibit urinary dilution, whereas loop diuretics inhibit urinary concentration and dilution.[482] Indeed, thiazides are 12-fold more likely than loop diuretics to cause hyponatremia.[483] The mechanism of thiazide-induced hyponatremia has long remained elusive. Although one could postulate that the natriuretic effect causes plasma volume depletion with AVP release, patients with thiazide-induced hyponatremia actually gain weight.[484] Clark and colleagues have shown that older age and thiazide diuretics are additive in impairing maximal free water excretion following a water load.[485] Some 80% of thiazide-induced hyponatremia occurs in females,[486] most of whom are older and with low body mass.[487,488] Hyponatremia can develop during rechallenge with a thiazide.[484,489,490] It often develops within the first 2 weeks of thiazide therapy.[483,489] A recent study that combined phenotypic and pharmacogenetic data has integrated these previous observations into a more consistent pathophysiologic mechanism.[491] Patients with thiazide-induced hyponatremia displayed increased free water reabsorption independently of AVP and increased urinary PGE2 excretion (Fig. 50.18). Pharmacogenetic analysis has identified a variant in *SLCO2A1*, which encodes a prostaglandin transporter in the distal nephron. In vitro, the variant of *SLCO2A1* displayed loss of function. A reduced or absent

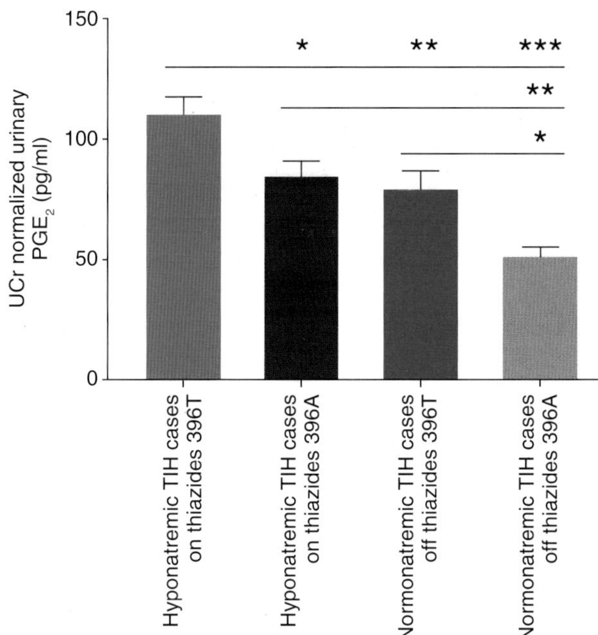


**Fig. 50.18** Urinary prostaglandin E2 *(PGE2)* concentration in thiazide-induced hyponatremia *(TIH)* cases, compared with normonatremic thiazide- and non–thiazide-treated controls, stratified according to their genotype at position 396 of the prostaglandin transporter gene, *SLCO2A1.* TIH cases who carry at least one copy of the risk allele (396T) have significantly elevated urinary PGE2 levels relative to those homozygous for 396A, whereas no such effect was observed in normonatremic controls. Data are represented as mean ± SEM. *$P < .05$; **$P < .01$; ***$P < .001$. *UCr,* Urinary creatinine. (From Ware JS, Wain LV, Channavajjhala SK, et al. Phenotypic and pharmacogenetic evaluation of patients with thiazide-induced hyponatremia. *J Clin Invest.* 2017;127(9):3367–3374.)

prostaglandin transporter in the apical plasma membrane allows PGE2 to stimulate $EP_4$ receptors, which can subsequently insert AQP2 water channels, increasing water reabsorption (Fig. 50.19).

Mild hyponatremia can be treated by withdrawal of diuretics, restriction of the daily intake of free water to 1.0 to 1.5 L, increasing solute intake, restoration of any $K^+$ and $Mg^{2+}$ losses, and replenishment of NaCl if the patient is clearly volume-depleted.[483,492]

It is becoming increasingly clear that even mild and chronic hyponatremia can produce symptoms.[493] Therefore, the development of diuretic-induced hyponatremia should probably be regarded as a contraindication to continue using the agent responsible. Despite the importance of diuretic-induced hyponatremia (and hypokalemia; see later) for individual cases, these side effects are relatively mild on a population basis and should therefore not discourage prescription of these effective drugs. For example, in a study of 3000 patients starting antihypertensive monotherapy, serum sodium and potassium values were only marginally lower in thiazide users, with more than 90% of patients maintaining normal levels.[494]

## HYPOKALEMIA

Four mechanisms have been identified that increase renal $K^+$ elimination during therapy with thiazides or loop diuretics (Fig. 50.20)—increased tubular flow, secretion of AVP, secretion of aldosterone, and alkalosis. Flow-dependent $K^+$ secretion by the distal nephron provides a universal mechanism for increased $K^+$ secretion in response to diuretics that act more proximally.[172] The basal and flow-dependent components of $K^+$ secretion have been shown to be largely mediated by distinct channels. Whereas basal secretion traverses ROMK channels, flow-dependent $K^+$ secretion is mediated

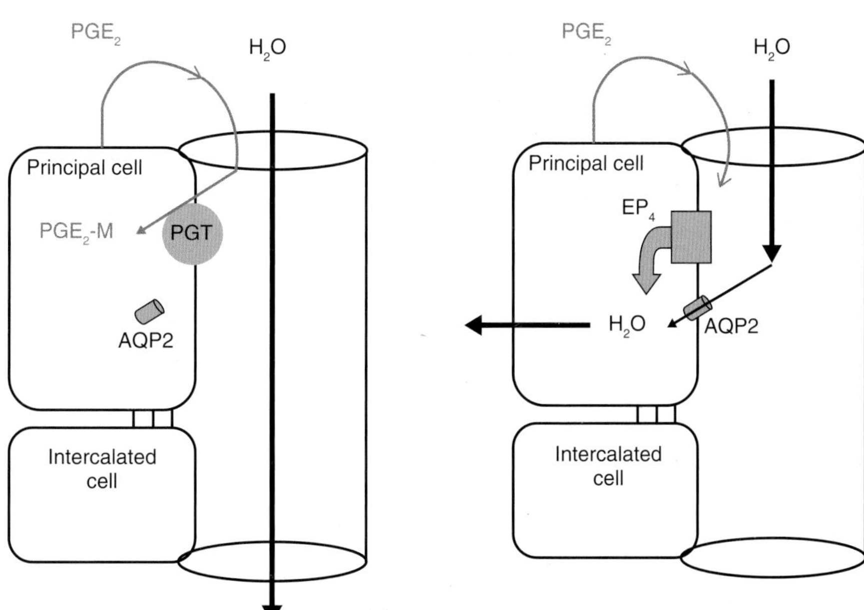


**Fig. 50.19** Hypothesis for the role of SLCO2A1 in contributing to TIH in individuals carrying the *SLCO2A1 A396T* variant. *Left,* Under low ADH conditions, apical PGT in the renal collecting duct scavenges PGE2 from the lumen, resulting in AQP2 internalization and minimal osmotic water reabsorption. *Right:* With reduced or absent apical PGT, PGE2 reaching the lumen is able to stimulate apical $EP_4$ receptors, resulting in the insertion of AQP2 and osmotic water reabsorption. *ADH,* Antidiuretic hormone; *AQP2,* aquaporin-2; *PGE2,* prostaglandin E2; *PGT,* phosphate glucuronyl transferase; *TIH,* thiazide-induced hyponatremia.

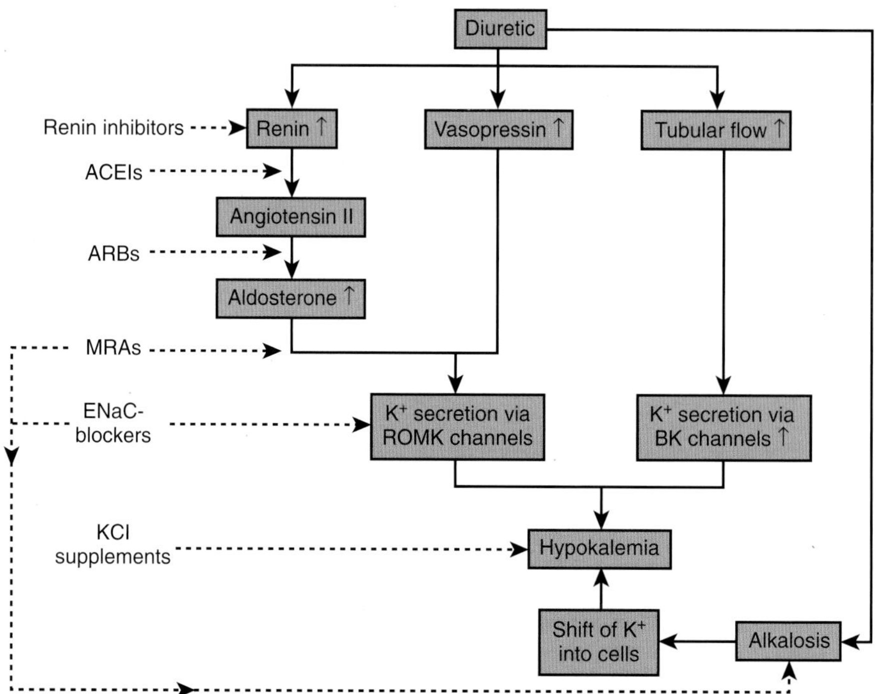


**Fig. 50.20** Diagrammatic representation of mechanisms that increase (↑) $K^+$ excretion by the collecting ducts or partition $K^+$ into cells during therapy with a thiazide or loop diuretic, and strategies for prevention or treatment (*dashed lines*) with direct renin inhibitors, angiotensin-converting enzyme inhibitors *(ACEIs)*, angiotensin receptor blockers *(ARBs)*, mineralocorticoid receptor antagonists (*MRAs*; e.g., spironolactone), epithelial $Na^+$ channel *(ENaC)* blockers (amiloride or triamterene), or KCl supplements. Diuretics stimulate the renin-angiotensin-aldosterone system (RAAS), increase distal tubule flow and release of arginine vasopressin, and generate a metabolic alkalosis, all of which enhance $K^+$ secretion in the collecting ducts. Two distinct mechanisms are responsible for $K^+$ secretion in the collecting ducts, one mediated by the renal outer medulla $K^+$ *(ROMK)* channels, and the other by big $K^+$ *(BK)* channels.

by calcium-activated maxi or big $K^+$ (BK) channels.[495,496] Normally, a flow-dependent rise in $K^+$ secretion during increased water intake is offset by a drop in AVP concentration that diminishes distal $K^+$ secretion. Diuretic therapy, however, is unusual because it combines increased distal tubule flow with maintained or increased AVP release due to nonosmotic stimulation, the second mechanism contributing to kaliuresis. Indeed, inhibition of AVP release in normal subjects undergoing a furosemide diuresis inhibits the kaliuresis.[277] Nonosmotic AVP release is common in edematous subjects.[492] Therefore, enhanced release of AVP and increased distal tubule fluid delivery combine to promote ongoing $K^+$ losses during diuretic therapy for edema. Diuretic-induced aldosterone secretion also promotes distal $K^+$ secretion.[172,295,497] The effects of flow and aldosterone on distal $K^+$ secretion are normally counterbalanced during changes in salt intake, just as the effects of flow and AVP induced by changes in water intake (see Fig. 50.20). Diuretic treatment, however, uncouples the two because it enhances the secretion of aldosterone and AVP but increases distal flow, thereby accounting for the particular importance of aldosterone and AVP in promoting $K^+$ loss with diuretics.[277] Finally, diuretic-induced alkalosis enhances the distal secretion of $K^+$.[172]

The serum potassium concentration in patients not receiving KCl supplements falls by an average of 0.3 mmol/L with furosemide and 0.6 mmol/L with thiazides.[498] This 20% fall in serum potassium level is accompanied by a fall in total body $K^+$ that averages less than 5%.[498] Moreover, in normal subjects receiving daily doses of loop diuretics, there is no detectable change in $K^+$ balance, despite a reproducible fall in serum potassium level of about 0.5 mmol/L.[277] This finding implies that the primary cause of hypokalemia during diuretic administration is a redistribution of $K^+$ into cells, likely related to the accompanying metabolic alkalosis.[70,123]

Mild, diuretic-induced hypokalemia (serum potassium, 3.0–3.5 mmol/L) increases the frequency of ventricular ectopy.[499] Some investigators have shown that thiazide-induced hypokalemia does not pose a risk of clinically significant cardiac dysrhythmia, even in large populations of hypertensive patients.[381,500] In contrast, others have reported a dose-dependent risk of cardiac arrest in patients receiving thiazides that is prevented by therapy with a $K^+$-sparing diuretic such as amiloride.[501] In one study in rats, thiazide-induced hypokalemia was associated with hypomagnesemia, hypertriglyceridemia, insulin resistance, hyperaldosteronism, and renal injury, all of which were absent in rats with a similar degree of hypokalemia due to a dietary potassium depletion.[502] Although of concern, these data may be species-specific and may also be ascribed to the dose given (10 mg/kg).[503] In a large population-based study of older adults, chlorthalidone was shown to be as effective in reducing cardiovascular outcomes as hydrochlorothiazide but more often resulted in hospitalization for hypokalemia or hyponatremia.[504]

Adverse effects of hypokalemia are clearly important in certain cases:

1. Severe hypokalemia (serum potassium < 3.0 mmol/L) requires treatment because it is associated with a doubling

of serious ventricular dysrhythmias, muscular weakness, and rhabdomyolysis.[505]

2. Mild hypokalemia can precipitate dangerous dysrhythmias in patients with cardiac dysfunction due to left ventricular hypertrophy, coronary ischemia, HF, prolonged QT interval, anoxia, or ischemia, as well as in patients with known dysrhythmias.
3. Hypokalemia enhances the toxicity of cardiac glycosides by diminishing the renal tubule secretion of digoxin and by enhancing its binding to cardiac $Na^+$-$K^+$-ATPase, thereby exaggerating its actions on the heart.
4. Hypokalemia stimulates renal ammoniagenesis. This effect is dangerous for patients with cirrhosis and ascites who are prone to the development of hepatic encephalopathy due to hyperammonemia. Moreover, the accompanying diuretic-induced alkalosis partitions ammonia into the brain.
5. Catecholamines partition $K^+$ into cells and lower serum potassium levels. Myocardial infarction provokes sufficient catecholamine release to lower serum potassium levels by approximately 0.5 mmol/L, which is potentiated in patients who have received prior thiazide therapy.[506]
6. Hypokalemia impairs insulin release and predisposes to hyperglycemia.[507]
7. Hypokalemia limits the antihypertensive action of thiazides.[508] In a placebo-controlled study of hypokalemic subjects receiving thiazide diuretics, coadministration of KCl that restored serum potassium levels also reduced BP significantly.[508]

Therefore, it is prudent to prevent even mild degrees of hypokalemia. Hypokalemia can be prevented by increasing the intake of $K^+$ with $Cl^-$ (see Fig. 50.20) but doing so often requires 40 to 80 mmol daily. Moreover, in the presence of alkalosis, hyperaldosteronism, or $Mg^{2+}$ depletion, hypokalemia is quite unresponsive to dietary KCl. A more effective, convenient, and predictable strategy is to prescribe a combined therapy with a distal $K^+$-sparing agent such as amiloride or triamterene, which maintains serum potassium levels during short- or long-term hydrochlorothiazide therapy (see Fig. 50.20).[509,510] It also prevents diuretic-induced alkalosis and provides further natriuresis and antihypertensive efficacy. An alternative strategy is to administer an ACE inhibitor, ARB, or MRA to counter angiotensin II–induced hyperaldosteronism, which would promote distal $K^+$ secretion. The fall in BP and the beneficial cardiovascular actions of these agents are clearly a further advantage. Finally, a small study has shown that combining torsemide with hydrochlorothiazide leads to a synergistic increase in sodium excretion but, surprisingly, reduces urinary potassium and magnesium losses in comparison with hydrochlorothiazide alone,[511] possibly owing to the antialdosteronic effects of torsemide.[512]

## HYPERKALEMIA

Diuretics acting in the ASDN decrease $K^+$ secretion and predispose to hyperkalemia.[497,513] As noted previously, this complication was observed more frequently after increased use of distal $K^+$-sparing diuretics in Canada,[211] although a later report from Scotland was not able to reproduce these findings.[514] The risk of hyperkalemia may rise, especially when spironolactone is combined with other drugs that interfere with renal potassium secretion, such as ACE inhibitors or the antibiotic trimethoprim-sulfamethoxazole.[515,516]

## HYPOMAGNESEMIA

Loop diuretics inhibit $Mg^{2+}$ reabsorption in the TAL[78,517] by reducing the transepithelial voltage that drives $Mg^{2+}$ and $Ca^{2+}$ paracellularly (see Fig. 50.4).[518] Thiazides first enhance $Mg^{2+}$ uptake in the DCT but, during prolonged therapy, there is enhanced renal $Mg^{2+}$ excretion.[156] Although this greater excretion has been attributed to a fall in cellular $[Na^+]$ that stimulates basolateral $Na^+$-$Mg^{2+}$ exchange,[518] later molecular data have suggested that long-term thiazide use leads to the downregulation of TRPM6, the predominant apical $Mg^{2+}$ channel of the distal nephron.[153,519] Distal $K^+$-sparing agents and spironolactone diminish $Mg^{2+}$ excretion. During prolonged therapy with thiazides and loop diuretics, serum $Mg^{2+}$ concentration falls by 5% to 10%. Diuretic-induced hyponatremia and hypokalemia cannot be reversed fully until any $Mg^{2+}$ deficit is replaced.[520] $Mg^{2+}$-depleted rats secrete $K^+$ inappropriately into the distal tubule, independently of aldosterone,[521] possibly because a decrease in intracellular magnesium releases the magnesium-mediated inhibition of ROMK channels.[522]

## HYPERCALCEMIA

Thiazides increase the serum concentrations of total and ionized calcium but rarely result in frank hypercalcemia. During established thiazide treatment, parathyroid hormone concentrations are inversely related to ionized serum calcium.[523] The increased serum calcium can be ascribed primarily to enhanced $Ca^{2+}$ reabsorption (the mechanism discussed previously). Persistent hypercalcemia should prompt a search for a specific cause—for example, an adenoma of the parathyroid glands.[523,524] A recent epidemiologic study from the United States has found an annual incidence of thiazide-associated hypercalcemia of 12/100,000.[525] Of the 221 subjects who were identified with thiazide-associated hypercalcemia, 53 (24%) had primary hyperparathyroidism.

## ACID-BASE CHANGES

Metabolic alkalosis induced by thiazides or loop diuretics is an important adverse factor in patients with hepatic cirrhosis and ascites, in whom the alkalosis may provoke hepatic coma by partitioning ammonia into the brain, and in those with underlying pulmonary insufficiency, in whom the alkalosis diminishes ventilation.[526] The generation of metabolic alkalosis with loop diuretics results from contraction of the extracellular $HCO_3^-$ space by the excretion of a relatively $HCO_3^-$-free urine.[70,527] The maintenance of metabolic alkalosis involves increased net acid excretion in response to hypokalemia-induced ammoniagenesis and mineralocorticoid excess during continued $Na^+$ delivery and reabsorption at the distal nephron sites of $H^+$ secretion.[528] Diuretic-induced metabolic alkalosis is best managed with the administration of KCl, but a distal $K^+$-sparing diuretic[529] or, occasionally, a CA inhibitor, should be considered.[19] Metabolic alkalosis impairs the natriuretic response to loop diuretics[123] (see Fig. 50.11) and may thereby contribute to diuretic resistance.

CA inhibitors produce metabolic acidosis. Spironolactone, eplerenone, amiloride, and triamterene can cause hyperkalemic metabolic acidosis, especially in older patients, patients with renal impairment, and those receiving KCl supplements.

## METABOLIC ABNORMALITIES

### HYPERGLYCEMIA

Diuretic therapy, especially with thiazides, impairs carbohydrate tolerance and occasionally precipitates diabetes mellitus.[530–532] This increase is attributed to decreased hepatic utilization of glucose.[533] Hyperglycemia persists[534] but is reversed rapidly after diuretic discontinuation, even after 14 years of thiazide therapy.[535] The increase in blood glucose levels provoked by thiazides is worsened by concurrent β-adrenergic receptor blockade.[533] A meta-analysis has shown that thiazide diuretics increase fasting blood glucose levels by approximately 30.4 mg/dL (1.69 mmol/L).[536]

Thiazides impair glucose uptake into muscle[537,538] and liver.[533] This effect is more pronounced during initiation of therapy. It has been ascribed to a diuretic-induced reduction in cardiac output with reflex activation of the SNS and catecholamine secretion, which lead to reductions in hepatic glucose uptake, muscle blood flow, and muscle glucose uptake (Fig. 50.21). During sustained thiazide therapy, there is decreased insulin release, which can be corrected by reversal of hypokalemia with KCl,[539] hypomagnesemia with magnesium oxide,[540] or administration of amiloride or spironolactone. Experimental $K^+$ deficiency causes glucose intolerance and impairs insulin secretion in the absence of diuretics.[541] Hydrochlorothiazide and ACE inhibitors have opposite effects on glucose disposal, which are attributed to their opposing effects on serum potassium levels.[538] The increase in serum glucose levels that occurs with thiazide therapy is more pronounced in obese patients and correlates with a fall in intracellular [$K^+$] or [$Mg^{2+}$].[542] It can be prevented by reducing the thiazide dosage[507] or by KCl replacement.[539] Therefore, care should be taken to monitor blood glucose levels during thiazide therapy, particularly in obese or diabetic patients, and to prevent hypokalemia.

Thiazide-induced hyperglycemia should be anticipated and prevented. Measures include coadministration of a distal $K^+$-sparing diuretic, ACE inhibitor, or ARB, prescribing extra KCl, or reducing the thiazide dosage.[510,543] Thiazide diuretics are not contraindicated in patients with diabetes mellitus. Indeed, diuretics produce an even greater reduction in the absolute risk for cardiovascular events in hypertensive patients who are diabetic.[544] Therefore, diabetes mellitus is an indication for close surveillance and attention to the coadministration of agents designed to prevent hypokalemia (see Fig. 50.21).

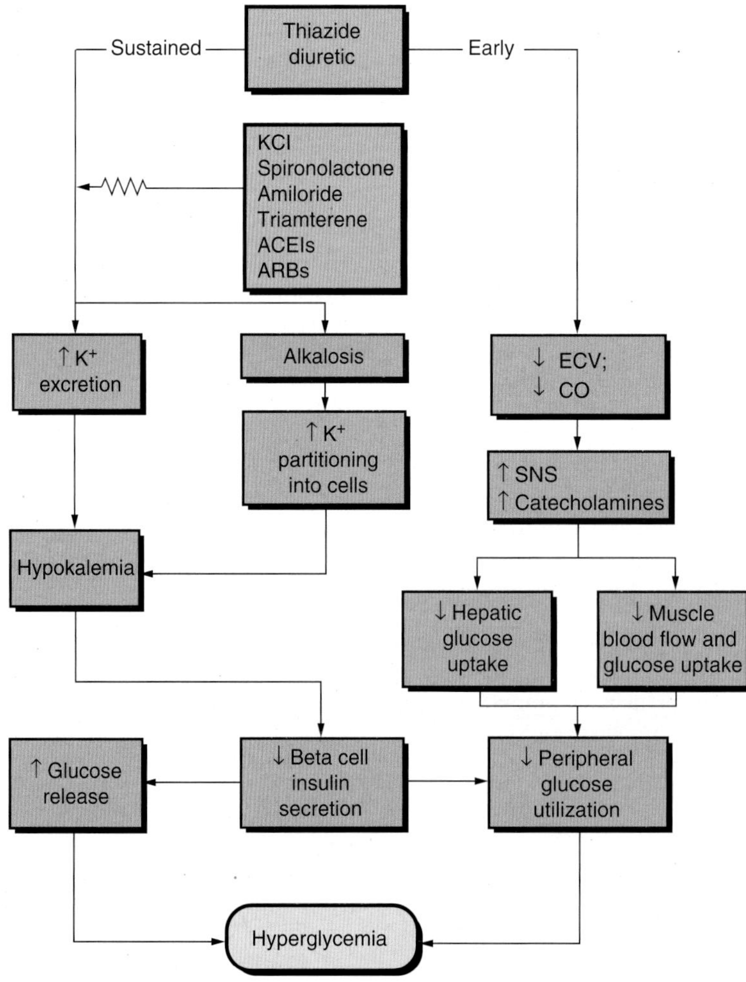


**Fig. 50.21** Hypothesis for the hyperglycemic actions of thiazide diuretics. *ACEI,* Angiotensin-converting enzyme inhibitor; *ARB,* angiotensin receptor blocker; *ECV,* extracellular fluid volume; *SNS,* sympathetic nervous system; *CO,* cardiac output; ↑, increase(d); ↓, decrease(d). (From Wilcox CS. Metabolic and adverse effects of diuretics. *Semin Nephrol.* 1999;19:557–568.)

### HYPERLIPIDEMIA

Administration of loop diuretics or thiazides raises the plasma concentrations of total cholesterol, triglycerides, and low-density lipoprotein cholesterol, but reduces the concentration of high-density lipoprotein cholesterol. These adverse changes average 5% to 20% during initiation of therapy.[545] The mechanism is uncertain; it may relate to ECV depletion because severe dietary NaCl restriction has similar metabolic effects,[546] whereas increasing NaCl intake lowers serum cholesterol levels. Alternatively, it may relate to hypokalemia, which impairs insulin secretion.[539,542] Importantly, most studies have shown that serum cholesterol levels return to baseline over 3 to 12 months of thiazide therapy.[545,547] In fact, when combined with lifestyle management, 4 years of thiazide therapy for hypertension is associated with a modest improvement in the lipid profile.[548,549]

### HYPERURICEMIA

Prolonged thiazide therapy for hypertension increases the serum urate concentration by approximately 35%. Renal urate clearance falls because of competition for secretion between urate and the diuretic[81] and ECV depletion–induced urate reabsorption (see Fig. 50.5).[82] Hyperuricemia is dose-related and can lead to gout. A very long-term outcome analysis of 3693 patients detected no adverse effects of diuretic-induced hyperuricemia in hypertensive subjects who did not have gout.[550] However, later studies have correlated raised serum urate levels with a higher cardiovascular death rate.[551] One possibility is to combine diuretic treatment with the ARB losartan, which has weak uricosuric properties.[552]

## OTHER ADVERSE EFFECTS

### IMPOTENCE

In the Medical Research Council trial involving 15,000 hypertensive subjects, impotence was much higher in those receiving a thiazide.[530] In the Treatment of Mild Hypertension Study, erection problems were twice as high in subjects receiving a thiazide as in those who were not.[553] A controlled trial has demonstrated the efficacy of sildenafil in reversing impotence in hypertensive patients receiving multiple antihypertensive agents, including diuretics.[554]

### OTOTOXICITY

Loop diuretics can cause deafness that may occasionally be permanent.[555] The risk is greater with ethacrynic acid than with other loop diuretics and is also greater when a loop diuretic is combined with another ototoxic drug (e.g., an aminoglycoside).[556] It is especially common during high-dose bolus intravenous therapy in patients with renal failure, in whom plasma levels are increased, and in hypoalbuminemic subjects.[557] In a crossover trial, no ototoxicity was noted in patients with severe HF when they were given an infusion of 250 to 2000 mg of furosemide over 8 hours, whereas reversible deafness occurred in 25% when the same dose was given as a bolus.[354]

### HAZARDS IN PREGNANCY AND NEWBORNS

Diuretics do not prevent preeclampsia. They have little effect on perinatal mortality.[558] Thiazide therapy can be continued during pregnancy in patients whose hypertension has been controlled by these agents or used to treat pulmonary edema.[559]

Intensive therapy with loop diuretics for neonates with respiratory distress syndrome increases the prevalence of patent ductus arteriosus because of the increased generation of prostaglandins,[560] cholelithiasis, secondary hyperparathyroidism, bone disease, and drug fever.[561] Prolonged furosemide therapy in preterm infants can cause renal calcification.[562] Diuretics can be transferred from the mother to the infant in breast milk,[562] in whom they can cause serious fluid and electrolyte abnormalities.[563]

### VITAMIN B DEFICIENCY

Diuretics increase the excretion of water-soluble vitamins.[564] Long-term diuretic therapy for HF reduces folate and vitamin $B_1$ (thiamine) levels[565] and increases plasma homocysteine levels. Thiamine can improve left ventricular function in some patients with HF being treated with furosemide.[566]

### DRUG ALLERGY

A reversible photosensitivity dermatitis occurs rarely during thiazide or furosemide therapy.[567] High-dose furosemide in renal failure can cause bullous dermatitis.[568] Diuretics may cause a more generalized dermatitis, sometimes with eosinophilia, purpura, or blood dyscrasia. Occasionally, they cause a necrotizing vasculitis or anaphylaxis.[569] Acute allergic reactions to sulfonamides are mediated via immunoglobulin E, whereas delayed-onset hypersensitivities are mediated by antibodies to specific protein epitopes.[570] Severe necrotizing pancreatitis is a rare complication.[571] Acute interstitial nephritis with fever, rash, and eosinophilia may develop abruptly some months after initiation of therapy with a thiazide or, less often, furosemide.[572,573] Ethacrynic acid is chemically dissimilar from other loop diuretics and can be a substitute.

### MALIGNANCY

Thiazide diuretics have been associated with both skin and lip cancers, possibly through their photosensitizing properties.[574,575] Although previous epidemiologic studies have suggested associations between diuretic use and cancer (renal cell carcinoma and colon carcinoma), a 2011 meta-analysis has refuted the suggestion of a higher risk of cancer or cancer-related death with use of any antihypertensive drugs.[576]

### ADVERSE DRUG INTERACTIONS

Hyperkalemia in patients receiving distal $K^+$-sparing diuretics, spironolactone, or eplerenone can be precipitated by concurrent therapy with KCl, ACE inhibitors, ARBs, heparin, ketoconazole, trimethoprim, or pentamidine. Therefore, these drugs should not normally be prescribed in combination, especially in patients with impaired renal function or diabetes. ACE inhibitors increase the risk of severe hyperkalemia in patients with decompensated HF receiving spironolactone.[577,578] Loop diuretics and aminoglycosides potentiate ototoxicity and nephrotoxicity.[557,579] Diuretic-induced hypokalemia increases digitalis toxicity fourfold.[580] Plasma lithium concentrations rise during loop diuretic therapy[581] because of increased proximal lithium reabsorption.[582] NSAIDs may impair the diuretic, natriuretic, antihypertensive, and venodilating responses to diuretics and predispose to renal vasoconstriction and a drop in the GFR (see earlier discussion, "Adaptation to Diuretic Therapy"). Used together, indomethacin and triamterene may precipitate renal failure.[583]

 Complete reference list available at ExpertConsult.com.

## KEY REFERENCES


1. Bleich M, Greger R. Mechanism of action of diuretics. *Kidney Int Suppl.* 1997;59:S11–S15.
2. Brater DC. Use of diuretics in cirrhosis and nephrotic syndrome. *Semin Nephrol.* 1999;19:575–580.
3. Brater DC. Pharmacology of diuretics. *Am J Med Sci.* 2000;319: 38–50.
4. Wilcox CS. New insights into diuretic use in patients with chronic renal disease. *J Am Soc Nephrol.* 2002;13:798–805.
83. Loon NR, Wilcox CS, Unwin RJ. Mechanism of impaired natriuretic response to furosemide during prolonged therapy. *Kidney Int.* 1989;36:682–689.
96. Ellison DH, Velazquez H, Wright FS. Thiazide-sensitive sodium chloride cotransport in early distal tubule. *Am J Physiol.* 1987;253: F546–F554.
104. Wilcox CS, Mitch WE, Kelly RA, et al. Response of the kidney to furosemide: I: effects of salt intake and renal compensation. *J Lab Clin Med.* 1983;102:450–458.
112. Vallon V, Rieg T, Ahn SY, et al. Overlapping in vitro and in vivo specificities of the organic anion transporters OAT1 and OAT3 for loop and thiazide diuretics. *Am J Physiol Renal Physiol.* 2008;294: F867–F873.
123. Loon NR, Wilcox CS. Mild metabolic alkalosis impairs the natriuretic response to bumetanide in normal human subjects. *Clin Sci.* 1998;94:287–292.
125. Pichette V, Geadah D, du Souich P. The influence of moderate hypoalbuminaemia on the renal metabolism and dynamics of furosemide in the rabbit. *Br J Pharmacol.* 1996;119:885–890.
128. Chennavasin P, Seiwell R, Brater DC. Pharmacokinetic-dynamic analysis of the indomethacin-furosemide interaction in man. *J Pharmacol Exp Ther.* 1980;215:77–81.
153. Nijenhuis T, Vallon V, van der Kemp AW, et al. Enhanced passive Ca2+ reabsorption and reduced Mg2+ channel abundance explains thiazide-induced hypocalciuria and hypomagnesemia. *J Clin Invest.* 2005;115:1651–1658.
202. Pitt B, Zannad F, Remme WJ, et al. The effect of spironolactone on morbidity and mortality in patients with severe heart failure. *N Engl J Med.* 1999;341:709–717.
211. Juurlink DN, Mamdani MM, Lee DS, et al. Rates of hyperkalemia after publication of the randomized aldactone evaluation study. *N Engl J Med.* 2004;351:543–551.
235. Heerspink HJ, Perkins BA, Fitchett DH, et al. Sodium glucose cotransporter 2 inhibitors in the treatment of diabetes mellitus: cardiovascular and kidney effects, potential mechanisms, and clinical applications. *Circulation.* 2016;134(10):752–772.
254. Ter Maaten JM, Rao VS, Hanberg JS, et al. Renal tubular resistance is the primary driver for loop diuretic resistance in acute heart failure. *Eur J Heart Fail.* 2017;19(8):1014–1022.
255. Kaissling B, Bachmann S, Kriz W. Structural adaptation of the distal convoluted tubule to prolonged furosemide treatment. *Am J Physiol.* 1985;248:F374–F381.
264. Almeshari K, Ahlstrom NG, Capraro FE, et al. A volume-independent component to post-diuretic sodium retention in man. *J Am Soc Nephrol.* 1993;3:1878–1883.
300. Hoorn EJ, Ellison DH. Diuretic resistance. *Am J Kidney Dis.* 2017;69(1):136–142.
304. Ellison DH. The physiologic basis of diuretic synergism: its role in treating diuretic resistance [see comments]. *Ann Intern Med.* 1991;114:886–894.
313. Brater DC. Diuretic therapy. *N Engl J Med.* 1998;339:387–395.
315. Anisman SD, Erickson SB, Morden NE. How to prescribe loop diuretics in oedema. *BMJ.* 2019;364:l359.
318. Ellison DH, Felker GM. Diuretic treatment in heart failure. *N Engl J Med.* 2017;377(20):1964–1975. doi:10.1056/NEJMra1703100.
352. Jentzer JC, DeWald TA, Hernandez AF. Combination of loop diuretics with thiazide-type diuretics in heart failure. *J Am Coll Cardiol.* 2010;56:1527–1534.
355. Rao VS, Planavsky N, Hanberg JS, et al. Compensatory distal reabsorption drives diuretic resistance in human heart failure. *J Am Soc Nephrol.* 2017;28(11):3414–3424.
372. Gines P, Cardenas A, Arroyo V, et al. Management of cirrhosis and ascites. *N Engl J Med.* 2004;350:1646–1654.
376. Runyon BA, AASLD. Introduction to the revised American Association for the Study of Liver Diseases Practice Guideline management of adult patients with ascites due to cirrhosis 2012. *Hepatology.* 2013;57:1651–1653.
427. Stewart RM, Park PK, Hunt JP, et al. Less is more: improved outcomes in surgical patients with conservative fluid administration and central venous catheter monitoring. *J Am Coll Surg.* 2009;208:725–735, discussion 735–727.
430. Voelker JR, Cartwright Brown D, Anderson S, et al. Comparison of loop diuretics in patients with chronic renal insufficiency. *Kidney Int.* 1987;32:572–578.
467. Blanchard A, Vargas-Poussou R, Vallet M, et al. Indomethacin, amiloride, or eplerenone for treating hypokalemia in Gitelman syndrome. *J Am Soc Nephrol.* 2015;26:468–475.
484. Friedman E, Shadel M, Halkin H, et al. Thiazide-induced hyponatremia: reproducibility by single dose rechallenge and an analysis of pathogenesis. *Ann Intern Med.* 1989;110:24–30.
491. Ware JS, Wain LV, Channavajjhala SK, et al. Phenotypic and pharmacogenetic evaluation of patients with thiazide-induced hyponatremia. *J Clin Invest.* 2017;127(9):3367–3374.
503. Ellison DH, Loffing J. Thiazide effects and adverse effects: insights from molecular genetics. *Hypertension.* 2009;54:196–202.
519. Alexander RT, Dimke H. Effect of diuretics on renal tubular transport of calcium and magnesium. *Am J Physiol Renal Physiol.* 2017;312(6):F998–F1015.
584. Sica DA, Gehr TW. Diuretic use in stage 5 chronic kidney disease and end-stage renal disease. *Curr Opin Nephrol Hypertens.* 2003;12: 483–490.

# SECTION VIII

# CONSEQUENCES OF CHRONIC KIDNEY DISEASE

# 51 Mechanisms of Progression in Chronic Kidney Disease

Maarten W. Taal

## CHAPTER OUTLINE



## KEY POINTS

- Although the usefulness of the term "chronic kidney disease" has been questioned, the concept of CKD is strongly supported by evidence that in response to nephron loss, a common pathway of mechanisms provokes a vicious cycle of progressive kidney damage that eventuates in further nephron loss and explains the progressive nature of CKD of diverse causes.
- Glomerular hemodynamic adaptations to nephron loss resulting in glomerular capillary hypertension and glomerular hyperfiltration are key factors that drive CKD progression. This hypothesis is strongly supported by trials showing that treatment with both RAAS inhibitors and SGLT2 inhibitors, drugs that act by different mechanisms to reduce glomerular capillary hydraulic pressure, affords renoprotection.
- Nonhemodynamic factors, including proteinuria, tubulointerstitial fibrosis, oxidative stress, acidosis,and renal hypertrophy, act in concert with hemodynamic factors to provoke progressive kidney damage.
- In human CKD, superimposed episodes of acute kidney injury likely play a significant role in accelerating nephron loss in many patients.
- A thorough understanding of the multiple factors that contribute to common pathway mechanisms of CKD progression is essential to inform strategies for achieving renoprotection. Because of the complexity of the interacting mechanisms, it is clear that to achieve optimal renoprotection, the common pathway must be blocked at multiple points.

## INTRODUCTION

The introduction of a definition for chronic kidney disease (CKD) by the National Kidney Foundation Kidney Disease Outcomes Quality Initiative (K/DOQI) and its adoption worldwide have made a valuable contribution to raising awareness of the global burden of disease due to CKD.[1] Importantly the adoption of a classification system for CKD that divides the spectrum of CKD into stages has emphasized the progressive nature of CKD and facilitated the development of stage-specific strategies for slowing progression. as well as treating the complications of chronic renal failure. These developments highlight the importance of understanding the mechanisms that contribute to CKD progression to inform strategies for slowing such progression. Central to these mechanisms are the adaptations observed in the kidney when nephrons are lost.

The kidney's primary function of maintaining constancy of the extracellular fluid (ECF) volume and composition is remarkably well preserved until late in the course of CKD. When nephrons are lost through disease or surgical ablation, those remaining or are least affected undergo remarkable physiologic responses, resulting in hypertrophy and hyperfunction that combine to compensate for the acquired loss of renal function. Effective kidney function requires close integration of glomerular and tubular functions. Indeed, the preservation of glomerulotubular balance seen until the terminal stages of CKD is fundamental to the intact nephron hypothesis of Bricker, which essentially states that as CKD advances, kidney function is supported by a diminishing pool of functioning (or hyperfunctioning) nephrons, rather than relatively constant numbers of nephrons, each with diminishing function.[2] This concept has important implications for the mechanisms of disease progression in CKD.

Several decades ago, clinical studies of patients with CKD established that once the glomerular filtration rate (GFR) fell below a critical level, a relentless progression to end-stage renal failure usually ensued, even when the initial disease activity had abated. The rate of decline of the GFR in a given individual often followed a near-constant linear relationship with time, enabling remarkably accurate predictions of the date at which end-stage renal failure would be reached and renal replacement therapy required. Among patients with diverse renal diseases, the slope of the GFR-time relationship was found to be a characteristic of individual patients rather than typical of their specific renal diseases. This observation suggested that the progressive nature of renal disease could be attributed to a final common pathway of mechanisms, independent of the primary cause of nephropathy.[3] Within this framework, Brenner and colleagues formulated a unifying hypothesis for renal disease progression based on the physiologic adaptations observed in experimental models of CKD.[4] The central tenets of the common pathway theory state that CKD progression occurs, in general, through focal nephron loss. and that the adaptive responses of surviving nephrons, although initially serving to increase single-nephron GFR and offset the overall loss in clearance, ultimately prove detrimental to the kidney. Over time, glomerulosclerosis and tubular atrophy further reduce nephron number, fueling a self-perpetuating cycle of nephron destruction, culminating in uremia. Although recent clinical studies have reported that the progression of CKD is variable and nonlinear in some persons,[5] these common pathway mechanisms remain relevant.

In this chapter, the functional and structural adaptations observed in remaining nephrons following substantial reductions in functioning renal mass and the mechanisms thought to be responsible for them are described in detail. How these changes may, in time, prove maladaptive and contribute to the progressive renal injury described earlier are then considered. Given the growing worldwide burden of CKD that causes substantial morbidity and mortality in individuals and threatens to overburden health care systems, it could be argued that the further elucidation of the mechanisms of CKD progression resulting in more effective interventions to slow its advance should remain among the highest priorities for nephrologists and health care systems today.

## STRUCTURAL AND FUNCTIONAL ADAPTATION OF THE KIDNEY TO NEPHRON LOSS

### ALTERATIONS IN GLOMERULAR PHYSIOLOGY

Glomerular hemodynamic responses to nephron loss have been studied largely in animals subjected to surgical ablation of renal mass. It was recognized several decades ago that unilateral nephrectomy in rats resulted in a rapid increase in function of the remaining kidney, detectable 3 days after nephrectomy, such that the GFR achieved a maximum of 70% to 85% of the previous two-kidney value after 2 to 3 weeks. More recent observations in conscious rats have reported a maximal increase of approximately 50% in the GFR of a single kidney at 8 days after uninephrectomy and a 300% increase in the GFR of the remnant kidney at 16 days after 5/6 nephrectomy (Fig. 51.1).[6] Because no new nephrons are formed in mature rodents, the observed rise in the GFR represents an increase in the filtration rate of remaining nephrons.

A detailed study of glomerular hemodynamics was facilitated by the identification of a rat strain, Munich-Wistar, which is unique in regularly bearing glomeruli on the kidney surface. This allowed micropuncture of the glomerulus and direct measurement of intraglomerular pressures, as well as sampling of blood from afferent and efferent arterioles. These techniques made possible the study of mechanisms underlying the compensatory rise in the GFR after renal mass ablation. Increases in whole-kidney GFR at 2 to 4 weeks after unilateral nephrectomy were attributable to an increase in the single-nephron GFR (SNGFR) averaging 83%, achieved in large part by a rise in the glomerular plasma flow rate ($Q_A$), which, in turn, resulted from dilation of afferent and, to a lesser extent, efferent arterioles. Although the systemic blood

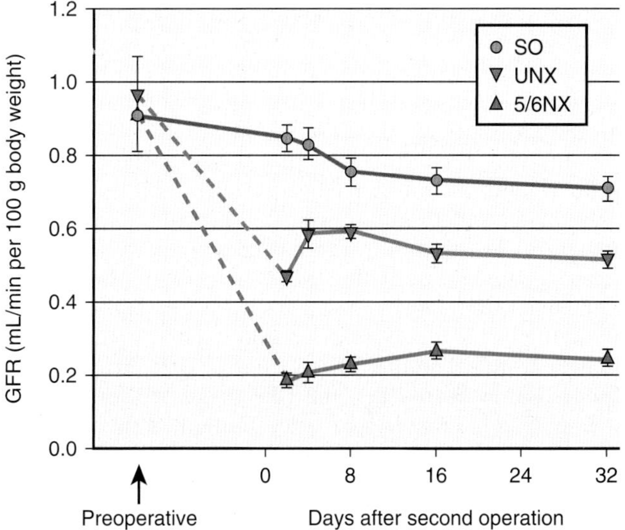


**Fig. 51.1** Glomerular filtration rate *(GFR)* in conscious rats before and after sham operations *(SO)*, uninephrectomy *(UNX)*, or 5/6 nephrectomy *(5/6NX)*. Values are mean ± standard error of the mean. (From Chamberlain RM, Shirley DG: Time course of the renal functional response to partial nephrectomy: measurements in conscious rats. *Exp Physiol.* 2007;92:251–262.)

pressure (BP) was not elevated, glomerular capillary hydraulic pressure ($P_{GC}$) and the glomerular transcapillary pressure difference ($\Delta P$) were increased significantly postuninephrectomy, accounting for an estimated 25% of the rise in SNGFR.[7] The glomerular ultrafiltration coefficient, $K_f$ (the product of glomerular hydraulic permeability and surface area available for filtration), was unaltered at this stage but may become elevated later.[8]

With more extensive nephron loss, even greater compensatory increases in SNGFR were observed. In Munich-Wistar rats studied 7 days after unilateral nephrectomy and infarction of 5/6 of the contralateral kidney, SNGFR in the remnant was more than double that of two-kidney controls. This increment was again attributable to large increases in $Q_A$ and a substantial rise in $P_{GC}$. Efferent and afferent arteriolar resistances were reduced but the decrease in afferent arteriolar resistance was again proportionately greater, accounting for the observed rise in $P_{GC}$.[9] Comparison of renal infarction versus surgical excision models of 5/6 nephrectomy subsequently found that changes in arteriolar resistance were similar, but that $P_{GC}$ was significantly more elevated in the infarction model, indicating that glomerular transmission of elevated systemic BP (absent in the surgical excision model) also contributes to the increase in $P_{GC}$.[10] Changes in $K_f$ after extensive renal mass ablation appeared to be time-dependent, with a decrease reported at 2 weeks after surgery[11] and an increase at 4 weeks.[12] Further studies have indicated that glomerular hemodynamic responses to nephron loss seem to be similar between the superficial cortical and juxtamedullary nephrons.[13] The rise in SNGFR associated with renal mass ablation is often referred to as *glomerular hyperfiltration* and the elevated $P_{GC}$ is termed *glomerular hypertension*. Together these terms encompass the central concepts underlying the hemodynamic adaptations in the remnant kidney.

Glomerular hemodynamic adaptations to nephron loss may show interspecies variation. In dogs, increases in SNGFR observed 4 weeks after 3/4 or 7/8 nephrectomy were attributable largely to increases in $Q_A$ and $K_f$. In contrast to the findings in rodents, $\Delta P$ in dogs was only modestly elevated, although after ablation of 7/8 of their renal mass, $P_{GC}$ did increase significantly, independent of arterial pressure, again as a result of relatively greater relaxation of afferent versus efferent arterioles.[14]

In humans, the effects of nephron loss on the physiology of the remnant kidney have been studied mainly in healthy individuals undergoing donor nephrectomy for kidney transplantation. Inulin clearance studies of the earliest kidney donors have revealed that the total GFR in the donor's remaining kidney had increased to 65% to 70% of the previous two-kidney value by 1 week postnephrectomy. A metaanalysis of data from 48 studies that included 2988 living kidney donors has estimated that the GFR decreased, on average, by only 17 mL/min/1.73 $m^2$ after uninephrectomy.[15] These observations imply that the single-kidney GFR (and therefore also the average SNGFR) increases by 30% to 40% after uninephrectomy in humans. There is currently no method for measuring SNGFR or $P_{GC}$ in humans, but detailed studies in 21 healthy kidney donors have reported that the observed 40% increase in single-kidney GFR could be accounted for by the observed increase in renal plasma flow and a rise in $K_f$ resulting from glomerular hypertrophy without the need for an increase in $P_{GC}$.[16]

## MEDIATORS OF THE GLOMERULAR HEMODYNAMIC RESPONSES TO NEPHRON LOSS

The specific factors that are sensed after renal mass ablation and serve as signals to initiate the adjustments in glomerular hemodynamics responsible for the increase in remnant kidney GFR remain to be identified. However, the effector mechanisms have been studied extensively; the hemodynamic changes can be attributed to the net effects of complex interactions of several factors, each having specific and sometimes opposing actions on the various determinants of glomerular ultrafiltration. Several vasoactive substances, including angiotensin II (Ang II), aldosterone, natriuretic peptides (NPs), endothelins (ETs) eicosanoids, and bradykinin, have been implicated. Moreover, sustained increases in the SNGFR also require resetting of the autoregulatory mechanisms that normally govern the GFR and renal plasma flow (RPF). For a detailed discussion of vasoactive peptides in the kidney, see Chapter 11.

### RENIN-ANGIOTENSIN-ALDOSTERONE SYSTEM

Ang II appears to play a critical role in the development of glomerular capillary hypertension following renal mass ablation and may also contribute to changes in $K_f$. The acute infusion of Ang II in normal rats results in a rise in $P_{GC}$ due to a greater increase in efferent than afferent resistance and reductions in $Q_A$ and $K_f$.[17,18] Chronic administration of Ang II for 8 weeks resulted in systemic hypertension, lowered single-kidney GFR and, with the exception of $K_f$, elicited similar glomerular hemodynamic changes to those observed after acute infusion in both normal and uninephrectomized rats.[8] The importance of the influence of endogenous Ang II on glomerular hemodynamics in remnant kidneys has been revealed by studies with pharmacologic inhibitors of the renin-angiotensin aldosterone system (RAAS). Chronic treatment of 5/6 nephrectomized rats with either an angiotensin-converting enzyme (ACE) inhibitor [19,20] or Ang II (subtype 1) receptor blocker (ARB)[21,22] results in normalization of $P_{GC}$ through a reduction in systemic BP and dilation of both afferent and efferent arterioles. SNGFR, however, remains elevated due to an increase in $K_f$. Furthermore, acute infusion of an ACE inhibitor or saralasin, a peptide analogue receptor antagonist of Ang II, was found to normalize $P_{GC}$ in 5/6 nephrectomized rats through efferent arteriolar dilation, without affecting the mean arterial pressure (MAP).[11,23] It is unclear why these findings could not be confirmed with the ARB losartan.[24]

These effects of RAAS inhibition imply that there is increased local activity of endogenous Ang II, yet plasma renin levels show only a transient increase following 5/6 nephrectomy.[10,25] This suggests differential regulation of the systemic versus intrarenal RAAS and that Ang II is formed locally. Detailed studies have identified that all components of the RAAS are expressed in the kidney.[26] Renin mRNA and protein levels are both increased in glomeruli adjacent to the infarction scar in 5/6 nephrectomized rats.[27–29] Furthermore renal renin mRNA levels are increased at day 3 and 7 after renal mass ablation by infarction but not when a renal mass is excised surgically, suggesting that renal infarction activates the RAAS by creating a margin of ischemic tissue around the organizing infarct and explaining the greater severity of hypertension and glomerulosclerosis associated with the infarction model.[10]

Detailed studies of intrarenal Ang II levels following 5/6 nephrectomy achieved by infarction have confirmed these findings by showing higher Ang II levels in the periinfarct portion of the kidney than the intact portion at all time points.[25] On the other hand, the studies also showed that the rise in intrarenal Ang II levels following 5/6 nephrectomy was transient. Whereas Ang II levels in the periinfarct portion were elevated compared with sham-operated controls at 2 weeks after surgery, they were not statistically different at 5 or 7 weeks. In the intact portion of the remnant kidney, Ang II levels were similar to controls at 2 and 5 weeks and were lower at 7 weeks.[25] Sustained increases in intrarenal Ang II levels are therefore not required to maintain the hypertension and progressive renal injury characteristic of this model. Nevertheless, subsequent studies have shown that the renoprotective effects of ACE inhibitor and ARB treatment are associated with a reduction in intrarenal Ang II levels in both the peri-infarct and intact portions of the remnant kidney.[30] In contrast, treatment with the dihydropyridine calcium antagonist, nifedipine, did not reduce proteinuria, despite lowering BP to the same levels as the RAAS antagonists and was associated with an increase in intrarenal Ang II.[30] Thus intrarenal Ang II appears to play a central role in the pathogenesis of hypertension and renal injury in this model, even in the absence of sustained increases in Ang II levels. Further research is required to explain these findings fully. It could be argued that apparently normal intrarenal Ang II levels are inappropriately high in the context of the hypertension and ECF volume expansion seen in these animals or that the total intrarenal Ang II levels measured may have failed to detect important local elevations of Ang II. Ongoing research has elucidated several novel aspects of the intrarenal RAAS, including regulation by several other factors, including prorenin receptor, prostaglandin E2, and Wnt/β-catenin (positive regulators), as well as Klotho, vitamin D receptor, and liver X receptor (negative regulators).[31]

Attention has focused on the potential role of aldosterone in progressive renal injury. In addition to evidence that aldosterone may exert profibrotic effects in the kidney (see later), these observations have suggested that it may also have important glomerular hemodynamic effects. Previous observations that the deoxycorticosterone (DOCA)–salt model of hypertension is associated with glomerular capillary hypertension prompted detailed studies of microperfused rabbit afferent and efferent arterioles; these found dose-dependent constriction of both arterioles in response to nanomolar concentrations of aldosterone, with greater sensitivity observed in efferent arterioles.[32] These effects were not inhibited by spironolactone and were still present with albumin-bound aldosterone, indicating that they may be mediated by specific membrane receptors rather than the intracellular receptors responsible for most of the actions of aldosterone. Interestingly aldosterone may also counteract rabbit afferent arteriolar vasoconstriction via a nitric oxide (NO)–dependent pathway, an action that would also be expected to increase $P_{GC}$.[33,34]

## ENDOTHELINS

ETs are potent vasoconstrictor peptides that act via at least two receptor subtypes, $ET_A$ and $ET_B$. ET receptors have been identified throughout the body and are most abundant in the lungs and kidneys. $ET_A$ receptors are primarily located on vascular smooth muscle cells and mediate vasoconstriction, as well as cellular proliferation. $ET_B$ receptors are expressed on vascular endothelial and renal epithelial cells and appear to pay a role as clearance receptors, as well as mediating endothelium-dependent vasodilation via NO.[35–37] Renal production of ETs is increased after 5/6 nephrectomy, raising the possibility that they may also contribute to the observed glomerular hemodynamic adaptations.[38,39] Acute and chronic infusion of ET elicits dose-dependent reductions in RPF and GFR in normal rats.[40–43]

Observations regarding the relative effects of ETs on afferent and efferent arterioles are to some extent contradictory, possibly reflecting different experimental conditions. Despite some differences, most studies in intact animals have reported greater increases in efferent than afferent arteriolar resistance, resulting in an increase in $P_{GC}$. The ultrafiltration coefficient ($K_f$) was significantly reduced, and thus the SNGFR was unchanged or decreased.[44–47] On the other hand, observations in microperfused arterioles have found that ETs cause greater constriction of the afferent than efferent arteriole. Studies with selective $ET_A$ and $ET_B$ receptor antagonists and $ET_B$ receptor knockout mice were somewhat contradictory, suggesting a complex interaction between $ET_A$ and $ET_B$ receptors in determining the response.[48,49] Comparative studies in rat juxtamedullary nephron preparations have shown that ET is a more potent vasoconstrictor of both afferent and efferent arterioles than Ang II, arginine vasopressin, norepinephrine, sphingosine-1-phosphate, and adenosine triphosphate (ATP).[50] In short-term studies of human subjects with CKD, ET receptor antagonists increased renal blood flow but had little effect on the GFR due to a decrease in filtration fraction, observations consistent with a greater vasodilatory effect on the efferent arteriole.[51,52] Interestingly these observations were made in subjects already receiving treatment with an ACE inhibitor or ARB. The potential interaction between ETs and other vasoactive molecules is further illustrated by observations that chronic infusion of Ang II results in increased production of ET[53] and that ET-1 transgenic mice are not hypertensive but show induction of inducible nitric oxide synthase (iNOS), resulting in increased NO production as a probable counterregulatory mechanism to maintain normal BP.[54] Furthermore some of the glomerular hemodynamic effects of ETs appear to be modulated by prostaglandins.[47] Detailed micropuncture studies to elucidate the role of endothelins in remnant kidney hemodynamics have not yet been published. These studies should be facilitated by the ongoing development of specific $ET_A$ and $ET_B$ receptor antagonists.

## NATRIURETIC PEPTIDES

Atrial natriuretic peptide (ANP) and other structurally related NPs mediate, in large part, the functional adaptations in tubular sodium reabsorption that maintain sodium excretion in 5/6 nephrectomized rats[55] but also exert important hemodynamic effects. Circulating ANP levels are elevated in 5/6 nephrectomized rats, and acute administration of an NP antagonist elicited profound decreases in the GFR and RPF in 5/6 nephrectomized rats on a high-salt (but not low-salt) diet, indicating that NP play an important role in the observed hemodynamic responses to 5/6 nephrectomy.[56]

In another study, brain natriuretic peptide (BNP) levels were found to be elevated after 3/4 nephrectomy in the absence of cardiac dysfunction or upregulation of myocardial BNP gene expression.[57] Further insights into the renal hemodynamic effects of NP have been gained from observations in normal rats infused with a synthetic ANP. Whole-kidney and single-nephron GFR increased by approximately 20% due entirely to a rise in $P_{GC}$, resulting from significant afferent arteriolar dilation and efferent arteriolar constriction.[58] In the previous experiments, some residual elevation in remnant kidney GFR appeared to persist, even after the NP system was suppressed by sodium restriction or a NP receptor antagonist, suggesting that factors other than NP contribute to glomerular hyperfiltration following renal mass ablation. The potential interaction between NP and other vasoactive molecules is illustrated by the observation that ANP infusion in normal rats induces an increase in renal nitric oxide synthase activity.[59]

## EICOSANOIDS

Eicosanoids, another family of potent vasoactive molecules present in abundance in the kidney, may also play a role in mediating glomerular hyperfiltration. Urinary excretion per nephron of both vasodilator and vasoconstrictor prostaglandins (PGs) is increased in rats and rabbits after renal mass ablation.[60–62] Infusion of PGE2, PGI2, or 6-keto-PGE1 into the renal artery elicits significant renal vasodilation.[63] Whereas acute inhibition of PG synthesis by infusion of the cyclooxygenase (COX) inhibitor indomethacin has no effect on GFR or glomerular hemodynamics in normal rats, indomethacin lowers both the SNGFR and $Q_A$ after 3/4 or 5/6 nephrectomy.[60,61] On the other hand, chronic treatment with a selective COX-2 inhibitor attenuates the systemic and glomerular hypertension observed in 5/6 nephrectomized rats but has no effect on the GFR.[64]

The relative effects of PG synthesis inhibitors on afferent and efferent arterioles may vary with time postnephrectomy. Afferent arteriolar constriction was the predominant finding reported at 24 hours postsurgery, whereas constriction of both afferent and efferent arterioles was observed at 3 to 4 weeks.[60,61] Some contribution of thromboxanes to glomerular hemodynamic adjustments after 5/6 nephrectomy in rats is suggested by the increase in the GFR seen after acute infusion of a selective thromboxane synthesis inhibitor.[62] Thus different eicosanoids appear to exert opposite effects, but the general impression is that the combined effects of vasodilator PGs outweigh those of the vasoconstrictors. This interaction is illustrated by the observation that perfusion of isolated glomeruli with bradykinin resulted in vasodilation of the efferent arteriole that was completely blocked by an indomethacin but that this blockade was reversed by a specific antagonist of 20-hydroxyeicosatetraenoic acid (20-HETE), a vasoconstrictor eicosanoid, indicating that the glomerulus produces both vasodilator and vasoconstrictor eicosanoids.[65]

## NITRIC OXIDE

The extremely short half-life of NO precludes direct measurement of NO levels or the administration of exogenous NO in experimental models. The actions of NO have thus been inferred from experiments with inhibitors of nitric oxide synthase (NOS). Intravenous infusion of NOS inhibitors results in systemic and renal vasoconstriction, as well as a reduction in the GFR, in normal rats.[66,67] Thus NO appears to exert a tonic effect on the physiologic maintenance of systemic BP and renal perfusion under resting conditions. It is unclear, however, whether NO plays a specific role in the adaptive hemodynamic changes that follow renal mass ablation. Indeed, renal expression of NOS and renal NO generation are reduced in 5/6 nephrectomized rats, whereas systemic production of NO is increased.[68,69] Mean arterial pressure and renal vascular resistance increase, whereas renal blood flow (RBF) and the GFR decrease to a similar extent after acute infusion of an endothelial NOS (eNOS) inhibitor, NG-monomethyl-L-arginine (L-NMMA), irrespective of whether given to normal rats or 3 to 4 weeks after unilateral or 5/6 nephrectomy.[67] Chronic NOS inhibition with nitro-L-arginine methyl ester (L-NAME) produces elevations in systemic BP and $P_{GC}$ in 5/6 nephrectomized rats without affecting the GFR,[70] whereas chronic treatment with aminoguanidine, an inhibitor of inducible NOS, has no effect on the GFR, RPF, or $P_{GC}$.[69]

Similarly, greater increases in BP and proteinuria were observed after 5/6 nephrectomy in eNOS knockout versus wild-type mice.[71] On the other hand, renal NOS expression and activity are increased early after unilateral nephrectomy, and pretreatment of rats with a subpressor dose of L-NAME prevents the early increase in RBF and decrease in renal vascular resistance usually observed after unilateral nephrectomy.[72,73] It therefore appears that NO plays a role in early hemodynamic adaptations to nephron loss, resulting in an increase in RBF, but in the longer term, NO retains a tonic influence on systemic and renal hemodynamics without being a specific determinant of the adaptive changes in glomerular hemodynamics.

## BRADYKININ

Bradykinin is a potent vasodilatory peptide that is elevated in the remnant kidney[25] and may therefore contribute to hemodynamic adaptations after nephron loss. Acute and chronic infusion of bradykinin result in increased RPF but have no effect on the GFR.[74,75] Micropuncture studies in intact animals are lacking, but studies of isolated perfused afferent arterioles have shown that bradykinin induces a biphasic response with vasodilation at low concentrations and vasoconstriction at higher concentrations. Both effects appear to be mediated by products of COX.[76] Similar experiments with efferent arterioles have found dose-dependent vasodilation (no biphasic response) that was dependent on cytochrome P450 metabolites but independent of COX products or NO.[77] When glomeruli were perfused with bradykinin, vasodilation of efferent arterioles was again observed but was inhibited by a COX inhibitor, indicating that bradykinin induces glomerular production of COX metabolites (PGs) that also contribute to efferent arteriolar dilation.[65] Further studies are required to elucidate the role of bradykinin after nephron loss.

## UROTENSIN II

Urotensin II (UII) is the most potent vasoconstrictor identified to date, but its actions appear to vary in different vascular territories and, in some vessels, it may even produce vasodilation. Infusion of exogenous UII has been reported to increase or decrease the GFR in normal rodents in different experiments (see Chapter 11). The vasoconstrictor effects of UII may be mediated, at least in part, by upregulation of renal renin and aldosterone synthase gene expression.[78] UII

**Table 51.1 Hemodynamic Effects of Vasoactive Molecules Mediating Glomerular Hemodynamic Adaptations After Partial Renal Mass Ablation**

| Parameter | $R_A$ | $R_E$ | $P_{GC}$ | $Q_A$ | $K_f$ | SNGFR | RPF | GFR |
|---|---|---|---|---|---|---|---|---|
| Angiotensin II | ↑ | ↑↑ | ↑ | ↓ | ↓↔ | ↓↔ | ↓ | ↔ |
| Aldosterone | ↑ | ↑↑ | ↑ | ? | ? | ? | ? | ? |
| Endothelins | ↑↔ | ↑ | ↑↔ | ↓ | ↓↔ | ↓↔ | ↓ | ↓↔ |
| Natriuretic peptides | ↓ | ↑ (?) | ↑ | ↔ | ↔ | ↑ | ↑↔ | ↑ |
| Prostaglandins | ↓ | ↓ | ↔ | ↑ | ↑ | ↑ | ↑ | ↑ |
| Bradykinin | ↓↑ | ↓ | ? | ? | ? | ? | ↑ | ↔ |
| Observed changes after partial renal ablation | ↓↓ | ↓ | ↑ | ↑ | ↑↓ | ↑ | – | ↓ |

*GFR,* Glomerular filtration rate; *$K_f$,* glomerular ultrafiltration coefficient; *$P_{GC}$,* glomerular capillary hydraulic pressure; *$Q_A$,* glomerular plasma flow rate; *$R_A$,* afferent arteriolar resistance; *$R_E$,* efferent arteriolar resistance; *RPF,* renal plasma flow; *SNGFR,* single-nephron GFR.

is produced in the kidney, and urotensin receptors have been localized to glomerular arterioles.[79] Increased renal expression of mRNA for urotensin-related protein (which also binds to the urotensin receptor) and urotensin receptor has been reported in rats after 5/6 nephrectomy,[80] but the potential role of UII in the hemodynamic adaptations that follow nephron loss has yet to be investigated.

### ADJUSTMENTS IN RENAL AUTOREGULATORY MECHANISMS

After extensive renal mass ablation, there is a marked readjustment of the autoregulatory mechanisms that control RPF and the GFR.[81–83] The role of myogenic mechanisms is uncertain, but detailed studies of afferent arteriolar myogenic responses have suggested that their primary role is to protect the glomerulus from elevations in SBP.[84] This notion has been supported by animal experiments that have reported that rat strains with impaired myogenic response show greater transmission of perfusion pressure to glomerular capillaries and are more susceptible to glomerular injury than strains with an intact myogenic response.[85] The tubuloglomerular feedback system is reset after renal mass ablation to permit and sustain the elevations in SNGFR and $P_{GC}$ described previously.[86,87] Studies have indicated that connecting tubule glomerular feedback mediated by the epithelial sodium channel (ENaC) plays a key role in this process after uninephrectomy.[88] Resetting appears to occur as early as 20 minutes after unilateral nephrectomy,[89] in proportion to the extent of renal ablation. The adjustments observed after uninephrectomy are of lesser magnitudes than those seen after 5/6 nephrectomy.[86]

### INTERACTION OF MULTIPLE FACTORS

As is readily appreciated from the previous discussion, the adjustments in glomerular hemodynamics seen after renal mass ablation represent the net effect of several endogenous vasoactive factors. Natriuretic peptides and vasodilator PGs dilate the preglomerular vessels, whereas bradykinin dilates both afferent and efferent arterioles. On the other hand, Ang II, vasoconstrictor PGs, and possibly ETs constrict both afferent and efferent arterioles, with a greater effect on the latter. A net fall in preglomerular vascular resistance is observed, whereas efferent arteriolar resistance decreases to a lesser extent. Together with greater transmission of the raised systemic BP to the glomerular capillary network, these alterations in microvascular resistances result in the observed elevations in $Q_A$, $P_{GC}$, ΔP, and SNGFR (Table 51.1). The importance of multiple vasoactive factors is illustrated by the observation that treatment of 5/6 nephrectomized rats with omapatrilat, an inhibitor of both ACE and neutral endopeptidase that results in reduced Ang II production, as well as increased NP and bradykinin levels, lowers $P_{GC}$ more than ACE inhibition alone.[90]

The complexity of factors involved is further illustrated by observations that other molecules involved in the modulation of progressive renal injury may exert hemodynamic effects by influencing the mediators discussed previously. Acute infusion of hepatocyte growth factor (HGF) has been shown to induce a decline in BP and GFR, an effect that is mediated by a short-term increase in ET-1 production.[91] In isolated perfused preparations, platelet-activating factor (PAF) at picomolar concentrations has been shown to induce glomerular production of NO, resulting in dilation of preconstricted efferent arterioles, whereas at nanomolar concentrations, PAF constricts efferent arterioles through local release of COX metabolites.[92] The potential role of other recently identified vasoactive molecules such as UII remains to be elucidated.

## RENAL HYPERTROPHIC RESPONSES TO NEPHRON LOSS

The notion that a single kidney enlarges to compensate for the loss of its partner has been entertained since antiquity. Aristotle (384–322 BC) noted that a single kidney was able to sustain life in animals, and that such kidneys were enlarged. In preparation for the first human nephrectomy in 1869, a German surgeon, Gustav Simon, uninephrectomized dogs and noted a 1.5-fold increase in the size of the remaining kidney at 20 days.[93] Compensatory renal hypertrophy has been studied in a variety of species, including toads, mice, rats, guinea pigs, rabbits, cats, dogs, pigs, and baboons. Most experimental work has been conducted in rodents subjected to uninephrectomy, but hypertrophic responses have also been studied in response to unilateral ureteric obstruction or after nephrotoxin administration.[94]

### WHOLE-KIDNEY HYPERTROPHIC RESPONSES

Among the earliest responses to unilateral nephrectomy are biochemical changes that precede cell growth. Increased incorporation of choline, a precursor of cell membrane phospholipid, has been detected as early as 5 minutes,[95,96] and increased choline kinase activity has been observed at 2 hours after nephrectomy.[97] Activity of ornithine decarboxylase, the enzyme catalyzing the first step of polyamine synthesis, is elevated at 45 to 120 minutes, and polyamine levels peak at 1 to 2 days postnephrectomy.[98–100] Early alterations in mRNA metabolism have also been observed. Although there are no changes in the half-life or cytoplasmic distribution of mRNA, a near-25% increase in the fraction of newly synthesized poly(A)-deficient mRNA occurs within 1 hour of uninephrectomy, and total RNA synthesis in the kidney increases by 25% to 100% relative to that in the liver.[101–103] Ribosomal RNA synthesis is increased by 40% to 50% at 6 hours.[104] The rate of protein synthesis is increased at 2 hours and is nearly doubled at 3 hours.[105] Data on cyclic nucleotide levels, which are thought to affect cell growth and proliferation, are conflicting. Some studies have reported elevated levels of cyclic guanosine monophosphate (cGMP) in the remaining kidney as early as 10 minutes after surgery,[106–108] whereas others have found no consistent changes in cyclic adenosine monophosphate (cAMP) or cGMP levels.[94,109] Genome-wide analysis of gene expression using cDNA microarrays in remaining rat kidneys up to 72 hours after uninephrectomy has revealed the dominant response to be suppression of the genes responsible for inhibition of growth and apoptosis.[110]

Early biochemical changes are followed by a period of rapid growth. DNA synthesis is increased at 24 hours, and increased numbers of mitotic figures are evident at 28 to 36 hours. Both reach a maximum five- to tenfold increase at 40 to 72 hours.[111–114] In rats, kidney weight is increased at 48 to 72 hours after uninephrectomy and increases by 30% to 40% at 2 to 3 weeks (Fig. 51.2).[73,94] The nephron number is fixed shortly before birth in most species, so this gain in kidney weight is attributable to increased nephron size. Growth is thought to occur largely through cell hypertrophy, accounting for 80% of the increase in renal mass seen in adult rats and, to a lesser extent, through hyperplasia.[105] Renal mass continues to rise for 1 to 2 months until a 40% to 50% increase is achieved. The degree of compensatory growth is a function of the extent of renal ablation. Uninephrectomy has been shown to provoke an 81% increase of residual renal mass at 4 weeks compared with an increase of 168% after 70% renal ablation. Normal controls gained 31% in kidney weight over the same period.[115]

Age diminishes renal hypertrophic responses. After uninephrectomy, greater increases in kidney weight and more extensive hyperplasia were observed in 5- versus 55-day-old rats,[116] and aging rats exhibited gains in kidney weight of only one-third to three-quarters of those seen in younger controls.[94,117–119]

In humans, assessment of renal hypertrophy after nephrectomy is dependent on radiologic studies. Ultrasound studies have reported increases of 19% to 100% in kidney volume,[120] and in computed tomography (CT) studies have found an increase of 30% to 53% in renal cross-sectional area after nephrectomy.[121,122] Contrast-enhanced CT has been used to measure renal parenchymal volume post–unilateral nephrectomy. One study reported increases of 12.1% and 8.9% at 1 week and 6 months, respectively.[123] The degree of hypertrophy correlated positively with the function of the kidney removed

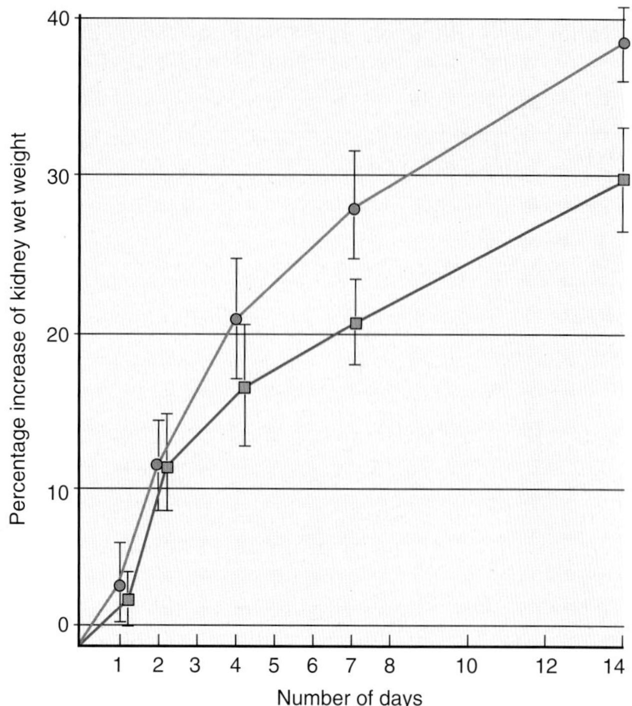


**Fig. 51.2** Rate of compensatory renal growth after unilateral nephrectomy *(circles)* and ureter ligation *(squares)*. (From Dicker SE, Shirley DG. Compensatory hypertrophy of the contralateral kidney after unilateral ureteral ligation. *J Physiol (Lond)*. 1972;220:199–210.)

and negatively with patient age. One relatively large study of living kidney donors observed a 27.6% ± 9.7% increase in the remaining kidney volume at 6 months post–donor nephrectomy,[124] and a recent detailed study has reported an increase in renal cortical volume of 27% at a median of 0.8 years postnephrectomy that increased to 35% after a median of 6.1 years.[16] Other studies using CT scans have reported increases in renal volume of 16.5 to 18.5% at 1 year after nephrectomy for renal cell carcinoma[125] and 22.4% ± 23.2% at 6 to 12 months after donor nephrectomy.[126] In a detailed study that used magnetic resonance imaging (MRI) to measure renal volume, an increase was observed from 198 ± 87 mL preoperatively to 329 ± 175 mL at 3 months postnephrectomy for renal cell carcinoma. The change in renal volume correlated positively with changes in renal blood flow at 1 week postnephrectomy ($r = 0.6$).[127] Differences among these studies are likely attributable to the relatively small number of subjects enrolled, wide variation in the time intervals between nephrectomy and assessment of renal size, and differing indications for nephrectomy.

## GLOMERULAR ENLARGEMENT

The principal morphometric change observed in glomeruli after uninephrectomy is an increase in volume. Glomerular enlargement appears to parallel whole-kidney growth and has been detected as early as 4 days after surgery.[128] The degree of enlargement of superficial and juxtamedullary glomeruli is similar. Proportionally similar increases in number and size of all cell types occur, with preservation of the relative volumes of different glomerular cells.[94] There is consensus that glomerular capillaries increase in length and number (i.e., more branching), but most studies have shown that diameter or cross-sectional surface area of the glomerular capillaries remains constant or increases only minimally.[129,130] Transplantation of hypertrophied kidneys into uninephrectomized rats has demonstrated regression of glomerular hypertrophy within 3 weeks, yet the increase in capillary length was maintained.[130]

Glomerular hypertrophy, as evidenced by elevated RNA/DNA and protein/DNA ratios, as well as by increased glomerular volume ($V_G$) on electron microscopy, has been detected at 2 days after 5/6 nephrectomy in rats.[131] The initial increase in $V_G$ was due almost entirely to increases in visceral epithelial cell volume, whereas at 14 days the increase in $V_G$ was largely accounted for by mesangial matrix expansion. Although several studies have reported glomerular capillary lengthening after 5/6 nephrectomy, few have detected any increase in cross-sectional area or diameter of the glomerular capillaries.[132–135] These observations should, however, be considered in the light of important technical considerations. In vitro perfusion of isolated glomeruli has demonstrated that $V_G$ increases as perfusion pressure is raised through physiologic and pathophysiologic ranges. Moreover, glomerular capillary "compliance" in these studies was a function of the baseline $V_G$, and glomeruli obtained from remnant kidneys post–5/6 nephrectomy had a higher compliance than those from control animals.[136] These findings have two important implications. First, although glomerular pressures are only minimally elevated after uninephrectomy, the glomerular capillary hypertension associated with more extensive renal ablation is likely to contribute significantly to the increase in $V_G$. Second, estimates of $V_G$ in tissues that have not been perfusion-fixed at the appropriate BP should be interpreted with caution. Direct comparison of $V_G$ in perfusion-fixed versus immersion-fixed kidney from the same rats yielded estimates of $V_G$ in immersion-fixed samples that were 61% lower than those from perfusion-fixed kidneys.[137]

## MECHANISMS OF RENAL HYPERTROPHY

Despite more than a century of research that identified a large number of mediators or modulators of renal hypertrophy, the identities of the specific factors that regulate hypertrophy and the stimuli to which these factors respond remained elusive until relatively recently. Renal innervation does not appear to play a role because kidneys transplanted into bilaterally nephrectomized rats exhibit the same degree of hypertrophy after 3 weeks as kidneys remaining after uninephrectomy.[138] The absence of any reduction in renal hypertrophy when rats are treated with an ACE inhibitor after uninephrectomy indicates that the renin-angiotensin system also does not play a major role.[139] Several hypotheses were advanced to account for the observed changes associated with renal hypertrophy and have been discussed in detail in other publications[93,94] but are summarized later.

### SOLUTE LOAD

The notion that hypertrophy after uninephrectomy is stimulated by the need for the remaining kidney to excrete larger amounts of metabolic waste products, necessitating more excretory "work," was proposed by Sacerdotti in 1896. Subsequently, it became apparent that urea excretion is largely a function of glomerular filtration, whereas the main energy-requiring function of the renal tubules is reabsorption of filtered electrolytes (principally sodium), and water. The hypothesis was therefore modified to view hypertrophy as a response to the increased demand for water and solute reclamation imposed by an increased SNGFR (solute load hypothesis). Several lines of evidence have supported the concepts underlying the solute load hypothesis. After uninephrectomy, RBF increased by 8% in the remaining kidney and preceded hypertrophy, and treatment with a subpressor dose of the NOS inhibitor L-NAME prevented the rise in RBF and substantially attenuated increases in renal weight, as well as glomerular and proximal tubule areas, at 7 days postnephrectomy.[73] In the remnant kidney, proximal tubule sodium absorption increased in parallel with GFR (glomerulotubular balance),[140] and tubules continued to display enhanced fluid reabsorption in vitro, implying that the adaptive changes were intrinsic to the tubular epithelial cells (TECs).[141,142] In chronic glomerulonephritis, a lesion characterized by marked heterogeneity in the SNGFR, there was preservation of the SNGFR to proximal fluid reabsorption ratio and a close correlation between glomerular and proximal tubule hypertrophy. Moreover, sustained increases in the GFR in the absence of renal mass ablation result in renal hypertrophy in some conditions, including pregnancy (in some but not all studies) and diabetes mellitus.[93]

On the other hand, experimental maneuvers dissociating renal solute load from hypertrophy appear to contradict the solute load hypothesis. Total diversion of urine from one kidney into the peritoneum by ureteroperitoneostomy was associated with an increase in the GFR in the contralateral kidney of similar magnitude to that seen after uninephrectomy, but no increase in renal mass or mitotic activity.[143] In another example, potassium depletion resulted in renal hypertrophy without any increase in GFR.[144] Moreover, the findings that some of the early biochemical changes associated with hypertrophy precede increases in glomerular filtration or sodium reabsorption argue against a causal association of hypertrophy and increased solute load. Despite these conflicting data, there is nevertheless considerable evidence of an association between the GFR and proximal tubule hypertrophy that may play a role in stimulating renal growth in the remnant kidney.[93]

### RENOTROPIC FACTORS

Failure of the solute load hypothesis to explain all the experimental data has led others to propose instead that the primary stimulus for renal hypertrophy is a change in renal mass, and that renal growth is under the control of specific growth and/or inhibitory factors. Evidence in support of this theory was derived from three types of experiments.[145]

In the first, a stable connection was established between the extracellular space and microcirculation of two animals (parabiosis), and the effects of renal mass ablation in one animal were assessed in the intact kidneys of its partner.[93] Despite some inconsistencies due to variations in methodology, these experiments generally found that uninephrectomy in one animal resulted in hypertrophy of the contralateral kidney and, to a lesser extent, of both kidneys of the parabiotic partner. Bilateral nephrectomy in one partner or a triple nephrectomy produced incremental degrees of hypertrophy in the remaining kidney(s). Furthermore, the hypertrophy was rapidly reversed following cessation of cross circulation.

A second strategy was to inject serum or plasma from uninephrectomized animals into intact subjects and then assess renal hypertrophy by radiolabeled thymidine uptake or mitotic count.[93] Although studies using single small intraperitoneal or subcutaneous doses were negative, the administration of repeated large doses by an intraperitoneal or intravenous route elicited renal hypertrophy in most subjects studied.

The data that most consistently supported the existence of a renotropic factor were derived from in vitro experiments in which renal tissues were incubated in the presence or absence of plasma or serum from rats subjected to renal mass ablation. Evidence for hypertrophy was generally assessed by the incorporation of radiolabeled thymidine or uridine into DNA or RNA, respectively. In general, these experiments showed increased uptake of radiolabeled nucleotides after incubation with serum from uninephrectomized animals. This effect appeared to be organ- but not species-specific. That a tissue factor produced by the kidneys and upregulated after nephrectomy may be required for the activity of a circulating renotropin was suggested by experiments in which kidney extract from rats taken 20 hours after uninephrectomy, in the presence of normal rat serum, was found to stimulate $^{3}$H-thymidine incorporation in normal renal cortex. However, addition of the same extract in the absence of the serum tended to depress $^{3}$H-thymidine uptake.[146] Serum taken from bilaterally nephrectomized animals lacked renotropic effects, but these were restored after dialysis of the serum, suggesting the presence of renotropin inhibitory factors that accumulated in the absence of renal function.[146] Although the specific identity of renotropin has remained elusive, several lines of evidence suggested that it was a small protein. Retention of activity after ultrafiltration, dialysis, and removal of albumin from serum implied that renotropin was a molecule of 12 to 25 kDa in size, with no significant binding to albumin.[93,94]

Several hypotheses were advanced to reconcile the previously observed effects and operation of a putative renotropic system.[93,94] The following were variously proposed: (1) renotropin is a circulating substance normally catabolized or excreted by the kidneys; (2) renal growth is regulated by a specific renotropin-producing tissue inhibited by a factor produced by normal kidneys; and (3) renal growth is tonically inhibited by a substance produced by normal kidneys, a decrease in the levels of which induce an enzyme in the renal cortex that cleaves a circulating precursor of renotropin to produce the active molecule.

## ENDOCRINE EFFECTS

Several of the major endocrine systems influence renal growth but each lacks selective effects on the kidney. There is little evidence that any of these systems represents the specific mediators of compensatory renal hypertrophy. Whereas early experiments suggested that hypophysectomy inhibits compensatory hypertrophy after uninephrectomy, later studies that controlled for the reduction in renal mass that usually accompanies hypopituitarism found a degree of hypertrophy comparable to that seen in normal rats.[147]

Nevertheless, specific renotropic activity has been identified in a subfraction of ovine pituitary extract associated with a lutropin-like substance.[93,94] Uninephrectomy is accompanied by a transient increase in the pulsatile release of growth hormone (GH) in male but not female rats, suggesting a role for this hormone in the early phase of hypertrophy in males.[148] When the increase in GH was prevented by the administration of an antagonist to GH-releasing factor or the effects of GH were blocked by a GH receptor blocker, renal hypertrophy was significantly attenuated.[149,150] Adrenal hormones appear to play only a small role in renal hypertrophy. Adrenalectomy does not inhibit compensatory growth after uninephrectomy.[151] Whereas renal weight relative to body weight is reduced in hypothyroidism and increased by excess thyroid hormone, compensatory hypertrophy still occurs in thyroidectomized rats.[152] Progesterone and estradiol in excess or ovariectomy has little effect on renal weight, but testosterone appears to play a role, as evidenced by a fall in kidney and body weight after orchidectomy and an increase in kidney weight with excess testosterone.[153,154] Whereas orchidectomy does not inhibit hypertrophy after uninephrectomy, exogenous testosterone does increase the degree of hypertrophy observed in some but not all studies.[93,94]

## GROWTH FACTORS

Of the numerous growth factors and their receptors that have been localized in the kidney, at least four are associated with renal hypertrophy.[155,156] Several lines of evidence suggest a role for insulin-like growth factor-1 (IGF-1). Renal tissue IGF-1 levels were elevated at 1 to 5 days after uninephrectomy and started to decline within days in some[157,158] but not all studies.[159] In one study, the level of renal IGF-1 expression correlated significantly with the extent of renal mass ablation.[160] On the other hand, Shohat and associates have found an increase in serum IGF-1 levels only at 10 days postnephrectomy, which was still present on day 60.[157] That IGF-1 may be induced independently of GH in the setting of renal hypertrophy is illustrated by preservation of the increase in renal IGF-1 in hypophysectomized[161] and GH-deficient rats.[162]

Other molecules related to IGF function are also upregulated. Renal IGF-1 receptor gene expression was increased two- to fourfold in female rats after uninephrectomy[148]; IGF-1 binding protein mRNA was upregulated in the remnant kidney at 2 weeks after 5/6 nephrectomy[163]; and analysis of the genome-wide transcriptional response to unilateral nephrectomy identified IGF-2 binding protein as one of the activated genes.[110] Further evidence has suggested that IGF-1 may in turn promote production of vascular endothelial growth factor (VEGF), implying that VEGF may be a downstream mediator of IGF-1 effects, at least in the pathogenesis of diabetic retinopathy.[164] That VEGF is important for compensatory renal hypertrophy has been confirmed by the observation that treatment of mice with VEGF antibodies after uninephrectomy completely prevents glomerular hypertrophy and inhibits renal growth at 7 days.[158] Epidermal growth factor (EGF) in the remaining kidney is increased on day 1 in mice[165] and by day 5 in rats.[166] In addition, EGF has been shown to induce IGF-I mRNA production in collecting duct cells in vitro, suggesting the existence of a local paracrine system.[167] Increased mRNA levels for both HGF and its receptor, c-met, have been demonstrated in the remaining kidney as early as 6 hours after uninephrectomy.[168,169] In another study, the rise in HGF message was found to be nonspecific, occurring in both liver and kidney, and also in sham-operated rats, whereas the increase in mRNA for c-met was specific for the outer renal medulla.[170]

Despite these associations, the timing of the changes in growth factor levels remains unclear. Whereas some investigators have reported early increases,[165,171] several others reported changes only at time points when significant hypertrophy is already present, thus failing to provide convincing evidence that they represent the proximal effectors in a renotropic system.[157,166]

## MESANGIAL CELL RESPONSES, A UNIFYING HYPOTHESIS

Mesangial cells play a central role in glomerular function, modulating glomerular capillary blood flow and ultrafiltration surface area. In addition, mesangial cells are both a source of and target for vasoactive molecules, growth factors, cytokines, and extracellular matrix proteins. Studies have suggested that they also play a major role in compensatory renal hypertrophy. In vitro experiments have found that when mesangial cells from a remaining kidney after uninephrectomy are cultured with serum obtained from rats after uninephrectomy, their conditioned medium induces hypertrophy in tubule cells.[172] Uninephrectomy induces significant transient proliferation of mesangial cells, reaching a peak at 24 hours and ceasing within 72 hours. This proliferation occurs in an environment of increased circulating as well as renal growth factors and cytokines, such as GH, IGF-1, and interleukin-10 (IL-10), as well as reduced levels of antiproliferative factors such as transforming growth factor-β (TGF)-β and ANP. A reduction in mesangial cell proliferation occurs in parallel with the onset of tubule cell hypertrophy. IL-10 and TFG-β have been identified as the major mediators of the mesangial regulation of tubule cell hypertrophy. Mesangial cells are the main source of IL-10 in the kidney, where it acts as an autocrine growth factor and induces the expression of TFG-β.[173] Mesangial cells are the only resident renal cells known to produce and activate TFG-β, a process that is regulated by multiple factors, including Ang II, IGF-1, HGF, basic fibroblast growth factor (bFGF), tumor necrosis factor-α (TNF-α), EGF, and platelet-derived growth factor (PDGF), all of which are produced by mesangial cells. IL-10 expression starts to increase in the remaining kidney within hours of uninephrectomy, peaks at 24 hours, and returns to normal within several days. In contrast, circulating and renal TFG-β levels fall in the first 24 hours after nephrectomy and start to rise from 72 hours, reaching a peak at 1 week.[173]

The importance of IL-10 was confirmed by experiments in which inhibition of IL-10 production resulted in lower TFG-β levels and reduced tubular hypertrophy, resulting in a 20% to 25% reduction in the weight of the remaining kidney.[173] IL-10 has no direct effect on tubule cells, whereas TFG-β has been identified as an important mediator of tubule cell hypertrophy.[174] The data presented are therefore consistent with the hypothesis that hyperfiltration after unilateral nephrectomy induces mesangial cell proliferation as well as the production of IL-10 and other growth factors that induce expression and activation of TFG-β in mesangial cells. TFG-β in turn stimulates tubule cell hypertrophy[175] (Fig. 51.3). This goes a long way to unifying the components of the solute load and renotropin hypotheses into a single paradigm to explain the mechanisms of compensatory renal hypertrophy.

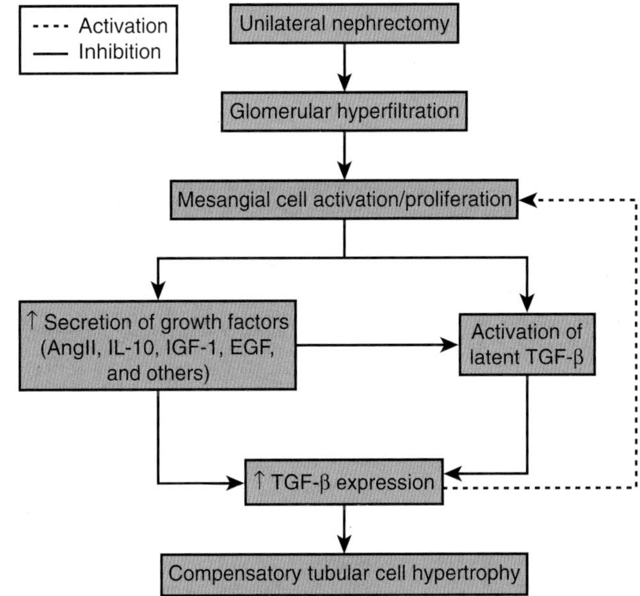


**Fig. 51.3** Possible mechanisms involved in compensatory renal growth after unilateral nephrectomy. *Ang II,* Angiotensin II; *EGF,* epidermal growth factor; *IGF-1,* insulin-like growth factor-1; *IL-1,* interleukin-1; *TGF- β,* transforming growth factor-β. (From Sinuani I, Beberashvili I, Averbukh Z, et al. Mesangial cells initiate compensatory tubular cell hypertrophy. *Am J Nephrol.* 2010;31:326–331.)

## TUBULE CELL RESPONSES

Detailed investigation of cellular responses to renal mass reduction has begun to elucidate some of the mechanisms involved in compensatory hypertrophy at the cellular level. Renal hypertrophy is achieved by modulation of the cell cycle, which becomes arrested in the late G1 phase and therefore does not progress to the S phase, resulting in cell hypertrophy instead of hyperplasia. This is achieved through activation of cyclin-dependent kinase (CDK) 4–cyclin D without subsequent engagement of CDK 2–cyclin E, a process thought to be regulated by TGF-β and CDK inhibitor proteins $p21^{Waf1}$, $p27^{kip1}$, and $p57^{kip2}$. Activity of CDK 4–cyclin D complexes increases at 4, 7, and 10 days postnephrectomy, and CDK 2–cyclin E increases at days 2, 4, and 7 to 14, implying that $p21^{Waf1}$, $p27^{kip1}$, and $p57^{kip2}$ may play an important role in regulating tubule cell hypertrophy.[176–178] The required increase in RNA and protein synthesis appears to be mediated by mammalian target of rapamycin (mTOR), a protein kinase that controls protein synthesis as well as cell growth and metabolism.

In cells, mTOR exists in two distinct multiprotein complexes, mTORC1 and mTORC2. mTORC1 acts through multiple mediators to regulate protein synthesis and cell size. Two important downstream effectors of mTORC1 are 4E-binding protein 1 and protein kinase p70S6 kinase 1 (S6K1). The importance of mTORC1 has been confirmed by the observation that pretreatment of rats with rapamycin, an inhibitor of mTORC1, inhibits renal hypertrophy after uninephrectomy.[179] Furthermore, experiments in S6K1 knockout mice have found inhibition of 60% to 70% of the hypertrophy observed after uninephrectomy, indicating that S6K1 plays a major role in compensatory hypertrophy.[180]

## ADAPTATION OF SPECIFIC TUBULE FUNCTIONS IN RESPONSE TO NEPHRON LOSS

As noted previously, the bulk of the increase in renal mass following uninephrectomy is due to hypertrophy of the proximal nephron. The more distal nephron segments also enlarge, but to a lesser extent. In uninephrectomized rats, the proximal convoluted tubule is increased on average by 17% in luminal diameter and 35% in length, yielding a 96% increase in total volume; the distal convoluted tubule is enlarged by 12% in luminal diameter and 17% in length, yielding a 25% increase in total volume.[181] Maintenance of homeostasis for various solutes in the presence of a declining GFR requires highly integrated responses from each tubule segment. Whereas some solutes, including creatinine and urea, are chiefly cleared by glomerular filtration and therefore rise gradually in plasma with a declining GFR, for others, the tubule solute handling adapts so that plasma levels remain constant, virtually until end-stage renal failure is reached (Fig. 51.4).

### ADAPTATION IN PROXIMAL TUBULE SOLUTE HANDLING

In renal ablation models, as with the increase in remnant kidney SNGFR, the extent to which the proximal tubule enlarges is inversely proportional to the remnant kidney mass. Proximal tubule enlargement is associated with an increase in proximal fluid reabsorption. In studies of animals and humans with reduced renal mass, the increase in proximal fluid reabsorption observed was found to be proportional both to the increase in the remnant kidney GFR and the increase in tubular volume.[182] Similarly, in proximal tubules isolated from remnant kidneys, the observed increase in transtubular fluid flux was proportional to the increases in size and protein content of the tubule epithelial cells.[141,183] Folding of the basolateral membrane of the proximal tubule epithelium was also found to increase, resulting in augmentation of the basolateral surface area, in proportion to the increase in cell volume.[184] This increase in surface area was accompanied by an increase in activity of $Na^+$-$K^+$-ATPase, the membrane pump that generates the main driving force for proximal tubule solute and water transport.[184]

Increases in proximal tubule size and surface area are not, however, the only determinants of increased transport activity in this nephron segment. Fluid reabsorption in isolated proximal tubule segments increases within 24 hours of nephrectomy—that is, when the GFR is already increasing, but well before significant hypertrophy occurs—implying an intrinsic TEC adaptation to nephron loss.[185] This observation also raises the possibility that the increase in proximal fluid reabsorption occurring in response to nephron loss is driven by the increase in the SNGFR.[93,94] Because solute reclamation is an energy-requiring process, it is not surprising that in uninephrectomized rabbits, the increase in proximal tubule volume is accompanied by a proportional increase in mitochondrial volume.[186] The observation that the increase in renal mass is outstripped by the rise in the GFR in models of progressive nephron loss implies that renal energy consumption per unit of remnant renal mass increases as renal function declines.[181]

The rise in the SNGFR that occurs in the remnant kidney presents increased loads of glucose, amino acids, and other solutes that should be reabsorbed entirely in the proximal tubule, provided that the maximal transport capacity was not exceeded. Maximal proximal tubular reabsorptive capacities for glucose and amino acids have been shown to increase in proportion to tubule mass after partial renal ablation.[187] Some metabolic functions of proximal tubules are also augmented in the remnant kidney to maintain adequate plasma levels of important metabolites, including citrulline, arginine, and serine.[188] Other proximal tubule functions, however, are not adjusted in proportion to proximal tubule mass; fractional phosphate reabsorption is decreased, whereas ammoniagenesis increases.[187,189,190] These adaptations are appropriate homeostatic responses that permit continued excretion of daily phosphate and acid loads as the number of functioning nephrons declines.

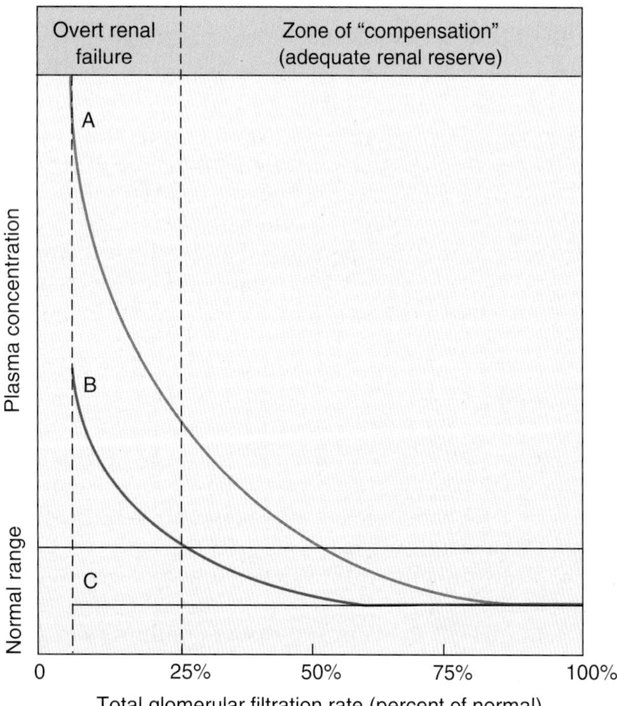


**Fig. 51.4** Representative patterns of adaptation for different types of solutes in body fluids in chronic renal failure. (A) Rise in serum concentration with each permanent reduction in the glomerular filtration rate (GFR) (e.g., creatinine). (B) Rise in serum concentration only after the GFR falls below a critical value due to adaptive increases in tubular secretion (e.g., phosphate). (C) Serum concentration remains normal throughout almost the entire period of progression of renal failure (e.g., sodium). (Modified from Bricker NS, et al. in Brenner BM, Rector FC, eds. *The Kidney,* 2nd ed. Philadelphia: WB Saunders; 1981.)

### LOOP OF HENLE AND DISTAL NEPHRON

Although there is little change in cross-sectional area in the thick ascending limb of the loop of Henle, fluid reabsorption in this segment also increases in proportion to the SNGFR.[181] In contrast, both the distal tubule and cortical collecting duct enlarge in response to nephron loss.[181] Unlike the proximal tubule, however, where the increased reabsorptive capacity is chiefly due to increased tubule dimensions, the increased reabsorptive capacity observed in the distal segments is far greater than would be expected for the corresponding increase in tubule volume, implying a major adaptive increase in active solute transport.[181] Levels of mRNA for the sodium-dependent *myo*-inositol cotransporter (SMIT) and $Na^+/Cl^-/$ betaine gamma-aminobutyric acid transporter (BGT-1) are increased in the cortex and outer medulla of remnant kidneys from 5/6 nephrectomized rats.[191] Likewise, potassium secretion by the distal nephron increases in compensation for nephron loss, facilitated by an increase in the basolateral surface area of cortical collecting duct principal cells and an increase in $Na^+$-$K^+$-ATPase activity.[192,193]

## GLOMERULOTUBULAR BALANCE

Micropuncture studies have confirmed that proximal fluid reabsorption remains proportional to glomerular filtration over a wide range of SNGFR values in both glomerular and tubulointerstitial diseases.[194,195] This glomerulotubular balance is critical to the physiologic integrity of remnant nephron function and hence ECF homeostasis. Compensatory increases in the SNGFR in surviving nephrons must be accompanied by similar increases in proximal tubular solute and water reabsorption to avoid overwhelming the distal nephron transport capacity and disrupting its regulation of the volume and composition of the final urine. Conversely, reductions in SNGFR in damaged nephrons must be matched by similar reductions in proximal fluid reabsorption to maintain adequate solute and water delivery to the distal tubule, again permitting excretion of urine of appropriate volume and composition.

Glomerulotubular balance is maintained as follows. The degree of single-nephron hyperfiltration occurring as a consequence of nephron loss determines the passive Starling forces operating in the postglomerular microcirculation, which, in turn, govern net transtubular solute reabsorption.[196] Increases in the SNGFR associated with an increased filtration fraction result in elevated postglomerular capillary protein concentrations, which determine nonlinear increases in oncotic pressure, $\Pi_E$, the major determinant of peritubular capillary reabsorptive force ($P_r$). Reductions in the SNGFR, in contrast, result in a lowered peritubular oncotic pressure, thereby reducing $P_r$. Thus the SNGFR and proximal fluid reabsorption remain in direct proportion to one another.

Prevention of hyperfiltration by dietary protein restriction has been shown to abrogate the increase in proximal fluid reabsorption in the remnant kidney, underscoring the dependence of proximal tubular function on the level of glomerular filtration.[196] In the remnant kidney of rats subjected to extensive renal mass ablation, absolute fluid reabsorption was found to be markedly increased in proximal portions of superficial and juxtamedullary nephrons, yet fluid delivery to the more distal segments of the nephron was also somewhat increased.[197] In the setting of nephron loss, sodium reabsorption by the loop of Henle has been shown to remain proportional to sodium delivery to that segment, indicating preservation of tubulotubular balance, a mechanism that maintains appropriate distal solute and water delivery in the presence of progressive nephron loss. Until the adaptive capacities of these mechanisms are finally exhausted, the operation of glomerulotubular balance and tubulotubular balance ensures that the distal tubule mechanisms that determine final urine volume and composition are not overwhelmed by unregulated distal delivery of water and solute.[198] In keeping with these physiologic observations, morphologic studies have shown that within the same kidney, nephrons associated with damaged glomeruli are usually atrophic and presumably hypo functioning or nonfunctioning, whereas those associated with healthier glomeruli are usually hypertrophic and hyperfunctioning.[199]

To maintain homeostasis in the presence of continued food and water intake, specific mechanisms that enhance single-nephron water and solute excretion must come into play, in addition to adjustments in the SNGFR and tubular reabsorption that occur in response to nephron loss. These mechanisms are not unique to the setting of renal insufficiency, however, and are also engaged when the normal kidney is challenged to excrete extraordinary loads of solute and water. In general, the adaptive physiology of the chronically injured kidney is adequate to preserve homeostasis for many solutes under baseline conditions, but the adaptive capacity may easily become overwhelmed by fluctuations in fluid intake, especially by increases in electrolyte and acid loads. Patients with chronic renal failure are therefore susceptible to develop volume overload, volume loss, hyperkalemia, and acidosis when the excretory capacity of the kidney is challenged by relatively modest changes in excretory demands.

## SODIUM EXCRETION AND EXTRACELLULAR FLUID VOLUME REGULATION

In chronic renal failure, ECF volume is often maintained very close to normal until end-stage is reached.[200] This remarkable feat is accomplished by an increase in fractional sodium excretion ($FE_{Na}$) in inverse proportion to decline in the GFR.[201] Many studies have attempted to identify which nephron segments are responsible for the decrease in sodium reabsorption:

- Micropuncture studies in uninephrectomized rats have shown that tubule fluid transit times, as well as the half-time for reabsorption of a stationary saline droplet in the proximal tubule lumen, were not different from controls.[181]
- In remnant kidneys of rats receiving high normal or low-sodium diets, absolute sodium reabsorption was found to increase, but fractional sodium and fluid reabsorption were found to decrease in all three uremic groups.[202]
- Micropuncture studies in dogs and rats have failed to detect significant reductions in fractional proximal tubule fluid and sodium reabsorption.[203]
- Distal sodium delivery was found to be markedly increased in the rat remnant kidney.[202]
- Increased solute transport activity has been demonstrated in the distal tubule of uninephrectomized rats.[181]
- Under conditions of hydropenia and salt loading, sodium reabsorption by the medullary collecting duct of the rat remnant kidney was markedly reduced.[204]

Investigators have also used a computational model of epithelial transport to investigate changes after nephron loss. Similar to experimental data, the simulations found that after uninephrectomy or 5/6 nephrectomy, fractional reabsorption of sodium and water remains normal from the proximal tubule to distal convoluted tubule but increases in the collecting tubule and collecting duct to maintain sodium balance.[205]

Taken together, these data suggest that proximal fractional reabsorption remains largely unchanged, and that in the setting of renal insufficiency, adjustments in sodium excretion occur predominantly in the loop and distal nephron segments.[206] These physiologic observations were supported by studies investigating changes in sodium transporters after 5/6 nephrectomy. At 4 weeks after surgery, a substantial increase in abundance of the $Na^+$-$K^+$-$2Cl^-$ and $Na^+$-$Cl^-$ cotransporters (expressed chiefly in the loop of Henle and distal tubule, respectively) was observed, whereas marked decreases were observed in both at 12 weeks.[207] The expression of ENaC alpha increased throughout the observation period.[207]

In addition to load-dependent tubular adaptations in sodium handling, sodium excretion is also modulated by hormonal influences. Levels of NPs are elevated in chronic renal failure as a result of reduced clearance and in response to alterations in sodium and volume status.[56,208] In rats with extensive renal mass ablation, plasma ANP levels may be restored toward normal levels by dietary sodium restriction but, in response to increases in sodium intake, they rise progressively along with sodium excretion.[209] The notion that ANP plays an important role in mediating adaptive changes in sodium excretion in the setting of renal ablation has been confirmed by observations that the administration of a NP receptor antagonist reduces both $FE_{Na}$ and GFR in 5/6 nephrectomized rats receiving normal or high- salt diets, but does not alter these variables in rats fed low-salt diets.[210] Significantly, NPs not only modulate sodium excretion but may also contribute to the attendant glomerular hyperfiltration and thereby further exacerbate renal injury (see previously).

Systemic hypertension has also been proposed by Guyton and associates to contribute to the increase in $FE_{Na}$ observed with renal insufficiency.[211] They hypothesized that a constant sodium intake in the presence of a reduced number of functioning nephrons leads to positive sodium balance as a result of reduced excretory capacity. Positive sodium balance leads to an increase in ECF volume and a rise in systemic BP that in turn leads to an increase in $FE_{Na}$ and reestablishes the steady state. In support of this hypothesis, salt intake has been shown to be critical to the development of hypertension in subtotally nephrectomized dogs,[212] and uremic patients have been found to exhibit marked sodium retention when treated with vasodilating antihypertensive agents.[213] On the other hand, a lowered salt intake in 5/6 nephrectomized rats does not prevent the development of systemic hypertension,[134] suggesting that sodium excretion and hypertension are not always interdependent in the setting of extensive renal mass ablation. Sodium conservation, on the other hand, is also impaired with renal insufficiency and, in response to an acute reduction in sodium intake, most patients were unable to reduce sodium excretion below 20 to 30 mEq/day.[214] The salt-losing tendency associated with CKD appears to be dependent on the salt load per nephron and may therefore be reversible with adequate dietary sodium restriction. Other factors modulating $FE_{Na}$ in the setting of renal insufficiency include changes in sympathetic nervous system activity, aldosterone, PGs, and parathyroid hormone (PTH) levels.[206,215] Sodium homeostasis and volume regulation are discussed in further detail in Chapters 6 and 10.

## URINARY CONCENTRATION AND DILUTION

ECF homeostasis is usually well maintained until renal insufficiency is far advanced, when the ability of the kidney to excrete a volume load becomes significantly reduced.[206] Normal generation of solute-free water is about 12 mL/100 mL of the GFR and is dependent on dilution of tubule fluid in the thick ascending limb, maintenance of low water permeability in the distal nephron segments in the absence of antidiuretic hormone (ADH), and decreased hypertonicity of the medullary interstitium during water diuresis. Although the single- nephron capacity to excrete free water per milliliter of the GFR is not reduced in patients with advanced renal disease,[216] the absolute reduction in the GFR reduces the overall capacity of the kidney to excrete a water load. Patients with chronic renal failure therefore cannot adequately dilute their urine and are prone to water intoxication and hyponatremia. Hypothetically, in addition to the excretion of the equivalent of 2 L of so-called isotonic urine per day (obligatory excretion of 600 mOsm/day), normal kidneys, with a GFR of 150 L/day, can excrete up to 18 L of free water/day, whereas failing kidneys, with a GFR of 15 L/day, can only excrete about 1.8 L of free water/day. The minimum urinary osmolality achievable by normal kidneys would therefore approach 30 mOsm/L (600 mOsm/20 L), whereas that of diseased kidneys would be 160 mOsm/L (600 mOsm/3.8 L).

Urinary concentration is also impaired in renal insufficiency. Normal urinary concentration requires preservation of the countercurrent mechanism to maintain hypertonicity of the medullary interstitium and normal water transport across the distal nephron segments in response to ADH. The maximal urinary osmolality in normal subjects is about 1200 mOsm/L. As the GFR decreases, however, maximal urinary osmolality falls and, with a GFR of 15 mL/min/1.73 $m^2$, s reduced to about 400 mOsm/L.[217] A normal individual can therefore excrete the obligatory daily 600 mOsm in as little as 0.5 L of urine, whereas the patient with a GFR of 15 mL/min/1.73 $m^2$ can excrete the same load in a minimum of 1.5 L. Part of the defect in urinary concentration observed with renal damage may be attributed to the high solute load imposed per surviving nephron. In patients with chronic renal failure, however, the osmotic effect of urea was shown to be inadequate to account fully for the reduction in maximal urine concentration, indicating that factors other than osmotic diuresis contribute to reduction in urine-concentrating ability in these patients.[217]

Furthermore, in patients with chronic glomerulonephritis, reduction in urine concentrating capacity was found to correlate significantly with the degree of medullary fibrosis on renal biopsy,[218] suggesting that disruption of the medullary architecture, with the consequent loss of medullary hypertonicity, may result in disproportionate impairment of urinary concentrating ability at any given level of the GFR. Consistent with this observation, patients with primary tubulointerstitial injury (e.g., analgesic nephropathy, sickle cell disease), have markedly impaired urine-concentrating abilities, even early in the course of their illness.[217,219,220] Similarly, in animal experiments, surgical exposure of the renal papilla in intact hydropenic rats was found to lead to a reduction in urinary osmolality because of the accompanying alterations in vasa recta flow and ensuing washout of medullary solutes.[221] Interestingly, similar exposure of papillae in rats with remnant kidneys did not affect urinary osmolality, presumably because medullary solute washout had already occurred due to the adaptive responses to nephron loss.

Urinary concentration also depends on water reabsorption in the distal nephron segments in the remnant kidney. Reduction in water reabsorption may be the result of several mechanisms in the failing kidney. A defective cAMP-mediated response to ADH may render the cortical collecting duct resistant to the effects of ADH, resulting in increased water delivery to the papillary collecting duct.[222] Urinary osmolality is inversely proportional to fractional water delivery to the papillary collecting duct in 5/6 nephrectomized rats, despite an increase in absolute water reabsorption per functioning collecting tubule when compared with controls.[221] Patients with renal insufficiency are therefore prone to volume depletion in the presence of water deprivation or impaired thirst mechanisms. More commonly, the inability to concentrate urine becomes manifest as nocturia, which develops as renal function deteriorates. Urinary concentrating and diluting mechanisms are discussed in further detail in Chapter 10.

## POTASSIUM EXCRETION

To maintain potassium homeostasis in the presence of continued dietary intake and a reduced number of functioning nephrons, potassium excretion per nephron must increase. In both normal and diseased kidneys, almost all the filtered potassium is reabsorbed in the proximal tubule and loop of Henle. Potassium excretion is therefore determined predominantly by distal secretion,[206] although a reduction in potassium reabsorption by the loop of Henle has been shown to contribute to increased potassium excretion in rats with reduced renal mass.[223] In both normal and partially nephrectomized dogs, urinary potassium excretion was found to correlate directly with serum potassium concentration.[224] Similarly, in intact and uninephrectomized rats, net potassium secretion in the distal convoluted tubule occurred only during potassium infusion, whereas potassium secretion by cortical collecting tubules (CCTs) occurred under all conditions and was greater after uninephrectomy.[225] Other studies have confirmed that the CCT is an important site of potassium secretion in the remnant kidney.[192,204] Secretion of potassium by CCTs isolated from remnant kidneys of rabbits fed normal or high-potassium diets was shown to persist in vitro and to be directly related to the dietary potassium content,[192] indicating an intrinsic tubular adaptation to potassium load. This adaptation was absent in CCTs from rabbits in which dietary potassium had been reduced in proportion to the amount of renal mass lost. In addition to variations with the dietary potassium load, the increase in potassium secretion by remnant CCTs was also found to correlate with plasma aldosterone levels, but not with intracellular potassium concentration or $Na^+$-$K^+$-ATPase.[192] In contrast, however, others have reported an increase in cortical and outer medullary $Na^+$-$K^+$-ATPase activity in homogenates from rat remnant kidneys that was abrogated when potassium intake was reduced in proportion to the reduction in the GFR.[226] These findings have been largely confirmed using a computational model of epithelial transport. In simulations of an acute potassium load and chronic high-potassium diet, potassium secretion increased in the connecting tubule, but the increase was less after uninephrectomy (18% less with acute and 13% less with chronic loads) and 5/6 nephrectomy (42% less with acute and 31% less with chronic loads) than in sham controls. The increase in potassium secretion per tubule failed to compensate fully for the decrease in nephron number.[227] Finally, the frequent occurrence of hyperkalemia in patients with chronic renal failure after treatment with an aldosterone antagonist or an ACE inhibitor, suggests that "normal" aldosterone levels are required to maintain adequate potassium excretion in this population.[228] In general therefore the increase in potassium secretion by surviving nephrons appears to be predominantly determined by the rise in plasma potassium levels after potassium ingestion and by intrinsic tubular adaptation to the increased filtered potassium load.[224,225] In both dogs and patients with chronic renal failure, however, the kaliuretic response to an oral potassium load is attenuated compared to normals, despite higher serum potassium levels.[224,229] The eventual complete excretion of a potassium load therefore occurs at the expense of a sustained increase in serum potassium levels. Control of potassium excretion is discussed further in Chapters 6 and 17.

## ACID-BASE REGULATION

Reduction of the GFR in patients with CKD is associated with the development of systemic metabolic acidosis due to a reduction in the serum bicarbonate concentration. Normal acid-base balance requires reabsorption of filtered bicarbonate, excretion of titratable acid, ammonia generation, and acidification of tubular luminal fluid by the distal nephron.[206] In chronic renal failure, acidosis develops as a result of varying degrees of impairment in each of these processes.[230]

A reduction in renal ammonia synthesis is the greatest limitation to acid excretion in CKD. Low serum bicarbonate levels result in maintenance of acidic urine, which stimulates proximal tubule ammoniagenesis and also promotes ammonia conversion, resulting in its entrapment as ammonium in the tubule lumen. Net ammonia production per hypertrophied proximal tubule has been shown to increase in response to nephron loss.[222] With a decreasing GFR, however, this increase becomes inadequate to compensate for further nephron loss, and absolute ammonia excretion falls.[190] In addition, disruption of the tubulomedullary ammonium concentration gradient because of structural injury may impair ammonia trapping and therefore reduce ammonium excretion.[190] Bicarbonate reabsorption by the nephron occurs predominantly in association with sodium reclamation in the proximal tubule and is dependent on the generation of a proton gradient in the distal nephron.

Conflicting data with respect to bicarbonate reabsorption in remnant kidneys may reflect species differences. In dogs with remnant kidneys, bicarbonate reabsorption was increased at both proximal and distal micropuncture sampling sites compared with intact controls.[231] In contrast, bicarbonate reabsorption per unit GFR is reduced in humans and rats with chronic renal failure,[206] and some patients with renal failure demonstrate bicarbonate wasting until the serum bicarbonate level drops below 20 mEq/L.[232] Bicarbonate reabsorption is also reduced in the setting of hyperkalemia, increased ECF volume, and hyperparathyroidism, all of which may be present in patients with chronic renal failure.[233–235] Distal urinary acidification tends to be relatively well preserved in patients with chronic renal failure, and urinary pH, although higher than in normal individuals with experimental acidosis, is usually around 5.[236] Urinary excretion of titratable acid is also generally well preserved in the setting of nephron loss as a consequence of increased fractional phosphate excretion.[187,190] As renal failure progresses, acid excretion becomes more dependent on the excretion of titratable acid. Renal acidification mechanisms are discussed more comprehensively in Chapters 9 and 16.

## CALCIUM AND PHOSPHATE

Derangements of calcium and phosphate metabolism occurring with renal insufficiency are the result of not only impaired urinary excretion of these solutes but also associated abnormalities in vitamin D metabolism and PTH secretion. With progressive renal dysfunction, 1α-hydroxylation of vitamin D by the kidney decreases, calcium absorption from the gut decreases, serum calcium level tends to decrease, serum phosphate level tends to increase, and PTH secretion increases. In response to increased PTH, calcium is mobilized from bone, renal phosphate excretion is enhanced, and the steady state becomes reestablished, with secondary hyperparathyroidism as the trade-off.[237] In chronic renal failure (CRF), the serum phosphate level does not increase until the GFR falls below 20 mL/min/1.73 m$^2$, and phosphate balance is maintained predominantly by an increase in fractional phosphate excretion.[238]

With moderate renal failure, therefore, filtered phosphate is not greatly increased, and the increase in phosphate excretion must be achieved by a reduction in phosphate reabsorption per nephron.[239] With more severe reductions in the GFR, however, phosphate excretion is maintained by an increase in serum phosphate levels as well as by reduced reabsorption per nephron. Sodium-dependent phosphate transport measured in proximal tubular brush border membrane vesicles prepared from the remnant kidneys of dogs was shown to be decreased when compared with that in vesicles derived from normal dogs.[187] Interestingly, however, this decrease was abolished if the partially nephrectomized dog had also undergone parathyroidectomy, indicating that PTH plays an important role in proximal tubular adaptation to phosphate excretion. Studies of isolated proximal tubules from euparathyroid uremic rabbits have shown a reduction in net phosphate flux per unit of reabsorptive surface area, and an increase in sensitivity to PTH.[189] The authors postulated that the number of PTH receptors per tubule must increase in the remnant kidney, concomitant with tubular hypertrophy. The levels of mRNA encoding the sodium-coupled phosphate transporter, NaPi-2, are reduced by approximately 50% in remnant kidneys from 5/6 nephrectomized rats.[240] In contrast, tubules from hyperparathyroid uremic rabbits demonstrated reduced PTH sensitivity, consistent with the downregulation or persistent occupancy of the PTH receptors.

On the other hand, studies in animals with reduced renal mass subjected to parathyroidectomy have shown that fractional excretion of phosphate remains inversely proportional to the reduction in the GFR,[241] indicating that phosphate excretion is not entirely dependent on the presence of PTH. Fibroblast growth factor 23 (FGF23) has been identified as a major mediator of increased phosphaturia after nephron loss.[242] First identified as the primary mediator of autosomal dominant hypophosphatemia, increased FGF23 expression has been shown in transgenic models to increase urinary phosphate excretion through the downregulation of NaPi-2a expression in proximal tubules.[243] Further experiments using gene deletion models have found that decreased expression of NaPi-2a and NaPi-2c by exogenous FGF23 is mediated predominantly by FGF receptor 1.[244] Activation of FGF receptors by FGF23 is critically dependent on binding with its coreceptor, Klotho.[242] After 5/6 nephrectomy in rats, investigators observed hyperphosphatemia after a high-phosphate diet, despite high levels of FGF23. This was explained by a marked reduction in levels of Klotho that was prevented by treatment with calcitriol. Further experiments in cultured cells have indicated that Klotho is suppressed by phosphaturia through Wnt/β-catenin signaling.[245] Circulating levels of FGF 23 become elevated early in the course of CKD, with levels rising once the GFR falls below 70 mL/min/1.73 m$^2$ in humans,[242] although this may depend to some extent on vitamin D status. In one study, FGF23 was elevated early in persons with CKD who were vitamin D–replete, but PTH was more frequently elevated than FGF23 in those with vitamin D insufficiency.[246] That FGF23 is important in mediating increased phosphaturia after nephron loss has been demonstrated by experiments in which the administration of neutralizing anti-FGF23 antibodies after renal mass reduction resulted in decreased fractional excretion of phosphate and increase in serum phosphate levels.[247] Whereas most of the reduction in phosphate reabsorption is achieved in the proximal tubule, there is also some evidence of increased fractional phosphate excretion by the distal tubule in uremic dogs and rats.[248]

As renal failure advances, renal 1α-hydroxylation of vitamin D decreases, and as a result, calcium absorption from the gut is reduced.[249] In addition to its effects on renal phosphate excretion, FGF23 inhibits renal 1α-hydroxylase activity, thereby reducing levels of 1,25-OH vitamin D.[243,247] In renal failure, fractional intestinal calcium absorption is inversely proportional to blood urea nitrogen levels.[249] Calcium excretion, on the other hand, varies widely in patients with renal disease, probably due to differences in diet, heterogeneity of vitamin D production, and predominance of glomerular versus tubulointerstitial injury.[250] In normal individuals, calcium excretion is mediated by the suppression of PTH-induced reabsorption in the distal nephron and by the suppression of PTH-independent mechanisms in the thick ascending limb. In patients with CRF, fractional calcium excretion remains unchanged until the GFR falls below 25 mL/min/1.73 m$^2$, when fractional excretion increases due to the obligatory solute diuresis.[206] Absolute calcium excretion, however, remains low. Hypocalciuria in patients with CRF has been shown to be due in part to the attendant hyperparathyroidism.[251] Similar findings were obtained in rats with reduced renal mass, in which parathyroidectomy resulted in increased calcium excretion compared with nonparathyroidectomized controls.[252] Renal calcium clearance is increased in patients with tubulointerstitial disease and in rats with surgical papillectomy, suggesting that regulation of calcium reabsorption depends on intact medullary structures and that regulation of calcium excretion may be largely modulated by the distal nephron segments.[206] The potential contributions of calcium and phosphate to renal disease progression are discussed below. Calcium and phosphate metabolism are also discussed in greater detail in Chapters 7 and 18.

## LONG-TERM ADVERSE CONSEQUENCES OF ADAPTATIONS TO NEPHRON LOSS

The functional and structural adaptations to nephron loss described previously may be regarded as a beneficial response that minimizes the resultant loss of the total GFR. It has been appreciated for several decades, however, that rats subjected to partial nephrectomy subsequently develop hypertension, albuminuria, and progressive renal failure. Detailed histopathologic studies in rat remnant kidneys after 5/6 nephrectomy have revealed mesangial accumulation of hyaline material that progressively encroaches on capillary lumina, obliterating Bowman's space and finally resulting in global sclerosis of the glomerulus. These findings, together with the observation that sclerosed glomeruli are a common finding in human CKD of diverse causes, have led to the hypothesis that glomerular hyperfiltration ultimately results in damage to the remaining glomeruli and contributes to a vicious cycle of progressive nephron loss. The 5/6 nephrectomy model has been extensively studied, and considerable progress has been made in elucidating how the physiologic adaptations of remaining nephrons, which initially permit greatly augmented function per nephron, ultimately produce a complex series of adverse effects that eventuate in progressive renal injury and an inexorable decline in function.[9]

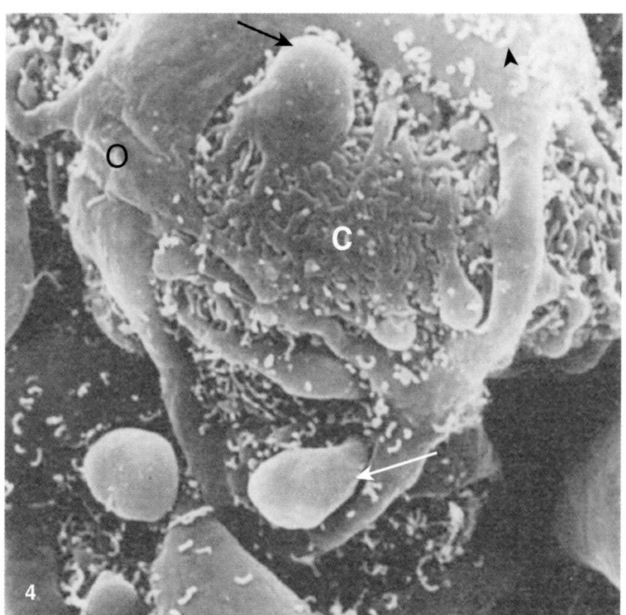


**Fig. 51.5** Scanning electron micrograph of a glomerulus from a rat following 5/6 nephrectomy; view from urinary space. Cytoplasmic blebs *(arrows)*, numerous microvilli *(arrowhead)*, focal obliteration (O), and coarsening (C) of foot processes are seen. (×3600.) (From Hostetter TH, Olson JL, Rennke HG, et al. Hyperfiltration in remnant nephrons: a potentially adverse response to renal ablation. *Am. J. Physiol.* 1981;241: F85–F93.)

## HEMODYNAMIC FACTORS

As early as 1 week after extensive renal mass ablation, glomerular hyperfiltration and glomerular capillary hypertension were found to be associated with morphologic changes in glomerular cells, including visceral epithelial cell cytoplasmic attenuation, protein reabsorption droplets and foot process fusion, mesangial expansion, and focal lifting of endothelial cells from the basement membrane (Figs. 51.5 and 51.6).[9] Evidence that these morphologic changes were a consequence of the glomerular hemodynamic alterations was provided by studies in rats fed a low-protein diet after 5/6 nephrectomy. This intervention prevented the hemodynamic changes, effectively normalizing $Q_A$, $P_{GC}$, and the SNGFR, and abrogated the structural lesions observed in rats on standard diet.[9] Similar findings were subsequently described in a variety of animal models of CKD, including diabetic nephropathy[253,254] and DOCA-salt hypertension.[255]

Together, these observations led Brenner and colleagues to propose that the hemodynamic adaptations following renal mass ablation ultimately prove injurious to glomeruli and initiate processes that result in glomerulosclerosis. The resulting obliteration of further glomeruli would induce hyperfiltration in remaining, less affected glomeruli, thereby establishing a vicious cycle of progressive nephron loss. These mechanisms constitute a common pathway for renal damage that could account for the inexorable progression of CKD, independent of the cause of the initial renal injury.[4] This hypothesis also explains the finding of both atrophic and hypertrophic nephrons typically encountered in chronically diseased kidneys. Further evidence supportive of the so-called hyperfiltration hypothesis was gleaned from the study of experimental diabetic nephropathy, in which glomerular hyperfiltration was also found to be a forerunner of glomerular pathology.[9,254] Maneuvers such as unilateral nephrectomy, which exacerbates hyperfiltration in the remaining kidney, were also found to exacerbate diabetic renal injury.[256] Furthermore, when the kidney was shielded from elevated perfusion pressure and from glomerular capillary hypertension by creating unilateral renal artery stenosis, the ipsilateral kidney was protected against the development of diabetic injury, which progressed unabated in the contralateral kidney.[257] In addition, when glomerular hyperfiltration was reversed in 5/6 nephrectomized rats by transplantation of an isogeneic kidney, hypertension and proteinuria were ameliorated, and glomerular injury was limited.[258]

Similarly, augmenting renal mass in the Fisher-Lewis rat transplant model normalized $P_{GC}$ and greatly reduced the development of chronic renal allograft injury.[259,260] Similarly, it is noteworthy that the phase of transition from an acute, nonhypertensive experimental injury, induced by puromycin aminonucleoside (PAN) administration, to a chronic nephropathy characterized by proteinuria and glomerulosclerosis, is also associated with the development of glomerular capillary hypertension.[261]

Direct evidence that similar mechanisms may operate in human kidneys has been derived from a study of 14 patients with solitary kidneys who had undergone varying degrees of partial nephrectomy of the remaining kidney for malignancy.[262] Before renal-sparing surgery, proteinuria was absent in all patients. Although serum creatinine levels remained stable after an initial rise of 50% in 12 patients, the 2 patients subjected to the most extensive nephrectomy (75% and 67%, respectively) developed progressive renal failure and required long-term dialysis. Moreover, among the remaining patients, 7 developed proteinuria, the levels of which were inversely related to the amount of renal tissue preserved. Renal biopsy

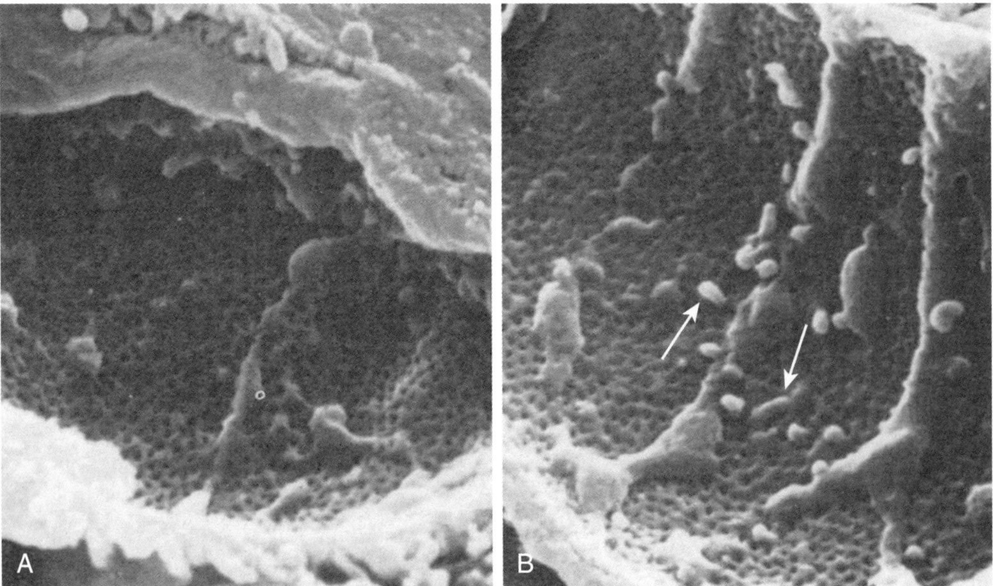


**Fig. 51.6** Scanning electron micrographs of glomerular capillaries. (A) Normal endothelial appearance. (B) Rats post–5/6 nephrectomy. Scattered endothelial blebs *(arrows)* are often present in this group. (×18,000.) (From Hostetter TH, Olson JL, Rennke HG, et al. Hyperfiltration in remnant nephrons: a potentially adverse response to renal ablation. *Am. J. Physiol.* 1981;241:F85–F93.)

specimens in 4 patients with moderate to severe proteinuria showed focal segmental glomerulosclerosis (FSGS),[262] which later morphometric analysis revealed involvement of virtually all glomeruli examined.[263] The importance of renal mass in humans was further illustrated by an observational study of 749 patients who underwent radical nephrectomy or nephron-sparing surgery for removal of a renal mass. Those who had nephron-sparing surgery had a significantly lower incidence of reduced the GFR (16.0% vs. 44.7%) and proteinuria (13.2% vs. 22.2%) compared with those who underwent radical nephrectomy.[264] Similarly, a large metaanalysis that included data from 31,729 people who had a radical nephrectomy and 9,281 people who had a partial nephrectomy for cancer found a 61% reduction in risk of developing CKD stages 3 to 5 after partial nephrectomy.[265]

Finally, whereas unilateral donor nephrectomy is associated with an excellent prognosis in most patients, two case-controlled studies have reported a small absolute increase in the long-term risk of end-stage kidney disease (ESKD).[266,267] One detailed study in 51 living donors has reported that hypertension in kidney donors 50 years of age and older was associated with a lower estimated number of functioning nephrons per kidney; it is therefore possible that donors with a low nephron number are at increased risk of subsequent kidney damage.[268]

The importance of glomerular hemodynamic factors in the development of progressive renal injury was further illustrated by studies that reported dramatic protective effects against the development of glomerulosclerosis after chronic inhibition of the RAAS with ACE inhibitor or ARB treatment in 5/6 nephrectomized rats.[19–22] Micropuncture studies have shown that like the low-protein diet, the renoprotective effects of RAAS inhibition are associated with near-normalization of the $P_{GC}$, yet, in contrast with the effects of dietary protein restriction, the SNGFR remained elevated.[269] This suggested that glomerular capillary hypertension, rather than hyperfiltration per se, was the key factor in the initiation and progression of glomerular injury.

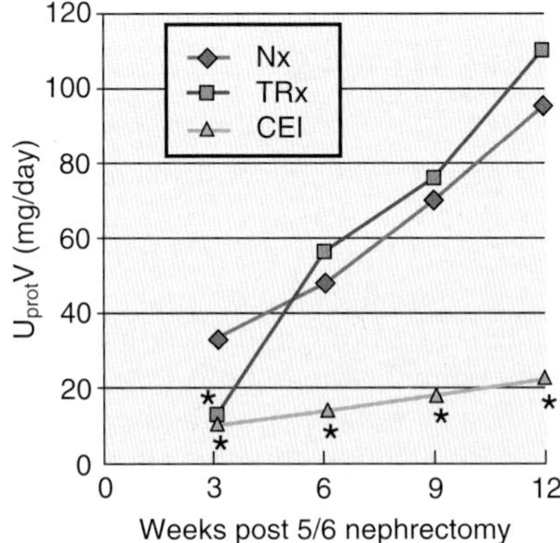


**Fig. 51.7** Proteinuria levels following 5/6 nephrectomy in untreated rats *(Nx)* versus treatment with triple therapy (reserpine, hydralazine, and hydrochlorothiazide *[TRx]*), Nx + TRx, or enalapril (NX + CEI). Despite equivalent levels of blood pressure control, enalapril therapy almost completely prevented proteinuria and glomerulosclerosis, whereas triple therapy afforded no renoprotection. $U_{prot}V$, 24-hour urine protein excretion; *$P < .05$ vs. Nx at the same time point. (From Anderson S, Rennke HG, Brenner BM. Therapeutic advantage of converting enzyme inhibitors in arresting progressive renal disease associated with systemic hypertension in the rat. *J Clin Invest.* 1986;77:1993–2000.)

Confirmation of this view has come from an experiment in which rats were treated with a combination of reserpine, hydralazine, and hydrochlorothiazide (triple therapy) to lower arterial pressure to levels similar to those obtained with an ACE inhibitor. In contrast to the glomerular hemodynamic effects of the ACE inhibitor, triple therapy did not alleviate glomerular hypertension or proteinuria, and glomerular injury progressed[20,21] (Fig. 51.7). Interestingly, within the context of pharmacologic inhibition of the RAAS, the level to which systemic BP is reduced remains a critical determinant of the extent of the renal protection conferred.[270] The effectiveness of both ACE inhibitor and ARB in lowering glomerular pressure and ameliorating glomerular injury has since been observed in several other animal models of chronic kidney disease, including diabetic nephropathy,[253,271,272] hypertensive kidney disease,[273,274] experimental chronic renal allograft failure (a model that lacks systemic hypertension but exhibits glomerular capillary hypertension),[275–277] age-related glomerulosclerosis,[278,279] and obesity-related glomerulosclerosis.[280]

That similar mechanisms are relevant in human CKD progression has been strongly suggested by the results of clinical trials showing substantial renoprotective effects with ACE inhibitor and ARB treatment.[281–285] The importance of glomerular capillary hypertension has been further illustrated by studies of the effects of omapatrilat, a vasopeptidase inhibitor. Micropuncture studies after 5/6 nephrectomy have shown an even greater lowering of $P_{GC}$ with omapatrilat than with ACE inhibitor treatment, despite equivalent effects on systemic BP. In subsequent chronic studies, omapatrilat produced more effective renoprotection than the ACE inhibitor.[90] Thus among the determinants of glomerular hyperfiltration, glomerular capillary hypertension has been identified as a critical factor in the initiation and progression of glomerular injury.

The development a new class of drug for the treatment of diabetes, the sodium glucose cotransporter 2 (SGLT2) inhibitors, has provided further evidence to support the importance of glomerular hemodynamic factors in CKD progression in the context of diabetes. These drugs act by inhibiting the reabsorption of filtered glucose and sodium in the proximal tubule, resulting in glycosuria that reduces hyperglycemia, and modest natriuresis. Importantly, it has been proposed that increased delivery of sodium chloride to the macula densa results in increased tubuloglomerular feedback, which reduces glomerular hyperfiltration by provoking the constriction of afferent arterioles.[286–288] In rats with streptozotocin-induced diabetes, treatment with an SGLT2 inhibitor resulted in a marked reduction in SNGFR that was inversely proportional to the distal tubular chloride concentration, indicating activation of tubuloglomerular feedback.[289] Similarly, in persons with type 1 diabetes, treatment with an SGLT2 inhibitor reduced glomerular hyperfiltration to normal levels in conjunction with a decrease in effective renal plasma flow and an increase in renal vascular resistance, observations consistent with preglomerular (afferent arteriole) vasoconstriction.[290]

Thus treatment with SGLT2 inhibitors ameliorates glomerular hyperfiltration and (by implication) glomerular hypertension in persons with diabetes. In large clinical trials in those with type 2 diabetes and the GFR greater than 30 mL/min/1.73 m$^2$, treatment with an SGLT2 inhibitor was associated with multiple renoprotective benefits, including reduced progression to macroalbuminuria, reduced doubling of serum creatinine levels, and a lower incidence of ESKD and death from renal causes,[291,292] confirming the importance of glomerular hyperfiltration (and glomerular hypertension) in CKD progression. Nevertheless, numerous other potential renoprotective effects of SGLT2 inhibitors have been identified, including lowering of systemic BP, reduction of albuminuria, weight loss, amelioration of arterial stiffness, reduction of renal oxygen demand, and induction of hypoxia-inducible factor 1 (HIF1).[286–288]

To investigate the potential benefit of SGLT2 inhibitors in persons with diabetes and CKD further, the CREDENCE trial enrolled 4,401 adults with type 2 diabetes, estimated GFR (eGFR) of 30 to 89 mL/min/1.73 m$^2$, and urine albumin-to-creatinine ratio (ACR) of 300 to 5000 mg/g, despite treatment with the maximum dose of an ACE inhibitor or ARB. In July 2018, the sponsors announced that the trial had been stopped early following an interim analysis that found benefit in the canagliflozin treatment arm with respect to the composite primary outcome of ESKD, doubling of serum creatinine levels, and cardiovascular or renal death,[293] although the results had not yet been published at the time of this writing. Further trials are now underway to evaluate the renoprotective potential of SGLT2 inhibitors across a broader spectrum of CKD, including nondiabetic CKD. Interestingly, however, treatment with an SGLT2 inhibitor (without the addition of an ACE inhibitor or ARB) did not afford renoprotection in rats after 5/6 nephrectomy.[294] The SGLT2 inhibitors are reviewed in more detail in relation to the treatment of diabetic kidney disease in Chapter 39.

## MECHANISMS OF HEMODYNAMICALLY INDUCED INJURY

### MECHANICAL STRESS

Several mechanisms have been proposed whereby glomerular hypertension and hyperperfusion may result in glomerular cell injury. Experiments in isolated perfused rat glomeruli have reported significant increases in glomerular volume, with increases in perfusion pressure over the normal and relevant abnormal range.[136] These increases in wall tension and glomerular volume likely result in stretching of glomerular cells. Experimental evidence has suggested that such stretching may have adverse consequences for all three major cell types in the glomerulus. Furthermore, advances in the study of cellular responses to mechanical stress raised the possibility that glomerular hyperperfusion may also promote the development of glomerulosclerosis through more subtle and complex pathways that induce profibrotic phenotypic alterations in glomerular cells.[295]

### ENDOTHELIAL CELLS

The vascular endothelium serves a number of complex functions, including acting as a dynamic barrier to leukocytes and plasma proteins, secretion of vasoactive factors (prostacyclin, NO, and endothelin), conversion of Ang I to Ang II, and expression of cell adhesion molecules. It is also the first cellular structure in the kidney that encounters the mechanical forces imparted by glomerular hyperperfusion. After 5/6 nephrectomy, endothelial cells are activated or injured, resulting in detachment and exposure of the basement membrane (Fig. 51.6). This in turn may induce platelet aggregation, deposition of fibrin, and intracapillary microthrombus formation.[9,296] It has been recognized for some time that segmental glomerulosclerosis is associated with focal obliteration of capillary loops[297] and that interstitial fibrosis is associated with a loss of peritubular capillaries.[298] Furthermore, it has been shown that this loss of capillaries in the remnant kidney is associated with a decrease in endothelial cell proliferation and reduced constitutive expression of VEGF by podocytes and renal tubule cells, as well as increased expression of the antiangiogenic factor, thrombospondin-1, by the renal interstitium.[299]

Because VEGF is an important endothelial cell angiogenic, survival, and trophic factor, these findings suggest that capillary loss may be caused in part by failure of recovery from hemodynamically mediated endothelial cell injury. Indeed inhibition of endothelial and mesangial cell proliferation by treatment with everolimus after 5/6 nephrectomy resulted in increased proteinuria, glomerulosclerosis, and interstitial fibrosis associated with reduced glomerular expression of VEGF.[300] Furthermore, short-term treatment of rats with VEGF ameliorated both glomerular and peritubular capillary loss after 5/6 nephrectomy.[301] This preservation of capillaries was associated with a trend toward less glomerulosclerosis and significantly less interstitial deposition of type III collagen, as well as better preservation of renal function. Further evidence of the importance of endothelial cells in the preservation of function after nephron loss has been provided by experiments in which bone marrow–derived endothelial progenitor cells (EPCs) were administered to mice after 5/6 nephrectomy. EPC-treated mice showed better preservation of renal function, less proteinuria, and relatively preserved renal structure, as well as decreased expression of proinflammatory molecules and restored levels of the angiogenic molecules VEGF, VEGF receptor-2, and thrombospondin 1.[302] Long-term studies are required to evaluate further the potential benefits of improving renal angiogenesis in the setting of progressive renal injury.

Endothelial cells bear numerous receptors that allow them to detect and respond to changes in mechanical forces. Thus exposure of endothelial cells to changes in shear stress, cyclic stretch, or pulsatile barostress that result from glomerular hyperperfusion may induce changes in the expression of genes involved in inflammation, cell cycle control, apoptosis, thrombosis, and oxidative stress.[303] The in vitro responses of endothelial cells to mechanical forces have largely been studied in the context of vascular remodeling and atherosclerosis, but it can readily be appreciated that similar responses may affect the development of inflammation and fibrosis in the remnant kidney. Of particular interest are observations that shear stress can stimulate endothelial expression of adhesion molecules[304] and proinflammatory cytokines.[305] It is clear therefore why biomechanical activation has emerged as an important paradigm in endothelial cell biology,[306] but further studies focusing on glomerular endothelial responses to mechanical stress are required to elucidate the role of these mechanisms in progressive renal injury.

## MESANGIAL CELLS

Mesangial cells are closely associated with the capillaries in the glomerulus and are therefore also exposed to mechanical forces. Evidence from in vitro studies has indicated that mesangial cells respond to changes in these mechanical forces in ways that may promote inflammation and fibrosis. Subjecting mesangial cells to cyclical stretch or strain has been shown to induce the proliferation[307] and synthesis of extracellular matrix constituents.[308,309] Cyclic stretch also activates the transcription factor nuclear factor-kappa B (NF-κB),[310] stimulates protein (monocyte chemoattractant protein 1 [MCP-1]),[311] and TGF-β[312] and its receptor,[313] as well as connective tissue growth factor (CTGF).[314] Cyclic stretch also activates the RAAS in cultured mesangial cells,[315] and Ang II in turn may induce TGF-β synthesis.[316] In vitro studies have identified several signaling pathways responsible for stretch-induced signal transduction in mesangial cells.

Cyclic stretch activates the serine-threonine kinase Akt through a mechanism requiring phosphatidylinositol-3-kinase and transactivation of EGF receptor and is necessary for the increased synthesis of collagen type 1A1 observed in the mesangial cells. Furthermore Akt activation was observed in remnant kidney glomeruli, indicating that these mechanisms are also present in vivo.[317] The actin cytoskeleton is an important transmitter of mechanical signals, and the GTPase, RhoA, a central regulator of the cytoskeleton, is activated by cyclic stretch. Stretch-induced activation of the mitogen-activated protein kinase Erk, linked to increased matrix production, is dependent on the activation of RhoA.[318] Mesangial cells cultured at ambient pressures of 50 to 60 mm Hg (i.e., levels corresponding to glomerular capillary hypertension) also show enhanced synthesis and secretion of extracellular matrix when compared with cells grown at "normal" pressures of 40 to 50 mm Hg.[319] Exposure of mesangial cells to barostress, achieved by culture under increased barometric pressure, stimulates the expression of cytokines, including platelet-derived growth factor (PDGF)-B[320] and MCP-1.[321] Transduction of mechanical forces by mesangial cells has been associated with tyrosine phosphorylation[322] and protein kinase C–induced increases in S-6 kinase activity.[323]

## PODOCYTES

A growing body of evidence attests to the importance of podocyte injury in a variety of renal diseases and in CKD progression.[324] Podocytes display morphologic evidence of injury as early as 1 week after 5/6 nephrectomy (see Fig. 51.5)[9] and 6 months after uninephrectomy.[325] Increased numbers of podocytes have been observed in the urine from rats after 5/6 nephrectomy and in human CKD.[324] In 5/6 nephrectomized rats, the number of podocytes correlated with the severity of proteinuria, as well as mean arterial BP, suggesting that podocyte loss may contribute to CKD progression.[326] The importance of podocyte injury in CKD progression is further supported by the observation that amelioration of glomerular damage in 5/6 nephrectomized rats treated with 1,25-dihydroxyvitamin D3 is associated with preservation of podocyte number, as well as prevention of podocyte hypertrophy and injury.[327] Detailed in vitro studies have shown that early podocyte injury is associated with dysregulation of calcium homeostasis and disruption of the actomyosin contractile apparatus. The Rho family of small guanosine triphosphatases plays a key role in this process. Calcium influx via transient receptor potential canonical type 5 (TRPC5) channels results in the activation of Rac1 and is associated with increased podocyte migration and proteinuria, whereas calcium influx via TRCP type 6 activates RhoA, resulting in the preservation of stress fibres, prevention of podocyte migration, and maintenance of the filtration barrier.[328] However, subsequent experiments in TRCP6-deficient podocytes have found that TRCP6 is not required for mechanotransduction.[329] Rather, mechanical stretch was found to induce ATP release from podocytes by a process dependent on cholesterol and podocin. ATP release in turn activated the purinergic channel $P2X_4$, resulting in an influx of calcium and increased disorganization of the actin cytoskeleton.[329]

Thus purinergic channels appear to be key mechanotransducers in podocytes. Because podocytes are attached to the outer aspect of the glomerular basement membrane, it is reasonable to expect that they would be exposed to increased mechanical forces resulting from glomerular hypertension. Confirmation that podocytes respond to such physical forces has been derived from several in vitro experiments that examined podocyte responses to stretching. Activation of a voltage-sensitive potassium channels was observed in response to stretching of the podocyte cell membrane,[330] and culture of podocytes under constant stretch induced activation of the protein kinases Erk1/2 and JNK via the EGF receptor, as well as other changes in cell signaling.[331] Mechanical stretch inhibited podocyte proliferation[332] and, in common with TGF-β, reduced $\alpha_3\beta_1$-integrin expression and podocyte adhesion in vitro.[333] Exposure to cyclic stretching that mimics pulsatile strain within the glomerulus has been shown to cause reorganization of the actin cytoskeleton,[334] upregulation of COX-2, and E prostanoid (EP)-4 receptor expression,[335] as well as podocyte hypertrophy.[336] Subsequent experiments using mice with podocyte-specific depletion or overexpression of EP4 receptors have found that prostaglandin E2 acting via EP4 receptors contributes to the development of proteinuria after 5/6 nephrectomy and therefore probably contributes to podocyte injury.[337]

In another experiment, cyclic stretching of podocytes was associated with increased production of Ang II and TGF-β, as well as upregulation of angiotensin subtype 1 (AT1) receptors, resulting in increased Ang II–dependent apoptosis.[338] Cyclic stretch of podocytes also resulted in a 50% reduction of nephrin (a key component of the slit diaphragm) mRNA and protein levels via an Ang II–dependent mechanism that was inhibited by the peroxisome proliferator-activated receptor-gamma (PPAR-γ) agonist, rosiglitazone, which prevented AT1 receptor upregulation.[339] Taken together, these data suggest that stretch-induced podocyte injury is a further mechanism whereby glomerular hypertension contributes to glomerular injury.

## CELLULAR INFILTRATION IN REMNANT KIDNEYS

Despite the lack of an obvious immune stimulus, an inflammatory cell infiltrate composed predominantly of macrophages and smaller numbers of lymphocytes is observed in remnant kidneys after 5/6 nephrectomy.[340] Interestingly, similar observations have been reported in a rat model of spontaneous renal agenesis associated with a 60.2% reduction in nephron endowment.[341] As discussed earlier, it is possible that the glomerular hemodynamic adaptations to nephron loss may provoke an inflammatory cell response through the effects of mechanical forces on endothelial and mesangial cells. Thus upregulation of renal endothelial adhesion molecules may facilitate the egress of leukocytes from the circulation into the mesangium, where they may participate in further renal injury. The recruited cellular infiltrate may constitute an abundant source of potent pleiotropic cytokine products, which in turn influence other infiltrating leukocytes, dendritic cells, and kidney cells, stimulating cell proliferation, elaboration of extracellular matrix components, and increased endothelial adhesiveness.[342]

Evidence is emerging that these proposed mechanisms, based largely on in vitro observations, are indeed relevant in vivo. In the two-kidney, one-clip model of renovascular hypertension, upregulated expression of adhesion molecules and TGF-β, as well as cell infiltration, is observed only in the nonclipped kidney that is exposed to the hypertensive perfusion pressure.[343,344] In the 5/6 nephrectomy model, coordinated upregulation of a variety of cell adhesion molecules, cytokines, and growth factors in association with macrophage infiltration has been observed at time points that precede the development of severe glomerulosclerosis.[345,346] Furthermore, the renoprotection afforded by an ACE inhibitor or ARB treatment in this model was associated with inhibition of cytokine upregulation and prevention of renal infiltration by macrophages.[346,347]

Infiltrating macrophages, although present in the glomeruli of remnant kidney, are chiefly distributed in the tubulointerstitial regions,[340,346] suggesting that they play a role in the development of the TIF that accompanies glomerulosclerosis. Further analysis of the cellular infiltrate has also identified mast cells in close proximity to areas of TIF.[348] It is possible that interstitial infiltrates are recruited as the result of tubulointerstitial cell activation by the downstream effects of cytokines released in the glomeruli. Alternatively, it has been proposed that excessive uptake of filtered proteins by tubule epithelial cells stimulates expression of cell adhesion and chemoattractant molecules that recruit macrophages and other monocytic cells to tubulointerstitial areas[349] (see later for further discussion). The chemokine receptor CCR-1 has been shown to be important in interstitial but not glomerular recruitment of leukocytes. Treatment with a nonpeptide CCR-1 antagonist has been shown to reduce interstitial macrophage infiltration and ameliorate interstitial fibrosis in the unilateral ureteric obstruction (UUO) model, but data are still lacking in the 5/6 nephrectomy model.[350] Furthermore, antagonism of MCP-1 signaling through gene therapy—induced production of a mutant form of MCP-1 by skeletal muscle resulted in reduced interstitial macrophage infiltration and amelioration of interstitial fibrosis in mice after UUO.[351]

The identification of renal tubule cells expressing alpha smooth muscle actin after 5/6 nephrectomy has raised the possibility that tubule cells may undergo transdifferentiation to a myofibroblast phenotype that contributes to interstitial fibrosis.[352] Furthermore the renoprotection observed with mycophenolate treatment in 5/6 nephrectomized rats is associated with reductions in interstitial myofibroblast infiltration and collagen type III deposition.[353] There is, however, ongoing debate regarding the origin of interstitial myofibroblasts in CKD. Fate-mapping studies have indicated that mesenchymal cells called *pericytes* are the predominant source of myofibroblasts, and that epithelial to mesenchymal transdifferentiation is not a source of myofibroblasts or accounts for only a small minority.[354] Other cells that may give rise to interstitial myofibroblasts include resident fibroblasts, endothelial cells, and bone marrow–derived cells.[355,356]

Several lines of evidence have suggested that this cellular infiltrate contributes to renal injury and is not merely a consequence of it.[357] In one study, multiple linear regression analysis identified glomerular macrophage infiltration in the remnant kidney as a major determinant of mesangial matrix expansion and adhesion formation between Bowman's capsule and glomerular tufts.[340] Furthermore, depletion of leukocytes by irradiation in rats delayed the onset of glomerular injury after renal ablative surgery.[358] Several studies have reported amelioration of the cellular infiltrate and renal injury in the 5/6 nephrectomy model following treatment with the immunosuppressive agent mycofenolate mofetil.[359–362] One study has found that mycophenolate also lowers $P_{GC}$, which may account for some of its renoprotective effects.[363] Several other antiinflammatory interventions have been shown to ameliorate renal injury after 5/6 nephrectomy. Treatment with the antiinflammatory agent nitroflurbiprofen, also a NO donor, was associated with moderate renoprotection.[364] Rats treated with a PPAR-γ receptor agonist evidenced significant attenuation of the proteinuria and glomerulosclerosis observed in untreated rats, despite the failure of treatment to lower BP.[365] This renoprotection was observed in association with marked reductions in glomerular cell proliferation, glomerular macrophage infiltration, and renal expression of plasminogen activator inhibitor-1 (PAI-1), as well as TGF-β. The authors speculated that some of these effects may have resulted from the known actions of PPAR-γ receptor activation to antagonize the activities of the transcription factors activator protein-1 (AP-1) and NF-κB.

Administration of a sphingosine-1-phosphate (S1P) receptor agonist, a novel immunosuppressant that inhibits the egress of T cells and B cells from lymph nodes, attenuated the increase in chemokine receptor expression observed in untreated rats and tended to normalize regulated on activation, normal T cell–expressed and secreted (RANTES) and MCP-1 gene expression.[366] Glomerular and interstitial inflammation, as well as fibrosis, were also reduced. Overexpression of the antiinflammatory cytokine interleukin-10 (IL-10) in rats was associated with reduced interstitial inflammation and lower levels of MCP-1, RANTES, interferon-γ (IFN-γ), and IL-2 expression, as well as attenuation of proteinuria, glomerulosclerosis, and TIF.[367] Finally, overexpression of the gene for angiostatin, an antiangiogenic factor that also inhibits leukocyte recruitment as well as neutrophil and macrophage migration, was associated with the inhibition of macrophage and T cell infiltrates in glomeruli, as well as the interstitium, reduced MCP-1 expression, and attenuation of glomerulosclerosis and interstitial fibrosis.[368] Taken together, these findings strongly support the hypothesis that in addition to direct glomerular cell injury, glomerular hemodynamic adaptations to nephron loss provoke a complex series of proinflammatory and profibrotic responses that further contribute to renal damage. Treatments that antagonize the mediators of these responses may therefore be of benefit in slowing the rate of CKD progression.

## NONHEMODYNAMIC FACTORS IN THE DEVELOPMENT OF NEPHRON INJURY FOLLOWING EXTENSIVE RENAL MASS ABLATION

The weight of evidence in support of the hypothesis that glomerular hemodynamic adaptations are central to progressive renal injury does not exclude the possibility that the kidney may also be affected by a variety of factors not directly attributable to hemodynamic changes. These nonhemodynamic factors have been extensively studied in recent years and may offer new therapeutic targets for future renoprotective interventions.

### PROTEINURIA

***Clinical Relevance***

**Proteinuria**

Reduction of proteinuria should be regarded as a key therapeutic goal. Specifically, the dose of RAAS inhibitor treatment should be titrated up until proteinuria has been minimized or the maximum dose has been reached. If required, additional antihypertensive drugs should be added to RAAS inhibitor treatment to achieve blood pressure targets and minimize proteinuria.

Abnormal excretion of protein in the urine is the hallmark of experimental and clinical glomerular disease. Whereas immune complex deposition and resulting inflammation account for abnormal permeability of the glomerular filtration barrier to proteins in glomerulonephritis, studies in rats subjected to extensive renal ablation have shown loss of glomerular barrier function to proteins of similar molecular size, yet in the apparent absence of primary immune-mediated renal injury or inflammatory response. Sieving studies using dextrans and other macromolecules in rats 7 or 14 days after 5/6 nephrectomy have revealed the loss of both size and charge selectivity of the glomerular filtration barrier. Ultrastructural examination of the remnant kidneys has revealed detachment of glomerular endothelial cells and visceral epithelial cells from the glomerular basement membrane. In addition, protein reabsorption droplets and attenuation of cytoplasm resulting in bleb formation was observed in podocytes. The authors concluded that the altered permselectivity may be caused in part by the separation of endothelial cells from the glomerular basement membrane, allowing access of macromolecules and, in part, to loss of anionic sites in the lamina rara externa, resulting in loss of charge selectivity and detachment of podocytes.[369]

Studies have identified decreased nephrin expression in podocytes as a further mechanism contributing to proteinuria after 5/6 nephrectomy,[370] and in vitro studies have reported a 50% reduction in nephrin expression when podocytes were exposed to cyclic stretching.[339] A direct role for Ang II in modulating glomerular capillary permselectivity has been suggested by the observation of marked increases in urinary protein excretion during infusion of Ang II in normal rats. Although some investigators have attributed this to a direct effect of Ang II on the cellular components of the glomerular filtration barrier, resulting in the opening of interendothelial junctions and epithelial cell disruption, others have shown that the increase in proteinuria may be accounted for almost completely by the associated hemodynamic changes, principally a reduction in $Q_A$ and an increase in filtration fraction.[371] On the other hand, the notion that Ang II may mediate changes in glomerular permselectivity, independent of its effects on glomerular hemodynamics, has been supported by studies in an isolated perfused rat kidney preparation in which infusion of Ang II augmented urinary protein excretion and enhanced the clearance of tracer macromolecules, independently of any change in filtration fraction.[372] Furthermore, Ang II and aldosterone have been shown to reduce nephrin expression in podocytes and may therefore directly affect glomerular permselectivity.[339,373,374]

Proteinuria, long considered simply a marker of glomerular injury, has also been implicated as an effector of injury processes involved in renal disease progression, especially those resulting in tubulointerstitial fibrosis.[375] In rats with aminonucleoside-induced nephrotic syndrome, the proteinuric phase of the disease was associated with an acute interstitial nephritis, the intensity of which correlated closely with the severity of the proteinuria.[349] Furthermore, in an overload proteinuria model induced by daily intraperitoneal administration of bovine serum albumin to uninephrectomized rats, proximal tubule cell injury and interstitial infiltration of macrophages and lymphocytes were evident after 1 week.[376] The severity of the proteinuria showed a positive correlation with the intensity of the infiltrate. At 4 weeks, focal areas of chronic interstitial inflammation were noted.[376] Other experiments have identified mast cells as a component of the inflammatory infiltrate observed after protein overload. The number of mast cells correlated with the severity of interstitial inflammation, as well as with levels of stem cell factor (SCF) and TGF-β.[377] A causative association between excessive proteinuria and interstitial inflammation has been suggested by in vitro studies of proximal tubule epithelial cells cultured in media supplemented with high concentrations of albumin, immunoglobulin G (IgG), or transferrin. Cellular uptake of these proteins by endocytosis was observed to increase secretion of ET-1,[378] MCP-1,[379] RANTES,[380] IL-8,[381] and fractaline.[382] Electrophoretic mobility shift assay of cell nucleus extracts has revealed intense activation of the transcription factor NF-κB that was dependent on the concentration of protein in the medium.[380] Furthermore, the liberation of these molecules was noted to be predominantly from the basolateral aspect of the cells. This would be in keeping with secretion into the renal interstitium in vivo, thereby contributing to the development of tubulointerstitial inflammation and fibrosis.

On the other hand, secretion of TGF-β by tubule cells in response to albumin was not inhibited by inhibitors of endocytosis, implying that a different mechanism must be responsible.[383] Exposure of tubule cells to albumin has also been shown to result in increased levels of intracellular reactive oxygen species and activation of the signal transducer and activator of transcription (STAT) signaling pathway.[384] The STAT pathway, in turn, mediates a variety of cellular responses, including proliferation and induction of cytokines, as well as growth factors. Preliminary evidence has suggested that exposure of tubule cells to albumin may also induce apoptosis.[385]

Other experiments have found apoptosis in tubule cells exposed to high-molecular-weight plasma proteins but not smaller proteins.[386] Albumin and transferrin exposure also induced complement activation in tubule cells and reduced binding of factor H, a natural inhibitor of the alternative complement pathway.[387] The involvement of immune cells in the processing of absorbed proteins has been shown in studies in which tubule cells were found to cleave albumin into an N-terminal, 24–amino acid peptide that was further processed by dendritic cells (DCs) into antigenic peptides, with binding sites for major histocompatibility complex (MCH) class I molecules that were capable of activating CD8+ T cells.[388] After 5/6 nephrectomy, DCs were found in the interstitium, peaking at 1 week and decreasing at 4 weeks, coinciding with their appearance in renal lymph nodes. DCs from the lymph nodes were able to activate CD8+ T cells in culture.

Despite the previous evidence, other investigators have raised concerns regarding the interpretation of these observations.[389] They pointed out that the concentrations of plasma proteins used in vitro were nonphysiologic and far exceeded those observed in proximal tubule fluid from experimental models of nephrotic syndrome. Furthermore, many of the experiments were performed in cells that were routinely cultured in the presence of high concentrations of protein (serum) that could significantly alter their phenotype. Not all investigators have been able to confirm these observations, however. In particular, some have found proliferative or profibrotic responses when proximal tubule cells are exposed to serum or serum fractions, but no response after exposure to purified forms of albumin or transferrin, suggesting that factors other than albumin or transferrin may be involved.[390,391] Furthermore experiments in mice with tubules deficient in megalin, the key molecule responsible for the endocytosis of filtered proteins by tubule cells, have found that tubulointerstitial inflammation is not inhibited in the absence of megalin, implying that it is not dependent on endocytosis.[392] It was proposed instead that tubulointerstitial inflammation is provoked by misdirection of protein-rich glomerular filtrate into the interstitium due to the formation of adhesions between the glomerular tuft and Bowman's capsule or, in the case of crescentic glomerulonephritis, encroachment of the crescent onto the proximal tubule, resulting in occlusion and tubule degeneration.[393] Moreover, it was proposed that the increase in cytokine and adhesion molecule production observed in tubule cells that have endocytosed excess protein may actually be a protective response.[392]

Several lines of evidence have suggested that filtered molecules other than albumin or immunoglobulin may play a role in the progression of chronic nephropathies. It has been proposed that free fatty acids (FFAs) bound to albumin may play an important role in provoking a proinflammatory response in tubule cells. In one experiment, albumin-bound fatty acids stimulated macrophage chemotactic activity, whereas delipidated albumin did not.[394] Albumin-bound FFAs have also been shown to activate PPAR-γ and induce apoptosis in proximal tubule cells.[395] High-density lipoprotein (HDL) and low-density lipoprotein (LDL) have been identified in the urine, renal interstitium, and tubule cells in renal biopsies of patients with nephrotic syndrome. In vitro, cultured human proximal TECs take up LDL and HDL.[396]

Oxidized LDL may cause tubular cell injury, and exposure of TECs to HDL is associated with increased synthesis of ET-1.[396,397] A role has also been proposed for other compounds bound to filtered proteins, such as IGF-1, which has been detected in increased amounts in the proximal tubular fluid of rats with adriamycin nephrosis.[398] Proximal TECs cultured in the presence of proximal tubular fluid from nephrotic rats exhibit enhanced cell proliferation and increased secretion of types I and IV collagen. Both effects were inhibited by neutralizing IGF-1 receptor antibodies. Other growth factors in plasma, including HGF and TFG-β, may also appear in glomerular ultrafiltrates with proteinuria and exert effects on tubule cells.[399] Furthermore, cytokines produced in injured glomeruli may have downstream proinflammatory effects. Whereas complement components are normally absent from tubular fluid, C3 and C5b-9 neoantigen were observed along the luminal border of TECs in the protein overload proteinuria model.

To examine the role of filtered complement in renal injury, rats with puromycin aminonucleoside nephrosis were subjected to complement depletion with cobra venom factor or inhibition of complement activation by the administration of soluble recombinant human complement receptor type 1, before the onset of proteinuria.[400] In control rats, proximal tubular degeneration, interstitial leukocyte infiltrate, and renal impairment (as assessed by inulin and *para*-aminohippurate [PAH] clearances) occurred at 7 days, together with positive staining for C3 and C5b-9 along the proximal tubule brush border. Both interventions were associated with significantly less tubulointerstitial pathology and greater clearance of PAH but not inulin; the severity of the proteinuria was unaffected, suggesting that filtered complement plays a significant role in the tubulointerstitial injury associated with proteinuria. A more selective approach, using recombinant complement inhibitory molecules targeted to proximal tubule cells with carrier antibodies to brush border antigen, resulted in a significant reduction of interstitial fibrosis in the same model.[401] Similarly, mice with C3 deficiency were protected against interstitial inflammation after protein overload, and wild-type kidneys transplanted into C3-deficient mice were protected, whereas kidneys from C3-deficient mice were not protected when transplanted into wild-type mice. This implies that filtered rather than locally synthesized C3 is important in the pathogenesis of interstitial inflammation associated with proteinuria.[402]

In experimental models of proteinuric renal disease, filtered proteins have also been found to accumulate in the glomerular mesangium[369] and may therefore contribute to glomerular a tubulointerstitial injury. Further support for this notion has been obtained from a metaanalysis of 57 studies of experimental CKD, which found a consistent positive correlation between the severity of proteinuria and the extent of glomerulosclerosis.[403] Lipoproteins, in particular, accumulate in the glomeruli of patients with glomerulonephritis.[404,405] Furthermore, LDL stimulates mesangial cells to proliferate in vitro[406,407] and enhances mesangial cell synthesis of the extracellular matrix protein fibronectin.[408] LDL exposure is also associated with increased mesangial cell mRNA levels for MCP-1[408] and PDGF.[407] Oxidation of LDL by mesangial cells or macrophages may enhance its toxicity.[406] Thus accumulation of proteins in the mesangium may stimulate a number of different mechanisms that contribute to glomerulosclerosis.

The relevance of these findings to the processes occurring in vivo has been borne out by studies in rats. In the protein overload model, the development of proteinuria at 1 week was associated with significant increases in TGF-β at both protein and mRNA levels in interstitial and proximal tubule cells.[376] Similarly, renal cortical mRNA levels encoding the macrophage chemoattractant, osteopontin, were increased on day 4, and immunofluorescence localized increased osteopontin staining to cortical tubules at day 7. MCP-1 and osteopontin mRNA and protein levels were elevated at 2 and 3 weeks.

Furthermore, a significant effect of proteinuria on molecules involved in extracellular matrix (ECM) protein turnover was observed. Although mRNA levels for various renal matrix proteins were variable, staining for the proteins in the cortical interstitium increased progressively. Levels of mRNA for the protease inhibitors PAI-1 and tissue inhibitor of metalloproteinases-1 (TIMP-1) were elevated at 2 weeks, at which time significant renal fibrosis was present.[376] Gene expression profiling has identified over 100 genes that are upregulated in the proximal tubule cells of mice exposed to overload proteinuria.[409] Consistent with the hypothesis that protein-bound FFAs are important, rats receiving FFA-replete bovine serum albumin (BSA) developed more severe tubulointerstitial injury and more extensive macrophage infiltration than those receiving FFA-depleted BSA.[410,411]

In other models of proteinuric renal disease, including 5/6 nephrectomy and passive Heymann nephritis, accumulation of albumin and IgG by proximal tubule cells occurred before infiltration of the interstitium by macrophages and MHC-II positive mononuclear cells.[412] The infiltrates localized to areas where proximal tubule cells stained positive for intracellular IgG or where luminal casts were present. Furthermore, proximal tubule cells that stained positive for IgG also showed evidence of increased osteopontin production. The IgG staining in proximal tubule cells was subsequently associated with the peritubular accumulation of macrophages and alpha smooth muscle actin-positive cells, as well as upregulation of TFG-β mRNA in the tubular and infiltrating cells.[413]

The importance of inflammatory factors in the development of interstitial fibrosis is illustrated by the observation that treatment of rats with experimental membranous nephropathy with rapamycin is associated with reduced expression of profibrotic and proinflammatory genes, as well as amelioration of interstitial inflammation and fibrosis.[414] Further studies in the 5/6 nephrectomy model have suggested that tubulointerstitial injury may play an important role in the decline of the GFR, especially in the late stages of progressive renal injury.[415] By examining serial sections of remnant kidneys, the investigators have shown that in association with a doubling in serum creatinine levels, there was a substantial increase in the proportion of glomeruli no longer connected to tubules (atubular glomeruli) or to atrophic tubules. Most of these glomeruli were not globally sclerosed, implying that the tubular injury was responsible for the final loss of function in these nephrons. The authors speculated that the absorption of excess filtered protein may play an important role in this tubular injury.[415] Finally, evidence has been accumulating for the role of proteinuria in the development of interstitial damage in human CKD. Among 215 patients with CKD, the urine ACR correlated with urinary MCP-1 levels and interstitial macrophage numbers.[416] Furthermore, urine ACR and interstitial macrophage numbers independently predicted renal survival.

Establishing a cause and effect relationship between proteinuria and renal damage in humans is difficult but several clinical studies have provided evidence to support this. A metaanalysis of 17 clinical studies of CKD has revealed a positive correlation between the severity of proteinuria and the extent of biopsy-proven glomerulosclerosis,[403] and data from a metaanalysis that included over 1 million participants identified albuminuria as a strong independent risk factor for progression to ESKD.[417] Observations from the Modification of Diet in Renal Disease (MDRD) trial have also suggested that proteinuria is an independent determinant of CKD progression. Greater levels of baseline proteinuria were strongly associated with more rapid declines in the GFR and reduction of proteinuria, independently of reduction in BP, was associated with lesser rates of decline in the GFR. Furthermore, the degree of benefit achieved by lowering BP below usual target levels was highly dependent on the level of baseline proteinuria.[418]

The severity of proteinuria at baseline has been shown to be the most important independent predictor of renal outcomes in randomized trials of ACE inhibitor or ARB treatment in those with diabetic nephropathy[419] and nondiabetic CKD.[282] Furthermore the percentage reduction in proteinuria over the first 3 to 6 months, as well as the absolute level of proteinuria at 3 or 6 months, are strong independent predictors of the subsequent rate of decline in the GFR among patients with diabetic nephropathy[419] and nondiabetic CKD.[420] A metaanalysis that included data from 1860 patients with nondiabetic CKD has confirmed these findings and has shown that during antihypertensive treatment, the current level of proteinuria is a powerful predictor of the combined endpoint of doubling of baseline serum creatinine levels or onset of ESKD (relative risk, 5.56 for each 1.0 g/day of proteinuria).[421] Similarly a metaanalysis of 21 randomized trials of drug treatment in CKD that included 78,342 participants has found that for each 30% initial reduction in albuminuria with treatment, the risk of ESKD decreased by 23.7% (95% confidence interval [CI], 11.4%– 34.2%) independently of the class of drug used for treatment.[422]

The Renoprotection of Optimal Antiproteinuric Doses (ROAD) study has provided the most direct evidence of the clinical benefit of proteinuria reduction to date. Subjects with proteinuric CKD were randomized to standard therapy with an ACE inhibitor or ARB (separate groups) or to ACE inhibitor or ARB therapy titrated to the maximum antiproteinuric dose (two further groups). Despite comparable BP control, subjects in the groups randomized to maximum antiproteinuric doses had 51% and 53% relative risk reductions in the combined primary endpoints of creatinine level doubling, ESKD, or death.[423]

Taken together, the evidence from experimental and clinical studies provides support for the hypothesis that impaired glomerular permselectivity results in excessive filtration of proteins and/or protein-bound molecules that contribute to kidney damage, but many questions regarding the tubulotoxic potential of filtered plasma proteins and the identity of the specific molecules involved remain unanswered. Despite these uncertainties, the close association between the severity of proteinuria and renal prognosis implies that reduction of proteinuria should be regarded as an important independent therapeutic goal in clinical strategies seeking to slow the rate of progression of CKD. The mechanisms and consequences of proteinuria are discussed further in Chapter 30.

## TUBULOINTERSTITIAL FIBROSIS

Together with secondary FSGS, TIF constitutes a major component of the progressive renal injury observed in CKD. TIF is characterized by inflammatory cell and fibroblast infiltration, accumulation of ECM, tubule cell loss, and rarefaction of peritubular capillaries. Fibrogenesis starts at small sites of inflammation and then expands if a profibrotic milieu persists. The inflammatory infiltrate is composed of lymphocytes, macrophages, detritic cells, and mast cells.[424] Lymphocytes are recruited early in the process, and their importance is highlighted by the protection from fibrosis observed in Rag-2 null mice, which lack B and T lymphocytes.[425] Monocytes are recruited and transdifferentiate into macrophages and fibrocytes. The profibrotic role of macrophages is illustrated by observations that the extent of macrophage accumulation correlates closely with the severity of fibrosis,[426] and macrophage depletion attenuates fibrosis.[427] Nevertheless, it has been proposed that alternatively activated M2 macrophages exert antiinflammatory actions, and the infusion of cells enriched for M2 macrophages has been shown to reduce renal fibrosis in mice.[428] Myofibroblasts are the chief source of ECM production, and the accumulation of interstitial myofibroblasts is central to the pathogenesis of TIF.

There has been considerable controversy regarding the cellular origins of interstitial myofibroblasts in TIF. Different investigators have identified resident fibroblasts,[429] transdifferentiation from tubule epithelial cells and endothelial cells,[430,431] bone marrow–derived fibrocytes,[432] and pericytes[354] as possible sources.[356] Fate-mapping studies have subsequently indicated that pericytes are the predominant source of myofibroblasts and that epithelial to mesenchymal transdifferentiation (EMT) is not a source of myofibroblasts or accounts for only a small minority.[354] Further studies have helped resolve the controversy by showing that TECs undergo partial EMT, expressing both epithelial and mesenchymal markers, but remain attached to the tubular basal membrane. Moreover, prevention of EMT substantially ameliorated renal fibrosis in animal models, confirming that partial EMT of TECs contributes to the pathogenesis of renal fibrosis.[433,434]

The excess ECM is composed largely of collagen types I and II, as well as fibronectin. Investigators have sought to identify the relative contribution of different cell types to the production of collagen I using cell type–specific knockouts. Experiments have revealed that bone marrow–derived cells (fibrocytes) contribute 38% to 50% of collagen deposition in a UUO model. Furthermore, initial collagen I synthesis was attributable to resident mesenchymal fibroblasts and was beneficial in preserving renal function in this model, whereas bone marrow–derived cells were responsible for later collagen I production that did not affect renal function.[435] TECs were found not to contribute directly to collagen I production. Bone marrow–derived cells were similarly shown to contribute substantially to collagen I production in an adenine-induced nephropathy model and, in this case, greater deposition of collagen was associated with lower the GFR at all time points.[435] Targeting of bone marrow–derived cell collagen I production therefore represents an attractive therapeutic option to ameliorate renal fibrosis.

Matrix accumulation has been proposed to commence with the appearance of collagen nucleators in the interstitial fluid that act as a scaffold for the deposition of fibrillar collagens. Fibroblasts use collagen fibrils as a scaffold to move through damaged tissue along chemoattractant gradients. Fibrogenesis is promoted by the expression of key growth factors, principally TFG-β.[436] The role of tissue proteases in TIF is complex and has not been fully characterized. Whereas matrix metalloprotease (MMP) types 2 and 9 degrade collagen type IV (and possibly type I and III) in vitro, they do not consistently abrogate TIF in vivo.[437,438] Indeed, in some models, MMPs appear to exert profibrotic effects.[438]

Rarefaction of peritubular capillaries is a hallmark of TIF. In the early stages, capillaries may be damaged by transient ischemia that promotes apoptosis.[439] Further capillary loss is attributable to an imbalance between pro- and antiangiogenic factors[440,441] or loss of peritubular endothelial cells through endothelial-mesenchymal transdifferentiation.[430] Detailed studies have identified changes in peritubular capillary endothelium in animal models of CKD, including the development of subendothelial spaces, loss of fenestrations, and generation of caveolae and vesicles, as well as increased permeability and degeneration of the microvascular tree.[442] Tissue hypoxia results from the rarefaction of peritubular capillaries and accumulation of ECM, requiring oxygen to diffuse over greater distances to reach cells. Hypoxia contributes to TIF by promoting EMT and apoptosis of tubule cells, as well as fibroblast activation and ECM production.[443,444] The importance of hypoxia in provoking interstitial (and glomerular) injury has been demonstrated by studies in which induction of hypoxia-inducible factor, a key mediator of protective responses to hypoxia, was associated with amelioration of proteinuria, glomerulosclerosis, and TIF, as well as decreased macrophage infiltration and expression of type IV collagen and osteopontin.[445,446] Tubulointerstitial inflammation and fibrosis are discussed in more detail in Chapter 35.

## MOLECULAR MEDIATORS OF RENAL FIBROSIS

TGF-β is associated with chronic fibrotic states throughout the body and is the central mediator of renal fibrosis.[447] Three isoforms of TGF-β have been described in mammals, but the focus of most research has been on TGF-β1. The active form of TGF-β is a dimer that binds to a transmembrane receptor, which is a heterodimer comprised of TGF-β receptor types I and II. Intracellular signaling occurs via Smad-dependent and Smad-independent pathways. Smad2 and Smad3 have been identified as the most important intracellular mediators of the actions of TGF-β, with Smad3 having profibrotic effects and Smad2 proposed to have counter-regulatory antifibrotic effects. In response to TGF-β receptor signaling, Smad2 and Smad3 are phosphorylated and form a complex with Smad4 that translocates into the nucleus and binds to DNA to modulate the transcription of multiple target genes. Smad3 has been shown to promote transcription of multiple genes involved in fibrosis, including PAI-1, proteoglycans, integrins, CTGF, TIMP-1, and collagen types 1, 5, and 6. SMAD 3 also plays a role in EMT.[448] In addition, TGF-β/Smad3 modulates the production of micro RNA molecules that promote fibrosis; levels of profibrotic miR-21, miR-192, and miR-433 are increased, whereas antifibrotic miR-29 and miR-200 are decreased.[449] Smad4 is a key modulator of the profibrotic actions of TGF-β and reduces the profibrotic actions of Smad3 by inhibiting its binding to the promoter regions of profibrotic genes. Smad7 is an important negative feedback regulator of TGF-β signaling, which acts by preventing the recruitment and phosphorylation of Smad2 and Smad3. Smad7 also increases the expression of inhibitor of kappa B (IκBα), an inhibitor of NF-κB, and may therefore be important in mediating the antiinflammatory actions of TGF-β. Finally, Smad signaling may also be activated by TGF-β–independent mechanisms that are relevant to CKD progression, including Ang II and advanced glycation end products (AGEs).[448]

In vitro TGF-β elicits overproduction of ECM constituents by mesangial cells, and its expression is increased in several experimental models of renal disease. These include diabetic nephropathy,[450] anti–Thy-1 glomerulonephritis,[451] adriamycin-induced nephropathy,[452] and chronic allograft nephropathy,[453] as well as human glomerulonephritis,[454,455] HIV nephropathy,[456] diabetic nephropathy,[457] and chronic allograft nephropathy.[458] The role of TGF-β in renal fibrosis has been further illustrated by experiments in which transfection of the gene for TGF-β into one renal artery produced ipsilateral renal fibrosis.[459] In 5/6 nephrectomized rats, a two- to threefold increase in remnant kidney mRNA levels for TGF-β was observed, and in situ hybridization revealed elevations in TGF-β mRNA throughout the glomeruli, tubules, and interstitium. Treatment with an ACE inhibitor or ARB resulted in substantial renal protection and prevented upregulation of TGF-β.[346,347] Furthermore, in rats treated with an ACE inhibitor or ARB, the extent of glomerulosclerosis correlated closely with remnant kidney TGF-β mRNA levels.[270]

Several interventions that inhibit the effects of TGF-β have been shown to afford renoprotection in animal models of renal disease. Transfection of the gene for decorin, a naturally occurring inhibitor of TGF-β, into skeletal muscle limited the progression of renal injury in anti–Thy-1 glomerulonephritis.[460] Administration of anti–TGF-β antibodies to salt-loaded, Dahl salt–sensitive rats ameliorated the hypertension, proteinuria, glomerulosclerosis, and interstitial fibrosis typical of this model.[461] Treatment with tranilast (N-[3′,4′-dimethoxycinnamoyl]-anthranilic acid; Pharm Chemical, Shanghai Lansheng, Shanghai, China), an inhibitor of TGF-β–induced ECM production, significantly reduced albuminuria, macrophage infiltration, glomerulosclerosis, and interstitial fibrosis in 5/6 nephrectomized rats.[462] Transfer of an inducible gene for Smad 7, which blocks TGF-β signaling by inhibiting Smad 2/3 activation, inhibited proteinuria, fibrosis, and myofibroblast accumulation after 5/6 nephrectomy.[463] Two weeks of treatment with a polyamide compound designed to suppress transcription of the TGF-β gene significantly reduced proteinuria and prevented upregulation of TGF-β, CTGF, collagen type I α1, and fibronectin mRNA in the renal cortex. This also suppressed urinary TGF-β excretion and staining for TGF-β by immunofluorescence in salt-loaded, Dhal salt–sensitive rats.[464] Another fibrogenic molecule, CTGF, has also been observed to be overexpressed in kidney biopsies from patients with a variety of renal diseases.[465] The specific induction of CTGF expression by exogenous TGF-β in mesangial cells[314,466] and fibroblasts,[467] together with the finding that blocking antibodies to TGF-β inhibits increased CTGF expression in mesangial cells exposed to high glucose concentrations,[466] suggests that CTGF may serve as a downstream mediator of the profibrotic effects of TGF-β.[468] Further experiments have shown that the fibrotic effects of TGF-β in the remnant kidney are mediated, at least in part, by the induction of the micro RNAs miR-21, miR-192, and miR-433 via Smad 3.[449] In vitro overexpression of miR-192 promotes, but inhibition of miR-192, attenuates, TGF-β–induced production of collagen type I in rat tubule cells.[469]

It is clear that interventions to inhibit the multiple mechanisms of renal fibrosis show promise as treatments for slowing the progression of CKD. However, despite the promising results of many preclinical studies inhibiting the expression or actions of TGF-β discussed previously, a phase 2 randomized trial of anti–TGF-$\beta_1$ monoclonal antibody therapy—added to RAAS inhibitor treatment in persons with diabetic kidney disease, GFR of 20 to 60 mL/min/1.73 m$^2$, and urine polymerase chain reaction (PCR) value higher than 800 mg/g, found no benefit with respect to change in serum creatinine levels after a median of 315 days of therapy.[470] Secondary analyses also found no differences in proteinuria or biomarkers of renal injury between groups receiving anti–TGF-$\beta_1$ antibody versus placebo.

This negative result may have been in part attributed to the relatively short trial duration, inadequate dosing of the antibody, or selection of participants with relatively severe and advanced nephropathy. Other possible explanations include redundancy in fibrotic mechanisms and the fact that TGF-β has potentially beneficial antiinflammatory actions. Nevertheless, it is likely that the development of interventions to inhibit renal fibrosis will remain an area of active research and result in multiple potential novel therapies.[471]

## HEPATOCYTE GROWTH FACTOR

Investigations have shed light on the role of HGF as a potential antifibrotic factor in CKD. Initial studies focused on the property of HGF to ameliorate tubule cell injury in models of renal ischemia,[472,473] but studies in models of CKD have suggested that HGF may also ameliorate chronic renal injury through its mitogenic, motogenic, morphogenic, and antiapoptotic actions.[474] As discussed, HGF is upregulated in the remaining kidney after uninephrectomy and may play a role in compensatory renal hypertrophy.[168] Further studies have confirmed that HGF and its receptor, c-met, are also upregulated in the remnant kidney after 5/6 nephrectomy.[475] Furthermore, blockade of HGF action with anti-HGF antibodies resulted in a more rapid decline in the GFR and more severe renal fibrosis, which was associated with increased ECM accumulation and a greater number of myofibroblasts in the interstitium and tubules. Other studies have identified multiple mechanisms whereby HGF may contribute to renoprotection, including amelioration of podocyte injury and apoptosis, as well as proteinuria,[476] increased apoptosis of myofibroblasts,[477] decreased ECM accumulation in association with increased expression of MMP-9, decreased expression of endogenous inhibitors of MMPs, TIMP-1 and TIMP-2, in proximal tubule cell cultues,[475] disruption of NF-κB signaling in tubule cells,[478,479] and suppression of TGF-β–induced CTGF expression in tubule cells.[480]

Multiple experiments have confirmed the renoprotective effects of HGF. The renoprotective effects of ACE inhibitor and ARB treatment were associated with increased renal expression on HGF mRNA.[481]Treatment with anti-HGF antibodies resulted in increased TGF-β levels in a mouse model of chronic glomerulonephritis.[482] HGF treatment ameliorated the progression of chronic allograft nephropathy in a renal transplant model.[483] HGF blocked the TGF-β–induced transdifferentiation of tubule epithelial cells to myofibroblasts.[484] Exogenous HGF administration[484] or HGF overexpression[485] blocked myofibroblast activation and prevented interstitial fibrosis in the unilateral ureteric obstruction model. HGF gene transfer into skeletal muscle ameliorated glomerulosclerosis and interstitial fibrosis after 5/6 nephrectomy.[486] HGF treatment suppressed CTGF expression and attenuated renal fibrosis after 5/6 nephrectomy.[487] In contrast, other studies have reported adverse renal effects associated with excess HGF exposure. Transgenic mice that overexpressed HGF developed progressive renal disease characterized by tubular hypertrophy, glomerulosclerosis, and cyst formation,[488] and HGF administration resulted in more rapid deterioration of creatinine clearance, as well as increased albuminuria in obese db diabetic mice.[489] Available evidence thus has suggested that HGF may play a role in ameliorating chronic renal injury but inappropriate or excessive exposure to HGF may have adverse renal effects.

## BONE MORPHOGENETIC PROTEIN-7

Bone morphogenetic protein (BMP)-7, also termed *osteogenic protein-1*, is a bone morphogen involved in embryonic development and tissue repair. Preliminary evidence has suggested that BMP-7 may also play a role in renal repair. BMP-7 is downregulated after acute renal ischemia,[490] early in the course of experimental diabetes,[491] and after 5/6 nephrectomy.[492] Furthermore, the administration of exogenous BMP-7 increased tubular regeneration after 5/6 nephrectomy,[492] attenuated interstitial inflammation and fibrosis after UUO,[493] and ameliorated glomerulosclerosis in rats with diabetic nephropathy.[494] In one model of diabetic nephropathy, BMP-7 was noted to be most effective at inhibiting tubular inflammation and TIF.[495] In vitro experiments have identified several potential renoprotective effects attributable to BMP-7, including inhibition of proinflammatory cytokine, as well as endothelin expression in tubule cells exposed to TNF-α,[496] reversal of renal tubule EMT,[497] antagonism of the fibrogenic effects of TGF-β in mesangial cells,[498] and protection from injury in podocytes exposed to high levels of glucose.[499] In a mouse model of UUO, administration of exogenous BMP-7 was associated with reduced accumulation of collagen type I, an effect attributed to reduced phosphorylation of Smad3 (canonical signaling of TGF-β) and Akt (noncanonical signaling TGF-β).[500] The renoprotective effect of BMP-7 was further illustrated by the observation that expression of a transgene for BMP-7 in podocytes and proximal renal tubule cells was associated with the prevention of podocyte dropout, as well as amelioration of albuminuria, glomerulosclerosis, and interstitial fibrosis after the induction of diabetes.[501] Further studies evaluating the effects of chronic treatment with BMP-7 or small- molecule BMP-7 agonists are still awaited.

## MICRO RNAS

Micro RNAs (miRNAs) are small noncoding RNAs that have been shown to have important posttranscriptional gene regulatory function. Attention has been focused on the potential role of miRs to modulate renal fibrosis. miR-21 and miR-214 have been shown to be upregulated in several experimental models of CKD,[502,503] and miR-21 has been reported to be upregulated in human transplant kidneys with nephropathy.[502] Deletion of miR-21 or treatment with anti–miR-21 oligonucleotides was associated with amelioration of interstitial fibrosis in animal models.[502] Similarly, deletion of miR-214 and treatment with anti–miR-214 were each associated with attenuation of interstitial fibrosis in the unilateral ureteric obstruction model. Importantly, the effects of miR-214 appear to be independent of TGF-β signaling, and TGF-β blockade had an additive antifibrotic effect with miR-214 deletion.[504] As discussed previously, TGF-β/Smad3 signaling increases the production of profibrotic miRs and decreases the production of antifibrotic miRs. Multiple other miRs have been implicated in the pathogenesis of different forms of CKD, including miRs 23b, 29b, 29c, and 129 in diabetic nephropathy and miRs 30c,129-5p, 145, 196a, 196b, 200b, 200c, 215, and 433 in renal fibrosis.[505] Studies have also identified that miRs can be transferred between cells in extracellular vesicles to exert autocrine or paracrine effects.[505] The potential to administer beneficial miRs or antagonize the effects of pathogenic miRs with antagomirs represents a further potential therapeutic strategy for CKD.

## OXIDATIVE STRESS

CKD is associated with increased oxidative stress that likely contributes to the progression of renal damage, as well as the pathogenesis of the associated cardiovascular disease.[506] Superoxide is the primary reactive oxygen species (ROS) that accounts for oxidative stress. Its major source is production by nicotinamide adenine dinucleotide phosphate (NADPH) oxidase, and it is removed (by conversion to hydrogen peroxide by superoxide dismutase (SOD). Following 5/6 nephrectomy, significant upregulation of NADPH oxidase and downregulation of SOD were observed in the liver and kidneys, indicating that the increase in superoxide is due to a combination of increased production and decreased removal.[507] Similarly, in a mouse model of proteinuric CKD induced by the administration of doxorubicin (ADR), NADPH oxidase was upregulated, and extracellular (EC-SOD) was downregulated. Furthermore, EC-SOD knockout mice showed greater albuminuria and more renal fibrosis after doxorubicin than wild-type mice, confirming that the antioxidant effects of EC-SOD protect against kidney damage.[508] Examination of human kidney biopsies confirmed that EC-SOD is similarly downregulated in human CKD.[508] BP was elevated, and nitrotyrosine levels were increased, whereas urine nitric oxide metabolites were decreased, observations consistent with increased NO inactivation by superoxide. The effects of increased levels of ROS are further compounded by the reduced abundance and activity of antioxidant enzymes (e.g., catalase, glutathione peroxidase, glutathione),[509] as well as reduced HDL, apolipoprotein A-1, and thiols.[510]

Adverse consequences of oxidative stress that may contribute to CKD progression include hypertension (due to inactivation of NO and oxidation of arachidonic acid to generate vasoconstrictive isoprostanes),[511] inflammation (due to activation of NF-κB),[509] fibrosis, and apoptosis,[510] as well as glomerular filtration barrier damage.[512] Inflammation may in turn increase oxidative stress due to the generation of ROS by activated leukocytes, thus establishing a vicious cycle of oxidative stress and inflammation.[506]

Other factors that may contribute to increased ROS production in CKD include Ang II,[513] reduced production of NO,[71] and hypertension.[514] The importance of ROS in the progression of CKD has been shown by experiments in which antioxidant therapies, including melatonin,[515] niacin,[516] and omega-3 fatty acids,[517] have reduced oxidative stress and ameliorated renal damage in the 5/6 nephrectomy model. On the other hand, treatment with tempol, an SOD mimetic, reduced plasma malondialdehyde levels and the number of superoxide-positive cells but did not reduce overall renal oxidative stress, inflammation, or renal damage.[518]

## ACIDOSIS

As the GFR declines, the ability of kidneys to excrete hydrogen ions becomes impaired, and a new steady state is achieved that allows excretion of acid at the cost of a persistent metabolic acidosis (see earlier, "Acid-Base Regulation"). Acidosis is present in most patients when the GFR falls below 20% to 25% of normal.[519] Chronic metabolic acidosis has multiple adverse consequences, including increased protein catabolism, increased bone turnover, induction of inflammatory mediators, insulin resistance, and increased production of corticosteroids and PTH.[519,520] These observations make it reasonable to consider whether acidosis may also contribute to progressive renal damage in CKD. Early experiments found no persisting renal damage after dietary acid loading in rats with normal renal function and no renoprotection associated with sodium bicarbonate treatment in the 5/6 nephrectomy model, suggesting that acidosis does not initiate or exacerbate renal damage.[521]

Later experiments, however, have found that an acid-generating diet of casein protein induces tubulointerstitial injury in rats with normal renal function, whereas a non–acid-inducing diet of soy protein does not.[522] Furthermore, dietary acid supplementation with $(NH_4)_2SO_4$ in soy protein–fed rats was associated with tubulointerstitial injury. Similarly, in the 5/6 nephrectomy model, a casein-rich diet was associated with metabolic acidosis and a progressive decline in the GFR and increasing albuminuria, whereas a soy protein diet was not.[523]

Dietary acid supplementation with $(NH_4)_2SO_4$ in soy protein–fed rats provoked a decline in the GFR and albuminuria. Treatment with sodium bicarbonate or $Ca(HCO_3)_2$, but not sodium chloride, was renoprotective in the casein-fed rats but only if the resultant hypertension—in sodium bicarbonate but not $Ca(HCO_3)_2$–treated rats—was adequately treated. Furthermore, when rats were subject to 2/3 rather than 5/6 nephrectomy, a level of renal mass reduction not associated with metabolic acidosis, microdialysis identified tissue acid accumulation in muscle and kidney that correlated with the subsequent GFR decline.[524] Amelioration of tissue acid accumulation by a low acid-generating diet or alkali supplementation was associated with abrogation of the GFR decline, whereas dietary acid supplementation was associated with exacerbation of the GFR decline. Treatment with calcium citrate has also been shown to improve acidosis and reduce glomerular as well as interstitial injury in the 5/6 nephrectomy model.[525] Mechanisms whereby acidosis may contribute to renal damage after nephron loss include activation of the alternative complement pathway by increased ammoniagenesis,[526] increased levels of plasma and kidney Ang II,[527] and induction of ET, as well as aldosterone production.[528]

Observational clinical studies have identified acidosis as an independent risk factor for CKD progression,[529,530] but to date only relatively small studies have investigated the renoprotective potential of alkali supplementation in human subjects. In the first randomized study in adults with a creatinine clearance of 15 to 30 mL/min, randomization to treatment of acidosis (serum bicarbonate, 16–20 mmol/L) with sodium bicarbonate was associated with a lower decline in creatinine clearance (1.88 vs. 5.93 mL/min) and lower incidence of ESKD (6.5% vs. 33%).[531] The authors conceded, however, that the study was not blinded or placebo- controlled. In a second nonrandomized study, treatment of 30 subjects with sodium citrate was associated with reduced urinary excretion of ET-1 and *N*-acetyl-β-D-glucosaminidase (a marker of tubulointerstitial injury), as well as a lower rate of estimated

GFR decline than that observed in 29 untreated controls who were unwilling or unable to take sodium citrate.[532] One study has reported renoprotective effects following sodium bicarbonate treatment in early CKD. In a randomized placebo-controlled trial in subjects with a mean estimated GFR of 75 mL/min/1.73 $m^2$, treatment with sodium bicarbonate for 5 years was associated with a slower reduction in the estimated GFR (derived from plasma cystatin C measurements) than placebo or treatment with sodium chloride.[533]

Further studies have reported that correction of acidosis with a diet rich in fruit and vegetables is as effective in ameliorating kidney damage in early (CKD stage 1 or 2)[534] and more advanced (CKD stage 4) disease.[535] In a further trial, people with CKD stage 3 and a serum bicarbonate level of 22 to 24 mmol/L were randomized to oral bicarbonate supplementation, a diet rich in fruit and vegetables, or usual care. All participants received treatment with RAAS inhibition (RAASi), and SBP was controlled to less than 130 mm Hg. Both interventions achieved an increase in serum bicarbonate levels and were associated with a decrease in urinary angiotensinogen. After 3 years, both interventions were associated with less albuminuria and GFR decline than the usual care group.[536] Bicarbonate supplementation is already recommended for patients with levels below 22 mEq/L, but further studies are required to further investigate whether it is beneficial in the setting of less severe acidosis.[537]

## HYPERTROPHY

The consistent observation of renal, and in particular glomerular, hypertrophy after renal mass reduction has prompted investigators to propose that processes involved in, or resulting from, hypertrophy may contribute to progressive renal injury in CKD.[538] The well- documented observation that renal and glomerular hypertrophy precede the development of diabetic nephropathy and the finding of a positive association between glomerular size and early sclerosis in rats subjected to renal mass ablation[539] further suggests that hypertrophy may play a direct role in the pathogenesis of glomerulosclerosis. Several clinical observations have also supported an association between glomerular hypertrophy and renal injury. Oligomeganephronia, a rare congenital condition with a nephron number 25% of normal or less, is characterized by marked hypertrophy of the remaining glomeruli and the development of proteinuria and renal failure in adolescence, with FSGS as the typical renal biopsy finding.[540] In children with minimal change disease, a glomerulopathy generally associated with spontaneous remission and lack of progression to renal failure, investigators have noted an association between glomerular size and the risk of developing FSGS and renal failure.[541]

Several interventions have been used in experiments to interrupt the development of glomerular hypertrophy after renal mass reduction and thereby assess its role in renal disease progression, but have produced contradictory results. Rats subjected to 5/6 nephrectomy were compared with rats in which 2/3 of the left kidney was infarcted and the right ureter drained into the peritoneal cavity, an intervention that apparently results in decreased renal clearance without compensatory renal hypertrophy.[538] Micropuncture studies confirmed similar degrees of elevation of $P_{GC}$ and SNGFR in both models. At 4 weeks, however, the maximal planar area of the glomerulus was significantly less, and glomerular injury, as assessed by sclerosis index, was significantly reduced in ureteroperitoneostomized rats versus 5/6 nephrectomized controls. Accordingly, the authors have concluded that glomerular hypertrophy is more important than glomerular capillary hypertension in the progression of glomerular injury in this model.

Dietary sodium restriction has also been used to inhibit renal hypertrophy after 5/6 nephrectomy. Although sodium restriction had no effect on glomerular hemodynamics, glomerular volume was significantly reduced in 5/6 nephrectomized rats fed low versus normal sodium diets.[134] Moreover, urinary protein excretion was lower, and glomerulosclerosis was less severe, in rats on restricted sodium intake. These findings were extended by another study in which the effect of sodium restriction in preventing glomerular hypertrophy and ameliorating glomerular injury was confirmed, but which also found that these benefits were overcome by the administration of an androgen that stimulated glomerular hypertrophy, despite sodium restriction. Glomerular hemodynamics were similar among the groups.[542] On the other hand, treatment with seliciclib, a cyclin-dependent kinase inhibitor, reduced renal hypertrophy by 45% after 5/6 nephrectomy but had no effect on kidney damage.[543]

Glomerular hypertrophy may contribute to glomerulosclerosis through a number of different mechanisms. According to the law of Laplace, the increase in glomerular volume could result in an increase in capillary wall tension only if the capillary wall diameter were also increased (Fig. 51.8).

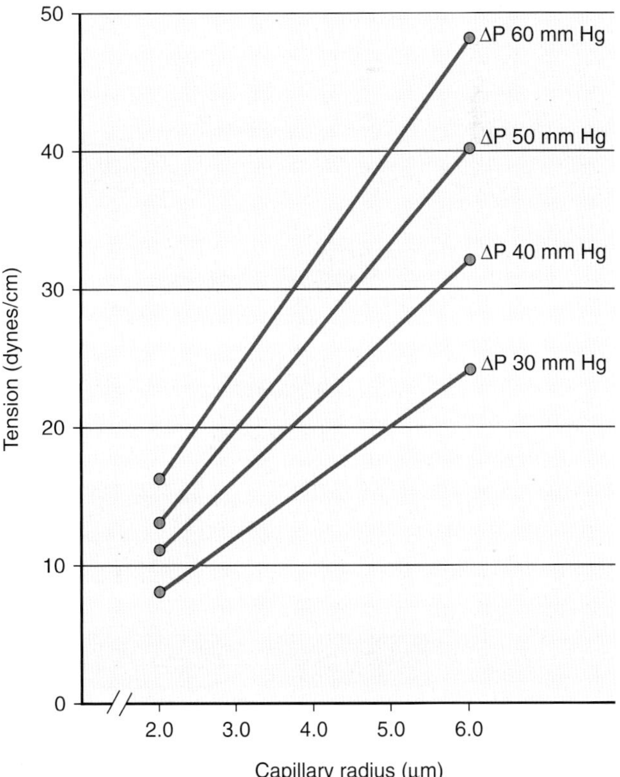


**Fig. 51.8** Illustration of the synergistic effects of changes in transcapillary hydrostatic pressure difference (ΔP, mm Hg) and mean glomerular capillary radius (μm) on the calculated capillary wall tension (dynes/cm). (From Bidani AK, Mitchell KD, Schwartz MM, et al. Absence of progressive glomerular injury in a normotensive rat remnant kidney model. *Kidney Int.* 1990;38:28–38.)

Cyclic stretch would then exert stress capable of damaging epithelial, mesangial, and endothelial cells, as described previously. Alternatively, glomerulosclerosis may be viewed as a maladaptive growth response following loss of renal mass and resulting in excessive mesangial proliferation and extracellular matrix production.[538] The identification of TGF-β as a key mediator of renal hypertrophy, as well as an important promoter of renal fibrosis, provides an obvious link between renal hypertrophy and fibrosis.[175]

Detailed studies of podocyte hypertrophy have found that impaired podocyte hypertrophy in response to glomerular enlargement is a further mechanism that may contribute to the development of proteinuria and FSGS. Using a transgenic rat model (dominant negative AA-4E-BP1 transgene) that resulted in impaired podocyte hypertrophy, the investigators observed a remarkable linear relationship among gain in body weight, proteinuria, and glomerulosclerosis that was accelerated after uninephrectomy. Dietary caloric restriction that prevented weight gain and glomerular enlargement also prevented the proteinuria. Analysis of the kidneys from rats with proteinuria demonstrated a mismatch between glomerular tuft volume and total podocyte volume, and electron microscopy revealed a pulling apart of podocyte foot process, resulting in exposed areas of glomerular basement membrane and adhesions to Bowman's capsule.[544] These findings were extended in the same model by showing that the prevention of glomerular hypertrophy after uninephrectomy by dietary caloric restriction, mTORC1 kinase pathway inhibition (with rapamycin), or treatment with an ACE inhibitor each prevented proteinuria and FSGS. Proliferation of glomerular cells other than podocytes was identified and has been proposed to contribute to the development of FSGS. Moreover, transcriptomic analysis of gene expression in isolated glomeruli from rats that developed FSGS evidenced a similar pattern of gene expression to that identified in glomeruli from human biopsies of persons with progressive CKD, suggesting that similar factors play a role in human CKD progression.[545]

## ANGIOTENSIN II

As noted, Ang II plays a central role in the glomerular hemodynamic adaptations observed after renal mass ablation. Ang subtype 1 receptors are, however, distributed on many cell types in the kidney, including mesangial, glomerular epithelial, endothelial, tubule epithelial, and vascular smooth muscle, cells suggesting multiple potential actions of Ang II in the kidney.[546] Experimental studies have revealed several nonhemodynamic effects of Ang II that may be important in CKD progression (Fig. 51.9). In isolated perfused kidneys, the infusion of Ang II results in loss of glomerular size permselectivity and proteinuria, an effect that has been attributed to both the hemodynamic effects of Ang II, resulting in elevations in $P_{GC}$, and a direct effect of Ang II on glomerular permselectivity.[372] Furthermore, overexpression of angiotensin subtype 1 receptors on podocytes resulted in albuminuria and FSGS in the absence of hypertension in transgenic rats.[547]

In vitro, Ang II has been shown to stimulate mesangial cell proliferation and induce expression of TGF-β, resulting in increased synthesis of ECM.[316] In vivo, transfection

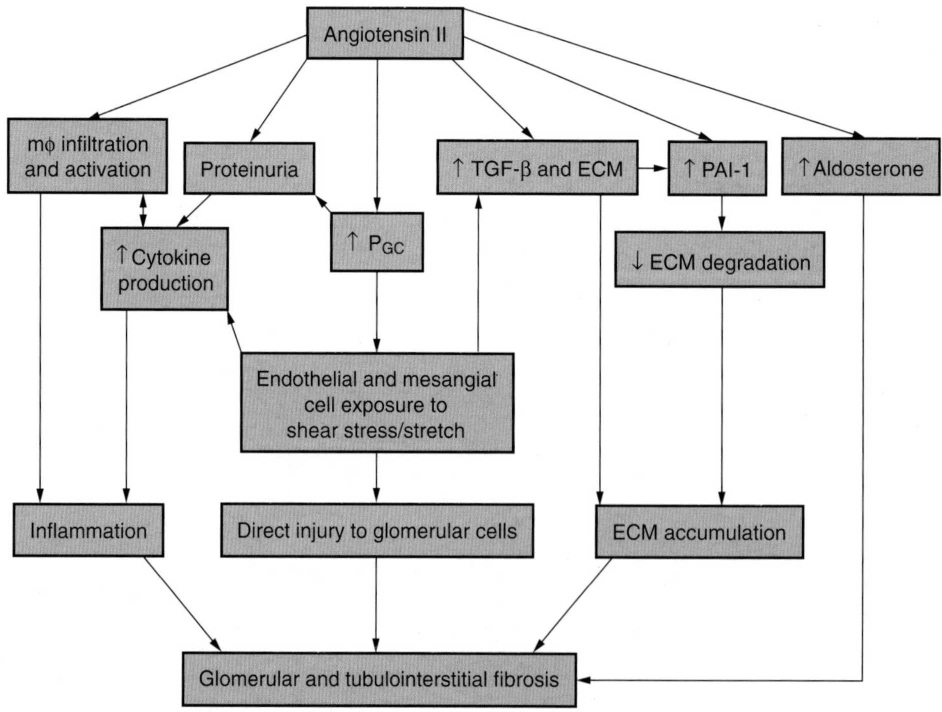


**Fig. 51.9** Schematic depicting the central role of angiotensin II through hemodynamic and nonhemodynamic effects in the pathogenesis of progressive renal injury and fibrosis following nephron loss. *ECM,* Extracellular matrix; *mϕ,* macrophage; *PAI-1,* plasminogen activator inhibitor-1; *$P_{GC}$,* glomerular capillary hydraulic pressure; *TGF-β,* transforming growth factor-β). (From Taal MW, Brenner BM. Renoprotective benefits of RAS inhibition: from ACEI to angiotensin II antagonists. *Kidney Int.* 2000;57:1803–1817,)

of rat kidneys with human genes for renin and angiotensinogen, resulted in glomerular ECM expansion within 7 days.[548] Ang II also stimulates the production of PAI-1 by endothelial cells and vascular smooth muscle cells[549–551] and may therefore further increase the accumulation of ECM through inhibition of ECM breakdown by MMPs that require conversion to an active form by plasmin. Other reports have indicated that Ang II may directly induce the transcription of a variety of cell adhesion molecules and cytokines, as well as activating the transcription factor NF-κB[552–554] and directly stimulating monocyte activation.[555] Ang II infusion provoked upregulation of COX-2 expression in rats that was not dependent on BP elevation,[556] and 5/6 nephrectomized rats evidenced Ang II-dependent upregulation of interstitial COX-2 expression.[557]

In other experiments, Ang II infusion has been shown to induce interstitial macrophage infiltration and increased expression of MCP-1 and TGF-β, effects that were sustained for up to 6 days after cessation of the infusion.[558] In cell culture and animal experiments, Ang II has been shown to promote tubule cell EMT by suppressing expression of miR-429, which inhibits EMT.[559] Finally, Ang II may have fibrogenic effects via mineralocorticoids (see below). Interestingly Ang II may also have antifibrotic effects via the angiotensin subtype 2 receptor ($AT_2$). Ang II appears to upregulate $AT_2$ receptor expression via an $AT_2$ receptor–dependent mechanism after 5/6 nephrectomy, and treatment with an $AT_2$ receptor antagonist exacerbates renal damage[560] and increased renal PAI-1 expression.[561] Furthermore, overexpression of $AT_2$ receptors in transgenic mice was associated with reduced albuminuria, as well as decreased glomerular expression of PDGF-BB chain and TGF-β after 5/6 nephrectomy.[562]

### ALDOSTERONE

Observations that aldosterone stimulates collagen synthesis in the myocardium, and that spironolactone treatment affords survival benefit in addition to that achieved with ACE inhibitor alone in heart failure patients,[563] have provided impetus to studies investigating the potential role of aldosterone in renal fibrosis. In the remnant kidney model, adrenal hypertrophy and markedly elevated plasma aldosterone levels have been reported. Furthermore, the administration of exogenous aldosterone during inhibition of the RAAS with combination ACE inhibitor–ARB therapy in the 5/6 nephrectomy model negates the renal protective effects of the latter.[564] Further evidence of the role of aldosterone has been provided by experiments in which rats subjected to adrenalectomy after 5/6 nephrectomy received replacement glucocorticoid but not mineralocorticoid therapy, resulting in less severe renal injury than rats with intact adrenal glands.[565]

Mechanisms whereby aldosterone may contribute to renal damage include hemodynamic effects (see previously), mesangial cell proliferation,[566] apoptosis,[567] hypertrophy and transdifferentiation,[568] podocyte injury and apoptosis associated with reduced expression of nephrin and podocin, resulting in proteinuria,[374,569,570] proximal tubule cell transdifferentiation and increased production of collagen types III and IV,[571] and increased renal production of ROS,[374,569] PAI-1,[572,573] TGF-β,[574] and CTGF.[575,576] Early experimental use of aldosterone receptor blockers in 5/6 nephrectomized rats has yielded only modest renoprotective effects,[564,577] but other studies have found significant amelioration of glomerulosclerosis in 5/6 nephrectomized rats treated with spironolactone, alone or in combination with triple antihypertensive therapy or an ARB.[572,578,579] In some rats, spironolactone was associated with the apparent regression of glomerulosclerosis. Furthermore, the observed renoprotection was associated with inhibition of PAI-1 mRNA expression in the renal cortex.[572]

In another experiment, renoprotection, achieved with combination ACE inhibitor and spironolactone treatment, was associated with abrogation of the increase in mesangial cells and decrease in podocytes observed in untreated rats. Combination treatment also attenuated the increase in expression of type IV collagen, TGF-β, and desmin.[578] Spironolactone has also been shown to ameliorate renal damage in other experimental models, including diabetic nephropathy,[575,580] Ren2 transgenic rats,[581] radiation nephritis,[582] and stroke-prone hypertension.[583] Several small clinical trials have reported an additional reduction of proteinuria by 15% to 54%, BP by approximately 40%, and the GFR by approximately 25% when aldosterone receptor blockers were added to ACE inhibitor or ARB treatment.[584]

More novel nonsteroidal aldosterone antagonists are also being evaluated. In one randomized trial that enrolled 336 subjects with hypertension, urine ACR of 30 to 599 mg/g, and an eGFR of 50 mL/min/1.73 $m^2$ or higher, treatment with eplerenone for 52 weeks, added to ACE inhibitor or ARB therapy, resulted in a 17.3% decrease in urine ACR, whereas a 10.3% increase was observed in those who received placebo ($P = .02$).[585] The serum potassium level was higher with eplerenone treatment, but no episodes of severe hyperkalemia (serum potassium >5.5 mmol/L) were observed. Nevertheless, large trials are required to assess the potential benefits of aldosterone antagonists in CKD fully; their use is currently limited by the associated risk of hyperkalemia.[586]

## A UNIFIED HYPOTHESIS OF CHRONIC KIDNEY DISEASE PROGRESSION

In the past, there has tended to be a dichotomy of viewpoints regarding the relative importance of hemodynamic and nonhemodynamic factors in the pathogenesis of glomerulosclerosis and TIF after nephron loss.[538,587] Proponents of the so-called hypertrophy hypothesis have pointed out that in some experiments, a dissociation between glomerular hemodynamic changes and glomerulosclerosis has been observed, and that in one study, antihypertensive therapy was renoprotective without lowering $P_{GC}$.[538] On the other hand, those favoring the hemodynamic hypothesis have noted that treatment with an ACE inhibitor[20] or ARB[22] in 5/6 nephrectomized rats results in renoprotection without preventing renal or glomerular hypertrophy, and that many of the studies purporting to show a positive association between glomerular hypertrophy and sclerosis failed to report glomerular hemodynamic data. Furthermore, rats subjected to ureteroperitoneostomy developed significantly more glomerulosclerosis than sham-operated controls, despite a lack of increase in glomerular size.[587]

Several other observations have suggested that hemodynamic factors override the potential role of hypertrophy in progressive renal damage. The renoprotection achieved after

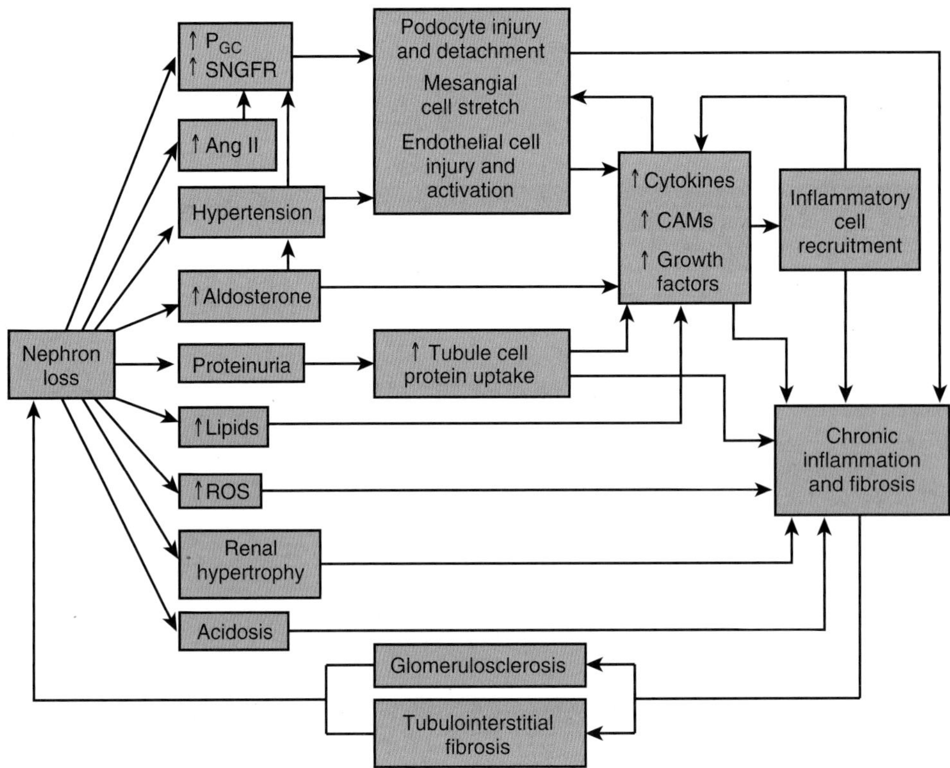


**Fig. 51.10** Schematic illustrating the hypothesized interaction of multiple hemodynamic and nonhemodynamic factors in the pathogenesis of progressive nephron injury in chronic kidney disease. *CAM,* Cell adhesion molecules; *GFR* Glomerular filtration rate; $P_{GC}$, glomerular capillary hydraulic pressure; *ROS,* reactive oxygen species; *SNGFR*, single nephron GFR.

5/6 nephrectomy by a low-protein diet (associated with prevention of glomerular hypertrophy) can be reversed by treatment with calcium channel blockers that inhibit renal autoregulation but have no effect on glomerular size.[588] Comparison of rats subjected to 5/6 nephrectomy by excision versus infarction of two-thirds of the remaining kidney has shown similar increases in glomerular volume, but the infarction model is associated with more severe glomerular hypertension and glomerulosclerosis.[10]

Despite these apparently conflicting views, it is clear from the earlier discussion that hemodynamic and nonhemodynamic mechanisms often overlap. For example, Ang II, a key mediator of glomerular hemodynamic adaptations after nephron loss, also exerts multiple nonhemodynamic deleterious effects. Furthermore, the inflammatory and profibrotic mechanisms that eventuate in glomerulosclerosis and tubulointerstitial fibrosis may be provoked by both hemodynamic and nonhemodynamic stimuli. A growing appreciation of the complexity of the multiple adaptations that follow nephron loss has facilitated the development of a consensus view that continues to regard raised glomerular capillary pressure as a central factor in initiating glomerulosclerosis, but also acknowledges that other nonhemodynamic pathogenic mechanisms may act in concert with hemodynamic factors in a complex interplay that results in a vicious cycle of progressive renal damage (Fig. 51.10). An appreciation of the many mechanisms involved in CKD progression is essential to inform strategies for achieving optimal renoprotection.

## INSIGHTS FROM MODIFIERS OF CHRONIC KIDNEY DISEASE PROGRESSION

*Clinical Relevance*

**Pharmacological Inhibition of the RAAS**

The treatment of hypertension with an optimal dose of a RAAS inhibitor is the mainstay of the approach to achieve renoprotection in proteinuric CKD. Blood pressure should be reduced to less than 130/80 mmHg and even lower targets should be considered in persons with persistent proteinuria, judged to be at low risk of adverse effects from lower blood pressue.

### PHARMACOLOGIC INHIBITION OF THE RENIN-ANGIOTENSIN- ALDOSTERONE SYSTEM

Experimental evidence showing a central role for Ang II in mechanisms of CKD progression through hemodynamic and nonhemodynamic effects has been borne out in randomized clinical trials of ACE inhibitor and ARB treatment in patients with all forms of CKD. ACE inhibitor treatment has been shown to be renoprotective in patients with microalbuminuria and type 2 diabetes mellitus,[589] type 1 diabetes, and overt nephropathy,[281] as well as nondiabetic CKD.[282,285,590,591] Treatment with an ARB affords renoprotection in patients with type 2 diabetes and microalbuminuria[592] or overt nephropathy.[283,284]

More complete inhibition of the RAAS with combination ACE inhibitor–ARB treatment was associated with additional lowering of proteinuria in several small clinical studies.[593] However, the largest randomized study of combination ACE inhibitor–ARB treatment versus monotherapy in CKD was withdrawn because of serious concerns regarding the integrity of the data.[594]

A large trial of combination therapy in patients with hypertension and increased cardiovascular risk has reported no additional benefit with respect to cardiovascular outcomes, but combination therapy was associated with greater reductions in proteinuria than monotherapy.[595] However, the trial reported an increase in the combined endpoint of creatinine doubling, ESKD, or death with combination therapy, indicating that combination ACE inhibitor–ARB therapy may be associated with adverse outcomes in some patient groups. It should be noted, however that subjects were selected on the basis of cardiovascular risk profile and that the majority did not have a reduced GFR or proteinuria. A similar study in 1448 people with type 2 diabetes and urine ACR of 300 mg/g or higher also found no benefit with respect to the primary outcome of CKD progression, ESKD, or death in participants randomized to combination ACE inhibitor–ARB therapy versus monotherapy. However, those receiving combination therapy evidenced a significantly higher incidence of acute kidney injury (AKI) and hyperkalemia.[596]

Thus in two large randomized trials, combination ACE inhibitor–ARB therapy did not confer additional benefit and was associated with an increased risk of adverse effects. Combination therapy should therefore not be used in the patient groups included in these studies. Further studies are required to assess the risks versus benefits of combination therapy in those with proteinuric nondiabetic CKD. The development of direct renin inhibitors (DRIs) has made it possible to inhibit the RAAS at its rate-limiting step—the conversion of angiotensinogen to angiotensin I—and thereby achieve more complete blockade. DRIs were effective as antihypertensive agents and reduced proteinuria in animal models.[597,598] Two early randomized trials have reported additional lowering of albuminuria in subjects with diabetic nephropathy receiving combination DRI and ARB therapy versus ARB therapy alone.[599,600] However, a large randomized trial that included 8561 people with type 2 diabetes and albuminuria or cardiovascular disease was stopped prematurely after the second interim efficacy analysis. Despite greater lowering of BP and albuminuria with combination DRI-ARB therapy, no benefit was observed with respect to the composite primary endpoint of cardiovascular events, CKD progression, ESKD, or death versus ARB monotherapy, but combination therapy was associated with a higher incidence of hyperkalemia and hypotension.[601] Taken together, published data from large randomized trials have to date failed to show additional renoprotective benefits with combination RAAS inhibitor therapy, and all have reported increased adverse effects. This implies that near-complete blockade of the RAAS may be undesirable in many patient groups, but this does not exclude the possibility that it may be beneficial in selected patients who are at high risk of CKD progression, are resistant to monotherapy, and are at a low risk of the reported adverse effects. Further studies are required to investigate this possibility before combination RAAS inhibitor therapy can be recommended in clinical practice.

One metaanalysis has called into question the importance of RAAS inhibition.[602] It should be noted that this study was dominated by data from the Antihypertensive and Lipid Lowering Treatment to Prevent Heart Attack (ALLHAT) study, which found no difference in fatal coronary heart disease or nonfatal myocardial infarction among hypertensive patients with at least one cardiovascular risk factor randomized to treatment with a thiazide diuretic, a calcium channel blocker, or an ACE inhibitor.[603] In a posthoc analysis, there was also no difference in the secondary outcome of ESKD or more than a 50% decrement in the GFR, although patients with a serum creatinine level higher than 2 mg/dL were specifically excluded, resulting in only a minority of patients (5662 of 33,357) having renal disease (eGFR <60 mL/min/1.73 m$^2$). Furthermore, there was no assessment of proteinuria.[604] Thus inclusion of the ALLHAT data was inappropriate and significantly affected the results of the metaanalysis.[605]

Other metaanalyses that did not include ALLHAT data have shown significant renoprotective benefits in patients receiving ACE inhibitor treatment.[606,607] In summary, there is now evidence from multiple randomized trails showing significant renoprotection associated with pharmacologic inhibition of the RAAS in a wide variety of forms of CKD. This confirms that Ang II is a critical mediator of mechanisms of CKD progression in humans and provides support for the consensus that RAAS inhibition should be central to treatment strategies for slowing CKD progression.[608] The role of RAAS inhibitor treatment in achieving optimal renoprotection is discussed further in Chapter 59.

## ARTERIAL HYPERTENSION

Malignant hypertension frequently leads to renal injury, but whether or not less severe forms of hypertension cause hypertensive nephrosclerosis remains a subject of debate.[609,610] An increased risk of developing progressive renal failure with higher levels of BP has been observed in several population-based studies[611–614] and is exemplified by findings from the Multiple Risk Factors Intervention Trial (MRFIT).[615] In a population of 332,544 men, there was a strong graded relationship between BP and the risk of developing or dying with ESKD over a 15- to 17-year follow-up period. Renal function was not assessed at screening or during follow-up, however, so it is not possible to establish with any certainty whether higher BP initiated renal disease or accelerated a nephropathy that was already present. In one study, the importance of hypertension as a risk factor for ESKD was further illustrated by the observation that lowering SBP by 20 mm Hg reduced the risk of ESKD by two-thirds.[612] Even small increases in BP, below the threshold usually used to define hypertension, are associated with an increased risk of ESKD.[611,613,616] Hypertension has also been identified as a risk factor for developing albuminuria or renal impairment among patients with type 2 diabetes mellitus.[617]

Whereas the role of hypertension in initiating renal disease requires further clarification, there is clear evidence that hypertension accelerates the rate of progression of preexisting renal disease, most likely through the transmission of raised hydraulic BP to the glomerulus, resulting in the exacerbation of glomerular capillary hypertension associated with nephron loss.[3] Among patients with diabetic nephropathy and nondiabetic CKD, the initiation of antihypertensive therapy results in

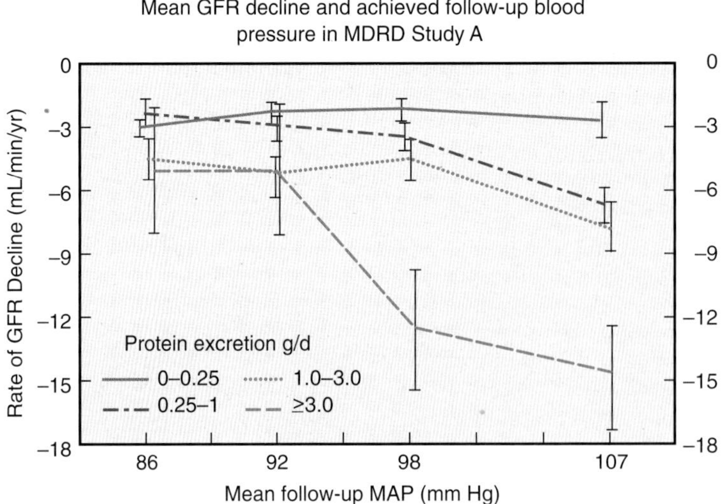


**Fig. 51.11** Interaction of blood pressure reduction and proteinuria at baseline on the rate of decline in the glomerular filtration rate. *GFR,* Glomerular filtration rate; *MAP,* mean arterial pressure; *MDRD,* Modification of Diet in Renal Disease trial. (From Peterson JC, Adler S, Burkart JM, et al. Blood pressure control, proteinuria, and the progression of renal disease. The Modification of Diet in Renal Disease Study. *Ann Intern Med.* 1995;123:754–762.)

significant reductions in rates of GFR decline, implying that hypertension, an almost universal consequence of impaired renal function, also contributes to the progression of CKD.[618] The potential impact of hypertension on the kidney has been exemplified by case reports of patients with unilateral renal artery stenosis who manifested diabetic nephropathy or FSGS only in the nonstenotic kidney and not in the stenotic side that was shielded from the hypertension.[619,620] Analysis of data from the Chronic Renal Insufficiency Cohort (CRIC) study has emphasized the importance of BP control over time. Time-updated SBP higher than 130 mm Hg was more strongly associated with an increased risk of CKD progression than a single baseline measurement.[621]

Uncertainty remains, however, as to the level of BP lowering that is required to achieve optimal renoprotection. Several randomized trials have sought to resolve this issue. In the Modification of Diet in Renal Disease (MDRD) study, patients with predominantly nondiabetic CKD were randomized to a target mean arterial pressure (MAP) of less than 92 mm Hg (equivalent to <125/75 mm Hg) versus less than 107 mm Hg (equivalent to 140/90 mm Hg). Whereas there was no difference between the overall rate of change in the GFR during a mean of 2.2 years follow-up, patients randomized to the low BP target evidenced an early rapid decrease in the GFR, likely attributed to associated renal hemodynamic effects, which obscured a later significantly slower rate of GFR decline. Furthermore the effect of BP control was strongly modulated by the severity of the proteinuria. Among patients with greater than 3 g/day of proteinuria at baseline, randomization to the low BP target was associated with a significantly slower rate of GFR decline.[622]

Secondary analysis also revealed significant correlations between the rate of GFR decline and achieved BP, an effect that was more marked among those with greater baseline proteinuria.[623] In study group 1 (patients with GFR of 25–55 mL/min/1.73 m$^2$), rates of the GFR decline increased above a MAP of 98 mm Hg among patients with baseline proteinuria of 0.25 to 3.0g/day, and above 92 mm Hg in those with baseline proteinuria more than 3.0g/day. In study group 2 (patients with GFR of 13–24 ml/min/m$^2$), higher achieved BP was associated with greater rates of GFR decline at all levels among patients with baseline proteinuria more than 1 g/day (Fig. 51.11). That the benefits of lower BP may become evident only over a longer period is illustrated by the observation that further follow-up (mean 6.6 years) of patients from the MDRD study revealed a significant reduction in the risk of ESKD (adjusted hazard ratio [HR]. 0.68; 95% CI. 0.57–0.82) or a combined endpoint of ESKD or death (adjusted HR. 0.77; 95% CI, 0.65–0.91) among patients randomized to the low BP target, even though treatment and BP data were not available beyond the 2.2 years of the original trial.[624]

In contrast, in the African American Study of Kidney Disease and Hypertension (AASK), no significant difference in the rate of GFR decline was observed between patients randomized to MAP goals of 92 mm Hg or lower versus 102 to 107 mm Hg. Even after prolonged follow-up of the randomized groups, no difference in the combined endpoints of creatinine doubling, ESKD, or death was observed.[625] It should be noted, however, that patients in AASK generally had low levels of baseline proteinuria (mean urine protein, 0.38–0.63 g/day)[591] and after prolonged follow-up, some reduction in the risk of the primary endpoint was observed among those with a baseline urine protein to creatinine ratio more than 0.22 mg/mg, a threshold chosen posthoc by the investigators to be roughly equivalent to 300 mg/day of protein excretion, a value commonly used to define proteinuria.[625] Thus the MDRD and AASK study results support the notion that lower BP targets afford additional renoprotection in patients with more severe proteinuria. Because not all the patients in the MDRD study received ACE inhibitor treatment, it remained unclear to what extent the level of BP attained is important in CKD patients receiving ACE inhibitor or ARB treatment.

Experimental studies have found SBP to be a major determinant of glomerular injury in rats receiving ACE inhibitor or ARB treatment.[270,626] Moreover, among patients with type 1 diabetes and established nephropathy receiving ACE inhibitor treatment, randomization to a low (MAP <92 mm Hg) versus usual (MAP = 100–107 mm Hg) BP target was associated with significantly lower levels of proteinuria after 2 years, although there was no significant difference in GFR decline.[627] Furthermore, secondary analysis of data from the Irbesartan Diabetic Nephropathy Trial (IDNT) showed greater renoprotection among patients who achieved lower BP targets, so that achieved SBP more than 149 mm Hg was associated with a 2.2-fold increased risk of developing ESKD or a doubling of serum creatinine levels versus achieved a SBP less than 134 mm Hg.[628] Importantly, the relationship between improved outcomes and lower achieved SBP persisted among those patients treated with irbesartan. Similarly, in a metaanalysis of data from 1860 nondiabetic patients with CKD, the lowest risk of progression was observed in patients with a SBP of 110 to 129 mm Hg.[629] The ESCAPE Trial investigated the optimal level of BP control for renoprotection in the setting of ACE inhibitor treatment. The study found that among children with CKD receiving treatment with an ACE inhibitor, those randomized to a lower BP target had a significantly reduced risk of reaching ESKD or doubling of serum creatinine levels.[630]

A further trial has reported significant benefit associated with a lower BP target in young people (age <50 years) with autosomal dominant polycystic kidney disease and GFR more than 60 mL/min/1.73 m$^2$. Participants randomized to a low BP target (110/75–95/60 mm Hg) in addition to RAAS inhibitor treatment showed a slower rate of increase in kidney volume, as well as a greater decrease in albuminuria and left ventricular mass index, than those randomized to usual BP control (120/70–130/80 mm Hg).[631] However, these findings cannot be applied to patients who do not meet the inclusion criteria for this study. On the other hand, additional BP reduction with a calcium channel blocker in patients with nondiabetic CKD on ACE inhibitor treatment failed to produce additional renoprotection, although the degree of additional BP reduction was modest (4.1/2.8 mm Hg) and may have been insufficient to improve outcomes in patients already receiving optimal ACE inhibitor therapy.[632]

Several lines of evidence have drawn attention to the possibility that aggressive BP lowering may be associated with adverse effects in some patients. In the IDNT study, an achieved SBP less than 120 mm Hg was associated with increased all-cause mortality and no further improvement in renal outcomes[628]; in the metaanalysis described earlier, achieved SBP less than 110 mm Hg was associated with a higher risk of CKD progression.[629] Furthermore, secondary analysis of data from the Ongoing Telmisartan Alone and in combination with Ramipril Global EndpoinT (ONTARGET) trial has found that subjects who achieved a SBP of less than 120 mm Hg had a significantly higher cardiovascular mortality than those who achieved a SBP of 120 to 129 mm Hg.[633] Similarly, the ACCORD study reported no additional benefit with respect to cardiovascular endpoints among patients with diabetes randomized to achieve a SBP less than 120 mm Hg (vs. conventional control to <130/80 mm Hg), but the lower BP target was associated with more treatment-related adverse events and a greater decline in the GFR.[634]

On the other hand, the largest randomized trial to date to compare the effects of different BP targets on cardiovascular and renal outcomes (The Systolic Blood Pressure Intervention Trial [SPRINT]) was stopped early due to evidence of significant benefit in the primary outcome of cardiovascular events (CVE) and all-cause mortality in the group randomized to a SBP target of less than 120 mm Hg versus less than 140 mm Hg.[635] Analysis of the main trial showed no evidence of effect modification by CKD status on the primary outcome of CVE or all-cause mortality.

A prespecified subgroup analysis was conducted in 2646 participants with CKD at baseline. There was no difference between BP target groups in the renal outcome of 50% decline in the GFR or ESKD after a median of 3.3 years. The lower BP target was associated with some initial decline in the eGFR, likely due to increased use of RAASi, whereas a small initial increase in the GFR was observed with the higher BP. After excluding the first 6 months of observation, the low BP target was associated with a slightly higher rate of GFR decline (0.47 vs. 0.32 mL/min/1.73 m$^2$ per year; $P < .03$). The lower BP target was associated with a lower urine ACR at all time points to 48 months. There was no difference in serious adverse events between the groups, but the low BP target was associated with a higher incidence of hyperkalemia, hypokalemia, and AKI.[636] The results of the SPRINT study therefore indicate survival and cardiovascular benefits but no renoprotective benefit with lower BP targets, and question the notion that the risk of lower BP targets outweighs the benefits in all older adults.

Whereas the results of randomized trials comparing low and usual BP targets among persons with CKD have not yielded unequivocal results, the overall picture is one of lower BP targets being associated with more effective renoprotection among those with more severe proteinuria. These observations have led to a consensus that BP should be lowered to less than 130/80 mm Hg in all patients with diabetic or proteinuric CKD and less than 140/90 mm Hg in patients without these risk factors,[637] although lower targets should be considered to optimize cardiovascular risk reduction in patients not judged to be at high risk of adverse effects from intensive BP lowering.

## DIETARY PROTEIN INTAKE

Increased dietary protein intake and intravenous protein loading in animals or humans with intact kidneys are associated with increases in renal mass, RBF, and GFR, as well as a decrease in renal vascular resistance. The magnitude of the increases in the GFR and RBF in response to a protein load is a function of renal reserve. In patients with a reduced GFR, some studies have shown that the percentage increase in the GFR in response to a protein meal is reduced in those with a lower baseline GFR,.[638] In contrast, a study comparing the renal response to an oral protein load in patients with moderate and advanced CKD found a similar percentage increase in the GFR over baseline in both groups, demonstrating that even with advanced renal disease, some renal reserve is still present, and that elevated intake of dietary protein may have undesirable effects on glomerular hemodynamics at all levels of renal function.[639]

To understand the mechanisms whereby protein loading acutely augments renal function, various components of protein diets have been examined individually. The administration of equivalent quantities of urea, sulfate, acid, and vegetable protein to dogs or humans all failed to reproduce a meat protein–induced rise in the GFR.[640–642] In contrast, feeding or infusion of mixed or individual amino acids (e.g., glycine, L-arginine) was shown to effect increases in the GFR of similar magnitude to those seen with meat ingestion.[643,644] Micropuncture experiments have demonstrated that amino acid infusion results in increases in glomerular plasma flow and transcapillary hydraulic pressure difference, thereby raising SNGFR without affecting the ultrafiltration coefficient.[643] Interestingly, however, perfusion of the isolated kidney with an amino acid mixture resulted in only a modest increase in the GFR.[645]

Taken together, these observations suggest that amino acids themselves do not have a major direct effect on renal hemodynamics, but their effects appear to be mediated by an intermediate compound generated only in the intact organism. Glucagon, the secretion of which is stimulated by protein feeding, has been proposed as such a mediator. The GFR and renal blood flow increase in response to glucagon infusion in dogs.[644] Furthermore, administration of the glucagon antagonist, somatostatin, consistently blocks amino acid–induced augmentation in renal function both in humans and rats.[643,646] Large protein meals are also rich in minerals, potassium, phosphate, and acids. Indeed, after feeding a protein meal to dogs, the excretions of sodium, potassium, phosphorus, and urea were found to increase in parallel to the increase in the GFR.[640] On the other hand, sodium chloride reabsorption in the proximal tubule and loop of Henle was found to be increased in rats maintained on a high-protein diet.[647] As result, less sodium and chloride would be delivered to the macula densa, thereby inhibiting tubuloglomerular feedback and adding a further stimulus to glomerular hyperperfusion. Because dietary protein does not affect systemic BP,[643] other factors have been suggested to contribute to the renal hemodynamic changes following a protein load. Administration of the nitric oxide inhibitor L-NMMA or nonsteroidal antiinflammatory drugs (NSAIDs) have been shown to blunt the renal hyperemic response to an oral protein load in both rats and humans, invoking a role for nitric oxide and PGs.[647,648] In addition, Ang II and ET have been proposed as mediators of protein-induced renal injury because low-protein diets have been shown to reduce renal ET-1, ET receptors A and B, and $AT_1$ receptor mRNA expression in PAN-injected and normal rats.[649,650]

It has been proposed that the augmented renal function induced by dietary protein may be an evolutionary adaptation of the kidney to the intermittent heavy protein intake of the hunter-gatherer.[4] Renal hyperfunction following a protein load would serve to facilitate excretion of the waste products of protein catabolism and other dietary components, thereby achieving homeostasis in the presence of an abrupt increase in consumption in times of nutritional plenty; the subsequent decline of the GFR to baseline during the intervals between meals would then favor mechanisms suited to conservation of fluid and electrolytes in times of scarcity. Persistent renal hyperfunction due to continuous excessive protein intake, however, leads to renal injury in experimental models. Laboratory animals with intact kidneys and ingesting food ad libitum become proteinuric and develop glomerulosclerosis with age.[4,196,651] This progression is significantly attenuated by feeding animals on alternate days only.[196]

Furthermore, aging rats fed a high-protein diet ad libitum showed accelerated and more severe renal injury compared with rats receiving a normal protein diet, whereas rats fed a low-protein diet were protected from renal injury.[651] Similarly, in diabetic rats, progression of nephropathy was markedly accelerated in the setting of a high-protein diet and substantially attenuated by a low-protein diet.[254] In this study, kidney weight in high-protein-diet-fed diabetic rats was significantly greater than in diabetic rats receiving normal protein diets, suggesting that protein-induced renal hypertrophy may itself contribute to acceleration of renal functional deterioration. As discussed earlier, the renoprotective effects of dietary protein restriction in experimental animals are associated with virtual normalization of $P_{GC}$ and SNGFR.[9]

Despite unambiguous evidence from experimental studies, confirmation of a beneficial effect of dietary protein restriction in clinical trials has proved elusive. Several small studies generally have suggested a beneficial effect from protein restriction, but suffered from deficiencies in design or patient compliance. A large, multicenter randomized study, the MDRD study, was therefore conducted to resolve the issue.[622] In this study, 585 patients with moderate chronic renal failure (GFR = 25–55 mL/min/1.73 m$^2$) were randomized to a usual (1.3 g/kg/day) or low (0.58 g/kg/day) protein diet (LPD; study 1), and 255 patients with severe chronic renal failure (GFR = 13–24 mL/min/1.73 m$^2$) were randomized to a to low (0.58 g/kg/day) or very low (0.28 g/kg/day) protein diet (VLPD; study 2), supplemented with keto–amino acids to prevent malnutrition. All causes of CKD were included, but patients with diabetes mellitus requiring insulin therapy were excluded. Patients were also assigned to different levels of BP control. After a mean of a 2.2-year follow-up, the primary analysis revealed no difference in the mean rate of GFR decline in study 1 and only a trend toward a slower rate of decline in the VLPD group in study 2.

Secondary analyses of the MDRD data, however, revealed that dietary protein restriction probably did achieve beneficial effects. In study 1, a LPD was associated with an initial reduction in the GFR that likely resulted from the functional effects of decreased protein intake and not from loss of nephrons. This initial reduction in the GFR obscured a later reduction in the rate of the GFR decline that was evident after 4 months in the LPD group, which may have resulted in more robust evidence of renoprotection had follow-up been continued for a longer period.[652] Disappointingly, long-term follow-up of 255 participants in study 2 of the MDRD trial found no renoprotective benefit associated with randomization to a VLPD in the original study but did report a higher risk of death in this group (HR, 1.92; 95% CI, 1.15–3.20).[653] In a more recent trial, 207 well-nourished persons without diabetes and with eGFR less than 30 mL/min/1.73 m$^2$ and urine PCR less than 1 g/g were randomized to a vegetarian VLPD (<0.3 g/kg/day) with ketoanalogue supplementation (ketoanalogue diet, KD) or a standard (nonvegetarian) LPD (<0.6 g/kg/day). After 15 months, the primary outcome of renal replacement therapy (RRT) or 50% reduction in eGFR was reached in 13% of those on a KD versus 42% of those on a LPD (adjusted HR 0.1; 95% CI, 0.05–0.2). Those on the KD also showed a 3.2-mL/min/year slower rate of eGFR decline. Metabolic factors were also improved by the KD; serum bicarbonate and calcium levels were higher and phosphate levels lower. There was no change in nutritional status in either group, and no adverse reactions were reported.[654]

Despite inconclusive findings in several of the individual studies, three metaanalyses have each concluded that dietary protein restriction is associated with a reduced risk of ESKD (odds ratio [OR] of 0.62 and 0.67, respectively)[655,656] as well as a modest reduction in the rate of eGFR decline (0.53 mL/min/1.73 $m^2$ per year).[657] A further recent metaanalysis included 16 randomized controlled trials (RCTs) of persons with relatively advanced CKD.(stages 4 and 5 in most cases). In studies comparing an LPD (<0.8 g/day) with higher protein intake, an LPD was associated with a small but significant absolute risk reduction for ESKD (4%) and higher serum bicarbonate level at 1 year (weighted mean difference 1.46 mEq/L) versus higher protein diets. Similarly, in studies comparing a VLPD to LPD, a VLPD was associated with an absolute risk reduction for ESKD (13%) and higher GFR at 1 year (weighted mean difference, 3.95 mL/min/1.73 $m^2$) versus LPD. No studies reported an increased risk of protein energy wasting or other safety concerns associated with dietary protein restriction.[658] An important caveat to these findings is that the proportion of the participants treated with RAAS inhibitors was variable. Although evidence suggests that LPD and RAAS inhibitors may have synergistic renoprotective effects, this has not yet been adequately evaluated in RCTs.

In summary, there is evidence from some small trials and several metaanalyses that dietary protein restriction may slow the progression of human CKD, particularly in more advanced and proteinuric disease. Whereas the renoprotective benefit appears modest, such dietary restriction is associated with other benefits, including improvement in acidosis, as well as a reduction in the phosphorus and potassium load. Thus comprehensive dietary intervention with a moderate restriction in dietary protein intake should be considered as part of the management of persons with CKD.[659] The potential benefit of VLPDs in advanced CKD requires further evaluation in RCTs. The role of dietary intervention in the management of CKD is discussed further in Chapter 60.

## GENDER DIFFERENCES

Laboratory studies have indicated that male animals appear to be at greater risk of developing renal disease and disease progression than females. Age-associated glomerulosclerosis is much more pronounced in male than in female rats, and it is notable that the male propensity for age-related glomerulosclerosis can be prevented by castration.[660] This gender difference was found to be independent of $P_{GC}$ or glomerular hypertrophy, suggesting a role for the sex hormones as modulators of renal injury. Ovariectomy had no effect on the development of glomerular injury in some animal models[660,661] but did accelerate progression in glomerulosclerosis-prone mice.[662]

In contrast, in the hypercholesterolemic Imai rat, the development of spontaneous glomerulosclerosis in males can be significantly reduced by castration or by the administration of exogenous estrogens.[663,664] These data suggest an important role for androgens in the development of renal injury and raise the possibility that estrogens may, to some extent, counteract the adverse effects of androgens. In an apparently conflicting observation, female Nagase analbuminemic rats developed more severe renal injury than males, a characteristic that is ameliorated by ovariectomy.[665] These rats may be unique, however, in that triglyceride levels, which are higher in females, may have an independent and overriding effect on renal disease propensity. Glomerulosclerosis also develops to a significantly greater extent in male versus female rats subjected to extensive renal ablation.[666] This difference was independent of BP and glomerular hypertrophy, but the degree of glomerulosclerosis and the extent of mesangial expansion were each found to correlate significantly with an increased expression of glomerular procollagen $\alpha_1$(IV) mRNA in males. Similarly, in aging Munich-Wistar rats, glomerular metalloproteinase activity was found to decrease with age in males but not in females or castrated rats, suggesting that suppression of metalloproteinase activity by androgens could account for the gender difference in disease susceptibility.[667] Finally, estrogens, but not androgens, possess antioxidant activity and have been shown to inhibit mesangial cell LDL oxidation,[668] a property that may contribute to renoprotection.

Clinical studies have suggest that a gender difference with respect to CKD progression also exists in humans. Data from the US Renal Data System (USRDS) have shown a substantially higher incidence of ESKD among males (413/million population in 2003) versus females (280/million population),[669] and several studies have reported worse renal outcomes in males. In a Japanese community-based mass screening program, the risk of developing ESKD (if baseline serum creatinine level was >1.2 mg/dL for males or >1 mg/dL for females) was almost 50% higher in men than in women.[670] In a large population-based study in the United States, male gender was associated with a significantly increased risk of ESKD or death associated with CKD.[613] Similarly, in France, studies of factors influencing the development of ESKD in patients with moderate and severe renal disease found that disease progression was accelerated in males versus females, especially in those with chronic glomerulonephritis or autosomal dominant polycystic kidney disease (ADPKD). Furthermore, the effect of hypertension as a risk factor for CKD progression appeared to be greater in males.[671,672] Other studies of patients with CKD have reported a lower risk of ESKD among females with CKD stage 3[673] and a shorter time to RRT among males with CKD stages 4 and 5.[674]

One metaanalysis of 68 studies that included 11,345 persons with CKD has reported a higher rate of decline of renal function in men,[675] but another metaanalysis of individual participant data from 11 randomized trials evaluating the efficacy of ACE inhibitor treatment in CKD did not show an increased risk of doubling the serum creatinine level or ESKD or ESKD alone in men.[676] On the contrary, after adjustment for baseline variables, including BP and urinary protein excretion, women had a significantly higher risk of these endpoints than men.[676] One limitation of these studies is that the menopausal status of the women was often not documented. Interestingly in one study, bilateral oophorectomy in 1653 premenopausal women was associated with a higher risk of developing CKD (defined by eGFR<60 mL/min/1.73 $m^2$ on two occasions >90 days apart) over a median of 14 years of observation when compared with age-matched women who did not undergo oophorectomy (adjusted HR, 1.42; 95% CI, 1.14–1.77; absolute risk increase, 6.6%).[677]

In general, the prevalence of hypertension and uncontrolled hypertension is higher among men. Men tend to consume more protein than women; the prevalence of dyslipidemias is greater in men than premenopausal women.

All these factors may contribute to the increased severity of renal disease observed in men but do not explain all the differences.[678,679] A recent review has also highlighted that disparities in access to health care between men and women in many regions may contribute to the observed differences in outcomes.[680] The impact of gender differences on the epidemiology of kidney disease is reviewed in more detail in Chapter 19.

## NEPHRON ENDOWMENT

Experimental and clinical studies have shown that the number of nephrons per kidney is variable and may be influenced by several factors during development in utero. Furthermore low nephron endowment predisposes individuals to hypertension and CKD. This has been confirmed in studies using a rat model of spontaneous renal agenesis. Rats born with a single kidney had 19% fewer nephrons per kidney than their two-kidney littermates, resulting in a 60.2% reduction in nephron endowment that was associated with subsequent renal and glomerular hypertrophy, proteinuria, glomerular sclerosis, and TIF.[341] It has been proposed that reduced nephron endowment results in an increase in the single-nephron GFR and therefore a reduction in renal reserve.[681] Whereas the glomerular hemodynamic changes associated with mild to moderate congenital nephron deficiencies may not in themselves be sufficient to provoke renal injury, they could be predicted to compound the effects of an acquired nephron loss and predispose an individual to progressive renal damage. Thus CKD should be viewed as a multihit process, in which the first hit may be reduced nephron endowment.[682] The impact of developmental programming on nephron endowment, BP, and kidney function is discussed in detail in Chapter 21.

## RACE AND ETHNICITY

Data from the USRDS have shown a substantially higher incidence of ESKD among African Americans, Hispanics, and Native Americans versus Caucasians. In 2015, the adjusted ESKD incidence rate ratios for Native Hawaiians/Pacific Islanders, African Americans, Native Americans/Alaska Natives, and Asians as compared with Caucasians were 8.4, 3.0, 1.2, and 1.0, respectively. Interestingly, these represent reductions in the relative risk of ESKD for these minorities compared with Caucasians over the past 15 years (Fig. 51.12). The rate ratio for Hispanics versus non-Hispanics was 1.3. Similarly, in 2015, the prevalence of ESKD per million population (pmp) was 14,448 among Native Hawaiians/Pacific Islanders, 5705 among African Americans, 2315 among Native Americans/Alaska Natives, 1905 among Asians, and 1519 among Caucasians.[683] The reasons for these obvious discrepancies are complex and include both social and biologic factors.[684,685] Interestingly, data from the Reasons for Geographic and Racial Differences in Stroke (REGARDS) Cohort Study have shown a lower prevalence of eGFR 50 to 59 mL/min/1.73 m$^2$, among African American versus Caucasian subjects but a higher prevalence of eGFR, 10 to 19 mL/min/1.73 m$^2$, suggesting that African Americans have a lower risk of developing CKD but a higher risk of progression of CKD to ESKD.[686]

African Americans appear to be more susceptible to FSGS. One retrospective analysis of 340 routine kidney biopsies

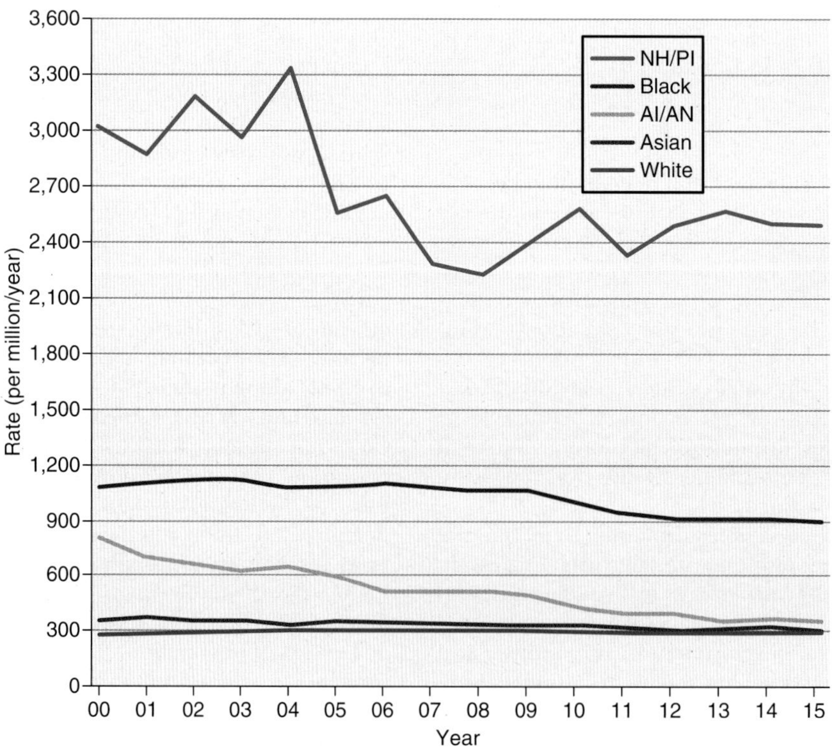


**Fig. 51.12** Trends in adjusted incidence rate of end-stage kidney disease (ESKD), by race, in the US population, 2000–2015. *AI/AN,* American Indian/Alaska Native; *NH/PI,* Native Hawaiian/Pacific Islander. (From the US Renal Data System. Annual Data Report 2017, Chapter 1: Incidence, Prevalence, Patient Characteristics, and Treatment Modalities. https://www.usrds.org/2017.)

has detected a significantly higher prevalence of FSGS and a significantly lower prevalence of membranous glomerulonephritis, IgA, and immunotactoid nephropathies among African American versus Caucasian patients.[687] Similarly, among pediatric transplant recipients, a higher proportion of African American and Hispanic children had FSGS as a primary diagnosis versus Caucasians.[688] The same investigators found that despite similar treatment modalities and similar durations of nephrotic syndrome, African American children with FSGS reached ESKD almost twice as frequently as Caucasian children.[688]

More significant in terms of patient numbers and morbidity, however, are the racial discrepancies in the incidence of ESKD due to hypertensive and diabetic nephropathies. One longitudinal study that examined data from 1,306,825 Medicare beneficiaries has reported substantially increased risks of developing ESKD in African American versus Caucasian participants in all categories—among persons with diabetes, a 2.4- to 2.7-fold increase; among hypertensive persons, a 2.5- to 2.9-fold increase; and among persons with neither hypertension or diabetes, a 3.5-fold increase.[689] MDRD study data showed the prevalence of hypertension to be higher in African Americans versus Caucasians among persons with CKD, despite a higher mean GFR in the African American participants.[679] Hypertensive persons were found to have had more rapid progression of renal disease prior to entry into the study, suggesting that the higher prevalence of hypertension in African American patients is likely to be a significant contributor to the accelerated progression of CKD. On the other hand, both higher MAP and African American race/ethnicity were independent predictors of a faster decline in the GFR in the MDRD study.[690]

In a large community-based epidemiologic study, African Americans were found to have a 5.6 times higher unadjusted incidence of hypertensive ESKD.[691] This increased incidence was directly related to the prevalence of hypertension, severe hypertension, and diabetes in the study population and was inversely related to age at diagnosis of hypertension and socioeconomic status. After adjustment for these factors, the risk of hypertensive ESKD remained 4.5 times greater among African Americans compared with Caucasians, providing further evidence that African Americans have an increased susceptibility to renal disease beyond that attributable to their increased prevalence of hypertension and diabetes. Salt-sensitive hypertension, in particular, is more prevalent in the African American population than in the Caucasian population.[692] Comparing renal responses to a high sodium intake in salt-sensitive versus salt-resistant persons, RBF was found to decrease in the presence of an increased filtration fraction (implying an increased $P_{GC}$) in salt-sensitive patients, whereas the converse occurred in salt-resistant patients.[609]

These observations are consistent with the notion that salt loading injures the glomerulus through glomerular capillary hypertension and that salt-sensitive individuals, and African American subjects in particular, are at added risk of this form of injury. The incidence of ESKD due to diabetic nephropathy is fourfold higher in African Americans than among Caucasian Americans.[693] It is notable that after controlling for the higher prevalence of diabetes and hypertension, as well as age, socioeconomic status, and access to health care, the excess incidence of ESKD due to diabetes in African Americans versus Caucasians was confined to type 2 diabetics.[694] Among type 1 diabetics, African Americans were not found to be at higher risk than Caucasians. Indeed, most African Americans with diabetic ESKD (77%) had type 2 diabetes, whereas most Caucasians with diabetic ESKD (58%) had type 1 diabetes.[695] African American race/ethnicity was also found to be associated with a threefold higher risk of early renal function decline (increase in serum creatinine of ≥0.4 mg/dL) among adults with diabetes.[696]

Several potential factors contributing to the different prevalence and severity of renal disease among population groups have been analyzed. Adjustment for socioeconomic factors reduces, but does not eliminate, the increased risk of African Americans to develop ESKD.[685,693,696] African Americans generally have lower birth weights than their Caucasian counterparts and may therefore have programmed or genetically determined deficits in nephron number, rendering them more susceptible to hypertension and subsequent ESKD.[697,698] Finally, 40% of African American patients with hypertensive ESKD and 35% with type 2 diabetes-associated ESKD have a first-, second-, or third-degree relative with ESKD, implying a strong familial susceptibility to ESKD and therefore a genetic predisposition.[699]

Evidence of a genetic explanation for the high incidence of ESKD observed in African Americans was provided by research that identified a strong association between ESKD and two coding variants of the gene for apolipoprotein L1 (*APOL1*).[700] These gene variants confer resistance to infection with *Trypanosoma brucei rhodesiense*, which causes sleeping sickness, providing an explanation for how selection likely resulted in a high prevalence of these variants in the population.[701] Subsequent studies have identified associations between *APOL1* risk variants and several renal pathologies, including FSGS, HIV-associated nephropathy (HIVAN), sickle cell kidney disease, and severe lupus nephritis. *APOL1* risk variants have also been associated with HIVAN in black South Africans.[702] Moreover, cohort studies have reported associations between *APOL1* risk variants and the risk of progression to ESKD. The risk of progression was the lowest in European Americans (with no risk variants), intermediate in African Americans with no or one risk variant, and highest in African Americans with two risk variants.[703] It is estimated that *APOL1* variants account for 40% of disease burden due to CKD in African Americans.

The biologic role of *APOL1* in the progression of CKD remains to be fully elucidated. Expression of the *APOL1* risk variants in divergent species, *Drosophila* and *Saccharomyces* (a yeast), has identified impairment of conserved core intracellular endosomal trafficking processes as a key mechanism of cellular injury.[704] The APOL1 protein is expressed in the kidney but is also secreted and is bound to circulating HDL particles. Current evidence suggests that it is the locally expressed form of APOL1 that is involved in CKD pathogenesis.[705] Despite the strong association between the inheritance of two *APOL1* risk variants and ESKD, only a minority of people with this genotype actually develop kidney disease, suggesting that the action of a second factor is required to cause disease in genetically susceptible individuals. HIV is one example of such a second hit, but it has been proposed that other viruses and other gene variants may also be important.[701]

Other ethnic and racial minority groups, including Asians,[617,706] Hispanics,[707] Native Americans,[708] Mexican

Americans,[709] and Australian Aborigines,[710] have also been found to be at increased risk of developing CKD and ESKD. See Chapter 19 for a further discussion of ethnicity and the epidemiology of CKD and Chapters 43 and 44 for a detailed discussion of genetic factors in the pathogenesis of CKD.

## OBESITY AND METABOLIC SYNDROME

Obesity may directly cause a glomerulopathy characterized by proteinuria and histologic features of focal and segmental glomerulosclerosis,[711] but it is likely that it also exacerbates the progression of other forms of CKD. Micropuncture studies have confirmed that obesity is another cause of glomerular hypertension and hyperfiltration that may contribute to the progression of CKD.[712,713] Griffin and colleagues have pointed out that whereas obesity is widespread, only a minority of obese individuals develop obesity-related glomerulopathy.[714] They have proposed that low nephron endowment (associated with low birth weight, which is also associated with an increased risk of later life obesity) or acquired nephron loss constitute a necessary additional factor that increases glomerular hypertrophy and preglomerular vasodilation and transmission of elevated systemic BP to the glomerulus, leading to glomerulosclerosis. A detailed investigation of adipocyte function has revealed that they are not merely storage cells but produce a variety of hormones and proinflammatory molecules that may contribute to progressive renal damage.[715,716] In addition, adiponectin, an adipokine produced by adipocytes, may exert a protective effect on podocyte function. Adiponectin levels are reduced in obesity and are inversely correlated with the magnitude of albuminuria.[717] Moreover, adiponectin knockout mice develop albuminuria associated with podocyte foot process effacement that is corrected by the administration of exogenous adiponectin.[718]

Obesity is also associated with increased production of aldosterone and expanded extracellular volume, both of which may contribute to progressive renal damage.[719]

In humans, severe obesity is associated with increased renal plasma flow, glomerular hyperfiltration, and albuminuria, abnormalities that are reversed by weight loss.[720] Several large population-based studies have identified obesity as an independent risk factor for developing CKD,[614,721] and one study has found a progressive increase in relative risk (RR) of developing ESKD associated with increasing body mass index (BMI; RR, 3.57; 95% CI, 3.05–4.18 for BMI 30.0–34.9 kg/m$^2$ vs. BMI 18.5–24.9 kg/m$^2$) among 320,252 subjects with no evidence of CKD at initial screening.[722]

On the other hand, analysis of data from the Framingham Heart Study has confirmed an increased risk of developing CKD stage 3 associated with obesity but found that this was no longer significant after adjustment for known cardiovascular risk factors. Nevertheless, the increased risk of incident proteinuria persisted in multivariable models.[723]

Change in body weight has also been identified as a risk factor for incident CKD. In one study of 8792 previously healthy men, an increase in body weight of 0.75 or more kg/year (and a decrease of <0.75 kg/year) was associated with an increased risk of developing CKD in previously obese and nonobese subjects.[724] The metabolic syndrome (insulin resistance) defined by the presence of abdominal obesity, dyslipidemia, hypertension, and fasting hyperglycemia is also associated with an increased risk of developing CKD. Analysis of the Third National Health and Nutrition Examination Survey (NHANES) data has revealed a significantly increased risk of CKD and microalbuminuria in subjects with the metabolic syndrome, as well as a progressive increase in risk associated with the number of components of the metabolic syndrome present.[725] Furthermore, a longitudinal study of 10,096 patients without diabetes or CKD at baseline has identified metabolic syndrome as an independent risk factor for the development of CKD over 9 years (adjusted OR, 1.43; 95% CI, 1.18–1.73). Again, there was a progressive increase in risk associated with the number of traits of the metabolic syndrome present (OR, 1.13; 95% CI, 0.89–1.45 for one trait versus OR, 2.45; 95% CI, 1.32–4.54 for five traits).[726] The metabolic syndrome has also been identified as a risk factor for incident CKD among Native Americans[727] and in Taiwan.[728] The waist-hip ratio (WHR), a marker of central fat distribution and insulin resistance, was independently associated with impaired renal function, even in lean individuals (BMI <25 kg/m$^2$) among a population-based cohort of 7676 subjects.[729] Furthermore, analysis of data from the Atherosclerosis Risk in Communities (ARIC) study has found that WHR but not BMI is associated with an increased risk of incident CKD and mortality,[730] suggesting that accumulation of visceral fat is more important as a risk factor than obesity per se.

The effect of obesity on progression in cohorts of patients with established CKD has been less well documented. In one study, increased BMI was an independent predictor of CKD progression among 162 patients with IgA nephropathy,[731] and BMI was independently associated with more rapid CKD progression in a cohort of CKD subjects (predominantly CKD stage 3).[732] On the other hand, obesity may be less relevant for progression in more advanced stages of CKD, as evidenced by the observation that BMI was unrelated to the risk of ESKD among a cohort of patients with CKD stages 4 and 5.[674] The association of obesity with CKD and increased risk of CKD progression suggests that weight loss may represent an important intervention for achieving renoprotection. Sustained weight loss is notoriously difficult to achieve, but a metaanalysis of several small, short-duration studies has found that weight loss achieved through diet or medication is associated with a reduction in proteinuria and BP. Surgical procedures to achieve weight loss in the morbidly obese were associated with normalization of glomerular hyperfiltration and reductions in microalbuminuria and BP.[733] A more recent systematic review has analyzed the effects of weight loss achieved by bariatric surgery, medication, or diet in 31 studies and found that in most studies, weight loss is associated with reductions in proteinuria. In people with glomerular hyperfiltration, the GFR tended to decrease with weight loss and, in those with a reduced GFR, it tended to increase.[734]

> ***Clinical Relevance***
> **Obesity and Metabolic Syndrome**
>
> Weight loss, because it is difficult to achieve, is an underutilized intervention to improve renoprotection. Nevertheless, available evidence indicates that in persons with obesity, weight loss affords renoprotection. In persons with severe obesity who are unable to achieve adequate weight loss with diet and exercise, bariatric surgery should be considered.

The increasing use of bariatric surgery to manage obesity has allowed investigation of the impact of surgically induced weight loss on CKD. In a long-term study of 2144 persons who underwent bariatric surgery, change in CKD risk category, as defined by the KDIGO classification, was assessed after 7 years. Among those with moderate risk at baseline, the risk category improved in 53% and deteriorated in 5% to 8%, in the high-risk group, improvement was observed in 56% and deterioration in 3% to 10%, and, in the very-high-risk group, 23% improved. The eGFR initially improved, with a peak at 2 years, and then gradually declined. Albuminuria showed large and sustained decreases in the moderate- (median urine ACR decreased from 48 to 14 mg/g) and high-risk groups (median urine ACR decreased from 326 to 26 mg/g).[735]

In another study comparing outcomes in persons with CKD stages 3 and 4 undergoing bariatric surgery with similarly obese propensity-matched persons who did not undergo surgery, the eGFR was significantly higher in the surgery group after 3 years by a mean of 9.84 mL/min/1.73 m$^2$.[736] In a metaanalysis that included 23 cohort studies and 3015 persons who underwent all forms of bariatric surgery, small but statistically significant improvements were observed in serum creatinine levels (mean decrease, 0.08 mg/dL) and proteinuria (mean decrease, 0.04 g/day).[737] Obesity therefore appears to be a modifiable risk factor for CKD progression.

## SYMPATHETIC NERVOUS SYSTEM

Overactivity of the sympathetic nervous system has been observed in patients with CKD, and several lines of evidence have suggested that this may be a factor contributing to progressive renal injury.[738] The kidneys are richly supplied with afferent sensory, and efferent sympathetic innervation and may therefore act as both a source and target of sympathetic activation. That the former is true has been suggested by a study that compared postganglionic sympathetic nerve activity (SNA) measured via microelectrodes in the peroneal nerve in normal individuals and hemodialysis patients who retained their native kidneys with those who had undergone bilateral nephrectomy.[739] SNA was 2.5 times higher in non-nephrectomized dialysis patients compared with both normals and nephrectomized patients in whom SNA was similar. Furthermore, increased SNA was associated with increased vascular tone and mean arterial BP in nonnephrectomized patients. SNA did not vary as a function of age, BP, antihypertensive agents, or body fluid status. The authors speculated that intrarenal accumulation of uremic compounds stimulates renal afferent nerves via chemoreceptors, leading to reflex activation of efferent sympathetic nerves and increased SNA. Other studies, however, have observed increased SNA in the absence of uremia in patients with renovascular disease,[740] hypertensive ADPKD,[741] and nondiabetic CKD[742] or increased noradrenaline secretion in patients with nephrotic syndrome[743] and ADPKD.[741,744] Furthermore, correction of uremia by renal transplantation does not abrogate the increased SNA.[745] Interestingly, investigation of eight living kidney donors found no increase in SNA after donor nephrectomy, suggesting that the rise in SNA is related to renal damage rather than nephron loss.[742]

Together, these findings suggest that that a variety of forms of renal injury may provoke increased SNA and that uremia is not required for this response. Evidence from experimental studies has indicated that sympathetic overactivity resulting from renal disease may also accelerate renal injury. Ablation of afferent sensory signals from the kidneys by bilateral dorsal rhizotomy in 5/6 nephrectomized rats prevented the expected rise in systemic BP, attenuated the rise in serum creatinine levels, and reduced the severity of glomerulosclerosis in the remnant kidneys when compared with sham rhizotomized controls.[746] Moreover, the renoprotective effects of rhizotomy were found to be additive to that of ACE inhibitor treatment.[747]

To investigate further whether the benefits of rhizotomy were solely attributable to the prevention of hypertension, 5/6 nephrectomized rats were treated with nonhypotensive doses of the sympatholytic drug moxonidine.[748] Despite the lack of effect on BP, moxonidine treatment was associated with lower levels of proteinuria and less severe glomerulosclerosis in treated compared with untreated rats. In a similar study, 5/6 nephrectomized rats were treated with the alpha blocker phenoxybenzamine, the beta blocker metoprolol, or a combination.[749] As in the previous study, the doses used did not lower BP, but all three treatments significantly lowered albuminuria and almost normalized the reductions in capillary length density (an index of glomerular capillary obliteration) and podocyte number. Metoprolol and combination therapy significantly lowered the glomerulosclerosis index versus untreated controls. Taken together, these results indicate that increased SNA accelerates renal injury independently of its effect on BP and that the adverse effects are mediated by catecholamines.[750] Furthermore, sympathetic nerve overactivity has been proposed to contribute to the development of tubulointerstitial injury by reducing peritubular capillary perfusion to the extent that tubular and interstitial ischemia result.[751]

Preliminary evidence has suggested that sympathetic overactivity may also be important in the progression of human CKD. Among patients with type 1 diabetes mellitus and proteinuria, evidence of parasympathetic dysfunction—which permits unopposed sympathetic tone—was associated with an increase in serum creatinine levels over the next 12 months.[752] Analysis of data from the Atherosclerosis Risk in Communities (ARIC) study has found that a higher resting heart rate and reduced heart rate variability, markers of autonomic dysfunction, are each independently associated with an increased risk of developing ESKD or a CKD-related hospital admission during 16 years of follow-up.[753] Several drug treatments may improve sympathetic overactivity in CKD patients. Among 15 normotensive type 1 diabetics, 3 weeks of treatment with moxonidine significantly lowered albumin excretion rates without affecting BP.[754] In other studies, chronic treatment with an ACE inhibitor or ARB, of proven benefit in renoprotection, was associated with reduction but not normalization of sympathetic overactivity.[755–757] In contrast, treatment with amlodipine was associated with increased SNA. Because ACE inhibitors and ARBs do not readily enter the central nervous system (CNS), it is possible that RAAS inhibition modulates neurotransmitter release in the kidney and reduces afferent signaling.

Finally, renal denervation achieved by radiofrequency catheter ablation through the renal artery has been proposed as an intervention to treat resistant hypertension and possibly slow CKD progression. Following several small studies that reported reductions in BP following renal denervation, a large randomized trial was undertaken in which 535 participants were randomly assigned to renal denervation or a sham procedure. After 6 months, a significant reduction in office BP was observed in both groups, but there was no difference between groups. There was also no difference in 24-hour ambulatory BP between groups.[758]

Several questions remain to be answered regarding the role of increased SNA in CKD progression. Whereas the renoprotective effects of sympatholytic drugs appear to be independent of effects on systemic BP, it is as yet unknown what effect they have on glomerular hemodynamics. Further studies are also required to determine the extent to which chronic inhibition of sympathetic overactivity may be beneficial in a variety of forms of human CKD and whether this benefit is additive to that derived from inhibition of the RAAS.

## DYSLIPIDEMIA

Moorhead and colleagues advanced the hypothesis that abnormalities in lipid metabolism may contribute to the progression of CKD.[759] Glomerular injury, accompanied by an alteration in basement membrane permeability, was envisaged as the initiator of a vicious cycle of hyperlipidemia and progressive glomerular injury. They proposed that urinary losses of albumin and lipoprotein lipase activators result in an increase in circulating LDLs, which in turn bind to the glomerular basement membrane, further impairing its permselectivity. Filtered lipoproteins accumulate in the mesangium, stimulating extracellular matrix synthesis and mesangial cell proliferation; filtered LDL is taken up and metabolized by the tubules, leading to cell injury and interstitial disease. Notably, this hypothesis did not propose hyperlipidemia as an initiating factor in renal injury, but rather as a participant in a self-sustaining mechanism of disease progression.

Several lines of experimental evidence have confirmed the association between dyslipidemia and renal injury. Both intact and uninephrectomized rats with dietary-induced hypercholesterolemia developed more extensive glomerulosclerosis than their normocholesterolemic controls, and the severity of glomerulosclerosis correlated with serum cholesterol levels[760]; aging female Nagase analbuminemic rats (NARs) have endogenous hypertriglyceridemia and hypercholesterolemia and develop proteinuria and glomerulosclerosis by 9 and 18 months of age, respectively, whereas male NARs have lower lipid levels and no glomerulosclerosis by 22 months of age.[665] Interestingly, ovariectomy in female NARs lowers triglyceride levels and reduces their renal injury. In seeming contradiction, however, young and aging male Sprague-Dawley rats developed more extensive glomerulosclerosis than age- and gender-matched NARs, despite higher cholesterol levels in the NARs.[761] Triglyceride levels, however, were lower in the NARs, again suggesting an independent role for triglycerides in lipid-mediated renal injury.

Whereas data regarding the role of lipids in initiating renal disease are conflicting, several studies have supported the notion that dyslipidemia may promote renal damage. Cholesterol feeding has been shown to exacerbate glomerulosclerosis in uninephrectomized rats, prediabetic rabbits, rats with puromycin aminonucleoside nephropathy, and in the unclipped kidney of rats with two-kidney, one-clip (2-K,1C) hypertension. When hypertension and dyslipidemia are superimposed, a synergistic effect that dramatically accelerates renal functional deterioration is observed.[762,763] In the 5/6 nephrectomy model, progressive renal damage is associated with renal tissue accumulation of lipids as well as upregulation of pathways involved in the tubular reabsorption of protein-bound lipids and downregulation of pathways involved in lipid catabolism.[764]

In humans, the role of lipids in the initiation and progression of renal disease remains unclear. At autopsy, a highly significant correlation was found between the presence of systemic atherosclerosis and the percentage of sclerotic glomeruli in normal individuals, fostering speculation that the development of glomerulosclerosis may be analogous to that of atherosclerosis.[765] A study designed to identify the clinical correlates of hypertensive ESKD has found a strong association between atherosclerosis and hypertensive ESKD among older Caucasian patients.[766] Furthermore, dyslipidemia has been identified in several large studies as a risk factor for the subsequent development of CKD in apparently healthy individuals.[614,767,768] The common forms of primary hypercholesterolemia are not associated with an increased incidence of renal disease in the general population, but renal injury has been described in association with rare inherited disorders of lipoprotein metabolism.[769,770]

Whereas primary lipid-mediated renal injury is rare among patients with CKD, the latter is frequently accompanied by elevations in serum lipid levels as a result of urinary loss of albumin and lipoprotein lipase activators, defective clearance of triglycerides, modification of LDLs by advanced glycation end products, reduced plasma oncotic pressure, adverse effects of medication, and underlying systemic diseases.[771,772] Among a cohort of adult patients with CKD, the most frequent lipid abnormalities noted were hypertriglyceridemia, low HDL levels, and increased apolipoprotein levels.[773] Furthermore, in a study of 631 routine renal biopsies, lipid deposits were detected in nonsclerotic glomeruli in 8.4% of kidneys, and staining for apolipoprotein B was positive in approximately 25% of biopsies, suggesting that lipid deposition is not infrequent in diverse renal diseases.[404] Several epidemiologic studies have found a strong association between CKD progression and dyslipidemia.

- In the MDRD study, low serum HDL cholesterol was found to be an independent predictor of more rapid rates of decline in the GFR.[774]
- Elevated total cholesterol, LDL cholesterol, and apolipoprotein B have been found to correlate strongly with the GFR decline in CKD patients.[775]
- Hypercholesterolemia was shown to be a predictor of loss of renal function in type 1 and 2 diabetes.[776,777]
- Among nondiabetic patients, CKD advanced more rapidly in patients with hypercholesterolemia and hypertriglyceridemia, independently of BP control.[778]
- Among patients with IgA nephropathy, hypertriglyceridemia was independently predictive of progression.[779]

However, not all studies have confirmed these findings:

- In the Multiple Risk Factor Intervention Trial (MRFIT), dyslipidemias were not associated with a decline in renal function.[780]

- After 10 years of follow-up in the MDRD study, measures of dyslipidemia were not predictive of cardiovascular events or ESKD.[781]
- In a retrospective analysis of patients with nephrotic syndrome, hypercholesterolemia at diagnosis was not found to be a predictor of renal disease progression.[782]
- In the CRIC study. no association was observed between total or LDL cholesterol and the risk of ESKD or a 50% reduction in the eGFR.[783]

Interpretation of these data is complicated by the fact that in patients with renal insufficiency, dyslipidemias do not occur in isolation and are associated with other factors that also affect renal disease progression, including hypertension, hyperglycemia, and proteinuria. Levels of serum cholesterol and triglycerides have been found to correlate with BP and circulating Ang II levels in type 1 and 2 diabetes with renal disease and to rise with increasing proteinuria in patients with nephrotic syndrome.[770]

The possible mechanisms whereby hyperlipidemia may contribute to renal injury have not been fully elucidated. Cholesterol feeding has been associated with an increase in mesangial lipid content,[760] glomerular macrophages, and TGF-β, as well as fibronectin mRNA levels.[784,785] Furthermore, reduction of glomerular macrophages by whole-body x-irradiation in the setting of nephrotic syndrome significantly reduced albuminuria without affecting serum lipid levels, indicating that macrophages play a central role in hyperlipidemic glomerular injury.[785] Mesangial cells express receptors for LDL, and uptake is stimulated by vasoconstrictor and mitogenic peptides such as ET-1 and PDGF.[407] Metabolism of LDL by mesangial cells leads to increased synthesis of fibronectin and MCP-1, which may contribute to mesangial matrix expansion and the recruitment of circulating macrophage/monocytes into the glomerulus.[408] Moreover, triglyceride-rich lipoproteins (very-low-density lipoprotein, [VLDL] and intermediate-density lipoprotein [IDL]) induce mesangial cell proliferation and elaboration of IL-6, PDGF, and TGF-β in vitro.[786] Mesangial cells, macrophages and renal tubule cells all have the capacity to oxidize LDL via the formation of ROS, a step that may be inhibited by antioxidants and HDL.[396,787,788] Oxidized LDLs may induce dose-dependent mesangial cell proliferation or mesangial cell death, as well as production of TNF-α, eicosanoids, monocyte chemotaxins, and glomerular vasoconstriction. These pathways, together with free radicals generated during LDL oxidation, may each contribute to renal inflammation and injury.[786,787]

Hyperlipidemia is also associated with elevated $P_{GC}$, raising the possibility of a further pathway to glomerulosclerosis via hemodynamic injury.[760] The elevated $P_{GC}$ appears to be mediated, in part, by an increase in renal vascular resistance that occurs in the context of increased plasma viscosity. In diabetic patients, circulating Ang II levels have been found to correlate with serum cholesterol,[789] and both oxidized LDLs and lipoprotein(a) have been shown to stimulate renin production by juxtaglomerular cells in vitro.[788] Moreover, oxidized LDL has been found to reduce nitric oxide synthesis by endothelial cells,[788] raising the possibility that alterations in activity of the RAAS and nitric oxide metabolism could also contribute to the increase in $P_{GC}$ observed with hyperlipidemia.

It would follow that if hyperlipidemia exacerbates renal injury, interventions designed to lower serum lipid levels should ameliorate disease progression. Treatment with a 3-hydroxyl-3-methylglutaryl coenzyme A (HMG-CoA) reductase inhibitor (statin) or clofibric acid in the obese Zucker rat, a strain with endogenous hyperlipidemia and spontaneous glomerulosclerosis, and 5/6 nephrectomized rats, which develop hyperlipidemia secondary to renal insufficiency, resulted in lowering of serum lipid levels, reduction in albuminuria, reduction in mesangial cell DNA synthesis, and attenuation of glomerulosclerosis, despite a lack of effect on either systemic BP or $P_{GC}$.[12,790] Indeed, statin treatment resulted in additional lowering of proteinuria, regression of glomerulosclerosis, normalization of podocyte number, and abrogation of tubulointerstitial injury when added to combination ACE inhibitor and ARB treatment.[791] In rats in the nephrotic phase of PAN, statin treatment resulted in reduction of albuminuria and serum cholesterol levels, reduction of MCP-1 mRNA expression, and a 77% reduction in glomerular macrophage accumulation.[792] The statins may therefore exert beneficial effects on renal disease progression, not only by reducing serum lipid levels, but also by inhibiting mesangial cell proliferation and mechanisms for the recruitment of macrophages due to the decreased expression of chemotactic factors and cell adhesion molecules.[793] Cholesterol-fed rats with puromycin aminonucleoside nephropathy, treated with the antioxidants probucol or vitamin E, showed significant reductions in proteinuria and glomerulosclerosis compared with untreated controls.[794] Furthermore, plasma VLDL and LDL from the treated animals were less susceptible to in vitro oxidation and less renal lipid peroxidation was evident, implying that lipid peroxidation plays an important role in renal injury associated with hyperlipidemia.

Niacin treatment after 5/6 nephrectomy resulted in lower BP, less proteinuria, less renal tissue accumulation of lipids, and attenuation of tubulointerstitial injury. This indicates that lipid lowering through strategies other than statins may also be renoprotective.[795]

In some clinical studies, dietary or pharmacologic lowering of serum lipid levels has also been associated with a reduction in proteinuria and lower rates of decline in renal function, but other studies have failed to demonstrate similar benefits, despite adequate therapeutic reductions in serum lipid levels. A metaanalysis of 13 small studies that included both diabetic and nondiabetic renal disease has found that lipid-lowering therapy significantly reduces the rate of decline in the GFR (mean reduction of 1.9 mL/min/1.73 $m^2$ per year).[796] Several secondary analyses of data from clinical trials have suggested that lipid-lowering therapy may slow progression in human CKD, but these data should be interpreted with caution.[797,798] In a placebo-controlled open-label study, atorvastatin treatment in patients with CKD, proteinuria, and hypercholesterolemia was associated with preservation of creatinine clearance, whereas those receiving placebo evidenced a significant decline.[799] In a metaanalysis of studies in which predialysis patients with CKD were randomized to therapy with a statin, and analysis of data from a relatively small subgroup in which renal endpoints were available, statin therapy was associated with a reduction in proteinuria but no improvement in creatinine clearance.[800]

Whereas these renoprotective effects were associated with cholesterol lowering, it is possible that they may also be due to the direct pleiotropic effects of HMG-CoA reductase inhibitors. This notion is further supported by the observation that lipid lowering with fibrates was not associated with preservation of renal function,[801,802] although one study did show reduced progression to microalbuminuria among type 2 diabetics receiving fenofibrate.[803] The Study of Heart and Renal Protection (SHARP) investigated the cardiovascular and renoprotective effects of lipid lowering with simvastatin and ezetimibe in 9438 subjects with CKD and ESKD.[804] Whereas the treatment arm showed a mean reduction of 43 mg/dL in LDL cholesterol and a 17% reduction in major atherosclerotic events, no significant effect was observed on the incidence of the renal endpoints in ESKD (risk ratio, 0.97; 95% CI, 0.89–1.05) and ESKD or creatinine doubling (risk ratio, 0.93; 95% CI, 0.86–1.01). It should be noted, however, that the subjects with CKD had relatively advanced disease (mean eGFR, 27 ± 13 mL/min/1.73 $m^2$), and these observations therefore do not exclude the possibility that lipid lowering may have renoprotective effects in less advanced CKD. However, a metaanalysis of 38 studies that included 37,274 participants with CKD has found that statin therapy is associated with a reduction in mortality and cardiovascular events but no clear effect on CKD progression.[805]

Inhibitors of the enzyme, proprotein convertase subtilisin/kexin type 9 (PCSK9), a key regulator of hepatic LDL receptor recycling, have been developed as novel potent treatments to lower cholesterol levels in persons with familial hyperlipidemias or those resistant to treatment with statins. Randomized trials to assess the renoprotective effects of PCSK9 inhibitors have not yet been published, but a pooled analysis of participants with CKD (eGFR, 30–59 mL/min/1.73 $m^2$; mean eGFR, 51 mL/min.1.73 $m^2$) in eight trials evaluating a monoclonal antibody to PCSK9, alirocumab, reported that treatment was associated with substantial reductions in LDL cholesterol and triglyceride levels, as well as other lipids versus placebo or ezetimibe. Alirocumab treatment was not associated with increased adverse events versus control groups, and no difference in eGFR was observed between groups at 24 or 104 weeks.[806] It should be noted, however, that the GFR was monitored for safety and not to assess renoprotection. Ongoing long-term trials will investigate the potential benefits of PCSK9 inhibitors on cardiovascular outcomes and will likely include participants with CKD.

## CALCIUM AND PHOSPHATE METABOLISM

As is the case with many of the adaptations that follow nephron loss, evidence has been accumulating that alterations in calcium and phosphate metabolism may also contribute to progressive renal damage. A retrospective analysis of 15 patients with nonprogressing CKD (GFR, 27–70 mL/min/1.73 $m^2$, followed for up to 17 years) revealed that the single feature common to all these patients was an enhanced capacity to excrete phosphate when compared with patients with a similar GFR but progressive renal disease.[807] In all the nonprogressors, serum phosphate and calcium levels remained within normal limits without the use of phosphate binders, calcium supplementation, or vitamin D. It is not yet clear which factors are most important, but evidence suggests that hyperphosphatemia, renal calcium deposition, hyperparathyroidism, and activated vitamin D deficiency may each play a role. FGF23 has recently been identified as a key mediator of bone mineral and vitamin D metabolism in CKD and may emerge as the dominant factor.

### HYPERPHOSPHATEMIA

Uninephrectomized rats receiving a high-phosphate diet (1%) developed renal calcium and phosphate deposition and tubulointerstitial injury within 5 weeks of nephrectomy.[239] Similar changes were observed in a proportion of intact rats fed a 2% phosphate diet. In clinical studies, serum phosphate has been identified as an independent risk factor for CKD progression[808] that may also attenuate the efficacy of ACE inhibitor treatment in the context of proteinuric nephropathies.[809] Phosphate excess therefore does appear to have some intrinsic nephrotoxicity that is enhanced in the setting of reduced nephron number. A high-phosphate diet has also been associated with the development of parathyroid hyperplasia and hyperparathyroidism in remnant kidney rats.[810] Conversely, in both animals and humans with renal insufficiency, dietary phosphate restriction or treatment with oral phosphate binders has been associated with reductions in proteinuria and glomerulosclerosis and attenuation of disease progression, as well as prevention of hyperparathyroidism.[811–814] A further mechanism whereby hyperphosphatemia may contribute to kidney damage has been suggested by the observation that a high-phosphate diet increases, and phosphate binder therapy decreases, renal expression of ACE after 5/6 nephrectomy.[815] Dietary phosphate restriction, however, almost inevitably also imposes dietary protein restriction. It is therefore not clear whether the benefit was derived directly from the reduced phosphate intake or indirectly from protein restriction. One study in humans has reported additional renoprotection when phosphate restriction is superimposed on protein restriction.[816]

### RENAL CALCIUM DEPOSITION

Calcium phosphate deposition is a frequent histologic finding in end-stage kidney biopsies, irrespective of the underlying cause of renal failure.[249,817] Calcium levels in end-stage kidneys have been found to be approximately nine times greater than levels in control kidneys.[817] Histologically, deposits were seen in cortical tubule cells, basement membranes, and the interstitium.[817,818] Furthermore, the severity of renal parenchymal calcification has been found to correlate with the degree of renal dysfunction, implicating calcium phosphate deposition in disease progression.[811,819] To determine whether the calcium deposits observed in end-stage kidneys precede or follow renal parenchymal fibrosis, rats with a reduced renal mass were maintained on a high-phosphate diet, thus ensuring a high calcium phosphate product. A subgroup was treated with 3-phosphocitrate, an inhibitor of calcium phosphate deposition.[819] Treatment with 3-phosphocitrate led to a significant reduction in renal injury compared with controls, indicating that calcium phosphate deposition in the kidney occurs during the evolution of renal injury and may exacerbate nephron loss. Calcium deposition in the renal parenchyma is associated with ultrastructural evidence of mitochondrial disorganization and calcium accumulation[818] and may therefore contribute to renal injury via the uncoupling of mitochondrial respiration and generation of ROS.[820] Mitochondrial calcium deposition was reduced by dietary protein restriction or calcium channel blocker therapy.[818,820] Other potential roles for calcium in renal disease progression include effects on vascular smooth muscle tone, mesangial cell contractility, cell growth and proliferation, extracellular matrix synthesis, and immune cell modulation.[821]

### HYPERPARATHYROIDISM

Podocytes express a unique transcript of PTH receptor, and PTH has been shown to have several effects on the kidney, including decreasing SNGFR (without change in $Q_A$, $P_{GC}$, or $\Delta P$), lowering $K_f$, and stimulating renin production.[814] Furthermore, increased PTH levels may exacerbate renal damage through effects on BP,[822] glucose intolerance, and lipid metabolism.[823,824] Two experimental studies have provided evidence that PTH may contribute to CKD progression. In the first study, parathyroidectomy was shown to improve survival, ameliorate the increase in renal mass, as well as renal calcium content, and attenuate the rise in serum creatinine levels observed in 5/6 nephrectomized rats fed a high-protein diet.[825] In the other, calcimimetic treatment and parathyroidectomy after 5/6 nephrectomy each abrogated TIF and glomerulosclerosis.[826] Interpretation of these data are, however, complicated by the observation in the latter study that both interventions also lowered BP.

### ACTIVATED VITAMIN D DEFICIENCY

It is perhaps not surprising that vitamin D, normally 1-hydroxylated in the kidney and therefore reduced in CKD, has several potentially beneficial effects on the kidney. Several experiments have reported amelioration of renal damage in rats treated with $1,25(OH)_2D_3$ or vitamin D analogue after 5/6 nephrectomy.[827–829] Interestingly, a further study found that $1,25(OH)_2D_3$ treatment also preserved podocyte number, volume, and structure after 5/6 nephrectomy.[327] In other experimental models, vitamin D or vitamin D analogues have been shown to abrogate interstitial inflammation by promoting the sequestration of NF-κB signaling,[830] inhibit renal hypertrophy after uninephrectomy,[831] reduce renin[814,832] and TGF-β expression,[829] and restore glomerular filtration barrier structure as well as slit diaphragm protein expression.[832] Several small trials have reported reductions in proteinuria among patients with diabetic[833] and nondiabetic CKD[834,835] randomized to treatment with the vitamin D analogue paricalcitol, but larger long-term studies are required to evaluate the potential renoprotective effects of vitamin D replacement further.

### FIBROBLAST GROWTH FACTOR 23

FGF23 has been identified as a key regulator of the bone mineral and vitamin D changes observed in CKD and may also contribute to CKD progression, as well as mediate some of the adverse cardiovascular consequences associated with CKD. It is produced by osteoblasts and osteocytes; levels rise early in the course of CKD. FGF23 is stimulated chiefly by $1,25(OH)_2D_3$ and dietary phosphate intake.[836] Its chief actions are to reduce phosphate reabsorption in the proximal tubule by downregulating sodium phosphate cotransporters and reduce $1,25(OH)_2D_3$ levels by inhibiting renal $25(OH)D_3$ 1α-hydroxylase, as well as stimulating the catabolic $25(OH)D_3$ 24-hydroxylase.[836] Thus decreased phosphate excretion early in the course of CKD stimulates FGF23 production, which increases phosphate excretion to prevent hyperphosphatemia until late in the course of CKD. This response is achieved at the expense of low $1,25(OH)_2D_3$ levels, which in turn facilitate the development of secondary hyperparathyroidism.[247,837] In addition to its role in bone mineral metabolism, longitudinal studies have identified FGF23 as an independent risk factor for mortality in hemodialysis patients[838,839] and in persons with earlier stage CKD,[840] although one group has suggested that the relationship may not be causal.[841]

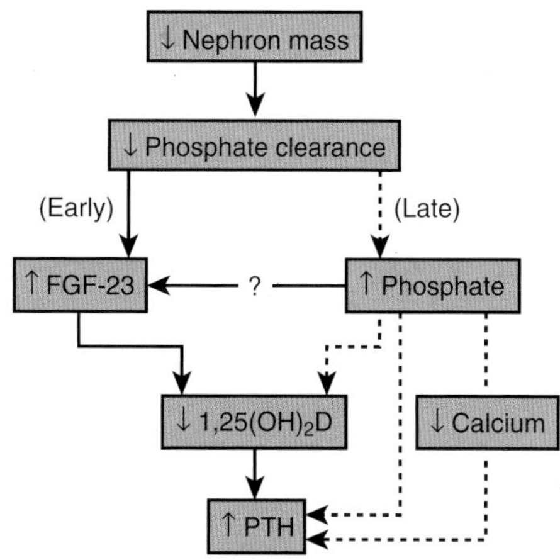


**Fig. 51.13** Schematic explaining the possible interactions among phosphate, vitamin D ($1,25(OH)_2D$), fibroblast growth factor 23 (FGF-23), and parathyroid hormone *(PTH)* in regulating serum phosphate and calcium levels after nephron loss. (From Gutierrez OM: Fibroblast growth factor 23 and disordered vitamin D metabolism in chronic kidney disease: updating the "trade-off" hypothesis. *Clin J Am Soc Nephrol.* 2010;5: 1710–1716.)

Several studies have also identified FGF23 as an independent risk factor for CKD progression in diabetics[842] and nondiabetics,[843] including African Americans[844] and children with CKD.[845] Whether FGF23 contributes directly to CKD progression or is simply a risk marker remains to be elucidated. Indeed, overexpression of mutant FGF23 in the Thy1 model of glomerulonephritis resulted in lowering of serum phosphate levels and amelioration of glomerulosclerosis.[846] Possible mechanisms whereby FGF23 may contribute to CKD progression include exacerbation of $1,25(OH)_2D_3$ deficiency and secondary hyperparathyroidism (Fig. 51.13; see sections earlier).

## ANEMIA

Anemia is a frequent consequence of CKD but may also influence its progression. Both acute and chronic anemia are associated with reversible increases in renal vascular resistance and a normal or reduced filtration fraction in animals and humans. Conversely, an increase in hematocrit is associated with an increase in filtration fraction. Thus hematocrit may influence renal hemodynamics and thereby affect the rate of progression of CKD. The effects of anemia on glomerular hemodynamics have been studied in rats subjected to 5/6 nephrectomy, DOCA-salt hypertension, and diabetes.[847–849] Irrespective of the model, anemia was associated with significant amelioration of glomerulosclerosis and a reduction in $P_{GC}$.

Reduced $P_{GC}$ resulted predominantly from reductions in efferent arteriolar resistance in rats with renal ablation, lowered SBP in DOCA-salt rats, and increased afferent arteriolar resistance in diabetic rats. Similarly, in the MWF/Ztm rat, which develops spontaneous glomerulosclerosis with age, anemia induced by dietary iron deficiency was associated with lower BP, reduced urinary protein excretion, and less extensive glomerulosclerosis compared with controls fed diets of normal iron content.[850] In contrast, prevention of anemia by the administration of erythropoietin to remnant kidney rats to maintain a normal hematocrit resulted in increased systemic and glomerular BPs, as well as markedly increased glomerulosclerosis.[847] In another apparently contradictory study, treatment with epoetin delta after 5/6 nephrectomy was associated with slower rates of decline in renal function, decreased renal fibrosis, and less interstitial macrophage accumulation.[851] Interestingly, these effects were observed at subhemopoietic doses, indicating that they may have resulted from direct actions of the epoetin rather than anemia correction.

Despite the apparently favorable hemodynamic effects of anemia in experimental models of CKD, humans studies have suggested that anemia may accelerate CKD progression. In patients with inherited hemoglobinopathies, chronic anemia is associated with glomerular hyperfiltration that eventuates in proteinuria, hypertension, and ESKD.[852,853] Furthermore, reduced hemoglobin level was an independent predictor of increased risk of developing ESKD among patients with diabetic nephropathy in the RENAAL trial.[854] Several longitudinal studies of patients with other forms of CKD have identified lower hemoglobin levels as a risk factor for progression.[855,856]

Further confirmation that anemia has an adverse effect of CKD progression has been derived from two small randomized studies that reported renoprotective benefit when anemia is corrected with erythopoietin.[857,858] On the other hand, two other studies that had effects on left ventricular mass as their primary endpoint,[859,860] as well as the Trial to Reduce Cardiovascular Events with Aranesp Therapy (TREAT),[861] found no effect of high versus low hemoglobin target on rate of decline in the GFR. In the Cardiovascular Risk Reduction by Early Anemia Treatment with Epoetin Beta (CREATE) study, randomization to a higher hemoglobin target (13–15 mg/dL) was associated with a shorter time to initiation of dialysis than the lower target (10.5–11.5 mg/dL).[862]

The reasons for the apparent contradiction between the beneficial hemodynamic effects of anemia in experimental models, and the identification of anemia as a risk factor for CKD progression in clinical studies, are unknown. It is possible that the benefit of the hemodynamic effects is outweighed by other factors, such as increased renal hypoxia and ROS formation, which may contribute to progressive renal damage.[863] Nevertheless, several recent studies have indicated that normalization of hemoglobin in CKD may be associated with several serious adverse effects, including increased risk of stroke[861] and death.[864] Issues related to the treatment of anemia in CKD are discussed further in Chapter 55.

## TOBACCO SMOKING

Smoking produces acute sympathetic nervous system activation resulting in tachycardia and an increase in SBP of up to 21 mm Hg.[865] Vasoconstriction occurs in several vascular beds, including the kidneys. Among healthy nonsmoking volunteers, acute exposure to cigarette smoke caused an 11% increase in renovascular resistance accompanied by a 15% reduction in the GFR and an 18% decrease in filtration fraction. These effects appear to be mediated, at least in part, by nicotine, because similar responses were observed after chewing nicotine gum.[866] The renal hemodynamic effects of smoking can be blocked by pretreatment with a beta blocker, indicating that β-adrenergic stimulation is also involved.[867]

The effects of chronic smoking on the normal kidney are less well defined. Renal plasma flow but not the GFR is reduced in chronic smokers, and plasma endothelin levels are elevated. In one population-based study, chronic smoking was associated with a small increase in creatinine clearance, implying that smoking may cause glomerular hyperfiltration.[868] That these functional abnormalities may result in structural changes to blood vessels is suggested by the observation of abnormal intrarenal vasculature in smokers.[869,870] Moreover, epidemiologic studies have found smoking to be an important predictor of albuminuria in the general population.[868,871] In one study, heavy smoking (>20 cigarettes/day) was associated with a relative risk for albuminuria of 1.92.[871]

Furthermore, in other epidemiologic studies, smoking has been identified as a significant risk factor for CKD[614,872,873] and the development of ESKD.[613] Smoking was associated with an increased risk of developing of glomerular hyperfiltration (eGFR ≥117 ml/min/1.73 m$^2$; OR, 1.32 vs. nonsmokers), as well as proteinuria (OR, 1.51 vs. nonsmokers) in one longitudinal study of 10,118 middle-aged Japanese workers.[874] Two other similar longitudinal studies from Japan have confirmed that smoking is associated with an increased risk of developing proteinuria but with a higher mean eGFR than in nonsmokers.[875,876] In one of the studies, smoking was associated with a reduced risk of developing CKD stage 3.[876]

Whereas more studies are required to elucidate the effects of smoking on healthy kidneys, several studies have suggested that smoking is a risk factor for disease progression in a variety of forms of CKD, including diabetic kidney disease,[877–884] autosomal dominant polycystic kidney disease, IgA nephropathy,[885] lupus nephritis,[886] primary glomerulonephritis,[887] and general population cohorts.[888–890] On the other hand, two large cohort studies of persons with CKD have reported no association between smoking status and CKD progression.[891,892]

Mechanisms whereby cigarette smoking may result in renal injury are the subject of ongoing research but are thought to include sympathetic nervous system activation, glomerular capillary hypertension, endothelial cell injury, and direct tubulotoxocity.[893] Furthemore, nicotine administration in Thy1 rats increased mesangial cell accumulation, and in vitro nicotine increased COX-2 expression and mesangial cell proliferation.[894] Similarly, in a mouse model of diabetic nephropathy, nicotine increased proteinuria, glomerular hypertrophy, and mesangial area. NOX4, nitrotyrosine, and Akt were also increased. In vitro nicotine and high glucose levels were found to have additive effects in stimulating the generation of ROS and Akt phosphorylation in mesangial cells.[895] Nicotine administration after 5/6 nephrectomy in rats was associated with a small increase in BP, as well as increased proteinuria (but not albuminuria). The glomerular injury score at 12 weeks was exacerbated by nicotine in association with increased expression of fibronectin, NADPH oxidase, and TGF-β.[896] Among patients with CKD, the hemodynamic effects of smoking were variable, but smoking was associated with a consistent increase in the urine ACR.[866] Analysis of urine from smokers and nonsmokers has revealed significantly higher excretions of thromboxane- and prostacyclin-derived products in smokers.[897] The authors have suggested that increased synthesis of thromboxanes and prostacyclins may have pathologic importance for vascular injury, given the biologic effects of these compounds on platelets and smooth muscle cells. An important role for sympathetic nervous system activation has been suggested by an experimental study in which sympathetic denervation abrogated renal injury induced by exposure to cigarette smoke condensate.[898] A growing body of evidence thus supports the notion that the kidney is yet another organ that is adversely affected by smoking, and that smoking cessation may contribute to slowing the rate of progression of CKD.[844,899]

## ACUTE KIDNEY INJURY

A growing body of evidence has indicated that recovery from AKI is associated with a substantially increased risk of CKD, and AKI superimposed on CKD has been proposed as a previously underappreciated mechanism for CKD progression. Following publication of several individual cohort studies, a metaanalysis of 13 studies reported a significantly increased risk of developing CKD and ESKD in patients who had survived an episode of AKI versus participants without AKI (pooled adjusted HR for CKD, 8.8; 95% CI, 3.1–25.5; pooled HR for ESKD, 3.1; 95% CI, 1.9–5.0).[900]

Studies in animal models of AKI have identified failure of dedifferentiation of tubule cells as a key mechanism associated with progressive TIF after AKI. After acute tubular necrosis, regeneration of tubules is achieved by dedifferentiation of remaining tubule cells, followed by proliferation to replace lost cells and redifferentiation. If this process fails, tubules become arrested in the dedifferentiated state and continue to produce proinflammatory and profibrotic cytokines that drive progressive interstitial fibrosis. Activation of pericytes results in differentiation into myofibroblasts that contribute to fibrosis. The loss of pericytes contributes to loss of endothelial integrity and capillary rarefaction that exacerbates tissue hypoxia and fibrosis.[901] The specific factors that provoke progressive kidney damage after AKI remain to be elucidated. It has been proposed that a single episode of AKI normally heals without progressive kidney damage but that repeated episodes of AKI, a single very severe episode of AKI, or AKI superimposed on preexisting CKD may provoke the above mechanisms.[902] The interaction between AKI and CKD progression has been demonstrated by a study of 39,805 patients with eGFR less than 45 mL/min/1.73 m$^2$ before hospitalization.[903] Those who survived an episode of dialysis-requiring AKI had a very high risk of developing ESKD within 30 days of hospital discharge—that is, nonrecovery of AKI that was related to preadmission eGFR. For an eGFR of 30 to 44 mL/min/1.73 m$^2$, the incidence of ESKD was 42%, and for an eGFR of 15 to 29 mL/min/1.73 m$^2$, it was as high as 63%, whereas the incidence of ESKD was only 1.5% among those who did not have dialysis-requiring AKI. Among patients who survived more than 30 days after hospital discharge without ESKD, the incidence of ESKD and death at 6 months were 12.7% and 19.7%, respectively, versus 1.7% and 7.4% in the comparator group with CKD but no AKI. After adjustment for multiple risk factors AKI was associated with a 30% increase in long-term risk for death or ESKD (adjusted HR, 1.30; 95% CI 1.04–1.64).

The interaction between AKI and CKD has been explored in multiple animal models.[904] In rats subjected to renal ischemia 2 weeks after 3/4 nephrectomy, uninephrectomy, or sham operation, ischemia after 3/4 nephrectomy was associated with a sustained increase in serum creatinine levels and more tubules that failed to redifferentiate, associated with more severe capillary rarefaction and TIF. Furthermore, rats that were initially normotensive after 3/4 nephrectomy developed hypertension and proteinuria at 2 to 4 weeks after ischemia.[905] The investigators proposed that loss of autoregulation results in greater transmission of elevated systemic BP to the glomerulus that exacerbates glomerular damage and contributes to CKD progression.[902] In another animal model, investigators observed that moderate ischemia reperfusion injury resulted in AKI with transient activation of Wtn/β-catenin signaling and renal recovery, but severe ischemia reperfusion injury caused a sustained and exaggerated activation of Wtn/β-catenin signaling associated with progressive renal fibrosis.[906] Moreover, overexpression of Wtn1 accelerated the progression of AKI to CKD, and blockade of Wnt/β-catenin ameliorated the progression of AKI to CKD. Proposed interactions between mechanisms of kidney injury post AKI and mechanisms of CKD progression are illustrated in Fig. 51.14.

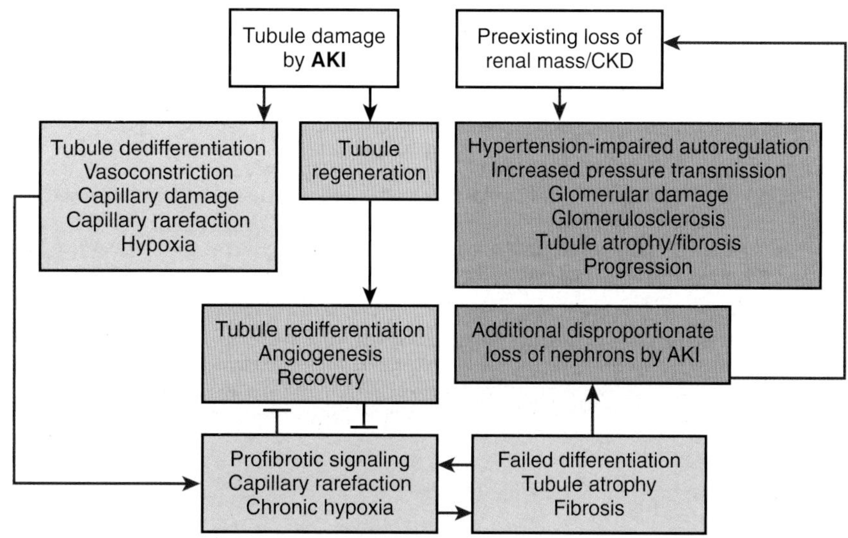


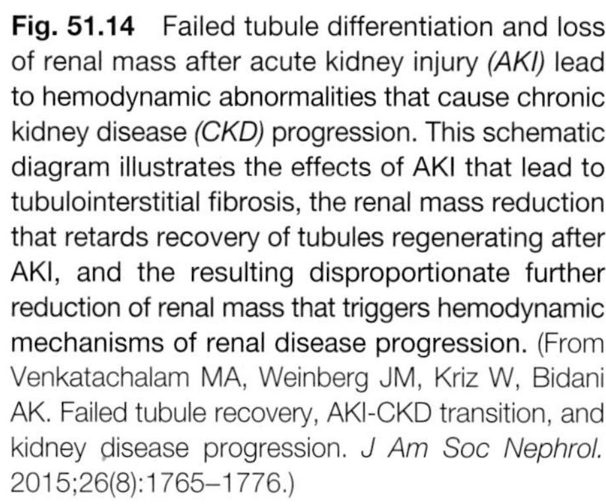

**Fig. 51.14** Failed tubule differentiation and loss of renal mass after acute kidney injury *(AKI)* lead to hemodynamic abnormalities that cause chronic kidney disease *(CKD)* progression. This schematic diagram illustrates the effects of AKI that lead to tubulointerstitial fibrosis, the renal mass reduction that retards recovery of tubules regenerating after AKI, and the resulting disproportionate further reduction of renal mass that triggers hemodynamic mechanisms of renal disease progression. (From Venkatachalam MA, Weinberg JM, Kriz W, Bidani AK. Failed tubule recovery, AKI-CKD transition, and kidney disease progression. *J Am Soc Nephrol.* 2015;26(8):1765–1776.)

## FUTURE DIRECTIONS

The development of pharmacologic inhibitors of the RAAS has provided powerful and incisive tools to explore renal hemodynamic and other associated adaptations in the setting of progressive renal injury. These insights have paved the way for clinical studies that provided clear evidence for the use of ACE inhibitor and ARB treatment as the mainstay of renoprotective strategies. Nevertheless, these studies have shown, at best, a 50% decrease in the rate of CKD progression. Ongoing research involving cell biology and molecular cloning, as well as genomics and proteomics, continues to yield novel insights into the mechanisms of progressive renal injury that promise to direct researchers to potential new molecular targets for renoprotective interventions. The development of the means to inhibit molecular targets specifically may provide new forms of therapy for those with CKD and enable physicians to realize the ultimate goal of achieving remission of progressive renal injury in most patients, and even regression of renal damage in some.

 Complete reference list available at ExpertConsult.com.

### KEY REFERENCES


4. Brenner BM, Meyer TW, Hostetter TH. Dietary protein intake and the progressive nature of kidney disease: the role of hemodynamically mediated glomerular injury in the pathogenesis of progressive glomerular sclerosis in aging, renal ablation and intrinsic renal disease. *N Engl Med J.* 1982;307:652–659.
5. Weldegiorgis M, de Zeeuw D, Li L, et al. Longitudinal estimated the GFR trajectories in patients with and without type 2 diabetes and nephropathy. *Am J Kidney Dis.* 2018;71(1):91–101.
9. Hostetter TH, Olson JL, Rennke HG, et al. Hyperfiltration in remnant nephrons: a potentially adverse response to renal ablation. *J Am Soc Nephrol.* 2001;12(6):1315–1325.
16. Lenihan CR, Busque S, Derby G, et al. Longitudinal study of living kidney donor glomerular dynamics after nephrectomy. *J Clin Invest.* 2015;125(3):1311–1318.
31. Yang T, Xu C. Physiology and pathophysiology of the intrarenal renin-angiotensin system: an update. *J Am Soc Nephrol.* 2017;28(4): 1040–1049.
50. Guan Z, VanBeusecum JP, Inscho EW. Endothelin and the renal microcirculation. *Semin Nephrol.* 2015;35(2):145–155.
83. Carlstrom M, Wilcox CS, Arendshorst WJ. Renal autoregulation in health and disease. *Physiol Rev.* 2015;95(2):405–511.
88. Monu SR, Ren Y, Masjoan-Juncos JX, et al. Connecting tubule glomerular feedback mediates tubuloglomerular feedback resetting after unilateral nephrectomy. *Am J Physiol Renal Physiol.* 2018;315(4): F806–F811.
90. Taal MW, Nenov VD, Wong W, et al. Vasopeptidase inhibition affords greater renoprotection than angiotensin-converting enzyme inhibition alone. *J Am Soc Nephrol.* 2001;12:2051–2059.
205. Layton AT, Edwards A, Vallon V. Adaptive changes in the GFR, tubular morphology, and transport in subtotal nephrectomized kidneys: modeling and analysis. *Am J Physiol Renal Physiol.* 2017;313(2): F199–F209.
227. Layton AT, Edwards A, Vallon V. Renal potassium handling in rats with subtotal nephrectomy: modeling and analysis. *Am J Physiol Renal Physiol.* 2018;314(4):F643–F657.
245. Munoz-Castaneda JR, Herencia C, Pendon-Ruiz de Mier MV, et al. Differential regulation of renal Klotho and FGFR1 in normal and uremic rats. *FASEB J.* 2017;31(9):3858–3867.
266. Mjoen G, Hallan S, Hartmann A, et al. Long-term risks for kidney donors. *Kidney Int.* 2014;86(1):162–167.
291. Neal B, Perkovic V, Mahaffey KW, et al. Canagliflozin and cardiovascular and renal events in type 2 diabetes. *N Engl J Med.* 2017;377(7):644–657.
292. Wanner C, Inzucchi SE, Lachin JM, et al. Empagliflozin and progression of kidney disease in type 2 diabetes. *N Engl J Med.* 2016;375(4):323–334.
293. Jardine MJ, Mahaffey KW, Neal B, et al. The canagliflozin and renal endpoints in diabetes with established nephropathy clinical evaluation (CREDENCE) study rationale, design, and baseline characteristics. *Am J Nephrol.* 2017;46(6):462–472.
329. Forst AL, Olteanu VS, Mollet G, et al. Podocyte purinergic P2X4 channels are mechanotransducers that mediate cytoskeletal disorganization. *J Am Soc Nephrol.* 2016;27(3):848–862.
339. Miceli I, Burt D, Tarabra E, et al. Stretch reduces nephrin expression via an angiotensin II-AT(1)-dependent mechanism in human podocytes: effect of rosiglitazone. *Am J Physiol Renal Physiol.* 2009;298(2):F381–F390.
341. Wang X, Johnson AC, Williams JM, et al. Nephron deficiency and predisposition to renal injury in a novel one-kidney genetic model. *J Am Soc Nephrol.* 2014;26(7):1634–1646.
355. Duffield JS. Cellular and molecular mechanisms in kidney fibrosis. *J Clin Invest.* 2014;124(6):2299–2306.
422. Heerspink HJ, Kropelin TF, Hoekman J, et al. Drug-induced reduction in albuminuria is associated with subsequent renoprotection: a meta-analysis. *J Am Soc Nephrol.* 2015;26(8):2055–2064.
433. Grande MT, Sanchez-Laorden B, Lopez-Blau C, et al. Snail1-induced partial epithelial-to-mesenchymal transition drives renal fibrosis in mice and can be targeted to reverse established disease. *Nat Med.* 2015;21(9):989–997.
434. Lovisa S, LeBleu VS, Tampe B, et al. Epithelial-to-mesenchymal transition induces cell cycle arrest and parenchymal damage in renal fibrosis. *Nat Med.* 2015;21(9):998–1009.
435. Buchtler S, Grill A, Hofmarksrichter S, et al. Cellular origin and functional relevance of collagen I production in the kidney. *J Am Soc Nephrol.* 2018;29(7):1859–1873.
436. Rosenbloom J, Castro SV, Jimenez SA. Narrative review: fibrotic diseases: cellular and molecular mechanisms and novel therapies. *Ann Intern Med.* 2010;152(3):159–166.
442. Hohenstein B, Hugo C. Peritubular capillaries: an important piece of the puzzle. *Kidney Int.* 2017;91(1):9–11.
500. Higgins DF, Ewart LM, Masterson E, et al. BMP7-induced-Pten inhibits Akt and prevents renal fibrosis. *Biochim Biophys Acta Mol Basis Dis.* 2017;1863(12):3095–3104.
504. Denby L, Ramdas V, Lu R, et al. MicroRNA-214 antagonism protects against renal fibrosis. *J Am Soc Nephrol.* 2014;25(1):65–80.
508. Tan RJ, Zhou D, Xiao L, et al. Extracellular superoxide dismutase protects against proteinuric kidney disease. *J Am Soc Nephrol.* 2015; 26(10):2447–2459.
536. Goraya N, Simoni J, Jo CH, et al. Treatment of metabolic acidosis in patients with stage 3 chronic kidney disease with fruits and vegetables or oral bicarbonate reduces urine angiotensinogen and preserves glomerular filtration rate. *Kidney Int.* 2014;86(5):1031–1038.
545. Nishizono R, Kikuchi M, Wang SQ, et al. FSGS as an adaptive response to growth-induced podocyte stress. *J Am Soc Nephrol.* 2017; 28(10):2931–2945.
585. Ando K, Ohtsu H, Uchida S, et al. Anti-albuminuric effect of the aldosterone blocker eplerenone in non-diabetic hypertensive patients with albuminuria: a double-blind, randomised, placebo-controlled trial. *Lancet Diabetes Endocrinol.* 2014;2(12):944–953.
631. Schrier RW, Abebe KZ, Perrone RD, et al. Blood pressure in early autosomal dominant polycystic kidney disease. *N Engl J Med.* 2014;371(24):2255–2266.
636. Cheung AK, Rahman M, Reboussin DM, et al. Effects of intensive BP control in CKD. *J Am Soc Nephrol.* 2017;28(9):2812–2823.
654. Garneata L, Stancu A, Dragomir D, et al. Ketoanalogue-supplemented vegetarian very low-protein diet and CKD progression. *J Am Soc Nephrol.* 2016;27(7):2164–2176.
658. Rhee CM, Ahmadi SF, Kovesdy CP, et al. Low-protein diet for conservative management of chronic kidney disease: a systematic review and meta-analysis of controlled trials. *J Cachexia Sarcopenia Muscle.* 2018;9(2):235–245.
677. Kattah AG, Smith CY, Gazzuola Rocca L, et al. CKD in patients with bilateral oophorectomy. *Clin J Am Soc Nephrol.* 2018.
703. Parsa A, Kao WH, Xie D, et al. APOL1 risk variants, race, and progression of chronic kidney disease. *N Engl J Med.* 2013;369(23):2183–2196.
704. Kruzel-Davila E, Shemer R, Ofir A, et al. APOL1-mediated cell injury involves disruption of conserved trafficking processes. *J Am Soc Nephrol.* 2017;28(4):1117–1130.

735. Friedman AN, Wahed AS, Wang J, et al. Effect of bariatric surgery on CKD risk. *J Am Soc Nephrol.* 2018;29(4):1289–1300.
737. Bilha SC, Nistor I, Nedelcu A, et al. The effects of bariatric surgery on renal outcomes: a systematic review and meta-analysis. *Obes Surg.* 2018.
758. Bhatt DL, Kandzari DE, O'Neill WW, et al. A controlled trial of renal denervation for resistant hypertension. *N Engl J Med.* 2014; 370(15):1393–1401.
804. Haynes R, Lewis D, Emberson J, et al. Effects of lowering LDL cholesterol on progression of kidney disease. *J Am Soc Nephrol.* 2014;25(8):1825–1833.
809. Zoccali C, Ruggenenti P, Perna A, et al. Phosphate may promote CKD progression and attenuate renoprotective effect of ACE inhibition. *J Am Soc Nephrol.* 2011;22(10):1923–1930.
841. Marthi A, Donovan K, Haynes R, et al. Fibroblast growth factor-23 and risks of cardiovascular and noncardiovascular diseases: a meta-analysis. *J Am Soc Nephrol.* 2018;29(7):2015–2027.
845. Portale AA, Wolf MS, Messinger S, et al. Fibroblast growth factor 23 and risk of CKD progression in children. *Clin J Am Soc Nephrol.* 2016;11(11):1989–1998.
891. Bundy JD, Bazzano LA, Xie D, et al. Self-reported tobacco, alcohol, and illicit drug use and progression of chronic kidney disease. *Clin J Am Soc Nephrol.* 2018;13(7):993–1001.
892. Staplin N, Haynes R, Herrington WG, et al. Smoking and adverse outcomes in patients with CKD: the study of heart and renal protection (SHARP). *Am J Kidney Dis.* 2016;68(3):371–380.
900. Coca SG, Singanamala S, Parikh CR. Chronic kidney disease after acute kidney injury: a systematic review and meta-analysis. *Kidney Int.* 2012;81(5):442–448.
904. Fu Y, Tang C, Cai J, et al. Rodent models of AKI-CKD transition. *Am J Physiol Renal Physiol.* 2018.
906. Xiao L, Zhou D, Tan RJ, et al. Sustained activation of Wnt/beta-catenin signaling drives AKI to CKD progression. *J Am Soc Nephrol.* 2016;27(6):1727–1740.

# 52 The Pathophysiology of Uremia

Timothy W. Meyer | Thomas H. Hostetter

**CHAPTER OUTLINE**



The word "uremic" is generally used to describe those ill effects of kidney failure that we cannot yet explain. Hypertension caused by volume overload, tetany caused by hypocalcemia, and anemia caused by erythropoietin deficiency were once considered uremic signs, but were removed from this category as their causes were discovered. Uremia may thus now be defined as the illness that would remain if the extracellular volume and inorganic ion concentrations were kept normal and the known renal synthetic products were replaced in patients without kidneys (Box 52.1).

Some features of uremia, thus defined, could reflect the lack of unidentified renal synthetic products. We presume, however, that uremia is caused largely by the accumulation of organic waste products that are normally cleared by the kidneys. In general, the study of renal organic waste removal lags far behind the study of inorganic ion excretion. A major problem is the multiplicity of waste solutes. The first comprehensive review prepared by the European Uremic Toxin Work Group (EUTox[1,2]) listed >80 uremic solutes, and further studies have increased this number to >250.[3–7] Untargeted mass spectrometry has revealed that the true number is much greater, and that the majority of uremic solutes cannot be found in standard databases of known biological compounds. With so many substances to study, it is hard to establish which ones are toxic. Bergstrom[8] suggested criteria for identifying uremic toxins that are analogous to Koch postulates for identifying infectious agents. According to these criteria, a uremic toxin must have a known chemical structure and the following features:

- Its plasma and/or tissue concentrations should be higher in patients with kidney failure than in normal persons.
- The high concentrations should be related to specific uremic symptoms that are ameliorated when the concentration is reduced.
- The effects observed in uremic patients should be replicated by raising the solute concentration to similar levels in normal persons, experimental animals, or in vitro systems.

No uremic solute has so far been shown to fully satisfy these criteria. Given the complexity of uremia, it is unlikely that the accumulation of a single solute in isolation could recapitulate uremia or that removal of the same could eliminate uremia; therefore progress in uremia research has been relatively slow. Most solutes that accumulate with advanced chronic kidney disease (CKD) are probably not toxic. Others that are toxic may exert their ill effects only when administered in combination. The difficulty imposed by the multiplicity of solutes is compounded by the multiplicity of ill effects encountered in uremia. Investigators of uremic toxicity thus face the daunting task of matching a solute or group of solutes to an appropriate endpoint. Many of the effects of uremia are hard to quantify, which makes the problem even more difficult. This is particularly true of major uremic symptoms, especially fatigue, anorexia, and diminished mental acuity.

A related problem encountered in studies of uremia is distinguishing the effects of uremia from those of related conditions. Paradoxically, the widespread availability of dialysis has made uremia more difficult to study. The severity of the classic uremic symptoms is attenuated, and patients now suffer from a new illness, which Depner[9] has named the "residual syndrome," which is composed of partially treated uremia and the side effects of dialysis. In most patients, features of the residual syndrome are further combined with the effects of age and of systemic diseases responsible for kidney failure. Disturbances of inorganic ion metabolism, including acidemia and hyperphosphatemia, although excluded from our definition of uremia, undoubtedly also contribute to untoward clinical manifestations of kidney failure. Given these difficulties, it is not surprising that although we have identified many uremic solutes, we know relatively little about their toxicity. In a few cases, uremic abnormalities

**Box 52.1 Metabolic Effects, Symptoms, and Signs of Uremia**

**Metabolic**

Increased oxidant levels
Reduced resting energy expenditure
Reduced body temperature
Insulin resistance
Muscle wasting
Amenorrhea and sexual dysfunction

**Neural and Muscular**

Fatigue
Loss of concentration ranging to coma and seizures
Sleep disturbances
Restless legs
Peripheral neuropathy
Anorexia and nausea
Diminution in taste and smell
Itching
Cramps
Reduced muscle membrane potential

**Other**

Serositis (including pericarditis)
Hiccups
Granulocyte and lymphocyte dysfunction
Platelet dysfunction
Shortened erythrocyte life span
Albumin oxidation

**Box 52.2 Uremic Abnormalities Transferable With Uremic Serum or Plasma**

Inhibition of $Na^+,K^+$-ATPase
Inhibition of platelet function
Leukocyte dysfunction
Loss of erythrocyte membrane lipid asymmetry
Insulin resistance

*ATPase,* Adenosine triphosphatase.

have been reproduced by the transfer of uremic serum or plasma to normal animals or addition of these factors to the media of cultured cells (Box 52.2). However, the role of particular solute(s) in causing the abnormalities remains uncertain.

## SOLUTES CLEARED BY THE KIDNEY AND RETAINED IN UREMIA

The long list of solutes retained in uremia has been assembled in two ways. Initially, biochemists would find a substance in the urine and then look for it in the blood of uremic patients. Several dozen uremic solutes were identified in this way as the biochemical pathways of intermediary metabolism were worked out. Beginning about 1970, improved analytic techniques, including gas chromatography, mass spectroscopy, and high-performance liquid chromatography, were used to identify additional uremic solutes.[3,10] Recent technical advances, including proteomic and metabolomic screening methods, are lengthening the list of putative uremic solutes. However, the problem is to determine which solutes are toxic. In general, the compounds that are present in the highest concentrations, and therefore had been identified first, have been studied most extensively. Experiments showing that uremic signs and symptoms can be replicated by raising solute levels in normal persons or animals to equal those observed in uremic patients are, for the most part, lacking. When attempted, such experiments have generally demonstrated that the solutes being studied are more toxic than urea, but that the levels required to produce toxic effects are higher than those measured in patients. Because so little is known about their toxicity, the discussion of uremic solutes is usually organized on the basis of their structure and not their contribution to disease.

## INDIVIDUAL UREMIC SOLUTES

### UREA

Urea is quantitatively the most abundant solute excreted by the kidney, and its levels rise higher than those of any other solute when the kidney fails. Early studies indicated that urea causes only a minor part of uremic illness.[11–13] In the most often cited of these studies, Johnson and colleagues[12] dialyzed patients with kidney failure against bath solutions containing urea. They found that initiation of hemodialysis improved uremic symptoms, including weakness, fetor, and gastrointestinal upset, even when urea was added to the dialysate to maintain the blood urea nitrogen (BUN) level at approximately 90 mg/dL (32 mmol/L). In patients already on dialysis, increasing the BUN level to 140 mg/dL (50 mmol/L) did not cause recurrence of uremic symptoms. Increasing the BUN level >140 mg/dL caused nausea and headaches, and increasing the BUN level >180 mg/dL (64 mmol/L) caused weakness and lethargy. However, symptoms in dialyzed patients whose BUN values were increased to these levels were less severe than symptoms in undialyzed patients with high BUN values. Studies in patients without kidney failure suggest that urea by itself does not cause uremia. Uremic symptoms have not been observed in patients in whom BUN levels are maintained at approximately 60 mg/dL (21 mmol/L) by high protein intake or increased tubular urea absorption.[14–16] Similarly, patients on high-dose glucocorticoids or those with heart failure, conditions commonly seen in modern medical practice, do not experience uremia when kidney function, estimated by other solutes (typically serum creatinine), is not severely impaired.

The finding that uremia is not replicated by an isolated elevation of the plasma urea concentration does not mean that urea has no toxic effects.[17] The full expression of uremia may require accumulation of urea plus other solutes. Johnson and associates[12] noted that patients dialyzed against solutions of urea exhibited increased bleeding, and subsequent studies suggested that urea promotes bleeding by promoting synthesis of guanidinosuccinic acid (GSA), which impairs platelet

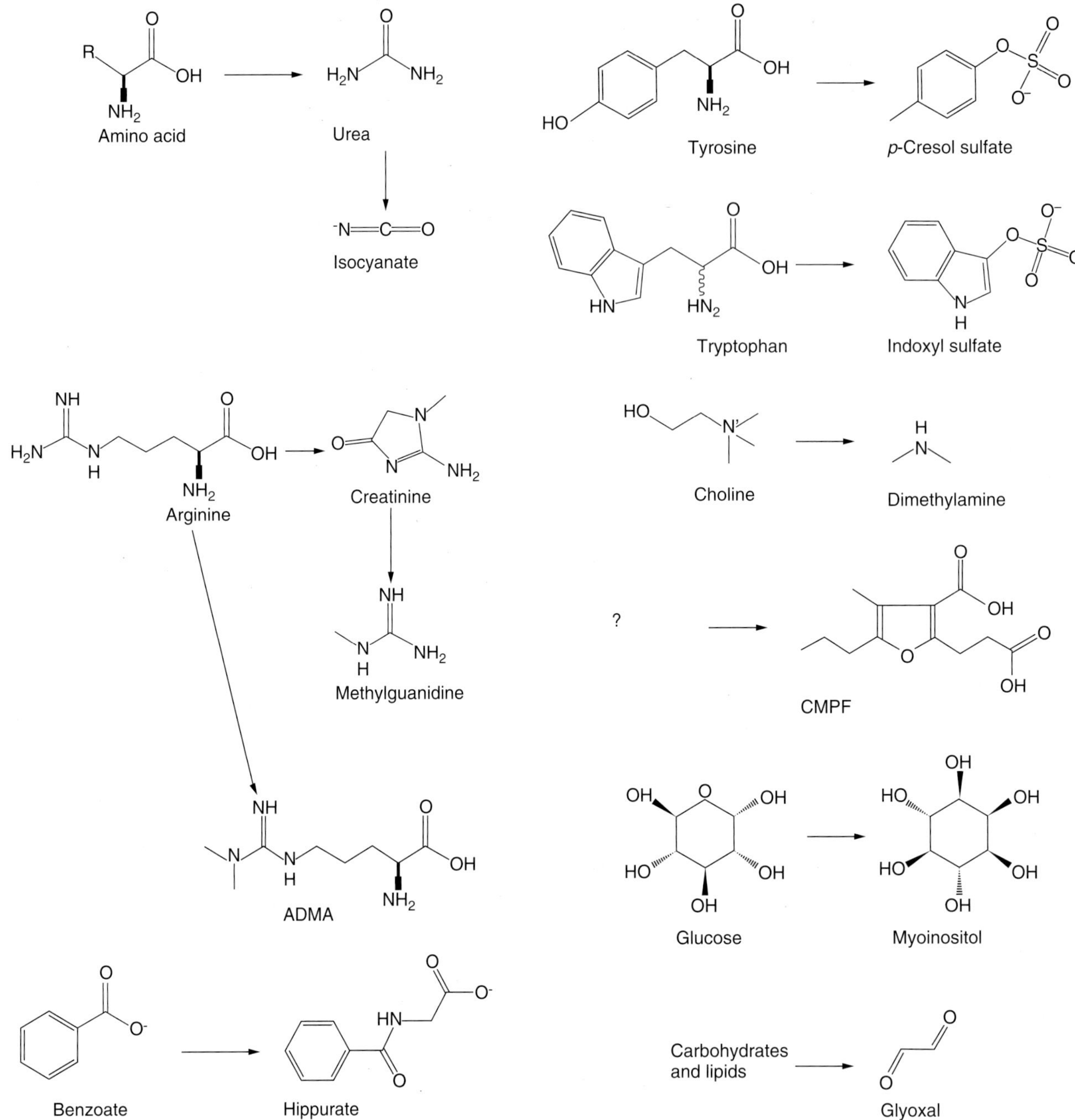


**Fig. 52.1** Generation of potential uremic toxins. The substances in the *right column* of each panel are metabolites that are normally excreted by the kidney and therefore accumulate in the extracellular fluid when kidney function is lost. The *left column* shows the substances from which these potential "uremic toxins" are derived. In some cases, the biochemical derivation of the potential toxins is uncertain. For example, it is not known what fraction of the dimethylamine normally excreted is derived from choline, and the source of 3-carboxy-4-methyl-5-prophy-2-furanpropanoic acid (CMPF) is obscure. See text for details. *ADMA,* Asymmetric dimethyl arginine.

function.[18,19] Increased plasma urea concentrations may cause other ill effects by increasing isocyanate concentration and thereby promoting protein carbamylation (Fig. 52.1).[20–24] Isocyanate can also combine reversibly with –OH and –SH groups of amino acids, and the various isocyanate-induced alterations in structure could impair protein function. A prominent contribution of urea to uremic toxicity would, however, be difficult to reconcile with the lack of benefit detected when urea levels were reduced by more intensive dialysis in the Hemodialysis (HEMO) study.[25]

## D-AMINO ACIDS

In comparison with urea, we know much less about most other potential uremic toxins. The D–amino acids exemplify this problem. Aggregate plasma concentrations of D–amino acids increase as kidney function declines.[26,27] However, the source, clearance, and toxicity of the D–amino acids found in the plasma are not well defined. D–Amino acids can be synthesized by mammalian cells, as well as derived from food, or produced by colonic bacteria.[28] Circulating D–amino acids are filtered by the glomerulus and then, in varying proportion, reabsorbed intact, degraded by D–amino acid oxidase (DAO) or D–aspartic acid oxidase in the proximal straight tubule, or excreted unaltered in the urine.[29,30] The liver can also clear D–amino acids, but the relative importance of renal and hepatic clearance is unknown. Aggregate D–amino acid concentrations have been found to increase almost in proportion to the serum creatinine level in kidney failure, suggesting that renal clearance predominates.[26,31,32] However, measured concentrations of individual D–amino acids, such as D-serine, increase less than creatinine.[31,32] This discrepancy remains unexplained. Of interest, D-serine is an endogenous coagonist of the synaptic *N*-methyl-D-aspartate receptor. It is tempting to speculate that D–amino acids are cleared rapidly from the extracellular fluid (ECF) because they have toxic effects. In addition, it has long been presumed that high levels of D–amino acids could impair protein synthesis or function.[28] D–amino acid accumulation could also interfere with the effects of endogenous D-serine and D-alanine on neuronal function,[33] but no major ill effects of D–amino acid accumulation have been observed in DAO-deficient mice, which have higher D–amino acid levels than humans with impaired kidney function.[34,35] Exogenous D–amino acids have so far been shown to be toxic only when administered in large quantities.[34,36]

## PEPTIDES AND PROTEINS

The kidney clears circulating dipeptides and tripeptides, which may comprise a significant portion of the extracellular amino acid pool.[37] Filtered dipeptides and tripeptides can be broken down by brush-border peptidases and reabsorbed as amino acids or reabsorbed by a brush-border peptide transporter and then hydrolyzed within proximal tubule cells.[38] Peritubular uptake, again followed by hydrolysis to amino acids, makes the renal clearance of many peptides higher than the glomerular filtration rate (GFR).[37,39] Small peptides are also taken up by other organs and generally do not accumulate in kidney failure. Peptides containing altered amino acids, which are normally cleared by the kidney, may be an exception to this rule.[39]

The kidney plays a proportionally larger role in the clearance of larger peptides. Proteins with a molecular weight of 10 to 20 kDa, such as $\beta_2$-microglobulin and cystatin C, are normally filtered by the glomerulus and then endocytosed and hydrolyzed in the lysosomes of proximal tubular cells.[40,41] Their plasma concentrations therefore rise in parallel with the plasma creatinine level as kidney function declines. Indeed, the plasma concentration of cystatin C, which is released at a near-constant rate by nucleated cells, may yield a more reliable estimate of GFR than the concentration of creatinine.[42] The role of the kidney in the removal of peptides with molecular weight between 500 Da and 10 kDa is less well defined. Peptides in this range are also filtered by the glomerulus and then hydrolyzed by brush-border peptidases or endocytosed, depending on their size and structure. Biologically active peptides such as insulin may also be cleared by peritubular uptake. Studies in patients with inherited dysfunction of proximal tubular endocytosis suggest that the normal kidney clears approximately 350 mg/day of peptides with molecular weights of 5 to 10 kDa from the circulation.[43] The relative importance of renal to extrarenal clearance has not been defined for most substances in this size range. The

**Box 52.3 Low-Molecular-Weight Proteins and Protein Fragments That Accumulate in Uremia**

$\alpha_1$-Microglobulin
$\beta_2$-Microglobulin
β-Trace protein (also known as prostaglandin D2 synthase)
Clara cell protein
Chromogranin A
Cystatin C
Free immunoglobulin light chains
Natriuretic peptides
Procalcitonin
Retinol-binding protein
Transcobalamin
Leptin
Ghrelin
Resistin
Troponin I

extent to which circulating levels of such peptides are increased in kidney failure is therefore unpredictable. Even less is known about the kidneys' contribution to the clearance of peptides in the range of 500 Da to 5 kDa.

Although the aggregate peptide levels in kidney failure remain ill defined, we have some knowledge of individual peptides that are retained in uremia. The best known are small proteins or fragments of large proteins for which immunoassays have been developed.[44–58] Box 52.3 provides a partial list of these substances. Retinol-binding protein, $\alpha_1$-microglobulin, and β-trace protein (also known as prostaglandin $D_2$ synthase) are members of the lipocalin superfamily, and future studies may identify elevated levels of other proteins of this group. Lipocalins are a family of proteins that transport small hydrophobic molecules and have an eight-stranded, antiparallel, symmetrical β-barrel fold. This reflects a β sheet that has been rolled into a cylindrical shape. A ligand-binding site is present in this cylinder. Studies using proteomic techniques have yielded a more complete picture of individual peptides that are retained in uremia.[59–61] These studies have shown that, as expected, uremic plasma contains a vast array of protein fragments that are normally cleared by the kidney. Many of these are derived from fibrinogen and the complement cascade.[61,62] One study has identified >1000 peptides with molecular weights from 800 Da to 10 kDa in the plasma of patients undergoing dialysis.[63] The toxicity of these peptides and low-molecular-weight proteins, like that of smaller molecular uremic solutes, is largely unknown. It has been widely speculated that retained peptides can cause inappropriate activation of various hormone or cytokine receptors. For example, retained complement protein D (molecular weight, 24 kDa) could contribute to the systemic inflammation and accelerated vascular disease observed in patients receiving dialysis.[64] Such hypotheses remain, however, to be proven. $\beta_2$-Microglobulin amyloidosis is the only disease attributable with certainty to a retained peptide, and its prevalence among the dialysis population appears to have declined over the past 30 years.[65] Plasma levels of peptides such as procalcitonin, troponin I, N-terminal brain natriuretic peptide, and chromogranin A are, however, increasingly used as diagnostic markers. And "false-positive" results may be obtained if criteria are not adjusted for the elevation of their plasma levels which normally accompanies loss of renal function.

## GUANIDINES

Among the compounds most frequently considered uremic toxins are guanidines, which, like urea, are derived from arginine (see Fig. 52.1).[66–68] One group of guanidines that accumulate in uremia includes creatinine and its breakdown products. Creatinine is produced by nonenzymatic degradation of creatine, which in turn is made from guanidinoacetic acid.[69] Creatinine itself appears nontoxic, and levels have been increased transiently to >100 mg/dL (8800 μmol/L) in subjects undergoing clearance studies. Instead, interest has been focused on the potential toxicity of various creatinine metabolites, especially creatol and methylguanidine (MG).[70,71] Creatol is a product resulting from the reaction of creatinine with the hydroxyl radical and is identified as a precursor of MG. Creatol and MG levels normally approximate 1% of creatinine levels. The production of these substances increases as plasma creatinine concentrations rise and may be stimulated by increased levels of intracellular oxidants.[67,69,70] MG is also produced by colonic bacteria, and its production may be increased by augmented dietary intake of protein or creatinine.[72] Another guanidine that has attracted interest is GSA, a substance formed not from creatinine but from the urea cycle intermediate argininosuccinate.[73,74] Rising plasma urea concentrations impede the conversion of argininosuccinate to urea and increase the production of GSA. The production of GSA thus depends on dietary protein intake as well as on kidney function, and may also be stimulated by increased concentrations of intracellular oxidants.[74,75]

Creatol, MG, and GSA share the interesting property that their plasma concentrations rise out of proportion to urea and creatinine levels as the GFR declines. This is because they are cleared largely by the kidney, and their production rates increase when plasma creatinine and urea concentrations are elevated.[67,69,70] In addition, relative to creatinine, large volumes of distribution, combined with restricted intercompartmental diffusion, limit the removal of creatol, MG, and GSA by intermittent hemodialysis.[66] In patients undergoing conventional hemodialysis, these compounds therefore exhibit high concentrations relative to normal.[1] The finding that they are present in relatively high concentrations does not prove that they are toxic. However, the evidence for toxicity of various guanidines, although incomplete, is stronger than that for most other solutes. Administration of MG aggravates uremic symptoms in dogs, whereas GSA contributes to uremic platelet dysfunction, and a number of guanidines impair neutrophil function.[18,76,77] In addition, various guanidines have been shown to accumulate in the brain and cerebrospinal fluid in uremia and may contribute to central nervous system dysfunction.[78]

The methylated arginines, asymmetric dimethyl arginine (ADMA) and symmetric dimethyl arginine (SDMA), also accumulate in kidney failure (Fig. 52.1). The metabolism of methylated arginines is quite different from that of the other uremic guanidines. ADMA and SDMA are formed by the methylation of arginine residues in nuclear proteins and released when these proteins are degraded. Interest has focused largely on ADMA because it inhibits nitric oxide (a potent local vasodilator) synthesis by the endothelial nitric oxide synthase (eNOS). The enzyme eNOS converts L-arginine to nitric oxide and L-citrulline and is an endothelial-enriched messenger RNA and protein. ADMA inhibits eNOS enzymatic activity.[79,80] SDMA has been less extensively considered as a toxin, but recent evidence has associated its plasma levels with cardiovascular risk.[80] The urinary clearance of ADMA is similar to that of creatinine, but most plasma ADMA is taken up and degraded in various tissues, including the kidney.[79,81] The presence of nonrenal clearance limits the rise in plasma ADMA concentrations observed as kidney function declines, so that ADMA concentrations rise to approximately two times normal early in the course of CKD and then do not increase much further as patients advance to end-stage renal disease (ESRD).[81,82] Increases in plasma ADMA concentration, although modest in proportion to other uremic solutes, have been associated with an increased risk for cardiovascular disease and death in patients with CKD.[80] It should be noted that differences in assay methods and reported reference ranges for ADMA greatly complicate the interpretation of these studies.

## PHENOLS AND OTHER AROMATIC COMPOUNDS

Phenols are compounds that have one or more hydroxyl groups attached to a benzene ring. In discussions of uremia, phenols are usually considered together with other aromatic compounds, such as hippurates, and the term "phenols" is sometimes used loosely to include these other substances. The aromatic compounds normally found in ECF are, for the most part, derived from the amino acids tyrosine and phenylalanine or from aromatic compounds contained in dietary vegetables. Medications provide an additional source in patients. The compounds in ECF are mostly metabolites; these are derived from their parent compounds by a combination of methylation, dehydroxylation, oxidation, reduction, and/or conjugation. Many of these reactions take place in colonic bacteria. The final step, which is usually conjugation with sulfate, glucuronic acid, or an amino acid, may take place in the liver, intestinal wall, or, to a lesser extent, kidney.[83,84] In general, conjugation tends to make the aromatic compounds both less toxic and more polar, thus facilitating their excretion by various organic ion transport systems.

These metabolic processes produce a bewildering array of aromatic compounds that are normally excreted in the urine or feces. The aggregate urinary excretion of aromatics is about 1000 mg/day and varies widely with the diet. The compounds normally excreted by the kidney accumulate in uremia and contribute to elevation of the anion gap, because most aromatic conjugates are negatively charged.[85] The concentration of individual aromatic compounds in uremic patients ranges from barely detectable up to 500 μM.[1,86–88] The relatively few compounds that have been studied extensively, including the examples described later, are among those found in the highest concentration. Interest in the contribution of phenols and other aromatic compounds to uremic toxicity has been encouraged by reports that uremic symptoms are better correlated with plasma concentration of these compounds than with those of other solutes.[13,89–91] Evidence obtained so far on the toxicity of individual aromatic compound is incomplete.

The most extensively studied aromatic uremic solute is hippurate (see Fig. 52.1). Because it is the aromatic waste compound normally excreted in the largest quantity, the concentration of free hippurate rises higher than those of other aromatic solutes in the plasma of patients with kidney failure. Hippurate is the glycine conjugate of benzoate, derived largely from vegetable foods, with only a small amount formed endogenously from the amino acid phenylalanine.[92,93] Diet therefore determines hippurate production, and hippurate excretion in aboriginal people eating vegetable diets may exceed hippurate excretion in people from industrialized nations by many fold.[94] In persons with normal kidneys, active tubular secretion maintains a plasma hippurate concentration much lower than it would be if hippurate were cleared solely by glomerular filtration. There is a clinical correlate of this property of hippurate. Aminohippuric acid or *para*-aminohippuric acid (PAH), a derivative of hippuric acid, is a diagnostic agent used in the measurement of renal plasma flow. PAH is completely removed from the blood that passes through the kidneys given that PAH undergoes both glomerular filtration and tubular secretion. Therefore the rate at which the kidneys can clear PAH from the blood reflects total renal plasma flow. By itself, hippurate is not toxic. The plasma hippurate concentration in a normal person can be increased to equal that of a uremic patient, without apparent ill effect.[95] Moreover, increasing the hippurate concentration by benzoate feeding in a patient with kidney failure does not aggravate uremic symptoms.[96] A further clinical correlate addresses the potential toxicity of aromatics, in this case an exogenous source. Toluene is a widely abused inhaled drug (e.g., glue sniffing) due, in part, to its acute neurologic effects of euphoria and hallucinations. Toluene is metabolized by cytochrome P-450 into benzoic acid and hippuric acid. The hallmarks of acute toluene intoxication are hypokalemic paralysis and metabolic acidosis due to distal renal tubular acidosis. Patients can also have hippurate crystals appear in the urine.

Another extensively studied aromatic compound is *p*-cresol. In contrast to hippurate, which is derived from aromatic compounds in plants, *p*-cresol is formed by the action of colonic bacteria on tyrosine and phenylalanine. The portion of amino acids that escapes absorption in the small intestine may be increased in uremic patients, leading to increased production of *p*-cresol and other bacterial metabolites.[97,98] Studies have shown that *p*-cresol circulates largely as *p*-cresol sulfate with a much lesser portion in the form of *p*-cresol glucuronide. Reports of unconjugated *p*-cresol in the plasma of uremic patients now appear to have been the result of inadvertent hydrolysis of *p*-cresol sulfate during sample processing.[99,100] *p*-Cresol sulfate binds avidly to serum albumin, and the effect of different renal replacement therapies on albumin-bound solutes has often been tested by measuring plasma *p*-cresol sulfate concentrations.[101–103] High concentrations of *p*-cresol sulfate (often measured as *p*-cresol) have been associated with cardiovascular death in patients undergoing hemodialysis, and *p*-cresol sulfate has been related to indices of endothelial injury, including endothelial microparticle production.[104–106] While the results of clinical studies are not uniform, these findings, along with in vitro evidence of *p*-cresol sulfate toxicity, have increased the focus on *p*-cresol sulfate as a potential uremic toxin.[105–107]

Other aromatic uremic solutes have been identified in great numbers but studied less extensively.[8,87,88] Metabolites of tyrosine and phenylalanine, which accumulate in uremia, include phenlylacetylglutamine, *para*-hydroxyphenylacetic acid, and 3,4-dihydroxybenzoic acid, as well as *p*-cresol.[108–110] Phenylacetylglutamine, like *p*-cresol sulfate, has been associated with cardiovascular disease and mortality in dialysis patients.[111] The structural relationship of the aromatic amino acid metabolites to neurotransmitters has stimulated interest in their potential role as uremic toxins. So far, 3,4-dihydroxybenzoate has been shown to cause central nervous system dysfunction in rats, but only at levels higher than those encountered in patients with kidney failure.[109] Increased levels of 4-hydroxyphenylacetate were associated with impaired cognitive function in patients maintained on hemodialysis.[112] The work of identifying toxic aromatic uremic solutes, however, remains daunting. Relatively little progress has been made, and caution is appropriate, particularly when interpreting studies relating levels of specific compounds to poor outcomes. Associations have necessarily been identified only for the few compounds extensively studied. Even if a positive association has been correctly identified, correlations of poor outcomes with abnormal blood levels could be confounded by associations with other unmeasured aromatic substance(s) evidencing related production and/or clearance rates.

## INDOLES AND OTHER TRYPTOPHAN METABOLITES

Indoles are compounds containing a benzene ring fused to a five-membered nitrogen-containing pyrrole ring (Fig. 52.1). Many similarities are encountered when considering the indoles and phenols in uremia. As with phenols, some indoles are derived from plant foods, and others are produced endogenously. However, the endogenous indoles are derived mostly from tryptophan, whereas the phenols are derived from phenylalanine and tyrosine. As with the phenols, minor chemical modifications in various combinations yield a remarkable variety of structures, with more than 600 indoles derived from tryptophan.[113] Those with known physiologic function include the neurotransmitter 5-hydroxytryptamine (serotonin) and melatonin. Other indoles are considered to be waste products and are often conjugated prior to urinary excretion. These uremic indoles accumulate when kidney function is impaired.

The most extensively studied of the uremic indoles is indoxyl sulfate; this is produced from tryptophan in a manner reminiscent of the production of *p*-cresol sulfate from tyrosine and phenylalanine. Gut bacteria convert tryptophan to indole, which is then oxidized to indoxyl and conjugated with sulfate in the liver. There is evidence that indoxyl sulfate is toxic in vitro, but early studies of indoxyl sulfate infusion failed to replicate uremic symptoms.[13,114–116] Like *p*-cresol sulfate, indoxyl sulfate is extensively bound to plasma albumin. It has also been suggested that indoxyl sulfate is toxic to renal tubular cells and the rising indoxyl sulfate levels accelerate the progression of renal disease.[117] Controlled trials to lower indoxyl sulfate levels, however, have not been found to slow progression.[118]

Other indoles that accumulate in uremia include indoleacetic acid, indoleacrylic acid, and 5-hydroxyindoleacetic acid.[1,119,120] As with the phenols, indoles are structurally related to potent neuroactive substances, including serotonin and (famously) D-lysergic acid diethylamide. This structural similarity has stimulated interest in the potential role of indoles as neurotoxins, but few uremic indoles have been administered to normal animals, and none have convincingly been shown to alter CNS function at the levels encountered in patients with kidney failure. There is, however, increasing evidence that indoxyl sulfate contributes to vascular disease and particularly to thrombosis.[106,121] Some effects of indoxyl sulfate have been shown to be mediated by activation of the aryl hydrocarbon receptor, a transcription factor originally identified as upregulating xenobiotic disposal pathways.[121,122] This work puts our knowledge of the mechanisms by which indoxyl sulfate acts ahead of that for other putative uremic toxins.

Only a minor portion of dietary tryptophan is excreted as indoles. Most is metabolized by the kynurenine pathway, which allows tryptophan to be converted to glutarate and oxidized or, when necessary, used in the synthesis of nicotinamide. Kidney failure causes members of the kynurenine pathway, including L-kynurenine and quinolinic acid, to accumulate in the plasma.[123,124] Knowledge that these substances play a physiologic role in the modulation of CNS function has stimulated interest in their possible contribution to uremic toxicity. As usual, however, evidence that they are toxic at the levels encountered in patients has not been obtained.

## ALIPHATIC AMINES

The methylamines monomethylamine (MMA), dimethylamine (DMA), and trimethylamine (TMA) are among the simplest compounds that have been considered to be uremic toxins. Reported serum levels are twofold to threefold higher in patients with ESRD compared with persons with normal or near-normal kidney function.[125,126] However, available data and predictions based on their chemistry suggest that the methylamines are poorly removed by dialysis, and early data suggest that they may even be produced in excess in those with uremia.[125–127]

A large volume of distribution may contribute to poor removal of the methylamines by dialysis. These compounds are bases, with a $pK_a$ ranging from 9 to 11. Thus they exist as positively charged species at a physiologic pH. The lower intracellular pH compared with extracellular pH should lead to their preferential intracellular sequestration, with volumes of distribution exceeding total body water. Indeed, measurements in experimental animals and humans have confirmed these predictions for DMA and TMA.[126,128,129]

Because they circulate as small organic compounds that are not protein bound, these three amines are likely freely filtered. However, because they exist as organic cations, they also have the potential to be secreted by one or another of the family of organic cation transporters and may also travel through Rh channels.[130,131] Hence they may achieve clearances that are higher than the GFR. The chemically similar exogenous compound, tetraethyl ammonium, has long been a prototype test solute for organic cation secretion and is cleared at rates up to (and in one study higher than) the renal plasma flow.[132,133] Although formal renal clearances of DMA and TMA are not available, the total metabolic clearance of DMA and TMA by plasma disappearance of labeled compounds in rats approaches that of renal plasma flow.[128] By contrast, the urinary clearance of MMA in normal subjects is about one-third that of creatinine, indicating no net secretion for this amine.[127]

The biochemical pathways leading to MMA, DMA, and TMA are not well delineated. Both the host's mammalian tissues and resident gut flora have been thought to contribute to the net appearance of these amines. However, plasma MMA and DMA concentrations were not different among patients with ESRD with and without colons.[134] The dietary precursors for MMA, DMA, and TMA include choline and trimethylamine oxide (TMAO).[135–137] Production of these compounds may actually be increased with kidney failure, perhaps caused by overgrowth of intestinal bacteria.[127,129,138] Thus production of aliphatic amines may be increased in the face of impaired renal removal.

Incomplete data also implicate the amines as toxic. Reported effects of MMA include a variety of neural toxicities, hemolysis, and inhibition of lysosomal function.[139] MMA has also been shown to be a potent anorectic agent when administered into the cerebrospinal fluid in mice.[140] Despite toxicities in cells and animals, however, MMA and DMA were not associated with all-cause mortality in a cohort of patients with ESRD.[141] Although of utmost importance, mortality is obviously a blunt metric of uremic toxicity. Other signs of toxicity of MMA and DMA should be explored.

The uremic fetor or fishy breath noted in uremic patients is attributable to TMA.[142] Although the malodor may be of no major consequence in itself, the potentially important and well-described diminutions in taste (dysgeusia) and smell (dysosmia) among patients with kidney failure (which may contribute to poor nutritional status) may also be related to the amines. Plasma MMA concentrations were not related to olfactory defects in ESRD.[143]

TMA can be both a precursor to TMAO and, as noted, a product of dietary TMAO.[144] TMAO is cleared by secretion in the normal kidney; its levels rise as the GFR falls and, like those of many other secreted solutes, are increased out of proportion to urea levels in dialysis patients.[145] TMAO was initially identified as a risk factor for cardiovascular disease in persons with normal renal function.[144,146] TMAO is a gut microbial metabolite that has been shown to be directly atherogenic. TMAO arises from gut microbiota metabolism following ingestion of diets rich in phosphatidylcholine (lecithin), the major dietary source of choline, and carnitine, an abundant nutrient in red meat. Recent studies employing microbial transplantation into recipients confirmed a direct causal role for gut microbes in transmitting atherosclerosis susceptibility and overall TMAO production. Subsequent studies showed that accumulation of TMAO is also associated with atherosclerosis burden and cardiovascular events in patients with renal insufficiency and in patients maintained on dialysis.[147,148]

## OTHER UREMIC SOLUTES

A wide variety of other compounds accumulate in kidney failure. One group is the polyols, of which the most extensively studied is myoinositol (Fig. 52.1).[149,150] Myoinositol is different from most other uremic solutes in that it is normally oxidized by the kidney. Its accumulation in uremia therefore reflects impaired degradation and not impaired excretion. Evidence that myoinositol causes nerve damage, although stronger than most of the evidence for the toxicity of uremic solutes, is far from conclusive.[151]

The purine metabolite uric acid is the only known organic substance with a plasma level actively regulated by variation of its renal excretion. With advanced CKD, the capacity of the kidney to increase the fractional excretion of uric acid is exceeded, and uric acid levels increase, along with those of its precursor molecules, xanthine and hypoxanthine.

Observational studies have shown that high uric acid levels are associated with increased survival in dialysis patients, perhaps because the plasma uric acid is a marker of nutritional status.[152] Other nucleic acid metabolites excreted by the kidney are produced in much lesser quantities. Many are derived from the modified nucleosides contained in transfer RNAs.[153] They appear to be cleared largely by filtration and to accumulate in the plasma as the GFR falls. Pseudouridine is an isomer of the nucleoside uridine in which the uracil is attached via a carbon–carbon instead of a nitrogen–carbon glycosidic bond. It has been suggested that pseudouridine, which is the most abundant of these variant nucleic acid metabolites, contributes to insulin resistance and altered CNS development but, as usual, the demonstration of its toxicity is not conclusive.[153,154]

Oxalate is also excreted by the kidney and accumulates in kidney failure. Oxalate is derived from catabolism of endogenous substances, including vitamin C, as well as from plant foods.[155,156] The potential for oxalate deposition in tissues may limit our ability to maintain normal plasma vitamin C concentrations in patients receiving dialysis.[157,158] Additional substances excreted by the kidney that accumulate in kidney failure include various pteridines, dicarboxylic acids, isoflavins, and furancarboxylic acids, including 3-carboxy-4-methyl-5-prophy-2-furanpropanoic acid.[102,153,159–162] Recently completed studies continue to add new solutes to the list, and the number reported will likely soon rise >1000, including many compounds that are at present identified only by their molecular mass and do not appear in standard databases of human metabolites as yet. The possibility of toxicity is invariably considered when new solutes are identified, but experiments to test the solute toxicity are rarely performed.

## SOLUTE REMOVAL BY DIFFERENT FORMS OF RENAL REPLACEMENT THERAPY

Although investigators have not succeeded in replicating uremic illness by administering uremic solutes to normal humans or animals, reversing illness by removing solutes has become a part of everyday practice. Because renal replacement therapies remove solutes indiscriminately, the improvement they effect cannot be attributed to removal of specific compounds. However, different forms of renal replacement therapy do clear solutes at different rates based on some characteristics, including molecular size, protein binding, and sequestration within cells or other body compartments. The demonstration that different therapies have different effects on some features of uremia might therefore reveal properties of the responsible toxin(s).

### ORIGINAL MIDDLE MOLECULE HYPOTHESIS

The suggestion that the nature of uremic toxins could be deduced by comparing the effects of different renal replacement methods was first advanced by Babb and colleagues.[163] In the 1960s, hemodialysis was performed with membranes that provided very limited clearance of solutes with molecular weight >1000 Da. Treatment with these membranes wakened patients from coma, relieved vomiting, and partially reversed other uremic symptoms. This provided evidence, which remains convincing, that some important uremic toxins are small. Babb and coworkers were impressed that patients on peritoneal dialysis were healthier than patients on hemodialysis who had the same plasma urea and creatinine concentrations. They further observed that increasing the dialysis duration from 6.5 to 9 hours three times weekly prevented neuropathy. These observations led them to conclude that important toxins were >300 Da because, as compared with contemporary hemodialysis membranes, the peritoneal membrane afforded greater relative permeability in this size range and because increasing the hemodialysis session length was expected to reduce the plasma concentration of larger molecules more than the concentrations of creatinine and urea. Based on their further impression that no additional benefit was obtained using membranes that provided superior clearance for solutes >2000 Da, they concluded that some important toxins were “middle molecules,” with a molecular weight >300 Da but <2000 Da.[164]

### LARGE SOLUTES—CHANGING DEFINITION OF "MIDDLE MOLECULES"

Studies during the 1970s provided only equivocal evidence that increasing the clearance of solutes with a molecular weight between 350 and 2000 Da improved the health of uremic patients.[163] The proposition that no benefit could be obtained by increasing the clearance of solutes with molecular weight >2000 Da was never prospectively tested. The original middle molecule hypothesis was thus never proven to be correct. And although the phrase “middle molecules” remains in use, its meaning has gradually shifted to include larger solutes. The 2003 report of the EUTox work group[1] thus defined middle molecules as those with a size ranging from 500 Da to <60,000 Da. The adoption of new membrane materials, which was in part a response to the original middle molecule hypothesis, ended the investigation of the relative toxicity of solutes that fall into different parts of the size range <1000 Da. The question of whether solutes with molecular weight >1000 Da exert toxic effects remains under investigation. Henderson and colleagues[165] showed that such solutes can be cleared more effectively by hemofiltration than by hemodialysis. The results of recent large trials combining hemofiltration with hemodialysis to increase the clearance of large solutes have been equivocal. One problem is that the concentration of putative high-molecular-weight toxins may not decline in proportion to the increase in clearance during treatment because they are cleared by extrarenal mechanisms and they move slowly from the interstitial fluid to the ECF during treatment.[166,167]

### PROTEIN-BOUND SOLUTES

Other solutes that are poorly removed by standard hemodialysis include those that bind to albumin.[102,168] Their dialytic clearance is low, not because they are large molecules, but because only the free, unbound solute concentration contributes to the gradient-driving solute across the dialysis membrane. In the normal kidney, the combination of protein binding and tubular secretion allows molecules to be excreted while keeping their concentrations in the ECF very low.[5] This presumably represents an evolutionary adaptation to excrete toxic substances, and there is indeed suggestive evidence that some important uremic toxins are protein bound.[169] The clearance of protein-bound solutes can be increased by raising dialysate flow and membrane size above the levels used in conventional hemodialysis or by combining a high hemofiltration rate with dialysis in hemodiafiltration treatment.[170,171] The aggregate toxicity of protein-bound solutes could thus theoretically be assessed by comparing the effects of different renal replacement prescriptions, but this has not been attempted do date. Other methods of improving bound solute removal including the use of sorbents, infusion of compounds that displace bound solute from albumin, and manipulation of the ionic strength of the dialysate remain to be tested. Studies carried out raise the possibility that levels of protein-bound solutes, like levels of large solutes, may not decline in proportion to the increase in clearance during treatment.[167] Peritoneal dialysis clears protein-bound solutes at a very low rate, and the total clearance of protein-bound solutes in patients maintained on peritoneal dialysis therefore depends heavily on the level of residual kidney function.[172,173] Surprisingly, however, plasma concentrations of the bound solutes *p*-cresol sulfate and indoxyl sulfate are not much higher in patients undergoing peritoneal dialysis without residual kidney function than in those with residual kidney function, suggesting that production of these solutes may diminish as residual kidney function is lost.[173] Besides, plasma concentration of *p*-cresol sulfate and indoxyl sulfate did not fall in proportion to the increase in time-averaged clearance in the more aggressively dialyzed patient groups in either the HEMO or Frequent Hemodialysis Network (FHN) studies.[174,175] The HEMO study assessed the effect of a higher dialysis dose (target equilibrated Kt/V 1.45) and a high-flux dialyzer membrane on all-cause mortality in patients undergoing hemodialysis three times per week compared with standard dose (target equilibrated Kt/V 1.05) and a low-flux membrane. The FHN trial aimed to determine whether increasing the frequency of in-center hemodialysis would result in beneficial changes in left ventricular mass, self-reported physical health, and other intermediate outcomes among patients undergoing maintenance hemodialysis.

### SEQUESTERED SOLUTES

Some solutes are sequestered, or held in compartments where their concentration does not equilibrate rapidly with that of the plasma.[176] Application of a high dialytic clearance may rapidly lower the plasma concentration of such solutes while removing only a small portion of the total body content. When this happens, intermittent dialysis treatment will be followed by a rebound in the plasma solute concentration toward predialysis levels.[66,177] Theoretically, the contribution of sequestered solutes to uremic toxicity, like the contribution of large solutes or protein-bound solutes, could be assessed by comparing the efficacy of different dialysis prescriptions. When treatment is intermittent, the removal of sequestered relative to freely equilibrating solutes can be increased by lengthening the treatment while simultaneously reducing the plasma clearance. To date, however, while prolonged treatment has been shown to lower plasma levels of phosphate, its effect on levels of organic uremic solutes has not been assessed.[159]

## EFFECTS OF DIET AND GASTROINTESTINAL FUNCTION

It may be possible to identify uremic toxins by comparing the effect of different diets as well as by comparing the effect of different renal replacement therapies. Patients with kidney failure tend to reduce their intake of protein spontaneously.[179] Before dialysis was available, physicians found that the protein restriction could ameliorate uremic symptoms.[180] These findings suggest that important uremic toxins are derived from protein catabolism. They call into question current recommendations that patients undergoing dialysis ingest a higher protein intake than what has been recommended for the general population.[181] Uremic solutes whose production depends on protein intake include urea, MG, GSA, and the indoles and phenols produced by the action of gut bacteria on tryptophan, phenylalanine, and tyrosine.[75,86,182–184] This group overlaps with the large group of uremic solutes made by colon microbes.[134] The production of such solutes may depend not only on dietary intake but also on gut function. Impaired small bowel function may increase the delivery of peptides to the colon in uremia, and the composition of the colon microbiome may also be altered.[185,186] If colonic bacteria produce uremic toxins, uremic symptoms could theoretically be relieved by altering the delivery of substrates to the colon or adding sorbents to the diet. Only limited studies of such maneuvers have so far been performed, with success most often obtained with the use of dietary fiber to reduce the production of selected colon-derived solutes.[187–189] Historically, once hemodialysis became widely available, attempts to modify uremic solute production were largely abandoned. However, interest in this area has been revived by the imperfect efficacy of conventional dialysis and by the relatively disappointing results to date of trials evaluating more intensive dialysis treatment.[98] Interest has also been stimulated by new knowledge of the microbiome, and the promise that if toxic solutes were better known, the microbiomes composition or enzymatic function could be manipulated to reduce their production.[190]

## SOLUTE CLEARANCE BY ORGANIC TRANSPORT SYSTEMS

The cloning of transporters, which move organic solutes into the lumen of the proximal tubule, has provided a potential new means to identify potential uremic toxins. To the extent that uremia is caused by accumulation of organic solutes, knocking out these transporters would be expected to recapitulate uremic symptoms. To date, knocking out individual transporters has been found not to cause detectable illness, likely because of redundancy of the transport systems.[191,192] The accumulation of uremic solutes may interfere with organic solute transport important for detoxification at other sites, most notably the liver and blood–brain barrier.[193–195]

# METABOLIC EFFECTS OF UREMIA

The loss of kidney function has numerous metabolic effects. Some of the most prominent are listed in Box 52.1. A few can be related to the loss of specific renal processes, such as the hydroxylation of vitamin D. However, most have no clear cause, and can at present only be attributed to the retention of uremic solutes.

## OXIDANT STRESS AND THE MODIFICATION OF PROTEIN STRUCTURE

Studies have suggested that loss of kidney function increases oxidant stress.[196] The term "oxidant stress" is acknowledged to be vague, although a wealth of evidence points to increased oxidant effects in uremia. Increased levels of primary oxidants cannot be documented because they are evanescent species, which act locally, such as superoxide anion, hydrogen peroxide, hydroxyl radical, and hypochlorous acid. The accumulation of various by-products of oxidant reactions is therefore taken as evidence of increased oxidant activity. Although the accumulation of these markers of oxidant activity is well documented, there is at present no explanation as to why the production of oxidants should be increased in uremia. Leukocyte activation leading to increased production of hypochlorous acid has been described in patients undergoing dialysis and may be especially prominent when uremia is accompanied by systemic inflammation.[197]

Among the most commonly measured markers of oxidant activity have been oxidized amino acids and related compounds and substances that react with thiobarbituric acid, including malondialdehyde.[198] The accumulation of these low-molecular-weight compounds could reflect reduced renal clearance as well as increased production. More convincing evidence of oxidant stress is the accumulation of intact proteins containing oxidized amino acids.[199,200] The accumulation of these larger markers of oxidation cannot be attributed to reduced renal clearance. Further potential evidence of oxidative stress in uremia is the loss of extracellular reducing substances. The extracellular compartment is normally provided with several reducing substances, of which the reduced forms of ascorbic acid and plasma albumin are considered to be the most important. In uremia, the portion of ascorbic acid and albumin circulating in the oxidized form is increased. The case of albumin, which undergoes oxidation at its single free cysteine thiol (SH) group, is particularly interesting. Plasma albumin in patients with kidney failure is rapidly restored to the reduced form during hemodialysis.[201] The shift to oxidized albumin in untreated uremia is associated with the accumulation of cystine, which is the oxidized form of the thiol amino acid cysteine, and the shift back to reduced albumin during hemodialysis is associated with a lowering of cystine levels toward normal. One explanation for these phenomena is that normal kidney function is required to accomplish the steady reduction of cystine and albumin, which must take place to offset normal oxidant production.

The major ill effect of increased oxidant activity in uremia is thought to be modification of proteins. Proteins are modified not only by direct oxidation of amino acids but also by the combination of amino acid side chains with carbonyl (C=O) compounds. The terminology in this area is confusing. The first carbonyl compounds shown to react with proteins were sugars, and the modified proteins formed after several reaction steps were therefore referred to as advanced glycosylation end products (AGEs). Elevated sugar concentrations could account for the increased concentrations of AGEs found in persons with diabetes mellitus, but not for the subsequent findings of similarly increased AGE concentrations in patients with ESRD. Studies have shown that the high levels of active nonsugar carbonyls are responsible for the increased production of these modified proteins when renal function is reduced.[202] The active carbonyls have not been fully characterized, but they include compounds such as glyoxal (Fig. 52.1), which can be produced by oxidation of sugars and lipids. It has therefore been suggested that the protein end products of carbonyl modification in uremia should be referred to not as AGEs but as advanced glycoxidation and lipoxidation end products. Terminology aside, interest in both directly oxidized and carbonyl-modified proteins has centered on the possibility that alterations in protein structure contribute to uremia.[203,204] The hypothesis that oxidant stress contributes to adverse health consequences in ESRD has prompted trials of various antioxidants. So far, administration of vitamin C, various forms of vitamin E, folate, and α-lipoic acid has failed to reverse plasma indices of oxidant stress in patients undergoing dialysis.[205–210]

## EFFECTS OF UREMIA

### ON RESTING ENERGY EXPENDITURE

Resting energy expenditure has been reported as increased, decreased, and normal in patients with kidney failure.[211–215] The choice of control populations and other methodologic issues, such as corrections for altered body composition, have probably contributed to this uncertainty. The effect of dialysis treatment, which may transiently increase energy expenditure, must also be considered. Uremia, apart from dialysis, likely reduces resting energy expenditure.[213,215] Lower energy expenditure accords with observations of lower body temperatures in those with uremia, although additional factors may be at play in thermoregulation.[13] However, dialysis treatment may itself speed metabolism and increase energy expenditure.[214] Effects of inflammation in patients with ESRD add further complexity to the assessment of energy requirements.[216] Using anthropometric techniques in patients with ESRD on chronic hemodialysis who were maintained for 3 months on carefully constructed diets, the energy requirements were found not to differ from those reported for similarly sedentary normal subjects.[217] The energy requirements in ESRD were, however, more variable than in normals.

Knowledge of the physiologic control mechanisms for appetite, fat metabolism, and energy expenditure is potentially relevant to uremic energy metabolism. Studies have focused on the signaling molecules ghrelin, produced by the stomach, and leptin, produced by adipose tissue along with other adipose tissue–derived hormones (adipokines). Levels of these small proteins tend to rise in kidney failure because of reduced clearance by the kidney and possibly because of increased production.[54,218]

### ON CARBOHYDRATE METABOLISM

Insulin resistance is the most conspicuous derangement in uremic carbohydrate metabolism.[219] The defect is clearly present in ESRD, but in cross-sectional studies, impairment can be detected when the GFR falls below 50 mL/min/1.73 $m^2$, with a graded relation to GFR.[220,221] There are probably several causes of this phenomenon.[222] Surprisingly, some obvious possibilities do not seem to contribute. Insulin binds normally to its receptor in uremia, and receptor density is unchanged.[223,224] Moreover, excess levels of glucagon or fatty acids do not account for the disorder.[225] As is the case with overall energy metabolism, interest has recently focused on the contribution of adipokines, including leptin, resistin, and adiponectin to insulin resistance. Adipose tissue has also been identified as a source of inflammatory cytokines that impair insulin action in various experimental systems and circulate at increased levels in many patients with advanced renal insufficiency.

However, correlations among levels of individual substances with measures of insulin resistance are poor, and the extent to which adipose tissue products contribute to uremic insulin resistance remains uncertain.[55,225,226]

Because dialysis, transplantation, and low-protein diets tend to restore insulin responsiveness, it has also been suggested that unidentified nitrogenous product(s) mediate insulin resistance.[225] Acidosis has been shown to provoke insulin resistance and accumulation of acid, as well as nitrogenous wastes, may contribute to insulin resistance in uremia.[227] 11-β-Hydroxysteroid dehydrogenase type 1 provokes insulin resistance by regenerating glucocorticoids. In experimental uremia, liver and fat tissues express increased activity of this enzyme as well as insulin resistance. The insulin resistance associated with 11-β-hydroxysteroid dehydrogenase can be mitigated with an inhibitor of the enzyme, all suggesting a role for this steroid pathway in insulin resistance.[228] The cause for increased enzymatic activity is unknown. Resistin is a protein capable of inducing insulin resistance, and its levels are high when kidney function is impaired. However, the plasma concentrations of resistin are not associated with insulin resistance if the GFR is taken into account.[55] Retinol-binding protein is also associated with insulin resistance (and also rises in ESRD) but is not related to markers of glucose control.[229] Finally, physical inactivity and deconditioning may contribute to insulin resistance. Exercise programs have been shown to mitigate insulin resistance but must be relatively protracted and intensive to be effective.[230,231]

Insulin resistance may have several adverse effects. Most importantly, it has been recognized as a risk factor for cardiovascular disease.[232] The connections between insulin resistance and vascular disease are not clear. A tendency to hyperglycemia is one presumably toxic effect. Some investigators have suggested that the sodium retentive effect of insulin on the kidney remains intact, whereas other tissues become insulin resistant in uremia. Increased plasma insulin concentrations could thus contribute to arterial hypertension in patients with impaired kidney function.[233,234] Outside of vascular disease, the loss of insulin's anabolic action may contribute to uremic muscle wasting.[225,235]

Even though insulin resistance is the rule in uremia, hypoglycemia can be a significant effect of renal insufficiency.[236] Hypoglycemia is likely to occur, despite insulin resistance, for two main reasons. First, the kidney is a major site of insulin catabolism. Patients with diabetes mellitus treated with insulin, or insulin secretagogues (e.g., sulfonylureas), frequently become hypoglycemic if doses are not adjusted downward as the GFR declines. Second, the kidney is a major site of gluconeogenesis.[236] The liver produces the bulk of glucose in postabsorptive and starvation states, but even in these situations, the kidney produces some glucose. With prolonged fasting, the kidney is responsible for approximately half of the total glucose production.[237,238] Thus advanced CKD may predispose to hypoglycemia, both by prolonging insulin action and by reducing gluconeogenesis. These effects may become particularly apparent when other hypoglycemic factors, such as ethanol ingestion or liver disease, are also evident.

## ON LIPID METABOLISM

Nephrotic syndrome and even lower-grade proteinuria are regularly associated with hyperlipidemia.[239] However, lipid abnormalities are modest when kidney function is impaired without significant proteinuria.[240] Indeed, total cholesterol falls on average as the GFR drops below about 30 mL/min/1.73 m$^2$.[179] Metabolite profiling in plasma of patients with ESRD using liquid chromatography and tandem mass spectrometry has revealed that lipid products deviate from normal levels far less than polar compounds. However, lower-molecular-weight triacylglycerols were generally decreased, and an increase in intermediate-weight triacylglycerols was observed.[3] The causes and consequences of these changes in lipids are uncertain. The decline in total cholesterol is taken to reflect, at least in part, progressive reduction in food intake. Numerous hypotheses have been advanced to account for the finding that atherosclerosis is accelerated but lipid levels are not markedly elevated in renal failure. Even though total lipid levels are not significantly elevated, there may be an increase in oxidized forms due to oxidant stress and reduced lipoprotein clearance rates.[241] The high prevalence of cardiovascular disease patients with ESRD has prompted several randomized clinical trials of statin agents. The largest trials performed to date have identified no clear benefit of statins in patients on dialysis, in sharp contrast to persons with normal or near-normal kidney function and, in one study,[242] to patients with advanced, non–dialysis-requiring CKD.[243–245] These trials are discussed in more detail in the chapter on cardiovascular disease (Chapter 54). Furthermore statins seem to provide no benefit in slowing the progression of kidney disease.[246]

## ON AMINO ACID AND PROTEIN METABOLISM

The normal kidney participates in the metabolism of several amino acids.[8,247–250] For example, the kidney converts citrulline to arginine. Loss of this function likely contributes to the increasing ratio of citrulline to arginine as the GFR declines below 50 mL/min/1.73 m$^2$.[248,249] Similarly, reduced renal production of serine from glycine probably underlies the rise in the plasma glycine-to-serine ratio. Increased concentrations of the sulfur-containing amino acids—cystine, taurine, and homocysteine—are especially intriguing. Cystine and homocysteine accumulate in the oxidized form, consistent with the concept that uremia is a state of oxidant stress, and homocysteine levels have been associated with the progression of cardiovascular disease.[248,249,251] Administration of folate to lower homocysteine levels neither restores the plasma redox state toward normal nor reduces the frequency of cardiovascular events.[207,252] The mechanism responsible for the accumulation of oxidized cystine and homocysteine remains unclear, but this change can be detected as the GFR drops below roughly half of normal and becomes more extreme at ESRD approaches.

Tissue protein loss reflected by muscle wasting is a major concern in patients with kidney failure. Factors that predispose to protein wasting include reduced appetite, along with insulin resistance and altered amino acid metabolism, as described earlier. Dialysis also results in some protein loss, with amino acids lost in the hemodialysate and plasma proteins and amino acids lost in the peritoneal dialysate. In the absence of other complications, the effect of uremia at the levels now seen clinically on protein metabolism is usually modest, at least over the short term.[235] Patients with advanced CKD can maintain nitrogen balance on low-protein diets as long as acidosis and inflammation are minimal. Several factors may combine with defects in insulin resistance and altered amino acid and adipose metabolism to produce muscle wasting. The best studied of these is acidosis, which has been shown to stimulate the ubiquitin–proteasome pathway of intracellular protein degradation. Activation of caspase-3 seems to be an important step in proteolysis, which is followed by disposal of protein cleavage fragments through the proteasome.[253] In addition to these effects, acidosis contributes to insulin resistance and thereby attenuates protein anabolic actions of insulin.[254] Base supplements can mitigate the catabolic effects of acidosis, but a long-term study establishing the value of normalizing bicarbonate levels in patients with impaired kidney function is lacking.[227,255–257]

Inflammation may be an even more important contributor to protein wasting than acidosis in patients with kidney failure. Muscle loss in patients with ESRD has been linked to an inflammatory state, characterized by increased serum concentrations of C-reactive protein and various cytokines. How these inflammatory mediators trigger net protein degradation in muscle and other tissues remains to be elucidated, although their presence is regularly accompanied by muscle loss. High levels of inflammatory mediators are also associated with lower serum albumin concentrations, which have been attributed largely to reduced hepatic production of albumin. Both muscle loss and reduced albumin concentration predict early death. The exact cause(s) of inflammation remains elusive. In some cases, inflammation can be ascribed to known episodes of infection or other intercurrent illness. In many cases, however, no cause can be identified. Occult inflammatory stimuli in these cases may include subclinical infection at hemodialysis catheter or arteriovenous graft sites, exposure to dialysate and various synthetic materials, and accelerated vascular injury that is common in ESRD.[258–260] Oxidant stress has also often been invoked. Attempts to reduce inflammation with free radical scavengers and other agents, however, have been largely unsuccessful.[261–263] An interesting possibility is that organic solutes retained in kidney failure, although they do not regularly trigger inflammation over the short term, cause the late appearance of inflammation in a subset of patients with ESRD. Some evidence has suggested that accumulation of proteins modified by glycation and oxidation can trigger a self-perpetuating inflammatory loop in these cases.[264,265]

Another factor contributing to muscle wasting is inactivity. Johansen and associates have shown that self-reported physical activity in patients starting dialysis is at, or below, the first percentile for population reference range,[266] and lower levels of physical activity are strongly associated with mortality.[267] In these patients, inactivity may be caused by fatigue and loss of energy, which are invariable although difficult-to-measure features of uremia, and by depression and other comorbid illnesses,[268] which are common in the ESRD population.

## OVERALL NUTRITION

As emphasized by Depner,[9] the condition of patients undergoing dialysis reflects a combination of residual uremia, side effects of dialysis mixed with the effects of comorbid conditions, and increasing age. Most patients starting on dialysis in Europe and the United States are overweight. This reflects population-wide overeating, which can contribute to, and accelerate the progression of, CKD. The protein wasting exhibited by a subset of patients undergoing dialysis is thus not malnutrition in the sense of limited nutrient availability. It is often accompanied by anorexia and reduced food intake, particularly when inflammation is prominent. It cannot, however, be reversed simply by increasing food intake.[269] Other measures of restoring body protein and muscle mass toward normal, including exercise, appetite stimulants, and newer anabolic and antiinflammatory agents, are under study.

# SIGNS AND SYMPTOMS OF UREMIA

Frequently identified signs and symptoms of uremia are listed in Box 52.1. That a fundamental metabolic disturbance such as uremia should have such a wide variety of consequences is not remarkable. The complications of untreated diabetes or hyperthyroidism are similarly extensive. However, uremia is different in that we cannot trace all its complications to dysregulation of a single key compound. And, except for renal transplantation, current therapy for uremia cannot return patients as close to normal as thyroid hormone or insulin replacement.

The level of renal function at which uremia can be said to appear is obscure. Furthermore, the diminution of functions other than solute clearance likely contributes to the symptoms and signs of uremia. In general, these other functions, such as ammoniagenesis, erythropoietin, and 1,25-dihydroxyvitamin D synthesis, urine-concentrating capacity, and tubular secretion, tend to decline in parallel with GFR, but not always. Nevertheless, defining the level of kidney function solely by GFR may be misleading. For example, certain potentially toxic solutes depend more on tubular secretion than on glomerular filtration for their excretion, and renal synthetic processes are probably linked to GFR only by virtue of the loss of functioning renal tissue. However, until particular renal dysfunctions are attached to specific aspects of the uremic syndrome, GFR will remain the principal index of kidney function.

Most of the clinical and biochemical characteristics of uremia have been defined in ESKD or at a level of GFR very near to ESKD. Thus, as noted at the beginning of this chapter, uremic characteristics may be hard to dissect from complications of the dialysis procedure. Other morbidities considered separate from the uremia also commonly interact with it. For example, the cardiovascular disease suffered especially by patients with diabetes and hypertension appears to be accelerated by CKD. However, the myocardial infarctions, strokes, and peripheral vascular diseases suffered by these patients have not traditionally been considered features of the uremic syndrome. These conditions nevertheless add to patients' disabilities in ways that are often not easily distinguishable from uremia or the residual syndrome of ESKD. Similarly, the peripheral neuropathy and gastroparesis of diabetes are difficult to disentangle from uremic neuropathy and uremic anorexia, nausea, and vomiting.

## WELL-BEING AND PHYSICAL FUNCTION

Given the list of signs and symptoms in Box 52.1, it is not surprising that health-related quality of life (HRQOL) tends to decline in patients with CKD. The point in the course of

CKD at which quality of life begins to decline has not been dissected in great detail, but some data exist. The authors of the National Kidney Foundation Kidney Disease Outcomes Quality Initiative (NKF KDOQI) guidelines have concluded that notable reductions in well-being appear when the GFR is <60 mL/min/1.73 m$^2$. Dialysis undoubtedly imposes a burden on patients. Interestingly, however, comparisons of HRQOL in patients on dialysis and patients with advanced CKD who are not on dialysis have yielded discordant results.[270–273] Other, often neglected features of treatment, such as pill burden and frailty, may also contribute to reduction in the quality of life.[274] Patients with ESKD are on average more depressed than healthy controls. However, it is difficult to distinguish the extent to which depression is caused by uremic solutes as compared with the effects of comorbid disease and the knowledge of ill health and limited life expectancy. Not surprisingly, transplantation has been found to consistently improve quality of life.[275] However, early versus later initiation of chronic hemodialysis does not seem to influence quality of life.[276]

Physical functioning in patients treated with dialysis is decidedly below normal.[277] The self-reported activity of people initiating dialysis is below the fifth percentile for healthy people.[266] Treatment of anemia improves this situation but does not normalize it.[278,279] The most detailed studies have identified multiple defects that are associated with fatigability.[280] These include muscle energetic failure and neural defects. The degree to which they are attributable to the uremic environment itself, deconditioning, and/or comorbid conditions such as diabetes mellitus is difficult to establish. Even highly functional patients on dialysis display notable physical limitations. Blake and O'Meara[281] have reported that middle-aged patients undergoing dialysis, with good nutrition and no significant comorbidities, exhibit a wide range of quantifiable deficiencies. For example, balance, walking, speed, and sensory function in these patients were clearly below those of matched controls.

## NEUROLOGIC FUNCTION

A particularly interesting group of uremic signs and systems reflects altered nerve function. Classic descriptions emphasized that uremic patients could appear alert, despite defects in memory, planning, and attention.[13,282] As kidney function worsened, patients progressed to coma or catatonia, which could be relieved by dialysis. Today, patients maintained on dialysis exhibit more subtle cognitive defects.[283] A difficulty in identifying the effects of uremia in these patients is that the hemodialysis procedure and/or associated factors (e.g., hypotension) may transiently impair cognitive function.[284] Studies in patients with CKD have suggested that cognitive impairment can be detected when the GFR falls below 60 mL/min/1.73 m$^2$ and worsens as the GFR declines.[285–287] As with other signs and symptoms of uremia, the degree to which cognition is influenced by uremia, as opposed to other comorbidities, especially cerebrovascular disease, is difficult to ascertain. Imaging studies suggest that subclinical cerebrovascular disease is common in CKD, and its role in poor cognition needs further definition.[288–290] The finding that kidney transplantation improves cognitive function suggests, however, that at least some of the impairment observed in ESRD patients is reversible and, perhaps, due to solute accumulation.[291–293] Impaired cognitive function has so far been associated with accumulation of one specific uremic solute, 4-hydroxyphenylacetate, and been shown to be partly reversed by acute dialysis treatment.[112,294] A further reflection of altered CNS function in uremia is impaired sleep.[295,296] Sleep is fragmented by brief arousals and apneic episodes, which are often associated with bursts of repetitive leg movement. When awake, patients may feel a need to move their legs continuously, termed the "restless legs syndrome."[297,298]

Sensorimotor neuropathy was a recognized component of the uremic syndrome decades ago.[13] Studies of conduction velocity and other nerve functions have since repeatedly found that most patients with uremia have peripheral neuropathy, albeit often subclinical.[282,299,300] Morphologic studies have shown that these functional changes are associated with axonal loss, and therefore may not be reversible in some patients. The extent to which peripheral nerve function is impaired earlier in the course of CKD is not certain. Autonomic neuropathy also develops in ESRD, but has been less extensively studied than peripheral neuropathy.[300] As with other uremic disturbances, the cause of neuropathy is unknown. Parathyroid hormone, multiple retention solutes, and more recently potassium have been associated with peripheral neuropathy, but without definitive proof of causality.[282,299]

## APPETITE, TASTE, AND SMELL

Loss of appetite is a common uremic symptom and presumably contributes to malnutrition in patients with advanced renal failure. A large number of causes have been proposed. Acidosis and inflammatory cytokines, including tumor necrosis factor and various interleukins, have been identified as contributing factors.[301] As with the uremic defects in energy metabolism, attention has been focused on the accumulation of small proteins produced by the gut and adipose tissue and acting on the brain to regulate appetite in normal people.[302,303] Levels of leptin, an anorexigen produced by adipose tissue, are elevated in ESKD. Antagonism of leptin in mice with experimental CKD attenuates a number of the molecular markers of proteolysis.[304] An interesting feature of uremic anorexia that remains to be explained is a disproportionate reduction in the intake of protein.[179] Along with overall loss of appetite, erosion of taste and smell has long been recognized in the ESRD population.[305,306] As with most defects, transplantation reverses the blunted smell.[305] Some studies have reported that odor threshold declines gradually with creatinine clearance, whereas others have found that even in patients undergoing dialysis, odor detection remains normal unless malnutrition is present.[143,305] Taste acuity has been reported as lower in patients undergoing dialysis than in those with renal insufficiency, and self-reported altered taste is associated with poor nutritional status.[307,308] The factors responsible for these defects are again unknown.

## CELLULAR FUNCTIONS

The most general cellular abnormality reported has been the inhibition of sodium–potassium adenosine triphosphatase ($Na^+$,$K^+$-ATPase). Decreased $Na^+$,$K^+$-ATPase activity in red cells of uremic patients was reported in 1964.[309] In general, subsequent reports have confirmed the observation, noted the same effect in other cell types, and emphasized that the inhibition was attributable to some factor in uremic serum.[310] The evidence for a circulating inhibitor includes the findings that dialysis reduces the inhibitory activity and uremic plasma can acutely suppress the pump activity.[310] However, the factor or factors have remained elusive. A number of candidates have been considered. Much attention has focused on digitalis-like substances. Several such compounds have been found in excess in humans with ESRD. These include marinobufagenin and telocinobufagin, which have a structure related to that of digitalis.

## WHY IS THE GLOMERULAR FILTRATION RATE SO LARGE?

Glomerular filtration, the initial step in urine formation, is quantitatively huge, with a volume equaling that of the entire ECF filtered every 2 hours. At rest, approximately 10% of the body's energy consumption is devoted to reabsorption of valuable solutes and water necessitated by this massive filtration rate. The rate of fluid processing clearly exceeds that required to rid the body of the daily intake of water and inorganic ions. Theoretically, the large tubular flow rate provided by the GFR could supply a sink into which organic solutes are secreted more favorably than at lower tubular flows. This hypothesis accounts for the presence of a large GFR but leaves unanswered the question of which solutes must be handled by secretion and thereby maintained at a low level in the ECF.

Homer Smith (1895–1962) recognized that the mammalian GFR was large in proportion to the kidney's known functions. He suggested that our high GFR was an evolutionary residual of the mechanism that allowed early vertebrates living in freshwater seas to excrete large volumes of water. If this were correct, the superfluity of GFR would constitute an expensive vestige in land-dwelling mammals, and the value of tubular secretion would remain unaccounted for. An alternate explanation for the apparent superfluity of kidney function is that it provides a safety factor, similar to the capacity of bone to withstand greater than usual mechanical loads. In the case of the kidney, the ingestion of toxins could constitute an analogous increase in load. It is noteworthy, however, that the proportion of GFR and kidney size to metabolic rate appears to be nearly constant across mammalian species, including herbivores and carnivores.[311,312] This suggests that the substances with excretion that necessitate a large kidney are products of common metabolic pathways rather than specific foodstuffs. The remarkable ability of bears to reduce kidney function and net protein breakdown to near zero during winter denning further suggests that these substances are end products of protein catabolism.[313,314]

We can further suppose that kidney capacity appears excessive because our clinical criteria are too coarse to detect the consequences of mild impairment in kidney function. Fitness in an evolutionary sense may require the concentrations in body water of some excreted solutes to be maintained below the levels at which we detect disease. That is, our clinical criteria for uremic illness may be too coarse to detect the consequences of mild impairment of renal function. One might speculate that disturbances in an important but sensitive parameter, perhaps fertility, growth in children, or peak physical performance, would occur with less than a twofold increase of some retained toxin. A particularly interesting finding has been the identification of similar transport systems in the kidney tubule and blood–brain barrier.[194,315] This finding suggests that the kidney, together with the liver, may be designed to keep organic waste levels in the ECF sufficiently low so that a second-stage pumping system in the blood–brain barrier can keep the brain interstitium exquisitely clean.

 Complete reference list available at ExpertConsult.com.

## KEY REFERENCES


1. Vanholder R, De Smet R, Glorieux G, et al. Review on uremic toxins: classification, concentration, and interindividual variability. *Kidney Int.* 2003;63:1934–1943.
2. Duranton F, Cohen G, De Smet R, et al. Normal and pathologic concentrations of uremic toxins. *J Am Soc Nephrol.* 2012;23:1258–1270.
5. Sirich TL, Aronov PA, Plummer NS, et al. Numerous protein-bound solutes are cleared by the kidney with high efficiency. *Kidney Int.* 2013;84:585–590.
8. Bergstrom J. Uremic toxicity. In: Kopple JD, Massry SG, eds. *Nutritional Management of Renal Disease.* Baltimore: Williams & Wilkins; 1997:97–190.
9. Depner TA. Uremic toxicity: urea and beyond. *Semin Dial.* 2001;14: 246–251.
12. Johnson WJ, Hagge WW, Wagoner RD, et al. Effects of urea loading in patients with far-advanced renal failure. *Mayo Clin Proc.* 1972;47:21–29.
13. Schreiner G, Maher J. Biochemistry of uremia. In: *Uremia.* Springfield, IL: Charles C Thomas; 1960:55–85.
21. Koeth RA, Kalantar-Zadeh K, Wang Z, et al. Protein carbamylation predicts mortality in ESRD. *J Am Soc Nephrol.* 2013;24:853–861.
40. Verroust PJ, Birn H, Nielsen R, et al. The tandem endocytic receptors megalin and cubilin are important proteins in renal pathology. *Kidney Int.* 2002;62:745–756.
43. Norden AG, Sharratt P, Cutillas PR, et al. Quantitative amino acid and proteomic analysis: very low excretion of polypeptides >750 Da in normal urine. *Kidney Int.* 2004;66:1994–2003.
55. Axelsson J, Bergsten A, Qureshi AR, et al. Elevated resistin levels in chronic kidney disease are associated with decreased glomerular filtration rate and inflammation, but not with insulin resistance. *Kidney Int.* 2006;69:596–604.
59. Richter R, Schulz-Knappe P, Schrader M, et al. Composition of the peptide fraction in human blood plasma: database of circulating human peptides. *J Chromatogr B Biomed Sci Appl.* 1999;726:25–35.
66. Eloot S, Torremans A, De Smet R, et al. Kinetic behavior of urea is different from that of other water-soluble compounds: the case of the guanidino compounds. *Kidney Int.* 2005;67:1566–1575.
69. Wyss M, Kaddurah-Daouk R. Creatine and creatinine metabolism. *Physiol Rev.* 2000;80:1107–1213.
95. Cathcart-Rake W, Porter R, Whittier F, et al. Effect of diet on serum accumulation and renal excretion of aryl acids and secretory activity in normal and uremic man. *Am J Clin Nutr.* 1975;28:1110–1115.
96. Mitch WE, Brusilow S. Benzoate-induced changes in glycine and urea metabolism in patients with chronic renal failure. *J Pharmacol Exp Ther.* 1982;222:572–575.
98. Meyer TW, Hostetter TH. Uremic solutes from colon microbes. *Kidney Int.* 2012;81:949–954.
103. Sirich TL, Luo FJ, Plummer NS, et al. Selectively increasing the clearance of protein-bound uremic solutes. *Nephrol Dial Transplant.* 2012;27:1574–1579.
105. Meijers BK, Van Kerckhoven S, Verbeke K, et al. The uremic retention solute *p*-cresyl sulfate and markers of endothelial damage. *Am J Kidney Dis.* 2009;51:891–901.
126. Ponda MP, Quan Z, Melamed ML, et al. Methylamine clearance by haemodialysis is low. *Nephrol Dial Transplant.* 2010;25:1608–1613.
130. Wright SH, Dantzler WH. Molecular and cellular physiology of renal organic cation and anion transport. *Physiol Rev.* 2004;84:987–1049.
132. Roch-Ramel F, Besseghir K, Murer H. Renal excretion and tubular transport of organic anions and cations. In: Windhager EE, ed. *Handbook of Physiology: Renal Physiology.* Oxford, England: Oxford University Press; 1992:2189–2262.

134. Aronov PA, Luo FJ, Plummer NS, et al. Colonic contribution to uremic solutes. *J Am Soc Nephrol.* 2011;22:1769–1776.
142. Simenhoff ML, Burke JF, Saukkonen JJ, et al. Biochemical profile of uremic breath. *N Engl J Med.* 1977;297:132–135.
144. Tang WH, Wang Z, Levison BS, et al. Intestinal microbial metabolism of phosphatidylcholine and cardiovascular risk. *N Engl J Med.* 2013;368:1575–1584.
165. Henderson LW, Colton CK, Ford CA, et al. Kinetics of hemodiafiltration. II. Clinical characterization of a new blood-cleansing modality. 1975. *J Am Soc Nephrol.* 1997;8:494–508.
166. Ward RA, Greene T, Hartmann B, et al. Resistance to intercompartmental mass transfer limits beta2-microglobulin removal by post-dilution hemodiafiltration. *Kidney Int.* 2006;69:1431–1437.
171. Luo FJ, Patel KP, Marquez IO, et al. Effect of increasing dialyzer mass transfer area coefficient and dialysate flow on clearance of protein-bound solutes: a pilot crossover trial. *Am J Kidney Dis.* 2009;53:1042–1049.
176. Schneditz D, Daugirdas JT. Compartment effects in hemodialysis. *Semin Dial.* 2001;14:271–277.
177. Eloot S, Torremans A, De Smet R, et al. Complex compartmental behavior of small water-soluble uremic retention solutes: evaluation by direct measurements in plasma and erythrocytes. *Am J Kidney Dis.* 2007;50:279–288.
180. Giovannetti S, Maggiore Q. A low-nitrogen diet with proteins of high biological value for severe chronic uraemia. *Lancet.* 1964;37:1000–1003.
181. Uribarri J. The obsession with high dietary protein intake in ESRD patients on dialysis: is it justified? *Nephron.* 2000;86:105–108.
192. Eraly SA, Vallon V, Vaughn DA, et al. Decreased renal organic anion secretion and plasma accumulation of endogenous organic anions in OAT1 knock-out mice. *J Biol Chem.* 2006;281:5072–5083.
193. Nolin TD. Altered nonrenal drug clearance in ESRD. *Curr Opin Nephrol Hypertens.* 2008;17:555–559.
196. Himmelfarb J. Uremic toxicity, oxidative stress, and hemodialysis as renal replacement therapy. *Semin Dial.* 2009;22:636–643.
201. Himmelfarb J, McMenamin E, McMonagle E. Plasma aminothiol oxidation in chronic hemodialysis patients. *Kidney Int.* 2002;61:705–716.
204. Thornalley PJ, Rabbani N. Highlights and hotspots of protein glycation in end-stage renal disease. *Semin Dial.* 2009;22:400–404.
214. Ikizler TA, Wingard RL, Sun M, et al. Increased energy expenditure in hemodialysis patients. *J Am Soc Nephrol.* 1996;7:2646–2653.
215. Avesani CM, Draibe SA, Kamimura MA, et al. Decreased resting energy expenditure in non-dialysed chronic kidney disease patients. *Nephrol Dial Transplant.* 2004;19:3091–3097.
240. Kwan BC, Kronenberg F, Beddhu S, et al. Lipoprotein metabolism and lipid management in chronic kidney disease. *J Am Soc Nephrol.* 2007;18:1246–1261.
248. Laidlaw SA, Berg RL, Kopple JD, et al. Patterns of fasting plasma amino acid levels in chronic renal insufficiency: results from the feasibility phase of the Modification of Diet in Renal Disease Study. *Am J Kidney Dis.* 1994;23:504–513.
252. Jamison RL, Hartigan P, Kaufman JS, et al. Effect of homocysteine lowering on mortality and vascular disease in advanced chronic kidney disease and end-stage renal disease: a randomized controlled trial. *JAMA.* 2007;298:1163–1170.
253. Rajan VR, Mitch WE. Muscle wasting in chronic kidney disease: the role of the ubiquitin proteasome system and its clinical impact. *Pediatr Nephrol.* 2008;23:527–535.
266. Johansen KL, Chertow GM, Kutner NG, et al. Low level of self-reported physical activity in ambulatory patients new to dialysis. *Kidney Int.* 2010;78:1164–1170.
274. Abdel-Kader K, Unruh ML, Weisbord SD. Symptom burden, depression, and quality of life in chronic and end-stage kidney disease. *Clin J Am Soc Nephrol.* 2009;4:1057–1064.
282. Blake C, O'Meara YM. Subjective and objective physical limitations in high-functioning renal dialysis patients. *Nephrol Dial Transplant.* 2004;19:3124–3129.
285. Murray AM, Pederson SL, Tupper DE, et al. Acute variation in cognitive function in hemodialysis patients: a cohort study with repeated measures. *Am J Kidney Dis.* 2007;50:270–278.
312. Singer MA, Morton AR. Mouse to elephant: biological scaling and Kt/V. *Am J Kidney Dis.* 2000;35:306–309.
315. Ohtsuki S. New aspects of the blood-brain barrier transporters; its physiological roles in the central nervous system. *Biol Pharm Bull.* 2004;27:1489–1496.

# 53

# Chronic Kidney Disease–Mineral Bone Disorder

Marta Christov | Stuart M. Sprague

## CHAPTER OUTLINE



## KEY POINTS

- Changes in mineral metabolism parameters occur as early as stage 2 chronic kidney disease (CKD), most commonly with increased serum fibroblast growth factor 23 (FGF-23) concentrations.
- Pi bioavailability depends on the food source, with plant-based sources such as legumes having less bioavailable Pi due to human's inability to digest phytate, the major Pi storage form in plants.
- The commonly used albumin-corrected total calcium values misclassify the true hypercalcemia or hypocalcemia in 20% of patients with CKD, thus whenever possible, ionized calcium concentrations should also be obtained, particularly when starting or modifying therapies for CKD-MBD (mineral bone disease).
- Vascular calcification of the medial layer of elastic arteries is extremely common in patients with CKD, although the pathophysiology may be similar to that of intimal calcifications associated with atherosclerosis.
- There is no definitive noninvasive way (by imaging or bloodwork) to assess bone physiology parameters such as turnover and mineralization.
- The new system for renal osteodystrophy classification focuses on abnormalities in bone turnover, mineralization, and volume, all of which impact bone strength.
- Dual-energy X-ray absorptiometry (DXA) may be used for assessment of fracture risk in patients with CKD, although clinical trials linking changes in DXA to relevant outcomes, including fracture, are lacking.
- There are no randomized controlled trials in CKD or end-stage kidney disease to show that treatment to a specific parathyroid hormone target leads to improved outcomes.
- Patients on dialysis have higher rates of hip fracture than in the general population in all age groups, and have a higher mortality when they experience a fracture.
- Fractures, especially in the appendicular skeleton, are common in kidney transplant recipients.

In persons with healthy kidneys, normal serum levels of phosphorus and calcium are maintained through the interaction of three hormones: parathyroid hormone (PTH); calcitriol [1,25-dihydroxyvitamin $D_3$ 1,25$(OH)_2$D], which is the active metabolite of vitamin D; and fibroblast growth factor 23 (FGF-23). Circulating or soluble klotho also plays a role in mineral homeostasis. These hormones act on four primary target organs: bone, kidney, intestine, and parathyroid glands. The kidneys play a critical role in the regulation of normal serum calcium and phosphorus concentrations and of the three hormones. Thus, derangements in mineral homeostasis are common in patients with chronic kidney disease (CKD). Abnormalities begin early in the course of CKD and are nearly universally observed at a glomerular filtration rate (GFR) less than 30 mL/min. With progression of CKD, the body attempts to maintain normal serum concentrations of calcium and phosphorus by altering the production of calcitriol, PTH, FGF-23, and klotho. Eventually these compensatory responses become unable to maintain normal mineral homeostasis, resulting in (1) altered serum concentrations of calcium, phosphorus, PTH, calcitriol, FGF-23, and klotho; (2) disturbances in bone remodeling and mineralization (often referred to as "renal osteodystrophy") and/or impaired linear growth in children; and (3) extraskeletal calcification in soft tissues and arteries. In 2006, the term chronic kidney disease–mineral and bone disorder (CKD-MBD) was developed to describe this triad of abnormalities in biochemical measures, skeletal abnormalities, and extraskeletal calcification (Table 53.1).[1] These abnormalities that constitute CKD-MBD are interrelated in both the pathophysiology of the disease and the response to treatment. All three components of CKD-MBD are associated with increased risk of fractures, cardiovascular disease, and mortality in patients with CKD stages 4 through 5D. However, to enhance understanding of the complex integration of these abnormalities in CKD, each component is first discussed independently.

**Table 53.1 Kidney Disease Improving Global Outcomes Classification of Chronic Kidney Disease–Mineral Bone Disease and Renal Osteodystrophy**

| | |
|---|---|
| Definition of chronic kidney disease–mineral bone disease (CKD-MBD) | A systemic disorder of mineral and bone metabolism due to CKD manifested by one or a combination of the following:<br>Abnormalities of calcium, phosphorus, parathyroid hormone, or vitamin D metabolism<br>Abnormalities in bone turnover, mineralization, volume, linear growth, or strength<br>Vascular or other soft tissue calcification |
| Definition of renal osteodystrophy | Renal osteodystrophy is an alteration of bone morphology in patients with CKD. It is one measure of the skeletal component of the systemic disorder of CKD-MBD that is quantifiable by histomorphometry of bone biopsy. |

From Moe S, Drüeke T, Cunningham J, et al. Definition, evaluation, and classification of renal osteodystrophy: a position statement from Kidney Disease: Improving Global Outcomes (KDIGO). *Kidney Int.* 2006;69:1945–1953.

# PATHOPHYSIOLOGY OF CHRONIC KIDNEY DISEASE-MINERAL AND BONE DISORDER

## PHOSPHORUS AND CALCIUM HOMEOSTASIS

### PHOSPHORUS BALANCE AND HOMEOSTASIS

Inorganic phosphorus is critical for numerous physiologic functions, including skeletal development, mineral metabolism, cell membrane phospholipid content and function, cell signaling, platelet aggregation, and energy transfer through mitochondrial metabolism. Because of the importance of phosphorus in these functions, normal homeostasis maintains serum phosphorus concentrations between 2.5 and 4.5 mg/dL (0.81 and 1.45 mmol/L). Serum concentrations are highest in infants and decrease throughout growth, reaching adult levels in the late teens. Total adult body stores of phosphorus are approximately 700 g, of which 85% is contained in bone in the form of hydroxyapatite $[(Ca)_{10}(PO_4)_6(OH)_2]$. Of the remainder, 14% is intracellular, and only 1% is extracellular. Of this extracellular phosphorus, 70% is organic (phosphate) and contained within phospholipids, and 30% is inorganic. The inorganic fraction is 15% protein bound, and the remaining 85% is either complexed with sodium, magnesium, or calcium or circulates as the free monohydrogen or dihydrogen form. It is this inorganic fraction that is freely circulating and measured. At a pH of 7.4, inorganic phosphates are in a ratio of about 4: 1 $HPO_4^{-2}$ to $H_2PO^{-1}$. For that reason, the serum phosphorus concentration is usually expressed in mmol/L rather than mEq/L. Thus serum measurements reflect only a minor fraction of total body phosphorus and therefore do not accurately reflect total body stores in the setting of the abnormal homeostasis that occurs in CKD. Furthermore, there is considerable diurnal variation in serum phosphorus concentrations in healthy persons[2] as well as in patients with advanced CKD.[3] The terms phosphorus and phosphate are often used interchangeably, but strictly speaking, "phosphate" means the inorganic freely available form ($HPO_4^{-2}$ and $H_2PO^{-1}$). However, most laboratories report phosphate, the measurable inorganic component of total body phosphorus, as "phosphorus." For simplicity we use the abbreviation Pi to represent phosphate and/or phosphorus throughout this chapter.

Pi is contained in almost all foods and is generally associated with a food's protein content or phosphate-containing additives. In most commonly ingested foods without additives, the mean Pi content ranges from 9.0 to 14.6 mg per gram of protein, with many foods having up to a 28% higher Pi content because of additives, which are used as preservatives, acidifying agents, acidity buffers, and emulsifying agents.[4] Although the recommended daily allowance for Pi is 800 mg/day, the average American diet contains approximately 1000 to 1400 mg Pi and that amount does not necessarily include inorganic Pi added as a preservative, a common practice.[5] The source of Pi has a significant impact on bioavailability. Pi in the form of preservatives or additives is nearly 100% bioavailable, whereas Pi bound to phytate, as in legumes, is less bioavailable owing to the lack of the enzyme phytase in humans.[6] In studies, the source of Pi directly affects Pi homeostasis.[3] As a result, it is challenging to balance dietary Pi restriction against the need for adequate protein intake in patients with CKD, especially with malnutrition present in up to 50% of patients undergoing dialysis. Pi balance in earlier stages of CKD (stage 3–4) is generally neutral because of the phosphaturic effects of PTH and FGF-23[7]; as these compensatory mechanisms begin to fail and particularly when patients have little to no residual kidney function, however, positive Pi balance likely ensues.

Approximately 60% to 70% of dietary Pi is absorbed by the gastrointestinal tract, predominantly in the small intestine, although transport can occur in all intestinal segments. Pi absorption occurs via passive sodium-independent transport and active sodium-dependent transport. Although it can vary depending on the study and experimental design, active transport is approximately 50% of total transport (Fig. 53.1).[8] Passive transport occurs down electrochemical gradient through paracellular tight junctions; claudins and occludins appear to be involved and to control transport rates and ion specificity.[9] Active absorption occurs via the epithelial brush border type II (solute carrier A34) transporters, specifically the sodium-Pi cotransporter (NaPi-IIb) utilizing energy from the basolateral sodium-potassium ATPase transporter. Complete ablation of the *NaPi-IIb* gene in mice demonstrates that this transporter is responsible for 90% of sodium-dependent transport but only 50% of total intestinal Pi transport.[10] In animals with CKD induced by adenine, ablation of the *NaPi-IIb* gene lowers serum Pi, with additional lowering by the Pi binder sevelamer, suggesting that both active transport and passive transport are important in CKD.[11] The NaPi-IIb transporter is predominantly stimulated by high dietary Pi and calcitriol.[8] In addition, studies suggest that the phosphatonins, matrix extracellular phosphoglycoprotein (MEPE),[12] and FGF-23[13] may play a role in intestinal transport. Tenapanor, an inhibitor of the gut sodium/hydrogen exchanger, also affects Pi transport in the intestine. Tenapanor decreases paracellular absorption by increasing resistance to Pi transport at tight junctions, and it decreases NaPi-IIb expression, thereby decreasing active Pi transport.[14] However, dietary Pi appears the most important regulator of intestinal absorption.

The kidneys are responsible for maintaining Pi balance by excreting the net amount of Pi absorbed (see Chapter 7). Most inorganic Pi is freely filtered by the glomerulus with approximately 70% to 80% reabsorbed in the proximal tubule, which serves as the primary regulated site of the kidney. The remaining 20% to 30% is reabsorbed in the distal tubule. Pi transport across the apical lumen occurs via an active transport

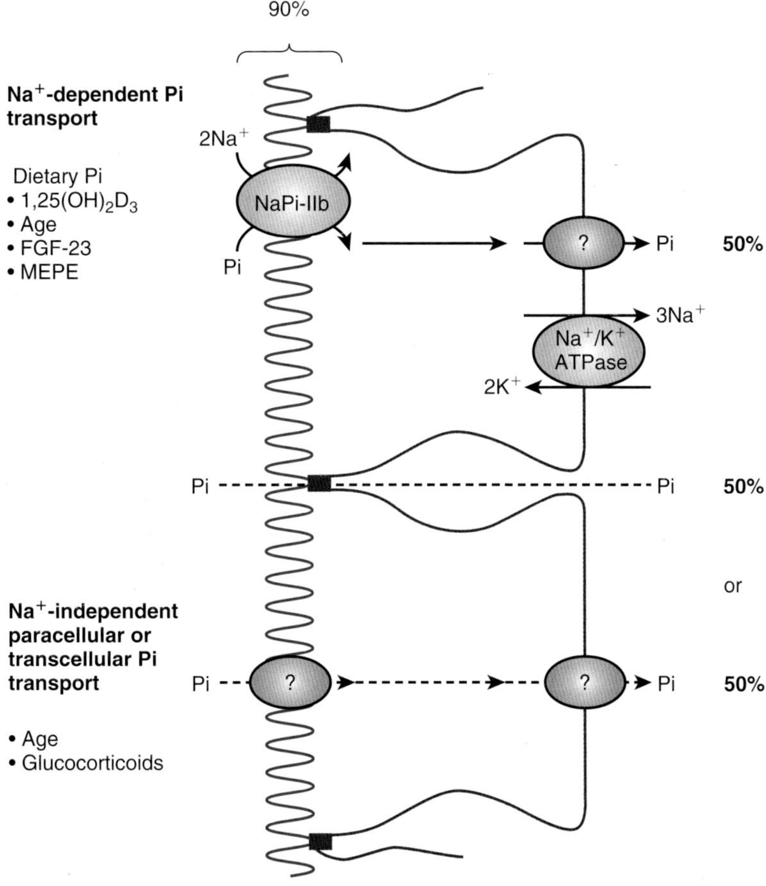


**Fig. 53.1** Intestinal phosphate transport. Approximately 50% of phosphate (Pi) transport is sodium ($Na^+$) dependent, due to active transport, and regulated by a number of factors. The remaining phosphate transport is sodium independent and due to paracellular or transcellular transport. *FGF-23,* Fibroblast growth factor 23; *MEPE,* matrix extracellular phosphoglycoprotein; *$Na^+/K^+$ ATPase,* sodium-potassium adenosine triphosphatase; *NaPi-IIb,* the sodium Pi cotransporter. (From Lee GJ, Marks J. Intestinal phosphate transport: a therapeutic target in chronic kidney disease and beyond? *Pediatr Nephrol.* 2015;30:363–371. With permission.)

process that is driven by active sodium transport on the basolateral side by the sodium-potassium adenosine triphosphatase ($Na^+$-$K^+$-ATPase). The primary transporters on the luminal surface are NaPi-IIa (SLC34A1) and NaPi-IIc (SLC34A3), with a minor component via the type III sodium-dependent Pi cotransporter Pit-2 (SLC20A2). PTH and FGF-23 both downregulate these NaPi transporters, but through different signaling mechanisms. FGF-23 stimulates endocytosis of the transporters after signaling through the FGF receptor (FGFR)–klotho complex, described later. PTH, after binding to PTHR1 receptor, leads to increased cyclic adenosine monophosphate/protein kinase A (cAMP/PKA) signaling with the scaffolding protein $Na^+$-$H^+$ exchanger regulatory factors 1 and 3 (NHERF1 and NHERF3) playing an important role. FGF-23 also decreases calcitriol production by reducing the conversion of 25(OH)D to calcitriol and increasing its catabolism. The reduction in calcitriol results in further reduction of intestinal Pi absorption.

## CALCIUM BALANCE AND HOMEOSTASIS

Serum calcium concentrations are tightly controlled within a relatively narrow range, usually 8.5 to 10.5 mg/dL (2.1 to 2.6 mmol/L). However, the serum calcium concentration is a poor reflection of overall total body calcium, because serum concentrations are less than 1% of total body calcium. The remainder of total body calcium is stored in bone. Ionized calcium, generally 40% of total serum calcium, is physiologically active, whereas the nonionized calcium is bound to albumin or anions such as citrate, bicarbonate, and Pi. In the presence of hypoalbuminemia, there is a relative increase in the ionized calcium relative to the total calcium; thus total serum calcium measurement may underestimate the physiologically active (ionized) serum calcium. A commonly utilized formula for estimating the ionized calcium from the total calcium value is to add 0.8 mg/dL for every 1-mg decrease in serum albumin below 4 mg/dL. However, in a study in patients with CKD stages 3 to 5 not undergoing dialysis, total calcium concentration and albumin-corrected total calcium values failed to correctly classify 20% of patients as either hypocalcemic or hypercalcemic whose state was documented by ionized calcium measurement.[15] The sensitivity to detect true hypocalcemia or hypercalcemia was only 40% and 21% for total serum calcium, and 36% and 21% for albumin-corrected serum calcium, respectively.[15] The primary causes of this discordance are thought to be albumin, PTH, and pH, although the last has been questioned.[16] Thus, whenever possible, ionized calcium measurement should be utilized. Serum concentrations of ionized calcium are maintained within the normal range by the secretion of PTH, as discussed later.

In normal individuals, the net calcium balance (intake–output) varies with age. Children and young adults are usually in a slightly positive net calcium balance to enhance linear growth; beyond ages 25 to 35 years, when bones stop growing, calcium balance tends to be neutral. Normal individuals have protection against calcium overload by virtue of their ability to increase renal excretion of calcium and reduce intestinal absorption of calcium through the actions of PTH and calcitriol. However, in CKD the ability to maintain normal homeostasis, including a normal serum ionized calcium level and appropriate calcium balance for age, is diminished, and lost completely when kidney function is absent. Two studies in patients with CKD stages late 3 to 4 demonstrate that 1000 mg per day of dietary or calcium supplement/binder leads to near-neutral calcium balance (reviewed in Chapter 19).[7,17]

Calcium absorption across the intestinal epithelium occurs via a vitamin D–dependent, saturable (transcellular) pathway and a vitamin D–independent, nonsaturable (paracellular) pathway. In states of adequate dietary calcium, the paracellular mechanism prevails, but the vitamin D–dependent pathways are critical in calcium-deficient states. The transcellular absorption occurs via three steps: (1) calcium enters from the lumen into the cells via transient receptor potential vanilloid (TRPV) channels, of which TRPV6 is most important in the intestine[18]; (2) the intracellular calcium associates with calbindin-D9K to be "ferried" to the basolateral membrane; and (3) calcium is removed from the enterocytes predominantly via the calcium-ATPase, with the $Na^+$-$Ca^{2+}$ exchanger playing a minor role. The duodenum is the major site of calcium absorption, although the other segments of the small intestine and the colon also contribute to net calcium absorption. All of the key regulatory components of active calcium transport—TRPV, calbindin, the $Ca^{2+}$-ATPase (PMCA1b), and the $Na^+$-$Ca^{2+}$ exchanger (NCX1)—are upregulated by calcitriol.[19] Mice with intestinal knockdown of the vitamin D receptor (VDR) are still able to maintain normal calcium levels because of PTH-induced increased bone resorption; by contrast, global knockdown of VDR leads to hypocalcemia. Hypocalcemia with VDR knockdown can be corrected with either a high-calcium diet (and presumed intestinal paracellular calcium transport) or the administration of calcitriol.[20] Thus bone and kidney can compensate for impaired responsiveness of the intestinal VDR, and diet alone can compensate for a total lack of vitamin D. The 1α-hydroxylase enzyme (CYP27B1) is also located throughout the intestine; to date, however, conversion of 25(OH)D to calcitriol has been identified only in the colonic epithelial cells in inflammation.[21]

The renal transport of calcium is further detailed in Chapter 7. In the kidney, the majority (60%–70%) of calcium is reabsorbed passively in the proximal tubule, a process driven by a transepithelial electrochemical gradient that is generated by sodium and water reabsorption. In the thick ascending limb, another 10% of calcium is reabsorbed via paracellular transport. Calcium-sensing receptor (CaSR) activation in this segment inhibits calcium absorption. This paracellular reabsorption also requires the specific protein paracellin-1, and genetic defects in paracellin-1 lead to a syndrome of hypercalciuria and hypomagnesemia.[22] However, the more regulated aspect of calcium reabsorption occurs via transcellular pathways in the distal convoluted tubule and connecting tubule (Fig. 53.2). The mechanism is similar to intestinal transport: Calcium enters these cells via TRPV5 calcium channels down electrochemical gradients. In the cells, calcium binds with calbindin-D28k and is transported to the basolateral membrane, where calcium is actively reabsorbed by the NCX1 and/or PMCA1b. As in the intestinal epithelial cell, calcitriol upregulates all of these transport proteins.[23] PTH has an indirect effect on renal calcium handling via stimulating the synthesis of calcitriol and increases TRPV5 activity.[24] The enzymatic activity of circulating klotho has been shown to cleave the extracellular domain of TRPV5 channels, keeping these channels at the cell membrane and thereby facilitating calcium reabsorption.[25]

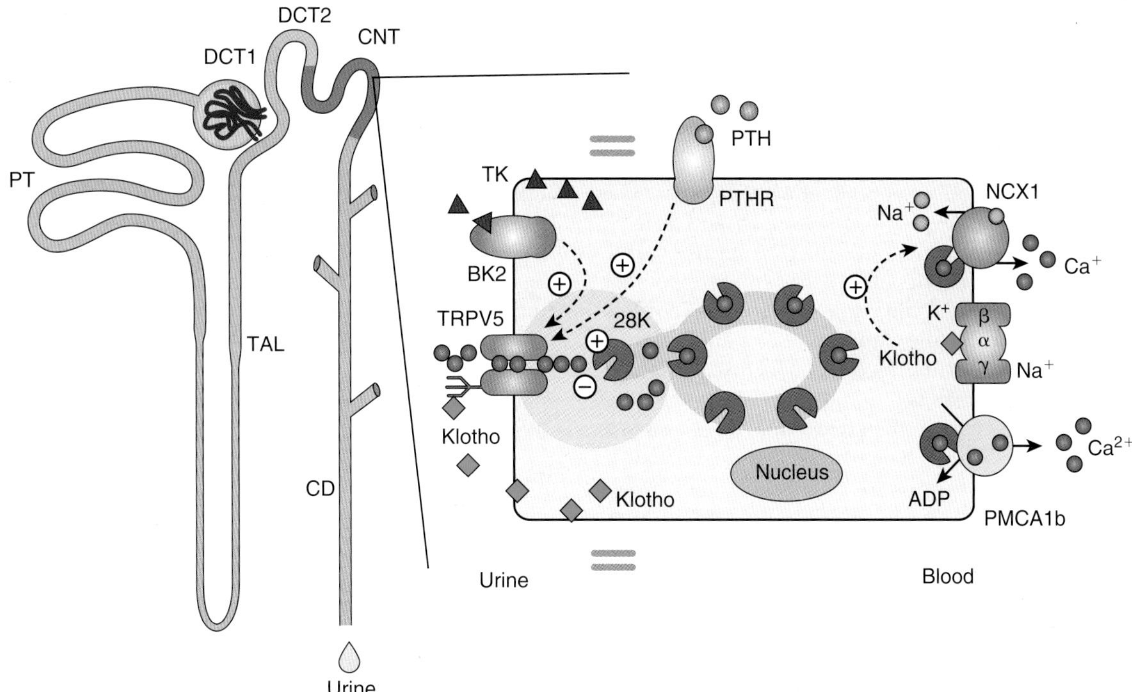


**Fig. 53.2** Epithelial calcium active transport. The late part of the distal convoluted tubule *(DCT)* and connecting tubule *(CNT)* play an important role in fine-tuning renal excretion of $Ca^{2+}$. The epithelial $Ca^{2+}$ channel (TRPV5) is primarily expressed apically in these segments and colocalizes with calbindin-$D_{28K}$ (28K), $Na^+/Ca^{2+}$ exchanger (NCX1), and the plasma membrane adenosine triphosphatase (ATPase; PMCA1b). Upon entry via TRPV5, $Ca^{2+}$ is buffered by 28K and diffuses to the basolateral membrane, where it is released and extruded by a concerted action of NCX1 and PMCA1b. In addition, the basolateral membrane exposes a parathyroid hormone *(PTH)* receptor *(PTHR)* and the $Na^+/K^+$-ATPase consisting of the α, β, and γ subunits. PTHR activation by PTH stimulates TRPV5 activity, and entered $Ca^{2+}$ can subsequently control the expression level of the $Ca^{2+}$ transporters. At the apical membrane, there is a bradykinin receptor *(BK2)* that is activated by urinary tissue kallikrein *(TK)* to activate TRPV5-mediated $Ca^{2+}$ influx. In the cell, entered $Ca^{2+}$ acts as a negative feedback on channel activity, and 28K plays a regulatory role by association with TRPV5 under low intracellular $Ca^{2+}$ concentrations. Extracellular urinary klotho directly stimulates TRPV5 at the apical membrane by modification of the N-glycan, whereas intracellular klotho enhances $Na^+/K^+$-ATPase surface expression, which in turn activates NCX1-mediated $Ca^{2+}$ efflux. *ADP,* Adenosine diphosphate; *DCT1,* early part of distal convoluted tubule; *PT,* proximal tubule; *TAL,* thick ascending limb of Henle. (From Boros S, Bindels RJM, Hoenderop JGJ. Active $Ca^{2+}$ reabsorption in the connecting tubule. *Pflügers Arch Eur J Physiol.* 2009;458:99–109.)

## CALCIUM-SENSING RECEPTOR

Physiologic studies in animals and humans in the 1980s demonstrated the rapid release of PTH in response to small reductions in blood ionized calcium, lending support to the existence of a CaSR in the parathyroid gland that was subsequently cloned in 1993.[26] The CaSR was shown to belong to the superfamily of G protein–coupled receptors and is a glycosylated protein with a very large extracellular domain, seven membrane-spanning segments, and a relatively large cytoplasmic domain. The primary ligand for the CaSR is $Ca^{2+}$, but it also senses other divalent and polyvalent cations, including $Mg^{2+}$, $Be^{2+}$, $La^{3+}$, $Gd^{3+}$, and polyarginine.[27] Extracellular calcium binds to multiple sites, leading to conformational changes that result in activation of phospholipases C, $A_2$, and D as well as inhibition of cAMP production.[28] Activation of the CaSR stimulates phospholipase C, leading to an increase in inositol 1,4,5-triphosphate ($IP_3$), which mobilizes intracellular calcium and decreases PTH secretion (Fig. 53.3). By contrast, inactivation of the CaSR reduces intracellular calcium and increases PTH secretion. CaSR messenger RNA (mRNA) is widely expressed in multiple tissues, including organs responsible for CKD-MBD (parathyroid, kidney, thyroid, bone, intestine, vasculature). Studies have demonstrated a diverse role for the CaSR in disease, including in the gastrointestinal

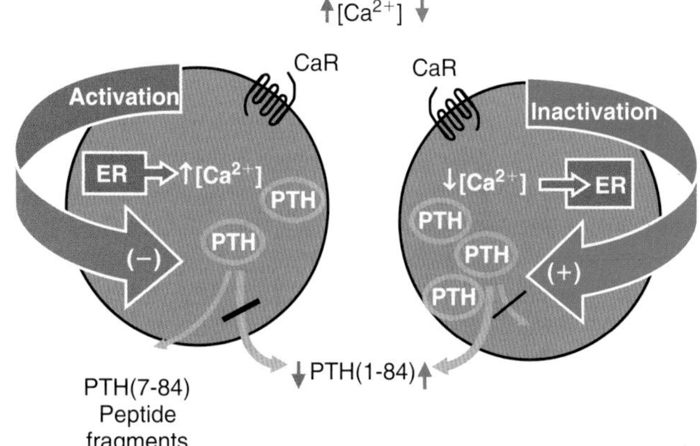


**Fig. 53.3** Calcium-sensing receptor *(CaR).* Activation of the CaR by calcium stimulates phospholipase C, leading to increased inositol 1,4,5-triphosphate ($IP_3$), which mobilizes intracellular calcium and inhibits parathyroid hormone *(PTH)* synthesis. A decrease in serum calcium ($Ca^{2+}$) inhibits intracellular signaling, leading to increased PTH synthesis and secretion. *ER,* Endoplasmic reticulum. (From Friedman PA, Goodman WG. PTH(1-84)/PTH(7-84): a balance of power. *Am J Physiol Renal Physiol.* 2006;290:F975–F984.)

tract, where it regulates gastrin, glucagon-like peptide-1, acid, and hormone secretion and is involved in taste, gastrointestinal fluid transport, and cell turnover.[29]

CaSR$^{-/-}$ mice die shortly after birth owing to hypercalcemia, hypocalciuria, and hyperparathyroidism. If the *PTH* gene is also ablated, the mice survive and most organs appear histologically normal, with healing of bone mineralization defects but no change in hypocalciuria.[30] However, these CaSR$^{-/-}$/PTH$^{-/-}$ mice demonstrate hypercalcemia in response to oral calcium, infusion of PTH, or administration of calcitriol, whereas the CaSR$^{+/+}$/PTH$^{-/-}$ mice are able to decrease gastrointestinal calcium absorption and increase renal calcium excretion to maintain normal levels of serum calcium.[31,32] These data indicate that CaSR activation corrects hypocalcemia by increasing PTH, whereas in hypercalcemia, the CaSR acts independent of PTH by increasing renal calcium excretion. In uremic animals, the expression of CaSR in the parathyroid gland is downregulated by a high-Pi diet and upregulated by magnesium[33] and calcimimetics. In parathyroid glands from patients with secondary hyperparathyroidism, the expression of the CaSR is downregulated in comparison with expression in nonuremic patients[34] but can be upregulated with the administration of cinacalcet.[35]

The CaSR is expressed throughout the kidney, where it is found in diverse locations and performs multiple physiologic functions: podocyte (cytoskeleton changes), proximal tubule (phosphate reabsorption, calcitriol synthesis, acidification/fluid reabsorption), macula densa (renin secretion), thick ascending loop of Henle (calcium, sodium, potassium, and chloride handling), distal convoluted tubule/connecting tubule (calcium transport), and connecting duct (acid/base, water handling).[36] Diverse functions in the kidney signify how important calcium homeostasis is to normal kidney function and vice versa. Furthermore, many of these functions avoid renal calcium precipitation. Most notably, activation of the luminal CaSR in the collecting duct by elevated urine calcium values leads to urinary acidification and polyuria,[37] a common clinical symptom in hypercalcemia, and prevents calcium-Pi precipitation.

There is some disagreement as to the role of the CaSR in bone and whether or not this role depends on PTH. Clearly bone cells respond to calcium. The CaSR is important in fetal bone development; conditional deletion of the CaSR in early osteoblasts leads to altered bone phenotype, although the results vary depending on the construct used.[38] Studies suggest that the CaSR modulates both bone resorption and formation induced by PTH.[39] In vitro, mesenchymal stem cells appear to require CaSR for differentiation,[40] but in more differentiated cells, calcium channels appear more involved in calcium transport.[41] An initial report found that calcium also regulates FGF-23 synthesis in bone, although this effect does not appear to be mediated via the CaSR.[42] Calcimimetics, allosteric activators of the CaSR, are used to treat secondary hyperparathyroidism as discussed in Chapter 63.

Data also suggest a role for the CaSR in vascular calcification. Immunohistochemical staining demonstrates expression of CaSR on normal human arteries with downregulation in areas of calcification.[43] The CaSR is expressed on cultured vascular smooth muscle cells (VSMCs), and calcimimetics inhibit in vitro calcification.[43,44] The calcimimetic R-568 reverses calcitriol-induced arterial calcification[45] and inhibits proliferation of VSMCs and endothelial cells in the 5/6 nephrectomy rat model.[46] Calcimimetics also retard uremia-enhanced vascular calcification and atherosclerosis in the ApoE$^{-/-}$ mouse[47] and prevent arterial and myocardial calcification in the Cy/+ model of slowly progressive CKD-MBD.[48] Calcimimetics also upregulate a potential local inhibitor of arterial calcification, matrix gla protein.[49] A trial of cinacalcet in patients with end-stage kidney disease (ESKD) treated with calcium-based phosphate binders showed amelioration in calcification relative to placebo (and active vitamin D analogs).[50] These data support a role for the CaSR in all three components of CKD-MBD.

## HORMONAL REGULATION OF CHRONIC KIDNEY DISEASE-MINERAL AND BONE DISORDER

### PARATHYROID HORMONE

The primary function of PTH is to maintain calcium homeostasis (Fig. 53.4) by (1) increasing bone mineral dissolution, thus releasing calcium and Pi; (2) increasing renal reabsorption of calcium and excretion of Pi; (3) increasing the activity of the renal CYP27B1 enzyme to convert 25(OH)D to calcitriol; and (4) enhancing the gastrointestinal absorption of both

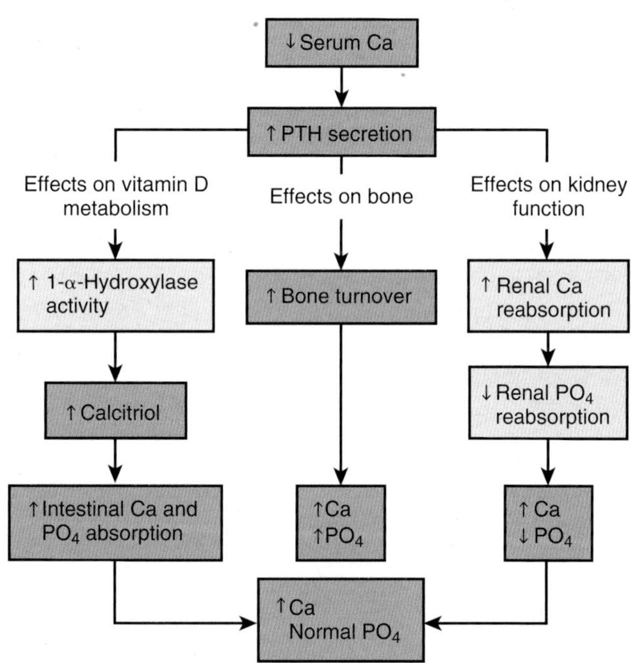


**Fig. 53.4** Normalization of serum calcium by multiple actions of parathyroid hormone *(PTH)*. Serum levels of ionized calcium *(Ca)* are maintained in the normal range by induction of increases in the secretion of PTH. PTH acts to increase bone resorption, renal calcium reabsorption, and the conversion of 25(OH)D to calcitriol in the kidney, thereby increasing gastrointestinal calcium absorption. The *blue boxes* indicate processes that are abnormal in chronic kidney disease, leading to altered calcium homeostasis. *$PO_4$*, Phosphate. (From Moe SM. Calcium, phosphorus, and vitamin D metabolism in renal disease and chronic renal failure. In: Kopple JD, Massry SG, eds. *Nutritional Management of Renal Disease.* Philadelphia: Lippincott Williams & Wilkins; 2004:261–285.)

calcium and Pi indirectly through its effects on the synthesis of calcitriol. In healthy persons, the increase in serum PTH concentration in response to hypocalcemia effectively restores serum calcium and maintains serum Pi concentrations. The kidneys are critical to this normal homeostatic response; thus patients with more severe CKD may lose the capacity to maintain calcium homeostasis.

PTH is cleaved to an 84–amino acid protein in the parathyroid gland, where it is stored as fragments in secretory granules for release. Once released, the circulating 1–84–amino acid protein has a half-life of 2 to 4 minutes and is further metabolized in the liver and kidney. PTH secretion occurs in response to hypocalcemia, hyperphosphatemia, and calcitriol deficiency. The extracellular concentration of ionized calcium is the most important determinant of minute-to-minute secretion of PTH from stored secretory granules. The CaSR mediates the rapid response in PTH secretion, which occurs within seconds of changes in ionized calcium concentration. Inactivating mutations of the CaSR have been associated with neonatal severe hyperparathyroidism and benign familial hypocalciuric hypercalcemia. Affected patients have asymptomatic elevations of serum calcium in the presence of nonsuppressed PTH. Activating mutations have been found in patients with autosomal dominant hypocalcemia resulting in inhibition of PTH secretion at relatively lower serum calcium concentrations. PTH is released as both an intact (1–84) protein and carboxy (C)-terminal fragments (often called PTH [7–84]; see Fig. 53.3). C-terminal PTH has the opposite effect on calcium release from bone in animals and cultured calvariae from that of PTH with an intact N terminus.[51] In addition, the C-terminal PTH inhibits apoptosis in osteoblasts, whereas the N-terminal PTH induces apoptosis.[51] Regulators of PTH secretion act by changing the proportion of intact 1–84 and C-terminal fragments.

PTH binds to the PTH1 receptor (PTH1R), which is a member of the G protein–linked seven membrane–spanning receptor family and is widely expressed. PTH-related peptide (PTHrp) shares homology with the first few amino acids of PTH and also binds the PTH1R. Activation of the PTH1R stimulates heterodimeric G proteins $G_s$ (leading to stimulation of cAMP and PKA signaling) and $G_{\alpha q}$ (leading to activation of $IP_3$ and protein kinase C), ultimately resulting in changes in intracellular calcium.[52] PTH1R activation may vary in response to time exposure, secondary conformational changes after binding, and which cell signaling mechanism is preferentially activated. In general, the effects of PTH are systemic and those of PTHrp are autocrine.

The interrelationship of calcium, Pi, FGF-23, and calcitriol in the development of secondary hyperparathyroidism in CKD is complex and nearly impossible to fully evaluate in humans, because changes in one lead to rapid changes in the others. The response to a decrease in ionized calcium mediated by the CaSR is likely the most potent stimulus for PTH release. Pi increases PTH production by enhancing the stability of PTH mRNA.[53] FGF-23 directly stimulates PTH release in a klotho-independent manner.[54] Calcitriol suppresses PTH release via the VDR to lead to direct suppression of the gene. Other vitamin D compounds that bind to the VDR with lower affinity still reduce PTH release if given in high enough quantities.[55] Although PTH-induced signaling predominantly affects mineral metabolism, there are also many extraskeletal manifestations of PTH excess in CKD. These include encephalopathy, anemia, extraskeletal calcification, peripheral neuropathy, cardiac dysfunction, hyperlipidemia, bone and muscle pain, pruritus, and impotence.[56]

In the kidney, PTH facilitates calcium reabsorption and Pi excretion, as noted earlier. In bone, PTH receptors are located on osteoblasts, with a time-dependent effect. PTH administered long term inhibits osteoblast differentiation and mineralization. By contrast, the administration of PTH to osteoblasts in a pulse rather than a continuous manner stimulates osteoblast proliferation, forming the basis for the administration of PTH as an anabolic therapy for osteoporosis.[57] PTH also interacts with wnt/β-catenin signaling, as discussed in the bone section.

## VITAMIN D

Cholesterol is synthesized to 7-dehydrocholesterol, which in turn is metabolized in the skin to vitamin $D_3$ (Fig. 53.5). This reaction is facilitated by ultraviolet light (ultraviolet B) and higher temperature, and is therefore reduced in individuals with high skin melanin content and inhibited by sunscreen containing sun protection factor 8 or higher. In addition, there are dietary sources of vitamin $D_2$ (ergocalciferol) and vitamin $D_3$ (cholecalciferol). The difference between $D_2$ (plant source) and $D_3$ (animal source) compounds is the presence of a double bound ($D_2$) between carbon numbers 22 and 23 in the side chain. Once in the blood, both $D_2$ and $D_3$ bind with vitamin D–binding protein (DBP) and are carried to the liver, where they are hydroxylated by CYP27A1 (25-hydroxylase) in an essentially unregulated manner to yield 25(OH)D, often called calcidiol. Once they are converted to calcidiol, there appears to be no difference between the biologic activities of $D_2$ and $D_3$. Calcidiol is then converted in the kidney (or other cells) to calcitriol by the action of CYP27B1. This active metabolite is also degraded by other kidney enzymes, 24,25-hydroxylase (CYP24A1), and CYP3A4, providing the primary metabolism of the active compound.

Vitamin D–binding protein is a 58-kDa protein synthesized in the liver. Its serum levels in humans are between 4 and 8 mM, and the protein has a half-life of 3 days. Both the parent vitamin D, 25(OH)D, and calcitriol are carried in the circulation by DBP, but its greater affinity is for 25(OH)D. Targeted gene disruption studies show that DBP-null mice have a marked reduction in both circulating and tissue distributions of calcitriol and yet are normocalcemic, indicating that the primary role of DBP is to maintain stable serum stores of vitamin D metabolites.[58] At the cellular level, both 25(OH)D and calcitriol are endocytosed. Inside the cell, calcitriol can be inactivated by mitochondrial 24-hydroxylase (CYP24A1) or can bind to the VDR in the cytoplasm. Once the VDR-ligand binding has occurred, the VDR translocates to the nucleus, where it heterodimerizes with the retinoid X receptor. This complex binds the vitamin D response element of target genes and recruits transcription factors and corepressors/coactivators that modulate the transcription.[59] These corepressors and coactivators appear to be specific for the ligand, and thus different forms and analogs of vitamin D may produce different effects at each tissue, forming the basis for the pharmacologic development of analogs. Degradation of calcidiol is believed to occur principally in the kidney, from side cleavage and oxidation, to form $24,25(OH)_2D$.[59]

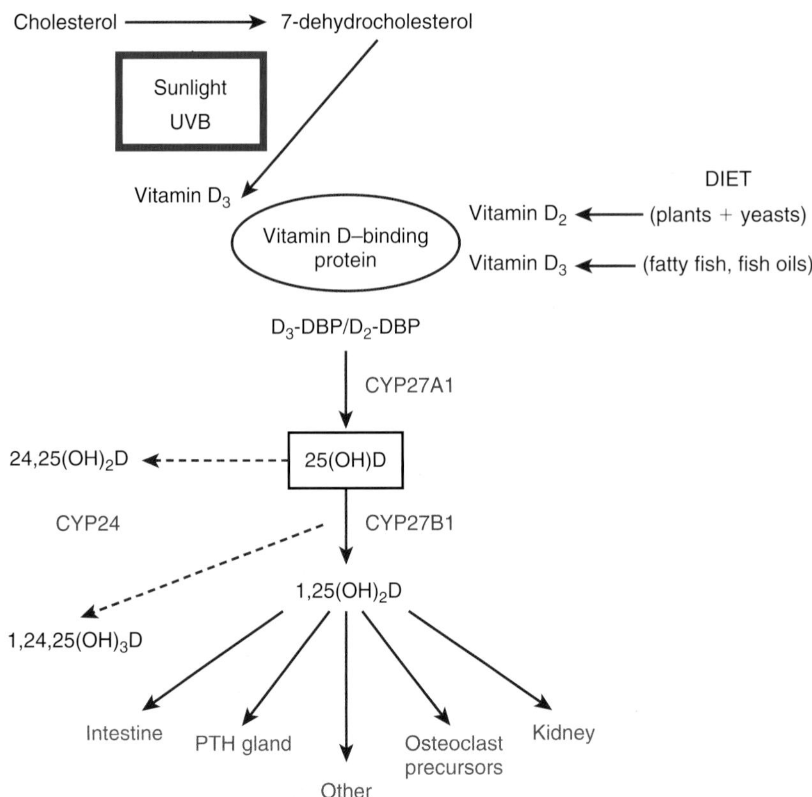


**Fig. 53.5** Overview of vitamin D metabolism. Vitamin D is obtained from dietary sources and is metabolized via ultraviolet light (ultraviolet B *[UVB]*) from 7-dehydrocholesterol in the skin. Both sources (diet and skin) of vitamin $D_2$ and vitamin $D_3$ bind to vitamin D–binding protein *(DBP)* and circulate to the liver. In the liver, vitamin D is hydroxylated by CYP27A1 *(25-hydroxylase)* to 25(OH)D, commonly referred to as calcidiol. Calcidiol is then further metabolized to calcitriol by the 1α-hydroxylase enzyme *(CYP27B1)* at the level of the kidney. The active metabolite $1,25(OH)_2D$ (calcitriol) acts principally on the target organs of intestine, parathyroid *(PTH)* gland, bone cell precursors, and the kidney. Calcitriol is metabolized to the inert $1,24,25(OH)_3D$ through the action of the 24,25-hydroxylase enzyme *(CYP24)*. Calcidiol is similarly hydroxylated to $24,25(OH)_2D$. (Modified from Moe SM. Renal osteodystrophy. In: Pereira BJG, Sayegh M, Blake P, eds. *Chronic Kidney Disease: Dialysis and Transplantation.* 2nd ed. Philadelphia: Elsevier Saunders; 2004.)

It is generally accepted that the major source of the circulating levels of calcitriol is the kidney. There is evidence that both 25(OH)D and calcitriol have local tissue effects because the VDR, CYP27B1, and CYP24A1 are found in many cells throughout the body.[60] While the kidneys are the predominant site of conversion of 25(OH)D to calcitriol, there is evidence of conversion in other organs, associated with CYP27B1 expression and/or activity in normal and abnormal cells. Other cell types active in conversion of 25(OH)D to calcitriol include osteoblasts, breast epithelial cells (normal and cancerous), prostate gland (normal and cancerous), alveolar and circulating macrophages, pancreatic islet cells, synovial cells, and arterial endothelial cells. Some of these cells may directly take up calcitriol, and others may endocytose the DBP–25(OH) D complex in a megalin-mediated manner (Fig. 53.6), after which the 25(OH)D is hydroxylated by CYP27B1 to act on that specific cell. The presence of CYP24A1 in cells also indicates that the metabolism of calcitriol may be regulated at a cellular level. Circulating concentrations of 25(OH)D are 1000 times higher than those of calcitriol, and thus 25(OH)D exhibits a local, or autocrine/paracrine, effect on many cell types.[60]

Circulating calcitriol mediates its cellular function via nongenomic and genomic mechanisms. Calcitriol facilitates the uptake of calcium in intestinal and renal epithelium by increasing the activity of the voltage-dependent calcium channels TRPV5 and TRPV6. Calcitriol then enhances the transport of calcium through and out of cells, by upregulating the calcium transport protein calbindin (calbindin-D9k in intestine, and calbindin-D28k in kidney) and the basolateral calcium-ATPase as detailed earlier. The CYP27B1 in the kidney is the site of regulation of calcitriol synthesis by numerous other factors, including serum calcium, serum Pi, estrogen, prolactin, growth hormone, FGF-23, and calcitriol itself. Studies show that FGF-23 and inflammatory mediators such as interferon regulate CYP27B1 at nonrenal sites.[61] In vitamin D knockout animals, parathyroid gland hyperplasia is consistently observed despite normalization of serum calcium. However, gland growth can be blunted by exogenous administration of calcitriol even in the absence of VDR, demonstrating a role for calcitriol in regulation of parathyroid gland growth.[62] In the rat, a single small dose of calcitriol decreases PTH secretion by nearly 100%. Studies in the 1970s demonstrated that oral calcitriol, but not the precursor hormone vitamin $D_3$, suppressed PTH in patients undergoing dialysis, leading to widespread use of calcitriol or its analogs in the management of secondary hyperparathyroidism. However, later studies in animals have demonstrated efficacy

ROLE OF EXTRARENAL 1α-HYDROXYLASE

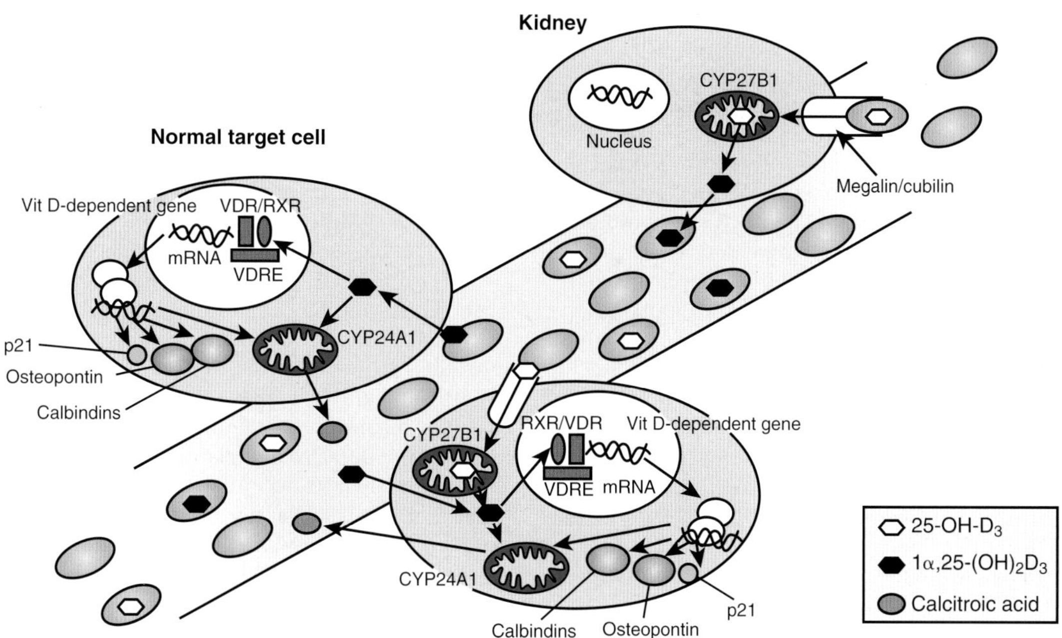


**Fig. 53.6** Concept of the role of the extrarenal 1α-hydroxylase. The metabolism of vitamin D in the context of the cells involved is shown. *Upper right,* Proximal tubular cell showing the key elements in the uptake of $25(OH)D_3$ and its conversion to $1\alpha,25(OH)_2D_3$. Megalin/cubilin are cell surface receptors that execute endocytosis of the vitamin D–binding protein (DBP)–$25(OH)D_3$ complex, and CYP27B1 is the main component of the 1α-hydroxylase, responsible for making $1\alpha,25(OH)_2D_3$. *Middle left,* Simple target cell that takes up 1α,25(OH, the vitamin D response element [VDRE])$_2D_3$ as the free ligand originally ferried to the target cell bound to DBP. The picture shows the key elements of the transcriptional machinery as well as some representative gene products, including the cell division protein p21, the bone matrix protein osteopontin, the calcium transport protein calbindin, and the autoregulatory protein CYP24A1. *Lower right,* Target cell expressing extrarenal 1α-hydroxylase, which possesses megalin/cubilin machinery to take up the DBP–$25(OH)D_3$ complex and also expresses CYP27B1, enabling it to make $1\alpha,25(OH)_2D_3$ intracellularly and also to respond in a likewise manner to the simple target cell because it also possesses the vitamin D receptor *(VDR)* and other transcriptional machinery. The expectation is that cells involved in cell differentiation or in control of cell division require higher concentrations of $1\alpha,25(OH)_2D_3$ in order to modulate a different set of genes, and that the CYP27B1 boosts local production to augment "circulating" $1\alpha,25(OH)_2D_3$ arriving from the kidney in the bloodstream. With normal physiologic processes, locally produced $1\alpha,25(OH)_2D_3$ would not enter the general circulation, although in pathologic conditions (e.g., sarcoidosis) it might. At this time, it is not clear how many cell types can be considered simple target cells and how many possess the CYP27B1 and megalin/cubilin to allow for local production of hormone. *mRNA,* Messenger RNA; *RXR,* retinoid X receptor. (From Jones G. Expanding role for vitamin D in chronic kidney disease: importance of blood 25-OH-D levels and extra-renal 1α-hydroxylase in the classical and nonclassical actions of 1α,25-dihydroxyvitamin $D_3$. *Semin Dial.* 2007;20:316–324. With permission.)

of 25(OH)D in suppression of PTH, but the doses required are much greater than for calcitriol. Studies in humans have shown efficacy of 25(OH)D in suppressing PTH in patients with advanced CKD, but direct comparison studies are lacking.[63]

Calcitriol has multiple effects on many cells that are important in bone remodeling; therefore it is not surprising that bone defects are well described in vitamin D–deficient states. However, the direct effects of the vitamin D system on bone have been difficult to differentiate from the secondary effects of hypocalcemia and hyperparathyroidism in vitamin D–deficient models. Transgenic animals, including 1α-hydroxylase$^{-/-}$/VDR$^{-/-}$ and 1α-hydroxylase$^{-/-}$/VDR$^{-/-}$, have impaired bone mineralization. In these animals, mineralization can be corrected with normalization of serum calcium; even exogenous calcitriol does not fully correct mineralization in the 1α-hydroxylase$^{-/-}$ animals unless serum calcium concentrations are also restored. Studies evaluating bone remodeling also demonstrate an important role for the calcitriol/VDR system. If hypocalcemia is not corrected (leading to secondary hyperparathyroidism), there is increased osteoblast activity and bone formation from the anabolic effects of PTH. The activation of osteoclasts by PTH is blunted, suggesting a synergistic effect of vitamin D and PTH. Supporting this suggestion is the finding that when serum calcium concentrations are corrected by "rescue" diets and secondary hyperparathyroidism is prevented, osteoblast numbers, mineralization activity, and bone volume are still reduced. Comparison studies of 1α-hydroxylase$^{-/-}$ and PTH$^{-/-}$ mice demonstrate a predominant role for PTH in appositional bone growth and for vitamin D in endochondral bone formation. Thus the calcitriol/VDR system has anabolic bone effects that are necessary for bone formation and are supplemental to the effect of PTH.[64]

## FGF-23 AND KLOTHO

"Phosphatonins" are circulating factors that regulate urinary Pi excretion. Two main phosphatonins have been described:

FGF-23 and MEPE. Various forms of rickets have now all been found to be due to abnormalities in FGF-23. Autosomal dominant hypophosphatemic rickets is rare and is associated with a mutation that limits normal degradation of FGF-23. Autosomal recessive hypophosphatemic rickets is also rare and is due to a mutation in dentin matrix protein (DMP), a locally produced inhibitor of FGF-23. X-linked hypophosphatemic rickets is the most common form of rickets due to a mutation in *PHEX* (phosphate-regulating gene with homologies to endopeptidases located on the X chromosome). Mutations in *PHEX* have been found to have deficient degradation of FGF-23 in the osteocyte, leading to inappropriately high serum concentrations of FGF-23.[65] Thus what previously was thought to be disorders of different etiologies are now all linked to FGF-23.

FGF-23 is a 251–amino acid hormone predominantly produced from bone cells (osteocytes and osteoblasts) during active bone remodeling, but its mRNA is also found in the heart, liver, thyroid/parathyroid, intestine, and skeletal muscle.[66] FGF-23 production in the osteocyte is stimulated by PTH[67] and calcitriol.[68] Elevated Pi or Pi load and hypercalcemia may also stimulate FGF-23 but this stimulation appears to be indirect. In the osteocyte, both DMP1 and PHEX protein degrade FGF-23 such that mutations in their corresponding genes lead to excess FGF-23.[65] In turn, calcitriol increases PHEX and FGF-23 inhibits calcitriol, completing a feedback loop. Regulation of NaPi-IIa by FGF-23 is independent of PTH; FGF-23 also inhibits the conversion of 25(OH)D to calcitriol by inhibition of CYP27B1 in the renal tubules[69] and at extrarenal sites,[61] and increases catabolism of calcitriol by activation of CYP24,[69] leading to hypophosphatemia and inappropriately normal or low serum calcitriol concentrations. An overview of the FGF–klotho axis is shown in Fig. 53.7.

FGF-23 is a member of a diverse family of 18 FGFs that bind to one of four receptors (FGFRs) via a heparan sulfate cofactor– or klotho coreceptor–dependent manner, leading to diverse biologic effects.[70] Identification of klotho as a coreceptor for FGF-23 was due to nearly identical phenotypes of the knockout mice, including hyperphosphatemia, hypercalcemia, and excess calcitriol levels associated with early mortality, growth retardation, vascular calcification, cardiac hypertrophy, and osteopenia.[71] Klotho was originally identified as an aging suppressor gene. α-Klotho is expressed in the kidney and parathyroid gland and forms complexes with FGFR1 and FGFR4 to enhance FGF-23 signaling. β-Klotho is expressed in the liver and fat, forms complexes with FGFR1 and FGFR4, and supports FGF-15/19 and FGF-21 signaling. γ-Klotho increases FGF-19 activity and is expressed in the eye, fat, and kidney. All three klothos are transmembrane proteins, with short intracellular domains and large extracellular domains that have β-glucosidase cleavage sites. In animals, α-klotho expressed in the distal tubule can be cleaved to release the extracellular domain into the circulation.

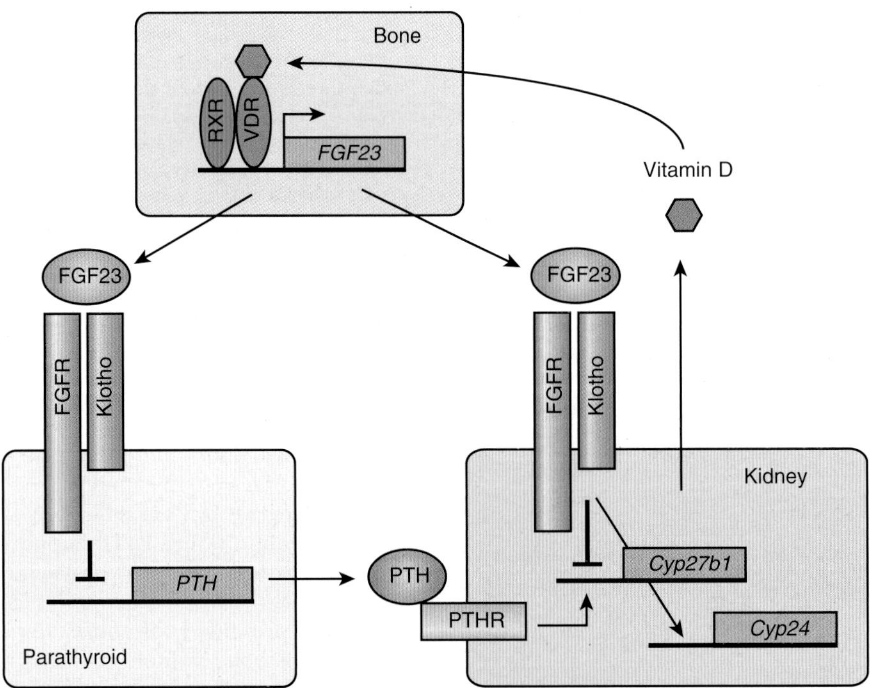


**Fig. 53.7** The bone–kidney–parathyroid endocrine axes mediated by fibroblast growth factor 23 *(FGF-23)* and klotho. Active form of vitamin D (calcitriol) binds to vitamin D receptor *(VDR)* in the bone (osteocytes). The ligand-bound VDR forms a heterodimer with a nuclear receptor *(RXR)* and transactivates expression of the FGF-23 gene. FGF-23 secreted from bone acts on the klotho–FGF receptor *(FGFR)* complex expressed in the kidney (the bone-kidney axis) and parathyroid gland (the bone-parathyroid axis). In the kidney, FGF-23 suppresses synthesis of active vitamin D by downregulating expression of the *Cyp27b1* gene and promotes its inactivation by upregulating expression of the *Cyp24* gene, thereby closing a negative feedback loop for vitamin D homeostasis. In the parathyroid gland, FGF-23 suppresses production and secretion of parathyroid hormone *(PTH)*. PTH binds to the PTH receptor *(PTHR)* expressed on renal tubular cells, leading to upregulation of *Cyp27b1* gene expression. Thus suppression of PTH by FGF-23 reduces expression of the *Cyp27b1* gene and serum levels of calcitriol. This step closes another long negative feedback loop for vitamin D homeostasis. (From Kuro-o M. Overview of the FGF23-Klotho axis. *Pediatr Nephrol.* 2010;25:583–590. With permission.)

Further, alternative splicing of the α-klotho gene produces only the extracellular domain that is released from cells and is called circulating or soluble klotho.[72] The soluble α-klotho acts as a coreceptor at nonrenal sites, and prevents FGF-23-induced cardiac hypertrophy.[71] The kidney regulates both renal production of soluble klotho and renal excretion.[72]

In the kidney, tissue klotho is downregulated[72] and FGF-23 is upregulated early in the course of CKD.[73] Klotho is shed from the distal convoluted tubule to serve as a coreceptor with FGF-23 on the proximal tubule, where it inhibits reabsorption of Pi that is regulated by NaPi-IIa, NaPi-IIc, and Pit-1 (similar to PTH but via different signaling mechanisms), and suppresses CYP27B1 to inhibit calcitriol production (opposite of PTH).[74] α-Klotho also increases calcium reabsorption by stimulating TRPV5,[75] decreases potassium excretion through effects on the ROMK1 (renal outer medullary potassium 1) channel,[76] protects against kidney injury and fibrosis,[77] and decreases insulin resistance.[74] Table 53.2 demonstrates the parallel changes in klotho deficiency and CKD.

**Table 53.2 Comparison of Phenotypes of Klotho Deficiency and Chronic Kidney Disease**

| | Klotho Deficiency | Chronic Kidney Disease |
|---|---|---|
| **Blood Chemistry:** | | |
| Phosphate | ↑↑↑↑ | ↑ or ↑↑↑[a] |
| Calcium | ↑ | ↔ or ↓↓ |
| Creatinine | ↑ | ↑↑↑ |
| Calcitriol | ↑↑↑ | ↓↓↓ |
| Parathyroid hormone | ↔ or ↓ | ↑↑ |
| Fibroblast growth factor 23 | ↑↑↑ | ↑↑ |
| Klotho | ↓↓↓ or disappears | ↓↓ at ESKD[b] |
| **Gross Phenotypes:** | | |
| Body weight | ↓↓↓ | ↓↓ |
| Growth retardation | ↓↓↓↓ | ↓↓ in children |
| Physical activity | ↓↓↓ | ↓ |
| Fertility | ↓↓↓↓ | ↓↓ |
| Life span | ↓↓↓↓ | ↓↓ |
| **Cardiovascular Disease:** | | |
| Cardiac hypertrophy | ↑↑ | ↑↑↑ |
| Cardiac fibrosis | ↑↑ | ↑↑↑ |
| Vascular calcification | ↑↑↑↑ | ↑↑ |
| Atherosclerosis | ↑↑ | ↑↑↑ |
| Blood pressure | ↑ | ↑↑↑↑ |
| Hematocrit levels | ↓ | ↓↓↓↓ |
| Bone disease | ↓↓↓ | ↓↓↓ |

[a]During early chronic kidney disease, blood phosphate level is in the normal range.

[b]Blood klotho may be increased in early chronic kidney disease.

*ESKD*, End-stage kidney disease; ↓, decreases; ↑, increases; ↔, unchanged.

Modified from Hu MC, Kuro-o M, Moe OW. Renal and extrarenal actions of Klotho. *Semin Nephrol.* 2013;33: 118–129.

In addition to klotho's role in mineral metabolism, klotho and FGF-23 are implicated in cardiovascular disease. FGF-23 can induce cardiac hypertrophy and increases intracellular calcium in a klotho-independent manner.[71,78,79] Klotho is localized in the heart at the sinoatrial node, and klotho deficiency may lead to arrhythmias.[80] Klotho suppresses cardiomyocyte apoptosis[81] and downregulates TRPC6 (transient receptor potential cation 6) calcium channel in the cardiomyocyte.[82] Both klotho and FGFR1 and FGFR3, but not FGF-23 and FGFR4, are expressed in human arteries.[83,84] In human arteries from patients with CKD, klotho and FGFR1 and FGFR3 are downregulated in the presence of calcification. VDR activators upregulate klotho, leading to an anticalcific effect on FGF-23-induced calcification.[84] Decreased klotho impairs endothelial function.[85] Activation of the renin–angiotensin–aldosterone system reduces renal klotho expression.[86] The pace of discovery of the systemic effects of FGF-23 and klotho has revolutionized our understanding of CKD-MBD.

## BONE BIOLOGY

The majority of the total body stores of calcium and Pi is located in bone and therefore bone plays an integral role in homeostasis. Trabecular (cancellous) bone is located predominantly in the epiphyses of the long bones, is 15% to 25% calcified, and serves a metabolic function, with a relatively short turnover time as shown by calcium[45] studies. By contrast, cortical (compact) bone is located in the shafts of long bones and is 80% to 90% calcified. This bone serves primarily a protective and mechanical function and has a calcium turnover time of months. Bone consists principally (90%) of highly organized cross-linked fibers of type I collagen; the remainder consists of proteoglycans and "noncollagen" proteins such as osteopontin, osteocalcin, osteonectin, and alkaline phosphatase. Hydroxyapatite—$Ca_{10}(PO_4)_6(OH)_2$—is the primary bone crystal.

The cellular components of bone are cartilage cells, which are critical to bone development; osteoblasts, which are the bone-forming cells; and osteoclasts, which are the bone-resorbing cells. Osteoblasts are derived from progenitor mesenchymal cells located in the bone marrow. They are then induced to become osteoprogenitor cells, then endosteal or periosteal progenitor cells, then mature osteoblasts. The control of this differentiation pathway is complicated and involves integration of circulating hormones, locally produced factors from the mesenchymal–hematopoietic cell niche, and transcription factors. Once bone formation is complete, osteoblasts may undergo apoptosis or may become quiescent cells trapped within the mineralized bone in the form of osteocytes.[87] The osteocytes are interconnected through a series of canaliculi and serve as mechanoreceptors. Osteocytes detect and respond to mechanical loading and initiate bone remodeling by regulating local osteoclastogenesis via paracrine signals. Osteoclasts are derived from hematopoietic precursor cells that differentiate and are signaled to arrive at a certain place in the bone through the osteoprotegerin (OPG)/RANKL (receptor activator of nuclear factor κB ligand) system detailed later. Once there, they fuse to form the multinucleated cells known as osteoclasts, which become highly polarized, reabsorbing bone through the release of derivative enzymes. These cells move along a resorption surface via changes in the cytoskeleton. PTH, cytokines, and calcitriol are all important in inducing the fusion of the committed osteoclast precursors.

The control of bone remodeling is highly complex, but appears to occur in very distinct phases, as follows: (1) osteoclast recruitment and activation, (2) osteoclast resorption, (3) preosteoblast migration and differentiation, (4) osteoblast deposition of matrix (osteoid or unmineralized bone), (5) mineralization, and (6) quiescence. At any one time, less than 15% to 20% of the bone surface is undergoing remodeling, and this process in a single bone remodeling unit can take 3 to 6 months.[88] How or why a certain segment of bone undergoes a remodeling cycle is not completely clear. The three main systems that interact to regulate remodeling are OPG/RANKL, sclerostin/Wnt/β-catenin, and PTH/PTHR1, which are discussed separately.

The identification of the OPG and RANK system in the 1980s sheds new light on the control of osteoclast function and the long observed coupling of osteoblasts and osteoclasts. RANK is located on osteoclasts, and RANK ligand (RANKL) is secreted by osteoblasts. Osteoblasts also synthesize the decoy protein OPG, which can bind to RANK ligand and inhibit the subsequent binding of RANKL to RANK on osteoclasts, thus inhibiting bone resorption (Fig. 53.8). Alternatively, if OPG production is decreased, RANKL can bind with RANK on osteoclasts and induce osteoclastic bone resorption. This control system is regulated by nearly every cytokine and hormone thought important in bone remodeling, including PTH, calcitriol, estrogen, glucocorticoids, interleukins, prostaglandins, and members of the transforming growth factor-β superfamily of cytokines.[89] OPG has been successful in preventing bone resorption in models of osteoporosis as well as hormone- and cytokine-induced bone resorption,[89] and denosumab, an anti-RANKL antibody, is an approved anabolic drug for the treatment of osteoporosis.[90] Interestingly, abnormalities in the OPG/RANKL system have been found in kidney disease,[91] and early animal models suggest that treatment with OPG may have a protective role in hyperparathyroid bone disease.[92] Initial studies in patients receiving dialysis have demonstrated hypocalcemia as a severe adverse effect of denosumab.[93] More information is required to understand how this system regulates bone remodeling in the context of CKD.

Genetic defects in the gene *SOST* have been identified in rare bone disorders. Sclerostin, the protein product of this gene, binds to low-density lipoprotein receptor–related proteins 5 and 6 (LRP5/LRP6) on the osteocyte to competitively inhibit the binding of the protein wnt (Fig. 53.9). Normally, wnt binding to LRP5/LRP6 leads to stabilization of β-catenin (canonical pathway) and regulation of normal bone accrual via osteoblast differentiation. In the presence of sclerostin, the β-catenin is degraded and mesenchymal stem cell differentiation to mature bone cells is inhibited. In animal models, sclerostin deletion enhances bone accrual,[94] and in early human trials, treatment with an antibody to sclerostin was found to be anabolic.[95,96] Given that sclerostin concentrations are elevated in the blood and bone of patients with CKD[97] and bone in animals with CKD,[98] the anabolic agent antisclerostin antibody may be efficacious in the treatment of renal osteodystrophy. However, initial studies in animals found that antisclerostin antibody was not efficacious in the setting of elevated PTH, although it did improve bone

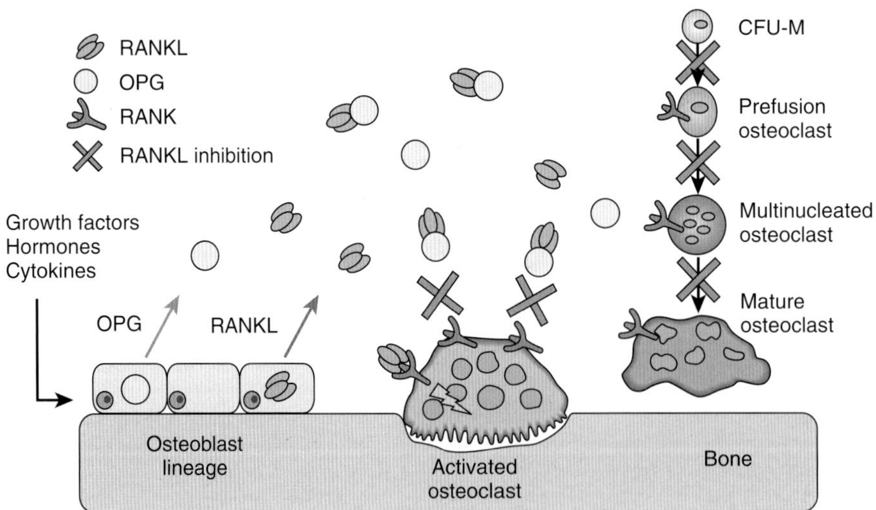


**Fig. 53.8** Role of osteoprotegerin *(OPG)*/receptor activator of nuclear factor kappaB ligand *(RANKL)* in bone remodeling. Mechanisms of action for OPG, RANKL, and RANK (receptor activator of nuclear factor kappaB) are depicted in this diagram. RANKL is produced by osteoblasts, bone marrow stromal cells, and other cells under the control of various proresorptive growth factors, hormones, and cytokines. Osteoblasts and stromal cells produce OPG, which binds to and thereby inactivates RANKL. The major binding complex is likely to be a single OPG homodimer interacting with high affinity with a single RANKL homotrimer. In the absence of OPG, RANKL activates its receptor, RANK, found on osteoclasts and preosteoclast precursors. RANK–RANKL interactions lead to preosteoclast recruitment, fusion into multinucleated osteoclasts, osteoclast activation, and osteoclast survival. Each of these RANK-mediated responses can be fully inhibited by OPG. *CFU-M,* Macrophage colony-forming unit. (From Kearns AE, Khosla S, Kostenuik PJ. Receptor activator of nuclear factor kappaB ligand and osteoprotegerin regulation of bone remodeling in health and disease. *Endocr Rev.* 2008;29:155–192.)

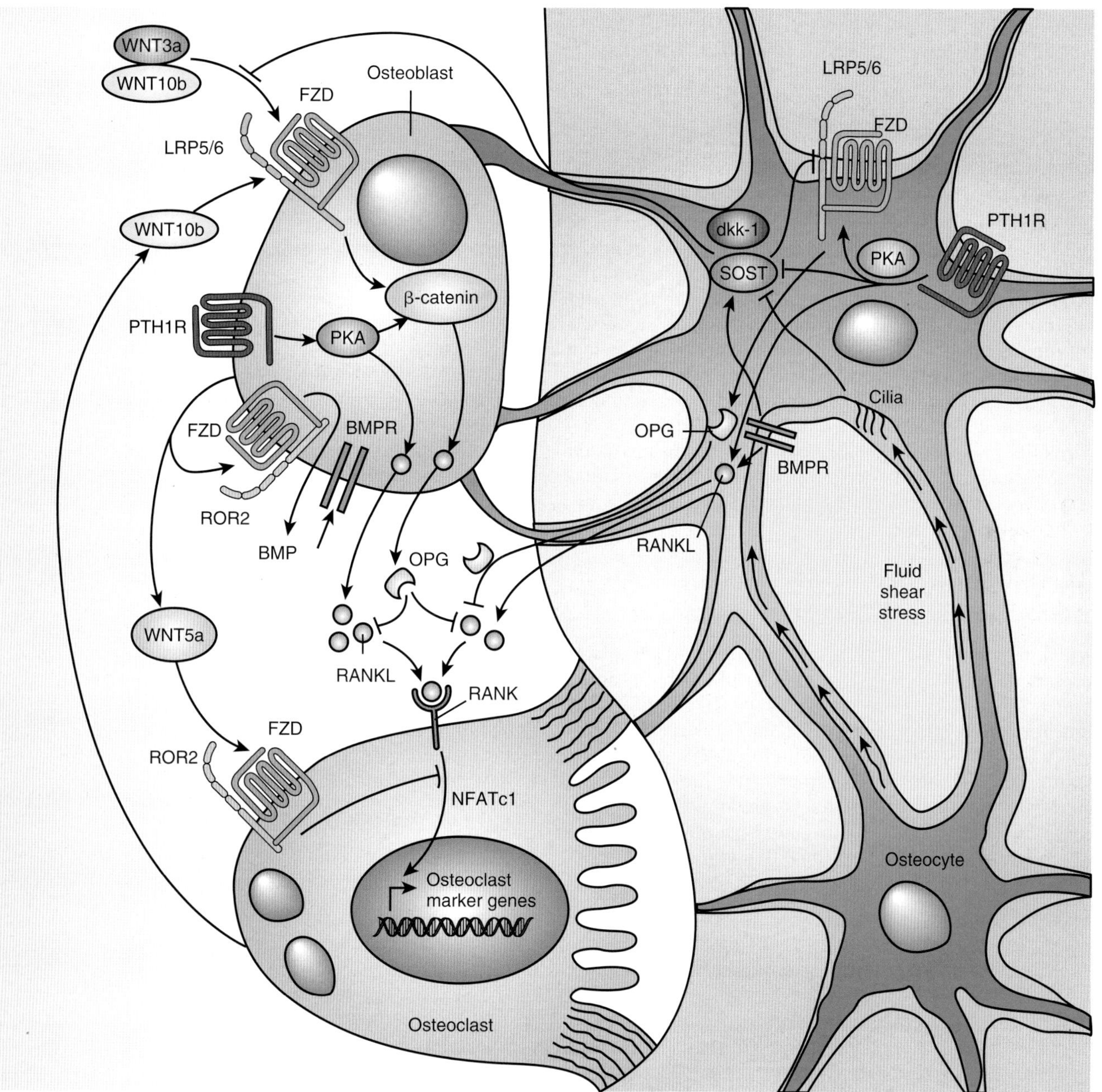


**Fig. 53.9** Parathyroid hormone *(PTH)* and β-catenin signaling in bone remodeling. Osteocytes control bone formation through the secretion of the WNT antagonists sclerostin *(SOST)* and Dickkopf WNT signaling pathway inhibitor 1 *(dkk-1),* the expression of which is regulated by mechanosignals and by signaling of PTH and bone morphogenetic protein *(BMP)*. PTH represses expression of these antagonists, whereas BMP signaling, which is mediated by BMP receptor 1A *(BMPR1A),* induces their expression. Moreover, WNT signaling in osteocytes controls the production of osteoprotegerin *(OPG)*, which is the decoy receptor for the key osteoclast differentiation factor RANKL (receptor activator of nuclear factor kappaB ligand). Osteoblast-expressed WNT5a stimulates differentiation of osteoclast precursors as a result of binding to the FZD–ROR2 (frizzled and receptor tyrosine kinase–like orphan receptor 2) receptor complex. In a feedback loop for bone remodeling, osteoclasts stimulate the local differentiation of osteoblasts at the end of the resorption phase by secreting WNT ligands. In addition, activation of parathyroid hormone 1 receptor *(PTH1R)*–mediated signaling in osteoblasts and osteocytes leads to stabilization of β-catenin and, thus, activation of WNT signaling. *LRP5/6,* Low-density lipoprotein (LDL) receptor–related proteins 5 and 6; *PKA,* protein kinase signaling. (From Baron R, Kneissel M. WNT signaling in bone homeostasis and disease: from human mutations to treatments. *Nat Med.* 2013;19:179–192. With permission.)

volume when PTH was suppressed.[99] Dickkopf-related protein 1 (dkk-1) also inhibits wnt binding to LRP5/LRP6, and an antibody to this circulating inhibitor of wnt signaling improved bone remodeling in a model of early CKD.[100] In osteocytes, PTH directly suppresses sclerostin and dkk-1 secretion[67,101] and thus inhibits the production of circulating inhibitors of wnt signaling.

In bone, PTH binds to its receptor, PTH1R, and activates β-catenin signaling via multiple mechanisms (Fig. 53.9): (1) direct activation through cAMP signaling; (2) indirect activation via osteoclast activation, which then increases β-catenin activity in osteoblasts; and (3) by binding to LRP6 to activate LRP5/LRP6 signaling even in the absence of wnt ligands.[94] Thus PTH can activate β-catenin through non–wnt-mediated pathways and through pathways not regulated by sclerostin or dkk-1. There are also differences in responses to continuous and intermittent PTH exposures. Mice expressing a constitutively active PTH1R or animals receiving continuous infusion of PTH(1–84) (analogous to secondary hyperparathyroidism) also have wnt-dependent remodeling with increased osteoclast bone resorption via the OPG/RANKL system, leading to osteoblast activation and β-catenin activation.[102,103] Hyperphosphatemia also activates β-catenin signaling.[104] Thus in CKD with hyperphosphatemia and secondary hyperparathyroidism, there is activation of β-catenin by PTH-mediated inhibition of circulating inhibitors of wnt signaling (sclerostin and dkk-1), PTH-mediated effects independent of wnt signaling, and phosphorus-mediated effects, all leading to enhanced mesenchymal differentiation to osteoblasts, increased RANKL-induced osteoclast activation, and increased bone resorption.

## PATHOPHYSIOLOGY OF VASCULAR CALCIFICATION

Vascular disease may be due to a variety of different pathologic processes in different arterial segments, all of which can be calcified. Atherosclerotic disease is characterized by fibro-fatty plaque formation, and on the basis of autopsy data and animal models, calcification had been thought to occur late in the disease course. These plaques can protrude into the arterial lumen, leading to a filling defect on angiography (Fig. 53.10A). However, advances in imaging, especially intravascular ultrasonography, have demonstrated that atherosclerosis can also be a circumferential lesion (without an obstructed lumen) with calcification earlier in the course of the disease.[105] The medial layer may also be affected in arteriosclerosis, leading to thickening commonly found in elastic arteries (Fig. 53.10B). In addition to the larger elastic arteries, smaller elastic arteries may be affected by medial thickening and calcification, classically described as Mönckeberg calcification, or medial calcinosis. This condition is more common in advanced age, and in patients with diabetes mellitus and/or CKD, and is associated with all-cause and cardiovascular mortality in patients with diabetes with and without CKD, as well as in patients with CKD with or without diabetes.

Although initially believed to be related to spontaneous precipitation in the setting of high serum concentrations of calcium and Pi, vascular calcification is now known to be a tightly regulated process that resembles mineralization in bone, a process kept “in check” through the actions of inhibitors of calcification. The current hypothesis accepted by most investigators is that VSMCs dedifferentiate or transform to osteocyte/chondrocyte-like cells (Fig. 53.11). These cells then lay down an extracellular matrix of collagen and noncollagenous proteins and make matrix vesicles that attach to the extracellular matrix to initiate and propagate mineralization. This process is regulated by the cells, the extracellular matrix proteins, and inhibitors that may act locally or systemically. In advanced CKD, there is abnormal bone remodeling and reduced renal clearance of phosphate, generating a positive calcium and Pi balance that “feeds” the mineral composition of matrix vesicles and augments the ability of existing calcification to expand. The evidence for each of these steps is discussed in the following sections.

### CELLULAR TRANSFORMATION

VSMCs, osteoblasts, chondrocytes, and adipocytes differentiate from mesenchymal precursors with normal differentiation

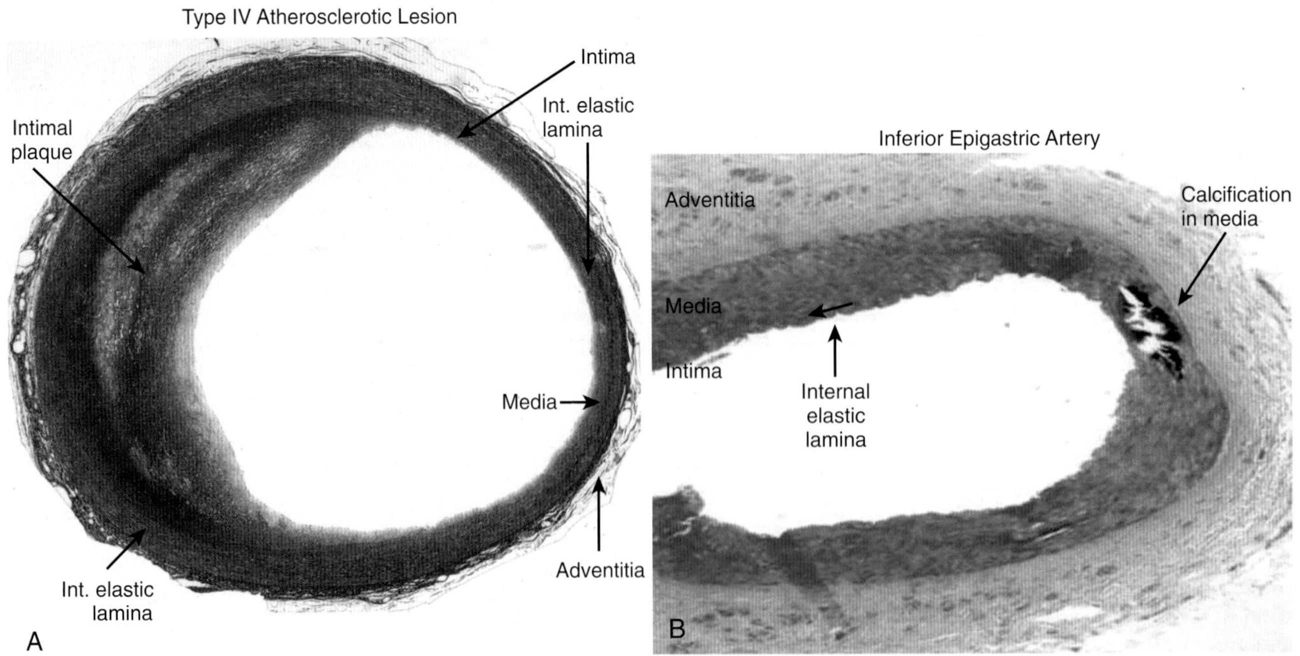


**Fig. 53.10** Arterial calcification. Histologic differences between atherosclerotic, or intimal, calcification (A) and medial calcification (B). *Int.,* Internal.

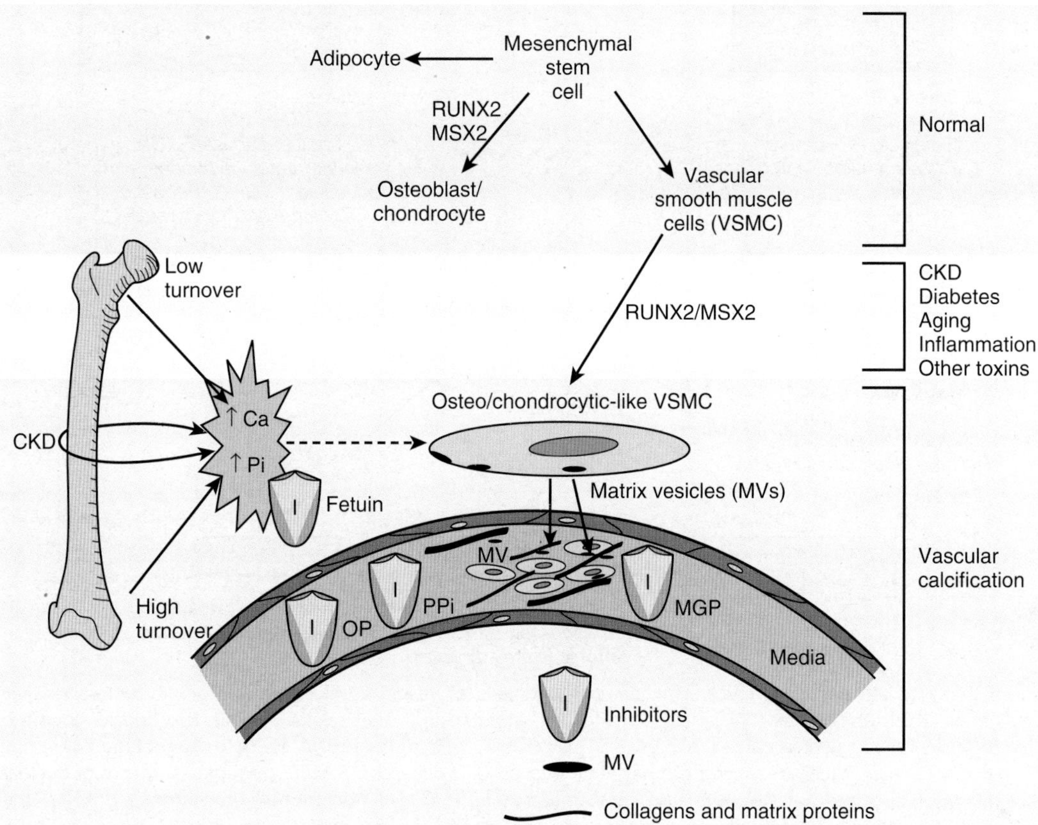


**Fig. 53.11** Overview of the pathophysiology of vascular calcification. Normally, mesenchymal stem cells differentiate to adipocytes, osteoblasts, chondrocytes, and vascular smooth muscle cells *(VSMCs)*. In the setting of chronic kidney disease *(CKD)*, diabetes, aging, inflammation, and the presence of multiple other toxins, these VSMCs can dedifferentiate or transform to chondrocyte/osteoblast-like cells by upregulation of transcription factors such as runt-related transcription factor 2 *(RUNX-2)* and homeobox protein MSX2. These transcription factors are critical for normal bone development, and thus their upregulation in VSMCs is indicative of a phenotypic switch. These osteocyte/chondrocyte-like VSMCs then become calcified in a process similar to bone formation. The cells lay down collagen and noncollagenous proteins in the intima or media and incorporate calcium (Ca) and phosphorus (Pi) into matrix vesicles to initiate mineralization and further grow the mineral into hydroxyapatite. The overall positive calcium and phosphorus balance of most patients undergoing dialysis feeds both the cellular transformation and the generation of matrix vesicles *(MVs)*. In addition, the extremes of bone turnover in CKD (low and high turnover or adynamic and hyperparathyroid bone, respectively) increases the available calcium and phosphorus by altering the bone content of these minerals. Ultimately, whether an artery calcifies or not depends on the strength of the army of inhibitors (Is) standing by in the circulation (fetuin-A) and in the arteries – for example, pyrophosphate *(PPi)*, matrix gla protein *(MGP)*, and osteopontin *(OP)*. (From Moe SM, Chen NX. Mechanisms of vascular calcification in chronic kidney disease. *J Am Soc Nephrol.* 2008;19:213–216. With permission.)

and in transformation (dedifferentiation), which are controlled by various transcription factors (Fig. 53.12). Expression of the osteoblast differentiation factor core binding factor α-1 (Cbfα1), now called Runx-2, has been identified in the inferior epigastric artery of adults undergoing kidney transplantation[106] and in sections from the brachial arteries of children undergoing dialysis.[107] Runx-2 is essential for normal bone development, in that Runx-2 knockout mice fail to form a skeleton.[108] Genetic techniques have confirmed that VSMCs give rise to osteochondrogenic-like cells in calcified blood vessels (as opposed to circulating cells).[109] Osteoclast-like cells can also be seen, more commonly in intimal lesions, and as in bone, they appear to arise from circulating precursors.[110]

In vitro, VSMCs upregulate Runx-2 in response to elevated Pi mediated by the type III sodium-dependent Pi cotransporters Pit-1 and Pit-2.[111] In addition, VSMCs incubated with uremic serum (pooled from anuric patients undergoing dialysis), in comparison with normal serum, express Runx-2 and its downstream protein osteopontin via a non–Pi-mediated mechanism.[112] Excess calcium can also induce mineralization in vitro, and the effects of calcium are additive to those of increased Pi.[113] Lastly, FGF-23 enhances Pi-induced vascular calcification in rat aortic rings and rat aorta VSMCs by promoting osteoblastic differentiation.[114] Numerous traditional and nontraditional cardiovascular risk factors in CKD can induce the transformation of VSMCs into osteoblast-like cells, with subsequent calcification in vitro (Fig. 53.12). Given these data, it is not surprising that arterial calcification is so common in patients with CKD.

In animal models of CKD, secondary hyperparathyroidism develops spontaneously with loss of kidney function and can be associated with vascular calcification.[48,115,116] Unfortunately, it is difficult to distinguish between the effects of Pi and PTH. However, one study found that vascular calcification developed in nephrectomized animals achieving supraphysiologic PTH

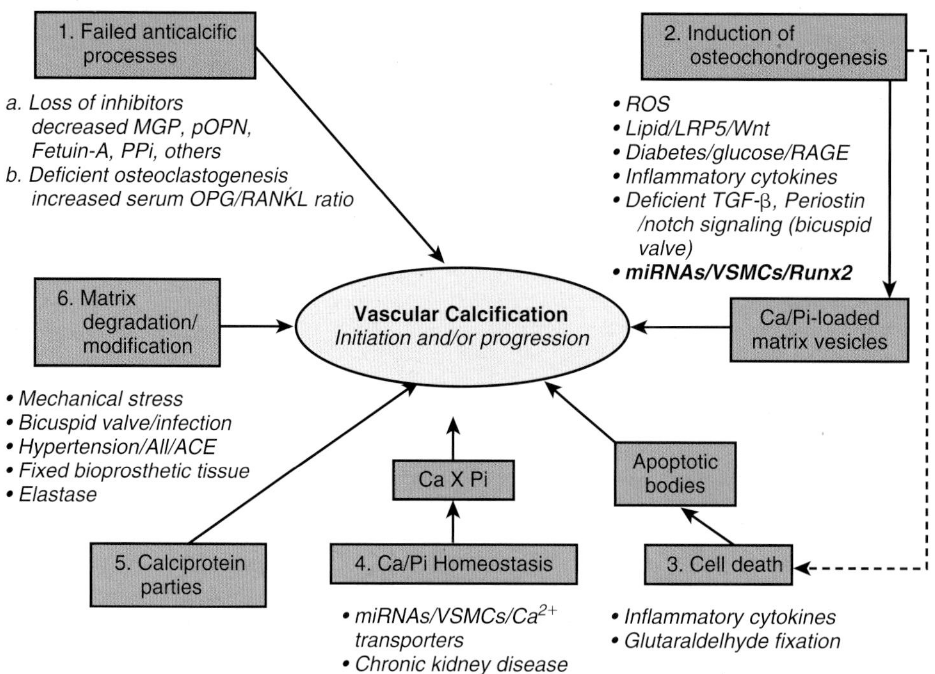


**Fig. 53.12** Factors that regulate pathways involved in the pathogenesis of vascular calcification. Multiple factors regulate each step of extraskeletal calcification. *ACE,* Angiotensin-converting enzyme; *AII,* angiotensin II; *Ca,* calcium; *LRP5,* low-density lipoprotein (LDL) receptor–related protein 5; *MGP,* matrix gamma-carboxyglutamate (Gla) protein; *miRNA,* microRNA; *OPG,* osteoprotegerin; *Pi,* phosphate; *pOPN,* osteopontin; *PPi,* pyrophosphate; *RAGE,* advanced glycosylation end product receptor; *RANKL,* receptor activator of nuclear factor kappaB ligand; *ROS,* reactive oxygen species; *Runx2,* runt-related transcription factor 2; *TGF-β,* transforming growth factor β; *VSMCs,* vascular smooth muscle cells; *Wnt,* wingless-type MMTV integration site family member. (From Wu M, Rementer C, Giachelli CM. Vascular calcification: an update on mechanisms and challenges in treatment. *Calcif Tissue Int.* 2013;93:365–373. With permission.)

levels by infusion, regardless of the Pi intake.[117] In a similar study, Runx-2 was upregulated in animals in three of the four Pi/PTH intake groups—those fed normal PTH + high Pi, high PTH + high Pi, and high PTH + low Pi—indicating that both Pi and PTH may lead to Runx-2 upregulation in arteries. However, the animals given high PTH + low Pi did not demonstrate arterial calcification,[118] suggesting that Pi is needed to provide the substrate for calcification to progress.

Arterial calcification and mineralization of bone are inversely related. In animal models of excessive bone resorption, treatments aimed at decreasing bone remodeling by inhibition of osteoclast activity (i.e., bisphosphonates, calcimimetics) have been found helpful in preventing vascular calcification in some[119–121] but not all studies.[122] Correction of low-turnover bone disease also appears to improve arterial calcification in animals.[123,124] The role of vitamin D has been controversial, but data now suggest that it is only when the circulating levels of calcitriol are increased (and thus induce hypercalcemia or hyperphosphatemia) that calcification is observed.[125] Treatment studies in humans are reviewed in Chapter 63.

## MATRIX VESICLES AND APOPTOSIS

In chondrocytes and osteoblasts, normal mineralization is initiated when matrix vesicles are released into the extracellular space from the cell surface via polarized budding with subsequent attachment to extracellular matrix proteins. Matrix vesicles are characterized by both their appearance as small (50–200 nm), electron-dense spherical particles on electron microscopy and the biochemical presence of calcium and Pi, alkaline phosphatase, and the membrane protein annexins. Matrix vesicles have been identified in nearly all forms of mineralization/calcification in human tissues, including bone, cartilage, tendon, calciphylaxis, and atherosclerosis. Cultured VSMCs incubated with elevated concentrations of calcium and Pi release matrix vesicles into the media, and the presence of fetuin-A (AHSG or α-2-Heremans-Schmid glycoprotein), the circulating inhibitor of mineralization (see later), decreases calcium uptake of the matrix vesicles.[126] Collagenase digestion of VSMCs has been found to lead to two populations of matrix vesicles, a secreted form in the media that had high fetuin-A and low annexin II content and could not mineralize type I collagen, and cellular matrix vesicles that had low fetuin-A and high annexin II content and could mineralize.[127] Matrix vesicles are similar to exosomes, which are known to transfer microRNAs from cell to cell and thus may play a role in calcification.[128] MicroRNAs have been found to regulate the phenotypic switch from contractile to synthetic VSMCs[129] and are involved in the regulation of arterial calcification in vitro in animal models.[128,130] These results suggest that the cellular regulation of the content of matrix vesicles may regulate the type and mineralizing capacity of the vesicle.

In addition to matrix vesicles, apoptotic bodies can induce calcification in vitro in VSMCs. Apoptotic bodies stimulated by calcium-Pi crystals of approximately 1 μm or less in diameter cause a rapid rise in intracellular calcium concentration and apoptosis, an effect triggered by lysosomal degradation.[131] Apoptosis has been identified in arterial segments with calcification obtained from children with ESKD.[107]

Activation of the DNA damage response by prelamin A accelerates arterial calcification.[132] Autophagy, a regulated process of cell survival, counteracts Pi-induced calcification by reducing matrix vesicle release.[133] By contrast, atorvastatin protects against calcification by inducing autophagy via suppression of the β-catenin pathway.[134] Thus cells appear to guard against calcification when able via a number of pathways.

## INHIBITORS OF VASCULAR CALCIFICATION

Vascular calcification, although prevalent in patients with CKD and particularly in patients receiving dialysis, is not uniform. Approximately 20% (depending on the published series) of patients undergoing dialysis have no vascular calcification and continue to have no calcification on follow-up despite risk factors similar to those in patients who do have calcification. These data support the concept of calcification inhibitors. Knockout animal models have demonstrated that selective deletion of many genes leads to vascular calcification.[135] These studies imply that mineralization (or calcification) of arteries will occur, at least in some species or individuals, unless inhibited. This concept, that the regulation of calcification in blood vessels occurs principally via inhibition rather than promotion, may also be true in bone.[136] Inhibitors can be circulating or locally produced and site specific. Three inhibitors that have been well characterized in the arterial calcification of CKD are fetuin-A, matrix gamma-carboxyglutamate (Gla) protein (MGP), and OPG.

Many other inhibitors of calcification exist. In aggregate, the data discussed in this section support the diversity and abundance of naturally occurring inhibitors of calcification. Thus vascular calcification in CKD represents a state of increased calcification promoters and decreased calcification inhibitors.

### Fetuin-A

Fetuin-A is a circulating inhibitor of calcification, abundant in plasma, and mainly produced by the liver in adults. The transcription and synthesis of fetuin-A are downregulated during inflammation and thus it is also a reverse acute phase reactant, like serum albumin and other hepatic proteins. Fetuin-A binds to both calcium and Pi in the serum, forming small "calciparticles" that are removed through the reticuloendothelial system. Fetuin-A inhibits the de novo formation and precipitation of the apatite precursor mineral basic calcium-Pi but does not dissolve it once the basic calcium-Pi is formed.[137] Therefore fetuin-A could be viewed as acting as a host defense to "cleanse the blood" of unwanted calcium and Pi and to prevent undesirable calcification in the circulation without causing bone demineralization. Fetuin-A has been found in matrix vesicles from VSMCs, and its presence renders the vesicles incapable of mineralization.[127,138] Fetuin-A is abundant in serum and is a major factor in the calcification propensity of serum,[139] a measure of which has been shown to reflect all-cause mortality in patients with CKD.[140]

Targeted disruption of fetuin-A leads to diffuse and profound soft tissue calcification and to arteriolar calcification of muscle, kidney, and lung but not large arteries.[141] When $Ahsg^{-/-}$ mice were crossed with $ApoE^{-/-}$ mice, the latter known to have increased cholesterol and atherosclerosis, both aorta and coronary artery calcification developed in the double-deficient $Ahsg^{-/-}/ApoE^{-/-}$ mice with high-Pi diet alone and were accelerated by CKD.[142] Thus extensive and multisite arterial calcification in this animal model required genetic predisposition to atherosclerosis (Apo $E^{-/-}$), a genetic defect in an inhibitor of mineralization ($Ahsg^{-/-}$), and hyperphosphatemia that was further accelerated by CKD. These data support the redundancy of the inhibitor system, in which multiple local regulators compensate for the absence of the circulating inhibitor fetuin-A. In patients with ESKD, lower serum fetuin-A concentrations are associated with mortality.[143,144] Serum concentrations of fetuin-A in patients undergoing dialysis were found to be inversely correlated with coronary artery calcification assessed by spiral computed tomography (CT),[145] with carotid artery plaques,[146] and, in children undergoing dialysis, arterial stiffness.[107] Fetuin-A deficiency in CKD is likely due to chronic inflammation, although gene polymorphisms may also play a role. It is also possible that there is inappropriate upregulation, leading to a relative deficiency of fetuin-A in the setting of elevated calcium and Pi.

## MATRIX GAMMA-CARBOXYGLUTAMATE (GLA) PROTEIN

MGP is a vitamin K–dependent protein expressed in a number of tissues but highly expressed in arteries and bone, where it acts predominantly as a local regulator of vascular calcification. MGP knockout mice have excessive cartilage and growth plate mineralization and arterial medial calcification, resulting in early mortality.[147] In MGP-deficient mice, calcification depends on elastin fragmentation due to increased elastase production.[148] Warfarin use and/or nutritional vitamin K deficiency result in undercarboxylation of MGP and impaired function.[149] Warfarin use is also a known risk factor for calcific uremic arteriolopathy (also referred to as calciphylaxis) and can induce calcification in an animal model of CKD.[150] The administration of vitamin K can prevent calcification, although definitive trials are underway in CKD.[149] Serum concentrations of carboxylated MGP were found to be nearly undetectable in patients undergoing dialysis and in patients with atherosclerotic disease.[149] Furthermore, lower levels of carboxylated MGP were associated with coronary artery calcification, arterial stiffness, and higher serum Pi in patients undergoing dialysis.[151] Lower serum concentrations of relative carboxylated MGP as well as vitamin K deficiency were also found in 20 patients with calcific uremic arteriolopathy compared with matched controls.[152] Progression of coronary calcification was more pronounced in patients taking warfarin.[153] Supplementation of vitamin $K_2$ in patients undergoing dialysis can restore carboxylated MGP,[154] and studies to determine whether such supplementation reduces calcification and cardiovascular events are underway.[149]

### Pyrophosphate

Another naturally occurring inhibitor of mineralization is pyrophosphate, which inhibits the formation of calcium-Pi crystals in vitro. Pyrophosphate is produced by VSMCs and inhibits arterial calcification. Pyrophosphate is inhibited by tissue-nonspecific alkaline phosphatase (TNAP), and TNAP activity is increased in calcified arteries from uremic animals[155] and patients with stage 5 CKD.[107] Pyrophosphate is also inhibited by another enzyme, ectonucleotide pyrophosphate/phosphodiesterase I (NPPI). Children deficient in NPPI have infantile arterial calcification.[156] Circulating levels of pyrophosphate are decreased in patients undergoing dialysis[157] and are negatively associated with arterial calcification in patients with CKD.[158] The intraperitoneal administration of pyrophosphate reduced vascular calcification in a rodent model of CKD.[159]

#### Osteoprotegerin

Osteopenia and arterial calcification develop in mice null for OPG, implying that OPG is an important direct inhibitor of vascular calcification, but it is not clear whether this development was due to abnormalities in bone[160] or a direct arterial effect. Studies in the low-density lipoprotein receptor null mice, a model of atherogenesis, demonstrated that the administration of OPG did not prevent atherosclerotic lesions but did prevent calcification of those lesions.[161] Bone marrow and vessel wall OPG reduces atherosclerosis and calcification,[162] via regulation of the procalcific effects of RANKL on VSMCs.[163] Such procalcification effects appear related to inflammation[164] and may explain mechanisms of calcification in areas of macrophage-laden atherosclerotic plaques.

### INTEGRATED REGULATION OF PHOSPHORUS AND CALCIUM

The four hormones PTH, FGF-23, calcitriol, and Klotho work together to maintain normal Pi and calcium homeostasis to achieve appropriate balance in the blood and urine of these ions so as to avoid extraskeletal calcification and ensure adequate availability of these ions for bone that is growing (modeling) or remodeling. A summary of the integrated physiologic response to hyperphosphatemia is depicted in Fig. 53.13. This response is a very complex system of multiple integrated feedback loops and is easier to understand if broken into loops that regulate calcitriol, Pi, and calcium.

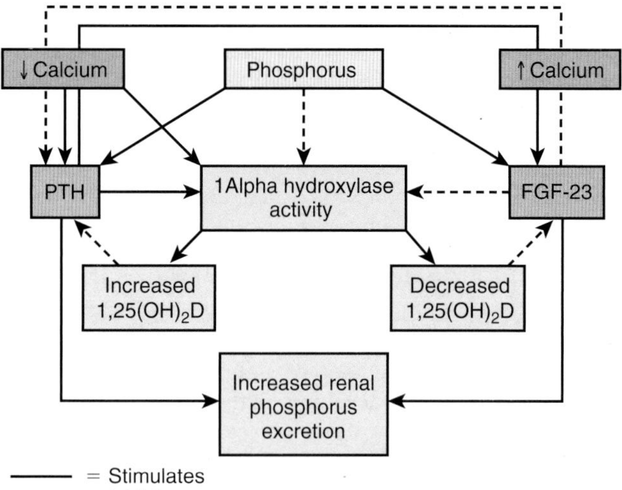


**Fig. 53.13** Regulation of serum phosphorus levels. As phosphorus levels increase (or there is a long-term phosphorus load), levels of both parathyroid hormone *(PTH)* and fibroblast growth factor 23 *(FGF-23)* are increased. Both of these elevations in turn increase urinary phosphate (Pi) excretion. The two hormones differ in respect to their effects on the vitamin D axis. PTH stimulates 1α-hydroxylase activity, thereby increasing the production of calcitriol, which in turn negatively feeds back on the parathyroid gland to decrease PTH secretion. By contrast, FGF-23 inhibits 1α-hydroxylase activity, thereby decreasing the production of calcitriol, thus feeding back to stimulate further secretion of FGF-23. FGF-23 and PTH also regulate each other. Finally, low calcium levels stimulate PTH, whereas high calcium levels stimulate FGF-23. Lastly, there is some evidence that FGF-23 also inhibits PTH secretion.

#### PTH–FGF-23–Calcitriol Loop

PTH and FGF-23 have similar effects in stimulating Pi excretion. However, these hormones differ in their effects on the vitamin D axis. PTH stimulates CYP27B1 activity, thus increasing the production of calcitriol, which in turn negatively feeds back on the parathyroid gland to decrease PTH secretion. By contrast, FGF-23 inhibits CYP27B1 and stimulates CYP24, thereby decreasing the production of calcitriol and feeding back to limit further secretion of FGF-23—as normally calcitriol stimulates FGF-23 production.

#### Pi–PTH–FGF-23 Loop

As Pi levels increase (or more likely there is a long-term Pi load), both PTH and FGF-23 are increased, the latter from bone. Both the elevated PTH and FGF-23 increase urinary Pi excretion through downregulation of NaPi transporters. The effect of FGF-23 in the kidney is klotho dependent. PTH increases renal calcium reabsorption, minimizing the possibility of high calcium and Pi concentrations in urine at a time when there is a desire to increase Pi urinary excretion. PTH stimulates the secretion of FGF-23 from osteocytes, and increased FGF-23 inhibits PTH by decreasing both *PTH* gene expression and PTH secretion.[165,166]

#### Calcium–PTH–FGF-23 Loop

Hypocalcemia, a potent stimulator of PTH, blunts FGF-23 release.[167] The latter would therefore "remove" both the FGF-23 inhibition of PTH and the FGF-23 inhibition of calcitriol synthesis during times of hypocalcemia. This process would maximize both the PTH effects to increase renal calcium reabsorption, increase bone resorption, and enhance calcitriol stimulation of intestinal calcium absorption with the goal of normalizing serum calcium concentrations. Hypercalcemia has opposing effects: it stimulates FGF-23[168] (which reduces PTH and calcitriol synthesis) and directly inhibits calcitriol synthesis and PTH secretion. The result is decreased intestinal calcium absorption, renal reabsorption of calcium, and bone resorption.

## DIAGNOSIS OF CHRONIC KIDNEY DISEASE-MINERAL AND BONE DISORDER

### MEASUREMENT OF THE BIOCHEMICAL ABNORMALITIES IN CKD-MBD

The measurement of calcium and Pi were discussed earlier in this chapter. Table 53.3 summarizes currently measured biomarkers used for the diagnosis and management of CKD-MBD.

### PARATHYROID HORMONE

PTH concentration in plasma or serum serves not only as an indicator of abnormal mineral metabolism in CKD-MBD but also as a noninvasive biochemical sign for the initial diagnosis of osteitis fibrosa cystica, the most common form of renal osteodystrophy in CKD-MBD. PTH measurement

**Table 53.3 Biomarkers for Chronic Kidney Disease–Mineral Bone Disease**

| | Affected by Sample Processing | Assay Validity | Renally Excreted | Diurnal Variation | Seasonal Variation | Variation With Meals | Variation With Dialysis Time |
|---|---|---|---|---|---|---|---|
| Parathyroid hormone | Yes | No; some assays pick up fragments | No | Yes | No | No | Yes |
| 25(OH)D (calcidiol) | No | Good (uncertain importance of differentiating $D_2$ from $D_3$) | No | No | Yes | No | No |
| 1,25$(OH)_2$D (calcitriol) | No | Good | No | Yes | No | No | ? |
| Fibroblast growth factor 23 | No | Intact versus C terminal | No | ? | ? | Yes | No |
| Soluble α-klotho | ? | Uncertain | Yes | ? | ? | ? | ? |
| Sclerostin | ? | Uncertain, likely valid | No | ? | ? | ? | ? |
| Bone-specific alkaline phosphatase | No | Good | No | No | No | ? | No |

"Assay validity" indicates that the measurement is of the biologically active hormone or marker, not fragments.
?, Indicates insufficient data.

also can be a useful index for monitoring the evolution of renal osteodystrophy and can serve as a surrogate measure of bone turnover in patients with CKD. Although the sensitivity and specificity of PTH as a marker of bone remodeling are not ideal, it is the best marker available at the current time.[169] However, the definitive method for establishing the specific type of renal osteodystrophy in individual patients requires bone biopsy, an invasive diagnostic procedure, and access to specialized laboratory personnel and equipment capable of providing assessments of bone histology.

PTH circulates not only in the form of the intact 84–amino acid peptide but also as multiple fragments of the hormone, particularly from the middle and C-terminal regions of the PTH molecule. These PTH fragments arise from direct secretion from the parathyroid gland as well as from metabolism of PTH(1–84) by peripheral organs, especially liver and kidney. The biologically active hormone produced (PTH[1–84]) exerts its effects through the interaction of its first 34 amino acids with PTHR1. PTH(1–84) has a plasma half-life of 2 to 4 minutes. In comparison, the half-life of C-terminal fragments, which are cleared principally by the kidney, is five to ten times longer with normal kidney function and even longer in the presence of CKD. There is also a diurnal variation in the secretion of PTH and the release is oscillatory, further complicating measurement.

Assays for PTH have undergone a number of improvements over the years (Fig. 53.14). In the early 1960s, radioimmunoassays were developed for measurement of PTH. However, these assays proved to be unreliable owing to different characteristics of the antisera used and are referred to as "first-generation" assays; consequently, two-site immunometric assays (IMAs) are referred to as "second- and third-generation" assays. The typical second-generation IMAs (known as intact PTH assays) measure PTH(1–84) and other large C-terminal PTH fragments because the antibodies do not bind to amino acid 1. These assays are most commonly used in clinical practice. By contrast, third-generation assays (bioactive, whole, or bio-intact PTH assays) use capture antibody similar to that of the intact PTH assays but also use detection antibodies directed against epitopes at the extreme N-terminal end (epitopes 1–4) of the molecule, and therefore are believed to detect exclusively the biologically active PTH(1–84) (Fig. 53.14). This difference may be important because C-terminal fragments (lacking small or large portions of the N terminus) are most abundant, representing approximately 80% of circulating PTH in healthy persons and 95% in patients with CKD.[170] This finding may in part explain why elevated PTH concentrations are "normal" in CKD, yet are increased relative to values observed in patients without CKD. The second-generation intact assays are commonly used on automated platforms. Although each assay has a reasonable coefficient of variation, the standards for the commercially available assays are not uniform and the detection antibodies do not all bind at the same sites. Thus the kit-to-kit variability can be high.[171] This is the reason the Kidney Disease Improving Global Outcomes (KDIGO) guidelines recommended using the same assay every time and evaluating trends rather than targeting precise PTH values.[172]

## VITAMIN D

Serum calcidiol concentrations are generally measured by immunoassay, although the gold standard for calcidiol measurement is high-performance liquid chromatography, which is not widely available clinically. Unlike in PTH assays, sample handling in calcidiol IMAs has little impact on results. However, vitamin D circulates as both $D_2$ and $D_3$, and some laboratory kits measure only $D_2$, others measure only $D_3$, and still others measure both (expressed as 25-hydroxyvitamin D). The rationale for distinguishing $D_2$ from $D_3$ is controversial, because it is unclear how differentiating the forms of vitamin D affects management or patient level outcomes. As with PTH, there is some assay-to-assay variability, which could affect the classification of insufficiency/deficiency or sufficient levels of calcidiol.[173] Fortunately, current initiatives are underway to standardize these assays.[174] The half-life of calcidiol is long and thus represents total body stores.

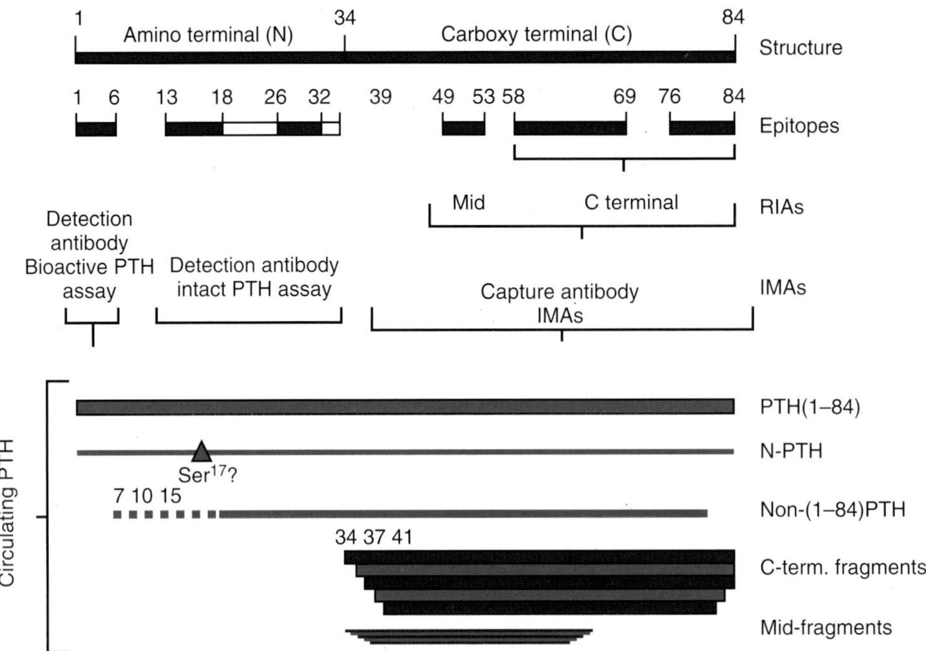


**Fig. 53.14** Parathyroid hormone *(PTH)* assays. Schematic presentation of PTH(1–84) and the relationship between PTH assays, PTH assay epitopes, and PTH molecular forms detected in the circulation. The *upper panel* depicts the structure of human PTH and the epitopes detected by various PTH assays. First-generation PTH assays detect full-length PTH (1–84) in addition to PTH fragments. These assays include radioimmunoassays *(RIAs)* that use antisera specific to the amino-terminal (N-RIA), middle (MID-RIA), or carboxyl-terminal (C-RIA) regions of PTH. Second-generation "intact PTH" assays detect full-length PTH (1–84) and non(1–84)–PTH fragments. Third-generation PTH assays (bio-intact PTH) detect only full-length PTH (1–84). The *bottom panel* depicts PTH molecular forms present in the circulation. *IMA,* Immunometric assay; *N-PTH,* amino-terminal PTH; *term.,* terminal. (From Henrich LM, Rogol AD, D'Amour P, Levine MA, Hanks JB, Bruns DE. Persistent hypercalcemia after parathyroidectomy in an adolescent and effect of treatment with cinacalcet HCl. *Clin Chem.* 2006;52:2286–2293.)

By contrast, calcitriol levels are generally measured only in the setting of hypercalcemia. The half-life is comparatively short, and the assay more expensive and difficult. Interpretation also requires consideration of clinical context. In other words, a patient with stage 4 or 5 CKD and hypercalcemia may have high normal serum calcitriol, which may be distinctly abnormal given the CKD stage and serum calcium concentration, and should prompt consideration of an extrarenal source of calcitriol.

## FGF-23

FGF-23 is currently measured primarily with two different assays (Fig. 53.15). The first uses two antibodies directed against the C-terminal end and thus measures the intact as well as C-terminal fragments (results are reported in relative unit/mL). The second assay uses one antibody directed against an epitope within the N-terminal region and a second antibody directed against an epitope within the C-terminal region of the molecule, and thus detects intact molecules (results are reported in picograms per milliliter). Although these two assays appear comparable in the association with clinical events at this time, they have poor agreement because of differences in FGF-23 fragment detection, antibody specificity, and calibration. Such analytical variability does not permit direct comparison of FGF-23 measurements made with different assays, a fact that probably, at least in part, accounts for some of the inconsistencies noted among observational studies.[175] FGF-23 can be detected in the urine, although at this time it is unclear how much, if any of the hormone is cleared by the kidneys.[176,177] From a clinical perspective, more data are required prior to the use of FGF-23 measurements for routine clinical management.

## SOLUBLE KLOTHO

It is unclear whether the circulating or soluble α-klotho levels reflect tissue level expression of klotho. Some studies have found that low circulating levels were associated with progression of CKD,[178] but other studies have failed to confirm this finding.[179] Klotho can be detected in urine,[180] suggesting its levels may be altered by residual renal function. Different assay kits give variable results.[72,181]

## SCLEROSTIN

Circulating sclerostin concentrations are elevated in CKD[182] and rise with progressive disease. However, sclerostin does not appear to be renally excreted,[183] suggesting that the rising levels reflect underlying biology. The role of sclerostin in clinical diagnosis of CKD remains exploratory, although elevated sclerostin values are associated with arterial calcification[184] and increased osteoblast number in human bone biopsy specimens.[185]

## BONE-SPECIFIC ALKALINE PHOSPHATASE

Bone-specific alkaline phosphatase (BALP) is not cleared renally. BALP concentration has relatively good correlation with bone formation in CKD and may be additive to the interpretation of PTH measurements.[172] However, its concentration has limited ability as an independent measurement.[169,186]

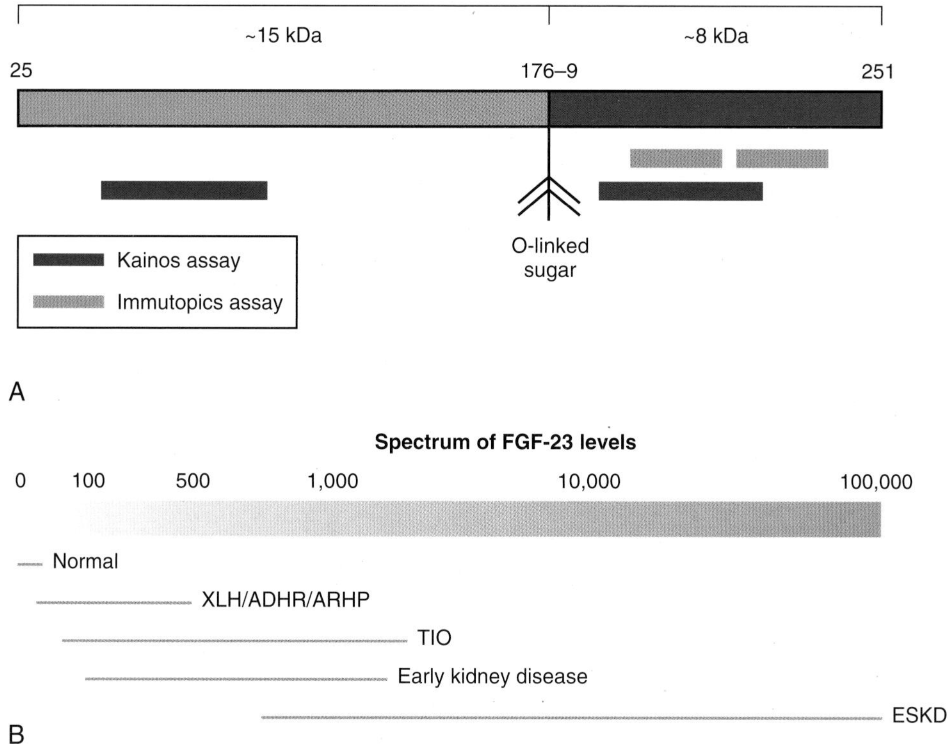


**Fig. 53.15** Fibroblast growth factor 23 *(FGF-23)* assays. (A) FGF-23 O-glycosylation site and epitopes recognized by antibodies used in current assays. (B) Spectrum of serum FGF-23 levels in early chronic kidney disease and end-stage kidney disease *(ESKD)* compared with the normal reference range and levels associated with different disorders affecting FGF-23. *ADHR,* Autosomal dominant hypophosphatemic rickets; *ARHP,* autosomal recessive hypophosphatemia; *TIO,* tumor-induced osteomalacia; *XLH,* X-linked hypophosphatemia. (From Block GA, Ix JH, Ketteler M, et al. Phosphate homeostasis in CKD: report of a scientific symposium sponsored by the National Kidney Foundation. *Am J Kidney Dis.* 2013;62:457–473. With permission.)

### COLLAGEN-BASED BONE BIOMARKERS

Osteoblasts secrete C- and N-terminal cleavage products of type I procollagen called secreted procollagen type IN propeptide (s-PINP) and secreted procollagen type IC propeptide (s-PICP), which are markers for bone formation. By contrast, serum C-terminal cross-linking telopeptide of type 1 collagen (s-CTX) and serum N-terminal cross-linking telopeptide of type I collagen (s-NTX) are measured as fragments of cross-links that are released when bone is resorbed. With the exception of the s-PICP, all of these markers are renally excreted, making interpretation of their measurements difficult.[187] In cross-sectional analyses, higher serum concentrations are associated with higher odds of fracture.[188]

### TARTRATE-RESISTANT ACID PHOSPHATASE 5B

Tartrate-resistant acid phosphatase 5b is released by osteoclasts during bone resorption and thus may be a good marker of bone resorption.[189] However, studies relating this biomarker to bone in patients with CKD-MBD are limited.[187]

## BONE BIOPSY ASSESSMENT OF BONE IN CHRONIC KIDNEY DISEASE-MINERAL AND BONE DISORDER

Abnormalities of bone quality and quantity are common in CKD-MBD (Fig. 53.16), leading to fractures and impaired growth in children. "Renal osteodystrophy" is defined as an alteration of bone morphology in patients with CKD that is quantifiable by bone histomorphometry.[1]

### HISTOMORPHOMETRY IN PATIENTS WITH CKD

The clinical assessment of bone remodeling is best performed with a bone biopsy of the trabecular bone, usually at the iliac crest. The patient is given a tetracycline derivative approximately 3 to 4 weeks prior to the bone biopsy and a different tetracycline derivative 3 to 5 days prior. Tetracycline binds to hydroxyapatite and emits fluorescence, thereby serving as a label for the bone. A core of predominantly trabecular bone is collected and embedded in a plastic material, and then sectioned. The sections can be visualized with special stains under fluorescent microscopy to determine the amount of bone between administrations of the two tetracycline labels, or that formed in the interval. This dynamic parameter assessed with bone biopsy is the basis for evaluating bone turnover, which is key in discerning types of renal osteodystrophy. In addition to dynamic indices, bone biopsies can be analyzed by quantitative histomorphometry for static parameters as well. The nomenclature for these assessments has been standardized.[190]

Clinically, bone biopsies are most useful for differentiating bone turnover as well as bone volume and mineralization. However, with the advent of several new markers of bone turnover, the use of bone biopsy has been reserved primarily for the diagnosis of renal osteodystrophy and for research purposes. Sherrard and colleagues proposed a classification

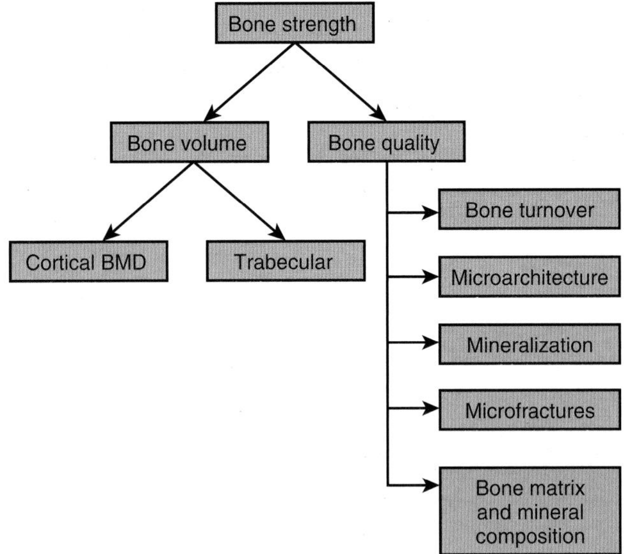


**Fig. 53.16** Determinants of bone strength. Bone strength comprises both bone density and bone quality. "Bone quality" refers to bone turnover, microarchitecture, microfractures, and mineralization as well as the composition of the mineral matrix. "Trabecular microarchitecture" involves trabecular thickness, the ratio of plates and rods, and their connectivity and spacing. "Cortical microarchitecture" consists of cortical thickness, porosity, and bone size. Composition of the mineral matrix includes changes in the cross-linking of type I collagen and alterations in the size and structure of bone mineral. Bones accumulate microfractures over time even with normal physical activity. The ability to repair them affects bone quality. *BMD,* Bone mineral density. (From Moorthi R, Moe S. Recent advances in the noninvasive diagnosis of renal osteodystrophy. *Kidney Int.* 2013;84:866–894. With permission.)

system for renal osteodystrophy that utilized the parameters of osteoid (unmineralized bone) area as a percentage of total bone area and fibrosis.[191] These two static parameters, together with the dynamic bone turnover assessed by bone formation rate or activation frequency, have been used to distinguish the various forms of renal osteodystrophy over the past 30 years[191]; however, this evaluation has been replaced by the KDIGO TMV (turnover, mineralization, volume) system (discussed later).[1]

Fig. 53.17 illustrates bone histology utilizing the original classification scheme. Normal bone is illustrated in Fig. 53.17A. The histologic features of high-turnover disease (predominant hyperparathyroidism or osteitis fibrosa cystica) are characterized by increased rate of bone formation, increased bone resorption, extensive osteoclastic and osteoblastic activity, and progressive increase in endosteal peritrabecular fibrosis (Fig. 53.17B). High osteoblast activity is manifested by an increase in unmineralized bone matrix. The number of osteoclasts is also increased as well as the total resorption surface. There may be numerous dissecting cavities through which the osteoclasts tunnel into individual trabeculae. In osteitis fibrosa cystica, the alignment of strands of collagen in the bone matrix has an irregular woven pattern, unlike the normal lamellar (parallel) alignment of strands of collagen in normal bone. Although woven bone may appear to be thicker, the disorganized collagen structure may render the bone physically more vulnerable to stress.

Low-turnover (adynamic) bone disease (Fig. 53.17C) is characterized histologically by absence of cellular (osteoblast and osteoclast) activity, osteoid formation, and endosteal fibrosis. It appears to be essentially a disorder of decreased bone formation accompanied by a secondary decrease in bone mineralization. Although low-turnover disease is common in the absence of aluminum, it was initially described as a result of aluminum toxicity. Aluminum bone disease is diagnosed with special staining that demonstrates the presence of aluminum deposits at the mineralization front (Fig. 53.17D). Frequently, aluminum disease is associated with osteomalacia. Osteomalacia is characterized by an excess of unmineralized osteoid, which manifests as wide osteoid seams and a markedly decreased mineralization rate (Fig. 53.17E). The presence of increased unmineralized osteoid per se does not necessarily indicate a mineralizing defect, because larger quantities of osteoid appear in conditions associated with high rates of bone formation when mineralization lags behind the increased synthesis of matrix. Other features of osteomalacia are the absence of cellular activity and the absence of endosteal fibrosis.

> ***Clinical Relevance***
> Patients with adynamic or low-turnover bone disease are at risk for fractures and vascular calcification. Common therapies for osteoporosis such as bisphosphonates and denosumab inhibit bone turnover and can result in adynamic bone disease in chronic kidney disease (CKD) and end-stage kidney disease patients. Therefore these drugs are not recommended for CKD patients unless workup reveals a high-turnover state.

"Mixed uremic osteodystrophy" is the term that has been used to describe bone biopsies that have features of secondary hyperparathyroidism together with evidence of a mineralization defect (Fig. 53.17F). There is extensive osteoclastic and osteoblastic activity and increased endosteal peritrabecular fibrosis coupled with more osteoid than expected, and tetracycline labeling uncovers a concomitant mineralization defect. Unfortunately, mixed uremic osteodystrophy, in particular, and high- and low-turnover bone diseases have been inconsistent and poorly defined.

## THE SPECTRUM OF BONE HISTOMORPHOMETRY IN CKD

The prevalence of different forms of renal osteodystrophy has changed over the past decade. Whereas osteitis fibrosa cystica due to severe hyperparathyroidism had previously been the predominant lesion, the prevalence of mixed uremic osteodystrophy and adynamic bone disease has increased. However, the overall percentage of patients with high bone formation compared with low bone formation has not changed dramatically over the last 20 to 30 years, although osteomalacia has been essentially "replaced" by adynamic bone disease. There are differences in prevalence of mixed uremic osteodystrophy in patients not yet undergoing dialysis, which appears to depend on the level of GFR and the country in which the study was performed.[192] Two large analyses of

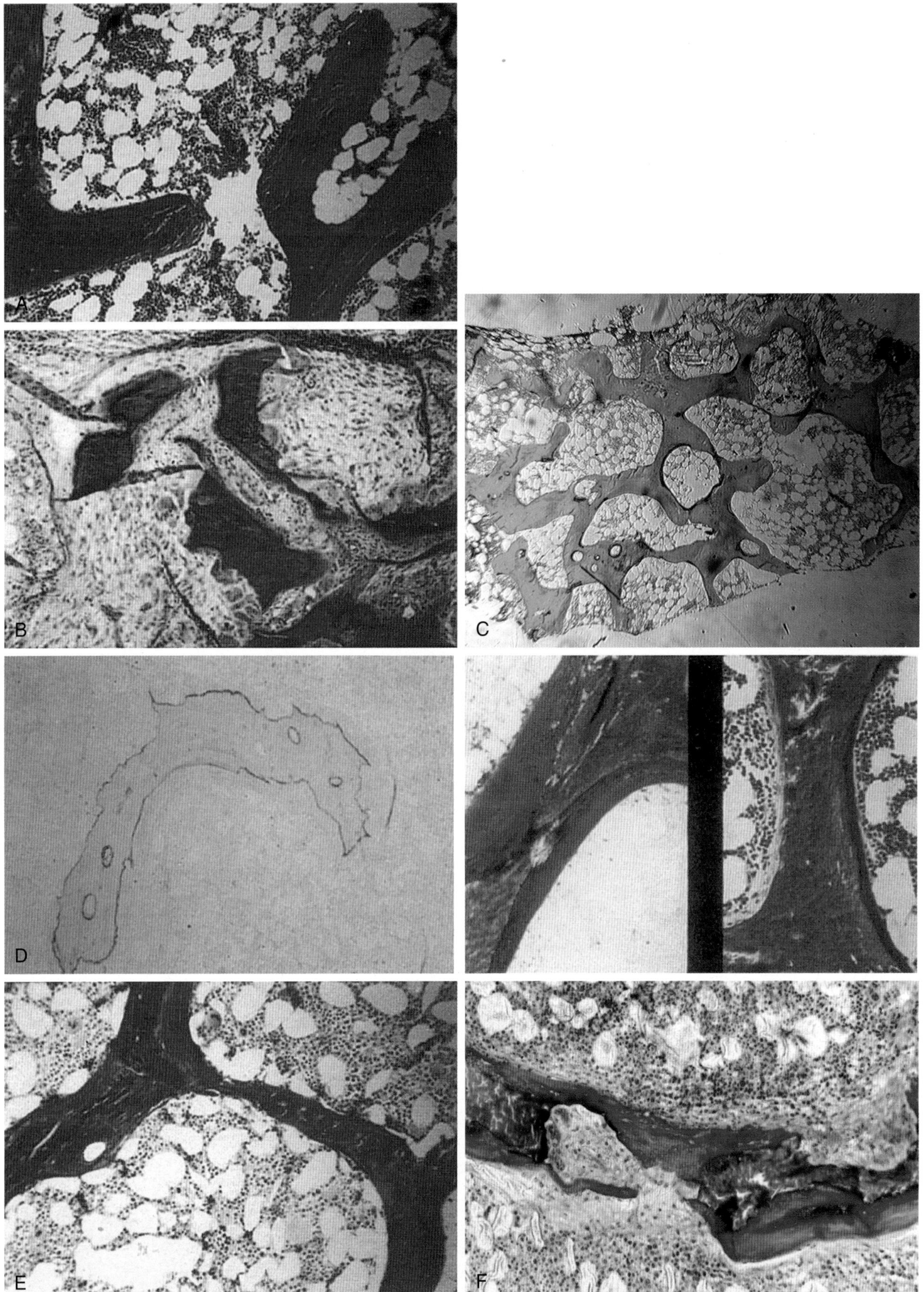


**Fig. 53.17** Bone histology. (A) Normal bone. (B) Hyperparathyroid bone (increased osteoclast and osteoblasts and fibrosis). (C) Adynamic bone (no cellular activity and no osteoid). (D) Aluminum bone disease (left aluminum staining at mineralization front) and right two panels show accumulation of osteoid *(orange-red stain).* (E) Osteomalacia (increased unmineralized osteoid in *pink/red*). (F) Mixed uremic osteodystrophy presence of increased osteoid *(orange red)* indicating mineralization defect, and increased osteoclast activity. (A, B, D *(right)*, and E, courtesy S.L. Teitelbaum, MD; D *(left)*, courtesy D. J. Sherrard, MD.)

patients undergoing long-term dialysis revealed a relatively high incidence of low bone turnover; one study of 489 biopsy specimens in predominantly Caucasian patients revealed low turnover in 59%,[169] whereas in another study of 630 patients, low-turnover disease was noted in 62% of Caucasian but only in 32% of African-American patients.[193] The prevalence of mineralization defect or osteomalacia was relatively low at only 3%.[193] Thus these data demonstrate that histologic abnormalities of bone begin very early in the course of CKD and that differences in bone turnover may be based on racial differences.

By contrast, low-turnover bone disease has diverse pathophysiology. In the 1980s, aluminum-induced osteomalacia was common. The potential toxicity of aluminum was initially recognized by Alfrey, who identified a fatal neurologic syndrome in patients receiving dialysis consisting of dyspraxia, seizures, and electroencephalographic abnormalities in association with high brain aluminum levels on autopsy.[194] The source of aluminum in these severe cases was believed to be elevated concentrations in dialysate water. Subsequently, aluminum-containing phosphate binders were also identified as a source. The additional symptoms of fractures, myopathy, and microcytic anemia were described several years after the initial reports of the neurologic syndrome.[194,195] Fortunately, exposure to aluminum is limited in the modern era, and the incidence of aluminum bone disease is relatively rare. However, the diagnosis of aluminum-induced bone disease can be difficult, because aluminum toxicity is due to tissue burden, not serum concentrations. Thus if aluminum bone disease is suspected, bone biopsy remains the gold standard for making the diagnosis.[195,196]

In adynamic bone disease, there is a paucity of cells with resultant low bone turnover (Fig. 53.17C). Unlike in osteomalacia, in adynamic bone there is no increase in osteoid or unmineralized bone. The lack of bone cell activity led to the initial description of the disease as "aplastic" bone disease. Early investigators believed that the disease was due to aluminum, but it was later identified in the absence of aluminum. The etiology of adynamic bone disease is likely multifactorial, and major contributory factors include diabetes mellitus, aging, and malnutrition.[197]

Proposed pathophysiologic mechanisms of low bone turnover are listed in Table 53.4. Increases in both sclerostin and dkk-1, which are soluble inhibitors of wnt signaling that inhibit osteoblastic bone formation, likely play a role in development of adynamic bone disease.[97,198,199] Circulating fragments of PTH (7–84–amino acid fragments) may also be antagonists to PTH,[200] resulting in an effective resistance to 1–84 amino acid at the level of bone. There is evidence that markedly elevated concentrations of FGF-23 may be associated with decreased osteoblastic activity.[201] Furthermore, abnormal regulation of cell differentiation in the presence of renal failure may explain, in part, the relative paucity of cells in adynamic bone, although this possibility remains to be proven. In rats, the administration of bone morphogenetic protein-7 can restore normal cell function, supporting that a failure of normal cell differentiation, likely due to a number of causes, may be critical.[202] Although most patients with low-turnover bone disease are asymptomatic, they are at increased risk of fracture owing to impaired remodeling[201,203,204] and at risk of vascular calcification because of the inability of bone to buffer a sudden calcium load.[201,205,206]

**Table 53.4 Causes and Proposed Mechanisms of Decreased Bone Formation in Patients With Chronic Kidney Disease**

| | Mechanism of Decreased Osteoblast Activity |
|---|---|
| Low serum calcitriol | ↓ Osteoblast differentiation<br>↓ Osteoblast life span |
| Metabolic acidosis | ↓ Calcitriol production<br>↓ Collagen synthesis |
| High serum phosphate | ↓ Calcitriol production |
| Calcium loading/ hypercalcemia | ↓ Calcitriol production and ↑calcitriol degradation (mediated by calcium-sensing receptor) |
| High serum interleukins 1 and 6, tumor necrosis factor | ↓ Osteoblast life span |
| Low serum insulinlike growth factor-I (IGF-I) activity | ↓ IGF-I and IGF binding protein 5 (IGFBP5) levels<br>↑ Inhibitory IGFBP (2, 4, 6) levels<br>↓ Osteoblast life span |
| Sclerostin | ↓ Wnt/β-catenin signaling<br>↓ Osteoblastic activity |
| Dickkopf-1 (dkk-1) | ↓ Wnt/β-catenin signaling<br>↓ Osteoblastic activity |
| Malnutrition, proteinuria | ↓ IGF-I; 25-hydroxyvitamin D levels |
| Diabetes | ↓ 25-Hydroxyvitamin D and calcitriol levels<br>↑ Advanced glycation end products (AGEs)<br>↓ Osteoblast life span |
| Age-related | ↑ AGEs<br>↓ Osteoblast life span |
| **Hypogonadal** | |
| Women (↓ estrogen and ↑ sex hormone–binding globulin [SHBG]) | ↓ Osteoblast life span |
| Men (↓ testosterone and ↑SHBG) | ↓ Osteoblast life span |
| Uremic toxins (uric acid) | ↓ Calcitriol production<br>↓ Vitamin D receptor activity<br>↓ Osteoblast proliferation |
| Aluminum toxicity | ↓ Osteoblast activity |

↓, Decreased; ↑, increased.

## TMV CLASSIFICATION

As previously noted, KDIGO recommends that the definition of renal osteodystrophy be limited to describing the alterations of bone morphology in patients with CKD and is one measure of the skeletal component of the systemic disorder of CKD-MBD that can be quantifiable by histomorphometry.[1] Historically, "renal osteodystrophy" often included disorders of bone mineral metabolism in addition to histomorphometric changes in bone. As our understanding of bone biology progresses, there is greater appreciation of the diverse physiologic processes leading to similar bone biopsy findings. In addition, information on bone volume as an independent

**Table 53.5 Turnover, Mineralization, Volume Classification System for Renal Osteodystrophy**

| Turnover | Mineralization | Volume |
|---|---|---|
| Low | | Low |
| | Normal | |
| Normal | | Normal |
| | Abnormal | |
| High | | High |

From Moe S, Drüeke T, Cunningham J, et al. Definition, evaluation, and classification of renal osteodystrophy: a position statement from Kidney Disease: Improving Global Outcomes (KDIGO). *Kidney Int.* 2006;69:1945–1953.

parameter is available.[207] Thus the previous classification was updated by KDIGO to use three key histologic descriptors – bone turnover, mineralization, and volume (TMV system), with any combination of each of the descriptors possible in a given specimen (Table 53.5).[1] The TMV classification scheme provides a clinically relevant description of the underlying bone pathology as assessed by histomorphometry, which in turn helps define the pathophysiology and thereby guide therapy.

Turnover reflects the rate of skeletal remodeling, which is normally the coupled process of bone resorption and bone formation. Turnover is assessed with histomorphometry by dynamic measurements of osteoblast function using double-tetracycline labeling, as previously described. Bone formation rate and activation frequency represent acceptable parameters for assessing bone turnover. Bone turnover is affected mainly by hormones, cytokines, mechanical stimuli, and growth factors that influence the recruitment, differentiation, and activity of osteoclasts and osteoblasts. It is important to clarify that although bone formation rate is frequently similar to bone resorption rate, which cannot be measured directly, it is not always so. Imbalance in these processes can affect bone volume. For example, if resorption exceeds formation, negative bone balance and decreased bone volume result.

Mineralization reflects how well bone collagen becomes calcified during the formation phase of skeletal remodeling. It is assessed with histomorphometry by static measurements of osteoid volume and osteoid thickness and by dynamic, tetracycline-based measurements of mineralization lag time and osteoid maturation time. Causes of impaired mineralization include inadequate vitamin D nutrition, mineral (calcium or Pi) deficiency, acidosis, and aluminum toxicity.

Volume indicates the amount of bone per unit volume of tissue. It is assessed with histomorphometry by static measurements of bone volume in cancellous bone. Determinants of bone volume include age, sex, race, genetic factors, nutrition, endocrine disorders, mechanical stimuli, toxicities, neurologic function, vascular supply, growth factors, and cytokines.

The KDIGO classification is consistent with the historically used classification system[191] but provides more information on parameters other than turnover. Two large-scale analyses utilizing the updated TMV system suggested that the newer TMV classification system provides clinically relevant information.[169,193] Low bone volume and low bone turnover are more common than heretofore appreciated, whereas defective mineralization is relatively rare in adult patients with ESKD.

Clinically, serum PTH concentration is used as a surrogate biomarker to predict bone turnover. However, as detailed earlier, studies evaluating the ability of the serum concentration of (intact) PTH to predict low- and/or high-turnover bone diseases have been disappointing. The ability to reliably predict the presence of high-turnover bone disease is poor until serum PTH concentrations exceed 500 pg/mL.[169,193] Primarily on the basis of earlier studies utilizing the Allegro intact PTH assay, the Kidney Disease Outcomes Quality Initiative (KDOQI) guidelines recommend a target-intact PTH level of 150 to 300 pg/mL.[195] Unfortunately, studies that correlate intact PTH with bone histology were performed with an assay no longer available. Use of currently available assays have shown that the intact PTH value between 150 and 300 pg/mL is not predictive of underlying bone histology.[208] However, an analysis of 610 biopsy specimens found that although the intact PTH value could not predict underlying bone histology, it was able to discriminate low-turnover from non–low-turnover bone diseases and high-turnover from non–high-turnover bone diseases.[169]

## NONINVASIVE ASSESSMENT OF BONE

### DUAL-ENERGY X-RAY ABSORPTIOMETRY

Dual-energy X-ray absorptiometry (DXA) measures areal bone mineral density (aBMD or simply BMD) in g/cm$^2$ using minimal radiation and rapid scan times. BMD assessment by DXA has good reproducibility (<1%–2% coefficient variation) and reliable reference ranges for age, sex, and race. In the general population, BMD measured by DXA can be used clinically to define osteoporosis and is an accepted surrogate endpoint after prospective studies demonstrated an age-dependent predictive value of DXA for fractures.[209] However, the discordance between changes in DXA findings and the efficacy of drugs at preventing fracture has led to appreciation of the importance of bone "quality," which is not assessed by DXA. This observation has forced the use of fractures as endpoints for approval of new therapeutics for the treatment of osteoporosis.

The KDIGO CKD-MBD guideline recommends DXA to assess fracture risk in patients with stage 1 through early stage 3 CKD, as long as biochemical testing does not suggest CKD-MBD.[172] However, for patients with CKD stages 3b through 5, the guideline did not recommend DXA owing to the lack of definitive data demonstrating that DXA predicts fracture in CKD-MBD. A meta-analysis was performed to determine whether DXA measurements at the femoral neck, spine, and radius were associated with spine and/or nonspine fractures in patients undergoing dialysis.[210] On the basis of results of six studies with 683 patients, lower BMD in the spine and distal radius, but not in the femoral neck, was associated with fractures. Although BMD may have been lower in patients with CKD and a history of fracture, there is considerable overlap in BMD such that BMD provides poor fracture discrimination in individuals. In addition, for lumbar spine assessment of BMD by DXA, existing aortic calcification may confound the measurement. Since the publication of KDIGO guidelines, studies have demonstrated fracture prediction value of DXA in CKD subjects at least equivalent to that in the general population.[211,212] These data therefore support that DXA can predict fracture risk in patients with CKD. However, DXA cannot make a specific diagnosis as to why there is low BMD. Unlike patients with normal kidney function and low BMD by DXA being classified as having osteoporosis, patients with CKD and low bone density should not be routinely treated with antiosteoporosis therapies.[213] DXA is an inexpensive and widely available technique that can be easily standardized among sites, so it may be a good tool in longitudinal CKD research studies for the serial assessment of BMD in response to interventions. Unfortunately, to date, treatment studies utilizing DXA as an endpoint in patients with CKD are limited.

### QUANTITATIVE COMPUTERIZED TOMOGRAPHY TECHNIQUES

Quantitative CT (QCT) allows three-dimensional imaging of cross sections of the central and axial skeleton to provide spatial or volumetric BMD (vBMD). It also allows distinction between cortical and trabecular compartments. In CKD, QCT measures of trabecular bone density at the spine have been correlated with trabecular bone volume histomorphometry.[214] Peripheral QCT (pQCT) avoids the large dose of ionizing radiation exposure for patients by focusing on the tibia and distal radius, and in one study, was associated with fracture.[215] Although derived from a single study, these results are in line with expected associations between loss of bone quality and fracture risk in patients undergoing dialysis.

High-resolution peripheral computerized tomography (HRpQCT) has greater resolution than pQCT and allows evaluation of trabecular microarchitecture (bone volume fraction, trabecular thickness, separation, and number). HRpQCT of the radius and tibia was found to discriminate among patients with CKD with and without fracture.[216,217] However, the discriminatory power of the various HRpQCT parameters to individually discriminate between those with and without fractures by receiver operating curve analyses was less than 0.75. When patients with the longest duration of CKD were considered, the area under the receiver operating curve improved to more than 0.8 for multiple parameters, including radial cortical thickness, radial total vBMD, and cortical vBMD. Interestingly, aBMD by DXA of the ultra-distal radius performed similarly in its ability to discriminate prevalent fractures in this subpopulation with the longest duration of kidney disease.[218] In another study, areal BMD by DXA at the ultra-distal radius was superior to HRpQCT measures for fracture discrimination.[219] Therefore high-resolution CT techniques do provide assessment of bone architecture, but their use at this time is limited to research centers and their additive value over distal radius DXA has not yet been proven.

### MICROCOMPUTED TOMOGRAPHY AND MICROMAGNETIC RESONANCE IMAGING

Resolution of microtechniques is as low as 8 mm, compared with about 100 μm for HRpQCT, thus providing spatial resolution almost that of an actual bone biopsy. Micro-CT was used to assess the effects of severe high-turnover renal osteodystrophy on trabecular and cortical architecture in growing rats. The technique demonstrated irregular trabecular thickening and loss of trabecular connectivity in the femoral neck and greater endocortical porosity in the femoral shaft, consistent with biopsy findings in high-turnover osteodystrophy.[220] Unfortunately, this technique is currently limited to in vitro studies. In an evaluation of 17 patients undergoing hemodialysis who had secondary hyperparathyroidism, micromagnetic resonance imaging (micro-MRI) demonstrated disruptions of the distal tibial trabecular network.[221] There have not been subsequent confirmatory studies or studies comparing this technique with other imaging methods in the ability to predict fractures in CKD.

## ASSESSMENT OF VASCULAR CALCIFICATION

Arterial calcification can be detected in humans through a number of techniques. Plain radiographs can be used to assess the presence or absence, and thus prevalence, of vascular calcification. Scoring methods utilizing the number of aorta segments calcified along the lumbar spine can also allow reproducible quantification during longitudinal follow-up,[222] although the sensitivity is less than with CT-based imaging. Although some distinction can be made between medial and intimal calcification on plain radiographs,[223] the reproducibility among multiple research sites of this method for differentiation of calcification type has not been evaluated. Ultrasonography of the carotid arteries can be used to assess intimal–medial thickness, which correlates well with atherosclerosis and cardiovascular events. In a later study, intravascular ultrasonography of the coronary arteries was able to detect atherosclerotic lesions and calcification. This technique, although invasive, can detect circumferential lesions, and external remodeling of atherosclerosis—lesions that invade the internal elastic artery into the medial layer rather than protrude into the vessel lumen. The latter luminal lesion is all that is detected on angiography, leading some to question the use of angiography as the "gold standard."[224] Finally, technologic advances have led to ultra-fast CT scans—electron beam CT (EBCT) and multislice CT—that use electrocardiography gating to allow imaging only in diastole, thus avoiding motion artifact of the heart. These techniques have allowed reproducible quantification of coronary artery and aorta calcification and therefore serve as excellent intermediate endpoints for CKD-MBD interventions that might alter progression of vascular calcification. Unfortunately, these techniques do not allow differentiation of medial from intimal calcification, and the radiation dose with their use is large.

A study in each of 140 prevalent patients undergoing hemodialysis compared a lateral radiograph of the lumbar abdominal aorta, an echocardiogram, and measurement of pulse pressure with EBCT results.[225] Calcification of the abdominal aorta was scored as 0 through 24 divided into tertiles; echocardiograms were graded as 0 through 2 for absence or presence of calcification of the mitral and aortic valves; and pulse pressure was divided in quartiles. The researchers found that the likelihood ratio (95% confidence interval [CI]) of coronary artery calcification score on EBCT of 100 or higher was 1.79 (1.09–2.96) for calcification of either valve on echocardiography and 7.50 (2.89–19.5) for participants with a lateral abdominal radiographic score greater or equal to 7. Verbeke and colleagues confirmed this predictive value of lateral abdominal radiographs in more than 1000 patients receiving dialysis.[226]

On the basis of observational studies, calcification detected on all of these imaging studies is associated with mortality in patients with CKD. Bellasi and Raggi analyzed multiple such studies and calculated the positive predictive value to be between 19% and 52% and the negative predictive value to be between 68% and 100%.[227] The addition of the clinical variables age and dialysis vintage to abdominal calcification, termed the "cardiovascular calcification index," was linearly associated with death, with a 12% increase in hazard ratio for each point increase in the cardiovascular calcification index.[228]

## CLINICAL CONSEQUENCES OF THE ABNORMALITIES IN CHRONIC KIDNEY DISEASE-MINERAL AND BONE DISORDER

### BIOCHEMICAL ABNORMALITIES

#### PHOSPHORUS AND CALCIUM

Epidemiologic data suggest that serum Pi levels above the normal range are associated with increases in morbidity and all-cause and cardiovascular mortality in patients with CKD. These studies differ in their sample size, analyses, and chosen reference ranges, and most evaluate only patients undergoing dialysis. In patients with CKD stages 2 to 5, higher levels of serum Pi, even within the normal range, have been associated with increased risk of all-cause or cardiovascular mortality in one study[229] but not in other studies.[230,231] However, in patients undergoing dialysis, nearly all studies demonstrate an association of elevated Pi with mortality, although there are slight differences in the inflection point or range at which Pi becomes significantly associated with increased all-cause mortality. Furthermore, several retrospective studies have demonstrated that treatment of patients undergoing dialysis with Pi binders is associated with a 20% to 40% lower risk of death.[232–234] However, there are no prospective studies that have demonstrated a survival benefit of lowering serum phosphate concentrations, and there is no specific target serum phosphate that has been identified as conferring a clinically relevant benefit. In patients with CKD stages 3 to 5, there are no data to support an increased risk of mortality or fracture with elevated serum calcium concentrations. However, as with Pi, there are several studies in patients receiving dialysis demonstrating higher mortality with higher serum calcium concentration and in some studies, among patients with very low serum calcium concentrations, as the latter may reflect more severe vitamin D deficiency and secondary hyperparathyroidism.

#### PARATHYROID HORMONE

Although PTH has long been considered a surrogate marker for bone disease, it also has systemic effects, including effects on endothelial, cardiac, and skeletal health. As with other biochemical measures of CKD-MBD, observational studies have found an association of all-cause mortality with various levels of PTH, with inflection points ranging from more than 400 to 600 pg/mL. On the basis of these observational data and the assay limitations, the KDIGO guidelines consider serum concentrations of intact PTH within two and nine times the upper limit of normal for the PTH assay (<130 and >585 pg/mL for most kits with an upper normal limit of 65 pg/mL) as a reasonable target range, and that values within that range should be interpreted by evaluation of trends. Intervention should occur if the trends are consistently going up or down.[172] However, it is important to recognize that there are no randomized clinical trials demonstrating that treatment to achieve specific PTH concentrations results in improved outcomes, with the exception of the Evaluation Of Cinacalcet Hydrochloride (HCl) Therapy to Lower CardioVascular Events (EVOLVE) trial discussed in Chapter 63.

A Cochrane meta-analysis found that serum Pi and calcium concentrations, but not PTH, were associated with cardiovascular and all-cause mortality.[235]

#### COMBINATION OF ABNORMALITIES OF CALCIUM, PHOSPHORUS, AND PARATHYROID HORMONE

The relationship of calcium, Pi, and PTH with outcomes is further complicated by the clinical reality that these laboratory parameters do not respond in isolation from one another, but rather change depending on the levels of other parameters and treatments. For example, Stevens and colleagues assessed various biochemical combinations and found that the relative risk for mortality was highest when serum concentrations of calcium and Pi were elevated and the serum PTH concentration was low and mortality was lowest when serum concentrations of calcium and Pi were normal and the serum PTH concentration was high.[236] In addition, results were modified by vintage (time since initiation of dialysis). A Dialysis Outcomes and Practice Patterns Study (DOPPS) trial also evaluated combinations of serum parameters of mineral metabolism and reached slightly different conclusions.[237] The DOPPS researchers found that in the setting of an elevated serum PTH (>300 pg/mL), hypercalcemia (>10 mg/dL) was associated with higher mortality risk even with normal serum Pi. Block and associates, analyzing average values over 4 months from more than 26,000 patients undergoing dialysis, categorized them according to whether serum concentrations of calcium, Pi, and PTH were below, within, or above target ranges. In only 20% of patients were all three variables within target ranges. Those patients with high PTH and high serum calcium had consistently higher mortality.[238] It is important to remember that abnormalities in mineral metabolism are common. Ultimately, we need quality evidence (i.e., from prospective randomized controlled trials using approaches that target specific biochemical endpoints) to determine whether these treatments—despite having been commonly administered in some cases for decades—are truly safe and efficacious.

#### FIBROBLAST GROWTH FACTOR 23

Serum concentrations of FGF-23 (>100 RU/mL) were observed in 70% and 100% of patients with estimated GFRs of 50 and less than 20 mL/min/1.73 m$^2$, respectively, in the Chronic Renal Insufficiency Cohort (CRIC) study.[73] Serum FGF-23 concentrations continue to rise throughout progressive CKD, presumably to maintain hemostasis vis-à-vis Pi and calcium. In CKD, elevations of serum FGF-23 are associated with death,[239] progression of CKD,[239,240] left ventricular hypertrophy,[78,241,242] and cardiovascular events,[243,244] independent of serum concentrations of Pi and PTH. Once patients reach levels of kidney function poor enough to require dialysis, serum concentrations of FGF-23 can be 1000-fold greater, and these have been associated with poorer survival in incident patients in some studies[245] but not others.[246,247] In prevalent patients receiving dialysis, serum FGF-23 was also associated with mortality[248] and directly correlated with left ventricular mass index.[247] In a secondary analysis of nearly 2000 hemodialysis patients treated with cinacalcet, a reduction of serum FGF-23 concentrations by 30% or more was associated with reduced risks of death and cardiovascular events.[249]

## NUTRITIONAL VITAMIN D DEFICIENCY

Although traditionally the term "vitamin D" has been used to indicate the active metabolite, calcitriol, the correct use of the term is for the precursor molecule, calcidiol or 25(OH) D. In the general population, serum calcidiol concentrations are accepted as the standard measures of nutritional uptake because they correlate best with end-organ effects. The conversion of vitamin $D_2$ and vitamin $D_3$ to 25(OH)D by CYP27A1 is essentially unregulated, and therefore levels of 25(OH)D are a reliable indicator of the vitamin D status of a given individual. However, what constitutes adequate stores remains a controversy. Although there is no absolute level of calcidiol that defines deficiency, a level less than 10 ng/mL (25 nmol/L) is typically used, because it is associated with rickets in children and osteomalacia in adults. The term "vitamin D insufficiency" has been used to describe less severe calcidiol-deficient states. Although controversial, the typical range of "insufficient" calcidiol levels is 10 to 30 ng/mL (25–75 nmol/L). In contrast to the severity of bone disease observed with deficiency, insufficiency is associated with elevated PTH and osteoporosis.[250] Unfortunately, despite supplementation of calciferol in various foods such as milk, calcidiol insufficiency is relatively common in the general population, particularly in some at-risk groups such as African-Americans, hospitalized patients, nursing home residents, and people living in northern climates.[251] The Institute of Medicine convened a panel whose report, released in November 2010, recommended that serum vitamin D concentrations of 20 ng/mL are adequate and that the adult-recommended dietary allowance is 600 IU/day, with an upper level intake of 4000 IU/day.[252] The Endocrine Society has subsequently recommended a vitamin D level higher than 30 ng/mL, further suggesting that 40 to 60 ng/mL is ideal and that up to 100 ng/mL is safe.[253] Either vitamin $D_2$ or vitamin $D_3$ can be used for vitamin D supplementation. Although there has been controversy regarding the use of $D_3$ or $D_2$ for achieving and maintaining higher serum vitamin D levels, most analyses have found them to be equally effective in raising and maintaining serum vitamin D levels in patients without CKD.[254]

The importance of vitamin D in health and disease is suggested by a number of observational studies, with the effects of local cellular (autocrine) conversion thought responsible for the purported nonendocrine benefits. Vitamin D deficiency (<20 ng/mL) is likely to be an important etiologic factor in the pathogenesis of many chronic diseases, including autoimmune diseases (e.g., multiple sclerosis, type 1 diabetes), inflammatory bowel disease (e.g., Crohn disease), infections, immune deficiency, cardiovascular diseases (e.g., hypertension, heart failure, sudden cardiac death), cancer (e.g., colon cancer, breast cancer, non-Hodgkin lymphoma), and neurocognitive disorders (e.g., Alzheimer disease).[253,255–260] The association between serum vitamin D concentrations and all-cause mortality was inverse and nonlinear, with increased risk evident at serum vitamin D concentrations below 30 ng/mL. Vitamin D deficiency was also associated with significantly higher rates of death due to cancer and respiratory diseases.[260] However, the only prospective study of vitamin D versus placebo was unable to demonstrate that vitamin D supplementation resulted in a lower incidence of invasive cancer or cardiovascular events.[261]

The results of randomized trials testing the safety and efficacy of vitamin D supplementation on fractures and falls have been mixed. Among the reasons put forth to explain mixed results is the concomitant use of calcium in most studies, and another is the wide range in dose of vitamin D utilized. According to the latest update of the Cochrane Review analysis of vitamin D and vitamin D analogs for prevention of fractures in postmenopausal women and older men, vitamin D alone is unlikely to prevent fractures in the doses and formulations tested so far. However, supplementation of vitamin D and calcium may prevent hip or any type of fracture. In this meta-analysis, vitamin D and calcium in combination resulted in a small but significant increase in gastrointestinal symptoms and kidney disease. The researchers found no evidence that calcium and vitamin D increased (or decreased) the risk of death.[262]

Vitamin D deficiency (<20 ng/mL) and insufficiency (<30 ng/mL) are common in patients with CKD, with only 29% and 17% of those with stage 3 and 4 disease, respectively, having sufficient levels in one study.[263] This prevalence of vitamin D deficiency and insufficiency in an ambulatory CKD population is similar to that in non-CKD nursing home residents, hospitalized patients, and elderly women with hip fractures. However, frank vitamin D deficiency (<10 mg/mL) was observed in 14% and 26% of patients with stage 3 and 4 CKD, respectively.[263] Several other investigators have also found widespread vitamin D insufficiency in patients with CKD, although not all investigators have identified a graded relation with CKD stage.[263–266]

Evidence from epidemiologic studies suggests that vitamin D deficiency and supplementation of vitamin D are associated with survival in patients with CKD regardless of dialysis status, although these analyses are heavily confounded, prohibiting causal inference.[267–272] A meta-analysis of prospective studies demonstrated a significant decrease, 14%, in mortality risk for every 10-ng/mL increase in serum vitamin D concentration.[273] Furthermore, the association of vitamin D supplementation and survival appears to be independent of changes in serum calcium, Pi, and PTH concentrations. There are several plausible mechanisms that could explain the connection between vitamin D deficiency and insufficiency and mortality; for example, serum vitamin D concentrations are inversely correlated with multiple cardiovascular risk factors, including plasma renin activity, blood pressure, left ventricular mass, markers of inflammation, markers of insulin resistance and type 2 diabetes mellitus, and albuminuria.[274–278]

In animal studies, activated vitamin D inhibits renin production.[279,280] Several trials in patients with CKD reported that the use of an active vitamin D analog, paricalcitol, resulted in a significant reduction in proteinuria.[281–283] Evaluation of patients with nondialysis-requiring CKD found an inverse correlation between serum vitamin D concentrations and brachial artery flow–mediated dilation as a marker of endothelial dysfunction.[284] Other studies have demonstrated that patients undergoing hemodialysis who have received cholecalciferol supplements have lower inflammatory parameters, as indicated by higher serum albumin and lower C-reactive protein and interleukin-6 concentrations, as well as improved cardiac function, as reflected by lower brain natriuretic peptide and left ventricular mass index.[285,286] In a prospective placebo-controlled trial in patients who had not started dialysis, paricalcitol failed to reduce left ventricular mass after 48 weeks in patients with mild-to-moderate left ventricular hypertrophy. There was, however, a decrease in hospitalizations, a secondary endpoint.[287] The lack of effect may have been a function of the relatively high dose of paricalcitol, which may have increased serum FGF-23 concentrations, as multiple studies have shown a direct link between FGF-23 and left ventricular hypertrophy.[78,241,287,288] Despite multiple observational studies and several clinical trials, additional controlled trials are required to determine the safety and efficacy of (nutritional and active) vitamin D supplementation in patients with CKD.

## FRACTURE

The incidence of fractures was reported to be significantly higher in patients with nondialysis-requiring CKD compared with persons with normal or near-normal kidney function, although lower than the risk of fractures in patients receiving dialysis,[172,289–291] suggesting that kidney disease is associated with progressive bone deterioration. However, not all studies have confirmed increased rates of hip, wrist, and vertebral fractures in patients with CKD independent of age and sex.[292] More recent studies have suggested that fracture rates in ESKD patients are declining compared with historical data.[293]

In patients undergoing dialysis, the studies are consistent and demonstrate a markedly higher incidence of hip fracture among all age groups.[203,294] Patients undergoing hemodialysis may have a 50% higher rate of hip fractures than patients undergoing peritoneal dialysis.[295] Furthermore, hip fractures in patients on dialysis were associated with a doubling of mortality observed after hip fracture in patients not on dialysis.[203,296] Depending on the study, 10% to 52% of prevalent patients undergoing dialysis have had fractures.[172] Unfortunately, most of these studies are of cross-sectional design or were cohort studies with limited follow-up.

Hyperparathyroidism is known to cause abnormal bone remodeling, especially of cortical bone. Serial studies using HRpQCT show a rapid decline in cortical bone in patients on dialysis.[297] In prevalent patients undergoing dialysis who have secondary hyperparathyroidism, clinical fractures are predominantly cortical in location.[298] However, the association of PTH with fracture has been inconsistent,[172] perhaps because both high and low PTH values are associated with fractures. Other risk factors for hip fracture include older age, female sex, low serum albumin, prior kidney transplantation, and peripheral vascular disease.[188,299–301] Falls are also more common in patients with CKD and predispose to fracture. Falls in patients undergoing dialysis may be related to peripheral vascular disease,[294] low muscle strength, impaired neuromuscular function,[302] and the administration of psychoactive medications.[300]

In summary, the abnormalities of bone, in terms of both quality and quantity, variable biochemical abnormalities, and multiple comorbid conditions likely all contribute to the pathogenesis of fractures in ESKD. This complexity also may limit generalizability of therapies routinely used in the general population to patients with the disease.

## EXTRASKELETAL CALCIFICATION

Arterial calcification has a multitude of clinical manifestations. Intimal calcification (in association with atherosclerotic disease) can lead to myocardial infarction from stenosis and acute thrombus or to ischemia in both coronary and peripheral arteries. Medial calcification (or circumferential calcification) can lead to arterial stiffening, with reduced compliance of the artery and an inability to appropriately dilate in the setting of increased stress. In the coronary arteries, similar symptoms of ischemia can develop, and in theory could lead to arrhythmias and sudden death. In the larger arteries such as the aorta, calcification can lead to increased pulse wave velocity and elevated pulse pressure and is commonly associated with systolic hypertension in the elderly, a known risk factor for cardiovascular disease in the general population. In addition, the premature return of wave reflections during systole (instead of diastole) can lead to altered coronary perfusion, especially in the setting of left ventricular hypertrophy. Lastly, calcification of the arterioles of the skin and other organs can lead to localized infarction and ischemia, including ischemic bowel and calcific uremic arteriolopathy (calciphylaxis).

### VASCULAR CALCIFICATION IN PATIENTS WITH CHRONIC KIDNEY DISEASE

The high prevalence of vascular calcification in patients with CKD is not a new observation. In 1979, Ibels and colleagues demonstrated that both renal and internal iliac arteries of patients undergoing renal transplantation had greater atherogenic/intimal disease and increased calcification (detected by biochemical methods) than transplant donors.[303] In addition, the medial layer was thicker and more calcified in uremic patients than in the donors. A study comparing histologic changes in coronary arteries from patients undergoing dialysis at autopsy were compared with nondialysis, age-matched patients who had died from a cardiac event found similar magnitudes of atherosclerotic plaque burden and intimal thickness, but with more calcification in the patients who had received dialysis.[304] In addition, morphometry of the arteries demonstrated increased medial thickening. When these same investigators evaluated more distal segments of the coronary arteries, they found medial calcification.[305] Studies of the inferior epigastric artery of patients undergoing kidney transplantation demonstrated calcification in 31% of patients, with histology demonstrating isolated medial calcification without evidence of atherosclerotic or intimal changes, and both medial and intimal calcification in the same artery without disruption of the internal elastic lamina.[306] Thus there is histologic evidence of (1) increased arterial calcification in coronary, renal, and iliac arteries of patients who undergo dialysis than in those who do not and (2) the presence of both intimal and medial calcification in patients undergoing dialysis, and this can occur independently of each other, suggesting unique inciting factors. As noted previously, it is likely that calcification of plaque (atherosclerosis) and calcification of medial layer occur by similar mechanisms. However, the initiating event is clearly different.

Braun and colleagues first demonstrated that coronary artery calcification as detected by EBCT increased with advancing age in patients on dialysis and that the calcification scores were twofold to fivefold higher in patients on dialysis than in age-matched persons with normal kidney function and angiographically proven coronary artery disease.[307] Nearly 50% to 60% of patients starting hemodialysis have evidence of coronary artery calcification,[308] with higher prevalence in patients with diabetes.[309] The prevalence of detectable coronary or peripheral artery calcification is 51% to 93% in prevalent patients undergoing dialysis and 47% to 83% in patients with CKD stages 3 through 5. Valvular calcification is similarly common, occurring in 20% to 47% of patients on dialysis.[172] Studies that have evaluated the natural history of coronary calcification demonstrate that once present, the course is progressive. By contrast, many patients without calcification remain free of calcification for several years.[172,310,311] The presence of calcification in the coronary arteries, valves, and peripheral arteries is associated with mortality.[227] Given the high prevalence of calcification, it is currently uncertain whether routine imaging offers clinical utility or whether it can help stratify patients whose calcification will and will not respond to specific therapies.

There is an inverse relationship between bone mineralization and vascular calcification in patients on dialysis. There are several different, not mutually exclusive, mechanisms by which disturbances in the bone metabolism may cause or accelerate vascular calcification.[307,312] Interestingly, it appears to be low-turnover bone disease that leads to greatest risk of vascular calcification. London and colleagues evaluated patients on hemodialysis who underwent assessment of vascular calcification by ultrasonography with semiquantitative scoring and by bone biopsy with histomorphometry. Those patients with lowest bone formation rates and decreased osteoblast surfaces had the most prominent degree of peripheral artery calcification, and this relation held true in patients with and without previous parathyroidectomy.[313] Another study found that patients with low-turnover bone disease on biopsy were more likely to have progression of coronary artery calcification over 1 year as assessed by serial multislice CT than those with high-turnover bone disease.[208] Abnormalities in cortical and trabecular bone on HRpQCT were associated with coronary artery calcification.[314] The likely mechanism relates to a reduced ability to mineralize bone in ESKD, especially in the setting of low-turnover bone disease, leading to dystrophic calcification in the setting of calcium (and vitamin D) intake; actively remodeling bone, by contrast, is able to mineralize, as demonstrated by Kurz and associates.[205] In contrast to evidence in low-turnover bone disease, data are less robust as to the effects of high-turnover bone disease on vascular calcification, perhaps because the treatments for high-turnover bone disease confound the effects of calcification.

## CHRONIC KIDNEY DISEASE-MINERAL AND BONE DISORDER IN KIDNEY TRANSPLANT RECIPIENTS

Bone and mineral disorders are universal complications in patients with CKD prior to transplantation. Ideally, all of these complications would be improved with successful kidney transplantation. Unfortunately, in many cases, kidney transplantation achieves milder forms of CKD (as opposed to normal kidney function), and thus kidney transplant recipients still suffer from disorders associated with CKD-MBD. In addition, disorders of mineral metabolism occur following successful transplantation, including the effects of medications (steroids and calcineurin inhibitors), persistence of underlying disorders (hyperparathyroidism and vitamin D deficiency), development of hyperphosphaturia with hypophosphatemia (especially with persistent hyperparathyroidism).

### BIOCHEMICAL CHANGES AFTER TRANSPLANTATION

Biochemical changes of mineral metabolism are common in patients after kidney transplantation.[315–318] Decreased calcidiol levels are common in kidney transplant recipients, with reported prevalence of up to 81%.[316] The causes are multifactorial, and may include nutritional deficiency, malabsorption, and decreased sun exposure. However, the improvement in kidney function results in an increase in CYP27B1 activity, resulting in greater conversion of calcidiol to calcitriol, which subsequently causes a gradual decrease in PTH concentrations during the first 3 to 6 months after transplantation. However, persistent hyperparathyroidism exists in about 33% and 20% of patients at 6 and 12 months, respectively.[319] Serum FGF-23 concentrations decrease immediately after transplantation, although they remain inappropriately elevated for the prevailing serum Pi concentration. By about 3 months after transplantation, serum FGF-23 concentrations are reduced by 89%, and at 12 months FGF-23 concentrations appear to be similar to those in patients without transplantation who have comparable stages of CKD.[316] The elevated FGF-23 inhibits CYP27B1 and contributes to the low calcitriol concentrations observed in the early post-transplantation period, likely contributing to the persistent hyperparathyroidism seen after transplantation. Thus elevated FGF-23 and PTH concentrations combined with low calcitriol concentrations likely contribute to hypophosphatemia observed in many transplant recipients.[319,320]

Serum calcium concentrations typically drop very early after transplantation, as a result of cessation of therapy with calcitriol and its analogs and/or calcium-containing phosphate binders. After that initial drop, however, calcium concentrations progressively increase, with hypercalcemia developing in a substantial number of patients during the first to third month after transplantation. Hypercalcemia can be transient, resolving by 6 to 8 months in some cases but lasting for many years in others. Hypercalcemia is typically associated with hyperparathyroidism and results from enhanced renal tubular reabsorption of calcium under the influence of PTH in the functioning allograft, the effects of calcitriol on the gastrointestinal absorption of calcium, and, potentially, a direct effect of PTH in causing calcium efflux from bone. Low bone turnover with relatively low PTH may also result in hypercalcemia because the bone is not able to act as a buffer for the circulating calcium pool.[315,316]

### BONE CHANGES AFTER TRANSPLANTATION

Disorders of mineral metabolism and associated bone disease lead to fractures following transplantation, which occur after up to 44% of successful kidney transplants.[315] This fracture risk appears to be less than that observed with other solid organ transplants.[315] The combination of kidney–pancreas transplantation raises fracture risk above that associated with kidney transplantation alone.[321,322] In a retrospective analysis of 68,814 patients, fracture developed in 22.5% within 5 years.[323] In a study of first-time kidney transplant recipients between 1997 and 2010, the incidence of hip fracture was 3.8 per 1000 person-years. The risk of fracture in 2010 was 0.56 (95% CI, 0.47–0.77) in comparison with that in 1997, indicating a decrease over the 13-year period, presumably due to changes in immunosuppression therapy.[324] Factors associated with higher fracture risk during the first 5 years included female sex, age older than 45 years, Caucasian race, recipient of a deceased donor kidney, increased human leukocyte antigen mismatches, diabetes, pretransplantation dialysis, steroid use, and an aggressive induction regimen.[323] Importantly, even with the use of steroid-sparing regimens, total (all sites) fractures have occurred in up to 50% of kidney transplant recipients at 6 years.[324,325] By contrast, a Canadian study evaluated 4821 kidney transplant recipients and found that the 10-year cumulative incidence of hip fracture was 1.7%.[326]

Studies evaluating bone histology in recipients of kidney transplants are limited. The main alteration is an uncoupling of bone remodeling, which results in a decrease of bone formation with persistent bone resorption and net bone loss. In a small cohort of young patients who underwent preemptive transplantation and were treated predominantly with corticosteroids, bone biopsies revealed a mineralization defect as early as 6 months after transplantation.[327] Another study evaluating the early histologic changes after transplantation revealed that osteoid volume, osteoid thickness, osteoid resorption surface, and osteoclast surface were elevated above the normal range before transplantation and remained increased approximately 35 days afterward. However, osteoid and osteoblast surfaces, which also were increased before transplantation, were significantly decreased approximately 35 days after transplantation.[328] Both bone formation and mineralization were also inhibited after transplantation. An important observation was that although none of the pretransplantation biopsy specimens showed evidence of apoptosis, 45% of posttransplantation specimens showed significant apoptosis after an average of only 35 days. Thus early posttransplantation apoptosis and a decrease in osteoblast number and osteoblast surface play a role in the pathogenesis of posttransplantation bone disease that may be related directly to the use of glucocorticoids. The few evaluations that examined the longer-term effect of transplantation on bone histology generally demonstrate low bone turnover and histology consistent with adynamic bone disease.[329,330] Lehmann and colleagues performed a retrospective study of 57 patients after approximately 54 months after kidney transplantation.[330] Seven histologic subgroups were identified: normal, osteitis fibrosa cystica, mild osteitis fibrosa, mixed uremic bone disease, osteomalacia, adynamic bone disease, and osteoporosis. Given the limited number of patients in the study, no significant correlations between the histological subgroups and PTH or alkaline phosphatase levels were observed. However, this study did show a variable degree of histologic abnormalities following transplantation that could not have been predicted by biochemical testing and confirmed that preexisting bone disease lesions persist in the posttransplantation period.

The effects of other immunosuppressive agents on bone histology have also been examined. Bone biopsies performed approximately 10 years after transplantation in patients whose treatment included cyclosporine monotherapy, azathioprine and prednisone, or triple therapy revealed no differences among the immunosuppressant regimens.[331,332] A subgroup analysis of 21 patients with normal serum PTH concentrations showed that cyclosporine monotherapy was associated with a more pronounced decrease in bone thickness than the other regimens.[332] In addition, the cyclosporine group showed a lower trabecular appositional rate than the azathioprine and prednisone group. Multiple regression analysis showed that sex and time after transplantation were the most significant factors predicting bone volume and mineralizing surface. Predictive factors for eroded bone surface and osteoclast number included age and time on dialysis before transplantation.[331,332]

Initial studies examining BMD by DXA showed severe and rapid bone loss after kidney transplantation.[327] However, later studies have not found the dramatic decrease initially described, perhaps because of the current practice of using lower steroid dosages or steroid-free immunosuppression regimens.[315,333] The use of corticosteroids is the major determinant of low BMD, because these agents impair calcium absorption from the gastrointestinal tract and inhibit bone cell recruitment and function. Cueto-Manzano and associates also evaluated BMD as a function of immunosuppressive therapy.[331,332] In comparison with age- and sex-matched controls, none of the treated groups showed a significant reduction in BMD in the lumbar spine or femoral neck. However, in comparison with young normal controls, osteopenia was detected in the femoral neck, except in premenopausal women. There was no significant difference in BMD related to immunosuppressant regimen, sex, or menopausal status.

Although reductions in BMD have been associated with an increased fracture rate in postmenopausal women and in men treated with glucocorticoids, as well as in heart or liver transplant recipients, very little data support its role in predicting fractures after kidney transplantation. In the one study that demonstrated low BMD to be predictive of fracture risk, 283 kidney transplant recipients with varying degrees of kidney function underwent 670 examinations of bone density at the hip. An absolute BMD value less than 0.9 g/cm$^2$ was associated with an increased risk of fracture.[334] A study evaluating patients with early steroid withdrawal after kidney transplantation found preservation of BMD by DXA but continued loss at the ultra-distal radius. The latter finding was confirmed by HRpQCT to be predominantly cortical loss, which was associated with persistent hyperparathyroidism.[335] As indicated earlier, abnormal bone turnover may alter the predictive value of BMD testing in patients with CKD, and thus preexisting rate of bone turnover likely affects the assessment and outcomes of bone disease in transplant recipients.

## VASCULAR CALCIFICATION CHANGES AFTER TRANSPLANTATION

Most transplant recipients enter their posttransplant course with a preexisting burden of vascular calcification; as in patients with CKD, vascular calcification strongly predicts cardiovascular events and all-cause mortality. Unfortunately there are few studies of the nature and consequences of vascular calcification in kidney transplant recipients. Although preexisting calcifications progress after transplantation, they appear to do so at a much slower rate than prior to transplantation.[336,337] A review of 13 clinical studies of the role of vascular calcifications in kidney transplant recipients shows that as in the CKD population, the associations of traditional and nontraditional risk factors with outcomes are variable in transplant recipients.[338] There is a strong association between baseline coronary artery calcification score and progression of coronary artery calcification. A significant improvement in secondary hyperparathyroidism after transplantation is associated with slowing the progression of coronary artery calcification. Independent risk factors of coronary artery calcification in kidney transplant recipients include low serum concentrations of calcidiol, fetuin-A, and MGP. Although diabetes is a risk factor for the presence of coronary artery calcification in transplant recipients, it has not been independently associated with progression of coronary artery calcification. Data on the effects of immunosuppressive drugs as factors in progression are few and inconclusive; however, it does appear that mycophenolate mofetil may have a beneficial effect because its antiproliferative action may inhibit smooth muscle cell proliferation, thus having a favorable effect on endothelial cell activity.[338] In the general population and in patients with ESKD, there is an inverse relation between coronary artery calcification and bone density. This association has not been shown in kidney or kidney–pancreas transplant recipients.[339]

## SUMMARY

In summary, some abnormalities of CKD-MBD persist after kidney transplantation, and other conditions unique to transplantation frequently develop. With changing immunosuppressive protocols and persistence of CKD, treatment of these conditions can be particularly challenging. Recent studies have highlighted the importance of management of CKD-MBD before transplantation. Additional studies are required to determine the safety and efficacy of established and novel therapies in patients with CKD and ESKD and after kidney transplantation.[317,318,340]

 Complete reference list available at ExpertConsult.com.

## KEY REFERENCES


1. Moe S, et al. Definition, evaluation, and classification of renal osteodystrophy: a position statement from Kidney Disease: Improving Global Outcomes (KDIGO). *Kidney Int.* 2006;69(11):1945–1953.
7. Hill KM, et al. Oral calcium carbonate affects calcium but not phosphorus balance in stage 3-4 chronic kidney disease. *Kidney Int.* 2013;83(5):959–966.
23. Bindels RJ. 2009 Homer W. Smith Award: Minerals in motion: from new ion transporters to new concepts. *J Am Soc Nephrol.* 2010; 21(8):1263–1269.
27. Brennan SC, et al. Calcium sensing receptor signalling in physiology and cancer. *Biochim Biophys Acta.* 2013;1833(7):1732–1744.
33. Rodriguez-Ortiz ME, et al. Magnesium modulates parathyroid hormone secretion and upregulates parathyroid receptor expression at moderately low calcium concentration. *Nephrol Dial Transplant.* 2014;29(2):282–289.
50. Raggi P, et al. The ADVANCE study: a randomized study to evaluate the effects of cinacalcet plus low-dose vitamin D on vascular calcification in patients on hemodialysis. *Nephrol Dial Transplant.* 2011;26(4):1327–1339.
56. Sprague SM, Moe SM. The case for routine parathyroid hormone monitoring. *Clin J Am Soc Nephrol.* 2013;8(2):313–318.
60. Jones G. Extrarenal vitamin D activation and interactions between vitamin D(2), vitamin D(3), and vitamin D analogs. *Annu Rev Nutr.* 2013;33:23–44.
61. Chanakul A, et al. FGF-23 regulates CYP27B1 transcription in the kidney and in extra-renal tissues. *PLoS ONE.* 2013;8(9):e72816.
72. Hu MC, et al. Renal production, uptake, and handling of circulating alphaKlotho. *J Am Soc Nephrol.* 2016;27(1):79–90.
73. Isakova T, et al. Fibroblast growth factor 23 is elevated before parathyroid hormone and phosphate in chronic kidney disease. *Kidney Int.* 2011;79(12):1370–1378.
74. Hu MC, Kuro-o M, Moe OW. Renal and extrarenal actions of Klotho. *Semin Nephrol.* 2013;33(2):118–129.
78. Faul C, et al. FGF23 induces left ventricular hypertrophy. *J Clin Invest.* 2011;121(11):4393–4408.
86. de Borst MH, et al. Cross talk between the renin-angiotensin-aldosterone system and vitamin D-FGF-23-klotho in chronic kidney disease. *J Am Soc Nephrol.* 2011;22(9):1603–1609.
94. Baron R, Kneissel M. WNT signaling in bone homeostasis and disease: from human mutations to treatments. *Nat Med.* 2013;19(2): 179–192.
103. Rhee Y, et al. Resorption controls bone anabolism driven by parathyroid hormone (PTH) receptor signaling in osteocytes. *J Biol Chem.* 2013;288(41):29809–29820.
135. Giachelli CM. The emerging role of phosphate in vascular calcification. *Kidney Int.* 2009;75(9):890–897.
143. Ketteler M, et al. Association of low fetuin-A (AHSG) concentrations in serum with cardiovascular mortality in patients on dialysis: a cross-sectional study. *Lancet.* 2003;361(9360):827–833.
149. Ketteler M, et al. The K-factor in chronic kidney disease: biomarkers of calcification inhibition and beyond. *Nephrol Dial Transplant.* 2014;29(7):1267–1270.
166. Lavi-Moshayoff V, et al. PTH increases FGF23 gene expression and mediates the high-FGF23 levels of experimental kidney failure: a bone parathyroid feedback loop. *Am J Physiol Renal Physiol.* 2010;299(4):F882–F889.
167. Rodriguez-Ortiz ME, et al. Calcium deficiency reduces circulating levels of FGF23. *J Am Soc Nephrol.* 2012;23(7):1190–1197.
169. Sprague SM, et al. Diagnostic accuracy of bone turnover markers and bone histology in patients with CKD treated by dialysis. *Am J Kidney Dis.* 2016;67(4):559–566.
172. Kidney Disease: Improving Global Outcomes, C.K.D.M.B.D.W.G. KDIGO clinical practice guideline for the diagnosis, evaluation, prevention, and treatment of Chronic Kidney Disease-Mineral and Bone Disorder (CKD-MBD). *Kidney Int Suppl.* 2009;113:S1–S130.
187. Moorthi RN, Moe SM. Recent advances in the noninvasive diagnosis of renal osteodystrophy. *Kidney Int.* 2013;84(5):886–894.
191. Sherrard DJ, et al. The spectrum of bone disease in end-stage renal failure–an evolving disorder. *Kidney Int.* 1993;43(2):436–442.
194. Alfrey AC. Aluminum and renal disease. *Contrib Nephrol.* 1993;102: 110–124.
195. National Kidney, F. K/DOQI clinical practice guidelines for bone metabolism and disease in chronic kidney disease. *Am J Kidney Dis.* 2003;42(4 suppl 3):S1–S201.
201. Ott SM. Bone disease in CKD. *Curr Opin Nephrol Hypertens.* 2012;21(4):376–381.
208. Barreto DV, et al. Association of changes in bone remodeling and coronary calcification in hemodialysis patients: a prospective study. *Am J Kidney Dis.* 2008;52(6):1139–1150.
218. Nickolas TL, et al. Bone mass and microarchitecture in CKD patients with fracture. *J Am Soc Nephrol.* 2010;21(8):1371–1380.
223. London GM, et al. Arterial media calcification in end-stage renal disease: impact on all-cause and cardiovascular mortality. *Nephrol Dial Transplant.* 2003;18(9):1731–1740.
228. Bellasi A, et al. Integration of clinical and imaging data to predict death in hemodialysis patients. *Hemodial Int.* 2013;17(1): 12–18.
235. Palmer SC, et al. Serum levels of phosphorus, parathyroid hormone, and calcium and risks of death and cardiovascular disease in individuals with chronic kidney disease: a systematic review and meta-analysis. *JAMA.* 2011;305(11):1119–1127.

239. Isakova T, et al. Fibroblast growth factor 23 and risks of mortality and end-stage renal disease in patients with chronic kidney disease. *JAMA*. 2011;305(23):2432–2439.
245. Gutierrez OM, et al. Fibroblast growth factor 23 and mortality among patients undergoing hemodialysis. *N Engl J Med*. 2008;359(6):584–592.
252. Ross AC, et al. The 2011 report on dietary reference intakes for calcium and vitamin D from the Institute of Medicine: what clinicians need to know. *J Clin Endocrinol Metab*. 2011;96(1):53–58.
266. Levin A, et al. Prevalence of abnormal serum vitamin D, PTH, calcium, and phosphorus in patients with chronic kidney disease: results of the study to evaluate early kidney disease. *Kidney Int*. 2007;71(1):31–38.
272. Zheng Z, et al. Vitamin D supplementation and mortality risk in chronic kidney disease: a meta-analysis of 20 observational studies. *BMC Nephrol*. 2013;14:199.
283. de Zeeuw D, et al. Selective vitamin D receptor activation with paricalcitol for reduction of albuminuria in patients with type 2 diabetes (VITAL study): a randomised controlled trial. *Lancet*. 2010;376(9752):1543–1551.
297. Nickolas TL, et al. Rapid cortical bone loss in patients with chronic kidney disease. *J Bone Miner Res*. 2013;28(8):1811–1820.
305. Gross ML, et al. Calcification of coronary intima and media: immunohistochemistry, backscatter imaging, and x-ray analysis in renal and nonrenal patients. *Clin J Am Soc Nephrol*. 2007;2(1):121–134.
316. Alshayeb HM, Josephson MA, Sprague SM. CKD-mineral and bone disorder management in kidney transplant recipients. *Am J Kidney Dis*. 2013;61(2):310–325.
317. Haffner D, Schuler U. Metabolic bone disease after renal transplantation. *Curr Opin Pediatr*. 2014;26(2):198–206.

# 54 Cardiovascular Aspects of Kidney Disease

Richard Haynes | David C. Wheeler | William G. Herrington | Martin J. Landray | Colin Baigent

CHAPTER OUTLINE



## INTRODUCTION

The expanding availability of dialysis and kidney transplantation in developed countries has led to improvements in the prognosis of patients with end-stage kidney disease (ESKD). However, the life expectancy of patients receiving such renal replacement therapy (RRT) remains considerably lower than that of age- and gender-matched healthy controls, and the risks of both cardiovascular and noncardiovascular causes of mortality are increased at all ages.[1] This chapter will focus on the pathology, epidemiology, and treatment of cardiovascular disease in the chronic kidney disease (CKD) population.

The first description of a link between diseases of the kidneys and the cardiovascular system is attributable to Richard Bright, who described cardiac hypertrophy in patients with small kidneys at postmortem over 170 years ago.[2] The problem became more obvious with the advent of dialysis, because patients survived long enough after ESKD to develop clinical manifestations of cardiovascular disease. In the early 1970s, clinicians were alarmed at the high incidence of cardiovascular events in young patients receiving RRT and presumed that either kidney disease or the dialysis process itself led to accelerated atherosclerosis.[3]

Twenty years later, a task force report published by the U.S. National Kidney Foundation focused the attention of the nephrology community on the problem of increased cardiovascular disease risk associated with CKD.[4] Research over the last 10 years or so has improved our understanding of the cardiovascular consequences of impaired kidney function and has helped suggest appropriate treatment strategies. For example, the nature of the cardiac and arterial changes that complicate CKD are now better described. Although atherosclerosis contributes to arterial pathology in advanced CKD, nonatherosclerotic changes, including arterial wall thickening and calcification, are the dominant pathologic feature.[5] Whereas an increased risk of cardiovascular events associated with atherosclerotic plaque rupture is recognized in patients with CKD,[6] the clinical consequences of structural heart disease (heart failure and sudden dysrhythmic death) appear to be a more important cause of morbidity and mortality than the complications of atherosclerotic disease.[7] However, our understanding remains incomplete.

Although the problem of premature cardiovascular disease was first recognized in dialysis populations, patients with lesser degrees of impaired kidney function are also at increased risk of cardiovascular events.[8] Numerous studies have shown an inverse association between estimated glomerular filtration rate (eGFR) and cardiovascular risk.[9] The nature of both cardiac and arterial disease may change with declining kidney function, and this might have implications for the development of optimal management strategies. It has also become clear that albuminuria is associated with an increased risk of cardiovascular disease, whether or not the GFR is reduced.[9,10]

It follows that the assessment and management of cardiovascular diseases should start early in the course of CKD in an effort to reduce morbidity and mortality, bearing in mind that most patients in whom CKD is diagnosed early do not progress to ESKD. Those who do may have well-established structural cardiac and vascular damage by the time they commence RRT.[11,12] This is particularly important when considering a patient's suitability for transplantation, and most clinicians will screen such patients (or at least those they consider to be at high risk) for cardiovascular disease before transplant listing in an effort to reduce perioperative morbidity and mortality and optimize the results of organ allocation.[13] Despite such screening strategies, patients who receive a kidney transplant remain at higher risk than age- and gender-matched controls without kidney disease.[4]

At present, there is much uncertainty about how to reduce cardiovascular risk in patients with CKD. Epidemiologic relationships among recognized cardiovascular risk factors and particular clinical outcomes are often confounded by other factors associated with ill health in CKD, such as inflammation and malnutrition,[14,15] and it may not be possible to account for them accurately or completely. Consequently, it may be more appropriate to approach the problem of preventing cardiovascular disease in CKD by defining the types of pathology observed in patients with CKD and then considering what is known about the treatment or prevention of such pathologies from studies among individuals without CKD. These provide more reliable information on the effectiveness of particular drugs in specific disease processes. Another possible strategy, which is applicable when treatments that modify a particular risk factor are available, is to conduct randomized trials of such treatments, which can yield unbiased assessments of the causal relevance of that risk factor for a particular type of cardiovascular disease.

**Box 54.1 Characteristics of Cardiovascular Diseases in Chronic Kidney Disease**

**Arteries**

Increased wall thickness
Arterial stiffness
Endothelial dysfunction
Arterial calcification

**Heart**

Altered cardiac geometry
Myocardial fibrosis
Left ventricular dysfunction
Valvular disease
Dysrhythmia and conduction defects

## SPECTRUM OF CARDIOVASCULAR PATHOLOGY IN CHRONIC KIDNEY DISEASE

Cardiovascular changes observed in patients with CKD can be divided broadly into those that involve the blood vessels (specifically the arteries) and those that involve the heart (Box 54.1). Although a wide spectrum of cardiovascular pathologies is recognized in CKD, much less is known about the association between particular pathologies and specific cardiovascular risk factors in the CKD population. It is likely that any associations between a given risk factor and particular cardiovascular pathologies will vary in their strength (and possibly direction), so careful phenotyping of cardiovascular outcomes is essential in epidemiologic studies.

### ARTERIAL DISEASE

The term *arteriosclerosis* (derived from the Greek, meaning hardening of the arteries) is generally used to describe a range of pathologic processes. Strictly speaking, arteriosclerosis encompasses three different lesions—atherosclerosis, arteriolosclerosis, and Mönckeberg medial calcific sclerosis (or Mönckeberg sclerosis).[16] Atherosclerosis, a word derived from the Greek "atheroma" (gruel-like material), is characterized by the development of lipid-enriched plaques in the intimal layer of the artery. Calcification is an important feature of atherosclerosis, and its presence or absence is relevant in determining the stage of the lesion.[17] Distinct from atherosclerosis, the phenomenon of noncalcified, nonatheromatous stiffening of smaller muscular arteries was first described in patients with Bright disease in 1868 and soon came to be known as "arteriolosclerosis." Then, 35 years later, in 1903, Mönckeberg reported what he considered to be a third distinct form of arterial disease involving the media of the artery, characterized by medial thickening and heavy calcification, without the presence of atheroma.[18]

Patients with CKD may exhibit all the previous features of arteriosclerosis. The exact nature of arterial disease in any given individual patient is likely to depend on multiple factors, including age, exposure to risk factors, and cause and duration of CKD. For example, a patient with preexisting atherosclerosis who develops CKD as a result of atherosclerotic renovascular disease may have a rather different spectrum of arterial pathology than a patient with a similar level of kidney function caused by kidney damage from glomerulonephritis. The various structural and functional arterial abnormalities associated with CKD are covered in more detail later.

#### ARTERIAL WALL THICKENING

One of the few autopsy studies examining arterial pathology in ESKD has reported that there is more pronounced medial thickening in sections of coronary artery than in equivalent sections from age- and gender-matched, non-CKD patients known to have had coronary artery disease (CAD).[5] Thickening of the arterial wall can be measured noninvasively by assessing the combined width of the intima and media of the carotid artery on ultrasound (carotid intima-media thickening [CIMT]) and has been found to be increased in populations at high risk of cardiovascular disease, such as older adults[19] and patients with type 2 diabetes mellitus.[20] Studies in patients on hemodialysis dating back to the mid-1990s have indicated higher arterial intima-media thickness values for carotid and femoral sites as compared with healthy controls.[21] More recent studies have suggested that increased CIMT is also found in patients with less advanced CKD, indicating that eGFR independently predicts carotid diameter, which increases wall stress.[22] Carotid IMT has also been shown to be a strong predictor of death from cardiovascular causes in patients with CKD, independent of other risk factors.[23,24]

### ARTERIAL STIFFENING

Stiffening is thought to be a functional consequence of artery wall thickening (and calcification) and is readily assessed noninvasively by measuring the velocity of propagation of a pulse wave through the arterial tree (pulse wave velocity [PWV]).[25] Stiffening may represent an early feature of CKD-associated arterial disease and can be detected in pediatric populations receiving dialysis as early as the first decade of life.[26] Stiffness has prognostic significance; both carotid[27] and aortic[28] stiffness independently predict death in adult patients on hemodialysis, as in other high-risk groups, such as patients with diabetes mellitus[29] and older adults.[30]

Another method of measuring arterial stiffness is to assess the pulse waveform in an accessible artery (e.g., the carotid artery). A parameter derived from the pulse waveform, the augmentation index, provides a measure of the interaction between outgoing and reflected pulse waveforms at the point of measurement and, in part, reflects the stiffness of the arterial tree.[31] The augmentation index assessed at the common carotid artery has been found to predict mortality in one study of ESKD,[32] but not in another.[33] A further study comparing different methods of measuring arterial stiffness has found that a higher PWV, but not the augmentation index, predicts an increased risk of cardiovascular disease outcomes in patients with CKD.[34]

A third method, the measurement of carotid artery stiffness parameter β, which is determined by monitoring pulsatile changes in the artery during echo-tracking sonography,[35] was used in a prospective cohort study examining the independent predictive value of arterial stiffness in 423 patients on hemodialysis. This measurement of stiffness independently predicted cardiovascular events, even after adjustments had been made for arterial thickness, possibly implicating distinct roles for stiffening and thickening in the development of arterial complications in patients with CKD.[36]

### ENDOTHELIAL DYSFUNCTION

The vascular endothelium plays a key role in maintaining arterial tone, predominantly through the continuous production of nitric oxide. Nitric oxide is a vasoactive compound that contributes to the resting tone of the artery and protects against the development of arterial disease by inhibiting vascular smooth muscle cell proliferation, platelet aggregation, and monocyte adhesion.[37] The production of nitric oxide is stimulated by hypoxia, increased sheer stress, or by locally released mediators such as acetylcholine.

Endothelial function can be measured by assessing the vasodilatory response of an artery to endothelial stimulation. This can be achieved by directly infusing compounds into an artery (usually the brachial) or by monitoring the response to reactive hyperemia following temporary arterial occlusion. Arterial vasodilation can be assessed by measuring changes in forearm size using strain gauge plethysmography, which works on the principle that the rate of distention of a forearm is proportional to the rate of arterial inflow, or by measuring the diameter of the arterial lumen using high-resolution ultrasonography.[38]

Studies in patients with stage 4 or 5 CKD have consistently demonstrated impairment of endothelial function by both invasive[39] and noninvasive approaches.[40] One possible mechanism for endothelial dysfunction in the context of CKD is the accumulation of asymmetric dimethylarginine (ADMA), an endogenous inhibitor of the enzyme nitric oxide synthetase.[41] ADMA inhibits nitric oxide synthetase and thereby limits the bioavailability of nitric oxide, which is essential for normal endothelial function.[42] Blood concentrations of ADMA are elevated in CKD, are inversely proportional to GFR,[41,43] and appear to be associated with an increased risk of cardiovascular disease in the general population in some but not all studies.[44] At present, there is no intervention that can selectively reduce ADMA concentrations, so the causal relationship (and clinical relevance) of this risk factor remain(s) unclear.

### ARTERIAL CALCIFICATION

Arterial calcification is a recognized feature of two of the pathologic processes that are prevalent in patients with CKD—namely, atherosclerosis[17] and Mönckeberg sclerosis (see earlier).[18] The pattern observed in atherosclerosis is of patchy intimal calcification in association with lipid deposits, whereas in Mönckeberg disease there is a linear pattern of medial calcium deposition (Fig. 54.1).[45] Both are closely linked to disturbances in calcium and phosphate homeostasis and to associated abnormalities in bone mineral metabolism (see Chapter 53).

Autopsy studies have indicated a greater degree of arterial calcification in patients with ESRD than controls with known CAD.[5] In life, calcification can be detected by both ultrasound- and x-ray–based techniques.[46] Studies using electron beam computed tomography, a technique that allows rapid image acquisition, thereby “freezing” the heart during diastole,[47] have indicated that, compared with patients known to have cardiovascular disease, patients on dialysis have much higher calcification scores.[48] Furthermore, calcification develops at a younger age in CKD than in non-CKD populations,[49] being detectable even in children and adolescents.[50]

Some investigators have attempted to distinguish the two patterns of arterial calcification on the basis of imaging studies.[51] Although they may represent a continuum of the same pathologic process,[52] patchy calcium deposition (suggestive of an atherosclerotic pattern) was more common in older patients with a clinical history of cardiovascular events prior to starting dialysis.[51] The physiologic consequences of arterial calcification may include stiffening of the artery,[53] but it is unclear whether calcification has a positive or negative impact on plaque stability.[54]

## CARDIAC DISEASE

Echocardiographic studies performed in the mid-1990s indicated a high prevalence of structural heart abnormalities in patients starting dialysis, with 74% having increased left ventricular mass in one study.[11] Left ventricular remodeling occurs well before the initiation of dialysis[55] and is detectable even in patients with stage 2 or 3 CKD.[56,57] Although adaptive in the early stages, such structural changes may eventually lead to functional impairment, including reduced compliance of the left ventricular wall during diastole (diastolic dysfunction), impaired myocardial contractility (systolic dysfunction), or both.[58] In addition to these changes in left ventricular geometry, histologic changes such as fibrosis and calcification occur in the myocardium,[59] and valvular calcification is also frequently observed.[60]

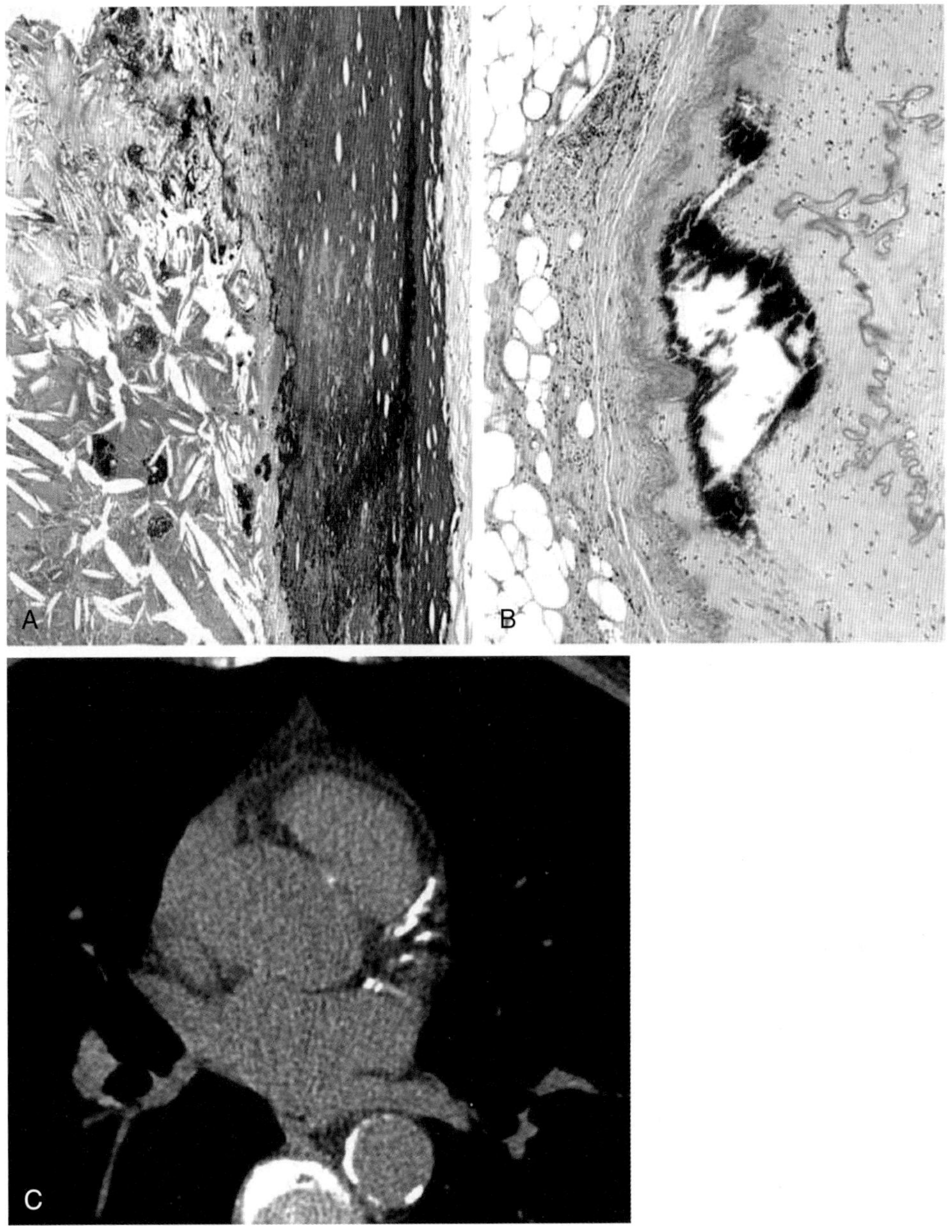


**Fig. 54.1** Arterial calcification in chronic kidney disease (CKD). Shown are cross-sections of medium-sized arteries from a patient with CKD showing deposition of calcium *(black)* in the intima (A) and media (B) in association with atherosclerosis (von Kossa stain). Calcium deposits may be visible on CT scanning of the heart as depicted in (C), where calcification is visible in the left anterior descending and left circumflex coronary artery, as well as the descending aorta. (Courtesy AJ Howie.)

## ALTERED CARDIAC GEOMETRY

Left ventricular hypertrophy is generally classified according to the predominant pattern of abnormality on echocardiogram. In one study of 3487 patients with CKD, the prevalence of left ventricular hypertrophy was 32%, 48%, 57%, and 75% for eGFR categories 60 or higher, 45–59, 30–44, and less than 30 mL/min/1.73 $m^2$ (Fig. 54.2).[56] After adjustment for numerous potential confounders, the odds of having left ventricular hypertrophy were more than double among patients with an eGFR less than 30 mL/min/1.73 $m^2$ compared with those with an eGFR 60 or higher mL/min/1.73 $m^2$ (odds ratio, 2.2; 95% confidence interval [CI] 1.4 to 3.4). Left ventricular hypertrophy is also recognized in children in whom other confounding diseases are less common (see Fig. 54.2).[61]

Recognizing that categorization is complicated by volume changes related to dialysis, Foley and associates found that 44% of patients had predominantly left ventricular wall thickening (concentric hypertrophy), and 30% had predominantly increased cavity volume (eccentric hypertrophy) in a study of patients starting dialysis.[11] Such changes are likely to represent adaptations to volume and pressure overload.[62] Volume overload increases left ventricular filling pressure and thereby stretches the ventricular wall. The heart adapts by lengthening existing myocytes, thus enlarging the internal dimensions of the left ventricular cavity. This process is usually accompanied by wall thickening, a further adaptive response that reduces wall stress. Thus volume overload results in a ventricle with a thickened wall and enlarged cavity, but with a normal wall thickness–to–internal diameter ratio (eccentric hypertrophy). In contrast, pressure overload increases wall stress during systole, leading to myocyte proliferation and wall thickening, with preservation or reduction of cavity volume (concentric hypertrophy; Fig. 54.3). The previous adaptive responses, which may be reversible in the early stages, are essentially beneficial, at least initially. Dilation permits increased cardiac output for a similar level of energy expenditure, whereas wall thickening redistributes increased tension over a larger area and reduces energy consumption/myocyte.[63] Nevertheless, despite such adaptation, volume overload has recently been shown to be associated with poor outcomes (independently of any effect on blood pressure) in a large cohort of hemodialysis patients.[64]

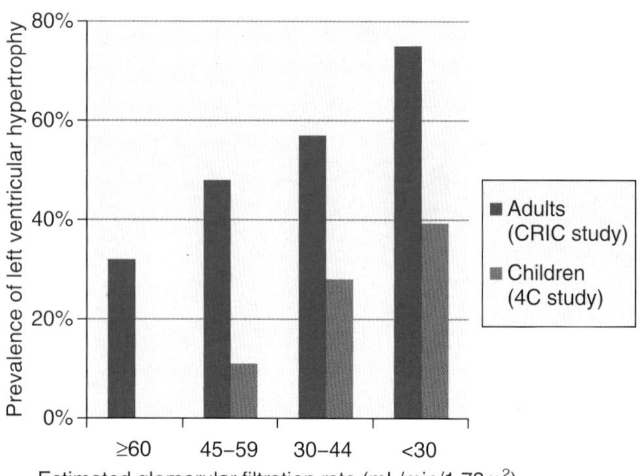


**Fig. 54.2** Prevalence of left ventricular hypertrophy in adults and children by estimated glomerular filtration rate. (From Park M, Hsu CY, Li Y, et al. Associations between kidney function and subclinical cardiac abnormalities in CKD. *J Am Soc Nephrol* 2012;23:1725-1734; Schaefer F, Doyon A, Azukaitis K, et al. Cardiovascular phenotypes in children with CKD: The 4C Study. *Clin J Am Soc Nephrol* 2017;12:19-28.)

Cardiac magnetic resonance studies have allowed the geometry of the heart to be assessed in a volume-independent manner. Such studies have identified two major types of cardiomyopathy in patients with advanced CKD.[65] Gadolinium-based contrast studies have shown that over two-thirds of patients have left ventricular hypertrophy, with preserved systolic volume and function, which is associated with diffuse myocardial fibrosis. Left ventricular dilation and impaired systolic function were observed in another 15% of patients but, by contrast, this was associated strongly with traditional atherosclerotic risk factors and a higher burden of CAD on angiography.[65] However, the recognition of gadolinium-induced nephrogenic systemic fibrosis has meant that such studies can no longer be conducted until a safer contrast agent has been identified.

## IMPAIRED ANGIOGENESIS

Maintaining perfusion to a hypertrophied left ventricle requires capillary angiogenesis, but this is disturbed in CKD—hence the term "impaired angio-adaptation." In the rat model of subtotal nephrectomy, capillary rarefaction begins

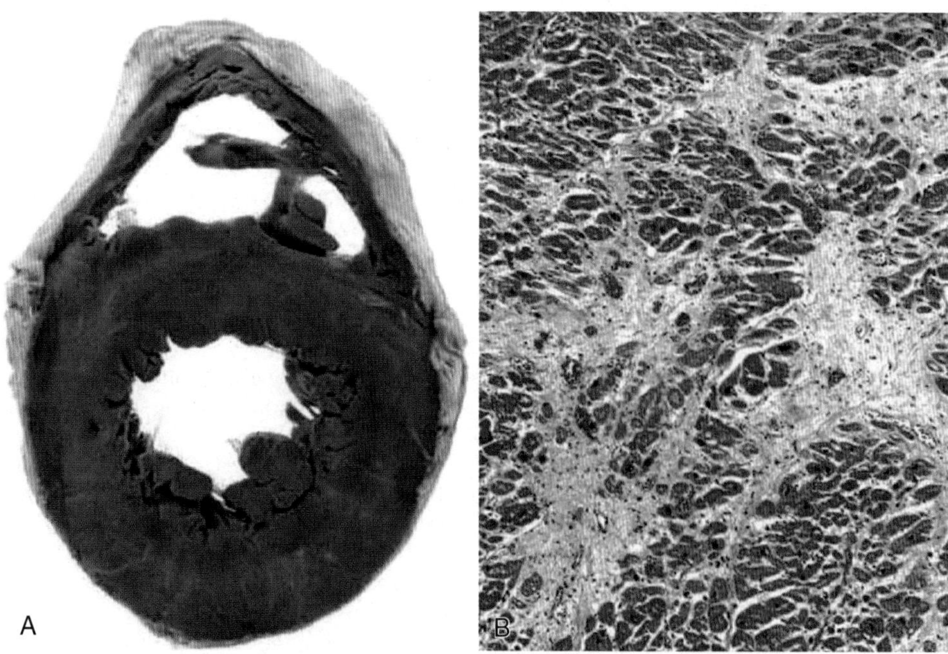


**Fig. 54.3** Myocardial disease in chronic kidney disease (CKD). (A) A cross-section of a postmortem heart from a patient with long-standing CKD showing concentric left ventricular hypertrophy. (B) Histologic analysis often reveals myocardial fibrosis (pale staining) disrupting the normal architecture of cardiac myocytes. (A, Courtesy AJ Howie; B, Courtesy Dr. M. Rubens.)

at about 8 to 12 weeks after induction and is progressive.[66] Consequently, such myocardium is more susceptible to an ischemic insult, as demonstrated by the increased volume of myocardium that infarcts in this rat model compared with a healthy rat with a similar ischemic insult.[66] Patients with CKD demonstrate more ischemia on stress than patients with preserved kidney function, and this difference is not simply explained by the burden of traditional cardiovascular risk factors or of coronary atheroma.[67] The cause of the reduced angiogenesis is unclear, although the fact that other tissues such as skeletal muscle and the skin are similarly affected suggests an imbalance in systemic angiogenic factors, such as vascular endothelial growth factor (VEGF) and its receptors, in particular soluble fms-like tyrosine kinase-1 (sFlt-1).[68]

## MYOCARDIAL FIBROSIS

In the longer term, excess myocyte work leads to cell death and interstitial cardiac fibrosis.[59] Such maladaptive changes may be exacerbated by ischemia. Even in the absence of occlusive coronary artery lesions, there may be a reduction in capillary density to hypertrophied cardiac myocytes, which exacerbates local hypoxia.[69] Furthermore, stiffening of conduit arteries leads to a fall in diastolic pressure, which in turn may compromise coronary artery perfusion during diastole. Finally, it is possible that repetitive myocardial ischemia induced by hemodialysis exacerbates myocyte injury.[70] A mismatch in oxygen supply and demand to the myocardium might explain the well-recognized clinical observation that patients on dialysis are prone to develop angina, even in the absence of occlusive lesions in the major epicardial coronary arteries (i.e., demand ischemia).[71]

An alternative explanation for the changes described is that patients develop a distinct uremic cardiomyopathy, defined as a primary disease of cardiac muscle associated with CKD and causing systolic dysfunction.[72] Characteristic histologic changes include interstitial myocardial fibrosis. Such pathologic changes may occur early in the course of CKD[73] and could be the result of metabolic changes (e.g., elevations in fibroblast growth factor 23 [FGF23] concentrations; see later, "Fibroblast Growth Factor 23") or neurohormonal adaptations (e.g., activation of the renin-angiotensin system), rather than a response to changes in left ventricular geometry.[74]

## CHANGES TO LEFT VENTRICULAR FUNCTION

In the early stages of left ventricular remodeling, indices of systolic function may be preserved by the Starling mechanism and increased sympathetic activity.[59] However, in the longer term, impaired myocardial contractility ensues, together with a reduction in ejection fraction (or systolic dysfunction). Echocardiographic studies have suggested that systolic dysfunction is present in approximately 20% of patients on maintenance dialysis.[75] The disease is clinically silent in the early stages, but in due course patients may develop symptoms suggestive of congestive cardiac failure. Furthermore, symptoms may result from diastolic dysfunction (see later) in patients with a well-preserved ejection fraction.[76] Severe systolic dysfunction may lead to a fall in systolic blood pressure in a previously hypertensive patient, a phenomenon that may help explain the association between lower systolic pressure and mortality in patients on dialysis (see "Blood Pressure").[77] Observational studies have suggested that systolic dysfunction improves following successful kidney transplantation, even in patients with severe disease.[78] Thus the practice of excluding such individuals from transplant waiting lists should be questioned, particularly if prolonged dialysis or CKD exacerbates myocardial dysfunction.[79]

The histologic changes to the myocardium described previously undoubtedly contribute to diastolic dysfunction, which is characterized by impaired ventricular relaxation and reduced ventricular compliance. Compared with systolic dysfunction, diastolic dysfunction is more likely to lead to clinical manifestations such as heart failure. A patient with a stiff left ventricle may be particularly sensitive to tachyarrhythmia (e.g., atrial fibrillation) or an increase in intravascular volume and pulmonary edema, whereas intravascular volume depletion results in reduced ventricular filling (with a risk of syncope) and hemodynamic instability on dialysis.[80] Diastolic dysfunction is more common than systolic dysfunction in patients on dialysis, being present in approximately 50% of prevalent patients,[81] and may be associated with an even worse prognosis than systolic dysfunction.[82]

## VALVULAR DISEASES

Calcification of the mitral and/or aortic valve is four times more common in patients on dialysis than in matched controls and is associated with increased intima-media thickening and arterial calcification, perhaps suggesting a common pathogenic mechanism.[60] Consequences of valvular calcification include acceleration of aortic sclerosis—and possible progression to symptomatic aortic stenosis and consequent pressure overload of the left ventricle[83]—and incompetence of the mitral valve (exacerbated by left ventricular dilation), which, if present, further contributes to volume overload of the left ventricle.

## DYSRHYTHMIA

Chronic kidney disease is associated with impaired intracardiac conduction, manifest as prolongation of the PQ and QRS intervals.[84] In critically ill patients[85] and infarct survivors[86] an eGFR less than 60 mL/min/1.73 m$^2$ has been consistently associated with two- to threefold increases in the risk of arrhythmias, such as atrial fibrillation, ventricular tachycardia, and ventricular fibrillation. The prevalence of arrhythmias is high among dialysis patients, with one study identifying nonsustained and sustained ventricular tachycardia in 25% and 57% of hemodialysis patients, respectively.[87] The contribution that these abnormalities make to the increased risk of sudden death among patients on dialysis and after transplantation is not known.

Most of the studies of electrophysiology in patients with CKD have been conducted in the hemodialysis population and therefore represent one extreme of the CKD phenotype. Hemodialysis is associated with particular risk factors that are known to trigger dysrhythmias, such as large changes in extravascular volume and rapid electrolyte shifts.[88] The excess of deaths around the first dialysis session of the week (i.e., after the typical longer interdialytic interval) also suggest these hemodialysis-specific factors are important[89] but perhaps not generalizable to other patients with CKD. However, other findings in this population do suggest that features associated with CKD per se, such as the presence of autonomic neuropathy (most marked among patients with diabetes) and reduced heart rate variability,[90,91] predispose to dysrhythmias.

Atrial fibrillation is also more common among patients with CKD.[92,93] The development of atrial fibrillation can reduce cardiac output in patients with left ventricular hypertrophy, who may rely on atrial contraction to fill the left ventricle. Furthermore, CKD is also a risk factor for thromboembolic complications of atrial fibrillation.[94] However, there is uncertainty about anticoagulation because the absolute excess of bleeding events is larger, so the risk-benefit balance is unproven (see discussion in Chapter 55). Furthermore, synthesis of matrix Gla protein (an important endogenous calcification inhibitor) is vitamin K–dependent; thus vitamin K antagonists may lead to excess vascular calcification.[93]

## CLINICAL MANIFESTATIONS OF CARDIOVASCULAR DISEASE IN CHRONIC KIDNEY DISEASE

Whereas CAD explains over half of cardiovascular mortality in the general population,[95] studies have shown that CAD accounts for less than 20% of cardiovascular mortality in dialysis patients.[96–98] At some point therefore in the natural history of CKD, nonatherosclerotic cardiovascular disease evolves to become the dominant pathology.

As the GFR falls, there is an increasing burden of arterial stiffness and structural heart disease.[56,62,99] The clinical picture in patients with structural heart disease but normal kidney function includes heart failure, arrhythmias, and sudden cardiac death (SCD).[100] Similar syndromes are also observed in patients with advanced CKD. Data from the United States have suggested that the annual incidence of SCD in the CKD population is 2.8%, which is five times that in the general population.[101] In the dialysis population, SCD accounts for over half of all cardiovascular mortality.[101,102] Strategies that target nonatherosclerotic cardiac disease are required, and randomized trials of these strategies should be a high priority.

Although atherosclerotic disease may account for a smaller proportion of cardiovascular events among persons with advanced CKD, the absolute risk of atherosclerotic events is high: the risk of myocardial infarction among such patients is around 2% to 3% annually.[96,97] Strategies that target atherosclerotic disease may therefore be effective at reducing the burden of cardiovascular disease in those with advanced CKD.[101]

## EPIDEMIOLOGY OF CARDIOVASCULAR DISEASE IN CARDIOVASCULAR DISEASE

Although the association between CKD and cardiovascular disease first became apparent from observations in young patients on dialysis, it is now recognized that the increased risk starts much earlier in the natural history of CKD.

### ASSOCIATION BETWEEN KIDNEY FUNCTION AND CARDIOVASCULAR DISEASE

Numerous studies have shown that there is an inverse association between kidney function (at least as measured by the GFR or an estimate thereof) and cardiovascular risk.[8,104–110] Studies that have assessed the relationship between kidney function and cardiovascular risk generally fall into three categories—community-based prospective epidemiologic studies, observational data from randomized controlled trials, and analyses of health care management databases. Despite differences in the populations studied and adjustment for confounding variables, the results are surprisingly consistent. A metaanalysis of 19 creatinine-based studies (including over 160,000 events) has shown that for each 30% reduction in eGFR, the risk of major vascular events, which includes nonfatal and fatal events, increases by about 30%.[111]

The Chronic Kidney Disease Prognosis Consortium has combined the results of 21 studies in the general population.[9] After adjustment for age, gender, ethnicity, diabetes, blood pressure, total cholesterol, smoking, and history of cardiovascular disease, a lower eGFR was associated with an increased risk of death from any cardiovascular cause as compared with the reference group (eGFR, 90–104 mL/min/1.73 m$^2$; Fig. 54.4).

However, very few of the available studies have sought to assess the nature of any associations between reduced eGFR and particular types of cardiac events, such as coronary artery disease, heart failure, and cardiac arrhythmia. A community-based prospective study from Iceland has demonstrated an inverse relationship between eGFR and coronary artery disease specifically, but few participants had CKD and, if present, it was mild (mean eGFR in the CKD group, 58.7 mL/min/1.73 m$^2$).[110] Such information will be essential if we are to develop a better understanding of the reasons why reduced kidney function is associated with an excess risk of the aggregate of deaths from any cardiovascular cause.

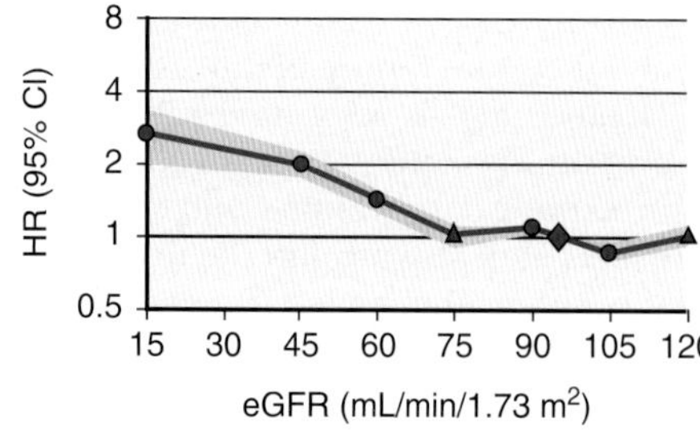


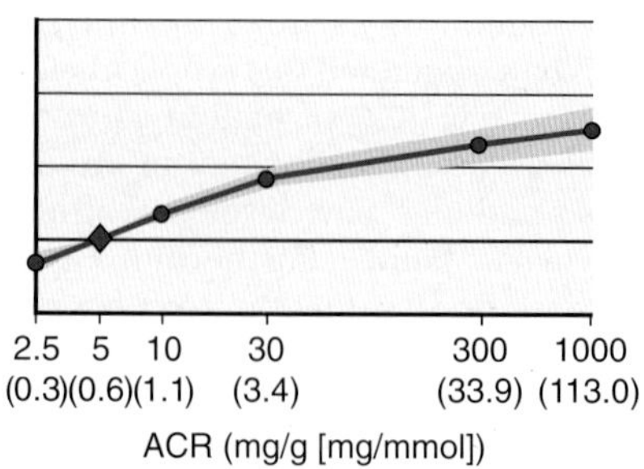


**Fig. 54.4** Association between the estimated glomerular filtration rate (eGFR; *left panel*) and albuminuria *(right panel)* and cardiovascular mortality. This meta analysis included data from 1,234,182 participants in 21 cohorts from the general population. The albumin-to-creatinine ratio (ACR) was available from 14 studies of 105,872 participants.[9]

## ASSOCIATION BETWEEN ALBUMINURIA AND CARDIOVASCULAR DISEASE

Data from the Chronic Kidney Disease Prognosis Consortium have indicated that among persons without known kidney disease, a higher level of albuminuria is associated with an increased risk of cardiovascular disease, and there is no apparent threshold below which lower albuminuria is not associated with lower risk (see Fig. 54.4).[9] In another meta-analysis of 26 cohorts with over 7000 coronary events, there was a continuous association between the degree of albuminuria and risk of coronary artery disease.[112] Compared with "normal" levels of albuminuria (i.e., <2.5 mg/mmol in men or <3.5 mg/mmol in women), microalbuminuria (i.e., <30 mg/mmol) was associated with a 50% increase in risk of coronary artery disease (HR, 1.47; 95.% CI, 1.30–1.66), and macroalbuminuria (≥30 mg/mmol) was independently associated with a doubling of risk (HR, 2.17; 95% CI, 1.87–2.52). The association between albuminuria and cardiovascular risk appears to be independent of the GFR.[9,10,113]

Because leakage of albumin into the extravascular space may occur as a result of endothelial dysfunction, it has been suggested that some albuminuria may represent a renal manifestation of progressive, diffuse arterial disease.[114,115] If true, this could imply that some or all of the observed association between albuminuria and cardiovascular disease is attributable to residual "confounding by disease," in which unmeasured vascular disease (manifest as endothelial dysfunction) is both a cause of albuminuria and of cardiovascular events. Because available treatments that reduce albumin leakage also exert other salutary effects on cardiovascular risk, it is unlikely that the multiple benefits of these therapies could be disentangled. It therefore remains unclear whether reducing albuminuria per se will reduce the risk of vascular disease. Indeed, trials of more -intensive versus less intensive albuminuria reduction strategies (e.g., adding angiotensin-converting enzyme or direct renin inhibitors to angiotensin receptor blockers) have not shown additional cardiovascular protection, although their statistical power to do so was limited.[116,117]

## KIDNEY DISEASE AS A CAUSE OF CARDIOVASCULAR DISEASE

As described in earlier chapters, the kidneys are responsible for a wide variety of physiologic processes, including clearance of metabolic waste products, salt and water balance, blood pressure regulation, and hormone production. Even mild kidney disease has direct effects on the regulation of these processes and could therefore potentially lead to disturbed function and metabolism in other systems, including the cardiovascular system. It is of considerable interest therefore to consider to what extent the excess risk of cardiovascular disease in CKD could be explained by such disturbances.

In this section and later (Indirect Risk Factors: Causes of Both Kidney and Cardiovascular Disease) we suggest a framework for considering the evolution of cardiovascular risk in CKD, as illustrated in Fig. 54.5. We consider two main types of risk factors:

1. Direct risk factors (e.g., hypertension) that arise as a direct consequence of kidney damage and are associated with one or more types of cardiovascular disease (Table 54.1)

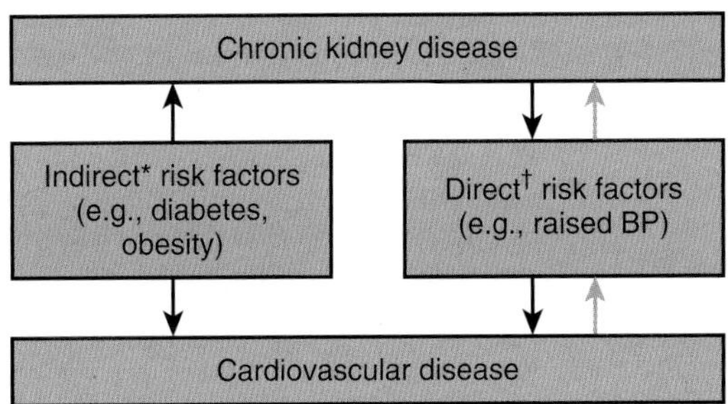


**Fig. 54.5** The relationship between chronic kidney disease (CKD) and cardiovascular disease is mediated by direct and indirect risk factors. *Indirect risk factors are those that cause both renal disease and one or more types of cardiovascular disease; †Direct risk factors are those that arise as a direct consequence of kidney damage and are associated with one or more types of cardiovascular disease.

2. Indirect risk factors (e.g., diabetes mellitus, obesity) that cause both kidney disease and one or more types of cardiovascular disease (see later)

In general, observational studies of particular risk factors among persons with kidney disease may not provide quantitatively reliable information about any associations that might exist because of the difficulty of adjusting for confounding by disease, also known as "reverse causality."[15] For example, reduced left ventricular function in patients on dialysis may lead to lower blood pressure, yielding an apparent association between lower blood pressure and cardiovascular mortality, which is not one of cause and effect.[15,118] Paradoxically therefore it may be more appropriate to rely chiefly on epidemiologic studies performed in nonrenal populations when assessing the potential relevance of particular risk factors to the cause of the various types of cardiovascular disease observed in CKD.

## BLOOD PRESSURE

The kidney is centrally involved in blood pressure regulation. Even relatively mild kidney damage can raise blood pressure, mediated by salt and water retention (and hence intravascular volume expansion), sympathetic overactivity, activation of the renin-angiotensin system, and accumulation of endogenous vasopressors.[119] In turn, hypertension can damage the kidneys further, leading to a vicious cycle of rising blood pressure (with arterial hyalinosis and vascular stiffening) and declining GFR. Evidence from kidney donors, who are selected for being healthy and in particular having preserved kidney function, have suggested that a 10-mL/min/1.73 m$^2$ reduction in GFR leads directly (i.e., causally) to a 5-mm Hg increase in systolic blood pressure. However, this may be an underestimate because elevations in blood pressure are likely to be treated in this population.[113]

Hypertension is strongly associated with several different types of cardiovascular disease in the general population. Prospective epidemiologic studies have indicated that there is a log-linear association between higher blood pressure and an increased risk of coronary artery disease, ischemic and hemorrhagic stroke, and congestive heart failure. The Prospective Studies Collaboration, in a meta analysis of 61 prospective studies (which included a total of 1,000,000 adults without prior cardiovascular disease and 56,000 cardiovascular

**Table 54.1 Direct Risk Factors Linking Chronic Kidney Disease and Cardiovascular Disease[a]**

| Risk Factor | Estimated Change (for each 10-mL/min/1.73 $m^2$ lower eGFR[b]) | Approximate Stage of Chronic Kidney Disease at Which Abnormality Manifests | Approximate Relative Risk[c] | Causal? | Comments |
|---|---|---|---|---|---|
| **Coronary Artery Disease** | | | | | |
| Systolic blood pressure | ↑5 mm Hg | 1–2 | 1.2 | Yes | Reliable data from large-scale observational[120] and RCTs[121] support a causal relationship. |
| HDL cholesterol | ↓0.2–0.4 mmol/L | 3 | 1.2 | Possible | Large-scale observational studies support an inverse association with coronary disease.[128] Genetic studies and randomized trials are inconclusive. |
| Lipoprotein(a) | ↑0.2–0.4 µmol/L | 3 | <1.5 | Possible | Genetic studies support a causal association with coronary disease and aortic valve disease.[138,203] Most of excess risk is in the top fifth of lipoprotein(a) distribution—that is, individuals with smaller apolipoprotein(a) particles; requires confirmation in trials. |
| Triglycerides | ↑0.1 mmol/L | 3 | 1.1 | Possible | Classical observational studies are unclear, but genetic data support a causal association; requires confirmation in trials. |
| Phosphate | ↑0.3 mmol/L | 3b–4 | 1.4 | Possible | Observational studies in general population[170] suggest possible causal link; requires confirmation in trials. |
| PTH | ↑3 pmol/L | 3 | 1.3 | Possible | Observational studies in general population suggest possible causal link.[190,204] |
| Anemia | ↓0.2–0.5 g/dL | 3b–4 | — | No | RCTs in CKD population do not show that correcting anemia improves cardiac outcomes.[205] |
| Homocysteine | ↑0.5 µmol/L | 3 | <1.5 | No | RCTs do not demonstrate reduced CHD risk with reduction in homocysteine.[161] |
| Uric acid | 10-15 µmol/L | 2–3 | 1.1 | No | Mendelian randomization studies suggest observed associations are probably confounded.[202] |
| **Congestive Heart Failure** | | | | | |
| Systolic blood pressure | ↑5 mm Hg | 1 | 1.2 | Yes | Reliable data from large-scale observational[120] and RCTs[121] support causal relationship. |
| Phosphate | ↑0.3 mmol/L | 3b–4 | 1.4 | Possible | Observational studies in general population[170] suggest possible causal link; requires confirmation in trials. |
| PTH | ↑3 pmol/L | 3 | 1.3 | Possible | Observational studies in general population (and secondary outcomes of trials) suggest possible causal link.[190,204,206] |
| Anemia | ↓0.2–0.5 g/dL | 3b–4 | — | No | Although observational data support link between anemia and structural heart disease,[147] randomized trials do not show that correcting anemia improves cardiac outcomes.[205] |
| FGF23 | ↑10 RU/mL (varies across range of GFR) | 1–2 | <1.5 | Possible | Supportive experimental and observational data in CKD and general population.[180] |
| **Stroke** | | | | | |
| Systolic blood pressure | ↑5 mm Hg | 1–2 | 1.3 | Yes | Reliable data from large-scale observational[120] and RCTs[121] support causal relationship. |
| HDL cholesterol | ↓0.2–0.4 mmol/L | 3 | 1.1 | Possible | Weak inverse association in observational studies.[128] |
| Phosphate | ↑0.3 mmol/L | 3b–4 | 1.4 | Possible | Observational studies in general population[170] suggest possible causal link. |

**Table 54.1 Direct Risk Factors Linking Chronic Kidney Disease and Cardiovascular Disease[a] (Cont'd)**

| Risk Factor | Estimated Change (for each 10-mL/min/1.73 m² lower eGFR[b]) | Approximate Stage of Chronic Kidney Disease at Which Abnormality Manifests | Approximate Relative Risk[c] | Causal? | Comments |
|---|---|---|---|---|---|
| Anemia | ↓0.2–0.5 g/dL | 3b–4 | — | No | No supportive observational data in general population.[207] RCTs in CKD population suggest that correcting anemia with ESA may cause stroke.[208] |
| Homocysteine | ↑0.5 μmol/L | 3 | <1.5 | No | RCTs do not demonstrate reduced stroke risk with reduction in homocysteine.[161] |

[a]The table shows typical differences in risk factors for coronary artery disease, stroke, and congestive heart failure between patients with mild renal impairment and middle-aged healthy general population.
[b]Associated with change in risk factor induced by a 10-mL/min reduction in the GFR.
[c]Associated with change in risk factor induced by 10 mL/min reduction in GFR.
*CHD*, Coronary heart disease; *eGFR*, estimated glomerular filtration rate; *ESA*, erythropoiesis-stimulating agent; *PTH*, parathyroid hormone; *RCT*, randomized controlled trial.

deaths), has shown that a prolonged 20-mm Hg increment in usual systolic blood pressure is associated with a more than twofold higher risk of stroke-related death and a twofold higher risk of death due to coronary artery disease and of death from heart failure.[120]

That these associations are causal has been established reliably by randomized trials showing that lowering systolic blood pressure reduces the risk of stroke, coronary artery disease, and of other cardiovascular diseases, with every 5-mm Hg reduction associated with a reduction of about 29% in risk.[121] The results are broadly similar for different classes of antihypertensive treatment, although there is some evidence to suggest that inhibitors of the renin-angiotensin system may have particularly beneficial effects on the risk of heart failure.[122]

Because hypertension appears very early in the natural history of CKD, a patient who has progressed to stage 3 CKD will generally have been exposed to a prolonged increase in blood pressure, which, depending on the degree of treatment received, would be expected to contribute substantially to the subsequent risk of nonatherosclerotic and atherosclerotic cardiovascular disease. For example, a 5-mm Hg difference resulting from a mild reduction in GFR (e.g., from 90 to 80 mL/min/1.73 m$^2$) could translate into an increase of about 25% for the risk of stroke death and 20% for the risks of coronary artery disease–associated death and other cardiovascular death. These relative risks may be substantially larger in younger individuals, in whom the association between blood pressure and cardiovascular death is stronger than in older individuals.[120]

## DYSLIPIDEMIA

The characteristic lipid profile resulting from impaired kidney function beyond about stage 3 CKD is an accumulation of partially catabolized, triglyceride-rich, very-low-density lipoprotein (VLDL) and intermediate-density lipoprotein (IDL) particles, leading to an elevated serum triglyceride concentration, with lower high-density-lipoprotein (HDL) cholesterol concentrations. LDL cholesterol concentration in CKD is similar or lower than the population average, except that nephrotic-range proteinuria leads to an increase in LDL cholesterol.[123] Cholesterol continues to be progressively removed from these particles, and triacylglycerol is added, leading to an excess of small, dense, LDL particles, which may be more atherogenic.[124] HDL function may also be impaired in CKD.[125] In addition, lipoprotein(a)—Lp(a)—concentrations are increased in association with CKD; again, this abnormality is a direct result of impaired kidney function because it can be normalized by kidney transplantation.[126,127]

Based on what is known from epidemiologic studies in persons without CKD, it remains unclear whether the typical dyslipidemia seen in CKD would be expected to result in a large increase in the risk of atherosclerotic events in patients with (nonnephrotic) CKD. Although it is clear from epidemiologic studies[95,128] and large-scale randomized trials[129] that elevated LDL cholesterol is a contributing cause of atherosclerotic events, the observed incidence of atherosclerotic events in CKD cannot be caused chiefly by increased LDL cholesterol concentrations because such an abnormality occurs in a minority of patients, usually in association with severe proteinuria.

The relevance of the increased triglyceride concentrations is unclear. Traditional observational epidemiologic studies have suggested that the positive association between triglyceride concentration and cardiovascular risk is confounded and does not persist once adjustment is made for HDL cholesterol and other confounders.[128] However, more recent genetic epidemiologic studies have shown that single-nucleotide polymorphisms (SNPs) associated with higher triglyceride concentrations are also associated with higher cardiovascular risk, and that this association is attenuated by adjustment for triglyceride concentration, suggesting that triglycerides are causally associated with cardiovascular risk.[130] In cross-sectional studies, triglyceride concentrations increase as the GFR falls, so that a 10-mL/min/1.73 m$^2$ reduction in the eGFR is associated with about a 0.1-mmol/L increase in triglyceride concentration.[131]

HDL cholesterol is generally reduced in CKD. In one study, for example, patients on hemodialysis had a mean HDL cholesterol of 0.89 mmol/L compared with 1.4 mmol/L in healthy controls.[132] Prospective studies have shown that a 0.4-mmol/L (15-mg/dL) higher HDL cholesterol is associated with a 20% reduction in coronary events (HR, 0.78; 95% CI, 0.74–0.82),[128] whereas the association with ischemic stroke is less clear.[128,133] However, trials of drugs that can raise HDL cholesterol have so far not shown clear benefit, and genetic studies have also been inconclusive.[134–137] Thus it remains unclear whether reduced HDL cholesterol is a cause of coronary heart disease (CHD) in the general or CKD population.

It is also possible that an elevated Lp(a) might contribute to an increase in risk of CHD. Modest reductions in the GFR are associated with an increase of 0.2 to 0.4 μmol/L in Lp(a) concentrations,[126] and genetic data have strongly suggested that there is a causal association between Lp(a) concentration and coronary artery disease in the general population.[138] However, most of the excess risk attributable to Lp(a) occurs among individuals with smaller apolipoprotein(a)—apo(a)—moieties, which is largely genetically determined by the number of kringle(IV) repeats,[139] whereas most of the increase in Lp(a) among patients with CKD occurs in patients with larger apo(a) moieties.[126] It is therefore uncertain how much of the excess risk of CHD observed in CKD can be attributed to altered Lp(a) metabolism.[140]

In summary, it is unclear to what extent the dyslipidemia typically found in association with CKD contributes materially to the excess risk of atherosclerotic cardiovascular disease observed in CKD. However, in the general population, reducing LDL cholesterol reduces the risk of atherosclerotic events, even among people with average or low LDL cholesterol values,[129] and this strategy has also proven effective in reducing atherosclerotic risk in CKD (see "Cardiovascular risk prevention: Dislipidemia").

## OTHER DIRECT RISK FACTORS

In addition to increased blood pressure, which has an established association with cardiovascular disease in the general population, several other metabolic disturbances caused by kidney disease may contribute to some of the increased risk of cardiovascular disease.

### COAGULATION DEFECTS

Chronic kidney disease is associated with raised fibrinogen concentrations, which in turn would increase plasma viscosity and modulate coagulation in a procoagulant direction.[141,142] Chronic kidney disease also increases factor VIII and von Willebrand factor concentrations.[143] Although increases in fibrinogen are not well characterized in CKD, a 1-g/L increase in fibrinogen concentration has been reported in one study.[143] Epidemiologic studies in the general population have suggested that after adjustment for potential confounders, such an increase is associated with a 1.8-fold excess risk of coronary disease, stroke, and other cardiovascular events.[144] However, the lack of an association between genetic variants that determine fibrinogen concentrations and cardiovascular risk make it less plausible that raised fibrinogen itself is a cause of atherosclerotic disease, so the relevance of any such increase in CKD is uncertain.[145]

### ANEMIA

Anemia in CKD is caused by a combination of factors, which include erythropoietin deficiency, functional iron deficiency, and chronic inflammation (see Chapter 55). The effects of chronic anemia on the cardiovascular system are not well studied in the general population because anemia is generally associated with disease. In CKD, however, anemia is associated with left ventricular hypertrophy, in one study, a 0.5-g/dL lower hemoglobin concentration was associated with a 30% higher frequency of increased left ventricular mass (defined as 20% greater than baseline).[146] In another study of dialysis patients, each 1-g/dL decrease in hemoglobin was associated with a 50% increased risk of left ventricular dilation and a 25% increased risk of cardiac failure.[147]

Although some small nonrandomized studies have suggested that partial correction of anemia reduces left ventricular mass index in patients with CKD,[148,149] randomized trials have not shown that complete correction of anemias, compared with partial correction, leads to a reduction in left ventricular mass.[150–152] It is therefore unclear whether anemia is a cause of structural heart disease in CKD but, because it does not appear until a significant amount of kidney function is lost (e.g., eGFR < ≈40 mL/min/1.73 m²),[153] it seems unlikely that it could contribute substantially to the excess risk of cardiovascular disease observed among those with a higher eGFR. The results of randomized trials of treatments to increase hemoglobin that involved assessment of cardiovascular endpoints are discussed later ("Cardiovascular risk prevention: Anemia") and reviewed in the context of treatments of anemia in Chapter 55.

### HOMOCYSTEINE

The observation that homocystinuria, which results in very large increase in plasma homocysteine concentrations is associated with premature cardiovascular disease led to interest in whether more moderate increases in homocysteine might be associated with an increased risk of coronary artery disease.[154] Homocysteine concentrations have a strong inverse association with the GFR and, because they are reduced by kidney transplantation, the rise in the homocysteine level is a direct result of impaired kidney function.[155] However, the mechanism(s) underlying hyperhomocysteinemia in CKD are complex and not fully understood. They are not attributable to reduced clearance, because renal homocysteine excretion accounts for less than 1% of its elimination, so it must instead involve metabolic disturbances in remethylation and transsulfuration pathways.[156] Moderate reductions in the GFR are associated with a 5-μmol/L increase in total plasma homocysteine.[157]

A meta analysis of prospective observational studies has shown that a 25% lower usual homocysteine concentration (≈3 μmol/L) is associated with an 11% lower risk of coronary disease and a 19% lower risk of stroke.[158] The earliest genetic studies of *MTHFR* mutations appeared consistent with this association being causal,[159] but subsequent metaanalysis of all available genetic data have indicated that such an association is unlikely to reflect causality.[160] Large-scale randomized trials of folate and B vitamins, which reduce plasma homocysteine concentration, have also failed to demonstrate a benefit of lowering homocysteine (see later, "Cardiovascular risk prevention: Homocysteine").[161–163]

## CHRONIC KIDNEY DISEASE AND MINERAL BONE DISORDERS

In regard to chronic kidney disease and mineral bone disorders (CKD-MBD), impaired kidney function causes a complex disorder of calcium and phosphate metabolism, including effects on vitamin D and parathyroid hormone (see Chapter 53 for a detailed description), which become especially marked after stage 3b CKD. Because such abnormalities are uncommon in persons without CKD, the information we have available is therefore derived mostly from observational studies conducted in patients with CKD, which, because of the likelihood of residual confounding, severely limits their interpretation.

### Phosphate

Serum phosphate concentrations rise once the kidney's ability to excrete the dietary phosphate load is exceeded.[153] Multiple homeostatic processes are in place to maintain serum phosphorus concentrations in the normal range, despite diminished excretion with impaired kidney function, and hence a serum phosphate concentration within the reference range does not necessarily imply normal phosphate metabolism.[164] Higher serum phosphate concentrations are associated with increased arterial stiffness[165,166] and calcification,[167,168] perhaps because hyperphosphatemia can induce vascular smooth muscle cells to develop an osteoblastic phenotype.[169] Such arterial stiffness could plausibly increase the risk of structural heart disease and thereby of heart failure and cardiac arrhythmias[76]

At least within the range of concentrations observed in the general population, there is an association between higher serum phosphate levels and increased risk of cardiovascular events and mortality.[170,171] In the Framingham Offspring Study, for example, a 1-mg/dL (0.32-mmol/L) increment in the serum phosphate level was associated with an increase in the risk of cardiovascular disease—namely, coronary artery disease, stroke, peripheral arterial disease, or heart failure—of about one-third (HR, 1.30; 95% CI, 1.05–1.63) after adjustment for conventional cardiovascular risk factors and the eGFR.[170] However, there were too few events to allow the association with heart failure to be assessed separately from typical atherosclerosis-related events.

Randomized trials of treatments that lower serum phosphate levels (e.g., phosphate binders) are required to determine whether hyperphosphatemia, or the counterregulatory processes that are activated in CKD, are causally related to cardiovascular disease. The issue is complicated by the possibility of adverse effects of calcium-containing phosphate binders; these may contribute to vascular calcification by inducing a positive calcium balance, which results in the deposition of calcium in the vasculature rather than bone.[172]

### Fibroblast Growth Factor 23

FGF23 concentrations rise earlier in CKD than the serum concentrations of phosphate or even parathyroid hormone[173] and help maintain a normal serum phosphate concentration via a phosphaturic effect. The association of FGF23 with mortality was first demonstrated in patients on maintenance hemodialysis[174] and, since then, other studies have found associations between FGF23 concentrations and all-cause and cardiovascular mortality in patients with CKD.[175–177] More recently, FGF23 was studied in a population without prior cardiovascular disease and over 10 years of follow-up. In this study, it was again independently associated with all-cause mortality (HR, per doubling 1.25; 95% CI, 1.14–1.36) and incident heart failure events (697 events; HR, 1.41; 95% CI, 1.23–1.61) but not incident atherosclerotic events (797 events; HR, 1.12; 95% CI, 0.98–1.29).[178]

Unlike phosphate, serum FGF23 concentrations do not correlate with arterial calcification.[179] Experimentally, FGF23 has been shown to induce left ventricular hypertrophy in the absence of its coreceptor klotho; furthermore, FGF23 and left ventricular mass are positively associated among patients with CKD and those with normal renal function.[180,181] Assuming that these associations are causal, the biologic mechanisms linking FGF23 with cardiovascular diseases may be different from those for serum phosphate.

### Vitamin D

As discussed in more detail in Chapter 53, vitamin D is activated (via 1α-hydroxylation) by the kidney, and therefore fully active 1,25-dihydroxy vitamin D concentrations decline early in the progression of CKD.[153,182] In addition, rising FGF23 concentrations also inhibit the activation of vitamin D. There is also an association between "native" vitamin D (usually measured as 25-hydroxy vitamin D) concentration and the GFR.[182] However, this may reflect poorer nutrition in patients with chronic disease. Vitamin D deficiency (and subsequent hypocalcaemia) removes negative feedback from the parathyroid glands, and parathyroid hormone (PTH) concentrations therefore rise as GFR falls.[153]

Some observational studies in the general population have suggested that there is an inverse association between 25-hydroxy vitamin D concentrations and subsequent cardiovascular events, whereas others have not.[183] A metaanalysis has demonstrated inverse associations between 25-hydroxy vitamin D and all-cause mortality (and its components including vascular, cancer and other non-vascular causes).[184] Randomized trials of vitamin D supplementation in the general population have not demonstrated a reduction in cardiovascular events.[183] However, it is possible that these trials used doses of vitamin D that were too low to induce a potent enough effect. Some studies have suggested that vitamin D deficiency predisposes patients to diabetes mellitus and raises blood pressure, but again these data are not conclusive.[183] It is unclear whether disturbed vitamin D metabolism could plausibly contribute to the observed excess risk of cardiovascular disease in CKD.

### Parathyroid Hormone

PTH concentrations rise as a direct result of declining GFR early in the progression of CKD; secondary hyperparathyroidism (sHPT) can be found in 20% of patients with CKD stages 1 and 2.[153] PTH rises because of a lack of negative feedback from declining 1,25-hydroxy vitamin D and calcium concentrations and rising concentrations of serum phosphate, even within the population reference range. Parathyroid hormone has been implicated in atherogenesis (and in calcification of atherosclerotic lesions) and also in modifying cardiac fibrosis in animal models.[185,186] There have been case reports of improved myocardial metabolism and structure after parathyroidectomy, suggesting that high concentrations of PTH may damage the heart.[187] There does not appear to be a clear association between PTH and all-cause and cardiovascular mortality in patients with CKD,[188] although one study has reported an association between elevated PTH and all-cause mortality in a cohort of persons with CKD stage 3.[189] Studies in the general population, which may be less prone to confounding, have suggested that there is an independent association between elevated PTH concentrations and fatal and nonfatal cardiovascular disease.[190] A metaanalysis of 12 such studies has shown that the risk of cardiovascular disease is 50% (HR, 1.50; 95% CI, 1.18–1.92) higher among patients in the groups with highest PTH concentration compared with those in the lowest.[190]

### OXIDATIVE STRESS AND INFLAMMATION

Oxidative stress is defined as tissue injury resulting from an excess of oxidant compounds; it is important in protecting against infection and tissue repair. Oxidative stress leads to a reduction in nitric oxide bioavailability and thus to endothelial dysfunction[191] and may also contribute to left ventricular remodeling and fibrosis and oxidation of lipoproteins.[192] Chronic kidney disease is associated with oxidative stress,[193] although precise quantification is difficult. In the general population, dietary intake or plasma concentrations of antioxidant vitamins (vitamin A [beta-carotene], C, and E) are inversely related to cardiovascular disease incidence and mortality,[194] but randomized trials of antioxidant treatments have indicated that at least in the doses studied, use of these drugs does not reduce the risk of cardiovascular disease.[195]

Patients with CKD have increased measures of inflammation compared with age- and gender-matched controls.[141] Genetic data from the general population have suggested that inflammation is causally associated with coronary disease, although the mechanism remains unclear.[196,197] A recently completed trial of canakinumab (an interleukin-1 β [IL-1β] antagonist) in persons with previous myocardial infarction and high-sensitivity C-reactive protein (hs-CRP) greater than 2 mg/L has reported a 15% relative risk reduction (HR, 0.85; 95% CI, 0.74–0.98; $P = .021$)) in nonfatal myocardial infarction or stroke or cardiovascular death observed in the group receiving a dose of 150 mg every 3 months, supporting the hypothesis that inflammation mediated via IL-1β does contribute to atherosclerotic cardiovascular events.[198,199]

### URIC ACID

Uric acid is cleared by the kidney, and its concentration rises as GFR falls (so that each 10- mL/min/1.73 $m^2$ lower eGFR is associated with a 10–15 μmol/L increase in uric acid concentration). Positive associations between uric acid concentration and the risk of CHD have been reported, which would suggest that a 10- to 15-μmol/L increase in uric acid would increase the risk of CHD by about 10%.[200,201] However, mendelian randomization experiments that took account of the pleiotropic effects of genetic variants have cast doubt on whether such associations are causal.[202]

## INDIRECT RISK FACTORS: CAUSES OF KIDNEY AND CARDIOVASCULAR DISEASE

### DIABETES MELLITUS

Diabetes mellitus is a common disease that affects about 150 million people worldwide. The overall prevalence is increasing—driven in part by a rise in the prevalence of obesity and an aging population—and it has been estimated that there will be over 300 million persons globally with type 2 diabetes by 2025.[209] A metaanalysis of 23 studies, including 21, 237 cardiovascular deaths, has found that the risk of cardiovascular death at a given eGFR or urine albumin-to-creatinine ration (UACR) was 1.2 to 1.9 times higher among individuals with diabetes than in those without, with no evidence of an interaction.[210]

Diabetic nephropathy is caused by the hemodynamic effects of chronic hyperglycemia and glycation of structural proteins within the kidney, beginning with the glomerular basement membrane but later causing mesangial and interstitial matrix expansion (see Chapter 39). Approximately 40% of patients new to dialysis in the United States have diabetic nephropathy, and diabetes mellitus is present as a comorbid illness in an additional 10% of patients; in other words, diabetes mellitus is present but is thought not to be the primary cause of ESKD.[101] Strict glycemic control and blood pressure control (with renin-angiotensin system inhibitors) both appear to retard the progression (and perhaps the development) of diabetic nephropathy.[211–215] Patients with diabetes (type 1 or 2) are at increased risk of mortality, and about two-thirds of deaths can be attributed to cardiovascular causes.[216]

Prospective data from a meta analysis of 102 studies with information on fatal and nonfatal outcomes have demonstrated that the presence of diabetes mellitus doubles the risk for coronary heart disease (HR, 2.00; 95% CI, 1.83–2.19).[217] The risk of ischemic stroke was increased by about half (HR, 1.56; 95% CI, 1.56–2.09), hemorrhagic stroke by around four-fifths (HR, 1.84; 95% CI, 1.54–2.13), and other vascular deaths (including heart failure) by about three-quarters (HR, 1.73; 95% CI, 1.51–1.98). These estimates were not significantly affected by adjustment for traditional cardiovascular risk factors (e.g., lipid levels and blood pressure), but were also unaffected by adjustment for kidney function.[217] Among patients with CKD therefore the presence of diabetes mellitus seems likely to contribute additional risk over and above any risk arising from direct risk factors associated with impaired kidney function (see Fig. 54.5).

### OBESITY

In the general population, observational studies have shown that obesity is associated with an increased risk of cardiovascular disease above a body mass index (BMI) of 25 kg/$m^2$, with each 5 kg/$m^2$ associated with an increase in risk of cardiovascular mortality of around 40% (HR, 1.41; 95% CI, 1.37–1.45).[218] This association is probably causal and mediated by the known adverse effects of adiposity on blood pressure, lipoprotein levels, and glucose intolerance.

Obesity is also known to increase the risk of death from nonneoplastic kidney disease by about 60% (HR, 1.59; 95% CI, 1.27–1.99) per 5 kg/$m^2$ above a BMI of 25 kg/$m^2$.[218] A systematic review has indicated that as compared with a BMI of 18 to 25 kg/$m^2$, being overweight (BMI $\geq$ 25 but < 30 kg/$m^2$) is associated with a 40% (HR, 1.40; 95% CI, 1.30–1.50) increase in the risk of kidney disease, whereas being obese (BMI $\geq$ 30 kg/$m^2$) is associated with an 80% increased risk (HR, 1.83; 95% CI, 1.57–2.13).[219] This association may be partly mediated by effects on blood pressure and diabetes, but these do not explain all the excess risk observed.[220] Kidney biopsies of overweight individuals (without diabetes or hypertension) may show typical features of glomerular hyperfiltration, a known mechanism of premature decline in kidney function.[221] Furthermore, weight loss can reduce blood pressure and proteinuria.[222]

## CARDIOVASCULAR RISK PREDICTION

Risk prediction models in the CKD population are desirable because they may help target therapies for those most at risk. Most people with stage 4 or 5 CKD are at high risk of atherosclerotic disease and so would be suitable candidates for effective treatments, but at earlier stages of CKD, the risk of cardiovascular events may be lower, so models are needed to assess who should be treated. Models that involve demographic variables (e.g., age, gender), basic clinical measurements (e.g., blood pressure, anthropometric measurements), and simple blood and urine biomarkers (e.g., lipid fractions, albuminuria) have now been developed, and there are also versions that incorporate imaging or other measurements (e.g., pulse wave velocity).

### BASIC RISK PREDICTION SCORES

Equations have been developed in the general population that can be used to predict cardiovascular events based on knowledge of a few basic parameters. For example, the Framingham risk score requires knowledge of the patient's age, gender, smoking status, total and HDL cholesterol, and systolic blood pressure.[223,224] However, such equations are inaccurate and generally underestimate the incidence of cardiovascular events in patients with CKD.[225]

### ROLE OF ESTIMATED GFR IN RISK PREDICTION

Estimated GFR equations were developed to assess kidney function without the need for invasive direct measurements. Since their introduction, the association between eGFR and cardiovascular risk has been the subject of much research. The most widely used filtration marker is creatinine, but its inadequacies in terms of measuring kidney function are well-recognized (including dependence on muscle mass and significant tubular secretion at low GFR). However, nonrenal determinants of creatinine and other filtration markers such as cystatin C may improve cardiovascular risk prediction[226] because they incorporate information on other cardiovascular risk factors such as diabetes mellitus.[227] Indeed, combining filtration markers may lead to better risk prediction.[228]

### USE OF IMAGING AND OTHER ASSESSMENTS OF CARDIOVASCULAR FUNCTION IN RISK PREDICTION

Blood markers of myocardial damage and dysfunction, such as cardiac troponin and brain natriuretic peptide (B type), strongly predict cardiovascular risk among patients with CKD,[229] including those on dialysis.[230,231] Furthermore, numerous studies have demonstrated that echocardiographic measures can provide useful prognostic information. This includes both static measures (e.g., left ventricular mass) and dynamic measures (e.g., dobutamine stress echocardiography). For example, left ventricular mass predicts mortality in patients on dialysis,[72,232–234] and the presence of systolic dysfunction can provide further information.[235] Echocardiography is therefore recommended for routine use in patients on dialysis,[236] but its additional value over more simple risk stratification tools has not been studied in detail.

CIMT has been used in the general population to predict the risk of cardiovascular events, but variation in the technique used makes comparison of studies difficult. Although CIMT appears to predict the risk of coronary and cerebrovascular events in the general population, it does not appear to provide additional prognostic information to a standard score, such as that derived from the Framingham equation.[237] In the CKD population, it is unclear whether CIMT provides independent prognostic information; one study of 203 Chinese patients with stage 3 or 4 CKD has found that CIMT is independently associated with outcome,[238] whereas another study of 315 stages 4 or 5 CKD patients did not find this relation.[34]

Vascular calcification can also be assessed using x-ray–based methods, and its presence is independently associated with subsequent cardiovascular events.[239,240] However, in the general population, the value of coronary calcification scores is uncertain because it may not add useful information to traditional scores.[241] The incremental predictive value of arterial calcium scoring has not been studied in detail in CKD populations. Similarly, the functional equivalent of calcification (i.e., arterial stiffness) independently predicts the risk of subsequent cardiovascular events in some studies,[34] but the method used may be important (see earlier, "Arterial Stiffening").

The purpose of risk prediction is to identify a high-risk group of patients who will benefit most from interventions. It is important to note that treatment decisions should not be based solely on the risk factor that will be modified by the treatment in question. For example, decisions on whether to lower LDL cholesterol should not be based on measured LDL cholesterol, but rather should be a holistic risk assessment that considers all available data. Treatment decisions based on single risk factors would lead to the undertreatment of the highest-risk patients. The next section will discuss the available evidence from randomized trials of treatments for cardiovascular disease in the CKD population.

## CARDIOVASCULAR RISK PREVENTION

In general, individual treatments for the prevention of cardiovascular events are at best only moderately effective, yielding relative risk reductions of at most 25%, so the detection of such effects can only be reliably achieved through large-scale randomized trials.[242] Observational studies are prone to at least moderate biases that may obscure or mimic treatment effects.[243] Because the pathophysiology of cardiovascular disease may be qualitatively different once patients reach stages 3 to 5 CKD, with a higher proportion of events attributable to structural heart disease, extrapolation of the results of trials conducted in the general population may not be appropriate. It is necessary therefore to consider what information is available from subgroup analyses of large trials, as well as from trials conducted exclusively among patients with CKD, before determining whether to extrapolate results obtained in studies in the general population to patients in varying stages of CKD.

## SMOKING CESSATION

In the general population, cigarette smoking is associated with an increased risk of cardiovascular disease,[244] and the beneficial effects of smoking cessation provide strong evidence that the association is one of cause and effect.[224,245] Substantial numbers of patients with CKD smoke tobacco,[246,247] and recent data have demonstrated that the hazards are similar in patients with CKD to those in the general population.[248] As a consequence, the absolute excess cardiovascular (and noncardiovascular) risks attributable to smoking are likely to be greater in smokers with CKD than in similarly aged smokers without CKD, and therefore the potential benefits of cessation are substantial.

## BLOOD PRESSURE

Among persons without CKD, randomized trials have shown clearly that lowering blood pressure reduces the risk of subsequent cardiovascular events.[121] Although there may be subtle differences in efficacy among different antihypertensive regimens, the major determinant of benefit is the absolute magnitude of any blood pressure reduction that is achieved.[122] After standardizing for the amount of blood pressure reduction, the relative reduction in risk appears to be approximately independent of the initial blood pressure level. This suggests that antihypertensive treatments will reduce the risk of cardiovascular events, even in those without obviously elevated blood pressure, but in those who are at increased risk for other reasons.[249]

Information about the effects of lowering blood pressure among persons with CKD stages 1 to 3 is available from trials conducted largely in people without known kidney disease. For example, the Perindopril Protection Against Recurrent Stroke (PROGRESS) study included 1757 participants with stage 3 or higher CKD among the 6105 participants with prior cerebrovascular disease who had been enrolled.[250] Assignment to active therapy was associated with a 35% reduction in the risk of stroke in subjects with CKD (HR, 0.65; 95% CI, 0.50–0.83), which was similar to the risk reduction observed in the whole study population. Because subjects with CKD had a higher background risk of cardiovascular events, the absolute treatment effect was 1.7-fold greater than for patients without CKD.[251]

Similarly, in a posthoc analysis of the Heart Outcomes and Prevention Evaluation (HOPE) study, 980 patients with impaired kidney function (serum creatinine level >124 μmol/L [1.4 mg/dL]) were studied,[252] and the proportional reduction in cardiovascular death, myocardial infarction, and stroke resulting from allocation to ramipril, 10 mg daily, was similar in patients with impaired kidney function and those without (HR, 0.79 vs. HR, 0.80; $P > .2$ for heterogeneity). An individual patient data metaanalysis of 26 trials, which included 152,290 participants, has shown that the benefits of reducing blood pressure among patients with eGFR less than 60 mL/min/1.73 m$^2$ were similar to those among patients with a higher eGFR.[253] However, most participants with CKD had stage 3A, and only 1% of participants had an eGFR less than 30 mL/min/1.73 m$^2$. An individual patient data metaanalysis has confirmed that the proportional effects of blood pressure lowering in patients with an eGFR less than 60 mL/min/1.73 m$^2$ are similar to those observed in patients with preserved kidney function.[253]

SPRINT (Systolic Blood Pressure Intervention Trial) compared a systolic blood pressure target of less than 120 mm Hg versus less than 140 mm Hg among 9361 participants at risk of cardiovascular disease, of whom 2646 had CKD at baseline. The trial was terminated early because the primary outcome (acute coronary syndrome, stroke, heart failure, or cardiovascular death) occurred significantly less frequently among those participants assigned the more intensive blood pressure target (5.2% vs. 6.8%; HR, 0.75; 95% CI, 0.64–0.89).[254] The effect was similar among participants with and without CKD.

However, most patients with CKD had relatively mild disease (average eGFR, 47 mL/min/1.73 m$^2$). A subsequent subgroup analysis of participants with CKD has confirmed that the lower systolic blood pressure target is associated with a reduction in all-cause mortality (HR, 0.72; 95% CI, 0.53–0.99) and cardiovascular events (HR, 0.81; 95% CI, 0.63–1.05), with no overall increase serious adverse events, although there was a greater decrease in GFR after 6 months (−0.47 vs. −0.32 mL/min/1.73 m$^2$ per year), and AKI, hypokalemia, and hyperkalemia were increased.[255]

Less information is available about the effects of lowering blood pressure on cardiovascular outcomes among patients with more advanced CKD, with most studies involving CKD stages 3b to 5 and primarily assessing kidney endpoints. The Irbesartan Diabetic Nephropathy Trial compared the effects of irbesartan, 300 mg daily, amlodipine, 10 mg daily, and placebo among 1715 subjects with type 2 diabetes mellitus and serum creatinine level of 1.0 to 3.0 mg/dL in women and 1.2 to 3.0 mg/dL in men, principally to assess the effects of each regimen on CKD progression. Irbesartan was shown to be effective at preventing the composite kidney outcome of doubling the serum creatinine level, dialysis, or death.[214] However, neither irbesartan nor amlodipine was superior to placebo in preventing the composite cardiovascular outcome of cardiovascular death, myocardial infarction, congestive heart failure, stroke, or coronary revascularization, despite a 6/3-mm Hg reduction in blood pressure in the irbesartan group and a 4/3-mm Hg reduction in the amlodipine group.[214]

Similarly, the Reduction in Endpoints in non–insulin-dependent diabetes mellitus (NIDDM) with the Angiotensin 2 Antagonist Losartan (RENAAL) study failed to demonstrate a reduction in cardiovascular morbidity and mortality, defined as myocardial infarction, stroke, first hospitalization for unstable angina or heart failure, arterial revascularization, or cardiovascular death.[215] Both these studies had limited power for detecting moderate effects on cardiovascular outcomes, but additional information on the effects of lowering blood pressure among people with advanced CKD is available from metaanalyses of trials conducted exclusively among patients on dialysis, with one including a total of 1202 patients from five trials[256] and the other 1679 patients from eight trials.[257] Both analyses have concluded that blood pressure–lowering therapy reduces cardiovascular event rates and cardiovascular death in patients on dialysis when compared with controls. In the more complete meta analysis, a reduction of 4 to 5 mm Hg in mean systolic and 2 to 3 mm Hg in diastolic blood pressure was associated with a 29% reduction in both cardiovascular events and cardiovascular mortality when compared with control regimens (HR, 0.71; 95% CI, 0.55–0.92).[257] This is comparable to the effect that would be expected from a blood pressure reduction of this magnitude in the general population.

Although a number of randomized controlled trials of blood pressure–lowering interventions have been conducted in kidney transplant recipients, these have almost exclusively examined transplantation-related outcomes such as graft loss, change in glomerular filtration rate, and proteinuria and have not assessed cardiovascular endpoints.[258]

> ***Clinical Relevance***
> Blood pressure is likely to be a key causal risk factor for cardiovascular disease among patients with CKD. Because patients with CKD typically have higher blood pressure, treatment may well be associated with significant risk reductions. Although uncertainties about precise details of how intensively to treat blood pressure among patients with CKD remain, it is likely that significant gains could be made with treatment to current targets, and further gains may be possible with more intensive treatment.

Thus, based on our present knowledge, it is sensible to treat hypertension in patients with CKD, although there is still much to be learned about the optimal timing of blood pressure measurements, the thresholds for treatment, and the safest method to achieve the largest possible reduction in blood pressure.[259] Older guidelines, including those published by the U,S. National Kidney Foundation, have recommended a target blood pressure of less than 130/80 mm Hg in patients with CKD.[260] However, because there are few studies that have addressed the optimal blood pressure goal in CKD, this target is largely based on data from other high-risk groups, such as patients with diabetes mellitus or congestive heart failure. A systematic review of 11 trials that assessed different targets in patients with advanced CKD has suggested that achieving a blood pressure less than 140/90 mm Hg may be adequate in nonproteinuric patients, with no additional benefits associated with tighter blood pressure control.[261] In observational studies, current targets are achieved in fewer than 50% of CKD patients, possibly in part because more intensive blood pressure control is associated with an increased number of adverse events.[262]

An international guideline published by the Kidney Disease: Improving Global Outcomes (KDIGO) study in 2012 has recommended aiming for a blood pressure less than 140/90 mm Hg in nonproteinuric patients with CKD who are not undergoing dialysis.[263] If proteinuria (UACR >3 mg/mmol) is present, the guideline recommends a lower blood pressure target of less than 130/80 mm Hg, although this is based on posthoc analyses and long-term follow-up of cohorts previously randomized to different blood pressure targets. Data from the general population support more intensive blood pressure lowering and suggest that the potential benefits among patients with CKD are substantial. Therefore the uncertainty surrounding the optimal target should not distract nephrologists from making efforts to reduce blood pressure in patients (especially the very large number of patients with systolic blood pressures well above 140 mm Hg) who frequently are undertreated and are therefore left at unnecessary risk.[262]

## DYSLIPIDEMIA

Other than in the presence of nephrotic range proteinuria, the blood LDL cholesterol concentration is not normally raised in patients with CKD. Nevertheless, randomized trials in the general population have clearly shown that reducing LDL cholesterol reduces the risk of myocardial infarction (MI) or death from coronary artery disease, ischemic stroke, and coronary revascularization, even among people with average or low blood cholesterol levels.[129] Therefore even though dyslipidemia is probably not the main contributor to an increased risk of atherosclerosis in CKD as compared with persons without CKD (see earlier, "Dyslipidemia"), reducing the blood LDL cholesterol level may be an effective strategy for reducing such risk, and a number of randomized trials have addressed this hypothesis.

Among persons without established kidney disease, posthoc analyses of randomized trials conducted in the general population have shown that the proportional reduction in the risk of a MI or CAD death, stroke, or coronary revascularization is independent of kidney function.[129] As discussed earlier, however, by the time patients reach stages 4 and 5 CKD, the pathophysiology of cardiovascular disease may have been modified by the "uremic" milieu and, as well as an increased risk of atherosclerotic events, there is an increased risk of cardiac arrhythmia and heart failure related to arteriosclerosis.

Two randomized trials have examined the effects of lowering the LDL cholesterol level with statin therapy on cardiovascular outcomes, specifically among patients receiving dialysis. In the 4D (Die Deutsche Diabetes Dialyse Study) randomized trial of atorvastatin, 20 mg daily, versus placebo among 1255 patients on maintenance hemodialysis with type 2 diabetes, lowering the LDL cholesterol level by an average of about 39 mg/dL (1.0 mmol/L) for a median of 4 years yielded a nonsignificant 8% reduction in the prespecified primary outcome of cardiac death, nonfatal MI, or stroke.[97] In the AURORA (A study to evaluate the Use of Rosuvastatin in subjects On Regular hemodialysis: an Assessment of survival and cardiovascular events) randomized trial of rosuvastatin, 10 mg daily, versus placebo among 2776 patients on maintenance hemodialysis (≈25% of whom had diabetes mellitus), lowering the LDL cholesterol level by an average of about 43 mg/dL (1.1 mmol/L) for a median of 4 years yielded a nonsignificant 4% reduction in the primary outcome of cardiovascular death, nonfatal MI, or stroke.[96] A high proportion of cardiac deaths in these trials were not attributable to CAD, and there was no evidence in either trial of a reduction in the risk of such deaths (Fig. 54.6).[96,97] However, although lowering the LDL cholesterol level with statin therapy among patients with ESKD did not yield statistically significant reductions in the primary outcomes in these trials, there were promising proportional reductions of 18% (risk ratio [RR], 0.82; 95% CI, 0.68–0.99; $P$ = .03) in major cardiac events in the 4D trial and of 16% (RR 0.84; 95% CI, 0.64–1.11; $P$ = .2) in nonfatal MI in the AURORA trial.[96,97] These findings raised the possibility of small, but meaningful, proportional

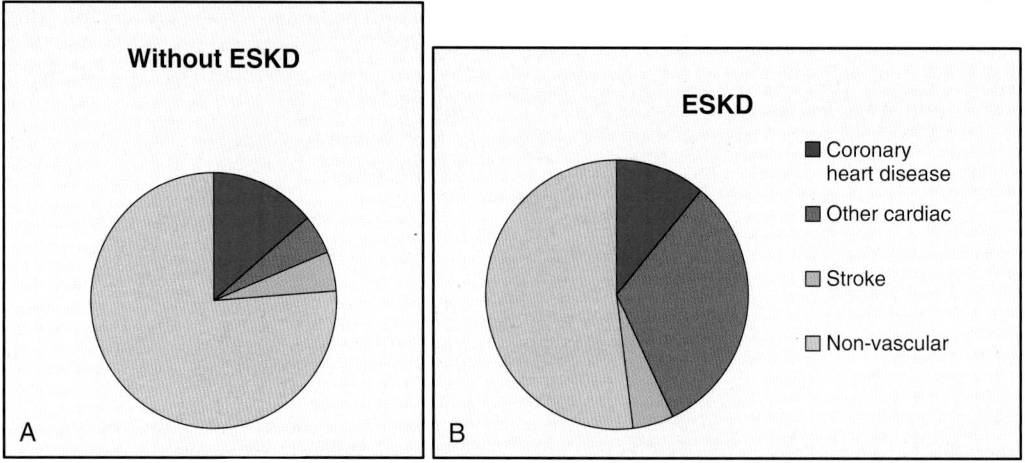


**Fig. 54.6** Causes of death in individuals with and without end-stage kidney disease (ESKD). (A) Shown is a group of patients without overt kidney disease recruited into trials of statin therapy (CTT; Cholesterol Treatment Trialists' collaboration) compared with patients with ESKD (B) as recorded by the US Renal Data System (USRDS) or recruited into the Die Deutsche Diabetes Dialyse (4D) trial or into A study to evaluate the Use of Rosuvastatin in subjects On Regular haemodialysis: an Assessment of survival and cardiovascular events (AURORA). Note the declining contribution of coronary artery disease and increasing proportion of other cardiac disease in the ESKD population. (From Baigent C, Keech A, Kearney PM, et al. Efficacy and safety of cholesterol-lowering treatment: prospective meta analysis of data from 90,056 participants in 14 randomised trials of statins. *Lancet* 2005;366:1267-1278; US Renal Data System. USRDS 2009 Annual data report: Atlas of chronic kidney disease and end-stage renal disease in the United States. Bethesda: National Institutes of Health, National Institute of Diabetes and Digestive and Kidney Diseases; 2009; Wanner C, Krane V, Marz W, et al. Atorvastatin in patients with type 2 diabetes mellitus undergoing hemodialysis. *N Engl J Med* 2005;353:238-248; Fellstrom BC, Jardine AG, Schmieder RE, et al. Rosuvastatin and cardiovascular events in patients undergoing hemodialysis. *N Engl J Med* 2009;360:1395-1407.)

benefits on atherosclerotic outcomes among patients on dialysis.

Subsequently, the SHARP (Study of Heart and Renal Protection) trial assessed the safety and efficacy of reducing the LDL cholesterol level among patients with stages 3 to 5 CKD, including many who were receiving dialysis. To achieve an average reduction in LDL cholesterol of about 1 mmol/L without using high statin doses (which are associated with an increased risk of myopathy,[264] especially in patients with impaired renal function[265]), a low dose of a statin (simvastatin, 20 mg daily) was combined with a cholesterol absorption inhibitor[9] (ezetimibe, 10 mg daily); the biochemical efficacy and tolerability of this regimen were first confirmed in the UK-HARP pilot studies.[266,267] Overall, 9270 patients were randomized to ezetimibe or simvastatin versus placebo, and allocation to ezetimibe or simvastatin yielded an average LDL cholesterol difference of 0.85 mmol/L (with about two-thirds adherence) during a median follow-up of 4.9 years, and produced a 17% proportional reduction in major atherosclerotic events (526 [11.3%] ezetimibe or simvastatin vs. 619 [13.4%]; RR, 0.83; 95% CI, 0.74–0.94; log rank $P = .0021$; Fig. 54.7).[98]

There was a nonsignificant reduction in nonfatal myocardial infarction or coronary death (213 [4.6%] vs. 230 [5.0%]; RR, 0.92; 95% CI, 0.76–1.11; $P = .37$), and significant reductions in nonhemorrhagic stroke (131 [2.8%] vs. 174 [3.8%]; RR, 0.75; 95% CI, 0.60 – 0.94; $P = .01$) and revascularization procedures (284 [6.1%] vs 352 [7.6%]; RR, 0.79; 95% CI, 0.68–0.93; $P = .0036$). Allocation to ezetimibe or simvastatin was not associated with a significant excess risk of myopathy, hepatitis, or gallstones, and there were no significant excesses of any type of cancer, death from cancer, or death from other noncardiovascular causes.

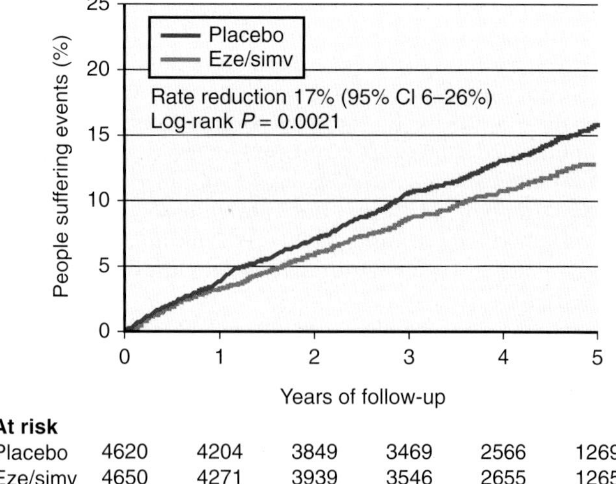


| At risk | | | | | | |
|---|---|---|---|---|---|---|
| Placebo | 4620 | 4204 | 3849 | 3469 | 2566 | 1269 |
| Eze/simv | 4650 | 4271 | 3939 | 3546 | 2655 | 1265 |

**Fig. 54.7** Life table plot of effects of allocation to ezetimibe (eze) or simvastatin (simv) on major atherosclerotic events. *CI*, Confidence interval.

Within SHARP, there was no statistical heterogeneity between those participants on dialysis at baseline and those who were not (*P* for heterogeneity = .25 for the primary outcome). This finding may at first seem to be discrepant with the earlier studies among dialysis patients. An individual patient data metaanalysis of 28 trials, including over 180,000 participants, showed a significant trend, such that the proportional reduction in major vascular events decreased as renal function declined (see Fig. 54.8).[103] However, it is not possible to determine whether the proportional effect

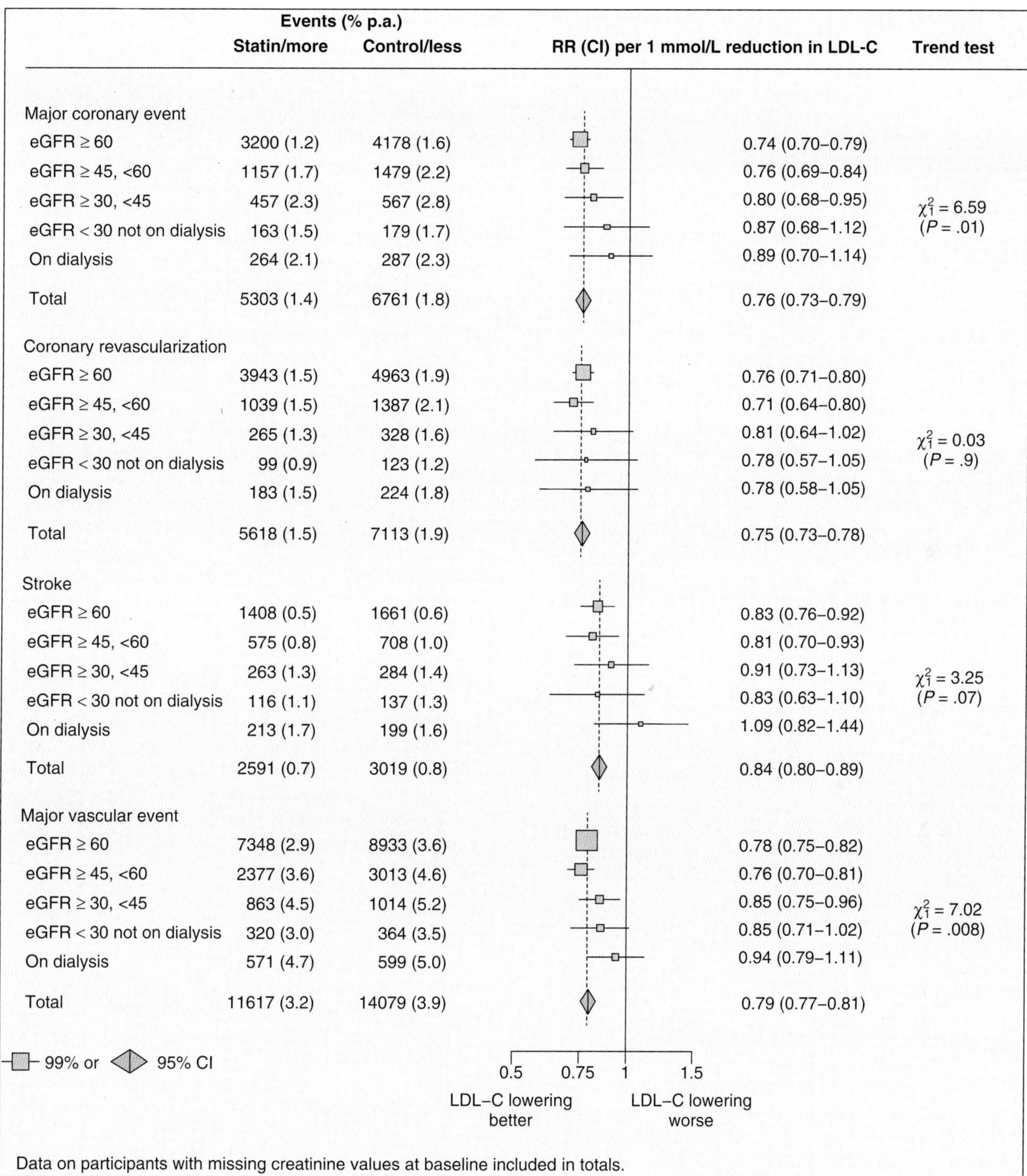

Events (% p.a.)
Statin/more
Control/less
RR (CI) per 1 mmol/L reduction in LDL-C
Trend test
Major coronary event
eGFR ≥ 60 3200 (1.2) 4178 (1.6) 0.74 (0.70–0.79)
eGFR ≥ 45, <60 1157 (1.7) 1479 (2.2) 0.76 (0.69–0.84)
eGFR ≥ 30, <45 457 (2.3) 567 (2.8) 0.80 (0.68–0.95)
eGFR < 30 not on dialysis 163 (1.5) 179 (1.7) 0.87 (0.68–1.12)
On dialysis 264 (2.1) 287 (2.3) 0.89 (0.70–1.14)
Total 5303 (1.4) 6761 (1.8) 0.76 (0.73–0.79)
$\chi^2_1$ = 6.59 (P = .01)
Coronary revascularization
eGFR ≥ 60 3943 (1.5) 4963 (1.9) 0.76 (0.71–0.80)
eGFR ≥ 45, <60 1039 (1.5) 1387 (2.1) 0.71 (0.64–0.80)
eGFR ≥ 30, <45 265 (1.3) 328 (1.6) 0.81 (0.64–1.02)
eGFR < 30 not on dialysis 99 (0.9) 123 (1.2) 0.78 (0.57–1.05)
On dialysis 183 (1.5) 224 (1.8) 0.78 (0.58–1.05)
Total 5618 (1.5) 7113 (1.9) 0.75 (0.73–0.78)
$\chi^2_1$ = 0.03 (P = .9)
Stroke
eGFR ≥ 60 1408 (0.5) 1661 (0.6) 0.83 (0.76–0.92)
eGFR ≥ 45, <60 575 (0.8) 708 (1.0) 0.81 (0.70–0.93)
eGFR ≥ 30, <45 263 (1.3) 284 (1.4) 0.91 (0.73–1.13)
eGFR < 30 not on dialysis 116 (1.1) 137 (1.3) 0.83 (0.63–1.10)
On dialysis 213 (1.7) 199 (1.6) 1.09 (0.82–1.44)
Total 2591 (0.7) 3019 (0.8) 0.84 (0.80–0.89)
$\chi^2_1$ = 3.25 (P = .07)
Major vascular event
eGFR ≥ 60 7348 (2.9) 8933 (3.6) 0.78 (0.75–0.82)
eGFR ≥ 45, <60 2377 (3.6) 3013 (4.6) 0.76 (0.70–0.81)
eGFR ≥ 30, <45 863 (4.5) 1014 (5.2) 0.85 (0.75–0.96)
eGFR < 30 not on dialysis 320 (3.0) 364 (3.5) 0.85 (0.71–1.02)
On dialysis 571 (4.7) 599 (5.0) 0.94 (0.79–1.11)
Total 11617 (3.2) 14079 (3.9) 0.79 (0.77–0.81)
$\chi^2_1$ = 7.02 (P = .008)
99% or 95% CI
0.5 0.75 1 1.5
LDL–C lowering better
LDL–C lowering worse
Data on participants with missing creatinine values at baseline included in totals.


**Fig. 54.8** Effects of low-density lipoprotein (LDL)–lowering therapy on particular vascular outcomes in 28 trials by baseline kidney function. *eGFR,* Estimated glomerular filtration rate; *LDL-C,* LDL cholesterol.

gradually diminishes once the eGFR falls below 30 mL/min/1.73 m$^2$ or whether it is consistent until patients require dialysis, when the proportional effect reduces substantially. A gradual diminution could be explained by the proportion of cardiac deaths that are attributable to coronary disease, which becomes smaller as CKD progresses, and potential misclassification (despite careful clinical outcome adjudication) caused by the atypical presentation of acute coronary syndromes in patients with advanced CKD, especially those on dialysis.

Note that although the proportional benefit may decline as CKD progresses, the absolute risk of atherosclerotic disease increases. Previous metaanalyses have suggested that the risk of a major vascular event increases by 29% for every 30% reduction in eGFR, so a reduction in the eGFR from 60 to 10 mL/min/1.73 m$^2$ would be associated with a fourfold increased risk of a major vascular event. This is of a similar magnitude to the reduction in the proportional effect of lowering the LDL cholesterol level by 1 mmol/L so that the absolute benefits of doing so would be similar among patients with an eGFR of 10 mL/min/1.73 [2] as those with an eGFR of 60 mL/min/1.73 m.[2] These estimates are based on the results of trials that typically lasted 3 to 5 years, but long-term follow-up of some of these trials has shown that the benefits may accrue beyond this within-trial period.[268,269]

Recent guidelines have emphasized the importance of treating overall risk rather than individual risk factors.[270,271] An international guideline published by KDIGO in 2013 recommended using statins or statin-based lipid lowering regimens in patients with stages 3 to 5 CKD who were older than 50 years and in those younger than 50 years, with additional risk factors.[270] Given the safety and current costs of generic statin-based therapy, the risk threshold at which LDL-lowering therapy should be considered has fallen (to 7.5% over 10 years in recent U.S. guidelines[271]). Although most risk calculators have not been validated in CKD populations, most patients with CKD will have an atherosclerotic risk that warrants treatment, even if their LDL cholesterol level is average or even below average. The potential benefits are substantial, and suggest that widespread use of LDL-lowering therapy in patients with CKD would result in a worthwhile reduction in cardiovascular disease complications.

*Clinical Relevance*

Reducing the LDL cholesterol level with statin-based therapy should be considered in most patients with CKD. Although the LDL cholesterol level might not be substantially elevated, reducing it will reduce the risk of atherosclerotic disease. To achieve a useful reduction in the LDL cholesterol level, it may be necessary to combine moderate doses of statins with other treatments (e.g., ezetimibe) that lower the LDL cholesterol level.

## TIGHT GLYCEMIC CONTROL

Among patients without established CKD, strict glycemic control has been shown in randomized trials to reduce the risk of microvascular disease outcomes (including the development of albuminuria). In type 1 diabetes, a strategy of more intensive glycemic control reduced the development of microalbuminuria by 39% (95% CI, 21%–52%).[211] In type 2 diabetes, the use of a gliclazide-based strategy to reduce hemoglobin A1c (HbA1c) below 6.5% was associated with a reduction in the development of nephropathy (HR, 0.79; 95% CI, 0.66–0.93, $P = .003$).[212] A recent individual patient data metaanalysis has shown that intensive glucose lowering (which reduced HbA1c by 0.9% on average) reduced the risk of nephropathy by 20% (HR, 0.80; 95% CI, 0.72–0.88) and retinopathy by 13% (HR, 0.87; 95% CI, 0.76–1.00).[272] Individual trials in the general population have not shown a clear benefit in terms of cardiovascular risk reduction with stricter glycemic control in type 1 or type 2 diabetes and, indeed, some have even suggested a hazard.[273] However, a metaanalysis of the available randomized trials has supported the hypothesis that stricter glycemic control (with HbA1c lower, on average, by 0.9%) reduces the risk of cardiovascular events, albeit modestly (OR, 0.85; 95% CI, 0.77–0.93).[274]

There is now evidence that certain glucose-lowering mechanisms may be particularly effective at reducing cardiovascular risk. Inhibitors of the sodium-glucose cotransporter 2 (SGLT2i) have been shown to reduce the risk of cardiovascular death among patients with diabetes, with similar effects observed in patients with and without CKD.[275,276] This class of drugs is of particular interest because there is some preliminary evidence to suggest that they may also slow the progression of diabetic kidney disease, which in turn may reduce the risk of cardiovascular disease.[277] Glucagon-like peptide-1 (GLP1) agonists have also been shown to reduce the risk of cardiovascular disease among patients with diabetes,[278,279] so it seems possible that the mechanism of glucose lowering may be important, in addition to the degree of glucose lowering.

It is very likely that the existing trials included a significant proportion of patients with diabetic kidney disease, but the results among such patients have not been reported as a specific subgroup analysis. Therefore the available data suggest that it would be reasonable to aim for tight glucose control among patients with CKD, but with due regard for the potential hazards of too rapid a reduction in HbA1c and hypoglycemia,[273,280] as well as the altered pharmacokinetics of hypoglycemic agents in CKD.[281]

## ANEMIA

As noted in the earlier section on anemia, a lower hemoglobin level is associated with an increased risk of structural heart disease. Some nonrandomized studies have suggested that the correction of anemia with recombinant human erythropoietin might lead to improvements in cardiac structure and function,[282,283] which led to the hypothesis that such treatment might improve cardiovascular outcomes among patients with renal anemia. A metaanalysis of nine small trials has suggested that erythropoiesis-stimulating agent therapy might reduce the risk of hospitalization for heart failure, but there were only 114 events among 734 participants in this meta analysis.[284] Four large trials have assessed the impact on mortality and cardiovascular events of partial or full correction of anemia. The first three of these studies investigated whether using two different erythropoietin regimens, normalization of hemoglobin, rather than partial correction, would improve cardiovascular outcomes. Only the more recent TREAT trial (see later) was placebo controlled.

The first study randomized 1233 patients on hemodialysis with clinical features suggestive of ischemic heart disease or heart failure. The trial was stopped early (after a median follow-up of 14 months) predominantly because of an excess risk of vascular access thrombosis with higher hemoglobin concentrations. At this point, 33% of patients had died or experienced a nonfatal MI in the group randomized to a hemoglobin target of 14.0 g/dL as compared with 27% of those randomized to the 10.0-g/dL target (RR, 1.3; 95% CI, 0.9–1.9).[285] The Correction of Haemoglobin and Outcomes in Renal Insufficiency (CHOIR) study, which recruited 1432 patients with CKD not undergoing dialysis and naïve to erythropoiesis-stimulating agent therapy, supported this observation. The trial was terminated because patients randomized to achieve a hemoglobin value of 13.5 g/dL were more likely to reach a primary endpoint—death, myocardial infarction, hospitalization to treat heart failure—than those in the 11.3-g/L target group (HR, 1.34; 95% CI, 1.03–1.74).[286]

The findings of the Cardiovascular Risk Reduction by Early Anemia Treatment with Epoetin Beta (CREATE) trial conducted among patients with stage 3 or 4 CKD were similar; no benefit was demonstrated for targeting a normal hemoglobin (13.0–15.0 g/dL) compared with a subnormal hemoglobin (10.5–11.5 g/dL) and, numerically, more cardiovascular events occurred in the normal hemoglobin group.[287] It has long been recognized that erythropoiesis-stimulating agents (ESAs) can increase blood pressure and blood viscosity (particularly when hemoglobin changes are rapid), and it was predicted over 20 years ago that hemodynamic and rheologic effects may offset the cardiovascular benefits of correcting anemia.[288] Thus in the Trial to Reduce Cardiovascular Events with Aranesp Therapy (TREAT), the first large randomized-controlled trial (RCT) to compare an erythropoiesis-stimulating agent with placebo, the protocol was designed to avoid rapid changes to hemoglobin concentrations.[208] In this study, 4038 patients with type 2 diabetes, CKD, and anemia received either darbepoietin alfa in an effort to achieve a target hemoglobin of 13 g/dL or a placebo with "rescue" therapy if hemoglobin fell below 9 g/dL. The primary endpoint of death or nonfatal cardiovascular event occurred in 31.4% of patients assigned to the active treatment and 29.7% of patients assigned to placebo (HR, 1.05; 95% CI, 0.94–1.17). There was a statistically significant twofold increase in the risk of stroke in the darbepoietin alfa-treated group (101 vs. 53 strokes; HR, 1.92; 95% CI, 1.38–2.68).

Taken together, the results of these four key trials do not support the concept that correction of anemia using ESAs reduces cardiovascular risk in patients with CKD, whether or not on dialysis.[205] However, the current data do not exclude the possibility that small corrections in hemoglobin (e.g., fixed, low-dose, ESAs) are beneficial in the context of CKD. The use of ESAs probably improves health-related quality of life among patients with debilitating symptoms of anemia, although the trials to date are inconclusive on this[205] and, by reducing transfusion requirements, also reduce the risk of sensitizing potential transplant recipients to nonself human leukocyte antigens (discussed in more detail in Chapters 55 and 70).

## HOMOCYSTEINE

Randomized trials of folate and B vitamins in both the general population and patients with CKD have shown that reducing the homocysteine level does not reduce the risk of cardiovascular events.[161] The HOST (Homocysteinemia in Kidney and End-Stage Renal Disease) trial randomized 2056 adults with an eGFR less than 30 mL/min/1.73 m$^2$ ($n$ = 1305) or ESKD ($n$ = 751) to a regimen of folic acid and B group vitamins or placebo.[289] Despite a 25.5% reduction in the plasma homocysteine level, there was no difference in mortality (448 deaths in the treated group vs. 436 in the placebo group; HR, 1.04; 95% CI, 0.91–1.18) nor was there a reduction in cardiovascular events, including MI, stroke, and amputation of the lower extremity, which were all components of the secondary endpoint. In addition, the Folic Acid for Vascular outcomes in Transplantation (FAVORIT) trial randomized 4110 kidney transplant recipients with elevated homocysteine levels and an eGFR of 30 mL/min/1.73 m$^2$ or higher to a multivitamin tablet containing folic acid, vitamin $B_6$, and vitamin $B_{12}$ or to a low-dose vitamin $B_6$ and $B_{12}$ regimen.[290] Despite the expected reduction in homocysteine levels in the treated group, there was no difference in a composite cardiovascular endpoint (adjusted HR, 1.0). A meta analysis of all trials of folic acid in CKD populations has found a similar null result.[163] These results are consistent with the totality of evidence in the general population.[161]

## CHRONIC KIDNEY DISEASE AND MINERAL BONE DISORDERS

Although interventions aimed at correcting the biochemical and endocrinologic manifestations of CKD-MBDs were initially driven by the need to prevent the associated debilitating bone pathologies, the suggestion that there might be a link between bone and vascular health in CKD has led to a greater focus on assessing the effects of interventions on cardiovascular outcomes.

### Reducing Serum Phosphate

Numerous observational studies have demonstrated a link between increased serum phosphate levels and mortality. However, there have been no placebo-controlled trials investigating the benefits of lowering phosphate levels.[291] It is therefore impossible to know whether current guideline recommendations to maintain serum phosphate concentrations *below* certain targets are beneficial or harmful. Current therapies only reduce the serum phosphate level modestly, although the effects on phosphate balance (as indicated by changes in urinary phosphate excretion) may be larger than suggested by the serum phosphate level alone.[292]

The most widely used phosphate binders are calcium-based, and there are some data to suggest that their use contributes to vascular calcification. Patients with advanced CKD and ESKD taking calcium-based phosphate binders are in positive calcium balance; only patients with ample residual kidney function on loop diuretic agents remain in neutral or possibly negative calcium balance. The availability of non–calcium-based phosphate binders (e.g., sevelamer, lanthanum, newer iron-based compounds) has allowed this hypothesis to be tested, but trials designed to assess whether sevelamer retards the progression of vascular calcification as compared with calcium-based phosphate binders have yielded conflicting results.[172,293,294,295] The Dialysis Clinical Outcomes Revisited (DCOR) trial compared sevelamer and calcium-based binders among 2103 patients on maintenance hemodialysis.[294] The primary outcome was all-cause mortality and was similar in both arms (HR, 0.93; 95% CI, 0.79–1.10), although nearly half of the trial participants discontinued their assigned treatment before the end of the trial, and over 200 were lost to follow-up. It is therefore unclear whether to treat elevated serum phosphorus concentrations and, if so, with what agent and to what target.

Reducing the serum phosphate level might be expected to reduce FGF23 concentrations. However, a randomized trial comparing sevelamer, lanthanum, and calcium-based phosphate binders found that overall (i.e., data pooling all binders ["active therapy"] vs. placebo), reducing the serum phosphate level by 0.3 mg/dL had no effect on FGF23 concentration.[292] However, whereas FGF23 increased in patients assigned calcium-based binders (median increase, 28 pg/mL; $P = .03$), it decreased in patients assigned sevelamer (median decrease, 24 pg/mL), and was unchanged in patients assigned lanthanum.

Niacin also reduces the serum phosphate level by about 0.4 mg/dL via inhibition of the intestinal sodium-phosphate transporter.[296] However, recent randomized trials have shown that niacin does not reduce cardiovascular risk, despite multiple potentially beneficial effects—lipid modification and blood pressure reduction, in addition to effects on phosphate balance—and, indeed, has a number of harmful effects.[136,297] These trials do not therefore provide support for the use of niacin for reducing the serum phosphate level or for other indications to reduce cardiovascular risk in CKD or ESKD.

#### Vitamin D

1,25-dihydroxyvitamin D (calcitriol) and its synthetic analogues (collectively termed "active vitamin D derivatives") have been used to correct vitamin D deficiency in the context of CKD for many years. These compounds replenish calcitriol, which is produced by the kidney and suppress levels of PTH, preventing the development of sHPT.[298] More recently, attention has focused on deficiency of parent vitamin D (usually measured indirectly as 25(OH)- vitamin D [25(OH)D], the hydroxylated compound produced in the liver). Over 80% of patients with CKD have vitamin D insufficiency or frank deficiency.[299] In patients not undergoing dialysis, low levels of 25(OH)D are more strongly associated with progression to ESKD and death than calcitriol (1,25-$(OH)_2D$) levels.[300] Two small trials of paricalcitol (an active vitamin D compound) have failed to demonstrate any effect on cardiac structure assessed by cardiac MRI.[301,302] To date, no trials of vitamin D (in any form) have been designed specifically to investigate clinical outcomes such as fractures, cardiovascular events, or mortality among patients with CKD, and a meta analysis of 76 randomized trials of vitamin D has found that insufficient data are available on cardiovascular outcomes to assess any possible reduction in the risk of such events.[303] Despite observational data suggesting that vitamin D supplementation may be beneficial, there is no randomized trial evidence to support recommending such treatment for the reduction of cardiovascular events among patients with CKD.

#### Calcimimetics

Calcimimetic treatment reduces serum PTH and calcium concentrations.[304] The Evaluation of Cinacalcet Hydrochloride Therapy to Lower Cardiovascular Events (EVOLVE) trial has compared a cinacalcet-based regimen with a non–cinacalcet-based regimen (including a placebo) in 3883 patients undergoing hemodialysis with moderate to severe sHPT.[305] The primary composite outcome was time to death, nonfatal MI, hospitalization for unstable angina, heart failure, or a peripheral vascular event. In the intention to treat analysis, allocation to cinacalcet was associated with a nonsignificant 7% reduction in the primary outcome (HR, 0.93; 95% CI, 0.85–1.02; $P = .11$).[206] However, the randomization process was only stratified for country and diabetes status and, by chance, the two groups were imbalanced for age (median age, 55.0 years, among those allocated cinacalcet vs. 54.0 years in those allocated placebo). After adjustment for age, allocation to cinacalcet was associated with a nominally significant reduction in the primary outcome (HR, 0.88; 95% CI, 0.79–0.97; $P = .008$) and all-cause mortality alone (HR, 0.86; 95% CI, 0.78–0.96; $P = .006$).

The treatment effect was similar for all components of the primary outcome and on vascular and nonvascular mortality. Taking all fatal and nonfatal cardiovascular events combined, randomization to cinacalcet was associated with a 16% lower hazard of nonatherosclerotic cardiovascular events(95% CI, 4%–26%). Although the hazard of atherosclerotic events was also numerically lower in patients randomized to cinacalcet (95% CI, −1%–24%), this difference was not significant. Although derived from posthoc analyses, these data support the hypothesis that mineral bone disease disturbances contribute to nonatherosclerotic cardiovascular disease.

Cinacalcet reduces PTH in patients with CKD not on dialysis.[306] However, the associated reduction in the serum calcium level is more marked than in patients undergoing dialysis (with 62% of those assigned cinacalcet having a serum calcium < 8.4 mg/dL compared with 6% of those assigned placebo). This has led to safety concerns that have limited the provision of cinacalcet to patients on dialysis or, rarely, to patients with other parathyroid disorders (e.g., parathyroid carcinoma, primary hyperparathyroidism (HPT) in a patient unsuitable for surgery).[306]

### ANTIPLATELET THERAPY

Antiplatelet therapy reduces the risk of occlusive cardiovascular disease among patients at high risk of such disease, and these benefits greatly outweigh any risks of bleeding,[307] but patients with CKD are at increased risk of bleeding.[308] Thus it is unclear whether the balance of benefit and hazard remains beneficial among such patients. The Anti-Thrombotic Treatment (ATT) trialists' collaborative metaanalysis of trials of antiplatelet therapy among patients at high risk of occlusive vascular disease included 14 trials conducted among 2632 patients on maintenance hemodialysis after placement of a dialysis graft or fistula. Overall, antiplatelet therapy yielded a 41% proportional reduction in the risk of nonfatal MI, nonfatal stroke, or vascular death, which was consistent with the proportional benefit observed among other high-risk patients studied, but there was insufficient data on bleeding risk to assess safety.[307] Based on event rates among patients receiving dialysis in SHARP (and applying the summary risk ratios for aspirin from the ATT metaanalysis),[309] treating 1000 patients on dialysis with vascular disease with aspirin for 5 years has been projected to cause an additional 19 intracranial bleeds and 53 serious extracranial bleeds. There is therefore substantial uncertainty about the relative benefits and harms of antiplatelet therapy in ESKD.

There have been no appropriately sized trials of aspirin with clinical endpoints in patients with CKD not requiring dialysis treatment. Among patients with early-stage CKD, posthoc analysis of the Hypertension Optimal Treatment trial has shown that the benefits of aspirin were similar in the 470 patients with a serum creatinine level higher than 117 μmol/L (1.5 mg/dL) than those with a lower serum creatinine level, but did not report information on any additional bleeding risks.[310] However, there is very little information about the effects of aspirin among those with more severe CKD. One pilot study has demonstrated that aspirin increases the risk of minor bleeding in patients with CKD, but there was no detectable increase in the risk of major bleeding.[266,307] Randomized trials will be required to evaluate the relative risks and benefits of antiplatelet therapy at different stages of CKD.

### MINERALOCORTICOID ANTAGONISM

Mineralocorticoid antagonists (MRAs) have been shown to reduce cardiovascular mortality and morbidity among patients with heart failure and reduced ejection fraction.[311–313] It is also likely that MRA treatment improves these outcomes among patients with heart failure and preserved ejection fraction, although the evidence is less clear.[314,315] Given the phenotypic similarity between heart failure and cardiovascular disease in CKD, there is a good rationale to test MRAs among patients with CKD. However, MRAs are known to increase potassium concentrations, so the safety of this among patients with reduced GFR is uncertain. However, patients on dialysis are at high risk of heart failure and at reduced risk of hyperkalemia because of their regular dialysis and lack of functioning nephrons to conserve potassium.[316] The outcomes of large trials of MRAs in dialysis patients are therefore of considerable interest.[317]

### DIALYSIS DELIVERY

For patients with CKD who are undergoing hemodialysis, there has been interest in whether modifying the dialysis technique could ameliorate the associated cardiovascular risk. Most hospital-based hemodialysis is delivered on a thrice-weekly schedule, which includes a long gap of 3 days each week. Observational studies have shown that the risk of death is highest at the end of this long gap, most likely due to the accumulation of fluid and toxins during this period.[89] Trials of more frequent dialysis have suggested a benefit on surrogate outcomes such as left ventricular mass, but have not been large enough to determine effects on clinical outcomes.[318] The HEMO study tested high- versus low-flux hemodialysis and more versus less intensive dialysis (i.e., a $Kt/V_{urea}$ target of 1.45 vs. 1.05), but did not demonstrate a benefit of either intervention on clinical outcomes.[319] High-flux dialysis did not demonstrate a benefit in other trials.[320] On-line hemodiafiltration (OL-HDF, which offers very high-flux dialysis) was reported to be associated with a reduced mortality risk in a metaanalysis,[321] but when further trials were included in an updated metaanalysis, this apparent benefit was no longer apparent.[322] The clinical benefit of the improved removal of so-called middle molecules by OL-HDF (compared with standard hemodialysis) therefore remains to be proved.

## CONCLUSIONS

Patients with CKD are at increased risk of atherosclerotic and nonatherosclerotic heart disease, as well as stroke and peripheral arterial disease. The increased risk of cardiovascular disease begins early in the natural history of CKD, so an understanding of that excess risk should begin with an assessment of the magnitude of any early changes in known causal risk factors. Hypertension seems likely to be the most important such risk factor because its control is disturbed early in the development of CKD. With CKD progression, other abnormalities, including disorders of mineral metabolism (elevated FGF23, PTH, and altered calcium and phosphate metabolism) appear and may contribute to the rising risk of cardiovascular disease, but there is a lack of evidence about the mechanism whereby these processes might occur.

Observational studies of particular risk factors among patients with advanced CKD cannot be expected to produce reliable information because, as in other sick populations (e.g., very old adults), the observed associations are distorted by confounding and may yield findings that are misleading. For example, there have been numerous observational studies suggesting that cholesterol is inversely associated with major outcomes among patients on dialysis, and yet in the randomized SHARP trial, an unconfounded assessment of the effects of reducing cholesterol has indicated that reducing the LDL cholesterol level is beneficial. For many of the risk factors considered in this chapter, whether established as causal (e.g., hypertension) or of uncertain relevance (e.g., disorders of mineral metabolism), there are no adequately powered randomized trials that assess whether currently available (and often widely used) treatments that modify these abnormalities can safely reduce the risk of cardiovascular events. Studies such as SHARP, TREAT, and EVOLVE have shown that international collaboration can yield really large and informative trials, but many more of comparable size are now needed if effective strategies for reducing the risk of cardiovascular disease are to be identified.

Complete reference list available at ExpertConsult.com.

### KEY REFERENCES


4. Foley RN, Parfrey PS, Sarnak MJ. Clinical epidemiology of cardiovascular disease in chronic renal disease. *Am J Kidney Dis.* 1998;32:S112–S119.
9. Matsushita K, van der Velde M, Astor BC, et al. Association of estimated glomerular filtration rate and albuminuria with all-cause and cardiovascular mortality in general population cohorts: a collaborative meta-analysis. *Lancet.* 2010;375:2073–2081.
15. Baigent C, Burbury K, Wheeler D. Premature cardiovascular disease in chronic renal failure. *Lancet.* 2000;356:147–152.
42. Vallance P. Importance of asymmetrical dimethylarginine in cardiovascular risk. *Lancet.* 2001;358:2096–2097.
65. Mark PB, Johnston N, Groenning BA, et al. Redefinition of uremic cardiomyopathy by contrast-enhanced cardiac magnetic resonance imaging. *Kidney Int.* 2006;69:1839–1845.
70. Burton JO, Jefferies HJ, Selby NM, et al. Hemodialysis-induced repetitive myocardial injury results in global and segmental reduction in systolic cardiac function. *Clin J Am Soc Nephrol.* 2009;4:1925–1931.
89. Foley RN, Gilbertson DT, Murray T, et al. Long interdialytic interval and mortality among patients receiving hemodialysis. *N Engl J Med.* 2011;365:1099–1107.
95. Lewington S, Whitlock G, Clarke R, et al. Blood cholesterol and vascular mortality by age, sex, and blood pressure: a meta-analysis of individual data from 61 prospective studies with 55,000 vascular deaths. *Lancet.* 2007;370:1829–1839.
96. Fellstrom BC, Jardine AG, Schmieder RE, et al. Rosuvastatin and cardiovascular events in patients undergoing hemodialysis. *N Engl J Med.* 2009;360:1395–1407.
97. Wanner C, Krane V, Marz W, et al. Atorvastatin in patients with type 2 diabetes mellitus undergoing hemodialysis. *N Engl J Med.* 2005;353:238–248.
98. Baigent C, Landray MJ, Reith C, et al. Randomised trial of the effects of lowering LDL-cholesterol with ezetimibe/simvastatin in patients with chronic kidney disease: the Study of Heart and Renal Protection (SHARP). *Lancet.* 2011.
109. Go AS, Chertow GM, Fan D, et al. Chronic kidney disease and the risks of death, cardiovascular events, and hospitalization. *N Engl J Med.* 2004;351:1296–1305.
120. Lewington S, Clarke R, Qizilbash N, et al. Age-specific relevance of usual blood pressure to vascular mortality: a meta-analysis of

individual data for one million adults in 61 prospective studies. *Lancet.* 2002;360:1903–1913.

121. Turnbull F. Effects of different blood-pressure-lowering regimens on major cardiovascular events: results of prospectively-designed overviews of randomised trials. *Lancet.* 2003;362:1527–1535.
129. Baigent C, Blackwell L, Emberson J, et al. Efficacy and safety of more intensive lowering of LDL cholesterol: a meta-analysis of data from 170,000 participants in 26 randomised trials. *Lancet.* 2010; 376:1670–1681.
137. HPS2-THRIVE Collaborative Group. Effects of extended-release niacin with laropiprant in high-risk patients. *N Engl J Med.* 2014;in press.
160. Clarke R, Bennett DA, Parish S, et al. Homocysteine and coronary heart disease: meta-analysis of MTHFR case-control studies, avoiding publication bias. *PLoS Med.* 2012;9:e1001177.
174. Gutierrez OM, Mannstadt M, Isakova T, et al. Fibroblast growth factor 23 and mortality among patients undergoing hemodialysis. *N Engl J Med.* 2008;359:584–592.
175. Isakova T, Xie H, Yang W, et al. Fibroblast growth factor 23 and risks of mortality and end-stage renal disease in patients with chronic kidney disease. *JAMA.* 2011;305:2432–2439.
176. Scialla JJ, Xie H, Rahman M, et al. Fibroblast growth factor-23 and cardiovascular events in CKD. *J Am Soc Nephrol.* 2013.
180. Faul C, Amaral AP, Oskouei B, et al. FGF23 induces left ventricular hypertrophy. *J Clin Invest.* 2011;121:4393–4408.
188. Palmer SC, Hayen A, Macaskill P, et al. Serum levels of phosphorus, parathyroid hormone, and calcium and risks of death and cardiovascular disease in individuals with chronic kidney disease. *JAMA.* 2011;305:1119–1127.
189. Shardlow A, McIntyre NJ, Fluck RJ, et al. Associations of fibroblast growth factor 23, vitamin D and parathyroid hormone with 5-year outcomes in a prospective primary care cohort of people with chronic kidney disease stage 3. *BMJ Open.* 2017;7(8): e016528.
190. van Ballegooijen AJ, Reinders I, Visser M, et al. Parathyroid hormone and cardiovascular disease events: a systematic review and meta-analysis of prospective studies. *Am Heart J.* 2013;165:655–664, 64.e1–64.e5.
195. Vivekananthan DP, Penn MS, Sapp SK, et al. Use of antioxidant vitamins for the prevention of cardiovascular disease: meta-analysis of randomised trials. *Lancet.* 2003;361:2017–2023.
199. Ridker PM, Everett BM, Thuren T, et al. Antiinflammatory therapy with canakinumab for atherosclerotic disease. *N Engl J Med.* 2017;377(12):1119–1131.
202. White J, Sofat R, Hemani G, et al. Plasma urate concentration and risk of coronary heart disease: a Mendelian randomisation analysis. *Lancet Diabetes Endocrinol.* 2016;4:327–336.
206. Chertow GM, Block GA, Correa-Rotter R, et al. Effect of cinacalcet on cardiovascular disease in patients undergoing dialysis. *N Engl J Med.* 2012;367:2482–2494.
208. Pfeffer MA, Burdmann EA, Chen CY, et al. A trial of darbepoetin alfa in type 2 diabetes and chronic kidney disease. *N Engl J Med.* 2009;361:2019–2032.
210. Fox CS, Matsushita K, Woodward M, et al. Associations of kidney disease measures with mortality and end-stage renal disease in individuals with and without diabetes: a meta-analysis. *Lancet.* 2012;380:1662–1673.
228. Shlipak MG, Matsushita K, Arnlov J, et al. Cystatin C versus creatinine in determining risk based on kidney function. *N Engl J Med.* 2013;369:932–943.
245. Pirie K, Peto R, Reeves GK, et al. The 21st century hazards of smoking and benefits of stopping: a prospective study of one million women in the UK. *Lancet.* 2013;381:133–141.
248. Staplin N, Haynes R, Herrington WG, et al. Smoking and adverse outcomes in patients with CKD: the Study of Heart and Renal Protection (SHARP). *Am J Kidney Dis.* 2016;68(3):371–380.
253. Blood Pressure Lowering Treatment Trialists C, Ninomiya T, Perkovic V, et al. Blood pressure lowering and major cardiovascular events in people with and without chronic kidney disease: meta-analysis of randomised controlled trials. *BMJ.* 2013;347:f5680.
254. SPRINT Research Group, Wright JT Jr, Williamson JD, et al. A randomized trial of intensive versus standard blood-pressure control. *N Engl J Med.* 2015;373:2103–2116.
255. Cheung AK, Rahman M, Reboussin DM, et al. Effects of intensive BP control in CKD. *J Am Soc Nephrol.* 2017;28(9):2812–2823.
257. Heerspink HJ, Ninomiya T, Zoungas S, et al. Effect of lowering blood pressure on cardiovascular events and mortality in patients on dialysis: a systematic review and meta-analysis of randomised controlled trials. *Lancet.* 2009;373:1009–1015.
272. Zoungas S, Arima H, Gerstein HC, et al. Effects of intensive glucose control on microvascular outcomes in patients with type 2 diabetes: a meta-analysis of individual participant data from randomised controlled trials. *Lancet Diabetes Endocrinol.* 2017;5:431–437.
275. Zinman B, Wanner C, Lachin JM, et al. Empagliflozin, cardiovascular outcomes, and mortality in type 2 diabetes. *N Engl J Med.* 2015; 373:2117–2128.
276. Neal B, Perkovic V, Mahaffey KW, et al. Canagliflozin and cardiovascular and renal events in type 2 diabetes. *N Engl J Med.* 2017.
277. Wanner C, Inzucchi SE, Lachin JM, et al. Empagliflozin and progression of kidney disease in type 2 diabetes. *N Engl J Med.* 2016; 375:323–334.
278. Marso SP, Daniels GH, Brown-Frandsen K, et al. Liraglutide and cardiovascular outcomes in type 2 diabetes. *N Engl J Med.* 2016; 375:311–322.
279. Marso SP, Bain SC, Consoli A, et al. Semaglutide and cardiovascular outcomes in patients with type 2 diabetes. *N Engl J Med.* 2016;375:1834–1844.
292. Block GA, Wheeler DC, Persky MS, et al. Effects of phosphate binders in moderate CKD. *J Am Soc Nephrol.* 2012;23:1407–1415.
301. Thadhani R, Appelbaum E, Pritchett Y, et al. Vitamin D therapy and cardiac structure and function in patients with chronic kidney disease: the PRIMO randomized controlled trial. *JAMA.* 2012;307: 674–684.
303. Palmer SC, McGregor DO, Macaskill P, et al. Meta-analysis: vitamin D compounds in chronic kidney disease. *Ann Intern Med.* 2007;147: 840–853.
309. Baigent C, Blackwell L, Collins R, et al. Aspirin in the primary and secondary prevention of vascular disease: collaborative meta-analysis of individual participant data from randomised trials. *Lancet.* 2009;373:1849–1860.
310. Jardine MJ, Ninomiya T, Perkovic V, et al. Aspirin is beneficial in hypertensive patients with chronic kidney disease: a post-hoc subgroup analysis of a randomized controlled trial. *J Am Coll Cardiol.* 2010;56:956–965.

# Hematologic Aspects of Kidney Disease

55

Carlo Brugnara | Kai-Uwe Eckardt

CHAPTER OUTLINE



KEY POINTS

- Anemia is relatively uncommon in earlier stages (stages G1–3) of CKD.
- The prevalence begins to increase significantly with an eGFR below 60 mL/min/1.73 $m^2$, but anemia is generally not a frequent or severe complication of CKD until the GFR is below 30 mL/min/1.73 $m^2$.
- Anemia is a more significant problem for younger women, older men, and blacks.
- Anemia occurs earlier in the course of disease and is often more severe among patients with CKD and diabetes mellitus.
- Screening for anemia (measurement of Hgb) should generally begin at CKD stage G3.
- Serum EPO concentrations are generally equal to or higher than those in patients without CKD.
- Mean serum EPO concentrations increase with worsening anemia in mild to moderate CKD, although to an insufficient degree.
- Mean serum EPO concentrations become more a function of GFR than of Hgb concentration when the GFR drops below around 40 mL/min/1.73 $m^2$.
- Even with advanced CKD, the ability to produce EPO is preserved. and some degree of responsiveness to lower Hgb is retained.

## ANEMIA OF KIDNEY DISEASE

Reduced erythrocyte mass, or anemia, is one of the regular consequences of chronic kidney disease (CKD), because of the central role played by erythropoietin (EPO) in the regulation of erythropoiesis. Anemia can manifest itself early in the course of CKD, and its severity and prevalence go together with the progression of kidney disease. Given the significant effect of severe anemia on quality of life among patients with kidney failure, anemia is considered as one of the most clinically significant complications of this disease. Nevertheless, the direct consequences of CKD-related anemia and the degree to which anemia should be corrected in patients with CKD remain controversial.[1]

### DEFINITION AND PREVALENCE OF ANEMIA IN CHRONIC KIDNEY DISEASE

Anemia is a state characterized by a reduced mass of red blood cells (RBCs) and hemoglobin (Hgb) concentration in blood, resulting in reduced oxygen-carrying capacity and delivery to the body's tissues and organs.[2–4] Because direct measurements of red cell mass are cumbersome and not readily available, anemia is defined as a reduction below the normal range for Hgb concentration and hematocrit (Hct); these values depend on gender, race, and age, with an increased prevalence of anemia in older adults.[5–8] The definition of anemia is somewhat arbitrary. The World Health Organization (WHO) defines anemia as an Hgb concentration below 13.0 g/dL for adult men and below 12.0 g/dL for adult women.[9] This definition has been adopted in the clinical practice guideline for anemia in CKD developed by Kidney Disease: Improving Global Outcomes (KDIGO),[10] whereas previous guidelines proposed a slightly higher threshold in men (13.5 g/dL).[11,12] Persons living at higher altitudes are characterized by a larger red cell mass and reduced Hgb oxygen affinity, compensatory changes required to maintain tissue oxygen delivery, given the reduced ambient oxygen tension at such altitudes.[13–19] Normal ranges for subjects living at high altitude are not well developed, resulting in potential misclassification of anemia.[20]

The prevalence of anemia in patients with CKD has been widely studied. In general, anemia is more frequent at lower levels of kidney function, becoming almost universal in those with end-stage kidney disease (ESKD; Figs. 55.1 and 55.2).[21,22] The prevalence reported in different studies depends on the definition of anemia and the target population. The most useful analyses are those that were community-based, avoiding biases inherent in studies of clinic-based populations. Hsu and coworkers have studied 12,055 adult ambulatory subjects from health clinics in Boston using the Cockcroft-Gault equation to estimate creatinine clearance and the Modification of Diet in Renal Disease (MDRD) formula to estimate the glomerular filtration rate (GFR) indexed to body surface area.[23] They found that mean Hct values were progressively lower with creatinine clearance below 60 mL/min/1.73 m$^2$ in men and below 40 mL/min/1.73 m$^2$ in women. Moderately severe anemia (Hct <33%) was present in more than 20% of patients when the GFR was below 30 mL/min/1.73 m$^2$ in women and below 20 mL/min/1.73 m$^2$ in men.[23] Similar results have been obtained in different populations. In Japan, a study of 54,848 subjects identified an estimated GFR (eGFR) threshold of 60 mL/min/1.73 m$^2$ for both genders, below which anemia prevalence increased significantly and a threshold of 45 mL/min/1.73 m$^2$ for the association of anemia with complications.[24] Hsu and coworkers conducted a second study, using the third National Health and Nutrition Examination Survey (NHANES III; 1988–1994) of 15,971 adults older than 18 years, with measurements of serum creatinine and Hgb values and iron indices. Creatinine clearance was estimated using the Cockcroft-Gault formula.[25] A statistically significant lower mean Hgb was found in men and women with creatinine clearances below 70 mL/min and 50 mL/min, respectively, than in those with creatinine clearances more than 80 mL/min. However, a mean decrease of 1.0 g/dL was found only for those with a creatinine clearance less than 30 mL/min. Astor and colleagues[22] studied the same NHANES III data as Hsu and coworkers but restricted analysis to a different age range, selecting 15,419 participants 20 years of age and older. Anemia according to the WHO definition was present in 7.3% of all participants (see Fig. 55.1). Functional iron deficiency and absolute iron deficiency were found to be important predictors of anemia.[22] Another study on the same dataset has shown that Hgb values below 11 g/dL were present in 42.2% of subjects with an eGFR below 30 mL/min/1.73 m$^2$ and in 3.5% of subjects with an eGFR between 30 and 60 mL/min/1.73 m$^2$ (MDRD formula).[26] Stauffer and Fan, using the 2007–2008 and 2009–2010 NHANES dataset, have estimated that 14.0% of the US adult population have CKD, with anemic individuals having a twofold greater prevalence of CKD than the general population (15.4% vs. 7.65%).[27]

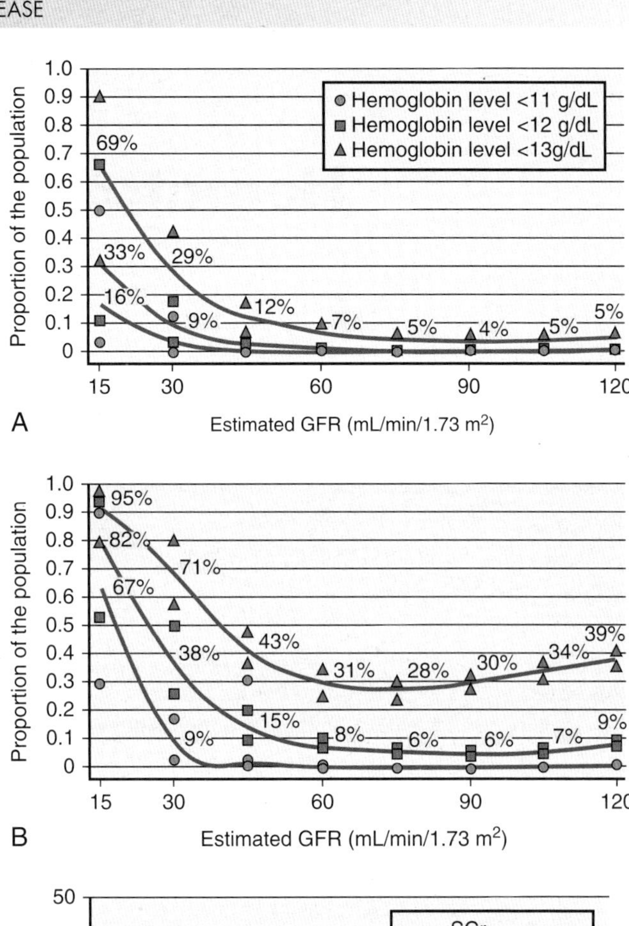


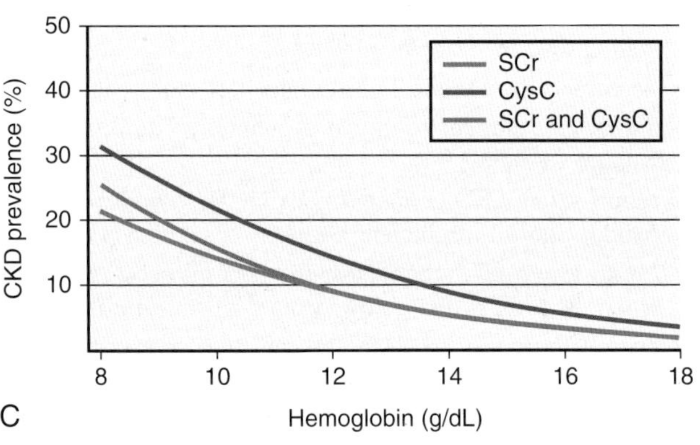


**Fig. 55.1** Prevalence of hemoglobin (Hgb) value less than 11 g/dL, 12 g/dL, and 13 g/dL among men (A) and women (B) 20 years of age and older from the Third National Health and Nutrition Examination Survey (NHANES III; 1988–1994). All values are adjusted to the age of 60 years. (C) Predicted prevalence of chronic kidney disease *(CKD)*. This is defined as an estimated glomerular filtration rate *(eGFR)* of 1 to 59 mL/min/1.73 m$^2$ using different GFR-estimating methods in US adults age 20 years or older by hemoglobin. The eGFR values are based separately on serum creatinine *(SCr)*, serum cystatin C *(CysC)*, and combined serum creatinine and cystatin C (SCr and CysC). Prevalence curves are truncated when the number of relevant participants is less than 30. (A and B modified from Astor B, Muntner P, Levin A, et al. Association of kidney function with anemia. Arch Intern Med. 2002;162:1401–1408; C from Estrella MM, Astor BC, Köttgen A, et al. Prevalence of kidney disease in anaemia differs by GFR-estimating method: the Third National Health and Nutrition Examination Survey [1988-94]. Nephrol Dial Transplant. 2010;25:2542–2548.)

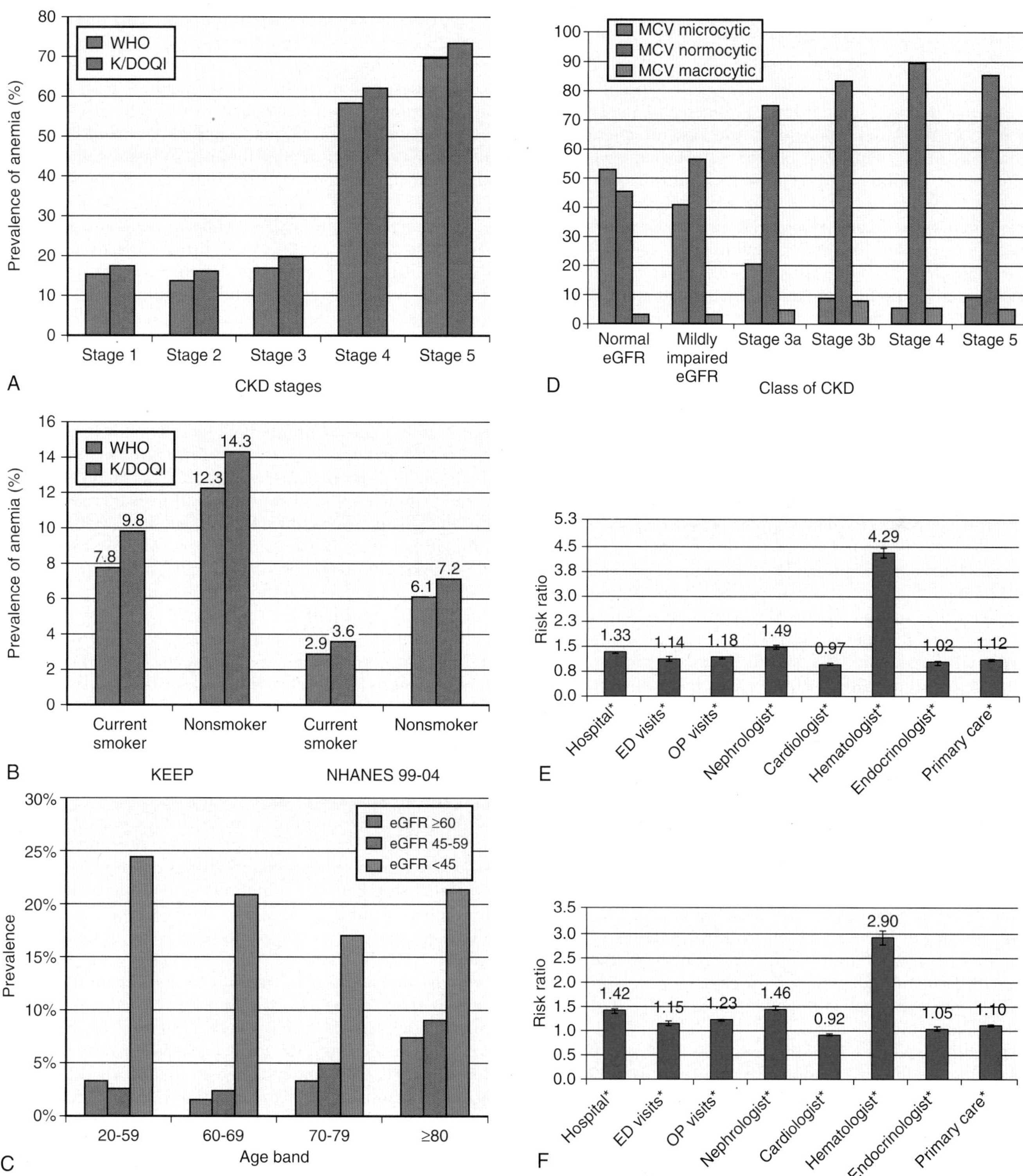


**Fig. 55.2** (A) Prevalence of anemia by stage of chronic kidney disease *(CKD)* in the Kidney Early Evaluation Program *(KEEP)*. (B) Prevalence of anemia by smoking status. (C) Age-specific prevalence of anemia in CKD according to estimated glomerular filtration rate *(eGFR)*. (D) Rates of microcytic, normocytic, and macrocytic anemia for each stage of CKD. Shown are adjusted hazard ratios of health care utilization in stage 3–5, non–dialysis-dependent CKD patients with and without anemia. (E) Medicare-covered patients aged 66–85 years. (F) Commercially insured patients aged 18 to 63 years. Results were from Poisson regression models, with the number of each type of health service as the dependent variable adjusting for patient demographics, baseline comorbidities, inflammatory conditions, and CKD stage. *$P < .05$. *ED,* Emergency department; *K/DOQI,* Kidney Disease Outcomes Quality Initiative; *MCV,* mean corpuscular volume; *NHANES,* National Health and Nutrition Examination Survey; *OP,* outpatient; *WHO,* World Health Organization. (A and B from McFarlane SI, Chen SC, Whaley-Connell AT, et al. Prevalence and associations of anemia of CKD: Kidney Early Evaluation Program [KEEP] and National Health and Nutrition Examination Survey [NHANES] 1999–2004. Am J Kidney Dis. 2008;51[Suppl]:S46–S55, 2008; C and D from Dmitrieva O, de Lusignan S, Macdougall IC, et al. Association of anaemia in primary care patients with chronic kidney disease: cross-sectional study of quality improvement in chronic kidney disease [QICKD] trial data. BMC Nephrol. 2013;14:24; E and F from St Peter WL, Guo H, Kabadi S, et al. Prevalence, treatment patterns, and healthcare resource utilization in Medicare and commercially insured non-dialysis-dependent chronic kidney disease patients with and without anemia in the United States. BMC Nephrol. 2018;19:67)

The worldwide prevalence of anemia associated with CKD rose from 1990 to 2010. CKD is currently the sixth leading cause of anemia in women and the ninth in men worldwide.[28]

Anemia is more common among women and non-Hispanic blacks. In the latter population, the risk for anemia was generally more than twice that in non-Hispanic whites in one study.[25] Another study reported a 3.3-fold higher prevalence of anemia in blacks than in whites, with CKD being less common in anemic blacks than in anemic whites (22% vs. 34%), suggesting a higher prevalence of non–CKD-related anemia as well.[29] The investigators extrapolated the data to the general US population and estimated that approximately 1,590,000 Americans with a creatinine clearance less than 50 mL/min are anemic, with an Hgb concentration lower than 12 g/dL.[25] A targeted community-based screening program for CKD has confirmed a threefold higher likelihood of anemia in blacks than in whites, as well as a twofold higher prevalence of anemia in this higher risk population compared with NHANES population survey[30]; the same study reported a lower prevalence of anemia in smokers than in nonsmokers, which has been attributed to enhanced stimulation of erythropoiesis due to relative hypoxia (see Fig. 55.2).

It has been advocated that the traditionally accepted eGFR threshold of 60 mL/min/1.73 m$^2$ to define CKD should be modified to higher values in blacks, in whom metabolic abnormalities and anemia are more common and are present at higher eGFR values than in whites.[31] In a large retrospective analysis, anemia was associated equally among blacks and whites with ESKD.[32] However, in patients on dialysis, the Hgb threshold below which higher mortality rates are observed is higher in blacks than in whites (11 g/dL vs. 10 g/dL).[33] In any case, observations on race and ethnicity cannot be interpreted in isolation, but must take into consideration socioeconomic status and cultural and behavioral differences.[34]

For people with an eGFR of 30 to 59 mL/min/1.73 m$^2$, low concentrations of 25-hydroxyvitamin D—25(OH)D—and elevations in C-reactive protein (CRP) were independently associated with Hgb concentrations below 12 g/dL.[35] A similar association has been described in ESKD patients who had undergone kidney transplantation.[36] Other studies have also reported an independent association of high-sensitivity CRP results with anemia in patients with an eGFR less than 60 mL/min/m$^2$.[37]

Anemia develops earlier in the course of CKD in patients with diabetes mellitus, and its magnitude tends to be more severe in patients with diabetes mellitus than in patients without diabetes.[8,38–46] El-Achkar and colleagues have studied 5380 community-dwelling patients surveyed as part of the Kidney Early Evaluation Program (KEEP), a community-based screening initiative for patients at high risk for kidney disease.[44] Anemia was more prevalent among patients with diabetes and developed earlier than in patients without diabetes mellitus. In patients with CKD stage G3 (GFR, 30–59 mL/min/1.73 m$^2$), 22.2% of those with diabetes were anemic; in patients with CKD stage G4 (GFR, 15–29 mL/min/1.73 m$^2$), the prevalence was 52.4%. The difference among patients with and without diabetes was most prominent in patients with CKD stage G3, in whom the prevalence of anemia was nearly threefold greater in those with diabetes. Men with diabetes were particularly prone to anemia, more so than women.

The prevalence of anemia in persons with diabetes and normal kidney function can be as high as 32%, with aggravating factors being advanced age and thiazolidinedione (glitazone) therapy.[47] Symeonidis and associates have explored the mechanism for anemia in diabetes by studying 694 anemic individuals, of whom 237 had diabetes.[45] Serum EPO concentrations were found to be lower in subjects with diabetes, particularly in relation to the degree of anemia present, with a significant inverse correlation between serum EPO value and the fraction of glycosylated Hgb. Thomas and associates have studied the contribution of proteinuria to anemia in 315 Australian patients with type 1 diabetes.[43] The prevalence of anemia was found to be higher in patients with macroalbuminuria than in those with microalbuminuria or with no albuminuria (52% vs. 24% vs. 8%, respectively).

A large study of 79,985 adults with diabetes mellitus has shown a higher risk of anemia in black subjects and a lower one in Asian subjects in comparison with white subjects.[48] A recent study in a large number of Medicare and commercially insured US patients has confirmed the greater prevalence of anemia in older patients, women, blacks (Medicare only), in the presence of comorbidities, and with increased CKD severity.[49] In anemic patients, RBC transfusion, erythropoiesis-stimulating agents (ESAs), and IV iron were used in 11.7%, 10.8%, and 9.4%, respectively, in younger patients (ages 18–63 years; $n = 15{,}716$); corresponding figures were 22.2%, 12.7%, and 6.7% in older patients (ages 66–85 years; $n = 109{,}251$), highlighting the fact that in this 2012 dataset, RBC transfusion was the most common therapy for anemia.[49] Anemic patients were also more likely to use health resources (see Fig. 55.2).

With aging, kidney function tends to decline progressively. The interaction of aging and loss of kidney function might be expected to raise the prevalence of anemia. In actuality, the relation is more complex.[50] Men with CKD tend to have a higher prevalence of anemia with older age, but among women with CKD, anemia is more frequent at a younger age.[25] It is likely that the high prevalence of iron deficiency in menstruating women accounts for this difference. However, if the analysis is limited to older men and women, the association between older age and anemia is clearer. Ble and colleagues have studied 1005 community-living older adults in Italy (InCHIANTI study).[51] The prevalence of anemia was found to increase with age in both genders. By multivariable analyses, much of the risk for anemia segregated to individuals with a creatinine clearance less than 30 mL/min, who also had lower mean serum EPO concentrations. Another InCHIANTI analysis has shown that lower than normal total and bioavailable testosterone concentrations resulted in a significantly higher risk for the development of anemia at 3-year follow-up for men and women.[52] In a study of 6200 nursing home residents (mostly white women), the prevalence of anemia and CKD were 60% and 43%, respectively.[53] Age was an important determinant of anemia in the absence of CKD, whereas this effect was lost in the presence of CKD, which became the strongest determinant of anemia.[53,54] One-third of the anemias found in older adults (>65 years) may be unexplained, but significant associations are present between anemia and low EPO concentrations and low lymphocyte counts.[55]

Hemoglobin values in patients with advanced CKD are frequently confounded by the use of ESAs (see later) and iron. Although there had been an increase in ESA use before

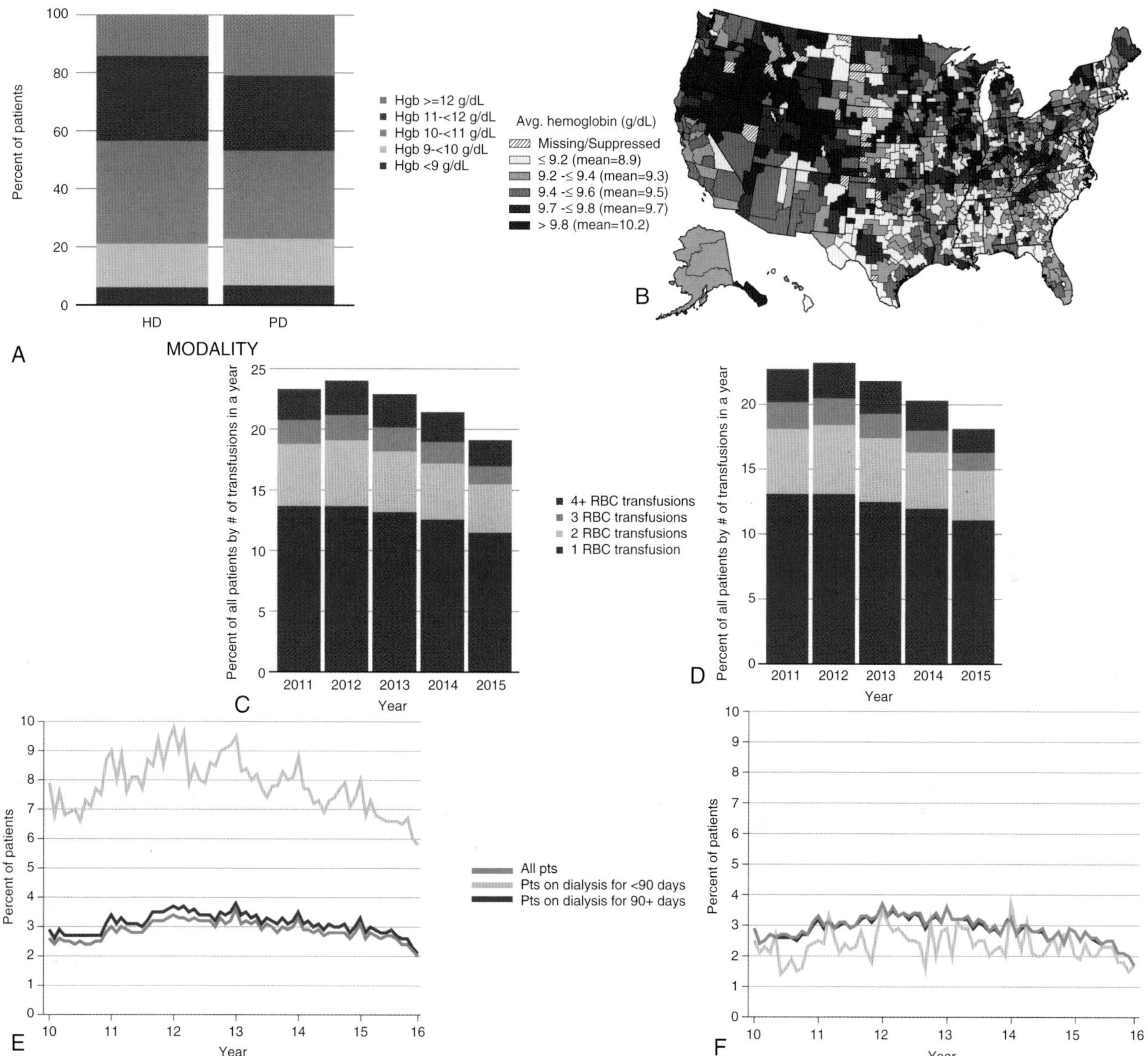


**Fig. 55.3** Anemia and treatment in end-stage kidney disease. (A) Percentage distribution of Hgb levels among prevalent hemodialysis and peritoneal dialysis patients. (B) Map of average hemoglobin level at initiation of renal replacement therapy, by health service area, 2011–2015. (C) Percentage of all adult hemodialysis patients by number of red blood cell transfusions received in a year. (D) Percentage of all adult peritoneal dialysis patients by number of red blood cell transfusions received in a year. (E) Percentage of all patients, patients on dialysis less than 90 days, or patients on dialysis 90 days or more who had one or more claims for a red blood cell transfusion in a month. (F) Percentage of all adult peritoneal dialysis patients with one or more claims for a red blood cell transfusion in a month. (From United States Renal Data System, 2017 annual data report. National Institutes of Health, National Institute of Diabetes and Digestive and Kidney Diseases, Bethesda, MD, 2017. A from CROWNWeb data, May 2016 vol 2 Figure 2.1.b; B from vol 2 Figure 1.20; C from Medicare claims data 2011-2015, vol 2 Figure 2.7.a; D from Medicare claims data 2010-2015, vol 2 Figure 2.13.a; E from Medicare claims data 2011-2015, vol 2 Figure 2.7.b; F from Medicare claims data 2010-2015, vol 2 Figure 2.13.b.)

the initiation of dialysis and in patients on dialysis in the past, this trend has reversed after publication of the results of randomized controlled trials (RCTs)—changes in prescribing instructions and new guidelines (see later). In fact, there has now been a steady decline in the use of ESAs before the initiation of dialysis (Fig. 55.3). The Hgb concentration at the initiation of dialysis has been declining since 2007 and, in most patients beginning hemodialysis in the United States, the Hgb value is now below 10 g/dL.[56,57]

## PATHOBIOLOGY OF ANEMIA IN CHRONIC KIDNEY DISEASE

### NORMAL ERYTHROPOIESIS

The delivery of oxygen to peripheral tissues is a highly regulated process; a crucially important determinant is the red blood cell mass, which is determined by the dynamic balance between the removal of older cells from the circulation and the production of newer cells by the bone marrow.

Under normal conditions, approximately 1% of circulating erythrocytes is replaced daily, corresponding to about 250 billion erythrocytes, with 2.5 to 3.0 million erythrocytes being produced each second.[58] The control of red blood cell mass is based on a classic negative feedback loop, mediated by changes in the production of the hormone EPO. EPO is mainly produced in the kidney and regulates the production of erythrocytes by interaction with specific EPO receptors (EPO-Rs) on bone marrow erythroid progenitors. For this mechanism to function properly, several other cofactors such as iron, vitamin $B_{12}$, and folic acid are also required.

### Erythropoietin

EPO, the major regulatory hormone of erythrocyte production, is a 30.4-kDa glycoprotein. Its production in the kidney is modulated by the delivery of oxygen from the circulating erythrocytes. When the mass of the circulating erythrocytes decreases because of decreased production, enhanced destruction, or loss of erythrocytes, the reduction in oxygen delivery results in increased production of this hormone. The first recognition of the linkage between hypoxia and erythrocyte quantity arose from astute 19th century observations on the effects of living at a higher altitude.[59,60] Carnot and Deflandre first postulated that a humoral factor (a so-called hemopoietin) might regulate erythropoiesis.[61] They injected serum from anemic rabbits into normal animals, resulting in increased reticulocyte counts; they termed the circulating factor "hematopoietin." However, in retrospect, this observation was probably an artifact because the amount of serum transferred was too low, and attempts to confirm their results were unsuccessful.[62]

44 years later, Reissmann rekindled interest in the field with ingenious experiments in parabiotic rats (artificial conjoined animals).[63] In this model, rats were joined by skin and muscle, ear to tail, living for 3 months in parabiosis. When one animal breathed air with low oxygen tension and the other breathed normal air, both animals demonstrated increased bone marrow erythropoiesis. This finding provided strong evidence that a humoral factor was the stimulus for erythropoiesis. In 1953, Erslev definitively demonstrated the erythropoietic role of the serum factor, now termed "erythropoietin."[64] He infused 100 to 200 mL of plasma from bled anemic rabbits into normal rabbit recipients. The reticulocyte count increased rapidly, with a fourfold increase in cell count within 4 days of infusion.[64,65] In 1957, Jacobson and coworkers provided indirect evidence to suggest that the kidneys were the primary source of EPO.[66] After demonstrating that removal of a variety of different organs did not affect EPO production after phlebotomy, they showed that nephrectomized rats and rabbits failed to increase EPO production (incorporation of iron-59 into erythrocytes) after blood loss.[66] Further studies by Koury and Lacombe and associates have demonstrated that the cells responsible for EPO production are peritubular interstitial cells,[67,68] which were subsequently identified as peritubular fibroblasts, located in the renal cortex.[69–71] Although the nature of these cells has still not been fully clarified, they have been suggested to be derived from the neural crest[72] and share characteristics of pericytes.[73,74]

It has also been shown that with the growing severity of anemia, the number of EPO-producing peritubular cells increases. This recruitment was found mostly in the inner cortex, but appeared also throughout the renal cortex when the anemia was particularly severe.[75,76] EPO production is regulated by a specific hypoxia-sensing mechanism based on transcription factors stabilized by hypoxia, called "hypoxia-inducible factors" (HIFs; Fig. 55.4).[74] This regulatory mechanism is not unique to EPO and is based on the capability of two separate helix loop–helix components, HIF-α and HIF-β, to bind as a complex to specific hypoxia-responsive DNA elements, which regulate the transcription of hypoxia-inducible genes.[77] The concentrations of the beta subunit do not respond to hypoxia.[78,79] The alpha subunits (1α, 2α, and 3α) are produced constitutively but are rapidly degraded in the presence of oxygen by the ubiquitin-proteasome system.[80–83] In hypoxic conditions, degradation of the alpha subunits is inhibited, leading to rapid increases in HIF-α concentrations and to the formation of the HIF transcription complex. For EPO regulation HIF-2 appears to be the important HIF isoform.[84–89] Renal HIF-2 is required for hypoxia-driven EPO production; in the absence of renal HIF-2, hepatic HIF-2 becomes the main regulator of EPO production.[74,84] HIF-2α, together with HIF-ß, hepatocyte nuclear factor-4 (HNF-4), and p300 bind to a 120-bp enhancer, which is located at the 3' end of the human EPO polyadenylation signal.[58,79,90–92] This interaction results in rapid EPO transcription, followed by translation and secretion of the EPO glycoprotein.[93–96]

The rapid degradation of HIF-α in the presence of oxygen depends on binding of the tumor suppressor protein von Hippel-Lindau (VHL), a process that results in tagging of the molecule for proteasomal degradation via polyubiquitination by ubiquitin ligase.[97,98] This regulatory mechanism is based on the hydroxylation of two proline residues, which are critical for the recognition of HIF-α by VHL. An additional hydroxylation of one asparagine residue is required for HIF binding with p300.[99–103] Hydroxylation at these three sites depends on the presence of oxygen as a molecular substrate for specific hydroxylase enzymes, placing these enzymes in a central role for sensing oxygen and detecting hypoxia. A mutation in the VHL protein that impairs the degradation of HIF-α, and increases EPO production causes the so-called Chuvash congenital polycythemia, an autosomal recessive disorder that is endemic in the mid–Volga River region.[104] HIF-2α but not HIF-1α displays a typical iron response element (IRE) in its 5′ untranslated region (UTR), which has been shown in mice to constitute an important regulatory loop for HIF-2α messenger RNA (mRNA) translation in the presence of hypoxia or iron loading.[105] This regulatory system in conditions of reduced iron availability would allow iron response protein 1 (IRP1) to bind with high affinity to IRE, inhibit mRNA translation, and decrease HIF-2α synthesis and EPO production. When cellular iron is abundant, IRP1 loses its RNA binding activity and becomes a cytosolic aconitase, resulting in derepression of mRNA translation, which increases HIF-2α synthesis and EPO production.

Purification and identification of EPO is credited to Miyake and colleagues.[106] From 2550 L of urine from patients with aplastic anemia, and using multiple isolation steps, they obtained a small quantity of pure glycoprotein.[106] Purification of human EPO led to successful cloning of the gene, reported in 1985 by Lin and associates.[107] They found that the gene encodes a protein of 193 amino acids, including a 27–amino acid leader sequence and a terminal single amino acid that are cleaved during processing, resulting in a 165–amino acid mature EPO molecule. When these investigators introduced

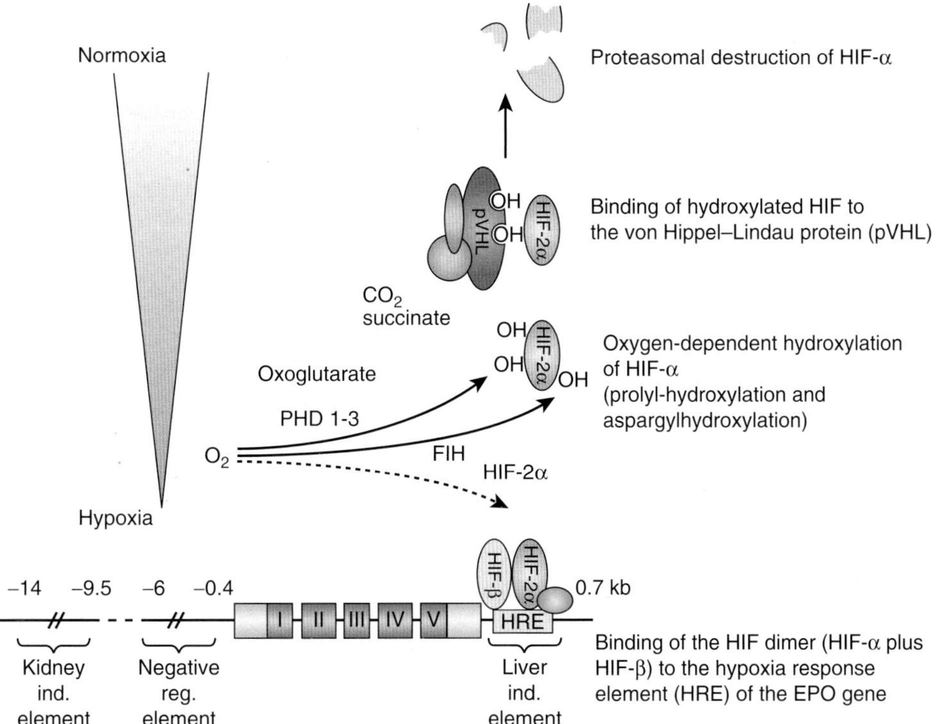


**Fig. 55.4** Schematic presentation of hypoxia-inducible factor *(HIF)* signaling and the oxygen-dependent control of erythropoietin *(EPO)* gene expression. HIF consists of one of two oxygen-dependent alpha subunits, HIF-1α and HIF-2α, and a constitutive beta subunit. For EPO regulation, HIF-2α is the relevant isoform. In the presence of oxygen (normoxia), HIF-α is hydroxylated at two prolyl and one asparagyl residues through prolyl hydroxylases (PHDs 1–3) and an asparagyl hydroxylase (factor-inhibiting HIF *[FIH]*), enzymes that require oxoglutarate as a cosubstrate. Hydroxylation of the asparagyl residue inhibits binding of the transcriptional coactivator p300, and hydroxylation of the prolyl residues enables binding to the von Hippel-Lindau protein, which represents the recognition component of an E3 ubiquitin ligase. Thus, hydroxylated HIF-α is targeted for proteasomal destruction, and hydroxylated HIF that escapes destruction is not transcriptionally active. Under hypoxia, there is no substrate (oxygen) for the hydroxylation reactions, and thus HIF-α is stabilized, can bind to hypoxia-responsive elements of its target genes, and can induce or enhance their transcription. The hypoxia response element *(HRE)* of the EPO gene is located at 5′ of the gene; other regulatory elements determine the tissue specificity of its expression, limiting EPO expression mainly to liver and kidneys. *ind.,* Inducible; *reg.,* regulatory.

the gene into Chinese hamster ovary cells, EPO with full biologic activity was produced.[107] These findings were confirmed by an almost simultaneous report by Jacobs and colleagues.[108] The results led in short order to the development of techniques to produce recombinant human EPO (rhEPO). By 1989, clinical trials of rhEPO had demonstrated its remarkable efficacy,[109–112] leading to regulatory approval and routine clinical use of EPO as replacement treatment.

EPO itself is a member of the family of class 1 cytokines.[113] The carbohydrate moiety is important for molecular stability, whereas the 165–amino acid protein component is critical for receptor binding.[114–116] There are four discrete carbohydrate chains, three *N*-linked and one *O*-linked, each of them having two to four branches, most of which end with a negatively charged sialic acid.[114,117–121] The physiologic role of the carbohydrate chains is complex. They seem to be required for the in vivo biologic activity of EPO, but are not essential for in vitro receptor binding or growth stimulation of cells in culture.[122] There is considerable heterogeneity in the glycosylation of EPO, resulting in multiple isoforms with different numbers of sialic acid residues. Isoforms with higher sialic content have a prolonged half-life in the circulation and induce greater stimulation of erythropoiesis, despite having a lower affinity for the EPO receptor.[123] A hyperglycosylated recombinant EPO, called "novel erythropoiesis-stimulating protein" (NESP) or darbepoetin, carries two additional *N*-linked carbohydrate chains with up to 22 sialic acid residues; the endogenous EPO has a maximum of 14.[124] Despite a lower (approximately fivefold) affinity for the EPO-R, darbepoetin exhibits a half-life in the circulation approximately three times longer than that of EPO.[125,126] Gross and Lodish have developed an in vitro model accounting for the prolonged bioactivity of darbepoetin.[123] They found that darbepoetin and EPO have similar rates of internalization when bound to the EPO-R, with similar degradation and resecretion, but that EPO dissociates at a much slower rate from the EPO-R than darbepoetin, so more EPO is internalized and degraded.

EPO is produced primarily by the liver in the fetal period; after birth, the kidneys become the major source of production.[69,70,113,127–130] Clearance of circulating EPO occurs by mechanisms that have not yet been fully elucidated. The liver, kidneys, and bone marrow have all been studied as possible sources of EPO elimination. A small fraction of endogenous or exogenous EPO appears to be cleared by filtration into the urine.[131] EPO degradation products can be found in urine, but the location and mechanisms responsible for this degradation are not known.[118]

An important determinant of the fate of the circulating EPO is its binding to the EPO-R on erythroid cells[132]; the relative abundance of erythroid precursors (i.e., the size of the pool of erythroid progenitors) is known to modulate serum EPO concentrations.[133] The EPO-R is a 55-kDa transmembrane protein that belongs to the cytokine receptor superfamily.[134–139] It is present on erythroid progenitors from the colony-forming unit erythroid (CFU-E) stage to late basophilic erythroblasts.[134] The number of receptors has been estimated to be around 1000/cell. The molecular signaling cascade activated on binding of EPO to EPO-R has been studied in great detail. The first event seems to be the homodimerization of the receptor, which also undergoes a conformational change. This is followed by the generation of the intracellular signal by clathrin-mediated endocytosis and proteolysis of the whole ligand receptor complex, which ultimately determines the clearance of EPO from the circulation.[123,140–145]

Rather than intrinsic enzymatic activity, the EPO-R signal transduction pathway depends on the activation of Janus tyrosine kinase 2 (JAK2), which is physically associated with the receptor, and become phosphorylated when the conformation of the receptor is changed by the binding of EPO.[146–153] Activated JAK2 phosphorylates several of the eight tyrosine molecules of the cytoplasmic side of the EPO-R, exposing SH2 (src homology 2) binding sites for key signaling proteins.[154,155] The result is a cascade of signal transduction, with the activation of multiple pathways, including Ras/MAP kinase, JNK/p38 MAP kinase, JAK/STAT, the p85 regulatory subunit of phosphoinositide 3-kinase (PI3K), and protein kinase B (AKT).[156–161] Both JAK2 and the tyrosines on the cytoplasmic portion of the EPO-R seem to play a role in the internalization process.[162] Familial and genetic forms of polycythemia due to truncations in the EPO-R with absence of key tyrosines such as Y429 and Y431 have been shown to result in defective internalization of the EPO-R complex, prolonged signal transduction, and increased EPO sensitivity.[162] The EPO-R endocytic machinery is critically dependent on a Cbl/p85/epsin-1 pathway, which ultimately leads to receptor downregulation.[163]

The interaction of JAK2 with important intermediaries in signal transduction, STATs (signal transducers and activators of transcription), has been extensively studied. After phosphorylation, STAT5 becomes activated and undergoes homodimerization; it may translocate to the nucleus, where it activates EPO-inducible genes.[164] In transgenic mice lacking both STAT5a and STAT5b, fetal anemia develops, with increased apoptosis of erythroid progenitors due to decreased survival of early erythroblasts.[165,166]

The signaling induced by the binding of EPO to the EPO-R eventually results in an increased number of erythroid progenitors and precursors, in particular CFU-E[167] and, at the same time, in the activation of parallel molecular pathways that eventually suppress the signaling of the receptor via tyrosine phosphatases, which dephosphorylate and inactivate JAK2, downregulate the EPO-R on the cell surface, and induce negative regulators such as CIS/SOCS (cytokine-inducible, SH2-containing protein-suppressor of cytokine signaling).[168–176]

An important aspect of the overall mechanism of action of EPO has been elucidated by Koury and Bondurant,[167] who demonstrated that EPO does not directly stimulate erythroid proliferation but rather prevents the programmed death (apoptosis) of the erythroid progenitors (Fig. 55.5).[177–179] Burst-forming units-erythroid (BFU-Es), named for their capacity to generate multiclustered colonies of cells, are the earliest cell type exclusively committed to the erythrocyte line.[180] It is believed that these cells are produced stochastically from pluripotent stem cells. Only a minority of BFU-Es, 10% to 20%, are in a cell cycle at any given time; the rest remain an inert reserve of progenitor cells. Cells then begin to take on the characteristics of CFU-Es.[181] BFU-Es contain only small quantities of GATA-1, a key transcription factor for erythroid development, whereas CFU-Es have much higher concentrations.[182,183] CFU-Es begin to express some attributes of mature erythrocytes, including blood group and Rh antigens.[184,185] It is at the CFU-E stage that EPO exerts its greatest influence; CFU-E cells express the highest surface concentration of EPO-Rs of any erythrocyte precursor.[180,186,187] Without EPO present, these cells are rapidly lost to programmed cell death.[188–190] EPO is an essential survival factor for erythroid progenitors, beginning from the CFU-E stage all the way to basophilic erythroblasts. There is substantial heterogeneity in the responsiveness of erythroid progenitors to EPO in a certain tissue and differentiation stage, possibly related to the number of EPO-Rs, their functional status, or both.[191] This diversity in EPO-responsiveness corresponds to the 3-log units' range of serum EPO concentrations that can be measured in human patients.

The quantity of EPO is traditionally expressed in units, with 1 unit (U) representing the same erythropoietic effect in animals as occurs after stimulation with 5-mmol cobalt chloride.[113] Steady-state production of small amounts of EPO maintains the serum EPO concentration at approximately 10 to 30 U/L, enough to stimulate sufficient production of erythrocytes to replace those lost to senescence.[90,113] When anemia or hypoxia is present, serum EPO concentrations increase rapidly, to as much as 10,000 U/L.[93–95] Human studies have indicated a sustained increase in serum EPO concentrations after phlebotomy, with values remaining elevated for several weeks.[192,193] With chronic anemia, as occurs with pure red cell aplasia (PRCA) and aplastic anemia, serum EPO values remains chronically elevated, with values as much as 1000-fold higher than normal in those with very severe aplastic anemias.[194–198]

Koury and Bondurant and other associates have incorporated these basic physiologic concepts into a model, which explains how EPO regulates erythropoiesis in a variety of pathologic conditions (see Fig. 55.5).[58,167,199] In this model, the EPO-dependent phase of erythropoiesis encompasses three generations (from CFU-E through early erythroblasts), with each generation having a certain proportion of surviving cells and the remaining cells being lost by apoptosis. Owing to their reduced EPO responsiveness (or greater EPO dependence) most of the cells at the CFU-E stage become victims of apoptosis, so the erythropoietic production flow in a normal subject is produced by a relatively small fraction of progenitors that have escaped apoptosis. When EPO concentrations increase in response to hypoxia, blood loss, or hemolysis, additional progenitors are allowed to escape apoptosis and, a few days later, result in the generation of an increased absolute number of reticulocytes and ultimately of RBCs. If this response is sufficient to compensate for the decreased oxygen-carrying capacity of blood, EPO concentrations decline and so does erythropoiesis. When EPO production is impaired, such as in CKD, a much greater number of cells become apoptotic, and EPO concentrations are

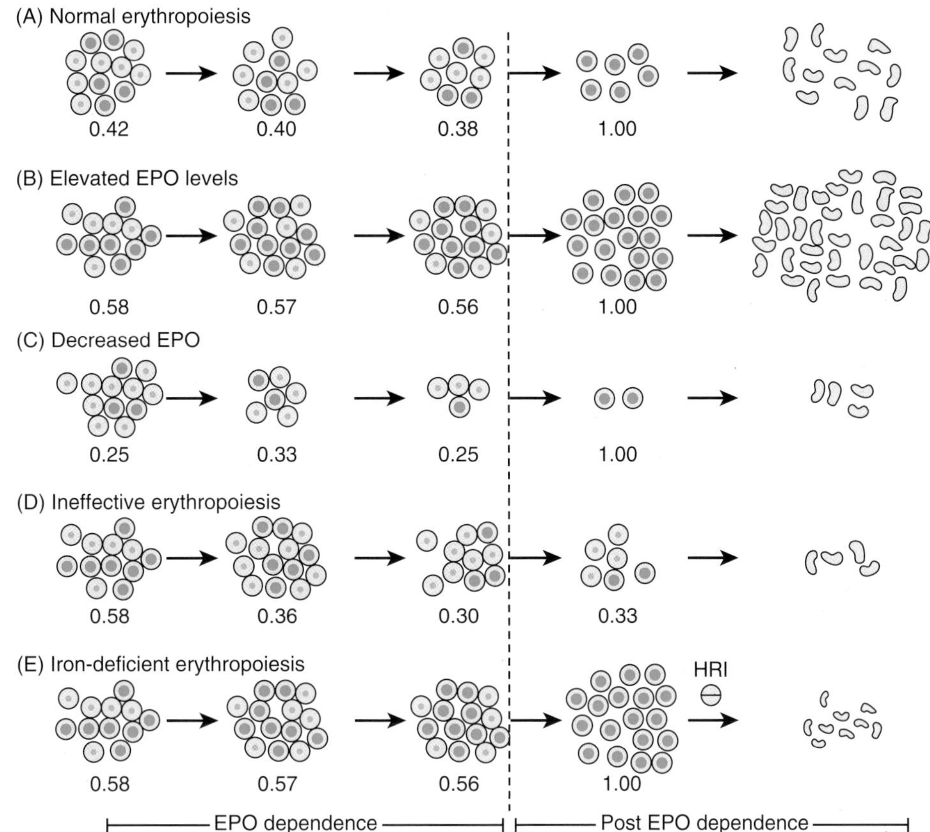


**Fig. 55.5** Model of erythropoiesis based on suppression of programmed cell death (apoptosis) by erythropoietin *(EPO)* and heterogeneity in EPO dependence among erythroid cells. (A) Normal erythropoiesis with an average survival rate of 40% in each of the EPO-dependent generations. Normal erythropoiesis produces about 250 billion new erythrocytes daily, even though a minority of all potential erythroid cells survive the EPO-dependent period. (B) Elevated EPO values as found after acute blood loss or hemolysis, increase average survival rates to 55% in each EPO-dependent generation. Daily erythrocyte production increases to three times the normal amount. (C) Decreased EPO values as found in renal failure, decrease the average survival rate to 28% in each EPO-dependent generation. Daily erythrocyte production is one-third of normal. (D) Ineffective erythropoiesis with high EPO values increases rates of apoptosis caused by a pathologic process such as folate or vitamin $B_{12}$ deficiency. High EPO values are the response to decreased erythrocyte production and expand surviving cells in the early EPO-dependent generation, but the increased rates of apoptosis in the late EPO-dependent and post–EPO-dependent stages decrease daily erythrocyte production to one-third normal. (E) Iron-deficient erythropoiesis with elevated EPO Values resulting in a similar increase to an average of 55% survival, as seen in B, but in the post–EPO-dependent period, when hemoglobin is synthesized, heme-regulated inhibitor *(HRI)* prevents apoptosis by inhibiting protein synthesis. The inhibited protein synthesis decreases the size of the erythrocytes produced and reduces daily erythrocyte production to 75% of the normal numbers. (From Koury M: Red cell production and kinetics. In Simon T, Snyder EL, Solheim BG, et al, eds. Rossi's Principles of Transfusion Medicine. Hoboken, NJ: Blackwell Publishing; 2009.)

insufficient to maintain an adequate pool of differentiating progenitors, with resulting impaired reticulocyte production and ultimately anemia.

It has become apparent that erythropoiesis does not happen in a vacuum and thus critically depends on the interaction of erythroblasts with the macrophages at the center of the erythroblastic island in the marrow.[200] A still undetermined fraction of basal and EPO-stimulated erythropoiesis requires contact between erythroblasts and central macrophages.[201,202] Macrophages play a role not only in the proliferation and final enucleation of erythroblasts, but also possibly in supplying ferritin and iron to the erythroblast.[203] In chronic inflammatory conditions, negative regulation of erythropoiesis may be mediated locally by macrophage-produced cytokines such as tumor necrosis factor-α (TNF-α), transforming growth factor-β (TGF-β), interferon-γ (INF-γ), and interleukin-6 (IL-6). Osteoblasts are another important component of the hematopoietic microenvironment in bone. They are able to produce EPO, and this local production can modulate the response to systemic anemia.[204]

## The Roles of Iron, Folate, and Vitamin $B_{12}$ in Erythropoiesis

Because of the continuous proliferative activity of the erythroid tissue and the associated production of large amounts of hemoglobin, adequate nutritional supplies of folate, vitamin $B_{12}$, and iron are essential for proper erythropoietic function. If any of these three components is inadequate, erythropoiesis becomes unable to meet both baseline and stimulated demands.

Inefficient erythropoiesis is a distinguishing feature of megaloblastic anemias, with the inability of erythroid progenitors to progress through the cell cycle and escape apoptosis owing to impaired DNA synthesis and repair. Studies by Koury and associates have shown that the erythroid differentiation stage that is most affected by folate or $B_{12}$ deficiency is the one coinciding with the end of the EPO-dependent effects and initiation of Hgb synthesis.[205,206] The expansion of erythroid progenitors induced by EPO creates a large pool of progenitors (CFU-Es and pro-erythroblasts), which are extremely susceptible to apoptosis. The inefficient erythropoiesis of megaloblastic anemias is characterized by a reduced number of reticulocytes, increased serum bilirubin and lactic dehydrogenase (LDH), and accelerated iron turnover. In the case of vitamin $B_{12}$ deficiency, thymidine and purine synthesis are impaired because of the unavailability of methylenetetrahydrofolate and formyltetrahydrofolate, respectively, and the trapping of folate as methyltetrahydrofolate.[207] Folate deficiency affects several key coenzymes that are involved in the transfer of single carbon units for the synthesis of pyrimidines and, for purines, and amino acid metabolism.

A regulated iron supply capable of matching the iron needs of the erythroid marrow is key for proper erythropoiesis. Intracellular availability of iron, heme, and globin chains have to be perfectly matched because excess of any of these constituents is toxic for the cell. Iron, 1 mg, can be adsorbed daily from the intestine, approximately 5% to 10% of the 14 mg of iron found in the average daily Western diet. The large majority of iron used for erythropoiesis comes from recycling of iron contained in aged RBCs via macrophages. Each milliliter of blood contains, on average, 0.5 mg of iron. Small, long-term blood losses result eventually in the depletion of the body iron stores and development of iron-deficient erythropoiesis and anemia. Iron deficiency partially suppresses the anemia-induced HIF-2α synthesis, which in turn reduces EPO production, resulting in decreased erythropoiesis and inappropriately low reticulocyte counts for the degree of anemia.[105,208,209] Heme-regulated eukaryotic initiation factor 2 (eIF-2α) kinase (HRI) is a key master controller of globin synthesis based on iron/heme availability.[210] In iron-sufficient states, free heme binds to HRI and inhibits the phosphorylation of eIF-2α, allowing globin synthesis to proceed. In iron-deficient states, HRI phosphorylates eIF-2α and suppresses mTORC1, leading to a numerically increased production of microcytic erythrocytes, without ineffective erythropoiesis.[211] In macrophages, HRI acts as a positive modulator of cytokine and hepcidin production, thus affecting both inflammation and iron metabolism.[212]

## ANEMIA OF CHRONIC KIDNEY DISEASE

Anemia in CKD can develop because of any of the diseases or deficiencies that may affect individuals without kidney disease, such as iron deficiency, vitamin $B_{12}$[213,214] or folic acid deficiency,[213] and chronic blood loss.[215] However, the form of anemia most common in CKD is a normocytic, normochromic, or slightly hypochromic[216] anemia, with insufficient production of erythrocytes (see Fig. 55.2).[217–220] The cause is multifactorial, with contributors such as relative EPO deficiency, iron deficiency, blood loss, hemolysis, chronic inflammation,[221] drugs such as nonsteroidal antiinflammatory drugs (NSAIDs), and other factors, which may include circulating inhibitors of erythropoiesis.[220,222–224] The preponderance of evidence has demonstrated that EPO deficiency is the major cause of anemia in those with CKD.[225–228] Ultimately, the greatest proof of the primacy of EPO deficiency in the pathogenesis of renal anemia has been the consistent success of treatment with rhEPO or its derivatives. Other contributing causes to anemia should be considered if the severity of anemia is much greater than expected, if higher than usual doses of rhEPO are needed, and in the presence of leukopenia or thrombocytopenia.

### ERYTHROPOIETIN PRODUCTION AND KIDNEY DISEASE

In normal persons, serum EPO concentrations rise in response to a reduction in red cell mass—in other words, anemia. In patients with CKD, EPO concentrations are inappropriately low for the degree of anemia, but may still be similar to or even higher than those in normal nonanemic subjects.[229–233] The adequacy of EPO production in response to anemia appears to decline in rough proportion to the degree of reduction in nephron mass.[234–236] Radtke and coworkers measured serum EPO in 135 patients with CKD and 59 normal subjects.[237] At all stages of CKD, serum EPO values were found to be higher than in nonanemic normal subjects, but the relationship between Hgb and serum EPO depended on the severity of the CKD. Among patients with mild to moderate CKD, the correlation was inverse, with lower Hgb concentrations being associated with higher serum EPO concentrations. However, among patients with creatinine clearances below 40 mL/min, mean serum EPO concentrations were severely depressed and uncorrelated with the degree of anemia, but directly correlated with creatinine clearance, indicating a parallel loss of renal excretory and endocrine function.[237] Fehr and associates have studied 395 patients undergoing coronary angiography, 84% of whom had reduced creatinine clearance values.[238] Like Radtke and colleagues, they found that serum EPO concentrations were higher in patients with lower Hgb, except when creatinine clearance was below 40 mL/min.[237,238]

Why EPO production by diseased kidneys is inadequately low remains incompletely understood. Some evidence has suggested that EPO production is reduced because of the transformation of peritubular fibroblasts into myofibroblasts.[239,240] On the other hand, it has been demonstrated that pharmacologic stabilization of HIF with inhibitors of the prolyl hydroxylases results in significant EPO secretion from renal and extrarenal tissues, even in patients undergoing dialysis.[241] On the basis of these findings and other circumstantial evidence, it appears that a disturbed oxygen-sensing mechanism rather than destroyed production capacity for EPO is the primary cause of renal anemia. In fact, despite the severely diminished EPO response with advanced CKD, some degree of sustained feedback remains. In the 6 months before starting dialysis, Radtke and colleagues found that as anemia worsened, serum EPO concentrations increased, and in the 6 months after the start of dialysis, the opposite occurred.[237] This continued response to anemia in patients with advanced CKD was also demonstrated by Walle and coworkers, who found that serum EPO values increased after hemorrhage and declined after blood transfusion in patients on dialysis.[242] Others have also reported that hypoxia can increase EPO production significantly in anemic patients with CKD.[243,244] Consistent with such observations and a relevant capacity for endogenous EPO secretion in patients with CKD, a large analysis in the United States has revealed that with increasing altitude—and thus lower blood oxygen content for any given Hgb concentration—higher achieved Hgb values were observed, even though lower doses of ESAs were used.[245]

The pronounced breakdown of EPO production in response to anemia when creatinine clearance is below 40 mL/min fits well with the observation that clinically relevant anemia becomes common only with moderate to advanced CKD (see earlier discussion and Figs. 55.1 and 55.2).[22,25]

## SHORTENED RED CELL SURVIVAL

Although there have been several published reports on reduced red cell survival in CKD,[21,218,246] it is not clear how much it contributes to the anemia of CKD. Several abnormalities have been described in uremic erythrocytes, which may result in their increased premature destruction. An abnormal externalization of phosphatidylserine (PS), a phospholipid normally present only on the inside of the RBC membrane, has been associated with increased erythrophagocytosis and anemia in CKD.[247] Uremic red cells have been reported to become more fragile in response to osmotic stimuli,[248] although this finding was not confirmed in pediatric patients undergoing peritoneal dialysis.[249] The rheologic properties of uremic erythrocytes are altered owing to changes in RBC shape and decreased deformability.[250] Uremic erythrocytes may not be able to mount an effective response to oxidative stress,[251–253] possibly because of glutathione deficiency,[254] and may benefit from the antioxidant effects of vitamin E bound to dialysis membranes.[253,255] Carnitine deficiency may also contribute to the reduced survival of uremic erythrocytes.[256,257] An abnormal deposition of complement onto erythrocytes in CKD could also play a role in their premature removal from the circulation.[258] Because the contribution to shortened RBC life span of each of these factors is variable from patient to patient and is not easily quantifiable, and because there are no simple reliable methods to measure RBC survival, it is extremely difficult to identify anemic patients who are particularly affected, unless they have a preexisting RBC disorder.

## BLOOD LOSS

Excessive bleeding has long been recognized as a common and significant complication of CKD.[259] The coagulopathy of CKD is discussed in the final section of this chapter and is thought to play a major role in the occult blood loss via gastrointestinal bleeding of patients with CKD.[260] In addition, blood loss due to the dialysis procedure and associated laboratory studies is also significant. A classic paper published 30 years ago estimated the blood loss due to hemodialysis to be between 1 and 3 L/year.[261] Subsequent improvements in dialysis techniques and clinical laboratory testing methodology have reduced this loss considerably. Later estimates of the blood lost in the whole extracorporeal circuit for each dialysis session vary from a range of 0.5 to 0.6 mL[262] to a median of 0.98 mL (range, 0.01–23.9 mL).[263] Each milliliter of blood contains approximately 0.5 mg of iron, so an important consequence of blood loss is the loss of iron and the development of iron deficiency (see below).

## UREMIC "INHIBITORS" OF ERYTHROPOIESIS

Although a variety of uremic toxins have been identified in CKD,[264,265] including some with hematologic effects, such as quinolinic acid[266] and *N*-acetyl-seryl-aspartyl-lysyl-proline (AcSDKP),[267] there is no convincing demonstration that any of them plays a significant role in the anemia of CKD. Nevertheless, the response to ESAs can be improved with dialysis, and the EPO doses used to treat patients with anemia in CKD are much higher than the amounts endogenously produced in normal individuals, indicating reduced responsiveness. Apart from factors associated with anemia, it is likely that inhibition of erythropoiesis in CKD also occurs through the concomitant chronic inflammatory state, which is characteristic for the anemia of chronic disease (ACD). Contributing factors include decreased EPO production or responsiveness plus hepcidin-induced reduction in iron availability or absorption.[268,269] No significant reduction in the dose of ESAs used to manage anemia was observed for patients undergoing frequent hemodialysis (six times/week) in comparison with those on the conventional three times/week schedule.[270]

## IRON METABOLISM, HEPCIDIN, AND ANEMIA OF CHRONIC DISEASE

During the last decade, we have witnessed an unprecedented explosion of our knowledge on the regulation of iron metabolism.[271] This has not only profoundly affected our understanding of iron metabolism in CKD but has also opened the door to novel therapeutic opportunities.[272] Although iron deficiency and functional iron deficiency have been a major focus of clinical and basic research in the iron metabolism of CKD, more attention is now being paid to patients in a positive iron balance and possible negative consequences of iron overload.[259]

Patients with CKD are in negative iron balance due to increased blood loss (see earlier), which frequently cannot be adequately compensated. In the absence of chronic inflammation, blood loss leads to a reduction of serum ferritin and serum iron values and a progressive increase in the desaturation of transferrin, below the 16% threshold that guarantees a normal supply of iron to the erythroid marrow.[273] Some studies have reported a reduced intestinal iron absorption in patients on maintenance dialysis,[274,275] mostly due to the concomitant inflammation. However, other studies have shown it to be upregulated by EPO administration and not substantially impaired in comparison with that in normal subjects.[276,277] The chronic inflammatory state frequently accompanying CKD creates additional constraints to the proper absorption and utilization of iron.[268]

The identification of hepcidin as a key regulator of iron homeostasis in normal conditions and in the ACD has redefined our understanding of iron homeostasis in CKD (Fig. 55.6).[278–286] Hepcidin, a 25–amino acid peptide produced and secreted by the liver,[287] modulates iron availability by promoting the internalization and degradation of ferroportin,[288] a key iron transporter (so far the only identified mammalian iron exporter) that is essential for iron absorption in the duodenum and recycling of iron/iron efflux by macrophages.[289,290]

High hepcidin concentrations turn off both duodenal iron absorption and release of iron from macrophages; low hepcidin concentrations promote iron absorption and heme iron recycling and iron mobilization from macrophages. Thus, hepcidin concentrations are expected to be high in iron overload states and decreased in iron deficiency states. In normal subjects, an oral iron load produces a measurable increase in hepcidin concentrations.[291] A hepcidin knockout mouse model has shown increased iron absorption, increased liver iron concentration, and decreased reticuloendothelial

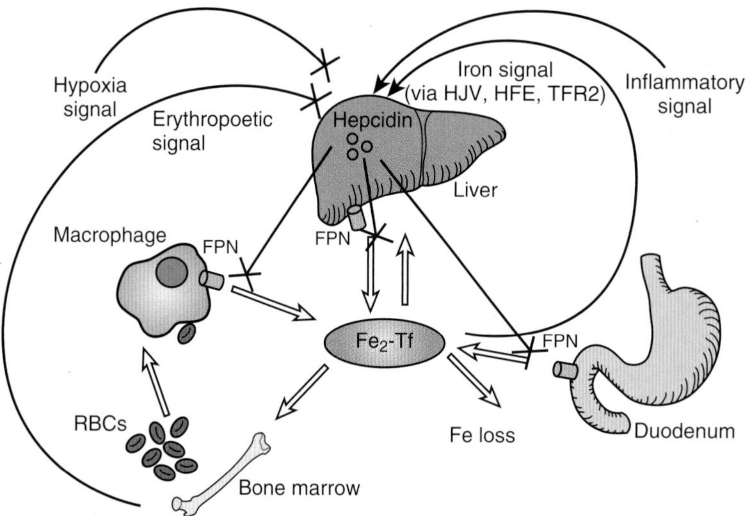


**Fig. 55.6** Hepcidin is a central regulator of systemic iron homeostasis. Serum iron concentrations are determined by the balance of iron entry from intestinal absorption, macrophage iron recycling, and mobilization of hepatocyte stores versus iron utilization, primarily by erythroid cells in the bone marrow. A peptide hormone secreted by the liver, hepcidin controls iron release into the plasma by downregulating cell surface expression of the iron export protein ferroportin *(FPN)* on absorptive enterocytes, macrophages, and hepatocytes. Hepcidin production is inhibited by the erythropoietic drive and hypoxia to ensure iron availability for erythropoiesis. Hepcidin production is stimulated by iron (through human hemochromatosis protein *[HFE]*, hemojuvelin *[HJV]*, and transferrin receptor 2 *[TFR2]*) as a negative feedback loop to maintain steady-state iron concentrations. Hepcidin production also is stimulated by inflammation, thereby sequestering iron from invading pathogens in the setting of infection but also causing the hypoferremia of anemia of chronic disease. *$FE_2$-Tf,* Transferrin-bound iron; *RBC,* red blood cell. (From Babitt JL, Lin HY: Molecular mechanisms of hepcidin regulation: implications for the anemia of CKD. Am J Kidney Dis. 2010;55:726–741.)

iron stores.[279] Hepcidin overexpression in mice leads to severe iron deficiency.[292] Some of the genetic forms of hemochromatosis, like juvenile hemochromatosis, are caused by mutations in the hepcidin gene.[293] Hepcidin production can be induced by type II acute inflammatory reactions, which are mediated by IL-6 but not IL-1 or TNF-α,[294,295] thus providing a mechanism for inflammation to affect iron availability and causing the ACD. Anemia, EPO administration, and hypoxia increase iron absorption and mobilization by decreasing hepcidin production,[296,297] although hepcidin is not a direct target gene of HIF.[298] Erythroferrone (ERFE) has been identified as the key mediator of the erythropoietic regulation of iron metabolism. ERFE production rises with increased erythropoietic activity, leading to hepcidin suppression and mobilization of the iron stores.[299,300]

Urinary and serum concentrations of hepcidin have been measured with mass spectrometry.[301–303] An immunoassay for serum human hepcidin has been developed, with a lower limit of detection of 5 ng/mL, yielding a normal range for serum hepcidin of 29 to 254 ng/mL in men and 16 to 288 ng/mL in women.[291] The assay has enough sensitivity to detect changes in serum hepcidin values due to diurnal variation and in response to oral iron. Measurements of prohepcidin, the precursor of the biologically active 25–amino acid hepcidin, seem to be poorly correlated with those of hepcidin and are unresponsive to known hepcidin regulators.[304] Several studies have measured hepcidin concentrations in CKD, but have at times produced conflicting results.[305] A proper interpretation of these studies' findings must consider the following caveats. First, in the presence of anemia, hepcidin concentrations are reduced in persons with normal kidney function; thus, a normal hepcidin concentration in CKD can be still inappropriately high for the level of anemia. Second, hepcidin concentrations in healthy persons are reduced by 70% to 75% 24 hours after EPO administration.[306]

Residual kidney function, iron stores, erythropoiesis status, and inflammation all seem to be related to the hepcidin concentrations observed in CKD.[307] Hepcidin concentrations were found in one study to be elevated in patients on dialysis, but were not correlated with IL-6 concentrations or responsiveness to treatment, although they decreased after initiation of EPO therapy.[308] Progression or severity of anemia in patients with nondialysis-requiring CKD (ND-CKD) seems to be associated with higher serum hepcidin concentrations.[309,310] Elevated serum hepcidin has also been observed in anemic patients with combined renal (GFR, 20–70 mL/min/1.73 $m^2$) and cardiac failure[311] and in association with fatal and nonfatal cardiovascular events in patients undergoing maintenance hemodialysis.[312] EPO therapy leads to a reduction in serum hepcidin values that correlates with the bone marrow response.[311] Elevated serum hepcidin concentrations in pediatric and adult patients with CKD have been found to be associated with elevated ferritin and/or CRP concentrations and with stage 5 CKD.[291,313] Serum hepcidin assessment by surface-enhanced laser desorption/ionization–time-of-flight (SELDI-TOF) mass spectrometry did not seem to offer any advantage as a predictor of iron needs over the established traditional markers for adult patients on hemodialysis and maintenance ESA therapy.[314] Serum hepcidin concentrations are reduced following dialysis treatment.[315,316] Hepcidin concentrations also may vary in patients on hemodialysis carrying concomitant *HFE* gene mutations, the presence of which results in reduced hepcidin production.[317] Other studies have reported normal concentrations of hepcidin in CKD, but did not address the caveats mentioned previously.[315,318] Although it has been suggested that hepcidin may improve the identification of iron deficiency in CKD prior to transplantation,[319] more work is needed to define the role of hepcidin in the assessment of iron status in CKD. In iron-deficient persons without CKD, elevated hepcidin values have been shown to predict unresponsiveness to oral iron therapy.[320] These findings have not been confirmed in non–dialysis-dependent CKD.[321] Baseline values or changes over treatment time of serum hepcidin did not predict a response to iron therapy in 61 patients with ND-CKD.[321]

ERFE is an EPO-driven negative regulator of hepcidin production.[299] A study in 148 patients with CKD has shown that endogenous EPO values in serum or weekly rhEPO doses positively correlate with serum ERFE values.[322] However, ERFE values did not seem to influence serum hepcidin values suggesting the influence of other regulatory mechanisms in determining hepcidin values in CKD. In another study, on 59 hemodialyzed patients, treatment with ESAs was associated with increased values of ERFE and reduced values of hepcidin in serum.[323]

Given the central role played by hepcidin in the ACD, pharmacologic modulation of its production or bioavailability has potential as a new therapeutic modality.[324] In particular, the use of antihepcidin compounds may restore iron availability in ACD and improve the effectiveness of ESA therapy.[325] Strategies targeting hepcidin production, neutralizing hepcidin with specific peptides, or interfering with the binding of hepcidin to ferroportin or with the hepcidin-induced endocytosis of ferroportin are under consideration.[324] For conditions of iron overload, hepcidin mimetics (minihepcidin) have shown effectiveness in vivo in animal models,[326] and stimulators or hepcidin production are also under study.[272]

Another regulator of iron homeostasis, growth differentiation factor 15 (GDF15), is induced by hypoxia and iron depletion[327] and downmodulates hepcidin, thus contributing to iron overload in conditions with significant expansions of the bone marrow and inefficient erythropoiesis, such as severe beta thalassemias.[328] However, in patients with ACD, there seems to be no association between GDF15 and hepcidin concentrations, suggesting that this regulatory loop may not be active in the presence of inflammation.[328] Serum values of GDF15 were strongly correlated with the risk of progression to CKD in two separate patient cohorts ($n = 224$ and $n = 297$).[329]

Transmembrane serine protease 6 (TMPRSS6) may act as a cell membrane sensor of iron deficiency, which in turn suppresses hepcidin production and allows increased intestinal absorption of iron.[330] Mutations in TMPRSS6 have been associated with iron-refractory iron deficiency anemia (IRIDA),[331] and population studies have identified a TMPRSS6 allele associated with lower serum iron and Hgb concentrations.[332–337] It is likely that iron metabolism in patients with CKD may be similarly affected by genetic polymorphism of TMPRSS6.

## INFLAMMATION AND ANEMIA OF CHRONIC DISEASE

Inflammation may also have an impact on erythropoiesis, independent of its effects on iron metabolism and RBC survival. Responsiveness to EPO declines in patients with CKD in the presence of acute inflammation, bacterial infections, and cancer.[338] A chronic inflammatory state with elevated serum cytokine concentrations and decreased lymphocytes and CD4+ T cell counts has been described in patients on dialysis.[339] Serum CRP has been used to monitor or predict the hematologic consequences of inflammation.[340] Inflammatory cytokines can induce anemia via impaired production of EPO, impaired erythropoietic response to EPO, with suppression of erythroid progenitor differentiation and proliferation, and possibly also reduced RBC survival. TNF-α is known to inhibit erythropoiesis directly[341] and to reduce EPO production.[342] Antibody-mediated blockade of TNF-α produces an improvement of anemia in rheumatoid arthritis[343] and inflammatory bowel disease.[344] Cytokines such as TNF-α, IL-1, IL-8, IL-12, and INF-γ may impair erythroid proliferation via multiple mechanisms, including cytokine-induced apoptosis,[345] downregulation of EPO-Rs, impaired production of other factors, such as stem cell factor, and direct toxic effects on progenitors.[346,347] It has also been proposed that inflammation may promote the release of soluble EPO-Rs, which may inhibit EPO signaling and increase EPO resistance.[348] Sotatercept and luspatercept, two novel therapeutic agents that target activin A and possibly other receptors of the TGF-β superfamily, have been under investigation for prevention of vascular calcification and improvement of anemia in CKD.[349,350]

## FOLIC ACID, VITAMIN D, AND ZINC DEFICIENCY

A net loss of folate is associated with dialysis, although the deficit is typically compensated for by a normal diet and/or routine supplementation of water-soluble vitamins. Folate status is best assessed by measuring RBC folate because the plasma assay is affected by recent dietary intake and overestimates the true prevalence of folate deficiency.[351] Changes in RBC parameters (e.g., increases in mean corpuscular cell volume [MCV] and mean corpuscular cell hemoglobin [MCH] from baseline) are helpful in identifying folate deficiency in patients on dialysis.[352,353]

Vitamin D deficiency is an independent predictor of anemia in early CKD,[35,354] as well as in normal subjects,[355] but whether vitamin D directly affects erythroid proliferation[356] or is just a marker remains to be demonstrated.[357] Vitamin D supplementation (50,000 IU/month) in patients on dialysis did not result in changes in Hgb concentrations in one study, although a possible EPO-sparing effect was reported.[358] Similar negative findings were reported for adult patients in stage 3 or 4 CKD,[359] ESKD,[360] and pediatric ND-CKD patients.[361]

Low plasma zinc (Zn) concentration has been reported, with variable incidences in patients undergoing hemodialysis.[362–364] A Zn supplementation trial has shown measurable improvements in Hgb concentrations.[365]

## ALUMINUM OVERLOAD

Formerly, aluminum was commonly used in patients on dialysis for its effects as a potent intestinal binder of phosphate. Although calcium-containing and non–calcium-containing phosphate binders have largely supplanted aluminum, the effects of aluminum toxicity on hematopoiesis are of historic interest. Parenteral aluminum exposure, either via dialysate contamination[366] or another route,[367] is still observed. The erythropoietic effects of aluminum toxicity are characterized by altered iron metabolism,[368] direct inhibition of erythropoiesis,[369,370] and disruption of red cell membrane function and rheology.[371–373] In dialyzed patients, the most notable hematologic effect of aluminum overload is microcytic anemia,[374,375] which improves with the use of deionized water to reduce the aluminum content of the dialysate[376] or chelation therapy with desferrioxamine.[377] EPO responsiveness is reduced in patients undergoing dialysis who have higher serum aluminum concentrations at baseline or after a deferoxamine challenge[378] and can be restored with deferoxamine treatment.[379] Improvement of anemia has also been shown in patients with the use of chelation therapy with deferoxamine, even in the absence of overt aluminum toxicity.[380,381] Interestingly, HIF destabilization requires iron as a cofactor, and iron chelation with deferoxamine can induce HIF, providing a possible alternative explanation for an improvement of anemia.

### HORMONES, PARATHYROID HORMONE, AND MARROW FIBROSIS

Elevated serum values of adiponectin have been reported in CKD; a large prospective study has shown a negative correlation of adiponectin with Hb values and a significant association with the risk of developing anemia in 1227 nonanemic patients at baseline.[382] Because multiple associations have been reported between adiponectin and a variety of markers of disease severity in CKD, the precise relevance and mechanistic implications of this finding remain unexplained.

Intact fibroblast growth factor has been shown to be an important determinant of anemia and iron deficiency in mouse models of renal failure.[383] Fibroblast growth factor 23 (FGF23) values in serum exhibited a negative correlation with Hb values in 3869 subjects with mild to severe CKD,[384] with high values being associated with a risk of developing anemia in a cohort of 1164 nonanemic patients[385] and a reduction in serum values after IV iron therapy.[386] However, FGF23 values showed no association with anemia in a cohort of 282 patients on hemodialysis.[387]

The inhibitory effects of parathyroid hormone (PTH) on erythropoiesis are primarily indirect and are a consequence of myelofibrosis.[388] Secondary hyperparathyroidism is associated with diminished responsiveness to EPO.[389] Moreover, PTH values were identified as effect modifiers of the erythropoietic response to EPO in adult CKD patients on hemodialysis.[390] In 979 patients with nondialysis CKD, a significant inverse association has been reported between PTH and hemoglobin.[391] However, in pediatric patients, no association was found between serum intact PTH and Hgb concentrations.[392] Racial differences have been reported for serum PTH levels, with higher values in blacks versus whites.[393] An increase of EPO values and improvement of anemia have been reported after parathyroidectomy.[394,395]

### DRUGS

Use of renin-angiotensin-aldosterone system (RAAS) inhibitors may induce or worsen anemia[396] for several reasons. Angiotensin II has direct facilitating effects on erythroid progenitor cells, which are inhibited by these compounds.[397] AcSDKP, an endogenous inhibitor of erythropoiesis, accumulates in patients treated with angiotensin-converting enzyme (ACE) inhibitors.[267] Endogenous EPO production may also be reduced through the hemodynamic effects of angiotensin II inhibition. Because angiotensin II leads to preferential constriction of efferent glomerular arterioles, it increases the ratio of filtered sodium—the main determinant of renal oxygen consumption—to peritubular blood flow and thus oxygen supply, thereby presumably lowering peritubular oxygen tension. RAAS inhibitors reverse these effects, and therefore have the potential to mitigate renal hypoxia and the signal for EPO production.[398] It has also been postulated that RAAS inhibitors may promote anemia and EPO resistance via a reduction in testosterone serum concentrations in men younger than 60 years.[399] Myelosuppressive effects of immunosuppression may further contribute to anemia, especially in the posttransplantation setting.[400–402]

## ASSOCIATION OF ANEMIA WITH ADVERSE OUTCOMES

The availability of rhEPO greatly increased interest in the role that anemia plays with respect to health-related quality of life (HRQOL) and prognosis of patients with CKD. A large number of observational studies have consistently shown that even modest reductions in Hgb concentrations are associated with adverse outcomes. This statement applies to mortality in patients on dialysis,[11,403] and patients with CKD not on dialysis,[404] as well as individuals in the general population[405] or with another complex chronic disease, such as heart failure.[406] A large study of 159,720 patients undergoing hemodialysis and receiving epoetin therapy has shown that the duration of anemia, rather than the Hgb concentration per se, is the most powerful predictor of short-term mortality, with Hgb concentrations less than 11 g/dL for 3 months or longer being associated with an increased risk of death.[407,408] However, there is no agreement on how best to study Hgb variability effects on mortality, with various methods having been applied to describe Hgb variability[409] and with significant confounding attributable to variations in Hgb concentrations among dialysis centers[410] and the effects of ESA dosing and iron therapy.[411] Hb values less than 10 g/dL and more than 12 g/dL prior to ESKD have been associated with values higher all-cause mortality and cardiovascular mortality, whereas Hb less than 10 g/dL was associated with increased hospitalization rates in a study of more than 31,000 US veterans.[412]

A systematic review has supported the notion that Hgb concentrations below a formerly established reference range (Hgb 9–10 g/dL in some studies and Hgb 11–12 g/dL in others) are generally associated with increased all-cause mortality in dialysis recipients. Similar findings have been reported in pediatric patients on peritoneal dialysis.[413] In ND-CKD patients, the severity of anemia is also associated with the rate of decline in kidney function,[414] consistent with the concept that anemia may aggravate intrarenal hypoxia.[415–417] Moreover, anemia was also found to be a strong risk factor for the development of left ventricular hypertrophy,[418,419] an established surrogate for mortality and cardiovascular events. An increase in cardiac output as part of the compensatory mechanisms that maintain oxygen delivery in anemia has been considered as a possible reason for the link between anemia and cardiac geometry.[418]

Other specific complications, such as proliferative retinopathy in patients with diabetes, were found to be associated with anemia.[420] In a relatively large (21,899) cohort of dialyzed patients in the United States, an Hgb concentration below 8 g/dL were associated with a twofold increase in the odds of death in comparison with those for an Hgb concentration between 10 and 11 g/dL; several laboratory parameters related to iron status and nutrition, as well as dose of dialysis, were also associated with Hgb concentration.[216] There was no association with mortality when Hgb was above 11 g/dL in this cohort study, but other studies have suggested that the relationship among Hgb, comorbidities, and outcomes extends into the normal range of Hgb, leading to the hypothesis that normalization of Hgb might be associated with best outcomes. However, RCTs have failed to confirm this suggestion (see later). Therefore, although it is undisputable that anemia is a sensitive risk marker for adverse outcomes, its role as a causal risk factor has not been established.

## ERYTHROCYTOSIS OF PATIENTS WITH KIDNEY DISEASES

Although anemia is a typical complication of advanced CKD, irrespective of its cause, there are few circumstances under which disorders of renal structure and function can also result in abnormally high rates of RBC production—that is, erythrocytosis. The pathogenesis of these disorders remains incompletely understood, but they probably all result from increased production of renal EPO.

### (POLY)CYSTIC KIDNEY DISEASE

The degree of anemia in patients with autosomal dominant polycystic kidney disease (ADPKD) is usually somewhat less severe than for other causes of CKD, although patients with ADPKD on dialysis usually require treatment with ESAs. Occasionally patients with ADPKD may become polycythemic.[421] Erythrocytosis may also develop in patients on hemodialysis with acquired renal cysts and single cysts.[422,423] Serum EPO concentrations in patients with ADPKD are, on average, up to twofold higher than in patients with CKD from other causes,[244,424,425] and significant arteriovenous concentration differences for EPO have been found in polycystic kidneys.[426] In the cyst walls of patients with ADPKD, interstitial cells have been shown to express EPO mRNA, and cysts derived from proximal but not distal tubules contain increased concentrations of bioactive erythropoietin.[426] In a later study, continuous activation of HIF was demonstrated in cyst walls of patients with ADPKD and in a rat model of cystic kidney disease.[427] The physiologic distinction between HIF-1α expression in tubular cells and HIF-2α expression in peritubular cells is maintained in the cyst walls. The genetic defects underlying ADPKD do not lead to HIF activation. However, cyst expansion results in pericystic hypoxia, and hypoxic stimulation of pericystic angiogenesis is believed to play an important role in cyst progression.[428,429] Therefore, the enhanced production of EPO in cystic kidneys is probably due to local hypoxia and mediated via HIF activation. It is possible that factors other than EPO, induced through this pathway, contribute to cyst growth. Regional hypoxia also appears to stimulate cyst growth, primarily via increased fluid secretion into the cyst lumen.[430]

### POSTTRANSPLANTATION ERYTHROCYTOSIS

Kidney transplantation is usually followed by full correction of renal anemia.[406,431,432] Interestingly, a regular increase of EPO production is not related to the presence of the transplant, but does correlate with the onset of graft function,[433] providing further evidence for the role of excretory kidney function in EPO regulation. Some 10% to 20% of patients manifest overcorrection and demonstrate erythrocytosis, usually within the first 6 months following transplantation.[434–436] Graft failure is associated with anemia, and therefore polycythemia is more likely to occur in patients with normal kidney function.[406,424]

Increased plasma EPO concentrations have been reported in patients with posttransplantation erythrocytosis.[437] Selective venous catheterization studies and the response to removal of the native kidneys have suggested that the native kidneys are the main source of increased EPO production.[437,438] Although this suggestion clearly indicates that a sufficient production capacity for EPO may be preserved in diseased kidneys, it is unclear how the secretion rate is enhanced after transplantation. Improvement of the uremic state has been speculated to play a role. Moreover, given that inflammatory cytokines can inhibit erythropoietin production, the application of immunosuppressive agents could theoretically enhance EPO formation. Interestingly, the prevalence of posttransplantation erythrocytosis seems to be elevated in combined kidney and pancreas transplantation,[439] but whether the erythrocytosis is related to enhanced EPO formation or to insulin-stimulated pathways remains unclear. In some patients with posttransplantation polycythemia, the circulating EPO concentrations are normal or reduced, and it may be that in these cases there is an increased sensitivity of the erythroid progenitor cells to EPO or loss of other feedback control mechanisms.

The most effective therapy of posttransplantation erythrocytosis consists of agents blocking the RAAS.[435,440–442] There is no evidence that angiotensin acts directly on EPO- producing cells, but there are several ways through which RAAS blockade may inhibit erythropoiesis (see earlier). Alternative therapeutic strategies to reduce increased RBC concentrations after transplantation include the discontinuation of diuretics, application of theophylline,[441] and phlebotomy, which, however, can lead to iron deficiency.

### RENAL ARTERY STENOSIS

Although renal artery stenosis reduces the oxygen supply to the kidneys, it is only rarely associated with erythrocytosis.[443–446] The data on EPO production in this case are contradictory. In experimental animals, enhancement of EPO production after renal artery stenosis has been demonstrated by some, but not all, investigators.[447] A study performed in rats has shown that graded reduction of renal blood flow to 10% of the control value caused a maximal threefold increase in serum EPO concentrations.[448] Therefore, renal EPO production appears rather insensitive to changes in renal blood flow. Because the ratio of oxygen demand and delivery determines local oxygen tension in the area of EPO-producing cells, it is possible that the two are equally reduced after a reduction in renal blood flow, thus not resulting in sufficient hypoxia to stimulate EPO gene expression. It has been argued that the indirect coupling of oxygen demand to supply makes the kidney an ideal site for the oxygen sensing that controls RBC production.[449]

### RENAL TUMORS

Up to 5% of patients with renal carcinomas have erythrocytosis[450] and, conversely, approximately one-third of tumor-associated erythrocytosis is caused by renal cancer.[451] Conflicting data have been reported concerning serum EPO concentrations in patients with renal tumors but, at least in some patients, raised values have been found.[452] Furthermore, overexpression of EPO mRNA has been demonstrated in renal tumors.[453] In situ hybridization has revealed that accumulation of EPO mRNA occurs in epithelial tumor cells, but not in interstitial cells of the tumor stroma.[453] Most clear cell renal carcinomas, the most frequent type of renal cancer, are associated with mutations of the VHL gene that interfere with its ability to target HIF for proteasomal degradation (see earlier).[454] Indeed, clear cell renal carcinomas contain high concentrations of HIF.[455–458]Although stabilized HIF in renal tumors appears to be functionally active in inducing HIF-target genes, it is as yet unclear why overexpression of EPO is confined to about one-third of these tumors.[459] Although activation of HIF appears necessary for EPO gene expression in renal cell carcinoma, it is clearly not the only determinant. The fact that erythrocytosis occurs far less frequently than overexpression of EPO in renal cancer is probably due to a variety of mechanisms causing anemia in patients with cancer, which include inhibition of the effect of EPO and reduced iron availability. There is some albeit controversial evidence suggesting that EPO has autocrine or paracrine tumor growth-promoting effects.[460,461]

> ***Clinical Relevance***
>
> When using ESAs, always consider the possibility of functional iron deficiency, especially in women and men with normal or borderline normal iron stores. Serum ferritin values are not indicative of iron stores in the presence of inflammation and in most patients with CKD or ESKD. Functional iron deficiency is less likely to occur when serum ferritin values are >100 for ND-CKD, and >200 for patients on dialysis. Monitor hematologic response and assess iron adequacy based on Hb increase and presence of normal reticulocyte Hb content (CHr or Ret-He).

## TREATMENT OF RENAL ANEMIA

### ERYTHROPOIESIS-STIMULATING AGENTS

Recombinant human erythropoietin was developed in the 1980s, with support from an orphan drug program. At that time, it was unclear to what extent the anemia of patients with kidney disease could be influenced by application of the hormone, as well as how many patients might benefit from this type of therapy. The initial clinical studies revealed an unexpected efficacy in patients undergoing dialysis, with both high response rates and evidence that hemoglobin concentrations could not just be increased to some extent, but could virtually be normalized.[110,112] In the subsequent years, the use of rhEPO in patients on maintenance dialysis became routine in most parts of the world. The indication was subsequently extended to the much larger group of patients with ND-CKD, as well as to several other patient groups with anemia, including those whose cancer was treated with chemotherapy.

Over the years, the efficacy of the therapy and presumed benefits led to a gradual increase in Hgb concentrations in virtually all treated patient groups (see Fig. 55.3). Data from the US Renal Data System have indicated a substantial increase in the use of these agents (as well as intravenous [IV] iron and blood transfusion) in older (≥67 years) adults with ESKD.[462] Not surprisingly, the expanded clinical use resulted in an extraordinary commercial success. Investigators originally intended to copy the endogenous molecule as closely as possible, but patent and marketing considerations, together with concepts for improving patient management, resulted in the development of a number of derivatives of the EPO molecule with altered pharmacokinetic properties and, later, the development of different molecules that can directly or indirectly stimulate the EPO-R. Discussions about the appropriate terminology for all these compounds have not been settled, but the term "erythropoiesis-stimulating agents" (ESA) is commonly used to describe the heterogeneous class of drugs that stimulate erythropoiesis through stimulation of the erythropoietin receptor.

#### Epoetin

The term *epoetin* is usually applied to rhEPO preparations, produced by means of overexpression of the human EPO gene in mammalian cell lines. Production in mammalian cells rather than bacteria is required because EPO is a highly glycosylated molecule, and bacteria lack the ability to generate glycoproteins. Epoetin alfa and epoetin beta are the two compounds first developed by two different companies. Both are produced in Chinese hamster ovary (CHO) cells and show a high degree of similarity, with identical protein backbones of 165 amino acids and one *O*-linked and three *N*-linked glycosylation sites each, but with subtle differences in their carbohydrate composition.[463]

Although the amino acid sequence unequivocally determines glycosylation sites, the precise composition of the sugar side chains is also determined by the repertoire and activity of glycating enzymes, which may vary among cell lines and under different tissue culture conditions. Glycosylation of the EPO molecule is not required for binding or activation of its receptor[122]; in fact, the in vitro activity of deglycosylated erythropoietin is enhanced.[464] However, in vivo deglycosylated EPO is inactive because of rapid clearance from the circulation, and the carbohydrate chains are thus responsible for its pharmacokinetic properties.

Early clinical trials in patients on hemodialysis used IV epoetin administered three times weekly; subsequently, the intraperitoneal (IP), subcutaneous (SC), and intradermal routes of administration were also investigated.[465,466] After IV administration, plasma EPO concentrations decay monoexponentially, with an elimination half-life of approximately 4 to 11 hours.[467] The apparent volume of distribution of EPO is about one to two times the plasma volume, and the total body clearance is lower than for other protein hormones, such as insulin, glucagon, and prolactin. The IP route was investigated as a potential means of administering EPO to patients on peritoneal dialysis but the bioavailability of intraperitoneal epoetin is disappointingly low, 3% to 8%. This application has therefore not been pursued.[465,468,469]

With SC administration, peak serum concentrations of about 4% to 10% of an equivalent IV dose are obtained at around 12 hours, and thereafter they decay slowly, so that concentrations greater than baseline are still present at 4 days.[466,467] The bioavailability of SC epoetin is around 20% to 25%. Nevertheless, SC application is even more efficient than

IV application, allowing a dose reduction of approximately 30% to maintain the same hemoglobin concentration.[470,471] Presumably, the early peak concentrations of epoetin after IV injection are inefficient, and the more prolonged elevation of hormone levels following SC application allows a more sustained stimulation of RBC production. Thrice-weekly administration has remained the most popular dosage frequency for both IV and SC administration, although once-weekly,[472] twice-weekly, and seven times weekly (once-daily) dosing have all been used.[473] With IV epoetin, once-weekly administration is associated with much lower efficacy, and twice- or thrice-weekly dosing is required. In 2015, the mean weekly dose of EPO in adult HD and peritoneal dialysis patients in the United States was below 10,000 U/week, a substantial reduction when compared with 2010 values (Fig. 55.7).

A number of additional epoetin preparations have been developed worldwide. Some have distinct differences in the

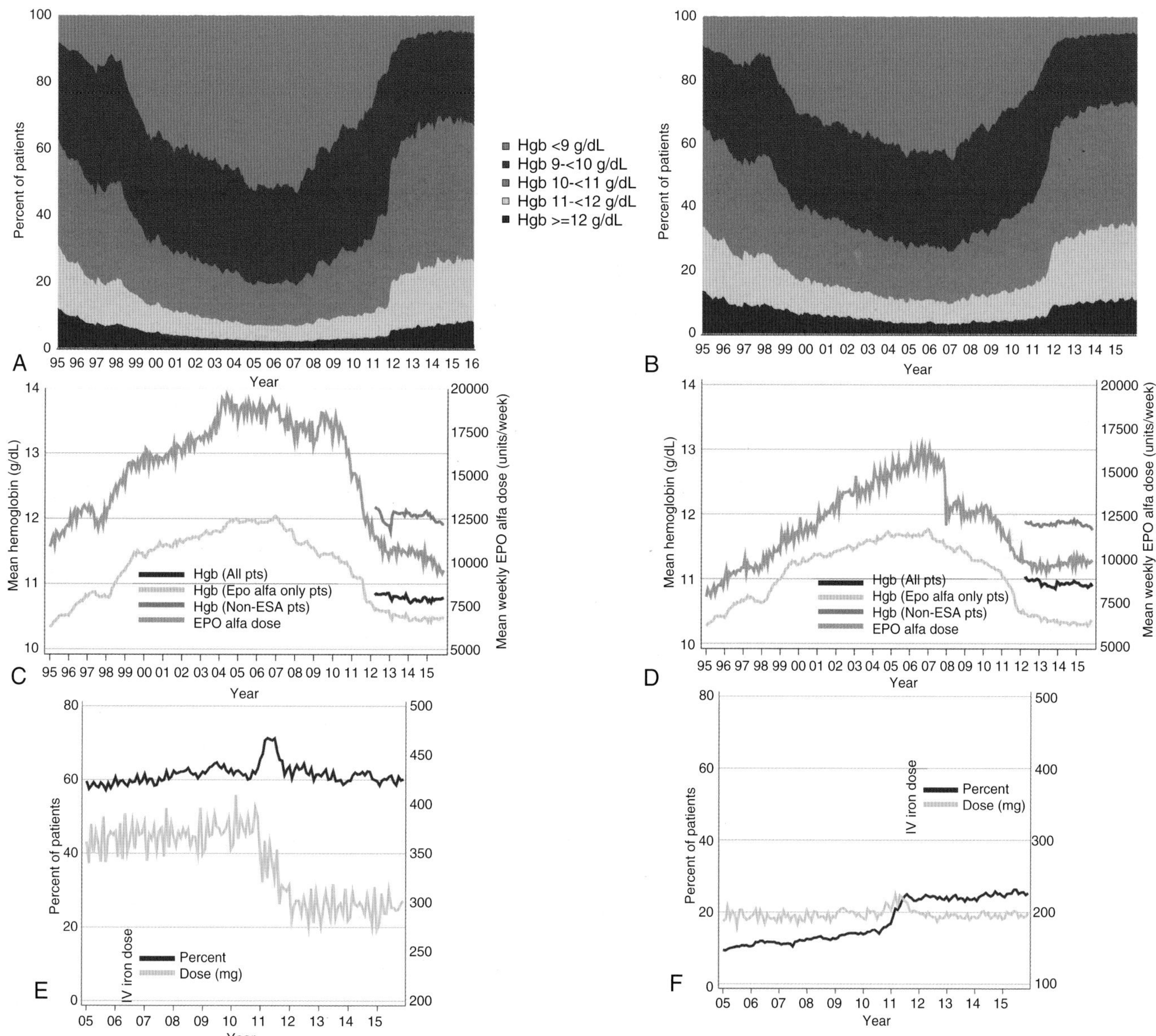


Fig. 55.7 Anemia, erythropoiesis-stimulating agents (ESAs), and IV iron in hemodialysis and peritoneal dialysis patients. (A) Distribution of monthly Hgb values in ESA-treated adult hemodialysis patients on dialysis ≥90 days, from Medicare claims; time trend from 1995–2015. (B) Distribution of monthly Hgb values in ESA-treated adult peritoneal dialysis patients on dialysis ≥90 days, from Medicare claims 1995–2015. (C) Anemia measures among adult hemodialysis patients on dialysis ≥90 days, 1995–2015. (D) Anemia measures among adult peritoneal dialysis patients on dialysis ≥90 days, mean monthly Hgb value and mean weekly EPO alfa dose (averaged over 1 month), from Medicare claims data 1995–2015. (E) Monthly percentages of IV iron use and mean monthly IV iron dose in adult hemodialysis patients on dialysis ≥90 days, from Medicare claims 2005–2015. (F) Monthly IV iron use and mean monthly IV iron dose in adult peritoneal dialysis patients on dialysis ≥90 days, from Medicare claims 2005–2015. *EPO,* erythropoietin. (From US Renal Data System. 2017 Annual Data Report. Bethesda, MD: National Institutes of Health, National Institute of Diabetes and Digestive and Kidney Diseases; 2017.)

production process—for example, epoetin delta was produced in a human cell line through increased transcription of the endogenous EPO gene,[474] but this product is currently not being distributed. Other epoetins are so-called "biosimilar" generic drugs designed as copies of epoetin alfa or beta; these are being licensed on the basis of a more limited clinical trial program after expiration of the patents for the originator compounds in Europe.[475] Additional epoetins are available in other parts of the world, which are not necessarily produced to the same regulatory standards as the preparations marketed in the United States and Europe and may show variable product characteristics.[476] Various studies in CKD patients have compared biosimilar and originator ESAs, with no significant difference in effectiveness or outcomes.[477–483]

The importance of the formulation of epoetins was highlighted in 2002 with an upsurge in cases of antibody-mediated, pure red cell aplasia (PRCA) in association with the SC use of epoetin alfa marketed outside the United States after a change to an albumin-free formulation. Patients affected by this complication develop neutralizing antibodies against both rhEPO and the endogenous hormone, resulting in severe anemia and transfusion dependence.[484] The cause of this serious complication remains obscure, although circumstantial evidence suggested that rubber stoppers of prefilled syringes used for the albumin-free epoetin alfa formulation may have released organic compounds that act as immunologic adjuvants.[485] Factors such as breach of the cold storage chain may also have played a role. In anti-EPO antibody cases observed so far, the SC application route was usually a prerequisite. Although the unfortunate combination of adverse factors leading to a temporary increase in antibody-induced PRCA was specific for one product, a low baseline rate of PRCA also occurs with use of epoetin beta and darbepoetin alfa (see later).[486]

#### Darbepoetin Alfa

Darbepoetin alfa is an EPO derivative with a further two *N*-linked glycosylation sites, created by site-directed mutagenesis to prolong its plasma survival time (as discussed earlier).[124] Each of these glycosylation sites can carry an additional four sialic acid residues. Thus, this molecule (called "darbepoetin alfa" or "novel erythropoiesis-stimulating protein" [NESP]) contains five *N*-linked and one *O*-linked glycosylation chains and has the capacity to carry up to 22 sialic acid residues, compared with a maximum of 14 sialic acid residues for original rhEPO. The additional glycosylation on darbepoetin alfa results in a molecule weighing 37.1 kDa compared with 30.4 kDa for epoetin. As intended, darbepoetin alfa has a longer half-life in vivo than rhEPO—25.3 hours versus 8.5 hours after IV administration.[126] The elimination half-life after SC administration is about 48 hours, which is approximately twice that previously reported for epoetin alfa or beta. A number of studies have examined once-weekly and once every other week dosing.[487,488] Darbepoetin alfa can both correct and maintain Hgb at these dosing frequencies, and its side effect profile is very similar to that of epoetin alfa or beta.[465,489] Several "conversion" studies have suggested that an appropriate conversion factor for switching patients on epoetin alfa or beta to darbepoetin alfa is 200 U of epoetin to 1 µg of darbepoetin alfa. In contrast to epoetin alfa or beta, the dose requirements for darbepoetin alfa do not differ significantly between the IV and SC administration routes.

#### Methoxypolyethylene Glycol Epoetin Beta

Alternative bioengineering techniques to prolong the half-life of EPO further have resulted in the development of methoxypolyethylene glycol epoetin beta (also called "continuous erythropoietin receptor activator" [CERA]), a PEGylated derivative of epoetin beta with an elimination half-life of about 130 hours when administered IV or SC.[490–492] A methoxypolyethylene glycol polymer chain is integrated through amide bonds between the N-terminal amino group or the ε-amino group of lysine (predominantly lysine-52 or lysine-45), with a single succinimidyl butanoic acid linker. The molecular weight of CERA is twice that of epoetin (~60 kDa). Phase III studies have shown that because of the longer half-life time of CERA, less frequent injections are sufficient to maintain stable hemoglobin values CERA given IV once every 2 weeks was found to be as safe and effective as epoetin given thrice weekly for correcting anemia in patients on hemodialysis.[493] A larger study has also shown that CERA given at 4-week dosing intervals was not inferior to epoetin given three times weekly in terms of maintaining Hbg concentrations.[494] So far, no significant differences in outcomes or complications have emerged for CERA compared with other ESAs.[495] Conversion factors have been established and tested for switching from other ESAs to CERA.[496]

#### Other Erythropoiesis-Stimulating Agents

Several other ESAs have been developed or are currently in clinical development.[497–499] These include EPO polymers, EPO fusion proteins, EPO mimetic molecules and the so-called HIF stabilizers, which induce endogenous EPO formation.[500] The ability of molecules that are structurally unrelated to EPO to dimerize the EPO-R and activate the intracellular signaling cascade was first described 20 years ago.[501] Peginesatide is an EPO mimetic peptide that was subsequently developed for the treatment of anemia. Its amino acid sequence was completely unrelated to that of native or rhuEPO, although it shares the same biologic properties with EPO with respect to EPO-R activation.[502,503] The potential advantages of this compound included greater ex vivo stability, allowing storage at room temperature, prolonged pharmacodynamic action, allowing once-monthly administration, and a simple manufacturing process involving synthetic peptide chemistry. In addition, because peginesatide was structurally unrelated to EPO, it did not cross-react with anti-EPO antibodies, allowing effective treatment of anti-EPO antibody-mediated PRCA.[504] Two phase 3 studies have demonstrated that peginesatide is not inferior to conventional epoetin for correcting anemia in CKD.[505,506] However, for reasons that remain unclear, peginesatide increased the risk of a combined cardiovascular endpoint in patients with ND-CKD.[505] Accordingly, it was only approved in the United States for use in patients on dialysis only. Only slightly more than 6 months after its introduction, the drug was recalled as a result of postmarketing reports of serious hypersensitivity reactions—including fatal reactions in approximately 0.02% of patients—that occurred within 30 minutes after the first IV dose and had not been reported during clinical trials.[507] Currently, no EPO mimetic is available for rescue therapy in patients with anti-EPO, antibody-mediated PRCA.

#### Hypoxia-Inducible Factor Stabilizers

The HIF stabilizers are competitive inhibitors of HIF prolyl hydroxylases and asparagyl hydroxylase, enzymes involved in the degradation of HIF and suppression of its transcriptional activity, respectively (as discussed earlier).[74,508,509] The HIF stabilizers, therefore, cause an increase in endogenous EPO production.[510] These drugs are orally active. They have been shown to stimulate erythropoiesis effectively in monkeys[511] and are currently being tested in phase 2 and 3 studies in patients with CKD.[512,513] A phase 1/2 single-dose study comparing erythropoietin formation in small groups of patients on dialysis with native kidneys and after bilateral nephrectomy has provided evidence that EPO production can be stimulated in extrarenal sites (presumably the liver) and the diseased, nonfunctioning, fibrotic kidneys.[241] These data provide proof for the concept that a disturbance of the renal oxygen-sensing mechanism, rather than a loss of EPO-producing cells, is the main cause of renal anemia. There has been much discussion about whether HIF stabilizers will upregulate not only EPO gene expression but also other HIF target genes, such as those involved in iron metabolism and neoangiogenesis. Although some of these effects may facilitate an increase in hemoglobin concentration, the long-term consequences, good or bad, of these other effects have not been established.[508] Roxadustat (FG-4592) and vadadustat (AKB-6548) have been tested with positive results in CKD (dialysis and nondialysis), with phase 3 studies ongoing.[514–517] Daprodustat and molidustat are also in advanced clinical development.[517a–517d]

Interestingly, genetic causes of impaired degradation of HIF, potentially comparable to long-term pharmacologic inhibition of HIF degradation, have been identified as causes of rare polycythemias.[104,518,519]

#### Initiation and Maintenance of Therapy

Following commencement of regular therapy with ESAs, a significant increase in the reticulocyte count to around two to three times baseline is usually evident at 1 week, and an increase in Hgb concentration is seen by 2 to 3 weeks. The increase is dose-dependent, and most physicians aim for an increment of not more than 1 g/dL/month to minimize the risk of adverse effects. In most patients, ESA therapy is initiated at the outset of dialysis therapy and, according to the US Renal Data System report, peak doses of ESA are being administered at month 2 after the initiation of dialysis (see Fig. 55.7). Only 0.3% of US CKD patients in the predialysis stage are treated with ESAs; these patients are usually older, with more advanced disease and significant comorbidities, resulting in high rates of death and cardiovascular complications.[520]

The increase in Hgb concentration following ESA therapy is associated with an increase in RBC count. No significant changes in leukocyte or platelet counts are usually seen, although a moderate increase in the platelet count has been documented in some studies. There is usually a marked decline in the serum ferritin concentration and/or the transferrin saturation value after the initiation of ESA therapy, unless iron stores are being replenished in parallel, because large quantities of iron are used up in the manufacture of new RBCs (see later).

Radioisotope blood volume studies have confirmed that there is an increase in RBC mass after treatment with ESAs, associated with a compensatory reduction in plasma volume so that the whole blood volume remains unchanged. Early ferrokinetic studies have indicated that epoetin therapy induces a twofold increase in marrow erythropoietic activity, as evidenced by a doubling of marrow and RBC iron turnover.[243,521] There is little or no change in mean RBC life span after epoetin therapy; thus, the increased RBC mass is largely accounted for by the production of greater numbers of RBCs, rather than by any significant change in their survival.

### IRON MANAGEMENT

Iron is the fourth most common element—after oxygen, silicon, and aluminum—in the earth's crust and the most abundant transitional metal in the human body. Although it plays an essential role in multiple biologic processes, such as transport of oxygen, transfer of electrons, DNA synthesis, and heme-based enzymatic reactions, iron is also highly susceptible to undergoing transition from the ferrous state ($Fe^{2+}$) to the ferric ($Fe^{3+}$) state and to generate reactive oxygen species (ROS) via the Haber-Weiss-Fenton reaction, thus requiring the presence of multiple systems to prevent or control this potentially harmful transition.[522]

The metabolism of iron is geared toward conservation and recycling, with the gastrointestinal absorption of iron in adults being tightly regulated to compensate for the daily losses and to keep the total iron pool in the body constant, in the range of 35 to 45 mg per kilogram of body weight. Of the iron pool, approximately two-thirds is contained in the RBC pool as Hgb, with the remaining fraction stored in macrophages and reticuloendothelial system (RES), liver, and muscle (myoglobin).

Multiple factors induce a negative iron balance in patients with CKD, including reduced intake and absorption, chronic losses due to occult and overt blood loss, and reduced bioavailability of iron due to the chronic inflammatory state and increased hepcidin production (see previously).[523] Iron losses in patients with CKD can be up to 5 to 6 mg iron daily (1 mg iron daily in normal subjects) and cannot be adequately compensated with oral iron supplements because gastrointestinal absorption is limited by the chronic inflammatory state and hepcidin. In addition, in patients with CKD treated with ESAs, insufficient amounts of iron are released from the body stores to meet the greater demand of ESA-driven erythropoiesis.[524] Similar evidence has been provided for normal subjects when erythropoiesis is increased by an intensive blood donation schedule and EPO, or EPO alone, despite concomitant oral iron supplementation.[525–527]

#### Markers of Iron Status

When hematologic signs of iron-deficient erythropoiesis—reduced Hgb value, with abnormally low MCV and MCH values inadequate reticulocyte response, and low reticulocyte Hgb content—are associated with biochemical markers of low iron stores (abnormally low serum ferritin), the diagnosis of absolute iron deficiency is straightforward. However, straightforward determination of iron deficiency is the exception rather than the rule in patients with CKD, in whom iron may be present in storage form but not readily available for erythropoiesis, and serum ferritin concentrations are increased owing to the concomitant inflammatory state. Thus, the diagnosis of iron deficiency in CKD must rely on a variety of markers, biochemical and hematologic and, in the most challenging cases, on the erythroid response to IV iron (see later for the significant limitations of bone marrow biopsy).

These markers are determined in individual patients over time; markers with high biologic and analytic variability, such as transferrin saturation and ferritin, are less suitable to assess iron status than markers with low variability such as Hgb, Hct, and reticulocyte Hgb content.[528,529]

**Serum Ferritin.** Serum ferritin values higher than 200 μg/L are recommended for patients on dialysis,[11,12] and values of 100 μg/L should be considered the lower limit of normal for ND-CKD patients.[530] The sensitivity for ruling out iron deficiency was reported to be 90% for a ferritin cutoff of 300 μg/L and 100% for 500 μg/L.[531,532] Concerns about iron toxicity and overload have resulted in several guidelines setting an upper limit for ferritin of 500 μg/L,[10–12,530] above which IV iron is not recommended. However, this recommendation is not evidence-based.[533] Additional factors that elevate serum ferritin are hyperthyroidism, liver disease (associated with hepatitis C virus [HCV] or other conditions), alcohol consumption, and oral contraceptives, whereas vitamin C deficiency and hypothyroidism decrease ferritin concentrations.[534] More than 50% of US patients on hemodialysis have serum ferritin values higher than 800 ng/mL, and more than 20% have values greater than 1200 ng/mL (see later; Fig. 55.8E).

**Serum Iron, Transferrin, and Transferrin Saturation.** The biochemical markers serum iron, transferrin, and transferrin saturation (TSAT) are routinely used in the diagnosis of iron deficiency but have some important limitations. Serum iron concentrations and TSAT values are sensitive to diurnal variations and to dietary intake, with serum iron concentrations being higher early in the day. These are increased by greater iron intake with food or dietary supplements and decreased in the presence of infection and inflammation.[535] Some biochemical methods used to measure iron are sensitive to hemolysis and will produce falsely elevated iron values,[536] whereas other serum iron assays have been shown to perform poorly in patients on dialysis.[537] Serum transferrin can be elevated by the use of oral contraceptives and reduced with inflammation or infection. Several studies have shown that these traditional biochemical iron parameters perform poorly in CKD and are inferior to some of the newer hematologic parameters (described later).[538–541] However, a lower serum iron concentration has been shown to be an independent predictor of mortality and hospitalization in dialysis recipients,[542] and a higher TSAT value has been associated with lower mortality.[543] A TSAT of 20% is generally considered a threshold value below which iron therapy is indicated.[11,12] In one study using data from NHANES, more than 50% of the noninstitutionalized adult US population was found to have values below the CKD threshold for ferritin (100 ng/mL) and TSAT (20%)[544] Overall, women were more likely to have laboratory-based evidence of iron deficiency. Men with CKD had a higher prevalence of iron deficiency than men without CKD, whereas the prevalences in women with and without CKD were similar (Fig. 55.8). Serum transferrin and total iron-binding capacity (TIBC) are dual markers of iron status and of nutritional status and protein balance: A lower baseline TIBC value or its decrease over time in dialyzed patients is associated with higher mortality and with the presence of protein-energy wasting and inflammation.[545] Approximately half of US patients on chronic hemodialysis have TSAT values of 30% or greater (see Fig. 55.8D).

**Serum Transferrin Receptor.** Serum transferrin receptor (sTfR) concentration is a marker of iron status that has shown promise in the evaluation of iron deficiency in patients with CKD. Transferrin receptors are shed from the membrane of maturing erythroblasts and reticulocytes, either in soluble form or as vesicles.[546–548] The concentration of sTfR is abnormally elevated in iron deficiency and has been shown to be a valuable parameter in several different clinical conditions, including ACD.[549–553] Although the sTfR concentration is not affected by inflammation, it is an expression of the size of the pool of maturing erythroblasts; also, independent of iron status, this parameter increases in hyperproliferative anemias and with the use of ESAs.

The sTfR assay is not yet widely available, and a single reference standard has been established only rather recently,[554] with different methods still reporting different units and normal ranges. A study in patients on dialysis with anemia has shown that an sTfR concentration lower than 6 mg/L (which rules out iron deficiency; normal value, 3.8–8.5) was associated with responsiveness to the initiation of EPO therapy.[555] However, because increased erythropoiesis by itself raises the sTfR concentration, sTfR measurement could not reliably detect functional iron deficiency in patients on maintenance EPO therapy. Other studies have failed to show a predictive value for sTfR in CKD anemia management.[556,557] A decline in sTfR concentration may reflect increases in iron availability when IV ascorbic acid is used to mobilize iron stores.[558] Race and ethnicity, smoking, alcohol consumption, and body mass index have been shown to be associated with sTfR values.[559,560] One can correct the sTfR value for the value of iron stores by also accounting for serum ferritin: The sTfR/ferritin ratio provides an accurate assessment of iron status and the need for iron supplementation.[547,561,562] However, to date, there is limited evidence to support the clinical use of this or similar ratios in patients on dialysis.[563–565]

***Clinical Relevance***

Although oral iron may be effective in ND-CKD patients, the response is generally suboptimal, and most patients do not display a hematologic response. Adherence is poor due to side effects. Side effects for the different IV iron preparations available in the United States and European markets (e.g., iron sucrose, ferric gluconate, ferric carboxymaltose, ferumoxytol, ferric isomaltoside) are usually rare and limited to mild to moderate hypersensitivity reactions. Many of these reactions are due to premedication with diphenhydramine. In approximately 1:200 administrations of IV iron, arthralgias, myalgias, or flushing appear at the beginning of the infusion in the absence of associated hypotension, tachypnea, tachycardia, wheezing, stridor, or periorbital edema. No intervention is necessary except for a temporary halt in the IV infusion. After symptoms abate, IV infusion can be restarted.

### Erythrocyte Ferritin Concentration

Some studies in the 1990s had suggested a potential value for using the erythrocyte ferritin concentration as a marker

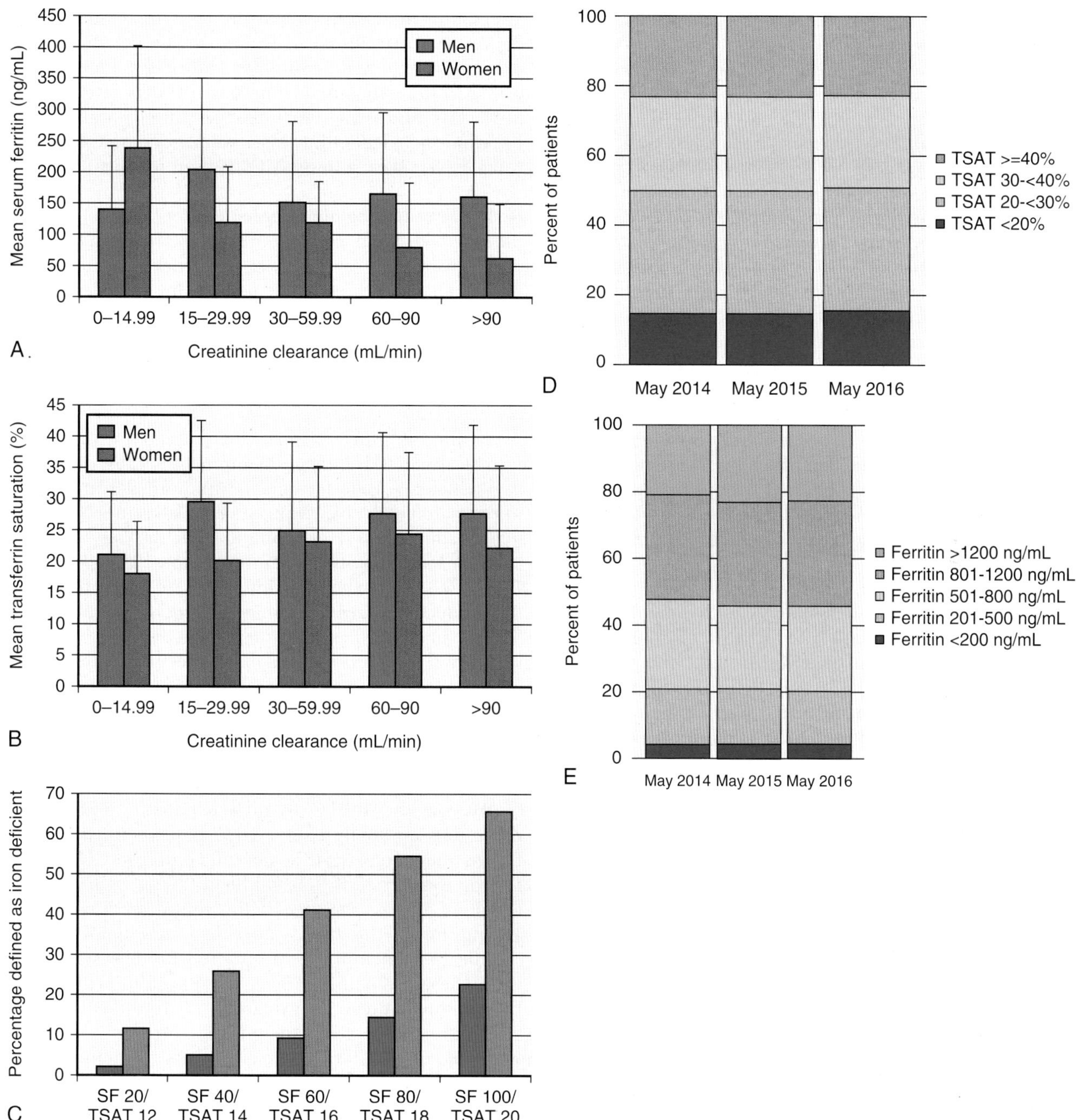


**Fig. 55.8** Mean (A) serum ferritin and (B) transferrin saturation *(TSAT)* as a function of creatinine clearance (CrCl) for the combined National Health and Nutrition Examination Survey (NHANES) cohorts (*error bars* are standard deviation [SD]). The trends for both TSAT and ferritin are not significant (NS) for men but, for women, $P < .0001$ for serum ferritin and $P < .02$ for TSAT. National Kidney Foundation (NKF) chronic kidney disease (CKD) stages relative to CrCl (mL/min) are stage 5, 0 to 14.99; stage 4, 15 to 29.99; and stage 3, 30 to 59.99. Patients with CrCl 60 to 90 mL/min and patients with CrCl greater than 90 mL/min may have CKD stage 1 or 2, respectively, if other renal abnormalities are present. (C) Percentage of individuals defined as iron deficient with the use of different threshold combinations of serum ferritin *(SF)* and TSAT. The NKF Kidney Disease Outcomes Quality Initiatives (KDOQI) thresholds of serum ferritin, 100 ng/mL, and TSAT, 20%, are different from indices of iron deficiency in the non-CKD population, in which lower thresholds are generally used. The *green bars* indicate "and logic," with both test results below the specified threshold, and the *yellow bars* indicate "or logic," with either test result being below the threshold. (D) Distribution of TSAT values in adult hemodialysis patients on dialysis for at least 90 days, May 2014, 2015, and 2016. (E) Distribution of the most recent value of serum ferritin taken between March and May in adult hemodialysis patients on dialysis for at least 90 days, 2013–2016. (A–C from Fishbane S, Pollack S, Feldman HI, et al. Iron indices in chronic kidney disease in the National Health and Nutritional Examination Survey 1988–2004. Clin J Am Soc Nephrol. 2009;4:57–61; D and E from US Renal Data System. 2017 Annual Data Report. Bethesda, MD: National Institutes of Health, National Institute of Diabetes and Digestive and Kidney Diseases; 2017.)

of iron status in patients on dialysis.[532,566–568] Although this assay can be run on automated analyzers using the regular serum ferritin methodology,[569] the method is cumbersome, requires complete removal of white blood cells to avoid measuring leukocyte ferritin,[570] is insensitive to dynamic changes in iron status, and is rarely available to clinicians.

**Erythrocyte Zinc Protoporphyrin Concentration.** The determination of erythrocyte zinc protoporphyrin (ZPP) concentrations has shown some promise to identify patients on maintenance dialysis who require iron replacement therapy.[571–574] This marker is elevated in the presence of iron-deficient erythropoiesis, with Zn replacing iron in the heme precursor protoporphyrin.[575] The erythrocyte ZPP concentration is also elevated in the presence of lead poisoning. However, the diagnostic value of erythrocyte ZPP concentration appears to be inferior to that of RBC or reticulocyte parameters.[539,576] In addition, because the whole-blood ZPP concentration is falsely elevated in patients undergoing dialysis and in the presence of bilirubin and various drugs, careful washing of the RBCs is required to remove these interferences, rendering this assay not suitable for routine clinical care.[577,578]

**Percentage of Hypochromic Red Blood Cells.** A distinguishing characteristic of iron-deficient erythropoiesis is the production of hypochromic microcytic erythrocytes. Iron-deficient erythropoiesis results in an increase in the percentage of hypochromic erythrocytes (%HYPO), defined as the percentage of erythrocytes with a mean corpuscular hemoglobin concentration (MCHC) lower than 28 g/dL, for hematology analyzers produced by Siemens Medical Solutions.[579,580] Similar parameters (low hemoglobin density, [LHD%], and DF-Hypo XE, respectively) are available when using Beckman-Coulter and Sysmex instruments.[581,582] A classic study by Macdougall and colleagues has shown that functional iron deficiency induced by epoetin treatment and the response to IV iron could be detected by changes in %HYPO.[524]

Several studies have confirmed that an increased %HYPO is a sensitive and early indicator of iron deficiency.[539,583–587] A European study has found %HYPO to be the only independent predictor of mortality among various iron status parameters, with a twofold higher mortality risk for values higher than 10% than for values lower than 5%.[588] According to the European Best Practice Guidelines for the Management of Anaemia in Patients with Chronic Renal Failure, patients with %HYPO values higher than 6% are most likely to show response to IV iron therapy.[530] A clinical study has tested these guidelines for anemia management; they recommended a %HYPO target of less than 10% by prospectively raising the delivered dose of IV iron to 228 patients to achieve a %HYPO lower than 2.5% and a serum ferritin concentration of 200 to 500 ng/mL.[587] In this study, the median %HYPO value decreased from 8% to 4%, the median serum ferritin concentration increased from 188 to 480 ng/mL, and the median rhEPO dose decreased from 136 to 72 IU/kg per week, showing that a strategy aimed at achieving %HYPO values much lower than 10% could be cost-effective. However, it also resulted in serum ferritin values in some patients much higher than those recommended by guidelines.

Contrary to the European studies, North American studies have failed to show value for %HYPO in assessing iron availability in dialysis patients.[589,590] The reasons for this discrepancy are not clear. It is worth noting that %HYPO progressively increases with storage of the blood sample, owing to the concomitant increase in MCV and reduction in MCHC, and is therefore best measured within 4 hours. In addition, %HYPO increases with reticulocytosis because reticulocytes have a lower MCHC than mature RBCs.[591]

**Reticulocyte Hemoglobin Content.** After being released from the marrow, reticulocytes spend 18 to 36 hours in the circulation before becoming mature erythrocytes. Studies of the cellular characteristics of reticulocytes thus provide a real-time assessment of the functional state of the bone marrow. Automated analyzers can determine not only the absolute number of reticulocytes with great precision, but also their size and Hgb concentration and content.[592,593] The reticulocyte Hgb content[594] (CHr or RetHe; in pg/cell) has been extensively studied, especially in patients treated with rhEPO.[595] A reduction in CHr is the most sensitive indicator of functional iron deficiency. Healthy subjects with normal iron stores who were treated with rhEPO produced a substantial fraction of hypochromic, low Hgb content reticulocytes when their baseline serum ferritin values were below 100 µg/L.[526] When IV iron was used in conjunction with EPO in normal subjects, the production of hypochromic reticulocytes was abolished.[596] Several small studies have described the value of CHr in identifying iron deficiency in dialysis recipients, mostly based on the subsequent response to IV iron.[541,589,590,597] A sensitivity of 100% and specificity of about 70% to 80% were reported in one study,[590] although other studies have reported lower values.[541,597] These initial studies led to additional large clinical trials that tested the values of CHr in managing the dosing of IV iron and rhEPO in dialysis patients. Fishbane and colleagues randomly assigned 157 patients to two different IV iron management strategies, one based on CHr, in which IV iron was started if CHr fell below 29 pg/cell, and one in which IV iron was started if the serum ferritin fell below 100 ng/mL or the TSAT values decreased below 20%.[540] A significant reduction in exposure to IV iron was obtained in the CHr-based management, with no differences in weekly EPO dosing between the two groups.[540] Tessitore and coworkers[539] have compared the diagnostic precision of a variety of hematologic and biochemical markers to identify subjects who exhibit an increase in Hgb values in response to IV iron. A combination of %HYPO higher than 6% and CHr less than 29 pg/cell has shown the best diagnostic efficiency for iron deficiency (80%) based on the Hgb response to IV iron. Other studies have provided additional confirmation of the diagnostic value of CHr,[598,599] although one has questioned its superiority to TSAT,[600] and only one study has shown that the use of IV iron in patients with low CHr resulted in decreased weekly usage of rhEPO.[601] A normal reticulocyte Hgb content may be used to optimize and reduce, if needed, the use of IV iron.[602]

Several studies have also validated reticulocyte Hgb measurements (RET-He and Ret-Hb) generated by analyzers produced by Sysmex.[528,582,603–606] The current availability of the reticulocyte Hgb parameter on several analytic platforms may allow a wider utilization of this parameter. Guidelines on the diagnosis and management of iron deficiency have included reticulocyte Hgb among those recommended.[529,607] A limitation of reticulocyte Hgb is that it cannot be used to assess iron availability in the presence of thalassemia traits (alpha or beta) or megaloblastic erythropoiesis.

**Bone Marrow Iron.** Although iron staining of a bone marrow biopsy is regarded as the gold standard method of assessing iron stores, widely divergent estimates of the prevalence of iron deficiency have been generated by this invasive, potentially painful procedure.[608–611] A study in 100 patients with ND-CKD has shown that evaluation of iron stores by iron staining of a bone marrow sternal aspirate was no better than TSAT or ferritin in correctly identifying responders to IV iron therapy.[612,613] Some patients with CKD have been found to have no stainable iron evident on sternal bone marrow biopsy, despite the presence of normal to elevated serum ferritin concentrations.[611,614] Bone marrow studies also have no value in identifying patients at risk for the development of functional iron deficiency with EPO therapy.

**Liver Magnetic Resonance Imaging.** Hepatic magnetic resonance imaging (MRI) provides a noninvasive tool to estimate liver iron deposition and is regarded as the gold standard methodology for monitoring patients with iron overload disorders. However, the number of studies applying this technology in CKD is still very limited.[615–618] In the largest of these studies, conducted in 119 patients undergoing hemodialysis and receiving IV iron in a single center, according to current guidelines, 84% had evidence of hepatic iron deposition, and 30% had hepatic MRI findings consistent with severe iron overload.[617] These data raise concerns that the use of IV iron and current thresholds for laboratory parameters may be too liberal, especially considering the increased use of IV iron in the United States since 2011 (see Fig. 55.7). On the other hand, contrary to cardiac iron MRI assessments,[619] it has not yet been demonstrated that the observed increases in hepatic iron are of any functional significance and/or are associated with clinically relevant adverse outcomes.[259,620]

**Iron Balance Considerations.** As noted, 1 mL of blood normally contains 0.5 mg of iron and proportionately less when the Hgb concentration is reduced. An estimated annual blood loss of 2 L in a dialysis recipient with moderate anemia (20% reduction in Hgb) therefore corresponds roughly to 0.8 g of iron loss. Irrespective of all parameters of iron metabolism, IV iron supplementation in excess of this amount results in positive iron balance unless blood loss (and thereby iron loss) is more pronounced than anticipated. When patients were categorized according to their level of hepatic iron deposition, the average monthly iron doses were 150 and 283 mg in those with signs of mild and moderate iron overload, respectively, compared with 100 mg in those without.[617] The functional consequences of a positive iron balance, and in particular whether it carries risk, however, are still unclear.[259]

### Intravenous Iron Therapy

There is general agreement that oral iron therapy is insufficient to support the functional needs of EPO-stimulated erythropoiesis in patients with ESKD properly. A systematic review and meta-analysis have shown that the Hgb response is much more potent with IV iron than with oral iron, with this effect being more substantial in patients on dialysis and of a lower magnitude in patients with ND-CKD.[621,622] A systematic Cochrane analysis has identified significant associations of IV iron therapy with increased Hgb, ferritin, and transferrin saturation values, as well as reduced ESA requirements, with no differences in mortality.[623]

These findings have been confirmed in a recent meta-analysis, which showed a 23% dose reduction in ESA with the use of IV iron.[624] The cost-effectiveness of IV iron therapy has also been demonstrated under the assumption that a higher mortality risk is associated with Hgb values less than 9.0 g/dL.[625]

Nevertheless, oral iron may be effective with ND-CKD patients.[624] The FIND CKD study (Ferinject assessment in patients with iron deficiency anemia and Non-Dialysis-dependent Chronic Kidney Disease) compared the efficacy and safety of oral iron with the IV administration of ferric carboxymaltose targeting two different serum ferritin ranges, 100 to 200 and 400 to 600 µg/L.[626] Although the IV therapy targeting the higher ferritin range showed greater efficacy, there was no difference in Hgb concentration or the need to switch to another anemia therapy between the IV arm targeting the lower ferritin range and the oral iron therapy arm. However, the response to oral iron was suboptimal in many patients, with only 21.6% showing an Hgb increase of at least 1 g/dL after 4 weeks of oral iron therapy, and more than half of the patients never achieving this level of response throughout the trial.[627] A recent systematic review and meta-analysis of trials comparing oral and IV iron therapy in CKD has shown significant benefit for IV iron use in CKD stages 3 to 5.[628]

Several IV iron preparations are available for clinical use, with most of them containing iron associated with a carbohydrate shell. The strength or lability of this association is crucial for dosing, with the most stable preparations, such as iron dextran, being suitable for large dose replacements, and the more labile preparations, such as iron gluconate, requiring multiple dosing, with a single-dose maximum of approximately 100 mg. Intravenous iron infusion may lead to some immediate binding of the infused iron to transferrin, resulting in its complete saturation and the generation of free iron, which has vasoactive effects and can produce hypotensive and/or anaphylactoid reactions. This risk involves mainly semilabile iron-sugar complexes such as iron sucrose and iron gluconate, and not more stable complexes, such as ferric carboxymaltose, ferumoxytol, and iron dextran.

Several preparations of IV iron are available in the US and European markets (Table 55.1).

**Lower Molecular Weight Iron Dextran.** This is produced by PharmaCosmos (Holbaek, Denmark) and is in use in the United States (INFeD, Actavis, Dublin Ireland) and Europe (Cosmofer, Pharmacosmos, Holbaek; Ferrisat, HAC Pharma, Caen, France). It has a significant better tolerability and fewer side effects than the higher molecular weight product, which has now been removed from the US and European markets.[629–635]

**Iron Sucrose.** Called Venofer, this is produced by Vifor (St. Gallen, Switzerland) and marketed in the United States by American Regent Laboratories (Shirley, NY). It is used worldwide for the treatment of renal anemia and is the most used parenteral iron preparation in the United States.[636]

**Table 55.1 Intravenous Iron Preparations**

| | FDA-Approved | | | | | Non–FDA- Approved |
|---|---|---|---|---|---|---|
| **Generic Name** | Iron Dextran | Iron Sucrose | Na Ferric Gluconate | Ferric Carboxymaltose | Ferumoxytol | Iron Isomaltoside 1000 |
| US trade name (marketed by) | INFed (Actavis) | Venofer (American Regent, Luitpold Pharmaceuticals) | Ferrlecit (Sanofi-Aventis); Nulecit (Actavis) | Injectafer (Luitpold, American Regent) | Feraheme (AMAG Pharmaceuticals) | Monofer (Pharmacosmos A/S) |
| Trade name, Europe | Cosmofer, Uniferon, Ferrisat | Venofer, Idafer, FerroLogic, Ferion, Venotrix, Fermed, Netro-Fer | Ferrlecit/Ferlixit | Injectafer, Ferinject | Rienso | Monofer, Monover, Monoferro, Diafer |
| Carbohydrate | Dextran polysaccharide (LMW) | Sucrose | Gluconate | Carboxymaltoside | Polyglucose sorbitol carboxymethylether | Isomaltoside |
| Molecular weight | 165 kDa | 34–60 kDa | 289–444 kDa | 150 kDa | 750 kDa | 150 kDa |
| Iron, mg/mL | 50 | 20 | 12.5 | 50 | 30 | 50 or 100 |
| Hemodialysis, mg/session | 100 | 100 | 125 | — | 510 | 100–200 (UK) |
| Peritoneal dialysis | 100 | 1 × 300 mg; 1 × 300 mg after 14 days; 1 × 400 mg after 14 days | | — | 510 | |
| CKD, nondialysis | 100 mg | 200 or 500 mg | | 750 mg | 510 mg | |
| TDI possible | Yes | No | No | Yes | No | Yes |
| Maximum approved dose | 100 mg | 400 mg | 125 mg | 750 mg for body weight >50 kg | 510 mg | Up to 20 mg/kg (UK) |
| Max safe dose | TDI over 1–4 hrs | 300 mg over 2 hrs | 250 mg over 1 hr | 750 mg over 15 min | 510 mg in >15 min | 20 mg/kg over 15 min |
| Premedication | No | No | No | No | No | No |
| Test dose required | Yes | No | No | No | No | No |
| Black box warning (FDA)[a] | Yes | No | No | No | Yes | Na |
| Adverse reactions | | | | Hypophosphatemia | Alteration of MRI scan | |
| Preservative | None | None | Benzyl alcohol | None | None | None |

[a]FDA warnings—iron dextran and ferumoxytol, fatal allergic reactions.

*CKD,* Chronic kidney disease; *FDA,* U.S. Food and Drug Administration; *LMW,* low molecular weight; *MRI,* magnetic resonance imaging; *NA,* not applicable; *TDI,* tolerable daily intake.

"All intravenous iron medicines have a small risk of causing allergic reactions, which can be life-threatening if not treated promptly." European Medicines Agency. New recommendations to manage risk of allergic reactions with intravenous iron-containing medicines.

http://www.ema.europa.eu/ema/index.jsp?curl=pages/news_and_events/news/2013/06/news_detail_001833.jsp&mid=WC0b01ac058004d5c1.

Allergic reactions have been reported in fewer than 1/100,000 infusions. IV injection into rats of three different commercial preparations of iron sucrose have resulted in different degrees of inflammation and oxidative stress, suggesting that the stability of the iron complex may differ from one iron sucrose preparation to another.[637]

**Ferric Gluconate.** This is marketed in the United States by Sanofi Aventis US (Bridgewater, NJ) as Ferrlecit. It is the second most commonly prescribed IV iron preparation in the United States and is frequently used worldwide in patients on hemodialysis.[638]

**Ferric Carboxymaltose.** This is marketed as either Ferinject (Vifor, St. Gallen, Switzerland) or Injectafer (American Regent, Luitpold Pharmaceuticals, Shirley, NY). It is the newest iron preparation registered in Europe and the United States.[639] A significant advantage of this preparation is the possibility of infusing up to 750 mg of iron in a short time (15 minutes), with minimal side effects.[640,641] Transient hypophosphatemia has been reported in patients without CKD and in those with ND-CKD treated with ferric carboxymaltose, possibly mediated by a decreased tubular reabsorption of phosphate.[642,643] FGF23 plays an important role in the hypophosphatemia observed with iron carboxymaltose administration. In iron deficiency, increased FGF23 production is associated with increased cleavage within osteocytes, with unchanged FGF23 plasma values and elevated values of FGF23 c-terminal fragments. Administration of iron carboxymaltose is associated with a large increase in plasma FGF23 values, possibly due to reduced cleavage. Low serum phosphate, increased phosphate fractional excretion, and decreased serum 1,25 vitamin D values are observed for 1 to 2 weeks following IV administration of 750 mg of iron carboxymaltose at week 0 and 1.[643a] In non–dialysis-dependent CKD cases, with serum ferritin values between 400 and 600 ng/mL (FIND-CKD trial), ferric carboxymaltose was better than oral iron in delaying and/or reducing ESA requirements.[626] There was no evidence of IV iron-related renal toxicity or decreased renal function in the FIND-CKD trial.[644]

**Ferumoxytol.** This is marketed by AMAG Pharmaceuticals (Lexington, MA) as Feraheme. It is an iron oxide nanoparticle with a polyglucose sorbitol carboxymethylether coating designed to minimize immunologic sensitivity and release of free iron, allowing a rapid injection of a large dose (510 mg) of iron, which can be repeated after 3 to 8 days.[645–648] Because infusion times of 17 to 60 seconds were associated with significant side effects, the US Food and Drug Administration (FDA) has demanded that infusion times be longer than 15 minutes.

Efficacy and adverse events in patients with CKD were found to be similar to those of iron sucrose.[649] Ferumoxytol is the only IV iron preparation possessing super magnetic properties, similar to MRI contrast agents, which may alter MRI imaging for up to 3 months owing to its uptake into the reticuloendothelial system.[646] On the basis on the studies used for FDA registration, 0.2% of treated subjects experienced anaphylaxis or anaphylactoid reactions, 3.7% had hypersensitivity-type reactions (e.g., pruritus, rash, urticaria, wheezing), 1.9% of patients had hypotension, and three patients experienced serious hypotensive reactions.[646] However, studies of larger datasets have not shown an increased incidence of adverse reactions for ferumoxytol compared with other IV iron preparations in CKD patients.[650] There were no significant differences between ferumoxytol and ferric carboxymaltose regarding hypersensitivity reactions or hypotension post-IV infusion, whereas the incidence of hypophosphatemia was greatly increased for ferric carboxymaltose (38.7% vs. 0.4%).[651] The Ferumoxytol for Anemia of CKD Trial (FACT) showed that ferumoxytol had similar efficacy and safety profile to iron sucrose in the treatment of iron deficiency anemia in patients with CKD undergoing hemodialysis.[652]

The development of nephrogenic systemic fibrosis following gadolinium use has prompted the use of ferumoxytol as an alternative MRI contrast agent in patients with CKD stage 4 or 5 and in dialysis-dependent CKD.[653,654]

**Ferric Isomaltoside.** This is marketed by Pharmacosmos A/S (Holbaek) as Monofer. It is based on a nonbranched carbohydrate, which does not form the typical spheroidal iron carbohydrate nanoparticle like other IV iron preparations and seems to be associated with lower immunogenic potential. Monofer can be administered in a single dose, with dosages up to 20 mg/kg, and has been shown to be equivalent to iron sucrose in CKD patients on dialysis.[655] Monofer is currently approved and marketed in 28 countries, including 21 European Union members, but not in the United States.

A US study on IV iron use for 1994 through 2002 has indicated that iron sucrose and ferric gluconate are the predominant forms of IV iron used in CKD, with 84.4% of hemodialysis and 19.3% of peritoneal dialysis patients having some form of IV iron therapy.[656] Parenteral iron administration has increased substantially in the United States, most likely because of a shift in reimbursement practices toward a bundled capitated model (see Fig. 55.7). Data from the Dialysis Outcomes and Practice Patterns Study (DOPPS) have shown IV iron use increasing from 55% to 68% of patients on hemodialysis between 2010 and 2012.[657] Similar trends have been reported for European countries, Japan, Australia, and New Zealand.[658] A ferritin threshold of 800 ng/mL is now commonly used for prompt withholding of IV iron therapy in patients on maintenance dialysis.

### Side Effects of Intravenous Iron

Iron sucrose, lower molecular weight iron dextran, and ferric carboxymaltose have excellent track records for safety and tolerability. Hypersensitivity reactions (e.g., erythematous rash, urticaria) are rare, and their intensity is usually mild or moderate. Lack of recurrence after rechallenge indicates that most of these events are not due to immunologic reactions. Severe life-threatening allergic reactions have been a major problem with the higher molecular weight iron dextran, prompting its removal from the European and US markets. The use of a test dose is still required for iron dextran in the United States, but the European Medicines Agency no longer recommends it.[659] A retrospective study by Chertow and colleagues examining more than 50 million doses of IV iron has demonstrated the higher risk of reactions with higher molecular weight iron dextran; they found that rates of serious events associated with lower molecular weight iron dextran were similar to those seen with the other forms of IV iron (~1/200,000).[630,631] A study from the FDA using data obtained from the administration's Adverse Event Reporting System (AERS) and other US databases, was unable to provide firm data on the relative safety of the four IV preparations marketed in the United States owing to incomplete brand information on these reports, but it did confirm that allergic reactions have been reported for all brands.[660,661] Chertow and colleagues estimated absolute rates of life-threatening reaction per million doses of 0.6 for iron sucrose, 0.9 for sodium ferric gluconate complex, 3.3 for lower molecular weight iron dextran, and 11.3 for higher molecular weight iron dextran.[631] However, a later systematic review has highlighted the lack of properly conducted and powered studies comparing adverse event rates between lower molecular weight iron dextran and iron sucrose.[662] The amount of labile iron, which differs among the various IV iron preparations, is likely an important determinant of possible oxidative and nitrosative stress.[663]

In ND-CKD patients, the FIND-CKD study observed no adverse effects of IV ferric carboxymaltose as compared with oral iron.[664] The REVOKE trial aimed to assess the effect of IV iron on the progression of CKD by comparing IV iron sucrose, 200 mg once a week for 2 weeks, with oral iron sulfate. Although there was no difference in the slope or GFR, the authors reported a higher number of SAEs in the IV iron arm and concluded that the risk for infections and cardiovascular events was increased.[665] This unexpected result was not confirmed in FIND-CKD, and the difference between the outcomes of both studies remains unexplained so far.[666,667]

**Infection Risk and Intravenous Iron Therapy.** In vitro data seem to support the notion that iron can promote bacterial growth and, at the same time, impair leukocyte function.[576,668–671] IV injection of iron sucrose in dialyzed patients has been associated with the dose-dependent appearance of markers of oxidant damage in lymphocytes and a decrease in plasma ascorbate and alpha-tocopherol in some studies[672] but not in others.[673–675] In addition, studies have not accounted for the fact that the capability of leukocytes to cope with oxidant damage is markedly affected by polymorphisms in glutathione S-transferase M1 (GST M1).[676] Although there is indirect and inconclusive evidence for an association between iron stores and bacteremia,[668] most studies have failed to show an association of IV iron therapy with an increased risk of infection in dialyzed patients.[576,669–671] Many studies attempting to link iron status and risk of bacterial infection have used serum ferritin, an unreliable marker of iron status in CKD, as discussed previously.[668,677–681] One study has shown that in patients receiving more than 10 vials of 100 mg iron dextran over 6 months, there was an increased risk of death and hospitalization.[682] One uncontrolled retrospective study has reported a higher incidence of bacteremia with iron sucrose than with ferric gluconate.[683] Other studies have failed to show a significant effect of IV iron dosing or iron status (using serum ferritin) on bacteremia, mortality, infection, or hospitalization.[576,671,684,685] On the other hand, a later observational study using a very large database has found that bolus administration of higher doses of IV iron is associated with higher risks for infection-related hospitalizations and death, particularly in patients undergoing dialysis with catheters, rather than arteriovenous fistulas or grafts.[686] Higher doses of IV iron have not been shown to be associated with higher mortality risk or infections.[687]

Despite the lack of proof of significant effects on the rates of infections, cardiac events, and mortality, long-term toxicities and, in particular, the possible consequences of oxidant damage due to free radical generation are still a concern.[604,688] Unfortunately, no large outcome studies have been performed so far to test the efficacy and safety of iron replacement strategies prospectively, either in the short or long term.[689] A trial in the United Kingdom (PIVOTAL) has compared proactive high-dose IV iron sucrose therapy with reactive low-dose therapy in 2141 patients new to dialysis, and assessed the impact of both regimens on mortality and cardiovascular events.[690] The high-dose IV sucrose regimen yielded a significant decrease in ESA monthly dose, with similar effects on mortality, cardiovascular events, and infection rates.[690]

**Iron Therapy in Patients With Chronic Kidney Disease.** Iron therapy in CKD should be guided by iron status test results and clinical considerations and needs to take into account the potential benefits of avoiding or minimizing blood transfusions, ESA use, and anemia-related symptoms against the risk of potential harm[10] (Table 55.2). Iron tests should be performed monthly in the initial phase of ESA treatment and every 3 months thereafter.[11,12] As discussed in detail previously, a target of serum ferritin concentration higher than 200 ng/mL and TSAT value greater than 20% or CHr value greater than 29 pg/cell has been used for patients on dialysis.[11,12] The KDIGO guideline recommends using IV iron if an increase in Hgb concentration or a decrease in ESA requirements is sought if the serum ferritin value is 500 ng/mL or less and TSAT is 30% or less.[10] For patients with ND-CKD and those undergoing peritoneal dialysis, target values of more than 100 ng/mL for serum ferritin and higher than 20% for TSAT should be used. The objective of iron therapy in CKD is to abolish overt and/or functional iron deficiency because this reduces the erythropoietic response to and effectiveness of ESAs. The response to ESAs can be optimized by the simultaneous use of IV iron, which enables a significant reduction in ESA dosing.[691] Several studies conducted in the early and late 1990s have demonstrated that IV iron therapy is associated with significant ESA dose reductions.[623,674,692–700] The DRIVE (Dialysis Patients Response on IV Iron with Elevated Ferritin) study has shown that an intensive IV iron administration protocol (125 mg ferric gluconate with each of eight hemodialysis sessions) can significantly reduce ESA dosing requirements.[701,702] A Cochrane systematic review has provided additional support to the ESA-sparing effects of IV iron.[623] Shirazian and associates have noted that the ESA-sparing effects of IV iron could easily be demonstrated when there is a high prevalence of iron deficiency and low usage of IV iron.[691] However, they have suggested that most of the benefits of IV iron in reducing ESA use have already been achieved, given that 60% to 80% of US patients on dialysis are being treated with IV iron, and that it is not clear how much additional ESA dose reduction could be obtained with more intensive IV iron regimens.

Given the potential adverse effects of ESAs (see later), the latest KDIGO anemia guideline mentions explicitly that the desire to avoid or minimize ESAs can influence the decisions about iron use[10] (see Table 55.2).

As shown in Table 55.1, several forms of IV iron are available worldwide. Although they have important differences in formulation and dosing, no convincing evidence has been

**Table 55.2 Current Anemia Guidelines and Position Statements Regarding Iron Administration**

| Guideline | Comments |
|---|---|
| KDIGO Clinical Practice Guideline (International) | 2.1.1: When prescribing iron therapy, balance the potential benefits of avoiding or minimizing blood transfusions, ESA therapy, and anemia-related symptoms against the risks of harm in individual patients (e.g., anaphylactoid and other acute reactions, unknown long-term risks) (not graded)<br>2.1.2: For adult CKD patients with anemia not on iron or ESA therapy, we suggest a trial of IV iron (or in CKD ND patients, alternatively, a 1–3 month trial of oral iron therapy) if (2C):<br>• An increase in Hb concentration without starting ESA treatment is desired[b] *and*<br>• TSAT is ≤30% and ferritin is ≤500 ng/mL (≤500 μg/L)<br>2.1.3: For adult CKD patients on ESA therapy who are not receiving iron supplementation, we suggest a trial of IV iron (or in CKD ND patients, alternatively, a 1–3 month trial of oral iron therapy) if (2C):<br>• An increase in Hb concentration[c] or a decrease in ESA dose is desired[d] *and*<br>• TSAT is ≤30% and ferritin is ≤500 ng/mL (≤500 μg/L) |
| KDOQI Commentary (United States) | • We believe that the degree of caution expressed by KDIGO is not supported by the available evidence and could have negative effects, such as sustained iron deficiency anemia, higher ESA dose requirements, and increased blood transfusions.<br>• We therefore believe that a therapeutic trial of IV iron could be considered when TSAT is low (≤30%), even if ferritin concentration is above 500 ng/mL.<br>• There is insufficient evidence on which to base a recommendation for an upper ferritin limit above which IV iron must be withheld.<br>• A decision to administer iron in the setting of high ferritin would require weighing potential risks and benefits of persistent anemia, ESA dosage, comorbid conditions, and health-related QoL. In accordance with KDIGO recommendations, Hb response to iron therapy, TSAT, and ferritin should be monitored closely and further iron therapy titrated accordingly. |
| CSN Commentary (Canada)[a] | • There is good evidence (1B) to support the administration of iron in adult CKD patients when the TSAT and ferritin thresholds are above 20% and 200 ng/mL. A therapeutic trial of iron can be considered in those where an increase in Hb or reduction of ESA or avoidance of ESA and transfusion is desired, while recognizing that an increase in hemoglobin is less likely when TSATs are >30% and ferritin values are >500 ng/mL.<br>• However, as opposed to the KDIGO anemia guideline, the CSN anemia work group believes that the current evidence does not permit a clear delineation for an upper limit of TSAT or ferritin values. |

[a]Quoted material is excerpted to focus on hemodialysis; ferritin units for CSN commentary converted to ng/mL.
[b]Based on patient symptoms and overall clinical goals, including avoidance of transfusion, improvement in anemia-related symptoms, and after exclusion of active infection.
[c]Consistent with recommendations 3.4.2 and 3.4.3.
[d]Based on patient symptoms and overall clinical goals, including avoidance of transfusion and improvement in anemia-related symptoms and after exclusion of active infection and other causes of ESA hyporesponsiveness.
*CKD,* Chronic kidney disease; *CKD ND,* non–dialysis-dependent CKD; *CSN,* Canadian Society of Nephrology; *ESA,* erythropoiesis-stimulating agent; *Hb,* hemoglobin; *IV,* intravenous; *KDIGO,* Kidney Disease: Improving Global Outcomes; *KDOQI,* Kidney Disease Outcomes Quality Initiative; *QoL,* quality of life; *TSAT,* transferrin saturation.
(Modified from Weiner DE, Winkelmayer WC. Commentary on "The DOPPS practice monitor for US dialysis care: update on trends in anemia management 2 years into the bundle": iron(y) abounds 2 years later. *Am J Kidney Dis.* 2013;62:1213–1220; quoted material from Kidney Disease Improving Global Outcomes (KDIGO) Anemia Work Group: KDIGO clinical practice guideline for anemia in chronic kidney disease. *Kidney Int Suppl.* 2012;2:279–335, 2012; Kliger AS, Foley RN, Goldfarb DS, et al. KDOQI US Commentary on the 2012 KDIGO clinical practice guideline for anemia in CKD. *Am J Kidney Dis.* 2013;62:849–859; and Moist LM, Troyanov S, White CT, et al. Canadian Society of Nephrology commentary on the 2012 KDIGO clinical practice guideline for anemia in CKD. *Am J Kidney Dis.* 2013;62: 860–873.)

provided about the superiority of one form over the others in the setting of CKD. The REPAIR-IDA trial has demonstrated the a regimen of two doses of 750 mg of ferric carboxymaltose in 1 week was not inferior to up to five infusions of iron sucrose in 14 days for anemic subjects with NK-CKD.[643] The use of larger doses of IV iron, rather than lower maintenance doses, does not appreciably affect cardiovascular morbidity and mortality in hemodialyzed patients.[703]

Some studies have suggested that the addition of ascorbic acid to the therapeutic regimen of patients treated with ESA and iron has beneficial effects, although none of these studies was rigorously conducted to provide definitive evidence.[704,705] Limited evidence has suggested that ascorbic acid may be pro-oxidant and may increase cytokine values.[706] A systematic review and meta-analysis has concluded that there is evidence in a limited number of small studies that the use of ascorbic acid results in increased Hgb concentrations, improves transferrin saturation, and reduces EPO utilization.[707] However, the use of ascorbic acid is not recommended in the KDOQI or KDIGO guidelines.[10–12]

## EFFICACY AND SAFETY OF ANEMIA MANAGEMENT WITH ERYTHROPOIESIS-STIMULATING AGENTS AND IRON

The change in the condition of patients on maintenance dialysis following the advent of rhEPO has been impressive

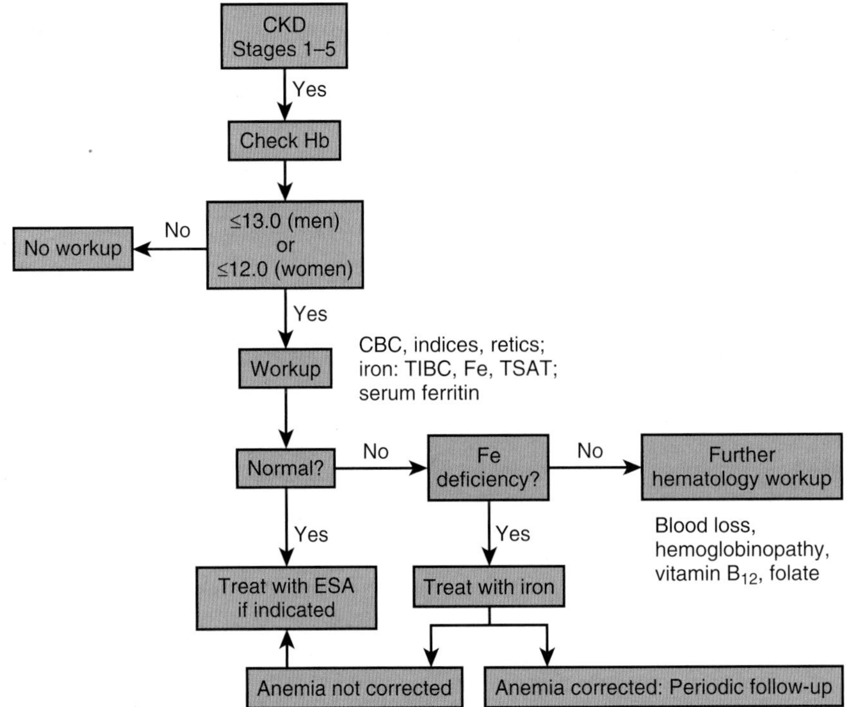


**Fig. 55.9** Flow chart for the evaluation of the patient with chronic kidney disease *(CKD)* and anemia. *CBC,* Complete blood count; *ESA,* erythropoiesis-stimulating agent; *Fe,* iron; *Hb,* hemoglobin; *TIBC,* total iron-binding capacity; *TSAT,* transferrin saturation. (Modified from Lankhorst CE, Wish JB. Anemia in renal disease: diagnosis and management. Blood Rev. 2010;24:39–47.)

and obviously advantageous. Transfusion requirements declined, iron overload due to previous RBC transfusions gradually resolved, and patients could easily be maintained at Hgb values above those that had to be accepted when RBC transfusions were the only viable option of anemia management. Androgen therapy, which had been associated with significant side effects, could also be abolished. Because of these obvious benefits, the use of epoetin soon became routine, and the workup for anemia is now considered part of the management program of patients in all stages of CKD (Fig. 55.9). If the workup reveals no reasons for anemia other than EPO deficiency associated with CKD, and in particular has ruled out iron deficiency, ESA therapy provides an option to correct anemia in almost all patients. However, despite the apparent advantages, formal evidence of a positive long-term benefit has never been established.

Several lines of indirect evidence have suggested that correcting or ameliorating anemia could reduce or at least mitigate the rate of left ventricular hypertrophy, a frequent complication in CKD, that is clearly associated with poor prognosis (see preceding discussion). Together with the apparent lack of adverse effects of ESA therapy, and the contention that higher Hgb concentrations might lead to improved HRQOL and physical function, this evidence led to an increase in Hgb target values. In addition, treatment was expanded to those patients not yet on dialysis, in whom anemia is generally less severe than in those on dialysis, because avoidance of anemia rather than late correction was intuitively considered the most appropriate strategy to improve prognosis and quality of life.

Unfortunately, however, the true nature of the relationship between long-term reductions in Hgb concentrations and adverse outcomes was not adequately tested in prospective interventional trials for a long time. Few studies have actually compared ESAs against placebo, and those trials, testing two different Hgb target ranges, have usually been inadequately powered. Subsequently evidence from several RCTs has become available, suggesting that normalization of Hgb concentrations with ESAs is associated with limited benefit and relevant harm.

#### Trial Overview

Since 1989, slightly more than 25 RCTs using ESAs in patients with CKD have been published, in which either different target Hgb concentrations were compared or ESA treatment was compared with placebo. Approximately 50% of these trials were conducted in patients on dialysis and the other half in patients with ND-CKD. Overall, approximately 11,000 patients have been enrolled in these trials, more than 4000 of whom were involved in one study, the Trial to Reduce Cardiovascular Events with Aranesp Therapy (TREAT).[708] The number of patients in the other trials varied from less than 20 to approximately 1400.[11,12] Several small trials conducted until 1997 compared ESA therapy with placebo. Thereafter, only treatment strategies testing two different ESA regimens were performed until TREAT was designed as the first large trial to compare ESA therapy with placebo in patients with diabetes and CKD who were not undergoing dialysis.

#### Large Randomized Controlled Trials

The US Normal Hematocrit Trial was the first study to test whether normalization of Hgb concentrations improves the prognosis of patients on dialysis.[709] It was hypothesized that any presumed benefit would be most obvious in patients with cardiac disease; therefore the trial enrolled slightly more than 1200 hemodialysis recipients who had congestive heart failure or ischemic heart disease. The target Hct in the higher arm was 42% and, in the lower arm, was 30%. The primary endpoint was a composite of death and first nonfatal myocardial infarction. The study was terminated early after 29 months because more patients in the higher arm had reached the primary endpoint. Although the difference did not reach statistical significance, study termination was recommended because it was obvious that the original hypothesis—that the higher Hct target was of benefit—could not be proven. In addition, the incidence of vascular access thrombosis was significantly higher in the higher target Hct arm. Self-reported physical function score improved at higher Hct values but, importantly, there was no significant difference between the two treatment arms for this parameter. A later analysis, which included endpoint events that the data safety monitoring committee had not yet considered when recommending termination of the study, also did not reveal a significant difference, and the rates of events occurring during 1-year of follow-up after study termination were similar in the two treatment arms.[710]

A second large trial in ESKD included almost 600 patients new to hemodialysis without symptomatic heart disease and left ventricular dilation.[711] Patients were randomly assigned in a double-blind fashion to an Hgb treatment target of either 13.5 to 14.5 g/dL or 9.5 to 11.5 g/dL. The primary endpoint was a change in left ventricular volume index on the assumption that raising the Hgb concentration would prevent the progression of left ventricular hypertrophy. However, changes in left ventricular volume index were similar for the two treatment groups. The only difference among a number of secondary outcomes was a better 36-Item Short Form Health Survey (SF-36) vitality score in the higher Hgb than in the lower Hgb group. Adverse event rates were also similar, except that rates of skeletal pain, surgery, and dizziness were higher in the lower arm, whereas those of headache and cerebrovascular events were slightly higher in the higher arm.

Thus, neither trial provided any evidence in favor of normalization of Hgb concentrations in patients on dialysis. However, because the prognosis, extent of comorbidities, and hemodynamic and metabolic milieu of patients undergoing dialysis are so different from those of patients with ND-CKD, the benefit of anemia correction was further tested in ND-CKD in three larger studies.

The CREATE (Cardiovascular Risk Reduction by Early Anemia Treatment with Epoetin Beta) trial was conducted in Europe, Mexico, and Taiwan.[712] It enrolled approximately 600 patients with an eGFR of 15 to 35 mL/min/1.73 $m^2$ and an Hgb concentration of 11 to 12.5 g/dL. Patients were randomly assigned to a treatment arm in which epoetin beta therapy was started immediately to achieve Hgb concentrations of 13 to 15 g/dL or to an arm in which treatment with epoetin was not initiated before Hgb had dropped to below 10.5 g/dL; the target Hgb in this second arm was 10.5 to 11.5 g/dL. The primary endpoint was a composite of eight cardiovascular events, which included the following:

*....the time to a first cardiovascular event, including sudden death, myocardial infarction, acute heart failure, stroke, transient ischemic attack, angina pectoris resulting in hospitalization for 24 hours or more or prolongation of hospitalization, complication of peripheral vascular disease (amputation or necrosis), or cardiac arrhythmia resulting in hospitalization for 24 hours or more.*"[712]

The study did not show a significant difference in the time to event between the treatment arms. Some dimensions of HRQOL were improved in the arm with earlier treatment and higher target, but, unexpectedly, time to dialysis was significantly shorter in this treatment arm. One of the limitations of the trial was that the observed event rate was much lower than the anticipated event rate, yielding lower than expected statistical power.

The CHOIR (Correction of Hemoglobin and Outcomes in Renal Insufficiency) study, conducted in the United States, had a similar design, but enrolled patients with more comorbid disease and yielded different conclusions.[713] More than 1400 patients with eGFR values of 15 to 50 mL/min/1.73 $m^2$ and Hgb concentrations below 11 g/dL were randomly allocated to receive epoetin alfa to achieve one of two different target Hgb values, 13.5 or 11.3 g/dL. The primary endpoint was a composite of death, myocardial infarction, hospitalization for congestive heart failure, and stroke. The trial was terminated when significantly more patients in the higher Hgb arm experienced at least one cardiovascular event. Separate analyses of the four components of the combined endpoint revealed trends for more frequent hospitalizations for heart failure and more frequent deaths but no difference in the rates of myocardial infarction or stroke. In addition, there was a trend toward more rapid progression of kidney disease in the higher Hgb target group. However, a meta-analysis of 19 trials did not support an effect of higher Hb targets on the progression of CKD, adverse events, or mortality.[714] Unlike in the CREATE trial, twofold to threefold higher doses of epoetin were needed in the CHOIR study to achieve and maintain similar Hgb values. Interestingly, a posthoc analysis has shown that the risks associated with the higher Hgb target are not apparent among subgroups with a higher mortality risk.[715]

In contrast to the other four large trials, the TREAT study was designed to test the effect of ESA in comparison with placebo in a sufficiently powered study. More than 4000 patients with CKD (eGFR = 20–60 mL/min/1.73 $m^2$), type 2 diabetes, and an Hgb concentration below 11 g/dL were randomly assigned to receive darbepoetin, with a treatment target of 13 g/dL, or placebo.[708] To avoid development of severe anemia in the placebo-treated group, a rescue protocol was established, according to which darbepoetin was administered when Hgb fell below 9 g/dL. The study was double-blinded. There were two primary endpoints—a cardiovascular composite endpoint and a renal composite endpoint, including death or initiation of maintenance dialysis. The trial showed no difference in the composite renal or cardiovascular endpoints, but analysis of the components of the primary endpoint revealed a significant, twofold higher risk of stroke in the darbepoetin arm. As an additional safety signal, the number of deaths attributed to cancer tended to be higher in the treatment arm, albeit not significantly and, in a subgroup of approximately 350 patients with a history of malignancy, all-cause mortality tended to be higher, and significantly more deaths were attributed to cancer. These findings were consistent with some findings in ESA RCTs in patients with cancer, which showed higher mortality and more rapid progression of malignancy in patients treated with ESA for chemotherapy-related anemia.[716] Patients in the darbepoetin arm of the TREAT study received fewer transfusions and showed a larger mean change in the Functional Assessment of Cancer Therapy: Fatigue (FACT) score.

### Risk-Benefit Relationship and Target Hemoglobin Recommendations

In summary, evidence from well-designed, larger RCTs has indicated that raising Hgb to normal or near-normal values with ESAs does not enhance survival or reduce the rate of cardiovascular events in patients with ND-CKD or ESKD, but is associated with risk for harm.[717] These results are also consistent with another large trial in patients with heart failure, many of whom had CKD.[633] Almost all studies showed increased rates of thromboembolic events but, for unknown reasons, other risks are not consistent across different studies. Although the CHOIR study, for example, suggested a mortality risk,[713] this finding was not confirmed in TREAT.[708] Also, a negative impact on the time to dialysis, as found in the CREATE trial,[712] was not found in TREAT. TREAT, on the other hand, found an increased incidence of stroke[708] and, although another study had previously reported a slightly higher number of strokes in a higher Hgb treatment arm,[718] neither the CREATE trial nor the CHOIR study found differences in stroke rates.[712,713] These inconsistencies may indicate important yet unrecognized factors that determine the side-effect profile of ESAs. Despite intensive investigation, it has not been possible so far to identify characteristics that distinguish patients in whom stroke developed during ESA therapy in TREAT.[719] Whether any of the observed adverse events is related to the actual achieved Hgb values, to indirect effects of an increase in erythropoiesis, or to direct, Hgb-independent effects of ESAs is unknown.[715]

Any benefit of higher Hgb values for HRQOL appears modest, on average, once Hgb concentrations above about 10 g/dL are reached. Transfusion rates are lower with higher Hgb values[720,721] but it is also clear that attempts to normalize Hgb by no means eliminate transfusion requirements. Moreover, the actual benefit from avoiding RBC transfusions is difficult to determine in individual patients, although the risk of sensitization in prospective transplant recipients should be strongly considered.[722]

Whether the balance of the risks and benefits of ESA therapy depends on the patient's responsiveness remains unclear. In treatment protocols driven by a target Hgb range, hyporesponsiveness leads to the use of higher doses and is associated with a greater likelihood of adverse events, but whether ESAs play a causal role remains unclear. A secondary analysis of the CHOIR study has suggested that high ESA doses rather than high Hgb concentrations are associated with poor outcomes.[411,715] In TREAT, the response to the first two weight-based doses of darbepoetin was a significant predictor of poor prognosis, with patients in the lowest quartile of ESA responsiveness having higher rates of the composite cardiovascular endpoint or death.[723] However, because "hyporesponders" could be identified only among the treated patients, it is unclear whether their poor prognosis was affected by ESA therapy.

The global KDIGO anemia guideline for anemia in CKD takes these considerations into account.[10] Careful balancing of the risks and benefits of ESA and iron therapy is an overarching recommendation. In patients not undergoing dialysis, the guideline recommends that a decrease of Hgb values to less than 9 g/dL be avoided by the initiation of ESA when Hgb is between 9 and 10 g/dL. In general, ESAs should not be used to maintain Hgb concentrations above 11.5 g/dL, and there is a strong recommendation against intentionally raising Hgb above 13 g/dL. However, individualization appears appropriate because some patients may have improvements in quality of life with Hgb values above 11.5 g/dL and are prepared to accept an increased risk.[724]

In the United States, a major change in payment for dialysis and related services has resulted in bundling of payments for laboratory services and IV medications and their oral equivalents. Together with the previously mentioned results from clinical trials and subsequent changes in drug labelling from the FDA, these payment changes have produced measurable reductions in the use of ESAs and Hgb values and have resulted in higher rates of transfusion in patients on maintenance dialysis.[57,725] The US experience may not be directly applicable to other countries.[726] A European study in 1679 patients on hemodialysis has identified weekly ESA doses more than 8000 IU as an independent risk factor for all-cause mortality and hospitalization.[727]

### Ferric Citrate–Based Phosphate Binding and Iron Metabolism in Chronic Kidney Disease

Ferric citrate (Zerenex, Keryx Biopharmaceuticals, NY), an iron-containing phosphate binder, has been shown to reduce serum phosphate values increase TSAT values, and moderately increase Hgb values in comparison with placebo in patients with ND-CKD, providing further support for the potential use of this product as an oral iron supplement in this patient group.[728–730] However, the FDA has approved use of the product only as a phosphate binder and placed a safety warning for a potentially excessive elevation of iron stores, suggesting regular monitoring with serum ferritin and TSAT values.[731] An increased incidence of gastrointestinal side effects was also noted for ferric citrate compared with placebo.[732] Control of serum phosphorus with another ferric citrate–based phosphate binder has been shown to be associated with lower ESA requirements and lower use of IV iron.[733] Sucroferric oxyhydroxide, another recently FDA-approved phosphate binder, has shown no significant effects on IV iron metabolism and anemia.[734]

## RED BLOOD CELL TRANSFUSION

When large RCTs questioned the safety and overall benefit of ESAs and of targeting higher Hgb concentrations, an appreciable increase was observed in the proportion of patients having Hgb values less than 10 g/dL, which, in conjunction with stable transfusion rates for this patient subgroup, translated into an increase in the absolute number of transfusions.[720] As shown in Fig. 55.10 (and Fig. 55.3), transfusion rates for US patients on maintenance dialysis were 2.9% in 2011 and 3.0% in 2012. Interestingly, transfusion rates in ND-CKD patients also rose significantly from 2002–2003 to 2008 (see Fig. 55.10).[721]

Transfusion is associated with the development of alloantibodies and human leukocyte antigen (HLA) sensitization,[735] which has important negative consequences for donor matching of patient candidates for a renal transplantation.

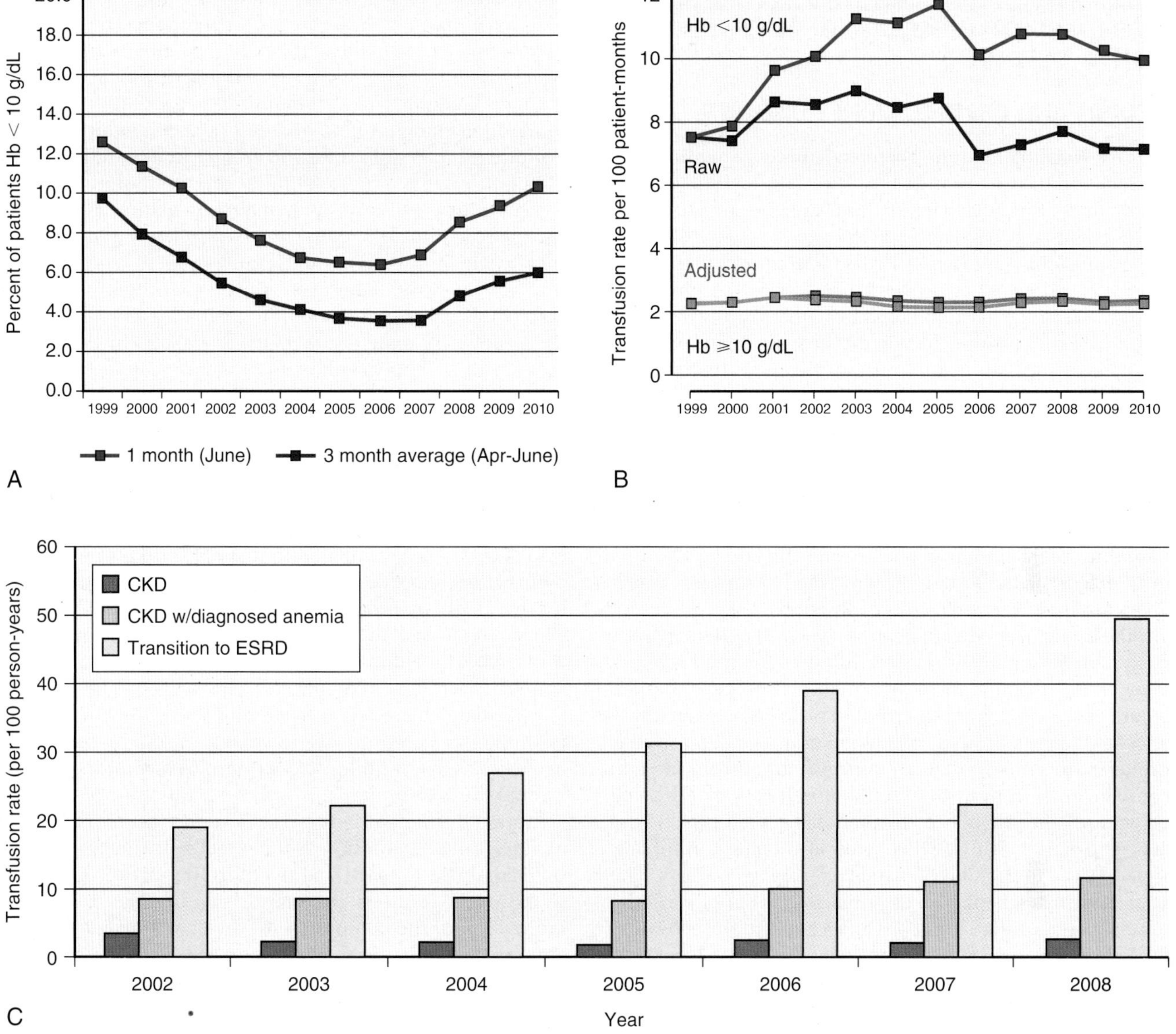


**Fig. 55.10** Red blood cell transfusion in chronic kidney disease *(CKD)*. (A) Proportion of patients with a single monthly or 3-month average hemoglobin *(Hb)* concentration less than 10 g/dL, 1999–2010. (B) Unadjusted and adjusted (for age, gender, race, primary cause of end-stage kidney disease, hospitalization days, and dose of erythropoiesis-stimulating agent) 6-month transfusion rates for patients with Hb values less than 10 and 10 g/dL or more (1999–2010). (C) Annual red blood cell transfusion rates/100 person-years (2002–2008) for patients with CKD, patients with CKD and diagnosed anemia, and patients with CKD transitioning to end-stage kidney disease (ESKD) during each follow-up year. *ESRD,* End-stage renal disease. (A and B from Gilbertson DT, Monda KL, Bradbury BD, et al. RBC transfusions among hemodialysis patients (1999–2010): influence of hemoglobin concentrations below 10 g/dL. Am J Kidney Dis. 2013;62:919–928; C from Gill KS, Muntner P, Lafayette RA, et al. Red blood cell transfusion use in patients with chronic kidney disease. Nephrol Dial Transpl. 2013;28:1504–1515.)

HLA sensitization also increases graft rejection and diminishes graft survival. It is unlikely that blood transfusion has any benefit on subsequent allograft function. Although the published literature seems to indicate mixed results, patients who received transfusions and developed alloantibodies were less likely to undergo transplantation. It is unreasonable and potentially misleading to compare patients who received transfusion and did not develop alloantibodies with all patients who did not receive a transfusion. We agree with the current consensus that blood transfusion should be avoided, if possible.[722] Because transplantation waiting times exceed life expectancy throughout most of the United States and much of the developed world, patients can ill afford a procedure (i.e., transfusion) that offers modest if any benefit and that can further lower the likelihood of ever receiving a kidney transplant.

Relatively common complications of RBC transfusions are febrile, urticarial, and/or allergic (immediate hypersensitivity) reactions. Less common complications include acute and delayed hemolytic transfusion reactions, hypotensive transfusion reactions, transfusion-associated dyspnea, transfusion-associated circulatory overload, transfusion-related acute lung injury, posttransfusion purpura, and transfusion-associated graft versus host disease. Additional complications of RBC transfusion include potential transmission of known and unknown infectious agents and iron overload.

## DISORDERS OF HEMOSTASIS IN CHRONIC KIDNEY DISEASE

### BLEEDING AND CHRONIC KIDNEY DISEASE

Excessive bleeding has long been recognized as an important complication of the uremic state.[736–738] This was particularly true prior to the advent of dialysis and the availability of rhEPO. Events may be as minor as epistaxis, excessive bleeding with toothbrushing, or easy bruisability. More severe, clinically relevant bleeding episodes tend to occur with trauma or after invasive procedures, rather than spontaneously.[739] Before the availability of routine dialysis, catastrophic gastrointestinal hemorrhage was the major cause of death with uremia.[736] Bleeding is frequently a predictor of increased mortality risk or complications.[740,741]

#### PATHOPHYSIOLOGY

Traumatic disruption of the endothelial lining of blood vessels results in a complex and coordinated response aimed to maintain vascular integrity and prevent bleeding. The first line of defense in hemostasis is represented by platelets, which specifically interact with ligands exposed as a consequence of endothelial damage. These ligands, which include collagen, fibronectin, laminin, thrombospondin, and von Willebrand factor (vWF) promote the adhesion of platelets to subendothelium and their activation. Activated platelets further release adhesive ligands stored in their alpha granules, such as vWF, fibrinogen, thrombospondin, fibronectin, and vitronectin and promote the activation of additional platelets by releasing aggregating agents such as thromboxane A2 (TXA2) and adenosine diphosphate (ADP). An occlusive plug is eventually formed by the deposition of platelets on collagen fibers. The surfaces of platelets play an essential role in supporting the coagulation cascade in plasma, which results in the activation of thrombin, conversion of fibrinogen to fibrin, and formation of the fibrin plug, which is stabilized by factor XIIIa. The generation of thrombin further enhances the activation of platelets and upregulates glycoprotein (GP) receptors, such as those for GPIb-IX-V and GPIIb/IIIa. Several systems play an important role in limiting the extent of coagulation activation and thrombus formation. Nitric oxide (NO) and prostacyclin limit the activation of platelets. Tissue factor pathway inhibitor (TFPI), the protein C and S system, and antithrombin turn off activated coagulation factors at various steps of the coagulation cascade. The fibrinolytic system is also crucial in both limiting the growth of thrombi and promoting their organization and removal. Fibrin digestion is mediated by plasmin, which is circulating in plasma as plasminogen, an inactive precursor. Conversion of plasminogen to plasmin is promoted by tissue plasminogen activator (tPA) and inhibited by plasminogen activator inhibitors (PAI-1 and PAI-2).[742,743]

Several factors contribute to increase the risk of bleeding in patients with CKD (Fig. 55.11).[744] It has long been noted that bleeding in uremic patients occurs despite normal or elevated circulating values of coagulation factors.[736] This observation has suggested that platelet abnormalities are the primary cause of the bleeding diathesis. The function of platelets is often impaired (thrombasthenia), whereas the number of circulating platelets is generally normal, with perhaps a tendency to decrease the longer that patients have been undergoing dialysis.[745] Thrombopoietin values are elevated in patients who are on maintenance hemodialysis and being treated with rhEPO but do not correlate with platelet counts.[745,746] Evidence for platelet dysfunction includes elevated bleeding time,[736] diminished aggregation response to ADP and epinephrine,[747] reduced ristocetin-induced platelet agglutination,[748] and prolonged closure time with the Platelet Function Analyzer (PFA, Siemens Medical Solutions).[749–751]

The most consistent abnormality in platelet function in uremia is an impaired interaction of platelets with the vascular subendothelium.[736] As a result, platelet adhesion and aggregation are hindered. The cause of this dysfunction is incompletely understood and could be related to abnormalities of the vessel wall, platelets, or plasma constituents. As for the vessel wall, it appears that its function may be altered in uremia. In particular, endothelial production of NO, a powerful platelet inhibitor, has been noted to be increased,[752–754] resulting in higher concentrations of cyclic guanosine monophosphate (cGMP) and reduction of platelet responsiveness. In uremic rats, treatment with an NO inhibitor partially restores platelet function.[755] Interestingly, guanidinosuccinic acid (GSA), long postulated to play a role in uremic platelet dysfunction, has been found to upregulate NO production by the vascular endothelium.[756] Prostaglandin I2 (PGI2), which is released by endothelium, is increased in patients with CKD who exhibit increased bleeding times[757] and probably plays a role in reducing platelet aggregability.[757]

The platelet itself is intrinsically altered in uremia. For example, the content of serotonin and ADP is reduced in uremic platelet granules.[747] Secretion of mediators may also be impaired, although this may be a function of repeated activation during hemodialysis.[758] Platelet receptors that play a critical role in adhesion to the vessel wall and aggregation, such as those for GP1b and GPIIb-IIIa, are probably not significantly reduced in quantity in uremia.[759] However, interaction of the receptors with vessel wall proteins may be abnormal.[760] In particular, activation of GPIIb-IIIa to facilitate its adhesion to vWF may be impaired.[761] The platelet cytoskeleton may be altered, with diminished actin incorporation and suboptimal intracellular trafficking of molecules.[762–764]

Although the platelet itself is not entirely normal in uremia, it appears that a more important pathogenic factor in platelet dysfunction may be the effect of uremic plasma on platelet responsiveness. Platelets from normal individuals develop impaired adhesive function on exposure to uremic plasma.[765] In contrast, platelets from uremic subjects regain some function on exposure to normal plasma.[765] Certain molecules with molecular weights that preclude adequate clearance with hemodialysis accumulate in uremia and may contribute to platelet dysfunction.[766] A variety of toxins, including quinolinic acids and guanidine substances, have been implicated.[736] In addition, a role for hyperparathyroidism has been suggested. Benigni and colleagues have found that PTH impairs platelet aggregation induced by a variety of substances.[767] Hyperparathyroidism may affect platelet function by elevating intracellular calcium concentrations via channels that are sensitive to calcium channel blockers such as nifedipine.[768]

It is generally accepted that dialysis reduces uremic platelet dysfunction and the risk for bleeding. However, dialysis does not completely eliminate the problem. Moreover, hemodialysis may induce a transient worsening in platelet function. Sloand

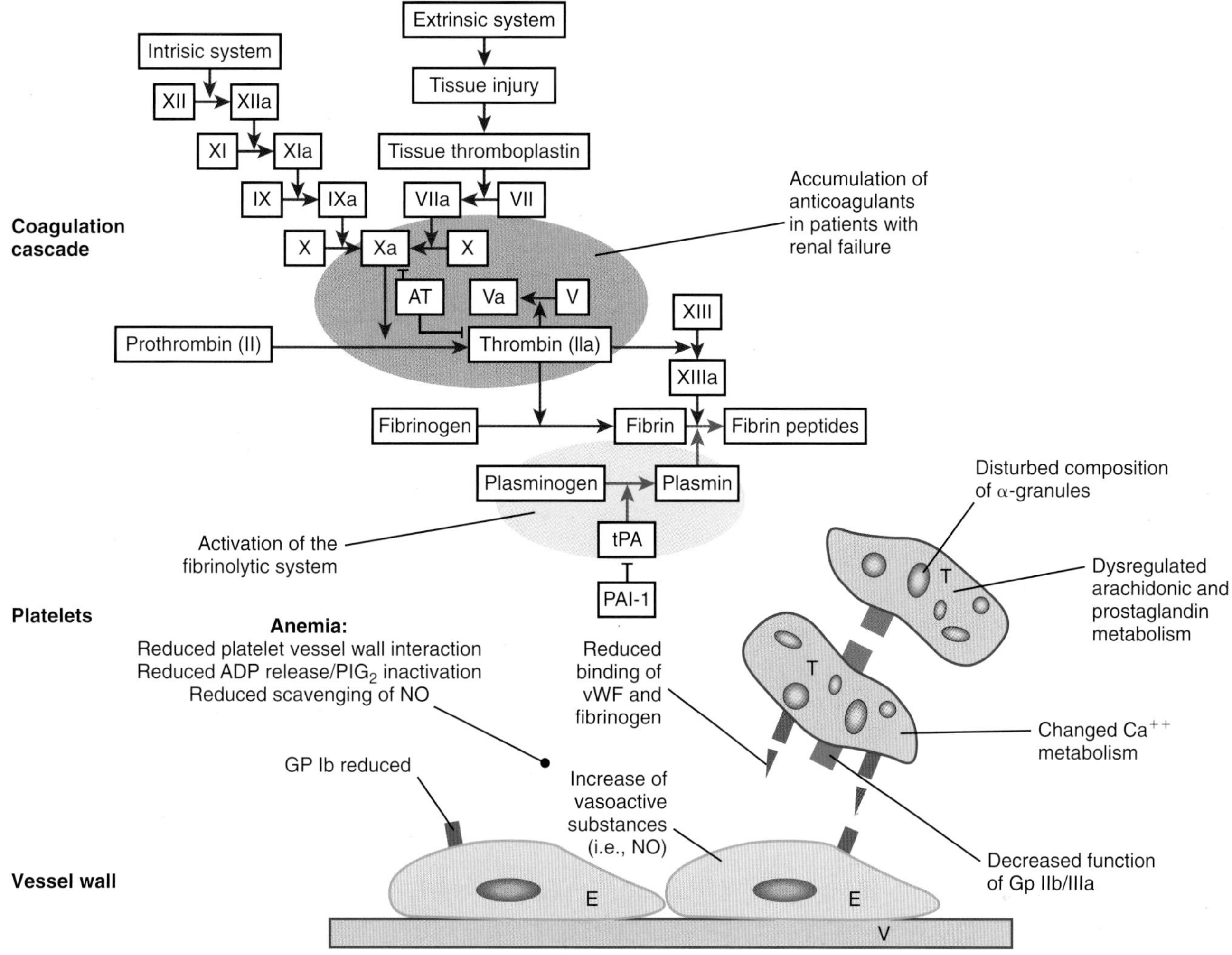


**Fig. 55.11** Factors involved in the increased risk of bleeding in patients with renal failure. *Roman numerals with or without lower case letters indicate clotting factors; ADP,* Adenosine diphosphate; *AT,* antithrombin; *$Ca^{2+}$,* calcium ion; *E,* endothelium; *GP,* glycoprotein; *NO,* nitric oxide; *PGI2,* prostaglandin I2; *T,* thrombocyte; *tPA,* tissue-type plasminogen activator; *V,* vessel; *vWF,* von Willebrand factor. (From Lutz J, Menke J, Sollinger D, et al. Haemostasis in chronic kidney disease. Nephrol Dial Transpl. 2014;29:29–40.)

and Sloand have measured a variety of indicators of platelet function immediately before and after treatments and noted a transient decrease of platelet membrane expression of GPIb after hemodialysis.[769] Ristocetin responsiveness was impaired after hemodialysis and normalized the day after treatment. Other potential detrimental consequences of hemodialysis include the enervating effect of repeated platelet activation,[770,771] removal of younger platelets with greater function,[772–774] and impairment of platelet function from a secondary effect of activated leukocytes.[775]

Anemia is an important contributor to uremic platelet dysfunction.[776] During normal circulation, erythrocytes tend to force the flow of platelets radially, away from the center of flow and toward the endothelial surfaces. When vascular injury occurs, platelets are in closer apposition to the vessel wall, facilitating platelet adherence and activation by vessel wall constituents such as collagen. With anemia, more platelets circulate in the center of the vessel, further from endothelial surfaces, hindering efficient platelet activation.[776] In addition, anemia may contribute to platelet dysfunction because release of ADP by erythrocytes normally stimulates platelet interaction with collagen.[777,778] Anemia has also been associated with increased urinary platelet activation markers in patients with CKD stages 1 to 4.[779] Treatment of anemia may help reverse platelet dysfunction because both transfusion of blood[776,780] and rhEPO therapy[781] have been found to be beneficial. Anemia is an important risk factor for hemorrhagic stroke—but not ischemic stroke—in patients undergoing hemodialysis.[782]

The plasma content of the major adhesive proteins, vWF and fibrinogen, are normal in uremia. One study has shown a normal distribution of vWF multimers,[748] but another reported a reduction in high-molecular-weight vWF multimers.[783] The functional properties of vWF are altered, however, mostly at the level of the interaction with the GPIb/IX-V platelet receptors, a key step in the signaling pathways, which ultimately lead to TxA2 production.[784–787]

Platelet-derived procoagulant microparticles have been described in CKD,[788,789] but inconsistent and unreliable measurement methodologies have hampered the assessment of their clinical relevance. Circulating endothelial microparticles are increased in CKD, and their baseline values (but not longitudinal changes) show an association with mortality risk.[790]

## DIAGNOSTIC STUDIES

Despite abundant evidence that the bleeding time is an unreliable test, with limited value in predicting bleeding complications,[791] use of this test is still reported in studies of CKD.[744] More reliable tests are available, such as platelet aggregation and platelet function analyser (PFA), although their value in predicting and managing bleeding complications has been questioned.[792] Thrombin generation assays may help in assessing both hypocoagulable and hypercoagulable states, but so far there are only limited studies in patients with CKD.[793]

## TREATMENT

The treatment of patients with renal failure experiencing bleeding episodes requires the following:

1. An assessment of the severity of blood loss
2. Hemodynamic stabilization
3. Replacement of blood products as needed
4. Identification of the bleeding source and cause
5. Correction of platelet dysfunction and other factors contributing to the bleeding diathesis (Fig. 55.12).

The first four factors are routine components of clinical care and are not discussed further here; the fifth extends from the previous discussion on the pathobiology of uremic bleeding. It should be clear, however, that the intensity of interventions to correct uremic platelet dysfunction hinges on the degree of bleeding severity.

The first aspect of treatment to correct uremic platelet dysfunction is provision of adequate dialysis. Initiation of dialysis will lead to some improvement in thrombasthenia and bleeding risk.[747,794] The PFA closure time improves in 25% of patients after a dialysis session.[795] No studies have fully elucidated the relative effectiveness of hemodialysis versus other dialytic modalities, but platelet activation measured by CD62 expression was increased by hemodiafiltration, whereas platelet degranulation products were increased in hemodialysis.[796] In any case, anticoagulation must be minimized. The

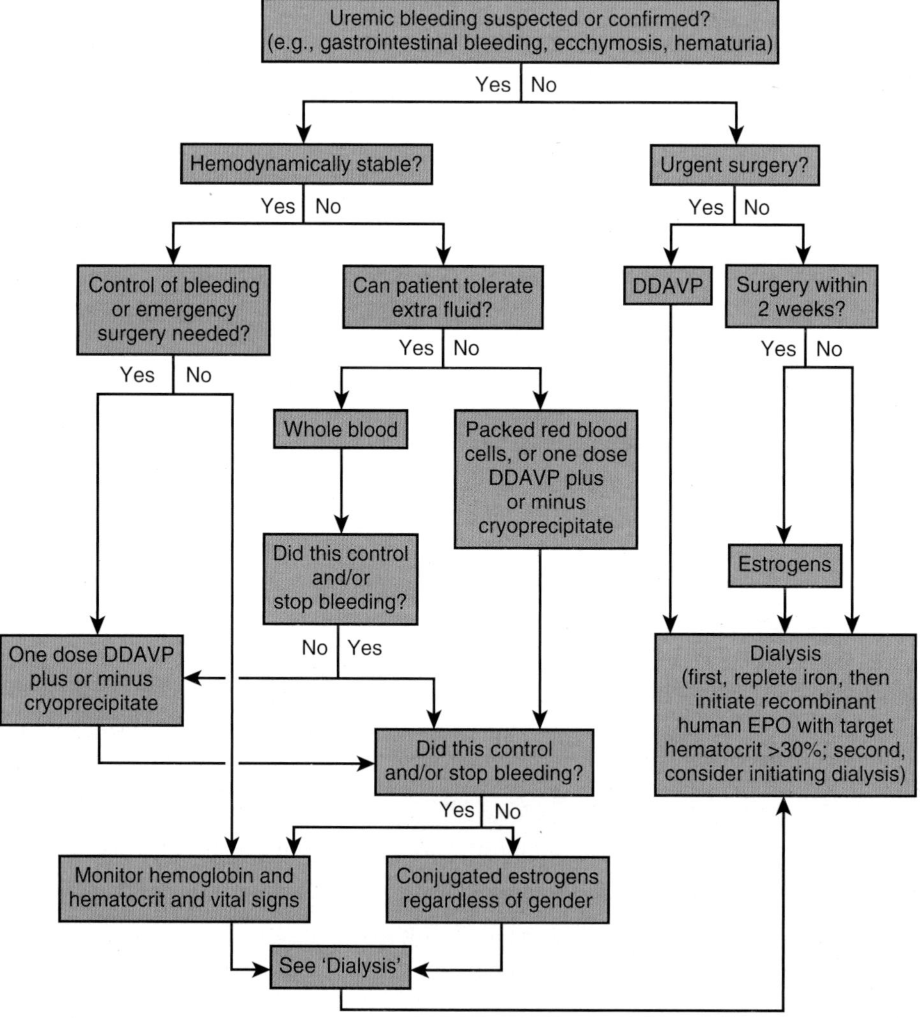


**Fig. 55.12** Algorithm for the management of patients with uremic platelet dysfunction. If at any stage in the algorithm the patient with uremic platelet dysfunction starts to bleed actively, the clinician should return to the top of the algorithm. This algorithm is not intended to replace sound clinical judgment or prevent additional consideration of patient factors that could influence management decisions. *DDAVP,* Desmopressin (1-deamino-8-D-arginine vasopressin; single doses of 0.3–0.4 µg/kg body weight IV); *EPO,* erythropoietin. (From Hedges SJ, Dehoney SB, Hooper JS, et al: Evidence-based treatment recommendations for uremic bleeding. Nat Clin Pract Nephrol. 2007;3:138–153.)

relationship of dose of dialysis with improvement of platelet function has not been well studied.

Treatment of anemia with rhEPO may be the most effective treatment of uremic platelet dysfunction (see earlier). Cases and associates have found that treatment with epoetin alfa, 40 U/kg IV, results in improvement in several parameters of platelet function as Hgb increases.[797] Others have found the same salutary effect of ESA treatment.[110,781] Improved platelet function following EPO treatment is most likely related to the associated changes in blood flow, with platelets moving closer to the vessel walls. However, it is also possible that EPO treatment itself may directly affect platelet function. Tassies and colleagues have found that platelet function improves in some patients after epoetin treatment is initiated, before Hgb values increase.[798] They attributed this effect to an increase in young circulating forms of platelets, with improved functional characteristics. Other potential direct beneficial effects of ESA include improved platelet intracellular calcium mobilization,[799] increased expression of GPIb,[736,800] and repaired platelet signal transduction.[801]

Desmopressin (1-deamino-8-D-arginine vasopressin; DDAVP) is a synthetic form of antidiuretic hormone that is often used to treat uremic bleeding. The drug has little vasopressor activity and only rarely induces hyponatremia. The mechanism of improved platelet function is not completely known, but enhanced release of larger vWF multimers by endothelial cells probably plays an important role.[802,803] Other factors may include improved platelet aggregation on contact with collagen[804] and increased concentrations of platelet GPIb/IX.[805] Given the unreliability of the bleeding time, it is no surprise that IV infusion of DDAVP (0.3 μg/kg [3.0 μg/kg subcutaneously]) produced inconsistent results.[802,806–808] DDAVP infusion improves platelet function in vitro and increases plasma concentrations for both vWF and factor VIII.[749] DDAVP may also be administered by the intranasal route, at a dose approximately tenfold greater than that given intravenously.[809–811] Repeated administrations of DDAVP may result in a diminished response, with the development of tachyphylaxis caused by the depletion of the endothelial stores of vWF multimers.[812,813]

Other treatments for uremic bleeding include infusion of cryoprecipitate, a plasma product rich in vWF and fibrinogen.[814,815] There has been very little published evidence to support the use of cryoprecipitate, and responses appear to be highly variable. In one study of five patients with active bleeding, only two had normalization of bleeding time and a favorable clinical outcome after treatment.[816] Cryoprecipitate use should be reserved for life-threatening bleeding due to the risk for infectious complications and limited availability.

Estrogens improve platelet function in men and women.[817–819] After IV infusion, Livio and associates have found the beneficial effect of conjugated estrogens to begin early and last for up to 2 weeks.[820] The mechanism of action of estrogen treatment is not fully known, but it may be related to the inhibition of vascular NO production by decreasing production of its precursor, L-arginine.[821] Transdermal estrogens at low doses (≤50 μg/day) are recommended for long-term therapy to balance the hemostatic benefit with thrombotic risks and are preferable to oral ones.[822,823]

Short-term (6 days) and long-term (3 months) treatments with the fibrinolytic inhibitor tranexamic acid have been associated with a reduction in bleeding time and improved platelet function.[824,825] Tranexamic acid may also be beneficial in the treatment of acute upper gastrointestinal bleeding episodes.[826]

## HYPERCOAGULABILITY AND CHRONIC KIDNEY DISEASE

Although bleeding is the most clinically relevant manifestation of the effects of advanced CKD on hemostasis, several lines of evidence indicate the presence of a prothrombotic, hypercoagulable state, which may play a role in the atherosclerotic/cardiovascular complications. Deep venous thrombosis (DVT) seems to affect predominantly CKD patients in younger age, of African-American or Hispanic background, in association with cardiovascular disease and prior surgical interventions.[827] The incidence of symptomatic venous thromboembolism is moderately increased in mild-to-moderate CKD (based on eGFR and albuminuria) as shown by a study pooling three European and two U.S.-based community cohorts,[828,829] as well as by a large population-based study in Denmark[830] and by smaller patient series.[831] The incidence of pulmonary embolism in CKD and ESKD is not precisely known (it may be particularly common after vascular access procedures – see Chapter 65), but mortality rates for pulmonary embolism are substantially higher in patients on dialysis than in the general population.[832] As described above, ESA therapy may further increase thromboembolic complications. Vascular calcification and cutaneous necrosis are the key features of calciphylaxis, a serious cutaneous disease affecting 1% to 4% of ESKD patients, which has been linked to a hypercoagulable state.[833]

### EVIDENCE FOR HYPERCOAGULABILITY IN CHRONIC KIDNEY DISEASE

As outlined in Fig. 55.13, several pathways are altered—toward hypercoagulability and increased risk of thrombosis in CKD.[744] Activated hypercoagulable platelets have been reported in patients with impaired or declining kidney function,[834,835] whereas other studies have shown increases in soluble markers of activated coagulation and fibrinolysis.[836,837] The values of several markers for thrombin activation (prothrombin fragment F1.2 and thrombin-antithrombin complex) and fibrinolysis (D-dimer and plasmin-antiplasmin complex) are abnormally elevated in dialyzed CKD patients, with erythrocyte membrane phosphatidylserine externalization possibly playing a role in this procoagulant state.[838–841] Phosphatidylserine externalization may be mediated by uremic toxins because it improves after dialysis treatment.[842]

Despite the functional platelet defects described previously, abnormalities in the soluble coagulation cascade and in some of the natural anticoagulant systems (e.g., fibrinolysis) generate a hypercoagulable state, which may facilitate cardiovascular and thrombotic complications in patients undergoing dialysis.[843,844] Complement activation may take place during dialysis, with increased expression of tissue factor on peripheral neutrophils and increased production of granulocyte colony-stimulating factor (G-CSF) resulting in a hypercoagulable state.[845] Increased prothrombotic markers and platelet activation have been reported following dialysis,[846] with some variability based on the type of membranes used.[847] Thromboelastography has shown delayed clot formation and

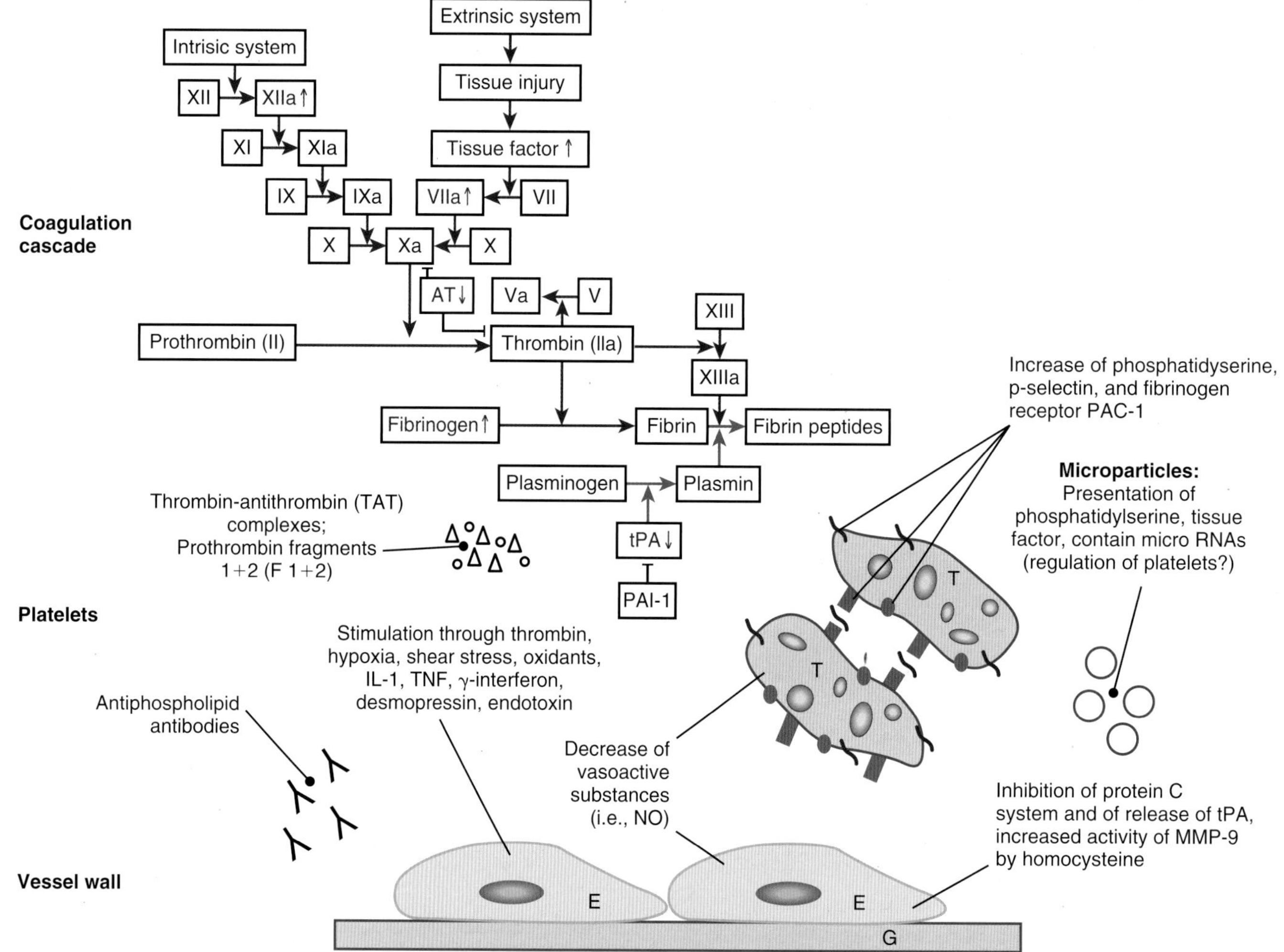


**Fig. 55.13** Factors involved in the increased risk of thrombosis in patients with renal failure. *Roman numerals with/without lower case letters* indicate clotting factors; *AT,* Antithrombin; *E,* endothelium; *G,* subendothelial connective tissue; *IL-1,* interleukin-1; *MMP-9,* matrix metalloproteinase 9; *NO,* nitric oxide; *PAC-1,* monoclonal antibody specific for the activated form of GPIIb-IIIa; *PAI-1,* plasminogen activator inhibitor-1; *T,* thrombocytes; *TNF,* tumor necrosis factor; *tPA,* tissue-type plasminogen activator; *↓,* decreased; *↑,* increased. (From Lutz J, Menke J, Sollinger D, et al. Haemostasis in chronic kidney disease. Nephrol Dial Transpl 29:29–40, 2014.)

decreased clot breakdown in patients with CKD, with increased plasma fibrinogen values playing a potential role.[848] Indolic uremic solutes have also been implicated in the procoagulant phenotype of uremia in animal models[849] and in patients with CKD.[850] Oxidized plasma albumin has also been implicated in generating a prothrombotic state via CD-36-mediated platelet activation.[851]

## PHARMACOLOGIC INTERVENTIONS

Treatment of hypercoagulability may expose patients to additional bleeding complications. A systematic review of bleeding rates in patients with CKD treated with antiplatelet drugs has shown that these agents are effective in reducing arteriovenous fistula and central venous catheter, but not arteriovenous graft thrombosis.[852] No firm conclusions could be reached about possible increases in bleeding rates in patients treated with a single agent, whereas there was an apparent increase in bleeding risk for combination therapy.[852] In patients treated for ischemic stroke, the presence of CKD was associated with a twofold increased frequency of clopidogrel resistance (by the VerifyNow P2Y12 Assay, Instrumentation Laboratory, Bedford, MA).[853]

Atrial fibrillation is a relatively common occurrence in patients with CKD and ESKD. The optimal approach to prevention of stroke and other embolic complications is unknown. There are concerns that chronic treatment with vitamin K antagonists may worsen vascular calcification.[854] Warfarin dosing is complicated in CKD and ESKD by drug-drug interactions, variability in dietary intake, and frequent administration of antibiotics, resulting in poor anticoagulation control.[855] The risk-benefit balance of warfarin for stroke prevention in advanced CKD and ESKD is unknown. The increased bleeding risk should be carefully considered,[856,857] especially in view of conflicting effects observed in older patients with atrial fibrillation and an eGFR less than 45 to 50 mL/min/1.73$^2$, which showed lower mortality despite a higher incidence of hemorrhage and higher or unchanged risk of ischemic stroke.[858,859]

One study has shown no reduction in the risk of stroke and higher bleeding risk in dialyzed CKD patients with atrial fibrillation treated with warfarin.[860] However, warfarin use to treat atrial fibrillation in patients with CKD post–myocardial infarction (MI) was associated with lower mortality and a lower incidence of MI and ischemic stroke, with no substantial higher risk of bleeding complications.[861] A Danish registry study has shown that in high-risk CKD patients, treatment of atrial fibrillation with warfarin results in measurable reductions in all-cause mortality and in hospitalization for stroke and bleeding.[862] This was contradicted by a small retrospective study that showed a substantially higher risk of death, bleeding, and MI for patients with CKD stages 3 to 5 and ESKD treated with warfarin.[863] A meta-analysis study has shown that warfarin therapy for atrial fibrillation in patients with CKD fails to reduce the risk of stroke and mortality, but it moderately increased the risk of bleeding.[864] A similar study in patients on chronic dialysis with atrial fibrillation and treated with warfarin has shown neither clear benefit nor clear harm.[865]

Novel oral anticoagulants (NOACs) have been approved for use in the general population; studies included a variable fraction (7%–21%) of subjects with impaired kidney function (eGFR <50 mL/min/1.73 m$^2$).[866] A systematic review and meta-analysis has shown no significant differences in thromboembolic or hemorrhagic complications in CKD patients treated with warfarin or NOACs.[867] Compared with warfarin, a similar study has shown a significant reduction for bleeding complications in patients with impaired renal function only for agents with lower renal excretion (<50%; e.g., apixaban, rivaroxaban, edoxaban).[866] In a primary care setting, bleeding risks and occurrence of stroke were similar in CKD patients with atrial fibrillation treated with an NOAC or warfarin.[868] Large randomized trials have included patients with reduced renal function and have shown efficacy for stroke prevention, with no increased bleeding risk.[856,869] However, due to the lack of specific trials in patients with CKD or ESKD, recommendations have been made to use NOAC in CKD stage G3,[870] not to use NOAC in advanced CKD.[871] and to perform proper studies in CKD.[872]

Dabigatran,[873] a direct thrombin inhibitor and apixaban[874] and rivaroxaban,[875] two factor Xa inhibitors, have been used in patients with CKD. Limited experience is available for newer agents, such as the indirect factor Xa inhibitor fondaparinux.[876,877] Although low-molecular- weight (LMW) and unfractionated heparin (UFH) can be reversed with the administration of protamine sulfate, newer agents such as fondaparinux have no specific antidotes, although recombinant factor VIIA and antithrombin have been used to reverse novel anticoagulant overdoses.[878–880] Table 55.3 provides some suggestions for the selection of an oral anticoagulant in patients with atrial fibrillation and CKD.[856] An essential part of this approach is the proper identification of stroke risk and bleeding risk using established tools such as the CHA2DS2-VASc and HAS-BLED scores, respectively,[856] although their utility has been questioned by a large Canadian study.[881]

The safety of omitting heparinization when dialyzing patients on chronic anticoagulation therapy with vitamin K antagonists has been demonstrated.[882] The PROMETHEUS study has shown no clinically significant difference in outcomes between prasugrel and clopidogrel treatment in patients with CKD undergoing percutaneous coronary intervention; it confirmed a higher adjusted risk for major adverse cardiac events and bleeding complications in the presence of CKD.[883]

### HEPARIN-INDUCED THROMBOCYTOPENIA

Heparin-induced thrombocytopenia (HIT) can be seen in patients undergoing hemodialysis due to their repeated and frequent exposure to heparin.[884,885] The presence of antibodies to the platelet factor 4–heparin (PF4-H) complex has been associated with arterial and venous thrombosis and increased mortality,[886,887] but other studies have found no correlation between the presence of these antibodies and reduction in platelet counts,[888] clinical complications,[885,889] or vascular access thrombosis.[890] An acute thrombotic event in a thrombocytopenic patient on maintenance hemodialysis or unexpected occlusions of the extracorporeal circuit[891] should prompt a search for possible HIT. However, the isolated presence of PF4-H antibodies should not by itself lead to a diagnosis of HIT or institution of specific anti-HIT therapies. The presence of oversulfated chondroitin sulfate as a purposeful contaminant of heparins produced in China, which resulted in a large number of adverse events, has also been associated with an increased prevalence of PF4-H antibodies but no thrombocytopenia.[892] If the presence of HIT is confirmed based on established criteria,[885] all heparin-based therapies should be discontinued, and the use of direct thrombin inhibitors or factor Xa inhibitors should be considered. Warfarin should not be considered until the resolution of thrombocytopenia and neither should prophylactic platelet transfusions.

## WHITE CELL FUNCTION IN CHRONIC KIDNEY DISEASE

CKD is accompanied by a chronic inflammatory state of complex pathogenesis, which is believed to be at least, in part, due to an increased generation of oxygen radicals and associated activation of monocytes. Uremic toxins have been blamed as a likely cause of this dysfunctional state, but with no specifically proven connections.[264,265,893,894] For more specific information on the biologic significance of uremic toxins; also, the European Uremic Solutes database (EUTox-db) can be found at http://eutoxdb.odeesoft.com/index.php. The use of particular dialyzers and dialysates has been associated with intradialytic leukocyte activation and enhanced oxidant stress, which may exacerbate the underlying activated inflammatory state. Activation of platelets adhering to dialysis membranes may contribute to leukocyte activation and the production of ROS.[895–901] Different types of synthetic dialysis membranes have been shown to induce different degrees of oxidative stress (measured in serum with the surrogate marker malondialdehyde or as ROS).[902,903]

### LEUKOCYTE (MONOCYTE) ACTIVATION

Several studies have shown elevations in markers of leukocyte and monocyte activation in patients undergoing dialysis,[900,904–906] as well as increased heterotypic aggregation for leukocytes and lymphocytes.[907] Advanced oxidation protein products (AOPPs) carried mostly by serum albumin have been identified in the serum of patients undergoing dialysis.[908] These AOPPs

**Table 55.3 Selection of Appropriate Oral Anticoagulant for Patients With Atrial Fibrillation and Chronic Kidney Disease**

| Drug (Renal Excretion[a]) | CrCl (mL/min)[b] ≥50 | 30–49 | 15–29 | <15 | ESKD on RRT |
|---|---|---|---|---|---|
| Preferred class | NOAC | NOAC | VKA or NOAC | VKA or NOAC (use with caution) | VKA or NOAC (use with caution) |
| VKA (NA) | Maintain TTR ≥70% | Maintain TTR ≥70% | Maintain TTR ≥70% | Maintain TTR ≥70% | Maintain TTR ≥70% |
| Dabibatran (80%) | 150 mg bid or 110 mg bid if patient is ≥80 years or receiving veraparamil or at increased bleeding risk | 150 mg bid or 110 mg bid if patient is ≥80 years or receiving verapamil or at increased bleeding risk | United States, 75 mg; other country, do not use. | Do not use. | Do not use. |
| Rivaroxaban (35%) | 20 mg once daily | 15 mg once daily | 15 mg once daily | Do not use. | Do not use. |
| Apixaban (27%) | 5 mg bid or 2.5 mg bid if two or more of the following criteria are fulfilled: age ≥80 years, body weight ≤60 kg, and sCr ≥1.5 mg/dL (133 µmol/L) | 5 mg bid or 2.5 mg bid if two or more of the following criteria are fulfilled: age ≥80 years, body weight ≤60 kg and sCr ≥1.5 mg/dL (133 µmol/L) | 2.5 mg bid | United States, 5 mg bid; other country, do not use. | United States, 5 mg bid; other country, do not use. |
| Edoxaban (50%) | 60 mg once daily or 30 mg once daily if two or more of the following criteria are fulfilled: body weight ≤60 kg; CrCl, 30–50 mL/min, and concomitant therapy with verapamil, dronedarone, or quinidine | 30 mg once daily | 30 mg once daily | Do not use. | Do not use. |

[a]Fraction of absorbed dose.
[b]Estimated using the Cockcroft-Gault criteria.
*CrCL,* Creatinine clearance; *NA,* not available; *NOAC,* non–vitamin K antagonist oral anticoagulant; *sCr,* serum creatinine; *TTR,* time in therapeutic range; *VKA,* vitamin K antagonist.
Adapted from January CT, Wann LS, Alpert JS, et al. 2014 AHA/ACC/HRS guideline for the management of patients with atrial fibrillation: a report of the American College of Cardiology/American Heart Association Task Force on Practice Guidelines and the Heart Rhythm Society. *J Am College Cardiol.* 2014; 64:e1–e76; Kirchhof P, Benussi S, Kotecha D, et al. 2016 ESC guidelines for the management of atrial fibrillation developed in collaboration with EACTS *Eur. Heart J.* 2016; 37:2893–2962; and Heidbuchel H, Verhamme P, Alings M, et al. Updated European Heart Rhythm Association practical guide on the use of non-vitamin K antagonist anticoagulants in patients with non-valvular atrial fibrillation. *Europace.* 2015; 17:1467–1507.

are believed to be end products of protein oxidation. Their concentration is correlated with the severity of uremia, extent of monocyte activation (assessed by serum neopterin),[909,910] and generation of myeloperoxidase by neutrophils in dialysis patients but not in predialysis conditions.[911] AOPPs can trigger neutrophil activation and respiratory burst, which can be reduced in vitro by N-acetylcysteine.[912] Leukocyte 8-hydroxy-2′-deoxyguanosine (8-OHdG) is a marker of oxidant-induced DNA damage, which is particularly elevated in patients carrying a GST M1 polymorphic dysfunctional variant.[676] Unique functional features of monocytes collected from patients on hemodialysis include increased transendothelial migration and induction of multiple activation markers on cultured human endothelial cells, which depend on superoxide generation.[913]

Evidence for leukocyte activation and ROS generation has also been found in patients with ND-CKD.[914] Degranulation of neutrophils results in release of a variety of enzymes and proinflammatory mediators[915,916]; some of these mediators, such as heparanase,[917] an endoglycosidase involved in the degradation of extracellular matrix, have been linked to the generation of atherosclerotic lesions; others, such as myeloperoxidase, generate hypochlorous acid, a potent microbicidal and oxidant compound. Hypochlorous acid may play a role in activating monocytes, which produce a whole array of inflammatory cytokines (e.g., IL-6, TNF-α, IL-1β).

## LEUKOCYTE FUNCTIONAL IMPAIRMENT

Granulocytes of patients undergoing hemodialysis exhibit impaired adhesion to fibronectin, especially in conditions of malnutrition.[918] Prominent apoptosis is observed in monocytes of patients with CKD,[919] and changes in monocyte subpopulations (CD16+) are associated with increased, soluble, proinflammatory markers, such as chemokine (C-X3-C motif) ligand 1 or CX(3)CL1.[920] Increased production of ROS and the accumulation of toxic products associated with uremia[264,265] are likely but not yet proven culprits in the generation of a dysfunctional immune response in patients with CKD. Phagocytosis by neutrophils is also impaired in patients on hemodialysis and is associated with increased serum endotoxin values.[921] Enhanced susceptibility to bacterial or viral infections and reduced response to hepatitis B vaccine have also been described.[922] Functional abnormalities in monocytes and T lymphocytes,[923–925] as well as in natural killer (NK) cells,[926] have been reported. It has been suggested that such abnormalities may be representative of a myeloid shift of erythropoiesis, similar to that observed with aging.[927] New dialysis membranes designed to reduce immune dysfunction are being developed, with encouraging but still preliminary results.[928]

## MARKERS OF LEUKOCYTE ACTIVATION

Elevations in serum CRP or myeloperoxidase have been associated with a higher mortality risk in hemodialyzed patients.[929] Expression studies with oligonucleotide microarray chips have identified distinct patterns of inflammatory and oxidative stress responses in dialyzed patients,[930] with some evidence suggesting a possible pathogenetic role of an impairment of the mitochondrial respiratory system.[931] IV administration of vitamin C in a small cohort of patients has produced changes in markers of oxidant stress.[932] Vitamin C supplementation in hemodialysis is a controversial issue because of the requirements for IV administration, prolonged therapy, and risk of hyperoxaluria.[933]

A better identification of the pathogenesis and clarification of disease modifier genes will allow us to design better focused and more personalized treatment approaches for the inflammatory state associated with CKD.[934,935]

 Complete reference list available at ExpertConsult.com.

## KEY REFERENCES


10. KDIGO clinical practice guideline for anemia in chronic kidney disease. *Kidney Int Suppl.* 2012;2:279–335.
21. Eschbach JJ, Funk D, Adamson J, et al. Erythropoiesis in patients with renal failure undergoing chronic dialysis. *N Engl J Med.* 1967;276:653–688.
22. Astor B, Muntner P, Levin A, et al. Association of kidney function with anemia. *Arch Intern Med.* 2002;162:1401–1408.
30. McFarlane SI, Chen SC, Whaley-Connell AT, et al. Prevalence and associations of anemia of CKD: Kidney Early Evaluation Program (KEEP) and National Health and Nutrition Examination Survey (NHANES) 1999-2004. *Am J Kidney Dis.* 2008;51:S46–S55.
49. St Peter WL, Guo HF, Kabadi S, et al. Prevalence, treatment patterns, and healthcare resource utilization in Medicare and commercially insured non-dialysis-dependent chronic kidney disease patients with and without anemia in the United States. *BMC Nephrol.* 2018;19.
69. Bachmann S, Le Hir M, Eckardt KU. Co-localization of erythropoietin mRNA and ecto-5'-nucleotidase immunoreactivity in peritubular cells of rat renal cortex indicates that fibroblasts produce erythropoietin. *J Histochem Cytochem.* 1993;41:335–341.
76. Eckardt KU, Koury ST, Tan CC, et al. Distribution of erythropoietin producing cells in rat kidneys during hypoxic hypoxia. *Kidney Int.* 1993;43(4):815–823.
74. Haase VH. Hypoxic regulation of erythropoiesis and iron metabolism. *Am J Physiol Renal Physiol.* 2010;299(1):F1–F13.
106. Miyake T, Kung CK, Goldwasser E. Purification of human erythropoietin. *J Biol Chem.* 1977;252:5558–5564.
109. Eschbach JW, Kelly MR, Haley NR, et al. Treatment of the anemia of progressive renal failure with recombinant human erythropoietin. *N Engl J Med.* 1989;321:158–163.
167. Koury MJ, Bondurant MC. Erythropoietin retards DNA breakdown and prevents programmed death in erythroid progenitor cells. *Science.* 1990;248:378.
199. Koury MJ, Bondurant MC. Control of red cell production: the roles of programmed cell death (apoptosis) and erythropoietin. *Transfusion.* 1990;30:673–674.
216. Madore F, Lowrie EG, Brugnara C, et al. Anemia in hemodialysis patients: variables affecting this outcome predictor. *J Am Soc Nephrol.* 1997;8:1921–1929.
220. Dmitrieva O, de Lusignan S, Macdougall IC, et al. Association of anaemia in primary care patients with chronic kidney disease: cross sectional study of quality improvement in chronic kidney disease (QICKD) trial data. *BMC Nephrol.* 2013;14:24.
240. Souma T, Yamazaki S, Moriguchi T, et al. Plasticity of renal erythropoietin-producing cells governs fibrosis. *J Am Soc Nephrol.* 2013;24:1599–1616.
241. Bernhardt WM, Wiesener MS, Scigalla P, et al. Inhibition of prolyl hydroxylase increases erythropoietin production in ESKD. *J Am Soc Nephrol.* 2010;21:2151–2156.
259. Wish JB, Aronoff GR, Bacon BR, et al. Positive iron balance in chronic kidney disease: how much is too much and how to tell? *Am J Nephrol.* 2018;47(2):72–83.
288. Nemeth E, Tuttle MS, Powelson J, et al. Hepcidin regulates cellular iron efflux by binding to ferroportin and inducing its internalization. *Science.* 2004;306:2090–2093.
299. Kautz L, Jung G, Valore EV, et al. Identification of erythroferrone as an erythroid regulator of iron metabolism. *Nat Genet.* 2014;46:678–684.
320. Bregman DB, Morris D, Koch TA, et al. Hepcidin levels predict nonresponsiveness to oral iron therapy in patients with iron deficiency anemia. *Am J Hematol.* 2013;88:97–101.
470. Kaufman JS, Reda DJ, Fye CL, et al. Subcutaneous compared with intravenous epoetin in patients receiving hemodialysis. Department of Veterans Affairs Cooperative Study Group on Erythropoietin in Hemodialysis Patients [see comments]. *N Engl J Med.* 1998; 339:578–583.
494. Levin NW, Fishbane S, Canedo FV, et al. Intravenous methoxy polyethylene glycol-epoetin beta for haemoglobin control in patients with chronic kidney disease who are on dialysis: a randomised non-inferiority trial (MAXIMA). *Lancet.* 2007;370:1415–1421.
495. Saglimbene VM, Palmer SC, Ruospo M, et al. Continuous erythropoiesis receptor activator (CERA) for the anaemia of chronic kidney disease. *Cochrane Database Syst Rev.* 2017;(8):CD009904.
525. Brugnara C, Chambers LA, Malynn E, et al. Red-blood-cell regeneration induced by subcutaneous recombinant erythropoietin—iron-deficient erythropoiesis in iron-replete subjects. *Blood.* 1993;81: 956–964.
535. Brugnara C. Iron deficiency and erythropoiesis: new diagnostic approaches. *Clin Chem.* 2003;49:1573–1578.
540. Fishbane S, Shapiro W, Dutka P, et al. A randomized trial of iron deficiency testing strategies in hemodialysis patients. *Kidney Int.* 2001;60:2406–2411.
544. Fishbane S, Pollack S, Feldman HI, et al. Iron indices in chronic kidney disease in the National Health and Nutritional Examination Survey 1988-2004. *Clin J Am Soc Nephrol.* 2009;4:57–61.
595. Brugnara C, Mohandas N. Red cell indices in classification and treatment of anemias: from M. M. Wintrobes's original 1934 classification to the third millennium. *Curr Opin Hematol.* 2013;20:222–230.
617. Rostoker G, Griuncelli M, Loridon C, et al. Hemodialysis-associated hemosiderosis in the era of erythropoiesis-stimulating agents: a MRI study. *Am J Med.* 2012;125:991, e1–999.e1.
626. Macdougall I, Bock A, Carrera F, et al. FIND-CKD: a randomized trial of intravenous ferric carboxymaltose versus oral iron in patients with chronic kidney disease and iron deficiency anaemia. *Nephrol Dial Transplant.* 2014;29:2075–2084.
687. Hougen I, Collister D, Bourrier M, et al. Safety of intravenous iron in dialysis: a systematic review and meta-analysis. *Clin J Am Soc Nephrol.* 2018;13(3):457–467.
701. Coyne DW, Kapoian T, Suki W, et al. Ferric gluconate is highly efficacious in anemic hemodialysis patients with high serum ferritin and low transferrin saturation: results of the Dialysis Patients' Response to IV Iron with Elevated Ferritin (DRIVE) Study. *J Am Soc Nephrol.* 2007;18:975–984.
708. Pfeffer MA, Burdmann EA, Chen CY, et al. A trial of darbepoetin alfa in type 2 diabetes and chronic kidney disease. *N Engl J Med.* 2009;361:2019–2032.
709. Besarab A, Bolton WK, Browne JK, et al. The effects of normal as compared with low hematocrit values in patients with cardiac disease who are receiving hemodialysis and epoetin. *N Engl J Med.* 1998;339:584–590.
711. Parfrey PS, Foley RN, Wittreich BH, et al. Double-blind comparison of full and partial anemia correction in incident hemodialysis

patients without symptomatic heart disease. *J Am Soc Nephrol.* 2005;16:2180–2189.

712. Drueke TB, Locatelli F, Clyne N, et al. Normalization of hemoglobin level in patients with chronic kidney disease and anemia. *N Engl J Med.* 2006;355:2071–2084.
713. Singh AK, Szczech L, Tang KL, et al. Correction of anemia with epoetin alfa in chronic kidney disease. *N Engl J Med.* 2006; 355:2085–2098.
723. Solomon SD, Uno H, Lewis EF, et al. Erythropoietic response and outcomes in kidney disease and type 2 diabetes. *N Engl J Med.* 2010;363:1146–1155.
729. Fishbane S, Block GA, Loram L, et al. Effects of ferric citrate in patients with nondialysis-dependent CKD and iron deficiency anemia. *J Am Soc Nephrol.* 2017;28(6):1851–1858.
747. Di Minno G, Martinez J, McKean ML, et al. Platelet dysfunction in uremia: multifaceted defect partially corrected by dialysis. *Am J Med.* 1985;79:552–559.
782. Yotsueda R, Tanaka S, Taniguchi M, et al. Hemoglobin concentration and the risk of hemorrhagic and ischemic stroke in patients undergoing hemodialysis: the Q-cohort study. *Nephrol Dial Transplant.* 2018;33(5):856–864.
820. Livio M, Mannucci PM, Vigano G, et al. Conjugated estrogens for the management of bleeding associated with renal failure. *N Engl J Med.* 1986;315:731–735.
828. Mahmoodi BK, Gansevoort RT, Næss IA, et al. Association of mild to moderate chronic kidney disease with venous thromboembolism: pooled analysis of five prospective general population cohorts. *Circulation.* 2012;126:1964–1971.
852. Hiremath S, Holden RM, Fergusson D, et al. Antiplatelet medications in hemodialysis patients: a systematic review of bleeding rates. *Clin J Am Soc Nephrol.* 2009;4:1347–1355.
855. Esteve-Pastor MA, Rivera-Caravaca JM, Roldan-Rabadan I, et al. Relation of renal dysfunction to quality of anticoagulation control in patients with atrial fibrillation: the FANTASIIA Registry. *Thromb Haemost.* 2018;118(2):279–287.
856. Potpara TS, Ferro CJ, Lip GYH. Use of oral anticoagulants in patients with atrial fibrillation and renal dysfunction. *Nat Rev Nephrol.* 2018;14(5):337–351.
858. Kumar S, de Lusignan S, McGovern A, et al. Ischaemic stroke, haemorrhage, and mortality in older patients with chronic kidney disease newly started on anticoagulation for atrial fibrillation: a population based study from UK primary care. *BMJ.* 2018;360:10.
860. Shah M, Tsadok MA, Jackevicius CA, et al. Warfarin use and the risk for stroke and bleeding in patients with atrial fibrillation undergoing dialysis. *Circulation.* 2014;129:1196–1203.
861. Carrero JJ, Evans M, Szummer K, et al. Warfarin, kidney dysfunction, and outcomes following acute myocardial infarction in patients with atrial fibrillation. *JAMA.* 2014;311:919–928.
913. Kliger E, Kristal B, Shapiro G, et al. Primed polymorphonuclear leukocytes from hemodialysis patients enhance monocyte transendothelial migration. *Am J Physiol Heart Circ Physiol.* 2017;313(5): H974–H987.

# 56 Endocrine Aspects of Chronic Kidney Disease

Juan Jesús Carrero | Peter Stenvinkel | Bengt Lindholm

CHAPTER OUTLINE



The kidney is a potent endocrine organ, a key modulator of endocrine function, and an important target for hormonal action. Thus alterations in signal feedback mechanisms and in production, transport, metabolism, elimination, and protein binding of hormones occur rather commonly in conditions affecting the kidney. As a direct consequence, chronic kidney disease (CKD), end-stage kidney disease (ESKD), and kidney transplantation are all associated with abnormalities in the synthesis or action of many hormones. The purpose of this chapter is to present an overview of specific endocrine abnormalities that manifest as a consequence of kidney disease.

## PANCREATIC HORMONAL DISORDERS: INSULIN RESISTANCE

Insulin resistance (IR) is a common feature of CKD—regardless of underlying cause—that describes a clinical condition in which there is a reduced biologic effect for any given blood concentration of insulin.[1] The body's resistance to the actions of insulin results in a compensatory increase in the production and secretion of insulin by the pancreas and leads to hyperinsulinemia to maintain euglycemia. If there is a concomitant inadequate secretion of insulin, this condition is manifested as abnormal glucose tolerance and, if severe, as diabetes mellitus. In CKD, both hyperparathyroidism and vitamin D deficiency may mediate insulin secretory abnormalities. Indeed, treatment of hyperparathyroidism[2] and pharmacologic doses of vitamin D[3] have been reported to correct glucose tolerance. The gold standard for determining IR is the euglycemic hyperinsulinemic clamp method.[4] However, because the clamp method is complex, expensive, and impractical to perform in large population studies, several surrogate methods (e.g., the homeostasis model assessment [HOMA]) have been developed. Unfortunately, all surrogate methods of determining insulin resistance suffer from important limitations, including poor precision, and oral glucose tolerance test (OGTT)–derived insulin sensitivity indices may be preferred to fasting sample–derived indices.[5] Insulin resistance is seen as the common denominator for a number of metabolic disturbances, including hyperinsulinemia, impaired glucose tolerance, fatty liver, abdominal obesity, hyperuricemia, elevated triglyceride levels, low high-density-lipoprotein (HDL) cholesterol levels, and hypertension.[6]

### CAUSES OF UREMIC INSULIN RESISTANCE

The seminal study by DeFronzo and colleagues has demonstrated that impaired tissue sensitivity to insulin is the primary cause of insulin resistance in uremia, implying a postreceptor defect in peripheral skeletal muscle.[7] Still, the molecular site of the postreceptor defect in humans has not been clearly established.[8] A recent study using the method of metabolic phenotyping and controls has confirmed that uremic patients exhibit IR with a compensatory increase in insulin secretion.[9] A reduced level of insulin receptor phosphorylation mediated by inflammation has been observed, both in animal models of diabetes and in patients with type 2 diabetes.[10] Whether the same mechanism is operative in CKD is unknown. Studies in animal models of uremia have reported downregulation of GLUT-4 in muscle,[11] failure of insulin to activate pyruvate dehydrogenase,[12] downregulation of insulin receptor substrate 1 (IRS-1)–associated phosphoinositol 3-kinase (PI3K), and upregulation of IRS-2–associated PI3K activity.[13] Recent studies based on hyperinsulinemic-euglycemic-euaminoacidemic clamp and $^{14}$Na–magnetic resonance imaging (to measure the concentration of $Na^+$ in the skin and muscle) in hemodialysis (HD) patients and controls have indicated that excessive muscle $Na^+$ content might also be a determinant of IR in HD patients.[15] Thus in the uremic milieu, the cause of IR is multifactorial, and many metabolic alterations may contribute concurrently (Table 56.1).

One feature of advanced CKD is low levels of 1,25-dihydroxyvitamin D (1,25[OH]$_2$D), a pleiotropic vitamin with multiple noncalcemic functions. Evidence of an important role for vitamin D in uremic IR was provided in an international study of patients undergoing dialysis in whom 1,25(OH)$_2$D infusion corrected glucose intolerance and IR

**Table 56.1 Multiple Causes and Consequences of Insulin Resistance and Abnormalities of Insulin Secretion in Chronic Kidney Disease**

| Causes | Consequences |
|---|---|
| Insulin secretion abnormalities: | Dyslipidemia |
| Hyperparathyroidism | Sodium retention |
| Vitamin D deficiency | Vascular calcification |
| Insulin resistance: | Muscle wasting |
| Uremic toxins | Hyperuricemia |
| Anemia | Renin activation |
| Metabolic acidosis | Hypertension and cardiovascular disease |
| Inflammation | |
| Oxidative stress | |
| Muscle loss and excessive muscle sodium | |
| Increased fat mass | |
| Physical inactivity | |

in the absence of changes in parathyroid hormone (PTH).[16] Although many studies in the general population have demonstrated that low serum 25-hydroxyvitamin D concentrations are associated with IR and diabetes risk,[17] the precise mechanism(s) whereby vitamin D supplementation improves IR is unknown. Metabolic acidosis is another common complication in uremia, also associated with IR, and 2 weeks of oral sodium bicarbonate supplementation in patients undergoing dialysis have been found to improve insulin sensitivity.[16] As in the general population without kidney disease, fat mass seems to be an important risk factor for IR in those with CKD.[18] Considering the obesity epidemic, the possible role of high fructose intake in the development of metabolic syndrome, and possibly CKD, definitely needs to be highlighted. Fructose may not only induce metabolic syndrome, hyperuricemia, and weight gain[19] but also exerts direct adverse effects on renal tubular cells.[20]

Persistent inflammation and protein-energy wasting (PEW) are two frequent and interrelated features of the uremic milieu that also may mediate IR. Loss of skeletal muscle mass results in abnormal glucose disposal, so it seems logical that treatment of PEW with intravenous nutrition improved IR in a study of surgical patients.[21] Elevated circulating proinflammatory cytokine values may also mediate IR.[22] Indeed, metabolic syndrome seems to be associated with inflammatory markers[23] and leukocyte count[24] in CKD. Among inflammatory mediators, tumor necrosis factor (TNF; partially produced by fat tissue) especially influences the ability of insulin to stimulate glucose transport.[25] Blockade of interleukin-1 (IL-1) with anakinra (an IL-1 receptor antagonist) in patients with type 2 diabetes is associated not only with less inflammation but also with improved glycemic control.[26] It has been shown that the suppressors of cytokine signaling (SOCS) family of proteins not only exacerbate IR but also inhibit insulin signaling and insulin-like growth factor (IGF) signaling.[14] On the basis of these findings, and from the fact that SOCS-1 knockout mice have a low blood glucose level and increased insulin signaling,[14] the SOCS proteins have been suggested to represent an important link between elevations of cytokine levels and IR. In patients with type 2 diabetes, high IL-6 levels are associated with increased SOCS-3 expression in skeletal muscle, and IL-6–induced SOCS-3 expression inhibits insulin signaling in human differentiated myotubes grown in vitro.[27] In CKD, few studies have yet examined the links between inflammation and IR. However, an inflammatory response during HD is linked to elevated SOCS-3 values and IR.[28]

In uremic mice, urea-induced generation of reactive oxygen species (ROS) has been suggested to induce IR,[29] although the mechanism thereof remains to be proven in humans. Additional factors that may contribute to uremic IR include physical inactivity and anemia. Correction of anemia by erythroid-stimulating agents (ESAs) has been reported to reverse IR in patients undergoing HD, independently of iron overload.[30] Furthermore, a small study in nonobese, nondiabetic, stable patients undergoing dialysis has demonstrated the beneficial effect of ESA treatment on IR.[31] The observation that IR is associated with reduced responsiveness to ESA in patients undergoing dialysis may, in part, be attributed to the presence of persistent inflammation in both conditions.[32] Finally, IR in patients receiving peritoneal dialysis (PD) merits discussion because the dialysis procedure itself, in addition to the uremic state, appears to modulate the magnitude of the IR.[33] IR may be exacerbated by the intraperitoneal presence of glucose-containing dialysate.[34,35] PD has significantly higher IR than HD, which may reflect the presence of glucose-based dialysate in the peritoneal cavity.[36,37]

## INSULIN RESISTANCE AS A RISK FACTOR FOR CHRONIC KIDNEY DISEASE

Whether IR (and metabolic syndrome) is an antecedent of CKD or merely a consequence of impaired kidney function has been debated. Large population-based studies have shown that the metabolic syndrome is associated with an increased risk for incident CKD.[38,39] A dose-response relationship has been documented between the number of metabolic syndrome traits and the prevalence of microalbuminuria.[39] Furthermore, a smaller scale study of nondiabetic patients with CKD has shown that IR estimated by HOMA is 2.5 times more prevalent in patients with CKD than in controls. Finally, a Japanese study in nondiabetic patients with hypertension and stage 3 CKD has shown that IR (estimated by both HOMA and the IR index) is a significant risk factor for the deterioration of kidney function.[40] The cross-sectional design of these studies precludes causal inferences, and mechanistic and intervention studies are needed to resolve whether the metabolic syndrome is a cause, consequence, or both of CKD. However, insulin has potent growth-stimulating properties and may have proliferative effects on glomerular and mesangial cells, and it also stimulates transforming growth factor-β (TGF-β) and the renin- angiotensin-aldosterone system (RAAS). Although insulin may also promote fibrosis,[41] it is not clear whether therapy directed to tackle the metabolic syndrome will delay, or even halt, the progression of CKD.

## INSULIN RESISTANCE AND CARDIOVASCULAR RISK

In a prospective observational study of nondiabetic patients with ESKD, IR was associated with cardiovascular mortality (Fig. 56.1) independently of Quételet's index (body mass index, BMI), hypertension, and dyslipidemia.[42] Thus as in the general population, IR and ensuing hyperinsulinemia

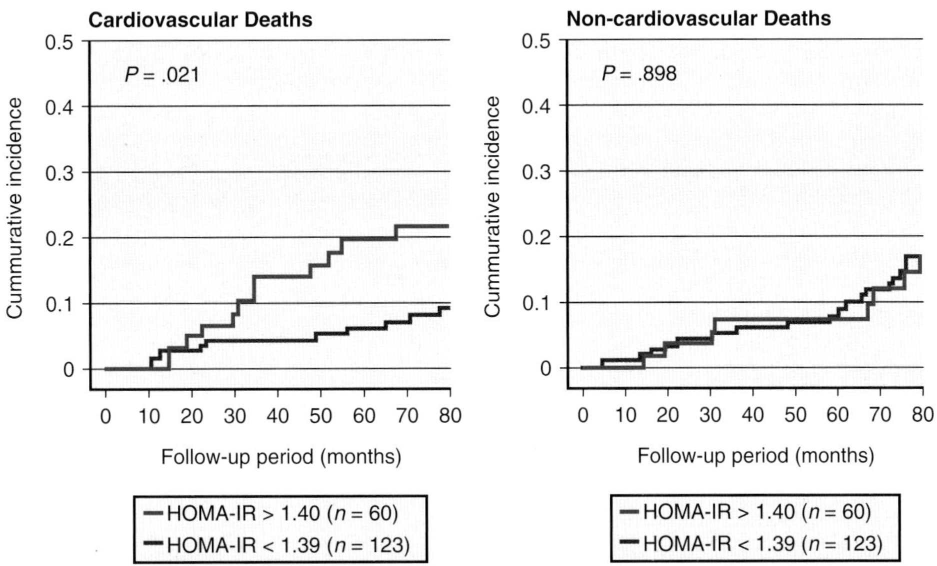


**Fig. 56.1** Kaplan-Meier curves showing the association between the homeostasis model assessment (HOMA)–estimated insulin resistance (HOMA-IR) and mortality in 183 nondiabetic patients with end-stage kidney disease (ESKD) treated with maintenance hemodialysis. (Modified from Shinohara K, Shoji T, Emoto M, et al: Insulin resistance as an independent predictor of cardiovascular mortality in patients with end-stage renal disease. *J Am Soc Nephrol.* 2002;13:1894-1900.)

may be independent risk factors for cardiovascular complications in patients with ESKD. A recent study based on the CRIC (Chronic Renal Insufficiency Cohort) cohort with 6.3 years of follow-up has shown that in addition to anemia, inflammation, and poor glycemic control, IR also was an independent predictor of congestive heart failure in CKD.[43]

Hyperinsulinemia promotes tubular sodium retention,[44] decreases urinary uric acid clearance, and upregulates the RAAS,[45] all established risk factors for hypertension. Another atherogenic link between IR and CVD is uremic dyslipidemia, typically characterized by hypertriglyceridemia, reduced HDL cholesterol, increased very low-density-lipoprotein (VLDL), and small dense low-density-lipoprotein (LDL) particles. Of note, uremic lipid abnormalities improve concomitantly with the correction of IR and glucose intolerance after the intravenous administration of $1,25(OH)_2D$ therapy.[16]

Because insulin accelerates calcium deposition in human vascular smooth muscle cells,[46] it has been speculated that although the beneficial metabolic and vasomotor effects of insulin are impaired in IR, the mitogenic signals are enhanced, and the resulting imbalance can promote vascular calcification.[47] Finally, the role of insulin in protein turnover merits attention, particularly given that altered protein turnover may have a role in CKD, cardiovascular disease (CVD), and PEW. Animal models of insulin deficiency have suggested that the effect of insulin on protein turnover is mediated through the activation of the ubiquitin proteasome pathway.[48] In accordance, uremic patients with type 2 diabetes who are undergoing dialysis have increased skeletal muscle protein breakdown in comparison with their nondiabetic counterparts.[49]

## TREATMENT OF INSULIN RESISTANCE IN CHRONIC KIDNEY DISEASE

Management of IR in uremia should be multifaceted. In addition to attention to and treatment of the many uremic metabolic alterations that may lead to IR and/or impaired insulin secretion, other more specific treatment options should be discussed with the patient. Regular exercise and lifestyle modification should be an integral part of the management of IR. Whereas a small interventional trial in patients receiving HD did not show IR improvements after 3 months of aerobic exercise training,[50] a study has shown that a 12-week lifestyle modification program in 295 diabetic and nondiabetic Japanese patients reduced albuminuria, maintained their estimated glomerular filtration rate (eGFR) and reduced fasting glucose levels in patients with the metabolic syndrome.[51] Because angiotensin-converting enzyme (ACE) inhibitor treatment appears to improve insulin sensitivity and may reduce the risk of type 2 diabetes mellitus in patients with essential hypertension,[52] the effect of ACE inhibitors or angiotensin receptor blockers (ARBs) on IR needs to be tested in CKD patients. The Diabetes REduction Assessment with ramipril and rosiglitazone Medication (DREAM) trial,[53] involving participants without CVD but with impaired levels of fasting glucose, has shown that ramipril does not reduce the incidence of diabetes or death but that it does facilitate the regression of glucose level elevations to normoglycemia.

In the evaluation of new users of oral hypoglycemic medication monotherapy in patients with type 2 diabetes mellitus, a higher risk of mortality was associated with glibenclamide, glipizide, and rosiglitazone than with metformin.[54] Because rosiglitazone was found to reduce the incidence of type 2 diabetes mellitus substantially and also increase the likelihood of regression to normoglyemia,[55] thiazolidinedione (glitazone) treatment was thought to be an attractive treatment option for patients with CKD. However, subsequent studies have provided conflicting results. A cross-sectional evaluation has shown significantly higher cardiovascular and all-cause mortality in rosiglitazone users,[56] consistent with a systematic review of trials in patients with type 2 diabetes mellitus that showed an increased risk of myocardial infarction and a borderline increased risk of death from cardiovascular causes.[57] In any case, thiazolidinedione treatment in ESKD cannot currently be advocated until its efficacy has been demonstrated in randomized controlled trials. A later randomized clinical trial in patients with CKD has shown that short-term rosiglitazone therapy reduces IR but has no effect on arterial function and stiffness.[58]

The insulin sensitizer metformin is a first-line pharmacologic agent for obesity and type 2 diabetes that has been widely used for over 5 decades. It is associated with a reduction in hemoglobin A1c (HbA1c) and improvements in micro- and macrovascular complications. Of note, this pleiotropic biguanide also has interesting additional outcomes, such as anticancer and life extension effects.[59] However, metformin is cleared by the kidneys, so there is a risk of metformin accumulation and associated lactic acidosis in CKD. Clinical practice guidelines have suggested that the drug should be used with caution when the estimated glomerular filtration rate (eGFR) is less than 60 mL/min/1.73 $m^2$, and the advisory board of European Renal Best Practice and the European Medicines Agency have concluded that metformin can be used with a GFR as low as 30 mL/min/$m^2$.[60,61] Some believe, however, that there is a disproportionate fear surrounding the safety of metformin in CKD that may not be valid if patients are counseled and monitored carefully.

A retrospective comparative effectiveness study of oral antidiabetic drugs has shown that in comparison with metformin, treatment with sulfonylureas increases the risks of a decline in eGFR, ESKD, and death.[62] Many of the sulfonylureas should be avoided in CKD owing to the risk of hypoglycemia; others should be used with caution. Newer approaches to improving IR, such as the provision of sodium glucose cotransporter 2 (SGLT-2) inhibitors and/or incretin-based therapies, provide novel strategies for diabetic kidney disease. Because recent large randomized trials have shown that empagliflozin, an inhibitor of SGLT-2, decreases the risk for composite cardiovascular events[63] and slows the progression of diabetic kidney disease,[64] this new class of drugs seems promising and may be a valuable addition to the current armamentarium of strategies to prevent the progression of diabetic kidney disease. Although dipeptidyl peptidase IV inhibitors are well tolerated in general, dosage adjustments according to kidney function are needed to avoid side effects.

## HYPOTHALAMOPITUITARY AXIS

### THYROID HORMONAL ALTERATIONS

Although thyroid hormones are necessary for the growth and development of the kidney and for the maintenance of water and electrolyte homeostasis, the kidney is involved in the metabolism and clearance of these hormones. Thus a decline of kidney function is accompanied by a characteristic disturbance in thyroid physiology (Table 56.2).

**Table 56.2 Thyroid Abnormalities in Chronic Kidney Disease**

| Site | Abnormality |
|---|---|
| Hypothalamus | Normal or high TSH<br>Altered TSH circadian rhythm<br>Altered TRH and TSH clearance |
| Pituitary gland | Increased thyroid volume<br>Higher prevalence of goiter and hypothyroidism<br>Low or normal total $T_3$ and total $T_4$<br>Low or normal free $T_3$ and free $T_4$<br>Impaired $T_3$ conversion from $T_4$<br>Normal total $rT_3$ and elevated free $rT_3$<br>Alteration in binding proteins<br>Elevated serum iodine due to reduced renal excretion |
| Cell | Reduced thyroid hormone cell uptake<br>Impaired binding of thyroid hormone receptor to DNA |

*$rT_3$,* Reverse triiodothyronine level; *$T_3$,* triiodothyronine; *$T_4$,* thyroxine; *TRH,* TSH-releasing hormone; *TSH,* thyroid-stimulating hormone.

#### CAUSES OF THYROID HORMONE DISTURBANCES IN CHRONIC KIDNEY DISEASE

The kidney contributes to the clearance of iodide. Plasma iodide retention in CKD favors thyroidal iodide uptake and potentially blocks thyroid hormone production by a negative feedback mechanism.[65,66] Serum free triiodothyronine ($T_3$) concentrations in uremia may also be low, serving as an appropriate compensatory response aimed at reducing energy expenditure and minimizing protein catabolism in the presence of PEW.[67] Metabolic acidosis[68,69] and systemic inflammation[70–72] are additional features of uremia that can contribute further. Medications that are able to suppress thyroid hormone metabolism include corticosteroids, amiodarone, propranolol, and lithium.[73,74]

Serum thyrotropin (thyroid-stimulating hormone [TSH]) concentrations are usually normal or elevated in CKD, but the response to TSH-releasing hormone (TRH) is generally diminished.[75] Both TSH circadian rhythm and TSH glycosylation are altered in CKD. The latter may compromise TSH bioactivity. Because serum TSH concentrations are frequently in the normal range, uremic patients are often considered euthyroid. Free and total thyroxine ($T_4$) concentrations may be normal or slightly reduced, mainly as a result of impaired hormone binding to serum carrier proteins. Circulating thyroid hormones are normally bound to thyroid hormone-binding globulin (TBG) and, to a lesser extent, to prealbumin (transthyretin) and albumin. Retained substances in CKD may inhibit hormone binding to these proteins. For example, urea, creatinine, indoles, and phenols all strongly inhibit protein binding of $T_4$. The transient elevation in plasma $T_4$ levels that occurs during the HD procedure may be due to the effect of the heparin used to prevent clotting in the hollow-fiber dialyzer and associated tubing, because heparin inhibits binding of $T_4$ to its binding proteins.[76] Most patients with ESKD have decreased plasma levels of free $T_3$ (low $T_3$ syndrome), which primarily reflects diminished conversion of $T_4$ to $T_3$ in the periphery.[77] This peculiar hormonal profile, however, is not associated with the increased conversion of $T_4$ to the metabolically inactive reverse $T_3$ ($rT_3$) because plasma $rT_3$ levels are typically normal in uremia. Such a finding differentiates the uremic patient from patients with other chronic illnesses.

In addition, the bioavailability and cell uptake of thyroid hormones may be partially blunted in uremia, leading to a state of thyroid resistance. This possibility is important to take into consideration because the serum TSH level may not be an accurate measure of the cellular action of thyroid hormone. In normal rat hepatocytes, treatment with serum from uremic patients reduced $T_4$ uptake by 30%.[78] Uremic plasma from patients undergoing HD inhibited the binding of thyroid hormone receptor to DNA and impaired $T_3$-dependent transcriptional activation.[79] Because dialysis per se corrected these abnormalities, the investigators suggested that a dialyzable substance was involved.[79]

As a consequence, CKD is associated with a higher prevalence of primary hypothyroidism, often subclinical.[80,81] Among incident dialysis patients, 18% of peritoneal dialysis and 22% of hemodialysis patients had hypothyroidism. The prevalence of the low $T_3$ syndrome (reduced $T_3$ in the presence of normal levels of TSH and $T_4$) is, in comparison, remarkably high, being reported in more than 70% of patients with ESKD.[82,83]

### CLINICAL IMPLICATIONS AND CONSEQUENCES OF THYROID HORMONE ALTERATIONS IN CHRONIC KIDNEY DISEASE

Because kidney function in hypothyroid patients was reported to be maintained or improved after thyroid hormone supplementation,[84–86] it has been speculated that thyroid disorders may impair kidney function and vice versa. Two observational studies with longitudinal design in patients with subclinical hypothyroidism and preexisting CKD have shown that $T_4$ supplementation attenuated the decline in kidney function over time.[87,88] The previously mentioned studies may be limited by confounding by indication, but their findings justify the need to explore this interesting possibility.

Hypothyroidism-associated outcomes has recently been the subject of investigation in various studies of dialysis patients. These studies reported an increased risk of mortality[89–92] and impaired health-related quality of life across energy, fatigue, physical function, and pain domains.[93]

Subclinical hypothyroidism, or the low $T_3$ syndrome, on the other hand, may constitute an intermediate link between the inflammatory stress, subsequent PEW, and impaired cardiovascular response in CKD. A number of studies have consistently shown that low $T_3$ concentrations are inversely correlated with markers of systemic inflammatory response and are an independent predictor of mortality in euthyroid patients with ESKD (Fig. 56.2)[94] and in dialysis populations,[95–97] having a stronger association with cardiovascular death.[98,99] A low $T_3$ level has also been linked to impaired cardiac function and geometry,[100,101] coronary artery calcification,[102,103] increased intima-media thickness,[103] flow-mediated vasodilation (FMD),[104] and measures of systemic arterial stiffness.[105] Low $T_3$ levels before kidney transplantation are associated with decreased graft survival.[106] The observational nature of the studies reporting these results emphasizes the importance of verifying whether uremic patients without primary thyroid dysfunction would benefit from thyroid hormone therapy. So far, there is insufficient evidence to recommend routine provision of thyroid hormone replacement in CKD with low $T_3$ alone. Because of potential unfavorable effects of thyrotoxicosis, such as tachycardia and loss of skeletal muscle and bone, the key therapeutic approach for the successful management of nonthyroidal illness in CKD might be simply to restore thyroid hormone deficiencies and maintain thyroid hormones within the normal range.

An early interventional study has shown that the intake of physiologic doses of $T_3$ (50 mcg/day) decreases thyrotropin levels and results in a borderline negative nitrogen balance (increased protein catabolism) in patients with ESKD.[107] This may be the natural consequence of restoring thyroid function and, in our opinion, may be easily counteracted by increasing protein intake. Before trials are conducted, other indirect approaches that may serve as proofs of concept include correcting acidosis,[108] oxidative stress,[109] or selenium deficiency.[110] In a placebo-controlled study of 30 euthyroid patients undergoing HD, exogenous $T_4$ administration over 3 months reduces lipoprotein(a) and total and low-density-lipoprotein cholesterol levels, without evidence of thyrotoxicosis.[111] However, in a large observational study of patients with ESKD, hypothyroid patients receiving exogenous thyroid hormones were at the same risk for death compared with those without medication.[112]

## GROWTH HORMONE

The growth hormone (GH)/insulin-like growth factor 1 (IGF-1) system is of key importance for anabolism, body growth, and body composition. It regulates a range of metabolic processes that are needed for the growth of cells and tissues in the body during all phases of life, but with the most profound effects during childhood. The metabolism and secretion of GH, a 22-kDa, 191–amino acid protein produced in the pituitary gland, are inhibited by somatostatin and stimulated by GH-releasing hormone, but many other factors are also involved, such as fatty acids and other nutrients and factors linked to nutrient intake, such as ghrelin, leptin, and neuropeptide Y. In general, nutrient intake regulates GH secretion so that body protein stores rather than fat tissue are preserved, especially during energy restriction. Fasting, as well as insulin-induced hypoglycemia, increases GH secretion, whereas a glucose load decreases circulating GH by reducing somatostatin release. On the other hand, the supply of protein and amino acids, especially arginine, increases GH secretion. During CKD, many of these pathways may be disturbed.[113–115]

GH is an anabolic hormone stimulating protein synthesis, bone growth, calcium retention, bone mineralization, and lipolysis, with decreases in body fat (Fig. 56.3). Although the effects of GH may vary according to whether the patient is fasting or fed, GH reduces hepatic glucose uptake and promotes gluconeogenesis and lipolysis, thereby opposing the glucose-lowering actions of insulin. GH released from the pituitary acts in an endocrine fashion on hepatic GH receptors to trigger the synthesis and release of IGF-1 from the liver. IGF-1 circulates free (biologically active) or bound to proteins (IGF-binding proteins [IGFBPs] 1–6). The binding of IGF-1 to specific muscle receptors induces muscle synthesis, inhibits muscle proteolysis, promotes the delivery of amino acids and glucose to myocytes, and stimulates myoblast proliferation.[113–115] Disturbances in the GH/IGF-1 system may therefore contribute to many complications in CKD, such as growth retardation, PEW and sarcopenia, and progression (i.e., loss of kidney function in CKD). GH deficiency is associated with decreases in GFR and renal plasma flow. Low circulating levels of IGF-1 are associated with increased

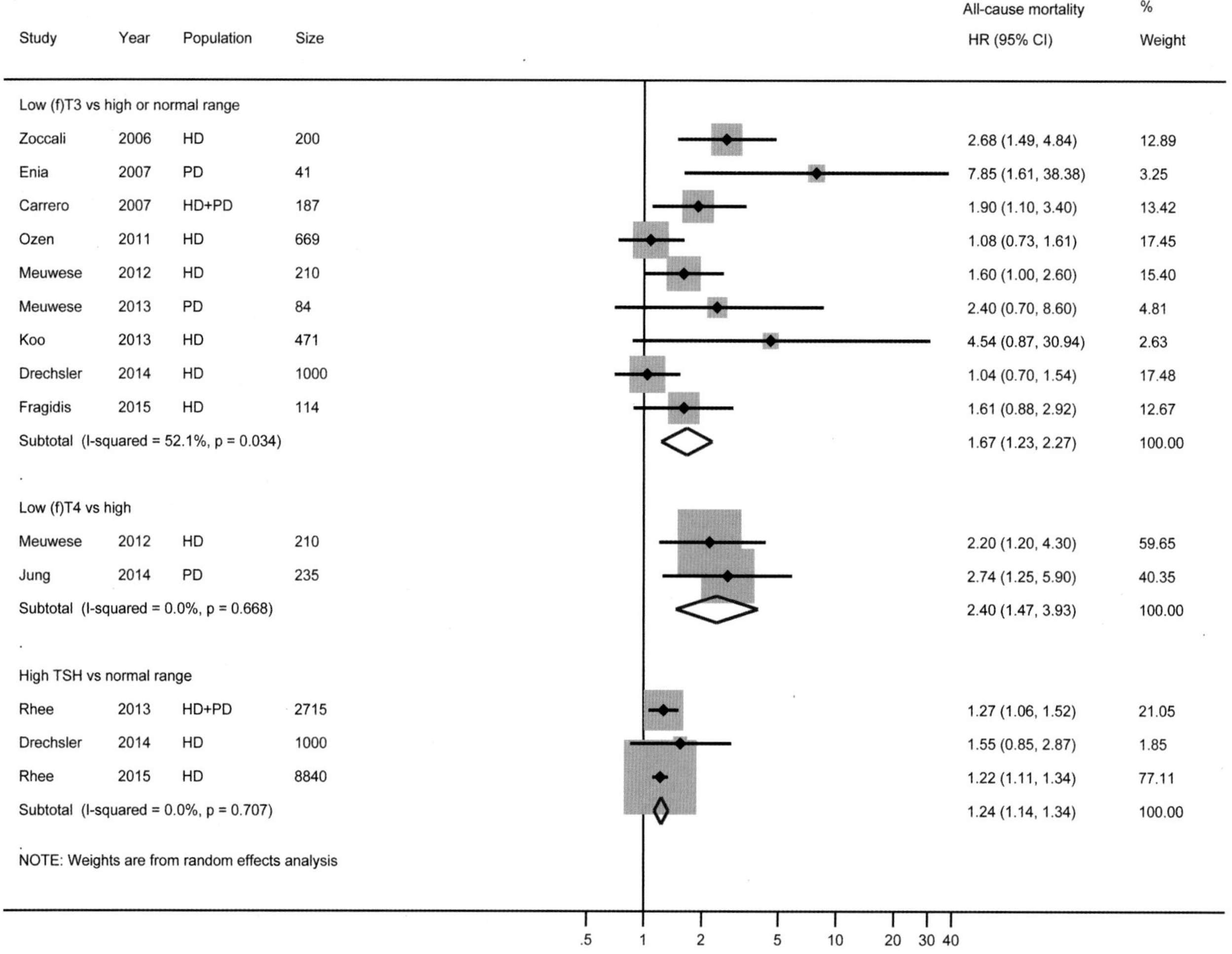


**Fig. 56.2.** Thyroid alterations and mortality. This Forest plot depicts the association between various forms of thyroid function test result derangements and risk for all-cause mortality, with a meta-analysis using the DerSimonian and Laird random-effects model. All hazard ratios (HRs) are based on the most fully adjusted reported model. *CI,* Confidence interval; *(f)T3,* free triiodothyronine; *(f)T4,* free thyroxine; *HD,* hemodialysis; *PD,* peritoneal dialysis; *TSH,* thyrotropin. (From Xu H, Brusselaers N, Lindholm B, et al. Thyroid function test derangements and mortality in dialysis patients: a systematic review and meta-analysis. *Am J Kidney Dis.* 2016;68[6]:923-932.)

mortality in patients with CKD stage 5 at the time of dialysis initiation.[116] Whereas the therapeutic use of GH to promote growth in growth-retarded children with advanced CKD is an accepted therapy, the administration of GH or IGF-1 might also improve nutritional status in adults with CKD. Furthermore, increased circulating levels of GH and IGF-1 may acutely improve kidney function in children and adults.[117–119] New therapeutic tools such as IGF-1 receptor inhibitors provide the possibility for modulating the IGF system to treat patients with kidney disease—for example, those with diabetic nephropathy[120] However, it should be noted that experimental studies in mice have suggested that GH and IGF-1 may increase the risk of glomerular sclerosis and could thereby contribute to the progression of CKD.[121,122]

## RESISTANCE TO GROWTH HORMONE IN CHRONIC KIDNEY DISEASE

Because growth retardation is common even though serum GH concentrations are normal or even elevated in children with CKD, a state of GH resistance and possibly also IGF-1 resistance has been proposed.[113,123,124] Insensitivity to GH is the consequence of multiple defects in the GH/IGF-1 system including, at the molecular level, a defect in JAK/STAT phosphorylation that may be due in part to concurrent inflammation.[125,126] One clinical implication of this resistance to GH and IGF-1 is that children with advanced CKD whose growth has been impaired often require very large doses of GH to achieve normal or near-normal body growth.

Resistance to the actions of GH and IGF-1 is also typically present in adult patients with advanced CKD.[114] This may be due to decreased GH receptors and/or post–GH receptor defects, as well as to decreased IGF-1 synthesis. Whereas serum IGF-1 levels in general are low, the circulating concentrations of IGFBPs are often elevated.[120] IGF-1 bioavailability may be reduced, because of the following: (1) reduced synthesis of IGF-1 receptors in the muscle[127]; (2) inactivation of IGF-1 due to increased binding to IGFBPs; and (3) increased hepatic production of IGFBPs (IGFBP-1 and IGFBP-2) and reduced excretion of IGFBPs in general, leading to a larger proportion of inactive IGF-1, despite normal total serum IGF-1 concentrations.[128,129] Newer treatment modalities targeting GH resistance with recombinant human IGF-1 (rhIGF-I),

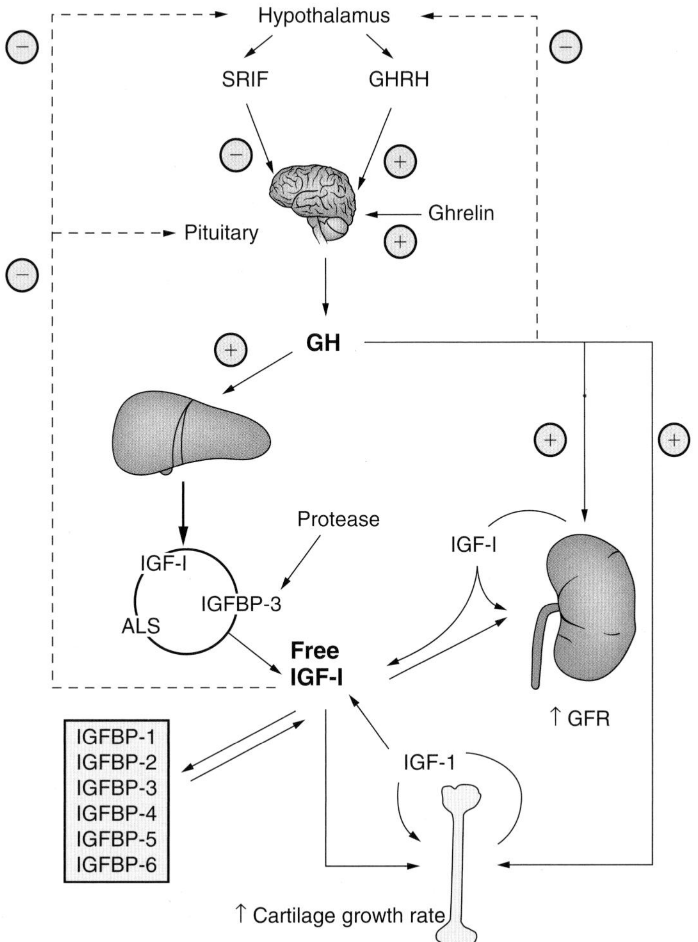


**Fig. 56.3** Deranged somatotropic axis in chronic renal failure. The growth hormone/insulin-like growth factor-1 (GH/IGF-1) axis in chronic kidney disease (CKD) is markedly different from the normal axis. In CKD, the total concentrations of the hormones in the GH/IGF-1 axis are not reduced, but there is reduced effectiveness of endogenous GH and IGF-I, which probably plays a major role in reducing linear bone growth. The reduced effectiveness of endogenous IGF-1 likely is due to decreased levels of free, bioactive IGF-1 as levels of circulating inhibitory IGF binding proteins (IGFBPs) are increased. *ALS,* Acid-labile subunit protein; *GFR,* glomerular filtration rate; *GHRH,* growth hormone–releasing hormone; *SRIF,* somatotropin release-inhibiting factor. (Modified from Roelfsema V, Clark RG: The growth hormone and insulin-like growth factor axis: its manipulation for the benefit of growth disorders in renal failure. *J Am Soc Nephrol.* 2001;12:1297–1306.)

recombinant human IGFBP3 (rhIGFBP3), and IGFBP displacers may prove to be more effective in treating growth failure in CKD.[114] Finally, it has been elegantly shown that resistance to pharmacologic doses of GH may be related not to uremia per se, but rather to an increased inflammatory state associated with uremia.[130] Abnormalities in the interaction of these pathways with those that involve other molecules, such as ghrelin, myostatin, and the SOCS family, may also be important.[113]

## GROWTH FAILURE IN CHILDREN WITH CHRONIC KIDNEY DISEASE

Recombinant human GH (rhGH) is an approved treatment for growth failure in children with kidney failure that has proven to be safe and efficacious. Identifying and addressing growth failure early on is an important component in the treatment of children with CKD. Treatment with rhGH is used in approximately 15% of all children undergoing dialysis in the United States.[131] Unfortunately, many children with CKD and growth retardation still do not receive adequate GH treatment for their growth failure. GH therapy should be considered in children with CKD who have a height less than 2 standard deviations (SDs) below the mean. Unusual causes for poor growth, such as hypothyroidism, should be investigated. Early institution of GH therapy is likely to improve the final achieved height. rhGH is administered as a daily subcutaneous injection. Once treatment is initiated, monitoring of growth, pubertal stage, nutritional state, funduscopic examination (to detect papilledema due to intracranial hypertension), and blood examination should occur every 3 to 4 months to determine whether growth is adequate and whether dose adjustments are needed. In patients younger than 3 years, the head circumference should be routinely monitored as well. Later studies have shown that rhGH treatment is most effective when started at an early age, and that the growth response is affected by the degree of impairment of kidney function.[132]

Even though rhGH has been shown to improve "catch-up" growth, the final adult height may still be below the genetic target. After kidney transplantation, growth retardation may persist because of multiple factors, such as corticosteroid use, decreased kidney function, and an abnormal GH/IGF-1 axis.[114] Although there have been concerns that long-term therapy with rhGH may have various adverse effects, rhGH is generally very well tolerated and does not seem to be associated with an increased incidence of glucose intolerance, pancreatitis, progressive deterioration of kidney function, acute allograft rejection, or fluid retention.[133–135] Newer formulations of rhGH have been undergoing experimental testing with the hope that adverse effects could be further reduced and efficacy increased, and the administration schedule might be more convenient in comparison with currently available formulations.

### GROWTH HORMONE TREATMENT IN ADULT PATIENTS WITH CHRONIC KIDNEY DISEASE

Many studies have explored a possible therapeutic role of rhGH and rhIGF-1 therapy in the CKD population. Among patients undergoing dialysis, evidence has suggested that rhGH stimulates protein synthesis, decreases urea generation, and improves nitrogen balance,[123] effects that appear to be dose-dependent.[136] IGF-1 enhances the intracellular transport of glucose and amino acids, stimulates protein synthesis, suppresses protein degradation, and stimulates bone growth and enlargement of many organs.[115,137] Whereas the use of rhGH or rhGH plus rhIGF-1 in patients undergoing dialysis has been generally well tolerated,[136–138] and long-term GH replacement may even improve cardiovascular mortality and morbidity in GH-deficient adults,[139,140] rhGH treatment in patients with an acute critical illness may result in increased mortality.[141] Among reported adverse reactions to GH treatment are a higher risk of benign intracranial hypertension, hyperglycemia, and fluid retention. In obese adults, rhGH therapy leads to a decrease in visceral adiposity and increase in lean body mass, as well as beneficial changes in the lipid profile, without inducing weight loss, despite increases in fasting plasma glucose and insulin levels.[142]

### GROWTH HORMONE/INSULIN-LIKE GROWTH FACTOR-1 SYSTEM AND KIDNEY FUNCTION

Disordered regulation of the IGF system is found in a number of kidney diseases, including polycystic kidney disease (PKD); IGF-1 stimulates the proliferation of cyst-lining cells from patients with PKD, an effect inhibited by rosiglitazone.[120] Receptors for GH and IGF-1 are expressed in the kidney and influence kidney structure and function,[117] and short-term rhGH treatment in CKD has been linked to a general improvement of capillary blood flow.[143]

Regarding kidney function, GH may increase renal hemodynamics and filtration rate, whereas rhIGF-1 can enhance GFR and renal plasma flow when administered short term to humans with ESKD.[118] In connection with this, the GFR and renal plasma flow rates are elevated in patients with acromegaly, whereas kidney function is usually low in GH-deficient states. GH increases the GFR with a delay of many hours, up to 1 day, consistent with the induction of IGF-1 synthesis. Endogenous IGF-1 may contribute to the physiologic regulation of GFR.[144]

Several studies have assessed the potential of rhGH and/or rhIGF-1 administration to improve kidney function. Whereas GH resulted in no or only a modest and transitory increase of the GFR in adults with advanced CKD and in children with growth failure,[117] IGF-1 produced a more sustained increase in GFR and renal plasma flow.[118] A regimen using rhIGF-1 in patients with advanced CKD was well tolerated and resulted in a sustained improvement in kidney function.[119] Transgenic mice expressing GH developed increased mesangial proliferation followed by progressive mesangial sclerosis, which was not seen in transgenic mice expressing IGF-1,[121,122] and there has been a concern that GH/IGF-1 therapy could contribute to the progression of CKD. However, prolonged treatment with GH in children with CKD has not been reported to lead to more rapid progression of CKD.[133,134]

## PROLACTIN

Prolactin's normal function in women is to promote lactation, but its function in men has not been fully established. Serum prolactin concentrations are usually elevated in patients with CKD, and the prevalence of hyperprolactinemia in ESKD ranges between 30% and 65%.[145–147] Hyperprolactinemia in CKD is understood as a consequence of reduced renal clearance[147] and increased production due to suppressed dopaminergic activity.[148] Thus antidopaminergic medications (e.g., neuroleptics, metoclopramide, cimetidine), which can further stimulate prolactin production, should be minimized or avoided if possible. The consequences of hyperprolactinemia in CKD and ESKD are reflected in the commonly observed reproductive abnormalities resulting from the associated inhibition of gonadotropin secretion. Hyperprolactinemic patients eventually experience galactorrhea and infertility due to the inhibition of gonadotropin secretion; in women, amenorrhea may concur, whereas in men, erectile dysfunction and hypogonadism often appear concomitantly. Although bromocriptine treatment has been proven to decrease prolactin levels in uremic men and women,[149] the previously mentioned symptoms do not fully disappear, suggesting that other factors may contribute in parallel. Therapy with ESAs has been suggested to decrease serum prolactin levels[150] and improve sexual function.[151] Thus it has been postulated that prolactin may contribute to the severity of anemia associated with CKD.

It is possible that prolactinemia may have previously underrecognized effects independent of its effects on the gonads. Studies in patients with CKD have reported a strong association among prolactinemia, endothelial dysfunction, arterial stiffness, and cardiovascular outcomes in men and in women.[152] These associations may be explained as a consequence of the following: (1) the inhibition of gonadotropic hormones, which may be linked per se to increased cardiovascular risk (discussed later); (2) decreased dopaminergic activity; (3) other risk factors affecting prolactin production, such as hypercytokinemia[153]; or (4) yet unknown mechanisms. Advancement in the understanding of prolactin physiology reveals additional functions, such as regulating the immune system and serving as a growth and antiapoptotic factor. As a growth factor, prolactin influences hematopoiesis, angiogenesis, and blood clotting. Prolactin modulates the inflammatory response, stimulates the adhesion of mononuclear cells to endothelium, and enhances vascular smooth muscle cell proliferation.[154–157] Prolactin also induces regional vasoconstriction through $\beta_2$-adrenergic and nitric oxide mechanisms.[158] Some small studies have evaluated the effects of bromocriptine therapy in CKD, describing a reduction in blood pressure and the regression of left ventricular hypertrophy in patients undergoing dialysis.[159–161] Another randomized-controlled trial in patients with diabetes mellitus and stage 4 CKD tested bromocriptine supplementation for 6 months versus placebo[162]; decreases in blood pressure and left ventricular mass index were observed. Whether these effects were, at least partly, mediated by prolactin reduction is unknown.

## ADRENAL GLANDS

Because symptoms of hypercortisolism and hyperaldosteronemia are common in CKD, it has been proposed that the hypothalamic-pituitary-adrenal (HPA) axis may be upregulated.[163] This proposal is plausible, given that both glucocorticoid and aldosterone metabolites are excreted by the kidneys and that cortisol metabolism is partly regulated by the kidneys. Nonetheless, few studies to date have addressed adrenal gland disorders in CKD, an issue in part hampered by the prescription of medication interfering with the RAAS and cortisol system.

### ADRENOCORTICOTROPIC HORMONE

Adrenocorticotropic hormone (ACTH) was used 60 years ago for the treatment of nephrotic syndrome in children but was gradually replaced by synthetic glucocorticoid analogs. In addition to its role in controlling steroidogenesis, ACTH stands as a physiologic agonist of the melanocortin system. Clinical and experimental evidence suggests that ACTH may have antiproteinuric, lipid-lowering, and renoprotective properties, which are not fully explained by its steroidogenic effects.[164,165]

### ALDOSTERONE AND CORTISOL

Over and above the classical effect on sodium reabsorption, aldosterone may exert other effects on renal and cardiovascular damage. Aldosterone increases oxidative stress and promotes vascular inflammation[166,167] and impairs vascular reactivity by limiting the bioavailability of nitric oxide.[168] In the presence of salt overload, aldosterone causes hypertrophy and fibrosis in the heart, both of which are prevented by the administration of mineralocorticoid receptor (MR) antagonists.[169] The MR binds aldosterone and cortisol with similar affinities. Under normal conditions cortisol is incapable of activating the MR because cortisol is converted into the inactive metabolite cortisone by 11β-hydroxysteroid dehydrogenase type 2 (11β-HSD2).[170] Thus it may be hypothesized that the beneficial effects of MR antagonists may result from blocking the action of both aldosterone and cortisol. In an observational analysis in patients with type 2 diabetes mellitus undergoing maintenance HD,[171] the joint presence of high serum aldosterone and high serum cortisol concentrations was associated with sudden cardiac death. Whether the use of MR antagonists decreases the risk of sudden death in such patients must be examined in future trials.

### ADRENAL ANDROGENS

Dehydroepiandrosterone (DHEA) and dehydroepiandrosterone sulfate (DHEA-S) are secreted from the zona reticularis of the adrenal gland. DHEA and DHEA-S are interconverted, and DHEA serves as a precursor of sex hormones. In a population-based study of young adults, serum DHEA concentrations were inversely associated with kidney function.[172] Low circulating serum concentrations of DHEA-S were also associated with the progression of glomerular injury in men with type 2 diabetes mellitus.[173] This finding is in line with those of two studies showing that serum DHEA-S was significantly reduced in male patients on maintenance HD and was associated with all-cause and CVD-related mortality.[174,175] Like concentrations of other hormones, the reduced DHEA-S concentration may be a surrogate of disease severity, being suppressed in critical illness. However, DHEA-S may have protective functions against atherosclerosis and CVD, given that DHEA supplementation improves endothelial function and insulin sensitivity in men.[176] DHEA-S may have other functions as a peroxisome proliferator–activated receptor α (PPARα) activator that can modulate immune function, inflammation, and oxidative stress.[177] Finally, one should not forget that DHEA-S may be an intermediate in the pathways of both prolactin (upstream) and testosterone (downstream), thus mediating the risk.

## GONADAL DYSFUNCTION

Disturbances in the hypothalamic-pituitary-gonadal axis are common in patients with CKD and play an important role in the development of sexual dysfunction (Table 56.3). Sexual dysfunction in these patients should be thought of as a multifactorial problem that is affected by a variety of physiologic and psychological factors, as well as comorbid conditions. In addition to a number of endocrine alterations described later, diabetes and vascular disease, for example, can interfere with the ability of the male patient to achieve an erection and the female patient to achieve sexual arousal. Various psychological factors, such as depression, can significantly and adversely affect sexual function in both men and women.

### IN WOMEN

#### Endocrine Abnormalities

Elevated serum concentrations of prolactin (see earlier discussion), follicle-stimulating hormone (FSH), and luteinizing hormone (LH) are usual findings in uremic women.

**Table 56.3 Endocrine Abnormalities Leading to Sexual Dysfunction in Chronic Kidney Disease**

| Gender Affected | Endocrine Abnormality |
|---|---|
| Men | Decreased production of testosterone<br>Blunted increase in serum luteinizing hormone (LH)<br>Decreased amplitude of LH secretory burst<br>Variable increase in follicle-stimulating hormone (FSH)<br>Increased prolactin |
| Women | Anovulatory menstrual cycles<br>Lack of midcycle surge in LH<br>Increased prolactin |

Disturbances in menstruation and fertility are commonly encountered, usually leading to amenorrhea by the time the patient is diagnosed with ESKD. The menstrual cycle typically remains irregular after the initiation of dialysis. Ovarian dysfunction in women undergoing dialysis is characterized by the absence of cyclic gonadotropin and estradiol release, which result in the lack of progestational changes in the endometrium.[178] A midcycle LH surge cannot be mitigated with the endogenous administration of estrogen, confirming a central hypothalamic derangement.[179] As a consequence, anovulation and subsequent infertility are probably the major menstrual abnormalities in uremic women, together with decreased libido and reduced ability to reach orgasm.[180] Therefore, successful conception with pregnancy is rare in women with ESKD. Pathologic endometrium morphology is very common in uremic women of reproductive age undergoing HD, with proliferative changes in 30% and atrophic changes in almost 25%. However, it seems that the endometrium has preserved normal reactivity to circulating estrogens.[181]

### Clinical Manifestations

Young uremic women usually experience premature menopause, approximately 4.5 years earlier on average than their healthy counterparts. Hypogonadism in women has been linked with sleep disorders, depression, urinary incontinence and, in the long term, osteoporosis, impaired cognitive function, and increased cardiovascular risk.[182] Up to 65% of women undergoing dialysis report problems with sexual function, and up to 40% no longer engage in sexual intercourse.[183] Loss of libido may also contribute to infertility.

Finally, megestrol acetate has successfully been used in patients with ESKD as an effective therapy to treat PEW.[184–187] This finding, together with the observation of an attenuation of the symptoms associated with uremic anorexia in women in comparison with men,[188] suggests the existence of a yet uncharacterized pleiotropic role for sex hormones in the regulation of nutrient homeostasis in uremia.

### Treatment

General principles of treatment include education about sexual function in the setting of CKD, adequate dialysis delivery, and treatment of underlying depression. Changes in lifestyle, such as smoking cessation, strength training, and aerobic exercises, may decrease depression, enhance body image, and have positive effects on sexuality.[179] Limited evidence has indicated that CKD alters the pharmacokinetics of estradiol. Free and total estradiol plasma concentrations are higher in women with ESKD after an oral estradiol dose, but no change occurs in estrone concentrations. Neither estradiol nor estrone is removed in the dialysate.[189] Steady-state pharmacokinetics of oral estradiol has shown that women with ESKD should receive approximately 50% of the typically prescribed dosages.[190] No information is available on the pharmacokinetics of any of the progestins in CKD.

Chronic anovulation and lack of progesterone secretion in uremic women may be treated with oral progesterone. Because ongoing menses can contribute to the anemia of CKD, particularly in patients with menorrhagia, administration of progesterone at the end of the menstrual cycle is preferred. At present, it is not clear whether unopposed estrogen stimulation (due to anovulatory cycles) predisposes women with CKD to endometrial hyperplasia or endometrial cancer. Thus routine gynecologic follow-up is recommended for such patients. Low estradiol levels in amenorrheic women undergoing dialysis can lead to vaginal atrophy and dyspareunia; topical estrogen cream and vaginal lubricants may be helpful in these patients. Uremic women who are menstruating normally should be encouraged to use birth control. Estradiol hormonal replacement therapy was able to restore regular menses and improve sexual function in premenopausal, estrogen-deficient women undergoing dialysis[191] and to improve bone histomorphometry in animal models of uremia.[192] Estrogen administration may positively affect sexual desire and prevent bone mass loss in postmenopausal women with ESKD.[193,194] Hypoactive sexual desire disorder is the most commonly reported sexual problem in women with CKD, and testosterone replacement therapy has shown effectiveness in patients without renal disease.[195,196] Nonetheless, successful kidney transplantation is clearly the most effective means to restore normal sexual desire in women with CKD.

### Female Sex Hormones and Progression of Chronic Kidney Disease

Because the progression rate of renal disease is in general faster for men than for women,[197] it has been suggested that this gender dimorphism may be explained by the interaction of circulating steroids with specific receptors in the kidney. In experimental animal models, endogenous estrogens have shown antifibrotic and antiapoptotic effects in the kidney,[198,199] and exogenous estradiol in ovariectomized rats attenuated glomerulosclerosis and tubulointerstitial fibrosis[200] by protecting podocytes against injury through the upregulation of estrogen receptor β.[201] A direct extrapolation from these animal studies would suggest that exogenous estrogen administration may slow CKD progression. However, clinical evidence in this regard has been elusive, with evidence suggesting that both estrogen replacement therapy and oral contraceptives are associated with albuminuria, increased creatinine clearance, and loss of kidney function.[202–206] The implications of these studies need to be carefully considered in the context of their observational and, in most of the cases, retrospective nature. It should also be noted that in general, hormone replacement therapy is prescribed less frequently to postmenopausal patients with ESKD than to the general population,[207] possibly incurring a selection and underrepresentation bias.

## IN MEN

### Endocrine Abnormalities

The occurrence of testosterone deficiency is estimated to vary from 6% to 9.5% in community-dwelling men aged 40 to 75 years, rising to 15% to 30% in diabetic or obese men.[208,209] In men with CKD, this prevalence is much higher, ranging between 50% and 75%.[210–213] This deficiency is true for both free and total serum testosterone, although the binding capacity and levels of sex hormone–binding globulin seem within normal range. Causes of hypogonadism in CKD are multiple and must be sought within hyperprolactinemia (see preceding discussion), comorbid conditions (e.g., PEW, obesity, diabetes mellitus, hypertension), and medications that may influence gonadal function (e.g., ACE inhibitors, ARBs, spironolactone, ketoconazole, glucocorticoids, statins, cinacalcet).

The plasma concentration of LH is typically elevated in men with uremia, mainly owing to changes in the pulsatile release of gonadotropin-releasing hormone and LH itself, diminished feedback inhibition of LH production (because of low testosterone levels), and impaired renal clearance. FSH secretion is also increased in men with CKD, although to a more variable degree, so that the LH/FSH ratio is typically increased. Feedback inhibition of FSH is impaired because of a decrease in the peptide inhibin, which is produced by the Sertoli cells.[179] All these disturbances can be detected with only moderate reductions in the GFR and progressively worsen in parallel with the progression of CKD. These disorders rarely normalize with the initiation of dialysis. Instead, they often progress. A well-functioning kidney transplant is likely to restore normal sexual activity, although some features of reproductive function may remain impaired.

### Clinical Manifestations

Symptoms and signs of hypogonadism in men depend on the stage in life at which hypogonadism develops and its duration. In adults with ESKD, hypogonadism, low testosterone levels, and hyperprolactinemia are likely responsible for decreased libido, erectile dysfunction, oligospermia and infertility, osteopenia and, to some extent, osteoporosis and anemia. Erectile dysfunction has been reported in 70% to 80% of men with CKD and ESKD.[214] Additional risk factors that increase the probability of erectile dysfunction are advanced age, diabetes, hypertension, dyslipidemia, smoking, and anxiety. Semen analysis typically shows a decreased volume of ejaculate, either a low sperm count or complete azoospermia, and a low percentage of motility. Medications frequently used in treating patients with CKD, such as diuretics, antihypertensive and antidepressant agents, and histamine $H_2$ blockers, can contribute to erectile dysfunction. Other drugs, such as spironolactone, ketoconazole, glucocorticoids, and cimetidine, can interfere directly with the synthesis of sex hormones.[215] Autonomic nervous system dysfunction, a frequent finding in patients with CKD (especially those with diabetes mellitus), likely also contributes to sexual abnormalities in CKD.[216] Disturbances in the pelvic autonomic nervous system can decrease sensation and arousal of stimuli during sexual activity. Autonomic neuropathy can also interfere with the complex neurologic axis that is necessary for the achievement of an adequate erection.

Uremic hypogonadism may contribute to sarcopenia. In physiologic conditions, testosterone is an anabolic hormone that plays an important role in inducing skeletal muscle hypertrophy by promoting nitrogen retention, stimulating fractional muscle protein synthesis, inducing myoblast differentiation, and augmenting the efficiency of amino acid reuse by skeletal muscles.[217] Consequently, positive associations between serum free and total testosterone levels with creatinine and hand grip strength have been reported in men undergoing dialysis,[218,219] and endogenous testosterone in men with CKD stages 3 to 4 emerged as an important determinant of both muscle mass and strength.[220] Interventional studies with nandrolone decanoate (a testosterone synthetic agonist) in dialysis populations have shown significant improvements in muscle mass and strength, as well as in nutritional status.[221,222]

Testosterone is known to exert a stimulatory effect on erythropoiesis[223] by inducing the growth of differentiated stem cells and enhancing the sensitivity of erythroid progenitors to circulating erythropoietin (EPO).[224,225] Because CKD is more common in older men, it is likely that both an age-associated decline in testosterone and the endocrine CKD abnormalities that encompass male hypogonadism contribute to some extent to a decline in erythroid mass and may contribute to anemia. For this reason, testosterone deficiency has been proposed as an additional cause of anemia in ESA-naïve nondialyzed male patients with CKD and as an additional cause of resistance to ESAs in men treated with ESA undergoing HD.[226] Before the clinical introduction of recombinant human EPO (rhEPO) in 1989, androgens were the main pharmacologic intervention for correcting the anemia of ESKD. Reciprocally, anemia in patients with ESKD has been associated with a reduction of libido and endothelial dysfunction,[227] and rhEPO therapy has led to an increase in sexual desire and performance and an improvement in erectile function in some, but not all, patients.[228,229] Correction of anemia, improved sense of well-being, and direct endocrine effects may play a role in this result.[180] In addition, studies evaluating changes in the health-related quality of life in response to rhEPO therapy have noted significant improvements in physical and social functioning, overall mental health, and satisfaction with sexual activity.[230]

Finally, hypogonadism in men with non–dialysis-requiring CKD has been associated with arterial stiffness, endothelial dysfunction, and risk of cardiovascular events.[231] In patients undergoing dialysis, hypogonadism has also been linked to increased mortality risk[213,218,232] (Fig. 56.4), arterial stiffness,[233] worse quality of life,[210] and heightened inflammation.[212] The links between testosterone and cardiovascular complications may be explained by its association with risk factors such as dyslipidemia, obesity, diabetes mellitus, and metabolic syndrome, which may contribute to endothelial dysfunction and atherosclerosis per se. However, testosterone may also have direct atheroprotective effects in the cardiovascular system.[123] Transdermal testosterone therapy improved exercise-induced myocardial ischemia during an exercise stress test in men with stable angina,[124] and men with prostate cancer undergoing androgen deprivation therapy experienced an increase in central arterial pressure.[125] In animal models, testosterone supplementation inhibits neointimal plaque development,[126] stimulates endothelial progenitor cells,[127] increases nitric oxide release from vascular endothelial cells,[128] and enhances myocardial perfusion.[129,130]

The gonadal axis is suppressed by inflammatory cytokines,[234,235] and therefore any inflammatory disease may induce testosterone deficiency. Thus low testosterone levels could be considered a biomarker of chronic inflammatory disease. In support of this contention, studies have depicted a strong inverse association between endogenous testosterone and surrogates of inflammation in various CKD populations.[212,218,232,233] However, it is also possible that testosterone has immunomodulatory actions per se, as suggested by the suppression of cytokine production in hypogonadal men with diabetes mellitus, coronary heart disease, and/or metabolic syndrome after supplementation with testosterone.[236–238]

### Treatment

General principles of treatment of hypogonadism in men include optimal delivery of dialysis and adequate nutritional intake, as well as screening for depressive symptoms. A study

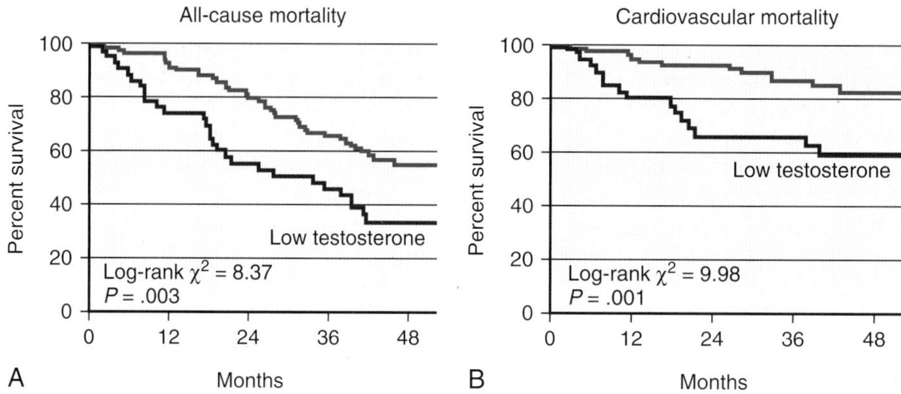


**Fig. 56.4** Sex hormone alterations and outcome of chronic kidney disease (CKD). Reduced testosterone levels in male patients undergoing hemodialysis have been linked to increased mortality risk, especially that from cardiovascular causes. (Modified from Carrero JJ, Qureshi AR, Parini P, et al: Low serum testosterone increases mortality risk among male dialysis patients. *J Am Soc Nephrol.* 2009;20:613–620.)

has compared the pharmacokinetics of a testosterone patch in patients with ESKD and in hypogonadal men with normal kidney function.[239] The researchers found that the half-life of testosterone after withdrawal of the patch was not different between the groups, nor was the minimum or maximum serum testosterone concentration during the period of patch application. Thus it is likely that usual doses of testosterone replacement can be used in men with ESKD, with the usual monitoring of serum testosterone concentrations, with dose adjustments as needed. Data on the use of testosterone in ESKD are limited; some studies have suggested that erectile function in ESKD does not improve with testosterone supplementation,[240] and others have indicated that normalization of endogenous testosterone by topical gels in hypogonadal men with advanced CKD improve sexual function.[241] The daily administration of 100 mg of 1% testosterone gel for 6 months in 40 hypogonadal men with ESKD neither increased serum testosterone concentrations nor had an effect on ESA requirements.[242] It is possible that higher testosterone dosages may be required to achieve a clinical benefit in this patient group. Alternative modes of administration, such as intramuscular injection, may ease compliance and bioavailability. The response of testosterone in this setting may be modulated by the patient's nutritional status, activity level, and GH (and GH-binding protein) status. Because psychosocial factors may also take part in the pathophysiology of erectile dysfunction, nocturnal penile tumescence testing may be used to differentiate organic and psychological causes of impotence.

Whether testosterone deficiency may constitute a new pathophysiologic pathway in CKD-related complications such as anemia, PEW, and cardiovascular risk deserves further attention. Androgen therapy in supraphysiologic dosages has been linked to adverse effects.[28,160] Isolated cases of increase in blood pressure and clinically significant edema in healthy older men have been reported,[28,151,152] as has fluid retention in men undergoing HD.[75] Treated patients must be closely monitored but, again, restoration of deficiencies and maintenance of total and free testosterone concentrations within the normal range may be the key to successful treatment.

### Male Sex Hormones and Progression of Chronic Kidney Disease

In line with the finding that CKD progression is faster in men than in women, animal models of kidney injury have shown that orchidectomy attenuates glomerular and tubular damage, kidney fibrosis, and proteinuria.[243,244] Furthermore, animal studies have described proinflammatory, proapoptotic, and profibrotic effects of supraphysiologic dosages of testosterone during acute and chronic kidney injury.[199,245,246] On the other hand, it is difficult to reconcile such experimental findings with clinical observations, given that testosterone production decreases with progressive CKD, and that both the incidence and progression of CKD occur mainly in older men, who have lower testosterone concentrations on average. In line with this thinking, a population-based study of men has reported that impaired kidney function and low serum testosterone concentrations are additive (and independent) mortality risk factors.[247] Thus evidence has accumulated suggesting that testosterone may be protective to the kidney.

A large case-control study involving more than 10,000 men newly diagnosed with nonmetastatic prostate cancer has demonstrated that androgen deprivation therapy increases the risk of acute kidney injury.[248] Potential protective mechanisms include inducing vasodilation in renal vessels and enhancing the production of nitric oxide.[249] Thus the use of androgen deprivation therapy might antagonize testosterone, raising the risk of damage to the glomerulus. An additional explanation for the role of hypogonadism on kidney injury has been demonstrated in male rats subjected to renal ischemia followed by reperfusion.[250] In this setting, testosterone concentrations decreased dramatically after only 3 hours. Infusion of testosterone 3 hours after reperfusion attenuated the 24-hour increase in plasma creatinine and urinary kidney injury molecule-1 (KIM-1), prevented the reduction in outer medullary blood flow, and attenuated the 48-hour increase in intrarenal inflammation. Castration caused greater rises in plasma creatinine levels and KIM-1, and treatment with anastrozole (an aromatase inhibitor) plus testosterone almost normalized these markers.[250]

## VITAMIN D, PARATHYROID HORMONE, AND KIDNEY DISEASE

The endocrine system of vitamin D and PTH is crucial for the homeostasis of calcium and phosphorus and for maintaining a healthy bone status. Altered levels of serum phosphate, calcium, vitamin D, PTH, and fibroblast growth factor 23

(FGF23) contribute to the complex multiorgan syndrome of CKD–mineral and bone disorder (CKD-MBD), which leads to osteoporosis, fractures, CVD, and other complications.[251–253] Whereas abnormalities in PTH and the consequences of hyperparathyroidism are well recognized clinical problems in the management of CKD-MBD,[254] the awareness of the importance of vitamin D deficiency has also increased.[251–253] Indeed, the expression of vitamin D receptors (VDRs) by many different tissues and cells suggests a multifaceted role for this system.[255,256] Physiology and management of these hormonal alterations are discussed in more detail in Chapter 53.

## VITAMIN D AND PARATHYROID HORMONE: METABOLISM AND ACTIONS IN CHRONIC KIDNEY DISEASE

The vitamin D family includes the biologically inert fat-soluble prohormones—vitamin $D_2$ (ergocalciferol) and vitamin $D_3$ (cholecalciferol). These prohormones are obtained mainly from sun exposure—by photochemical conversion of 7-dehydrocholesterol in the skin, food (especially fatty fish), and nutritional supplements. These prohormones are converted by hydroxylation in the liver to 25-hydroxyvitamin D and by a second hydroxylation step (performed by the 1α-hydroxylase) to its active form, 1,25-dihydroxyvitamin D (calcitriol). The kidney is the most abundant source (but not exclusive) of 1α-hydroxylase in the body, and therefore CKD coincides with natural deficiencies in calcitriol.[252,253]

In normal conditions, the renal production of calcitriol is tightly regulated by PTH and by serum calcium and phosphorus levels. FGF23, which is secreted from the bone, suppresses calcitriol synthesis, as does metabolic acidosis. Extrarenal calcitriol is converted in other tissues, including the skin, colon, prostate, and macrophages, but the regulatory processes for this conversion are not well understood. Calcitriol has a half-life of only 4 to 6 hours, and the circulating levels are low. Calcitriol, which is transported to various target organs by the vitamin D–binding protein (VDBP), mobilizes calcium into the bloodstream by promoting the absorption of calcium and phosphorus from food in the intestines and reabsorption of calcium in the kidneys. Calcitriol also promotes bone mineralization, bone growth, and bone remodeling by osteoblasts and osteoclasts and prevents hypocalcemia. Vitamin D deficiency has been linked to multiple disorders, including growth retardation, skeletal abnormalities (e.g., osteopenia, osteoporosis, increased risk of fractures), muscle weakness, left ventricular hypertrophy, and increased susceptibility to cancer, diabetes, and autoimmune and infectious diseases.[254,257–259] The effects of vitamin D goes beyond those linked to calcium and bone homeostasis. In patients with CKD who display a combination of bone metabolism disorder, muscle wasting, and muscle weakness, vitamin D is thought to contribute to maintain musculoskeletal health.[260] In the kidney, vitamin D may be important for maintaining podocyte function, preventing epithelial to mesenchymal transformation, and suppressing renin gene expression and inflammation.[261] Vitamin D also appears to be protective in models of diabetic nephropathy through targeting of the RAAS and the nuclear factor-kappa B (NF-κB) pathway.[262]

PTH has a key role in calcium and phosphate homeostasis. It stimulates excretion of phosphate by the renal tubular cells and indirectly modulates intestinal calcium absorption by stimulating the activation of calcitriol synthesis. As vitamin D deficiency progresses, the parathyroid glands are maximally stimulated, causing secondary hyperparathyroidism. Thus levels of 25-hydroxyvitamin D are inversely associated with PTH levels, and calcitriol inhibits PTH expression. PTH increases the metabolism of 25-hydroxyvitamin D to calcitriol, further exacerbating the vitamin D deficiency. Hyperparathyroidism has been implicated in left ventricular hypertrophy, as well as in the metabolic syndrome contributing to impaired glucose tolerance and dyslipidemia.[263] PTH and serum phosphate are well-established biomarkers of CKD-MBD, and FGF23 has been gaining increased attention.[264] However, the value of PTH[265] and FGF23 in clinical monitoring,[266] among others, has been questioned owing to their wide (and assay-dependent) biologic variability.

## VITAMIN D DEFICIENCY IN CHRONIC KIDNEY DISEASE

Insufficient to deficient levels of 25-hydroxyvitamin D have been reported in most individuals with CKD, including patients undergoing maintenance dialysis and others with non–dialysis-requiring CKD.[267,268] Vitamin D deficiency seems to be more pronounced in blacks.[269] The circulating levels of 25-hydroxyvitamin D and calcitriol decrease with diminishing kidney function.[268,270] Because 25-hydroxyvitamin D has a longer half-life than calcitriol (≈3 weeks), it is considered the best measure of vitamin D status.[271] On these premises, vitamin D insufficiency is commonly defined as 25-hydroxyvitamin D levels lower than 30 ng/mL, whereas deficiency starts at the threshold of less than 15 ng/mL. Although there are known seasonal, geographic, ethnic, and age-related variations, the desirable level of vitamin D in patients with CKD has not yet been defined; nevertheless, it is recommended to maintain serum concentrations of 25-hydroxyvitamin D above 30 ng/mL.[254] Most commercial assays for 25-hydroxyvitamin D are thought to be acceptable for detecting vitamin D deficiency.[252] However, it should be noted that there are considerable between-laboratory and interassay variations in tests for the measurement of circulating concentrations of 25-hydroxyvitamin D and PTH.[272] The 1,25-dihydroxyvitamin D assay should not be used to detect vitamin D deficiency in CKD because 25-dihydroxyvitamin D levels are usually low as a consequence of reduced 1α-hydroxylase activity in this disease, but they could also be normal, or even elevated, as a result of secondary hyperparathyroidism.

## VITAMIN D SUPPLEMENTATION IN CHRONIC KIDNEY DISEASE

Providing children and adults with at least 800 IU of 25-hydroxyvitamin $D_3$/day or its equivalent should guarantee vitamin D sufficiency. Unless a person eats oily fish frequently, it is difficult to provide that much vitamin $D_3$ on a daily basis from dietary sources. Thus moderate sun exposure and/or provision of supplements are needed to fulfill the vitamin D requirement in patients with CKD.[267] Pharmacologic doses of vitamin D can be administered in the form of nutritional supplements or active vitamin D agents. The National Kidney Foundation Kidney Disease Outcomes Quality Initiative (K/DOQI) guidelines have recommended starting with nutritional vitamin D supplements before using activated vitamin D derivatives in patients with concurrent hyperparathyroidism associated with vitamin D insufficiency.[267,271] Although some studies have shown that vitamin D supplementation may improve physical performance and protect against the development of of hyperparathyroidism, evidence is still insufficient.[260] Six months of therapy with calcitriol or cholecalciferol in CKD patients did not improve vascular endothelial function or inflammation.[273] whereas in another study, 6 months of supplemental vitamin D analogues achieved a reduction of pulse wave velocity in patients with advanced CKD.[274] Although epidemiologic studies have generally indicated a survival benefit associated with the provision of activated vitamin D derivatives in all CKD stages[267,275–278] and a 27% lower associated mortality risk has been found in patients receiving calcitriol or analogues,[279] the studies are subject to confounding by indication, and recommendations regarding nutritional vitamin D supplements are thus largely opinion-based. However, existing randomized-controlled trials do not provide sufficient or precise evidence that vitamin D supplementation lowers the mortality of patients with CKD.[267,280]

 Complete reference list available at ExpertConsult.com.

## KEY REFERENCES


7. DeFronzo RA, Alvestrand A, Smith D, et al. Insulin resistance in uremia. *J Clin Invest.* 1981;67:563–568.
23. Beddhu S, Kimmel PL, Ramkumar N, et al. Associations of metabolic syndrome with inflammation in CKD: results from the Third National Health and Nutrition Examination Survey (NHANES III). *Am J Kidney Dis.* 2005;46:577–586.
28. Raj DS, Dominic EA, Pai A, et al. Skeletal muscle, cytokines, and oxidative stress in end-stage renal disease. *Kidney Int.* 2005;68:2338–2344.
39. Chen J, Muntner P, Hamm LL, et al. The metabolic syndrome and chronic kidney disease in U.S. adults. *Ann Intern Med.* 2004;140:167–174.
42. Shinohara K, Shoji T, Emoto M, et al. Insulin resistance as an independent predictor of cardiovascular mortality in patients with end-stage renal disease. *J Am Soc Nephrol.* 2002;13:1894–1900.
49. Pupim LB, Flakoll PJ, Majchrzak KM, et al. Increased muscle protein breakdown in chronic hemodialysis patients with type 2 diabetes mellitus. *Kidney Int.* 2005;68:1857–1865.
50. Mustata S, Chan C, Lai V, et al. Impact of an exercise program on arterial stiffness and insulin resistance in hemodialysis patients. *J Am Soc Nephrol.* 2004;15:2713–2718.
56. Ramirez SP, Albert JM, Blayney MJ, et al. Rosiglitazone is associated with mortality in chronic hemodialysis patients. *J Am Soc Nephrol.* 2009;20:1094–1101.
62. Hung AM, Roumie CL, Greevy RA, et al. Comparative effectiveness of incident oral antidiabetic drugs on kidney function. *Kidney Int.* 2012;81:698–706.
94. Carrero JJ, Qureshi AR, Axelsson J, et al. Clinical and biochemical implications of low thyroid hormone levels (total and free forms) in euthyroid patients with chronic kidney disease. *J Intern Med.* 2007;262:690–701.
95. Zoccali C, Mallamaci F, Tripepi G, et al. Low triiodothyronine and survival in end-stage renal disease. *Kidney Int.* 2006;70:523–528.
102. Meuwese CL, Carrero JJ, Cabezas-Rodriguez I, et al. Nonthyroidal illness: a risk factor for coronary calcification and arterial stiffness in patients undergoing peritoneal dialysis? *J Intern Med.* 2013;274:584–593.
113. Mak RH, Cheung WW, Roberts CT Jr. The growth hormone-insulin-like growth factor-I axis in chronic kidney disease. *Growth Horm IGF Res.* 2008;18:17–25.
114. Mahesh S, Kaskel F. Growth hormone axis in chronic kidney disease. *Pediatr Nephrol.* 2008;23:41–48.
124. Ding H, Gao XL, Hirschberg R, et al. Impaired actions of insulin-like growth factor 1 on protein synthesis and degradation in skeletal muscle of rats with chronic renal failure: evidence for a postreceptor defect. *J Clin Invest.* 1996;97:1064–1075.
126. Sun DF, Zheng Z, Tummala P, et al. Chronic uremia attenuates growth hormone-induced signal transduction in skeletal muscle. *J Am Soc Nephrol.* 2004;15:2630–2636.
127. Wang H, Casaburi R, Taylor WE, et al. Skeletal muscle mRNA for IGF-IEa, IGF-II, and IGF-1 receptor is decreased in sedentary chronic hemodialysis patients. *Kidney Int.* 2005;68:352–361.
130. Garibotto G, Russo R, Sofia A, et al. Effects of uremia and inflammation on growth hormone resistance in patients with chronic kidney diseases. *Kidney Int.* 2008;74:937–945.
133. Fine RN, Ho M, Tejani A, et al. Adverse events with rhGH treatment of patients with chronic renal insufficiency and end-stage renal disease. *J Pediatr.* 2003;142:539–545.
136. Feldt-Rasmussen B, Lange M, Sulowicz W, et al. Growth hormone treatment during hemodialysis in a randomized trial improves nutrition, quality of life, and cardiovascular risk. *J Am Soc Nephrol.* 2007;18:2161–2171.
137. Guebre-Egziabher F, Juillard L, Boirie Y, et al. Short-term administration of a combination of recombinant growth hormone and insulin-like growth factor-I induces anabolism in maintenance hemodialysis. *J Clin Endocrinol Metab.* 2009;94:2299–2305.
152. Carrero JJ, Kyriazis J, Sonmez A, et al. Prolactin levels, endothelial dysfunction, and the risk of cardiovascular events and mortality in patients with CKD. *Clin J Am Soc Nephrol.* 2012;7:207–215.
162. Mejia-Rodriguez O, Herrera-Abarca JE, Ceballos-Reyes G, et al. Cardiovascular and renal effects of bromocriptine in diabetic patients with stage 4 chronic kidney disease. *Biomed Res Int.* 2013;2013:104059.
165. Gong R. The renaissance of corticotropin therapy in proteinuric nephropathies. *Nat Rev Nephrol.* 2012;8:122–128.
171. Drechsler C, Ritz E, Tomaschitz A, et al. Aldosterone and cortisol affect the risk of sudden cardiac death in haemodialysis patients. *Eur Heart J.* 2013;34:578–587.
174. Kakiya R, Shoji T, Hayashi T, et al. Decreased serum adrenal androgen dehydroepiandrosterone sulfate and mortality in hemodialysis patients. *Nephrol Dial Transplant.* 2012;27:3915–3922.
179. Anantharaman P, Schmidt RJ. Sexual function in chronic kidney disease. *Adv Chronic Kidney Dis.* 2007;14:119–125.
180. Palmer BF. Sexual dysfunction in uremia. *J Am Soc Nephrol.* 1999;10:1381–1388.
189. Anderson GD, Odegard PS. Pharmacokinetics of estrogen and progesterone in chronic kidney disease. *Adv Chronic Kidney Dis.* 2004;11:357–360.
193. Hernandez E, Valera R, Alonzo E, et al. Effects of raloxifene on bone metabolism and serum lipids in postmenopausal women on chronic hemodialysis. *Kidney Int.* 2003;63:2269–2274.
203. Agarwal M, Selvan V, Freedman BI, et al. The relationship between albuminuria and hormone therapy in postmenopausal women. *Am J Kidney Dis.* 2005;45:1019–1025.
211. Carrero JJ, Stenvinkel P. The vulnerable man: impact of testosterone deficiency on the uraemic phenotype. *Nephrol Dial Transplant.* 2012;27:4030–4041.
212. Carrero JJ, Qureshi AR, Nakashima A, et al. Prevalence and clinical implications of testosterone deficiency in men with end-stage renal disease. *Nephrol Dial Transplant.* 2011;26:184–190.
214. Palmer BF. Outcomes associated with hypogonadism in men with chronic kidney disease. *Adv Chronic Kidney Dis.* 2004;11:342–347.
218. Carrero JJ, Qureshi AR, Parini P, et al. Low serum testosterone increases mortality risk among male dialysis patients. *J Am Soc Nephrol.* 2009;20:613–620.
221. Johansen KL, Painter PL, Sakkas GK, et al. Effects of resistance exercise training and nandrolone decanoate on body composition and muscle function among patients who receive hemodialysis: a randomized, controlled trial. *J Am Soc Nephrol.* 2006;17:2307–2314.
222. Johansen KL, Mulligan K, Schambelan M. Anabolic effects of nandrolone decanoate in patients receiving dialysis: a randomized controlled trial. *JAMA.* 1999;281:1275–1281.
226. Carrero JJ, Barany P, Yilmaz MI, et al. Testosterone deficiency is a cause of anemia and reduced responsiveness to erythropoiesis stimulating agents in men with chronic kidney disease. *Nephrol Dial Transplant.* 2012;27:709–715.

254. Kidney Disease: Improving Global Outcomes (KDIGO) CKD-MBD Work Group. KDIGO clinical practice guideline for the diagnosis, evaluation, prevention, and treatment of chronic kidney Disease-Mineral and bone disorder (CKD-MBD). *Kidney Int Suppl.* 2009;113:S1–S130.
261. Agarwal R. Vitamin D, proteinuria, diabetic nephropathy, and progression of CKD. *Clin J Am Soc Nephrol.* 2009;4:1523–1528.
265. Garrett G, Sardiwal S, Lamb EJ, et al. PTH—a particularly tricky hormone: why measure it at all in kidney patients? *Clin J Am Soc Nephrol.* 2013;8:299–312.
268. Ravani P, Malberti F, Tripepi G, et al. Vitamin D levels and patient outcome in chronic kidney disease. *Kidney Int.* 2009;75:88–95.
279. Duranton F, Rodriguez-Ortiz ME, Duny Y, et al. Vitamin D treatment and mortality in chronic kidney disease: a systematic review and meta-analysis. *Am J Nephrol.* 2013;37:239–248.

# 57 Neurologic Aspects of Kidney Disease

Manjula Kurella Tamura

CHAPTER OUTLINE



Neurologic aspects of chronic kidney disease (CKD) encompass a diverse spectrum of clinical disorders and syndromes. Indeed, clinical uremia was first described principally as a neurologic illness manifested by disturbances of cognitive, somatosensory, neuromuscular, and autonomic dysfunction.[1] Renal replacement therapy attenuates these features of the uremic syndrome, suggesting a central role for a retained solute (or solutes) in the pathogenesis of the neurologic manifestations of uremia. However, identification of the responsible solute(s) has proven difficult, in part due to the vast array of solutes that are retained in CKD. Earlier recognition and treatment of CKD and aging of the CKD population have changed the clinical presentation of neurologic illness in kidney disease, further complicating efforts to identify causative factors. Dialysis therapy itself is also associated with neurologic complications, including dialysis disequilibrium, a syndrome of delirium rarely associated with the initiation of dialysis therapy, and dialysis dementia, a progressive disorder linked to parental exposure to aluminum. Fortunately, these disorders have sharply decreased in incidence over the past 30 years.

Cerebrovascular disease, now recognized as a major cause of morbidity and mortality in patients with CKD, is an equally important part of the spectrum of neurologic illness associated with CKD. Stroke rates are increased sixfold to tenfold and stroke mortality twofold to threefold in patients on dialysis. While there has been substantial progress in the identification, treatment, and prevention of stroke in the general population, evidence-based treatment strategies for patients with CKD are still lacking. Interestingly, subclinical cerebrovascular disease is not only a major risk factor for stroke and a marker for future cardiovascular events, but may also play an important role in the cognitive manifestations of CKD.

This chapter reviews the epidemiology, pathophysiology, and treatment approach for stroke, disorders of cognitive function and sleep, and neuropathy in patients with kidney disease.

## STROKE

Stroke is the third leading cause of death and a major cause of disability in the United States.[2] Acute stroke is characterized by a sudden onset of focal neurologic symptoms, such as dysphasia, dysarthria, hemianopia, weakness, ataxia, sensory loss, and neglect, resulting from an interruption in blood supply to a corresponding area of the brain. Symptoms are typically unilateral, and consciousness is generally preserved except in the case of some posterior circulation strokes. By convention, neurologic deficits persisting longer than 24 hours are classified as stroke, whereas deficits persisting less than 24 hours are classified as transient ischemic attack (TIA). With widespread use of brain imaging, it is now apparent that 15% to 20% of persons with symptoms lasting less than 24 hours have evidence of a brain infarct; thus some authorities have proposed modifying the TIA definition to clinical symptoms lasting less than 1 hour and without evidence of infarction.[3] Over 30% of persons with TIA subsequently suffer from stroke; most occur within weeks of the TIA event.[4]

Strokes can be classified as ischemic, resulting from occlusion of a blood vessel, and hemorrhagic, resulting from rupture of a blood vessel. In the United States and European general population, 80% of strokes are caused by ischemia, and 20% of strokes are caused by hemorrhage.[5] It is useful to classify ischemic strokes based on the mechanism of injury—large artery atherosclerosis, cardiogenic embolism, small vessel occlusive disease, and other or undetermined cause,[6] and the location of infarct—anterior circulation versus posterior circulation, because these distinctions have important therapeutic implications. In the general population, cardiogenic embolism accounts for 25% of ischemic stroke, followed by large artery atherosclerosis and small vessel occlusive disease; however, these rates vary by sex and race/ethnicity. Men and whites are reported to have a higher incidence of large artery atherosclerosis as compared with women and blacks, respectively.[7–9] Hemorrhagic stroke can also be divided into two subtypes: intracerebral hemorrhage, accounting for the majority of hemorrhagic strokes, and subarachnoid hemorrhage. Intracerebral hemorrhage is most frequently attributed to hypertension, amyloid angiopathy, septic embolism, mycotic aneurysm, and bleeding diatheses, whereas subarachnoid hemorrhage is most often due to rupture of an arterial aneurysm or vascular malformation.

The presence of CKD, defined as an estimated glomerular filtration rate (eGFR) of less than 60 mL/min/1.73 m$^2$, has several important implications for the detection, management, and prevention of stroke. Persons with CKD have a different risk factor profile and stroke epidemiology compared with persons in the general population, and they are at higher risk for stroke events and stroke-related mortality. Furthermore, several stroke detection, management, and prevention strategies may have lower efficacy and/or safety in patients with CKD.

## EPIDEMIOLOGY OF STROKE IN PATIENTS WITH CHRONIC KIDNEY DISEASE AND END-STAGE KIDNEY DISEASE, AND IN KIDNEY TRANSPLANT RECIPIENTS

Stroke is the third leading cause of cardiovascular disease death among persons with end-stage kidney disease (ESKD) on dialysis.[10] As compared with the general population, stroke event rates and stroke mortality rates are increased sixfold to tenfold among patients on dialysis (Fig. 57.1).[11,12] As in the general population, ischemic stroke is more common than hemorrhagic stroke,[11,13] though the excess risk is higher for hemorrhagic stroke.[14] Among US patients on dialysis, cardioembolic stroke is the most common cause of ischemic stroke, followed by small vessel occlusion, and then by large artery stroke (Table 57.1).[12] Among Japanese patients, small vessel occlusion is more common, followed by cardioembolic stroke.[13] Posterior circulation strokes involving the vertebrobasilar system occur more commonly in patients on dialysis than in the general population.[13] This distribution pattern suggests screening for carotid artery disease may not be as effective as stroke prevention strategy in patients on dialysis relative to the general population. Kidney transplantation is associated with 30% lower risk for stroke or TIA compared with patients remaining on the transplant waiting list, whereas allograft failure increases the risk for stroke or TIA by 150%.[15]

The extent to which less advanced stages of CKD increase stroke risk independent of traditional risk factors remains unclear, and most guidelines from professional societies do not include CKD as a stroke risk factor. In a meta-analysis of 33 cohort studies, CKD was associated with a 1.4-fold higher risk for stroke.[16] One limitation of this analysis is that it did not account for proteinuria. Some, but not all, studies have reported racial variation in stroke risk, with CKD being associated with a heightened risk for stroke among blacks more so than among whites.[17] Relative to the general population, CKD is associated with a twofold to threefold increase in the risk for death and disability following stroke.[18]

Neuroimaging studies suggest that persons with CKD and ESKD have a substantial burden of cerebrovascular disease

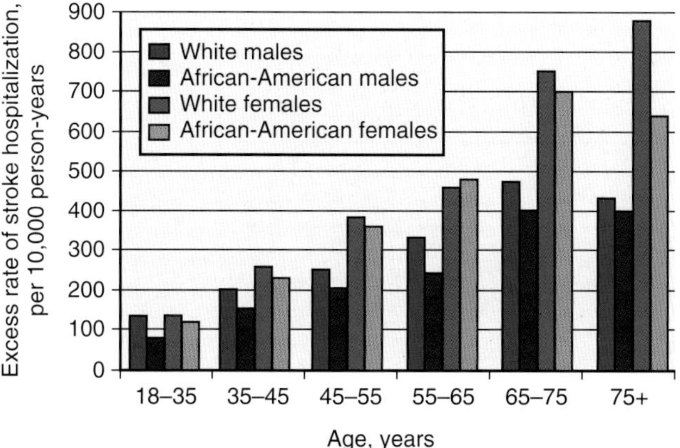


**Fig. 57.1** Excess rate of stroke hospitalization in patients on dialysis compared with the general population (per 10,000 person-years). (Modified from Seliger SL, Gillen DL, Longstreth Jr WT, et al. Elevated risk of stroke among patients with end-stage renal disease. *Kidney Int.* 2003;64:603–609. With permission.)

**Table 57.1 Stroke Subtypes in the General Population and in the Incident Dialysis Population**

| | US General Population | US Incident Dialysis Population (*n* = 176) | |
|---|---|---|---|
| **Stroke Subtype** | Prevalence (%) | Prevalence (%) | Case Fatality Rate (%) |
| Ischemic stroke | 80 | 87 | 28 |
| Large artery | 7–18 | 10 | 29 |
| Cardioembolism | 15–27 | 24 | 36 |
| Small vessel occlusion | 11–21 | 17 | 17 |
| Multiple causes | 3–7 | 16 | 41 |
| Other/undetermined | 35–42 | 20 | 19 |
| Hemorrhagic stroke | 20 | 13 | 90 |

Data for US general population modified from Zimmerman D, Sood MM, Rigatto C, Holden RM, Hiremath S, Clase CM. Systematic review and meta-analysis of incidence, prevalence and outcomes of atrial fibrillation in patients on dialysis. *Nephrol Dial Transplant.* 2012;27:3816–3822; Locatelli F, Choukroun G, Truman M, Wiggenhauser A, Fliser D. Once-monthly continuous erythropoietin receptor activator (C.E.R.A.) in patients with hemodialysis-dependent chronic kidney disease: pooled data from phase III trials. *Adv Ther.* 2016;33:610–625; Yamada S, Tsuruya K, Taniguchi M, et al. Association between serum phosphate levels and stroke risk in patients undergoing hemodialysis: the Q-cohort study. *Stroke.* 2016;47:2189–2196. Data for incident dialysis population modified from Panwar B, Jenny NS, Howard VJ, et al. Fibroblast growth factor 23 and risk of incident stroke in community-living adults. *Stroke.* 2015;46:322–328.

even in the absence of clinical stroke. For example, up to 50% of patients receiving dialysis without a history of clinical stroke have evidence of an infarct with brain magnetic resonance imaging (MRI), and these patients are at increased risk for future cardiovascular events.[19,20] Brain white matter lesions, a marker of small vessel disease, are also highly prevalent among patients on dialysis,[21,22] as well as among patients with mild or moderate CKD not requiring dialysis.[23–25] Among patients who experienced an intracerebral hemorrhage, patients with CKD had a twofold to threefold higher likelihood of cerebral microbleeds, a marker of lipohyalinosis or amyloid angiopathy, compared with patients without CKD.[26] This association was stronger among blacks than among whites.

## STROKE PREVENTION IN CHRONIC KIDNEY DISEASE AND END-STAGE KIDNEY DISEASE

The vascular beds of the kidney and the brain are quite similar—both are low-resistance end organs that receive a high blood volume.[27] The pathologic correlates of brain white matter disease (or microbleeds) and nondiabetic CKD, namely, arteriolar intima–media thickening and hyalinosis, are also quite similar. Thus the high prevalence of cerebrovascular disease in CKD may reflect a shared risk factor or factors and the similarity of their vascular supply. Differences in stroke risk between the CKD and non-CKD population might be explained by a higher prevalence or higher cumulative exposure to traditional stroke risk factors, such as hypertension and hyperlipidemia. Genome-wide association studies suggest a shared genetic component between CKD and large artery atherosclerotic stroke.[28] Traditional stroke risk factors such as hypertension and hyperlipidemia may be altered by CKD or confounded by the presence of protein energy wasting, heart failure, and other comorbid conditions, whereas nontraditional CKD-related factors may also contribute to stroke risk. Modifiable risk factors for stroke in patients with CKD and ESKD are discussed in the following sections.

### HYPERTENSION

Hypertension is a major risk factor for both ischemic and hemorrhagic stroke. In the general population, stroke risk doubles for each 20-mm Hg increase in systolic blood pressure or 10-mm Hg increase in diastolic blood pressure above 115/75 mm Hg.[29] Treatment of hypertension in the general population reduces stroke risk by an average of 40%; this benefit has been confirmed in a number of large randomized controlled trials.[2,30–32]

In the dialysis population, each 10-mm Hg increase in mean blood pressure is associated with an 11% increased risk for stroke.[33] A J-shaped association of systolic blood pressure with stroke incidence has been reported in some, but not all, studies of CKD and ESKD.[33–35] For example, in a community-based sample of persons with CKD, systolic blood pressure of less than 120 mm Hg was associated with a doubling of stroke risk as compared with individuals with systolic blood pressure of 120 to 129 mm Hg.[34] However, this finding has not been replicated in clinical trials.

For example, in post hoc analyses of the Perindopril Protection Against Recurrent Stroke Study (PROGRESS),[35] blood pressure lowering with an angiotensin-converting enzyme (ACE) inhibitor was associated with a 25% risk reduction for stroke events among the subgroup of persons with CKD (Fig. 57.2). These findings were consistent for both systolic and diastolic blood pressure lowering and for both ischemic and hemorrhagic stroke. In the Action to Control Cardiovascular Risk in Diabetes (ACCORD) BP trial, which randomly assigned patients with type 2 diabetes to a target systolic blood pressure of greater than 120 mm Hg versus less than 140 mm Hg, patients in the lower blood pressure target group had a 40% reduction in stroke events compared with standard blood pressure target.[36] This trial included patients with albuminuria but it had few participants with moderate-to-advanced CKD. In the Systolic Pressure INtervention Trial (SPRINT), which compared the same blood pressure targets among nondiabetic patients at high

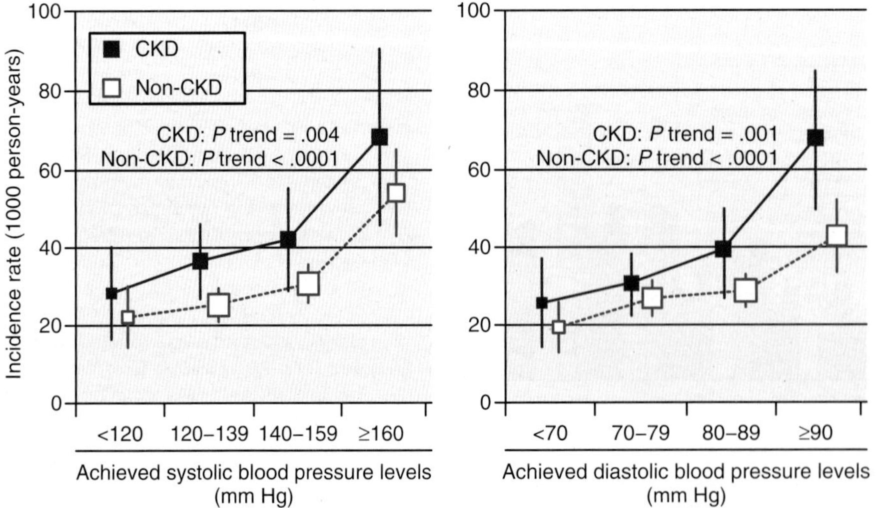


**Fig. 57.2** Age- and sex-adjusted incidence rate of total stroke, according to follow-up blood pressure levels and chronic kidney disease *(CKD)* status in the Perindopril Protection Against Recurrent Stroke Study. (Modified from Ninomiya T, Perkovic V, Gallagher M, et al. Lower blood pressure and risk of recurrent stroke in patients with chronic kidney disease: PROGRESS trial. *Kidney Int.* 2008;73:963–970. With permission.)

cardiovascular risk, there was no significant difference in stroke risk for patients assigned to the lower compared with standard blood pressure target.[37] Similarly, among the sizable subgroup of patients with CKD in SPRINT, there was also no difference in stroke risk, though the number of events was low.[38] No clinical trials have evaluated blood pressure targets in patients with ESKD receiving dialysis.

Several antihypertensive drug classes, including ACE inhibitors, angiotensin receptor blockers (ARBs), β-blockers, calcium channel blockers, and thiazide diuretics, reduce stroke risk.[39] However, there are few data comparing drug classes head to head. In the Losartan Intervention for Endpoint Reduction in Hypertension Study (LIFE), which included 9193 patients with hypertension and left ventricular hypertrophy, the relative risk (RR) for stroke was reduced by 26% (95% confidence interval [CI], 0.63–0.88) when comparing losartan with atenolol, despite similar reductions in blood pressure.[40] Aside from the isolated findings observed in the LIFE trial, there is a lack of compelling evidence favoring one drug class over another vis-à-vis stroke reduction. Thus other indications should be taken into account when choosing initial therapy. For example, ACE inhibitors or ARBs are preferred in the setting of proteinuria, reduced ejection fraction, or diabetes. To achieve blood pressure targets, most patients with CKD will require treatment with two or more agents.[41]

Dietary modification is an overlooked but efficacious strategy for lowering blood pressure. For example, the Dietary Approaches to Stop Hypertension (DASH) diet, rich in vegetables, fruits, and low-fat dairy products, when combined with reduced sodium intake, can lower blood pressure by an average of 11.5 mm Hg systolic in hypertensive persons.[42] In persons without CKD, the Institute of Medicine and clinical practice guidelines recommend less than 2300 mg sodium (5.8 g sodium chloride) intake.[43] Whether intake of sodium should be lower (<1500 mg sodium [3.8 g sodium chloride]) in subpopulations with salt-sensitive hypertension, including persons with CKD, is controversial.[44]

### DIABETES MELLITUS

Diabetes mellitus increases the risk for a first stroke by roughly twofold to sixfold in the general population,[2] and this relation appears to be similar in the CKD and ESKD populations. For example, in analyses of a community-based sample of US adults, diabetes was associated with an 89% increased risk for stroke among persons with CKD.[45] Among patients starting dialysis, diabetes was associated with a 35% increased risk for stroke.[33]

Multicomponent interventions targeting hypertension, dyslipidemia, proteinuria, and behavioral risk factors reduce stroke risk in persons with diabetes by 50%.[46] Although intensive glycemic control conclusively reduces microvascular complications, a similar benefit has not been demonstrated for macrovascular diseases, including stroke, a conclusion confirmed by two large randomized trials in patients with type 2 diabetes comparing standard glycemic control (glycosylated hemoglobin [$HbA_{1c}$] = 7% to 7.9%) with more intensive glycemic control ($HbA_{1c}$ <6%–6.5%).[47–50] Notably, fewer than 30% of participants in these studies had CKD, and most with CKD had at most mild-to-moderate reductions in GFR (CKD stage 3).

### PROTEINURIA

In a meta-analysis of stroke cohort studies involving more than 140,000 participants from several continents, proteinuria was associated with a 50% to 70% increased risk for stroke, independent of traditional stroke risk factors such as hypertension and diabetes.[51] The link between proteinuria and stroke was consistently observed across categories of sex, ethnicity, and diabetes subgroups, and for stroke subtypes. In a later study of 30,000 black and white adults in the United States, albuminuria was associated with an increased risk for incident stroke among blacks but not among whites. This association was independent of traditional stroke risk factors and present at levels of albuminuria below 30 mg/g.[52] In a pooled analysis of four cohort studies, reduced eGFR was significantly associated with the risk for ischemic stroke, whereas proteinuria was associated with an increased risk for ischemic and hemorrhagic stroke.[53] Furthermore, in one study, proteinuria largely explained the higher risk for death and disability following stroke among patients with CKD.[54] Thus the presence and degree of proteinuria may be a more important determinant of stroke risk (and stroke outcomes) than solute clearance. It is not known whether interventions which target proteinuria per se (vs. interventions targeting blood pressure) reduce stroke risk.

### ATRIAL FIBRILLATION

In the general population, atrial fibrillation is a potent risk factor for stroke, especially among older adults. The presence of nonvalvular atrial fibrillation increases the risk for stroke by 2.5- to 4.5-fold.[55] In patients with atrial fibrillation associated with valvular heart disease, stroke risk and prevention strategies depend on the underlying type of valvular lesion. Among patients with ESKD receiving dialysis, atrial fibrillation has been associated with an increased risk for stroke in meta-analyses, but there was considerable variability across individual studies.[56] The safety and efficacy/effectiveness of anticoagulation strategies are discussed in detail in Chapter 55.

### DYSLIPIDEMIA

In patients with preexisting cerebrovascular or coronary artery disease, 3-hydroxy-3-methylglutaryl–coenzyme A reductase inhibitor (statin) therapy reduces the risk for stroke by 25% to 30%.[57–59] Many of the large randomized trials of lipid lowering for primary or secondary prevention of cardiovascular events largely excluded, or attempted to exclude, individuals with CKD.[60] Nevertheless, some patients with mild-to-moderate CKD were included in these trials, because exclusion was typically based on serum creatinine rather than eGFR criteria. A subsequent meta-analysis of statin trials evaluating results in patients with moderate (stage 3) CKD concluded that statins appear to have a beneficial effect for reducing cardiovascular event rates in patients with CKD, with no greater risk for adverse events such as elevated liver enzyme levels or rhabdomyolysis.[61] Stroke event rates were not analyzed separately. Nonstatin lipid-lowering agents such as niacin or gemfibrozil appear to have similar benefits as in the general population,[62] though there are fewer data regarding use of these agents for stroke prevention.

Since these studies were published, results from several randomized trials in patients with CKD or ESKD or in kidney transplant recipients have been reported. In the Die Deutsche

Diabetes Dialyse Studie (4D study) of 1255 patients with type 2 diabetes on maintenance hemodialysis, atorvastatin resulted in no difference in the primary cardiovascular composite endpoint as compared with placebo, despite lowering low-density lipoprotein cholesterol by an average of 42%.[63] There was a twofold increase in fatal stroke events in the atorvastatin group (RR, 2.03; 95% CI, 1.03 to 3.93), primarily attributable to an increase in ischemic stroke events. There was no difference in the rate of nonfatal strokes. In A Study to Evaluate the Use of Rosuvastatin in Subjects on Regular Hemodialysis: An Assessment of Survival and Cardiovascular Events (AURORA), a trial of 2776 patients on hemodialysis, rosuvastatin yielded no benefit on the composite cardiovascular endpoint compared with placebo,[64] despite favorable changes in lipid and inflammatory surrogate markers. Unlike the 4D study, there was no increase in the incidence of stroke in AURORA.

In the Study of Heart and Renal Protection (SHARP), involving over 9000 persons with CKD, including approximately one-third who were receiving dialysis, treatment with ezetimibe plus simvastatin resulted in a statistically significant 17% reduction in the primary composite cardiovascular endpoint, incidence of first major vascular event, and a 28% reduction in the incidence of ischemic stroke, one of the secondary endpoints.[65] There was a nonsignificant increase in the rate of hemorrhagic stroke. In a trial of 2102 kidney transplant recipients treated with fluvastatin or placebo, active treatment yielded no significant effect on the primary composite cardiovascular endpoint (RR, 0.83; 95% CI, 0.64–1.06).[66] There was no statistically significant (or nominally significant) effect on stroke reduction.

## NUTRITIONAL FACTORS

In the general population, higher sodium and lower potassium intakes are linked to a heightened risk for stroke in epidemiologic studies. These associations appear to be mediated in part by blood pressure, as higher sodium intake tends to increase blood pressure in a dose-dependent manner, whereas higher potassium intake blunts the pressor effects of sodium.[42,67,68] Some evidence suggests that dietary sodium and potassium intake affect stroke risk through blood pressure–independent mechanisms.[69]

In addition to specific dietary factors, the syndrome of malnutrition and inflammation is strongly linked with atherosclerosis and cardiovascular events in patients on dialysis, but the association of malnutrition or inflammation syndromes with stroke is not as clear. For example, in a large sample of US patients on dialysis, subjective assessment of malnutrition was associated with an increased risk for hemorrhagic and ischemic stroke,[33] whereas serum albumin concentration and body weight have not yielded consistent associations with stroke risk. In a large community sample of adults with CKD, lower serum albumin concentration, lower body weight, and other markers of inflammation were associated with a significantly higher risk for stroke.[45]

## ANEMIA

Anemia is a common complication of CKD and linked with increased risk for cardiovascular events, including stroke, in many epidemiologic studies of CKD. One study noted a fivefold increased risk for stroke in CKD when accompanied by anemia; conversely, stroke risk was modestly and not significantly increased in CKD in the absence of anemia.[70] In another study of patients on dialysis, anemia was associated with a 22% increased risk for stroke.[33]

In several large randomized controlled trials in patients with CKD and anemia (including those on and not on dialysis), complete or partial correction of anemia with erythropoiesis stimulating agents (ESAs) increased adverse events and did not reduce mortality or cardiovascular events, including in subgroup analyses of stroke events.[71–73] Similarly, in a trial comparing darbepoetin and placebo in patients with type 2 diabetes, CKD, and hemoglobin less than 11 g/dL, darbepoetin resulted in no difference in the primary composite cardiovascular outcome and a twofold increase in the risk for stroke, one of the secondary outcomes.[74] Post hoc analysis failed to identify factors associated with the increase in stroke events, including blood pressure, dose of darbepoetin, or baseline hemoglobin. An observational study of US Veterans found that a higher risk for stroke among patients with CKD starting erythropoietin was primarily observed among patients with cancer, who required significantly higher doses of erythropoietin compared with patients with CKD without cancer.[75] Based on these data, Kidney Disease Improving Global Outcomes (KDIGO) 2012 guidelines recommend using ESAs with caution, if at all, in patients with CKD with a history of stroke.[76] Preliminary data suggest that continuous erythropoietin receptor activators have a similar safety profile compared with erythropoietin or darbepoetin.[77]

## DISORDERED MINERAL METABOLISM

Disordered mineral metabolism is characterized by abnormalities in calcium, phosphorus, parathyroid hormone, vitamin D, and fibroblast growth factor 23 (FGF-23) metabolism. In the general population, there are inconsistent associations between serum phosphate concentrations and stroke risk. Among patients with CKD, elevated serum phosphate concentrations have been associated with an increased risk for hemorrhagic stroke, whereas low serum phosphate concentrations have been associated with an increased risk for ischemic stroke.[78] Elevated levels of FGF-23 have been associated with an increased risk for stroke in several, but not all studies, independent of other markers of mineral metabolism.[79,80] The most commonly reported association is between elevated FGF-23 and hemorrhagic stroke[79,80]; another study has reported an association between elevated FGF-23 and cardioembolic stroke.[81] The efficacy of interventions targeting serum phosphate, FGF-23, or other components of the mineral metabolism axis for lowering stroke risk has not been studied.

## HOMOCYSTEINE

Numerous observational studies in the general population have identified hyperhomocysteinemia as a risk factor for stroke.[82–84] A single-nucleotide polymorphism in the gene methylenetetrahydrofolate reductase (*MTHFR*) reduces activity of the enzyme that metabolizes homocysteine, resulting in an increase in serum homocysteine concentration and a corresponding increase in stroke risk among persons with the homozygous genotype.[2] Serum homocysteine concentrations are increased in the setting of CKD, and up to 90% of patients on dialysis have elevated serum homocysteine concentrations.[85] The causes for elevated homocysteine levels in CKD and ESKD are thought to be altered homocysteine metabolism (either renal or nonrenal) and folate deficiency, as renal elimination of homocysteine appears to have a minor contribution to plasma concentrations.[85,86]

Despite substantial encouraging data in observational studies, clinical trials of homocysteine lowering with B vitamin supplementation yielded definitively null results. In the Vitamin Intervention for Stroke Prevention trial conducted in patients with a previous stroke, high-dose vitamin B failed to reduce the risk for recurrent stroke.[87] In three trials involving patients with CKD, including two trials among patients receiving dialysis and one among kidney transplant recipients, homocysteine lowering with B vitamin supplementation did not reduce mortality or cardiovascular events,[88,89] including analyses limited to stroke events. Thus high-dose folic acid and vitamin B in patients with CKD and ESKD with hyperhomocysteinemia are not recommended to reduce stroke risk.

## ANTIPLATELET AGENTS

In patients with noncardioembolic stroke or TIA, guidelines recommend antiplatelet agents to reduce the risk for recurrent stroke. Four antiplatelet agents have been approved by the US Food and Drug Administration for this indication—aspirin, dipyridamole plus aspirin, ticlopidine, and clopidogrel. Guidelines for the general population recommend aspirin for primary prevention of stroke when the risk for stroke is sufficiently high (10-year incidence > 6%) such that benefits outweigh risks of treatment.[2] Studies of aspirin for secondary prevention of stroke indicate RR reductions of 20% to 30%.[90] High and low doses of aspirin appear to have similar efficacy, though higher doses have increased rates of adverse events.

The KDIGO 2012 guidelines on management of CKD recommend offering antiplatelet agents to adults with CKD at risk for atherosclerotic events unless there is an increased risk for bleeding. These recommendations are based on post hoc analysis of the Hypertension Optimal Treatment trial. In this analysis it was estimated that for every 1000 persons with eGFR of less than 45 mL/min/1.73 $m^2$ treated with aspirin for 3.8 years, 54 all-cause deaths and 76 major cardiovascular events would be prevented, while 27 excess episodes of major bleeding would occur.[91]

Similarly, in one observational study of patients with ESKD, aspirin use was associated with an 18% reduction in cerebrovascular events[92] and no significant increase in the risk for hemorrhagic complications.[92,93] Short-term studies of aspirin use in the setting of acute coronary syndromes also seem to confirm the safety of aspirin in patients with CKD and ESKD.[94,95] Nevertheless, prescription rates for aspirin among patients with ESKD and a previous cerebrovascular event are relatively low (19%–30%).[92]

In the Clopidogrel versus Aspirin in Patients at Risk for Ischaemic events (CAPRIE) trial, clopidogrel reduced the risk for recurrent vascular events with a similar or better safety profile compared with aspirin[96]; however, patients with CKD were not included in this trial. In post hoc analyses of patients receiving clopidogrel versus placebo after percutaneous coronary intervention, participants with CKD receiving clopidogrel had no increased risk for bleeding compared with participants with normal kidney function, but also no benefit.[97] In a study of clopidogrel plus aspirin for prevention of arteriovenous graft thrombosis in patients with ESKD, combination therapy increased the risk for bleeding by twofold.[98] In a subsequent larger study of clopidogrel alone versus placebo to facilitate maturation of arteriovenous fistulas, treatment with clopidogrel did not increase the risk for hemorrhage.[99] The combination of dipyridamole plus aspirin has been evaluated in several studies for stroke prevention. Combination therapy reduces the rate of recurrent stroke by 23% to 38% when compared with either agent alone or placebo.[100] In a study of dipyridamole plus aspirin versus placebo for prevention of graft thrombosis in persons with ESKD, active therapy did not increase the risk for adverse events[101]; thus this combination appears to be relatively safe for use in patients with ESKD. American Stroke Association guidelines recommend selection of antiplatelet agents for stroke prevention based on evaluation of individual risk factors and comorbid conditions. For persons with CKD or ESKD, aspirin alone because of its low cost, safety, and over-the-counter availability is a reasonable choice. Aspirin plus dipyridamole may be considered in high-risk patients, and clopidogrel may be considered for those intolerant to aspirin or with a recent acute coronary syndrome or stenting.

## CAROTID STENOSIS

In the general population, carotid endarterectomy (CEA) has been demonstrated to be beneficial in patients with symptomatic atherosclerotic carotid stenosis of 70% or greater.[102–104] Uncertainty exists about the benefits of CEA among patients with symptomatic stenosis of 50% to 69%, and several studies indicate no benefit of surgery in patients with stenosis of less than 50%. In a post hoc analysis of the North American Symptomatic Carotid Endarterectomy Trial, which randomized patients with symptomatic high-grade stenosis (70%–99%), including 524 patients with CKD, to CEA versus medical management, event rates were higher in patients with CKD relative to those without CKD. Notably, the risk for ipsilateral stroke was reduced by 82% in patients with CKD who underwent CEA. Perioperative stroke and death risk were not increased. In analyses of US veterans undergoing CEA, veterans with CKD had increased risks for cardiovascular and pulmonary complications following CEA surgery compared with patients without CKD, as well an increased risk for postoperative mortality among those with stage 4 CKD. A limitation is that postoperative stroke rates were not reported.[105] Thus CEA should be considered for most patients with CKD with symptomatic severe carotid stenosis after optimization of their cardiac risk factors.

## DIALYSIS-ASSOCIATED FACTORS

A number of dialysis-associated factors have been speculated to increase the risk for stroke. Even absent intradialytic hypotension, hemodialysis has been shown to cause cerebral hypoperfusion. In a study utilizing noninvasive cerebral oxygenation monitoring during hemodialysis, absolute and relative changes in mean arterial pressure were associated with cerebral ischemia, whereas systolic blood pressure was unrelated to ischemia.[106] Importantly, the lower limit of cerebral autoregulation varied widely across patients. Taken together, these observations may explain why there are inconsistent associations between systolic blood pressure and stroke risk in epidemiologic studies. Overcorrection of anemia, especially in the setting of ultrafiltration, is another factor that is speculated to contribute to stroke by causing vascular stasis and thrombosis. Conversely, anticoagulation used for hemodialysis has also been speculated to contribute to hemorrhagic stroke risk during dialysis. Clinical evidence supporting these hypotheses is conflicting. Some studies note an increased risk for stroke during or immediately after hemodialysis treatments,[13] and one study found an increased rate of stroke during the months immediately before and after dialysis initiation compared with the prior year.[107] However, others have found no association between hemodialysis treatments and timing of stroke events[12] or the type of stroke events. Similarly, there is a paucity of data regarding dialysis modality (hemodialysis vs. peritoneal dialysis) and stroke risk.

## MANAGEMENT OF ACUTE STROKE IN CHRONIC KIDNEY DISEASE AND END-STAGE KIDNEY DISEASE

### INITIAL EVALUATION

The first step in the diagnostic evaluation of stroke is to confirm that the patient's symptoms are due to stroke, and not another systemic or neurologic illness, and to distinguish ischemic from hemorrhagic stroke. Presentation with severe headache, vomiting, coma, a systolic blood pressure above 220 mm Hg, or history of anticoagulant use is associated with a higher likelihood of hemorrhage,[108] but symptoms alone do not have sufficient diagnostic accuracy, and brain imaging is warranted to definitively distinguish hemorrhagic stroke from ischemic stroke. The next step is to determine the appropriateness of thrombolytic therapy. Timing of symptom onset, history of recent medical events (especially any history of trauma, surgery, or cardiovascular events), and use of antiplatelet agents or anticoagulants should be ascertained. The National Institutes of Health Stroke Scale can be used to estimate prognosis and determine the risk for hemorrhage with thrombolytic therapy, although it should be emphasized that the scale has not been validated in patients on dialysis and is likely to underestimate hemorrhage risk.[109]

### NEUROIMAGING

Neuroimaging plays a central role in the acute management of stroke in the era of thrombolytic therapy. Neuroimaging provides information on the size, location, and vascular distribution of the infarction, as well as the presence of bleeding, and, depending on the technique used, may also provide information on the degree of reversibility and the integrity of intracranial vessels. Noncontrast media–enhanced computed tomography (CT) of the brain is the most common neuroimaging modality used for the initial diagnostic evaluation because it can usually be performed urgently, it reliably distinguishes infarction from hemorrhage, and it identifies other causes for neurologic symptoms, with the caveat that CT is relatively insensitive for detecting small cortical or subcortical infarctions, especially in the posterior fossa. Administration of intravenous radiocontrast is usually unnecessary for acute stroke evaluation but in some cases may be indicated, if there is a high suspicion for brain tumors or infection. In these cases the risk for radiocontrast media–associated nephropathy must be weighed against the potential benefits of enhanced imaging. The American Stroke Association recommends that candidates for thrombolytic therapy have a completed CT scan within 25 minutes of arrival at the emergency department.[110]

Standard MRI techniques are not sufficiently sensitive to detect the acute changes of ischemic stroke, and therefore MRI is not usually indicated in routine evaluation. Imaging of the cerebral vasculature with angiography, CT angiography, or MR angiography is not usually a standard part of the initial evaluation but may become more common if intraarterial thrombolysis is more widely adopted. In these cases, the risks for radiocontrast media–associated nephropathy or nephrogenic systemic fibrosis (associated with gadolinium-enhanced MR angiography) must be carefully weighed against the potential benefits of the imaging procedure.

### INTRAVENOUS THROMBOLYSIS

In carefully selected patients in the general population treated within 3 hours of symptom onset, intravenous administration of recombinant tissue plasminogen activator (rt-PA) improves stroke outcomes[110]; however, the safety, efficacy, and practicality of thrombolytic therapy in the setting of CKD and ESKD remain unclear. Despite frequent contact of patients on dialysis with health care professionals, the median time from symptom onset to presentation among patients on dialysis is 8 hours, thus precluding consideration for thrombolytic therapy for most patients.[12] In trials of thrombolytic therapy conducted in the setting of acute myocardial infarction, patients with CKD were two to four times as likely to experience major bleeding, including intracranial hemorrhage, compared with those without CKD, with hemorrhage rates of 3% to 4% depending on the severity of CKD.[111,112] Similar findings have been noted in patients with stroke who received thrombolytic therapy.[113,114] The same study noted a high rate of recurrent ischemic stroke among patients with CKD receiving rt-PA, calling into question the efficacy of intravenous thrombolytics for acute ischemic stroke in this population. Based on these findings, caution should be exercised before considering thrombolysis in a patient with advanced CKD or ESKD. If utilized, anticoagulants or antiplatelet agents should be withheld for 24 hours following rt-PA administration.

### SUPPORTIVE CARE

Hypertension is common preceding and following acute stroke, but optimal management remains unclear. In ischemic stroke, overly aggressive treatment of hypertension is thought to lead to reduced perfusion and infarct expansion, but there is a lack of definitive data supporting this contention. In patients without CKD, hypertension typically resolves spontaneously; however, spontaneous resolution of hypertension may be less likely to occur in patients with CKD, as hypertension in patients with CKD tends to be more severe and difficult to control than in persons with normal or near-normal kidney function. In patients who are not candidates for thrombolytic therapy, consensus guidelines recommend blood pressure lowering for systolic blood pressure above 220 mm Hg or diastolic blood pressure above 120 mm Hg, or if there is other evidence for end-organ damage.[110] The threshold for treatment is lowered to above 185 mm Hg systolic or above 110 mm Hg diastolic in candidates for thrombolytic therapy. For patients with hemorrhagic stroke due to intracerebral hemorrhage, the threshold for treating hypertension is lower. When indicated, the use of parenteral agents that can be titrated easily, such as nicardipine or labetalol, is recommended. The timing of hemodialysis treatments in the setting of acute stroke should be individualized based on consideration of fluid and metabolic control. It seems prudent to avoid aggressive ultrafiltration during hemodialysis or to consider slower rates of ultrafiltration if fluid overload is present in the acute stroke period. Dialysis-related anticoagulation should be held after hemorrhagic stroke and held or minimized following ischemic stroke.

## DISORDERS OF COGNITIVE FUNCTION

Changes in modern ESKD epidemiology and practice have greatly altered the presentation, significance, and risk factor profile for cognitive disorders among persons with ESKD. Neurocognitive symptoms were among the first described symptoms of the uremic syndrome and were later proposed as sensitive indicators of dialysis adequacy or, in some cases, side effects of dialysis therapy. However, with the aging of the population with ESKD and changes in dialysis practice, including earlier initiation of dialysis and elimination of aluminum contamination of dialysate water, the relation between neurocognitive disorders and uremia per se is less clear. Patients with neurocognitive disorders are at higher risk for death, hospitalization, and dialysis withdrawal. Neurocognitive disorders are also likely to reduce health-related quality of life and hinder adherence with the complex dietary and medication regimens prescribed to patients with CKD. This section will review the evaluation and management of delirium, dementia, and chronic cognitive impairment among persons with CKD and ESKD.

### DELIRIUM SYNDROMES

Delirium is an acute confusional state characterized by a recent onset of fluctuating awareness, impairment of memory and attention, and disorganized thinking that can be attributable to a medical condition, intoxication, or medication side effect. Delirium is typically precipitated by an acute or subacute event such as a neurologic disorder, infection, electrolyte disorder, or intoxication (Box 57.1). Older patients with cognitive or sensory impairment, chronic diseases, or those taking multiple medications are thought to be most vulnerable for delirium; thus it is not surprising that delirium would occur commonly in patients with ESKD. Several syndromes of delirium specific to patients with ESKD are described in more detail in the following section.

**Box 57.1 Differential Diagnosis of Delirium in End-Stage Kidney Disease**

- Cerebrovascular disorder (stroke, subdural hematoma, hypertensive encephalopathy)
- Seizure
- Infection (sepsis, meningitis)
- Electrolyte disorder (hypoglycemia, hyponatremia or hypernatremia, hypercalcemia)
- Intoxication (alcohol, drugs, aluminum, star fruit, sugihiratake mushrooms)
- Alcohol withdrawal
- Nutritional deficiency (thiamine)
- Hepatic encephalopathy
- Uremic encephalopathy or inadequate dialysis
- Dialysis disequilibrium
- Dialysis-associated hypotension

### UREMIC ENCEPHALOPATHY

#### Clinical Features

Uremic encephalopathy is a syndrome of delirium seen in untreated or inadequately treated ESKD. It is characterized by lethargy and confusion in early stages and can progress to seizures and/or coma. It may be accompanied by other neurologic signs, such as tremor, myoclonus, or asterixis. Electroencephalographic abnormalities correspond with clinical symptoms and improve with treatment of uremia.[1,115] Conversely, the degree of azotemia alone correlates poorly with the presence or degree of encephalopathy.

Radiologic and pathologic studies in the setting of uremic encephalopathy are sparse. While available studies report white matter lesions suggestive of small vessel cerebrovascular disease (see previous section), it is unclear whether these pathologic abnormalities play a role in the development of uremic encephalopathy because most studies did not conduct simultaneous neurophysiologic or neuropsychiatric testing. In a study of 30 patients on hemodialysis and controls without CKD, cognitive impairment was associated with more extensive enlargement of the third ventricle and temporal horns, but not with the presence of cerebrovascular disease lesions.[21] Brain perfusion studies have demonstrated reduced perfusion in the frontal cortex among patients on hemodialysis compared with controls, although these findings did not correlate with cognitive performance.[116] MRI studies utilizing diffusion-weighted imaging to detect changes in brain water have noted findings consistent with brain edema in uremic encephalopathy.[117,118]

#### Pathophysiology

A number of biochemical changes have been reported in acute and chronic uremic encephalopathy, including alterations in water transport and brain edema, disturbances of the blood–brain barrier, and changes in cerebral metabolism.[119–124] The significance of these changes on neurotransmitter release and neuronal function is unclear.

Studies contrasting animal models of uremic encephalopathy in acute kidney injury with hepatic encephalopathy have demonstrated an increase in brain inflammation in conjunction with vascular permeability in uremic encephalopathy.[125] Kidney injury may activate cytokines that cross the blood–brain barrier or activate other messengers that contribute to neuronal dysfunction. Alternatively, the retention of uremic solutes may trigger both the inflammatory reaction and the neuronal dysfunction. A large number of solutes are retained in uremia (Chapter 52), and several may have direct neurotoxicity or contribute indirectly to the pathogenesis of uremic encephalopathy by altering the blood–brain barrier. For example, the guanidine compounds are low-molecular-weight solutes with deleterious effects on immune and neurologic function in vivo. Levels of guanidinosuccinic acid and methylguanidine are increased 100-fold in uremic brain tissue and cerebrospinal fluid,[126] and several guanidine compounds, including guanidinosuccinic acid, methylguanidine, and homoarginine, induce seizures, possibly through their effects on *N*-methyl-D-aspartate (NMDA) receptors and/or by modulating calcium channels.[127–129] Solutes derived from gut microbial metabolism have also been linked with impaired cognitive function in human studies. For example, metabolites related to phenylalanine, benzoate, and glutamate metabolism have been linked with impaired cognitive function among patients receiving dialysis.[130]

In addition to uremic retention solutes, anemia and secondary hyperparathyroidism are proposed risk factors for uremic encephalopathy. In uncontrolled short-term studies, administration of erythropoietin is associated with improved performance on cognitive function and electrophysiologic testing.[131–133] Parathyroid hormone is known to have central nervous system effects in persons with primary hyperparathyroidism,[134] and cognitive function has been reported to improve after parathyroidectomy in persons with primary hyperparathyroidism and normal kidney function.[135,136] Animal models of uremia have noted an increase in brain calcium content and electroencephalographic abnormalities with administration of parathyroid hormone, a finding that can be prevented by parathyroidectomy.[123] These alterations in brain calcium content may in turn disrupt cerebral function by interrupting neurotransmitter release or cerebral metabolism.

#### Treatment

Once other causes of delirium have been ruled out, prompt treatment of uremic encephalopathy with initiation or intensification of renal replacement therapy is indicated. Resolution of symptoms typically occurs within days. Dietary protein restriction is another adjunctive measure used to delay the development of uremic symptoms, though there are few published data supporting its use for the purpose of improving cognitive function. With proper instruction and follow-up, modest dietary protein restriction may be appropriate in certain settings.

### DIALYSIS DISEQUILIBRIUM

#### Clinical Features

This syndrome of delirium is attributable to the dialysis procedure itself and seen during or shortly after the first several dialysis treatments. It is most likely to occur in pediatric or older adult patients, patients with severe azotemia, and patients undergoing high-efficiency hemodialysis; however, it has also been reported in patients undergoing peritoneal dialysis and maintenance hemodialysis.[137,138] Dialysis disequilibrium is characterized by symptoms of headache, visual disturbance, nausea, or agitation, and, in severe cases, delirium, lethargy, seizures, and even coma. The incidence and severity of this syndrome are felt to be declining because of earlier initiation of dialysis and institution of preventative measures in high-risk patients, including reducing the efficiency dialysis, increasing the dialysate sodium concentration, and administering mannitol.[139] Symptoms are usually self-limited.

#### Pathophysiology

The clinical features of dialysis disequilibrium syndrome are primarily attributable to brain edema, although the nature and cause of the edema remain uncertain. Two hypotheses have been suggested to explain the development of brain edema. In the first, rapid removal of urea (and other water-soluble, rapidly diffusible solutes) by dialysis leads to a solute gradient between the blood and brain, in turn leading to influx of water into the brain. This theory is supported by animal studies in which the brain-to-plasma urea gradient induced by rapid hemodialysis accounted for the increase in brain water.[140] In the second theory, a decrease in intracellular pH and formation of idiogenic osmoles (osmolytes) within the brain contributes to the development of cerebral edema when an osmolar gradient develops during dialysis.[119]

## SYNDROMES OF CHRONIC COGNITIVE IMPAIRMENT

Dementia is a chronic confusional state characterized by impairment in memory and at least one other cognitive domain, such as language, orientation, reasoning, or executive functioning. The impairment in cognitive function must represent a decline from the patient's baseline level of cognitive function and must be severe enough to interfere with daily activities and independence. "Dialysis dementia" is a term reserved to describe a syndrome of progressive dementia related to aluminum intoxication and first described several decades ago in the setting of aluminum contamination of dialysate. While aluminum-based phosphate binders were often blamed for this syndrome, the aluminum moiety is so inefficiently absorbed and only parenteral exposure was likely relevant. There is growing awareness that many patients with CKD have a syndrome of chronic cognitive impairment unrelated to aluminum intoxication. This entity has various names in the literature, including "mild cognitive impairment," "subclinical dementia," "residual syndrome,"[141] and "chronic dialysis-dependent encephalopathy," reflecting an unknown but probable multifactorial origin.

### DIALYSIS DEMENTIA

Dialysis dementia was first described in the 1970s, and among adults it occurred almost exclusively among patients on hemodialysis rather than peritoneal dialysis.[142,143] Epidemic, sporadic, and childhood forms of dialysis dementia have been reported. Epidemic forms occur in geographic clusters and are strongly associated with aluminum contamination of dialysate. The relation of aluminum intoxication to the sporadic and childhood forms of dialysis dementia is less clear. Some early studies revealed an increase in brain aluminum content 11-fold higher than in healthy persons and threefold to fourfold higher than in patients requiring hemodialysis without dementia[144] and speculated that use of aluminum-containing phosphate binders might be involved. Clinical manifestations include a variety of neuropsychiatric symptoms, osteomalacia, myopathy, and anemia. Symptoms may be exacerbated by hemodialysis or by administration of chelating agents such as deferoxamine or desferrioxamine, presumably due to mobilization and redistribution of tissue aluminum into the brain. If aluminum intoxication is confirmed, the dialysate should be checked for aluminum contamination, and any other sources of parenteral aluminum exposure should be explored. Chelation therapy is indicated despite the caveats noted earlier because there is no other effective method for removal of aluminum.[145]

## CHRONIC COGNITIVE IMPAIRMENT

### Epidemiology

The epidemiology of chronic cognitive impairment among patients with CKD remains only partly defined, owing to the lack of a standard definition of cognitive impairment and relatively few longitudinal studies of cognition. Fukunishi and associates were among the first investigators to describe an increased incidence of dementia in ESKD. In their study the annual incidence of dementia was 2.5% among patients with ESKD, double than that of the general population.[146] Among US patients the incidence of dementia is estimated at 1% to 2% for patients under age 65 years, reaching up to 6% to 8% for patients over age 85 years.[147] The prevalence of moderate-to-severe cognitive impairment based on neurocognitive testing ranges from 16% to 38% depending on the sample and the definition of impairment (Fig. 57.3A).[148–151]

The incidence and prevalence of cognitive impairment are also increased among patients with CKD that does not require dialysis. The prevalence of cognitive impairment rises relatively early in the course of CKD and is higher at lower eGFR, reaching 20% for persons with an eGFR of less than 20 mL/min/1.73 m$^2$ (Fig. 57.3B).[152] Neurocognitive deficits have also been described among children with CKD and ESKD. For example, among children with CKD not requiring dialysis, 21% to 40% fall below normative values for academic achievement, attention regulation, and executive function, though GFR is not a consistent correlate of cognitive performance.[153] In a cohort of community-dwelling older adults, CKD was associated with a 37% increased risk for dementia, attributable to an increased incidence of vascular dementia.[154] Similarly, several other studies, primarily in older adult cohorts, have described an independent association between CKD and cognitive decline.[155] However, not all studies have confirmed such an association.[156,157] Whether this is due to

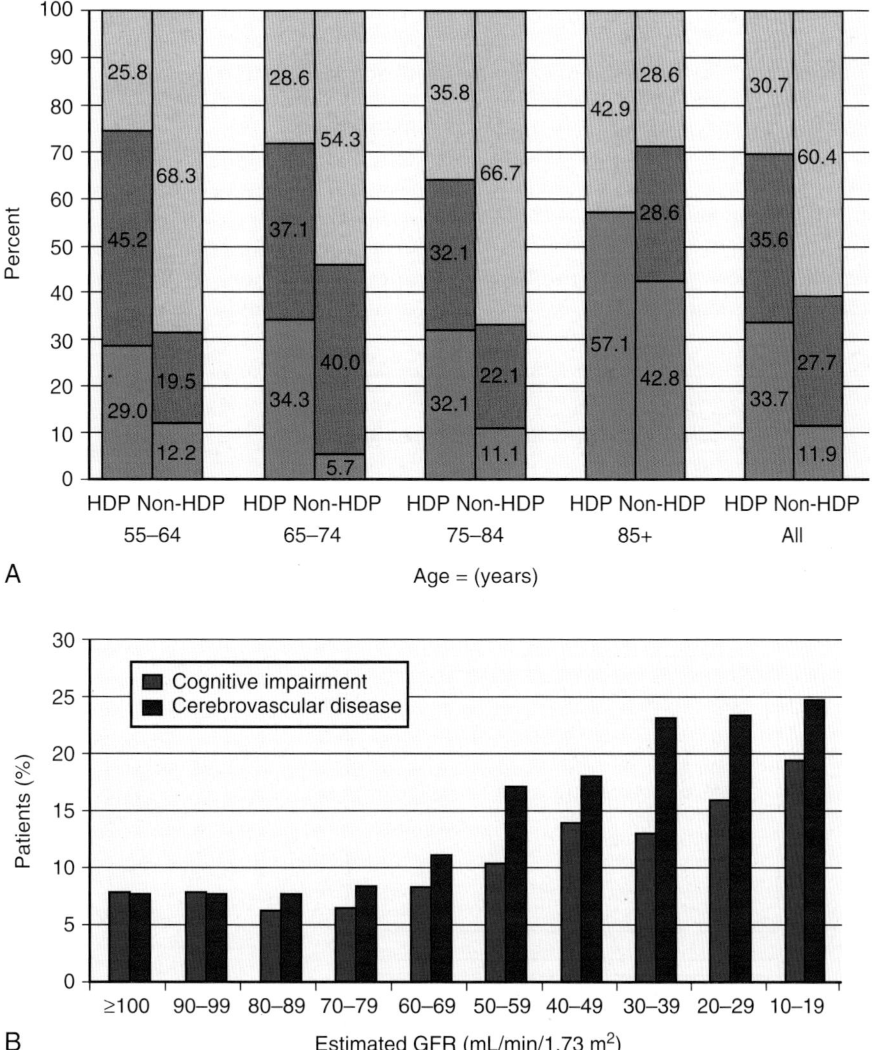


**Fig. 57.3** (A) Frequency of cognitive impairment in 101 hemodialysis patients *(HDPs)* and 101 nonhemodialysis patients (non-HDPs) according to age group. *Yellow bars* indicate normal to mild impairment, *red bars* indicate moderate impairment, and *blue bars* indicate severe cognitive impairment. (B) Unadjusted prevalence of cognitive impairment in 23,405 black and white US adults, according to estimated glomerular filtration rate *(GFR).* (A, modified from Murray AM, Tupper DE, Knopman DS, et al. Cognitive impairment in hemodialysis patients is common. *Neurology.* 2006;67:216–223; B, modified from Kurella Tamura M, Wadley V, Yaffe K, et al. Kidney function and cognitive impairment in US adults: the Reasons for Geographic and Racial Differences in Stroke [REGARDS] Study. *Am J Kidney Dis.* 2008;52:227–234. With permission.)

differences in cohort risk for dementia, misclassification of CKD, or confounding factors, such as proteinuria, remains unclear. For example, cystatin C, a purportedly more sensitive marker of CKD in patients with low muscle mass, is associated with an increased risk for cognitive decline among patients with normal creatinine-based eGFR.[158] In some studies, albuminuria, but not eGFR, has been associated with an increased risk for cognitive decline.[156]

### Risk Factors and Mechanisms

Microvascular disease appears to be a major contributing factor to chronic cognitive impairment in CKD. Patients with CKD and ESKD have a high prevalence of subclinical stroke, white matter hyperintensities (thought to represent chronic ischemia), and cerebral microbleeds identified by neuroimaging. In the general population these lesions are linked with a higher risk for dementia and cognitive decline. Among patients with CKD or ESKD, stroke and symptoms of stroke have been linked with poorer cognitive function.[148,151,159] Finally, changes in kidney function appear to parallel changes in cognition,[156] suggesting shared risk factors for the decline in kidney function and cognition (Fig. 57.4).

Novel factors may also contribute to chronic brain ischemia and cognitive decline in patients with CKD. For example, anemia, vitamin D deficiency, vascular calcification, inflammation, and oxidative stress are common among patients with CKD and have been linked with cognitive decline in the general population, though further study is needed to confirm their importance in patients with CKD.[160–162]

Retention of uremic solutes may contribute to chronic cognitive impairment despite the fact that dialysis appears "adequate" by conventional criteria (usually urea kinetics). Support for the "uremic solute" hypothesis comes from studies demonstrating improvement in cognitive function among children and middle-aged adults who undergo transplantation compared with matched patients on the transplant waiting list and studies linking uremic solutes to impaired cognitive function among patients receiving dialysis.[130,163,164] Recurrent brain ischemia from circulatory stress induced by the hemodialysis process has also been implicated as a contributing factor to chronic cognitive impairment. In one study utilizing intradialytic cerebral oxygenation measurements, intradialytic cerebral ischemia was associated with absolute and relative changes in mean arterial pressure, and with prospective decline in cognitive function.[106] In a small clinical trial, dialysis treatment with cooled dialysate reduced hemodynamic instability and abrogated brain ischemic changes.[165]

In addition to cooled dialysate, the effect of frequent hemodialysis on cognitive function has been assessed in two small clinical trials. In a randomized clinical trial of frequent in-center hemodialysis, and a parallel trial of frequent home-based nocturnal hemodialysis, there were no improvements in several cognitive domains compared with conventional thrice weekly dialysis.[166]

### Evaluation

History taking, ideally from the patient and caregiver, should focus on the duration and severity of cognitive and behavioral deficits, as well as use of medications that might interfere with cognitive function such as antihistamines, antipsychotics, and anticholinergics. The value of routine screening for dementia in the general population is controversial. Given

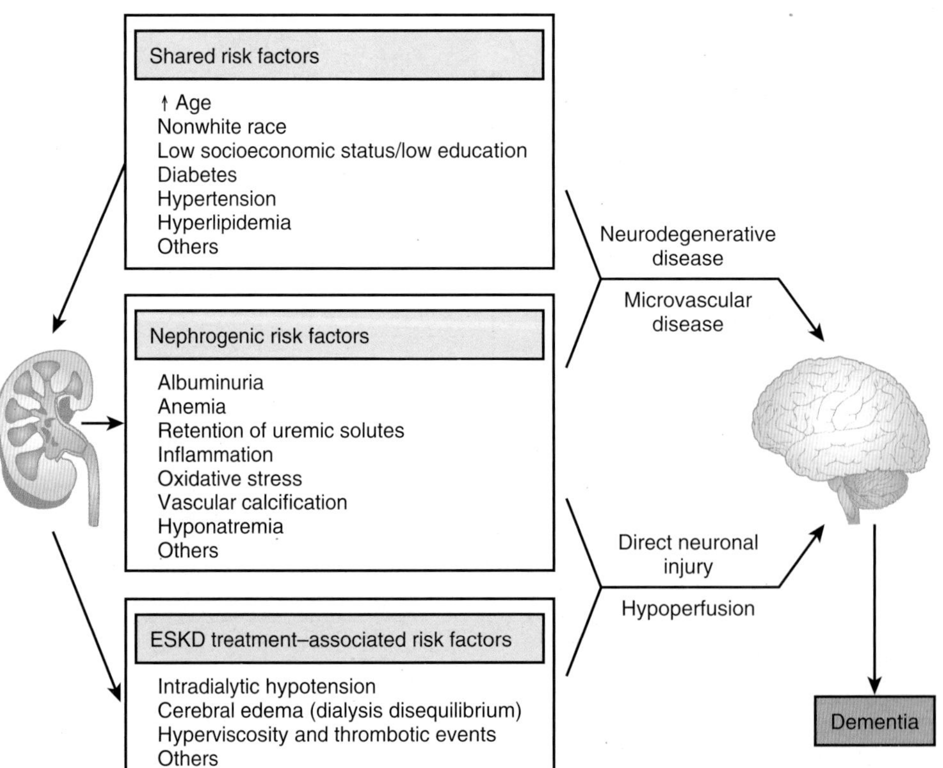


**Fig. 57.4** Proposed mechanisms of chronic cognitive impairment in chronic kidney disease. *ESKD,* End-stage kidney disease. (Modified from Kurella Tamura M, Yaffe K. Dementia and cognitive impairment in end-stage renal disease: diagnostic and therapeutic strategies. *Kidney Int.* 2011;79:14–22.)

the high prevalence of cognitive impairment in the CKD population and its implications for disease management, screening for cognitive impairment in older patients with CKD seems warranted. A large number of screening tests are available with a range of administration times and diagnostic accuracy; thus there is no single best screening test. Impairments in executive function are most commonly observed, and may be particularly important to identify, because impairments in this domain are strongly linked with adherence to therapy, and ability to live independently. Screening tests of cognitive function may also be useful for identifying patients who lack capacity to provide informed consent for medical procedures.

Delirium and depression frequently coexist with dementia; however, it is important to exclude these conditions as the sole cause of cognitive impairment before establishing a diagnosis of dementia. In practice, differentiating delirium and depression from dementia can be difficult, because unresolved uremia and subtle dialysis disequilibrium can contribute to temporal fluctuations in cognitive function.[167,168] Neuropsychologic testing on a nondialysis day can be useful if the diagnosis is uncertain or when testing is performed to establish capacity or potential reversibility (e.g., before kidney transplantation). In addition to cognitive function testing, laboratory testing for vitamin $B_{12}$ deficiency and hypothyroidism is recommended for all patients with suspected dementia. In patients with ESKD, inadequate dialysis, severe anemia, and aluminum toxicity should be ruled out. There are conflicting recommendations from guideline panels regarding the routine use of structural neuroimaging in the work-up of chronic cognitive impairment.[169] The role of testing for genetic markers of dementia risk (e.g., apolipoprotein E variants) is controversial.

#### Management

The management of patients with CKD and ESKD with chronic cognitive impairment not meeting criteria for dementia is uncertain. While kidney transplantation is an optimal therapy for most patients with ESKD, many patients with chronic cognitive impairment may not be eligible for transplantation due to coexisting illness. Further, the extent to which transplantation reverses cognitive impairment, especially in frail patients with coexisting illness, is uncertain. Some studies report improvements in cognitive function after transplantation among young or middle-aged patients,[170] but a few cross-sectional studies note high rates of cognitive impairment even after transplantation.[163] Intensification of the dialysis regimen is not routinely recommended due to nondefinitive findings from two clinical trials. There may be a subset of patients with cognitive impairment who benefit from these strategies, such as those without underlying microvascular disease; however, this remains speculative. Homocysteine lowering with B vitamin supplementation has failed to show benefit for reducing the risk for cognitive decline in the general population and in patients with CKD or ESKD.[171]

For patients with dementia, two classes of medications are now available for treatment of both Alzheimer type and vascular dementia. Cholinesterase inhibitors are approved for treatment of mild-to-moderate dementia, whereas memantine, an NMDA receptor antagonist, is approved for treatment of moderate-to-severe Alzheimer dementia and may also have some efficacy in treatment of vascular dementia. The clinical benefit of both classes of agents appears to be modest, and the effect of treatment on long-term outcomes such as nursing home placement remains unclear. Limited pharmacokinetic data suggest that the cholinesterase inhibitors donepezil and rivastigmine do not require dose modification for patients with CKD or ESKD.[172] Dose modification for the cholinesterase inhibitor galantamine is suggested for patients with "moderate" kidney disease and its use is not recommended for patients with ESKD. Dose modification is also suggested for the NMDA receptor antagonist memantine for patients with a creatinine clearance less than 30 mL/min, including those with ESKD. Given the limited data on safety or efficacy of these agents in patients with advanced CKD, therapy decisions should be individualized.

Behavioral symptoms such as agitation or hallucinations should be treated with a stepped approach, beginning with nonpharmacologic approaches such as removal of precipitating factors (e.g., pain, excessive noise), followed by psychosocial interventions (e.g., caregiver education), and pharmacologic therapy as a last step. A key aspect of dementia management is the assessment of patient safety and ability to perform self-care functions, comply with medical regimens, and participate in medical decision making. Patients on dialysis with dementia have a higher incidence of all-cause mortality and withdrawal from dialysis[173]; therefore goals of care should be discussed early in the course of disease when possible.

## SEIZURES

### EPIDEMIOLOGY OF SEIZURES IN PATIENTS WITH ESKD

Seizures are caused by paroxysmal, disorganized electrical activity in the brain. Seizures may manifest as motor, sensory, autonomic, or psychic symptoms with or without impairment in cognition. Epilepsy is a group of related disorders affecting approximately 1% of the US population, characterized by recurrent seizures.

There is limited contemporary information regarding the incidence and prevalence of seizures among patients with ESKD. Among children receiving maintenance dialysis, seizures have been reported in 7% to 8%.[174] Risk factors in these studies included a prior history of seizure and hemodialysis versus peritoneal dialysis as treatment modality. In adults with ESKD receiving maintenance dialysis, seizures are reported to affect between 2% and 10%.[175,176]

### DIFFERENTIAL DIAGNOSIS OF SEIZURE IN PATIENTS WITH END-STAGE KIDNEY DISEASE

The differential diagnosis of de novo seizure in patients with ESKD includes acute intracranial events such as subarachnoid hemorrhage or head trauma, intracranial tumor, systemic illness such as meningitis, drug intoxication, and metabolic disorders such as hypoglycemia, hypocalcemia, and hypomagnesemia. Uremia lowers the seizure threshold. That is, a central nervous system insult alone might not produce seizure, but in the presence of uremia may result in seizure activity. Conditions associated with seizure that require special consideration in patients with ESKD are discussed in the following sections.

### UREMIC ENCEPHALOPATHY

Seizures resulting from advanced uremia are often described as generalized tonic-clonic or myoclonic seizures.[174] Partial motor seizures have also been reported. Definitive treatment involves the institution of renal replacement therapy. Antiepileptic drugs (AEDs) with low dialytic clearance may also be used as adjunctive therapy.

### DIALYSIS DISEQUILIBRIUM

Seizures may be a severe manifestation of dialysis disequilibrium syndrome. As discussed in the preceding section, pediatric or elderly patients with severe azotemia recently initiated on hemodialysis therapy are at greater risk. Seizures characteristically occur during or immediately after hemodialysis treatment.

### POSTERIOR REVERSIBLE ENCEPHALOPATHY SYNDROME

Posterior reversible encephalopathy syndrome (PRES) is characterized by headache, altered mental status, visual disturbance, and seizures. Seizures are reported in up to 90% of patients with PRES. The diagnosis of PRES is made radiographically based on the presence of vasogenic edema predominantly affecting white matter in the posterior cerebral hemispheres.[177,178] The condition often, though not invariably, occurs in association with hypertensive crisis. It may also occur with eclampsia, vasculitis, thrombotic microangiopathy, and with immunosuppressive drugs including calcineurin inhibitors, rituximab, and sirolimus.

PRES has been described in children and adults with ESKD receiving dialysis.[179,180] In addition, erythropoietin has also been described as a cause of PRES, typically accompanied by hypertension.[181] Although the exact pathogenesis of PRES is unknown, failure of cerebral autoregulatory mechanisms and endothelial dysfunction are implicated. In patients with ESKD, fluid overload is felt to play a central role. In this way, erythropoietin treatment, which expands plasma volume, may also contribute to PRES. Whether the risk of PRES is also related to the rate of rise in hemoglobin concentration or the dose of erythropoietin is unknown. The clinical manifestations of PRES are usually reversible with appropriate volume and blood pressure management.

## DRUGS AND INTOXICATIONS

A number of drugs and/or their metabolites may lower the seizure threshold in patients with ESKD, including meperidine, acyclovir, penicillin, cephalosporins, theophylline, metoclopramide, and lithium. Ingestion of star fruit has been linked with seizures in patients with ESKD.[182]

## USE OF ANTIEPILEPTIC DRUGS

### FIRST-GENERATION ANTIEPILEPTIC DRUGS

The first-generation AEDs—carbamazepine, phenytoin, phenobarbital, valproic acid, and ethosuximide—undergo extensive hepatic metabolism and most have minimal clearance by the kidney. These drugs have complicated pharmacokinetic profiles, narrow therapeutic windows, and significant drug–drug interactions and/or adverse effects.

Phenytoin is highly protein bound and only the unbound fraction is active.[183] Both uremia and hypoalbuminemia can affect the free phenytoin concentration. In both circumstances, the total phenytoin concentration may not be a reliable indicator of the free phenytoin concentration. Patients with hypoalbuminemia and/or uremia will have a higher free phenytoin concentration with similar total phenytoin concentration compared with patients without these conditions. Where available, direct measurement of free phenytoin concentrations is preferred for patients with ESKD. Similarly, phenobarbital also has significant protein binding which can be affected by uremia and hypoalbuminemia.

Dose reduction is not recommended for most first-generation AEDs in the setting of reduced kidney function. Phenobarbital and primidone are partially cleared by the kidneys, and may require longer dosing intervals. The dialytic clearance of phenytoin, carbamazepine, and valproic acid is thought to be minimal and therefore supplemental dosing after dialysis is not routinely recommended. Phenobarbital, ethosuximide, and primidone are removed by dialysis[183]; therefore supplemental dosing based on therapeutic monitoring of drug levels is suggested.

### SECOND-GENERATION ANTIEPILEPTIC DRUGS

Newer AEDs, in contrast to first-generation AEDs, have more predictable pharmacokinetic profiles and fewer drug–drug interactions or serious adverse effects. Several of the second-generation agents are cleared by the kidney, and require dose modification in the setting of CKD or ESKD. Dose adjustment is recommended for gabapentin, levetiracetam, topiramate, and felbamate when eGFR falls below 60 mL/min/1.73 $m^2$, whereas adjustment is recommended for oxcarbazepine when eGFR falls below 30 mL/min/1.73 $m^2$.[23] No dose adjustment is suggested for tiagabine, and there are insufficient data for lamotrigine.[23]

## NEUROPATHY

### UREMIC POLYNEUROPATHY

Uremic neuropathy is a distal, symmetric, mixed sensorimotor polyneuropathy. It typically involves the lower extremities more than the upper extremities, and sensory symptoms typically precede motor symptoms. Motor involvement usually indicates advanced disease. Some authorities consider restless legs syndrome (RLS) part of the clinical spectrum of uremic polyneuropathy. Differentiating uremic polyneuropathy from other systemic diseases that contribute to ESKD and also affect nerve function, such as diabetes, amyloidosis, and systemic lupus erythematosus, can be difficult. Abnormalities in motor nerve conduction velocity parallel the decline in GFR and improve substantially after kidney transplantation.[184,185] Nerve conduction abnormalities have been reported in up to 60% of patients receiving dialysis.[186] Other manifestations of uremic polyneuropathy include symmetric muscle weakness, areflexia, and loss of vibratory sense. Similar to uremic encephalopathy, retention of a number of uremic solutes, including parathyroid hormone, myoinositol, and other "middle molecules," has been correlated with motor nerve conduction velocity. Nerve excitability studies demonstrate alterations in membrane potential and have suggested that hyperkalemic depolarization may underlie the development of uremic neuropathy rather than middle molecules.[187]

## MONONEUROPATHY

Mononeuropathy syndromes typically involve compression or ischemia of the ulnar or median nerves and are most often attributable to dialysis-related ($\beta_2$-microglobulin) amyloidosis or ischemic mononeuropathy associated with an arteriovenous fistula.

## AUTONOMIC NEUROPATHY

The existence of an autonomic neuropathy attributable to uremia is controversial. Manifestations include orthostatic or dialysis-associated hypotension and impotence. A study of 25 patients with ESKD who were not on dialysis and eight healthy controls conducted extensive testing of autonomic function. Function of the efferent sympathetic pathway was similar in patients with ESKD who were not on dialysis and in controls. By contrast, functions of the efferent parasympathetic pathway and baroreceptor sensitivity were abnormal in patients with ESKD who were not on dialysis compared with controls.[188] Among the eight patients who initiated hemodialysis, autonomic function was unchanged after 6 weeks of dialysis. By contrast, among the 12 patients who underwent kidney transplantation, autonomic function improved a mean of 24 weeks after transplantation.

# SLEEP DISORDERS

## PREVALENCE OF SLEEP COMPLAINTS

Sleep complaints are common among patients on dialysis with and without associated sleep disorders. In some series, sleep complaints are present in more than 80% of patients on dialysis.[189] Disruption of the sleep–wake cycle is a characteristic feature of uremia, with both excessive daytime sleepiness and insomnia noted in clinical studies.[190,191] Complaints of daytime sleepiness are present in 30% to 67% of patients on dialysis,[189,192,193] whereas complaints of insomnia are reported in 50% to 73%.[192,194] Using multiple sleep latency testing, an objective measure of daytime sleepiness, the prevalence of daytime sleepiness is lower than prevalence estimates using sleep questionnaires, but still abnormally elevated.[192-194] Sleep disorders (e.g., sleep apnea, RLS, and periodic limb movements of sleep [PLMS]) have been correlated with complaints of excessive daytime sleepiness in some but not in all studies, and therefore other factors associated with uremia, such as altered melatonin metabolism or disrupted regulation of body temperature related to use of dialysate, have been suggested as potential etiologic mechanisms.[195]

## SLEEP APNEA

Sleep apnea is characterized by the repetitive cessation of respiration during sleep, resulting in oxygen desaturation and arousal. Apnea associated with continued respiratory effort is classified as obstructive, whereas apnea associated with an absence of respiratory effort is classified as central. Clinical symptoms include loud snoring, repetitive awakening from sleep with feelings of breathlessness, nocturia, excessive daytime sleepiness, and cognitive impairment.

### EPIDEMIOLOGY

Utilizing polysomnography to diagnose sleep apnea, the prevalence of this disorder in the ESKD population is estimated at 50%, substantially higher than the recently estimated 10% to 20% in the US population.[196] Some of this difference is explained by differences in age and other chronic diseases that predispose to sleep apnea. In one study the prevalence of sleep apnea was fourfold higher in patients on dialysis compared with age-, sex-, race-, and body mass index–matched controls, suggesting factors specific to ESKD may be implicated in the pathogenesis of this condition.[197] While obstructive sleep apnea is the predominant presentation in the general population, the presentation varies in patients with ESKD with a broad distribution of obstructive, central, and mixed types of apnea.

### PATHOPHYSIOLOGY

Based on the distribution of apnea subtypes in this population, both upper airway occlusion and disturbances of central ventilatory control have been implicated in the pathophysiology of sleep apnea in ESKD. Pharyngeal narrowing has been demonstrated in patients on dialysis compared with healthy controls, which in turn may predispose to upper airway occlusion.[198] Upper airway occlusion has been attributed to pharyngeal water content and rostral overnight fluid shifts, as well as to impaired upper airway muscle tone resulting from uremic neuropathy.[199] Impairment of central ventilatory control may be a consequence of hypocapnia resulting from adaptation to chronic metabolic acidosis. In a study of 58 patients requiring hemodialysis, patients with sleep apnea demonstrated augmented responsiveness of central and peripheral chemoreflexes, which in turn may destabilize ventilatory control.[200] Infusion of branched-chain amino acids, which are depleted in ESKD, may improve ventilation and sleep architecture.[201]

### TREATMENT

In the general population, continuous positive airway pressure (CPAP) is the primary therapy for sleep apnea, and small studies suggest that this therapy has similar efficacy in patients with ESKD.[202] CPAP therapy improves symptoms of daytime sleepiness, quality of life, and hypertension and may also attenuate other cardiovascular risk factors in the general population[203,204]; however, compliance with CPAP is often less than optimal, and up to one-third of patients will not tolerate CPAP. Nonpharmacologic approaches, such as weight loss, have noted limited success. Several clinical studies have suggested that nocturnal hemodialysis or kidney transplantation may have salutary effects on sleep apnea. For example, in a study of 14 patients requiring hemodialysis before and after conversion from conventional thrice-weekly dialysis to nocturnal dialysis, sleep apnea severity improved substantially.[205] Subsequent studies have suggested that improvements in sleep apnea severity associated with nocturnal dialysis are associated with improvements in pharyngeal narrowing and chemoreflex responsiveness.[206,207]

## RESTLESS LEGS SYNDROME

RLS is characterized by an urge to move the legs associated with feelings of discomfort or paresthesias. Symptoms occur during periods of inactivity and are alleviated by movement. The diagnosis of RLS is based on clinical criteria (Box 57.2). The reported prevalence of RLS in ESKD varies widely.[189,194,208,209] The clinical consequences are substantial. RLS impairs health-related quality of life and is associated with an increased risk for all-cause mortality and dialysis withdrawal.[209,210]

The pathogenesis of RLS is associated with disrupted dopaminergic function in the brain. Iron is a cofactor for dopamine production in certain brain regions, and iron deficiency has been implicated as an important contributing factor. Comorbid conditions, immobility, and specific medications may also contribute to the development of RLS in patients with ESKD. To date, no specific uremic risk factors have been identified.

For patients with mild or moderate symptoms, lifestyle modification, such as the practice of good sleep hygiene and elimination of exacerbating substances such as antidepressant medications, caffeine, nicotine, and alcohol, is recommended. For patients with more severe symptoms, dopaminergic therapy is recommended as first-line therapy. Levodopa and the dopamine receptor agonists pramipexole and ropinirole are effective in reducing symptoms of RLS.[211] These agents appear to be safe and effective in short-term studies of patients on dialysis,[212–215] although side effects such as daytime worsening of symptoms may occur with continuous use. Anticonvulsants, such as carbamazepine or gabapentin, and benzodiazepines may be second-line agents for RLS treatment but, with the exception of gabapentin, have not been studied as extensively. Intravenous iron infusion is associated with improvement in RLS symptoms in ESKD.[216,217] Kidney transplantation and short daily hemodialysis, but not conventional dialysis, appear to have a beneficial effect on symptoms.[218,219] Finally, in a clinical trial of 25 patients requiring hemodialysis, RLS symptoms were reduced with intradialytic exercise.[220]

**Box 57.2 The International Restless Legs Syndrome Study Group Criteria**

1. An urge to move the legs, usually accompanied or caused by uncomfortable and unpleasant sensations in the legs.
2. The urge to move or unpleasant sensations begin or worsen during periods of rest or inactivity, such as lying or sitting.
3. The urge to move or unpleasant sensations are partially or totally relieved by movement, such as walking or stretching, for at least as long as the activity continues.
4. The urge to move or unpleasant sensations are worse in the evening or night than during the day or only occur in the evening or night.

All four criteria are required for the diagnosis.

From Allen RP, Picchietti D, Hening WA, et al. Restless legs syndrome: diagnostic criteria, special considerations, and epidemiology. A report from the restless legs syndrome diagnosis and epidemiology workshop at the National Institutes of Health. *Sleep Med.* 2003;4:101–119.

## PERIODIC LIMB MOVEMENTS OF SLEEP

PLMS are characterized by sudden and repetitive jerking movements of the lower extremities during sleep. This disorder is diagnosed by sleep testing. Like other sleep disorders, PLMS are common among patients on dialysis and associated with daytime sleepiness, low quality of life, and, in one study, an increased risk for mortality.[221] The pathogenesis of PLMS remains unknown; however, kidney transplantation has been reported to reduce the frequency of PLMS and improve symptoms of daytime sleepiness.[222]

 Complete reference list available at ExpertConsult.com.

## KEY REFERENCES


1. Teschan PE, Ginn HE, Bourne JR, et al. Quantitative indices of clinical uremia. *Kidney Int.* 1979;15(6):676–697.
11. Seliger SL, Gillen DL, Longstreth WT Jr, et al. Elevated risk of stroke among patients with end-stage renal disease. *Kidney Int.* 2003;64(2):603–609.
12. Sozio SM, Armstrong PA, Coresh J, et al. Cerebrovascular disease incidence, characteristics, and outcomes in patients initiating dialysis: the Choices for Healthy Outcomes in Caring for ESRD (CHOICE) Study. *Am J Kidney Dis.* 2009;54:468–477.
14. Masson P, Kelly PJ, Craig JC, et al. Risk of Stroke in Patients with ESRD. *Clin J Am Soc Nephrol.* 2015;10(9):1585–1592.
18. Yahalom G, Schwartz R, Schwammenthal Y, et al. Chronic kidney disease and clinical outcome in patients with acute stroke. *Stroke.* 2009;40(4):1296–1303.
23. Seliger SL, Longstreth WT Jr, Katz R, et al. Cystatin C and subclinical brain infarction. *J Am Soc Nephrol.* 2005;16(12):3721–3727.
35. Ninomiya T, Perkovic V, Gallagher M, et al. Lower blood pressure and risk of recurrent stroke in patients with chronic kidney disease: PROGRESS trial. *Kidney Int.* 2008;73(8):963–970.
38. Cheung AK, Rahman M, Reboussin DM, et al; Group SR. Effects of intensive BP control in CKD. *J Am Soc Nephrol.* 2017.
51. Ninomiya T, Perkovic V, Verdon C, et al. Proteinuria and stroke: a meta-analysis of cohort studies. *Am J Kidney Dis.* 2009;53(3):417–425.
53. Mahmoodi BK, Yatsuya H, Matsushita K, et al. Association of kidney disease measures with ischemic versus hemorrhagic strokes: pooled analyses of 4 prospective community-based cohorts. *Stroke.* 2014;45(7):1925–1931.
65. Baigent C, Landray MJ, Reith C, et al. The effects of lowering LDL cholesterol with simvastatin plus ezetimibe in patients with chronic kidney disease (Study of Heart and Renal Protection): a randomised placebo-controlled trial. *Lancet.* 2011;377(9784):2181–2192.
74. Skali H, Parving HH, Parfrey PS, et al. Stroke in patients with type 2 diabetes mellitus, chronic kidney disease, and anemia treated with darbepoetin alfa: the Trial to Reduce Cardiovascular Events with Aranesp Therapy (TREAT) experience. *Circulation.* 2011;124(25):2903–2908.
75. Seliger SL, Zhang AD, Weir MR, et al. Erythropoiesis-stimulating agents increase the risk of acute stroke in patients with chronic kidney disease. *Kidney Int.* 2011;80(3):288–294.
105. Sidawy AN, Aidinian G, Johnson ON 3rd, et al. Effect of chronic renal insufficiency on outcomes of carotid endarterectomy. *J Vasc Surg.* 2008;48(6):1423–1430.
106. MacEwen C, Sutherland S, Daly J, et al. Relationship between Hypotension and Cerebral Ischemia during Hemodialysis. *J Am Soc Nephrol.* 2017.
107. Murray AM, Seliger S, Lakshminarayan K, et al. Incidence of stroke before and after dialysis initiation in older patients. *J Am Soc Nephrol.* 2013;24(7):1166–1173.
119. Arieff AI, Massry SG, Barrientos A, et al. Brain water and electrolyte metabolism in uremia: effects of slow and rapid hemodialysis. *Kidney Int.* 1973;4(3):177–187.
130. Kurella Tamura M, Chertow GM, Depner TA, et al. Metabolic profiling of impaired cognitive function in patients receiving dialysis. *J Am Soc Nephrol.* 2016;27(12):3780–3787.
148. Murray AM, Tupper DE, Knopman DS, et al. Cognitive impairment in hemodialysis patients is common. *Neurology.* 2006;67(2):216–223.

153. Hooper SR, Gerson AC, Butler RW, et al. Neurocognitive functioning of children and adolescents with mild-to-moderate chronic kidney disease. *Clin J Am Soc Nephrol.* 2011;6(8):1824–1830.
154. Seliger SL, Siscovick DS, Stehman-Breen CO, et al. Moderate renal impairment and risk of dementia among older adults: the Cardiovascular Health Cognition Study. *J Am Soc Nephrol.* 2004;15(7):1904–1911.
164. Harciarek M, Biedunkiewicz B, Lichodziejewska-Niemierko M, et al. Continuous cognitive improvement 1 year following successful kidney transplant. *Kidney Int.* 2011;79(12):1353–1360.
165. Eldehni MT, Odudu A, McIntyre CW. Randomized clinical trial of dialysate cooling and effects on brain white matter. *J Am Soc Nephrol.* 2015;26(4):957–965.
166. Kurella Tamura M, Unruh ML, Nissenson AR, et al. Effect of more frequent hemodialysis on cognitive function in the frequent hemodialysis network trials. *Am J Kidney Dis.* 2013;61(2):228–237.
185. Bolton CF, Baltzan MA, Baltzan RB. Effects of renal transplantation on uremic neuropathy. A clinical and electrophysiologic study. *N Engl J Med.* 1971;284(21):1170–1175.
191. Perl J, Unruh ML, Chan CT. Sleep disorders in end-stage renal disease: "markers of inadequate dialysis"? *Kidney Int.* 2006;70(10):1687–1693.
197. Unruh ML, Sanders MH, Redline S, et al. Sleep apnea in patients on conventional thrice-weekly hemodialysis: comparison with matched controls from the Sleep Heart Health Study. *J Am Soc Nephrol.* 2006;17(12):3503–3509.
205. Hanly PJ, Pierratos A. Improvement of sleep apnea in patients with chronic renal failure who undergo nocturnal hemodialysis. *N Engl J Med.* 2001;344(2):102–107.
216. Sloand JA, Shelly MA, Feigin A, et al. A double-blind, placebo-controlled trial of intravenous iron dextran therapy in patients with ESRD and restless legs syndrome. *Am J Kidney Dis.* 2004;43(4):663–670.
217. Benz RL, Pressman MR, Hovick ET, et al. A preliminary study of the effects of correction of anemia with recombinant human erythropoietin therapy on sleep, sleep disorders, and daytime sleepiness in hemodialysis patients (the SLEEPO study). *Am J Kidney Dis.* 1999;34(6):1089–1095.
219. Jaber BL, Schiller B, Burkart JM, et al. Impact of short daily hemodialysis on restless legs symptoms and sleep disturbances. *Clin J Am Soc Nephrol.* 2011;6(5):1049–1056.

# 58 Dermatologic Conditions in Kidney Disease

Christine J. Ko | Shawn E. Cowper

**CHAPTER OUTLINE**



**KEY POINTS**

- Skin manifestations of end-stage renal disease are diverse, with pruritus being very common.
- Calciphylaxis may lead to high morbidity and mortality. Skin lesions range morphologically from a broken-up, lacelike pattern of pink to purple erythema early on (reticulated vascular pattern) to ulcers, with black eschars in later stages.
- Pseudoporphyria and porphyria cutanea tarda may have very similar clinical presentations. Normal levels of plasma uroporphyrin and red blood cell protoporphyrin are typical of the former.

Many patients with end-stage renal disease (ESRD) have associated skin manifestations.[1,2] In addition, skin findings may specifically direct an astute clinician to check for concomitant renal dysfunction. This chapter summarizes different dermatologic conditions that may be seen in patients with kidney disorders. Because of the large number of diseases falling into this category (Boxes 58.1 to 58.4 and Table 58.1), emphasis is placed on the more commonly encountered entities.

## SKIN MANIFESTATIONS SECONDARY TO KIDNEY DYSFUNCTION

See Box 58.1.

### SIGNS AND SYMPTOMS

#### PRURITUS

Pruritus is more common in patients with ESRD disease than in those with acute kidney injury (AKI). Up to 90% of patients undergoing hemodialysis may experience pruritus, and patients undergoing hemodialysis are more commonly affected than patients undergoing peritoneal dialysis.[2] In one of the largest trials (the Dialysis Outcomes and Practice Patterns Study [DOPPS]), pruritus was noted in 42% of hemodialysis patients. Sleep and mood are negatively affected.[3] Patients with severe pruritus have a poor outcome compared with patients undergoing hemodialysis without severe pruritus.[4]

Patients complaining of pruritus may or may not have skin changes. Pruritus can be defined as at least three episodes of itch in a 2-week period that cause difficulty for the patient or as itch that occurs over a 6-month period in a regular pattern.[3] Pruritus can be localized or generalized.[5] When present, skin manifestations are secondary, with excoriations being the main finding (Fig. 58.1). Lichenified skin, prurigo nodularis, and koebnerization (the appearance of skin lesions on lines of trauma) may also be seen. Pruritus tends to be prolonged, frequent, and intense.[3] Exacerbating factors include heat, nighttime dry skin, and sweat.[3]

The cause of pruritus in renal failure is unclear and may be multifactorial. Risk factors include male gender and high levels of urea, $\beta_2$-microglobulin, calcium, and phosphate.[4,6] Patients treated with angiotensin-converting enzyme inhibitors are more likely to have pruritus than those receiving furosemide.[3] Decreasing urine output, secondary hyperparathyroidism, abnormal levels of magnesium and aluminum, increased levels of histamine and vitamin A, increased numbers of mast cells,[7] xerosis,[8] and iron deficiency anemia are other proposed factors.[9,10]

Pruritus is transmitted through C fibers in the skin.[11] C group fibers are unmyelinated and have a small diameter and low conduction velocity. They represent one of three

**Box 58.1 Skin Manifestations Secondary to Renal Disease**

**Nonspecific**

Pruritus
Xerosis
Acquired ichthyosis
Pigmentary alteration
- Pallor (secondary to anemia)
- Hyperpigmentation
- Dyspigmentation (yellow tint)

Infections (fungal, bacterial, viral)
Purpura

**Somewhat Specific**

Acquired perforating dermatosis
Calciphylaxis
Metastatic calcification
Blistering disorders
- Porphyria cutanea tarda
- Pseudoporphyria

Eruptive xanthomas
Pseudo–Kaposi sarcoma

**Specific**

Nephrogenic systemic fibrosis
Dialysis-associated steal syndrome
Metastatic renal cell carcinoma
Dialysis-related amyloidosis
Arteriovenous shunt dermatitis
Uremic frost

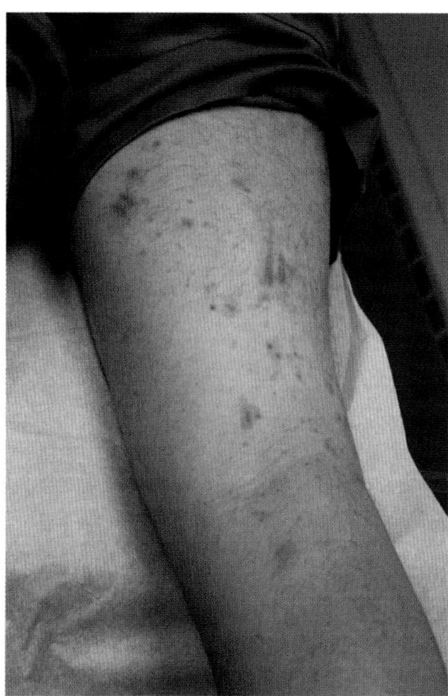

**Fig. 58.1 Pruritus.** Shown is a patient with linear excoriations. (Courtesy Dr. Oscar Colegio.)

classes of nerve fibers in the peripheral nervous system and carry sensory information. They are afferent fibers, sending input signals from the periphery to the central nervous system (CNS). Known stimulants of C fibers include cytokines, histamine, serotonin, prostaglandins, neuropeptides,[5] and enzymes.[12] Because cytokines can stimulate nerve fibers,[12] one major theory regarding the pathogenesis of pruritus in renal failure is that it involves systemic inflammation.[13] Markers of inflammation, such as C-reactive protein and interleukin-6, show elevated levels in pruritus associated with renal disease.[13,14] An imbalance of inflammatory proteins may somehow lead to pruritus. This theory is supported by the fact that ultraviolet light treatments, which can decrease the levels of inflammation markers,[15] often ameliorate pruritus.

Another major theory focuses on the opioid system. Opioids can stimulate C fibers.[12] Central μ-opioid receptor stimulation in mice leads to scratching, and this can be prevented by central κ-opioid receptor stimulation.[16] Successful treatment of patients with opioid antagonists also supports the involvement of the opioid system in pruritus.[17–19] Other potentially pathogenic factors include xerosis, elevated histamine, excess uremic toxins, peripheral neuropathy, and hyperparathyroidism.[2]

Treatment of pruritus must be tailored to the individual patient. In general, antihistamines are not effective.[20] Any condition that can exacerbate pruritus, such as xerosis, should be treated.[21] Symptoms may be alleviated by optimization of hemodialysis[1] and administration of erythropoietin.[22] For more localized areas of pruritus, topical corticosteroids, pramoxine (also known as pramocaine),[23] and capsaicin[5,24] may be used. In addition, twice-weekly ultraviolet light phototherapy is effective.[25] Oral treatments include gamma-linoleic acid,[26] naltrexone,[17,18] cholestyramine,[27] gabapentin,[28,29] pregabalin,[30] thalidomide,[31] and activated charcoal.[32] κ-Opioid receptor agonists such as nalfurafine[19] and nalbuphine[33] may be helpful. Kidney transplantation may effectively "cure" patients,[34] as may parathyroidectomy.[35]

A therapeutic ladder has been proposed, based on efficacy and safety considerations.[34] The first rung of the ladder consists of emollients and capsaicin. If pruritus is not relieved, ultraviolet light treatments can be added. Phototherapy with ultraviolet B (UVB; 280–320 nm) is effective in reducing pruritus in dialysis patients and may act by suppressing histamine release or vitamin A levels in the epidermis, which are known pruritogenic substrates. Importantly, the risk of skin cancer should be balanced with decision making, especially in patients who are on immunosuppressive therapy. UVB radiation is absorbed in the epidermis and superficial dermis by molecules called "chromophores," which include DNA, urocanic acid, keratin, and melanin. UVB radiation induces the release of a variety of proinflammatory and immunosuppressive cytokines from keratinocytes and T cells. If light treatments fail or are not feasible for the patient, oral gabapentin or intravenous nalfurafine may be considered.

## XEROSIS

Xerosis, or dry skin, is quite common in the general population. The skin appears dry, rough, or shiny. It may be scaly or fissured, with a cracked appearance. Xerotic skin may or may not be pruritic.[21] If it is pruritic, there may be excoriations. Skin involvement may be diffuse but is often most prominent over the extensor surfaces of the lower extremities (Fig. 58.2).[1]

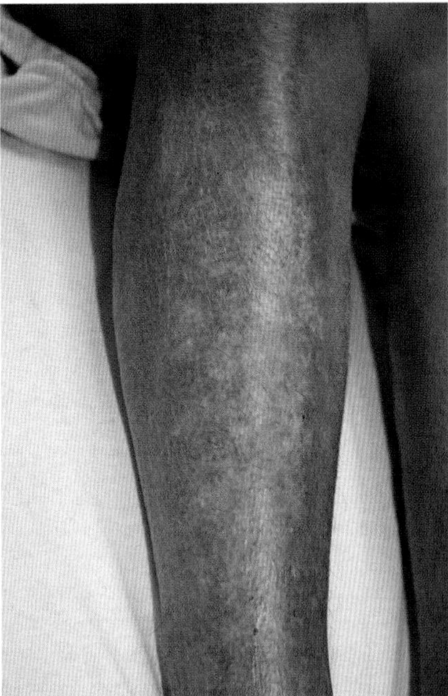

**Fig. 58.2** Xerosis and dyspigmentation. (Courtesy Dr. Marcus McFerren.)

The cause of xerosis is unknown. Decreased stratum corneum hydration[21] and abnormal eccrine gland function[36] are two proposed mechanisms. The mainstay of treatment is hydration of the skin. For pruritic cases, direct treatment of the pruritus may be helpful.

### ACQUIRED ICHTHYOSIS

Ichthyosis is related to xerosis but is more than just dry skin because the skin develops patterned scale. Histopathologic features include hyperkeratosis and occasionally epidermal hypogranulosis. The pathogenesis of acquired ichthyosis in renal failure is unknown. Treatment consists of hydration of the skin.

### PIGMENTARY ALTERATION

Of patients undergoing dialysis, 70% or more may have pigmentary changes of the skin.[2,37] The most common alteration is the development of a yellowish tint. This is more common among patients undergoing hemodialysis than those on peritoneal dialysis.[2] Hyperpigmentation may be secondary to increased melanin production as a result of elevated levels of β-melanocyte–stimulating hormone.[38] Pallor of the skin secondary to anemia has also been described.[1]

## MANIFESTATIONS SOMEWHAT SPECIFIC TO KIDNEY DISEASE

### ACQUIRED PERFORATING DERMATOSIS

An umbrella term for perforating disorders in adults with kidney dysfunction and/or diabetes mellitus is "acquired perforating dermatosis." This term is often used in place of older nomenclature (e.g., perforating folliculitis, Kyrle disease, reactive perforating collagenosis). Some authors consider this disorder to be a variant of prurigo nodularis.[39] Pruritus is generally severe.[40] Lesions are distributed predominantly on the legs and arms, although the trunk and head may also be involved. Individual lesions are crateriform, umbilicated, or centrally hyperkeratotic papules and nodules (Fig. 58.3). They may develop in crops and commonly resolve with scarring after 6 to 8 weeks. Histopathologic evidence of extrusion of dermal material through an epidermal channel is necessary for the diagnosis (Fig. 58.4).

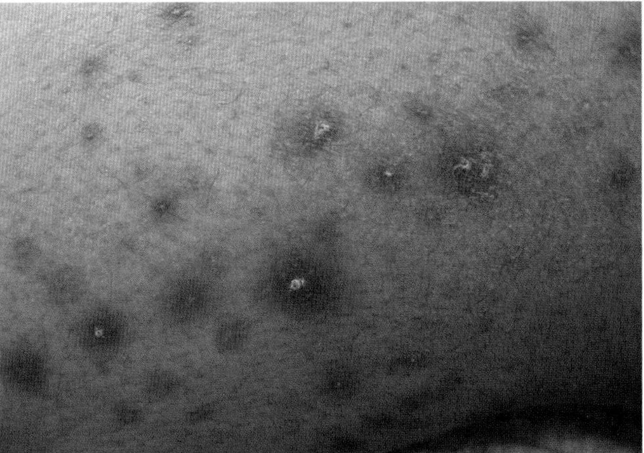

**Fig. 58.3** Acquired perforating dermatosis. (Courtesy Yale Residents' Collection.)

The pathogenesis of this disorder is unknown. Proposed factors include increased fibronectin,[41] pruritus and scratching,[40] epidermal dysmaturation, and dermal deposition of substances not excreted in renal failure.[42,43] Patients with diabetes and renal failure are more likely to manifest acquired perforating dermatosis than patients without diabetes.[1,40] Other associations include hepatitis and hypothyroidism.[43] Patients who are otherwise healthy may also develop acquired perforating dermatosis.[43] Treatment of this disorder is difficult, with some relief afforded by topical steroids, keratolytics, lubrication, and topical or oral retinoids.[42] Narrow-band UVB light may also be helpful.[44] Patients with severe and generalized pruritus may benefit from treatments specifically directed at pruritus.

### CALCIPHYLAXIS (CALCIFIC UREMIC ARTERIOLOPATHY)

Calciphylaxis is most often seen in patients with ESRD who are on hemodialysis, generally with associated hyperparathyroidism or an elevated calcium phosphate product. Although rare, calcific uremic arteriolopathy (CUA) can also present in chronic kidney disease (CKD). An incidence of approximately 4% of patients/year at one dialysis center has been reported.[45] Morbidity and mortality are high, especially once ulceration develops.[45] Involvement of the trunk and buttocks is associated with high mortality.[46] Other risk factors include female gender,[45] diabetes,[45] obesity, hypoalbuminemia,[47] malignancy, administration of systemic steroids, iron usage, warfarin use,[47] chemotherapy, systemic inflammation, hepatic cirrhosis, rapid weight loss, protein C or S deficiency, and infection.[48]

The precise mechanism of calciphylaxis is unclear. The classic model, as described by Selye in rats, hypothesized a predisposing factor, with a secondary inciting factor.[49] This model has been criticized as not being fully reflective of calciphylaxis in humans, because Selye rats displayed only

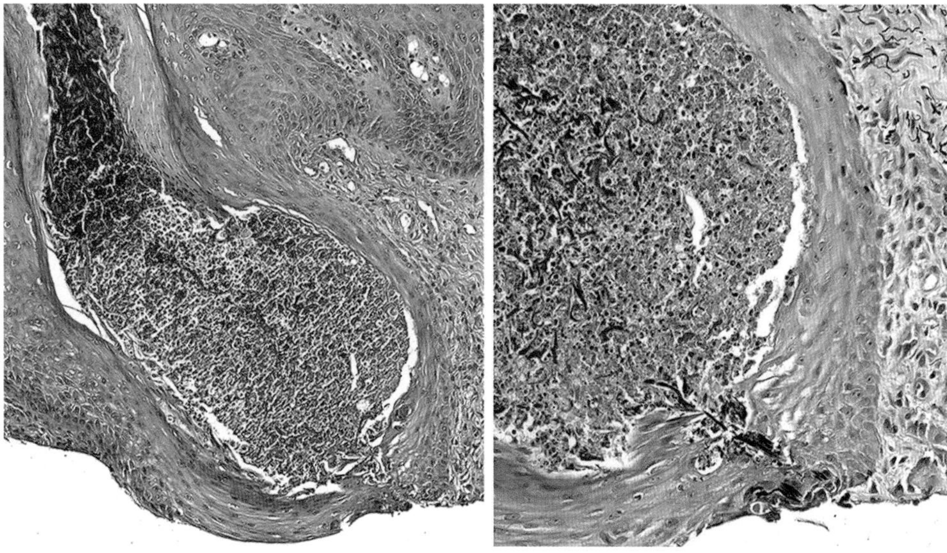

**Fig. 58.4 Acquired perforating dermatosis.** There is an epidermal channel with extrusion of dermal elastic material and inflammatory cells. (*Left,* Hematoxylin and eosin stain, ×40; *right,* elastic van Gieson stain, ×100.)

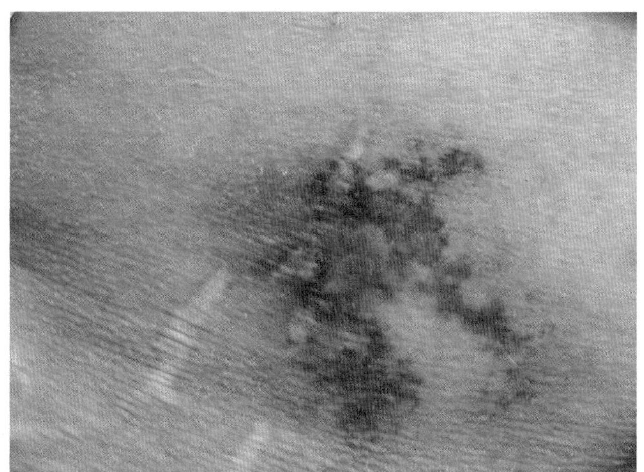

**Fig. 58.5 Calciphylaxis.** Shown is an early lesion with a retiform purpuric appearance.

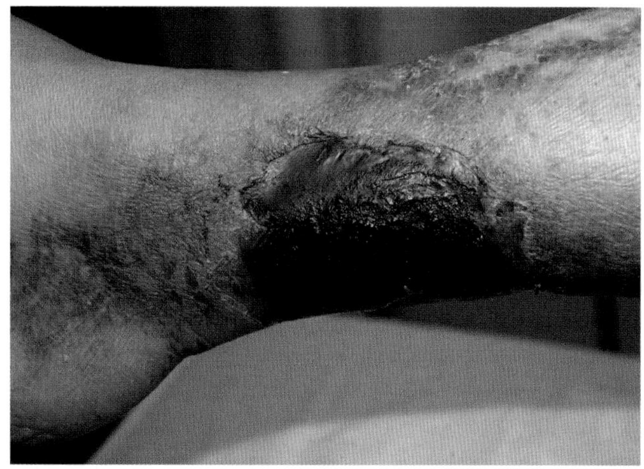

**Fig. 58.6 Calciphylaxis.** Shown is an ulcerated lesion with black eschar. (Courtesy Yale Residents' Collection.)

soft tissue calcification and not skin necrosis.[50,51] Although prior literature focused on calcium, phosphate, and inhibitors and inducers of vascular calcification,[51] hypercoagulability may play a more important role.[52]

Clinically, calciphylaxis usually affects the fatty areas of the thighs, abdomen, and buttocks symmetrically. Lesions may also affect the lower extremities.[45] Early lesions may be pink-violaceous, broken-up circles, firm plaques, solid purple-pink or mottled, retiform purpura, erosions, or subcutaneous nodules (Fig. 58.5).[53] Occasionally, bullae may be seen. Early lesions may progress to painful ulcers with a black eschar (Fig. 58.6). Surrounding the ulcers, there may be skin mottling, with reticulate dyspigmentation. The skin may be tender. Histopathologic findings supportive of calciphylaxis include medial calcification of medium-sized vessels (Fig. 58.7), with intimal hyperplasia and thrombosis. Special stains, such as von Kossa or alizarin red, may be required to detect early calcification. Radiographic studies and tissue mammography may also show linear calcium deposits

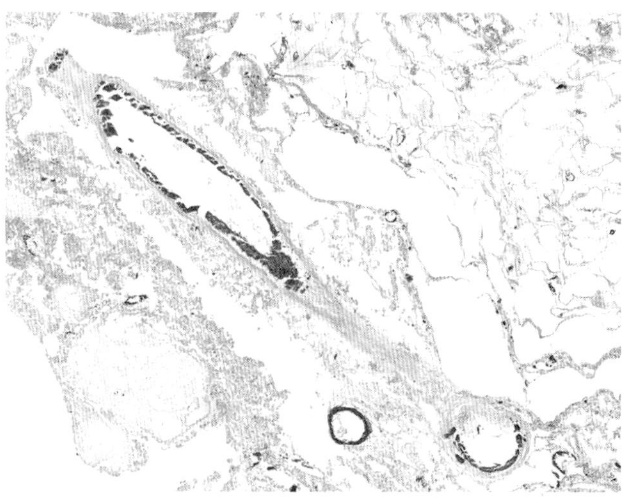

**Fig. 58.7** Calciphylaxis. Shown are medium-sized vessels with extensive calcium deposition. (Hematoxylin and eosin stain, ×40.)

in the skin. Laboratory evaluation should include renal function, evaluation of parameters related to bone mineralization (e.g., calcium, phosphate, parathyroid hormone), workup for thrombophilia, liver function, assessment for any infections based on the patient's presentation, and evaluation for autoimmune diseases, as clinically indicated. Deficiencies in inhibitors of vascular calcifications may play a role in CUA pathogenesis, especially fetuin-A and vitamin K–dependent matrix Gla protein. Polymorphisms in ecto-5′-nucleotidase CD73, vitamin D receptor, and fibroblast growth factor-23 (FGF-23) have been suggested to play a role in calciphylaxis development.[54]

Supportive and preventive measures are the mainstay of treatment, including wound care, pain management, and modification of any risk factors. For nonulcerated lesions, systemic steroids may lead to rapid healing.[45] Ulcers should be kept clean, débrided if necessary, with the addition of hyperbaric oxygen therapy[55] and/or antibiotics, depending on clinical factors and the response. Potentially associated factors such as elevated calcium and phosphate levels can be addressed with intravenous sodium thiosulfate,[56] parathyroidectomy,[45,50] oral cinacalcet and phosphate binders,[57] use of low-calcium dialysate and non–calcium-based phosphate binders,[58] and bisphosphonates.[59] If there is a hypercoagulable state, anticoagulation may be considered. If the patient is on warfarin, it is worthwhile to consider changing to another anticoagulant.[51,52]

## METASTATIC CALCIFICATION

An abnormal calcium phosphate product, with or without hyperparathyroidism, can lead to metastatic calcification of the skin. Clinically, lesions are hard, yellow to bluish papules and nodules, which usually affect periarticular areas and the fingertips.[58] A biopsy specimen from a nodule should reveal calcium deposits in the tissue. Importantly, not all calcification in the skin is secondary to metastatic calcification. Trauma may result in so-called dystrophic calcification. Some systemic diseases, such as dermatomyositis, may be associated with calcification of the skin. Calcification may also be idiopathic.

Treatment of metastatic calcification focuses on normalizing calcium and phosphate levels. If hyperparathyroidism is present, parathyroidectomy may be beneficial. Use of phosphate binders and reduction of dietary phosphate are important. Foods that should be avoided include milk and milk products, certain vegetables (e.g., broccoli, Brussels sprouts), oysters, salmon, beer, nuts, and wheat germ.[58] If particular lesions are symptomatic, surgical removal may be considered.

## PORPHYRIA CUTANEA TARDA

Up to 18% of patients with renal failure may have porphyria cutanea tarda, with a deficient activity of the heme biosynthetic enzyme uroporphyrinogen decarboxylase (UROD) in the liver. These patients have elevated levels of urinary uroporphyrin (if not anuric) and fecal isocoproporphyrin. The pathogenesis of porphyria cutanea tarda in renal patients is unclear, yet reduced UROD activity is responsible for the accumulation of porphyrinogens that are auto-oxidized to photosensitizing porphyrins. These cause photodamage on exposure to light with a wavelength near 400 nm. Heterozygosity for a UROD mutation may predispose some patients, with acquired functional UROD deficiency being superimposed. The serum aluminum level may also be a contributing factor.[60] Other risk factors for the development of porphyria cutanea tarda include hepatitis B and C, estrogen administration, excess alcohol intake, and human immunodeficiency virus (HIV) infection.

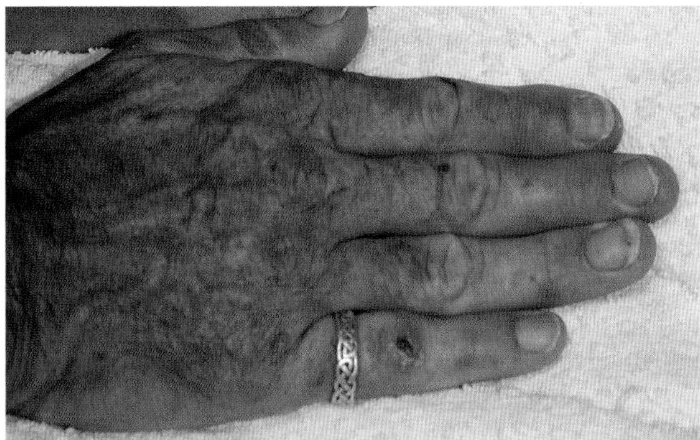

**Fig. 58.8 Porphyria cutanea tarda.** Shown are eroded blisters and crusts. (Courtesy Yale Residents' Collection.)

Cutaneous findings include noninflamed blisters, erosions, and crusts (Fig. 58.8), especially those involving the dorsal hands and forearms. Blisters may heal with scarring or milia. There may be notable hypertrichosis on the face. Hyperpigmentation and sclerodermoid plaques have also been described. Biopsy findings typically include a subepidermal cleft, with minimal inflammation. There may be festooning of the papillary dermis at the base of the cleft. Thickened vessel walls may be present. Direct immunofluorescent findings in porphyria cutanea tarda include granular to linear staining of immunoglobulin G (IgG) and C3 at the dermoepidermal junction and sometimes around vessels.

Treatment includes sun avoidance and sun protection. Concomitant exacerbating factors (e.g., alcohol, estrogens, iron, hepatitis) should be avoided or treated. Because iron overload can exacerbate the disease, small-volume phlebotomy may be helpful, although anemia needs to be carefully monitored. Desferoxamine, an iron chelator, is also sometimes used. If a patient is not anuric, chloroquine may be used cautiously.[58]

## PSEUDOPORPHYRIA

In pseudoporphyria, patients have a presentation similar to that in porphyria cutanea tarda, with noninflamed blisters on the extremities, especially the hands and forearms and other sun-exposed areas. Milia, scarring, and hyperpigmentation may result.[61] Hypertrichosis is seen in a minority of patients.[61] Plasma uroporphyrin and red blood cell protoporphyrin levels rarely are elevated.[60] The separation of pseudoporphyria from porphyria cutanea tarda is clearer when these levels are normal.[61] Concomitant use of drugs such as tetracycline, furosemide, naproxen, amiodarone, and nalidixic acid may be involved in the development of pseudoporphyria.[61] Histologic findings are similar to those of porphyria cutanea tarda.[61] Although the pathogenesis of pseudoporphyria is unclear, elevated aluminum levels were found in a small study.[60]

### ERUPTIVE XANTHOMAS

Eruptive xanthomas are yellow-orange smooth papules and plaques (Fig. 58.9) that rapidly appear on the buttocks and proximal extremities. Histopathologic examination of a lesion reveals extracellular lipid and foamy macrophages (Fig. 58.10). These lesions are associated with hyperlipidemia, either familial or due to other causes, such as hypothyroidism and nephrotic syndrome. In nephrotic syndrome, the xanthomas are likely secondary to various lipid abnormalities, including elevated levels of cholesterol and triglycerides, elevated lipoprotein synthesis, diminished level of lipoprotein lipase, and elevated apolipoprotein B-100 level, with diminished hepatic uptake of lipoproteins.[62] Generally, eruptive xanthomas resolve spontaneously once lipid levels are normalized.

### PSEUDO–KAPOSI SARCOMA

Very rarely, patients may develop a vascular proliferation that mimics Kaposi sarcoma near or over an arteriovenous shunt.[63]

### IODODERMA

Often, in the setting of renal insufficiency or failure, patients who receive iodide in the form of intravenous contrast may develop translucent papulonodular or vegetative lesions of iododerma (Fig. 58.11).[64] Histopathologically, there is marked epidermal hyperplasia, with intraepidermal pustules of neutrophils and sometimes eosinophils (Fig. 58.12). Clinical and histopathologic exclusion of infectious causes is required.

## MANIFESTATIONS SPECIFIC TO KIDNEY DISEASE

See Box 58.1.

### NEPHROGENIC SYSTEMIC FIBROSIS

The first case of nephrogenic systemic fibrosis (NSF), originally described under various terms, including "scleromyxedema-like changes in renal failure" and "nephrogenic fibrosing

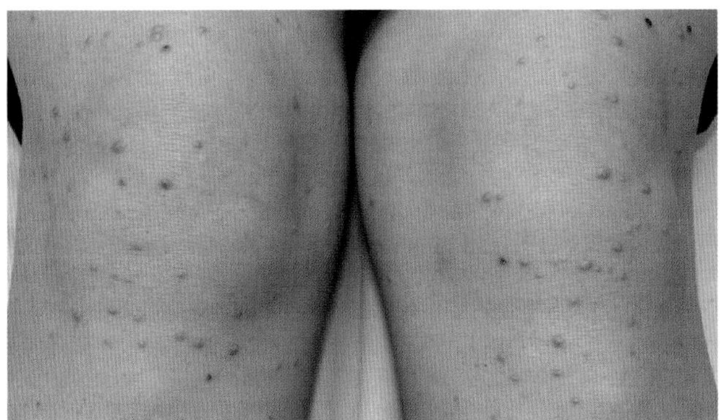

**Fig. 58.9 Eruptive xanthomas.** Shown are small, yellow-orange papules over the knees. (Courtesy Yale Residents' Collection.)

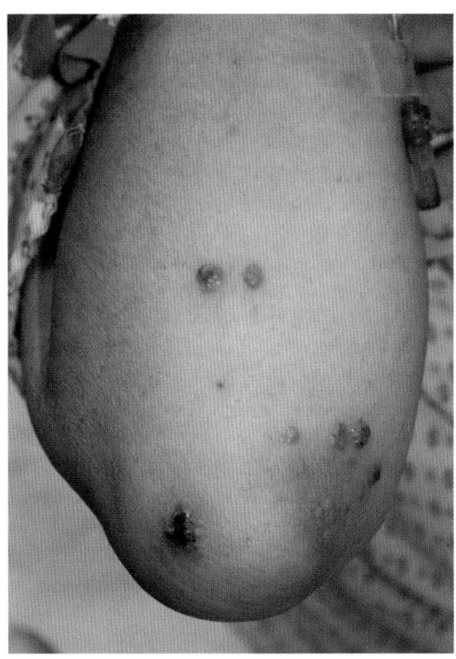

**Fig. 58.11 Iododerma.** Shown are translucent papules and crusted plaques on the elbow. (Courtesy Dr. Oscar Colegio and Dr. Christine Warren.)

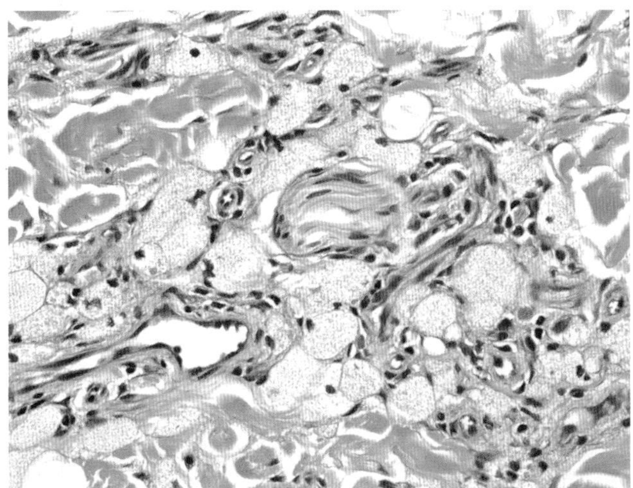

**Fig. 58.10 Eruptive xanthoma.** Shown are lipid-containing foamy macrophages within the dermis. (Hematoxylin and eosin stain, ×40.)

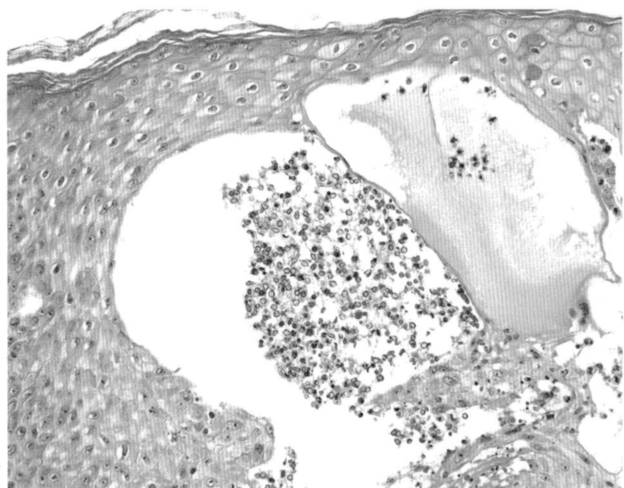

**Fig. 58.12 Iododerma.** Shown is epidermal hyperplasia with intraepidermal pustules. (Hematoxylin and eosin stain, ×200.)

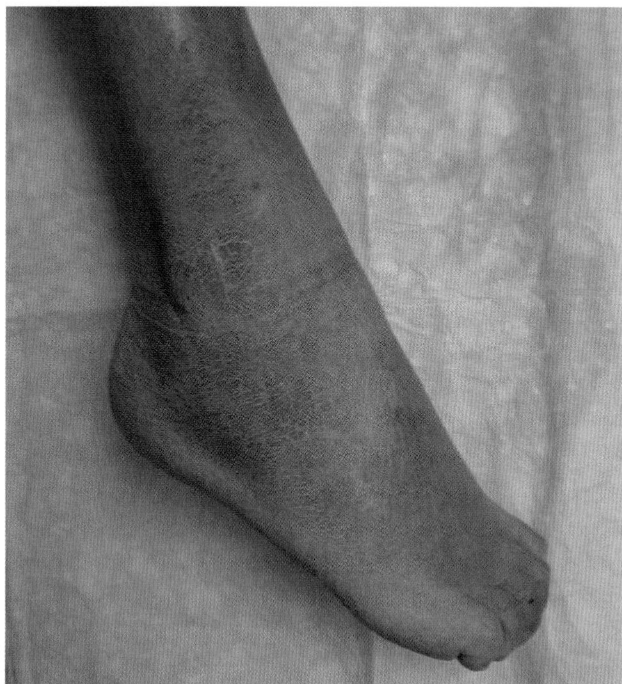

**Fig. 58.13 Nephrogenic systemic fibrosis.** The lower leg has indurated, bound-down skin and contractures of the toes. (From Cowper SE, Rabach M, Girardi M. Clinical and histological findings in nephrogenic systemic fibrosis. *Eur J Radiol.* 2008;66[2]:191–199.)

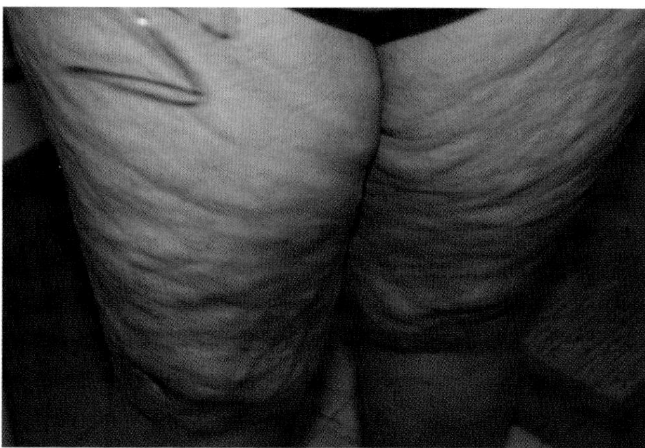

**Fig. 58.14 Nephrogenic systemic fibrosis.** The legs have the cobblestone appearance of indurated skin. (From Girardi M. Nephrogenic systemic fibrosis: a dermatologist's perspective, *J Am Coll Radiol.* 2008;5[1]:40–44.)

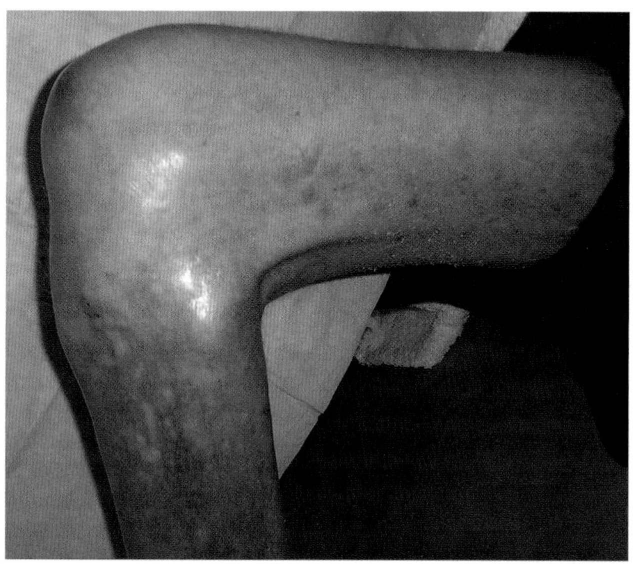

**Fig. 58.15 Nephrogenic systemic fibrosis.** Shown is a joint contracture. (From Girardi M. Nephrogenic systemic fibrosis: a dermatologist's perspective, *J Am Coll Radiol.* 2008;5[1]:40–44.)

dermopathy,"[65] was identified in 1997. Although the cause of NSF was long debated, exposure to gadolinium-based magnetic resonance imaging (MRI) contrast agents in patients with abnormal renal function is now considered the precipitating factor.[66,67] The U.S. Food and Drug Administration (FDA) recommends caution when using gadolinium in patients with an estimated glomerular filtration rate (eGFR) less than 30 mL/min/1.73 m$^2$, undergoing dialysis, or with AKI. The latter is especially important given that it is difficult to predict eGFR in a non–steady-state setting. Gadolinium, an element highly toxic to tissues in its unbound state, is present in a chelated form in contrast agents such as gadodiamide (Omniscan; GE Healthcare, Piscataway, NJ) and gadopentetate dimeglumine (Magnevist; Bayer HealthCare, Whippany, NJ). Gadolinium is a nonradioactive paramagnetic element in the lanthanide series. Impaired excretion of gadolinium-based contrast may allow more time for gadolinium atoms to dissociate from their proprietary ligand molecule. Unbound gadolinium is theorized to bind to other available anions (chiefly phosphates) and deposit peripherally, perhaps inducing long-standing effects on local tissue fibroblasts and/or circulating matrix stem cells termed "circulating fibrocytes." Gadolinium has been detected in tissues of patients with NSF and in in vivo animal studies, findings that corroborate the postulated effects of prolonged gadolinium exposure.[68]

Clinically, patients with NSF have bound-down, indurated skin on the extremities (Fig. 58.13), although truncal involvement has also been reported. The skin may have a cobblestone appearance (Fig. 58.14). Early in NSF, patients may have edema and erythema that mimics cellulitis. Joint contractures (Fig. 58.15; see Fig. 58.13) and yellow scleral plaques (Fig. 58.16) are common. Histopathologically, increased dermal and/or subcutaneous fibroblast-like cells are seen (Fig. 58.17). A deep biopsy may be needed because the fibrotic lesions can extend into the subcutaneous tissue. The cells stain with procollagen I and CD34 by immunohistochemical methods. It is postulated that these cells are circulating fibrocytes.[69] Mucin deposition may also be observed. The prevalence of systemic involvement is unknown, but a number of different organ system manifestations have been described (e.g., heart, muscle, lung). Patients with systemic disease may have marked elevations in their erythrocyte sedimentation rate and serum C-reactive protein level. The clinical and histopathologic differentials are broad and overlap with some more common entities, such as lipodermatosclerosis and morphea. Clinicopathologic correlation is essential to reach an accurate diagnosis.[70]

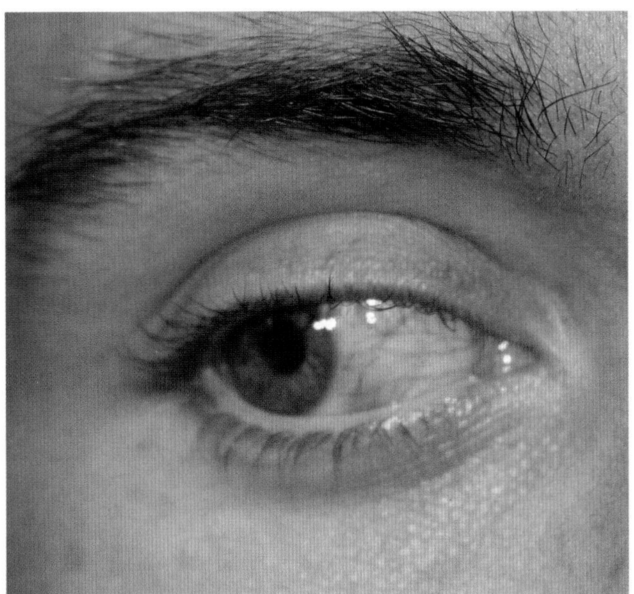

**Fig. 58.16 Nephrogenic systemic fibrosis.** Shown is a scleral plaque. (From Cowper SE, Rabach M, Girardi M. Clinical and histological findings in nephrogenic systemic fibrosis. *Eur J Radiol.* 2008;66[2]:191–199.)

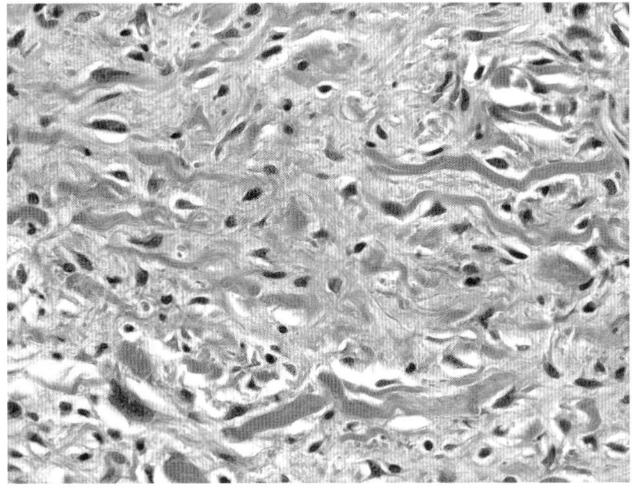

**Fig. 58.17 Nephrogenic systemic fibrosis.** There are increased numbers of fibroblast-like cells, preserved elastic tissue, and increased space between collagen bundles, suggestive of mucin deposition. (Hematoxylin and eosin stain, ×200.)

Prevention of NSF by avoiding the administration of gadolinium-containing agents to patients with CKD or ESKD is key because there is no reliable treatment for the disease. There is evidence that a dose-response relationship exists. The risk in individuals with eGFR of 15 to 59 mL/min/1.73 $m^2$ remains unclear, but cases have been reported. Changes in the labeling of gadolinium-containing contrast agents and careful screening of patients for underlying kidney disease have been successful preventive measures. In patients who develop the disorder, renal transplantation is sometimes helpful in halting progression and occasionally reverses the disease.[71] Extracorporeal photopheresis may also be useful. Physical therapy may ameliorate some symptoms for patients. Reports of imatinib treatment are encouraging.[72]

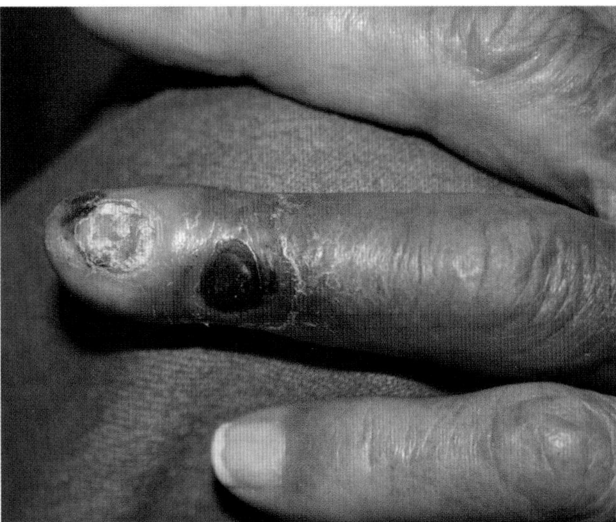

**Fig. 58.18 Dialysis-associated steal syndrome.** Shown is an ulcer with overlying crust, with surrounding erythema, distal pallor, and nail atrophy. (From Kravetz JD, Heald P. Bilateral dialysis-associated steal syndrome, *J Am Acad Dermatol.* 2008;58:888–891,2008.)

## DIALYSIS-ASSOCIATED STEAL SYNDROME

Dialysis-associated steal syndrome is a rare complication of fistula construction.[73] This syndrome usually involves the brachial area in patients with diabetes. There may be associated pallor or a reticulated pink to blue discoloration of the skin surrounding necrosis, ulceration, or gangrene (Fig. 58.18). Altered hemodynamics secondary to the fistula result in decreased distal perfusion. Associated risk factors are diabetes, vascular stenosis, neuropathic disease, and calcifying sclerosis. Effective treatment involves fistula ligation and/ or banding.

## METASTATIC RENAL CELL CARCINOMA

Although approximately 4.6% of cutaneous metastases originate from the kidney, only 3% to 4% of renal cell carcinomas metastasize to the skin.[74] Metastases may occasionally precede the diagnosis of the primary tumor, but often they are a late manifestation.[75] The prognosis is poor, with a 5-year survival of less than 5%. Common cutaneous sites for metastatic renal cell carcinoma are the trunk and scalp.[75] Nodules may be flesh-colored, violaceous, or pink-red. Histopathologic examination often shows a tumor with clear cells and prominent hemorrhage. The latter is a feature of the highly vascular nature of von Hippel–Lindau (VHL)-deficient clear cell renal cell carcinoma.

## DIALYSIS-RELATED AMYLOIDOSIS

Dialysis-related amyloidosis is secondary to $\beta_2$-microglobulin deposition. Unlike AL amyloid, skin involvement is unusual, and the more common presentations involve carpal tunnel syndrome and destructive arthropathy. However, there have been rare reports of immobile dermal nodules secondary to $\beta_2$-microglobulin deposition, most often affecting the buttocks.[76,77]

## ARTERIOVENOUS SHUNT DERMATITIS

In one study, 7 of 88 patients on long-term hemodialysis developed an irritant contact dermatitis over their shunts.[78]

None of the patients had an allergic component to the rash. Substituting normal saline for the cleansers (soaps, disinfectants, and alcohol) used to clean the skin before hemodialysis was helpful in alleviating the skin rash. Use of a mild topical steroid was also helpful.

## NAIL CHANGES ASSOCIATED WITH KIDNEY DISEASE

See Box 58.2.

### LINDSAY (HALF-AND-HALF) NAIL

Up to 40% of patients with renal dysfunction have half-and-half nails (Fig. 58.19).[2] The condition may resolve spontaneously and is likely secondary to melanin deposition in the nail bed and plate. Fingernails are affected more commonly than toenails. The nails have a white to normal proximal half and a red-brown distal half.

## SELECTED CONDITIONS WITH SKIN AND RENAL INVOLVEMENT

See Box 58.3.

### LUPUS ERYTHEMATOSUS

The skin manifestations of lupus erythematosus are varied. Acute skin changes include the classic malar rash. Annular plaques and papules with scale and erythema are typical of subcutaneous lupus erythematosus. These lesions generally resolve without scarring. In discoid lupus erythematosus, coin-shaped to oval plaques heal with dyspigmentation and scarring. There is often adherent scale within the lesions that, when lifted off, has a "carpet tack" appearance on the underside. Such discoid lesions in the conchal bowl of the ear are characteristic of lupus erythematosus (Fig. 58.20). Neonates with lupus erythematosus may occasionally have annular, erythematous plaques in sun-exposed areas. In addition to these skin lesions, patients may complain of photosensitivity, oral ulcers, or alopecia.

The different skin manifestations of lupus look similar histopathologically. There are vacuolar changes at the dermoepidermal junction, with a variable infiltrate of lymphocytes. There is often a superficial and deep perivascular and periadnexal lymphocytic infiltrate as well. Mucin may be increased. Direct immunofluorescence testing may show a discontinuous linear band of IgG, C3, IgA, and/or IgM at the dermoepidermal junction.

The pathogenesis of lupus erythematosus involves autoantibodies that can form immune complexes that deposit

**Box 58.2 Nail Changes Associated With Kidney Disease**

- Lindsay (half-and-half) nail
- Triangular lunulae (nail patella syndrome)
- Splinter hemorrhages
- Onychomycosis
- Koilonychia
- Onycholysis
- Mees lines
- Muehrcke lines
- Beau lines

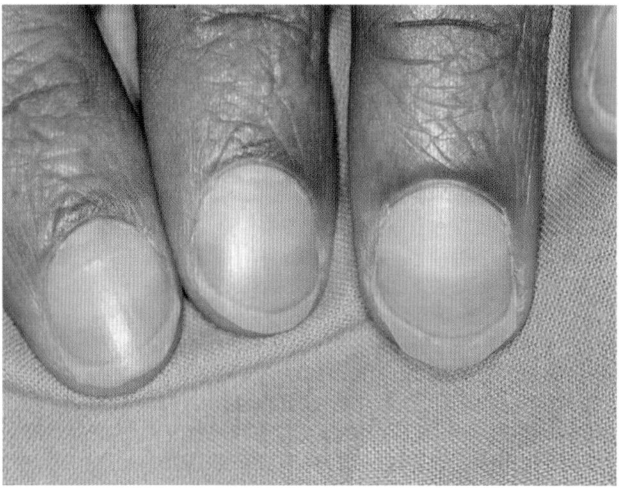

**Fig. 58.19 Lindsay (half-and-half) nail.** (From Butler DF. Pruritus. In Schwarzenberger K, Werchniak A, Ko C, eds. *General Dermatology*. Philadelphia: Saunders; 2009:17–22.)

**Box 58.3 Selected Conditions With Concurrent Skin and Renal Involvement**

**More Common**

- Lupus erythematosus
- Leukocytoclastic vasculitis
- Henoch–Schönlein purpura
- Mixed cryoglobulinemia
- Diabetes mellitus
- Systemic vasculitis

**Less Common**

- Nail–patella syndrome
- Hemolytic-uremic syndrome
- Toxic shock syndrome
- Mixed connective tissue disease
- Dermatomyositis
- Rheumatoid arthritis
- Sjögren syndrome
- Dermatitis herpetiformis
- Sarcoidosis
- Systemic sclerosis
- Ulcerative colitis
- Amyloidosis
- Toxic epidermolysis
- Hypothyroidism
- Graves disease
- Fabry disease
- Neurofibromatosis
- Hurler syndrome
- Castleman disease
- Infectious endocarditis
- Staphylococcal scalded skin syndrome (in adults)

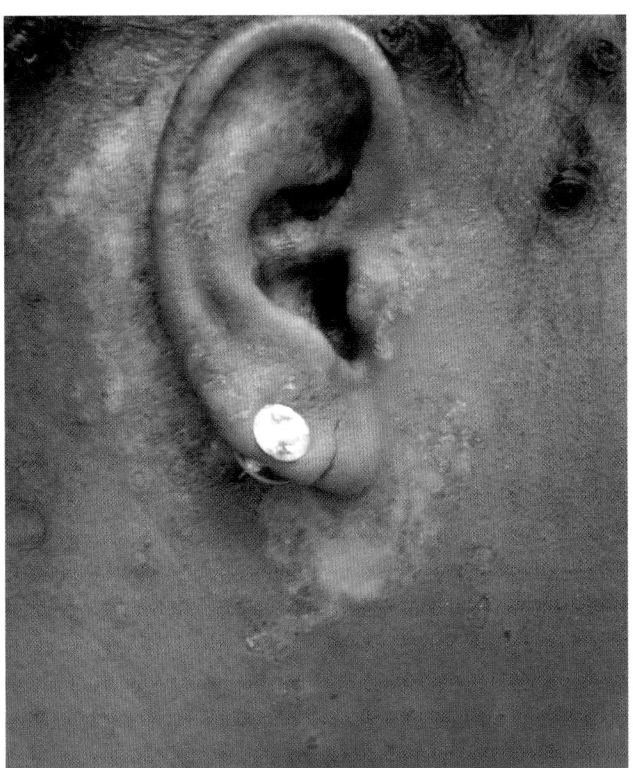

**Fig. 58.20 Discoid lupus erythematosus.** (Courtesy Yale Residents' Collection.)

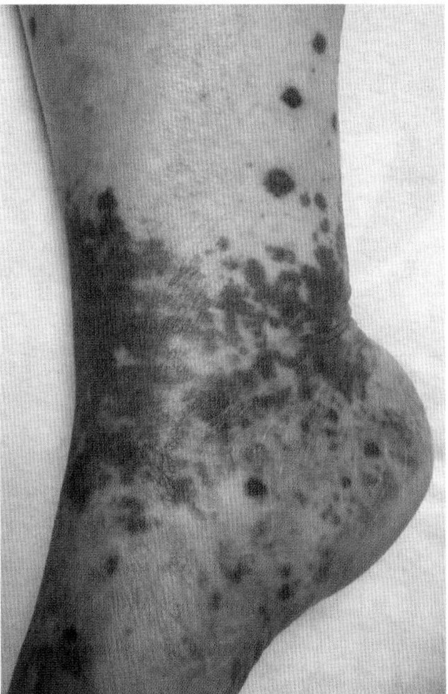

**Fig. 58.21 Leukocytoclastic vasculitis.** (Courtesy Yale Residents' Collection.)

in end-organs, causing damage.[79] Animal models of lupus have suggested that inhibition of oxidative stress and production of nitric oxide via inactivation of the nuclear factor-κB pathway may be important in modulating disease.[80]

Skin manifestations of lupus erythematosus are treated with steroids (oral or topical), antimalarials, and/or other immunosuppressants.

## LEUKOCYTOCLASTIC VASCULITIS

Leukocytoclastic vasculitis, clinically known as "palpable purpura," may be seen in a variety of clinical situations. Characteristically, the lesions are found on the lower extremities as nonblanching to partially blanching papules and plaques (Fig. 58.21). Histopathologically, there is leukocytoclasia, fibrin thrombi within vessels, extravasated erythrocytes, and swollen endothelial cells. If direct immunofluorescence testing is performed on the skin, deposits of IgG, IgM, and/or C3 may be seen around the vessels.

Associated diseases include Henoch–Schönlein purpura, infections (e.g., streptococcal, mycoplasmal, viral), systemic vasculitis (granulomatosis with polyangiitis [formally designated as Wegener granulomatosis], eosinophilic granulomatosis with polyangiitis [formally designated as Churg-Strauss syndrome], polyarteritis nodosa), inflammatory bowel disease, and malignancy.[81] Lesions may also be drug-induced. In Henoch–Schönlein purpura, the skin lesions are often seen in association with gastrointestinal pain, joint pain, and renal involvement. Mixed cryoglobulinemia is another disorder that can present with palpable purpura in the skin, hypocomplementemia, and a membranoproliferative glomerulonephritis.[82] Other skin manifestations include ulcers and dyspigmentation. Many cases of mixed cryoglobulinemia are associated with hepatitis C infection; however, a variety of other infections, systemic diseases, or lymphoproliferative processes may also be associated.

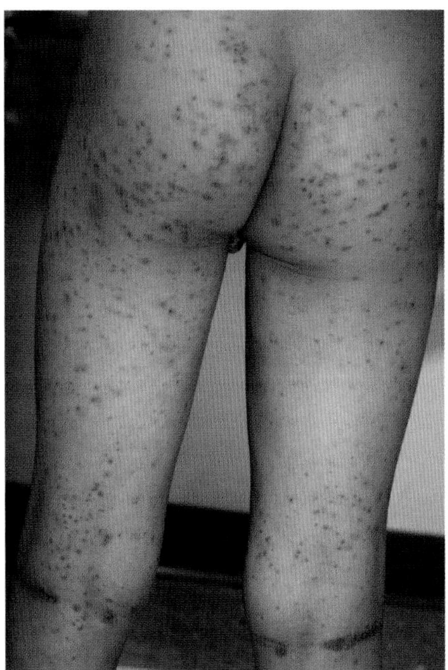

**Fig. 58.22 Henoch–Schönlein purpura.** Nonblanchable macules and papules are distributed over the buttocks and lower extremities.

## HENOCH–SCHÖNLEIN PURPURA

Henoch–Schönlein purpura typically involves the skin (Fig. 58.22), joints, gastrointestinal tract, and kidneys.[83] Children between the ages of 3 and 10 years are most commonly affected. In one series, 82% of affected children had joint pain, 63% had abdominal pain, 33% had gastrointestinal bleeding, and 40% had nephritis.[84] In a cohort of 250 adults, 61% had arthritis, 48% had gastrointestinal involvement, and 32% had proteinuria or hematuria.[85]

Skin involvement is manifested as palpable purpura involving the lower extremities and, occasionally, the upper extremities, buttocks, and trunk. Biopsy specimens from skin lesions show leukocytoclastic vasculitis, and direct immunofluorescence testing may reveal deposits of IgA, and sometimes C3 and IgG within vessel walls. The skin findings generally fade without treatment. Ankles and knees tend to be more painful than other joints. Pain, nausea, vomiting, melena, and hematochezia herald gastrointestinal involvement, especially intussusception.

Kidney involvement may manifest only as microscopic hematuria and proteinuria, although some patients develop nephrotic syndrome. Renal involvement can be the most severe aspect of Henoch–Schönlein purpura.[84] In children, renal function generally returns to normal with treatment,[86] but in a cohort of 250 adults, 11% developed ESRD and another 27% developed chronic moderate to severe renal insufficiency.[85] A retrospective study of patients with Henoch–Schönlein purpura has shown increased renal morbidity to be associated with nephrotic syndrome, decreased factor XIII levels, hypertension, and certain biopsy findings (e.g., crescents, mesangial macrophages, tubulointerstitial fibrosis). Kidney biopsy specimens generally show glomerulonephritis, often with IgA deposits in the mesangium and vessel walls.[87] The association of IgM deposition in the skin with renal involvement in adults is unclear.[88,89]

The pathogenesis of Henoch–Schönlein purpura is unknown. In one series, 62% of affected children had increased serum IgA levels.[84] Abnormal antigenic stimulation, possibly due to an infectious agent, may be a factor.[84] Elevated levels of vascular endothelial growth factor and endothelin have been reported,[90,91] as have decreased levels of factor XIII.[92] Abnormal cytokine levels (elevated tumor necrosis factor-α and interleukin-1β) have been described.[93] High titers of IgA anti–endothelial cell antibodies are seen in patients with more severe renal involvement.[94]

Most patients do not need treatment because the disease is self-limited. Joint pain may be ameliorated with analgesics. Severe gastrointestinal pain may benefit from systemic steroid treatment. Plasmapheresis and administration of steroids, intravenous immunoglobulin, and other immunosuppressants may decrease morbidity from renal involvement.[83,84]

## GENODERMATOSES

Several genodermatoses have prominent skin and renal findings (see Table 58.1). In Birt-Hogg-Dubé syndrome,[95,96] patients have numerous flesh-colored to slightly tan, smooth papules on the face (Fig. 58.23) that histopathologically are fibrofolliculomas or trichodiscomas. Skin tag–like lesions may also be seen in the axillary areas.[97] Angiofibromas and perifollicular fibromas are other potential cutaneous lesions.[98] This autosomal dominant disorder is associated with renal cell carcinoma (e.g., chromophobe, hybrid, oncocytic and, rarely, clear cell types) and cysts, with a defect in folliculin, a product of the *BHD* gene on chromosome 17. Folliculin likely functions as a tumor suppressor, and haploinsufficiency may be sufficient to lead to skin tumor formation.[99] Other manifestations include spontaneous pneumothorax.

**Table 58.1 Genodermatoses With Associated Skin and Kidney Tumors**

| Syndrome | Skin Findings | Renal Findings |
|---|---|---|
| Birt-Hogg-Dubé syndrome | Fibrofolliculoma<br>Trichodiscoma<br>Skin tag–like lesion | Renal cell carcinoma<br>Cysts |
| Tuberous sclerosis | Adenoma sebaceum | Angiomyolipoma<br>Cysts |
| Von Hippel–Lindau syndrome | Port-wine stain | Clear cell renal cell carcinoma<br>Cysts |
| Muir-Torre syndrome | Sebaceous neoplasia | Genitourinary carcinoma, including renal |
| Hereditary leiomyomatosis and renal cell carcinoma syndrome | Leiomyoma | Renal cell carcinoma |

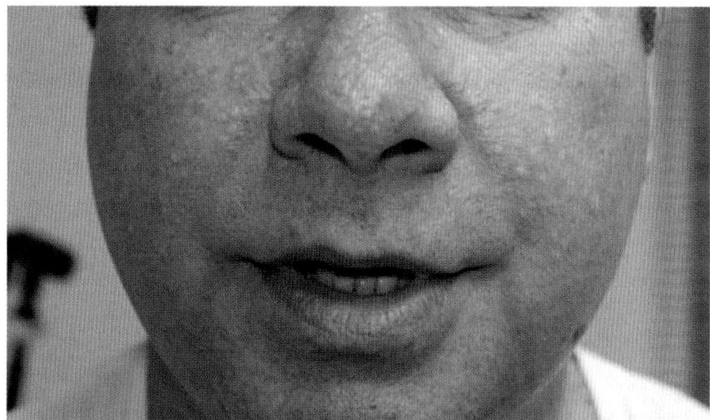

**Fig. 58.23 Birt-Hogg-Dubé syndrome.** Multiple whitish, smooth-surfaced papules (identified as fibrofolliculomas on biopsy) are present on the face. (Courtesy Yale Residents' Collection.)

In tuberous sclerosis,[100] another autosomal dominant disorder that is sometimes sporadic, there are also numerous facial papules clustered in the nasolabial areas and over the nose—so-called adenoma sebaceum or angiofibromas. Lesions are erythematous and smooth and may resemble acne. These lesions have histopathologic features similar to those of fibrous papules of the nose, with dilated vessels, stellate fibroblasts, and onion skin fibrosis around vessels and adnexal structures. Other skin findings include ash leaf–shaped hypopigmented macules and patches, small hypopigmented macules in a confetti-like pattern in the axillary areas, and periungual fibromas. Renal angiomyolipomas, cysts, or carcinoma may be seen. Patients may also have seizures or mental retardation. Genetic mutations are found in tuberin and hamartin, tumor suppressor proteins.

In von Hippel–Lindau syndrome, port-wine stains of the skin (seen in a minority of patients) are associated with ocular, cerebellar, medullary, and spinal hemangioblastomas, clear

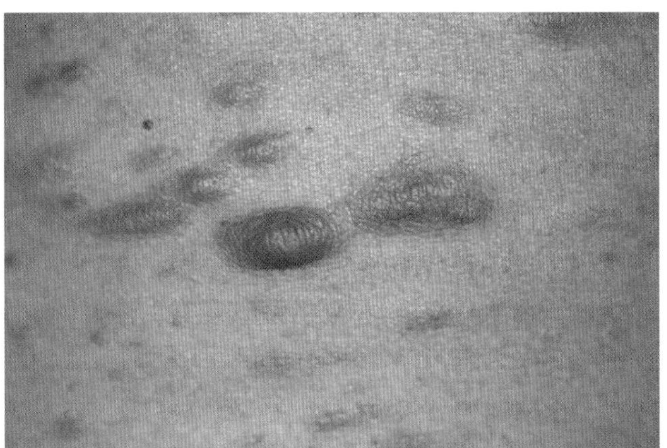

**Fig. 58.24** Multiple piloleiomyomas in a patient with Reed syndrome. (Courtesy Yale Residents' Collection.)

cell renal cell carcinoma and cysts, pheochromocytoma, pancreatic tumors and cysts, and testicular cysts. The disease has an autosomal dominant inheritance pattern, and ocular evaluation should begin at birth. Neurologic, otologic, and endocrine evaluation with abdominal ultrasonographic screening may be initiated at the age of 8 years or earlier if symptoms are present. The defective gene is *VHL,* a tumor suppressor gene on chromosome 3.[101] The VHL protein regulates hypoxia-inducible factors 1α and 2α, and dysregulation leads to augmented angiogenesis in tumors.

In hereditary leiomyomatosis and renal cell carcinoma syndrome, cutaneous (Fig. 58.24) and uterine leiomyomas are associated with an aggressive renal cell carcinoma. Inheritance may be autosomal dominant, and mutations are in fumarate hydratase, a Krebs cycle enzyme that when defective, may lead to dysregulation of the same hypoxia-inducible factors as those in von Hippel–Lindau syndrome.[102]

In Fabry disease,[103] numerous bright red, sometimes hyperkeratotic, papules are seen distributed in the bathing suit–trunk area. Such lesions may also be a manifestation of other genetic disorders, such as fucosidosis and other lipid storage disorders. Histopathologically, these lesions, termed "angiokeratomas," are composed of dilated vessels that abut the undersurface of the epidermis. Other associated findings include paroxysmal pain, cornea verticillata, strokes, seizures, heart disorders, and chronic kidney failure. The defect is in α-galactosidase A, a product of the *GAL* gene on the X chromosome.

In Muir–Torre syndrome, multiple keratoacanthomas or a single sebaceous neoplasm (adenoma, carcinoma, or epithelioma) is associated with an internal malignancy. Usually, patients have a colorectal carcinoma, but carcinomas of the renal pelvis, ureter, and bladder are also associated. Muir–Torre syndrome is an autosomal dominant disorder with mutations described in *MSH2, MSH1* and, rarely *MSH6.*[104]

Alport syndrome is the association of hematuric nephropathy, hearing defects, and ocular abnormalities. Although there are no skin findings, it is important to note that a simple skin biopsy can aid in the diagnosis. In Alport syndrome, there are mutations in the genes encoding type IV collagen. An absence of collagen IV may be seen in skin biopsy specimens from patients with X-linked Alport syndrome.[105]

**Box 58.4 Dermatologic Conditions That May Later Involve the Kidneys**

Impetigo and streptococcal skin infection
Metastatic melanoma

## DERMATOLOGIC CONDITIONS THAT MAY LATER INVOLVE THE KIDNEYS

See Box 58.4.

### IMPETIGO AND STREPTOCOCCAL SKIN INFECTION

Although poststreptococcal glomerulonephritis is usually associated with a preceding streptococcal pharyngitis, streptococcal skin infections can be the initiating event. The renal symptoms may present 2 to 3 weeks or more after the skin infection, by which time the skin findings have generally resolved.

 Complete reference list available at ExpertConsult.com.

### KEY REFERENCES


3. Zucker I, Yosipovitch G, David M, et al. Prevalence and characterization of uremic pruritus in patients undergoing hemodialysis: uremic pruritus is still a major problem for patients with end-stage renal disease. *J Am Acad Dermatol.* 2003;49:842–846.
4. Narita I, Alchi B, Omori K, et al. Etiology and prognostic significance of severe uremic pruritus in chronic hemodialysis patients. *Kidney Int.* 2006;69:1626–1632.
12. Etter L, Myers SA. Pruritus in systemic disease: mechanisms and management. *Dermatol Clin.* 2002;20:459–472, vi–vii.
13. Kimmel M, Alscher DM, Dunst R, et al. The role of micro-inflammation in the pathogenesis of uraemic pruritus in haemodialysis patients. *Nephrol Dial Transplant.* 2006;21:749–755.
14. Melo NC, Elias RM, Castro MC, et al. Pruritus in hemodialysis patients: the problem remains. *Hemodial Int.* 2009;13:38–42.
17. Peer G, Kivity S, Agami O, et al. Randomised crossover trial of naltrexone in uraemic pruritus. *Lancet.* 1996;348:1552–1554.
18. Pauli-Magnus C, Mikus G, Alscher DM, et al. Naltrexone does not relieve uremic pruritus: results of a randomized, double-blind, placebo-controlled crossover study. *J Am Soc Nephrol.* 2000;11:514–519.
19. Wikström B, Gellert R, Ladefoged SD, et al. Kappa-opioid system in uremic pruritus: multicenter, randomized, double-blind, placebo-controlled clinical studies. *J Am Soc Nephrol.* 2005;16:3742–3747.
20. Weisshaar E, Dunker N, Rohl FW, et al. Antipruritic effects of two different 5-HT3 receptor antagonists and an antihistamine in haemodialysis patients. *Exp Dermatol.* 2004;13:298–304.
21. Morton CA, Lafferty M, Hau C, et al. Pruritus and skin hydration during dialysis. *Nephrol Dial Transplant.* 1996;11:2031–2036.
22. De Marchi S, Cecchin E, Villalta D, et al. Relief of pruritus and decreases in plasma histamine concentrations during erythropoietin therapy in patients with uremia. *N Engl J Med.* 1992;326:969–974.
23. Young TA, Patel TS, Camacho F, et al. A pramoxine-based anti-itch lotion is more effective than a control lotion for the treatment of uremic pruritus in adult hemodialysis patients. *J Dermatolog Treat.* 2009;20:76–81.
24. Tarng DC, Cho YL, Liu HN, et al. Hemodialysis-related pruritus: a double-blind, placebo-controlled, crossover study of capsaicin 0.025% cream. *Nephron.* 1996;72:617–622.
25. Gilchrest BA, Rowe JW, Brown RS, et al. Relief of uremic pruritus with ultraviolet phototherapy. *N Engl J Med.* 1977;297:136–138.
34. Patel TS, Freedman BI, Yosipovitch G. An update on pruritus associated with CKD. *Am J Kidney Dis.* 2007;50:11–20.

35. Jovanovic DB, Pejanovic S, Vukovic L, et al. Ten years' experience in subtotal parathyroidectomy of hemodialysis patients. *Ren Fail.* 2005;27:19–24.
36. Park TH, Park CH, Ha SK, et al. Dry skin (xerosis) in patients undergoing maintenance haemodialysis: the role of decreased sweating of the eccrine sweat gland. *Nephrol Dial Transplant.* 1995;10:2269–2273.
37. Lai CF, Kao TW, Tsai TF, et al. Quantitative comparison of skin colors in patients with ESRD undergoing different dialysis modalities. *Am J Kidney Dis.* 2006;48:292–300.
40. Hong SB, Park JH, Ihm CG, et al. Acquired perforating dermatosis in patients with chronic renal failure and diabetes mellitus. *J Korean Med Sci.* 2004;19:283–288.
43. Saray Y, Seckin D, Bilezikci B. Acquired perforating dermatosis: clinicopathological features in twenty-two cases. *J Eur Acad Dermatol Venereol.* 2006;20:679–688.
45. Fine A, Zacharias J. Calciphylaxis is usually non-ulcerating: risk factors, outcome and therapy. *Kidney Int.* 2002;61:2210–2217.
48. Kalajian AH, Malhotra PS, Callen JP, et al. Calciphylaxis with normal renal and parathyroid function: not as rare as previously believed. *Arch Dermatol.* 2009;145:451–458.
51. Weenig RH. Pathogenesis of calciphylaxis: Hans Selye to nuclear factor kappa-B. *J Am Acad Dermatol.* 2008;58:458–471.
60. Gafter U, Mamet R, Korzets A, et al. Bullous dermatosis of end-stage renal disease: a possible association between abnormal porphyrin metabolism and aluminium. *Nephrol Dial Transplant.* 1996;11:1787–1791.
61. Schanbacher CF, Vanness ER, Daoud MS, et al. Pseudoporphyria: a clinical and biochemical study of 20 patients. *Mayo Clin Proc.* 2001;76:488–492.
62. Tsimihodimos V, Dounousi E, Siamopoulos KC. Dyslipidemia in chronic kidney disease: an approach to pathogenesis and treatment. *Am J Nephrol.* 2008;28:958–973.
63. Goldblum OM, Kraus E, Bronner AK. Pseudo–Kaposi's sarcoma of the hand associated with an acquired, iatrogenic arteriovenous fistula. *Arch Dermatol.* 1985;121:1038–1040.
65. Cowper SE, Su LD, Bhawan J, et al. Nephrogenic fibrosing dermopathy. *Am J Dermatopathol.* 2001;23:383–393.
67. Grobner T. Gadolinium—a specific trigger for the development of nephrogenic fibrosing dermopathy and nephrogenic systemic fibrosis? *Nephrol Dial Transplant.* 2006;21:1104–1108.
68. Bucala R. Circulating fibrocytes: cellular basis for NSF. *J Am Coll Radiol.* 2008;5:36–39.
70. Girardi M, Kay J, Elston DM, et al. Nephrogenic systemic fibrosis: clinicopathologic definition and workup recommendations. *J Am Acad Dermatol.* 2011;65:1095–1106.
73. Kravetz JD, Heald P. Bilateral dialysis-associated steal syndrome. *J Am Acad Dermatol.* 2008;58:888–891.
76. Shimizu S, Yasui C, Yasukawa K, et al. Subcutaneous nodules on the buttocks as a manifestation of dialysis-related amyloidosis: a clinicopathological entity? *Br J Dermatol.* 2003;149:400–404.
78. Goh CL, Phay KL. Arterio-venous shunt dermatitis in chronic renal failure patients on maintenance haemodialysis. *Clin Exp Dermatol.* 1988;13:379–381.
79. Bagavant H, Fu SM. Pathogenesis of kidney disease in systemic lupus erythematosus. *Curr Opin Rheumatol.* 2009;21(5):489–494.
82. Ferri C. Mixed cryoglobulinemia. *Orphanet J Rare Dis.* 2008;3:25.
84. Saulsbury FT. Henoch-Schönlein purpura in children. Report of 100 patients and review of the literature. *Medicine (Baltimore).* 1999;78:395–409.
85. Pillebout E, Thervet E, Hill G, et al. Henoch-Schönlein purpura in adults: outcome and prognostic factors. *J Am Soc Nephrol.* 2002;13:1271–1278.
87. Kawasaki Y, Suzuki J, Sakai N, et al. Clinical and pathological features of children with Henoch-Schoenlein purpura nephritis: risk factors associated with poor prognosis. *Clin Nephrol.* 2003;60:153–160.
95. Adley BP, Smith ND, Nayar R, et al. Birt-Hogg-Dubé syndrome: clinicopathologic findings and genetic alterations. *Arch Pathol Lab Med.* 2006;130:1865–1870.
98. Toro JR, Wei MH, Glenn GM, et al. BHD mutations, clinical and molecular genetic investigations of Birt-Hogg-Dubé syndrome: a new series of 50 families and a review of published reports. *J Med Genet.* 2008;45:321–331.
100. Rosser T, Panigrahy A, McClintock W. The diverse clinical manifestations of tuberous sclerosis complex: a review. *Semin Pediatr Neurol.* 2006;13:27–36.
101. Seizinger BR, Rouleau GA, Ozelius LJ, et al. Von Hippel–Lindau disease maps to the region of chromosome 3 associated with renal cell carcinoma. *Nature.* 1988;332:268–269.
102. Sudarshan S, Pinto PA, Neckers L, et al. Mechanisms of disease: hereditary leiomyomatosis and renal cell cancer—a distinct form of hereditary kidney cancer. *Nat Clin Pract Urol.* 2007;4:104–110.
103. Masson C, Cisse I, Simon V, et al. Fabry disease: a review. *Joint Bone Spine.* 2004;71:381–383.
104. Abbas O, Mahalingam M. Cutaneous sebaceous neoplasms as markers of Muir-Torre syndrome: a diagnostic algorithm. *J Cutan Pathol.* 2009;36(6):613–619.
105. Heidet L, Gubler MC. The renal lesions of Alport syndrome. *J Am Soc Nephrol.* 2009;20:1210–1215.

SECTION IX

# MANAGEMENT OF CHRONIC KIDNEY DISEASE

# 59 Classification and Management of Chronic Kidney Disease

Maarten W. Taal

## CHAPTER OUTLINE



## KEY POINTS

- The 2012 Kidney Disease Improving Global Outcomes (KDIGO) classification system for chronic kidney disease (CKD) provides simple risk stratification and serves as a convenient framework for guiding management through different stages.
- Lifestyle measures including smoking cessation, weight loss, and dietary sodium restriction should form part of any strategy to achieve renoprotection and reduce cardiovascular risk in persons with CKD.
- Antihypertensive therapy with angiotensin-converting enzyme inhibitors or angiotensin receptor blockers as "first line" in persons with albuminuria is the mainstay of treatment to achieve optimal renoprotection.
- Evidence from The Systolic Blood Pressure Intervention Trial (SPRINT) indicates that a lower target for the treatment of systolic blood pressure may afford improved cardiovascular risk reduction but may also be associated with some increase in risk of acute kidney injury and hyperkalemia. The risks versus benefits of a lower blood pressure target should be evaluated in each individual.
- To achieve optimal renoprotection careful attention should be paid to addressing all modifiable aspects of CKD to achieve target blood pressure, minimize proteinuria, and slow glomerular filtration rate decline.
- All persons with CKD should be regarded as having a high risk of cardiovascular disease and management offered to reduce this risk, including treatment with a statin.

## INTRODUCTION

Chronic kidney disease (CKD) is a collective term covering all primary disease processes that result in structural or functional kidney abnormalities, or both, persisting for at least 3 months. Abnormal urinalysis results identifying proteinuria or hematuria and abnormal kidney structure or histologic features, with or without a decreased glomerular filtration rate (GFR), are the defining manifestations.[1] The rationale for having a single term that encompasses a wide range of kidney pathologies is that damage to the kidneys results in shared pathophysiological features and that many of the interventions to slow the progression of CKD or reduce the associated cardiovascular risk should be applied regardless of the etiology of the CKD. The aforementioned formal definition of CKD was proposed relatively recently in 2002 and has had a profound impact on the specialty of nephrology. Prior to this it was difficult to compare the results of epidemiological and clinical studies because each used a different definition. In addition, there was no unified terminology and several imprecise terms such as chronic renal disease, impairment, insufficiency, and failure were used by different authors. Epidemiological research based on the unified definition has revealed that CKD is common, affecting on average 13.4% of the adult population globally,[2] and CKD has been identified as a leading cause of death in global burden of disease studies,[3] though it should be noted that most epidemiological studies rely on only a single abnormal GFR value for the diagnosis of CKD and therefore probably overestimate the true prevalence. Nevertheless, nephrology has changed from a specialty that focused largely on the treatment of rare and advanced kidney diseases as well as renal replacement therapy (RRT) to one that is now concerned with a condition, CKD, that affects a substantial proportion of the general population. Of necessity, this has also resulted in the need for healthcare workers who are not nephrologists to gain knowledge of CKD and its management. Importantly, most of the treatments required for CKD are relatively cheap and simple to apply and can therefore be delivered in healthcare settings where diagnostic services are limited and provision of RRT is inadequate. Thus education of healthcare workers on the management of CKD has the potential to reduce the burden of disease and the need for RRT without the need for sophisticated diagnostics or expensive drugs. This chapter will review in detail the classification of CKD and the evidence-based treatments that should be offered to persons with CKD regardless of the underlying kidney pathology. Within this context, there are four broad aims:

1. Attenuate GFR decline and thus prevent or delay the need for dialysis. It is perhaps self-evident, but the earlier that CKD progression can be halted, the greater is the possibility of maintaining kidney function as close to normal as possible.
2. Prevent premature cardiovascular death at all stages of CKD.
3. Recognize and manage complications of CKD as they arise, particularly in stages 4 and 5.
4. Timely preparation for RRT or conservative and palliative care.

Because the pathophysiology associated with CKD changes as the condition progresses, we also propose a stepped care approach and consider how primary and secondary care clinicians should cooperate to provide optimal care for the large number of persons now identified to have CKD.

## CLASSIFICATION OF CHRONIC KIDNEY DISEASE

The original classification proposed in 2002 subdivided CKD into five stages according to the GFR, reflecting the observation that in the majority of cases, CKD progresses slowly through the stages before reaching end-stage kidney disease (ESKD). In 2008, a National Institute for Health and Care Excellence (NICE) guideline proposed that stage 3 (GFR 59–30 mL/min/1.73 $m^2$) be subdivided into stages 3a (GFR 59–45 mL/min/1.73 $m^2$) and 3b (GFR 44–30 mL/min/1.73 $m^2$), reflecting a broad consensus that there are important differences in clinical aspects and prognosis between these groups. The CKD staging system has two important implications: First, it suggests that if CKD is detected at an early stage, intervention may be possible to prevent or slow progression to more advanced stages.[4] Second, it reflects the observation that as GFR declines, the risk profile of persons and associated complications changes. Thus the staging system provides a useful framework for structuring therapy and prioritizing interventions to produce a comprehensive strategy for the management of CKD. Although universally adopted, this classification system was limited by not reflecting the risk status of those classified, a feature that is present in the many other disease classification systems. Following extensive epidemiological investigations that identified reduced GFR and albuminuria as independent risk factors for adverse outcomes, the CKD classification system was revised by Kidney Disease Improving Global Outcomes (KDIGO) in 2012. The GFR stages were preserved, though now termed categories G1 to G5, and new categories were added for albuminuria; categories A1 to A3, corresponding to the previously used descriptions of "normoalbuminuria," microalbuminuria," and "macroalbuminuria." In addition, it was emphasized that the etiology of the CKD should be included in the classification, giving rise to the term "CGA" classification (cause, GFR, albuminuria; Fig. 59.1).[5,6] According to this system, a person with immunoglobulin A (IgA) nephropathy, a GFR of 34 mL/min/1.73 $m^2$, and a urine albumin-to-creatinine ratio (UACR) of 367 mg/g would be classified as "IgA nephropathy, category G3b A3". Implementation of the CGA classification has been greatly aided by the global adoption of equations to derive an estimated GFR (eGFR) from the serum creatinine concentration and use of UACR on a random sample to quantitate albuminuria (see Chapter 23). Importantly, in this classification system each category reflects a risk status for multiple adverse outcomes including ESKD, progression of CKD, cardiovascular events (CVEs), and all-cause mortality as indicated in the accompanying heat map. Thus the category is useful to guide the therapeutic approach at each stage and prompt referral for specialist care when indicated.

Despite its global adoption, some commentators have questioned the utility of the CKD definition and classification, suggesting that the high prevalence of CKD reflects a normal aging process and pointing out that mildly reduced GFR (category G3a) in the absence of albuminuria is associated with minimal increase in risk, particularly in older persons.[7,8] Various solutions have been proposed to address this issue, including the introduction of an age-adjusted GFR threshold for defining CKD or a modification of the classification for different age groups, but to date no consensus has been reached and the KDIGO classification is used worldwide.

## MECHANISMS OF DISEASE PROGRESSION AND THE RATIONALE FOR INTERVENTIONS TO ACHIEVE RENOPROTECTION

It has long been appreciated that regardless of the primary renal disease, kidney damage tends to progress toward ESKD, especially if more than half of glomeruli have been lost. This suggests that a common pathway of mechanisms may promote

Prognosis of CKD by GFR and Albuminuria categories: KDIGO 2012

| GFR categories (mL/min/1.73 m²) Description and range | | | | Persistent albuminuria categories Description and range | | |
|---|---|---|---|---|---|---|
| | | | | A1 | A2 | A3 |
| | | | | Normal to mildly increased | Moderately increased | Severely increased |
| | | | | <30 mg/g <3 mg/mmol | 30–300 mg/g 3–30 mg/mmol | >300 mg/g >30 mg/mmol |
| | G1 | Normal or high | ≥90 | | | |
| | G2 | Mildly decreased | 60–89 | | | |
| | G3a | Mildly to moderately decreased | 45–59 | | | |
| | G3b | Moderately to severely decreased | 30–44 | | | |
| | G4 | Severely decreased | 15–29 | | | |
| | G5 | Kidney failure | <15 | | | |

Green: low risk (if no other markers of kidney disease, no CKD)
Yellow: moderately increased risk
Orange: high risk
Red: very high risk

**Fig. 59.1** Current classification system and nomenclature proposed by the Kidney Disease Improving Global Outcomes *(KDIGO)* in 2012. Chronic kidney disease *(CKD)* is defined as abnormalities of kidney structure or function, present for 3 months, with implications for health. CKD is classified based on cause, glomerular filtration rate *(GFR)* category, and albuminuria category. (From Kidney Disease: Improving Global Outcomes CKD Work Group. KDIGO 2012 clinical practice guideline for the evaluation and management of chronic kidney disease. *Kidney Int.* 2013;3(Suppl):1–150. With permission.)

kidney damage and establish a vicious cycle of nephron loss. In research efforts since the 1960s, investigators have identified glomerular hemodynamic factors (glomerular hypertension and hyperfiltration), multiple effects of angiotensin II, proteinuria, and proinflammatory and profibrotic molecules as key elements of this pathway (discussed in detail in Chapter 51). A common pathway underlies progressive kidney damage from kidney diseases of diverse causes, and recognition of this pathway has been vital in informing strategies to achieve renoprotection. Thus the interventions to slow CKD progression discussed in the following sections are each aimed at attenuating mechanisms of progression. In view of the redundancy that is characteristic of most biologic systems, it has become clear that to achieve optimal renoprotection, attempts should be made to inhibit the vicious cycle of common pathway mechanisms at multiple points (Fig. 59.2).

## INTERVENTIONS FOR SLOWING PROGRESSION OF CHRONIC KIDNEY DISEASE

### LIFESTYLE INTERVENTIONS

All guidelines support healthy lifestyle advice for persons with CKD, citing the substantial literature that exists largely for the general population. A major issue for nephrologists and physicians managing CKD is that the available randomized controlled trials (RCTs) of the effect of lifestyle interventions rarely enrolled persons with CKD. Moreover, lifestyle changes require considerable effort from persons and may take years to be effective. In the prospective observational Chronic Renal Insufficiency Cohort (CRIC) study, regular physical activity, nonsmoking, and a body mass index (BMI) 25 kg/m$^2$ or higher were associated with lower risk of adverse outcomes, including a 50% decrease in eGFR or ESKD, atherosclerotic events, and all-cause mortality,[9] but there are potential biases in such observational studies because cardiovascular diseases and CKD may themselves result in low physical activity (reverse causality). Evidence does exist for the value of lifestyle intervention with regard to treating hypertension and preventing CVEs. Although specific studies of lifestyle interventions in persons with CKD are still lacking, it is reasonable to expect that a similar relative (and greater absolute) benefit might be gained.

### SMOKING CESSATION

Tobacco use is the most common cause of avoidable cardiovascular mortality worldwide; therefore, not surprisingly, smoking cessation is one of the most promoted methods in management of cardiovascular risk in the general population and in persons with CKD. Evidence that smoking cessation

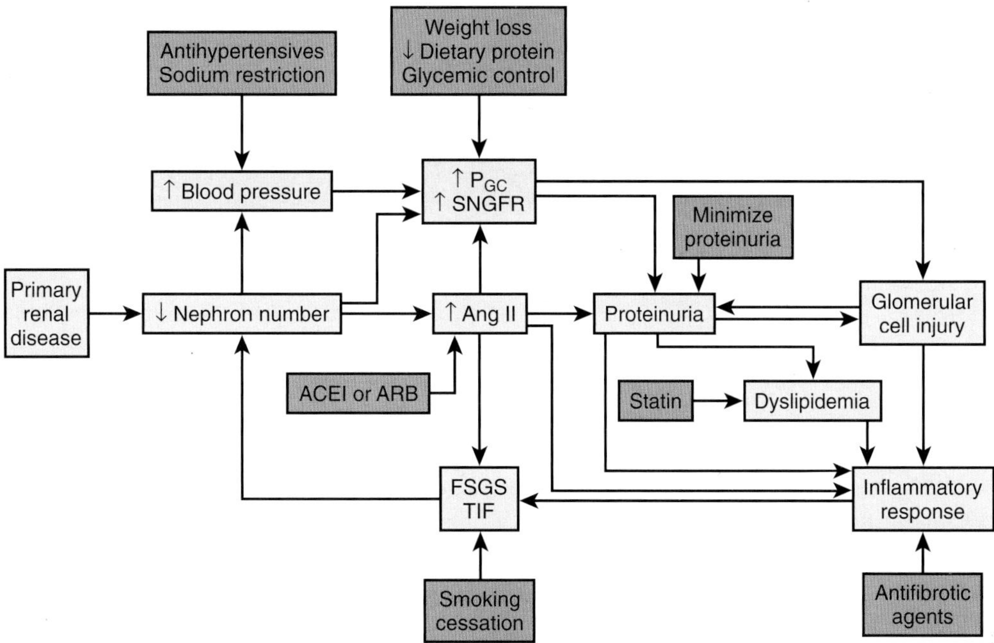


**Fig. 59.2** A common pathway of mechanisms that result in a vicious circle of nephron loss in chronic kidney disease (CKD). Interventions (in *red*) for achieving renoprotection are directed at inhibiting the common pathway at multiple points to slow CKD progression. *ACEI,* Angiotensin-converting enzyme inhibitor; *Ang II,* angiotensin II; *ARB,* angiotensin receptor blocker; *FSGS,* focal segmental glomerulosclerosis; $P_{GC}$, glomerular capillary hydraulic pressure; *SNGFR,* single nephron glomerular filtration rate; *TIF,* tubulointerstitial fibrosis.

helps prevent CKD progression is emerging.[10] In the Multiple Risk Factor Intervention Trial (MRFIT), smoking was significantly associated with an increased risk for ESKD[11]; in the Prevention of Renal and Vascular End-stage Disease (PREVEND) study, the rate of urine albumin excretion was correlated with the number of cigarettes smoked.[12] Smoking has been identified as a risk factor for the development of microalbuminuria and overt proteinuria and for the progression of CKD in persons with type 1 and type 2 diabetes.[13–15] In a large Swedish study, the risk for disease-specific types of CKD among smokers was compared with that among people who had never smoked. Overall, the association was modest, but an important finding was that the risk increased with high daily consumption (>20 cigarettes/day), long duration (>40 years), and a high cumulative "dose" (>30 pack-years) in comparison to participants who had never smoked. Smoking increased risk most strongly for persons with CKD classified as nephrosclerosis and also glomerulonephritis.[16] In the Jackson Heart Study, smoking was associated with a higher risk of rapid GFR decline (>30% decline from baseline) in a dose-dependent manner[17] and in a combined analysis of five large US cohort studies ($n$ = 954,029), smoking was associated with a doubling in the risk of death from ESKD.[18] Finally, a meta-analysis of 15 community-based cohort studies observed an increase in the risk of developing CKD in former (hazard ratio [HR], 1.15; 95% confidence interval [CI], 1.08–1.23) and current smokers (HR, 1.34; 95% CI, 1.23–1.47) as well as an increased risk of ESKD in former (HR, 1.44; 95% CI, 1.00–2.09) and current smokers (HR, 1.91; 95% CI, 1.39–2.64), though smoking was not associated with the development of proteinuria.[19]

Smoking has been described as a risk factor for progression in various forms of nondiabetic CKD. Of persons with adult polycystic kidney disease, immunoglobulin A (IgA) nephropathy, and lupus nephritis, those who were smokers had a substantially increased risk of progression to ESKD in comparison with nonsmokers.[15,20] Two large cohort studies have reported detailed data on the impact of smoking on CKD progression. In the CRIC study, smoking was associated with increased all-cause mortality as well as the combined endpoint of all-cause mortality and CKD progression, though not with CKD progression alone.[21] In an analysis of data from the Study of Heart and Renal Protection (SHARP) trial, current and former smoking were associated with higher levels of proteinuria but not with CKD progression during a median follow-up 4.9 years. Smoking was associated with significantly increased risks of CVEs, cancer, and all-cause mortality.[22] RCTs on the effect of smoking cessation on CKD progression have yet to be published, and few prospective data are available, but in one study of persons with diabetes, smoking cessation was associated with less progression to macroalbuminuria (proteinuria) and a slower rate of GFR decline in comparison to persons who continued smoking.[23] In addition, the intermediate risk for adverse outcomes reported for ex-smokers versus current smokers in several of the aforementioned studies provides indirect evidence of benefit from smoking cessation. Further prospective studies are required, but published evidence strongly supports smoking cessation as an intervention to reduce the incidence and progression of CKD.

Pharmacotherapy to assist in smoking cessation is now well established. A meta-analysis of RCTs in the general population (69 trials involving a total of 32,908 persons) showed that varenicline, bupropion, and five nicotine replacement therapies were all more efficacious than placebo at promoting smoking abstinence at 6 and 12 months. In comparison with persons taking placebo, persons treated with these agents were 1.5 to 2.5 times more likely to quit smoking, depending on the specific agent.[24] Indeed, combining varenicline and a nicotine replacement patch achieved an impressive higher continuous abstinence rate at 12 weeks (55.4% vs. 40.9%) and 6-month point prevalence abstinence rate of 65.1% versus 46.7% compared with varenicline treatment alone.[25] An important finding is that people who smoke are more likely to stop smoking if offered a combination of interventions, such as behavioral support and pharmacotherapy. Multicomponent interventions are now part of many public health guidelines. We see no reason to exclude people with CKD from this advice.

## WEIGHT LOSS

Obesity is the dominant risk factor for type 2 diabetes and is also a major risk factor for hypertension and progression of CKD. Evidence linking the metabolic syndrome and CKD has emerged; each element of the metabolic syndrome is associated with increased prevalence of CKD and microalbuminuria. In animal models (obese Zucker rats with type 2 diabetes), early progressive podocyte damage and macrophage infiltration are associated with hyperlipidemia and antedate both the development of glomerulosclerosis and tubulointerstitial damage.[26,27] In humans, there was a graded relationship between the number of components of the metabolic syndrome present and the corresponding prevalence of CKD or microalbuminuria.[28]

Epidemiologic studies have identified obesity as a risk factor for CKD,[29,30] and in one study, obesity was an independent risk factor for progression of IgA nephropathy.[31] Furthermore, the largest such study to assess risk of CKD in association with obesity demonstrated a very strong biologic gradient: Increasing BMI was associated with increasing risk of ESKD. In comparison to persons with an "ideal" BMI (18.5–24.9 kg/m$^2$), the relative risk (RR) of ESKD was 3.6-fold for those with a BMI of 30 to 34.9 kg/m$^2$, sixfold for those with BMI of 35 to 39.9 kg/m$^2$, and sevenfold for those with BMI of 40 kg/m$^2$ or higher. Controlling for baseline blood pressure and presence of diabetes attenuated the associations, but the gradient between increasing body size and ESKD risk remained strong.[32]

Because these components are major factors in the initiation and progression of CKD, respectively, persons with CKD would probably benefit from weight loss and reversal of the features of the metabolic syndrome, as observed in the general population.[33] Results of early studies support this assertion, inasmuch as weight loss in humans with obesity demonstrated reversal of glomerular hyperfiltration and albuminuria.[34]

Moreover, there is evidence that weight loss of as little as 10 lbs (4.5 kg) reduces blood pressure, prevents hypertension, or does both in a large proportion of overweight persons, although the ideal is to maintain normal body weight.[35] In the Framingham Heart Study, weight loss of 5 lbs (2.25 kg) or more was associated with reductions in cardiovascular risk of about 40%[36] for both men and women, and thus should be a clear goal for persons with CKD who are overweight. It also appears that the degree of weight loss, regardless of method (lifestyle changes or bariatric surgery), dictates the benefits of lowering of blood pressure and reduction in glycemic markers.[37] However, according to longer-term studies of lifestyle modification and of persons after bariatric surgery, the blood pressure–lowering benefits regress somewhat over time, although the vascular outcomes continue to be better than those in control groups.[33,38,39]

Renoprotective effects associated with weight loss interventions (dietary caloric restriction, exercise, antiobesity medications, and bariatric surgery) were reported in a meta-analysis of data from 522 participants in five controlled and eight uncontrolled trials.[40] In persons undergoing intervention to lose weight, those with proteinuria had a mean reduction of urine protein levels of 1.7 g/day; even among persons with microalbuminuria, mean reduction of urinary albumin excretion was 14 mg/day. Although these reductions were modest in comparison with those in persons with overt proteinuria, results of other studies of blood pressure and glycemic control interventions on microalbuminuria suggest that they will have long-term benefit in such persons.[40] This was confirmed by a secondary analysis of the Look AHEAD trial in which 5145 overweight or obese persons with type 2 diabetes were randomly assigned to an intensive lifestyle intervention (ILI) or diabetes support and education (DSE). The trial was stopped early due to lack of any difference in the primary outcome, CVEs, but analysis of renal outcomes showed a 31% reduction in the incidence of "high-risk CKD" as defined by the KDIGO classification system (HR, 0.69; 95% CI, 55 to 0.87) in the ILI versus DSE group, mediated in part by weight loss and improvements in hypertension and glycemic control.[41] A systematic review of 31 studies analyzed the effects of weight loss achieved by bariatric surgery, medication, or diet and found that in the majority of studies, weight loss was associated with reductions in proteinuria. In people with glomerular hyperfiltration, GFR tended to decrease with weight loss, and in those with reduced GFR, it tended to increase.[42]

Increasing use of bariatric surgery to manage obesity has resulted in several studies evaluating impact on kidney function and incidence of CKD. In one long-term study of 2144 persons who underwent bariatric surgery, renal outcomes were assessed after 7 years as change in CKD risk category as defined by the KDIGO classification. Among those with moderate risk at baseline, the risk category improved in 53% and deteriorated in 5% to 8%; in the high-risk group, improvement was observed in 56% and deterioration in 3% to 10%; in the very-high-risk group, 23% improved. eGFR initially improved with a peak at 2 years and then gradually declined. Albuminuria showed large and sustained decreases in moderate (median UACR 48–14 mg/g) and high-risk groups (median UACR 326–26 mg/g).[43] In another study that included only persons with CKD stage 3 and 4 and propensity score matching with similarly obese persons who did not undergo bariatric surgery, eGFR was significantly higher by a mean of 9.84 mL/min/1.73 m$^2$ in the surgery group after 3 years.[44] These studies are limited by relying on eGFR to assess kidney function but the finding that benefit was sustained over several years provides reassurance that improvement was not simply an artifact due to early decrease in serum creatinine secondary to weight loss after surgery. In a meta-analysis that included 23 cohort studies and 3015 persons who underwent all forms of bariatric surgery, small but statistically significant improvements were observed in serum creatinine (mean decrease 0.08 mg/dL) and proteinuria (mean decrease 0.04 g/day).[45]

Further large randomized studies of weight loss in persons with CKD are required because gastric bypass surgery is associated with renal risks including increased risk of renal calculi[46,47] and treatment with orlistat is associated with increased risk of acute kidney injury (AKI) as well as CKD.[48] On the basis of the available data, we recommend weight loss in obese persons with CKD through a combination of increased exercise and reduced caloric intake, and consideration of bariatric surgery if these are not successful.

## DIETARY SODIUM RESTRICTION

There is substantial evidence from epidemiologic, migration, intervention, genetic, and animal studies that salt intake plays an important role in regulating blood pressure. Essential hypertension is observed primarily in societies in which the average sodium intake exceeds 100 mEq/day (2.3 g sodium or ≈6 g sodium chloride) and is rare in societies in which the average sodium intake is less than 50 mEq/day (1.2 g sodium or 3 g sodium chloride).[49] This relationship between sodium intake and population levels of hypertension is strong and consistent. Of importance is that sodium restriction produces a significant reduction in blood pressure.[50,51] Salt (sodium chloride) intake in many countries is 9 to 12 g/day. The World Health Organization's current recommendation for adults is to reduce salt intake to 5 g/day or less.

A meta-analysis of RCTs with a duration of at least 4 weeks concluded that reducing salt intake by 3 g/day is predictive of a linear fall in blood pressure of, on average, 3.6 to 5.6 mm Hg (systolic blood pressure [SBP]) and 1.9 to 3.2 mm Hg (diastolic blood pressure [DBP]) in hypertensive persons and of 1.8 to 3.5 mm Hg (SBP) and 0.8 to 1.8 mm Hg (DBP) in normotensive participants.[52] The effect may be doubled with a 6 g/day reduction, and estimates suggest that reducing salt intake by 9 g/day (e.g., from 12 to 3 g/day) would reduce strokes by approximately 33% and ischemic heart disease by 25%. Weight loss and reduced sodium intake are particularly beneficial in older people. In the Trial of Nonpharmacologic Interventions in the Elderly (TONE), reducing sodium intake to 80 mEq (2 g) per day reduced blood pressure over 30 months, and about 40% of participants on the low-salt diet were able to discontinue their antihypertensive medications.[53]

In many persons with CKD, especially those with glomerular disease and severe proteinuria, hypertension behaves in a salt-sensitive manner. In one large observational study of persons without CKD at baseline, both high (>4.03 g/day of sodium) and low (<2.08 g/day of sodium) dietary sodium intake were associated with an increased incidence of CKD during follow-up of over 10 years in 3106 hypertensive participants, but no association with sodium intake was observed in those without hypertension ($n$ = 4871).[54] This supports that salt sensitivity is important in the association between sodium intake and CKD. The reason for the association with low sodium intake is unknown but may be confounded by associations between sodium intake and several other nutritional factors including potassium, total calorie, fat, protein, and carbohydrate intake, though the analysis was adjusted for these factors. A systematic review of 16 small studies that investigated the association of dietary sodium intake and CKD progression concluded that marked heterogeneity between the studies precluded meta-analysis.[55] Nevertheless, the general trend observed was that increasing sodium intake is associated with worsening albuminuria. An analysis of 3757 participants with CKD from the CRIC study found that after 15,807 person-years of follow-up, the highest quartile of urinary sodium excretion (≥195 mmol/day) was associated with a significantly increased risk of CKD progression (HR, 1.54; 95% CI, 1.23–1.92) and all-cause mortality (HR, 1.45; 95% CI, 1.08–1.95) compared with the lowest quartile (<117 mmol/day).[56]

High dietary sodium intake has also been shown to negate the antiproteinuric effects of treatment with angiotensin-converting enzyme (ACE) inhibitors.[57] In a prospective, randomized, placebo-controlled crossover study, dietary sodium restriction increased the antihypertensive and antiproteinuric effects of therapy with angiotensin receptor blockers (ARBs), as monotherapy or in combination with a thiazide diuretic, in persons with nondiabetic CKD (Fig. 59.3).[58] Whereas the protocol aimed to restrict dietary salt intake to less than 50 mEq/day (1.2 g of sodium or 3 g of sodium chloride), these impressive results were observed with achieved sodium restriction of only 92 mEq/day.[58] Furthermore, a post hoc analysis of data from the first and second Ramipril Efficacy In Nephropathy (REIN) trials found that medium and high sodium intake were associated with significant increases in the incidence of ESKD versus low sodium intake. Each 100-mEq/g increase in 24-hour urinary sodium/creatinine excretion was associated with a 1.61-fold (95% CI, 1.15–2.24) higher risk of ESKD, independent of blood pressure.[59]

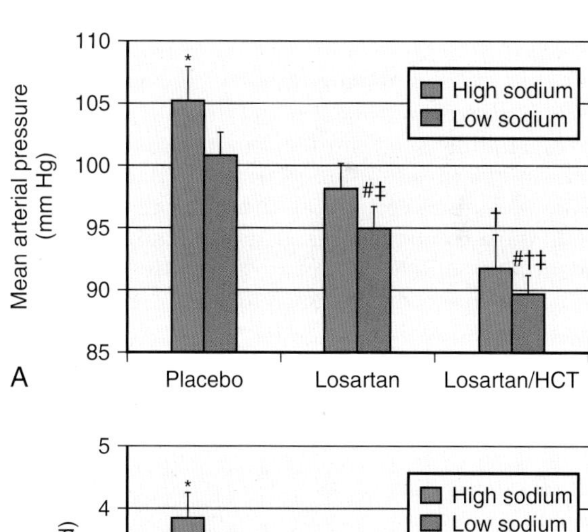


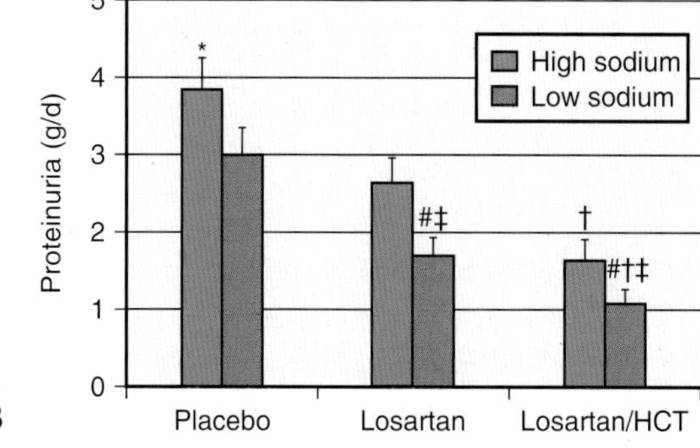


**Fig. 59.3** Results of a prospective randomized crossover trial showing the effect of dietary sodium restriction on the (A) antihypertensive and (B) antiproteinuric effects of treatment with an angiotensin receptor blocker as monotherapy or in combination with a thiazide diuretic. *$P$ < .05 versus all periods; #$P$ < .05 versus same treatment on high-salt diet (effect of low-salt diet); †$P$ < .05 versus losartan treatment on same diet [effect of hydrochlorothiazide (*HCT*)]; ‡$P$ < .05 versus placebo on same diet. (From Vogt L, Waanders F, Boomsma F, et al. Effects of dietary sodium and hydrochlorothiazide on the antiproteinuric efficacy of losartan. *J Am Soc Nephrol.* 2008;19:999–1007.)

Several small prospective studies have investigated the impact of dietary sodium restriction on blood pressure and proteinuria in persons with CKD. In a randomized placebo-controlled crossover study (achieved using low-sodium diet of 60 to 80 mmol/day plus sodium chloride tablets [120 mmol/day] or placebo) in 20 people with stage 3 or stage 4 CKD, low sodium intake was associated with an average 10/4 mm Hg reduction in blood pressure as well as reductions in albuminuria and proteinuria.[60] In a similar randomized crossover study dietary sodium restriction to less than 2 g/day for 4 weeks in persons with CKD stage 3 and 4 was associated with an average reduction in extracellular volume of 1.02 L, weight loss of 2.3 kg, and mean reduction in ambulatory SBP of 10.8 mm Hg but no improvement in albuminuria.[61] By contrast, another study in persons with CKD stage 1–3 and persistent albuminuria greater than 300 mg/day despite treatment with ramipril 10 mg/day reported that dietary sodium restriction for 8 weeks was associated with a reduction in arterial pressure from a mean of 95 to 90 mm Hg and a significant decrease in albuminuria from a mean of 1060 to 717 mg/day. Creatinine clearance also decreased slightly from a mean 101 to 91 mL/min.[62] Another study illustrated the challenges associated with achieving sustained reduction in sodium intake. In an RCT, persons with CKD assigned to a 3-month intervention of education and coaching as well as self-monitoring achieved a modest mean reduction in urinary sodium excretion of 30 mmol/day associated with a mean reduction in ambulatory DBP of 3.4 mm Hg and mean reduction in proteinuria of 0.4 g/day, but at 3 months after completion of the intervention there was no difference in urinary sodium excretion or ambulatory BP compared with controls, although proteinuria remained 0.3 g/day lower.[63] Further long-term randomized trials are needed to define the role of sodium restriction in renoprotective strategies, but even the incomplete evidence available supports a recommendation for moderate dietary sodium restriction to less than 5 g/day of salt in persons with CKD.

Food processing drastically changes the cationic content of natural foods, increasing sodium content and decreasing potassium content. On average, approximately 10% of dietary sodium chloride originates naturally in foods, whereas approximately 80% is the result of food processing, the remainder being discretionary (added during cooking or at the table). We advocate assessment of salt intake in individuals with CKD and advise reducing salt intake with the assistance of a dietitian to less than 5 g/day (<90 mmol/day of sodium) as recommended by KDIGO.[5]

## DIETARY PROTEIN RESTRICTION

Dietary protein restriction as a renoprotective strategy is based on the notion that reducing the excretory burden on the kidneys would slow the rate of progressive injury. Accordingly, dietary protein restriction was among the first interventions proposed to slow CKD progression. Experimental studies showed that a low-protein diet (LPD) normalized glomerular hemodynamics in the remnant kidney model[64] and resulted in effective long-term renoprotection.[65] Unfortunately, clinical studies to date have failed to provide unambiguous evidence to support the use of protein restriction in human CKD. The proposal of nomenclature and diagnostic criteria for protein-energy wasting in AKI and CKD was an important step in planning future studies.[66] The suggested criteria for diagnosing protein-energy wasting include the presence of reduced body mass (specifically muscle mass) and serum evidence of low albumin, prealbumin, or cholesterol levels.

The Modification of Diet in Renal Disease (MDRD) study was designed to provide a definite answer to the question of whether dietary protein restriction slows the progression of CKD. The study had two components: In study A, 585 persons with mostly nondiabetic CKD (GFR, 25–55 mL/min/1.73 $m^2$) were randomly assigned to follow either a diet with "usual" protein levels (1.3 g/kg/day) or LPD (0.58 g/kg/day); in study B, 255 persons with GFRs of 13 to 24 mL/min/1.73 $m^2$ were randomly assigned to follow either LPD (0.58 g/kg/day) or "very low" protein diet (VLPD; 0.28 g/kg/day) with keto-amino acid supplementation to prevent malnutrition. After a mean follow-up period of 2.2 years, there was no difference in the rate of GFR decline in study A and only a trend toward slower decline in the VLPD group in study B.[67] Further analysis indicated, however, that the desired protein intake was not achieved in the randomized groups, and secondary analysis based on achieved dietary protein intake demonstrated that a reduction in protein intake of 0.2 g/kg/day was correlated with a 1.15-mL/min/year reduction in the rate of GFR decline, equivalent to a 29% reduction in mean rate of GFR decline.[68] In addition, a post hoc two-slope analysis, in which presumptive acute effects of dietary protein restriction were taken into account, suggested a modest long-term benefit. Long-term follow-up of the cohort in MDRD study A yielded disappointingly inconclusive results.[69] In a more recent trial, 207 well-nourished persons without diabetes and with eGFR less than 30 mL/min/1.73 $m^2$ and urine protein-to-creatinine ratio (PCR) less than 1 g/g were randomized to a vegetarian VLPD (<0.3 g/kg/day) with ketoanalog supplementation (ketoanalog diet [KD]) or standard (nonvegetarian) LPD (<0.6 g/kg/day). After 15 months the primary outcome of RRT or 50% reduction in eGFR was reached in 13% of those on KD versus 42% on LPD (adjusted HR, 0.1; 95% CI, 0.05–0.2). Those on the KD also evidenced a 3.2 mL/min/year slower rate of eGFR decline. Metabolic factors were also improved by the KD; serum bicarbonate and calcium were higher and phosphate lower. There was no change in nutritional status in either group and no adverse reactions were reported.[70] However, it is unclear what proportion of the benefit was attributable to the vegetarian VLPD versus the ketoanalog supplementation.

The effect of dietary protein restriction has been examined in several meta-analyses of smaller randomized studies. Pedrini and associates[71] summarized findings on 1413 persons with nondiabetic CKD from five studies (including those from study A of the MDRD trial). LPD was associated with an RR of 0.67 (95% CI, 0.50–0.89) for ESKD or death. Similarly, among 108 persons with type 1 diabetes from five studies, LPD significantly slowed the increase in albuminuria or the decline in GFR or creatinine clearance (RR, 0.56; 95% CI, 0.40–0.77). Kasiske and colleagues[72] pooled the results of 13 RCTs (1919 persons) and found that dietary protein restriction reduced the rate of decline in eGFR by 0.53 mL/min/year.

Larger effects were observed in participants with diabetes, and so the findings of a meta-analysis of LPD in persons with diabetes are important. In this study, Pan and colleagues[73] assessed eight RCTs. In contrast to a previous meta-analysis, they found that in comparison with a normal-protein diet, treatment with an LPD was not associated with a significant improvement in kidney function (assessed by GFR). However, in only two of these trials, there was a significant but marginal decrease in proteinuria or albuminuria in the participants following the LPD. Of importance was that persons following the LPD had lower serum albumin levels and poorer glycemic control, both of which are relevant to outcomes and their assessment.

Fouque and Laville[74] performed a Cochrane Database systematic review of all randomized studies, comparing two different levels of protein intake in adult persons suffering from moderate to severe CKD. A total of 2000 nondiabetic persons were identified in 10 studies (of a total of 40 studies) in which follow-up lasted at least 1 year. There were 281 renal deaths (progression to ESKD) recorded, 113 among participants following the LPD and 168 among those following the higher protein diet (RR, 0.68; 95% CI, 0.55–0.84; $P = .0002$). The authors concluded that reducing protein intake in persons with CKD reduces the occurrence of renal death by 32% in comparison with higher or unrestricted protein intake. The most recent meta-analysis included 16 RCTs of persons with relatively advanced CKD (stage 4 and 5 in most cases) not receiving RRT. Inclusion required at least 30 participants per study. In studies comparing LPD (<0.8 g/day) with higher protein intake, LPD was associated with a small but significant absolute risk reduction for ESKD (4%) and higher serum bicarbonate at 1 year (weighted mean difference [MD], 1.46 mEq/L) versus higher protein diets. Similarly, in studies comparing VLPD with LPD, VLPD was associated with an absolute risk reduction for ESKD (13%) and higher GFR at 1 year (weighted MD, 3.95 mL/min/1.73 $m^2$) versus LPD. No studies reported increased risk of protein energy wasting or other safety concerns associated with dietary protein restriction.[75]

The caveats for these trials are that most were of short duration, the largest trial (MDRD) mostly excluded persons with diabetes, and compliance with LPDs was a factor in interpretation in some of the results. Furthermore, the proportion of the participants treated with renin–angiotensin–aldosterone system inhibitors (RAASi) was variable. Available evidence suggests that LPD and RAASi may have synergistic renoprotective effects but this has not yet been adequately evaluated in an RCT.[76] In addition to possible renoprotective effects, dietary protein restriction results in reduced intake of sodium, phosphate, and acid all of which may be beneficial in CKD.[77]

In summary, published data indicate that there is likely some renoprotective benefit from dietary protein restriction but conclusive evidence is lacking, in particular for additional benefit in persons already treated with RAASi. The benefits are more apparent in persons with proteinuria and lower GFR, and the risks are greater in those at risk of malnutrition, such as elderly persons (age >75 years); those with below-average BMI (<20 kg/$m^2$), muscle wasting, or myopathic symptoms; and those with evidence of protein-energy wasting. We therefore recommend that the potential benefits and risks should be considered carefully on an individual basis and with the assistance of a trained renal dietitian. The 2012 KDIGO guideline recommends reducing dietary protein intake to less than 0.8 g/kg/day in adults with stages 4 and 5 CKD, and avoiding a high-protein diet (>1.3 g/kg/day) in adults with CKD who are considered to be at risk of progression.[5] By contrast, the 2014 NICE guideline recommends against dietary protein restriction for all persons with CKD.[78] For further discussion of dietary aspects in kidney disease, see Chapter 60.

## GLYCEMIC CONTROL IN PERSONS WITH DIABETES

The role of glycemic control in protecting the kidneys in persons with diabetes is discussed fully in Chapter 39. In summary, the benefit of tight glycemic control in ameliorating diabetic nephropathy seems to decrease as CKD progresses; the greatest benefits are observed in stages 1 and 2. In addition to the renoprotective effects, however, there is clear evidence that improving glycemic control can reduce the risk of developing other microvascular and macrovascular complications such as blindness and cardiovascular disease.[79] Of importance is that these benefits were maintained for up to 10 years after the trial, even though intensive control regressed to standard control levels.[80] Achieving optimal glycemic control should therefore be an important goal for all persons with diabetes and CKD, but should be balanced against the risk of developing hypoglycemia, which may be increased in the elderly and those with more advanced CKD. The KDIGO guidelines recommend a target hemoglobin $A_{1c}$ of 7.0% (53 mmol/mol) to prevent or delay progression of microvascular complications, including diabetic kidney disease, unless persons have multiple comorbidities, have reduced life expectancy, or are at risk of hypoglycemia.[5]

### ANTIHYPERTENSIVE THERAPY

The treatment of systemic hypertension was the first intervention shown to significantly slow the rate of CKD progression and remains fundamental in renoprotective strategies. Mogensen[81] and Parving and colleagues[82] pioneered the role of blood pressure control in studies of persons with type 1 diabetes, in whom the initiation of antihypertensive therapy significantly slowed the rate of GFR decline.

Similar observations were subsequently reported among persons with nondiabetic forms of CKD.[83–85] In one of the earliest meta-analyses in nephrology, Kasiske and colleagues[86] studied 100 controlled and uncontrolled studies that provided data on kidney function, proteinuria, or both before and after treatment with an antihypertensive agent in people with diabetes. Multiple linear regression analysis indicated that ACE inhibitors decreased proteinuria independently of changes in blood pressure, treatment duration, type of diabetes or stage of nephropathy, and study design. Reductions in proteinuria from other antihypertensive agents could be attributed entirely to changes in blood pressure. Furthermore, blood pressure reduction was associated with a relative increase in GFR (3.70 ± 0.92 mL/min for each 10-mm Hg reduction in mean arterial pressure [MAP]; $P = .0002$), but in comparison with other agents, ACE inhibitors had an additional favorable effect on GFR that was independent of blood pressure changes (3.41 ± 1.71 mL/min; $P = .05$).

### ANTIHYPERTENSIVE DRUGS

Data from the Antihypertensive and Lipid-Lowering Treatment to Prevent Heart Attack Trial (ALLHAT) have been misinterpreted by some as implying that the choice of antihypertensive drug does not affect renal outcomes in persons with

CKD. Note that ALLHAT was designed to investigate the effect of antihypertensive drugs on cardiovascular rather than renal outcomes in persons who had hypertension and at least one cardiovascular risk factor. There was no significant difference in the incidence of the primary outcome of fatal or nonfatal myocardial infarction among persons randomly assigned to receive treatment with a thiazide diuretic, a calcium channel blocker, or an ACE inhibitor.[87] Whereas a post hoc analysis also showed no difference in the secondary outcome of ESKD or more than a 50% decrease in GFR, persons with serum creatinine levels exceeding 2 mg/dL (>170 μmol/L) were specifically excluded from the study, and therefore only a minority (5662 of 33,357) had CKD, mostly in stages 1 to 3. Furthermore, the presence of proteinuria was not assessed.[88] By contrast, a large body of evidence supports the use of ACE inhibitors or ARB agents as first-line antihypertensive therapy in persons with CKD (see the "Pharmacologic Inhibition of the Renin–Angiotensin–Aldosterone System" section under "Interventions for Slowing Progression of Chronic Kidney Disease").

Despite the importance of ACE inhibition and ARB therapy in achieving renoprotection, thiazide and other diuretics are valuable and sometimes essential as additional antihypertensive agents to achieve optimal blood pressure control. Studies have shown that high dietary sodium intake may abrogate the antiproteinuric effect of ACE inhibitor treatment, but addition of a thiazide diuretic restores the antiproteinuric effect despite ongoing high sodium intake.[57] Similarly, addition of a thiazide diuretic to ARB treatment reduced blood pressure and proteinuria in persons with IgA nephropathy.[89] We therefore recommend a thiazide diuretic as second-line antihypertensive therapy in persons who have not achieved adequate blood pressure control with an ACE inhibitor or an ARB alone. In persons with advanced CKD, thiazide diuretics are considered less likely to be effective, although a recent review of published literature suggests that they may still be beneficial in stage 4 CKD.[90] In those who do not respond to a thiazide diuretic, a loop diuretic should be considered instead.

There is some evidence that, despite their efficacy as antihypertensive drugs, dihydropyridine calcium channel blockers (DCCBs) may have adverse effects with regard to CKD progression. In experimental studies, DCCB treatment was observed to allow greater transmission of systemic blood pressure to glomerular capillaries and was associated with more rapid progression of renal injury than was ACE inhibitor treatment in the 5/6 nephrectomy model.[91] Whereas one relatively small study revealed no difference between the renoprotective effects of the DCCB nifedipine and the ACE inhibitor captopril,[92] two larger studies demonstrated adverse outcomes associated with the use of DCCB agents.

A secondary analysis of data from the REIN study revealed that among participants not randomly assigned to receive ACE inhibitor treatment who failed to achieve a MAP of less than 100 mm Hg, the DCCB agents nifedipine and amlodipine were associated with a higher magnitude of proteinuria and more rapid GFR decline than were other antihypertensives.[93] Observations from the African American Study of Kidney Disease and Hypertension (AASK) provoked even greater concern.[94] In this study, persons with CKD and hypertension were randomly assigned to receive either treatment with an ACE inhibitor or amlodipine (DCCB) or treatment with a β-blocker and diuretic in combination. The amlodipine arm of the study was stopped prematurely because recipients exhibited a more rapid decline in GFR than did participants receiving the β-blocker or ACE inhibitor, particularly among those with urine protein levels higher than 1 g/day. The Ramipril Efficacy In Nephropathy-2 (REIN-2) study revealed no additional renoprotection when a DCCB was added to ACE inhibitor treatment in persons with nondiabetic CKD, but there was also no adverse effect.[95] By contrast, treatment with nondihydropyridine calcium channel blockers (NDCCBs) ameliorated glomerular hypertension, reduced proteinuria, and afforded renoprotection in some experimental studies.[96] In one clinical study, the combination of ACE inhibition and NDCCB treatment resulted in greater reduction of proteinuria than did either of these treatments alone in persons with type 2 diabetes and overt nephropathy.[97] Furthermore, a meta-analysis of data from 28 RCTs revealed a 2% increase in proteinuria with DCCB treatment, in contrast to a 30% reduction with NDCCB treatment, despite similar effects on blood pressure in hypertensive persons with proteinuria.[98]

On the basis of the evidence discussed, we recommend that DCCBs be avoided in persons with CKD unless they are used in combination with ACE inhibition or ARB treatment to achieve adequate blood pressure control. If possible, NDCCBs should be used in preference over DCCBs. Most of the trials in persons with CKD have established that between two and four agents is the median number of antihypertensive agents required for the respective target blood pressures. Therefore third-line agents are needed by a substantial proportion of persons with CKD. We recommend that the choice of third- and fourth-line agents be based on factors other than renoprotection. Therefore in addition to RAASi, diuretic therapy, and NDCCBs, we suggest use of β-blockers, α-blockers, and central nervous system agents, depending on comorbid conditions, side-effect profile, drug interactions (in particular, NDCCBs should not be used in combination with β-blockers due to increased risk of cardiac conduction abnormalities), convenience, and cost.

## TRIALS OF LOW VERSUS USUAL TARGETS FOR LOWERING BLOOD PRESSURE

Despite the importance of blood pressure control in achieving renoprotection, the optimal blood pressure remains uncertain, particularly in elderly persons and those with mild proteinuria. In several RCTs, researchers have investigated whether blood pressure targets lower than previously recommended levels afford greater renoprotection than "usual" blood pressure control, but these studies have not provided a conclusive answer. In the MDRD study, primary analysis showed no significant difference in the rate of GFR decline between participants aged 18 to 60 years randomly assigned to achieve a target MAP of less than 92 mm Hg (equivalent to <125/75 mm Hg), or MAP less than 98 mm Hg or participants aged 61 years or older assigned a MAP target of less than 107 mm Hg (equivalent to 140/90 mm Hg), or MAP less than 113 mm Hg. Participants assigned to achieve the lower blood pressures, however, evidenced an early rapid decrease in GFR, probably as a result of associated renal hemodynamic effects, that obscured a later slower rate of GFR decline. Furthermore, secondary analysis did show benefit associated with the lower blood pressure target among persons with more severe baseline proteinuria (urine protein level >1 g/

day). Further secondary analysis revealed that lower achieved blood pressure was also associated with a slower GFR decline, an effect that was more marked among persons with more severe baseline proteinuria.[67] The authors concluded by recommending a blood pressure goal of less than 125/75 mm Hg (MAP, 92 mm Hg) for persons with CKD whose urine protein levels exceed 1 g/day, and a goal of less than 130/80 mm Hg (MAP, 98 mm Hg) for those with urine protein levels of 0.25 to 1.0 g/day.[99]

Findings of prolonged follow-up of the participants in the MDRD study suggest that the benefits of lower blood pressure may become evident only over a longer period. Analysis after almost 10 years revealed a significant reduction in the risk of ESKD (adjusted HR, 0.68) and a combined endpoint of ESKD or death (adjusted HR, 0.77) among persons randomly assigned to achieve the lower blood pressure targets. An important caveat is that treatment and blood pressure data were not available beyond the 2.2 years of the original trial.[100] In the AASK, no significant difference in the rate of GFR decline was observed among participants randomly assigned to achieve a MAP goal of 92 mm Hg or lower versus a goal of 102 to 107 mm Hg. One possible explanation for this outcome is that participants in the AASK generally had milder baseline proteinuria (mean urine protein excretion, 0.38–0.63 g/day).[101] The results are therefore consistent with those of the MDRD study, which showed benefit only in persons with significant proteinuria. Likewise, in the REIN-2 trial, additional blood pressure reduction (blood pressure of <130/80 mm Hg vs. DBP of <90 mm Hg, regardless of SBP) failed to provide additional renoprotection in persons with nondiabetic CKD who were already receiving ACE inhibitor treatment.[95] Possible explanations are that the degree of additional blood pressure reduction was modest (4.1/2.8 mm Hg) and that in the group undergoing intensive blood pressure reduction, the number of participants with moderate to heavy proteinuria was small.

The Systolic Blood Pressure Intervention Trial (SPRINT) is the largest randomized trial to date to compare the effect of different BP targets on cardiovascular and renal outcomes in persons with CKD. The study included 9361 participants aged 50 years and over with BP 130 to 180 mm Hg and increased cardiovascular risk (including all with CKD) who were randomly allocated to a systolic BP target of less than 120 mm Hg or less than 140 mm Hg. Persons with diabetes, proteinuria of greater than 1 g/day, adult polycystic kidney disease, previous stroke, and cardiac failure were excluded. The main trial was stopped early due to evidence of significant benefit in the primary outcome of CVE and all-cause mortality in the lower BP group.[102] A prespecified subgroup analysis was conducted in 2646 participants with CKD at baseline. Analysis of the main trial showed no evidence of effect modification by CKD status on the primary outcome of CVE or all-cause mortality. In addition, in the CKD subgroup, participants in the lower BP group evidenced a lower incidence of CVE (HR, 0.81; 95% CI, 0.63–1.05) and all-cause mortality (HR, 0.72; 95% CI, 0.53–0.99; Fig. 59.4). Importantly, these benefits were also observed in participants aged 75 years and older. There was no difference between groups in the renal outcome of 50% decline in GFR or ESKD after a median of 3.3 years. The lower BP target was associated with some initial decline in eGFR, likely due to increased use of RAASi, whereas a small initial increase in GFR was observed with the higher BP. After excluding the first 6 months of observation the low BP target was associated with a slightly higher rate of GFR decline (0.47 mL/min/year vs. 0.32 mL/min/year; $P < .03$). The lower BP target was associated with lower UACR at all time points to 48 months. There was no difference in serious adverse events between the groups but the low BP target was associated with a higher incidence of hyperkalemia, hypokalemia, and AKI[103] (predominantly stage 1 and 2 and most had recovery of kidney function).[104] In summary, this largest randomized trial to date found that a lower BP target than previously recommended was associated with a significant reduction in CVE and all-cause mortality. There was no benefit in renal outcomes but also no evidence of harm (apart from a small increase in incidence of AKI). It should be remembered that persons with advanced or severe CKD (evidenced by proteinuria >1 g/day) as well as those with diabetes were excluded. The findings are therefore consistent with those of the MDRD and AASK studies, confirming that there is little renoprotective benefit associated with low BP targets in mild and nonproteinuric CKD. However, the results do indicate significant survival and cardiovascular benefit with lower BP targets and question the notion that the risk of lower BP targets outweighs the benefits in all older people.

Because not all the persons in the aforementioned trials received ACE inhibitor treatment, it remained unclear how important the level of blood pressure attained was in persons with CKD who were receiving an ACE inhibitor or an ARB. Several studies have sought to address this issue. Among persons with type 1 diabetes and established nephropathy who were receiving ACE inhibitor treatment, attainment of a "low" (MAP, 92 mm Hg) versus "usual" (MAP, 100–107 mm Hg) target blood pressure was associated with significantly milder degrees of proteinuria after 2 years, but there was no significant difference in GFR.[105] The Effect of Strict Blood Pressure Control and ACE Inhibition on the Progression of Chronic Renal Failure in Pediatric Patients (ESCAPE) trial was conducted to investigate the role of blood pressure control in children with CKD who were receiving treatment with an ACE inhibitor. Attainment of a lower blood pressure target was associated with a significantly reduced risk of reaching ESKD or doubling of serum creatinine concentration.[106] This is an important trial inasmuch as the primary endpoint (time to 50% decline in GFR or progression to ESKD) was not as affected by the competing mortality effects that complicate studies in older persons. A total of 30% of the participants who received intensified treatment for blood pressure control reached the primary endpoint, in comparison with 42% of those who received conventional treatment for blood pressure control (HR, 0.65; 95% CI, 0.44–0.94; $P = .02$). Urine protein excretion gradually rebounded during ongoing ACE inhibition after an initial 50% decrease, despite persistently good blood pressure control. Achievement of blood pressure targets and a decrease in proteinuria were significant independent predictors of delayed progression of CKD.

Results of secondary analyses of other studies also indicate that lower blood pressure is associated with more effective renoprotection in persons receiving ACE inhibitors or ARB treatment. In the Irbesartan in Diabetic Nephropathy Trial (IDNT), greater renoprotection was observed in persons who achieved lower blood pressure: Achieved SBP greater than 149 mm Hg was associated with a 2.2-fold increased risk of

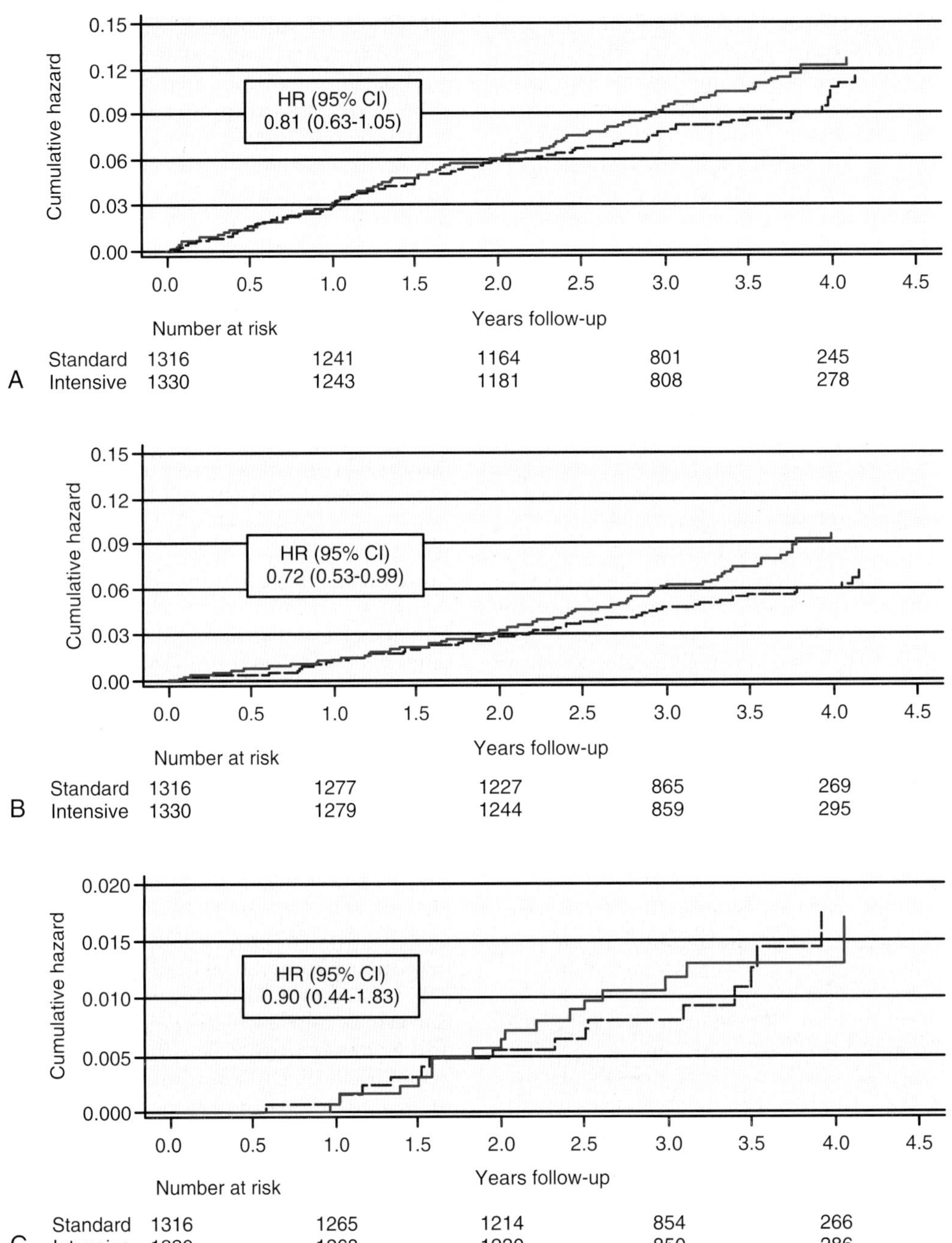


**Fig. 59.4** Kaplan–Meier curves for prespecified outcomes in the Systolic Blood Pressure Intervention Trial (SPRINT) participants with chronic kidney disease. (A) The primary cardiovascular outcome, defined as the composite of myocardial infarction, acute coronary syndrome, stroke, acute decompensated heart failure, and death from cardiovascular causes. (B) The all-cause death outcome. (C) The main kidney outcome, defined as the composite of a decrease in estimated glomerular filtration rate of 50% or more from baseline (confirmed by repeat testing ≥90 days later) or the development of end-stage kidney disease. The *broken lines* depict the intensive blood pressure treatment group [systolic blood pressure (SBP) less than 120 mm Hg]; the *solid lines* depict the standard blood pressure treatment group (SBP <140 mm Hg). *CI,* Confidence interval; *HR,* hazard ratio. (From Cheung AK, Rahman M, Reboussin DM, et al. Effects of intensive BP control in CKD. *J Am Soc Nephrol.* 2017;28:2812–2823.)

developing ESKD or of serum creatinine doubling, in comparison with an achieved SBP less than 134 mm Hg, independent of ARB treatment.[107] Progressive lowering of SBP to 120 mm Hg was associated with improved renal outcome and improved rates of patient survival, an effect independent of baseline GFR. However, the lower blood pressure observed was not a primary aim of these studies, and it cannot be assumed that this observed association (between lower blood pressure and improved renal and patient outcomes) is causative.

Several meta-analyses have combined data from multiple trials to examine the potential benefit of lower BP targets in persons with CKD. In one study that included 11 randomized trials with 1860 participants who had nondiabetic CKD

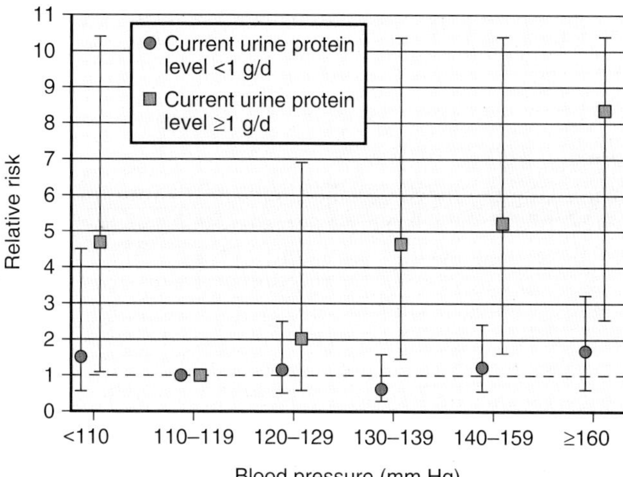


**Fig. 59.5** Results of a meta-analysis of 11 randomized trials that included 1860 persons with nondiabetic chronic kidney disease, showing the relationship between relative risk for kidney disease progression (doubling of serum creatinine level or end-stage kidney disease) and achieved systolic blood pressure in two groups according to the magnitude of proteinuria. (From Jafar TH, Stark PC, Schmid CH, et al. Progression of chronic kidney disease: the role of blood pressure control, proteinuria, and angiotensin-converting enzyme inhibition: a patient-level meta-analysis. *Ann Intern Med.* 2003;139:244–252.)

and proteinuria greater than 1 g/day, the lowest risk of progression was associated with an achieved SBP of 110 to 129 mm Hg, independent of ACE inhibitor treatment (Fig. 59.5).[108] A more recent analysis that included 8127 participants from nine trials (including SPRINT) did not show a significant difference between intensive and usual BP control on the annual rate of change in GFR (MD, 0.07; 95% CI, −0.16 to 0.29 mL/min/year), doubling of serum creatinine concentration or 50% reduction in GFR (RR, 0.99; 95% CI, 0.76–1.29), ESKD (RR, 0.96; 95% CI, 0.78–1.18), composite renal outcome (RR, 0.99; 95% CI, 0.81–1.21), or all-cause mortality (RR, 0.81; 95% CI, 0.64–1.02). Intensive BP control did reduce mortality (RR, 0.78; 95% CI, 0.61–0.99) in a sensitivity analysis that excluded participants with diabetes. In addition, a trend toward a slower rate of GFR decline was observed in those with proteinuria greater than 1 g/day.[109] By contrast, another recent meta-analysis of 18 randomized trials involving 15,924 participants with and without diabetes reported a 14.0% lower risk of all-cause mortality associated with intensive BP lowering (odds ratio [OR], 0.86; 95% CI, 0.76–0.97; $P = .01$). These findings remained similar when data were reanalyzed without the data from SPRINT.[110] The difference in results between meta-analyses is likely attributable to the inclusion of different trials in each, but they are broadly in keeping with the findings of the individual trials discussed earlier.

By contrast, several sources indicate that excessive lowering of blood pressure may be associated with adverse effects in some persons with CKD. In one meta-analysis,[108] an achieved SBP lower than 110 mm Hg was associated with an increased risk of CKD progression (RR, 2.48; 95% CI, 1.07–5.77; see Fig. 59.5), and in IDNT, an achieved SBP lower than 120 mm Hg was associated with increased rates of all-cause mortality and no further improvement in renal outcomes.[107] In addition, secondary analysis of data from the Ongoing Telmisartan Alone and in Combination with Ramipril Global Endpoint Trial (ONTARGET) revealed that hypertensive persons with risk factors for cardiovascular disease who achieved an SBP of less than 120 mm Hg had a significantly higher rate of cardiovascular mortality than did those who achieved an SBP of 120 to 129 mm Hg.[111] Similarly, the Action to Control Cardiovascular Risk in Diabetes (ACCORD) blood pressure study reported no difference in primary cardiovascular outcomes (nonfatal myocardial infarction, nonfatal cerebrovascular accident, or cardiovascular death) among persons with diabetes randomly assigned to achieve an SBP target of less than 120 mm Hg, in comparison with a conventional control target of less than 140/80 mm Hg. During follow-up, the mean SBP was 119.3 mm Hg in persons undergoing intensive therapy and 133.5 mm Hg in those undergoing standard therapy. Persons undergoing intensive therapy demonstrated a slightly lower stroke rate (annual rates of 0.32% vs. 0.53%) but a higher rate of treatment-related adverse events (3.3% vs. 1.3%). Specifically, there were significantly more instances of an eGFR of less than 30 mL/min/1.73 m$^2$ among persons receiving intensive therapy than among those receiving standard therapy (99 vs. 52 events; $P < .001$) and no difference in the primary cardiovascular composite outcome.[112]

The randomized trials in which "low" and "usual" blood pressure targets were compared among persons with CKD have not yielded unequivocal results, but overall, lower blood pressure targets were associated with more effective renoprotection, particularly among persons with significant proteinuria, and lower risk of CVE and/or all-cause mortality. By contrast, there is also an increase in adverse events in some but not all studies. Starting with the observation that persons most likely to benefit from lower BP targets are likely different from those most at risk of adverse events, Basu et al. developed a model for predicting those who would most likely benefit from lower BP targets using data from SPRINT and validated this using data from ACCORD. Older age, black race, higher diastolic BP, and higher lipids were associated with greater cardiovascular risk reduction and current smoking was associated with less cardiovascular risk reduction (C-statistic, 0.71; 95% CI, 0.68–0.74), whereas male sex, current smoking, statin use, elevated creatinine, and higher lipids were associated with higher risk of adverse events (C-statistic, 0.71; 95% CI, 0.69–0.73). In the SPRINT cohort, 4.7% of participants were in the highest two benefit subgroups but the lowest subgroup of harm and 25.7% were in the lowest benefit subgroup (no significant benefit) but the highest two harm subgroups. By contrast, in the ACCORD cohort only 1.5% of participants were in the highest benefit subgroup but the lowest subgroup of harm and 60.9% were in the two lowest benefit subgroups (no significant benefit) but the highest two harm subgroups.[113] An online risk assessment tool has been developed to facilitate the assessment of benefit versus risk.[114]

Current guidelines differ somewhat in their recommendations for blood pressure targets. The KDIGO guidelines (which predate the publication of SPRINT) recommend an SBP of 140 mm Hg or less and DBP of 90 mm Hg or less for diabetic and nondiabetic adults with CKD and urine albumin excretion of less than 30 mg/day (or equivalent). For adults with diabetic or nondiabetic CKD and albumin excretion of at least 30 mg/day, the target values are 130 mm Hg or lower and 80 mm

Hg or lower, respectively.[5] The 2017 American College of Cardiology/American Heart Association guidelines did not adopt the low systolic BP target of less than 120 mm Hg supported by SPRINT but did recommend a target of less than 130/80 mm Hg for persons with increased cardiovascular risk, including those with diabetes and/or CKD.[115] We support these recommendations with a caveat that treatment should be individualized and that low BP targets should be avoided in those at increased risk of adverse effects.

*Clinical Relevance*

Evidence from the Systolic Blood Pressure Intervention Trial (SPRINT) indicates that a lower target for the treatment of systolic blood pressure may afford improved cardiovascular risk reduction but may also be associated with some increase in risk of acute kidney injury and hyperkalemia. The risks versus benefits of a lower blood pressure target should be evaluated in each individual.

## PHARMACOLOGIC INHIBITION OF THE RENIN–ANGIOTENSIN–ALDOSTERONE SYSTEM

A large number of published clinical trials and meta-analyses provide clear evidence to support the use of pharmacologic inhibitors of the RAAS as an essential component of any strategy aiming to achieve maximal renoprotection in persons with CKD (Table 59.1).

### ANGIOTENSIN-CONVERTING ENZYME INHIBITORS

#### Diabetic Kidney Disease

In 1993 the Captopril Collaborative Study Group published results of the first large prospective RCT to clearly show specific renoprotection attributable to ACE inhibitor treatment, a landmark event in the development strategies for achieving renoprotection in persons with diabetes and CKD.[116] Persons ($n$ = 409) with type 1 diabetes and established nephropathy (urine protein excretion >0.5g/day; serum creatinine levels <2.5 mg/dL) were randomly assigned to receive captopril or placebo, and a blood pressure goal of less than 140/90 mm Hg was set for both groups. After a median follow-up period of 3 years, captopril treatment was associated with a 50% reduction in the risk of the combined endpoint of death, dialysis, and renal transplantation and a 48% reduction in the risk of serum creatinine doubling (Fig. 59.6). Because blood pressure control was not statistically different between the groups, the additional renoprotection was not attributable simply to the antihypertensive effects of ACE inhibitors.

These results prompted several further studies to investigate whether ACE inhibitors may also benefit persons with early stage nephropathy characterized by microalbuminuria. A meta-analysis of 12 such studies, including 689 persons with

**Table 59.1 Summary of Studies Showing the Renoprotective Effects of Angiotensin-Converting Enzyme Inhibitors and Angiotensin Receptor Blockers in Diabetic and Nondiabetic Persons With Chronic Kidney Disease**

| CKD Type | Trial Outcome | Reference |
|---|---|---|
| **Angiotensin-Converting Enzyme Inhibitors** | | |
| Type 1 DM + CKD | ↓ Risk of dialysis or death | Lewis et al.[116] |
| Type 1 DM + microalbuminuria | ↓ Risk of overt nephropathy | Mathiesen et al.[116a]<br>Laffel et al.[116b]<br>Viberti et al.[116c] |
| Type 1 DM + normoalbuminuria | No significant benefit | Mauer et al.[132]<br>EUCLID Study Group[116d] |
| Type 2 DM + CKD | Benefit in 1 study only | Bakris et al.[118] |
| Type 2 DM + microalbuminuria | ↓ Risk of overt nephropathy | Ravid et al.[125,126]<br>Sano et al.[122]<br>Trevisan and Tiengo[122]<br>Agardh et al.[124]<br>Ahmad et al.[127]<br>Ruggenenti[130] |
| Type 2 DM + normoalbuminuria | ↓ Risk of developing microalbuminuria | Ravid et al.[128] |
| Nondiabetic CKD | ↓ Doubling of creatinine level/ESKD | Ruggenenti et al.[138,139] |
| **Angiotensin Receptor Blockers** | | |
| Type 1 DM + normoalbuminuria | Small ↑ in albuminuria or no benefit | Mauer et al.[132]<br>Bilous et al.[147] |
| Type 2 DM + normoalbuminuria | ↓ Risk of developing microalbuminuria (small ↑ in rate of cardiovascular mortality) | Bilous et al.[147]<br>Haller et al.[148] |
| Type 2 DM + microalbuminuria | ↓ Risk of overt nephropathy | Parving et al.[146] |
| Type 2 DM + CKD | ↓ Risk of doubling of creatinine level<br>↓ Risk of ESKD | Lewis et al.[145]<br>Brenner et al.[144] |

*CKD,* Chronic kidney disease; *DM,* diabetes mellitus; *ESKD,* end-stage kidney disease.

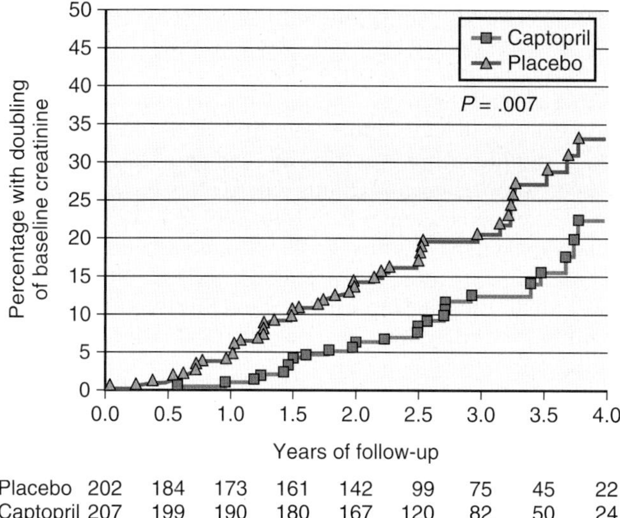


**Fig. 59.6** Results of the first randomized controlled trial to show the renoprotective effects of angiotensin-converting enzyme inhibitor treatment, independent of blood pressure lowering. Persons with type 1 diabetes and nephropathy were randomly assigned to receive treatment with captopril or placebo, and blood pressure was matched between the groups. The graph shows that the cumulative incidence of the primary endpoint, doubling of serum creatinine level, was significantly lower in the persons who received captopril treatment. (From Lewis EJ, Hunsicker LG, Bain RP, et al. The effect of angiotensin-converting-enzyme inhibition on diabetic nephropathy. *N Engl J Med.* 1993;329:1456–1462.)

type 1 diabetes who were monitored for at least 1 year, revealed that ACE inhibitor treatment was associated with a significant reduction in the risk of progression to overt nephropathy (OR, 0.38) and three times the incidence of normalization of microalbuminuria.[117]

Data regarding the renoprotective effects of ACE inhibitors in persons with type 2 diabetes are, to some extent, equivocal. Comparisons of ACE inhibitors and other antihypertensives among persons with overt nephropathy have included relatively small numbers of participants, and only one[118] demonstrated greater reduction in GFR decline in association with ACE inhibitor treatment.[119–121] Evidence of renoprotective benefit at earlier stages of nephropathy is more consistently supportive. Several studies, including the diabetic subgroup analysis of the Heart Outcomes Prevention Evaluation (HOPE) study, demonstrated beneficial effects of ACE inhibitor treatment among persons with type 2 diabetes in decreasing microalbuminuria[122–124] or in reducing the number of persons progressing from microalbuminuria to overt proteinuria (risk reduction, 24% to 67%).[125–128] In addition, the HOPE study reported a 25% reduction in the combined primary endpoint of myocardial infarction, stroke, or cardiovascular death in ramipril-treated persons with type 2 diabetes and risk factors for cardiovascular disease.

Two studies revealed a beneficial role for ACE inhibitor treatment in primary prevention of nephropathy in persons with type 2 diabetes. Among 156 normotensive, normoalbuminuric persons, ACE inhibitor treatment was associated with a 12.5% absolute risk reduction for microalbuminuria,[128,129] and in 1204 hypertensive normoalbuminuric persons, the addition of ACE inhibitor treatment to verapamil was associated with a lower incidence of microalbuminuria than was placebo plus verapamil.[130] By contrast, one relatively large study demonstrated no renoprotective benefit of ACE inhibitors over β-blocker treatment among hypertensive persons with type 2 diabetes with normoalbuminuria or microalbuminuria,[131] and another revealed no reduction in the incidence of microalbuminuria in persons with type 1 diabetes randomly assigned to receive treatment with an ACE inhibitor versus placebo.[132] Three meta-analyses were conducted to investigate the effect of ACE inhibitor treatment in persons with diabetic nephropathy. One analysis included only studies of type 2 diabetes with albuminuria or proteinuria as an outcome; it revealed statistically significant reductions in albuminuria in association with ACE inhibitor treatment versus placebo.[133] A second, larger analysis combined data from studies of type 1 and type 2 diabetes and revealed weak evidence of a reduced risk of serum creatinine doubling (RR, 0.60; 95% CI, 0.34–1.05) or reduced incidence of ESKD (RR, 0.64; 95% CI, 0.40–1.03) and stronger evidence of reduced risk of progression of microalbuminuria to macroalbuminuria (RR, 0.45; 95% CI, 0.28–0.71) with ACE inhibitor treatment versus placebo. All-cause mortality was significantly reduced in persons receiving ACE inhibitors (RR, 0.79; 95% CI, 0.63–0.99).[134] A third meta-analysis involved data from 16 studies of the effect of ACE inhibitor treatment on reducing the risk of microalbuminuria in type 1 and type 2 diabetes. This meta-analysis revealed a significantly reduced risk of developing microalbuminuria with ACE inhibitors in comparison with placebo (RR, 0.60; 95% CI, 0.43–0.84) or calcium channel blocker treatment (RR, 0.58; 95% CI, 0.40–0.84).[135]

On the basis of the data just described, we recommend ACE inhibitor treatment as first-line therapy for all persons with type 1 diabetes and microalbuminuria or overt nephropathy. At present, data are insufficient to support the use of ACE inhibitors to prevent nephropathy in normoalbuminuric persons with type 1 diabetes, but it seems reasonable to recommend them as the treatment of choice in those with hypertension. There is, however, sufficient evidence to recommend the use of ACE inhibitors to reduce progression to overt nephropathy in persons with type 2 diabetes and microalbuminuria or to prevent microalbuminuria in those with hypertension. There is no clear evidence of specific benefit associated with ACE inhibitors in slowing the progression of overt nephropathy in persons with type 2 diabetes; this lack of evidence may be ascribable to the lack of adequately powered studies. Finally, because cardiovascular disease is the most common cause of morbidity and mortality among persons with type 2 diabetes, ACE inhibitor treatment should be considered for the reduction of cardiovascular risk. The KDIGO guidelines recommend treatment with an ACE inhibitor or ARB in all adults with diabetes and urine albumin excretion 30 mg/day or more (or equivalent).[5] For further discussion of the management of diabetic nephropathy, see Chapter 39.

### Nondiabetic Chronic Kidney Disease

After reports of renoprotection with ACE inhibitor treatment in diabetic nephropathy, further studies sought to investigate the renoprotective potential of ACE inhibitors in nondiabetic forms of CKD. One early study demonstrated a 53% reduction in risk of the composite endpoint (serum creatinine doubling or ESKD) in association with ACE inhibitor treatment, but a significantly lower blood pressure in persons receiving ACE inhibitors versus placebo made it impossible to separate the beneficial effects of lowering blood pressure from any unique effects of ACE inhibitor treatment.[136] By contrast, in the REIN study of 352 persons with nondiabetic CKD and urine protein levels exceeding 1 g/day, similar control of blood pressure was achieved in the participants randomly assigned to receive an ACE inhibitor or placebo. Among persons with at least 3 g/day of urine protein at baseline, the study was stopped early because the rate of decline in GFR in participants receiving the ACE inhibitor was significantly lower (0.53 vs. 0.88 mL/min/month)[137]; further analysis showed a significantly lower risk of the combined endpoint (serum creatinine doubling or ESKD) in the participants taking ACE inhibitors (RR, 1.91; 95% CI, 1.10–3.33) for the placebo recipients; Fig. 59.7).

One hundred eighty-six persons from the REIN study who had less than 3 g/day of urine protein were monitored for a median of 31 months after randomization. In findings similar to those of participants with more severe proteinuria, ACE inhibitor treatment significantly reduced the incidence of ESKD (for placebo recipients, RR, 2.72; 95% CI, 1.22–6.08), particularly among those with a GFR of less than 45 mL/min at baseline.[138] After the randomized phase of the study, persons who had received placebo were switched to ACE inhibitors, and those taking ACE inhibitors continued treatment. In a finding consistent with those of the first phase of the study,

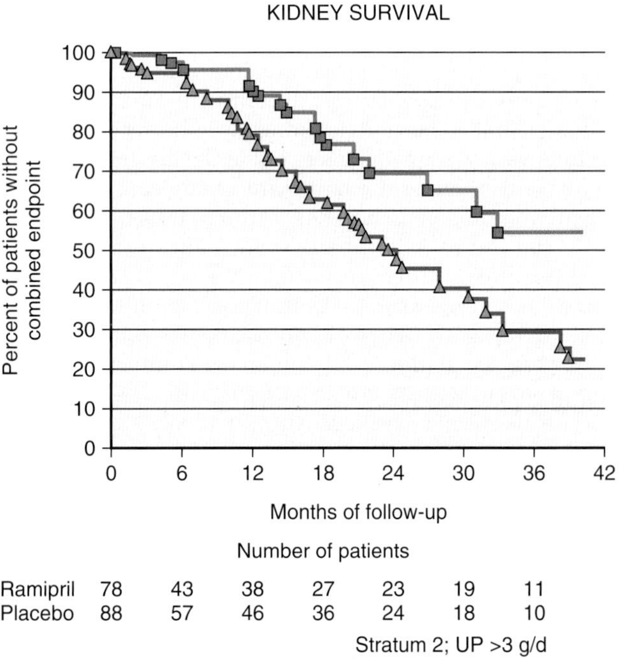


**Fig. 59.7** Kaplan–Meier plot showing the cumulative incidence of the primary endpoint of doubling of serum creatinine level or end-stage kidney disease in persons with nondiabetic chronic kidney disease and urine protein levels exceeding 3 g/day. Persons were randomly assigned to receive treatment with ramipril *(squares)* or placebo *(triangles)*; the graph shows improved renal survival in the ramipril recipients. (From Gruppo Italiano di Studi Epidemiologici in Nefrologia [GISEN]. Randomised placebo-controlled trial of effect of ramipril on decline in glomerular filtration rate and risk of terminal renal failure in proteinuric, non-diabetic nephropathy. *Lancet* 1997;349:1857–1863.)

there was a significant reduction in the rate of decline in GFR of persons switched to ACE inhibitors. In addition, persons continuing with ACE inhibitor treatment showed a further reduction in the rate of GFR decline. Persons who had received ACE inhibitors from the start of the REIN study had a significantly lower risk of reaching ESKD than did those who switched to ACE inhibitors after the initial phase (for placebo recipients, RR, 1.86; 95% CI, 1.07–3.26). In fact, from 36 to 54 months of follow-up, no additional persons in the former group experienced ESKD.[139] Of interest is that a small number of persons who continued taking ACE inhibitors exhibited an increase in GFR after prolonged treatment.[140]

One RCT confirmed that the renoprotective benefits of ACE inhibitor treatment may be observed even in advanced stages of CKD. Among 244 persons with a serum creatinine level of 3.1 to 5.0 mg/dL at baseline, random assignment to ACE inhibitor treatment was associated with a 52% reduction in urine protein levels and a 43% reduction in the risk of the primary endpoint (serum creatinine doubling, ESKD, or death).[141] A meta-analysis of 11 studies that included 1860 persons with nondiabetic CKD[142] revealed that ACE inhibitor treatment was associated with significantly lower risks of ESKD (RR, 0.69; 95% CI, 0.51–0.94) and with the composite endpoint of serum creatinine doubling or ESKD (RR, 0.70; 95% CI, 0.55–0.88). Moreover, the benefits of ACE inhibitor treatment were greater in persons with more severe baseline proteinuria but were inconclusive in persons with urine protein levels of less than 0.5 g/day. A further analysis restricted to persons with autosomal dominant polycystic kidney disease showed greater reduction in proteinuria with ACE inhibitor treatment, but overall evidence of slowing CKD progression was inconclusive and was limited to persons with more severe proteinuria.[143]

In addition to the renoprotective benefits of ACE inhibitor treatment, the HOPE study reported substantial reductions in overall mortality (RR, 0.84) and cardiovascular mortality (RR, 0.74) among 9297 participants who were at increased risk of cardiovascular disease receiving an ACE inhibitor versus placebo.[142a] Although the HOPE study did not include large numbers of persons with nondiabetic CKD, cardiovascular disease remains the most widespread cause of morbidity and mortality among these persons, and the data therefore provide further support for the use of ACE inhibitor therapy in persons with CKD.

In view of the unequivocal data regarding renoprotection and the probable reduction in cardiovascular risk, we recommend ACE inhibitor treatment for all persons with CKD and urine protein levels greater than 0.5 g/day (ACR >30 mg/mmol; PCR >50 mg/mmol) unless there are specific contraindications. The KDIGO guidelines similarly recommend treatment with an ACE inhibitor or ARB in adults with CKD and urine albumin excretion exceeding 300 mg/day (or equivalent).[5]

## ANGIOTENSIN RECEPTOR BLOCKERS

### Diabetic Kidney Disease

ARBs inhibit the RAAS by blocking angiotensin II subtype 1 receptors. Although ACE inhibitors and ARBs differ significantly in their effects on the RAAS in ways that may be therapeutically relevant, experimental studies indicate that both treatments produce similar changes in glomerular hemodynamics (for a given blood pressure change) and afford equivalent renoprotection in a variety of CKD models.[143a] Three large RCTs published simultaneously established a clear role for ARB therapy in achieving renoprotection for persons with type 2 diabetes. In the Reduction of Endpoints in NIDDM with the Angiotensin II Antagonist Losartan (RENAAL) trial, 1513 persons with overt diabetic nephropathy were randomly assigned to receive ARB treatment or placebo and were monitored for a mean of 3.4 years.[144] ARB treatment was associated with significant reductions in the incidence of serum creatinine doubling (RR reduction, 25%) and in ESKD (RR reduction, 28%; Fig. 59.8).

In IDNT, 1715 persons with overt diabetic nephropathy were randomly assigned to receive treatment with the ARB irbesartan, amlodipine, or placebo.[145] After a mean of 2.6 years, the risk of serum creatinine doubling was 33% lower with irbesartan than with placebo and 37% lower with irbesartan than with amlodipine. ARB treatment was associated with a 23% reduction in the risk of ESKD in comparison with placebo and amlodipine, but this reduction was not statistically significant (Fig. 59.9). Of importance is that close matching of achieved blood pressure between groups in both these trials implies that, as with the ACE inhibitor studies, the additional renoprotective effects of ARB treatment could not be attributed merely to their antihypertensive effects.

In a third study, investigators examined the renoprotective effects of an ARB (irbesartan) in 590 persons with type 2 diabetes, hypertension, and microalbuminuria.[146] Persons were randomly assigned to receive irbesartan at one of two different dosages (300 or 150 mg/day) or placebo. After 2 years, there were significant differences in the incidence of overt proteinuria (5.2%, 9.7%, and 14.9%), and the higher dose of irbesartan was associated with substantial reduction in the risk of overt nephropathy (HR, 0.30; 95% CI, 0.14–0.61) in comparison with placebo. This dose-dependent effect indicates that when ARBs are used to treat diabetic microalbuminuria, the dose should be titrated up to the maximum antihypertensive dose.

A meta-analysis confirmed the results of individual trials by showing significant reductions in the risk of ESKD (RR, 0.78; 95% CI, 0.67–0.91) and in doubling of serum creatinine level (RR, 0.79; 95% CI, 0.67–0.93), as well as a reduction in risk of progression from microalbuminuria to macroalbuminuria

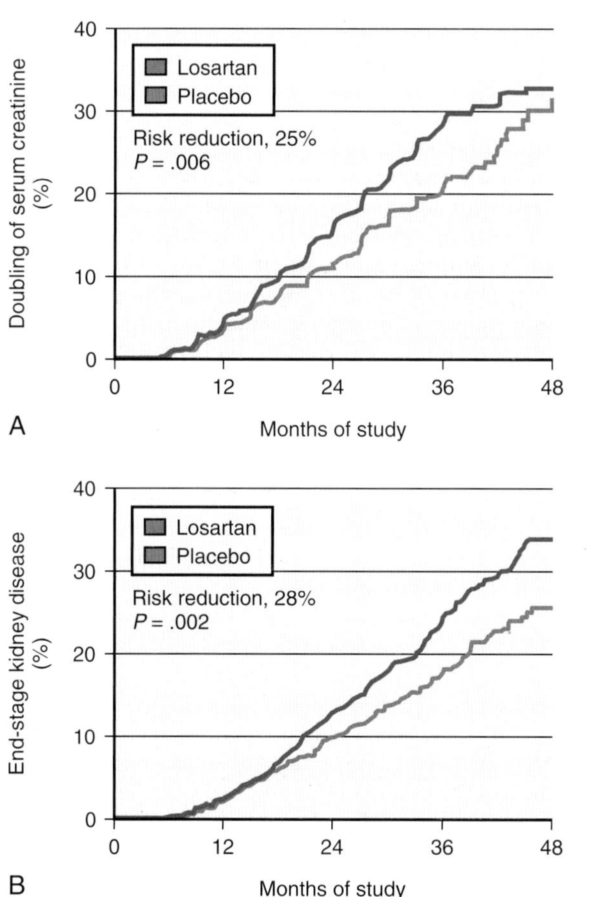


**Fig. 59.8** Kaplan–Meier curves showing the incidence of (A) doubling of serum creatinine level and (B) end-stage kidney disease in persons with type 2 diabetes and nephropathy who were randomly assigned to receive treatment with losartan or placebo. (From Brenner BM, Cooper ME, de Zeeuw D, et al. Effects of losartan on renal and cardiovascular outcomes in persons with type 2 diabetes and nephropathy. *N Engl J Med.* 2001;345:861–869.)

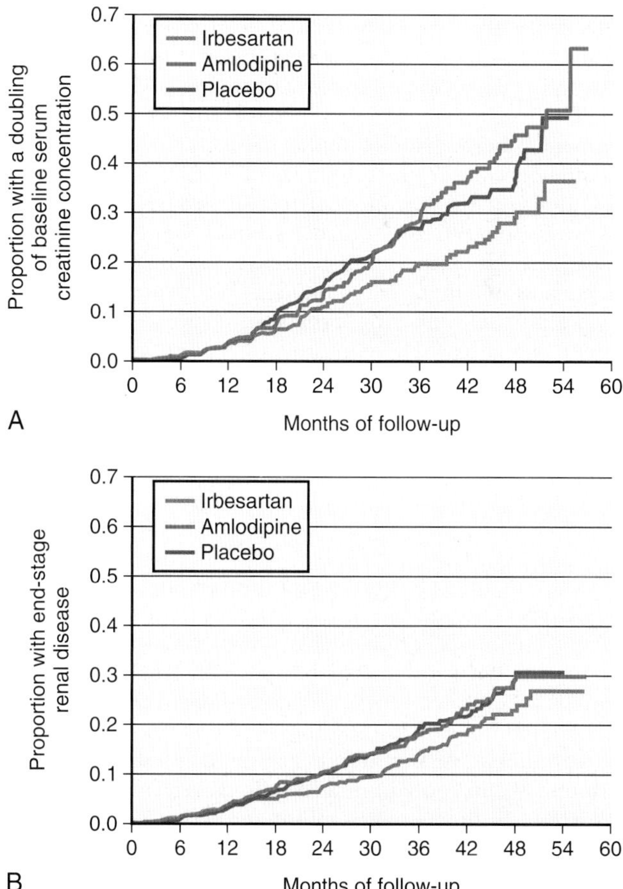


**Fig. 59.9** Kaplan–Meier curves showing the incidence of (A) doubling of serum creatinine levels and (B) end-stage kidney disease in persons with type 2 diabetes and nephropathy who were randomly assigned to receive treatment with irbesartan, amlodipine, or placebo. (From Lewis EJ, Hunsicker LG, Clarke WR, et al. Renoprotective effect of the angiotensin-receptor antagonist irbesartan in persons with nephropathy due to type 2 diabetes. *N Engl J Med.* 2001;345:851–860.)

(RR, 0.49; 95% CI, 0.32–0.75) among diabetic persons treated with ARB versus placebo.[134] Of interest is that there was no reduction in all-cause mortality.

Several RCTs have been conducted to investigate the potential role of ARB treatment to prevent the development of microalbuminuria in persons with diabetes. In the Renin Angiotensin System Study (RASS), normotensive persons with type 1 diabetes randomly assigned to receive treatment with losartan evidenced a significantly higher incidence of microalbuminuria than did the participants receiving placebo (17% vs. 6%; $P = .01$),[132] and in the Diabetic Retinopathy Candesartan Trials (DIRECT), mainly normotensive persons with type 1 or type 2 diabetes randomly assigned to receive treatment with candesartan evidenced no reduction in the incidence of microalbuminuria in comparison with participants receiving placebo.[147] By contrast, when hypertensive persons with type 2 diabetes were studied in the Randomized Olmesartan and Diabetes Microalbuminuria Prevention (ROADMAP) trial, those who received treatment with olmesartan evidenced a 23% delay in the time to onset of microalbuminuria in comparison with participants who received placebo. A small but significantly higher incidence of death from cardiovascular causes was observed, particularly in persons with a previous history of cardiovascular disease and in those with the greatest reduction in blood pressure.[148]

In summary, there is sufficient evidence to support the use of ARB treatment to achieve renoprotection in persons with type 2 diabetes and overt nephropathy. ARB treatment is also effective in preventing progression from microalbuminuria to overt diabetic nephropathy in persons with type 2 diabetes. Data from the ROADMAP trial show that ARB treatment delays the onset of microalbuminuria in hypertensive persons with type 2 diabetes, but the associated increase in death from cardiovascular disease remains a concern. It seems reasonable to recommend ARB treatment for hypertensive persons with type 2 diabetes in the absence of cardiovascular disease. By contrast, no renoprotective benefit is associated with ARB treatment in normotensive persons with type 1 or 2 diabetes. The KDIGO guidelines recommend treatment with an ACE inhibitor or ARB in all adults with diabetes and urine albumin excretion 30 mg/day or higher (or equivalent).[5]

### Nondiabetic Chronic Kidney Disease

No large RCTs have investigated the renoprotective effects of ARBs versus other antihypertensive drugs in nondiabetic kidney disease. As will be discussed later, published evidence indicates that it is reasonable to expect that ARBs will provide similar renoprotective benefits in nondiabetic CKD to those observed in diabetic kidney disease. Based on the evidence, we recommend ACE inhibitor treatment as first-line therapy for nondiabetic, proteinuric CKD but ARBs provide a valuable alternative in persons who are intolerant to ACE inhibitors. The KDIGO guidelines recommend treatment with an ACE inhibitor or ARB in adults with all forms of CKD and albuminuria greater than 300 mg/day (or equivalent).[5]

## ANGIOTENSIN-CONVERTING ENZYME INHIBITORS VERSUS ANGIOTENSIN RECEPTOR BLOCKER TREATMENT

Despite differences in their mode of action, the renoprotective effects of ACE inhibitors and ARB treatment have been directly compared in few studies. In a mixed group of persons with type 2 diabetes and microalbuminuria or macroalbuminuria, there was no significant difference between ACE inhibitors and ARB treatment in the primary outcome of change in GFR or a secondary outcome of UACR.[149] According to a meta-analysis of small trials in which ACE inhibitors were compared with ARB treatment in persons with diabetic CKD, benefits were similar with regard to incidence of ESKD, serum creatinine doubling, and progression of microalbuminuria to macroalbuminuria.[150] Similarly, in ONTARGET, there was no difference in cardiovascular or renal endpoints between persons randomly assigned to receive treatment with an ACE inhibitor and those assigned to receive an ARB.[151] By contrast, in the RASS, ARB treatment was associated with a higher incidence of microalbuminuria than was placebo in persons with type 1 diabetes, whereas ACE inhibitors were not significantly different from placebo in this regard.[132]

Most national and international guidelines therefore recommend ACE inhibitor or ARB treatment for all forms of diabetic and nondiabetic CKD and leave the choice to individual physicians. One advantage of ARBs over ACE inhibitors is their more favorable side-effect profile.[152] In clinical trials, ARBs have been reported to have side-effect profiles similar to those of placebo[153,154] and, in particular, are not associated with the cough that may occur in up to 20% of persons receiving an ACE inhibitor. Among persons who switched from ACE inhibitors to ARB therapy, cough recurred significantly less often than in persons rechallenged with an ACE inhibitor.[155,156]

In choosing between ACE inhibitor and ARB therapy for persons with type 2 diabetes and diabetic nephropathy, physicians have to consider evidence of proven renoprotection with ARB treatment versus a mortality benefit associated with ACE inhibitor treatment (in persons without established diabetic nephropathy). One meta-analysis suggested a modestly increased risk of new cancer occurrence in persons on ARB treatment; this finding has created some controversy.[157] However, two long-term antihypertensive cohort studies linked to cancer registries, which can explore competing risk, showed no increased cancer risk from long-term hypertension therapy and RAAS blockade.[158,159] A large network meta-analysis of 70 RCTs of antihypertensive therapy in 324,168 persons recorded no difference in risk of cancer between the participants receiving treatment (including ARBs) and control participants.[160]

Some meta-analyses have called into question the value of RAAS inhibition for renoprotection. In one study, trials of ACE inhibitor and ARB treatment were pooled, and when studies of diabetic and nondiabetic CKD were considered together, the analysis revealed a benefit in reducing the risk of ESKD (RR, 0.87; 95% CI, 0.75–0.99) and albuminuria (mean urine albumin level, −15.7 mg/day; 95% CI, −24.7 to −6.7 mg/day) but no significant benefit in reducing the risk of serum creatinine doubling (RR, 0.71; 95% CI, 0.49–1.04). When data from studies of diabetic and nondiabetic CKD were considered separately, no significant benefits were evident with regard to incidence of ESKD or serum creatinine doubling, but the benefit for albuminuria reduction persisted. The authors concluded that the renoprotective effects of ACE inhibitor or ARB therapy probably result only from their antihypertensive effects.[161] This meta-analysis is, however, flawed in our opinion, and its conclusions have been rejected by many other investigators.[162] The principal weaknesses were inclusion of data from the large ALLHAT study, in which only a minority of persons (5662 of 33,357) actually had CKD[88]; heterogeneity across trials that should not have been pooled; and lack of patient-level data.[163] A more recent meta-analysis focused on the potential benefits of RAAS inhibitors in persons with diabetes. The analysis included 19 RCTs that enrolled 25,414 participants and reported no significant difference between groups receiving RAASi inhibitors or other antihypertensives for risk of death, cardiovascular death, and CVE apart from heart failure, which was reduced with RAAS inhibitor treatment (HR, 0.78; 95% CI, 0.70–0.88). In addition, no difference was observed in incidence of ESKD, the only renal outcome evaluated.[164] These findings should, however, be interpreted in light of several substantial limitations. First, only a minority of the included trials enrolled participants with CKD and the findings are therefore not necessarily applicable to persons with diabetes and CKD. Second, median follow-up was relatively short at 3.8 years, which is too short to expect any impact of RAAS inhibitor treatment on the incidence of ESKD in the populations studied. Third, the analysis excluded placebo-controlled trials, ignoring the fact that in many of these trials other antihypertensive medication was prescribed to achieve similar control of blood pressure between groups.

By contrast, a large-network meta-analysis included data from 43,256 participants with diabetes and CKD from 157 randomized trials that compared one blood pressure treatment with another or placebo or control. No drug treatment was more effective than placebo in reducing all-cause mortality but ARB treatment was associated with a significant reduction in incidence of ESKD (OR, 0.77; 95% CI, 0.65–0.92) and combination ACE inhibitor and ARB was similarly effective (OR, 0.62; 95% CI, 0.43–0.90). The effect of ACE inhibitor monotherapy was of borderline statistical significance (OR, 0.71; 95% CI, 0.51–1.01). Endothelin inhibitors, ACE inhibitors, and ARBs significantly reduced the risk of serum creatinine doubling. All regimens that included an ACE inhibitor or ARB were associated with regression of albuminuria. No treatment significantly increased the risks of hyperkalemia or AKI, though for combination ACE inhibitor and ARB therapy this was of borderline significance. Interestingly some other treatments were associated with adverse outcomes when used as monotherapy: Calcium channel blockers did not improve albuminuria and tended to increase doubling of serum creatinine; β-blockers were associated with reduced survival; renin inhibitors increased the risk of serum creatinine doubling.[165]

## COMBINATION TREATMENT WITH ANGIOTENSIN-CONVERTING ENZYME INHIBITORS AND ANGIOTENSIN RECEPTOR BLOCKERS

The differing mechanisms of ACE inhibitors and ARBs on the RAAS imply that in combination, they may have additive or synergistic effects. The added antihypertensive effects of combination therapy have, however, made it difficult to separate the benefits of additional blood pressure lowering from added renoprotection directly attributable to dual blockade of the RAAS. In several small studies, researchers reported additional lowering of urine protein excretion with combination therapy of ACE inhibitors and ARBs, in comparison with monotherapy; when pooled in three meta-analyses, all data indicate that there is greater antiproteinuric effect with combination RAAS inhibition therapy.[166–168] Only one RCT yielded results indicating benefit associated with ACE inhibitor and ARB combination therapy in CKD with respect to serum creatinine doubling or ESKD incidence. Publication of that study was, however, withdrawn because of concerns about the conduct of the study and integrity of the data.[169]

Furthermore, the results of the ONTARGET trial cast doubt on the benefit of dual therapy.[151] In ONTARGET, 25,620 persons with hypertension and additional cardiovascular risk factors were randomly assigned to receive therapy with an ACE inhibitor alone, an ARB alone, or a combination of both.[170] The primary analysis revealed no difference in CVEs between the randomized groups, but the number of events for the composite renal outcome—need for dialysis, doubling of serum creatinine level, and death[151]—was increased with combination therapy ($n$ = 1233, or 14.5%; HR, 1.09; 95% CI, 1.01–1.18; $P$ = .037) versus monotherapy (ARB: $n$ = 1147, or 13.4%; ACE inhibitor: $n$ = 1150, or 13.5%). This excess was attributable predominantly to more acute dialysis and to the combination of all types of dialysis and serum creatinine doubling. In addition, hyperkalemia (K >5.5 mmol/L) was more frequent with combination therapy (ACE inhibitor, 3.2%; ARB, 3.3%; combination, 5.6%; $P <$ .001 for combination versus ACE inhibitor). However, participants were recruited on the basis of cardiovascular risk profile, and the majority did not have reduced GFR (mean baseline eGFR, 74 mL/min/1.73 $m^2$) or proteinuria (13% had microalbuminuria and 4% had macroalbuminuria). In addition, participants were elderly (mean age 66.5 years) and predominantly male (73%). They had substantial vascular disease: coronary artery disease (75%), previous myocardial infarction (50%), angina (35%), unstable angina (15%), and peripheral vascular disease (13%). Angiographic studies[171] suggest that approximately 10% to 15% of this cohort would be expected to have atheromatous renal vascular disease in large vessels, and many more would have small vessel disease.

Several other studies have provided evidence of the potential risks of combination therapy. A population-based observational study reported a significantly higher incidence of the combined endpoint of serum creatinine doubling, ESKD, or death in elderly persons (older than 65 years) receiving combination therapy with ACE inhibitors and ARBs than among those receiving monotherapy (5.2 vs. 2.4 events per 1000 persons per month; adjusted HR, 2.36; 95% CI, 1.51–3.71). The incidence of hyperkalemia was also higher with combination therapy (2.5 vs. 0.9 events per 1000 persons per month; adjusted HR, 2.42; 95% CI, 1.36–4.32).[172] A further RCT (VA NEPHRON-D) in 1448 people with type 2 diabetes and UACR of at least 300 mg/g was stopped early due to safety concerns. Analysis of available data found no benefit with respect to the primary outcome of CKD progression, ESKD, or death in participants randomized to combination versus monotherapy, though early termination of the trial reduced the potential to observe benefit. Of concern, those receiving combination therapy evidenced a significantly higher incidence of AKI (12.2 vs. 6.7 events per 100 person-years; $P <$ .001) and hyperkalemia (6.3 vs. 2.6 events per 100 person-years; $P <$ .001).[173]

In a meta-analysis of 59 RCTs comparing the efficacy and safety of combination versus single RAAS inhibitor therapy in CKD, combination therapy was associated with significant improvement in urine albumin and protein excretion as well as blood pressure control. These beneficial effects, however, were associated with a net 1.8 mL/min/1.73 m$^2$ decline in GFR, a significant increase in serum potassium level (3.4% higher rate of hyperkalemia), and a 4.6% higher rate of hypotension. There was no effect on doubling of the serum creatinine level, hospitalization, or mortality.[174]

The KDIGO guidelines do not recommend the use of combination ACE inhibitor and ARB therapy for renoprotection[5] and NICE guidelines[78] as well as the 2017 American College of Cardiology/American Heart Association guidelines[115] recommend against combination therapy. Nevertheless, as discussed earlier, there is some evidence of potential benefit, particularly in nondiabetic, proteinuric CKD and it may be possible to reduce the risk of harm by avoiding combination therapy in high-risk groups, such as those with extensive atherosclerosis. It has been proposed that using lower doses of ACE inhibitor and ARB in combination may achieve benefit while reducing harm and this hypothesis is currently being tested in an RCT.

### ALDOSTERONE ANTAGONISM

Aldosterone has been identified as an important factor in the pathogenesis of hypertension, cardiovascular disease, and progressive kidney injury through hemodynamic and profibrotic actions. Treatment with spironolactone and other aldosterone antagonists has produced renoprotective effects in experimental[175] and small clinical studies.[176] One meta-analysis of their use in comparison with other RAAS-inhibiting agents included data from 10 trials and 845 participants. In comparison with ACE inhibitor or ARB plus placebo, nonselective aldosterone antagonists added to ACE inhibitor or ARB treatment significantly reduced proteinuria (weighted MD, −0.80 g/day; 95% CI, −1.23 to −0.38) and blood pressure, but these developments did not translate into an improvement in GFR (weighted MD, −0.70 mL/min/1.73 m$^2$; 95% CI, −4.73 to 3.34). There was a significant increase in the risk of hyperkalemia with the addition of an aldosterone antagonist (RR, 3.06; 95% CI, 1.26–7.41).[177] A more recent meta-analysis of 27 studies confirmed that treatment with a nonselective aldosterone antagonist (spironolactone) alone or in combination with an ACE inhibitor or ARB was associated with reduction in proteinuria (standardized MD, −0.61 g/day; 95% CI, −1.08 to −0.13) and blood pressure (MD, −3.44 mm Hg; 95% CI, −5.05 to −1.83) but provided no data on reduction in CVEs or ESKD. In addition, aldosterone antagonist treatment was associated with an increased risk of hyperkalemia (RR, 2.00; 95% CI, 1.25–3.20) and gynecomastia compared with ACE inhibitor or ARB (or both) (RR, 5.14; 95% CI, 1.14–23.23).[178] The renoprotective potential of the more novel nonsteroidal aldosterone antagonists is also starting to be evaluated. In one RCT that enrolled 336 persons with hypertension, UACR 30 to 599 mg/g, and eGFR of 50 mL/min/1.73 m$^2$ or above, treatment with eplerenone for 52 weeks, added to ACE inhibitor of ARB therapy, resulted in a 17.3% decrease in UACR, whereas a 10.3% increase was observed in those who received placebo ($P$ = .02). Serum potassium was higher with eplerenone treatment but no episodes of severe hyperkalemia (serum potassium > 5.5 mmol/L) were observed.[179]

Aldosterone antagonists are recommended as part of the management of heart failure and resistant hypertension, but their use is often limited by the development of hyperkalemia, particularly in persons with reduced GFR. The use of novel potassium-binding agents has been proposed as a strategy to prevent hyperkalemia and facilitate aldosterone antagonist treatment and clinical trials are underway to evaluate this in the context of CKD.[180] Until the results of further RCTs are published, treatment with an aldosterone antagonist cannot be recommended for the management of CKD, though it may be beneficial to improve control of resistant hypertension, provided that care is taken to monitor and avoid hyperkalemia. Further studies are required to evaluate the long-term effects of aldosterone antagonists on renal outcomes, mortality, and safety.

### DIRECT RENIN INHIBITORS

Direct renin inhibitors inhibit the RAAS at its rate-limiting step (the conversion of angiotensinogen to angiotensin I) and may therefore achieve more complete blockade of the RAAS than do ACE inhibitors or ARBs. Direct renin inhibitors are effective antihypertensive drugs and reduced proteinuria in experimental models of CKD[181,182] and RCTs.[183,184] However, a large randomized trial that included 8561 people with type 2 diabetes and albuminuria or cardiovascular disease was stopped prematurely after the second interim efficacy analysis. Despite greater lowering of blood pressure and albuminuria with a combination of direct renin inhibitor and ARB therapy, no benefit was observed with respect to the composite primary endpoint of CVE, CKD progression, ESKD, or death versus ARB monotherapy, but combination therapy was associated with a higher incidence of hyperkalemia and hypotension.[185,186] There is currently, therefore, no evidence that direct renin inhibitor therapy, alone or in combination with ACE inhibitor therapy, affords more effective renoprotection than ACE inhibitor or ARB therapy alone.

***Clinical Relevance***

Antihypertensive therapy with angiotensin-converting enzyme inhibitors or angiotensin receptor blockers as "first line" in persons with albuminuria is the mainstay of treatment to achieve optimal renoprotection. Treatment should be started at a low dose and titrated upward. Serum creatinine and potassium should be checked approximately 1 week after initiation or dose titration.

## SODIUM GLUCOSE COTRANSPORTER 2 (SGLT2) INHIBITORS

The sodium glucose cotransporter 2 (SGLT2) inhibitors block the reabsorption of glucose and sodium in the proximal tubule and were developed primarily as a treatment for type 2 diabetes mellitus. RCTs in persons with diabetes and normal or moderately reduced GFR found that these drugs improved glycemic control but importantly also afforded significant reductions in fatal and nonfatal CVE, all-cause mortality, and multiple measures of diabetic kidney disease progression.[187] These renoprotective effects have been attributed to multiple mechanisms including lowering of system blood pressure and intraglomerular hydraulic pressure, amelioration of glomerular hyperfiltration, reduction of albuminuria, weight loss, amelioration of arterial stiffness, and induction of hypoxia-inducible factor 1.[188] At present, the SGLT2 inhibitors are indicated only in persons with type 2 diabetes and normal or mildly reduced GFR (eGFR ≥45 mL/min/1.73 m$^2$ for some drugs) but further trials are investigating whether these drugs may afford renal protection in persons with more advanced CKD. The CREDENCE trial enrolled 4401 adults with type 2 diabetes, eGFR 30 to 89 mL/min/1.73 m$^2$, and UACR 300 to 5000 mg/g despite treatment with the maximum dose of an ACE inhibitor or ARB. The study was stopped early due to evidence of benefit in a planned interim analysis. The risk of the composite primary outcome of ESKD, doubling of serum creatinine, and cardiovascular or renal death, was reduced by 30% in participants who received canagliflozin (HR, 0.70; 95% CI, 0.53 to 0.81; $p < 0.001$) and the risk of ESKD was reduced by 32% (HR, 0.68; 95% CI, 0.54 to 0.86; $p = 0.002$).[189] Furthermore, trials are now underway to evaluate the renoprotective potential of SGLT2 inhibitors across a broader spectrum of CKD including nondiabetic CKD. The SGLT2 inhibitors are reviewed in more detail in relation to the treatment of diabetic kidney disease in Chapter 39.

## HYPERURICEMIA

A number of studies have highlighted evidence that elevated serum uric acid concentration is a risk factor for the development and progression of CKD.[190,191] It has also been associated with excess cardiovascular risk and hypertension in a cohort of community-based persons.[192] Whether it is an independent risk factor for these outcomes in CKD or a marker of more severe renal and cardiovascular outcomes is an issue of ongoing debate.[193] In animal studies, elevated serum uric acid decreases nitric oxide production, which provokes endothelial dysfunction, increases blood pressure, promotes fibrosis, and causes the release of proinflammatory cytokines and thereby results in T-cell activation. A meta-analysis of eight small trials investigating the potential benefits of lowering uric acid in CKD with allopurinol included data from 476 participants. In three studies that reported serum creatinine concentration, allopurinol treatment was associated with a lower serum creatinine than was placebo, but in five studies that reported eGFR, there was no significant difference between groups treated with allopurinol or placebo. In five trials that measured proteinuria, no benefit was observed. Progression to ESKD was reported in only two studies and was not different between treatment groups, although the incidence was too low to allow robust conclusions to be made.[194] A more recent meta-analysis included nine trials of all xanthine oxidase inhibitors (febuxostat and topiroxostat in addition to allopurinol) in persons with CKD and hyperuricemia.[195] In three studies the risk of the combined outcome of 50% reduction in eGFR, doubling of serum creatinine, or initiation of dialysis was significantly reduced by xanthine oxidase inhibitor treatment (204 participants; RR, 0.42; 95% CI, 0.22–0.80). Better preservation of eGFR was observed in data pooled from RCTs of minimum 3 months' duration (4 studies, 357 patients; MD, 6.82 mL/min/1.73 m$^2$; 95% CI, 3.50–10.15) and in trials of high methodological quality (blind design; 3 studies, 400 patients; MD, 2.61 mL/min/1.73 m$^2$; 95% CI, 0.23–4.99). However, no benefits were observed with respect to serum creatinine or proteinuria.[195]

One randomized trial of allopurinol in 113 persons with CKD (included in the aforementioned meta-analysis) reported a 47% reduction in risk of CKD progression (defined as decrease in eGFR of >0.2 mL/min/month) in participants treated with allopurinol after multivariable Cox proportional hazards analysis, as well as a 71% reduction in risk of new CVEs and 62% reduction in risk of hospitalization.[196] Long-term follow-up of these participants reported further benefit with a 68% reduction in risk of a renal event (initiation of RRT or 50% reduction in GFR or doubling of serum creatinine) and a 57% reduction in risk of CVE.[197] One observational study compared outcomes in 874 persons with CKD and hyperuricemia treated with benzbromarone, allopurinol, or febuxostat using Cox proportional hazards models. Febuxostat was more effective in lowering serum uric acid concentration than the other treatments. Benzbromarone was associated with a lower risk of ESKD (defined by initiation of dialysis) than allopurinol (HR, 0.50; 95% CI, 0.25–0.99), which evidenced similar lack of benefit to febuxostat. Participants who achieved the target for lowering serum uric acid concentration with febuxostat or benzbromarone also had a reduced risk of ESKD.[198]

Despite the aforementioned evidence suggesting renoprotective benefit, the trials published to date are of insufficient size to recommend uric acid lowering as part of the management of CKD unless there is clinical evidence of gout.

## TREATMENT OF METABOLIC ACIDOSIS

As the number of functioning nephrons declines, CKD leads to net retention of hydrogen ions, which begins when GFR falls below 40 to 50 mL/min/1.73 m$^2$.[199] Among persons in whom GFR decreases from 90 to less than 20 mL/min/1.73 m$^2$, the prevalence of metabolic acidosis rises from 2% to 39% and is higher among younger persons and those with diabetes.[200] As the patient approaches ESKD, the plasma bicarbonate concentration tends to stabilize between 15 and 20 mEq/L. Chronic metabolic acidosis has multiple adverse consequences, including increased protein catabolism, increased bone turnover, induction of inflammatory mediators, insulin resistance, and increased production of corticosteroids and parathyroid hormone. Several observational studies, including the CRIC study, have identified low serum bicarbonate as a risk factor for CKD progression,[201] although post hoc analysis of data from persons with diabetic kidney disease enrolled in the RENAAL and IDNT studies found that an association between lower serum bicarbonate and renal outcomes was not maintained after adjustment for baseline GFR.[202]

The first study to show convincing renoprotection with bicarbonate supplementation was from a single center and involved 134 persons with advanced CKD (creatinine clearance rates between 15 and 30 mL/min/1.73 m$^2$) and baseline serum bicarbonate concentrations of 16 to 20 mEq/L. The participants were randomly assigned to receive treatment with oral bicarbonate or no treatment.[203] After 2 years of follow-up, there was a lower mean rate of decline in creatinine clearance (1.88 vs. 5.93 mL/min/1.73 m$^2$) and a lower risk of ESKD among the persons who received the bicarbonate treatment than among the controls (6.5% vs. 33%). In a subsequent randomized, placebo-controlled trial in persons with a mean eGFR of 75 mL/min/1.73 m$^2$, treatment with sodium bicarbonate for 5 years was associated with a slower rate of decline in eGFR (derived from plasma cystatin C measurements) compared with placebo or treatment with sodium chloride.[204] Western diets are typically acid producing, but the addition of significant portions of fruits and vegetables can move this to a base-producing state. Further studies have reported that correction of acidosis with a diet rich in fruits and vegetables was as effective as sodium bicarbonate in ameliorating kidney damage in early (stage 1 or 2 CKD)[205] and more advanced (stage 4 CKD) disease.[206] Furthermore, a recent trial has reported benefit even in people with mild acidosis. People with stage 3 CKD and serum bicarbonate 22 to 24 mmol/L were randomized to oral bicarbonate supplementation, a diet rich in fruits and vegetables, or "usual care." All participants received treatment with an RAAS inhibitor, and SBP was controlled to lower than 130 mm Hg. Both interventions achieved an increase in serum bicarbonate and were associated with a decrease in urinary angiotensinogen. After 3 years, both interventions were associated with less albuminuria and GFR decline than the "usual care" group.[207] The KDIGO guidelines recommend bicarbonate supplementation for persons with levels below 22 mEq/L,[3] but further studies are required to further investigate whether this may also be beneficial in the setting of less severe acidosis.

## PROTEINURIA AS A THERAPEUTIC TARGET

Proteinuria is a marker of glomerular filtration barrier integrity, and the magnitude of proteinuria has therefore been used as an indicator of the severity of glomerulopathy. This view has been confirmed by several observations that the severity of proteinuria at baseline is the most important independent predictor of renal outcomes in randomized trials of persons with diabetic nephropathy[208,209] and nondiabetic nephropathy.[210–212] In addition, it has been proposed that proteinuria per se contributes to progressive renal injury[213] and that amelioration of proteinuria should therefore be viewed as a therapeutic goal.

Support for this hypothesis is derived from a number of sources. In the MDRD study, reduction in urine protein levels, independent of blood pressure, was associated with slower progression of CKD, and the degree of benefit achieved through blood pressure lowering was dependent on the extent of baseline proteinuria.[99] Furthermore, several other investigators have observed that the percentage reduction in urine protein level after initiation of ACE inhibitor or ARB treatment and the magnitude of proteinuria during treatment (residual proteinuria) are strong independent predictors of the subsequent rate of decline in GFR among persons with diabetic and nondiabetic CKD.[208,209] A meta-analysis that included data from 1860 persons with nondiabetic CKD confirmed these findings and showed that during antihypertensive treatment, the achieved level of urine protein was a powerful predictor of the combined endpoint of serum creatinine doubling or onset of ESKD (RR, 5.6 for each 1.0-g/day increase in achieved level of proteinuria).[142] A further meta-analysis of 21 randomized trials of drug treatment in CKD that included 78,342 participants found that for each 30% initial reduction in albuminuria on treatment, the risk of ESKD decreased by 23.7% (95% CI, 11.4%–34.2%) independent of the class of drug used for treatment.[214]

One RCT provided direct evidence that the extent to which proteinuria is lowered determines subsequent prognosis. In the Renoprotection of Optimal Antiproteinuric Doses (ROAD) study, 360 nondiabetic persons with proteinuria and CKD were randomly assigned to receive a conventional dosage of benazepril (10 mg/day), a conventional dosage of losartan (50 mg/day), an upward titration of benazepril (range of 10–40 mg/day), or an upward titration of losartan (range of 50–200 mg/day).[215] In upward titration, the dosage of the RAAS-inhibiting agent was increased to maximize the antiproteinuric effect. After a median of 3.7 years, titration of benazepril and losartan to the maximum antiproteinuric dose, in comparison with the fixed conventional dosages, reduced the risk of serum creatinine doubling by 49% and 50%, respectively, and the risk of ESKD by 47% in both groups (Fig. 59.10). Both agents provided similar overall RR reductions at optimal antiproteinuric dosages. Reduction of urine protein levels at 3 months (approximately 50% decrease with the upward-titration strategy) was closely correlated with the subsequent rate of GFR decline. Participants in all groups of the study had similar reductions in blood pressure. Regardless of whether proteinuria contributes directly to renal injury, the strong association between achieved reduction in urine protein and renoprotection in clinical studies implies that amelioration of proteinuria should be regarded as an important therapeutic goal in renoprotective strategies. We recommend a goal of reducing proteinuria to less than 0.5 g/day (equivalent UACR of ≈300 mg/g or 30 mg/mmol).

> ***Clinical Relevance***
> Proteinuria should be regarded as a therapeutic target and renin–angiotensin–aldosterone system inhibitor therapy should be escalated and other antihypertensive therapy added to achieve blood pressure targets with the aim of reducing proteinuria to less than 0.5 g/day.

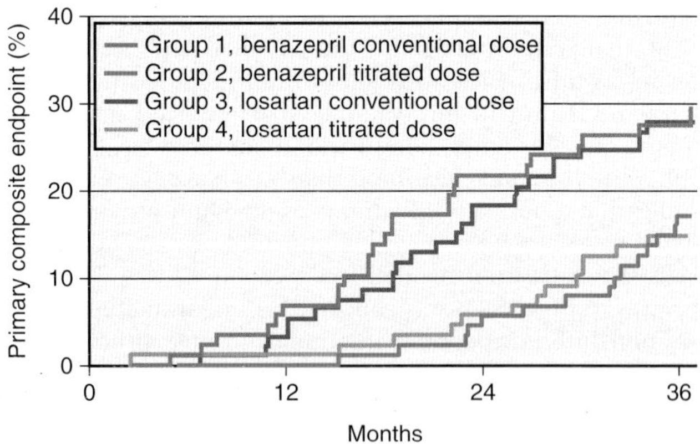


**Fig. 59.10** Kaplan–Meier curves showing the incidence of the combined endpoint of doubling of serum creatinine level or end-stage kidney disease in persons with nondiabetic chronic kidney disease and urine protein levels exceeding 1 g/day. Persons in group 1 were randomly assigned to receive standard doses of angiotensin-converting enzyme (ACE) inhibitors; those in group 3 received standard doses of angiotensin receptor blockers (ARBs); those in group 2 received ACE inhibitors titrated upward to the maximum antiproteinuric levels; and those in group 4 received ARBs titrated upward similarly. (From Hou FF, Xie D, Zhang X, et al. Renoprotection of Optimal Antiproteinuric Doses [ROAD] study: a randomized controlled study of benazepril and losartan in chronic renal insufficiency. *J Am Soc Nephrol.* 2007;18:1889–1898.)

## TIME COURSE FOR PROTEINURIA RESPONSE

In most persons, the reduction of proteinuria takes several weeks to achieve its maximal effect, which should be considered when dosages are titrated.[216] In persons in earlier stages of CKD (with diabetes and microalbuminuria, for instance) the effects are observed more promptly and tend to parallel the time course and fall in blood pressure.[217]

## MONITORING AND SAFETY CONSIDERATIONS

Regular monitoring is essential for optimizing therapeutic interventions to slow CKD progression and ensure safety. Kidney function is best assessed with the use of eGFR, derived from a serum creatinine measurement with the Chronic Kidney Disease Epidemiology Collaboration (CKD-EPI) equation, recommended by KDIGO.[5] This strategy allows direct monitoring of the rate of GFR decline and assessment of the therapeutic goal to reduce this decline to less than 1 mL/min/year, a rate associated with normal aging. The majority of laboratories now facilitate this monitoring by reporting eGFR with every serum creatinine measurement. In addition, monitoring allows for the detection of side effects of drug treatment and, in particular, of electrolyte disorders (hyperkalemia and hyponatremia), as well as acute changes in kidney function related to volume depletion.

### RENAL DYSFUNCTION AND HYPERKALEMIA INDUCED BY INHIBITORS OF THE RENIN–ANGIOTENSIN–ALDOSTERONE SYSTEM

The appropriate frequency for monitoring of persons with CKD should depend on the CKD stage, previous rate of GFR decline, risk of future GFR decline, and use of medication that may cause acute deteriorations in GFR or electrolyte disorders (especially RAAS inhibitors and diuretics). Despite clear trial evidence of the renoprotective and cardioprotective effects of ACE inhibitors and ARBs, some physicians remain cautious about prescribing these drugs to persons with stages 3 and 4 CKD. This caution results from concerns about renal dysfunction induced by these drugs, with a potential rise in serum creatinine or potassium level (reviewed by Schoolwerth et al.[218] and Palmer[219]). General guidance on risk factors for AKI and frequency of monitoring are given in Tables 59.2 and 59.3.

The initiation of therapy with RAAS inhibition may provoke an acute decline in GFR or hyperkalemia in persons with CKD, particularly in those with volume depletion, poor cardiac status, elderly persons, those with stage 4 or 5 disease, and persons with atherosclerotic renovascular disease. GFR and electrolytes should therefore be checked before and approximately 1 week after treatment is started or dosage is increased. Based on a review (but not a meta-analysis) of data for 12 RCTs, it has previously been recommended that an acute increase in serum creatinine of up to 30% after initiation of RAAS inhibitor therapy is acceptable because it is attributable to glomerular hemodynamic effects and correlates with slower subsequent annual decline in GFR.[220] This advice has recently been questioned by analysis of data from a large database of 122,363 persons initiating RAAS inhibitor therapy in primary care. The analysis confirmed that a greater than 30% increase in serum creatinine within 2 months after initiation of RAAS inhibitors (observed in 1.7% of participants) was associated with a significant increase in risks of ESKD, myocardial infarction, cardiac failure, and death, although the incidence rate ratio decreased with time after starting treatment. Importantly the study also reported a graduated relationship between all of these adverse outcomes and acute increase in serum creatinine at all values ≥10% (Fig. 59.11).[221] An important limitation of this analysis is that data on proteinuria were not available. Nevertheless, these data indicate that a more cautious approach is warranted, although it is not clear whether the increase in serum creatinine is a biomarker of risk or if there is a causal relationship between the rise in serum creatinine and adverse outcomes. A rapid initial rise in serum creatinine level or a more gradual progressive increase should prompt discontinuation of therapy and consideration of further investigation to exclude renovascular disease (see Chapter 47).

It should be remembered that AKI can occur even if RAAS inhibition therapy has been successful for months or years, usually when provoked by factors such as volume depletion or nephrotoxic medications. In the Studies of Left Ventricular Dysfunction (SOLVD), a rise in serum creatinine level of 0.5 mg/dL (44 µmol/L) from baseline was noted in 16% of persons randomly assigned to receive enalapril, in comparison with 12% of persons receiving placebo. This absolute 4% excess of GFR decline was associated with older age, diuretic therapy, and diabetes. A progressive rise in serum creatinine level is much less common in persons younger than 70 years and in those without renovascular disease. As evidence for this, persons in the second Evaluation of Losartan in the Elderly (ELITE II) study of heart failure (average age of 73.5) showed relatively high rates of creatinine elevation during the 50-week follow-up period.[222] The incidence of persistent elevated serum creatinine did not differ between the losartan and captopril recipients (both 10.5%), and less than 2% of persons discontinued the RAAS agent for this reason. However, slightly more than 25% of the losartan and captopril recipients experienced at least one rise in creatinine level of 26.5 µmol (0.3 mg). These findings indicate that vigilance is needed for older persons with other comorbid conditions.

ACE inhibitor or ARB treatment should be started at a low dose and titrated upward, with monitoring of creatinine and potassium levels 5 to 7 days after each increase. To avoid compromise from intravascular volume depletion, persons should be counseled to omit ACE inhibitor or ARB treatment during vomiting or diarrheal illnesses and to seek medical advice if these illnesses do not resolve within 48 hours. Likewise, it is important to ensure adequate hydration, to omit or reduce diuretics for 48 to 72 hours if clinically appropriate, and to avoid nonsteroidal antiinflammatory drugs (NSAIDs) before starting an RAAS inhibitor. In general, we strongly advise discontinuation of NSAIDs because these are potent causes of AKI in persons with CKD.

Discontinuation of therapy because of uncontrolled hyperkalemia has been reported in only up to 4% of persons with CKD in trials, and the overall incidence was no different from that among persons taking ACE inhibitors versus non–ACE inhibitor treatment when data from six studies were combined.[223] However, the participants were highly selected persons in trials and therefore generally have a lower risk of hyperkalemia than is observed in the general population. This important issue was highlighted by the observation

**Table 59.2 Overview of Chronic Kidney Disease Management by Stage**

| Features | Stages 1 and 2 | Stage 3a | Stage 3b | Stage 4 | Stage 5 |
|---|---|---|---|---|---|
| Estimated GFR | ≥60 mL/min/1.73 $m^2$ + albuminuria or hematuria or structural kidney damage | 45–59 mL/min/1.73 $m^2$ | 30–44 mL/min/1.73 $m^2$ | 15–29 mL/min/1.73 $m^2$ | <15 mL/min/1.73 $m^2$ |
| Frequency of Monitoring | Annual | 6–12 months | 3–6 months | 3–4 months | 1–3 months |
| Laboratory testing | Annual electrolytes and estimated GFR<br>Annual urine ACR (or other estimate of proteinuria)<br>Baseline anemia and mineral and bone profiles<br>Glucose, lipids, and $HbA_{1c}$<br>See Table 59.3 for causes of AKI after initiation of ACE inhibitor or ARB therapy. | | | | Check electrolytes and estimated GFR 1 week after new use or higher doses of ACE inhibitors or ARBs; otherwise, assess electrolytes/estimated GFR, mineral and bone, and anemia profiles every 3–6 months, depending on GFR decline. |
| Blood pressure targets | BP target <130/80 mm Hg with proteinuria<br>BP target <140/90 mm Hg without proteinuria if no clinical or radiologic evidence of ARVD or previous episodes of AKI | | | | Risk of AKI is increased in elderly persons (>75 years), those with CHF, and those with ARVD; 140/90 mm Hg may be more appropriate for these groups. |
| Blood pressure agents | ACE inhibitor or ARB if urine ACR ≥30 mg/g<br>Most persons need two to four agents in total to achieve these targets, in a combination of ACE inhibitors or ARBs and one or more of the following: a diuretic (all classes), a calcium channel blocker, and a β-blocker. | | | | Loop diuretics are now usually required for BP and edema control. |
| Cardiovascular prevention | Statin if CVD risk ≥10% over 10 years<br>$HbA_{1c}$ <7.0% unless at risk for severe hypoglycemia | | | Consider statin for all persons. | Continue statin. |
| Bone and anemia complications | If PTH level rises progressively, commence phosphate restriction and then consider therapy with vitamin D or analog.<br>If anemia is out of keeping with GFR, confirm or rule out gastrointestinal blood loss. | | | | Give intravenous iron before ESA if hemoglobin count <10 g/dL.<br>Maintain target hemoglobin count of 10–11.5 g/dL. |
| Lifestyle and nutritional management | Smoking cessation<br>Moderate exercise up to 30–60 min/day 4 to 7 days/wk<br>Target weight with BMI <25 kg/$m^2$<br>Reduced salt intake as per DASH diet <5 g/day | | | | Limit dietary potassium excess.<br>Weigh at each clinic and assess fluid overload, anorexia, physical function. |
| Specific RRT planning steps | Education regarding progression and role of conservative management with regard to blood pressure targets and specific primary renal disease treatment if indicated<br>Hepatitis B vaccination if risk of progression is high | | | Education on RRT types and palliative care if CKD is progressing or patient is at high risk of progression.<br>Hepatitis B vaccination. | AVF creation<br>PD catheter insertion<br>Enter on list for transplant |
| Referral guidance from primary care physician to nephrologist | Progressive or abrupt fall in estimated GFR<br>Proteinuria (urine protein levels >0.5 g/day; ACR >300 mg/g or >30 mg/mmol) | | | Refer unless patient is terminally ill | Refer unless patient is terminally ill |

*ACE,* Angiotensin-converting enzyme; *ACR,* albumin-to-creatinine ratio; *AKI,* acute kidney injury; *ARB,* angiotensin receptor blocker; *ARVD,* atherosclerotic renovascular disease; *AVF,* arteriovenous fistula; *BMI,* body mass index; *BP,* blood pressure; *CHF,* congestive heart failure; *CKD,* chronic kidney disease; *CVD,* cardiovascular disease; *DASH,* Dietary Approaches to Stop Hypertension; *ESA,* erythropoietin-stimulating agent; *GFR,* glomerular filtration rate; *$HbA_{1c}$,* hemoglobin $A_{1c}$; *PD,* peritoneal dialysis; *PTH,* parathyroid hormone; *RAAS,* renin–angiotensin–aldosterone system; *RRT,* renal replacement therapy.

**Table 59.3 Causes of Acute Kidney Injury After Initiation of Therapy With Angiotensin-Converting Enzyme Inhibitor or Angiotensin Receptor Blocker**

| |
|---|
| **Blood Pressure Insufficient for Adequate Renal Perfusion** |
| Poor cardiac output |
| Low systemic vascular resistance (e.g., as in sepsis) |
| Volume depletion (gastrointestinal loss, poor oral intake, excess diuretic use) |
| **Presence of Renal Vascular Disease**[a] |
| Bilateral renal artery stenosis |
| Stenosis of dominant or single kidney |
| Afferent arteriolar narrowing (caused by hypertension and cyclosporine) |
| Diffuse atherosclerosis in smaller renal vessels |
| **Vasoconstrictor Agents (Nonsteroidal Antiinflammatory Drugs, Cyclosporine)** |

[a]Clinical features of renal vascular disease include vascular bruits (areas of the epigastric, femoral, and carotid arteries), prior rise in serum creatinine level of more than 30%, fall in estimated glomerular filtration rate of more than 20% after beginning of treatment with an angiotensin-converting enzyme inhibitor or angiotensin receptor blocker, and a history of flash pulmonary edema.

of higher rates of hyperkalemia after publication of results of the Randomized Aldactone Evaluation Study (RALES), in which spironolactone was used in addition to ACE inhibitors for heart failure.[224,225] The risks associated with hyperkalemia and hypokalemia have been investigated in a large meta-analysis that combined data from 27 general population and CKD cohort studies to include 1,217,986 participants. The lowest risk of adverse outcomes was observed when serum potassium was in the range 4.0 to 4.5 mmol/L. Compared with a reference value of 4.2 mmol/L, serum potassium concentration greater than 5.5 mmol/L or less than 3.0 mmol/L was associated with significantly increased risk of all-cause mortality (HR, 1.22; 95% 1.15–1.29 and HR, 1.49; 95% CI, 1.26–1.76, respectively). A similar pattern was observed for the outcomes of cardiovascular mortality and ESKD.[226] Randomized trials are required to establish whether correction of abnormal serum potassium is associated with improved outcomes. The discontinuation of potassium supplements, avoidance of potassium-sparing diuretics, and dietary advice to avoid high-potassium foods may all help reduce the incidence of hyperkalemia. Trials are underway to evaluate the use of novel oral potassium binding drugs to prevent hyperkalemia and facilitate RAAS inhibitor treatment for persons with CKD.[180]

## STRATEGY FOR MAXIMAL RENOPROTECTION: AIMING FOR REMISSION OF CHRONIC KIDNEY DISEASE

The earlier that interventions to slow CKD progression start, the more kidney function there is to protect and preserve. The best chance of achieving maximal renoprotection is therefore when therapy is established as early as possible, preferably in stage 1 or 2 disease. The concepts of "remission" and "regression" have been applied to renoprotection. "Remission" indicates that therapy has been optimized to the point that there is no evidence of active disease and GFR declines by no more than expected with aging. "Regression" implies that there is recovery of renal function with improving GFR.

The fact that remission of kidney disease can be achieved was demonstrated in one of the first follow-up studies from the Captopril Collaborative Study Group in 1994.[227] Of the 409 persons recruited into that study, 108 had nephrotic-range proteinuria (urine protein levels >3.5 g/day) at study entry. Remission of nephrotic-range proteinuria occurred in seven of 42 persons randomly assigned to receive captopril (16.7%) and in one of 66 persons randomly assigned to receive placebo (1.5%). Of importance is that over the follow-up period, those achieving remission had the largest initial fall in mean urine protein levels (from 5.0 g/day to 0.9 g/day, in contrast to 6.2 g/day to 5.1 g/day in participants who did not reach remission), lower SBP (135–119 mm Hg in the persons in remission; 145–143 mm Hg in those not in remission), and stable serum creatinine levels (baseline vs. final serum creatinine measurement: 1.5–1.6 mg/dL for persons in remission; 1.5–3.2 mg/dL for those not in remission). Similarly, Hovind and colleagues[228] reported remission in 31% and regression (in this case, defined as GFR decline similar to that in normal aging) in 22% of 301 consecutive persons with type 1 diabetes and nephropathy who were monitored with annual measurements of isotopic GFR for 7 years. Hovind and colleagues also reported increasing prevalence of remission and regression with lower achieved blood pressure (Fig. 59.12).

Nevertheless, it is clear that even in the setting of a randomized trial, treatment with the most active agents (RAAS inhibitor therapy) is no guarantee that remission will occur; each renoprotective intervention discussed slows the rate of CKD progression by 50% at best. To achieve maximal long-term renoprotection, it is therefore necessary to use a comprehensive strategy with multiple interventions directed at different aspects of the pathogenesis of progressive renal injury (Fig. 59.2).[229–231] Moreover, once treatments have been introduced, frequent monitoring of blood pressure, proteinuria, and GFR is essential so that therapy can be escalated until therapeutic goals have been achieved (see Tables 59.2 and 59.4). In this regard, our approach is analogous to that applied in modern oncology chemotherapeutic strategies, in which multiple agents are used and treatment is directed toward correcting all signs of disease activity until the patient is said to be in "remission."

Data from a small number of persons suggest that if remission can be maintained over the long term, some recovery of kidney function or regression of kidney disease may be achieved.[140] Limited data indicate that significant improvements in renoprotection can be achieved with this strategy. Among 160 persons with type 2 diabetes and microalbuminuria, intensive therapy resulted in a marked reduction in the risk of overt nephropathy (OR, 0.27; 95% CI, 0.1 to 0.75)[229] as well substantial reductions in cardiovascular events and survival as well as progression of CKD during long term follow-up for up to 21 years.[230–233] Similarly, 26 of 56 persons with resistant nephrotic-range proteinuria and CKD who were referred to a "remission clinic" achieved reduction of urine

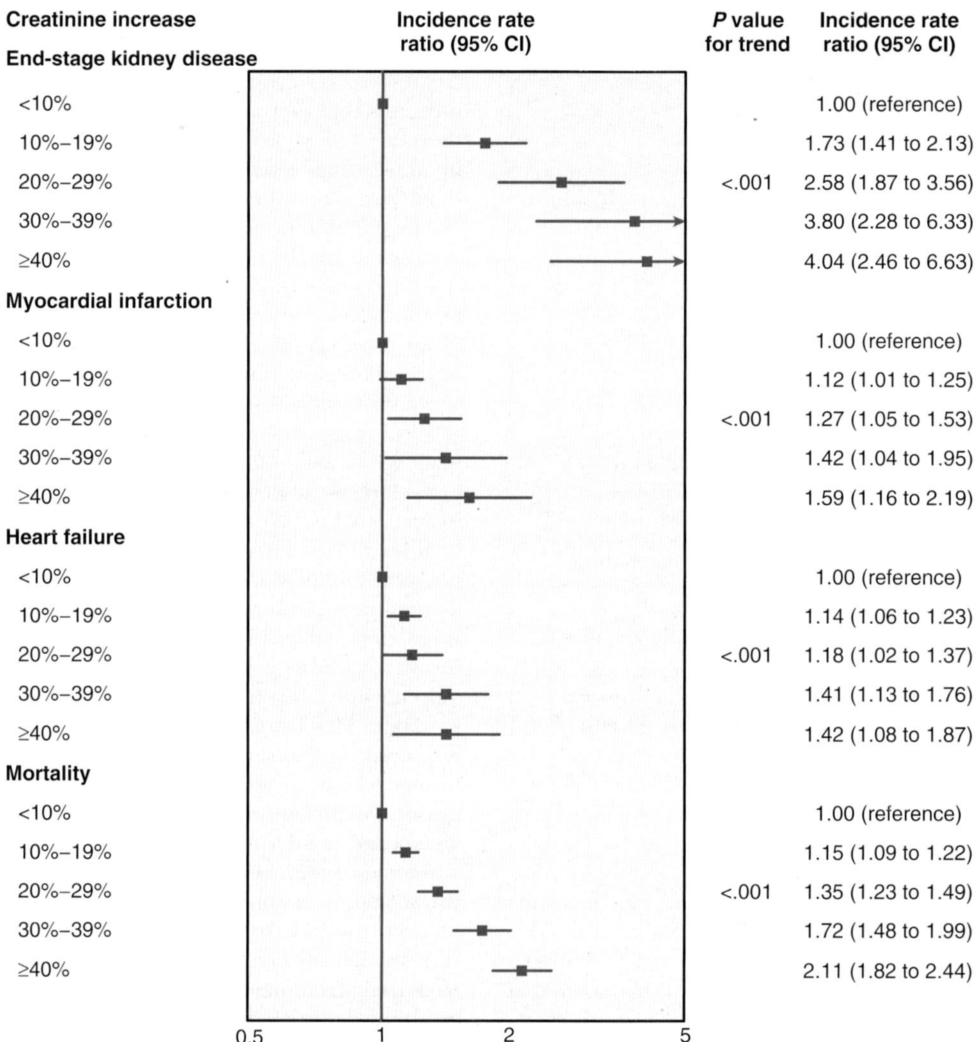


**Fig. 59.11** Cardiorenal risks associated with levels of serum creatinine increase within 2 months after initiating treatment with renin–angiotensin–aldosterone system inhibitors. *CI,* Confidence interval. (From Schmidt M, Mansfield KE, Bhaskaran K, et al. Serum creatinine elevation after renin-angiotensin system blockade and long term cardiorenal risks: cohort study. *BMJ.* 2017;356:j791.)

protein levels to less than 1 g/day and stabilization of renal function after application of a similar intensive therapy protocol. Furthermore, the rate of GFR decline was significantly slower than that observed in 56 matched historical controls, and only 3.6% reached ESKD, in contrast to 30.4% of the controls.[234] This strategy is based on currently available interventions, and the measurements required for monitoring are already widely used. Thus a comprehensive approach to renoprotection is an achievable goal for all persons with CKD. Although it has been argued that there is a need for new renoprotective agents, it is also true that these available therapies are not yet applied to all persons with CKD.[235,236] If widely implemented, a comprehensive renoprotective strategy may not only delay the need for dialysis in many persons but may also substantially reduce the number of persons progressing to ESKD.

The different incidence rates of ESKD across the similarly developed nations, Norway and the United States,[237] despite similar CKD prevalence rates, suggest that lower rates of progression to ESKD is a realistic goal of CKD treatment. The risk for progression in general was higher for US white persons than for Norwegians. Of a population of 100,000 with stage 3 or 4 CKD, 610 progressed to ESKD in the United States and 240 in Norway, a 2.5-fold excess that, after adjustment, was twofold higher among nondiabetic US persons and 2.8-fold higher among diabetic US persons with stages 3 and 4 CKD. In addition, white US persons were referred later to a nephrologist. These results also underscore the need for public health systems to target or screen populations at high risk. In the United Kingdom, a pay-for-performance system for primary-care family physicians has had dramatic impacts on the screening and management of diabetes; both levels of care for diabetes and testing rates for nephropathy have increased.[238,239] In addition, pay for performance was associated with improved control of blood pressure in persons with CKD.[240] Regrettably this system has subsequently been discontinued. Patient self-management is a further strategy that should be pursued, as highlighted by an RCT showing improved blood pressure control in participants with hypertension and cardiovascular disease, diabetes, or CKD randomized to self-management versus usual care.[241] Reports of a decline in the incidence of new persons starting

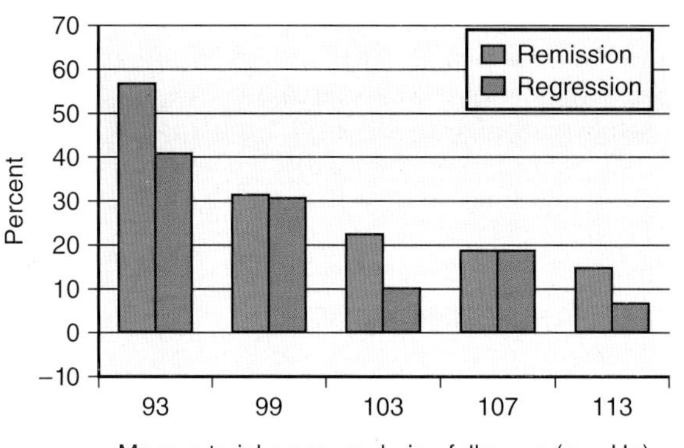


**Fig. 59.12** Results from a prospective observational cohort study in which 301 consecutive persons with type 1 diabetes and diabetic nephropathy were monitored with isotopic glomerular filtration rate (GFR) measurements annually and who underwent aggressive lowering of blood pressure. Thirty persons (10%) remained normotensive (blood pressure <140/90) during this period and did not receive prolonged antihypertensive agents. 17% of the persons received monotherapy, 47% received two agents, 30% three agents, and 6% four or more agents. "Remission" was defined in this study as urine albumin levels lower than 200 μg/min sustained for at least 1 year and a decrease of at least 30% from levels before remission (surrogate endpoint). "Regression" was defined as a rate of decline in GFR equal to that in the natural aging process: less than 1 mL/min/year during the entire observation period (principal endpoint). Remission and regression may have occurred in the same persons. (Modified from Hovind P, Rossing P, Tarnow L, et al. Remission and regression in the nephropathy of type 1 diabetes when blood pressure is controlled aggressively. *Kidney Int.* 2001;60:277–283.)

**Table 59.4 Comprehensive Strategy and Therapeutic Goals for Achieving Maximal Renoprotection in Persons With Chronic Kidney Disease**

| Intervention | Goals |
|---|---|
| ACE inhibitor or ARB treatment | Urine protein level <0.5 g/day<br>GFR decline <1 mL/min/year |
| Additional antihypertensive therapy | BP <130/80 mm Hg if urine albumin excretion > 30 mg/day<br>BP <140/90 mm Hg if urine albumin excretion < 30 mg/day |
| Weight loss if patient is obese | Aim for 5% weight loss |
| Dietary salt restriction | <5 g/day (equivalent to 90 mEq sodium/day) |
| Dietary protein restriction | Avoid high protein intake >1.3 g/kg/day<br>In stages 4 and 5 CKD, consider reducing intake to 0.8 g/kg/day |
| Tight glycemic control | $HbA_{1c}$ <7.0% unless considered high risk for hypoglycemia |
| Smoking cessation | Complete cessation |
| Lipid-lowering therapy | Total cholesterol <200 mg/dL (5.2 mmol/L)<br>LDL cholesterol <100 mg/dL (2.6 mmol/L) |

*ACE,* Angiotensin-converting enzyme; *ARB,* angiotensin receptor blocker; *BP,* blood pressure; *CKD,* chronic kidney disease; *GFR,* glomerular filtration rate; *$HbA_{1c}$,* hemoglobin $A_{1c}$; *LDL,* low-density lipoprotein.

dialysis therapy in the United States indicate that strategies to improve renoprotection may be starting to have an effect (Table 59.4).[242,243]

## INTERVENTIONS TO REDUCE CARDIOVASCULAR RISK ASSOCIATED WITH CHRONIC KIDNEY DISEASE

Following a seminal report in the early 1970s describing accelerated atherosclerosis in persons receiving maintenance hemodialysis,[244] a large body of research has focused on the relationship between CKD and cardiovascular disease. It is now clear that increased cardiovascular mortality is expressed early in the course of CKD, for example, in the setting of microalbuminuria in persons with diabetes[245] and when the GFR starts to decline[246] in stage 3 CKD. Furthermore, the rate of CVEs associated with CKD is substantial, so that reduced eGFR is now regarded as an effective marker (or "risk equivalent") of premature cardiovascular disease, similar to diabetes. For this reason, any strategy for the management of CKD should also include interventions to reduce the associated risk of cardiovascular disease.

The pathogenesis and management of cardiovascular disease associated with CKD are discussed in detail in Chapter 54 and are therefore reviewed only briefly here. As discussed throughout the text earlier, the interventions recommended for optimal renoprotection also contribute to reducing the risk of adverse CVEs. Thus lifestyle measures including smoking cessation, weight loss, and dietary sodium restriction afford both renal and cardiovascular protection. In addition, the treatment of hypertension with RAAS inhibitors and a lower blood pressure target of 130/80 mm Hg, central to achieving renoprotection, also reduces cardiovascular risk. One exception to the principle that most interventions afford renal and cardiovascular protection is treatment with statins. The largest RCT to date found a 17% RR reduction in atherosclerotic CVEs in participants randomly assigned to statin (with or without ezetimibe) therapy[247] but no benefit with respect to CKD progression.[248] The 2013 KDIGO guideline for lipid management in CKD recommends treating all persons aged 50 years and older with CKD not treated with dialysis or renal transplant with a statin or statin and ezetimibe, regardless of low-density lipoprotein cholesterol levels. For persons with CKD younger than 50 years, the guideline recommends similar treatment for persons with a 10-year risk of CVE greater than 10%.[249]

***Clinical Relevance***

All persons with chronic kidney disease should be regarded as having a high risk of cardiovascular disease and management offered to reduce this risk, including treatment with a statin.

## INTERVENTIONS TO MANAGE COMPLICATIONS OF CHRONIC KIDNEY DISEASE

### ANEMIA

The anemia of CKD results from a combination of reduced renal erythropoietin production (a presumed reflection of the reduction in functioning renal mass), shortened red blood cell survival, and functional iron deficiency. Anemia—defined as a hemoglobin count lower than 13 g/dL in men and lower than 12 g/dL in women[5]—can develop well before the onset of uremic symptoms. Among over 15,000 participants in the Third National Health and Nutrition Examination Survey (NHANES III), the prevalence of anemia increased from 1% at an eGFR of 60 mL/min/1.73 $m^2$ to 9% at an eGFR of 30 mL/min/1.73 $m^2$ and from 33% to 67% at an eGFR of 15 mL/min/1.73 $m^2$.[250]

If left untreated, the anemia of CKD is associated with several adverse effects. These include deterioration in cardiac function, decreased cognition and mental acuity, and fatigue. In cross-sectional studies, associations between anemia and an increased risk of morbidity and mortality, caused principally by cardiac disease and stroke, have been described in persons on dialysis.[251] In addition, anemia may influence the progression of CKD. The effects of anemia on glomerular hemodynamics have been studied in various rat models of CKD.[252] In each of these models, anemia was associated with a reduction in hydraulic pressure in the glomerular capillaries ($P_{GC}$) and amelioration of glomerulosclerosis. By contrast, prevention of anemia in the remnant kidney model by administration of erythropoietin resulted in increased systemic and glomerular blood pressures and markedly increased glomerulosclerosis (see Chapter 51 for more detailed discussion).

Despite the apparently favorable hemodynamic effects of anemia in experimental models of CKD, some human studies suggest that anemia may in fact accelerate CKD progression. In persons with inherited hemoglobinopathies, chronic anemia is associated with glomerular hyperfiltration that eventuates in proteinuria, hypertension, and ESKD.[253] In several longitudinal studies, lower hemoglobin value was identified as a risk factor for CKD progression[254,255] and ESKD.[256] Whether this reflects more severe kidney disease in persons with lower hemoglobin values or more rapid progression secondary to low hemoglobin value and oxygen carriage per se is unclear.

Two small randomized studies revealed renoprotective benefit when anemia was corrected with erythropoietin.[257,258] By contrast, enthusiasm for the normalization of hemoglobin has been tempered by the results of several large RCTs that revealed no benefit or adverse effects. In two studies in which effect on left ventricular mass was the primary endpoint, as well as the Trial to Reduce Cardiovascular Events with Aranesp Therapy (TREAT),[259] there was no effect of higher versus lower hemoglobin target on rate of decline in GFR.[260,261] Moreover, in the Cardiovascular Risk Reduction by Early Anemia Treatment with Epoetin Beta (CREATE) study, achievement of a higher hemoglobin target (13–15 mg/dL) was associated with a shorter time to initiation of dialysis than was achievement of the lower target (10.5–11.5 mg/dL).[262] Further concern was provoked by serious adverse effects associated with higher hemoglobin targets, including increased rate of mortality[263] and increased risk of stroke.[259] Current KDIGO recommendations are therefore to treat symptomatic anemia in CKD with erythropoietin or iron supplementation, or both, to partially correct the hemoglobin and achieve a range of 10 to 11.5 mg/dL.[264] Hemoglobin value should not exceed 13 g dL.[264] The pathogenesis and treatment of anemia in CKD are discussed further in Chapter 55.

### MINERAL AND BONE DISORDER

Numerous cohort studies have shown strong associations between disorders of mineral metabolism and fractures, cardiovascular disease, and mortality (reviewed by the KDIGO CKD-MBD work group[265] (see also Chapter 53). Some of caveats are relevant here. Most of the studies reporting observational data and relationships between individual parameters and clinical outcomes have been performed in dialysis populations. The limited data regarding the prevalence of biochemical and hormonal abnormalities in stages 3 to 5 CKD often do not include analyses by primary disease, which can influence the natural history of mineral and bone disorder.

Changes in mineral metabolism and bone structure are detectable much earlier in CKD than had previously been considered. There is a slow decline in levels of 1,25-dihydroxyvitamin D and 25-hydroxyvitamin D, starting once the GFR is in the range of 60 to 70 mL/min. 1,25-Dihydroxyvitamin D values were correlated positively with GFR and negatively with the log of plasma parathyroid hormone and serum phosphorus concentrations. The plasma parathyroid hormone concentration rises later in the progression of CKD but more exponentially when GFR falls below 45 mL/min/1.73 $m^2$.[266] Calcium and phosphorus values do not generally become abnormal until GFR falls below 40 mL/min/1.73 $m^2$, and this occurs more commonly below 20 mL/min/1.73 $m^2$.[267]

In the community-based Kidney Early Evaluation Program (KEEP) and NHANES cohorts, there is evidence that parathyroid hormone levels increased early in persons with stage 3 CKD, typically while calcium and phosphorus levels remained normal.[267,268] These findings highlight the importance of monitoring parathyroid hormone along with calcium and phosphorus in individuals with eGFR less than 60 mL/min/1.73 $m^2$. Investigators have also described an earlier biomarker of altered mineral and bone disorder in persons with CKD. Fibroblast growth factor-23 (FGF-23) regulates phosphorus metabolism and is associated with mortality in persons on dialysis.[269] High levels of this growth factor, defined as being above 100 reference units/mL, were more common than secondary hyperparathyroidism and hyperphosphatemia at all levels of eGFR in a cohort of almost 4000 persons with stages 2 to 4 CKD.[270] Further analysis in the same cohort identified elevated FGF-23 levels as an independent risk factor for progression to ESKD and mortality.[271] However, testing for this early marker is not routinely available, and so we recommend monitoring according to the KDIGO guidelines.[272]

Thus monitoring of serum levels of calcium, phosphorus, and parathyroid hormone and of alkaline phosphatase activity should begin in stage 3 CKD. Few persons with mineral and bone disorder in CKD develop symptomatic disease until they have stage 5 CKD; therefore the main reason for monitoring is to implement early preventive treatment to suppress secondary hyperparathyroidism. In the majority of persons with CKD who do not require dialysis, treatment of mineral and bone disorder is based initially on dietary phosphate restriction, followed by oral phosphate binders in order to maintain phosphorus in the normal range, although there is no evidence from RCTs that this affects clinical outcomes.

In persons with stages 3 to 5 CKD who are not on dialysis, the optimal level of parathyroid hormone is unknown. However, it is suggested that persons with levels of intact parathyroid hormone above the upper normal limit of the assay be first evaluated for hyperphosphatemia, hypocalcemia, and vitamin D deficiency.[5] If parathyroid hormone level is progressively rising and remains persistently above the upper limit of normal for the assay despite correction of modifiable factors, treatment with calcitriol or vitamin D analogs (once phosphate is under control) may be considered. Treatment with the vitamin D analog paricalcitol has been reported to reduce albuminuria in persons with diabetic nephropathy already receiving treatment with an ACE inhibitor or an ARB,[273] but further studies are needed to investigate the renoprotective potential of vitamin D therapies. Detailed discussion of the pathogenesis and treatment of mineral and bone disorder in CKD are beyond the scope of this chapter and are presented in Chapter 53.

## A STEPPED CARE APPROACH TO CHRONIC KIDNEY DISEASE

In addition to being useful for risk stratification, the KDIGO classification of CKD serves as a convenient framework to identify differing priorities for management at different stages. This "stepped care" approach is discussed in the following sections and summarized in Table 59.2.

### STAGES 1 AND 2

At these stages of CKD, the diagnosis is based on the presence of albuminuria, hematuria, or structural kidney disease, and an eGFR above 60 mL/min/1.73 $m^2$. Stage 1 disease is defined by a GFR greater than 90 mL/min/1.73 $m^2$ (5.7% of the total US population) and stage 2 by a GFR between 60 and 89 mL/min/1.73 $m^2$ (5.4% of the US population).[274] These statistics indicate that CKD of all stages affected an estimated 16.8% of adults aged 20 years during the period 1999 to 2004, an increase from the recalculated NHANES III (1988–1994) estimate of 14.5%.[275]

Persons with stages 1 and 2 disease do not have specific symptoms or complications of renal failure such as anemia or bone and mineral disorder. Those with symptoms may have a multisystem disease with secondary glomerular or interstitial disease (see Chapters 32 and 35). The majority of persons with stages 1 and 2 CKD are detected by routine or health care insurance–mandated screening and are visiting primary care or other physicians; in many countries only a small proportion are ever evaluated by a nephrologist. With increased access to radiologic imaging, more persons are now identified with structural abnormalities such as polycystic kidney disease or single kidney.

The emphasis at these early stages should be on identification of specific renal diseases when present, appropriate referral to a nephrologist, and reduction of cardiovascular risk. A detailed family history is important because persons with a positive family history need more detailed investigation to allow early detection of inherited renal disease and, in particular, adult polycystic kidney disease. The following initial investigations are appropriate for assisting with risk assessment and for informing decisions about referral to a nephrologist or urologist (see also Chapter 23):

1. Estimation of urinary albumin or protein excretion by measurement of ACR or PCR on a random urine sample. Persons with a urine protein measurement equivalent to 0.5 g/day (UACR, 300 mg/g or 30 mg/mmol) or greater should be referred for investigation by a nephrologist.[5]
2. Further urinalysis is needed to detect hematuria. For painless but visible hematuria, serious urologic causes—such as bladder, renal cell, and, less often, prostatic cancers—must be confirmed or ruled out, particularly in persons older than age 50 years, smokers, and those with a family history of renal tract malignancy. They should generally be assessed by a urologist or nephrologist who has experience in screening for these conditions. Painless microscopic hematuria (nonvisible hematuria) is much more likely to be caused by glomerular disease, but referral to a urologist may be necessary to confirm or rule out renal tract malignancy in persons at increased risk.[276] There are several national guidelines for the investigation of hematuria.[276,277] Initial blood tests include measurements of creatinine, eGFR, urea, electrolytes ($Na^+$, $K^+$, $HCO_3^-$, $Cl^-$), bone and liver profiles, blood glucose, glycosylated hemoglobin, blood cell count, erythrocyte sedimentation rate, and (in men) prostate-specific antigen. Serologic screening for underlying myeloma, antineutrophil cytoplasmic antibody (ANCA)–associated vasculitis, antiglomerular basement membrane disease, and systemic lupus erythematosus may be indicated, depending on symptoms and the results of other investigations.
3. Abdominal ultrasonography to exclude structural abnormalities and determine the bipolar diameter of the kidneys is indicated if urinalysis results are abnormal, if there is a strong family history of CKD, or if there is significant hypertension. Asymmetry with regard to renal size may be suggestive of atherosclerotic renovascular disease, and angiography (computed tomography or magnetic resonance angiography) may therefore be helpful if this is suspected.

In general, persons with stages 1 and 2 CKD, who do not have a specific renal disease or significant proteinuria, require only annual monitoring of blood pressure, eGFR, and proteinuria. Those who develop an abrupt or sustained decline in GFR or worsening proteinuria should be referred to a nephrologist for further investigation and optimization of therapy.[5]

### STAGE 3

In stage 3 CKD, GFR is between 30 and 59 mL/min/1.73 $m^2$. This is a significant stage because it represents the majority of persons in whom CKD is identified (stages 1 and 2 often

**Table 59.5 Recommended Frequency of Monitoring by Stage of Chronic Kidney Disease**

| Variable | Stage 1 and 2 | Stage 3 | Stage 4 | Stage 5 |
|---|---|---|---|---|
| GFR and electrolytes | Every 12 months | Every 3–12 months | Every 3–6 months | Every 1–3 months |
| Proteinuria with ACR or PCR testing | Every 12 months | Every 3–12 months | Every 3–6 months | Every 3–6 months |
| Blood pressure | Each visit | Each visit | Each visit | Each visit |
| Calcium and phosphate levels | Every 12 months | Every 12 months | Every 3–6 months | Every 3 months |
| Parathyroid hormone level | — | Every 12 months | Every 3–6 months | Every 3–6 months[a] |
| Hemoglobin | Every 12 months | Every 12 months | Every 3–6 months | Every 1–3 months[a] |

Monitoring should be individualized according to previous rate of GFR decline, risk assessment of future GFR decline (particularly high if heavy proteinuria, >1 g/day or equivalent), and current drug therapy.

[a]Monitoring of parathyroid hormone and anemia should depend on the previous results and specific treatment, if any, for these conditions. Stable values with no specific treatment require less monitoring as indicated.

*ACR,* Albumin-to-creatinine ratio; *GFR,* glomerular filtration rate; *PCR,* protein-to-creatinine ratio.

remain undetected unless urinalysis is performed) and because many of the complications start to manifest once the GFR drops below 45 mL/min/1.73 m$^2$. In addition, the rate of cardiovascular mortality increases substantially among persons with a GFR lower than 45 mL/min/1.73 m$^2$.[2,246,278] Some national guidelines and the KDIGO guidelines have therefore split this stage into two: 3A, defined by reduced GFR of 45 to 59 mL/min/1.73 m$^2$, and 3B, defined by reduced GFR of 30 to 44 mL/min/1.73 m$^2$.[2,5,279,280] Depending on the underlying etiology, Stage 3 CKD may be appropriately managed by a collaboration of primary care with a nephrology service. One study that employed mathematical modeling techniques reported that multidisciplinary care for CKD is a cost-effective model that could help to reduce the need for dialysis and prolong life expectancy.[281] The aims of management at this stage are to identify specific renal disease, correct reversible causes of renal dysfunction, prevent or slow the progression of CKD, reduce cardiovascular risk, and treat the complications of CKD (usually in stage 3B CKD). Referral criteria are the same as for earlier stages of CKD, with the addition of anemia and mineral and bone disorder, which may necessitate specialist treatment. Monitoring of blood pressure, eGFR, and serum biochemistry profile, as well as complete blood cell count and evaluation for proteinuria, should be performed every 3 to 12 months, depending on risk profile and clinical circumstances (Table 59.5).

## STAGE 4

Persons with stage 4 CKD have a high cumulative risk of cardiovascular death and progression to ESKD. Almost 66% of such persons experience either a renal event or a CVE over 5 years after diagnosis. In a population-based study,[282] the proportions of persons who needed RRT during a 5-year observation period were 1.1%, 1.3%, and 19.9%, respectively, for stages 2, 3, and 4, and the respective mortality rates were 19.5%, 24.3%, and 45.7%. Not surprisingly, persons with stage 4 disease often make up a large proportion of those attending outpatient nephrology clinics. Achieving renoprotection remains an important goal to delay the onset of RRT for as long as possible, as does minimizing cardiovascular risk. Blood pressure, eGFR, and serum biochemistry profile, including level of parathyroid hormone as well as complete blood cell count, should be monitored every 3 to 6 months.

As the GFR declines to below 20 mL/min/1.73 m$^2$, the focus should change to treating the complications of CKD and planning for RRT.[283] Effective preparation for RRT requires input from multiple staff disciplines (medical, nursing, pharmacy, dietetics, psychology, and social work) and is best delivered in a multidisciplinary clinic. There is emerging evidence that persons prefer this approach to preparation and that such clinics are associated with better outcomes, at least in observational studies.[284,285]

It is clear that late referral (less than 3 months before initiation of dialysis) for dialysis preparation is associated with significantly higher rates of mortality[286] and lower quality of life.[287] Results of a Canadian study also indicated that even when referral was appropriately timed, there was a 53% higher rate of reaching the composite endpoint of death, need for transfusion, or subsequent hospitalization in those without an optimal start to RRT.[288]

The need for timely preparation for dialysis is clear and is emphasized in the majority of national guidelines. However, not all persons with stage 4 CKD progress to stage 5, and unnecessary preparation may do harm. Persons with stage 4 CKD should therefore undergo a formal assessment of their risk of progression to ESKD (see Chapter 20). This is particularly relevant in older persons, in whom the competing risk of death is an important consideration. A comprehensive approach to assessing the risk of ESKD versus death to assist decision-making about RRT has been proposed by the European Renal Best Practice (ERBP) group.[289] Preparation for initiation of dialysis requires multiple interventions to deal with both medical and psychosocial aspects. Persons require adequate counseling to assist them in the choice of dialysis modality and in coping with the psychosocial effects of starting dialysis. Elderly persons are often more accepting of dialysis than are younger persons, who may still be working or have family commitments. One large US study confirmed that social support is important for persons on hemodialysis and peritoneal dialysis in terms of greater satisfaction, higher quality of life, and fewer hospitalizations.[290] Timely formation of vascular access, ideally a forearm arteriovenous fistula, is important to allow adequate maturation, modification if necessary, and repeat surgery in case of primary site failure. Peritoneal catheter insertion requires less maturation time but should be performed early enough to allow time for adequate training for peritoneal dialysis. See Chapters 63,

64, and 68 for further discussion of preparation for dialysis and vascular access.

### HEPATITIS B VACCINATION

Persons on hemodialysis have a small but significantly increased risk of exposure to hepatitis B and other bloodborne viruses. Severe outbreaks of hepatitis B in hemodialysis units have resulted in considerable morbidity and even mortality among susceptible persons and staff. Therefore persons with CKD in whom dialysis is anticipated should be screened for hepatitis B and C, as well as human immunodeficiency virus infection. Persons who are seronegative for hepatitis B surface antigen and hepatitis B surface antibody should be immunized and their antibody levels measured after vaccination. Because seroconversion rates decrease with GFR,[291] immunization should ideally occur in stage 3 in persons with a high risk of progression; however, in view of the large number of persons and lack of precision in predicting outcomes, it is usually delayed until stage 4. Seroconversion rates are low once dialysis has commenced, particularly in older persons.[292] Results of a meta-analysis of 12 studies indicated that increased seroconversion rates can be achieved by administering multiple doses of vaccine and preferably by the intradermal route.[293] The mechanism is unclear, but this finding is consistent with the observed increased immunogenicity of other vaccinations after intradermal administration in persons with CKD and the rare cases of pure red blood cell aplasia after subcutaneous administration of recombinant erythropoietin.[294,295]

### PREEMPTIVE RENAL TRANSPLANTATION

Assessment and preparation for possible kidney transplantation should be undertaken before initiation of dialysis. The increase in death rates among waitlisted persons in comparison with transplant recipients is consistent although still debated in view of methodologic issues, such as lead-time bias and unmeasured differences confounding these analyses.[296] The clear benefits to recipients and the potential reduced demand for dialysis make a strong case for strategies to increase preemptive transplantation. Many countries and centers now permit kidney transplantation when the recipient's GFR is less than 15 to 20 mL/min/1.73 $m^2$ and if renal function has decreased progressively over the previous 6 to 12 months.[297] The optimal timing of preemptive kidney transplantation remains unclear. Neither higher nor lower pretransplantation GFR appears to be associated with superior allograft survival.[298]

## STAGE 5

Once GFR declines to below 15 mL/min/1.73 $m^2$, priorities include maintaining optimal health and function as well as achieving a planned and uncomplicated initiation of RRT. If persons have been referred in a timely manner, preparation for RRT should already be complete, but ongoing psychosocial support is often necessary as persons come to terms with the imminent need to start therapy. The optimal time to initiate RRT remains a topic of debate.[299] A retrospective analysis of data from 896,546 persons commencing dialysis revealed a higher mortality rate among those commencing dialysis "early" (GFR >15 mL/min/1.73 $m^2$) and a lower mortality rate among those commencing "late" (GFR <5 mL/min/1.73 $m^2$), although the authors conceded that the results may have been affected by unaccounted confounding and selection, as well as lead-time bias.[300] In a landmark RCT, persons with stage 5 CKD were randomly assigned to "early" (GFR = 10–14 mL/min/1.73 $m^2$) or "late" (GFR = 5–7 mL/min/1.73 $m^2$) initiation of dialysis. After a median of 3.59 years of follow-up, there was no difference in rate of survival or adverse events (CVEs, infections, or complications of dialysis) between the groups.[301]

We therefore recommend that the initiation of RRT should be individualized but in general should occur when the GFR falls below 10 mL/min/1.73 $m^2$ but before significant uremic symptoms or malnutrition occurs. In order to facilitate this timing, the frequency of monitoring of GFR, serum biochemistry, and hemoglobin, together with clinical assessment, should increase to every 1 to 3 months. Persons who decline RRT should continue to be treated for complications of CKD to optimize their quality of life and, if necessary, be referred to a palliative care service to allow adequate planning of their care once they develop symptomatic uremia.

 Complete reference list available at ExpertConsult.com.

## KEY REFERENCES


2. Hill NR, Fatoba ST, Oke JL, et al. Global prevalence of chronic kidney disease—a systematic review and meta-analysis. *PLoS ONE.* 2016;11(7):e0158765.
3. Global Burden of Disease Collaborators. Global, regional, and national age-sex specific mortality for 264 causes of death, 1980-2016: a systematic analysis for the Global Burden of Disease Study 2016. *Lancet.* 2017;390(10100):1151–1210.
5. Kidney Disease: Improving Global Outcomes CKD Working Group. KDIGO 2012 clinical practice guideline for the evaluation and management of chronic kidney disease. *Kidney Int Suppl.* 2013;3:1–150.
17. Hall ME, Wang W, Okhomina V, et al. Cigarette smoking and chronic kidney disease in African Americans in the Jackson Heart Study. *J Am Heart Assoc.* 2016;5(6):e003280.
18. Carter BD, Abnet CC, Feskanich D, et al. Smoking and mortality–beyond established causes. *N Engl J Med.* 2015;372(7):631–640.
21. Bundy JD, Bazzano LA, Xie D, et al. Self-reported tobacco, alcohol, and illicit drug use and progression of chronic kidney disease. *Clin J Am Soc Nephrol.* 2018;13(7):993–1001.
22. Staplin N, Haynes R, Herrington WG, et al. Smoking and adverse outcomes in patients with CKD: the study of heart and renal protection (SHARP). *Am J Kidney Dis.* 2016;68(3):371–380.
41. Look AHEAD Research Group. Effect of a long-term behavioural weight loss intervention on nephropathy in overweight or obese adults with type 2 diabetes: a secondary analysis of the Look AHEAD randomised clinical trial. *Lancet Diabetes Endocrinol.* 2014;2(10):801–809.
43. Friedman AN, Wahed AS, Wang J, et al. Effect of bariatric surgery on CKD risk. *J Am Soc Nephrol.* 2018;29(4):1289–1300.
44. Imam TH, Fischer H, Jing B, et al. Estimated GFR before and after bariatric surgery in CKD. *Am J Kidney Dis.* 2017;69(3):380–388.
54. Yoon CY, Noh J, Lee J, et al. High and low sodium intakes are associated with incident chronic kidney disease in patients with normal renal function and hypertension. *Kidney Int.* 2018;93(4):921–931.
56. He J, Mills KT, Appel LJ, et al. Urinary sodium and potassium excretion and CKD progression. *J Am Soc Nephrol.* 2016;27(4):1202–1212.
58. Vogt L, Waanders F, Boomsma F, et al. Effects of dietary sodium and hydrochlorothiazide on the antiproteinuric efficacy of losartan. *J Am Soc Nephrol.* 2008;19(5):999–1007.
59. Vegter S, Perna A, Postma MJ, et al. Sodium intake, ACE inhibition, and progression to ESRD. *J Am Soc Nephrol.* 2012;23(1):165–173.
61. Saran R, Padilla RL, Gillespie BW, et al. A randomized crossover trial of dietary sodium restriction in stage 3-4 CKD. *Clin J Am Soc Nephrol.* 2017;12(3):399–407.

62. Keyzer CA, van Breda GF, Vervloet MG, et al. Effects of vitamin D receptor activation and dietary sodium restriction on residual albuminuria in CKD: the ViRTUE-CKD trial. *J Am Soc Nephrol.* 2017;28(4):1296–1305.
63. Meuleman Y, Hoekstra T, Dekker FW, et al. Sodium restriction in patients with CKD: a randomized controlled trial of self-management support. *Am J Kidney Dis.* 2017;69(5):576–586.
70. Garneata L, Stancu A, Dragomir D, et al. Ketoanalogue-supplemented vegetarian very low-protein diet and CKD progression. *J Am Soc Nephrol.* 2016;27(7):2164–2176.
78. National Institute for Health and Care Excellence (NICE). *Early identification and management of chronic kidney disease in adults in primary and secondary care.* Clinical Guideline 182. 2014. https://www.nice.org.uk/guidance/cg182. Accessed September 18, 2018.
102. Group SR, Wright JT Jr, Williamson JD, et al. A randomized trial of intensive versus standard blood-pressure control. *N Engl J Med.* 2015;373(22):2103–2116.
103. Cheung AK, Rahman M, Reboussin DM, et al. Effects of intensive BP control in CKD. *J Am Soc Nephrol.* 2017;28(9):2812–2823.
108. Jafar TH, Stark PC, Schmid CH, et al. Progression of chronic kidney disease: the role of blood pressure control, proteinuria, and angiotensin-converting enzyme inhibition: a patient-level meta-analysis. *Ann Intern Med.* 2003;139(4):244–252.
109. Tsai WC, Wu HY, Peng YS, et al. Association of intensive blood pressure control and kidney disease progression in nondiabetic patients with chronic kidney disease: a systematic review and meta-analysis. *JAMA Intern Med.* 2017;177(6):792–799.
110. Malhotra R, Nguyen HA, Benavente O, et al. Association between more intensive vs less intensive blood pressure lowering and risk of mortality in chronic kidney disease stages 3 to 5: a systematic review and meta-analysis. *JAMA Intern Med.* 2017;177(10):1498–1505.
112. ACCORD Study Group, Cushman WC, Evans GW, et al. Effects of intensive blood-pressure control in type 2 diabetes mellitus. *N Engl J Med.* 2010;362(17):1575–1585.
113. Basu S, Sussman JB, Rigdon J, et al. Benefit and harm of intensive blood pressure treatment: derivation and validation of risk models using data from the SPRINT and ACCORD trials. *PLoS Med.* 2017;14(10):e1002410.
114. Basu S, Sussman JB, Rigdon J, et al. *Risk calculator for benefit and harm from intensive blood pressure treatment*, 2017. http://sanjaybasu.shinyapps.io/intbp. Accessed July 13, 2019.
115. Whelton PK, Carey RM, Aronow WS, et al. 2017 ACC/AHA/AAPA/ABC/ACPM/AGS/APhA/ASH/ASPC/NMA/PCNA guideline for the prevention, detection, evaluation, and management of high blood pressure in adults: executive summary: a report of the American College of Cardiology/American Heart Association task force on clinical practice guidelines. *J Am Coll Cardiol.* 2018;71(19):2199–2269.
116. Lewis EJ, Hunsicker LG, Bain RP, et al. The effect of angiotensin-converting-enzyme inhibition on diabetic nephropathy. The Collaborative Study Group. *N Engl J Med.* 1993;329(20):1456–1462.
134. Strippoli GF, Craig M, Deeks JJ, et al. Effects of angiotensin converting enzyme inhibitors and angiotensin II receptor antagonists on mortality and renal outcomes in diabetic nephropathy: systematic review. *BMJ.* 2004;329(7470):828.
137. Randomised placebo-controlled trial of effect of ramipril on decline in glomerular filtration rate and risk of terminal renal failure in proteinuric, non-diabetic nephropathy. The GISEN Group (Gruppo Italiano di Studi Epidemiologici in Nefrologia). *Lancet.* 1997;349(9069):1857–1863.
138. Ruggenenti P, Perna A, Gherardi G, et al. Renoprotective properties of ACE-inhibition in non-diabetic nephropathies with non-nephrotic proteinuria. *Lancet.* 1999;354(9176):359–364.
144. Brenner BM, Cooper ME, de Zeeuw D, et al. Effects of losartan on renal and cardiovascular outcomes in patients with type 2 diabetes and nephropathy. *N Engl J Med.* 2001;345(12):861–869.
145. Lewis EJ, Hunsicker LG, Clarke WR, et al. Renoprotective effect of the angiotensin-receptor antagonist irbesartan in patients with nephropathy due to type 2 diabetes. *N Engl J Med.* 2001;345(12):851–860.
146. Parving HH, Lehnert H, Brochner-Mortensen J, et al. The effect of irbesartan on the development of diabetic nephropathy in patients with type 2 diabetes. *N Engl J Med.* 2001;345(12):870–878.
151. Mann JF, Schmieder RE, McQueen M, et al. Renal outcomes with telmisartan, ramipril, or both, in people at high vascular risk (the ONTARGET study): a multicentre, randomised, double-blind, controlled trial. *Lancet.* 2008;372(9638):547–553.
164. Bangalore S, Fakheri R, Toklu B, et al. Diabetes mellitus as a compelling indication for use of renin angiotensin system blockers: systematic review and meta-analysis of randomized trials. *BMJ.* 2016;352:i438.
165. Palmer SC, Mavridis D, Navarese E, et al. Comparative efficacy and safety of blood pressure-lowering agents in adults with diabetes and kidney disease: a network meta-analysis. *Lancet.* 2015;385(9982):2047–2056.
173. Fried LF, Emanuele N, Zhang JH, et al. Combined angiotensin inhibition for the treatment of diabetic nephropathy. *N Engl J Med.* 2013;369(20):1892–1903.
183. Parving HH, Persson F, Lewis JB, et al. Aliskiren combined with losartan in type 2 diabetes and nephropathy. *N Engl J Med.* 2008;358(23):2433–2446.
187. Heerspink HJL, Kosiborod M, Inzucchi SE, et al. Renoprotective effects of sodium-glucose cotransporter-2 inhibitors. *Kidney Int.* 2018;94(1):26–39.
188. Wanner C. EMPA-REG OUTCOME: the Nephrologist's point of view. *Am J Cardiol.* 2017;120(1S):S59–S67.
189. Perkovic V, Jardine MJ, Neal B, et al. Canagliflozin and renal outcomes in type 2 diabetes and nephropathy. *N Engl J Med.* 2019;380(24):2295–2306.
221. Schmidt M, Mansfield KE, Bhaskaran K, et al. Serum creatinine elevation after renin-angiotensin system blockade and long term cardiorenal risks: cohort study. *BMJ.* 2017;356:j791.
226. Kovesdy CP, Matsushita K, Sang Y, et al. Serum potassium and adverse outcomes across the range of kidney function: a CKD Prognosis Consortium meta-analysis. *Eur Heart J.* 2018;39(17):1535–1542.
231. Gaede P, Lund-Andersen H, Parving HH, et al. Effect of a multifactorial intervention on mortality in type 2 diabetes. *N Engl J Med.* 2008;358(6):580–591.
234. Ruggenenti P, Perticucci E, Cravedi P, et al. Role of remission clinics in the longitudinal treatment of CKD. *J Am Soc Nephrol.* 2008;19(6):1213–1224.
247. Baigent C, Landray MJ, Reith C, et al. The effects of lowering LDL cholesterol with simvastatin plus ezetimibe in patients with chronic kidney disease (Study of Heart and Renal Protection): a randomised placebo-controlled trial. *Lancet.* 2011;377(9784):2181–2192.
281. Lin E, Chertow GM, Yan B, et al. Cost-effectiveness of multidisciplinary care in mild to moderate chronic kidney disease in the United States: a modeling study. *PLoS Med.* 2018;15(3):e1002532.
289. Farrington K, Covic A, Nistor I, et al. Clinical Practice Guideline on management of older patients with chronic kidney disease stage 3b or higher (eGFR<45 mL/min/1.73 m2): a summary document from the European Renal Best Practice Group. *Nephrol Dial Transplant.* 2017;32(1):9–16.

# 60

# Dietary Approaches to Kidney Diseases

Nimrit Goraya | Donald Everett Wesson

## CHAPTER OUTLINE



## KEY POINTS

- Diet is an underused strategy by clinicians in their goal to prevent or slow progression of chronic kidney disease (CKD) to end-stage kidney disease (ESKD) and in the management of CKD-related complications.
- Diet is a cornerstone strategy in the prevention and management of the two syndromes that are the major contributors to CKD in developed societies, diabetes mellitus and hypertension.
- Predominantly plant-based diets are associated with reduced overall mortality risk in CKD, an important consideration for clinicians given that CKD patients suffer higher mortality than patients without CKD.
- Diets low in acid production and that promote a gut microbiome with low levels of nephrotoxic metabolites are associated with reduced risk for initiation and progression of CKD.
- Diet modifications can reduce uremic complications due to accumulation of nitrogenous wastes. Such modifications include limiting the amount of, and focusing on the character of, ingested dietary protein.
- Predominantly plant-based diets appear to have an important role in CKD management, and CKD patients with reduced but comparatively well-preserved glomerular filtration rate appear able to tolerate the increased potassium load of predominantly plant-based diets better than once thought.
- Public policy approaches to implementation of "healthy" diet components for populations might prevent CKD and reduce its incidence, particularly in high-risk populations, in addition to provision of these diet components to individuals by their clinicians.

## INTRODUCTORY POINTS

### DIET IS A KEY COMPONENT OF THE MANAGEMENT OF CHRONIC KIDNEY DISEASE

Analysis of US data showing that diet is the single largest CKD-related risk factor for death and disability in individuals with chronic kidney disease (CKD) show the importance of diet in CKD management.[1] Furthermore, a "healthy" diet in CKD patients is associated with reduced mortality.[2,3] These data support that diet can enhance the length and quality of life of individuals with CKD and should encourage clinicians to know and recommend food patterns which accomplish these goals. Additional reasons for clinicians to consider diet as the cornerstone of CKD management include the following:

- Diet is a cornerstone component of the management of diabetes, the major cause of CKD in developed societies.[4] Individuals with diabetes-related CKD must have their diabetes properly managed along with their CKD. Importantly, the "healthier" (we will subsequently detail the components of a "healthy" diet) the diet in CKD due to type 2 diabetes (T2D) the lower the mortality and the lower the risk for CKD progression.[5]
- Diet is recommended as first-line management of hypertension,[6] a comorbid condition present in more than 90% of individuals with CKD.[4] Consequently, diet will help control hypertension in CKD and long-term studies support that better hypertension control yields lower mortality in CKD.[7,8]
- Diet helps control some of the metabolic complications of CKD.
- Diet also helps ameliorate some of the organ dysfunction associated with CKD.
- Properly applied, diet can limit body accumulation of waste products ordinarily excreted by the kidney that cause harm, thereby delaying the need for kidney replacement therapy in the form of dialysis or kidney transplantation. The accompanying imbalance in acid-base, fluid, electrolytes, and mineral bone disease decreases the quality of life of patients with CKD. Ameliorating these metabolic complications by skillful application of effective food patterns that successfully delay the need for kidney replacement therapy can improve patient life quality and reduce societal costs for CKD management.
- Diet might also be used to help slow CKD progression, as will be discussed.

Together, these data support that diet in CKD plays an important role in its prevention, its progression once it is established, and in management of its complications. Although the focus of our discussion will be strategies and tactics available to clinicians caring for CKD patients, the data will support that changes in food policy will facilitate some interventions, particularly when considering strategies for CKD prevention. The data to be discussed support diet as the foundational, "food first"[9] approach to the management of individuals with CKD as well as those at risk for it, with pharmacologic therapy as adjunctive to diet. This is the reverse of the current approach in which pharmacologic therapy is foundational to CKD management. We will begin our discussion with the contributions of diet to the major disease entities responsible for CKD, diabetes and hypertension, which account for 72% of incident end-stage kidney disease (ESKD) cases in the US.[4]

## DIETARY CONTRIBUTIONS TO THE MAIN SYNDROMES WHICH CAUSE CKD: DIABETES AND HYPERTENSION

### DIABETES

Diabetes mellitus remains the single largest contributor to ESKD in the US with T2D being responsible for greater than 90% of the cases and type 1 (T1D) contributing the remainder.[4,10] Although US incidence of T2D is decreasing, its prevalence is increasing,[11] likely due to T2D individuals living longer which unfortunately exposes them to greater risk of developing CKD. Ten years following T2D diagnosis, 5.3% had macroalbuminuria (i.e., greater than 300 mg of daily urine albumin excretion [4]), indicative of established nephropathy.[12] Unfortunately, many T2D patients already have signs of CKD at the time of diagnosis,[13] possibly because they had experienced an indeterminate period of the abnormal metabolic state known as "pre-diabetes" which can be associated with signs of kidney injury, like albuminuria.[14] More concerning, about one third of US adults have "prediabetes"[11] and such individuals have a higher prevalence of reduced eGFR compared to the general population.[14] In the past quarter century, both cardiovascular and kidney disease have become highly prevalent in adults with prediabetes, irrespective of the definition used to define prediabetes.[14] It is therefore important to consider dietary approaches to CKD, particularly strategies intended to prevent CKD onset and its progression, within the context of dietary contributions to this major health condition that leads to CKD in developed societies.

**Dietary contributions to T2DM.** Overweight is the single most important modifiable risk factor for T2DM[15] and so the dietary factors that contribute to it provide the context for diabetes-related CKD. Observational studies support that adherence to a "healthy" as opposed to an "unhealthy" diet, including the "Mediterranean" diet that emphasizes fresh fruits and vegetables, olive oil, fish as the source of animal protein, and de-emphasizes simple sugars and red meat as a protein source, is associated with reduced T2D risk.[16,17] Dietary components that appear to influence T2D risk include:

- *Character of ingested carbohydrates.* High intake of the indigestible component of complex carbohydrate known as fiber is associated with reduced T2D risk.[18,19] Increased fiber intake enhances the growth of gut bacteria whose fermentation of the ingested fiber produces short chain fatty acids that promote improved glycemic control.[20] Whole grain foods are particularly high in fiber. Fruits and vegetables, in general, are fiber sources. On the other hand, chronically high ingestion of foods with greater propensity to increase blood glucose levels when ingested (i.e., foods with a high glycemic index such as simple sugars) is associated with increased T2D risk.[21–23] The glycemic index is a relative ranking of carbohydrate in foods according to how they affect blood glucose levels. It is a number from 0 to 100, with pure glucose arbitrarily given the value of 100. Carbohydrates with a low glycemic index value (55 or less) are more slowly digested, absorbed and metabolized and cause slower rise in blood glucose, often to lower levels.
- *Character of ingested fat.* Although high intake of saturated fat appears not to affect the risk for T2D,[24] high intake of the polyunsaturated fats omega 6[25,26] and omega 3[27] appear to reduce the risk for T2D.
- *Character of ingested protein.* High intake of animal-based protein is associated with increased risk for T2D,[28,29] particularly increased intake of red meat.[28–31] On the other hand, diets proportionally high in plant-based protein are associated with reduced T2D risk.[32]

**Table 60.1 Dietary Approaches to Reduce Incidence of Type 2 Diabetes**

| Strategy | Tactic |
|---|---|
| Emphasize carbohydrates that promote healthy glucose metabolism | • Promote foods with dietary fiber<br>◦ Whole grains<br>◦ Fruits and vegetables<br>• Minimize foods with high glycemic index<br>◦ Simple sugars<br>◦ Fructose |
| Emphasize fats that promote healthy fat metabolism | • Promote polyunsaturated fats, including omega 6s and omega 3s |
| Emphasize dietary protein that is less likely to increase insulin resistance | • Promote plant-based foods<br>• Minimize animal-based foods, particularly red meat |
| Emphasize an overall diet that minimizes net endogenous acid production | • Promote base-producing fruits and vegetables<br>• Minimize animal-based foods<br>• Minimize NaCl ("salt") |
| Reduce obesity risk | • Promote a healthy caloric intake<br>◦ Maximize foods with high nutrition/low calorie ratio like fruits and vegetables<br>◦ Minimize processed foods<br>• Promote omega 3 polyunsaturated fats |

**Table 60.2 Dietary Approaches to Reduce Incidence of Hypertension**

| Strategy | Tactic |
|---|---|
| Emphasize a "healthy" profile of electrolyte intake | • Minimize NaCl ("salt")<br>◦ Fresh rather than processed foods<br>◦ Fresh fruits and vegetables<br>• Promote potassium intake as tolerated<br>◦ Fruits and vegetables<br>• Promote magnesium intake as tolerated<br>◦ Fruits and vegetables |
| Emphasize proteins that promote healthy blood pressure | • Promote plant-based foods<br>• Minimize animal-based foods |
| Emphasize an overall diet that minimizes net endogenous acid production | • Promote base-producing fruits and vegetables<br>• Minimize animal-based foods<br>• Minimize NaCl ("salt") |
| Reduce obesity risk | • Promote a healthy caloric intake<br>• Maximize foods with high nutrition/low calorie ratio like fruits and vegetables<br>• Minimize processed foods |

- *Dietary effects on endogenous acid production.* Animal-based protein is metabolized to yield acid but most plant-based protein is metabolized to yield base or is metabolized to yield neither.[33] In addition, a high salt (NaCl) diet increases endogenous acid production.[34] Whether ingested diets are acid-producing or base-producing is determined to large degree by the balance of acid-producing and base-producing dietary components. High acidogenic diets increase insulin resistance,[35] their chronic ingestion is associated with increased T2D risk,[36–38] and insulin resistance in T2D is associated with hypertension and microalbuminuria.[36]

Together, these data guide dietary strategies to prevent diabetes, particularly in individuals and populations at risk (Table 60.1). In addition, they help guide dietary management of CKD patients with concomitant diabetes.

## HYPERTENSION

Hypertension is the second largest contributor to ESKD in the US and is a comorbid factor in more than 90% of patients with CKD.[4] As discussed for diabetes, it is important to consider dietary approaches to CKD, particularly strategies intended to prevent CKD, its progression, and the effect of CKD on mortality, within the context of dietary contributions to hypertension. This is particularly important given that better blood pressure control in CKD is associated with lower mortality.[7,8]

**Dietary contributions to hypertension**. As described for diabetes, adherence to a "healthy" as opposed to an "unhealthy" diet is associated with lower incidence of hypertension in populations.[39,40] Other observational studies support that population adherence to the previously described Mediterranean diet is associated with lower blood pressure.[41] Furthermore, current guidelines recommend the Dietary Approaches to Stop Hypertension (DASH) diet as first-line therapy for hypertension[6] because it effectively reduces blood pressure.[42] This diet emphasizes fruits and vegetables, whole grains and nuts, and limits consumption of animal-based protein, such as red meat, in preference for moderate intake of fish and poultry. The DASH diet reduces blood pressure in hypertensive patients.[42] Dietary components that appear to contribute to hypertension risk are summarized in Table 60.2, and include:

*Electrolyte intake.* Multiple studies highlight the important role of sodium (NaCl or "salt") in the initiation and maintenance of hypertension, noting that hypertension is rare in societies with very low dietary sodium intake, even in individuals of advanced age.[43] In addition, there is a direct relationship between population sodium intake and blood pressure,[43,44] and dietary sodium restriction reduces blood pressure in patients with hypertension.[45] As noted, the DASH diet reduces blood pressure[42] but sodium restriction further reduces blood pressure in patients eating this diet.[46] By contrast, high dietary sodium appears to abrogate the blood pressure-lowering effects of a "healthy diet".[47] On the other hand, urine potassium excretion, which is reflective of dietary potassium intake, is inversely associated with blood pressure.[48,49] Dietary potassium appears to have a number of blood pressure-lowering benefits, including facilitating urine sodium excretion.[50] The dietary sodium and potassium combination that appears to reduce hypertension risk best is low sodium combined with high potassium intake.[48,49] In addition, some studies suggest that dietary magnesium intake is inversely associated with hypertension risk[51,52] and some others show that magnesium supplements can slightly decrease blood pressure in those with hypertension.[53]

- A plant-based diet, including fresh fruits and vegetables is naturally low in sodium and high in potassium,[48] and is a good source of magnesium[52]
- *Character of ingested protein.* Components of "unhealthy" diets, which have been associated with augmented hypertension risk, include increased intake of animal-based protein such as cheese and processed red meat.[54] In contrast, food components associated with lower hypertension risk include plant-based protein, like fruits and vegetables.[55,56] Epidemiologic studies show that strict vegetarians have a lower incidence of hypertension than those who are not[57] and that the blood pressure of vegetarians is less likely to increase with aging as is typically the case in most individuals eating the standard diets of developed societies.[58] Such studies suggest that reduced dietary intake of particular components of our standard diet was not the responsible factor for this blood pressure difference but that lower blood pressure in vegetarians was due instead larger intake of potentially beneficial nutrients from the increased intake of vegetables (and fruits).[59] In support of this contention, supplemental addition of fruits and vegetables to the Mediterranean diet, one that is similar in make-up to the DASH diet and is already higher in vegetables than diets typical of developed societies, was associated with a lower risk for development of hypertension.[60] Furthermore, reduction of red meat consumption and substitution with vegetable protein reduced blood pressure in prehypertensive, post-menopausal women.[61]
- *Dietary effects of endogenous acid production on hypertension.* As indicated, the body metabolizes animal-based protein in a way that increases endogenous acid production whereas most plant-based protein is metabolized in a way that either decreases endogenous acid production or has no net effect on it.[33] In addition, as indicated, high salt (NaCl) diets increase endogenous acid production.[34] Indeed, dietary NaCl intake has approximately 50% to 100% of the acidosis-producing effect of the diet net acid load.[34] Studies in children[62] and adults[63,64] support that diets that increase endogenous acid production increase blood pressure. Because dietary sodium increases,[34] dietary potassium decreases,[33] animal-based protein increases,[33] and plant-based protein decreases[33] endogenous acid production, dietary effect on endogenous acid production might be a common mechanism through which these and possibly other dietary components influence blood pressure and the risk for hypertension.
- *Obesity.* There are, of course, strong dietary contributions to obesity and population studies show that obesity is associated with increased risk for hypertension.[65,66] In addition, weight loss in obese patients with hypertension reduces their blood pressure.[67]

Strategies to reduce CKD incidence in populations can begin by reducing the incidence of its two major causes, diabetes (particularly T2D) and hypertension. Data presented support strong dietary contributions to both and suggest that dietary strategies instituted for individual at-risk patients and, more broadly, populations as a whole, hold promise to reduce CKD incidence through reducing the incidence of diabetes and hypertension. Such interventions might be more effectively instituted at an overall population, rather than on an individual, level, particularly when focused on population segments at particularly high CKD risk. Furthermore, because diabetes is the single largest contributor to CKD in developed societies and because more than 90% of CKD patients have hypertension, these data support effective dietary strategies in individual CKD patients to manage concomitant diabetes and/or hypertension in CKD patients.

## DIETARY CONTRIBUTIONS TO CKD INCIDENCE AND PROGRESSION

### DIETARY FACTORS ASSOCIATED WITH INITIATION OF CKD

Similar to what has been described for the two syndromes that are the main contributors to CKD, observational studies support that adherence to a "healthy" as opposed to an "unhealthy" diet is associated with reduced risk for CKD.[68–71] Although the components of a "healthy" diet that mediate reduced CKD risk remain to be clearly identified, observations that adherence to the "Mediterranean" diet which emphasizes fresh fruits and vegetables, olive oil, and fish as the source of animal protein and de-emphasizes red meat and simple carbohydrates is associated with reduced CKD risk[72–75] offers some dietary elements to consider.

Plant-based diets are high in fiber and such diets, particularly those with a high ratio of fiber to animal-based protein, are associated with reduced CKD risk,[75,76] possibly in part because diets with a high proportion of animal-based protein are associated with high levels of gut-derived substances that are putative kidney toxins.[77] As indicated, most plant-based protein is metabolized to yield base after ingestion as opposed to animal-based protein which yields acid.[33] Low acid diets are associated with reduced, and high acid diets with increased, CKD risk.[78,79] High intake of red meat, in particular, is associated with increased CKD risk.[80,81] High dietary acid diets, caused largely by disproportionately high intake of animal-based protein, might contribute to kidney injury that initiates CKD by causing chronic hyperfiltration,[82] a phenomenon linked to hemodynamically-induced kidney injury.[83]

Other potential kidney protective benefits of the Mediterranean diet might derive from its oily fish and other plant-based foods which contain omega 3 polyunsaturated fatty acids, high intake of which has been associated with reduced CKD risk.[84] Omega 3 polyunsaturated fatty acids are also associated with reduced risk of obesity[85] and obesity itself is associated with increased CKD risk,[86,87] even independent of diabetes and hypertension.[88,89]

### DIETARY FACTORS ASSOCIATED WITH PROGRESSION OF ESTABLISHED CKD

Individuals with albuminuria, even with initially normal eGFR, have increased risk for subsequent eGFR decline[4] whether due to diabetes[90] or to nondiabetic CKD associated with primary hypertension.[91] As has been described for diabetes, hypertension, and initiation of CKD, adherence to a "healthy" as opposed to an "unhealthy" diet is associated slower eGFR decline of established CKD.[5,92,93] These "healthy" diets have high content of plant-based protein[68–71] and increasing the proportion of dietary plant-based protein decreases urine indices of kidney injury[94] and slows CKD progression.[95–97] Because, as indicated, plant-based protein is largely metabolized to yield base, at least part of the benefit of plant-based diets might be their effect to reduce dietary acid[33,94] because correction of metabolic acidosis[96–99] and dietary acid reduction even without underlying metabolic acidosis[100] slows the rate of eGFR decline in CKD. Other mechanisms contributed by plant-based protein might be promotion of a gut microbiome that yields reduced metabolism of diet components delivered to the gut into kidney toxic substances.[101] Diets with high intake of plant-based components are comparatively lower in sodium than diets high in animal-based components, particularly processed meats, and high sodium diets have been associated with progression of CKD.[102]

### POTENTIAL MECHANISMS FOR DIET-RELATED KIDNEY INJURY

- **Hyperfiltration.** When a substantial number of functioning nephrons is lost, remaining functioning nephrons increase filtration above that when they were part of a normal contingent of nephrons, a process known as hyperfiltration.[83] Animal models of CKD support that the high glomerular filtration pressure associated with hyperfiltration is injurious to kidneys in the long term and contributes to progressive GFR decline.[103] High intake of animal-based protein contributed to hyperfiltration with increased glomerular capillary pressure in these animal models of CKD and these diets high in animal-based proteins induced greater kidney injury in animals with reduced compared to those with intact nephron mass.[103,104] Chronically high intake of animal-based dietary proteins also appears to cause hyperfiltration in humans.[82] Hormonal systems that appear to contribute to hyperfiltration in these animal models of CKD include glucagon, insulin, insulin-like growth factor-1, angiotensin II, prostaglandins, and kinins.[105–108]
- **Oxidative stress.** Oxidative metabolism yields molecules that are potentially injurious to surrounding tissue and innate systems normally remove or detoxify them. These oxygen-related molecules can cause tissue injury if their production exceeds normal detoxifying mechanisms or if the normal detoxifying mechanisms are compromised by a phenomenon known as oxidative stress. The reduced nephron mass animal model of CKD is associated with oxidative stress that is exacerbated by increased intake of animal-based dietary protein.[109,110]
- **Inflammation.** Progressive nephropathy is characterized by inflammation, including fibrosis, particularly of the kidney tubule interstitium.[111] Diets high in animal-based protein increase kidney production of transforming growth factor β-1 and fibronectin, two substances that mediate kidney fibrosis.[112] Furthermore, high-intake of animal-based protein increased kidney levels of endothelin-1, aldosterone, and angiotensin II, each of which mediates progressive GFR decline and tubule-interstitial fibrosis in the reduced kidney mass model of CKD in animals. Conversely, increased intake of plant-based dietary protein ameliorated GFR decline and caused less tubule-interstitial fibrosis.[113–116]
- **Acid-induced kidney injury.** As noted, high dietary acid is associated with increased CKD incidence[78,79] but is also associated with its progression.[117] Animal studies show that high acid diets increase kidney levels of substances such as endothelin-1, aldosterone, and angiotensin II, all of which help mediate increased kidney tubule acidification in response to these acid diets[118–120] but also cause kidney injury that contributes to progressive GFR decline.[113–116,121] Correction of metabolic acidosis in CKD patients with amelioration of nephropathy progression is associated with reduced urine excretion of these substances.[96,99,100] Together, these data support that high dietary acid causes acid-induced kidney injury through increased kidney levels of these, and possibly other, cytokines.

The data support that a plant-based diet is associated with less kidney injury or can ameliorate kidney injury by each of the diet-related mechanisms of kidney injury described.

### DIETARY CONTRIBUTIONS TO INCREASED CKD-RELATED MORTALITY

Reduced eGFR is associated with increased mortality,[122] due particularly to increased cardiovascular mortality,[123] and was associated with 4% of worldwide deaths in 2013.[124] The appearance of reduced GFR significantly shortens life expectancy in patients with diabetes compared those with diabetes and normal GFR.[125] Diet is the single largest CKD-related risk factor for death and disability[1] and a "healthy" diet is associated with reduced mortality in CKD.[2] Excess animal-based protein to fiber intake is associated with increased mortality in CKD patients[126] but increases in dietary fiber were associated with reduced CKD-related inflammation and mortality.[127]

Together, these data support dietary strategies as front-line management of individuals at increased risk for or with established CKD in an effort to reduce their risk for developing CKD, for progression of established CKD, and to reduce the excess mortality associated with CKD.

## COMPONENT CONSIDERATIONS IN THE DIETARY MANAGEMENT OF CKD

### NUTRITIONAL COMPONENTS TO CONSIDER WHEN DESIGNING DIETARY MANAGEMENT OF CKD PATIENTS

- **Energy requirements.** Most studies support that energy requirements for CKD patients are not different from non-CKD patients but energy requirements did not decrease in response to decreased caloric intake as it did non-CKD patients,[128] suggesting that CKD patients do not respond normally to a reduction in caloric intake. Some studies support a slight increase in energy requirements in hemodialysis patients due to uremic factors that cause insulin resistance.[129] Although CKD patients might have steady-state levels of energy intake below the recommended 30-35 kcal/kg body weight/day,[130] most studies support the 30-35 kcal/kg body weight/day recommendation when prescribing a protein-restricted diet for kidney protection to avoid protein energy wasting.[131,132] Carbohydrates can account for 5% to 15% of energy requirements for CKD patients[133] but practitioners must exercise caution when including foods with high fructose content because it is associated with increased insulin resistance[134] and with increased all-cause and CVD mortality.[135] Additional reasons to limit or avoid dietary fructose as an energy source for CKD patients is that it increases serum uric acid levels,[135] which are associated with exacerbated nephropathy progression.[136,137] Furthermore, lowering serum uric acid improves kidney outcomes and reduces the risk for cardiovascular events in CKD patients.[138]

**Protein requirements.** Empiric observations support minimum dietary protein requirements as 0.6 g/kg of ideal body weight per day; adding 2 standard deviations for a general recommendation to theoretically encompass the dietary protein needs of 97.5% of individuals yields the standard recommendation of 0.75 g/kg bw/day[139] which is often rounded up to 0.8 g/kg/bw/day. This recommendation applies to both vegetarians and non-vegetarians.[140] These guidelines suggest that dialysis patients increase this amount to 1.2 g/kg bw/day because of their high protein catabolism and/or loss.[141] Unlike that described for energy requirements, CKD patients can adapt to dietary protein restriction by reducing amino acid oxidation and protein degradation.[142] Naturally occurring amino acids contain nitrogen, which when metabolized yield nitrogenous wastes that increase blood urea and possibly adversely affect kidney function.[143] Symptoms of uremia are associated with breakdown products of protein catabolism. Therefore, restriction in dietary protein can delay the need to start kidney replacement therapy despite a decline in GFR by ameliorating uremic symptoms. This confounds, by potentially introducing bias favoring dietary protein restriction, defining mechanisms that protect renal function directly. Dietary animal protein will reduce measured GFR, as defined by creatinine, unrelated to changes in true GFR.

Low protein diets (0.6-0.8 g/kg bw/day), sometimes supplemented with non-nitrogen ketoanalogs, have been associated with slower GFR decline[143,144] and with lower levels of gut-derived uremic toxins[145] in non-dialysis CKD patients. Nevertheless, the largest study to date that examined the impact of total dietary protein restriction on nephropathy progression, the Modification of Diet in Renal Disease (MDRD) study, showed that GFR decline at three years was no different between subjects given a low protein diet (0.58 g/kg/day) and a usual protein diet (1.3 g/kg/day).[146] The MDRD study was the largest randomized clinical trial to test the hypothesis that protein restriction over a 2- to 3-year period slows the progression of chronic kidney disease. However, the primary results published in 1994 were not conclusive with regard to the efficacy of this intervention. Long-term follow-up of the cohort also remained inconclusive. Furthermore, despite the benefit of low protein diets to reduce the rate of GFR decline shown in some studies, some patients with intakes below 0.8 g/kg/bw/day, even the described minimum level of 0.6 g/kg/bw/day, develop protein energy wasting[147] and increased mortality.[144] Even so, some studies show that CKD patients can safely eat these diets without compromising nutritional status.[143,148] Because of the described benefits of primarily plant-based diets, investigators have studied these diets in CKD patients and show similar nutritional status in such patients compared to those ingesting similar amounts of a primarily animal-sourced protein diet.[149] Controversy still exists about the potential for a beneficial effect of reduction in dietary protein on the rate of progression of loss of kidney function. The level of residual kidney function at the time of initiation of therapy and the heterogeneity of etiologies of CKD in the populations tested are some of the factors that confound interpretation of collective studies.

Individuals living in developed societies typically ingest dietary protein in excess of requirements, averaging about 60% more,[140] and most of this ingested protein is animal-based.[33] As noted, animal-based protein increases intrinsic acid production when metabolized[33] and increased dietary acid has been associated with increased risk for CKD appearance[78,79] and progression.[96–100] Also as noted, animal-based dietary protein is associated with the production of high levels of gut-derived substances which are putative kidney toxins.[77] For these reasons, many guidelines recommend restricting dietary protein intake for those living in developed societies to that necessary to satisfy requirements, typically 0.7 to 0.8 g/kg of ideal body weight daily.[133]

Ingested dietary protein that is not converted into protein is converted to urea, the major waste product derived from protein catabolism,[150] which can accumulate and contribute to uremic symptoms. Steady-state blood urea levels directly parallel levels of all nitrogen-containing waste products that contribute to uremic symptoms,[151] so following urea levels is a helpful guide to the accumulation of these substances. Steady-state concentration of urea is a function of dietary protein intake that contributes to urea production of the comparatively small amount of urea degradation and extra-kidney clearance,[150] and of how well the kidney excretes urea, the latter being directly related to GFR and the tubular handling of urea. It follows that reducing dietary protein is an effective strategy to reduce urea and the associated blood levels of nitrogenous wastes in patients with declining GFR.

Metabolic acidosis, a comorbid condition that appears when eGFR is comparatively low (typically, less than 40% of normal),[152] increases protein catabolism[153] mediated through the adenosine triphosphate-dependent ubiquitin-proteasome system.[154] Correction of the metabolic acidosis of CKD with alkali decreases protein catabolism, improves protein balance with increased muscle mass, and decreases induction of the ubiquitin-proteosome system.[155,156] Metabolic acidosis also decreases protein anabolism, manifest by decreased albumin synthesis[157] that is improved with correction of the metabolic acidosis.[158] Because diets in developed societies are typically acidogenic[33] and can contribute to metabolic acidosis, particularly in individuals with low GFR,[159] modifying diet can help prevent or treat metabolic acidosis in CKD and thereby ameliorate its untoward effects on protein metabolism. Options to accomplish this modification include reducing the amount of animal-based protein in the diet and/or adding base-producing fruits and vegetables, the latter of which effectively treats metabolic acidosis in CKD.[96,160]

Guidelines for dietary protein in CKD have most often focused on the amount of dietary protein but less so on character of the ingested protein. The 2013 Kidney Disease: Improving Global Outcomes (KDIGO)[161] guideline 3.1.13 for CKD patients suggests "lowering protein intake to 0.8 g/kg body weight/day in adults with diabetes ("2C" level of strength, meaning that this is a suggestion and that the true effect of this suggestion might be substantially different from the estimated effect) or without diabetes ("2B" level of strength, meaning that this is a suggestion and that its true effect is likely to be close to the estimated effect but there is a possibility that it is substantially different) and GFR < 30 mi/min/1.73 $m^2$ (GFR categories G4-G5) with appropriate education." The guidelines suggest that the recommended protein be of "high biologic value" but do not discuss if this includes plant-based protein. Guideline 3.1.14 reads "we suggest avoiding high protein intake (> 1.3 g/Kg/body weight/day) in adults with CKD at risk of progression" ("2C" level of strength, as explained above). The qualifications for these two suggestions reflect the need for additional research to develop more concrete dietary protein recommendations for patients with very low (< 30 mL/min/1.73 $m^2$) GFR. In particular, further studies will elucidate importance of the protein's character compared its amount, particularly with respect to the acid-producing or base-producing protein ability. In addition to the aforementioned potential advantages of plant-based compared to animal-based protein in CKD, carnitine and lecithin in animal-based protein are metabolized by gut microbes to trimethylamine, which in turn is metabolized by liver flavin monoxygenases to trimethylamine-N-oxide (TMAO).[162] High blood levels of TMAO strongly correlate with CVD and are associated acute clinical events of CKD.[162,163] Together, these data support considering the character, in addition to the amount, of dietary protein recommended for CKD patients, particularly plant-based protein for those able to tolerate the increased potassium that accompanies plant-based diets.

- **Sodium.** Adults in the United States consume an average of 3400-3600 mg (148-156 mmol) of sodium per day,[164,165] an amount in great excess of dietary recommendations.[140] Processed foods comprise the majority of sodium consumed in the United States, which industry typically adds to increase shelf life of and enhance palatability for consumers.[166] Foods eaten outside of homes typically have even higher sodium content.[166] Higher dietary sodium in CKD is associated with higher blood pressure whereas its reduction is associated with reduced blood pressure and reduced albuminuria.[167,168] In addition, high sodium diets are associated with CKD progression.[102] Together, these data support some level of dietary sodium restriction below current dietary intake in CKD patients but there are not enough data to determine the optimal level of dietary sodium intake. The 2015 report of the American Dietary Guidelines Advisory Committee[169] recommends a daily sodium intake for adults of less than 2300 mg (100 mmol). The KDIGO recommendation (3.1.19)[161] for adult CKD patients is a daily sodium intake of less than 2000 mg (90 mmol) unless otherwise contraindicated. Despite that this recommendation is of "1 C" quality (i.e., most clinicians would agree but the true effect may be substantially different from the estimated effect), it seems to be reasonable until more definitive studies determine a more specific level of dietary sodium restriction.
- **Potassium.** Patients with CKD appear to benefit from diets high in plant-based components, including fruits and vegetables, as discussed but the high potassium content of these diets historically has made practitioners reluctant to prescribe them because of the reduced potassium excretory capacity of CKD patients with reduced GFR.[161] Nevertheless, only limited data to support that dietary potassium restriction improves outcomes in CKD and most of the recommendations are opinion based. Relatedly, some reports question the historic admonition to limit intake of plant-based foods in CKD patients, including fruits and vegetables.[170] Enhanced kidney excretion mediated by increased serum potassium, increased serum aldosterone, and increased distal urine flow, and enhanced $Na^+$-$K^+$-ATPase activity can help maintain potassium balance in CKD.[171] Patients with CKD stage 4 who had fruits and vegetables added to their ad lib diets increased urine aldosterone excretion and exhibited urine hormonal changes consistent with lower urine 11β-hydroxysteroid dehydrogenase type 2 activity.[160] The latter response to this increment in dietary potassium due to added fruits and vegetables indicates greater glucocorticoid access to the mineralocorticoid receptor, which along with aldosterone, yields added stimulation of distal nephron potassium excretion.[172] Importantly, potassium in plant-based food is predominantly in the form of non-chloride ions, a form that facilitates urine potassium excretion.[173] Additionally, CKD patients have increased potassium secretion into the gastrointestinal tract with increased fecal potassium losses.[174] Together, these data support that CKD patients have the capacity to increase potassium excretion in response to an increment in dietary potassium.

A comprehensive analysis of 36,000 CKD 3-4 patients reported a U-shaped mortality risk for both higher (> 5 mEq/L) and lower (< 3.5 mEq/L) serum potassium levels.[175] Additionally, a secondary analysis of 840 patients from the MDRD cohort found that higher urine potassium excretion, a surrogate marker for higher dietary potassium intake, was associated with a lower risk for all-cause mortality.[176] This higher potassium intake was unlikely due to pharmacologic potassium administration to these CKD patients known to have reduced ability to excrete potassium; more likely, the higher potassium intake was due to higher intake of potassium-containing foods like plant-based food components that these patients tolerated without untoward effects. In support of this supposition, patients with CKD stages 3-4 tolerated diets high in plant-based food components given to improve calcium/phosphate metabolism[177,178] and to treat metabolic acidosis[96,160] without developing hyperkalemia. In addition, patients in these studies tolerated these plant-based diets despite their taking inhibitors of the renin-angiotensin-aldosterone system (RAAS), which can limit urine potassium excretion, given for kidney protection. Limiting other drugs that can also reduce urine potassium excretion, such as nonsteroidal antiinflammatory drugs (NSAIDs) as was done in these studies,[96,160,177,178] might help CKD patients eating a potassium-rich diet avoid hyperkalemia.

The 2015 report of the American Dietary Guidelines Advisory Committee[169] recommends a daily potassium intake for the general population of adults of 4700 mg (121 mmol). Nevertheless, average daily potassium intake for US adults is 2155 mg (55 mmol), likely being lower than recommended due to poor intake of fruits and vegetables.[169] The NKF-KDOQI initiative has recommended potassium intake identical to the general population in patients with CKD stages 1 and 2 (> 4 g/day or > 102 mmol/day) and reduced intake of potassium to 2 to 4 g/day (51-102 mmol/day) in patients with CKD 3 and 4.[179] Because of the described benefits of plant-based diets, recommendations to restrict potassium should ideally be tailored to allow CKD patients 1) with hypertension to eat the DASH diet with its high plant-based content[42] for hypertension control; 2) the added plant-based food components for effective management of the disturbed calcium/phosphate metabolism of CKD[177,178]; and 3) with metabolic acidosis to receive base-producing fruits and vegetables for management of their metabolic acidosis.[96,160] To date, published studies have not defined a clear role for potassium binding agents that might allow for liberalization of dietary potassium intake in patients with CKD, particularly when given with RAAS blockers.[180]

- **Phosphorus.** Patients with CKD and reduced GFR are in positive phosphorus balance yet can maintain phosphorus levels in the normal range until advanced CKD stages (i.e., stages 4-5) through phosphaturia induced by increases in fibroblast growth factor-23 and parathyroid hormone.[181] Phosphorus metabolism is linked to increase CVD, vascular calcifications, and morbidity in CKD patients.[182] Nevertheless, dietary phosphate intake measured by 24-hour urine phosphate excretion was not associated with ESKD incidence or with cardiovascular mortality as long as the resulting serum phosphate levels were within the normal range.[183] Historically, practitioners have limited dietary phosphate intake by limiting intake of phosphate-containing foods, particularly processed foods that often have elemental phosphate-added preservatives.[133] The elemental phosphates added to processed foods are of particular concern because they are quickly and completely absorbed from the gastrointestinal tract when ingested.[184] By contrast, phosphate in plant-based food is in the form of phytates (phytic acid) that have much lower gastrointestinal tract absorption than the elemental phosphate in food additives.[178,185] This helps explain the lower levels of serum phosphate and FGF23 in CKD patients eating a primarily plant-based diet in comparison to those eating a diet more typical of developed societies in which the protein source was primarily an animal-based based diet.[177,178] In addition, CKD patients eating the plant-based diet had need for fewer phosphate-binding medications with a resulting lower pill burden in these patients with advanced CKD.[178]

Together, these data support the recommendation for restricted phosphorus intake in CKD patients, specifically to less than 800 mg/day[133] in comparison to the average of 1000 mg/day for the average US adult.[140] Importantly, this requires limited or no intake of processed food that contains elemental phosphate additives. Relatedly, fresh and home-prepared foods yielded better phosphate control than processed foods without compromising nutritional status.[186] Dietary phosphate restriction can also be helped by restricting intake of animal-based protein and/or by adding plant-based protein with its less absorbable phosphate[178,185] and/or substituting plant-based for animal-based dietary protein.

- **Calcium.** Recommendations for daily dietary calcium intake are 1000 mg (23 mmol) for adults age 19 to 50 years, 1200 mg (28 mmol) for females 51 to 70 years old, and 1200 mg for all adults older than 70 years for the general population.[187] Published data are insufficiently robust to offer a specific recommendation for dietary calcium intake for CKD patients beyond that for the general population.[188] Recognizing the potential benefits of a plant-based compared to an animal protein-based diet in CKD patients, such diets affect overall calcium metabolism. Individuals eating a primary animal-based protein diet have higher urine calcium excretion than those eating a primary plant-based diet.[189] Earlier studies supported that this higher urine calcium excretion was due to bone buffering of acid produced from metabolism of the ingested animal-based protein with resorption of bone mineral and release of calcium into extracellular fluid.[190] Studies that are more recent support that a likely greater contributor to the increased urine calcium excretion observed with the diets high in animal-based protein is that such diets are typically very low in oxalate that binds to calcium in the gastrointestinal tract, thereby preventing calcium absorption and promoting its fecal excretion.[191] Greater gastrointestinal calcium absorption promoted by these low oxalate diets leads to greater calcium transport into the extracellular fluid with greater increased urine calcium excretion.[192] On the other hand, diets high in plant-based protein have high amounts of calcium-binding oxalate that yield decreased gastrointestinal calcium absorption with subsequent lower urine calcium excretion.[191,192]
- **Dietary fiber.** Advanced CKD patients appear to have a "leaky gut" with translocation of endotoxins and bacterial DNA with untoward downstream untoward consequences including increased inflammation and increased CVD morbidity.[193] Diets typical of developed societies drive a milieu of metabolic abnormalities including uremic toxin production, inflammation, and immunosuppression that ultimately promotes progressive kidney failure and cardiovascular disease.[193,194] Some dietary components are metabolized in the colon by fermentation, with the two predominant types being saccharolytic (carbohydrate) and proteolytic (protein). Saccharolytic fermentation is beneficial with generation of short chain fatty acids such as butyrate, propionate and acetate, whereas proteolytic fermentation produces uremic toxins such as p-cresyl sulfate and indoxyl sulphate.[195] Furthermore, diets with higher animal-based protein-to-fiber ratio are associated with higher serum levels of p-cresyl sulfate and indoxyl sulphate.[195] p-Cresol sulfate is a microbial metabolite that is found in urine and likely derives from secondary metabolism of p-cresol. Indoxyl sulfate, also known as 3-indoxylsulfate, is a metabolite of dietary l-tryptophan. Indole is produced from l-tryptophan in the human intestine via tryptophanase-expressing gastrointestinal bacteria. Whereas indoxyl is produced from indole via

enzyme-mediated hydroxylation in the liver. *SULT1A1* appears to be the primary sulfotransferase enzyme involved in the conversion of indoxyl into indoxyl sulfate in the liver. On the other hand, analysis of 14,543 NHANES participants demonstrated that increases in dietary fiber intake were associated with reductions in inflammation and mortality in patients with CKD.[196] Increased dietary fiber was associated with decreased mortality in CKD patients[196] and with reduced serum levels of creatinine and urea.[197] The many discussed benefits of increasing the dietary intake of plant-based dietary components in CKD patients include increasing their fiber intake that is generally lower than that of the general population.[197]

Mean daily fiber intake in the general US population is 16 grams, much lower than the recommended daily intake of 25 to 30 grams.[198] On the other hand, mean daily fiber intake for CKD patients was 12 grams,[199] showing even lower intake than the general population, likely due to the historic limitation of plant-based foods in CKD patients. The American Heart Association recommends daily fiber intake greater than 25 grams to help reduce CVD risk.[200] Because of the comparably high CVD risk in CKD patients,[4] it seems prudent to follow this recommendation for patients with CKD. Increased intake of plant-based foods is an effective strategy to increase dietary fiber but this intervention should be limited to CKD patients who can tolerate the associated increased potassium load without developing hyperkalemia.

- **Micronutrients.** Unfortunately, there have been few published studies regarding the micronutrient status of CKD patients and their need for trace elements and vitamins required for energy production, cell and organ function, and for growth. Although some studies show that many hemodialysis patients have dietary intakes of trace elements and vitamins that fall below recommended values,[201] plasma levels of these substances in hemodialysis patients are typically not low.[202] Other studies in a general population show that high intake of several micronutrients was associated with a reduced CKD risk.[203] Despite most guidelines that recommend multivitamin supplements for dialysis patients,[133] a comprehensive examination of the literature found insufficient evidence to support routine multivitamin use in hemodialysis patients.[204] This is in stark contrast to the need for water-soluble vitamin supplementation when kidney replacement therapy is initiated, especially for folate.

Nevertheless, because both peritoneal and hemodialysis patients are routinely exposed to dialysates without trace elements and because many predialysis CKD patients are frequently prescribed diuretic agents, practitioners have understandable concerns that CKD patients are at risk for being deficient in water-soluble vitamins. Some studies report low vitamin C levels in peritoneal dialysis patients[205] and vitamin C supplements reduced dosage requirements for erythropoiesis-stimulating agents in other studies.[206] Still others report that L-carnitine supplement reduced resistance to erythropoietin-induced red blood cell production.[207] Relatedly, half or more of nondialysis CKD patients had plasma studies consistent with iron deficiency.[208] Accordingly, dietary guidelines for CKD patients often include supplement for the water-soluble vitamins including $B_1$, $B_6$, $B_{12}$, C, folate, and niacin.[133] Vitamin D is commonly prescribed to CKD patients and its appropriate use is discussed elsewhere in this book. The paucity of published studies regarding the status of other fat-soluble vitamins in CKD patients do not allow an evidence-base recommendation for them.

Because of the disproportionately high contribution of coronary artery calcification (CAC) to the increased CVD risk of CKD[209] and the contribution of vitamin K-dependent matrix Gla protein to the physiologic prevention of CAC,[210] vitamin K status of CKD patients has attracted attention. Dietary intake of vitamin K was low in hemodialysis patients in comparison to the general population[211,212] and was inversely related to CVD-related mortality in non-dialysis CKD patients.[213] Because many fruits and vegetables contain vitamin K,[211] their addition to the diets of CKD patients would appear to help provide vitamin K and possibly ameliorate CAC.

Regarding micronutrients in CKD, it seems that a reasonable approach would be to recommend the previously-described components of a "healthy" diet as tolerated, emphasizing plant-based proteins, with a smaller proportion of animal-based protein to provide micronutrients that are more abundant in animal-based compared to plant-based food components such as riboflavin.

## OVERALL DIET CONSIDERATIONS IN THE MANAGEMENT OF CKD

### DIETARY APPROACHES TO PREVENTION OF THE CONDITIONS THAT MOST COMMONLY CAUSE CKD IN DEVELOPED SOCIETIES, DIABETES AND HYPERTENSION

As indicated, prevention of CKD importantly focuses on prevention of the two major syndromes leading to CKD in developed societies, diabetes (predominantly T2D) and hypertension. Tables 60.1 and 60.2 list strategic considerations in this approach for T2D and hypertension, respectively, and tactics to execute these strategies. Strategies common to both T2D and hypertension include diets that reduce net endogenous acid production, contain a high proportion of plant-based components, limit dietary NaCl, and reduce the risk for obesity. Institution of a predominately plant-based diet can achieve each of these strategies common to prevention of T2D and hypertension. This common thread of a dietary approach designed to prevent both T2D and hypertension supports a population approach emphasizing increased intake of plant-based foods that holds promise to reduce the incidences of these two syndromes that contribute significantly to early death and increased disability in developed societies.[1] Such interventions, including this focus on increased intake of plant-based foods, are best applied at the level of overall populations if they are to reduce the incidences of T2D and hypertension and thereby CKD incidence. Doing so at the population level will likely require policy changes combined with public marketing. Practitioners can also consider these approaches for their individual patients deemed to be at increased risk for T2D and hypertension as suggested by family history, ethnic history, and/or their socioeconomic circumstance.

**Table 60.3 Dietary Approaches to Reduce the Risk for Initiation of CKD in Susceptible Individuals**

| Strategy | Tactic |
|---|---|
| Emphasize an overall diet that minimizes net endogenous acid production | • Promote base-producing fruits and vegetables<br>• Minimize animal-based foods<br>• Minimize NaCl ("salt") |
| Emphasize an overall diet with a high ratio of fiber to animal-based protein | • Promote plant-based foods<br>• Minimize animal-based foods, particularly red meat |
| Emphasize fats that enhance kidney health | • Promote polyunsaturated fats, including omega 3's |

**Table 60.4 Dietary Approaches to Reduce the Risk for Progression of Established CKD**

| Strategy | Tactic |
|---|---|
| Emphasize an overall diet that minimizes net endogenous acid production | • Promote base-producing fruits and vegetables as tolerated<br>• Minimize animal-based foods<br>• Minimize NaCl ("salt") |
| Emphasize an overall diet which yields a gut microbiome that promotes kidney health | • Promote plant-based foods as tolerated<br>• Minimize animal-based foods, particularly red meat |

## DIETARY APPROACHES TO MINIMIZING THE RISK FOR INITIATION OF CKD IN SUSCEPTIBLE INDIVIDUALS/POPULATIONS

Practitioners can consider dietary approaches for individuals who presently have no CKD but are at increased risk for it (Table 60.3). Their increased risk might be because they have diabetes (T2D or T1D) and/or hypertension, have other systemic conditions associated with CKD, or because of a strong family history. Again, these strategies might be applied to overall populations considered to be at increased CKD risk, e.g., US ethnic minorities concentrated in low-income communities or Native Americans living on reservations.[4] Primary care providers can also consider these interventions in patients that they manage with T2D and/or hypertension.

## DIETARY APPROACHES TO MINIMIZING THE RISK FOR PROGRESSION OF ESTABLISHED CKD TO ESKD

Table 60.4 depicts approaches that practitioners might consider to reduce the risk for progression to ESKD for individuals with established CKD, particularly those with reduced eGFR at presentation. Successful prevention of, or delay of, ESKD adds to the quality of life to CKD patients and reduces their management costs.[4] Practitioners currently underuse dietary strategies designed to prevent or slow CKD progression.[9]

**Table 60.5 Dietary Approaches to Reduce Mortality in Established CKD**

| Strategy | Tactic |
|---|---|
| Emphasize an overall diet with a high ratio of fiber to animal-based protein | • Promote plant-based foods<br>• Minimize animal-based foods, particularly red meat |
| Minimize dietary NaCl ("salt") | • Promote fresh fruits and vegetables as tolerated<br>• Minimize processed foods |

## DIETARY APPROACHES TO REDUCING MORTALITY IN ESTABLISHED CKD

Practitioners might consider the approaches listed in Table 60.5 in an effort to reduce the mortality risk for individuals with established CKD, especially those with reduced eGFR because mortality in CKD is inversely associated with eGFR.[122] Practitioners managing CKD patients often focus on CKD-related complications and less so on strategies to reduce mortality.[122] Currently, when the management focus includes mortality reduction, the focus is typically on pharmacologic strategies[4] with less focus on the effectiveness of dietary strategies.[2] As described for strategies to reduce CKD progression, dietary strategies designed to reduce mortality appear to be underused.

## GENERAL DIETARY MANAGEMENT OF PATIENTS WITH CKD

Table 60.6 lists general management approaches to CKD patients, distinguished by important nutritional components.

## DIETARY APPROACHES TO MANAGING SOME CKD-RELATED COMPLICATIONS

Table 60.7 lists some effective dietary strategies for management of the indicated CKD-related complications. Practitioners might use these dietary strategies along with appropriate pharmacologic interventions.

## CONSIDERATIONS FOR ENABLING CKD PATIENTS TO EAT A MORE PLANT-BASED DIET

Many of the dietary recommendations for CKD patients supported by published studies include increasing the plant-based component of their diets. Nevertheless, diets typical of developed societies are comprised predominantly of animal-based components.[33] Facilitating CKD patients eating these diets requires practitioners, health system leaders, and even government leaders to address real and perceived barriers for patients to acquire and consume such diets, including expense (e.g., fresh fruits and vegetables are generally more expensive that packaged, processed foods) and accessibility (many low-income communities have limited access to fresh fruits and vegetables).[214] Once CKD patients gain access to these foods, practitioners must simplify the

**Table 60.6 General Approach for a Dietary Recommendation for an Individual With CKD and Reduced GFR**

| Dietary Consideration | Recommendation |
|---|---|
| Energy | • 30-35 kcal/kg body weight/day<br>• 5%-15% from carbohydrates<br>• Avoid fructose |
| Protein | • 0.7-0.8 g/ideal body weight/day for non-dialysis patients<br>• 1.2 g/ideal body weight/day for dialysis patients<br>• Non-nitrogen keto-analogues might be substituted for a portion of recommended dietary protein<br>• Plant-based protein can be considered for patients able to tolerate the additional potassium load |
| Sodium | • <2g (90 mmol)/day unless otherwise contraindicated |
| Potassium | • >4 g (102 mmol)/day for CKD stages 1 and 2<br>• 2-4 g (51-102 mmol)/day for CKD stages 3 and 4<br>• As instructed by provider for CKD stage 5 |
| Phosphorous | • < 800 mg/day<br>• Promote plant-based sources over animal-based sources<br>• Minimize processed foods |
| Calcium | • 1000 mg (23 mmol)/day for adults age 19-50 years<br>• 1200 mg (28 mmol)/day for adult females age 51-70 years<br>• 1200 mg (28 mmol)/day for adults >70 years |
| Fiber | • ≥25 g/day |
| Micronutrients | • Promote a primary plant-based diet<br>• Multivitamin supplement for dialysis patients |

**Table 60.7 Dietary Interventions That Help in the Management of CKD-Related Complications**

| Strategy | Tactic |
|---|---|
| Nephropathy progression | • Reduce net endogenous acid production<br>• Promote a "kidney friendly" gut microbiome |
| Hypertension | • Minimize NaCl ("salt")<br>• Promote plant-based food as tolerated<br>  • Potassium as tolerated<br>  • Magnesium as tolerated |
| Disturbed calcium/ phosphate metabolism | • Promote plant-based food as tolerated<br>• Minimize processed foods |
| Metabolic acidosis | • Promote base-producing fruits and vegetables as tolerated<br>• Minimize animal-based protein<br>• Minimize NaCl ("salt") |
| Increased protein catabolism | • Treat metabolic acidosis with the described dietary approaches |

approach to healthy food patterns such that patients have a variety of food options to achieve food patterns that achieve intended goals.[215] This simplified approach must include culturally sensitive instructions for food preparation.[96] In addition, gaining support of all members of a patient's household helps facilitate successful dietary interventions for CKD patients whose recommended diet often contrasts with that of remaining household members.[96]

## FUTURE RESEARCH DIRECTIONS

Despite published data that support effective dietary approaches to the management of patients with CKD, many areas require further examination. For example, the benefits to CKD patients of a plant-based diet on mortality, progression of underlying nephropathy, and on some CKD-related co-morbid conditions support such diets as first-line treatment of CKD patients with pharmacologic therapy as adjunctive.[9] Future studies will determine, however, if this suggested approach will become standard of care for CKD management. In addition, future research will better determine in what circumstances these diets are most effective and how best to facilitate their implementation by CKD patients. In the meantime, it is imperative that clinicians, importantly those providing primary care, recognize the kidney protection benefits of the discussed dietary interventions for CKD patients.

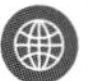 Complete reference list available at ExpertConsult.com.

## KEY REFERENCES


1. US Burden of Disease Collaborators. The state of US health, 1990-2010: burden of diseases, injuries, and risk factors. *JAMA.* 2013;310:591–608.
3. Kelly JT, Palmer SC, Wai SN, et al. Healthy dietary patterns and risk of mortality and ESRD in CKD: a meta-analysis of cohort studies. *Clin J Am Soc Nephrol.* 2017;12:272–279.
4. US Renal Data System. USRDS 2016. *Annual Data Report: The National Institutes of Health, National Institute of Diabetes and Digestive and Kidney Diseases,* Bethesda, MD; 2017.
7. Ku E, Gassman J, Appel LJ, et al. Blood pressure control and long-term risk of ESRD and Mortality. *J Am Soc Nephrol.* 2017;28: 671–677.
13. Gatwood J, Chisholm-Burns M, Davis R, et al. Evidence of chronic kidney disease in veterans with incident diabetes mellitus. *PLoS ONE.* 2018;13(2):e1092712. doi:10.1371/journal.pone.0192712.
14. Ali MK, McKeever K, Saydah S, et al. Cardiovascular and renal burdens of prediabetes in the USA: analysis of data from serial cross-sectional surveys, 1988-2014. *Lancet Diabetes Endocrinol.* 2018; doi:10.1016/S2213-8587(18)30027-5.
34. Frassetto LA, Morris RC Jr, Sebastian A. Dietary sodium chloride intake independently predicts the degree of hyperchloremic metabolic acidosis in healthy humans consuming a net acid-producing diet. *Am J Physiol Renal Physiol.* 2007;293:F521–F525.
56. Borgi L, Muraki I, Satija A, et al. Fruit and vegetable consumption and the incidence of hypertension in three prospective cohort studies. *Hypertension.* 2016;67:288–293.
57. Sacks FM, Kass EH. Low blood pressure in vegetarians: effects of specific foods and nutrients. *Am J Clin Nutr.* 1988;48:795–800.
68. Gopinath B, Harris DC, Flood VM, et al. A better diet quality is associated with a reduced likelihood of CKD in older adults. *Nutr Metab Cardiovasc Dis.* 2013;23:937–943.
70. Rebholz CM, Anderson CAM, Grams ME, et al. Relationship of the American Heart Association's impact goals (Life's Simple 7) with risk of chronic kidney disease: results from the Atherosclerosis Risk in Communities (ARIC) cohort study. *J Am Heart Assn.* 2016;5:e003192. doi:10.1161/JAHA.116.003192.

72. Chrysohoou C, Panagiotakos DB, Pitsavos C, et al. Adherence to the Mediterranean diet is associated with renal function among health adults: the ATTICA study. *J Ren Nutr.* 2010;20:176–184.
73. Khatri M, Moon YP, Scarmeas N, et al. The association between a Mediterranean-style diet and kidney function in the Northern Manhattan study cohort. *Clin J Am Soc Nephrol.* 2014;9:1868–1875.
77. Rossi M, Johnson DW, Xu H, et al. Dietary protein-fiber ratio associates with circulating levels of indoxyl sulfate and p-cresyl sulfate in chronic kidney disease patients. *Nutr Metab Cardiovasc Dis.* 2015;25:860–865.
78. Banerjee T, Crews DC, Wesson DE, et al. Dietary acid load and chronic kidney disease in the United States. *BMC Nephrol.* 2014; 15:137–149.
79. Rebholz CM, Coresh J, Grams ME, et al. Dietary acid load and incident chronic kidney disease: results from the ARIC study. *Am J Nephrol.* 2015;42:427–435.
80. Lew QL, Jafar T, Koh HWL, et al. Red meat intake and ESRD risk. *J Am Soc Nephrol.* 2017;28:304–312.
84. Gopinath B, Harris DC, Flood VM, et al. Consumption of long-chain n-3. PUFA, alpha linolenic acid and fish is associated with the prevalence of chronic kidney disease. *Br J Nutr.* 2011;105:1361–1368.
88. Hsu CY, McCulloch CE, Iribarren C, et al. Body mass index and risk for end-stage renal disease. *Ann Intern Med.* 2006;144:21–28.
94. Goraya N, Simoni J, Jo C-H, et al. Treatment of metabolic acidosis in individuals with stage 3. CKD with fruits and vegetables or oral $NaHCO_3$, reduces urine angiotensinogen and preserves GFR. *Kidney Int.* 2014;86:1031–1038.
97. Garneata L, Stancu A, Dragomir D, et al. Ketoanalogue-supplemented vegetarian very low-protein diet and CKD progression. *J Am Soc Nephol.* 2016;27:2164–2176.
98. de Brito-Ashurst I, Varagunam M, Raferty MJ, et al. Bicarbonate supplementation slows progression of CKD and improves nutritional status. *J Am Soc Nephrol.* 2009;20:2075–2084.
101. Evenepoel P, Meijens BKI, Mammens BRM, et al. Uremic toxins originating from colonic microbial metabolism. *Kidney Int.* 2009; 76(suppl 114):S12–S19.
102. Smyth A, O'Donnell MJ, Yusef L, et al. Sodium intake and renal outcomes: a systematic review. *Am J Hypertens.* 2014;27(10):1277–1284.
117. Banerjee T, Crews D, Wesson DE, et al. High dietary acid load predicts ESRD among US adults with CKD. *J Am Soc Nephrol.* 2015; 26:1693–1700.
121. Wesson DE, Simoni J. Increased tissue acid mediates progressive GFR decline in animals with reduced nephron mass. *Kidney Int.* 2009; 75:929–935.
123. Hu X, Matsushita K, Sang Y, et al. CKD and cardiovascular disease in the Atherosclerosis Risk in Communities (ARIC) Study: interactions with age, sex, and race. *Am J Kidney Dis.* 2013;62:691–702.
124. Global Burden of Diseases 2013, GFR Collaborators. CKD prognosis consortium, and global burden of Disease Genitourinary Expert Group. *J Am Soc Nephrol.* 2017;28:2167–2179.
126. Xu H, Rossi M, Campbell KL, et al. Excess protein intake relative to fiber and cardiovascular events in elderly men with chronic kidney disease. *Nutr Met Cardiovasc Dis.* 2016;26:597–602.
127. Krishnamurthy VM, Wei G, Baird BC, et al. High dietary fiber intake is associated with decreased inflammation and all-cause mortality in patients with chronic kidney disease. *Kidney Int.* 2012;81:300–306.
143. Jiang Z, Zhang X, Yang L, et al. Effect of restricted protein diet supplemented with keto analogues in chronic kidney disease: a systematic review and meta-analysis. *Int Urol Nephrol.* 2016;48:409–418.
144. Cirillo M, Cavallo P, Bilancio G, et al. Low protein intake in the population: low risk of kidney function decline but high risk of mortality. *J Ren Nutr.* 2017;doi:10.1053/j.jrn.2017.11.004.
146. Klahr S, Levey AS, Beck GJ, et al. Modification of Diet in Renal Disease Group: the effects of dietary protein restriction and blood-pressure control on the progression of chronic renal disease. *N Engl J Med.* 1994;330:877–884.
147. Noce A, Vidiri MF, Moriconi E, et al. Is low-protein diet a possible risk factor of malnutrition in chronic kidney disease patients? *Cell Death Discov.* 2016;doi:10.1038/cddiscovery.2016.2016.26.
149. Soroka N, Silverberg DS, Greemland M, et al. Comparison of a vegetable-based (soya) and animal-based low-protein diet in predialysis chronic renal failure patients. *Nephron.* 1998;79:173–180.
154. Bailey JL, Wang XN, England BK, et al. The acidosis of chronic renal failure activates muscle proteolysis in rats by augmenting transcription of genes encoding proteins of the ATP-dependent ubiquitin-proteosome pathway. *J Clin Invest.* 1996;97:1447–1453.
156. Papadoyannakis NJ, Stefanidis CJ, McGeown M. The effect of correction of metabolic acidosis on nitrogen and protein balance of patients with chronic renal failure. *Am J Clin Nutr.* 1984;40:623–627.
157. Ballmer PE, McNarlan MA, Hulter HN, et al. Chronic metabolic acidosis decreases albumin synthesis and induces negative nitrogen balance in humans. *J Clin Invest.* 1995;95:39–45.
158. Verove C, Maisonneuve N, El Azouzi A, et al. Effect of the correction of metabolic acidosis on nutritional status in elderly patients with chronic renal failure. *J Ren Nutr.* 2002;12:224–228.
160. Goraya N, Simoni J, Jo C-H, et al. Comparison of treating the metabolic acidosis of CKD stage 4. hypertensive kidney disease with fruits and vegetables or sodium bicarbonate. *Clin J Am Soc Nephrol.* 2013;8:371–381.
161. KDIGO Guidelines. Chapter 3: management of progression and complications of CKD. *Kidney Int.* 2013;(suppl 3):73–90.
167. McMahon E, Campbell K. A randomized trial of dietary sodium restriction in CKD. *J Am Soc Nephrol.* 2013;24:2096–2103.
168. Saran R, Padilla RL, Gillespie BW, et al. A randomized crossover trial of dietary sodium restriction in stage 3-4. CKD. *Clin J Am Soc Nephrol.* 2017;12:399–407.
170. St-Jules DE, Goldfarb DS, Sevick MA. Nutrient non-equivalence: does restricting high potassium plant foods help to prevent hyperkalemia in hemodialysis patients? *J Ren Nutr.* 2016;26:282–287.
177. Moe SM, Zidehsarai MP, Chambers MA, et al. Vegetarian compared with meat dietary protein source and phosphorous homeostasis in chronic kidney disease. *Clin J Am Soc Nephrol.* 2011;6:257–264.
178. Moorthi RN, Armstrong CLH, Janda K, et al. The effect of a diet containing 70% protein from plants on mineral metabolism and musculoskeletal health in chronic kidney disease. *Am J Nephrol.* 2014;40:582–591.
186. De Fornasari MLL, dos Santos Sens YA. Replacing phosphorous-containing food additives with foods without additives reduces phosphatemia in end-stage renal disease patients: a randomized clinical trial. *J Ren Nutr.* 2017;27:97–105.
195. Rossi M, Johnson DW, Xu H, et al. Dietary protein-fiber ratio associates with circulating levels of indoxyl sulfate and p-cresyl sulfate in chronic kidney disease patients. *Nutr Metab Cardiovasc Dis.* 2015;25:860–865.
214. Johnson AE, Boulware LE, Anderson CAM, et al. Perceived barriers and facilitators of using dietary modification for CKD prevention among African Americans of low socioeconomic status: a qualitative study. *BMC Nephrol.* 2014;15:194–202.

61

# Drug Dosing Considerations in Patients With Acute Kidney Injury and Chronic Kidney Disease

Gary R. Matzke | Frieder Keller | Marisa Battistella

## CHAPTER OUTLINE



## KEY POINTS

- Chronic kidney disease (CKD) results in alterations in the absorption, volume of distribution ($V_D$), metabolism, and elimination of most drugs.
- The $V_D$ of many drugs is increased in the presence of acute and CKD as a consequence of volume expansion and/or reduced protein binding.
- In addition to the expected decrement in renal clearance, nonrenal clearance (i.e., gastrointestinal and hepatic drug metabolism) of several drugs is also reduced in CKD patients.
- Individualization of a drug dosage regimen for a patient with reduced kidney function is based on the pharmacodynamic/pharmacokinetic characteristics of the drug, the patient's degree of residual renal function, and his or her overall clinical condition.
- Patient covariates, disease covariates, and pharmacogenetics all contribute to variability in drug disposition.
- The drug dosing guidelines for CKD patients in many drug information resources are highly variable and many are not optimal for clinical use.
- The effect of hemodialysis, peritoneal dialysis, and continuous renal replacement therapy on drug elimination is dependent on the characteristics of the drug and the dialysis prescription.
- Prospective monitoring of serum concentrations is often warranted, especially for narrow therapeutic index drugs.

It is estimated that 10% to 15% of the global population had chronic kidney disease (CKD) and the number of deaths from CKD has risen by more than 80% in the past 2 decades.[1–3] The prevalence varies widely across the world, in part, because of differences in the prevalence of CKD; heterogeneity of the laboratory methods used to detect CKD; and environmental factors, public health policies, and genetics.[3] The incidence of CKD has more than doubled in the past 20 years in adults older than 65 years.[4] This is due to age-related reductions in kidney function, multiple medical comorbidities, increases in the prevalence of older individuals who have survived cardiovascular disease, and an increased use of medications that alter kidney function, among others.[5] CKD can affect multiple organ systems, and the associated pathophysiologic changes can profoundly alter the pharmacokinetics (PK) and pharmacodynamics (PD) of many drugs.[5–7] Clinicians must assess kidney function and consider how it alters the disposition of drugs and their active or toxic metabolites to optimize the health outcomes of their patients.

The epidemiology of acute kidney injury (AKI) varies widely due to the variability in the criteria used to evaluate the patient.[8] A the disorder has a frequency of 2% in hospitalized patients, its prevalence among the critically ill is up to 30 times greater.[9–13] The number of patients with AKI has increased in the past 10 years in most regions of the world.[13] The development of some degree of CKD and/or need for chronic renal replacement therapy (RRT) are increasingly common among some survivors of AKI.[14] The widespread use of renal replacement therapies for treating patients with AKI (e.g., continuous venovenous hemodiafiltration) and end-stage kidney disease [ESKD; hemodialysis (HD) or hemodiafiltration] during the past decade mandates an understanding of their influences on drug disposition in the high-risk patients.[15,16] The advances in dialyzer technology and delivery systems have resulted in enhanced efficiency of dialysis treatments for many patients. Unfortunately, rarely have these advances been accompanied by reevaluations of the influence of dialysis on drug disposition.[6,7,17] Although innovation in peritoneal dialysis has been more modest, few studies have examined the effects of newer adequacy targets, or the use of non-dextrose–containing peritoneal dialysates on drug disposition.

Medications that are predominantly eliminated unchanged (fractional extraction [FE]) by the kidney may accumulate in CKD patients, which can increase the risk of adverse effects. As a general concept, if 30% or more of a drug is eliminated unchanged in the urine, it will have a high likelihood of requiring dosage regimen adjustment in CKD patients, especially those with stage 3 to 5 disease.[5,7,18] The PK of drugs with an FE less than 30% also may be affected and thus require a dose adjustment. In fact, 32.2% of such drugs approved in the United States from 1998 to 2010 had a dosage-adjustment recommendation for CKD patients in the product labeling.[19] Despite an increasing number of renal studies by the pharmaceutical and biotechnology industry and improvements in approved product labeling language, challenges remain for dose adjustments in CKD patients, especially for oncology and antiretroviral agents.[20]

Although PK and PD studies in CKD patients are done for an increasing percentage of drugs, for up to 70+% in the United States in the past decade the results are often not published in a timely fashion, if at all.[19] Regulatory authorities have not yet responded to the challenge of ensuring robust data for patients with impaired kidney function by requiring a PK and PD investigation plan as a routine part of drug development.[6] Furthermore, patients with moderate to severe CKD are typically excluded from participation in major safety and efficacy studies required for drug registration. Therefore the usefulness of the dosage recommendations, if developed early, cannot be evaluated in those with the disease or condition for which they are intended. Data on the use of many drugs in patients with CKD, as well as the impact of dialysis, are often limited or absent for years after regulatory approval. If there is no official dosage regimen recommendation in the product labeling, an adjustment may be calculated on the basis of the drug's FE and the ratio of the patient's residual renal function relative to an age and gender normal value for estimated creatinine clearance (eCrCl) or estimated glomerular filtration rate (eGFR).[21,22]

The pharmaceutical industry began to investigate the relationship of kidney function to the PK and PD of the drugs they had in development in the 1970s. Regulatory guidance or clinical consensus on when investigations should be conducted and with what degree of rigor, however, did not appear until the late 1990s and they continue to evolve.[23] Thus much of the data on the PK of drugs in patients with kidney disease were the result of clinician-initiated, postmarketing studies. Significant differences exist with respect to the means of assessment of kidney function and classification of the degree of impaired kidney function in those studies that have been conducted.[18] Studies conducted to meet global regulatory expectations have resulted in the generation of conflicting results for some drugs, in part, because of the differences in the ethnic composition of the patient population, the study design (single dose vs. multiple dose), and the data analysis methods that were used. This has contributed to marked variability among common sources for renal drug dosage recommendations.[24–27] The availability of robust and reliable information to guide prescribing for patients with kidney disease remains challenging. Despite the availability of this extensive collection of published evidence, dosing errors in CKD patients still occur at an alarming rate.[20,28–30] The expanded use of electronic medical records has not resolved the need for clinician proactivity to optimize the use of medications in CKD patients; in these studies, up to 85% of the medications ordered had nephrotoxic potential and greater than 20% of the drugs ordered were not dose adjusted for the patient's kidney function.[28,31–33] Thus the optimization of therapy for AKI and CKD patients is ultimately dependent on the clinicians' utilization of the data that are available and in many cases presented to them via electronic medical record system alerts at the time of prescribing.

In this chapter, the influence of AKI and CKD on drug PK properties is characterized, and a guide for individualizing drug therapy in patients with AKI and CKD is presented. We also present dosage recommendations for many commonly used drugs. The role of PK measures alone, their use in combination with PD, and pharmacogenetic testing in drug dosage regimen design are all discussed. The impact on drug disposition on either maintenance dialysis for ESKD or continuous RRT (CRRT) for patients with AKI is discussed. Again, dosage recommendations for many critical drugs are presented.

## EFFECTS OF AKI AND CKD ON DRUG DISPOSITION

PK describes the time course of drug absorption, distribution, metabolism, and elimination. PD provides a characterization of the complex interaction of drug concentrations, receptor–drug interactions, mechanism of action, and clinical factors, such as concurrent diseases and degree of organ dysfunction on patients' response to drug therapy. The combination of PK and PD drug characteristics allows clinicians with foundational information to make rational prescribing decisions.

When given intravenously (IV), a rapid decrease in the plasma concentration follows an initial high drug concentration. This decrease occurs as the drug distributes from the

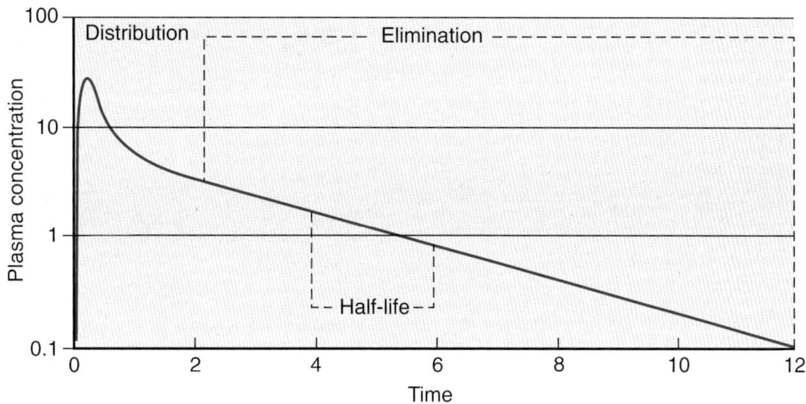


**Fig. 61.1** Distribution and elimination of a drug after intravenous administration.

plasma into the extravascular space and beyond. During the terminal elimination phase, drug concentrations in plasma are in equilibrium with concentrations in body tissues (Fig. 61.1). The rate and extent of drug absorption and distribution and rate of drug elimination may be ascertained by mathematical analysis of the serum or plasma concentration data collected over an appropriate time interval. The terminal elimination half-life of a drug is the time required for the plasma concentration to decline by 50%; this can be determined from the slope during the elimination phase of the plot of serum or plasma drug concentration versus time after the drug is ingested or injected. By comparing PK data from patients with normal kidney function with PK data from patients with impaired kidney function, rational drug dosing regimens may be proposed.[21,22]

## ABSORPTION

Drugs given IV enter the central circulation directly and generally have a rapid onset of action. Drugs given by other routes must first pass through important organs of elimination before entering the systemic circulation; thus a smaller proportion of the drug reaches the systemic circulation. In many cases, only a fraction of the administered dose may reach the circulation and become available at the site of drug action. Even drugs given IV and by inhalation must pass though the lungs before reaching arterial blood. Similar to other organs, the lungs remove substantial amounts of some agents (e.g., removal of IV administered adenosine by passage through the pulmonary circulation). For drugs administered orally, the rate and extent of gastrointestinal (GI) absorption are important considerations. Absorption has been characterized by determining the maximum attained serum or plasma concentration ($C_{max}$), as well as the time after ingestion when the $C_{max}$ was observed ($T_{max}$). Differences in these two parameters among patient groups were historically considered evidence of altered GI absorption when actually the bioavailability may have been unchanged.[34] The bioavailability of a drug depends on the extent of metabolism during its first pass through the intestinal wall and liver before reaching the systemic circulation. The absolute bioavailability is determined by comparing the area under the serum/plasma concentration–time curve (AUC) after oral administration with that observed after IV administration. When this measure of bioavailability was assessed, there were very few drugs shown to be affected by the presence of CKD or AKI.[7,35]

First-pass biotransformation may also occur in the gut; bioflavonoids in grapefruit juice can inhibit cytochrome P450 (CYP) 3A4 and noncompetitively inhibit the metabolism of drugs metabolized by this enzyme. This grapefruit juice–CYP3A4 interaction was first noted with the calcium channel blocker felodipine.[36] This interaction also increases the bioavailability of cyclosporine by as much as 20%.[37] A wide variety of other drugs are similarly affected, including several medications used for depression and anxiety (e.g., selective serotonin reuptake inhibitors, serotonin–norepinephrine reuptake inhibitors) and statins.[38] Herbal medicine (e.g., hypericin, one of the constituents of St. John's wort) can activate the adenosine triphosphate–binding cassette transporter or P-glycoprotein (multidrug resistance) transporter in gut mucosa, leading to reduced drug absorption.[39]

Although GI symptoms are common in patients with ESKD, little specific information about alimentary function is available. The salivary concentration of urea increases when urea accumulates in plasma. Ammonia forms from urea in the presence of gastric urease and buffers gastric acid, increasing gastric pH. The ammonia is absorbed and converted to urea again by the liver. The gastric alkalinizing effect of this internal urea–ammonia cycle decreases the absorption of drugs that are best absorbed in an acidic environment. Drug malabsorption may be further aggravated by the increased use of various therapies to reduce gastric acidity and/or reduce phosphate absorption, especially in patients who are dialysis dependent.[40,41] The resultant chelation and formation of nonabsorbable complexes reduce the bioavailability of some drugs, including several antibiotics and digoxin.

The processes of GI drug absorption are complex, may be saturable and dose dependent, and are more variable in patients with ESKD than in those with normal kidney function. Gastroparesis, commonly observed in patients with diabetes mellitus, many of whom also have CKD, prolongs gastric emptying and delays drug absorption (i.e., $T_{max}$ is observed to be delayed). Conversely, diarrhea decreases gut transit time ($T_{max}$ is shortened and diminishes drug absorption by the small bowel). Gut mucosal integrity becomes impaired across the spectrum of CKD, as evidenced by increasing levels of circulating translocated endotoxins.[42]

## DISTRIBUTION

The volume of distribution ($V_D$) of a drug does not necessarily correspond to a specific anatomic space. Rather, the $V_D$ is a mathematical construct based on the plasma concentration achieved following the IV administration of a given dose of a drug. Agents that are highly protein bound and those that are water soluble tend to be restricted to the vascular compartment and extracellular fluid (ECF) space, respectively, and thus have volumes of distribution less than 0.20 L/kg. Highly lipid-soluble drugs and those extensively bound to tissues often exhibit volumes of distribution in excess of 1 L/kg. The drug distribution volume of highly water-soluble or protein-bound drugs may be increased in patients with AKI or CKD if edema and/or ascites is present (Table 61.1).[5,7,35,43] Drug distribution is one of the most important and complicated factors to quantify in patients with AKI. There is a fine balance between detrimental fluid overload and adequate hydration to preserve and optimize perfusion and function. Critically ill patients should be managed in a slightly negative fluid balance after initial adequate fluid resuscitation has been achieved.[44–46] If patients are volume expanded, the administration of the usual doses of many drugs will result in inadequately low plasma concentrations.

The distribution volume of drugs may be altered by fluid removal during dialysis. Changes in body cell mass (nonfat, nonwater, nonbone mineral mass) commonly occur over time in patients on dialysis, resulting in sarcopenia.[47] Failure to detect a reduction in body cell mass may lead to inappropriate maintenance of the same dry weight and drug dosage regimen, despite a real increase in total body water (and thus the distribution volume of several drugs).[48] Finally, the method used to calculate the $V_D$ may be influenced by impaired kidney function. The three most commonly used $V_D$ terms are volume of the central compartment ($V_c$), volume of the terminal phase ($V_\beta$ and $V_{area}$), and $V_D$ at steady state ($V_{ss}$). The $V_c$ for many drugs approximates ECF volume and thus may be increased or decreased by acute changes. Oliguric acute renal failure is often accompanied by fluid overload and a resultant increased $V_c$ for many drugs. The $V_{area}$ or $V_\beta$ represents the proportionality constant between plasma concentrations in the terminal elimination phase and the amount of drug remaining in the body. $V_\beta$ is affected by distribution characteristics and by the terminal elimination rate constant. $V_\beta$ and $V_{ss}$ will often be similar in magnitude, with $V_\beta$ being slightly larger. Because $V_{ss}$ has the advantage of being independent of drug elimination, it is the most appropriate volume term to use when it is desirable to compare drug distribution volumes between patients with renal insufficiency and those with normal renal function.[49]

Alterations of plasma protein binding in patients with CKD can also affect drug distribution and elimination. The $V_D$ of a drug, quantity of unbound drug available for action, and the degree to which the agent is eliminated by hepatic or renal excretion are all influenced by protein binding. Drugs that are protein bound attach reversibly to albumin or $\alpha_1$-glycoprotein in plasma (Fig. 61.2). Whereas organic acids bind to a single binding site, organic bases probably have multiple sites of attachment.[50–53]

Protein-bound organic acids such as hippuric acid, indoxyl sulfate, and 3-carboxy-4-methyl-5-propyl-2-furanpropionic acid accumulate in advanced CKD and decrease the protein binding of many acidic drugs.[53,54] A combination of decreased serum albumin concentration and reduction in albumin affinity for the drug reduces protein binding in dialysis-dependent patients. Even when the plasma albumin concentration is normal, the protein-binding defect of

**Table 61.1 Volume of Distribution of Selected Drugs in Patients With Normal Kidney Function and Those on Dialysis**

| Drug | Normal (L/kg) | Stage 5 Chronic Kidney Disease (L/kg) | Change From Normal (%) |
|---|---|---|---|
| **Increased** | | | |
| Amikacin | 0.20 | 0.29 | 45 |
| Cefazolin | 0.13 | 0.17 | 31 |
| Cefoxitin | 0.16 | 0.26 | 63 |
| Ceftriaxone | 0.28 | 0.48 | 71 |
| Cefuroxime | 0.20 | 0.26 | 30 |
| Doripenem | 0.25 | 0.47 | 88 |
| Dicloxacillin | 0.08 | 0.18 | 125 |
| Erythromycin | 0.57 | 1.09 | 91 |
| Furosemide | 0.11 | 0.18 | 64 |
| Gentamicin | 0.20 | 0.32 | 60 |
| Isoniazid | 0.6 | 0.8 | 33 |
| Minoxidil | 2.6 | 4.9 | 88 |
| Naproxen | 0.12 | 0.17 | 42 |
| Phenytoin | 0.64 | 1.4 | 119 |
| Trimethoprim | 1.36 | 1.83 | 35 |
| Vancomycin | 0.64 | 0.85 | 33 |
| **Decreased** | | | |
| Atenolol | 1.2 | 0.9 | –25 |
| Chloramphenicol | 0.87 | 0.60 | –31 |
| Ciprofloxacin | 2.5 | 1.95 | –22 |
| Digoxin | 7.3 | 4.0 | –45 |
| Ethambutol | 3.7 | 1.6 | –57 |
| Methicillin | 0.45 | 0.3 | –33 |
| Metoprolol | 5.6 | 1.0 | –82 |
| Pindolol | 2.1 | 1.1 | –48 |
| Propranolol | 4.4 | 3.6 | –18 |

Data from Matzke GR, Nolin TN. Drug dosing in renal disease. In: Bomback A, Gilbert S, Perazella M, et al., eds. *National Kidney Foundation Primer on Kidney Diseases*. 7th ed. Philadelphia: Elsevier; 2017; Heintz BH, Matzke GR, Dager WE. Antimicrobial dosing concepts and recommendations for critically ill adult patients receiving continuous renal replacement therapy or intermittent hemodialysis. *Pharmacotherapy* 2009;29:562–577; Thummel KE, Shen DD, Isoherranen N. Appendix II. Design and optimization of dosage regimens: pharmacokinetic data. In: Brunton LL, Chabner BA, Knollmann BC, eds. *Goodman & Gilman's The Pharmacological Basis of Therapeutics*. 12th ed. New York: McGraw-Hill; 2011; Murphy JE. *Clinical Pharmacokinetics Pocket Reference*. 5th ed. Bethesda, MD: American Society of Health-System Pharmacists; 2015; Verbeeck RK, Musuamba FT. Pharmacokinetics and dosage adjustment in patients with renal dysfunction. *Eur J Clin Pharmacol.* 2009;65:757–773; and Olyaei AJ, Steffl JL. A quantitative approach to drug dosing in chronic kidney disease. *Blood Purif.* 2011;31:138–145.

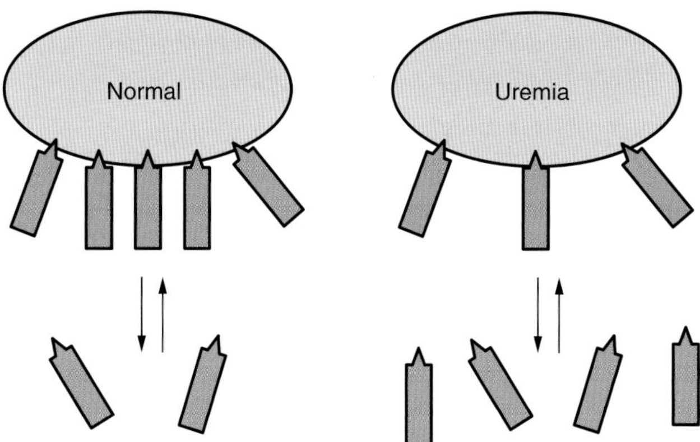


**Fig. 61.2 Protein-binding defect in uremia.** Displacement of the drug from its binding site by an accumulation of undefined uremic toxins or a uremia-induced conformational change in the binding-site geometry results in more free drug in the plasma.

some drugs correlates directly with the level of azotemia and may be corrected with dialysis.[5,7,55] Binding affinity is influenced by changes in the structural orientation of the albumin molecule or by the accumulation of endogenous inhibitors of protein binding that compete with drugs for their binding sites.[50]

The unbound fraction of several acidic drugs is increased in CKD because of impaired plasma protein binding. Toxicity can occur if the total plasma concentration of these drugs is pushed into the therapeutic range by increasing the dose, wherein the free (active) concentration may be in the supratherapeutic range. For such drugs, unbound plasma concentrations should be measured to guide therapy. The need to measure unbound drug concentrations applies especially to drugs with very narrow therapeutic ranges, such as phenytoin.[55] Predicting the clinical consequences of altered protein binding is difficult. Although decreased binding results in more unbound drug being available at the site of drug action or toxicity, the distribution volume is increased, resulting in lower plasma concentrations after a given dose. More unbound drug is available for metabolism and excretion, which increases the clearance and decreases the half-life of the drug in the body. Drugs with decreased protein binding in patients on dialysis are listed in Table 61.2.

## METABOLISM

The disposition of drugs metabolized by the liver may be altered by changes in plasma protein binding. The systemic clearance of a highly protein-bound drug with a low hepatic extraction ratio depends on the simultaneous effects of AKI or CKD on protein binding and intrinsic metabolic drug clearance. Because the effects of severe CKD on these two factors offset each other in terms of total systemic clearance, the lowest total systemic clearance is not seen in patients with ESKD but rather occurs in patients with moderate to severe CKD. The systemic clearance of drugs with a high hepatic extraction ratio is not thought to be as susceptible to the effect of CKD as that of drugs with a low extraction ratio.[56]

**Table 61.2 Unbound Fraction of Selected Drugs in Patients With Normal Kidney Function and End-Stage Kidney Disease (ESKD)**

| Drug | Normal Patient | ESKD Patient | Change From Normal (%) |
|---|---|---|---|
| **Acidic Drugs** | | | |
| Abecarnil | 4 | 15 | 275 |
| Azlocillin | 62.5 | 75 | 20 |
| Cefazolin | 16 | 29 | 81 |
| Cefoxitin | 27 | 59 | 119 |
| Ceftriaxone | 10 | 20 | 100 |
| Clofibrate | 3 | 9 | 200 |
| Dicloxacillin | 3 | 9 | 200 |
| Diflunisal | 12 | 44 | 267 |
| Doxycycline | 12 | 28 | 133 |
| Furosemide | 4 | 6 | 50 |
| Methotrexate | 57.2 | 63.8 | 12 |
| Metolazone | 5 | 10 | 100 |
| Moxalactam | 48 | 64 | 33 |
| Pentobarbital | 34 | 41 | 21 |
| Phenytoin | 10 | 21.5 | 115 |
| Salicylate | 8 | 20 | 150 |
| Sulfamethoxazole | 34 | 58 | 71 |
| Valproic acid | 8 | 23 | 188 |
| Warfarin | 1 | 2 | 100 |
| **Basic Drugs** | | | |
| **Decreased** | | | |
| Bepridil | 0.3 | 0.1 | −67 |
| Clonidine | 55.6 | 47.6 | −14 |
| Disopyramide | 32 | 28 | −13 |
| Propafenone | 3.4 | 2.4 | −29 |
| **Increased** | | | |
| Amphotericin B | 3.5 | 4.1 | 17 |
| Chloramphenicol | 45 | 64 | 42 |
| Clonazepam | 13.9 | 16 | 15 |
| Diazepam | 2 | 8 | 300 |
| Fluoxetine | 5.5 | 6.5 | 18 |
| Ketoconazole | 1 | 1.5 | 50 |
| Prazosin | 6 | 10.1 | 68 |
| Rosiglitazone | 0.16 | 0.22 | 38 |
| Triamterene | 19 | 43 | 126 |

Data from Matzke GR, Nolin TN. Drug dosing in renal disease. In: Bomback A, Gilbert S, Perazella M, et al., eds. *National Kidney Foundation Primer on Kidney Diseases*. 7th ed. Philadelphia: Elsevier; 2017; Heintz BH, Matzke GR, Dager WE. Antimicrobial dosing concepts and recommendations for critically ill adult patients receiving continuous renal replacement therapy or intermittent hemodialysis. *Pharmacotherapy* 2009;29:562–577; Thummel KE, Shen DD, Isoherranen N. Appendix II. Design and optimization of dosage regimens: pharmacokinetic data. In: Brunton LL, Chabner BA, Knollmann BC, eds. *Goodman & Gilman's The Pharmacological Basis of Therapeutics*. 12th ed. New York: McGraw-Hill; 2011; Murphy JE. *Clinical Pharmacokinetics Pocket Reference*. 5th ed. Bethesda, MD: American Society of Health-System Pharmacists; 2015; and Verbeeck RK, Musuamba FT. Pharmacokinetics and dosage adjustment in patients with renal dysfunction. *Eur J Clin Pharmacol.* 2009;65:757–773.

**Table 61.3 Drugs With Pharmacologically Active Metabolites That May Affect Efficacy or Toxicity in Patients With Severe Chronic Kidney Disease**

| Parent Drug | Metabolite | Pharmacologic Activity of Metabolites |
|---|---|---|
| Acetaminophen | *N*-Acetyl-*p*-benzoquinoneimine | Responsible for hepatotoxicity |
| Allopurinol | Oxipurinol | Metabolite primarily responsible for suppression of xanthine oxidase |
| Azathioprine | Mercaptopurine | All immunosuppressive activity resides in the metabolite |
| Cefotaxime | Desacetyl cefotaxime | Similar antimicrobial spectrum, but 10% to 25% as potent |
| Chlorpropamide | 2-Hydroxychlorpropamide | Similar in vitro insulin-releasing activity |
| Clofibrate | Chlorophenoxyisobutyric acid | Primarily responsible for hypolipidemic effect and direct muscle toxicity |
| Codeine | Morphine-6-glucuronide | Possibly more active than parent compound; may contribute to prolonged narcotic effect in renal failure patients |
| Imipramine | Desmethylimipramine | Similar antidepressant activity |
| Ketoprofen | Ketoprofen glucuronide | Accumulation of acyl glucuronide may worsen toxic effects (GI disturbances, impairment of kidney function) |
| Meperidine | Normeperidine | Less analgesic activity than parent, but more central nervous system stimulatory effects, epileptogenic |
| Morphine | Morphine-6-glucuronide | Possibly more active than parent compound; may contribute to prolonged narcotic effect in ESKD |
| Mycophenolic acid | Mycophenolic acid glucuronide | Lacks pharmacologic activity but may be associated with dose-limiting (GI) side effects |
| Procainamide | *N*-Acetyl procainamide | Distinct antiarrhythmic activity; mechanism different from that of parent compound |
| Sulfonamides | Acetylated metabolites | Devoid of antibacterial activity; elevated concentrations associated with increased toxicity |
| Theophylline | 1,3-Dimethyl uric acid | Cardiotoxicity has been demonstrated |
| Zidovudine | Zidovudine triphosphate | Primarily responsible for antiretroviral activity |

*ESKD,* End-stage kidney disease; *GI,* gastrointestinal.

Data from Matzke GR, Nolin TN. Drug dosing in renal disease. In: Bomback A, Gilbert S, Perazella M, et al., eds. *National Kidney Foundation Primer on Kidney Diseases*. 7th ed. Philadelphia: Elsevier; 2017; Thummel KE, Shen DD, Isoherranen N. Appendix II. Design and optimization of dosage regimens: pharmacokinetic data. In: Brunton LL, Chabner BA, Knollmann BC, eds. *Goodman & Gilman's The Pharmacological Basis of Therapeutics*. 12th ed. New York: McGraw-Hill; 2011; Naud J, Nolin TD, Leblond FA, et al. Current understanding of drug disposition in kidney disease. *J Clin Pharmacol.* 2012;52:10S–22S; and Batistellia M, Matzke GR. Drug dosing in renal failure. In: DiPiro J, Talbert R, Yee G, et al, eds. *Pharmacotherapy: A Pathophysiologic Approach*. 10th ed. New York: McGraw-Hill; 2017.

Many active or toxic metabolites depend on the kidneys for their removal from the body. The accumulation of these metabolites in patients with impaired kidney function (AKI and CKD) can explain, in part, the high incidence of adverse drug reactions in this patient population. For example, although the liver usually rapidly metabolizes morphine, it is categorized to be excreted mainly in the urine because its active metabolites, morphine-3-glucuronide (M3G) and morphine-6-glucuronide (M6G), readily cross the blood–brain barrier and bind to opiate receptors, exerting strong analgesic effects. In patients with CKD, morphine itself is metabolized more slowly, and these active metabolites increase, making prolonged narcosis and respiratory depression more likely.[57,58] Similarly, the biotransformation of meperidine results in the production of normeperidine, a more polar metabolite that is normally rapidly excreted in the urine. Normeperidine has little to no analgesic activity but lowers the seizure threshold. In patients with impaired kidney function, repeated doses of meperidine may result in the accumulation of this potentially toxic metabolite, with resultant seizures.[59] Table 61.3 lists some drugs that form active or toxic metabolites in CKD patients and have been associated with adverse outcomes.

## ALTERATIONS OF CYTOCHROME P450 ENZYME ACTIVITY

A decrease in the renal clearance ($Cl_R$) of drugs in patients with CKD is well appreciated. However, there is now preclinical and emerging clinical evidence suggesting that advanced CKD (stages 4 and 5) may lead to reductions in the nonrenal clearance of many medications as the result of alterations in the activities of uptake and efflux transporters, as well as CYP enzymes, in the liver and other organs (Table 61.4).[60–62] The effect(s) of AKI and CKD on nonrenal drug clearance appear to depend on whether the reduction in renal function is acute or chronic in nature—and based on recent evidence the dialysis modality (i.e., HD or peritoneal).[63]

Preservation of nonrenal metabolic clearance has been observed early in the course of AKI,[64–66] and thus drug dosing schemes extrapolated from those with stable CKD may therefore result in ineffectively low drug concentrations. Furthermore, failure to appreciate that changes in serum creatinine (sCr) levels are not an accurate marker of the GFR early in AKI may lead to further dosing errors. The first reports of nonrenal clearance of drugs being affected by AKI came from the observation that the residual nonrenal clearances of vancomycin, ceftriaxone, meropenem, and

**Table 61.4 Major Pathways of Nonrenal Drug Clearance ($Cl_{NR}$)**

| $Cl_{NR}$ Pathway | Selected Substrates |
|---|---|
| **Oxidative Enzymes** | |
| CYP1A2 | Polycyclic aromatic hydrocarbons, caffeine, imipramine, theophylline |
| CYP2A6 | Coumarin |
| CYP2B6 | Nicotine, bupropion |
| CYP2C8 | Retinoids, paclitaxel, repaglinide |
| CYP2C9 | Celecoxib, diclofenac, flurbiprofen, indomethacin, ibuprofen, losartan, phenytoin, tolbutamide, *S*-warfarin |
| CYP2C19 | Diazepam, *S*-mephenytoin, omeprazole |
| CYP2D6 | Codeine, debrisoquine, desipramine, dextromethorphan, fluoxetine, paroxetine, duloxetine, nortriptyline, haloperidol, metoprolol, propranolol |
| CYP2E1 | Ethanol, acetaminophen, chlorzoxazone, nitrosamines |
| CYP3A4/5 | Alprazolam, midazolam, cyclosporine, tacrolimus, nifedipine, felodipine, diltiazem, verapamil, fluconazole, ketoconazole, itraconazole, erythromycin, lovastatin, simvastatin, cisapride, terfenadine |
| **Conjugative Enzymes** | |
| UGT | Acetaminophen, morphine, lorazepam, oxazepam, naproxen, ketoprofen, irinotecan, bilirubin |
| NAT | Dapsone, hydralazine, isoniazid, procainamide |
| **Transporters** | |
| OATP1A2 | Bile salts, statins, fexofenadine, methotrexate, digoxin, levofloxacin |
| OATP1B1 | Bile salts, statins, fexofenadine, repaglinide, valsartan, olmesartan, irinotecan, bosentan |
| OATP1B3 | Bile salts, statins, fexofenadine, telmisartan, valsartan, olmesartan, digoxin |
| OATP2B1 | Statins, fexofenadine, glyburide |
| PGP | Digoxin, fexofenadine, loperamide, irinotecan, doxorubicin, vinblastine, paclitaxel, erythromycin |
| MRP2 | Methotrexate, etoposide, mitoxantrone, valsartan, olmesartan |
| MRP3 | Methotrexate, fexofenadine |

Data from Naud J, Nolin TD, Leblond FA, et al. Current understanding of drug disposition in kidney disease. *J Clin Pharmacol.* 2012;52:10S–22S; Yeung CK, Shen DD, Thummel KE, et al. Effects of chronic kidney disease and uremia on hepatic drug metabolism and transport. *Kidney Int*. 2014;85:522–528; Kagaya H, Niioka T, Saito M, et al. Effect of hepatic drug transporter polymorphisms on the pharmacokinetics of mycophenolic acid in patients with severe renal dysfunction before renal transplantation. *Xenobiotica* 2017;47:916–922; Thomson BK, Nolin TD, Velenosi TJ, et al. Effect of CKD and dialysis modality on exposure to drugs cleared by nonrenal mechanisms. *Am J Kidney Dis.* 2015;65:574–582; Joy MS, Frye RF, Nolin TD, et al. In vivo alterations in drug metabolism and transport pathways in patients with chronic kidney diseases. *Pharmacotherapy* 2014;34:114–122; Lee W, Kim RB. Transporters and renal drug elimination. *Annu Rev Pharmacol Toxicol.* 2004;44:137–166; Masereeuw R, Russel FGM. Therapeutic implications of renal anionic drug transporters. *Pharmacol Ther.* 2010;126:200–216; and Hsueh CH, Yoshida K, Zhao P, et al. Identification and quantitative assessment of uremic solutes as inhibitors of renal organic anion transporters, OAT1 and OAT3. *Mol Pharm.* 2016;13:3130–3140.

imipenem were higher in patients with AKI compared with patients with CKD, who had comparable CrCl.[64–67]

Most of the direct evidence on metabolism in the presence of AKI has been derived from investigations in animal models. A number of drugs have been studied in a variety of AKI models. AKI is a heterogenous insult that is often part of multisystem failure of cellular respiration, which can have protean consequences.[68–71] CYP enzymes are affected by AKI, and the extent of these effects may depend on the mechanism of experimental AKI. Definitive conclusions on the PK of metabolized medications in AKI remain hampered by the clinical complexity and potential confounders (hypoxia, decreased protein synthesis, competitive inhibition from concomitant medications, and decreased hepatic perfusion).

In humans with CKD, the activities of CYPs appear to be relatively unaffected.[60,72] It has been reported that CYP3A4 activity is reduced,[60] but recent studies have indicated that organic anion transporting polypeptide uptake activity is decreased.[72] Thus, the perceived changes in CYP3A4 activity were likely due to altered transporter activity, not to an alteration in CYP activity. The reduction of nonrenal clearance of several drugs that exhibit overlapping CYP and transporter substrate specificity in patients with stage 4 or 5 CKD supports this premise. These studies must be interpreted with caution, however, because concurrent drug intake, age, smoking status, and alcohol intake were often not taken into consideration. Furthermore, pharmacogenetic variations in drug-metabolizing enzymes that may have been present in the individual before the onset of AKI or CKD must also be considered.

## RENAL EXCRETION

Renal clearance ($Cl_R$) of a drug is the composite of the GFR, tubular secretion, metabolism, and reabsorption, where $f_u$ is the fraction of the drug unbound to plasma proteins.

$$Cl_R = (GFR \times f_u) + (Cl_{secretion} + Cl_{metabolism} - Cl_{reabsorption})$$

Drug elimination by filtration occurs by a pressure gradient, whereas tubular secretion and reabsorption are bidirectional processes that involve carrier-mediated renal transport systems.[60,73,74] Renal transport systems have been broadly classified on the basis of substrate selectivity into anionic and cationic renal transport systems, which are responsible for the transport of a number of organic acidic and basic drugs, respectively.[51,60] Several drugs are actively secreted by one or more of these transporter families, including organic cationic (e.g., famotidine, trimethoprim, dopamine), organic anionic (e.g., ampicillin, cefazolin, furosemide), nucleoside (e.g., zidovudine), and P-glycoprotein transporters (e.g., digoxin, *Vinca* alkaloids, steroids).[7,73,74] Alterations in filtration, secretion, or reabsorption secondary to CKD may have a dramatic effect on drug disposition.[75] For drugs that are primarily filtered, a reduction in GFR will result in a proportional decrease in renal drug clearance. However, recent evidence indicates that the clearance of cationic secreted drugs correlates poorly with measured GFR[76] and that uremic solutes inhibit OAT1 and OAT3 transporters and contribute to the decline in renal drug clearance in CKD patients.[75] OAT1 and 3 are multispecific exchangers or antiporters that transport predominantly anionic substrates against a concentration gradient from the blood into proximal tubule cells for subsequent elimination into the urine. The clinical impact of these findings limits the utility of eGFR for dosage regimen adjustment in CKD patients.

## PHARMACOGENOMICS

Over the past 2 decades, genome-wide analyses have identified genetic variants that are associated with either a relative increased or decreased risk of several diseases.[77,78] Most confer a low relative risk, are common alleles, and have low discriminatory and predictive values.[79,80] The combined effect of a number of common weak variants seems to more relevant. For example, the activity of different enzymes involved in warfarin and vitamin K metabolism has produced varying effects on anticoagulation. Genotyping data on two genes, the warfarin metabolic enzyme CYP2C9 and warfarin target enzyme vitamin K epoxide reductase complex 1 (VKORC1), confirmed that each can influence warfarin maintenance dose.[81] Two genome-wide association studies also found a weak, but significant, effect of CYP4F2 on warfarin dosing.[82,83] The presence of *CYP2C9*2* or *CYP2C9*3* variant alleles, which results in decreased metabolic enzyme activity, is associated with a significant decrease in the mean warfarin dose,[84] whereas *VKORC1* single-nucleotide polymorphisms identify *VKORC1* haplotypes accounting for a large fraction of the interindividual variation in warfarin dose.[85] The combination of both *VKORC1* and *CYP2C9* polymorphisms is associated with severe over-anticoagulation.[86] In contrast to these common but weak effect genetic variants, some DNA sequence variants are rare but have a strong effect; one example would be azathioprine. Polymorphisms in the gene that encodes thiopurine S-methyltransferase (*TPMT*) lead to reduced activity of this metabolizing enzyme, and patients with low activity (10% prevalence) or absent activity (0.3% prevalence) are at higher risk of bone marrow depression because of drug accumulation.[87,88] The variability in how patients respond to drug treatments is clearly a consequence of alterations in PK and PD, as well as differences in their genotypes and/or phenotypes.[78,89–94] In general, DNA sequence code variants affect prodrug activation (i.e., clopidogrel), drug metabolism and degradation (i.e., warfarin), or predisposition to adverse drug effects (i.e., azathioprine).

The validity of phenotyping cocktails and their correlation with genotyping data are still in need of clarification.[95] Genotyping information is becoming more widely available than phenotyping data and this increases demands for a more individualized approach to pharmacotherapy. A key question now arises—Will patients be willing to pay for these tests?[96] Genotypic characterization now serves as the basis for dosing recommendations for some drugs, and >120 U.S. Food and Drug Administration (FDA)–approved drugs have pharmacogenomic information in their labeling, including fluoropyrimidines, codeine, selective serotonin reuptake inhibitors, tricyclic antidepressants, β-blockers, opiates, neuroleptics, antiarrhythmic agents, and statins.[97–101]

However, the promise of pharmacogenomics has not always translated into improvements in patient care because of the inaccuracy of results and the complexities involved. In late 2013, the FDA approved four diagnostic, high-throughput, gene-sequencing devices, which represents a significant step forward in the ability to generate genomic information that will ultimately improve patient care.[102,103] As Collins and Hamburg[102] from the National Institutes of Health and FDA have stated, "There are many challenges ahead before personalized medicine can be considered truly embedded in health care. We need to continue to uncover variants within the genome that can be used to predict disease onset, affect progression, and modulate drug response." Their identification of challenges to clinical utilization has been answered, in part, with the recent publication of the implementation plans of several U.S. hospitals that have launched clinical services to guide clopidogrel and warfarin.[104] With the increase in the number of clinical genetic tests requested by health care providers, there has been an increase in direct-to-consumer advertising of genetic tests, including at-home tests and those provided by private companies.

Although similar to direct-to-consumer advertising of prescription drugs, marketing of genetic testing raises additional concerns and considerations. These include limited knowledge among patients and health care providers regarding accuracy and reliability of available genetic tests, difficulty in interpretation of genetic testing results, lack of governmental oversight of companies offering genetic testing, and issues of privacy and confidentiality. New genomic findings need to be validated before they can be integrated into medical decision making. Physicians and other health care professionals will need support in interpreting genomic data, integrating these into clinical decision making, and applying the results to individual patients. With the right information and support, patients will be able to participate with their physicians in making more informed decisions.

An example of the complexity of individualizing drug therapy on the basis of genomic information is illustrated with the anticoagulant warfarin. Two published trials raised significant questions regarding the value of genomic data to guide the initial dosing of this agent.[105,106] A genotype-guided approach to warfarin dosing failed to improve anticoagulation control during the first 4 weeks of treatment, according to the first of the articles.[105] Among 1015 patients assigned to usual care or usual care plus genotype, international normalized ratio (INR) results showed that the mean percentage of time in the therapeutic range at 4 weeks was 45.2% in the genotype-guided group and 45.4% in the usual care group. Moreover, rates of the combined outcome of an inappropriately high INR of 4 or more, major bleeding, or thromboembolism did not differ significantly according to dosing strategy.

The second study reported conflicting results in that pharmacogenetic-based dosing was associated with a slightly but significantly higher percentage of time in the therapeutic INR range, with significantly fewer incidences of excessive anticoagulation (INR ≥ 4.0) in the genotype-guided group.[106] Thus, at present, the use of genomic information to guide warfarin dosing in persons with normal kidney function, which is much less than dosing for patients with CKD or AKI, remains controversial.[107] There are, however, published guidelines on the use of *TPMT* genotyping for azathioprine dosing in clinical practice.[108,109] Several TPMT variant alleles exist, which vary in frequency among ethnic populations. In African and Asian individuals, *TPMT*3C* is the most frequent deficient allele (6.5% and 2.5%, respectively), whereas in white individuals *TPMT*3A* is the most frequently found variant (4.5%).[110] *TPMT* testing before the prescription of azathioprine is one of the few examples of a pharmacogenetic test that has definitively made the transition from research into clinical practice. This testing improves safety by avoiding full-dose treatment in patients with a (partial) enzyme deficiency. The future of pharmacogenetics will be in treatment models in which patient characteristics such as CKD or AKI are combined with polymorphism information regarding relevant genes.

## PHARMACODYNAMICS

The fundamental concept of PD is described by the Hill equation. This model has been extensively used to optimize the effects of many antimicrobial agents.[111] The principles are applicable to guide the dosing of medications in patients with CKD, as well as those with normal kidney function. In the patient with CKD, the concentration–time profile of many drugs is altered, so the dosage regimen predicted will likely be different than the normal regimen. This is because of the prolonged elimination half-life, which results in an increased AUC. Only rarely has there been evidence of an alteration in the PD concentration–effect relation in patients with AKI or CKD; PK changes predominantly contribute to the need for a modified dosing regimen.

The concentration (C) is the primary driving force that obligates altered dosage regimens to achieve the desired PD targets. The actual effect is a function of the maximum effect and the concentration producing the half-maximum effect. The Hill coefficient (H) is a measure of the sigmoidicity of the effect–concentration correlation:

$$E = \frac{E_{max}}{1 - \left(\frac{CE_{50}}{C}\right)^{H}}$$

From this equation, the threshold concentration, which produces 5% of the maximum effect, and the ceiling concentration, which is associated with 95% of the maximum effect, can be derived. The higher the Hill coefficient, the higher the threshold concentration and the narrower is the range of lower and upper target concentrations; this is because

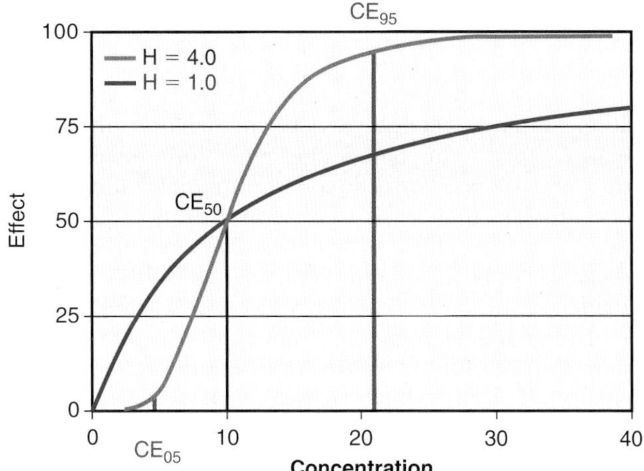


**Fig. 61.3 Threshold concentration, $CE_{05}$, producing 5% of the maximum effect and ceiling concentration, $CE_{95}$, producing 95% of the maximum effect.** With a Hill coefficient of H = 1.0, $CE_{05}$ = 0.5 and $CE_{95}$ = 190, whereas for H = 4.0, the threshold is higher, with $CE_{05}$ = 6.0, but the ceiling is much less, with $CE_{95}$ = 21 mg/L.

the ceiling concentration comes down close to the concentration producing the half-maximum effect (Fig. 61.3):

$$CE_{05} = 19^{\frac{-1}{H}} \bullet CE_{50}$$

$$CE_{95} = 19^{\frac{1}{H}} \bullet CE_{50}$$

The difference between the ceiling and threshold concentrations can be measured by multiples of the respective elimination half-life. The ceiling concentration is the upper limit of the targeted peak concentration ($C_{peak} < CE_{95}$), whereas the threshold concentration marks the lower limit of effective trough concentration ($C_{trough} > CE_{05}$). For a drug with a short half-life ($t_{1/2}$) and a high Hill coefficient, the therapeutic range of target concentrations can be very small (Fig. 61.3):

$$CE_{05} = CE_{95} \bullet \exp\left[-\frac{\ln(2)}{t_{1/2}} \bullet t\right]$$

$$t_{ceiling-threshold} = t_{1/2} \bullet \frac{2}{H} \bullet \frac{\ln(19)}{\ln(2)}$$

$$t_{ceiling-threshold} = t_{1/2} \bullet \frac{8.5}{H}$$

For the β-lactam ceftazidime, with a short half-life of 2.1 hours in patients with normal kidney function but with a high Hill coefficient of 3.7,[112] the peak to trough or ceiling to threshold time of 5 hours indicates that ceftazidime should be given at least every 6 hours to maximize efficacy. By contrast, and in agreement with the postulated postantibiotic effect, the maximum peak to trough time is estimated as 13 hours for gentamicin, with a half-life of 2 hours but a Hill coefficient of 1.3.[112]

The most important progress in antiinfective dosing has been achieved with the differentiation of drugs with time-dependent actions from drugs with concentration-dependent actions.[113,114] Specific examples are the β-lactam antibiotics and antiviral drugs with a known time-dependent effect, whereas aminoglycosides and quinolones have a concentration-dependent activity. The threshold and ceiling concentrations are specific functions of the concentration producing the half-maximum effect and the Hill coefficient. Both can be used to explain the observation that antiinfective drugs with a time-dependent effect have a significantly higher Hill coefficient than those with a concentration-dependent action.[112] A high Hill coefficient is associated with a high threshold concentration but, simultaneously, with a relatively low ceiling concentration. Thus, it makes no sense to increase the dose of time-dependent antiinfective drugs above the ceiling concentration. By contrast, a low Hill coefficient is associated with a high ceiling concentration and low threshold concentration. Thus it might increase the effect of concentration-dependent antiinfective drugs to give a high single dose but it is not so critical to extend the administration interval, as proposed for aminoglycosides.[115] Practically, it is necessary to administer antiinfective drugs with a time-dependent action more frequently, whereas antiinfective drugs with a concentration-dependent action should be given with a higher maintenance dose to increase efficacy (Fig. 61.4).

Usual measures of the antimicrobial effect, such as the minimal inhibitory concentrations (MICs), AUC over MIC, time over MIC (T > MIC), or peak over MIC, can be unified to the following concept. The target concentration should not be less than the threshold concentration for time-dependent effects, but it could be as high as the ceiling concentration for concentration-dependent effects. A close correlation of the MIC and concentration producing the half-maximum effect has been postulated.[112] It was obvious, however, that for concentration-dependent antimicrobial action, the MIC could fall considerably below the concentration producing the half-maximum effect ($MIC \ll CE_{50}$). Consequently, it might be more reasonable to compare the bacteriologic MIC with the PD parameter of a threshold concentration:

$$CE_{threshold} = CE_{05} = MIC$$

From the Hill coefficient, one can postulate that the time-dependent action and concentration-dependent action are only the extreme positions of a continuum. Every drug can be considered as concentration dependent and time dependent. To overcome resistance, a higher dose might be necessary, because relative resistance can be seen in cases in which a high concentration is required to produce the half-maximum effect. The potency is the inverse concentration producing the half-maximum effect:

$$\text{Potency} = \frac{1}{CE_{50}}$$

This concept distinguishes a relative resistance from an absolute drug resistance. A pathogen with a relative resistance can be made sensitive by increasing the dose.[116–118] Thus, for example, it has been recommended to treat severe infections with resistant strains by increasing the standard meropenem dose from 1000 mg/day, 3 times daily, to 2000 mg/day, 3 times daily,[119] or the daptomycin dose from 4–6 mg/kg/day to >8 mg/kg/day,[120] with careful monitoring of side effects.

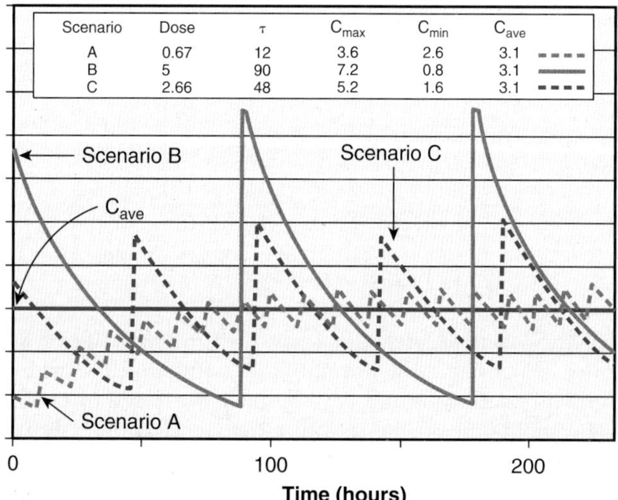


**Fig. 61.4** Although the average steady-state concentrations *($C_{ave}$)* are identical regardless of which dosage adjustment strategy one decides to use, the concentration–time profile will be markedly different if one changes the dose and maintains the dosing interval *(τ)* constant *(Scenario A)*, versus changing the dosing interval and maintaining the dose constant *(Scenario B)*, or changing both *(Scenario C)*.

> ***Clinical Relevance***
> Pharmacogenetic factors predicting therapeutic response and toxicity in patients with kidney disease are emerging. However, the unpredictable changes in pharmacokinetic pathways of absorption, distribution, and elimination (metabolism, transport, and excretion) of prescribed drugs observed in patients with acute kidney injury and chronic kidney disease can confound the outcomes of personalized therapeutic interventions.

## ASSESSMENT OF KIDNEY FUNCTION

The standard measure of kidney function for decades has been the GFR. GFR can be measured using many exogenous substances; however, the administration of exogenous substances is not practical for routine individual drug dose calculations in clinical practice because the procedures are not timely and not uniformly available.

### CHRONIC KIDNEY DISEASE

Although GFR has been estimated based on the measured urinary clearance of creatinine (mCrCl) derived from a 24-hour urine collection, the eCrCl or eGFR (Table 61.5) is predominantly determined in clinical practice for calculation from the sCr and/or cystatin C (CysC) concentrations and patient factors.[121–127] After years of quiescence it seems like there is a new renal function assessment tool published every few months for the past several years. The introduction of these new GFR predictive methodologies, some focused on

**Table 61.5 Equations for Estimation of Creatinine Clearance or Glomerular Filtration Rate in Adults With Stable Renal Function[a,b]**

| Reference | Equation |
|---|---|
| Cockcroft and Gault (1976) | Men: CrCl = (140 − age)IBW/(sCr × 72)<br>Women: CrCl × 0.85 |
| Jelliffe (1973) | Men: CrCl = 98 − [0.8 (age − 20)]/sCr<br>Women: CrCl × 0.9 |
| MDRD6 (1999) | eGFRCr = 170 × $(sCr)^{-0.999}$ × $(age)^{-0.176}$ × (0.762 if patient is female) × (1.180 if patient is black) × $(BUN)^{-0.170}$ × $(Alb)^{0.318}$ |
| MDRD4 (2000) | eGFRCr = 186 × $(sCr)^{-1.154}$ × $(age)^{-0.203}$ × (0.742 if patient is female) × (1.210 if patient is black) |
| MDRD4-IDMS (2007) | eGFRCr = 175 × $(sCr)^{-1.154}$ × $(age)^{-0.203}$ × (0.742 if patient is female) × (1.210 if patient is black) |
| CKD-EPI (2009) | eGFRCr = 141 × $\min(sCr/\kappa, 1)^{\alpha}$ × $\max(sCr/\kappa, 1)^{-1.209}$ × $0.993^{age}$ × (1.018 if patient is female) × (1.159 if patient is black)<br>• κ is 0.7 for females and 0.9 for males.<br>• α is −0.329 for females and −0.411 for males.<br>• min is the minimum of sCr/κ or 1.<br>• max is the maximum of sCr/κ or 1. |
| Larsson et al. (2004) | eGFRCys = 77.24 × $(CysC\ [in\ mg/L])^{-1.2623}$ |
| Macdonald et al. (2006) | $\text{Log}_{10}\ eGFRCys = 2.222 + (-0.802 \times \sqrt{CysC\ in \frac{mg}{L}}) + (0.009876 \times LM)$ |
| CKD-EPI cystatin C Eq. (2012) | eGFRcys = 133 × min(sCys/0.8, 1) − 0.499 × max (sCys/0.8, 1) − 1.328 × $0.996^{age}$ (× 0.932 if female)<br>• sCys is serum cystatin C.<br>• min is the minimum of sCys/0.8 or 1.<br>• max indicates the maximum of sCys/0.8 or 1. |
| CKD-EPI creatinine–cystatin C Eq. (2012) | eGFRCr-Cys = 135 × min(sCr/κ, 1)α × max(sCr/κ, 1) − 0.601 × min(sCys/0.8, 1) − 0.375 × max(sCys/0.8, 1) − 0.711 × $0.995^{age}$ (× 0.969 if female) (× 1.08 if black)<br>• κ is 0.7 for females and 0.9 for males.<br>• α is −0.248 for females and −0.207 for males.<br>• min indicates the minimum of sCr/κ or 1.<br>• max indicates the maximum of sCr/κ or 1. |

[a]For SI conversion purposes, serum or plasma creatinine is converted from μmol/L to mg/dL by multiplying by 0.0113; conversion from creatinine clearance conventional units of mL/min to SI units of mL/s requires multiplication by 0.0167.
[b]Equations compiled from references 121–138.
*Alb,* Albumin; *BUN,* blood urea nitrogen; *CKD-EPI,* Chronic Kidney Disease Epidemiology Collaboration; *CrCl,* creatinine clearance in mL/min; *CysC,* cystatin C; *eGFR,* estimated glomerular filtration rate; *IBW,* ideal body weight (kg); *IDMS,* isotope dilution mass spectroscopy; *LM,* lean mass; *MDRD,* Modification of Diet in Renal Disease; *sCr,* serum or plasma creatinine (mg/dL).

children or ethnicity, has made it challenging to ascertain their place and relative value in clinical practice. The advantages of several of these methods are that timely results are available for routine clinical practice and for many patients they provide a reasonable approximation of measured GFR or mCrCl. The variation in sCr assays, as described in the past decade, led to differences in reported sCr values among as well as within laboratories.[128] To address this issue the U.S. National Institute of Standards and Technologies released materials that are traceable to the certified reference materials for creatinine, whose roughly 5% lower values were assigned using isotope dilution mass spectroscopy (IDMS).[122,129] It is now estimated that most laboratories currently report creatinine values traceable to this reference method. The use of IDMS creatinine assays will likely lead to less variation in kidney function estimates and theoretically more consistent drug dosing recommendations across institutions and clinical settings. Estimated GFRs based on current creatinine assays are likely to yield different CKD diagnostic categorization as well as drug dosage recommendations from those intended by the original study, even if the same estimating equation is used due to this change in analytic methodology.[130] It is not possible or practical to repeat all the PK studies with standardized creatinine-determined eCrCl or eGFR, and therefore it is still reasonable to use drug dosing adjustments that appear in FDA- and European Medicines Agency (EMA)-approved product labeling.

Traditionally, drug dosing was based on eCrCl using the Cockcroft and Gault (CG) formula.[5,7,18,19] For implementation in the chemical laboratory report, the CG equation is not suitable because body weight is usually not available in the electronic health record. The Modification of Diet in Renal Disease (MDRD) equations, which do not require body weight, were developed from an extensive sample of patients with CKD, all of whom had a measured GFR (i.e., iothalamate clearance) of <90 mL/min/1.73 m$^2$.[131,132] They were initially used by clinical laboratories, although they were only validated for patients with a GFR < 60 mL/min. Therefore, the new Chronic Kidney Disease Epidemiology Collaboration (CKD-EPI) equation was developed to allow estimation of GFR throughout the full range of the CKD.[125] The CKD-EPI eGFR equation has recently replaced the MDRD equation as the primary index for the staging of CKD, and values are now reported throughout the GFR range by Quest and LabCorp, the two largest laboratory service providers in the United States. For classifying kidney function into one of the five stages of CKD, the standardized CKD-EPI formula is currently preferred.[132] Both the MDRD and CKD-EPI equations estimate the GFR for a standard 1.73-m$^2$ body surface area (BSA); thus for an individual patient, the BSA must be determined separately so that the eGFR can be expressed in milliliters per minute (mL/min).

$$\text{BSA} = \frac{\sqrt{\text{weight (kg)} \bullet \text{height (m)}}}{60}$$

$$\text{GFR} = \text{eGFR} \bullet \frac{\text{BSA}}{1.73\ (\text{m}^2)}$$

Serum cystatin C has been proposed as an alternative marker to estimate GFR, rather than sCr. Multiple equations have been proposed to estimate GFR from age, weight, gender, race, and muscle mass based on serum cystatin C measurements.[133] The combined use of both serum markers, cystatin C and creatinine, allows an even more accurate estimate of kidney function than either of them alone.[134] Adjusting drug doses based on the measurement of cystatin C appears to be an effective and valid tool in the limited number of applications (mainly relating to chemotherapy and antibiotic dosing) for which it has been studied.[135–138]

The automated reporting of eGFR in the clinical setting has led some practitioners to consider substituting eGFR in place of eCrCl for renal dose adjustments. Others argue that use of the MDRD and CKD-EPI equations for drug dosing is not appropriate given that the PK studies were performed using eCrCl via the CG equation.[18,126] Furthermore, many studies have highlighted discordance between drug dosing recommendations based on these equations.[139–147] These studies have compared dosing recommendations based on three or more different equations for commonly used drugs in CKD patients. Average discordance rates for the MDRD Study and CG equations were between 20% and 30%.[139–144] Another study that evaluated eight antimicrobial dosing regimens based on CKD-EPI, MDRD, and CG equations demonstrated that overall discordance rates were 15%–25% between CG and CKD-EPI and 7%–12% between MDRD and CKD-EPI.[145] Two recent reports highlight the challenge of choosing the best eGFR method to project aminoglycoside clearance and attainment of the desired PD endpoint.[146,147] Major limitations with these studies include equations were not compared with a gold standard such as measured GFR and the studies did not assess drug concentrations or clinical outcomes. Although Stevens et al.[148] described average concordance rates for the MDRD Study and CG equations to measured GFR to be 88% and 85%, respectively; this was a simulation study and they did not evaluate drug concentrations or patient outcomes. Therefore none of these equations for estimating GFR should be used as the primary determinant for drug dosing decision making. Potential discrepancies in kidney function estimates and corresponding drug dosing regimens necessitate careful consideration of the risk–benefit ratio of each approach within the context of the complete clinical picture of the patient.

## PEDIATRICS

The original equation to estimate GFR, as described by Schwartz and colleagues,[149] is dependent on the child's age and length:

$$\text{GFR} = (\text{length [cm]} \times \text{k})/\text{sCr (in mg/dL)},$$

where k is defined by age group: infant (1 to 52 weeks) = 0.45; child (1 to 13 years) = 0.55; adolescent male = 0.7; and adolescent female = 0.55. The sCr level in µmol/L can be converted to mg/dL by multiplication using 0.0113 as the conversion factor. A newer version of the Schwartz equation[150] was developed from a population of 349 children (age 1–19 years) with mild to moderate CKD enrolled in the Chronic Kidney Disease in Children (CKiD) study:

$$\text{GFR} = 0.41 \times (\text{length in cm})/\text{sCr in mg/dL}$$

Lee and associates[151] have recently reported that this new Schwartz equation performed better than the original Schwartz equation for patients with moderate CKD, but was less accurate in patients with mild CKD. In pediatric patients, methods incorporating cystatin C have several advantages for evaluating kidney function.[152] The most recent eGFR equation evaluated in pediatrics includes use of cystatin C, blood urea nitrogen (BUN), sCr level (in mg/dL) and demographic data derived from over 600 pediatric patients enrolled in the CKiD study[153]:

$$\begin{aligned}\text{eGFR (mL/min/1.73 m}^2) &= 39.8 \times (\text{ht [m]/sCr})^{0.456} \times (1.8/\text{cystatin C})^{0.418} \\ &\quad \times (30/\text{BUN})^{0.079} \times 1.076^{\text{male}} \times (\text{ht [m]}/1.4)^{0.179}\end{aligned}$$

This equation had the highest $R^2$ value (0.863) and the highest frequency of values within 30% of iohexol-measured GFR (91.3%) when compared with seven other GFR estimating equations.

## ACUTE KIDNEY INJURY

At present, the staging of AKI is based on sequential measurement of the sCr level and urine output.[154–158] Because the GFR is inferred from the sCr or cystatin C, all estimates of kidney function are delayed and lag the real-time GFR. Although several methods have been proposed to estimate GFR in this patient population, none have been rigorously evaluated, and their use in clinical practice is extremely limited.[159–162] The latest proposed method to estimate GFR in patients with AKI is the kinetic GFR (kinetGFR), which is based on age (years), weight (kg), and sCr (µmol/L) and holds true for increasing and decreasing kidney function.[163]

$$\text{kinetGFR} = \frac{[150 - \text{age (years)}] \bullet \text{weight (kg)}}{\text{Cr}_1\ (\mu\text{mo/L})} \bullet \left[1 - \frac{\text{Cr}_2 - \text{Cr}_1}{t_2 - t_1} \bullet \frac{24\ (\text{hours})}{200\ (\mu\text{mol/L})}\right]$$

This approach is based on an estimate of the creatinine production similar to the CG equation.[121] The kinetic eGFR incorporates changing creatinine values over specified time intervals as well as the actually measured sCr values. It relates the increase in sCr within a specified time interval to the maximum increase in creatinine level in 1 day. Because creatinine excretion in the urine corresponds to creatinine production, the maximum increase in sCr is about 200 μmol/L if the patient's actual GFR is 0. The kinetic eGFR predicts what subsequently will be measurable, but in fact is already the case with kidney function. The kinetic eGFR solves the problem that there is always a delay between rapidly changing kidney function and measurable variables—namely, sCr or urine output. The calculation of a patient's kinetic eGFR may allow one to use the eCrCl- or eGFR-based dose adjustment recommendations derived from patients with CKD and be applicable in part for those with AKI.[163] Rigorous independent studies will be needed to confirm its validity and utility in clinical practice.

## PATIENTS RECEIVING DIALYSIS

Some ESKD patients on dialysis as well as those with AKI on CRRT have residual kidney function that substantially contributes to better patient outcomes and the elimination of drugs and their metabolites.[164] Unfortunately, estimating residual kidney function in patients undergoing dialysis is challenging because the sCr concentration reflects not only residual kidney function, but also the efficiency of dialysis and role of muscle mass in creatinine generation. CrCl measurements are less reliable as a measure of GFR in patients on HD or CRRT than in those with earlier stages of CKD because of the following: (1) the volume of urine output is heavily influenced by changing effective arterial blood volume during the cyclic changes that are inherent as a result of intermittent ultrafiltration; (2) the sCr concentration changes over the duration of the clearance measurement; and (3) tubular secretion of creatinine contributes to its clearance. Estimation of residual kidney function in patients on HD or CRRT is often done by calculating the mean of a measured urea and mCrCl. Measuring the elimination of iohexol after an IV dose has been reported to be an accurate and safe measure of residual kidney function in patients on dialysis and can inform drug dosing.[166,167] Recently Vilar et al.[168] and Shafi and colleagues[169] have reported that measurement of beta trace protein, also known as the enzyme prostaglandin $H_2$ D-isomerase, or $\beta_2$-macroglobulin serum concentrations provides clinically useful estimates of residual renal function that can be used to individualize dialysis dose and perhaps could be used to individualize drug dosing.

Which one of the many eCrCl or eGFR equations should be used to determine the degree of adjustment of drug dosage regimens for patients with AKI or CKD? The pros and cons of the various GFR estimating equations are reviewed earlier. The MDRD and CKD-EPI equations significantly overestimated CrCl (mCrCl and CG) in older individuals.[141,166] This has led to dose calculation errors for many drugs, particularly in the elderly and in individuals with severe CKD. It is an advantage of the CG equation that body weight is considered as a determinant of drug distribution volume. The choice of the optimal GFR estimating equation is of utmost importance for drugs with a narrow therapeutic index for which dosing individualization is often continuous rather than categorical. Finally, because most PK studies in patients with CKD conducted over the past 40 years have used eCrCl or mCrCl as the estimate of GFR, the CG method in adults and the latest Schwartz method in children remain the criteria to be used.[18]

Thus we have concluded that current evidence does not support the use of eGFR equations in place of the CG equation in older adults for the purpose of renal dosage adjustments. However, for patients with AKI, there is no obvious best choice for GFR estimation to guide drug dosing.

# DRUG DOSING CONSIDERATIONS

## PATIENTS WITH CHRONIC KIDNEY DISEASE

Despite the availability of numerous guidelines regarding drug dosing for patients with impaired kidney function, there is insufficient evidence as to which, if any, is preferred.[6,19,51,170–176] Occasionally, recommendations derived from postmarketing studies conflict with the information in these reports, as well as the official FDA or EMA product labeling. Prior to 1998, there were no official guidelines regarding when and how to characterize the relationship between the PK and PD of a drug and kidney function. The FDA guidelines issued in May 1998[177] and the 2010 proposed revision,[178] and the EMA guidelines of 2015[179] have provided frameworks for which drugs should be evaluated and guidance regarding study design, data analysis, interpretation of study results, and recommendations for the incorporation of data into product labeling.

### GOALS OF THERAPY

The desired goal is typically the maintenance of a similar peak, trough, or average steady-state drug concentration or, for antibiotics, an optimized PD measure, such as the peak over MIC, the time above the MIC, or the ratio of the drug area under the AUC to the MIC, as would be optimal for persons with normal kidney function (see the "Pharmacodynamics" section for more detail). When there is a significant relationship between drug concentration and clinical response[112] (e.g., aminoglycosides) or toxicity[55] (e.g., phenytoin), attainment of the specific target values becomes critical. If, however, no specific PK or PD target values have been reported, a regimen goal of attaining and maintaining the same average steady-state concentration may be appropriate.

FDA-approved drug labels, and commonly used drug information sources such as American Hospital Formulary Service Drug Information, Goodman and Gilman's *The Pharmacological Basis of Therapeutics*, the *British National Formulary*, and *Drug Prescribing in Renal Failure* are excellent sources of information about a drug's PK characteristics, goals of therapy, and the dosing regimens to achieve the goals (i.e., adequate drug concentrations or PD target values, in various patient populations).[173–176] However, in the digital era, many clinicians rely on drug information via their smartphone or personal digital assistant. Commonly used programs that answer frequent bedside drug questions, such as the proper dosing, pharmacology, adverse side effects, drug–drug interactions, and pregnancy safety, are Epocrates Rx,[180] Medscape Mobile,[181] Micromedex Drug Information,[182] and mobilePDR.[183] There are more specific applications for renal drug dosing but they require payment to access the information: KidneyCalc[184] and ABX Dosage–Adjustments in Renal Failure.[185] Regardless of dosing recommendations by the various sources, the design of the optimal dosage regimen is dependent on the availability of an accurate characterization of the relationship between the PK parameters of the drug and renal function and an accurate assessment of the patient's renal function.

## INDIVIDUALIZATION OF THE DRUG DOSAGE REGIMEN

Most dosage adjustment guidelines have proposed the use of a fixed dose or interval for patients with broad ranges of kidney function.[51,170–175] The mild, moderate, and severe CKD categories vary among reference sources, so the recommended regimen may not be "optimal" for all patients whose kidney function lies within the range, especially for agents with a narrow therapeutic index.[18] The approach to developing drug dosage adjustment recommendations for the patient with CKD is predicated on attainment of the desired exposure goal at steady state. To achieve the desired goal in a timely fashion, a stepwise approach that includes multiple considerations (Table 61.6) for each individual drug should be considered.[172] The following considerations may help guide individualization of therapy.

The initial or loading dose (LD), which in many patients with AKI will be larger than the typical maintenance dose, should be calculated to achieve the desired $C_{max}$ therapeutic drug concentration. An LD should be used for most patients with stage 4 or 5 CKD to achieve the desired steady-state concentration rapidly and in which the $V_D$ of a drug is significantly increased in extracellular volume-expanded patients with AKI and/or CKD relative to those with normal kidney function. If the relationship between $V_D$ and CrCl has been characterized, then the $V_D$ should be estimated from that relationship. If no LD is prescribed, four to five half-lives of the drug will pass before the desired steady-state plasma concentration is achieved; however, doing so may contribute to therapeutic failure. The proportion of the LD given affects the magnitude of the steady-state plasma concentration and how rapidly plasma concentrations are achieved. An LD equivalent to the dose given to a patient with normal kidney function should be given to patients with impaired kidney function if the drug's half-life is especially long and if the physical examination suggests normal ECF volume. If the patient has marked volume expansion or evidence indicates that the $V_D$ of the drug is larger in patients with CKD, then a higher dose can be calculated from the following expression:

$$LD = V_D \times C_{max} \times \text{actual weight/IBW},$$

where $V_D$ is the drug's volume of distribution (in liters per kilogram of IBW in those with CKD), IBW is the patient's ideal body weight (in kilograms), and $C_{max}$ is the desired steady-state maximum plasma drug concentration.

The primary reference for information regarding the maintenance dose for patients with CKD should be the FDA and/or EMA official product labeling. If no official drug dosing guidance is available, one may need to search the literature to find a recommendation strategy derived from nonregulatory or postmarketing clinical investigations. If no such resource is found, one can consult online or published tertiary references that have developed dosing recommendations based on the Dettli or Tozer method, initially published in 1974.[21,22] They used similar foundational PK characteristics and approaches to calculate the maintenance dose for a patient with a given eCrCl. In essence, either the dose (D) should be reduced or the interval (τ) extended. When the dose is reduced, the $C_{max}$ will be lower and the trough concentrations will be higher than those observed in persons with normal kidney function. When the administration interval is extended, the peak and trough concentrations are kept constant but the dosing frequency decreases (Fig. 61.4).

To maintain the normal dose interval in patients with impaired kidney function, the amount of each dose after the LD can be estimated from the following equation:

$$D_f = D_n \times Q,$$

where $D_f$ is the dose for the patient with impaired kidney function to be given at the normal dosing interval, $D_n$ is the normal dose, and Q is the dosage adjustment factor. The dosage adjustment factor (Q) can be calculated as

$$Q = 1 - (FE[1 - KF]),$$

where FE is the fraction of the drug eliminated unchanged renally in a patient with normal renal function and KF is the ratio of the patient's CrCl or GFR to the assumed normal value of 120 mL/min (equivalent to 2.00 mL/sec). Thus, for a drug that is 85% eliminated unchanged by the kidneys, the Q factor in a patient who has a CrCl of 10 mL/min (0.17 mL/sec) would be as follows:

$$\begin{aligned} Q &= 1 - \left(0.85\left[1 - \frac{10}{120}\right]\right) \\ &= 1 - (0.85[0.92]) \\ &= 1 - 0.78 \\ &= 0.22 \end{aligned}$$

**Table 61.6 Stepwise Approach to Adjust Drug Dosage Regimens for Patients With Impaired Kidney Function**

| Step | Process | Assessment |
|---|---|---|
| 1 | Obtain history and relevant demographic and clinical information | Record demographic information, obtain past medical history (including history of renal disease), and record current laboratory information (e.g., serum creatinine). |
| 2 | Estimate creatinine clearance | Use Cockcroft–Gault equation to estimate creatinine clearance, or calculate creatinine clearance from timed urine collection. |
| 3 | Review current medications | Identify drugs for which individualization of the treatment regimen will be necessary |
| 4 | Calculate individualized treatment regimen | Determine treatment goals (see text); calculate dosage regimen based on pharmacokinetic characteristics of the drug and patient's renal function. |
| 5 | Monitor | Monitor parameters of drug response and toxicity; monitor drug levels if available or applicable. |
| 6 | Revise regimen | Adjust regimen based on drug response or change in patient status (including renal function), as warranted. |

Adapted from Battistella M, Matzke GR. Drug dosing in renal failure. In: DiPiro J, Talbert R, Yee G, et al., eds. *Pharmacotherapy: A Pathophysiologic Approach*. 10th ed. New York: McGraw-Hill; 2017.

If one desires to give the same maintenance dose, a factor that may be required because of the limited availability of alternative formulations, the dosing interval at which the normal dose should be administered can be calculated as follows:

$$\tau_f = \tau_n / Q$$

The decision to extend the dosing interval beyond a 24-hour period should be based on the need to maintain therapeutic peak or trough levels. The dosing interval may be prolonged if the peak level is most important. Prolonging the dose interval in patients on dialysis is frequently a convenient method to modify the drug dosage regimen. This method is particularly useful for drugs with a long plasma half-life. In general, drugs removed by dialysis given once daily should be given after the dialysis treatment, with aminoglycosides being a controversial exception.[186–190]

A third alternative that is especially helpful when the calculated dose or dosing interval is impractical is to select the administration interval according to the target trough concentration while the peak is kept constant:

$$\tau_{target} = \left(t_{1/2}/0.693\right) \times \ln(C_{peak}/C_{trough-target})$$

$$D = LD \times (1 - C_{trough-target}/C_{peak})$$

Alternatively, one can calculate the adjusted dose ($D_p$) to be given at the predetermined practical dosage interval ($\tau_p$ or $\tau_{ptarget}$) as follows:

$$D_p = (D_n \times \tau_p \times Q)/\tau_n,$$

where $\tau_p$ is the estimated dosing interval, as calculated from the aforementioned equation for $\tau_{ptarget}$, or the clinically practical value for the renally impaired patient (e.g., 12, 18, 24, 36, and 48 hours). These approaches, which use a combination of the dose reduction and interval prolongation methods, are often the most clinically practical. When in doubt, clinicians should consult an experienced pharmacist, preferably one with extensive experience in evaluating patients with CKD and altered body composition (e.g., fluid overload).

## MEASUREMENT OF THERAPEUTIC DRUG LEVELS

Measuring drug concentrations is one way to optimize therapeutic regimens and account for changes among and within individuals. Therapeutic drug monitoring requires availability of rapid, specific, and reliable assays and known correlations of drug concentration to therapeutic and toxic outcomes. Indications for therapeutic drug monitoring include an experimentally determined relationship between plasma drug concentration and the pharmacologic effect, medications with a narrow therapeutic window, knowledge of the drug level influences management, potential patient compliance problems, and the drug dose cannot be optimized by clinical observation alone. Examples of drugs analyzed by therapeutic drug monitoring include digoxin, lithium, phenytoin, theophylline, valproic acid, warfarin, tacrolimus, sirolimus, aminoglycosides, vancomycin, and clozapine. Unless therapeutic drug monitoring is being used to forecast a dose or there are concerns about toxicity, samples should be taken at steady state (four to five half-lives after starting therapy). The timing of the collection of the sample is important as the drug concentration changes during the dosing interval. The least variable point in the dosing interval to collect a blood sample is just before the next dose is due. The drug concentration is complementary to and not a substitute for clinical judgment, so it is important to treat the individual patient and not the laboratory value. Drug concentrations may be used as surrogates for drug effects so therapeutic drug monitoring may assist with dose individualization. It can also be used to detect toxicity, so therapeutic drug monitoring can optimize patient management and improve clinical outcomes.[191]

Hypoalbuminemia may influence interpretation of drug concentrations because the total drug concentration may be reduced, even when the active unbound drug concentration generally is not. Unbound drug concentrations are often not clinically available, so clinicians must empirically consider the influence of hypoalbuminemia in their interpretation of measured total drug concentrations, as in the case of phenytoin and several antibiotics (e.g., ceftriaxone, daptomycin).[55,192,193]

# PATIENTS WITH ACUTE KIDNEY INJURY

Critically ill patients frequently develop AKI, depending on the definition, from 5% to 15% of all non–same-day hospitalization care is complicated by AKI.[9–13] In most cases, drug dosing is based on drug disposition information derived from studies in stable patients with CKD. Unfortunately, there are large gaps in knowledge of drug metabolism and disposition in patients with AKI; thus patients may be at significant risk for underdosing as well as overdosing. More than 30 definitions of AKI have been published in the literature.[155–158] The lack of a consensus definition and classification of AKI reflects the wide range of causes and severity with which it presents. The presentation can vary from part of multiorgan dysfunction in critically ill patients to isolated AKI.[194] As a result, AKI-related, in-hospital mortality rates vary from 70% in intensive care unit (ICU) patients[195] to 35% in other hospitalized patients.[196]

The potential effects of AKI on drug dosing are of major consequence because AKI patients are often critically ill and require multiple drug therapies, some of which may be nephrotoxic or require dose modification in the setting of AKI. The PK changes in absorption, distribution, metabolism, and excretion presented earlier in this chapter, and in other sources, are foundational to optimal patient care.[7,51,172,197,198] The clinician needs to appreciate these factors and realize that they may worsen and improve over the period of evolution or recovery of the AKI episode. Critically ill patients with AKI typically have minimal oral intake of food and liquids and commonly require parenteral administration of drugs otherwise given orally (e.g., antihypertensives, immunosuppressives).

There is a paucity of dosing algorithms to guide pharmacotherapy, derived from investigations of the PK and PD of multiple dose studies in patients with AKI. Most of the critical care literature and almost all FDA or EMA product labeling contain drug dosage recommendations derived from observations of patients with CKD and ESKD. The limited data available in the setting of AKI have predominantly been developed by clinicians; rarely is this information incorporated into official product labeling. The principles of drug dosage regimen modification described earlier for use in CKD thus remain the foundation for therapy optimization in patients with AKI.

### LOADING DOSE

Many patients with AKI are overhydrated, and the distribution volume is much larger than under normal conditions. Thus, the LD may need to be higher than the normal starting dose for persons with normal kidney function. Because the $V_D$ of many drugs, especially hydrophilic antibiotics, including β-lactams, cephalosporins, and carbapenems, is significantly increased in the presence of AKI, the administration of proactive LDs (25% > normal) is highly recommended.

### MAINTENANCE DOSE

Forecasting the degree and rate of change in kidney function and fluid volume status is extremely challenging. Thus maintenance dosing regimens for many drugs, especially antimicrobial agents, should be initiated at normal or near-normal dosage regimens and adjustments made based on the relationship between drug PK characteristics and kidney function, as described earlier. Prospective measurement of serum drug concentrations and analysis using state-of-the-art PK and PD approaches should be used whenever possible.

## PATIENTS UNDERGOING HEMODIALYSIS

The optimization of pharmacotherapy for patients receiving maintenance HD and emergent HD are both critically dependent on the availability of reliable information from well-designed PK studies.[7,17,25,199–204] The impact of HD on drug therapy is dependent on the drug characteristics and dialysis prescription. Drug-related factors include molecular weight (MW) or size, degree of protein binding, and distribution volume.[172,201] The vast majority of HD filters in use up until the mid-1990s was generally impermeable to drugs with an MW > 1 kDa.[199–201] Dialysis membranes in the 21st century are predominantly composed of semisynthetic or synthetic materials, which have larger pore sizes, and this allows the ready passage of drugs that have an MW up to 20 kDa.

Drug clearance during dialysis can occur by three different processes.[7,201] Drug removal by conventional HD occurs primarily by diffusion down a concentration gradient from the plasma to the dialysate. Removal of low-MW drugs is enhanced by increasing blood and dialysate flow rates and by using large-surface-area dialyzers. Larger molecules require more porous membranes for increased removal. The clearance of a drug by conventional HD can be estimated from the unbound fraction ($f_u$) and the following relationship:

$$Cl_{HD} = f_u \times Cl_{urea} \times (60/MW_{drug}),$$

where $Cl_{HD}$ is the drug's clearance by HD, $Cl_{urea}$ is the dialyzer clearance of urea, and $MW_{drug}$ is the MW of the drug. The urea clearance for most conventional dialyzers varies between 150 and 200 mL/min and is comparable with values reported with high-flux hemodialyzers.[201] With high-flux HD, the $V_D$ and degree of protein binding of the drug become more important determinants of dialyzer clearance. The hemodialyzer clearance of drugs that are not highly protein bound and have relatively small volumes of distribution runs in parallel to urea clearance, despite their large molecular mass.[205] The convective transport and removal of drugs during high-flux HD depends primarily on filtration pressure gradient, treatment time, blood, and dialysate flow rates. Despite the widespread adoption of high-flux HD in certain parts of the world, there are sparse quantitative data on drug clearance.

Total daily small solute removal is more efficient if the frequency of HD is increased. Daily and nocturnal dialysis therapies yield different clearance values compared with thrice-weekly, high-flux, in-center HD, and also differ from each other. Although there is an increase in dialysis hours, which would suggest an increase in drug removal, the blood and dialysate flow rates are slower and thus drug clearance per unit of time is less. There has been little investigation of the effects of sustained low-efficiency hemodialysis (SLED) regimens on drug disposition or comparison among modalities.[206–209] Only a few agents have been evaluated during the delivery of one of these dialytic variants. Slow nocturnal dialysis required a significant increase in gentamicin dosage to achieve therapeutic levels compared with conventional thrice-weekly dialysis.[206,207] The variability in drug clearance was high and did not correlate with small solute clearance. Similar findings were reported with cefazolin.[208] The cefazolin clearance during NHD was slightly lower (Cl = 1.65 L/hr) than during high-flux intermittent HD (Cl = 1.85 L/hr). However, a greater percentage of cefazolin was removed in 8 hours of NHD (80%) than conventional 4-hour high-flux HD (60%). The investigators concluded that a dosing regimen of a 2-g LD followed by 1-g IV dose after each NHD was sufficient to achieve concentrations 6 × MIC for *Staphylococcus* species for at least 70% of the dosing interval. As a result, though drug dosing in patients receiving one of these dialytic variants may be empirically increased, drug dosing regimens should be guided by drug-level monitoring when feasible. Drugs with a molecular size of 500 to 5000 Da appear to be particularly likely to have an increased clearance with this modality. Studies of modeled clearance have suggested that frequent HD regimens would be associated with enhanced clearance (and thereby the potential of under dosing) of daptomycin.[210,211] This enhanced clearance was confirmed in the setting of AKI when the PK associated with extended daily dialysis (EDD) was investigated.[192] These findings should be transferable to maintenance HD, with a degree of caution about the effects on distribution volumes that might arise in the setting of septic shock.[212] One of the other effects of prolonged HD appears to be a reduction in rebound of drug concentrations after the termination of dialysis.[213,214] This is probably because the rate of transfer from the peripheral to central compartment relative to the rate of diffusive removal is lower.

There were >100 different dialysis or hemofilters available in the United States in 2013, and at least four distinct variants of HD are currently being used.[201] The effect of HD or hemofiltration on the disposition of a drug may vary markedly and, because dialyzer or hemofilter clearance is rarely evaluated more than once, clinicians have to extrapolate data from one procedure to another.[215–217] The enhanced efficiency of 21st century dialyzers means that most of the literature for medications developed prior to 2000 probably reflects an underestimation of the impact of HD.[200] Consequently, the dosage may need to be empirically increased by 25% to 50%. Therapeutic drug monitoring should be used for drugs with narrow therapeutic indices to optimize safety and efficacy.

## ASSESSMENT OF THE IMPACT OF HEMODIALYSIS

The most commonly used means for assessing the effect of HD is to calculate the dialyzer clearance of a drug ($Cl^p_D$) from plasma, as follows:

$$Cl^p_D = Q_p([A_p - V_p]/A_p),$$

where $Q_p$ is plasma flow through the dialyzer, $A_p$ is the concentration of drug in plasma going into the dialyzer, and $V_p$ is the plasma concentration of drug leaving the dialyzer.[199,214] This equation tends to underestimate HD clearance for drugs that readily partition into and out of erythrocytes. In addition, venous plasma concentrations may be artificially high if extensive ultrafiltration is performed, so $Cl^p_D$ will be lower than it really is. Because of these limitations, the recovery clearance approach remains the benchmark for the determination of dialyzer clearance and can be calculated as follows[175,199–201]:

$$Cl^r_D = R/AUC_{0-t},$$

where R is the total amount of drug recovered unchanged in the dialysate and $AUC_{0-t}$ is the area under the predialyzer plasma concentration–time curve during the period that the dialysate was collected. The HD clearance values reported in the literature may vary significantly, depending on which of these methods were used.[200]

It is common practice in most HD units to administer drugs after dialysis to minimize the loss of drug that would result from the additional clearance during HD. However, performing HD immediately after dosing has been proposed as an option for removal of toxic antibiotics[187–189,212,217] and chemotherapeutic agents.[218–240] For anticancer drugs, the predialysis administration of a normal dose makes sense when the patient undergoes HD 2 to 12 hours later. This strategy delivers the desired maximum plasma concentration effect while minimizing the toxic drug or metabolic effects (Table 61.7). Emerging PK and PD considerations suggest that administration after HD may not be the optimal approach for some antibacterial agents, such as aminoglycosides and vancomycin.[187–189,212,217] High-bolus dosing immediately before or during the last hour of dialysis has been proposed for some antibiotics, but there have been few clinical studies.

If the drug is given after dialysis, the postdialysis dose ($D_{HD}$) should first replace the amount eliminated during the interval between dialysis sessions ($D_{fail}$) that is the result of clearance by the patient's residual renal function and nonrenal clearance. Furthermore, the fraction of drug removed by HD (FR) should be estimated and a supplementary dose calculated ($D_{suppl}$). The dose the patient should receive after HD would thus be the sum of these two doses (Fig. 61.5):

$$D_{HD} = D_{fail} + D_{suppl} = D_{fail} + (FR \times (D_{start} - D_{fail}))$$

## PATIENTS RECEIVING CONTINUOUS RENAL REPLACEMENT THERAPY

CRRT and hybrid RRTs are commonly used to manage patients with AKI in intensive care units.[241] CRRT seems to

**Table 61.7 Drugs Best Administered Prior to Hemodialysis**

| Drug Class | Examples | Drug Fraction Removed by One Dialysis Session | Reference |
|---|---|---|---|
| Anticancer | Carboplatin | 20% dose post-HD; 84% dose prior to HD | Chatelut et al.[218]; Kamata et al.[219]; Yoshida et al.[220]; Oguri et al.[221] |
| | Cisplatin | 85% | Watanabe et al.[222] |
| | Oxaliplatin | 65% | Katsumata et al.[223] |
| | Cyclophosphamide | 22% (M % unknown) | Haubitz et al.[224] |
| | Ifosfamide | 70%–87% (M, 72%–77%) | Carlson et al.[225] |
| | Capecitabine | FBAL 50% | Walko and Lindley[226] |
| | Gemcitabine | dFdU 50% | Koolen et al.[227] |
| | Methotrexate | (M, 36%) | Garlich and Goldfarb[228] |
| | Cytosine arabinoside | 39% (M, 52%–63%) | Radeski et al.[229] |
| | Topotecan | 50% | Herrington et al.[230] |
| | Bleomycin | 30%–60% | Kamidono et al.[232] |
| | Lenalidomide | 30% | João et al.[233] |
| | Pemetrexed | 30% | Izzedine[234] |
| | Tegafur = S-1 | 60% | Tomiyama et al.[235] |
| | Carboplatin | 84% | Oguri et al.[236] |
| | Fludarabine | 2F-Ara-A 25% | Kielstein et al.[237] |
| | Fluorouracil = 5-FU infusion | FBAL 60% | Rengelshausen et al.[238] |
| | Iodine 131 | 50% | Fofi et al.[239] |
| | Irinotecan | SN-38 50% | Koike et al.[240] |
| Aminoglycoside | Gentamicin | 75% | Veinstein et al.[212] |
| | Tobramycin | 80% | Kamel et al.[189] |
| Contrast agent | Gadolinium | 65%–74% | Rodby[231] |

*dFdU*, 2′,2′-Difluorodeoxyuridine; *FBAL*, alpha-fluoro-beta-alanine; *HD*, hemodialysis; *M*, metabolite.

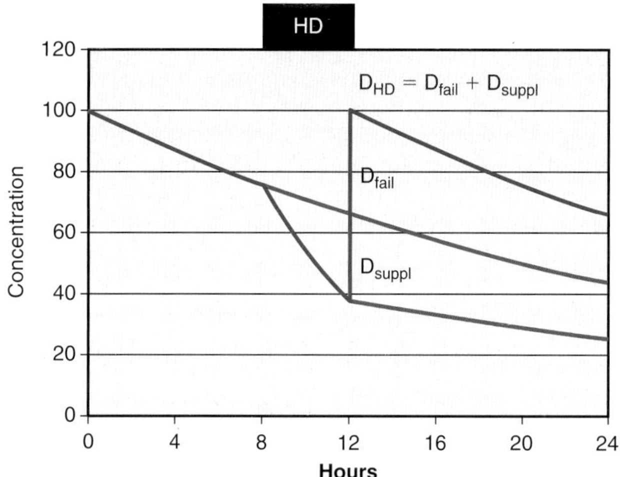


**Fig. 61.5 Supplementary dose after hemodialysis *(HD)*.** To maintain therapeutic target concentrations, a supplementary dose must be given after hemodialysis to replace the removed fraction of the dose. The dose after dialysis *($D_{HD}$)* combines both the adjusted maintenance dose *($D_{fail}$)* and the supplementary dose *($D_{suppl}$)*.

provide less of a challenge for drug dosing than intermittent HD because its continuous nature is analogous with drug removal by native kidneys and potentially amenable to the use of standard, first-order drug clearance equations to calculate dosing. However, in practice, CRRT rarely proves as continuous as planned. The CRRT modality and details of the therapy prescription can also have significant effects on drug clearance. MW, membrane characteristics (highly variable between systems), blood flow rate, and dialysate flow rate determine the rate and extent of drug removal.[242] Because most drugs have MWs < 1.5 kDa, drug removal by CRRT does not depend greatly on MW. The use of higher hemofiltration volumes, especially if infused prefilter, can also affect clearance. The removal of urea, creatinine, and vancomycin was increased by 15% to 25% by the predilution modality.[243,244]

CRRT clearances have been noted to decline because the time the hemofilter has been in use increases due to the accumulation of protein on the dialysis membrane. Clotting within the hemofilter's hollow fibers also reduces the overall surface area for clearance. Although these factors have received little direct investigation, it appears that they do affect drug clearance.[245,246]

Drug protein binding also affects how much is removed during CRRT because only unbound drug is available for elimination by CRRT. Protein binding of >80% provides a substantial barrier to drug removal by convection or diffusion. During continuous venovenous hemofiltration, drug clearance generally approximates the ultrafiltration rate. The addition of diffusion by continuous venovenous hemodiafiltration increases drug clearance and is dependent on the ultrafiltration and dialysate flow rates. As is the case during high-flux dialysis, drug removal often parallels the removal of urea and creatinine. Thus the simplest method for estimating drug removal during CRRT is to estimate the total urea or CrCl.[7,245,246]

Hybrid RRTs, including sustained or slow low-efficiency dialysis (SLED), EDD, continuous SLED, slow low-efficiency daily dialysis, and slow low-efficiency daily hemodiafiltration, which use higher dialysate flow rates and shorter treatment periods (6–12 hours in duration), are frequently used as well.[247–250] As of 2011, hybrid RRT PK data have been published for fewer than 20 drugs.[6] The improvement of RRT machines and filters has rendered old dosing guidelines for drugs, especially antibiotics, obsolete and potentially hazardous because they are underdosed. Although there are only a few FDA or EMA official drug dosing recommendations for patients receiving CRRT, several published dosing guidelines are widely used.[17,216,245,246] Unfortunately, these recommendations have generally not been prospectively evaluated and their influence on patient outcomes is largely unknown.

In the absence of FDA or EMA recommendations, tertiary reference sources, or any published studies relating to the handling of a drug by CRRT (common with agents that are new to the market), it may be necessary for the clinician to formulate a dosing regimen using the PK principles presented in this chapter. The lack of PK data for antibiotics during prolonged RRT and intermitted HD in critically ill patients has made the attainment and maintenance of effective concentrations a major challenge.[250,251] If the $V_D$ is large (>1 L/kg), there is a low likelihood that CRRT will substantially remove the drug. The use of a high-flux dialyzer or hemofilter allows for drugs with an MW < 20 kDa to be readily removed. If the clearance of the drug by CRRT or hybrid RRT is <25% of the patient's estimated total body clearance, a further dosing adjustment is probably unnecessary. By contrast, if CRRT or hybrid RRT results in an augmentation of drug clearance by 25% to 50%, an LD based on the patient's estimated volume status should be given, and maintenance doses similar to those given to a patient with a CrCl of 30 to 50 mL/min can be used. Such estimates obviously have to take into account changing volume status and be supplemented by regular drug concentration measurements, if technically feasible.

## PATIENTS UNDERGOING PERITONEAL DIALYSIS

Peritoneal dialysis, as practiced in 2018, is very unlikely to enhance total body clearance of any drug by >10 mL/min because most typical peritoneal dialysis prescriptions can achieve a urea clearance of about ≤10 mL/min. As most drugs are larger than urea, their clearance is even less; thus it is very likely to be from 5 to 7.5 mL/min or less. Many studies performed in the 1970s and 1980s showed that drug clearances by peritoneal dialysis were in this very low range, so one can conclude that peritoneal dialysis does not enhance drug removal to a degree that would require a special dosage regimen modification.[252–254] Accordingly, when given only once a day with the first dialysis bag, antibiotics are well absorbed from the peritoneum into the systemic circulation. The systemic drug concentrations will persist for the rest of the day during the three subsequent changes of peritoneal fluid. Thus oral or IV drug therapy recommendations for patients with an eCrCl or eGFR <15 mL/min are likely clinically useful.

Intraperitoneal drug administration is well accepted for the treatment of peritoneal dialysis–associated peritonitis and other infections.[254,255] Administration intervals depend on the half-life of the drug, which is mainly determined by residual renal and extrarenal metabolic clearance. Long-standing experience with intermittent antibiotic administration exists for the glycopeptides vancomycin and teicoplanin, which can be administered at 5- to 7-day intervals, as well as for aminoglycosides and cephalosporins, which are suitable for once-daily dosing.[256,257]

Patients treated by automated peritoneal dialysis (APD), with frequent short-dialysis cycles, may achieve higher plasma concentrations as compared with antibiotic loading in a single extended dwell period in patients on continuous ambulatory peritoneal dialysis (CAPD). Conversely, the higher dialysate flow and small-molecule clearance achieved with APD regimens may lead to a greater peritoneal clearance of antibiotic in the intervals between dosing.[256]

Because most PK studies establishing peritoneal antibiotic doses have used 4- to 8-hour loading periods, it is recommended to perform antibiotic loading by an extended cycle in both CAPD and APD patients. For intermittent maintenance dosing, a long nighttime dwell time should be used in CAPD patients and a long daytime dwell time in APD patients. In clinical practice, intraperitoneal antibiotic dosing has not been unequivocally successful in eradicating bacterial growth, partially questioning the concept of antibiotic back diffusion into the peritoneal cavity. Thus antibiotics may need to be administered IV to enhance the antimicrobial effect.

*Clinical Relevance*

Hemodialysis removal of therapeutic drugs can dramatically impact the clinical outcomes of patients. High rates of removal can lead to therapeutic failures, morbidity, and even death. The advances in dialyzer membrane technology continue to increase the efficiency of the dialysis process and thus therapeutic failures become more common, especially if clinicians base their prescribing practices on data derived from low-efficiency dialyzers that are no longer clinically available.

## CLINICAL BOTTOM LINE

Recommendations for dosing selected drugs in patients with CKD and AKI are given in Table 61.8. These are meant only as a guide and do not imply the safety or efficacy of a recommended dose in an individual patient. An LD equivalent to the usual dose in patients with normal kidney function should be considered for drugs with half-lives >12 hours. No controlled clinical trials have established the efficacy of these dosage recommendations. The effect on drug removal of HD, ambulatory peritoneal dialysis, and CRRT is variable and the values in the table are more qualitative than quantitative. Most of these recommendations were established before high-efficiency HD treatments were practical, continuous cycling nocturnal peritoneal dialysis was common, and diffusion was added to hemofiltration in CRRT.

 Complete reference list available at ExpertConsult.com.

**Table 61.8** Recommendations for Dosing Selected Drugs in Patients With Chronic Kidney Disease or Acute Kidney Injury

| | Degree of Drug Dose Reduction or Interval Prolongation | | | Dosage Recommendations for Patients Receiving Renal Replacement Therapy | | |
|---|---|---|---|---|---|---|
| **Drug** | GFR > 50 mL/min | GFR = 10–50 mL/min | GFR < 10 mL/min | HD | CAPD | CRRT |
| Acebutolol | 100% | 50% | 25% | Dose as GFR < 10 | Dose as GFR < 10 | Dose as GFR 10–50 |
| Acetaminophen | q4h | q6h | q8h | Dose as GFR < 10 | Dose as GFR < 10 | Dose as GFR 10–50 |
| Acetazolamide | q6h | q12h | q24h | Dose as GFR < 10 | Dose as GFR < 10 | Dose as GFR 10–50 |
| Acetohexamide | Avoid | Avoid | Avoid | Avoid | Avoid | Avoid |
| Acetohydroxamic acid | 100% | 100% | Avoid | Unknown | Unknown | Unknown |
| Acetylsalicylic acid | q4h | q4–6h | Avoid | As normal GFR | As normal GFR | Dose as GFR 10–50 |
| Acrivastine | 8 mg q6h | 8 mg q8–12h | 8 mg q12–24h | Dose as GFR < 10 | Dose as GFR < 10 | Dose as GFR 10–50 |
| Acyclovir | 5 mg/kg q8h | 5 mg/kg q12–24h | 2.5–5 mg/kg q24h | Dose as GFR < 10 | Dose as GFR < 10 | Dose as GFR 10–50 |
| Allopurinol | 100% | 50% | 33% | Dose as GFR < 10 | Dose as GFR < 10 | Dose as GFR 10–50 |
| Amantadine | q24h | q48–72h | q7days | Dose as GFR < 10 | Dose as GFR < 10 | Dose as GFR 10–50 |
| Amikacin[a] | 5–6 mg/kg q12h | 3–4 mg/kg q24h | 2 mg/kg q24–48h | 5 mg/kg after HD | 15–20 mg/L/day | 7.5 mg/kg q24h |
| Amiloride | 100% | 50% | Avoid | NA | NA | NA |
| Amlodipine | 100% | 100% | 100% | Dose as GFR < 10 | Dose as GFR < 10 | Dose as GFR < 10 |
| Amoxapine | 100% | 100% | 100% | Unknown | Unknown | Dose as GFR 10–50 |
| Amphotericin | q24h | q24h | q24h | Dose as GFR < 10 | Dose as GFR < 10 | Dose as GFR 10–50 |
| Amphotericin B | q24h | q24h | q24h | Dose as GFR < 10 | Dose as GFR < 10 | Dose for GFR 10–50 |
| Amphotericin B lipid | q24h | q24h | q24h | Dose as GFR < 10 | Dose as GFR < 10 | Dose as GFR 10–50 |
| Ampicillin | 250 mg–2 g q4–6h | 250 mg–2 g q6h | 250 mg–1 g q6h | Dose as GFR < 10 | Dose as GFR < 10 | Dose as GFR 10–50 |
| Apixaban | 100% | 25–50 mL/min: 100%<br><25 mL/min: Not recommended | Not recommended | 5 mg BID;<br>2.5 mg BID if age >79 years or body weight <61 kg | Unknown | Unknown |
| Aripiprazole | 100% | 100% | 100% | Dose as GFR < 10 | Dose as GFR < 10 | Dose as GFR < 10 |
| Atenolol | 100% q24h | 50% q24h | 25% q24h | Dose as GFR 25–50 | Dose as GFR < 10 | Dose as GFR 10–50 |
| Auranofin | 6 mg q24h | 3 mg q24h | Avoid | Avoid | Avoid | Dose as GFR 10–50 |
| Azathioprine | 100% | 75%–100% | 50%–100% | Dose as GFR < 10 | Dose as GFR < 10 | Dose as GFR 10–50 |
| Aztreonam | 100% | 50% | 25% | Dose as GFR < 10 | Dose for GFR < 10 | Dose as GFR 10–50 |
| Benazepril | 100% | 50%–75% | 25%–50% | Dose as GFR < 10 | Dose as GFR < 10 | Dose as GFR 10–50 |
| Bezafibrate | 50%–100% | 25%–50% | Avoid | 200 mg q72h | 200 mg q72h | 200 mg q24–48h |
| Bisoprolol | 100% | 100% | 50% | Dose as GFR < 10 | Dose as GFR < 10 | Dose as GFR 10–50 |
| Bleomycin | 100% | 75% | 50% | Dose as GFR < 10 | Dose as GFR < 10 | Dose as GFR 10–50 |
| Bretylium | 100% | 25%–50% | 25% | Dose as GFR < 10 | Dose as GFR < 10 | Dose as GFR 10–50 |
| Bumetanide | 100% | 100% | 100% | Dose as GFR < 10 | Dose as GFR < 10 | Dose as GFR < 10 |
| Bupropion | 100% q24h | 100% q24h | 100% q24h | Dose as GFR < 10 | Dose as GFR < 10 | Dose as GFR 10–50 |
| Butorphanol | 100% | 75% | 50% | Unknown | Unknown | Dose as GFR 10–50 |
| Canagliflozin | 100% | 30–50 mL/min: Not Recommended<br><30 mL/min: Avoid | Avoid | Avoid | Unknown | Unknown |
| Capreomycin | q24h | q24h | q48h | Dose as GFR < 10 | Dose as GFR < 10 | As normal GFR |
| Captopril | 100% q8–12h | 75% q12–18h | 50% q24h | Dose as GFR < 10 | Dose as GFR < 10 | Dose as GFR 10–50 |
| Carboplatin | 100% | 50% | 25% | Dose as GFR < 10 | Dose as GFR < 10 | Dose as GFR 10–50 |

| | | | | | | |
|---|---|---|---|---|---|---|
| Carteolol | 100% | 50% | 25% | Dose as GFR < 10 | Dose as GFR < 10 | Dose as GFR 10–50 |
| Cefaclor | 100% | 100% | 50%–100% | 250–500 mg q8h | 250 mg q8–12h | Dose as GFR 10–50 |
| Cefadroxil | q12h | q12h | q24h | 0.5–1.0 g after HD | 0.5 g/day | Dose as GFR 10–50 |
| Cefamandole | q6h | q6–8h | q8–12h | 0.5–1.0 g q12h | 0.5–1.0 g q12h | Dose as GFR 10–50 |
| Cefazolin | q8h | q12h | 50% q24–48h | 15–20 mg/kg after HD | Dose as GFR 10–50 | Dose as GFR 10–50 |
| Cefepime | q12h | 50%–100% q24h | 25%–50% q24h | Dose as GFR < 10 | Dose for GFR < 10 | 1–2 g q12h |
| Cefixime | 100% | 75%–100% | 50% | Dose as GFR < 10 | Dose for GFR < 10 | Dose as GFR 10–50 |
| Cefotaxime | q6h | q6–12h | 1 g q8–12h | Dose as GFR < 10 | Dose as GFR < 10 | 1–2 g q12h |
| Cefotetan | q12h | q24h | q48h | 1 g after HD | 1 g q24h | Dose as GFR 10–50 |
| Cefoxitin | q6–8h | q8–12h | q24–48h | 1 g after HD | 1 g q24h | Dose as GFR 10–50 |
| Cefpodoxime | 100% | 100% | 100–200 mg q24–48h | Dose as GFR < 10 | Dose as GFR < 10 | As normal GFR |
| Cefprozil | 100% | 50% q12h | 50% q12h | 250 mg after HD | Dose as GFR < 10 | Dose as GFR < 10 |
| Ceftazidime | 100% | 1–2 g q24h | 0.5–1 g q48h | 1 g after HD | 0.5–1 g q24h | 1–2 g q12h |
| Ceftibuten | 100% | 50% | 25% | 400 mg after HD | Dose as GFR < 10 | Dose as GFR 10–50 |
| Ceftizoxime | q8h | q12h | q24h | 1 g after HD | 0.5–1.0 g q24h | Dose as GFR 10–50 |
| Cefuroxime (IV) | 100% q8h | q8–12h | 750 mg q12h | Dose as GFR < 10 | Dose as GFR < 10 | Dose as GFR 10–50 |
| Celiprolol | 100% | 100% | 75% | Dose as GFR < 10 | Dose as GFR < 10 | As normal GFR |
| Cephalexin | 250–500 mg q6h | 250–500 mg q8–12h | 250–500 mg q12–24h | Dose as GFR < 10 | Dose as GFR < 10 | Dose as GFR 10–50 |
| Cephradine | 100% | 50% | 25% | Dose as GFR < 10 | Dose for GFR < 10 | As normal GFR |
| Cetirizine | 100% | 100% | 50% | Dose as GFR < 10 | Dose as GFR < 10 | As normal GFR |
| Chloroquine | 100% | 100% | 50% | Dose as GFR < 10 | Dose as GFR < 10 | As normal GFR |
| Chlorpropamide | 50% | Avoid | Avoid | Avoid | Avoid | Avoid |
| Chlorthalidone | q24h | Avoid | Avoid | Avoid | Avoid | Unknown |
| Cibenzoline | 100% q12h | 100% q12h | 66% q24h | Dose as GFR < 10 | Dose as GFR < 10 | Dose as GFR 10–50 |
| Cidofovir | 50%–100% | Avoid | Avoid | No data | No data | Avoid |
| Cilazapril | 75% q24h | 50% q24–48h | 10%–25% q72h | Dose as GFR < 10 | Dose as GFR < 10 | Dose as GFR 10–50 |
| Cimetidine | 100% | 50% | 50% | Dose as GFR < 10 | Dose as GFR < 10 | Dose as GFR 10–50 |
| Ciprofloxacin | 100% | 50%–100% | 50% | 250 mg q12h | 250 mg q8h | 200 mg IV q12h |
| Cisplatin | 100% | 75% | 50% | Dose as GFR < 10 | Dose as GFR < 10 | Dose as GFR 10–50 |
| Clarithromycin | 100% | 75% | 50%–75% | Dose as GFR < 10 | Dose as GFR < 10 | Dose as GFR 10–50 |
| Clodronate | 100% | 50% | Avoid | Dose as GFR < 10 | Dose as GFR < 10 | Dose as GFR 10–50 |
| Clofazimine | 100% | 100% | 100% | Dose as GFR < 10 | Dose as GFR < 10 | Dose as GFR 10–50 |
| Clofibrate | q6–12h | q12–18h | Avoid | Dose as GFR < 10 | Dose as GFR < 10 | Dose as GFR 10–50 |
| Clomipramine | 100% | Start at lower dose, monitor effect | Start at lower dose, monitor effect | Dose as GFR 10–50 | Dose as GFR 10–50 | Dose as GFR 10–50 |
| Clonidine | q12h | q12–24h | q24h | As normal GFR | As normal GFR | As normal GFR |
| Clopidogrel | 100% | 100% | 100% | Dose as GFR < 10 | Dose as GFR < 10 | Dose as GFR 10–50 |
| Codeine | 100% | 75% | 50% | As normal GFR | As normal GFR | As normal GFR |
| Colchicine | 100% | 100% | 50% | Dose as GFR < 10 | Dose as GFR < 10 | Dose as GFR 10–50 |
| Cyclophosphamide | 100% | 75%–100% | 50%–75% | 50% | 75% | 100% |
| Cycloserine | q12h | q12–24h | q24h | Dose as GFR < 10 | Dose as GFR < 10 | Dose as GFR 10–50 |
| Dabigatran | 100% | 15–50 mL/min: 75 mg BID | Not Recommended | Not Recommended | Unknown | Unknown |
| Dapsone | 100% | 100% | 50% | Dose as GFR < 10 | Dose as GFR < 10 | Dose as GFR 10–50 |
| Daunorubicin | 100% | 75% | 50% | Dose as GFR < 10 | Dose as GFR < 10 | Dose as GFR 10–50 |
| Didanosine | 50%–100% | 33%–50% | 25% | Dose as GFR < 10 | Dose as GFR < 10 | Dose as GFR 10–50 |
| Diflunisal | 100% | 50% | 50% | Dose as GFR < 10 | Dose as GFR < 10 | Dose as GFR 10–50 |
| Digitoxin | 100% | 100% | 50%–75% | Dose as GFR < 10 | Dose as GFR < 10 | Dose as GFR 10–50 |
| Digoxin[a] | 100% q24h | 25%–50% q24h | 10%–25% q24–48h | Dose as GFR < 10 | Dose as GFR < 10 | Dose as GFR 10–50 |
| Disopyramide | q8h | q12h | q48h | Dose as GFR < 10 | Dose as GFR < 10 | Dose as GFR 10–50 |

*Continued on following page*

**Table 61.8 Recommendations for Dosing Selected Drugs in Patients With Chronic Kidney Disease or Acute Kidney Injury (Cont'd)**

| | Degree of Drug Dose Reduction or Interval Prolongation | | | Dosage Recommendations for Patients Receiving Renal Replacement Therapy | | |
|---|---|---|---|---|---|---|
| **Drug** | GFR > 50 mL/min | GFR = 10–50 mL/min | GFR < 10 mL/min | HD | CAPD | CRRT |
| Dobutamine | 100% | 100% | 100% | As normal GFR | As normal GFR | As normal GFR |
| Doxacurium | 100% | 50% | 50% | Unknown | Unknown | Dose as GFR 10–50 |
| Dyphylline | 75% | 50% | 25% | Dose as GFR < 10 | Unknown | Dose as GFR 10–50 |
| Emtricitabine | q24h | q48–72h | q96h | Dose as GFR < 10 | Dose as GFR < 10 | Dose as GFR 10–50 |
| Enalapril | 100% | 50%–100% | 25% | Dose as GFR < 10 | Dose as GFR < 10 | Dose as GFR 10–50 |
| Ertapenem | 100% | 100% | 50% | Dose as GFR < 10 | Dose as GFR < 10 | Dose as GFR 10–50 |
| Erythromycin | 100% | 100% | 50%–75% | Dose as GFR < 10 | Dose as GFR < 10 | As normal GFR |
| Ethambutol | q24h | q24–36h | q48h | Dose as GFR < 10 | Dose as GFR < 10 | Dose as GFR 10–50 |
| Ethchlorvynol | 100% | Avoid | Avoid | Dose as GFR < 10 | Dose as GFR < 10 | NA |
| Ethionamide | 100% | 100% | 50% | Dose as GFR < 10 | Dose as GFR < 10 | Dose as GFR 10–50 |
| Ethosuximide | 100% | 100% | 75%–100% | As normal GFR | As normal GFR | As normal GFR |
| Etoposide | 100% | 75% | 50% | Dose as GFR < 10 | Dose as GFR < 10 | Dose as GFR 10–50 |
| Famciclovir | 100% | q12–24h | 50% q24–48h | Dose as GFR < 10 | Dose as GFR < 10 | Dose as GFR 10–50 |
| Famotidine | 100% | 50% | 20 mg q24h | Dose as GFR < 10 | Dose as GFR < 10 | Dose as GFR 10–50 |
| Fentanyl | 100% | 75% | 50% | Dose as GFR < 10 | Dose as GFR < 10 | Dose as GFR 10–50 |
| Fexofenadine | q12h | q12–24h | q24h | Dose as GFR < 10 | Dose as GFR < 10 | Dose as GFR 10–50 |
| Flecainide | 100% | 50% | 50% | Dose as GFR < 10 | Dose as GFR < 10 | Dose as GFR 10–50 |
| Fluconazole | 100% | 100% | 50% | Dose as GFR < 10 | Dose as GFR < 10 | As normal GFR |
| Flucytosine | 50 mg/kg q12h | 50 mg/kg q24h | 50 mg/kg q24–48h | Dose as GFR < 10 | Dose as GFR < 10 | Dose as GFR 10–50 |
| Fludarabine | 75%–100% | 75% | 50% | Dose as GFR < 10 | Dose as GFR < 10 | Dose as GFR 10–50 |
| Foscarnet | 28 mg/kg/q8h | 15 mg/kg/q8h | 6 mg/kg/q8h | Dose as GFR < 10 | Dose as GFR < 10 | Dose as GFR 10–50 |
| Fosinopril | 100% | 100% | 75%–100% | Dose as GFR < 10 | Dose as GFR < 10 | Dose as GFR 10–50 |
| Gabapentin | 300–600 mg q8h | 200–700 mg q12h | 100–300 mg q24h | LD: 300 mg<br>MD: 100–300 mg q24h | As normal GFR | As normal GFR |
| Gallamine | 75% | Avoid | Avoid | NA | NA | Avoid |
| Ganciclovir | 2.5–5 mg/kg q12h | 1.25–2.5 mg/kg q24h | 1.25 mg/kg q24h | Dose as GFR < 10 | Dose as GFR < 10 | 2.5 mg/kg q24h |
| Gemfibrozil | 100% | 75% | 50% | Dose as GFR < 10 | Dose as GFR < 10 | Dose as GFR 10–50 |
| Gentamicin[a] | 5–7 mg/kg/day | 2–3 mg/kg/day by levels | 2 mg/kg q48–72h by levels | 3 mg/kg after HD by levels | 3–4 mg/L/day by levels | Dose as GFR 10–50 by levels |
| Gliclazide | 50%–100% | 20–40 mg/day | 20–40 mg/day | Dose as GFR < 10 | Dose as GFR < 10 | Dose as GFR 10–50 |
| Glipizide | 100% | 50% | 50% | Dose as GFR < 10 | Dose as GFR < 10 | Dose as GFR < 10 |
| Guanadrel | q12h | q12–24h | q24–48h | Unknown | Unknown | Dose as GFR 10–50 |
| Guanethidine | q24h | q24h | q24–36h | Dose as GFR < 10 | Dose as GFR < 10 | Dose as GFR 10–50 |
| Hydralazine | q8h | q8h | q8–12h | Dose as GFR < 10 | Dose as GFR < 10 | Dose as GFR 10–50 |
| Hydroxyurea | 100% | 50% | 20% | Dose as GFR < 10 | Dose as GFR < 10 | Dose as GFR 10–50 |
| Hydroxyzine | 100% | 50% | 50% | Dose as GFR < 10 | Dose as GFR < 10 | Dose as GFR 10–50 |
| Idarubicin | 100% | 75% | 50% | Dose as GFR < 10 | Dose as GFR < 10 | Dose as GFR 10–50 |
| Ifosfamide | 100% | 75% | 50% | Dose as GFR < 10 | Dose as GFR < 10 | Dose as GFR 10–50 |
| Iloprost | 100% | 100% | 50% | Dose as GFR < 10 | Dose as GFR < 10 | Dose as GFR 10–50 |
| Imipenem | 100% | 50% | 25% | Dose as GFR < 10 | Dose as GFR < 10 | Dose as GFR 10–50 |
| Indapamide | 100% | 100% | 50% | Dose as GFR < 10 | Dose as GFR < 10 | NA |
| Indobufen | 100% | 50% | 25% | Unknown | Unknown | Unknown |
| Isoniazid | 100% | 100% | 75%–100% | Dose as GFR < 10 | Dose as GFR < 10 | As normal GFR |

| | | | | | | |
|---|---|---|---|---|---|---|
| Kanamycin[a] | 7.5 mg/kg q12h | 7.5 mg/kg q24–72h | 7.5 mg/kg q48–72h | 50% the normal dose | 15–20 mg/L/day | Dose as GFR 10–50 |
| Ketorolac | 100% | 50% | 50% | Dose as GFR < 10 | Dose as GFR < 10 | Dose as GFR 10–50 |
| Lamivudine | 100% | 50–150 mg q24h | 25–50 mg q24h | Dose as GFR < 10 | Dose as GFR < 10 | 50 mg q24h |
| Lenalidomide | 100% | 10 mg q24h for 30–60 mL/min<br>15 mg q48h for 10–29 mL/min | Avoid | 5 mg q24h after HD | Avoid | Avoid |
| Lepirudin | 100% | 25%–50% | Avoid | Avoid | Avoid | Avoid |
| Levofloxacin | 100% | 50% | 25%–50% | Dose as GFR < 10 | Dose as GFR < 10 | Dose as GFR 10–50 |
| Lincomycin | q6h | q6–12h | q12–24h | Dose as GFR < 10 | Dose as GFR < 10 | Dose as GFR 10–50 |
| Lisinopril | 100% | 50%–75% | 25%–50% | Dose as GFR < 10 | Dose as GFR < 10 | Dose as GFR 10–50 |
| Lithium carbonate[a] | 100% | 50%–75% | 25%–50% | Dose as GFR < 10 | Dose as GFR < 10 | Dose as GFR 10–50 |
| Lomefloxacin | 100% | 50%–100% | 50% | Dose as GFR < 10 | Dose as GFR < 10 | Dose as GFR 10–50 |
| Loracarbef | q12h | q24h | q3–5days | Dose as GFR < 10 | Dose as GFR < 10 | Dose as GFR 10–50 |
| Melphalan | 100% | 75% | 50% | Dose as GFR < 10 | Dose as GFR < 10 | Dose as GFR 10–50 |
| Meperidine | 100% | 75% | 50% | Avoid | Avoid | Avoid |
| Meprobamate | q6h | q9–12h | q12–18h | Dose as GFR < 10 | Dose as GFR < 10 | Dose as GFR 10–50 |
| Meropenem | 500 mg–2 g q8h | 500 mg–1 g q12h | 500 mg–1 g q24h | Dose as GFR < 10 | Dose as GFR < 10 | Dose as GFR 10–50 |
| Metformin | 100% | 30–50 mL/min: 25%–50%<br>10–29 mL/min: 25% | Avoid | Avoid | Avoid | Avoid |
| Methadone | 100% | 100% | 50%–75% | Dose as GFR < 10 | Dose as GFR < 10 | Dose as GFR 10–50 |
| Methotrexate | 100% | 50% | Avoid | Avoid | Avoid | Dose as GFR 10–50 |
| Methyldopa | q8h | q8–12h | q12–24h | Dose as GFR < 10 | Dose as GFR < 10 | Dose as GFR 10–50 |
| Metoclopramide | 100% | 75% | 50% | Dose as GFR < 10 | Dose as GFR < 10 | Dose as GFR 10–50 |
| Metocurine | 75% | 50% | 50% | Unknown | Unknown | Dose as GFR 10–50 |
| Mexiletine | 100% | 100% | 50%–75% | Dose as GFR < 10 | Dose as GFR < 10 | As normal GFR |
| Midazolam | 100% | 100% | 50% | Dose as GFR < 10 | Dose as GFR < 10 | As normal GFR |
| Midodrine | 5–10 mg q8h | 5–10 mg q8h | 2.5–10 mg q8h | Dose as GFR < 10 | Dose as GFR < 10 | Dose as GFR 10–50 |
| Milrinone | 100% | 100% | 50%–75% | No data | No data | Dose as GFR 10–50 |
| Mitomycin C | 100% | 100% | 75% | Dose as GFR < 10 | Dose as GFR < 10 | As normal GFR |
| Mivacurium | 100% | 50% | 50% | Dose as GFR < 10 | Dose as GFR < 10 | Dose as GFR 10–50 |
| Morphine | 100% | 75% | 50% | Dose as GFR < 10 | Dose as GFR < 10 | Dose as < 10 |
| Mycophenolate mofetil | 100% | 50%–100% | 50%–100% | Dose as GFR < 10 | Dose as GFR < 10 | As normal GFR |
| *N*-Acetylcysteine | 100% | 100% | 75% | Dose as GFR < 10 | Dose as GFR < 10 | Dose as GFR 10–50 |
| Nadolol | q24h | q24–48h | q48h | Dose as GFR < 10 | Dose as GFR < 10 | Dose as GFR 10–50 |
| Nalidixic acid | 100% | Avoid | Avoid | Avoid | Avoid | Avoid |
| Neostigmine | 100% | 50% | 25% | Dose as GFR < 10 | Dose as GFR < 10 | Dose as GFR 10–50 |
| Netilmicin[a] | 4–7.5 mg/kg/day | 3–7.5 mg/kg/day | 2 mg/kg Q24h | 2 mg/kg after each HD | IV: 2 mg/kg Q48h | Dose as GFR 10–50 |
| Nicotinic acid | 100% | 50% | 25% | Dose as GFR < 10 | Dose as GFR < 10 | Dose as GFR 10–50 |
| Nitroprusside | 100% | 100% | Avoid | Avoid | Avoid | Dose as GFR 10–50 |
| Nitrosoureas | 100% | 75% | 25%–50% | Dose as GFR < 10 | Dose as GFR < 10 | Unknown |
| Nizatidine | 75%–100% | 50% | 25% | Dose as GFR < 10 | Dose as GFR < 10 | Dose as GFR 10–50 |
| Norfloxacin | q12h | q12–24h | q24h | Dose as GFR < 10 | Dose as GFR < 10 | Dose as GFR 10–50 |
| Ofloxacin | 100% | 50% | 25% | Dose as GFR < 10 | Dose as GFR < 10 | Dose as GFR 10–50 |
| Oxcarbazepine | 100% | 75%–100% | 50% | Dose as GFR < 10 | Dose as GFR < 10 | Dose as GFR 10–50 |
| Pancuronium | 100% | 50% | 25% | Dose as GFR < 10 | Dose as GFR < 10 | Dose as GFR 10–50 |
| Paroxetine | 100% | 50%–75% | 50% | Dose as GFR < 10 | Dose as GFR < 10 | Dose as GFR 10–50 |

*Continued on following page*

**Table 61.8 Recommendations for Dosing Selected Drugs in Patients With Chronic Kidney Disease or Acute Kidney Injury (Cont'd)**

| | Degree of Drug Dose Reduction or Interval Prolongation | | | Dosage Recommendations for Patients Receiving Renal Replacement Therapy | | |
|---|---|---|---|---|---|---|
| **Drug** | GFR > 50 mL/min | GFR = 10–50 mL/min | GFR < 10 mL/min | HD | CAPD | CRRT |
| *p*-Aminosalicylic acid | 100% | 50%–75% | 50% | Dose as GFR < 10 | Dose as GFR < 10 | Dose as GFR 10–50 |
| Penicillamine | 100% | Avoid | Avoid | Avoid | Avoid | Avoid |
| Penicillin G | 100% | 75% | 20%–50% | Dose as GFR < 10 | Dose as GFR < 10 | Dose as GFR 10–50 |
| Pentamidine | q24h | q24h | q24–36h | Dose as GFR < 10 | Dose as GFR < 10 | Dose as GFR 10–50 |
| Pentazocine | 100% | 75% | 50% | Dose as GFR < 10 | Unknown | Dose as GFR 10–50 |
| Pentopril | 100% | 50%–75% | 50% | Dose as GFR < 10 | Dose as GFR < 10 | Dose as GFR 10–50 |
| Pentoxifylline | q8–12h | q12–24h | q24h | Dose as GFR < 10 | Dose as GFR < 10 | Dose as GFR 10–50 |
| Perindopril | 2 mg q24h | 2 mg q24–48h | 2 mg q48h | Dose as GFR < 10 | Dose as GFR < 10 | Dose as GFR 10–50 |
| Phenobarbital | q8–12h | q8–12h | q12–16h | Does as GFR < 10 | Dose as GFR < 10 | Dose as GFR 10–50 |
| Phenylbutazone | 100% | 50% | Avoid | Dose as GFR < 10 | Dose as GFR < 10 | Dose as GFR 10–50 |
| Pipecuronium | 100% | 50% | 25% | Avoid | Avoid | Dose as GFR 10–50 |
| Piperacillin | q6h | q6–12h | q12h | Dose as GFR < 10 | Dose as GFR < 10 | Dose as GFR 10–50 |
| Plicamycin | 100% | 75% | 50% | Unknown | Dose as GFR < 10 | Dose as GFR 10–50 |
| Pomalidomide | 100% | Avoid | Avoid | Unknown | Unknown | Unknown |
| Pravastatin | 100% | 30–50 mL/min: 100%<br>10–30 mL/min: 10 mg q24h | 10 mg q24h | Dose as GFR < 10 | Unknown | Unknown |
| Pregabalin | 100% q8–12h | 50% q8–12h | 25% q24h | Dose as GFR < 10 | Dose as GFR < 10 | Dose as GFR 10–50 |
| Primidone | q12 | q12–24h | q24h | Dose as GFR < 10 | Dose as GFR < 10 | Dose as GFR 10–50 |
| Probenecid | 100% | Avoid | Avoid | Avoid | Avoid | Avoid |
| Procainamide | q4h | q6–12h | q8–24h | Follow levels | Dose as GFR < 10 | Dose as GFR 10–50 |
| Propoxyphene | 100% | 100% | Avoid | Avoid | Avoid | Avoid |
| Propylthiouracil | 100% | 75% | 50% | Dose as GFR < 10 | Dose as GFR < 10 | Dose as GFR 10–50 |
| Pyrazinamide | 100% | 100% | 50%–100% | Dose as GFR < 10 | Dose as GFR < 10 | Dose as GFR 10–50 |
| Pyridostigmine | 100% | 35% | 20% | Dose as GFR < 10 | Dose as GFR < 10 | Dose as GFR 10–50 |
| Quinapril | 100% | 2.5–5 mg q24h | 2.5 mg q24h | Dose as GFR < 10 | Dose as GFR < 10 | Dose as GFR 10–50 |
| Quinine | q8h | q8–12h | q24h | Dose as GFR < 10 | Dose as GFR < 10 | Dose as GFR 10–50 |
| Ramipril | 100% | 50% | 25% | Dose as GFR < 10 | Dose as GFR < 10 | Dose as GFR 10–50 |
| Ranitidine | 100% | 150 mg q24h | 75 mg q24h | Dose as GFR < 10 | Dose as GFR < 10 | Dose as GFR 10–50 |
| Ribavirin | 100% | Avoid | Avoid | Avoid | Avoid | Avoid |
| Rifampin | 100% | 50%–100% | 50%–100% | Dose as GFR < 10 | Dose as GFR < 10 | As normal GFR |
| Rivaroxaban | 100% | 15–50 mL/min 15 mg q24h | Avoid | Avoid | Avoid | Avoid |
| Simvastatin | 100% | 100% | 5 mg q24h | Dose as GFR < 10 | Dose as GFR < 10 | As normal GFR |
| Sitagliptin | 100% | 30–50 mL/min: 50%<br>10–30 mL/min: 25% | 25% | Dose as GFR < 10 | Dose as GFR < 10 | Dose as GFR 10–50 |
| Sotalol | 100% | 25%–50% | 25% | Dose as GFR < 10 | Dose as GFR < 10 | Dose as GFR 10–50 |
| Spironolactone | 100% | Usual dose q12–24h | Avoid | Avoid | Dose as GFR < 10 | Dose as GFR 10–50 |
| Stavudine | 100% | 50% q12–24h | 50% q24h | Avoid | Avoid | Avoid |
| Streptomycin[a] | q24h | q24–72h | q72–96h | Dose as GFR < 10 | 20–40 mg/L/day | Dose as GFR 10–50 |
| Streptozocin | 100% | 75% | 50% | Unknown | Unknown | Unknown |
| Sulfamethoxazole | q12h | q18h | q24h | 1 g after dialysis | 1 g/day | Dose as GFR 10–50 |
| Sulfinpyrazone | 100% | 100% | Avoid | Avoid | Avoid | Dose as GFR 10–50 |
| Sulfisoxazole | q6h | q8–12h | q12–24h | 2 g after dialysis | 3 g/day | NA |
| Sulindac | 100% | 50%–100% | 50%–100% | Dose as GFR < 10 | Dose as GFR < 10 | Dose as GFR < 10 |

| | | | | | | |
|---|---|---|---|---|---|---|
| Sulotroban | 50% | 30% | 10% | Unknown | Unknown | Unknown |
| Tazobactam | 100% | 75% | 50% | Dose as GFR < 10 | Dose as GFR < 10 | Dose as GFR 10–50 |
| Teicoplanin | q24h | q24–48h | q48–72h | Dose as GFR < 10 | Dose as GFR < 10 | Dose as GFR 10–50 |
| Temocillin | q12–24h | q24h | q48h | Dose as GFR < 10 | Dose as GFR < 10 | Dose as GFR 10–50 |
| Terbutaline | 100% | 50% | Avoid | Dose as GFR < 10 | Dose as GFR < 10 | Dose as GFR 10–50 |
| Tetracycline | 100% | 100% | 50% | Dose as GFR < 10 | Dose as GFR < 10 | Dose as GFR 10–50 |
| Thiazides | 100% | 100% | Avoid | Dose as GFR < 10 | Dose as GFR < 10 | NA |
| Thiopental | 100% | 100% | 75% | NA | NA | NA |
| Ticarcillin | 50–75 mg/kg q6h | 50–75 mg/kg q8h | 50–75 mg/kg q12h | Dose as GFR < 10 | Dose as GFR < 10 | Dose as GFR 10–50 |
| Tobramycin[a] | 5–7 mg/kg/day | 2–3 mg/kg/day | 2 mg/kg q48–72h | 3 mg/kg after HD | 3–4 mg/L/day | Dose as GFR 10–50 |
| Tolvaptan | 100% | 100% | Avoid | Avoid | Avoid | Avoid |
| Topiramate | 100% | 50% | 25% | Dose as GFR < 10 | Dose as GFR < 10 | Dose as GFR 10–50 |
| Topotecan | 75% | 50% | 25% | Dose as GFR < 10 | No data | No data |
| Tramadol | 100% | 50–100 mg q8h | 50 mg q8h | Dose as GFR < 10 | Dose as GFR < 10 | Dose as GFR 10–50 |
| Tranexamic acid | 50% | 25% | 10% | Dose as GFR < 10 | Dose as GFR < 10 | Dose as GFR 10–50 |
| Trazodone | 100% | 100% | Avoid/50% | Dose as GFR < 10 | Dose as GFR < 10 | Dose as GFR 10–50 |
| Triamterene | 100% | Avoid | Avoid | Avoid | Avoid | Avoid |
| Trimethoprim | q12h | q12h | q24h | Dose as GFR < 10 | Dose as GFR < 10 | Dose as GFR 10–50 |
| Trimetrexate | 100% | 50%–100% | Avoid | No data | No data | Dose as GFR 10–50 |
| Tubocurarine | 75% | 50% | Avoid | Unknown | Unknown | Dose as GFR 10–50 |
| Valganciclovir | 50%–100% | 450 mg q24–48h | 450 mg q72–96h | Avoid | Avoid | 450 mg q48h |
| Vancomycin[a] | 1 g q12–24h | 1 g q24–96h | 1 g q4–7days | Dose as GFR < 10 | Dose as GFR < 10 | Dose as GFR 10–50 |
| Venlafaxine | 100% | 25%–50% | 25%–50% | Dose as GFR 10–50 | Dose as GFR < 10 | Dose as GFR 10–50 |
| Vigabatrin | 100% | 50% | 25% | Dose as GFR < 10 | Dose as GFR < 10 | Dose as GFR 10–50 |
| Zalcitabine | 100% | q12h | q24h | Dose as GFR < 10 | No data | Dose as GFR 10–50 |
| Zidovudine (AZT) | 100% q8h | 100% q8h | 50% q8h | Dose as GFR < 10 | Dose as GFR < 10 | Dose as GFR 10–50 |
| Zileuton | 100% | 100% | 100% | Dose as GFR < 10 | Unknown | Dose as GFR 10–50 |
| Zopiclone | 100% | 3.75–5 mg daily | 3.75–5 mg daily | Dose as GFR < 10 | Dose as GFR < 10 | Dose as GFR < 10 |

[a]Adjust dose to achieve desired serum concentrations using measured serum concentrations and pharmacokinetic modeling principles.

*AZT,* Azidothymidine; *BID,* two times a day; *CAPD,* continuous ambulatory peritoneal dialysis; *CRRT,* continuous renal replacement therapy; *GFR,* glomerular filtration rate; *HD,* hemodialysis; *IV,* intravenous; *LD,* loading dose; *MD,* maintenance dose; *NA,* not applicable; q*n*days, every *n* days; q*n*h, every *n* hours.

## KEY REFERENCES


6. Matzke GR, Aronoff GR, Atkinson AJ Jr, et al. Drug dosing consideration in patients with acute and chronic kidney disease—a clinical update from Kidney Disease: Improving Global Outcomes (KDIGO). *Kidney Int.* 2011;80:1122–1137.
7. Matzke GR, Nolin TN. Drug dosing in renal disease. In: Bomback A, Gilbert S, Perazella M, et al, eds. *National Kidney Foundation Primer on Kidney Diseases.* 7th ed. Philadelphia: Elsevier; 2017.
8. Zeng X, McMahon GM, Brunelli SM, et al. Incidence, outcomes, and comparisons across definitions of AKI in hospitalized individuals. *Clin J Am Soc Nephrol.* 2014;9:12–20.
15. Chan CT, Covic A, Craig JC, et al. Novel techniques and innovation in blood purification: a clinical update from Kidney Disease: Improving Global Outcomes. *Kidney Int.* 2013;83:359–371.
16. Hoste EA, Dhondt A. Clinical review: use of renal replacement therapies in special groups of ICU patients. *Crit Care.* 2012;16:201–211.
17. Heintz BH, Matzke GR, Dager WE. Antimicrobial dosing concepts and recommendations for critically ill adult patients receiving continuous renal replacement therapy or intermittent hemodialysis. *Pharmacotherapy.* 2009;29:562–577.
18. Dowling TC, Matzke GR, Murphy JE, et al. Evaluation of renal drug dosing: prescribing information and clinical pharmacist approaches. *Pharmacotherapy.* 2010;30:776–786.
19. Matzke GR, Dowling TC, Marks SA, et al. Influence of kidney disease on drug disposition: an assessment of industry studies submitted to the FDA for new chemical entities 1999–2010. *J Clin Pharmacol.* 2016;56:390–398.
20. Chang F, O'Hare AM, Miao Y, et al. Use of renally inappropriate medications in older veterans: a national study. *J Am Geriatr Soc.* 2015;63:2290–2297.
25. Khanal A, Castelino RL, Peterson GM, et al. Dose adjustment guidelines for medications inpatients with renal impairment: how consistent are the drug information sources? *Intern Med J.* 2014;44(1):77–85.
27. Czock D, Spitaletta M, Keller F. Suboptimal antimicrobial drug exposure in patients with renal impairment. *Int J Clin Pharm.* 2015;37:906–916.
28. Awdishu L, Coates CR, Lyddane A, et al. The impact of real-time alerting on appropriate prescribing in kidney disease: a cluster randomized controlled trial. *J Am Med Inform Assoc.* 2016;23:609–616.
30. Muller C, Mimitrov Y, Imhoff O, et al. Oral antidiabetics use among diabetic type 2 patients with chronic kidney disease. Do nephrologists take account of recommendations? *J Diabetes Complications.* 2016;30:675–680.
39. Borst P, Schinkel AH. P-glycoprotein ABCB1: a major player in drug handling by mammals. *J Clin Invest.* 2013;123:4131–4133.
51. Verbeeck RK, Musuamba FT. Pharmacokinetics and dosage adjustment in patients with renal dysfunction. *Eur J Clin Pharmacol.* 2009;65:757–773.
61. Yeung CK, Shen DD, Thummel KE, et al. Effects of chronic kidney disease and uremia on hepatic drug metabolism and transport. *Kidney Int.* 2014;85:522–528.
63. Thomson BK, Nolin TD, Velenosi TJ, et al. Effect of CKD and dialysis modality on exposure to drugs cleared by nonrenal mechanisms. *Am J Kidney Dis.* 2015;65:574–582.
67. Vilay AM, Churchwell MD, Mueller BA. Drug metabolism and clearance in acute kidney injury. *Crit Care.* 2008;12:235–243.
72. Joy MS, Frye RF, Nolin TD, et al. In vivo alterations in drug metabolism and transport pathways in patients with chronic kidney diseases. *Pharmacotherapy.* 2014;34:114–122.
75. Hsueh CH, Yoshida K, Zhao P, et al. Identification and quantitative assessment of uremic solutes as inhibitors of renal organic anion transporters, OAT1 and OAT3. *Mol Pharm.* 2016;13:3130–3140.
78. Godman B, Finlayson AE, Cheema PK, et al. Personalizing health care: feasibility and future implications. *BMC Med.* 2013;11:179–202.
89. Drozda K, Müller DJ, Bishop JR. Pharmacogenomic testing for neuropsychiatric drugs: current status of drug labelling, guidelines for using genetic information, and test options. *Pharmacotherapy.* 2014;34:166–184.
91. Becker ML, Pearson ER, Tkáč I. Pharmacogenetics of oral antidiabetic drugs. *Int J Endocrinol.* 2013, doi:10.1155/2013/686315.
92. Needham M, Mastaglia FL. Statin myotoxicity: a review of genetic susceptibility factors. *Neuromuscul Disord.* 2014;24:4–15.
93. Kawaguchi-Suzuki M, Frye RF. The role of pharmacogenetics in the treatment of chronic hepatitis C infection. *Pharmacotherapy.* 2014;34:185–201.
103. Patel HN, Ursan ID, Zueger PM, et al. Stakeholder views on pharmacogenomic testing. *Pharmacotherapy.* 2014;34:151–165.
111. Czock D, Markert C, Hartman B, et al. Pharmacokinetics and pharmacodynamics of antimicrobial drugs. *Expert Opin Drug Metab Toxicol.* 2009;5:475–487.
114. Eyler RF, Mueller BA. Antibiotic dosing in critically ill patients with acute kidney injury. *Nat Rev Nephrol.* 2011;7:226–235.
122. Earley A, Miskulin D, Lamb EJ, et al. Estimating equations for glomerular filtration rate in the era of creatinine standardization. *Ann Intern Med.* 2012;156:785–795.
126. Steffl JL, Bennett W, Olyaei AJ. The old and new methods of assessing kidney function. *J Clin Pharmacol.* 2012;52:63S–71S.
127. Dowling TD. Quantification of renal function. In: DiPiro J, Talbert R, Yee G, et al, eds. *Pharmacotherapy: A Pathophysiologic Approach.* 10th ed. New York: McGraw-Hill; 2017.
130. Lee E, Collier CP, White CA. Interlaboratory variability in plasma creatinine measurement and the relation with estimated glomerular filtration rate and chronic kidney disease diagnosis. *Clin J Am Soc Nephrol.* 2017;12:29–37.
147. Lim AK, Mathanasenarajah G, Larmour I. Assessment of aminoglycoside dosing and estimated glomerular filtration rate in determining gentamicin and tobramycin are under the curve and clearance. *Intern Med J.* 2015;45:319–329.
153. Schwartz GJ, Schneider MF, Maier PS, et al. Improved equations estimating GFR in children with chronic kidney disease using an immunonephelometric determination of cystatin C. *Kidney Int.* 2012;82:445–453.
162. Bouchard J, Macedo E, Soroko S, et al. Comparison of methods for estimating glomerular filtration rate in critically ill patients with acute kidney injury. *Nephrol Dial Transplant.* 2010;25:102–107.
163. Chen S. Retooling the creatinine clearance equation to estimate kinetic GFR when the plasma creatinine is changing acutely. *J Am Soc Nephrol.* 2013;24:877–888.
164. Matthew AT, Fishbane S, Obi Y, et al. Preservation of residual kidney function in hemodialysis patients: reviving an old concept. *Kidney Int.* 2016;90:262–271.
165. Lee MJ, Park JT, Park KS, et al. Prognostic value of residual urine volume, GFR by 24-uhour urine collection, and eGFR in patients receiving dialysis. *Clin J Am Soc Nephrol.* 2017;12:426–434.
169. Shafi T, Michels WM, Levey AS, et al. Estimating residual kidney function in dialysis patients without urine collection. *Kidney Int.* 2016;89:1099–1110.
179. European Medicines Agency. Note for guidance on the evaluation of the pharmacokinetics of medicinal products in patients with impaired renal function. Available at: http://www.ema.europa.eu/docs/en_GB/document_library/Scientific_guideline/2016/02/WC500200841.pdf Accessed April 25, 2017.
190. Zhuang L, He Y, Xia H, et al. Gentamicin dosing strategy in patients with end-stage renal disease receiving hemodialysis: evaluation using a semi-mechanistic pharmacokinetic/pharmacodynamics model. *J Antimicrob Chemother.* 2016;71:1012–1021.
198. Lewis SJ, Mueller BA. Antibiotic dosing in patients with acute kidney injury: "enough but not too much." *J Intensive Care Med.* 2016;31(3):64–76.
201. Daugirdas JT, Blake PG, Ing TS. *Handbook of Dialysis.* 5th ed. Philadelphia: Lippincott Williams & Wilkins; 2014.
202. Tieu A, Leither M, Urquhart BL, et al. Clearance of cardiovascular medications during hemodialysis. *Curr Opin Nephrol Hypertens.* 2016;25:257–267.
209. Mei JP, Ali-Moghaddam A, Mueller BA. Survey of pharmacists' antibiotic dosing recommendations for sustained low-efficiency dialysis. *Int J Clin Pharm.* 2016;38:127–134.
236. Oguri T, Shimokata T, Ito I, et al. Extension of the Calvert formula to patients with severe renal insufficiency. *Cancer Chemother Pharmacol.* 2015;76:53–59.
251. Jamal JA, Mueller BA, Choi GYS, et al. How can we ensure effective antibiotic dosing in critically ill patients receiving different types of renal replacement therapy? *Diagn Microbiol Infect Dis.* 2015;82:92–103.
252. Janknegt R, Nube MJ. A simple method for predicting drug clearances during CAPD. Available at: http://www.pdiconnect.com/content/5/4/254.2.full.pdf+html. Accessed March 15, 2015.
254. Ballinger AE, Palmer SC, Wiggins KJ, et al. Treatment for peritoneal dialysis-associated peritonitis. *Cochrane Database Syst Rev.* 2014;(4):CD005284, doi:10.1002/14651858.CD005284.pub3.
255. Li PKT, Szeto CC, Piraino B, et al. ISPD Peritonitis recommendations: 2016 update on prevention and treatment. *Perit Dial Int.* 2016;36:481–508.

62

# Supportive Care in Advanced Chronic Kidney Disease

Sara Davison

CHAPTER OUTLINE



KEY POINTS

- "Kidney supportive care" is replacing the term "kidney palliative care" and encompasses services aimed at improving the quality of life (QOL) for chronic kidney disease (CKD) patients, at any age, throughout the continuum of illness, regardless of life expectancy. It can be provided together with therapies intended to prolong life, such as dialysis, and requires culturally sensitive shared decision making to prioritize the components of medical care most important to the patient. This includes careful attention to physical and emotional symptom management and advance care planning.
- Dialysis treatment may address some symptoms, such as fatigue, anorexia, nausea, and vomiting, especially for more robust individuals with less comorbidity, but it may do little to address symptom burden in more frail patients or those with multimorbidity. When taken as a whole, symptom burden is similar in predialysis G5 CKD patients, those treated with conservative kidney management (i.e., those who have chosen nondialysis care), and those on chronic dialysis.
- The Edmonton Symptom Assessment System: Renal (ESAS-r: Renal) is a simple tool to screen for 12 commonly experienced symptoms in CKD using 0–10 visual analog scales.
- The aim of symptom management is to ameliorate symptoms that are burdensome and adversely impact the patient's QOL as it is not always necessary or possible to resolve them completely. This usually requires that symptoms be treated to ≤3/10.
- Gabapentin can be used to effectively treat neuropathic pain, restless legs, pruritus, and insomnia if used carefully in low doses and titrated slowly to effect.
- Dialysis is unlikely to benefit patients with significant preexisting functional or cognitive impairment and high levels of comorbidity. These patients are often better cared for with conservative kidney management and careful attention to the principles of kidney supportive care.

Despite advances in predialysis care and dialysis technology, people with advanced chronic kidney disease (CKD) continue to have a shortened life expectancy and poor outcomes, including physical, emotional, and spiritual suffering, and low quality of life (QOL).[1] The majority of patients die in acute care facilities, with aggressive care plans in place[2] and without accessing palliative care services.[3–6] Current end-of-life care practices are not consistent with patients' preferences.[7,8]

Supportive care is central to the provision of patient-centered care for patients with chronic diseases. Many countries are placing increased emphasis on the provision of supportive and end-of-life care by "generalist" and community providers as a component of usual care.[9] Kidney supportive care, therefore is increasingly being recognized as a core clinical competency for the care of patients with advanced CKD. Unfortunately, nephrologists are often not trained adequately to address multifactorial suffering and address many of the end-of-life challenges inherent in the care of their patients.[10] Consequently, patients with advanced CKD experience significant unmet care needs.[7,11,12] Training in supportive care for clinicians treating CKD patients is an urgent priority. This chapter aims to serve as an introduction to kidney supportive care and provide some of the foundations for understanding and delivering the key components of kidney supportive care.

## DEFINING KIDNEY SUPPORTIVE CARE

The modern hospice movement began in Britain by Dame Cicely Saunders in the 1960s and was concerned with terminal care, predominantly for cancer patients. Dr. Balfour Mount, a Canadian physician, who opened one of the first two hospice programs in Canada in 1975, coined the term "palliative care" to replace the word "hospice," which in Canada was commonly considered a place of last resort for the derelict. However, these programs continued to focus predominantly on the care of imminently dying cancer patients. Palliative medicine has undergone many developments since then and has extended the range of services, the timing of services within the illness trajectory, and the eligible patient groups such that palliative care is no longer limited to terminal care focused primarily on those dying with cancer. The WHO defines palliative care as "an approach that improves the QOL of patients and their families facing the problems associated with life-threatening illness, through the prevention and relief of suffering by means of early identification and impeccable assessment and treatment of pain and other problems, physical, psychosocial and spiritual."[13]

Unfortunately, despite the evolution of palliative care over the past several decades, the belief that "palliative care" and "terminal care" are synonymous, such that only patients at the end of life are appropriate for palliative care, remains prevalent among patients, family, and health–care providers.[14,15] This is not appropriate for patients with CKD who frequently have high palliative care needs for years before death. For this reason, the term "supportive care" has emerged as yet another term to describe noncurative treatments focused on improving QOL and is increasingly being used to replace the term "palliative care," until the more terminal phase of life. Both patients and health–care professionals appear to prefer this.[16–18] The international kidney community, therefore, is increasingly using the term, "kidney supportive care," rather than "kidney palliative care."[1] The term "kidney supportive care" is used throughout this chapter, with the understanding that it conceptually presents the World Health Organization (WHO) definition for palliative care. Kidney supportive care, therefore, is defined as services aimed at improving the QOL for patients with established CKD, at any age, throughout the continuum of illness, regardless of life expectancy and can be provided together with therapies intended to prolong life, such as dialysis.[1] Kidney supportive care is not restricted to withdrawal of dialysis or conservative (nondialysis) kidney management. End-of-life care (sometimes referred to as "terminal care" or "hospice care") is under the umbrella of supportive care but is typically limited to the care of patients who are believed to be within months of death (Fig. 62.1). Ideally, supportive care should be started early so that issues of suffering are addressed as they present. As illness progresses, the need for supportive care services is likely to increase and may progress into terminal, end-of-life care.

## KEY COMPONENTS OF KIDNEY SUPPORTIVE CARE

Kidney supportive care is patient-centered care that integrates culturally sensitive shared decision making to (1) prioritize the components of medical care most important to the patient and (2) ensure those priorities guide clinical decisions.[19–23] Kidney supportive care includes relief of suffering through meticulous symptom assessment and management; emotional, social and spiritual support; patient-specific estimates of prognosis; advance care planning; and the consideration of treatment options such as conservative kidney management (CKM)—that is, nondialysis care—and the appropriate and timely withdrawal of dialysis. Recent patient engagement has highlighted many of these issues as top priorities for people with advanced CKD.[24] A comprehensive approach to kidney supportive care must also integrate a way to identify patients most likely to benefit from supportive care interventions (Fig. 62.2). Each of these components of kidney supportive care is discussed within the context of CKD.

## CULTURALLY COMPETENT SHARED DECISION MAKING

Culturally competent shared decision making is the foundation of kidney supportive care and must be incorporated into all components from assessment and management of suffering, sharing prognosis, advance care planning, through to delivery of end-of-life care and bereavement support (see Fig. 62.2). To relieve suffering and provide care aligned to the preferences and goals of the individual patient, care teams must understand and incorporate the patient's needs and perspective and adapt the care plan to facilitate integration of the patient's lifestyle, including his or her family and social community. This means allowing the components of medical care deemed most important to the patient to be prioritized.[19–23] This may require balancing the management of symptoms (e.g., dizziness and fatigue) with optimal control of blood pressure or serum chemistry with greater emphasis

Curative/remittive care
Kidney supportive care
Terminal/
end-of-life
care
Bereavement
Presentation of illness
Death
Based on supportive care needs
rather than prognosis
Patient is identified as dying
(usually with a prognosis ≤ 6 months)

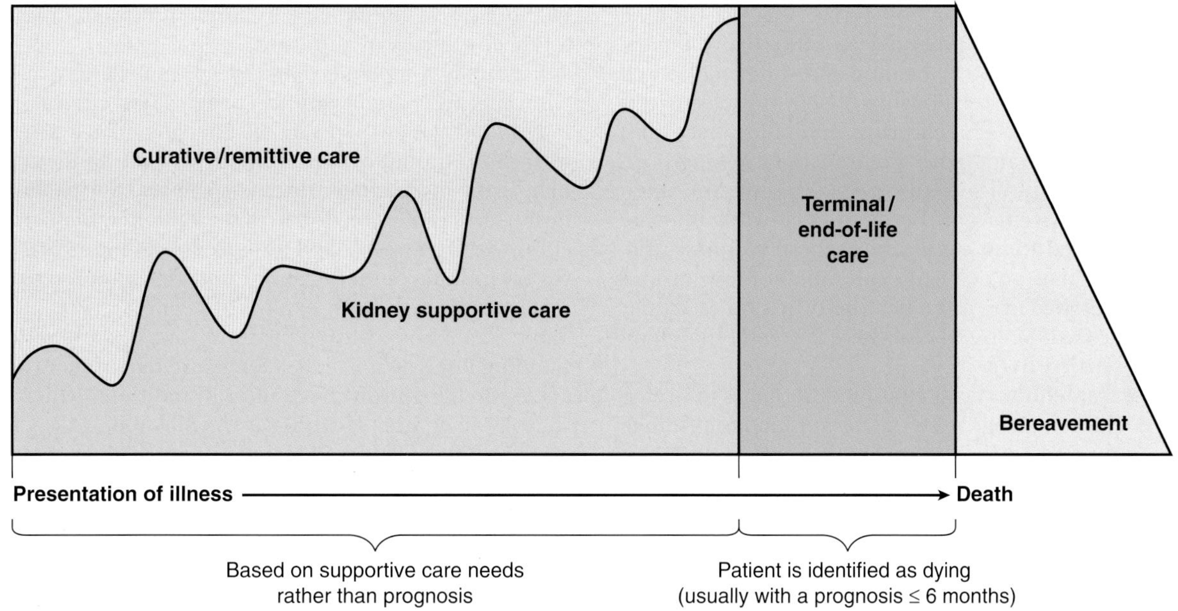

**Fig. 62.1** Conceptual framework for kidney supportive care.

Identification of patients most likely to benefit from supportive care
Patients at high risk for death within the next year
If you answer "No" to the Surprise Question.
"Would you be surprised if the patient died in the next 12 months?"
General indicators of decline
Functional or cognitive decline
Repeated unplanned admissions
Specific clinical indicators
Poor tolerance of dialysis with a change in modality
High physical or psychosocial symptom burden
CKM or withdrawal of dialysis
Poor or decreasing QOL
Decision making
Difficulty determining goals of care
Considering withdrawal from dialysis or CKM
Assess
Key components of kidney supportive care
Symptom management and relief of suffering
Physical symptom management
Emotional and psychosocial support
Includes anticipatory grief
Spiritual support
Address cultural domains of care where relevant
Prognostication
Consider all clinically relevant outcomes of importance to patients, for example:
Survival
Physical function
Quality of life
Cognitive function
Advance care planning
Goals of care
Identify surrogate decision-maker
Special considerations:
Conservative management or initiation of dialysis
Initiation of/or transition to palliative dialysis
Withdrawal of dialysis
Death
Bereavement support
Culturally competent shared decision

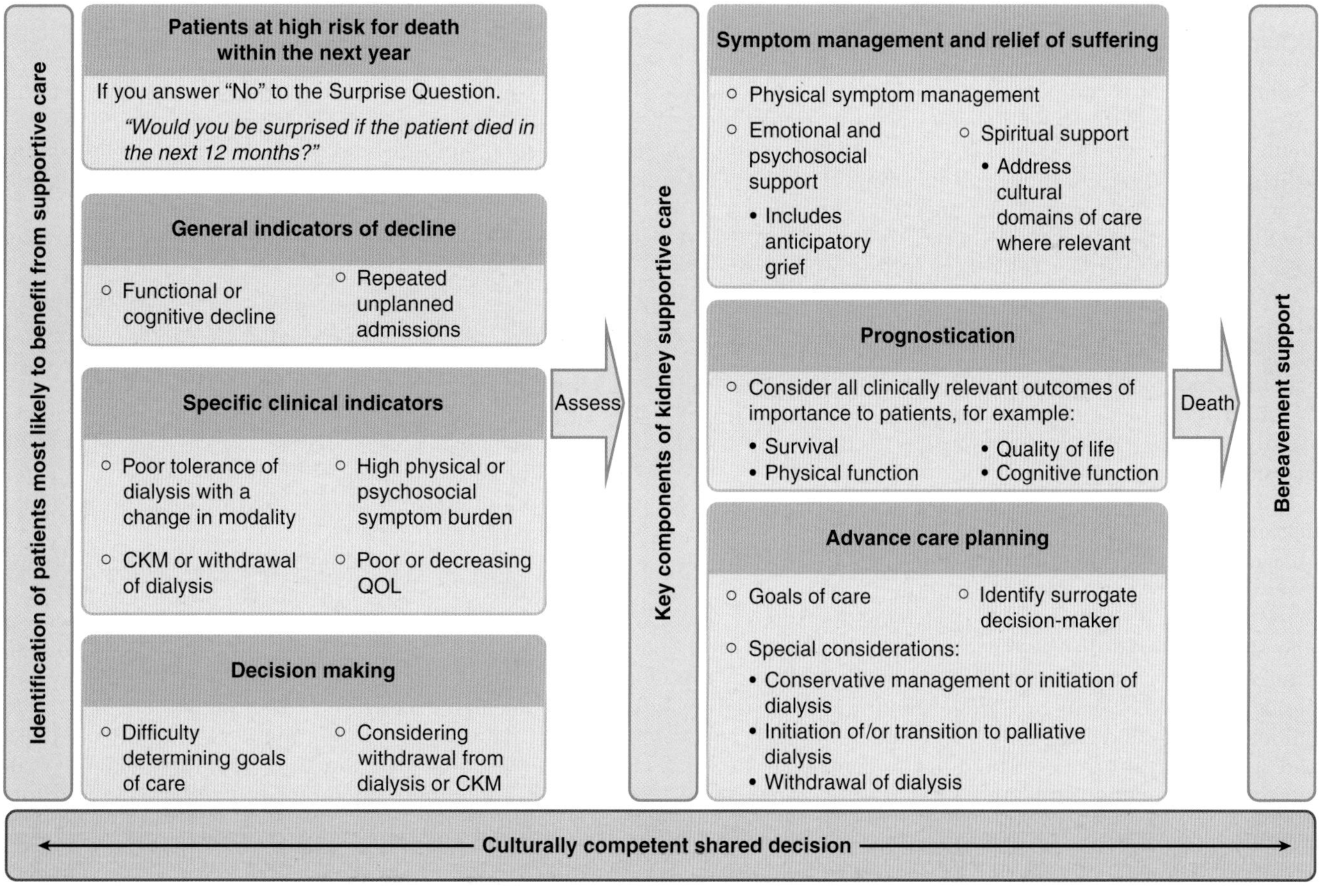

**Fig. 62.2** An approach to kidney supportive care. *CKM,* Conservative kidney management; *QOL,* quality of life. (Adapted from Davison SN. Integrating palliative care for patients with advanced chronic kidney disease: recent advances, remaining challenges. *J Palliat Care* 2011;27:53–61.)

being placed on managing bothersome symptoms rather than maximizing long-term health outcomes such as survival. As disease progresses, patients' goals of care often shift to focus almost exclusively on QOL rather than survival, with a strong emphasis on emotional, social, and family support.[7,25] The ethical imperatives of shared decision are discussed further in Chapter 82.

All cultures generate explanatory models that attempt to account for the phenomenon of illness; to define what a disease is, how it occurs, what measures can prevent or control it, and why some people and not others are affected. Culture, therefore, has enormous potential to influence patients' beliefs around life and death, healing and suffering, as well as the physician–patient relationship.[26] Cultural sensitivity is particularly important in delivering end-of-life care and cultural variations in end-of-life preferences have long been noted.[27] In multicultural societies, very different, and often divergent, value systems may be at work and health–care providers will need to be cognizant of these cultural influences. Although a more detailed exploration of how various cultural perspectives may influence the provision of kidney supportive care can be found elsewhere,[26] several high-level issues are discussed here.

There are tremendous cross-cultural differences in preferences for decision making. Western cultures tend to promote "patient autonomy," where the patient is viewed as the best person to make health–care decisions. However, many cultures are characterized by strong communal and social bonds where the person is viewed as a "relational-self," where social relationships, rather than individualism, provide the basis for moral judgments.[26] From this perspective, an insistence on self-determination erodes the value placed on personal interconnectedness and challenges the assumption that the patient should make his or her own medical decisions in isolation from their community. In practice, this might mean that the family or community receive and disclose information, even when the patient is competent.

In many parts of the world, the cultural norm is protection of the patient from the truth. This often involves cultural beliefs surrounding the cause and meaning of illness. This can complicate decision making, especially in the context of sharing prognosis. For example, some Aboriginal and Asian cultures prohibit explicit references to dying based on an interpretative framework in which language has the capacity to create reality.[28] Positive thinking is felt to promote health, whereas the delivery of bad news could shorten the life of the patient. Family members may prefer to communicate prognostic information themselves in such a way as to "balance" hope with the bad news. Health–care providers need to understand that in some contexts, this may be appropriate.

Cultural views can impact how patients want care to be delivered. Many cultures possess little knowledge of, or have little exposure to, palliative care and may be reluctant to receive this care without understanding the direct benefit to them. Cultural values may also determine who should and who should not be directly involved in providing physical care, with many cultures strongly preferring that family be directly involved.[29] Many non-Western cultures such as Traditional Chinese and indigenous cultures view the body, soul, and spirit as an integrated whole in the context of strong interpersonal relationships and may require access to a traditional healer. This may be viewed as similar to access to a hospital chaplain in a Western context.[30]

Many people from rural and remote areas wish to die at home connected to land and family for strong cultural reasons, yet are relocated for end-of-life care. For indigenous people, relocation at the end of life is an extremely frightening experience.[31] Culture also plays a role in the expression of suffering and grief, with many cultures being reluctant to complain of pain. Others are not comfortable with frank, direct styles of communication and therefore may not express suffering or grief overtly as this may be seen as inappropriate. In these cases, emotional containment does not mean indifference or a lack of suffering.

Culturally competent shared decision making requires that clinicians and patients jointly consider best clinical evidence in light of a patient's specific health characteristics and values within the framework of the patient's and family's cultural beliefs. In increasingly diverse societies, the challenge for health–care professionals is to understand how these numerous cultural differences shape the care for an individual patient. Cross-cultural communication strategies required to address this have recently been explored[32,33] and are summarized in Table 62.1. Cross-cultural communication starts with understanding one's own beliefs, values, and experiences and then acknowledging individual cultural traditions, which may be sharply divergent. Health–care professionals also need to recognize the diversity of beliefs and practices within cultural groups. The process of acculturating may complicate this and many people will hold blended cultural perspectives. Health–care professionals, therefore, must be careful not to assume the preferences of individuals based on their cultural group. When uncertain about how a patient or family perceives a situation, it is best simply to ask.[32,33]

## PROGNOSTICATION

Estimating and communicating prognosis to patients and family, balancing biomedical facts with relevant emotional, social, cultural, and spiritual issues, are required for shared decision making and providing supportive care.[1] Being able to prognosticate accurately helps health–care professionals identify high-risk patients, facilitate discussions regarding the need for targeted supportive care services, and align care pathways to best meet patients' needs. Given that supportive care focuses on the patient's priorities, patient-specific prognoses for relevant outcomes beyond survival, such as the impact of treatments on QOL, physical function, hospital-free survival, and symptoms, are needed. This would facilitate recommendations such as dialysis services to those most likely to benefit or CKM for those unlikely to benefit. For further discussions on appropriateness of initiating or forgoing dialysis, see Chapters 82 and 84.

Studies have shown that despite patients wanting to discuss their prognosis, it is often not done.[7,34] Prognostication is challenging in CKD given the great variation in individual illness trajectories.[35] Accurate prognostic models are limited, and nephrologists struggle to explain illness complexity and predict clinical trajectories.[36,37] Although there is a large volume of data on prognostic markers, individually these factors are often of little practical relevance. Only a small number of studies have attempted to combine these factors into clinically useful prognostic tools. A recent review highlights the limits and deficiencies of currently available prognostic tools,[38] which are outlined in Table 62.2. These tools are limited to progression of kidney failure and survival on dialysis. They do not prognosticate outcomes with non-dialysis (CKM) care, nor do they address patient or family concerns of QOL, function, and symptom burden.

As the field of prognostication moves forward, new markers may enhance current approaches. These may include identifying a decline in physical function using tools such as gait speed, a modified Karnofsky activity scale, activities of daily

**Table 62.1 Strategies for Culturally Competent Shared Decision Making**

| Task | Communication Strategy | Additional Considerations |
|---|---|---|
| Understand one's own beliefs, values, and experiences | Having an awareness of individual differences from that of the patient is important to create a respectful and nonbiased dialog. It will also help resolve conflict when differences with patients' beliefs and wishes arise. | Consider one's perspective as a clinician and the influence of the health–care system and institution within which one delivers care. |
| Understand the patient's experience | Ask about the patient as a person, where they are from and degree of integration within the ethnic community. Assess how the patient interprets his or her condition (i.e., the cause and impact). | This includes asking what their most important concerns are now that they have this illness. This establishes the groundwork for negotiating mutually acceptable goals for care. |
| Acknowledge individual cultural traditions | Ask about the patient's health beliefs, values, practices, and cultural communication etiquette. This includes attitudes toward truth telling. Avoid generalizing a patient's beliefs or values based on cultural norms. | The "RISK" reduction assessment is a helpful strategy to ascertain the level of cultural influence for a patient.[33] |
| Giving information | **Ask–Tell–Ask** (this strategy can extend to many of the tasks described here):<br>**Ask** the patient's understanding of his or her illness, what kind of information the patient and/or family needs, and how they want the information told.<br>**Tell** (give) information concisely, avoid jargon, and disclose only one to three pieces of information at any given time.<br>**Ask** what the patient understands or will take away from the conversation. | The final ask ensures the information has been understood and invites the patient and family to share concerns or explore lingering questions. Are there language barriers or low health literacy barriers that may hinder understanding and shared decision making? |
| Determine the level of patient engagement in decision making | Assess preferences for decision making and who will be involved. | Explicitly explore preferences for family-centered versus individual-centered decision making. |
| Address trust concerns | Be nonjudgmental, transparent, and avoid defensiveness. | The goal is to create an atmosphere of mutual respect and avoid misunderstanding. |
| Address resources needs | Ask what tangible resources they need to navigate the health–care system. Ask if assistance is available to them and their family in their community. | This may be influenced by language, level of education, socioeconomic status, and their social support networks. |

From Brown EA, Bekker HL, Davison SN, et al. Supportive care: communication strategies to improve cultural competence in shared decision making. *Clin J Am Soc Nephrol*. 2016;11:1902–1908.

living, or frailty scores.[39–45] Repeat hospitalizations,[46] a decline in QOL scores,[47] reduced nutritional scores,[48] reduced appetite,[49] and lower body weight[50,51] may all be simple and reliable means for independently identifying CKD patients at risk for early death or poor health outcomes. Ideally, these prognostic tools would be used alongside patient decision aids to help in the shared decision making process. Well-designed decision aids can improve people's knowledge regarding treatment options, reduce their decisional conflict related to feeling uninformed or unclear about their personal values, and can improve accurate risk perceptions.[52] Accurate prognostication will likely provide better opportunities to meet patients' and families' needs in the final years and months of life. New models, however, will need to be evaluated in different clinical and cultural contexts.

## SYMPTOM ASSESSMENT AND MANAGEMENT

Symptom assessment and management are integral components of kidney supportive care. Advanced CKD is associated with a high symptom burden and patients often experience complex clusters of symptoms, such as pruritus, pain, restless legs, fatigue, anorexia, nausea, insomnia, anxiety, and depression.[53–55] Although dialysis treatment may address some symptoms, such as fatigue, anorexia, nausea, and vomiting, especially for more robust individuals with less comorbidity, it may do little to address these and other symptoms in more frail patients, and may add to their overall symptom burden. When taken as a whole, symptom burden is similar in predialysis G5 CKD patients and chronic dialysis patients. Research suggests that symptom burden is more important than objective clinical parameters in determining QOL in CKD patients.[56] Symptom burden was shown to account for 29%–38.5% of the impairment in dialysis patients' physical QOL scores and 39%–42.5% of their impairment in mental QOL scores.[53] Moreover, changes in symptom burden were shown to account for 34%–44.6% of the change in physical QOL and 46%–48.7% of the change in mental QOL.[54,55] Kidney Disease Improving Global Outcomes recommends incorporating regular global symptom screening using validated tools such as the Edmonton Symptom Assessment System: Renal (ESAS-r: Renal)[57] into routine clinical practice, and the incorporation of systematic, stepwise approaches to managing these symptoms.[1]

**Table 62.2 Prognostic Tools Relevant to Kidney Supportive Care**

| Data Source | Population Studied | Parameter | C-Statistic |
|---|---|---|---|
| **Progression of CKD to ESKD Defined as Need for Dialysis or Preemptive Kidney Transplantation: Kidney Failure Risk Equation** | | | |
| Two Canadian cohorts[93,94] A total of 31 multinational cohorts from the CKD Prognosis Consortium[71] | Development and initial validation with 3449 and 4942 Canadian patients with G3–5 CKD, respectively. Additional validation in 721,357 multinational participants with G3–5 CKD | Four-variable model: age, gender, eGFR, and ACR Currently available for free online (https://www.qxmd.com/calculate/calculator_308/kidney-failure-risk-equation-4-variable) | Pooled data from the 31 multinational cohorts 2-year prediction: 0.9 (95% CI 0.89–0.92) 5-year prediction: 0.88 (95% CI 0.86–0.90) |
| | | Eight-variable model: age, gender, eGFR, ACR, calcium, phosphate, bicarbonate, and albumin | Pooled data from the 31 multinational cohorts 2-year prediction: 0.89 (95% CI 0.88–0.91) 5-year prediction: 0.87 (95% CI 0.85–0.88) |
| **3 Months' Survival After Dialysis Start** | | | |
| USRDS[95] | 69,441 incident patients aged ≥ 67 years | Age, albumin, assistance with ADL, nursing home, cancer, heart failure, and hospitalization Currently available for free online (https://qxmd.com/calculate/3-month-mortality-in-incident-elderly-esrd-patients) | 0.681 (95% CI 0.676–0.686) |
| | | A more comprehensive version adds gender, race, central vein dialysis catheter use, early nephrology referral, albumin, creatinine, peripheral vascular disease, and alcohol abuse | 0.712 (95% CI 0.706–0.718) |
| French REIN registry[96] | 28,496 incident patients aged ≥ 75 years | Gender, age, congestive heart failure, severe peripheral vascular disease, dysrhythmia, severe behavioral disorders, active malignancy, serum albumin, and impaired mobility | 0.749 (95% CI 0.743–0.755) |
| Catalan[97] renal registry | 1365 incident diabetic adult patients | Age, functional autonomy, heart disease, and central catheter as vascular access | 0.77 (95% CI 0.742–0.798) |
| **6 Months' Survival After Dialysis Start** | | | |
| French REIN[98] registry | 4142 incident patients aged ≥ 75 years | BMI, diabetes, congestive heart failure, peripheral vascular disease, dysrhythmia, active malignancy, severe behavioral disorder, dependency for transfers, and initial context of dialysis start | 0.70 (95% CI 0.671–0.729) |
| **6 Months' Survival on Hemodialysis** | | | |
| New England HD clinics[99] | 1026 adult-prevalent patients on maintenance hemodialysis | Age, dementia, peripheral vascular disease, serum albumin, and the "surprise question" Currently available for free online (https://qxmd.com/calculate/calculator_135/6-month-mortality-on-hd) | 0.80 (95% CI 0.73–0.88) |

*ACR,* Urine albumin-to-creatinine ratio; *ADL,* activities of daily living; *BMI,* body mass index; *CI,* confidence interval; *CKD,* chronic kidney disease; *C-statistic,* concordance (C)-statistic (which corresponds to the area under receiver operating characteristic curve, ranges from 0 to 1 depending on accuracy of discrimination); *eGFR,* estimated glomerular filtration rate; *ESKD,* end-stage kidney disease; *G3–5,* estimated glomerular filtration rate category 3–5; *HD,* hemodialysis; *REIN,* Renal Epidemiology and Information Network; *USRDS,* United States Renal Data System.

Many global symptom assessment tools of varying length have been used in CKD studies.[58] For clinical utility it is important that these tools are not only valid and reliable but that they are also sufficiently short and simple to minimize patient and staff burden. They must be appropriate for use in high-risk patients who are often frail with cognitive impairment. In the case of pain, 0–100-mm visual analog scales (VASs) or 0–10 numerical rating scales (NRSs) are advised based on extensive literature around what constitutes clinically important differences in pain intensity.[59] Core domains that should be assessed when managing pain include pain intensity, function, QOL, and adverse events.[59,60]

Several self-reported QOL measures have also been used for CKD patients. Some are generic measures, whereas others are disease specific such as the Kidney Dialysis Quality of Life (KDQOL) Questionnaire and the shorter version (KDQOL-SF).[61] These multidimensional tools focus on physical and emotional symptoms, burden of disease and effects on daily life, cognitive function, work status, sexual function, quality of social interaction and social support, staff encouragement, and patient satisfaction. Unfortunately, they are burdensome. They typically require interviewer assistance and take substantial time to complete, especially for elderly, frail patients. Although such tools provide comprehensive QOL information, they are perhaps more suited to a research environment where dedicated staff can help with the administration and complex scoring. To embed a QOL measure into routine clinical care, simple tools that can be interpreted easily by staff will most likely be required.[62,63] Generic and disease-specific measures have been shown to perform similarly in assessing changes in QOL in hemodialysis patients,[64] and a recent Oxford review of patient-reported outcome measures in CKD recommended EQ-5D-5L for use in this patient population.[65] Recommendations for symptom assessment tools that can be used in routine clinical care are outlined in Table 62.3.

The aim of treatment is to ameliorate symptoms that are burdensome and adversely impact the patient's QOL as it is

**Table 62.3 Recommendations for Clinical Symptom Assessment Tools for Use in Patients With Advanced CKD**

| Description | Clinical Utility |
|---|---|
| **Global Symptom Assessment** | |
| Edmonton Symptom Assessment System-Revised: Renal (ESAS-r: Renal)[57] | |
| A 0–10 NRS for 12 symptoms: pain, activity, nausea, depression, anxiety, drowsiness, appetite, well-being, shortness of breath, pruritus, sleep, and restless legs. It also has a place to capture "other problems." The scale for each symptom is anchored by the words "no" and "severe" at 0 and 10, respectively. The sum of all scores makes up the overall symptom distress score ranging from 0 to 120. | This is a short, practical tool for global symptom screening, which can be rapidly and repeatedly completed by patients and therefore incorporated easily into routine clinical care, even for patients who are preterminal. It has been translated into several languages. It uses the 0–10 NRS advised for the assessment of pain intensity. |
| Palliative Care Outcome Scale-Renal (POS-Renal)[100] | |
| Assesses 17 symptoms: pain, shortness of breath, weakness or lack of energy, nausea, vomiting, poor appetite, constipation, mouth problems, drowsiness, poor mobility, itching, difficulty sleeping, restless legs or difficulty keeping legs still, anxiety, depression, changes in skin, and diarrhea. These are rated in terms of their impact on the patient over the last week using a 0 (not at all) to 4 (overwhelmingly) Likert scale. | This tool is slightly longer that the ESAS-r: Renal but is simple to use. It has been translated into several languages. A disadvantage is that is does not use the 0–10 NRS that is advised for assessing pain. |
| **Multidimensional Pain Assessment** | |
| The Brief Pain Inventory (BPI)[101] | |
| Assesses the location, type (nociceptive vs. neuropathic), and intensity of pain. It also evaluates the impact of pain on the core domains of function and QOL. Specifically, it explores the impact of pain on general activity, mood, walking ability, work, relationships, sleep, and enjoyment of life. The standard 32-question instrument has been condensed to a nine-question- short–form. | This tool has been used successfully in clinical and research settings internationally to assess pain once identified as problem. The short–form is simple to use with minimal respondent burden and seriously ill patients have been successful in completing it. The Interference Scale of the BPI has been recommended by IMMPACT for the assessment of physical functioning, one of the core pain assessment domains.[102] A change of 1 point on the Interference Scale is considered the minimally clinically important change.[59,60] It has been translated into several languages. |
| **Quality of Life Assessment** | |
| 5-Level EuroQol 5 Dimension (EQ-5D-5L)[65] | |
| This generic QOL measure has two parts: (1) EQ-5D descriptive system and (2) EQ VAS. The descriptive system comprises five dimensions: mobility, self-care, usual activities, pain/discomfort, and anxiety/depression. Each dimension has five levels: "no problems," "slight problems," "moderate problems," "severe problems," and "extreme problems." The EQ VAS records the patient's self-rated health on a vertical 0–100-mm VAS, where the endpoints are labeled "The best health you can imagine" and "The worst health you can imagine." | This is a short, practical tool for assessing QOL. It is available in more than 130 languages. |

*CKD,* Chronic kidney disease; *IMMPACT,* Initiative on Methods, Measurement, and Pain Assessment in Clinical Trials; *NRS,* numerical rating scale; *QOL,* quality of life; *VAS,* visual analog scale.

not always necessary or possible to resolve them completely. It is important to acknowledge this and negotiate with the patient an acceptable level of symptom control. For pain, there is good evidence to suggest that targeting a final pain state of less than 33/100 mm on a VAS or 3/10 on an NRS or a change in pain intensity of at least 30% (moderate benefit) or 50% (substantial benefit) will deliver worthwhile QOL benefits.[60,66] Given the synergistic and interrelated nature of symptoms experienced in advanced CKD, an approach to care that addresses overall symptom burden is likely to improve QOL even if each individual symptom has not resolved completely. For example, a moderate reduction in pain may be sufficient to improve sleep, improve mood, and increase the ability to cope with health challenges, resulting in a substantial improvement in function and QOL. Recommendations for the management of common symptoms in CKD are outlined in Table 62.4. These recommendations are appropriate for patients with G5 CKD who have yet to start dialysis, patients who have chosen CKM, and for dialysis patients.[67,68] A general stepwise approach to symptom management involves (1) ruling out contributing factors, (2) maximizing the use of nonpharmacologic-interventions, and finally (3) considering pharmacologic interventions if symptoms continue to impact adversely the patient's QOL.

## CHRONIC PAIN MANAGEMENT

Although detailed information on the management of chronic or persistent pain is beyond the scope of this chapter, some

**Table 62.4 Symptom Management for Patients With Advanced Chronic Kidney Disease[67]**

| Address Possible Contributing Factors | Nonpharmacologic Management | Pharmacologic Management | Additional Considerations |
|---|---|---|---|
| **Restless Legs Syndrome** | | | |
| • Anemia<br>• Iron deficiency<br>• Hyperphosphatemia<br>• Medications such as dopamine antagonists, antidepressants, and opioids (some of these drugs are commonly prescribed at end of life, e.g., haloperidol and opioids) | • Abstinence from stimulants (e.g., alcohol, caffeine, and nicotine)<br>• Mental alerting activities (e.g., puzzles or games)<br>• Good sleep hygiene<br>• Exercise | First line: gabapentin (50–300 mg daily) 2–3 hours before sleep, especially if concomitant pruritus, insomnia, and/or neuropathic pain are reported<br>Second line: nonergot-derived dopamine agonists (pramipexole 0.125 mg daily, ropinirole 0.25 mg daily, rotigotine transdermal patch 1–3 mg) given 2 hours before sleep<br>At the end of life if swallowing is problematic: consider midazolam 1 mg subcutaneously q4h PRN | The most common side effects of gabapentin are drowsiness, dizziness, confusion, fatigue, and occasionally peripheral edema<br>Nonergot-derived dopamine agonists have shown success in reducing symptoms in idiopathic RLS, but there are very limited data in uremic RLS. Side effects might include headache, insomnia, and nausea. Augmentation may occur with long-time use. Benzodiazepines are not a first-line treatment for RLS but there is some limited evidence for their use. If the patient is experiencing refractory RLS causing significant sleep disturbance, or if benzodiazepines may potentially treat concurrent symptoms (e.g., anxiety), they could be considered. |
| **Uremic Pruritus** | | | |
| **Address Possible Contributing Factors** | **Nonpharmacologic Management** | **Pharmacologic Management** | **Additional Considerations** |
| • Anemia<br>• Iron deficiency<br>• Hyperphosphatemia<br>• Hypercalcemia<br>• Other: xerosis, drug hypersensitivities, allergies, infestations, contact dermatitis, or inflammation | • Good skin care and moisturizers (e.g., baths with lukewarm water, pat dry and moisturize within 2 minutes; gentle soaps with no fragrances or additives)<br>• Keep skin cool<br>• Humid environment<br>• Avoid scratching—keep fingernails short, encourage gentle massage, wear gloves at night<br>• Consider complimentary therapies: e.g., phototherapy (UVB) 3 times weekly for a 3-week trial; acupuncture. Very little evidence exists for these alternative therapies. | Topical<br>• Capsaicin 0.025% or 0.03% ointment<br>• Pramoxine 1%<br>• Menthol/camphor/phenol – 0.3% each<br>• γ-Linolenic acid cream 2.2%<br>Systemic<br>First line: gabapentin (50–300 mg daily) 2–3 hours before sleep.<br>Second line: tricyclic antidepressant such as doxepin 10 mg daily at night | Topical<br>These agents can be applied two times daily (four times daily for capsaicin). Capsaicin may cause burning to the area initially.<br>Menthol, camphor, and phenol are separate products that can be added to most creams. All three may be added together, commonly with a 0.3% concentration for each.<br>Systemic<br>The most common side effects of gabapentin are drowsiness, dizziness, confusion, fatigue, and occasionally peripheral edema.<br>Potential adverse effects of tricyclic antidepressants include dizziness, blurred vision, constipation, and urinary retention. There is an increased risk of confusion and sedation, particularly in older adults. |

**Table 62.4 Symptom Management for Patients With Advanced Chronic Kidney Disease[67] (Cont'd)**

| Address Possible Contributing Factors | Nonpharmacologic Management | Pharmacologic Management | Additional Considerations |
|---|---|---|---|
| **Nausea and Vomiting** | | | |
| • Metabolic disturbances (e.g., uremia)<br>• Medications (e.g., opioids, SSRI antidepressants)<br>• Gastrointestinal disturbances (e.g., constipation, delayed gastric emptying) | • Manage constipation<br>• Encourage good oral hygiene<br>• Smaller, more frequent meals; eat meals slowly<br>• Avoid alcohol<br>• Avoid foods that are greasy, spicy, or excessively sweet<br>• Minimize aromas (e.g., cooking odors, perfumes, smoke)<br>• Encourage relaxed, upright position after eating to facilitate digestion<br>• Loose-fitting clothing<br>• Consider complementary therapies (e.g., relaxation techniques, acupressure, the use of ginger) | First line: Ondansetron 4–8 mg every 8 hours as needed<br>Second line: metoclopramide 2.5 mg every 4 hours as needed<br>Third line: olanzapine 2.5 mg every 8 hours as needed OR haloperidol 0.5 mg every 8 hours as needed<br>Fourth line: for persistent and severe nausea, consider increasing haloperidol to 1.0 mg (maximum 5 mg in 24 hours) OR replacing with methotrimeprazine 5 mg orally or 6.25 mg subcutaneously every 8 hours as needed | Ondansetron can be constipating.<br>Haloperidol, metoclopramide, and olanzapine are all dopamine antagonists: avoid prescribing them together. They can also exacerbate RLS. They all cross the blood–brain barrier and extrapyramidal symptoms are possible. Haloperidol has a higher risk of extrapyramidal symptoms than metoclopramide and olanzapine.<br>Increasing the dose of methotrimeprazine may lead to levels of drowsiness that the patient may find unacceptable and should be discussed with the patient and/or family. |
| **Breathlessness** | | | |
| **Address Possible Contributing Factors** | **Nonpharmacologic Management** | **Pharmacologic Management** | **Additional Considerations** |
| • Anxiety<br>• Anemia<br>• Infection<br>• Volume overload leading to pulmonary edema | • Sit in an upright position (e.g., 45°)<br>• Position by a window or use a fan to blow air gently across the face<br>• Maintain a humid environment<br>• Pursed lip breathing<br>• Supplemental oxygen<br>• Complementary therapies (e.g., relaxation techniques, music)<br>• Consider role of diet such as sodium and fluid restriction if patient is volume overloaded | If patient is intravascularly volume overloaded: diuretic such as a loop diuretic—furosemide.<br>Occasionally patients may require combination diuretic therapy—consider adding metolazone.<br>Near the end of life: low doses of opioids are the most effective treatment.<br>**For breathlessness that is episodic** and primarily associated with a specific activity, consider fentanyl 12.5 μg subcutaneously or sublingually PRN.<br>**For shortness of breath that is more constant or unpredictable** in nature, consider hydromorphone 0.5 mg PO (0.2 mg subcutaneously) every 4 hours around the clock and every hour as needed. | Due to the accumulation of metabolites, opioids should always be started at a low dose and monitor closely for adverse effects.<br>Due to its fast action, fentanyl works well in cases where breathlessness is predictable. |

*Continued on following page*

**Table 62.4 Symptom Management for Patients With Advanced Chronic Kidney Disease[67] (Cont'd)**

**Fatigue and Sleep Disturbances**

| Address Possible Contributing Factors | Nonpharmacologic Management | Pharmacologic Management | Additional Considerations |
|---|---|---|---|
| Fatigue<br>• Vitamin D deficiency<br>• Metabolic acidosis<br>• Hyperphosphatemia<br>• Secondary hypothyroidism<br>• Anemia<br>• Malnutrition<br>• Mood disorders<br>• Sleep disturbances<br>Sleep Disturbances<br>• Other symptoms (e.g., restless legs, pruritus, pain, breathlessness)<br>• Cognitive impairment<br>• Medications<br>• Generalized insomnia<br>• Mood disorders<br>• Sleep apnea | Fatigue<br>• Exercise<br>• Nutrition and hydration management<br>• Energy-conservation strategies<br>• Good sleep hygiene (e.g., avoid stimulants before bed, avoid napping during the day, save the bedroom for sleep)<br>• Cognitive and psychological approaches (e.g., relaxation therapy, delegating, and setting limits)<br>• Complementary treatments (e.g., acupressure, massage, acupuncture) | Sleep Disturbances<br>First line: consider low-dose gabapentin (50–300 mg at night), especially if the patient has concomitant neuropathic pain, RLS, or uremic pruritus<br>Second line:<br>Doxepin 10 mg at bedtime, especially if concomitant pruritus or neuropathic pain reported<br>Third line: cautiously consider mirtazapine 7.5 mg or zopiclone 3.75–5 mg at night or melatonin 2–5 mg at night | Reassess medications after 2–4 weeks. Avoid over-the-counter sleep aids and benzodiazepines if possible. Specifically, avoid mirtazapine if taking tramadol or antidepressants. Monitor doxepin for anticholinergic side effects (e.g., dizziness, blurred vision, constipation, urinary retention, and cardiac arrhythmias). Evidence for melatonin is limited and inconclusive. Ideally, all of these medications should be prescribed for short-term use only. |

**Nociceptive Pain**

| Address Possible Contributing Factors | Nonpharmacologic Management | Pharmacologic Management | Additional Considerations |
|---|---|---|---|
| • Determine cause for pain and consider appropriate investigations | • Physical therapies (e.g., physical therapy, aerobic exercise, stretching, massage, acupressure, acupuncture)<br>• Behavioral therapies (e.g., cognitive behavioral therapy—most commonly used behavioral therapy), biofeedback, relaxation techniques, psychotherapy/individual or group counselling, guided imagery, mindfulness-based stress reduction<br>• Interventional and surgical (e.g., ablative techniques, nerve blocks, trigger point injections) | Step 1: Acetaminophen/paracetamol, maximum of 3 g daily. If pain is localized to a small joint, consider a topical NSAID (e.g., diclofenac gel 5% or 10% two to three times daily).<br>Step 2: There are no safe step 2 analgesics for nociceptive pain.<br>Step 3: ADD a strong opioid to step 1 in very low doses. Hydromorphone starting at 0.5 mg PO (0.2 mg subcutaneously) every 4–6 hours; buprenorphine/fentanyl/methadone. | Trial each step for 1–4 weeks before progressing, depending on pain severity.<br>Before starting a strong opioid, consider completing an opioid risk tool and order a bowel routine to avoid constipation (e.g., PEG 3350). All opioids should be started at low doses, monitored carefully for adverse effects and overall benefit, and titrated slowly (see Table 62.5). |

**Table 62.4 Symptom Management for Patients With Advanced Chronic Kidney Disease[67] (Cont'd)**

**Neuropathic Pain**

| Address Possible Contributing Factors | Nonpharmacologic Management | Pharmacologic Management | Additional Considerations |
|---|---|---|---|
| • Determine cause for pain and consider appropriate investigations | • As for nociceptive pain | Start with adjuvant therapy.<br>First line: gabapentin, pregabalin (calcium channel alpha 2–delta ligands)<br>Second line: tricyclic antidepressants, amitriptyline starting at 10–25 mg daily or doxepin starting at 10 mg daily.<br>If additional analgesia is required **in addition** to adjuvant therapy, add a nonopioid and then proceed low dose of a strong opioid and titrate as described for nociceptive pain. | Methadone may be effective for severe neuropathic pain because of its activity against the NMDA receptor antagonism. |

*NMDA,* *N*-methyl-D-aspartate; *NSAID,* nonsteroidal antiinflammatory drug; *PO,* per os; *q4h,* every 4 hours; *PRN,* as needed; *RLS,* restless legs syndrome; *SSRI,* selective serotonin reuptake inhibitor; *UVB,* short-wave ultraviolet B.

general principles are worth highlighting. Chronic pain can be defined as any painful condition that persists for more than 3 months.[69] Dialysis patients may also experience recurring episodes of acute pain, such as pain from needling fistulas or intradialytic steal syndrome, intradialytic headaches, and cramps. These acute pains tend to be associated with tissue damage but typically have no progressive pattern, last a predictable period, subside as healing occurs, and are episodic with periods without pain. By contrast, chronic pain is present for long periods and is often out of proportion with the extent of the originating injury. It is more likely to result in functional impairment and disability, psychological distress, sleep deprivation, and poor QOL.

Nonpharmacologic therapies have become a vital part of managing chronic pain and are often required to augment pharmacologic treatments to achieve adequate relief (i.e., multimodal therapy). They may also be used as stand-alone therapies. Examples are outlined briefly in Table 62.4. Core principles in developing a treatment plan for chronic pain include explaining the nature of the chronic pain condition, setting appropriate goals, and developing a comprehensive treatment approach and plan for adherence. Medication should not be the sole focus of treatment and should only be used when needed, in conjunction with other treatment modalities, to meet treatment goals. Optimal patient outcomes often require multiple approaches used in concert, coordinated via a multidisciplinary team.

There are five essential principles for the pharmacologic management of pain. These are described in Table 62.5. Of particular importance is the careful selection of analgesics when prescribing for patients with advanced CKD. Many analgesics and their metabolites are excreted by the kidney through glomerular filtration, tubular secretion, or both and are at risk for accumulation of toxic metabolites if not monitored carefully. The choice of an appropriate initial therapeutic strategy is dependent on an accurate evaluation of the cause of the pain and the type of chronic pain syndrome. In particular, neuropathic pain should be distinguished from nociceptive pain (Table 62.6). For most patients with advanced CKD, the initial treatment of neuropathic pain involves calcium channel alpha 2–delta ligands (e.g., gabapentin and pregabalin) or a tricyclic antidepressant (see Table 62.4). Opioid medications are second-line agents for most patients with neuropathic pain. By contrast, the pharmacologic approach to nociceptive pain primarily involves nonnarcotic and opioid analgesics if nonpharmacologic strategies are insufficient. The strong opioids that are generally considered safer for use in patients with advanced CKD are hydromorphone, buprenorphine, fentanyl, and methadone, with doses started low, titrated slowly, and the patient monitored carefully for analgesia, adverse effects, overall function, and QOL (Table 62.4).

## SPECIAL CONSIDERATIONS AT THE END OF LIFE

As a patient's condition deteriorates, certain nonpharmacologic interventions will become less realistic (e.g. exercise). Energy conservation and restoration will become of utmost importance. Ensure that appropriate supports are in place to assist with activities of daily living and that nursing care is available as needed. Drowsiness may increase as the end-of-life approaches due to disease progression (and/or

**Table 62.5 Five Principles of Pain Management in Advanced CKD**

| Principle | Description | Specific Considerations in Advanced CKD |
|---|---|---|
| "By mouth" | • Oral administration is the safest and therefore preferred.<br>• Patient comfort and effectiveness must be considered. If ingestion or absorption is uncertain, analgesics need to be given by alternative routes, such as transdermal, rectal, or subcutaneous. | • Hemodialysis patients have easy intravenous access. However, this is to be avoided as the route of administration for analgesics to optimize safety and minimize the risk of abuse and addiction. |
| "By the clock" | • For continuous or predictable pain, analgesics should be given regularly. Additional "breakthrough" or "rescue" medication should be available on an "as needed" (PRN) basis in addition to the regular dose. | • Some patients with mild pain may achieve adequate pain relief with analgesic dosing posthemodialysis only. An example would be mild neuropathic pain dosed with gabapentin postdialysis. |
| "By the ladder" | • Pharmacologic management proceeds stepwise from nonopioids (step 1) to very low doses of strong opioids (step 3) using the WHO analgesic ladder. There are no good options for step 2 analgesics for patients with advanced CKD. | • Careful selection of analgesics for each step of the ladder, taking into account degree of kidney failure, is critical (see Table 62.4).<br>• Sustained-release preparations are generally not recommended in patients with advanced CKD. |
| "For the individual" | • There is large variability in patients' response to analgesics. The "correct" dose is the amount needed to relieve the pain without producing intolerable side effects.<br>• Evaluation and recording of benefit and toxicity are essential. | • Chronic pain is often experienced in the context of numerous other physical, psychosocial, and spiritual concerns, including end-of-life issues. Close attention to these other issues must not be forgotten as part of the pain management strategy. |
| "Attention to detail" | • Pain changes over time; therefore there is the need for ongoing reassessment.<br>• Side effects should be explained and managed actively (e.g., constipation). | • There are no studies on the long-term use of analgesics in patients with CKD. Careful attention must be paid to efficacy and safety.<br>• The impact on overall symptom burden, physical function, emotional state, cognition, and QOL should be assessed routinely. |

*CKD,* Chronic kidney disease; *QOL,* quality of life; *WHO,* World Health Organization.

**Table 62.6 Categories of Pain**

| | Neuropathic Pain | Nociceptive Pain |
|---|---|---|
| Description | Pain that results from damage to the nervous system resulting in either dysfunction or pathological change. | Pain that results from tissue damage in the skin, muscle, and other tissues, causing stimulation of sensory receptors. |
| Pain Characteristics | • Common descriptors include burning, tingling, and shooting.<br>• May be associated with episodes of spontaneous pain, hyperalgesia, and allodynia. The presence of the latter is pathognomonic.<br>• The pain may be felt at a site distant from its cause, in the distribution of a nerve, for example. | • Pain may be described as sharp, like a knife–often felt at the site of damage.<br>• Pain may also be experienced as dull, aching, and poorly localized (as with stimulation of visceral nociceptors). |
| Response to Analgesics | Generally responds poorly to analgesics and requires the use of adjuvant therapy. | Generally responds well to analgesics. |

medications). Some patients and families may even prefer increased sleepiness if the patient remains comfortable. Symptoms should be anticipated with the appropriate prescriptions in place to address a patient's symptoms as they appear, including an alternative route to oral as swallowing becomes compromised. Fig. 62.3 outlines a terminal care algorithm for pain, which can also be used for breathlessness.[67] As a general rule, benzodiazepines should be avoided in patients with advanced CKD, especially those who are functionally impaired and/or more frail. Benzodiazepines can carry significant risks, including an increased risk of falls, fractures, and decreased cognition. However, they may be the only option for a patient who can no longer swallow and may be beneficial for restless legs, anxiety, and agitation near the end of life. Fig. 62.4 describes a terminal care approach to restlessness, agitation, and delirium.[67]

## ADVANCE CARE PLANNING

The unpredictable nature of CKD progression and the associated complications make it particularly important for patients and families to plan for end-of-life care needs.[35] Advanced care planning (ACP) is a process that involves

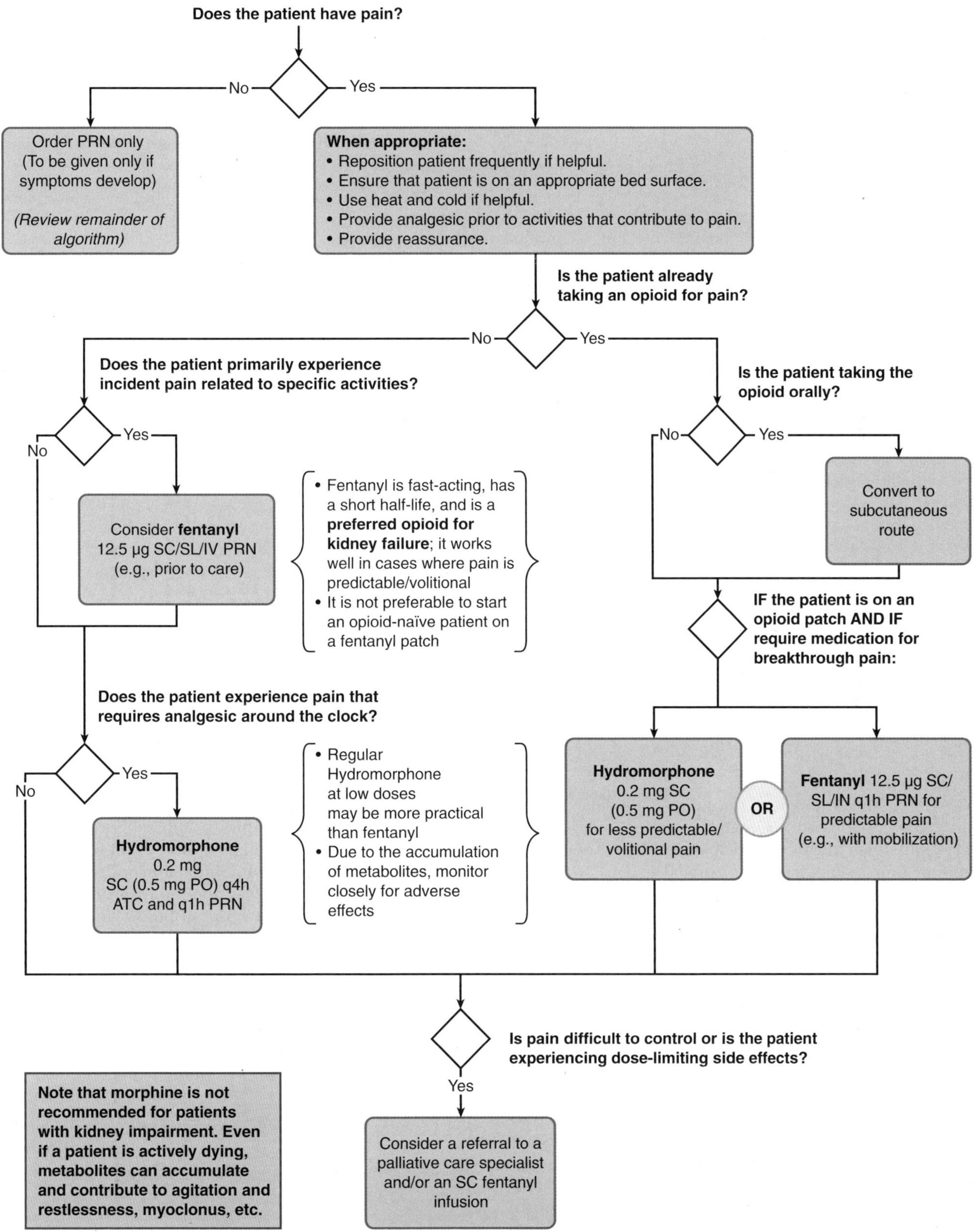


**Fig. 62.3** Algorithm for the management of pain at the end of life for patients with advanced chronic kidney disease. *ATC,* Around the clock; *PO,* per os; *q1h,* every 1 hour; *q4h,* every 4 hours; *SC,* subcutaneous; *SL,* sublingual. (Adapted with permission from Sara N. Davison, Kidney Supportive Care Research Group. *Conservative Kidney Management Care Pathway*. 2016. Available from: www.ckmcare.com. Last accessed September 20, 2017.)

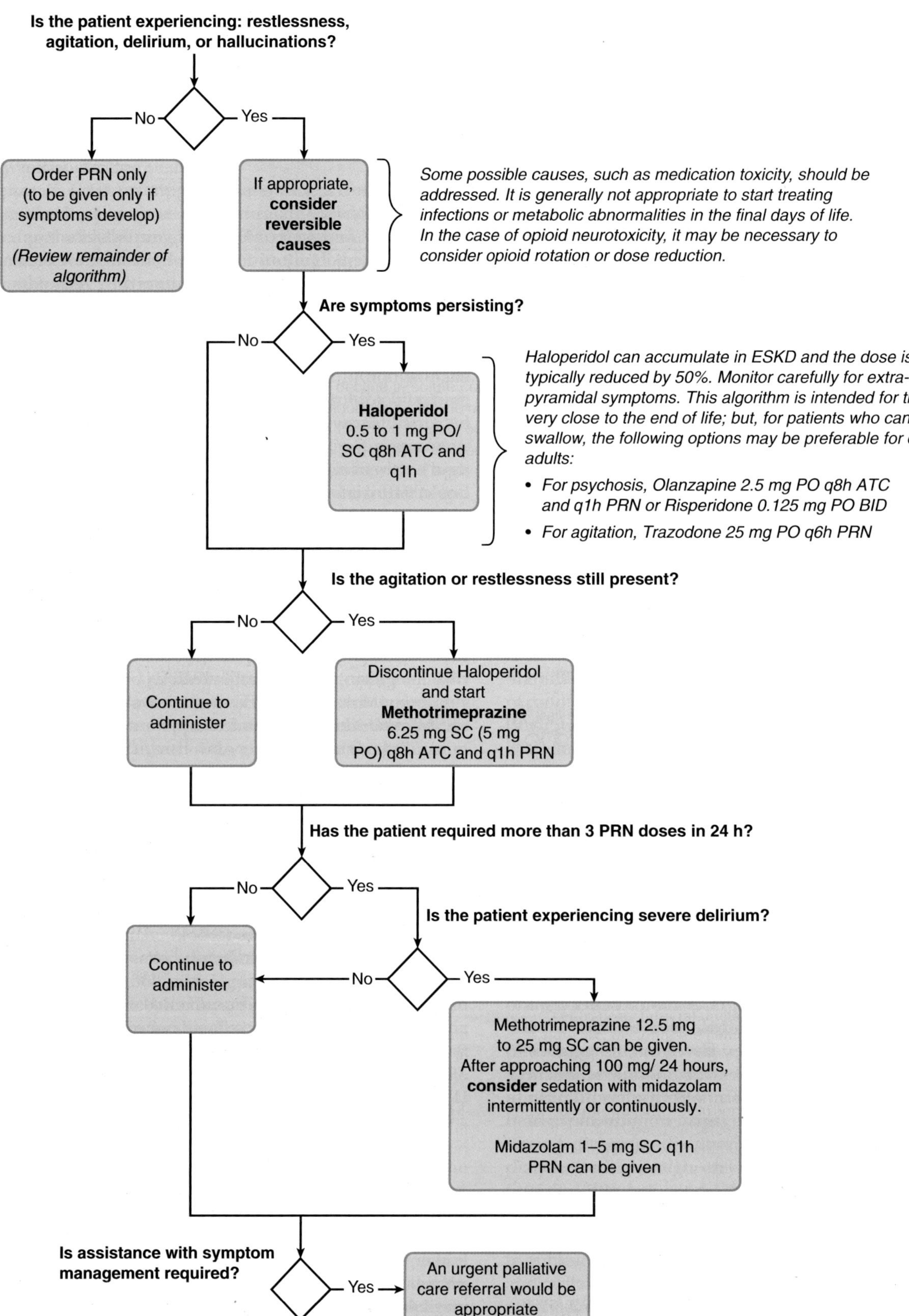


**Fig. 62.4** Algorithm for the management of restlessness, agitation, and delirium at the end of life for patients with advanced chronic kidney disease (CKD). *ATC,* Around the clock; *BID,* twice a day; *ESKD,* end-stage kidney disease; *PO,* per os; *PRN,* as needed; *q1h,* every 1 hour; *q6h,* every 6 hours; *q8h,* every 8 hours; *SC,* subcutaneous. (Adapted with permission from Sara N. Davison, Kidney Supportive Care Research Group. *Conservative Kidney Management Care Pathway*. 2016. Available from: www.ckmcare.com. Last accessed September 20, 2017.)

understanding, communication, and discussion between a patient, the family (or other caregiver), and health–care providers, for the purpose of clarifying preferences for end-of-life care. It lays out a set of relationships, values, and processes for approaching end-of-life decisions for individual people when they can no longer speak for themselves, including attention to ethical, psychosocial, and spiritual issues relating to starting, continuing, withholding, and stopping dialysis.[1,70] The unique circumstances around treatment options for patients with advanced CKD, such as palliative dialysis, CKM, and dialysis withdrawal, are discussed in greater detail later and further perspectives are also discussed in Chapters 82 and 84. When goals for care have not been established, patients often experience unnecessary hospitalizations, unwanted invasive treatments, a prolonged dying process, and ultimately the type of death they would not have wanted.[2]

An approach to ACP for patients with advanced CKD was developed based on the perspectives of patients with advanced CKD[70,71] and is illustrated in Fig. 62.5. ACP is a health behavior and these conversations need to be tailored to the readiness of the individual.[71] Behavior change theories such as the

**Identification of patients most likely to benefit from ACP** (see identification of patients most like to benefit from supportive care, **Fig. 2**)

**Determine patient and family readiness for participation in ACP**

- Cognitive capacity
- Mental health: anxiety, depression
- Language and literary barriers
- Cultural, religious, or spiritual issues
- Adequate family/social support

**Introduce ACP**

- Explore the patient's understanding of ACP
- Normalize the topic
  - Benefits for all adults, including those who are healthy as well as those who have a serious illness
- Help patient understand the value of ACP in their situation
- Ask for permission to continue the conversation
- Identify whom the patient wishes to include in ACP conversations
  - Is there a role for facilitated ACP?

**Facilitation of ACP: Key elements**

- **Explore current health condition**
  - What does the patient know about their disease and treatment options?
  - How do they feel about their illness?
  - What do they expect may happen in the future?
- **Explore values, goals, and beliefs on living well**
  - What is important to the patient?
  - What makes them happy or gives their life purpose or meaning?
  - What are their fears?
  - What are their beliefs, including cultural, religious, or spiritual, that might impact their end-of-life care?
- **Explore past health experiences**
  - This includes their experiences and others' close to them.
  - What defines a good death for the patient?

**Patient-led ACP**

Not all patients want to talk extensively with their health–care team about ACP. Some patients view conversations with their loved ones as more valuable.

**Decision making**

- **Care decisions**
  - Determine goals of care
  - Clarify preferences for end-of-life care, including the use of life-sustaining treatments
  - Decisions should include issues such as CKM vs. initiation of dialysis; withdrawal of dialysis
- **Identify an appropriate substitute decision–maker**
  - Ensure this individual has the appropriate knowledge of the patient's wishes, is willing to take on the role, is able to honor the patient's wishes, and is able to make decisions under stressful circumstances
  - Determine leeway of substitute decision–maker
- **Summarize and close the conversation**
  - Ensure mutual understanding.
  - Make a follow-up plan to continue, complete, or review ACP

**Documentation and development of a follow-up plan**

- Advance directive
- Physician order (POLST, GCD)
- In many U.S. and Canadian centers, the above documents are placed in a green sleeve and given to the patient.
  - Documents travel with patient between health–care settings.
  - The green sleeve is easily identifiable to emergency medical and hospital staff.
  - Copies of documents can be given to loved ones and placed in medical records.
- Involve other professionals as necessary to address knowledge gaps and provide appropriate support.

**Fig. 62.5** A framework for facilitating advanced care planning *(ACP)* in patients with advanced chronic kidney disease. *CKM,* Conservative kidney management. (Adapted from Davison SN. Facilitating advance care planning for patients with end-stage renal disease: the patient perspective. *Clin J Am Soc Nephrol.* 2006;1:1023–1028; Davison SN, Torgunrud C. The creation of an advance care planning process for patients with ESRD. *Am J Kidney Dis.* 2007;49:27–36.)

trans-theoretical model or the "stages of change" model provide a useful framework for assessing patient readiness to engage in ACP.[72] Patients go through the stages of precontemplation (no intention of engaging in ACP in the near future), to contemplation, to preparation, and finally to action. This framework takes into account an individual's weighing of the pros and cons of engaging in ACP and assesses their attitudes about barriers to and facilitators of behavior change. A patient who is cognitively impaired or who is depressed or extremely anxious may have limited ability to participate meaningfully in ACP. The evidence suggests that a patient is much more likely to engage actively in ACP when he or she understands the personal relevance and perceived benefit.[71] Cultural, spiritual, and religious beliefs and variances around the concepts of autonomy, decision-making authority, communicating prognosis, and views around care at the end of life may influence attitudes toward ACP.[73–75] Clinicians should address any misconceptions the patient may have toward ACP and highlight the value of these conversations as it relates to that specific individual.

There are several key elements to ACP conversations that involve exploring the patient's understanding of their illness, past health–care experiences, and values and beliefs (see Fig. 62.5). It is only through this exploration and understanding that the clinician will be able to align treatment options and end-of-life care with the patient's personal goals for living and dying well. It is not necessary that all elements be addressed in a single conversation, but rather that over time both the patient and the clinician gain a full understanding of the patient's beliefs, values, and overall goals for care. In routine clinical practice it is common for these conversations to build on each other in subsequent visits. Although many clinicians feel they lack the skills and confidence to have ACP conversations with their patients,[34] effective ACP communication skills can be learned,[76,77] especially when using the strategies for culturally sensitive shared decision making outlined in Table 62.1.

Ideally, ACP should be integrated into routine kidney care early and readdressed throughout the patient's illness. This helps to normalize the process; to afford patients the time to think, reflect, and make well-informed choices for future care; and to ensure care plans remain aligned with their preferences and prognosis as their health state declines. This often proves challenging as patients may feel that ACP is not yet relevant for them early in their disease. However, sudden illness or complications can occur without warning. At a minimum, however, high-risk patients should be identified through regular supportive care assessments as outlined in Fig. 62.2, to facilitate timely conversations with those most in need.

## CONSERVATIVE KIDNEY MANAGEMENT

There is growing recognition that dialysis is unlikely to benefit and may even harm some patients, particularly those with significant preexisting functional or cognitive impairment and high levels of comorbidity.[78–81] Frail patients often experience accelerated functional and cognitive decline after starting dialysis.[82,83] Patients residing in long-term care facilities at the time of starting dialysis have especially poor outcomes.[82] CKM is an appropriate alternative to chronic dialysis for patients unlikely to benefit from dialysis (see also Chapter 84).

CKM can be defined as holistic patient-centered care for patients with G5 CKD that through shared decision making emphasizes QOL, active symptom management, and advance care planning. It includes interventions to delay progression and minimize complications of CKD but it does not include dialysis.[1] Some elderly patients managed conservatively live as long as patients who choose to start dialysis with better preservation of function, fewer admissions to acute care settings, while avoiding the burdens of dialysis and remaining in their home communities, resulting in a better QOL.[78–81] The international nephrology community recognizes that for patients unlikely to benefit from dialysis, dialysis should not be the default therapy and advocates strongly for the provision of quality CKM.[1]

Choosing CKM does not mean imminent death. Many patients live for months or years with G5 CKD. Nor does CKM imply a "no care" philosophy. In fact, CKM requires highly integrated communication and care that involves tailor-made combinations of structures, processes, and interventions to address unique patient needs and unique system-community circumstances. Careful planning is necessary to link and transition patients at various points along the continuum of care, such as between primary, secondary, and tertiary care; between community-based and institutional care; and between acute care and long-term care. It may require involvement of mental health–care and social services and should assist with referral to specialist supportive/palliative care and hospice services as available and appropriate. Multidisciplinary care teams will be required to deliver CKM. How best to implement CKM throughout complex, multisector health–care systems is unclear. One method of implementation is through a clinical pathway that operationalizes best-practice guidelines into "how to" steps for care delivery. A successful example of this is the interactive, online Canadian CKM pathway that includes an integrated plan of communication and care and a CKM patient decision aid that has been implemented across the province of Alberta and has shown to be effective in both increasing uptake of evidence-based care and optimizing patient management and outcomes (Fig. 62.6).[67]

Until recently, there were no clear recommendations for managing the metabolic complications of CKD. Current CKD guidelines were established for optimizing long-term health outcomes and do not address the priorities of care for patients who have chosen CKM. CKM-specific recommendations for both CKD management and symptom control (as outlined in Table 62.4) have recently been suggested to assist with the standardization and evaluation of high-quality CKM care.[68] These recommendations and their associated rationales are outlined in Table 62.7. The illness trajectory of patients on a CKM pathway can be highly variable and is anticipated to pass through several stages. Patients with an estimated glomerular filtration rate (eGFR) of 10–15 mL/min/1.73 $m^2$ may remain relatively functional and stable for many months to years, whereas a patient who spends much of their time lying down with an eGFR of 5 mL/min/1.73 $m^2$ likely has a life expectancy measured in weeks to a couple of months. Comprehensive CKM guidelines need to take the patient's general condition, prognosis, and goals of care into account. Earlier in the disease trajectory, maximizing QOL likely

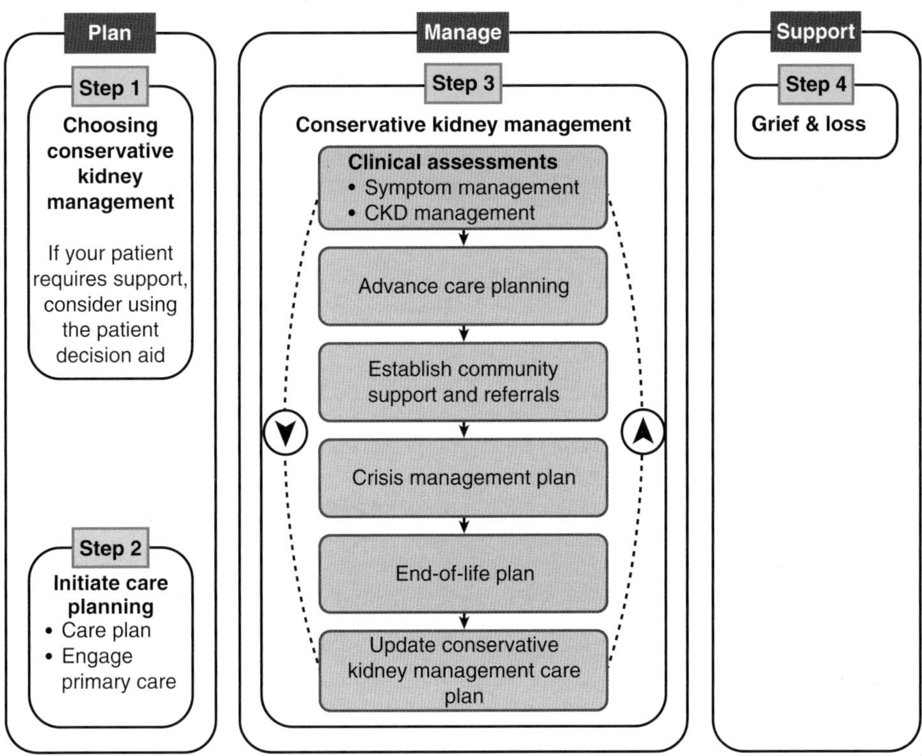


**Fig. 62.6** An integrated approach to the care of patients who have chosen conservative kidney management.[67] *CKM,* Conservative kidney management. (Reproduced with permission from Dr. Sara Davison, Kidney Supportive Care Research Group.)

**Table 62.7 Summary of CKD Management Recommendations for Patients Who Have Chosen CKM[67,68]**

| Guideline | Treatment Rationale | Recommended Interventions |
|---|---|---|
| Dyslipidemia | Patients are unlikely to benefit from treating dyslipidemia in the last few years of life. Patients may gain improvement in QOL from stopping statin medications.[103,104] | Care providers, in discussion with the patient, can discontinue statin medications. |
| Blood Pressure | The primary goal of blood pressure management is to optimize physical and cognitive function and minimize the risk of falls, while avoiding very high readings. Decisions about specific medications would depend on the patient's comorbidities. Diuretics are a unique consideration and are aimed primarily at the treatment of volume overload that causes breathlessness or symptomatic peripheral edema. | Blood pressure targets can be relaxed for most CKM patients to ≤160/90 mm Hg.[104–106] This applies to patients with diabetes as well. |
| Sodium Restriction | High sodium intake may be associated with volume overload leading to breathlessness and symptomatic peripheral edema.<br>Because sodium restriction can influence palatability, strategies should balance symptom management and the patient's priorities for care and other issues such as appropriate nutrition. | Diuretics and dietary sodium restriction to assist with volume control if volume overload is contributing to symptom burden. |
| Anemia | Anemia can contribute to fatigue and breathlessness. The purpose of treating anemia would be to reduce these symptoms as opposed to reducing cardiac mortality or morbidity. When a patient starts spending most of his or her time lying down and/or the end of life is near, it is no longer appropriate to manage fatigue and breathlessness by addressing anemia and anemia treatment can be stopped. | Erythropoiesis-stimulating agents and iron supplementation.<br>Anemia-related bloodwork every 3–6 months is appropriate but should be based on patient preference and symptoms.<br>It is appropriate to stop managing anemia in the last weeks or days of life. |
| Hyperkalemia | Hyperkalemia predisposes patients to cardiac arrhythmias and sudden death. Acute treatment of hyperkalemia is appropriate if consistent with the patient's goals.<br>If patients wish to liberalize their potassium intake, the risks of lifting the restriction must be explained clearly. | Interventions include a potassium-restricted diet and the use of potassium-binding resins such as sodium polystyrene sulfonate.<br>For those aiming to maintain normal potassium levels, it is reasonable to monitor potassium levels monthly. It is appropriate to stop monitoring and managing potassium levels in the last weeks or days of life. |

*Continued on following page*

**Table 62.7 Summary of CKD Management Recommendations for Patients Who Have Chosen CKM[67,68] (Cont'd)**

| Guideline | Treatment Rationale | Recommended Interventions |
|---|---|---|
| Acidosis | Metabolic acidosis can contribute to fatigue, bone loss, and muscle wasting[107]; Treatment is aimed at managing these symptoms. If the patient finds the pill burden too great, or when the patient can no longer swallow, treatment should be stopped. | The primary intervention is the use of sodium bicarbonate. It is reasonable to monitor bicarbonate every 3–6 months if patients are being treated.<br>It is appropriate to stop monitoring and managing bicarbonate levels in the last weeks or days of life. |
| Calcium/ Phosphorus | We recommend promoting QOL through liberalizing diet and maintaining adequate nutrition rather than normalizing biochemistry as it is not clear that there are benefits to normalizing in patients being cared for conservatively in the last few years of life. Rather, there is a possibility of harm in promoting lower protein intake in patients already at high risk for protein malnutrition.<br>Hyperphosphatemia may contribute to RLS; calcium and phosphorous depositions can lead to myalgias, arthralgias, and pseudogout.<br>Interventions to partially normalize biochemistry should only be considered to minimize these symptoms. | If the patient is experiencing symptoms, interventions include a phosphorus-restricted diet (being careful to maintain adequate nutrition) and the use of phosphate binders such as calcium carbonate.<br>Bloodwork every 3–6 months is appropriate if patients are being treated but should be based on patient preference and symptoms. |
| Vitamin D | Vitamin D may have a role in the symptoms of fatigue, weakness, and muscle loss. | Low-dose active vitamin D (vitamin D analog) may be beneficial. There is no additional benefit in monitoring parathyroid hormone levels. |

*CKD,* Chronic kidney disease; *CKM,* conservative kidney management; *QOL,* quality of life; *RLS,* restless legs syndrome.

requires a careful balance between promoting function and addressing symptom burden, whereas comfort and control of symptoms generally take precedence in the last weeks and days of life. Although there is minimal level I–III evidence specific to CKM patients, these recommendations have incorporated both geriatric and palliative care principles and serve as a starting point for standardization of care that will need to be refined as evidence for best practice accumulates. Many CKM patients present with complex health scenarios and recommendations have to be individualized. By explaining the rationale and possible benefits and drawbacks of interventions, patients can become active participants in the shared decision-making process, ensuring that all interventions remain aligned appropriately with their prognosis, values, and preferences.

Shared decision making for CKM versus dialysis is not integrated routinely into practice and patients continue to enter dialysis care pathways that are aligned poorly with their preferences and prognosis. The substantial regional variations in rates of kidney failure treated with dialysis for older patients suggest that decisions to start dialysis are influenced by factors other than clinical outcomes and may be more reflective of physician preferences.[84] Recent studies report that most elderly patients feel they have no choice in the decision to start dialysis; are not informed fully of their options or the risks of dialysis; experience distress over unexpected complications and burdens of dialysis; desire more conversation about the decision; and rarely recall being given the option for CKM.[85,86] Many patients feel a sense of resignation to dialysis, especially when decisions are framed incorrectly as choosing between life and death.[37] Physicians conceded that they struggle to explain illness trajectory and complexity and do not discuss prognosis unless prompted. There are currently extremely limited comparative prognostic data on CKM and dialysis. However, a recent systematic review of survival of CKM versus dialysis for elderly patients demonstrated a broadly similar 1-year survival.[80] Patients who choose CKM tend to have stable symptom burden and QOL until the last 1 or 2 months of life, and symptoms are amenable to supportive care interventions.[81] Given the degree of uncertainty about benefits and risks, and the potentially profound impact on QOL, patient values must be paramount in the decision about whether or not to have dialysis.

There has been great interest in the development of patient decision aids to help with renal replacement therapy decisions, including CKM. Patient decision aids are tools designed to facilitate people's ability to make reasoned decisions about care, which are compatible with their goals, values, and prognosis. These tools help supplement and guide the shared decision-making process and can be developed in multiple media forms, such as written materials, audiotapes, videos, Web-based formats, and oral presentations.[87] Two Cochrane reviews evaluating the use of patient decision aids have shown them to be effective[52,88] and can improve peoples' knowledge regarding options, reduce their decisional conflict, improve understanding of the relative risks and benefits, increase their participation in decision making, and improve values–choice concordance.[89] However, most decision aids for dialysis treatment options either do not mention CKM or address it only in a peripheral way. The main decision support is around which form of dialysis (or transplantation) to choose. These decision aids also do not include patient-specific risks and benefits so are not positioned to weigh QOL versus survival advantage, which patients require to make the decision that is best for them. New CKM decision aids are currently under development and evaluation to address these deficits.[67,90] These tools, however, must be used with caution. They are educational tools only and should not be used to mandate certain care pathways over others.

## PALLIATIVE DIALYSIS

As disease progresses, patients' goals of care may shift to focus almost exclusively on QOL rather than survival, with a strong emphasis on symptom control; advance care planning; and emotional, social, and family support. Palliative dialysis is an approach to dialysis that "prioritizes" QOL over survival and requires full integration of kidney supportive care (Fig. 62.7). Palliative dialysis is often, incorrectly, perceived as being equivalent to less dialysis or a precursor to withdrawal of dialysis. Although adaptation of dialysis timings or eventual withdrawal from dialysis may be a component, this alone will rarely ameliorate symptoms or suffering for patients.[25] This care pathway has recently been explored in greater detail elsewhere.[25] Dialysis patients may transition to a palliative approach to their dialysis care near the end of their life (see Chapter 84). Patients also may start dialysis with this palliative approach to their care. The dialysis guidelines and standards of care will need to permit flexibility so that care can be tailored appropriately for each patient and will look more like the CKM guidelines in Fig. 62.6.

## WITHDRAWAL OF DIALYSIS

Withdrawal from dialysis remains a leading cause of death for dialysis patients, although there are significant differences in reported rates across studies and national renal registries[91] and in practice patterns between countries.[92] Likely many of these differences relate to variations in culture, policy and physician perceptions, and attitudes toward withdrawal. For most cultures, withdrawal of dialysis is ethically and clinically acceptable, when based on shared decision making that balances the patient's interests with local cultural norms.[1]

Potential situations in which it is appropriate to withdraw dialysis are described in Box 62.1. It is incumbent upon all providers caring for a patient contemplating stopping dialysis to address potentially remedial factors contributing to the decision, such as depression or other symptoms such as pain, as well as potentially reversible social factors (discussed further in Chapter 82). Ensuring access to appropriate supportive care is an integral part of the care following a decision to withdraw dialysis.

**Box 62.1 Situations in Which It Is Appropriate to Consider Withdrawal from Dialysis[1,23]**

1. Patients with decision-making capacity, who being fully informed and making voluntary choices, refuse dialysis or request that dialysis be discontinued.
2. Patients who no longer possess decision-making capacity who have previously indicated refusal of dialysis through appropriate advance care planning.
3. Patients who no longer possess decision-making capacity and whose properly appointed legal agents/surrogates refuse dialysis or request that it be discontinued.
4. Patients with irreversible, profound neurologic impairment such that they lack signs of thought, sensation, purposeful behavior, and awareness of self and environment.

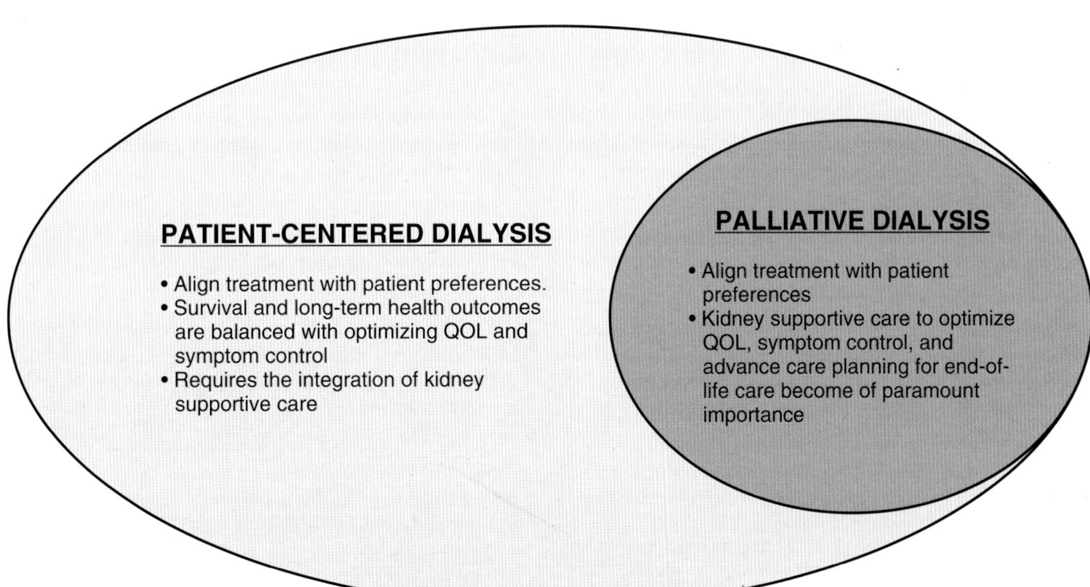


**Fig. 62.7** Conceptualizing palliative dialysis. *QOL,* Quality of life. (Adapted from Davison SN, Jassal SV. Supportive care: integration of patient-centered kidney care to manage symptoms and geriatric syndromes. *Clin J Am Soc Nephrol.* 2016;11:1882–1891.)

## EARLY IDENTIFICATION OF PATIENTS MOST LIKELY TO BENEFIT FROM SUPPORTIVE CARE SERVICES

A systematic approach to identify patients most likely to benefit from supportive care is critical in integrating kidney supportive care. Patients need to be identified based on need, not just poor prognosis. Not all patients require ongoing supportive care services, and requirements may fluctuate over the course of their illness trajectory (Fig. 62.1). However, most patients transition to a trajectory of progressive functional decline and/or experience complex clusters of physical and psychological symptoms. Early recognition of needs helps with planning, results in fewer hospital admissions and crises as patients approach the end of life, avoids needless suffering, and ultimately improves both patient and health system outcomes. Once the key elements of kidney supportive care are understood, it becomes clearer how to screen for patients in need. Fig. 62.2 highlights key issues that should be considered when screening patients for supportive care needs. At a minimum, this would include patients at a high risk of early death, those whose condition is deteriorating, patients with a high symptom burden or poor QOL, and those who are struggling with decision making and goals of care.

## SUMMARY

Addressing supportive care needs is a high priority for patients with advanced CKD.[24] The international kidney community recognizes that access to supportive care services should be available to all patients with advanced CKD, although the extent and form of these services will depend on local resources. For optimal delivery, multidisciplinary teams will need to work collaboratively across health–care sectors. There will also need to be an increased emphasis on education in kidney supportive care that recognizes this as a core competency in nephrology. Integrating kidney supportive care will also require recognition that our current models of care, policies, and clinical standards do not consistently meet the needs of our patients. Ongoing work will help determine best practices, including appropriate quality of kidney supportive care metrics.

 Complete reference list available at ExpertConsult.com.

### KEY REFERENCES


1. Davison SN, Levin A, Moss AH, et al. Executive summary of the KDIGO Controversies Conference on Supportive Care in Chronic Kidney Disease: developing a roadmap to improving quality care. *Kidney Int.* 2015;88:447–459.
7. Davison SN. End-of-life care preferences and needs: perceptions of patients with chronic kidney disease. *Clin J Am Soc Nephrol.* 2010;5:195–204.
8. Tong A, Cheung KL, Nair SS, et al. Thematic synthesis of qualitative studies on patient and caregiver perspectives on end-of-life care in CKD. *Am J Kidney Dis.* 2014;63:913–927.
9. Quill TE. Perspectives on care at the close of life. Initiating end-of-life discussions with seriously ill patients: addressing the "elephant in the room." *JAMA.* 2000;284:2502–2507.
10. Combs SA, Culp S, Matlock DD, et al. Update on end-of-life care training during nephrology fellowship: a cross-sectional national survey of fellows. *Am J Kidney Dis.* 2014.
11. Culp S, Lupu D, Arenella C, et al. Unmet supportive care needs in U.S. dialysis centers and lack of knowledge of available resources to address them. *J Pain Symptom Manage.* 2015;51:756–761.
12. Davison S, Jhangri GS. Existential and supportive care needs among patients with chronic kidney disease. *J Pain Symptom Manage.* 2010;40:838–843.
13. Organization WH. WHO definition of palliative care. World Health Organization; 2008. http://www.who.int/cancer/palliative/definition/en/. Accessed April 5, 2016.
15. Davison SN, Jhangri GS, Koffman J. Knowledge of and attitudes towards palliative care and hospice services among patients with advanced chronic kidney disease. *BMJ Support Palliat Care.* 2014;6:66–74.
22. Brown EABH, Davison SN, Koffman J, et al. Supportive care: religious and multicultural aspects of advance care planning and shared decision-making including the role for decision science. *Clin J Am Soc Nephrol.* 2016;11:1915–1920.
23. Renal Physicians Association. In: Association, ed. Shared decision-making in the appropriate initiation of and withdrawal from dialysis. Renal Physicians Association and American Society of Nephrology; 2010. https://www.renalmd.org/catalogue-item.aspx?id=682. Accessed April 5, 2016.
24. Manns B, Hemmelgarn B, Lillie E, et al. Setting research priorities for patients on or nearing dialysis. *Clin J Am Soc Nephrol.* 2014;9:1813–1821.
25. Davison SN, Jassal SV. Supportive care: integration of patient-centered kidney care to manage symptoms and geriatric syndromes. *Clin J Am Soc Nephrol.* 2016.
32. Brown EA, Bekker HL, Davison SN, et al. Supportive care: communication strategies to improve cultural competence in shared decision making. *Clin J Am Soc Nephrol.* 2016.
33. Kagawa-Singer M, Kassim-Lakha S. A strategy to reduce cross-cultural miscommunication and increase the likelihood of improving health outcomes. *Acad Med.* 2003;78:577–587.
36. Chiu HH, Tangri N, Djurdjev O, et al. Perceptions of prognostic risks in chronic kidney disease: a national survey. *Can J Kidney Health Dis.* 2015;2:53.
37. Schell JO, Patel UD, Steinhauser KE, et al. Discussions of the kidney disease trajectory by elderly patients and nephrologists: a qualitative study. *Am J Kidney Dis.* 2012;59:495–503.
38. Couchoud C, Hemmelgarn B, Kotanko P, et al. Supportive care: time to change our prognostic tools and their use in CKD. *Clin J Am Soc Nephrol.* 2016.
42. Walker SR, Gill K, Macdonald K, et al. Association of frailty and physical function in patients with non-dialysis CKD: a systematic review. *BMC Nephrol.* 2013;14:228.
47. Johnstone S, Dombro L, Garza GSCK, et al. Declines in hemodialysis patients' physical and mental component scores before death. *J Am Soc Nephrol.* 2014;25.
48. Thijssen S, Wong MM, Usvyat LA, et al. Nutritional competence and resilience among hemodialysis patients in the setting of dialysis initiation and hospitalization. *Clin J Am Soc Nephrol.* 2015;10:1593–1601.
50. Kotanko P, Kooman J, van der Sande F, et al. Accelerated or out of control: the final months on dialysis. *J Ren Nutr.* 2014;24:357–363.
52. Stacey D, Legare F, Col NF, et al. Decision aids for people facing health treatment or screening decisions. *Cochrane Database Syst Rev.* 2014;(1):CD001431.
53. Davison SN, Jhangri GS, Johnson JA. Cross-sectional validity of a modified Edmonton symptom assessment system in dialysis patients: a simple assessment of symptom burden. *Kidney Int.* 2006;69:1621–1625.
54. Davison SN, Jhangri GS, Johnson JA. Longitudinal validation of a modified Edmonton symptom assessment system (ESAS) in haemodialysis patients. *Nephrol Dial Transplant.* 2006;21:3189–3195.
55. Davison SN, Jhangri GS. Impact of pain and symptom burden on the health-related quality of life of hemodialysis patients. *J Pain Symptom Manage.* 2010;39:477–485.
57. Edmonton Zone Palliative Care Program and Northern Alberta Renal Program. 2016. http://www.palliative.org/tools.html. Accessed March 31, 2018.
58. Davison SN, Koncicki H, Brennan F. Pain in chronic kidney disease: a scoping review. *Semin Dial.* 2014;27:188–204.
59. Dworkin RH, Turk DC, Wyrwich KW, et al. Interpreting the clinical importance of treatment outcomes in chronic pain clinical trials: IMMPACT recommendations. *J Pain.* 2008;9:105–121.

60. Andrew Moore R, Eccleston C, Derry S, et al. "Evidence" in chronic pain—establishing best practice in the reporting of systematic reviews. *Pain.* 2010;150:386–389.
63. Antunes B, Harding R, Higginson IJ. Implementing patient-reported outcome measures in palliative care clinical practice: a systematic review of facilitators and barriers. *Palliat Med.* 2014;28:158–175.
67. Kidney Supportive Care Research Group. *Conservative Kidney Management Care Pathway*, 2016. www.ckmcare.com. Accessed September 20, 2017.
68. Davison SN, Tupala B, Wasylynuk BA, et al. *Recommendations for the care of patients receiving conservative kidney management: focus on management of chronic kidney disease and symptoms. Clin J Am Soc Nephrol.* 2018 (in press).
71. Davison SN, Torgunrud C. The creation of an advance care planning process for patients with ESRD. *Am J Kidney Dis.* 2007;49:27–36.
74. Chambers EJ, Brown E, Germain M. *Supportive Care for the Renal Patient.* Oxford University Press; 2010.
77. Schell JO, Green JA, Tulsky JA, et al. Communication skills training for dialysis decision-making and end-of-life care in nephrology. *Clin J Am Soc Nephrol.* 2013;8:675–680.
80. Foote C, Kotwal S, Gallagher M, et al. Survival outcomes of supportive care versus dialysis therapies for elderly patients with end-stage kidney disease: a systematic review and meta-analysis. *Nephrology (Carlton).* 2016;21:241–253.
81. Murtagh FE, Burns A, Moranne O, et al. Supportive care: comprehensive conservative care in end-stage kidney disease. *Clin J Am Soc Nephrol.* 2016.
82. Tamura MK, Covinsky K, Chertow G, et al. Functional status of elderly adults before and after initiation of dialysis. *N Engl J Med.* 2009;361:1539–1547.
83. Jassal SV, Chiu E, Hladunewich M. Loss of independence in patients starting dialysis at 80 years of age or older. *N Engl J Med.* 2009;361:1612–1613.
85. Ladin K, Lin N, Hahn E, et al. Engagement in decision-making and patient satisfaction: a qualitative study of older patients' perceptions of dialysis initiation and modality decisions. *Nephrol Dial Transplant.* 2016.
86. Song MK, Lin FC, Gilet CA, et al. Patient perspectives on informed decision-making surrounding dialysis initiation. *Nephrol Dial Transplant.* 2013;28:2815–2823.
90. Davis JL, Davison SN. Hard choices, better outcomes: a review of shared decision-making and patient decision aids around dialysis initiation and conservative kidney management. *Curr Opin Nephrol Hypertens.* 2017;26:205–213.
91. Murphy E, Germain MJ, Cairns H, et al. International variation in classification of dialysis withdrawal: a systematic review. *Nephrol Dial Transplant.* 2014;29:625–635.
94. Tangri N, Grams ME, Levey AS, et al. Multinational assessment of accuracy of equations for predicting risk of kidney failure: a meta-analysis. *JAMA.* 2016;315:164–174.
95. Thamer M, Kaufman JS, Zhang Y, et al. Predicting early death among elderly dialysis patients: development and validation of a risk score to assist shared decision making for dialysis initiation. *Am J Kidney Dis.* 2015;66:1024–1032.
99. Cohen LM, Ruthazer R, Moss AH, et al. Predicting six-month mortality for patients who are on maintenance hemodialysis. *Clin J Am Soc Nephrol.* 2010;5:72–79.
102. Dworkin RH, Turk DC, Farrar JT, et al. Core outcome measures for chronic pain clinical trials: IMMPACT recommendations. *Pain.* 2005;113:9–19.
103. Kutner JS, Blatchford PJ, Taylor DH Jr, et al. Safety and benefit of discontinuing statin therapy in the setting of advanced, life-limiting illness: a randomized clinical trial. *JAMA Intern Med.* 2015;175:691–700.
106. Musini VM, Tejani AM, Bassett K, et al. Pharmacotherapy for hypertension in the elderly. *Cochrane Database Syst Rev.* 2009;CD000028.

# SECTION X

# DIALYSIS AND EXTRACORPOREAL THERAPIES

# 63 Hemodialysis

Jane Y. Yeun | Brian Young | Thomas A. Depner | Andrew A. Chin

CHAPTER OUTLINE



Hemodialysis (HD) sustains life for more than 1 million patients throughout the world. Without it, most would die within a few weeks.[1,2] This vital aspect of the treatment highlights the need among caregivers to gain an in-depth understanding of all aspects of HD, including its target, the uremic syndrome (see Chapter 52). This chapter reviews the history of dialysis, the epidemiology of the HD patient population, the physical, chemical, and clinical principles of HD as they relate to the treatment of patients with uremia, and the complications associated with this treatment.

HD has been applied routinely to preserve life in patients with end-stage kidney disease (ESKD) only for the past 40 years. Several early pioneers laid the foundation. Graham (1805–1869), a Scottish professor of chemistry, invented the fundamental process of separating solutes in vitro using semipermeable membranes and coined the word "dialysis."[3] In 1916, Abel dialyzed rabbits and dogs with a so-called *vividiffusion* device using celloidin membranes and a leech extract, hirudin, as an anticoagulant.[4] He was the first to dialyze a living organism and to use the term "artificial kidney." In 1924, in Germany, Haas was the first to dialyze a human[5] but was only marginally successful because of toxicity from his crude anticoagulant.

In 1944, Willem Kolff succeeded in using extracorporeal dialysis to support patients with acute kidney failure.[6] His success was partly attributable to the invention of cellophane, the discovery of antibiotics, and the availability of heparin. Kolff was often called the "father of hemodialysis," and his method became the standard for temporary replacement of kidney function in patients with short-lived acute renal failure.[7,8] However, HD could not support patients with prolonged or permanent loss of kidney function because of the difficulty with vascular access, subsequently solved by the creation of the arteriovenous (AV) fistula (see "Vascular Access").

Although it had become technically feasible, HD remained expensive and inefficient and was offered only to those who were free of comorbid conditions, gainfully employed, and better educated. Because dialysis was so successful in preventing death from kidney failure, Congress, after much debate, passed a law in 1973 approving public funding for dialysis and kidney transplantation, regardless of the patient's means, education, employment, or comorbidities.[9] This law paved the way to life-sustaining kidney replacement for all US patients.

## THE HEMODIALYSIS POPULATION

### INCIDENCE AND PREVALENCE

According to the US Renal Data System (USRDS), 124,114 patients developed ESKD in the United States in 2015, with an unadjusted incidence rate of 378/million population. Of these, 2.5% were transplanted preemptively, 87.7% were started on HD, and 9.6% on peritoneal dialysis.[10] Fig. 63.1A shows that the adjusted incidence rate of ESKD in the United States steadily increased from 1987 to 2002, most likely as a result of aging of the population and increasing acceptance of dialysis for older patients as part of their Medicare entitlement. This leveled off in 2002 and has declined since 2006, with the largest decrease of 3.8% in 2011, and has leveled off again since 2013 (see Fig. 63.1B).

In contrast, both the prevalent count and prevalence rate of ESKD continue to rise in the United States (see Fig. 63.1C).[10] At the end of 2015, 703,243 patients had ESKD, with an adjusted prevalence of 2203/million population. Of these patients, 30% had functioning transplants, and the remainder were maintained by dialysis, with 11.7% of patients undergoing dialysis on home modalities (10% on peritoneal dialysis; 1.7% on home hemodialysis). Although the prevalent number of patients with ESKD continues to grow, the annual growth rate in the prevalent count of 3.3% to 3.6% and in adjusted prevalence of 1.2% to 1.6% since 2011 represent the lowest in 35 years.

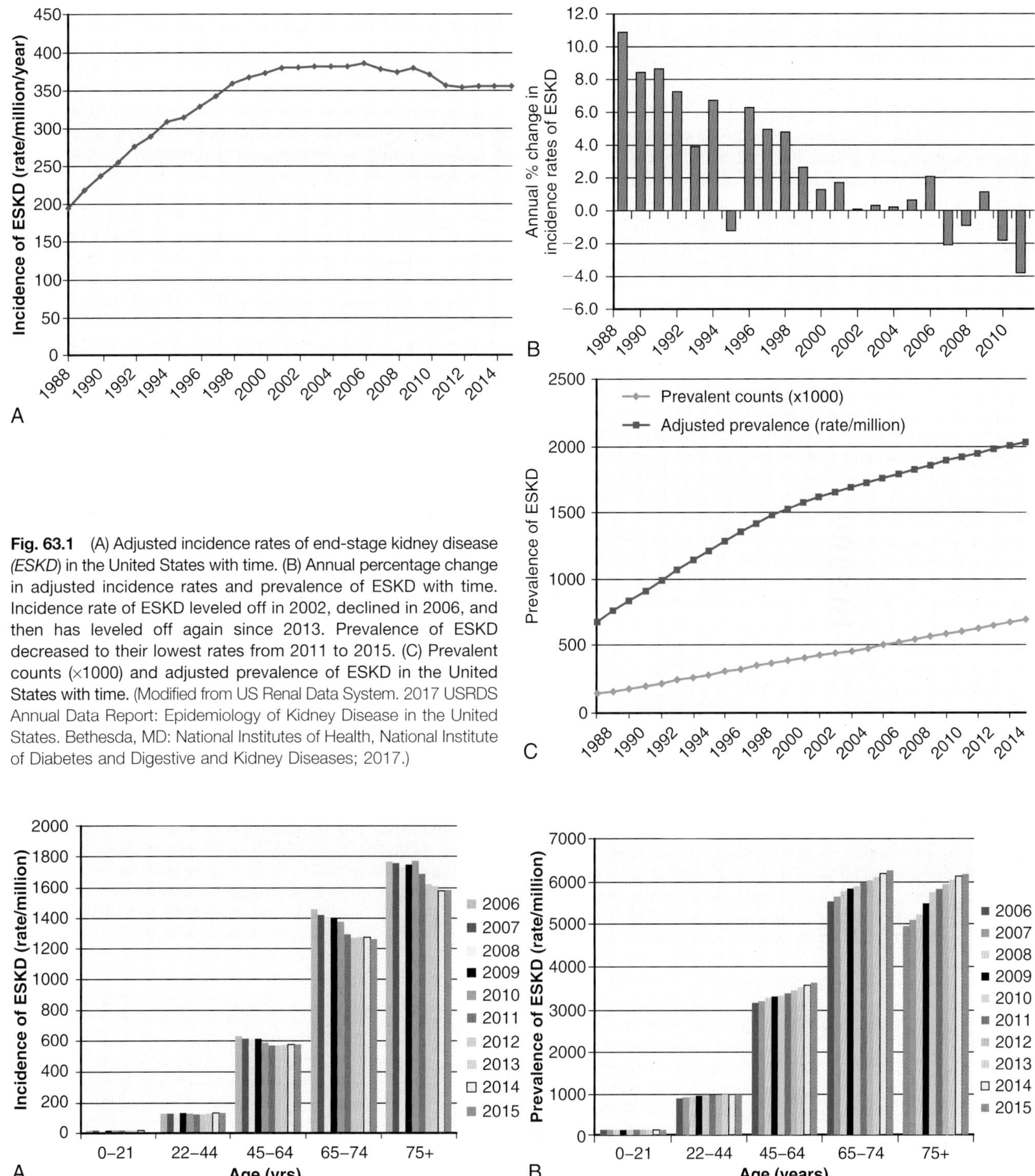


**Fig. 63.1** (A) Adjusted incidence rates of end-stage kidney disease (*ESKD*) in the United States with time. (B) Annual percentage change in adjusted incidence rates and prevalence of ESKD with time. Incidence rate of ESKD leveled off in 2002, declined in 2006, and then has leveled off again since 2013. Prevalence of ESKD decreased to their lowest rates from 2011 to 2015. (C) Prevalent counts (×1000) and adjusted prevalence of ESKD in the United States with time. (Modified from US Renal Data System. 2017 USRDS Annual Data Report: Epidemiology of Kidney Disease in the United States. Bethesda, MD: National Institutes of Health, National Institute of Diabetes and Digestive and Kidney Diseases; 2017.)



**Fig. 63.2.** Incidence (A) and prevalence (B) of end-stage kidney disease (rate/million per year) with age from 2006 to 2015. (Modified from US Renal Data System. 2017 USRDS Annual Data Report: Epidemiology of Kidney Disease in the United States. Bethesda, MD: National Institutes of Health, National Institute of Diabetes and Digestive and Kidney Diseases; 2017.)

Both the prevalence and incidence of ESKD vary widely with age (Fig. 63.2), gender (Fig. 63.3), and race and ethnicity (Fig. 63.4), with a predilection for older age, men, African-Americans, Native Hawaiians, and Pacific Islanders.[10] Over the past few years, the incidence of ESKD has declined in persons older than 45, African-Americans, Hispanics, and American Indians and Alaskan natives, but has continued to rise in Native Hawaiians and Pacific Islanders (see Figs. 63.2A and 63.4A). In contrast, the prevalence of ESKD has continued to rise, suggesting improved survival in those on dialysis.

Worldwide, in 2014, Taiwan, the Jalisco region in Mexico, and the United States had the highest incidence rates for ESKD at 455, 421, and 370 per million population (pmp), respectively, followed by Thailand (299 pmp), Singapore (294 pmp), and Japan (285 pmp).[11] Thailand experienced the highest percentage rise in ESKD incidence rates from 2002 to 2014 at 1009%, followed by Bangladesh (643%), Russia (291%), the Philippines (190%), and Malaysia (162%). In contrast, the ESKD incidence rates decreased in Austria, Denmark, Sweden, Scotland, Finland, and Iceland by 3% to 14%. The prevalence rate for ESKD continues to rise in all countries, with the highest rates in Taiwan at 3219 pmp (2014 data), followed by Japan (2505 pmp) and the United States (2076 pmp). The median increase in prevalence rates from 2002 to 2014 was 48%, ranging from 18% to 1092%, with the largest proportionate increase in prevalence rates in the Philippines, Thailand, and the Jalisco region of Mexico (343%–1092%). However, the worldwide prevalence of ESKD varies greatly, with the lowest rates reported in the Philippines, Russia, South Africa, Indonesia, and Bangladesh at less than 300 pmp. The broad ranges of reported ESKD prevalence likely result from variable access to treatment and to preventive and maintenance health care.

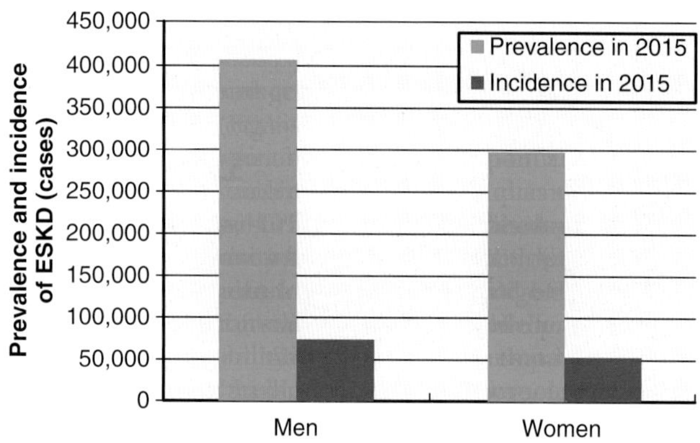


**Fig. 63.3.** Incidence and prevalence of end-stage kidney *(ESKD)* disease with gender. (Modified from US Renal Data System. 2017 USRDS Annual Data Report: Epidemiology of Kidney Disease in the United States. Bethesda, MD: National Institutes of Health, National Institute of Diabetes and Digestive and Kidney Diseases; 2017.)

## CAUSES OF END-STAGE KIDNEY DISEASE

The causes of ESKD in the United States are listed in Table 63.1. Since 1980, the percentage of patients with diabetic kidney disease starting dialysis has increased from near 0% to 45% of patients starting dialysis in 2015 (Fig. 63.5), primarily because of increased acceptance of patients with diabetes into dialysis programs, but with a potential contribution from improved survival of these patients so that they live long enough to develop ESKD. Although the incidence rate of ESKD from diabetes in the United States has declined since 2006 (172.9 pmp in 2006 compared with 162.7 pmp in 2015; see Fig. 63.5), diabetes remains the most common cause of ESKD in the United States and in many other countries,[11] exceeding 40% in Israel, the Republic of Korea, Hong Kong, Taiwan, the Philippines, Japan, the United States, New Zealand, Thailand, Chile, and Kuwait, and reaching as high

**Table 63.1 Causes of End-Stage Kidney Disease in Incident and Prevalent Patients[a]**

| Primary Kidney Disease | Incident Patients No. | Incident Patients % of Total | Prevalent Patients No. | Prevalent Patients % of Total |
|---|---|---|---|---|
| Diabetes mellitus | 56,218 | 45.4 | 267,956 | 38.2 |
| Hypertension | 34,727 | 28.1 | 178,875 | 25.5 |
| Glomerulonephritis | 9198 | 7.4 | 112,235 | 16.0 |
| Cystic kidney disease | 2833 | 2.3 | 33,194 | 4.7 |
| Other | 20,856 | 16.8 | 109,092 | 15.6 |
| Total | 123,832 | 100 | 701,352 | 100 |

[a]In the United States in 2015.

Data from US Renal Data System. 2017 USRDS Annual Data Report: Epidemiology of Kidney Disease in the United States. Bethesda, MD: National Institutes of Health, National Institute of Diabetes and Digestive and Kidney Diseases; 2017.

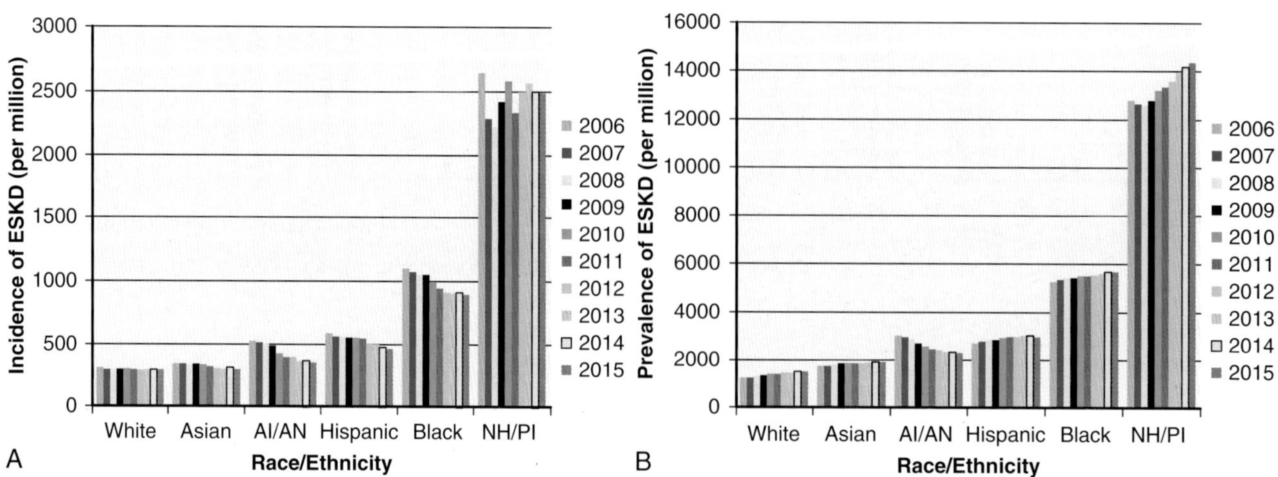


**Fig. 63.4.** Incidence (A) and prevalence (B) of end-stage kidney disease *(ESKD)* with race and ethnicity. *AI/AN,* American Indian or Alaska Native; *Black,* black or African-American; *NH/PI,* Native Hawaiian or Pacific Islander. (Modified from US Renal Data System. 2017 USRDS Annual Data Report: Epidemiology of Kidney Disease in the United States. Bethesda, MD: National Institutes of Health, National Institute of Diabetes and Digestive and Kidney Diseases; 2017.)

as 58% to 66% in Singapore, Malaysia, and the Jalisco region of Mexico. Remarkably, diabetes accounted for less than 20% of new ESKD cases in Italy, Switzerland, the Netherlands, Belgium, Estonia, Norway, Romania, and Iceland.

## MORTALITY

The survival of patients undergoing dialysis in the United States has slowly improved in the past 20 years, despite increasing comorbidities, with the largest gains in the last 10 years. The adjusted mortality rate for prevalent hemodialysis patients has decreased by 29% from 1996 to 2014, with a 4% reduction from 1996 to 2003 and 24% from 2004 to 2014 (Fig. 63.6).[11] Although 5-year survival rates have increased from 30% in the 1998 cohort to 42% in the 2010 cohort (Fig. 63.7), mortality remains very high. Patients starting hemodialysis in 2010 have a 78% 1-year survival, 66% 2-year survival, and 42% 5-year survival (see Fig. 63.7).[11] Compared with age-matched persons without kidney disease, patients undergoing dialysis have a markedly reduced life expectancy (Fig. 63.8A).[10] At age 60 years, a healthy person can expect to live for about 20 years, but the median life expectancy of a 60-year-old patient starting HD is only 4 to 5 years (see Fig. 63.8A). Remarkably, mortality rates of patients with ESKD undergoing dialysis is higher than that of patients with AIDS, most forms of cancer, and heart failure (see Fig. 63.8B). Patients older than 65 years were faring better in 2014 than in 1996, with a 39% decline in adjusted mortality rate, compared with a 37% drop in mortality rate for cancer and 21% for heart failure.[11]

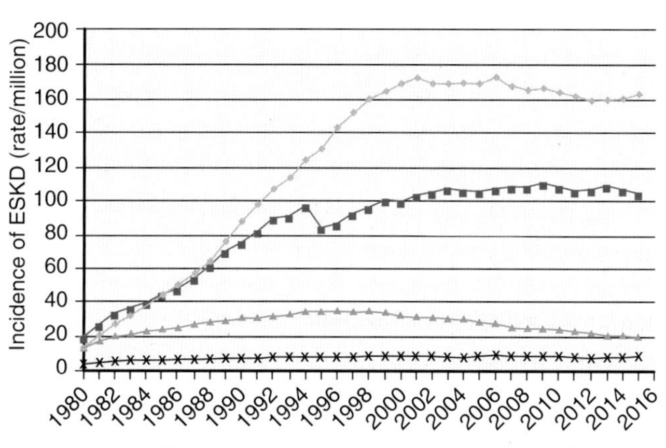


**Fig. 63.5** Causes of end-stage kidney disease *(ESKD)* in the United States. (Modified from US Renal Data System. 2017 USRDS Annual Data Report: Epidemiology of Kidney Disease in the United States. Bethesda, MD: National Institutes of Health, National Institute of Diabetes and Digestive and Kidney Diseases; 2017.)

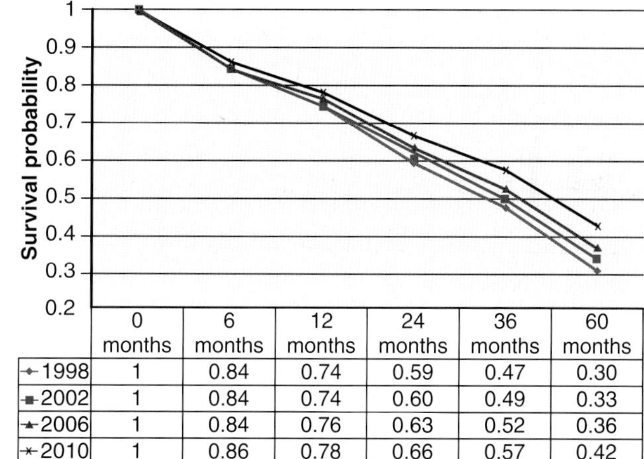


| | 0 months | 6 months | 12 months | 24 months | 36 months | 60 months |
|---|---|---|---|---|---|---|
| 1998 | 1 | 0.84 | 0.74 | 0.59 | 0.47 | 0.30 |
| 2002 | 1 | 0.84 | 0.74 | 0.60 | 0.49 | 0.33 |
| 2006 | 1 | 0.84 | 0.76 | 0.63 | 0.52 | 0.36 |
| 2010 | 1 | 0.86 | 0.78 | 0.66 | 0.57 | 0.42 |

**Fig. 63.7** Probability of survival for hemodialysis patients. The likelihood for survival of hemodialysis patients has improved slightly over the past 10 years. (Modified from US Renal Data System. 2017 USRDS Annual Data Report: Epidemiology of Kidney Disease in the United States. Bethesda, MD: National Institutes of Health, National Institute of Diabetes and Digestive and Kidney Diseases; 2017.)

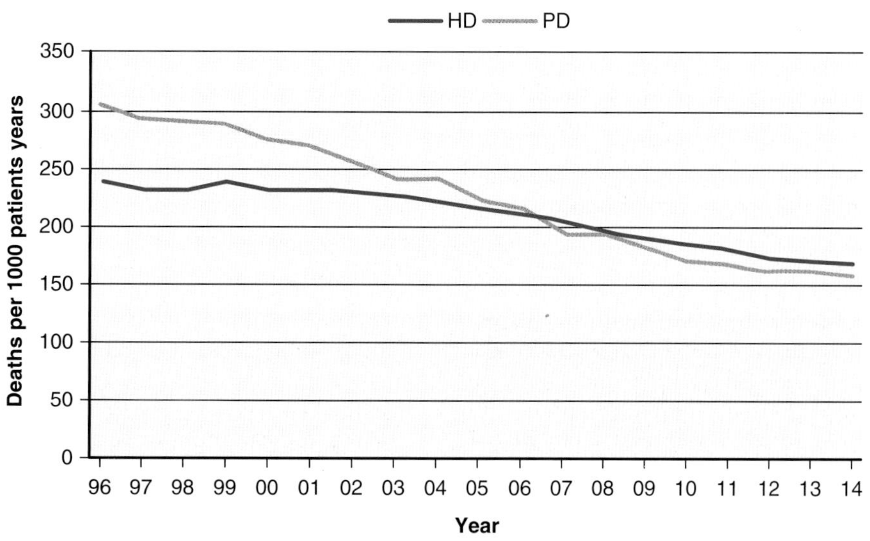


**Fig. 63.6** Mortality rates for patients on hemodialysis. Mortality rates for patients on hemodialysis (HD) as well as peritoneal dialysis (PD) have declined steadily. (Modified from US Renal Data System. 2017 USRDS Annual Data Report: Epidemiology of Kidney Disease in the United States. Bethesda, MD: National Institutes of Health, National Institute of Diabetes and Digestive and Kidney Diseases; 2017.)

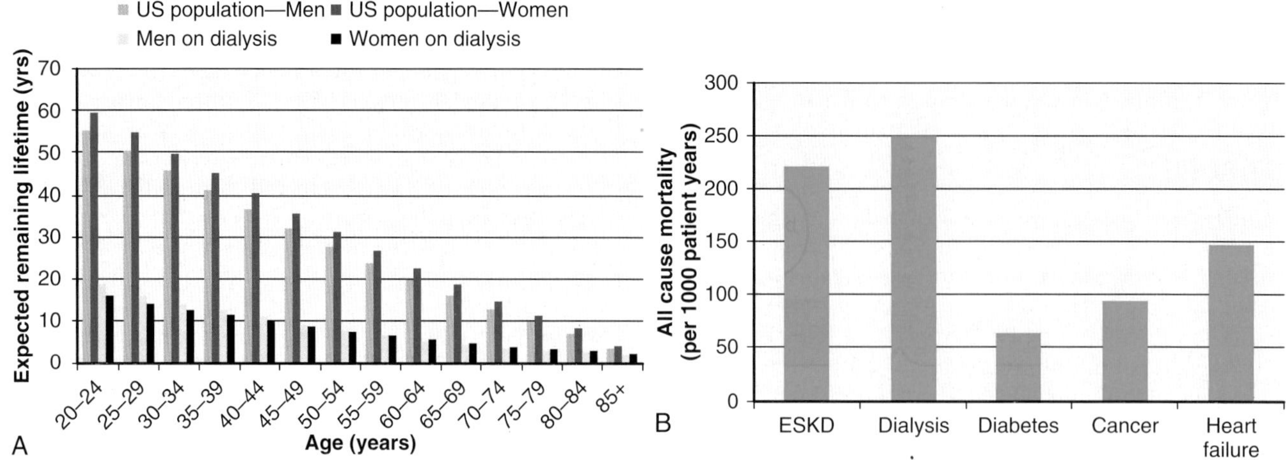


**Fig. 63.8.** Life expectancy and adjusted all-cause mortality rates for end-stage kidney disease *(ESKD)* patients in 2014. (A) Patients with ESKD or on dialysis have a markedly reduced life expectancy compared with the general population. (B) Their mortality rate is even higher than that of patients with diabetes, cancer, and heart failure. (Modified from US Renal Data System. 2017 USRDS Annual Data Report: Epidemiology of Kidney Disease in the United States. Bethesda, MD: National Institutes of Health, National Institute of Diabetes and Digestive and Kidney Diseases; 2017.)

**Table 63.2 Causes of Death for Prevalent Hemodialysis Patients (2013)**

| Cause of Death | % of Total |
|---|---|
| Cardiovascular disease | 41% |
| • Arrhythmia, cardiac arrest | 29% |
| • Myocardial infarction | 4% |
| • Other | 8% |
| Infection | 8% |
| Withdrawal from dialysis | 13% |
| Other causes | 14% |
| Missing causes | 24% |

Data from US Renal Data System. 2017 USRDS Annual Data Report: Epidemiology of Kidney Disease in the United States. Bethesda, MD: National Institutes of Health, National Institute of Diabetes and Digestive and Kidney Diseases; 2017.

Causes of death are listed in Table 63.2. Deaths from cardiovascular disease were 41%, with 29% from arrhythmia or cardiac arrest and only 4% from myocardial infarction.[10] The cause(s) for the high burden of cardiovascular disease in patients undergoing dialysis remain a source of debate, but it appears that the dialysis process itself may play a significant role through the long interval between dialysis over the weekend, excessive rates of ultrafiltration during dialysis, and aggressive correction of electrolyte and acid-base abnormalities during dialysis[12] (see Chapter 54 and "Dialysate Composition," later). Infections accounted for another 8% of deaths.[10,13] Overall, voluntary withdrawal from dialysis accounted for another 13% of deaths, a 3% increase compared with 2009 to 2011 data. Patients who withdraw from dialysis tend to be older, women, and white and have higher rates of medical events and higher levels of morbidity in the period preceding withdrawal.[14] In addition, a nonuniform approach to advanced care planning in patients with multiple comorbidities and poorer quality of life and insufficient exploration of goals of care in this population before embarking on maintenance dialysis may contribute toward the rising incidence of voluntary withdrawal.[15,16]

## TRANSITION FROM CHRONIC KIDNEY DISEASE, STAGE 5

The high mortality of patients undergoing HD results in part from many associated comorbid conditions, including cardiovascular disease, diabetes, and hypertension. These comorbid conditions extract a toll on patients with chronic kidney disease (CKD) before they develop ESKD and require dialysis. The relative risk of death is two to three times higher in patients with CKD, diabetes, and cardiovascular disease than in patients without these conditions; patients with CKD stage 4 or 5 experience the highest mortality risk.[11] A patient with stage 4 or 5 CKD who has an acute myocardial infarction (MI) has a 2-year mortality rate of 47% compared with 20% in the absence of CKD. Reducing or improving comorbidities, then, is critical in caring for patients with CKD (see Chapter 59).

In addition, close attention to replacing hormone deficiencies such as erythropoietin (see Chapter 55) and calcitriol (see Chapter 53) and preventing complications of uremia such as malnutrition (see Chapter 60) and CKD–mineral bone disorder (Chapter 53) are essential. Another critical element in preparing patients with CKD for ESKD care is preemptive planning for potential transplantation as well as for a permanent vascular access to support hemodialysis (see later), beginning when the estimated glomerular filtration rate (eGFR) has declined to 20 to 25 mL/min/1.73 m$^2$.

Psychological support is another important but often overlooked and poorly understood part of caring for a patient on hemodialysis. Depression, disabling fatigue, severe restless legs syndrome, insomnia, anxiety, and prolonged recovery time after dialysis are common in patients undergoing HD.[17–33] Their presence is associated with poorer quality of life, malnutrition, poor quality of sleep, low level of physical function, presence of inflammation, hospitalization, and death.[17,19,20,22,25,26,29,30,34–42]

Despite the profound impact of these factors on the quality of life and outcome of patients on dialysis, little is known about their true epidemiology, pathogenesis, and effective treatment. Diagnosing depression may be difficult in patients on dialysis because some of the symptoms used to make the diagnosis may be present due to uremia.[17–19] Once the diagnosis is made, patients and their providers may be resistant to treatment because of increased pill burden, potential toxicity of medications, and lack of mental health resources.[43] Some studies have suggested that certain selective serotonin reuptake inhibitors (SSRIs), intensive hemodialysis, cognitive-behavioral therapy, and may be effective in reducing depressive symptoms, anxiety, sleep disturbances, postdialysis recovery time, and quality of life, but others debate the effectiveness of SSRIs and intensive dialysis, likely because many studies are small and/or uncontrolled.[17,31,35,44–58] Dopamine agonists, gabapentin, and exercise may ameliorate restless legs syndrome.[26,42,59,60] Larger and more rigorous studies are needed and are underway.[45,61]

Because of the multifaceted care required before starting HD, timely referral to a nephrologist is essential. Studies have documented higher hospitalization rates,[62,63] more symptoms of depression,[64] worse anemia and biochemical disturbances (e.g., hypoalbuminemia, hyperphosphatemia, hypocalcemia, acidosis, hyperkalemia),[62,63,65–67] lesser use of peritoneal dialysis,[63] higher use of dialysis catheters,[63,68] and higher mortality[62,63,67–73] when nephrology referral is delayed, but other studies have found no difference in mortality risk and in ESKD risk.[71,74–76] Potential confounders may be the reasons underlying late referral such as patient nonadherence, multiple comorbidities, advanced age, and rapid decline in kidney function.[67,77,78] The widely varying definitions of early referral, ranging from more than 1 to 6 months before starting dialysis to CKD stage 3 (eGFR <60 mL/min/1.73 m$^2$), may have also contributed to the disparate findings. Studies of patients with nondialysis-requiring CKD followed by nephrologists have suggested that death occurs more frequently than ESKD in patients with CKD 3a (eGFR 45–60 mL/min), whereas the opposite is true in patients with CKD 5 (eGFR <15 mL/min).[63,67,68,71,73–76,79,80]

The competing risks of death or ESKD reach parity at CKD stage 3b (eGFR 30–45 mL/min/1.73 m$^2$) to CKD stage 4 (eGFR 15–30 mL/min/1.73 m$^2$).[67,79–81] In patients managed only by primary care physicians, the mortality rate for patients with CKD stage 3a is comparable to those with CKD stages 1 to 2 and rises progressively with more advanced stages of CKD.[81] Referral to nephrologists at CKD stage 3a or 3b was not associated with a change in the risk for death and/or progression to ESKD,[75,76] whereas referral at CKD stage 4 was associated with a lower mortality risk but not with risk of progression to ESKD.[67] It is unclear why nephrology care was not associated with the risk for ESKD, but these findings have suggested that the most appropriate early referral to nephrology for established CKD may be at stage 3b or 4.

Current clinical practice guidelines have suggested that dialysis be initiated when patients become symptomatic from uremia, often occurring at an eGFR between 5 and 10 mL/min/1.73 m$^2$.[82] In some patients, volume overload and hyperkalemia not responsive to conservative medical management with diuretics and dietary potassium restriction and/or unexplained progressive decline in nutritional status, despite aggressive dietary intervention, may dictate earlier initiation of dialysis. The goal for patients with kidney failure is a smooth transition from CKD to ESKD, avoiding the complications of overt uremia. The results of several studies have supported these clinical practice guidelines.[83–86] The IDEAL (Initiating Dialysis Early and Late) study,[83] the only randomized controlled trial, has reported comparable survival and clinical outcomes in patients randomized to early start (eGFR >10 mL/min/1.73 m$^2$ by the Cockcroft-Gault equation) versus late start of dialysis (eGFR = 5–7 mL/min/1.73 m$^2$). However, 75% of the patients randomized to a late start of dialysis initiated dialysis when the eGFR was above 7 mL/min/1.73 m$^2$ because of intervening symptoms attributed to uremia, volume overload, or nutritional decline. A potential weakness of the IDEAL study was use of the Cockcroft-Gault equation to estimate the GFR. However, secondary analysis of the trial data using the MDRD (Modification of Diet in Renal Disease) and the CKD-EPI (Chronic Kidney Disease–Epidemiology) formula to estimate GFR also demonstrated no significant effect of timing of dialysis initiation on survival.[87] Earlier initiation of dialysis is not cost-effective[88] and may be harmful,[89–91] possibly because of an accelerated loss of residual kidney function, more use of dialysis catheters, myocardial stunning, depression, and provider inexperience at a time when lifesaving benefits from dialysis are low.[91,92] Current guidelines have suggested a patient-centered approach in determining when to initiate dialysis, balancing the prevention of uremic complications with quality of life and patient preferences.[82,93–97]

## VASCULAR ACCESS

Establishing and maintaining a reliable and trouble-free vascular access, which is often seen as the weakest and most troublesome aspect of hemodialysis, is paramount for the successful long-term application of HD. Vascular access planning, placement and trouble shooting require a multidisciplinary team approach, which traditionally has included surgeons and interventional radiologists, in addition to the nephrologist. Interventional nephrology, a procedurally oriented subspecialty in nephrology, has been increasing its presence in many health markets. The field of interventional nephrology has allowed nephrologists to intervene in dysfunctional HD vascular accesses directly (see Chapter 68). Nonetheless, a large proportion of patients with advanced CKD begin HD with a catheter. Therefore, much work is still needed to optimize vascular access in both incident and prevalent patients.

### BACKGROUND

Innovative techniques in vascular surgery have allowed the widespread use of maintenance HD as a viable approach to the management of ESKD. Although external constant flow arteriovenous (AV) devices, such as the Quinton-Scribner shunt, have led to more reliable and repeatable access to the circulation, thrombosis and infection have limited the longevity of these devices, and the procedure permanently damaged major arteries and veins.[98] In 1966, Brescia and colleagues[99] developed the procedure to create an endogenous

AV fistula which allowed for long-term HD. This procedure was relatively simple, was totally subcutaneous, and preserved arterial flow to the hand.

The advent of procedures using AV grafts allowed patients who were not candidates for a fistula to receive a durable subcutaneous access.[100,101] The 1970s brought the development of vascular conduits made of expanded polytetrafluoroethylene (ePTFE) and biologically processed bovine carotid arteries, which greatly expanded AV access for patients whose natural veins were not suitable for an AV fistula. In recent years, the use of polyurethane self-sealing materials in AV grafts, as well as a hybrid graft with a catheter venous outflow device, have expanded vascular access options for patients with suboptimal native vasculature.[102,103]

The arm is clearly the preferred site for fistulas or grafts; however, in some patients, the leg becomes an alternative when necessary.[104] It is nearly always preferred to use the most distal vein feasible for an AV shunt to preserve more proximal vessels for future HD accesses. Nephrologists should champion a "preserve the vein" program in patients with advanced CKD who will likely require HD in the future. Such a program includes the avoidance of a peripherally inserted central catheter (PICC line) in patients who may later require HD. PICC lines are often placed from the antecubital vein through the cephalic or basilic vein and into the central venous system. Used to facilitate medication infusions or blood draws, these catheters are associated with a high rate of venous stenosis,[105] and loss of these veins essentially prohibits that arm from serving as a site (or sites) for future HD vascular access.

Historically, the use of synthetic graft material does not provide the same long-term success as a Brescia-Cimino or other autogenous AV fistula with respect to duration of function and incidence of complications (see later). However, recent studies using more contemporary patient cohorts have indicated that the gap in key clinical outcomes between AV fistulas and AV grafts may not be as wide as previously described.[106,107] Rather than a fistula-first approach for all patients, nephrologists should call for a catheter-last approach to HD access.

Procedures that allowed the safe placement of wide-bore catheters in large-diameter veins were developed in the 1970s. First, single-lumen and then double-lumen catheters led to the use of these devices to support patients on maintenance HD who lacked AV access. The creation of more flexible plastics and the advent of cuffed catheters inserted through subcutaneous tunnels have led to the use of so-called permanent catheters, offering longevity of use that make them practical for maintenance HD. In the United States, the availability of these catheters has allowed patients to undergo maintenance HD, despite inadequate vasculature to support endogenous AV access. However, there is growing concern that these catheters are used for longer periods of time than necessary and, in some cases, in lieu of AV fistulas or grafts. Around 80% of patients in the United States start dialysis with a catheter access and, even among patients with CKD seen by a nephrologist prior to the development of ESKD, a large proportion of patients begin with a catheter.[10] By comparison, other countries where HD serves most patients have much lower incident catheter rates.[108] However, there will always be patients undergoing HD in whom a catheter will be the appropriate or only feasible long-term vascular access.

Characteristics of an ideal HD vascular access and how the present types of accesses compare with each other are listed in Table 63.3. The fact that no single type of vascular access fulfills all these desired requirements is what makes a reliable vascular access the Achilles' heel of long-term HD.[109] There are well-recognized associations among type of vascular access, mortality, and cost of care in ESKD.[110] The 2010 Annual Report of the US Renal Data Service (USRDS) has outlined the annual direct vascular access event costs per patient by access type (Fig. 63.9A), as well as the total annual health care expenditures per patient per year based on the type of HD vascular access (see Fig. 63.9B). Although the annual direct vascular access–related costs of an AV graft are higher than those for both catheter and fistula, the total annual health care expense is highest for a patient with a catheter.

## TYPES OF VASCULAR ACCESS

### ARTERIOVENOUS FISTULAS

This preferred type of vascular access is created by connecting a vein to an artery, which requires that the two vessels be in proximity to each other. An ideal mature (ready to use)

**Table 63.3 Characteristics of Ideal Hemodialysis Vascular Access Compared With Commonly Available Types**

| Desired Characteristic | Autogenous AV Fistula | AV Graft | Central Venous Catheter |
|---|---|---|---|
| High primary patency rate | ★ | ★★ | ★★★ |
| Instant usability | ★ | ★★ | ★★★ |
| Long survival | ★★★ | ★★ | ★ |
| Low thrombosis rate | ★★★ | ★★ | ★ |
| Low infection rate | ★★★ | ★★ | ★ |
| High blood flow rate on hemodialysis | ★★★ | ★★★ | ★ |
| Patient comfort | ★ | ★ | ★★★ |
| Patient bathing/hygiene | ★★★ | ★★★ | ★ |
| Minimize needles | ★ | ★ | ★★★ |
| Minimal cosmetic affect | ★ | ★★ | ★★ |

*AV*, Arteriovenous.

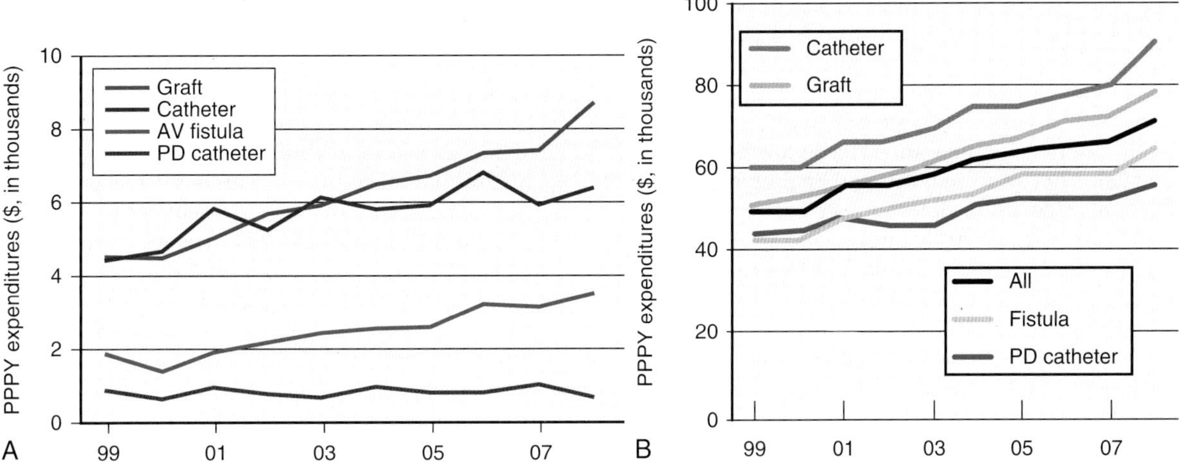


**Fig. 63.9** Health cost of varying types of vascular access. (A) Direct expenditures of access events per person per year *(PPPY)* varies with the type of hemodialysis (HD) vascular access. The graft is most expensive to maintain, whereas the fistula is the least expensive form of vascular access. (B) Total health care expenditures PPPY vary with the type of HD vascular access. Patients with a catheter are the costliest, whereas the patient with a fistula is the least expensive. *AV,* Arteriovenous; *PD,* peritoneal dialysis. (Modified from US Renal Data System. 2017 USRDS Annual Data Report: Epidemiology of Kidney Disease in the United States. Bethesda, MD: National Institutes of Health, National Institute of Diabetes and Digestive and Kidney Diseases; 2017.)

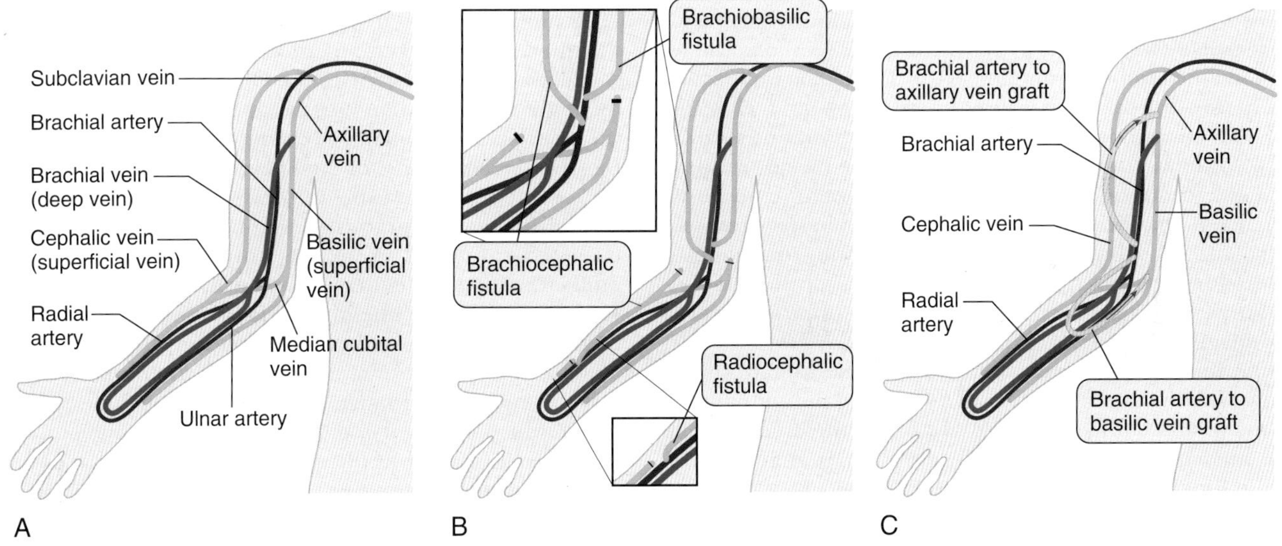


**Fig. 63.10** (A) Vasculature of the right upper limb outlining superficial and deep veins and major arteries. (B) Location of anatamoses for typical wrist (radiocephalic) and upper arm (brachiocephalic and brachiobasilic) arteriovenous (AV) fistulae. (C) Location of typical AV grafts.

fistula should be easily accessible by physical examination and provide a robust blood flow of at least 400 mL/min, with enough distance between the cannulation of two needles to allow for dialysis machine blood pump flow rates of 400 mL/min without developing recirculation. The "rule of 6" serves as an easy way to remember physical examination guidelines to determine if an AV fistula is ready for use: (1) at least 6 mm in diameter; (2) at least 6 cm of overall needle-accessible length; and (3) no more than 6 mm below the skin surface.

At this point in time, fistula creation is a surgical procedure that can often be done with just local or regional block anesthesia. In general, both the artery and vein must have adequate lumens for the procedure to be successful. The original procedure described by Brescia and colleagues[99] was a side to side AV fistula using the radial artery and the cephalic vein at the wrist and has become the preferred access when these vessels are adequate. Recent studies in upper arm AV fistulas have suggested similar patency rates of side to side versus end to side anastomoses, but with a higher incidence of arterial steal phenomenon with the side to side technique.[111] An additional advantage of the end to side procedure is the avoidance of venous hypertension that can occur distally with the side to side approach. Data supporting the benefit of a fistula have created some concern that perhaps radiocephalic fistulas are being attempted in patients with known higher failure rates, such as women and persons with diabetes and obesity.[112] Typical vascular anatomy of the arm and the location of commonly placed fistulas are shown in Fig. 63.10A and B.

Systematic use of preoperative ultrasonographic imaging to examine vascular anatomy is often used in the preoperative evaluation to decide on the type and location of fistula placement and may increase the success rate of AV fistulas.[113,114] Commonly and inappropriately termed "vein mapping," this study should interrogate veins and arteries. Commonly used lower limits for artery and vein internal diameters are 2 mm and 2 to 3 mm, respectively. However, even in situations where blood vessel size appears to be appropriate, maturation of the AV fistula—the increase in vein blood flow rate, size, and wall strength that allows it to be used for HD—may still not occur. There is now better understanding that issues such as intimal hyperplasia not readily seen by imaging techniques or arterial lesions that limit augmentation of flow after fistula creation are probably additional factors in the unsuccessful AV fistula.[115,116] Surgical technique is also a well-recognized variable in AV fistula outcomes.[117]

The upper arm veins provide alternatives when a distal fistula has failed or when distal vessels are inadequate. With incident patients now older and with more extensive comorbidities, more first-time AV fistulas are being placed using the upper arm veins when vein mapping reveals small lower arm wrist vessels. The cephalic and basilic veins are considered superficial veins of the arm and lend themselves to fistula creation. The basilic vein courses up the arm and perforates the deep fascia to join the brachial vein somewhere between the midbiceps and the axilla. The basilic vein fistula often uses the brachial artery as its inflow and typically requires an additional procedure of transposition because of its location along the medial side of the biceps, making it an awkward location for cannulation in its native position. The brachiobasilic fistula can be performed in stages, which is particularly advantageous in children, with anastomosis first followed by the transposition surgery after the vein has matured.[118] Even in adults, this procedure appears to have advantages over an AV graft in terms of longevity.[119] The basilic vein has also been transposed to the forearm, with successful outcomes.[120] Alternatives to using the cephalic or basilic vein as outflow for an AV fistula are the brachial vein and median antecubital vein. The former is anastomosed to the brachial artery and requires a second procedure to superficialize and transpose, whereas the latter (variants of the Gracz fistula) has potential dual outflow through both the cephalic and basilic veins.[121] These AV fistulas have purported advantages and disadvantages that are beyond the scope of this chapter.

Focus on the superiority of fistulas versus other forms of vascular access appears to have successfully increased the prevalence of fistulas in the United States. In Europe, the prevalence of fistulas for maintenance HD has long been greater than in the United States. Data from the Dialysis Outcomes and Practice Patterns Study (DOPPS) have demonstrated a marked difference in the training of surgeons in Europe compared with those in the United States.[122] The much greater volume of procedures completed by European surgeons in training may lead to more expertise or comfort in performing fistula procedures.

The dogmatic placement of fistulas in all patients, however, has its disadvantages. A recent meta-analysis of over 12,000 patients has found that the failure rate for fistulas may be increasing, casting concern about overly aggressive "fistula-first" approaches.[123] The major disadvantages of the AV fistula are the high failure to mature rate—around 25%—and the need for surgical or percutaneous balloon angioplasty to assist in maturation in an additional 25% of patients.[115,124] These high incidences and the tradition of waiting months for the AV fistula to mature prolong the duration of and need for catheters. Although some data have shown that early cannulation of the AV fistula is associated with higher failure rates,[125] lack of change on physical examination of the fistula within the first 4 to 6 weeks after surgery may also be prognostic of nonmaturation and dictate sooner interventions.[126]

## ARTERIOVENOUS GRAFTS

Vascular access using ePTFE conduits had become the most prominent type of AV vascular access in the United States in the 1980s and 1990s, at least partly due to the ease of placement, the short time required between the placement of an AV graft and initiation of cannulation, and possibly factors related to reimbursement. Placement of an AV graft is perceived as advantageous by many nephrologists and surgeons because it does not require maturation of the native vein and allows for a forearm site for access placement (see Fig. 63.10C). Although the recognized low primary failure rate for grafts is an early advantage, the primary patency rate at 12 months is only around 50%.[127] The graft material has a higher risk for development of infection compared with the native vessel of an AV fistula. Other approaches to placement are available when vascular anatomy or previous access prohibits placement in the forearm. The thigh often becomes the only remaining site for graft placement but poses a higher risk of infection; however, an observational report has suggested that a thigh graft may be a better alternative than a tunneled catheter.[128] Regardless of location, most ePTFE grafts require about 4 weeks of time after placement before cannulation is recommended. This allows time for the graft material to scar or incorporate into the surrounding soft tissue and for endotheliazation of the intraluminal surface.

More recent alternative graft materials include polyurethane, which has a self-sealing characteristic at the puncture site when the dialysis needle is removed. This property obviates the need for graft incorporation into the surrounding soft tissue, allowing for early cannulation after its surgical placement, and plays a role in limiting or avoiding a dialysis catheter. Although seemingly ideal, the clinical experience with these types of grafts has been mixed, with some reports of increased infections, although some retrospective series have found noninferior results to traditional grafts.[129,130]

A new hybrid device for patients with limited venous outflow options uses a typical graft at the point of the arterial anastomosis, transitions to a large-bore, single-lumen catheter at the venous outflow end, and is tunneled up the arm and placed into the central venous circulation, much like a typical catheter, to achieve central venous drainage. This Hemodialysis Reliable Outflow (HeRO) device (Merit Medical, South Jordan, UT) has a potential role in some patients as an AV access of last resort.[131]

A complex biologic response develops within the lumen of the graft and in the distal native vein after an AV graft is surgically placed. Possibly stimulated by areas of turbulent blood flow or changes in wall shear stress, a host of immune responses occur. The resulting hyperplasia leads to a high incidence of stenosis, which is the leading cause of graft failure.[132] The vast majority of stenoses that develop are at the venous anastomosis or beyond, within the native outflow vein. As discussed later, the high incidence of stenosis certainly is a rationale for monitoring graft flow in an effort to allow preemptive intervention before thrombosis. The documented inflammatory response and hyperplasia in grafts have focused attention on devices and drugs that may prevent or reduce the eventual stenosis. In addition to angioplasty, stents are frequently used as a tool to prevent restenosis and maintain patency. Whether drug-eluting stents will have a role in AV graft survival has yet to be determined. Use of drug elution from the graft material itself is also under investigation in animals and may offer promise in the future.[133] One study has redefined the concept of grafts by constructing totally biologic grafts, using artificial materials as the initial skeleton for a conduit over which autologous fibroblasts are grown. Then the lumen is seeded with autologous endothelial cells.[134] This technology may eventually offer biologic grafts that are less vulnerable to thrombosis and infection than conventional ePTFE grafts.

An access plan that is often overlooked, but has potential of combining the merits of the graft and fistula, is the creation of a secondary AV fistula after graft placement. In this scenario, an AV graft is placed to minimize or avoid catheter time. However, when the patient encounters the first episode of graft dysfunction, the outflow vein is evaluated for conversion to a traditional AV fistula. Theoretically, the outflow vein will already have arterialized due to its exposure to high flow and pressure from the prior graft and possibly allow for cannulation at the time of, or soon after, the creation of the new surgical anastomosis to the artery.[135]

### Central Venous Catheters

Technology has greatly advanced the use of external connections for HD, providing HD with venous access alone and eliminating the need to sacrifice an artery, as required with the use of AV shunts. Initially, large single-lumen catheters supported HD through single veins. Later, improved plastic materials allowed the construction of large double-lumen catheters that greatly improved HD efficiency over single-lumen catheters. Further advances resulted in catheters made of softer materials that are also more resistant to degradation by cleansing solutions such as alcohols. Most importantly, the development of the subcutaneous cuff provided catheters that could be used for markedly longer durations. Clearly, this technology has been a blessing and a curse because the ease of insertion and duration of use have resulted in the cuffed catheter's being a viable vascular access for patients on maintenance HD.

Some patients would face death from kidney failure without the availability of this catheter technology. However, the data have suggested an inappropriately high utilization of catheters as a means of vascular access. Observational studies such as those using data from DOPPS have suggested that the high prevalence of catheter use in the United States may explain a large fraction of the higher US mortality in the HD population compared with similar patients in Europe.[136] However, other recent, well-done studies have suggested that much of the mortality risk is related to noncatheter patient factors.[137] Regardless, the elevated mortality risk and frequent complications with catheters create major challenges for nephrologists.[138]

Thrombosis with loss of catheter function is a frequent complication leading to the need for intervention. No uniform solution to prevent these events has been established. Catheters are routinely locked, with the installation of high-dose heparin solutions injected into both lumens, but this procedure does not completely prevent the problem. The use of heparin for locking may occasionally result in bleeding through an error in dose, failure or inability to remove the heparin solution before use, and/or leakage of heparin between dialysis treatments. Even the addition of systemic therapy with low-dose warfarin did not prevent thrombosis in a clinical trial setting and led to an increase in complications.[139] Small studies have explored alternatives to heparin, such as locking catheters with citrate-containing solutions.[140] One such study has demonstrated that locking the catheter with recombinant tissue plasminogen activating factor once a week and heparin the other 2 days compared with heparin 3 days a week reduces both thrombosis and the incidence of bacteremia.[141,142] However, the cost of implementing this strategy would be prohibitive in the United States.

Infection isolated to the catheter itself or systemic infection with the catheter as a source is a substantial complication of catheter use resulting in morbidity, costly hospitalizations, and mortality. The frequency of bacteremia associated with HD catheters has been estimated to be two to four episodes/1000 patient-catheter days,[143] a frequency 10- to 20-fold higher than rates of infection estimated in patients with AV fistulas. These catheter-related infections can result in more complex infections such as osteomyelitis, endocarditis, or septic arthritis, despite antibiotic therapy.

Careful management of catheter-related infection is critical, including an adequate duration of antibiotic treatment, an aggressive approach to catheter removal and replacement, and delayed replacement until the patient is symptom free (so-called "line holiday").[144–146] When the infection is isolated to the exit site or does not involve the tunnel, studies have suggested that catheter exchange can be successfully undertaken. Attempting to treat infected catheters with antibiotics alone usually results in failure, although some organisms (e.g., *Staphylococcus epidermidis*) may clear. The combined use of antibiotic installation into catheter lock solutions, in addition to systemic antibiotics, may increase success in preserving the existing catheter.

Several approaches to the prevention of infection with catheters have demonstrated potential promise. The use of mupirocin ointment at the exit site may reduce the incidence of infection.[147,148] Locking catheters with antibiotic-containing solutions as a routine after all HD treatments may also be helpful in reducing the incidence of catheter-related infections.[146,148–150] With the prophylactic use of antibiotics to minimize bacterial catheter infections, the issue of antibiotic-resistant bacterial selection is always a concern. The use of catheters impregnated with antibacterial agents so far has not been as promising in preventing infection.[151]

Even if the thrombotic and infectious complications could be solved, catheters may not support the blood flow rates needed to achieve an adequate HD dose in some patients. Additionally, long-term catheter use results in vascular damage that often leads to central vein stenosis and in situ thrombosis.[152] In the end, catheters must remain an interim solution or the access of last resort in the patient on maintenance HD.

## MAINTENANCE OF VASCULAR ACCESS FUNCTION

After some form of long-term vascular access is achieved, maintaining patency and adequate function is paramount. Numerous strategies have been explored to accomplish this goal. Cannulation methods have received some attention, with speculation that methods such as the buttonhole technique might provide advantages over other methods. One nonrandomized study has compared the rope ladder technique (70 patients), in which cannulation occurs along the entire length of the fistula, with the buttonhole procedure (75 patients), where repeated cannulation occurs in the exact spot over 9 months.[153] Unsuccessful cannulation occurred more frequently in the buttonhole group, but there were fewer complications, including hematoma and aneurysm formation, compared with the rope ladder group. More recent data have suggested that the buttonhole technique is associated with a higher rate of infection, without evidence of improved fistula survival.[154] At present, the buttonhole technique has fallen out of favor due to its higher rate of bacteremia, but is still an important option for patients doing their own cannulation for home HD. Guidelines for needle insertion were created through the National Kidney Foundation's effort to develop management standards, but these guidelines did not include definitive recommendations regarding this question of cannulation methodology.[82] However, clinical experience has suggested that good cannulation technique, such as using the entire length of the AV fistula or graft, and careful post-HD needle site care are both important for access longevity.

Other strategies to extend access life span include methods of AV graft and fistula monitoring for early signs of potential failure, treatments to prevent access dysfunction or loss, and interventions to fix problems found during monitoring or when shunt thrombosis occurs. There is an accepted nomenclature for access failure that categorizes access as having primary or secondary patency. The definition of primary access patency is an access capable of supporting adequate HD without any intervention since the time of original placement. After an intervention has occurred for any reason (e.g., reduced flow, total thrombosis), secondary patency is then invoked to characterize the status of the vascular access.

### MONITORING AND SURVEILLANCE

The natural history of vascular access loss has suggested that observable and physiologic changes in access venous pressure or total blood flow occur before and predict impending loss of function. If detectable change in either pressure or flow were observed reliably, an intervention to prevent emergent loss of access function would be possible theoretically. The question is whether salvaging the access before total loss of function occurs offers any advantage.

A consistently applied program of AV shunt monitoring is recommended by most dialysis guidelines. Although there are many techniques and devices available to accomplish this, a good physical examination of the AV shunt remains the most important monitoring technique.[155] This can be taught to dialysis technicians, nurses, and nephrologists. For example, if an AV fistula has a bounding pulsation with increasing aneurysm size or does not flatten when the fistula arm is raised above the head, then a venous outflow or central venous stenosis should be suspected.

Other hints to access dysfunction may come from information gathered from the monthly blood tests, as well as through feedback from the dialysis staff. For example, if a decline in HD urea clearance cannot be readily explained, a poor access flow rate may be the root cause. Also, if the dialysis nurse or technician is experiencing difficulty in cannulation, or the staff reports prolonged hemostasis time (or even bleeding from the AV shunt at home reported by the patient), arterial inflow or venous outflow stenosis may be the respective culprits.

Currently, vascular access shunt pressure can be monitored by measuring static or dynamic venous pressures using several standardized methods. To detect stenosis adequately, these procedures must be done serially using consistent techniques; the change or trend in measurements over time is more important in predicting a stenosis than an absolute threshold value. Shunt blood flow measurement that uses indictor flow detection by ultrasound (sometimes termed the "ultrasound dilution method using the Transonic device" [Transonic, Ithaca, NY]) can be done routinely and easily. Regardless of method, monitoring of HD access should be championed by a member of the dialysis clinic and be part of continuous quality improvement.

Despite the theoretic advantage of access monitoring, the impact of aggressive surveillance programs on maintenance of vascular access has been controversial.[156] In lending support to regular monitoring, a nonrandomized report comparing three monitoring schemes in a single dialysis program has demonstrated significant improvement in short-term AV graft and fistula survival using blood flow monitoring versus dynamic pressure monitoring or no monitoring.[157] In addition to access survival, there were fewer missed HD sessions and reduced overall patient costs when using the blood flow monitoring protocol. The overall goal of surveillance protocols, however, is to prolong the function of an AV access. The unfortunate natural history of access failure, especially with AV grafts, is the occurrence of restenosis after intervention procedures such as angioplasty (venoplasty). There may be no difference in eventual access survival whether preemptive intervention is practiced versus simply responding to a thrombosis event when it occurs. A review of surveillance trials did not definitively support routine monitoring of HD access.[158] Therefore, access surveillance is a topic of ongoing research.

Whether the additional intervention of stent placement improves access survival has received a great deal of attention. A randomized trial of 190 HD patients has provided evidence that use of a stent is superior to balloon dilation alone with stenosis at the venous end of an AV graft.[159] New materials for manufacturing stents are under investigation, and the place for drug-eluting stents, although well studied in other vascular systems, needs to be addressed in regard to AV access.[156] The subspecialty of interventional nephrology has emerged in the field of nephrology as a result of the need for timely treatment of vascular access dysfunction and prevention of associated complications. Supported by the creation of the American Society of Diagnostic and Interventional Nephrology, reports have documented the quality and safety of the care delivered by these physicians.[160,161] Interventional nephrologists have been reporting experience with AV access, as well as additional experience with related arterial disease, such as subclavian and renal artery stenosis and peripheral vascular disease.[162] No longer just responsible for monitoring the vascular access, suitably trained nephrologists have tools at their disposal to intervene on behalf of their patients. See Chapter 68 for a further discussion of interventional nephrology.

### PROPHYLACTIC THERAPY FOR ACCESS MAINTENANCE

Access loss occurs from the combined pathologic events of thrombosis and hyperplasia leading to stenosis. Strategies to prevent these pathologic processes have been used with the goal of prolonging access survival, so far with no clear prevention regimen established. Thrombosis may be the final pathway to access failure but, so far, agents well known to prevent thrombosis in other vascular diseases have not consistently enhanced vascular access survival. A multicenter trial in the Veterans' Affairs Heath System with clopidogrel plus aspirin had to be discontinued because of bleeding problems in the treatment group.[163] The Dialysis Access Consortium (DAC) Study Group has reported that although clopidogrel reduces the early thrombosis rate of new AV fistulas, it does not increase the number of usable fistulas.[164] Some small randomized trials have suggested that agents such as fish oil may be effective in reducing thrombosis in grafts, but this approach has yet to receive further study or widespread use.[165,166] The DAC graft study has provided support for the use of dipyridamole and low-dose aspirin started immediately after placement of an AV graft,[167] although the practice has not been widely adopted.

The myointimal proliferation and resulting stenosis that occur, particularly with AV grafts, have also been a focus of prevention, especially because this process may be the ultimate final pathway of access failure.[168] Strategies to prevent cell proliferation in AV grafts have been adapted from studies of other vascular diseases, such as cardiac disease. For example, a retrospective study using angiotensin-converting enzyme (ACE) inhibitors in patients with AV grafts has suggested a reduced risk for graft loss compared with patients not receiving this class of medication.[169] Interventions that have been shown to reduce proliferation in other vascular diseases are being studied. Brachytherapy has been used for some time and has been shown to be safe and have promise in reducing stenosis in AV grafts.[170] Far-infrared light therapy, which improves endothelial function, was shown in a randomized trial to improve patency rates of new AV fistulas when administered repeatedly[171] and may become a future tool to improve AV graft survival.[172] Experimental grafts created by biologic autologous materials, as already described, may eventually provide one solution for access maintenance.

Finally, personalized medicine may eventually be integrated into vascular access protocols as genetic studies uncover possible predictors of risk for access loss. One such study has suggested that polymorphism in the methylenetetrahydrofolate reductase gene *(C677T)* may be a predictor of access thrombosis, presumably through its effect on homocysteine.[173] Another study has suggested that the complex relationship between transforming growth factor beta 1 (TGF-β1) and polymorphisms in the plasminogen activator inhibitor type 1 gene may predict patients who are at risk for access thrombosis.[174] Preknowledge of genetic determinants may allow tailored prophylactic therapy to be administered in the future to patients at risk.

### VASCULAR ACCESS TIMING AND DECISION MAKING

In an ideal world, discussion, planning, and placement of HD vascular access would be done with a nephrologist in a structured and orderly manner. Unfortunately, the reality is that 36% of patients starting HD in the United States have little or no pre-ESKD nephrology care.[10] Even in those individuals whose care is managed by a nephrologist, the decline in kidney function in CKD is rarely a linear predictable process and is often characterized by abrupt changes.[175] Therefore, even the best laid-out plans for timely HD access may be foiled, with the patient starting dialysis with a catheter. On the other hand, an unwavering adherence to dialysis guidelines, which suggest consideration of HD vascular access placement when the eGFR falls below 20 mL/min/1.73 m$^2$, would certainly result in unnecessary surgery and procedures in some patients who will never need or want dialysis.

Although registry data and retrospective studies using large databases have consistently found AV fistulas associated with best outcomes, the right access for the individual patient is much more than simply placing an AV fistula in all patients. The decision is complex, because clinical outcomes and cost analysis must take into account the morbidity and mortality of each access type, success rate of the access, and cost of maintaining patency, as well as the cost of alternative access types. A detailed model incorporating many of these variables was recently published and provides insight into the decision-making process that must also take into account patient factors such as age, gender, comorbidities, and competing risk of death.[176] Recent studies examining older adults who have started dialysis also found that a single-minded, fistula-first approach to HD vascular access may not be optimal.[177]

## GENERAL PRINCIPLES OF HEMODIALYSIS: PHYSIOLOGY AND BIOMECHANICS

Therapeutic HD removes solutes principally by diffusion and, to a lesser extent, by convection across a semipermeable membrane. The driving force for solute diffusion is the transmembrane concentration gradient (Fig. 63.11A), and the driving force for convection, commonly called "ultrafiltration," is the transmembrane hydrostatic pressure (see Fig. 63.11B). Selective removal of solutes is achieved by restricting the pore size in the membrane to admit small molecules and reject large molecules and by including desirable solutes in the dialysate, effectively preventing their removal (and often prompting their influx).

### NATIVE KIDNEY VERSUS ARTIFICIAL KIDNEY

The native kidney's glomerular filter separates solutes based on molecular size, a function that the dialyzer attempts to mimic. Most of the soluble large molecules found in the blood are the products of complex intracellular synthetic processes that require energy. Most continue to be active, serving to signal and regulate processes in distant organs. Their loss by filtration through the kidneys would be a liability best avoided. Loss is

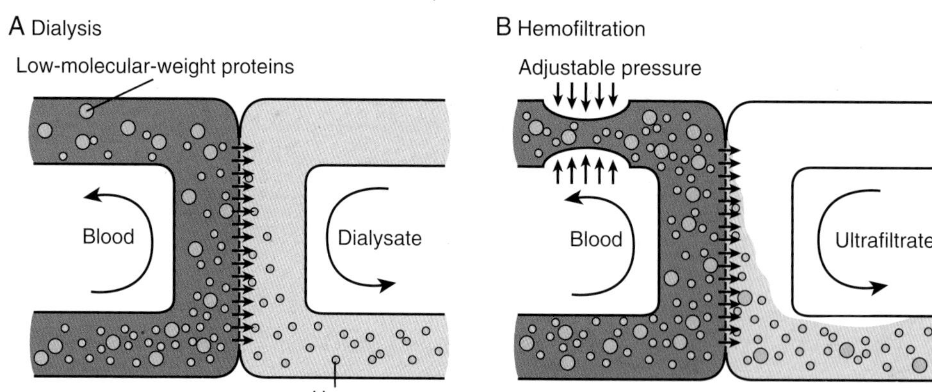


**Fig. 63.11** Diffusion versus convection. (A) Diffusion across a semipermeable membrane. The driving force for solute diffusion is the transmembrane concentration gradient. Small solutes with higher concentrations in the blood compartment, such as potassium, urea, and small uremic toxins, diffuse through the membrane into the dialysate compartment. Dialysis dissipates this concentration gradient (i.e., the molecular concentration gradient decreases with dialysis). Larger solutes and low-molecular-weight proteins such as albumin diffuse poorly across the semipermeable membrane. (B) Convection across a semipermeable membrane. The driving force for convection, commonly called ultrafiltration, is the transmembrane hydrostatic pressure. When applied to the blood compartment, solvent flows across the membrane into the dialysate compartment, bringing along solutes. For solutes with a sieving coefficient close to 1, there is no change in concentrations in the blood compartment with time. (From Meyer TW, Hostetter TH. Uremia. *N Engl J Med.* 2007;357(13):1316–1325.)

first prevented by the bilipid cell membrane barrier that keeps precious molecules sequestered intracellularly. Those that are secreted or leak out of the cell are often bound to serum macromolecules, most notably serum albumin, a well-known transport protein. Although the glomerular membrane is highly permeable when compared with cell membranes in general, albumin and its bound ligands, as well as other macromolecules, are poorly filtered and thus protected from loss. Small proteins and peptides that leak through the filter are efficiently reabsorbed by the proximal tubule where they are broken down and their subunits reused.

Smaller molecules are often end products of metabolism or ingested intruders that the kidney effectively eliminates by filtration without reabsorption. Precious small molecules are reclaimed after filtration by selective reabsorptive mechanisms in the renal tubules. Dialyzers lack the latter vital functions, so losses are prevented by including the measurable, desirable small solutes in the dialysate, effectively eliminating the gradient for diffusive loss. Fortunately, most of these small solutes are abundant and relatively inexpensively added to the dialysate.

Although both the native and artificial kidney are excretory organs, and both use semipermeable membranes to separate small from large particles, each operates on a different principle. The natural kidney is a selective filtration or convection device driven by blood pressure generated by the heart, with highly selective reabsorption and secretion downstream. In contrast, the dialyzer separates molecular species primarily by simple diffusion, without the need for pressure generation or reabsorption. Urea, for example, is highly reabsorbed after filtration by the glomerulus, but selective reabsorption plays no role in hemodialyzers. The rapid equilibration of urea across red blood cell (RBC) membranes facilitates urea removal during dialysis but plays no role during glomerular filtration. In contrast, creatinine and most other water-soluble compounds are poorly reabsorbed by the native kidney and exhibit slow or no transport across RBC membranes within the short time frame that blood transits through the dialyzer. Consequently, clearance rates of creatinine by the native kidneys are higher, and by the dialyzer lower, than their respective urea clearances. The artificial hollow fiber kidney contains 8000 to 10,000 fibers, each with an internal diameter of approximately 200 μm and length of 250 mm, providing a surface area for exchange of about 1.5 $m^2$. Each of the 1 to 2 million functioning nephrons in the two native kidneys has a proximal tubule diameter of about 40 μm and a length of about 14 mm, providing a minimum surface area for proximal reabsorption of approximately 3 $m^2$ (ignoring microvilli).

Another major difference between the native kidney and artificial filter is active tubular excretion. Just as the native kidneys reabsorb desired substances, they also actively secrete waste products that are filtered poorly by the glomerulus because of significant protein binding. For example, the native kidney clearance of hippurate, which is 56% protein-bound, in HD patients with residual kidney function is 6.6 times that of native urea clearance, suggesting active tubular secretion of the substance.[178] Other metabolic functions of the native kidney, many of which are performed by the tubular and interstitial cells, are also not found in the artificial kidney. Known native kidney synthetic functions include the synthesis of erythropoietin and the 1-hydroxylation of 25-hydroxy vitamin D.

For endogenous solutes, the first pathway on the route to elimination by native or artificial kidneys is diffusion through intracellular and extracellular pathways, including passive or facilitated diffusion across membranes. Thus, diffusion is a vital transport mechanism for native kidney and artificial kidneys. Because removal of small solutes appears to be the major function of both excretory methods, dialyzer clearance of small solutes can be compared with similar clearances by the native kidney as a reasonable first step toward assessing hemodialyzer adequacy.

## CLEARANCE

The goals of dialysis are straightforward—removal of accumulated fluid and retained solutes, some of which are toxic. With respect to toxins, the ultimate goal is to maintain concentrations below the threshold at which uremic symptoms and signs begin to appear. However, the levels of retained toxic solutes are not used as performance measures for dialysis because their identities are unknown, and their generation rates probably vary from patient to patient and from time to time (see later). Instead, performance of dialysis is judged by the clearance of representative solutes.

As already noted, most targeted solutes are small, so the clearance of a small representative solute can be used to measure the most important dialyzer function, which is to lower the concentration of small toxic solutes in the patient. This is an inescapable conclusion based on the observation that dialysis works extremely well to reverse life-threatening uremia rapidly. The mechanism for this lifesaving property of dialysis is not mysterious; it is simply the result of solute removal by diffusion across the semipermeable dialysis membrane. Earlier cellulose-based dialyzer membranes removed solutes with molecular weights above 3000 Da very poorly, yet were effective in reversing uremia, so small solutes are the obvious primary culprits accounting for the life-threatening aspects of the uremic syndrome. It is therefore reasonable to use the clearance of a representative small solute as a measure of this fundamental dialysis function.

Clearance is recognized as the best measure of first-order processes such as diffusion and filtration. A zero-order process such as urea generation by the liver is not influenced by the solute concentration, but first-order removal processes, such as diffusion, are driven by the concentration, rendering the removal rate directly proportional to the concentration. Clearance (K) is the proportionality constant, as shown in this equation:

$$K = \text{removal rate}/\text{concentration} \quad [1]$$

K has value as an expression of a first-order process that is independent of the solute removal rate or its concentration. For intermittent dialysis, the main advantage of the clearance expression is that it tends to remain constant, despite rapid changes in both the solute concentration and removal rate during the procedure.

In a simple flowing system, the removal rate is the difference between the inflow concentration ($C_{in}$) and the outflow concentration ($C_{out}$) multiplied by flow (Q). From the first equation, clearance can also be expressed as the extraction ratio (E) multiplied by flow:

$$E = (C_{in} - C_{out})/C_{in} \quad [2]$$

$$K = Q \times E \quad [3]$$

For a constant-flow system, the extraction ratio is also constant over time, despite marked changes in concentration. E is the fraction of total inflow (Q), and K is the absolute flow that is completely cleared of the solute; both tend to remain constant during dialysis. Clearance is affected by the flow of both blood and dialysate, as well as other variables, such as the convective filtration rate (see later), but is independent of concentration.

Although clearance is independent of solute concentration, the converse is not true (i.e., concentrations depend on clearance, and solute concentrations are used to measure clearance). During a period of steady-state kinetics, in which generation equals removal, the concentration of a solute is inversely proportional to its clearance if its generation rate is fixed. Because dialysis is simpler than native kidney function and removes solutes primarily by diffusion, the calculation of clearance is nearly the same for all easily dialyzed substances if one assumes that these solutes are distributed in a single mixed pool in the patient. Application of this principle allows selection of an easily measured solute (e.g., urea) to assess dialyzer performance, with the expectation that the measured clearance will correlate inversely with patient levels of similar, easily dialyzed solutes. The measured solute need not be toxic, but its removal must occur in parallel with removal of the toxic solutes. Generation rates of various solutes differ, but if each is relatively constant from week to week (e.g., creatinine generation), then the measured clearance of a representative solute can be used to reflect the effectiveness of the dialysis for clearing all easily dialyzed solutes. This principle, which forms the basis of established standards for measuring and prescribing HD, has logical merit, but its applicability has been challenged and may require modification for solutes that are strongly sequestered in remote body compartments (see later).[82,179–181] In addition, after adjustment for body size and possibly sex (see later), all patients appear to require the same weekly clearance. Furthermore, the dose requirement or need for dialysis does not seem to vary from time to time in the same (anuric) patient, provided a minimum threshold clearance is delivered during each treatment.

Native kidneys appear to clear small solutes at a rate far above the minimum required to sustain life. For example, removal of a kidney for transplantation can be done without major adverse consequences in the donor. Although the reason for this surplus function is unknown, it helps explain how modern intermittent HD, which achieves a continuous equivalent small solute clearance that is only about 10% to 15% of the normal GFR of normal kidneys, is able to sustain life (see discussion of continuous equivalent clearance).

## CLEARANCE VERSUS REMOVAL RATE

The clearance of a solute must be distinguished from its absolute removal rate. Clearance is best envisioned as a measure of removal expressed as a fraction of the remaining solute and is therefore independent of the concentration. Two substances may have the same clearance, but if one is present at half the concentration of the other, the removal rate will also be half of the other's. In practical terms, it is impossible to compare dialyzers by measuring removal rates alone because removal depends on the solute concentration. Measurement of clearance eliminates this requirement, allowing use of a single term to make valid comparisons among purgative instruments.

Similarly, finding a lower concentration of a solute in a patient does not indicate that the clearance is higher; it may simply reflect a lower generation rate. If a steady state exists where input equals output, the removal rate of a substance is simply a measure of its generation rate, revealing little about the effectiveness of the dialyzer. If the clearance decreases, and the generation rate does not change, the patient's solute concentration will increase until a new steady state is reached, when the removal rate again matches the generation rate.

## SERUM UREA CONCENTRATION VERSUS UREA CLEARANCE

The serum urea concentration has proven to be a poor surrogate for uremic toxicity. The determinants of urea

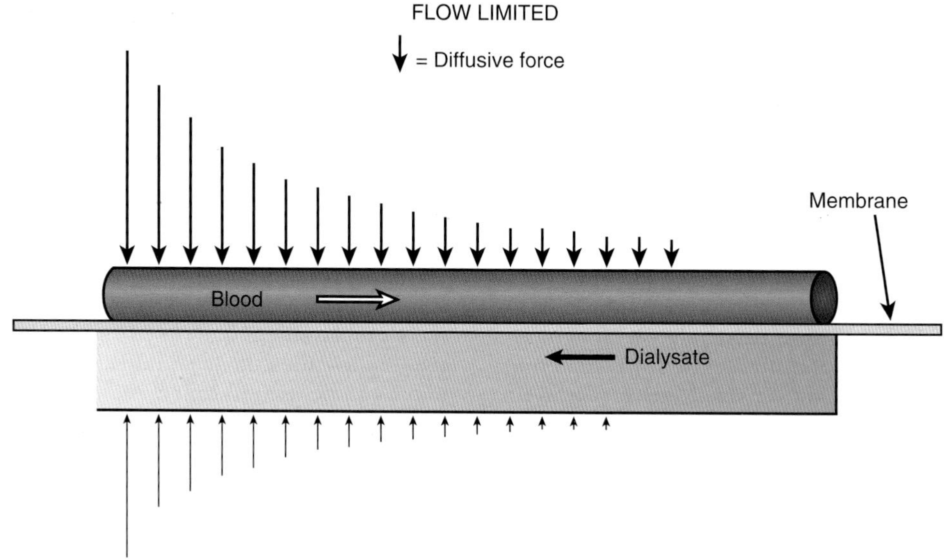


**Fig. 63.12** Flow-limited clearance. A logarithmic decline in solute concentrations, indicated by the *arrows* on either side of the membrane, is depicted from the dialyzer inlet at the *left* to the blood outlet on the *right*. This predictable decline is attributable to relatively rapid diffusion of solute across the membrane and forms the basis for Eq. 5. Flux is equal to the product of membrane-solute $K_0A$ and the log mean gradient. Solute flux and removal are maximized by countercurrent flow of blood and dialysate.

concentration are generation and clearance. Whereas urea clearance by the dialyzer should correlate with the clearance of other small (dialyzable) solutes that are presumably responsible for uremic toxicity, the generation of urea as an end product of protein catabolism correlates poorly with uremic toxicity, despite cell culture and animal studies that have suggested that urea disrupts cellular function and promotes metabolic disturbances.[182] In fact, patients with higher urea generation rates have better outcomes, probably as a reflection of better appetite and higher protein intake.[183] It is difficult to dissect the clearance factor from the generation factor in a single blood urea nitrogen (BUN) measurement but, as explained later, this can be differentiated by modeling the change in BUN during a dialysis treatment. For purposes of measuring the dose of dialysis and dialysis adequacy, only the relative change in urea concentration during dialysis is used to model clearance; the absolute concentrations are ignored. Thus, despite its lack of intrinsic toxicity and the poor correlation with overall uremic toxicity, urea measurements during dialysis can be used to assess dialysis effectiveness and adequacy. The change in urea concentration during dialysis, which reflects its clearance, is used as a surrogate for the clearance of other small, easily dialyzed solutes, some of which must be toxic, or conventional diffusive dialysis would not reverse the life-threatening component of uremia. This logic justifies the use of urea clearance as an index of dialysis adequacy while acknowledging that isolated urea concentrations cannot be used for this purpose.

## FACTORS THAT AFFECT CLEARANCE IN A FLOWING SYSTEM

Diffusive clearance in a flowing system depends on the rates of blood and dialysate flow, as well as the targeted solute membrane permeability. The biomaterials used to make the hollow fiber dialyzer, together with the pore size and thickness of the membrane, determine its clearance, or the membrane permeability constant ($K_0$), for a given solute. Multiplying $K_0$ by the surface area for diffusion (A) yields the permeability, or mass transfer area coefficient ($K_0A$), of an entire dialyzer. $K_0A$ is expressed in milliliters per minute and is independent of solute concentration, similar to clearance. The predictable exponential decline in concentration gradient along the dialyzer membrane from blood inflow to outflow (Fig. 63.12) is the basis for the calculation of $K_0A$ from the blood and dialysate flow rates and is widely used in mathematical models of solute kinetics. For countercurrent dialysate and blood flow,[184] where $K_d$ is dialyzer clearance, the following equation is applicable:

$$K_0A = (Q_bQ_d/[Q_b - Q_d])\ln(Q_d[Q_b - K_d]/Q_b[Q_d - K_d]) \quad [4]$$

Analogous to clearance, which expresses the dialyzer removal rate normalized to the inflow solute concentration, $K_0A$ is an expression of dialyzer performance normalized to blood ($Q_b$) and dialysate flow rates ($Q_d$). $K_0A$ is sometimes called the "intrinsic clearance" of a dialyzer and can be viewed as the maximum clearance possible for a particular solute and dialyzer at infinite $Q_b$ and $Q_d$. Note that $K_0A$ is both dialyzer- and solute-specific. It is the best parameter for comparing dialyzers, with higher values indicating more efficient solute removal.

A useful rearrangement of this equation provides a measure of clearance at any blood and dialysate flow rate, as shown in the following:

$$K_d = Q_b \left[ \frac{e^{K_0A\left(\frac{Q_d - Q_b}{Q_dQ_b}\right)} - 1}{e^{K_0A\left(\frac{Q_d - Q_b}{Q_dQ_b}\right)} - \frac{Q_b}{Q_d}} \right] \quad [5]$$

The preceding expression of clearance does not include the contribution of convective solute removal by ultrafiltration ($Q_f$) during therapeutic HD. Convective clearance results from bulk movement of solute across the membrane driven by hydrostatic pressure. Simultaneous filtration across the same membrane used for dialysis removes additional solute, but the amount removed is inversely related to the efficiency of the dialysis. For example, if the dialyzer removes solute very efficiently by diffusion, with an extraction ratio approaching 100%, addition of ultrafiltration adds very little or nothing to the removal rate, which cannot exceed 100% of the inflow. The effect of ultrafiltration on clearance is expressed as follows[185]:

$$K_d = Q_b([C_{in} + C_{out}]/C_{in}) + Q_f(C_{out}/C_{in}) \qquad [6]$$

where $Q_b$ is the blood inflow rate, $C_{in}$ is the inflow concentration, $C_{out}$ is the outflow concentration, and $Q_f$ is the ultrafiltration rate, in millimeters per minute. As $C_{out}$ approaches zero, the dialysis component of clearance maximizes, and the $Q_f$ component extinguishes.

## DIALYSANCE

For peritoneal dialysis (PD), after the infusion of fresh dialysate, solute begins to accumulate in the peritoneal fluid. As the level increases, the concentration gradient from blood to dialysate decreases, which causes the removal rate and clearance to decrease, both eventually falling to zero as equilibrium is reached. However, the flux of solute per unit of concentration gradient, also known as "dialysance" (D), remains constant:

$$D = (\text{removal rate})/(\text{concentration gradient}) \qquad [7]$$

Dialysance can be formulated as the initial clearance when the dialysate concentration is zero or, in a flowing HD system, as the solute removal rate per mean solute gradient along the membrane (blood minus dialysate concentration), and is equivalent to the dialyzer's $K_0A$ for the measured solute.

## DETERMINANTS OF CLEARANCE

A number of variables affect clearance during dialysis (Table 63.4). Solute-related variables include the physical and chemical properties of the substance to be removed (e.g., size, charge, protein binding) and its distribution in the body (e.g., intracellular, extracellular, interstitial). Treatment-related variables include the permeability of the membrane to solutes of various sizes, dialysis treatment time, membrane surface area, and flow rates of blood and dialysate (see preceding equations).

Molecular size and membrane permeability together limit the rate of movement for individual molecular species. In flowing systems, the concentrations of larger molecules tend to remain constant along the length of the dialyzer, uninfluenced by blood and dialysate flow. Their clearances, which are low because of their large size, are limited by the size and permeability of the membrane alone and independent of flow rates (Fig. 63.13). Smaller molecules tend to be cleared at the proximal end of the dialyzer, leaving the more distal end for further enhancement of clearance as flow is increased (see Fig. 63.12). In this situation, clearance is said to be flow-limited. Note that flow-limited clearance for small solutes and membrane-limited clearance for larger solutes may occur at the same time in a dialyzer. The relation between flow and clearance is shown graphically in Fig. 63.14 for both limiting scenarios.

The molecular activity of a solute determines its capacity for movement across the dialysis membrane. Because water-soluble solutes are active only in the water phase of the blood, only the water component (~90% of normal blood

**Table 63.4 Factors Influencing Effective Clearance**

| | Treatment-Related (in Order of Importance) | |
|---|---|---|
| **Solute-Related** | **Small Molecules** | **Large Molecules** |
| Molecular size<br>Molecular charge<br>Macromolecular binding<br>Body distribution and sequestration | Blood and dialysate flow<br>Membrane surface area<br>Treatment time<br>Membrane permeability | Membrane permeability<br>Treatment time<br>Membrane surface area<br>Blood and dialysate flow |

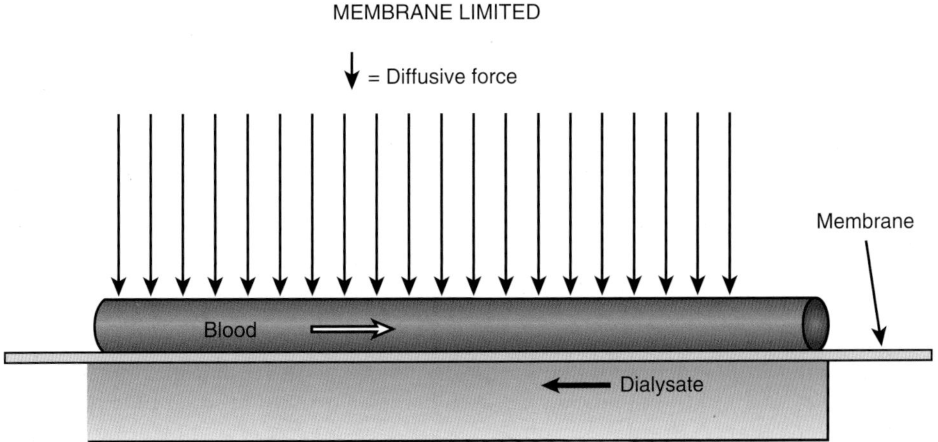


**Fig. 63.13** Membrane-limited clearance. The diffusive force is the solute concentration gradient. Solute concentrations along the membrane from dialyzer inflow to outflow for both blood and dialysate are relatively constant because transport across the membrane is limiting and relatively low.

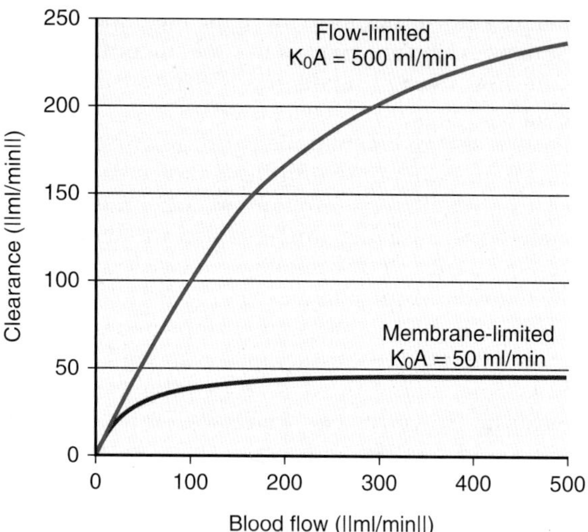


**Fig. 63.14** Flow-limited versus membrane-limited clearances. Flow limits clearance when the membrane is not fully exposed to inflow solute concentrations (see Fig. 63.12). This typically occurs for small, easily dialyzed solutes. In contrast, larger solutes tend to saturate the membrane along its entire length at lower blood (or dialysate) flow rates (see Fig. 63.13). For these less easily dialyzed solutes, further increases in flow have no influence on clearance. *$K_oA$,* Mass transfer area coefficient.

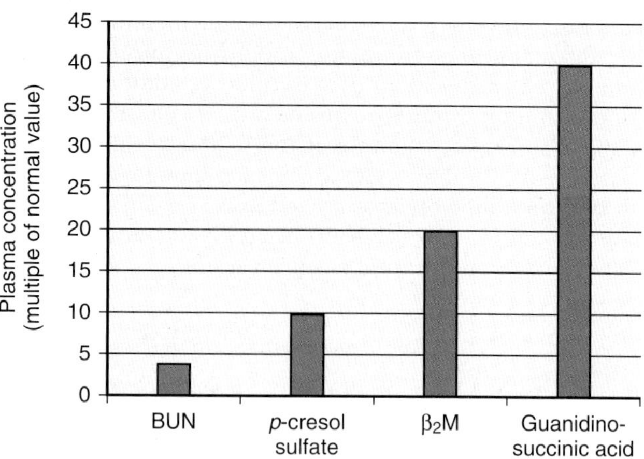


**Fig. 63.15** Effect of protein binding, molecular weight, and sequestration on solute concentrations in hemodialysis (HD) patients. Conventional thrice-weekly dialysis is very effective at removing blood urea nitrogen *(BUN)*, resulting in an average urea level of about four times the normal value in a patient undergoing HD. Binding of *p*-cresol to albumin and the large molecular size of beta-2 microglobulin limit their removal with conventional dialysis, resulting in levels about 10 to 20 times that of normal, respectively. Plasma guanidinosuccinic acid levels are even higher (≈40 times normal) because of increased production in kidney failure and intracellular sequestration, making it difficult to remove during dialysis. Although the plasma levels of these other solutes are several orders of magnitude higher than normal, their absolute levels are much lower than that of urea, and it is unclear if they exert any toxicity. (Modified from Meyer TW, Hostetter TH. Uremia. *N Engl J Med.* 2007;357(13):1316–1325.)

volume) participates in the dialysis process. Blood flow through the dialyzer for water-soluble solutes (nearly all) should be expressed as blood water flow, or about 90% of whole blood flow. Similarly, blood concentrations should be expressed as blood water concentrations, which are about 7% higher than whole serum concentrations. Note that BUN is a misnomer; serum urea nitrogen is actually measured. For charged molecules, the Donnan effect acts in the opposite direction, reducing the effective blood activity.[186] Correcting for this reduced activity, the effective sodium concentration on the blood side of the membrane is about 3 mEq/L lower than its actual concentration. The Donnan effect for blood equilibrated with dialysate is attributable to nondialyzable plasma proteins, mostly albumin, which has a net negative charge (≈17 mEq/mmol albumin). The asymmetric charge distribution across the membrane effectively "captures" a small fraction of the positively charged sodium ions on the plasma side, reducing their potential for diffusion.

The size of the molecule is the most important intrinsic physical feature governing its removal (Fig. 63.15). In general, the rate of movement, or flux (J), of smaller molecules is higher than the flux of larger molecules. Other factors such as binding to plasma proteins, shape, charge, and sequestration in the intracellular compartment must be considered when predicting clearance (see Fig. 63.15).

## DIALYZER CLEARANCE VERSUS WHOLE-BODY CLEARANCE

A distinction must be made between clearance across the dialyzer and clearance across the patient. For each of these, the removal rate (first equation) is the same, but the denominator differs. Dialyzer clearance is an expression of solute removal as a fraction of the blood concentration (adjusted for blood water content) at the dialyzer inflow port. In contrast, whole-body clearance is an expression of removal as a fraction of average concentrations throughout the body. The average whole-body concentration is substituted for dialyzer inflow concentration in the denominator of the standard clearance formula (first equation). Whole-body concentrations are higher than serum concentrations during dialysis because of solute disequilibrium, or nonuniform distribution of solutes, so whole-body clearances are always lower than dialyzer clearances. Higher concentrations throughout the body result from solute sequestration or a delay in the diffusive movement of solute from remote body compartments to the patient's blood, which is the immediately dialyzed compartment.

Typical solutes that exhibit disequilibrium distribute preferentially in the intracellular compartment and diffuse slowly across the cell membrane to the extracellular compartment. Such solutes are sometimes labeled as "difficult to dialyze." For example, therapeutic dialysis is not recommended for removal of digoxin in patients with digoxin intoxication,[187] even though it is water-soluble and easily removed in vitro, with a high clearance across the dialyzer membrane. Removal in vivo, however, is limited by sequestration in remote tissue compartments. Solutes such as digoxin have an apparent large distribution, often larger than total body water volume.

Even urea, one of the most diffusible solutes, in normal physiologic conditions is often termed an "ineffective osmole" and exhibits disequilibrium during HD. Whole-body urea clearance can be calculated by substituting the equilibrated postdialysis BUN (Fig. 63.16) for the immediate postdialysis BUN in the modeling equations. Experience has shown that urea sequestration can be predictable from the rapidity or rate of solute removal. This observation has led to the

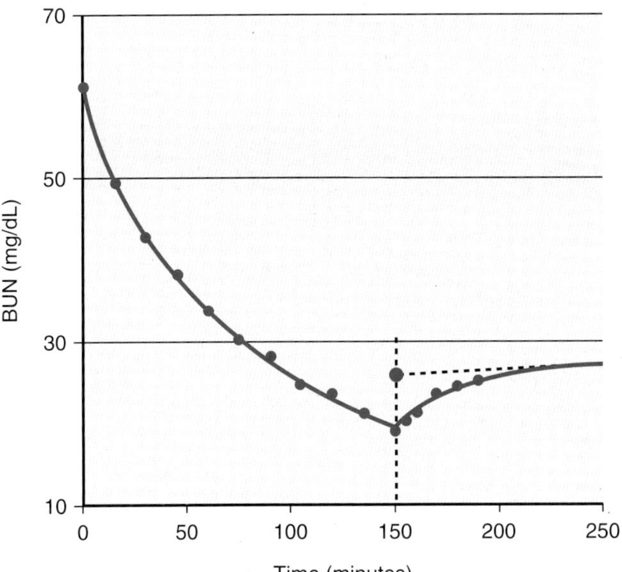


**Fig. 63.16** Equilibrated postdialysis blood urea nitrogen *(BUN)*, the basis for eKt/V. Precise measurements of BUN every 15 minutes during a typical patient's 2.5-hour hemodialysis shows a logarithmic decrease in concentration during the treatment and a rapid rebound that is complete approximately 1 hour later. The double-pool model shown in Fig. 63.21 and the *solid line* in the graph predict the concentrations accurately. The equilibrated postdialysis BUN is an extrapolated value shown as the *large solid circle*.

development of simplified equations to estimate the equilibrated Kt/V (eKt/V) from single-pool Kt/V (spKt/V),[188,189] where Kt/V is dialyzer clearance × time over volume:

$$eKt/V = spKt/V - 0.6(spK/V) + 0.03 \quad [8]$$

$$eKt/V = spKt/V[t/(t+35)] \quad [9]$$

When eKt/V is the chosen standard of care measure of hemodialysis adequacy, these equations allow its calculation without requiring the patient to wait 30 to 60 minutes after dialysis has stopped to measure the equilibrated BUN.

### EFFECT OF RED BLOOD CELLS PASSING THROUGH THE DIALYZER

In the blood compartment, solutes may diffuse slowly or not at all out of RBCs during transit through the dialyzer.[190,191] Water content of red blood cells is about 64% by volume, so this may account for the additional transport of water-soluble toxins during dialysis.[192] Clearances of solutes depend on how readily they move out of RBCs. For example, creatinine and uric acid are small molecules with clearances similar to that of urea when measured in a saline solution in vitro. Measured in vivo, however, their clearances are lower than urea clearance because movement out of the RBCs as it passes through the dialyzer is much slower than that of urea, limited by lack of specific urea-like transporters in the RBC membrane.[193–195]

### SEQUESTRATION IN REMOTE COMPARTMENTS

Other solutes such as potassium and phosphorus are cleared easily in vitro, but their removal is limited by cellular and bone sequestration in patients, explaining the need for dietary restriction and for the use of intestinal binders to diminish absorption and, ultimately, the serum concentration of these solutes. Phosphorus is rapidly removed from the intravascular compartment, causing hypophosphatemia during HD in most conventionally treated patients. However, for 2 to 4 hours after dialysis, the serum phosphorus concentration increases relatively rapidly, returning to near-predialysis levels (Fig. 63.17). Thus, sequestration and its consequent postdialysis rebound account for the failure of conventional HD alone to normalize interdialytic concentrations. Low blood phosphate generated during dialysis may also account for at least part of the postdialysis disequilibrium syndrome, discussed elsewhere in this chapter. A pseudo–one-compartment model has been proposed to explain the behavior of phosphorus with HD.[196] Extrapolating further, one can speculate that the magnitude of sequestration for the toxic solutes responsible for the reversible life-threatening aspect of uremia cannot be as pronounced as for phosphorus; otherwise, HD would not be successful.

## COMPONENTS OF THE EXTRACORPOREAL CIRCUIT

The HD system for a single patient in the 1940s was about the size of a twin bed. Modern HD machines are about the size of a three- to four-drawer filing cabinet. Central to the dialysis delivery system is the artificial kidney or dialyzer, which acts as the point of exchange between blood and the dialysate. The system is designed to deliver blood and properly constituted dialysate to the dialyzer, where diffusion and convection occur. Technologic advances have allowed the development of online monitors that accurately monitor and regulate the blood flow and dialysate flow rates, circuit pressures, and dialysate composition and temperature. Additional advances include automated safety mechanisms designed to detect blood leaks and air in the circuit and online devices that monitor vascular access, hematocrit, and dialysis adequacy during each treatment.

### BLOOD CIRCUIT

During dialysis, the steady flow of blood required may be obtained from a central venous catheter or from an AV fistula or graft. If a catheter is used, blood enters the extracorporeal circuit from the ports along the sides of the double-lumen catheter (arterial lumen) and returns through the port at the distal tip (venous lumen). Alternatively, the graft or fistula is cannulated with two needles, with blood flowing from the arterial needle into the blood tubing and dialyzer and returning to the patient through the venous needle. The driving force for the blood circuit is a peristaltic roller pump, which sequentially compresses the pump segment of the tubing against a curved rigid track, forcing blood from the tubing. Elastic recoil refills the pump tubing after the roller has passed, readying it for the next roller. Because of the elastic recoil, and because most pumps have only two or three rollers, blood flow through the dialyzer is pulsatile. Increasing the number of rollers makes the flow less pulsatile but increases the risk of hemolysis and damage to the pump segment.

An alternative configuration of the dialysate delivery system allows the use of a single needle in the vascular access or a

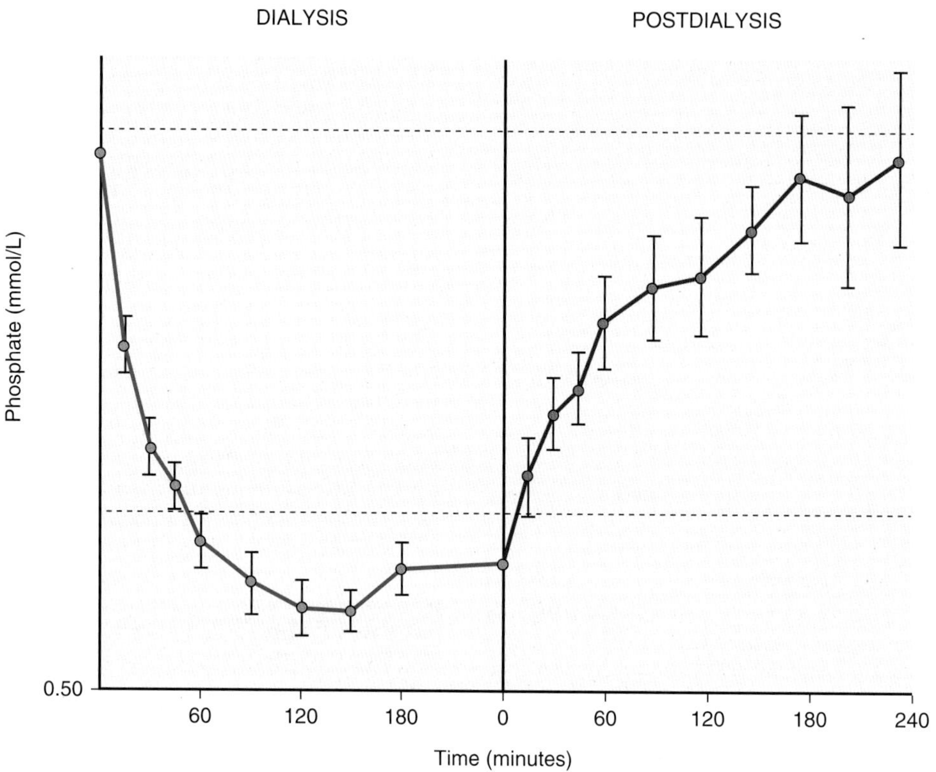


**Fig. 63.17** Effect of sequestration on serum phosphate levels and removal during dialysis. Measurements of serum inorganic phosphorus concentrations were taken at 15-minute intervals during both high flux and standard hemodialysis. The rapid flux of phosphorus due to its relatively high mass transfer area coefficient caused levels to fall into the hypophosphatemic range (below the lower *dotted line*) during most of the 4-hour dialysis. A marked rebound continued for 4 hours after dialysis ended. (Modified from DeSoi CA, Umans JG. Phosphate kinetics during high-flux hemodialysis. *J Am Soc Nephrol.* 1993;4:1214–1218.)

single-lumen catheter for dialysis.[197,198] This arrangement uses one blood pump and two pressure-controlled blood line clamps or two pressure-controlled blood pumps. The advantage is reduced trauma to the vascular access, especially during initial cannulation of a new fistula, and potentially reduced dialysis catheter use after surgical revision of a vascular access.[198] However, recirculation and hemolysis may be increased, and efficiency (adequacy) may be compromised.[197,199,200] Increasing the effective blood flow rate to 250 mL/min, increasing the length of the dialysis session, or using a larger dialyzer may improve the efficiency of solute clearance, but careful monitoring of adequacy and for complications is essential.[199]

Pressure monitors are located proximally to the blood pump and immediately distal to the dialyzer. The proximal or arterial pressure monitor guards against excessive suction on the vascular access site by the blood pump. Accepted ranges for arterial inflow pressures are −20 to 80 mm Hg, but may be as low as −200 mm Hg when the blood flow rate ($Q_b$) is high. The distal or venous pressure monitor gauges the resistance to blood return in the vascular access; acceptable values range from +50 to +200 mm Hg. When the upper or lower limits of arterial or venous pressures are exceeded, an alarm sounds, and the blood pump turns off. Excessively low arterial pressures may be caused by kinks in the tubing, improper arterial needle position, hypotension, or arterial inflow stenosis. Blood clotting in the dialyzer, kinking or clotting in the venous blood lines, improperly positioned venous needles, infiltration of a venous needle, or venous outflow stenosis can cause high venous pressures. Accurate measurements of the arterial and venous pressures are essential to determining the transmembrane pressure (TMP), which partly determines the ultrafiltration rate. Excessively high pressures anywhere in the blood compartment may rupture the dialyzer membrane or disconnect the blood circuit, leading to an abrupt decrease in pressure in the blood circuit. The automatic shutoff of the blood pump in this circumstance is potentially lifesaving.

Two additional safety devices, the venous air trap and air detector, are located in the blood line distal to the dialyzer. Air may enter the blood circuit through loose connections, improper arterial needle position, or the saline infusion line. The venous air trap prevents any air that may have entered the blood circuit from returning to the patient. If air is detected in the venous line after the air trap, the machine sounds an alarm, and a relay switch turns off the blood pump. Excessive foaming of blood also triggers the air detector. These safety features prevent air embolism, which can lead to stroke, cardiac and/or respiratory failure, and death if not immediately recognized.[201] However, microbubbles formed during dialysis may escape detection and lodge in organs such as the brain and lungs, possibly contributing to the higher incidence of pulmonary hypertension and cognitive decline observed in dialysis patients.[202,203] Ensuring a high blood level in the venous air trap, avoiding extremely high blood flow rates, and adequately priming a dry-packed dialyzer may reduce the incidence of such microemboli.[201,204]

## HEMODIALYZERS

A hemodialyzer, or dialyzer, is often called an "artificial kidney." Its configuration allows blood and dialysate to flow, preferably in opposite directions, through individual compartments separated by a semipermeable membrane. By convention, blood entering the hemodialyzer is designated arterial, and blood leaving the hemodialyzer is venous. The many available hemodialyzers differ mainly in the composition, configuration, and surface area of the membrane. Hemodialyzers influence the efficiency and quality of dialysis through their membranes, which determine their $K_0A$ value, and through the blood and dialysate flow rates, which determine the clearance values (see also $K_0A$; Table 63.5).

Virtually all commercial dialyzers available in the United States are hollow fiber dialyzers. These hemodialyzers are constructed with a cylindric plastic casing (usually polycarbonate) that encloses several thousand hollow fiber semipermeable membranes stretched from one end to the other and anchored at each end by a plastic potting compound, usually polyurethane. The blood compartment or fiber bundle volume of the hollow fiber dialyzer ranges from 60 to 150 mL and, in contrast to older dialyzer designs, does not expand during dialysis. Each fiber has an inner diameter of approximately 200 μm. Along with the semipermeable membrane, the potting material separates the blood compartment from the dialysate compartment, where dialysate flows between and around each fiber. Blood flows to or from the open end of each fiber through a removable header attached to the blood tubing. Apart from lowering blood priming volume, the hollow fiber design also improves the efficiency of solute exchange by increasing the contact area between blood and dialysate. Additional maneuvers to maximize surface area include insertion of spacer yarns between fibers and a wavy moiré configuration[205] of the fibers to prevent loss of surface area through fiber to fiber contact. The arterial port design also influences the distribution of blood flow through the hollow fibers and can reduce dialysis efficiency.[206] Thrombosis and the need for potting compound are major disadvantages of the hollow fiber design. The potting compound absorbs chemicals used to disinfect newly manufactured dialyzers (e.g., ethylene oxide) or reprocessed dialyzers (e.g., formaldehyde, peracetic acid, glutaraldehyde) and acts as a reservoir for these chemicals, allowing them to leach out slowly during dialysis into the patient's blood.[207]

**Table 63.5 Key Factors That Affect the Solute Clearance of a Hemodialyzer**

| Parameter | Key Factors | Clearance |
|---|---|---|
| Properties of the membrane | Membrane porosity | ↑ |
| | Membrane thickness | ↓ |
| | Membrane surface area | ↑ |
| | Membrane charge | Varies |
| | Membrane hydrophilicity | ↑ |
| Properties of the solute | Molecular weight and size | ↓ |
| | Charge | Varies |
| | Lipid solubility | ↓ |
| | Protein binding | ↓ |
| Blood side | Unstirred blood layer | ↓ |
| | Blood flow | ↑ |
| Dialysate side | Dialysate channeling and unstirred layer | ↓ |
| | Dialysate flow | ↑ |
| | Countercurrent direction of flow | ↑ |

### MEMBRANE COMPOSITION

The biomaterials used to make the hollow fiber dialyzer dictate its clearance and ultrafiltration characteristics, as well as its biocompatibility. Two major classes of membrane material are available commercially: (1) cotton fiber, or cellulose-based membranes; and (2) synthetic membranes. Unmodified cellulose-based membranes contain many free hydroxyl groups, which activate white blood cells, platelets, and serum complement via the alternate pathway (see later).[208] Treating the cellulose polymer with acetate and tertiary amino compounds improves membrane biocompatibility, presumably through the covalent binding of the hydroxyl groups to form acetylated cellulose and laminated cellulose, such as Cellosyn or Hemophan.[209,210]

The major polymers in synthetic membranes are polyacrylonitrile, polysulfone, polycarbonate, polyamide, polyether sulfone, and polymethylmethacrylate. Although these membranes are thicker, they can be rendered more permeable than the cellulose membranes, yielding greater fluid and solute removal. The larger pore sizes in the synthetic membranes remove higher molecular weight substances, such as beta-2 microglobulin, more efficiently.[211–213] Some membranes, such as polyacrylonitrile, polyamide, and polymethylmethacrylate membranes, have low hydrophilicity, providing significant protein adsorption and enhancing their removal.[214]

### MEMBRANE BIOCOMPATIBILITY

Dialyzer membranes may interact with blood components during dialysis to activate white blood cells, platelets, and the complement cascade via the alternative pathway with generation of the anaphylatoxins C3a and C5a.[208,213–216] The degree to which the membrane activates blood components determines what is called its "biocompatibility." Through activation of white blood cells, platelets, and the complement cascade, bioincompatible membranes may cause allergic reactions, hypoxemia, transient neutropenia (due to leukosequestration), altered immunity, tissue damage, anorexia, protein catabolism, or an inflammatory state. Because dialysis is repetitive, the effects of low-grade subclinical membrane interactions during each treatment may be cumulative, eventually resulting in adverse clinical outcomes such as infection, accelerated atherosclerosis, frequent hospitalization, and death.

In addition to the capability of the membrane to activate blood elements, its absorptive capacity also can influence its biocompatibility. Some synthetic membranes, such as polyacrylonitrile, are more hydrophobic, bind proteins to a greater extent, and may ameliorate bioincompatible inflammatory reactions through their ability to bind anaphylatoxins such as C3a and C5a and cytokines.[213,214] Therefore, measurements of these elements in blood may not reflect accurately the true capability of a membrane for inciting the complement cascade, producing cytokines, and inducing an inflamed state.[213] In general, however, synthetic membranes and modified or substituted cellulose membranes are more biocompatible than unmodified cellulose membranes,[208,213,214] but issues may still arise, as in a recent report of increased blood levels of bisphenol A in patients treated with a polysulfone membrane.[217]

Because bacterial contaminants in product water (see "Water Treatment") also can activate complement and leukocytes if they are in contact with blood, it is difficult to determine the relative contribution from bioincompatible membrane versus nonsterile or inadequately purified water to the inflamed state seen in dialysis patients. With increasing use of modified cellulose and synthetic membranes and closer attention to water quality, the distinction has become even more difficult. Studies evaluating the relative biocompatibility of substituted cellulose versus synthetic membranes have reported no difference.[210,218,219] Ongoing efforts to improve biocompatibility include coating the membrane with heparin or vitamin E.[220,221]

## MEMBRANE PERMEABILITY AND SURFACE AREA

Dialyzers perform two important functions, elimination of unwanted solutes and removal of excess fluid. The thickness, porosity, composition, and surface area of a membrane determine its ability to clear solutes and remove water. In general, the thinner the membrane and the more porous the membrane, the more efficient is the transport of solutes and fluid across the membrane. The urea $K_0A$ (or clearance) of the dialyzer describes its ability to eliminate low-molecular-weight substances, the vitamin $B_{12}$ and beta-2 microglobulin ($B_2M$) $K_0A$ (or clearance) capacity to remove higher molecular weight substances, and the ultrafiltration coefficient ($K_{Uf}$) ability to remove water (Table 63.6).

Most hemodialyzers have a membrane surface area of 0.8 to 2.1 $m^2$. The desirable increase in solute transport associated with larger membranes can be achieved by increasing the length, increasing the number, or decreasing the diameter of the hollow fiber,[222] but each maneuver has undesirable effects when carried too far. Lengthening the fiber increases the shear rate and resistance to blood flow, magnifying the pressure decrease between blood entering and exiting the dialyzer. Increasing the shear rate can damage RBCs, and the increased pressure can increase the ultrafiltration rate. However, the higher filtration rate at the arterial inflow end of the dialyzer is partially offset by the dissipation of pressure at the venous end, reducing the contribution of ultrafiltration to solute clearance and offsetting this potential advantage of greater surface area.[205] Increasing the number of hollow fibers increases surface area but expands the extracorporeal blood volume, which can compromise the patient's hemodynamic stability. Smaller diameter fibers can offset this disadvantage but, as the fiber diameter decreases, resistance to blood flow increases, enhancing not only filtration but also backfiltration and clotting.[223] As fibers thrombose, the effective surface area for diffusion decreases, and solute clearances decrease. Because of these adverse effects, the minimal acceptable internal fiber diameter is 180 μm.[223] The design and geometry of the hollow fiber dialyzer represent a delicate balance among these factors.

**Table 63.6 Characteristic Values for Standard, High-Efficiency, and High-Flux Dialyzers[a]**

| | Standard | High Efficiency | High Flux |
|---|---|---|---|
| Blood flow rate (mL/min) | 250 | ≥350 | ≥350 |
| Dialysate flow rate (mL/min) | 500 | ≥500 | ≥500 |
| $K_0A$ urea | 300–500 | ≥600 | Variable |
| Urea clearance (mL/min) | <200 | >210 | Variable |
| Urea clearance/body weight (mL/min/kg) | < 3 | >3 | Variable |
| Vitamin $B_{12}$ clearance (mL/min) | 30–60 | Variable | >100 |
| Beta-2 microglobulin clearance (mL/min) | <10 | Variable | >20 |
| Ultrafiltration coefficient (mL/hr/mm Hg) | 3.5–5.0 | Variable | >20 |
| Membrane | Cellulose | Variable | Variable |

[a]See text.

## HIGH-EFFICIENCY AND HIGH-FLUX DIALYZERS

Historically, low dialyzer membrane permeability has limited the efficiency of HD, requiring more than 6 hours for each treatment. As dialyzer design improved, treatment times were shortened progressively. In the late 1980s, with the advent of more permeable dialyzer membranes, improved techniques to reduce bacteriologic contamination of bicarbonate dialysate (see later), more precise ultrafiltration control, and more reliable vascular access to achieve adequate blood flow, treatment times decreased to 2 to 3 hours three times weekly in the United States. These substituted cellulose and synthetic membranes ushered in the era of high-efficiency and high-flux dialysis.

The distinction between high-efficiency and high-flux dialyzers is imprecise, and sometimes these terms are used interchangeably. Both types of dialyzers have improved solute and fluid clearance compared with standard hemodialyzers and take advantage of higher blood and dialysate flow rates to reduce dialysis time while maintaining an adequate dose. High-efficiency dialyzers have a high $K_0A$ and a high clearance of small molecules, such as urea, compared with standard dialyzers (see Table 63.6). High-flux dialyzers have a highly permeable membrane for larger molecules, such as vitamin $B_{12}$ and $B_2M$, and have a higher $K_{Uf}$ than high-efficiency dialyzers, but not necessarily high urea clearances (see Table 63.6). As evident from the foregoing discussion, the two dialyzer designs frequently overlap—hence, the imprecision (see Table 63.6).

High-efficiency and high-flux dialyzers contain a substituted cellulose or synthetic membrane. Both membranes improve dialyzer permeability because substituted cellulose membranes can be made thinner to increase porosity and surface area, and synthetic membranes can be manufactured with more and larger pores. Both high-efficiency and high-flux dialysis require the use of bicarbonate dialysate and volume-controlled filtration. When acetate was used as the prominent base in dialysate, its rate of diffusion into blood exceeded the metabolic capacity of the body, leading to acidosis, vasodilation, and intradialytic hypotension (see "Dialysate Composition"). The high $K_{Uf}$ of these dialyzers creates the potential for hemodynamic instability with pressure-controlled filtration;

hence, the need for volume-controlled filtration (see "Dialysate Circuit").

Because of their relative porosity, high-flux dialyzers can remove larger molecules such as $B_2M$, which are not removed at all by standard cellulosic dialyzers.[211–213] $B_2M$ removal reduces the risk of carpal tunnel syndrome and other complications in long-term patients.[211,224,225] Initial results have suggested that removal of other large molecules may offer additional benefits, such as an enhanced response to erythropoietin,[226] higher leptin removal, possibly leading to a better appetite,[227] and perhaps lower mortality and hospitalization rates.[225,228] However, potential adverse consequences include more efficient removal of amino acids,[229] albumin,[230] and drugs such as vancomycin.[231] Theoretically, the backfiltration that occurs during high-flux dialysis can increase the exposure of patients to endotoxin from dialysate, but this theoretic concern has not been verified clinically.[232,233]

Despite early promise in patients undergoing maintenance hemodialysis, randomized controlled or crossover trials comparing high-flux dialysis with standard dialysis have found no difference in the incidence of hypotension and intradialysis symptoms,[211,234] control of blood pressure,[235] neuropsychological function,[236] hemoglobin concentration, and use of erythropoiesis-stimulating agents (ESA)s[237–239] or markers of inflammation, oxidative stress, and nutritional status.[238] Three large randomized controlled trials, the Hemodialysis (HEMO) Study,[240,241] the Membrane Permeability Outcome (MPO) Study,[242] and the EGE Study (Multiple Interventions Related to Dialysis Procedures in Order to Reduce Cardiovascular Morbidity and Mortality in Hemodialysis Patients)[243] detected no significant difference in mortality or morbidity between patients treated with standard versus high-flux membranes. Post hoc subgroup analyses have demonstrated that high-flux dialysis reduces cardiovascular events in patients with longer dialysis vintage in the HEMO Study,[240,241] reduces mortality in patients with low serum albumin concentrations (<4.0 g/dL) and diabetes in the MPO Study,[242] and reduces cardiovascular mortality in patients with an AVF or diabetes in the EGE study.[243] A meta-analysis of available data has concluded that high-flux hemodialysis may reduce cardiovascular mortality by 15% but does not alter infection-related or all-cause mortality.[244]

### Convection Versus Diffusion

Further increases in dialyzer flux may not lead to improved middle molecule clearance or outcomes because some solutes that accumulate in kidney failure are protein-bound or sequestered inside the cell.[245] Because of slow diffusion caused by low free concentrations of protein-bound solutes and delayed diffusion across cell membranes, the removal of such solutes remains time-dependent. Initial experience has suggested that hemofiltration (HF) and hemodiafiltration (HDF) may augment the removal of larger molecules and protein-bound solutes through increased convective clearance.[245–247] However, randomized controlled studies comparing HF and HDF with HD have found no difference in hemoglobin or ESA resistance,[248,249] serum phosphate levels,[250] health-related quality of life,[251] cardiovascular parameters such as left ventricular mass and pulse wave velocity,[252] and intradialytic hypotension,[253,254] although some studies have reported less intradialytic hypotension with HDF.[255,256] Two of the three largest randomized controlled studies, the Convective Transport Study (CONTRAST)[257] and Turkish Online Haemodiafiltration Study (OL-HDF),[254] have reported no difference in cardiovascular and all-cause mortality, but subgroup analyses have suggested a benefit in patients treated with greater convective and replacement volumes (>22 L and 17.4 L, respectively, so-called "high efficiency" HDF). The ESHOL (Estudio de Supervivencia de Hemodiafiltracion On-Line) Study,[256] which achieved about 23 L of convective volume per session, reported lower cardiovascular mortality, all-cause mortality, and hospitalization in patients randomized to HDF. Recent meta-analyses have concluded that convective therapies may reduce intradialytic hypotension[247,258,259] and cardiovascular mortality,[247,259] but additional high-quality randomized and controlled studies addressing the effect of convective volume on outcomes are needed.[260]

Further technologic advances have allowed the development of high-retention onset or mid- or high-cutoff hemodialyzer membranes, which have larger but more homogenous pore sizes that will clear molecules up to 45 kDa in size yet prevent the excessive loss of albumin.[261–263] Preliminary clinical data have suggested that HD with these membranes allows the clearance of larger middle molecules, such as advanced glycation end products and inflammatory mediators, comparable to that achieved with HDF, and may improve the residual syndrome (symptoms that remain in patients despite adequate dialysis) and reduce cardiovascular risk.[261–265]

## DIALYSATE CIRCUIT

Another major function of the HD system is the preparation and delivery of dialysate to the dialyzer. Most dialysis clinics use a single-pass delivery system, which discards the dialysate after a single passage through the dialyzer, and a single-patient delivery system, which prepares dialysates individually and continuously at each patient station by mixing liquid concentrates with a proportionate volume of purified water. To ensure that the dialysate concentrates are diluted safely and accurately, the delivery system has many built-in safety monitors. Some clinics use a central multipatient delivery system. The dialysate is mixed in an area separate from patient care and then piped into each patient station, or the concentrate is piped to each station before mixing. These centralized systems lower patient care costs and reduce staff back injuries from carrying the individual concentrate jugs. However, a disadvantage is the additional effort and cost required to modify the dialysate concentration of electrolytes such as calcium and potassium for individual patients.

The dialysis machine warms purified water to physiologic temperatures and then deaerates it under vacuum. Because the patient is exposed to 100 to 200 L of dialysate during each treatment, the dialysate must be warmed to avoid hypothermia. In practice, the dialysate temperature is maintained at 35° to 37°C. If the dialysate is too hot, protein denaturation (>42°C) and hemolysis (>45°C) occur. To ensure safety, the temperature monitor in the dialysate circuit sounds an alarm, and a bypass valve diverts the dialysate directly to the drain, automatically bypassing the dialyzer if the dialysate temperature is outside the limits of 35° to 42°C. Without deaeration, dissolved air will come out of solution as negative pressure is applied during dialysis, creating air bubbles in the dialysate, which leads to malfunction of the blood leak detector and conductivity detector, increased channeling, masking parts of the membrane, and reduced surface area.

The heated and deaerated product water is then mixed proportionately with the concentrate to produce dialysate. Improperly proportioned dialysate may cause severe electrolyte disturbances in the patient and lead to death. Because the primary solutes in the dialysate are electrolytes, the electrical conductivity of the dialysate varies directly with the concentration of solutes. Based on this principle, the conductivity monitor downstream from the proportioning pump continuously measures the electrical conductivity of the product solution to ensure proper proportioning. It has a narrow range of tolerance, is usually redundant, and must be calibrated periodically using standardized solutions or by laboratory measurements of electrolytes in the dialysate. Changes in temperature, the presence of air bubbles, or malfunction of the sensor (usually an electrode) can alter the dialysate conductivity.

The dialysate pump, located downstream from the dialyzer, controls dialysate flow and dialysate pressure. Although many dialyzers require a negative dialysate pressure for filtration, the circuit also must be able to generate positive dialysate pressures within the dialyzer because positive pressure is required to limit filtration when using dialyzers with a high $K_{Uf}$ or under conditions that increase pressure in the blood compartment. The dialysate circuit regulates the pressure by controlled constriction of the dialysate outflow tubing while maintaining a constant flow rate. In addition, the dialysate delivery system controls the filtration rate, either indirectly by altering the TMP (pressure-controlled ultrafiltration) or directly by modifying the actual filtration rate (volume-controlled ultrafiltration). Earlier systems used manual pressure-controlled filtration, requiring dialysis personnel to calculate and enter the TMP, closely monitor the filtration rate, and recalculate and adjust the TMP as needed. For dialyzers with a $K_{Uf}$ greater than 6 mL/hr/mm Hg, dialysate delivery systems with built-in balance chambers and servomechanisms that accurately control the volume of the fluid removed during dialysis (volume-controlled filtration)[266] are mandatory to prevent excessive fluid gain or removal.

When blood is detected in the dialysate, the blood leak monitor located in the dialysate outflow tubing sounds an alarm and shuts off the blood pump. Blood in the dialysate usually indicates membrane rupture and may be caused by a TMP exceeding 500 mm Hg or by a damaged dialyzer membrane from the bleach and heat disinfection used to reprocess dialyzers for repeated use. Although a rare complication, membrane rupture can be life-threatening because it allows blood to come into contact with nonsterile dialysate.

## ONLINE MONITORING

In addition to delivering dialysate to the dialyzer and the many built-in safety features described previously, modern dialysis machines also record and store such varied, real-time data as patient vital signs, blood and dialysate flows, arterial and venous pressures, delivered dialysis dose, plasma volume, thermal energy loss, and access recirculation. Linking computerized medical information systems with dialysis delivery systems can facilitate and improve patient care by allowing the integration of patient data while maintaining treatment records. These capabilities may be most important among patients receiving in-center self-care or home-based HD, where there are fewer personnel present at the point of care.

### MONITORING CLEARANCE

Online monitoring of clearance may provide the best assessment of dialysis adequacy.[267–271] Online monitors record urea clearances by measuring the urea concentration in the dialysate, either continuously or periodically,[267,271,272] determining dialyzer sodium clearance by pulsing the dialysate with sodium and measuring dialysate conductivity at the dialyzer inlet and outlet (ionic dialysance),[267,268,273,274] or determining clearance of uremic solutes by measuring ultraviolet light absorbance of spent dialysate.[267,275,276] Most online methods for monitoring urea or sodium kinetics provide Kt/V based on whole-body clearance in addition to dialyzer clearance.[268,273] Online urea monitoring has not gained popularity, possibly because of the need for repeated calibration and the added expense for additional disposable supplies. Online clearance monitoring removes the expense and risks of blood sampling, reduces dialysis personnel time, allows more frequent determination of delivered dose, and provides real-time measurements for instant feedback.[268–270] However, reported clearance values may differ, depending on the online equipment used and adjustments applied by the instrument's software to match the urea Kt/V more closely.[274,275] Drawbacks of online clearance monitoring include the need for multiple measurements of $K_d$ to obtain an average for the entire dialysis, accurate monitoring of treatment time, the need for blood urea sampling to allow determination of protein catabolic rate (a marker of nutrition), and the need to measure or estimate V to allow the calculation of Kt/V from the online $K_d$ measurements.[277]

### MONITORING HEMATOCRIT AND RELATIVE BLOOD VOLUME

The hematocrit can be measured online during dialysis using an ultrasound determination of plasma protein concentration[278] or an optical measure of hemoglobin concentration or hematocrit.[267,269,270,279] Of these, the optical technique is most widely available. In theory, patients treated with dialysis who are prone to hypotension and cramping may benefit from online monitoring of hematocrit because their symptoms are usually caused by a decrease in circulating blood volume when the ultrafiltration rate exceeds intravascular refilling from the interstitium and intracellular spaces.[267,269,270,279,280] The degree of hemoconcentration reflects the immediate magnitude of intravascular volume depletion and allows determination of changes in the blood volume or relative blood volume. Theoretically, monitoring the hematocrit online and altering the filtration rate during dialysis to minimize excessive hemoconcentration may reduce the occurrence of symptoms during dialysis and optimize the dry weight.[267,270,281–283] In practice, using just the relative blood volume to guide the filtration rate has not been very successful in ameliorating symptoms, likely because of inaccuracies in the measurements, the varied compensatory cardiovascular responses to volume depletion within and among individual patients, and a dialysis-induced reduction in arteriolar tone and left ventricular function (myocardial stunning).[267,270,279,280,284–289]

Online determination of relative blood volume varies significantly among devices and underestimates the true decline in blood volume because of intravascular translocation of blood from the microcirculation (capillaries and venules), which has a lower hematocrit, to the larger vessels.[279,280,282] Because of the previous limitations, identifying the pattern of the relative blood volume decline and using a computer-controlled biofeedback system to modify the filtration rate continuously during dialysis (see later), in combination with clinical assessment such as symptoms and bioimpedance spectrometry, have shown more promise.[267,269,270,290–292] The absolute or total blood volume may be more predictive of intradialytic symptoms; automated online monitoring of absolute blood volume is not currently available, although mathematical models may allow derivation of the total blood volume from relative blood volume.[280,293–296]

## COMPUTER CONTROLS

Solute removal during HD reduces plasma osmolarity, favoring fluid shift into the cells and thwarting efforts to achieve net fluid removal.[297–299] Raising the dialysate sodium concentration (sodium ramping) helps preserve plasma osmolarity and may allow continued fluid removal but leads to increased thirst, excessive interdialytic weight gain (IDWG), and hypertension, although the latter is not a consistent finding.[269,297–303] Computer-controlled sodium modeling changes the dialysate sodium concentration automatically during dialysis, usually starting at 150 to 155 mEq/L and stepping down to 135 to 140 mEq/L near or at the end of dialysis, and offers the theoretic benefit of reducing intradialytic symptoms (hypotension and cramps) while minimizing thirst, IDWG, and hypertension. In practice, however, thirst, increased IDWG, and hypertension persist because of predialysis hyponatremia (on average, 134–136 mEq/L) and an overall positive sodium balance during dialysis, despite the step-down.[269,300,304,305] Instead, individualizing dialysate sodium to maintain a sodium gradient of 0 to −2 mEq/L with respect to the predialysis plasma sodium concentration results in less thirst, lower IDWG, improved blood pressure control, and perhaps diminished intradialytic symptoms because of lower ultrafiltration requirements.[297–300,306] Such individualization may be accomplished through the use of online conductivity monitoring or by estimating each patient's inherent plasma sodium concentration (sodium set point) using an average predialysis sodium concentration. This can be measured with direct potentiometry or mathematically corrected for the Gibbs-Donnan effect—sodium that is not available for diffusion because of trapping by negatively charged proteins.[297–300,305] To complicate matters further, data from DOPPS have suggested a differential effect of dialysate sodium on outcome; HD patients with the lowest predialysis plasma sodium levels have a lower mortality when dialyzed against a high-dialysate sodium, despite an increase in IDWG.[302] In addition, measured dialysate sodium levels deviate significantly from prescribed levels in over 40% of assays, ranging from 13 mEq/L higher to 6 mEq/L lower than prescribed,[307–309] making it difficult to interpret studies evaluating the clinical effects of varying dialysate sodium concentrations.[297–299,310] Given our incomplete understanding of the effects of altering dialysate sodium levels on morbidity and mortality, the indiscriminate use of dialysate sodium ramping and sodium modeling in its current form should be abandoned, and individualization of dialysate sodium should be done cautiously.[289,297–299,311,312]

Ultrafiltration modeling provides a variable rate of fluid removal during dialysis according to a preprogrammed profile (e.g., linear decline, stepwise changes, exponential decline of filtration rate with time). Theoretically, altering the filtration rate during dialysis allows time for the blood compartment to refill from the interstitial compartment, leading to less hypotension and cramping. As with sodium modeling, standalone ultrafiltration modeling is relatively crude, and altering the ultrafiltration rate in response to blood volume monitoring may be of more benefit (see earlier, "Monitoring Hematocrit and Relative Blood Volume"). The effects of sodium and ultrafiltration modeling may be difficult to separate because they are often used together.[267,269,270,304]

Recent technologic advances include the development of dialysis machines with biofeedback systems, allowing for computer-controlled adjustments of treatment parameters based on real-time input from the online monitors. The most common system in use monitors the blood volume (see earlier) and adjusts the ultrafiltration rate and dialysate conductivity to prevent it from decreasing below a preset value during dialysis. Small studies have demonstrated that this device ameliorates symptoms in hypotension- and nonhypotension-prone patients.[267,269,270,282,283,290,313,314]

Although the ability to monitor plasma conductivity throughout dialysis may ensure sodium balance, despite constant modifications to the dialysate conductivity, and may reduce the problem of thirst, IDWG, and hypertension,[267] most authorities have advised against sodium modeling, even with a feedback control system (see previous discussion).[181,269,270,313,315] Instead, automated control of the dialysate temperature to maintain isothermic dialysis (constant body temperature) has shown promise and is superior to thermoneutral dialysis (using lower but constant dialysate temperature) in reducing intradialytic hypotension without incurring a sodium load.[267,270,316–319] Other recent studies have suggested that individualized dialysate cooling (0.5°C lower than body temperature, averaged over six preceding treatments) reduces episodes of intradialytic hypotension by 70%, raises mean arterial blood pressure during HD by 12 mm Hg, and abrogates both HD-associated cardiomyopathy and brain white matter changes.[320,321] Although these online monitors and automated biofeedback systems are expensive, they have the potential to reduce hypotension, detect vascular access dysfunction, and increase dialysis efficiency while minimizing blood sampling.[271,282,283,322,323] By improving patient care, they may prove not to be cost-prohibitive in the long run.

# DIALYSATE

During HD, blood flows in the blood compartment in one direction, and iso-osmotic dialysate flows in the opposite direction in the dialysate compartment (see Fig. 63.12). This countercurrent flow optimizes the concentration gradient for solute removal. Preparation of the dialysate and its composition is critical to the success of dialysis. The solution must be prepared from properly treated water (see later) that includes reducing the concentration of endotoxins to prevent pyrogenic reactions in the patient. Sterility is not required because the semipermeable membrane excludes large particles such as bacteria and viruses. The concentrations of vital solutes added to the dialysate reflect those normally maintained in the body by the native kidneys (Table 63.7).

The dialysate is essentially a physiologic salt solution that creates a gradient for removal of unwanted solutes and maintains a constant physiologic concentration of extracellular electrolytes (see later).

## WATER TREATMENT

Because HD patients are exposed to as much as 600 L of dialysate water/week, treating the water used to generate dialysate is essential to avoid exposure to harmful substances such as aluminum, chloramines, fluoride, endotoxins, and bacteria.[324–328] Technical advances such as high-flux dialyzers, reuse or reprocessing of dialyzers, and bicarbonate-based dialysate have made high water quality even more imperative. To avoid these complications, tap water is softened, exposed to charcoal to remove contaminants such as chloramine, filtered to remove particulate matter, and then filtered again under high pressure (reverse osmosis) to remove other dissolved contaminants (Fig. 63.18). A complete review of this topic is beyond the scope of this chapter, and readers are referred to reviews on the topic.[324–329] Highlights are discussed later.

### Hazards Associated With Dialysis Water

Improperly treated water contains potentially harmful substances and can cause patient injury or death.[324–330] Accumulation of aluminum in the body may cause osteomalacia, microcytic anemia, and dialysis-associated encephalopathy (dialysis dementia and movement disorders).[331–333] Treating water to keep aluminum levels below 10 mg/L has markedly reduced aluminum-associated diseases.[334,335] Chlorine is added to municipal water as a bactericidal agent and interacts with organic material in the water to form chloramines. Alternatively, chloramine may occur naturally or may be added directly to municipal water as a bactericidal agent. Unfortunately, in contrast to chlorine, direct exposure of the blood to chloramine causes acute hemolysis and methemoglobinemia.[327,328,336–338] Fluoride can cause cardiac arrhythmias and death acutely[339,340] and osteomalacia chronically.[341] Excess calcium and magnesium have been linked to the hard water syndrome with a constellation of symptoms, including nausea, vomiting, weakness, flushing, and labile blood pressures.[342] Close communication with water suppliers is critical to anticipate changes in feed water quality from added chemicals and environmental conditions such as flooding or contamination, because alterations in the water purification process may be required.[327,329] With the advent of large-pore, high-flux membranes, efforts at improving water purity have focused on further reducing bacterial endotoxins, which can cause febrile reactions, hypotension, and chronic inflammation (see later).[325,327–329]

**Table 63.7 Solutes Present in the Dialysate**

| Solute | Concentration (mEq/L) |
|---|---|
| Sodium | 135–145 |
| Potassium | 0–4.0 |
| Chloride | 102–106 |
| Bicarbonate | 30–39 |
| Acetate | 2–4 |
| Calcium | 0–3.5 |
| Magnesium | 0.5–1.0 |
| Dextrose | 11 |
| pH | 7.1–7.3 |

### Essential Components of Water Purification

Temperature-blending valves proportion incoming hot and cold tap water to yield a water temperature of about 77°F, the optimal temperature for the carbon tank and most reverse osmosis membranes. Water temperature below 77°F reduce the flow rate and thus the efficiency of the reverse osmosis system, and temperature above 100°F may damage the membrane. Multimedia depth filters then remove particulate matter from the water (see Fig. 63.19). Using cation exchange resins that contain sodium, the water softener then removes calcium, magnesium, and other polyvalent cations from the feed water, preventing these cations from depositing on and damaging the reverse osmosis membrane. Next, granular

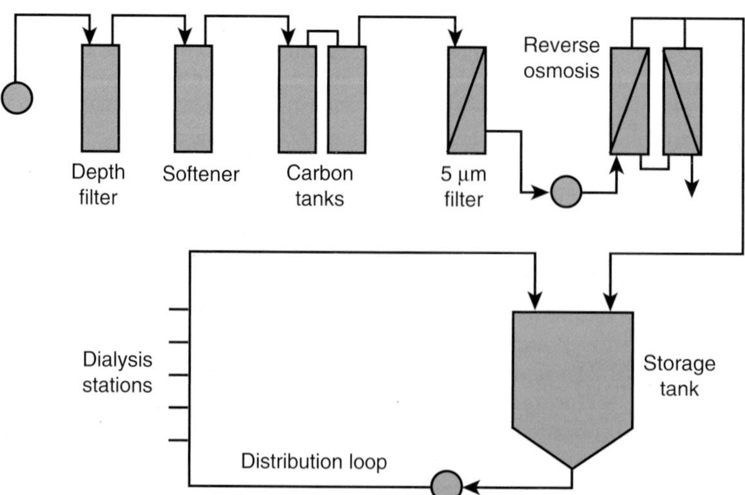


**Fig. 63.18** Schematic of a typical configuration of a reverse osmosis water treatment system. Tap water undergoes filtration to remove gross particulate matter and then is softened before exposure to charcoal (carbon tanks) to remove contaminants such as chloramine. A second filtration process removes particulate matter, as well as microbiologic organisms. Finally, water is filtered under high pressure to remove dissolved contaminants such as aluminum (reverse osmosis). Product water is then either stored in a water tank or piped directly to each dialysis station.

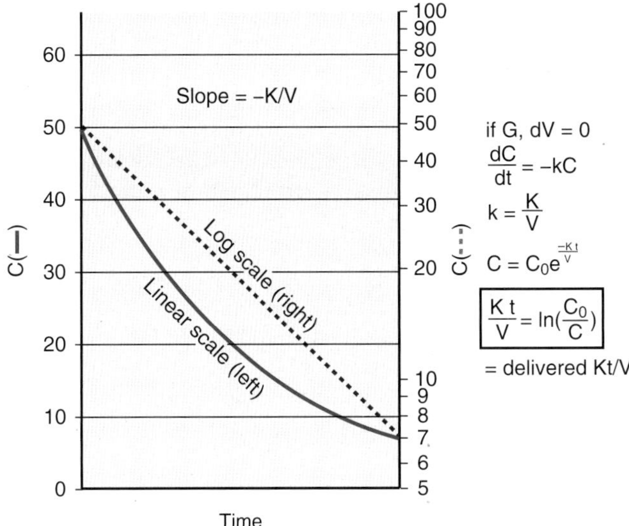


**Fig. 63.19** Intradialysis urea kinetics: origin of Kt/V. *Left,* The nonlinear decrease in blood urea nitrogen during dialysis (*solid line*) becomes a straight line when plotted on a log scale (*dashed line*). The fractional rate of decrease is a constant, k = K/V, where k is the elimination constant, K is the clearance, and V is the urea distribution volume. *Right,* The solution to the equation describing first-order kinetics shows that delivered Kt/V primarily depends on the predialysis and postdialysis blood urea nitrogen values (see text and legend for Fig. 63.20 for definition of variables shown). This oversimplified equation is expanded in Fig. 63.20 to include the other important variables.

activated carbon in the carbon filtration tank absorbs chlorine, chloramines, and other organic substances from the water. Activated carbon is very porous and has a high affinity for organic material but, if not serviced properly or exchanged frequently, it can be contaminated with bacteria. Downstream, the water is then filtered through a 5-μm cartridge filter to prevent carbon particles from fouling up the reverse osmosis pump and membrane. Finally, the water is delivered to the reverse osmosis unit, which applies high hydrostatic pressure to force water through a highly selective semipermeable membrane that rejects 90% to 99% of monovalent ions, 95% to 99% of divalent ions, and microbiologic contaminants larger than 200 daltons. The water exiting the reverse osmosis unit is termed the "permeate" or "product water" and, in most clinics, can be used safely for dialysis.

When there is heavy ionic contamination of feed water, however, the product water from the reverse osmosis unit is further polished with a mixed bed ion exchange system (deionization system) and then passed through an ultrafilter to remove any bacterial contamination from the ion exchanger. The cationic resin exchanges hydrogen ions for other cations in descending order of affinity—calcium, magnesium, potassium, sodium, and then hydrogen. The anionic resin exchanges hydroxyl ions for other anions in decreasing order of affinity—nitrites, sulfates, nitrates, chloride, bicarbonate, hydroxyl, and fluoride. When the resin is exhausted, previously adsorbed ions, especially those of lower affinity, can elute into the effluent and result in levels that are more than 20 times their usual concentration in tap water, causing severe toxicity and even death.[339,343] Because of this danger, the deionization system is rarely used alone in treating water for dialysis and requires stringent monitoring of product water.

## Microbiology of Hemodialysis Systems

Despite municipal treatment of tap water and the extensive water treatment system described previously, water used for dialysis still can become contaminated with bacteria and endotoxins,[324,325,327–330,344–346] mainly with water-borne, gram-negative bacteria and nontuberculous mycobacteria. Such contamination arises because the system removes the normally protective chlorine and chloramine described previously, and low flow and stagnation points in the water treatment circuit predispose to biofilm deposition. Although nontuberculous mycobacteria do not produce endotoxins, they are more resistant to germicides than gram-negative bacteria and can survive and multiply in product water that contains little organic matter.[347–350] In 1984, the Centers for Disease Control and Prevention (CDC) found nontuberculous mycobacteria in the water of 83% of surveyed dialysis centers.[348]

In addition to treating water to remove potentially harmful chemicals, routine disinfection and surveillance of the water treatment equipment, product water, and dialysate are also critically important to optimize dialysis water quality.[324,327–330,345] Because of dialyzer reprocessing and the use of high-flux dialyzers, the patient may be exposed to bacterial and endotoxin contaminants in improperly handled product water, either through direct contact of product water with the blood compartment during reprocessing or through backleak of endotoxin into the blood compartment during dialysis. Therefore, high-level disinfection to kill all microorganisms (except bacterial spores) is necessary, as well as stricter standards for water quality. In 2009, the Association for the Advancement of Medical Instrumentation (AAMI) adopted the International Organization for Standardization (ISO) guidelines for dialysis water quality, recommending a lower maximal level of 100 colony-forming units (CFU)/mL for bacteria and a maximal concentration of less than 0.25 endotoxin units (EU)/mL for endotoxin (compared with 200 CFU/mL and 2 EU/mL previously), with action levels of 25 CFU/mL and 0.125 EU/mL, respectively.[351,352] In addition to routine scheduled disinfection, the water treatment equipment and system and affected dialysis machines must be disinfected when action levels are detected on scheduled monitoring. For ultrapure dialysate, even more stringent criteria are in place, including a bacterial count of less than 0.1 CFU/mL and endotoxin level of less than 0.03 EU/mL.[353] A meta-analysis has reported that ultrapure dialysate use is associated with less inflammation and oxidative stress, higher serum albumin and hemoglobin levels, and lower ESA requirement.[354] The only randomized controlled trial to evaluate the effect of ultrapure dialysate on fatal and nonfatal cardiovascular events has found no benefit, although its power to detect a difference may have been reduced by a lower than expected endotoxin level (0.15 ± 0.22 EU/mL) in the conventional dialysate group.[243] Despite the absence of large randomized controlled trials, ultrapure dialysate use may be desirable because of these potential benefits, the potential to reduce overall cost of dialysis through decreased ESA use, and the necessity of ensuring water quality with the advent of high-cutoff dialyzer membranes.[261,263,355,356]

Water contaminated with bacteria and endotoxins can lead to pyrogenic reactions, characterized by shaking chills, fever, and hypotension in a previously afebrile and asymptomatic patient.[324,326,328,345,357] Headache, myalgia, nausea, and vomiting also may be present. Typically, the symptoms begin 30 to 60 minutes into the dialysis treatment. The source of the reaction is unlikely to be the microorganisms per se because they are too large to cross an intact dialyzer membrane. Instead, bacterial pyrogens such as lipopolysaccharide, peptidoglycans, exotoxins, and their fragments are thought to be responsible.[324,326,328,345,358] Pyrogenic reactions are typically seen in association with reprocessing of dialyzers because contaminated water gains direct access to the blood compartment during reprocessing.[207,357,359,360] In the absence of reuse, pyrogenic reactions are rare and occur only with high-level bacterial contamination of the dialysate or bicarbonate. Although the larger pore size in high-flux dialyzers may increase backfiltration and allow endotoxins to enter the blood compartment from the dialysate, synthetic membranes also adsorb endotoxins, thereby attenuating the effect of imperfectly processed dialysate.[207,324,345] However, even in the absence of pyrogenic reactions, low levels of dialysate contamination with microbes may result in chronic inflammation, manifested as higher serum C-reactive protein levels, increased oxidative stress, lower serum albumin and hemoglobin levels, and ESA resistance,[354–356] reversed by the use of ultrapure dialysate (see earlier).

#### Monitoring Water Quality

Because of the potential complications that can occur when improperly treated water is used for dialysis, monitoring of water quality is crucial. The source water and product water must be assayed routinely to ensure that product water meets the standards for heavy metal and other ionic contaminants. In the United States, the Association for the Advancement of Medical Instrumentation (AAMI) has adopted ISO water standards for dialysis (see previously). The frequency of scheduled testing depends on the quality of the water source, type of water treatment system used, and seasonal variation in chemicals added to municipal water to ensure its potability.

Samples of source water, water obtained from critical points in the water treatment system, product water, dialysate, and bicarbonate solution must be cultured at least monthly to ensure that bacterial contamination is below the limits set forth by AAMI standards. In addition, water is tested with the Limulus amebocyte lysate (LAL) assay to determine the degree of endotoxin contamination. Although the most common test used, the LAL assay may not detect smaller endotoxin fragments that are small enough to cross even low-flux membranes to cause pyrogen reactions. The cytokine induction assay using mononuclear cells may allow improved detection of these low-molecular-weight substances.[325,345,361]

## HEMODIALYSIS ADEQUACY

### HISTORICAL PERSPECTIVES

In 1973, when Medicare in the United States began to fund dialysis for any citizen with a modest record of employment, regardless of age, little attention was paid to the adequacy of dialysis. If the patient was awake and functioning at any level, the dialysis was deemed successful. As dialysis evolved and the prophylactic aspect of dialysis was better appreciated, concerns raised about the adequacy of dialysis therapy led to a meeting in Monterey, California, in 1974 that served to launch the National Cooperative Dialysis Study (NCDS).[362] Sponsored by the National Institutes of Health (NIH), this first clinical trial of HD adequacy aimed to control the average BUN level at 50 mg/dL versus 100 mg/dL, but the ultimate finding was a strong association between $Kt/V_{urea}$ and outcome.[363] Subsequent observational studies have repeatedly confirmed the higher risk of mortality when the fractional clearance during each dialysis, expressed as Kt/V, falls below 1.2.[364–366] Another controlled trial of dialysis dose and adequacy sponsored by the NIH in the late 1990s (the HEMO Study) showed no further benefit from increasing the dialyzer single-pool Kt/V above 1.3/treatment three times weekly.[241] This study also showed that previously reported benefits from doses above 1.3 observed in uncontrolled studies were subject to bias from regression to the mean and from a newly recognized dose targeting bias.[367–369] Failure to achieve the targeted dose is apparently a risk factor in itself, independent of the actual dose. Together, these findings have led the medical community and the Medicare sponsor to issue guidelines for HD adequacy that have become standards of care in the United States and later in other countries.[94,370–372] The persistently high mortality rate in the dialysis population, although often unrelated to the dialysis itself, has spurred interest in dialysis adequacy and its methods of measurement over the years. This section reviews the rationale and methods for measuring dialysis adequacy, focusing on mathematical models of solute kinetics that have been effectively put into clinical practice in nearly all HD clinics.

In view of recent discussions about the scope of dialysis adequacy, it is important to distinguish the adequacy of the treatment itself (i.e., removal of accumulated solutes and water) from global kidney replacement therapy. The clinician must treat the whole patient, including providing treatments such as psychotherapy for depression, management of anemia, nutrition, minimizing infection risks, treatment of cardiovascular disease risk factors and, above all, maintaining a good quality of life for the patient.

However, it is important to put proper emphasis on the primary reason for the patient's attendance at the dialysis clinic, the dialysis itself. Clearly, not all compounds that accumulate in kidney failure are readily removed with dialysis, such as those that are highly protein-bound or tightly sequestered. Although it remains possible that some aspects of dialysis (e.g., high-molecular-weight solute flux) may affect conditions found in kidney failure that are not directly related to the dialysis process (e.g., anemia, cardiovascular disease) but may be considered part of dialysis adequacy, it is intuitive that erythropoietin replacement or parathyroidectomy cannot cure uremia. Although discussions focused on the role of nontraditional toxins in patient outcomes are worthwhile,[373,374] they should not distract from what is still the most critical part of maintaining health on dialysis—the treatment itself. The focus of the following discussion is on solute and water removal; standards established for other aspects of kidney replacement are discussed later (see "Management of Patients on Maintenance Hemodialysis").

### UREMIA: THE SYNDROME REVERSED BY DIALYSIS THERAPY

The clinical syndrome resulting from kidney failure is a toxic state caused by the accumulation of solutes normally excreted by the kidney (see also Chapter 52). These include water-soluble, freely filtered solutes, as well as protein-bound substances, which may require active renal tubular transport for final excretion. The relationship between the syndrome and kidney disease was not obvious in antiquity and, even after the relationship was known, loss of nonexcretory functions of the kidney could be equally implicated as the cause, especially because urine volume and content, which reflect oral intake, differ little from normal as the disease progresses. When urea was discovered more than 200 years ago, investigators began to find elevated concentrations of urea and other organic solutes in patients' serum that are normally found in urine. This finding confirmed suspicions of an accumulation disease, but it was not until dialysis reversed the syndrome that this hypothesis could be considered proven. Clinicians can be confident that the immediate, life-threatening aspect of uremia is a toxic state caused by small-molecule accumulation because it is rapidly reversed by HD, a process that does little else than to remove small solutes by diffusion across a semipermeable membrane (therefore, fulfilling Koch's postulates).

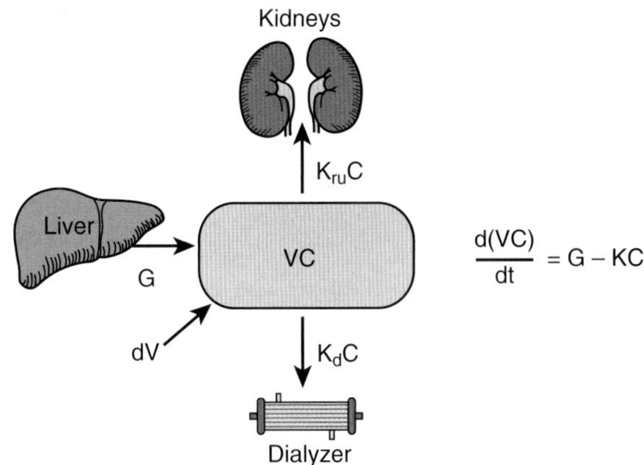


**Fig. 63.20** Single-pool model of urea mass balance in a hemodialysis (HD) patient. When the patient is not undergoing dialysis (most of the time for conventional HD), $K_d$ is 0, and removal is determined solely by $K_{ru}$. V is the urea distribution volume, equated to body water space; C is urea concentration; and dV is the rate of fluid gain (negative during dialysis, positive between dialyses). During HD, total clearance (K) is the sum of $K_d$ and $K_{ru}$. An explicit solution is available to the differential equation that describes the rate of urea accumulation or loss (dVC/dt) as the difference between generation *(G)* and removal *(KC)*.

## MEASURING HEMODIALYSIS ADEQUACY

As noted in the discussion of the general principles of hemodialysis, measuring dialyzable solute levels in the blood as a method for assessing the effectiveness or adequacy of dialysis treatments has been replaced by measuring the clearance of the marker solute urea. Clearance can be measured instantaneously across the dialyzer or as an integrated parameter over time. For native kidney function, the latter is achieved by collecting timed urine specimens. For intermittent HD, collection of dialysate is impractical, so advantage is taken of the perturbations in serum urea concentrations that allow estimation of the urea clearance simply by sampling blood before and after dialysis. The magnitude of the reduction in urea concentrations during each HD session can be translated to a urea clearance much like the decrease in drug levels after a loading dose can be used to measure the drug's clearance. Application of well-established pharmacokinetic principles to urea kinetics provides an estimate of the elimination constant for urea (K/V), which is essentially the slope of the decrease in concentration expressed on a logarithmic scale, as shown in Fig. 63.19. K is the urea clearance and V is the volume of urea distribution, which is the patient's total body water volume. If one incorporates the treatment time element and ignores fluid removal and the generation of urea during dialysis, the log of the ratio of predialysis to postdialysis BUN values can be simply translated to Kt/V (see Fig. 63.19).

Because substantial fluid volume is removed as part of therapeutic HD, and a significant amount of urea is generated, especially during longer treatments, a more formal model of urea mass balance, shown in Fig. 63.20, is required to measure Kt/V accurately. In addition to the change in urea volume and urea generation, this model can be extended to include the interdialysis interval and the effects of residual kidney function (residual kidney urea clearance, $K_{ru}$). The latter, in contrast to the dialyzer clearance, is a continuous clearance that has minimal effect on urea removal during intermittent dialysis but provides a marked benefit between treatments when the dialyzer clearance is zero. In addition,

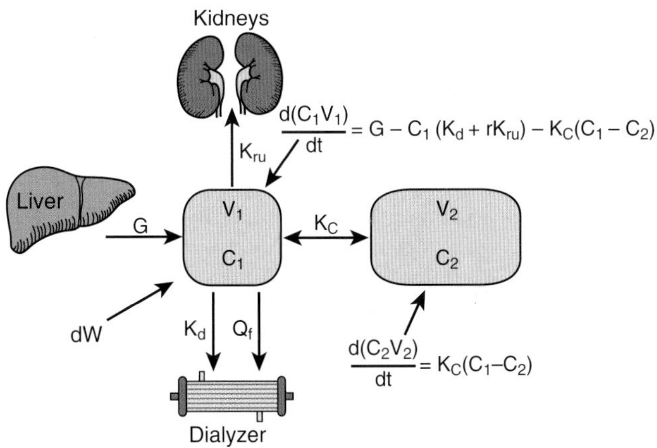


**Fig. 63.21** Double-pool model of urea mass balance in a hemodialysis patient. Addition of a second compartment to the diffusion model of urea mass balance shown in Fig. 63.20 accounts for the postdialysis rebound in urea concentration shown in Fig. 63.16 and, in general, is considered a more accurate model. $K_c$ is the coefficient of mass transfer between compartments, analogous to dialyzer $K_0A$. Solution of the differential equation requires numeric analysis and is not commonly applied in dialysis clinics.

solute sequestration or delayed transport of dialyzed solutes in the patient during dialysis, as discussed before, causes postdialysis rebound (see Fig. 63.17) and can be incorporated in the model if a second compartment is included, as shown in Fig. 63.21. The single-compartment model shown in Fig. 63.20, however, remains the standard for measuring dialysis in most dialysis clinics, primarily because of the complexities of the two-compartment model, which requires numeric analysis to solve, but also because the errors in the single-compartment model caused by ignoring two-compartment effects tend to cancel out.[185] The two models give similar results for Kt/V in the usual clinical range of Kt/V when dialysis is provided three times weekly.[185,375] A two-compartment model with formal numeric analysis is available on the Internet and may become useful for measuring nonstandard dialysis schedules, such as daily or nocturnal dialysis or for more prolonged treatments given three times weekly.[376,377]

## IMPORTANCE OF THE POSTDIALYSIS CONCENTRATION

Accurate measures of predialysis and postdialysis BUN are required to measure the delivered dose of dialysis reliably (see Fig. 63.19). Predialysis sampling of blood is straightforward, but the postdialysis BUN can vary significantly, depending on when it is drawn (see Fig. 63.16), and measurement errors are more significant when the BUN level is low.[378,379] Although it decreases more slowly toward the end of dialysis, the BUN level rebounds rapidly as soon as the blood pump is stopped (see Fig. 63.16). The early rapid phase of upward rebound is determined by both access recirculation and cardiopulmonary recirculation. Efforts should be made to sample after access-related rebound is complete but before cardiopulmonary rebound begins. The Kidney Disease Outcomes Quality Initiative (KDOQI) guidelines recommend slowing the blood pump to 100 mL/min for 15 seconds (to permit access rebound) or stopping the dialysate flow for 3 minutes and then drawing the sample from the dialyzer inflow port.[380] Access recirculation dilutes the postdialysis BUN level, causing a falsely high Kt/V, which can endanger the patient because of inadequate dialysis. Sampling after cardiopulmonary rebound has begun gives a falsely low Kt/V.

## SOLUTE GENERATION

In addition to measuring the dose of dialysis, urea modeling allows the measurement of two patient parameters that independently influence the patient's risk of mortality—urea generation (G) and the patient's volume of urea distribution (V). Accumulation of urea in the patient results from both amino acid catabolism, a measure of protein nutrition, and failure of renal excretion. Although these dual effects on urea concentrations complicate the interpretation of any single measured level, mathematical modeling of urea mass balance allows separation of the two and an estimate of urea distribution volume. Both higher urea generation rates and higher urea volumes have been associated with lower patient mortality.[381,382] For patients dialyzed three times weekly, diurnal variations in urea generation have little effect but, for nocturnal dialysis, the reduction in urea generation at night can cause a significant error, an overestimation of Kt/V and underestimation of V if G is modeled as a constant.[383]

Blood concentrations are the net effect of solute generation and elimination. If one attributes uremic toxicity to the concentrations of accumulated solutes (concentration-dependent toxicity), it might seem logical that the clearance (Kt/V) should sufficiently balance the generation rate to maintain a safe low concentration. However, during the NCDS, attempts to demonstrate this relationship by reducing the dose of dialysis in patients who ate poorly caused an unfortunate vicious cycle of uremia-induced anorexia and malnutrition that eventually led to early discontinuation of the study.[384,385] Similarly, observational studies have shown consistently enhanced survival in patients who eat more, even when Kt/V is held constant, and patients who generate more creatinine have a similar higher rate of survival.[183,386] It appears that the relationship between diet and uremic toxin generation and elimination is complex and poorly understood. Control of solute concentrations by dialysis clearly improves outcomes, but control by limiting dietary intake is often ill-advised. Consuming a vegetarian or high-fiber diet may alter intestinal flora and reduce the generation of gut-derived toxins[387–392]; many of these purported uremic toxins are not removed well with dialysis. Although altering gut microbiome or diet may benefit the patient and reduce the residual syndrome, it does not obviate the importance of assessing what the dialysis treatment is accomplishing in terms of quantification of urea clearance as a surrogate for small, water-soluble toxin removal.

## UREA VOLUME

Urea modeling essentially provides a measure of the urea elimination constant, which can be considered as the fractional rate of urea disappearance during HD (K/V). To calculate K, one must know V or vice versa. Because the prescribed K should be the same as the delivered K, and prescribed K can be determined from Eq. 5, modeled V is easily determined. By convention, V is expressed after dialysis because it is less variable. Comparison of modeled V from dialysis to dialysis can be used as a quality assurance measure, and values should not differ by more than 15%.[185,393] Causes of a discrepancy include access recirculation, dialyzer malfunction (e.g., from clotting or fouling of hollow fibers), blood pump variances, and blood sampling and measurement errors.[394,395]

Several studies have shown that various measures of body size, including V, are associated independently with mortality (Fig. 63.22).[381,382,396,397] Survival rates in larger patients are higher than in smaller patients for reasons that are not entirely clear but may be related to nutrition and the caloric buffer afforded by muscle and fat. Because body size expressed as V is the size-normalizing factor for urea clearance in the Kt/V expression, larger patients require higher clearances and are therefore at higher risk for underdialysis. However, correction for the favorable influence of large size on mortality tends to mitigate this risk, as shown in Fig. 63.23A.[382] Kt/V is a more powerful predictor of mortality than body size, and correction of Kt/V for the independent (and opposing) risk associated with body size renders it an even more powerful predictor of mortality (see Fig. 63.23B).

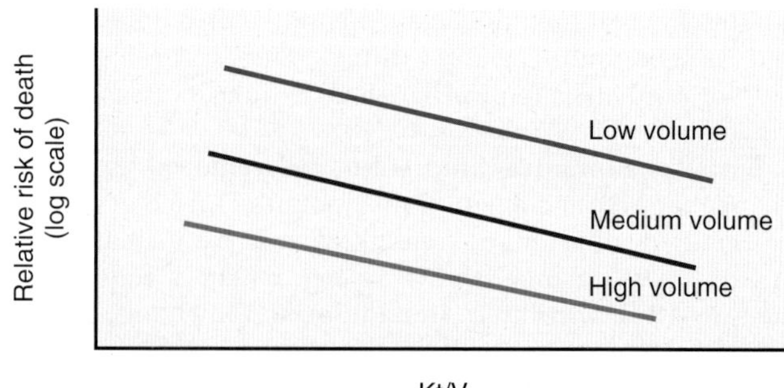


**Fig. 63.22** Risk of death as a function of dialysis dose and body size. The risk of death in hemodialysis patients decreases with increased dialysis dose *(Kt/V)* and may be further stratified by urea volume as a measure of body size. Larger patients, in general, have a lower death risk.

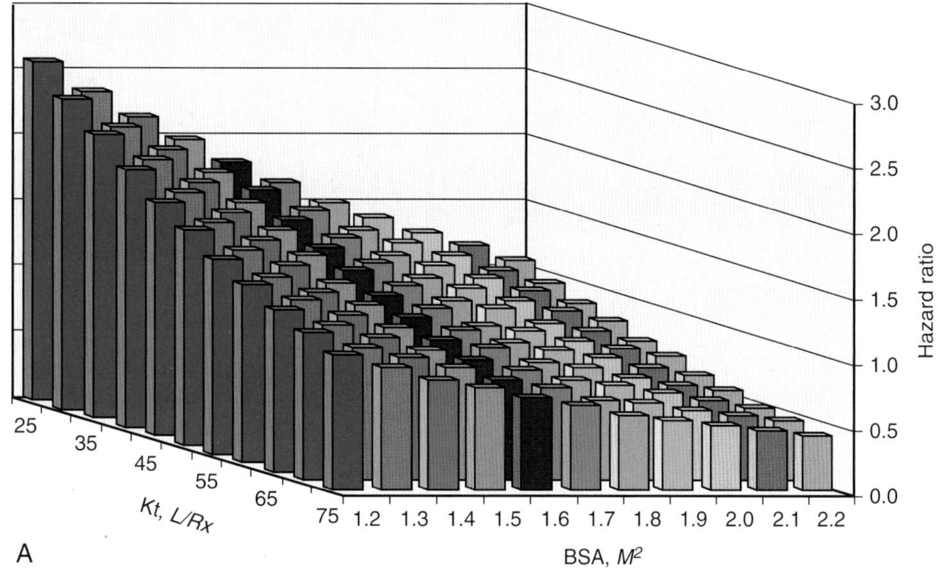


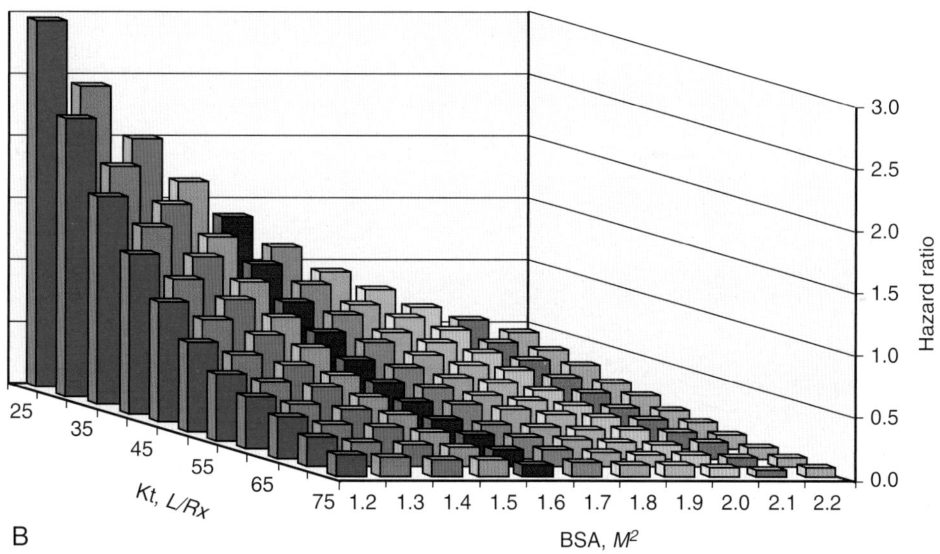


**Fig. 63.23** Risk of mortality related to body size and dialysis dose. These data were obtained from a large observational study of 43,334 patients. (A) Hazard ratio analysis was adjusted for case mix. (B) Hazard ratio analysis included an interaction term between Kt and body mass index and was adjusted for case mix. *BSA,* Body surface area; *L/Rx,* liters per treatment. (From Lowrie EG, Li Z, Ofsthun N, Lazarus JM. Body size, dialysis dose and death risk relationships among hemodialysis patients. *Kidney Int.* 2002;62:1891–1897.)

The HEMO study has uncovered a potentially size-independent effect of sex on the response to higher doses of Kt/V. Although mortality was not affected by administering a higher dialysis dose for the 1846 randomized patients as a whole, when women were analyzed separately, a borderline significant improvement in outcomes was seen at the higher dose.[398] The counterbalancing effect was a nonsignificant higher mortality in men, especially African-American men. However, sex was difficult to separate from size because the two are so closely linked, especially with regard to V. If body surface area is considered to be the more appropriate denominator for dosing dialysis,[399] women, and perhaps smaller men, would clearly require more dialysis than larger men when the dose is measured as Kt/V (Fig. 63.24).[400–403] Similarly, malnourished patients who lose weight have an automatic increase in Kt/V unrelated to the effort of dialysis, but simply because the denominator in the Kt/V expression decreases. This dose increase in patients at higher risk of death may explain the reverse J-shaped relationship between Kt/V and survival in observational studies.[404] Although the latest update of the KDOQI guidelines for dialysis adequacy raises the idea of normalizing Kt by body surface area, use of body weight (V) to normalize dialysis dose still predominates currently.[380]

## TREATMENT TIME

Attempts by patients to shorten their HD treatment times reflect the discomfort they experience toward the end of

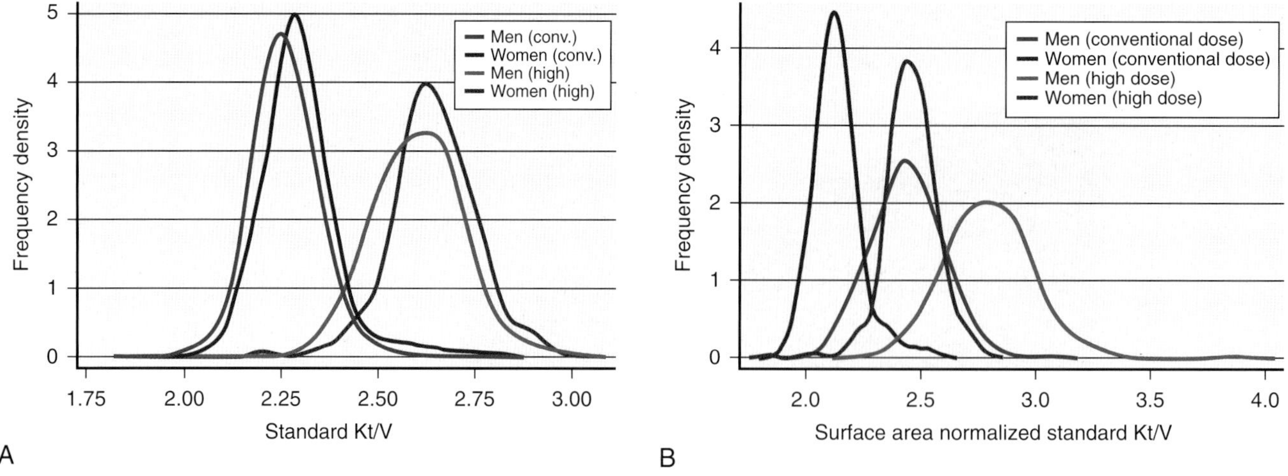


**Fig. 63.24** (A) Standard Kt/V in the conventional and high-dose HEMO study subjects, by gender. (B) Surface area normalized standard Kt/V in the conventional and high-dose HEMO study subjects, by gender. Conversion to surface area was based on an anthropometric estimate of V in each patient.[403,417] *V*, Urea distribution volume. (From Daugirdas JT, Greene T, Chertow GM, Depner TA: Can rescaling dose of dialysis to body surface area in the HEMO study explain the different responses to dose in women versus men? *Clin J Am Soc Nephrol.* 2010;5(9):1628–1636.)

the procedure. Muscle cramps, fatigue, and general malaise increase in intensity as more fluid and solute are removed. Paradoxically, shortening the treatment typically accentuates these symptoms because the rate of removal must increase if the patient is to remain in solute and water balance. Extending treatment time (Td) or increasing the dialysis frequency tends to alleviate these symptoms. Many hours have been spent by nephrologists and dialysis nurses in attempts, often unsuccessful, to convince patients that extending Td would be beneficial. Sometimes a temporary trial of either an extended Td or increased frequency is sufficient to persuade the patient.

Although the NCDS has shown only a borderline significant effect of Td, most population studies have shown that a longer Td is associated with enhanced survival.[405–408] Like the NCDS, the HEMO study failed to show a significant benefit from a longer Td but it also did not specifically target Td, and the range of treatment times in the study was limited.[241] No clinical trials specifically targeting long versus short conventional treatments has been done, but prospective observational studies and clinical experience favor prolonged treatments, including slower ultrafiltration rates.[369,407,409–411]

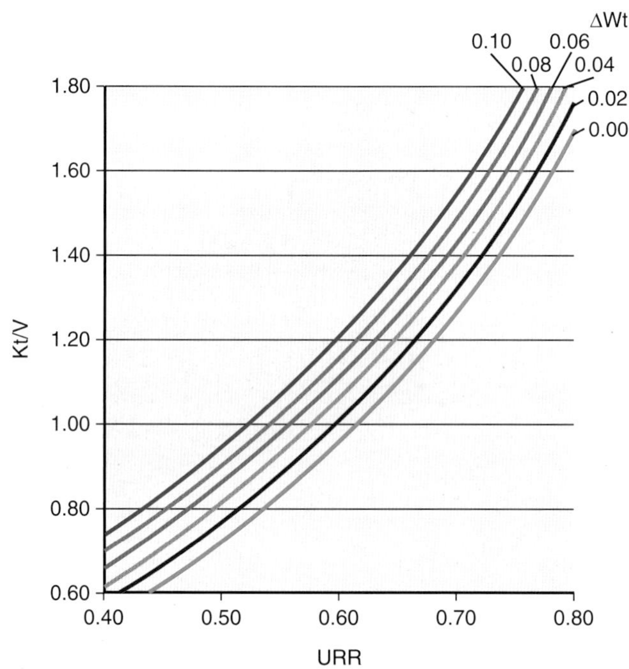


**Fig. 63.25** Curvilinear relationship between urea reduction ratio *(URR)* and Kt/V, stratified by degree of ultrafiltration during dialysis. Whereas the URR (see text) falls with increasing fluid removal during dialysis (ΔWt) from 0% to 10% of body weight, Kt/V increases. The latter more appropriately accounts for the increase in clearance caused by ultrafiltration. Curves are derived from formal urea modeling.

## ALTERNATIVE MEASURES OF DIALYSIS

### UREA REDUCTION RATIO

In the past, the US Centers for Medicare and Medicaid Services required participating dialysis clinics to report the monthly urea reduction ratio (URR), as defined here, for each patient:

$$URR = (C_0 - C)/C_0 \quad [10]$$

where $C_0$ is the predialysis BUN and C the postdialysis BUN level. Currently, Kt/V (using formal kinetic urea modeling or the Daugirdas II equation) is the standard reporting metric.

URR has the advantage of simplicity, but it is the least accurate measure of HD. For example, as the frequency of dialysis increases, and presumably its efficiency improves, URR decreases. It is not possible to add URR values to show a cumulative weekly effect and, as the frequency extends to continuous dialysis, URR extinguishes to zero. URR is also reduced by interdialysis fluid accumulation, urea generation, and residual renal function, and the additional clearance afforded by fluid removal during dialysis is not incorporated in URR. On the positive side, however, in addition to its simplicity, URR has a curvilinear relationship with Kt/V, as shown in Fig. 63.25, paralleling the relationship between outcome and Kt/V. For example, if Kt/V doubles from 1.5 to 3.0/dialysis three times a week, URR increases only from 0.75 to 0.85.

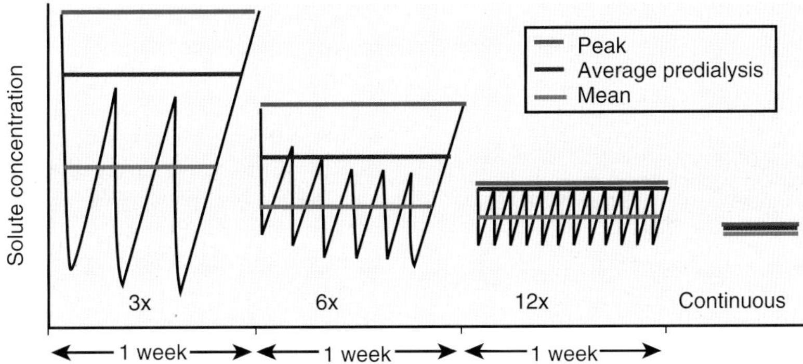


**Fig. 63.26** Effect of frequency on peak and average solute concentrations. Two-compartment formal kinetic modeling of a solute with low $K_c$ predicts that both peak and mean concentrations decrease significantly as the frequency of treatments increases, despite no change in the weekly dialyzer clearance × treatment time (Kt).

Although efforts have been made to convert Kt/V to a URR equivalent[412] or to use the solute removal index, a more reliable index of dialysis dose,[413] these approaches have not been popular. Other efforts to report the reciprocal of Kt/V as a concentration equivalent,[414] targeting low concentrations instead of high clearances, has not been applied, partly because Kt/V has become ingrained in the practice of dialysis quantification. URR is mathematically inexact because it is the ratio of postdialysis to predialysis BUN values (URR = $1 - C_{post}/C_{pre}$) instead of predialysis to postdialysis values. However, it correlates better than Kt/V with small (toxic) solute concentrations, and its relationship with the outcome is more linear.

### CONDUCTIVITY CLEARANCE

The average clearance of small (dialyzable) solutes is easily derived from measurement of the predialysis and postdialysis BUN levels, as explained earlier. The instantaneous clearance of small solutes is also easily measured from the dialyzer inlet and outlet BUN, but it can also be derived by measuring the change in electrical conductivity of dialysate before and after an abrupt change in the dialysate concentration (conductivity clearance).[415,416] Because the major electrically conducting ion in the dialysate is sodium, conductivity clearance is primarily a measure of sodium clearance, which is nearly equivalent to urea clearance. This method requires multiple measurements during dialysis to obtain the treatment average, as well as an adjustment for cardiopulmonary recirculation, but it has the advantage that no blood specimens are required, and the result is available immediately because all measurements are done via the conductivity monitor on the dialysate side of the machine. The clearance is expressed in milliliters per minute and must be adjusted to body size using an estimate of V for comparison with Kt/V or an estimate of surface area.[399,400,417,418] Surface area as a denominator is more consistent with measures of native kidney clearance and may reduce or eliminate the potential gender error discussed previously.[397,401,403]

## COMPARISON OF HEMODIALYSIS AND PERITONEAL DIALYSIS DOSES

The minimum recommended weekly dose of peritoneal dialysis (PD) expressed as Kt/V is 1.7 (see Chapter 64 for discussion of PD adequacy). This dose compares with a cumulative 3.6/week for HD (1.2/dialysis three times weekly). Although the minimum HD dose is more than twice the minimum PD dose, outcomes are similar or better, even when adjusted for the lower average comorbidity in PD patients.[419–421] Furthermore, solute kinetic analyses have shown that the dialysis efficiency improves with increased frequency of treatments (Fig. 63.26). These observations, together with acknowledgment of little or no benefit from more intense or more prolonged intermittent dialysis[241] have led to the conclusion that intermittent treatments are less efficient than continuous treatments and have stimulated efforts to define a continuous equivalent clearance expression for HD.

## STANDARD CLEARANCE AND STANDARD KT/V

These efforts have produced a continuous equivalent expression for urea clearance as G/TAC,[185,422] where TAC is the time-averaged urea concentration and a more profound adjustment defined as "standard K" and "standard Kt/V."[413,423] The latter redefines clearance as the removal rate factored for the predialysis concentration, placing more emphasis on the predialysis BUN level as a risk factor for uremia. Because the predialysis BUN level is always higher than the mean BUN, the standard Kt/V is always lower than the continuous urea clearance and is comparable to fractional clearances achieved with continuous PD. Despite its somewhat arbitrary definition, the matching of doses with PD has generated interest in standard Kt/V (stdKt/V) as an expression of dialysis dose that is independent of frequency. Increasing interest in clinical applications of HD given more frequently than three times/week has generated a need for quantification that accounts for the improved efficiency of more frequent treatments. For patients in a steady state of urea, mass balance in which generation equals removal and dialyzed according to any schedule of treatments, stdKt/V is defined as follows:

$$\begin{aligned} \text{stdKt/V} &= (\text{urea removal rate})/(\text{peak concentration}) \\ &= \text{G}/(\text{average predialysis BUN}) \end{aligned} \quad [11]$$

where G is the patient's urea generation rate derived from formal urea modeling. KDOQI guidelines call for a minimum stdKt/V of 2.0/week, significantly higher than the minimum PD dose but considered safe in the absence of controlled

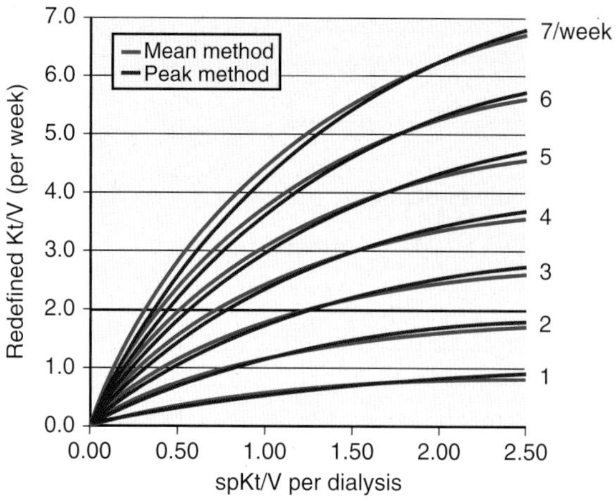


**Fig. 63.27** Effect of increased dose versus increased frequency on effective clearance. The effective clearance, expressed as "standard Kt/V" on the vertical axis, tends to plateau, despite increases in dialyzer clearance, expressed as single-pool Kt/V (spKt/V) on the horizontal axis. Two different models of solute kinetics show similar diminishing returns as the delivered dose increases. A marked increase in effective clearance can be achieved only by increasing the frequency of treatments.

trials of dialysis frequency.[181] An explicit mathematical formula for calculating standard Kt/V based on spKt/V[424] has greatly simplified the calculation, and subsequent refinements have allowed inclusion of the effects of ultrafiltration during dialysis and the patient's residual native kidney clearance[425]:

$$\text{stdKt/V} = \frac{10080([1 - e^{-\text{eKt/V}}]/t)}{([1 - e^{-\text{eKt/V}}]/\text{eKtV}] + [10080/\text{Nt}] - 1)} \qquad [12]$$

where Nt is the number of dialysis treatments per week.

Because urea is relatively nontoxic, peak levels probably do not mediate uremic toxicity, so an alternative explanation for the inefficiency of infrequent HD was developed based on the sequestration of compartmentalized solutes other than urea. A two-compartment model that accounts for sequestration gives a pattern of average clearances that closely match stdKt/V values,[426] as shown in Fig. 63.27, providing further theoretic support for the clinical application of stdKt/V in recipients of frequent dialysis.

## NOCTURNAL HEMODIALYSIS AND HOME HEMODIALYSIS

An alternative to thrice-weekly, in-center HD is nocturnal dialysis. As the term implies, dialysis is performed during the night, usually while the patient sleeps. Nocturnal dialysis can be performed in-center, three times weekly, with the major advantage of increased dialysis treatment duration of 6 to 8 hours. Observational studies have found regression of left ventricular mass, better bone mineral indices, and improved quality of life with this approach to HD.[427,428]

Home HD, which can be applied during the waking hours for 2 to 4 hours a treatment, five or six times weekly, provides more frequent HD treatments while controlling costs and patient burden.[429–433] Nocturnal home HD is a variant of this, with longer treatment times and perhaps only three or four treatments/week. The advantage of more frequent and/or longer treatments includes patient freedom during the day to conduct normal life activities unfettered by dialysis and associated symptoms. Several studies have shown improvements in blood pressure, nutrition, stamina, and health-related quality of life, which are presumably responsible for patient acceptance of a procedure that requires considerably more patient effort and time than standard in-center HD.[430,434,435] Controlled trials have confirmed improvements in left ventricular mass, blood pressure, need for phosphate binders, and some aspects of quality of life.[434,436–438] However, recruitment of patients for home training was difficult, more vascular access interventions were required, and the nocturnal group of patients in one study experienced a more rapid decline in residual kidney function.[431,437–439] Observational studies have reported similar patient and treatment survival rates, regardless of the home modality.[440]

## SHORT DAILY HEMODIALYSIS

The incentive to shorten the Td is often patient-generated, as noted but, when combined with an increase in frequency, outcomes might be improved, as suggested in Fig. 63.27. Controlled studies of short daily dialysis have shown improvements in cardiac hypertrophy, health-related quality of life, and cardiac function.[434,436,437] All studies of short daily dialysis have shown decreases in interdialysis weight gain and predialysis blood pressure, but such changes are to be expected when the interdialytic interval is shortened to nearly half that of thrice-weekly dialysis. The NIH-sponsored daily in-center HD study, the largest randomized and controlled trial to date, has shown a reduction in left ventricular mass, an improvement in self-reported physical health, a reduction in predialysis serum phosphate concentration, and a reduction in predialysis systolic blood pressure relative to conventional thrice-weekly dialysis.[437] However, the trial was unable to demonstrate improvements in survival, hospitalization rates, predialysis serum albumin level (a marker of nutrition and inflammation), or a reduction in the dose of erythropoiesis-stimulating agents required to control anemia.

## ACCOUNTING FOR NATIVE KIDNEY FUNCTION

Clearance of small solutes, the principal metric of dialyzer function, is augmented by clearance of the same solutes by the patient's remnant native kidney. Addition of the two urea clearances ($K_d$ and $K_{ru}$) seems reasonable except for intermittently dialyzed patients in whom the two clearances do not occur simultaneously. Because, as noted previously, continuous clearances are more efficient than intermittent clearances, an adjustment is required before the two clearances can be summed. This adjustment consists either of inflating $K_{ru}$ or deflating $K_d$. As noted previously, conversion to stdKt/V effectively deflates $K_d$ to the equivalent of a continuous clearance, allowing simple addition. For example, if the patient's stdKt/V determined by Eq. 12 is 2.2/week, the native kidney urea clearance is 4 mL/min, and the patient's urea volume is 35 L, the two can be added to yield a continuous urea clearance:

$$\begin{aligned} &2.2/\text{week} \times (35{,}000 \text{ mL}/10{,}080 \text{ min/week}) + 4 \text{ mL/min} \\ &= 11.6 \text{ mL/min} \end{aligned} \qquad [13]$$

or

$$4\ \text{mL/min} \times (10{,}080\ \text{min/week}/35{,}000\ \text{mL}) + 2.2/\text{week} = 3.4\ \text{weekly stdKt/V} \quad [14]$$

If the dialyzer stdKt/V is determined by formal urea modeling, care must be taken to avoid inappropriate deflation of $K_{ru}$ when calculating stdKt/V from the predialysis and postdialysis BUN values.[425] Alternatively, $K_{ru}$ can be inflated to add to $K_d$ as originally described by Gotch and associates[440a] and later outlined in the KDOQI guidelines.[181]

Residual kidney function confers a survival advantage far in excess of that associated with the dialyzer's urea clearance.[440b] Despite near-complete destruction by the patient's disease, the native kidney continues to eliminate by secretion solutes that are eliminated poorly, if at all, by dialysis, helps maintain salt and water balance, and may supply synthetic functions.[178,440c,440d] Recent studies have suggested that residual kidney function may last longer than realized, prescribing HD to complement the amount of $K_{ru}$ may slow its decline,[440e] and incorporation of $K_{ru}$ in the prescription of dialysis is underused in many incident HD patients.[440f] Preservation of $K_{ru}$ is therefore an important goal of kidney replacement therapy.

**Box 63.1 Components of the Dialysis Prescription**

- Duration
- Frequency
- Vascular access
- Dialyzer (membrane, configuration, surface area, sterilization method)
- Blood flow rate
- Dialysate flow rate
- Ultrafiltration rate
- Dialysate composition (see Table 63.7)
- Anticoagulation
- Dialysate temperature
- Intradialytic medications

## THE DIALYSIS PRESCRIPTION

### GOALS OF HEMODIALYSIS

The goal of HD is to replace the kidneys' excretory function. To accomplish this goal, blood and dialysate are circulated in opposite directions (countercurrent) on opposite sides of a semipermeable membrane in the dialyzer (see Fig. 63.12), allowing unwanted solutes such as potassium, urea, and phosphorus to diffuse from the blood into the dialysate and permitting addition of solutes such as bicarbonate and calcium from the dialysate into blood. The concentrations of the solutes added to the dialysate mirror those normally maintained in the body by the native kidneys (see Table 63.6). An additional goal is the elimination of excess volume via ultrafiltration, accomplished by controlling the hydrostatic pressure gradient across the semipermeable membrane (see "Dialysate Circuit").

The rate of accumulation of solutes and fluid in each patient varies and depends on his or her nutritional and metabolic status and adherence to dietary restrictions. Thus, the HD prescription must be individualized to achieve these goals for each patient. The separate components of the HD prescription that may be individualized after clinical assessment are listed in Box 63.1.

### HEMODIALYSIS SESSION LENGTH AND FREQUENCY

The clearance of any solute, such as urea, can be increased by lengthening the session length or increasing its frequency. After optimizing blood and dialysate flows and selecting a dialyzer with a large mass transfer coefficient, the time during which the patient receives dialysis can be lengthened to augment solute clearance. However, because diffusive solute clearance depends on solute concentration on the blood side, the efficiency of solute removal declines over the course of the dialysis procedure, leading to diminishing returns for total solute removal, as suggested by urea concentrations with dialysis treatments longer than 4 to 5 hours (see "Hemodialysis Adequacy"). Conversely, reducing session length below 3 hours accentuates the effects of intermittence, exacerbates solute disequilibrium (see "Dialyzer Clearance Versus Whole-Body Clearance" and Fig. 63.18), reduces the clearance of larger molecules such as beta-2 microglobulin, for which removal is more time-dependent, increases the ultrafiltration (UF) rate, and increases the potential for hypotension and myocardial stunning.[12,211,212,441–446] Providing HD more frequently lessens the impact of declining solute concentrations and improves clearance but incurs added expense, resources, vascular access dysfunction, and potentially patient and caregiver burnout.[12,32,441,442,445–449]

Additional benefits of longer or more frequent HD sessions include optimal volume homeostasis and enhanced removal of high-molecular-weight, sequestered, or protein-bound solutes (see "Hemodialysis Adequacy").[32,441,442,448,450–456] Longer or more frequent HD allows the accumulated fluid to be removed over a longer period of time and may reduce intradialytic symptoms such as nausea, vomiting, cramping, and hypotension (see "Complications for Patients on Maintenance Hemodialysis"), decrease postdialysis fatigue, improve blood pressure control, and ameliorate myocardial stunning.[436–438,457,458] Sequestered solutes such as phosphate have more time to equilibrate among the various volume compartments, leading to improved total removal and lower serum concentrations. More frequent HD also may mitigate the higher cardiovascular morbidity and mortality rate observed at the end of the long interdialytic interval in patients receiving conventional thrice weekly dialysis.[451,458–461] The Frequent Hemodialysis Network (FHN) Daily Trial, the largest randomized controlled study to compare thrice-weekly, in-center HD with 6 days/week, in-center HD, has confirmed that more frequent HD improves blood pressure and phosphate control, decreases left ventricular mass and left ventricular end-diastolic volume, and results in favorable effects on the composite endpoints of death or change in left ventricular mass and death or change in self-reported physical health.[437,457] However, more frequent HD did not significantly improve several tests of cognitive function, measures of depressive symptoms, serum albumin level, or utilization of ESAs. The FHN and Canadian studies comparing frequent nocturnal HD with thrice-weekly HD, hampered by the small number of trial participants, only demonstrated beneficial effects on blood pressure and phosphate control and possibly left ventricular mass.[436,438] Because of the increased burden and cost of longer or more frequent HD sessions, along with concerns regarding the adverse effects of more frequent HD on the provision of vascular accesses procedures and (in the smaller, nocturnal trial) on residual kidney function,[439,447,449] more frequent HD has not been routinely adopted. The current conventional practice in the United States is to prescribe HD three times/week for 3 to 4 hours each session.[441] Longer duration or more frequent dialysis is often used for larger patients, patients with severe hypertension not responding to maximal antihypertensive treatment, or those with volume overload and intradialytic hypotension preventing fluid removal. Current session lengths average about 3.5 hours in the United States, about 3.25 hours for women and 3.75 hours for men on average, depending on body size. Prolonging session length and/or including one additional session of HD or UF to avoid the long interdialytic interval can help patients who are struggling to maintain their health and well-being on a conventional thrice-weekly HD schedule, possibly mitigating risks that might develop with daily or near-daily (five or six times weekly) therapy.[441,442,449]

## DIALYZER CHOICE

In choosing a dialyzer, the most critical determinants are as follows: (1) its capacity for solute clearance; (2) its capacity for fluid removal; and (3) the potential of the dialyzer membrane to interact with components of the blood or the degree of biocompatibility.[209] The ideal hemodialyzer membrane would have high clearance of low-molecular-weight and mid-molecular-weight uremic toxins, adequate UF, high biocompatibility, and low blood volume compartment to maximize the efficiency of and reduce the adverse metabolic and hemodynamic effects from the HD procedure.

Urea is the solute most often used to evaluate dialyzer solute clearance characteristics because of its relevance to kinetic models of dialysis adequacy (see earlier). In clinical practice, physicians rely on industry-derived determinations of in vitro dialyzer clearance of low-molecular-weight and mid-molecular-weight solutes. Gibbs-Donnan effects, membrane adsorption of solute, protein binding of solute, and solute aggregation are not taken into account in determining in vitro dialyzer clearances and will reduce in vivo clearances. The variable relation between the diffusive and convective clearance of a solute further complicates the determination of solute clearance of different dialyzers. Solutes larger than 300 Da have lower diffusive clearance than smaller solutes such as urea and potassium and may rely primarily on convective clearance. For patients with large interdialytic weight gains requiring more UF during each dialysis session, simple comparisons of the in vitro diffusive solute clearances may be misleading.

Another factor in the selection of a hemodialyzer is its UF coefficient, which describes the capacity of a dialyzer to remove fluid (in units of mL/min/mm Hg). As with solute clearances, the manufacturer performs in vitro tests to determine the UF coefficient of each dialyzer model. In vivo values may vary by as much as 10% to 20%.

As already discussed, dialyzer membranes vary in their capacity to activate the coagulation cascade and formed blood elements, with synthetic membranes, in general, being the most inert and hence the most biocompatible,[210,213–216] but even synthetic membranes vary in the degree of biocompatibility.[217,462,463] In addition to the issues of biocompatibility and cytokine release, activated thrombin is adsorbed on the dialyzer membrane, creating a nidus for platelet adhesion and further thrombin deposition.[464] The propensity of a dialyzer for thrombogenesis may be another important factor in selecting a dialyzer, especially when anticoagulation during dialysis is not feasible. It is unclear whether dialyzers bonded with heparin will reduce the incidence of thrombosis during heparin-free dialysis. A randomized crossover study has suggested that such dialyzers are superior to both saline flushes and infusion in preventing intradialytic thrombosis,[465] whereas others have found comparable thrombotic rates with the use of saline flushes or a polysulfone memebrane.[466,467]

An additional consideration in hemodialyzer selection is whether it will be reused for subsequent dialysis sessions because the chemicals used in reprocessing dialyzers may damage some of the membranes.[207] Bleach, which is commonly used to strip protein off the membrane and improve the appearance of the dialyzer, may increase the pore size of some synthetic membranes after repeated use. This results in the loss of plasma proteins during each dialysis session, rivaling that seen in nephrotic patients. Heat disinfection may result in cracks in the headers of the dialyzers.

## BLOOD AND DIALYSATE FLOW RATES

Configuring the dialysate flow countercurrent to blood flow maximizes the concentration gradient between the two throughout the length of the dialyzer (see Fig. 63.12A and Table 63.5). When flows are in the same direction (cocurrent), small solute clearance decreases by about 10%. Increasing the dialysate flow ($Q_d$) reduces the accumulation of waste products in the dialysate and provides a higher solute gradient between blood and dialysate for optimal diffusion. Higher $Q_d$ also decreases boundary layers and streaming effects in the dialysate. Dialysate flowing along the membrane tends to adhere to it to create an unstirred layer, or boundary layer, which reduces the rate of diffusion across the membrane.[214,468] Dialysate also tends to move along the path of least resistance or channel (streaming effect), resulting in nonuniform flow and bypassing some of the membrane area. As dialysate flow increases or turbulence is produced at the membrane surface, the unstirred layer becomes thinner, channeling is minimized,[469] and $K_0A$ increases,[470] although the effect is less in vivo than in vitro.[471,472] These findings prompted an increase in $Q_d$ from 500 to 800 mL/min when the dialyzer blood flow rate ($Q_b$) was prescribed at 350 to 500 mL/min. Advances in hemodialyzer technology have led to modification of the hollow fiber shape and insertion of inert spacer yarns, reducing channeling and unstirred layers and further improving dialyzer performance.[205,473] With these new dialyzers, increasing $Q_d$ above 600 mL/min has yielded minimal increases in urea, phosphate, and beta-2 microglobulin clearance,[474,475] but may still have a significant impact on the clearance of protein-bound solutes.[476,477]

Dialyzer blood flow ($Q_b$) is driven by a roller pump and usually ranges from 200 to 500 mL/min, depending on the type of vascular access. Blood flow influences the efficiency of solute removal (see Table 63.5). As $Q_b$ increases, more solute is presented per minute to the membrane, and solute removal increases. Urea removal increases steeply as $Q_b$ increases to 300 mL/min, but the rate of increase is less steep as $Q_b$ approaches 400 to 500 mL/min because of increased resistance to and turbulence of flow within the hollow fibers, resulting in nonlinear flow and reduced clearance. Unlike dialysate, the boundary layer and streaming effects are less prominent on the blood side of hollow fibers because of the geometric advantages of flow in hollow fibers, the scrubbing effects of RBCs, and less variance in $Q_b$. For larger molecules, sequestered solutes and protein-bound solutes, removal is slower and more time-dependent rather than flow-dependent because of limited diffusion across the membrane and protein binding, as discussed previously.[440d,441,442,454–456]

## ANTICOAGULATION

Blood clotting during dialysis results in patient blood loss and reduces solute clearance through decreasing the dialyzer surface area.[479,480] To prevent clotting, an anticoagulant is usually delivered into the blood circuit before the dialyzer via a peristaltic pump or syringe pump.

Heparin, the most commonly used anticoagulant, may be given as a bolus at the start of dialysis (fixed dose 1000–5000 U or weight-based dose 50-U/kg bolus) followed by a continuous infusion (1000–1500 U/hr) until 15 to 60 minutes before the end of dialysis or as intermittent boluses as needed during dialysis.[479–483] Disadvantages of the bolus method include an increase in nursing time and episodic over- and underanticoagulation. In patients at risk of bleeding (Table 63.8), low-dose heparin (500–1000 U bolus followed by 500–750 U/hr), regional anticoagulation, dialyzers coated with heparin, or no anticoagulation may be appropriate.[479,482,483]

In regional anticoagulation, the anticoagulant is infused into the blood circuit (arterial line) before the hemodialyzer, followed by infusion of a neutralizing agent into the venous line (after the dialyzer). Regional citrate anticoagulation, a common strategy in the acute dialysis setting, uses citrate as the anticoagulant and calcium as the neutralizing agent, with the dialysate being calcium-free.[482–485] Citrate binds calcium in the blood, an important cofactor in the coagulation cascade, thereby inhibiting clotting in the dialyzer. Infusion of calcium after the dialyzer restores the ability of blood to clot. Regional anticoagulation also may be accomplished with heparin as the anticoagulant and protamine as the reversing agent.[486,487] Both methods are labor-intensive and prone to error in inexperienced hands, requiring frequent monitoring of ionized calcium or partial thromboplastin time, respectively, when using the citrate-calcium or heparin-protamine combination. Citrate anticoagulation also may result in hypocalcemia if calcium replacement is inadequate and metabolic alkalosis as citrate is metabolized.[483–485] However, in intermittent short-duration HD, metabolic alkalosis may not be an issue.[484] Rebound in anticoagulation may be seen after the completion of dialysis with regional heparinization because heparin has a longer half-life than protamine. Because of the close monitoring required and the risk of serious complications, regional anticoagulation is not commonly used in the outpatient dialysis setting and is used more in the intensive care unit for continuous renal replacement therapy. However, if a simplified treatment protocol can be perfected, regional citrate anticoagulation may become more feasible and desirable in the outpatient setting because citrate may reduce inflammation, lower bleeding risk, and improve clearance from less dialyzer clotting when compared with heparin.[485,486,489–492] Currently, low-dose heparin and anticoagulation-free HD remain more commonly used strategies in outpatients.

During anticoagulation-free dialysis, several strategies may help prevent clotting, such as the following: (1) rinse the circuit before dialysis with heparinized saline; (2) use a less thrombogenic dialyzer; (3) flush the circuit with 100 to 200 mL of 0.9% sodium chloride every 30 minutes during dialysis; (4) avoid blood or platelet transfusions through the circuit; (5) maintain a high blood flow rate to decrease sludging of blood in the hollow fibers; and (6) limit UF as feasible because hemoconcentration in the hollow fibers increases thrombotic risk. In a patient with a hypercoagulable state or the situation in which higher blood flow rates and limited UF are not possible, these measures are unlikely to prevent clotting. Remaining options, then, are regional citrate anticoagulation or the use of heparin-coated dialyzers,[483,493] although heparin-coated dialyzers may be inferior to citrate in reducing dialyzer clotting.[467,493]

Alternative anticoagulants include low-molecular-weight heparin (LMWH), hirudin, prostacyclin, dermatan sulfate, and argatroban.[480–483,494–501] Of these, LMWH is more widely used in Europe,[483,496–498] but the complexity of use, expense, lack of sufficient experience, and equivalency to heparin have deterred the widespread use of the other anticoagulants. For the rare patient with confirmed heparin-induced thrombocytopenia, lepirudin, bivalirudin, argatroban, and citrate anticoagulation are viable alternatives.[483,501–503] Finally, substituting citric acid for acetic acid in the dialysate may augment the effect of heparin use, improve clearance, and increase dialyzer reuse, presumably because of decreased clotting, but may increase cramps and hypotension.[504–507]

**Table 63.8 Guidelines for Anticoagulation in Hemodialysis Patients at High Risk for Serious Bleeding**

| Anticoagulation for Hemodialysis | Clinical Condition |
|---|---|
| No anticoagulation or regional anticoagulation | Actively bleeding<br>Significant risk for bleeding<br>Major thrombostatic defect<br>Major surgery within 7 days<br>Intracranial surgery within 14 days<br>Biopsy of visceral organ within 72 hours<br>Pericarditis |
| Low-dose heparin | Major surgery beyond 7 days<br>Biopsy of visceral organ beyond 72 hours<br>Minor surgery 8 hours prior<br>Minor surgery within 72 hours |
| Low-dose heparin or no anticoagulation | Major surgery 8 hours prior |

## DIALYSATE COMPOSITION

The composition of dialysate is crucial to attaining the desired blood purification and to achieving body fluid and electrolyte homeostasis.[508–511] To reach these endpoints, dialysate contains the solutes listed in Box 63.1 in concentrations comparable to those of plasma. Addition of electrolytes and glucose to the dialysate reduces or eliminates their concentration gradients and prevents excessive removal during dialysis. Potassium is nearly always individualized; sodium, calcium, and bicarbonate concentrations may also be individualized, although they may be standardized for most patients in a facility where centralized dialysate production and distribution are used (see Table 63.7). Because the dialysate glucose concentration is comparable to plasma, osmotic forces do not drive fluid removal, unlike PD.

### SODIUM

Because sodium is the major determinant of tonicity of extracellular fluids, the dialysate sodium concentration influences cardiovascular stability during HD. Historically, the dialysate sodium concentration was kept lower than blood sodium concentration (130–135 mEq/L) to facilitate diffusive sodium loss during dialysis and prevent interdialytic hypertension, exaggerated thirst, and excessive interdialytic weight gain.[297–299] However, with the advent of high-flux dialyzers and more efficient solute removal, headaches, nausea, vomiting, seizures, hypotension, and cramps became more common and were attributed to the hyponatric dialysate[297–299,310,508] but were more likely caused by the use of acetate as a source of base (see later). This development prompted the progressive increase in dialysate sodium concentration—first to that of plasma and subsequently to higher than plasma—with an improvement in symptoms.[297–299,310,508] The pendulum now has swung back, with some, but not all studies, demonstrating that a high-sodium dialysate leads to thirst with polydipsia, increased weight gains, and hypertension, leading to a resurgent interest in reducing dialysate sodium concentrations and abandoning the use of sodium modeling or "ramping" (see previously) in most patients. [297–299,301,302,306,313,508,512,513]

However, some studies have suggested that the use of a high-sodium dialysate may reduce mortality in a subset of patients whose predialysis serum levels are low.[301,302] The ongoing debate and uncertainty regarding the optimal dialysate sodium concentration are due to multiple confounding factors, such as lack of randomized and controlled studies, inaccuracy of dialysate sodium delivery compared with prescribed, differences in dietary sodium intake and urinary sodium excretion, varying tissue sodium stores, which affect vascular stiffness, and disparate predialysis plasma osmolarity not due to blood sodium concentrations that results in hypotension during dialysis as the osmolarity decreases.[297–299,307–310,514] The conflicting data have suggested that one size does not fit all, leading to a growing interest for an individualized approach. Although a computer-controlled biofeedback system using conductivity to lower the plasma sodium level to 135 mEq/L may offer the added benefits of decreased extracellular water, improved blood pressure control, and lower interdialytic weight gains without sacrificing hemodynamic stability, these methods add complexity and/or increase demand on staff time.[297–300,310,513,515] A reasonable alternative may be to apply a constant dialysate sodium of 136 to 138 mEq/L empirically or align the dialysate sodium with the average predialysis serum sodium concentration to achieve the same ends, because many dialysis patients tend to be hyponatremic.[297–299,305,515]

### POTASSIUM

Unlike sodium, only 2% of the 3000 to 3500 mEq of potassium is distributed in the extracellular space. Although colonic elimination of potassium increases threefold in patients with ESKD and accounts for about 30% of dietary intake,[511] the remaining potassium accumulates in between dialysis treatments and can become life-threatening. By using a dialysate potassium concentration lower than that of plasma, excess potassium is removed during dialysis, mainly through diffusion down its concentration gradient.[269,508,510,515,516] However, potassium flux from the intracellular to extracellular compartment is usually slower than the efflux of potassium into the dialysate, and use of a high dialysate bicarbonate concentration and/or creating a large bicarbonate gradient during HD may enhance potassium shift into the intracellular compartment, potentially creating significant intradialytic hypokalemia; this is followed by a 30% rebound in the potassium concentration 3 to 4 hours after completion of dialysis.[511,516–518] Life-threatening levels of hypokalemia typically occur during the first 2 hours of dialysis, when a high predialysis potassium level favors efficient removal and a precipitous decline in its concentration, leading to arrhythmias through hyperpolarization of cardiac membrane potential, QT prolongation, and increase in ventricular late potentials.[508,510,511,516,518]

Minimizing the risk for intradialytic hypokalemia and postdialysis rebound is made even more complex by the highly variable efficiency of potassium removal among patients (≤70% variability) and between treatments for each patient (≤20%), despite an identical dialysis prescription.[519] The intracellular distribution of potassium leads to a variable volume of distribution such that the greater the total body potassium content, the lower the volume of distribution and the higher the fractional decline in potassium concentration during dialysis. During dialysis, amelioration of acidosis, stimulation of insulin release by dialysate glucose, release of catecholamines in response to hemodynamic events, and decline of plasma tonicity all favor the shift of potassium into cells, thus reducing the gradient for its removal.[508,510,511,516,518] The degree to which each of these factors is present varies considerably among patients.

Several large epidemiologic studies have sought to clarify the risks associated with varying dialysate potassium concentrations.[461,520–522] The optimal predialysis serum potassium level appears to be 4.6 to 5.3 mEq/L,[521] with poor nutritional status contributing to death at lower potassium levels and fatal arrhythmias at predialysis potassium levels higher than 5.6 to 6 mEq/L. Dialyzing against a dialysate potassium concentration lower than 2 or 3 mEq/L appears to increase the risk for sudden death, especially in patients with a predialysis potassium level less than 5 mEq/L.[461,522] A more recent DOPPS study did not find a difference in risk for sudden death between dialysate potassium concentrations of 2 mEq/L versus 3 mEq/L and was unable to interpret data for dialysate potassium lower than 2 mEq/L because of the small number of patients in this category, likely reflecting changes in practice since the previous studies.[520] Although some studies have suggested a survival benefit in hyperkalemic patients dialyzed against a low-potassium dialysate,[461,521] other studies have found no difference in survival, even in patients with predialysis serum potassium levels higher than 6.5 mEq/L.[520,522] In addition, lower dialysate potassium concentrations seem to have little effect on predialysis serum potassium, given the 2- to 3-day interval in between dialysis.[520] Individualizing the dialysate potassium concentration, depending on the unique situation of each patient, may be crucial in navigating between increased mortality from predialysis hyperkalemia and sudden death from hypokalemia during and after each dialysis session.[510,511,516]

The prescribed dialysate potassium concentration is guided by the serum concentration before dialysis and the previous considerations.[510,511,516,518] Because of the increased incidence of sudden death during and after dialysis, presumably due to a rapid decline in serum potassium levels, dialysate potassium concentration of 0 mEq/L should be abandoned. Most patients should dialyze against a dialysate potassium of 2 to 3 mEq/L. Patients with increased total body potassium from diet, medications, hemolysis, tissue breakdown, catabolism, or gastrointestinal bleeding may require a lower dialysate potassium concentration. However, concentrations of 1 mEq/L should be used only when a compelling reason exists because of the higher risk for arrhythmias and death and only after exhausting all efforts targeting dietary potassium restriction and discontinuing medications that interfere with aldosterone production and gastrointestinal elimination of potassium (e.g., ACE inhibitor, angiotensin receptor blocker [ARB], aldosterone antagonist). In particular, patients on digoxin must dialyze against a dialysate potassium level of at least 2 mEq/L because of the greater propensity for digoxin toxicity and death with predialysis potassium levels less than 4.3 mEq/L[523] and intradialytic hypokalemia. Potassium modeling, with a gradual stepdown in dialysate potassium concentration, thus keeping the blood to dialysate potassium gradient constant, during each dialysis session may optimize potassium removal and minimize the risk for arrhythmias.[508,510,511,516,524] However, experience with and data for this approach are scant and consist of small studies using electrocardiography to detect repolarization abnormalities (e.g., prolonged QT interval or QT dispersion) as surrogate markers for sudden death. The validity of these tools as surrogate markers has been questioned in the cardiology literature.[525,526] Randomized trials are needed to inform this dilemma.

The use of oral sodium polystyrene sulfonate to control hyperkalemia remains controversial, although data from DOPPS have suggested that it may be safe and effective, associated only with increased IDWG and higher serum bicarbonate and phosphorus levels.[527] New oral agents to control hyperkalemia—patiromer and sodium zirconium cyclosilicate—are now available and may help solve the potassium conundrum.[528,529]

## CALCIUM

Historically, patients with ESKD were dialyzed against a higher calcium (Ca) concentration (3–3.5 mEq/L [1.5–1.75 mmol/L]) to help control hyperparathyroidism and prevent Ca and subsequent bone mineral loss.[510,511] However, increased use of Ca-containing phosphate binders and vitamin D analogs has led to more frequent hypercalcemia and concern for accelerated vascular calcification in HD patients, prompting the KDOQI committee to recommend reducing the dialysate Ca concentration to 2.5 mEq/L (1.25 mmol/L).[530] In contrast, international guidelines have recommended a concentration of 2.5 to 3 mEq/L (1.25–1.5 mmol/L).[530] The differing opinions reflect limited understanding of Ca mass balance in patients undergoing dialysis.[510,511,530–532] Data from retrospective and small randomized studies have suggested that 2.5 mEq/L is the fulcrum for dialysate Ca, below which Ca is removed from the patient and above which Ca diffuses into the patient during dialysis, although there is wide variability among patients.[510,511,531,532] Patients whose dialysate Ca concentration was reduced from 3 to 3.5 mEq/L to 2.5 mEq/L or lower had lower serum Ca and higher parathyroid hormone concentrations, correction of low bone turnover (adynamic bone disease), and improvement in vascular calcification, although other studies have reported unchanged or worsening vascular calcification with lower dialysate Ca concentration.[532–540] Vascular calcification was assessed variably with measures of aortic calcification, coronary artery calcification, arterial stiffness, carotid intimal media thickness, and carotid femoral pulse wave pressures. None of the studies addressed interdialytic Ca mass balance, which may be variable, given the selection of available phosphorus binders, vitamin D analogues, and calcimimetic agents, and its contribution to vascular calcification.

Dialysate Ca concentration may also affect hemodynamic stability during dialysis through lowering ionized Ca concentrations, resulting in impaired left ventricular contractility and peripheral vasoconstriction.[508,532,541] Levels less than 2.5 mEq/L or a higher serum to dialysate Ca gradient are associated with an increased risk of intradialytic hypotension,[510,511,532,533,541] potentially placing patients at risk of myocardial stunning and increased risk of sudden death. Using a higher dialysate bicarbonate concentration may exacerbate intradialytic hypotension because an increase in pH during dialysis may further reduce ionized Ca concentration, as well as affect the proportioning of dialysate Ca from concentrate.[510,511,532]

Whether or how vascular calcification and intradialytic hypotension relate to morbidity and mortality is not clear. Reports from studies of patients treated with lower dialysate Ca concentration (≤2.5 mEq/L) have ranged from an increased risk for hospitalization for congestive heart failure, enhanced survival, and no difference in survival to an increased risk for sudden death.[533,535,537,541] Most of these studies were small; the largest study involved over 43,000 patients but used a case-control methodology using retrospective data, with potential for residual confounding.[541] Phosphorus (P) is a potential confounder that likely contributes to vascular calcification, yet has not been adequately addressed in studies on dialysate calcium. Rat aortic rings incubated with the Ca and P concentrations found in patients before (Ca, 2.1 mmol/L; P, 2.5 mmol/L) and after hemodialysis (Ca, 2.4 mmol/L; P, 1.5 mmol/L) against a 3-mEq/L Ca dialysate concentration demonstrated increased calcification. This was not seen when aortic rings were incubated with Ca and P concentrations found in postdialysis serum with neutral Ca flux (Ca, 2.1 mmol/L; P, 1.5 mmol/L; Ca is unchanged but P is reduced).[542]

Given the complexities discussed and the observed wide variations in predialysis Ca concentration, individualizing dialysate Ca concentration may be ideal. Patients prone to hypotension or at risk for sudden death may benefit from increasing the dialysate Ca concentration to 3 to 3.5 mEq/L at the expense of increased risk for hypercalcemia, vascular calcification, and low bone turnover.[510,511,532] Until a Ca kinetic model accounting for the various factors discussed is available to guide an optimal dialysate Ca prescription, one rational approach would be to maintain near-neutral Ca mass balance during dialysis, which can be accomplished with a 2.5-mEq/L dialysate Ca in patients with predialysis Ca less than 8.75 mEq/L and a 3-mEq/L dialysate Ca in those with predialysis Ca more than 9.15 mEq/L.[542]

## MAGNESIUM

As observed with potassium, only 1% to 2% of magnesium (Mg) is in the extracellular compartment.[543] Because two-thirds is in bone, Mg flux during HD is difficult to predict. With current practice in the United States of using a dialysate Mg concentration of 0.5 to 1 mEq/L, up to one-third of HD patients have low serum Mg concentrations, sometimes exacerbated by concurrent proton pump inhibitor use.[543] Raising the dialysate Mg to 1.5 mEq/L will normalize predialysis Mg levels in most patients and will make some mildly hypermagnesemic.[543,544] Traditionally, nephrology practice has been to avoid Mg supplementation in patients with advanced CKD because of their reduced ability to eliminate Mg, placing them at risk of life-threatening hypermagnesemia with attendant bradyarrhythmias and neurotoxicity (decreased deep tendon reflexes and muscle weakness). However, higher Mg levels may also inhibit vascular calcification, suppress parathyroid hormone concentrations, and reduce bone mineralization; some of these may be beneficial.[543] Low serum Mg concentrations may predispose to intradialytic hypotension, increase osteoclast activation, and enhance the propensity for ventricular arrhythmias through depolarizing resting membrane potentials.[543] Epidemiologic studies have suggested that low serum Mg concentrations are associated with mortality, but the absolute level differed among the studies and ranged from less than 1.6 to less than 2 mg/dL, with one study suggesting that the optimal serum Mg level may be between 2.7 and 3.1 mg/dL.[544–546] Adjusting for comorbidities and indices of malnutrition, inflammation, and atherosclerosis syndrome markedly attenuated the risk conferred by low serum Mg levels, but residual increased risk persisted in malnourished and/or inflamed HD patients.[544–546] Only one study found an increased risk of death with high serum Mg levels, more than 3.1 mg/dL.[546] Whether supplementing the dialysate with higher levels of Mg would reduce mortality risk is unclear. For now, consider the use of higher dialysate Mg concentration for patients with persistent intradialytic hypotension and/or at risk for cardiac arrhythmias or vascular calcification and lower dialysate Mg if adynamic bone disease is a concern.[543]

## BICARBONATE

Correction of metabolic acidosis during dialysis is achieved through increasing the dialysate concentration of a base equivalent to promoting its diffusion into the blood.[510,547,548] Historically, bicarbonate was introduced into the dialysate by bubbling carbon dioxide through it to lower the pH and prevent the precipitation of Ca and Mg salts. In the 1960s, acetate was introduced as a source of bicarbonate and became the standard for 2 decades. Acetate offered the advantages of a low incidence of bacterial contamination, lack of precipitation with Ca and Mg, and ease of storage. However, it became a hemodynamic stressor when high-efficiency and high-flux dialysis was introduced in the 1980s because the higher rate of acetate diffusion into blood exceeded the metabolic capacity of the liver and skeletal muscle. Acetate accumulation led to acidosis, vasodilation, and hypotension. These complications prompted a resurgence of bicarbonate-based dialysate, which has been sustained.

The major complications of bicarbonate dialysate are bacterial contamination and the precipitation of Ca and Mg salts.[510,547,548] Gram-negative halophilic rods thrive in bicarbonate dialysate because they require sodium chloride or sodium bicarbonate to grow.[549,550] With regular disinfection of bicarbonate containers, these bacteria have a latency period of 3 to 5 days, an exponential growth phase at 5 to 8 days, and maximal growth rate at 10 days,[549] which compare favorably with a latency of 1 day, exponential growth at 2 to 3 days, and maximal growth by 4 days in a contaminated container. Thus, disinfecting the containers and mixing the bicarbonate daily help prevent bacterial contamination. The use of commercially available dry powder cartridges offers an alternative solution to this problem.[547–550]

To minimize the formation of insoluble Ca and Mg salts with bicarbonate, bicarbonate and the acid concentrate, which contains all solutes other than bicarbonate, are separated until use.[510,547,548] The acid concentrate derives its name from the small amount of acetic acid (4–8 mEq/L in the final dilution, depending on the preparation) used to ensure the solubility of divalent cations. The dialysate delivery system draws up the two components separately and mixes them proportionately with purified water to form the final dialysate. This technologic advance allowed the widespread reintroduction of bicarbonate as a dialysate buffer in the 1970s. Because some precipitation of Ca and Mg salts still occur, the dialysate delivery system must be rinsed periodically with an acid solution to eliminate any buildup.

In many dialysis centers, the bicarbonate concentration is fixed at 32, 35, or 38 mEq/L to accommodate the use of a central bicarbonate delivery system in which the bicarbonate concentrate is piped from a centrally located tank to the individual patient stations. The advantage of a centralized delivery system is fewer back injuries in the dialysis personnel, but a major disadvantage is the inability to individualize the dialysate bicarbonate concentration. As noted, dry powder cartridges placed in line at each patient station or individual bicarbonate containers at each station will allow individualized dialysate bicarbonate prescriptions.

Although correction of metabolic acidosis is desirable to reduce protein catabolism, bone demineralization, inflammation, and insulin resistance, overcorrection to generate metabolic alkalosis during dialysis may predispose patients to hemodynamic instability, reduced cerebral blood flow, paresthesias, muscle twitching, and cramping, possibly through alkalosis-induced lowering of the serum potassium and ionized Ca levels, as well as increased tissue calcium phosphate deposition.[547,548,551–553] Several large observational studies have reported that very low (<17 mEq/L) and very high (>27 mEq/L) predialysis bicarbonate levels were associated with mortality and hospitalization but, after adjusting for case mix and markers of inflammation and malnutrition, only the association between very low bicarbonate levels and adverse outcomes remained.[553–555] A higher predialysis bicarbonate level is likely a marker for poorer nutritional status. Patients with mild to moderate acidosis (bicarbonate, 20–23 mEq/L) appear to have the best survival, perhaps reflecting more robust dietary protein intake, although more recent studies have found no association between serum bicarbonate levels and mortality.[551–556] Instead, a predialysis serum pH of 7.40 or higher and a higher dialysate bicarbonate concentration are associated with death from cardiovascular causes for pH and, unexpectedly, infectious causes for the latter.[547,551,553,556] It is difficult to reconcile these findings, and no large-scale, event-driven randomized trials have compared higher versus lower dialysate bicarbonate concentrations or oral bicarbonate supplementation in ESKD.

Although lowering dialysate bicarbonate levels for patients with predialysis hyperbicarbonatemia is prudent, especially if postdialysis metabolic alkalosis is present, it may not improve outcomes. Instead, causes of malnutrition and inflammation should be identified and corrected if possible.[552,553] Whether patients with very low serum bicarbonate concentrations would benefit from raising dialysate bicarbonate levels is unclear.[551] In addition, kinetic studies have indicated that raising dialysate bicarbonate levels increases serum bicarbonate levels at the end of and 2 hours after HD, but do not affect predialysis levels.[557] Postdialysis metabolic alkalosis and its effect on serum potassium and ionized calcium levels, however, could explain a fraction of the excess mortality observed after the first HD treatment of the week.[547,553]

Residual confounding from inaccurate reporting of comorbidities, variability of serum bicarbonate measurements, disparity between prescribed and delivered dialysate bicarbonate concentration, and incomplete accounting of total base (acetate or citrate in the acid bath are converted to bicarbonate in the body) may have contributed to the disparate findings discussed previously.[547,553] Recent data have suggested that the base equivalent in the acid bath has negligible influence on the serum bicarbonate level.[557–559] If increased mortality risk is related to a high dialysate-to-blood bicarbonate gradient and abrupt changes in serum bicarbonate levels, bicarbonate modeling and individualizing dialysate bicarbonate may be of benefit, in theory.[558,560] Until a definitive answer is available, oral bicarbonate supplementation may be preferable to raising the dialysate bicarbonate to correct very low predialysis serum bicarbonate levels (<18 mEq/L).

### Glucose

Historically, dialysate glucose concentrations were high (>320 mg/dL) to provide osmotic pressure for fluid removal and prevent hypoglycemia. However, a high dialysate glucose concentration can lead to hyperglycemia and reduce potassium removal through stimulation of insulin production and a consequent potassium shift to the intracellular space.[508] With technologic advances to allow alteration of hydrostatic pressure to enhance UF, using a glucose-free or lower glucose dialysate concentration of 100 to 200 mg/dL has become the current standard.[508,509] Glucose-free dialysis resulted in more episodes of hypoglycemia in diabetic patients during HD, especially in those with better glycemic control.[561] However, patients with diabetes undergoing HD against a dialysate glucose level of 200 mg/dL had more frequent episodes of hyperglycemia and evidence for increased vagal tone, which may increase the risk for intradialytic hypotension (IDH).[562] Given the paucity of available data regarding the optimal dialysate glucose concentration, continued use of physiologic dialysate glucose concentrations (100–200 mg/dL) seems reasonable.[508,563]

## DIALYSATE TEMPERATURE

The dialysate temperature is generally maintained between 35° and 37°C at the inlet of the dialyzer (see "Dialysate Circuit"). If the dialysate temperature is kept constant at 37°C or at the patient's core body temperature at the start of dialysis (thermoneutral dialysis, where no heat energy is transferred through the dialysis circuit), the patient's core temperature increases during dialysis. The average predialysis core body temperature in patients undergoing dialysis is around 36.6°C[564] and increases by 0.7°C during HD when the dialysate temperature is set at 37°C.[565] The pathogenesis is incompletely understood, but may in part be due to vasoconstriction in response to fluid removal and blood volume contraction and consequent reduced heat loss from the skin.[315,564] With progressive heat accumulation, a reflex dilation of the peripheral blood vessels occurs and leads to intradialytic hypotension.

Isothermic dialysis (no intradialytic change in core temperature) using a blood temperature monitor with computer-controlled modulation of dialysate temperature improves hemodynamic stability in hypotension-prone patients.[315,318,319,564,566] If such technology is not available, cooling the dialysate temperature empirically to 35° to 36° C or 0.5° to 1°C below predialysis core body temperature also alleviates IDH but may increase patient discomfort from cold and reduce clearance through inducing flow disequilibrium and impeding solute diffusion across membranes. The hemodynamic effects of dialysate cooling appear similar to those of sodium modeling and high dialysate sodium levels but without the undesirable side effects of positive sodium balance.[267,270,318,319,564,565,567]

However, a small randomized crossover trial in 80 patients has suggested that dialysate cooling may be less effective than sodium modeling in ameliorating IDH.[568]

Small mechanistic studies have suggested that dialysate cooling ameliorates IDH through increased baroreceptor variability, with an attendant rise in systemic vascular resistance, cardiac output, and stroke volume during HD.[564,565,567] Dialysate cooling does not seem to improve vascular refilling.[569] Regardless of the mechanism, dialysate cooling in hypotension-prone patients is associated with a lower risk for cardiovascular mortality, preserved left ventricular function, and reduced injury of brain white matter, but does not appear to affect risks for hospitalization, cardiovascular events, and all-cause mortality.[320,321,564,570]

## ULTRAFILTRATION RATE AND DRY WEIGHT

Another main goal of HD is to maintain fluid balance, accomplished through establishing a dry weight and applying UF during each dialysis to remove the interdialytic weight gain. UF, or fluid removal, occurs when hydrostatic pressure in the blood compartment is higher than that in the dialysate compartment, accomplished through a combination of positive pressure in the blood compartment and "negative" pressure created in the dialysate compartment. Adjusting the amount of negative pressure within the dialysate compartment controls the total level of TMP (the difference between the two pressures); the higher the TMP, the greater the UF rate.

Traditionally, dry weight is defined as the lowest body weight a patient can tolerate without becoming hypotensive, using clinical examination and evaluation as a crude estimate.[282,446,571] A more rigorous definition is the body weight at which extracellular volume is physiologic because both volume depletion and volume overload are associated with significant morbidity and mortality.[282,446,571] However, a physiologically appropriate extracellular volume and body weight are difficult to assess clinically, especially because patients undergoing dialysis vary widely in their response to fluid removal.

Although healthy individuals can tolerate a loss of 20% of their circulating blood volume before becoming hypotensive, HD patients are highly variable; some become symptomatic with as little as a 2% decline of their blood volume.[315] This wide patient variability likely results from the differing response to blood volume depletion and the disparate rate of vascular refilling from the interstitial and intracellular spaces, as well as a myriad of other factors.[315,446,572–574] Autonomic dysfunction, diastolic dysfunction, increased core temperature, and intradialytic hypocalcemia, hypokalemia, alkalosis (see previously), and myocardial stunning may all lead to an impaired cardiac response and impaired constriction of resistance and capacitance vessels during volume depletion. Dialytic removal of solutes, malnutrition, and inflammation may retard vascular refilling through decreased osmotic pressure, reduced oncotic pressure, and increased vascular permeability. Hence, patients on HD may become symptomatic before their physiologic weight is reached, and clinically determined dry weight is an unreliable measure of physiologic weight. Even the presence or absence of pedal edema and hypertension are unreliable tools to assess dry weight because they correlate poorly with volume status estimated by multifrequency bioimpedance.[282,571,575]

Newer technologies to help determine the optimal dry weight and improve tolerance of dialysis include continuous online blood volume determination during dialysis coupled with computer-controlled UF rates and UF modeling (see "Online Monitoring") and bioimpedance analysis (BIA).[575–577] Although continuous blood volume determination may reduce hypotensive episodes during dialysis, it is unable to assess the extracellular volume compartment accurately and detect patients with impaired vascular refilling; therefore, it is less useful for determining an optimal dry weight.[282,578,579]

BIA shows promise in establishing dry weight and in reducing intradialytic symptoms but is not widely used because of the underlying complex principles and lack of a gold standard method for determining dry weight to allow full validation.[576,577,580,581] Briefly, an electrical current is applied to the body, and the resistance (opposition to flow of the current) and reactance (opposition to passage of the current) are measured. The resistance is used to estimate the volume of extracellular fluid; the reactance is used to estimate the volume of intracellular compartments. Two small randomized controlled studies have suggested that multifrequency bioimpedance spectroscopy is superior to clinical evaluation in determining physiologic dry weight, as evidenced by improvements in blood pressure control, left ventricular mass index and arterial stiffness, and lower mortality.[582,583] Cases of intradialytic hypotension and access thrombosis were comparable, but the percentage of patients with residual kidney function declined from 20% to 10% in the bioimpedance group.[582] Although promising, the small number of patients studied and the potentially deleterious effects from loss of residual kidney function require further study to help define the role of BIA in optimizing volume status.[576,577]

Recent data have linked a greater rate of fluid removal during HD (UF rate [UFR]) with higher mortality, although the threshold has been debated; it ranges from more than 10 to 13 mL/kg/hour.[311,446,572,584,585] Some studies have suggested that a continuum exists with incremental risk, starting at 6 mL/kg/hour.[584,585] Strategies to reduce the UFR include reducing interdialytic weight gain through dietary sodium restriction and isonatric to hyponatric dialysis, judicious use of diuretics in patients with residual kidney function, extending session length, and/or increasing frequency of dialysis.[446,572,586] Although a higher UFR, greater interdialytic weight gain, and shortened session length are closely intertwined, each may independently confer mortality risk through mechanisms that are poorly understood.[446,587] The HD treatment itself may induce left ventricular dysfunction, independently from the hemodynamic effects of UF.[588]

Current strategies to determine dry weight rely on clinical evaluation and maintaining a high index of suspicion for volume overload, with periodic empiric challenges of the patient's end-dialysis weight by 0.2 to 0.3 kg/session when excess volume is suspected. Subtle clinical indicators include persistence of hypertension despite escalation of antihypertensive medications, reduced appetite, and very low intradialytic weight gains.[446,571] In hypotension-prone dialysis patients, UF modeling, avoiding intradialytic hypocalcemia, hypomagnesemia, and alkalosis, lowering dialysate temperature, increasing the duration or frequency of dialysis, reducing dietary sodium intake, and possibly separating UF from diffusive clearance during dialysis may be of benefit.[510,572–575] Sequential UF and diffusive clearance provides initial isolated UF with iso-osmotic removal of fluid, followed by diffusive clearance with or without additional fluid removal. Maintaining constant plasma osmolarity during UF prevents further depletion of the blood volume from fluid shifts into the interstitial and intracellular spaces, although sequential UF was found to be inferior to sodium modeling and dialysate cooling in preventing intradialytic hypotension.[589]

## REUSE

Hemodialyzer reuse peaked in the 1990s, primarily because of the potential benefits of improved biocompatibility and reduced cost.[207,590,591] Reprocessing dialyzers for repeated use took advantage of dialyzer membrane coating with plasma proteins that occurs during the first treatment, effectively camouflaging hydroxyl groups that can activate complements, white blood cells, and platelets. It also reduced the incidence of first-use syndrome, thought to be mediated in part by ethylene oxide, a commonly used sterilant that is absorbed by the potting compound of the dialyzer that can induce an immunoglobulin E (IgE)-mediated anaphylactic reaction (see "Hemodialyzers").

Automated devices that reprocess the dialyzers are safer and result in lower incidences of febrile reactions compared with manual reprocessing.[207] During the cleaning process, bleach or hydrogen peroxide is used to improve the aesthetics. However, bleach also strips proteins off the membrane and can damage the membrane, thereby negating the improved biocompatibility afforded by the protein-coated membrane, reducing phosphorus clearance through increased negative membrane charge, and increasing loss of albumin.[592,593] After cleaning, dialyzer integrity is assessed by measuring the volume of the fiber bundle in the blood compartment (fiber bundle volume) and by pressurizing the dialyzer to ensure that the fibers are structurally intact (pressure test). For a dialyzer to be accepted for reuse, the fiber bundle volume must be greater than 80% of the initial value, and the dialyzer should hold more than 80% of the maximal operating pressure. The dialyzer is then packed with chemical disinfectants such as peracetic acid or formaldehyde or subject to heat disinfection, with or without citrate. Over the decades, peracetic acid has gained popularity over formaldehyde, increasing from 5% in 1983 to 72% in 2002 of centers that practice reuse; formaldehyde use fell from 95% to 20% by 2002.[594]

Close scrutiny of the safety of dialyzer reuse practices has yielded conflicting results when comparing reuse with nonreuse and when comparing the various disinfectants, largely because the studies were nonrandomized and uncontrolled.[207,591,595–597] Overall, however, data have suggested that when reuse is applied meticulously and complies with AAMI standards, risk-adjusted mortality rates are similar, and the various disinfectants are comparable.

Since the peak of 80% in 1997, the prevalence of reuse declined to 40% in 2005, with an even lower rate of 24% in 2012.[598,599] This sharp decline is largely due to a change in practice patterns in some large dialysis chain providers favoring single use, the wide availability and lower cost of dialyzers constructed with synthetic and more biocompatible membranes, lingering concerns that long-term exposure to chemical disinfectants may be detrimental to the health of patients and health care staff, and the potential for infectious or pyrogenic reactions from flawed reuse practices.[207,590,591,595,598,599]

However, abandoning reuse would result in an estimated 903,000 tons of dialyzer-related polymer waste worldwide, compared with 45,000 tons if each dialyzer were reused 20 times.[591,600–602] Research on best management of the medical waste associated with dialysis is needed, with the decline in reuse and potential rise in more frequent dialysis.

## MANAGEMENT OF PATIENTS ON MAINTENANCE HEMODIALYSIS

### END-STAGE KIDNEY DISEASE

ESKD is considered the level of kidney function that requires renal replacement therapy to sustain a patient's life. If HD is the therapy of choice, the patient begins a therapy that removes numerous solutes and water, as described in detail in this chapter. In some respects, the process of HD can be viewed as the glomerular component of kidney function, during which water and smaller solutes cross a membrane, limited in part by its molecular size. Unfortunately, the analogy ends because the filtering surface in HD is an artificial membrane without biologic function. For example, dialysis lacks an active tubular transport component to reclaim or further eliminate specific solutes. Beneficial solutes such as amino acids may cross the dialysis membrane and are "excreted," but larger or protein-bound substances that may be toxic are not removed at all. Furthermore, HD does not replace the metabolic capacity of the kidneys to synthesize critical proteins. Some of the renally synthesized proteins can be exogenously provided (e.g., erythropoietin), but others may not be recognized. HD remains a lifesaving therapy but is far from full renal replacement, and thus it is not surprising the general care of an HD patient is broad and complicated. This section provides an overview of the medical management of patients undergoing HD.

### ANEMIA

The kidney is the major source of endogenous erythropoietin. (See Chapter 55 for a full discussion of anemia in advancing CKD and its management; in this chapter, we focus on the management of anemia in patients undergoing maintenance HD.) Before the advent of recombinant erythropoietin in 1989, severe anemia with hemoglobin (Hgb) levels below 7 g/dL was common in patients undergoing HD, leading to frequent transfusions and iron overload in many patients. HD by itself only partially corrected the anemia, presumably by improving erythrocyte survival and reducing erythropoietin resistance. Currently, with erythropoietin and optimal management of CKD, patients generally begin and undergo HD therapy with Hgb concentrations in an acceptable range.

#### PRINCIPLES OF ERYTHROPOIESIS-STIMULATING AGENT USE

Recombinant human erythropoietin (EPO) is extremely effective in increasing Hgb concentrations in the vast majority of patients.[603] The positive clinical effects are numerous—enhanced exercise capability, presumably in part from improved cardiac function with reduction in ventricular hypertrophy, a better quality of life, with improved physical performance, work capacity, and cognitive capacity, improved sexual function and, because of fewer transfusions, reduced rates of hepatitis, iron overload, and alloantibody production precluding transplant.[604–614]

Several preparations of EPO are produced and available worldwide (e.g., epoetin alpha, epoetin beta, epoetin omega, epoetin zeta). They differ from each other and the native hormone with respect to production methods and glycosylation. These differences may contribute to the development of neutralizing anti-EPO antibodies and pure red cell aplasia (PRCA), characterized by severe anemia due to the absence of bone marrow erythroid precursors. Reports of PRCA first surfaced in 1998, peaked in 2002, and continue to appear periodically.[615,616] Potential mechanisms for anti-EPO antibody development include immunogenic aggregation of inappropriately stored EPO—for example, at a high temperature, various organic compounds are leached from syringe components by polysorbate 80, a stabilizer substituted for albumin. Unfortunately, these neutralizing antibodies appear to react to native EPO and all forms of EPO, including epoetin zeta and darbepoetin.[617,618] Diagnosis should include a bone marrow biopsy and evaluation for anti- EPO antibodies. Affected patients are treated with withdrawal of EPO and immunosuppression, yet they largely remain transfusion-dependent. Fortunately, the incidence of PRCA appears to be on the decline. PRCA has predominantly been reported with subcutaneous administration of an older formulation of Eprex, an epoetin alfa product produced outside the United States. Newer preparations of EPO appear to have less risk of PRCA,[619] although a small number of cases may still occur.[620]

At present, HD patients with anemia are generally treated with EPO or one of its longer acting analogues such as darbepoetin (created by the addition of *N*-linked carbohydrates) or methoxy polyethylene glycol-epoetin beta (formed by adducts with polyethylene glycol). However, as discussed in Chapter 55 and later in this section, controversy exists about the safety of EPO because high doses or higher Hgb targets are associated with adverse effects, including increased risks of cardiovascular and cerebrovascular events. Thus, several novel drugs that act on alternate pathways of red cell production have recently been studied or are under development. EPO and these newer agents are collectively referred to as erythropoiesis-stimulating agents (ESAs). Further research is needed to determine the efficacy and safety of the different ESAs. As a cautionary example, peginesatide, a synthetic EPO receptor agonist, corrected anemia as well as EPO, and was approved for use by the US Food and Drug Administration (FDA) in 2012.[619] Unfortunately, postmarketing reports of serious hypersensitivity reactions, including anaphylaxis causing death, resulted in its withdrawal from the market in 2014. Prolyl hydroxylase inhibitors that increase erythropoiesis through the transcription pathway of hypoxia-inducible factor have been shown to be efficacious in anemia management,[621–624] although they remain in development, with ongoing trials necessary to determine their safety and efficacy relative to ESAs.

The optimal route of administration of ESAs remains controversial. Studies have demonstrated that subcutaneous dosing may reduce EPO requirements by approximately 30% and, possibly because of reduced EPO exposure, may be associated with less cardiovascular and cerebrovascular events.[625,626,630,631] However, intravenous administration has been favored historically in HD due to less patient discomfort, readily available blood access, and concern about the increased risk of anti-EPO antibodies with subcutaneous administration.

## HEMOGLOBIN TARGET

The optimal goal for Hgb concentrations in patients with ESKD has received substantial attention since the advent of ESAs. Goals of therapy should be to minimize symptoms attributable to anemia while also reducing the need for transfusion. ESAs may mitigate symptoms at lower Hgb concentrations than formerly thought. A systematic review of randomized controlled trials up to 2015 comparing higher versus lower Hgb concentrations has shown no substantial improvement in health-related quality of life with the higher targets.[627] More importantly, multiple clinical trials have shown that Hgb targets more than 13 g/dL, in attempts to "normalize" the Hgb level in patients with CKD, are associated with adverse outcomes. The best data in ESKD have come from a large randomized trial of more than 1200 HD recipients with underlying cardiovascular disease comparing a higher versus lower hematocrit target (42% vs. 30%).[628] The trial was terminated early because of safety concerns about a trend toward worse mortality and more vascular access thrombosis in the higher hematocrit target group. Three large randomized controlled studies in the predialysis CKD population have reported that compared with an Hgb level less than 11.5 g/dL, normalization of Hgb increases risks for cardiovascular and cerebrovascular events, hypertension, and headaches.[629–631] Careful reviews have concluded that in patients undergoing HD, no data support an Hgb goal above 12 g/dL due to these risks.[632–634] These conclusions led the Kidney Disease: Improving Global Outcomes (KDIGO) group to recommend initiating an ESA when the Hgb level is less than 10 g/dL while avoiding a target Hgb greater than 11.5 g/dL.[634] A large meta-regression analysis of more than 12,000 patients has suggested that higher doses of ESAs may increase mortality risk independently of the Hgb concentration.[635]

## IRON THERAPY

The role of iron in the management of anemia for patients on maintenance HD has been a fascinating saga. Before ESAs, frequent transfusion requirements in severely anemic patients resulted in iron overload and hemosiderosis, requiring iron chelation with deferoxamine to prevent hemochromatosis and other complications. The complex protocols required to ensure intradialytic removal of the chelated iron and the increased risk of infection further complicated the delivery of dialysis.[636] However, the widespread use of ESAs has completely transformed the problem from a risk of iron overload to one of insufficient iron stores limiting response to ESAs.

Patients on HD who are receiving ESAs have substantial requirements for iron, typically 1 to 2 g/year, due to loss of blood from dialysis, laboratory testing, vascular procedures, and gastrointestinal bleeding.[634] The challenge is to identify the markers that would indicate the need for iron replacement most accurately.[637] The most commonly used markers to define iron status are serum ferritin, which mirrors iron stores, and transferrin saturation, which is a surrogate for iron availability. However, these markers may have limited sensitivity and specificity, particularly because the ferritin level is frequently elevated in the setting of inflammation, independently of iron stores. A multicenter trial of patients with serum ferritin concentrations higher than 500 ng/mL, transferrin saturation less than 25%, and anemia despite ESAs has demonstrated that empiric intravenous iron replacement increases Hgb.[638] These patients are thought to have functional iron deficiency, recognition of which may be as important to anemia management as identifying absolute iron deficiency, especially with the current interest in avoiding high ESA doses. However, the long-term clinical benefits and safety of intravenous iron dosing in patients with high ferritin levels is unknown (see later).

Among patients undergoing hemodialysis, intravenous iron is more effective than oral iron in increasing Hgb and markers of iron availability.[639] Multiple formulations exist, with varying potential for side effects, including allergic reactions, such as rash, flushing, hypotension, and anaphylaxis. A large retrospective study using Medicare claims data has found the highest anaphylactic risk with iron dextran and substantially lower risk with agents such as iron sucrose and sodium ferric gluconate.[640] Newer forms of supplemental iron have garnered interest. Ferric pyrophosphate citrate was approved by the FDA in 2015 as a water-soluble iron salt that can be administered via dialysate. Small randomized trials have suggested that this form of delivery can help maintain Hgb levels.[641,642] Additionally, novel iron-based phosphorus binders may also allow for the maintenance of iron stores, reducing or eliminating the need for intravenous iron.[643,644]

Theoretically, excess iron may increase the risk of cardiovascular disease and infection by exacerbating oxidative stress, enhancing bacterial growth, and impairing phagocytic cell function.[645–647] However, whether these effects translate into clinically relevant events is unknown. Observational data have been conflicting, with some studies suggesting increased hospitalization and mortality associated with high doses of intravenous iron[648] and others finding no significant associations.[649–651] Of note, these studies were not randomized or controlled, and the dosing of iron may be affected by various confounders. Comparative studies of intravenous iron sucrose, ferric gluconate, and ferumoxytol also have shown mixed results, with mostly small observational differences between the formulations.[652–654]

### Hyporesponsiveness to Erythropoiesis-Stimulating Agent Therapy

ESA hyporesponsiveness describes patients who do not achieve or maintain a target Hgb concentration, despite high and/or increasing ESA doses. Resistance to ESAs may be due to inadequate iron stores, presence of inflammation, hyperparathyroidism, inadequate dialysis, nutrient deficiencies, or underlying bone marrow diseases.[655,656] Inflammatory states are common in patients undergoing HD and may interfere with erythropoiesis and the response to ESAs beyond their effect on iron availability.[657] The use of hemodialysis catheters is associated with chronic inflammation,[658] even when not overtly infected. Occult infections in thrombosed AV grafts and inflammation from a failed kidney transplantation also should be considered in patients with ESA hyporesponsiveness. Maneuvers that reduce inflammation, such as the use of ultrapure water, may improve the response to ESAs.[656] Although more frequent dialysis was thought to improve ESA response in early trials, a randomized trial did not confirm this finding.[659]

## NUTRITION

The complex relationship between protein metabolism and body composition in kidney disease is discussed elsewhere (see Chapter 60). Nutrition in HD patients is influenced by factors related to kidney failure and the HD treatment itself (Box 63.2). There is strong evidence that nutrition affects overall morbidity and mortality in the dialysis population, highlighting the need to look for and treat patients with malnutrition. Growing evidence has suggested that the problem is not simply protein malnutrition but protein energy wasting (PEW), similar to the cachexia seen with inflammation.[660–663] Hence, simply adding protein supplements will not reverse the wasting.

**Box 63.2 Factors Causing Malnutrition in Hemodialysis Patients[a]**

Inadequate protein or calorie intake
Increased energy expenditure
Metabolic acidosis
Hormonal alterations
Comorbidities or hospitalizations
Dialytic nutrient losses
Dialysis-induced catabolism
Infection

[a]For a comprehensive discussion on the factors causing malnutrition, see Chapter 60.

### MARKERS OF NUTRITION

A global approach to nutritional assessment should include an evaluation of dietary history, physical findings, and laboratory testing. Patients should be questioned monthly about their appetite, gastrointestinal symptoms, and weight changes. Monthly trends of postdialysis dry weight should be monitored. Unintentional weight loss over time, particularly in patients with low body weight or body mass index (BMI), likely reflects PEW and is associated with increased mortality.[664,665]

No single laboratory assessment of nutrition is adequate. Low predialysis BUN concentrations are associated with mortality. However, the predialysis BUN level is also affected by residual kidney function and adequacy of dialysis. The normalized protein catabolic rate (nPCR), calculated using predialysis and postdialysis BUN levels adjusted for interdialytic interval and body habitus, is likely a better surrogate for dietary protein intake.[666] However, the nPCR calculation assumes a steady state from day to day, which may overestimate nutritional status in patients with active catabolism such as inflammation or infection and underestimate nutrition in anabolic states such as a maturing child or pregnancy. The association of nPCR with serum albumin levels and survival may be strengthened after accounting for residual renal urea clearance,[667] an important factor to consider when assessing nPCR values.

The serum albumin concentration is a strong predictor of mortality in observational studies,[668] yet it is difficult to determine whether the nutritional component or other factors are responsible for the association. Albumin is increased by nutritional protein intake but also may fall due to nonnutritional factors such as acute illness, inflammation, acidemia, urinary loss, and volume overload.[669–671] Because of its shorter half-life, serum prealbumin (transthyretin) has been studied as another nutritional marker. However, the kidneys are the primary source of clearance for prealbumin, rendering interpretation of its level difficult in the setting of a low GFR.[662] The serum creatinine level also may reflect dietary protein intake and muscle mass, but is unreliable as a marker for PEW because other factors may affect its level. Other laboratory markers such as insulin-like growth factor 1 (IGF-1) and ghrelin have been studied but are neither readily available nor validated.[672–675]

Body composition techniques may be useful in assessing nutrition. Anthropometric measurements, such as midarm muscle circumference and skinfold thickness, appear deceptively easy to perform but must be taken carefully by a trained technician. They also may be inaccurate because of varying tissue hydration and because standardization was undertaken in healthy volunteers.[676,677] Therefore, changes over time may be more reliable than isolated values. Additional methodologies to estimate body composition, such as dual-energy x-ray absorptiometry (DEXA) and BIA are available.[678–680] However, DEXA does not differentiate intracellular from extracellular water, and extracellular fluid is counted as part of the lean (nonfat) body mass, potentially overestimating lean body mass in edematous patients. In addition, DEXA is relatively expensive and requires travel to a facility with dedicated equipment.

Although BIA has been available for years, it remains mainly a research tool. As the technology has progressed from single-frequency to multifrequency, its accuracy in estimating total body water and lean body mass has improved, but equipment cost and complexity have increased as well, making multifrequency BIA less practical.[679] Results obtained with BIA correlate with those from DEXA[680] but, as with other body composition technologies, are most reliable when completed after dialysis.[681] The increased use of BIA in clinical trials may eventually inform its optimal use in the clinical setting.[583,682] Protocols using multifrequency BIA to estimate changes in extracellular fluid in the calf during HD may become a tool for establishing an optimal dry weight (see also "Ultrafiltration and Dry Weight" section).[581,683]

### MANAGEMENT OF PROTEIN ENERGY WASTING

Several criteria have been proposed for diagnosing PEW. Each assigns a score to multiple nutritional measures and designates a threshold above which the diagnosis of PEW is made.[684–687] Each of these PEW criteria correlates strongly with clinical outcomes, including mortality, yet it is not clear how these criteria, and which one, will be incorporated into future clinical management strategies across wide groups of patients. At present, the diagnosis of PEW is suspected clinically in patients with a progressive trend of weight loss, low albumin level, and declining nPCR.

If PEW is present, increased nutritional support is critical. Use of the enteral route in patients with adequate gastrointestinal function can improve serum albumin and prealbumin concentrations and other measures of nutritional status such as the subjective global assessment,[663] even when oral supplements are only provided during dialysis.[688,689] In fact, intradialytic oral protein supplementation in patients with low albumin levels has been associated with reduced hospital stays and better survival in observational studies.[690–692] When oral supplementation is unsuccessful, tube feeding has been attempted in some cases, especially in young children for whom nutrition is critical for growth and development.[689,693] Parenteral nutrition has been considered when enteral feeding is not possible, mainly during each HD session to ameliorate the challenge of large volume infusions. Providing intradialytic parenteral nutrition (IDPN) to patients with hypoalbuminemia has increased serum albumin concentrations.[689,694] However, the only randomized controlled trials evaluating the efficacy of IDPN was in comparison to oral protein supplementation rather than placebo[695] and did not find a difference between the two interventions with respect to serum albumin, weight, or mortality. Thus, IDPN is generally reserved for patients with intestinal malabsorption or other types of dysfunction, in which oral or enteral supplementation is unsafe or poorly tolerated, particularly because of its expense.

Pharmacologic intervention to reverse the anorexia and muscle loss often seen in patients on maintenance HD has received increased attention.[696] Providing specific replacement of deficient branched-chain amino acids or ghrelin may improve appetite and nutritional status.[674,697,698] Agents such as megestrol acetate, used in other chronic diseases, have led to weight gain and an improved ability to exercise in a small pilot study.[699] Other hormonal therapies such as human growth hormone, IGF-1, and anabolic steroids have also been used and are associated with increased lean muscle mass.[696] Further investigation is needed to determine if these interventions are sufficiently safe to warrant administration.

### VITAMINS AND TRACE ELEMENTS

Water-soluble vitamins are recommended for patients on HD because intake of these vitamins is low as a result of dietary restriction and because the dialysis process itself removes these vitamins, especially folic acid, pyridoxine, and vitamin C.[700] Vitamin supplementation has been associated with lower mortality risk in observational studies,[701,702] although the direct mechanism of benefit is unclear, and these analyses suffered from confounding by indication. B vitamins play important diverse roles as coenzymes and cofactors in various cellular metabolic processes, although vitamin B supplementation alone does not alter cardiovascular risk or mortality in randomized trials.[703,704] Vitamin C is an antioxidant involved in collagen formation, wound healing, hormone regulation, resistance to infections, and iron metabolism.[700] Intravenous vitamin C supplementation may reduce ESA dose requirements while improving transferrin saturation without changes in ferritin,[705] although its use has been limited due to lack of long-term safety data related to oxalic acid production and effects on oxidative stress. Regardless, prescribing oral, water-soluble vitamin supplementation is advocated to prevent nutritional deficiency and its adverse effects.

Vitamin D is covered in detail in Chapter 53, along with the complex interactions among the kidney, bone, and Ca and phosphorus metabolism. Retrospective studies have suggested that vitamin 25(OH)D deficiency may be associated with cardiovascular mortality and is a growing problem in the general population, as well as in ESKD.[706,707] However, two small trials evaluating ergocalciferol supplementation in patients undergoing HD with vitamin D deficiency have found no difference in effects on Ca, phosphorus, parathyroid hormone, other bone medication use, ESA use, hospitalizations, or death.[708,709]

Because most trace elements are excreted by the kidneys, their levels rise as kidney function declines and may contribute to uremic toxicity. Exceptions are selenium and zinc, which are the most common elements found at low serum concentrations.[710–714] Selenium is an important cofactor in certain antioxidant enzymes, and its deficiency is associated with cardiovascular disease in patients without kidney disease. However, selenium supplementation is controversial because it has a narrow therapeutic index and may result in selenosis, with nausea, vomiting, peripheral neuropathy, and loss of hair or nails.[710,711,714] Zinc deficiency is associated with immunodeficiency, ESA resistance, anorexia, dysgeusia, and impotence. Limited data have shown that zinc supplementation in deficient HD patients may improve appetite, nutritional status, and ESA responsiveness.[715–717]

## MINERAL METABOLISM–RELATED ISSUES

The complex influence of kidney disease on bone and mineral metabolism is covered in detail in Chapter 53. Although maintaining a normal or near-normal serum phosphorus concentration may be one of the most challenging goals for patients on maintenance HD, growing evidence has suggested its importance because serum phosphorus concentrations correlate directly with mortality.[718] Several complications thought to be related to Ca and phosphorus perturbations in kidney failure present challenging management issues in patients undergoing HD and are highlighted here briefly.

### VASCULAR CALCIFICATION

Although atherosclerosis is a major cause of cardiovascular mortality in the general population, growing evidence has suggested that diffuse vascular calcification may be an equally or more important contributor to cardiovascular mortality and morbidity in the HD population. Vascular calcification in advanced CKD appears to differ from "garden variety" atherosclerosis and disproportionately involves the medial portion of the vessel in association with disorganized vascular smooth muscle cells (VSMCs) and expression of bone matrix protein.[719–721] This process is evident even in children and adolescents.[722] The molecular mechanisms underpinning vascular calcification involve a complex balance among inhibitors and potentiators of calcification.[720,723–727] Inhibitors of calcification, such as fetuin-A and matrix Gla protein, are reduced or inactivated in vessel walls.[723,728] A careful study of blood vessels in patients with CKD and ESKD has suggested that although significant Ca loading of vessels is present, dialysis appears to trigger an increased rate of apoptosis of VSMCs, which then leads to vascular calcification.[729]

The exact signals responsible for inducing VSMC apoptosis have yet to be identified. Serum phosphorus, Ca, and parathyroid hormone (PTH) concentrations correlate with the degree of vascular calcification, making control of phosphorus and PTH and avoidance of Ca logical targets for reducing cardiovascular risk.[721,725] To date, studies have yielded conflicting results. Use of Ca-free phosphorus binders has ameliorated vascular calcification in some studies but not in others and did not appear to be associated with lower rates of all-cause or cause-specific (infectious or cardiovascular) mortality in HD patients compared with calcium-containing binders.[730–735] A prospective cohort study of more than 10,000 patients has found that those who received phosphorus binders during the first 90 days of HD therapy had a lower 1-year all-cause mortality than those not taking binders,[736] regardless of the type of binder and serum phosphorus concentration. However, improved control of hyperparathyroidism with cinacalcet in patients undergoing dialysis[737] and with paracalcitol in patients with nondialysis-requiring CKD[738] did not reduce mortality or morbidity, although off-protocol use of the study drug in control subjects may have reduced the power of these studies to detect significant differences.[739] Additional controlled trials addressing the effect of phosphorus and/or PTH control with different classes of phosphorus binders and PTH-lowering agents on hard clinical endpoints are needed.

### CALCIFIC UREMIC ARTERIOLOPATHY

Calcific uremic arteriolopathy (CUA), previously referred to as *calciphylaxis*, is a devastating condition characterized by painful ischemia of the skin and subcutaneous tissues, manifesting as symmetric, violaceous patches early on and usually progressing to subcutaneous plaques as a result of infarction[740] and less so to necrotizing, nonhealing skin ulcers.[741–743] The name suggests a connection to substantial kidney impairment but, rarely, cases are seen in nonuremic patients.[744] Lesions tend to occur in areas of high adipose content and usually involve the abdominal wall, breasts, buttocks, and thighs, but they can also develop at more distal sites such as the calves, forearms, hands, feet, and face. Pathologically, the presence of diffuse calcification of the media and internal elastic lamina of dermal and subcutaneous small arteries and arterioles, with atrophy of smooth muscle cells leading to cutaneous ischemia, is an important diagnostic finding.[742,743] Imaging modalities such as plain radiography, computed tomography (CT), mammography, and bone scanning may provide supportive information, although none of these modalities has been systematically evaluated.[745–747] Skin biopsy provides a definitive diagnosis, allowing the exclusion of other potential causes of skin necrosis with secondary calcification, although it requires extreme care because of the increased risk of poor healing and infection associated with CUA.[740,743,748]

The pathogenesis of CUA is controversial.[741,742,747] Recognized risk factors include diabetes mellitus, obesity, female gender, white race, hypercalcemia, hyperphosphatemia, use of Ca-containing phosphorus binders and vitamin D, hyperparathyroidism, chronic inflammatory states, and the use of vitamin K antagonists (e.g., warfarin). Skin trauma may provide an inciting event because diabetics requiring insulin injections appear more likely to develop CUA than those not on insulin injections.[749] The extent to which disorders of mineral metabolism contribute to CUA is unclear because severe CUA cases appeared to resolve after parathyroidectomy in some reports but not in others,[750–754] and hyperparathyroidism did not appear to be critical for CUA development in some observational reports.[755] Analyses of pathologic specimens from a small number of patients with CUA have demonstrated deposits of iron and aluminum in the lesions but none in adjacent normal tissue or in tissue from CKD controls, suggesting a potential role for metal deposition in the pathogenesis.[756,757] Histologic studies have also revealed the presence of an active osteogenic process in CUA lesions, including increased expression of bone morphogenic protein 2 and osteopontin.[719,758]

Therapy for CUA is focused on reducing Ca and phosphorus concentrations and controlling high PTH levels,[741,742,747,759] although the role of parathyroidectomy remains controversial.[750–754] Discontinuing or avoiding Ca-containing phosphorus binders and vitamin D, along with a prescription of a physiologic or slightly lower calcium dialysate, seem prudent. When ulcerations occur, aggressive local wound care and antibiotics to prevent wound infections are important. Case reports and small case series have introduced novel therapies that may aid in healing—hyperbaric oxygen, cinacalcet, bisphosphonates, and sodium thiosulfate, with many authors advocating a multimodal treatment approach to include optimization of and potentially more frequent dialysis.[747,748,760–770] Sodium thiosulfate therapy appears to be the most promising and may offer benefit through both chelation of Ca and amelioration of inflammation.[761,764,770] Reports of intralesional sodium thiosulfate have also shown promise for localized CUA.[771]

## CARDIOVASCULAR DISEASE

Cardiovascular disease is the leading cause of mortality in patients undergoing HD, accounting for roughly half of known causes of death.[10] The complex relationships between CKD and cardiovascular biology are described in detail in Chapter 54. In general, the interplay of traditional cardiac risk factors with nontraditional cardiac risk factors unique to patients undergoing HD, such as inflammation, oxidative stress, retained metabolites (e.g., advanced glycation end products), and PEW combine to lead ultimately to severe cardiomyopathy, ischemic heart disease, and death.[772]

## TRADITIONAL CARDIOVASCULAR RISK FACTORS

Atherosclerotic cardiovascular risk factors such as diabetes, hypertension, low physical activity, left ventricular hypertrophy, and low high-density lipoprotein (HDL) levels are substantially more common in HD patients than in the general population.[773] Risk factors such as obesity and high low-density lipoprotein (LDL) cholesterol levels are less frequent. When present, obesity seems to confer a paradoxically protective effect and elevated serum concentrations of LDL are not associated with mortality.[774–776] These findings suggest that the pathogenic relationship of traditional cardiovascular risk factors and adverse cardiovascular outcomes differs in ESKD compared with the general population.

One possible explanation is that lipoproteins are modified in the setting of ESKD. LDL appears to undergo uremia-induced modification and carbamylation, resulting in a more dense form that better predicts cardiac events than total LDL.[777,778] In particular, elevated levels of lipoprotein(a)—Lp(a)—a modified LDL that has a highly glycosylated apolipoprotein A (apo A) linked to apolipoprotein B100 (apo B100), appears to be a key predictor.[779–782] Lp(a) has atherogenic properties, accumulates in the wall of atherosclerotic lesions, and is increased in HD possibly because the kidney degrades Lp(a). An in vivo turnover study has suggested that elevated levels of Lp(a) in the HD population are caused by decreased clearance rather than overproduction.[783] Moreover, low levels of HDL exist, and those particles have lost their antiinflammatory and antiatherogenic components, potentially due to reduced activity of HDL-associated enzymes—paraoxonase 1, nitric oxide synthase, and lecithin-cholesterol acyltransferase.[777,784]

Left ventricular hypertrophy (LVH) is a risk factor for cardiovascular events in the general population.[785] It is prevalent in most patients on HD and may represent a major risk factor for cardiac events, not specifically related to traditional atherosclerosis.[786] Multiple factors have been invoked for the high prevalence of LVH in the HD population, including volume overload, hypertension, age, anemia, and hypoalbuminemia. AV HD access with prolonged high cardiac output may also contribute to the frequency of left ventricular disease,[787,788] although this has been debated.[789] Assessment of LVH by echocardiography is optimal when the patient is at her or his dry weight. Cardiac magnetic resonance imaging (CMRI) may be better for measuring left ventricular mass than traditional echocardiography because it abrogates confounding by volume overload,[790,791] and LVH demonstrated by CMRI has been associated with higher systolic blood pressure, predialysis pulse pressure, and calcium × phosphorus products.[791]

## NONTRADITIONAL CARDIOVASCULAR RISK FACTORS

Inflammation has gained appreciation as an important factor in cardiovascular disease in both the CKD and general populations.[792–794] Plasma levels of C-reactive protein (a marker of inflammation) and interleukin-6 (a proinflammatory cytokine) are strong predictors of cardiovascular and all-cause mortality in the ESKD population.[774,775,795] Numerous factors predispose patients undergoing HD to the burden of endogenous inflammation compared with the general population. Kidney failure, the dialysis process, genetic predisposition, chronic periodontitis, type of vascular access, and other as yet unidentified factors act in concert to contribute to oxidative stress, endothelial dysfunction, carbonyl stress, and accumulation of advanced glycation end products.[110,774,792,796] The critical role of inflammation in cardiovascular disease has led to the hope that statins, which lower lipid levels and reduce vascular inflammation,[797] would ameliorate cardiovascular risk in dialysis patients, but several large randomized controlled studies have yielded disappointing results (see later, "Diagnosis and Treatment").[798]

Homocysteine levels are elevated in ESKD and correlate with cardiovascular risk,[799–801] presumably through inducing endothelial dysfunction and a prothrombotic state. Because homocysteine is largely protein-bound, poor nutritional status may confound the relationship between homocysteine concentrations and cardiovascular disease.[801] Although small studies in the HD population have suggested a potential benefit from folic acid and methylcobalamin administration to lower homocysteine levels and cardiovascular risk, most data in the general population and patients with CKD and ESKD have suggested that lowering homocysteine levels with folic acid and B vitamins does not reduce the risk of cardiovascular events.[703,704,800,802–806] Nonetheless, oral supplementation with folic acid and B vitamins is recommended to prevent nutritional deficiencies and support hematopoiesis, as discussed earlier.

Oxidative stress from kidney failure or the dialysis process itself may contribute to the high risk of cardiovascular disease.[807,808] Biomarkers of oxidative stress in HD patients are difficult to quantify accurately but seem to correlate with carotid intimal thickness (CIMT), a surrogate marker for cardiovascular disease.[809] Strategies to reduce oxidative stress include oral administration of antioxidants such as vitamin E, which reduce the composite rate of cardiac events but not individual endpoints or all-cause mortality in small controlled trials.[807,810–812] These findings were not replicated in larger trials of antioxidant therapy. One randomized trial of oral tocopherols and alpha-lipoic acid that included 353 patients on HD has shown no effect on markers of inflammation (e.g., high-sensitivity C-reactive protein. [hsCRP], interleukin-6 [IL-6], F2 isoprostane, and isofuran concentrations), EPO responsiveness, hospitalization, or mortality.[813] A large randomized trial of vitamin E–impregnated membranes, a novel method targeting intradialytic oxidative stress, did not improve response to ESAs,[814] although smaller studies have suggested that these dialyzers lower biomarkers of oxidative stress and reduce CIMT.[221,815,816] Coenzyme Q10 appears to reduce plasma isoprostanes and isofurans, both markers of oxidative stress and endothelial dysfunction.[817,818] Use of ultrapure dialysate produced by filtering standard dialysis fluid through an added bacteria- and endotoxin-retentive filter reduced markers of inflammation and oxidative stress.[354,819,820] Whether reducing inflammatory mediators and oxidative stress translates to improved cardiovascular outcomes is unclear.

Novel biomarkers such as the proteins paraoxonase (PON1), fibroblast growth factor 23 (FGF-23), and indoxyl sulfate also are associated with cardiovascular disease. HDL-associated PON1 protects LDLs against oxidation. Reduced

PON1 activity, determined by genetic factors in concert with several environmental factors, including smoking, correlates inversely with markers of inflammation and cardiovascular mortality in patients on HD.[821,822] Elevated levels of FGF-23 in CKD may directly influence LVH and cardiovascular risk, independent of its relationship to phosphorus.[823,824] Indoxyl sulfate appears to be a powerful inducer of oxidative stress. It is derived from dietary protein metabolism by intestinal bacteria, accumulates in ESKD, and is poorly removed, even with more frequent dialysis, due to protein binding.[825,826] Heightened interest in extradialytic methods of indoxyl sulfate removal has included intensification of dietary fiber to alter the gut microbiome.[390]

## DIAGNOSIS AND TREATMENT

Unique factors in the HD population complicate the diagnosis and treatment of cardiovascular disease. A classic example is the reduced rate of symptoms, especially in patients with diabetes, despite substantial angiographic evidence for coronary disease.[827,828] There are conflicting data regarding the utility of the various screening tests for coronary artery disease in HD patients.[828–830] In general, tests that require the patient to exercise or that rely on electrocardiographic (ECG) findings for diagnosis are less reliable because of reduced exercise tolerance and abnormal resting ECG findings in HD patients. Dobutamine stress echocardiography and pharmacologic nuclear stress imaging have better sensitivity and specificity in HD patients,[831] although their predictive value remains lower than for the general population. Angiography remains the gold standard for the detection of coronary artery disease and should be considered in patients with positive stress tests or acute coronary syndromes.

Studies have suggested that patients on HD with acute coronary syndromes are managed less aggressively than the general population. They are less likely to receive thrombolytic therapy[832,833] or undergo diagnostic coronary angiography and revascularization,[834] despite epidemiologic data suggesting that revascularization improves survival.[833,835] Part of the reluctance in pursuing aggressive interventions in HD patients may stem from the five- to sixfold increase in early mortality (9%–12% vs. 2%–3%) and 5-year mortality (>50% vs. 10%) after coronary revascularization compared with the general population.[836–840] Optimal management of HD recipients with coronary artery disease remains controversial[839,841] because no randomized trials have been published that compare interventional strategies.[842] Several epidemiologic studies and meta-analyses have reported better long-term outcomes—lower risks of late cardiac deaths, sudden death, myocardial infarction, and repeat coronary revascularization—with coronary artery bypass grafting (CABG) compared with percutaneous intervention, but at the cost of a higher risk of mortality and stroke within the initial 3 months.[837,838,840,843–847] In the absence of definitive data, the decision to select CABG versus percutaneous intervention may be influenced by individual patient characteristics and center-specific factors. If a percutaneous approach is chosen, drug-eluting stents appear to be superior to bare metal stents.[845,848,849]

Strategies for the secondary prevention of cardiovascular disease in ESKD are largely based on evidence from the general population. Randomized controlled trials in ESKD have been limited in size and number, and those that have been undertaken have often yielded disappointing conclusions. For example, despite the promise of statins to reduce LDL, atherosclerotic burden, and perhaps inflammation in the HD population, two large randomized, placebo-controlled trials of statins in HD patients have reported no improvement in rates of cardiovascular deaths and nonfatal cardiovascular events despite a greater than 40% reduction in LDL cholesterol levels.[850–853] Reviews of these trials have highlighted the presence of underlying cardiomyopathy, increased incidence of sudden death, and altered lipid profile with higher levels of Lp(a) and modified LDL particles, all of which may, in part, explain the lack of benefit from statins in this population.[850,854] A subsequent trial randomizing patients to simvastatin plus ezetimibe has demonstrated that statins reduce the risk of major atherosclerotic events in the total CKD study population, but not in the subgroup of over 3000 patients with ESKD, although the study was not specifically powered for this subgroup.[855]

The growing emphasis on health has focused attention on behavioral interventions that may reduce cardiovascular risk by modifying traditional risk factors. For example, smoking is a risk predictor even in the HD population.[512,856] However, little is known regarding the impact of smoking cessation on cardiovascular risk in patients on HD because the only data available in this patient population only explored the pharmacokinetics of various smoking cessation aids in the setting of kidney impairment.[857] Exercise has received growing attention. Intradialytic exercise may improve adherence and self-reported physical function measures,[858] as well as cardiac functional measures such as aerobic capacity, heart rate variability, late potentials, and T wave alternans.[859] A home-based exercise program managed by the dialysis staff is another example of a simple personalized intervention that improves physical performance and measures of quality of life.[860] Although physical activity is associated with survival in observational studies,[861,862] evidence that increasing exercise lowers mortality is still lacking. However, for patients on HD who have undergone a cardiac intervention such as CABG, exercise through a cardiac rehabilitation program is beneficial and cost-effective.[863] Finally, substantial epidemiologic data have linked poor oral health and the presence of periodontal disease to systemic inflammation and cardiovascular risk in the general population,[864] and some data for the link exist in patients on HD,[796,865,866] but causality has not been established. Whether diminishing the periodontal disease burden would reduce mortality remains to be seen.[865]

As mentioned previously, sudden cardiac death appears to be the leading cause of mortality among HD patients.[867–869] A myriad of factors may increase the risk for arrhythmias and sudden death in patients on dialysis, with the presence of LVH being one of the most prominent and coronary artery diseases playing a minor role.[289,450,870–873] Reducing LVH remains a major therapeutic focus, but without clear evidence that doing so will improve survival. The dialysis prescription itself poses additional risks for sudden death (see also "Dialysis Duration and Frequency" and "Dialysate Composition"), including short treatment time, large UF volume, and low dialysate potassium, which are potentially modifiable practices that may improve outcomes.[461] The timing of sudden death appears to cluster around the long interdialytic interval in patients on three times/week dialysis or less (either Monday or Tuesday),[460,874] a pattern not seen with more frequent therapy or PD.[875] The high incidence of sudden death has focused attention on the role of implantable defribrillators to improve survival in the dialysis population, but indications for implantation may differ from those in the general public, risks may be higher, and benefit is uncertain.[867,876,877]

In the general population, LVH is a cardiovascular risk factor that may be modified by treatment to reduce ventricular mass, such as with an ACE inhibitor.[878,879] For the HD population, an extensive review has found very limited evidence to support the use of pharmacologic treatment for cardioprotection.[880] The only reported controlled trial for ACE inhibitors and ARBs in patients on HD has demonstrated improved blood pressure control but did not reduce cardiovascular risk.[881,882] Patients with a recent MI may benefit more specifically from classic cardioprotective medications such as ACE inhibitors and beta-blockers.[880] More frequent HD reduces LVH significantly,[436,457] but whether this will translate into lower mortality is not clear.

Cardiovascular disease remains the number one cause of death in patients on HD, despite substantial progress in understanding the natural history of this disease through all the stages of CKD. Part of the reason for the lack of success in preventing cardiovascular deaths in this population may be that the vast burden of disease already exists at the initiation of HD. Another contribution is the complex interplay among inflammation, oxidative stress, malnutrition, retention of uremic solutes, the dialysis process itself, and cardiovascular disease that remains poorly understood, but renders traditional cardiac risk factors and treatment less effective in predicting and ameliorating cardiovascular mortality and morbidity in the HD population.[839,850,852,883] Finally, the transition from the high incidence of atherosclerosis-induced cardiovascular events in CKD patients (for whom traditional therapies such as statins do improve outcomes) to the predominance of sudden cardiac deaths in dialysis patients likely accounts in part for the persistently high cardiovascular mortality once patients start dialysis. For now, applying established therapeutic approaches to ameliorating traditional risk factors earlier in the course of CKD while awaiting more evidence to support altering HD management and treating nontraditional risk factors in the HD population would seem prudent. Increasing the frequency of dialysis, prolonging treatment times, limiting rapid ultrafiltration, and modifying dialysate potassium, bicarbonate, and calcium concentrations may reduce the rate of intradialytic myocardial stunning and the risk for sudden death. [436,444,445,457,843,884]

## HYPERTENSION

The complex relationship between blood pressure (BP) and the kidneys is discussed in detail in Chapters 46 and 54. Here we provide a brief discussion of the unique challenges in patients receiving HD.

The evaluation and management of BP in the HD population are complicated by the many variations in predialysis, intradialytic, postdialysis, and interdialytic BPs in any given patient and their clinical significance.[885–887] Combining intradialytic BP values with both predialysis and postdialysis BP measures have traditionally been used as surrogates of overall BP status.[888] However, peridialysis BPs are influenced significantly by volume status and correlate less well with mortality than interdialytic BPs.[889] Ambulatory BP monitoring may yield a more realistic picture of BP control and offer more prognostic information,[890,891] but its use is limited by cost and availability to patients.

Complicating matters further, several studies have shown that excessively low BPs rather than high BPs measured in the dialysis clinic are associated with mortality.[892,893] An explanation for this U-shaped curve may be that low BP acts as a potential indicator of underlying cardiac disease, poor nutritional status, and risk for dialysis-associated events. This phenomenon was illustrated in a recent prospective study that compared the utility of dialysis clinic BPs with home BPs.[894] Whereas a U-shaped association of dialysis clinic systolic BP was shown to nadir from 140 to 170 mm Hg, home BP readings showed a linear association with cardiovascular risk and death, suggesting that BPs outside the dialysis clinic may be a better measure to target.

The pharmacologic approach to managing BP has been presented (see Chapter 49) and applies to the HD population, with several unique caveats. Volume expansion is a major cause of hypertension in HD patients, with high BPs that persist, even posttreatment.[895] The challenge for nephrologists is to determine the optimal dry weight for each patient at which the BP is controlled with the fewest medications and the patient can tolerate the UF required to achieve that goal weight.[896] Achieving optimal dry weight through more frequent HD treatments per week[437] or through a gradual, protocol-driven reduction in weight for patients receiving conventional thrice-weekly HD[897] markedly improves BP control and supports volume regulation as a critical element in BP management (see also "Dialysis Duration and Frequency" section). The optimal antihypertensive regimen in ESKD has not been established.[887] The only controlled trial comparing antihypertensive agents in an HD population randomized 200 patients with LVH to atenolol versus lisinopril, with each administered thrice weekly. The findings have suggested that atenolol is superior to lisinopril in reducing cardiovascular morbidity and all-cause hospitalization.[898] Other studies have suggested that the use of ACE inhibitors and ARBs may reduce left ventricular mass[899,900] but does not seem to have an effect on cardiovascular events or mortality.[882,900,901] Drugs that are removed poorly with HD (e.g., losartan, fosinopril, ramipril, carvedilol, bisoprolol, propranolol) may improve BP control, but appear to have variable effects on cardiovascular mortality, likely through the competing effects of improved overall BP control but higher risk for intradialytic hypotension.[902–906] No definitive conclusions are possible because the studies have been few, retrospective and, when randomized, small. BPcontrol continues to be important, although the best method for establishing dry weight, optimal use of antihypertensives, target for BP control, and observed BP paradox in dialysis require further research.[885–887,896]

## IMMUNE DISORDERS AND INFECTION

Infection is the second leading cause of death and hospitalization for patients on maintenance HD after cardiovascular disease, accounting for nearly 25% of deaths and one-third of hospitalizations.[907,908] The mortality rate from sepsis may be as high as 300 times that of the general population.[909,910] Of these infections, 20% are access-related, with pulmonary, soft tissue, and genitourinary infections accounting for the remainder.[907,908] Likely reasons for the increased infection risk can be divided into two categories—those related to the

HD treatment itself and those endogenous to the patient and the uremic milieu.

## ROLE OF THE VASCULAR ACCESS AND HEMODIALYSIS PROCEDURE

A leading factor related to the HD treatment is the universal presence of some form of vascular access. As discussed earlier, the use of catheters is a significant cause of sepsis in the HD population (see "Vascular Access" section).[147,907] Biofilm, which seems to develop on all indwelling artificial surfaces, appears to play an important role in the pathogenesis of these infections.[911] Although indwelling catheters are clearly the major source of vascular access infection, the repeated percutaneous needle insertions required with AV access also contribute, with AV grafts implicated more frequently than AVF.[110] Infections in AV grafts often require removal of the graft.

The HD treatment itself presents a risk of bacterial or viral infection from the dialysis machine, dialyzer, or dialysate because of exposure to nonsterile water in the dialysate and through dialyzer reuse (see "Water Treatment"). In addition, microbe-generated impurities such as endotoxins in water may cross the dialyzer membrane and stimulate an endogenous inflammatory response. As noted, strict standards have been established for purifying water, disinfecting HD machines, and handling dialyzers, particularly if reuse is practiced. Growing evidence has suggested that impurities in the water may be a significant cause of the inflammatory responses in patients on HD,[330] and efforts are underway to find more sensitive assays and improved methods of treating water to allow for the detection and removal of these impurities.[345,354,361]

## UREMIA-INDUCED IMMUNE DISORDER

The uremic milieu gives rise to both immune activation and immunodeficiency, which contribute to the high risk and severity of infections, the reduced response to vaccines, a state of chronic inflammation and, indirectly, to cardiovascular disease.[912–914] Both innate and adaptive immune systems are altered. Monocytes, neutrophils, and dendritic cells exhibit decreased endocytosis and impaired maturation but enhanced production of interleukin-12p70 (a T cell–stimulating factor) and allogeneic T-cell proliferation.[915] The expression of Toll-like receptor 4, which detects lipopolysaccharides (LPSs) from gram-negative bacteria and leads to activation of the innate immune system, is reduced constitutively in infection-prone CKD patients not yet on HD.[916] Monocytes from these patients, when challenged with LPS, demonstrate reduced synthesis of tumor necrosis factor-α and several interleukins. This relative acquired immunodeficiency state from chronic immune activation leads to inflammation and may explain the high failure rates for vaccinations in the HD population, as well as the viral infections endemic in this population.[913,914,917]

## INFECTIONS AND RESPONSE TO VACCINATION

Hepatitis viruses have presented management challenges for the HD population since maintenance therapy became available. The risk of hepatitis B transmission has been greatly reduced by a lesser need for blood transfusions (through the use of ESAs and intravenous iron), strict isolation procedures, and vaccination, although the hepatitis vaccine is less effective than in the general population, especially if administration is delayed until after the initiation of dialysis.[913,914,918] With the declining incidence of hepatitis B, hepatitis C has become a major concern in HD clinics since the discovery that this virus explained much of the non-A, non-B hepatitis in patients on HD. The prevalence of hepatitis C is extremely variable, depending on the location of the dialysis clinic, and ranges from 4% to 70% worldwide.[919] The natural history of the disease is also variable and depends on the severity of underlying liver disease and the presence or absence of known complications, such as hepatocellular carcinoma. In a large meta-analysis, the presence of anti–hepatitis C antibodies was associated independently with a 34% increase in all-cause mortality.[920] Current recommendations to control hepatitis C transmission in the dialysis clinic include strict adherence to universal precautions, careful attention to hygiene and sterilization of dialysis machines, and routine serologic testing and surveillance for hepatitis C infection, but they do not require isolation of the affected patient or dialysis machine.[921] In the past, hepatitis C treatment in HD patients with a pegylated interferon–based regimen was complicated by lower response rates and more side effects, particularly because the use of ribavirin was limited due to the risk of drug accumulation and hemolysis.[922–924] Fortunately, newer direct-acting antivirals have become available, which have already begun to transform hepatitis C treatment in patients with CKD and ESKD.[925] These drugs are safer, better tolerated, and provide a dramatic virologic response, particularly for genotype 1, the most prevalent genotype in the United States.[926,927]

The prevalence of human immunodeficiency virus (HIV) in the HD population remains unknown because routine screening is not practiced. Estimates by the CDC of rates of HIV infection and acquired immunodeficiency syndrome (AIDS) in HD patients were about 1.5% and 0.4%, respectively.[928] The survival of HD patients infected with HIV improved significantly during the latter half of the 1990s as experience treating HIV and AIDS in the HD population increased.[929,930]

Pneumonia is a particularly common infection in the HD population. A recent observational study of Medicare patients found an incidence rate of 21.4 events/100 patient-years, with over 90% requiring hospitalization and more than 10% dying within 1 month of the event.[931] Hospital stays were almost five times longer compared with nondialysis patients and were associated with substantial cost.[931,932] Administering the pneumococcal vaccine to patients undergoing HD is recommended and is associated with decreased mortality.[933] Because of the reduced acquired immunity, patients on HD may have an impaired antibody response to vaccines, and measurable antibody levels may decrease quickly,[934] raising questions about the best approach for revaccination.

Current recommendations are for all patients on dialysis to receive the full vaccine series for hepatitis B, pneumococcal vaccine, and the appropriate seasonal influenza vaccine. The observed poor response rate to hepatitis B vaccine in the HD population mandates vaccination as early in the course of CKD as possible, careful follow-up, and revaccination when indicated. Appropriate surveillance for hepatitis B should continue, with booster vaccination for low titers of anti–hepatitis B surface antigen. Caution should be given to avoid surveillance of hepatitis B surface antigen within 3 weeks of vaccination because false- positives may occur.[935] Vaccination for herpes zoster infection is now available to minimize the impact of zoster infections in adults older than 60 years, and it appears to be most effective when given near the time of dialysis initiation.[936] Special consideration should be given to provide zoster vaccination in older pretransplantation candidates because posttransplantation immunosuppression precludes live vaccination.

## PRIMARY CARE MANAGEMENT

Patients undergoing HD still need routine health care for non-dialysis problems, just like the general population. Although opinions differ widely on its practicality and effectiveness,[937] the nephrologist will frequently find himself or herself as the sole care provider for a patient on HD, particularly those receiving in-center treatment. Of 158 patients surveyed in a suburban HD clinic, only 56 had a primary care physician. Patients just starting HD were more likely to have a primary care physician than those on HD for more than 1 year.[938] A Canadian survey has demonstrated the importance of communication among family physicians, nephrologists, and patients because excess use, duplication, and/or omission of important health care services was common.[939]

Based on limited survival benefit, routine preventive cancer screening may not be cost-effective in the average HD patient.[940,941] Instead, efforts should be made to direct age-appropriate tests to HD patients with a longer expected survival or are transplantation candidates while limiting screening in patients with significant baseline comorbidities. A recent study of colon cancer screening of Medicare beneficiaries from 2007 to 2012 reflected this, although high usage rates across all risk groups suggested persistent over-screening in the HD population.[942]

Serious clinical depression is an underrecognized illness in HD patients and correlates strongly with mortality and morbidity (see also "Transition from Chronic Kidney Disease Stage V").[30,37–39] Hence, depression is another important health care issue that should be addressed by the primary care physician, nephrologist or, optimally, both. In a review of a national Taiwanese database, it was found that HD patients are three times more likely to commit suicide than controls, with many events occurring within the first 3 months of starting dialysis.[943] It is paramount that nephrologists know if each patient has a primary care physician and communicate regularly with this physician.

# COMPLICATIONS FOR PATIENTS ON MAINTENANCE HEMODIALYSIS

Hemodialysis is a complex, life-sustaining procedure provided to patients with comorbidities. Despite the significant physiologic events that occur during the process, HD has become a relatively safe procedure. Advances in water treatment, more physiologic dialysate, technologic advances, and detailed treatment policies and protocols have contributed to its safety. However, with more than 400,000 patients undeergoing over 60 million HD sessions/year in the United States alone,[10] complications are rare but inevitable. This section will highlight important complications of maintenance HD that a clinician may encounter.

## HYPOTENSION

KDOQI guidelines define intradialytic hypotension (IDH) as a decrease in systolic BP of 20 mm Hg or more or a decrease in mean arterial pressure of 10 mm Hg or more, provided the decrease is associated with clinical events and a need for staff intervention.[944] IDH occurs in 15% to 30% of all HD sessions, with subsets of patients experiencing IDH in more than 50% of their sessions, strongly associated with large interdialytic weight gains.[575,945] Interdialytic weight gain depends principally on the difference between residual urine output and intake of sodium and fluid. Excess fluid must be removed during HD to maintain balance. Large weight gains contribute to the frequency of IDH, particularly in female patients and those with diabetes, longer dialysis vintage, older age, and underlying heart disease.[946]

### ULTRAFILTRATION

For successful UF, refilling the intravascular compartment from the extravascular space must occur. Heart rates and systemic vascular resistance increase during UF to help compensate for the decline in vascular volume. IDH occurs when these physiologic responses are unable to compensate for imbalances in vascular refilling, particularly in the setting of aggressive UF. Importantly, high UF rates (e.g., >10–13 mL/kg per hour) may increase cardiovascular morbidity and mortality.[311,572,947]

Complicating matters, solute diffusion during HD will transfer heat from dialysate to the patient (see later). A physiologic response to heat transfer is vasodilation, which counteracts the corrective response to intravascular volume reduction. Furthermore, solute diffusion will reduce intravascular osmolality and can therefore reduce the osmotic drive for vascular refilling.

### DIALYSATE FACTORS

During HD, solute removal decreases plasma osmolality and favors a shift in volume from the intravascular to extravascular space. This osmolar shift may be reduced by using a high dialysate sodium of more than 140 mEq/L. Unfortunately, the consequence is a sodium gain in most patients because predialysis serum sodium levels tend to be less than 140 mEq/L, leading to thirst, worsening of hypertension, and larger interdialytic weight gains. For these reasons, high fixed dialysate sodium concentrations are discouraged. Sodium modeling protocols, with the dialysate sodium programmed to start at a high level and decrease during treatment, were designed to reduce positive sodium balance. However, they still resulted in higher interdialytic weight gains and hypertension.[303–305,948] Individualized dialysis prescriptions with dialysate sodium approximating the endogenous sodium level may be preferred.[297–300,305]

Calcium plays a crucial role in cardiac myocyte and vascular smooth muscle contractility. A high dialysate calcium concentration of 3.5 mEq/L or higher can reduce the incidence of IDH but may accelerate vascular calcification.[510,511] In the United States, dialysate calcium concentration is typically set between 2.25 and 2.5 mEq/L to minimize calcium loading. Dialysate calcium concentrations lower than this range are associated with more frequent hypotensive episodes and cardiac arrhythmia.[541]

Although infrequently discussed, intracellular magnesium is also important for myocardial and vascular stability. Lower dialysate magnesium concentrations and hypomagnesemia may result in IDH.[543] Dialysate magnesium concentrations in the United States are usually from 0.5 to 1 mEq/L to prevent intradialytic hypomagnesemia.

As discussed in the "Dialysate Composition" section, replacement of acetate with bicarbonate as base in the dialysate may greatly reduce the incidence of IDH.

### MANAGEMENT

The first approach to managing hypotension during HD is to establish the pattern of the hypotensive episodes. Isolated episodes of hypotension may not require any alteration in the dialysis prescription other than treating the acute event. Modest declines in BP are addressed by temporary reduction in the UF rate alone or in combination with placing the patient in a supine or Trendelenburg position. For significant hypotension, these maneuvers should be combined with fluid replacement, usually 100 to 250 mL of normal saline every few minutes. On occasion, albumin or mannitol is used, although availability of these agents is limited. Saline is preferred and may be just as effective, at less expense.[949] When an episode does not reverse quickly, the dialysis staff should administer oxygen, reduce the blood flow rate, and consider more complex causes such as myocardial injury or pericardial disease. Persistent hypotension or suspicion of a dangerous clinical event requires discontinuation of the HD treatment.

Preventing further episodes of hypotension becomes the goal after the acute episode has resolved (Box 63.3). The timing of the episode within the treatment may provide some insight into a prevention strategy. Hypotension that occurs late in the treatment course may reflect a fluid removal goal that is incorrect or excessive, and patients should be carefully evaluated to determine whether postdialysis weight should be increased. There is no simple method to determine the ideal dry weight, and physical examination findings such as edema may not correlate well with intravascular volume.[575,950] Thus, careful and frequent adjustments while monitoring hemodynamics are required when reestablishing goal weight. Promising technical tools such as bioelectrical impedance analysis and lung ultrasound to estimate fluid status are under review,[582,951–953] although are not readily available at this time.

**Box 63.3 Interventions to Consider in Recurrent Intradialytic Hypotension**

Reassess dry weight.
Reduce interdialytic sodium gain.
Reduce intradialytic sodium gain.
Assess intradialytic hypocalcemia, hypokalemia, and hypomagnesemia.
Avoid food intake during dialysis.
Adjust antihypertensive medications and their timing.
Assess cardiac function.
Cool dialysate.
Extend dialysis time or add sessions per week.
Use sequential ultrafiltration or ultrafiltration modeling.
Prescribe midodrine.

Meal ingestion during dialysis may also make patients prone to IDH by lowering the peripheral vascular resistance.[954,955] Susceptible patients, particularly diabetics, should be asked to eat meals after dialysis. Antihypertensive medications also render patients more susceptible to hypotension during HD.[575] If possible, shorter acting antihypertensive medications should be avoided before HD. Longer acting antihypertensives are preferred and should be taken daily at the same time, selecting a time that would allow the scheduled antihypertensives to be given after dialysis on treatment days.

Reducing the dialysate temperature may improve hemodynamic stability by increasing vascular resistance and cardiac contractility via cold-induced sympathetic nervous system activation and may ameliorate dialysis-induced left ventricular dysfunction, myocardial stunning, and brain ischemia.[316,317,319–321,956,957] Empiric reductions of dialysate temperature by 0.5° to 1°C below body temperature, staying above 35°C, may be considered while monitoring the patient for cold-induced symptoms that could limit this intervention.

Often, the target weight may be correct but the interdialytic fluid gain is too large to remove during a single HD treatment. In this case, IDH may occur earlier in the treatment because vascular refilling cannot match the required UF rate. The focus for these patients must be on the reduction of sodium and water intake. Lowering the dialysate sodium concentration as previously described to match the patient's serum sodium level may prevent a positive sodium balance and help limit interdialytic weight gains.[297–300,305,515] In some cases, prolonging the treatment duration or providing more frequent dialysis[32,958] is required to ameliorate IDH, mainly by increasing the time available for UF in patients with large interdialytic fluid gains. Other tools to improve UF tolerance include sequential UF[589,959] and computer-controlled UF modeling. Separating filtration from diffusion may improve hemodynamic tolerability[959] but is difficult to achieve in the outpatient setting because of time constraints. Advances in technology now allow continuous monitoring of intravascular volume and/or sodium concentration with automated control of the UF rate but as yet have not solved this complication in HD. This is because most methods monitor relative and not absolute blood volume (see earlier discussion).[279,280,284,291,960]

Assessment of primary cardiac disease should also be considered. IDH may be a manifestation of heart failure, ischemic heart disease, or a pericardial effusion. Echocardiography or stress testing may help elucidate any potential underlying cardiac factors.

A meta-analysis of the literature concluded that patients with resistant IDH despite the interventions described or with autonomic insufficiency may respond to midodrine, an oral $\alpha_1$-adrenergic agonist, at a dose of 2.5 to 10 mg given 15 to 30 minutes before HD.[961] Side effects include supine hypertension, urinary retention, pilomotor reactions, and gastrointestinal complaints.[956,962] Peak levels occur at 60 minutes; it is partially removed by HD, so a second smaller dose may be required partly through the HD session.

## MUSCLE CRAMPS

Muscle cramps occur during or after approximately 60% of HD treatments, are quite painful, reduce quality of life, and are a common reason for early session termination.[963]

Pathogenic mechanisms may relate to vasoconstriction and impaired oxygen delivery to muscle in the setting of hypotension, as well as muscle cell osmotic and fluid shifts during HD. The accumulation of as yet unidentified uremic solutes may predispose to interdialytic muscle cramps, along with a deficiency of various nutritional substances.

When muscle cramps accompany hypotensive episodes on HD, giving careful attention to UF rates, reassessing dry weight, increasing the frequency or duration of dialysis, and educating the patient to reduce interdialytic fluid gains can prevent cramps in many cases. The strategies described earlier to prevent IDH may also be applicable to dialysis-associated cramps. Acute management may include cessation of UF in conjunction with small boluses of normal saline to treat both cramps and IDH. Hypertonic (23%) saline and 50% dextrose solution have occasionally been used in small volumes for acute management of cramps,[964] although they will predispose to interdialytic weight gain and hyperglycemia, respectively, and are thus less desirable agents.

No agent is universally effective in preventing HD-associated cramps. Vitamin E before bedtime may be considered, although its effectiveness has only been examined in a few small studies.[965–968] L-Carnitine deficiency has been proposed as a cause of muscle cramping, but a meta-analysis of L-carnitine supplementation was inconclusive as to its benefit.[969] In the past, quinine was prescribed to treat intradialytic and nocturnal cramps. However, due to controversy over its efficacy and adverse events such as drug-induced thrombotic microangiopathy, QT prolongation, and hypersensitivity reactions, its use has largely been abandoned. The FDA has placed a black box warning against quinine use for muscle cramps and has removed it from the over-the-counter market.

## DIALYSIS DISEQUILIBRIUM SYNDROME

Severe dialysis disequilibrium syndrome (DDS) is characterized by mental status changes, generalized seizures, and coma. Its occurrence has declined, in part because of increased awareness and earlier initiation of maintenance HD.[970,971] A milder form of DDS, manifesting with nausea and vomiting, headaches, fatigue, and restlessness, is still evident. Risk factors include first dialysis treatment, a markedly elevated predialysis BUN level, severe metabolic acidosis, extremes of age, and preexisting neurologic conditions.[970] However, there is no set BUN value above which patients predictably develop DDS nor a BUN value below which uremic patients are safe from developing DDS.

The pathogenesis for DDS is likely multifactorial, but the major suspect is the rapid reduction in solute levels over a relatively short time frame.[971,972] Animal studies have suggested that a transient urea concentration gradient may be created between plasma and the cerebrospinal fluid (CSF) during dialysis.[970,971] Uremia may potentiate this gradient by reducing urea transporter expression and increasing aquaporin expression in the brain.[973] Cerebral edema during dialysis may occur due to the resulting delay in urea egress and enhancement of water uptake into brain cells. In addition, provision of bicarbonate in the dialysate may lead to paradoxic acidosis in the CSF through diffusion of carbon dioxide across the blood-brain barrier, further compromising the ability of the brain to regulate solute and water transport.[970,971]

Timely initiation of dialysis and careful attention in crafting the initial dialysis prescription are the keys to preventing DDS. Several maneuvers can be used to reduce clearance and hence the risk for DDS during the first two or three HD treatments: (1) prescribing shorter treatment times of 1.5 to 2 hours; (2) lowering blood flow rates to 200 to 250 mL/min; (3) reducing dialysate flow rate and using concurrent rather than countercurrent flow; and (4) choosing a dialyzer with a small surface area. Increasing the dialysate sodium concentration or administering intravenous mannitol may also help prevent disequilibrium.[970,971] If an acute event with significant mental status changes or seizures occurs, immediate termination of treatment and the use of mannitol or hypertonic saline are recommended.

## CARDIAC EVENTS

### ARRHYTHMIAS, MYOCARDIAL STUNNING, AND DEATH

According to USRDS data, arrhythmia and cardiac arrest account for 40% of identifiable deaths among patients with ESKD, an alarmingly high number.[10] Underlying cardiac disease with LVH, coronary vascular disease, and disordered calcium and phosphate metabolism, with possible calcific deposits in the conduction system, predispose patients to arrhythmias and cardiac arrest during HD.[445] The high propensity for arrhythmias is partly attributable to the interdialytic accumulation and subsequent HD-induced removal of solute and fluid, especially when the removal rate exceeds diffusion out of the extravascular and intracellular compartments. Cardiac arrest events appear to cluster around the long interdialytic interval in patients undergoing three or fewer HD sessions/week (either Monday or Tuesday),[460,874] a pattern that is not seen with more frequent therapy or PD.[875]

Alterations in serum potassium during dialysis may be the major factor, although changes in Ca, magnesium, and pH may also be contributing factors (see "Dialysate Composition"). Large observational studies have shown associations between arrhythmia and low-potassium baths (<2 mEq/L).[461,522,974] Many patients in these studies were prescribed low potassium dialysate concentrations despite normal predialysis serum potassium levels, supporting the need to be vigilant in adjusting potassium prescriptions. No difference in risk was seen in a recent observational study comparing potassium baths of 2 versus 3 mEq/L.[520]

Cardiac arrest may be the most concerning occurrence in an outpatient HD clinic. One center has reported 102 cardiac arrests over a 14-year period, with the vast majority occurring during treatment; 72 of the episodes were related to ventricular tachycardia.[975] Although the availability of easy to use external defibrillators may have a positive impact on the outcomes of such arrests, the 1-year survival rate is poor at 15%.[975] An implantable cardioverter defibrillator (ICD) may reduce cardiac arrest rates in high-risk patients, but still leave HD patients with a 2.7-fold higher risk of death compared with nondialysis ICD recipients.[976,977] The use of ICDs for primary prevention does not appear to provide a survival benefit.[978,979] Furthermore, there is a risk of central venous stenosis and infectious complications from intravascular ICD leads.[980] Newer leadless devices, such as subcutaneous implantable and wearable external defibrillators, may be promising alternatives in the future.

In addition to ventricular arrhythmias, atrial arrhythmias may occur during HD. Atrial fibrillation is common in patients on HD, with a prevalence rate of over 20%.[10] Compared with the general population, patients with ESKD have a risk factor profile that could theoretically benefit from anticoagulation because of enhanced stroke risk.[981–984] However, patients on HD also experience more bleeding complications, making management decisions difficult and requiring an individualized risk-benefit analysis.[985–989] Most studies of anticoagulation in patients undergoing HD have evaluated the efficacy of warfarin and are observational.[982,983,990] The outcomes of patients treated with newer, non–vitamin K-dependent oral anticoagulants are presently being evaluated in clinical trials.

Finally, ischemia may occur during HD, even in the absence of chest pain, as demonstrated by the release of troponin during HD, the onset of regional left ventricular dysfunction on the echocardiogram, and reduced myocardial blood flow by positron emission tomography.[289,870,871,991,992] Ultimately, such changes in myocardial blood flow lead to myocardial stunning, and the HD procedure itself may contribute significantly to overall cardiac mortality.[12]

### PERICARDIAL DISEASE

Pericardial disease is a well-recognized complication in patients with ESKD. Occasionally, pericarditis develops in patients with stage 5 CKD before they start dialysis, likely because of an inappropriate delay in therapy. Patients may present with typical findings of fever, pleuritic chest pain worse when recumbent, and a pericardial rub, although a fair proportion of patients may be asymptomatic and without physical findings.[993] Pericarditis that occurs within 8 weeks of initiation of dialysis is arbitrarily considered uremic disease, presumed to be due to the accumulation of as yet unidentified uremic toxins. Pericarditis in patients already on maintenance HD is likely multifactorial and not attributable to uremia because most of these patients are undergoing adequate and consistent dialysis. However, HD patients with a catheter as access, vascular access malfunction (e.g., stenosis at the venous anastomosis, with recirculation), larger body size, or poor adherence with treatment are at risk of having poor solute clearance and, hence, uremic pericarditis. Patients with uremic disease are managed with intensification of dialysis via longer or more frequent sessions.[994] Pericarditis in a well-dialyzed patient does not respond to intensifying dialysis and is likely related to another condition, such as a viral infection or autoimmune disease.[994] Complications of pericarditis in patients undergoing HD include cardiac tamponade and constrictive disease. Systemic anticoagulation, including during HD, should be avoided to reduce the risk of pericardial hemorrhage. Approaches to treating pericarditis that does not improve with intensification of dialysis range from antiinflammatory medication (both systemic and intrapericardial) to surgery when pericardial disease leads to hemodynamic compromise.[994]

## REACTIONS TO DIALYZERS

Historically, reactions to hemodialyzer membranes or residual sterilants frequently occurred during the HD treatment. Dialyzer reactions were classified as types A and B.[201,995] Type A reactions occur within 5 to 20 minutes and present with pruritus, urticaria, bronchospasm, or anaphylactic shock. The classic "first use" syndrome, when a patient is exposed to a particular dialyzer for the first time, can resemble an anaphylactic episode and result in profound hypotension and death. These reactions are likely caused by IgE antibodies to membrane material or ethylene oxide, a sterilizing agent that is rarely used now (see also "Hemodialyzers" section).[996]

Type B reactions are complement-mediated, occur later in the dialysis session, and are associated with less severe symptoms, such as chest and back discomfort. The advent of more biocompatible membrane material, careful rinsing of the dialyzer before each session, and nonchemical methods such as the use of steam, gamma rays, and electron beams to sterilize dialyzers, has greatly reduced the frequency of these events. Newer synthetic membrane materials such as polyacrylonitrile and polysulfone cause less complement activation and are better tolerated than older cellulose membranes. However, one specific membrane, polyacrylonitrile (AN69), confers a unique risk when used in patients receiving ACE inhibitors. Bradykinin that is stimulated by AN69-induced activation of Hageman factor accumulates in the presence of ACE inhibitors (ACE degrades bradykinin) and predisposes to episodes of hypotension.[997,998]

The differential diagnosis for an allergic event during HD includes reactions to dialyzers, dialyzer sterilants or disinfectants (e.g., ethylene oxide, formaldehyde, bleach), or administered medications (e.g., heparin, intravenous iron).[201] Treatment of patients suspected of having a severe allergic reaction includes saline for hypotension, epinephrine for anaphylaxis or severe hypotension, urgent cessation of HD without blood return, and possibly corticosteroid use. Other complications that can mimic an allergic reaction should also be ruled out, such as exposure to contaminated water used to prepare the dialysate (see "Water Treatment" section), pyrogenic reaction, hemolysis, and air embolism.

## OTHER COMPLICATIONS

When the dialyzer membrane separating blood from the dialysate is disrupted, the patient's blood is contaminated with nonsterile dialysate, and pyrogenic reactions may ensue. The HD machine is designed to detect such blood leaks, signal an alarm, and turn off the blood pump to stop dialysis. The dialysis staff must then test the dialysate directly to confirm the blood leak. Administration of cyanocobalamin may trigger a false blood leak alarm in some dialysis machines.[999,1000]

Hemolysis likely occurs to some degree during every HD treatment because of mechanical trauma to RBCs.[1001] More profound acute hemolysis during dialysis may result from mechanical problems such as defective dialysis tubing and roller pumps, with excessive RBC fragmentation, improper proportioning of the dialysate concentrate with osmotically induced hemolysis, overheating of the dialysate, and contamination of the dialysate with chemicals such as formaldehyde, bleach, chloramines, zinc, and copper.[201,1002] This degree of hemolysis will likely trigger the blood alarm, and patients may experience chest tightness, back pain, and shortness of breath, with acute pigmentation of the skin and port wine appearance of the blood in the venous line.[1003] In such an event, treatment should be discontinued immediately without returning the blood to the patient, and the serum potassium concentration should be determined. The diagnosis can be confirmed by assaying for free hemoglobin and examining the peripheral smear. The dialysate should be screened for its composition and contaminants, and the blood tubing should be inspected to determine the proximate cause.

Air embolism is another complication of the dialysis procedure that can lead to death unless quickly detected.[201] Air may enter the circuit due to a loose prepump connection or residual air left in the tubing or dialyzer from poor priming; this manifests as foam in the venous line. Fortunately, air detectors in HD machines have made air embolism a rare occurrence while on treatment, but air entry during disconnection may still occur, particularly with a catheter access. Immediate treatment of suspected air embolism includes stopping the blood pump, clamping the venous dialysis line to prevent further air entry, administering oxygen to reduce air bubble size, performing volume resuscitation, and placing the patient supine to preserve hemodynamic stability and reduce the potential for cerebral edema..[201,1004]

Hemorrhage during dialysis is an obvious risk, given the typical dialysis blood flow of 300 to 500 mL/min into an extracorporeal circuit. Mechanical events such as blood tubing disconnection and needle dislodgement are usually detected by safety technology in the HD machine (see "Components of the Extracorporeal Circuit" section). However, venous needle dislodgement may be unnoticed until significant loss of blood has occurred because venous pressure thresholds, and subsequent alarms, may vary with needle and tubing sizes, blood flow and viscosity, access characteristics, and patient positioning.[201] Proper taping of access needles, adequate tightening of connections, and loose looping of lines all help prevent such events. Exposure of the access during HD should be the practice in every clinic, increasing the likelihood that the dialysis staff will promptly identify and address bleeding from the vascular access or blood circuit.

Hypoglycemia is a rare event during HD because of the common use of dialysate with a glucose concentration of 200 mg/dL.[1005] When observed, it is often in a diabetic patient on an antiglycemic agent and warrants adjusting the dose or time of administration of the drug. Studies have suggested that dialysate glucose concentrations higher than 100 mg/dL predispose to hyperglycemia and increased vagal tone in patients with diabetes, possibly contributing to intradialytic hypotension.[562,563]

 Complete reference list available at ExpertConsult.com.

## KEY REFERENCES


12. Loutradis C, Sarafidis PA, Papadopoulos CE, et al. The Ebb and Flow of Echocardiographic Cardiac Function Parameters in Relationship to Hemodialysis Treatment in Patients with ESKD. *J Am Soc Nephrol.* 2018;29:1372–1381.
26. Giannaki CD, Hadjigeorgiou GM, Karatzaferi C, et al. Epidemiology, impact, and treatment options of restless legs syndrome in end-stage renal disease patients: an evidence-based review. *Kidney Int.* 2014;85:1275–1282.
30. Goh ZS, Griva K. Anxiety and depression in patients with end-stage renal disease: impact and management challenges - a narrative review. *Int J Nephrol Renovasc Dis.* 2018;11:93–102.
46. Hedayati SS, Gregg LP, Carmody T, et al. Effect of sertraline on depressive symptoms in patients with chronic kidney disease without dialysis dependence: the CAST randomized clinical trial. *JAMA.* 2017;318:1876–1890.
67. Fung E, Chang TI, Chertow GM, et al. Receipt of nephrology care and clinical outcomes among veterans with advanced CKD. *Am J Kidney Dis.* 2017;70:705–714.
97. Rivara MB, Mehrotra R. Timing of dialysis initiation: what has changed since IDEAL? *Semin Nephrol.* 2017;37:181–193.
110. Ravani P, Palmer SC, Oliver MJ, et al. Associations between hemodialysis access type and clinical outcomes: a systematic review. *J Am Soc Nephrol.* 2013;24:465–473.
123. Al-Jaishi AA, Oliver MJ, Thomas SM, et al. Patency rates of the arteriovenous fistula for hemodialysis: a systematic review and meta-analysis. *Am J Kidney Dis.* 2014;63:464–478.
137. Brown RS, Patibandla BK, Goldfarb-Rumyantzev AS. The survival benefit of "fistula first, catheter last" in hemodialysis is primarily due to patient factors. *J Am Soc Nephrol.* 2017;28:645–652.
144. Allon M. Treatment guidelines for dialysis catheter-related bacteremia: an update. *Am J Kidney Dis.* 2009;54:13–17.
152. Krishna VN, Eason JB, Allon M. Central venous occlusion in the hemodialysis patient. *Am J Kidney Dis.* 2016;68:803–807.
176. Drew DA, Lok CE, Cohen JT, et al. Vascular access choice in incident hemodialysis patients: a decision analysis. *J Am Soc Nephrol.* 2015;26:183–191.
177. Hall RK, Myers ER, Rosas SE, et al. Choice of hemodialysis access in older adults: a cost-effectiveness analysis. *Clin J Am Soc Nephrol.* 2017;12:947–954.
201. Saha M, Allon M. Diagnosis, treatment, and prevention of hemodialysis emergencies. *Clin J Am Soc Nephrol.* 2017;12:357–369.
260. Locatelli F, Karaboyas A, Pisoni RL, et al. Mortality risk in patients on hemodiafiltration versus hemodialysis: a 'real-world' comparison from the DOPPS. *Nephrol Dial Transplant.* 2018;33:683–689.
282. Ekinci C, Karabork M, Siriopol D, et al. Effects of Volume Overload and Current Techniques for the Assessment of Fluid Status in Patients with Renal Disease. *Blood Purif.* 2018;46:34–47.
295. Kron S, Schneditz D, Czerny J, et al. Adjustment of target weight based on absolute blood volume reduces the frequency of intradialytic morbid events. *Hemodial Int.* 2018;22:254–260.
299. Flythe JE, McCausland FR. Dialysate sodium: rationale for evolution over time. *Semin Dial.* 2017;30:99–111.
328. Coulliette AD, Arduino MJ. Hemodialysis and water quality. *Semin Dial.* 2013;26:427–438.
374. Vanholder RC, Eloot S, Glorieux GL. Future avenues to decrease uremic toxin concentration. *Am J Kidney Dis.* 2016;67:664–676.
440. Tennankore KK, Na Y, Wald R, et al. Short daily-, nocturnal- and conventional-home hemodialysis have similar patient and treatment survival. *Kidney Int.* 2018;93:188–194.
441. Hakim RM, Saha S. Dialysis frequency versus dialysis time, that is the question. *Kidney Int.* 2014;85:1024–1029.
445. Makar MS, Pun PH. Sudden cardiac death among hemodialysis patients. *Am J Kidney Dis.* 2017;69:684–695.
480. Kessler M, Moureau F, Nguyen P. Anticoagulation in chronic hemodialysis: progress toward an optimal approach. *Semin Dial.* 2015;28:474–489.
510. McGill RL, Weiner DE. Dialysate composition for hemodialysis: changes and changing risk. *Semin Dial.* 2017;30:112–120.
520. Karaboyas A, Zee J, Brunelli SM, et al. Dialysate potassium, serum potassium, mortality, and arrhythmia events in hemodialysis: results from the Dialysis Outcomes and Practice Patterns Study (DOPPS). *Am J Kidney Dis.* 2017;69:266–277.
529. Sterns RH, Grieff M, Bernstein PL. Treatment of hyperkalemia: something old, something new. *Kidney Int.* 2016;89:546–554.
531. Langote A, Ahearn M, Zimmerman D. Dialysate calcium concentration, mineral metabolism disorders, and cardiovascular disease: deciding the hemodialysis bath. *Am J Kidney Dis.* 2015;66:348–358.
543. Alhosaini M, Leehey DJ. Magnesium and dialysis: the neglected cation. *Am J Kidney Dis.* 2015;66:523–531.
553. Abramowitz MK. Bicarbonate Balance and Prescription in ESKD. *J Am Soc Nephrol.* 2017;28:726–734.
564. Larkin JW, Reviriego-Mendoza MM, Usvyat LA, et al. To cool, or too cool: is reducing dialysate temperature the optimal approach to preventing intradialytic hypotension? *Semin Dial.* 2017;30:501–508.
571. Sinha AD, Agarwal R. Setting the dry weight and its cardiovascular implications. *Semin Dial.* 2017;30:481–488.
572. Kramer H, Yee J, Weiner DE, et al. Ultrafiltration rate thresholds in maintenance hemodialysis: an NKF-KDOQI controversies report. *Am J Kidney Dis.* 2016;68:522–532.
573. Chou JA, Kalantar-Zadeh K, Mathew AT. A brief review of intradialytic hypotension with a focus on survival. *Semin Dial.* 2017;30:473–480.

577. Tabinor M, Davies SJ. The use of bioimpedance spectroscopy to guide fluid management in patients receiving dialysis. *Curr Opin Nephrol Hypertens.* 2018.
586. Trinh E, Bargman JM. Are diuretics underutilized in dialysis patients? *Semin Dial.* 2016;29:338–341.
591. Upadhyay A, Jaber BL. Reuse and biocompatibility of hemodialysis membranes: clinically relevant? *Semin Dial.* 2017;30:121–124.
600. Agar JW. Green dialysis: the environmental challenges ahead. *Semin Dial.* 2015;28:186–192.
639. Shepshelovich D, Rozen-Zvi B, Avni T, et al. Intravenous versus oral iron supplementation for the treatment of anemia in CKD: an updated systematic review and meta-analysis. *Am J Kidney Dis.* 2016;68:677–690.
696. Kovesdy CP. Malnutrition in dialysis patients–the need for intervention despite uncertain benefits. *Semin Dial.* 2016;29:28–34.
709. Miskulin DC, Majchrzak K, Tighiouart H, et al. Ergocalciferol supplementation in hemodialysis patients with vitamin D deficiency: a randomized clinical trial. *J Am Soc Nephrol.* 2016;27:1801–1810.
759. Nigwekar SU, Thadhani R, Brandenburg VM. Calciphylaxis. *N Engl J Med.* 2018;378:1704–1714.
846. Wang Y, Zhu S, Gao P, et al. Comparison of coronary artery bypass grafting and drug-eluting stents in patients with chronic kidney disease and multivessel disease: a meta-analysis. *Eur J Intern Med.* 2017;43:28–35.
887. Miskulin DC, Weiner DE. Blood pressure management in hemodialysis patients: what we know and what questions remain. *Semin Dial.* 2017;30:203–212.
894. Bansal N, McCulloch CE, Lin F, et al. Blood pressure and risk of cardiovascular events in patients on chronic hemodialysis: the CRIC study (Chronic Renal Insufficiency Cohort). *Hypertension.* 2017;70:435–443.
902. Assimon MM, Brookhart MA, Fine JP, et al. A comparative study of carvedilol versus metoprolol initiation and 1-year mortality among individuals receiving maintenance hemodialysis. *Am J Kidney Dis.* 2018.
954. Agarwal R, Georgianos P. Feeding during dialysis-risks and uncertainties. *Nephrol Dial Transplant.* 2018;33:917–922.
984. McCullough PA, Ball T, Cox KM, et al. Use of oral anticoagulation in the management of atrial fibrillation in patients with ESKD: pro. *Clin J Am Soc Nephrol.* 2016;11:2079–2084.
985. Keskar V, Sood MM. Use of oral anticoagulation in the management of atrial fibrillation in patients with ESKD: con. *Clin J Am Soc Nephrol.* 2016;11:2085–2092.

# 64 Peritoneal Dialysis

Ricardo Correa-Rotter | Rajnish Mehrotra | Anjali Bhatt Saxena

## CHAPTER OUTLINE



## PERITONEAL MEMBRANE ANATOMY AND STRUCTURE

The peritoneum is a serous, semipermeable membrane constituted of a thin layer of connective tissue covered by a mesothelial cell monolayer, which covers most of the abdominal wall and intraabdominal organs. This mesothelium derives from mesenchymal cells which form a basement membrane, develop tight junctions, and desmosomes.[1] At the peritoneal cavity side, the mesothelial cells have abundant microvilli, which have anionic fixed charges and play a role in the transmembrane transfer of small charged molecules as well as plasma proteins.[1–4] The surface area of the human adult peritoneum is variable and ranges from 1.6 to 2.0 $m^2$, yet microvilli increase total peritoneal surface up to 40 $m^2$.[5] Loss of microvilli is a common morphological change of the peritoneal membrane in patients receiving peritoneal dialysis (PD). When the peritoneal membrane is injured and mesothelial cells are undergoing apoptosis, surface anionic charges are reduced.[6]

The peritoneal microvessels and mesothelium are thought to function by either a two- or three-pore size model of capillary permeability.[7,8] The three pore model pore sizes are: more than 150 Å for large pores, up to 40 to 45 Å for small pores, and 2 to 5 Å for ultra-small pores. The main pathway for exchanges across the microvascular wall is the junctions between capillary endothelial cells.

Mesothelial cells of the peritoneum have glucose transporters which play an active role in solute transport.[9] In addition, mesothelial cells express aquaporin channels, which correspond physiologically to the "ultra-small pores." These channels may be modulated by diverse stimuli, including stimuli that are osmotic and nonosmotic.[8] Desmosomes have also been observed near the cellular luminal front and gap junctions.[10]

The presence of mesothelial cells with stomata of 4 to 12 μm that communicate between the abdominal cavity and the submesothelial diaphragmatic lymphatics have been demonstrated.[11] Movement through this pathway of very large particles, as large as red blood cells, malignant cells, bacteria, and others have been demonstrated.[12,13] Acti-like filaments of stomatal mesothelial cells, their channels, and lymphatic endothelial cells induce cell contraction and allow the passage of macromolecules and cells.

Under the mesothelial cell layer of the peritoneum there is a mono-layered structure denominated by the basement membrane, which has anionic charges along both the lamina rara externa and lamina rara interna.[1,3] After long-term treatment with PD this basement membrane may duplicate and this phenomenon may be induced by cell death and by local exposure to high glucose concentration.[14]

The peritoneal interstitium (variable in thickness from 1 to 30 μm) is composed mainly of fibroblasts, collagen fibers, and by an amorphous proteinaceous substance (glycosaminoglycans, mainly hyaluronic acid), which displays anionic charges. Additionally, macrophages and mast cells are often, and monocytes rarely, present in this structure.[3,15] Solute movement across the interstitial tissue is modified by diverse factors including thickness of the interstitium in that specific site as well as molecular weight, shape, and electric charge of the molecule.[16] To modulate the flow of water from plasma to lymph and to prevent interstitial edema, the local interstitial pressure is usually low and, at times, negative (0 to −4 mm Hg).[17] Transfer of small solutes along the interstitium that is in general diffusive yet convective transport also contributes in the parietal peritoneum.[18] Intraabdominal pressure plays an important role in the movement of fluid from the cavity to the interstitium. During PD, a positive intraabdominal pressure from 4 to 10 cm of $H_2O$ drives fluid and solutes from the cavity to the interstitium and fluid loss is directly proportional to intraabdominal pressure.[19]

A thin basement membrane of the endothelial capillaries separates them from the connective tissue of the interstitium. Capillaries with fenestrae are present in the peritoneum and these structures as well as intercellular junctions play an important role in their permeability.[20] Tight junctions (zonula occludens) link the endothelial cells in a monolayer structure.[21] In addition, the arteriolar endothelium typically exhibits gap junctions. There is significant controversy on which is the main pathway for water as well as small and large solutes across the peritoneal membrane. While some consider the intercellular cleft as the main pathway, others believe that tight junctions offer a paracellular barrier that regulates movement of water, solutes, and even immune cells between the interstitial space and the microvascular compartment.[22,23]

When the presence of aquaporin-1 channels was demonstrated, it was clear that water transport occurs through several pathways. In addition to its transport via the paracellular pathway through intercellular junctions at the endothelial level, transcellular water transport was confirmed and a significant proportion of water transport flows through these ultra-small transcellular pores.[24,25]

## PERITONEAL TRANSPORT PHYSIOLOGY

In PD, solute transport occurs through both diffusion and convection. Diffusion takes place given the presence of a concentration gradient across a semipermeable membrane. The first law of Fick (the transfer rate of a solute is determined by the diffusive permeability of the membrane to that solute, the surface area available for transport, and the concentration) governs diffusion across the peritoneal membrane. A second mechanism involved in solute transport is convection, which takes place during ultrafiltration. This type of transport is determined by the mean concentration of the solute, water flux, and the specific solute reflection coefficient of the membrane.[26] A factor that influences transport across the peritoneal membrane is the effective surface area available for this process to happen and is strongly determined by the number of capillaries and the proportion of the peritoneal membrane in contact with the dialysate. In addition, the peritoneal membrane has a defined intrinsic permeability, which determines the features of solutes to be transported.[27]

The peritoneum poses several barriers to solute transport.[28] Peritoneal capillaries are the main barrier. A two-pore theory proposes the presence of abundant small pores of 40 to 50 Å and few larger pores of up to 150 Å.[29] With the confirmation of the presence of transcellular (endothelial cells) ultra-small pores (aquaporin-1 channels, 3 to 5 Å) it has been shown that around 50% of the transcapillary ultrafiltration occurs through them.[25,30] This led investigators to propose a three-pore model, which has shown that around 50% of the transcapillary ultrafiltration occurs through aquaporin-1 channels and the remaining mostly through small pores.[31,32] The interstitium constitutes a significant barrier to water and solute transport across the peritoneal membrane.[33–35] In order to describe the kinetics of water and solute movement during PD, several distributed models have been proposed.[34,36–38]

Solute transport along time is highly dependent on the ultrastructural characteristics of peritoneal capillaries. Transport of low and medium molecular weight solutes depends mostly on their size and the surface area available for transport and to a lesser degree to changes of permeability of the, and peritoneum.[39] Transport of larger molecules is size-selective therefore depends on several factors including effective membrane surface area, permeability of the membrane itself, and on the molecular size of the solute.[31,40] While in animal models the anionic negative charge at the peritoneal barrier may restrict macromolecular clearance, this phenomenon has not been demonstrated in humans.[40,41] In order to calculate the mass transfer area coefficient (MTAC), which is the theoretical instantaneous maximal clearance at time 0 without ultrafiltration, models of variable complexity have been proposed.[38,42] For PD clinical practice, simple procedures that correlate appropriately with MTAC have been developed. For example, a 24-hour clearance or a 4-hour dialysate/plasma (D/P) ratio of low molecular weight solutes is clinically used to evaluate dialysis efficiency.[43] As described above, diffusive transport accounts for the majority of low molecular weight removal (e.g., potassium, urea, and creatinine) and convection represents a small proportion of solute transport.[44,45]

Peritoneal water transport is mostly driven through an osmotic gradient generated by additives of the PD solution, generally glucose or icodextrin. The normal peritoneal membrane also presents a small and continuous amount of transcapillary ultrafiltration to the peritoneal cavity through differences in hydrostatic and colloid osmotic pressures and via small and ultra-small pores. Coupled to this transcapillary ultrafiltration there is reabsorption of water from the peritoneal cavity through transcapillary back-filtration and peritoneal lymphatics.[46] Given these physiologic pathways of water transport, the net ultrafiltration achieved in a PD exchange is the balance between the transcapillary ultrafiltration into the cavity and back absorption through capillaries and lymphatics.

As described above, the osmotic reflection coefficient of a given dialysate solution determines its effectiveness to induce ultrafiltration. Large molecules such as proteins are not permeable and have a reflection coefficient of 1, while very small solutes have a reflection coefficient close to 0. The reflection coefficient may be different according to the size of the pores; therefore glucose through "small pores" is very low and close to 0, while it is very high (value of 1 and impermeable) through aquaporin-1 ultra-small pores.[47–49]

Water transport during a standard glucose-based dialysate can be described as follows[44,46]: When dialysate is infused (time 0), glucose concentration in the dialysate is highest and therefore, crystalloid osmotic pressure and ultrafiltration rate are also highest. Glucose is absorbed from the dialysate over time (almost two thirds of glucose content of a solution over a 4-hour period), and the crystalloid pressure and ultrafiltration diminish.[50] Ultrafiltration volume accumulates within the peritoneal cavity and will peak at the time there is osmotic equilibrium between serum and dialysate. This process will take place along with a progressive reduction of transcapillary ultrafiltration rate, to the point in which it is equal to the rate of lymphatic and back absorption of the capillaries. From then on, and if the lymphatic and back absorption rates exceed the transcapillary ultrafiltration rate, intraperitoneal volume will diminish. Patients will display individualized transport characteristics that can be explored with a clinical peritoneal transport test (see the following section).[44]

## EVALUATION OF PERITONEAL SOLUTE AND WATER TRANSFER RATE

In patients with end-stage renal disease, maintenance dialysis allows for the removal of solutes and water that would otherwise be excreted by the kidneys. The efficiency of solute and water removal depends, in part, on the characteristics of the dialysis membrane. In patients treated with PD, the naturally occurring peritoneal barrier serves as the dialysis membrane. It has long been recognized that there is a large inter-individual variability in the efficiency of transfer of solutes and water across the peritoneal barrier and in a significant proportion of individuals the efficiency and other transport characteristics change over time with exposure to PD solutions.[44,51] Hence, it is imperative to characterize the peritoneal solute and water transfer rate to individualize the dialysis prescriptions. This testing is often performed at the time of initiation of dialysis or soon thereafter and repeated if clinically indicated.

Several approaches have been developed to characterize the rate of solute and water transfer in patients undergoing PD. These include the Peritoneal Equilibration Test (PET), Standard Permeability Analysis (SPA), Peritoneal Dialysis Capacity (PDC), and Dialysis Adequacy and Transport Test (DATT).[44,50,52,53] Each of these tests allow for a standardized assessment of solute transfer and ultrafiltration capacity of the peritoneum, information that is critical to fashion an effective PD prescription (Table 64.1). Often, the solute transfer function and ultrafiltration capacity as assessed by each of these tests is not the same as a precise measure of diffusion and convection across the peritoneum. Common to these approaches is that each step of the procedure is performed in a standardized way. This standardization is critical in ensuring the reproducibility of the results, essential for its clinical application.

**Table 64.1 Parameters Obtained From Standardized Tests to Evaluate Peritoneal Membrane Function**

| Test | Solute | Fluid Removal |
|---|---|---|
| Peritoneal equilibration test | D/P creatinine<br>D/D0 glucose | Drain volume |
| Standard permeability analysis | Mass transfer area coefficient, creatine | Drain volume<br>D/P sodium |
| Peritoneal dialysis capacity | Area parameter | Ultrafiltration coefficient |
| Dialysis adequacy and transport test | 24-hour D/P creatinine | 24-hour drain volume |

The PET is the most widely used measure of assessment of peritoneal solute and water transfer rates because of overall ease of use and interpretation in day-to-day clinical practice. The key elements of the process that were standardized when the test was first described included having a long preceding overnight exchange (8-12 hours), method to completely drain the overnight exchange prior to start of test (sitting position, over 20 minutes), volume and concentration of dialysate instilled (2L of 2.5% dextrose), rate of infusion (400 mL/2 minutes; total infusion time, 10 minutes), total dwell time (240 minutes), timing of collection of dialysate (0, 30, 60, 120, 180, and 240 minutes), time for venipuncture (120 minutes), and the way the results of the test are expressed (4-hour dialysate to 2-hour plasma creatinine, "D/P" creatinine, or similarly for other solutes; 4-hour to 0-hour dialysate glucose, D/D0 glucose; and ultrafiltration volume).[44] Since the first description of the test, the standardized test has been modified for collection of dialysate at 0, 120, and 240 minutes (modified PET). A large number of other variations to this initial description of the modified PET have been described and include variation in length of preceding exchange, dwell time (60 minutes), tonicity of dialysate (4.25% dextrose), or the use of biocompatible PD solutions.[54–60] Still, the overwhelming majority of patients starting treatment undergo the modified PET with 2 L 2.5% dextrose.

As noted above, there is a large inter-individual variability in the rate of transfer of solute and water across the peritoneum, requiring assessment of peritoneal function in each patient. Even though the PET can describe the rate of transport of virtually any solute, the 4-hour D/P creatinine is the parameter most widely used both for clinical and research purposes. Large population-based studies suggest that, on average, the dialysate concentration of creatinine at four hours is about two thirds that in the blood (or 4-hour D/P creatinine, 0.67).[44] It is conventional to assign patients a "transport" type based on the results of the PET as low, low-average, high-average, or high (or slow, slow-average, fast-average, and fast) transporters.[44] Individuals assigned as having an average transport are the ones that are within one standard deviation of the mean and the ones with slow or fast transport are more than one standard deviation below or above the mean, respectively.

Variability in the peritoneal solute transfer rate likely reflects, for the most part, the density of peritoneal capillaries per unit surface area. Simply, the 4-h D/P creatinine could be considered as a measure of the effective peritoneal surface area. The reason for the large inter-individual variability in peritoneal solute transfer rate is not clear. Demographic and clinical variables (such as age, sex, race, diabetes, cardiovascular disease) explain only a very small fraction of this variability.[61] Preliminary studies indicate that some of this variability is, in part, genetically determined.[62–68] There is also compelling evidence for intra-peritoneal inflammation as measured by dialysate IL-6 levels as an important determinant of peritoneal solute transfer rate; this may, in part, be also genetically determined.[62,69,70] Large population-based genome wide association studies are presently underway that could help clarify the genetic underpinnings in the variability of peritoneal solute transfer rate; this, in turn, could help us better understand peritoneal biology and pathobiology.

The information obtained from a PET could be used as a guide to optimize PD prescription; several validated software programs based upon urea kinetic modeling have been developed that use data from the PET to optimize prescriptions.[71,72] The slower the peritoneal solute transfer rate, the greater is the challenge with solute removal particularly in large, muscular anuric individuals; inadequate ultrafiltration is rarely, if ever, a concern. These individuals need longer dwell times to achieve adequate solute removal, which can be done both with continuous ambulatory or automated PD. In contrast, the faster the solute transport, the greater is the challenge with fluid removal, particularly with loss of residual kidney function; achieving an adequate dose of dialysis is rarely, if ever, a concern. These individuals generally need shorter dwell times with a cycler at night and extreme care in limiting long dwell times with dextrose-based solutions. The long dwell times can be optimized with either complete or partially "dry" days in individuals with significant residual kidney function (RKF), or with the addition of daytime exchange or icodextrin in individuals without RKF.

In addition, a large number of studies have examined the association of peritoneal solute transfer rate with meaningful patient outcomes. The preponderance of evidence seems to suggest that patients with higher peritoneal solute transfer rates have a higher risk for death.[73–78] Evidence linking peritoneal solute transfer rate with other meaningful outcomes, such as risk for transfer to hemodialysis or protein-energy wasting, is inconsistent. Several hypotheses have been put forth to explain the higher risk for death in high/fast transporters and include a higher prevalence of protein-energy wasting from greater protein losses and/or suppression of appetite from greater absorption of glucose, systemic inflammation, or comorbidity. However, there is an emerging consensus that the higher risk for death in high/fast transporters is from inadequate ultrafiltration with conventional PD prescriptions, particularly with continuous ambulatory PD.[79] Even though the risk is mitigated with use of automated PD with shorter nighttime dwells, the risk is not abrogated.[78] Thus, it is imperative that care be observed when designing prescriptions that optimize fluid removal in high/fast transporters.

## THE PERITONEAL CATHETER AND ACCESS

Successful PD therapy depends upon permanent and safe access to the peritoneal cavity. A well-functioning catheter provides obstruction-free access to the peritoneum. Mechanical catheter problems cause transfer to HD in nearly 20% of prevalent PD patients; peritoneal infections, which are often catheter-related, are responsible for another 30% to 50% of PD technique failures.[80,81] Therefore, proper catheter selection and placement is imperative to the success of PD.

Globally, the most widely used catheter is the standard Tenckhoff catheter followed by the swan-neck catheter.[82] Catheters are made either of polyurethane or silicone rubber. Polyurethane, a stronger material than silicone rubber, allows creation of a thinner catheter wall resulting in a larger catheter lumen, which in turn allows faster flow rates (3.1 mm polyurethane vs. 2.6 mm internal diameter traditional silicone). More recently, some manufacturers have begun offering larger diameter silicone catheters in some countries (e.g., Flex-neck catheter, Cardiomed). Polyurethane catheters are most often found outside of the US and can degrade with the routine use of ointments and povidone-iodine at the exit site, whereas silicone catheters have been reported to degrade with exposure to povidone-iodine but not ointments such as mupirocin.[83]

PD catheters have essentially three segments: the intraperitoneal, tunneled, and extraperitoneal segment. The intraperitoneal segment is the portion of the catheter that resides inside the peritoneal cavity; side holes along the length of the intraperitoneal portion deliver and drain dialysate. The extraperitoneal segment passes through a subcutaneous tunnel within the abdominal wall (intramural), exits through the skin, and has an external (outside the body) segment. The catheter may contain one or two polyester cuffs, typically 1 cm long, referred to as the internal (pre-peritoneal) and external (subcutaneous) cuffs. Fig. 64.1 shows different intraperitoneal and extraperitoneal designs of currently available peritoneal catheters.

The straight double-cuff Tenckhoff catheter is available in variable lengths but is most often used in either the 42 cm or 47 cm length, with an intraperitoneal segment length of 15 cm in the former and 20 cm in the latter; both have an intramural segment about 5 to 7 cm long, and an external segment about 20 cm long.[84,85] The intraperitoneal segment has multiple 0.5-mm side openings along its course, the length of which measures 10-15 cm depending on the total catheter

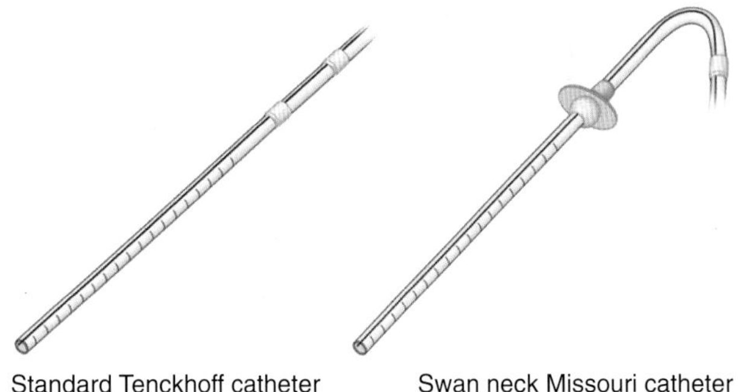


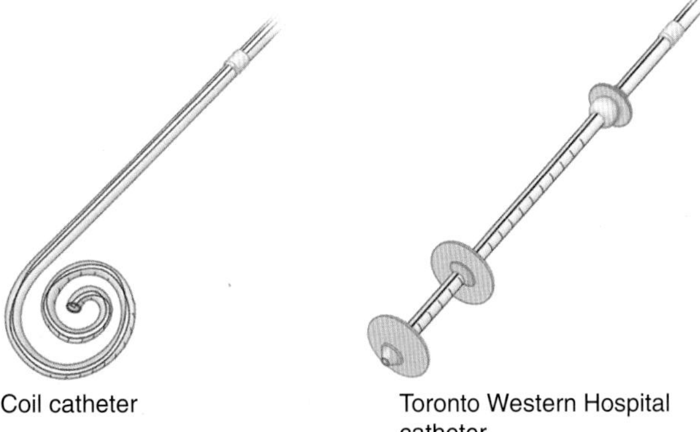


**Fig. 64.1** Intraperitoneal and extraperitoneal designs of currently available peritoneal catheters.

length. The coiled Tenckhoff catheter is also available in variable lengths between 57 cm and 72 cm with a coiled, perforated intraperitoneal end that is 19.5 cm long for all coiled catheters. It is important to select the proper catheter length for each patient individually to avoid malposition of the catheter in the peritoneum; too-short catheters are at risk for incomplete drainage and entrapment from hanging omentum while too-long catheters can lead to inflow pain most often in the rectal or perineal region. Most Tenckhoff catheters have a barium-impregnated radiopaque stripe throughout the catheter length to assist in radiologic visualization.

Several different configurations of peritoneal catheters exist beyond the straight and coiled-tip Tenckhoff catheter. The swan-neck catheter, a modified Tenckhoff catheter, features a preformed 180-degree bend between the two cuffs.[82,86] These catheters can be placed in an arcuate tunnel such that both external and internal segments of the tunnel can easily be directed downward. The preformed angle between cuffs eliminates the risk of the catheter straightening over time due to rubber "shape memory," thus potentially reducing the risk for internal catheter tip migration and external cuff extrusion.[87] Swan-neck catheters are available with three different intraperitoneal configurations: straight, coiled, and straight with two intraperitoneal silicone discs (also called the Toronto-Western or Oreopoulos-Zellerman catheter). The coiled and silicon-disk configurations were each developed to help reduce omental wrapping and to maintain catheter position in the pelvis. The Toronto-Western and Missouri catheters also differ from the Tenckhoff catheter because they replace the internal cuff with a felt disc-silicone bead combination; the disk is sutured to the rectus muscle just outside the peritoneum and serves as an anchor for the catheter while the bead is placed just inside the peritoneum and serves as a physical barrier to prevent peritoneal fluid leakage. All of the aforementioned catheters are available with the traditional subcutaneous cuff that is optimally placed 2 cm proximal to the catheter exit site.

Presternal catheters, another modification of catheter design, enter the peritoneum in the traditional location and are then tunneled subcutaneously and ipsilaterally up to the chest wall, where they finally exit the skin. The unique design of the presternal catheter offers several benefits over standard abdominal catheters in certain settings. Presternal exit sites are easily visible even in the obese patient who has a large pannus, or other visual obstruction to the lower abdominal skin. Patients with limited flexibility who cannot easily bend to see a traditional exit site also benefit from the easy visibility of a presternal exit site. The presternal catheter allows patients with abdominal ostomies and pediatric patients in diapers to utilize PD without risk of exit-site cross-contamination. Presternal catheters potentially reduce the risk of catheter trauma (a risk factor for exit-site infection) because the chest is a rather rigid structure with minimal wall motion. A long catheter tunnel, combined with three cuffs, may reduce pericatheter bacterial contamination of the peritoneal cavity and hence reduce the incidence of peritonitis.[88]

The presternal catheter is composed of two silicone rubber tubes, cut to an appropriate length and connected end to end at the time of implantation. The intraperitoneal tube is available in the dual cuff or the Missouri catheter configuration while the upper tube is a variation on the swan-neck catheter. A titanium connector connects the two components at the time of implantation. The catheter should be tunneled ipsilaterally to the peritoneal insertion point so that implantation directly over the sternum is avoided, therefore preventing catheter damage during any cardiac surgery that would necessitate sternotomy. Outcomes with the presternal catheter have been favorable in experienced hands.[88]

The Moncrief-Popovich (embedded) catheter is a modified swan-neck coiled catheter with a longer subcutaneous cuff (2.5 cm instead of 1 cm) that is implanted normally except that the external portion of the catheter is buried subcutaneously at the time of placement. This catheter is inserted months before it is needed, typically before the patient requires dialysis. The embedded catheter heals in a sterile environment thus there is low risk for early bacterial catheter colonization, in turn reducing the risk for exit site or peritoneal infection.[89,90] When dialysis is needed, the external portion of the catheter is exteriorized and connected to an external catheter extender in a short outpatient procedure. Full inflow volumes can be used immediately without increased risk of catheter leak because the catheter has healed fully over the preceding months while embedded. A futility rate of approximately 10% has been reported with embedded catheters (due to transplantation, death, or treatment with hemodialysis instead of PD); nevertheless, overall embedded catheters that are needed tend to work well. Early catheter drain problems have been reported to occur in 5% to 29% of exteriorized embedded catheters, are most often due to fibrin, and can be readily corrected without catheter removal.[91–94]

Rigid catheters for acute dialysis, rarely used in developed nations, are still used in some countries. Complications of rigid catheter insertion include minor bleeding, leakage of dialysis solution, extravasation of fluid into the abdominal wall, particularly in patients who have had a previous abdominal surgery or multiple catheter insertions, and inadequate drainage as a result of omental wrapping, loculation, or misplaced catheter in the upper abdomen. Loss of a part or the entire rigid catheter after manipulation of a poorly functioning rigid catheter has been reported. The incidence of peritonitis varies widely with rigid catheters; the rate may be dependent on the duration of dialysis and history of catheter manipulation among other factors.[95,96]

For long-term use, standard non-rigid PD catheters can be inserted by nonsurgical or surgical methods. PD catheter placement can occur at the patient's bedside by using Seldinger technique (blind insertion); however this method incurs a nontrivial risk of bowel trauma. Peritoneoscopic-assisted catheter placement, often used by nephrologists, allows visualization of the peritoneum before catheter insertion, thus limiting the risk of bowel trauma, but does not allow simultaneous visualization while the catheter is physically inserted. A modified percutaneous approach with fluoroscopic and ultrasound guidance at the time of catheter placement allows both avoidance of bowel and confirmation of catheter placement.[97] An experienced (interventional) nephrologist, interventional radiologist, or surgeon should be the operator in such cases. Surgical catheter placement was historically performed using open surgical techniques (mini-laparotomy) but technological advances have led to increased utilization of laparoscopic catheter placement techniques that offer the advantage of direct peritoneal visualization. Basic laparoscopic-guided PD catheter placement allows proper catheter placement in the lower pelvis. Surgical placement via open mini-laparotomy has been increasingly replaced by surgical laparoscopic catheter placement because the latter allows visualization and correction of hernia, adhesions, and low-hanging omentum at the time of catheter insertion; additionally, laparoscopy ensures correct catheter tip placement in the pelvis.[98,99] Advanced laparoscopic techniques such as rectus sheath tunneling, selective prophylactic omentopexy, and selective prophylactic adhesiolysis provides additional benefits at the time of catheter placement and in experienced hands has resulted in a 2-year catheter survival rate of 99.5%.[98,100,101]

## CATHETER-RELATED COMPLICATIONS

The most common complications of PD catheters include exit site and tunnel infection, impaired flow, external cuff extrusion, dialysate leaks, and infusion pain. Catheter-related infections can result from improper catheter placement, poor wound healing at the exit site, external catheter trauma, interference of the normal healing process during and after catheter placement, and inadequate routine exit-site care. Exit-site infections have been shown to be a result of sinus tract bacterial colonization; therefore it is imperative for a new exit site to heal in a sterile environment for as long as possible. One way to achieve this is by keeping the original post-surgical dressing in place for 5 to 7 days after catheter placement, removing it only in the case of frank bleeding or drainage; trained PD personnel should be the first to uncover the original catheter dressing and they should always wear masks while inspecting the exit site. After the exit site is well healed, trauma to the external segment of the catheter predisposes to infection by allowing bacterial colonization of the sinus tract and exit site and impairing normal tissue regeneration.[102–106] Certain cleansing agents can also impair normal skin cell turnover and should be avoided (e.g., iodine, bleach, alcohol).

Impaired dialysate flow can be seen either during drainage, inflow, or both. Impaired catheter drainage is often associated with constipation, when stool-filled bowel loops either obstruct catheter side holes or cause loculated fluid collections that are not readily accessible for drainage. A successful laxative regimen, over the course of one day, is often successful in restoring proper catheter drainage; abdominal radiographs can confirm constipation when the clinical picture is unclear. Abdominal radiographs are also useful to detect PD catheter tip migration, which is another cause of impaired dialysate drainage. Catheter repositioning can be attempted noninvasively using guidewire manipulation under fluoroscopy, and if unsuccessful, laparoscopic catheter repositioning is typically successful in improving catheter function when performed by an experienced surgeon. As described earlier, the swan-neck catheter configuration may reduce the risk of catheter migration over time.[107]

Entrapment, or "capture," of the catheter by the active omentum may cause outflow obstruction in the post implantation period. Omental "capture" as a late event is rare. From time to time in some patients, drainage slows as a result of catheter translocation, obstruction by omentum, or fibrin clot formation. Laxatives or addition of heparin, 500 U per liter of dialysis solution, or both may be successful in restoring good dialysate flow. In some patients, catheters have migrated out of the true pelvis. If the catheter continues to function appropriately, it is not necessary to reposition it. If the catheter fails to function after simple maneuvers are implemented, more aggressive measures (e.g., laxatives, forced flushing) may be tried. When these measures fail, laparoscopic repositioning of the catheter tip back to the true pelvis and anchoring may be necessary. The Toronto Western catheter has two silicone discs in the intraperitoneal segment of the catheter that hinder the free movement of catheter tip out of the pelvis after placement.[102]

The catheter tip, as it rests against the pelvic wall or intraabdominal organs, may cause localized pain from irritation.[105] The jet effect of rapidly flowing dialysis solution may also cause abdominal pain. In some rare instances, compartmentalization from adhesion formation around the catheter may cause severe abdominal pain.[108] Coiled catheters are designed to reduce infusion-related abdominal pain by avoiding a direct jet effect of solution against the bowel.

The extrusion of the external synthetic cuff can be prevented by creating the tunnel in a shape similar to the shape of the catheter and placing this cuff approximately 2 to 3 cm from the skin. In the absence of catheter infection, shaving off the extruded external cuff may help prolong the life of the catheter.[104]

Insertion of the deep cuff into the center of the rectus muscle, as opposed to midline placement, has significantly reduced the incidence of early leakage of pericatheter dialysis solution.[102,105] Pericatheter leaks are rare with catheters that have a bead and polyester flange at the deep cuff (Toronto Western Hospital catheter, Swan Neck Missouri catheter, Swan Neck Presternal Peritoneal catheter). In contrast to the early leaks, which are usually external, the late leaks infiltrate the abdominal wall through prior healed incisions. PD catheters may cause hemoperitoneum by causing minor tears of small vessels. On occasion, a peritoneal catheter erodes into the mesenteric vessels, leading to hemoperitoneum. In rare cases, a peritoneal catheter damages the internal organs, which leads to intraabdominal bleeding. Transvaginal leakage of peritoneal fluid is rare, but the possibility should be considered in an appropriate clinical setting.[102–105]

## PERITONEAL DIALYSIS SOLUTIONS

The dialysate used to perform PD can be considered to have three components: (1) an osmotic agent to induce ultrafiltration; (2) buffer to correct uremic metabolic acidosis; and (3) a combination of electrolytes to optimize diffusive removal of solutes. The various options for each of these components among the solutions that are commercially available are listed in Table 64.2. The most widely used formulation comprises dextrose as an osmotic agent (1.5%, 2.5%, or 4.25%), lactate as the buffer (usually 40 mEq/L), physiologic concentration of calcium (2.5 mEq/L), at a pH of 5.4. Even though several decades of use support the general efficacy and safety of conventional PD solutions for the long-term treatment of end-stage kidney disease (ESKD), concerns about the limitations or concerns about each of these components has driven the quest for better solutions.

Conventional PD solutions contain dextrose (or glucose monohydrate) as the **osmotic agent**; three different strengths of solution are commercially available as 1.5%, 2.5%, or 4.25%

**Table 64.2 Components of Different Peritoneal Dialysis Solutions Available Commercially**

| | Osmotic Agent | Buffer | pH |
|---|---|---|---|
| Conventional | Dextrose | Lactate | 5.2 |
| Low-glucose degradation product | Dextrose | Lactate or bicarbonate | 7.0-7.4 |
| | Dextrose | Lactate and bicarbonate | 7.4 |
| Icodextrin | Icodextrin | Lactate | 5.2 |
| Amino acids | Amino acids | Lactate | 6.4 |

dextrose (or 1.36%, 2.25%, and 3.86% glucose, respectively). The supraphysiologic concentration of glucose in PD solutions exerts a high osmotic force across the peritoneal barrier to generate brisk ultrafiltration.[46] Yet, there are two major limitations. First, glucose is absorbed across the peritoneum and this reduces the osmotic force driving ultrafiltration over the course of an intraperitoneal dwell. Hence, ultrafiltration volume is often inadequate with glucose-based PD solutions with longer dwell times such as the overnight dwell in patients undergoing continuous ambulatory PD or the day dwell in patients treated with automated PD.[109] Second, a wide range of glucose degradation products form during heat sterilization of glucose-based PD solutions.[110,111] Many of these degradation products are either directly cytotoxic or accelerate the formation of advanced glycosylation end-products and are thought to underlie the structural and functional changes seen in the peritoneum with long-term PD.[112] These limitations have led to development of solutions that contain either an osmotic agent better suited for longer dwell times (such as icodextrin), or glucose-based solutions with undetectable concentrations of glucose degradation products (biocompatible PD solutions). A 1% amino acid solution can also be used as an osmotic agent – alone, or in combination with 1.5% dextrose – and may be a useful adjunct in patients with protein-energy wasting (see below).

Lactate is the most commonly used **buffer** in PD solutions. During PD, bicarbonate in the blood moves into the dialysate, and lactate is absorbed systemically, each along its concentration gradient. Lactate is metabolized in the liver into bicarbonate and leads to correction of uremic metabolic acidosis. There are few, if any, adverse consequences from the use of lactate as a buffer. However, with the recognition that lactate is not a physiologic buffer, bicarbonate-based solutions have been developed. Such solutions have two compartments that separate calcium and magnesium from bicarbonate; this precludes precipitation of bicarbonate salts during heat sterilization of PD solutions. The two compartments are separated by a thin membrane that is disrupted prior to infusion of dialysate into the peritoneal cavity. The resultant solution has a physiologic pH, unlike the solution in single chamber bags such as dextrose- or icodextrin-based solutions.

Conventional PD solutions also have a combination of other **electrolytes** such as sodium, calcium, magnesium, and chloride. The concentration of sodium in PD solutions (132 mEq/L) is lower than in the dialysate used for HD (138-142 mEq/L); this allows for a somewhat greater diffusive removal of sodium. In order to further enhance sodium removal, PD solutions with significantly lower concentrations of sodium (102-125 mEq/L) have been tested. Such low sodium PD solutions may require higher concentration of glucose to ensure an adequate osmotic force across the peritoneal barrier and result in greater sodium removal with resultant better control of blood pressure than conventional PD solutions.[113,114] However, a recent multicenter trial has raised concern about lower residual kidney function in patients randomized to low-sodium dialysate (125 mEq/L).[114] As such, low-sodium dialysate remains experimental thus far and is not commercially available.

Older formulations of PD solutions contained a higher concentration of calcium (3.5 mEq/L). Supraphysiologic calcium concentrations can help to control hyperparathyroidism in some patients, but can place others at risk for hypercalcemia and oversuppression of parathyroid hormone, especially if treated with calcium-based phosphate binders and/or calcitriol of active vitamin D analogs. In order to mitigate this risk, most PD solutions used in contemporary clinical practice contain physiologic concentrations of calcium (2.5 mEq/L).[115,116]

The following paragraphs provide an overview of three different PD solutions available commercially in different parts of the world (icodextrin, low-glucose degradation product solution, and bicarbonate-based solution) and the role for glucose-sparing regimens; the clinical experience with amino acid solutions is discussed along with other considerations for management of protein energy wasting.

## ICODEXTRIN PD SOLUTION

Icodextrin is a polymer in which molecules of glucose are linked by alpha (1-4) bonds.[117] It is derived from hydrolysis of corn starch, each chain has variable number of molecules of glucose, and the average molecular weight is about 16,000 daltons.[117] It is available commercially as a 7.5% solution with lactate as a buffer, calcium concentration of 3.5 mEq/L, and pH of 5.4. The solution is isoosmotic to normal plasma and icodextrin exerts oncotic pressure across the peritoneum to induce ultrafiltration through the small pores, but not through aquaporins.[118] Given the large molecular weight, icodextrin is not absorbed across the peritoneal barrier but is removed slowly from the peritoneal cavity via the lymphatics. Only about one third of the icodextrin is absorbed, on average, over 12 hours. This, in turn, maintains the oncotic pressure for ultrafiltration for longer dwell periods and is optimally suited for use during either the overnight dwell of patients treated with continuous ambulatory PD or a day dwell for patients undergoing nighttime automated PD.[119] The icodextrin that is absorbed is metabolized by circulating amylase into oligosaccharides of varying length, with maltose being the dominant circulating compound in patients treated with icodextrin-based dialysate.[120] Maltose readily enters the cells and is metabolized by maltase found in lysozymes of many cells into glucose.

A large number of clinical trials have tested the efficacy of icodextrin.[121–128] In patients with high-average or high peritoneal membrane transport characteristics, icodextrin generates greater ultrafiltration volume than either 2.5% or 4.25% dextrose during the long dwells of either continuous ambulatory or automated PD, an advantage that persists during episodes of peritonitis.[121,122,126,129] Relative to 2.5% or 4.25% dextrose, the use of icodextrin is associated with higher ultrafiltration efficiency, i.e., a larger volume per gram of absorbed carbohydrate.[121,126] The greater ultrafiltration volume results in a reduction in total body water and a higher likelihood of euvolemia than patients treated with dextrose-based solutions.[127] Perhaps as a result of achieving euvolemia, patients undergoing continuous ambulatory PD treated with icodextrin have been shown to have regression left ventricular hypertrophy compared to 1.5% dextrose.[123] Despite a reduction in total body water and claims to the contrary, there appears to be no meaningful effect of treatment with icodextrin on RKF.[130,131]

In addition to improved control of hypervolemia, there is evidence that the use of icodextrin can exert beneficial metabolic effects, including enhanced insulin sensitivity, glycemic control and correction or attenuation of dyslipidemia.[132,133] An observational study also suggested potentially beneficial effects on maintaining peritoneal membrane function (i.e., maintenance of the peritoneal solute transport rate) when compared with conventional PD solutions.[134] Moreover, a small clinical trial has demonstrated that patients with diabetes mellitus treated with icodextrin have a lower probability for transfer to in-center HD.[125] Finally, an observational study has shown a lower risk for death in patients treated with icodextrin.[135]

Based on the accumulated body of evidence, it is recommended that icodextrin be used as a single exchange during the long dwell in patients with inadequate ultrafiltration with dextrose-based solutions; a phenomenon most likely to be present in individuals with high-average and high transport. At least two studies have examined the use of two daily exchanges with icodextrin and demonstrated a higher ultrafiltration volume and improvement in other clinically relevant parameters.[136,137] However, such use remains investigational. Hybrid solutions containing both icodextrin and glucose have also been tested and shown to have substantially higher ultrafiltration volumes; however, none such hybrid solutions are commercially available.[138]

Skin rash is the most commonly reported adverse effect with the use of icodextrin.[122,130] The rash is typically an exfoliating rash that involves the palms and soles, is reported to occur 2 to 3 weeks from the start of exposure to the solution, and resolves after cessation of exposure. In addition, glucometers that use glucose dehydrogenase pyrroloquinolinequinone overestimate the blood glucose levels secondary to the accumulation of maltose.[139] Extreme caution should be exercised to ensure that insulin or other hypoglycemic agents are not administered because of a falsely elevated glucose test. Episodes of aseptic peritonitis have also been reported in patients treated with icodextrin. These episodes have been traced to the presence of peptidoglycan in the solution from hydrolysis of corn starch; the problem has been substantially minimized with change in manufacturing processes such that the commercially available solution has no detectable peptidoglycan.[140]

## LOW GLUCOSE-DEGRADATION PRODUCT GLUCOSE-BASED SOLUTIONS

This dual-chamber PD solution, commercially available in some parts of the world, comprises glucose as the osmotic agent, lactate as the buffer, but has a physiologic pH and undetectable levels of glucose degradation products. Several clinical trials have examined the potential clinical benefits with such biocompatible solutions but results are mixed.[141–152]

The primary impetus for the development of these solutions were laboratory studies that demonstrated that glucose-degradation products contributed to damage to the integrity the long-term health of the peritoneum and precluded long-term treatment with PD. Post hoc analyses of data from the BalANZ study suggests that the peritoneal solute transfer rate does not change over time in patients treated with these solutions compared to a progressive increase in peritoneal solute transfer rate with an associated decrease in ultrafiltration capacity in patients treated with conventional PD solutions.[153] However, evidence to date has not shown that these effects translate into a clinically meaningful benefit such as a lower likelihood of modality failure (i.e., transfer to in-center hemodialysis).[151]

An early crossover study demonstrated that patients had a higher urine volume when treated with a biocompatible PD solution, which decreased upon restarting treatment with conventional PD solutions.[154] Even though some have proposed a hemodynamic effect of such solutions with lower ultrafiltration volume and consequent volume expansion leading to natriuresis, the mechanism for higher urine volume with biocompatible PD solutions is currently not known.[155] Results of studies examining the effects of these solutions on RKF are heterogenous, but the totality of evidence suggests that these solutions result in a higher urine volume and a slower decline in RKF, particularly with long-term treatment.[151,156]

At least one large clinical trial has shown a significantly lower risk for peritonitis in patients treated with a PD solution with low concentration of glucose degradation products[147]; however, this finding has not been validated in other clinical trials.[149,152,157–159] While observational studies have shown a lower risk for death in patients treated with biocompatible PD solutions, no such benefit was evident in a systematic review of clinical trials,[151,160] raising the possibility of publication bias, and equally as likely, confounding by indication. Nevertheless, there is no evidence for harm with the use of these solutions and the decision to use them is driven by availability and cost.

## BICARBONATE-BASED PD SOLUTION

This dual-chamber PD solution commercially available in some parts of the world contains glucose as the osmotic agent and bicarbonate as the buffer, has a physiologic pH, and has low concentrations of glucose degradation products. The development of this solution was also driven by the laboratory evidence demonstrating risk to the health and integrity of the peritoneum with the use of bio-incompatible PD solutions. There is no evidence for better preservation of structural or functional integrity of the peritoneum in humans with bicarbonate-based solutions. However, these solutions result in a more complete correction of metabolic acidosis and reduce infusion pain when compared to conventional solutions.[161,162] A single observational study demonstrated a lower risk for death in patients treated with this solution[135]; however, such a finding has not be demonstrated in a prospective clinical trial.

## GLUCOSE-SPARING REGIMENS

A large number of studies have raised concern about the local and systemic effects of glucose in patients treated with PD.[163] Thus, many studies have examined the safety and efficacy of PD regimens that systematically reduce exposure to glucose with PD solutions through the course of the day. Central to such glucose-sparing regimens is substitution of one glucose-based exchange with icodextrin for the long dwell. The glucose exposure can be further reduced by substituting a second glucose-based exchange with amino acid solution. Such glucose-sparing regimens have been shown to result in improvement in glycemic control in individuals with diabetes treated with PD along with improvement in lipid parameters.[128,132,164–166] However, there is a higher risk for adverse events in patients treated with these regimens,[132] thought to result from a greater risk of volume overload with reduction in glucose exposure. Moreover, it remains unclear if glucose-sparing regimens reduce cardiovascular risk in patients treated with PD.[167] Given the higher cost of glucose-sparing regimens, the decision to use them should be made on a on a case-by-case basis.

## PERITONEAL DIALYSIS MODALITIES

PD allows flexibility in regimen such that the prescription can be individualized to meet the lifestyle considerations of each patient while reducing the burden of treatment. Broadly speaking, PD prescriptions can be (1) continuous or intermittent, and (2) involve manual exchanges or be automated using a cycler. Continuous regimens are the ones in which there is intraperitoneal dialysate 24 hours a day, 7 days a week. Continuous regimens may involve only manual exchanges [continuous ambulatory PD (CAPD) and continuous cyclic peritoneal dialysis (CCPD)]. The most widely used intermittent regimens comprise the use of a cycler to deliver PD for a part of the day – either at night (nocturnal intermittent PD; NIPD), or day (diurnal intermittent PD). On occasion, patients doing CAPD may be prescribed a "dry night". Such intermittent regimens are appropriate only for individuals with significant RKF.[168] Rarely, intermittent PD is delivered by performing frequent exchanges over 10 to 36 hours every few days. This is used either as a bridge for individuals in the immediate postoperative period (such as "urgent start" PD) or as palliative therapy for patients as part of end-of-life care.[169,170]

Arguably, patients with slower peritoneal solute transfer rates (slow or low transporters) would require longer dwell periods to achieve adequate solute removal. In contrast, patients with faster peritoneal solute transfer rates (fast or high transporters) could benefit with shorter nighttime dwells to optimize daily ultrafiltration. However, most patients can be successfully treated with either continuous ambulatory or automated PD, particularly in the presence of RKF.

A large number of observational studies have examined the potential effects of treatment with continuous ambulatory or automated PD on clinically meaningful outcomes; the evidence has recently been summarized in a narrative review.[171] In the early days of PD, use of the cycler reduced the number of connections and disconnections that needed to be made during the course of the day when compared to patients treated with continuous ambulatory PD. Studies from this period showed a lower risk for peritonitis in patients treated with automated PD. However, there has been a widespread adoption of flush-before-fill, twin-bag systems and disconnect systems for automated PD such that in contemporary practice, there is no difference in risk for peritonitis in patients treated with continuous ambulatory or automated PD.[171]

Concern has been raised that the total daily sodium and water removal may not be adequate in patients treated with automated PD.[172–175] This phenomenon has been attributed to sodium sieving during short nighttime dwells and fluid reabsorption during the long day dwell that are typical for automated PD prescriptions. Sodium sieving refers to the exclusion of sodium when water is transported across ultrasmall aquaporin pores, leading to disproportionately less sodium removal. This occurs early in the dwell, but is compensated by diffusive equilibration of plasma sodium with the dialysate, if the dwell continues for long enough. However, comparative studies of CAPD with automated PD have typically not taken into account overfill for flush-before-fill that is common in bags used for continuous ambulatory PD.[176] As a result, these studies may have overestimated the sodium and water removal with continuous ambulatory PD. This explanation is consistent with the observed results in comparative studies, showing no difference in the prevalence of volume overload or hypertension control in patients treated with continuous ambulatory or automated PD.[177]

Despite a reduction in burden of treatment, there is no evidence that patients treated with automated PD have lower mortality, enhanced health-related quality of life, or lower risk for transfer to in-center hemodialysis.[178–182] The differential use of the two PD modalities is likely to continue to be driven by lifestyle and cost considerations with a likely greater use of automated PD in many countries such as the United States or Western Europe.

## DIALYSIS ADEQUACY

The concept of an "adequate" PD dialysis dose has been strongly influenced by randomized controlled trials and better understanding of the multiplicity of factors affecting PD patients with little or no RKF.[183–186] Before the Adequacy of Peritoneal Dialysis in Mexico (ADEMEX) study and the HD Study (HEMO), the notion that prevailed was that a continuous increase in small solute clearances would lead to better clinical results and patient survival.[183,184,187] The present concept of an adequate dialysis now encompasses attention to a multiplicity of clinical and nonclinical variables (multidimensional concept), including RKF, cardiovascular effects of blood pressure control, ultrafiltration and volume overload, mineral metabolism, nutrition, and individual psychologic and nonphysiologic (i.e., those related to other domains of health status) indicators (Table 64.3).[183,187–189]

*Adequate dialysis* is defined as the administration of an effective dosage of dialysis solution, capable of keeping a patient clinically asymptomatic and active and maintaining sufficient correction of the altered metabolic and homeostatic components secondary to the loss of kidney function.[188] *Optimal dialysis* is defined as either (1) the dose capable of reducing morbidity and mortality associated with ESKD and with the dialytic procedure itself or (2) the dose above

**Table 64.3 Considerations for Adequate Dialysis**

Clinical manifestations: fluid balance, systemic blood pressure control, and cardiovascular risk
Residual kidney function
Acid-base homeostasis
Nutritional status
Calcium-phosphorous metabolism homeostasis
Inflammation
Small solute clearance
Middle molecule clearance
Psychologic and quality-of-life indicators

which an increase does not justify the increased burden of treatment.[190–192]

## INDICATORS TO EVALUATE DIALYSIS ADEQUACY

The dialysis dose prescribed is often based on clinical evaluations as the presence or absence of symptoms related to uremia (e.g., nausea, vomiting, dysgeusia, sleeping disorders). Nevertheless, this may be highly subjective and prone to dosage underestimation and while clinical indicators should not be ignored, therapeutic decisions should not be based solely on them.[186] Clearance of urea is at present still employed as a marker of dialysis dose, in conjunction with other indicators described above. Residual kidney function tends to be maintained in PD for a longer period than in HD and may account for a significant proportion of the total clearance.[191,193,194]

Urea is the traditional solute to quantitate dialysis as its concentration is increased in CKD and has a low molecular weight (60 kDa), which allows rapid diffusion between body compartments and therefore application of a single-pool model for approximation. In addition, its volume of distribution is the total body water, it easily diffuses across the dialysis membrane, and is easy to measure.[188–194] After the National Cooperative Dialysis Study (NCDS) results were published in the early 1980s, the urea kinetic model took on a prominent role in dosage prescription in PD as well, notwithstanding the fact that it was created for HD and that its application to PD was accomplished only with inferences and analogies.[195]

The fractional clearance of urea is expressed as $Kt/V_{urea}$, which is the clearance of urea (K) per time unit (t) in relation to its volume of distribution or total body water (V). Peritoneal Kt is calculated by collecting a 24-hour amount of effluent dialysate and determining its urea concentration; this in turn is divided by the plasma urea concentration ($D/P_{urea}$). To compare clearance values among patients, these values are normalized to a function of patient size: For urea, the metric is typically the volume of urea distribution (V). In PD practice, $Kt/V_{urea}$ is expressed as a total (sum of peritoneal $pKt/V_{urea}$ and renal urea clearances). Renal Kt is calculated similarly, with a 24-hour urine collection. $Kt/V_{urea}$ may be expressed as a daily value but is usually multiplied by 7 and expressed as a weekly value. This was done to compare PD and HD delivered dosages, yet these comparisons are not logical, given the intermittent nature of HD and the continuous nature of PD (Table 64.4).[196] The urea kinetic model, repeatedly validated for HD prescription, has been applied to PD, but its validity is questionable. If the same dosing principles employed for HD were used for CAPD, then patients on PD would be considered grossly underdialyzed because their $Kt/V_{urea}$ values would be much lower in absolute numbers; nevertheless, most patients on PD do not have more uremic manifestations, higher rates of morbidity, or mortality than do patients on HD.

**Table 64.4 Calculations for Dosage of Dialysis Solution**

Fractional Urea Clearance ($Kt/V_{urea}$)
Daily total $Kt/V_{urea}$ = peritoneal $Kt/V_{urea}$ + renal $Kt/V_{urea}$
Weekly $Kt/V_{urea} = 7 \times ([(24\text{-hr urea } D/P \times 24\text{-hr } EV)/V] + [(U_{urea}/P_{urea}) \times 24\text{-hr } UV)])$
Total Body Water (Watson's Formula)[a]
Male: $V = 2.447 - (0.3362 \times \text{weight}) - (0.1074 \times \text{height}) - (0.09516 \times \text{age})$
Female: $V = -2.097 + (0.2466 \times \text{weight}) + (0.1069 \times \text{height})$

[a]In Watson's formula, age is in years, height is in centimeters, and weight is in kilograms.

**Table 64.5 Determinants of Solute Clearance and Fluid Removal in Peritoneal Dialysis**

| Patient-Related Factors | Prescription-Related Factors |
|---|---|
| Residual kidney function | Dialytic modality |
| Body mass index | Frequency of exchanges per day |
| Peritoneal transport type | Volume of each exchange |
| | Dwell time |
| | Dialysis fluid tonicity |

## DETERMINANTS OF SOLUTE CLEARANCE AND FLUID REMOVAL IN PERITONEAL DIALYSIS

The initial PD prescription is defined empirically; a series of factors that influence clearance of solutes and fluid removal are considered. Some of these factors are modifiable and others are nonmodifiable (Table 64.5).[192,197,198]

### PATIENT-RELATED FACTORS

Residual kidney function contributes significantly to fluid removal and variably to solute clearance in PD patients. In these patients, RKF is best estimated by measuring the weekly renal component of the $Kt/V_{urea}$. Each milliliter per minute of urea clearance accounts for an additional 0.25 L to the total weekly $Kt/V_{urea}$.[199] Estimation of RKF enables physicians to plan the PD prescription and during follow-up, RKF should be evaluated periodically as it tends to decrease over time; thus, the dialysis prescription should be modified to compensate. A faster decline in RKF is associated with lower survival in PD patients.[200]

## VOLUME OF DISTRIBUTION AND BODY SURFACE AREA

The volume of distribution of urea is equivalent to the total body water, which can be estimated by the Watson or Hume formula, but these formulas may underestimate total body water in patients on dialysis and potentially overestimate dialysate dosage.[201] An equation has specifically been developed for patients undergoing maintenance dialysis and has been validated to provide superior prediction of total body water in HD and, potentially, also in patients on PD.[202]

## PERITONEAL TRANSPORT TYPE

Fig. 64.2 displays the $D/P_{Cr}$ versus dwell time of a dialytic exchange in patients with high and low (or fast and slow) peritoneal transport. The $D/P_{Cr}$ equilibrium (ratio of 1.0) is achieved earlier in high peritoneal transport; therefore, a shorter dwell time is preferred for patients with higher peritoneal transport rates, and a longer dwell time is required to augment solute clearance in patients with lower transport rates (Fig. 64.2). In comparison, patients with lower peritoneal transport rates achieve higher ultrafiltration volumes, whereas patients with higher peritoneal transport rates reabsorb larger quantities of glucose, an occurrence that reduces the gradient for ultrafiltration and generates net fluid reabsorption with longer dwell times (Fig. 64.3).[44] Patients with higher peritoneal transport rates obtain better ultrafiltration and adequate clearance of small molecules with techniques that promote shorter dwell times, such as APD, prescribed with multiple short exchanges. In contrast, patients with lower peritoneal transport rates benefit from longer exchange dwell times to augment removal of small molecules while preserving the ultrafiltration capability. It is noteworthy that most patients have intermediate transport rates; therefore, individualized evaluation is required to prescribe the best regimen.[44]

In addition to the discussed relation between transport type with ultrafiltration and solute clearance, is important to consider that the smaller the solute, the faster is the diffusive equilibrium reached. Urea, with a molecular weight of 60 Da, reaches equilibrium much faster than does creatinine (molecular weight of 112 Da). Conditions influencing small-molecule solute clearance may not be relevant to clearance of large molecules, charged, or protein-bound solutes. A more detailed discussion of uremic solutes and the limitations of using urea as a solute marker are provided in Chapter 52.

## PRESCRIPTION-RELATED FACTORS

The main modifiable factors in the PD prescription are: frequency of exchanges, volume of PD fluid exchanges, and tonicity of solutions.

### Frequency of Exchanges

Traditional CAPD prescription is based on four exchanges of 1.5-3.0 L every day. Yet some patients with small body surface area or significant RKF may start their treatment with three or fewer exchanges per day; this approach has been defined as incremental, as with time patients are expected to require an increase in dosage.[203,204] As creatinine is a larger molecule than urea, an increase in exchange frequency is less effective than an increase in fluid volume per exchange for removal of creatinine, particularly in patients with low peritoneal transport rates.[199] In APD, an increase in frequency of exchanges also induces an increase in solute clearance as the concentration gradient between dialysate and blood is maximized, but an increase in exchange frequency obligates a larger proportion of the total treatment time be dedicated to infusion and drainage. Therefore, there is a point at which the number of exchanges may be counterproductive in relation to clearance attained (and in relation to costs). The "break even" point is variable from patient to patient and is related in part to the peritoneal transport rate.[197] A recent addition to dialysis prescription that may add important benefits is the possibility of remote monitoring of dialysis performance in patients with APD, which may help to personalize, and thus improve individual dialysis prescription.[205]

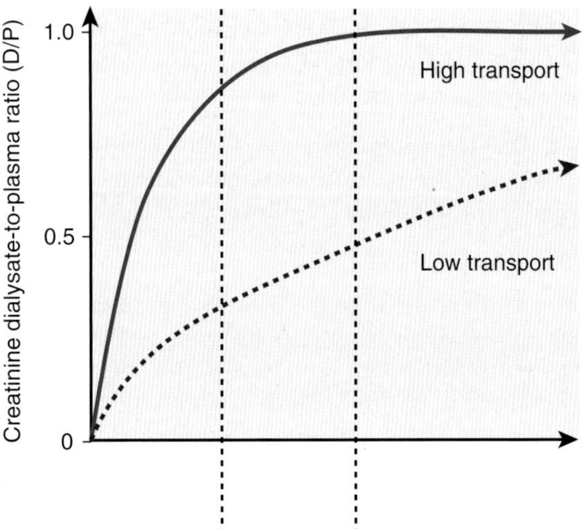


**Fig. 64.2** The ratio of dialysate-to-plasma ratio for creatinine ($D/P_{Cr}$) plotted against dwell time of a dialytic exchange in conditions of high and low peritoneal transport.

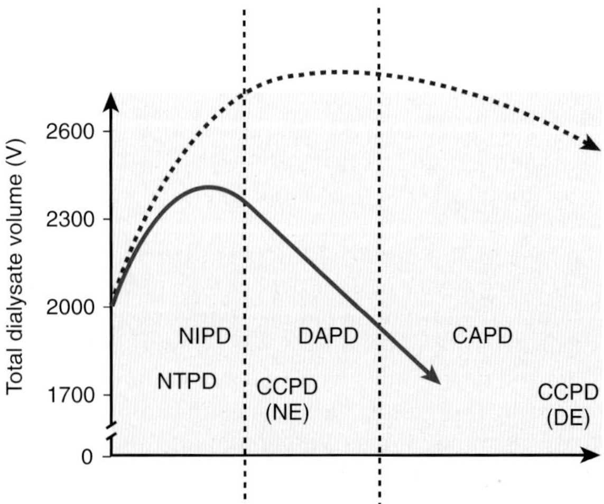


**Fig. 64.3** Differences in ultrafiltration and net fluid reabsorption between patients with lower peritoneal transport *(red line)* and patients with higher peritoneal transport *(blue line). CAPD,* Continuous ambulatory peritoneal dialysis; *CCPD,* continuous cycling peritoneal dialysis; *DAPD,* daytime ambulatory peritoneal dialysis; *DE,* daytime exchanges; *NE,* nocturnal exchanges; *NIPD,* nocturnal intermittent peritoneal dialysis; *NTPD,* nightly tidal peritoneal dialysis.

The best way to increase clearance in NIPD is to add a daytime exchange. The daytime exchange increases $Kt/V_{urea}$ by approximately 25%. The main drawback is that a long daytime exchange often leads to net fluid reabsorption, particularly in patients with high and high-average peritoneal transport rates. A way to avoid this problem is to individually tailor the daily exchange time for each patient according to the clinical response. In some patients, additional clearance may be obtained by adding a second or third daytime exchange or by switching to CAPD.

### Increase in Volume Exchange

An increase in fill volume is generally a more effective means of increasing small-molecule solute clearance than is an increase in exchange frequency. Therefore, it is one of the main prescription actions to achieve goals for CAPD, as well as for APD. Volume exchange is limited by patient body surface area and tolerance of higher fill volumes, and complications such as PD fluid leaks, and hernias of the abdominal wall.[192,197,198]

### Increase in Solution Osmolality

A dialysate with a higher tonicity induces an increase in ultrafiltration volume, and is employed mainly to avoid or control hypervolemia, often present in patients without RKF independent of their transport type, and in patients with high and high-average transport rates and in nonadherent patients that ingest large amounts of salt or water. These dialysates may also induce a convection-driven, quantifiable increase in solute clearance. It is important to point out that use of hypertonic glucose solutions has potential adverse metabolic consequences, as addressed below. The use of polyglucose solutions (icodextrin) allows for increased ultrafiltration with a lower risk of inducing metabolic complications.[197]

## CLEARANCE TARGETS AND CLINICAL OUTCOMES

When outcomes of patients on PD were assessed in the prospective Canada-USA cohort study of adequacy in PD (CANUSA), there was an inverse correlation between $Kt/V_{urea}$ and mortality.[193] This finding led to the implementation of "evidence-based" recommendations by the Kidney Disease Outcomes Quality Initiative (KDOQI) that the weekly dose of CAPD be at least $Kt/V_{urea}$ of 2.0 for all patients and that the total creatinine clearance rate be at least 60 L/week/1.73 $m^2$ for high and high-average transporters and 50 L/week/1.73 $m^2$ for low and low-average transporters. In a reanalysis of CANUSA, the same authors noted that one conclusion was erroneous[206]: In CANUSA's first analysis, the equivalence of renal and peritoneal clearances was assumed, and therefore they were merely added. For every 5-L/week/1.73 $m^2$ higher residual creatinine clearance, there was a 12% lower relative risk of death; no such association with peritoneal creatinine clearance was evident. The observed survival advantage associated with higher small solute clearances could be accounted for by RKF.[206] This fact was further supported by the findings of other investigators who have stressed the greater importance of RKF. Other studies were unsuccessful in evaluating the effect of peritoneal clearance on patients.[207–209]

The ADEMEX study was a prospective, randomized clinical trial to evaluate the effect of higher peritoneal clearance on patient survival.[183] The trial included 960 patients with incident and prevalent kidney disease (>50% anuric) who were receiving CAPD with four 2-L exchanges, and had peritoneal creatinine clearance rates of less than 60 L/week/1.73 $m^2$ at 24 centers in Mexico. Trial participants were monitored for more than 2 years. A control group received a standard prescription (four 2-L exchanges), and for the experimental group the prescription was changed to achieve a peritoneal creatinine clearance of 60 L/week, by increasing dwell volumes and, when necessary, adding a fifth automated night exchange. The control group achieved a weekly peritoneal creatinine clearance rate of 46 L and a peritoneal $Kt/V_{urea}$ of 1.62, whereas the experimental group achieved a peritoneal creatinine clearance rate of 56 L and a $Kt/V_{urea}$ of 2.13 per week; thus, substantial group separation was achieved. No differences were observed between the two groups in primary (risk of death) and secondary (technique failure, hospitalization, nutritional status) outcomes.[183] These results support the hypothesis that increases in creatinine and urea clearance with higher PD dosage, within the studied ranges, do not enhance patient survival.

Data from several subgroups—including younger and older patients, those with or without RKF, those with or without diabetes, and those with larger and smaller body surface areas—were analyzed and, again, showed no differences in mortality or other outcomes by randomized group among these subgroups. Control participants were more likely to drop out of the study due to uremia. The results of the study may not be fully generalizable as patients in the ADEMEX trial were smaller in size, younger, and had more pronounced protein-energy wasting than other PD populations.[210] However, these arguments do not preclude the external validity of the trial, inasmuch as comorbid conditions, general survival rates, and causes of mortality were similar to those observed in all other studies, including CANUSA.[193]

Results of ADEMEX were supported by those of Li and colleagues in a randomized clinical trial of 320 patients with incident kidney disease who were receiving CAPD and whose baseline renal $Kt/V_{urea}$ values were less than 1.0.[185] Patients were randomly assigned to three target groups: In group A, $Kt/V_{urea}$ ranged from 1.5 to 1.7; in group B, $Kt/V_{urea}$ ranged from 1.7 to 2.0; and in group C, $Kt/V_{urea}$ exceeded 2.0. Total $Kt/V_{urea}$ values of the three groups were significantly different, and this difference was mostly attributable to peritoneal $Kt/V_{urea}$. There was no difference in patient survival, serum albumin concentration, and hospitalization rates among the three groups; however, more patients from group A required erythropoietin and were withdrawn from the study by their physicians. Thus, patients with total $Kt/V_{urea}$ values below 1.7 had more anemia and clinical complications, and yet there was no difference in survival or other outcomes for groups B and C; i.e., patients targeted to $Kt/V_{urea}$ between 1.7 and 2.0 or above 2.0. Results from these two clinical trials support the notion that a total $Kt/V_{urea}$ of 1.7 or higher is an appropriate target for small solute clearance in PD.[185] In addition, Lo and colleagues performed a 10-year retrospective survival analysis of 150 anuric patients on PD, according to the baseline peritoneal $Kt/V_{urea}$ at time of documentation of anuria and at the latest PD prescription (based on $Kt/V_{urea}$).[211] Baseline $Kt/V_{urea}$ was not independently associated with patient survival;

**Table 64.6 Adequacy Targets in Peritoneal Dialysis**

| Index Measure | Adequacy Index | | |
|---|---|---|---|
| | European Renal Association (2005) | Kidney Disease Dialysis Outcomes Quality Initiative (2006) | International Society of Peritoneal Dialysis (2006) |
| **Total $Kt/V_{urea}$** | | | |
| CAPD | 1.7 | 1.7 | 1.7 |
| APD | 1.7 | 1.7 | 1.7 |

nevertheless, patients with peritoneal $Kt/V_{urea}$ values lower than 1.67 had poorer survival rates. Survival rates did not differ among patients with $Kt/V_{urea}$ either higher or lower than 1.80. The survival rate was best among female patients with $Kt/V_{urea}$ of 1.67 to 1.86, followed by those with $Kt/V_{urea}$ higher than 1.86, and was lowest in those with $Kt/V_{urea}$ lower than 1.67. Peritoneal $Kt/V_{urea}$ below 1.67 was consistently associated with lower survival rates. These observational results could be confounded by protein energy wasting, with "shrinkage" of the total body water (largely housed within skeletal muscle) space. Parallel controlled trials of dialysis dose in APD are lacking.

Given the current body of evidence, clinical practice guidelines recommend that $Kt/V_{urea}$ is still the best available index of "adequacy" and that a value of total $Kt/V_{urea}$ of 1.7 or more can be considered adequate (Table 64.6).[182,186,195,198,212] Overemphasis on urea kinetic modeling has resulted in the neglect of several relevant issues. Chronic overhydration has major negative consequences, and cardiovascular disease is the most frequent cause of morbidity and mortality in patients with ESKD in general and in those on PD specifically.[212] The adverse effects of overhydration may counterbalance the marginal benefits of higher solute clearance if the latter is solely attended to in lieu of the former. Salt and water overload have to be closely monitored and corrected through dietary restrictions, ultrafiltration, pharmacologic interventions (i.e., use of oral diuretics in patients with RKF), or a combination thereof.

Renal clearance is not equivalent to peritoneal clearance, inasmuch as the kidney provides benefits that are not achieved with PD, including better middle molecule clearance, volume control, and metabolic and endocrine benefits. Hyperphosphatemia and other abnormalities of mineral metabolism are strongly associated with cardiovascular morbidity and mortality.[213] Protein-energy wasting should also receive close attention because it is present in many patients with CKD (see Chapter 60). Protein-energy wasting is a negative prognostic indicator to be considered even before the need of dialysis and is discussed in the "Nutritional Counseling and Nutrient Supplements" section. Attention to nontraditional risk factors, particularly inflammation, almost always present in patients with kidney disease, is important; inflammation is also discussed in more detail in the "Inflammation and Peritoneal Dialysis" section. Social and psychologic factors are also important for the care of the patient on PD.

Volume status constitutes an important determinant for PD patient survival and for an adequate prescription. Volume overload has an impact on cardiovascular morbidity as well as mortality in PD patients. Therefore, it is of upmost importance to consider normovolemia (achieved via "adequate" ultrafiltration) as a major target of dialysis adequacy.[192,198,214] Determination of optimal volume status is a complex issue and recent studies with bioimpedance spectroscopy have proven useful for this purpose.[215,216]

## NUTRITION AND PERITONEAL DIALYSIS

Protein-energy wasting is often present in patients on PD, and correlates directly with time on PD.[217–219] A deficient nutritional status in the PD patient is strongly associated with morbidity and mortality.[220–222] Multiple variables are employed to assess nutritional status, including serum albumin and prealbumin concentrations, body cell mass, total body nitrogen, creatinine excretion, anthropometric indices, subjective global assessment (which ironically, is neither fully subjective nor global), bioimpedance vector analysis, and composite nutritional scores. In order to better evaluate and monitor the nutritional status of a patients receiving PD, the use of multiple tools is required, as no single measure provides a complete evaluation.[223,224]

The cause of protein-energy wasting in PD patients is multifactorial and complex (Table 64.7). Nutrient losses during dialysis, low nutrient intake, comorbid conditions, chronic inflammation, metabolic acidosis, loss of RKF, uncorrected uremia, peritoneal transport type, aging, and a variety of endocrine disorders contribute to the deficient nutritional status.[225–229] Some studies have shown that patients with high peritoneal membrane permeability could be at higher risk for protein-energy wasting; however, studies examining the links between peritoneal transport and nutritional status have yielded contradictory results.[229–231] It has been long described that patients on dialysis may have at least two different types of protein-energy wasting.[232] The first one related to low nutrient intake and a second form associated with inflammation and cardiovascular disease, not unlike the classic definitions of marasmus and kwashiorkor; the latter form is more common in PD, as the modality often contributes to the delivery of adequate (or sometimes in conjunction with intake, excessive) calories. These types of protein-energy wasting often coexist in the clinical setting.

A diversity of therapeutic strategies to treat or prevent declining nutritional status in the PD patient has been suggested. These include: nutritional counseling for adequate nutrient intake, treatment of reversible causes of anorexia, and correction of catabolic factors (inflammation, correctable comorbidities, uremia, and acidosis; see Table 64.7).

**Table 64.7 Etiology of Protein-Energy Wasting in Patients on Peritoneal Dialysis**

| Causes of Protein-Energy Wasting | Possible Management Strategies |
|---|---|
| **Nutrient Losses** | |
| Amino acids<br>Peptides<br>Proteins<br>Water-soluble vitamins<br>Other bioactive compounds | Nutritional counseling<br>30-35 kcal/kg/day<br>1.2 g of protein/kg/day<br>Nutrient and vitamin supplements<br>Dialysis solutions with amino acids |
| **Low Nutrient Intake** | |
| Anorexia | Treatment of reversible causes of anorexia |
| Impaired gastric emptying | Increasing the dosage of dialysis solution |
| Altered taste sensation | Prokinetic agents |
| Unpalatable diet | Nutritional counseling |
| Inadequate clearance of anorexigens | 30-35 kcal/kg/day |
| Intercurrent illness | 1.2 g of protein/kg/day |
| Emotional distress | Nutrient and vitamin supplements |
| Impaired ability to procure, prepare, or ingest food | Dialysis solutions with amino acids |
| **Comorbidity** | Treatment of comorbid illnesses |
| **Chronic Inflammation** | Extracellular fluid volume control<br>Antiinflammatory drugs (in the future) |
| **Metabolic Acidosis** | Correction of acidosis |
| **Loss of Residual Kidney Function** | Renin angiotensin system inhibitors<br>High-dose furosemide (urine volume)<br>Avoidance of nephrotoxins |
| **Possible Role** | |
| Endocrine disorders of uremia<br>Fast peritoneal membrane transport<br>Occult gastrointestinal bleeding | Recombinant growth hormone<br>Correction of anemia and comorbid conditions |

## NUTRITIONAL COUNSELING AND NUTRIENT SUPPLEMENTS

Nutritional counseling is the first-line intervention to achieve adequate nutrient intake.[233] The usual recommended daily energy intake for patients on maintenance PD is 35 kcal per kilogram of body weight per day for those younger than 60 years of age and 30 to 35 kcal/kg/day for those aged 60 years or older.[223] Nevertheless, the presence of obesity may modify our prescription accordingly, as in some patients a lower intake is preferred in order to limit weight gain or even to induce weight loss. Energy intake in patients on PD, in addition to dietary intake, should take into account glucose absorbed from the dialysate, which is dependent on several factors such as peritoneal transport, volume, dwell time, and glucose concentration. Energy from dialysate on average is around 20% of the total energy intake, corresponding to 3 to 13 kcal/kg/day.[234] In relation to protein intake, no less than 1.2 g/kg (≥50% of proteins with high biologic value) is the daily recommendation for adults on PD, and in some specific instances of severe protein-energy wasting it should be higher[223]; nevertheless, it is important to point out there is a significant lack of evidence from randomized trials to confirm optimal protein intake in this population.[235] It is important to point out that actual protein and energy intake of PD patients is often considerably lower than recommended and anorexia, dysgeusia, and gastrointestinal symptoms could be contributing to this situation.[223,236]

Intensive nutritional support may be of value during hypercatabolic conditions, including episodes of peritonitis. However, the effect of counseling on the nutritional status of affected patients remains largely untested. One report suggested that nutritional counseling, as an isolated measure, may maintain nutritional status despite a decrease in RKF and higher rates of systemic inflammation.[237] Administration of oral nutritional supplements may contribute to improvement of nutritional status. Few controlled clinical trials have involved commercially available supplements, dry egg albumin-based supplements, and whey-protein supplements as a nutritional intervention, with results that are positive, suggesting the benefit of this approach.[238–243]

## DIALYSIS SOLUTIONS WITH AMINO ACIDS

Management of protein-energy wasting with the available PD solutions has been poorly explored and seems to require a personalized prescription.[244] The use of amino acids has been explored and in few randomized trials conducted to date, anthropometric and biochemical measures have been better preserved in some but not all treated patients.[245,246]

## REVERSIBLE CAUSES OF ANOREXIA

Increasing dialysis dose to correct anorexia is an approach often attempted but found to be ineffective in large randomized trials.[183,209,217] Gastroparesis is a frequent complication in patients on PD, particularly, but not exclusively, among those with diabetes[247]; correction of gastroparesis may increase dietary intake and reduce nausea and vomiting. The use of prokinetic agents has been reported to increase serum albumin concentration in hypoalbuminemic patients on dialysis with delayed gastric emptying.[248]

## METABOLIC ACIDOSIS

Given that acidosis induces protein catabolism, correction of acidosis with oral alkali has been a measure to improve nutritional status (see Chapter 60). In a randomized trial conducted among patients on PD, oral sodium bicarbonate supplementation resulted in a significant increase in the plasma bicarbonate concentration, along with improvements in some anthropometric measurements and nutritional status (evaluated by subjective global assessment); this in turn was associated with shorter hospitalization period and reduced morbidity.[249] A recent study demonstrated that oral bicarbonate administration may decelerate the loss of RKF in PD patients.[250]

### ANABOLIC HORMONES

An anabolic strategy is to administer recombinant growth hormone. Its administration has been reported to be effective in improving nutritional parameters in short-term studies in children; however, its use is limited by cost and the development of hyperglycemia and other side effects.[251] Similar results have been observed with the use of insulin-like growth factor-I.[252] In addition, in small randomized trials, androgenic (anabolic) steroids have been shown to improve some parameters of nutritional status, yet significant risks and side effects preclude their use in clinical practice.[253] Ghrelin is a hormone synthesized by gastric endocrine cells and is involved in regulation of food ingestion and energy metabolism. Patients on PD have lower ghrelin concentrations than patients on HD or controls.[254] Although ghrelin, administered subcutaneously, enhances short-term food intake in patients with mild to moderate protein-energy wasting, further studies are necessary to determine the therapeutic role of this hormone.[255] Other hormones and cytokines such as leptin, TNFα, and IL-6, all of which have been found to be elevated in patients undergoing maintenance dialysis, could participate in the loss of appetite present in patients on PD.[256]

### L-CARNITINE

Advanced chronic kidney disease is associated with abnormal L-carnitine metabolism. At present, data demonstrating a beneficial effect of L-carnitine on nutritional status in PD patients are insufficient to recommend routine use.[257–259]

## INFLAMMATION AND PERITONEAL DIALYSIS

An inflammatory phenomenon evidenced by increased proinflammatory cytokines and acute phase reactants is observed in 12% to 65% of patients with advanced CKD before they start dialysis, and it is aggravated with both PD and HD.[260,261] Systemic inflammation is strongly related to atherosclerosis and protein-energy wasting.[260,261] Local intraperitoneal inflammation induces important structural alterations, including thickening and cubic transformation of mesothelial cells, fibrin deposition, fibrous capsule formation, perivascular bleeding, and interstitial fibrosis, and is associated with peritoneal solute transfer rate.[70] These structural alterations induce clinical and functional changes, including ultrafiltration failure, which can occur in a large proportion of longstanding PD patients.[262]

In the stable patient on PD without active peritonitis or other infection, several conditions may be implicated in the origin of systemic inflammation, including the use of bioincompatible dialysis solutions. Additional factors, such as rapid peritoneal membrane transport, low RKF, and overhydration, have also been associated with inflammation.[263] It is clear and a universal consensus that systemic inflammation, independently or in combination with all the variables mentioned previously, is an important factor associated with morbidity and mortality.[226,264–266]

There is a strong association among fluid overload, cardiac natriuretic hormones, and proinflammatory cytokines.[267] Adequate control of the hypervolemia may reduce a heightened inflammatory state, particularly in patients with high transport rates. When hypervolemia was ameliorated in high and high-average transport PD patients with NIPD, a reduction of serum C-reactive protein and IL-6 was observed.[268]

Results of small studies indicate that agents such as thiazolidinediones and statins may have relevant antiinflammatory effects, but these effects are modest.[269,270] Angiotensin-converting enzyme inhibitors may suppress C-reactive protein and oxidized low-density lipoprotein (LDL) cholesterol in patients with diabetes, but they do not appear to reduce inflammation in patients on HD.[271,272] In contrast, some evidence has been generated to support the idea that inhibition of the renin-angiotensin system may have an anti-inflammatory effect on the peritoneal membrane.[273]

At present, there are no studies testing the impact of treatment for chronic nondialysis-related infections (*Chlamydia pneumoniae, Helicobacter pylori,* dental-gingival infections, or viral hepatitis) on the inflammatory status of PD patients. The development of drugs targeting specific mediators of the inflammatory response, such as IL-6 or tumor necrosis factor may hold promise for the future.

## RESIDUAL KIDNEY FUNCTION AND PERITONEAL DIALYSIS

Peritoneal dialysis is associated with preservation of RKF, and PD has been shown to preserve RKF longer than hemodialysis.[274] PD may preserve RKF better than HD in part because, in comparison to HD, PD is associated with less hemodynamic instability, less frequent volume depletion, and avoidance of the extracorporeal system of hemodialysis that serves as sources of systemic inflammation, oxidative stress, and subsequent kidney injury. Several factors have been associated with loss of RKF in patients receiving PD, including female sex, diabetes mellitus, and nonwhite race, as well as comorbid conditions including congestive heart failure, poorly controlled hypertension, coronary artery disease, and aminoglycoside use.[275–278]

Multiple cohort studies have confirmed a positive association between the presence and degree of RKF and survival in PD patients.[206,279,280] Subsequent studies have consistently shown an association between loss of RKF and higher risk for volume overload, left ventricular hypertrophy, and congestive heart failure, all of which are meaningful to patients, and associate with survival.[281,282] These observations of greater survival in PD patients with better preserved RKF has been postulated to result from several factors including: renal clearance of circulating proinflammatory cytokines, middle molecular weight uremic toxins and protein-bound toxins (e.g., p-cresol), which are otherwise poorly removed with dialysis alone; improved anemia management due to persistent endogenous erythropoietin production; and preserved renal salt and water excretion allowing better maintenance of euvolemia and normotension.[281,282] Additionally, preserved RKF allows for better maintenance of normal bone mineral metabolism; RKF loss in PD patients is associated with higher serum phosphate concentrations and higher serum FGF-23 levels (independent of serum phosphorus), both of which have been implicated in causing increased arterial stiffening and valvular calcification, and hence increased cardiovascular mortality.[283] Loss of RKF per se is associated with increased valvular calcification and cardiac hypertrophy.[284]

Nutritional status, which is strongly related to the presence of inflammation, is better maintained in the presence of RKF.[226,285] Appetite, macro- and micronutrient intake are linked to better preserved RKF.[226,266] Moreover, anuric patients seem to have higher resting energy expenditure compared to patients with RKF, which may partially explain the superior nutritional status seen in the latter group.[286] Better nutrition has been linked to a stronger immune system, and indeed incident PD patients with RKF have been shown to have lower rates of peritonitis and peritonitis-related mortality, compared with anuric patients.[285,287] The strategy of preferentially using PD as the initial dialysis modality in patients with RKF is intriguing and deserves additional investigation; small studies seem to show a better survival in patients who initiate PD therapy and subsequently transfer to hemodialysis therapy compared with matched hemodialysis-only patients, particularly those who begin hemodialysis with a central venous catheter.[288–290]

### MEASURES TO PRESERVE RESIDUAL KIDNEY FUNCTION

The effect of PD modality (i.e., CAPD versus APD) on RKF preservation has been investigated in numerous studies.[171] While some reports suggest that APD is associated with a more rapid decline of RKF than CAPD in spite of similar peritoneal UF volumes, the preponderance of evidence suggests that PD modality has no effect on change in RKF.[171]

High-dose furosemide has been shown to preserve urinary volume, increase sodium removal and decrease weight gain better than placebo, without an independent effect on solute clearances per se.[291] On the other hand, hypovolemia and hypotension have been shown to be independently associated with a more rapid loss of RKF, thus special care is needed to achieve a safe balance between extracellular fluid volume overload and hypovolemia caused by overzealous diuresis and ultrafiltration.

Biocompatible PD fluids have been hypothesized to be less glomerulotoxic than conventional glucose-based solutions; the effect of low glucose-degradation product glucose-based PD solutions and icodextrin is discussed in more detail above. In summary, evidence suggests that low-glucose degradation product glucose-based PD solutions are associated with slower decrease in urine volume and solute clearance in the long-term. In contrast, there is no meaningful effect of icodextrin on the rate of loss of residual kidney function.

Inhibitors of the renin-angiotensin-aldosterone system blockade slow the progression of chronic kidney disease of multiple etiologies, with the preponderance of evidence accumulated in type 2 diabetes. In two small trials of prevalent patients receiving PD, angiotensin converting enzyme inhibitors and angiotensin receptor blockers promote preserved RKF relative to control antihypertensive agents.[292,293]

## CARDIOVASCULAR DISEASE IN PERITONEAL DIALYSIS

Cardiovascular disease—including new-onset congestive heart failure, peripheral vascular disease, ischemic heart disease, sudden cardiac death, and stroke—is common among patients with ESKD.[294] Moreover, patients on PD have a remarkably high risk of dying from myocardial infarction, arrhythmias, valvular disease, and sudden cardiac death.[295] Vascular and valvular calcification, volume overload with resultant left ventricular hypertrophy, inflammation and accelerated atherosclerosis all contribute to cardiovascular mortality in patients with ESKD.[296]

The interplay of many pathways underlie the development of cardiovascular disease in patients on PD. These pathways include traditional risk factors (diabetes mellitus, hypertension, dyslipidemia, sedentary lifestyle, left ventricular hypertrophy, smoking, male sex, insulin resistance), uremia-specific factors (anemia, phosphate retention, vascular calcification, uremic toxins, volume overload, hyperparathyroidism), novel risk factors (inflammation, oxidative stress, endothelial dysfunction, activation of the sympathetic nervous system, protein-energy wasting, carbamylation of proteins, epigenetic changes), and genetic factors.[297] Additionally, there are factors specific to PD that increase cardiovascular risk, e.g., hypokalemia (more common with PD than HD) has been demonstrated to confer a higher risk of death in patients receiving PD[298]; similarly, overhydration and loss of RKF have each been associated with higher risk for cardiovascular disease.[183,206,279,299–301]

### MANAGEMENT OF CARDIOVASCULAR DISEASE IN PERITONEAL DIALYSIS

Hypertension is a well-recognized risk factor for cardiovascular disease in the general population. The relationship between hypertension per se and cardiovascular disease in dialysis patients is complex due to the myriad comorbidities seen in the ESKD population. While short-term studies have found a weak or even inverse relation between hypertension and cardiovascular disease in ESKD, longer-term studies have found benefit to control of hypertension.[302–304] Volume overload is a major cause of hypertension in patients receiving PD, particularly when ultrafiltration capacity is insufficient to maintain normotension after RKF declines. Therefore, it is of utmost importance to monitor urine volumes over time and to adjust PD prescriptions when needed to compensate for loss of RKF. Patients with higher peritoneal membrane transport rates should be evaluated for cycler therapy and/or icodextrin use during the long dwell period, to reduce the risk of volume overload due to long dwell times.

Glucose-containing PD solutions may contribute to cardiovascular disease by increasing a patients' exposure to GDPs (and hence, circulating AGEs) and by possibly inducing insulin resistance, which is associated with cardiovascular morbidity.[305,306] Thiazolidinediones can be used to modulate insulin resistance, but published evidence in favor of their use is scarce.[307] Exercise including strength training may improve glucose tolerance in ESKD with impaired glucose tolerance.[308,309] Nonglucose PD solutions are another potential solution to this problem; lower serum insulin levels and increased insulin sensitivity have been reported with icodextrin.[133,310,311] The role of glucose sparing regimens is discussed above.

Hyperlipidemia due to systemic glucose absorption and peritoneal protein losses potentially contribute to the observation of higher levels of total and LDL cholesterol, apolipoprotein B, lipoprotein (a), and triglycerides as well as lower levels of high-density lipoprotein cholesterol in patients on PD than in patients on hemodialysis.[312] As in the general population, statins safely decrease serum cholesterol concentrations in patients receiving dialysis but their efficacy in decreasing cardiovascular mortality has not yet been proven.[313] The Study of Heart and Renal Protection (SHARP) included patients who were receivingh PD at the time of enrollment or who had imitated therapy with the modality during the course of the trial.[314] The study demonstrated a lower risk for cardiovascular events in patients treated with simvastatin-ezetemibe, without a beneficial effect on cardiovascular mortality.[314] Further studies should provide more insight about the efficacy of statins in reducing mortality among patients receiving dialysis, particularly among those on PD, for whom virtually no information is available.

Vascular calcification, affecting the arterial media, atherosclerotic plaques, myocardium, and heart valves, is a common feature in patients with ESKD and is associated with cardiovascular disease and mortality in patients on dialysis, including those treated with PD.[315] Moreover, cardiac valve calcifications are more frequent in patients on PD who have inflammation, and are associated with a 6-fold higher risk of cardiovascular death.[316] In patients on hemodialysis, therapy with sevelamer, a non–calcium phosphate binder, attenuates the progression of vascular calcification scores relative to calcium-based binders; effects on survival are uncertain.[317] Newer, non-calcium binders are now available and future studies with these agents may help elucidate the matter further.

Genetic factors may also affect the risk of vascular complications and outcome in the PD population. Examples are (1) the finding that a single nucleotide polymorphism in the IL-6 gene is associated with higher plasma levels of IL-6, higher diastolic blood pressure, and higher left ventricular mass and (2) the finding that non–BB allele variants of the BsmI polymorphism of the vitamin D receptor gene are associated with increased risk of hypercalcemia.[318,319] The clinical relevance of these associations, however, remain uncertain.

## PERITONITIS

### DEFINITION, DIAGNOSIS, AND CLINICAL COURSE

The presence of a cloudy peritoneal effluent is often the earliest sign of peritonitis, although abdominal pain precedes it in some patients. A diagnosis of peritonitis can be established when at least two of the following manifestations are present: abdominal pain, positive result of a peritoneal fluid culture, and more than 100 white cells/mm$^3$ in the dialysis effluent.[320,321] A bacterial peritonitis typically presents with more than 50% of its WBC as polymononuclear cells. Although turbid effluent is not always associated with peritonitis, its presence should always be considered a sign of possible infection until proven otherwise. When the peritoneal fluid culture is negative and the effluent leukocyte count is normal, other causes for the cloudy effluent should be considered, including the following: fibrin, chylous ascites, malignancy, chemical or eosinophilic peritonitis, and a specimen taken from a dry peritoneum.[321–326] The presence of more than 10% eosinophils in a cloudy effluent is diagnostic of eosinophilic peritonitis. The condition may manifest early after catheter placement, or it may be associated with mycotic infections, allergic reactions, and exposure to drugs such as vancomycin.[327,328]

The most frequent pathway for invasion of the peritoneal cavity by infectious agents is through the catheter's lumen; the next most frequent pathway is the pericatheter route.[329] Transmural bacterial migration has been implicated as another cause of PD-related peritonitis in patients with constipation, diarrhea, recent colonoscopy, diverticulitis, or other bowel pathology. Carriage of *Staphylococcus aureus* in the nasal mucosa and skin is linked to exit-site and catheter-related infections, both of which are risk factors for peritonitis.[330] When purulent exudate is present at the exit site, a swab culture should be performed. Other less common routes of peritonitis are hematogenous spread, either due to active bacteremia or transient bacteremia after periodontal procedures and ascending bacterial spread from the female genital tract. The incubation period of a peritonitis episode is variable depending on the route of infection and the specific organism; for example, touch contamination has been reported to cause symptoms between 6 and 48 hours later.[331] The severity of clinical manifestations is also variable between episodes of peritonitis and may be related to the specific causal agent. *Staphylococcus epidermidis* infections in general cause milder symptoms than gram-negative organisms, *S. aureus,* and mycotic organisms.[320,332] In comparison to surgical or spontaneous peritonitis, PD-related peritonitis is rarely associated with bacteremia.

Bacterial peritonitis typically presents with a peritoneal effluent leukocyte count exceeding 100/mm$^3$ with a leukocyte predominance (effluent neutrophils comprise >50% of the total leukocyte count). Adequate cultures of peritoneal effluent samples should yield positive results in more than 80% of cases. If a high rate of culture-negative peritonitis is present, peritoneal culture methods should be reviewed and optimized. The simplest way to obtain peritoneal fluid cultures is by inoculating 5 to 10 mL of effluent directly into a blood culture bottle; the sample should be sent to the lab within 6 hours or less for best results. Another culture method involves inoculating 50 mL of centrifuged dialysate into a solid culture media; conflicting reports are unable to confirm which method leads to lower rates of culture-negative peritonitis.[333–335]

Gram stains of PD effluent are notoriously insensitive methods of detecting bacteria, and are useful mainly for early identification of yeast (see fungal peritonitis, below).[331] Inadequate effluent collection can cause low leukocyte counts despite clinical symptoms of peritonitis; this occurrence is more common in APD due to short dwell times. If indicative symptoms are present without effluent leukocytosis, cultures and cell counts should be repeated after a dwell period of at least 2 hours. The differential diagnosis of culture-negative peritonitis with dialysate leukocytosis includes inadequate sample collection or laboratory processing, previous antibiotic treatment, or the presence of fungi or mycobacteria.[320]

In spite of double-bag systems substituting spike connection in the PD exchange procedure, the most prevalent organism in most reported series is still gram-positive bacteria, particularly *S. epidermidis* acquired through touch contamination. Pathogenic flora may vary significantly according to geographic and other environmental circumstances.[329,336,337] The second most frequent bacterial cause of PD-peritonitis is *S. aureus*, often associated with tunnel or exit-site infection; compared with *S. epidermidis*, *S. aureus* peritonitis may cause more severe disease and more often lead to catheter loss and the need to transfer temporarily or permanently to hemodialysis.[338,339] *Enterococci* are the third most commonly encountered agents of gram-positive peritonitis; they typically respond to antimicrobial treatment but care must be taken to review bacterial sensitivity patterns because vancomycin-resistant strains are not uncommon.[340] Constipation and other bowel pathology may predispose to *Enterococcal* infections, which frequently cause recurrent and relapsing peritonitis.[341]

Although gram-positive organisms are the most common cause of PD-peritonitis, the proportion (but not total number) of infections due to gram-negative organisms has increased over the past 20 years.[342,343] A variety of organisms derived from bowel, skin, urinary tract, water sources, and animal contact have been reported to cause gram-negative peritonitis. Peritonitis from *Escherichia coli* strains and other *Enterobacteriaceae* such as *Klebsiella* or *Proteus* organisms pose serious problems particularly in developing nations, but in most cases, they respond to antibiotic regimens. *Pseudomonas* peritonitis accounts for approximately 8% to 10% of gram-negative peritonitis cases and can frequently necessitate catheter removal. Early catheter removal, temporary transfer to hemodialysis with peritoneal cavity rest, and dual-antipseudomonal antibiotic coverage are all associated with better outcomes, oftentimes allowing a patient to return to PD therapy. *Pseudomonas* species are also commonly associated with exit-site and tunnel infection.[331,344–346]

Multiorganism gram-negative peritonitis should prompt consideration of a primary abdominal pathologic process, such as diverticulitis or an intraabdominal abscess; however, most patients with polymicrobial peritonitis do not have an underlying abdominal catastrophe.[347] In cases of bowel perforation, fecal effluent may be evident and anaerobes are often present. The mortality rate in cases secondary to an abdominal catastrophe may be as high as 50% and is correlated with the primary event, as well as with delayed diagnosis and surgery.[348]

Fungal peritonitis occurs rarely but is always feared because of high mortality rates; early peritoneal catheter removal is required.[349] The species most frequently involved is *Candida albicans*; the concurrent presence of bowel obstruction and abdominal pain portend worse outcomes. It has been postulated that current or recent antibacterial treatment may increase the risk for fungal peritonitis; systemic antibiotics (for peritonitis or even non-PD infections) are thought to suppress normal bowel flora, thus allowing intestinal overgrowth of fungi; fungal peritonitis then can result due to fungal mural transmigration from the intestine into the peritoneum.[350]

Peritonitis caused by mycobacteria is very rare; in most instances, it is initially diagnosed as culture-negative peritonitis. Diagnosis requires adequate culture techniques and a high index of suspicion. In mycobacterial infections, leukocyte counts generally exhibits a predominance of polymorphonuclear leukocytes in the peritoneal effluent.[320,351] Acid-fast smears are notoriously insensitive and mycobacterial cultures require days to weeks of incubation time. Polymerase chain reaction techniques have been useful in detecting tuberculous gene products in peritoneal fluid, and there are reports of retrospective diagnosis either after peritoneal biopsy (at the time of catheter removal) or after empiric anti-mycobacterial therapy led to a clinical resolution of the infection. In areas that are endemic for tuberculosis, tuberculosis peritonitis may comprise up to 4% of all infections and carries a high morbidity, particularly in patients with protein-energy wasting.[352,353]

## PERITONITIS TREATMENT

Empirical antibiotic treatment should be started as soon as infectious peritonitis is diagnosed, i.e., within hours. Peritoneal fluid leukocytosis is sufficient cause to initiate antimicrobial therapy, and treatment should start immediately without delay even if culture results are pending.[320] Initial empiric antibiotic regimens should include both gram-negative and gram-positive coverage. Thereafter, antibiotic regimens should be tailored to culture and sensitivity reports once available; center-specific bacterial sensitivity patterns should be taken into consideration when choosing antimicrobial therapy. Cloudy effluent and abdominal pain usually improve early in the course of treatment and may disappear within 48 to 72 hours. Persistent clinical manifestations of peritonitis may indicate a nonresponding bacterial organism, and necessitates prompt change in antibiotic treatment or consideration of catheter removal.[320] Follow-up effluent cell counts, preferably within the first 5 days, are a useful tool to evaluate treatment response because prolonged peritoneal fluid leukocytosis is associated with a higher rate of treatment failure and need for catheter removal.[354–356]

### INITIAL EMPIRIC THERAPY

Ideal empirical peritonitis treatment should provide broad antimicrobial coverage for the most frequent causes, should be convenient to administer, and should not favor the development of resistant organisms.[357] Such a perfect regimen does not exist. Selection of empirical therapy should be center-specific, depending on the local history of sensitivities of organisms. Empirical antibiotics must cover both gram-positive and gram-negative organisms. The latest international guidelines, based on evidence when available, include a regimen containing a cephalosporin or vancomycin for gram-positive bacteria together with either a third-generation cephalosporin, such as ceftazidime or cefepime, or an aminoglycoside.[320] Vancomycin is highly effective against most gram-positive bacteria, but its use has raised discussions about whether it favors the appearance of vancomycin-resistant staphylococci and enterococci.[358] Drug-resistant *S. aureus* and *Enterococcus* strains may necessitate administration of newer agents such as linezolid, quinupristin/dalfopristin, carbapenems, or daptomycin.[359]

Changing microbiologic features, toxic effects of drugs, or difficulties administering therapy may lead individual clinical groups to tailor their initial antimicrobial regimen to their own patients' needs. Evidence exists from several prospective studies that monotherapy with different agents (aztreonam, oral quinolones, cefepime) may be efficacious, but results are controversial.[359]

Antibiotic dosages should be determined based on the patient weight and RKF; when not adjusted for patient weight and RKF there is a considerable risk for underdosing with the result of an increased risk of treatment failure.

## ROUTE AND SCHEDULE OF ADMINISTRATION

Antibiotics can be administered by different routes (e.g., oral, intraperitoneal, intravenous). Intraperitoneal (IP) administration is much preferred to intravenous infusion; IP administration produces a greater concentration of antibiotics locally at the infection site, it is easy to administer, and has been demonstrated to be superior in a meta-analysis of randomized controlled trials (Table 64.8).[359] According to this analysis, intermittent (once a day in a long dwell of at least 6 hours) and continuous (antibiotics with each exchange) administration of antibiotics are equally efficacious in CAPD, and there is no benefit for routine peritoneal lavage or use of urokinase.[360] Antibiotic dosing and interval of administration in APD has not been sufficiently studied for all available regimens. The most recent guidelines acknowledge the lack of evidence for adequate antibiotic prescription in APD and guidelines are available for intermittent dosing of antibiotics for such patients (Table 64.9); nevertheless, they propose continuous dosing particularly of cephalosporins for this modality.[320] Cephalosporins and aminoglycosides could be administered intermittently in the long-dwell daytime exchange.[361,362] Vancomycin is administered intermittently every 3 to 5 days based upon the patient's own drug metabolism, and blood levels may be monitored to guide therapy, at least initially. Since vancomycin efficacy is time-dependent, care should be taken to maintain therapeutic blood levels above the bacteria's minimum inhibitory concentration (MIC) for as long as possible during the entire dosing interval. Researchers recommend keeping the peak value 5 to 8 times the MIC and that the trough value should be 1 to 2 times the MIC in order to reduce the risk for the development of resistance.[363]

## SPECIFIC ANTIBIOTIC TREATMENT

Once the results of the peritoneal effluent culture are known, if the initial empirical treatment is inadequate, it should be adjusted and the response monitored.

### Gram-Positive Bacteria

Coagulase-negative staphylococci usually respond rapidly to treatment and are adequately eradicated with the initially prescribed cefazolin or vancomycin, subsequently administered for 2 weeks.[320] Treatment of *S. aureus* peritonitis can continue with a first-generation cephalosporin if the organism is methicillin sensitive, or with vancomycin if it is methicillin resistant. In the rare occurrence of vancomycin-resistant *S. aureus,* linezolid, daptomycin, or quinupristin/dalfopristin should be prescribed. *S. aureus* infections should be treated for 3 weeks, even if a clinical response is seen early in the infection course. In the presence of an exit-site infection by the same microorganism, the catheter often must be removed.[320,338–340] If enterococcal peritonitis is diagnosed, intraperitoneal ampicillin and an aminoglycoside are indicated, or vancomycin in the case of ampicillin-resistant enterococci for 3 weeks.[320]

### Gram-Negative Bacteria

Non-pseudomonal gram-negative enterobacteria usually respond to third-generation cephalosporins or aminoglycosides; dual-antibiotic coverage may reduce the relapse and recurrence rate of certain gram-negative peritoneal

**Table 64.8 Intraperitoneal Antibiotic Dosing Recommendations for Patients on CAPD[a]**

| Drug | Intermittent (Per Exchange, Once Daily) | Continuous (mg/L[b]; All Exchanges) |
|---|---|---|
| **Aminoglycosides** | | |
| Amikacin | 2 mg/kg | LD 25, MD 12 |
| Gentamicin, netilmicin, or tobramycin | 0.6 mg/kg | LD 8, MD 4 |
| **Cephalosporins** | | |
| Cefazolin, cephalothin, or cephradine | 15 mg/kg | LD 500, MD 125 |
| Cefepime | 1000 mg | LD 500, MD 125 |
| Ceftazidime | 1000-1500 mg | LD 500, MD 125 |
| Ceftizoxime | 1000 mg | LD 250, MD 125 |
| **Penicillins** | | |
| Amoxicillin | ND | LD 250-500, MD 50 |
| Ampicillin, oxacillin, or nafcillin | ND | MD 125 |
| Azlocillin | ND | LD 500, MD 250 |
| Penicillin G | ND | LD 50,000 U, MD 25,000 U |
| **Quinolones** | | |
| Ciprofloxacin | ND | LD 50, MD 25 |
| **Others** | | |
| Aztreonam | ND | LD 1000, MD 250 |
| Daptomycin[115] | ND | LD 200, MD 20 |
| Linezolid[41] | Oral 200-300 mg qd | |
| Teicoplanin | 15 mg/kg | LD 400, MD 20 |
| Vancomycin | 15-30 mg/kg every 5-7 days | LD 1000, MD 25 |
| **Antifungals** | | |
| Amphotericin | NA | 1.5 |
| Fluconazole | 200 mg IP every 24-48 hours | |
| **Combinations** | | |
| Ampicillin/sulbactam | 2 g every 12 hours | LD 1000, MD 100 |
| Imipenem/cilastatin | 1 g bid | LD 250, MD 50 |
| Quinupristin/dalfopristin | 25 mg/L in alternate bags[c] | |
| Trimethoprim/sulfamethoxazole | Oral 960 mg bid | |

[a]For dosing of drugs with renal clearance in patients with residual kidney function (defined as >100 mL/day urine output), dosage should be empirically increased by 25%.
[b]Except as noted.
[c]Given in conjunction with 500 mg intravenous twice daily.
From Li PK-T, Szeto CC, Piraino B, et al: Peritoneal dialysis-related infections recommendations: 2010 update. *Perit Dial Int* 30:393-423, 2010.

**Table 64.9 Intermittent Administration of Antibiotics in Automated Peritoneal Dialysis**

| Drug | Intraperitoneal Dosage |
|---|---|
| Cefazolin | 20 mg/kg every day, in long daytime dwell[114] |
| Cefepime | 1 g in one exchange per day |
| Fluconazole | 200 mg in one exchange per day every 24-48 hours |
| Tobramycin | LD, 1.5 mg/kg in long dwell; then 0.5 mg/kg each day in long dwell[114] |
| Vancomycin | LD, 30 mg/kg in long dwell; repeat 15 mg/kg in long dwell every 3-5 days (aim to keep serum trough levels above 15 µg/mL) |

infections.[344,346] *Pseudomonas aeruginosa* peritonitis should be treated with two antibiotics for three weeks; if clinical improvement is not seen promptly, catheter removal is indicated. In individuals with coexisting exit-site infection with the same organism, catheter removal is recommended because of a high incidence of relapse even if there is clinical improvement with antibiotics alone.[320] Intraperitoneal aminoglycosides and third-generation cephalosporins, oral quinolones, and intravenous piperacillin have been employed with success in pseudomonal peritonitis.[348] Aminoglycosides should be used with caution; in addition to effects on RKF, aminoglycosides can result in serious vestibulotoxicity. Given the lower efficiency of solute clearance in PD, higher time-averaged exposure to aminoglycosides may be seen, placing patients at higher risk of adverse effects.

### Polymicrobial Peritonitis

In the presence of multiple enteric organisms, catastrophic intraabdominal pathologic processes such diverticulitis or appendicitis should be considered and, if diagnosed, surgery performed.[348] Antibiotic treatment should include an aminoglycoside, a third-generation cephalosporin or carbapenem, and anaerobic coverage with metronidazole or clindamycin. Treatment should continue for at least 3 weeks.

### Fungal Peritonitis

Fungal peritonitis is a potentially lethal infection that responds poorly to antifungal agents if the catheter is not removed because the organism forms biofilm on the catheter, thus resulting in a permanent reservoir for the fungus.[349,350] Occasionally, patients with fungal peritonitis may be too ill for surgery or may refuse catheter removal. Small case reports describe successful treatment of fungal peritonitis without catheter removal by using a combination of systemic and IP antifungal therapy plus continuous high-dose intracatheter amphotericin B.[364] With respect to selection of antifungal agents, a combination of flucytosine and amphotericin B has traditionally been recommended; development of resistance is high with flucytosine so this agent should never be used alone. Newer, less toxic antifungal agents (e.g., voriconazole, fluconazole, or caspofungin) may be successful when chosen according to fungal culture results and antifungal sensitivity reports; infectious disease consultation can be helpful in choosing proper antifungal therapy in complicated situations.[320,350] Treatment typically continues for 2 to 4 weeks once the catheter is removed.[320] There is a high mortality rate associated with keeping the catheter in situ; therefore fungal peritonitis should always require catheter removal.[349] Intraperitoneal abscess and adhesion formation are the most common reasons patients cannot return to PD after microbiologic cure.[365] Some have advocated keeping the catheter in place for a short period of time in order to administer IP antifungals, in an attempt to reduce the chance of adhesion formation.

### Mycobacterial Peritonitis

Treatment of mycobacterial peritonitis requires a complex antibiotic regimen including isoniazid, pyrazinamide, ofloxacin, and intraperitoneal rifampicin. Catheter removal may be required and treatment with four agents should commence as soon as possible, but definitely within 4 to 6 weeks of initial presentation to produce the best outcomes. Treatment should continue for 6 to 9 months, incorporating an initial intense treatment with four drugs followed by a maintenance period with two antimycobacterial agents.[351,352]

## CATHETER REMOVAL IN PERITONITIS

In addition to fungal peritonitis, intraabdominal disease, and refractory tunnel and/or exit-site infections, two other conditions warrant catheter removal: (1) relapsing peritonitis, defined as an episode with the same organism that caused the preceding episode of peritonitis, or one sterile peritonitis within 4 weeks after the end of the initial course of antibiotics, or (2) refractory peritonitis, defined as the failure to respond within 5 days of appropriate antibiotics. Catheter removal and simultaneous placement of a new catheter is most successful for exit-site or tunnel infections, or in relapsing infections once the effluent cell count and future have normalized; it should not be done in refractory peritonitis or in severe peritoneal infections[366]; success is most common in infections that do not involve *S. aureus*, *Pseudomonas*, mycobacteria, or fungi – in these cases the patient should be placed on hemodialysis until peritonitis is resolved (usually 3 to 4 weeks) before the placement of a new catheter.[320]

## PERITONITIS PREVENTION

Adequate catheter placement is relevant for peritonitis prevention. Exit-site placement and prophylactic antibiotic therapy at the time of placement, usually with a first-generation cephalosporin, is used to prevent postoperative infections. Only when the exit site is healed should the patient take over care of the exit site. Mupirocin cream applied to the exit site has proved useful in preventing local *S. aureus* infection. Mupirocin applied to the nares 5 days a month is also effective in reducing *S. aureus* exit-site infection, however it is ill-tolerated and requires monthly therapy. The use of local gentamicin has been shown to reduce *Pseudomonas* and other gram-negative infections at the exit site, as well as peritonitis rates.[367] The training of patients should include teaching them how to identify and notify the dialysis facility that contamination has occurred; episodes of contamination can be managed with change of transfer set with/without administration of prophylactic antibiotics depending upon whether a minor or major contamination occurred.[368] The use of double-bag systems in ambulatory patients and a flush-before-fill step after connection of the tubing to the solution bags in automated procedures are highly efficacious in preventing peritonitis episodes.[368–372]

## NONINFECTIOUS COMPLICATIONS OF PERITONEAL DIALYSIS

### MECHANICAL COMPLICATIONS

Intraperitoneal instillation of dialysate causes an increase in intraabdominal pressure, and the amount of intraabdominal pressure varies depending upon several factors including age, body mass index, volume of dialysate, and patient position, where intraabdominal pressure is highest in the sitting position, less when standing, and least in the supine position.[373,374] Additionally, certain maneuvers such as coughing, straining during defecation, and lifting may further increase intraabdominal pressure. The major risks associated with increased intraperitoneal pressure are the development of hernia, pericatheter leaks, diaphragmatic leaks, restriction of pulmonary expansion with resultant dyspnea, gastroesophageal reflux, abdominal discomfort, and pain.[375]

Hernias occur in more than 10% of patients on peritoneal dialysis. Many hernias, particularly in the inguinal or periumbilical region, are present prior to start of PD and become more apparent with the intraperitoneal instillation of dialysate. Hernias manifest as several different types including umbilical, abdominal (ventral), incisional, and indirect inguinal hernia. A preexisting but previously undetected patent processus vaginalis can suddenly become apparent as an inguinal hernia after initiation of PD due to new dialysate flow into the hernia, causing genital swelling.[376] New hernia can form de novo at the catheter incision site, umbilicus, ventral abdominal wall, or inguinal areas. Most hernia require surgical repair; however, conservative treatment may be indicated for some, particularly in elderly patients. Surgical repair may be performed successfully without temporary transfer to hemodialysis if the patient can be treated with low-volume supine exchanges for 2 to 4 weeks postoperatively.[377] For cases requiring mesh placement, surgical techniques have been described wherein the mesh can be placed extraperitoneally.[378] Ultimately, however, the need for surgery must be judged and decided on an individual basis.[376–378]

Pericatheter leaks may occur after dialysis initiation and are more common in obese patients. They may manifest as an external dialysate leak or as abdominal or genital edema. Conservative treatment, often successful, includes reduction of inflow volume per exchange, nocturnal intermittent PD, or temporary PD postponement and, if needed, temporary transfer to hemodialysis.[375,376,378–382] If leakage recurs, the catheter may require reinsertion.[378,348] A 3- to 4-week break-in period, defined as the time between catheter insertion and initial use, significantly reduces the risk of pericatheter leaks.[375,378]

Diaphragmatic leaks, due to preexisting diaphragmatic stoma, are uncommon and become typically clinically apparent soon after initiation of PD. The diagnosis of pleuro-peritoneal fistula may be made using imaging techniques whereby contrast dye or radioactive isotope is instilled into the dialysate solution, and later found in the pleural space. Upright daytime-only dialysis (with an empty peritoneum at night) can be performed for very temporary relief, and ultimately surgical correction or pleurodesis is needed to continue PD.

### METABOLIC COMPLICATIONS

The most relevant metabolic complications associated with PD are related to the consequences of systemic glucose absorption. Absorption of glucose from PD solutions may provide 500 to 800 kcal/day.[382–386] Glucose absorption may induce hyperglycemia in previously nondiabetic PD patients with impaired glucose tolerance.[386] Treatment of hyperglycemia may be a complex clinical problem. Biguanides are contraindicated, as in all patients with ESKD, but other hypoglycemic agents, including some sulfonylureas and thiazolidinediones, may be used.[384] The latter have been associated with reduction of fibrosis by inhibiting inflammation and regulating the transforming growth factor/SMAD signaling pathway.[387] Intraperitoneal insulin has been used in diabetic patients with CAPD because it appears convenient and physiologically beneficial, but it poses an important risk of contamination in the process of bag injection. Use of non-dextrose containing PD fluids has been associated with improved glycemic control.

A second metabolic condition highly prevalent in patients on PD is the presence of hyperlipidemia, accompanied by high levels of LDL cholesterol and apolipoprotein B; this lipid profile may be atherogenic and potentially contribute to the high cardiovascular mortality among patients on PD, although direct evidence of a link is lacking.[388] Patients may be treated with fibrates if hypertriglyceridemia is severe; statins are also used to lower levels of low-density lipoprotein cholesterol.[389] Combined use of these two agents is not recommended because of risk for rhabdomyolysis and/or hepatotoxicity.

Abnormalities in mineral metabolism are frequently present in patients on PD. Hypercalcemia may occur in PD due to vitamin D use, high calcium levels in some peritoneal fluids (i.e., 3.5 mEq/L), and ingestion of calcium-based phosphate binders; this in turn may induce suppression of parathyroid hormone secretion resulting in adynamic bone disease, a condition which has been reported to occur more frequently in PD than in hemodialysis.[367,390,391] The increased use of lower calcium dialysate (i.e., 2.5 mEq/L) and the use of non–calcium phosphate binders has reduced the incidence of hypercalcemia with PD. Phosphate control tends to be better in PD than in hemodialysis, probably from better adherence to diet and/or binders in patients who have additionally assumed the responsibility for their own dialysis, the continuous nature of the dialytic procedure, and longer maintenance of RKF.[390–392] Nevertheless, similar associations of hyperphosphatemia and mortality have been observed among patients on PD and HD.[393]

Among all patients receiving dialysis, those on PD are far more likely than those on HD to experience hypokalemia. Hypokalemia is not uncommon in PD, owing to the continuous nature of PD and the use of dialysate devoid of potassium; additionally, low potassium intake and/or high dose of loop diuretic therapy can also contribute to hypokalemia. Fortunately, nearly all patients on PD can achieve normal serum potassium concencentrations by increasing dietary intake of potassium-containing foods and/or oral potassium supplements. Hyperkalemia is less commonly encountered in PD than hypokalemia and is usually related to renin-angiotensin system blockade, missed dialysis or dietary excess. It is usually self-limited and not severe, as long as the patient is adherent with the dialysis prescription.

Hyponatremia is a common finding in patients on PD, partly because of fluid overload and the low dialysate sodium concentration, usually 132 mmol/L. Severe hyponatremia is infrequent and may be associated with hyperglycemia, protein-energy wasting, or water overload.[394,395] Hypernatremia is very rarely observed but may be present in older patients who have lost the sense of thirst or have limited access to water; a long series of frequent exchanges with very short dwell periods using hypertonic dialysate can also lead to hypernatremia through the mechanism of sodium-sieving, discussed above. Sodium sieving is easily avoided by allowing some longer dwell periods throughout the 24-hour cycle, thus allowing sodium to re-equilibrate between blood and dialysate.

## ENCAPSULATING PERITONEAL SCLEROSIS

Encapsulating peritoneal sclerosis (EPS), one of the most feared complications of PD, is an uncommon but serious entity that is most often associated with longer time on PD; the cumulative incidence varies between 0.5% to 4.4%.[396,397] In this condition, massive sclerosis of the peritoneal membrane ensues, resulting in encapsulation of the intestines. Encapsulating peritoneal sclerosis is responsible for severe disturbances of intestinal function, manifesting as motility disorders that cause impaired nutrient absorption, obstructive ileus, hemorrhagic ascites, anorexia, weight loss, and progressive clinical deterioration. Systemic inflammation is usually present, manifested by low-grade fever, hypoalbuminemia, elevated levels of serum C-reactive protein, and other inflammatory markers. The diagnosis requires clinical features of intestinal obstruction or disturbed gastrointestinal function and evidence of bowel encapsulation, either radiologically or pathologically. Computed tomography (CT) scanning is a reliable tool and can be used to confirm a diagnosis of EPS in an appropriate clinical setting.[398–402] Pathologic confirmation is available when patients are subjected to surgery for treatment or catheter removal.[403–405] However, care should be exercised because accidental injury to bowel may result in the formation of entero-cutaneous fistula.

The cause of encapsulating peritoneal sclerosis is unknown, but a number of factors that may contribute or predispose to its development have been identified. Contributing factors can be divided into those directly related to PD (time on PD, peritonitis, plasticizers, bio-incompatible dialysate, discontinuation of PD) and those that are not (idiopathic, β-blockers, autoimmune diseases, cancer, talc or other particulate substances, genetic predisposition).[403,404] Unknown factors render some patients more susceptible, inasmuch as some never develop encapsulating peritoneal sclerosis even after continuous exposure to multiple predisposing conditions. The reported incidence is higher in some countries, particularly Japan and Australia and an apparent increase in incidence has been reported in the European Union.[403,404,406] This increase may be related to ethnic or genetic factors, increased longevity of PD technique in certain areas, longer waiting times for kidney transplantation, or due to improved diagnosis and awareness of the disease. Among patients with a confirmed diagnosis, the mortality rate is very high, varying from 20% to more than 90%.[404,406] However, the survival in recent cohorts appears considerably higher than the earlier reports,[457] possibly related to a greater recognition of the disease entity and diagnosis at an early stage than in previous years.

Treatment for encapsulating peritoneal sclerosis is often unsuccessful and could even be described as ineffective, particularly if it is not implemented early in the course of the disease. There is no defined treatment of choice. Surgical treatment involves releasing or lysing adhesions of the small bowel, and requires precision and expertise to avoid morbid outcomes such as enterocutaneous fistula.[407] Medical treatments are either supportive or therapeutic, the latter aimed at ameliorating the inflammatory and pro-fibrotic processes in EPS. Total parenteral nutrition and discontinuation of PD with subsequent transfer to hemodialysis are often required; in some (but not all) instances, such treatment may induce regression of the pathogenic process.[403,404,406,408,409] One promising therapeutic option in EPS is the antifibrotic agent tamoxifen.[410,411] Prevention of encapsulating peritoneal sclerosis is not yet possible because clinicians do not understand the process that leads to this condition; nevertheless, early identification may be of great importance because early intervention is more effective than treatment later in the disease process.[403,406,408,409]

## PATIENT OUTCOMES WITH PERITONEAL DIALYSIS

Optimal comparison of two therapies, such as HD and PD, requires adequately powered randomized controlled clinical trials. One such trial had been attempted in the Netherlands but had to be abandoned as over 90% of eligible patients refused to be randomized.[412] A more recent clinical trial in China has been closed for recruitment without achieving its target enrollment and results are awaited (clinicaltrials.gov identifier: NCT01413074). Up until the results of this trial is available, the information available is based on national registries and a few prospective cohorts from around the world.[413–424]

Results of these studies are not conclusive and discrepancies can be attributed to multiple factors, including methodological issues such as use of intent-to-treat versus as-treated analysis, degree of case-mix adjustments, use of proportional versus nonproportional hazards models, assessment of prevalent versus incident patients, among others.[425–427] In general, when these differences are accounted for, similar results are found among registry studies and, to a lesser degree, among prospective cohort studies.[420,422,423]

Nondiabetic and younger patients treated with PD have an equal or lower risk for death compared to those treated with HD; among older diabetic patients, results vary by country.[425] For example, the Canadian registry showed no difference in risk for death between PD and HD among older diabetic patients and similar results were reported in Korea,[428] whereas in the United States, older diabetic patients treated with HD had a lower risk for death than those treated with PD.[420] In Danish and Norwegian populations, recent studies demonstrate a similar or lower risk for patients undergoing PD, which could be related to a cohort effect and to the mode of dialysis initiation.[429,430] Another Korean study demonstrated that patients with cardiovascular disease or diabetes on PD had a lower survival than those undergoing HD.[431] A recently published analysis of the REIN Registry demonstrated that patients with heart failure treated with HD had a lower risk for death than the patients treated with PD.[432] Similarly, the study of Wang and coworkers demonstrated that PD was associated with poorer survival among patients with cardiovascular disease or diabetes mellitus.[431] Despite disparate findings, it remains unclear whether the differences in risk for death are a result of differences in patients treated with the two modalities, or a direct benefit (or harm) of the therapy itself.[426,427] Hence, at present, these studies should inform but not be central to the selection of dialysis modality for an individual patient.[433]

Multiple studies have demonstrated a time-dependent trend in the relative risk of death, whereby PD is generally associated with equivalent or better survival rates during the first 1 or 2 years of dialysis. A European study reported that patients on PD had better survival during the first year and HD patients had better survival in the next 2 years of dialysis, yet overall survival comparing HD and PD was similar and influenced by age, diabetes mellitus, and center size.[434] Recent studies suggest that some of these differences are because of bias: many patients who start treatment with HD have had inadequate preparation for dialysis, which in turn, is an independent risk factor for death. When accounting for this source of bias, there does not seem to be significant differences in early survival among patients treated with PD or HD.[420,435]

When long-term survival is analyzed, results vary according to the nature of the study and to different subgroups within studies. Although subgroup analyses in the cohort studies have the advantages of being prospective and provides more clinical and laboratory details, they are usually limited by smaller numbers of patients in comparison with larger registry-based studies.[417,436,437] Large registry-based studies, although offering adequate statistical power for subgroup analyses, may be "overpowered" for detecting differences between the whole population of subjects on PD and those on HD. For instance, the overall relative risk of death in PD versus HD was 1.04 (95% confidence interval = 1.03 to 1.06, $P < 0.001$) for U.S. Medicare recipients who initiated dialysis between 1995 and 2000[414]; this difference was statistically significant in being powered by nearly 400,000 patients studied. However, this relative risk of 1.04 translates into an adjusted 3-year survival difference between HD and PD of 1 month.[425] A general improvement in survival among patients with renal replacement therapy has been observed; these improvements seem to be greater for patients undergoing PD than those treated with HD.[419,438,439] According to the 2013 United States Renal Data System (USRDS) Annual Data Report, there is a continued trend to an improvement in survival in patients who begin either HD or PD as compared to data between 1993 and 1997 as well as data from 1998 and 2002.[440] Data from other countries of the world, in particular Europe and Japan, have demonstrated better survival than data from the USRDS, results initially attributed to higher quality of treatment yet multiple factors including patients' comorbidities, age, and other factors undoubtedly play an important role in these differences, which make comparisons quite difficult.

As noted above, most studies demonstrate similar survival between PD and conventional HD. Therefore, modality choice must be individualized and tailored to maximize patient-reported outcomes including health-related quality of life.[441]

Patients on PD experience technique failure, most often due to peritonitis, catheter malfunction, "burn-out", and in some long-term patients, ultrafiltration failure; such patients are transferred to HD.[442,443] This fact should not be regarded as a limitation of PD, as in an appropriate renal replacement therapy program, patients must be requiring to be transferred from one modality (PD, HD, or transplantation) to another according to medical and other needs.

In summary, there is no conclusive evidence that one modality is superior to the other in terms of survival rate for all patients with ESKD, yet some subpopulations seem to perform better than others in PD and others in general do better in HD. It is important to point out that an individualized and educated decision is essential in deciding renal replacement modality and may play a role in survival.[441,444] Appropriate clinical judgment, consideration of cultural factors and informed patient choice are factors that should be always taken into account in deciding which dialytic modality will be chosen.

## ECONOMICS AND COST EFFECTIVENESS OF PERITONEAL DIALYSIS

ESKD is a constantly growing problem worldwide, and its treatment is extremely expensive. According to the 2015 USRDS report, the overall Medicare expenditure for ESKD treatment was $33.9 billion in the United States.[445] The economics of dialysis is very complex, and dialysis cost may threaten the health care systems of many countries.[446] In the industrialized world, PD has been shown to be less expensive than HD.[447–449] Most of the studies are either limited cost analyses or considerations of costs in relation to survival. Some studies have also shown that the cost-utility ratio is most favorable for PD.[450] In general, the cost continuum, from most to least expensive, is as follows: in-center HD, out-of-center HD (satellite-, or self-care HD) similar to APD, home HD, and CAPD.

Several reasons may explain the lower cost of PD, including the fact that the patient or a helper administers dialysis, whereas HD must be performed by trained staff, which is relatively expensive. In addition, PD requires fewer physical resources than does HD. Therefore, in countries with predominantly public dialysis providers such as government-run hospitals (Great Britain, Canada, New Zealand, Hong Kong, and Mexico), the use of PD is much higher than in countries with mainly private providers, such as physicians' offices or dialysis chains (United States, France, Germany, and Japan) in order to constrain ESKD expenditure.

The question that arises next is: If PD is less costly, why do private providers continue to prescribe it in a small percentage of cases? Several factors may explain this phenomenon, but the underlying argument is that the economic drivers of modality selection in countries with mainly private providers are determined by the local economic features of the system and not by actual costs (HD is more profitable).[451,452] In this situation, it is important to consider the following: (1) Once an HD unit is set up, there is economic pressure to maximize its efficiency by operating it at full capacity; (2) PD may cost less, but the payer (frequently the government) may reimburse expenses at a correspondingly lower level; and (3) in many countries with mainly private providers, HD offers more opportunity to bill for additional procedures (e.g., provision and administration of intravenous erythropoietin, vitamin D analogs, and iron).[451] An analysis of reimbursement policies and regulations in seven developed nations gives further insight to the complexity and diversity of factors that may influence dialysis modality selection and further stresses the need for better research in this area.[453] Changes implemented in 2010 in ESKD reimbursement policies in the United States, in which a bundled payment per person is considered, independent of modality chosen, continues to promise an increase in the use of PD.[452,454] A factor that significantly reduces the use of PD in some regions is a lack of adequate PD education and training in some nephrology programs, as a result of lack of expertise, interest, or economic incentive to promote PD growth. This has been reported as a significant factor limiting the increase of PD in the United States.[455]

The economics of dialysis in developing nations differs from that of industrialized nations.[446] In developing nations, where labor is relatively inexpensive and the cost of imported equipment and solutions is high, PD could be more expensive than HD. A further negative aspect for PD therapy in developing nations is that treatment may still entail outdated intermittent systems, and sometimes transfer sets are even reused, with high rates of peritonitis, increased costs, and high dropout rates. Several published analyses disavow this perception, showing that PD treatment may be less expensive than HD in developing nations[456]; in fact, the local production of PD fluids and competition between different providers may influence the lowering of PD costs. Thus, the perception that PD is not a viable option for developing countries is clearly inappropriate. In countries where the cost of PD is lower than that of HD, an increased use of clinically appropriate PD provides an opportunity to substantially lower overall the cost of ESKD treatment, as is being demonstrated in some nations.

 Complete reference list available at ExpertConsult.com.

## KEY REFERENCES

50. Pannekeet MM, Imholz AL, Struijk DG, et al. The standard peritoneal permeability analysis: a tool for the assessment of peritoneal permeability characteristics in CAPD patients. *Kidney Int.* 1995;48(3):866–875.
55. Mujais S, Nolph K, Gokal R, et al. Evaluation and management of ultrafiltration problems in peritoneal dialysis. International Society for Peritoneal Dialysis Ad Hoc Committee on Ultrafiltration Management in Peritoneal Dialysis. *Perit Dial Int.* 2000;20 Suppl 4:S5–S21.
70. Lambie M, Chess J, Donovan KL, et al. Independent effects of systemic and peritoneal inflammation on peritoneal dialysis survival. *J Am Soc Nephrol.* 2013;24(12):2071–2080.
78. Mehrotra R, Ravel V, Streja E, et al. Peritoneal equilibration test and patient outcomes. *Clin J Am Soc Nephrol.* 2015;10(11):1990–2001.
97. Abdel-Aal AK, Dybbro P, Hathaway P, et al. Best practices consensus protocol for peritoneal dialysis catheter placement by interventional radiologists. *Perit Dial Int.* 2014;34(5):481–493.
99. Morelle J, Sow A, Fustin CA, et al. Mechanisms of Crystalloid versus Colloid Osmosis across the Peritoneal Membrane. *J Am Soc Nephrol.* 2018;29(7):1875–1886.
101. van Laanen JHH, Cornelis T, Mees BM, et al. Randomized controlled trial comparing open versus laparoscopic placement of a peritoneal dialysis catheter and outcomes: the CAPD I trial. *Perit Dial Int.* 2018;38(2):104–112.
112. Perl J, Nessim SJ, Bargman JM. The biocompatibility of neutral pH, low-GDP peritoneal dialysis solutions: benefit at bench, bedside, or both? *Kidney Int.* 2011;79(8):814–824.
114. Rutkowski B, Tam P, van der Sande FM, et al. Low-sodium versus standard-sodium peritoneal dialysis solution in hypertensive patients: a randomized controlled trial. *Am J Kidney Dis.* 2016;67(5):753–761.
115. Weinreich T, Passlick-Deetjen J, Ritz E. Low dialysate calcium in continuous ambulatory peritoneal dialysis: a randomized controlled multicenter trial. The Peritoneal Dialysis Multicenter Study Group. *Am J Kidney Dis.* 1995;25(3):452–460.
116. Kang SH, Cho KH, Park JW, et al. Low-calcium dialysate as a risk factor for decline in bone mineral density in peritoneal dialysis patients. *Scand J Urol Nephrol.* 2012;46(6):454–460.
123. Takatori Y, Akagi S, Sugiyama H, et al. Icodextrin increases technique survival rate in peritoneal dialysis patients with diabetic nephropathy by improving body fluid management: a randomized controlled trial. *Clin J Am Soc Nephrol.* 2011;6(6):1337–1344.
127. Chow KM, Szeto CC, Kwan BC, et al. Randomized controlled study of icodextrin on the treatment of peritoneal dialysis patients during acute peritonitis. *Nephrol Dial Transplant.* 2014;29(7):1438–1443.
130. Li PKT, Ariza A, Culleton BF, et al. Randomized controlled trial of glucose-sparing peritoneal dialysis in diabetic patients. *J Am Soc Nephrol.* 2013;in press.
131. de Moraes TP, Andreoli MC, Canziani ME, et al. Icodextrin reduces insulin resistance in non-diabetic patients undergoing automated peritoneal dialysis: results of a randomized controlled trial (STARCH). *Nephrol Dial Transplant.* 2015;30(11):1905–1911.
132. Davies SJ, Brown EA, Frandsen NE, et al. Longitudinal membrane function in functionally anuric patients treated with APD: data from EAPOS on the effects of glucose and icodextrin prescription. *Kidney Int.* 2005;67(4):1609–1615.
147. Johnson DW, Brown FG, Clarke M, et al. Effects of biocompatible versus standard fluid on peritoneal dialysis outcomes. *J Am Soc Nephrol.* 2012;23(6):1097–1107.
149. Cho Y, Johnson DW, Badve SV, et al. The impact of neutral-pH peritoneal dialysates with reduced glucose degradation products on clinical outcomes in peritoneal dialysis patients. *Kidney Int.* 2013.
151. Johnson DW, Brown FG, Clarke M, et al. The effect of low glucose degradation product, neutral pH versus standard peritoneal dialysis solutions on peritoneal membrane function: the balANZ trial. *Nephrol Dial Transplant.* 2012;27(12):4445–4453.
154. Yohanna S, Alkatheeri AM, Brimble SK, et al. Effect of neutral-pH, low-glucose degradation product peritoneal dialysis solutions on residual renal function, urine volume, and ultrafiltration: a systematic review and meta-analysis. *Clin J Am Soc Nephrol.* 2015;10(8):1380–1388.
169. Bieber SD, Burkart J, Golper TA, et al. Comparative outcomes between continuous ambulatory and automated peritoneal dialysis: a narrative review. *Am J Kidney Dis.* 2014.
177. Michels WM, Verduijn M, Grootendorst DC, et al. Decline in residual renal function in automated compared with continuous ambulatory peritoneal dialysis. *Clin J Am Soc Nephrol.* 2011;6(3):537–542.
181. Paniagua R, Amato D, Vonesh E, et al. Effects of increased peritoneal clearances on mortality rates in peritoneal dialysis: ADEMEX, a prospective, randomized, controlled trial. *J Am Soc Nephrol.* 2002;13(5):1307–1320.
186. Perl J, Dember LM, Bargman JM, et al. The use of a multidimensional measure of dialysis adequacy–moving beyond small solute kinetics. *Clin J Am Soc Nephrol.* 2017;12(5):839–847.
187. Akonur A, Firanek CA, Gellens ME, et al. Volume-based peritoneal dialysis prescription guide to achieve adequacy targets. *Perit Dial Int.* 2016;36(2):188–195.
208. Churchill DN. The ADEMEX Study: make haste slowly. *J Am Soc Nephrol.* 2002;13(5):1415–1418.
210. Lo WK, Bargman JM, Burkart J, et al. Guideline on targets for solute and fluid removal in adult patients on chronic peritoneal dialysis. *Perit Dial Int.* 2006;26(5):520–522.
214. Van Biesen W, Williams JD, Covic AC, et al. Fluid status in peritoneal dialysis patients: the European Body Composition Monitoring (EuroBCM) study cohort. *PLoS ONE.* 2011;6(2):e17148.
233. Naylor HL, Jackson H, Walker GH, et al. British Dietetic Association evidence-based guidelines for the protein requirements of adults undergoing maintenance haemodialysis or peritoneal dialysis. *J Hum Nutr Diet.* 2013;26(4):315–328.
288. Lukowsky LR, Mehrotra R, Kheifets L, et al. Comparing mortality of peritoneal and hemodialysis patients in the first 2 years of dialysis

therapy: a marginal structural model analysis. *Clin J Am Soc Nephrol.* 2013;8(4):619–628.

296. Torlen K, Kalantar-Zadeh K, Molnar MZ, et al. Serum potassium and cause-specific mortality in a large peritoneal dialysis cohort. *Clin J Am Soc Nephrol.* 2012;7(8):1272–1284.
298. Brown EA, Davies SJ, Rutherford P, et al. Survival of functionally anuric patients on automated peritoneal dialysis: the European APD Outcome Study. *J Am Soc Nephrol.* 2003;14(11):2948–2957.
302. Shen JI, Mitani AA, Saxena AB, et al. Determinants of peritoneal dialysis technique failure in incident US patients. *Perit Dial Int.* 2013;33(2):155–166.
318. Li PK, Szeto CC, Piraino B, et al. Peritoneal dialysis-related infections recommendations: 2010 update. *Perit Dial Int.* 2010;30(4):393–423.
364. Mehrotra R, Singh H. Peritoneal dialysis-associated peritonitis with simultaneous exit-site infection. *Clin J Am Soc Nephrol.* 2013; 8(1):126–129, discussion 129–130.
374. Garcia-Urena MA, Rodriguez CR, Vega Ruiz V, et al. Prevalence and management of hernias in peritoneal dialysis patients. *Perit Dial Int.* 2006;26(2):198–202.
376. Crabtree JH. Rescue and salvage procedures for mechanical and infectious complications of peritoneal dialysis. *Int J Artif Organs.* 2006;29(1):67–84.
377. Stuart S, Booth TC, Cash CJ, et al. Complications of continuous ambulatory peritoneal dialysis. *Radiographics.* 2009;29(2):441–460.
378. Rabindranath KS, Adams J, Ali TZ, et al. Continuous ambulatory peritoneal dialysis versus automated peritoneal dialysis for end-stage renal disease. *Cochrane Database Syst Rev.* 2007;(2):CD006515.
380. McCormick BB, Bargman JM. Noninfectious complications of peritoneal dialysis: implications for patient and technique survival. *J Am Soc Nephrol.* 2007;18(12):3023–3025.
394. Johnson DW, Cho Y, Livingston BE, et al. Encapsulating peritoneal sclerosis: incidence, predictors, and outcomes. *Kidney Int.* 2010;77(10):904–912.
408. Guest S. Tamoxifen therapy for encapsulating peritoneal sclerosis: mechanism of action and update on clinical experiences. *Perit Dial Int.* 2009;29(3):252–255.
416. Chang YK, Hsu CC, Hwang SJ, et al. A comparative assessment of survival between propensity score-matched patients with peritoneal dialysis and hemodialysis in Taiwan. *Medicine (Baltimore).* 2012;91(3):144–151.
417. Mehrotra R, Chiu YW, Kalantar-Zadeh K, et al. Similar outcomes with hemodialysis and peritoneal dialysis in patients with end-stage renal disease. *Arch Intern Med.* 2011;171(2):110–118.
420. Weinhandl ED, Foley RN, Gilbertson DT, et al. Propensity-matched mortality comparison of incident hemodialysis and peritoneal dialysis patients. *J Am Soc Nephrol.* 2010;21(3):499–506.
440. Htay H, Cho Y, Pascoe EM, et al. Multicenter registry analysis of center characteristics associated with technique failure in patients on incident peritoneal dialysis. *Clin J Am Soc Nephrol.* 2017;12(7): 1090–1099.
441. Kurella Tamura M, Li S, Chen SC, et al. Educational programs improve the preparation for dialysis and survival of patients with chronic kidney disease. *Kidney Int.* 2014;85(3):686–692.
450. Vanholder R, Davenport A, Hannedouche T, et al. Reimbursement of dialysis: a comparison of seven countries. *J Am Soc Nephrol.* 2012;23(8):1291–1298.
456. Chang YT, Hwang JS, Hung SY, et al. Cost-effectiveness of hemodialysis and peritoneal dialysis: a national cohort study with 14 years follow-up and matched for comorbidities and propensity score. *Sci Rep.* 2016;6:30266.

# Critical Care Nephrology

# 65

Ron Wald | Kathleen Liu

## CHAPTER OUTLINE



## KEY POINTS

- In the setting of acute liver failure, continuous renal replacement therapt (CCRT) is the preferred renal replacement therapy (RRT) modality to mitigate the risks of cerebral edema and herniation.
- Permissive hypercapnia can occur with lung-protective low tidal volume ventilation, indicated for the management of the acute respiratory distress syndrome; with concomitant acute kidney injury (AKI), a severe mixed acidosis may arise.
- There is no benefit to early goal-directed therapy for the management of sepsis, either with regard to mortality or the prevention of AKI.
- The use of balanced crystalloids for resuscitation may reduce the risk of AKI.
- Although there is no definitive evidence favoring a particular RRT modality, it is reasonable to use intermittent and continuous modalities in the context of the patient's hemodynamic status.
- The optimal timing of dialysis initiation in severe AKI remains controversial; although the preemptive initiation of RRT in the absence of any emergent indications has conceivable benefits, it may expose patients who might otherwise recover kidney function without a need for RRT to undue risk.
- In critically ill patients with AKI receiving CRRT, effluent flow should be targeted to 25 mL/kg/hour.
- In critically ill patients with AKI, frequent and careful review of medications is warranted, with close attention to the avoidance of nephrotoxins and agents that accumulate in AKI while tailoring dosing and frequency of medication administration to the RRT modality in use.

Studies now suggest that up to 60% of patients in intensive care units (ICUs) experience an episode of acute kidney injury (AKI).[1-3] In the most severe cases, renal replacement therapy (RRT) is commenced. Short-term mortality among critically ill patients with acute AKI who receive RRT is in excess of 50%[4] and, among survivors, longevity and health-related quality of life are often poor.[5] AKI, as well as electrolyte and acid-base abnormalities, occurs on the background of multiple conditions that necessitate critical care. In this chapter, we first discuss AKI in the context of conditions that are frequently encountered in the ICU—acute liver failure, acute respiratory distress syndrome, acute decompensated heart failure, and sepsis. This is followed by a discussion of fluid management and its relevance to the care of patients with AKI. We then review the principles of RRT delivery to critically ill patients with AKI. We do not discuss acute brain injury in the ICU setting, which is associated with dysnatremias (including the syndrome of inappropriate secretion of antidiuretic hormone, cerebral salt wasting, and central diabetes insipidus). The reader is referred to Chapter 15 for further discussion of these disorders.

## ACUTE KIDNEY INJURY IN THE CONTEXT OF CRITICAL ILLNESS

### LIVER FAILURE

In the setting of acute liver failure, a major cause of death is cerebral edema, resulting in elevated intracranial pressure and, if severe or sustained, brain stem herniation.[6] Elevated intracranial pressure occurs in up to 35% of patients with grade III and 75% of patients with grade IV encephalopathy.[7] Continuous RRT (CRRT) is often used for meticulous control of volume status in these patients, given the high risk of cerebral edema in hepatic failure and frequent high obligate intake in the form of infusions (*N*-acetylcysteine, vasopressors, and blood products, including fresh-frozen plasma). CRRT can also be used to manage hyponatremia, a common complication of liver failure that may further exacerbate cerebral edema.

Patients with acute liver failure are at risk of developing AKI from hepatorenal syndrome or acute tubular necrosis. Acute tubular necrosis may be caused by profound hypotension, concomitant sepsis (a common complication of acute liver failure), or ingestion of a substance that is both hepatotoxic and nephrotoxic (e.g., acetaminophen, *Amanita* mushrooms).

### ACUTE RESPIRATORY DISTRESS SYNDROME

The mainstay of supportive care for patients with acute respiratory distress syndrome (ARDS) is low tidal volume, lung-protective ventilation, which has led to a significant reduction in mortality and is associated with decreased levels of proinflammatory cytokines.[8] As part of the lung-protective ventilation strategy, permissive hypercapnia is encouraged to minimize ventilator-associated lung injury. In the setting of normal kidney function, compensatory metabolic alkalosis will ensue. However, in the setting of impaired kidney function (acute or chronic), the metabolic acidosis that arises and the inability to compensate for associated respiratory acidosis may prompt the administration of bicarbonate-containing infusions or trigger the initiation of RRT for correction of the acid-base imbalance. In patients with severe ARDS in whom ventilation is markedly impaired because of alveolar injury (as reflected by a high dead space fraction and impaired respiratory carbon dioxide excretion), bolus doses of bicarbonate may worsen arterial pH through an abrupt increase in $Pa{CO_2}$ and conversion to carbonic acid.[9] Therefore, CRRT may be the preferred modality to correct pH slowly and compensate for respiratory acidosis. A fluid conservative management strategy has been associated with improved outcomes and no adverse kidney consequences, although patients with dialysis-requiring AKI at the time of study enrollment were excluded from the study.[10]

Studies in animal models have suggested that there is significant cross-talk between the kidney and lung—that is, injury to one organ results in injury to the other.[11-14] For example, kidney injury is associated with elevations of proinflammatory cytokines and worse lung injury in mice[15]; in one study, concentrations of interleukin-6 and interleukin-8 were higher in children with AKI after cardiopulmonary bypass surgery than in controls (children without AKI) and were associated with a longer duration of mechanical ventilation.[16]

### HEART FAILURE

Because cardiac function affects kidney function and vice versa, the following five clinical subtypes of the cardiorenal syndrome (CRS) have been proposed:[17,18]

1. Acute CRS (type 1), in which acute worsening of heart function leads to AKI
2. Chronic CRS (type 2), in which chronic abnormalities in heart function result in impaired kidney function
3. Acute renocardiac syndrome (type 3), in which AKI precedes impaired cardiac function
4. Chronic renocardiac syndrome (type 4), in which CKD leads to impaired cardiac function
5. Secondary CRS (type 5), in which systemic conditions such as sepsis result in simultaneous impairment in cardiac and kidney function

With type 1 CRS in particular, volume overload and consequent venous congestion may result in kidney dysfunction via several mechanisms, including profound hypotension compromising kidney perfusion, kidney venous hypertension, the development of ascites with intraabdominal hypertension, and perhaps inflammation.[19] Consequently, the use of diuretics to improve volume overload in acute decompensated heart failure may actually improve kidney function by relieving renal venous hypertension. On the other hand, excessive diuresis may lead to volume depletion and cause or exacerbate AKI.

There has been significant interest in the optimal management of volume overload in the context of acute decompensated heart failure. Several studies have compared the use of continuous versus intermittent bolus dosing of loop diuretics[20,21] on the basis of the hypothesis that continuous infusion results in more effective diuresis by avoiding periods of "rebound" sodium retention between bolus doses. However, the incremental benefit of continuous infusions over bolus dosing has not been demonstrated to date.

Extracorporeal ultrafiltration has been proposed as an alternative to diuretic management for volume overload in acute decompensated heart failure and has been tested in a number of randomized clinical trials. The Cardiorenal Rescue Study in Acute Decompensated Heart Failure (CARESS-HF) trial compared the safety and efficacy of ultrafiltration (with a target fluid removal of 200 mL/hour) to stepped pharmacologic therapy (target urine output of 3–5 L/day) in patients with acute CRS type 1 (Fig. 65.1).[22] The primary endpoint was the bivariate change from baseline in serum creatinine concentration and body weight. The trial was terminated early owing to a lack of benefit in the ultrafiltration group (serum creatinine level increased slightly compared with the pharmacologic group, and weight change was similar in both groups), combined with an increased

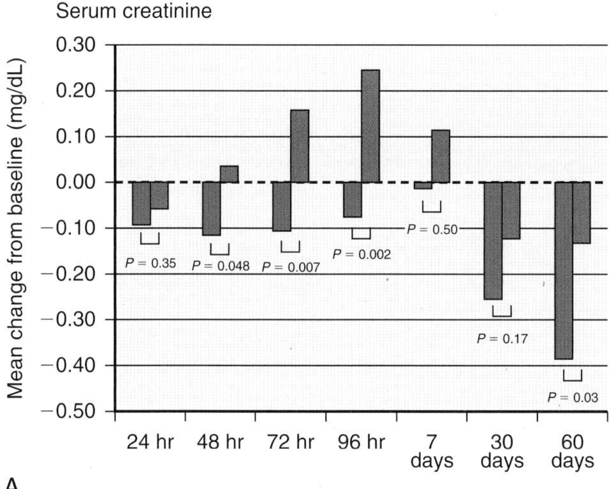


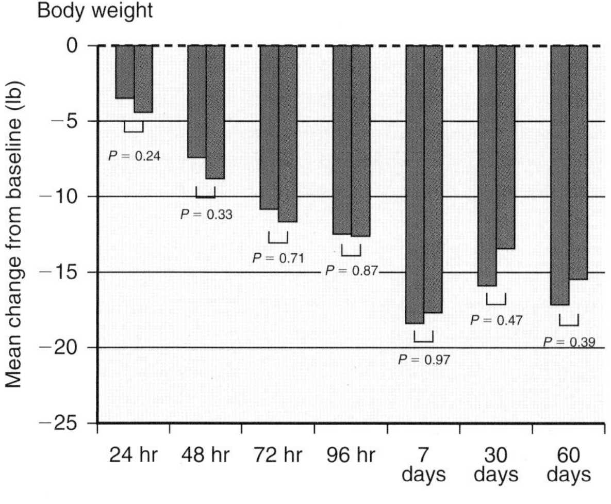


**Fig. 65.1** Role of ultrafiltration in decompensated heart failure. Changes from baseline in (A) serum creatinine level and (B) body weight at various time points, according to treatment group. The *P* values were calculated with the use of a Wilcoxon test. (From Bart BA, Goldsmith SR, Lee KL, et al. Heart Failure Clinical Research Network: ultrafiltration in decompensated heart failure with cardiorenal syndrome. *N Engl J Med.* 2012;367:2296–2304.)

risk of adverse events, including bleeding and catheter-related complications. On the basis of this experience, ultrafiltration is no longer favored as a first-line therapy for patients with acute decompensated heart failure. Nonetheless, ultrafiltration may be required in patients with acute decompensated heart failure that fails to respond to maximal doses of intravenous diuretics and other pharmacotherapy (e.g., cardiac inotropic agents), particularly in the presence of acute kidney injury (CKD) and/or acute kidney injury (AKI).

## SEPSIS

AKI is a common complication of sepsis and occurs via multiple mechanisms, including hypotension leading to hypoperfusion, inflammation, and oxidative stress.[23,24] There are no specific treatments for AKI or for sepsis itself, apart from source control and treatment with appropriate antimicrobials. With regard to inflammatory mediators in sepsis, there has been interest in the use of high-volume hemofiltration and adsorptive (e.g., polymyxin B) columns to remove proinflammatory cytokines, but studies to date have not shown any benefit.[25,26]

With regard to the early management of sepsis, publication of the pivotal study by Rivers and colleagues[27] has stimulated a major shift in clinical practice toward early "goal-directed therapy," in which inotropes and packed red blood cell transfusions are used in addition to early volume resuscitation and vasopressors in patients with septic shock. However, the results of three subsequent large randomized clinical trials have suggested no benefit of early goal-directed therapy over standard therapy.[28-30] The ProCESS (Protocol-Based Care for Early Septic Shock) trial randomly allocated 1341 patients in the United States to protocol-based early goal-directed therapy, protocol-based standard therapy, or usual care. There was no difference in 60-day, 90-day, or 1-year mortality among the treatment arms (60-day mortality 21% in the protocol-based early goal-directed therapy arm, 18.2% in the protocol-based standard therapy arm, and 18.9% in the usual care arm). There was also no impact on the rate of AKI after enrollment (40.3% in the protocol-based early goal-directed therapy arm, 34.9% in the protocol-based standard therapy arm, and 38.1% in the usual care arm).[31] Patients in the protocol-based standard therapy and usual care arm received fewer packed red blood cell transfusions and less dobutamine than patients in the other two arms, suggesting that these interventions are of limited benefit in a general population with sepsis. These findings have been further supported by the ProMISe (Protocolised Management in Sepsis) and ARISE (Australasian Resuscitation in Sepsis Evaluation) trials. An ongoing clinical trial, CLOVERS (Crystalloid Liberal or Vasopressors Early Resuscitation in Sepsis), is comparing the impact of early fluid resuscitation versus early vasopressor use in patients with septic shock.[32]

## FLUID MANAGEMENT AND ITS IMPACT ON ACUTE KIDNEY INJURY

There has been an increasing appreciation of the potentially deleterious effects of fluid overload in critically ill patients, particularly in the context of AKI. Fluid excess has been associated with a number of adverse consequences, including decreased gastrointestinal absorption and impaired wound healing.[33] In patients with AKI, fluid overload has been independently associated with an increased risk of new sepsis, as well as with increased short- and long-term risks of death.[34-37] However, the observational nature of these studies makes it difficult to determine if the relationship between fluid overload and mortality is causal. Specifically, it is unclear whether fluid overload directly mediates adverse outcomes or if sicker patients who are hemodynamically unstable—and who have an inherently worse prognosis—are more likely to receive fluid boluses and other infusions that generate a more positive fluid balance. Furthermore, total body fluid overload may dilute serum creatinine concentration and mask AKI.[38,39]

An adverse consequence of fluid overload that has gained significant interest is intraabdominal hypertension and the abdominal compartment syndrome.[40] Intraabdominal hypertension is defined as an intraabdominal pressure greater than 12 mm Hg. This pressure is typically measured by instilling a fixed volume of water (30 mL) into the urinary bladder via a Foley catheter and using pressure tubing to transduce a bladder pressure. The abdominal compartment syndrome is defined as an intraabdominal pressure greater than 20 mm Hg with associated end-organ dysfunction. Intraabdominal hypertension may mediate AKI through direct compression of the inferior vena cava, which results in impaired venous return and venous stasis throughout the abdominal cavity, including the renal veins.[41,42] Impaired venous return leads to decreased cardiac output and increased sympathetic and renin-angiotensin-aldosterone system (RAAS) signaling, resulting in renal vasoconstriction. The result is a functional prerenal state, characterized by low urinary sodium concentration and oliguria. Decompression of the abdominal compartment (typically via a surgical approach) may lead to an improvement of kidney function.[40] However, identification of patients whose kidney function will benefit from decompression remains elusive.

There has also been significant interest in the type of fluid administered and its impact on kidney function. It has been suggested that chloride-rich solutions may cause renal vasoconstriction and exacerbate renal medullary hypoxia.[43] In a small crossover study of human volunteers, administration of chloride-rich solutions was associated with greater fluid retention and reduced kidney perfusion than administration of balanced salt solutions.[44] A number of observational studies have suggested that the use of chloride-rich solutions is associated with a higher risk of AKI than balanced salt solutions.[45,46] The largest of these studies was a single-center, prospective, open-label sequential study.[46] During the 6-month control period, patients received normal saline (chloride concentration, 154 mmol/L, or chloride-rich colloids) for resuscitation. During the intervention period that commenced six months thereafter, patients received Plasma-Lyte (chloride concentration, 98 mmol/L) or chloride-restricted colloids for resuscitation. The incidence of AKI was 14% in the control period and 8.4% in the intervention period ($P < .001$). This was accompanied by a lower use of RRT (10% and 6.3%; $P = .005$) during the control and intervention periods, respectively). Challenges to the interpretation of these findings include the larger than expected effect size, concurrent changes made to other aspects of fluid management, and other practice changes that may have reduced the risk of AKI. One potential explanation for this difference is that the concomitant hyperchloremic metabolic acidosis from chloride-rich fluid administration may have triggered earlier RRT initiation.

The Saline vs Plasma-Lyte 148 for ICU fluid Therapy (SPLIT) trial[47] compared 0.9% Saline vs Plasma-Lyte 148 using a double-blind, double-crossover cluster design in four ICUs in New Zealand. Participating units were randomized to administer one of the study solutions to all admitted patients in two alternating 7-week blocks. Plasma-Lyte 148 did not lower the risk of acute kidney injury, the primary outcome of the trial, nor did it affect the receipt of RRT or any other marker of ICU resource utilization. A key limitation of this trial was the high number of patients who were enrolled postcardiac surgery, which may limit generalizability. More recently, two very large, pragmatic, single-center clinical trials have been published: SALT-ED (Saline against Lactated Ringer's or Plasma-Lyte in the Emergency Department, $N =$ 13,347)[48] and SMART (Isotonic Solutions and Major Adverse Renal Events Trial, $N = 15{,}082$).[49] Patients admitted to the emergency department or ICU, respectively, at Vanderbilt University Medical Center were allocated to receive a balanced salt solution (selected by the clinician—e.g., lactated Ringer's or Plasma-Lyte) or normal saline in alternating months. Although clinicians could choose to break the allocation and prescribe the opposite fluid, protocol compliance was excellent, at greater than 88% across the two arms of both studies. Both SALT-ED and SMART demonstrated a reduction in a composite endpoint of Major Adverse Kidney Events at 30 days (MAKE-30, which is comprised of a persistent doubling of serum creatinine level, new RRT, or death) with the use of balanced salt solutions (14.3% vs. 15.4% in SMART, $P =$ 0.04; 4.7% vs. 5.6% in SALT-ED, $P = .01$). Thus these two studies add strength to the argument that there is no benefit to the use of normal saline and possibly some potential harm. The ongoing Plasma-Lyte 148 versUs Saline (PLUS) trial, with a planned recruitment of 8800 critically ill patients and a primary outcome of 90-day mortality, may provide more definitive guidance on this question.[50]

## RENAL REPLACEMENT THERAPY IN THE INTENSIVE CARE UNIT

### GOALS OF CARE

Severe AKI frequently prompts discussions about the initiation of RRT. The broad goal of RRT revolves around management of the fluid and metabolic abnormalities of AKI in a manner that facilitates and promotes recovery from the underlying illness. RRT should ideally be performed with minimal disruption to the broader care received by the patient. One may debate whether RRT is merely supportive or confers an additional therapeutic benefit that may enhance survival. At present, there are no data on any specific RRT-related maneuver that improves patient survival. A further goal of RRT is maximizing the likelihood of recovery of kidney function among surviving patients. This objective is driven by the growing recognition that AKI survivors are at high risk for CKD.[51,52] RRT protocols should be designed to minimize iatrogenic injury to the kidney (e.g., injury due to hypotension and/or hypovolemia) in the hope that dialysis independence can be achieved, with an eventual return to the level of kidney function that preceded the acute illness (or almost to this level).

## INDICATIONS FOR COMMENCING RENAL REPLACEMENT THERAPY

The decision to initiate RRT is unambiguous when AKI is complicated by hyperkalemia, pulmonary congestion refractory to medical maneuvers, or concomitant intoxication with a dialyzable toxin.[53] However, even in the absence of a life-threatening AKI complication, some have argued in favor of a strategy of early or preemptive RRT initiation. Proponents of this approach have cited the mitigation or reversal of volume overload and tempering the toxicity of uncontrolled uremia as justifications for the earlier initiation of RRT.[54,55] On the other hand, a preemptive approach to RRT initiation has conceivable shortcomings. Even in patients with severe AKI, spontaneous kidney recovery is frequently observed, and the widespread adoption of earlier RRT could result in the potentially unnecessary exposure of patients to the risks associated with vascular access placement and the RRT procedure itself (e.g., hypotension, arrhythmia, electrolyte abnormalities, ineffective antibiotic concentrations). Furthermore, if a strategy of earlier RRT initiation does not confer any meaningful patient benefits, adoption of a more conservative approach to RRT initiation and commencing RRT only when an overt complication develops could lead to resource savings.

The controversy surrounding the optimal circumstances for RRT initiation in AKI was addressed in two recently completed randomized trials.[56,57] The Artificial Kidney Initiation in Kidney Injury (AKIKI) trial was a multicenter trial of 620 critically ill adults with Kidney Disease Improving Global Outcomes (KDIGO) stage 3 AKI conducted in France. The investigators hypothesized that a delayed strategy of RRT initiation (RRT only after 72 hours of persistent oligoanuria, serum urea > 40 mmol/L, or development of an AKI-related emergency) would confer better patient survival at 60 days compared with a strategy of early initiation, defined as commencing RRT within 6 hours of patients meeting criteria for stage 3 AKI. Patients in the delayed arm commenced RRT 55 hours later than those in the early arm but, importantly, only half the participants allocated to the delayed arm started RRT. The trial did not show an appreciable difference in mortality between the two strategies (60-day mortality in early and delayed groups was 48.5% and 49.7%, respectively; $P = .79$).

A single-center trial in Germany, Effect of Early vs Delayed Initiation of Renal Replacement Therapy on Mortality in Critically Ill Patients with Acute Kidney Injury (ELAIN), was designed to test the hypothesis that an early strategy of RRT initiation confers improved survival. The trial recruited 231 patients with stage 2 AKI who had a blood neutrophil gelatinase-associated lipocalin (NGAL) greater than 150 ng/mL and at least one other element of severe illness (e.g., one or more of sepsis, catecholamine dependence, hypoxemia, fluid overload, or progressive nonrenal organ injury). In the early RRT arm, RRT was started within 8 hours of fulfilling KDIGO stage 2 AKI, whereas in the delayed arm, RRT was deferred until KDIGO stage 3 criteria were met, or if an absolute indication became apparent. All patients in the early initiation arm received RRT at a median of 6 (interquartile range [IQR], 4–7) hours from meeting stage 2 AKI criteria; almost all (91%) patients in the late initiation arm attained a trigger for RRT initiation, which in most cases was achievement of KDIGO stage 3 AKI. These individuals started RRT at a median of 25.5 (IQR, 18.8–40.3) hours from reaching stage 2 AKI. Mortality was significantly lower in the early initiation arm compared with the delayed initiation arm (39.3% vs. 54.7%; $P = .03$; hazard ratio [HR], 0.66; 95% confidence interval [CI], 0.45–0.97). Secondary endpoints such as duration of RRT, mechanical ventilation days, and length of hospitalization were all markedly lower in the early arm. Table 65.1 provides a more detailed summary of the AKIKI and ELAIN trials.

The divergent findings in the AKIKI and ELAIN trials have not settled the controversy surrounding the optimal timing of RRT initiation in AKI. Moreover, both trials were

**Table 65.1 Comparison of Artificial Kidney Initiation in Kidney Injury and Effect of Early Versus Delayed Initiation of Renal Replacement Therapy on Mortality in Critically Ill Patients With Acute Kidney Injury**

| Parameter | AKIKI | ELAIN |
|---|---|---|
| Principal hypothesis | Delayed RRT reduces 60-day mortality by 15% | Early RRT reduces 90-day mortality by 18% |
| No. of patients enrolled | 620 | 231 |
| Centers | 31 | 1 |
| Age | 66 | 66 |
| SOFA | 11 | 16 |
| CKD, % | 10 | 43 |
| Mechanical ventilation, % | 86 | 88 |
| Pressor requirement, % | 85 | 88 |
| Septic shock, % | 67 | 32 |
| Criteria for early RRT | KDIGO stage 3 AKI | KDIGO stage 2 AKI |
| Criteria for delayed RRT | Clinical indications | KDIGO stage 3 AKI |
| sCr at RRT initiation in early group (SD), mg/dL | 1.9 (0.6) | 3.3 (1.4) |
| sCr at RRT initiation in delayed group (SD), mg/dL | 2.4 (1.0) | 5.3 (2.3) |
| RRT modality | IHD, SLED, or CRRT | CVVHDF only for 7 days |
| Received RRT in early arm, % | 98 | 100 |
| Received RRT in delayed arm, % | 51 | 91 |

*AKI,* acute kidney injury; *AKIKI,* Artificial Kidney Initiation in Kidney Injury; *CKD,* chronic kidney disease; *CRRT,* continuous renal replacement therapy; *CVVHDF,* continuous venovenous hemodiafiltration; *ELAIN,* Effect of Early vs Delayed Initiation of Renal Replacement Therapy on Mortality in Critically Ill Patients with Acute Kidney Injury; *IHD,* intermittent hemodialysis; *KDIGO,* Kidney Disease Improving Global Outcomes; *RRT,* renal replacement therapy; *sCr,* serum creatinine; *SD,* standard deviation; *SLED,* sustained low-efficiency dialysis; *SOFA,* Sequential Organ Failure Assessment Score.

likely underpowered for the detection of a realistic difference in mortality that could be plausibly conferred by any RRT initiation strategy. Ongoing and recently completed studies will hopefully shed further light on this issue.[58,59]

## RENAL REPLACEMENT THERAPY MODALITY

A variety of RRT modalities are available for the treatment of critically ill patients, each with a unique set of advantages and shortcomings (Table 65.2). However, no single modality has been shown to confer improved survival. As a result, logistic factors such as costs, local availability, and staff expertise can be justified as factors that determine modality choice.

### INTERMITTENT HEMODIALYSIS

Intermittent hemodialysis (IHD) can be broadly defined as the application of a prescription designed for patients with end-stage kidney disease to individuals with AKI. However, some key modifications are needed for patients with AKI. Due to the lower blood flow rates typically achieved with temporary dialysis catheters and the high catabolic rates of critically ill patients, session durations up to 5 hours may be required.[60] Heparin is often omitted owing to the bleeding risks that are frequently seen in critically ill patients (see later discussion of anticoagulation). Blood flow ranges from 200 to 400 mL/min, with lower blood flows used in initial sessions for patients who are believed to be at risk for dialysis disequilibrium. In hemodynamically unstable patients, the use of a hypertonic dialysate sodium concentration (e.g., 145 mmol/L) may promote stability by enhancing fluid movement from the intracellular to extracellular space. Although hyperkalemia is often a trigger for RRT initiation, excessive potassium removal may result in hypokalemia-mediated arrhythmias. A dialysate potassium concentration less than 2 mmol/L should be avoided when possible.

To achieve euvolemia in a population that is generally fluid-overloaded,[35,37] the prescribed ultrafiltration volume must address the patient's expected intake from infusions and nutrition while achieving net fluid removal. The key challenge of IHD is the need to ultrafilter relatively large volumes in a short time in patients who are frequently hemodynamically compromised and have a tendency to poor vascular refilling from the interstitium. In addition to modification of the dialysate sodium concentration, intradialytic hypotension can be prevented or attenuated by lowering the dialysate temperature or initiating or escalating vasopressor doses. However, if a patient develops intradialytic hypotension or requires escalating doses of vasopressors to tolerate fluid removal via IHD, conversion to modalities (see later) that permit a slower rate of fluid removal should be considered. The introduction of more frequent IHD sessions (e.g., daily) or supplemental sessions devoted exclusively to ultrafiltration, may permit a lower ultrafiltration volume per session, thereby enabling the achievement of euvolemia with greater hemodynamic tolerability.

### CONTINUOUS RENAL REPLACEMENT THERAPY

CRRT enables the slow removal of fluid and solutes using hemodialysis and/or hemofiltration, either exclusively or in combination (see later section on clearance mode). On a unit-time basis, CRRT is an inefficient form of RRT and thus would not be considered optimal when the goal is the rapid removal of a dangerous solute (e.g., potassium, ingested toxin). The efficacy of CRRT, and its putative benefits, is thus realized only when it is applied throughout the 24-hour period, with minimal interruption. Technical factors (e.g., frequent clotting) and time away from the ICU for procedures may hamper delivery that is truly continuous. Clinical practice guidelines from KDIGO have suggested using CRRT and intermittent forms of RRT in a complementary fashion.[61] A frequent approach is to use CRRT for patients who are hemodynamically unstable and IHD for patients who are more stable, with the understanding that intermodality changes will occur as the clinical picture evolves.

The administration of CRRT should be carefully protocolized. Ordering clinicians must determine the optimal intensity of RRT to be administered (see later section on dose and intensity). Fluid balance is frequently managed on an hourly basis; because volume overload is virtually ubiquitous in the critically ill patient with AKI, achievement of a net fluid removal mandates that hourly ultrafiltration exceeds the patient's overall fluid balance during the preceding hour. As an example, one may consider a desired net ultrafiltration goal of 50 mL/hour being prescribed to an anuric patient. If the patient received 30 mL from parenteral nutrition and 40 mL from a variety of infusions and lost 30 mL from a variety of postoperative drains (net balance + 40 mL), the

**Table 65.2 Advantages and Shortcomings of Renal Replacement Therapy Modalities**

| Advantage or Shortcomings | Intermittent Hemodialysis | Sustained Low-Efficiency Dialysis | Continuous Renal Replacement Therapy |
|---|---|---|---|
| Advantage | Familiarity to nursing staff<br>Widespread availability<br>Low cost of disposables<br>Delivery with no anticoagulation feasible | Low cost of disposables<br>Delivery with no anticoagulation feasible<br>Reasonable hemodynamic tolerability | Greater hemodynamic tolerability<br>Ability to adjust prescription rapidly to patient's evolving needs<br>Possibility of improved kidney survival among survivors |
| Shortcomings | Challenges with hemodynamic instability<br>Limitations of fluid removal | Limited data on appropriate dosing of antimicrobials<br>Lack of randomized controlled trials comparing efficacy with that of other modalities | High cost of disposables<br>Greater logistic complexity<br>Challenging to administer without anticoagulation |

actual ultrafiltration volume needs to be 90 mL to achieve a net loss of 50 mL in the subsequent hour. CRRT offers the unique flexibility of tailoring ultrafiltration volumes on an hourly basis according to the variability of intake/losses and the patient's dynamic hemodynamic picture.

### SUSTAINED LOW-EFFICIENCY DIALYSIS

Sustained low-efficiency dialysis (SLED), also known as prolonged intermittent renal replacement therapy (PIRRT), is a hybrid modality that uses conventional hemodialysis devices with an extension of therapy to 8 to 12 hours in the hope of achieving some of the putative hemodynamic benefits of CRRT. SLED has gained popularity owing to the absence of a survival benefit with CRRT when compared with IHD, the high costs associated with the application of CRRT,[62,63] and the concomitant desire to provide safe RRT to hemodynamically unstable patients. Initial reports have shown that SLED is associated with reasonable solute control and an achievement of planned ultrafiltration goals.[64-66] SLED was also associated with acceptable hemodynamic stability as compared with CRRT.[66-68] Further practical advantages of SLED include the delivery of therapy without anticoagulation and the potential for administration overnight to minimize interruptions by clinical procedures and investigations that occur during daytime hours.

### IMPACT OF MODALITY ON CLINICAL OUTCOMES

#### CONTINUOUS RENAL REPLACEMENT THERAPY VERSUS INTERMITTENT HEMODIALYSIS

Despite the theoretic benefits attributed to CRRT, randomized trials have not demonstrated enhanced survival in comparison with IHD. The largest of such trials randomly allocated 360 patients (the vast majority of whom were catecholamine-dependent and mechanically ventilated) to IHD or CRRT and demonstrated a 60-day survival of approximately 32% in both groups.[69] A recent meta-analysis of trials and cohort studies comparing the two modalities has shown no benefit of CRRT as compared with IHD (relative risk [RR], 1.00; 95% CI, 0.92–1.09] for mortality and RR of 0.90 [95% CI, 0.59–1.38] for dialysis dependence).[70]

If the putative advantages of CRRT are based on more favorable hemodynamics and the prevention of iatrogenic kidney ischemia, one would expect that better kidney function would be observed in survivors of the acute phase of illness. A meta-analysis of predominantly observational studies has demonstrated a lower risk of dialysis dependence among recipients of CRRT as compared with those who received IHD.[71] A study from Ontario, Canada, has shown that among patients who survived to 90 days after the initiation of acute RRT, the risk of long-term dialysis dependence over 2 years of follow-up was 25% lower among recipients of CRRT than in matched controls whose initial modality was IHD.[72] The possible nephroprotective benefits seen with CRRT are potentially relevant because the cost utility of applying RRT in AKI is closely tied to patients who achieve dialysis independence and survive for longer than 1 year.[73] Although the in-hospital costs of CRRT are higher than for IHD, this initial cost increment may be neutralized if CRRT reduces the risk of long-term dialysis among surviving patients.[62]

#### CONTINUOUS RENAL REPLACEMENT THERAPY VERSUS SUSTAINED LOW-EFFICIENCY DIALYSIS

The increasing utilization of SLED has been accompanied by limited evidence. A single-center trial randomly assigned 232 patients with AKI admitted to a surgical ICU to SLED (target, 12 hours/session) or CRRT.[74] The primary outcome of 90-day mortality did not differ between the groups (49.6% vs. 55.6% in SLED and CRRT recipients, respectively; $P = .43$). However, inferences from these results are limited by the small sample size and limited statistical power of this trial. Furthermore, the mean duration of SLED treatments was longer than expected (15 hours), and the mean duration of CRRT sessions was shorter than expected (16 hours). Two studies have evaluated recipients of SLED compared with historical controls comprised of patients treated with CRRT prior to an institutional policy in which SLED replaced CRRT. In one study, the introduction of SLED was associated with improved outcomes compared with patients who were previously treated with CRRT[75] and, in the other, outcomes were comparable.[76] Thus, the limited available data have suggested that SLED is reasonably tolerated by critically ill patients with hemodynamic compromise and appears to be a safe alternative to CRRT.

## MODE OF CLEARANCE

As in chronic RRT, solute removal in patients with AKI may be mediated by diffusive and/or convective mechanisms. The relative contributions of diffusive versus convective clearance to the administered therapy may vary and ultimately define the clearance mode—hemodialysis, hemofiltration, or hemodiafiltration. In hemodialysis, a concentration gradient is maintained by the countercurrent flow of dialysate and blood across a semipermeable membrane. The diffusive clearance that ensues is the essence of hemodialysis. With convective clearance, the ultrafiltration of large volumes of plasma water down a pressure gradient forces the concomitant "drag" of solutes through the membrane pores. In hemofiltration, a balanced electrolyte solution devoid of the unwanted solutes then replaces the ultrafiltrate. Hemodialysis and hemofiltration are equally effective in the removal of low-molecular-weight substances (e.g., creatinine, urea, electrolytes). However, because diffusion is size-related, slower moving larger molecules are less efficiently cleared by dialysis. With hemofiltration, in contrast, the clearance of a solute is related to the size of the molecule in relation to the size of the membrane's pores. Thus, depending on the porosity of the membrane, larger molecules, which include potentially toxic cytokines, are more efficiently removed by hemofiltration than by hemodialysis.

Hemofiltration may be provided in tandem with hemodialysis (hemodiafiltration) or as the exclusive mode of clearance. It can be applied in the context of continuous (as in continuous venovenous hemofiltration [CVVH] or continuous venovenous hemodiafiltration [CVVHDF]) or intermittent forms of RRT.[77] Despite its theoretic benefits, there is no evidence that hemofiltration ameliorates clinical outcomes.[78] The largest trial to date on this topic, a comparison of CVVH and CVVHDF, enrolled only 75 patients and did not find a difference in 60-day mortality.[79]

## INTENSITY OF RENAL REPLACEMENT THERAPY

Small clinical trials have suggested that the escalation of RRT intensity or dose, defined as increased effluent volume in CRRT[80] or increased session frequency in IHD,[81] could lead to enhanced survival. These findings stimulated two large-scale trials to address definitively whether dialysis intensification could improve survival in AKI. The Acute renal failure Trials Network (ATN) trial randomly assigned 1124 critically ill patients with AKI to two strategies of RRT intensity; in this study, RRT modality varied with in each group, depending on a patient's evolving hemodynamics (Fig. 65.2).[60] Intensive therapy consisted of CVVHDF at 35 mL/kg/hour or SLED, 6 days/week, when the patient was hemodynamically unstable and IHD, 6 days/week, when the patient was hemodynamically stable; the less intensive strategy was CVVHDF at 20 mL/kg/hour or SLED, 3 days/week, when hemodynamically unstable, and IHD, 3 days/week, during periods of hemodynamic stability. For patients receiving IHD or SLED, the dialysis prescription targeted a $Kt/V_{urea}$ of 1.2 to 1.4. The intensive RRT strategy was not associated with lower mortality at 60 days (53.6% vs. 51.5% in the less intensive arm) or a higher likelihood of kidney recovery. The Randomized Evaluation of Normal Versus Augmented Level of Replacement Therapy (RENAL) trial enrolled 1508 critically ill patients with AKI in Australia and New Zealand and compared CVVHDF at

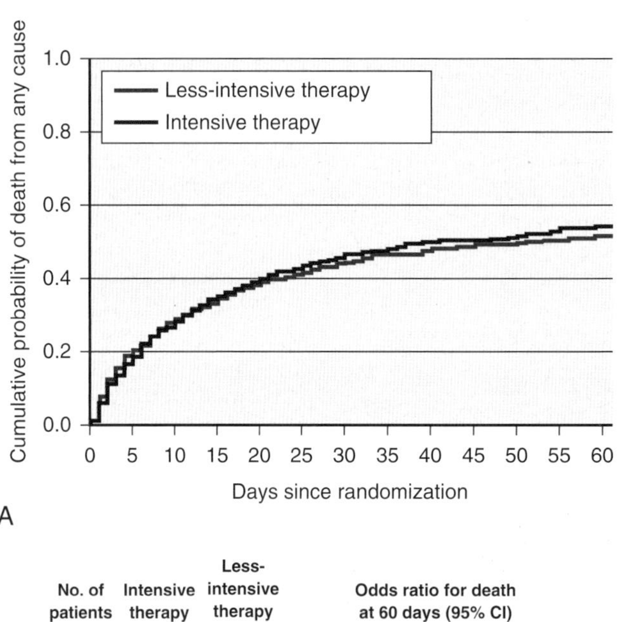


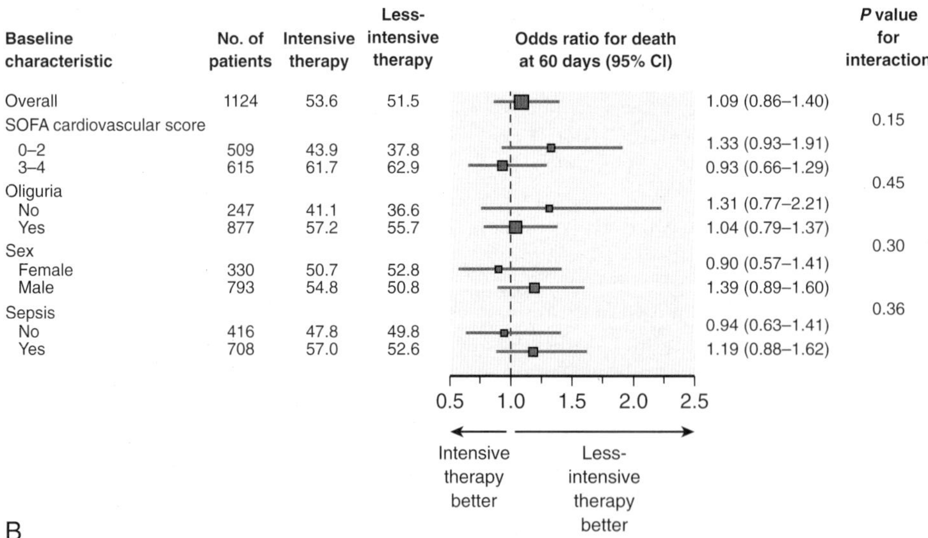


**Fig. 65.2** Effect of intensity of renal support in critically ill patients with acute kidney injury. (A) Kaplan-Meier plot of cumulative probabilities of death and odds ratios for death at 60 days, according to baseline characteristics (B) from the VA/NIH Acute Renal Failure Trial Network. (A) shows the cumulative probability of death from any cause in the entire study cohort. (B) shows odds ratios (and 95% confidence intervals [CIs]) for death from any cause by 60 days in the group receiving the intensive treatment strategy, in comparison with the group receiving the less intensive treatment strategy, as well as *P* values for the interaction between the treatment group and baseline characteristics. *P* values were calculated with the use of the Wald statistic. Higher Sequential Organ Failure Assessment (SOFA) scores indicate more severe organ dysfunction. There was no significant interaction between treatment and subgroup variables, as defined according to the prespecified threshold level of significance for interaction ($P$ = .10). (From Palevsky PM, Zhang JH, O'Connor TZ, et al. Intensity of renal support in critically ill patients with acute kidney injury. *N Engl J Med.* 2008;359:7–20.)

doses of 40 and 25 mL/kg/hour.[82] Higher CRRT intensity did not confer improved survival at 90 days. No specific advantage of intensive therapy was observed in either trial with respect to prespecified patient subgroups, such as those with sepsis. Studies of ultrahigh CRRT doses (i.e., up to 70–85 mL/kg/hour) have similarly shown no benefit.[25,83] Ultimately, it remains unclear whether the improved control of harmful solutes afforded by high-intensity RRT is counterbalanced by the removal of beneficial solutes such as essential nutrients, endogenous antiinflammatory cytokines, and vital drugs, especially antibiotics. The results of these trials have informed clinical practice guidelines, which currently recommend a target RRT dose of 20 to 25 mL/kg/hour in CRRT and a Kt/V of 3.9/week for patients receiving SLED or IHD.[61]

## ANTICOAGULATION

Anticoagulation of the extracorporeal circuit is widely prescribed to counter the propensity of blood to clot when it comes in contact with an artificial membrane in the chronic setting. Other factors that must be considered in the selection of an anticoagulant for RRT include the presence of concomitant indications for anticoagulation, the patient's propensity for bleeding and thrombosis, and the chosen RRT modality.

Regional citrate anticoagulation (RCA) has emerged as an effective and safe anticoagulation strategy and the default strategy for anticoagulation of the CRRT circuit at many centers.[84,85] When infused into the extracorporeal circuit, citrate chelates calcium, a required cofactor in the clotting cascade, and the resulting extracorporeal hypocalcemia (0.25–0.45 mmol/L) prevents circuit clotting. The systemic serum calcium concentration is maintained in the normal range through a concurrent calcium infusion. There are also custom solutions that deliver citrate as part of the replacement solution, thereby obviating the need for a dedicated citrate solution. When compared with unfractionated heparin, RCA confers a lower risk of bleeding.[86,87] There is also accumulating evidence to suggest that RCA prolongs filter life as compared with heparin-based anticoagulation strategies.[88-91] Because citrate is converted to bicarbonate in the liver, RCA often leads to metabolic alkalosis, which can be corrected by reducing the bicarbonate content of the replacement solution or dialysate. In the setting of impaired hepatic function, citrate accumulation may occur, manifesting as a wide anion gap and hypocalcemia. With judicious monitoring, however, RCA can be safely used in some patients with hepatic failure.[92,93]

For patients who require anticoagulation for alternative indications (e.g., mechanical heart valves, deep vein thrombosis), or for those who experience metabolic complications with RCA, unfractionated heparin provides adequate anticoagulation of the RRT circuit. In patients with heparin-induced thrombocytopenia, systemically infused argatroban is an appropriate alternative.[94]

RRT can also be readily administered without anticoagulation. SLED and IHD treatments are more likely to be successfully completed with no anticoagulation owing to the typically higher blood flows and shorter session durations. CRRT may also be administered with no anticoagulation, with an expectation that clotting will necessitate more frequent changing of the extracorporeal circuit. Acceleration of blood flow (e.g., ≥250 mL/min) and the use of hemofiltration with administration of replacement solution in the prefilter position can lower the risk of clotting.

## FLUID BALANCE, ULTRAFILTRATION, AND MAINTENANCE OF HEMODYNAMIC STABILITY

The achievement of euvolemia is one of the central goals of any RRT strategy, especially in light of emerging data suggesting the harm of fluid overload.[33] Extracellular volume expansion is often substantial at RRT initiation and has been associated with adverse outcomes.[34-37] In addition, persistent fluid overload while patients are receiving RRT is associated with higher mortality. Although the relationship between fluid overload and death is likely confounded by a variety of factors, an effective ultrafiltration strategy may have many benefits, including reduction in pulmonary edema (which may facilitate ventilator weaning) and mitigation of peripheral edema (which might help the mobilization process).

Effective ultrafiltration entails two challenges. The first is performing a reliable assessment of the patient's volume status. Standard physical examination maneuvers (e.g., assessment of the jugular venous pressure, chest auscultation, peripheral edema) may be difficult to apply in the critical care setting and may be complemented by a search for pulmonary congestion on chest radiographs or information gleaned from a transduced central venous pressure. However, given the limitations of all these tools,[95,96] emerging technologies such as bedside point of care ultrasonography (for assessment of lung fluid[97] and inferior vena cava diameter[98,99]) and bioelectric impedance analysis[100] may prove to be useful adjuncts to standard volume assessment techniques.

A second challenge is the achievement of net fluid removal while avoiding RRT-associated hypotension. Such hypotension occurs, even in patients with bona fide extracellular volume expansion, through inadequate refilling of the intravascular space from the interstitium to compensate for fluid that was removed. The proclivity for hypotension is further enhanced by impairment of vascular tone, which may result from the underlying illness, medications, or dialysis-induced rise in core body temperature.[101] Continuous therapies have been advocated in patients with hemodynamic instability who might derive particular benefit from the low yet consistent ultrafiltration rate afforded by this modality. For patients receiving intermittent modalities, modifications to the dialysis prescription, as described previously, can mitigate iatrogenic hypotension.[102] In addition, novel biofeedback technology, including blood volume monitoring, appears promising but has not been definitively proven to reduce intradialytic hypotension.[103]

## VASCULAR ACCESS CONSIDERATIONS

The initiation of acute RRT mandates placement of a dedicated dual-lumen central venous catheter with the goal of sustaining an adequate blood flow with minimal recirculation to ensure adequate solute clearance. To maximize RRT efficiency, the distal catheter tip should reside in a large vein, necessitating the use of a catheter of adequate length. An internal jugular catheter tip should be at the atriocaval junction, thereby requiring a catheter length of 15 to 20 cm; a catheter placed in the femoral veins must reach the inferior vena cava and must have an optimal length of at least 20 to 25 cm.[104] To minimize mechanical and infectious complications of central venous catheters, ultrasound-guided insertion[105] is recommended, and adherence to strict aseptic technique[106] is required.

Although subclavian catheters may be associated with a lower rate of infection,[107] they are generally avoided, owing to the risk of pneumothorax with insertion (especially among patients on mechanical ventilation) and the higher rate of central vein stenosis relative to internal jugular catheters, which might preclude the future creation of a permanent vascular access in the ipsilateral arm in those who will require maintenance hemodialysis.[108,109] The tortuosity of the subclavian vein makes it more likely for the catheter to abut the vessel wall, also increasing the likelihood of endothelial damage and subsequent stenosis.

A randomized clinical trial has shown similar rates of catheter colonization among those receiving internal jugular and femoral catheters overall and no difference in catheter associated-bacteremia.[110] A secondary analysis of these data has suggested a trend for less catheter dysfunction among catheters placed in the right internal jugular vein than in the femoral vein; however, the rate of dysfunction was highest for catheters in the left internal jugular vein.[111] Accordingly, the KDIGO Clinical Practice Guidelines for AKI suggest the right internal jugular vein (which flows in a direct path to the superior vena cava) as the preferred access site for patients with AKI, followed by the femoral veins, left internal jugular vein, and, as a last resort, subclavian vein on the dominant side.[61] Because of their ease of insertion at the bedside, temporary noncuffed catheters are preferred in critically ill patients with AKI. However, even well-functioning, nontunneled catheters should be replaced with cuffed tunneled catheters, which are associated with a lower risk of infection, if a prolonged need for RRT is anticipated.

## DRUG DOSING CONSIDERATIONS

In critically ill patients with AKI, medications must be reviewed frequently and meticulously. There are three principal issues of concern:

1. Exacerbation or perpetuation of kidney injury through the administration of nephrotoxins
2. Accumulation of nonnephrotoxic drugs that cause extrarenal toxicity in the setting of impaired kidney function
3. Clearance of vital drugs when patients are receiving RRT

In patients with established AKI, irrespective of cause, avoidance of nephrotoxic medications is a fundamental component of any AKI management strategy. Nephrotoxic agents that are frequently used in the ICU include antimicrobials such as aminoglycosides and amphotericin B, phosphate-based enemas, and radiocontrast agents.[112] Later trials have highlighted the potential nephrotoxicity of hydroxyethyl starches used as volume expanders.[113,114] Alternative agents and imaging strategies should be considered.

Because the glomerular filtration rate (GFR) abruptly declines during AKI, drugs that depend on kidney excretion may rapidly accumulate, with dangerous consequences.[115] Specific examples include morphine, which has an active metabolite that accumulates in the setting of a decreased GFR.[116] The oral anticoagulant dabigatran, a thrombin inhibitor, may rapidly accumulate in the setting of AKI, with dangerous implications for bleeding.[117,118] The accumulation of the sulfonylurea agents used in the treatment of type 2 diabetes mellitus may precipitate hypoglycemia, and metformin might contribute to lactic acidosis.[119] Finally, the accumulation of gabapentin and pregabalin, agents commonly used in the treatment of neuropathy, can cause sedation and myoclonus.[120,121]

Dosing adjustments in the setting of AKI are fraught with challenges because much of the available data about adjustments in drug dosing has been derived from patients with CKD. Even in the setting of a comparable GFR, critical illness and AKI have unique implications for pharmacokinetics. Volume overload may markedly inflate the volume of distribution, necessitating higher loading doses. Once a drug is in the bloodstream, its concentration may be altered by fluctuations in hepatic and kidney metabolism. Finally, drug excretion, predominantly of water-soluble drugs, is impaired in the setting of AKI. Thus, although published recommendations can be used as a starting point for drug dosing, careful monitoring, by following drug levels when available or by clinical assessment for evidence of toxicity, is warranted.

When RRT is initiated, dosing strategies must further account for the extracorporeal clearance of medications. Drug characteristics (e.g., volume of distribution, molecular weight, extent of protein binding), RRT prescription (e.g., blood flow, session duration, proportion of convective and diffusive clearances) and dialyzer features (e.g., porosity or flux, surface area) are important determinants of medication clearance. In some cases, RRT may have a more subtle impact on drug clearance by enhancing extrarenal drug metabolism, perhaps through the removal of uremic toxins.[115] For recipients of intermittent dialysis, medications should be administered after dialysis or a postdialysis supplemental dose should be considered. With the predominant use of high-flux filters, which enhance drug clearance, dosing recommendations that were derived for use with low-flux filters typically need to be increased by 25% to 50%.[115]

The advent of SLED poses a further challenge because extracorporeal clearance is augmented by this modality as compared with IHD. This may result in increased drug removal and compromise blood concentrations of vital medications, including antibiotics. To date, drug dosing guidance with SLED is available for only a few agents.[122] As a general rule, drug doses should probably be higher than those administered to patients receiving standard IHD and, where feasible, their use should be accompanied by careful drug level monitoring.[123] A "top-up" dose following the conclusion of a SLED session is advisable for agents that are likely to be dialyzable. In patients receiving CRRT, total effluent flow and the relative breakdown of convective and diffusive therapy will affect drug removal and subsequent dosing changes. The initiation of CRRT at usual doses, assuming that there are no interruptions to the therapy, will begin to approximate endogenous kidney function, and more frequent drug dosing is generally required than with IHD or SLED. For a more detailed discussion of this topic, the reader is referred to Chapter 61.

 Complete reference list available at ExpertConsult.com.

## KEY REFERENCES


2. Hoste EA, Bagshaw SM, Bellomo R, et al. Epidemiology of acute kidney injury in critically ill patients: the multinational AKI-EPI study. *Intensive Care Med.* 2015;41:1411–1423.
8. The ARDS Network. Ventilation with lower tidal volumes as compared with traditional tidal volumes for acute lung injury and the acute respiratory distress syndrome. *N Engl J Med.* 2000;342:1301–1308.
10. Wiedemann HP, Wheeler AP, Bernard GR, et al. Comparison of two fluid-management strategies in acute lung injury. *N Engl J Med.* 2006;354:2564–2575.
13. Grams ME, Rabb H. The distant organ effects of acute kidney injury. *Kidney Int.* 2012;81:942–948.
17. Ronco C, Haapio M, House AA, et al. Cardiorenal syndrome. *J Am Coll Cardiol.* 2008;52:1527–1539.
22. Bart BA, Goldsmith SR, Lee KL, et al. Ultrafiltration in decompensated heart failure with cardiorenal syndrome. *N Engl J Med.* 2012;367:2296–2304.
23. Gomez H, Kellum JA. Sepsis-induced acute kidney injury. *Curr Opin Crit Care.* 2016;22:546–553.
28. Angus DC, Yealy DM, Kellum JA, et al. Protocol-based care for early septic shock. *N Engl J Med.* 2014;371:386.
29. Mouncey PR, Osborn TM, Power GS, et al. Trial of early, goal-directed resuscitation for septic shock. *N Engl J Med.* 2015;372:1301–1311.
30. Peake SL, Delaney A, Bailey M, et al. Goal-directed resuscitation for patients with early septic shock. *N Engl J Med.* 2014;371:1496–1506.
31. Kellum JA, Chawla LS, Keener C, et al. The effects of alternative resuscitation strategies on acute kidney injury in patients with septic shock. *Am J Respir Crit Care Med.* 2016;193:281–287.
33. Prowle JR, Echeverri JE, Ligabo EV, et al. Fluid balance and acute kidney injury. *Nat Rev Nephrol.* 2010;6:107–115.
36. Mehta RL, Bouchard J, Soroko SB, et al. Sepsis as a cause and consequence of acute kidney injury: program to Improve Care in Acute Renal Disease. *Intensive Care Med.* 2011;37:241–248.
39. Liu KD, Thompson BT, Ancukiewicz M, et al. Acute kidney injury in patients with acute lung injury: impact of fluid accumulation on classification of acute kidney injury and associated outcomes. *Crit Care Med.* 2011;39:2665–2671.
40. Kirkpatrick AW, Roberts DJ, De Waele J, et al. Intra-abdominal hypertension and the abdominal compartment syndrome: updated consensus definitions and clinical practice guidelines from the World Society of the Abdominal Compartment Syndrome. *Intensive Care Med.* 2013;39:1190–1206.
46. Yunos NM, Bellomo R, Hegarty C, et al. Association between a chloride-liberal vs chloride-restrictive intravenous fluid administration strategy and kidney injury in critically ill adults. *JAMA.* 2012;308:1566–1572.
47. Young P, Bailey M, Beasley R, et al. Effect of a buffered crystalloid solution vs saline on acute kidney injury among patients in the intensive care unit: the SPLIT randomized clinical trial. *JAMA.* 2015;314:1701–1710.
48. Self WH, Semler MW, Wanderer JP, et al. Balanced crystalloids versus saline in noncritically ill adults. *N Engl J Med.* 2018;378:819–828.
49. Semler MW, Self WH, Wanderer JP, et al. Balanced crystalloids versus saline in critically ill adults. *N Engl J Med.* 2018;378:829–839.
51. Chawla LS, Eggers PW, Star RA, et al. Acute kidney injury and chronic kidney disease as interconnected syndromes. *N Engl J Med.* 2014;371:58–66.
52. Chawla LS, Kimmel PL. Acute kidney injury and chronic kidney disease: an integrated clinical syndrome. *Kidney Int.* 2012;82:516–524.
53. Tolwani A. Continuous renal-replacement therapy for acute kidney injury. *N Engl J Med.* 2012;367:2505–2514.
54. Kellum JA, Bellomo R, Ronco C. Kidney attack. *JAMA.* 2012;307:2265–2266.
56. Zarbock A, Kellum JA. Timing of initiation of renal replacement therapy in critically ill patients with acute kidney injury-reply. *JAMA.* 2016;316:1214.
57. Gaudry S, Hajage D, Schortgen F, et al. Initiation strategies for renal-replacement therapy in the intensive care unit. *N Engl J Med.* 2016;375:122–133.
58. Wald R, Adhikari NK, Smith OM, et al. Comparison of standard and accelerated initiation of renal replacement therapy in acute kidney injury. *Kidney Int.* 2015;88:897–904.
59. Barbar SD, Binquet C, Monchi M, et al. Impact on mortality of the timing of renal replacement therapy in patients with severe acute kidney injury in septic shock: the IDEAL-ICU study (initiation of dialysis early versus delayed in the intensive care unit): study protocol for a randomized controlled trial. *Trials.* 2014;15:270.
60. Palevsky PM, Zhang JH, O'Connor TZ, et al. Intensity of renal support in critically ill patients with acute kidney injury. *N Engl J Med.* 2008;359:7–20.
61. Kidney Disease: Improving Global Outcomes (KDIGO) Acute Kidney Injury Work Group. KDIGO clinical practice guideline for acute kidney injury. *Kidney Int Suppl.* 2012;2:1–138.
64. Marshall M, Golper T, Shaver M, et al. Sustained low-efficiency dialysis for critically ill patients requiring renal replacement therapy. *Kidney Int.* 2001;60:777–785.
69. Vinsonneau C, Camus C, Combes A, et al. Continuous venovenous haemodiafiltration versus intermittent haemodialysis for acute renal failure in patients with multiple-organ dysfunction syndrome: a multicentre randomised trial. *Lancet.* 2006;368:379–385.
71. Schneider AG, Bellomo R, Bagshaw SM, et al. Choice of renal replacement therapy modality and dialysis dependence after acute kidney injury: a systematic review and meta-analysis. *Intensive Care Med.* 2013;39:987–997.
72. Wald R, Shariff SZ, Adhikari NK, et al. The association between renal replacement therapy modality and long-term outcomes among critically ill adults with acute kidney injury: a retrospective cohort study. *Crit Care Med.* 2014;42:868–877.
76. Marshall MR, Creamer JM, Foster M, et al. Mortality rate comparison after switching from continuous to prolonged intermittent renal replacement for acute kidney injury in three intensive care units from different countries. *Nephrol Dial Transplant.* 2011;26:2169–2175.
78. Friedrich JO, Wald R, Bagshaw SM, et al. Hemofiltration compared with hemodialysis for acute kidney injury: systematic review and meta-analysis. *Crit Care.* 2012;16:R146.
82. RENAL Replacement Therapy Study Investigators, Bellomo R, Cass A, et al. Intensity of continuous renal-replacement therapy in critically ill patients. *N Engl J Med.* 2009;361:1627–1638.
84. Morabito S, Pistolesi V, Tritapepe L, et al. Regional citrate anticoagulation for RRTs in critically ill patients with AKI. *Clin J Am Soc Nephrol.* 2014.
85. Tolwani A, Wille KM. Advances in continuous renal replacement therapy: citrate anticoagulation update. *Blood Purif.* 2012;34:88–93.
87. Liu C, Mao Z, Kang H, et al. Regional citrate versus heparin anticoagulation for continuous renal replacement therapy in critically ill patients: a meta-analysis with trial sequential analysis of randomized controlled trials. *Crit Care.* 2016;20:144.
104. Wilson P, Lertdumrongluk P, Leray-Moragues H, et al. Prevention and management of dialysis catheter complications in the intensive care unit. *Blood Purif.* 2012;34:194–199.
106. Pronovost P, Needham D, Berenholtz S, et al. An intervention to decrease catheter-related bloodstream infections in the ICU. *N Engl J Med.* 2006;355:2725–2732.
110. Parienti JJ, Thirion M, Megarbane B, et al. Femoral vs jugular venous catheterization and risk of nosocomial events in adults requiring acute renal replacement therapy: a randomized controlled trial. *JAMA.* 2008;299:2413–2422.
111. Parienti JJ, Megarbane B, Fischer MO, et al. Catheter dysfunction and dialysis performance according to vascular access among 736 critically ill adults requiring renal replacement therapy: a randomized controlled study. *Crit Care Med.* 2010;38:1118–1125.
112. Perazella MA. Drug use and nephrotoxicity in the intensive care unit. *Kidney Int.* 2012;81:1172–1178.
114. Perner A, Haase N, Guttormsen AB, et al. Hydroxyethyl starch 130/0.42 versus Ringer's acetate in severe sepsis. *N Engl J Med.* 2012;367:124–134.
115. Matzke GR, Aronoff GR, Atkinson AJ Jr, et al. Drug dosing consideration in patients with acute and chronic kidney disease-a clinical

update from Kidney Disease: improving Global Outcomes (KDIGO). *Kidney Int.* 2011;80:1122–1137.

116. Trainor D, Borthwick E, Ferguson A. Perioperative management of the hemodialysis patient. *Semin Dial.* 2011;24:314–326.
118. Ghannoum M, Nolin TD. What is the role of renal replacement therapy in the setting of dabigatran toxicity? *Semin Dial.* 2014;27:223–226.
122. Bogard KN, Peterson NT, Plumb TJ, et al. Antibiotic dosing during sustained low-efficiency dialysis: special considerations in adult critically ill patients. *Crit Care Med.* 2011;39:560–570.
123. Heintz BH, Matzke GR, Dager WE. Antimicrobial dosing concepts and recommendations for critically ill adult patients receiving continuous renal replacement therapy or intermittent hemodialysis. *Pharmacotherapy.* 2009;29:562–577.

# 66 Plasmapheresis

Ernesto Sabath | Bradley M. Denker

**CHAPTER OUTLINE**



**KEY POINTS**

- TPE can be effective in removing large toxins and pathogenic antibodies when combined with immunosuppression.
- TPE is considered first-line treatment in the management of patients with pulmonary hemorrhage in the setting of anti-GBM disease or vasculitis.
- TPE is indicated in patients with anti-GBM disease (without advanced kidney failure), and RPGN (with advanced renal failure).
- The evidence for using TPE in cast nephropathy is controversial, but TPE is indicated in patients with hyperviscosity syndrome.
- The only drug for which TPE is indicated is ticlopidine.
- TPE is indicated in renal transplantation for patients with antibody-mediated rejection, desensitization, and recurrent FSGS posttransplantation.
- TPE is effective in nonrenal diseases such as fulminant Wilson disease, familial hypercholesterolemia, and neurologic diseases, including Guillain-Barré syndrome, demyelinating polyneuropathies, and myasthenia gravis.

## CLINICAL RELEVANCE

Therapeutic plasma exchange (TPE) permits removal of high-molecular-weight substances such as antibodies, immune complexes, and toxic proteins. When used in combination with other therapies, TPE has been shown to improve patient outcomes in specific diseases significantly.

Although randomized controlled trials are often lacking, TPE has a role in the treatment of several kidney diseases, including antiglomerular antibody disease, rapidly progressive glomerulonephritis, thrombotic microangiopathies, and kidney transplantation. In addition, TPE is first-line therapy for nonrenal diseases such as Guillain-Barré syndrome, dymyelinating polyradiculopathy, and familial hypercholesterolemia. The procedure is generally well-tolerated, with few side effects, but usually requires central venous catheter placement.

TPE is an extracorporeal therapeutic procedure in which blood from a patient is separated into plasma and other blood components. The plasma is removed and replaced with another solution. The term "plasmapheresis" refers to the same procedure but does not use a replacement solution. In this chapter, TPE will be used instead of plasmapheresis according to the most recent guidelines of the American Society for Apheresis.[1] This chapter will review the history of plasmapheresis, the major conditions for which it has therapeutic benefit, and technical aspects of the TPE process.

## HISTORICAL PERSPECTIVE

The word "apheresis" is derived from the Greek word that means "taking away" or "separation." It is unclear when the notion of therapeutic removal of blood components first originated, but it was flourishing even before Hippocrates in the fifth century BC. Bloodletting to remove evil humors was a commonplace medical practice, in part due to a lack of understanding of disease processes and the paucity of effective therapies. By the Middle Ages, surgeons and barbers were specializing in this bloody and often painful practice and, even as late as the 19th century, bloodletting was used for nearly every infectious and malignant malady afflicting patients in the United States and Europe.[2] The first true therapeutic plasma exchange involving the removal of the bad blood and replacement with a clean solution was performed in 1914 by Abel, Rowntree, and Turner at the John Hopkins Hospital. The procedure was called "vividiffusion" and demonstrated the principle that the blood of a living animal could be dialyzed outside the body and then returned to the circulation.[3] In 1960, Schwab and Fahey performed the first therapeutic manual plasmapheresis to reduce elevated globulin levels in a patient with Waldenstrom macroglobulinemia.[4]

In the early days, the utility of TPE was based on anecdotal or uncontrolled studies but, in recent years, the number of clinical indications for this procedure has been growing. However, the number of clinical conditions that have been rigorously studied with prospective and randomized controlled trials remains small, and decisions for the implementation of TPE still rest on anecdotal and uncontrolled studies in most cases. A summary of disorders treated with TPE and the evidence supporting its use for each condition can be found in the recent therapeutic apheresis guidelines.[1]

## GENERAL PRINCIPLES OF THERAPEUTIC PLASMA EXCHANGE

The mechanism(s) for clinical improvement of kidney diseases by TPE depends on the pathophysiology of the underlying disease. TPE should be considered when the pathogenic factor is a high-molecular-weight substance or when the patient is deficient in a plasma component. However, hemodialysis and hemofiltration are more efficient procedures for the removal of small molecules and toxins with large volumes of distribution. The success of TPE in treating any disease characterized by accumulation of toxic proteins or antibodies depends on two variables: (1) the rate of production of the abnormal protein or antibody; and (2) the efficiency of removal with TPE. This balance will determine whether an abnormal component can be removed sufficiently rapidly to provide clinical benefit. This occurs in parallel to the end-organ damage, so the ultimate benefit of the procedure depends on the efficiency of toxin reduction and the rate of end-organ damage. As a result, TPE is rarely used in isolation, but is most often used in combination with immunosuppressive strategies to decrease production and reduce inflammation. In addition to the removal of toxic proteins or replacement of deficient ones (Box 66.1) with plasma exchange, other benefits may include reversal of impaired splenic function to remove immune complexes, removal of fibrinogen, replacement of humoral factors, changes in natural killer cell numbers and activity, decline in B cells, an increase in T cells, an increase in T-suppressor cell function, and a shift from a T helper 2 (Th2)-predominant pattern to a Th1-predominant pattern.[5]

**Box 66.1 Pathologic Factors Removed by Plasmapheresis**

ADAMTS 13 (metalloproteinase)
Autoantibodies
Complement products
Cryoglobulins
Immune complexes
Lipoproteins
Myeloma proteins
Protein-bound toxins

## PLASMAPHERESIS USE IN RENAL DISEASE

The clinical indications of TPE for renal diseases according to category are summarized in Table 66.1.

### ANTI–GLOMERULAR BASEMENT MEMBRANE DISEASE

Anti–glomerular basement membrane (anti-GBM) disease is a disorder in which circulating antibodies are directed against the noncollagen (NC)-1 domain of the $\alpha_3$ chain of type IV collagen, resulting in rapidly progressive glomerulonephritis (RPGN). Goodpasture syndrome is classically defined by the triad of pulmonary hemorrhage, RPGN, and circulating anti-GBM antibodies. A recent study has suggested that environmental factors, including infection, may trigger disease in genetically susceptible individuals. More than 90% of patients have circulating anti-GBM antibodies, and the titer of circulating antibodies correlates with disease activity. Approximately 60% to 70% of patients will have pulmonary disease in addition to RPGN and, rarely, a patient may present with pulmonary hemorrhage and no renal involvement.[6]

Before the use of TPE and immunosuppression, the mortality rate exceeded 90%, with a mean survival time of less than 4 months. The use of TPE was introduced for the treatment of anti-GBM disease in 1975,[7] and numerous uncontrolled studies and case series published in the last 40 years have suggested the beneficial effect of TPE on overall survival and renal survival. Currently, with the combination of TPE, corticosteroids, and cyclophosphamide, the mortality rate has been reduced to less than 20%. The role of TPE in anti-GBM disease is the rapid removal of the pathogenic antibodies, whereas the cyclophosphamide and corticosteroids are essential to prevent additional antibody synthesis and reduce inflammation. A rapid reduction in anti-GBM antibody titers is necessary in view of the speed of glomerular damage, and this cannot be achieved by drug therapy alone.

Rapid initiation of treatment is critical because recovery of kidney function is much more likely in the early phase of disease, before oliguria develops or dialysis is required. Albumin is the replacement fluid of choice but fresh-frozen plasma (FFP) will be needed in patients with pulmonary hemorrhage or at increased risk for bleeding (after kidney biopsy).[8] Some of the major studies[9–16] are summarized in Table 66.2; although none are prospective randomized trials, the use of TPE is now considered standard therapy (category I[1] if not presenting with dialysis dependence; category III if

**Table 66.1 Summary of Renal Diseases Treated With Plasmapheresis**

| Disease | Category[a] |
|---|---|
| Anti–glomerular basement membrane disease | |
| Dialysis dependence, No DAH | III |
| DAH | I |
| Renal failure; not requiring dialysis | I |
| Rapidly progressive glomerulonephritis (ANCA) | |
| Dialysis dependence | I |
| DAH | I |
| Renal failure; not requiring dialysis | III |
| Thrombotic thrombocytopenia purpura | I |
| Thrombotic microangiopathy, drug associated | I |
| Ticlopidine | III-IV |
| All others | I |
| Thrombotic microangiopathy, complement | III |
| mediated | III |
| Factor H autoantibodies | |
| Complement gene mutations | |
| Thrombotic microangiopathy, Shiga toxin–mediated (formerly called hemolytic-uremic syndrome [HUS]) | |
| Renal transplant rejection | |
| Antibody-mediated rejection (ABO compatible) | I |
| Antibody-mediated rejection (ABO | II |
| incompatible) | I |
| Desensitization, living donor (ABO compatible) | III |
| Desensitization, deceased donor (ABO | I |
| compatible) | |
| Desensitization, living donor (ABO incompatible) | |
| Recurrent focal and segmental glomerulosclerosis | |
| Recurrent in transplanted kidney | I |
| Steroid resistant, native kidney | III |
| Cryoglobulinemia | II |
| Systemic lupus erythematosus (severe) | II |
| Systemic lupus nephritis | IV |
| Myeloma cast nephropathy | II |
| Hyperviscosity in monoclonal gammopathy | I |
| Nephrogenic systemic fibrosis | III |

[a]Category I, standard primary therapy; category II, supportive therapy; category III, when evidence of benefit is unclear; category IV, when there is no current evidence of benefit or for research protocols.

dialysis-dependent and no pulmonary hemorrhage). Levy et al.,[14] in an uncontrolled study, have reported the long-term outcomes in 71 patients with anti-GBM disease. All patients received a standard immunosuppressive regimen of oral prednisolone and oral cyclophosphamide plus TPE. Plasma exchange (50 mL/kg, to a maximum of 4 L) was performed by using a centrifugal cell separator daily for at least 14 days or until anti-GBM antibody was undetectable. Human albumin (5%) with added calcium and potassium was used as replacement fluid, and fresh frozen plasma (FFP) (150–300 mL at the end of the exchange) was used in patients with recent surgery or renal biopsy and those with pulmonary hemorrhage. Overall patient survival was 81% at 1 year of follow-up (95% in those with a creatinine level less than 5.7 mg/dL and 65% in those who presented with dialysis-dependent renal failure). In patients who presented with a serum creatinine concentration more than 5.7 mg/dL (but did not require immediate dialysis), renal survival was 82% at 1 year and 69% at last follow-up. There was only 8% renal survival in patients presenting with dialysis-dependent kidney failure, and all patients who required immediate dialysis and had 100% crescents on kidney biopsy remained dialysis-dependent. The conclusion was that all patients with anti-GBM antibody disease and severe kidney failure who do not require immediate dialysis should be treated with aggressive immunosuppression and intensive TPE. Because pulmonary hemorrhage is associated with high mortality, TPE should be initiated in patients with anti-GBM disease, regardless of the severity of the kidney failure.

A retrospective review[16] of 221 patients with anti-GBM disease from a single center in China comparing corticosteroids alone and corticosteroids plus cyclophosphamide with corticosteroids plus cyclophosphamide and TPE found overall 72.7% patient survival and 25% renal survival at 1 year. The combination therapy of TPE plus corticosteroids and cyclophosphamide had an overall beneficial effect on patient survival (hazard ratio [HR] for mortality, 0.31 [0.16–0.63]; $P$ = .001) and renal survival (HR for renal failure, 0.60 [0.37–0.96]; $P$ = .032). In 96 patients with kidney-limited disease (no hemoptysis), the risk factors for end-stage kidney disease (ESKD) were oliguria or anuria (HR, 3.34; 95% confidence interval [CI], 2.03–5.50; $P < .001$), initial serum creatinine (doubling from 1.5 mg/dL; HR, 2.13; 95% CI, 1.65–2.76; $P < .001$), and the percentage of crescents (increased by 20%; HR, 1.83; 95% CI, 1.34–2.48; $P < .001$). Only the combination therapy of TPE plus corticosteroids and cyclophosphamide had a beneficial effect on renal survival (HR for renal failure, 0.41; 95% CI, 0.23–0.73; $P$ = .002). Only 2 of 63 patients (3%) with serum creatinine more than 6.8 mg/dL remained dialysis-independent at 1 year (see Table 66.2). To date, there has only been one randomized trial in anti-GBM disease,[17] which compared the addition of TPE to cyclophosphamide and corticosteroids on the clinical course of 17 patients with anti-GBM disease. Only 2 of 8 patients who received TPE became dialysis-dependent compared with 6 of 9 in the immunosuppression-alone group, suggesting a trend toward better outcomes in the TPE group. However, the initial serum creatinine concentration and number of crescents were associated with outcome.

After kidney transplantation, allograft survival rates are comparable between patients with anti-GBM disease and those with ESKD due to other causes, although up to 50% may show linear immunoglobulin G (IgG) staining of the glomerular basement membrane. Kidney transplantation in patients with anti-GBM disease should be delayed at least 12 months after antibody levels have returned to normal. The immunosuppression used to prevent allograft rejection and the sustained disappearance of anti-GBM antibodies are thought to be the main reasons why recurrences in the allograft are rare.[18,19]

## RAPIDLY PROGRESSIVE GLOMERULONEPHRITIS

RPGN is characterized by rapid deterioration in kidney function occurring over a few days to a few weeks. Untreated RPGN usually leads to ESKD. RPGN is characterized by severe

**Table 66.2 Renal Recovery in Patients With Anti–Glomerular Basement Membrane Antibody Disease[a]**

| | | Patients With Independent Renal Function at 1 Year | | |
|---|---|---|---|---|
| Study (Year) | No. of Patients in Study | Initial Cr Concentration < 5.7 mg/dL | Initial Cr Concentration ≥ 5.7 mg/dL[b] | Treatment |
| Bouget et al. (1990)[9] | 13 | 50% | 0% | Most patients received PE. |
| Herody et al. (1993)[10] | 29 | 93% | 0% | Most patients received PE. |
| Merkel et al. (1994)[11] | 32 | 64% | 3% | 25 patients received PE. |
| Andrews et al. (1995)[12] | 15 | NA | 7% | All patients had Cr concentration ≥600 mmol/L; only 8 patients received treatment. |
| Daly et al. (1996)[13] | 40 | 20% | 0% | 23 patients received PE. |
| Levy et al. (2001)[14] | 71 | 94% | 15% | All patients received PE, C, and CFM. |
| Saurina et al. (2003)[15] | 32 | 71% | 18% | 24 patients received treatment with C, CFM, and PE. |
| Cui et al. (2011)[16] | 176 | 25%[c] | 3% | 76 patients C, CFM and PE, 59 PE + C, 41C |

[a]According to initial creatinine concentration.
[b]Or dialysis-dependent.
[c]This study used a 6.8-mg/dL cutoff.
*C*, Corticosteroids; *CFM*, cyclophosphamide; *Cr*, creatinine; *PE*, plasmapheresis.

inflammation and necrosis of most glomeruli and, frequently, by fibrocellular crescents (crescentic glomerulonephritis, GN). There are three major subgroups of RPGN: (1) anti-GBM disease and Goodpasture syndrome (discussed previously); (2) immune complex–mediated processes where there is immune deposition usually resulting from autoimmune diseases such as systemic lupus erythematosus (SLE), postinfectious processes, mixed cyroglobulinemia, and IgA nephropathy; and (3) pauci-immune diseases that are usually (~80% of patients) associated with antineutrophil cytoplasmic antibodies (ANCA), including granulomatosis with polyangiitis (GPA) or microscopic polyangiitis (MPA). There are limited data for the role of TPE in immune complex–mediated processes (see later).

The rationale for using TPE in pauci-immune ANCA-associated diseases (e.g., GPA, MPA) was initially based on the similarity of the renal pathology of these disorders with anti-GBM disease, and some patients will have both anti-GBM and ANCA-related disease. The first use of TPE for the treatment of RPGN associated with GPA was reported in 1977 when the combination of plasmapheresis, oral prednisolone, and cyclophosphamide was associated with rapid recovery of kidney function in five of nine patients.[20] However, several studies throughout the 1990s did not demonstrate an additional benefit for the use of TPE in the treatment of ANCA-associated diseases. For example, the Hammersmith Hospital reported a controlled trial of TPE in focal necrotizing glomerulonephritis on 48 patients randomized to conventional treatment with oral steroids, cyclophosphamide followed by azathioprine, with or without intensive TPE (at least five exchanges in the first 7 days). There was no benefit in patients with moderate or severe kidney disease who were not dialysis-dependent at presentation.[21] However, this study was the first to suggest that some patients who were dialysis-dependent may be able to discontinue dialysis after treatments that included TPE (10/17 in the TPE group vs. 3/8 in the conventional group).

The Canadian Apheresis Study Group randomized 32 patients with RPGN to receive intravenous methylprednisolone, followed by oral prednisolone, and azathioprine with or without TPE (10 exchanges in the first 16 days). Again, there was no demonstrable benefit of TPE in non–dialysis-dependent patients; however, 3 of 4 dialysis-dependent patients who received TPE were able to come off dialysis compared with only 2 of 7 patients who did not receive TPE.[22]

In one of the largest studies to date, Jayne et al.[23] reported on 137 patients with ANCA-associated systemic vasculitis confirmed by kidney biopsy and serum creatinine concentrations higher than 5.7 mg/dL. Patients were randomized to receive seven TPE procedures ($n = 70$) or 3 g of methylprednisolone in divided doses ($n = 67$). Both groups received oral cyclophosphamide and oral prednisolone as maintenance therapy. Dialysis independence at 3 months was the primary endpoint, and 33/67 (49%) of methylprednisolone-treated patients were alive and independent of dialysis compared with 48/70 (69%) of patients who received TPE ($P = .02$). When compared with methylprednisolone, TPE was associated with a 24% reduction in risk of progression to ESKD at 1 year.

A recent meta-analysis has supported the concept that TPE may reduce dialysis dependence, although there was no benefit on survival. Randomized controlled trials for treating renal vasculitis were included in the analysis (31 trials), and 8 included adjuvant plasma exchange. At 12 months, there was a significant reduction in the provision of dialysis in six trials with 235 patients (relative risk, 0.45; 95% CI, 0.29–0.72); the number needed to treat was 4 to 10.[24] In conclusion, although patient numbers are relatively small, and the provision of TPE cannot be blinded, available data in aggregate support a beneficial role for TPE in the treatment of patients with ANCA-associated vasculitis and severe kidney disease (sCr > 500 μmol or 5.7 mg/dL) at presentation or relapsing disease. In patients with ANCA- and anti-GBM–associated disease presenting with diffuse pulmonary alveolar hemorrhage, TPE is beneficial for recovery and reduction of risk of progression to dialysis.[25–27] Therefore, TPE is, at present, the best adjunct to immunosuppressive therapy for patients with advanced kidney disease from these mechanisms of injury. Nevertheless, the use of TPE for less severe kidney disease is still not sufficiently investigated.[28]

Data on the safety and efficacy of TPE are even more sparse in other forms of vasculitis and in children. In patients with Churg-Strauss syndrome or polyarteritis nodosa, TPE does not appear to be of benefit in addition to cyclophosphamide and steroids.[29] In children with ANCA-associated vasculitis, the removal of circulating ANCA through TPE is a short-term measure reserved for severe or refractory disease.[30] There is little evidence for or against TPE in other causes of RPGN, although there has been one report of benefit in children with rapidly progressive glomerulonephritis from Henoch-Schönlein purpura (HSP).[31] A recent study has suggested that TPE may be beneficial in kidney transplant recipients with recurrent HSP nephritis, but there have been no prospective studies or protocols indicating the optimal therapeutic regimen in this group of patients.[32]

## LUPUS NEPHRITIS

Acute and chronic kidney disease are common and potentially serious complications of SLE. Management of patients with active lupus nephritis (LN) comprises an induction treatment followed by long-term maintenance therapy. Treatment of LN is based on the use of corticosteroids plus cyclophosphamide (IVC) or mycophenolate mofetil[33] in patients with active proliferative disease. The use of biologic agents such as rituximab[34] has also been considered as an alternative in the treatment of proliferative LN, but recent data have suggested that rituximab offers no additional benefit to conventional treatment.

The use of TPE for patients with proliferative LN was first reported in the 1970s but it was not until the results of the Lupus Nephritis Collaborative Study Group in 1992 that there was a randomized study to examine the safety and efficacy of TPE systematically. The Lupus Nephritis Collaborative Study Group[35] was a large, randomized, controlled multicenter trial comparing a standard therapy regimen of prednisone and cyclophosphamide with a regimen of standard therapy plus TPE in patients with severe LN. In this study, 46 patients were randomized to the standard therapy group and 40 were randomized to the TPE group. Histologic categories included LN types III, IV, and V. TPE was carried out three times per week for 4 weeks, and drug therapy was standardized. The mean follow-up was 136 weeks and, although patients treated with TPE experienced more rapid reduction of antibodies to double-stranded DNA and cryoglobulins, the addition of TPE did not improve clinical outcomes. Kidney failure developed in 8 of 46 patients (17%) in the standard therapy group compared with 10 of 40 patients (25%) in the TPE group, and 6 of 46 (13%) died in the standard therapy group compared with 8 of 40 (20%) in the TPE group. Results were similar in magnitude and direction after an extended follow-up of 277 weeks.

Another small trial has confirmed these findings. Wallace et al.[36] randomly assigned 18 patients to receive either 6 months of intravenous cyclophosphamide and prednisone or TPE prior to each infusion of cyclophosphamide. In each group, 2 of 9 patients developed ESKD, and 3 of 9 patients went into renal remission at 24 months. Taken together, these studies suggest that the addition of TPE to conventional treatment for LN does not improve the prognosis of LN, despite more rapid reduction in circulating autoantibodies.

In contrast to the studies of the Lupus Nephritis Collaborative Study Group and Wallace et al., some smaller studies have suggested a benefit of TPE in a select group of patients with aggressive LN. Euler et al.[37] used TPE and pulse intravenous cyclophosphamide followed by oral cyclophosphamide and prednisone in an uncontrolled study of 14 patients with severe lupus; all 14 patients responded, and 8 remained off therapy for 5 to 6 years. One patient had a major relapse, and two others had a minor relapse at 2 and 3 years. The main adverse effect was herpes zoster; in addition, 4 of 14 women developed irreversible amenorrhea. Danieli et al.[38] compared two groups of patients with proliferative LN at 4 years of follow-up. Group I (12 patients) received synchronized therapy with TPE and cyclophosphamide, whereas group II (16 patients) received intermittent cycles of cyclophosphamide. At the end of the follow-up, the patients who received synchronized therapy had a faster remission than the other group, but renal outcomes were not superior to conventional therapy at long-term follow-up.

Although TPE does not demonstrate clear benefits in severe LN, immunoadsorption using protein A, C1q, or dextran sulfate cellulose columns was shown to be useful for refractory LN with antiphospholipid syndrome in a small case series.[39] Li et al.[40] have shown in a series of 9 patients that additional TPE above and beyond conventional induction therapy may benefit patients with LN and severe thrombotic microangiopathy. Thus, the current literature does not support a benefit for the addition of TPE to immunosuppressive therapy for LN, although it may be considered for select patients with severe disease and no response to conventional treatment. As a result, the American Society for Apheresis considers TPE for LN as category IV (no evidence),[1] but TPE should be considered in patients with catastrophic antiphospholipid antibody syndrome in patients with lupus (category II; accepted second-line therapy).[1]

## MIXED CRYOGLOBULINEMIA

Cryoglobulinemia refers to the presence of serum proteins that precipitate at temperatures below 37°C and redissolve on rewarming. More than 80% of patients with mixed cryoglobulinemia are infected by hepatitis C virus (HCV), although cryoglobulinemia can also be seen in plasma cell dyscrasias and with vasculitis. The glomerular injury is the consequence of glomerular deposition of immune complexes, and the kidney's manifestations may range from isolated proteinuria to overt nephritic or nephrotic syndrome, with variable progression toward ESKD.[41,42] There have been no randomized, controlled studies of TPE for cryoglobulinemia; however, the goal of removing pathogenic cryoglobulins is rational, and there have been numerous anecdotal case reports and uncontrolled studies showing that TPE may benefit

**Table 66.3 Randomized Controlled Trials of Plasmapheresis in Treatment of Multiple Myeloma**

| Study (Year) | Renal Biopsy | No. of Patients | Dialysis (%) | PE Sessions | Chemotherapy | Outcome | Results |
|---|---|---|---|---|---|---|---|
| Zucchelli et al. (1988)[49] | 17 | 29 | 82.8 | 5 -7 | Melphalan and PDN or VAD | Recovery—renal function | 13/15 PE group 2/14 control group |
| Johnson et al. (1990)[50] | 21 | 21 | 57.1 | 3–12 | Melphalan and PDN | Recovery—if dialysis-independent | 3/7 PE group; 0/5 control group |
| Clark et al. (2005)[51] | Not stated | 104 | 29.9 | 5–7 | Melphalan and PDN or VAD | Death or dialysis at 6 mo | 33/57 PE group; 27/39 control group |

*PDN,* Prednisone; *PE,* plasmapheresis; *VAD,* vincristine, Adriamycin, dexamethasone.

patients with severe active disease manifested by progressive kidney failure, severe or malignant hypertension, purpura, and advanced neuropathy.[43,44] Uncontrolled studies with more than five patients have shown that TPE induces rapid reduction in the "cryocrit" (the proportion of plasma comprised of cryoglobulin), improved kidney function in 55% to 87% of patients, and improved survival (~25% mortality rate) compared with historical data (~55% mortality rate).[45] Plasma exchange does not prevent the formation of new cryoglobulins or treat the underlying disease, and rebound production can occur after cessation of TPE without therapy directed at the cryoglobulin-producing B cell clones or treatment of the underlying disease process. The unique characteristics of cryoglobulins have led to modifications of the TPE technique to enhance their removal. Cryofiltration is a modified technique that reduces circulating levels of cryoproteins. In this technique, the plasma is cooled in the extracorporeal circuit to precipitate the proteins, allowing a more efficient removal of the pathogenic proteins.[46]

The treatment of hepatitis C has been revolutionized with the introduction of direct antiviral agents, but few data are available on the safety and efficacy of antiviral therapy with direct-acting antivirals in the treatment of HCV-related cryoglobulinemia. Recently, some trials have shown that patients treated with sofosbuvir-based, direct-acting antiviral therapy experience improvement in kidney function.[47]

## KIDNEY FAILURE ASSOCIATED WITH MULTIPLE MYELOMA AND OTHER HEMATOLOGIC DISORDERS

Kidney impairment in patients with multiple myeloma (MM) is defined as an acute decompensation of kidney function that results in a serum creatinine level of 2.0 mg/dL or higher. Kidney biopsy is currently not required for diagnosis, but can help distinguish the various myeloma-related kidney diseases and aid in the treatment plan. Kidney disease is a common finding in MM, affecting 20% to 50% of patients at diagnosis, and 10% to 15% will develop ESKD. Impaired kidney function can be caused by a variety of factors, including precipitation of myeloma light chains in renal tubules (Bence Jones proteins) that can lead to direct tubular toxicity. Other factors frequently implicated in MM-associated kidney failure include hypercalcemia, hyperuricemia, amyloidosis, hyperviscosity, infections, and chemotherapeutic agents.[48]

TPE could be of benefit in preventing tubular damage by the removal of nephrotoxic Bence Jones proteins; these studies are summarized in Table 66.3. An early study of 29 patients with MM and acute kidney injury (AKI) included 24 patients on dialysis and 5 with serum creatinine concentrations more than 5 mg/dL. Patients were randomly divided into two groups: 15 patients received TPE plus standard therapy and 14 patients had standard therapy alone. In the TPE group, 13 of 15 patients recovered kidney function (defined as serum creatinine <2.5 mg/dL) versus 2 of 14 in the control group.[49] However, Johnson et al. have reported no difference in patient survival or recovery of kidney function in a study of 21 patients who were randomly assigned to TPE plus chemotherapy or to chemotherapy alone. The mortality at 6 months was 20% in each group, which increased to 60% to 80% at 12 months.[50] In the largest study to date, 97 patients with MM and AKI were randomly assigned to conventional therapy plus five to seven plasma exchanges of 50 mL/kg of body weight of 5% human serum albumin for 10 days or conventional therapy alone. The primary endpoint (death, dialysis, or estimated glomerular filtration rate [eGFR] <30 mL/min/1.73 m$^2$) occurred in 33 of 58 (56.8%) patients in the TPE group and in 27 of 39 (69.2%) patients in the control group.[51]

In aggregate, these studies leave the role of TPE in the management of cast nephropathy unresolved. Questions remain about subgroups of patients who may benefit. In general, these studies have suggested caution in considering TPE for the AKI associated with MM.[52,53] Novel agents are associated with excellent disease response, and bortezomib is a first-line drug in the treatment of patients with severe acute and chronic kidney disease.[54]

Waldenström macroglobulinemia (WM) is a B cell disorder resulting from the accumulation of clonally related IgM-secreting lymphoplasmacytic cells. The morbidity associated with WM is typically mediated by tissue infiltration by neoplastic cells and by the physicochemical and immunologic properties of the monoclonal IgM. In patients with symptomatic hyperviscosity, cryoglobulinemia, or moderate to severe cytopenias, emphasis should be placed on achieving rapid reduction in the burden of plasma paraproteins. In these circumstances, TPE of two or three sessions will be effective in reducing serum IgM levels by 30% to 60%. Treatment should be initiated as soon as possible, with a regimen including bortezomib, dexamethasone, and rituximab to achieve more rapid disease control.[55]

TPE has been widely used in hematologic and oncologic diseases; however, only the following disorders are considered category I by the American Society for Apheresis: (1)

TTP (discussed later); (2) polycythemia vera with severe erythrocytosis; (3) sickle cell disease (red cell exchange); (4) ABO-incompatible bone marrow transplantation (red cell removal from the marrow; TPE in the recipient to eliminate ABO antibodies is considered category II); (5) hyperviscosity in monoclonal gammopathies; and (6) cutaneous T cell lymphoma (photopheresis).[1]

## SYNDROMES OF THROMBOTIC MICROANGIOPATHY

The thrombotic microangiopathies (TMAs) are multisystem disorders that can affect children and adults, may be hereditary or acquired, and share a spectrum of abnormalities in numerous organ systems. The hallmark clinical features of this syndrome include microangiopathic hemolytic anemia, thrombocytopenia, and organ (including kidney) injury. The pathologic features are vascular damage manifested by arteriolar and capillary thrombosis. Common causes of this syndrome include toxins from bacteria or drugs, abnormal complement activation that can be genetic or autoantibody-induced, production of procoagulant factors (antiphospholipid antibodies), loss of anticoagulants (defects on ADAMTS13), and severe hypertension.[56,57] According to the most recent ASFA guidelines, the TMA diseases with class I recommendation for TPE procedures are thrombotic thrombocytopenic purpura (TTP), complement-mediated TMA when it is associated with factor H antibodies, and ticlopidine-associated TMA.[1]

TTP, also known as TMA-ADAMTS13 deficiency, is a systemic thrombotic illness affecting mostly small vessels. Presenting clinical features of acquired TTP are weakness, gastrointestinal symptoms, purpura, and transient focal neurologic abnormalities. Clinical presentation is diverse, because some patients have minimal abnormalities, whereas others are critically ill. Diagnostic criteria are the presence of microangiopathic hemolytic anemia and thrombocytopenia without another apparent cause; an ADAMTS13 level of less than 10% of normal activity supports the clinical diagnosis of acquired TTP.[58,59] Multimers of von Willebrand factor (VWF) normally accumulate on the endothelial cell membrane and are rapidly cleaved into normal-sized multimers by the ADAMTS13 protease. TTP results from the accumulation of unusually large VWF (ULVWF) due to insufficient ADAMTS13 activity. The accumulation of UVWF multimers results in platelet microthrombi formation and subsequent microangiopathic hemolytic anemia. An inhibitory autoantibody to the ADAMTS13 metalloproteinase has been found at varying titers among a high percentage of patients with the idiopathic form of this disease.[60–62]

Prior to the introduction of plasma infusion and TPE, the disease rapidly progressed and was almost uniformly fatal (90% mortality). In 1977, it was discovered that infusion of FFP or TPE with FFP replacement was able to reverse the course of disease.[63,64] Currently, daily TPE is the mainstay treatment by removing the inhibitory autoantibody and repletion ADAMTS13 with FFP. Plasma exchange with FFP is more effective than plasma infusion alone; at 6 months, the remission rate is 78% versus 31%, and the survival rate with these two procedures is 78% versus 50%.[65] If there is a delay in initiating TPE, large-volume plasma infusions are indicated as initial therapy.[66]

The optimal duration of TPE is not known but, in TTP, TPE is performed daily until the platelet count has risen to near-normal and evidence for hemolysis (schistocytes, lactate dehydrogenase [LDH] elevation) has resolved. There is a wide range of reported exchanges (3–145), with an average of 7 to 16 daily exchanges necessary to induce remission.[59,67] The ASFA guidelines recommend daily TPE until the platelet count is above 150,000/L for 2 or 3 consecutive days, and the LDH level is close to normal.[1] When present, neurologic symptoms usually improve rapidly, and the serum LDH level tends to improve over the first 1 to 3 days. Improvement in the platelet count may not be seen for several days, however, and improvements in kidney function often take longer. Patients requiring dialysis at presentation may be able to recover enough function to discontinue dialysis, but many patients have residual chronic kidney disease (CKD). When a normal platelet count has been achieved, plasma exchange is gradually tapered by increasing the interval between treatments. Many patients (one-third to one-half) will abruptly develop recurrent thrombocytopenia and increased evidence of hemolysis when daily plasma exchanges are tapered or stopped. Some of these patients may benefit from the addition of prednisone or other immunosuppressive therapy (e.g., cyclosporine, rituximab), although there are sparse data evaluating the safety, efficacy, and effectiveness of these agents.

Although there is no evidence for a beneficial role of TPE in patients with hemolytic-uremic syndrome (HUS), TTP is secondary to most drugs, including cancer chemotherapy and calcineurin inhibitors or when associated with bone marrow transplantation.[68] There is a single uncontrolled report of 60 patients with ticlopidine-associated TMA, suggesting that TPE enhances survival (50% vs. 24% mortality).[69] One well-defined cause of HUS (now called TMA–Shiga toxin-mediated) is the syndrome associated with hemorrhagic diarrhea caused by *Escherichia coli* O157:H7. In this disease, the enterotoxin induces colonic vascular injury, leading to systemic absorption and activation of numerous pathways, causing endothelial cell damage over several days. Platelet microthrombi are particularly prominent in the glomerular capillaries and often lead to severe AKI. Supportive care with fluid resuscitation and timely renal replacement therapy are the mainstay of therapy, glucocorticoids are not indicated, and there is no compelling evidence from the literature that TPE benefits patients with this syndrome. However, patients with severe bloody diarrhea or neurologic involvement may respond to TPE. During the 2011 outbreak in Germany, TPE was carried out in 87% patients, yet evidence of benefit was not seen, and improvement in general medical care rather than the frequent and early use of TPE was the potential explanation of the better outcome in comparison to historic controls. A group of patients with more severe disease received TPE plus eculizumab, but survival was not enhanced with addition of this agent.[70]

## KIDNEY TRANSPLANTATION

TPE has been used in several different clinical scenarios involving kidney transplantation. These include recurrent primary focal glomerulosclerosis (FSGS) in the transplant, ABO blood group–incompatible transplants, positive T-cell crossmatch, and acute humoral rejection.

## RECURRENT FOCAL SEGMENTAL GLOMERULOSCLEROSIS

Primary FSGS is a common cause of end-stage renal failure, and recurrent primary FSGS occurs at a rate of 20% to 30% in kidney transplant recipients. In addition, the risk of relapse is higher (80%–90%) in patients with a prior history of allograft loss due to recurrent FSGS. Additional factors associated with an increased risk of recurrence are rapid progression to ESKD, heavy proteinuria, mesangial hypercellularity, and younger age.

The mechanisms of recurrent FSGS and early detection of proteinuria after kidney transplantation are unclear, but the early reappearance of proteinuria suggests the presence of a nondialyzable circulating factor that alters glomerular permeability. Removal of a circulating factor by immunoadsorption or plasma exchange may account for the remission of the disease in some patients. To date, several circulating factors have been proposed to be the triggers of FSGS, including the soluble urokinase plasminogen activating receptor (suPAR), anti-CD40 autoantibody, and cardiotrophin-like cytokine factor-1 (CLCF1). suPAR represents a soluble (circulating) form of an otherwise membrane-bound, three-domain receptor for urokinase that mediates extracellular proteolysis. The suPAR signaling protein has been shown to be expressed on a variety of cells, including active leukocytes, endothelial cells, podocytes, and immature myeloid cells.[71–73] In renal transplantation patients, serum concentrations of suPAR were not associated with recurrence, but urine concentrations were (odds ratio [OR], 2.67; 95% CI, 1.23–5.77; $P = .013$].[74]

No consistently effective therapeutic approach has yet emerged. Treatment options include immunosuppressive drugs (e.g., cyclophosphamide, methylprednisolone, high-dose cyclosporine, rituximab) and TPE.[75] TPE has been used as a first-line treatment for recurrent FSGS, but there are few randomized controlled studies, and most reports have been retrospective reviews of a single center, often without controls.[76] Nevertheless, TPE has been widely applied in the prevention and treatment of recurrent FSGS recurrence since the initial 1985 report by Zimmerman.[77] Since then, numerous systematic reviews have shown that TPE promotes partial or complete remission in 70% of children and 63% of adults with recurrence of prior FSGS.[78] The addition of rituximab has been useful for treating recurrent FSGS in small case series.[79,80] Rituximab is now widely used as a treatment for recurrent FSGS in cases of incomplete remission or TPE dependence, despite conflicting results, with some studies showing a transient or absent response.

Preemptive treatment of high-risk individuals with TPE in the pretransplantation or perioperative period may alter or even prevent disease recurrence. Ohta et al.[81] have reported the recurrence rate of primary FSGS in patients who received preoperative TPE. TPE was performed in 15 patients and recurrence developed in 5 (33%), whereas 4 of 6 (66%) without preoperative TPE developed recurrence. Gohh et al.[82] have reported on 10 patients at high risk for FSGS recurrence because of rapid progression to renal failure ($n = 4$) or prior transplantation recurrence of FSGS ($n = 6$). Patients underwent a course of 8 TPE treatments in the perioperative period; 7 patients, including all 4 with first grafts and 3 of 6 with prior recurrence were free of recurrence at follow-up (238–1258 days). Final serum creatinine concentrations in the 8 patients with functioning kidneys averaged 1.53 mg/dL. Therefore, the use of preoperative and prophylactic postoperative TPE appears promising in high-risk patients, but controlled multicenter trials are lacking. An alternative approach has been to use immunoadsorption columns.[79] In a recent multicenter French study, the use of early immunoadsorption showed a remission rate of 83%.[83]

## ABO-INCOMPATIBLE KIDNEY TRANSPLANTATION

The ABO blood group antigen system was discovered on red blood cells by Landsteiner in 1901; these antigens are expressed throughout the body and, in the kidney, are found in the distal tubules, collecting tubules, and vascular endothelium of peritubular and glomerular capillaries. The ABO antibodies (isoagglutinins) are produced in the first years of life by sensitization to environmental substances such as food, bacteria, and viruses and are usually of the IgM type. These antibodies against ABO antigens generally prohibit kidney transplantation across ABO barriers and are key mediators of antibody-mediated rejection.

In the early days of kidney transplantation, results with ABO-incompatible (ABOi) transplants were disappointing, but a major breakthrough came with the first large study on ABOi kidney transplantation reported by Alexandre et al.[84,85] Recipients received two to five TPE sessions, pretransplantation immunosuppression, and splenectomy. Graft survival rates were better in younger patients (89% at 5 years in patients <15 years old compared with 77% in older patients).

In Japan, ABOi renal transplantation flourished in the 1990s, and the outcomes to date have been excellent. In the first report of 441 ABOi kidney transplantations performed at 55 centers across Japan from 1989 to 2001, graft survival was 84% in the first year and 59% at 9 years of follow-up. Allograft survival was not significantly lower than in historical controls who received ABO-compatible living donor organs. For the period of 2001 to 2010, patient and graft survival rates for the 1427 analyzed patients were an excellent 98% and 96% for the first year and 83% and 91% after 9 years, respectively.[86] The protocol to prepare recipients consisted of four components: (1) extracorporeal immunomodulation to remove AB antibodies before the transplantation; (2) use of immunosuppressive drugs; (3) splenectomy; and (4) anticoagulation. TPE and immunoadsorption were the two techniques performed to remove the AB antibodies, and the goal with either technique was to decrease pretransplantation serum AB titers by 8- to 16-fold. Antibody removal was usually not performed after transplantation.

Splenectomy was more recently replaced by the anti-CD20 antibody rituximab.

The Johns Hopkins group has established a preconditioning protocol of TPE, cytomegalovirus (CMV) hyperimmune globulin (CMVIg), and anti-CD20 (rituximab) to allow ABOi kidney transplantation without splenectomy. The treatment protocol requires four to five preoperative TPE sessions to remove anti-A/B antibodies, and each session is followed by the administration of CMVIg. After achieving a pretransplant A/B-antibody titer less than 1:16, a single dose of rituximab is given 1 or 2 days prior to transplantation. Thereafter, immunosuppression with tacrolimus and mycophenolate mofetil is initiated, followed by steroids and daclizumab after transplantation. Postoperative treatment included another three TPE-CMVIg sessions on days 1, 3, and 5. The 5-year graft survival rate for the cohort of 60 consecutive patients was 88.7%.[87,88] Data from the Scientific Registry of Transplant Recipients on the outcomes of 738 ABOi kidney transplantations performed between 1995 and 2010 in the United States have shown a cumulative incidence of graft loss during the first year of 5.9% in ABOi (vs. 2.9% in ABO-compatible recipients). This occurred mainly during the first 2 weeks after surgery due to rejection.[89]

## POSITIVE T CELL CROSSMATCH

High sensitization to human leukocyte antigen (HLA) indicates positive T cell crossmatches against multiple potential donors. The degree of sensitization is quantified as the percentage of the donor pool against which the serum of the patient has positive T cell crossmatches—the panel-reactive antibody (PRA) status. Patients with a PRA persistently higher than 50% are generally considered as highly sensitized; primary sensitization results from exposure to foreign HLA antigens via transplantation, transfusion, or pregnancy, although infection and other conditions can also alter sensitization status. Patients with preformed antibodies against HLA antigens have a lower probability of receiving a matched kidney from a deceased or living donor. Furthermore, presensitized recipients enjoy less favorable outcomes after deceased donor kidney transplantation and are at increased risk for hyperacute or acute antibody-mediated rejection and graft loss. Successful transplantation in these patients requires a desensitization protocol of the recipient to a specific donor to reduce the risk of hyperacute rejection and immediate graft loss.[90,91]

The general approach in HLA antibody reduction protocols involves the use of low-dose IgG and TPE. TPE is used to remove anti-HLA antibodies and is followed by infusion of low doses of IgG during hemodialysis. The rationale is that low-dose IgG will have beneficial immunomodulating effects. Concurrent with TPE initiation, patients are treated with tacrolimus, mycophenolate mofetil, steroids, and antimicrobial prophylaxis. TPE is continued three times weekly until the T cell crossmatch is negative, and transplantation usually takes place within 24 hours. TPE and low-dose IgG are usually repeated several times during the first 2 posttransplantation weeks to remove any rebounding antibody.[92] TPE-based protocols are usually not suitable for highly sensitized patients awaiting deceased donor transplantation because the availability of suitable organs is unpredictable, and TPE is both difficult and very expensive to continue indefinitely. If TPE is stopped, anti-HLA antibody titers will rebound.[93]

## ACUTE HUMORAL REJECTION

Acute humoral rejection (AHR) is characterized by a severe allograft dysfunction associated with the presence of circulating donor-specific antibodies. The primary aims of therapeutic modalities for AHR are to remove existing antibodies and inhibit their redevelopment. Very poor outcomes are seen with AHR, and treatment with pulse steroids and antilymphocyte therapy is often ineffective. There are few randomized controlled studies using TPE, and most of them were conducted before current high-potency immunosuppression regimens were available.[94,95] Removal of the donor-specific antibodies with TPE has been successful when combined with tacrolimus and mofetil mycophenolate.[96] It is now proposed that the combination of TPE and IVIG may lead to short-term recovery from acute antibody-mediated rejection in more than 80% of cases.[97] Lefaucheur and colleagues[98] have compared outcomes of 12 patients with a TPE + intravenous immunoglobulin (IVIg) + rituximab regimen versus 12 patients with IVIg alone, and found better outcomes using TPE + rituximab (91.7% vs. 50% graft survival at 36 months).

Immunoadsorption allows more specific and effective clearance of circulating immunoglobulins, and some authors have proposed that this technique may provide a more effective and selective antibody depletion in few hours. It has been considered as an effective strategy for rapid desensitization in deceased donor transplantation.[99,100]

## OTHER RENAL DISEASES

Dialysis-related amyloidosis is a serious complication of long-term hemodialysis, and it has been considered that accumulation of $\beta_2$-microglobulin in tissues is involved in its pathogenesis. Treatment with direct hemoperfusion column for adsorption of $\beta_2$-microglobulin has been shown to improve symptoms and/or prevent the progression of dialysis-related amyloidosis in most patients.[101]

Nephrogenic systemic fibrosis (NSF) is a rare but severe systemic disorder that has been rarely observed in patients with acute or chronic kidney disease (more commonly in ESKD), yet it is strongly associated with exposure to select gadolinium-based contrast agents using in magnetic resonance imaging (MRI). Fortunately, the incidence of NSF has declined sharply since 2013. Case reports were published, with moderate treatment success using TPE when symptoms progressed[102,103]; photopheresis has also been used, with some reported success.

Catastrophic antiphospholipid syndrome (CAPS) is a rapidly progressive and life-threatening disease that results in thromboses in multiple organs in the presence of antiphospholipid antibodies. Rapid-onset thromboses in multiple organs and extensive small and medium vessel involvement in atypical locations are the general characteristics of CAPS. Treatment with anticoagulation, corticosteroids, and TPE or IVIg can be initiated. TPE can remove pathologic antiphospholipid antibodies as well as cytokines, tumor necrosis factor-α (TNF-α), and complement products. Although TPE improves outcomes in patients with CAPS, note that most reported CAPS patients received TPE FFP as the replacement fluid. FFP contains natural anticoagulants (e.g., antithrombin III and protein C), as well as clotting factors, so it is unknown if TPE per se or the FFP replacement provides the benefits to patients with CAPS. There are currently no randomized controlled trials evaluating the safety and efficacy/effectiveness of TPE in CAPS.[104,105]

# THERAPEUTIC PLASMA EXCHANGE AND NONRENAL DISEASE

According to several national registries, TTP, myasthenia gravis, chronic inflammatory demyelinating polyneuropathy, WM, and Guillain-Barré syndrome (GBS) are the most frequent indications for plasmapheresis, and there are randomized controlled trials indicating benefits for these disorders.[106] There are now nearly 100 rational indications for TPE, and an exhaustive review of the experimental data supporting the different indications for TPE has recently been published by the ASFA.[1] In many clinical settings, it is the nephrologist who is called for initiation of TPE; therefore, it is essential that nephrologists be generally familiar with the literature supporting the use of this procedure in nonrenal diseases.

Plasma exchange is a well-established therapeutic procedure commonly used in many neurologic disorders of autoimmune cause. It is thought that the beneficial effects of TPE occur through the removal of inflammatory mediators, including autoantibodies, complement components, and cytokines. GBS, myasthenia gravis, chronic inflammatory demyelinating polyneuropathy, and demyelinating polyneuropathy with IgG/IgA are considered as indication category I by the ASFA.[1,107]

## GUILLAIN-BARRÉ SYNDROME

GBS has emerged in the 25 years as the most frequently occurring clinical paralytic disorder, with an annual incidence of two cases/100,000 persons. GBS is dangerous, with 10% to 23% of patients requiring mechanical ventilation; up to 1 in 20 patients may die from complications of the disease. In about 60% of cases, GBS develops shortly after an infection, most commonly caused by *Campylobacter jejuni*. A large number of diverse antibodies against different glycolipids, including GM1, GD1a, and GQ1b, have been described.[108] The disorder is characterized by symmetric weakness, paralysis, and distal paresthesias that usually start with the lower limbs, followed by rapid progression to the proximal limbs and trunk over several days. A typical diagnostic feature is the finding of an increased concentration of protein in the absence of a pleocytosis (albumin-cytologic dissociation) in the cerebrospinal fluid (CSF).[109]

TPE is a well-established treatment for GBS. Its benefits over and above supportive care have been demonstrated in two large randomized, controlled, nonblinded, multicenter trials.[110,111] Substantial benefit has been documented for the time to recover the ability to ambulate with assistance, reduction of the proportion of patients who needed assisted mechanical ventilation, a more rapid recovery of motor function, and time to walk with and without assistance. The French Cooperative Group on Plasma Exchange in Guillain-Barre Syndrome[110] has addressed the optimal number of TPE sessions for the treatment of GBS and established that two sessions for patients with mild disability and four sessions for patients with moderate and severe disability were the optimal number of sessions. TPE is considered equally efficacious to IVIg therapy; combined treatment of TPE and IVIg does not seem to provide an additional benefit.[111]

## CHRONIC INFLAMMATORY DEMYELINATING POLYNEUROPATHY

Chronic inflammatory demyelinating polyneuropathy (CIDP) is a common and potentially treatable disease, with an estimated prevalence of about 1 to 2 cases/100,000 adults. The occurrence of symmetric weakness in both proximal and distal muscles that progressively increases for more than 2 months is the pivotal symptom in the diagnosis of this disease. CIDP is associated with impaired sensation, absent or diminished tendon reflexes, an elevated protein level in CSF, demyelinating nerve conduction studies, and signs of demyelination in nerve biopsy specimens. The presence of autoantibodies against various proteins and glycolipids of the peripheral nerve in samples of serum and CSF from patients with CIDP may provide a rationale for the therapeutic use of TPE. The most widely used treatments for CIDP consist of IVIg, TPE, and corticosteroids. Therapy should be initiated early in the course of the disease to prevent continued demyelination and secondary axonal loss leading to permanent disability. According to published data, there appears to be no difference in efficacy among these three main therapies.[112,113]

## MYASTHENIA GRAVIS

Myasthenia gravis (MG) is an autoimmune-mediated disorder of the neuromuscular junction, clinically characterized by fluctuating muscle weakness and fatigability. The most common variant of the disease is mediated by circulating autoantibodies against the nicotinic acetylcholine receptor (AChR). Mechanisms responsible for the loss of functional AChR that compromise neuromuscular transmission include the degradation of the AChR, complement-mediated lysis of the AChR, and interference with neurotransmitter binding. In subgroups of patients negative for AChR antibody, antibodies against the receptor tyrosine kinase can be detected.[114]

The treatment of MG includes thymectomy, acetylcholine esterase inhibitors, corticosteroids, immunosuppressive agents, TPE, and IVIg. It is presumed that elimination of circulating AChR antibodies and other humoral factors account for the observed beneficial effects of TPE. TPE is indicated where there is a need for rapid clinical improvement, including myasthenic crisis, impending crisis, preoperative stabilization, and patients in whom long-term control of symptoms is suboptimal with other forms of therapy. Occasional patients require long-term outpatient exchange to achieve adequate control of MG symptoms. Treatment consists of four to six exchanges, each removing 3 to 5 L of plasma, performed daily or every other day. With this TPE regimen, MG symptoms improved within 2 to 3 weeks in 65% of patients but rarely lasted more than 10 weeks without other immunosuppressive therapy. Some patients may have a more prolonged response.[115–117]

## FAMILIAL HYPERCHOLESTEROLEMIA

For familial hypercholesterolemia (FH), the successful use of an apheresis procedure was first described in 1975. Clinical practice recommendations include lipid apheresis as a cornerstone in therapy for lipid lowering in homozygous familial hypercholesterolemia (HoFH) and severe heterozygous familial hypercholesterolemia (HeFH) when traditional lipid-lowering drugs are not sufficiently effective. It is now recommended that low-density lipoprotein (LDL) apheresis should be the treatment of choice for FH homozygotes from the age of 7 years unless their serum cholesterol level can be reduced by more than 50% or decreased to less than 9 mmol/L by drug therapy. It is also indicated for individual patients with heterozygous FH or a family history of premature cardiac death, progressive coronary disease, and where LDL cholesterol remains higher than 5.0 mmol/L or is decreased less than 40% with maximal drug therapy. Apheresis may also occasionally be indicated in patients with aggressive progressing coronary disease and lipoprotein (a)—Lp(a)—and LDL cholesterol higher than 60 mg/L and 3.2 mmol/L, respectively, despite maximal drug therapy.[118,119] The use of PCSK9 inhibitors may obviate the role of LDL pheresis in these patients; 11 patients were successfully transitioned to biweekly evolocumab (PMID no. 28926730).

### TOXINS AND DRUGS

TPE has also been used to remove toxins, depending on the effective clearance, plasma protein binding, and volume of distribution of the toxic substance. TPE is used to treat mushroom intoxications by *Amanita phalloides* but some reports have suggested that forced diuresis is the treatment of choice.[120] There is controversy about the beneficial effect of TPE for the treatment of life-threatening intoxications with tricyclic antidepressants, benzodiazepines, quinine, and phenytoin. Other drugs such as L-thyroxine, verapamil, diltiazem, carbamazepine, theophylline, and heavy metals are removed effectively by TPE but the overall change in total body toxin level is usually not clinically significant. Due to the lack of controlled studies, it is difficult to make recommendations for the treatment of poisonings and overdoses.[121]

## PREGNANCY AND THERAPEUTIC PLASMA EXCHANGE

TPE can be safely performed during pregnancy; introduction of this procedure during pregnancy for diseases requiring that procedure has improved maternal and fetal survival rates. TPE has been safely carried out in myasthenic crisis, Guillain-Barré syndrome, anti-GBM disease, acute fatty liver of pregnancy, and TTP. Until TPE was used for TTP during pregnancy, maternal survival was rare, and the fetal mortality rate approached 80%. In the last 2 decades, a series of reports have revealed the efficacy of plasma exchange, and TTP in pregnancy became a curable disease, with a response rate of about 80% and minimal or no sequelae. LDL apheresis has been tried with varied success in acute hypertriglyceridemia-induced pancreatitis in pregnancy and also as a prophylactic measure for the prevention of pancreatitis in pregnant women with known hypertriglyceridemia.

When maternal plasma contains an alloantibody against a red cell antigen carried by the fetus, hemolytic disease of the fetus and newborn (HDFN) occurs. The maternal IgG crosses the placenta and causes hemolysis of the fetal red cells. This leads to fetal anemia and, when severe enough, fetal death (hydrops fetalis). Usually HDFN is secondary to anti-D (previously termed “Rh disease”), but it can be caused by a variety of red cell alloantibodies—such as anti-K, anti-C, anti-PP1Pk, and anti-E. TPE removes the maternal red cell alloantibody that causes HDFN. Therefore, it is thought that TPE will decrease the maternal antibody titer and, in turn, the amount transferred to the fetus, thereby protecting it from HDFN. Survival in severe cases of HDFN with the use of TPE and/or IVIg prior to intrauterine transfusion is about 70%.

TPE can result in premature delivery because of the removal of hormones crucial in the maintenance of pregnancy. Other complications can occur due to hypovolemic reaction, allergy, transitory cardiac arrhythmias, nausea, and obscured vision. During the exchanges, hypotension must be carefully monitored and corrected and, in the second or third trimester, it is preferable to place the patient on her left side to avoid compression of the inferior vena cava by the gravid uterus.[56,122–124]

## TECHNICAL ASPECTS

The TPE technique involves the withdrawal of venous blood through a needle or central catheter to separate the plasma from blood cells by centrifugation or membrane filtration and reinfuse the cells, plus autologous plasma or another replacement solution. For most conditions, the aim of the procedure is the removal of pathologic autoantibodies or toxins; the initial treatment goal is to exchange 1 to 1.5 times the plasma volume per TPE procedure. This will lower plasma macromolecule levels by 60% to 75%, respectively. A formula that can be used to estimate plasma volume in an adult is as follows[125]:

$$\text{Estimated plasma volume (in L)} = 0.07\ \text{weight (in kg)} \times (1 - \text{hematocrit [Hct]})$$

For removal of components predominantly restricted to the plasma space, the use of higher exchange volumes will require significantly longer procedure times, without additional clinical benefit. The ultimate clinical success of the procedure depends on the abundance of the abnormal protein in plasma and its rate of production. Unless the removal of the protein by TPE is combined with additional therapies (usually immunosuppressive or cytotoxic) to eliminate or reduce the source of the abnormal protein(s), the procedure is unlikely to provide clinical benefit. The time required to suppress abnormal protein production can take several weeks, which is why TPE protocols often require daily apheresis (or near-daily) for prolonged times.

### PLASMA SEPARATION TECHNIQUES

The two major modalities to separate the plasma from the blood during a TPE procedure are centrifugation and membrane filtration (Fig. 66.1). The centrifugation method uses centrifugal force to separate whole blood into plasma and cellular fractions according to their density. The centrifugation process can be intermittent or continuous. In intermittent centrifugation, sequential volumes of whole blood are removed and centrifuged; the cellular fraction is returned to the patient, and the process is repeated until the desired volume of plasma is removed. The blood is pumped from the patient at a flow rate of up to 100 mL/min into the processing unit, which consists of a bell-shaped bowl that rotates at high speed. The denser cellular blood components are centrifuged against the lateral walls and the plasma is removed through a central outlet on the top of the bowl. Each cycle removes about 500 to 700 mL of plasma; usually it is necessary to perform the process five or six times to achieve the goal of 2.5 to 4.0 L (1–1.5 plasma volumes) during a session. At the conclusion of each segment, the packed

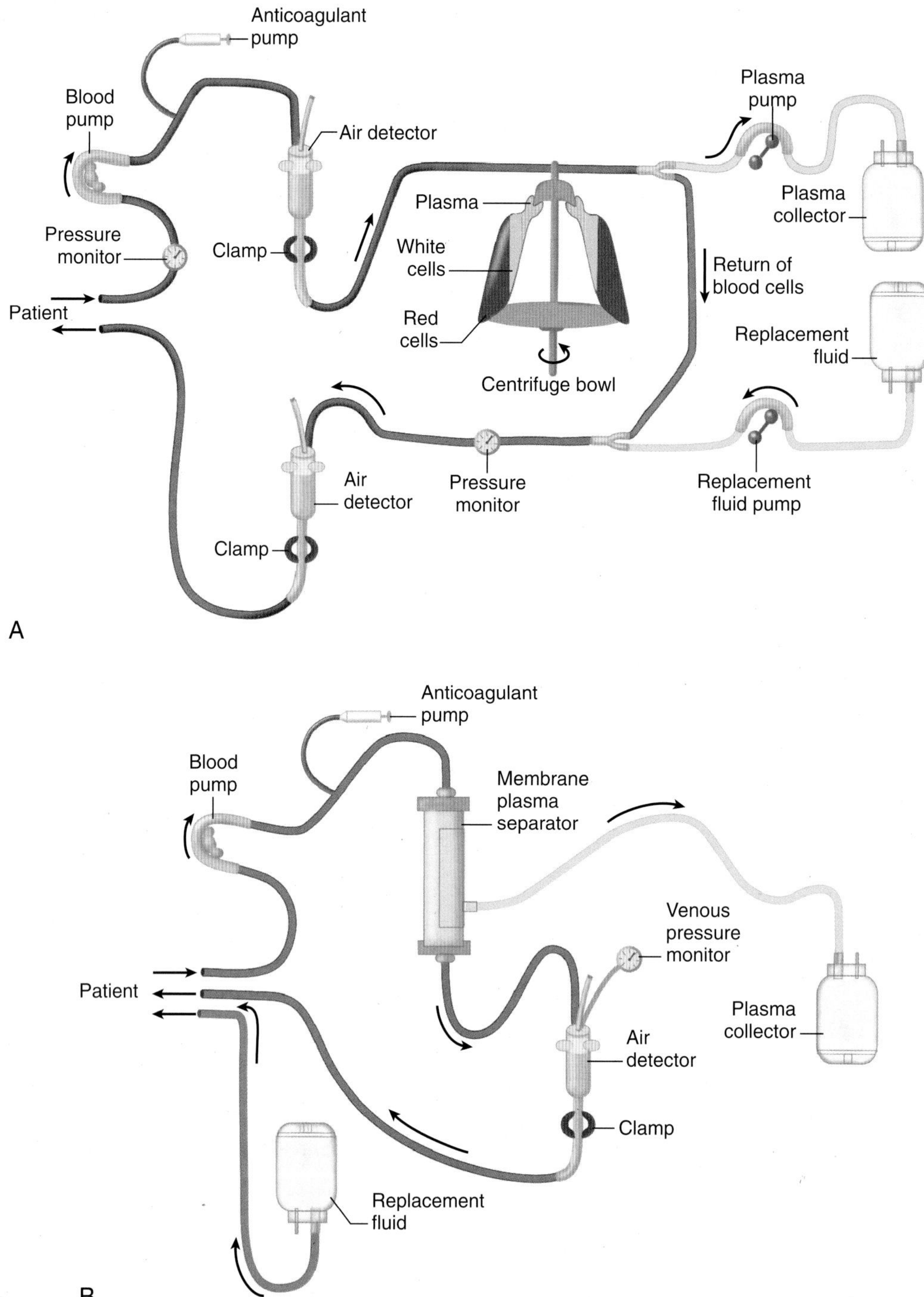


**Fig. 66.1** Centrifugal separator (A) and membrane filtration systems (B) for plasma exchange. (A) Blood is pumped into the separator container. As the centrifuge revolves, different blood components are separated into discrete layers, which can be harvested separately. Plasma is pumped out of the centrifuge into a collection chamber. Red blood cells, leukocytes, and platelets are returned to the donor, along with replacement fluid. (B) Blood is pumped into a biocompatible membrane that allows the filtration of plasma while retaining cellular elements. (From Madore F, Lazarus JM, Brady HR: Therapeutic plasma exchange in renal diseases, *J Am Soc Nephrol.* 1996;7:367–386.)

cells are emptied from the bowl and returned to the patient. The advantages of intermittent centrifugation include the relative simplicity of operation, portability of machines, and convenience of a single-needle peripheral venipuncture. The disadvantages include the time (the procedure typically takes >4 hours) and the relatively large extracorporeal volume removed each time. In the continuous flow centrifugation system, the blood is pumped continuously into a rapidly rotating bowl, where plasma and cells are separated. Plasma is removed at a specified rate, and the cells plus replacement fluid are returned to the patient in a continuous manner. This method is faster and is more suitable for hemodynamically unstable patients; however, it is more costly and requires two venipunctures or insertion of a dual-lumen central venous catheter.

The membrane filtration technique is based on a synthetic membrane filter composed of different pore sizes. Similar to a hemodialysis filter, the plasmapheresis filter is composed of many hollow fiber tubes made of a membrane material with relatively large pore sizes (0.2–0.6 μm in diameter) and arranged in parallel. Blood is pumped through the hollow fiber tubes, and the large pores are sufficient to allow passage of plasma (proteins and plasma water) while retaining cells within the hollow fiber lumen. The plasma is drained off while the cells are returned to the patient through a typical hemodialysis circuit. This technique can be done using conventional or continuous hemodialysis equipment, with a blood flow rate of 100 (±20) mL/min and an optimal transmembrane pressure less than 70 mm Hg. Plasma is removed at a rate of 30 to 50 mL/min, and the infusion rate of replacement fluid is adjusted to maintain intravascular volume. Potential disadvantages of membrane filtration include activation of complement and leukocytes by the artificial membrane and the need for a central catheter to obtain adequate blood flow rates. If severe kidney failure is present, and dialysis is required, the membrane filtration method can be done in combination with conventional hemodialysis. Both centrifugation and membrane filtration are safe and efficient TPE techniques; the main differences are the cost and expertise needed to operate.[126,127]

The double-filtration plasmapheresis (DFPP; also called "cascade filtration") is another variation of membrane plasmapheresis. In this technique, the plasma that has been separated by the membrane flows again through membranes with different pore diameters and filtration and adsorption characteristics, high-molecular-weight proteins are discarded, and low-molecular-weight substances, including valuable albumin, are returned to the patient. A small amount of substitution fluid such as albumin may be added.[128]

## OTHER SEPARATION MODALITIES

In recent years, these basic techniques have been modified and/or coupled to other separation modalities. Cytapheresis is the removal of leukocytes or platelets in hematologic conditions with hyperleukocytosis or thrombocytosis. Cytapheresis can also be performed for sickle cell crisis; in this setting, the goal is the removal of more than 50% of hemoglobin S and replacement with normal allogenic red cells.

When the plasma filtration is carried out above a normal physiologic temperature, the process is called "thermofiltration." This procedure is performed on patients with severe dyslipidemia, whereas cryofiltration is when the procedure is done with the temperature below normal and is used to remove immunoglobulin and immune complexes. Alternatively, plasma absorption and immunoabsortion procedures use affinity columns for processing the separated plasma. Adsorption columns such as protein A columns remove IgG antibodies and immune complexes; chemical affinity columns such as dextran sulfate have a negative charge and are used to remove antibodies or other positively charged plasma substances, such as LDLs and very-low-density lipoproteins (VLDLs).[129]

## VENOUS ACCESS

Successful implementation of the TPE procedure requires reliable venous access. The clinical scenario, especially the possibility for long-term venous access, and the type of TPE being used are important factors to consider when deciding on peripheral or central venous access. A peripheral vein allows a maximum flow of up to about 50 to 90 mL/min, so a single venous access is adequate for intermittent centrifugation, whereas continuous centrifugation techniques will require two venous access sites. For short-term procedures, this may be adequate but loss of venous access from recurrent intravenous catheters and phlebotomy in chronically ill patients is a major problem. If a long-term TPE is planned (>1–2 weeks), then a central venous catheter is required, preferably one that is tunneled beneath the skin; this generally reduces the likelihood of infection and allows for better catheter performance. When the membrane filtration technique is used, a central venous catheter is necessary to sustain blood flows over 70 mL/min. Central venous access can be achieved through the femoral, internal jugular, or subclavian vein; the femoral vein should be avoided if the treatment of the patient will be ambulatory.[130] In patients who require lifelong therapy, such as LDL apheresis, either an arteriovenous (AV) fistula or AV graft should be considered.

Central venous catheters have numerous long-term complications, including catheter thrombosis, catheter infection, pneumothorax, central vein thrombosis, and vein stenosis. These issues will not be discussed here; see Chapter 68 regarding the catheters used for maintenance hemodialysis.

## ANTICOAGULATION

To prevent activation of the coagulation system within the extracorporeal circuit, the TPE procedure requires anticoagulation. For centrifugation procedures, the acid-citrate-dextrose (ACD) solution (one-ninth the volume of solute/volume of solution), given as a continuous intravenous infusion, is the most frequently used anticoagulant. The infusion rate is adjusted according to the blood flow rate (target ratio ranges from 1:10 to 1:25). When the venous flux and infusion rate of citrate are slow, there is an increased risk for catheter clotting. In this case, heparin (if not contraindicated) can be used alone or in combination with citrate.

For membrane filtration TPE procedures, the use of standard unfractionated heparin is preferred; the required dose of heparin is about twice that needed for hemodialysis because a significant amount of infused heparin is removed along with the plasma. However, heparin may enhance systemic anticoagulation more than expected because of the additional effect of dilution of clotting factors by the nonplasma replacement solutions. The initial loading dose of heparin (40 U/kg) is usually administered intravenously, followed by a continuous infusion (20 U/kg per hour) adjusted to maintain an adequate anticoagulation in the circuit.[126,127]

For patients who are receiving standard oral anticoagulation—warfarin or one of the newer oral anticoagulants—additional low-dose anticoagulation with regional citrate or heparin should to be added to facilitate the treatment and prevent clotting during the procedure. The heparin dose can usually be reduced by at least 50% in this situation.[131] In critically ill patients with coagulation abnormalities, the use of regional citrate is recommended.[132] Hirudin and lepirudin (thrombin inhibitors) are effective and relatively safe alternatives for patients with increased risk for thrombosis but have contraindications for heparin administration (e.g., heparin-induced thrombocytopenia, thrombosis).[133,134]

## REPLACEMENT FLUID

The choice of replacement fluids includes 5% albumin, FFP (or other plasma derivatives such as cryosupernatant), crystalloids (e.g., 0.9% saline, Ringer's lactate), and synthetic plasma expanders (e.g., hydroxyethyl starch [HES]).[135] Albumin is the most commonly used solution in TPE and is generally combined with 0.9% saline on a 50:50 basis. Albumin does not contain calcium or potassium and also lacks coagulation factors and immunoglobulins. It is safe and has never been associated with transmission of hepatitis or HIV viruses.[136] FFP contains complement and coagulation factors and is the replacement fluid of choice in patients with TTP because the infusion of normal plasma may contribute to the replacement of the deficient plasma factor ADAMTS13 (discussed previously). Plasma may also be preferable in patients at risk of bleeding (e.g., those with liver disease, disseminated intravascular coagulation, after a renal biopsy) or those requiring intensive therapy (e.g., daily exchanges for several weeks) because frequent replacements with albumin solution will eventually result in post-TPE coagulopathy and a net loss of immunoglobulins. The disadvantages of using FFP include the risk of viral disease transmission and citrate overload.

Colloidal starch has been used for a replacement solution. It is well tolerated, drug interaction is minimal, the potential for disease transmission is absent and it is cost-effective when compared with human albumin.[137] HES is a polysaccharide colloid used as an agent for plasma volume expansion and for enhancement of granulocyte yields during leukapheresis. Its pharmacology and safety have been well studied and, when used in moderate amounts in humans and animals, HES produces relatively minor changes in coagulation tests, and overt bleeding rarely occurs. The exact mechanisms of these changes are unclear, but have been ascribed, at least in part, to hemodilution. In TPE procedures, the side effects of HES on coagulation factors and tests are comparable to those of other replacement fluids. HES can be safely used in the first two sessions of therapy in patients with an albumin level above 30 g/dL to perform short-term TPE[138]; longer HES exposure (130 L within 20 months) can lead to symptomatic effects (e.g., sensory polyneuropathy, weight loss) and diffuse tissue infiltration with HES-laden foamy macrophages.[139] Excessive HES exposure in patients with impaired renal function can result in acquired lysosomal storage disease, so HES should be avoided in chronic TPE procedures. Contraindications for using starches in TPE are congestive heart failure, renal or liver failure, coagulopathy, hyperviscosity, allergic reactions to starches, pregnancy, breastfeeding, and pediatric patients.[140]

## COMPLICATIONS

TPE is a well-tolerated and relatively safe procedure and, although adverse events are common, death is rare, occurring in less than 0.1% of all procedures.[141] There are fewer adverse reactions when albumin is administered as volume replacement than when using FFP (1.4% vs. 20%). The high-risk criteria for adverse reactions associated with TPE are unstable vital signs, hypotension, active bleeding, severe bronchoconstriction, severe anemia, pregnancy, and conditions requiring continuous nursing support.[142] Table 66.4 summarizes the most common complications related to the procedure.

**Table 66.4 Complications of Plasmapheresis**

| Modality | Complications |
|---|---|
| Vascular access | Hematomas<br>Pneumothorax<br>Catheter infections |
| Replacement fluids | Anaphylactoid reactions to fresh-frozen plasma<br>Coagulopathies<br>Transmission of viral infections<br>Hypocalcemia<br>Hypokalemia |
| Other modalities | Hypotension<br>Dyspnea<br>Thrombocytopenia<br>Removal of erythropoietin and drugs bound to plasma proteins |

The Swedish registry of therapeutic apheresis has reported more than 14,000 procedures from 1996 to 1999; adverse events occurred in 4.2% of procedures, and no fatalities were reported. Of all the apheresis procedures, 1% had to be interrupted due to an adverse event. The most common adverse effects reported were paresthesias (0.52%) hypotension (0.5%), urticaria (0.34%), shivering, and nausea. These adverse events were most frequent in patients with Goodpasture syndrome (12.5%), TTP-HUS (10.5%), and Guillain-Barré syndrome (11.0%).[143] Kiprov and associates,[144] in another report of 17,940 procedures performed on 3583 patients, had an occurrence rate of adverse events in 3.9% of all procedures. The following adverse reactions were documented: reactions related to citrate toxicity (3%), vasovagal reactions and hypotension (0.5%), vascular access–related complications (0.15%), reactions related to FFP (0.12%), hepatitis B from FFP (0.06%), arrhythmias (0.01%), hemolysis due to inappropriate dilution of 25% albumin (0.01%), and one death (from underlying disease) during a TPE procedure (0.006%). No significant bleeding complications were observed, and patients receiving FFP had significantly higher rates of adverse reactions than patients receiving other exchange fluids.

One of the most frequent complications of TPE is the hypocalcemia related with citrate infusion as anticoagulant for the extracorporeal system or in the FFP administered as a replacement fluid. Citrate binds to free calcium to form soluble calcium citrate, thereby lowering the free but not the total serum calcium concentration. Hypocalcemia may manifest with perioral and distal extremity paresthesias. Symptoms can be prevented and reduced by administration of intravenous or oral calcium if the TPE therapy will last longer than 1 hour. The administration of oral calcium carbonate or addition of calcium gluconate to the return fluid are useful maneuvers to prevent hypocalcemia.[145] The incidence of hypocalcemic symptoms is lowered with the prophylactic administration of calcium; without calcium prophylaxis, the incidence of symptoms was 9.1% (6 in 66 treatments), whereas with calcium prophylaxis the incidence was reduced to 1% (6 in 633 treatments). Marques and coworkers[146] have reported an incidence of hypocalcemia of 3% when calcium gluconate is infused in 5% albumin.

Another complication of citrate administration is the development of metabolic alkalosis, but serum concentrations of bicarbonate higher than 35 mEq/L are rarely seen. Risk factors more frequently associated with this complication are use of FFP and low GFR (e.g., patients with TTP); this is because the excess of citrate generates bicarbonate, the excretion of which is limited by impaired kidney function. Replacement regimens using saline and albumin solutions can result in a 25% reduction in the plasma potassium concentration in the postapheresis period, which can be minimized by adding 4 mEq potassium/L to the replacement solution. Hypokalemia is also a consequence of metabolic alkalosis.[146]

TPE can lead to a reduction in blood pressure that is usually due to a decrease in intravascular volume. Because the volume of extracorporeal whole blood is higher with intermittent centrifugation techniques, hypotension episodes are more common than with continuous modalities. Hypotension can also occur in response to complement-mediated reactions to the membrane filter or sensitivity to the ethylene oxide that is used to sterilize the membrane. Intravenous administration of FFP can rarely result in anaphylactoid reactions, themselves rarely resulting in death. FFP reactions are most often characterized by fever, rigors, urticaria, wheezing, and hypotension.

The development of dyspnea suggests the presence of pulmonary edema due to fluid overload; noncardiogenic edema can rarely occur as a component of anaphylactoid reactions. Rarely, massive pulmonary emboli can develop if the blood components that are reinfused are not adequately anticoagulated.

Plasma exchange with albumin replacement produces a predictable decrease in clotting factors that may predispose to bleeding (Table 66.5). A single plasma volume exchange increases the prothrombin time by 30% and the partial thromboplastin time by 100%; these changes return toward normal within several hours but, with repeated TPE sessions, these abnormalities can persist. In reported studies, the most significant change is on the fibrinogen. Keller and colleagues[147] have reported that fibrinogen levels decrease to 25% of pre-TPE levels and recover to baseline after 2 to 3 days. Therefore, 1 L or more of FFP (3–4 U/L) should be substituted as the replacement fluid each week or sooner in patients at risk for bleeding. Thrombocytopenia is also a consequence of plasma removal, with larger volumes removed associated with greater platelet loss; the mean platelet reduction following a TPE procedure ranges from 9.4% to 52.6%. Clinical bleeding associated with TPE is rarely reported and, when TPE-related hemorrhage is present, it is more likely a consequence of thrombocytopenia or inadequate heparin neutralization.[148,149]

Removal of immunoglobulins and complement can result in immunodeficiency, which can exacerbate immune effects of other therapeutic agents (e.g., corticosteroids, cyclophosphamide, rituximab). However, in a randomized controlled trial of TPE in patients with lupus nephritis, TTP, or multiple myeloma, patients receiving TPE were not more prone to infection than the other patients.[150] Nevertheless, repeated apheresis treatments with albumin replacement will deplete the patient's reserve of immunoglobulins for several weeks. If an infection occurs, a single infusion of IVIg (100–400 mg/kg) will restore the plasma immunoglobulin concentration toward normal. Although estimates for the risk of viral transmission by the use of FFP are low, the large volumes from multiple donors increase the risk in patients receiving long-term TPE therapy. Use of large-volume plasma units collected from a single donor and the use of hepatitis B vaccine may reduce the risk of the patient acquiring a virally transmitted infection.

Substantial drug removal by TPE occurs for those drugs that are highly protein-bound and therefore primarily limited to the vascular space. Among drugs used to treat renal diseases, prednisone is not substantially removed, whereas cyclophosphamide and azathioprine are removed to some extent. This potential problem can be circumvented by administering the drug after a plasma exchange treatment.

Flushing, hypotension, abdominal cramping, and other gastrointestinal symptoms have been reported during TPE

**Table 66.5 Decrease of Clotting Factors Following Plasmapheresis**

| | | Factor Level | |
|---|---|---|---|
| Factor | Decrease From Baseline (%) | 24 Hours After Plasmapheresis | 48–96 Hours After Plasmapheresis |
| V | 50–71 | RTB | RTB |
| VII | 69–82 | 62 | RTB |
| VIII | 50–82 | 62, RTB | RTB |
| IX | 26–55 | RTB | RTB |
| X | 67–84 | RTB | RTB |
| XI | 50–66 | | RTB |
| XII | 66 | | RTB |
| Antithrombin III | 58–84 | 70, RTB | 82%, RTB |
| Fibrinogen | 50–78 | 60 | 63%, RTB |

*RTB*, Return to baseline.

in patients receiving angiotensin-converting enzyme (ACE) inhibitors. In one report of 299 consecutive patients undergoing TPE, these atypical symptoms occurred in all 14 patients receiving an ACE inhibitor versus only 7% of those not treated with this medication.[151] The administration of an ACE inhibitor may prolong the half-life of bradykinin, thus permitting the attainment of a clinically significant concentration in the plasma, so it is recommended to withhold this type of drug for 24 hours prior to TPE.[152]

In conclusion, TPE is a relatively safe procedure, with most of complications being mild and reversible. However, moderate to severe reactions, even death, can occur, especially in patients with severe primary diseases.

## CONCLUSION

The use of TPE to treat a variety of conditions has grown significantly in recent years. In some cases, the rationale and benefit are supported by clinical studies, but in many cases the benefits have not been well established. Nevertheless, the concept of removing plasma containing pathogenic antibodies is now well established. Additional studies are needed to determine the potential benefits for TPE in these other conditions.

Complete reference list available at ExpertConsult.com.

### KEY REFERENCES


1. Schwartz J, et al. Guidelines on the use of therapeutic apheresis in clinical practice—evidence-based approach from the writing committee of the American Society for apheresis: the seventh special issue. *J Clin Apher.* 2016;31:149–162.
5. Reeves HM, et al. The mechanism of action of plasma exchange. *Br J Haematol.* 2014;164:342–351.
6. McAdoo S, et al. Anti-glomerular basement membrane disease. *Clin J Am Soc Nephrol.* 2017;12:1162–1172.
8. Henderson SR, et al. Diagnostic and management challenges in Goodpasture's (antiglomerular basement membrane) disease. *Nephrol Dial Transplant.* 2017;[Epub ahead of print].
16. Cui Z, et al. Antiglomerular basement membrane disease: outcomes of different therapeutic regimens in a large single-center Chinese cohort study. *Medicine (Baltimore).* 2011;90:303–311.
18. Tang W, et al. Anti-glomerular basement membrane antibody disease is an uncommon cause of end stage renal disease. *Kidney Int.* 2013;83:503–510.
23. Jayne DR, et al. Randomized trial of plasma-exchange or high dosage methylprednisolone as adjunctive therapy for severe renal vasculitis. *J Am Soc Nephrol.* 2007;18:2180–2188.
24. Walters G, Willis NS, Craig JC. Interventions for renal vasculitis in adults. *Cochrane Database Syst Rev.* 2015;(24):CD003232.
25. Yates M, et al. EULAR/ERA-EDTA recommendations for the management of ANCA-associated vasculitis. *Ann Rheum Dis.* 2016;75:1583–1594.
28. Szpirt WM. Plasma exchange in antineutrophil cytoplasmic antibody-associated vasculitis—a 25-year perspective. *Nephrol Dial Transplant.* 2015;30:146–149.
30. Plumb LA, et al. Paediatric anti-neutrophil cytoplasmic antibody (ANCA)-associated vasculitis: an update on renal management. *Pediatr Nephrol.* 2017;[Epub ahead of print].
34. Mok CC. Towards new avenues in the management of lupus glomerulonephritis. *Nat Rev Rheumatol.* 2016;12:221–234.
39. Kronbichler A, et al. Efficacy of plasma exchange and immunoadsorption in systemic lupus erythematosous and antiphospholipid syndrome: a systematic review. *Autoinmun Rev.* 2015;15:38–49.
40. Li QY, et al. Plasmapheresis is associated with better renal outcomes in lupus nephritis patients with thrombotic microangiopathy. *Medicine (Baltimore).* 2016;18:1–10.
41. Leung N, Drosou ME, Nasr SH. Dysproteinemias and glomerular disease. *Clin J Am Soc Nephrol.* 2017;[Epub ahead of print].
43. Ramos-Casals M, et al. The cryoglobulinemias. *Lancet.* 2012;379:348–360.
45. Ostojic P, Jeremic IR. Managing refractory cryoglobulinemic vasculitis: challenges and solutions. *J Inflamm Res.* 2017;8:49–54.
46. Taniyama Y, et al. Efficacy of cryofiltration for treatment of mixed cryoglobulinemia: a report of four cases. *Ther Apher Dial.* 2017;21:238–242.
47. Sise ME, et al. Treatment of hepatitis C virus-associated mixed cryoglobulinemia with direct-acting antiviral agents. *Hepatology.* 2016;63:408–417.
48. Leung N, et al. Myeloma-related kidney disease. *Adv Chronic Kidney Dis.* 2014;21:36–47.
53. Madore F. Plasmapheresis in cast nephropathy: yes or no? *Curr Opin Nephrol Hypertens.* 2015;24:177–182.
54. Yadab P, et al. Current trends of renal impairment in multiple myeloma. *Kidney Dis (Basel).* 2016;1:241–257.
56. George JN, et al. Syndromes of thrombotic microangiopathy. *N Engl J Med.* 2014;371:654–666.
57. Appel GB. Thrombotic microangiopathies: similar presentations, different therapies. *Cleve Clin J Med.* 2017;84:114–130.
59. Bérangére S, et al. Thrombotic thrombocytopenic purpura. *Blood.* 2017;129:2836–2846.
66. Scully M, et al. Guidelines on the diagnosis and management of thrombotic thrombocytopenic purpura and other thrombotic microangiopathies. *Br J Haematol.* 2012;158:323–335.
67. Mehmood T, et al. Management of thrombotic microangiopathic hemolytic anemias with therapeutic plasma exchange: when it works and when it does not. *Hematol Oncol Clin North Am.* 2016;30:679–694.
68. Al-Nouri ZL, et al. Drug-induced thrombotic microangiopathy: a systematic review of published reports. *Blood.* 2015;22:616–618.
70. Kielstein JT, et al. Best supportive care and therapeutic plasma exchange with or without eculizumab in Shiga-toxin-producing E. coli O104:H4 induced haemolytic-uremic syndrome: an analysis of the German STEC-HUS registry. *Nephrol Dial Transplant.* 2012;27:3807–3815.
71. Wei C, et al. Circulating urokinase receptor as a cause of focal segmental glomerulosclerosis. *Nat Med.* 2011;17:952–960.
72. Reiser J, et al. Permeability factors in focal and segmental glomerulosclerosis. *Adv Chronic Kidney Dis.* 2014;21:417–421.
73. Leca N. Focal segmental glomerulosclerosis recurrence in the renal allograft. *Adv Chronic Kidney Dis.* 2014;21:448–452.
74. Franco-Palacios CR, et al. Urine but not serum soluble urokinase receptor (suPAR) may identify cases of recurrent FSGS in kidney transplant candidates. *Transplantation.* 2013;96:394–399.
76. Trachmant R, et al. Recurrent focal segmental glomerulosclerosis after kidney transplantation. *Pediatr Nephrol.* 2015;30:1793–1802.
78. Mesina M, et al. Update on the treatment of focal segmental glomerulosclerosis in renal transplantation. *World J Transplant.* 2016;24:54–68.
83. Allard L, et al. Treatment by immunoadsorption for recurrent focal segmental glomerulosclerosis after pediatric kidney transplantation: a multicenter French cohort. *Nephrol Dial Transplant.* 2017;[Epub ahead of print].
86. Takahashi K, et al. ABO-incompatible kidney transplantation. *Transplant Rev.* 2013;27:1–8.
88. Morath C, et al. ABO-Incompatible kidney transplantation. *Front Immunol.* 2017;8:234.
89. Montgomery RA, et al. Outcomes of ABO-incompatible kidney transplantation in the United States. *Transplantation.* 2012;93:603–609.
94. Garces JC, et al. Antibody-mediated rejection: a review. *Ochsner J.* 2017;17:46–55.
95. Djamali A, et al. Diagnosis and management of antibody-mediated rejection: current status and novel approaches. *Am J Transplant.* 2014;14:255–271.
101. Gejyo F, et al. Survey of the effects of a column for adsorption of β2-microglobulin in patients with dialysis-related amyloidosis in Japan. *Ther Apher Dial.* 2013;17:40–47.
103. Poisson JL, et al. The treatment of nephrogenic systemic fibrosis with therapeutic plasma exchange. *J Clin Apher.* 2013;28:317–320.
107. Gwathmey K, et al. Neurologic indications for therapeutic plasma exchange: 2013 update. *J Clin Apher.* 2014;29:211–219.
109. Willison HJ, et al. Guillain – Barre syndrome. *Lancet.* 2016;388:717–727.

118. Steffanutti C, et al. Toward an international consensus-integrating lipoprotein apheresis and new lipid-lowering drugs. *J Clin Lipidol.* 2017;111:858–871.
137. Agreda-Vasquez GP, et al. Starch and albumin mixture as replacement fluid in therapeutic plasma exchange is safe and effective. *J Clin Apher.* 2008;23:163–167.
140. Auwerda JA, et al. Acquired lysosomal storage caused by frequent plasmapheresis procedures with hydroxyethyl starch. *Transfusion.* 2006;46:1705–1711.
142. Lu Q, et al. Standardized protocol to identify high-risk patients undergoing therapeutic apheresis procedures. *J Clin Apher.* 2008; 23:111–115.
145. Kankirakawana S, et al. Continuous infusion of calcium gluconate in 5% albumin is safe and prevents most hypocalcemic reactions during therapeutic plasma exchange. *J Clin Apher.* 2007;22:265–269.

# 67 Enhanced Elimination of Poisons

Marc Ghannoum | Darren M. Roberts | Josée Bouchard

CHAPTER OUTLINE



Poisonings are a major cause of morbidity and mortality, and their treatment is a significant contributor to health care expenditure worldwide. According to the National Poison Data System compiled by the American Association of Poison Control Centers, nearly 2.2 million human poisonings were reported in the United States in 2015.[1] Approximately 78% of reported cases were unintentional (e.g., therapeutic error, bites, stings), 18% were intentional (e.g., deliberate self-poisoning, misuse, abuse), and the remaining were adverse reactions or related to other reasons. Although most reported exposures occurred in children, most fatalities involved adults. Unfortunately, over the past 15 years, human exposures associated with more serious outcomes have increased by 4.3% per year. The classes of drugs accounting for most fatal cases were sedatives, hypnotics, antipsychotics, cardiovascular agents, opioids, stimulants, and other recreational drugs. Table 67.1 shows the 2015 U.S. statistics of the incidence and outcomes related to various poisons that may require the care of a nephrologist.

All acute exposures to potentially toxic xenobiotics should be considered life-threatening until a complete risk assessment has been performed.[2] The general approach to the poisoned patient necessitates prompt resuscitation and stabilization, clinical and laboratory evaluation, antidote administration, and gastrointestinal decontamination, if appropriate, which are outlined elsewhere.[2,3] Although the prognosis of most toxic exposures is excellent with supportive measures, a minority of poisonings can benefit from treatments that actively enhance elimination (Fig. 67.1). Elimination enhancement modalities can be divided between corporeal treatments, which augment physiologic processes, and extracorporeal treatments (ECTRs), which require an artificial device located outside the body.[4]

Evidence-based treatment recommendations from randomized trials are lacking for many poisonings due to infrequent presentations, heterogeneous baseline characteristics, complexity with regard to consent in urgent conditions, and potential ethical issues comparing treatment by ECTRs with a control. The current evidence base is mostly derived from retrospective observational cohorts, human case reports, and animal studies, with each having significant limitations.

Fortunately, consensus-based expert recommendations derived from published data are now becoming available for both corporeal[5,6] and extracorporeal treatments[7–19] and have been endorsed by international toxicology and nephrology societies. To treat poisonings efficiently, attending physicians must know the characteristics of the poisons, their clinical effects, pharmacokinetics, and potential removal by various techniques. The purpose of this chapter is to review the fundamental concepts of poison elimination, available elimination enhancement modalities, and poisons for which the expertise of nephrologists is most likely needed.

## OVERVIEW OF CORPOREAL TREATMENTS FOR ENHANCED ELIMINATION OF POISONS

### FORCED DIURESIS

Physiologic mechanisms involved in the elimination of xenobiotics by the kidney include the following: (1) glomerular filtration; (2) active secretion in the proximal tubule; and (3) reabsorption in the distal tubule. The intended goal of forced diuresis is to induce a urine output in excess of what is considered physiologic (≥4–5 mL/kg per hour) to enhance the renal elimination of poisons. Historically, forced diuresis is performed through volume expansion with isotonic fluids (0.9% NaCl or lactated Ringer solution), with or without concomitant diuretics. Results of early studies have failed to

**Table 67.1 American Association of Poison Control Centers' Statistics for Exposures of Common Dialyzable Toxins**

| Poison | Total Exposures[a] | Deaths |
|---|---|---|
| Acetaminophen | 120,156 | 111 |
| Barbiturates | 1997 | 2 |
| Carbamazepine | 3574 | 0 |
| Ethylene glycol | 6178 | 22 |
| Gabapentin | 17,702 | 2 |
| Isopropanol | 16,538 | 2 |
| Lithium | 7306 | 4 |
| Metformin (biguanides) | 8733 | 8 |
| Methanol | 2117 | 16 |
| Paraquat | 113 | 3 |
| Phenytoin | 2556 | 2 |
| Salicylates | 29,504 | 21 |
| Theophylline | 146 | 2 |
| Valproic acid | 7928 | 4 |

[a]Includes coingestions and mixed formulations.

Adapted from Mowry JB, Spyker DA, Brooks DE, et al. 2015 Annual Report of the American Association of Poison Control Centers' National Poison Data System (NPDS): 33rd Annual Report. *Clin Toxicol (Phila).* 2016;54(10):924–109.

show any significant benefit of forced diuresis. Unfortunately, forced diuresis is also associated with complications, such as volume overload, pulmonary edema, cerebral edema, and electrolyte disturbances (e.g., hyponatremia, hypokalemia). At present, forced diuresis is never recommended in the management of acute poisonings. However, aggressive volume repletion remains warranted for some poisons to correct hypotension and/or to overcome tubular reabsorption of some offending agents (e.g., lithium) during volume contraction.

## URINARY ALKALINIZATION

Urinary alkalinization is based on the concept of what is termed "ion trapping." The goal of manipulating urinary pH is to create an ionized form of the poison, which is less amenable to passive reabsorption, because ionized particles are less lipid-soluble. The ionized poison then becomes "trapped" in the renal tubular lumen and is eliminated in the urine. The dissociation of a weak acid or base into its ionized state is determined by its dissociation constant ($pK_a$)—that is, the pH at which it is 50% ionized and 50% nonionized. For example, the $pK_a$ of salicylic acid is 3, so when the urinary pH is 3, salicylate exists in a 1:1 ratio of the ionized to nonionized form. Alkalinization of the urine

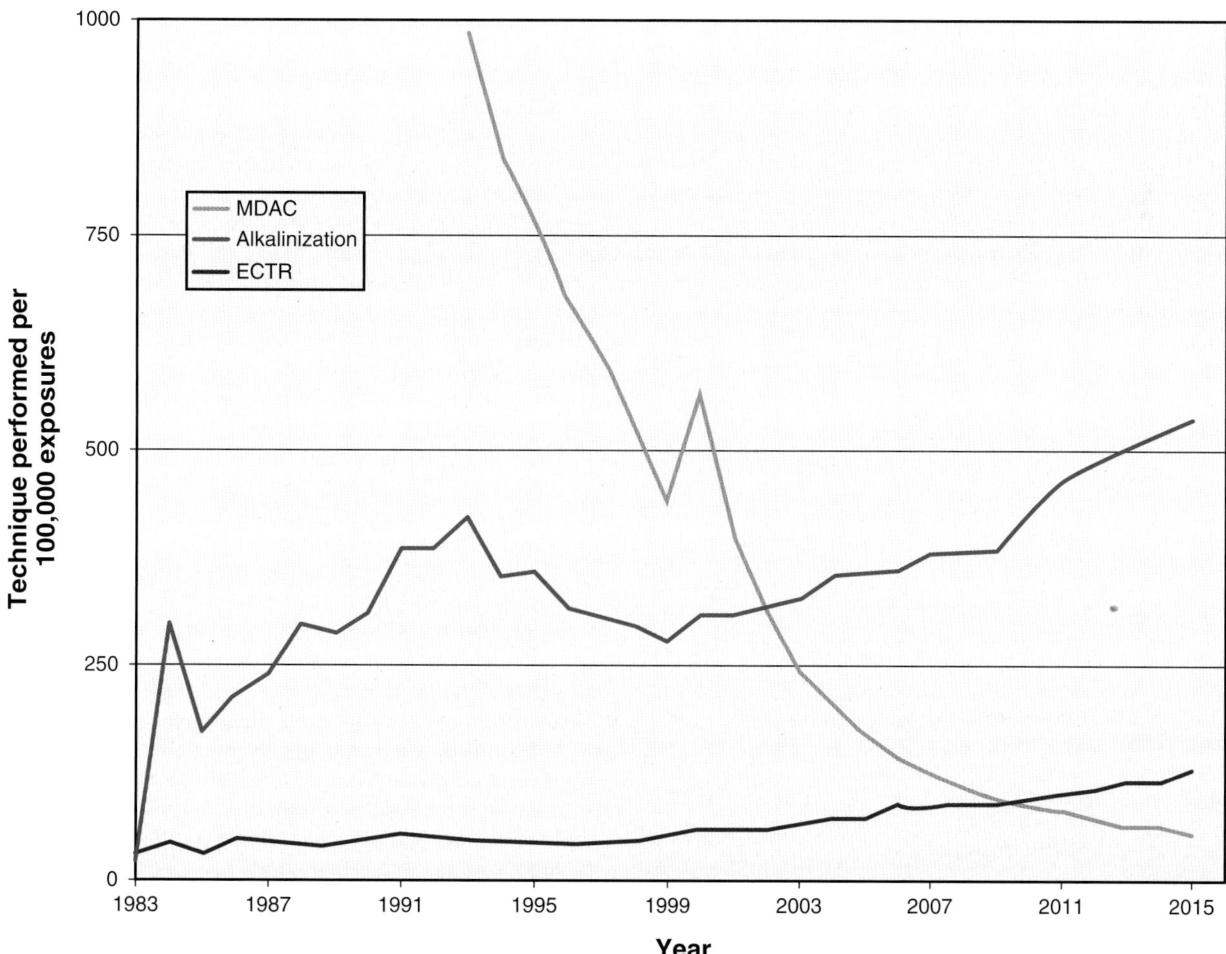


**Fig. 67.1** This figure illustrates how often these various elimination enhancement techniques were used in the United States from 1983 to 2015. *ECTR,* Extracorporeal treatment; *MDAC,* multiple-dose activated charcoal.

to a pH of 7.4 increases the ratio to 20,000:1 in favor of the ionized form, which is more readily eliminated in the urine.

The clinical efficacy of urine alkalinization depends on the relative contribution of kidney clearance to the total body clearance of active poison. If only 1% of the ingested poison is excreted unchanged in the urine, even a 10-fold increase in renal elimination will have no clinically significant effect.[6] Criteria that determine whether a poison is amenable to urinary alkalinization include the following: (1) it is eliminated unchanged by the kidneys; (2) it is not strongly protein-bound; (3) it is distributed primarily in the extracellular fluid compartment; and (4) it is weakly acidic (i.e., with a $pK_a$ of 3.0–7.0). Urine alkalinization is generally used to enhance the excretion of salicylates and phenobarbital, but can also be used for chlorpropamide, 2,4-dichlorophenoxyacetic acid, mecoprop (methylchlorophenoxypropionic acid), diflunisal, fluoride, and methotrexate (Table 67.2).[6] For salicylate poisoning, urine alkalinization reduces the elimination half-life from 19 to 5 hours.[20]

Urine alkalinization requires the administration of intravenous sodium bicarbonate by the infusion of a bolus of 1 or 2 ampoules of 50 mL of 8.4% sodium bicarbonate, followed by 2 or 3 ampoules added to each liter of 5% dextrose in water. The rate of infusion should be adapted to the volume status and cardiac condition of the patient but can be as high as 250 mL/h. Contraindications include severe kidney disease, pulmonary edema, and cerebral edema. Serum electrolytes and urinary pH must be closely monitored (every 4 hours). The target urine pH is between 7.5 and 8.5 while maintaining a serum blood pH no higher than 7.55. Complications of urine alkalinization include hypokalemia, hypocalcemia, hypernatremia, fluid overload, and pulmonary and cerebral edema, as well as metabolic alkalosis. The degree of hypokalemia may be profound because of intracellular potassium shifts and urinary potassium losses. Moreover, normokalemia is a prerequisite for urine alkalinization to be effective; in the setting of hypokalemia, potassium is reabsorbed at the collecting tubule in exchange for a hydrogen ion. Therefore, if hypokalemia remains uncorrected during urine alkalinization, not only is the nephron unable to produce alkaline urine, but the patient is also at a higher risk of developing alkalemia. Carbonic anhydrase inhibitors (e.g., acetazolamide) can alkalinize urine but also create metabolic acidosis; this can exacerbate toxicity by increasing the proportion of the poison that is nonionized in the blood, which increases its intracellular distribution and toxicity, and thus these are never recommended.

In the past, urinary acidification, aiming for a urinary pH less than 6.0, was used to enhance renal elimination of weak bases such as amphetamines, phencyclidine, and quinine. It is no longer recommended because of lack of efficacy and potential complications.

**Table 67.2 Poisons Whose Elimination May Be Enhanced by Corporeal Techniques**

| Urine Alkalinization | Multiple Doses of Activated Charcoal | Sodium Polystyrene Sulfonate | Prussian Blue |
|---|---|---|---|
| Chlorophenoxy herbicides (e.g., 2,4-D, MCPA, MCPP)[a] | Carbamazepine | Lithium | Radiocesium |
| Chlorpropamide | Colchicine | Potassium | Thallium |
| Diflunisal | Dapsone | | |
| Fluoride | Digoxin | | |
| Methotrexate | Phenobarbital | | |
| Phenobarbital | Phenytoin | | |
| Salicylates | Quinine | | |
| | Salicylates | | |
| | Theophylline | | |
| | Yellow oleander | | |

[a]*2,4-D,* 2,4-Dichlorophenoxyacetic acid; *MCPA,* 4-chloro-2-methylphenoxyacetic acid; *MCPP,* methylchlorophenoxypropionic acid (Mecoprop).

## FECAL ELIMINATION ENHANCEMENT

Activated charcoal, when given in multiple doses, can enhance the elimination of certain poisons. Ideal properties of poisons amenable to multiple-dose activated charcoal (MDAC) include a low intrinsic clearance, small volume of distribution, and prolonged half-life. MDAC promotes the clearance of poisons by interrupting their enterohepatic circulation, by promoting passive diffusion down a concentration gradient from the intestinal capillaries to the intraluminal gut space, a process often referred as "gut dialysis," and/or by limiting the absorption of controlled-release formulations. Multiple dosage regimens exist and usually include 50 g every 4 hours or 25 g every 2 hours until an improvement in clinical status is seen. Contraindications to the administration of MDAC include an altered level of consciousness with an unprotected airway, protracted vomiting unresponsive to antiemetic therapy, and impaired intestinal function, such as obstruction or ileus. Complications such as aspiration pneumonitis, appendicitis, and bowel obstruction due to charcoal bezoar are very rare, and their incidence increases with the number of doses given. Present guidelines recommend MDAC for poisoning due to carbamazepine, dapsone, phenobarbital, quinine, and theophylline.[5] MDAC is also recommended within 2 hours of salicylate poisoning. In addition, MDAC may be of benefit in select poisonings due to colchicine, cardiac glycosides,[21] or phenytoin (see Table 67.2).[22]

Ion exchange resins may also attract poisons from the gut capillaries to the lumen. Sodium polystyrene sulfonate is used to treat hyperkalemia, and there is current evidence that it can also reduce lithium's half-life.[23] Prussian blue can be used to enhance the fecal elimination of radiocesium and thallium (see Table 67.2).[24]

Whole-bowel irrigation (WBI) consists of the administration of electrolyte-balanced polyethylene glycol (macrogol) solution (up to 2 L/h) to induce diarrhea until the rectal effluent is clear to remove poisons from the gastrointestinal tract. WBI may be considered in specific circumstances, such as massive ingestions of sustained-release or enteric-coated drugs (e.g., salicylate) in a cooperative patient, massive ingestions of toxins not adsorbed by activated charcoal (e.g., iron or lithium tablets), or illicit drugs from body packers. Contraindications include intestinal perforation or obstruction, significant gastrointestinal hemorrhage, and protracted vomiting. WBI may interfere with the adsorptive effect of MDAC if administered concomitantly, but whether this compromises overall elimination is uncertain.

## PRINCIPLES AND FACTORS INFLUENCING POISON REMOVAL DURING EXTRACORPOREAL TREATMENTS

The elimination of a poison depends on its physicochemical and pharmacokinetic properties, as well as the extracorporeal technique used. Extracorporeal elimination of a poison is only significant if the following conditions are present: (1) it can be extracted from the plasma compartment, (2) extracorporeal clearance contributes to a significant proportion of total clearance; and (3) if the poison exerts its toxicity outside of the plasma compartment, a significant proportion of its body stores can be eliminated during the treatment. The first condition depends on the molecular size, water solubility, and protein binding of the poison because these correlate to its extraction ratio (ER) and extracorporeal clearance ($CL_{ECTR}$). ER can be calculated as (A – V)/A, where A represents the inflow (or prefilter) plasma concentration and V represents the outflow (or postfilter) plasma concentration. An extraction ratio of 1.0 implies complete removal of a substance from the plasma after a single pass through the extracorporeal circuit (i.e., V = 0). Extracorporeal plasma clearance may be calculated as

$$CL_{ECTR} = Q_B \times (1 - Hct) \times ER$$

where $Q_B$ is the blood flow and Hct is the hematocrit. $CL_{ECTR}$ can also be calculated by quantifying the amount of poison in the spent ultrafiltrate and/or dialysate over a period of time and dividing by its averaged plasma concentration during the same time frame. The second condition relates to its endogenous clearance, and the third depends on its volume of distribution ($V_D$; see later).

Modality-specific factors to consider include the process of poison removal (e.g., diffusion, adsorption, convection, centrifugation; Table 67.3), as well as the parameters chosen for a specific technique, such as the dialysis membrane (dialyzer surface area, membrane pore structure), blood flow rate, and effluent flow rate.[25] These are summarized later, after "Poison-Related Factors."

## POISON-RELATED FACTORS

### MOLECULAR SIZE

Poisons with a molecular weight below 1000 Da will be removed by any of the processes noted but are removed best by diffusion and convection. Solutes in excess of 1000 Da will be more easily removed by convection, adsorption, or centrifugation,[26] although modern intermittent hemodialysis (IHD) using diffusion alone can now clear poisons with an upper limit of approximately 10,000 Da (see Table 67.3). Convection from hemodiafiltration (HDF) and continuous renal replacement therapy (CRRT) can remove poisons with molecular weight up to 50,000 Da. Poisons with very high molecular weights (>100,000 Da) can only be removed by adsorption or centrifugation.

### PROTEIN BINDING

The degree of protein binding will also determine its removal. Hemofiltration and hemodialysis can remove only unbound poison because the poison–protein complex size exceeds the pore size of the hemofilter or dialyzer. Diffusion (IHD) and convection (HDF, CRRT) can remove poisons with protein binding up to 80%, with a few exceptions. Hemoperfusion, however, may be more effective in poisons with protein binding up to 90% to 95%, because binding to the adsorbent (activated carbon or, less commonly, a resin) competes with

**Table 67.3 Summary of Extracorporeal Treatments[a]**

| Treatment | Process | Molecular Weight Cutoff (Da) | Protein Binding Cutoff | Relative Cost | Complications | Comments |
|---|---|---|---|---|---|---|
| Albumin dialysis | Diffusion, adsorption | <60,000–100,000 | <95% | ++++ | ++ | Liver replacement support |
| CRRT | Convection and/or diffusion | <10,000–50,000 | <80% | ++ | + | Correction of uremia and acid-base and E+ disorders |
| Exchange transfusion | Centrifugation, separation, filtration | None | None | ++ | ++ | Easier than other ECTRs in neonates; correction of hemolysis |
| Hemodialysis | Diffusion | <10,000 | <80% | + | + | Correction of uremia and acid-base and E+ disorders |
| Hemofiltration | Convection | <50,000 | <80% | ++ | + | Correction of uremia and acid-base and E+ disorders |
| Hemoperfusion | Adsorption | <50,000 | <95% | ++ | +++ | Saturation of cartridge requires changes |
| Peritoneal dialysis | Diffusion | <500–5000 | <80% | ++ | ++ | Low efficacy |
| Plasma exchange | Centrifugation, separation, filtration | <1,000,000 | None | +++ | +++ | |

[a]All extracorporeal treatments above are less likely to be useful for poisons that have a high $V_D$ or a high endogenous clearance.
*CRRT,* Continuous renal replacement therapy, *E+,* electrolyte; *ECTR,* extracorporeal treatment; +, low; ++, moderate; +++, high; ++++, very high.

binding to plasma proteins. The clearance therefore depends on the affinity of the poison for the adsorbent.

The degree of protein binding can be influenced by acute alterations in poison or protein concentration and the presence of different pathologic states.[27] For example, in the context of hypoalbuminemia, there is less protein available to bind poison. As such, the concentration that is free (unbound) is higher with hypoalbuminemia, which will result in increased removal by ECTRs. Similarly, accumulation of organic acids in uremia leads to a reduction in binding sites for some xenobiotics (e.g., salicylates, warfarin, phenytoin), which also increases the unbound concentration and favors removal by ECTR. Furthermore, in toxic concentrations, there may be saturation of the protein binding sites (e.g., valproic acid, salicylate, 4-chloro-2-methylphenoxyacetic acid [MCPA]), increasing the fraction of poison that is unbound in relation to its total concentration, which also increases the amount that is amenable to removal by ECTR.[28]

### ENDOGENOUS CLEARANCE

Extracorporeal removal will not be useful if the endogenous clearance of a poison via its metabolism and native elimination routes far outweighs the clearance provided by an ECTR.[29] The endogenous clearance should usually be less than 4 mL/min per kg (or <200 mL/min) for extracorporeal removal to be considered potentially beneficial. This explains why hemodialysis is not indicated for poisons such as cocaine or toluene, which have very high endogenous clearances. Additionally, significant impairment in endogenous metabolic and/or elimination pathways may increase the relative efficacy of extracorporeal treatments; for example, the renal clearance of metformin decreases from 600 to 0 mL/min in anuric acute kidney injury (AKI).

### VOLUME OF DISTRIBUTION

The $V_D$ of a drug is the apparent volume into which a poison is distributed at equilibrium before clearance occurs. The $V_D$ is calculated by dividing the total drug in the body by its concentration. This mathematical relationship assumes that the body is a single homogenous compartment of water into which the drug is distributed.

Drugs that distribute extensively in tissues (e.g., tricyclic antidepressants) have a high $V_D$; conversely, drugs that distribute in total body water, such as methanol, have a low $V_D$ (<1 L/kg). Poisons exclusively confined to the blood compartment (e.g., mannitol) have a $V_D$ of 0.06 L/kg. Because ECTRs can only remove poisons in the intravascular space, they will not be useful to eliminate poisons with a high $V_D$. For example, due to its low protein binding (25%) and relatively low molecular weight (780 Da), digoxin easily crosses the dialyzer; however, because of its high $V_D$ (7 L/kg), less than 5% of the total body burden of digoxin will be removed in a 6-hour dialysis session. Many publications still erroneously conclude that a poison with a high $V_D$ is amenable to extracorporeal clearance, solely based on a high clearance or rapid reduction of serum concentrations.[30–32]

ECTR may be considered for very toxic xenobiotics with a high $V_D$ (e.g., thallium) only if a patient presents early after exposure. In this case, a high proportion of the poison has not yet distributed into various tissues or there may be ongoing absorption and so may successfully be removed by an ECTR.[33]

## AVAILABLE EXTRACORPOREAL TREATMENTS TO ENHANCE ELIMINATION OF POISONS

Numerous techniques can facilitate poison removal. These can be classified by their mechanism of removal: diffusion (hemodialysis, peritoneal dialysis), convection (hemofiltration), adsorption (hemoperfusion), and centrifugation (therapeutic plasma exchange).[34,35] The features of these treatments are summarized in Table 67.3.

## INTERMITTENT HEMODIALYSIS

During IHD, the poison diffuses from the blood compartment to a dialysate flowing in a countercurrent direction, separated by a semipermeable dialysis membrane. The principles that dictate solute removal in IHD also apply to poison elimination (see Chapter 63 for a detailed discussion). The characteristics of a xenobiotic that favor efficient poison removal by IHD are a low molecular weight (<5000–10,000 Da), low $V_D$ (<1–2 L/kg), low protein binding (<80%), and low endogenous clearance (<4 mL/min per kg).

Specific components of the dialysis system will influence poison clearance. These components include the type of dialysis membrane, its surface area, and the blood and dialysate flow rates (Box 67.1). Poison elimination is limited by the pore size of the dialysis membrane. However, even if the poison size is smaller than the cutoff of the membrane, larger molecules do not diffuse as freely as smaller ones, so clearance is reduced with larger molecules. New synthetic high-flux membranes and catheters now allow the removal of larger poisons considered nondialyzable 20 years ago.[26] Increasing the dialysate flow rate and, more importantly, the blood flow rate, will result in greater diffusion and elimination of the poison.[35] In poisoning, a filter with a large surface and maximal blood and dialysate flow rates should be used unless a contraindication is present (e.g., concern for disequilibrium syndrome).[35]

IHD has several distinct advantages over other extracorporeal modalities in the management of acute poisonings because it rapidly removes poisons and corrects metabolic disequilibria associated with severe poisonings, such as AKI, volume overload, acid–base abnormalities, electrolyte disturbances, and even hypothermia.[36] IHD is also the most available ECTR, the least expensive, and the quickest ECTR to implement.[37]

**Box 67.1 Factors That May Enhance Poison Clearance During Hemodialysis**

Larger surface area of dialysis membrane
High-flux dialyzer
High blood and dialysate flows
Increased ultrafiltration rate (with replacement solution)
Increased time on dialysis
Reduced recirculation
Two dialyzers in series
Two distinct extracorporeal circuits

The most common acute complication of IHD is systemic hypotension, and this is most relevant for patients with AKI or end-stage renal disease (ESRD) who require fluid removal. Because poisoned patients rarely require net ultrafiltration, the true incidence of dialytic hypotension in the toxicology setting is unknown but is more likely related to the effect of the poison, rather than to the dialysis treatment itself. Although hypotension itself is often a marker of toxin severity and can be an indication for ECTR, it is acknowledged that hypotension may limit the ECTR's performance.

## HEMOPERFUSION

During hemoperfusion (HP), blood circulates through an extracorporeal circuit equipped with a charcoal or resin cartridge onto which the poison can be adsorbed.[38] Compared with diffusion, adsorption is not as limited regarding the molecular size, lipid solubility, or protein binding of the poison. Alcohols and most metals, however, are poorly adsorbed to HP columns. Although certain exchange resins (e.g., XAD-4) are effective in the removal of organic solutes and nonpolar, lipid-soluble drugs, they are no longer available in the United States.

Current HP devices have improved their biocompatibility over the years; the coating of the sorbent material minimizes direct contact between the adsorbent and blood constituents, thereby greatly reducing the risk of embolization without impairing its adsorptive capacity. The circuit requires more generous systemic anticoagulation than dialysis. Blood flows are limited to 350 mL/min to minimize the risk of hemolysis.[39]

HP-associated complications are mostly related to the nonselective adsorption of certain cells and molecules, such as platelets (≅30%–50%), white blood cells (≅10%), serum fibrinogen, fibronectin, calcium, and glucose.[40,41] From a practical point of view, thrombocytopenia, hypoglycemia, and hypocalcemia can occur within hours after treatment initiation. Although these complications were more common with older devices and are reversible and treatable, HP still carries a higher risk of complications than IHD.[42] Furthermore, a cartridge costs several-fold more than a dialyzer and needs to be replaced every 3 to 4 hours due to saturation.

Twenty years ago, clearances of many poisons were higher with HP compared with IHD. However, with recent technologic advancements in IHD, these results have improved. For example, clearances of theophylline and phenobarbital by HP or IHD are now considered comparable.[38,42,43] In addition, HP does not correct electrolyte and acid–base disturbances, cannot remove fluid, and is less readily available. For these reasons, IHD is generally preferred in most settings where HP is indicated.[38] These considerations are reflected by recent trends in the choice of ECTR for poisonings (Fig. 67.2).[44–46]

## HEMOFILTRATION

During hemofiltration (HF), solute and solvent are removed by solvent drag, a process known as "convection," and replaced by a physiologic solution. Ultrafiltration is dependent on the sieving coefficient of the membrane. The sieving coefficient is the ratio of a solute concentration in the ultrafiltrate to its respective concentration in the plasma. A solute that freely crosses the membrane has a sieving coefficient of 1, whereas a sieving coefficient of 0 means that the solute cannot cross the membrane. Drug elimination by HF depends on factors similar to those regulating diffusion. However, convective

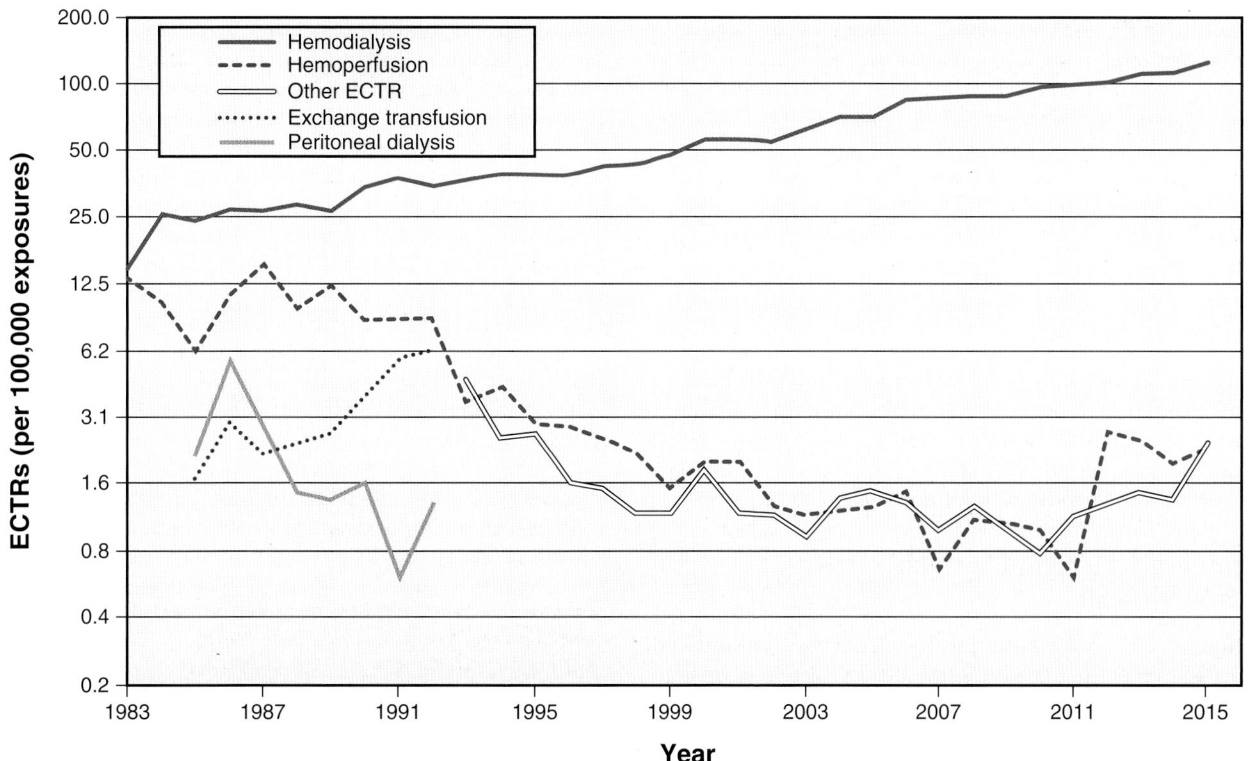


**Fig. 67.2** This figure illustrates how often extracorporeal treatments were used in the United States from 1983 to 2015. *ECTR,* Extracorporeal treatment.

transport also allows the removal of larger toxins—that is, having a molecular weight of up to 50,000 Da.[35] Because most poisons have a low molecular weight (<1000 Da), HF does not offer an advantage over IHD in the removal of most poisons.

## COMBINED THERAPIES

Clinicians sometimes combine more than one mechanism to optimize poison removal. For example, adsorption (HP) and diffusion (IHD) are sometimes used concurrently, in series, to maximize poison clearance. Although there is evidence that this combination approach may yield better results, the amount removed by the two procedures in series is usually not additive of the effect when either is used solely and may also increase the incidence of complications. Diffusion and convection (intermittent HDF) are also commonly combined.

## CONTINUOUS RENAL REPLACEMENT THERAPY

Most ECTRs can be offered intermittently or continuously. CRRTs are particularly popular in the critical care setting to manage AKI, and they are available in various forms (see Chapter 65): continuous venovenous hemodialysis (CVVHD), continuous venovenous hemofiltration (CVVH), and continuous venovenous hemodiafiltration (CVVHDF). Their role in the management of acute poisonings remains uncertain.[47] The solute clearance rate with continuous modalities is usually much lower than with intermittent modalities because of lower blood, dialysate, and ultrafiltrate flow rates. In AKI, continuous modalities are often chosen for fluid removal because of their better tolerability in hemodynamically unstable patients. However, in poisoned patients, because net ultrafiltration is rarely required, and because the removal of the offending agent is urgent, intermittent therapies are usually the modality of choice. CRRT may be used after IHD to avoid a sudden reincrease in poison concentration (so-called rebound); however, the benefit of this practice remains to be determined (see later).

Sustained low-efficiency dialysis (SLED) is a hybrid technique between IHD and CRRT.[48,49] Although used in anecdotal reports,[50] it provides a lower poison clearance than IHD over a same period of time.

## PERITONEAL DIALYSIS

Peritoneal dialysis (PD) clears substances by diffusion but has a limited role in acute poisoning because the maximum clearance obtainable is usually 10 to 15 mL/min (<10% of the clearance achievable by IHD).[34] PD has no advantages over other extracorporeal treatments in poisoning.

## THERAPEUTIC PLASMA EXCHANGE AND PLASMAPHERESIS

Plasmapheresis involves the withdrawal of venous blood and separation of plasma from blood cells by filtration or centrifugation and reinfusion of cells plus autologous plasma or another replacement solution (see Chapter 66). In therapeutic plasma exchange (TPE), the removed plasma is discarded and replaced by 5% albumin or fresh-frozen plasma. During TPE, clearance is limited by the plasma removal rate, which cannot exceed 50 mL/min.[34,51] The role of TPE in the treatment of acute poisoning is not well defined, but this method should only be considered for highly protein-bound (>95%) or very large poisons over the accepted cutoffs for HP or HF (>50,000 Da), if available. Drugs for which TPE may increase clearance in poisoning include cisplatin,[52] L-thyroxine,[53] and vincristine.[54] TPE has also been reported to treat near-fatal infusion reactions to rituximab.[55] Complications of TPE include those associated with installation of the vascular access, bleeding, hypocalcemia, and hypersensitivity reactions to the replacement solution.[56,57]

## EXCHANGE TRANSFUSION

During exchange transfusion (ET), there is removal of whole blood or red blood cells (by apheresis); this is used to remove the patient's red blood cells and replace them with transfused blood products. Its role in poisoning is unclear but may be considered in poisons causing massive hemolysis (e.g., sodium chlorate or nitrite poisoning in a patient with glucose-6-phosphate dehydrogenase [G6PD] deficiency) or in infants because it is technically less cumbersome to use than IHD in this population.

## EXTRACORPOREAL LIVER ASSIST DEVICES (ALBUMIN DIALYSIS)

Albumin dialysis is a relatively new extracorporeal treatment that can be used to replace liver function in fulminant hepatitis or severe cirrhosis, often as a bridge to transplantation. There are three different types of albumin dialysis. Single-pass albumin dialysis (SPAD) is a technique similar to IHD or CRRT but with albumin added in the dialysate. The albumin is discarded after its contact with the filter. The Molecular Adsorbents Recirculation System (MARS) is identical to SPAD, but the albumin-enhanced dialysate (with the adsorbed xenobiotics) is recycled after going through a dialysis filter, resin, and charcoal cartridge. The Prometheus system combines albumin adsorption with high-flux IHD after selective filtration of the albumin fraction through a polysulfone filter.

Theoretically, these devices can remove albumin-bound xenobiotics and endogenous substances (e.g., bile acids, bilirubin) better than the classic diffusive and convective techniques. However, preliminary data have not shown their superiority in terms of clearance of theophylline, valproic acid, or phenytoin.[58–60] An application of extracorporeal liver assist devices in toxicology may include toxin-induced hepatotoxicity, especially from *Amanita* mushroom or acetaminophen.[61–64] The precise role of liver assist devices in poisoning is currently unclear due to their relatively limited clearance, high cost, complication rates, and limited availability. Table 67.3 summarizes the various extracorporeal treatments available for poison removal.

# GENERAL INDICATIONS FOR EXTRACORPOREAL REMOVAL OF POISONS

The EXTRIP (EXtracorporeal Treatment In Poisoning; http://www.extrip-workgroup.org/) work group[65,66] has completed guidelines for the use of blood purification for several key toxins.[7–19] These recommendations help standardize management for these types of poisonings and propose directions for future research.[66] The decision to initiate any form of blood purification must take into account the clinical status, benefit expected from extracorporeal treatments, and poison-related factors.

Absolute indications for ECTR include the following (all must be present)[36]:

1. The poison exposure will result in severe toxicity. The exposure to a specific poison must be significant enough to warrant the cost and complications associated with ECTR. Obviously, a patient with life-threatening clinical signs (e.g., repeated seizures, respiratory depression, dysrhythmias) will be categorized as severe. A proper risk assessment of the exposure, which includes close collaboration with a poison control center, may help estimate the risk for any specific patient. In some cases, a poison exposure produces delayed effects (e.g., methanol, paraquat, acetaminophen), and monitoring of their concentration might predict future clinical compromise and would prompt prophylactic ECTR (i.e., before the appearance of toxic symptoms).
2. There is an absence of preferable alternative treatments. Antidotes may amend or prevent the apparition of toxicity related to a poison, so ECTR then becomes less crucial or indicated. This is the case for acetaminophen poisoning, when *N*-acetylcysteine is available. Because ECTR is somewhat invasive and may require transfer to a specialized center, its cost and benefit should be weighed against those of the antidote.
3. The ECTR must be able to remove the poison. (see earlier). To decide whether blood purification is indicated for a specific poisoning, the clinician must anticipate which benefits are expected from the procedure; some exposures can cause death (e.g., salicylates at high ingestions, paraquat), whereas others may cause irreversible tissue damage (e.g., blindness from methanol). The advantages of ECTR in those circumstances would largely outweigh the costs and complications of the procedure. In other situations, the poisoning itself may not cause irreversible injury, but the patient may be subjected to prolonged coma and immobilization, requiring mechanical ventilation and close surveillance in the intensive care unit (ICU), as seen in poisonings causing central nervous system (CNS) depression (e.g., barbiturates, anticonvulsants).
4. Finally, there may be situations in which ECTR will likely not affect outcomes but may reduce ICU or hospital length of stay and associated costs (e.g., dialysis versus fomepizole alone in a methanol-poisoned patient without metabolic acidosis).[67] The clinician should therefore assess the risks of the specific exposure and assess the cost-effectiveness of an ECTR in this context. Complications associated with ECTR are minimal and are usually limited to the insertion of a vascular access (which can be minimized with ultrasonographic guidance).[68] ECTR can also potentiate the elimination of certain antidotes (e.g., ethanol, *N*-acetylcysteine)[69] and precipitate withdrawal symptoms if drug concentrations fall below the therapeutic range (e.g., phenobarbital in a non-naïve patient).[70] Costs of a single dialysis, including equipment, nursing, and physician fees, are minor compared with the cost of a day in the ICU.[37] In the absence of any clinical outcome data, studies should demonstrate, at a minimum, significant drug removal.

## TECHNICAL CONSIDERATIONS

Patients presenting with poisonings are different from patients with AKI or ESRD. Therefore, the prescription of any extracorporeal treatment for the purpose of poison removal should reflect these differences.

### VASCULAR ACCESS

A double-lumen central catheter is required for administering most forms of ECTR. Because time is usually a concern, a temporary instead of a permanent catheter is preferred, using ultrasound guidance to reduce complications and ensure patency.[71] The femoral line is simpler for insertion and does not require X-ray placement confirmation but increases recirculation compared with subclavian or right jugular insertion sites.[72] However, there is less catheter malfunction with a femoral catheter than with a left jugular catheter.[73] There has been some experience on the use of dual-catheter sites and circuits to maximize poison clearance.[74,75]

### CHOICE OF HEMODIALYZER, FILTER, AND ADSORBER

For IHD, high-flux, high-efficiency dialyzers with the largest surface area should be used. The dialyzer or hemofilter should have a molecular size cutoff above that of the poison to be removed. With respect to HP, the only column available in the United States is the Gambro Adsorba 300C (Baxter Healthcare, Wayne, PA), a coated, activated, charcoal cartridge.[38]

### ANTICOAGULATION

Heparinization of the dialysis circuit is usually done with unfractionated heparin or low-molecular-weight heparin to prevent clotting and maintain patency of the circuit. In patients at high risk of bleeding, heparin can be substituted by saline flushes. For HP, heparin is also used to reduce the risk of hemolysis[39] and is usually required in larger quantities than for IHD.

### BLOOD, DIALYSATE, AND EFFLUENT FLOW

These should be maximized to increase clearance according to the capacities of the machine.[35]

### DIALYSATE COMPOSITION

As mentioned, poisoned patients may not present with the same metabolic disturbances as those with AKI or ESRD. The sodium, bicarbonate, potassium, calcium, and magnesium concentrations in the dialysate (or replacement fluid) need to be adjusted according to their serum concentrations. Phosphate may also be added to the dialysate or replacement fluid to avoid hypophosphatemia. It is also recommended that periodic measurements of serum biochemistry be performed and the content of the dialysate modified accordingly.

### DURATION OF EXTRACORPOREAL TREATMENT

A single 6-hour, high-efficiency ECTR will usually suffice for most poisonings for which ECTR is indicated. When significant toxicity is present or suspected to be prolonged, there is little risk to extend a treatment for several additional hours. However, HP cartridges usually need to be replaced after 3 to 4 hours because of saturation. Obviously, a longer period of treatment will be required if a less efficient therapy (e.g., CRRT, peritoneal dialysis, SLED) is used.

### PATIENT DISPOSITION

Many poisoned patients die prior to the initiation of dialysis.[76] If the risk assessment for a suspected toxic exposure suggests that a patient may require dialysis, prompt communication with a dialysis unit and preemptive transfer may be required, even if the patient does not yet meet the criteria for blood purification. Because a significant delay may occur between the time a decision is taken to perform ECTR and the time when it is initiated,[37] a dialysis nurse should be rapidly contacted and a temporary dialysis catheter installed as early as possible. Logistics and clinical status may require transfer of the patient to the ICU.[36]

### REBOUND

Rebound is defined as a sudden increase in poison concentration after the discontinuation of ECTR and usually occurs after the cessation of intermittent therapies. Rebound may either be due to the redistribution of poison from deep compartments (e.g., tissues and intracellular space) to the plasma (such as seen with lithium,[77] dabigatran,[78] and methotrexate[79]), especially in poisons with a large $V_D$, or due to ongoing absorption of the poison. In the former case, elevation of the serum concentration might reflect a concomitant decrease of the poison concentration from the toxic compartments (e.g., lithium) and so may even be beneficial.[80] In the latter situation, the increase in serum concentration can cause a recurrence of toxic symptoms. If rebound is thought to be worrisome, a clinician may choose to repeat an intermittent session, switch to a continuous therapy, or extend the intermittent therapy longer than the typical 4- to 6-hour treatment duration.[81] Following ECTR, serial poison concentrations and clinical status should be monitored for a period long enough to account for redistribution (≅12–24 hours) or ongoing absorption. The catheter should remain in place until the physician is convinced that additional sessions are unnecessary.

## POISONS AMENABLE TO EXTRACORPOREAL ELIMINATION

In the large majority of poisoning cases, ECTRs are not required. Drugs or poisons that are most commonly responsible for poisoning-related fatalities (e.g., tricyclic antidepressants, short-acting barbiturates, stimulants, "street drugs") are not effectively amenable to extracorporeal removal,[82] or severe toxicity and death occur rapidly, which limit the opportunity to initiate ECTR. The remainder of this chapter focuses on the clinical characteristics of key poisons for which ECTR may be considered. Physicochemical characteristics of major xenobiotics, including toxic alcohols, are shown in Table 67.4; the most common indications for ECTR in the context of poisoning are shown in Fig. 67.3 (U.S. data).

### TOXIC ALCOHOLS: ETHYLENE GLYCOL, METHANOL, ISOPROPANOL

Toxic alcohols share many similar molecular characteristics and toxicity and will therefore be considered together. They are all colorless. In its pure form, ethylene glycol (EG) is sweet-tasting, which makes it attractive to young children. It is commonly found in antifreeze, radiator fluid, solvents, hydraulic brake fluid, de-icing solutions, detergents, lacquers, and polishes. Methanol, also known as "wood alcohol," has an odor similar to ethanol. It is used as a solvent, as an intermediate of chemical synthesis during various manufacturing processes, or as an octane booster in gasoline. Products that contain methanol include windshield or glass-cleaning solutions, enamels, printing solutions, stains, dyes, varnishes, thinners, fuels, and antifreeze additives for gasoline. Isopropanol (isopropyl alcohol [2-propanolol]) has a bitter taste. It is commonly found in rubbing alcohol, skin lotion, hair tonics, aftershave lotion, denatured alcohol, solvents, cements, and cleaning products. Although the parent alcohols themselves cause minor toxicity (usually no more than moderate inebriation), their metabolites can induce life-threatening toxicity.

**Table 67.4 Physicochemical Characteristics and Toxicokinetics of Various Poisons**

| Poison | Molecular Weight (Da) | Protein Binding (%) | Volume of Distribution (L/Kg) | Endogenous Clearance in Healthy Adults (mL/min per kg) |
|---|---|---|---|---|
| Acetaminophen | 151 | 20 | 1 | 5 |
| Carbamazepine | 236 | 75 | 1.2 | 1.3 |
| Ethylene glycol | 62 | 0 | 0.6 | 1.8 |
| Isopropanol | 60 | 0 | 0.6 | 1.2 |
| Lithium | 7 | 0 | 0.8 | 0.4 |
| Metformin | 166 | 5 | 5 | 10 |
| Methanol | 32 | 0 | 0.6 | 0.7 |
| Methotrexate | 454 | 50 | 0.8 | 1.5 |
| Paraquat | 186 | 5 | 1.0 | 8 |
| Phenobarbital | 232 | 40 | 0.7 | 0.2 |
| Phenytoin | 252 | 90 | 0.6 | 0.4 |
| Salicylic acid | 138 | 80[a] | 0.2 | 1.5 |
| Theophylline | 180 | 60 | 0.5 | 0.7 |
| Valproic acid | 144 | 90[a] | 0.2 | 0.1 |

[a]Protein binding saturation occurs at high concentration.

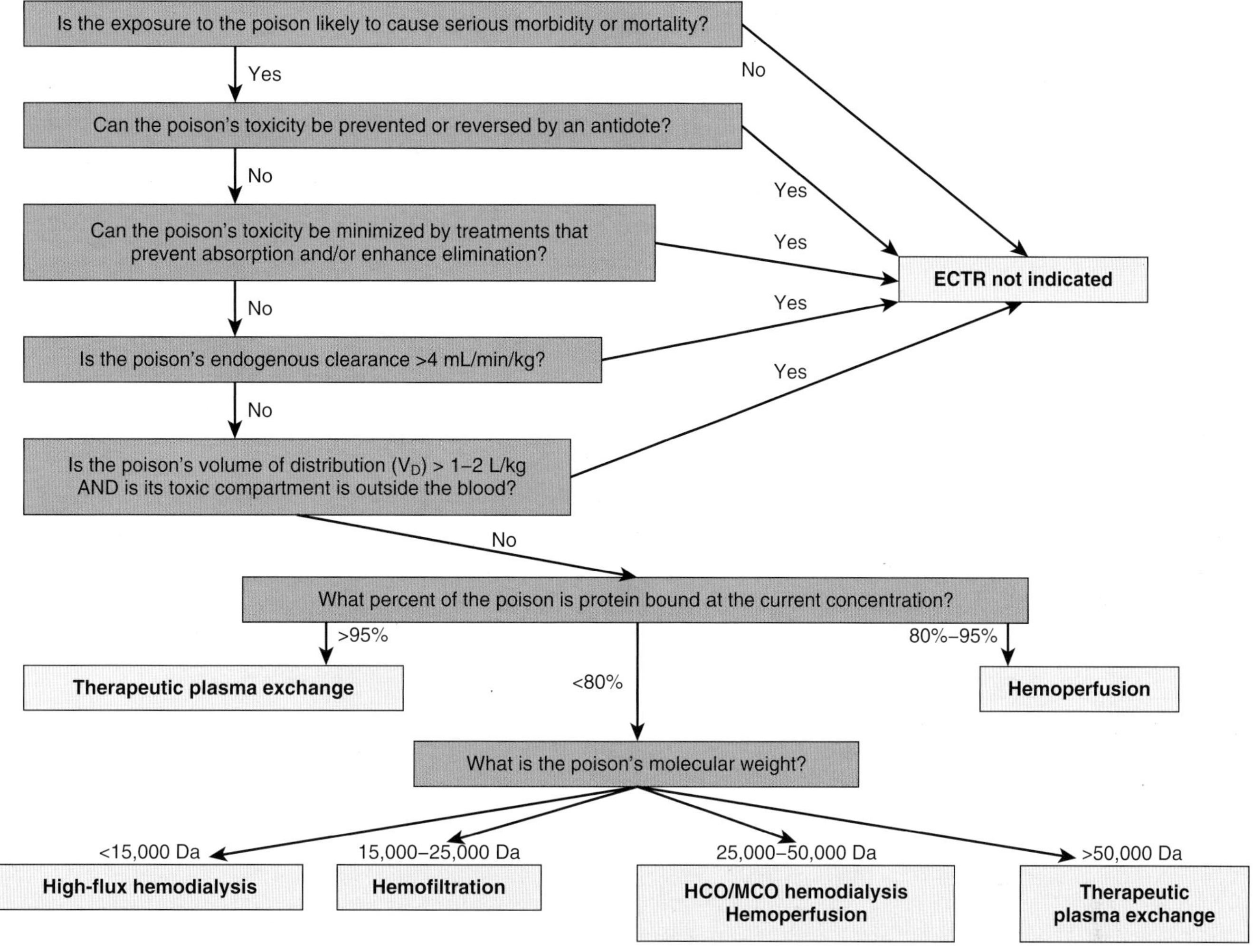


**Fig. 67.3** Most common toxin indications for extracorporeal treatments. *ECTR,* Extracorporeal treatment; *HCO,* high cut-off; *MCO,* medium cut-off; $V_D$, volume of distribution. (Adapted with permission from *Seminars* of dialysis.)

## TOXICOLOGY AND TOXICOKINETICS

EG, methanol, and isopropanol are all small unbound molecules that are distributed in total body water ($V_D = 0.6$ L/kg). Intoxication from these alcohols occurs rapidly after exposure and usually results from oral ingestion, although inhalation of vapors[83,84] and cutaneous absorption have been reported, especially in children.[85,86]

Approximately 30% of EG is excreted unmetabolized by the kidneys. The remaining 70% is oxidized to glycoaldehyde by alcohol dehydrogenase (ALDH) in the liver and then rapidly converted to glycolic acid by aldehyde dehydrogenase; this is followed by the slow conversion of glycolic acid to glyoxylic acid, the rate-limiting step (Fig. 67.4A). The end products include oxalic acid, glycine, and oxalomalic acid. Metabolic acidosis results from the formation and accumulation of glycolic acid and glyoxylic acid.[87,88] Lactic acidosis may also be present because the decrease in the $NAD^+$/NADH ratio promotes the reduction of pyruvate to lactate. However, glycolate also cross-reacts with the lactate assay on some point-of-care blood analyzers, which falsely elevates lactate concentrations. Another mechanism of toxicity of EG is the systemic deposition of precipitated calcium oxalate in various tissues, including the kidneys. Any pure EG ingestion > 0.1 mL/kg requires medical treatment. The potentially lethal dose of EG is approximately 1.4 mL/kg, but deaths have been reported with ingestions as low as 30 mL.

Methanol is metabolized principally by ALDH (85%) to formaldehyde and then rapidly oxidized by formaldehyde dehydrogenase to formic acid (see Fig. 67.4B). Small amounts are excreted unchanged by the lungs (10%) and the kidneys (5%). In a folate-dependent step, formic acid is then transformed to water and carbon dioxide.

Formic acid is the main metabolite responsible for methanol-related toxic symptoms because it induces cellular toxicity due to the inhibition of cytochrome *c* oxidase in cell's mitochondria, interfering with cellular oxidative metabolism.[89] The minimum lethal dose of methanol is estimated at 10 mL, although this is highly variable.[90]

Approximately 80% of isopropanol is metabolized to acetone via ALDH, and the remainder is eliminated unchanged in urine, with very small amounts excreted by the lungs (see Fig. 67.4).[91] Isopropanol displays first-order elimination kinetics, with an elimination half-life of 3 to 8 hours[92,93]; the half-life of acetone is 10 hours.[94,95] ALDH inhibitors markedly increase the half-life of isopropanol but have little effect on that of acetone.[96] Most CNS depressant effects are attributed to isopropanol, whereas acetone likely has a minor effect.[92] The potentially lethal dose of pure isopropanol is reported to be 100 to 250 mL.[97]

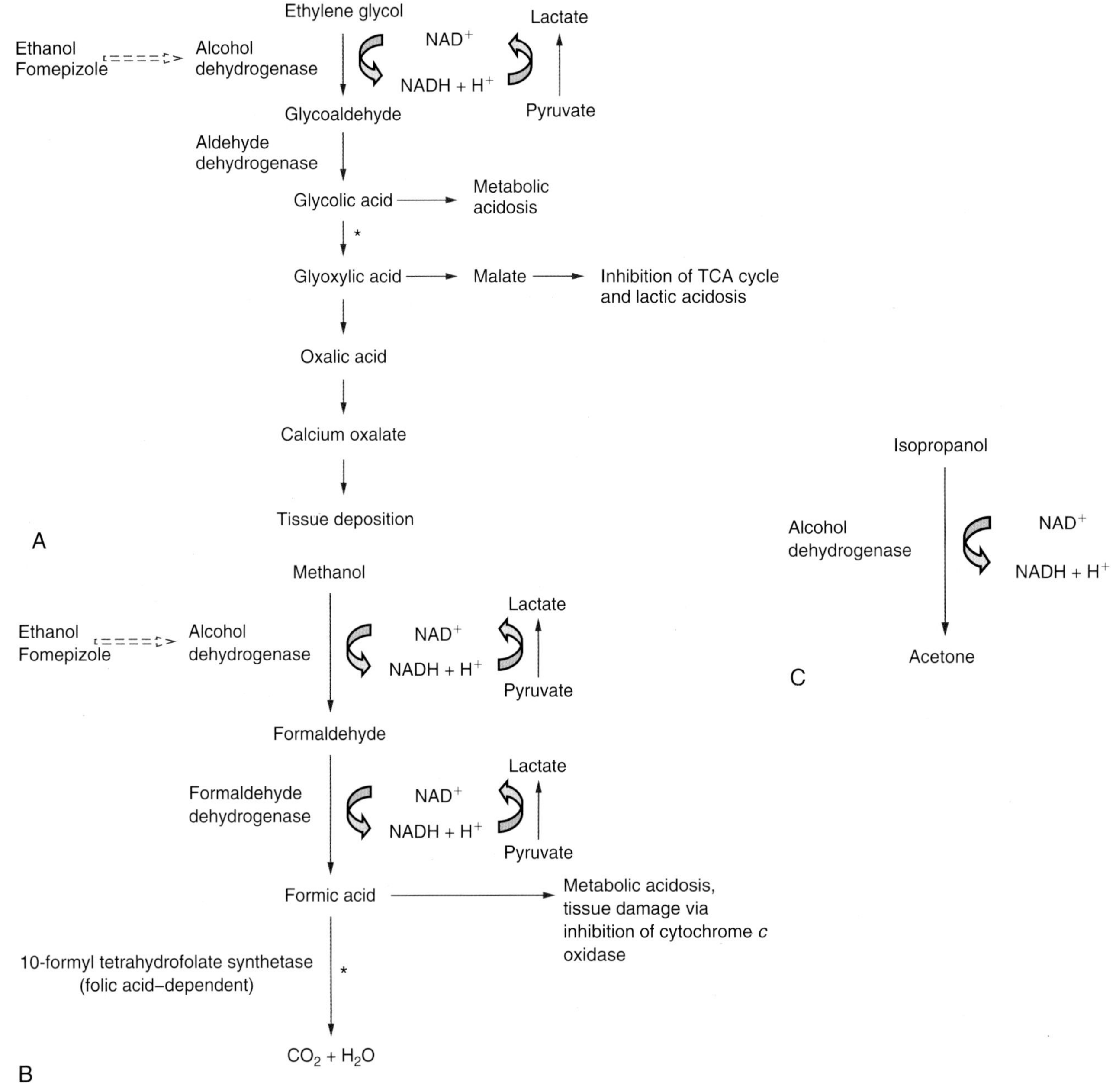


**Fig. 67.4 Metabolism of toxic alcohols.** (A) Ethylene glycol: The *broken arrow* points to inhibitors of alcohol dehydrogenase; the *asterisk* denotes the rate-limiting step. In the presence of the electron acceptor, nicotinamide adenine dinucleotide *($NAD^+$)*, ethylene glycol is oxidized to glycoaldehyde by alcohol dehydrogenase. Aldehyde dehydrogenase then rapidly converts glycoaldehyde to glycolic acid, which is followed by the slow conversion of glycolic acid to glyoxylic acid (the rate-limiting step). The final end products include oxalic acid, glycine, and oxalomalic acid, which are all effectively removed by IHD. (B) Methanol: The *broken arrow* points to inhibitors of alcohol dehydrogenase; the *asterisk* denotes the rate-limiting step. (C) Isopropanol: *IHD,* Intermittent hemodialysis; *4-MP,* fomepizole; *$NAD^+$,* nicotinamide adenine dinucleotide; *$NADH + H^+$,* reduced form of nicotinamide adenine dinucleotide; *TCA,* tricarboxylic acid.

## CLINICAL PRESENTATION

Following ingestion, the severity of the symptoms associated with EG poisoning depends on the ingested dose, concurrent ingestion of ethanol, and timing of treatment.[98] The first symptoms are neurologic and occur 0.5 to 12 hours after ingestion due to the parent alcohol causing inebriation, similar to ethanol but without the typical breath smell. A high osmol gap is present. Altered consciousness may progress to coma and seizures. Cerebral edema, nystagmus, ataxia, myoclonic jerks, and hyporeflexia have been described. New onset of cranial nerve (CN) defects (in particular CN VII) should make a clinician suspect EG ingestion. Gastrointestinal irritation may lead to vomiting, hematemesis, and aspiration pneumonia. Cardiopulmonary symptoms may occur 12 to 24 hours after ingestion; these result from the accumulation of newly formed organic acids. Calcium oxalate crystals deposit in the vasculature, myocardium, and lungs.[99] Hypertension or hypotension, dysrhythmias, myocarditis, pneumonitis, and noncardiogenic pulmonary edema have all been reported.

A severe high anion gap (AG) metabolic acidosis is present, and most deaths occur at this stage. Finally, 24 to 72 hours after ingestion, flank pain, hematuria, crystalluria, and AKI can occur due to the precipitation of calcium oxalate crystals in the kidneys. The pathogenesis of AKI is unclear but may relate to interstitial nephritis, cortical necrosis, direct renal cytotoxicity, or tubular obstruction. However, because the degree of renal injury does not correlate with the extent of calcium oxalate deposition in the kidney, it has been suggested that glycolic acid or other metabolites may be primarily responsible for the development of AKI.[100] Additionally, a low serum calcium concentration may occur and cause brisk deep tendon reflexes and QT interval prolongation.

Methanol intoxication should always be suspected in a patient presenting with neurologic, visual, and gastrointestinal symptoms in the presence of high AG metabolic acidosis with an increased osmol gap. The CNS presentation may include inebriation, headaches, dizziness, nausea, and seizures and may progress to cerebral edema. Methanol can produce a Parkinson-like syndrome by damage to the putamen and subcortical white matter of the basal ganglia.[101,102] Gastrointestinal symptoms include anorexia, nausea, vomiting, gastritis, and abdominal pain from acute pancreatitis. Metabolic acidosis, caused by the accumulation of formate and lactate, can be severe. Vision deficits are the hallmark of methanol poisoning and usually occur 6 to 30 hours after exposure, depending on how much ethanol has been coingested. Vision deficits include blurred vision (flashes or snowstorm), central scotoma, impaired papillary response to light, decreased visual acuity, photophobia, visual field defects, and progression to complete blindness.[103,104] The mechanisms of vision deficits are poorly defined but may relate to the inhibition of mitochondrial function in the optic nerve. Because the optic nerve cells possess few mitochondria and low cytochrome oxidase levels, they are extremely susceptible to the toxic effects of formic acid. Vision deficits are permanent in 25% of cases. Death is usually caused by cardiovascular shock and respiratory arrest.

The diagnosis of isopropanol overdose should be suspected in any patient with altered sensorium, a "fruity" acetone breath, an increased osmol gap without an increase in the AG, and the presence of acetonemia or acetonuria in the absence of hyperglycemia, glycosuria, or acidosis. Isopropanol poisoning mainly affects the CNS, with symptoms ranging from mild inebriation to lethargy, stupor, respiratory depression, and even coma. Isopropanol is also a gastrointestinal tract irritant and can cause nausea, vomiting, gastritis, and abdominal pain. Finally, isopropanol is directly toxic to myocytes and can induce severe hypotension, which is the strongest predictor of mortality in an isopropanol overdose.[90] Other systemic findings include hypoglycemia from impaired gluconeogenesis, hypothermia, and hemolytic anemia.

## DIAGNOSTIC TESTING

Because specific measurement of toxic alcohols (by colorimetric and enzymatic assays or chromatographic methods) is not widely available, treatment should begin immediately if exposure to toxic alcohols is suspected.[105] EG and methanol poisoning should be considered in any patient presenting with a high AG metabolic acidosis and/or a high osmol gap, even in the absence of symptoms.[106] In early presentations, the osmol gap is more prominent, whereas in later presentations the high AG predominates. Because toxic alcohols are osmotically active compounds, the osmol gap, calculated as the difference between measured osmolality (by freezing point depression) and calculated osmolality, can be used as an approximation of the toxic alcohol concentration (in mmol/L), which can then be converted to mg/dL (Table 67.5). This estimation can be monitored serially during admission, and especially during dialysis, when precise serum concentrations are unavailable.[107,108] The calculated osmolality is based on the concentrations of sodium, glucose, blood urea nitrogen, and ethanol (if coingested), as follows:

**Table 67.5 Conversion of Toxic Alcohol Concentration From mmol/L to mg/dL**

| Toxic Alcohol | Conversion From mmol/L to mg/dL |
|---|---|
| Acetone | ×5.81 |
| Diethylene glycol | ×10.61 |
| Ethanol | ×4.61 |
| Ethylene glycol | ×6.21 |
| Isopropanol | ×6.01 |
| Methanol | ×3.20 |
| Propylene glycol | ×7.61 |

$$\begin{aligned}&\text{Toxic alcohol concentration (in mmol/L)} \cong \text{osmol gap} =\\&\text{osmolality}_{\text{meas}} - \text{osmolality}_{\text{calc}} = \text{osmolality}_{\text{meas}} -\\&2\times\text{Na} + \text{gluc} + \text{urea} + 1.2\times\text{ethanol; in SI units}) =\\&\text{osmolality}_{\text{meas}} - (2\times\text{serum [Na]}) + (\text{glucose})/18 +\\&(\text{blood urea nitrogen})/2.8 + \text{ethanol}/4\text{; in Imperial units})\end{aligned}$$

The normal osmol gap is between 0 and 10 mOsm/kg. An osmol gap higher than 10 suggests the presence of EG, methanol, isopropanol, propylene glycol, or acetone.[109] In isopropanol poisoning, both isopropanol and acetone contribute to the osmol gap.[110] However, it is important to recognize that a "normal" osmol gap does not exclude the diagnosis of toxic alcohol poisoning; if a specific patient has a baseline gap of 0, an excess of 25.6 mg/dL (8 mmol/L) of methanol would not result in an elevated osmol gap but would be clinically significant and warrant treatment. Also, the osmol gap would remain normal if a patient presents late after ingestion, once the parent alcohol has undergone complete oxidation, because glycolic acid and formic acid do not contribute to the osmol gap.[111]

Similarly, the AG can be used to estimate the glycolic acid and formic acid concentrations. The AG is the difference between measured cations ($Na^+$ and $K^+$) and measured anions ($Cl^-$ and $HCO_3^-$), representing the difference between unmeasured anions and unmeasured cations (all values are in mmol/L). Lactate can also contribute to the AG and needs to be factored into the following equation:

$$\begin{aligned}&\text{Glycolic acid/formic acid concentration} = \Delta\text{AG} - \Delta\text{lactate} =\\&([\text{Na}+\text{K}] - [\text{Cl}+\text{HCO}_3] - 16\,[\text{AG upper reference limit}]) -\\&[\text{lactate}] - 2[\text{lactate upper reference limit}]) =\\&\text{Na}+\text{K}-\text{Cl}-\text{HCO}_3 - \text{lactate} - 14\end{aligned}$$

Studies have shown a good correlation between the concentration of metabolites and the calculated AG.[109] The absence of an AG suggests early presentation after EG or methanol exposure before metabolism into metabolites and coingestion of ethanol or another alcohol (e.g., isopropanol, propylene glycol).

Urinalysis can provide supporting evidence of EG exposure; calcium oxalate crystals (mono- and dihydrate forms) may be present in the urine sediment. These crystals appear 4 to 8 hours after ingestion and are found in approximately 50% of patients.[112,113] The presence of oxalate crystals is not specific for EG poisoning because it is also seen in individuals who ingest large amounts of vitamin C or a high-oxalate–containing food. Urine that fluoresces under Wood lamp illumination is another unique feature of EG poisoning. Many types of antifreeze contain sodium fluorescein, a fluorescent dye used as a marker to detect radiator leaks. Sodium fluorescein can be detected in the urine for up to 6 hours after ingestion.[114,115] Other laboratory abnormalities commonly found are hypocalcemia, leukocytosis, and an elevated protein concentration in cerebral spinal fluid.

Characteristic test findings of isopropanol exposure include increased osmol gap, the absence of metabolic acidosis (except if lactic acidosis is present), ketonemia, ketonuria, and normoglycemia. Acetonemia or acetonuria can be suspected by a positive sodium nitroprusside reaction in plasma or urine. A low concentration of serum ketones after 2 hours of isopropanol ingestion (in the absence of ALDH inhibition) generally excludes substantial ingestion.[92] Ketoacidosis from starvation, alcohol ingestion, or diabetes mellitus can be differentiated from isopropanol poisoning by the presence of metabolic acidosis.

## TREATMENT

In case of toxic alcohol poisoning, rapid decision making is critical because most clinicians have to proceed without a toxic alcohol concentration confirmation. Management can be divided into supportive care, correction of the acidemia, antidote therapy, and enhanced elimination with ECTRs, although many of these are performed concomitantly.

Initial management, as for all poisonings, is directed toward stabilization and providing appropriate supportive care, which may include airway management, volume resuscitation, seizure management, and vasopressors. High minute ventilation should be maintained if significant acidemia is present. Because toxic alcohols are rapidly absorbed from the gastrointestinal tract, and because mucosal irritation is often present, gastrointestinal decontamination is seldom performed in this context. Aspiration of the gastric contents using a nasogastric tube may be useful if the ingestion is very recent.

The cornerstone of treatment for EG or methanol poisoning is to prevent their metabolism into toxic metabolites using an antidote (e.g., ethanol or fomepizole), which inhibits ALDH.

Indications for the use of these antidotes are as follows[106,116]:

1. Serum concentration of EG > 20 mg/dL (3.2 mmol/L) or methanol > 20 mg/dL (6.3 mmol/L)
2. Documented recent (hours) ingestion of toxic amount of EG or methanol and osmol gap > 10 mOsm/kg
3. A history or strong clinical suspicion of EG or methanol poisoning and at least two of the following: arterial pH < 7.3, serum bicarbonate < 20 mEq/L, osmol gap > 10 mOsm/kg, or presence of oxalate crystals in urine

Antidote treatment is not recommended for isopropanol poisoning because the metabolite acetone does not cause metabolic acidosis and is eliminated by endogenous routes. If fomepizole were used, the CNS depressant effect of isopropanol could even be prolonged.[117] Because ALDH has a greater affinity for ethanol than for methanol or EG, ethanol has been the traditional antidote used to prevent the formation of toxic metabolites and can be given enterally, intravenously, or via the dialysate. The intravenous formulation has the advantages of immediate bioavailability and avoiding gastrointestinal distress. Target serum ethanol concentrations for ADLH competition are between 100 and 150 mg/dL (21.7 and 32.5 mmol/L)[118]; below this concentration, ADLH inhibition would not maximally inhibit metabolite formation, whereas above this range, ethanol can exacerbate CNS and respiratory depression.[116] More predictable serum ethanol concentrations can be obtained during IHD by adding 475 mL of 65% ethanol to the 4.5-L acid bath of the dialysate.[118]

Fomepizole (4-methylpyrazole; Antizol) is a newer U.S. Food and Drug Association (FDA)–approved antidote for EG and methanol poisoning and has largely replaced ethanol in the United States. Compared with ethanol, fomepizole has multiple advantages: (1) more potent ALDH inhibition; (2) simple dosing; (3) predictable pharmacokinetics; (4) no blood monitoring; (5) few side effects and no CNS depression; and (6) longer duration of action. Its main drawback is the cost ($1000/dose in the United States). Either antidote is usually continued until EG or methanol concentrations are below 20 mg/dL (EG < 3.2 mmol/L or methanol < 6.3 mmol/L), and the patient is asymptomatic, with a normal arterial pH. Table 67.6 lists dosages of ethanol and fomepizole during toxic alcohol poisonings.

Acidemia should be corrected with the administration of IV sodium bicarbonate,[119] which enhances the deprotonation of acid metabolites, making them less likely to penetrate in end-organ tissues (e.g., retina, kidney) and more likely to be excreted by the kidneys. An initial intravenous bolus (1–2 mEq/kg), followed by an infusion, if necessary, should be given to maintain an arterial pH no less than 7.35. Asymptomatic hypocalcemia is not routinely treated in the setting of EG poisoning because it can potentially exacerbate calcium oxalate crystal formation and deposition.

Pyridoxine, thiamine, and magnesium are cofactors in the metabolism of EG, and their supplementation is recommended in patients who may be malnourished (e.g., alcoholics) or in those with known deficits.[106] Because the rate-limiting step of methanol metabolism is mediated by 10-formyltetrahydrofolate synthetase, which is folic acid—dependent, folic acid supplementation is recommended for the treatment of methanol poisoning. The suggested dose is 50 mg IV every 4 hours for 5 doses and then once daily.

Extracorporeal treatments, especially IHD, are extremely efficient at removing alcohols and their toxic metabolites, as well as rapidly correcting metabolic acidosis. When dialysis parameters are optimized (see earlier), the rate of clearance of alcohols and metabolites can reach 250 mL/min.

The increasing availability of fomepizole has modified the indications and pertinence of ECTR because of its great efficacy at preventing metabolite formation.[120] For example,

**Table 67.6 Antidote Dosage During Toxic Alcohol Poisoning**

| Dose | Absolute Ethanol | 10% IV Ethanol[b] | Fomepizole |
|---|---|---|---|
| Loading dose[a] | 600 mg/kg | 7.6 mL/kg | 15 mg/kg IV |
| Maintenance dose | 66 mg/kg per hour (nondrinker)<br>154 mg/kg per hour (chronic drinker) | 0.8 mL/kg per hour (nondrinker)<br>2.0 mL/kg per hour (chronic drinker) | 10 mg/kg q12h × 4 doses, then 15 mg/kg q12h |
| Maintenance dose during IHD | 169 mg/kg per hour (nondrinker)<br>257 mg/kg per hour (chronic drinker) | 2.1 mL/kg per hour (nondrinker)<br>3.3 mL/kg per hour (chronic drinker) | Same dose but q4h or a constant infusion of 1.0–1.5 mg/kg per hour |

[a]Assumes initial ethanol concentration is zero; dose is independent of chronic drinking status.
[b]Equivalent to 7.9 g ethanol/dL.
*IHD,* Intermittent hemodialysis.

patients who are poisoned with EG but are neither acidotic nor have renal impairment may be treated with fomepizole alone, whatever the concentration of EG.[121] The same applies for methanol; however, the endogenous clearance of methanol is extremely low when fomepizole/ethanol is used. Assuming a methanol half-life of 54 hours under fomepizole,[122] a patient with an initial methanol concentration of 320 mg/dL (100 mmol/L) would need to be hospitalized 9 days until the methanol is at a safe concentration (<20 mg/dL, or 6.3 mmol/L). Dialysis might therefore be instituted to reduce hospitalization costs and antidote requirement for patients poisoned with EG or methanol.[67,123] However, IHD is mandatory when there is metabolic acidosis or an increased AG because these are suggestive of toxic metabolites accumulation.

Indications for ECTR for EG and methanol poisoning include the following[15]:

- Serum EG or methanol concentration > 50 mg/dL (8.0 mmol/L, or 15.6 mmol/L, respectively) if fomepizole is not used
- Metabolic acidosis (pH < 7.2) or an AG > 28 mmol/L
- Coma or seizures
- Vision deficits secondary to methanol
- AKI or chronic kidney disease (CKD)

The expected duration of dialysis in hours can be estimated using these formulas and using SI units:

$$4.7 \times (\text{Ln}\,[\text{initial EG concentration}/2])$$ [124]

or

$$3.5 \times (\text{Ln}\,[\text{initial methanol concentration}/4])$$ [125]

provided that the metabolic acidosis is corrected. However, serial monitoring of the toxic alcohol concentration or osmol gap is recommended to confirm the estimation.[126] IHD should be continued until the parent alcohol levels are < 20 mg/dL (EG < 3.2 mmol/L or methanol < 6.3 mmol/L), and the metabolic acidosis is corrected. Other modalities, such as CRRT, would offer lower clearance and require longer treatment but may be considered if IHD is unavailable.[127]

IHD can also effectively remove isopropanol and acetone, although it is only indicated when the isopropanol concentration is > 400 mg/dL (66.6 mmol/) or there is prolonged coma, hypotension, myocardial depression, tachydysrhythmias, or AKI.[128–130] Other modalities would not offer comparable clearances.[131]

Phosphate addition in the dialysate is often required during IHD. The use of heparin should be minimized or preferably avoided in methanol-poisoned patients due to the increased risk of intracerebral hemorrhage.

## SALICYLIC ACID

Salicylates are widely used as analgesics and antiinflammatory medications. Salicylic acid produces its antiinflammatory effects by suppressing the expression of cyclooxygenase (COX), thereby reducing the production of proinflammatory mediators such as prostaglandins. In overdose, salicylic acid also uncouples oxidative phosphorylation, which is a key contributor to toxicity and death. Aspirin (acetylsalicylic acid) is commonly prescribed as an antiplatelet therapy. Salicylic acid is used as a topical keratolytic agent and wart remover, bismuth subsalicylate (Pepto-Bismol; 236 mg of salicylate/15 mL) is used for reflux disease, and methyl salicylate (oil of wintergreen; 98% salicylate; 1 teaspoon contains 7 g of salicylates) is used for pain relief and as a flavoring agent.[132,133] Because there are many over-the-counter formulations, salicylates are among the substances most commonly involved in exposure calls to poison centers.[1] Fortunately, because of modification in packaging and the availability of nonsteroidal antiinflammatory drug (NSAID) alternatives, significant salicylate poisonings have become less frequent in the United States.

### TOXICOLOGY AND TOXICOKINETICS

Salicylates, in general, are rapidly absorbed by the gastrointestinal tract. Peak serum concentrations are reached within 1 hour, unless enteric-coated products are used. However, in an acute overdose, bezoar formation and pylorospasm may delay absorption and the appearance of symptoms.[134,135]

Within the therapeutic range, salicylic acid (molecular weight = 138.1 Da; $V_D$ = 0.2 L/kg) is 90% protein-bound and undergoes first-order hepatic metabolism. Normally, less than 10% of salicylate is excreted unchanged by the kidneys, and its elimination half-life is between 2 and 4 hours.[136,137] Salicylic acid is filtered at the glomerulus, actively secreted in the proximal tubule, and reabsorbed passively in the distal tubules. In case of an acute overdose, the protein binding falls to 50%, the $V_D$ increases, and major pathways of metabolism become saturated, so clearance changes from first-order to zero-order. Although more salicylic acid is eliminated by the kidneys in these circumstances, the other dose-dependent changes result in a marked increase in the elimination half-life (>30 hours).[138–140]

Salicylic acid is a weak acid, with a $pK_a$ of 3.0. It exists in an ionized and a nonionized state in the plasma:

$$H^+ + Sal^- \leftrightarrow HSal$$

Uncharged particles, such as unionized salicylic acid, cross the blood-brain barrier and other tissues more readily than the charged form. Acidemia drives the above equilibrium to the right, therefore causing more CNS toxicity.[141] Elimination is similarly influenced by the urinary pH, where an increase in tubular lumen pH drives the equilibrium toward the ionized form, limits its uptake by renal tubular cells, and favors its elimination in urine. This provides the rationale for urinary alkalinization to enhance the elimination of salicylates.

## CLINICAL PRESENTATION AND DIAGNOSTIC TESTING

Salicylate poisoning can be acute or chronic. Acute ingestions >150 mg/kg usually present with mild to moderate toxicity; >300 mg/kg, patients are at risk of severe poisoning, and exposures >500 mg/kg are potentially lethal. The therapeutic range is 10 to 30 mg/dL (0.7–2.2 mmol/L); concentrations > 40 mg/dL (2.9 mmol/L) can be associated with toxicity, and concentrations > 75 mg/dL (5.4 mmol/L) are associated with significant severe effects.

Acute salicylate ingestion often causes nausea and vomiting as a result of gastritis and direct stimulation of the chemoreceptor trigger zone in the medulla. Hemorrhagic ulcers, decreased gastric motility, and pylorospasm are also seen. A variety of acid–base abnormalities may occur with salicylate poisoning, but the classic finding is mixed respiratory alkalosis and high AG metabolic acidosis. Salicylate stimulates the respiratory center in the brainstem independently of the aortic and carotid chemoreceptors, leading to an early fall in $CO_2$ partial pressure and respiratory alkalosis.[142–144] Subsequently, metabolic acidosis is induced by the accumulation of salicylate and organic acids. Increased minute ventilation promotes lactic acid production.[142,145] In addition, salicylates uncouple mitochondrial oxidative phosphorylation and interrupt glucose and fatty acid metabolism in the Krebs cycle, leading to an increase in the production of tissue carbon dioxide, lactic acid, and ketoacids.[145]

Salicylates cause a variety of CNS effects, either directly or through the selective reduction of the brain glucose concentration. Cerebral edema, perhaps secondary to capillary leak, may also play a role in alterations in mental status.[145] Neurologic manifestations include tinnitus, central hyperthermia, vertigo, altered mental status (e.g., hyperactivity, agitation, delirium, hallucination), and coma.[146,147] As stupor progresses, there may be blunting of the respiratory response, which may further decrease the pH and increase salicylate entry into the CNS.[141,148] Tinnitus occurs at salicylate concentration of 30 mg/dL (2.2 mmol/L) and may lead to decreased auditory acuity and even deafness.[149] Early salicylate poisoning may present with hyperglycemia resulting from glycogenolysis, gluconeogenesis, and decreased peripheral use. Hypoglycemia occurs later, with heightened cellular energy demand and uncoupling of oxidative phosphorylation.[150]

Chronic poisoning may be seen in patients who receive prolonged salicylate therapy, often in the setting of reduced renal clearance. Symptoms in this setting are often more prominent than after an acute ingestion at the same salicylate concentration; such patients are often misdiagnosed as having delirium, encephalopathy, or fever of unknown origin, and they have a high mortality.[151,152] Noncardiogenic pulmonary edema, a classic albeit rare finding, may occur as a result of gastrointestinal local release of vasoactive peptides and increased capillary permeability, which further limits the application of urine alkalinization.[153,154]

The diagnosis of salicylate intoxication is usually suspected from the history, classic clinical findings, and metabolic abnormalities (described earlier). An elevated AG with concomitant respiratory alkalosis should prompt confirmation of salicylate exposure. Quantitative serum salicylate concentrations can generally be determined rapidly in many centers. Because absorption may be erratic or prolonged, serial measurements (every 2–4 hours) are initially required. The magnitude of the concentration is less important in patients with significant symptoms because treatment will be initiated regardless. In these cases, the salicylate concentration is most useful for monitoring the effectiveness and determining the duration of therapy. The Done nomogram, which was an attempt to correlate salicylate concentrations with toxicity, is no longer used in practice because of its poor predictive value.[155]

## TREATMENT

General principles of poisoning management apply to salicylates. Special consideration should be geared toward respiratory support. Patients are dependent on maintaining a high minute ventilation and high serum pH to reduce salicylate entry into the CNS. Endotracheal intubation should therefore only be performed if absolutely necessary, and by an experienced clinician, to avoid prolonged periods of apnea, during which many deaths have been reported.[156] Ventilator settings should try to replicate the patient's respiratory pattern prior to intubation, although this is usually difficult because of auto–positive end-expiratory pressure (PEEP).

Once the patient is stabilized, further therapy is aimed toward decreasing absorption and increasing elimination of salicylates. Activated charcoal remains the preferred decontamination technique.[157,158] MDAC can enhance the elimination of salicylates but is considered less efficacious and more cumbersome to perform compared with urine alkalinization.[5,6,159,160] Nevertheless, MDAC should be considered, especially for patients who may have a significant amount of unabsorbed salicylate in the gastrointestinal tract.

Serum and urine alkalinization is a crucial component of treatment. As mentioned previously, alkalinization will drive salicylate to be dissociated, which will reduce its diffusion through the blood-brain barrier and its tubular reabsorption (ion trapping). Because the ionization constant ($pK_a$) is a logarithmic function, small changes in urine will have a large effect on salicylate elimination.[161] Urinary clearance of salicylate is enhanced several-fold with alkalinization when compared with forced diuresis alone. In one small series, the percentage of the salicylate dose excreted in urine increased from 2% under acidic conditions to 30% under alkaline conditions.[162] The bicarbonate infusion is titrated to reach a urinary pH of 7.5 or until the salicylate concentration is below 30 mg/dL (2.2 mmol/L). An alkaline urine cannot be produced in the presence of severe hypokalemia because kidney reabsorption of potassium occurs via the $H^+/K^+$ exchange pump in the collecting tubule, so the potassium level should be monitored and aggressively corrected.

Alkalinization may be contraindicated in patients with AKI or pulmonary edema; in these cases, IHD may be preferred over the risk of precipitating respiratory failure and requiring mechanical ventilation. Acetazolamide induces urinary alkalinization but is absolutely contraindicated because it lowers the arterial pH, which promotes salicylate movement into the CNS and other tissues.

The first article ever published on diffusion-based techniques—in 1913, by John Abel—showcased the removal of salicylates from animal subjects.[163] Salicylate displays properties of a highly dialyzable compound because of its low $V_D$, small molecular size, and low protein binding at high concentrations.[164–166] IHD is the best extracorporeal treatment because it can remove salicylate while correcting the acid–base and volume status of salicylate-poisoned patients. Although peritoneal dialysis,[167,168] exchange transfusion,[155] HP,[169–171] and CRRT[172–174] all increase salicylate clearance, none of them achieve the efficacy of IHD. IHD remains underused in salicylate poisoning; the availability of alternative treatments (e.g., MDAC, urinary alkalinization) may lure the clinician into a false sense of security, so most deaths still occur before ECTR is initiated.[76]

Indications for ECTR include any of the following attributable to salicylate poisoning[16]:

- Neurologic symptoms (e.g., confusion, seizures, coma)
- Pulmonary edema
- pH < 7.25
- Serum salicylate concentration > 90 mg/dL (6.5 mmol/L)
- Acute kidney injury
- Clinical deterioration, despite appropriate treatment

Patients with chronic poisoning display more toxicity at lower salicylate concentrations. Therefore, in chronic poisoning, the initiation of ECTR is based largely on signs and symptoms. ECTR should be maintained until the salicylate concentration is below 19 mg/dL (1.4 mmol/L) and there has been a clinical improvement. Although some authors have suggested continuing urinary alkalinization during ECTR, dialysis would likely alkalinize a patient much more quickly and reliably than an intravenous infusion of bicarbonate.[175]

## LITHIUM

Lithium, the lightest metal on the periodic table, was used therapeutically for gout in the 19th century and later in soft drink preparations. Its use became widespread in the 1950s, when it became a first-line therapy for the treatment of bipolar disorder.[176] Although generally considered a safe drug, lithium has a narrow therapeutic range (0.7–1.0 mmol/L) and can induce major side effects when serum concentrations become supratherapeutic. Lithium may also cause long-term metabolic and renal effects, such as dysthyroidism, hyperparathyroidism, nephrogenic diabetes insipidus, and a progressive decline in the glomerular filtration rate (GFR), which are beyond the scope of this chapter.[177] Its mechanism of action and toxic effects are incompletely understood. Lithium is thought to stabilize cell membranes, reduce neural excitation, and reduce synaptic transmission. Potential mechanisms include depletion of CNS inositol,[178] inhibition of the intracellular signaling pathways involved in neuroprotection,[179,180] and modulation of nitric oxide, glutamate, and other neurotransmitters.[181]

### TOXICOLOGY AND TOXICOKINETICS

The pharmacokinetic parameters of lithium are well known. Lithium is a 7 Da monovalent cation, orally administered as a carbonate (capsule) or citrate (liquid). Oral absorption is rapid and complete at therapeutic doses, and its bioavailability is not affected by food. Peak blood concentrations with therapeutic dosing are reached within 1 to 2 hours for an immediate-release formulation and within 4 to 6 hours for the sustained-release form, but they are usually delayed severalfold in acute poisoning. Lithium is unbound to proteins and has a $V_D$ of 0.7 to 0.8 L/kg. Its distribution into various tissues is variable—lithium diffuses into the liver and kidneys rapidly, but its transfer into bone, muscle, and brain is much slower, which explains the delay in peak CNS concentrations relative to the serum concentration after an acute overdose.[182] Lithium also predominantly distributes into the intracellular compartments by active transport. It is eliminated almost exclusively by the kidney, where it is freely filtered; 80% of filtered lithium is reabsorbed (75% in the proximal tubule and 25% in the distal tubule). Total body clearance is therefore approximately 20% of the GFR. Lithium reabsorption follows that of sodium, and therefore sodium-avid states (e.g., volume depletion, NSAIDs, congestive heart failure, cirrhosis) markedly increase lithium retention. The half-life of lithium with therapeutic use is about 18 to 24 hours for normal subjects but can be prolonged in older adults, chronic lithium users, and CKD.[183,184] However, in patients with normal renal function, in an acute overdose the plasma elimination half-life is approximately 10 hours (largely due to distribution into extravascular tissues), whereas in a chronic overdose it is 30 to 40 hours.[185]

### CLINICAL PRESENTATION AND DIAGNOSTIC TESTING

Lithium overdose may be defined as acute when it occurs after a single massive exposure in a patient naïve to lithium and as chronic when it occurs after dosing or prescribing errors or in situations where lithium clearance becomes impaired.[186] The severity of symptoms does not correlate closely to the serum lithium concentration. Acutely poisoned patients may be completely asymptomatic at a lithium concentration of 4.0 mmol/L, whereas there may be evident clinical signs in chronic poisonings with concentrations near the therapeutic range.[184,187] Acute poisoning is predominantly manifested by gastrointestinal symptoms (e.g., nausea, vomiting, diarrhea) and by nonspecific cardiac conduction delay, although life-threatening dysrhythmias are uncommon. Neurologic findings are especially prominent in chronic poisoning and may range from mild symptoms (e.g., coarse tremor or dysarthria to a more severe presentation, such as lethargy, seizures, hyperthermia, coma, and death).[188,189] A protracted neurologic course is sometimes seen after severe poisoning,[183] and some patients develop a syndrome of irreversible lithium-effectuated neurotoxicity (SILENT), which relates to cerebellar and cognitive deficits that may last years. Causative factors and their relation to lithium is unknown.[190]

### TREATMENT

Therapy should not only be guided by lithium concentrations but also by symptoms, underlying kidney function, and a patient-specific risk assessment.[185,187] Initial supportive care should target the specific manifestations of lithium toxicity, including treatment of hyperthermia, dysrhythmias, and seizures. Volume contraction favors proximal lithium reabsorption and should therefore be promptly corrected. Although isotonic saline (0.9%) is preferred for volume resuscitation, it may need to be subsequently replaced by hypotonic solutions or free water if lithium-induced nephrogenic diabetic insipidus and hypernatremia become a concern.

Gastrointestinal decontamination may be required in massive oral ingestions, although oral activated charcoal does not bind lithium and has no role in isolated lithium poisoning.[191] Whole-bowel irrigation with polyethylene glycol can be considered for sustained release formulations.[192] Oral sodium polystyrene sulfonate (Kayexalate), a cation exchanger commonly used for the treatment of hyperkalemia, has been shown to bind unabsorbed lithium from the gastrointestinal tract and enhance elimination of absorbed lithium in animals and humans.[23,193,194] It should be considered in patients who have mild to moderate symptoms for whom dialysis is delayed or not considered as a treatment option.[23]

Lithium has ideal properties for extracorporeal removal—small size, negligible protein binding, small $V_D$, low endogenous clearance. However, it is unknown if enhancement of lithium removal by ECTR translates into clinical benefit; in one retrospective and underpowered comparative study, clinical outcomes were similar between groups treated or untreated with IHD, although cohorts were not comparable at baseline.[195]

IHD is the modality of choice when extracorporeal elimination is required. Clearances in excess of 180 mL/min can be obtained with modern filters.[196–199] Serum lithium concentrations often rebound after IHD termination,[183,200] but as mentioned earlier, this may not be concerning, because lithium CNS concentrations actually decrease during redistribution back to the circulation[80] unless there is ongoing absorption of lithium from the gut. CRRT provides inferior clearance and removal rates than IHD.[197,201–203] Lithium clearance with PD is inferior to that of functioning kidneys.[204,205]

Indications for ECTR include any of the following[12]:

- Severe neurologic features (central hyperthermia, seizures, and/or depressed consciousness)
- Serum [Li] > 5 mmol/L (although good outcomes have been noted from much higher concentrations in acute poisoning without ECTR)
- Kidney impairment with symptoms and serum [Li] > 4 mmol/L
- Life-threatening cardiac dysrhythmias

The threshold for dialysis initiation should be lower in patients who cannot tolerate volume repletion or those with impaired kidney function.[183,206]

## VALPROIC ACID

Valproic acid (VPA) is used for the treatment of absence seizures, complex partial seizures, migraine, and mood disorders. Although acute VPA intoxication often results in mild self-limiting CNS depression, serious toxic effects and death have been reported.[207,208]

### TOXICOLOGY AND TOXICOKINETICS

VPA (molecular weight, 144.21 Da; $V_D$, 0.2 L/kg) is available in immediate and sustained-release formulations, both of which have a high bioavailability. Serum concentrations typically peak 1 to 13 hours after ingestion, depending on the preparation.[209] Therapeutic serum concentrations range from 50 to 100 mg/L (347–693 μmol/L). Protein binding of VPA is saturable in overdose. Protein binding is typically 90% at therapeutic concentrations, but decreases to 35% at 300 mg/L (2079 μmol/L).[210]

VPA is rapidly metabolized by the liver. It undergoes glucuronic acid conjugation (70%) and beta and omega oxidation to various metabolites, whereas less than 3% is normally excreted unchanged in urine.[210] In overdose, more of its metabolism undergoes CYP450-mediated omega oxidation, the metabolites of which are thought to be responsible for some of the toxic effects of VPA, such as 5-OH-VPA and 4-en-VPA.

### CLINICAL PRESENTATION AND DIAGNOSTIC TESTING

Most VPA overdoses are well tolerated, but toxicity is more likely following ingestions over 200 mg/kg.[208,211] Acute poisoning is typically manifested by gastrointestinal distress (e.g., nausea, vomiting, diarrhea), CNS abnormalities (e.g., confusion, obtundation, coma with respiratory failure), hypotension, and elevated transaminase concentrations. Free (unbound) and total VPA serum concentrations are poorly correlated with severity of intoxication, but most patients with total concentrations greater than 180 mg/L (1247 μmol/L) develop some degree of CNS depression.[212]

Hyperammonemia is seen at therapeutic and toxic valproate concentrations[213] and does not usually cause toxicity but, when markedly elevated, it can cause encephalopathy, cerebral edema, and death. The mechanism of valproate-induced hyperammonemia is incompletely understood, but may relate to the inhibition of carbamoyl phosphate synthetase, *N*-acetylglutamate synthetase, or carnitine-dependent beta oxidation, which inhibits the urea cycle.[213]

At very high serum concentrations (>1000 mg/L [6930 μmol/L]), complications include high AG metabolic acidosis, elevated osmolality (VPA concentration > 1500 mg/L [10,395 μmol/L] may raise the osmol gap by 10 mOsm/kg or more), hypernatremia, hypocalcemia, pancreatitis, noncardiogenic pulmonary edema, bone marrow suppression, and AKI.[214,215] Diagnosis of VPA intoxication is based on a history of exposure, typical toxic symptoms, and an elevated serum valproate concentration.

### TREATMENT

Treatment consists of initial stabilization of respiratory and cardiovascular function. Gastrointestinal decontamination using activated charcoal should be administered, particularly if the patient presents within 1 hour of exposure. Due to the prolonged absorption noted in overdose, it may also be useful beyond that period. Urine elimination enhancement is ineffective because the excretion of VPA by the kidney is limited. L-Carnitine has been proposed as a treatment for hyperammonemic encephalopathy but supporting data are limited.[216] If used, intravenous L-carnitine should be administered with a loading dose of 100 mg/kg, followed by infusions of 50 mg/kg every 8 hours, until ammonia levels are decreasing.

The low molecular weight and $V_D$ of VPA are favorable for extracorporeal elimination. Although IHD has little effect on the elimination of VPA at usual serum concentrations because of its extensive protein binding, significant clearance can be obtained at supratherapeutic drug concentrations when binding to plasma proteins is saturated.[209,217] IHD has the added advantage of clearing ammonia and reversing metabolic acidosis.[209]

Indications for ECTR include any of the following attributable to valproate toxicity[14]:

- Serum valproate concentration > 900 mg/L (6250 μmol/L)
- Cerebral edema or shock
- Coma or respiratory depression requiring mechanical ventilation
- Acute hyperammonemia
- pH ≤ 7.10

Rebound of VPA concentrations is often observed 5 to 13 hours following cessation of high-flux IHD, requiring additional sessions.[210] Charcoal HP has been successfully used in some cases but is limited by early column saturation.[207] Tandem, or IHD-HP in series, may be the most effective technique but probably offers only a marginal advantage over IHD to offset the added cost and potential complications of the technique.[218] Intermittent HDF has been used successfully in two reports,[219,220] but there is insufficient evidence to determine whether this technique offers additional benefit over IHD alone. CRRT appears considerably less effective than intermittent alternatives and should only be used if IHD is unavailable.[14,221] Albumin dialysis, slow low-efficiency dialysis with filtration, TPE, and PD are inferior therapeutic options in valproate poisoning and have not been recommended.[222,223]

## CARBAMAZEPINE

Carbamazepine is a widely used anticonvulsant agent that is also being used increasingly for pain management and mood disorders.

### TOXICOLOGY AND TOXICOKINETICS

Carbamazepine (molecular weight, 236 Da) and tricyclic antidepressants have a similar chemical structure. Its therapeutic effect results from binding to sodium channels, inhibiting neuronal depolarization, and decreasing glutamate release. It also has anticholinergic effects at high concentrations.

Carbamazepine is available in immediate- and modified-release formulations and is characterized by erratic and incomplete absorption, which is exacerbated in overdose due to pharmacobezoar formation and ileus secondary to its anticholinergic properties.[224] It is lipophilic and has a $V_D$ of 1.2 L/kg and a protein binding of approximately 75%, which does not decrease much in overdose.[225] It undergoes hepatic metabolism, mainly through CYP450 3A4 into many metabolites, the most important being carbamazepine-10,11-epoxide, which is pharmacologically active. Carbamazepine induces its own metabolism, which increases endogenous clearance with chronic use. The therapeutic concentration range of carbamazepine is 4 to 12 mg/L (16.9–50.8 μmol/L).

### CLINICAL PRESENTATION AND DIAGNOSTIC TESTING

Carbamazepine toxicity frequently presents with neurologic, cardiovascular, and anticholinergic symptoms, which may be delayed in onset because of its erratic absorption. Mild toxicity (≅ 30 mg/L [127 μmol/L]) presents as drowsiness, nystagmus, tachycardia, hyperreflexia, or dysmetria. In more severe exposures (>40 mg/L [169 μmol/L]), lethargy, seizure, coma, QRS prolongation, hypotension, and pronounced anticholinergic symptoms (especially ileus) may develop; death is unusual. Agranulocytosis and syndrome of inappropriate antidiuretic hormone (SIADH) are associated with chronic use and are not typically seen in acute poisonings.

The diagnosis of carbamazepine toxicity relies on the history and presence of typical clinical findings and is confirmed by laboratory testing. Serial measurements of serum carbamazepine concentrations are required because the time to peak concentration may be significantly delayed, including beyond 24 hours. Concentrations should be obtained every 4 to 6 hours until a definite downward trend is seen.

### TREATMENT

Most patients poisoned with carbamazepine can be managed with supportive care alone, including fluids, ventilatory support, benzodiazepines for seizure control, vasopressors for hypotension, and sodium bicarbonate for sodium channel blockade. Gastrointestinal decontamination is administered, even if the patient presents late after ingestion due to the prolonged absorption phase, but is contraindicated if ileus is present. No antidote exists to reverse carbamazepine's toxicity. MDAC can enhance carbamazepine clearance and may even reduce the duration of coma and need for mechanical ventilation[5,226] but, again, is contraindicated in the presence of ileus.[5,226–229]

Severe carbamazepine poisonings can be treated using ECTR, which can provide better and more predictable clearance than MDAC, particularly when there is an ileus.[230–232] Historically, charcoal or resin HP was the ECTR of choice because of carbamazepine's extensive protein binding. However, with high-flux filters, high blood flows, and larger catheters, carbamazepine clearance with HP and IHD are comparable, exceeding 100 mL/min.[231–239] IHD is preferred due to its greater availability, lower cost, and lower complication rate compared with HP. There are limited data on the ECTR clearance of the toxic metabolite carbamazepine-10-11-epoxide, but it also appears to be dialyzable—its protein binding is less than that of carbamazepine (50% vs. 75%–90%).[225,236,240,241] CRRT, TPE, and albumin dialysis have been used in carbamazepine poisoning but do not provide comparable removal rates.[242,243]

Indications for ECTR include any of the following attributable to carbamazepine toxicity[11]:

- Prolonged coma
- Seizures, cardiovascular instability, symptoms unresponsive to supportive care
- Rising concentrations despite MDAC
- Serum carbamazepine concentration > 45 mg/L (190 μmol/L)

## BARBITURATES

Barbiturates are CNS-depressants used as sedatives, hypnotics, anxiolytics, and anticonvulsants. Barbiturates were extremely popular until the availability of benzodiazepines in the 1960s. Although their use has steadily decreased over the years, barbiturates, especially those that are long-acting agents, are still a concern.[1] Phenobarbital is the most commonly available barbiturate worldwide and is most often implicated in poisoning, although others are seen in developing countries.[244]

## TOXICOLOGY AND TOXICOKINETICS

Most barbiturates are weak acids, with a $pK_a$ of approximately 7. Their two principal mechanisms of action are potentiating the effect of the gamma-aminobutyric acid (GABA) receptor and blocking the α-amino-3-hydroxy-5-methyl-4-isoxazolepropionic acid (AMPA) receptor (a subtype of glutamate receptor); both contribute to the CNS effects.[245] They are usually categorized by their duration of action: short (>3–4 hours; pentobarbital, secobarbital), intermediate (>4–6 hours; amobarbital, butabarbital), or long-acting (≥6–12 hours; barbital, primidone, phenobarbital).[244] Absorption is variable and is influenced by the dose ingested, presence of an ileus, and concomitant ingestion of other drugs. The ability of a particular barbiturate to penetrate the blood-brain barrier reflects its lipophilicity and determines its clinical effects. Barbiturates are small molecules with a protein binding usually below 50%, although long-acting barbiturates are less protein-bound than short-acting ones. The metabolism of barbiturates is mostly hepatic, but there may be renal excretion for those that are less lipophilic, such as phenobarbital. There may be enzymatic induction and higher barbiturate clearance for patients on chronic therapy.

The following discussion focuses on phenobarbital because it is the most commonly encountered, although it shares properties similar to other long-acting and short-acting barbiturates. Recommendations also apply to primidone because it is metabolized to phenobarbital.[246] An oral dose of 1 g of most barbiturates will cause serious toxicity in most adults, whereas death can result with ingestions of more than 2 g[247] or with a concentration higher than 80 mg/L (345 μmol/L)[248] in the absence of supportive care.

## CLINICAL PRESENTATION AND DIAGNOSTIC TESTING

Phenobarbital has clinical effects that are prolonged.[249,250] In mild exposures, toxicity usually manifests as an altered level of consciousness. Moderate poisonings will produce apnea and hypotension. More severe cases present with areflexia, cutaneous bullae, circulatory collapse (although more common with short-acting barbiturates), hypothermia, and coma.[244,247] Concomitant AKI, cardiac, or pulmonary disease may increase the clinical sensitivity to barbiturates.[251] Early deaths after barbiturate ingestion are caused by respiratory and cardiovascular collapse, whereas delayed deaths are caused by acute lung injury, ventilator-acquired pneumonia, cerebral edema, or multiorgan system failure. Specific serum testing assays of barbiturates other than phenobarbital are not widely available.

## TREATMENT

Supportive measures, including rewarming, hydration, and vasopressors, are usually sufficient in most cases of barbiturate poisoning. Patients may be profoundly comatose and require prolonged mechanical ventilation. There is no antidote for barbiturates.

If an airway is secured, MDAC can facilitate the clearance of phenobarbital.[252] Because barbiturates are weak acids, urinary alkalinization can also increase phenobarbital renal clearance by at least two- to threefold.[253,254] However, because renal clearance of phenobarbital is already low (<3 mL/min), alkalinization would have little effect on total body clearance.[253] MDAC has a greater impact on clearance than alkalinization.[254,255] Surprisingly, the duration of coma was shown to be reduced by urine alkalinization in one study[256] but not by MDAC in a small randomized trial despite a decreased half-life.[257] Another controlled study has suggested that MDAC alone is superior to either urinary alkalinization alone or MDAC plus urinary alkalinization.[255] Therefore, MDAC is preferred to urine alkalinization in the absence of ileus.[5,6,244]

An animal study has shown a very significant and clear decrease in mortality in dogs and rats that underwent HP after a lethal phenobarbital infusion[164] compared with those who did not. No randomized studies have evaluated the effect of ECTR in humans, although the mortality rate appeared lower in an uncontrolled group that underwent HP.[258] HP and IHD are particularly appealing treatments for toxicity from long-acting barbiturates because the endogenous clearance is low, especially in patients who are naïve to barbiturates.[244] The endogenous elimination half-life for barbiturates other than phenobarbital, barbital, and primidone is short and therefore less likely to benefit from extracorporeal removal. Modern high-flux dialyzers provide clearances at least equal to those of HP.

Indications for ECTR include any of the following (in particular for phenobarbital poisoning)[244]:

- Coma with respiratory depression
- Hypotension not responding to vasopressors
- Inefficiency of MDAC at reducing serum concentrations

A caution with the treatment of barbiturate poisoning is the risk of precipitating barbiturate withdrawal in chronic users. This occurs when concentrations fall below the therapeutic range and can manifest as seizures and/or persistent delirium after approximately 48 to 72 hours of treatment.[70,259–261] This can be minimized by stopping ECTR and other treatments when the phenobarbital concentration is therapeutic; ongoing monitoring can promptly detect rebound toxicity or withdrawal, especially for short-acting barbiturates and chronic users. In the case of phenobarbital, it may also be prudent to reinitiate barbiturate treatment when the serum concentration is therapeutic and clinical recovery has been observed.

# PHENYTOIN

Phenytoin is used as a first-line treatment of epilepsy, both for status epilepticus and seizure prevention. Phenytoin toxicity is relatively frequent considering its narrow therapeutic range, although phenytoin-related deaths are rare.

## TOXICOLOGY AND TOXICOKINETICS

Phenytoin stabilizes neuronal membranes and decreases seizure activity, possibly by producing a voltage-dependent blockade of membrane sodium channels implicated in the action potential leading to seizures.[262] Phenytoin has a molecular weight of 252 Da and high protein binding (90%–95%), which decreases to 70% in the presence of renal failure or hypoalbuminemia, although surprisingly remains almost unchanged in overdose. Only the unbound fraction of phenytoin has a biologic effect.

Phenytoin is available in various dosing forms and has erratic oral bioavailability,[263] especially in overdose.[264] Phenytoin is metabolized predominantly by hepatic hydroxylation through CYP2C9 and is then eliminated in the bile as an inactive metabolite, reabsorbed from the intestinal tract and excreted in urine. Elimination is first-order at low serum concentrations but becomes zero-order (saturable) at higher concentrations, but within the reference range. The elimination half-life of oral preparations ranges from 14 to 22 hours. Therapeutic serum concentrations range between 10 and 20 mg/L (40–80 μmol/L). The lethal dose in adults is estimated at 2 to 5 g.

### CLINICAL PRESENTATION AND DIAGNOSTIC TESTING

Most of the toxic manifestations of phenytoin are neurologic; their severity is loosely correlated to its serum concentration; between 20 and 40 mg/L (80–160 μmol/L), symptoms include nystagmus, ataxia, dysarthria, and mild CNS depression.[265] Over 40 mg/L (160 μmol/L), lethargy, confusion, hypotension, coma, and seizures may be observed. Death is usually caused by respiratory or circulatory depression but is rare. Cardiovascular toxicity is unusual with oral formulations, but short-lived atrioventricular delays and bradycardia may be occasionally seen with rapid intravenous infusion.[265]

Total serum phenytoin concentrations should be determined in all suspected overdose cases. Some conditions may alter the protein-binding capacity, such as uremia, extremes of age, and concomitant use of agents that displace phenytoin from its albumin binding site (e.g., salicylates, sulfonamides, tolbutamide, VPA). The free phenytoin concentration can be determined in such cases and, in the context of hypoalbuminemia, can assist with interpretation; toxicity is apparent when its free level is more than 2.1 mg/L (8.3 μmol/L).[266]

### TREATMENT

Treatment of phenytoin poisoning is primarily supportive because most patients have an excellent outcome, although the duration of admission can be prolonged. Benzodiazepines can be given for seizures. Gastrointestinal decontamination can reduce the severity of toxicity and limit the systemic burden of phenytoin, MDAC significantly reduces the elimination half-life of phenytoin in healthy and poisoned patients[22,267,268] and is commonly used, particularly in patients in whom serum phenytoin concentrations are increasing or remain elevated.[5] There is no specific antidote for phenytoin poisoning.

Experience with ECTRs remains anecdotal and limited. In theory, given the high protein binding of phenytoin, HP or TPE has been historically favored, and they both has been used successfully in this context.[269–275] Surprisingly, despite phenytoin's high protein binding, there is some evidence that IHD may also enhance its elimination, perhaps due to its low binding constant to albumin, which ensures a constant pool of freely diffusible unbound phenytoin.[276–278] This finding is attributable to newer high-flux, high-efficiency dialyzers—older obsolete dialysis apparatus did not have any effect on phenytoin clearance.[279]

The combination of HP and IHD could potentially maximize clearance and has been used in a few studies,[274,280,281] although it remains unclear if the combination is superior to either technique used alone. Neither peritoneal dialysis nor CRRT has any role in phenytoin poisoning,[282–285] whereas the data are still uncertain for albumin dialysis.[59] In summary, the outcome of most phenytoin poisonings is favorable, although the duration of admission can be prolonged by many days. Supportive care alone is usually sufficient. In the case of actual or anticipated (e.g., persistently elevated phenytoin concentration) prolonged neurologic toxicity, IHD or HP can be considered.[18]

## METFORMIN

Metformin is a first-line drug for the treatment of non–insulin-dependent diabetes, particularly in overweight patients. Metformin improves insulin sensitivity in patients and is now the most popular antidiabetic drug in the world. The related biguanide, phenformin, was withdrawn in 1978 because of the high incidence of severe lactic acidosis.

### TOXICOLOGY AND TOXICOKINETICS

Metformin is a small unbound molecule (165 Da) that has a large volume of distribution (3 L/kg) due to its ability to diffuse into the intracellular compartment and bind to microsomes. Its bioavailability is incomplete. It does not undergo hepatic metabolism and is eliminated unchanged by renal tubular secretion (renal clearance ≅ 500 mL/min with normal renal function); hence, caution is required when prescribing it to patients with kidney impairment. The toxic dose in acute ingestions is not well established but is likely to exceed 100 mg/kg.

### CLINICAL PRESENTATION AND DIAGNOSTIC TESTING

Metformin toxicity can manifest in various ways—gastrointestinal symptoms (e.g., abdominal pain, diarrhea, nausea, vomiting), lactic acidosis, and hypotension are all hallmarks of metformin intoxication. Hypoglycemia, hypothermia, altered mental status, and acute pancreatitis have also been reported.[286,287] Metformin-associated lactic acidosis (MALA) usually occurs in the presence of underlying conditions, particularly AKI or CKD. MALA is defined as an arterial pH ≤ 7.35 and lactate concentration > 45 mg/dL (5 mmol/L)[288,289]; it can result from acute or chronic poisoning. There is controversy in regard to the association between metformin and lactic acidosis; some sources have claimed that the association is coincidental and due to other factors, such as sepsis and heart failure,[290,291] whereas others have suggested that metformin itself directly causes lactic acidosis.[292] The finding of asymptomatic patients who develop toxicity shortly after an acute toxic ingestion of metformin appears to give credence to the latter hypothesis[293–295] and is occasionally named "metformin-induced lactic acidosis" (MILA).[292] The true prevalence of MALA and MILA is unknown, but severe life-threatening acidosis is estimated at a rate of 0.05 cases/1000 patient-years.[296]

The physiopathology of MALA is not entirely understood but seems to be related to interference with hepatic gluconeogenesis and impaired lactate utilization. Metformin also binds to mitochondrial membranes, which in overdose can shift energy utilization toward anaerobic metabolism, leading to the production of lactate.[297] The increase in lactic acid production is then compounded by the defect in lactate clearance by the kidneys or liver (mentioned earlier).

Because serum metformin measurements are not usually available in a clinically useful time frame, the diagnosis must be suspected in every patient taking metformin who presents with severe lactic acidosis. Some studies have reported a correlation between metformin concentrations and markers of lactic acidosis,[290,292,298] but not all.[299] A range of factors may influence the relationship between metformin concentrations and clinical outcomes, which have been discussed elsewhere.[292,300]

### TREATMENT

Given the absence of a specific antidote to metformin, the management of metformin toxicity is supportive care—normalizing the acid–base status, reducing the metformin concentration, and treating concomitant and exacerbating conditions. Decontamination with activated charcoal should be considered after an acute large ingestion of metformin in patients presenting within 1 to 2 hours of ingestion. Patients who develop lactic acidosis, hypoglycemia, or other signs of metformin toxicity should be admitted to an intensive care unit to facilitate treatment.

Severely acidotic patients (pH ≤ 7.1) should receive intravenous sodium bicarbonate, although treatment can be limited by hypernatremia and volume overload. ECTRs have a definite role in the treatment of MALA because they can correct acidosis faster than intravenous bicarbonate, contribute to the clearance of lactate and metformin, and treat volume overload and uremia. A dramatic improvement from ECTR has been described in some acutely poisoned patients soon after dialysis initiation, suggesting that the benefit might be more attributable to pH correction than metformin removal.[301] One study compared patients who underwent dialysis with those who did not, and the mortality rate did not differ between the two groups. However, the IHD group was sicker at baseline.[288] There is some evidence that ECTRs can remove a significant amount of metformin, especially when kidney function is impaired,[302–304] and also because metformin distributes to a smaller apparent $V_D$ in AKI; thus it is more available for extracorporeal removal. In terms of case reports of ECTR in the treatment of poisoning, metformin is the leading intoxication reported in the recent literature.[305]

Indications for ECTR include any of the following attributable to metformin toxicity[19]:

- Lactate concentration > 180 mg/dL (20 mmol/L)
- Arterial pH ≤ 7.1
- Failure of supportive therapy in severe MALA
- The presence of shock, impaired kidney function, or coma

IHD is preferred over CRRT due to higher metformin and lactate clearances[19,74,306]—for example, lactate removal is greater following 6 hours of IHD compared with 24 hours of CVVHDF,[307] although it is likely that lactate removal by ECTR is much less than that by physiologic processes that are functioning normally.[308] Endpoints for ECTR cessation include normalization of blood pH and lactate level. Shortened sessions can result in a marked rebound in lactic acidosis,[309] which may possibly be reduced by using IHD initially, followed by CRRT.[310] HP is not recommended for treatment of MALA without IHD because it will not correct acid-base abnormalities.[310]

## PARAQUAT

Paraquat (1,1′-dimethyl-4-4′-bipyridylium dichloride) is a cheap, nonselective, fast-acting herbicide that is inactivated on contact with soil, which reduces environmental contamination. Because it is not readily absorbed across intact skin, and because the droplets generated from the aerosol spray are large, toxicity from direct contact or inhalation is rare. However, accidental or intentional oral ingestion of paraquat is extremely toxic, with high rates of morbidity and mortality (50%–90%). Its use and access are restricted in many parts of the world due to its high toxicity, but it is available in many developing countries.[311]

### TOXICOLOGY AND TOXICOKINETICS

Paraquat (molecular weight, 186 Da; protein binding, 5%) has an oral bioavailability that is less than 30%. Peak concentrations are generally reached 2 hours after ingestion, but maximal tissue distribution occurs during the next 6 hours.[312,313] Paraquat distributes to most organs, especially the lungs, kidneys, and liver, with a $V_D \cong 1.0$ L/kg. It is predominantly excreted by the kidneys, so that the elimination half-life is 12 hours with normal renal function, but it can increase to more than 48 hours with impaired renal function.[313,314]

Paraquat is directly toxic to mucosal membranes, causing corrosion and esophageal perforation. Paraquat catalyzes the formation of reactive oxygen species (ROS), in particular superoxide radicals, through redox cycling. Because this process can be sustained by the extensive supply of electrons and oxygen in the lungs, the resultant oxidative stress causes extensive cell injury and necrosis and a secondary inflammatory reaction.[312,315,316]

### CLINICAL PRESENTATION AND DIAGNOSTIC TESTING

The presentation and clinical course of paraquat poisoning depend largely on the dose ingested and timing of presentation to a health care facility after exposure. Ingestions < 20 mg/kg may not cause symptoms other than oral ulceration, vomiting, and diarrhea. Ingestions between 20 and 40 mg/kg will usually cause multiple organ failure, with death occurring between 1 and several weeks postexposure. Patients who ingest over 40 mg/kg usually die within 3 days from accelerated multiorgan failure and/or from the corrosive effects of paraquat.[317–320]

Most paraquat-related deaths are caused by respiratory failure. Types I and II alveolar epithelial cells take up paraquat via an energy-dependent polyamine transporter.[312,321] Patients develop an acute respiratory distress syndrome (ARDS)–like presentation, which ultimately progresses to irreversible pulmonary fibrosis. In the kidneys, paraquat causes acute tubular necrosis, which may be severe, but will resolve if the patient survives the acute phase of poisoning.[322,323] Other clinical manifestations include severe upper gastrointestinal tract ulcerations, hepatic injury, and shock. Paraquat does not readily cross the blood-brain barrier, and therefore does not typically cause CNS effects; seizures are rarely reported.

Serum paraquat concentration predicts the mortality risk, and nomograms have been validated to correlate with clinical outcome.[324–326] Unfortunately, few laboratories have the ability to perform a quantitative paraquat assay.[326–329] A rapid and inexpensive qualitative test for urine paraquat can be performed by adding sodium dithionite to urine. If the color of urine changes from yellow to blue, it confirms the presence of recent paraquat exposure (the more intense the blue, the higher the paraquat exposure).

### TREATMENT

Any suspected paraquat exposure warrants prompt assessment and aggressive management. After initial stabilization, volume resuscitation should be provided. Oxygen should be used only if required for hypoxemic patients because it may promote cellular toxicity from paraquat but, in such patients, the prognosis is likely to be very poor. Paraquat is absorbed quickly, which limits the efficacy of the usual decontamination techniques, although activated charcoal should be administered for presentations within 1 hour of ingestion; paraquat-induced caustic injury is not usually noted for many hours postingestion. Many paraquat formulations already contain a proemetic, and some contain an alginate to reduce absorption.[330] Forced diuresis does not increase the renal clearance of paraquat,[314] and no specific antidote is available.

Because paraquat is a small molecule, unbound to protein, and with a reasonably small volume of distribution, its content in plasma is removable by standard ECTRs (clearance > 120 mL/min). However, paraquat distributes quickly to tissues, especially to the lungs, where it is trapped and accumulates. Furthermore, once the toxic process of free-radical generation is established, it is unlikely that any elimination enhancement could lessen its progression. This concept has been confirmed in animal studies; 50% of the dogs exposed to a lethal dose of paraquat survived with HP when it was initiated 2 hours after exposure, whereas 100% mortality occurred when it was initiated at 12 hours.[331]

IHD or HP is mostly reserved for patients presenting early after ingestion, especially within 4 hours.[332] In that scenario, all resources should be pooled to initiate ECTR as quickly as possible.[333] Other ECTRs, including peritoneal dialysis, are of no use.[314] Rebound is usually observed following ECTR treatment.[314,334–339]

The poor prognosis related to paraquat poisoning has prompted the use of several experimental treatments, largely based on immunosuppression, or other types of antiinflammatories. Unfortunately, none has been proven to alter clinical outcomes significantly. Examples include vitamins C and E, superoxide dismutase, deferoxamine, selenium, niacin, *N*-acetylcysteine, thiosulfate, salicylate, corticosteroids, cyclophosphamide, and radiotherapy.

Of note, the combination of cyclophosphamide and corticosteroids failed to identify a statistically significant benefit,[340] although high-dose corticosteroids remain recommended. The palliative care team should also be integrated into the treatment plan early, given the disastrous outcome of most patients.

## THEOPHYLLINE

Theophylline is a methylxanthine bronchodilator used in the treatment of asthma, chronic obstructive pulmonary disease, and infant apnea. Its use has largely declined over the years in favor of inhaled corticosteroids, anticholinergics, and $\beta_2$-adrenergic agonists.[341]

### TOXICOLOGY AND TOXICOKINETICS

Theophylline (molecular weight, 180.2 Da; protein binding, 40%) acts as a nonselective inhibitor of phosphodiesterase and a nonselective antagonist of the adenosine receptor. This results in smooth muscle relaxation, catecholamine release, bronchodilation, peripheral vasodilatation, and inotropic and chronotropic activation.[342]

Theophylline is available in immediate- and slow-release formulations and is completely absorbed by the gastrointestinal tract. It distributes in a volume smaller than that of water (0.5 L/kg). Theophylline is predominantly metabolized in the liver by CYP1A2, and only 10% is excreted by the kidneys. Endogenous metabolism is generally slow, but the pharmacokinetics and metabolism of theophylline are influenced by age, gender, body weight, concurrent illness (e.g., congestive heart failure, liver disease, infection), cigarette smoking (increases clearance), and medications known to induce or inhibit the CYP1A2 isozyme.[343] At the therapeutic range (10–20 mg/L [55–110 μmol/L]), theophylline exhibits first-order kinetics; however, at toxic concentrations, the kinetics change to zero order, and a small increase in dosage can lead to a dramatic increase in serum concentration.[344]

### CLINICAL PRESENTATION AND DIAGNOSTIC TESTING

Theophylline intoxication may result from acute ingestion (e.g., deliberate self-poisoning or medication error) or chronic use (e.g., prescribing or dispensing error; decrease in clearance from a drug interaction, smoking cessation, or intercurrent illness). The distinction is important because for the same serum theophylline concentration, symptoms are more severe from chronic toxicity than those following acute intoxication.[345] The therapeutic index is very narrow; even at therapeutic concentrations, nearly one-third of patients may exhibit signs of mild intoxication. Patients are likely to demonstrate toxicity at serum concentrations > 30 mg/L (167 μmol/L), and severe toxicity is likely when it is >90 mg/L (500 μmol/L). Caffeine, which is an active metabolite of theophylline, shares many of its toxic effects.

Early symptoms of toxicity consist of transient caffeine-like effects, such as nausea, vomiting, diarrhea, irritability, tremor, headache, insomnia, and tachycardia. Patients with moderate intoxication may be lethargic and disoriented and may develop supraventricular tachycardia and frequent premature ventricular contractions. Severe intoxication is potentially life-threatening and includes symptoms such as seizures, hyperthermia, hypotension, ventricular tachycardia, rhabdomyolysis, and AKI. Irreversible brain injury may follow seizures if they are not prevented or treated rapidly. Death most often results from cardiorespiratory collapse or hypoxic encephalopathy following cardiac dysrhythmias or generalized seizures.[345–347] Hypokalemia, caused by $\beta_2$-adrenergic–induced transcellular potassium shifts, can be severe and is most often seen following acute overdose.[346,348]

### TREATMENT

Aggressive supportive measures are required for severe theophylline poisoning. Hypotension usually responds to volume repletion and vasopressors. Tachydysrhythmias can be corrected by β-adrenergic antagonists, such as propranolol or esmolol, but should be used with caution in patients susceptible to bronchospasm.[349,350] Theophylline-associated seizures can be particularly difficult to control; benzodiazepines are first-line therapy, but propofol, barbiturates, and even neuromuscular paralysis may be required in refractory cases, at which point the prognosis is poor. MDAC increases the clearance of theophylline but is sometimes limited by profound and intractable emesis in severely intoxicated patients.[351–353] Intubation and ventilation can be performed for the purpose of preventing vomiting to enable MDAC treatment.

Because of its low molecular weight, low protein binding, low endogenous clearance, and low $V_D$, theophylline is an ideal candidate for extracorporeal elimination. Extracorporeal clearances can surpass 150 mL/min.[354–356] There are numerous reports of successful treatment with HP and IHD. In one observational retrospective cohort study, a group treated with HP or IHD had a significantly shorter duration of clinical toxicity compared with a group managed with supportive care only, despite being sicker at presentation.[357] IHD was shown to provide similar clearance to HP, with fewer complications in one retrospective study[42] and, because it also corrects hypokalemia, IHD is the preferred treatment.

Continuous techniques have also been reported in the management of theophylline intoxication with acceptable results, despite their inferior clearances.[358,359] Peritoneal dialysis and TPE are not useful alternatives. Exchange transfusion is an option for neonates.[360]

Indications for ECTR include any of the following attributable to theophylline toxicity[13]:

- Clinical deterioration despite optimal therapy
- Serum theophylline concentration > 100 mg/L (555 μmol/L)
- Chronic poisoning with serum theophylline concentration > 60 mg/L (333 μmol/L)
- The presence of refractory seizures, shock, life-threatening dysrhythmias, inability to administer charcoal because of intractable vomiting, or extremes of age (<6 months or >60 years)
- A rising serum theophylline concentration despite optimal therapy, or if MDAC cannot be administered

The ECTR should be continued until clinical improvement is achieved, and the serum concentration is less than 15 μg/mL (83 μmol/L). Rebound is usually minor but should be monitored after ECTR in case there is also ongoing absorption.

## ACETAMINOPHEN

Acetaminophen (*N*-acetyl-*p*-aminophenol, also known as paracetamol) is an analgesic and antipyretic available without prescription in various forms and combinations. Acetaminophen is a major cause of deliberate self-poisoning.

### TOXICOLOGY AND TOXICOKINETICS

The actions of acetaminophen remain poorly defined, but may include the inhibition of COX in the brain. Analgesic and antipyretic activity occurs at serum acetaminophen concentrations between 10 and 20 mg/L (66–132 μmol/L).[361] Acetaminophen is available in immediate- and extended-release preparations and has high oral bioavailability. Serum concentrations usually peak within 4 hours of ingestion, but may be delayed by many hours with massive overdoses or from sustained-release formulations.

Protein binding (≅20%) and volume of distribution (0.8 L/kg) of acetaminophen are small and not known to change in overdose. Acetaminophen undergoes extensive hepatic metabolism, in which 90% is conjugated to inactive metabolites and the remainder is oxidized, mostly by CYP2E1 to *N*-acetyl-*p*-benzoquinoneimine (NAPQI). Glutathione combines with NAPQI to form a nontoxic complex that is eliminated in the urine. In overdose, however, there is an accumulation in NAPQI and glutathione depletion, allowing NAPQI to bind covalently to proteins in hepatocytes, inducing injury and liver cell necrosis.[362] The lowest toxic dose following acute poisoning is 10 g in a single dosing over 8 hours.[363]

### CLINICAL PRESENTATION AND DIAGNOSTIC TESTING

Acetaminophen poisoning cases are difficult to recognize at the early stages. Patients may experience nonspecific symptoms, including nausea, vomiting, anorexia, malaise, or abdominal pain, in the first 24 hours. Hepatic injury, according to an increase in transaminase levels, typically occurs 12 to 24 hours after ingestion, by which time the efficacy of *N*-acetylcysteine is reduced. The severity of hepatotoxicity varies with acetaminophen dose, nutrition, and other medical conditions and is usually detected by an elevation in serum transaminase levels (aspartate aminotransferase [AST] and alanine transaminase [ALT]), which peak 2 to 3 days after ingestion in mild to moderate poisoning but later in severe hepatotoxicity. Hepatotoxicity is defined as a peak AST above 1000 IU/L.[364] More severe cases can evolve to fulminant liver failure with encephalopathy, coagulopathy, hypoglycemia, and death for those who cannot undergo liver transplantation. AKI may also occur because of tubular susceptibility to NAPQI by various possible mechanisms, which include the CYP450 pathway, as well as prostaglandin synthetase and *N*-deacetylase enzymes.[365] AKI can persist beyond the duration of hepatotoxicity but generally recovers after 1 to 3 months.

The assessment of the risk associated with acute acetaminophen poisoning can be largely estimated by timing the exposure to a serum acetaminophen concentration using the Rumack-Matthew nomogram (or a locally applicable version).[366] A point below the treatment line indicates that the patient has a low risk of developing hepatotoxicity. This nomogram has been validated, despite some limitations (which are outside the scope of this chapter). For example, a serum acetaminophen concentration of 150 mg/L (1000 μmol/L) at 4 hours postingestion indicates the need for *N*-acetylcysteine (NAC) treatment.

### TREATMENT

A comprehensive management of acetaminophen toxicity is reviewed elsewhere.[367] Most cases are triaged and treated in the emergency department in collaboration with the regional poison control center and intensivists, without the involvement of a nephrologist. Management of acetaminophen toxicity is mainly focused on decontamination for early presentations and timely administration of the antidote, NAC.[368] NAC serves as a glutathione donor, increasing the capacity to detoxify NAPQI.[369] It is most efficacious when initiated within 8 hours of an acute overdose but is also useful if initiated later. NAC is prescribed if there is evidence of hepatic injury following a history of known or possible acetaminophen poisoning or if the acetaminophen concentration is above the treatment line on the Rumack-Matthew nomogram.

Although acetaminophen is amenable to extracorporeal removal (low $V_D$, small molecule, low protein binding), ECTR is rarely necessary, given the safety, low cost, efficacy, and availability of NAC. IHD or CRRT can be considered for patients with severe AKI according to the usual criteria or occasionally in those presenting following massive ingestions with a pattern of mitochondrial toxicity—coma, lactic metabolic acidosis, and/or cardiovascular instability.[8,370,371] These patients can be identified by early onset of these signs in the context of a massive exposure, as opposed to the features of hepatotoxicity due to the delayed presentation, as described earlier. In these cases, the potential risk of ECTR removing NAC and compromising its effect can be overcome by at least doubling its rate of infusion (some sources have suggested that an increased dose of NAC is required with massive acetaminophen poisoning anyway).[69,372] Liver replacement therapies such as the molecular adsorbents recirculating system (MARS) and single-pass albumin dialysis (SPAD) have been used for liver support as bridges to liver transplantation or pending native liver recovery.[373–377] However, limited availability of these techniques, as well as major bleeding complications associated with them and their high cost,warrant further investigation.

## METHOTREXATE

Methotrexate is a folate analog used to treat a variety of cancers and rheumatologic and dermatologic diseases. Methotrexate inhibits dihydrofolate reductase, an enzyme necessary for the synthesis and replication of RNA and DNA.

### TOXICOLOGY AND TOXICOKINETICS

The oral absorption of methotrexate is limited by a saturable intestinal absorption mechanism for doses over 30 mg/m$^2$. Recent research has suggested that a single acute oral ingestion of methotrexate is unlikely to have any toxic potential in patients with normal renal function.[378]

Methotrexate toxicity is most often related to dosing errors with parenteral administration or repeated supratherapeutic chronic dosing. Methotrexate (molecular weight, 454 Da) has a small $V_D$ (0.4–0.8 L/kg) and is 50% bound to plasma proteins, regardless of serum concentration. Methotrexate is primarily excreted unchanged (80%–90%) in the urine by passive glomerular filtration and active tubular secretion; its renal clearance varies greatly and decreases at higher doses. It also undergoes hepatic and intracellular metabolism into active metabolites.

In the presence of renal failure, methotrexate can rapidly accumulate in the serum and tissue cells. A toxic concentration of methotrexate is defined as greater than 5 to 10 μmol/L at 24 hours, 1 μmol/L at 48 hours, and 0.1 μmol/L at 72 hours.[379,380] These concentrations are predictive of renal, gastrointestinal, mucosal, and bone marrow toxicity in patients receiving chemotherapy. Methotrexate concentrations in patients being treated for indications other than cancer should not surpass 0.01 μmol/L.[381]

### CLINICAL PRESENTATION AND DIAGNOSTIC TESTING

At high concentrations, methotrexate and its metabolites can precipitate in renal tubules, causing crystal nephropathy and AKI. Methotrexate can also cause bone marrow suppression, mucositis and stomatitis, liver damage, and neurotoxicity. The onset of the toxicity is generally rapid; nausea and vomiting typically begin 2 to 4 hours after high-dose therapy (>1000 mg/m$^2$). CNS toxicity usually follows approximately 12 hours after high-dose intravenous methotrexate therapy or intrathecal administration. Mucositis and pancytopenia will manifest approximately 1 to 2 weeks after exposure.

### TREATMENT

Activated charcoal may be given early after presentation after an acute oral overdose, although toxicity in this scenario is unusual if kidney function is normal.[378] Aggressive hydration is indicated for patients presenting with methotrexate toxicity. Because methotrexate is a weak acid ($pK_a = 5$), and because it is eliminated largely unchanged in the urine, urinary alkalinization with intravenous sodium bicarbonate (target urine pH ≅ 8) will enhance methotrexate elimination and may help prevent AKI.[6,382]

Leucovorin (folinic acid, an active form of folate) can limit the bone marrow and gastrointestinal toxicity of methotrexate by bypassing the effects of methotrexate on dihydrofolate reductase. Leucovorin rescue is most beneficial when administered promptly after methotrexate exposure and should always be given to patients after a supratherapeutic exposure. Other supportive measures include transfusion of blood components for established cytopenias, antiemetics, and nutritional support for stomatitis. Dose recommendations and precise application are covered elsewhere.[383]

Glucarpidase (carboxypeptidase $G_2$; $CPDG_2$) is a recombinant bacterial enzyme that catabolizes methotrexate to inactive metabolites. It is used in combination with leucovorin because glucarpidase cannot access intracellular stores of methotrexate. It decreases the serum methotrexate concentration within 1 hour following administration. This FDA-approved antidote is used in patients with a serum methotrexate concentration > 1 μmol/L with prolonged methotrexate clearance (AKI) or under investigational protocol for intrathecal (IT) overdoses (100 mg IT methotrexate). Because it is expensive (>$50,000) and is unavailable or restricted in most countries, it may not be readily available for each case of methotrexate toxicity.

IT overdoses of methotrexate may require special measures, including cerebrospinal fluid drainage and exchange and administration of corticosteroids, in addition to leucovorin-glucarpidase. Methotrexate can be removed by extracorporeal treatments; high clearances can be achieved by various modalities, especially charcoal HP and high-flux IHD.[379] CRRT, as expected, provides lesser removal rates,[384] whereas PD and TPE are ineffective.[385–387] ECTR clearance is usually below endogenous clearance in patients with intact kidney function and is therefore most beneficial for patients with AKI. The indication for ECTR, especially with the arrival of glucarpidase, remains to be defined but may be related to cost and availability. ECTR seems to be indicated if serum methotrexate concentrations are above the following: 1600 to 2200 μmol/L at the end of infusion, 30 to 300 μmol/L at 24 hours, 3 to

30 μmol/L at 48 hours, and over 0.3 μmol/L at 72 hours. ECTR protocols are usually continued until methotrexate concentrations are less than 0.1 μmol/L.[388] Rebound in serum methotrexate concentrations, attributable to redistribution, often follows ECTR.

## OTHER FACTORS

There are other conditions and poisoning situations for which enhanced elimination using ECTR may reduce the duration of toxicity. Although we cannot present them in detail here, there have been reports of successful extracorporeal removal of the following poisons: aluminum,[389] *Amanita phalloides*,[390] baclofen,[391] barium,[392] bromate,[393] carambola,[394] cefepime,[395] cibenzoline,[396] dabigatran,[78,397,398] dapsone,[399] diethylene glycol,[400] fluoride,[401] gabapentin,[402] gentamicin,[403] isoniazid,[404] metronidazole,[405] pregabalin,[406] propylene glycol,[407] thallium,[7] and vancomycin.[408]

## CONCLUSION

General supportive care is sufficient to manage most poisoned patients. In a small selection of cases, extracorporeal blood purification, usually consisting of IHD, can help reduce the exposure of a patient to the toxic effects of a poison. An understanding of poison toxicokinetics can help a clinician discern the timely conditions and circumstances when ECTRs are most likely to be beneficial.

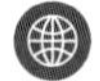 Complete reference list available at ExpertConsult.com.

## KEY REFERENCES

1. Mowry JB, Spyker DA, Brooks DE, et al. 2015 Annual report of the American Association of Poison Control Centers' National Poison Data System (NPDS): 33rd annual report. *Clin Toxicol (Phila)*. 2016;54(10):924–1109.
5. Vale J, Krenzelok EP, Barceloux VD. Position statement and practice guidelines on the use of multi-dose activated charcoal in the treatment of acute poisoning. American Academy of Clinical Toxicology; European Association of Poisons Centres and Clinical Toxicologists. *J Toxicol Clin Toxicol*. 1999;37(6):731–751.
6. Proudfoot AT, Krenzelok EP, Vale JA. Position paper on urine alkalinization. *J Toxicol Clin Toxicol*. 2004;42(1):1–26.
8. Gosselin S, Juurlink DN, Kielstein JT, et al. Extracorporeal treatment for acetaminophen poisoning: recommendations from the EXTRIP Workgroup. *Clin Toxicol (Phila)*. 2014;52(8):856–867.
9. Mactier R, Laliberte M, Mardini J, et al. Extracorporeal treatment for barbiturate poisoning: recommendations from the EXTRIP Workgroup. *Am J Kidney Dis*. 2014;64(3):347–358.
10. Yates C, Galvao T, Sowinski KM, et al. Extracorporeal treatment for tricyclic antidepressant poisoning: recommendations from the EXTRIP workgroup. *Semin Dial*. 2014;27(4):381–389.
11. Ghannoum M, Yates C, Galvao TF, et al. Extracorporeal treatment for carbamazepine poisoning: systematic review and recommendations from the EXTRIP workgroup. *Clin Toxicol (Phila)*. 2014;52(10):993–1004.
12. Decker BS, Goldfarb DS, Dargan PI, et al. Extracorporeal treatment for lithium poisoning: systematic review and recommendations from the EXTRIP Workgroup. *Clin J Am Soc Nephrol*. 2015;10(5):875–887.
13. Ghannoum M, Wiegand TJ, Liu KD, et al. Extracorporeal treatment for theophylline poisoning: systematic review and recommendations from the EXTRIP workgroup. *Clin Toxicol (Phila)*. 2015;53(4):215–229.
14. Ghannoum M, Laliberte M, Nolin TD, et al. Extracorporeal treatment for valproic acid poisoning: systematic review and recommendations from the EXTRIP workgroup. *Clin Toxicol (Phila)*. 2015;53(5):454–465.
15. Roberts DM, Yates C, Megarbane B, et al. Recommendations for the role of extracorporeal treatments in the management of acute methanol poisoning: a systematic review and consensus statement. *Crit Care Med*. 2015;43(2):461–472.
16. Juurlink DN, Gosselin S, Kielstein JT, et al. Extracorporeal treatment for salicylate poisoning: systematic review and recommendations from the EXTRIP Workgroup. *Ann Emerg Med*. 2015;66(2):165–181.
17. Mowry JB, Burdmann EA, Anseeuw K, et al. Extracorporeal treatment for digoxin poisoning: systematic review and recommendations from the EXTRIP Workgroup. *Clin Toxicol (Phila)*. 2016;54(2):103–114.
18. Anseeuw K, Mowry JB, Burdmann EA, et al. Extracorporeal treatment in phenytoin poisoning: systematic review and recommendations from the EXTRIP (Extracorporeal Treatments In Poisoning) Workgroup. *Am J Kidney Dis*. 2016;67(2):187–197.
19. Calello DP, Liu KD, Wiegand TJ, et al. Extracorporeal treatment for metformin poisoning: systematic review and recommendations from the Extracorporeal Treatments In Poisoning Workgroup. *Crit Care Med*. 2015;43(8):1716–1730.
22. Skinner CG, Chang AS, Matthews AS, et al. Randomized controlled study on the use of multiple-dose activated charcoal in patients with supratherapeutic phenytoin levels. *Clin Toxicol (Phila)*. 2012;50(8):764–769.
23. Ghannoum M, Lavergne V, Yue CS, et al. Successful treatment of lithium toxicity with sodium polystyrene sulfonate: a retrospective cohort study. *Clin Toxicol (Phila)*. 2010;48(1):34–41.
29. Schreiner GE. The role of hemodialysis (artificial kidney) in acute poisoning. *AMA Arch Intern Med*. 1958;102(6):896–913.
32. Lavergne V, Ouellet G, Bouchard J, et al. Guidelines for reporting case studies on extracorporeal treatments in poisonings: methodology. *Semin Dial*. 2014;27(4):407–414.
34. Ouellet G, Bouchard J, Ghannoum M, et al. Available extracorporeal treatments for poisoning: overview and limitations. *Semin Dial*. 2014;27(4):342–349.
35. Bouchard J, Roberts DM, Roy L, et al. Principles and operational parameters to optimize poison removal with extracorporeal treatments. *Semin Dial*. 2014;27(4):371–380.
36. Ghannoum M, Roberts DM, Hoffman RS, et al. A stepwise approach for the management of poisoning with extracorporeal treatments. *Semin Dial*. 2014;27(4):362–370.
37. Bouchard J, Lavergne V, Roberts DM, et al. Availability and cost of extracorporeal treatments for poisonings and other emergency indications: a worldwide survey. *Nephrol Dial Transplant*. 2017;32(4):699–706.
38. Ghannoum M, Bouchard J, Nolin TD, et al. Hemoperfusion for the treatment of poisoning: technology, determinants of poison clearance, and application in clinical practice. *Semin Dial*. 2014;27(4):350–361.
42. Shannon MW. Comparative efficacy of hemodialysis and hemoperfusion in severe theophylline intoxication. *Acad Emerg Med*. 1997;4(7):674–678.
45. Shalkham AS, Kirrane BM, Hoffman RS, et al. The availability and use of charcoal hemoperfusion in the treatment of poisoned patients. *Am J Kidney Dis*. 2006;48(2):239–241.
46. Ghannoum M, Lavergne V, Gosselin S, et al. Practice trends in the use of extracorporeal treatments for poisoning in four countries. *Semin Dial*. 2016;29(1):71–80.
57. Perino GC, Grivet V. Hemoperfusion and plasmapheresis complications. *Minerva Urol Nefrol*. 1987;39(2):161–163.
58. Dichtwald S, Dahan E, Adi N, et al. Molecular adsorbent recycling system therapy in the treatment of acute valproic acid intoxication. *Israel Medical Association Journal*. 2010;12(5):307–308.
65. Ghannoum M, Nolin TD, Lavergne V, et al. Blood purification in toxicology: nephrology's ugly duckling. *Adv Chronic Kidney Dis*. 2011;18(3):160–166.
66. Lavergne V, Nolin TD, Hoffman RS, et al. The EXTRIP (Extracorporeal Treatments In Poisoning) workgroup: guideline methodology. *Clin Toxicol*. 2012;50:403–413.
69. Ghannoum M, Kazim S, Grunbaum AM, et al. Massive acetaminophen overdose: effect of hemodialysis on acetaminophen and acetylcysteine kinetics. *Clin Toxicol (Phila)*. 2016;54(6):519–522.
71. Prabhu MV, Juneja D, Gopal PB, et al. Ultrasound-guided femoral dialysis access placement: a single-center randomized trial. *Clin J Am Soc Nephrol*. 2010;5(2):235–239.
73. Parienti JJ, Megarbane B, Fischer MO, et al. Catheter dysfunction and dialysis performance according to vascular access among 736

critically ill adults requiring renal replacement therapy: a randomized controlled study. *Crit Care Med.* 2010;38(4):1118–1125.
78. Bouchard J, Ghannoum M, Bernier-Jean A, et al. Comparison of intermittent and continuous extracorporeal treatments for the enhanced elimination of dabigatran. *Clin Toxicol (Phila).* 2015;53(3):156–163.
82. Lavergne V, Hoffman RS, Mowry JB, et al. Why are we still dialyzing overdoses to tricyclic antidepressants? A subanalysis of the NPDS database. *Semin Dial.* 2016.
106. Barceloux DG, Krenzelok EP, Olson K, et al. American Academy of Clinical Toxicology practice guidelines on the treatment of ethylene glycol poisoning. Ad hoc committee. *J Toxicol Clin Toxicol.* 1999;37(5):537–560.
107. Hoffman RS, Smilkstein MJ, Howland MA, et al. Osmol gaps revisited: normal values and limitations. *J Toxicol Clin Toxicol.* 1993;31(1): 81–93.
109. Hovda KE, Hunderi OH, Rudberg N, et al. Anion and osmolal gaps in the diagnosis of methanol poisoning: clinical study in 28 patients. *Intensive Care Med.* 2004;30(9):1842–1846.
116. Barceloux DG, Bond GR, Krenzelok EP, et al. American Academy of Clinical Toxicology practice guidelines on the treatment of methanol poisoning. *J Toxicol Clin Toxicol.* 2002;40(4):415–446.
119. Megarbane B, Baud F. What is the role of bicarbonate in the management of acidosis in the poisoned patient. *Clin Toxicol (Phila).* 2006;44(4):415–416.
120. Ghannoum M, Hoffman RS, Mowry JB, et al. Trends in toxic alcohol exposures in the United States from 2000 to 2013: a focus on the use of antidotes and extracorporeal treatments. *Semin Dial.* 2014;27(4):395–401.
124. Iliuta IA, Lachance P, Ghannoum M, et al. Prediction and validation of the duration of hemodialysis sessions for the treatment of acute ethylene glycol poisoning. *Kidney Int.* 2017.
125. Lachance P, Mac-Way F, Desmeules S, et al. Prediction and validation of hemodialysis duration in acute methanol poisoning. *Kidney Int.* 2015;88(5):1170–1177.
175. Dargan PI, Wallace CI, Jones AL. An evidence based flowchart to guide the management of acute salicylate (aspirin) overdose. *Emerg Med J.* 2002;19(3):206–209.
185. Baird-Gunning J, Lea-Henry T, Hoegberg LCG, et al. Lithium poisoning. *J Intensive Care Med.* 2017;32(4):249–263.
208. Isbister GK, Balit CR, Whyte IM, et al. Valproate overdose: a comparative cohort study of self poisonings. *Br J Clin Pharmacol.* 2003;55(4):398–404.
244. Roberts DM, Buckley NA. Enhanced elimination in acute barbiturate poisoning—a systematic review. *Clin Toxicol (Phila).* 2011;49(1):2–12.
292. Duong JK, Furlong TJ, Roberts DM, et al. The role of metformin in metformin-associated lactic acidosis (MALA): case series and formulation of a model of pathogenesis. *Drug Saf.* 2013.
345. Shannon M. Predictors of major toxicity after theophylline overdose. *Ann Intern Med.* 1993;119(12):1161–1167.
366. Rumack BH, Peterson RC, Koch GG, et al. Acetaminophen overdose. 662 cases with evaluation of oral acetylcysteine treatment. *Arch Intern Med.* 1981;141(3 Spec No):380–385.

# 68 Interventional Nephrology

Timmy Lee | Ivan D. Maya | Michael Allon

CHAPTER OUTLINE



## INTRODUCTION

During the lifetime of a hemodialysis patient, he/she will require many vascular access procedures including frequent placement of temporary or tunneled hemodialysis catheters, arteriovenous (AV) fistula and AV graft placements and revisions, surgical or percutaneous thrombectomies of AV fistulas and grafts, and other related endovascular procedures for AV access. For many years the majority of vascular access procedures were performed by surgeons and interventional radiologists. However, in recent years nephrologists have strived to improve the quality and timely provision of these vascular access services, and have formed a new subspeciality in nephrology: interventional nephrology. As a result, dialysis access procedures are increasingly being performed by appropriately trained nephrologists. Furthermore, in recent years interventional nephrologists have expanded the services they perform and many interventional nephrologists also are trained to create primary AV fistulas and grafts, insert peritoneal dialysis catheters, and perform native kidney biopsies. Issues relating to these procedures will be discussed in this chapter.

## OVERVIEW OF VASCULAR ACCESS FOR DIALYSIS

The majority of patients with end-stage kidney disease (ESKD) receive hemodialysis three times weekly to optimize their survival, minimize medical complications, and enhance quality of life.[1] Thus, vascular access is the lifeline for a patient receiving hemodialysis. A reliable and durable vascular access is a critical requirement for provision of adequate hemodialysis. The ideal vascular access would be easy to place, ready to use as soon as it is placed, deliver high blood flows indefinitely, and be free of complications. None of the existing types of vascular access achieves this ideal. Among the three types of vascular access currently available, native AV fistulas are superior to AV grafts, which in turn are superior to dialysis catheters.

Native AV fistulas are created by performing a direct anastomosis between a high-pressure artery and a low-pressure vein. Exposure of the vein to the high arterial pressure causes it to dilate and increase its blood flow. To be used reproducibly for dialysis, an AV fistula must have a large enough diameter to be safely cannulated with large-bore dialysis needles, and a sufficiently high access blood flow to permit blood flow ≥ 350 mL/min. It also must be superficial enough for the landmarks to be easily appreciated by the dialysis staff performing the cannulation. Increases in blood flow and draining vein diameter occur fairly rapidly following AV fistula creation. Whereas blood flow in a normal radial artery is only 20 to 40 mL/min, it increases more than 10-fold within a few weeks of fistula creation. In one study, the mean access blood flow in successful AV fistulas was 634 mL/min two weeks postoperatively[2]; in a second study it was 650 mL/min 12 weeks following AV fistula creation.[3] Moreover, the mean access blood flows and AV fistula diameters are not significantly different in the second, third, and fourth months following AV fistula creation.[4] This implies that determination of whether a new AV fistula is likely to be used successfully for dialysis should be possible within 4 to 6 weeks of the initial surgery. AV fistulas should not be cannulated immediately as the maturation process requires several weeks to months.

AV grafts are artificial connections between arteries and veins most commonly consisting of polytetrafluoroethylene (PTFE), which can be cannulated very early, ideally 3-4 weeks following surgical creation, once the AV artery and vein heal following the surgical procedure and the surrounding edema has settled.

Dialysis catheters include temporary large-bore venous catheters which are usually only used short-term, and tunnelled, cuffed permanent venous catheters. Of the long-term access options, tunneled catheters have the highest frequency of infection and thrombosis, but are a necessary evil, either as a bridge device in patients waiting for an AV fistula to mature or an AV graft to heal, or as an access of last resort in patients who have exhausted all AV fistula or graft options.[5,6] As compared to patients who continue to dialyze with catheters, those who switch from a catheter to an AV fistula or graft have a substantially lower mortality,[7,8] as well as improvements in serum albumin and erythropoietin responsiveness.[9]

Recognizing the relative merits of the type of vascular access, the 2006 Kidney Disease Outcomes Quality Initiative (K/DOQI) guidelines for vascular access recommended a target use of AV fistulas in at least 40% of hemodialysis patients and catheter use in only 10% of prevalent patients.[10] The proportion of U.S. patients using an AV fistula has increased progressively from 2003 to 2012 in response to the KDOQI guidelines and the Center for Medicare and Medicaid Service (CMS)'s Fistula First initiative (Fig. 68.1).[11] Unfortunately, there has been only a modest improvement in dialysis catheter reduction among prevalent hemodialysis patients from 27% in 2003 to 20% in 2012, well above the KDOQI target of 10%. More recently, the Fistula First initiative has raised the target goal to 66% AV fistula use in prevalent hemodialysis patients.[11] Distribution of vascular access types among prevalent patients in the United States is presently around 63% AV fistulas, 18% AV grafts, and 19% dialysis catheters (Fig. 68.1).[11] However, despite substantial improvements in the prevalent AV fistula rates, rates in incident patients have not improved in a similar fashion. The current distribution of vascular access types among patients initiating dialysis is 20% AV fistulas, 5% AV grafts, and 75% catheters.[11]

Patients with advanced chronic kidney disease (CKD) are regularly seen by their nephrologists and referred to different sub-specialists, including vascular surgeons and interventional radiologists, for vascular access placement for hemodialysis or peritoneal dialysis. For patients who choose hemodialysis, a vascular access plan becomes a very important aspect of care, ideally completed well before hemodialysis initiation. The goal is to have a functioning AV fistula in the large majority of patients at the time of hemodialysis initiation. Even with ongoing efforts to meet K/DOQI guideline targets, it is likely that all three types of vascular access will remain in use for the foreseeable future. Thus, substantially more clinical research will be necessary to learn how to minimize complications of, and optimize outcomes associated with, each type of vascular access, as well as basic research to elucidate the pathophysiology of vascular access dysfunction and failure to develop novel and targeted therapies.

## INTERVENTIONAL NEPHROLOGY IN MAINTENANCE OF HEMODIALYSIS VASCULAR ACCESS

During the course of their vascular access history, many patients undergo frequent placement of temporary or tunneled hemodialysis catheters, revision of a permanent access, surgical or percutaneous thrombectomies, and other related endovascular procedures. For many years, nephrologists took a passive role in this critically important area of dialysis care. However, during the past 20 years nephrologists have strived to improve the quality and timely provision of these services. As a consequence, dialysis access procedures are increasingly being performed by appropriately trained nephrologists who

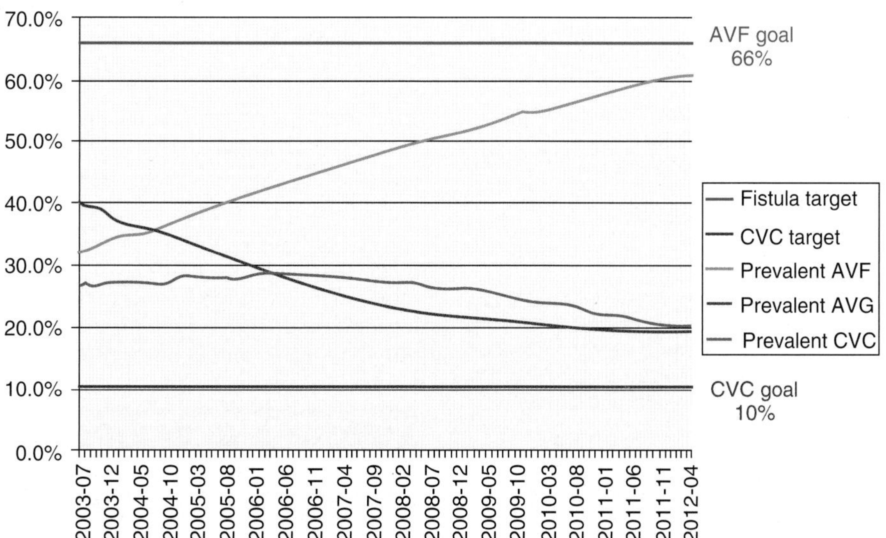


**Fig. 68.1** Impact of Fistula First Breakthrough Initiative (FFBI): Since initiation of FFBI there has been an increase AV fistula use (AVF) and reduction in AV graft (AVG) use. There has been only a modest reduction in central venous catheter (CVC) use. (Adapted from Fistula First Breakthrough Initiative Dashboard, www.fistulafirst.org.)

know the patients extremely well and are focused on these procedures.[12]

In the past, interventional techniques to address problems with vascular access were underutilized and care of the dysfunctional access was primarily surgical. However, since publication of the initial KDOQI guidelines in 1997 and its subsequent updates, nephrologists (and interventional radiologists) have become directly involved in providing vascular access procedures. Interventional nephrology was pioneered by Gerald Beathard,[13] and subsequently adopted by nephrologists at other medical centers.[14–19]

In 2000, a group of interventional nephrologists and radiologists, under the leadership of Dr. Beathard, formed the American Society of Diagnostic and Interventional Nephrology (ASDIN).[20] This organization provides certification to interventional nephrologists, as well as accreditation to the institutions involved in the practice and teaching of interventional procedures in the nephrology specialty.[17] Training, certification, and accreditation are given for diagnostic ultrasound, peritoneal dialysis catheter insertion, and endovascular procedures on AV fistulas and grafts and central venous catheters for hemodialysis.[21] Comprehensive training is required to achieve dexterity and knowledge. Several academic and nonacademic centers train practicing nephrologists and nephrology fellows in the techniques and procedures pertinent to interventional nephrology. These training centers are located either in a freestanding interventional facility or in a hospital-based radiology suite. Workshops and training are increasingly being supported in low and middle income countries by nephrology organizations worldwide to improve dialysis access competence and thereby dialysis quality.

Over the past 15 years, the profile of endovascular procedures performed at freestanding vascular access centers has evolved to include more procedures in AV fistula versus AV graft, a lower proportion of AV fistula thrombectomies versus elective angioplasties, and fewer catheter placements.[22] The approval of several new devices (mechanical thrombectomy devices, angioplasty balloons, hemodialysis catheters) over the past twenty years has expanded the repertoire of percutaneous interventions for vascular access.[23] A comprehensive list of procedures typically performed by interventional nephrologists is provided in Table 68.1. A given interventional

**Table 68.1 Procedures Performed by Interventional Nephrologists**

| |
|---|
| Placement of non-tunneled and tunneled dialysis catheters |
| Exchange of tunneled dialysis catheters |
| Implantation of subcutaneous dialysis devices |
| Preoperative vascular mapping |
| Surveillance for stenosis |
| Diagnostic fistulograms of grafts and fistulas |
| Angioplasty of peripheral and central stenosis |
| Deployment of endoluminal stents for peripheral and central stenosis |
| Thrombectomy of grafts and fistulas |
| Sonographic or angiographic assessment of immature fistulas |
| Salvage procedures for immature fistulas |
| Placement of peritoneal dialysis catheters |
| Diagnostic renal ultrasound |
| Percutaneous renal biopsy |

nephrology program may provide only a subset of these procedures, depending on the local needs and arrangements with radiology and surgical subspecialties. A solo nephrologist may decide to perform selected procedures necessary to provide an immediate dialysis access (such as insertion of dialysis catheters), thus eliminating delays resulting from scheduling difficulties. Other nephrology practices may include one or two nephrologists fully trained to perform a spectrum of interventional procedures.

When nephrologists perform interventional access procedures, hospitalizations for vascular access-related complications and missed outpatient hemodialysis sessions because of vascular access problems decrease.[19,24–26] Given the increasing numbers of chronic kidney disease patients worldwide, the role of the interventional nephrologist may need to expand more consistently from vascular maintenance to include AV access creation.

At University of Alabama at Birmingham, a unique multidisciplinary model has been adopted to streamline vascular access management. This model consists of a joint interventional radiology/nephrology program, with interventional nephrologists and interventional radiologists sharing the same radiology suites, and working side by side to perform all dialysis access procedures, profiting from the existing technical, clinical, imaging, and surgical competencies at the same institution.[27] Recent publications from other academic medical centers have also highlighted the opportunity for interventional nephrology to serve as a model for interdisciplinary training, research, and patient care.[28–30]

A key element of any successful interventional program, whether it involves radiologists or nephrologists, is active collaboration with nephrology and dialysis programs to track outcomes of the procedures, and implement timely quality improvement initiatives. This can be best accomplished by having dedicated vascular access coordinators who maintain prospective, computerized records of all procedures performed and follow patients up regularly.[27]

Vascular access procedures and their subsequent complications represent a major cause of anxiety, morbidity, hospitalization, and cost for patients on maintenance hemodialysis.[31–35] In an earlier publication from 1996, more than 20% of hospitalizations in US hemodialysis patients are vascular access-related, and the annual cost of vascular access morbidity is close to 1 billion U.S. dollars.[34] A more recent publication from Thamer et al. reported that Medicare paid 2.8 billion U.S. dollars for dialysis vascular access services in the United States.[36] Complications that occur commonly with AV fistulas and grafts are stenosis and thrombosis, and contribute to the rising costs of vascular access care. AV grafts are prone to recurrent stenosis and thrombosis, and often require multiple interventions to ensure long-term patency. AV fistulas have a much lower incidence of stenosis and thrombosis than AV grafts, and require fewer interventions.[34,35,37]

## BIOLOGY AND PATHOGENESIS OF VASCULAR ACCESS STENOSIS IN AV FISTULAS AND AV GRAFTS

Analysis of the multicenter Hemodialysis Fistula Maturation (HFM) study revealed a progressive increase in AV fistula diameter and blood flow in the 6-week period following AV fistula creation.[38] Incorporating data from the Dialysis Access Consortium (DAC) Fistula Trial, Dember et al. reported that AV fistula non-maturation rates in the U.S. are approximately 60% even among centers of excellence.[39] The magnitudes of postoperative AV fistula diameter and blood flow were directly associated with the preoperative arterial function, assessed by nitroglycerin-mediated dilation and flow-mediated dilation.[40] Recent investigations from experimental models have provided valuable insight into the downstream biology of AV fistula non-maturation.[41] These studies have shown that proper balance of expression of protective factors that regulate oxidative stress and endothelial function—such as heme-oxygenase-1 (HO-1) and nitric oxide synthase (eNOS) and inhibition of chemokines and mediators that modulate inflammation and vessel wall remodeling, such as monocyte chemoattractant protein-1 and matrix metalloproteinases (MMP-2 and MMP-9)—are crucial to increasing AV fistula blood flow and vasodilation and inhibiting venous neointimal hyperplasia and stenosis after AV fistula creation.[42–44] From clinical studies, gene polymorphisms in HO-1[45] and factor V Leiden[46] have been associated with AV fistula failure.

In recent years, the preexisting health of the vein and artery at the time of access creation and its impact on AV graft and fistula outcomes has emerged as an active area of research interest.[47] Several studies have shown that preexisting venous neointimal[48–51] and arterial neointimal hyperplasia[52] are present in the large majority of vessels collected at the time of new vascular access surgery. Preexisting arterial intimal hyperplasia and arterial microcalcification has been associated with early AV fistula failure.[52] A few studies have evaluated the association of preexisting venous neointimal hyperplasia and AV fistula outcomes. A recent study by Allon et al. demonstrated that preexisting venous neointimal hyperplasia was not associated with early postoperative AV fistula stenosis.[53] Another single-center study of patients undergoing a two-stage AV fistula, found no significant association between preoperative venous intimal hyperplasia and postoperative neointimal hyperplasia or clinical AV fistula survival.[54] Similarly, analysis of the HFM study observed only a weak association between the magnitude of preoperative venous intimal hyperplasia with postoperative AV fistula blood flow, stenosis, or clinical maturation.[55] This suggests the possibility that outward remodeling after AV fistula creation plays a more important role in the maturation process.

In AV fistulas, neointimal hyperplasia has been shown to be the most common histology in both early and late fistula failures[41,56–60] (Fig. 68.2). The predominant cellular phenotype present within the neointima are myofibroblasts.[56–60] However, in AV fistula non-maturation, inadequate vasodilation (poor outward remodeling), in addition to neointimal hyperplasia, play an important role.[58,61,62] The most common mechanism of vascular access dysfunction in AV grafts is development of venous neointimal hyperplasia at the vein-graft anastomosis[41,58,63] (see Fig. 68.2). Venous neointimal hyperplasia is characterized by myofibroblasts and extracellular matrix components within the neointima.[63] In addition, angiogenesis within the adventitia and a macrophage layer lining the perigraft region also develop.[63]

The pathogenesis of neointimal hyperplasia after AV fistula creation or graft creation placement involves a cascade of events that are best divided into upstream and downstream events[61] (Fig. 68.3). Upstream events are characterized as the initial injuries to the vascular endothelium and smooth muscle cells, which include: (1) surgical trauma at the time of AV access creation; (2) hemodynamic shear stress at the vein-artery or vein-graft anastomosis; (3) inflammatory

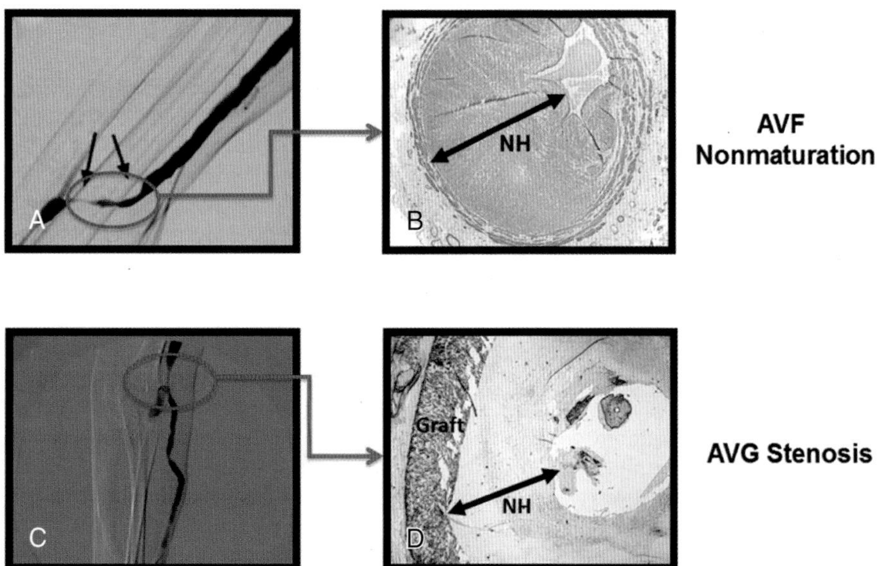


**Fig. 68.2** Histologic and angiographic lesions of venous stenosis in arteriovenous fistula (AVF) and arteriovenous graft (AVG). (A) Angiographic and (B) histologic features of AVF nonmaturation. Note aggressive venous neointimal hyperplasia (NH) at vein-artery anastomosis. (C) Angiographic and (D) histologic features of AVG stenosis. Note aggressive neointimal hyperplasia at graft–vein anastomosis. *Arrows* show the histologic features at the site of the angiographic venous stenosis in both AVF and AVG. Images are alpha-smooth muscle actin stain and magnification is 4X. (Adapted and reprinted from Lee T, Misra S. New Insights into Dialysis Vascular Access: Molecular Targets in Arteriovenous Fistula and Arteriovenous Graft Failure and Their Potential to Improve Vascular Access Outcomes. *Clin J Am Soc Nephrol.* 2016;11(8):1504–1512, with permission from the American Society of Nephrology.)

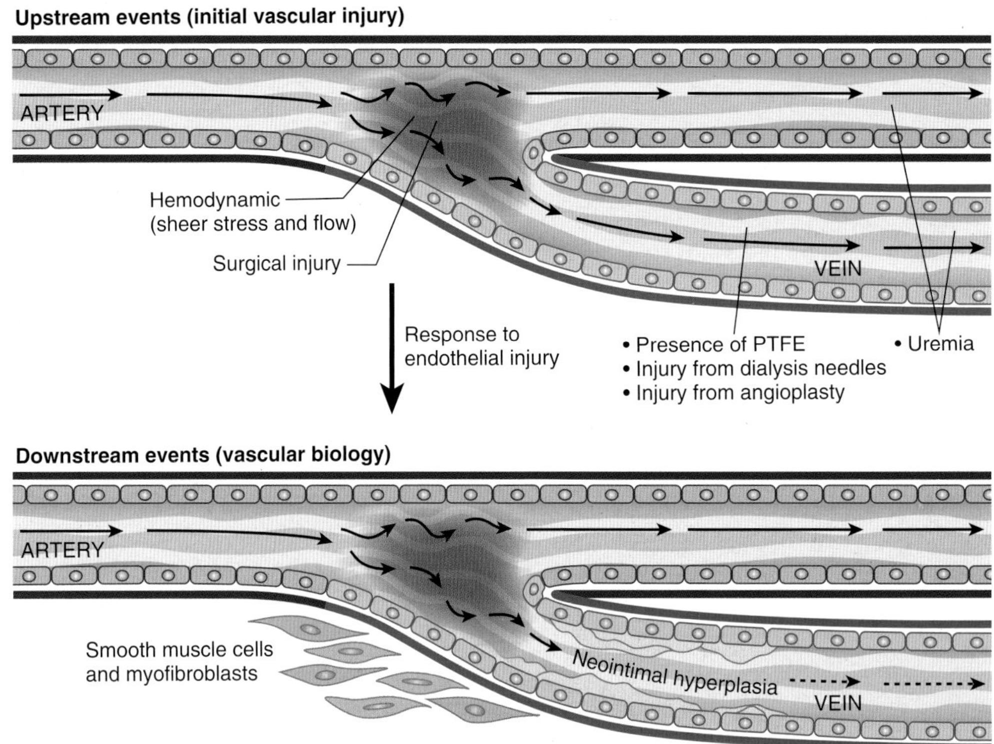


**Fig. 68.3** Upstream and downstream events in hemodialysis vascular access dysfunction. Upstream events result in initial vascular injury. Downstream events are the vascular biologic response to upstream injury. Downstream biology involves mediators of oxidative stress and inflammation that regulate activation, proliferation, and migration of fibroblasts, smooth muscle cells, and myofibroblasts. *PTFE,* polytetrafluoroethylene. (Adapted and reprinted from Lee T. Novel paradigms for dialysis vascular access: downstream vascular biology–is there a final common pathway? *Clin J Am Soc Nephrol.* 2013;8(12):2194–2201, with permission from the American Society of Nephrology.)

response to the PTFE grafts; (4) injury from vessel cannulation; (5) the effects of uremia on the veins and arteries leading to endothelial dysfunction; and (6) angioplasty-related injury.[58,59,61] Downstream events represent the vascular biological response to these upstream vascular injuries (Fig. 68.3). An inappropriate downstream response will lead to activation, proliferation, and migration of fibroblasts, smooth muscle cells, and myofibroblasts, ultimately leading to the development of neointimal hyperplasia.[58,59,61,62] In AV fistulas, vasodilation is a necessary downstream response for maturation, in addition to inhibition of neointimal hyperplasia[41,61,62] (Fig. 68.4).

## PREOPERATIVE VASCULAR MAPPING

The need to increase primary placement of native AV fistulas has been highlighted by the K/DOQI guidelines[64] and by the Fistula First initiative (www.fistulafirst.org). There is widespread consensus among nephrologists and surgeons about the importance of maximizing functional AV fistula prevalence in patients receiving hemodialysis. Achieving this goal, however, requires overcoming a number of hurdles, including timely referral of the patient with CKD to the nephrologist and access surgeon, timely placement of an AV fistula, adequate maturation of new AV fistulas, and successful cannulation of the AV fistula for dialysis.[35] In the past, the surgeon's decision about the type and location of vascular access placed was determined by a physical examination of the extremity, with and without a tourniquet. This approach was prone to substantial errors. The surgeon may not be able to adequately visualize the veins in obese patients. As a result, the surgeon might place an AV graft when an AV fistula could have been feasible. In other patients, the surgeon may decide to place a radiocephalic AV fistula after visualizing a large diameter cephalic vein at the wrist. However, an unsuspected stenosis or thrombosis in a proximal portion of that vein could doom the outcome of such an AV fistula.

The use of preoperative sonographic vascular mapping substantially increases the proportion of patients receiving an AV fistula rather than an AV graft. A prospective pilot study compared the surgeon's decision about access placement in 70 consecutive patients with CKD, before and after the results of preoperative vascular mapping were provided to the surgeon.[65] In almost one third of the patients, the surgeon changed his mind about the intended access procedure after receiving the mapping results. In most of these cases, the surgeon decided to place an AV fistula rather than an AV graft, or to place an AV fistula at a different location.[65] On the basis of these promising results, a program of routine preoperative vascular mapping was implemented. The results were dramatic: as compared to the historical control period, the proportion of patients having an AV fistula placed increased from 34% to 64%. Moreover, the proportion of patients dialyzing with an AV fistula doubled from 16% to 34%.[66] Similar increases in AV fistula placement following

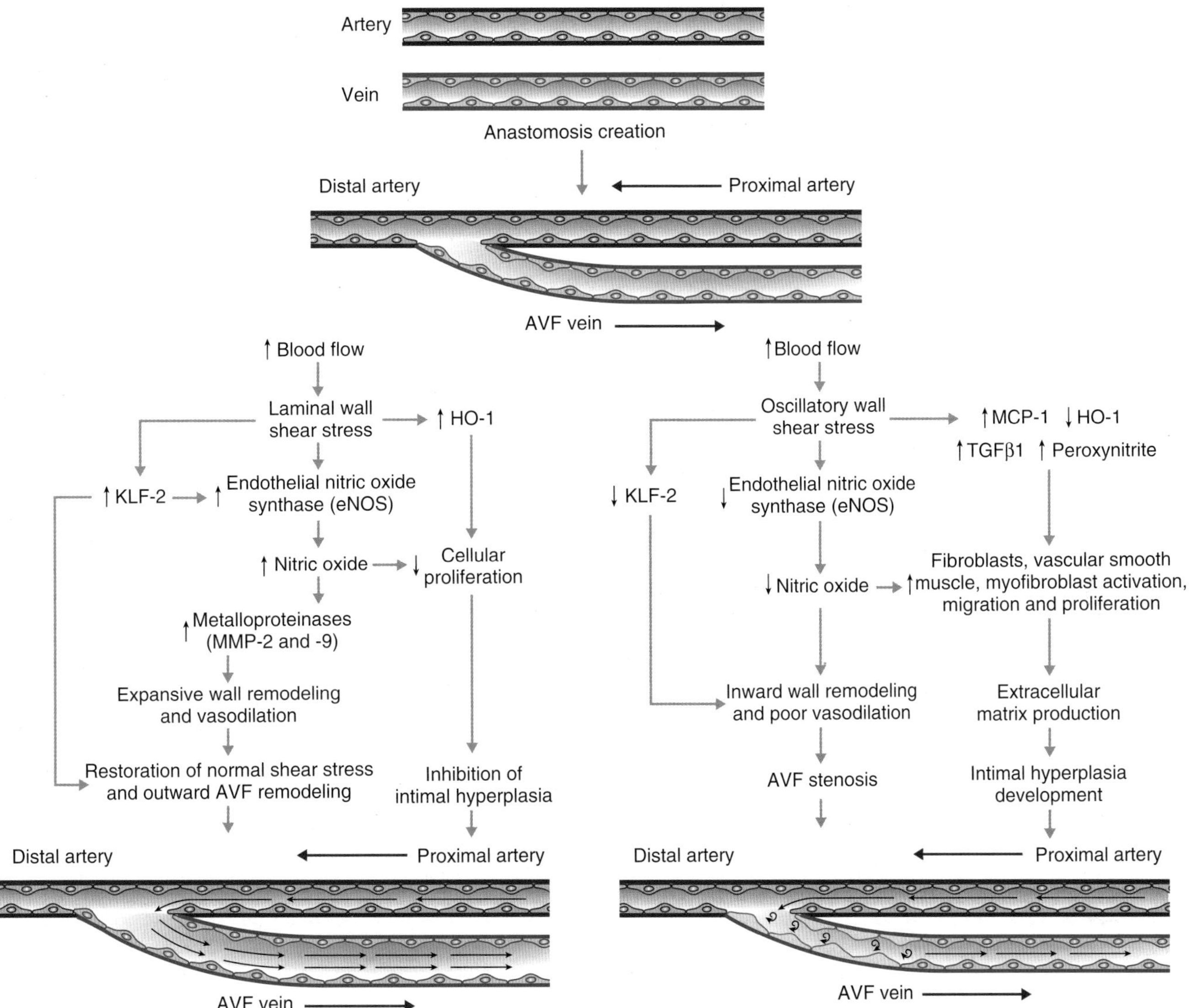


**Fig. 68.4** Pathophysiologic events of successful arteriovenous fistula (AVF) maturation and AVF maturation failure. Left panel describes events of successful AVF maturation and right panel describes events of AVF maturation failure. Successful AVF maturation is dependent on outward vascular remodeling and inhibition of neointimal hyperplasia, regulated through nitric oxide production and appropriate regulation of matrix metalloproteinases. Fibroblast, smooth muscle cell, and myofibroblast activation, migration, and proliferation play a key role in neointimal hyperplasia development and AVF maturation failure. Mediators such as heme-oxygenase-1 (HO-1), monocyte chemoattractant protein (MCP-1), kruppel-like factor-2 (KLF-2), transforming growth factor beta (TGFβ1), and high levels of local oxidant stress (e.g., peroxynitrite), play essential roles in regulating cellular proliferation and neointimal hyperplasia development. (Adapted and reprinted from from Lee T, Misra S. New Insights into Dialysis Vascular Access: Molecular Targets in Arteriovenous Fistula and Arteriovenous Graft Failure and Their Potential to Improve Vascular Access Outcomes. *Clin J Am Soc Nephrol.* 2016;11(8):1504–1512, with permission from the American Society of Nephrology.)

introduction of preoperative vascular mapping have been documented by other investigators (Table 68.2),[67] although a reduction in primary AV fistula failure has not been a consistent finding in all studies.[66,68–74] Two randomized clinical trials have compared outcomes of new AV fistulas placed after preoperative ultrasound vascular mapping, as compared to those placed after clinical evaluation alone. In a Turkish study of 70 patients, the two treatment groups had similar primary and secondary AV fistula survival.[75] In a British study of 218 patients, the patients undergoing a preoperative ultrasound had a lower incidence of immediate AV fistula failure (4% vs 11%, $p = 0.03$).[76] Primary (intervention-free) AV fistula survival was not different between the two groups (65% vs 56%, $p = 0.08$),[76] but the assisted primary (thrombosis-free) AV fistula survival was superior in the group undergoing preoperative ultrasound mapping (80% vs 65%, $p = 0.01$).

Although most centers have utilized sonographic vascular mapping, some have employed conventional venography.[77] In patients with stage 4 CKD, who have not yet started dialysis, there is a theoretical concern of radiocontrast-associated nephropathy precipitating the need for initiation of dialysis. However, in a series of 25 patients with a mean glomerular

**Table 68.2 Effect of Preoperative Vascular Mapping on Vascular Access Outcomes**

| | % Fistulas Placed | | % Primary Fistula Failure | | % Prevalence of Fistula Use | |
|---|---|---|---|---|---|---|
| **Reference** | Pre-VM | Post-VM | Pre-VM | Post-VM | Pre-VM | Post-VM |
| Silva, 1998[70] | 14 | 63 | 36 | 8 | 8 | 64 |
| Ascher, 2000[68] | 0 | 100 | N/A | 18 | 5 | 68 |
| Gibson, 2001[69] | 11 | 95 | 18 | 25 | N/A | N/A |
| Allon, 2001[66] | 34 | 64 | 54 | 46 | 16 | 34 |
| Sedlacek, 2001[72] | N/A | 62 | N/A | 25 | N/A | N/A |
| Mihmanli, 2001[73] | | | 25 | 6 | | |
| Miller, 1997[74] | N/A | 76 | | | | |
| Kakkos, 2011[71] | 12 | 53 | 32 | 18 | | |

*N/A,* Not available; *VM,* preoperative vascular mapping.
Adapted from Allon M, Robbin ML. Increasing arteriovenous fistulas in hemodialysis patients: problems and solutions. *Kidney Int.* 2002;62:1109–24.

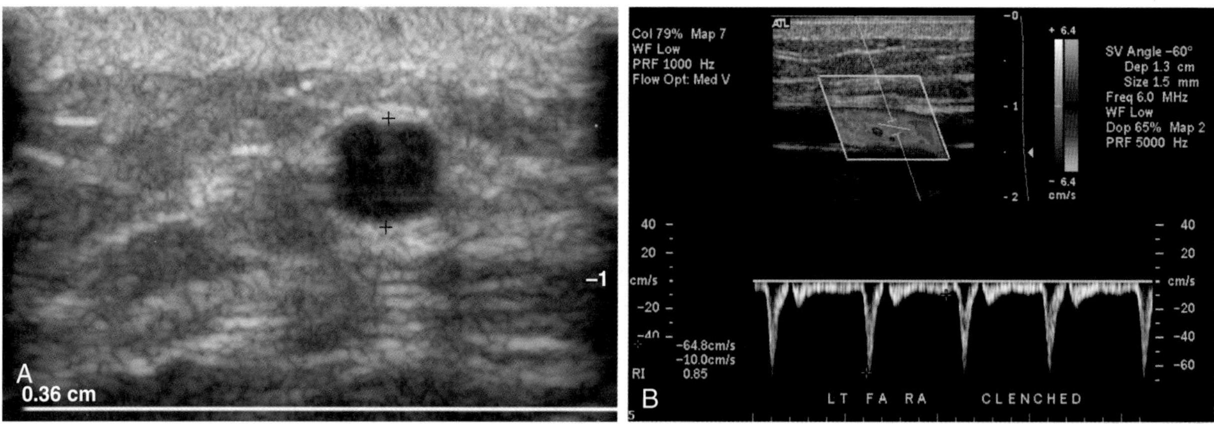


**Fig. 68.5** A, Venous mapping: Venous ultrasound showing a transverse section of a cephalic vein being measured (0.36 cm). B, Venous mapping: Doppler flow measurements and color Doppler ultrasound showing a longitudinal section of a left forearm radial artery that is 1.3 cm deep and 1.5 mm in diameter.

filtration rate of 13 mL/min, none developed acute kidney injury after undergoing angiography with 10 to 20 mL of low osmolality contrast material.[78] Another potential risk of venography is injury to the very vein required for future AV fistula creation. One advantage of venography over ultrasound is its superior ability to image the central vessels and exclude central vein stenosis. Venipuncture should be performed in the hand veins if at all possible, and the cephalic vein avoided. Prospective studies are needed to further define which preoperative vascular mapping techniques are most useful in optimizing fistula maturation and in which specific situations.

## TECHNICAL PROCEDURE: SONOGRAPHIC PREOPERATIVE VASCULAR MAPPING

Vascular measurements are performed with the patient in a seated position, with the arm resting comfortably on a Mayo stand. All measurements are performed in the anteroposterior dimension in the transverse plane (Fig. 68.5A, 68.5B). The minimum vein diameter for a native AV fistula is 2.5 mm.[79] The minimum vein diameter for AV graft placement is 4.0 mm.[79] The minimum arterial diameter for either AV fistula or graft placement is 2.0 mm.[79] Veins are assessed for stenosis, thrombus, and sclerosis (thickened walls).

First, the radial artery diameter at the wrist is measured. A tourniquet is then placed at the mid to upper forearm. The veins above the wrist are percussed for two minutes, with special emphasis on the cephalic vein area. Sequential measurements are made of the cephalic vein at the wrist, and mid and cranial forearm. Any other dorsal or volar veins at the wrist are also measured and followed up the arm, according to established diameter criteria. The tourniquet is sequentially moved up the arm, and cephalic, basilic, and brachial vein diameters are measured.

After the tourniquet is removed, the subclavian and jugular veins are assessed for stenosis and thrombus. Evidence of a more central stenosis is determined by analysis of the spectral Doppler waveform for respiratory phasicity and transmitted cardiac pulsatility. If there is a clinical or sonographic suspicion of central vein stenosis, a venogram or magnetic resonance venography (MRV) is obtained.

Measurements are recorded on a worksheet. The sonographic measurements are used by the surgeon to select the most appropriate vascular access, on the basis of the following list agreed upon by nephrologists, radiologists, and vascular surgeons, from most desirable to least desirable[79]:

1. Nondominant forearm cephalic vein AV fistula.
2. Dominant forearm cephalic vein AV fistula.
3. Nondominant, or dominant upper arm cephalic vein AV fistula.
4. Nondominant or dominant upper arm basilic vein transposition AV fistula.
5. Forearm loop AV graft.
6. Upper arm straight AV graft
7. Upper arm loop AV graft (axillary artery to axillary vein)
8. Thigh AV graft

## PROCEDURES INVOLVING AV GRAFTS

### SURVEILLANCE FOR GRAFT STENOSIS

About 80% of AV graft failures are due to thrombosis, whereas 20% are due to infection.[80,81] Thus, improving AV graft longevity requires implementing measures to reduce the frequency of AV graft thrombosis. Reports from United States Renal Data System (USRDS) showed that the number of angioplasties and thrombectomies ("declots") for AV grafts had substantially increased from 0.49 to 1.10 (rate per patient year) and 0.15 to 0.48, respectively, from 1998 to 2007.[1] Among AV grafts referred for thrombectomy, a significant proportion have underlying stenosis, most commonly at the venous anastomosis, the recipient/draining vein, or the central veins.[82–84] This observation suggests that prophylactic angioplasty of hemodynamically significant AV graft stenosis may reduce the frequency of AV graft thrombosis, and thereby increase cumulative AV graft survival.

A seminal study by Schwab et al. was the first to provide evidence supporting this approach.[85] This group of investigators measured dynamic venous pressures in AV grafts during consecutive hemodialysis sessions under carefully standardized conditions. A persistent elevation in the venous pressure measured at a low dialysis blood flow (200 mL/min) was associated with hemodynamically significant stenosis. The investigators then instituted a program of clinical monitoring for AV graft stenosis, with referral for prophylactic angioplasty if there was a suspicion of AV graft stenosis. As compared to the historical control period, a regimen of stenosis monitoring and prophylactic angioplasty reduced the frequency of AV graft thrombosis by about two thirds, from approximately 0.6 to 0.2 events per year. This landmark study stimulated a large volume of subsequent clinical research directed at two fundamental issues: (1) identifying a variety of noninvasive methods to screen for AV graft stenosis, and (2) evaluating whether stenosis surveillance and prophylactic angioplasty improved AV graft outcomes.

A variety of methods have been validated for detection of hemodynamically significant AV graft *stenosis* (Table 68.3). Clinical monitoring consists of using information that is readily available from physical examination of the AV graft, abnormalities experienced during the dialysis sessions (difficult cannulation or prolonged bleeding from the needle puncture sites), or unexplained decreases in the dose of dialysis, urea reduction ratio (URR), or the volume indexed clearance-time product (Kt/V).[82,83,86] The positive predictive value has been reported to be between 69% and 93% for clinical monitoring (Table 68.4).[82,86–89] AV graft surveillance uses noninvasive tests requiring specialized equipment or technician training that are not obtained as part of the routine dialysis treatment. These include measurement of static dialysis venous pressure (normalized for the systemic pressure), measurement of the access blood flow, or Duplex ultrasound to directly evaluate stenosis. Each of these monitoring or surveillance tools has been reported to have a positive predictive value for AV graft stenosis between 70% and 100% (Table 68.4).[89–92] The negative predictive value has not been studied systematically, as it would require obtaining routine angiography (fistulograms or "graft-o-grams") in patients whose screening test is negative. However, the negative predictive value can be inferred from the proportion of AV graft thromboses not preceded by abnormalities of AV graft surveillance, which is around 25%.[93]

**Table 68.3 Methods of Stenosis Monitoring**

| Clinical Monitoring |
|---|
| Physical examination (abnormal bruit, absent thrill, distal edema) |
| Dialysis abnormalities (prolonged bleeding from needle sites, difficult cannulation) |
| Unexplained decrease in Kt/V or URR |
| **Surveillance** |
| Static dialysis venous pressure (adjusted for systemic pressure) |
| Access blood flow |
| $Q_a$ < 600 mL/min |
| $Q_a$ decreased by >25% from baseline |
| Doppler ultrasound |

**Table 68.4 Positive Predictive Value of Monitoring Methods for Graft Stenosis**

| Surveillance Method | N of Measurements | Positive Predictive Value |
|---|---|---|
| **Clinical Monitoring** | | |
| Cayco, 1998[87] | 68 | 93% |
| Robbin, 1998[88] | 38 | 89% |
| Safa, 1996[86] | 106 | 92% |
| Maya, 2004[82] | 358 | 69% |
| Robbin, 2006[89] | 151 | 70% |
| **Static Venous Pressure** | | |
| Besarab, 1995[90] | 87 | 92% |
| **Flow Monitoring** | | |
| Schwab, 2001[91] | 35 | 100% |
| Moist, 2003[92] | 53 | 87% |
| **Ultrasound** | | |
| Robbin, 2006[89] | 122 | 80% |

In contrast, the predictive value of surveillance methods for AV graft *thrombosis* is much less impressive. Thus, when AV grafts with abnormal monitoring criteria suggestive of stenosis are observed without preemptive angioplasty, only about 40% of the AV grafts clot over the following three months.[94,95]

In practice, this means that in any program of AV graft monitoring, about half of preemptive angioplasties performed may be unnecessary. Unfortunately, there are no reliable tests to distinguish between the subset of AV grafts with stenosis that will progress to thrombosis from those that will remain patent without any intervention.

Several observational studies have documented that introduction of a monitoring or surveillance program for AV graft stenosis with preemptive angioplasty lowered the frequency of AV graft thrombosis by 40% to 80%, as compared to the historical control period during which there was no monitoring program (Table 68.5).[27,86,87,90,96,97] The promising findings from multiple observational studies led the K/DOQI Work Group to recommend implementing programs of graft surveillance and preemptive angioplasty in all dialysis centers, with the goal of reducing the frequency of AV graft thrombosis.[64]

Only in the last few years has the value of AV graft stenosis surveillance been subjected to rigorous testing in randomized clinical trials. To date, there have been six such trials, evaluating surveillance with access flow monitoring, static dialysis venous pressure, or ultrasound (Table 68.6).[89,92,98–101] Only one of the six randomized trials has demonstrated a benefit of ultrasound AV graft surveillance[101]; the other five showed no benefit of surveillance, despite a substantial increase in the frequency of preemptive angioplasty in the surveillance group.[89,92,98–100] For example, one study randomized patients with AV grafts to standard clinical monitoring alone or to a combination of clinical monitoring and ultrasound surveillance for stenosis. The patients in the ultrasound group underwent a 66% higher frequency of preemptive angioplasty, yet there was no difference between the two randomized groups in terms of frequency of AV graft thrombosis, time to first thrombosis, or likelihood of AV graft failure (Fig. 68.6A and 68.6B).[89] Because the randomized trials have been relatively small in size, it is possible they were inadequately powered to detect a modest benefit of AV graft surveillance. However, a recent meta-analysis of the randomized studies suggested that the benefit of surveillance with preemptive angioplasty, if present, is likely to be quite small, with a reduction of AV graft thrombosis not exceeding 23% and a reduction in AV graft failure no greater than 17%.[102] A large-scale, multi-center study trial, which takes into account multiple factors involved in access thrombosis, would be required to provide a definitive answer to this controversial question. In the meantime, the value of surveillance of AV graft stenosis and preemptive angioplasty in improving graft outcomes remains controversial.[103–106]

If underlying AV graft stenosis is an important predictor of AV graft thrombosis, why is preemptive angioplasty not

**Table 68.5 Effect of Surveillance on Graft Thrombosis: Observational Studies**

| | | Thrombosis Rate (Per Graft-Years) | | |
|---|---|---|---|---|
| **Reference** | **Surveillance Method** | Historical Control | Surveillance Period | Percent Reduction |
| Schwab, 1989[85] | Dynamic dialysis venous pressure | 0.61 | 0.20 | 67 |
| Besarab, 1995[90] | Static dialysis venous pressure | 0.50 | 0.28 | 64 |
| Safa, 1996[86] | Clinical monitoring | 0.48 | 0.17 | 64 |
| Allon, 1998[27] | Clinical monitoring | 0.70 | 0.28 | 60 |
| Cayco, 1998[87] | Clinical monitoring | 0.49 | 0.29 | 41 |
| McCarley, 2001[97] | Flow monitoring | 0.71 | 0.16 | 77 |

**Table 68.6 Randomized Clinical Trials of Graft Surveillance**

| | | # Subjects | | PTA/yr | | Thrombosis-Free Survival at 1 yr | | Cumulative Survival at 1 Year | |
|---|---|---|---|---|---|---|---|---|---|
| **Reference** | **Surveillance Method** | con | surv | con | surv | con | surv | con | surv |
| Lumsden, 1997[98] | Doppler US | 32 | 32 | 0 | 1.5 | 0.51 | 0.47 | N/A | N/A |
| Ram, 2003[99] | Access flow | 34 | 32 | 0.22 | 0.34 | 0.45 | 0.52 | 0.72 | 0.80 |
| | Doppler US | | 35 | | 0.65 | | 0.70 | | 0.80 |
| Moist, 2003[92] | Access flow | 53 | 59 | 0.61 | 0.93 | 0.74 | 0.67 | 0.83 | 0.83 |
| Dember, 2004[100] | Static DVP | 32 | 32 | 0.04 | 2.1 | N/A | N/A | 0.74 | 0.56 |
| Malik, 2005[101] | Doppler US | 92 | 97 | N/A | N/A | N/A | N/A | 0.73 | 0.93 |
| Robbin, 2006[89] | Doppler US | 61 | 65 | 0.64 | 1.06 | 0.57 | 0.63 | 0.83 | 0.85 |

*PTA,* Percutaneous transluminal angioplasty; *US,* ultrasound; *DVP,* dialysis venous pressure; *con,* control; *surv,* surveillance.

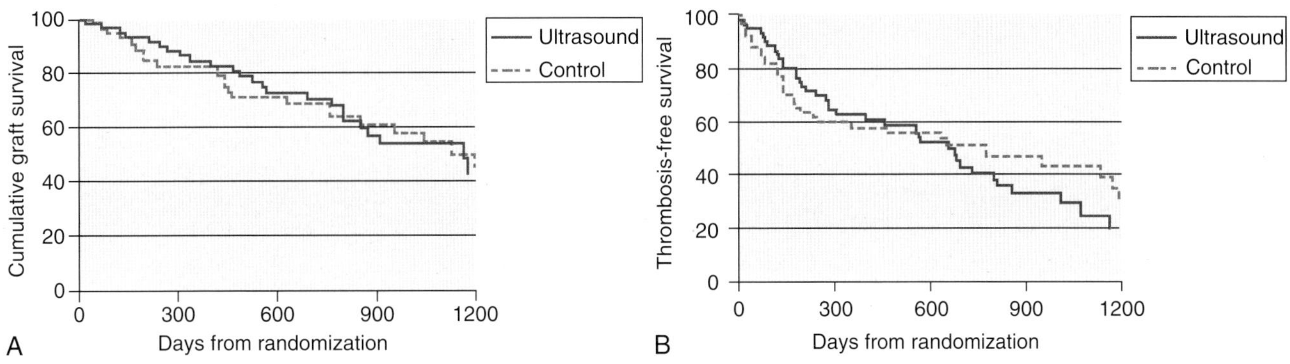


**Fig. 68.6** A, Comparison of cumulative graft survival between randomized patients with clinical monitoring versus clinical monitoring plus regular ultrasound surveillance of grafts. $P = 0.93$ by the log rank test. B, Comparison of thrombosis-free graft survival between randomized patients with clinical monitoring versus clinical monitoring plus regular ultrasound surveillance of grafts. $P = 0.33$ by the log rank test. (A and B, Reproduced from Robbin ML, Oser RF, Lee JY, et al. Randomized comparison of ultrasound surveillance and clinical monitoring on arteriovenous graft outcomes. *Kidney Int.* 2006;69(4):730–735.)

more successful in reducing AV graft thrombosis? The fundamental problem appears to be the short-lived efficacy of angioplasty to relieve AV graft stenosis. When serial access blood flows have been used as a surrogate marker of successful angioplasty, 20% of AV grafts have recurrent stenosis within one week of angioplasty, and 40% within one month of angioplasty.[91,92] In another study, the mean vascular access blood flow following angioplasty increased from 596 to 922 mL/min. However, three months later the mean flow had decreased to 672 mL/min.[107] In addition, there is published evidence suggesting that the injury from balloon angioplasty can actually accelerate neointimal hyperplasia, thereby resulting in recurrent stenosis.[108] Not surprisingly, patients undergoing angioplasty for AV graft stenosis require frequent re-interventions due to recurrent stenosis. The median intervention-free patency following AV graft stenosis is only about six months.[82,83] Finally, AV graft surveillance is likely to be most useful in new AV grafts (within three months of their creation).[109] Unfortunately, a large proportion of AV grafts fail before there has been adequate opportunity for surveillance to be performed and for hemodynamically significant stenosis to be detected and treated.[110] One study evaluated drug-coated balloon angioplasty with paclitaxel versus standard balloon angioplasty to evaluate the effects of minimizing endothelial injury following angioplasty.[111] The results from this study showed that cumulative target patency at 6 months, defined as angiographic evidence of a patent lesion or circuit with <50% angiographic restenosis and without requirement for repeat procedures during the follow-up period was significantly higher in the drug-coated balloon group (70% in drug-coated balloon group vs. 25% in standard balloon angioplasty group, $p < 0.0001$).[111] A recent multicenter, randomized controlled trial in 285 patients evaluated the safety and effectiveness of Lutonix® drug-coated balloon compared to standard balloon angioplasty in treating patients presenting with clinical and hemodynamic abnormalities in native AV fistulas located in the upper extremity.[112] The primary efficacy endpoint was target lesion primary patency at 6 months defined as no need for clinically driven reintervention on the target lesion or access thrombosis.[112] The 6-month endpoint was not met for target lesion primary patency (71% for the drug-coated balloon and 63% for the control group; $P = 0.06$).[112] However, both arms of the study demonstrated equivalent safety.[112]

The pathophysiology of AV graft stenosis involves proliferation of vascular smooth muscle cells (neointimal hyperplasia), with progressive encroachment of the lesion into the AV graft lumen.[113] To improve the patency of AV grafts following angioplasty, some investigators have attempted stent deployment. The rationale is that the rigid scaffold of the stent helps to keep open the vascular lumen.[114] There has also been an ongoing interest in pharmacologic approaches to prevention of neointimal hyperplasia. Two small, single-center, randomized clinical trials have documented a beneficial effect of dipyridamole and fish oil in preventing AV graft thrombosis.[115,116] A multicenter, randomized, double-blind study compared clopidogrel plus aspirin to placebo for prevention of AV graft thrombosis. The study was terminated early due to an excess of bleeding complications in the intervention group; there was no difference in the rate of AV graft thrombosis between the two randomized groups.[117] Similarly, a randomized clinical trial found that low-intensity warfarin posed a substantial risk of major hemorrhagic complications without reducing the frequency of AV graft thrombosis.[118]

The Dialysis Access Consortium was a larger multicenter, randomized, double-blinded clinical trial comparing long-acting dipyridamole + low-dose aspirin (Aggrenox™) to placebo in prevention of AV graft failure.[110] There was a modest but statistically significant improvement in primary unassisted AV graft survival in patients receiving dipyridamole-aspirin, as compared with those treated with placebo (28% vs 23%, at one year $P = 0.03$). Cumulative AV graft survival did not differ between the two treatment arms.[110] Most recently, a double-blind, randomized controlled study evaluating fish oil on PTFE AV graft patency and cardiovascular outcomes reported that fish oil did not decrease loss of native patency (time from creation to first intervention) of AV grafts at 12 months, but did show improvement in overall AV graft patency and cardiovascular outcomes.[119] More detailed discussion of pharmacologic approaches to prophylaxis of AV graft stenosis and thrombosis is beyond the scope of this chapter, but has been reviewed recently.[120]

## ANGIOPLASTY OF AV GRAFT STENOSIS

Patients with patent AV grafts are frequently referred for elective angioplasty when hemodynamically significant stenosis is detected either by clinical monitoring or by AV graft surveillance. The goal of elective angioplasty is to correct the stenotic lesion that impairs optimal delivery of dialysis, and hopefully delay AV graft thrombosis. The most common location of the stenosis localized by angiography is the venous anastomosis, followed by the peripheral draining vein, the central veins, and intra-graft (Table 68.7).[82–84] Inflow (arterial anastomosis) stenosis has been rare (<5%) in most series. However, one study, using retrograde angiography with manual occlusion of the venous limb, documented an inflow stenosis (> 50%) in 29% of grafts referred for diagnostic angiography, although all these patients also had venous anastomosis stenosis as well.[121]

A number of published series have documented the short-lived primary patency (time to next radiologic or surgical intervention) of AV grafts following elective angioplasty (Table 68.8),[82–84,86,122,123] with only 50% to 60% patency at 6 months and 30% to 40% at 1 year. This means that on the average, each AV graft requires two angioplasties per year. The primary patency is shorter after angioplasty of central vein stenosis, as compared with other stenotic locations. In one study, the primary patency at 6 months was only 29% for central vein stenosis, as compared with 67% for stenosis at the venous anastomosis.[84] Most studies have documented progressively shorter patency after each consecutive angioplasty, although one investigator found comparable primary patency for the first and subsequent AV graft angioplasties.[84]

The primary patency of AV grafts following elective angioplasty is not affected by patient age, race/ethnicity, diabetes, or peripheral vascular diseases.[82] However, the patency tends to be shorter in women than in men.[82] The primary patency after angioplasty is also not influenced by the location of the AV graft or the number of concurrent stenotic lesions found.[83]

The technical success of an angioplasty procedure may be assessed in several ways. The first is visual inspection of the fistulogram before and after the procedure to determine whether the magnitude of the stenosis (percent stenosis relative to the normal vessel diameter) has been reduced. The degree of stenosis of each lesion can be quantified with calipers, electronic quantitative analysis (QVA) or graded semi-quantitatively using the following scale: grade 1, no (<10%) stenosis; grade 2, mild (10% to 49%) stenosis; grade 3, moderate (50% to 69%) stenosis; and grade 4, severe (70% to 99%) stenosis.[82,83] A second approach is to measure the intra-graft pressure before and after the procedure, and normalize it for the systemic blood pressure. A third approach is to measure the change in access blood flow before and after the procedure. Each of these measures has been shown to be predictive of the primary patency of AV grafts following elective angioplasty. In one large series, following elective angioplasty, the median intervention-free survival of AV graft with no residual stenosis was 6.9 months, as compared with 4.6 months with any degree of residual stenosis.[83] Similarly, the median primary patency of AV grafts following angioplasty was inversely-related to the intra-graft to systemic pressure ratio, being 7.6, 6.9, and 5.6 months, when this ratio was < 0.4, 0.4 to 0.6, and >0.6, respectively.[83] Finally, a failure to significantly increase the access blood flow after angioplasty is observed in 20% of AV grafts at 1 week and in 40% by 1 month,[124,125] confirming the short-lived benefit of this intervention.

Measurements of the degree of stenosis are not always feasible, nor are they entirely objective. Caliper measurement or "eyeballing" are to various degrees, subjective. Even QVA is not reliable in detecting the various densities and edges of the normal vessels and requires operator adjustment of detected vascular edges (a subjective intervention). Arteriovenous graft loops originating from the brachial artery and anastomosis at a 90-degree angle with the basilic vein are hardest to image in profile, which is necessary in order to get an accurate measurement of stenosis. We routinely obtain intra-graft pressure measurement during angiography and

**Table 68.7 Location of Stenosis in Patients With Grafts Undergoing Angioplasty**

| | Percent of All Stenotic Lesions | | | | |
|---|---|---|---|---|---|
| **Reference** | **VA** | **VO** | **CV** | **IG** | **AA** |
| Beathard, 1992[84] | 42 | 34 | 4 | 20 | 0 |
| Lilly, 2001[83] | 55 | 22 | 15 | 6 | 2.5 |
| **Elective PTA** | | | | | |
| Lilly, 2001[83] | 60 | 14 | 9 | 10 | 7 |
| **Thrombectomy** | | | | | |
| Maya, 2004[82] | 62 | 16 | 8 | 12 | 1.5 |

*VA*, Venous anastomosis; *VO*, venous outflow; *CV*, central vein; *IG*, intragraft; *AA*, arterial anastomosis; *PTA*, percutaneous transluminal angioplasty.

**Table 68.8 Primary Graft Patency After Elective Angioplasty**

| | | Primary Patency at: | | |
|---|---|---|---|---|
| **Reference** | **N Procedures** | **3 Months** | **6 Months** | **12 Months** |
| Beathard, 1992[84] | 536 | 79 | 61 | 38 |
| Kanterman, 1995[122] | 90 | | 63 | 41 |
| Safa, 1996[86] | 90 | 70 | 47 | 16 |
| Turmel-Rodrigues, 2000[123] | 98 | 85 | 53 | 29 |
| Lilly, 2001[83] | 330 | 71 | 51 | 28 |
| Maya, 2004[82] | 155 | 79 | 52 | 31 |

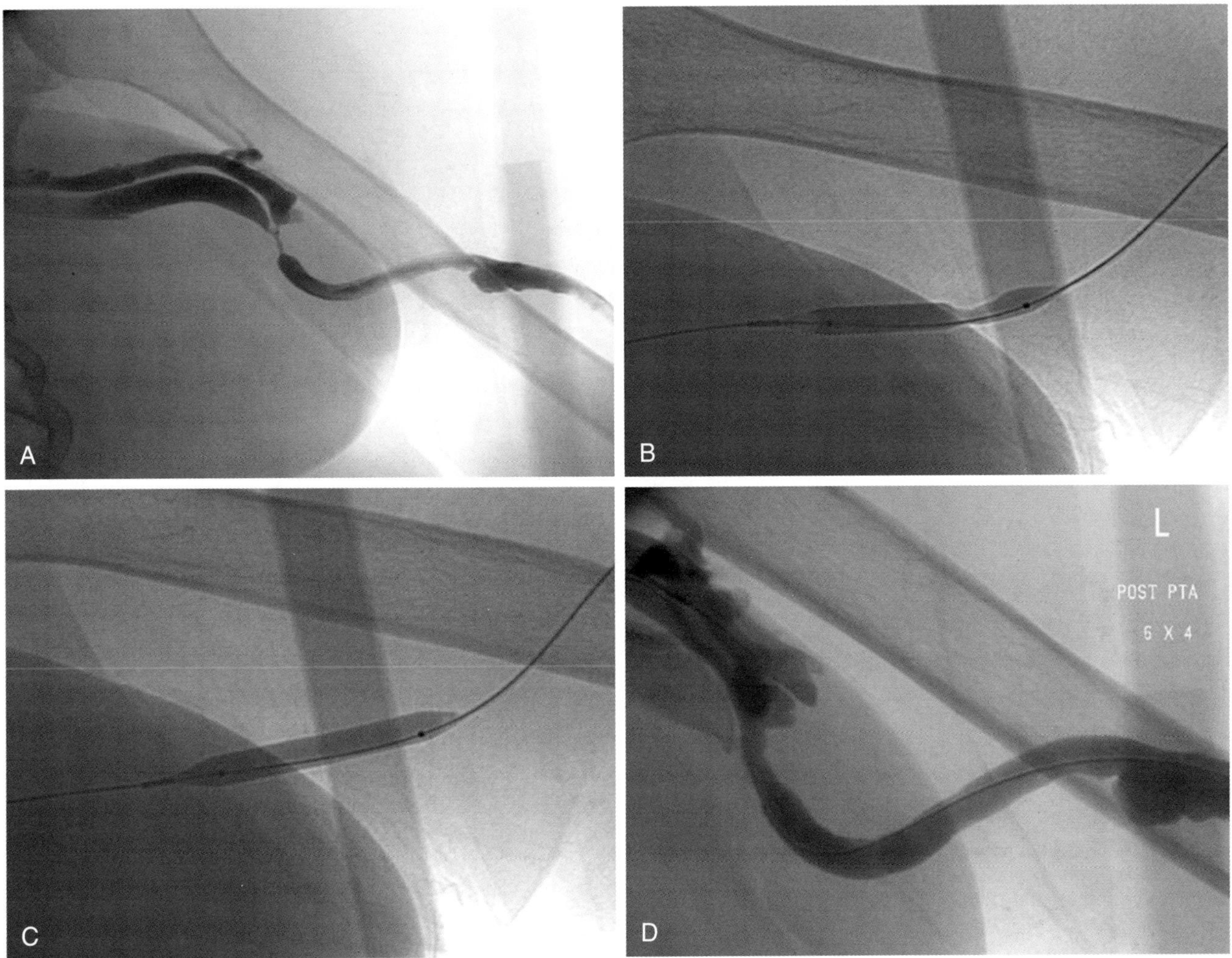


**Fig. 68.7** A, Left upper arm arteriovenous (AV) graft angiogram showing a severe (95%) stenotic lesion at the level of the venous anastomosis. B, Left upper arm AV graft stenotic lesion at the venous anastomosis with the angioplasty balloon partially inflated. C, Left upper arm AV graft stenotic lesion at the venous anastomosis with the angioplasty balloon fully inflated. D, Final post-angioplasty left upper arm AV graft angiogram showing a treated lesion with minimal residual stenosis.

PTA to add a hemodynamic parameter in addition to the visual assessment of fistulograms.

## TECHNICAL PROCEDURE: PERCUTANEOUS GRAFT ANGIOPLASTY

A digitally subtracted antegrade angiogram is performed to visualize the entire access circuit. The presence or absence of stenotic lesions and their number and location is assessed, and arterial anastomosis, intragraft, venous anastomosis, draining vein and central vein lesions are documented. The degree of stenosis of each lesion is quantified with calipers or graded semi-quantitatively.[82,83] Lesions with at least 50% stenosis are considered to be hemodynamically significant and undergo angioplasty. If a stenotic lesion is encountered, then an angioplasty of the lesion or lesions is performed. Angioplasty balloon sizes vary from 4 to 14 mm in diameter to 20 to 80 mm in length, depending on the vessel to be treated. The chosen balloon is usually selected to be 1 mm larger than the size of the AV graft or the vessel to be treated. The balloon is placed within the stenotic lesion, through a sheath, and inflated to its nominal pressure for 30 to 90 seconds (Fig. 68.7A, 68.7B, 68.7C, 68.7D) and (Fig. 68.8A, 68.8B, 68.8C). The majority of anastomotic lesions require higher pressure than those required for peripheral arterial angioplasty. Therefore, high pressure balloons with minimal burst pressure > 25 atmospheres are routinely used.[126] If a residual (>30%) stenosis is found, prolonged angioplasty (5-minute inflation), higher-pressure balloons (up to 30 atmospheres), and occasionally stent or covered stent deployment may be required to treat these lesions.

The major complication of this procedure is vessel extravasation and/or rupture of the vessel during angioplasty. Deploying a covered stent (wall-graft) can treat these complications. Surgical repair is indicated if the rupture is not corrected by stent placement.

## THROMBECTOMY OF ARTERIOVENOUS GRAFTS

The majority of AV graft failures are due to thrombosis, which occurs most commonly in the context of underlying stenosis at the venous anastomosis.[83,127] For this reason, successful graft thrombectomy requires both resolution of the clot and

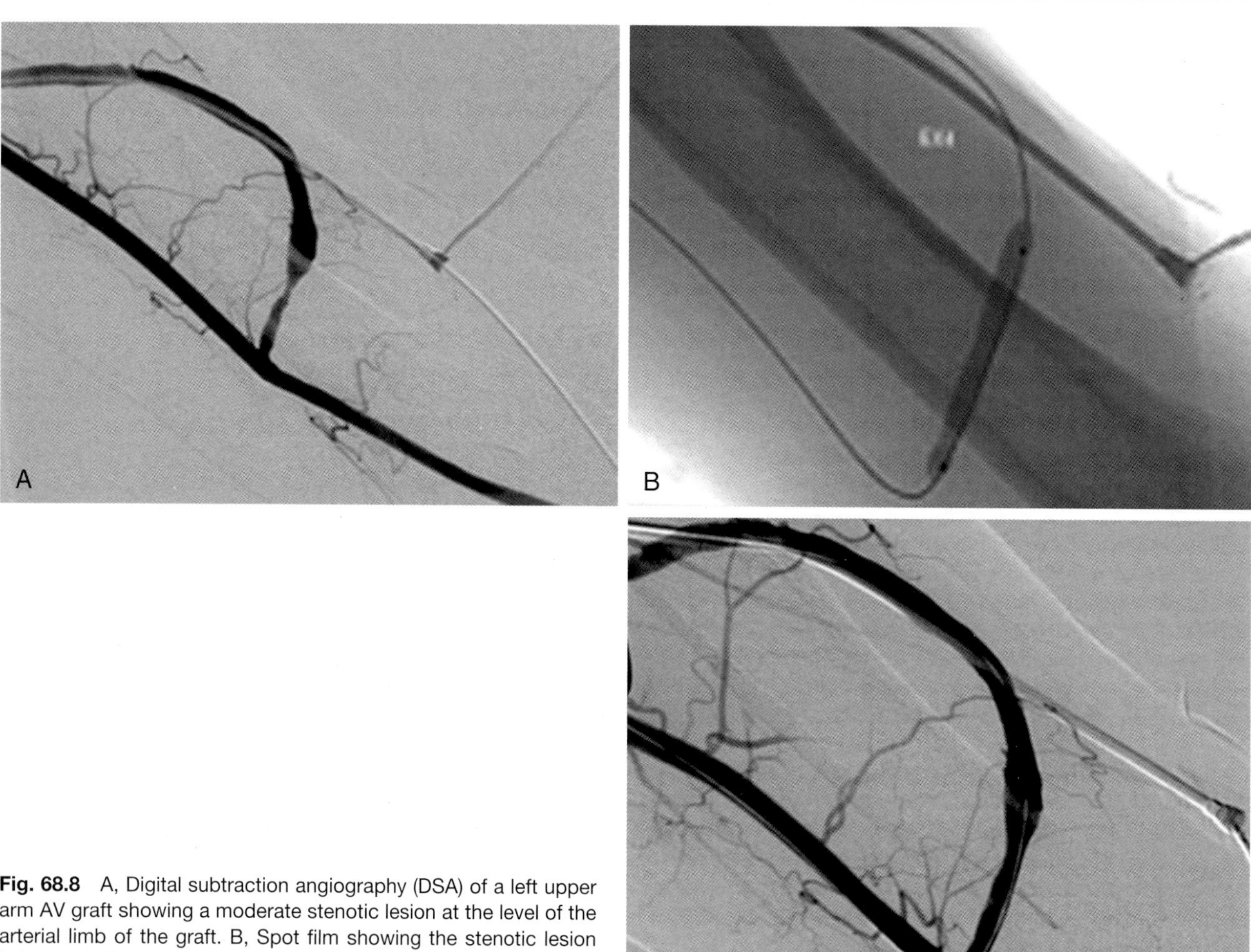


**Fig. 68.8** A, Digital subtraction angiography (DSA) of a left upper arm AV graft showing a moderate stenotic lesion at the level of the arterial limb of the graft. B, Spot film showing the stenotic lesion being angioplastied. C, Final post-angioplasty DSA showing excellent results.

correction of the underlying stenotic lesion. The primary patency of AV grafts after thrombolysis or thrombectomy and angioplasty (Table 68.9) ranges from 30% to 63% at 3 months and 11% to 39% at 6 months.[83,123,128–135] These outcomes are considerably worse than the primary patency observed after elective angioplasty (Table 68.8), which is 71% to 85% at 3 months and 47% to 63% at 6 months.[82–84,86,122,123]

The primary AV graft patency is similar for mechanical thrombectomy and pharmaco-mechanical thrombectomy.[130] A large series comparing the outcomes of both types of radiologic procedures at one institution found that the primary patency was only 30% at 3 months for clotted AV grafts, as compared with 71% for patent AV grafts undergoing elective angioplasty (Fig. 68.9A).[83] The discrepancy was still apparent when the analysis was restricted to the subset of procedures in which there was no residual stenosis, with a median primary patency of 2.5 months after thrombectomy, as compared with 6.9 months after elective angioplasty (Fig. 68.9B).[83]

The duration of AV graft patency following thrombectomy does not appear to differ among patients with and without diabetes mellitus. Arteriovenous graft patency is also generally unrelated by the AV graft location or the number of concurrent AV graft stenoses found.[83] However, similar to the

**Table 68.9 Primary Graft Patency After Thrombectomy**

| Reference | N Procedures | Primary Patency at: 3 Months | 6 Months |
|---|---|---|---|
| Valji, 1991[128] | 121 | 53 | 34 |
| Trerotola, 1994[129] | 34 | 45 | 19 |
| Beathard, 1994[130] | 55 mech | 37 | |
| | 48 pharm | 46 | |
| Cohen, 1994[131] | 135 | 33 | 25 |
| Sands, 1994[132] | 71 | | 11 |
| Beathard, 1995[133] | 425 | 50 | 33 |
| Beathard, 1996[134] | 1176 | 52 | 39 |
| Trerotola, 1998[135] | 112 | 40 | 25 |
| Turmel-Rodrigues, 2000[123] | 58 | 63 | 32 |
| Lilly, 2001[83] | 326 | 30 | 19 |

*Mech*, Mechanical; *pharm*, pharmacomechanical.

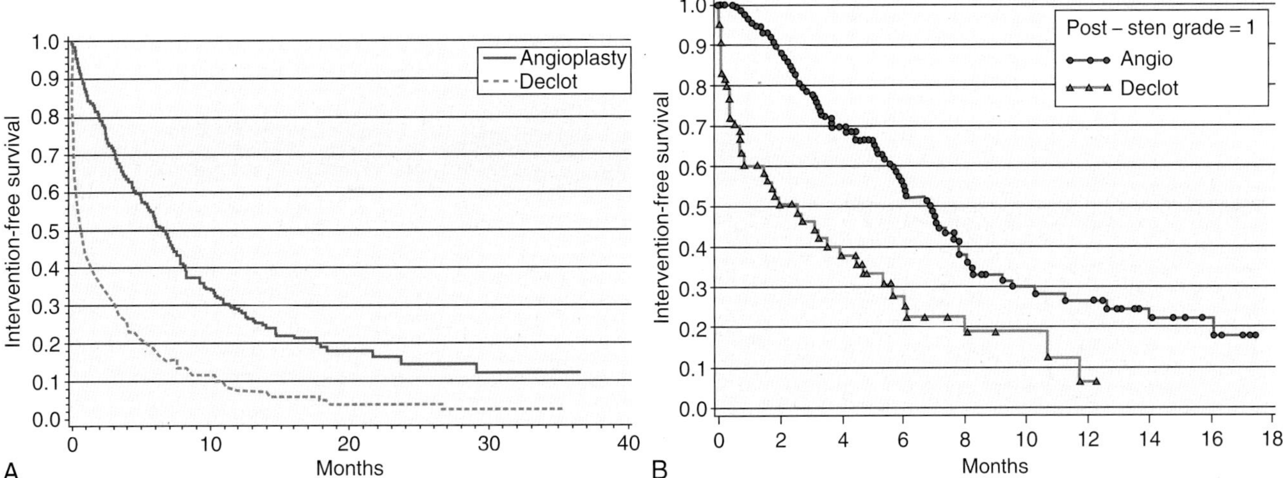


**Fig. 68.9** A, Intervention-free graft survival following elective angioplasty *(solid line)* or thrombectomy + angioplasty *(dotted line).* Graft survival was calculated from the date of the initial intervention to the date of the next intervention (angioplasty, declot, or surgical revision). $P < 0.001$ for the comparison between the two groups. B, Intervention-free graft survival following elective angioplasty *(circles)* or thrombectomy + angioplasty *(triangles)* in the subset of procedures with no residual stenosis. Graft survival was calculated from the date of the initial intervention to the date of the next intervention (angioplasty, declot, or surgical revision). $P < 0.001$ for the comparison between the two groups. (A and B, Reproduced from Lilly RZ, Carlton D, Barker J, et al. Predictors of arteriovenous graft patency after radiologic intervention in hemodialysis patients. *Am J Kidney Dis.* 2001;37(5):945–953.)

observations obtained after elective angioplasty, the primary patency of AV grafts after thrombectomy is inversely proportional to the magnitude of residual stenosis at the end of the procedure.[83]

## TECHNICAL PROCEDURE: PERCUTANEOUS ARTERIOVENOUS GRAFT THROMBECTOMY

The AV graft is initially accessed with a single-wall needle at level of the arterial limb of the graft. A guidewire is passed up to the venous outlet and the needle exchanged for a 6-French sheath. A catheter is placed beyond the clotted AV graft and a venogram is performed of the venous outflow and central circulation. Extreme caution is exercised not to pressure inject contrast into the AV graft, since it can dislodge clot and cause arterial emboli. Since more than 60% of the stenotic lesions are located at the venous anastomosis, an angioplasty of this area is performed, usually with an 8-mm balloon. Mechanical thrombectomy can be achieved by one of several methods: manual aspiration of the clots, infusion of a thrombolytic agent (tissue plasminogen activator [tPA], urokinase), use of a "clot buster" device (Angiojet, Arrow-Trerotola, Cragg thrombolytic brush, Hydrolyser, Prolumen, Amplatz thrombectomy device), or a combination of any of the above (Fig. 68.10A and 68.10B). Pure mechanical thrombectomy is generally sufficient, and thrombolysis is rarely necessary. Second, entry of the AV graft is performed toward the arterial anastomosis. A Fogarty balloon is passed beyond the arterial anastomosis and pulled back to dislodge the arterial plug, if present. Aspiration of the clots through both sheaths is performed. Finally, antegrade and retrograde angiograms of the AV graft are performed to assess for patency and look for other stenotic lesions. Intra-access pressure and systemic pressure (measured inside the AV graft by occluding the venous outflow) are measured. The ratio is calculated to confirm acceptable angioplasty results. High intragraft pressures indicate residual venous anastomotic obstruction, whereas extreme low pressures indicate obstruction at the arterial inflow.

Major complications of the thrombectomy procedure are vessel extravasations (Fig. 68.11) and rupture of the vein either because of wire manipulation or as a result of the angioplasty. Small extravasations are self-limited and could be observed; otherwise, stent deployment is the treatment of choice. Arterial emboli distal to the arterial anastomosis may occur and if encountered either intervention or surgical embolectomy is required. One interventional method to treat this complication is "back bleeding"; this refers to an occlusion of the artery before its anastomosis to the AV graft, causing retrograde blood flow that brings the clot into the AV graft. The use of a Fogarty balloon to remove the clot and the use of thrombolytic agents can also be performed to treat this complication.[136] There are very few published studies evaluating the frequency of pulmonary embolism following thrombectomy. One study has reported that pulmonary embolism is common (~35%) in patients undergoing AV graft thrombectomy.[137]

## DEPLOYMENT OF STENTS FOR AV GRAFT STENOSIS/THROMBOSIS

As discussed above, the primary patency of AV grafts following angioplasty is short-lived, and there is evidence that the vascular injury from angioplasty may actually accelerate neointimal hyperplasia.[108] In view of these considerations, there has been considerable interest in technical modifications to improve the patency of AV grafts following angioplasty. Endoluminal stents work by forming a rigid scaffold preventing elastic recoil and help to keep the vascular lumen open. Therefore, although neointimal hyperplasia recurs, a 1-mm thick layer on the wall of a stent is unlikely to cause a

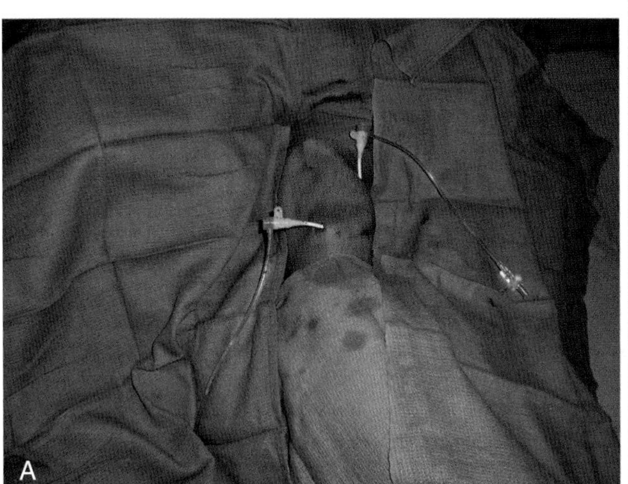


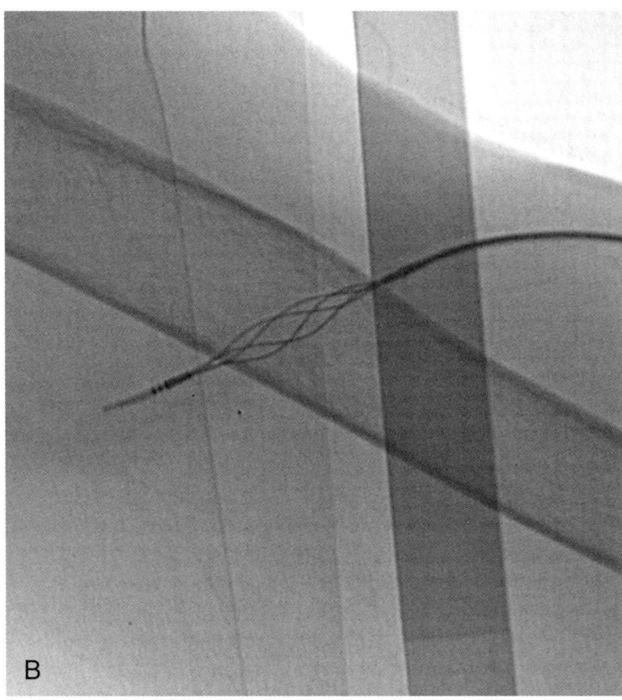


**Fig. 68.10** A, Percutaneous mechanical thrombectomy: A left upper arm arteriovenous graft site is prepared and two 6-French sheaths are in place. B, Percutaneous mechanical thrombectomy: Spot film showing the use of a percutaneous thrombectomy device. (Arrow-Trerotola-PTD).

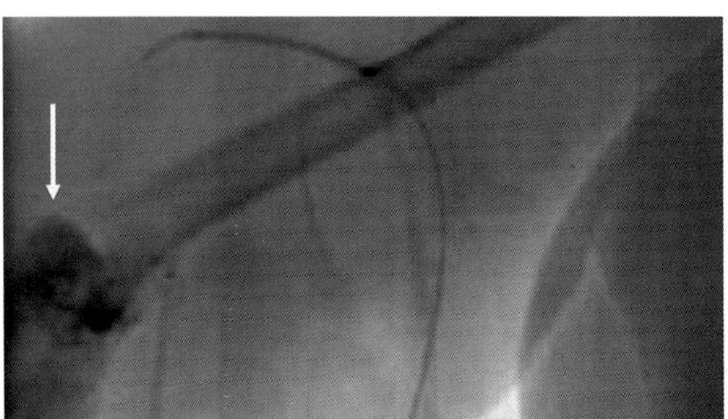

**Fig. 68.11** Mechanical thrombectomy complication: Extravasation of contrast *(white arrow)* at the middle portion of the arteriovenous graft.

significant stenosis of the vascular lumen of an 8-mm stent. Stent placement has been attempted for the treatment of rapidly recurring stenosis. A stenosis that is highly resistant to balloon angioplasty and cannot be expanded with a balloon is a contraindication for stent placement, because the stent will be as narrow as the original stenosis. On rare occasions, when trying to overcome such resistant stenoses with very high pressure, angioplasty may result in venous rupture and extravasation. Surgery is not necessary in these situations, as the complication can be converted to success by using stents or stent grafts (endograft).

The K/DOQI Clinical Practice Guidelines for Vascular Access recommend stent deployment only when there is acute elastic recoil of the vein (>50% stenosis) after angioplasty, when stenosis recurs within a 3-month period, or to treat vascular rupture complicating the angioplasty.[138]

Several small series have reported outcomes following stent deployment for refractory vascular access stenosis.[139–145] Most of these studies have been limited by retrospective data collection, absence of a suitable control group, lumping together of patent and thrombosed accesses, and combining grafts with fistulas.[146] A small randomized study comparing stents with conventional angioplasty found no difference in primary AV graft patency following the intervention.[140] However, this study enrolled a mixture of clotted and patent AV grafts, and the stenotic lesions were at a variety of locations, thus limiting the interpretation of the findings.

Since primary AV graft patency is particularly short-lived in clotted AV grafts undergoing thrombectomy, those AV grafts may experience better patency after stent deployment. One series reported the outcomes of 34 clotted AV grafts undergoing thrombectomy with stent placement at the venous anastomosis.[143] The primary patency following intervention in this homogeneous group of AV grafts was 63% at 6 months. Although there was no matched control group treated with angioplasty alone, the primary AV graft patency was much higher than that reported previously (11% to 39% at 6 months) (Table 68.9). A nonrandomized study comparing outcomes of clotted AV grafts treated with thrombectomy and stent placement at the venous anastomosis with matched control patients treated with only thrombectomy and angioplasty observed a significantly longer primary patency in AV grafts treated with a stent, as compared with those treated with angioplasty alone.[147] Similarly, a retrospective study with 48 patients observed longer AV graft patency after elective treatment of stenosis with stent deployment, as compared with angioplasty alone.[148] A definitive, randomized clinical trial is warranted to evaluate whether the patency of AV grafts following thrombectomy is enhanced by stent deployment.

There are a number of stent types available, including covered and noncovered stents, and either balloon or self-expandable. Balloon expandable are susceptible to be crushed under pressure if used peripherally and may only be used centrally. A variety of self-expanding Nitinol-based stents are available for use outside the coronary circulation. Although they appear similar, there are subtle differences, which may favor one stent over others in a particular circulation. However, there are no published clinical trials comparing the outcomes among stent types used for dialysis access. The advent of drug-eluting stents (DES) in the coronary circulation significantly reduced recurrent stenosis from 20% to 23% to less than 10%. Drug-eluting stents were implicated in cases of acute and late thrombosis, which led to the routine and obligatory administration of antiplatelet agents (aspirin and clopidogrel) for at least one year from stenting. It is also possible that the administration of antiplatelet agents after stent placement or employment of drug-eluting stents (DES) (e.g, sirolimus) or both may further improve the primary patency of AV grafts following angioplasty and/or thrombectomy for AV grafts, but there are no definitive data at this time. However, a recent randomized clinical trial in 119 patients with failing AV fistula or AV graft randomly assigned to a paclitaxel DES or standard balloon angioplasty reported prolongation of primary patency of dialysis access stenoses at 6 months and 1 year.[149] Future studies should help to resolve the question of whether DES are truly superior to balloon angioplasty in managing AV graft failure.

Finally stent grafts, which consist of a metallic stent covered with graft material, have been used to treat and exclude large pseudoaneurysms in the AV graft and complications such as rupture and extravasation successfully. However, a recent multicenter, randomized clinical trial allocated 190 patients with >50% AV graft stenosis at the venous anastomosis to treatment with stent-grafts or balloon angioplasty, with follow-up protocol angiograms performed at two and six months.[150] AV graft patency at six months was significantly higher in patients randomized to stent-grafts, but AV graft thrombosis was not different in the two treatment arms. Another recently published study evaluated 2-year data from a multicenter randomized controlled study comparing an expanded PTFE stent graft and percutaneous transluminal angioplasty for treatment of AV graft anastomotic stenosis.[151] Treatment area and overall access primary patency and time to subsequent intervention was longer in the stent graft group versus the angioplasty group.[151] Despite the cost of these endografts/covered stents, they may become quite valuable if long-term patency proves superior to angioplasty and bare metal stents.

### TECHNICAL PROCEDURE: PERCUTANEOUS DEPLOYMENT OF STENT

If a severe elastic recoil is seen on the final angiogram or a large residual stenosis (>50%) is seen at the level of the original stenotic lesion, a stent could be deployed.[136] Self-expanding stent sizes vary from 4 mm to 14 mm in diameter, and 10 to 80 mm in length. The most commonly used stents are nitinol or nitinol covered with expanded e-PTFE. The appropriate size and length is determined by grading the stenotic lesion at the time of placement. Usually the stent is selected to be 1 mm larger than the size of the AV graft or the vessel to be treated, and the length 5 mm longer than the stenotic lesion on each side. The stent comes already mounted in a device that is inserted through the sheath located at the arterial limb of the AV graft. A "road map" contrast injection of the stenotic lesion is performed. The stent is placed at the site of the stenotic lesion and deployed under fluoroscopic guidance (Fig. 68.12A, 68.12B, 68.12C). A post-deployment angioplasty with an appropriate size balloon is usually necessary to reexpand recoiled lesions. A final angiogram is performed to assess for patency and proper placement of the stent.

Complications of stent deployment include those related to angioplasty. In addition, underestimation of the required stent size may result in stent migration to the systemic circulation. If the stent is placed at a site where another vessel joins the main venous outlet, that vessel may be completely or partially occluded. The stent can fracture (Fig. 68.13) and occasionally thrombose (Fig. 68.14A, 68.14B, 68.14C). Finally, a potential long-term complication is intra-stent restenosis or thrombosis, which may require multiple frequent re-interventions. There has been a recently published multicenter randomized controlled trial assessing the safety and efficacy of an expanded PTFE stent graft versus balloon angioplasty for the treatment of in-stent restenosis in the venous outflow of AV grafts and fistulas.[152] Stent-graft use provided better access circuit primary patency and treatment area primary patency than balloon angioplasty when treating in-stent restenosis in patients receiving dialysis with AV grafts and fistulas.[152]

## PROCEDURES INVOLVING AV FISTULAS

### SALVAGE OF IMMATURE AV FISTULAS

As compared with AV grafts, AV fistulas require a much lower frequency of intervention (angioplasty or thrombectomy) to maintain their long-term patency for dialysis.[79] However, AV fistulas have a substantially higher primary failure rate (AV fistulas that are never usable for dialysis). Similar to AV grafts, the rate of angioplasty use from USRDS data has increased from 0.16 to 0.47 (rate per patient year) from 1998 to 2007,[1] likely due to the increasing frequency of treating primary AV fistula failures. The proportion of AV fistulas with primary failure has ranged from 20% to 50% in multiple recent series, even when routine preoperative vascular mapping has been employed.[35] A recent landmark multicenter randomized controlled trial reported a primary AV fistula failure rate of 60% in the United States.[39] Primary AV fistula failures fall into two major categories: early thrombosis and failure to mature.[153–155] Early thrombosis refers to AV fistulas that thrombose within three months of their creation, before they have been used for dialysis. Failure to mature refers to AV fistulas that never develop adequately to be cannulated reproducibly for dialysis. Non-maturation is less common with upper arm than forearm AV fistulas.[35] Among upper arm AV fistulas, non-maturation is less likely with transposed brachiobasilic AV fistulas than with brachiocephalic AV fistulas.[156]

In some patients, maturation of the AV fistula can be assessed easily by clinical evaluation by the nephrologist, surgeon, or an experienced dialysis nurse. In less straightforward cases, Duplex ultrasound may be useful in predicting

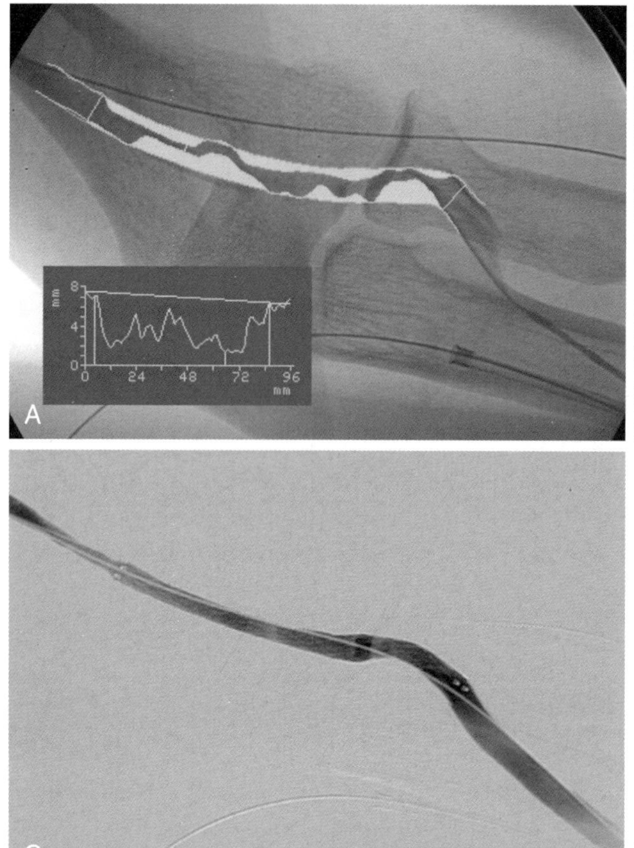


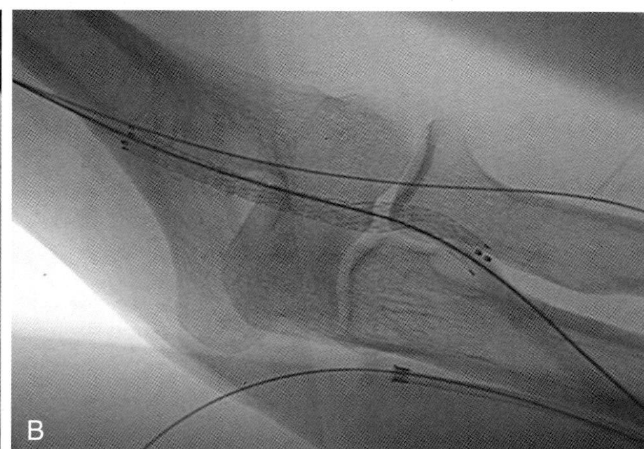


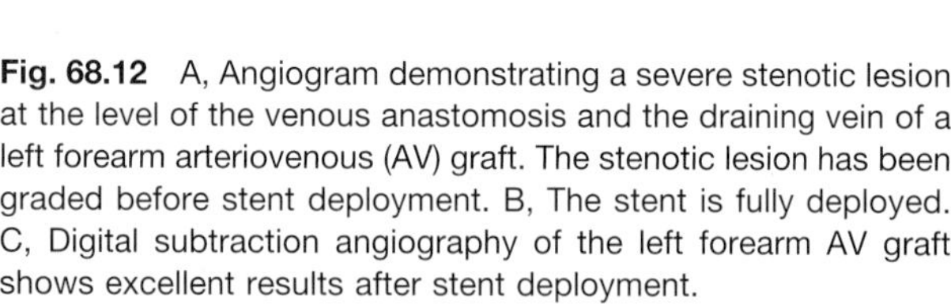

**Fig. 68.12** A, Angiogram demonstrating a severe stenotic lesion at the level of the venous anastomosis and the draining vein of a left forearm arteriovenous (AV) graft. The stenotic lesion has been graded before stent deployment. B, The stent is fully deployed. C, Digital subtraction angiography of the left forearm AV graft shows excellent results after stent deployment.

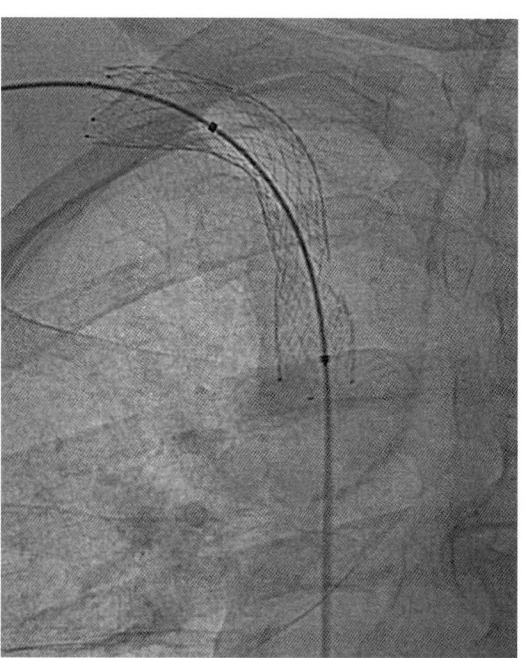

**Fig. 68.13** Stent fracture at the level of the right subclavian vein and right innominate vein.

whether a new AV fistula can be used successfully for hemodialysis. One pilot study used a combination of two simple sonographic criteria to assess AV fistula maturation: AV fistula diameter and access blood flow.[4] When the ultrasound documented a draining vein diameter ≥4 mm *and* an access blood flow ≥ 500 mL/min, 95% of the AV fistulas were subsequently usable for dialysis. In contrast, when neither criterion was met, only 33% of the AV fistulas achieved adequacy for dialysis. The likelihood of AV fistula adequacy for dialysis was intermediate (~70%) when only one of the two criteria was met.

Failure of an AV fistula to mature can be related to one of several anatomic defects, which can be identified either by sonography or angiography.[157] Stenosis at the anastomosis or in the draining vein is one such problem. Another possibility is that the draining vein has one or more large side branches. With these tributary veins, the arterial blood flow is distributed among two or more competing veins, thereby limiting the increase in blood flow in each. A third scenario may be observed in obese patients, in which the AV fistula has adequate caliber and blood flow, but is simply too deep to be cannulated safely by the dialysis staff. In most patients, these anatomic problems can be corrected by percutaneous or surgical interventions. Stenotic lesions can be treated by angioplasty or surgical revision. Superficial side branches can be ligated by a suture through the skin; deeper branches can be embolized. Finally, the surgeon can superficialize AV fistulas that are too deep to be cannulated safely.

In immature AV fistulas with one or more of these anatomic lesions, specific interventions to correct the underlying lesion

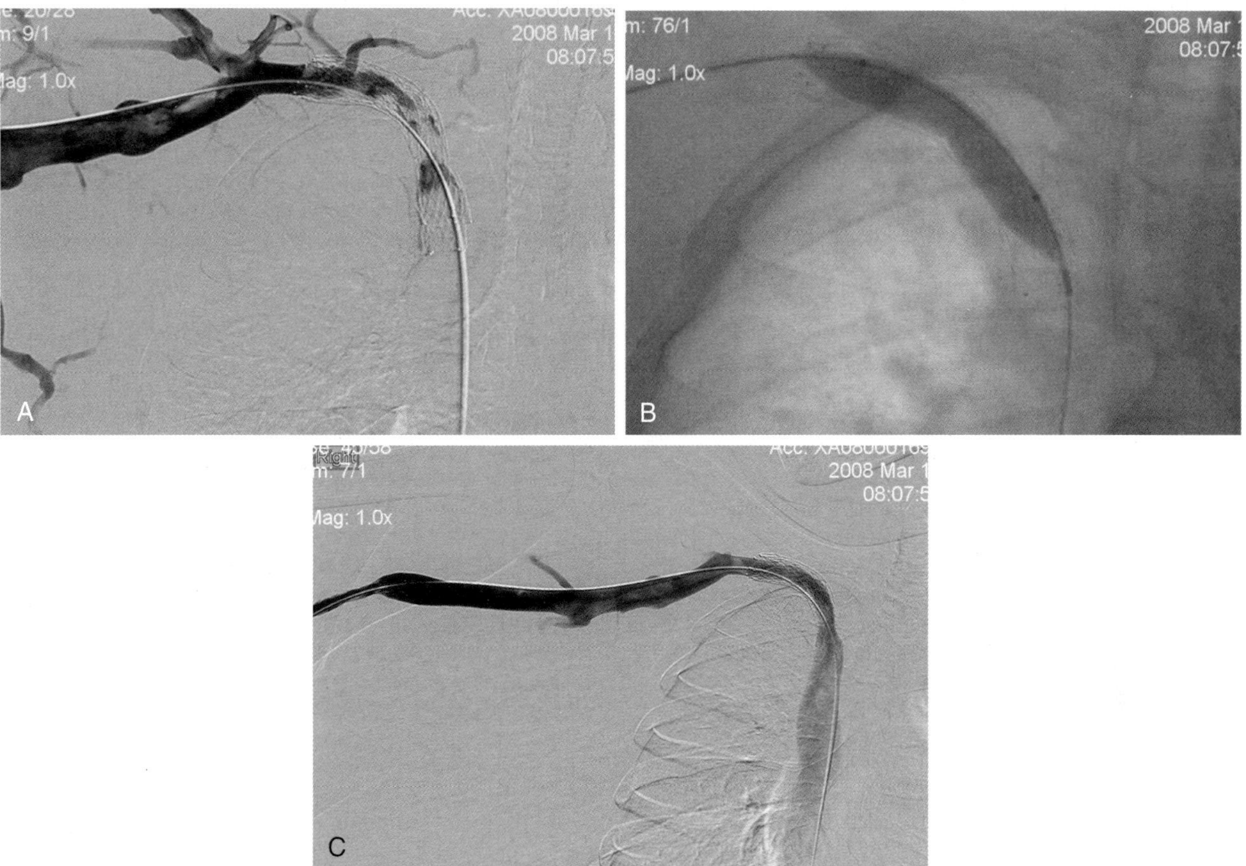


**Fig. 68.14** A, Thrombosed and fractured stent at the level of the right subclavian vein and right innominate vein. B, Angioplasty of the stenotic intra-stent lesion, which caused the thrombosis of the access circuit. C, Restoration of blood flow of the thrombosed stent.

may promote subsequent AV fistula maturation. Several published series have evaluated the ability to salvage immature AV fistulas such that they are subsequently usable for dialysis. A number of studies utilizing only radiographic procedures (angioplasty of stenotic lesions or obliteration of side branches) in immature AV fistulas have had a high success rate (Table 68.10).[77,158–162] An initial salvage (ability to use the AV fistula for dialysis) was accomplished in 80% to 90% of patients, with a subsequent 1-year primary patency of 39% to 75%. In another study utilizing a combination of radiologic and surgical salvage procedures in an unselected dialysis population, the salvage rate was more modest at 44%.[155] Of interest, the frequency of a salvage procedure for immature AV fistulas in that study was twice as high in women than in men. A recent retrospective study reported that immature AV fistulas with an anatomic abnormality that was corrected percutaneously or surgically were much more likely to achieve suitability for dialysis, as compared with similar fistulas that did not undergo a salvage procedure.[163] Recently, a novel approach to enhance AV fistula maturation, balloon assisted maturation (BAM), has been described.[164] In this procedure, repeated long-segment angioplasty procedures are used to sequentially dilate the peri-anastomotic venous segment, converting it at times into a collagen tube.[164] Other recent articles have described the use of intraoperative "primary balloon angioplasty" at the time of surgery ± BAM, which could allow for AV fistulas to be created in patients with small arteries and veins (artery, <2 mm; vein, <2.5 mm).[165,166] None of these studies have evaluated their techniques with a control group, and all have suggested that a large number of post-maturation angioplasties are needed to maintain patency. There are no randomized studies comparing different types of interventions or different timing of interventions in terms of their effect on AV fistula maturation. Two studies observed that immature AV fistulas requiring interventions to achieve maturity had significantly shorter cumulative patency and required more interventions to maintain patency, as compared with AV fistulas achieving maturation without interventions[167,168] (Fig. 68.15). In summary, proactive percutaneous or surgical interventions are worthwhile, as they can often convert immature AV fistulas to ones that are suitable for dialysis.

There has also been interest in pharmacologic interventions to promote AV fistula maturation. A randomized study of 877 US patients undergoing creation of a new AV fistula allocated patients to receive clopidogrel or placebo for the initial 6 weeks.[39] Clopidogrel significantly decreased the frequency of AV fistula thrombosis within 6 weeks. However, there was no improvement in the likelihood of clinical AV fistula maturation.[39] Subsequently, another randomized study from Australia and New Zealand of 567 patients reported that neither fish oil nor low-dose aspirin prevented new AVF failure.[169] There are several ongoing clinical trials evaluating novel therapies to improve AV fistula maturation. Perivascular elastase, topically

**Table 68.10 Effect of Salvage Procedures on Immature Fistulas**

| Reference | # Patients | Type of Intervention | Percent Usable for Dialysis | Primary Patency at 1 Year |
|---|---|---|---|---|
| Beathard, 1999[158] | 63 | PTA, Vein ligation | 82 | 75% |
| Turmel-Rodrigues, 2001[160] | 69 | PTA, Vein ligation | 97 | 39% |
| Miller, 2003[155] | 41 | PTA Vein ligation Surgical revision | 44 | N/A |
| Beathard, 2003[159] | 100 | PTA, Vein ligation | 92 | 68% |
| Asif, 2005[77] | 24 | PTA, Vein ligation | 92 | N/A |
| Nassar, 2006[161] | 119 | PTA, Vein ligation | 83 | 65% |
| Singh, 2008[163] | 32 | PTA Vein ligation Surgical revision | 78 | NA |
| Han, 2013[152] | 141 | PTA | 87 | 72% |

*NA,* Not available; *PTA,* percutaneous transluminal angioplasty.

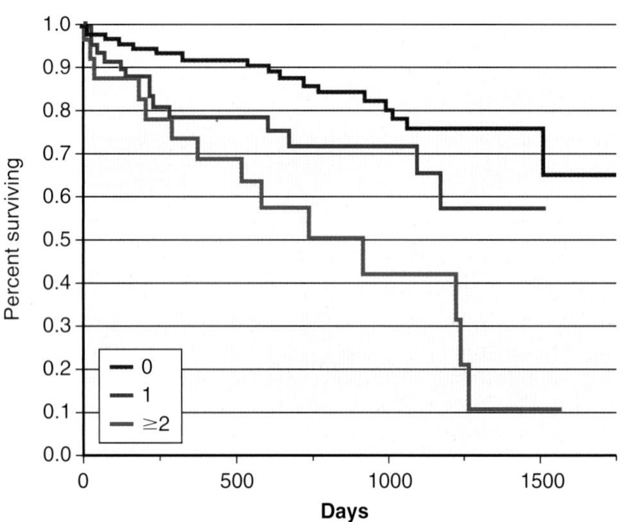


**Fig. 68.15** Interventions to Promote AV Fistula Maturation: Cumulative survival, defined from the time of access cannulation to permanent failure, is shorter in patients receiving two or more interventions before arteriovenous fistula maturation compared with those with zero interventions (HR, 2.07; 95% CI, 1.21 to 2.94; $P = 0.0001$). (Reproduced from Lee T, Ullah A, Allon M, et al: Decreased Cumulative Access Survival in Arteriovenous Fistulas Requiring Interventions to Promote Maturation. *Clin J Am Soc Nephrol.* 6:575–581, 2011 with permission from the American Society of Nephrology.)

applied over the AVF artery and vein anastomosis at the time of AV fistula, has been studied in early-phase clinical trials.[170,171] These early-phase studies of elastase to date have demonstrated safety and feasibility and have shown promising results with regard to improvement of physiologic maturation from ultrasound studies in radiocephalic AV fistulas. Given the promising results from early-phase studies, an ongoing phase III randomized controlled clinical trial is evaluating perivascularly delivered elastase administered at the time of new radiocephalic AVF creation (NCT02110901). Finally, an ongoing randomized controlled clinical trial is evaluating locally applied nitroglycerin ointment over the area of future AV fistula creation as a therapy to enhance local nitric oxide bioavailability and improve AV fistula maturation (NCT02164318). The goal of this therapy is to restore local endothelial function in patients with CKD and those with ESKD planned for AV fistula creation in order to promote outward AV fistula remodeling and maturation.

## TECHNICAL PROCEDURE: SALVAGE OF IMMATURE AV FISTULAS

### a. Angioplasty of Stenotic Lesions

The stenosis at the juxta arterial anastomosis can be treated with sequential balloon dilatations. This requires two to five treatments until the size of the anastomosis is appropriate. Long segments of stenotic lesions at the level of the most proximal part of the venous outlet near the anastomosis are amenable to balloon angioplasty and sometimes may require several follow-up interventions.

Immature AV fistulas are by definition small and could be difficult to access: therefore, it is best to evaluate the vessels with high-resolution ultrasound guidance to avoid repeated puncture, extravasation, and vein damage. Subtracted digital angiograms of the venous outlet, central circulation, and a reflux retrograde arteriogram are performed. Once the lesion is identified the proper technique is selected. The initial fistulogram could be avoided if reliable information is obtained from a surveillance ultrasound indicating the presence of a stenosis near or at the arterial anastomosis.

Depending on the severity of the stenosis a balloon is selected from sizes between 2 mm through 6 mm in diameter and from 10 mm through 40 mm in length. The angioplasty

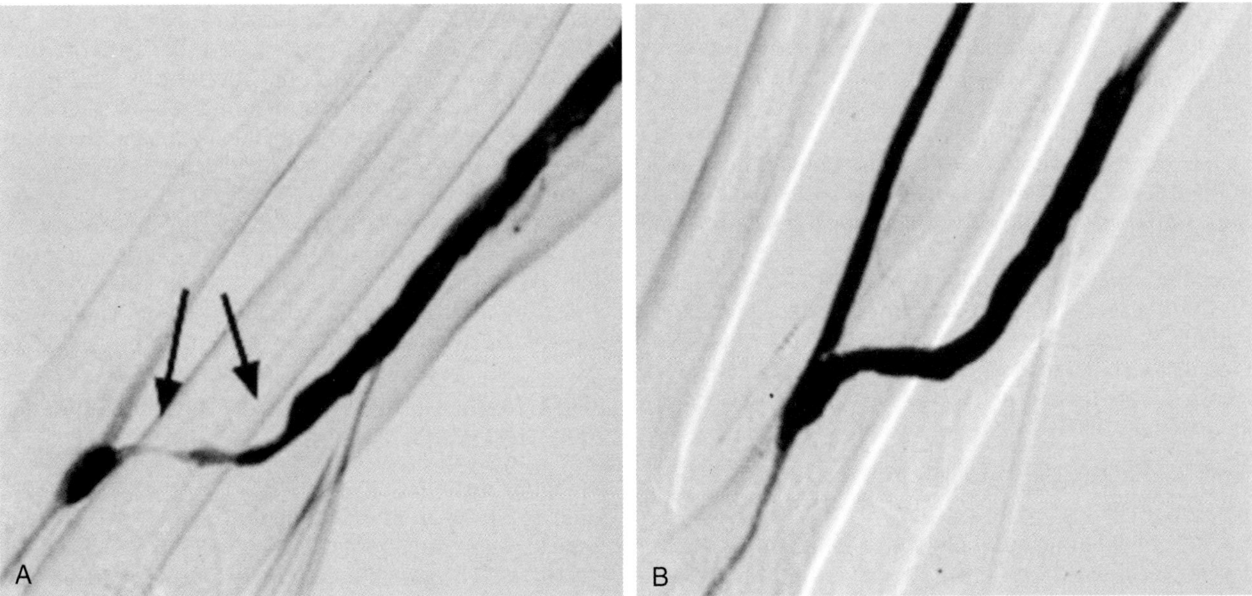


**Fig. 68.16** A, Fistula salvage: Digital subtraction angiography (DSA) of a radiocephalic arteriovenous fistula showing a severe stenotic lesion at the level of the juxta arterial anastomosis. B, Fistula salvage: Post-angioplasty DSA of a radiocephalic fistula showing radiologic improvement of the stenotic lesion at the level of the juxta arterial anastomosis.

balloon is introduced into the stenotic lesion and inflated carefully up to its nominal pressure. Subsequent angiograms are performed for post-angioplasty grading of the lesion (Fig. 68.16A, 68.16B). Patients are brought back to the intervention suite two to four weeks later for a second-look angiogram of the AV fistula.

Patients are followed at their local dialysis center and if the AV fistula does not mature or problems cannulating the AV fistula persist, a follow-up angiogram of the AV fistula is indicated.

### b. Ligation of Accessory Veins

Accessory veins can be treated either by surgical ligation or by endovascular coil deployment. Treatment of these lesions requires a well-trained interventionist due to the difficult technical approach to these lesions. Accessory veins are treated depending on size, location, and number (Fig. 68.17). Some interventionists advocate percutaneous ligation of superficial accessory veins at time of the initial angiogram of the AV fistula.[172] If the accessory vein is deep and has a large lumen size, then surgical ligation is indicated. If the accessory vein is deep but has a small lumen size then a coil deployment should be considered (Fig. 68.18).

The AV fistula is accessed and depending on its size, an appropriate sheath is introduced. A selective catheter is introduced in each accessory vein, and an appropriate size coil is deployed. A final angiogram of the AV fistula is taken to ascertain proper coil deployment and occlusion of all collateral veins.

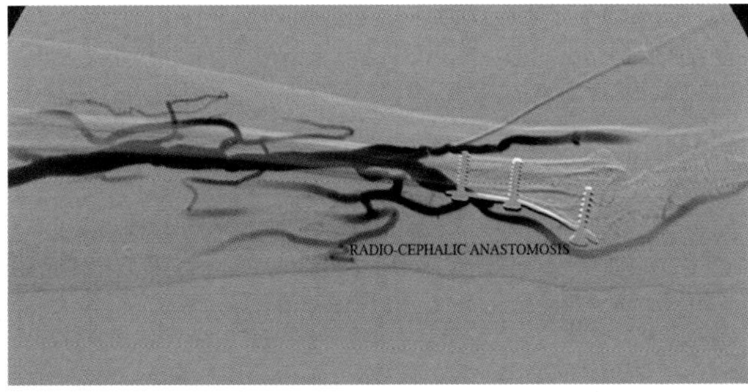


**Fig. 68.17** Digital subtraction angiography of a left radiocephalic arteriovenous fistula showing multiple collaterals. There is a metallic plate from a prior open reduction and internal fixation of a radius bone fracture.

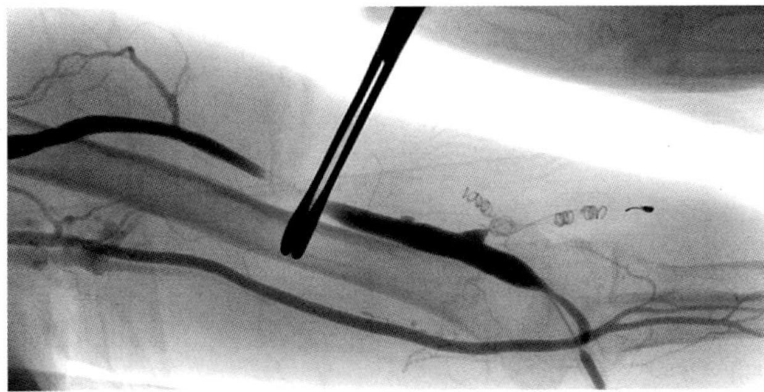

**Fig. 68.18** Coil deployed in a collateral vein of an upper arm arteriovenous fistula.

## PERCUTANEOUS TRANSLUMINAL ANGIOPLASTY (PTA) OF AV FISTULAS

Although the frequency of interventions is several-fold lower in AV fistulas than grafts,[35] fistulas are also susceptible to developing stenosis and thrombosis. Most studies have documented a comparable primary patency of fistulas and grafts following elective PTA (Table 68.11),[82,86,97,123] although one study observed a higher primary patency in fistulas.[173] As is the case with angioplasty of grafts, the primary patency of AV fistulas following PTA is inversely related to the magnitude of post-angioplasty stenosis, as well as the magnitude of the post-angioplasty intra-access to systemic pressure ratio.[82] It should be noted that highly matured and developed AV fistulas dilate and elongate significantly over the years, forming aneurysmal dilatation. With fixed points at the wrist and elbow or elbow and shoulder, they become tortuous and form significant kinks at certain points between dilated segments at certain intervals, which appear as significant stenoses. Many of these are not flowlimiting, while some are truly flow limiting but are unlikely to respond to PTA and may require surgical intervention. Clinical factors and major comorbidities such as age, race, diabetes, presence of peripheral vascular disease, access location, and number of stenotic sites have not been associated with the likelihood of vascular access patency after PTA.[82]

### TECHNICAL PROCEDURE: ANGIOPLASTY OF AV FISTULAS

Initial digitally subtracted angiogram of the AV fistula is performed including the venous outlet and central circulation. Lesions with more than 50% stenosis are considered hemodynamically significant and should undergo angioplasty. A final digitally subtracted angiogram is performed to assess for residual stenosis and requirement for further treatment of the stenotic lesion (Fig. 68.19A, 68.19B, 68.19C). The patient's intra-fistula pressure and systemic pressure are measured before and immediately after the intervention, and a reduction intra-fistula to systemic pressure ratio is used to confirm hemodynamic improvement.

The major complications of this procedure are vessel extravasations and rupture of the vessel after the angioplasty (Fig. 68.20A, 68.20B). Deploying a covered stent can treat these complications. Surgical repair is indicated if the rupture is not corrected by stent placement.

**Table 68.11 Primary Patency After Elective Angioplasty: Fistulas vs Grafts**

| | Primary Access Patency at 6 Months | |
|---|---|---|
| **Reference** | Grafts | Fistulas |
| Safa, 1996[86] | 43% | 47% |
| Turmel-Rodrigues, 2000[123] | 53% | 67% |
| McCarley, 2001[97] | 37% | 34% |
| Van der Linden, 2002[173] | 25% | 50% |
| Maya, 2004[82] | 52% | 55% |

## PERCUTANEOUS MECHANICAL THROMBECTOMY AND THROMBOLYSIS OF AV FISTULAS

Salvaging thrombosed AV fistulas is one of the most challenging aspects in interventional nephrology.[174] Thrombectomy of aneurysmally dilated AV fistulas is the most difficult technically. The most common cause of AV fistula thrombosis is an underlying stenotic lesion in the venous outflow circulation (either peripherally or centrally). Less common causes include needle infiltration,[175] excessive manual pressure for hemostasis at the needle insertion site, or severe and prolonged hypotension.[176] Successful restoration of patency in a thrombosed AV fistula requires expeditious thrombectomy within 48 hours of thrombosis. Several series have reported on the outcomes of radiologic thrombectomy of AV fistulas.[123,177–184] The immediate technical success has been fairly high, ranging from 73% to 93%. The primary patency of these AV fistulas following thrombectomy has ranged from 27% to 81% at 6 months, and 18% to 70% at 1 year (Table 68.12).[123,178,181–185] In one study primary patency following thrombectomy was lower in upper arm AV fistulas, as compared to those in the forearm.[123] However, with additional interventions, the secondary patency of these AV fistulas ranges from 44% to 93% at 1 year. A recent study evaluated

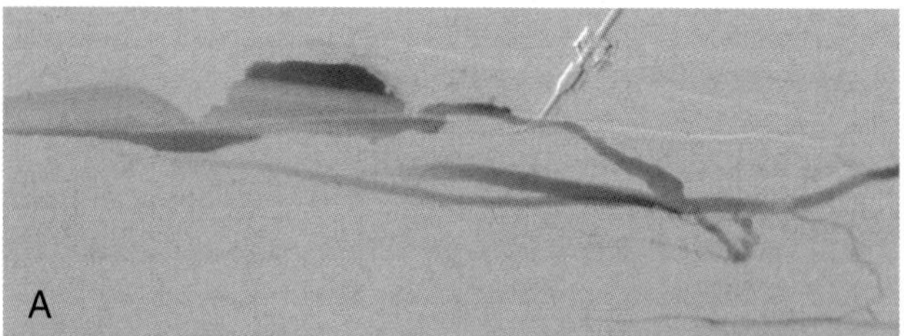


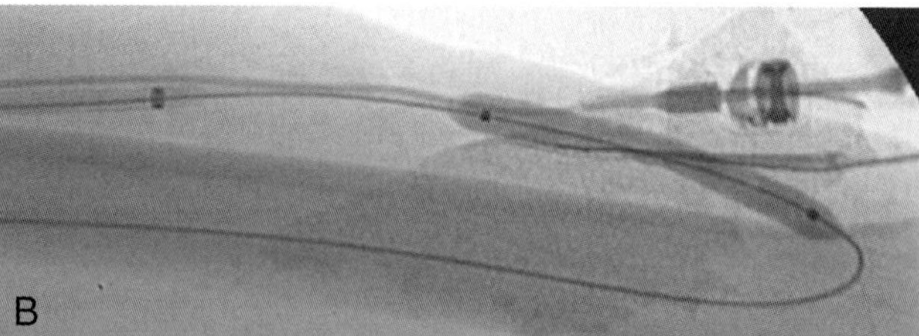


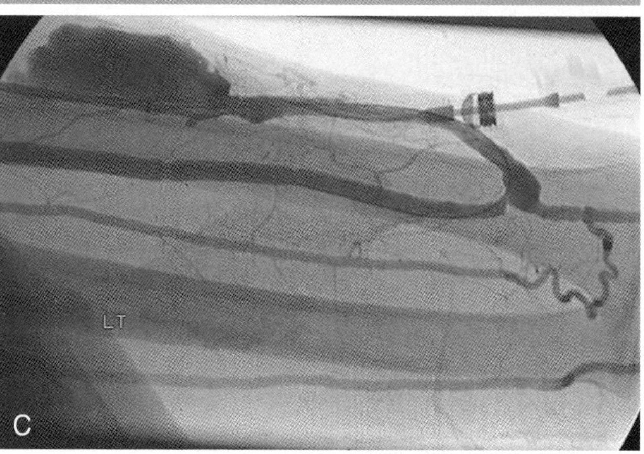


**Fig. 68.19** A, Digital subtraction angiography (DSA) of a left radiocephalic arteriovenous (AV) fistula showing a long severe segment of stenosis distal to the arterial anastomosis followed by a pseudoaneurysm of the fistula. B, Spot film of a left radiocephalic AV fistula showing the segment of stenosis being angioplastied. C, Post-angioplasty DSA shows a successful treatment, the pseudoaneurysm is unchanged.

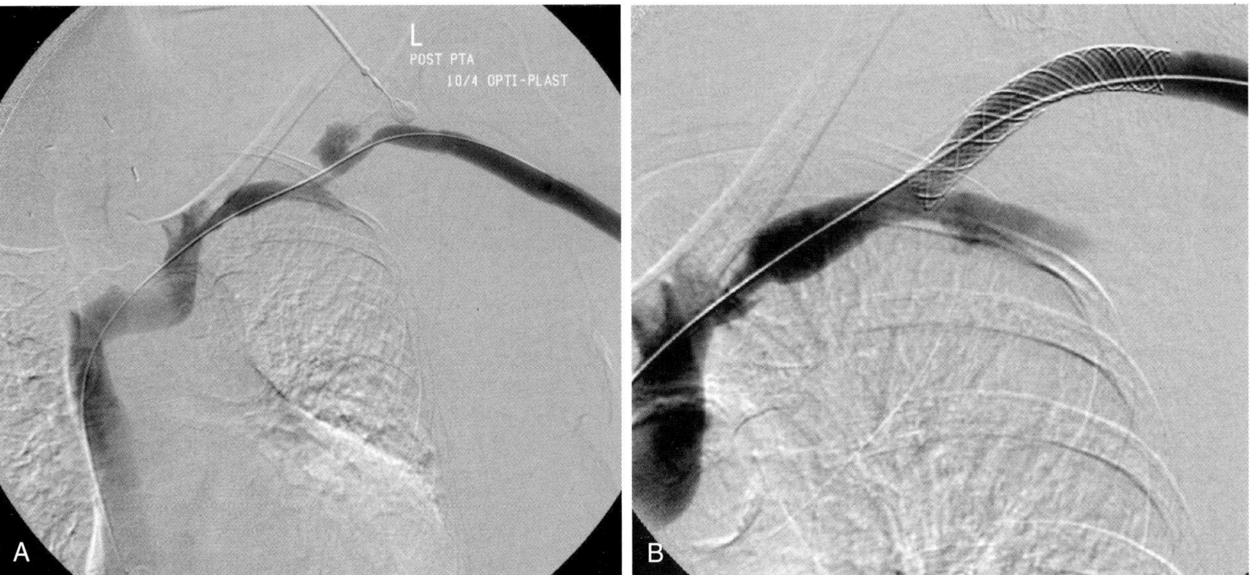


**Fig. 68.20** A, Angioplasty complication: Digital subtraction angiography (DSA) showing a rupture of the left cephalic vein after aggressive percutaneous transluminal angioplasty. There is a coexisting stenosis of the left subclavian. B, Angioplasty complication: DSA showing salvage and correction of the complication by deploying a covered stent (wall-graft).

**Table 68.12 Primary Fistula Patency After Thrombectomy**

| Reference | # Procedures | Primary Patency at: 6 Months | 12 Months |
|---|---|---|---|
| Haage, 2000[178] | 54 | | 27 |
| Turmel-Rodrigues, | 54 FA | 74 | 47 |
| 2000[123] | 9 UA | 27 | 27 |
| Rajan, 2002[182] | 30 | 28 | 24 |
| Liang, 2002[181] | 42 | 81 | 70 |
| Shatsky, 2005[183] | 44 | 38 | 18 |
| Jain, 2008[184] | 41 | 20 | – |
| Miller, 2011[185] | 140 | — | 59 |

Series with fewer than 25 procedures not included.
*FA*, Forearm; *UA*, upper arm.

140 consecutive patients, over a two-year period, with thrombosed immature AV fistulas, who underwent attempts at salvage via thrombectomy procedures.[185] All AV fistulas had thrombosed following access creation and had never been used for hemodialysis. Thrombectomy was successful in 119 (85%) immature clotted AV fistulas, and hemodialysis adequacy was achieved in 111 (79%) AV fistulas. The average maturation time from thrombectomy to cannulation for dialysis was 46.4 days, with an average of 2.64 interventions per patient. There were five (3.5%) cases of angioplasty-induced rupture, all of which were treated with stent placement. Clinically significant pseudoaneurysm formation occurred in four (2.8%) patients. At 12 months, secondary access patency of salvaged accesses was 90%. Considering that the alternative would be to abandon the thrombosed fistula and proceed with placement of a new AV fistula, concerted efforts to salvage thrombosed AV fistulas are extremely worthwhile.

### TECHNICAL PROCEDURE: PERCUTANEOUS THROMBECTOMY OF AV FISTULAS

Although more challenging than AV graft thrombectomy, AV fistulas can also be declotted successfully. There are few contraindications, including concurrent infection, fistula immaturity, and very large aneurysms. The technical challenges include difficulty in the initial cannulation of a thrombosed AV fistula, complete removal of large thrombi, and successful treatment of recalcitrant stenotic lesions.

A percutaneous thrombectomy, an interventional procedure of removing a blood clot (thrombus) using an over-the-wire device can be used (such as Angiojet). After successful thrombolysis (dissolving of the thrombus) of the AV fistula, a Fogarty balloon is passed beyond the arterial anastomosis and pulled back to dislodge the plugging clot. Once the thrombus is cleared and blood flow reestablished, a digitally subtracted angiogram of the AV fistula is performed to evaluate for stenotic lesions along the venous outlet track or central circulation.

The major complications of this procedure are vessel extravasations and rupture of the vessel after the angioplasty. Pulmonary embolism is generally of greater concern with AV fistula thrombectomy, as compared with AV graft thrombectomy, due to the larger volume of thrombus. Finally, arterial emboli distal to the arteriovenous anastomosis may occur with higher frequency than for AV grafts.

## NOVEL TECHNIQUES FOR TREATMENT OF SEVERE STENOTIC LESIONS

### CUTTING BALLOON

Despite the use of angioplasty with high-pressure balloons and prolonged inflations, some lesions remain severely stenotic. The use of cutting balloons has been advocated as a tool to treat these lesions by creating a controlled rupture of the vessel wall. The cutting balloon catheter is a balloon with four blades arranged along the balloon. When the balloon is inflated, it exposes the blades to the offending lesion; this will create a controlled rupture of the intima or hyperplastic fibrous tissue. A regular angioplasty balloon can be used afterwards to shape the vessel and expand it to the desired diameter. It has been used in lesions at all levels from intragraft to central lesions. Preliminary reports suggested that cutting balloons may result in superior outcomes as compared with conventional angioplasty.[186,187] In one series of nine patients, grafts with high-grade venous anastomosis stenosis were treated with cutting balloon plus stent deployment.[186] The patients maintained a functional graft during short-term follow-up (up to 20 months in one patient). However, a randomized, multicenter clinical trial comparing use of the cutting balloon with conventional angioplasty for treatment of AV graft stenosis observed no advantage to the cutting balloon.[188] The primary patency at 6 months was 48% in grafts treated with a cutting balloon, as compared with 40% for AV grafts treated with angioplasty.[188] Device-related complications occurred in 5% of the patients in the cutting balloon group (primarily vein rupture or dissection), as compared with none of the patients whose AV grafts were treated with angioplasty alone.[188] The considerable additional cost of cutting balloons is substantial, and precludes their routine use.

### CRYOPLASTY BALLOON

Cryotherapy with the cryo-balloon is a novel therapy for patients with intractable stenoses at the venous anastomosis of AV grafts. This technique utilizes cold temperatures at the balloon site to cause apoptosis of the intima layer. Rifkin et al. reported the outcomes of five patients with recurrent stenotic lesions at the venous anastomosis that were treated with the cryo-balloon.[189] The primary patency increased from 3 weeks after angioplasty alone to more than 16 weeks after cryoplasty. There are no published randomized trials comparing the outcomes of AV graft stenosis treated with cryoplasty compared with angioplasty alone.

### LOCAL PERIVASCULAR MODALITIES

Recent investigations have evaluated prophylaxis of access stenosis in animal models using local perivascular drug delivery to the site of neointimal hyperplasia. Antiproliferative drugs are injected locally during access creation, or introduced by drug-eluting stents or wraps. These novel pharmacologic therapies remain investigational, but offer promise for the future. Detailed discussion of these potential therapies is beyond the scope of this chapter, but this topic has been recently reviewed.[120,190]

## ENDOVASCULAR PROXIMAL FOREARM ARTERIOVENOUS FISTULA FOR HEMODIALYSIS ACCESS

Recently creation of an AV fistula using an endovascular approach has been evaluated in pilot studies.[191] The rationale is that creating an AV fistula using an endovascular approach may reduce vessel trauma and injury, leading to decreased intimal hyperplasia and AV fistula maturation failure. The endovascular approach for AV fistula creation uses a novel magnet-based endovascular technology (endovascular AV fistula [endoAVF]). The technical aspects have been detailed in two publications by Rajan et al.[192] and Lok et al.[193] Early results from a prospective, single-arm, multicenter study (Novel Endovascular Access Trial (NEAT) in 80 patients have demonstrated: (1) successful endovascular AV fistula creation in 98% of participants, (2) 87% physiologic suitability for dialysis (e.g., mean brachial artery flow, 918 mL/min; endoAVF vein diameter, 5.2 mm of cephalic vein), (3) EndoAVF functional usability of 64% in participants who received dialysis, and (4) 12-month primary and cumulative patency of 69% and 84%, respectively.[192]

## CENTRAL VEIN STENOSIS

Central vein stenosis is a frequent occurrence in patients on hemodialysis.[6,194,195] Acute or chronic trauma of the central vessels caused by either temporary or permanent dialysis catheters is the major cause.[196] Stenosis leads to impairment of venous return on the ipsilateral extremity, and may in turn result in malfunction or thrombosis of the vascular access.[197] Although it may be asymptomatic, patients with central vein stenosis most commonly present with ipsilateral upper extremity edema. In some patients, a previously unappreciated central vein stenosis becomes evident clinically following creation of an ipsilateral AV fistula or graft. The diagnosis can be confirmed by angiography, ultrasound, or magnetic resonance venography.

The most commonly encountered location of central vein stenosis is at the junction of the cephalic vein with the subclavian vein (not catheter injury related). Other central veins that may be affected (often related to injury from previous catheters) include the subclavian vein, brachiocephalic vein, and superior vena cava (Fig. 68.21). In patients with tunneled femoral catheters, central vein

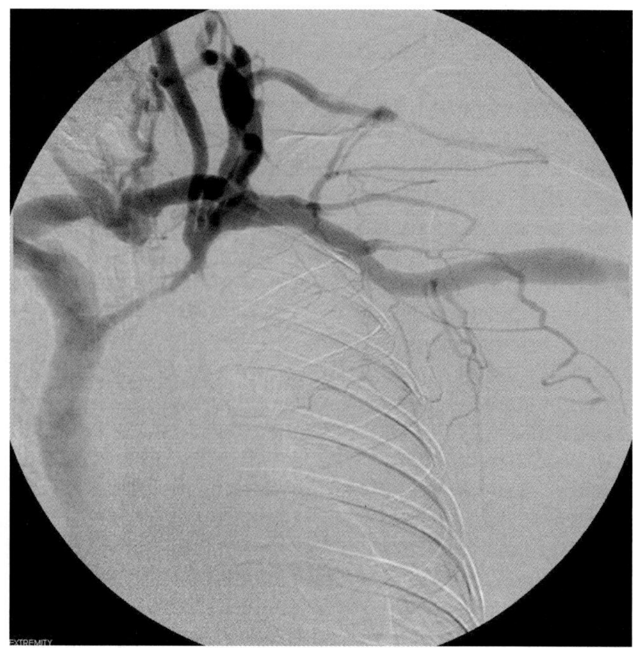

**Fig. 68.21** Digital subtraction angiography showing a severe stenosis of the left innominate vein. There are multiple ipsolateral and across the neck collaterals draining into a normal right innominate vein.

stenosis may occur in the external iliac vein, common iliac vein or inferior vena cava (Fig. 68.22), resulting in ipsilateral lower extremity edema. The stenotic lesion is an aggressive neointimal proliferation, or clot and fibrin sheath formed around an indwelling dialysis catheter that becomes organized and incorporated into the vessel wall. Stenoses may progress over time to complete occlusion of the venous circulation (Fig. 68.23). If left untreated, central vein stenosis will cause increased retrograde pressure and formation of venous collaterals (Fig. 68.24A, 68.24B). In some patients, the collaterals are sufficiently well developed to permit adequate venous drainage that prevents formation of edema (Fig. 68.25A, 68.25B)

The treatment of choice of symptomatic central vein stenosis is PTA of the stenotic lesion.[198–205] Unfortunately, the long-term success of PTA of central venous stensosis is quite poor, due to a combination of elastic recoil and aggressive neointimal hyperplasia. In one study, the primary patency was substantially shorter after angioplasty of central vein

**Fig. 68.22** Digital subtraction angiography showing a severe stenosis of the intrahepatic portion of the inferior vena cava with some intrahepatic collaterals.

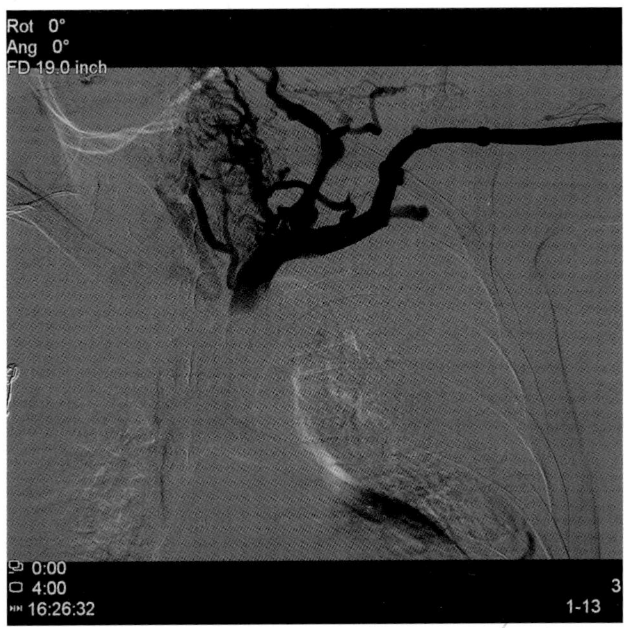


**Fig. 68.23** Digital subtraction angiography showing a complete occlusion of the left innominate vein.

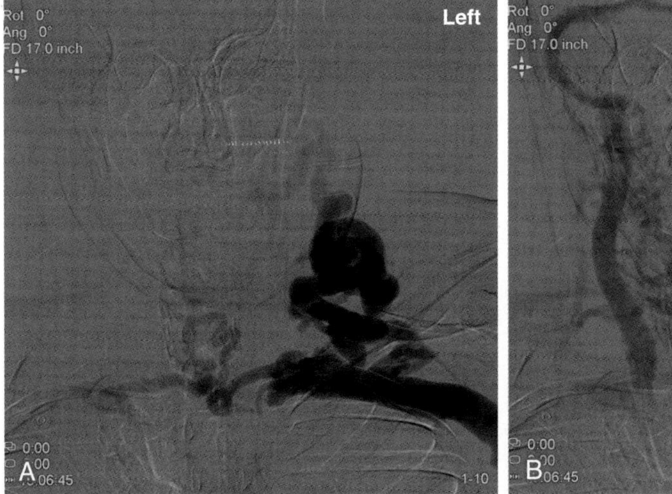


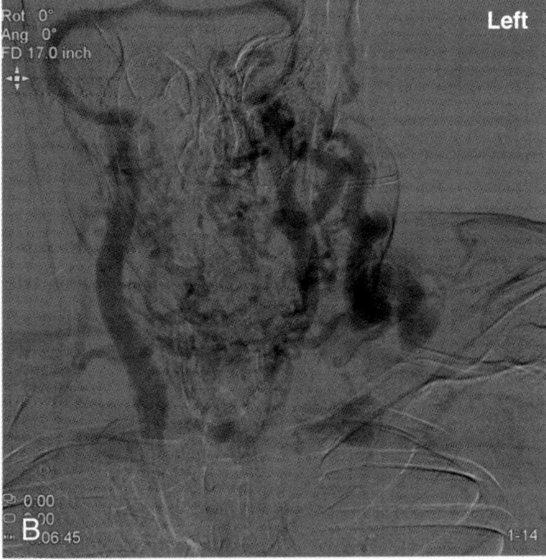


**Fig. 68.24** A, Digital subtraction angiography (DSA) showing a complete occlusion of the left innominate vein with severe enlargement of the left internal jugular and multiple ipsolateral and across the neck collaterals draining into a normal right innominate vein. B, DSA of the same patient showing the drainage of the left internal jugular to the right internal jugular across the cavernous veins.

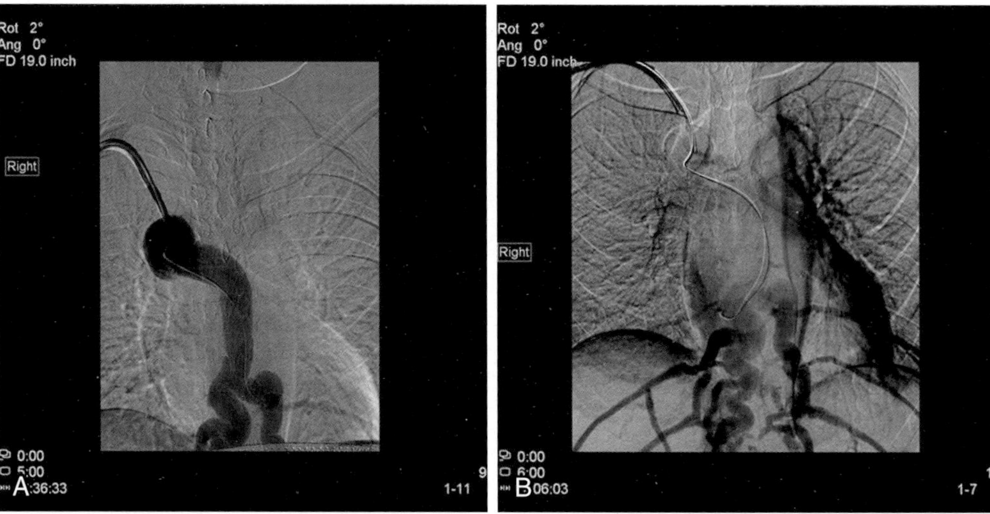


**Fig. 68.25** A, Digital subtraction angiography (DSA) showing a complete occlusion of the superior vena cava with severe augmentation of the Azigos vein. B, DSA of the same patient showing the drainage of the azigos vein into the lumbar and intercostal vein.

stenosis, as compared to stenoses at more peripheral locations.[84] As a result, patients with central vein stenosis may require multiple angioplasties to treat recurrent lesions.

Stent placement has been attempted in the management of refractory central vein stenosis due to elastic recoil (Fig. 68.26A, 68.26B, 68.26C). Several small series have reported the outcomes of stent placement for refractory central venous stenotic lesions. These studies have been limited by their retrospective study design, the small numbers of patients, and the absence of a control group. In two uncontrolled series, the primary patency following stent deployment for central vein stenosis was 42% to 50% at 6 months, and only 14% to 17% at 1 year.[198,201] Although there are no published randomized studies comparing stent deployment with angioplasty of central vein stenosis, the primary patency utilizing stents appears no better than that achieved with angioplasty alone.[206] In patients with ipsilateral vascular access and persistent upper extremity edema despite attempted angioplasty, the only recourse may be ligation of the vascular access, creation or placement of a contralateral arteriovenous access, transition to peritoneal dialysis, or urgent kidney transplantation.

## ACCESS-INDUCED HAND ISCHEMIA

The clinical manifestations of access-induced hand ischemia can vary widely, ranging from mild (hand pain) to severe (tissue necrosis with loss of digits). Vascular accesses have a normal retrograde blood flow, which does not cause hand ischemia. There are three recognized mechanisms for access-induced hand ischemia: (1) True arterial steal (with complete retrograde blood flow toward the graft or fistula); (2) Arterial stenosis distal to the arterial anastomosis, and (3) Generalized arterial calcification (most commonly seen in patients with diabetes mellitus) with distal digital occlusions (Fig. 68.27A, 68.27B, 68.27C). Since all three mechanisms may coexist in a single patient, "distal hypoperfusion ischemic syndrome" is the preferred term.[207] Other causes of hand pain, such as carpal tunnel syndrome, arthropathies, diabetic neuropathy, ischemic monomelic neuropathy and reflex sympathetic dystrophy syndrome, should be excluded before making a definitive diagnosis of vascular access-induced hand ischemia.

Physical examination is the most important tool to diagnose access-induced hand ischemia. Pale, cold digits during and between hemodialysis sessions are seen in almost 90% of the cases. There are several additional diagnostic tools including: digital brachial index measurement, digital plethysmography, duplex ultrasound, and transcutaneous oxygen saturation. If these noninvasive tests are suggestive of access-induced hand ischemia, then a complete angiogram of the vascular access, including the feeding artery, should be performed.

Management of access-induced hand ischemia is directed at alleviating the underlying etiology. Treatment options range from angioplasty of the stenosis distal to the anastomosis to ligation of the vascular access. Other interventions that have been successful in relieving the ischemia while maintaining patency of the AV fistula include banding or plication of the AV fistula, graft interposition, and distal revascularization with interval ligation (DRIL).[208]

## INDWELLING HEMODIALYSIS CATHETERS

### NON-TUNNELED TEMPORARY HEMODIALYSIS CATHETERS

Temporary hemodialysis catheters are indicated for acute dialysis treatments. They are made of polyurethane, polyethylene, or polytetrafluoroethylene; they have a double lumen, are semi-rigid, and relatively easy to place in the internal jugular (preferably on the right side), femoral, and rarely subclavian veins. Each site has its advantages and disadvantages, but if they are placed in the femoral vein, the catheter should not stay longer than 72 hours, and the internal jugular vein catheters not longer than 1 week, due to the high risk of bacteremia with longer dwell times.[209] The subclavian vein is usually used only if there is no other access available since it is more difficult and a higher risk puncture (pneumothorax) and there is an increased risk for central venous stenosis

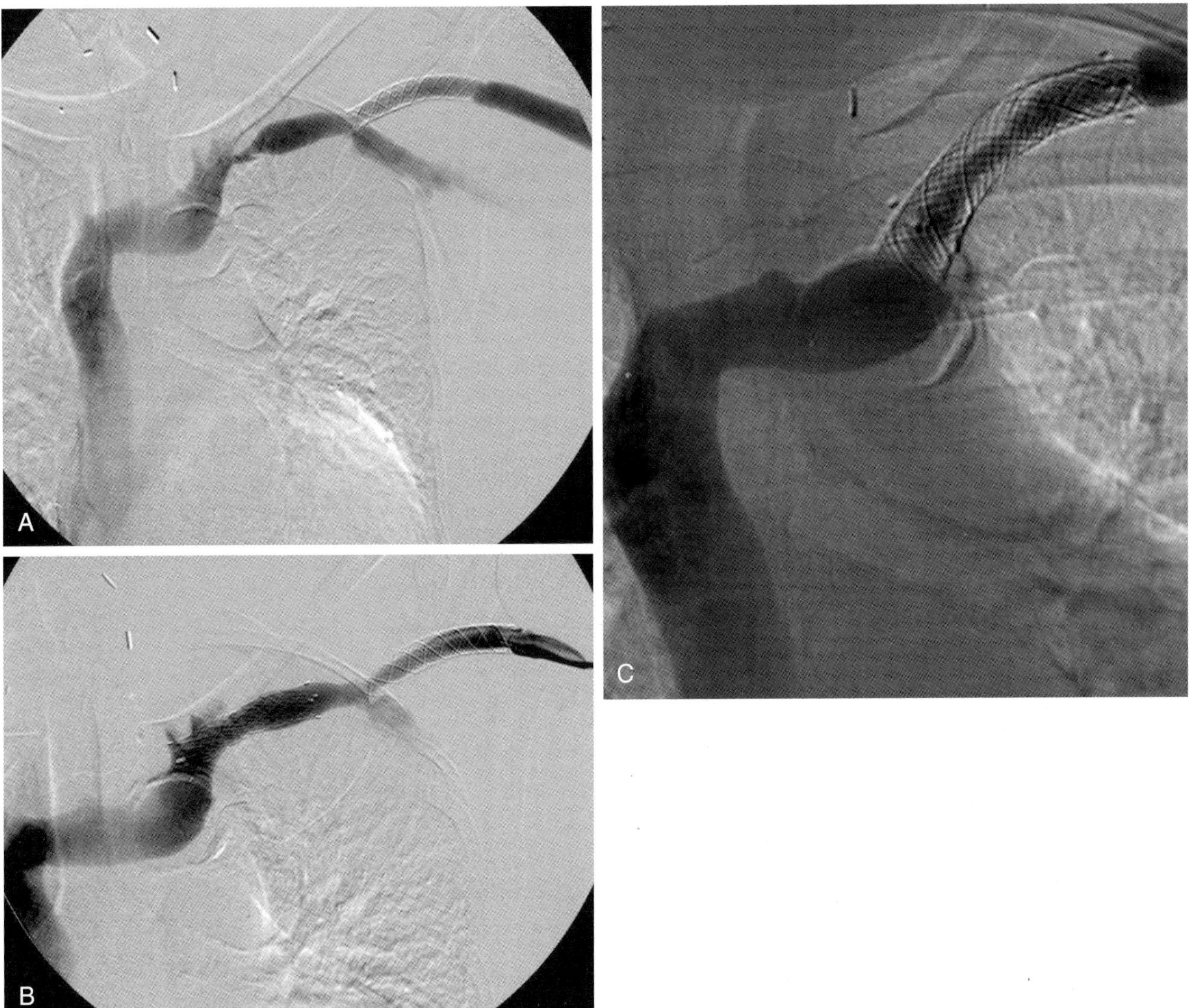


**Fig. 68.26** A, Digital subtraction angiography (DSA) showing a severe stenotic lesion of the left subclavian. There is also a stent in the left cephalic vein. B, DSA showing a stent deployed at the severe stenotic lesion of the left subclavian with excellent initial results. C, DSA taken 12 months after the initial placement of a stent in the left subclavian showing intra-stent stenosis due to significant myointimal hyperplasia.

with occlusion of the subclavian and central vessels, which can compromise creation or placement of future AV fistulas or grafts on the same side.[196] If the upper vessels are used, the catheter should be long enough to have its tip at the junction of the right atrium and superior vena cava; if the femoral vein is used, the catheter's tip should be located in the inferior vena cava. If the patient is expected to remain catheter-dependent for a longer time period, a tunneled catheter should be placed. Temporary hemodialysis catheters can be placed blindly, by ultrasound guidance or by fluoroscopic guidance. A chest radiograph should always be obtained immediately following placement of a central vein dialysis catheter before hemodialysis is initiated to confirm line placement and exclude pneumothorax; it is not needed after placement of a femoral dialysis catheter.

## TECHNICAL PROCEDURE: INSERTION OF TEMPORARY DIALYSIS CATHETERS

The procedure is usually performed at the patient's bedside, but occasionally performed in the interventional suite. The patient must be fully informed of the risks and benefits of the procedure. Strict sterile technique and use of local anesthesia is indicated. Access to the femoral or internal jugular vein may be done either blindly or by real-time ultrasound guidance. Real-time ultrasound is highly recommended, as it decreases the number of attempts at vein cannulation, and minimizes the risk of inadvertent arterial cannulation.

Potential complications at time of placement at the upper vessels include: pneumothorax, vein or arterial perforation, mediastinal or pericardial perforation with possibility of hemothorax and cardiac tamponade, air embolism, and local hematoma with possible extension into the soft subcutaneous tissue of the neck and possible external obstruction of the airways. The long-term complications include development of stenotic lesions along the trajectory of the catheter, which may preclude the use of the ipsilateral limb for future creation of a vascular access. If the patient already has a documented stenotic lesion of the central vessels, placement of an indwelling catheter may cause life-threatening acute central vessel

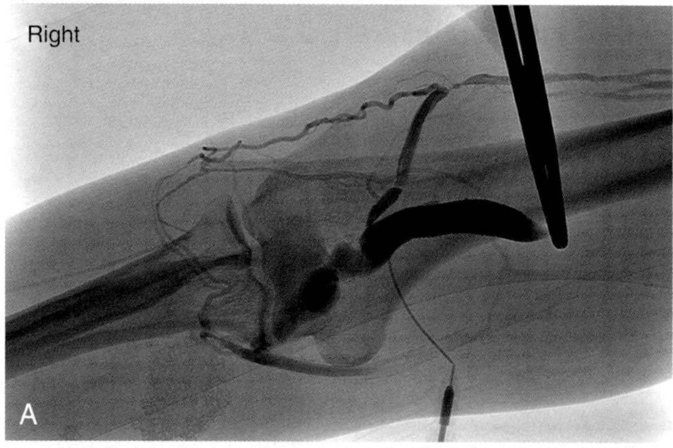


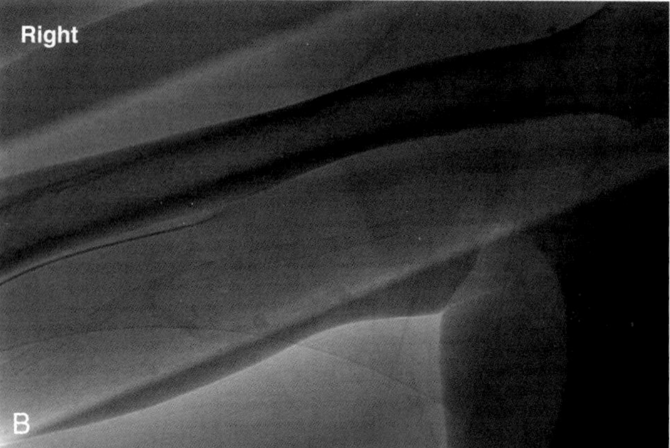


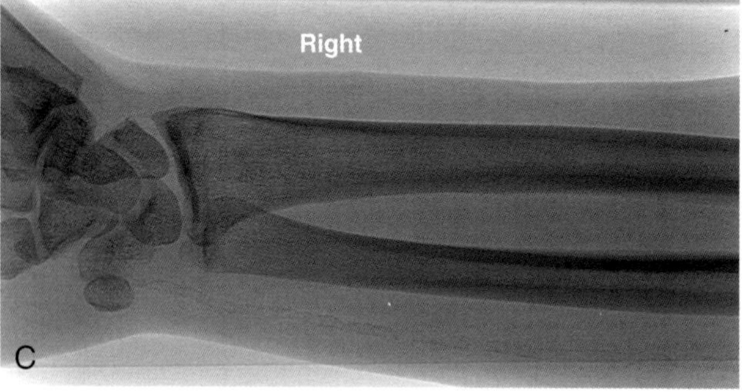


**Fig. 68.27** A, Angiogram of a right upper arm fistula demonstrating an arterial steal syndrome on a patient with generalized arterial disease. B, Spot film of the same patient showing a calcified braquial artery. C, Spot film of the same patient showing a calcified ulnar artery.

occlusion. Exit-site infections and catheter-related bacteremia are frequent complications of temporary dialysis catheters. Development of catheter-related bacteremia requires institution of systemic antibiotics and removal of the non-tunneled dialysis catheter.

The complications at the femoral site are less dramatic, but vein or arterial perforation and formation of arteriovenous fistula are possible. Deep vein thrombosis, (either related to the catheter itself, or immobilization related to prescribed bed rest) local hematomas, exit-site infections, and bacteremia are other important complications.

## TUNNELED HEMODIALYSIS CATHETERS

Tunneled hemodialysis catheters are also commonly used for vascular access in patients waiting for placement or

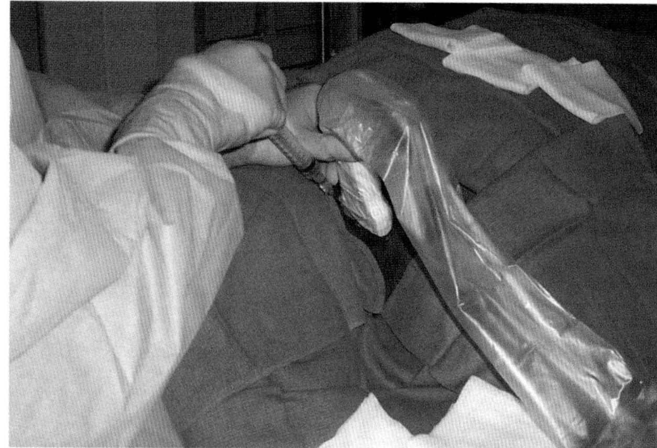

**Fig. 68.28** Access to the right internal jugular vein guided by real-time ultrasound.

maturation of a permanent vascular (AV fistula or graft). They are also required for long-term access in patients who have exhausted all options for placement of a permanent AV access in all four extremities. Tunneled dialysis catheters are usually placed in a central vein in the chest, most commonly through the internal jugular vein, and rarely in the subclavian vein. They have the same characteristics as temporary catheters, but are longer and have a Dacron cuff located in the tunneled portion of the catheter in the subcutaneous tissue. An inflammatory response around the cuff results in scar tissue, creating a mechanical barrier that prevents introduction of infection from the exit site into the bloodstream. As a result, the frequency of catheter-related bacteremia is lower with tunneled dialysis catheters as compared with acute non-tunneled catheters.[210,211]

### TECHNICAL PROCEDURE: INSERTION OF TUNNELED HEMODIALYSIS CATHETERS

Strict sterile technique, topical local anesthesia (1% Xylocaine), and frequently conscious sedation are used. Access to the internal jugular vein is guided by real-time ultrasound (Fig. 68.28). A 21-gauge needle is used for access. A wire is passed down into the IVC under fluoroscopy guidance. A skin pocket of about 1 cm is created at this location. The permanent indwelling hemodialysis catheter is attached to a tunneler device and a tunnel is created lateral, inferior, under the clavicle, approximately 5 to 7 cm from the initial needle insertion. (Fig. 68.29). The tip of the catheter is introduced and fed up to the junction of the superior vena cava and right atrium (Fig. 68.30). The cuff should be 2 cm from the exit site. A final X-ray is taken to assess for kinks of the catheter and for placement (Fig. 68.31). The catheters are 14.5 or 16 French with lengths from 24 cm for right internal jugular, 28 cm for left internal jugular, and from 36 to 42 cm for femoral veins.

Complications at the time of placement are similar to those associated with temporary catheters (Figs. 68.32, 68.33, 68.34, 68.35). Internal jugular thrombosis develops in about 25% of tunneled catheters, but is usually asymptomatic.[212] Other long-term complications include dysfunction due to intraluminal thrombosis or fibrin sheaths, exit-site infections, tunnel infections, and catheter-related bacteremia.[6]

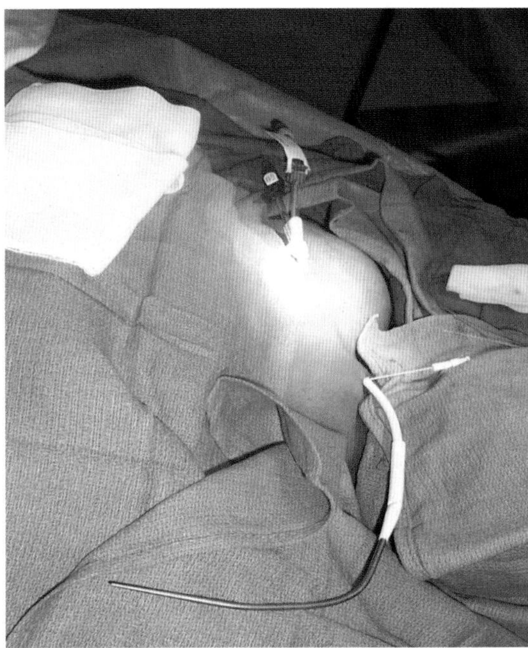

**Fig. 68.29** The catheter has been tunneled from the upper part of the chest to the internal jugular site entrance.

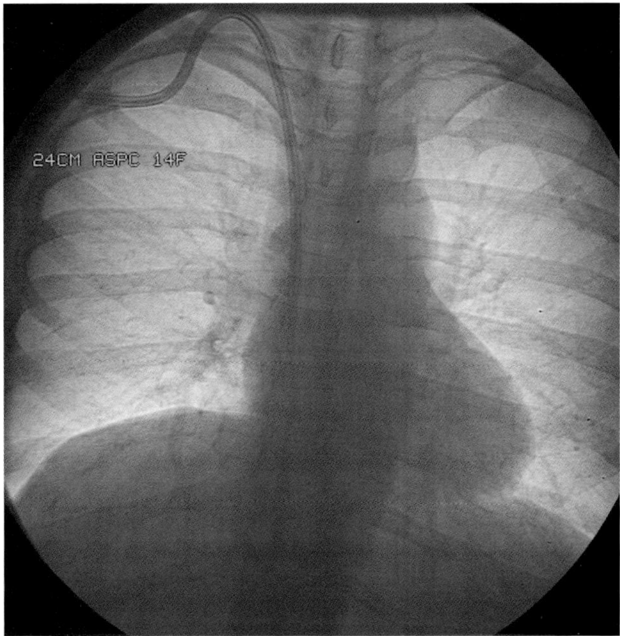


**Fig. 68.31** Spot film of an appropriate placement of a right internal jugular vein tunneled chronic dialysis catheter.

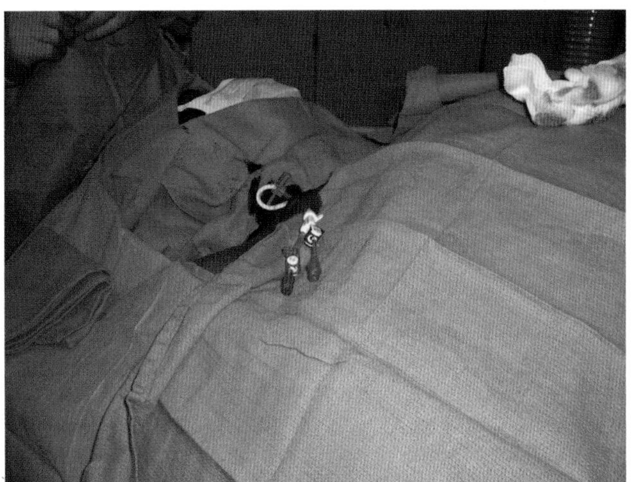

**Fig. 68.30** The catheter is introduced into the opening of the peel-away sheath and fed up to the junction of the superior vena cava and right atrium

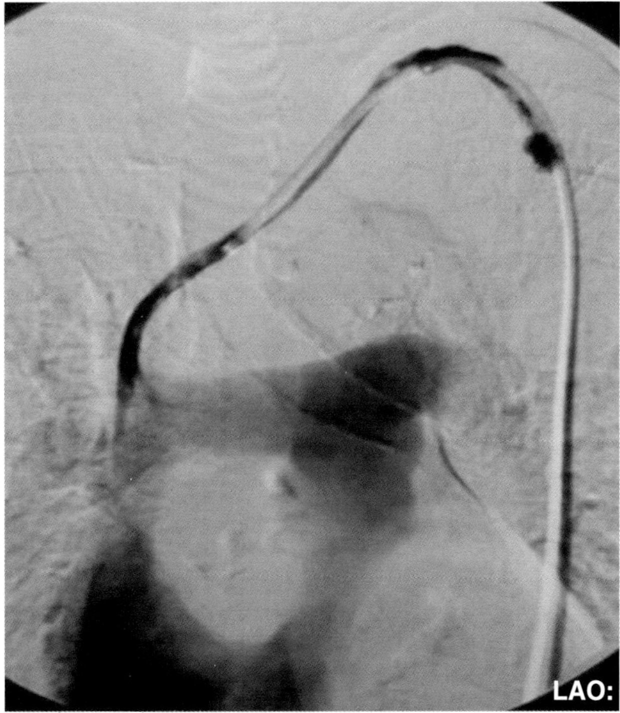


**Fig. 68.32** Tunneled catheter complication: Fibrin sheath around the left internal jugular vein catheter.

Tunneled dialysis catheters can be removed at bedside.[213] Fulop et al. have recently published a bedside procedure of tunneled dialysis catheter removal with safe and successful outcomes, providing a detailed description of supplies and procedure technique.[213] In brief, the precise location of the "cuff" is identified followed by cleansing of catheter exit area and the preparation of the sterile field.[213] Next, the subcutaneous tissue surrounding the dialysis catheter up to the cuff is bluntly dissected with a hemostat clamp in order to achieve mobilization of the dialysis catheter from the surrounding tissue.[213] Once the cuff and dialysis catheter are free from the surrounding connective tissue, the dialysis catheter should be pulled with a measured level of force.[213] Hemostasis should be achieved by applying direct pressure over the proximal *venous puncture* site (and not only the exit site) with a gauze for 10 to 15 minutes until bleeding is not detectable.[213]

## LESS COMMON LOCATIONS FOR TUNNELED HEMODIALYSIS CATHETERS

If prolonged use of upper extremity dialysis catheters leads to bilateral central vein occlusion, it becomes necessary to place

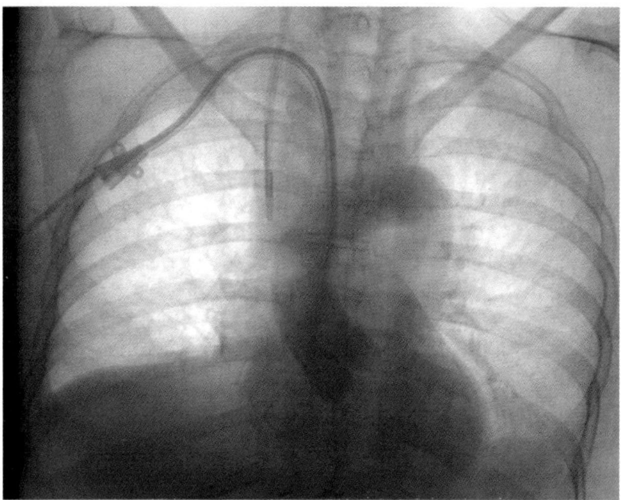

**Fig. 68.33** Tunneled catheter complication: The catheter was placed in the right carotid artery with the tip near the aortic valves. Contrast demonstrates the aortic arch.

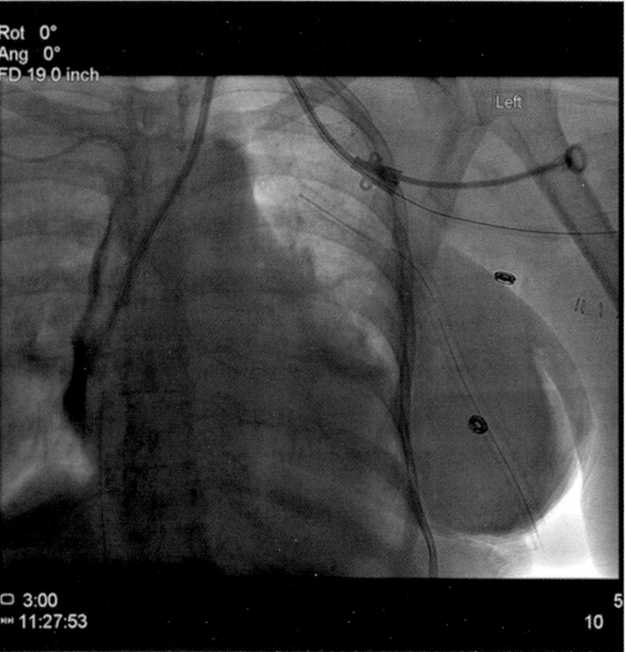


**Fig. 68.34** Tunneled catheter complication: Left internal jugular vein catheter with its tip located in the pericardial sac. Contrast demonstrates the outer lining filling defect that corresponds to the lower part of the adventitia of the superior vena cava and upper part of the pericardium.

a *tunneled catheter in the femoral vein.*[214,215] The procedure for placement of a tunneled femoral catheter is similar to that for a tunneled internal jugular vein catheter, except that a longer (36 to 42 cm) catheter is required, and the catheter tip is placed in either the proximal inferior vena cava or in the right atrium (Fig. 68.36A and 68.36B).[214] The subcutaneous tunnel is created in the anterior upper thigh. The primary patency of tunneled femoral catheters is significantly worse than that of tunneled internal jugular catheters.[214] Presumably, some failures are due to kinking of the catheter in the groin when the thigh is flexed. The frequency of catheter-related

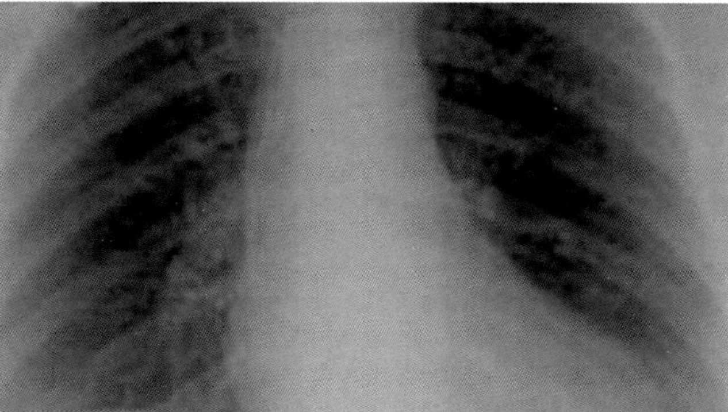

**Fig. 68.35** Tunneled catheter complication: Foreign body (metallic wire) that was left behind after an attempt for a internal jugular vein catheter placement.

bacteremia is similar for patients with femoral and internal jugular dialysis catheters. The likelihood of catheter-related bacteremia is proportional to the duration of catheter use.[197,216] There is high (~25%) frequency of symptomatic ipsilateral deep vein thrombosis after placement of a tunneled femoral catheter.[214] Fortunately, this complication can be treated with long-term anticoagulation, thereby permitting continued use of the catheter. In patients on hemodialysis in whom the central veins in the chest and groin have been exhausted, the placement of tunneled dialysis catheters at unconventional sites (translumbar and transhepatic) has been described. Catheters at these locations should be considered as last-resort options, as they are associated with a substantial risk for complications.

For *translumbar catheters* there are essentially two tunnels. One tunnel extends from the access site in the back toward the IVC and the second from the abdomen to the access site in the back. The patient is placed on the angiography table in a lateral position with his or her left side down. The initial access site is in the right lower back postero-laterally just above the iliac wing. The needle is directed toward the inferior vena cava under fluoroscopy guidance; once venous access is achieved a glide-wire is placed. A tunnel is created from a lower abdominal site approximately 10 cm from the initial needle access around the waist toward the initial needle access. The permanent hemodialysis catheter is advanced through the tunnel and the cuff is buried into the adjacent subcutaneous tissue (Fig. 68.37).[217,218] Dilation followed by peel-away sheath insertion is done from the back access to the IVC. The dialysis catheter is then inserted through the sheath to the IVC, preferably over the glide wire, which is passed in a retrograde fashion all the way through the catheter. The access site is sutured and catheter is secured in place.

Placement of tunneled trans-lumbar hemodialysis catheters requires greater expertise in interventional techniques than jugular or femoral access especially since ultrasound guidance is not possible. The risk of bleeding and retroperitoneal hematoma is considerably higher than that associated with tunneled femoral vein catheters. The most common complication of translumbar catheters in one series of 10 patients is partial dislodgment of the catheters.[218]

Interventional radiologists at some centers have placed *transhepatic catheters*. The right upper quadrant is prepped

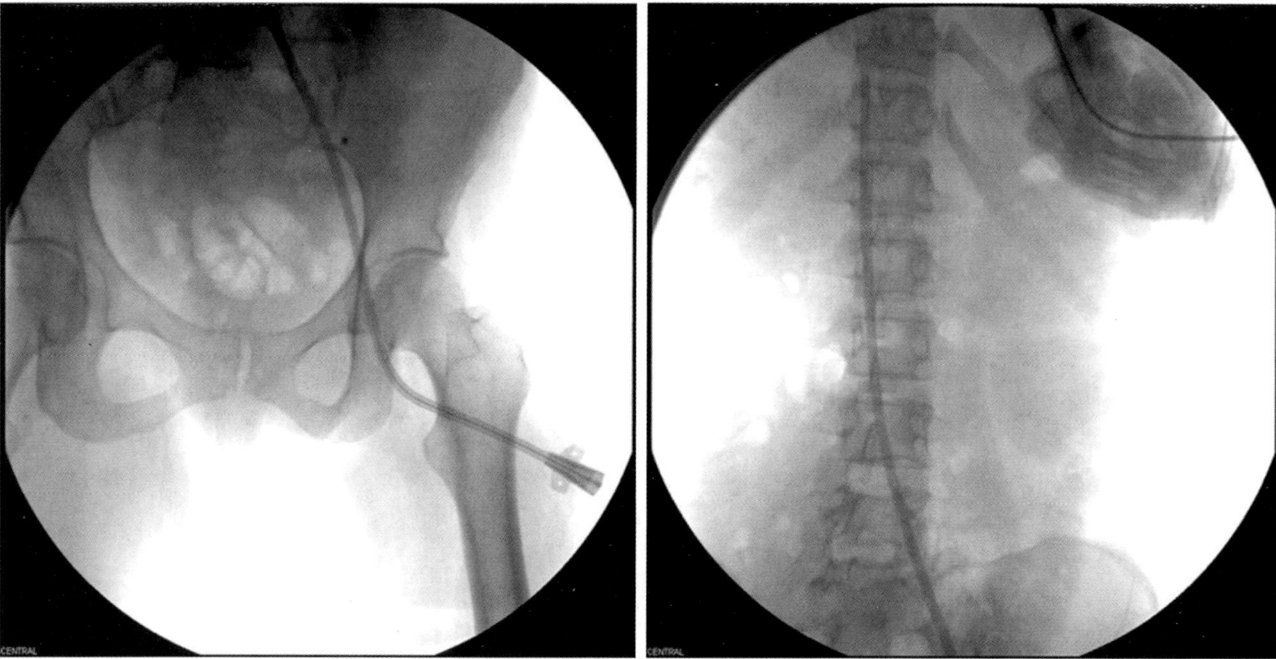

**Fig. 68.36** Spot films of an appropriate placement of a left femoral vein tunneled chronic dialysis catheter.

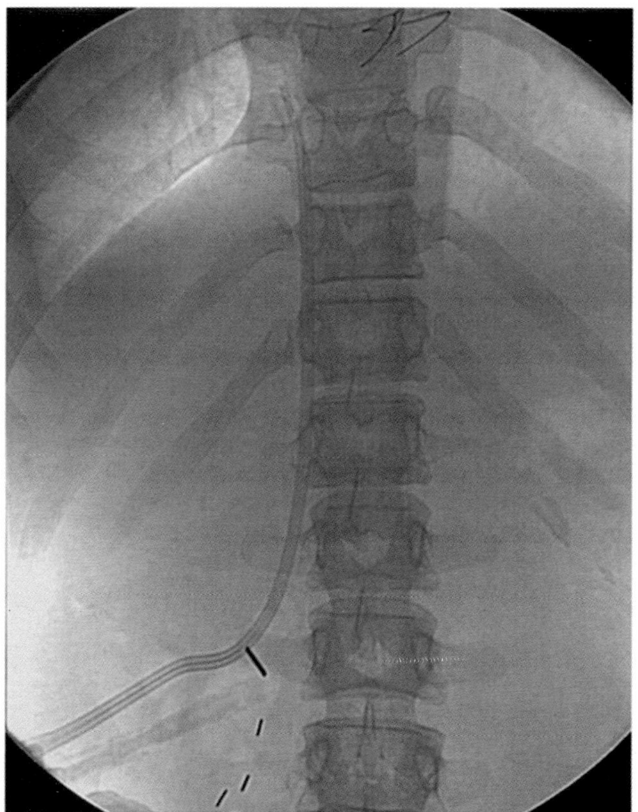

**Fig. 68.37** Spot film of an appropriate placement of a translumbar tunneled chronic dialysis catheter.

and draped in the usual manner; a 21-gauge needle is placed halfway through the liver in a direction parallel to the right of the middle hepatic veins under fluoroscopy guidance, contrast material is injected through the needle and the needle withdrawn until a hepatic vein is visualized. Once a suitable vein is accessed, a guidewire is placed and advanced to the right atrium. A subcutaneous tunnel is created inferiorly to the insertion site and a dual lumen cuffed hemodialysis catheter is placed.[219–221] The major complications are bleeding and peri-hepatic hematoma. Hepatic vein thrombosis is likely, and dislodgment of catheter due to liver excursion movement with breathing is frequent. Stavropoulos et al. reported a series of 36 transhepatic dialysis catheters placed in 12 patients.[220] The mean survival of these catheters was only 24 days. The thrombosis rate was 2.40 per 100 catheter-days, with the poor catheter patency rates being associated with a high rate of late thrombosis.

## EXCHANGE OF TUNNELED HEMODIALYSIS CATHETERS

There are two major indications for catheter exchange: dysfunction and infection. Catheter dysfunction is diagnosed when blood cannot be aspirated from the catheter lumen at the time of dialysis initiation, or more commonly, if it is not possible to consistently achieve a blood flow required to yield sufficient urea and other solute clearance (>250 mL/min). In catheters that were previously delivering an adequate blood flow intraluminal thrombus is the most common etiology for dysfunction, although a fibrin sheath may be the culprit in some patients. This problem is usually treated empirically in the dialysis unit by instilling t-PA into the catheter lumens.[222] Tissue plasminogen activator (tPA) instillation is successful in about 70% to 80% of catheters, but problems with poor flow frequently recur within 2 to 3 weeks. If the thrombolytic agent does not improve the catheter flow, the patient is referred for catheter exchange.

An exit-site infection alone usually resolves with topical antimicrobial agents or oral antibiotics, and is not usually an indication for catheter removal. However, if the patient has a tunnel track infection, catheter removal is mandatory. Catheter-related bacteremia (CRB) is a common indication for catheter replacement.[5] In one series, the cumulative risk of CRB among catheter-dependent patients was 35% at 3 months and 48% at 6 months.[216] Similar risks were observed in a larger prospective study of incident tunneled dialysis catheters.[197] Catheter-related bacteremia is suspected when a catheter-dependent patient experiences fever or chills, and is confirmed by blood cultures from the catheter and a peripheral vein (or the dialysis bloodline) growing the same organism.[5] When a single set of blood cultures is positive, CRB is still the most likely diagnosis, in the absence of clinical evidence of an alternative source of infection.

The clinical management of CRB has evolved in the past few years.[5] In the subset of patients whose fever persists after 48 to 72 hours despite appropriate systemic antibiotics (~10% to 15% of patients with CRB), removal of the infected catheter is mandatory. For the remaining patients, there are several management options. The first option is to continue systemic antibiotics without removal of the infected catheter. Unfortunately, infection is infrequently eradicated with this approach; once the course of systemic antibiotics has been completed, bacteremia recurs in 63% to 78% of patients.[223–227] Moreover, delays in removing an infected catheter may result in metastasic infection, such as endocarditis, septic arthritis, or epidural abscess.[228] The second option is therefore prompt removal of the catheter which removes the source of infection, although this necessitates placement of a temporary (non-tunneled) dialysis catheter, if possible a day or two later to avoid immediate contamination of the new catheter. Once the bacteremia has resolved, a new, tunneled catheter is placed. In an effort to reduce the number of required access procedures, a number of investigators have evaluated the strategy of exchanging the infected catheter for a new one over a guidewire. Several publications have documented the safety and efficacy of this approach.[226,229–232]

In the past few years, there has been a growing recognition of the central role of bacterial biofilms in causing CRB. Biofilms develop on the inner surface of the lumens of central vein catheters in as little as 24 hours, and are relatively refractory to conventional plasma concentrations of antibiotics.[233–235] The third option is instillation of a concentrated antibiotic solution into the catheter lumen after each dialysis session ("antibiotic lock") which can frequently kill the bacteria in the biofilm. This approach can potentially remove the source of the infection (the biofilm), while permitting catheter salvage. The use of antibiotic locks, in conjunction with systemic antibiotics, has been shown to eradicate infection, while salvaging the catheter, in about two thirds of the patients.[5,236–239] This strategy is not associated with an increased risk of metastatic infections, as compared to prompt catheter removal or exchange of the infected catheter over a guidewire. In our experience, implementation of an antibiotic lock protocol has dramatically reduced the frequency of catheter exchanges due to infection. The overall success rate with the addition of an antibiotic lock in conjunction with systemic antibiotics in curing an episode of catheter-related bacteremia is about 70%.[240] However, the success rate varies considerably depending on the bacterial organism, being highest for gram-negative infections, intermediate for *Staphylococcus epidermidis* and *Enterococcus* infections, and lowest for *Staphylococcus aureus* infections.[238,239,241–243] Catheter-related candidemia always requires catheter exchange, in conjunction with antifungal therapy.[244] If fever and/or bacteremia persist despite a trial of an antibiotic lock, the catheter should be removed or exchanged over a guidewire.[5]

Thrombus inside the catheter may act as a nidus for the catheter biofilm. Heparin coating of the catheters may prevent bacterial adherence.[245] Two randomized clinical trials with short-term, non-tunneled central vein catheters found a lower rate of catheter-related bacteremia in patients with heparin-coated catheters than those with non-coated catheters.[245,246] A recent retrospective study observed fewer infections in patients with heparin-coated tunneled dialysis catheters, as compared with those using an uncoated catheter.[247] A randomized clinical trial is needed to confirm this benefit. A recent study by Hemmelgarn et al. reported that instillation of rt-PA instead of heparin into the dialysis catheter lumen once weekly, as compared with the standard use of heparin locks three times a week, significantly reduced the incidence of catheter malfunction and bacteremia,[248] suggesting that rt-PA may prevent thrombosis as well as biofilm development.

## PERITONEAL DIALYSIS CATHETER PROCEDURES

Peritoneal dialysis (PD) is an alternative to hemodialysis in patients with ESKD. Although it is widely used in many countries, fewer than 10% of the US dialysis population is treated by this modality.[249] Peritoneal catheters can be placed into the abdominal cavity by surgeons,[250–252] interventional radiologists,[253] or interventional nephrologists.[254] There are several techniques: blind (Seldinger) technique,[255] surgical placement,[250] peritoneoscopic,[256] laparoscopic,[257] Moncrief-Popovich technique,[258] and fluoroscopic insertion.[254] Incorporation of PD catheter placement in an established interventional nephrology program increases the utilization of this dialysis modality.[259] A modified fluoroscopic technique, which adds real-time ultrasound visualization, avoids the risk of inadvertent epigastric artery injury.[260]

Peritoneal catheters are made of either silicone rubber or polyurethane. The Tenckhoff catheter is still the most common type of PD catheter placed. The intraperitoneal portion of the catheter can be either straight, coiled, Ash (T-Fluted), or with a silicone disc.[261] The extraperitoneal portion of the catheter may be straight or have a swan-neck design with single or double inner cuffs, or a combination of a single cuff and a silicone disc. The most widely used PD catheter is the double cuff, swan neck, coiled Tenckhoff design. This design has been shown to decrease mechanical complications, i.e., inflow and outflow problems. The coiled catheter design also decreases pain during infusion, and is less likely to migrate. The swan-neck design was introduced to avoid cuff extrusions.[262] The intraperitoneal portion of the catheter should be placed between the visceral and parietal peritoneum near the pouch of Douglas. The inner cuff should be inserted in the abdominal wall musculature (rectus muscle) to prevent leaks. The outer cuff should be located in the subcutaneous tissue to create a dead space in between the two cuffs, which it is believed would prevent migration of infections coming from the exit site. The subcutaneous tract and exit site should face downward and laterally to avoid exit-site infection. The exit site should be determined and marked prior to the insertion while the patient is in the upright position. The beltline, prior surgical sites and the abdominal midline should be avoided. Postoperative catheter care is very important. The catheter should be covered with a nonocclusive dressing, and should not to be used for 10 to 14 days. The catheter should be flushed at least two or three times per week with saline or dialysate solution until the patient is ready to start PD.[263] Usually PD is started between 2 to 4 weeks after placement of the catheter, to allow for wound healing, and securing of the catheter cuff. Providing sufficient time for healing helps to avoid leaks, which can increase the risk of infection and are discouraging to patients. Low-volume PD may be attempted within 24 hours of catheter placement, if no other dialysis access is available and an urgent start is required.[264]

Two studies comparing swan-neck and straight Tenckhoff catheters have shown a similar risk for peritonitis and exit infection, but less cuff extrusion with the swan-neck design. The lower incidence of cuff extrusion enhances the survival of the swan-neck catheters.[265–267] A modified technique, which places the swan-neck catheter in a presternal exit-site location, has been reported by Twardowski et al. and has shown an increase in access survival up to 95% at 2 years. The presternal exit-site modification has been shown to decrease the incidence of peritonitis as well as exit-site infection. The authors advocate the use of the presternal catheters in obese patients, patients with ostomies, and children wearing diapers and/or with fecal incontinence.[268,269] Gadallah et al. demonstrated that placement of PD catheters by peritoneoscopic approach had a longer survival rate (survival defined as inflow/outflow obstruction, persistent dialysate leak and persistent peritonitis, or exit-site/tunnel infection requiring catheter removal) than those placed surgically, and that the rates of exit infection and leak were lower.[270] Moncrief et al. described a technique in which the extraperitoneal portion of the catheter is buried in the abdominal subcutaneous tissue until the patient is ready for PD. It appears that the Montcrief modification may lower the risk of initial infection of the tract.[258]

A major complication during placement of the PD catheter is bowel perforation. It is infrequent with all techniques except for blind placement, but once identified it requires bowel rest, intravenous (IV) antibiotic therapy, and rarely surgical exploration.[250,259] Tip migration is a very common (up to 35%) late complication, which could cause problems with draining of the PD fluid. It can be fixed with either radiologic or surgical manipulation.[271,272] PD leaks around the catheter have been reported as high as 10%.[273] Perioperative infection and bleeding are very rare, as prophylactic antibiotics are usually given.[272]

### TECHNICAL PROCEDURE: INSERTION OF PERITONEAL CATHETERS BY FLUOROSCOPIC AND ULTRASOUND TECHNIQUE[274]

The abdomen is prepped and draped in a sterile fashion. Conscious sedation is administered with midazolam hydrochloride and fentanyl citrate in many facilities with these capabilities. A registered nurse obtains vital signs and administers conscious sedation during the procedure. The insertion site is selected to be 2 cm to the left or right and below the umbilicus. An ultrasound machine with a 5 to 12 MHz transducer and a sterile cover is used to guide a 21-guage needle into the peritoneum. Under ultrasound guidance the needle penetrates through the skin, the subcutaneous tissue, the outer fascia of rectus muscle, the muscle fibers, the inner fascia, and the parietal layer of peritoneum. Three to 5 mL of radiocontrast are injected into the peritoneal cavity under fluoroscopy to assure appropriate location: a radiologic pattern of outer bowel delineation is indicative of a good placement. A 0.018-inch cope-mandrel-wire is introduced through the needle. The needle is exchanged for a 6-French catheter sheath. A 2-cm incision is made on the skin and the subcutaneous tissue is digitally dissected up to the rectus muscle. A series of dilators (8-, 12-, and 14-French) are passed over a stiff glide-wire, and an 18-French peel-away sheath is placed. A double-cuff, swan-neck, Tenckhoff peritoneal dialysis catheter is introduced over the stiff glide-wire into the peritoneal cavity. The coiled intraperitoneal portion is placed in the lower intraabdominal area. The inner cuff is pushed into the muscle before removing the peel-away sheath. Alternatively, the tunnel can be created before catheter insertion into the peritoneum. A tunnel is created with an exit site located distal, lateral, and below the initial incision with the outer cuff buried in the subcutaneous tissue. A final fluoroscopic imaging is performed to verify placement of the Tenckhoff catheter (Fig. 68.38A, 68.38B, 68.38C). Inflow and outflow of the PD catheter is tested with 500 mL of normal saline. The PD catheter is flushed with 10 to 15 mL of heparin. The subcutaneous tissue and skin are sutured, and the site is dressed.

### TECHNICAL PROCEDURE: INSERTION OF PERITONEAL CATHETERS BY PERITONEOSCOPIC TECHNIQUE

Peritoneal catheters placed peritoneoscopically are implanted through the rectus muscle using the Y-TEC technique. It has the same initial preparation as for the fluoroscopic/ultrasound technique. Under local anesthesia, a 2-cm skin incision is made. The subcutaneous tissue is dissected up to the rectus muscle. A catheter guide is inserted into the abdomen and the Y-TEC peritoneoscope into the catheter to assess initial entry to the peritoneal cavity. The scope is removed and 500 mL of air infused into the cavity. The scope is again replaced and advanced to the pelvic area. This area is inspected for adhesions and bowel loops. The scope is again removed and the peritoneal catheter is introduced through the catheter with the help of a stainless steel stylette. The catheter is advanced to the pelvic area. The stylette is removed and the inner cuff is buried into the musculature. The exit location is determined and the catheter is tunneled to that location.

### TECHNICAL PROCEDURE: INSERTION OF PERITONEAL CATHETERS BY PRESTERNAL CATHETER PLACEMENT

The peritoneal catheter implantation technique is the same as the peritoneoscopic insertion, except that the PD catheter has a straight design instead of a swan neck. After the PD catheter is placed, then a second catheter is tunneled from the midabdomen up to the chest wall. The two catheters are connected by a titanium joint piece. The second catheter has the swan-neck design and two cuffs. The exit site is located lateral to the mid-sternal line.

## PERCUTANEOUS KIDNEY BIOPSY (SEE ALSO CHAPTER 26)

A percutaneous kidney biopsy is an important procedure in the diagnosis of acute and chronic kidney disease. The results

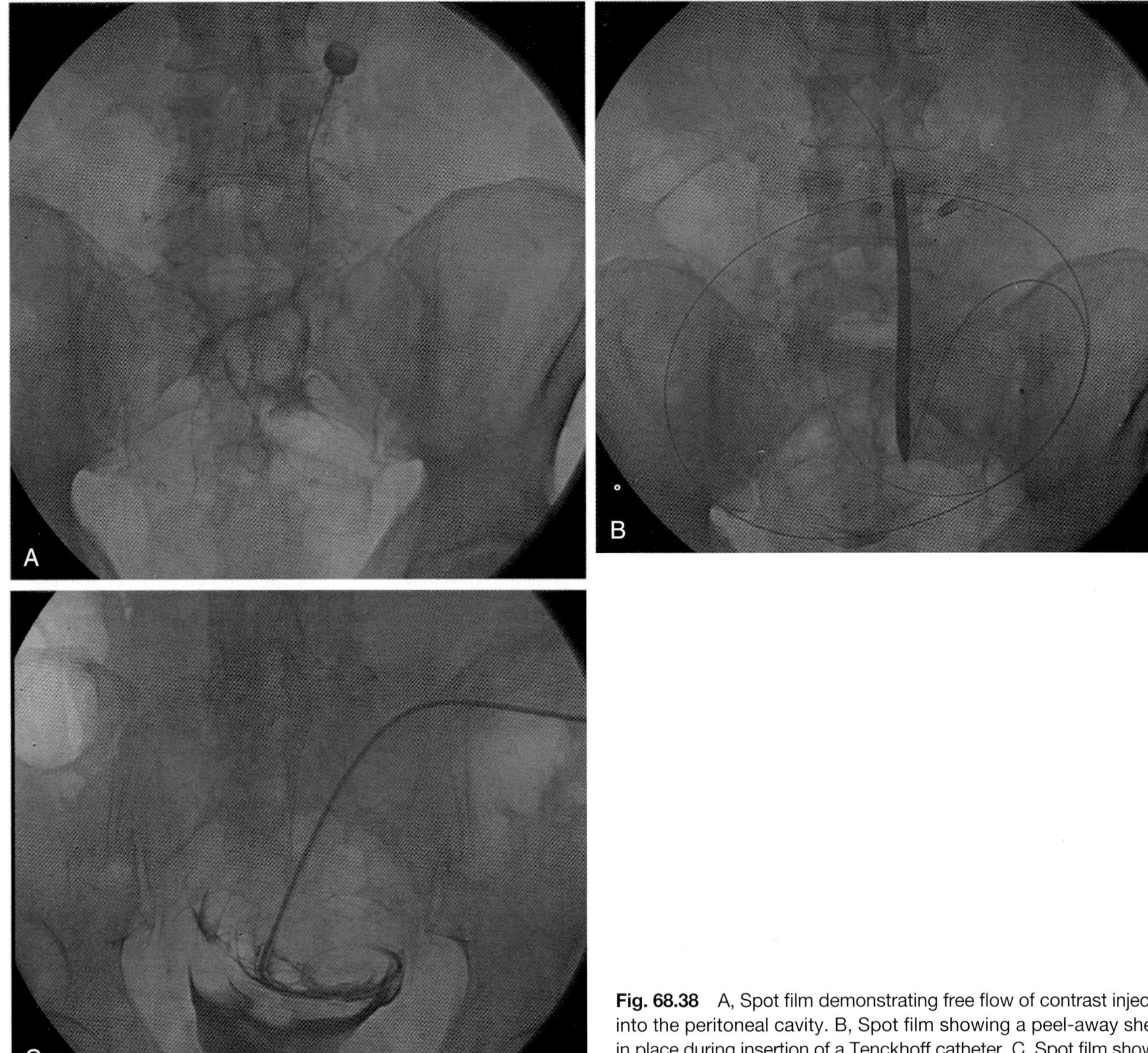


**Fig. 68.38** A, Spot film demonstrating free flow of contrast injection into the peritoneal cavity. B, Spot film showing a peel-away sheath in place during insertion of a Tenckhoff catheter. C, Spot film showing appropriate placement of a Tenckhoff catheter.

of a kidney biopsy are helpful in guiding medical therapy and providing a prognosis. The goal of a kidney biopsy should be to maximize the yield of adequate tissue while minimizing the risk of complications. Percutaneous kidney biopsies have evolved from a blind procedure to a real-time ultrasound-guided needle biopsy. At some institutions, radiologists perform kidney biopsies under ultrasound or CT guidance. Although some nephrologists still use the Franklin-Silverman needle and the Tru-cut needle for blind biopsy, several authors have documented that the use of real-time guided ultrasonography along with the use of an automatic biopsy gun minimizes complications and provides a high yield of adequate tissue for pathologic diagnosis (Table 68.13).[275–282] Cozens et al. retrospectively compared a 15-gauge Tru-cut renal biopsy with ultrasound localization and marking to use of an 18-gauge spring-loaded gun renal biopsy under real-time ultrasound guidance. They reported a 79% yield of adequate renal tissue with the blind technique (15 gauge), as compared with 93% with real-time ultrasound guidance (18 gauge).[280] Similarly, two other studies reported a higher mean number of glomeruli from biopsies obtained under real-time ultrasound, as compared to those performed blindly.[279,281]

Major complications of kidney biopsies, including gross hematuria or retroperitoneal hematoma requiring blood transfusion, invasive procedure, or surgical intervention have been reported in less than 1% of biopsies in some series, and 5% to 6% in others (Table 68.13). The likelihood of major complications was not associated with patient age, blood pressure, or serum creatinine in one large series.[281] Among those patients with major complications, the time interval from biopsy to diagnosis of the complication was ≤ 4 hours in 52%, ≤ 8 hours in 79%, and ≤ 12 hours in 100% of patients.[281] A recent prospective study of 100 consecutive patients showed that outpatient, real-time, ultrasound-guided percutaneous renal biopsy is safe and minimizes the need for post-biopsy hospitalization.[281] Minor complications, including transient gross hematuria or perinephric hematoma not requiring transfusion or intervention, occurred after 6.6% of biopsies in one series.[281] Either ultrasound or computerized tomography can be used to diagnose perinephric hematomas.[283] Most hematomas resolve spontaneously within a few weeks with no significant sequelae. Major bleeding complications that do not resolve with conservative measures require further intervention. In the past, this entailed urgent surgical nephrectomy. However, selective renal arteriogram with embolization of the bleeding arteriole is often able to stop the bleeding in most cases. A review article reported major complications in only 0.3% of cases, with death in fewer than 0.1% among 9595 percutaneous kidney biopsies performed over the last 50 years.[284]

For patients at high risk of bleeding complications or liver disease with coagulopathy in whom a kidney biopsy is indicated, a transjugular kidney biopsy may be performed by an interventional radiologist or nephrologist. Thompson et al. reported 91% adequate tissue retrieval with an average of nine glomeruli for light microscopy in 23 patients undergoing transjugular renal biopsy.[285] A capsular perforation was encountered in 17 (74%) patients, of whom six (26%) required coil embolization of the bleeding vessel. Two major complications were reported, one arterio-calyceal system fistula and one renal vein thrombosis six days after the biopsy.[285] Abbott et al. reported a series of nine patients undergoing transjugular renal biopsy.[286] Adequate tissue was obtained from all patients. Capsular perforation occurred in 90% of the patients, and two patients developed gross hematuria requiring transfusion.[286] The very high rate of capsular perforation casts real doubts on any advantage of transjugular over percutaneous kidney biopsy.

A bleeding disorder is an absolute contraindication to performing a percutaneous kidney biopsy. However, if it can be corrected medically, and if the potential benefit of doing a biopsy outweighs the potential risk, the biopsy can still be performed. Relative contraindications to kidney biopsy include a solitary kidney, pyelonephritis, perinephric abscess, uncontrolled hypertension, hydronephrosis, polycystic kidney disease, severe anemia, pregnancy, renal masses, and renal artery aneurysms.

**Table 68.13 Adequacy of Kidney Tissue Retrieval and Complications by Real-Time Ultrasound-Guided Percutaneous Renal Biopsy**

| Reference | Number of Biopsies | Adequate Tissue | Major Complications[a] |
|---|---|---|---|
| Dowd, 1991[275] | 23 | 95.5% | <0.5% |
| Doyle, 1994[276] | 86 | 99% | 0.8% |
| Hergesell, 1998[277] | 1090 | 98.8% | <0.5% |
| Donovan, 1991[278] | 192 | 97.8% | <1% |
| Burstein, 1993[279] | 200 | 97.5% | 5.6% |
| Cozens, 1992[280] | | 93% | N/A |
| Marwah, 1996[281] | 394 | | 6.6% |
| Maya, 2007[282] | 65 | 100% | 0% |

[a]Definitions of major complications differed among studies.

## TECHNICAL PROCEDURE: PERCUTANEOUS KIDNEY BIOPSY UNDER REAL-TIME ULTRASOUND GUIDANCE

A complete blood count, prothrombin time, and partial thromboplastin time are checked before the procedure, as well if the patient is taking medications such as antiplatelet agents, anticoagulants, and nonsteroidal antiinflammatory agents. The patient is taken to the ultrasound suite and placed in the prone position. An initial ultrasound examination is performed to confirm the presence of two kidneys. Sterile technique is observed and sterile cover placed over the ultrasound probe. The lower pole of the left kidney is preferred for right-handed operators. The skin and subcutaneous tissue are anesthetized with 1% lidocaine Under real-time ultrasound guidance, a biopsy needle gun is advanced up to the capsule of the kidney (Fig. 68.39A, 68.39B). The patient is asked to hold his breath, and the spring-loaded gun is activated. The gun is retrieved and the specimen placed in a container with media. There are different types of needle biopsy guns: full-core, half-core, or ¾ of a core. Sizes vary

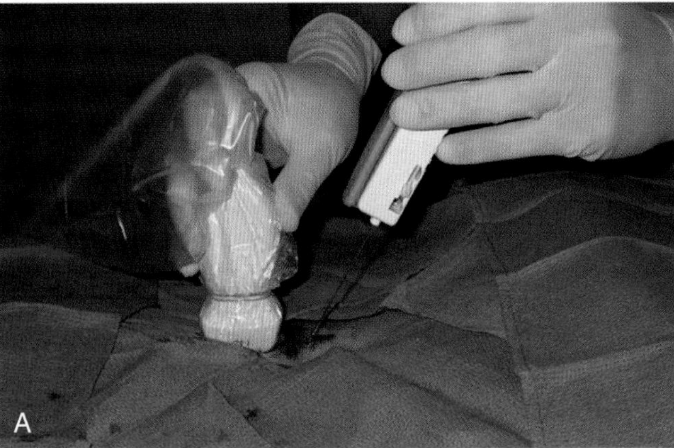


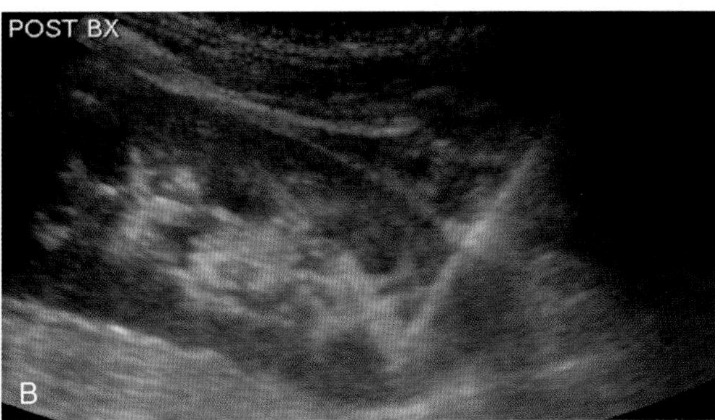


**Fig. 68.39** A, Operator showing the technique of a real-time ultrasound kidney biopsy. B, Kidney ultrasound image showing a biopsy needle located at the lower pole of the kidney.

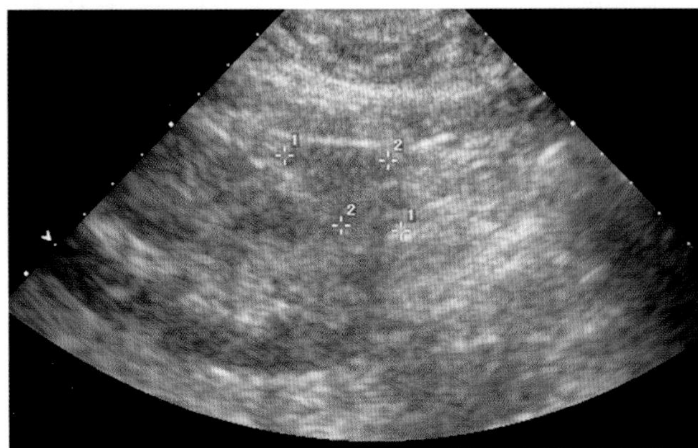

**Fig. 68.40** Post-biopsy kidney ultrasound image of a perinephric hematoma. The markers show the size if the perinephric hematoma as a complication of a kidney biopsy.

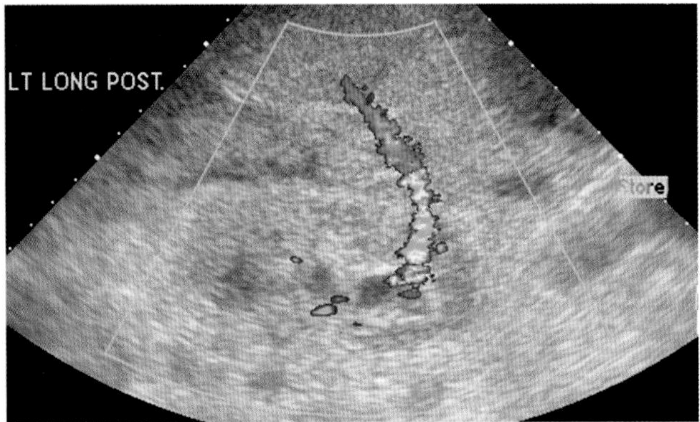


**Fig. 68.41** Post-biopsy kidney color Doppler ultrasound image showing active bleeding.

from 14 French to 18 French and lengths from 10 cm to 20 cm. Also, the throw (amount of tissue that the gun can obtain) of the device can be adjusted from 13 mm to 33 mm. Usually two or three biopsy samples are taken in one setting to provide enough tissue for light microscopy, immunofluorescence, and electron microscopy studies. After the biopsy is completed, a second-look ultrasound examination is performed to assess for perinephric hematomas (Fig. 68.40). A color Doppler ultrasound post-biopsy surveillance imaging examination is helpful to localize any active bleeding (Fig. 68.41). The patient remains on bedrest for 4 to 6 hours and vital signs are obtained frequently in the first hour and then hourly over 4 to 6 hours. Hematocrits are checked every 6 hours for the next 24 hours. However, some centers may have protocols for same-day observation and discharge may not need observation for 24 hours.

## RADIATION AND PERSONAL SAFETY

The understanding of basic radiation safety is very important to protect the patient, physician, and staff involved in the care of the patient in interventional nephrology. Unnecessary radiation exposure is harmful and can be easily prevented. The Food and Drug Administration (FDA) oversees the rules and regulations for use of X-ray equipment. The Occupational Safety and Health Administration (OSHA) regulates the radiation exposure of workers. Each state has its own regulatory office to ensure that workers do not exceed a predetermined radiation dose.

Exposure is the amount of ionizing radiation reaching a subject, and is measured in units of Roentgen. The amount of energy absorbed by a material when it is exposed to ionizing radiation is measured in Rads. The absorbed dose is always lower than the exposure, because the tissue does not absorb all the energy from the radiation. An absorbed dose equivalent is used to relate the amount of biological damage and is measured in Rem. The OSHA occupational dose limit for the whole body is 1.25 Rem/quarter; for the extremities it is 18.75 Rem/quarter. A dosimeter must be worn at all times on the outside of the lead apron, and the absorbed dose measured monthly. To protect against radiation the interventionist should minimize the time of exposure to radiation, minimize the use of magnification imaging, properly use collimators and field filters, maximize the distance between the source of radiation and personnel involved with the procedure, minimize the use of cineangiography and continuous fluoroscopy, and use proper shielding, including lead aprons, thyroid collars, leaded glasses, and lead shields.

Knowledge of these facts and application of appropriate safeguards is particularly important in hemodialysis access procedures, especially those involving vascular access interventions in the upper extremity. The operators' proximity to the x-ray tube and difficulty in shielding increases their radiation exposure.

 Complete reference list available at ExpertConsult.com.

## KEY REFERENCES


4. Robbin ML, Chamberlain NE, Lockhart ME, et al. Hemodialysis arteriovenous fistula maturity: US evaluation. *Radiology*. 2002;225:59–64.
7. Allon M, Daugirdas JT, Depner TA, et al. Effect of change in vascular access on patient mortality in hemodialysis patients. *Am J Kidney Dis*. 2006;47:469–477.
10. Clinical practice guidelines for vascular access. *Am J Kidney Dis*. 2006;48:S176–S273.
19. Mishler R, Sands JJ, Osfsthun NJ, et al. Dedicated outpatient vascular access center decreses hospitalization and missed outpatient dialysis treatments. *Kidney Int*. 2006;69:393–398.
22. Beathard GA, Urbanes A, Litchfield T. Changes in the Profile of Endovascular Procedures Performed in Freestanding Dialysis Access Centers over 15 Years. *Clin J Am Soc Nephrol*. 2017;12(5):779–786.
35. Allon M, Robbin ML. Increasing arteriovenous fistulas in hemodialysis patients: problems and solutions. *Kidney Int*. 2002;62:1109–1124.
36. Thamer M, Lee TC, Wasse H, et al. Medicare costs associated with arteriovenous fistulas among US hemodialysis patients. *Am J Kidney Dis*. 2018;72:10–18.
37. Schwab SJ. Vascular access for hemodialysis. *Kidney Int*. 1999;55:2078–2090.
39. Dember LM, Beck GJ, Allon M, et al. Effect of clopidogrel on early failure of arteriovenous fistulas for hemodialysis: a randomized controlled trial. *JAMA*. 2008;299(18):2164–2171.
41. Lee T, Misra S. New insights into dialysis vascular access: molecular targets in arteriovenous fistula and arteriovenous graft failure and their potential to improve vascular access outcomes. *Clin J Am Soc Nephrol*. 2016;11(8):1504–1512.
48. Alpers CE, Imrey PB, Hudkins KL, et al. Histopathology of veins obtained at hemodialysis arteriovenous fistula creation surgery. *J Am Soc Nephrol*. 2017;28(10):3076–3088.
56. Roy-Chaudhury P, Arend L, Zhang J, et al. Neointimal hyperplasia in early arteriovenous fistula failure. *Am J Kidney Dis*. 2007;50(5):782–790.

58. Roy-Chaudhury P, Sukhatme VP, Cheung AK. Hemodialysis vascular access dysfunction: a cellular and molecular viewpoint. *J Am Soc Nephrol.* 2006;17(4):1112–1127.
61. Lee T. Novel paradigms for dialysis vascular access: downstream vascular biology–is there a final common pathway? *Clin J Am Soc Nephrol.* 2013;8(12):2194–2201.
62. Rothuizen TC, Wong C, Quax PH, et al. Arteriovenous access failure: more than just intimal hyperplasia? *Nephrol Dial Transplant.* 2013;28(5):1085–1092.
63. Roy-Chaudhury P, Kelly BS, Miller MA, et al. Venous neointimal hyperplasia in polytetrafluoroethylene dialysis grafts. *Kidney Int.* 2001;59(6):2325–2334.
65. Robbin ML, Gallichio ML, Deierhoi MH, et al. US vascular mapping before hemodialysis access placement. *Radiology.* 2000;217:83–88.
66. Allon M, Lockhart ME, Lilly RZ, et al. Effect of preoperative sonographic mapping on vascular access outcomes in hemodialysis patients. *Kidney Int.* 2001;60:2013–2020.
84. Beathard GA. Percutaneous transvenous angioplasty in the treatment of vascular access stenosis. *Kidney Int.* 1992;42(6):1390–1397.
88. Robbin ML, Oser RF, Allon M, et al. Hemodialysis access graft stenosis: US detection. *Radiology.* 1998;208(3):655–661.
89. Robbin ML, Oser RF, Lee JY, et al. Randomized comparison of ultrasound surveillance and clinical monitoring on arteriovenous graft outcomes. *Kidney Int.* 2006;69(4):730–735.
101. Malik J, Slavikova M, Svobodova J, et al. Regular ultrasonographic screening significantly prolongs patency of PTFE grafts. *Kidney Int.* 2005;67(4):1554–1558.
102. Tonelli M, James M, Wiebe N, et al. Ultrasound monitoring to detect access stenosis in hemodialysis patients: a systematic review. *Am J Kidney Dis.* 2008;51:630–640.
105. Allon M, Robbin ML. Hemodialysis vascular access monitoring: current concepts. *Hemodial Int.* 2009;13:153–162.
106. Paulson WD, Moist L, Lok CE. Vascular access surveillance: an ongoing controversy. *Kidney Int.* 2012;81(2):132–142.
110. Dixon BS, Beck GJ, Vazquez MA, et al. Effect of dipyridamole plus aspirin on hemodialysis graft patency. *N Engl J Med.* 2009;360:2191–2201.
112. Trerotola SO, Lawson J, Roy-Chaudhury P, et al; Lutonix AV Clinical Trial Investigators. Drug coated balloon angioplasty in failing AV fistulas: a randomized controlled trial. *Clin J Am Soc Nephrol.* 2018;13(8):1215–1224.
114. Haskal ZJ, Trerotola S, Dolmatch B, et al. Stent graft versus balloon angioplasty for failing dialysis-access grafts. *N Engl J Med.* 2010;362(6):494–503.
119. Lok CE, Moist L, Hemmelgarn BR, et al. Effect of fish oil supplementation on graft patency and cardiovascular events among patients with new synthetic arteriovenous hemodialysis grafts: a randomized controlled trial. *JAMA.* 2012;307(17):1809–1816.
120. Li L, Terry CM, Shiu YTE, et al. Neointimal hyperplasia associated with synthetic hemodialysis grafts. *Kidney Int.* 2008;74:1247–1261.
123. Turmel-Rodrigues L, Pengloan J, Baudin S, et al. Treatment of stenosis and thrombosis in haemodialysis fistulas and grafts by interventional radiology. *Nephrol Dial Transplant.* 2000;15(12):2029–2036.
134. Beathard GA, Welch BR, Maidment HJ. Mechanical thrombolysis for the treatment of thrombosed hemodialysis access grafts. *Radiology.* 1996;200(3):711–716.
135. Trerotola SO, Vesely TM, Lund GB, et al. Treatment of thrombosed hemodialysis access grafts: Arrow-Trerotola percutaneous thrombolytic device versus pulse-spray thrombolysis. Arrow-Trerotola Percutaneous Thrombolytic Device Clinical Trial. *Radiology.* 1998;206(2):403–414.
136. Patel AA, Truite CM, Trerotola SO. Mechanical thrombectomy of hemodialysis fistulae and grafts. *Cardiovasc Intervent Radiol.* 2005;28:704–713.
146. Yevzlin AS, Asif A. Stent placement in hemodialysis access: historical lessons, the state of the art and future directions. *Clin J Am Soc Nephrol.* 2009;4:996–1008.
149. Irani FG, Teo TKB, Tay KH, et al. Hemodialysis arteriovenous fistula and graft stenoses: randomized trial comparing drug-eluting balloon angioplasty with conventional angioplasty. *Radiology.* 2018;289(1):238–247.
158. Beathard GA, Settle SM, Shields MW. Salvage of the nonfunctioning arteriovenous fistula. *Am J Kidney Dis.* 1999;33:910–916.
167. Lee T, Ullah A, Allon M, et al. Decreased cumulative access survival in arteriovenous fistulas requiring interventions to promote maturation. *Clin J Am Soc Nephrol.* 2011;6(3):575–581.
174. Turmel-Rodrigues L, Pengloan J, Rodrigue H, et al. Treatment of failed native arteriovenous fistulae for hemodialysis by interventional radiology. *Kidney Int.* 2000;57:1124–1140.
193. Lok CE, Rajan DK, Clement J, et al. Endovascular proximal forearm arteriovenous fistula for hemodialysis access: results of the prospective, multicenter novel endovascular access trial (NEAT). *Am J Kidney Dis.* 2017;70(4):486–497.
201. Lumsden AB, MacDonald MJ, Isiklar H, et al. Central vein stenosis in the hemodialysis patient: incidence and efficacy of endovascular treatment. *Cardiovasc Surg.* 1997;5:504–509.
205. Vesely TM, Hovsepian DM, Pilgram TK, et al. Upper extremity ventral venous obstruction in hemodialysis patients: treatment with Wallstents. *Radiology.* 1997;204:343–348.
237. Krishnasami Z, Carlton D, Bimbo L, et al. Management of hemodialysis catheter related bacteremia with an adjunctive antibiotic lock solution. *Kidney Int.* 2002;61:1136–1142.
244. Sychev D, Maya ID, Allon M. Clinical outcomes of dialysis catheter-related candidemia in hemodialysis patients. *Clin J Am Soc Nephrol.* 2009;4:1102–1105.
248. Hemmelgarn BR, Moist LM, Lok CE, et al. Prevention of dialysis catheter malfunction with recombinant tissue plasminogen activator. *N Engl J Med.* 2011;364(4):303–312.
273. Ash SR. Chronic peritoneal dialysis catheters: overview of design, placement, and review procedures. *Semin Dial.* 2003;16:323–334.
274. Maya ID. Ultrasound/fluoroscopy-assisted placement of peritoneal dialysis catheters. *Semin Dial.* 2007;20(6):611–615.
281. Marwah DS, Korbet SM. Timing of complications in percutaneous renal biopsy: what is the optimal period of observation? *Am J Kidney Dis.* 1996;28(1):47–52.
282. Maya ID, Maddela P, Barker J, et al. Percutaneous renal biopsy: comparison of blind and real-time ultrasound-guided technique. *Semin Dial.* 2007;20(4):355–358.
284. Korbet SM. Percutaneous renal biopsy. *Semin Nephrol.* 2002;22(3):254–267.

# KIDNEY TRANSPLANTATION

## SECTION XI

# 69 The Immunobiology of Transplantation

Marie Josée Hébert | Héloise Cardinal | Kathryn Tinckam

## CHAPTER OUTLINE



## KEY POINTS

- Allograft rejection occurs because the recipient's immune system recognizes the donor's human leukocyte antigens (HLA) as non-self through three pathways. In the direct pathway, recipient CD8+ T cells recognize intact donor HLA class I molecules on donor antigen presenting cells (APC) that migrate from the allograft to the recipient's lymph nodes. In the indirect pathway, donor peptides are processed by the recipient's APC and expressed on HLA class II molecules, where they are recognized by recipient CD4+ T lymphocytes. In the semidirect pathway, donor HLA molecules are transferred on recipient APC that can then interact with recipient CD8+ T lymphocytes.
- After alloantigen recognition by the T-cell receptor, cosignals must take place for T-cell activation to occur. Although many other cosignals exist, the interaction between B7 at the surface of APC and CD28 on the T-cell surface is one of the important stimulatory cosignals, while the interaction between B7 and CTLA4 is an important coinhibitory pathway.
- Following their activation and depending on signals provided by the inflammatory milieu, CD4 T cells can differentiate into at least five major subsets: Th1, Th2, Th17, follicular helper T (Tfh) cells, and regulatory T (Treg) cells. Three subtypes are involved in immunogenic responses and rejection: Th1, Th17, and Tfh. Two subtypes display tolerogenic roles: Th2 and Treg.
- B lymphocytes become activated when their B-cell receptor engages an alloantigen (soluble or presented by an APC) that they internalize, process, and re-express on HLA class II molecules. Through interactions with cognate CD4+ follicular helper T cells, B lymphocytes differentiate into antibody-producing plasmocytes or memory B cells.
- Important effector mechanisms of allograft rejection include T-lymphocyte (CD8+) cytotoxicity through the perforin-granzyme and the Fas/Fas-ligand pathways and donor-specific, anti-HLA antibody-mediated damage, which is secondary to complement activation through the classical pathway or antibody-dependent cytotoxicity.

Allograft rejection occurs because antigenic determinants present within the allograft are recognized by the recipient's immune system as non-self, dangerous, or both. In this chapter, we will first review the mechanisms involved in allorecognition. Then, we will discuss transplant-relevant antigens and antibodies. Finally, we will provide a mechanistic overview of acute kidney graft rejection and immunosuppressive drugs. The clinical aspects of acute kidney graft rejection are covered in greater depth in Chapter 70.

## MECHANISMS INVOLVED IN ALLORECOGNITION

T cells recognize foreign human leukocyte antigens (HLAs) through their T-cell receptors (TCR) after these antigens are presented by APCs. The TCR is expressed at the cell surface in conjunction with CD3, which is present on all mature T cells. Both cytotoxic (CD8+) and helper (CD4+) T cells are activated by the CD3-TCR complex. Different cells within the immune system, such as dendritic cells (DCs), monocytes, macrophages, and B cells, play important roles in presenting antigens to T cells. In 95% of cases, the TCR is composed of α and β chains while in 5% of cases, it is made up of γ and δ chains. The TCR is linked to the cell membrane CD3 complex, which comprises CD3ε/γ and CD3ε,/δ with a homodimer of a ζ-chain (Fig. 69.1). Upon TCR ligation, phosphorylation of the CD3 complex favors calcium release from the endoplasmic reticulum and calcium binding to calmodulin, leading to activation of the phosphatase activity of calcineurin. Calcineurin dephosphorylates nuclear factor of activated T cells (NFAT), allowing for its nuclear translocation and transcription of a series of effector genes, including interleukin-2 (IL-2) and the IL-2 receptor (IL-2R). Two major T cell subsets, CD4 and CD8 T cells, are central players in allograft rejection.

Antigen presentation is an integral component of the normal immune response that helps protect against infectious agents and maladapted cells, such as cancer cells. However, in transplantation, the immune system is activated by alloimmune triggers, that is, antigens that are genetically encoded to differ between two individuals of the same species, such as the HLA molecules, which are encoded by the major histocompatibility complex (MHC). Antigen presentation may follow one of two major pathways: direct antigens presentation by MHC class I (MHC I) molecules and indirect antigens presentation by MHC II molecules.

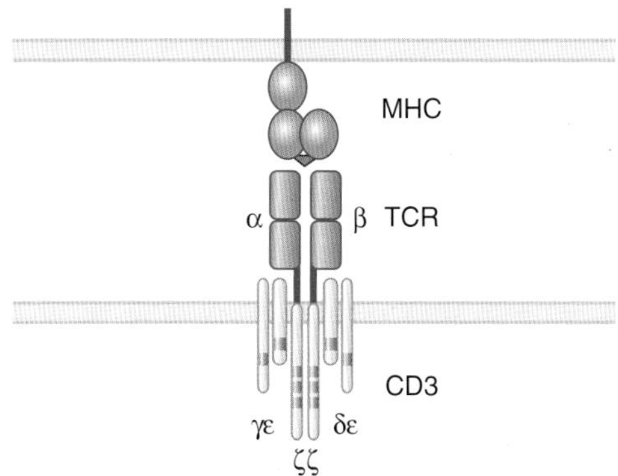


**Fig. 69.1 The T-cell receptor. T-cell receptors (TCR) alpha/beta heterodimers associate with the chains of the CD3 complex. This association is essential for expression of the TCR on the cell surface. The CD3 chains are also essential for signal transduction. The red dots represent immunoreceptor tyrosine-based activation motifs that can be phosphorylated when the TCR recognizes a peptide presented by a major histocompatibility complex molecule.** (Permission needed from: Stauss H, et al. Monoclonal T cell receptors: New reagents for cancer therapy. *Molecular Therapy*. 2007;15(10):1744–1750.)

## ANTIGEN PRESENTATION PATHWAYS

### DIRECT PATHWAY

In the transplantation setting, intact MHC I molecules expressed on donor cells can be recognized by alloreactive recipient T cells. This mode of recognition is referred to as direct allorecognition. Direct allorecognition[1,2] is thought to depend on the presence of donor DCs that traffic from the allograft to secondary lymph nodes, where they interact with recipient CD8 cytotoxic T cells. Large numbers of alloreactive T cells are present in all individuals, including transplant recipients, since thymic maturation of T cells deletes only autoreactive T cells without affecting alloreactive T cells.[3] The direct response is thought to be rapid and relatively short-lived owing to eventual destruction of donor DCs.[4]

MHC I molecules are expressed on all nucleated cells. In the normal nontransplanted host, MHC I molecules at the surface of APCs also interact with CD8 T cells. However, in the normal host, peptide antigens bound to MHC I molecules are being recognized rather than the MHC molecules themselves. Antigenic peptides presented by MHC I (HLA-A, B, C) usually originate from endogenous proteins that have been degraded to 8 or 9 amino acid peptides by the proteasome complex.[5] Proteasomes are composed of a barrel-shaped catalytic 20S complex capped at both ends by 19s regulatory complexes that control access to the catalytic core. Proteins that are damaged or dysfunctional are targeted for degradation by the addition of ubiquitin tags in a process called ubiquitination. Polyubiquitinated proteins are recognized by the 19S complex, allowing them to move toward the proteolytic core for degradation. This process is responsible for degradation of 75% to 95% of intracellular proteins.[6] Peptides are degraded down to 8 or 9 residues and loaded onto MHC I molecules in the endoplasmic reticulum by the transporter associated with antigen processing (TAP).[7] In the nontransplant setting, presentation of antigenic peptides by MHC I molecules plays an important role in the immunogenicity of mutant sequences with regard to cancer cells or proteins that stem from a viral infection. In the setting of transplantation, however, donor peptides presented within the MHC I groove of donor APCs can impact, either positively or negatively, the capacity to present allogeneic determinants to the recipient's immune system. They can alter the stability of the immunologic synapse (the site of physical interaction between APC and T cell), and therefore modulate the robustness of the response.

### INDIRECT PATHWAY

The indirect presentation pathway proceeds when allopeptides (fragments of donor HLA molecules) are loaded onto the

MHC II molecules expressed on the recipient's APCs. Non-MHC peptides can also be presented in this manner since, in the nontransplanted host, this pathway deals with the presentation of endocytosed antigens digested by the lysosomal pathway, which are re-expressed on the cell surface as peptides (≥15 amino acids) bound to MHC II molecules. MHC II-bound peptides are recognized by the TCR of CD4 T cells, leading to their activation when proper costimulatory signals are also provided. MHC II molecules are expressed on a restricted number of immune cells, such as DCs, monocytes, macrophages, and B cells. However, interferon-γ can induce the expression of MHC II on several cell types, including epithelial and endothelial cells, which can then acquire non-professional antigen-presenting capacity.

MHC II molecules are formed in the endoplasmic reticulum, where they associate with the invariant chain ''li'' that fills the peptide-binding groove.[8] The invariant chain targets MHC II for the endosomal pathway, where various degradation steps allow for the loading of MHC II with antigenic peptides. Once loaded and stabilized, the MHC II molecule moves to the plasma membrane. In the transplant setting, peptides derived from polymorphic regions of the donor MHC molecules can be taken up by recipient APCs, degraded within the endocytic compartment, and loaded onto recipient MHC II molecules for presentation to alloreactive recipient CD4 T cells. MHC II molecules expressed by DCs play an important role in initiating the indirect antigen presentation pathway through interactions with CD4 T cells. The indirect pathway is thought to be activated in the long term after transplantation and may play an important role in promoting alloantibody production and chronic antibody-mediated allograft rejection.

## SEMIDIRECT PATHWAY AND CROSS-DRESSING

The semidirect pathway was described more recently, and refers to the transfer of intact donor MHC molecules to the recipient's APCs.[9–12] The semidirect pathway is posited to play an important role in T-cell allosensitization after donor APCs have been eliminated by the host response, or when these cells are unable to migrate to secondary lymph nodes because of severed lymphatic vessels at the time of transplantation. In the semidirect pathway, intact donor HLA molecules can be picked up by recipient APCs and re-expressed on their surface, a mechanism termed *cross-dressing*. Directly alloreactive recipient T cells can then interact with cross-dressed APCs, leading to their activation.

The semidirect pathway helps explain the activation of naïve T cells in situations where donor DCs are not available for alloantigen presentation. In several transplantation models, donor DCs have been detected only at very low numbers in draining lymphoid organs, and they have been shown to be rapidly eliminated by natural killer (NK) cells.[13–15] Recipient DCs rapidly invade and replace donor DCs within a few days after transplantation. It is thought that the semidirect pathway is used by recipient DCs, in conjunction with the indirect pathway, to present alloantigens to naïve recipient T cells, explaining the long-term capacity to mount a rejection response even after donor DCs have been destroyed. Although different types of DCs have been implicated in alloantigen presentation, monocyte-derived DCs are thought to play a central role in the sensing of self and non-self antigens, and in the presentation of donor alloantigens through the semidirect pathway.[4,16] The mechanisms responsible for cross-dressing of donor MHC molecules on DCs are the subject of intense investigation. It was previously thought that MHC molecules shed from the allograft could be taken up by DCs and re-expressed on the cell surface. More recently, a potential role for extracellular vesicles in the transfer of intact donor MHC molecules was suggested. All cell types can release a wide array of extracellular vesicles that can serve as intercellular cargo for protein, mRNA, and microRNA. Exosomes—extracellular vesicles of endocytic origin—can carry MHC molecules and are thought to initiate cross-dressing of MHC molecules when engulfed by DCs.[17,18]

The antigen presentation capacity of DCs (whether allogenic or not) varies with their state of maturation and activation. Release of danger-associated molecular patterns (DAMPs) by the graft, in association with ischemia-reperfusion at the time of transplantation, favors maturation of DCs.[4] Exosomes released by the allograft can also promote inflammation and DC maturation.[19,20] Regardless of donor or recipient origin, DCs migrate to secondary lymphoid tissue to interact with naïve T cells. However, under certain inflammatory conditions, such as chronically rejecting allografts, structures reminiscent of lymphoid organs can form within allografts. These structures, called tertiary lymphoid organs, allow antigen presentation within the allograft, thus favoring the production of allo- and autoantibodies[19,21] that are important in rejection.

## T-CELL COSIGNALING PATHWAYS

The TCR is an octomeric complex of variable TCR receptor α and β chains with three dimeric signaling modules$^{\text{CD3}}\delta/\varepsilon$, CD3 $\gamma/\varepsilon$ and$^{\text{CD247}}\zeta/\zeta$ or $\zeta/\eta$ (Fig. 69.1). TCR ligation activates Signal 1. However, a second signaling pathway, Signal 2, needs to be triggered for T-cell activation and acquisition of effector function. Pathways that activate or inhibit Signal 2 are known as cosignaling pathways (Fig. 69.2).[22] These pathways have profound implications on T-cell responses to antigenic determinants, controlling activation, proliferation, differentiation, cytokine production, and effector functions.

The first and most well-characterized costimulatory pathway depends on interactions between the CD28 receptor, expressed on naïve T cells, and B7 ligands, expressed on APCs.[23–28] CD28 is constitutively expressed by naïve CD4 and CD8 T cells, and, upon ligation with B7.1 (CD80) or B7.2 (CD86), it activates cosignaling pathways that drive activation and survival of T cells. The expression of B7.1 and B7.2 by APCs is influenced by their activation state, which can be triggered by exposure to proinflammatory cytokines, such as interleukin-1β (IL-1β), interleukin-6 (IL-6), and tumor necrosis factor-alpha (TNF-α). Cytotoxic T-lymphocyte antigen-4 (CTLA4) was the first coinhibitory pathway to be described.[29–32] CTLA4 overexpression and concomitant downregulation of CD28 by endocytosis help prevent unregulated T-cell activation. Since the initial description of co-signaling pathways in the late 1980s, more than 25 different types of cosignaling pathways have been characterized. Most belong to the immunoglobulin superfamily (IgSF) and the tumor necrosis factor receptor superfamily (TNFRSF). Other costimulatory pathways that have emerged as important regulators of T-cell activation in transplantation include the CD40/CD154 (CD40 ligand) and CD278/CD275 pathways. CD40, a member of the TNFRSF expressed on most APCs, interacts with the CD40 ligand expressed on T cells, favoring their activation. This pathway impacts both T-cell activation and T- and B-cell interactions. Inducible T-cell costimulator (ICOS or CD278), a member of the IgSF, is expressed on activated T cells, and favors further proliferation, cytokine production, and effector functions upon interaction with CD275.[33]

## T-CELL PHENOTYPES

Following their activation and depending on signals provided by the inflammatory milieu, CD4 T cells can differentiate into at least five major subsets: Th1, Th2, Th17, follicular helper T (Tfh) cells, and regulatory T (Treg) cells. Three subtypes are involved in immunogenic responses and rejection: Th1, Th17, and Tfh. Two subtypes display tolerogenic roles: Th2 and Treg.

Th1 cells have long been considered the cornerstone of allograft rejection. Activated Th1 CD4 T cells produce IL-2 and express IL-2R, with their interaction prompting proliferation. The transcription factor T-bet, also present in Th1 cells, favors the expression of interferon-γ and TNF-α. Cytokines released by Th1 CD4 T cells promote the activation of CD8 cytotoxic T cells, which in turn recognize allograft cells through the direct pathway and use the perforin-granzyme cytolytic pathway to destroy them. Interferon-γ produced by Th1 cells also induces the production of complement-activating antibodies by B cells, therefore recruiting an additional mechanism of allograft rejection.

Th17 cells are induced under the combined actions of transforming growth factor-β (TGF-β), IL-6, and IL-1β. They produce interleukin-17 (Il-17), interleukin-21 (IL-21), and interleukin-22 (IL-22) following the activation of the transcription factors STAT3 and RORγt. Th17 cells have been implicated in many autoimmune diseases in addition to transplant rejection.[34]

Tfh cells secrete interleukin-4 (IL-4) and IL-21, and express CD40 ligand. The interaction between CD40 ligand and CD40, expressed on B cells, promotes the maturation of naïve B cells into memory B cells and antibody-secreting plasmocytes.

Th2 cells are considered anti-inflammatory and are characterized by the production of IL-4, interleukin-5 (IL-5), and interleukin-13 (IL-13). IL-4 produced by Th2 cells induces the differentiation of CD8 T cells into a noncytotoxic phenotype, and the production of non-complement fixing antibodies by B cells. Th2 cytokines can also prompt the emergence of Treg cells.

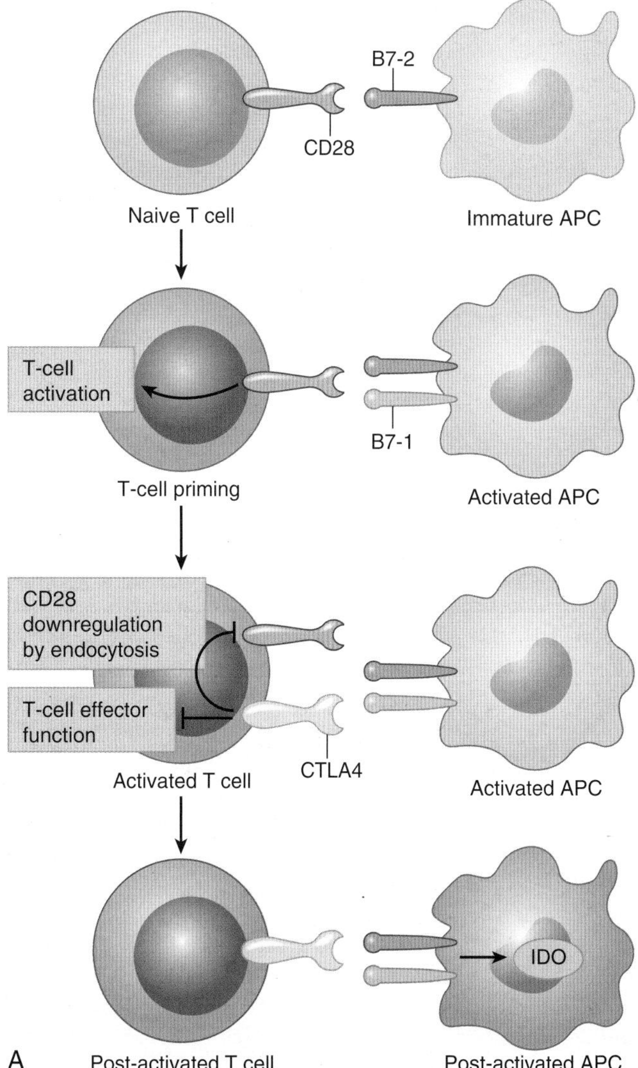


**Fig. 69.2 Cosignaling interactions in T cells. A, CD28 is constitutively expressed on the cell surface of naive CD4+ and CD8+ T cells and provides an essential costimulatory signal for T-cell growth and survival upon ligation by B7-1 and B7-2 on antigen-presenting cells (APCs). Cytotoxic T lymphocyte antigen 4 (CTLA4) is induced, following T-cell activation, and it suppresses T-cell responses. When CTLA4 is upregulated, CD28 expression is subsequently downregulated by endocytosis. Expression of B7-1 and B7-2 is modulated by the activation state of the APC. B7-2 is constitutively expressed on APCs at low levels, and infection, stress, and cellular damage recognition by innate receptors activate APCs and induce transcription, translation, and transportation of both B7-1 and B7-2 to the cell surface.** *Continued*

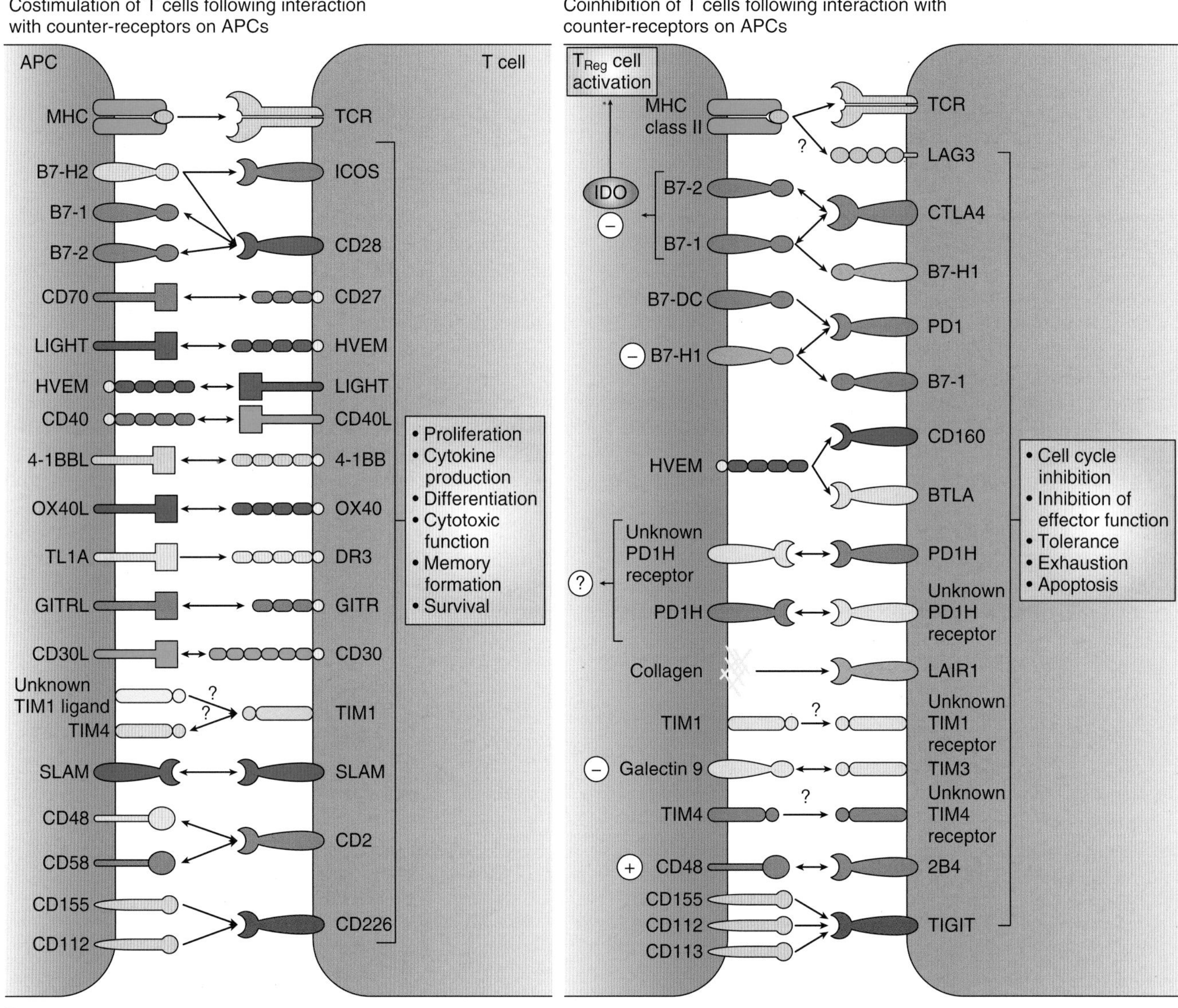


**Fig. 69.2, cont'd** B, *Left panel*, Costimulatory molecules deliver positive signals to T cells following their engagement by ligands and counter-receptors on APCs. Several costimulatory molecule interactions are bidirectional. *Right panel*, Coinhibitory molecules deliver negative signals into T cells. CTLA4 is involved in bidirectional interactions: It inhibits T-cell function after binding B7-1 and B7-2, and CTLA4-bound B7-1 and B7-2 may induce the expression of indoleamine 2,3-dioxygenase (IDO), which acts in *trans* to suppress activation of conventional T cells and promote the function of regulatory T cells. (From Chen L, Flies DB. Molecular mechanisms of T cell co-stimulation and co-inhibition. *Nat Rev Immunol*. 2013;13(4):227–242. With permission.)

Treg cells express CD4, CD25, and the transcription factor forkhead box P3 (FOXP3). They are considered the primary mediators of peripheral tolerance. Like effector T cells, Treg cells express a TCR that activates calcineurin-dependent pathways upon ligation with antigenic peptides presented by MHC II molecules. Their activation is dependent on two signals (Fig. 69.3).[35] However, unlike effector T cells, the second signal does not depend on interactions between CD28 and B7.1 or B7.2, since CTLA4 expressed on Treg cells inhibits CD28 signaling. Rather, the second signal is initiated by IL-2/IL-2R interactions, and thus tends to occur in the presence of high levels of IL-2. Treg cells have been shown to suppress the function of CD4 T cells, CD8 T cells, B cells, and macrophages. Their suppressive activity can inhibit a number of immunogenic reactions, including allograft rejection. This immunosuppressive function depends on at least 4 mechanisms of action:

- Secretion of inhibitory cytokines such as interleukin-10 (IL-10), TGF-β, and interleukin-35 (IL-35)
- Suppression by metabolic disruption: Treg cells express the ectoenzymes CD39 and CD73, therefore favoring extracellular ATP and ADP metabolism to adenosine. The latter interacts with the A2A adenosine receptor on effector T cells, thereby launching signaling pathways that inhibit effector T-cell activation[36]

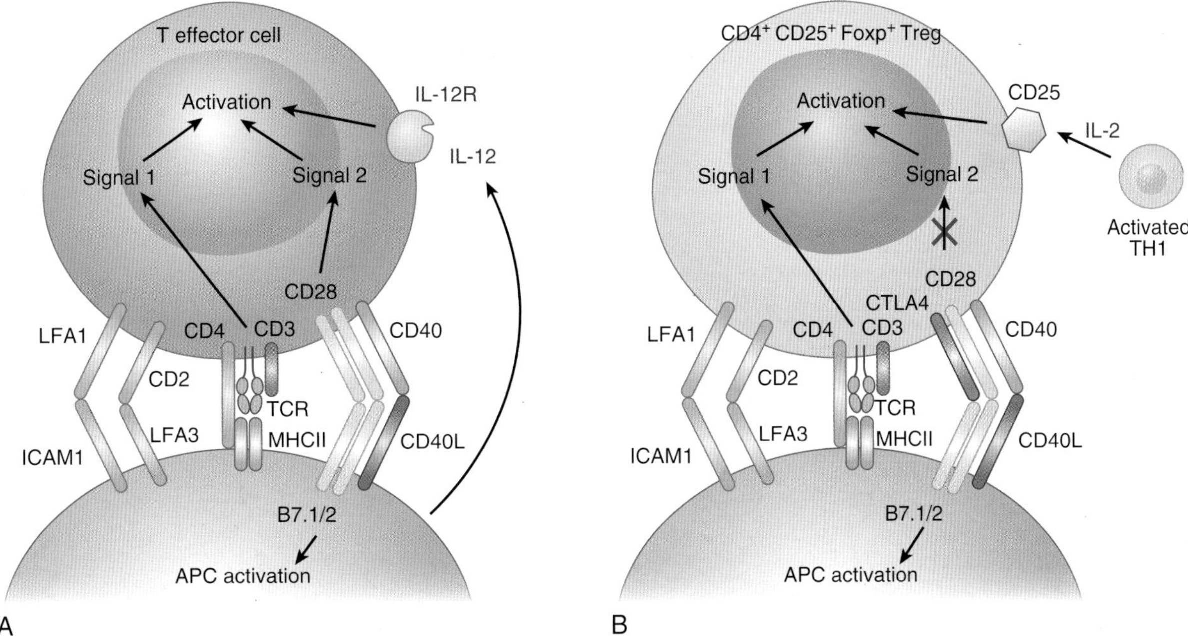


**Fig. 69.3 Activation of effector and regulatory T cells by antigen-presenting cells. Key surface molecules in activation of A, T effector cells and B, T regulatory cells (Tregs). The key molecules required for both cells are similar. The T-cell receptor complex includes CD3, CD2, CD4 or CD8, LFA1, and CD45R, and activation of T-cell receptor (TCR) by antigen results in Signal 1 for T effector cells and Tregs. In effector T cell-lineage T cells, CD28 on the T cells is activated by B7.1 and B7.2 on antigen-presenting cells (APCs) and generates Signal 2, which, combined with Signal 1, initiates effector T-cell activation. The activation of effector T cells is augmented by CD40L binding to CD40 and cytokines, such as IL-2 and IL-12, for generation of Th1 cells. With Tregs, CTLA4 binds to B7.1 and B7.2 and limits activation through CD28. Thus the effector T cells Signal 2 pathway is not required for Treg activation. The second signal for Treg activation is generated by IL-2 binding to the IL-2 receptor, which includes CD25.** (From Hall BM. T cells: soldiers and spies—the surveillance and control of effector T cells by regulatory T cells. *Clin J Am Soc Nephrol.* 2015;10(11):2050–2064. With permission.)

- Suppression by cytotoxicity: Treg cells employ the granzyme-perforin lytic system to kill activated NK cells and cytotoxic CD8 T cells
- Modulation of the activation and maturation of APCs, such as DCs

Following their activation, CD4 T cells initiate a proliferative response regulated by the mammalian target of rapamycin (mTOR) pathway, thus leading to clonal expansion. Depending on their phenotype, CD4 T cells can favor either activation or inhibition of other components of the adaptive immune response, including CD8 T cells and B cells. Activation of cytotoxic CD8 T cells can, in turn, directly damage and kill allograft cells through the release of perforin and granzyme B, whereas maturation of B cells into antibody-secreting plasmocytes can lead to the production of donor-specific antibodies and autoantibodies that are detrimental to the allograft.

## B CELLS AND ANTIBODY PRODUCTION

The humoral response, mediated by antibody-producing B cells, and leading to antibody-dependent damage to the allograft, is the other major component of the adaptive immune system that is of pivotal importance in allograft rejection. Hyperacute antibody-mediated rejection was described in the 1960s as an extremely severe and rapid form of rejection dependent on the presence of preformed anti-HLA antibodies that target the allograft endothelium as soon as reperfusion is established. The use of crossmatching to screen for the presence of preformed anti-HLA antibodies has resulted in a sharp decrease in the occurrence of hyperacute antibody-mediated rejection. Hence the importance of antibodies and B cells as mediators of rejection was forgotten or dismissed until the turn of the 21st century, when standardization of C4d staining for kidney allograft biopsies—a readout of complement activation by immune complexes—reactivated the field of antibody-dependent rejection. HLA typing and anti-HLA antibodies are discussed in later in this chapter.

B cells exert a number of important immunologic functions; the most studied is the production of antibodies that can bind protein, peptide, and carbohydrate antigens (as opposed to T cells that react exclusively to antigenic peptides). B cells are good APCs and play an important role in the architecture of secondary lymphoid organs. They are characterized by the surface expression of a B-cell receptor (BCR), composed of a membrane-bound immunoglobulin (Ig) molecule associated with an Ig $\alpha\beta$ heterodimer (CD79a and CD79b) that controls downstream signaling. B cells also express different surface markers depending on their state of maturation and differentiation. The B-cell lineage contains three major subsets: B1, B2, and regulatory B cells. (Fig. 69.4)[37] B1 cells are found in the peritoneal and pleural cavity. They express CD19 and CD5, produce low-affinity polyreactive natural antibodies, and do not require T-cell help. B2 cells are formed in the bone marrow and circulate to the spleen and lymph

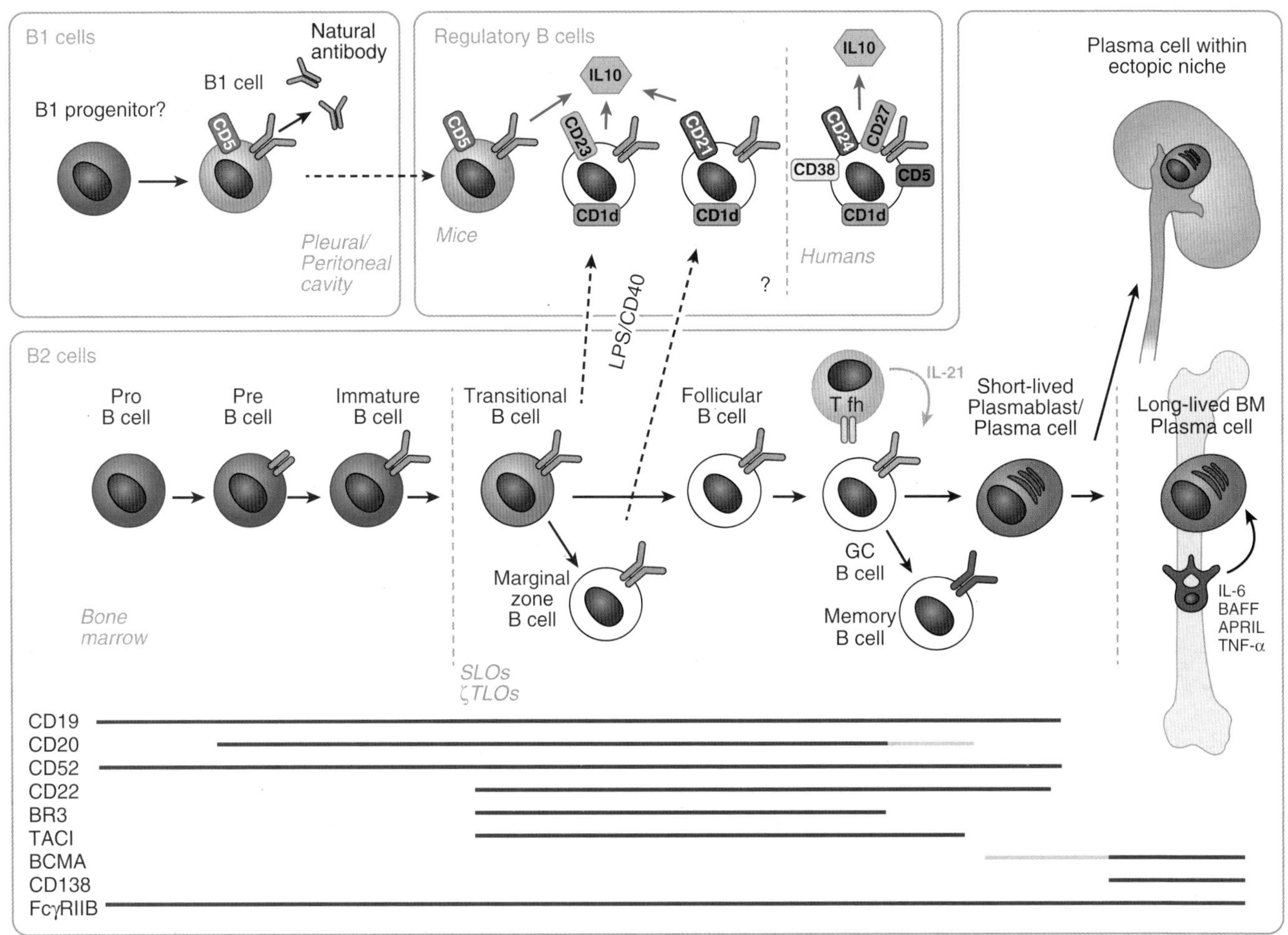


**Fig. 69.4 B-cell ontogeny and differentiation. Most peripheral B cells are produced in the bone marrow and referred to as B2 cells. A minor B-cell population, known as B1 cells, are found not only in the pleural and peritoneal cavities but also in small numbers in the spleen. B1 cells express CD19, high levels of CD5, and produce low-affinity natural antibody (mainly IgM), without T-cell help. It is currently unclear whether B1 cells arise from a unique progenitor or from a progenitor common to both B1 and B2 cells. B2 cells are formed in the bone marrow and develop from pro-B cells, to pre-B cells, to immature B cells, which are released into the periphery. Following antigen encounter, B cells obtain T-cell help and enter the germinal center. Here they undergo class switch recombination and affinity maturation, a process involving iterative cycles of somatic hypermutation and proliferation. A specific subset of T cells, known as T follicular helper cells (Tfh) are critical for germinal center formation and are thought to provide both contact and cytokine (IL-21) signals for germinal center B cells. Short-lived plasmablasts and memory cells arise from GC B cells. Some plasmablasts circulate (depending on the expression of CXCR3 and CXCR4), and a small proportion find a suitable niche for long-term survival within bone marrow and inflamed tissue, for example, rejecting allografts. A variety of molecules are expressed by B2 cells during their maturation and activation, as shown; Fcγ RIIB is expressed throughout development, whereas most other markers are expressed either on B cells or on antibody-producing plasma cells. Dark-blue bars represent high expression, light-blue bars intermediate expression. Regulatory B cells are a recently described subset, which inhibits T-cell responses via the production of IL10. These cells are likely to arise from multiple B-cell subsets (B1, transitional and marginal zone). Regulatory B cells have recently been described in humans and are characterized by surface expression of CD5, CD1d, CD24, CD27, and CD38. There are also thought to be regulatory B cells, which act independently of IL-10 (not shown).** (From Clatworthy MR. Targeting B cells and antibody in transplantation. *Am J Transplant*. 2011;11(7):1359–1367. With permission.)

nodes as immature B cells. They differentiate into either plasmablasts, memory B cells, or long-lived plasma cells following antigenic interaction and maturation within lymph nodes. Regulatory B cells with immune inhibitory functions are characterized by IL-10 secretion and the surface expression of CD24, CD38, CD5, and CD1d. Regulatory B cells represent approximately 5% of circulating B cells.

B cells become activated when their BCR engages an antigen, either soluble or presented by an APC, such as follicular DCs. This leads to phosphorylation of tyrosine residues within the cytoplasmic domains of CD79a and CD79b, and activation of downstream signaling pathways. Several receptors present on B cells, such as CD19 and toll-like receptors, or the presence of complement components, such as C3b and C3d, can lower the threshold of signaling initiation. The presence of cytokines, such as B-cell activating factor (BAFF), can also enhance B-cell activation and survival. Full B-cell activation and maturation occurs in the lymph nodes, which are composed of an outer portion or cortex of B-cell lymphoid follicles, and an inner portion rich in immature and mature T cells. Upon antigen recognition by the BCR, B cells internalize and process bound antigen, and re-express antigenic peptides on MHC II molecules. These B cells then move to the border between the follicle and the T-cell zone, where they present antigen to a cognate (i.e., matching) Tfh CD4 T cell. This first phase of activation can result in the differentiation of B cells into short-lived plasmablasts that produce low-affinity IgM antibodies, or the formation of a germinal center that will allow B-cell differentiation into either memory B cells or long-lived plasma cells that are responsible for the production of high-affinity antibodies. (Fig. 69.5)[38] Germinal centers are formed when B cells proliferate after BCR engagement, forcing naïve B cells to leave the follicle. B cells then present MHC II-bound antigens, in association with CD40 and CD80 or CD86, to Tfh cells for a second time. This leads to interactions with the TCR, CD40 ligand, and CD28 on follicular T cells. In addition, follicular T cells produce IL-21, which favors B-cell clonal expansion and antibody class switch recombination.

Antibodies are heterodimeric protein structures composed of a light chain and a heavy chain. There are five different human Ig isotypes (IgM, IgG, IgA, IgE, and IgD), which differ in the structure of the constant region. The antigen-binding site is composed of the variable regions of the heavy and light chains. Both chains contain a constant region and a variable region that undergoes recombination and somatic hypermutation. The variable (V), diversity (D), and joining (J) gene segments of the Ig heavy and light chain loci rearrange through DNA recombination to produce a diversified B-cell repertoire. However, BCRs with higher affinity confer enhanced capacity to interact with Tfh cells, therefore favoring the selection and expansion of the most effective B-cell clones.

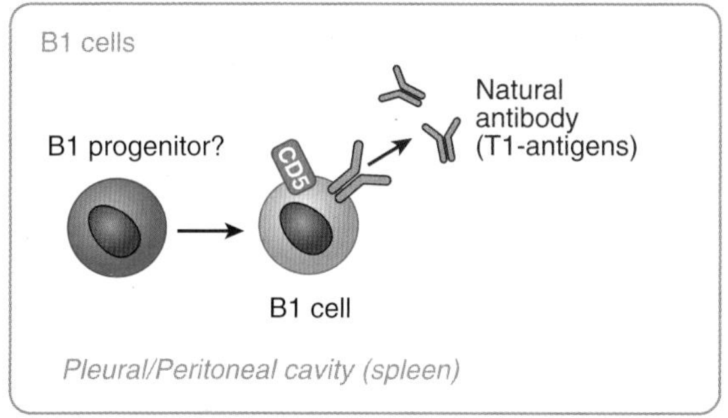


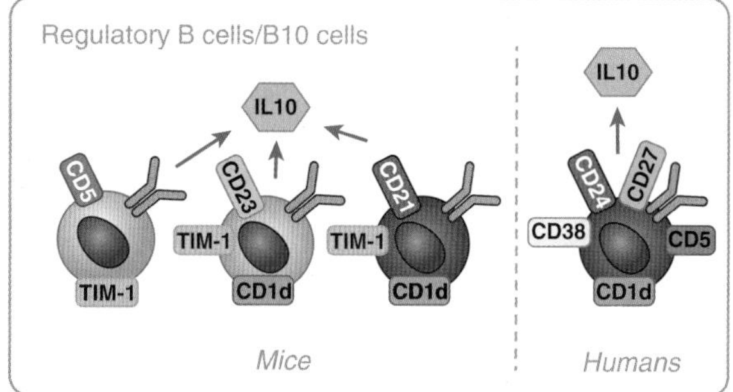


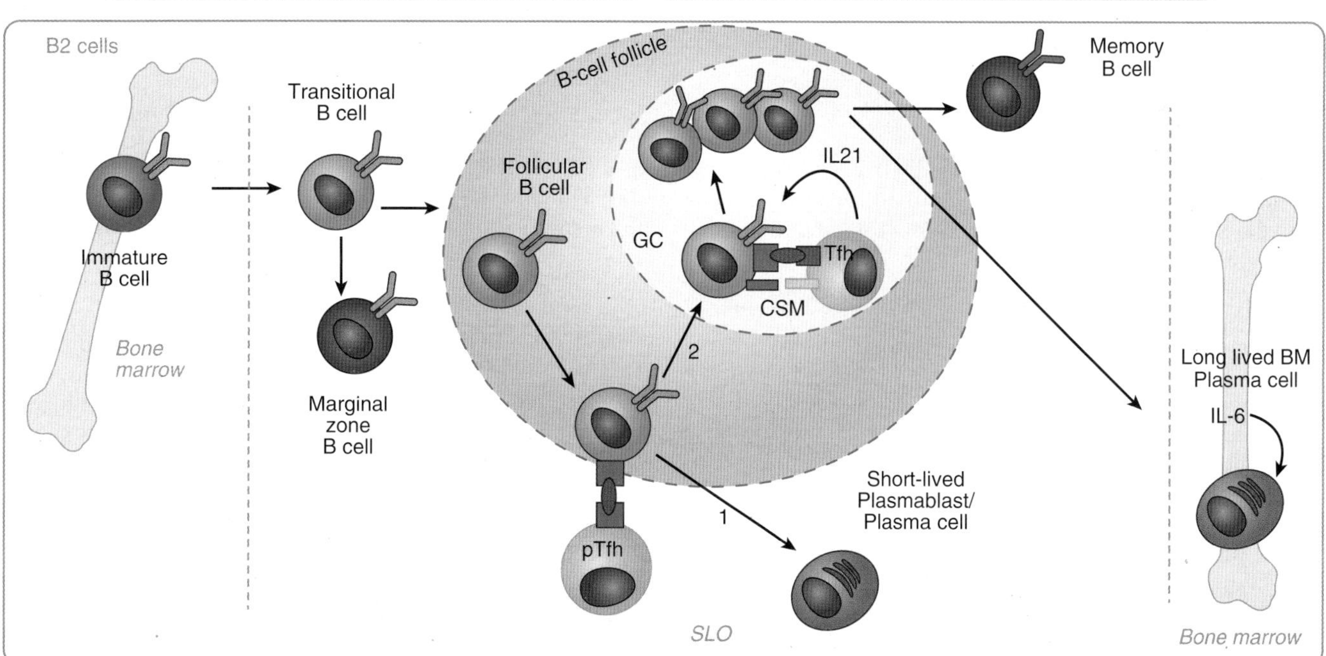


**Fig. 69.5 B-cell subsets. B1 cells reside within pleural and peritoneal cavities (and in smaller numbers in the spleen). They produce low-affinity natural antibody to T-independent antigens. B2 cells are formed in the bone marrow and develop from pro-B cells, to pre-B cells, through to immature B cells, which are released into the periphery. Following the antigen encounter, follicular B cells move to the T–B border within secondary lymphoid organs (SLO) and present antigen to a cognate CD4 T cell, known as a pre-T follicular helper cell (pTfh). Following this interaction, the fate of the B cell lies between two pathways: 1) To become a short-lived extrafollicular plasmablast or 2) to enter the germinal center, undergo rounds of somatic hypermutation and selection to generate class-switched memory B cells or plasma cells. This process requires the presence of IL-21-producing T follicular helper cells (Tfh). The interactions between Tfh and B cells also requires costimulatory molecule (CSM) interactions, including CD40L/CD40, ICOS/ICOS-L, and CD28/CD86. Some B cells have the capacity to produce the immunoregulatory cytokine IL10 and have been dubbed *regulatory B cells* or *B10 cells*.** (From Clatworthy MR. B-cell regulation and its application to transplantation. *Transpl Int*. 2014;27(2):117–128. With permission.)

While long-lived plasma cells home to the bone marrow to continuously produce high-affinity antibodies, memory B cells require antigen rechallenge to initiate antibody production.

Mounting evidence suggests that B-cell activation, maturation, and antibody production can also occur within tertiary lymphoid structures developing within allografts. These structures are found in association with chronic inflammatory conditions, including autoimmune disorders, infection, cancer, and transplantation. Tertiary lymphoid structures are reminiscent of germinal centers, with compartmentalization of T and B cells and the presence of DCs. They have been reported in animal models of rejection and in chronically rejected human renal and cardiac allografts. Mounting evidence suggests that anti-HLA antibodies and autoantibodies deleterious to the allograft are produced within tertiary lymphoid structures.[39–41] The production of lymphotoxin-β by B cells can favor the formation of tertiary lymphoid structures.

The current classification of rejection establishes a distinction between T-cell–mediated and antibody-mediated rejection episodes. However useful for histopathologic classification, it is important to remember that in most cases, the activation of naïve B cells leading to the production of donor-specific antibody (DSA) requires T-cell help. However, if the production of long-lived plasmablasts or memory B cells is established prior to transplantation because of allosensitizing events, such as pregnancy or prior transplantation, the need for T-cell help is bypassed. Autoantibodies have also been associated with either increased risk of acute rejection or reduced long-term allograft survival,[42] as will be discussed in detail later in this chapter. The role of T-cell help in the production of these autoantibodies remains unclear.

## ANTIHUMAN LEUKOCYTE ANTIGEN ANTIBODIES AND GRAFT INJURY

DSA can injure the allograft through various pathways, including complement activation, antibody-dependent cell-mediated cytotoxicity (ADCC), and induction of endothelial dysfunction.

### COMPLEMENT ACTIVATION

Complement is an important component of the innate immune response and plays a major role in clearing damaged cells and invading pathogens.[43,44] The complement pathway is composed of cell surface receptors, regulatory proteins, and soluble proteins that can interact and cleave one another to activate downstream components. The complement pathway consists of three distinct activating components: Classical, lectin, and alternate pathways (Fig. 69.6).[43] All three pathways converge into a common effector phase initiated by the formation of a C3 convertase, which results in the formation of the membrane attack complex C5b-9 that precipitates cell lysis. The classical pathway is activated when C1q binds to IgG or IgM antibodies present within immune complexes. The general order of complement fixing activity for antibodies is IgM>IgG3>IgG1>IgG2≫IgG4. IgE antibodies are non-complement fixing, whereas IgA can activate the alternative, but not classical pathway. The binding of C1q to complement-fixing antibodies leads to interactions with the serine proteases C1r and C1s, allowing for the cleavage of C4 and C2, and the formation of the multiprotein complex and C3 convertase, C4b2a. The classical pathway plays an important role in antibody-mediated rejection. C4d staining, as used in the diagnosis of antibody-mediated rejection, is a read-out of C4 cleavage, and is considered a good marker of classical pathway activation. The lectin pathway is activated by the interaction of mannose-binding lectin (MBL), ficolins, and collectin-11 with carbohydrate pathogen-associated molecular patterns (PAMPs) and DAMPs, which are expressed on the surface of pathogens or damaged cells. Like the classical pathway, the lectin pathway leads to the formation of the C4b2a C3 convertase and is therefore an additional source of positive C4d staining. The lectin pathway is thought to play an important role in ischemia-reperfusion injury.[43] Lastly, the alternative pathway is activated in circumstances where soluble inhibitors cannot keep basal C3 hydrolysis in check, therefore allowing for interactions between C3, factor B and factor D. This leads to the formation of the C3 convertase C3bBb. Increased activation of the alternative pathway occurs in the presence of various factors associated with tissue injury, including microparticles, platelet surfaces, and endotoxins. C3 convertases (either C4b2a or C3bBb) cleave C3 into C3a, which has proinflammatory and chemotactic functions, and C3b, which in turn cleaves C5. This leads to the formation of C5a, another potent chemotactic and proinflammatory mediator, and C5b. The latter interacts with distal complement components C6 to C9, leading to the formation of a lytic complex, C5b-9, that subsequently creates a pore in the plasma membrane of the target cell.

A number of soluble regulatory molecules can keep complement activation in check. Factor H accelerates degradation of key components of the alternative pathway and serves as a cofactor for factor I. The latter accelerates degradation of C3b and C4b. C1 esterase inhibitor and C4b binding protein interfere with the activation of the classical pathway. Cell membrane regulatory proteins include decay-accelerating factor (DAF, CD55), membrane cofactor protein (CD46), and CR1 (CD35). During antibody-mediated rejection, DSA and autoantibodies interact with antigens present on the microvascular endothelium, leading to activation of the classical complement pathway and lytic injury and inflammation of the microvasculature.

### ANTIBODY-DEPENDENT CYTOTOXICITY

Interactions between antibodies and cognate antigens, such as MHC molecules or autoantigens expressed on the allograft endothelium, can also favor the recruitment and activation of innate immune effectors that express Fc receptors, such as monocytes, macrophages, DCs, and NK cells.[45] There are three classes of Fc receptors, FcγRI (CD64), FcγRII (CD32), and FcγRIII (CD16), the latter two of which both have A and B isoforms. All Fc receptors, except FcγRIIIB, are activating. NK cells and innate types of lymphoid cells are considered central effectors of ADCC. They express FcγRIIIA in the absence of inhibitory FcγRIIIB.[46,47] Binding of antibodies to Fc receptors activates NK cells, leading to the release of cytotoxic granules such as perforin/granzyme B. Indeed, renal biopsies from transplant patients with DSA show higher NK cell transcripts and increased numbers of NK cells within peritubular capillaries.[48]

### ENDOTHELIAL ACTIVATION

Antibodies that target endothelial cells can also injure renal allografts by inducing endothelial activation and dysfunction.

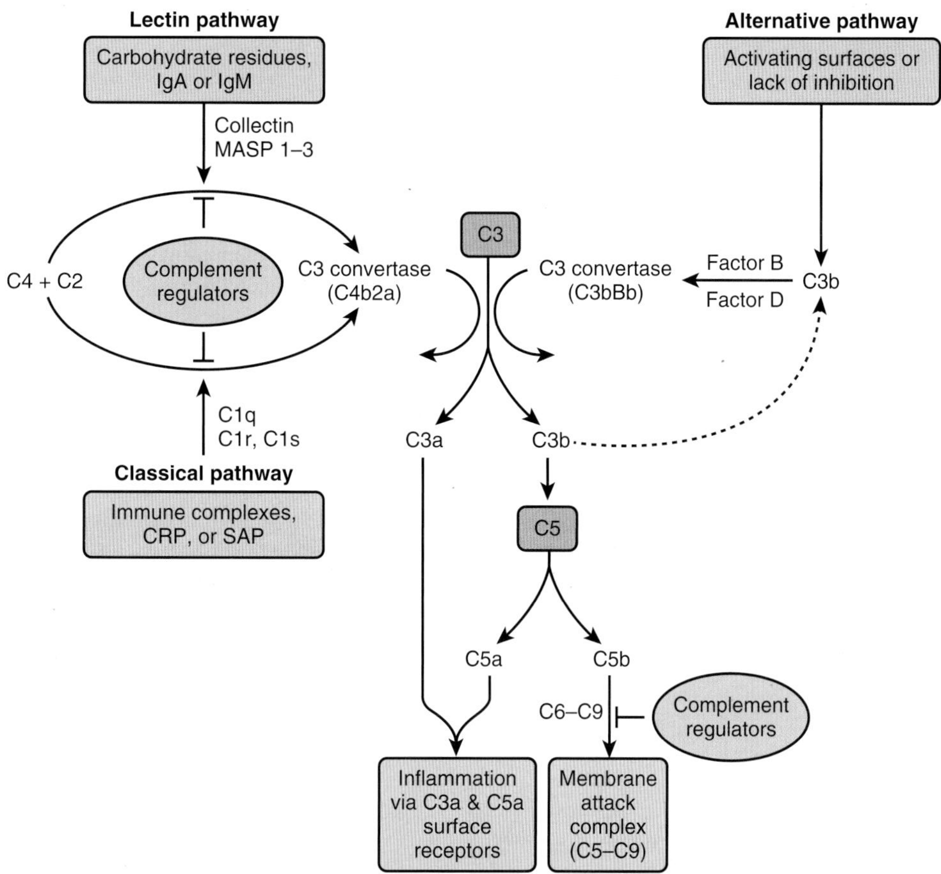


**Fig. 69.6 The complement cascade. The complement system is activated by one of three major pathways: classical, lectin, or alternative. The classical pathway is triggered by C1 binding to immune surveillance molecules, such as IgG, IgM, C-reactive protein (CRP), or serum amyloid protein (SAP), which are attached to the target sequence. The LP is triggered by the binding of collectins, such as MBL and collectin-11, or ficolins to carbohydrate residues on a pathogenic surface or IgA and IgM molecules. The alternative pathway is initiated by direct binding of C3b to activating surfaces. All three pathways converge at the production of the central complement component C3. That is, all pathways form enzyme complexes (classical or alternative convertases) that cleave either C3 (into C3a and C3b) or C5 (into C5a and C5b). C5b triggers the terminal pathway by creating a pore in the target cell membrane via the formation of the membrane attack complex (C5b-C9). Soluble complement effectors C3a and C5a are detected by specific cell receptors thereby promoting inflammation. Complement inhibition occurs via a variety of molecules ultimately inhibiting C3 and C5 convertase or blocking the formation of the membrane attack complex (C5b–C9).** (From Sacks S et al. Complement recognition pathways in renal transplantation *J Am Soc Nephrol.* 2017; 28: 2571–2578, Fig 1).

Anti-HLA antibodies cross-linking cognate HLA molecules at the surface of endothelial and vascular smooth muscle cells can initiate signal transduction pathways that favor cytoskeletal rearrangement, proliferation, activation, exocytosis, and recruitment of leukocytes. Activation of the SRC/FAK/PI3K/AKT pathway by integrin signaling, as triggered by anti-HLA antibodies, activates the mTOR signaling pathway, favoring proliferation and accumulation of vascular cells. Collectively, these changes are thought to favor neointimal thickening and mononuclear leukocyte infiltration.[49]

## OTHER TRANSPLANT-RELEVANT ANTIGENS AND ANTIBODIES

DSA have classically been involved in the majority of cases of acute and chronic antibody-mediated rejection (ABMR). However, ABMR has also been documented in patients who do not have circulating DSA.[50,51] Although DSA can be adsorbed within the allograft,[52] mounting evidence has pointed to the role of non-HLA antibodies as important contributors to ABMR. The most recent versions of the Banff classification system now recognize that, in addition to the presence of DSA, antibodies targeting other donor antigens can be considered as one of the diagnostic criteria for acute or chronic ABMR.[53,54]

The MHC I-related chain gene A (MICA) is located within the MHC I region of chromosome 6.[55] The MICA protein is highly polymorphic, has an extracellular domain, is constitutively expressed on endothelial cells, and its expression has been documented in kidney graft biopsies.[56–58] Taken together, these features make MICA an antigenic target of potential clinical relevance in solid organ transplantation. The demonstration that MICA was indeed a target for complement-dependent cytotoxicity[59] was followed by clinical studies showing that pretransplant MICA antibodies were associated with ABMR[60–62] and decreased graft survival.[61] However, two recent studies failed to show an association between pretransplant MICA status and ABMR or graft survival,[63,64] which may relate to differences in the strength of the immunosuppressive regimen used.[55] The detection of anti-MICA antibodies posttransplant has also been linked to an increased risk of ABMR,[65,66] chronic rejection,[67] and decreased graft survival[68,69] in some, but not all studies.[70] In addition to studies yielding discordant results, whether the anti-MICA antibodies identified are specific to the donor has rarely been assessed.[55] Hence the association between anti-MICA antibodies and graft outcomes remains controversial.

The proximity of donor endothelial cells to the recipient's immune system makes endothelial antigens likely targets for antibody-mediated injury. Anti-endothelial cell antibodies (AECA) have been detected in prekidney transplant patients, regardless of whether they are HLA-sensitized or desensitized.[71] Hyperacute rejections involving AECA but not anti-HLA DSA have been described, suggesting that these antibodies can be pathogenic.[72,73] The appearance of de novo, posttransplant AECA has been linked to adverse graft outcomes,[74,75] although the relevance of pretransplant AECA on graft outcomes is controversial.[61,72,74,76] These discrepancies may stem from the variability in the methods used to measure AECA and the lack of standardized assays,[77] given that the exact antigenic targets had not been uncovered when these studies were conducted. Recent progress on this issue stems from the identification of potential targets for AECA. Using a proteomic approach, novel endothelial antigenic targets (endoglin, Fms-like tyrosine kinase-3 ligand, EGF-like repeats, discoidin I-like domains 3, and intercellular adhesion molecule 4) have recently been characterized from antibody eluates in kidney transplant patients with DSA-negative ABMR. Reactivity of pretransplant serum to these antigens was associated with an increased risk of ABMR in a validation cohort.[78] Keratin 1 has also been identified as a potential antigenic target for AECA.[79]

In addition to alloantibodies, emerging evidence shows that autoantibodies are actively involved in acute and chronic rejection in kidney,[80–84] heart, and lung transplant recipients.[85,86] For instance, polyreactive, natural IgG autoantibodies against apoptotic Jurkat cells that can activate complement were isolated from the sera of kidney transplant recipients with ABMR.[84] In a retrospective cohort study, the presence of these antibodies before transplantation was associated with decreased graft survival.[87] Agonistic autoantibodies against angiotensin II receptor type 1 ($AT_1R$-Abs) have been associated with acute vascular rejection in DSA-negative renal transplant patients.[80] The passive transfer of these autoantibodies in an animal model reproduced the phenotype observed in transplant patients, demonstrating the pathogenic impact of these autoantibodies.[80] Multiple studies have shown that the presence of pretransplant $AT_1R$-Abs is associated with an increased risk of rejection and graft loss.[88–90] A recent study has questioned the association between $AT_1R$-Abs, rejection, and graft failure in the era of Luminex-based DSA screening.[91]

Autoantibodies against components of the vascular basement membrane such as the LG3 fragment of perlecan or agrin[42,81] have been associated with acute vascular rejection or transplant glomerulopathy.[83] Similarly, de novo and pretransplant levels of antifibronectin and anticollagen type 4 autoantibodies were linked to transplant glomerulopathy in kidney transplant patients.[82]

## INTERACTIONS BETWEEN ISCHEMIA-REPERFUSION AND AUTOANTIBODIES

Ischemia-reperfusion, a key feature of the solid organ transplantation process, seems to enhance both the impact and the production of autoantibodies. In contrast to HLA and MICA, which are constitutively expressed on the cell surface of the allograft endothelium, autoantigens are usually cryptic and only become exposed following ischemia-reperfusion-induced tissue damage.[42,92] In line with this concept, ischemia-reperfusion was found to enhance the contractile effect of $AT_1R$-Abs on isolated aortic rings and the impact of anti-LG3 on vascular rejection in an animal model of aortic transplantation.[81,93] In mice, passive transfer of anti-K-α-1 tubulin, an autoantibody associated with chronic lung rejection, increased airway inflammation in an animal model of autologous lung transplantation.[94] Taken together, these studies suggest that ischemia-reperfusion can increase the availability or affinity of antigenic targets, as well as enhance the deleterious impact of autoantibodies on the transplanted allograft.[42,81,93,94] Recent data also suggest that ischemia-reperfusion can fuel the production of autoantibodies in the context of transplantation. In a cohort of stable pediatric kidney transplant recipients, an enrichment in autoantibodies directed at antigenic targets from the renal pelvis and medulla, areas that are particularly sensitive to ischemia, was observed when pre- and posttransplant sera were compared.[95]

## INTERACTIONS BETWEEN ALLOANTIBODIES AND AUTOANTIBODIES

In addition to their interaction with ischemia-reperfusion, some transplant-relevant autoantibodies seem to promote the development of alloantibodies. In a cohort of kidney transplant patients, the presence of pretransplant $AT_1R$-Abs was an independent risk factor for the development of *de novo* DSA.[96] In lung transplant recipients, pretransplant positivity for autoantibodies against lung-restricted antigens, such as K-α-1 tubulin, was associated with the production of *de novo* DSA and chronic lung rejection.[86] This association could be explained by both autoantibody-mediated endothelial activation, which increases the expression of HLA targets on the graft endothelium, and by the recipient's overall propensity to mount an antibody response. Autoantibodies can also enhance the effect of alloantibodies. Indeed, kidney transplant patients with abnormal kidney biopsies who were positive for both $AT_1R$-Abs and DSA experienced a higher risk of graft loss compared with those who were only DSA positive.[97]

## MECHANISTIC EFFECT OF NON–HUMAN LEUKOCYTE ANTIGEN ANTIBODIES

Although mechanistic pathways for non-HLA antibodies have not been studied to the same extent as anti-HLA antibodies, they may also cause graft injury through the activation of endothelial cells or complement, and/or the promotion of leukocyte interaction/activation.[98] AECA activate endothelial cells, increase the expression of HLA class 1 and adhesion molecules (E selectin, ICAM1), and promote the production of inflammatory cytokines such as platelet-derived growth factor (PDGF).[78] $AT_1R$-Abs mediate endothelial cell activation and vasoconstriction by binding to the second extracellular loop of the angiotensin II receptor type 1 protein, therefore promoting the activation of NF-κB and downstream cytokines.[80] Anti-MICA, anti-LG3, and polyreactive antibodies to apoptotic cells mediate injury, at least in part, through complement activation.[42,59,81,84,99]

## HISTOCOMPABILITY TESTING FOR THE KIDNEY TRANSPLANT CANDIDATE AND RECIPIENT

In the previous section, we discussed mechanisms of allorecognition and effectors pathways inducing allograft rejection. Because HLA are the most important foreign antigens recognized on kidney allografts, this section will cover this topic in greater depth, focusing primarily on clinical translation of HLA basic science into clinical testing considerations. The Histocompatibility Laboratory (HLA Laboratory) can be considered as the site of applied transplant immunobiology. The HLA Laboratory offers clinical immunologic risk consultation, with the purpose of estimating immunologic risk throughout transplant assessment, consideration of potential donor(s), and the posttransplant period. Indeed, since the first clinical histocompatibility testing was defined in 1969,[100] the laboratory has grown to play a critical role in transplant decision making and allocation science. Histocompatibility testing (henceforth called HLA testing) focuses predominantly on assessing the humoral branch of the alloimmune response and does not routinely assess directly for activity within or risk associated with the cellular compartment of the immune response. Notwithstanding the clear interplay between cellular and humoral alloreactivity, there is a clear and strong association with measurement of both histocompatibility and the humoral response and clinical outcomes (ABMR, transplant glomerulopathy and premature graft loss). Hence precise and thorough delineation of the presence and risk of memory and de novo humoral alloreactivity to non-self HLA antigens is required. This section will focus on the most common platforms of testing utilized in the modern HLA laboratory, their strengths and limitations. We will describe how these platforms can support humoral immunologic risk assessment that can be translated into clinical action with the goals of increasing transplant access, and reducing allograft damage related to immunologic incompatibility, optimizing both equity and utility. As discussed in the previous section, antibodies to non-HLA antigens may also be correlated with worse allograft outcomes or augment the risk portended by HLA antibodies. At present, routine screening for these non-HLA antibodies is not common in clinical programs but may occur on a case by case basis.

Three testing platforms have formed the core of clinical transplant immunologic testing for more than 40 years: HLA typing (of alleles with determination of their corresponding antigen(s)); HLA antibody screening and identification, and donor-specific crossmatching. Clearly, there have been significant advances in the methods themselves but the foundational principles of using their results in context to quantify donor and recipient HLA antigen differences, as well as HLA antibody reactivity to potential donor(s), remain unchanged. We will focus on the most current methodologies here, with mention of historical, largely obsolete methods, only briefly for reference in the context of interpreting older literature based on these tests. This section will concentrate on the three core HLA testing methods, their interpretation considerations, their limitations and their practical utilization in clinical transplantation.

## HUMAN LEUKOCYTE ANTIGEN TYPING

### CONTEXT

Outside of transplantation, HLA antigens are themselves the antigen presenting molecules, alerting the immune system to foreign peptides (for example, infectious or malignancy derived peptides). Clearly significant diversity in the HLA repertoire is beneficial for ensuring effective vigilance against environmental threats within and between populations. However, it is this diversity that gives the HLA antigen its potent immunogenicity in transplantation, cognizant that the immune system cannot distinguish the threat potential of an infectious agent from that associated with a foreign HLA antigen on a transplanted organ. Indeed, there are more than 10,000 unique HLA alleles coding for more than 8000 distinct HLA proteins reported across the human repertoire, where each person has up to 18 unique HLA proteins on the surface of their nucleated cells. In sibling relationships HLA identity can occur by chance in 25% of pairs through Mendelian inheritance of the short arm of chromosome 6 where the HLA proteins are coded, but outside of this relationship, complete HLA identity between randomly selected donors and recipients is indeed rare. Hence, in most cases, the goal of HLA typing is not to find HLA identical donor–recipient pairs but to quantify the degree of difference between donors and recipients (as one estimate of the stimulus of the alloimmune response) and to determine if a recipient carries HLA antibodies specific to a given donor, driving clinical decision making accordingly. Indeed, any degree of mismatch between a donor and a recipient can stimulate an alloimmune response in the absence of enough immunosuppression, leading to subclinical and clinical rejection.[101–109]

### HUMAN LEUKOCYTE ANTIGENS

HLA class I molecules (HLA-A, B, C) are found on the surface of all nucleated cells, whereas the expression of HLA class II molecules (HLA-DR, DRw, DQ, DP) is limited to B cells, APCs, and endothelial cells. The expression of class II molecules on endothelial cells is particularly important in the transplanted organ[109–111] that may undergo injury during or after transplantation, upregulating these very important immune targets. Class I molecules are comprised of a polymorphic chain encoded by the HLA class I gene, supported by a monomorphic $\beta_2$-microglobulin. As such, the immunogenicity of the class I molecule is defined by the polymorphism in this single chain. Conversely, although the three-dimensional structure of class II antigens is similar to class I (Fig. 69.7), their amino acid configuration is different; the molecule is comprised of two distinct chains (alpha and beta), each with inherent polymorphism. The molecule's immunogenic potential in transplantation is therefore present within each amino acid chain, but also with additional immunogenicity potential at the interface of the alpha and beta chains. It

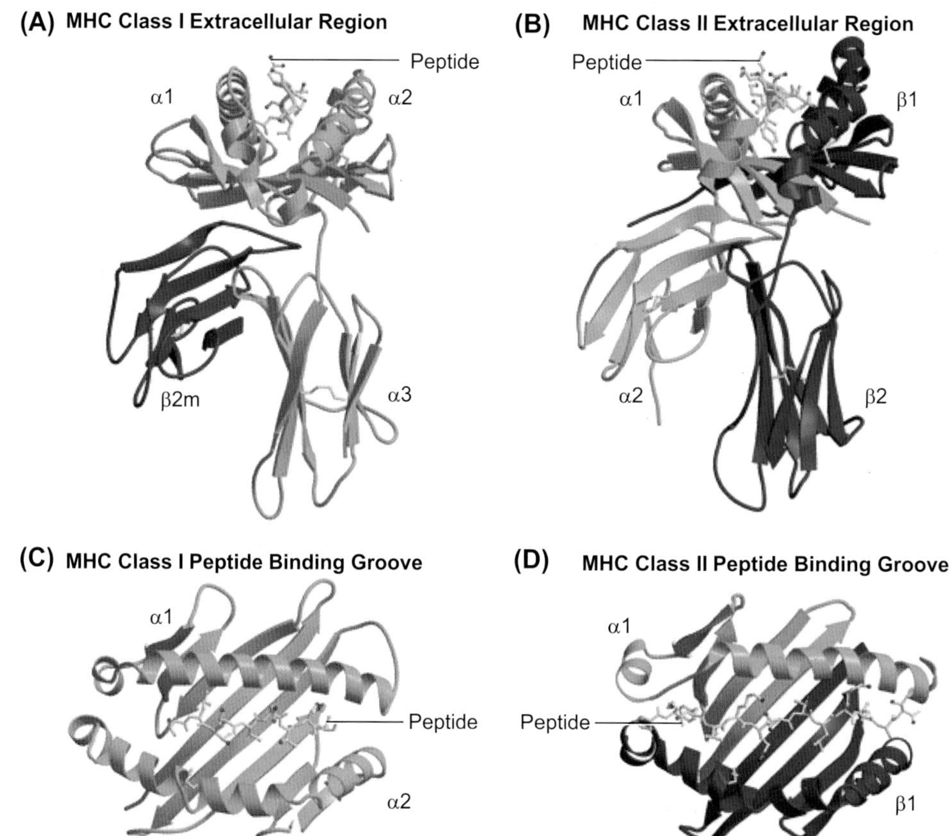


**Fig. 69.7 X-ray crystal structures of MHC Class I and II molecules in the mouse crystal structures showing the carbon backbone of murine MHC class I and II molecules. (A) and (B) show peptides bound to the extracellular regions of MHC class I or II, respectively. (C) and (D) show the view looking down at the peptide in the peptide-binding groove of MHC class I or II, respectively.** (Reproduced by permission of Bjorkman PJ. MHC restriction in three dimensions: A view of T cell receptor/ligand interactions. *Cell.* 1977;9:167–170.)

is in this complex and polymorphic structure of the HLA molecules that the immunologic challenges of transplantation begin: Even single amino acid differences between a donor and recipient HLA, if sufficiently different in charge, size or polarity, can trigger alloimmune pathways in the recipient.

## HUMAN LEUKOCYTE ANTIGEN TYPING METHODS

### SEROLOGIC METHODS

Historically, HLA antigens were identified using common serologic methods. Sera containing HLA antibodies of both single and multiple specificities to broad groups of HLA antigens were obtained from sensitized patients (usually multiparous women) and specifically chosen in combination in panels to cover the most common HLA antigen types in a population. The lymphocytes of the individual to be typed were then mixed with all serum samples in the panel in the presence of complement and a vital dye. If the sera in each reaction resulted in cell death with complement visualized by vital dye uptake, it could be inferred that the antibody(ies) in that serum had specificity(ies) to one or more HLA antigens on the cell surface. Careful examination of the pattern of positive reactions across the test sera would yield the predicted HLA antigens on the lymphocytes being tested.

### MOLECULAR METHODS

Several molecular methods have been developed to better characterize HLA antigens by determining more precisely the HLA alleles that encode them, and in doing so, more accurately identify the amino acid differences between different HLA antigens (and indeed even between different alleles within the same antigen group). Currently utilized methods use polymerase chain reaction (PCR) platforms, and options include the real time PCR (rtPCR), sequence-specific primer (SSP) method, the reverse sequence-specific oligonucleotide (R-SSO) probe method, Sanger-based sequencing, and, most recently, next-generation sequencing. It warrants mention that the sequencing methods are not suitable for deceased donor typing, as they can take several days to complete; these are more commonly employed for recipient typing and living donor typing when used. Conversely, rtPCR, SSP and SSO methods are more commonly used for deceased donor typing because their rapid turnaround times facilitate prompt transplant decision making in allocation. The details of each method will not be reviewed here, as methods are in rapid evolution and chosen in the context of what is appropriate for a given program's clinical needs. Readers are directed to their own HLA laboratory for a more complete review of the local methods used. Regardless of the specific molecular platform employed, molecular methods as a group allow for a more precise determination of HLA alleles and their corresponding immunogenicity, where serologic typing would fail to identify many of these small but important differences.

## INTERPRETING HUMAN LEUKOCYTE ANTIGENS TYPING RESULTS

### NOMENCLATURE—ALLELES AND ANTIGENS

Molecular methodology for HLA typing uses a precise nomenclature to identify HLA alleles; it uses a letter to identify the locus (A, B, C, DRB1, DRB3/4/5, DQA1, DQB1, DPA1, DPB1), an asterisk, which confirms that molecular methods were used, and then a series of numbers separated by colons (called field separators) to identify precisely the unique allele.[112]

For example, HLA-A*03:01:01:02N refers to a molecular defined allele at the A locus, followed by four unique fields, each of which has a precise meaning. Field 1 (in this example 03) identifies the allele group. Field 2 (in this example 01) identifies a precise allele, with at least 1 amino acid difference in the mature protein that distinguishes it from all other alleles in the allele group. Field 3 identifies if the genotype of the allele contains a synonymous DNA substitution in a coding region that does not alter the final protein structure, and field 4 indicates a difference in DNA sequence in a noncoding region of the gene. Additionally, a suffix may be appended to the allele name (in this example N) indicating a variant of expression of the final protein product, where N represents Null or No expression; L indicates Low expression; S indicates a molecule that is Secreted and Soluble but not present on cell surfaces; C is assigned to alleles producing products only detected in the Cytoplasm; A indicates Aberrant expression, where the expression is not confirmed; and Q is assigned to Questionable, where the impact of the mutation on expression is not confirmed but has been seen in other alleles.

For practical purposes in solid organ transplantation, only the first two fields have clinical impact in so far as they determine the protein to be considered in mismatching and antibody production. Additionally, the N or L suffix is important in transplantation, as where a protein has null or low expression it may not have any (null) or reduced (low) relevance in immunogenicity or antibody specificity considerations. Indeed, most commonly at the present time molecular typing in kidney transplantation is reported at only the first field level unless the specific allele is needed to quantify differences between a donor and recipient or to interpret a specific antibody pattern as donor specific or not.

Molecular typing nomenclature also permits a more accurate description of the complexity of the class II DQ and DP proteins, where the antigen is named only for the beta chain, but the immunologic relevance of the molecule requires identification of the alpha chain distinctly and in combination with the beta chain[113–117] (Fig. 69.7). Indeed, the authors recommend to always identify DQ and DP antigens by both their alpha and beta chains to properly describe the encoded final protein and any antigen–antibody interactions involving the alpha chain. The DRA1* chain is not sufficiently polymorphic such that naming the DR antigens in accordance to their beta chain allele is immunologically enough.

**Table 69.1 Common Human Leukocyte Antigen Genes With Multiple Human Leukocyte Antigens Associated**

| Human Leukocyte Antigen Gene | Antigens Encoded by Gene |
|---|---|
| HLA-B*14 | B64 or B65 |
| HLA-B*15 | B62, B63, B71, B72, B75, B76, or B77 |
| HLA-B*40 | B60 or B61 |
| HLA-C*03 | Cw9 or Cw10 |
| HLA-DRB1*03 | DR17 or DR18 |
| HLA-DQB1*03 | DQ, DQ8, or DQ9 |

By way of comparison, HLA antigens (serologically determined) are identified by the locus (with no asterisk) and a single number that indicates the specific protein being expressed; for example, A2 or B27. This format specifically indicates a protein rather than an allele and, in fact, represents the group of all A2 proteins; that is, the protein product of all the HLA-A*02 alleles. This nomenclature is particularly important because whenever HLA antibodies are identified (see later), the antibody is most typically named for its target antigen using antigen nomenclature. Generally, the gene group from the molecular name and the antigen number are both familiar and similar; for example, HLA-A*02 gene group codes for A2 proteins and HLA-B*27 group codes for B27 proteins. However, there are some exceptions noted (Table 69.1). Typically, in these cases the molecular typing is followed by the relevant antigen in parenthesis; for example, HLA-DQB1*03(7), where the DQB1*03 gene codes for DQ7 protein.

### MATCHING AND MISMATCHING OF ALLELES, ANTIGENS AND EPITOPES

Donors and recipients may be compared by identifying the differences between their HLA antigens and alleles; however, directionality is critical in describing this accurately. Biologically, the most relevant comparison in transplantation is to describe the donor differences to the recipient from the perspective of the recipient's immune system, and to describe the donor antigen or allele differences in terms of the number of mismatches in the host versus graft (HvG) direction. This is particularly important when either the donor or recipient is homozygous for one or more HLA antigens or alleles (Table 69.2). Newer analytic methods such as HLA Matchmaker[118–120] also allow laboratories now not only to compare allele and antigen differences from a donor to a recipient but also to identify and count the number of eplet (3–4 amino acid differences at positions with immunogenicity potential) and epitope (structure surrounding the eplet where the Fab' can bind) differences, typically expressed as the total number of eplet differences or eplet "load." Methods such as these can also identify specific eplets that are different between donor–recipient pairs that may have greater immunologic relevance.[121–126]

## LIMITATIONS OF HUMAN LEUKOCYTE ANTIGEN TYPING METHODS

Serologic methods identify only the broadest of HLA antigens at their most common and strongest humoral targets;

**Table 69.2 Human Leukocyte Antigens Mismatching Considered From the Perspective of the Recipient Immune System**

| Human Leukocyte Antigen Locus | A* | B* | Cw* | DRB1* | DQA1* | DQB1* | DPA1* | DPB1* | Total Mismatches |
|---|---|---|---|---|---|---|---|---|---|
| Recipient | 11 | 15(62) 15(75) | 04 | 12 | 06:01 | 03:01(7) | 01:03 | 02:02 | |
| | 24 | | 08 | 14 | – | – | 02 | 21:01 | |
| Donor | 2 | 46 | 01 | 09 | 03 | 03:03(9) | 02- | 05:01 | |
| | – | 52 | 14 | – | – | – | – | 09:01 | |
| Mismatch | 1 | 2 | 2 | 1 | 1 | 1 | 0 | 2 | 10 |
| Recipient | 2 | 46 | 01 | 09 | 03 | 03:03(9) | 02- | 05:01 | |
| | – | 52 | 14 | – | – | – | – | 09:01 | |
| Donor | 11 | 15(62) 15(75) | 04 | 12 | 06:01 | 03:01(7) | 01:03 | 02:02 | |
| | 24 | | 08 | 14 | – | – | 02 | 21:01 | |
| Mismatch | 2 | 2 | 2 | 2 | 1 | 1 | 1 | 2 | 13 |

Molecularly determined alleles at each human leukocyte antigen (HLA) locus in recipient and donor in two different scenarios (upper and lower section of table), showing the number of mismatches.

In the case where either a recipient or donor is homozygous for one or more antigens, there is a difference in mismatches depending on which direction the mismatches are considered. In the first example, considering the foreign HLA donor, antigen burden yields 10 mismatches in the host versus graft direction. However, if the donor and recipient had the opposing HLA typing, it would give a total of 13 mismatches from the perspective of this recipient.

*Clinical Relevance*

The authors encourage the reader to interpret any historical data limited to HLA-A, B, and DR typing with caution considering modern-era data supporting the immunogenic role of proteins from HLA loci in transplant outcomes. When interpreting molecular results, the clinician should be sure to note whether allele level typing (second field resolution) is in fact necessary to interpret immunologic risk either at the eplet mismatch level or antibody–antigen interaction level. Consultation with histocompatibility specialists should be sought to determine the level of resolution needed in any given case.

they do not distinguish, in most cases, between small but immunologically important differences that may be present at alleles within the same antigen group. This is particularly relevant when HLA antibodies (see later) have only a subset of allele-coded proteins within a group (allele-specific antibodies) as their target. Additionally, serologic methods only commonly identified with any accuracy A, B and DR proteins, giving rise to the (now recognized as incorrect) paradigm that these six antigens were the most significant in transplantation. The authors encourage the reader to interpret any historical data limited to HLA-A, B, DR typing with caution, considering modern era data supporting the immunogenic role of proteins from HLA loci in transplant outcomes. Molecular methods in general have advanced the understanding of HLA diversity and its contribution to alloimmunity, but different platforms have different levels of typing resolution and all are under rapid evolution such that any specific discussion of limitation would shortly be obsolete. At present, the major limitation to some methods that result in a high level of resolution is that several days may be required to obtain a result, which is prohibitive in deceased donor transplantation workup and allocation; this, however, is anticipated to change with the rapid improvement of methods and platforms. Rather, when interpreting molecular results, the clinician should be sure to note whether allele level typing (second field resolution) is in fact necessary to interpret immunologic risk, either at the eplet mismatch level or antibody-antigen interaction level. Consultation with Histocompatibility specialists should be sought out to determine the level of resolution needed in any given case.

## USING HUMAN LEUKOCYTE ANTIGEN TYPING RESULTS IN KIDNEY TRANSPLANTATION

### INTERPRETING THE TRANSPLANT CANDIDATE'S ANTIBODY PROFILE

The first step in evaluating a transplant candidate is to determine their own HLA allele and antigen profile using the highest resolution typing available in that center. This information is useful immediately, well before a donor is under consideration, as the recipient's HLA antibody profile must always be interpreted in the context of their own HLA typing to ensure that the antibodies identified are as accurate as possible (cognizant that one does not make HLA antibody to self-HLA antigens or self-epitopes). We note that antibodies can form to self-eplets,[126] but only when the surrounding epitope is non-self. These considerations are crucial for accurate antibody interpretation, and sufficient resolution of recipient HLA typing is thus of utmost importance. Furthermore, in very highly sensitized patients, understanding the population frequency of the candidate's own HLA alleles and haplotype can aid in the estimate of donor access (likelihood to receive a donor organ), with those patients who have rarer HLA alleles potentially having an even further reduced access compared with those with more common HLA phenotypes.

## CLINICAL ESTIMATE OF IMMUNOGENICITY OF HUMAN LEUKOCYTE ANTIGEN MISMATCHES

The number of HLA mismatches between donor and recipient was one of the first recognized predictors of transplant outcome as early as 3 years posttransplant, even in the early days of transplantation, when typing was only resolved at the serologic level and assessment was limited to only a few loci.[127–130] With improved immunosuppression, the impact of mismatching at the antigen level was reduced, and its role in allocation correspondingly diminished.[131,132] Studies using larger data sets and performed in the era of modern immunosuppression, with a view to longer-term clinically relevant outcomes, however, still show that donor–recipient HLA mismatching, even at the antigen level, can have a deleterious impact on graft survival.[133–136] Notably, however, all HLA antigens are not equally different at the eplet/epitope level, and simply considering the integer difference in mismatches is at best a crude estimate of immunogenicity (Table 69.3). Eplet analysis is a more granular and biologically relevant estimate of immune differences at the level of the HLA molecule. Early data support this strategy with HLA eplet load being strongly associated with both *de novo* DSA development[123,137] and clinically relevant outcomes, such as transplant glomerulopathy.[124] It is further recognized that not all HLA eplets are immunologically equivalent. As such, eplet load is itself also only an estimate of immune difference. There is much interest in determining which eplet differences carry the greatest risk of adverse outcome, but such data are currently not yet available.

As mentioned earlier, the role of HLA matching in allocation has been reduced in many jurisdictions. This is both because of the reduced impact on short- and medium-term outcomes, as well as concerns about creating biases against individuals of certain races/HLA phenotypes, where their group's HLA antigens are less commonly found among typical organ donors. There is insufficient evidence available at this time to allocate organs strictly based on eplet load or eplet matching. However, this may evolve with rapidly emerging data. How then should the clinician interpret HLA mismatch data at the antigen, allele, or eplet level? It is important to acknowledge that if the mismatches in a given pair are greater, then the immunologic potential for alloimmune recognition and response is also greater. The clinician should use this information to refine the risk assessment along a continuum. Higher-risk states may warrant greater vigilance in follow-up (lab tests, HLA antibody monitoring) or greater caution in reducing immunotherapy.

### AVOIDANCE OF UNACCEPTABLE DONOR ANTIGENS/ALLELES

Foundational to modern organ allocation is evaluating donor HLA typing in the context of a recipient's HLA to identify if there are any DSA. This is commonly referred to as virtual crossmatching (VXM), where positive DSA is interpreted as a positive VXM and the absence of DSA is a negative VXM. This is discussed in more detail in the section on virtual crossmatching later. From the perspective of HLA typing, it is critical that donor typing be performed at all loci to which a recipient has detectable anti-HLA antibodies, using enough resolution (up to 2 field) to evaluate allele-specific antibody relevance.

### DONOR DATA SUPPORTING CALCULATED PANEL REACTIVE ANTIBODY CALCULATORS

Foundational to the estimate of calculated panel reactive antibody (cPRA)[138,139] (see section later) is a database of many deceased donor HLA typings to which an antibody profile can be compared. It is essential that these data sets be large and as complete at all loci as possible so that the calculation

**Table 69.3 Quantifying Human Leukocyte Antigens Versus Eplet Mismatches**

| Human Leukocyte Antigen Locus | A* | B* | Cw* | DRB1* | DQA1* | DQB1* | Total Mismatches |
|---|---|---|---|---|---|---|---|
| Recipient | 01:01 | 07:02 | 07:01 | 03:01 | 01:03 | 02:01 | |
| | 03:01 | 08:01 | 07:02 | 13:09 | 05:01 | 06:03 | |
| Donor | 02:01 | 44:02 | 03:01 | 01:01 | 01:02 | 06:-2 | |
| | 11:01 | 54:01 | 05:01 | 04:05 | 03:01 | 03:02 | |
| HLA antigen mismatch | | 6 | | | 4 | | 10 |
| Eplet mismatch | | 35 | | | 51 | | 86 |
| Recipient | 01:01 24:02 | 51:01 35:01 | 07:01 01:02 | 03:02(18) | 03:01 | 02:02 | |
| | | | | 07:01 | 04:01 | 04:02 | |
| Donor | 23:01 36:01 | 52:01 53:01 | 15:02 18:01 | 03:01(17) | 05:01 | 02:01 | |
| | | | | 11:04 | – | 03:01 | |
| HLA antigen mismatch | | 6 | | | 4 | | 10 |
| Eplet mismatch | | 4 | | | 23 | | 27 |

HLA antigen mismatch is only a very crude estimate of the degree of mismatch between donors and recipients. In these examples, despite the same number of Class I and Class II antigen mismatches, the first pair has almost 3 times the number of eplet mismatches (not shown) representing a more potent alloimmune stimulus.

of cPRA is immunologically relevant and accurately representative of access.

## HUMAN LEUKOCYTE ANTIGEN ANTIBODY SCREENING AND IDENTIFICATION

### CONTEXT

Sensitization occurs when an individual is exposed to non-self HLA epitopes via pregnancy, prior transplant or blood transfusion. As a result of sensitization, a significant proportion of individuals can develop HLA antibodies: 50% to 74 % in pregnancy,[140–142] 1% to 20% of transfusion-exposed patients,[142–144] and 45% to 80% of patients with prior transplants.[145–148] A small percentage of patients also appear to have some HLA antibodies in the absence of a sensitizing event, but the clinical significance of these antibodies remains questionable.[149]

The detection of HLA antibodies prior to transplantation and their precise specificities (the exact antigens to which they are expected to bind) allows estimating the percentage of available donors to whom they may have DSA. Further, this allows estimating access to transplantation because of antibody profile. At the time of considering a potential donor, the recipient HLA antibody specificities can be examined for DSA to those of the donor in order to make a more informed and precise immunologic risk and transplant decision, as DSA portends a higher risk of humoral immune complications posttransplant.

After transplantation, the development of de novo DSA carries a particularly deleterious prognosis and is strongly associated with worse outcomes, both at the short and long term and with graft survival. Patently clear, however, is that both sensitive and specific antibody detection as well as identification methods are critical in guiding both the interventions and treatments for better outcomes, at all times during the transplant patient lifecycle.

### ANTIBODY DETECTION AND IDENTIFICATION METHODS

#### SEROLOGY

The term *panel reactive antibody* (PRA) is broadly used to describe the percentage of donors in a candidate donor population to whom a recipient may have DSA. The term *PRA* comes from the original serologic methods for detecting HLA antibodies. PRA testing involves exposing a panel of various cells from different donors (selected to represent the common HLA frequencies in a potential donor population) to a recipient's serum, to which complement, and a vital dye are added. The percentage of the cells in the panel which are lysed is an estimate of the percentage of donors from that population against whom the recipient has cytotoxic antibodies (IgG1 or IgG3 of sufficiently high titer to initiate the complement cascade).[150–152] Due to the limitations of serologic screening, including lack of sensitivity, limited specificity with high false-positive rates due to non-HLA antibodies, IgM and autoantibodies[153–155] (which are immunologically irrelevant) and volatility of the PRA estimate based on cell panel phenotype variation regardless of recipient serum changes, this method will not be further discussed.

#### SOLID-PHASE HUMAN LEUKOCYTE ANTIGEN ANTIBODY SCREENING

In these assays, purified HLA antigens are covalently bound to inert beads or less commonly to an ELISA platform.[156–158] The latter have been largely replaced with bead-based assays due to their increased sensitivity and capacity for high-volume testing and will not be further discussed. In screening solid-phase assays, beads carry the complete class I or class II HLA profile of an individual and can be detected when the antibody in serum binds, regardless of complement activation, with a secondary fluorescent anti–human IgG detector antibody on a flow cytometric platform. A bead is determined to be positive when its fluorescence is above the threshold level validated by the laboratory and manufacturer. The PRA estimate, in this case stratified by class, is similar in principle to serology methods as the percentage of total beads with positive fluorescence.[159–167]

#### SOLID-PHASE HUMAN LEUKOCYTE ANTIGEN ANTIBODY-SPECIFICITY TESTING

Although PRA testing yields a population-based estimate of the number of donors to whom a recipient may have DSA, for these to be used in transplant decision making and donor selection, greater detail is needed as to which precise antigens the antibodies are directed toward. Single antigen beads (SABs) are similar in platform to HLA solid-phase screening assays, but in this case each bead has only one distinct type of HLA antigen bound. Also analyzed on flow cytometric platforms, up to 100 unique beads per class can be tested simultaneously.[168] The output of this test is also fluorescence-based and defines a list of antibody specificities that then must be reverse engineered into a cPRA using a calculator informed by large numbers of donor genotypes.[138,139,169]

#### COMPLEMENT-BINDING SOLID-PHASE ASSAYS

These assays are derived from the classic SAB test, and instead of simply detecting any antibody bound to the bead's antigens, they are designed to detect the binding of C1q or C3d complement by HLA-specific antibody.[170] Complement-binding DSA are associated with an acute rejection phenotype that is more severe and with an increased risk of allograft failure compared with noncomplement-binding DSA.[171] These assays will only be positive if IgG 1/3 antibodies are also first bound in sufficient density (high concentration) to antigens on the bead surface.[171–173] If low-titer IgG 1/3 antibody is present or IgG 2/4 isotypes dominate the serum antibody profile, then the result will be negative. Isotype-specific assays can also be used to discriminate between all four isotypes within a given SAB reaction and infer similar complement-binding potential, but are not commonly used in routine clinical practice.[174,175] It is notable that almost all antibodies that are detectable on traditional SAB platforms are present in all four isotypes,[176,177] suggesting that complement activation is at least possible for all antibodies, and its detection is dependent largely on titer of the IgG1/3 components.[170,173]

#### NON-HUMAN LEUKOCYTE ANTIGEN ANTIBODIES

Though not yet routinely implemented in all labs as a part of standard testing, commercial assays are now available for several non-HLA antibodies, including endothelial antibodies,[178,179] MICA,[61,68] and angiotensin type 1 receptor antibodies[88,97] in renal transplantation. These assays are also solid-phase–based with correspondingly similar methodologies as other solid-phase assays. Although there have been studies detailing univariate associations with transplant outcomes, the incremental additional value of these tests for population screening remains uncertain[179,180] and their current utilization potential is determined at the individual patient level.

## INTERPRETING SOLID-PHASE HUMAN LEUKOCYTE ANTIGEN ANTIBODY TESTS

### GENERAL INTERPRETATION

The numerical output from both screening and SABs is mean fluorescence intensity (MFI), which is compared with both negative control bead and negative control serum fluorescence in order to identify whether a given bead is of sufficiently high fluorescence to be deemed positive. It is important to note that although MFI output is numerical, it should not be interpreted as quantitative or an equivalent to antibody titer (see Limitations later).[181–183] Other factors can and should be considered in determining the relevance of a given bead reactivity, including sensitization history (and HLA type(s) of the sensitizer(s), if available), a pattern of shared eplets or a known Cross Reactive Group (CREG) among beads deemed to be fluorescing that would support their positivity as biologically plausible from an antibody-eplet binding perspective, a change in reactivity pattern over time (where a bead representing an antigen of interest and previously lower ranked in the assay MFI is now relatively increased, even if below usual thresholds for positive), interval changes in immunosuppression treatments, the presence of autoimmune disease with antibody binding to denatured antigens in the SAB assay[184] and the administration of any agents that could increase background interference. Once the determination of the list of positive beads has been made, further analysis of these positive reactions is required to determine the list of antibody specificities.

### ANTIBODIES REPORTED AT THE ANTIGEN LEVEL

Antibodies are identified most commonly as specific to HLA antigens. These are reported as lists of serologic equivalents in nomenclature; for example, A2, B7, DR15, and so on. The interpretation by the clinician is correspondingly that the patient has an antibody that will bind all members of the antigen group regardless of specific allele. Biologically, it is inferred that the antibody is directed toward the epitope(s) that are common to all members of the antigen group and not at the epitope(s) that would distinguish unique alleles. Additionally, for class II, although not traditionally considered antigens in their own right, antibodies can form to the unique polymorphic alpha chains (coded by DQA1 and DPA1 genes). When these are identified, they will be listed with the alpha chain specified. For example, DQA1 or DPA2 antibody, distinct from DQ7 or DP3, which infers the antibody is to the beta chain.

### ALLELE-SPECIFIC ANTIBODIES

Although antibodies are most commonly identified toward antigen groups, it is recognized that there are multiple different alleles comprising each antigen group. Sometimes, an antibody may be directed to one of the eplet/epitopes unique to a certain allele, in which case it will typically be identified using up to four digits; for example, B5102 antibody, where this nomenclature implies an antibody binding to the protein encoded by HLA-B*51:02 allele but not the other alleles in the B51 chain, including B*51:01 (Fig. 69.8).

### ALPHA/BETA ANTIBODIES

Given the nature of class II molecules, it can occur that Fab' of the antibody can bridge the polymorphic alpha and beta chains of an antigen, resulting in an antibody that is specific to the unique combination of an alpha and beta chain. Wherever this occurs, the antibody is identified using some combination of the alpha and beta nomenclature; for example, DQA5-DQ2 (or similar).

### CALCULATED PANEL REACTIVE ANTIBODY (OR EQUIVALENT) DETERMINATION

A recipient's list of antibodies is inherently useful in determining toward which donors a recipient has antibodies. However, to estimate a better likelihood of access it is useful to understand to what percentage of donors in a population the recipient bears antibody. To determine this, the list of antibodies is compared with a database of donor typings specific to the population of interest. The percentage of donors to whom a recipient has one or more DSA represents the cPRA[139,185] or equivalent (e.g., calculated reaction frequency or cRF in the United Kingdom).[186] The cPRA varies based not only on the list of antibodies but also, and more importantly, to the loci included in the donor typing and frequency of target HLA antigens in the donor population of interest. This, in turn, is strongly related to population-based racial differences.[187] At the time of this publication, cPRA calculators most widely available do not incorporate allele-specific antibodies.

## LIMITATIONS OF HUMAN LEUKOCYTE ANTIGEN ANTIBODY TESTING

### DEFINING A POSITIVE BEAD

Although the output of the SAB assay is a numerical MFI on each bead, which has a unique antigen on it, the MFI alone is insufficient to determine whether or not the fluorescence on a bead represents a true antibody being detected, and no universal threshold for positive should ever be assigned.[188] There is a widely varying density of HLA antigens between beads, such that the maximum MFI on any given bead may be determined by antigen density rather than serum level of antibody. In the presence of very high levels of complement-binding antibody; C1q may be generated in vivo from soluble complement proteins and interfere with the binding of the antibody to the bead, significantly lowering the MFI of the beads, representing very high levels of antibody. Dilution of serum samples when this phenomenon occurs can clearly show that MFI increases with serum dilution, confirming its nonquantitative value on the undiluted serum. Very commonly, groups of HLA antigens share common epitopes to which antibodies are targeted, and when the antibody to a shared target is present at a subsaturating level, it can spread across the multiple beads with antigens sharing this target, thereby reducing the MFI of any given single

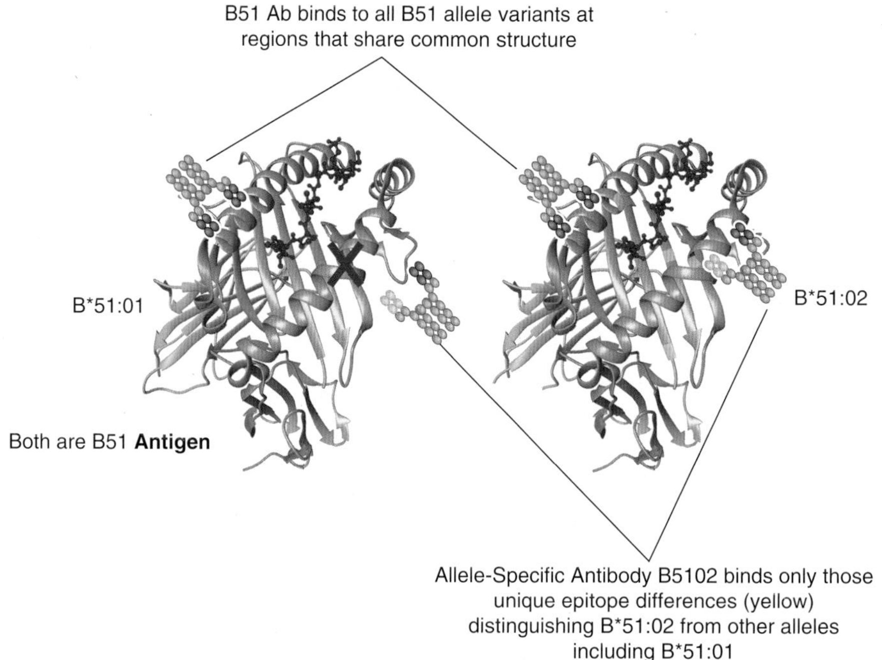
B51 Ab binds to all B51 allele variants at
regions that share common structure
B*51:01
B*51:02
Both are B51 **Antigen**
Allele-Specific Antibody B5102 binds only those
unique epitope differences (yellow)
distinguishing B*51:02 from other alleles
including B*51:01

**Fig. 69.8 Allele differences in protein structure can lead to different immunogenicity. Proteins coded by B*51:01 and B*51:02 alleles differ by a 3 amino acid substitution in the peptide-binding region. Both are referred to as B51 antigens. Antibodies that bind to regions common to all the B51 antigens will bind proteins coded by all alleles in the group. Some antibodies bind only to those specific epitope region(s) that distinguish one allele from the others. These allele-specific antibodies may be identified by their four-digit names, in this example, B5102 antibody.**

> ***Clinical Relevance***
> Although the output of the single-bead assays is a numerical mean fluorescence intensity on each bead, which has a unique antigen on it, the mean fluorescence intensity alone is insufficient to determine whether or not the fluorescence on a bead represents a true antibody being detected and no universal threshold for positive should be assigned. For multiple lab-specific validation and reagent-based reasons, it is strongly recommended that the readers consult with their own laboratory as to the analytic strategies employed to optimally identify antibodies and thresholds used for calling a positive test.

bead within the group. This single-bead MFI can be misleadingly low as an estimate of antibody. Similarly, some antigens that have several common alleles are represented on more than one bead in the SAB assay; again, an antibody to this antigen at an epitope shared by all alleles can be diluted across the multiple beads, lowering single-bead MFI estimate. For these and other lab-specific validation and reagent-based reasons, it is strongly recommended that the readers consult with their own laboratory as to the analytic strategies employed to optimally identify antibodies and thresholds for positive (Fig. 69.9).[181–183]

## DEFINING IMMUNOLOGIC RELEVANCE

A conundrum of the detection of antibody, as for all laboratory results, is that mere identification does not precisely determine relevance at that time or in the future. Whereas higher-titer antibodies, persistent (versus transient) antibodies, and class II antibodies may be associated with worse outcomes post-transplant, it would be misleading to classify these as absolute risk states. Rather the clinical relevance of an antibody is part of a multifactorial patient and donor assessment in the context of patient history, immunosuppression, sensitizing events, and current clinical status and organ function. There are no indisputable features that clearly discriminate antibodies with more deleterious or immediate consequences from those that portend a more benign course.

## NATURALLY OCCURRING ANTIBODIES

SAB assays are so sensitive that reactions may be detected in individuals without any history of sensitizing events.[149,184] The clinical consequences of these antibodies, the nature of their target antigen (denatured in assay versus intact in vivo) and whether they should be avoided or considered in donor selection still requires further study.

## ANTIBODY CAN BE BOUND TO THE ALLOGRAFT

The SAB assay detects circulating antibodies. However, it has been shown, in individuals with a failed allograft in place, that significant antibody may be removed from circulation and bound to the endothelium, reducing the sensitivity of the assay. Following nephrectomy, antibody levels may increase.[52,189] If an allograft remains in situ, the full antibody potential may be dampened.

## COMPLEMENT FIXING ASSAYS

Although some studies have shown that antibodies detected by complement fixing assays are associated with worse

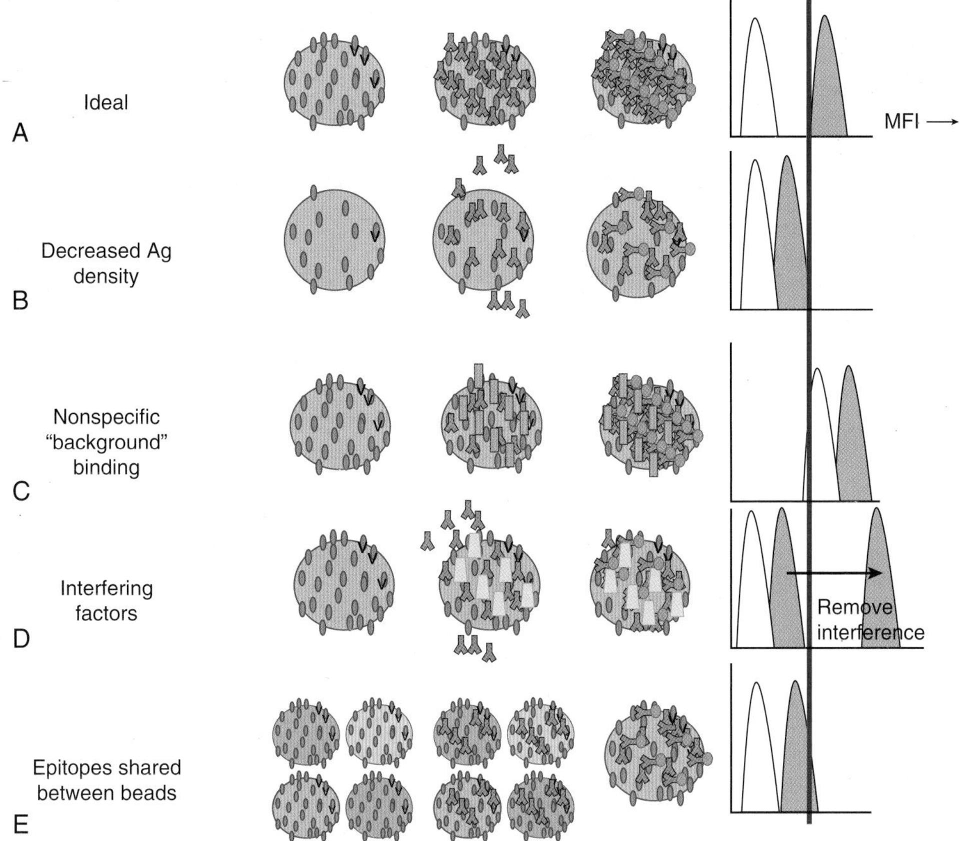


**Fig. 69.9 Median fluorescence intensity (MFI) of single antigen bead assays has analytic limitations and cannot be used as a quantitative metric of antibody amount. A, An ideal test should always be able to distinguish antibody binding *(blue signal)* from negative control *(white)* with a clear threshold and no overlap between the MFI distributions. B, Decreased density of antigen (Ag) on the surface of the bead will result in MFI measurement that underestimates the amount of the antibody present. C, In contrast, nonspecific binding to the bead can result in artificially high background and signal MFI, with overestimation of antibody. D, Interfering substances may prevent the detection of the antibody of interest with lower MFI. E, Epitopes shared between different beads can dilute the amount of antibody bound to any single bead, with an erroneously low MFI on the given bead of interest.** (From Konvalinka A, Tinckam K. Utility of HLA antibody testing in kidney transplantation. *J Am Soc Nephrol* 2015;26(7):1489–1502. With permission.)

outcomes, not all studies demonstrate this, and pretransplant routine SAB testing alone predicts posttransplant outcomes as well as complement assays. These assays do not detect specific deleterious antibodies, but rather higher-titer IgG1/3 in vitro.[172,190] If there are multiple low-titer IgG 1/3 antibodies in a sample, they may be C1q negative in vitro, but when present in vivo, they may nonetheless activate complement on the endothelium. Indeed, C1q positivity does not correlate with C4d presence in tissues,[191] and merely concentrating a C1q-negative serum can change results to C1q positive.[173] Finally, not all deleterious antibody-mediated pathways are complement-dependent; it is erroneous to surmise that antibodies that do not bind complement in vitro have less potential for harm in vivo.[170]

### GENERALIZABILITY OF CALCULATED PANEL REACTIVE ANTIBODY

For a cPRA to best estimate the percentage of potential donors to whom a recipient has DSA (and consequently higher immune risk to those donors), not only do the antibodies need to be accurately identified, but also the donor typings utilized must be representative of the donor population accessible to that individual. As such, a cPRA based on one donor population may not be an accurate assessment of donor access in other populations with different racial distribution and different associated HLA antigen frequencies.[187] Additionally, the cPRA may be systematically underestimated when donor typing is not complete at loci where HLA antibodies to those loci are utilized in donor decision making.[139]

## USING HUMAN LEUKOCYTE ANTIGEN ANTIBODY TESTING IN KIDNEY TRANSPLANTATION

### ON THE WAITLIST

In addition to HLA typing of the recipient, waitlist HLA antibody testing is foundational to ongoing patient immunologic assessment. The main goal of waitlist testing is to estimate the transplant candidate's access to donors from the perspective of avoiding donor antigens to whom they have antibodies. This estimate is quantified as the cPRA, where (100-cPRA) is the percentage of donors otherwise medically and ABO suitable that would be accessible to the recipient. If the candidate has a high cPRA, longer wait times and higher waitlist mortality are anticipated.[192–194] In that case, strategies to improve access to more donors should be sought. If no potential living donor is available, then desensitization,[195–197] or deceased donor acceptable mismatch allocation strategies,[198–200] should be considered. If a living donor is available, then desensitization or kidney paired donation programs[201] could improve access. A second goal of waitlist antibody testing is to compile a longitudinal immunologic profile of the candidate; antibodies can wax and wane over time, so repeated testing is indicated (usually every one to three months) to ensure the most complete list of antibody potential is compiled for use at the time of a potential donor evaluation. If a patient incurs a sensitizing event, repeat testing 6 weeks after the event is recommended to capture any memory responses or de novo antibodies. It is critical to remember that patients frequently have a long immunologic history predating their entrance to the waitlist, so even repeated HLA antibody testing may not identify all antibody potential; a thorough history of sensitizing events both prior to and while on the waitlist remains foundational to counselling patients as to their immunologic risk posttransplant. Finally, the cPRA and its contributing antibody specificities are, in and of themselves, not a measurement of immunologic risk (only risk of reduced access to donors); immunologic risk is a measurement unique to each donor-recipient pair under consideration.

#### At the Time of Transplant Offer: Virtual Crossmatching

In conjunction with donor HLA typing, the full history of recipient HLA antibodies may be compared with donor HLA antigens in what has come to be known as a virtual crossmatch (VXM). If any of the current or historical specificities correspond to donor antigens, these DSA confer a positive VXM. Under optimal circumstances, the VXM is intended to be a predictor for an actual cell-based crossmatch performed on the corresponding sera, in order to facilitate allocation and transplant decision making. However, the predictive values of VMX for actual crossmatch (XM) can vary widely depending on XM methodology[202–204] and the laboratory- and program-specific parameters for identifying antibodies. The current VXM reflects the most recent serum tested prior to donor offer and most closely reflects the antibodies likely to be present at the time of transplant and is associated with early and late rejections and reduced allograft survival. Conversely, the historical VXM reflects the cumulative history of DSA. When current VXM is negative but historical is positive, there is an increased risk for memory B-cell reactivity after transplant and corresponding adverse allograft outcomes. Despite historical and fewer recent reports of high PRA association with adverse transplant outcome, the ability to more precisely assess VXM/DSA has revealed that it is in fact DSA that drives adverse outcomes, regardless of the level of PRA directed toward third-party antibody, further improving treatment decision making.[200,205,206] In some jurisdictions where regulatory requirements allow, the VXM has replaced the actual XM for many transplant decisions, with comparable transplant outcomes.[207,208] Additionally, the virtual crossmatch is an important part of crossmatch interpretation to ensure that the cell-based crossmatch, if positive, is in fact immunologically relevant[165] (see Crossmatching later).

### POSTTRANSPLANT ANTIBODY MONITORING

Following transplantation, all HLA mismatched patients are at risk of de novo HLA DSA development. Landmark studies in 2005 and 2007 first identified that posttransplant HLA antibodies had higher rates of graft failure than those without antibody development.[68,69] In the years since, it has become clear that *de novo* HLA DSA development is a major risk factor for rejection and premature graft loss. Despite numerous studies, there is no consensus to date as to the optimal timing and frequency of monitoring.

Although associations of de novo DSA and the range of transplant-associated outcomes cannot be absolute or perfectly predictive, de novo DSA remain a strong independent risk factor for significant antibody-mediated outcomes. De novo DSA appear at a median of 3 to 68 months posttransplant and positive de novo DSA are found in 6% to 38% of patients 3 years after transplantation.[122] Class II antibodies predominate in most series. As a diagnostic tool the presence of DSA is supportive of a diagnosis of ABMR in the context of aligned pathology and dysfunction,[53,209–211] but ABMR may also occur in the absence of detectable HLA DSA, often dependent on timing of testing, with antibody bound in the failed allograft[52,189] or rarely to non-HLA antibody.[51,61,212] Late ABMR is associated with chronic pathology, Class II Ab and lower response rate to treatment.[213–215] DSA MFI thresholds do not reliably discriminate prognosis or treatment responsiveness,[213,216] nor is it a tool to determine duration of treatment as DSA frequently persist well beyond clinical and histopathologic resolution of ABMR.[214,216]

As a prognostic tool, when detected before graft dysfunction or pathology of ABMR, the role of de novo DSA role is not clearly defined. The interval between de novo DSA detection and clinical outcome can vary widely from months to years, as can the phenotype of the outcome itself, suggesting diverse pathways of injury at play with many effect modifiers.[191,217–223] Data do not presently support empirical treatment for de novo DSA in the absence of graft dysfunction and/or tissue injury. At this juncture, asymptomatic de novo DSA can best be considered a higher-risk state for future adverse events that may warrant closer patient follow-up.

## DONOR-SPECIFIC (CELL-BASED) CROSSMATCHING

### CONTEXT

Before the introduction of the complement-dependent cytotoxicity (CDC) crossmatch in 1969,[100] the phenotype of early graft loss (as hyperacute or accelerated rejection) was a recognized but largely unpredictable event. The introduction of the CDC crossmatch provided clinicians with a tool to predict early graft loss prior to transplantation and improved decision making. The cell-based crossmatch in general may be considered a "surrogate" transplant; rather than exposing the endothelial cells of the allograft to the recipient circulation at the time of operation, the donor lymphocytes (expressing the same HLA antigens as donor endothelium) are first exposed to recipient serum in vitro. Where HLA antibodies are detected on the surface of the lymphocytes, it is surmised that these antibodies would also bind to the allograft endothelium with deleterious consequence; the transplant can then be avoided, or immunosuppression modified. Although supplanted by

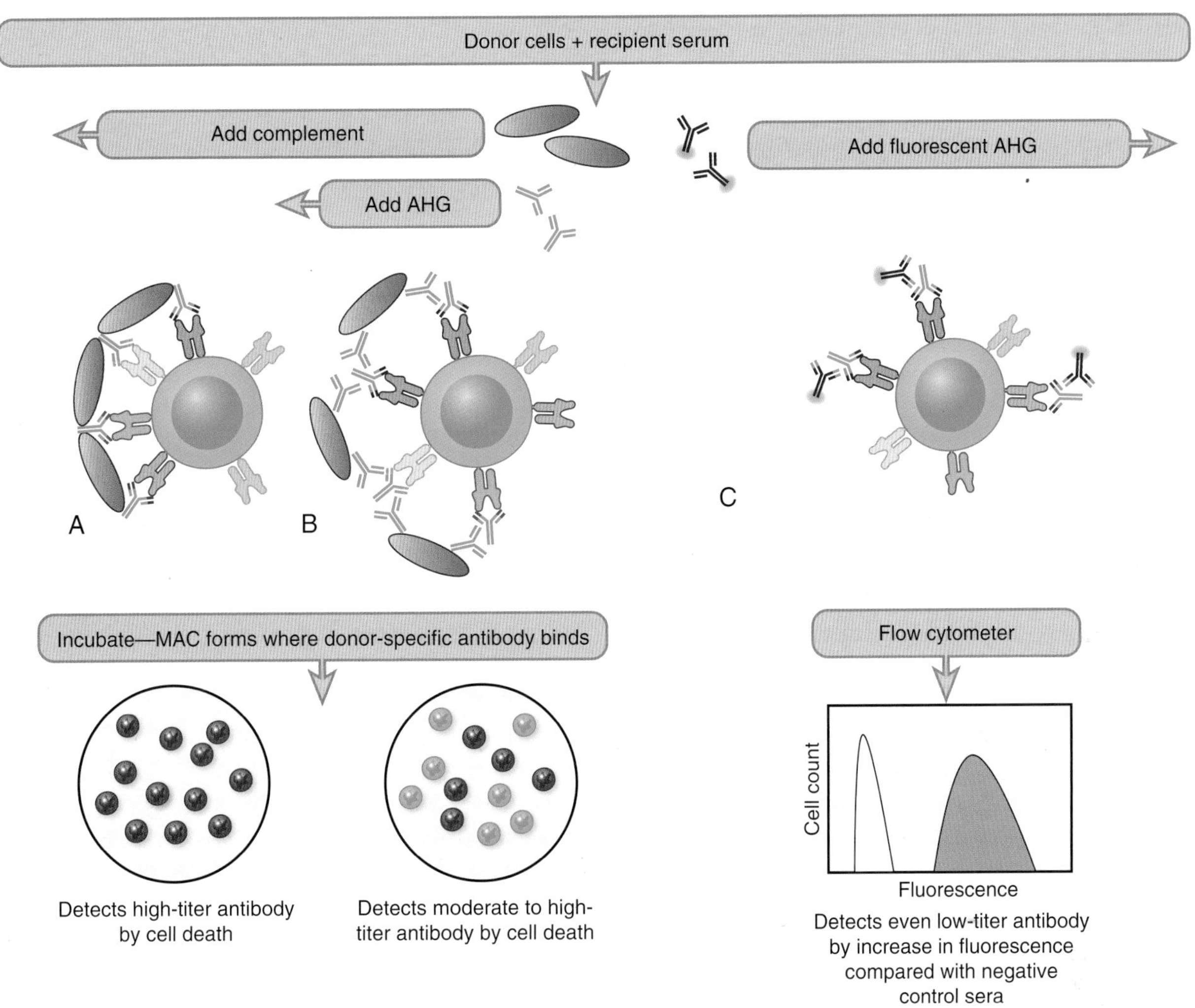


**Fig. 69.10 Crossmatch methods. A, The complement-dependent cytotoxicity (CDC) crossmatch detects high-titer donor-specific antibody (DSA) when it binds to the cell in sufficient density to activate the complement cascade. The resulting formation of the membrane attack complex (MAC) results in cell death, which can be detected via microscopy with a vital dye. A positive CDC crossmatch due to human leuckocyte antigen (HLA) antibody is associated with hyperacute or early accelerated rejection. B, The antihuman globulin (AHG)-enhanced CDC crossmatch increases sensitivity for moderate-titer antibody with the addition of AHG. AHG binds to donor-specific antibody (DSA) already bound to its target antigen, allowing for activation of complement at lower levels of original DSA. The MAC will form again and kill cells with antibody bound to it, deleted under microscopy. A positive AHG-CDC crossmatch due to HLA antibody is associated with hyperacute or early accelerated rejection. C, The flow cytometry crossmatch can detect even lower-level antibodies using fluorescence detection if the antibody is bound to the cell. Noncomplement-binding antibodies are also detected using this methodology. Positive flow cytometry crossmatches may vary in strength. Strongly positive results due to HLA antibodies are associated with not only higher rates of earlier antibody-mediated rejection (AMR) but also subclinical rejection and chronic AMR. However, not all positive flow cytometry crossmatches are clearly associated with an adverse outcome, and methods to distinguish pathologic from nonpathologic antibodies are needed.** (From Lapointe I, Tinckam K. *Histocompatibility testing for kidney transplantation risk assessment*. Scientific American Nephrology, Dialysis and Transplantation. ©Decker Intellectual Properties, Inc. 2017. With permission.)

virtual crossmatching in some clinical circumstances, the cell-based crossmatch remains an important test for donor recipient compatibility immediately prior to transplant.

## CROSSMATCH METHODS

### COMPLEMENT-DEPENDENT CYTOTOXICITY

This method employs the same serologic principles described for the earliest typing and antibody detection methods, where cells from the donor are mixed with recipient serum in the presence of complement and cell death detected by vital dye uptake is the marker of a positive test, detecting high-titer complement-binding antibodies likely to result in hyperacute rejection (Fig. 69.10).

### ANTIHUMAN GLOBULIN ENHANCED COMPLEMENT-DEPENDENT CYTOTOXICITY

By the early 1990s a more sensitive derivation of the CDC crossmatch was achieved by adding antihuman globulin (AHG) to the test, binding any antibody on the cell surface, increasing overall antibody density and increasing the probability that complement would become activated with lower levels of HLA antibody. These lower-titer HLA antibodies were nonetheless clinically relevant and associated with earlier antibody-mediated outcomes not predicted by the less sensitive CDC crossmatch.[224–229]

### FLOW CYTOMETRY CROSSMATCH

With the awareness that antibody-mediated adverse outcomes could still occur with negative AHG-CDC crossmatch, the flow cytometry crossmatch (FCXM) permitted detection of even very low-level and/or noncomplement-binding antibody on the cell surface, detected by fluorescent anti–human IgG rather than complement activation.[230–235]

### INTERPRETING CELL-BASED CROSSMATCH RESULTS

Crossmatches are performed separately on both T and B lymphocytes. T lymphocytes express Class I HLA antigens whereas B lymphocytes express both class I and Class II HLA antigens. Historically, it was thought that only the T-cell crossmatch representing Class I HLA antigens predicted antibody-mediated early outcomes, but it is now known that endothelium that has sustained injury (for example, ischemia-reperfusion as is common in transplantation) can also upregulate class II expression so that positive B-cell crossmatches, when due to HLA antibody, can result in early accelerated rejection even when the T-cell crossmatch is negative.

A positive cytotoxic crossmatch when due to HLA antibody, (see Limitations later), indicates high-titer complement-binding antibody and predicts hyperacute rejection. A positive AHG-CDC XM (with negative CDC XM) detects lower-titer, still complement-binding antibody, and may be associated less commonly with hyperacute rejection, and more commonly with early or accelerated rejection in the hours to days after transplant. Positive FCXM, on the other hand, detects both complement and noncomplement-binding antibodies, and where cytotoxic crossmatches are negative and tend to be associated with later rejection and graft loss outcomes, they are less likely to result in hyperacute or accelerated rejection as well.

## LIMITATIONS OF CELL-BASED CROSSMATCH

### COMPLEMENT DEPENDENCE FOR DETECTING HUMAN LEUKOCYTE ANTIGEN ANTIBODIES

The use of the CDC XM greatly reduced, but did not eliminate, early accelerated rejection (false-negative test),[236] which could result from antibodies below the level of detection by complement-dependence that still caused damage to the graft endothelium in the hours to days after transplantation.

### IMMUNOLOGICALLY IRRELEVANT NON–HUMAN LEUKOCYTE ANTIGEN TARGETS ON CELLS

False-positive results can occur from autoantibodies[150,153–155] or immunologically irrelevant antibodies (including IgM antibody) binding non-HLA targets.[155,207,237,238]

### DRUG INTERFERENCE

Drugs that bind to lymphocytes, such as Thymoglobulin, Alemtuzumab and Rituximab or that contain nonspecific antibodies (intravenous immunoglobulins) may result in false-positive XM.

### B-CELL FALSE-POSITIVE CROSSMATCH

The B-cell receptor includes constitutively expressed immunoglobulin that can increase the likelihood of a positive B cell crossmatch in the absence of donor-specific HLA antibody. Laboratories routinely account for this by setting cutoffs for positivity and by using Pronase in flow cytometry crossmatching, which can improve the crossmatch specificity.[239–243]

### INCREASING SENSITIVITY MAY REDUCE PREDICTIVE VALUE

With all methods that increase sensitivity, the strength of correlation with any clinical outcome of interest becomes less specific. Although higher rates of adverse outcomes occur with positive FCXM in isolation, a positive FCXM does not guarantee worse transplant results, and in some cases these transplants can be performed with short- to medium-term success in the context of augmented immunotherapy or desensitization.

### LABORATORY VARIABILITY

The cell-based crossmatch is not a commercially available assay but rather developed within HLA laboratories frequently using nonstandard incubation times and variable reagents and controls. As such, there are no standard cutoffs for positive results and considerable inter laboratory variability may occur at the lower limit of detection of antibody.[244]

### USING THE CELL-BASED CROSSMATCH IN THE MODERN ERA

The cell-based crossmatch (most commonly the FCXM in the modern era) remains in many programs the gold standard for immediate pretransplant decision making. Unlike single antigen bead assays, which may not be easily performed on serum collected on the day of transplantation, the flow crossmatch may be quickly performed with serum that is temporally reflective of the immediate transplant environment. Considering the limitations described previously, we encourage the simultaneous performance of autocrossmatches (to assess for autoantibody) as well as crossmatches on historical sera that have been thoroughly evaluated using solid-phase antibody platforms; the authors strongly recommend that optimal interpretation of a crossmatch includes the solid-phase antibody data to confirm or exclude HLA antibody as the cause of the positive crossmatch. This is more easily arranged for living donor transplants; for deceased donor transplantation, historical sera crossmatches with their corresponding solid-phase antibody data that are already known may provide additional context for interpretation of a positive current serum cell-based crossmatch, where a current solid-phase result is not immediately available.

If a positive cell-based crossmatch is interpreted as caused by an autoantibody or non-HLA antibody, the transplant may proceed in most circumstances, as the crossmatch is deemed immunologically irrelevant.

If a positive cell-based crossmatch is interpreted as caused by an HLA antibody or an HLA antibody cannot be reliably excluded, transplant may be relatively contraindicated or require significantly augmented immunotherapy.

It is now true that as the VXM has become more commonplace, it has replaced the pretransplant cell-based crossmatch in some centers, where regulations permit, without demonstrable negative impact on patient and graft outcomes, and where VXM results are unambiguous in the context of a reliable history excluding recent sensitizing events. Nonetheless, in circumstances where the antibody

**Table 69.4 Clinical Histocompatibility Testing Menu and Associated Interpretations and Actions**

| Timepoint | Clinical Question(s) Applicable | Tests Used | Interpretation and Potential Actions |
|---|---|---|---|
| Pretransplant | How sensitized is the patient? How difficult is it be to find a (HLA-based) suitable donor? | • HLA typing • HLA AB Screening and Identification | If reduced access to donors from high cPRA, then access to more donors is optimal (increased sharing for acceptable mismatches, kidney paired donation programs) or desensitization to reduce current burden of circulating antibody. |
| | What is the patient's risk of a memory response post-transplant? | • HLA typing • HLA AB screening • In the context of a good clinical history of sensitizing events | All patients with HLA antibodies as well as those with sensitizing events should be considered at higher risk of memory responses post-transplant; closer follow-up posttransplant may be warranted. |
| At Transplant | Is the patient PREDICTED to have HLA antibodies to the donor? Will the cell-based crossmatch prior to transplant be positive? | • The virtual crossmatch: Donor typing PLUS • HLA AB identification (current and historical results) | Positive HISTORICAL VXM: Patient is at higher risk of memory response. Some programs do not transplant; others augment immunotherapy or monitoring. Positive CURRENT VXM: Patient is at higher risk of ABMR. Transplant decision making depends on strength of antibody (AB test plus cell-based crossmatch). |
| Posttransplant | Has the patient developed de novo HLA antibodies? (no graft dysfunction) | Donor typing from transplant Posttransplant AB testing | If positive, may indicate risk of future or current subclinical) ABMR? Guides further diagnostics or monitoring noting certain HLA loci portend a worse prognosis (Class II). |
| | Does the patient have ABMR? (with or without graft dysfunction) | Donor typing Posttransplant AB testing In context of biopsy if available | HLA antibodies are supportive of a diagnosis of AMR but may not always be present. |

*AB*, antibody; *ABMR*, antibody-mediated rejection; *HLA*, human leukocyte antigen; *VXM*, virtual crossmatch.

testing is indeterminate, the cell-based crossmatch still may serve as additional information to adjudicate the relevance of the antibody result.

An additional conundrum exists when the cell-based crossmatch is negative but the VXM is positive, due to the increased sensitivity of SAB over cellular assays.[245–247] ABMR has been reported in up to 55% of these patients[207,246,248,249] (greater than VXM negative counterparts) impacting graft survival in some,[249,250] but not all[195,251–253] series.

Indeed, the decision to proceed with transplant in the face of a positive crossmatch or negative crossmatch in the presence of HLA DSA should usually consider center expertise and the patient-specific competing risks of not receiving the transplant (including chance for a future DSA negative offer, and risk of dialysis-associated mortality).[196,254] The exception is with the positive cytotoxic crossmatch, where HLA DSA are confirmed because this confers an unacceptably high risk of hyperacute rejection precluding immediate transplant.

## THE EVOLVING ROLE OF HISTOCOMPATIBILITY CONSULTATION

Over the almost 50-year history of histocompatibility testing, testing has gone from simple pretransplant serologic-based assays with dichotomous risk classifications guiding the most basic of transplant decision making to sensitive, specific, individualized, and dynamic testing throughout the duration of the transplant experience (Table 69.4). Indeed, the test platforms and their corresponding results have evolved to such a degree of complexity that significant and discipline-specific postgraduate training and expertise is required to render a thoughtful and informative opinion. Adding to the complexity is the awareness that all biologically based HLA testing has inherent strengths and limitations, and the understanding of the interpretation of these myriads of tests in the context of these limitations is highly nuanced and requires consideration of not only immunologic but also competing medical, surgical, infectious, and even socioeconomic risks to the patient.[250,255] Histocompatibility testing has evolved to such a state of complexity and expertise that ongoing patient-specific consultation with laboratory specialists beyond simply the passive receipt of testing results is a mandatory part of good clinical transplant care, pre, post and long after transplant has occurred.

## KIDNEY ALLOGRAFT REJECTION

### ACUTE CELLULAR AND ANTIBODY-MEDIATED REJECTION

With the advent of modern immunosuppressive regimens[256] and increased sensitivity of pretransplant anti-HLA screening,[257] the incidence of acute rejection has decreased substantially over the last few decades. Approximately 15%

to 20% of kidney transplant recipients now experience a first rejection episode in the first 5 years after transplantation.[258] Rejection episodes are classified histologically using the Banff classification system.[54] This system provides criteria for the diagnosis of acute cell-mediated and antibody-mediated rejection, which can coexist. The main histologic feature of acute T-cell–mediated rejection (TCMR) is a mononuclear leukocyte infiltrate located in the tubules, interstitium, and/or arteries of the graft.[54] The cellular infiltrate is classically composed of T cells and monocytes/macrophages. Acute cell-mediated rejections are classified as Banff grade 1A or 1B, depending on the extent of inflammation, when the cellular infiltrate affects only the tubules and the interstitium. When endarteritis is present, rejections are classified as Banff grade 2A, 2B, or 3 according to the severity of the vascular involvement. In acute cell-mediated rejection, vascular involvement has classically been regarded as portending a poor prognosis in terms of resistance to treatment and graft survival.[259] This may in part be due to the previously unrecognized coexistence of cell-mediated endarteritis with classical features of ABMR, such as DSA and microcirculatory inflammation.[260] In line with this observation, a recent cohort study showed that endarteritis did not increase the risk of graft loss compared with tubulointerstitial involvement alone in patients who were DSA negative.[261] In contrast, patients who had endarteritis and DSA experienced a risk of graft loss that was 9 times greater than that observed in patients with DSA-negative tubulointerstitial rejection.

In addition to the presence of circulating DSA or antibodies against other donor antigens, ABMR is characterized by acute tissue injury, as evidenced by either microvascular inflammation (glomerulitis, peritubular capillaritis), endarteritis, or, in the absence of other causes, thrombotic microangiopathy or acute tubular injury. Evidence of antibody interaction with the endothelium has long been recognized by diffuse C4d deposition in peritubular capillaries. However, as antibodies can target the endothelium through both complement-dependent and -independent cytotoxicity, the existence of C4d-negative ABMR has been well established in recent years.[53,262,263] Other markers of endothelial interaction with antibodies, such as increased endothelial gene transcripts[264] in the biopsy and at least moderate microvascular inflammation, are now also recognized as histologic features of ABMR.[54]

The use of microarray technology to analyze RNA transcripts from biopsies obtained from transplant rejection cases has provided novel insights on the mechanism of acute rejection in recent years. For instance, transcripts from NK cells and macrophages, as well as endothelial-associated transcripts, have been associated with DSA and ABMR.[48,264] Archetypal signatures of TCMR and various stages of ABMR have been found to correlate with graft survival and clinical judgment through transcript analysis, making this technology a promising tool to overcome some of the limitations of histologic analysis, such as poor reproducibility.[265,266] The clinical aspects of acute rejection are covered in detail in Chapter 70.

## CHRONIC ALLOGRAFT INJURY

The term chronic allograft nephropathy or, more recently, *chronic allograft injury* (CAI) has been used to describe the clinical presentation of relatively slow renal function decline, proteinuria, and/or hypertension occurring more than 3 months after renal transplantation, as accompanied by interstitial fibrosis and tubular atrophy (IFTA) on the graft biopsy.[267] Because these features are not specific, kidney graft biopsy should be performed to investigate the cause of deteriorating graft function.[268] Recent data show that specific causes for IFTA can be found in over 80% of cases through biopsy and/or clinical history.[269,270] Causes include recurrent glomerular disease, transplant glomerulopathy, polyomavirus nephropathy, and pyelonephritis.[269,270] Although chronic active TCMR or ABMR can result in IFTA, their diagnoses require other histologic criteria that are presented later.

Rather than being a disease per se, CAI and IFTA are the end result of both alloimmune and nonalloimmune injuries that can occur in transplanted kidneys. Moderate to severe IFTA is a predictor of adverse graft outcomes, being associated with both impaired function and poorer graft survival.[271,272] Studies performed in the early 2000s pointed to an important role for calcineurin inhibitor toxicity in the development of IFTA. A study of cyclosporine-treated pancreas-kidney transplant recipients showed moderate to severe IFTA and arteriolar hyalinosis in 66% and 90% of surveillance biopsies, respectively, at 5 years.[273] However, recent data show that the incidence of IFTA is lower among solitary kidney transplant recipients, with only 17% of 5-year surveillance biopsies showing moderate to severe IFTA, and no significant differences observed between patients maintained on calcineurin inhibitors versus those who were not.[274] Hence although calcineurin inhibitors are profibrotic and nephrotoxic, their contribution to the progression of IFTA, relative to other causes of graft injury, is unclear.[275]

One of the key factors that trigger the development of IFTA is inflammation. Processes such as acute and chronic ABMR and TCMR, recurrent glomerular diseases, BK polyomavirus, CMV nephritis, and bacterial acute or chronic pyelonephritis all involve the activation of macrophages and graft infiltration by leukocytes (mainly T cells). Under the influence of proinflammatory cytokines, T cells, macrophages, and tubular epithelial cells produce TGF-β, connective tissue growth factor (CTGF), and other profibrotic cytokines. In response to these cytokines, fibroblasts, fibrocytes and pericytes are activated and transform into matrix-producing contractile myofibroblasts, leading to allograft fibrosis.

Another important trigger of fibrosis is microvascular injury, which can occur during ischemia-reperfusion or acute and chronic ABMR. In kidney transplant patients, ischemia-reperfusion injury occurs at the time of transplantation. Acute kidney injury that occurs in the immediate posttransplant period is termed *delayed graft function.* Delayed graft function is associated with a moderately increased risk of graft loss[276] and with the degree of IFTA after transplantation.[275] In experimental models of ischemia-reperfusion injury, renal perfusion in peritubular capillaries is compromised within minutes of unclamping.[277,278] Endothelial dysfunction/injury and apoptosis compromise microcirculatory renal blood flow through decreased vasodilatory capacity, coagulation activation and the formation of microvascular thrombi, and increased rolling/adhesion of inflammatory cells.[279,280] Because the regenerative capacity of endothelial cells in peritubular capillaries appears limited, microvascular damage occurring during an episode of acute kidney injury can lead to permanent peritubular capillary rarefaction. Loss of peritubular capillaries favors chronic hypoxia, leading to overexpression of hypoxia inducible factor 1-α (HIF-1α). HIF-1α promotes the transcription of fibrogenic genes, such as TGF-β and CTGF, accumulation of α-smooth muscle actin-positive myofibroblasts, and the production of fibrogenic mediators by dying endothelial cells.[281] In transplanted kidneys, the magnitude of microvascular involution during the first 3 months following transplantation is a major negative predictor of long-term renal allograft function.[282] Recent studies using in vivo imaging and electron microscopy demonstrated a tight correlation between peritubular capillary dysfunction/rarefaction and renal fibrosis in both murine models of acute kidney injury and human kidney biopsy samples.[282–287]

### CHRONIC ACTIVE CELLULAR AND ANTIBODY-MEDIATED REJECTION

Allograft vascular involvement by cell- or antibody-mediated processes is the hallmark of chronic active TCMR and ABMR. Chronic allograft arteriopathy, defined as arterial intimal fibrosis with mononuclear cell infiltration and neointima formation, is a key feature of chronic active TCMR, but is also seen in chronic active ABMR.[54] Other histologic criteria for chronic active ABMR include the presence of circulating DSA, evidence of chronic vascular damage and remodeling of the graft microcirculation (double contours in glomerular capillaries or multilayered basement membrane in peritubular capillaries), diffuse C4d staining in peritubular capillaries, and gene transcripts of endothelial injury.[54] The presence of inflammation in zones of IFTA is associated with decreased graft survival,[288,289] and may be seen in chronic active TCMR.[54] The clinical aspects of chronic active ABMR and TCMR are discussed in Chapter 70.

## MECHANISMS OF ACTION OF IMMUNOSUPPRESSIVE DRUGS

To prevent the development of rejection, immunosuppressive drug regimens comprise induction and maintenance immunosuppressive agents. Induction agents are powerful immunosuppressants that are administered in the immediate perioperative period and discontinued in the early posttransplant period. These agents include polyclonal antibodies (anti-thymocyte globulins or ATG) and monoclonal antibodies (basiliximab, alemtuzumab). Maintenance immunosuppressive agents are also administered at the time of transplantation but are continued for the lifespan of the graft and sometimes beyond. They include calcineurin inhibitors (tacrolimus and cyclosporine), mycophenolate mofetil, rapamycin, azathioprine, and corticosteroids. The majority of American centers are currently using ATG (60%) or basiliximab (20%) for induction, and a combination of tacrolimus, mycophenolate mofetil, and corticosteroids for maintenance.[290] The first-line treatment of acute TCMR is steroid pulses, while ATG and alemtuzumab can be used as second-line therapy for steroid-resistant rejection. Some centers use antibodies in combination with corticosteroids as first-line therapy for Banff grade 2 TCMR or higher.[291] The clinical aspects of acute rejection management are covered in more detail in Chapter 70. Here, we will discuss the mechanism of action of immunosuppressive agents. Fig. 69.11 illustrates the action mechanisms of the most frequently used immunosuppressive drugs.

## INDUCTION AGENTS

### POLYCLONAL ANTIBODIES

Polyclonal ATG are produced by injecting animals, such as horses or rabbits, with human thymocytes to obtain the purified γ-globulin fractions of the resulting immune sera. Many preparations have been developed, marketed by different companies, but the one that is most commonly used in clinical practice is rabbit antithymocyte globulin (rATG-Thymoglobulin, Genzyme). Two other existing preparations are rATG-Fresenius, where rabbits are immunized with Jurkat T-cell leukemia lines instead of human thymocytes, and equine ATG (ATGAM, Pfizer), which is a result from the immunization of horses with human thymocytes. Because polyclonal antibodies originate from animals, antirabbit (or antiequine) antibodies can form after ATG administration, which can lead to decreased activity and serum sickness upon re-exposure.[292]

ATG targets multiple epitopes present on thymocytes, including immune response antigens and adhesion/cell trafficking molecules, which explains its various mechanisms of action.[293] Although its primary mode of action is T-cell depletion, ATG can also bind to B cells, DCs, and nonlymphoid cell lines, such as monocytes, neutrophils, platelets, and red blood cells.[294] ATG induces lymphocyte depletion in the peripheral blood primarily by complement-dependent cell lysis, although other mechanisms, such as ADCC and induction of apoptosis through Fas/Fas ligand interactions, have been documented.[294–296] Lymphocyte depletion also occurs in the spleen and axillary lymph nodes, mainly through T-cell apoptosis.[294] Although the T-cell count returns to baseline 10 days after a single dose of ATG,[297] about 40% of patients treated with a full course recover more than 50% of the initial lymphocyte count after 3 months.[298]

Another important mechanism of action of ATG is modulation, which occurs both in the peripheral blood and peripheral lymphoid tissues.[294] ATG binds to antigenic target molecules on the cell surface, including the TCR/CD3 complex. The antigen–antibody complex is then internalized, and the pathway through which the target cell surface molecule was acting remains inhibited for up to 4 weeks. This down-modulation affects not only molecules that regulate T-cell activation but also molecules that are involved in leukocyte–endothelial interactions, such as integrins, intercellular adhesion molecules, and chemokine receptors.[295,299] Hence ATG interferes with leukocyte–endothelial interactions that play a role in ischemia-reperfusion injury and can potentially decrease the inflammatory response in patients at risk of delayed graft function. Lastly, Thymoglobulin promotes the induction and proliferation of Treg cells, which play an important role in limiting the immune response to alloantigens.[300,301]

A recent meta-analysis concluded that ATG used as an induction agent prevents acute rejection, but increases the risk of CMV infection, thrombocytopenia, and leukopenia. However, the impact of ATG on death, graft survival, and malignancy are unclear.[302] ATG is also used as a treatment for acute rejection.[291]

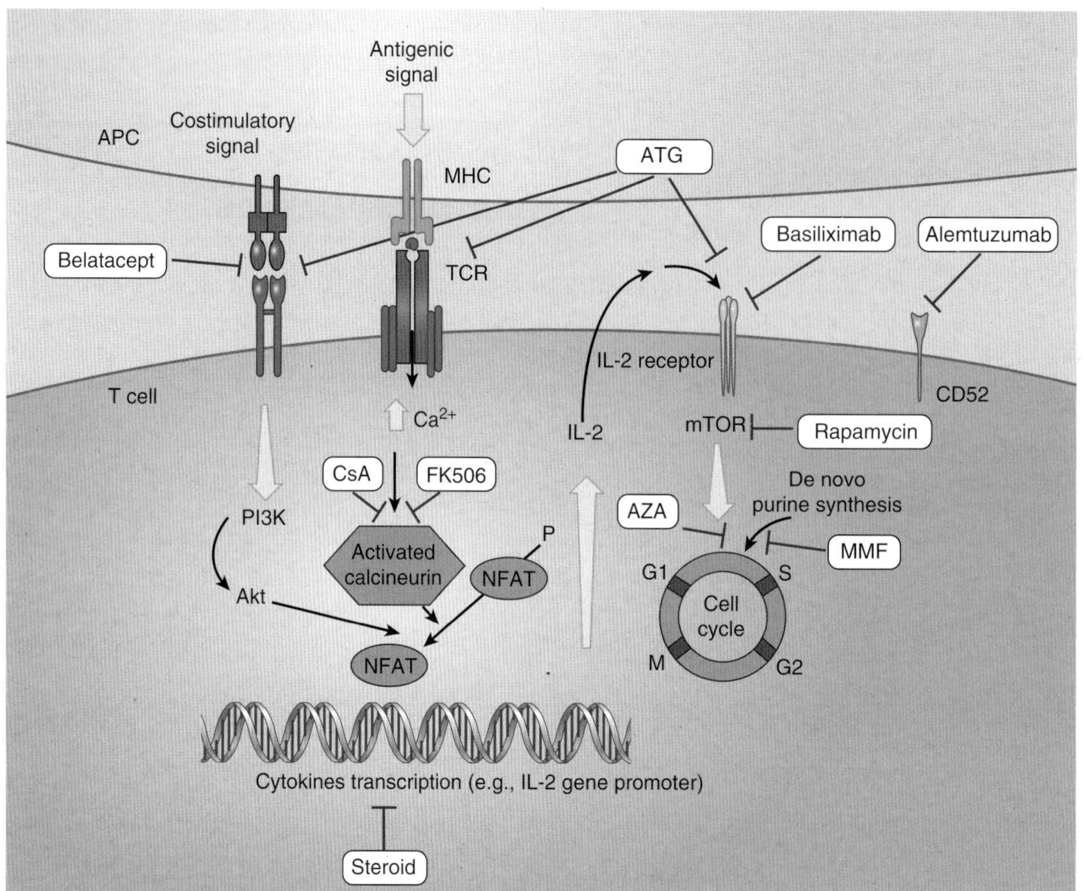


**Fig. 69.11 Mechanisms of action of immunosuppressive agents viewed as a function of inhibiting T-cell activation. Signal 1: The calcium-dependent signal induced by T-cell receptor (TCR) stimulation results in calcineurin activation, a process inhibited by cyclosporine (CsA) and tacrolimus. Calcineurin dephosphorylates nuclear factor of activated T cells (NFAT), enabling it to enter the nucleus and bind to the interleukin-2 (IL-2) promoter. Corticosteroids bind to cytoplasmic receptors, enter the nucleus, and inhibit cytokine gene transcription in both T cells and the antigen-presenting cells (APCs). Corticosteroids also inhibit nuclear factorκlight-chain enhancer of activated B cells (NF-κB) activation (not shown). Signal 2: Costimulatory signals are necessary to optimize T-cell IL-2 gene transcription, prevent T-cell energy, and inhibit T-cell apoptosis (belatacept target). Signal 3: IL-2 receptor stimulation induces the cell to enter the cell cycle and proliferate. Signal 3 may be blocked by IL-2 receptor antibodies (basiliximab) or by mammalian target of rapamycin (mTOR) inhibitors (such as rapamycin), which inhibits S6 kinase activation. Following progression into the cell cycle, azathioprine (AZA) and mycophenolate mofetil (MMF) interrupt DNA replication by inhibiting purine synthesis. Antithymocyte globulin (ATG) has multiple targets, including IL-2R, CD3, and CD28, leading to T-cell depletion. Alemtuzumab selectively targets CD52 receptor on T cells. *MHC*, Major histocompatibility complex; *PI3K*, phosphatidylinositol-3-kinase.**

## MONOCLONAL ANTIBODIES

### ANTI-IL-2R ANTIBODIES

In contrast to polyclonal antibodies and alemtuzumab, anti-IL-2R antibodies are nondepleting, chimeric, monoclonal antibodies targeted against CD25, or IL-2R, which is expressed on activated lymphocytes. Since daclizumab was withdrawn from the market because of lack of demand in 2009, basiliximab is currently the only agent in the anti-IL-2R class. Basiliximab is composed of mouse light and heavy chains and a human Fc portion. Activated T cells produce IL-2, which acts in an autocrine fashion on IL-2R to induce T-cell proliferation (Fig. 69.11).[303] Binding to the α subunit of IL-2R, basiliximab competitively inhibits IL-2–induced lymphocyte proliferation, therefore suppressing T-cell activity against the allograft. Internalization of IL-2R follows basiliximab administration and is associated with decreased counts of circulating CD25-expressing T cells.[296,304,305] Basiliximab induction achieves complete IL-2R saturation and T-cell suppression for 4 to 6 weeks.[305]

Anti-IL-2R antibodies are indicated in the prevention, but not the treatment, of rejection. Their use decreases rejection rates and early graft loss when compared with placebo.[306] Although randomized controlled trials have reported that ATG was superior to anti-IL-2R antibodies in the prevention of acute rejection in patients at high risk of delayed graft function or rejection,[307,308] graft survival was similar between the two treatment groups up to 5 years posttransplantation.[309] Despite the fact that severe hyperreactivity reactions have been described, anti-IL-2R antibodies are generally well tolerated.

### ALEMTUZUMAB

Alemtuzumab (Campath-1H) is a humanized, rat monoclonal IgG1 antibody directed against CD52. CD52 is a cell surface glycoprotein expressed on both B and T cells and on NK cells, monocytes, macrophages, and DCs. Recent data suggest that CD52 is involved in T-cell costimulation, migration, and adhesion, and may also induce T-reg cells.[310] Alemtuzumab acts though the depletion of B cells, T cells, and other cell lines expressing CD52. First, binding of alemtuzumab to CD52 on the cell surface can activate the complement cascade through the classical pathway, leading to formation of the membrane attack complex and target cell lysis. Second, through their IgG fragment C receptor (FcYR), NK cells and macrophages can recognize the Fc region of lymphocyte-bound alemtuzumab, favoring the release of perforins and granzymes, and leading to target cell lysis. Lastly, binding of alemtuzumab seems to induce a nonclassical, caspase-independent, apoptotic response in target cells.[311,312]

Alemtuzumab induces a rapid but long-lasting depletion of B and T cells in the peripheral blood and secondary lymphoid organs. After standard induction treatment, reconstitution occurs at a variable rate in kidney transplant patients, with B cells recovering after 12 months and T-cell counts recovering to approximately 50% of baseline after 36 months.[313] Furthermore, alemtuzumab treatment induces an increase in FoxP3+ Treg cells and an anti-inflammatory pattern in the immune system.[314,315] Although alemtuzumab is a humanized antibody, it contains regions originating from a rat IgG2 antibody, and the development of antidrug antibodies has been reported.[316]

Alemtuzumab is used off label as an induction agent for the prevention of rejection and as a rejection treatment in kidney transplant recipients. Systematic reviews show that when administered as an induction agent to prevent rejection, the efficacy of alemtuzumab is similar to that of ATG.[302,317] Nevertheless, some studies have reported an increased risk of formation of *de novo* DSA compared with basiliximab or ATG,[318] as well as an increase in the incidence of acute ABMR.[319–321] Alemtuzumab has also been used as a treatment for acute TCMR in patients with steroid-resistant rejection in observational studies. The efficacy of alemtuzumab appears similar to that of Thymoglobulin in this context,[310] although large randomized controlled trials are lacking.

## MAINTENANCE IMMUNOSUPPRESSIVE DRUGS

Maintenance immunosuppressive regimens usually consist of the concomitant administration of 3 agents that act through different pathways in a synergistic fashion, with the goal of avoiding allograft rejection. Although other combinations exist, the combination of tacrolimus, mycophenolate mofetil, and corticosteroids is most frequently used.

### CALCINEURIN INHIBITORS

Although tacrolimus and cyclosporine differ in origin, intracellular protein binding, and side effect profiles, they share a common final pathway in terms of mechanism of action: the inhibition of calcineurin. Calcineurin is a serine threonine phosphatase that dephosphorylates the cytosolic component of the nuclear factor of activated T cells (NFAT) (Fig. 69.11) After dephosphorylation, NFAT is translocated from the cytosol to the nucleus, where it forms a complex with other DNA-binding proteins, including FOS and JUN. This complex regulates gene transcription, including the gene for IL-2. During treatment with calcineurin inhibitors, the inhibition of the formation of the NFAT complex has been shown to prevent transcription of the *IL-2* gene, and a similar complex has been shown to regulate *TNF-α* gene transcription. The net result is a reduction in T-cell activation and, indirectly though decreased IL-2 production, decreased T-cell proliferation.

### DIFFERENCES BETWEEN TACCOLIMUS AND CYCLOSPORINE

Tacrolimus (FK506) is a macrolide antibiotic produced by fungi that binds to a family of cytosolic proteins, the FK binding proteins. In contrast, cyclosporine is a small cyclic peptide of fungal origin that binds to a family of cytoplasmic molecules termed *cyclophilins*. As mentioned previously, both medication-bound protein complexes then inhibit calcineurin. Tacrolimus is now generally preferred to cyclosporine, as randomized controlled trials have demonstrated superior efficacy in terms of acute rejection prevention and graft function 1 year and 3 years posttransplantation.[322–324] The side effect profiles of tacrolimus and cyclosporine are similar, with a few exceptions. Although hirsutism and gingival hyperplasia are caused by cyclosporine, tacrolimus is associated with alopecia instead. Neurotoxicity, diarrhea, and post-transplant diabetes are more frequent with tacrolimus, whereas dyslipidemia is more commonly seen with cyclosporine.[325] In contrast with cyclosporine, tacrolimus is now available as once-daily formulations.[326]

### MYCOPHENOLIC ACID

Mycophenolic acid (MPA) is a fermentation product of *Penicillium brevicompactum* fungi that inhibits the proliferation of human T and B cells.[327] The production of purines, which are subunits of nucleic acids, is necessary for DNA synthesis and cell proliferation. There are 2 routes for the synthesis of nucleotides: the de novo and the salvage pathways. The de novo pathway uses simple molecules, such as $CO_2$, amino acids, and tetrahydrofolate, to build novel purine molecules. In contrast, the salvage pathway recycles purine bases. While most cells use both pathways to synthesize purines, T and B cells are dependent on the de novo pathway. The main mechanism of action of MPA is the inhibition of inosine-5'-monophosphate dehydrogenase (IMPDH), an enzyme that limits the rate of guanosine nucleotide synthesis through the de novo pathway, thereby limiting DNA synthesis and cell proliferation. IMPDH has two isoforms. Although the type I isoform is expressed in most cell types, the type II isoform is preferentially expressed in T and B cells.[328] MPA inhibits the type II IMPDH isoform 5 times more potently than the type I isoform. The preferential expression of type II IMPDH in lymphocytes and the dependence of lymphocytes on the de novo pathway for purine synthesis may explain why MPA's antiproliferative effect is mostly observed in lymphocytes,[329] although monocytes can also be affected.[330] MPA has also been shown to decrease antibody responses to multiple alloantigens, including CMV[331] and equine proteins found in ATGAM preparations.[332] In addition, it is believed to suppress DSA production,[333] although this can still develop with the use of combinations of tacrolimus and MPA. MPA also suppresses autoantibody production through early inhibition of B-cell proliferation and differentiation,[329] and is now a recognized treatment for autoimmune diseases such as lupus nephritis.[268]

MPA has other mechanisms of action that are relevant in the context of organ transplantation. For instance, MPA can suppress the maturation of DCs and inhibit their capacity to present antigens.[334,335] MPA can also reduce the recruitment of monocytes into sites of graft rejection and inflammation, and induce apoptosis in these cells,[336] hence exerting an anti-inflammatory effect. Finally, MPA reduces the expression of adhesion molecules on endothelial cells[337] and decreases lymphocyte adhesion/infiltration of the allograft.[329]

MPA has superior efficacy in preventing acute rejection episodes and death-censored graft loss when compared with azathioprine,[338] and it is used in combination with calcineurin inhibitors and prednisone in most transplant centers.[256]

## AZATHIOPRINE

Azathioprine is a purine analog that is enzymatically converted in vivo to 6-mercaptopurine and other derivatives, which are molecules that function as antimetabolites. After metabolic conversion, it has multiple activities, including incorporation into DNA, inhibition of purine nucleotide synthesis, and alteration of RNA synthesis. The major immunosuppressive effect is thought to be caused by blocking of DNA replication, which prevents lymphocyte proliferation after antigenic stimulation. Although it is useful for inhibiting primary immune responses, azathioprine has little effect on secondary responses or the reversal of acute allograft rejections, which are not dependent on lymphocyte proliferation. Azathioprine also decreases the number of migratory mononuclear and granulocytic cells, while inhibiting proliferation of promyelocytes in the bone marrow. As a result, the number of circulating monocytes capable of differentiating into macrophages is decreased. Among the possible deleterious effects of azathioprine are leukopenia, thrombocytopenia, hepatotoxicity, and an increased risk of neoplasia. Pancreatitis is also a rare but serious side effect of azathioprine. Azathioprine can be used in combination with calcineurin inhibitors in patients who are intolerant to MPA. Azathioprine-treated patients are less likely to experience gastrointestinal disturbances but are more likely to have thrombocytopenia and elevated liver enzymes than those receiving MPA.[338]

## MAMMALIAN TARGET OF RAPAMYCIN INHIBITORS

Rapamycin, or sirolimus, is a macrolide antibiotic that blocks T-cell proliferation during the late G1 phase of the cell cycle and before the S phase, resulting in a mid-to-late G1 arrest of the cell cycle.[339] After binding to intracellular FK-binding proteins, rapamycin forms an effector complex that inhibits mTOR. Everolimus (RAD) is a rapamycin derivative that has a similar mode of action to sirolimus. mTOR inhibition prevents phosphorylation of the p70 S6 kinase, which reduces the translation of mRNAs that encode ribosomal proteins and elongation factors, ultimately decreasing protein synthesis.[339] In addition, rapamycin prevents the decline of p27 cyclin-dependent kinase (cdk) inhibitor that typically follows IL-2 stimulation. In turn, this leads to an inhibition of the enzymatic activity of the cdk2-cyclin E complex, a regulator of G1/S transition. In functional studies, activation of T cells by monoclonal antibodies against the TCR was inhibited by either cyclosporine or tacrolimus, but not rapamycin. Conversely, the activation of T cells by exogenous IL-2 plus protein kinase C stimulation with a phorbol ester was inhibited by rapamycin, but not cyclosporine or tacrolimus.[340] Similarly, T-cell activation by monoclonal antibodies against the CD28 costimulatory molecule plus protein kinase costimulation with a phorbol ester was also inhibited by rapamycin, but not cyclosporine or tacrolimus. In contrast, cyclosporine and tacrolimus inhibit an early signal in T-cell activation that is transduced by the TCR signal transduction pathway. Hence rapamycin exerts its effect by interfering with the CD28 costimulatory and IL-2R signal transduction pathways.

Even though rapamycin interacts with the same binding proteins as tacrolimus, there is no competitive inhibition between these drugs, because the binding proteins are present in great excess compared with tacrolimus and rapamycin. The mTOR inhibitors have been shown to be potent inhibitors of vascular endothelial growth factor, which may explain their role in preventing progression of many forms of cancer. mTOR inhibitors have been used in combination with calcineurin inhibitors to replace azathioprine or MPA, as well as in combination with MPA to replace calcineurin inhibitors, which are associated with nephrotoxicity. In a recent meta-analysis, kidney transplant recipients who received mTOR inhibitors were at a lower risk of neoplasia, but at higher risk of death.[341] Whereas conversion from calcineurin to mTOR inhibitors is associated with better short-term graft function,[342] enhanced long-term survival has never been demonstrated. Moreover, retrospective registry cohort studies have suggested an increased risk of graft loss with mTOR inhibitors in combination with, or in replacement of, calcineurin inhibitors[343] Additionally, increased de novo DSA have been reported in patients who switched from calcineurin to mTOR inhibitors.[344] mTOR inhibitors are not routinely administered in most transplant centers, but benefit may be derived from their use for selected populations, such as patients at high risk of cancer and those who are intolerant or show toxicity from calcineurin inhibitors. Nevertheless, side effects can be frequent, and may include dyslipidemia, peripheral edema, cytopenia, acne, proteinuria, and oral ulcers.[345]

## CORTICOSTEROIDS

Corticosteroids modulate the immune response by regulating gene expression. The steroid molecule enters the cytosol, where it binds to the steroid receptor and induces a conformational change in the latter. The complex then migrates to the nucleus and binds regulatory regions of DNA called glucocorticoid response elements, which regulate the transcription of many genes, including *IL-1, IL-2, IFN-γ, TNF-α,* and *IL-6.* Most immunosuppressive drug regimens include a corticosteroid, such as prednisone, in combination with other immunosuppressive agents. A recent meta-analysis showed that steroid avoidance (use of corticosteroids for less than 14 days posttransplant) or steroid withdrawal (discontinuation of corticosteroids after more than 14 days of use posttransplant) led to an increased risk of acute rejection, while there was no significant effect on graft loss or patient mortality up to 1 year posttransplant.[346] The risk of posttransplant diabetes and CMV infection were similar whether or not steroids were maintained. However, long-term data on the risk and benefits of steroid avoidance or discontinuation are lacking.

### BELATACEPT

Belatacept is a fusion protein composed of an Fc fragment of human IgG1 linked to an extracellular domain of cytotoxic T lymphocyte antigen-4 (CTLA-4), which is a molecule expressed on activated T cells.[347] As discussed earlier in this chapter, the CD28 molecule is constitutively expressed on naïve T cells. After binding with B7-1 and B7-2 (also called CD80 and CD86, respectively) on the surface of APCs, CD28 provides a costimulatory signal that is crucial for T-cell activation and proliferation via IL-2 secretion.[348] CD80 and CD86 also bind with CTLA-4, inducing a negative regulatory effect on T-cell activation.[349] The affinity of CD80/CD86 is much greater for CTLA-4 than for CD28.[350] Through its CTLA-4 domain, belatacept binds to CD80/CD86 on the surface of APCs, thus preventing the binding of CD80/CD86 to CD28. This then impedes the CD28-mediated costimulatory signal that is required for T-cell activation.[348]

Belatacept is the first intravenous maintenance immunosuppressive agent that has been marketed. It is not used for the treatment of acute rejection episodes. In de novo transplant recipients receiving standard or extended criteria donors, use of belatacept (versus cyclosporine) in combination with mycophenolate mofetil, prednisone, and basiliximab induction has resulted in higher graft function 1 year posttransplantation, although the rate of acute rejection episodes was higher.[351] Follow-up studies after 7 years have suggested that the benefit seen in graft function preservation may be maintained long term.[352,353] Cases of posttransplant lymphoproliferative diseases have been observed in patients with belatacept, especially in transplant recipients who were EBV-seronegative before transplantation, leading the US Food and Drug Administration (FDA) to issue a black box warning against the use of belatacept in EBV-seronegative recipients.[354] Conversion from calcineurin inhibitors to belatacept has resulted in an improvement in graft function up to 3 years after conversion.[355] Hence belatacept can be used as an alternative for recipients who are intolerant or have nephrotoxicity associated with calcineurin inhibitors.[55]

## OTHER IMMUNOSUPPRESSIVE AGENTS USED IN THE FIELD OF KIDNEY TRANSPLANTATION

### RITUXIMAB

Rituximab is a chimeric murine/human monoclonal antibody directed against CD20, a transmembrane protein expressed by B cells but not plasma cells or memory B cells.[296] Rituximab strongly depletes peripheral B-cell levels via complement-dependent cytotoxicity, ADCC, and caspase-dependent apoptosis.[356] Rituximab has been studied as an induction agent, as well as for the treatment of acute and chronic ABMR, but clinical benefits remain uncertain at present time.[302,357–359]

### BORTEZOMIB

Bortezomib is a reversible inhibitor of the 26S proteasome, a multicatalytic enzyme complex localized in the cell nucleus and cytosol. Since the proteasome is the principal pathway by which cellular proteins are degraded,[360] proteasome inhibition leads to the accumulation of misfolded proteins within the endoplasmic reticulum, leading to apoptosis. Due to their high rate of antibody synthesis, plasma cells are particularly sensitive to proteasome inhibition, and bortezomib has been shown to deplete plasma cell levels.[361]

Although bortezomib has successfully been used in desensitization protocols that also included rituximab and intravenous immunoglobulins in some small case series,[362,363] its benefits remain controversial.[364] Multiple case reports and case series have reported reversal of acute ABMR using bortezomib,[365–369] although its beneficial effect seems to be limited to ABMR episodes occurring in the early posttransplant period.[214] The impact of bortezomib on late ABMR is currently being investigated in a randomized controlled trial.[370]

### ECULIZUMAB

Eculizumab is a humanized monoclonal antibody that targets the complement C5a component and prevents its cleavage, thereby inhibiting the formation of the membrane attack complex and preventing complement-mediated injury.[296] Eculizumab prevents the recurrence of atypical hemolytic uremic syndrome after transplantation,[371,372] and has reversed acute ABMR in case reports and small case series,[296] sometimes in combination with splenectomy.[373] Meningococcal vaccination is recommended at least 2 weeks before administering the first dose of eculizumab if the risk of delaying therapy is not judged prohibitive. The use of antibiotic prophylaxis (2 weeks of ciprofloxacin followed by amoxicillin, for instance) can be considered for the duration of treatment with eculizumab, especially when vaccination has not taken place in a timely fashion.[374]

#### TOCILIZUMAB

Tocilizumab is a humanized monoclonal antibody directed at the soluble and membrane forms of IL-6R. IL-6 is a pleiotropic cytokine that is not expressed in healthy individuals but is rapidly synthesized during infection and tissue injury. Innate immune cells, such as monocytes and macrophages, release IL-6 after recognizing PAMPs or DAMPs. IL-6 stimulates B cells, promotes antibody synthesis and Tfh cell populations, and preferentially induces proinflammatory Th17 cell differentiation at the expense of Treg-cell induction.[296,375] Tocilizumab is FDA-approved for the treatment of severe rheumatoid arthritis and juvenile arthritis. Although not studied on a large scale in the field of transplantation, tocilizumab has shown promising results in desensitization protocols,[376,377] as well as for the treatment of chronic ABMR.[378]

## CONCLUDING REMARKS

The field of transplantation immunobiology has been the topic of abundant research efforts in the last decades. In this chapter, we have provided an overview of alloantigen recognition, HLA antigen/antibodies, and mechanisms of rejection and immunosuppressive agents focusing on their relevance to current clinical practice in kidney transplantation. Immunosuppression remains a double-edged sword for kidney transplant patients. Although current immunosuppressive regimen has yielded excellent results in terms of acute rejection prevention and increased short-term graft survival, the risk of infection and cancer remain problematic. While xenotransplantation and genetically engineered grafts are not ready to move to the bedside,[379] the induction of donor-specific tolerance by mixed chimerism[380,381] and regulatory cell therapy[382] are currently being studied in humans. Such initiatives represent future perspectives to decreased adverse effects of immunosuppressants while preserving long-term graft function.

 Complete reference list available at ExpertConsult.com.

## KEY REFERENCES


4. Alegre ML, Lakkis FG, Morelli AE. Antigen presentation in transplantation. *Trends Immunol.* 2016;37(12):831–843.
5. Eskandari SK, Seelen MAJ, Lin G, et al. The immunoproteasome: an old player with a novel and emerging role in alloimmunity. *Am J Transplant.* 2017.
11. Brown K, Sacks SH, Wong W. Extensive and bidirectional transfer of major histocompatibility complex class II molecules between donor and recipient cells in vivo following solid organ transplantation. *FASEB J.* 2008;22(11):3776–3784.
12. Brown K, Sacks SH, Wong W. Coexpression of donor peptide/recipient MHC complex and intact donor MHC: evidence for a link between the direct and indirect pathways. *Am J Transplant.* 2011;11(4):826–831.
18. Liu Q, Rojas-Canales DM, Divito SJ, et al. Donor dendritic cell-derived exosomes promote allograft-targeting immune response. *J Clin Invest.* 2016;126(8):2805–2820.
19. Dieude M, Bell C, Turgeon J, et al. The 20S proteasome core, active within apoptotic exosome-like vesicles, induces autoantibody production and accelerates rejection. *Sci Transl Med.* 2015;7(318):318ra200.
22. Chen L, Flies DB. Molecular mechanisms of T cell co-stimulation and co-inhibition. *Nat Rev Immunol.* 2013;13(4):227–242.
29. Brunet JF, Denizot F, Luciani MF, et al. A new member of the immunoglobulin superfamily–CTLA-4. *Nature.* 1987;328(6127):267–270.
35. Hall BM. T cells: soldiers and spies–the surveillance and control of effector T cells by regulatory T cells. *Clin J Am Soc Nephrol.* 2015;10(11):2050–2064.
37. Clatworthy MR. Targeting B cells and antibody in transplantation. *Am J Transplant.* 2011;11(7):1359–1367.
38. Clatworthy MR. B-cell regulation and its application to transplantation. *Transpl Int.* 2014;27(2):117–128.
39. Thaunat O, Field AC, Dai J, et al. Lymphoid neogenesis in chronic rejection: evidence for a local humoral alloimmune response. *Proc Natl Acad Sci USA.* 2005;102(41):14723–14728.
42. Cardinal H, Dieude M, Hebert MJ. The emerging importance of non-HLA autoantibodies in kidney transplant complications. *J Am Soc Nephrol.* 2017;28(2):400–406.
43. Nauser CL, Farrar CA, Sacks SH. Complement recognition pathways in renal transplantation. *J Am Soc Nephrol.* 2017;28(9):2571–2578.
48. Hidalgo LG, Sis B, Sellares J, et al. NK cell transcripts and NK cells in kidney biopsies from patients with donor-specific antibodies: evidence for NK cell involvement in antibody-mediated rejection. *Am J Transplant.* 2010;10(8):1812–1822.
49. Hickey MJ, Valenzuela NM, Reed EF. Alloantibody generation and effector function following sensitization to human leukocyte antigen. *Front Immunol.* 2016;7:30.
50. Dragun D, Catar R, Philippe A. Non-HLA antibodies in solid organ transplantation: recent concepts and clinical relevance. *Curr Opin Organ Transplant.* 2013;18(4):430–435.
53. Haas M, Sis B, Racusen LC, et al. Banff 2013 meeting report: inclusion of c4d-negative antibody-mediated rejection and antibody-associated arterial lesions. *Am J Transplant.* 2014;14(2):272–283.
54. Loupy A, Haas M, Solez K, et al. The Banff 2015 kidney meeting report: current challenges in rejection classification and prospects for adopting molecular pathology. *Am J Transplant.* 2017;17(1):28–41.
95. Li L, Wadia P, Chen R, et al. Identifying compartment-specific non-HLA targets after renal transplantation by integrating transcriptome and "antibodyome" measures. *Proc Natl Acad Sci USA.* 2009;106(11):4148–4153.
120. Duquesnoy RJ, Mulder A, Askar M, et al. HLAMatchmaker-based analysis of human monoclonal antibody reactivity demonstrates the importance of an additional contact site for specific recognition of triplet-defined epitopes. *Hum Immunol.* 2005;66(7):749–761.
123. Wiebe C, Pochinco D, Blydt-Hansen TD, et al. Class II HLA epitope matching—a strategy to minimize de novo donor-specific antibody development and improve outcomes. *Am J Transplant.* 2013;13(12):3114–3122.
126. Tambur AR, Claas FH. HLA epitopes as viewed by antibodies: what is it all about? *Am J Transplant.* 2015;15(5):1148–1154.
136. Williams RC, Opelz G, McGarvey CJ, et al. The risk of transplant failure with HLA mismatch in first adult kidney allografts from deceased donors. *Transplantation.* 2016.
137. Hricik DE, Formica RN, Nickerson P, et al. Adverse outcomes of tacrolimus withdrawal in immune-quiescent kidney transplant recipients. *J Am Soc Nephrol.* 2015.
139. Tinckam KJ, Liwski R, Pochinco D, et al. cPRA increases with DQA, DPA, and DPB unacceptable antigens in the Canadian cPRA calculator. *Am J Transplant.* 2015;15(12):3194–3201.
170. Lan JH, Tinckam K. Clinical utility of complement dependent assays in kidney transplantation. *Transplantation.* 2018;102(1S suppl 1):S14–S22.
171. Loupy A, Lefaucheur C, Vernerey D, et al. Complement-binding anti-HLA antibodies and kidney-allograft survival. *N Engl J Med.* 2013;369(13):1215–1226.
173. Yell M, Muth BL, Kaufman DB, et al. C1q binding activity of de novo donor-specific HLA antibodies in renal transplant recipients with and without antibody-mediated rejection. *Transplantation.* 2015;99(6):1151–1155.
174. Lefaucheur C, Viglietti D, Bentlejewski C, et al. IgG donor-specific anti-human HLA antibody subclasses and kidney allograft antibody-mediated injury. *J Am Soc Nephrol.* 2016;27(1):293–304.
175. Viglietti D, Loupy A, Vernerey D, et al. Value of donor-specific anti-HLA antibody monitoring and characterization for risk stratification of kidney allograft loss. *J Am Soc Nephrol.* 2016.
181. Konvalinka A, Tinckam K. Utility of HLA antibody testing in kidney transplantation. *J Am Soc Nephrol.* 2015.
185. Cecka JM, Kucheryavaya AY, Reinsmoen NL, et al. Calculated PRA: initial results show benefits for sensitized patients and a reduction in positive crossmatches. *Am J Transplant.* 2011;11(4):719–724.
191. Wiebe C, Gareau AJ, Pochinco D, et al. Evaluation of C1q status and titer of de novo donor-specific antibodies as predictors of allograft survival. *Am J Transplant.* 2016.
196. Orandi BJ, Luo X, Massie AB, et al. Survival benefit with kidney transplants from HLA-incompatible live donors. *N Engl J Med.* 2016;374(10):940–950.
205. Bray RA, Nolen JD, Larsen C, et al. Transplanting the highly sensitized patient: the emory algorithm. *Am J Transplant.* 2006;6(10):2307–2315.
206. Wehmeier C, Honger G, Cun H, et al. Donor specificity but not broadness of sensitization is associated with antibody-mediated rejection and graft loss in renal allograft recipients. *Am J Transplant.* 2017;17(8):2092–2102.
218. Wiebe C, Gibson IW, Blydt-Hansen TD, et al. Evolution and clinical pathologic correlations of de novo donor-specific HLA antibody post kidney transplant. *Am J Transplant.* 2012;12(5):1157–1167.
257. Tait BD, Susal C, Gebel HM, et al. Consensus guidelines on the testing and clinical management issues associated with HLA and non-HLA antibodies in transplantation. *Transplantation.* 2013;95(1):19–47.
260. Sis B, Einecke G, Chang J, et al. Cluster analysis of lesions in nonselected kidney transplant biopsies: microcirculation changes, tubulointerstitial inflammation and scarring. *Am J Transplant.* 2010;10(2):421–430.
261. Lefaucheur C, Loupy A, Vernerey D, et al. Antibody-mediated vascular rejection of kidney allografts: a population-based study. *Lancet.* 2013;381(9863):313–319.
264. Sis B, Jhangri GS, Bunnag S, et al. Endothelial gene expression in kidney transplants with alloantibody indicates antibody-mediated

damage despite lack of C4d staining. *Am J Transplant.* 2009;9(10): 2312–2323.

267. Shrestha B, Haylor J. Evolution of the concept and pathogenesis of chronic renal allograft injury: an updated review. *Exp Clin Transplant.* 2016;14(6):596–605.
274. Stegall MD, Park WD, Larson TS, et al. The histology of solitary renal allografts at 1 and 5 years after transplantation. *Am J Transplant.* 2011;11(4):698–707.
302. Hill P, Cross NB, Barnett AN, et al. Polyclonal and monoclonal antibodies for induction therapy in kidney transplant recipients. *Cochrane Database Syst Rev.* 2017;(1):CD004759.
317. Morgan RD, O'Callaghan JM, Knight SR, et al. Alemtuzumab induction therapy in kidney transplantation: a systematic review and meta-analysis. *Transplantation.* 2012;93(12):1179–1188.
322. Ekberg H, Tedesco-Silva H, Demirbas A, et al. Reduced exposure to calcineurin inhibitors in renal transplantation. *N Engl J Med.* 2007;357(25):2562–2575.
346. Haller MC, Royuela A, Nagler EV, et al. Steroid avoidance or withdrawal for kidney transplant recipients. *Cochrane Database Syst Rev.* 2016;(8):CD005632.
352. Vincenti F, Rostaing L, Grinyo J, et al. Belatacept and long-term outcomes in kidney transplantation. *N Engl J Med.* 2016;374(4):333–343.
362. Woodle ES, Shields AR, Ejaz NS, et al. Prospective iterative trial of proteasome inhibitor-based desensitization. *Am J Transplant.* 2015;15(1):101–118.

# 70 Clinical Management of the Adult Kidney Transplant Recipient

Colin R. Lenihan | Jane C. Tan

CHAPTER OUTLINE



## THE TRANSPLANT SURGERY PROCEDURE

The kidney allograft is placed in the extra peritoneal iliac fossa (Fig. 70.1). A curvilinear incision is made in the right or left lower quadrant, the retroperitoneal space is widened, and the iliac vessels exposed. The external iliac artery and vein are mobilized and surrounding lymphatic vessels are ligated and divided. End-to-side anastomoses are performed between the renal vein and the external iliac vein, followed by the renal artery and the external iliac artery. Alternate techniques for the renal artery are end-to-side to the common iliac artery or end-to-end to the mobilized internal iliac artery. The site of anastomosis is chosen after examining the length, size, and quality of the donor's and recipient's vessels. The Lich-Gregoir implantation of the ureter to the bladder, a technique designed to minimize urinary reflux into the ureter, has become the preferred technique for neo-ureterocystostomy. A double J ureteric stent can be inserted either routinely, or selectively for higher risk candidates. It is usually retrieved 2 to 4 weeks after transplantation in the outpatient setting. A Cochrane review suggested that the incidence of urine leak and ureteric stenosis were significantly reduced with prophylactic uretic stenting.[1,2] A low-pressure suction drain can also be used and retrieved within the first week after surgery. While the surgical techniques for deceased- and living-donor kidney transplant are similar, with deceased donor allografts attention is given to preserving longer stretches of the donor vessels. The renal artery or arteries are procured along with an aortic patch; this technique facilitates the vascular anastomosis and reduces the risk of renal artery stenosis.

### LIVE DONOR NEPHRECTOMY

Traditionally, the procurement of kidneys from live donors has been performed through a right or left flank incision. In 1995, a laparoscopic approach for kidney donation was introduced as an alternative that would reduce postoperative pain, wound morbidity, and reduce recovery time associated with the traditional donor nephrectomy.[3] The laparoscopic approach is now the procedure of choice, and is performed in over 90% of live kidney donations in the United States.[4] Initial concerns regarding ureteral complications and graft dysfunction have mostly subsided with improvements in surgical technique and experience.[5,6] Pure laparoscopic, hand-assisted, robotic-assisted, and single-port access are variants of the laparoscopic donor nephrectomy. All of these techniques avoid flank incision by intraabdominal mobilization of the kidney after establishing the pneumoperitoneum. A periumbilical or infra-umbilical small incision, which spares transection of muscle tissue, is used to retrieve the kidney. The hand-assisted variant is the most popular approach. A small periumbilical or infra-umbilical incision of 8 cm allows

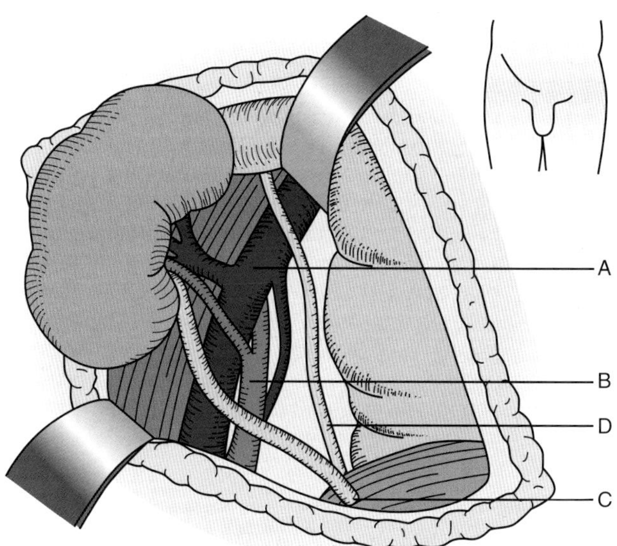


**Fig. 70.1** The anatomy of a typical first kidney transplant. A, external iliac artery, B, external iliac vein, C, implanted donor ureter, D, native ureter.

the surgeon to insert one hand inside the abdomen with the help of a device that seals the pneumoperitoneum. The hand is used to help with retraction of the kidney and also allows faster retrieval of the kidney, reducing the warm ischemia by 50% compared to a pure laparoscopic approach. The left kidney is preferred even more so than with the open nephrectomy, because the laparoscopic instrument used to secure the renal vein effectively reduces its length by ½ to 1 cm. When an open donor nephrectomy is performed, an incision is made from the rectus muscle in the direction of the twelfth right or left rib tip. This operation is retroperitoneal as opposed to the laparoscopic approach, which is transperitoneal. Smaller muscle sparing incisions are now used to improve the postoperative recovery.

## HANDLING AND PRESERVATION OF THE DONOR KIDNEY

The basic principle of organ preservation is to prevent damage from ischemia by replacing the circulating blood with a preservation solution, and retrieving and cooling the organs expediently. The composition of preservation solutions vary, but all have ingredients designed to a) minimize intracellular edema, b) preserve the integrity of cells and tissue, and c) buffer free radicals.

The two cold storage preservation solutions most widely used in the United States are the University of Wisconsin (Viaspan, UW) and the Histidine-Tryptophan Ketoglutarate (Custodiol, HTK) solutions. The UW solution has an electrolyte composition similar to that of the intracellular fluid, with a high concentration of potassium (120 mmol/L). Lactobionate and raffinose prevent cellular edema, and hydroxyethyl starch buffers free radicals. Its viscosity is three times that of water, making it relatively difficult to flush. The HTK solution is a low viscosity, low sodium (15 mmol/L) solution. The concentration of potassium is also low (15 mmol/L), and this reduced the risk of hyperkalemia after transplantation. Histidine serves as a buffer, and tryptophan and mannitol are free radical scavengers.

The UW solution had been the preservation solution of choice for multiorgan deceased donor recovery since its introduction in 1988. However, HTK is used by a growing number of Organ Procurement Organizations (OPO). One of the major advantages of HTK is its relatively low cost. Two small randomized studies comparing UW to HTK preservation solutions found no difference in delayed graft function or graft survival between groups.[7,8] However, a large retrospective (non-randomized) study comparing HTK to UW preservation solution found that HTK use was associated with an increased risk of late death-censored graft loss.[9] For living donor kidneys with short ischemia times, the use of simple and inexpensive solutions such as heparinized lactated Ringer's with procaine has been proposed; however, we prefer to use a preservation solution such as HKT.[10]

Hypothermic machine perfusion is an alternative to static cold preservation for deceased donor kidneys. Following standard retrieval and flushing of the kidney allograft, the renal artery is connected to a perfusion pump that circulates a preservation solution, maintained at 1°C to 10°C. Perfusion parameters can be used to determine the quality of the graft. Hypothermic machine perfusion is associated with a reduction in delayed graft function compared to static cold storage and some, but not all, studies have shown an improvement of graft survival at 1 year.[11] There is increasing interest in ex vivo normothermic perfusion as a preservation method; one potential advantage of this technique is that it allows ex vivo assessment of graft function.[12]

## SURGICAL COMPLICATIONS OF THE TRANSPLANT PROCEDURE

Advances in donor and recipient surgical technique, anesthesia, organ preservation, and perioperative care have all likely contributed to improvements in 1-year patient and graft survival rates.[13] However, early recognition and management of surgical complications remains important. Specific vascular and urologic complications are described more fully later in the section on Management of Allograft Dysfunction. A brief description of these complications is discussed here.

## VASCULAR COMPLICATIONS

### HEMORRHAGE

Acute and life-threatening hemorrhagic complications in the immediate postoperative period usually involve the anastomotic site. Bleeding can be brisk and immediate surgical exploration is required. Perirenal hematomas can result from either venous or small artery bleeding and may be related to the incision or retroperitoneal dissection. Unless small and stable, perirenal hematomas require surgical exploration to ensure adequate hemostasis. Large hematomas should be evacuated in order to reduce the risk for subsequent infection.[14]

### ARTERIAL THROMBOSIS

Renal artery thrombosis of the allograft is rare (0.5% to 1%). Acute thrombosis is usually related to an anastomotic problem or kink in the renal artery. Recipient arteriosclerosis, multiple arteries, vasospasm, and hypotension are risk factors. Sudden anuria is a clue to arterial thrombosis. Arterial thrombosis results in immediate warm ischemia. Delays inherently associated with confirming the diagnosis and preparing the patient for surgical exploration usually exceed the time required to reestablish arterial flow to the kidney, resulting in prolonged warm ischemia and hypoxia and often permanent loss of function.

### VENOUS THROMBOSIS

Renal vein thrombosis usually presents with local swelling, pain, and hematuria. Ultrasound shows decreased or absent blood flow in the renal vein and either absent or reversed diastolic arterial flow. The causes of venous thrombosis include problems with the surgical anastomosis, extrinsic compression by a lymphocele or a hematoma, and a deep venous thrombosis that extends in the iliac vein at the level of the venous anastomosis. Surgical exploration to attempt thrombectomy followed by anticoagulation can be performed; however, it is rarely successful. Contributing factors such as thrombophilia, should be evaluated and corrected if possible.[15]

Pseudoaneurysm of the arterial anastomosis is a rare infectious complication that leads almost invariably to graft loss and is associated with significant mortality and morbidity. Depending on the severity, noninvasive treatment with covered stenting has been attempted; however, transplant nephrectomy, vascular reconstruction and/or excision with extraanatomical bypass is usually required.[16] The loss of a lower limb due to distal thrombosis of the femoral artery or arterial dissection at the time of transplant is a very rare but devastating complication.

### LYMPHOCELE

A lymphocele is a lymphatic fluid collection originating from either the severed iliac lymphatics or lymphatic drainage of the renal allograft itself. Most lymphoceles are asymptomatic. However, some may compress the ureter causing hydronephrosis, or obstruct lower limb venous return resulting in unilateral edema. Large lymphoceles may present as an abdominal mass. Analysis of aspirated fluid will typically show a high lymphocyte count and a creatinine concentration similar to serum. This contrasts with a urinoma, which has a fluid creatinine concentration much higher than serum. Lymphoceles frequently reaccumulate following percutaneous drainage, although injection of sclerosing agent following aspiration may reduce the risk of recurrence. The preferred and more definitive treatment is internal drainage of the lymphocele into the peritoneal cavity. In many centers, a laparoscopic transabdominal approach has replaced the traditional open approach that utilizes the kidney transplant incision.[17]

## CURRENTLY USED IMMUNOSUPPRESSIVE AGENTS IN KIDNEY TRANSPLANTATION

### OVERVIEW

The immunosuppressive drugs commonly used in clinical transplantation are summarized in Table 70.1 and their mechanisms of action are illustrated in Fig. 70.2. T lymphocytes play a central role in the recognition of the allograft as foreign and in the initiation of the rejection process. The T-cell immune response is described as requiring three distinct signaling events (the three signal model). Briefly, antigen-presenting cells (APCs; dendritic cells, macrophages, activated endothelium), most likely of donor origin, migrate to the secondary lymphoid organs of the recipient where foreign antigen/major histocompatibility (MHC) complex is presented to the (recipient) T-cell receptor (**signal 1**). A co-stimulatory T cell-APC interaction (**signal 2**) is then required

**Table 70.1 Drugs Used in Maintenance Immunosuppression**

| Drug | Mechanism of Action | Adverse Effects |
|---|---|---|
| Corticosteroids | Block synthesis of several cytokines including IL-2; multiple antiinflammatory effects | Glucose intolerance, hypertension, hyperlipidemia, osteoporosis, osteonecrosis, myopathy, cosmetic defects; growth suppression in children |
| Cyclosporine | Inhibits calcineurin: synthesis of IL-2 and other molecules critical for T-cell activation thereby inhibited | Nephrotoxicity (acute and chronic), hyperlipidemia, hypertension, glucose intolerance, cosmetic defects |
| Tacrolimus | Similar to cyclosporine, although binds to different cytoplasmic protein (FKBP) | Broadly similar to cyclosporine; diabetes mellitus more common; hypertension, hyperlipidemia, and cosmetic defects less common |
| Azathioprine | Inhibits purine biosynthesis; lymphocyte replication therefore inhibited | Bone marrow suppression; rarely pancreatitis, hepatitis |
| Mycophenolate mofetil (MMF) | Inhibits de novo pathway of purine biosynthesis (relatively lymphocyte selective); lymphocyte replication therefore inhibited | Bone marrow suppression, gastrointestinal upset; invasive. CMV disease more common than with azathioprine |
| Sirolimus | Sirolimus-FKBP complex inhibits TOR blocking lymphocyte proliferative response | Bone marrow suppression, proteinuria, mouth ulcers, hyperlipidemia, interstitial pneumonitis; edema; enhanced nephrotoxicity of cyclosporine/tacrolimus |
| Belatacept | Blocks T-cell costimulation | PTLD in EBV seronegative, PML (rare), reactivation of TB |

*CMV,* Cytomegalovirus; *EBV,* Epstein-Barr virus; *FKBP,* FK-binding protein; *IL-2,* interleukin-2; *MMF,* mycophenolate mofetil; *PTLD,* posttransplant lymphoproliferative disorder; *TB,* tuberculosis; *TOR,* target of rapamycin.

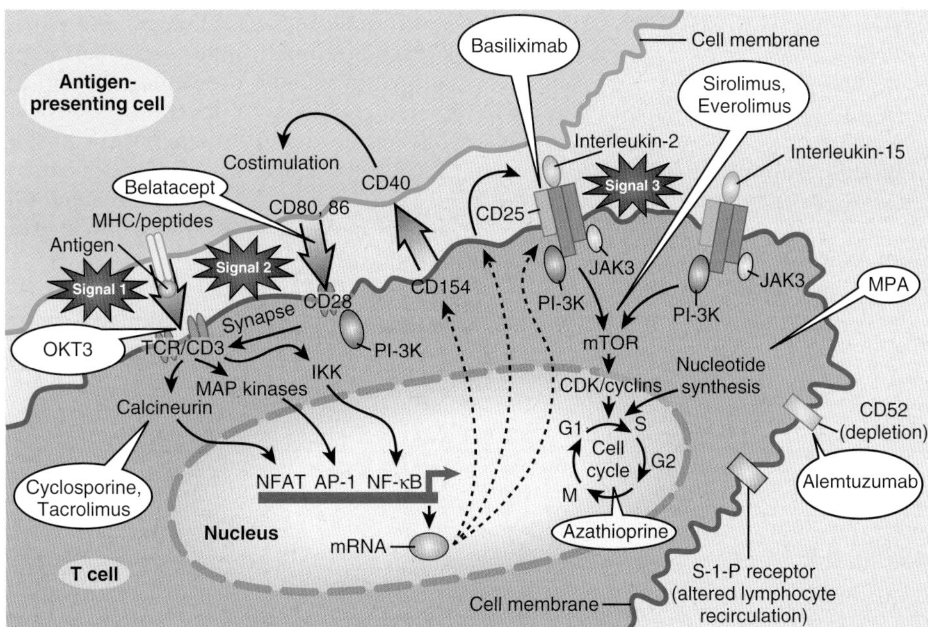


**Fig. 70.2** Stages of T-cell activation: multiple targets for immunosuppressive agents. Signal 1: The $Ca^{++}$-dependent signal induced by T-cell receptor (TCR) stimulation results in calcineurin activation, a process inhibited by the calcineurin inhibitors (CNIs). Calcineurin dephosphorylates nuclear factor of activated T cells (NFAT), enabling it to enter the nucleus and bind to the interleukin-2 (IL-2) promoter. Corticosteroids bind to cytoplasmic receptors, enter the nucleus, and inhibit cytokine gene transcription in both the T cell and antigen-presenting cell (APC). Corticosteroids also inhibit activation of the transcription factor, nuclear factor-κB (not shown). Signal 2: Costimulatory signals, such as that between CD28 on the T cell and B7 on the APC, are necessary to optimize T-cell transcription of the IL-2 gene, prevent T-cell anergy, and inhibit T-cell apoptosis. Signal 3: IL-2 receptor stimulation induces the cell to enter the cell cycle and proliferate. IL-2 and related cytokines have both autocrine and paracrine effects. Signal 3 may be blocked by IL-2 receptor antibodies or by sirolimus. Further downstream, azathioprine and mycophenolate mofetil (MMF) inhibit progression into the cell cycle by inhibiting purine and therefore DNA synthesis. (From Halloran PF: Immunosuppressive drugs for kidney transplantation. *N Engl J Med* 351:2715-2729, 2004.)

for downstream signal transduction to occur. The ensuing activation of the T-cell calcineurin-NFAT, MAP kinase and NFκB signaling pathways results in the production of cytokines (including interleukin-2, interleukin-15) and surface molecules (including the interleukin-2 receptor). Interleukin-2 (and other cytokines) then stimulate T-cell proliferation (**signal 3**) via the PI3K/Akt/mTOR, JAK3/STAT5 and MAP kinase signaling pathways.[18] Most immunosuppressive agents either deplete lymphocytes (depleting agents) or act at the level of, or downstream from, one or more of the three T-cell immune activation signals.

The B cell immune response is increasingly being targeted by newer therapies in kidney transplantation. Key roles for B cells in the alloimmune response include 1) the production of anti-HLA antibody, 2) differentiation into HLA-antibody producing plasma cells, 3) the development of long-lasting immune memory through the generation of B memory cells, 4) antigen presentation, and 5) cytokine production.[19]

Immunosuppressive strategies can also be divided into: 1) induction and 2) maintenance therapy. Induction of immunosuppression is defined as the rapid achievement of profound immunosuppression, usually at the time of transplant, with the use of depleting agents. Maintenance immunosuppression is achieved by the combination of oral agents that take advantage of additive or synergistic immunosuppressive effects of different drug categories to minimize their non-immunosuppressive side effects. Dosage is usually greater during the first three months after transplantation and decreases afterwards. A combination of calcineurin inhibitor (CNI), antiproliferative agent, and corticosteroids is the most common regimen.

## INDUCTION THERAPIES

### LYMPHOCYTE-DEPLETING AGENTS

Rabbit antithymocyte globulin (Thymoglobulin) and horse antithymocyte globulin (Atgam) are approved in the United States for treatment of acute rejection. Muromonab-CD3 (Orthoclone OKT 3) is no longer commercially available. Alemtuzumab (Campath) was initially approved for the treatment of B-cell chronic lymphocytic leukemia, but has been used off-label for the induction of immunosuppression.

## POLYCLONAL T-CELL DEPLETING ANTIBODIES

Polyclonal antibodies against human T cells, antithymocyte globulins (ATG), are prepared by immunization of animals with human lymphoid cells; available products include Thymoglobulin (globulin derived from rabbits inoculated with human thymocytes) ATG-Fresenius (globulin derived from rabbits inoculated with Jurkat T-cells, [not available in the United States]), and Atgam (gamma globulin derived from horses inoculated with human thymocytes). For Thymoglobulin, the resulting purified globulin includes antibodies that target more than 20 different T-cell epitopes. Antibodies at higher concentrations include TCR, CD2, CD3, CD5, CD6, CD8, CD11A, CD49, and β2 microglobulin.[20,21] The mechanism of T-cell depletion is thought to involve complement-dependent lysis, mostly in the blood compartment, and apoptosis and phagocytosis in the peripheral lymphoid tissue. Antibodies against adhesion molecules that are present in the ATG preparation may also play a role by modulating leukocyte function.[22]

A number of randomized controlled trials have compared ATG induction with other strategies. A study from the late 1970s compared a one-month induction using horse ATG with no induction treatment in patients treated with azathioprine and steroid-based immunosuppression regimen and found a significantly improved 2-year graft survival in the ATG treated group.[23] Rabbit ATG (ATG-Fresenius) induction resulted equivalent 1-year graft survival but a lower rate of acute rejection- and infection- and noninfection-related complications compared to OKT3 in patients treated with cyclosporine, azathioprine, and steroid maintenance immunosuppression.[24] A long-running randomized trial comparing horse ATG to rabbit ATG induction therapy demonstrated the superiority of rabbit ATG in terms of reduction of the composite of death, graft loss, or rejection.[25] In sensitized patients, defined as a current or peak PRA >30% or >50%, respectively, rabbit ATG induction was associated with significantly lower rate of biopsy proven acute rejection and steroid resistant rejection in the first year posttransplant but no difference in 1-year survival compared to daclizumab induction.[26] In another study of kidney transplant recipients with risk factors for delayed graft function or acute rejection, rabbit ATG resulted in a lower acute rejection rate than basiliximab induction but no difference in delayed graft function or 1-year graft survival; 5-year follow-up of this study showed sustained superiority of rabbit ATG in terms of acute rejection.[27,28] Notably, infectious complications were more common in the recipients of rabbit ATG (versus IL-2 receptor antibodies) in both aforementioned trials. In immunologically high-risk kidney transplant recipients randomly assigned to either rabbit ATG or alemtuzumab induction, no differences were seen in acute rejection rates between the groups followed out to 3-years posttransplant,[29] although infectious complications were more common in rabbit ATG-treated subjects. A recent retrospective analysis of US kidney transplant recipients that compared outcomes in matched patients receiving induction with 1) ATG versus alemtuzumab and 2) ATG versus basiliximab found that ATG use was associated with improved outcomes (death or allograft failure versus alemtuzumab and death *versus* basiliximab).[30]

ATG also has an important role in the treatment of severe or steroid-resistant acute cellular rejection. A randomized study showed rabbit ATG superior to horse ATG in the treatment of acute rejection in terms of rejection reversal and 90-day recurrence rates.[31] In another study, rabbit ATG and OKT3 were shown similarly efficacious in the treatment of steroid-resistant acute rejection; however, rabbit ATG had the advantage of a more favorable side-effect profile.[32] Given a more favorable side-effect profile, rabbit ATG has now replaced OKT3 as the second-line therapy for acute rejection.

Rabbit ATG is given at 1 to 1.5 mg/kg per day. The initial regimen of 7 to 14 days of treatment is rarely used nowadays, as a shorter course of treatment (5 days) has been demonstrated to be efficacious.[27] Infusion-related side effects, such as fever, chills, hypotension and, less frequently, cardiovascular events, are usually mild, particularly with adequate steroid and antihistamine premedication and a slow infusion rate. These reactions are more likely to occur during the first few infusions and become rare with subsequent infusions. Serum sickness, characterized by fever, rash and arthralgia, occurring 10 to 15 days after treatment have been reported as well, possibly more frequently in patients not receiving steroid prophylaxis.[33]

## MONOCLONAL T-CELL DEPLETING ANTIBODY

Muromonab-CD3 (Orthoclone OKT3) is a mouse anti-human monoclonal antibody against the T-cell receptor-associated CD3 antigen that was first approved for clinical use in 1985. OKT3 results in apoptosis and rapid depletion of T cells from the circulation. The cytotoxic effect is preceded by a transient antibody-induced T-cell activation and cytokine surge, an effect that is responsible for many of the undesired effects associated with OKT3. T-cell number and function usually return to normal limits one week after the completion of the treatment. Cytokine release syndrome is present usually after the first infusion. It is most frequently reported to be a mild, self-limited flu-like illness; however, severe life-threatening reactions, such as serious cardiovascular and central nervous system manifestations, have been reported.[34] Non-cardiac pulmonary edema has also been seen, particularly if the patient is fluid overloaded pretransplant. Patients may develop anti-mouse neutralizing antibodies rapidly, and this may limit the efficacy of the treatment and prevent retreatment.[35] The efficacy of OKT3 as an induction agent and in the treatment of acute rejection is well established.[34,36] As a result of its side effects, the use of OKT3 decreased considerably following the emergence of alternative immunosuppressive agents, such as ATG and IL-2 blockers.[37] OKT3 was the first monoclonal antibody to be approved by the U.S. Food and Drug Administration (FDA); however it role is now consigned to the history books as its manufacture was discontinued by Janssen-Cilag in 2010.

## ANTI-CD52 ANTIBODY

Alemtuzumab (Campath) is a humanized monoclonal antibody against CD52, and was originally developed to treat refractory B-cell chronic lymphocytic leukemia. Alemtuzumab treatment results in depletion of both T and B lymphocytes. Evidence for the efficacy of alemtuzumab as an induction agent was provided by a randomized controlled trial that compared a single 30-mg dose of alemtuzumab to induction with basiliximab in immunologically low-risk patients and with rabbit ATG in immunologically high-risk patients. Alemtuzumab treatment proved superior to basiliximab and equivalent to rabbit ATG in terms of biopsy-confirmed acute rejection followed out to 3 years posttransplant, although the overall rate of late biopsy-proven rejection (between 1 and 3 years posttransplant) was significantly higher in the alemtuzumab group.[29] Infectious complications were higher with alemtuzumab than basiliximab but lower with alemtuzumab than rabbit ATG. Alemtuzumab may cause an infusion first dose reaction, which can be avoided if the subcutaneous route is used.[38] Neutropenia and anemia are also seen. Concern about the development of autoimmune disease (especially thyroid-related) following alemtuzumab treatment was initially raised after publication of data from a study comparing the agent with interferon beta for the treatment of multiple sclerosis.[39] The development of autoimmune disease has also been reported in solid organ transplant recipients treated with alemtuzumab induction.[40,41] Potential advantages of alemtuzumab include the simplicity of a single dose treatment and lower cost compared to other induction agents. Since 2012, alemtuzumab has not been widely commercially available, although the manufacturer does offer ongoing access to the drug for use as induction immunosuppression through the 'Campath Distribution Program'.[42]

## INTERLEUKIN-2 RECEPTOR ANTAGONIST (IL-2-RA)

Daclizumab is a humanized monoclonal antibody and basiliximab is a chimeric monoclonal antibody. Both are IgG1 antibodies directed against the alpha chain of the IL-2 receptor (CD25 antigen), which is expressed on activated T-lymphocytes. Blockade of the IL-2 receptor inhibits a key T-lymphocyte proliferation signaling pathway, thereby blunting the cellular immune response. These agents reduce the rate of rejection by approximately 30% to 40% compared to placebo when used in combination with conventional immunosuppression.[43–45] Rabbit ATG and alemtuzumab are both more effective in reducing the rate of rejection, but incur a higher infectious risk than the IL-2 receptor blockers.[26,27,29] Advantages of IL-2 receptor blockers include minimization of injection-related side effects and lack of risk of infection or cancer compared to placebo.[44,45] Daclizumab was withdrawn from the market by the manufacturer in 2009 and thus basiliximab is the only IL-2 blocker available in the United States. The regimen of the treatment consists of two infusions of 20 mg; the first at the time of transplantation, and the second 3 to 4 days posttransplantation. The pharmacokinetics of that dose regimen provides prophylaxis for 30 days post-transplant. Few data exist regarding the use of IL-2 receptor antagonists in the treatment of acute rejection.

## ANTI-CD20 ANTIBODIES

Rituximab (Rituxan) is a chimeric anti-CD20 cytolytic monoclonal antibody that has been approved for the treatment of non-Hodgkin's lymphoma, chronic lymphocytic leukemia, and rheumatoid arthritis. Rituximab was initially used in the transplant population for the treatment of post-transplant lymphoproliferative disease.[46] It interferes with the humoral allo-response by targeting B-lymphocytes. Many transplant programs, ourselves included, now use rituximab as part of an induction regimen for selected immunologically high-risk patients based on evidence that rituximab treatment in such patients has a favorable safety profile and is associated with a reduction in rejection and antibody-mediated graft dysfunction.[47–49] Rituximab is commonly employed in protocols for the treatment of frequently in combination with steroids, plasmapharesis, and/or intravenous immunoglobulin (IVIg).[50,51] Rituximab is also an important element in many pretransplant desensitization protocols (see section on desensitization)[52,53] and has been used in the treatment of recurrent or de novo posttransplant glomerular diseases such as membranous glomerulonephritis and focal segmental glomerulosclerosis (FSGS).[54,55] In patients receiving rituximab, we routinely premedicate with steroid, acetaminophen and an anti-histamine in order to decrease infusion-related side effects. We very carefully weigh the risk-benefit of rituximab treatment in those patients with positive hepatitis B surface antigen/detectable hepatitis B DNA.[56] We initiate hepatitis B prophylaxis in all patients treated with rituximab who have evidence of prior hepatitis B infection (positive hepatitis core antibody/negative hepatitis surface antigen) irrespective of hepatitis surface antibody titer. Obintuzumab, a next generation anti-CD20 antibody, is currently under clinical trial for pre-transplant desensitization.[57]

## INTRAVENOUS IMMUNOGLOBULIN (IVIg)

Various pooled human immunoglobulin products are commercially available. The increasingly widespread use of IVIg in the kidney transplant population parallels a greater awareness in recent years of antibod-mediated rejection (ABMR) and its risk factors. IVIg is used pretransplant as part of both HLA- or ABO incompatible-desensitization protocols, at induction in patients with pre-formed donor-specific antibody (DSA) and for treatment of ABMR.[47,58–60] Its mechanism of action is not fully understood but may include neutralization of circulating (anti-HLA) antibody, inhibition of complement, modulation of B-cell and antigen presenting cell function, and cytokine inhibition.[57,61,62] IVIg has also been used in the treatment of posttransplant viral infections such as BK virus and parvovirus.[60] Side effects include infusion reaction, headache (common and troublesome), aseptic meningitis, hemolysis (especially in patients who are blood group A) and, rarely, thrombosis.

# MAINTENANCE IMMUNOSUPPRESSIVE AGENTS

## CALCINEURIN INHIBITORS (CNIS)

Calcineurin is a calcium dependent serine/threonine phosphatase that is involved in a diverse range of cellular functions including T-cell signal transduction.[63] Binding of foreign antigen to the T-cell receptor, when accompanied by a co-stimulatory signal, triggers the cytosolic influx of calcium and the downstream activation of calcineurin. Activated calcineurin dephosphorylates the transcription factor, nuclear factor of activated T-cells (NFAT), which then translocates to the nucleus and activates a host of target genes, including the cytokine IL-2.[64] IL-2 then binds to its receptor and initiates T-cell expansion.[18]

The excellent posttransplant outcomes seen with the advent of the CNIs in the 1980s made the widespread expansion of solid organ transplantation possible, heralding the modern era of transplantation. CNIs, first in the form of cyclosporine and then later tacrolimus, have remained the cornerstone of transplant immunosuppression. However, the CNIs are not without side effects. CNI-associated nephrotoxicity, first described in the heart transplant population certainly contributes to a reduction in long-term graft survival in a proportion of kidney transplant recipients.[65–67] However, the magnitude kidney transplant failure attributable to CNI toxicity remains hotly debated.

## CYCLOSPORINE

Cyclosporine is a lipophilic amino acid cyclic peptide that binds to cyclophilin, a cytoplasmic protein, and forms a complex that inhibits calcineurin. Cyclosporine came into clinical use in the early 1980s. Both European and American clinical trials demonstrated the superiority of cyclosporine either alone or with steroid over the standard immunosuppression regimen of azathioprine and steroid.[68,69] The original oil-based formulation of cyclosporine (Sandimmune) was associated with erratic gastrointestinal absorption and highly variable bioavailability. The subsequent development of a microemulsion formulation of cyclosporine (Neoral) significantly improved the drug's absorption and the pharmacokinetic profile.[70] Cyclosporine is now also available in a generic microemulsion formulation. Gengraf is an alternative water-based microemulsion that many patients find more palatable.[71] Care should be taken to avoid non-microemulsion generic cyclosporine formulations without the prescriber's knowledge, as they are associated with unpredictable absorption and may expose the patient to an increased risk of rejection or toxicity.

Therapeutic drug monitoring of cyclosporine is most commonly performed using 12-hour trough levels, although monitoring blood levels two hours after ingestion of cyclosporine (C2 level) actually has a better correlation with drug exposure.[72] The side effects of cyclosporine include hypertension, hyperlipidemia, gingival hyperplasia, hypertrichosis, tremors, and nephrotoxicity. Cyclosporine is also associated with the development of posttransplant diabetes mellitus (PTDM) and rarely hemolytic uremic syndrome.

## TACROLIMUS

Tacrolimus (Prograf) is a macrolide antibiotic that binds to the cytosolic FK506 binding protein (FKBP12). The resulting drug-protein complex inhibits calcineurin activity. Many trials have demonstrated reduced rates of rejection compared to cyclosporine,[73] particularly the original formulation of cyclosporine. The toxicity profile is slightly different than cyclosporine; tacrolimus is not associated with gingival hyperplasia, hypertrichosis, or hyperlipidemia. However, it is associated with greater neurotoxicity, a higher incidence of PTDM, and gastrointestinal toxicity. Hypertension and nephrotoxicity appear to be milder than with cyclosporine. Mycophenolate acid exposure is reduced by approximately 40% when combined with cyclosporine versus tacrolimus (see below), an effect that likely contributes to the relatively greater immunosuppressive potency of tacrolimus compared to cyclosporine-based CNI-MMF regimens.[74] Tacrolimus is now also available in generic formulation. Two extended-release formulations of tacrolimus (Astagraf and Envarsus XR) have also been approved in the US. Once daily tacrolimus may be beneficial in terms of compliance and may mitigate neurological side effects.[75,76] Close monitoring of levels, especially in patients early posttransplant, is recommended following formulation changeover.[77]

## CALCINEURIN-INHIBITOR TARGET LEVELS

In patients treated with CNIs, the dangers of drug overexposure must be weighed against those of underexposure. CNI overexposure puts the patient at heightened risk of opportunistic infections and cancer. In addition, good evidence exists that chronic exposure to CNI is itself nephrotoxic and may result in progressive graft failure, so-called calcineurin-inhibitor nephrotoxicity.[78] Concern regarding CNI nephrotoxicity has, in recent decades, led to a greater focus on strategies to minimize CNI exposure. Data from two randomized controlled trials from the late 2000s supported the efficacy and safety of lower dose cyclosporine and tacrolimus-based regimens in immunologically low-risk patients.[79,80] However, over the past decade antibody mediated allograft injury has been increasingly recognized as an important cause of late graft loss.[81] There is increasing awareness that chronic CNI underexposure may permit allorecognition and chronic ABMR to occur. Targeting very low CNI levels or CNI withdrawal does appear to increase the risk of de novo donor-specific antibody (DSA) formation.[82,83] The development of posttransplant de novo DSA is in turn associated with reduced graft survival.[84,85] To date, belatacept (see below) probably represents the best available option for calcineurin avoidance.[86]

## ANTIPROLIFERATIVE AGENTS

### AZATHIOPRINE

Azathioprine (Imuran) is a pro-drug whose metabolites exert a number of actions including 1) the incorporation of thioguanine purine analogues into DNA and RNA resulting in cell death, 2) inhibition of de novo purine synthesis by methylthioinosine monophosphate, and 3) T-cell apoptosis via inhibition of the Rho family GTPase, Rac1.[87] Azathioprine, in combination with prednisone, was the mainstay of transplant immunosuppression from the early 1960s until the introduction of cyclosporine in the early 1980s, at which point it maintained its role as an adjuvant medication to cyclosporine. Azathioprine has now been largely superseded by mycophenolate mofetil (MMF) in most new immunosuppressive protocols,[88] although many longer vintage kidney transplant recipients remain on the drug. Additionally, azathioprine is commonly substituted for MMF in female transplant recipients who are planning to conceive. The most important side effect of azathioprine is myelosuppression. Individuals with reduced thiopurine methyltransferase enzyme activity (TPMT) tend to accumulate active drug metabolites and are predisposed to hematologic toxicity. By some estimates, 10% of the population have reduced and 0.3% absent TPMT activity.[89] Notably, coadministration of allopurinol with azathioprine also shifts azathioprine metabolism toward the production of metabolically active substrates and may lead to potentially serious toxicity.

## MYCOPHENOLATE ACID

Mycophenolate mofetil (MMF) is a pro-drug that releases mycophenolate acid, an inhibitor of inosine monophosphate dehydrogenase (IMPDH), which is required for the de novo pathway synthesis of guanosine from inosine. The effects of MMF are relatively lymphocyte-specific as, lacking a purine salvage pathway, T and B cells rely exclusively on de novo purine synthesis. By limiting the pool of available guanine triphosphate, MMF prevents T and B lymphocyte replication and suppresses both the cellular and humoral immune responses. Clinical trials have demonstrated that MMF reduces acute rejection rates by 50% compared to azathioprine or placebo.[90] A meta-analysis of 19 trials has shown that MMF was associated with a reduction of acute rejection and improved graft survival compared to azathioprine.[88] Cyclosporine blocks the enterohepatic recirculation of MMF reducing the exposure of the drug by approximately 40%. In contrast, tacrolimus and sirolimus do not interfere with the metabolism of MMF.[74] The most troublesome MMF side effects are gastrointestinal: diarrhea, bloating, epigastric pain and nausea, and such side effects may require dose reduction. MMF can cause neutropenia and, less frequently, anemia. Alopecia may also occur with MMF treatment and can be very bothersome. However, it is not associated with nephrotoxicity or hypertension. MMF is associated with an increased risk of major fetal malformations and patients who are planning pregnancy should be switched to azathioprine at least 6 weeks before attempting to conceive.[91] Despite the high inter- and intra-individual variability of its pharmacokinetics, routine therapeutic drug monitoring of MMF has not been established. MMF is approved at a dose of 1 g bid when used in conjunction with a calcineurin inhibitor and steroids. The excellent results obtained with a standard dosing regimen and the poor correlation of a single time point to area under the curve (AUC) (particularly when used in combination with CsA) supports a fixed dose regimen.[18,92] Mycophenolate mofetil is now also available in generic formulation in the US.

Mycophenolate sodium (Myfortic) is an enteric-coated slow-release formulation of mycophenolic acid that was developed to decrease the gastrointestinal side effects of MMF. Randomized trials have demonstrated a similar efficacy and side effect profile to MMF.[93] The dose conversion for mycophenolate mofetil to mycophenolate sodium is 250 mg to 180 mg.

## TARGET-OF-RAPAMYCIN INHIBITORS

Sirolimus (Rapamune) is a macrocyclic antibiotic that has immunosuppressive properties. Even though it shares its cytoplasmic binding protein with tacrolimus (FKBP12), the resulting complex does not interfere with calcineurin. Rather, it binds with the mammalian target of rapamycin (mTOR). The resulting inhibition of mTOR prevents the propagation of IL-2-mediated cell proliferation signaling through the PI3K/AKT/mTOR pathway.[94] Sirolimus inhibits cellular proliferation of T and B lymphocytes and reduces antibody production.[18] Its immunosuppressive effects have been demonstrated in preclinical studies to be synergistic with CsA and tacrolimus.[95,96] Side effects of sirolimus include hyperlipidemia, thrombocytopenia, anemia, poor wound healing, diarrhea, pneumonitis, mouth ulcers, proteinuria, and peripheral edema. Indeed, high drug withdrawal rates due to side effects are a common theme in many of the sirolimus trials.

Sirolimus has been studied in a number of different immunosuppression protocols including as de novo maintenance immunosuppression in combination with either a CNI and steroid or an anti-metabolite and steroid, in early CNI withdrawal protocols or as replacement for a CNI in patients with chronic allograft dysfunction or cancer. Sirolimus/MMF versus cyclosporine/MMF combined with rabbit ATG induction and 6 months of steroids resulted in similar 12-month survival and rejection rates, although adverse drug events and discontinuation rates were significantly higher in sirolimus-treated subjects.[97] Another study that compared sirolimus/tacrolimus with tacrolimus withdrawn at 3 months, sirolimus/MMF and tacrolimus/MMF in patients treated with daclizumab induction and steroid maintenance reported significantly higher acute rejection rates with sirolimus/MMF treatment, prompting early withdrawal of the group from the trial; impaired wound healing and dyslipidemia were both more common in the sirolimus treated groups, as was drug withdrawal.[98] In another study, switching from tacrolimus to sirolimus at 3 months posttransplant (versus staying on tacrolimus) was associated with similar graft function but a higher rate of acute rejection.[99]

A randomized controlled trial with median follow-up of 8 years reported increased acute rejection rates and lower glomerular filtration rate (GFR) in cyclosporine/sirolimus and tacrolimus/sirolimus versus tacrolimus/MMF treated subjects. Tacrolimus/sirolimus treatment was also associated with an excess in death with a functioning graft compared to the other groups. A trend toward worse GFR in CNI/sirolimus treatment combinations (especially cyclosporine) is consistent with animal studies that show that sirolimus co-treatment potentiates CNI nephrotoxicity.[100,101]

Late conversion from CNI to sirolimus has shown some promise in improving/stabilizing kidney function in patients with chronic allograft dysfunction, with the caveat that the development of nephrotic or sub-nephrotic range proteinuria following conversion to sirolimus is relatively common and requires cessation of the treatment. The presence of proteinuria before conversion is predictive of a poor response and should be screened for prior to considering a switch to sirolimus.[102] Proposed mechanisms for sirolimus-associated proteinuria include reduced tubular protein reabsorption (often exacerbated by the glomerular hemodynamic effects of concurrent CNI withdrawal) and sirolimus induced podocyte injury.[103,104] Finally, conversion from CNI to sirolimus is associated with regression of Kaposi's sarcoma and reduction in the development of squamous cell skin cancers.[105,106] Sirolimus use peaked at just under 20% of kidney transplants in the early 2000s but its use has since declined to the low single digits.

Everolimus (Zortress) is derived from sirolimus and has a shorter half-life. It has been approved in the United States for prophylaxis against rejection in kidney and heart transplant recipients. A recent randomized controlled trial compared everolimus and low-dose tacrolimus (EVR/Tac) with MMF and standard dose tacrolimus (MMF/Tac) in de novo kidney transplant recipients. At 12-months posttransplant the EVR/Tac group was noninferior compared to MMF/Tac for the composite outcome of biopsy proven acute rejection or an eGFR < 50 mL/min. The rates of death, graft loss, and rejection were similar in the two groups at 12 months. CMV and BK infection occurred less frequently in EVR/Tac treated subjects. As with many mTor studies, drug discontinuation due to adverse events was more frequent in the everolimus vs MMF treatment groups (23% vs 12%).[107] Everolimus has also been approved for the treatment of advanced renal cell carcinoma (Affinitor).

## CO-STIMULATORY SIGNAL BLOCKERS

Belatacept is a selective co-stimulation blocker. This human fusion protein binds the ligands CD80 and CD86 on antigen presenting cells and prevents their interaction with the co-stimulation receptor on the T cells (CD28). Blockade of the co-stimulation signal (signal 2) prevents T-cell activation. Belatacept is given as an IV infusion. Two studies randomized recipients of living or standard deceased donor (BENEFIT) and expanded criteria deceased donor kidneys (BENEFIT-EXT) to higher dose belatacept, lower dose belatacept or cyclosporine, with all subjects receiving IL-2 antagonist induction, MMF, and steroid concurrently. One-year results showed similar graft and patient survival across the groups but significantly higher GFR in belatacept treated subjects. Acute rejection was significantly higher in those treated with belatacept in the BENEFIT study but not BENEFIT-EXT.[86,108] Estimated GFR remained approximately 25 and 19 mL/min higher with belatacept versus cyclosporine treatment at 7-year follow-up of the BENEFIT and BENEFIT-EXT studies, respectively.[109,110] In addition, graft and patient survival were significantly higher at 7 years posttransplant in the belatacept versus cyclosporine treated group in the BENEFIT Study.[109] A recent analysis of a subset of patients from the BENEFIT and BENEFIT-EXT trials showed a lower rate of development of de novo DSA in belatacept versus cyclosporine at 3 years posttransplant, a finding that may bode well for the long-term outcome of belatacept patients.[111] The incidence of (mostly central nervous system) PTLD was higher in patients treated with belatacept in both trials and was associated with pretransplant EBV seronegativity. The current package insert recommends use of belatacept only in kidney transplant patients who are documented anti-EBV antibody seropositive because of the risk of PTLD. Posttransplant conversion from CNI- to belatacept-based therapy is also a viable strategy and may help to preserve GFR.[112] While the BENEFIT studies certainly show belatacept to be a viable alternative to CNI-based immunosuppression regimens it must be remembered that these trials compared belatacept to cyclosporine and not to the modern era 'standard of care' CNI, tacrolimus; tacrolimus is itself associated with superior graft survival when compared to cyclosporine (see above).

## CORTICOSTEROIDS

Since the early days of clinical transplantation, corticosteroids have played an important role in the immunosuppressive management of transplant recipients. It remains the first line of treatment for acute rejection. Corticosteroids have both antiinflammatory and immunosuppressive properties. The antiinflammatory effects of steroids are mediated by reduction of pro-inflammatory molecules including the platelet activated factor (PAF), prostaglandins, and leukotrienes and reduction of the release of tumor necrosis factor-α (TNF-α). Immunosuppressive properties of steroids include prevention of T-cell proliferation, inhibition of cytokine production including IL-2 and interference with antigen presentation. Some of these effects are mediated through the inhibition of the transcription factor nuclear factor kappa B (NF-κB). Chronic use of steroids potentiates lymphocyte apoptosis and results in lymphopenia and interferes with the leukocyte trafficking.[14] These various mechanisms acting in concert make steroids a potent and versatile immunosuppressive drug. However, the side effects related to its chronic use are also extensive (e.g., diabetes, hypertension, hyperlipidemia, osteoporosis, avascular necrosis, truncal obesity, hypertrichosis, acne, and cataracts). The emergence of new, more potent immunosuppressive drugs has allowed the successful implementation of steroid sparing protocols (avoidance, minimization, or withdrawal).[113,114] This is reflected by a significant trend toward decreased steroid utilization, with just over 60% compared to 90% of US kidney transplant recipients maintained on the drug in the years 2011 and 1995, respectively.

The reported benefits of steroid sparing strategies are manifold and include improvements in blood pressure, glycemic and lipid control, reduced posttransplant weight gain, better bone mineral density, growth, and physical appearance.[115–118] A Cochrane review of 30 randomized trials of steroid avoidance (less than 2 weeks of exposure) and steroid withdrawal (greater than 2 weeks exposure) demonstrated that such steroid sparing strategies are not associated with an increase in mortality or all-cause graft loss but were associated with an increase in death censored graft loss and acute rejection. However, the increased risk of acute rejection was seen in those treated with cyclosporine but not tacrolimus-based immunosuppression regimens.[119] Steroid sparing strategies are a reasonable option for low immunological risk patients who are treated with modern era (tacrolimus/MMF) immunosuppression regimens. Most steroid withdrawal protocols wean steroids within 3 to 6 months of transplant. Late withdrawal from steroid (greater than 1 year post-transplant) has been associated with increased acute rejection rates and deterioration in graft function in studies from the cyclosporine/azathioprine era.[120,121] While late withdrawal may be safer in the tacrolimus/MMF era, ongoing caution is recommended with this approach.[122]

## IMMUNOSUPPRESSION AT OUR INSTITUTION

The vast majority of kidney transplant recipients in the US are maintained on tacrolimus and MMF and around two thirds of patients currently receive maintenance steroid.[123] The greatest source of intra-program variability in immunosuppressive regimen is in the choice of induction therapy and in patient selection for, and method of, steroid withdrawal.

At our institution, we aim to tailor the immunosuppressive regimen to strike the best balance between over- and under-immunosuppression based on patient characteristics detailed below. Our options for induction immunosuppression, used either alone or in various combinations, include intravenous glucocorticoid (methylprednisolone), IL-2 receptor antagonist (basiliximab), anti-thymocyte globulin (Thymoglobulin), IVIg and rituximab. Maintenance immunosuppression usually consists of tacrolimus and MMF with or without steroid. Around one third of our patients meet the criteria for early steroid withdrawal. We have a protocol for rapid steroid withdrawal (steroid free by hospital discharge) but most commonly employ a slower steroid taper that results in the patient being off steroid by around 6 months posttransplant. We take a number of factors into account when deciding about a patient's induction and maintenance immunosuppression.

**Flow crossmatch.** We consider a positive flow crossmatch (in the presence of a DSA) to be a contraindication to kidney transplantation in the absence of pretransplant desensitization (see desensitization section).

**Calculated panel reactive antibody (cPRA).** We consider those patients with a cPRA ≥20% to be sensitized and use

Thymoglobulin induction therapy. For 'hypersensitized' patients (cPRA >98%) or previously desensitized patients we additionally administer a single dose of rituximab (usually 500 mg) prior to discharge in the hope of preventing de novo DSA formation and acute rejection.[48,49,124] All sensitized patients (cPRA ≥20%) are maintained on lifelong triple immunosuppression with CNI, MMF, and steroid. For unsensitized patients we use either steroid alone or IL-2 receptor antagonist at induction. Many unsensitized patients are eligible for early steroid withdrawal.

## PREFORMED DONOR-SPECIFIC ANTIBODY WITH A NEGATIVE FLOW CROSSMATCH

The presence of preformed DSA (with or without high cPRA) versus a high cPRA (without DSA) has much greater prognostic significance for graft survival.[125] We try to avoid crossing immunological barriers; however, in the absence of a better alternative option, we do not consider the presence of low level preformed DSA to be a contraindication to transplant. Depending on the strength of the DSA at the time of transplant we either monitor the antibody closely posttransplant or administer high dose IVIg in the immediate posttransplant period and repeat another dose around 4 weeks posttransplant. We also take the presence of preformed 'historic' DSA, present on prior but not current HLA antibody screening sera, into account when planning the posttransplant immunosuppression and immune monitoring regimen.

**HLA mismatch.** We take donor-recipient HLA mismatch into account in assessing immunological risk in all patients. The recipients of two haplotype matched sibling donated kidney transplants merit a special mention as these patients can expect excellent outcomes with relatively little immunosuppression. Our practice for these patients has been to use steroid-only induction and low dose dual immunosuppression usually with a CNI and antimetabolite thereafter.

**Prior Kidney Transplant.** We treat these patients as sensitized irrespective of their cPRA and therefore give Thymoglobulin for induction and maintain on chronic triple immunosuppression.

**ESRD from Primary or Secondary GN.** We do not usually withdraw prednisone in patients with ESRD from lupus nephritis because of concern regarding a higher rejection risk and lupus nephritis recurrence.[126,127] We discuss the retrospective study that showed a significantly reduced risk of IgA recurrence in steroid-treated versus steroid-free transplant recipients with ESRD from IgA nephropathy. For each patient with IgA nephropathy, we weigh this potential benefit of remaining on steroid against the advantages of steroid withdrawal.[128] There is little firm evidence on what to do with steroid in patients with ESRD from other GNs, although we will continue steroid therapy if it was being taken chronically pretransplant.

**African-American Ethnicity.** We usually maintain African-American kidney transplant recipients on chronic maintenance steroid even if unsensitized. This stems from data showing that African-Americans, perhaps because of an intrinsically more robust alloimmune response, appear to be at higher rejection risk in the absence of steroid.[129] However, a newer study suggests that early steroid withdrawal may be safe in unsensitized African-American recipients when transplant is performed with lymphocyte depleting induction.[130]

Other important factors that must be taken into consideration are the baseline quality of the allograft, and the anticipated vulnerability profile to specific side effects of immunosuppression.

## DESENSITIZATION

Finding a compatible match for highly sensitized patients can be very challenging.[4,131] The last 15 years has seen significant growth in desensitization protocols that aim to lower anti-HLA antibody titers in sensitized kidney transplant candidates sufficiently to create an immunological window for successful transplantation. Desensitization protocols vary from center to center but fall into two broad categories 1) high-dose IVIg/anti-CD20-based,[53] and 2) low-dose IVIg/plasmapharesis-based[131] regimens. High-dose IVIg has been employed as a monotherapy and does effectively lower DSA titers and permit successful transplantation;[58] however, a number of studies have suggested that IVIg alone (versus IVIg plus plasmapharesis and rituximab or IVIg plus rituximab) is associated with a posttransplant rebound in DSA titres and increased incidence of ABMR.[132] More recent reports have also described successful desensitization using newer agents such as the anti-IL-6 receptor antibody, tocilizumab, and the IgG-degrading enzyme (IdeS).[133,134]

Desensitization may be performed in patients who have an identified living donor or may be timed to coincide with the candidate being positioned at the top of the deceased donor waiting list. Desensitization increases the prospect of highly sensitized patients receiving a transplant and is associated with good medium term graft survival rates and a survival advantage compared to remaining on dialysis.[52,131,135] However, ABMR rates are high[52,136] and few data are available about long-term graft survival in desensitized patients.

We believe that crossing immunological barriers in transplant should be a last resort. At our institution we explore alternative avenues to transplant before embarking on desensitization. Like most other transplant centers in the United States, we have had great success using donor exchange programs to help recipients with immunologically incompatible living donors get transplanted.[137] The new U.S. Kidney Allocation System, which offers significant allocation score bonuses (the equivalent of waiting time) and high priority access to kidney transplants across the country for the most sensitized patients on the list, was implement in December 2014. This has resulted in a significant increase in transplantation rates of highly sensitized patients (cPRA >98%).[138,139] Indeed, absent the new Kidney Allocation System, many of these highly sensitized patients would have lingered on the waiting list and perhaps been offered desensitization. There remains a group of hypersensitized patients (often with cPRAs of 99.8% and above) who in the absence of some intervention remain unlikely to get transplanted.[140] We believe that it is this select group of patients who should be offered desensitization therapy.

## ABO INCOMPATIBLE TRANSPLANTATION

The other important immunological barrier in kidney transplantation is the ABO blood group barrier. Blood group antigens are expressed on endothelial cells and, with certain exceptions, ABO-incompatible transplantation in the absence of desensitization will result in ABMR.[141] Much of the pioneering work on desensitization for ABO-incompatible transplant has been done in Japan where reliance on living donation created a need to eliminate ABO-incompatibility as a barrier to transplant.[142] ABO-incompatible protocols now mostly entail a relatively short but intensive pretransplant regimen consisting of rituximab, IVIg and plasmaphereis – continued until anti-A/B titres fall below a prespecified safe threshold (usually 1:8 or 1:16), some protocols also include additional posttransplant plasmapheresis or IVIg.[143–145] The long-term outcome of desensitized recipients of blood group incompatible organs is good although perhaps slightly inferior to that of ABO-compatible kidney transplant recipients, much of the excess risk associated with ABO-incompatible (versus compatible) kidney transplantation being concentrated in the early posttransplant period.[146,147] In patients with low baseline anti-A/B titers ABO-incompatible transplant has been shown to be safe with minimal pretreatment (1-2 weeks MMF).[148] The transplantation of blood group A2 donors (about 20% of the blood group A population who express A antigen at low level) into B donors with low anti-A titres is safe without desensitization.[148–150] The new Kidney Allocation System in the United States has permitted that A2 or A2B deceased donor kidneys be allocated to selected blood group B recipients in an attempt to reduce the long waiting times faced by blood group B patients.

## EVALUATION OF THE RECIPIENT IMMEDIATELY BEFORE THE TRANSPLANT

### ASSESSING COMPATIBILITY AND IMMUNOLOGICAL RISK

#### DONOR IMMUNE STATUS AND CROSSMATCH

The presence of preformed recipient antibody against either the donor ABO blood group or donor human leukocyte antigen (HLA) will frequently result in hyperacute rejection. The past 50 years has seen huge advances in the laboratory detection of recipient anti-HLA antibody. The complement dependent lymphocyte cytotoxicity (CDC) assay, where donor lymphocytes were incubated with recipient serum, was first developed in the 1960s.[151] Preformed recipient antibody to donor lymphocytes (subsequently identified as anti-HLA antibody) resulted in lymphocyte death in vitro and predicted rapid (hyperacute) graft failure in vivo. The test was subsequently refined and divided into two separate assays 1) with donor T lymphocytes, which exclusively express HLA class I antigen, and 2) with donor B lymphocytes, which express both HLA class I and II antigens. The addition of antihuman globulin to the assay increased its sensitivity.

A positive CDC T-cell crossmatch is an absolute contraindication to transplantation. A positive CDC B cell crossmatch (in the setting of a negative T-cell flow crossmatch) may indicate the presence of preformed antibody to class II HLA antigen or low level antibodies against class I antigens; however, this scenario (negative CDC T/positive CDC B crossmatch) is always best interpreted in combination with other HLA antibody detection techniques as the binding of (clinically irrelevant) non-HLA antibodies may result in a false positive B cell crossmatches. The CDC assays are now being phased out in many US laboratories having been largely supplanted by flow crossmatch and solid phase technologies.

The flow crossmatch (FCXM) is a more sensitive assay for detecting donor anti-HLA antibody. Donor T lymphocytes (T-cell flow) or B lymphocytes (B cell flow) are mixed with recipient serum and a fluorescent anti-IgG antibody. Any recipient antibody that binds to donor HLA will be tagged by the fluorescent IgG and subsequently detected using flow cytometry. Flow crossmatch detects low-titer and non-complement binding anti-HLA antibody and may be positive when a CDC crossmatch is negative. A negative CDC crossmatch but positive T-cell FCXM is associated with poor short-term transplant outcomes and is a (relative) contraindication to transplantation.[152]

Solid phase technologies such as the Luminex single antigen bead (SAB) anti-HLA antibody assay permit detection and quantification of a wide array of anti-HLA antibodies. Multiple color-coded beads coated with a broad range of HLA antigens are incubated with recipient serum. Binding of antibody to a bead coated with a specific HLA antigen results in a distinct fluorometric signal that is then detected by flow cytometry. Molecular (polymerase chain reaction) HLA typing techniques have now superseded serologic identification of HLA-type for both donors and recipients. Accurate molecular donor HLA-typing and SAB-based recipient anti-HLA antibody screening can be combined to perform a virtual crossmatch. Many centers (ours included) will now proceed with a deceased donor transplant in low immunological risk patients based on a negative virtual crossmatch. For high immunological risk donors, virtual crossmatching has assisted in the identification of potentially compatible donors and has improved transplant rates for sensitized donors.[153] Computerized virtual crossmatch algorithms have also been central to the success of kidney paired donor exchange and transplant chains.[154,155] In the US, wait-listed kidney transplant candidates usually have SAB-based HLA-antibody screening performed every three months. Transplant centers regularly update each candidate's antibody status on UNet, a centralized computer database that virtually matches candidates with potential donors. HLA antigens against which a candidate has antibody are listed as unacceptable HLA antigens or 'avoids' on the system.

The calculated panel reactive antibody (cPRA) replaced the measured PRA in the US in 2009 as the main measure of immune sensitization. The cPRA is calculated using an algorithm that correlates donor anti-HLA antibody (as measured by SAB assay) with the population frequency of HLA antigens to generate a percent score. A candidate with no anti-HLA antibody will have a cPRA of 0%. While a sensitized candidate with a cPRA of 85% will be immunologically incompatible with 85% of the donor population. The choice of predonation crossmatch depends mostly on a donor's immunological risk (see Table 70.2). Intended recipients should be specifically asked if they have recently received a blood transfusion because this could cause a surge in alloantibodies.[156]

Donor-specific anti-HLA antibody (DSA) may be present pretransplant or develop de novo posttransplant. De novo DSA development frequently follows TCMR and is also associated with patient noncompliance.[157] Preformed and de novo DSA are both associated with an increased risk

**Table 70.2 Recipient Risk Factors for Acute Rejection**

| |
|---|
| Previous blood transfusions, particularly if recent |
| Previous pregnancies, particularly if multiple |
| Previous allograft, particularly if rejected early |
| African-American ethnicity |
| cPRA > 20% |
| Donor-specific antibody (current or historic) |

*cPRA,* Calculated panel reactive antibody.

of ABMR and poor graft outcomes.[125,158] DSAs may also be measured using a variation on the SAB technique, the Luminex C1q assay, which detects anti-HLA antibodies that bind and activate complement. The development of post-transplant C1q-binding DSA is strongly associated with poor graft outcome.[159] DSA IgG subtyping also yields similarly helpful prognostic information with DSAs of the IgG3 subclass being associated with the worst clinical prognosis.[160]

The use of HLA epitope matching is a new way at looking at donor-recipient tissue matching, though not yet in widespread clinical use. Briefly, each HLA antigen can be broken into a series of epitopes – (3-dimensional) regions that are capable of binding antibody. These HLA epitopes may be shared across different HLA molecules. The regions of the epitope that are targets for antibody binding are short polymorphic (often nonlinear) amino acid sequences on the HLA molecule that are clustered together in the 3-dimensional structure of the HLA molecule and are known as 'eplets'.[161] Donor-recipient compatibility is expressed as the number of eplet-mismatches. Minimizing donor-recipient epitope mismatch reduces the number of viable 'foreign' targets to which the recipient may make antibody and represents a more relevant way quantify tissue mismatch. Certain eplet mismatches may be especially unfavorable and should be avoided if possible.

### MEDICAL STATUS

The potential recipient should be evaluated to ensure that there are no new contraindications to general anaesthesia, and transplant surgery. This is more relevant to recipients of deceased donor allografts, for whom the date of surgery cannot be planned. Special emphasis should be placed on cardiovascular and infectious risk. With longer waiting periods for transplantation, it is common for a potential recipient to have increased cardiovascular risks since the time of last evaluation. The need for hemodialysis prior to surgery should be assessed. In general, preoperative hemodialysis is advisable if the plasma K is greater than 5.5 mmol/L or severe volume overload is present. The threshold for preoperative dialysis should be lower when delayed or slow graft function is anticipated or in patients with higher cardiovascular risk. A short session of 1½ to 2 hours without anticoagulation usually suffices. Patients on peritoneal dialysis need only drain out instilled fluid before surgery; if the patient is hyperkalemic, several rapid exchanges can be performed.

## EVALUATION OF THE RECIPIENT IMMEDIATELY AFTER THE TRANSPLANT

The nephrologist should carefully review the donor history and the operating room records, noting all intraoperative fluids given, intra- and postoperative blood pressures and urine output, and any technical difficulties encountered. Warm and cold ischemia times should be established. Between donor nephrectomy and reperfusion there are two distinct 'warm ischemia' periods: 1) donor warm ischemia time/extraction time is the period during donor surgery between aortic cross clamping or asystole and the establishment of cold preservation and 2) graft warm ischemia time is the period between the removal of the kidney from cold storage to reperfusion of the graft in the recipient.[162,163] Cold ischemia time (CIT) is the time that the kidney spends in cold preservation and is sandwiched between the two warm ischemia periods. Prolonged warm and cold ischemia times increase the risk of ischemic graft injury and delayed graft function (DGF). Immediate excellent urine output, which should always be the case with living donor transplants, greatly simplifies management. The management of the oligoanuric recipient can be complicated and is discussed later.

## MANAGEMENT OF ALLOGRAFT DYSFUNCTION

In the current era of surgical technique and immunosuppression, major postoperative complications are rare. The focus of clinical management has shifted from improving short-term outcomes to long-term outcomes. Early detection and treatment of early graft dysfunction is an important factor in preserving long-term allograft function. Because early signs of graft dysfunction rarely manifest as detectable symptoms, routine surveillance laboratory testing is a key element of posttransplant management. Surveillance laboratory testing should be performed regardless of the difficulty of the immediate post-operative course. In general, surveillance is performed frequently in the early posttransplant period, and progressively less frequently with time. While there may be variations to this schedule among different centers, a typical schedule for routine surveillance laboratory testing is shown in Table 70.3.

Management is discussed here under three time periods: immediate, early, and late post-transplant.

### IMMEDIATE POSTTRANSPLANT PERIOD (FIRST WEEK)

Patients can be divided into three groups based on allograft function in the first posttransplant week: those with excellent graft function, DGF, and slow graft function (SGF). Excellent allograft function is manifest by an ample urine output and rapidly falling plasma creatinine concentration. Management of patients with excellent allograft function (almost all living donor recipients and a highly variable percentage of deceased donor allograft recipients) is relatively straightforward. Routine imaging studies are not required.

DGF is usually defined by the need for one or more dialysis treatments within the first posttransplant week. SGF defines

**Table 70.3 Routine Surveillance Laboratory Testing After Transplantation**

| | < 1 Month | 1-2 Months | 2-6 Months | 6-24 Months | >24 Months |
|---|---|---|---|---|---|
| CBC | Twice Weekly | Weekly | Every 2 weeks | Monthly | Every 2-3 months |
| BMP/glucose/phosphorus | Twice Weekly | Weekly | Every 2 weeks | Monthly | Every 2-3 months |
| Drug level[a] | Twice Weekly | Weekly | Every 2 weeks | Monthly | Every 2-3 months |
| Liver enzymes | Weekly | Weekly | Every 2 weeks | Monthly | Every 6-12 months |
| Urinalysis | Twice Weekly | Weekly | Every 2 weeks | Monthly | Every 2-3 months |
| Lipid profile | | | Annually | Annually | Annually |
| UPCR[b] | | | 3 Monthly | 6 Monthly | Annually |
| BK PCR | Monthly | Monthly | 3 Monthly | 3/6 Monthly | |
| PTH[c] | | | 3 Monthly[c] | 6 Monthly[c] | Annually[c] |
| DSA[d] | d | d | d | d | d |

[a]Depending on the immunosuppressive regimen, to include tacrolimus, cyclosporine, MPA.
[b]Frequent UPCR monitoring for patients with ESRD from FSGS.
[c]Posttransplant parathyroid hormone monitoring frequency determined by individual PTH and calcium levels.
[d]DSA monitoring frequency determined by patient risk profile.

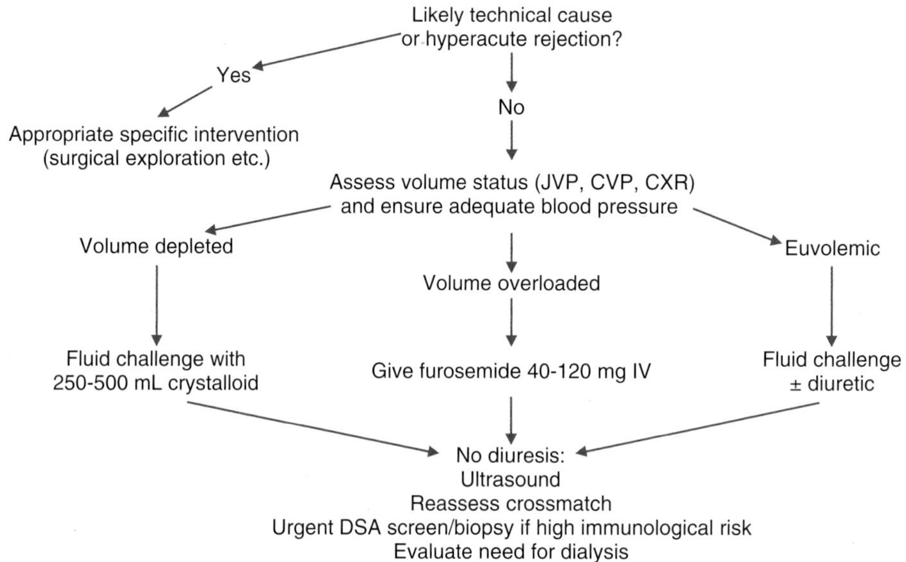


**Fig. 70.3** Management of kidney allograft non-function/oliguria immediately after transplant.

a group of recipients with moderate early graft dysfunction. One commonly employed definition of SGF is a plasma creatinine level greater than 3 mg/dL at 1 week post-transplant.[164] The causes, management, and outcomes of SGF are similar to those of DGF (see below).[164] Interventions that simply convert DGF to SGF appear to have little effect on allograft outcomes. A scheme for managing allograft dysfunction in the immediate post-transplant period is depicted in Fig. 70.3.

## DELAYED GRAFT FUNCTION

The definition of DGF as the requirement for dialysis within one week of transplantation is somewhat arbitrary. The designation excludes some patients with residual native kidney function, such as those undergoing preemptive transplantation, who have DGF per se, but do not require dialysis. There is also likely significant intra-center variation in the use of dialysis posttransplant. The incidence of DGF, by the conventional definition, varies widely depending on the donor source. Scientific Registry of Transplant Recipients data (up to 2012) shows a 3%, 23%, and 31% incidence of DGF in living donor, standard deceased donor, and expanded–criteria donor (ECD) allografts, respectively.[4] Although the causes of DGF include prerenal, intrarenal, and postrenal insults, ischemic acute tubular necrosis (ATN) is by far the most common cause of DGF.

Risk factors for DGF include recipient factors such as male sex, black race, longer dialysis vintage, higher panel-reactive antigen (PRA) status, and greater degree of HLA mismatching. Recipient hypotension requiring pretransplant midodrine use is associated with an increased risk of DGF, graft failure, and death.[165] Donor factors include use of deceased donor kidneys (especially with ECD or DCD), older donor age, and longer cold ischemia time. Most of these factors mediate their effects through ischemia-reperfusion injury as well as

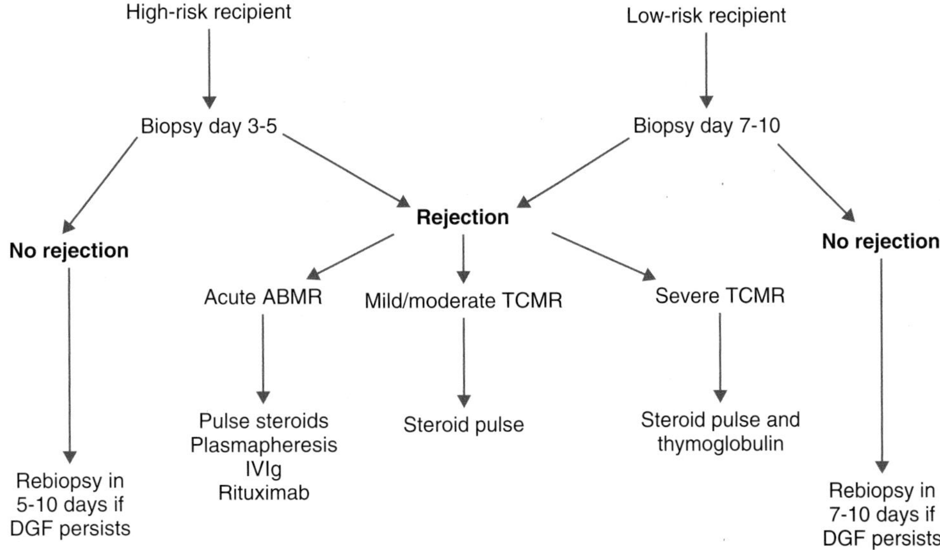


**Fig. 70.4** Algorithm for management of persistent delayed graft function. The presence of anti-donor human leukocyte antigen (HLA) antibodies should prompt immediate biopsy in this setting.

immunologic mechanisms. Older studies suggested that CNIs prolonged or worsened DGF; however, a French randomized controlled trial comparing delayed versus immediate introduction of cyclosporine posttransplant showed no difference in DGF rates or graft function at 3 months but did show a numerical trend toward increased acute rejection in the delayed cyclosporine group.[166]

The diagnosis of the underlying cause of DGF is based on clinical, radiologic, and histologic findings. Careful review of the donor history and of the retrieval and transplantation procedure provides clues about the etiology of DGF. Notably, the interpretation of posttransplant urine output requires knowledge of the residual (native) urine output. Prerenal and postrenal causes (such as volume depletion and urinary catheter malposition or obstruction) should be excluded. If such simple steps fail to improve urine output, further investigation is warranted. Standard ultrasonography is commonly used to assess potential surgical complications in the immediate postoperative period. Ultrasonography can be performed quickly, is inexpensive and noninvasive, and is usually effective in identifying postrenal causes of kidney failure. Duplex sonography is also useful in assessing the graft's arterial and venous blood flow. The resistive index (RI) is often reported in transplant kidney ultrasounds and is elevated in the setting of intrarenal graft dysfunction. However, a raised RI does not discriminate between ATN and rejection and is therefore of limited diagnostic utility.[167]

The evaluation and management of DGF is patient context dependent. Persistent oliguria in a living donor kidney is much more likely to be a major surgical complication than ATN. However, in many cases, both prerenal and postrenal causes of DGF are excluded in deceased donor kidney transplant recipients who are at high risk of ischemic ATN. In the absence of a high suspicion for an alternative diagnosis (such as rejection), expectant management for 7 to 10 days posttransplant is a reasonable approach. A typical algorithm for managing persistent DGF is shown in Fig. 70.4.

**Table 70.4 Risk Factors for DGF**

| |
|---|
| **Prerenal** |
| Severe hypovolemia/hypotension |
| Renal vessel thrombosis |
| **Intrarenal** |
| Ischemic ATN |
| Hyperacute rejection |
| Accelerated or acute rejection superimposed on ATN |
| Acute CNI nephrotoxicity superimposed on ATN |
| **Postrenal** |
| Urinary tract obstruction/leakage |

*ATN,* Acute tubular necrosis; *CNI,* calcineurin inhibitor; *DGF,* delayed graft function.

## CAUSES OF DELAYED GRAFT FUNCTION

### ISCHEMIC ACUTE TUBULAR NECROSIS

Ischemic ATN is the most common cause of DGF in deceased donor kidney recipients. At multiple steps during the surgical transplantation procedure, the allograft is at risk of ischemia-reperfusion injury (Table 70.4).[168]

There are no clinical or radiologic features unique to early posttransplant ATN. As is the case with acute kidney injury (AKI) in native kidneys, transplant ATN should be a diagnosis of exclusion. Several of the risk factors identified in Table 70.5 may be present. Intact allograft perfusion and the absence of obstruction should be confirmed with renal imaging. Histology, if available, shows tubular cell damage and necrosis. Patchy interstitial mononuclear cell infiltrates, but not tubulitis, may be present. The natural history of uncomplicated

**Table 70.5 Causes of Ischemic Damage to the Deceased Donor Kidney Allograft**

| |
|---|
| **Donor State Prior to Organ Procurement** |
| Shock syndromes<br>Endogenous and exogenous catecholamines<br>Brain injury[a]<br>Nephrotoxic drugs |
| **Organ Procurement Surgery** |
| Hypotension<br>Trauma to renal vessels |
| **Organ Transport and Storage** |
| Prolonged storage (cold ischemia time)<br>Pulsatile perfusion injury |
| **Transplantation of Recipient** |
| Prolonged second warm ischemia time<br>Trauma to renal vessels<br>Hypovolemia/hypotension |
| **Postoperative Period** |
| Cyclosporine/tacrolimus<br>Acute heart failure/venous congestion<br>Hemodialysis[a] |

[a]Some evidence.

ATN is spontaneous resolution. Usually, improvements in urine output begin from 5 to 10 days after transplant, but ATN may persist for weeks.

Management of the patient during this period is supportive. When early hemodialysis is required, minimal anticoagulation should be used to reduce the risk of postsurgical bleeding. Intradialytic hypotension should also be avoided in order to prevent further renal ischemic injury. Peritoneal dialysis may be successfully continued posttransplant, although should be avoided if the peritoneum was opened at the time of surgery. Early postoperative treatments should be performed with low volume exchanges.

A major concern in the management of the patient with posttransplant ATN is that the concurrent diagnosis of new surgical or medical complications involving the allograft is difficult. Rejection, for example, may be easily missed. In fact, acute rejection occurs more frequently in allografts with delayed as versus immediate function. The postulated mechanism is that ischemia-reperfusion injury increases the immunogenicity of the allograft, thereby predisposing to acute rejection. Indeed, experimental animal models have demonstrated that ischemic ATN is associated with increased expression/production of class I and II MHC molecules, co-stimulatory molecules, proinflammatory cytokines, and adhesion molecules within the kidney parenchyma.[168] Such an altered local milieu could amplify the alloimmune response. Therefore, a high degree of suspicion for additional complications related to the allograft must be maintained. The possibility of accelerated acute rejection must be considered, particularly in the high-risk recipient. We recommend a low threshold for performing a graft biopsy in patients with DGF. Radiologic evaluation of the graft should also be repeated if there is suspicion of new urinary or vascular complications.

## HYPERACUTE REJECTION

Hyperacute rejection has become a rare cause of immediate graft non-function because of improved tissue-typing technology. However, the increased prevalence of desensitization protocols has made this diagnosis regain clinical relevancy. Hyperacute rejection is caused by preformed recipient antibodies reacting with antigens on the endothelium of the allograft, resulting in activation of the complement and coagulation cascades. These antibodies are usually directed against antigens of the ABO blood group system or against HLA class I antigens. Anti-HLA class I antibodies are formed in response to previous transplantation, blood transfusion, or pregnancy. Less commonly, hyperacute rejection is caused by antibodies directed against donor HLA class II antigens or endothelial or monocyte antigens (the last two are not detected in the standard crossmatch). In classic hyperacute rejection, cyanosis and mottling of the kidney and anuria occur minutes after the vascular anastomosis is established. Disseminated intravascular coagulopathy may occur. Histology shows widespread small vessel endothelial damage and thrombosis, usually with neutrophils incorporated into the thrombus. There is no effective treatment and transplant nephrectomy is indicated. Screening for recipient-donor ABO or class I HLA incompatibility (the presence of the latter is often referred to as a "positive T-cell crossmatch") has ensured that hyperacute rejection is now uncommon. Rare cases occur because of clerical errors or due to the presence of the other preformed antibodies that are not detected by routine screening methods.

## ACCELERATED REJECTION SUPERIMPOSED ON ACUTE TUBULAR NECROSIS

Accelerated acute rejection refers to rejection occurring roughly 2 to 5 days after transplant. Accelerated rejection occurs in recipients with pretransplant sensitization to donor alloantigen and is frequently associated with the presence of historic or low-titer pretransplant anti-donor antibody. Rapid post-transplant antibody production by memory B cells may represent an important mechanism for this phenomenon.[169]

Accelerated acute rejection may be superimposed on ischemic ATN, in which case there may be no signs of rejection, or it may occur in an initially functioning allograft. Diagnosis is made by kidney biopsy in conjunction with crossmatch findings and DSA titers. Histology usually shows evidence of predominantly antibody rather than cell-mediated immune damage. The diagnosis and management of these two forms of rejection are discussed in detail below.

## ACUTE CYCLOSPORINE OR TACROLIMUS NEPHROTOXICITY SUPERIMPOSED ON ACUTE TUBULAR NECROSIS

Cyclosporine and tacrolimus, especially in high doses or by intravenous route of administration, may result in an acute decrease in GFR through renal vasoconstriction, particularly of the afferent glomerular arteriole. Potentially, such vasomotor effects could exacerbate ischemic ATN. Acute CNI toxicity is now rare with the targeting of lower CNI levels. Caution should, however, be taken in the context of drug interactions that raise CNI levels (discussed later).

### VASCULAR AND UROLOGIC COMPLICATIONS OF SURGERY

Renal vessel thrombosis, urinary leaks, and obstruction are rare but important causes of DGF. These complications may also cause allograft dysfunction in the early postoperative period and are discussed later in this chapter.

## OUTCOME AND SIGNIFICANCE OF DELAYED GRAFT FUNCTION

In most cases, recovery of kidney function is sufficient to become independent of dialysis. There is no renal recovery in less than 5% of cases, resulting in primary non-function (PNF). The majority of studies suggest that DGF has a negative impact on long-term kidney allograft survival.[168] Patients with DGF require longer hospitalization and more investigations, and are at higher risk of occult rejection. Postoperative fluid and electrolyte management is more difficult.

Therefore, measures that limit the incidence and duration of DGF are important. Graft injury may occur 1) prior to donation, 2) at retrieval, 3) during transport, 4) during transplant surgery, or 5) postoperatively. Prior to donation heart-beating donors are potentially exposed to various renal insults that may impact future graft function. Good ICU management of the potential deceased donor is of great importance in mitigating many of these factors. Treating the donor with dopamine prior to organ retrieval has been shown to reduce the rate of DGF.[170] However, other specific donor interventions, including desmopressin and steroids, have not been shown to improve subsequent graft function.[171,172]

Meticulous surgical technique, rapid transport of retrieved allografts and use of optimum preservation solutions are also of extreme importance. Data regarding machine perfusion has been somewhat conflicting. A study that randomly assigned one kidney from 336 consecutive deceased donors to machine perfusion and the other to cold storage, showed a reduction in DGF and an improvement in 1-year graft survival in the machine perfusion group.[173] However, machine perfusion was associated with no benefit compared to cold storage in kidneys donated after cardiac death in a UK study.[174] The major disadvantages of machine perfusion are its relative expense and complexity compared to standard cold perfusion techniques.

Cold ischemia time is an important risk factor for DGF.[175] Measures that may decrease CIT include faster identification of potential recipients, the establishment of a list of patients in each transplant region who would quickly accept ECD kidneys and a consensus on allocation and management of DCD organs.[176,177] Nationwide organ sharing of zero HLA-mismatched organs also results in prolongation of cold ischemia time in some cases. However, the small increase in CIT, associated with national organ sharing, is offset by the substantial immunologic benefits of zero-HLA mismatched transplantation.[178] Similarly, the new Kidney Allocation System in the United States has resulted in greater regional and national sharing of organs for highly sensitized patients at the expense of a longer CIT.[138]

Intraoperative mean arterial pressure should be maintained greater than 70 mm Hg in the recipient. In cases in which DGF is expected, antilymphocyte antibody preparations are often used and may have benefits beyond acute rejection prophylaxis. In experimental models, antithymocyte globulins directly ameliorate ischemia reperfusion injury through modulation adhesion molecule expression and the inflammatory response.[179] Indeed, intra-operative (versus postoperative) thymoglobulin administration was associated with reduced DGF in one randomized study.[180] Another study demonstrated reduced DGF with thymoglobulin over daclizumab.[26]

Despite theoretical benefits, peri-transplant erythropoitin treatment showed no effect on DGF in two randomized controlled trials.[181,182] Calcium channel blockers have been shown in experimental models to prevent ischemic injury and attenuate CNI-mediated renal vasoconstriction. These properties suggested that their administration to recipients or to the donor before organ retrieval might reduce the incidence and duration of ischemic ATN. A Cochrane review that included 13 trials suggested a reduced risk of ATN and delayed graft function associated with perioperative calcium channel blocker use but no difference in graft loss or mortality.[183] A number of interventional trials have attempted to target patients at risk of DGF with various treatments to prevent IRI in the immediate post-transplant period. Experimental treatments have included C1 esterase inhibition and p53 siRNA.[184,185] However, data are currently insufficient to recommend their inclusion into the transplant therapeutic repertoire.

## EARLY POSTTRANSPLANT PERIOD (FIRST SIX MONTHS)

Table 70.6 shows the causes of allograft dysfunction during the early post-transplant period. Despite its known limitations, the primary measure of early and late transplant function remains the plasma creatinine concentration. Prerenal and postrenal causes of graft dysfunction should be systematically excluded. An algorithm for the management of allograft dysfunction in the early posttransplant period is shown in Fig. 70.5.

**Table 70.6 Causes of Allograft Dysfunction in the Early Postoperative Period**

| |
|---|
| **Prerenal** |
| Hypovolemia/hypotension |
| Renal vessel thrombosis |
| Hemodynamic drug effects: ACE inhibitors, NSAIDs, acute CNI nephrotoxicity |
| Transplant renal artery stenosis |
| **Intrarenal** |
| Acute rejection – TCMR or ABMR |
| CNI-induced thrombotic microangiopathy |
| Recurrence of primary disease |
| Acute pyelonephritis |
| Acute interstitial nephritis |
| **Postrenal** |
| Urinary tract obstruction/leakage |

*ACE,* Angiotensin-converting enzyme; *CNI,* calcineurin inhibitor; *NSAIDS,* nonsteroidal antiinflammatory drugs.

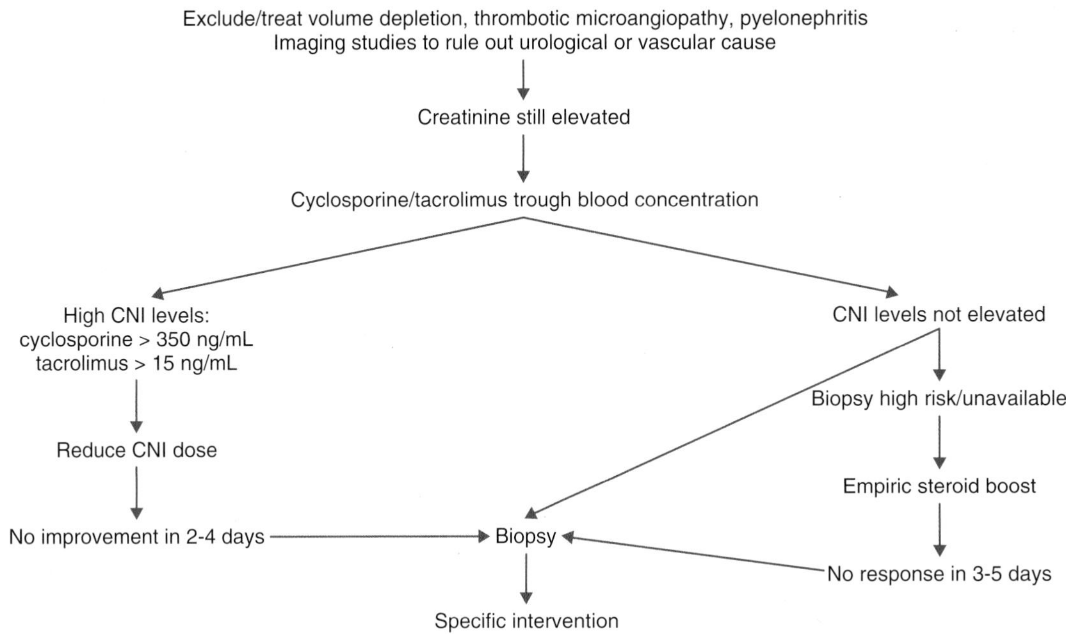


**Fig. 70.5** Algorithm for management of allograft dysfunction in early posttransplant period. *CNI,* Calcineurin inhibitor.

## PRERENAL RENAL DYSFUNCTION IN THE EARLY POSTTRANSPLANT PERIOD

### Hypovolemia and Drugs

Hypovolemia may develop after excessive diuresis from the transplanted kidney or from diarrhea. Diarrhea is a common adverse effect of the MMF, especially when used with tacrolimus. Angiotensin-converting enzyme (ACE) inhibitors (ACE-Is), angiotensin-receptor blockers (ARBs), and nonsteroidal antiinflammatory drugs (NSAIDs) should be avoided in the early posttransplant period because of the risk of functional prerenal failure, a risk that may be potentiated by the renal vasoconstrictive effects of CNIs.

### Renal Vessel Thrombosis

Transplant renal artery or renal vein thrombosis usually occurs in the first 72 hours but may be delayed for up to 10 weeks. Acute vascular thrombosis is the most common cause of allograft loss in the first week. Although surgical technique is a factor in some cases, there is now greater appreciation of the role of hypercoagulable states.[15]

Renal artery thrombosis presents with abrupt onset of anuria (unless there is a native urine output) and rapidly rising plasma creatinine, but often with negligible graft pain. Duplex studies show absent arterial and venous blood flow. Renography or magnetic resonance (MR) angiography shows absent perfusion of the transplanted kidney. Removal of the infarcted kidney is indicated.

Renal vein thrombosis also manifests with anuria and rapidly increasing plasma creatinine. Pain, tenderness, swelling in the graft, and hematuria are more pronounced than in renal artery thrombosis. Severe complications such as embolization or graft rupture and hemorrhage may occur. Duplex studies show absent renal venous blood flow and characteristic highly abnormal renal arterial waveforms. MR venography demonstrates thrombus in the vein. Transplant nephrectomy is usually indicated. If the venous thrombosis extends beyond the renal vein, anticoagulation is necessary to reduce the risk of embolization. There are reports of salvaging kidney function after early diagnosis of renal vessel thrombosis and its treatment with thrombolysis or thrombectomy. In almost all cases, however, infarction occurs too quickly to make this treatment worthwhile. Furthermore, thrombolysis is relatively contraindicated in the early posttransplant period because of the high risk of graft-related bleeding.

## INTRARENAL DYSFUNCTION IN THE EARLY POSTTRANSPLANT PERIOD

### Acute Rejection

Acute rejection is characterized by a decline in kidney function mediated by a recipient immune reaction against the allograft. Although acute rejection can occur at any time, it is most common in the first 6 months posttransplant. Fortunately, the incidence of acute rejection has decreased dramatically in the past 25 years; it is now around 10% in the first 12 months in the United States.[123]

In the era of modern immunosuppression, symptoms and signs of acute rejection are rarely pronounced, but low-grade fever, oliguria, and graft pain or tenderness may occur. Most cases of acute rejection are identified through surveillance monitoring of graft function. However, creatinine is a rather late and insensitive marker of renal injury. There is, therefore, a growing interest in development of early biomarkers of immune system activation. However, for now, the definitive diagnosis of acute rejection requires transplant biopsy.

Acute rejection involves both cellular and/or humoral immune mechanisms (TCMR and ABMR). Clinical transplantation has traditionally been focused on cell-mediated responses. However, ABMR has been receiving more attention because of improvements in diagnostic techniques and increased transplantation of immunological high-risk candidates. Differences between TCMR and ABMR are summarized in Table 70.7.

**Table 70.7 Differences Between Pure Forms of Acute TCMR and Active ABMR**

| | Acute TCMR | Active ABMR |
|---|---|---|
| Timing of clinical onset | >5 days | >0 days |
| Tubulitis/interstitial inflammation | Present | Absent |
| Microvasular inflammation: peritubular capillaritis and/or glomerulitis | Absent | Present |
| C4d staining of peritubular capillaries | Absent | Present |
| Donor-specific antibody in serum | Usually absent | Present |
| Therapy | Pulse steroids/ATG | Pulsed steroids, plasmapheresis, IVIg, rituximab steroids, rituximab |

**T-Cell Mediated Rejection.** The Banff classification[186,187] (Table 70.8) is a widely used schema for classifying rejection. Histologic findings characteristic of TCMR include 1) mononuclear cell infiltration of the interstitium, mainly with T cells but also with some macrophages and plasma cells; 2) tubulitis (infiltration of tubule epithelium by lymphocytes); and 3) arteritis which manifests as infiltration of mononuclear cells beneath the endothelium. Vascular involvement reflects more severe rejection.

Borderline TCMR, where histologic findings fall below the threshold for Banff 1A TCMR, is a fairly frequent finding. We usually treat borderline rejection.[188] Conversely, histologic evidence of rejection can also be seen in the presence of stable allograft function (subclinical TCMR). Some studies have reported improvement of graft function with treatment of subclinical TCMR,[189] but no benefit was found in a larger multicenter trial.[190] The presence of eosinophils in the infiltrate suggests severe rejection, but allergic interstitial nephritis should also be considered. Note that polyoma virus infection may also cause tubulointerstitial nephritis.

Uncomplicated TCMR is generally treated with a short course of high-dose steroids. There is a 60% to 70% response rate to this regimen, but the dose and duration of treatment has not been standardized. Typically, methylprednisolone 250 to 500 mg is given intravenously for 3 to 5 days. After completion of pulse therapy, the dose of oral steroids can be tapered back or resumed immediately to the maintenance dose. If the patient has been on a steroid-free regimen, adding a maintenance dose should be considered. An episode of acute rejection implies that prior immunosuppression has been inadequate. The patient's compliance with prescribed medications should be reviewed. If there are no contraindications, baseline immunosuppression should be increased or changed, at least in the short term. Lymphocyte-depleting antibodies are highly effective in treating first rejection episodes but because of toxicity and cost, these agents are usually reserved for steroid-resistant cases or when there is severe rejection on the initial biopsy.[191]

Steroid-resistant TCMR, defined somewhat arbitrarily as failure of improvement in urine output or plasma creatinine within 5 days of starting pulse treatment, is usually treated with depleting antibodies. If steroid treatment was based on an empiric rather than a histologic diagnosis, allograft biopsy should be performed to confirm this diagnosis before starting treatment with depleting antibody agents. A higher grade of TCMR with endothelial involvement (Banff II or III) is more likely to be steroid-resistant, and many centers use depleting antibody therapy as an initial treatment. The advantage of this approach is prompt and effective treatment of the TCMR in higher-risk patients. The disadvantage is cost, inconvenience, and exposure of the patients to potentially serious complications of therapy such as infection and cancer. However, in steroid-resistant rejection, the benefits of lymphocyte depleting agents outweigh their risks. ATG is the most commonly employed depleting agent.[32]

**Refractory T-Cell Mediated Rejection.** Refractory TCMR is generally defined as TCMR resistant to treatment with anti-lymphocyte antibody. By definition, the patient has already received aggressive immunosuppression; the risks and benefits of further amplifying immunosuppression should be very carefully considered. Renal histology is helpful in this regard. Therapeutic options include 1) continuing maintenance immunosuppression in the hope that kidney function will slowly improve, 2) repeating a course of antilymphocyte antibody therapy, or 3) switching from cyclosporine to tacrolimus if not already done.[192] If there is a component of active ABMR, this can be treated as discussed below.

**Active Antibody-Mediated Rejection.** ABMR is increasingly recognized as a cause of allograft dysfunction and is reported in 3.5% to 9% of for-cause biopsies.[193,194] Increased recognition of ABMR is partly a result of improved diagnostics (in particular, assays for C4d and DSA[195]) and in the expansion of immunologically high-risk and incompatible transplantation.[59] Diagnosis of active ABMR requires the presence of all of the following: 1) characteristic histological features which include microvascular inflammation (peritubular capillaritis and/or glomerulitis), intimal or transmural arteritis, thrombotic microangiopathy (TMA), and acute tubular necrosis; 2) evidence of recent antibody-endothelial interaction, usually identified using C4d staining of peritubular capillaries; and 3) serologic evidence of antibody against donor HLA or other antigens.[196] Active ABMR typically occurs early after transplantation but can also occur late, especially in the setting of reduced immunosuppression or noncompliance. Active ABMR may occur alone or with TCMR. In addition, subclinical active ABMR is commonly present on surveillance biopsies of immunologically high-risk kidney transplant recipients and is associated with poor graft outcome.[197]

The prognosis of active ABMR is poorer than TCMR. The optimal treatment of ABMR is as yet unestablished.[188,198] The most commonly employed regimens for active ABMR

**Table 70.8 Banff Diagnostic Categories for Kidney Transplant Histopathology (Including 2017 Update)**

*Category 1: Normal biopsy* or *nonspecific changes*

*Category 2: Antibody-mediated changes*

Active ABMR; all 3 criteria must be met for diagnosis

1. Histologic evidence of acute tissue injury, including 1 or more of the following:
   - Microvascular inflammation (g > 0 and/or ptc > 0), in the absence of recurrent or de novo glomerulonephritis, although in the presence of acute TCMR, borderline infiltrate, or infection, ptc ≥1 alone is not sufficient and g must be ≥1
   - Intimal or transmural arteritis (v > 0)c
   - Acute thrombotic microangiopathy, in the absence of any other cause
   - Acute tubular injury, in the absence of any other apparent cause
2. Evidence of current/recent antibody interaction with vascular endothelium, *including 1 or more of the following*:
   - Linear C4d staining in peritubular capillaries (C4d2 or C4d3 by IF on frozen sections, or C4d >0 by IHC on paraffin sections)
   - At least moderate microvascular inflammation ([g + ptc] ≥2) in the absence of recurrent or de novo glomerulonephritis, although in the presence of acute TCMR, borderline infiltrate, or infection, ptc ≥2 alone is not sufficient and g must be ≥1
   - Increased expression of gene transcripts/classifiers in the biopsy tissue strongly associated with ABMR, *if thoroughly validated*
3. Serologic evidence of donor-specific antibodies (DSA to HLA or other antigens). C4d staining or expression of validated transcripts/classifiers as noted above in criterion 2 may substitute for DSA; however, thorough DSA testing, including testing for non-HLA antibodies if HLA antibody testing is negative, is strongly advised whenever criteria 1 and 2 are met.

Chronic active ABMR; all 3 criteria must be met for diagnosis

1. Morphologic evidence of chronic tissue injury, including 1 or more of the following:
   - Transplant glomerulopathy (cg >0) if no evidence of chronic TMA or chronic recurrent/de novo glomerulonephritis; includes changes evident by electron microscopy (EM) alone (cg1a)
   - Severe peritubular capillary basement membrane multilayering (requires EM)
   - Arterial intimal fibrosis of new onset, excluding other causes; leukocytes within the sclerotic intima favor chronic ABMR if there is no prior history of TCMR, but are not required
2. Identical to criterion 2 for active ABMR, above
3. Identical to criterion 3 for active ABMR, above, including strong recommendation for DSA testing whenever criteria 1 and 2 are met

C4d staining without evidence of rejection; all 4 features must be present for diagnosis

1. Linear C4d staining in peritubular capillaries (C4d2 or C4d3 by IF on frozen sections, or C4d>0 by IHC on paraffin sections)
2. Criterion 1 for active or chronic, active ABMR not met
3. No molecular evidence for ABMR as in criterion 2 for active and chronic, active ABMR
4. No acute or chronic active TCMR, or borderline changes

*Category 3: Borderline changes*

Suspicious (borderline) for acute TCMR

Foci of tubulitis (t > 0) with minor interstitial inflammation (i0 or i1), or moderate-severe interstitial inflammation (i2 or i3) with mild (t1) tubulitis; retaining the i1 threshold for borderline with t > 0 is permitted although this must be made transparent in reports and publications

- No intimal or transmural arteritis (v = 0)

*Category 4: TCMR*

Acute TCMR

| | |
|---|---|
| Grade IA | Interstitial inflammation involving >25% of nonsclerotic cortical parenchyma (i2 or i3) with moderate tubulitis (t2) involving 1 or more tubules, not including tubules that are severely atrophic |
| Grade IB | Interstitial inflammation involving >25% of nonsclerotic cortical parenchyma (i2 or i3) with severe tubulitis (t3) involving 1 or more tubules, not including tubules that are severely atrophic |
| Grade IIA | Mild to moderate intimal arteritis (v1), with or without interstitial inflammation and/or tubulitis |
| Grade IIB | Severe intimal arteritis (v2), with or without interstitial inflammation and/or tubulitis |
| Grade III | Transmural arteritis and/or arterial fibrinoid necrosis of medial smooth muscle with accompanying mononuclear cell intimal arteritis (v3), with or without interstitial inflammation and/or tubulitis |

Chronic Active TCMR

| | |
|---|---|
| Grade IA | Interstitial inflammation involving >25% of the total cortex (ti score 2 or 3) and >25% of the sclerotic cortical parenchyma (i-IFTA score 2 or 3) with moderate tubulitis (t2) involving 1 or more tubules, not including severely atrophic tubules; other known causes of i-IFTA should be ruled out |
| Grade IB | Interstitial inflammation involving >25% of the total cortex (ti score 2 or 3) and >25% of the sclerotic cortical parenchyma (i-IFTA score 2 or 3) with severe tubulitis (t3) involving 1 or more tubules, not including severely atrophic tubules; other known causes of i-IFTA should be ruled out |
| Grade II | Chronic allograft arteriopathy (arterial intimal fibrosis with mononuclear cell inflammation in fibrosis and formation of neointima) |

*Category 5: Interstitial fibrosis and tubular atrophy*

Grade
- I. Mild interstitial fibrosis and tubular atrophy (≤25% of cortical area)
- II. Moderate interstitial fibrosis and tubular atrophy (26% to 50% of cortical area)
- III. Severe interstitial fibrosis and tubular atrophy (>50% of cortical area)

**Table 70.8 Banff Diagnostic Categories for Kidney Transplant Histopathology (Including 2017 Update) (Cont'd)**

*Category 6: Other changes not considered to be caused by acute or chronic rejection*

- BK virus nephropathy
- Posttransplant lymphoproliferative disorders
- Calcineurin inhibitor nephrotoxicity
- Acute tubular injury
- Recurrent disease
- De novo glomerulopathy (other than transplant glomerulopathy)
- Pyelonephritis
- Drug-induced interstitial nephritis

include some combination of pulsed steroids, plasmapheresis, intravenous immunoglobulins, and anti-CD20 monoclonal antibody to suppress/remove DSA.[199] Other therapies that have been used for active ABMR include C1 inhibition, eculizumab, bortezomib, and bortezomib plus conversion to belatacept.[198,200]

There is also a growing body of literature regarding non-HLA antibody-mediated ABMR.[201] The best studied non-HLA antibody implicated in graft injury is probably the angiotensin II type 1-receptor activating antibody, the effects of which may be mitigated by angiotensin receptor blockade blocker therapy.[202]

### Significance of Acute Rejection

Although acute rejection is frequently reversed, retrospective studies show that it is strongly associated with the development of chronic rejection and poorer allograft survival. Both increased severity (as evidence by histology and change in creatinine) and later timing (more than 6 months posttransplant) of acute rejection are associated with poorer long-term outcomes.[203] Whatever the outcome is in terms of allograft function, treatment involves exposing the patient to supplemental immunosuppression and its attendant risks.

**Acute Calcineurin Inhibitor Nephrotoxicity.** The CNIs, especially in high doses, cause an acute decrease in GFR by renal vasoconstriction, particularly of the afferent glomerular arteriole. This is manifested clinically as dose and blood concentration–dependent acute reversible increase in plasma creatinine. Because acute CNI nephrotoxicity is mainly hemodynamic in origin, histology is frequently normal. However, with prolonged CNI toxicity tubular cell vacuolization and hyaline arteriolar thickening may be seen.[204] The treatment of acute CNI nephrotoxicity is dose reduction.

**Distinguishing Acute Calcineurin Inhibitor Nephrotoxicity and Acute Rejection.** Distinguishing acute CNI nephrotoxicity and acute rejection clinically can be difficult. Low and high blood concentrations in the presence of rising creatinine suggest but do not imply rejection and drug nephrotoxicity, respectively. Both syndromes can coexist. Indicators of a diagnosis of acute CNI nephrotoxicity are severe tremor (neurotoxicity), a moderate increase in plasma creatinine (>25% over baseline), and high trough blood CNI concentrations (e.g., cyclosporine >350 ng/mL or tacrolimus levels >15 ng/mL). Indicators of a diagnosis of acute rejection are low-grade fever, allograft pain and tenderness (although with current drug regimens these symptoms or signs are uncommon), rapid, non-plateauing increases in plasma creatinine, and low drug concentrations. Fever and symptoms localized to the allograft do not occur with CNI toxicity but do not necessarily imply rejection; acute pyelonephritis must also be considered.

If acute CNI nephrotoxicity is suspected, our practice is to reduce the CNI dose and repeat a serum creatinine and drug level within 48 to 96 hours. If graft function has not improved or plateaued at this point we usually go on to kidney biopsy. The threshold for biopsy is lower in high-risk patients: those who are highly sensitized, have previously rejected an allograft, or are at high risk of early recurrent primary kidney disease (see later). In certain circumstances, where kidney biopsy is deemed high risk, we will empirically treat with a steroid pulse for a presumptive diagnosis of acute rejection. However, failure of graft function to rapidly improve with this strategy will usually prompt a biopsy.

Most transplant centers provide rapid biopsy and processing of tissue, with basic histology available within 5 to 6 hours. Since a delay of 6 hours in initiating specific therapy should not be detrimental to the graft, a biopsy-proven diagnosis is the preferred approach. In addition to determining the degree and type of rejection in the allograft, histology also occasionally reveals unexpected pathology such as TMA or polyoma virus infection. Biopsy results alone should not dictate management; rather, the combination of clinical and histologic findings should be used to shape a treatment plan.

**Monitoring.** Signs and symptoms of graft dysfunction often occur late, after significant graft injury. Thus, monitoring of serum electrolytes and immunosuppressive drug levels is an essential part of posttransplant management. Serum creatinine, basic chemistry panel, liver function tests, and CBC are routinely checked to screen for graft dysfunction and manifestations of drug toxicity. Drug levels for CNI, MMF, and mTORi are also monitored for adjustment of immunosuppressive drug dosing. The frequency of monitoring is greater immediately posttransplant, and gradually decreased. At our institution, we monitor routine blood levels twice weekly during the first month, once a week during the second month, and once every two weeks during the $3^{rd}$-$6^{th}$ months posttransplant. Thereafter, we require monitoring on a monthly basis. The frequency of monitoring is increased if there is graft dysfunction and subsequent treatment. BK plasma PCR monitoring is performed at set time points in the first two years posttransplant.

Most patients are on CNIs. Cyclosporine A (CsA) can be measured using trough (C0) levels, 2-hour post-dose (C2) or through abbreviated AUCs. C0 is the measured level after the dosing interval (e.g., 12 hours after dosing if given every 12 hours), C2 is the measured level 2 hours after dosing, and AUC is the area under the curve during the first 4 hours after dosing. C2 levels correlate more closely with AUC, but no significant differences have been found in the incidence of acute rejection, graft loss, or adverse events between patients monitored using C0 or C2 levels.[205] The standard target level for CsA is C0 of 150-300 ng/mL early and 100-200 ng/mL late posttransplant[206] or C2 1400-1800 ng/mL early and 800-1200 ng/mL later after transplantation.[207] Tacrolimus C0 levels correlate better with AUC[208,209] and measuring the C0 tacrolimus level is usual practice. The standard target level for tacrolimus C0 is 8-12 ng/dL in the early posttransplant months and 6-9 ng/dL in the first posttransplant year to year–and-a-half. We individualize our longer term tacrolimus targets aiming for a level at the lower or higher end of 5-8 ng/mL depending on immune risk, tolerability, and other clinical factors. For patients with evidence of CNI toxicity and who are otherwise stable, compliant, and at low immunological risk, a target of 3-7 ng/mL may be reasonable in the long term.[80,210]

There are two major weaknesses in transplant rejection monitoring and diagnosis in its current form. 1) Graft dysfunction (as evidenced by creatinine rise) may occur relatively late into a rejection episode, resulting in a delay in diagnosis and treatment. 2) Kidney biopsy, the gold standard for rejection diagnosis, is expensive, invasive and has real risks. The development of biomarkers that can aid in the early detection of graft dysfunction or even obviate the need for biopsy is therefore highly desirable. Biomarkers that have been investigated include cytokines, IL-2 receptor, CD30, adhesion molecules, and other inflammatory markers such as complement and acute-phase proteins.[211–213] A three-gene model of urinary 18S-normalized CD3ε messenger RNA, 18S-normalized IP-10 messenger RNA, and 18S ribosomal RNA showed good discrimination for acute rejection, with the test preempting acute rejection episodes by up to 10 days.[214]

Donor-derived cell-free DNA measurement is now commercially available. The technique utilizes the presence of single nucleotide polymorphisms (SNPs), which are nucleotides at specific positions in the human genome that commonly vary between individuals.[215,216] The most commonly used assay analyzes over 250 different SNPs, allowing the test to distinguish donor-form recipient cell-free DNA without a donor blood sample. The assay reports donor-derived cell-free DNA as a percentage of total cell-free DNA in the recipient's blood. A donor-derived cell-free DNA level in excess of 1% likely reflects underlying graft injury. The test is of limited utility in the diagnosis of TCMR, especially Banff 1A or less. However, testing appears more sensitive for microvascular inflammation and ultimately may prove useful in identifying those patients with subclinical ABMR.[217] The test cannot be reliably used in those patients with prior kidney transplants or other solid organ transplants.

Protocol posttransplant DSA monitoring is performed at many centers on all or select groups of patients. DSA may either be formed prior to transplant (preformed) or occur de novo posttransplant. De novo (versus preformed) DSA are associated with worse allograft outcomes.[218] DSA may be accompanied by 1) normal renal function and histology, 2) normal renal function and ABMR histology (subclinical ABMR), 3) overt ABMR, or 4) chronic active ABMR. DSA screening is certainly warranted in immunologically high-risk recipients and at the time of 'for clinical indication' biopsy. Treatment of DSA depends on accompanying clinical and histological findings. The detection of an isolated de novo DSA warrants intensification of immunosuppression, strong consideration for allograft biopsy (irrespective of graft function) and, in some centers, will trigger specific therapies such as IVIg. DSA may be further risk stratified by assessing their ability to bind complement (C1q assay) or by typing their (IgG) subclass. Treatment of DSA accompanied by ABMR is discussed separately.

The use of molecular diagnostic tools, such as the 'molecular microscope', which employs a microarray-based approach to measure differential gene expression in renal biopsy tissue, have promise, and may prove particularly useful in diagnosis and prognosis of ABMR.[219]

Many transplant centers perform elective protocol biopsies at set time points after transplant irrespective of graft function. The merits and demerits of such an approach are keenly debated.[220] To our knowledge, there are no data showing that widespread screening with protocol biopsies in the tacrolimus-MMF era results in better outcomes.[190] Protocol biopsies may, however, have a useful role in selected high immunological risk groups.[221]

### Acute Thrombotic Microangiopathy

Acute de novo TMA after kidney transplantation is a rare but serious complication.[222] It usually occurs in the early post-transplant period and is accompanied by increasing plasma creatinine and lactate dehydrogenase levels, thrombocytopenia, falling hemoglobin level, schistocytosis, and low haptoglobin concentrations. This diagnosis can be overlooked because thrombocytopenia and anemia occur commonly after transplantation in the setting for ATG induction therapy. The diagnosis is confirmed by allograft biopsy, which shows endothelial damage and, in severe cases, thrombosis of glomerular capillaries and arterioles.

Causes include CNIs,[223] OKT3, ABMR,[224] viral infections such as cytomegalovirus (CMV), and the recurrence of a previously undiagnosed primary disease. The presence of hepatitis C and anticardiolipin antibodies increases the risk.[225] Early diagnosis of TMA is essential to salvage kidney function. There are no controlled trials of therapy for de novo TMA after transplant. Our initial measure is to switch CNI (either from tacrolimus to cyclosporine or cyclosporine to tacrolimus). Another reasonable approach is to switch off treatment with the CNI drug class completely and move to a belatacept or mTori-based immunosuppression regimen. We concurrently look for other potential underlying etiologies including ABMR. If the syndrome fails to improve with the above measures we initiate plasma exchange.[226,227] Eculizumab has also been employed successfully.[228,229]

### Acute Pyelonephritis

Urinary tract infections (UTIs) may occur at any period but are most frequent shortly after transplantation because of catheterization, stenting, and aggressive immunosuppression.[230] Other risk factors for urinary tract infection (UTI) are anatomic abnormalities and neurogenic bladder. Fever, allograft pain and tenderness, and leukocytosis are usually more pronounced in acute pyelonephritis than in acute rejection. Diagnosis requires urine culture, but empiric antibiotic treatment should be started immediately. Delay in treatment can lead to rapid clinical decline in the immunosuppressed patient. The most commonly implicated microorganisms are gram-negative bacilli, coagulase-negative staphylococci, and enterococci. Kidney function usually returns to baseline quickly with antimicrobial therapy and volume expansion. Recurrent pyelonephritis requires investigation to exclude underlying urologic abnormalities. A voiding cystourethrogram (VCUG) should be considered to evaluate for reflux into the transplant allograft. High-grade reflux may warrant reimplantation of the transplanted ureter to the bladder.[231]

### Acute Allergic Interstitial Nephritis

In the setting of kidney transplantation, acute allergic interstitial nephritis is a diagnosis of exclusion. Distinguishing acute allergic interstitial nephritis and TCMR is very difficult. In fact, the pathogenesis is somewhat similar in both cases, involving mainly cell-mediated immunity. While fever and rash after ingestion of a new drug favor the former, these clinical features are rarely seen. Mononuclear cell and eosinophil infiltration of the transplanted kidney may occur with either condition, but endothelialitis implicates rejection. Polyomavirus infection must also be considered in the differential diagnosis. Both acute allergic interstitial nephritis and TCMR usually respond to steroids; of course, the suspected drugs must be stopped. SMX-TMP is the drug most commonly implicated in causing allergic interstitial nephritis in kidney transplant patients; other antibiotics including penicillins, cephalosporins, and quinolones can also be implicated.

### Early Recurrence of Primary Disease

Several kidney diseases may recur early and cause acute allograft dysfunction. These may be classified into three groups: 1) glomerulonephritides, 2) metabolic diseases such as primary oxalosis, and 3) systemic diseases such as hemolytic-uremic syndrome/thrombotic thrombocytopenia purpura (HUS/TTP). Primary focal segmental glomerulosclerosis (FSGS) is considered in more detail in the following section because of its relatively high frequency of recurrence and its propensity to cause severe graft injury.

**Primary Focal Segmental Glomerulosclerosis.** The recurrence of primary FSGS is variable. For the sporadic variety it is reported to be about 30%,[232] but recurrence of familial FSGS is rare. Risk factors for recurrence include white ethnicity, younger age, rapidly progressive FSGS in the recipient's native kidneys, and recurrence of disease in a previous allograft. Most cases become manifest (as proteinuria) hours to weeks after transplant. This rapidity of recurrence suggests the presence of a pathogenic circulating plasma factor.[233] Because of the poor prognosis of delayed treatment, patients with primary FSGS should be monitored after transplantation for new-onset proteinuria. Early biopsy is indicated in those who develop proteinuria; this may not show FSGS lesions per se, but the electron microscopic demonstration of diffuse foot process effacement. Treatment options include plasmapheresis or immunoadsorption, high-dose CNIs, ACE-inhibitors, high-dose corticosteroids, cyclophosphamide, adrenocorticotropic hormone gel and rituximab, but controlled studies are lacking.[234–237]

**Antiglomerular Basement Membrane Disease.** Before transplantation, patients with ESRD due to antiglomerular basement membrane (GBM) disease should generally be on dialysis for at least 6 months and have negative anti-GBM serology.[238] If these criteria are fulfilled, posttransplant recurrence is rare. De novo anti-GBM disease can occur in recipients with Alport syndrome. Here, the recipient with abnormal type IV collagen produces antibodies against the previously "unseen" normal α5 chain NC1 domain in the basement membrane of the transplanted kidney. Patients with allograft dysfunction should be treated with plasmapheresis and cyclophosphamide.[238]

**Hemolytic-Uremic Syndrome/Thrombotic Thrombocytopenia Purpura (HUS/TTP).** The causes of *de novo* TMA after kidney transplant have been discussed earlier. Recurrence of classic (diarrhea-associated) HUS/TTP is uncommon. However, transplantation should still be deferred until the disease is quiescent for at least 6 months. In contrast, recurrence of atypical (non–diarrhea-associated) HUS/TTP, particularly if inherited, has been reported to be as high as 80%.[239] Certain genetic disorders of complement regulation (such as of Factor H) are associated with high risks of severe recurrence, so it is very useful to define these risks, if possible, before proceeding with transplant.[240] One treatment option in patients with underlying mutations in the genes coding liver-produced proteins such as Factor H or Factor I is to perform dual liver kidney transplant, where the role of liver transplant is to supply functional factor H or I.[241] Eculizumab has been shown to successfully treat and prevent recurrent atypical HUS and post-kidney transplant 'prophylactic' eculizumab represents a viable, if expensive, option for preventing disease recurrence.[140,228]

## POSTRENAL DYSFUNCTION IN THE EARLY POSTTRANSPLANT PERIOD

Most urologic complications are secondary to technical factors at the time of transplant and manifest themselves in the early postoperative period, but immunologic factors may play a role in some cases.

### Urine Leaks

Leaks may occur at the level of the renal calyx, ureter, or bladder. Causes include infarction of the ureter due to perioperative disruption of its blood supply and breakdown of the ureterovesical anastomosis. Severe obstruction may also result in rupture of the urinary tract with leakage. Clinical features include abdominal pain and swelling; the plasma urea and creatinine levels increase due to resorption of solutes across the peritoneal membrane. If a perirenal drain is being used, however, a urine leak may present with high-volume drainage of fluid. Ultrasound may demonstrate a fluid collection (urinoma); aspiration of fluid from the collection (or from the drain bag) by sterile technique allows comparison of the fluid and plasma creatinine. When the excretory function of the kidney is good, the creatinine concentration in the urinoma greatly exceeds that in the plasma.

In cases in which ultrasound diagnosis is difficult, renal scintigraphy may be useful in demonstrating extravasation of tracer from the urinary system, provided there is adequate kidney function. Rough localization of the site of the leak is sometimes possible by this technique. Antegrade pyelography allows precise diagnosis and localization of proximal urinary leaks. Cystography is the best test to demonstrate a bladder leak.

The clinical features may mimic those of acute rejection. Whenever urine leakage is suspected, a bladder catheter should be immediately inserted to decompress the urinary tract. Selected patients may do well with a bladder catheter or endourologic treatment. Many cases, however, require urgent surgical exploration and repair. The type of repair depends on the level of the leak and the viability of involved tissues.

#### Urinary Tract Obstruction

Although urinary tract obstruction can occur at any time after transplantation, it is most common in the early postoperative period. Intrinsic causes include poor implantation of the ureter into the bladder, intraluminal blood clots or slough material, and fibrosis of the ureter due to ischemia or rejection. Extrinsic causes include an enlarged prostate in elderly men (causing bladder outlet obstruction) and compression by a lymphocele or other fluid collection. Rarely, calculi cause transplant urinary tract obstruction.

Urinary tract obstruction is often asymptomatic, and should always be considered in the differential diagnosis of allograft dysfunction in the early transplant period. Ultrasound often demonstrates hydronephrosis. However, some dilation of the transplant urinary collecting system is often seen in the early postoperative period, and serial scans showing worsening hydronephrosis may be needed to confirm the diagnosis. Renal scintiscan with diuretic washout is useful in equivocal cases. Percutaneous antegrade pyelography is the best radiologic technique for determining the site of obstruction and can be combined with interventional endourologic techniques. In expert hands, endourologic techniques (e.g., balloon dilation, stenting) may be effective in treating ureteric stenosis and stricture. More complicated cases require open surgical repair. Extrinsic compression requires specific intervention such as draining or fenestration of the lymphocele. Obstruction in the early postoperative period due to an enlarged prostate should be managed with bladder catheter drainage and drugs such as tamsulosin.

## LATE POSTTRANSPLANT PERIOD

### LATE ACUTE ALLOGRAFT DYSFUNCTION

The causes and evaluation of late acute allograft dysfunction (defined as occurring >6 months posttransplant) include those of early acute dysfunction. Acute prerenal failure and ATN may occur at any time, and the causes are similar to those seen with native kidneys, such as shock syndromes, and may be further exacerbated by the hemodynamic effects of concurrent ACE-I or nonsteroidal antiinflammatory drug (NSAID) use. Urinary tract obstruction must also be considered in the differential diagnosis. In contrast to the early posttransplant period, the causes of obstruction are similar to those associated with native kidney disease (e.g., stones, bladder outlet obstruction, and neoplasia). Ureteric obstruction due to BK virus infection has also been described. Several causes of late acute allograft dysfunction are reviewed in more detail below.

#### Late Acute Rejection

Acute rejection is less common after the first 6 months. Late acute rejection should alert the physician to prescription of inadequate immunosuppression or patient noncompliance.[242] Withdrawal of steroids or CNIs by the physician may be initiated due to side effects of these medications, but when carried out later in the posttransplant period, may be associated with a high risk of acute rejection;[243,244] therefore, plasma creatinine must be carefully monitored in this setting. ABMR is increasingly recognized as an important cause of late acute allograft dysfunction, especially many years posttransplant; in a recent study, over 50% of 173 subjects biopsied for acute graft dysfunction, a mean of 7 years posttransplant, had evidence of ABMR.[81]

Acute rejection can also occur when CNI levels are subtherapeutic in the setting of newly prescribed medications that are known to decrease CNI levels (Table 70.9). Common

**Table 70.9 Agents That May Interact With Transplant Medications**

| **Drugs That Interact With CNIs and Sirolimus** | | |
|---|---|---|
| Class of Drug | Increase Level | Decrease Level |
| **Ca channel blocker** | Diltiazem, verapamil | |
| **Antibiotics** | Erythromycin, azithromycin, clarithromycin | Nafcillin |
| **Antifungals** | Fluconazole, ketoconazole, itraconazole, voriconazole | |
| **Antituberculin** | | INH, Rifampin, Rifabutin |
| **Antiviral** | Ritonavir, nelfinavir, saquinavir | Efvirez, Nevirapine |
| **Anti-seizure** | | Phenytoin, phenobarbital, carbamazepine, primidone |
| **Antidepressant** | Fluoxitine, nefazodone, fluvoxamine | |
| **Foods and Herbal Preparations That Interact With CNIs** | | |
| **Food** | Grapefruit juice/pomegranate juice | |
| **Herbs** | | St. Johns's wort |

agents that decreased CNI levels include antituberculosis medications and anti-seizure medications. CNI levels should be measured more frequently and doseadjustments should be made when prescribing or withdrawing these medications.

Treatment is the same as for early acute rejection (whether TCMR or active ABMR or both) but responses are poorer with greater negative impact on allograft survival than early acute rejection or DGF. Risk factors for noncompliance include adolescence, more immunosuppressant adverse effects, lower socioeconomic status, and psychological stress or illness.[245] Closer monitoring, simplification of the drug regimen, and social worker assistance may aid in the management of patients with high-risk of nonadherence.

### Late Acute Calcineurin Inhibitor Nephrotoxicity

Although lower doses of CNIs are generally prescribed after the first 12 months, acute CNI toxicity may occur at any time after transplant. This occurs most often in the setting of taking new medications that impair metabolism of the CNIs (Table 70.9). Patients should be made aware of common medications that interact with CNI. CNI levels should be monitored closely and dose-adjustments should be made when such medications are prescribed.

### Transplant Renal Artery Stenosis

**Renal Artery Stenosis.** Transplant renal artery stenosis (TRAS) is the most common transplant vascular complication and is associated with reduced long-term allograft survival.[246,247] TRAS can arise at any time after transplantation, although the mean time to diagnosis is 0.83±0.81 years posttransplant.[248] The reported incidence varies widely.[247] TRAS may be a consequence of an inadequate arterial anastomosis, inherent vascular disease of the recipient, or preexisting renovascular disease of the donor. Immune-mediated or infection-related damage to the transplant renal artery also plays and important role in some patients; new posttransplant DSAs and CMV infection are both associated with the development of TRAS.[249,250]

Luminal narrowing of more than 70% is probably required to render a stenosis functionally significant. The stenosis may occur in the donor or recipient artery or at the anastomotic site. Stenosis of the recipient iliac artery may also compromise renal arterial flow. Worsening or difficult to control hypertension, an unexplained deterioration in kidney function, or azotemia associated with the introduction of an angiotensin-converting enzyme or angiotensin-receptor blocker should raise suspicion of TRAS.[247,251,252] Clinical examination may also reveal a new vascular bruit over the graft. Ultrasound with Doppler, magnetic resonance, and CT-angiography can support a diagnosis but direct angiogram is usually required for confirmation. $CO_2$ or minimal contrast angiography can be used to reduce the risk of radiocontrast injury.[253] Good outcomes have been reported with both primary angioplasty and with stent placement in terms of blood pressure control and renal function.[254,255] If the diagnosis is made in the early postoperative period, surgical approach with revision of the anastomosis may be preferred.[247]

### Infections Causing Late Acute Allograft Dysfunction

**Human Polyomavirus Infection.** The polyomaviruses are DNA viruses, the best known of which are BK virus, JC virus, and SV40 virus. BK virus causes a mild self-limiting upper respiratory tract infection in healthy individuals (mostly in childhood). Around 80% of the adult population have serological evidence of prior BK infection. Following primary infection, the virus remains dormant in the urothelium. In immunosuppressed states, the virus may reactivate and replicate. Viral reactivation may result in viral shedding into the urine, viremia, cystitis, ureteritis, or interstitial nephritis (BK nephropathy).

Over the past 25 years, BK virus has been increasingly recognized as an important cause of kidney allograft dysfunction and loss. This probably reflects both improved recognition and reporting of the disease and the increasing use of lymphocyte depleting induction therapies and more potent maintenance MMF- and tacrolimus-based immunosuppression regimens. BK nephropathy is most common in the first 2 years posttransplant. Around 30% to 40% of renal transplant recipients develop BK viruria, around 10% to 20% will become BK viremic, and about half of those BK viremic patients will manifest BK nephropathy on biopsy.[256] Because BK viruria and viremia almost always precede BK nephropathy, urine or plasma BK viral screening offers the opportunity to identify infection early and instigate measures to clear the virus before nephropathy occurs.[257] Many centers advocate biopsy when plasma viral titers reach a predefined threshold (usually >$10^4$ copies/mL), while others, such as our own, treat empirically and reserve biopsy for patients with evidence of new graft dysfunction. Caution is warranted in lowering immunosuppression without an allograft biopsy; underimmunosuppression may precipitate acute rejection especially in the early posttransplant period and patients with high risk for rejection.

Approaches to screening vary and are influenced by local prevalence and economic factors. Many transplant centers now screen all new transplant recipients at intervals over the first two years posttransplant. Protocols for screening include testing the urine by light microscopy for decoy (infected) cells or by polymerase chain reaction (PCR) quantification of urinary or plasma viral load. KDIGO guidelines recommend quantitative plasma PCR testing as follows: 1) monthly for the first 3-6 months after transplantation, 2) then every 3 months until the end of the first posttransplant year, 3) whenever there is an unexplained rise in serum creatinine, and 4) after treatment of acute rejection.[188]

Allograft biopsy is required for the diagnosis of BK interstitial nephritis. Adequate sampling is needed, as the interstitial nephritis can be patchy. The presence of intranuclear tubule cell inclusions by light microscopy should raise suspicion; diagnosis is confirmed by immunohistochemistry using antibodies against BK viral proteins (SV-40). The excellent performance of immunohistochemical stains and concurrent measurement of BK viral titers at the time of 'for-cause' biopsy mean that BK nephropathy is no longer frequently mistaken for and treated as TCMR.

The mainstay of treatment is reduction in immunosuppression.[257] Our usual practice has been to first discontinue the anti-metabolite (usually MMF) in response to significant viremia or biopsy evidence of nephropathy. If this measure fails to result in a favorable viral response, we reduce the dose of CNI by 30% to 50% and continue to monitor viral titers. There are a number of adjunct therapies that may be considered in subjects who either fail to respond to immunosuppression reduction or in whom very aggressive immunosuppression reduction is unattractive because of their high-risk immune risk status. Leflunomide is a tyrosine kinase inhibitor, approved for the treatment of rheumatoid arthritis, that has antiviral effects in vitro. A number of small series have suggested that treatment with leflunomide (usually as a substitute for an antimetabolite) results in enhanced BK viral clearing, although in the absence of clinical trials its efficacy remains contentious.[258,259] The antiviral cidofovir has also, by some reports, been associated with a reduction in BK viral load; prudent dosing is of importance in view of the drug's potential nephrotoxicity.[260] Successful treatment of BK virus with intravenous immunoglobulin has been reported.[261] Switching tacrolimus to cyclosporine or mTORi should also be considered (although this may simply represent a de facto reduction in immunosuppression).[107,262] Finally, hopes for fluoroquinolones as a therapy for BK virus were dashed by two randomized controlled trials that showed levofloxacin to be no better than placebo at 1) treating or 2) preventing BK viremia/viruria in kidney transplant recipients.[263,264]

**Hepatitis C.** Around 1% of the U.S. population is hepatitis C (HCV) positive. Left untreated, 10% to 20% of persons infected with HCV will develop end-stage liver disease (ESLD) over a period of 20 to 30 years. In the absence of advanced liver disease, the presence of hepatitis C is not considered a contraindication to kidney transplant. However, historically post-kidney transplant outcomes in HCV+ recipients have been significantly worse than those of HCV- recipients.[265] Prior to the emergence of the new direct-acting antiviral regimens, the options for treatment of HCV in patients with ESRD, either before or after transplant, were limited by relative contraindications to interferon-α therapy in kidney transplant recipients and to ribavirin treatment in patients on dialysis.[266–268] However, HCV treatment has undergone a revolution in the past five years.[269] The infection is now reliably curable in kidney transplant recipients with combination antiviral therapy, and we are optimistic that these new HCV therapies will translate into improved post-kidney transplant survival for HCV+ recipients.[270,271] Indeed, such is the confidence in the new HCV therapies that expansion of the deceased donor transplant pool by allowing HCV+ donor kidneys be transplanted into HCV- recipients is being investigated. A recent small study reported on 10 HCV- patients who received kidney transplants from HCV RNA positive donors. All recipients received HCV treatment, starting immediately before transplant and continuing for 12 weeks after transplant and had undetectable HCV RNA at 12 weeks.[272]

### Drug and Radiocontrast Nephrotoxicity

Drugs that cause nephrotoxicity in the native kidney will also adversely affect the kidney allografts. Drug-related nephrotoxic effects that are more common in the setting of transplantation are listed in Table 70.9. Special attention should be paid to drugs that interact with CNIs. CNIs are metabolized by the cytochrome P-450 isoenzyme CYP3A5, and drugs that interact with CYP3A5 will affect its plasma level. When prescribing diltiazem, verapamil, ketoconazole, and the macrolide antibiotics, particularly erythromycin and clarithromycin, the dose of CNI should be reduced and levels should be followed. Conversely, rifampicin, phenobarbital, and phenytoin lower the CNI level, so the CNI should be increased.

Drugs with known nephrotoxic effects such as aminoglycosides, amphotericin, and NSAIDs probably have enhanced toxicity when used concomitantly with a CNI. Nevertheless, they are sometimes required in transplant recipients. Use of the liposomal preparation of amphotericin is preferable because it is less nephrotoxic than the standard preparation (amphotericin B).

Plasma creatinine can be increased with high-dose SMX-TMP by inhibiting tubule secretion of creatinine (GFR per se is not compromised and plasma creatinine decreases within 5 days of stopping SMX-TMP). Rarely, SMX-TMP can provoke allergic interstitial nephritis.

Not surprisingly, ACE-inhibitors or ARBs have been implicated in precipitating AKI in the presence of transplant renal artery stenosis. Overall, if carefully prescribed, these agents are well tolerated. The use of ACE-inhibitors or ARBs in the immediate posttransplant period, when volume status and CNI dosages are fluctuating, is not recommended.

The risk of developing AKI after administration of radiocontrast to kidney transplant recipients has not been well defined. Single-center studies point toward a higher prevalence in kidney transplant recipients.[273] Presumably, risk factors for contrast nephrotoxicity are similar to those in patients who have not undergone transplant surgery. Thus, the same preventive measures should be used.

### Late Allograft Dysfunction and Late Allograft Loss

Preventing late allograft loss remains a major challenge. Death with a functioning graft accounts for approximately half of graft losses. Important causes of death-censored late graft loss include acute rejection, recurrent or de novo glomerular diseases, AKI related to sepsis or hypotension, and pyelonephritis.[274] The majority of the remaining late graft failures, with features of interstitial fibrosis and tubular atrophy (IF/TA) on histology, were conventionally attributed to an amalgam of immune and non-immune (CNI)-mediated fibrosis and vascular injury termed chronic/sclerosing allograft nephropathy. More recently improved pathologic and immunologic diagnostic tools (C4d stain and DSA) mean that underlying chronic ABMR is increasingly recognized in biopsies with IF/TA. Any biopsy with IF/TA may be further supplemented to include features suggestive of non-immune causes of IF/TA such as CNI toxicity, chronic hypertension, obstruction, pyelonephritis, viral infection, and recurrent or de novo glomerular disease (Table 70.8).

Fig. 70.6 illustrates factors that are thought to contribute to the development of late allograft failure, often referred to under the umbrella term 'chronic allograft injury'.

The causes of late dysfunction are summarized in Table 70.10 and further discussed in the following sections. Certain causes such as transplant renal artery stenosis and urinary tract obstruction have been discussed earlier.

**Chronic ABMR.** Several studies have shown that an antibody-mediated process is commonly implicated in late graft injury. In one study, 99 of 173 patients that underwent 'for-cause' biopsy, a mean of seven years posttransplant, had evidence of an ABMR, indicated by C4d positivity, DSA or both[81]. Another study that evaluated all death censored graft losses in 1317 kidney transplant recipients (KTRs), irrespective of time since

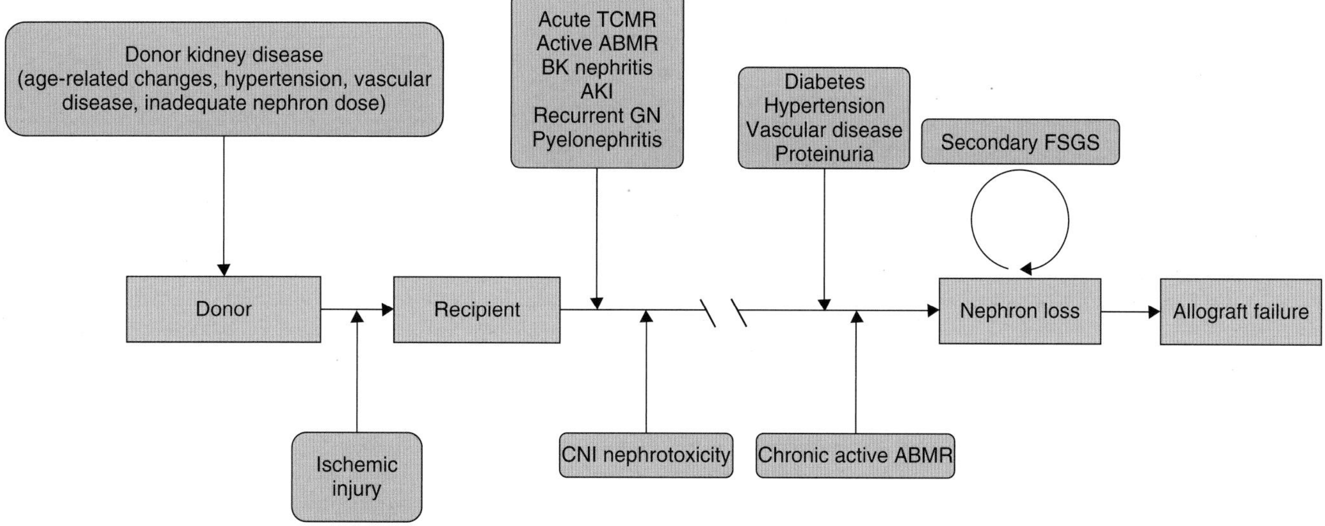


**Fig. 70.6** The multifactorial pathogenesis of chronic allograft injury.

**Table 70.10 Causes of Late Chronic Allograft Dysfunction**

| |
|---|
| **Prerenal** |
| Transplant renal artery stenosis |
| **Intrarenal** |
| Acute rejection - TCMR or ABMR<br>Chronic active ABMR<br>Chronic active TCMR<br>CNI nephrotoxicity<br>BK nephropathy<br>Recurrence of primary disease<br>De novo primary kidney disease |
| **Postrenal** |
| Urinary tract obstruction |

*CNI,* Calcineurin inhibitor.

transplant, found evidence for chronic ABMR in 18% (with histologic evidence of either transplant glomerulopathy or IF/TA). The probability of ABMR on 'for-cause' biopsies rises from around 10% at six months to 35% at five years posttransplant, is associated with medication nonadherence, and augurs poor graft survival.[275]

The Banff 2005 update added the term 'chronic active antibody-mediated rejection', currently requiring all three of the following 1) morphologic evidence of chronic tissue injury evidenced by transplant glomerulopathy, peritubular capillary basement membrane multilayering (on EM), and/or arterial intimal fibrosis of new onset; 2) evidence of recent endothelial-antibody interaction (peritubular capillary C4d staining); and 3) evidence of DSA.

Chronic active ABMR, most commonly accompanied by transplant glomerulopathy on histology, is clinically characterized by a slow decline in kidney function, hypertension, and (often heavy) proteinuria. Treatment options are limited. A single center study of 23 consecutive kidney transplant recipients with ABMR diagnosed at least 6 months post-transplant, nearly half of whom had some evidence of transplant glomerulopathy on biopsy, observed minimal benefit in response to therapies that included plasmapharesis, IVIg, rituximab and bortezomib.[276] A recent randomized controlled trial showed no benefit in terms of change in GFR or proteinuria for bortezomib treatment versus placebo in patients with chronic ABMR.[277] Another small randomized controlled trial showed no benefit for rituximab combined with intravenous immunoglobulin versus placebo for the treatment of chronic ABMR.[278] A recent small case series reported excellent allograft outcomes in patients with chronic ABMR treated with tocilizumab, suggesting that more rigorous studies of the IL-6 receptor antibody in this population are warranted.[279]

Our approach to patients with a diagnosis of chronic active ABMR is to optimize maintenance immunosuppression. We switch to a tacrolimus-MMF regimen if the patient has been taking CsA or AZA. We target tacrolimus levels around 8 ng/mL, maximize MMF dosing, and add low dose maintenance prednisone if the patient is not already on steroid.[280] We also add ACE-inhibitors or ARBs, control hypertension, and modify other cardiovascular risk factors. The lack of good treatment options for chronic ABMR underscores the importance of preventing de novo DSA formation and minimizing, to the greatest degree possible, the use of donors to whom the recipient has preformed DSA.

**Calcineurin Inhibitor Toxicity.** Over thirty years after CNI-associated nephropathy was first described in heart transplant recipients there remains debate about the importance of CNI in late graft failure.[67] Nankivell et al. reported longitudinal histologic data on 120 diabetic kidney transplant recipients [119 were simultaneous pancreas kidney (SPK) recipients] who underwent sequential kidney transplant biopsies from the time of transplant up to 10 years post-transplant. The study identified histologic evidence of CNI toxicity defined as the presence of 'striped cortical fibrosis or new-onset arteriolar hyalinosis (not from renal ischemia or preexisting hyalinosis in the allograft) supported by tubular microcalcification (without preceding acute tubular necrosis)' in over 50% of biopsies at five years and 100% of biopsies at 10 years posttransplant. Based on the pathological findings, the authors attributed the majority of late graft dysfunction to CNI toxicity.[65] In contrast, newer studies have suggested a much lower prevalence of interstitial fibrosis at five years post-biopsy and question the specificity of arteriolar hyalinosis for the diagnosis of CNI toxicity.[274,281] This, combined with increased evidence for immune-mediated injury in many cases of late allograft failure, has led many to deemphasize the importance of chronic CNI toxicity.

We remain believers in CNI toxicity as a cause of graft dysfunction. Indeed, the significant difference in GFR between belatacept- and cyclosporine-treated patients five years posttransplant in the BENEFIT trial lends credence to the nephrotoxic effects of CNIs and emphasizes the potential merits of developing CNI avoidance strategies.[282] If the clinical and histologic picture suggests a significant component of chronic CNI nephrotoxicity without evidence of rejection, we dose-reduce the CNI. Substituting CNI with either sirolimus or belatacept should also be given strong consideration.[102,112] mTORi treatment should probably be avoided in those with baseline proteinuria or GFR of less than 40 mL/min.[283]

## RECURRENCE OF PRIMARY DISEASE

Diseases that recur early in the posttransplant period are addressed above. The incidence of late recurrence is difficult to estimate: the original cause of ESRD is often unknown, transplant kidney biopsies are not always performed, and most relevant studies are small and retrospective with variable follow-up periods. An Australian study of patients with biopsy-proven glomerulonephritis found a 10-year incidence of graft loss from recurrence of 8.4%.[284] However, patients whose primary kidney disease was biopsy-proven glomerulonephritis had allograft survival that was comparable to patients with non-glomerulonephritis etiologies. As kidney allograft survival improves, recurrent or de novo disease is being increasingly diagnosed and is recognized as an important cause of late graft loss.[274] Recurrence can present as decreasing GFR, proteinuria, or hematuria.

### IgA Glomerulonephritis

Studies with longer follow-up times have shown that histologic recurrence of this condition is common. The reported incidence varies from 13% to 53%,[285] and likely reflects the varying threshold for biopsies among different centers. The estimated 10-year incidence of graft loss due to recurrence was 9.7%.[284] The risk of recurrence is higher if a previous graft was lost to recurrent disease.[286] In patients with proteinuria, ACE-inhibitors and ARBs should be initiated.[287] One large retrospective study showed an association between maintenance steroid use and a reduction in posttransplant IgA recurrence.[128] This should be taken into account when discussing the plan for maintenance immunosuppression with the patient.

### Lupus Nephritis

Allograft and patient survival overall have been thought to be similar in patients with ESRD due to lupus nephritis compared with those with ESRD from other causes,[288] but analysis of the United States Renal Data System (USRDS) database showed worse outcomes of deceased-donor transplant recipients with ESRD due to lupus nephritis.[289] Recurrence of severe systemic lupus erythematosus (SLE), either systemically or within in the graft, is uncommon. Low rates of recurrence in SLE probably reflect patient selection, disease activity "burning out" on maintenance dialysis, and the effects of powerful posttransplant immunosuppression. Indeed, a recent analysis of nearly 7000 kidney transplant recipients with ESRD from SLE suggested that acute rejection (affecting 26%) had a far more important impact on graft failure than recurrent disease (affecting 3%).[126] As with other glomerular diseases that may recur, transplantation should be deferred until SLE is clinically quiescent. Many centers prefer a 6 to 12 month period of clinical quiescence before proceeding with transplantation to reduce the risk of recurrence. If the patient is receiving anticoagulation for antiphospholipid syndrome (APS) before transplantation, anticoagulation should be resumed as soon as safely possible (initially with intravenous heparin) after transplant surgery. This procedure is used to reduce the risk of thrombosis of the allograft or other sites.

### Granulomatosis With Polyangiitis and Microscopic Polyangiitis

Renal and extrarenal recurrences of these diseases have been described. In a pooled series of 127 patients, antineutrophil cytoplasmic antibody (ANCA)–associated small vessel vasculitis recurred in 17% of cases; renal involvement recurred in 10% of cases.[290] A lower incidence (7%) of recurrence has been reported in a more recent study.[291] Positive ANCA serology at the time of transplant does not appear to predict relapse. However, patients with ESRD secondary to ANCA-associated vasculitis should not undergo transplant surgery until the disease is clinically quiescent. Treatment options for recurrence include cyclophosphamide and rituximab.[292]

### Membranoproliferative Glomerulonephritis (MPGN)

MPGN has recently been reclassified based on the deposition of C3 alone (the C3 nephritides) versus C3 and immunoglobulin on immunofluorescence.[293] The C3 nephritides (dense deposit disease and C3 nephritis) are driven by an underlying defect in the regulation of the alternative complement pathway. The recent classification change means that there are limited data on the recurrence rate of the C3 nephritides; however, five-year graft survival in 75 patients with ESRD from MPGN type II (now termed 'dense deposit disease') was reported to be significantly worse than other pediatric kidney transplant recipients and recurrence was documented in 12 of the 18 patients biopsied.[294] Limited success has been reported in treating posttransplant recurrence of the C3 nephritides with the complement inhibitor eculizumab.[295,296] Membranoproliferative glomerulonephritis associated with glomerular deposition of C3 and immunoglobulin should trigger the evaluation and treatment of underlying causes such as infection (especially hepatitis C), autoimmune diseases, and plasma-cell dyscrasias.

### Membranous Nephropathy

Membranous nephropathy may recur after transplant or arise de novo.[297] The associated clinical features vary from minimal proteinuria to nephrotic syndrome. As with native kidney disease, hepatitis B virus (HBV) infection and other conditions associated with membranous nephropathy such as malignancy should be excluded. A high proportion of patients with primary membranous nephropathy are positive for the anti-PLA2R1 antibody and monitoring antibody levels may be useful in tracking disease activity.[298–300] Management includes treatment of the underlying cause and RAAS inhibition. The recurrence of primary membranous nephropathy has been successfully treated with rituximab, and some investigators argue that treatment with rituximab (either 375 mg/m$^2$ x 4 doses or 1 g x 2 doses) should be offered to those patients with recurrent posttransplant membranous nephropathy whose proteinuria remains over 1 g/24 hours despite maximum tolerated ACEI/ARB therapy.[54,301]

#### Comparative Transplant Outcomes in Patients With ESRD From Glomerulonephritides

A recent study compared the posttransplant outcomes of U.S. patients with ESRD from different GN types. Using those patients with ESRD from IgA nephropathy as the referent group the adjusted hazard ratios for the 1) death and 2) allograft failure excluding death with a functioning graft, respectively, were 1.57 and 1.20 for FSGS, 1.52 and 1.27 for membranous nephropathy, 1.76 and 1.50, membranoproliferative GN, 1.82 and 1.11 for lupus nephritis, and 1.56 and 0.94 (not statistically significant) for vasculitis. [302]

#### Diabetic Nephropathy

Recurrence of diabetic nephropathy in the allograft has not been well studied. This reflects the relatively poor long-term survival of diabetic kidney transplant recipients; the duration of exposure to the diabetic milieu is often insufficient to allow development of severe diabetic nephropathy. PTDM can also result in diabetic nephropathy;[303] histologic evidence of this may occur surprisingly rapidly after transplant.[304]

## ASSESSING OUTCOMES IN KIDNEY TRANSPLANTATION

The most convenient and widely used method for assessing outcomes after kidney transplantation is measurement of allograft survival. Other important measures include allograft function (typically measured by plasma creatinine), patient survival, number of rejection episodes, days of hospitalization, and quality-of-life indices. Registry data from the USRDS, the Scientific Registry of Transplant Recipients, the Collaborative Transplant Study (CTS), and Australia and New Zealand Dialysis and Transplant Registry (ANZDATA) have all proved extremely useful in assessing these outcomes.

### ACTUAL AND ACTUARIAL ALLOGRAFT AND PATIENT SURVIVAL

Allograft survival is calculated from the day of transplantation to the day of reaching a defined end point (e.g., return to dialysis, re-transplantation, or death). The most widely accepted measure of outcome is the Kaplan-Meier probability estimate of patient and graft survival. One year, 5-year, and 10-year actuarial survival rates are frequently presented, but actual survival may ultimately not be as impressive as projected survival.[305] Another actuarial measure commonly used is allograft half-life (median allograft survival).

Traditionally, allograft survival is assessed under two distinct time phases: early and late. Early allograft loss refers to loss within the first 12 months, and late loss to any time thereafter. This distinction is empiric but makes clinical sense. In the first 12 months, allograft loss is relatively common, because of technical complications and rejection. After 12 months, the incidence is lower and generally stable over time. Usually, analysis of long-term survival is restricted to those allografts that have survived to 12 months after transplant. The causes of late allograft loss are also different and are discussed later. Patient death is in essence equivalent to allograft loss, but allograft survival is also sometimes calculated after censoring for patient death ("allograft failure excluding death with a functioning graft").

### SURVIVAL BENEFITS OF KIDNEY TRANSPLANTATION

Comparison of survival between the general dialysis population and transplanted patients is greatly affected by selection bias, as only relatively healthy patients are referred (and listed) for transplantation. Thus, comparisons among patients on the waiting list who do or do not receive a transplant are usually performed instead. Of course, such analyses assume that the two groups (those who have undergone transplant surgery or those still on the list) can otherwise be matched; this is not necessarily true.

One USRDS study found that during the first 106 days after transplantation, the risk of death after transplantation was higher than the corresponding risk while remaining on the waiting list (on dialysis). This mainly reflected the risks associated with the transplant procedure itself. Thereafter, however, transplantation conferred a survival benefit. On the basis of 3 to 4 years of follow-up, transplantation reduced the risk of death overall by 68%.[306]

### SHORT-TERM OUTCOMES IN KIDNEY TRANSPLANTATION

The acute rejection rate has fallen substantially over the past 25 years. The rate of acute rejection in the first year posttransplant is currently around 10%. Fig. 70.7 illustrates the decline in rate of acute rejection in the first posttransplant year between the years 1992 and 2010.[123] Short-term graft survival has improved. One-year graft survival in 2014 was 93% for deceased donor transplants and 97% for living donor transplants. Tables 70.11 and 70.12 illustrate one-year graft survival by donor type between 1998 and 2014.[13]

### LONG-TERM OUTCOMES IN KIDNEY TRANSPLANTATION

There has also been an improvement in long-term allograft survival (Tables 70.11 and 70.12). This improvement is seen most prominently in the recipients of living kidney donor transplants.[13]

Beyond the first posttransplant year, the principal causes of kidney allograft loss are death with a functioning graft and chronic allograft injury (CAI); less common causes are late acute rejection and recurrent disease.[274] The primary cause of death remains cardiovascular disease, followed by infection and malignancy (Fig. 70.8).[123] In children, death is a much less common cause of allograft loss; conversely in the elderly, death is more common.

## FACTORS AFFECTING KIDNEY ALLOGRAFT SURVIVAL

Prospective studies and analyses of registry data have shown that many variables influence kidney allograft survival. These can be considered as donor, recipient, or donor-recipient factors. Many of them contribute to the development of chronic allograft injury and have been discussed above.

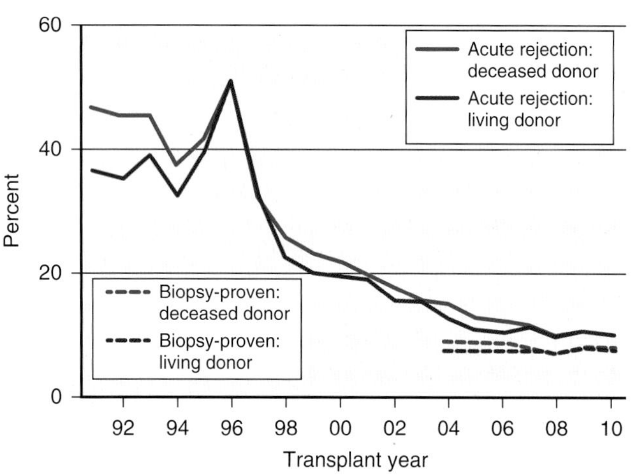


**Fig. 70.7** Secular trends in acute rejection in the first year posttransplant.

## DONOR-RECIPIENT FACTORS

### Delayed Graft Function

DGF is associated with poorer allograft and patient survival and poorer allograft function.[307] Registry data show that DGF reduces allograft half-lives by 30%, a larger effect than early acute rejection.[308] Even though cold ischemia time has been steadily decreased from 24 hours to 18 hours over the past 20 years, the incidence of DGF in deceased donor transplants has remained at approximately 25%.[4]

### Human Leukocyte Antigen Matching

The goal of HLA matching is to reduce the number of 'foreign targets' against which a recipient may develop an immune

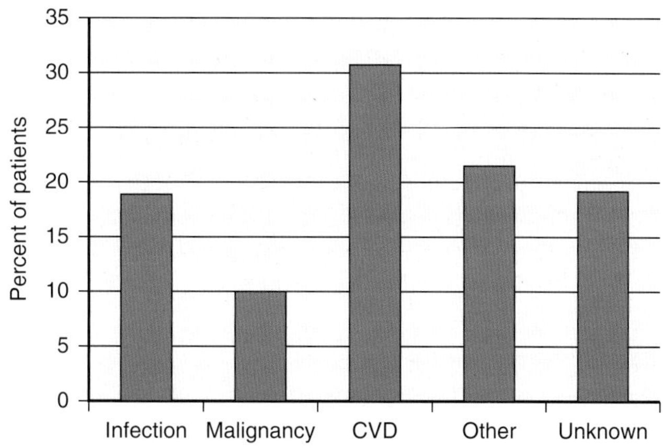


**Fig. 70.8** Causes of death with allograft function (2007-2011) taken from the United States Renal Data System 2013 Annual Data Report. *CVD*, Cardiovascular disease.

**Table 70.11 Secular Trends in 1-, 5-, and 10-Year Mortality and Graft Failure for Adult Deceased Donor Transplant Recipients in the United States**

| | 1 Year Posttransplant | | | 5 Years Posttransplant | | | 10 Years Posttransplant | | |
|---|---|---|---|---|---|---|---|---|---|
| Year | Probability of All-Cause Graft Failure (%) | Probability of Return to Dialysis or Repeat Transplant (%) | Probability of Death (%) | Probability of All-Cause Graft Failure (%) | Probability of Return to Dialysis or Repeat Transplant (%) | Probability of Death (%) | Probability of All-Cause Graft Failure (%) | Probability of Return to Dialysis or Repeat Transplant (%) | Probability of Death (%) |
| 1998 | 12.6 | 8.9 | 5.5 | 33.8 | 24.1 | 18.2 | 56.7 | 40.6 | 37.9 |
| 1999 | 13.2 | 8.8 | 5.9 | 33.6 | 23.0 | 18.8 | 56.3 | 39.3 | 38.1 |
| 2000 | 12.7 | 8.1 | 6.4 | 33.9 | 22.7 | 19.6 | 56.3 | 38.3 | 38.9 |
| 2001 | 12.2 | 8.0 | 5.7 | 33.1 | 21.3 | 19.7 | 55.3 | 36.7 | 38.5 |
| 2002 | 12.3 | 8.3 | 5.6 | 32.8 | 22.1 | 18.8 | 53.5 | 35.9 | 37.0 |
| 2003 | 11.8 | 7.3 | 5.6 | 31.7 | 20.3 | 18.4 | 54.4 | 35.7 | 37.6 |
| 2004 | 11.1 | 7.1 | 5.4 | 31.3 | 20.5 | 18.2 | 53.2 | 35.4 | 36.7 |
| 2005 | 11.2 | 6.9 | 6.0 | 29.9 | 19.0 | 17.8 | 52.4 | 33.4 | 36.5 |
| 2006 | 10.4 | 6.6 | 5.1 | 29.3 | 18.6 | 17.1 | | | |
| 2007 | 9.5 | 5.9 | 4.6 | 28.2 | 17.7 | 16.8 | | | |
| 2008 | 9.4 | 6.0 | 4.5 | 26.8 | 16.1 | 16.3 | | | |
| 2009 | 9.3 | 5.5 | 4.9 | 26.9 | 16.4 | 16.2 | | | |
| 2010 | 8.8 | 5.4 | 4.4 | 26.6 | 16.0 | 16.5 | | | |
| 2011 | 7.4 | 4.4 | 3.9 | | | | | | |
| 2012 | 7.8 | 4.7 | 3.8 | | | | | | |
| 2013 | 7.7 | 4.7 | 3.5 | | | | | | |
| 2014 | 6.9 | 3.8 | 3.7 | | | | | | |

**Table 70.12 Secular Trends in 1-, 5-, and 10-Year Mortality and Graft Failure for Adult Living Donor Transplant Recipients in the United States**

| | 1 Year Posttransplant | | | 5 Years Posttransplant | | | 10 Years Posttransplant | | |
|---|---|---|---|---|---|---|---|---|---|
| Year | Probability of All-Cause Graft Failure (%) | Probability of Return to Dialysis or Repeat Transplant (%) | Probability of Death (%) | Probability of All-Cause Graft Failure (%) | Probability of Return to Dialysis or Repeat Transplant (%) | Probability of Death (%) | Probability of All-Cause Graft Failure (%) | Probability of Return to Dialysis or Repeat Transplant (%) | Probability of Death (%) |
| 1998 | 6.5 | 4.8 | 2.3 | 21.3 | 15.0 | 10.1 | 42.4 | 30.8 | 23.2 |
| 1999 | 6.3 | 4.6 | 2.1 | 21.0 | 14.9 | 9.4 | 41.0 | 28.9 | 22.4 |
| 2000 | 7.0 | 5.0 | 2.6 | 22.3 | 15.2 | 10.6 | 42.1 | 29.2 | 23.7 |
| 2001 | 6.7 | 4.6 | 2.5 | 21.7 | 14.8 | 10.2 | 41.4 | 28.1 | 23.7 |
| 2002 | 6.3 | 4.4 | 2.4 | 20.8 | 14.1 | 10.2 | 39.9 | 26.4 | 24.3 |
| 2003 | 5.5 | 4.0 | 1.8 | 20.1 | 13.8 | 9.4 | 39.3 | 26.0 | 23.0 |
| 2004 | 5.2 | 3.6 | 2.1 | 18.8 | 12.7 | 8.8 | 38.3 | 24.6 | 22.4 |
| 2005 | 5.4 | 3.7 | 2.0 | 18.7 | 12.7 | 8.8 | 38.4 | 25.1 | 22.2 |
| 2006 | 4.5 | 3.1 | 1.7 | 16.8 | 11.2 | 8.0 | | | |
| 2007 | 3.8 | 2.5 | 1.4 | 16.7 | 10.5 | 7.9 | | | |
| 2008 | 4.3 | 2.9 | 1.6 | 15.4 | 10.1 | 7.4 | | | |
| 2009 | 4.1 | 2.8 | 1.3 | 15.2 | 9.4 | 7.6 | | | |
| 2010 | 3.7 | 2.4 | 1.4 | 15.3 | 9.6 | 7.3 | | | |
| 2011 | 3.5 | 2.0 | 1.8 | | | | | | |
| 2012 | 3.5 | 2.1 | 1.5 | | | | | | |
| 2013 | 2.6 | 1.5 | 1.2 | | | | | | |
| 2014 | 3.0 | 1.9 | 1.4 | | | | | | |

response. While modern era immunosuppression can undoubtedly 'overpower' HLA mismatching, good HLA matching nonetheless remains desirable and beneficial in terms of graft survival. In a recent study of nearly 200,000 deceased donor kidney transplant recipients between 1987 and 2013, each additional HLA donor-recipient mismatch (out of 6 HLA A, B and DR loci) was associated with a reduction in allograft survival. A similar, but somewhat diminished, association was observed between HLA mismatch and allograft in an analysis restricted to the more modern transplant era (2009-2013).[309,310] For living donor recipients the receipt of a two-haplotype matched kidney still confers a significant survival advantage, haplo-identical graft half-lives being over 25-years.[311] The advent of HLA epitope-matching may prove important in the coming years.

### Cytomegalovirus Status of Donor and Recipient

Registry data show a small but definite association of donor and recipient CMV serologic status with kidney allograft and recipient survival (hazard ratio 1.1).[312] Donor-negative–recipient-negative pairings have the best outcomes, whereas donor-positive–recipient-negative pairings have the worst. Cytomegalovirus probably affects graft outcomes through overt infection, but subclinical effects on immune function may also be important.

### Timing of Transplantation

There is evidence that preemptive (before initiation of dialysis) transplantation is associated with a lower risk of acute rejection and allograft failure.[313] Other retrospective studies have shown that longer time on dialysis is independently associated with poorer graft and patient survival.[314,315] Between 2003 and 2012, 17% of kidney transplants performed in the United States were preemptive.[316] Minimizing time on dialysis has many potential benefits; this strategy should thus be pursued whenever possible.[4,317]

### Center Effect

Not surprisingly, reported outcomes have varied from transplant center to center.[318] This reflects normal statistical variance as well as center expertise. Outcomes are confounded by many donor and recipient factors that differ across centers.[319] USRDS data suggest minimal difference in outcomes among small and large transplant centers in the United States.[320]

## DONOR FACTORS

The quality of the kidney immediately before transplantation has a major impact on long-term graft function and the risk of developing chronic allograft injury.

### Donor Source: Deceased Versus Living Donor

The donor source is one of the most important predictors of short- and long-term allograft outcomes. In general, living donor allografts are superior to deceased donor allografts (see Tables 70.11 and 70.12). This benefit applies across all degrees of HLA mismatching. The better outcomes reflect several factors: very healthy living donors, the absence of brain death, the benefits of elective as opposed to semi-urgent surgery, minimization of ischemia-reperfusion injury, higher nephron mass and the effects of a shorter waiting time on, or complete avoidance of, dialysis. This further emphasizes the importance of the "healthy transplant kidney" effect.

Allograft outcomes are superior from deceased donors with trauma as opposed to non-trauma being the cause of death.[321]

### Donor Age

Older kidney donor age is associated with reduced kidney transplant survival. A donor age effect is apparent among deceased and living donor transplants.[4,322,323] These results are thought to reflect a higher incidence of DGF and of nephron "underdosing." Allografts from older donors have fewer functioning nephrons because of the aging process[324] and donor-related conditions such as hypertension and atherosclerosis. However, because of the organ donor shortage, older deceased donor kidneys are being increasingly utilized. Donor age younger than 5 years is also associated with poorer outcomes, reflecting higher rates of technical complications and probably nephron underdosing (see later). En bloc transplantation (two kidneys) from donors aged 0 to 5 years significantly improves survival, however.

### Donor Sex

There is evidence that allografts from female donors have slightly poorer survival.[325] Again, this probably reflects a nephron underdosing effect (see later), because women have a smaller kidney mass than men. However, female recipients of male kidneys may have poorer graft survival that is related an immune response to antigens encoded by the Y-chromosome (H-Y antigens).[326–328]

### Donor Race/Ethnicity

Deceased donor kidneys from African-Americans are associated with reduced allograft survival compared to those donated by non–African-Americans.[329] There is increasing evidence that much of the increased risk of graft loss that is associated with African-American donated kidneys is attributable to the presence of the APOL1 high-risk variant (present in around 15% of African-American donors). African-American donated kidneys from donors lacking the APOL1 high-risk variant have outcomes comparable to non-African-American donated kidneys. Integration of APOL1 genotyping (instead of race) into clinical prediction models such as the KDPI is warranted.[330,331]

### Donor Nephron Mass

An imbalance between the metabolic/excretory demands of the recipient and the functional transplant mass has been postulated to play a role in the development and progression of chronic allograft injury (Fig. 70.6). Nephron underdosing, exacerbated by perioperative ischemic damage and postoperative nephrotoxic drugs, might lead to nephron overwork and eventual failure, similar to the mechanisms occurring in native progressive kidney disease. Thus, kidneys from small donors transplanted into recipients of large body surface area or large body mass index would be at highest risk of this problem. There is support for this hypothesis from animal[332] and retrospective human studies.[333–335]

### Cold Ischemia Time

Prolonged cold ischemia time is associated with higher risk of DGF and poorer allograft survival.[175,336] Registry data suggest that more than 24 hours is particularly deleterious to the graft.

### Expanded Criteria Donors and Kidney Donor Profile Index

As the discrepancy between the numbers of patients awaiting kidney transplant and available organs increases, many countries are now using ECD allografts. ECD kidneys are defined by donor characteristics that are associated with a 70% greater risk of allograft failure when compared to a reference group of non-hypertensive donors of age 10 to 39 years, whose cause of death was not cerebrovascular accident (CVA) and whose terminal creatinine is less than 1.5 mg/dL.[337] This includes donors who are 60 years or older and donors aged 50 to 59 with two of the following criteria: 1) CVA as cause of death, 2) history of hypertension, or 3) terminal creatinine > 1.5 mg/dL. Survival of ECD kidneys is, on average, shorter for two general reasons: first, the baseline GFR of these kidneys is likely lower, and second, ECD kidneys tend to be transplanted into older recipients, who have higher rates of posttransplant death. Older patients have higher risk of mortality while awaiting transplantation, and have been shown to benefit from ECD kidney transplantation.[338]

In the US, the new Kidney Allocation System has replaced the standard and expanded criteria deceased donor categories with a single pool of kidneys graded using the kidney donor profile index (KDPI). The KDPI score is calculated using 10 donor characteristics and is a modified version of the predictive tool first described by Rao et al.[329] The KDPI is expressed as a percentile score with 0% and 100% signifying excellent quality and marginal organs, respectively. In order to maximize the utility of the deceased donor organ supply, deceased donor kidneys with a KDPI < 20% are to be allocated to candidates with the highest posttransplant life expectancy, as judged by the 4-variable estimated posttransplant survival (EPTS) score. Older candidates, for whom long waiting times represent a barrier to transplantation, who would previously have agreed to receipt of an ECD kidney, may now choose to accept deceased donor kidneys with a high KDPI value (>85%).

### Donation After Cardiac Death

There has been significant increase in the use of donation after cardiac death (DCD) kidneys.[339] DCD donors can be sub-classified as 'uncontrolled' or 'controlled'. Uncontrolled donors are either unsuccessfully resuscitated or present dead on arrival to hospital, while controlled donors suffer a cardiac arrest following the withdrawal of life support in the intensive care unit or operating room immediately prior to donation. The duration of warm ischemia time is likely to be significantly greater in the setting of uncontrolled donation.[340] Protocols for managing DCD kidneys vary from center to center. In uncontrolled donation, isolated perfusion of the kidneys with cold preservation solution can be achieved using double-balloon aortic catheterization (with balloons inflated in the aorta above and below the renal arteries) to minimize warm ischemia time. Short-term outcomes (such as rates of DGF and primary nonfunction) are inferior to those seen with brain dead donors. However, long-term outcomes of DCD organs (from donors <50 years old) are similar to those from standard deceased donors.[341]

## RECIPIENT FACTORS

### Recipient Age

In general, allograft survival rates are poorer in those at the extremes of age, that is, younger than 18 or older than 65 years of age.[4,342] In the very young, technical causes of graft loss such as vessel thrombosis are relatively more common. Acute rejection is also a more common cause of allograft loss; conversely, death with a functioning graft is relatively rare. Death with a functioning allograft is a much more common cause of graft loss in the elderly (responsible for more than 50% of graft failures). Conversely, acute rejection may be less common. Thus, although randomized controlled trials are not available to definitively inform practice, it seems reasonable, in general, to use less aggressive immunosuppression in the elderly.[343]

### Recipient Race/Ethnicity

African-American recipients have poorer allograft survival compared with that of whites.[344] This probably reflects multiple factors including higher incidence of DGF, higher incidence of acute and late acute rejection, stronger immune responsiveness, a predominantly white donor pool (with resultant poorer matching of HLA and non-HLA antigens), altered pharmacokinetics of immunosuppressive drugs, and a higher prevalence of hypertension. In the United States, socioeconomic factors may also play a role.[345] Indeed, there is some evidence that African-Europeans have equivalent outcomes to whites in Europe.[346] Asian and Latino recipients have superior outcomes to whites; the reasons for this are unknown.[344] Strategies that may improve outcomes in African-American recipients include diligent use of higher doses of immunosuppression and the identification of barriers that may limit equitable access to healthcare.[347] Increasing living donation from African-American donors is also desirable. Pre-donation screening for the APOL1 high-risk genotype in donors of African descent may improve African-American living donor safety and recipient outcomes.[330] Further good data will hopefully come from the APOLLO Network research consortium, which has been recently established with a goal of prospectively identifying, genotyping, and following up African-American donors and recipients.[348]

### Recipient Sex

Registry studies of the association of recipient sex with transplant outcomes have yielded differing results. In the CTS database, female recipients had slightly better allograft survival than male recipients of deceased donor kidneys or HLA-identical living donor kidneys.[325] Data from US transplant centers has shown better allograft survival in male as opposed to female recipients of living donor kidneys.[349] An important difference between female and male transplant candidates is the higher degree of sensitization of the former to HLA antigens, as well as to non-HLA antigens. Women tend to be more sensitized because of pregnancy and possibly because of more blood transfusions because of anemia related to menstruation. An immune response to H-Y antigens by female recipients may play a role, although the generally larger nephron dose in male donors may be a confounding factor in registry analyses.

### Recipient Sensitization

Patients who are highly sensitized are generally considered at higher risk for adverse early and late graft outcomes compared with unsensitized recipients. We use pretransplant cPRA to help guide immunosuppression planning, although preformed DSA, rather than a high cPRA per se, probably has greater prognostic significance for graft outcome.[125] The principal reasons for sensitization are previous transplants, pregnancy, and blood transfusion. Indeed, allograft survival is poorer in recipients of subsequent transplants compared with recipients of a first transplant.[350] Highly sensitized patients have longer wait-times until transplantation and are usually given more intensive immunosuppression. Recent improvements made to the allocation system in the United States and the availability of desensitization protocols have offered such patients better access to transplantation.

### Acute Rejection

Acute rejection remains a significant risk factor for allograft loss. Even when acute rejection is successfully treated, some irreversible graft injury/scarring likely ensues. Acute rejection refractory to steroids, acute rejection with a humoral component, and late acute rejection have particularly negative impacts on allograft and patient outcomes.[305]

### Recipient Immunosuppression

Undoubtedly, improvements in the acute rejection rate and in allograft survival reflect the effectiveness of modern antirejection drugs such as the CNIs and MMF. The contribution of long-term CNI nephrotoxicity, particularly with currently used maintenance doses, to chronic kidney allograft dysfunction and loss remains controversial (see Late Allograft Dysfunction and Late Allograft Loss). For now, CNIs remain the cornerstone of immunosuppression.[351] Registry data show that the most immunosuppression regimens used at transplant centers in the United States include tacrolimus and MMF.

### Recipient Compliance

Poor compliance with the immunosuppressive regimen markedly increases the risk of acute rejection (particularly late acute rejection) and allograft loss.[352] Allograft loss has been reported to be seven-fold higher in nonadherent patients.[353] Efforts are being made to improve strategies to prevent nonadherence.[354] Noncompliance is a particularly difficult problem in the pediatric adolescent transplant population.[352,355]

### Recipient Body Size

Morbid (grade 2 or higher) obesity, corresponding to a Quételet's (body mass) index (BMI) of 35 kg/m$^2$ or greater, is associated with more transplant surgery–related complications, more DGF, and poorer allograft survival.[356,357] Indeed, even grade 1 obesity (BMI of 30 to 34.9 kg/m$^2$) is a risk factor for allograft failure. Poorer long-term graft survival probably reflects the effects of DGF, nephron overwork, and more difficult dosing of immunosuppressive drugs. Nevertheless, study of patients with BMI greater than 30 kg/m$^2$ suggest that transplantation provides a survival benefit over remaining on the waiting list (on dialysis), at least up to a BMI of 41 kg/m$^2$.[358] Bariatric surgery prior to transplantation is an option for morbidly obese patients.[359] The issue of nephron underdosing has been discussed in the donor factors above, but also relates to its interaction with the recipient's size. Body surface area has been used as a surrogate measure for both donor nephron mass, as well as recipient metabolic demand. Gross mismatch (i.e., low donor body surface area [BSA] and high recipient BSA) has been associated with poorer long-term allograft survival.[334,335]

#### Recipient Diabetes Mellitus

Diabetes mellitus as the primary cause of ESRD is a risk factor for allograft failure, due to death with a functioning graft.

#### Recipient History of Hepatitis C

Hepatitis C antibody positivity is a risk factor for allograft failure, due to both premature graft failure and death with a functioning graft.[265] The natural history of kidney transplantation in HCV+ recipients may, however, change (for the better) with the advent of new highly effective antiviral therapies.

## IMPROVING KIDNEY ALLOGRAFT OUTCOMES: MATCHING KIDNEY AND RECIPIENT RISK

Maximizing the life span of donated organs is a key goal in kidney transplantation. The criteria used for allocation of deceased donor allografts can have an important effect on overall allograft survival. A purely utilitarian approach (to maximize allograft survival) would direct organs only to the youngest and healthiest, maximizing the "life years from transplant" (LYFT) gained from transplantation.[360] In practice, a balance must be struck between utility and equity (ensuring that anyone medically fit for a transplant has a reasonable chance of obtaining one).[361] In the US, the New Kidney Allocation system was instituted in late 2014. This system matches the 20% highest quality deceased donor kidneys with the top 20% of candidates, in the hope of maximizing the utility of the best organs (see section on ECD and KDPI).

# MEDICAL MANAGEMENT OF THE TRANSPLANT RECIPIENT

More emphasis is being placed on the general medical management of transplant patients. Comprehensive practice guidelines on the care of kidney transplant recipients were published by both the American Society of Transplantation and the European Best Practice Guidelines Expert Group in 2000 and 2002, respectively.[362,363] KDIGO (Kidney Disease: Improving Global Outcomes) has more recently published its evidenced-based 2009 KDIGO Clinical Practice Guideline for the Care of Kidney Transplant Recipients.[188] Reflecting the paucity of quality evidence, only 25% of the KDIGO graded guidelines were level '1' ("we recommend") and 75% were level '2' ("we suggest"). The evidence supporting the guidelines was of low or very low quality in almost 85%. There is much opportunity for improving our understanding and management of transplant recipient care.

Transplantation is generally preferable to dialysis, but there is an increased appreciation that the posttransplant state is often one of chronic kidney disease and heightened cardiovascular risk. The management of common electrolyte, endocrine, and cardiovascular complications after transplant is discussed in the following sections.

## ELECTROLYTE DISORDERS

### HYPERCALCEMIA AND HYPOPHOSPHATEMIA

Hypercalcemia is common and is due mainly to persistent hyperparathyroidism or the overzealous administration of calcium and vitamin D. The management of posttransplant hyperparathyroidism is discussed later. Hypophosphatemia is also common in the early posttransplant period, particularly when allograft function is excellent. This is due to a combination of reduced phosphate absorption (vitamin D depletion is common) and urinary phosphate wasting which is a consequence of high fibroblast growth factor (FGF)-23 and PTH levels and the tubular effects of CNIs, sirolimus and high-dose steroids.[364] Rarely, phosphate depletion is severe enough to cause profound muscle weakness, including respiratory muscle weakness. Phosphate normalizes in the majority of patients by one year posttransplant, mirroring post-transplant declines in fractional excretion of phosphate, PTH, and FGF-23.[365] In the longer term, persistent negative phosphate balance likely contributes to posttransplant bone disease. Treatment involves a diet high in phosphorus (e.g., inclusion of low-fat dairy products) and vitamin D replacement. However, over-aggressive replacement of phosphate posttransplant can lower calcium and vitamin D levels and potentially exacerbate hyperparathyroidism.[366] In addition, acute phosphate nephropathy has been reported in posttransplant recipients on phosphate replacement.[367] Our practice is to reserve oral phosphate supplements for patients with a phosphate < 1-1.5 mg/dL or symptomatic hypophosphatemia.

#### Hyperkalemia

Mild hyperkalemia is common, even with good allograft function. The principal cause is CNI-induced impairment of tubular potassium secretion. Indeed, a recent study suggests that tacrolimus activates the thiazide sensitive renal sodium-chloride transporter resulting in hypertension and reduced renal potassium excretion.[368] Hyperkalemia may be exacerbated by poor allograft function, ingestion of excess potassium, hyperglycemia, and medicines such as ACE-inhibitors and β-blockers. Hyperkalemia can also be caused by an amiloride-like effect of trimethoprim, a component of TMP-SMX, frequently used for prophylaxis against *Pneumocystis jirovecii* (previously *carinii*). Because the hyperkalemia is usually not severe and typically improves with reduction in CNI dosage, additional treatment is often not required. Treatment with the mineralocorticoid fludrocortisone is usually effective in decreasing potassium (although sometimes at the expense of hypertension and edema) and may be considered in occasional cases.[369] Other medications that may be considered include a loop diuretic, a thiazide diuretic, sodium polystyrene sulfonate (Kayexalate), or patiromer.[370]

#### Metabolic Acidosis

Mild metabolic acidosis is also common and often associated with hyperkalemia. In most cases, it has the features of a distal (hyperchloremic) renal tubular acidosis. This reflects tubule dysfunction caused by CNIs, rejection, or residual hyperparathyroidism (and the effect of TMP, as above). Alkali repletion with oral bicarbonate may be necessary.

#### Other Electrolyte Abnormalities

Hypomagnesemia is common and due to a magnesuric effect of the CNIs, as well as to residual hyperparathyroidism, and is usually asymptomatic. Magnesium supplements are sometimes prescribed when the plasma magnesium level is less than 1.5 mg/dL. However, their effectiveness is limited, they can cause diarrhea, and they add more complexity to the multidrug regimen of the transplant recipient.

## BONE DISORDERS AFTER KIDNEY TRANSPLANTATION

Bone disease in the ESRD patient is multifactorial and involves varying degrees of hyperparathyroidism (osteitis fibrosa cystica), vitamin D deficiency, low bone turnover, aluminum intoxication (osteomalacia), and amyloidosis (see Chapter 53). Unfortunately, bone disease can remain a problem after transplantation owing to persistence of the conditions discussed above and to the superimposed effects of immunosuppressants on bone.

## HYPERPARATHYROIDISM

Residual hyperparathyroidism is very common in the first posttransplant year. However, hyperparathyroidism may persist for years; one study found elevated serum PTH in 23 (54%) of 42 normocalcemic patients more than two years after transplant who had plasma creatinine levels less than 2 mg/dL.[371] Not surprisingly, the main risk factors for posttransplant hyperparathyroidism are the degree of pretransplant hyperparathyroidism and the duration of dialysis.[372] Inadequate vitamin D stores and poor allograft function (de novo secondary hyperparathyroidism) probably contribute to persistence of the condition in some patients.

Typically, posttransplant hyperparathyroidism is manifest by a low plasma phosphate and a mild to moderate elevation in the plasma calcium. Serum PTH is inappropriately high for the level of plasma calcium. Posttransplant hyperparathyroidism is often asymptomatic and tends to improve with time. Posttransplant therapy with paricalcitol has been shown to increase the likelihood of resolution of hyperparathyroidism at 1 year posttransplant.[373] However, active vitamin D analogs must be used with caution and stopped if the plasma calcium rises above the normal range or complications of hypercalcemia occur. The calcimimetic, cinacalcet, has been shown safely and effectively lower serum PTH and calcium and raise serum phosphate concentrations in a placebo-controlled study of kidney transplant recipients with persistent hyperparathyroidism.[374]

There are two main indications for posttransplant parathyroidectomy: 1) severe symptomatic hypercalcemia (in the early posttransplant period, now rare, and usually managed medically with cinacalcet and/or bisphosphonate), and 2) persistent, moderately severe hypercalcemia (serum calcium 12.0–12.5 mg/dL or greater) for more than a year after transplantation or calcific uremic arteriolopathy (calciphylaxis), a rare complication following transplantation. Subtotal parathyroidectomy is the procedure of choice.

## GOUT

The most important cause of hyperuricemia and gout after transplant are the CNIs, particularly cyclosporine. The CNIs impair renal uric acid clearance. Approximately 80% of CNI-treated kidney transplant recipients develop hyperuricemia, and about 13% develop new onset gout.[375] Diuretic use may exacerbate hyperuricemia and precipitate a gout attack.

Acute gout should be treated with colchicine or high-dose steroids; NSAIDs should generally be avoided. Colchicine-induced myopathy and neuropathy is more common in patients with impaired kidney function and in cyclosporine-treated (and presumably tacrolimus-treated) patients, due to an increase in colchicine levels. Therefore, the lowest effective dose of colchicine should be used and patients should be monitored for muscle weakness. For prevention of further gouty attacks, allopurinol is usually employed. Note that the metabolism of azathioprine is inhibited by allopurinol. Ideally, these drugs should not be co-prescribed. If azathioprine must be used in conjunction with allopurinol, then the azathioprine dose should be reduced to one quarter of the original dose and the complete blood count closely monitored. A safer alternative is to change azathioprine to MMF; no adjustment of MMF is required. The newer xanthine oxidase inhibitor, febuxostat, has also been successfully employed in hyperuricemic kidney transplant patients.[376] The packaging insert for febuxostat warns against concurrent azathioprine use. In cases of severe recurrent gout, it may be worthwhile to stop CNIs altogether. The uricosuric agent, probenicid, may be cautiously employed in kidney transplant recipients with excellent renal function. The uricase, pegloticase, remains untested in the transplant population.

## CALCINEURIN INHIBITOR–ASSOCIATED BONE PAIN

A syndrome of severe bone pain in the lower limbs has been associated with CNI use. This is uncommon and thought to represent a vasomotor effect of the CNIs. Osteonecrosis and other common bone lesions should be excluded before the diagnosis is made. Symptoms usually respond to reduction in CNI dosage and administration of calcium channel blockers (especially nifedipine). Calcitonin has also been used successfully. Magnetic resonance imaging (MRI) of the involved bones may show bone marrow edema.[377]

## OSTEONECROSIS

Osteonecrosis (avascular necrosis) is a serious bone complication of kidney transplantation. The pathogenesis is not well understood, but high doses of steroids are one risk factor. Up to 8% of kidney transplant patients develop osteonecrosis of the hips;[378] this figure is falling with lower dose steroid protocols.[379] The most commonly affected site is the femoral head; other sites are the humeral head, femoral condyles, proximal tibia, vertebrae, and small bones of the hand and foot. Many patients have bilateral involvement at the time of diagnosis. The principal symptom is pain; signs are nonspecific. Diagnosis is made by imaging studies; MRI is the most sensitive, plain radiography is the least sensitive, and scintigraphy is intermediate. However, MRI abnormalities do not always imply clinically significant osteonecrosis. Treatment remains controversial. Options include resting the joint, decompression, or joint replacement.

## OSTEOPOROSIS

Osteoporosis is a common bone disorder characterized by a parallel reduction in bone mineral and bone matrix so that bone mass is decreased but is of normal composition.

The most commonly used definition is that based on the World Health Organization scoring system. Osteoporosis is defined as bone density greater than 2.5 SD below the mean of sex-matched young adults (T score); osteopenia, as 1.0 to 2.5 SD below the T score. The greater the reduction in bone density in the non-transplant population, the greater is the risk of fracture.

Reduction in bone mineral density is now recognized as a very common complication of kidney transplantation. Most bone loss occurs in the first 6 months after transplant.[380] Risk factors for posttransplant osteoporosis include steroid use, ongoing hyperparathyroidism, vitamin D deficiency or resistance, and phosphate depletion. Diabetes mellitus is also associated with an increased risk of posttransplant fracture. The risk of hip fracture in the kidney transplant population is high at 3.3 to 3.8 events per 1000 person-years; indeed, transplant recipients have a 34% increased risk of fracture early posttransplant when compared to transplant-waitlisted dialysis patients. The risk of hip fracture in transplant and waitlisted dialysis patients subsequently equalizes before 2 years posttransplant.[381]

Bone mineral density (BMD) as measured by dual X-ray absorptiometry has been shown to predict fractures in the general population.[382] Surprisingly, the effects of steroid avoidance and minimization protocols on BMD and fracture rates have been somewhat contradictory with some studies finding an association with reduced fracture rates[383,384] and improved bone mineral density while others have failed to identify a beneficial association.[379,385] Treatment with bisphosphonates early posttransplant has been shown to prevent bone loss when compared to control, but may exacerbate preexisting adynamic bone disease.[386] Perhaps as a consequence, bisphosphonates have not been shown to reduce fracture rates in the kidney transplant population.[387] Notably, bisphosphonates are not recommended in patients with a GFR < 30 mL/min/1.73 m$^2$. A number of studies have shown a favorable effect for vitamin D derivatives with or without calcium supplementation on BMD in kidney transplant recipients.[388,389] In patients with persistent posttransplant hyperparathyroidism and hypercalcemia, cinacalcet treatment may improve BMD, in addition to serum calcium and PTH levels.[390]

Current KDIGO guidelines recommend monitoring of calcium, phosphate, and PTH posttransplant. Dual-energy X-ray absorptiometry (DEXA) scanning is recommended in the first 3 months posttransplant for patients on steroid or with risk factors for osteoporosis and GFR > 30 mL/min/1.73 m$^2$. For kidney transplant recipients within a year of transplant, with GFR > 30 mL/min/1.73 m$^2$ and low BMD, treatment with vitamin D, calcitriol/alfacalcidiol, or bisphosphonate should be considered.[188]

## POSTTRANSPLANT DIABETES MELLITUS

Posttransplant diabetes mellitus, formerly referred to as new-onset diabetes after transplantation (NODAT) is common after kidney transplantation. First-time kidney transplant recipients in the US between the years 2004-2008 had a 3-year cumulative incidence of posttransplant diabetes of over 40%. Risk factors include older age, obesity, positive hepatitis C antibody, CMV infection status, non-white ethnicity, family history, steroids, CNIs (especially tacrolimus), and episodes of acute rejection. Strategies to prevent and treat PTDM include steroid minimization, avoidance of tacrolimus, and lifestyle modification. The adoption of steroid-free immunosuppression regimens at discharge after kidney transplantation has been shown to reduce the odds of PTDM.[391,392] A small Austrian study reported a reduction in PTDM at one year in patients whose blood glucose was strictly maintained with insulin immediately posttransplant versus those that received standard management of blood glucose.[393]

Unfortunately, PTDM is associated with reduced graft and patient survival.[394] PTDM may require treatment with oral agents or insulin. Metformin is probably the drug of choice in kidney transplant recipients with adequate GFR because it is the most effective in reducing complications of type 2 diabetes mellitus.[303] For most patients with type 2 diabetes mellitus the American Diabetes Association recommends an HbA1C target of 7%. There are certainly benefits of tight glycemic control, especially in terms of the reduction in microvascular complications.[395,396] However, these benefits must be weighed against the risks of overzealous glycemic control as evidenced by the ACCORD trial where intensive glycemic control (targeting a HbA1C <6%) was associated with an increased risk of mortality and severe hypoglycemia.[395,397] For most patients a 'personalized' HbA1C target based on carefully considered risks and benefits is a good strategy.

## CARDIOVASCULAR DISEASE

Cardiovascular disease is a leading cause of death in kidney transplant recipients.[398] Despite pretransplant screening, the cumulative incidence of myocardial infarction (MI), stroke, and de novo peripheral arterial disease are 11%, 7%, and 24%, respectively.[399,400,401] De novo congestive heart failure is also common.[402] The kidney transplant recipient population is enriched with traditional cardiovascular risk factors such as smoking, diabetes mellitus, and hypertension and are also burdened with nontraditional CKD-related and transplant-associated risk factors.[403,404] Aspirin is an effective therapy for secondary prevention of cardiovascular disease in the general population.[405,406] However, a recent study showed marked variability in the use of cardioprotective medications, including aspirin, in kidney transplant recipients.[407]

### SMOKING

Tobacco smoking should be strongly discouraged; there is evidence that it affects allograft function as well as recipient survival.[408]

## HYPERTENSION

The prevalence of hypertension in the CNI era is at least 60% to 80%.[188] Causes include use of steroids, CNIs, weight gain, allograft dysfunction, native kidney disease, and transplant renal artery stenosis. The complications of posttransplant hypertension are presumed to be a heightened risk of cardiovascular disease and allograft failure.[409] A post hoc analysis of the FAVORIT trial (which investigated the effect of lowering homocysteine levels on cardiovascular outcomes in kidney transplant recipients) found that each increase of 20 mm Hg in baseline systolic blood pressure was associated with 32% and 13% increases in the adjusted relative risks of cardiovascular events and death, respectively. In contrast, each 10 mmHg drop in diastolic blood pressure below 70 mm Hg was associated with a 31% increase in the relative risks of both cardiovascular events and death. The highest risk was seen in patients with a systolic blood pressure > 140 mm Hg and diastolic blood pressure < 70 mm Hg.[410]

There has been some controversy over blood pressure treatment targets in recent years. For transplant patients we follow the 2017 American College of Cardiology/American Heart Association Hypertension Guidelines for adults with CKD and hypertension to *initiate antihypertensive drug therapy at SBP ≥130 mm Hg or DBP ≥80 mm Hg and treat to goal of SBP <130 mm Hg and DBP <80 mm Hg.*[411]

Nonpharmacologic measures such as weight loss, reduced sodium intake, reduced alcohol intake, treatment of obstructive sleep apnea, and increased exercise should be encouraged. The dosage of steroids and CNIs should be minimized. However, antihypertensive drug therapy is still frequently required. There is little evidence for one antihypertensive drug class over another. In stable transplant recipients (good allograft function and more than 6 to 12 months out from transplant) we treat with the 2017 American College of Cardiology/American Heart Association Hypertension Guidelines recommended first-line antihypertensive drugs, namely thiazide diuretics, calcium channel blockers, and ACEIs or ARBs.

We routinely use ACEIs and ARBs, especially in patients with proteinuria, diabetes, or other cardiovascular indications. However, in the early posttransplant months, we generally avoid ACEIs or ARBs as they may exacerbate hyperkalemia or result in a creatinine increase that may be confused for rejection. Clinical factors that influence our choice of antihypertensive therapy in kidney transplant recipients are shown in Table 70.13.

## PROTEINURIA

Proteinuria, even when modest, is associated with poorer allograft survival.[412] We initiate ACEI or ARB treatment in our kidney transplant recipients with proteinuria, although we note that the only randomized controlled trial of ACEI or ARB therapy (Ramipril) in proteinuric kidney transplant patients was negative (no difference in doubling of creatinine, ESRD, or death compared to placebo). Indeed, the only between group difference at the end of the study was a significantly lower hemoglobin in the ramipril treated group.[413]

**Table 70.13 Antihypertensive Agents in the Transplant Recipient**

| Indication | β-Blocker | ACE-I/ARB | Ca-Channel Blocker | Thiazide Diuretic |
|---|---|---|---|---|
| Hypertension only | | X | X | X |
| CHF | X | X | | |
| Post-MI | X | X | | |
| CAD | X | X | | |
| Diabetes | | X | | |
| Proteinuria | | X | | |

*ACE-I*, Angiotensin-converting enzyme inhibitor; *ARB*, angiotensin receptor blocker; *CAD*, coronary artery disease; *CHF*, congestive heart failure; *MI*, myocardial infarction.

## HYPERLIPIDEMIA

The prevalence of hyperlipidemia after transplant is very high.[414] Steroids, CNIs (cyclosporine more than tacrolimus), and sirolimus are the principal causes. Some studies suggest that hyperlipidemia is associated with poorer allograft outcomes, although no causal relation has been established. The American Heart Association Guidelines (for the general population) have deemphasized the importance of cholesterol concentration on the decision to treat with statin and highlighted the importance of assessing cardiovascular risk. High-intensity statin is recommended for all patients over 21 years of age with 1) atherosclerotic cardiovascular disease, 2) LDL >190 mg/dL, and 3) persons aged 40 to 75 years with diabetes mellitus and an estimated 10-year cardiovascular risk > 7.5%. Moderate intensity statin is recommended for 1) persons aged 40 to 75 years with an estimated 10-year cardiovascular risk < 7.5% and diabetes mellitus and 2) non-diabetics 40 to 75 years of age with an estimated 10-year cardiovascular risk > 7.5%.[415] The application of a risk-guided statin treatment algorithm in the kidney transplant population seems like a reasonable approach. The only caveat is that the starting dose of a statin should be reduced in kidney transplant recipients as the CNIs (especially cyclosporine) increase statin blood levels and may predispose to statin-related toxicities.[416]

The main randomized controlled trial of statin therapy in kidney transplant recipients showed no benefit in the primary outcome (composite of cardiac death, nonfatal myocardial infarction or coronary intervention procedure).[417] However, follow-up after an additional two years of statin therapy showed a significantly reduced risk of major cardiac events.[418] As in the general population, statin use is associated with an increased risk hyperglycemia in kidney transplant recipients.[419]

Hypertriglyceridemia can be a problem posttransplant. Strategies for lowering triglyceride levels include, lifestyle modification, substitution of sirolimus for an alternative agent (e.g., MMF), and treatment with ezetimibe.

The high prevalence of metabolic syndrome, a consequence of dysregulation of glucose and vascular metabolism, is being increasingly recognized in kidney transplant recipients.[420] Better recognition and management of metabolic syndrome, including control of obesity, glucose, hyperlipidemia, and blood pressure, are expected to decrease the morbidity and mortality of transplant recipients.

## HYPERHOMOCYSTEINEMIA

As in the general population, hyperhomocysteinemia has been proposed as a risk factor for cardiovascular disease in kidney transplant recipients. Plasma homocysteine concentrations typically fall after transplant but do not normalize. Based on the results of well-performed randomized controlled trials in both the general and CKD populations, current interventions to lower homocysteine cannot be recommended.[421]

## CANCER AFTER KIDNEY TRANSPLANTATION

A number of recent studies have linked transplant and cancer registry data, giving good insight into posttransplant

**Table 70.14 Cancers Categorized by SIR for Kidney Transplant Patients and Cancer Incidence**

| | Common Cancers in Both General and Transplant Populations: Incidence ≥10 Per 100,000 People | Common Cancers in the Transplant Population: Incidence in General Population <10 Per 100,000, but Estimated Incidence in Transplant Population ≥10 Per 100,000 People | Rare Cancers Incidence in Both General and Transplant Populations <10 Per 100,000 People |
|---|---|---|---|
| High SIR >5 | Kaposi's Sarcoma (with HIV) | Kaposi's sarcoma<br>Vagina<br>Non-Hodgkin's lymphoma<br>Kidney<br>Non-melanoma skin<br>Lip<br>Thyroid<br>Penis<br>Small intestine | Eye |
| Moderate SIR (1-5) | Lung<br>Colon<br>Cervix<br>Stomach<br>Liver | Oro-nasopharynx<br>Esophagus<br>Bladder<br>Leukemia | Melanoma<br>Larynx<br>Multiple myeloma<br>Anus<br>Hodgkin's lymphoma |
| No Increased Risk | Breast<br>Prostate<br>Rectum | | Ovary<br>Uterus<br>Pancreas<br>Brain<br>Testis |

*SIR*, Standard Incidence Rate.
Adapted from the KDIGO practice gudelines.[183–188]

cancer incidence. Data from the US and UK show that kidney transplant recipients are at considerably greater risk for certain cancers when compared to the general population (Table 70.14).[422–424]

There are several reasons why reported cancer incidence has increased. First, immunosuppression inhibits normal tumor surveillance mechanisms, allowing unchecked proliferation of "spontaneously occurring" neoplastic cells. There is also experimental evidence that cyclosporine has tumor-promoting effects mediated by its effects on TGF-β production[425] and expression of the angiogenic cytokine vascular endothelial growth factor (VEGF).[426] Second, immunosuppression allows uncontrolled proliferation of oncogenic viruses (Table 70.15). Third, factors related to the primary kidney disease (analgesic abuse, certain herbal preparations, HBV or HCV infection) or the ESRD milieu (acquired renal cystic disease) might promote neoplasia.

It is believed that the cumulative amount of immunosuppression rather than a specific drug is the most important factor increasing the cancer risk. However, there is evidence that the routine use of CNIs has increased the risk of skin cancers,[427] fortunately, these are usually not fatal. The long-term impact of the currently employed powerful immunosuppression regimens on cancer incidence is unknown, but it is certainly of concern. The single most important measure to prevent cancers is to minimize excess immunosuppression. A general rule is that when cancer occurs, immunosuppression should be significantly decreased. In some cases, rejection of the allograft may result, but the risks and benefits of immunosuppression must be judged on a case-by-case basis.

**Table 70.15 Viral Infections Associated With Development of Cancers in Kidney Transplant Patients**

| Virus | Neoplasm |
|---|---|
| HBV | Hepatocellular cancer |
| HCV | Hepatocellular cancer |
| EBV | PTLD |
| HPV | Squamous cell cancers of anogenital area and of mouth |
| HHV-8 | Kaposi's sarcoma |

*HBV*, Hepatitis B virus; *HCV*, hepatitis C virus; *EBV*, Ebstein-Barr virus; *HPV*, human papillomavirus; *HHV-8*, human herpes virus-8, *PTLD*, posttransplant lymphoproliferative disorder.

## SKIN AND LIP CANCERS

Squamous cell carcinoma, basal cell carcinoma, and malignant melanoma are all more common in kidney transplant patients. The incidence of non-melanomatous skin cancer in kidney transplant recipients is 13 times greater than in the general population.[423] Risk factors include time after transplant, cumulative immunosuppressive dose, exposure to ultraviolet light, fair skin, and human papillomavirus infection. Primary and secondary prevention is important: Patients should be specifically counseled on minimizing exposure to ultraviolet light and to self-screen for skin lesions.[188] Retinoids are sometimes used in high-risk patients.[428] Suspicious skin lesions should be surgically excised. In patients with posttransplant squamous

**Table 70.16 Clinical and Pathologic Spectrum of PTLD and Summary of Its Management**

| | Early Disease (50%) | Polymorphic PTLD (30%) | Monoclonal PTLD (20%) |
|---|---|---|---|
| Clinical features/ symptoms | Infectious mononucleosis-type illness | Infectious mononucleosis-type illness ± weight loss, localizing symptoms | Fever, weight loss, localizing symptoms |
| Pathology | Preserved architecture, atypical cells infrequent | Intermediate transformed cells | High-grade lymphoma with confluent and marked atypia |
| Clonality | Polyclonal | Usually polyclonal | Monoclonal |
| Treatment | Reduce immunosuppression | Reduce immunosuppression ±rituximab | Reduce immunosuppression ± rituximab ± chemotherapy |
| Prognosis | Good | Intermediate | Intermediate/poor |

*PTLD,* Posttransplant lymphoproliferative disorder.

cell carcinoma, switching from a CNI to sirolimus reduces the risk of further such tumors developing by 44% (although places patients at risk for other important metabolic effects).[106]

## ANOGENITAL CANCERS

Cancers of the vulva, uterine cervix, penis, scrotum, anus, and perianal region are significantly more common in kidney transplant recipients. Furthermore, these cancers tend to be multifocal and more aggressive than in the general population. Infection with certain human papillomavirus strains is an important risk factor. Secondary prevention measures include yearly physical examination of the anogenital area and, in women, yearly pelvic examinations, and cervical histology. Suspicious lesions should be excised, and patients should be closely followed for recurrence.

## KAPOSI'S SARCOMA

The incidence of Kaposi's sarcoma in transplant and non-transplant patients depends greatly on ethnic background. Those of Jewish, Arab, and Mediterranean ancestry are at much higher risk. Other risk factors are cumulative immunosuppressive dose and human herpes virus-8 infection. Visceral (lymph nodes, lungs, gastrointestinal tract) and nonvisceral (skin, conjunctivae, oropharynx) involvement may occur. The prognosis for the former is poor, but for the latter it is good. Treatment involves various combinations of surgical excision, radiotherapy, chemotherapy, and immunotherapy. Immunosuppression, of course, should be reduced or modified. Substitution of sirolimus for CNIs has been reported to stop progression of the disease without sacrificing allograft function.[105]

## POSTTRANSPLANT LYMPHOPROLIFERATIVE DISORDER

Posttransplant lymphoproliferative disorder (PTLD) is one of the most feared complications of transplantation because it can occur early after transplant and it carries a high morbidity and mortality. The cumulative 3-year incidence of PTLD is 0.5% in adult and 1.5% in pediatric kidney transplant recipients. More than 90% are non-Hodgkin's lymphomas, and most are of recipient B cell origin.[429] Risk factors include 1) Epstein-Barr virus (EBV)–positive donor and EBV-negative recipient; 2) CMV-positive donor and CMV-negative recipient; 3) pediatric recipient (in part because children are more likely to be EBV naive); and 4) intensity of immunosuppression.[430]

Clinical trials of belatacept saw high rates of PTLD in EBV-negative subjects; the drug is now contraindicated in patients who are seronegative for EBV.[86]

Important in the pathogenesis of PTLD is the infection and transformation of B cells by EBV; transformed B cells undergo proliferation that is initially polyclonal, but a malignant clone may evolve. Thus, the clinical and histologic spectrum of PTLD at presentation and its treatment can vary greatly (Table 70.16). Extranodal, gastrointestinal tract, and central nervous system involvement is more common than in non-transplant lymphomas. The kidney allograft may be involved. Treatment options for PTLD include immunosuppression reduction, rituximab and CHOP [cyclophosphamide, doxorubicin (Adriamycin), vincristine, prednisone]. Screening high-risk patients (EBV+ donor/EBV- recipient) for EBV viremia in the first year posttransplant with institution of rituximab treatment for persistently viremic patients has been shown to reduce PTLD incidence in one small study.[431]

### CANCER SCREENING

Since life expectancy in the kidney transplant population is significantly improved compared to patients receiving dialysis, we recommend that patients follow cancer screening guidelines (cervical smear, mammogram, colonoscopy) for the general population. We also recommend annual dermatologic screening. Screening for kidney cancer is not advised in the most recent KDIGO guidelines.[188]

## INFECTIOUS COMPLICATIONS OF KIDNEY TRANSPLANTATION

The transplant procedure itself and subsequent immunosuppression increase the risk of serious infection. The principal factors determining the type and severity of infection are exposure (in the hospital and community) to potential pathogens and the state of immunosuppression.[432] Factors affecting the net state of immunosuppression include the cumulative amount of immunosuppression, recipient comorbidities (e.g., diabetes, UTIs), infection of viruses that affect the immune system (e.g., EBV, CMV, HIV, hepatitis C), and the integrity of mucocutaneous barriers.

The patterns of infection after kidney transplantation can be roughly divided into three time periods: 0 to 1 month, 1 to 6 months, and more than 6 months after transplant.[432] These divisions of time serve as guidelines only. Maintenance immunosuppressive regimens are becoming more powerful, and more elderly patients are undergoing transplant surgery;

on the other hand, antimicrobial prophylaxis is becoming more effective. An outline of the pattern of infection after transplantation according for time after transplantation is shown in Table 70.17.

A general point is that at any time when life-threatening infection occurs, immunosuppression should be reduced to an absolute minimum or stopped altogether (so-called stress-dose steroids often are required). Prompt diagnosis (e.g., bronchoscopy in patients with pneumonitis) and therapy are essential.[432]

**Table 70.17 Infections After Transplantation According to Time After Transplantation**

| Time After Transplant | Type of Infection |
|---|---|
| <1 month | Infection with antimicrobial-resistant species:<br>MRSA, VRE, Candida species (non-albicans)<br>Aspiration<br>Catheter infection<br>Wound infection<br>Anastomotic leaks and ischemia<br>*Clostridium difficile* colitis<br>Donor-derived infection (uncommon):<br>HSV, LCMV, Rhabdovirus (rabies), West Nile virus, HIV, *T. cruzi*<br>Recipient-derived infection (colonization):<br>Aspergillus, pseudomonas |
| 1-6 months | With PCP and antiviral (CMV, HBV) prophylaxis:<br>Polyomavirus, BK infection, nephropathy<br>*C. difficile* colitis<br>HCV infection<br>Adenovirus infection, influenza<br>*Cryptococcus neoformans* infection<br>*Mycobacterium tuberculosis* infection<br>Without prophylaxis:<br>Pneumocystis<br>Infection with herpesviruses (HSV, VZV, CMV, EBV)<br>HBV infection<br>Infection with Listeria, Nocardia, toxoplasma, stongyloides, leishmania, *T.cruzi* |
| >6 months | Community-acquired pneumonia, UTI<br>Infection with aspergillus, typical molds, mucor species<br>Infection with Nocardia, rhodococcus species<br>Late viral infections:<br>CMV infection<br>Hepatitis (HBV, HCV)<br>HSV encephalitis<br>Community-acquired (SARS, West Nile virus infection)<br>JC polyomavirus infection (PML)<br>Skin cancer, lymphoma (PTLD) |

*CMV,* Cytomegalovirus; *EBV,* Epstein-Barr virus; *HBV,* herpes virus B; *HCV,* herpes virus C; *HSV,* herpes simplex virus; *LCMV,* lymphocytic choriomeningitis virus; *MRSA,* methicillin-resistant Staphylococcus aureus; *PCP,* Pneumocystis carinii pneumonia; *SARS,* severe acute respiratory syndrome; *UTI,* urinary tract infection; *VRE,* vancomycin-resistant enterococcus.

Adapted from Fishman JA. Infection in solid-organ transplant recipients. *N Engl J Med* 2007;357:2601-2614.

## INFECTIONS IN THE FIRST MONTH

The majority of infections in the first month are standard infections, as would be seen in non-transplant patients after surgery. Thus, infections of surgical wounds, the lungs, and the urinary tract, and infections related to vascular catheters predominate. Bacterial infections are much more common than fungal ones. Preventive measures include ensuring that donor and recipient are free of overt infection before transplant, good surgical technique, and SMX-TMP prophylaxis to prevent UTIs.

## INFECTIONS FROM 1 TO 6 MONTHS AFTER TRANSPLANT

Weeks of intensive immunosuppression increase the risk of opportunistic infections. Infections with CMV, EBV, *Listeria monocytogenes, Pneumocystis jirovecii,* and *Nocardia* spp. are relatively common. Preventive measures include antiviral prophylaxis (for 3 to 6 months) and SMX-TMP prophylaxis (for 6 to 12 months).

## INFECTIONS MORE THAN 6 MONTHS AFTER TRANSPLANT

With gradual reduction in immunosuppression, the risk of infection long-term usually diminishes. However, patients can be roughly divided into two groups based on risk. Those with good ongoing allograft function and no need for late supplemental immunosuppression are at low risk for developing opportunistic infections unless exposure is intense (e.g., to *Nocardia* spp. from soil). In contrast, those with poor allograft function are at higher risk for opportunistic infection. This probably reflects both poor allograft function and that many of these patients have received large cumulative doses of immunosuppression.

Late amplification of immunosuppression may increase the risk of opportunistic infection in any patient. Therefore, any patient receiving a "late" steroid pulse or antithymoglobulin therapy should be restarted on SMX-TMP +/- anti-CMV prophylaxis (if donor or recipient were CMV positive). The role of EBV infection in causing PTLD has been discussed earlier; CMV and *P. jirovecii* pneumonia infection are discussed later.

## CYTOMEGALOVIRUS

Exposure to CMV (as evidenced by the presence in serum of anti-CMV IgG) increases with age; more than two thirds of adult donors and recipients are latently infected before kidney transplantation. Infection may arise from 1) reactivation of latent recipient virus, 2) primary infection with donor-derived virus (transmitted in the allograft or less commonly via blood products), or 3) reactivation of latent donor-derived virus. CMV *disease* means that there is infection with symptoms or with evidence of tissue invasion, or both. The risk of CMV infection or disease is highest in CMV-positive donor/CMV-negative recipient pairings, followed by CMV-positive donor/CMV-positive recipient pairings and then CMV-negative donor/CMV-positive recipient pairings. The risk is lowest with CMV-negative donor/CMV-negative recipient pairings. OKT3/polyclonal antibody therapy, particularly

**Table 70.18 Manifestations of CMV Disease in the Kidney Transplant Recipient**

| Tissue Affected | Clinical/Pathological Features | Comment |
|---|---|---|
| Viremia (blood) | Fever, malaise, myalgia | Nonspecific, may occur after cessation of prophylaxis |
| Bone marrow | Leukopenia | May require azathioprine or MMF dose reduction. Valganciclovir may also cause leukopenia |
| Lungs | Pneumonitis | May be life-threatening; exclude coinfection with other organisms |
| GI tract | Inflammation and ulceration of esophagus or colon | May be life-threatening. |
| Liver | Hepatitis | Rarely severe |
| Retina | Blurred vision, flashes, floaters | Relatively rare in kidney transplants; if occurs, usually late. |
| Kidney | Viral inclusions | Association with FSGS |

*CMV,* Cytomegalovirus; *GI,* gastrointestinal; *MMF,* mycophenolate mofetil.

when prescribed for treatment of rejection, significantly increases the risk of subsequent CMV disease.

CMV disease usually arises 1 to 6 months after transplantation, although gastrointestinal and retinal involvement often occur later. Typical clinical features are fever, malaise, and leukopenia; there may be symptomatic or laboratory evidence of specific organ involvement (Table 70.18). Urgent investigation and immediate empiric treatment are needed in severe cases. Confirmation of presumed CMV disease is by demonstration of the virus in body fluids or solid organs. CMV infection after transplantation is most commonly associated with viremia. CMV viremia may be detected by culture, antigenemia assay, or quantitative PCR. The PCR assay is fast, sensitive, and allows the monitoring of viral load in response to therapy. However, viremia may be absent in certain CMV infections, most notably the retina or gastrointestinal tract. In such instances the CMV infection may be diagnosed by ophthalmologic exam +/- vitreous humor CMV PCR and immunohistochemistry or culture of gastrointestinal tissue, respectively. Other procedures such as lumbar puncture and bronchoscopy should be aggressively pursued according to symptoms and signs. A "tissue diagnosis" is also required to exclude coinfection with other microbes such as *P. jirovecii.* In addition to its direct effects, CMV may have indirect effects after transplant, including an increased risk of infection, rejection, and PTLD.[433]

The treatment of posttransplant CMV infection depends on disease severity and organ systems involved. Low-grade CMV viremia usually responds to a reduction in immunosuppression (usually the antimetabolite). The VICTOR trial demonstrated that oral valganciclovir was non-inferior to intravenous ganciclovir in the treatment of non-life-threatening CMV infection in solid organ transplants.[434] Therefore, patients with symptomatic or significant viremia but relatively mild symptoms may be treated as an outpatient with oral valganciclovir. However, patients with severe systemic CMV infection or organ-specific disease [i.e., pneumonitis, gastrointestinal, or central nervous system (CNS)] should be treated initially with intravenous ganciclovir with a transition to oral valganciclovir as symptoms improve. CMV viral load should be monitored with therapy. For viremic patients with mild to moderate disease we generally advocate continuing maintenance treatment for 2 weeks after resolution of viremia. Treatment of severe or invasive disease may benefit from longer courses of induction treatment followed by maintenance dose therapy.[435] Dose adjustment is required in kidney dysfunction for both valganciclovir and ganciclovir. Although supportive data are unavailable, it is reasonable to add CMV hyperimmune globulin in severe cases.[436]

The prevention of CMV disease is of great clinical importance. One strategy is to give prophylaxis to all patients at risk (D+/R-, D-/R+, D+/R+). Another strategy is to monitor for CMV viremia and begin prophylaxis only when there is evidence of active viral replication.[433] Prophylactic and preemptive strategies using valganciclovir have been shown comparable in terms of cost and prevention of symptomatic CMV.[437] Valganciclovir has proven to be an excellent therapy both for the prophylaxis and treatment of CMV; however, myelosuppression, especially leukopenia/neutropenia, is a common and sometimes difficult to manage side effect. Letermovir is currently being trialled as CMV prophylaxis in kidney transplant patients and may prove to be a useful alternative agent.[438]

## PNEUMOCYSTOSIS

Antimicrobial prophylaxis is very effective in preventing pneumonia due to *P. jirovecii* (previously *carinii*). The preventive agent of choice is SMX-TMP: It is generally well tolerated and quite inexpensive; furthermore, it prevents UTIs and opportunistic infections such as nocardiosis, toxoplasmosis, and listeriosis. Alternative preventive agents include dapsone and pyrimethamine, atovaquone, and aerosolized pentamadine.[439] Typical symptoms of pneumonia due to *P. jirovecii* are fever, shortness of breath, and cough. Chest radiography characteristically shows bilateral interstitial-alveolar infiltrates. Diagnosis requires detection of the organism in a clinical specimen by colorimetric or immunofluorescent stains. Because the organism burden is usually lower than in human immunodeficiency virus (HIV)–infected patients, the sensitivity of induced sputum or bronchoalveolar lavage specimens is lower in kidney transplant recipients; tissue should be quickly obtained if these tests are negative and the clinical suspicion remains high.

The treatment of choice remains SMX-TMP.[439] High-dose SMX-TMP may increase the plasma creatinine without affecting GFR. There is no firm evidence to support the use of higher dose steroids during the early treatment phase of pneumocystosis in kidney transplant recipients.

**Table 70.19 Recommended and Contraindicated Vaccines in Transplant Recipients**

| Recommended | Comments | Contraindicated[a] |
|---|---|---|
| Influenza | Annually | Live varicella vaccine[b] |
| PCV13 | Once | BCG |
| PPSV23 | Repeat every 5 years, up to 3 doses/lifetime including one dose in those aged 65 years and older | Smallpox |
| Tdap/Td | Td booster every 10 years | Intranasal influenza |
| 9vHPV | Only for ≤ 26 years of age | Live Japanese B encephalitis |
| HepA | | Oral polio |
| HepB | Give 3-dose series if anti-HBS<10 mIUL/mL | MMR |
| **Asplenia or complement inhibitor therapy** | | Live oral typhoid Ty21a |
| MenACWY | 2-dose series with booster every 5 years | Yellow fever |
| MenB | 2-dose series, no booster | |
| Hib | If not already given | |

[a]Not an exhaustive list, all live vaccines are generally contraindicated.
[b]Awaiting data on the non-live 'Shingrix' (HZ/su) zoster vaccine.
*PCV13,* Pneumococcal conjugate vaccine (13-valent); *PPSV23,* pneumococcal polysaccharide vaccine (23-valent); *MenACWY,* meningococcal (quadrivalent) conjugate; *MenB,* serogroup B meningococcal vaccines; *Hib,* Haemophilus influenzae type b conjugate vaccine; *Tdap,* tetanus and reduced diphtheria toxoid, and acellular pertussis vaccine; *Td,* tetanus and reduced diphtheria toxoids; *HepA,* hepatitis A vaccine; *HepB,* hepatitis B vaccine; *9vHPV,* human papillomavirus vaccine; *MMR,* measles, mumps, and rubella vaccine.

## IMMUNIZATION IN KIDNEY TRANSPLANT RECIPIENTS

Important general rules concerning immunization in kidney transplant patients are the following: 1) Immunizations should be completed at least 4 weeks before transplantation; 2) live vaccines are generally contraindicated after transplantation. We follow the *IDSA clinical practice guideline for vaccination of the immunocompromised host.*[440] We pay special attention to pretransplant vaccination in asplenic patients and those who will or may require eculizumab therapy. Vaccines that are recommended and contraindicated are summarized in Table 70.19. We await further data on the Shingrix (HZ/su) non-live vaccine in kidney transplant recipients but expect that it may soon be recommended.[441] Household contacts of transplant recipients should receive yearly immunization against influenza.

## SUMMARY

Infections are a predictable complication of kidney transplantation. Minimizing infections requires meticulous surgical technique, antiviral prophylaxis for the first 3 to 6 months, SMX-TMP prophylaxis for the first 6 to 12 months, vaccination and, of course, avoidance of excess immunosuppression. A substantial increase in immunosuppression, no matter what the time period after transplant, should trigger resumption of SMX-TMP and probably antiviral prophylaxis.

# TRANSPLANT ISSUES IN SPECIFIC PATIENT GROUPS

## TRANSPLANTATION IN PATIENTS WITH DIABETES

Although the survival rate of diabetic patients after kidney transplantation is lower than that of nondiabetic patients, the benefits of transplantation versus staying on dialysis remain.[306] Cardiovascular disease is highly prevalent in the diabetic ESRD population and aggressive cardiovascular risk modification should be undertaken. A subset of diabetic ESRD patients is also suitable for kidney-pancreas transplantation (see the following discussion).

## KIDNEY-PANCREAS TRANSPLANTATION

The benefits of pancreas transplantation are 1) freedom from insulin therapy and the metabolic derangements of type 1 diabetes mellitus and 2) potentially slowing or reversal of the progression of end-organ damage from this condition. The disadvantage of pancreas transplantation is higher risk of surgical complications, and the need for higher levels of immunosuppression. Thus, patients must be carefully selected for this procedure. Although select patients with type 2 diabetes can undergo pancreas transplantation, the vast majority of pancreas transplantations are performed in patients with type 1 diabetes. For diabetic ESRD patients deemed suitable candidates for kidney plus pancreas transplantation, options include simultaneous kidney and pancreas (SPK) transplantation or pancreas after kidney (PAK) transplantation (the latter allows living donor kidney transplantation). Pancreas transplant alone (PTA) was also performed in a minority of patients without ESRD. In contrast to SPK transplantation, there is some concern as to whether pancreas transplant alone/later improves patient survival. However, PAK transplantation offers the advantages of preemptive living donor kidney transplantation and better kidney allograft outcomes. Rates of pancreas transplantation have decreased somewhat over the past decade from a peak of around 1500 procedures in 2004 to just over 1000 in 2017.

Complications of pancreatic transplantation include thrombosis, infection, rejection, and problems related to drainage of the exocrine secretions.[442] Safe drainage of the exocrine secretions is vital. Drainage of exocrine secretions into the bladder affords the advantages of sterility and of serial measurement of urinary amylase concentrations that can aid in early detection of pancreatic allograft dysfunction. Important disadvantages include severe cystitis, hypovolemia, and acidosis (the last two due to large losses of bicarbonate-rich fluid). Because rates of technical complications from enteric drainage have decreased, this technique is becoming more popular.[442]

The graft half-life for pancreas transplants is over 12 years in the US. Pancreas graft survival rates are better for recipients of SPK allografts than for PTA or PAK recipients.[443] The major causes of graft failure are technical (40%) and acute rejection (15%) in the early posttransplant period, and chronic rejection (25%) in the late posttransplant period.[444]

## KIDNEY TRANSPLANTATION IN PATIENTS WITH HUMAN IMMUNODEFICIENCY VIRUS INFECTION

HIV infection was traditionally considered an absolute contraindication to kidney transplantation. This reflected fears that immunosuppression would promote severe infections and that the short survival of HIV-positive patients undergoing transplant surgery would waste valuable allografts. With the introduction of antiretroviral agent therapy in 1996 and subsequent improvements in the survival of HIV-positive patients, many centers accept patients with HIV for transplantation. Indeed, very good allograft and recipient survival has been reported.[445,446] A recent study, which included 510 patients transplanted with HIV, found that HIV+ kidney transplant recipients had a lower 5- and 10-year graft and patient survival when compared to HIV- controls. Interestingly, when those 362 HIV+ patients not coinfected with HCV were compared to HIV- controls 5- and 10-year graft and patient survival were identical suggesting HCV coinfection was the driver of worse outcomes in the HIV+ group as a whole.[447] Interestingly HIV+ patients undergoing kidney transplant appear to be at higher risk of acute rejection and likely benefit from ATG induction.[448] Generally, HIV+ patients must be stable on HAART and have CD4+ T-cell counts of at least $200/m^3$ and undetectable HIV RNA levels before being considered for transplant. Patients with HIV should be referred to centers with specialized HIV+ transplant programs because of the complexity of posttransplant management; e.g., the potential for interactions between the multiple antiviral medicines, some of which inhibit and some of which induce the cytochrome P450 system. Successful transplantation of kidneys from HIV-positive donors to HIV-positive recipients has been reported.[449]

## PREGNANCY IN THE KIDNEY TRANSPLANT RECIPIENT

Fertility is often improved after kidney transplantation.[450] Although the risks of pregnancy and childbirth are greater in kidney transplant recipients compared to the general population, it is generally considered safe for the mother, fetus, and kidney allograft if the following criteria are met before conception: good general health for more than 18 months before conception, stable allograft function with a plasma creatinine level less than 2.0 mg/dL (preferably less than 1.5 mg/dL), minimal hypertension, minimal proteinuria, immunosuppression at maintenance doses, and no dilation of the pelvicalyceal system on recent imaging studies.[451]

A recent systematic review and meta-analysis of 50 studies that included data on 4706 pregnancies in 3570 KTRs, between the years 2000 and 2010, gives insight into the relative risks of pregnancy post-kidney transplant. The rate of live births was actually higher than that of the general population. However, KTR pregnancies were more likely to end with cesarean sections, preterm births (35.6 vs 38.7 weeks), and lower birth weights (2.4 kg vs 3.3 kg). Preeclampsia and gestational diabetes were both more common in KTRs than the general population. More than 50% of KTRs were hypertensive during pregnancy. Overall, pregnancy did not appear to associate with an increased risk of acute rejection or subsequent graft loss.[452]

All pregnant kidney allograft recipients should be managed as high-risk obstetric cases with nephrology involvement. Throughout the pregnancy, regular monitoring of blood pressure, proteinuria, kidney function, and urine cultures is advised. Significant kidney dysfunction occurs in a minority of cases; the principal causes are severe preeclampsia, acute rejection, acute pyelonephritis, and recurrent glomerulonephritis. Distinguishing these causes clinically may be difficult. Initial investigations should include plasma creatinine, creatinine clearance, 24-hour urinary protein excretion, urine microscopy, urine culture, and kidney ultrasound. Acute rejection should be confirmed by allograft biopsy before instituting antirejection therapy. Pulse steroids are used to treat rejection.

There are no transplant-specific reasons to perform cesarean section; if it is performed (for obstetric reasons), care should be taken to avoid damaging the transplant ureter. Kidney function should be monitored closely for 3 months postpartum because of the increased risk of HUS and possibly acute rejection.

Short-term and long-term data indicate that children born to transplant recipients using cyclosporine, steroids, or azathioprine do not have a significant increase in morbidity. Short-term data on tacrolimus are similarly reassuring. Dosages of cyclosporine and tacrolimus may need to be increased to maintain pre-pregnancy trough concentrations. CNI levels typically decrease during the first trimester due to increased volume of distribution. Therefore, CNI levels should be closely monitored and doses should be adjusted to avoid acute rejection from subtherapeutic levels. MMF is considered to be teratogenic, and it should not be used in women contemplating pregnancy.[453] Sirolimus should also be avoided.

## SURGERY IN THE KIDNEY TRANSPLANT RECIPIENT

### ALLOGRAFT NEPHRECTOMY

Allograft nephrectomy is not commonly required. Indications include 1) allograft failure with ongoing symptomatic rejection causing fever, malaise, and graft pain; 2) infarction due to thrombosis; 3) severe infection of the allograft such as emphysematous pyelonephritis; and 4) allograft rupture. The morbidity associated with allograft nephrectomy is relatively high. Ongoing rejection in a failed allograft can sometimes be controlled with steroids, but prolonged immunosuppression of a patient who is on dialysis is obviously not ideal. Rejection in this context is less likely to be controlled by small doses of steroids when it is acute and when the transplant is recent. Whether nephrectomy of the allograft after a patient returns to dialysis offers a survival advantage remains controversial. A retrospective analysis of registry data noted a survival advantage in transplant recipients who underwent allograft nephrectomy after returning to dialysis.[454] However, any potential benefits of nephrectomy must be weighed against the heightened risk of HLA-sensitization around the time of allograft nephrectomy.[455] This may be of great importance for those patients relisted repeat kidney transplant. We generally only perform nephrectomy for symptomatic late rejection.

## NONTRANSPLANT-RELATED SURGERY OR HOSPITALIZATION

Many kidney transplant recipients are hospitalized or undergo surgery for non-transplant reasons. Precautions for procedures and surgery in transplant recipients are listed in Table 70.20. Common-sense measures such as maintenance of adequate volume status, avoidance of nephrotoxic medicines (including NSAIDs), and proper dosing of immunosuppressive drugs are advised. Whenever possible, immunosuppressive drugs should be given by the enteral route. When not possible we use intravenous steroid and intravenous MMF or AZA, we prefer when possible to use sublingual tacrolimus, usually at half the oral dose, instead of intravenous tacrolimus. When necessary, intravenous tacrolimus should be started at one fifth of the total daily dose. Intravenous cyclosporine should be prescribed in slow infusion form at one third of the total daily oral dose.

## THE PATIENT WITH THE FAILING KIDNEY

As for native CKD, management of anemia, hyperparathyroidism, hypertension, preparation for dialysis, and creation of appropriate dialysis access are important. If there are no contraindications, patients should be relisted for transplant. Once the patient returns to dialysis, immunosuppression should be weaned gradually. In patients who are likely to be re-transplanted in the near future, we maintain immunosuppression to avoid HLA sensitization. Active communication between the primary nephrologist and the transplant physician is critical to ensuring a smooth transition for the patient. In cases where management of the patient has been primarily through a transplant center, early referral to a primary nephrologist is important for preparation and initiation of dialysis. Conversely, patients who are managed primarily by a general nephrologist should alert the transplant center to coordinate the modification and weaning of immunosuppressive medications.

**Table 70.20 Precautions for Procedures and Surgery in Kidney Transplant Recipients**

- Caution with radiocontrast exposure
- Maintain hydration
- Avoid nephrotoxic antibiotics and analgesic
- "Stress-dose steroids" is not always necessary
- If enteral route of medication is contraindicated, give CNI via IV route (1/3 total oral dose)
- Monitor allograft function, plasma potassium and acid-base balance daily
- Consider wound-healing impairment with sirolimus

## TRANSPLANTATION/ IMMUNOSUPPRESSION: THE FUTURE

Major areas of ongoing investigation include expansion of the donor pool,[456,457] optimization of immunosuppression regimens (with particular focus on individualizing immunosuppression), induction of tolerance,[458–460] and xenotransplantation. There is also growing interest in therapies that modulate B cell and plasma cell function, thus preventing or treating ABMR.

## CONCLUSION

Improvements in short- and long-term kidney allograft survival have been encouraging. This reflects multiple influences, including more effective immunosuppression, more frequent use of living donors, and better medical and surgical care. The focus is likely to shift somewhat toward improving other posttransplant outcomes such as complications of immunosuppression, chronic allograft dysfunction, and morbidity from cardiovascular disease. Availability of adequate numbers of organs for transplantation remains an ongoing problem.

Complete reference list available at ExpertConsult.com.

## KEY REFERENCES

18. Halloran PF. Immunosuppressive drugs for kidney transplantation. *N Engl J Med.* 2004;351:2715–2729.
25. Hardinger KL, Rhee S, Buchanan P, et al. A prospective, randomized, double-blinded comparison of thymoglobulin versus Atgam for induction immunosuppressive therapy: 10-year results. *Transplantation.* 2008;86:947–952.
28. Brennan DC, Schnitzler MA. Long-term results of rabbit antithymocyte globulin and basiliximab induction. *N Engl J Med.* 2008; 359:1736–1738.
30. Koyawala N, Silber JH, Rosenbaum PR, et al. Comparing outcomes between antibody induction therapies in kidney transplantation. *J Am Soc Nephrol.* 2017;28:2188–2200.
44. Nashan B, Moore R, Amlot P, et al. Randomised trial of basiliximab versus placebo for control of acute cellular rejection in renal allograft recipients. CHIB 201 International Study Group. *Lancet.* 1997;350:1193–1198.
52. Riella LV, Safa K, Yagan J, et al. Long-term outcomes of kidney transplantation across a positive complement-dependent cytotoxicity crossmatch. *Transplantation.* 2014;97:1247–1252.
55. Alasfar S, Matar D, Montgomery RA, et al. Rituximab and therapeutic plasma exchange in recurrent focal segmental glomerulosclerosis postkidney transplantation. *Transplantation.* 2018;102:e115–e120.
65. Nankivell BJ, Borrows RJ, Fung CL, et al. The natural history of chronic allograft nephropathy. *N Engl J Med.* 2003;349:2326–2333.
73. Webster AC, Woodroffe RC, Taylor RS, et al. Tacrolimus versus ciclosporin as primary immunosuppression for kidney transplant recipients: meta-analysis and meta-regression of randomised trial data. *BMJ.* 2005;331:810.
81. Gaston RS, Cecka JM, Kasiske BL, et al. Evidence for antibody-mediated injury as a major determinant of late kidney allograft failure. *Transplantation.* 2010;90:68–74.
85. Guidicelli G, Guerville F, Lepreux S, et al. Non-complement-binding de novo donor-specific anti-HLA antibodies and kidney allograft survival. *J Am Soc Nephrol.* 2016;27:615–625.

88. Knight SR, Russell NK, Barcena L, et al. Mycophenolate mofetil decreases acute rejection and may improve graft survival in renal transplant recipients when compared with azathioprine: a systematic review. *Transplantation.* 2009;87:785–794.
106. Euvrard S, Morelon E, Rostaing L, et al. Sirolimus and secondary skin-cancer prevention in kidney transplantation. *N Engl J Med.* 2012;367:329–339.
107. Pascual J, Berger SP, Witzke O, et al. Everolimus with reduced calcineurin inhibitor exposure in renal transplantation. *J Am Soc Nephrol.* 2018.
109. Vincenti F. Belatacept and long-term outcomes in kidney transplantation. *N Engl J Med.* 2016;374:2600–2601.
111. Everly MJ, Roberts M, Townsend R, et al. Comparison of De novo IgM and IgG anti-HLA DSA between Belatacept and Calcineurin Treated Patients: an Analysis of the BENEFIT and BENEFIT-EXT Trial Cohorts. *Am J Transplant.* 2018.
119. Pascual J, Zamora J, Galeano C, et al. Steroid avoidance or withdrawal for kidney transplant recipients. *Cochrane Database Syst Rev.* 2009;(1):CD005632.
125. Lefaucheur C, Loupy A, Hill GS, et al. Preexisting donor-specific HLA antibodies predict outcome in kidney transplantation. *J Am Soc Nephrol.* 2010;21:1398–1406.
130. Taber DJ, Hunt KJ, Gebregziabher M, et al. A comparative effectiveness analysis of early steroid withdrawal in black kidney transplant recipients. *Clin J Am Soc Nephrol.* 2017;12:131–139.
138. Hickey MJ, Zheng Y, Valenzuela N, et al. New priorities: analysis of the New Kidney Allocation System on UCLA patients transplanted from the deceased donor waitlist. *Hum Immunol.* 2017;78: 41–48.
151. Patel R, Terasaki PI. Significance of the positive crossmatch test in kidney transplantation. *N Engl J Med.* 1969;280:735–739.
159. Loupy A, Lefaucheur C, Vernerey D, et al. Complement-binding anti-HLA antibodies and kidney-allograft survival. *N Engl J Med.* 2013;369:1215–1226.
160. Lefaucheur C, Viglietti D, Bentlejewski C, et al. IgG donor-specific anti-human HLA antibody subclasses and kidney allograft antibody-mediated injury. *J Am Soc Nephrol.* 2016;27:293–304.
168. Perico N, Cattaneo D, Sayegh MH, et al. Delayed graft function in kidney transplantation. *Lancet.* 2004;364:1814–1827.
186. Haas M, Loupy A, Lefaucheur C, et al. The Banff 2017 Kidney Meeting Report: revised diagnostic criteria for chronic active T cell-mediated rejection, antibody-mediated rejection, and prospects for integrative endpoints for next-generation clinical trials. *Am J Transplant.* 2018;18:293–307.
188. Kasiske BL, Zeier MG, Chapman JR, et al. KDIGO clinical practice guideline for the care of kidney transplant recipients: a summary. *Kidney Int.* 2009.
198. Wan SS, Ying TD, Wyburn K, et al. The treatment of antibody-mediated rejection in kidney transplantation: an updated systematic review and meta-analysis. *Transplantation.* 2018;102:557–568.
210. Ekberg H, Tedesco-Silva H, Demirbas A, et al. Reduced exposure to calcineurin inhibitors in renal transplantation. *N Engl J Med.* 2007;357:2562–2575.
214. Suthanthiran M, Schwartz JE, Ding R, et al. Urinary-cell mRNA profile and acute cellular rejection in kidney allografts. *N Engl J Med.* 2013;369:20–31.
217. Bloom RD, Bromberg JS, Poggio ED, et al. Cell-free DNA and active rejection in kidney allografts. *J Am Soc Nephrol.* 2017;28: 2221–2232.
219. Halloran PF, Pereira AB, Chang J, et al. Microarray diagnosis of antibody-mediated rejection in kidney transplant biopsies: an international prospective study (INTERCOM). *Am J Transplant.* 2013;13:2865–2874.
228. Zuber J, Le Quintrec M, Krid S, et al. Eculizumab for atypical hemolytic uremic syndrome recurrence in renal transplantation. *Am J Transplant.* 2012;12:3337–3354.
257. Hardinger KL, Koch MJ, Bohl DJ, et al. BK-virus and the impact of pre-emptive immunosuppression reduction: 5-year results. *Am J Transplant.* 2010;10:407–415.
271. Saxena V, Khungar V, Verna EC, et al. Safety and efficacy of current direct-acting antiviral regimens in kidney and liver transplant recipients with hepatitis C: results from the HCV-TARGET study. *Hepatology.* 2017;66:1090–1101.
271. Saxena V, Khungar V, Verna EC, et al. Safety and efficacy of current direct-acting antiviral regimens in kidney and liver transplant recipients with hepatitis C: results from the HCV-TARGET study. *Hepatology.* 2017;66:1090–1101.
274. El-Zoghby ZM, Stegall MD, Lager DJ, et al. Identifying specific causes of kidney allograft loss. *Am J Transplant.* 2009;9:527–535.
276. Gupta G, Abu Jawdeh BG, Racusen LC, et al. Late antibody-mediated rejection in renal allografts: outcome after conventional and novel therapies. *Transplantation.* 2014;97:1240–1246.
278. Moreso F, Crespo M, Ruiz JC, et al. Treatment of chronic antibody mediated rejection with intravenous immunoglobulins and rituximab: a multicenter, prospective, randomized, double-blind clinical trial. *Am J Transplant.* 2018;18:927–935.
302. O'Shaughnessy MM, Liu S, Montez-Rath ME, et al. Kidney transplantation outcomes across GN subtypes in the United States. *J Am Soc Nephrol.* 2017;28:632–644.
306. Wolfe RA, Ashby VB, Milford EL, et al. Comparison of mortality in all patients on dialysis, patients on dialysis awaiting transplantation, and recipients of a first cadaveric transplant. *N Engl J Med.* 1999;341:1725–1730.
329. Rao PS, Schaubel DE, Guidinger MK, et al. A comprehensive risk quantification score for deceased donor kidneys: the kidney donor risk index. *Transplantation.* 2009;88:231–236.
330. Reeves-Daniel AM, DePalma JA, Bleyer AJ, et al. The APOL1 gene and allograft survival after kidney transplantation. *Am J Transplant.* 2011;11:1025–1030.
368. Hoorn EJ, Walsh SB, McCormick JA, et al. The calcineurin inhibitor tacrolimus activates the renal sodium chloride cotransporter to cause hypertension. *Nat Med.* 2011;17:1304–1309.
393. Hecking M, Haidinger M, Döller D, et al. Early basal insulin therapy decreases new-onset diabetes after renal transplantation. *J Am Soc Nephrol.* 2012;23:739–749.
413. Knoll GA, Fergusson D, Chassé M, et al. Ramipril versus placebo in kidney transplant patients with proteinuria: a multicentre, double-blind, randomised controlled trial. *Lancet Diabetes Endocrinol.* 2016;4:318–326.
423. Collett D, Mumford L, Banner NR, et al. Comparison of the incidence of malignancy in recipients of different types of organ: a UK Registry audit. *Am J Transplant.* 2010;10:1889–1896.
424. Engels EA, Pfeiffer RM, Fraumeni JF, et al. Spectrum of cancer risk among US solid organ transplant recipients. *JAMA.* 2011;306: 1891–1901.
434. Asberg A, Humar A, Jardine AG, et al. Long-term outcomes of CMV disease treatment with valganciclovir versus IV ganciclovir in solid organ transplant recipients. *Am J Transplant.* 2009;9:1205–1213.
446. Stock PG, Barin B, Murphy B, et al. Outcomes of kidney transplantation in HIV-infected recipients. *N Engl J Med.* 2010;363:2004–2014.
452. Deshpande NA, James NT, Kucirka LM, et al. Pregnancy outcomes in kidney transplant recipients: a systematic review and meta-analysis. *Am J Transplant.* 2011;11:2388–2404.
454. Ayus JC, Achinger SG, Lee S, et al. Transplant nephrectomy improves survival following a failed renal allograft. *J Am Soc Nephrol.* 2009;21:374–380.

# 71 Considerations in Living Kidney Donation

Ngan N. Lam | Steven Habbous | Amit X. Garg | Krista L. Lentine

## CHAPTER OUTLINE



## KEY POINTS

- The donor candidate evaluation should be completed efficiently but also comprehensively to meet the needs of the donor candidate, intended recipient, and health care system.
- Donor candidates should be provided with individualized estimates of short- and long-term risks, and risks should be considered with respect to predetermined program acceptance thresholds.
- Explicit recognition of perspectives of comparison is critical for drawing inferences about donor health outcomes (e.g., estimation of predonation risk, absolute postdonation risk, and donation-attributable risk).
- Recent studies grounded in comparison to healthy nondonor controls have identified small, donation-attributable increases in the long-term risks of kidney failure and gestational hypertension and preeclampsia in living kidney donors. This information should be shared with donor candidates.
- Simultaneous consideration of each donor candidate's profile of demographic and health characteristics advances a new framework for consistent and transparent risk assessment. New risk prediction tools are available to help apply this framework in practice.
- Accurate assessment of kidney function is central to the donor candidate evaluation and may be efficiently assessed by estimated glomerular filtration rate (GFR) screening, followed by confirmatory testing (e.g., measured GFR or creatinine clearance).
- If a donor candidate is of sub-Saharan African ancestry, testing for *APOL1* renal risk variants may be offered, and associated costs should be covered as part of the candidate evaluation. Candidates should be informed that the presence of two *APOL1* renal risk variants increases the lifetime chance of developing kidney failure even in the absence of donation; however, the effects of kidney donation on this risk are not currently known.
- Local laws and regulations on living donation must be followed and explained to donor candidates, and donor autonomy should be respected during all phases of evaluation and donation.

## INTRODUCTION

The first successful living donor kidney transplantation (LDKT) occurred on December 23, 1954, between identical twins, Ronald (donor) and Richard (recipient) Herrick.[1,2] The operation was performed by Dr. Joseph Murray at the Peter Bent Brigham Hospital in Boston and was recognized by the Nobel Prize in Medicine in 1990. Over the ensuing 60 years, advances in immunosuppression expanded opportunities for living donations from identical twins to other biologic relatives and then to unrelated persons with essentially equivalent outcomes, regardless of the donor-recipient relationship.[3,4] Opportunities for successful LDKT have expanded further over recent decades through the widespread access to laparoscopic donor nephrectomy, acceptance of donor candidates with medical complexities such as predonation hypertension, and the use of techniques to overcome immune incompatibility, such as kidney paired donation (KPD) programs.[5]

Worldwide, approximately 27,000 LDKT are performed each year.[6] Rates of LDKT vary across nations with the highest rates, per million population (pmp), in countries such as Saudi Arabia (32 pmp), Jordan (29 pmp), Iceland (26 pmp), Iran (23 pmp), and the United States (21 pmp). In many regions, the LDKT rates have increased over the last decade, with 62% of countries reporting at least a 50% increase, whereas in many other regions, rates have become stagnant or have steadily declined. Generally, LDKT represent almost 40% of all kidney transplantations performed; however, in some countries, such as Pakistan, India, Iran, and Japan, LDKT comprise over 80% of all kidney transplantations. Thus, considerations for the safe, effective, and ethical practices in living kidney donation have global significance, affecting over 90 countries worldwide.

## CONSIDERATIONS FOR THE KIDNEY TRANSPLANT RECIPIENT

For eligible patients with end-stage kidney disease (ESKD), kidney transplantation is the preferred treatment option compared with chronic dialysis because it is associated with superior long-term patient survival, improved quality of life, and lower health care costs.[7–10] Unfortunately, there is a shortage of organs to meet the need, resulting in a high proportion of patients dying while on the kidney transplant waiting list.[4] LDKT is a key strategy to help meet the growing demand for kidney transplants.

Compared with deceased donor kidney transplantation (DDKT), LDKT is also associated with superior patient and graft survival.[11] The 5-year, age-adjusted patient survival is higher for LDKT recipients (94%) than DDKT recipients (76%), and both are higher than remaining on the kidney transplant waiting list (60%).[11] Graft survival at 1, 5, and 10 years is also higher after LDKT versus DDKT (10-year graft survival, 63% vs. 47%).[4,12]

Other benefits for the recipient include the potential for preemptive transplantation or shorter waiting time until transplantation, allowing recipients to avoid or decrease the risks associated with chronic dialysis.[13,14] Furthermore, LDKT can be scheduled with advance notice at a time that works well for donors and recipients, compared with the urgent nature of DDKT. This may allow for better optimization of pretransplantation conditions prior to surgery. LDKT may provide additional opportunities for better genetic matching and a lower risk of rejection. Finally, with LDKT, the cold ischemia time is shortened, and the risk of delayed graft function is decreased. For all of these reasons, LDKT offers advantages to the recipient compared with DDKT.

Based on clear evidence of recipient benefit and surveys supporting positive public perceptions of living donation, a number of initiatives are underway to increase awareness of LDKT and reduce disincentives.[15] A 2015 American Society of Transplantation (AST) Live Donor Community of Practice consensus conference recognized LDKT as the "best treatment option" for eligible patients with kidney failure.[16] The importance of educating and supporting patients, families, and front-line renal health care providers to enable informed decisions about kidney transplantation and living kidney donation has been receiving greater attention. For example, education tools have been developed to provide individualized, risk-adjusted outcomes to help transplant candidates understand the relative benefits of LDKT and various types of DDKT compared with chronic dialysis.[17,18] Also, there have been greater efforts to support kidney patients finding living kidney donors.

## EVALUATION AND SELECTION OF THE LIVING KIDNEY DONOR CANDIDATE

The practice of LDKT is based on the principle that the benefits to the recipient (see "Considerations for the Kidney Transplant Recipient") outweigh the minimal risks to the carefully evaluated and selected living donor (see "Risks and Outcomes of Living Kidney Donation"). Living kidney donors should undergo a rigorous evaluation and selection process to ensure that the short- and long-term risks to the donor are minimized (Fig. 71.1). In addition to this, the benefits and risks to the intended recipient are also considered. From the recipient's perspective, an aim is to select donors who will provide adequate graft function while minimizing the transmission of any donor-derived diseases, such as infections or malignancy. To mitigate potential conflict of interest, it is recommended that the evaluations of the donor candidate and intended recipient be performed by separate, independent teams.[19–23] Moreover, the living donor evaluation process should be completed in a timely fashion to improve the donor candidate experience and optimize recipient outcomes.[13,14,24] One international multicenter study has reported that the median time from the beginning of the donor candidate evaluation until donor nephrectomy is 10 months.[24] Avoidable delays can lead to dialysis initiation for preemptive transplant candidates, lengthen dialysis time for patients on dialysis, and reduce donor satisfaction.[13,25] Opportunities to improve efficiency include the choice, timing, and sequence of evaluation tests and visits, use of navigators, and monitoring of evaluation timeliness as a quality metric.[26]

***Clinical Relevance***

An efficient living donor candidate evaluation is completed in as little time as possible and meets the needs of the donor candidate, intended recipient, and health care system. Avoidable delays can lead to dialysis initiation for preemptive transplant candidates, lengthen dialysis time for patients on dialysis, and reduce donor satisfaction. Opportunities to improve efficiency include the choice, timing, sequencing of evaluation tests, procedures and consults, use of navigators, and monitoring of evaluation timeliness as a quality metric.

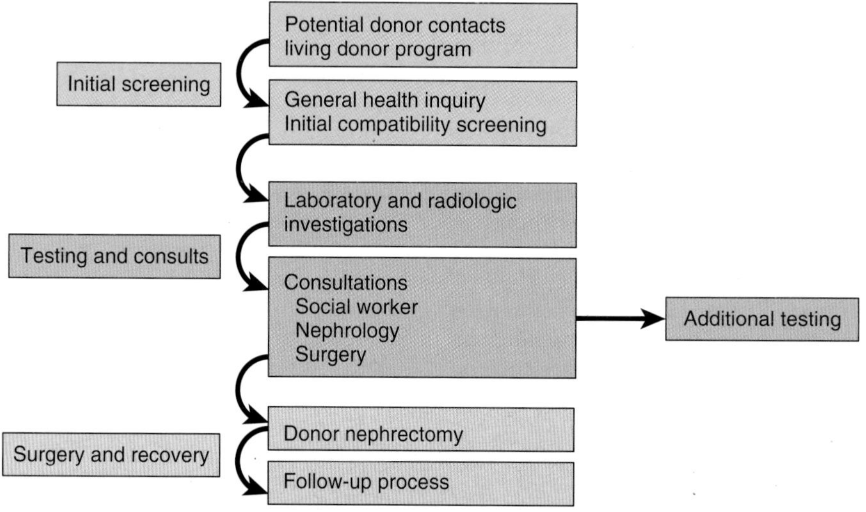


**Fig. 71.1** Overview of the living kidney donor evaluation process.

**Table 71.1 Existing Guidelines and Policies on the Evaluation of Living Kidney Donors**

| Guidelines | Year | National/ International |
|---|---|---|
| Kidney Disease: Improving Global Outcomes (KDIGO): Evaluation and Care of Living Kidney Donors[30] | 2017 | International |
| Organ Procurement and Transplantation Network (OPTN) Policy 14: Living Donation[23] | 2013<br>2015 (update) | United States |
| Kidney Paired Donation (KPD) Protocol for Participating Donors[137] | 2015 | Canada |
| European Renal Best Practice (ERBP) Guideline on Kidney Donor and Recipient Evaluation and Perioperative Care[22] | 2013 | Europe |
| British Transplantation Society (BTS): United Kingdom Guidelines for Living Donor Transplantation[21] | 2011 | United Kingdom |
| Caring for Australasians with Renal Impairment (CARI)[138] | 2010 | Australia/New Zealand |
| A Report of the Amsterdam Forum on the Care of the Live Kidney Donor: Data and Medical Guidelines[139] | 2005 | International |

Multiple guidelines have assisted clinicians in the complex process of donor evaluation and selection (Table 71.1). A systematic review of these clinical practice guidelines has found that although many recommendations were consistent, important variations exist, and many appeared to lack methodologic rigor.[27] The 2017 Kidney Disease: Improving Global Outcomes (KDIGO) "Clinical Practice Guideline on the Evaluation and Care of Living Kidney Donors" provides a comprehensive set of best practice recommendations based on a systematic evidence review, de novo evidence generation, and expert opinion when evidence is lacking.[19] When possible, the guideline recommends that transplantation programs establish numeric thresholds for short- and long-term post-donation risks, above which the program will not accept the candidate for donation (Fig. 71.2). It also demonstrates how tools can be developed to help estimate a donor candidate's risk of long-term complications such as ESKD based on their individualized set of predonation demographic and health characteristics.

A central goal of the KDIGO guideline is to promote "consistent, transparent and defensible decision-making" based on comparisons of individualized, quantitative estimates of donor risks "to a transplant program's acceptable risk threshold."[19] Risk threshold is defined as the upper limit of acceptable risk established by a program for donor candidate selection. Under this framework, when a candidate's estimated risk is above the acceptable threshold, the transplant program is justified in declining the candidate and can ground its decision in a quantitative framework. When a donor candidate's estimated risk is below the acceptable risk threshold, the transplant program should accept a donor candidate, and it should be the candidate's decision whether to proceed with living kidney donation after being informed of the risks. Once established, acceptable risk thresholds should be applied consistently and transparently for all donor candidates evaluated at a program. The KDIGO framework was informed by a systematic evidence review.[28] The KDIGO group also developed a tool to quantify a donor candidate's risk of postdonation complications such as ESKD. This tool projects the 15-year and lifetime risk of ESKD based on the level of the predonation glomerular filtration rate (GFR) and other baseline demographic and health factors.[29] For practical applications, the resulting risk models were incorporated into an online risk prediction tool (http://www.transplantmodels. com/esrdrisk). This tool serves as an example and can be improved with future research efforts for various types of living kidney donors worldwide.

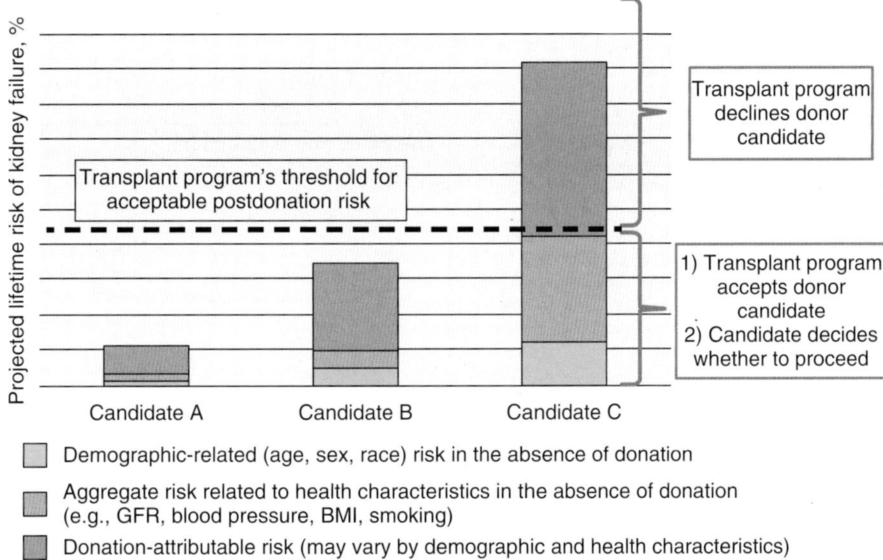


**Fig. 71.2** Kidney Disease: Improving Global Outcomes framework to accept or decline donor candidates based on a transplantation program's threshold of acceptable projected lifetime risk of kidney failure, quantified as the aggregate of risk related to demographic and health profile and donation-attributable risks. *BMI,* Body mass index; *GFR,* glomerular filtration rate. (From Lentine KL, Kasiske BL, Levey AS, et al. KDIGO clinical practice guideline on the evaluation and care of living kidney donors. *Transplantation.* 2017;101(8 Suppl 1):S7–S105.)

***Clinical Relevance***

Simultaneous consideration of each donor candidate's profile of demographic and health characteristics advances a new framework for consistent and transparent risk assessment. As demonstrations of proof of concept, online tools have been developed to estimate the risk of kidney failure in healthy persons based on 10 demographic and health traits (currently in the absence of donation), as well as postdonation risk based on a more limited set of factors. These tools can be refined and expanded with more precise risk information (e.g., risk based on longer follow-up, additional risk factors such as emerging genetic markers, and integration of predonation and postdonation risks). Estimation of risk using the best available data, and communication of risks and associated uncertainty in a manner easily understood by donor candidates, can support evidence-based donor selection and shared decision making.

The evaluation process should include a comprehensive history, physical examination, laboratory and radiologic investigations, and specialist consultations (Table 71.2). Aspects of the process may vary by region and transplantation center, including the order and timing of the components and what is considered required or additional testing. Depending on local resources and policies, transplantation programs may also choose to evaluate multiple donors for an intended recipient, either simultaneously or sequentially. The 2017 KDIGO living kidney donor guideline recommends that all donor candidates should be evaluated using the same criteria, regardless of the intended recipient.[19] Table 71.3 summarizes several contraindications to living kidney donation.

## KIDNEY FUNCTION

The purpose of evaluating GFR in kidney donor candidates is to detect kidney disease and project long-term outcomes for the candidate and the recipient should they go on to donation. Recommended methods for evaluating GFR in donor candidates are based on the 2012 KDIGO Chronic Kidney Disease (CKD) guideline.[30,31] Considering practicality, test availability, and costs, the 2017 KDIGO living donor guideline recommends an initial estimated GFR (eGFR) based on the serum creatinine level (eGFRcr) and confirmation using one or more of the following measurements according to their availability: measured GFR (mGFR) from clearance of exogenous radiolabeled filtration markers, measured creatinine clearance (mCrCl) based on collecting a timed (24-hour) urine specimen, eGFR based on serum creatinine and cystatin levels (eGFRcr-cys), or repeated eGFRcr, with the latter being the least preferred approach.[19,30,31] Although mGFR or mCrCl is required for donor evaluation in the United States according to Organ Procurement and Transplantation Network (OPTN) policy, a timed urine collection for the albumin excretion rate (AER) is not required—measurement of urine protein or albumin may be performed on a random "spot" urine sample. In countries where clearances are required for the assessment of GFR, an efficient strategy may be to omit timed urine collections and rely on the mGFR using clearance of an exogenous filtration marker and a random urine albumin-to-creatinine ratio (ACR). In countries where clearance measures are not required for the assessment of GFR, transplantation programs could obtain the eGFRcr, eGFRcr-cys, and urine ACR prior to a donor candidate's visit to the center (Fig. 71.3).[32]

An Internet-based application has been published to compute the probability of mGFR above or below clinically-appropriate thresholds based on the results of eGFR testing

**Table 71.2 Components of the Living Kidney Donor Evaluation**

| Medical and Surgical History | Examples |
|---|---|
| **Disease or Condition** | |
| Genitourinary disease | Hematuria |
| | Proteinuria |
| | Kidney stones |
| Cardiac disease | Coronary artery disease |
| | Myocardial infarction |
| | Heart failure |
| | Arrhythmia |
| Cardiac risk factors | Hypertension |
| | Impaired fasting glucose (IFG) |
| | Impaired glucose tolerance (IGT) |
| | Diabetes mellitus |
| | Hyperlipidemia |
| | Exercise tolerance |
| Peripheral vascular disease | Intermittent claudication |
| Pulmonary disease | Asthma |
| | Chronic obstructive pulmonary disease |
| | Obstructive sleep apnea |
| Gastrointestinal disease | Peptic ulcer disease |
| | Inflammatory bowel disease |
| Hematologic disease | Deep vein thrombosis |
| | Pulmonary embolism |
| | Bleeding disorders |
| | Blood transfusions |
| Neurologic disease | Stroke |
| | Parkinson disease |
| | Neurodegenerative disease |
| Autoimmune disease | Systemic lupus erythematosus |
| | Rheumatoid arthritis |
| Rheumatologic disease | Gout |
| Psychiatric conditions | Anxiety |
| | Depression |
| | Suicide attempts |
| Infections | Urinary tract infection |
| | Hepatitis B and C viruses (HBV, HCV) |
| | Human immunodeficiency virus (HIV) |
| | Syphilis |
| | Sexually transmitted infections |
| | Severe acute respiratory syndrome |
| | Meningitis, encephalitis |
| | Creutzfeldt-Jakob disease |
| | Tuberculosis |
| Cancer | Melanoma |
| | Renal cell carcinoma |
| | Breast cancer |
| | Lung cancer |
| | Colon cancer |
| | Hematologic cancer (e.g., leukemia, lymphoma) |
| | Monoclonal gammopathy |
| Pregnancy-related complications | Gestational hypertension |
| | Gestational diabetes |
| | Preeclampsia, eclampsia |
| | Future childbearing plans |
| **Allergies and Medications** | |
| Allergies | Anesthesia reactions |
| Nephrotoxic medications | Lithium |
| | Nonsteroidal antiinflammatory drugs (NSAIDs) |
| Chronic pain medications | Opioids |
| **Family History** | |
| Genitourinary disease | Alport syndrome |
| | Autosomal-dominant polycystic kidney disease (ADPKD) |
| | Kidney stones |
| Cardiac disease | Sudden cardiac death |
| | Early coronary artery disease |
| Cardiac risk factors | Hypertension |
| | Diabetes mellitus |
| Cancer | Renal cell carcinoma |
| | Breast cancer |
| | Colon cancer |
| **Social History** | |
| Smoking, alcohol, drug use | Abuse, dependency |
| | Intravenous drug use |
| Employment | Healthcare workers |
| | Veterinarians |
| Health insurance status | |
| Social supports | Marital status |
| | Living arrangements |
| Exposure history | Sexual history |
| | Tattoos |
| | Body piercings |
| | Travel or prolonged residency |
| | Country of origin, birth |
| | Incarceration |
| **Physical Examination** | |
| Vital signs | Blood pressure |
| | Heart rate and rhythm |
| | Body mass index (BMI) based on height and weight |
| Head and neck | |
| Cardiac examination | |
| Respiratory examination | |
| Abdominal examination | Prior surgeries, hernias, vascular bruits |
| Skin examination | Lymphadenopathy |
| | Mucocutaneous lesions |
| | Needle tracks |
| **Laboratory Studies** | |
| Compatibility | ABO blood group (including subtype A1, if indicated) |
| | Human leukocyte antigen (HLA) typing |
| | Crossmatch |

**Table 71.2 Components of the Living Kidney Donor Evaluation (Cont'd)**

| Medical and Surgical History | Examples |
|---|---|
| Renal | Serum creatinine level with estimation of glomerular filtration rate (eGFR)<br>Urinalysis<br>Urine microscopy<br>24-hour urine (creatinine clearance, protein excretion, metabolic stone panel,[a] including calcium, oxalate, uric acid, citric acid, sodium)<br>Protein-to-creatinine ratio (PCR)<br>Albumin-to-creatinine ratio (ACR) |
| Blood work | Complete blood count (hemoglobin, white blood cells, platelets)<br>International normalized ratio (INR)<br>Partial thromboplastin time (PTT)<br>Electrolytes (sodium, potassium, bicarbonate, calcium, phosphate, magnesium)<br>Fasting lipid profile (total cholesterol, high-density lipoprotein, low-density lipoprotein, triglycerides)<br>Pancreas enzymes (lipase, amylase)<br>Liver enzymes (aspartate aminotransferase, alanine aminotransferase, alkaline phosphatase, gamma-glutamyl transferase)<br>Bilirubin<br>Albumin<br>Uric acid<br>Thyroid function test[a]<br>Beta-human chorionic gonadotropin (β-hCG)[a] |
| Genetic renal disease[a] | Apolipoprotein L1 (*APOL1*) genotyping<br>ADPKD mutation analysis |
| Diabetes mellitus | Fasting blood glucose<br>Hemoglobin A1C<br>Oral glucose tolerance test (OGTT)[a] |
| Infection | Urine culture and sensitivity<br>Cytomegalovirus (CMV)<br>Epstein-Barr virus (EBV)<br>Hepatitis B (HBV surface antigen, HBV core antibody)<br>Hepatitis C (anti-HCV)<br>Human immunodeficiency virus (anti-HIV)<br>Human T-lymphotrophic virus (HTLV)<br>Herpes simplex virus (HSV)<br>Varicella zoster virus (VZV)<br>Treponema pallidum (syphilis)<br>*Mycobacterium tuberculosis* (purified protein derivative, interferon-gamma release assay)<br>Malaria[a]<br>*Trypanosoma cruzi*[a]<br>Schistosomiasis[a]<br>Human herpes virus (HHV8)[a]<br>Strongyloides[a]<br>Typhoid[a]<br>Brucellosis[a]<br>West Nile virus[a]<br>Zika virus[a]<br>Chagas disease[a]<br>Toxoplasmosis[a] |
| Cancer screening | Urine cytology<br>Fecal occult blood test (FOBT)<br>Fecal immunochemical test (FIT)[a]<br>Colonoscopy[a]<br>Prostate-specific antigen (PSA)[a]<br>Pap smear[a] |
| **Radiologic Studies** | |
| Renal system | Abdominal computed tomography (CTA) or magnetic resonance angiography (MRA)<br>Measured glomerular filtration rate (mGFR: iothalamate, ethylenediaminetetraacetic acid [EDTA], diethylenetriaminepentaacetic acid [DTPA])<br>Cystoscopy[a]<br>Renal biopsy[a] |
| Cardiac system | Electrocardiography<br>24-hour Holter monitor[a]<br>24-hour ambulatory blood pressure monitor (ABPM)[a]<br>Echocardiography[a]<br>Non-invasive myocardial perfusion study (exercise or pharmacological stress)<br>Coronary angiography[a] |
| Pulmonary system | Chest x-ray<br>Pulmonary function test (PFT)[a] |
| Cancer screening | Mammography[a]<br>Low-dose chest computed tomography (CT)[a] |
| **Specialist Consultation** | |
| Psychosocial specialist | Social worker<br>Psychologist<br>Psychiatrist |
| Nephrologist | |
| Surgeon | |
| Other specialists[a] | Cardiology<br>Infectious disease<br>Dietitian |

[a]If indicated, based on the donor demographic, history, physical examination, and/or laboratory or radiologic studies.

**Table 71.3 Contraindications to Living Kidney Donation**

| Absolute Contraindications | Relative Contraindications |
|---|---|
| • Both <18 years old and mentally incapable of making an informed decision<br>• High suspicion of donor coercion<br>• High suspicion of illegal financial exchange between donor and recipient<br>• ABO or HLA incompatibility, without a planned management protocol<br>• Impaired kidney function (e.g., eGFR <60 mL/min/1.73 m$^2$)<br>• Proteinuria (>300 mg/day)<br>• Diagnosis of IgA nephropathy or Alport syndrome<br>• Bilateral, recurrent kidney stones<br>• Uncontrolled hypertension or hypertension with evidence of end-organ damage<br>• Type 1 diabetes mellitus<br>• Acute symptomatic infection (until resolved)<br>• Chronic infection, without a management plan for donor and recipient<br>• Active cancer or incompletely treated cancer<br>• History of melanoma, testicular cancer, choriocarcinoma, hematologic cancer, monoclonal gammopathy, bronchial cancer, metastatic cancer<br>• Current pregnancy<br>• Uncontrolled psychiatric illness | • Two *APOL1* renal risk variants<br>• Chronic illness (cardiac, pulmonary, gastrointestinal, neurologic)<br>• Type 2 diabetes mellitus<br>• Morbid obesity (e.g., BMI >35 mg/m$^2$)<br>• Active substance use disorder |

Modified from Lentine KL, Kasiske BL, Levey AS, et al. KDIGO clinical practice guideline on the evaluation and care of living kidney donors. *Transplantation*. 2017;101(8S Suppl 1):S7–S105; and Organ Procurement and Transplantation/United Network for Organ Sharing (OPTN/UNOS). Policies. https://optn.transplant.hrsa.gov/media/1200/optn_policies.pdf# nameddest=Policy_14.

(http://ckdepi.org/equations/donor-candidate-gfr-calculator). The algorithm was based on demographic characteristics obtained from the National Health and Nutrition Examination Survey (NHANES) and the test performance of eGFR (categoric likelihood ratios) from the CKD Epidemiology Collaboration.[33] The algorithm can be applied to living donor candidates and has been tested in a French cohort of 311 living donor candidates.[34] If there is a high probability that the mGFR is greater than a threshold needed for donation, and if the urine ACR is low, these tests could be repeated for confirmation without mGFR, mCrCl, or timed AER.[35] Alternatively, donor candidates with a high probability of the mGFR less than 60 mL/min/1.73 m$^2$ or high urine ACR could be reliably excluded from donation, with any additional testing for the purposes of caring for the candidate's long-term health. Donor candidates with the eGFR or urine ACR in intermediate ranges would require confirmatory tests with mGFR, mCrCl, and/or urine AER. Determining the eGFR and urine ACR in advance of a visit to the transplantation center allows planning for confirmatory tests with fewer visits to the center.

The physiologic renal adaptive response to nephrectomy in the donor is reviewed elsewhere.[36] Nephrectomy in a healthy donor (removal of 50% of the nephron mass) is associated with a fairly consistent adaptive increase of the remaining kidney's GFR such that the postdonation GFR is around 60% to 70% of the predonation value.[36] This information is relevant in considering an acceptable baseline predonation GFR. The 2017 KDIGO living kidney donor guideline recommends a GFR of 90 mL/min/1.73 m$^2$ or higher as an acceptable level of kidney function for donation; donor candidates with a GFR less than 60 mL/min/1.73 m$^2$ should not donate. The decision to approve donor candidates with a GFR of 60 to 89 mL/min/1.73 m$^2$ should be individualized based on their demographic and health profile (see Fig. 71.3).

## ALBUMINURIA

Elevated protein in the urine (proteinuria) may suggest the presence or risk of developing kidney disease due to increased permeability of the glomeruli to protein and/or an inability of the renal tubules to reabsorb protein. Until acceptable standardization methods are available for quantifying deficiencies in tubular reabsorption, the urine albumin level remains the most reliable indicator of kidney disease, standardized to urinary creatinine as the ACR. The 2017 KDIGO living kidney donor guideline recommends an initial evaluation using the urine ACR in a random urine specimen, with confirmation by AER (from a timed urine specimen) or otherwise a second random urine ACR. Donor candidates with an AER more than 100 mg/day (or ACR >30 mg/mmol) should not donate. Such candidates have microalbuminuria and are at an elevated risk of developing CKD in their lifetime.[37] Candidates with an AER less than 30 mg/day (or ACR <3 mg/mmol or below the detectable limit of the assay) may be acceptable for donation; the decision to approve donor candidates with an AER of 30 to 100 mg/day should be individualized based on their demographic and health profiles in relationship to the transplantation program's acceptable risk threshold.

## HEMATURIA

Persistent blood in the urine (hematuria) is another indicator for the presence or risk of developing kidney disease. The presence of hematuria is established by visualizing 2 to 5 red blood cells/high-powered field on microscopic evaluation. "Persistence" is established if hematuria is observed in more than 50% of urine samples obtained on two or three occasions. When hematuria is persistent, further investigation is warranted, which many include urine culture for

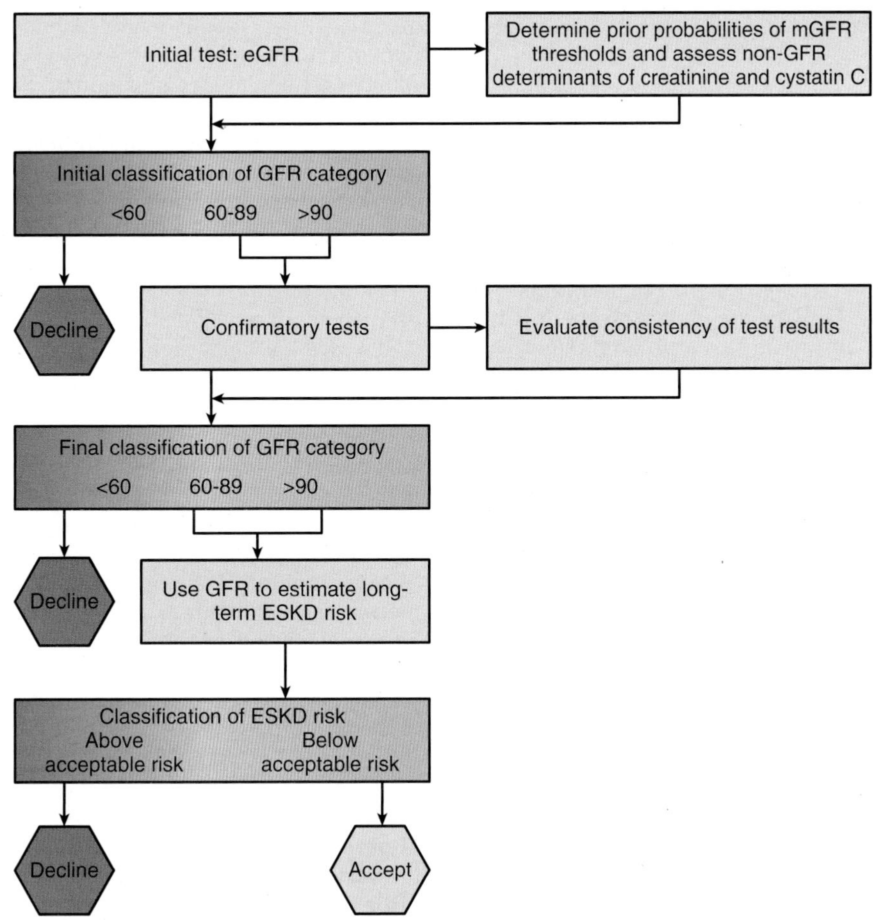


**Fig. 71.3** Assessment of glomerular filtration rate. *Initial test,* eGFRcr is the initial test in most candidates. eGFRcys may be the preferred initial test for candidates with variations in non-GFR determinants of serum creatinine—for example, variation in muscle mass or diet. Interpretation of eGFR should include consideration of the probability that mGFR is above or below the threshold for decision making (http://ckdepi.org/equations/donor-candidate-gfr-calculator). A high likelihood that eGFR less than 60 mL/min/1.73 $m^2$ is justification for a decision to decline without further consideration. *Confirmatory tests,* mGFR or mCrCl is required in the United States. Elsewhere, eGFRcr-cys can be acceptable if mGFR or mCrCl is not available and eGFRcys was not used as the initial test. Repeat eGFRcr can be acceptable if none of the other confirmatory tests are available, but is not preferred. Inconsistent test results suggest inaccuracy of one or more tests, which should be discarded or repeated. Very high likelihood that mGFR less than 60 mL/min/1.73 $m^2$ is justification for a decision to decline without further consideration. *Use GFR to estimate long-term ESKD risk,* Long-term estimated risk of ESKD is compared with the transplantation center's threshold for acceptable risk. Long-term risk in the absence of donation can be computed from demographic and clinical characteristics, including the GFR (http://www.transplantmodels.com/esrdrisk). Additional risk attributable to donation is likely to be 3.5 to 5.2 times higher than risk in the absence of donation, but there is substantial uncertainty, especially in younger donor candidates, and we suggest caution in decision making. Postdonation risk above the threshold is justification for a decision to decline. Candidates with risk below the threshold are acceptable to make their own decision about whether to donate. Colors are blended together to signify that the threshold for decision making is imprecise. *eGFR,* estimated glomerular filtration rate; *eGFRcr,* estimated glomerular filtration rate based on serum creatinine; *eGFRcr-cys,* estimated glomerular filtration rate based on serum creatinine and cystatin C; *eGFRcys,* estimated glomerular filtration rate based on cystatin C; *ESKD,* end-stage kidney disease; *GFR,* glomerular filtration rate; *mCrCl,* measured creatinine clearance; *mGFR,* measured glomerular filtration rate.

bacterial or fungal infection (this may be treated without affecting candidacy), 24-hour urine stone panel, cystoscopy, imaging to rule out a urinary tract malignancy, and a kidney biopsy to rule out underlying kidney disease (a thin basement membrane may not be a contraindication to donation).[38,39]

## KIDNEY STONES

A renal calculus in the donor's remaining kidney may affect kidney function if it results in ureteral obstruction. Reassuringly, living kidney donors do not appear to have an increased risk of kidney stones requiring treatment with surgical intervention compared with healthy, matched nondonor controls (median follow-up, 8 years).[40] Evaluation of kidney stones in living kidney donor candidates includes a history from the candidate, laboratory investigations, including urine samples for evaluation of persistent microscopic hematuria, and renal imaging, such as computed tomography (CT). If suspected, further investigations may be performed, including parathyroid hormone measurements and 24-hour urine collections for metabolic testing. A history of previous stones does not necessarily rule out donation, particularly small, unilateral, nonrecurrent stones.[19] There is also the option to remove small kidney stones at the time of procurement prior to transplantation.[41]

## HYPERURICEMIA, GOUT, AND METABOLIC BONE DISEASE

Compared with nondonor controls, living kidney donors have an increased risk of gout (3.4% vs. 2.0%) after a median of 8 years after donation.[42] This may be due to the reduced ability of a single kidney to excrete excess uric acid, a precursor to gout. Although a comprehensive gout assessment is not usually conducted for all candidates, a predonation serum urate level is frequently ordered, as well as other biochemical indicators of metabolic kidney disease, including inorganic phosphate, calcium, and parathyroid hormone levels. A living kidney donor nephrectomy may lower the concentrations of 1,25-dihydroxyvitamin D and phosphate and raise the concentration of parathyroid hormone, with no appreciable effect on the concentration of calcium. Whether these changes in bone mineral metabolism alter skeletal fracture risk in living kidney donors is unknown. To date, a single study of over 2000 living kidney donors (median age, 43 years) matched to a segment of the general population selected for good health found that after a median follow-up of 7 years (maximum, 18 years), the rate of fragility (osteoporotic) fractures was no higher in donors compared with nondonors.[43]

## BLOOD PRESSURE

Sustained elevated blood pressure is a common cause of kidney disease and, conversely, kidney disease may accelerate the development of high blood pressure. Candidates with hypertension are eligible for donation only if their blood pressure can be controlled with antihypertensive medications and they are without end-organ damage related to their hypertension.[19] The systolic and/or diastolic blood pressure thresholds and the nature of the antihypertensive medications used (e.g., number of agents, class of drugs, dosage used) to disqualify a candidate may vary across programs and according to other candidate characteristics. Trained personnel should perform blood pressure measurements on at least two separate occasions. An ambulatory (e.g., 24-hour) blood pressure monitor may be used if hypertension is suspected. Donor candidates with hypertension that can be controlled to less than 140/90 mm Hg using one or two antihypertensive agents, and who do not have evidence of target organ damage, may be acceptable for donation. The decision to approve donation in persons with hypertension should be individualized based on their demographic and health profiles in relationship to the transplantation program's acceptance risk threshold.

## METABOLIC AND LIFESTYLE RISK FACTORS

Obesity is a strong risk factor for diabetes mellitus, cardiovascular disease, and kidney disease.[44] Living donor nephrectomy is more difficult for patients with excess visceral fat, increasing the risk of perioperative complications, including infection, blood loss, and delayed wound healing.[45] Various body mass index (BMI) cut points have been reported in the literature as absolute or relative contraindications to donation. Elevated serum glucose levels or glucose intolerance are also strong risk factors for diabetes mellitus. Apart from personal and family history assessments of diabetes mellitus (childhood, adult-onset, gestational), glycosylated hemoglobin and serum and urinary glucose levels are typically measured early in the assessment of all candidates. Fasting glucose and oral glucose tolerance tests are recommended for high-risk candidates (e.g., high random glucose, positive family history). According to the 2017 KDIGO living kidney donor guideline, donor candidates with type 1 diabetes mellitus should not donate. The decision to approve donor candidates with prediabetes or type 2 diabetes mellitus should be individualized based on their demographic and health profiles in relationship to the transplantation program's acceptance threshold. Donor candidates with prediabetes and type 2 diabetes mellitus should be counseled that their condition may progress over time and may lead to end-organ complications.[19] Less evidence is available to comment on the influence of predonation lipid levels (e.g., cholesterol, triglycerides, high-density and low-density lipoproteins) and smoking on donor candidacy although, notably, smoking was a strong risk factor for ESKD in healthy persons.[29] Candidates should be educated and encouraged to modify their dietary and smoking habits, but eligibility based on these factors may vary across programs. Smoking should be considered as part of a comprehensive risk assessment.

## SCREENING FOR TRANSMISSIBLE INFECTIONS

To reduce the risk of viral transmission from the donor to the recipient, the evaluation should include assessment of prior history of infections, recent travel history, and virology screens early in the evaluation—and again within the 2 to 4 weeks of donation to minimize the window of infection.[46] The 2017 KDIGO living kidney donor guideline recommends screening for human immunodeficiency virus, hepatitis B and C, Epstein-Barr virus, cytomegalovirus, syphilis, urinary tract infection, and other potential infections based on geography and environmental exposures.[19] If a donor candidate is found to have a potentially transmissible infection, the donor candidate, intended recipient, and transplantation team should weigh the risks and benefits of proceeding with donation and develop a management plan if the decision is made to proceed with donation.

## CANCER SCREENING

All candidates should be up to date with local cancer screening guidelines according to age, gender, and family history. Donors with active cancer are generally not eligible to donate. Donors with a prior history of successfully treated cancer with a high risk of recurrence may be excluded from donation because antineoplastic agents may be nephrotoxic and transmission of cancer from the donor to the recipient can have serious consequences for the immunocompromised recipient.[47] Candidates with a prior history of cancer with a low risk of recurrence may be considered on an individual basis. In some cases, candidates with small renal tumors (high-grade Bosniak renal cysts [III or higher] or small [T1a] renal cell carcinoma curable by nephrectomy) may be acceptable for donation, and the donor and recipient provide consent for the cancer to be resected at the time of donor nephrectomy.[48,49]

## GENETIC KIDNEY DISEASES

If the donor candidate is biologically related to the intended recipient, the cause of the recipient's kidney disease should be well understood before accepting the candidate. Candidates with a genetic kidney disease generally are not eligible to become donors. If a candidate has a family history of a genetic kidney disease, the candidate may be eligible to donate if the risk of developing kidney disease after donation is acceptably low, and the risks are discussed with the candidate. Genetic diseases that may be assessed during the donor candidate evaluation include autosomal dominant polycystic kidney disease, *APOL1*-related kidney disease, atypical hemolytic uremic syndrome, Alport syndrome, Fabry disease, familial focal segmental glomerulosclerosis, and autosomal dominant tubulointerstitial kidney disease. If a donor candidate is of sub-Saharan African ancestry, testing for *APOL1* renal risk variants may be offered.[50,51] The presence of two *APOL1* renal risk variants increases the lifetime chance of developing kidney failure, even in the absence of donation. The effects of kidney donation on this risk are unknown but are a topic of active research including in the national '*APOL1* Long-Term Outcomes' (APOLLO) and "Living Donor Extended Time Outcomes" (LETO) studies in the United States.

## PREGNANCY

Although donation does not preclude future pregnancy and childbearing, candidates are not evaluated and/or do not donate while they are pregnant. A history of hypertensive disorders related to pregnancy (e.g., preeclampsia, gestational hypertension) increase the risk of developing kidney failure later in life, and the severity, timing, and frequency of these conditions should be considered before determining the potential donor's candidacy. The risk of adverse outcomes in subsequent pregnancies after kidney donation is increased, as discussed later (see "Maternal and Fetal Complications").

## PSYCHOSOCIAL ASSESSMENT

The 2017 KDIGO living kidney donor guideline recommends that a psychosocial assessment be conducted for all donors (regardless of relationship with the intended recipient), in the absence of the intended recipient (to reliably assess voluntariness), and by a professional who is not involved with the care of the intended recipient. A thorough psychosocial assessment should minimize the incidence of poor psychosocial outcomes postdonation by careful selection or treatment (e.g., counseling).[52] Quality of life is generally positive postdonation, but there have been cases of regret, depression, and financial hardships.[53,54]

# KIDNEY PAIRED DONATION AND INCOMPATIBLE LIVING DONOR TRANSPLANTS

Unintended ABO-incompatible transplants should be avoided, with duplicate blood typing of both the donor and intended recipient. If the intended recipient has anti-A antibodies and the donor candidate has A-type blood, the A subtype should be determined to establish compatibility instead of ruling it out at this stage (e.g., an A-type donor may donate to an O-type recipient if the donor is of the non-A1 subtype). Donor candidates and the intended recipient should also undergo allelotyping for human leukocyte antigen (HLA) types A, B, C, DP, DQ, and DR. The presence and strength of donor-specific anti-HLA antibodies should also be measured in the recipient; these are in addition to complement-dependent cytotoxicity or flow cytometry crossmatching and Luminex assays to determine the history of sensitization. If the intended recipient develops donor-specific, anti-HLA antibodies between the time of the initial crossmatch and donation (e.g., acquired by viral infections, pregnancy, or blood transfusion), a final crossmatch is required before donation.

For incompatible pairs, candidates should be informed of the availability, risks, and benefits of KPD, incompatibility management strategies, and waiting for a suitable deceased donor. The emergence of KPD, together with logistical advances (e.g., coordinating multiway exchanges, shipping organs rather than the donor), has increased the potential for KPD to substantially increase the number of living donor transplants performed.[55,56] Some programs even permit compatible donors to participate in KPD if they choose to wait for a living donor who is younger or has fewer donor-specific antibodies.[57]

# DONOR NEPHRECTOMY APPROACHES

The surgical approach to donor nephrectomy is based on the surgeon's experience, as well as the donor's history, physical examination, renal anatomy and function, and personal preference. Following an uncomplicated donor nephrectomy, most donors can expect to spend 2 to 7 days in hospital and return to work in 4 to 9 weeks.[58]

## LAPAROSCOPIC VERSUS OPEN DONOR NEPHRECTOMY

Laparoscopic donor nephrectomy has replaced the open technique as the standard of care, with the laparoscopic approach accounting for more than 90% of all living donor nephrectomies performed in the United States.[4,5] The conversion rate from laparoscopic to open donor nephrectomy ranges from 1% to 1.8%.[59] The average operative time for laparoscopic nephrectomy is longer compared with open nephrectomy (3–4 hours vs. 2–3 hours) and is associated with increased warm ischemia time (mean difference, 1.8 minutes; range, 2–17 minutes).[58,59] It is also associated with less perioperative blood loss (mean difference, −99.6 mL) and reduced postoperative pain and analgesic use.[58,59] Compared with open nephrectomy, the laparoscopic approach has other advantages, including shorter hospital stay (mean difference, −1.3 days), faster return to work (mean difference, −16.4 days), and improved cosmetic appearance due to the smaller incisions.[58] Thus, laparoscopic nephrectomy offers reduced surgical risk, pain, and cost, with no difference in ureteric complications, reoperations, delayed graft function, acute rejection, 1-year graft function, and early graft loss or 1-year graft loss.[59] Advances in surgical techniques, including the use of hand-assisted laparoscopic donor nephrectomy, aim to improve these donor experiences and outcomes. By doing so, potential donors, including older donors, may be more willing to undergo nephrectomy.[60]

## LEFT VERSUS RIGHT DONOR NEPHRECTOMY

The laterality of donor nephrectomy may be influenced by anatomic or functional factors. Multiple renal arteries, unilaterally or bilaterally, may be technically more complicated or may increase the risk of dissection and bleeding. Structural abnormalities, such as the presence of renal cysts or calculi, may result in the removal of the affected kidney, with or without additional bench excision, leaving the donor with the unaffected kidney. Similarly, for donors with significant differences in split kidney function (>55% vs. <45%), the recommendation is to leave the donor the kidney with better function.[19]

Beyond these considerations, left nephrectomy is generally preferred because it is technically easier due to the longer left renal vein compared with the right.[19,61] A systematic review and meta-analysis has found that compared with right laparoscopic donor nephrectomy, there is less delayed graft function and thrombosis with left laparoscopic donor nephrectomy.[62] However, there was no significant difference in other surgical outcomes, including operative times, blood loss, warm ischemia time, and length of stay.

# LIVING KIDNEY DONOR FOLLOW-UP

When the first living kidney donor, Ronald Herrick, completed his initial donor evaluation, he asked his surgeon whether the hospital would be responsible for his health care after donation.[1] The surgeon replied, "Ronald, do you think anyone in this room would ever refuse to take care of you if you needed help?" Since then, postdonation follow-up care continues to be an important consideration for living kidney donors.[63] A personalized plan for early- and long-term living kidney donor follow-up care should be discussed during the evaluation process.[19,64] This follow-up care plan may outline the timing and frequency of visits, as well as who will be providing the follow-up care (primary care provider vs. transplantation center). Early follow-up care (within 3–6 months) is routinely done, usually by the surgical team, as part of the postoperative care plan.[65]

The 2017 KDIGO living kidney donor guideline recommends lifelong annual assessment of kidney health, including blood pressure measurement, serum creatinine level testing for eGFR, and urine sample for albuminuria.[19] Currently, it is unclear how frequently living kidney donors are receiving follow-up care. In 2013, the United Network for Organ Sharing implemented mandatory reporting of clinical and laboratory data for living kidney donors at 6, 12, and 24 months after donation by the transplantation centers to the national transplant registry.[66] Although this led to improved rates of timely and complete donor follow-up data collection across the United States (from 33% prepolicy to 54% postpolicy), 43% of centers still did not meet the mandatory reporting threshold by 2015.[67,68] Donor follow-up data beyond 2 years, when medical conditions are more likely to develop, is not currently mandated in the United States.[69,70] Follow-up care at 1, 5, 10, and 15 years in Norway is achieved by 99%, 95%, 84%, and 77% of donors, respectively.[19] In a retrospective Canadian study of 534 living kidney donors from a single province, with a median follow-up of 6.5 years (maximum, 12.5 years), 25% of donors had all three markers of care—physician visit, serum creatinine level, albuminuria testing—performed on an annual basis.[71] The adherence to physician visits was higher than serum creatinine level or albuminuria testing (Fig. 71.4).

Unfortunately, there are barriers to follow-up for living kidney donors, including sociodemographic and geographic factors, perception of unnecessary need for follow-up due to excellent donor health, outdated donor contact information, cost of follow-up to the donor, and time constraints.[65,72–74] Donor factors associated with lack of follow-up includes younger age, black ethnicity, lack of insurance, lower educational attainment, and greater distance from the transplantation center.[67,75] Available resources and personnel may also limit monitoring by transplantation centers. Currently, there are no data to support the clinical and cost-effectiveness of lifelong follow-up of an otherwise healthy population. In addition to this, instead of providing reassurance of donor well-being, obligatory follow-up care may burden donors or give them an undue sense of concern about their health.[72]

However, there are numerous reasons to ensure adequate long-term follow-up care for living kidney donors. It allows the health care team to remain invested in the medical and psychosocial well-being of donors who have undergone an altruistic act for the benefit of another. Follow-up care may result in prevention, early detection, and treatment of diseases, particularly those associated with reduced kidney function and its complications. It also provides an opportunity to document medical and surgical complications that may be attributed to donation. This information can be used to develop interventions to mitigate these risks and can also improve the informed consent process for future living kidney donors. Follow-up care may also improve the living donor experience.[76] Lastly, ongoing follow-up care allows the health care team to update and educate prior donors on relevant outcomes as new research arises.

Recognizing the importance of living donor follow-up, the European Living Donation and Public Health project has mandated living donor registration and follow-up data collection through a centralized donor database.[77] In the United States, the Health Resources and Services Administration asked the Scientific Registry of Transplant Recipients (SRTR) to establish a national scientific registry for living donors, the Living Donor Collective.[78] This registry aims to collect follow-up data on living donors, including living donor candidates who undergo the evaluation process, but do not end up donating. Through staff contact and novel data linkages, the registry seeks to promote lifelong living donor follow-up.

Despite challenges in achieving it, most transplantation centers believe that living donor follow-up is a high priority and could mitigate adverse outcomes.[64] The transplant community has an obligation to promote the integrity, quality, and safety of the donation and transplantation system.[19] In doing so, transplantation programs may improve patient satisfaction and trust with the donation process, which could lead to increased rates of LDKT.

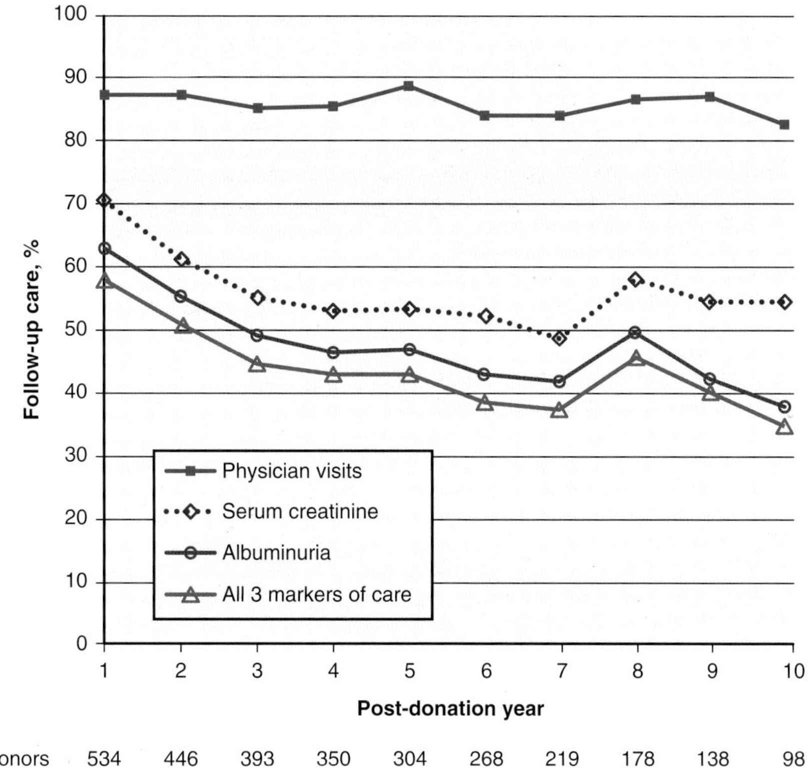


| # of donors | 534 | 446 | 393 | 350 | 304 | 268 | 219 | 178 | 138 | 98 |
|---|---|---|---|---|---|---|---|---|---|---|

**Fig. 71.4** Proportion of donors who have evidence of follow-up care during each postdonation year. (From Lam NN, Lentine KL, Hemmelgarn B, et al. Follow-up care of living kidney donors in Alberta, Canada. *Can J Kidney Health Dis.* 2018;5:1–11.)

## RISKS AND OUTCOMES OF LIVING KIDNEY DONATION

Although most living kidney donors will not experience major morbidity or mortality after donation, donation does carry some risk of surgical, medical, and psychosocial complications.[69] Unfortunately, comprehensive data on long-term outcomes for living kidney donors are limited due to single-center studies with small sample sizes, insufficient power to quantify rare events, significant missing data or data lost to follow-up, short duration of follow-up, lack of donor diversity in race, ethnicity, and comorbidities, and lack of a comparable control group.[72,73,78–80] Living kidney donors are carefully selected following a rigorous evaluation process (see "Evaluation and Selection of the Living Kidney Donor Candidate") and, as a result are inherently healthier than the general population. Comparing outcomes in donors with nondonors selected for comparable baseline health offers a perspective of risk that can better capture the attributable risk of donation (Fig. 71.5).[19,80] In addition to this, the characteristics of living kidney donors have evolved over time. Transplantation programs are now accepting donors who are older, with more comorbidities, including hypertension and obesity.[81] Such practices are defensible if the risks, based on the candidate's demographic and health profiles, are acceptably low. Ongoing work is needed to capture and quantify risks in groups with less aggregate follow-up to date, such as ethnic minorities and medically complex donors.[72,81]

> *Clinical Relevance*
>
> Explicit recognition of perspectives of comparison is critical for drawing inferences about donor health outcomes (e.g., estimation of predonation risk, absolute postdonation risk, and donation-attributable risk). Recent studies grounded in comparison to healthy nondonor controls have identified small, donation-attributable increases in the long-term risks of kidney failure and gestational hypertension and preeclampsia in living kidney donors. These observations emphasize the need for careful donor candidate evaluation, selection, and informed consent. Donor candidates should have adequate time to consider the information provided to them during the evaluation process, although the duration of adequate time is not well defined and may vary according to donor characteristics. Ongoing efforts to develop best practices for the disclosure of donor risks and verification of comprehension are important research priorities.

### PERIOPERATIVE MORTALITY AND COMPLICATIONS

In a study of 80,347 living kidney donors in the United States from 1994 to 2009, the 90-day surgical mortality rate was 3.1/10,000 donors.[82] This rate was higher in men than in women (5.1 vs. 1.7/10,000 donors; risk ratio, 3.0), in black

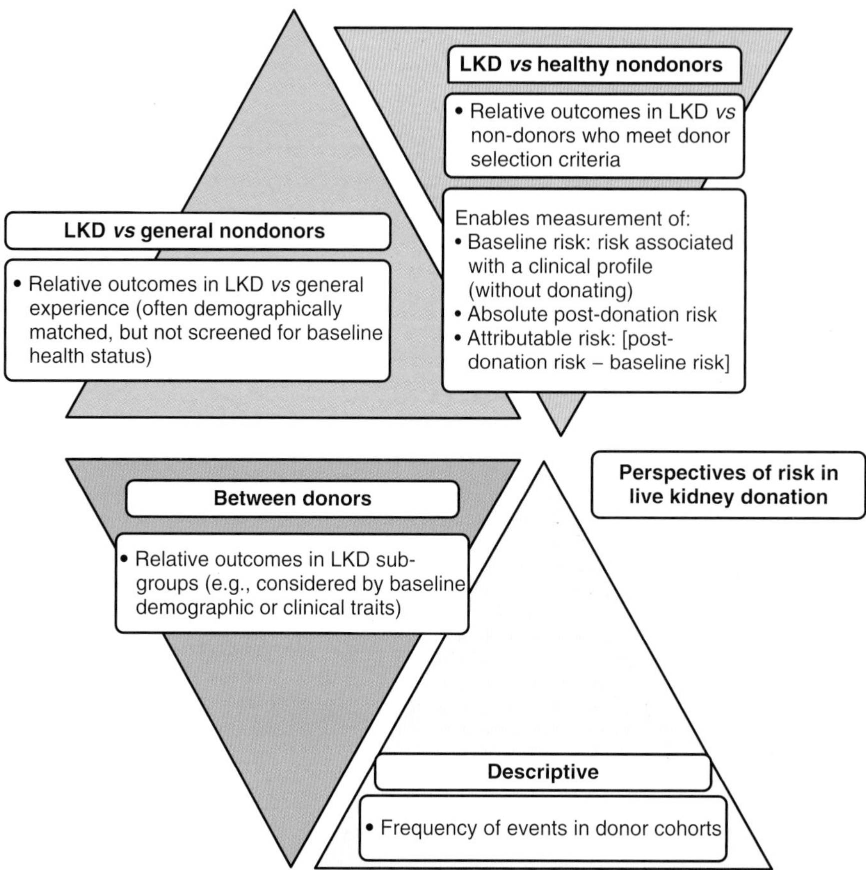


**Fig. 71.5** Perspectives of risk in living kidney donation *(LKD).* (Modified from Lentine KL, Kasiske BL, Levey AS, et al. KDIGO clinical practice guideline on the evaluation and care of living kidney donors. *Transplantation*. 2017;101(8 Suppl 1):S7–S105; and Lentine KL, Segev DL. Understanding and communicating medical risks for living kidney donors: a matter of perspective. *J Am Soc Nephrol.* 2017;28(1):12–24.)

versus white and Hispanic donors (7.6 vs. 2.6 and 2.0/10,000 donors; risk ratio, 3.1), and in donors with hypertension versus those without (36.7 vs. 1.3/10,000 donors; risk ratio, 27.4). In comparison, the 90-day surgical mortality following donor nephrectomy was much lower compared with laparoscopic cholecystectomy (18/10,000 cases) and nondonor nephrectomy (260/10,000 cases).[83,84]

The incidence of perioperative morbidity has been reported to be 18% to 22% for minor complications and less than 3% to 6% for major complications.[80,81,85–88] A study integrating national donor registry data in the United States from 2008 to 2012 with administrative records from a consortium of 98 academic hospitals found that 16.8% of living kidney donors ($n$=14,964) experienced a perioperative complication, usually gastrointestinal (4.4%), bleeding (3.0%), respiratory (2.5%), and surgical and anesthesia-related injuries (2.4%).[85] Major complications, defined as Clavien severity level 4 or 5, were identified in 2.5% of donors. After adjustment for demographic, clinical (including comorbidities), procedural, and center factors, compared with white donors, black donors had significantly higher risks of experiencing any complication (18.2% vs. 15.5%) and of experiencing major complications (3.7% vs. 2.2%). Other significant correlates of major complications included obesity, predonation blood disorders, psychiatric conditions, and robotic nephrectomy, whereas greater annual hospital volume predicted lower risk. Another study has reported that procedure-related complications were similar for living donor nephrectomies, as they were for cholecystectomies or appendectomies, and all were significantly lower than nondonor nephrectomies.[81]

## LONG-TERM MORTALITY

A meta-analysis of 19 studies involving 8098 living kidney donors has reported that the pooled mortality is 3.8%.[89] The risk of all-cause mortality is lower in living kidney donors compared with the general population, likely due to the rigorous evaluation and selection process.[90–93] When compared with age- and comorbidity-matched participants in the third National Health and Nutrition Examination Survey (NHANES), Segev and associates reported that the long-term mortality for living kidney donors in the United States, after a median follow-up of 6 years, was similar or lower, even when stratified by age, gender, and race (Table 71.4).[82] One study from Norway has reported that in the first decade of follow-up, the risk of all-cause mortality is similar in donors ($n$=1901) compared with healthy matched nondonors from the Health Study of Nord Trøndelag ($n$=32,621); however, at 25 years of follow-up, the cumulative incidence of all-cause mortality was higher in donors compared with nondonors (~18% vs. ~13%; adjusted hazard ratio [HR], 1.3; 95% confidence interval [CI], 1.1–1.5).[70] The most common cause

**Table 71.4 Long-Term Medical Outcomes in Living Kidney Donors Compared With Selected Healthy Controls**

| Reference | Living Kidney Donors (n) | Healthy Matched Nondonors (n) | Median Donor Follow-up Time (years) | Donor Age at Donation (years)[a] | No. of Donor Events (%) [Event Rate] | No. of Healthy Nondonor Events (%) [Event Rate] | Event Rate Hazard Ratio (95% Confidence Interval) | *P* Value |
|---|---|---|---|---|---|---|---|---|
| **End-Stage Kidney Disease** | | | | | | | | |
| Mjøen[70] | 1901 | 32,621[b] | 15.1 | 46 (11) | 9 (0.47%) | 22 (0.067%) | 11.38 (4.37–29.63) | *P* < .001 |
| Muzaale[115] | 96,217 | 96,217 | 7.6 | 40 (11) | 99 (0.10%) [30.8/10,000] | 36 (0.037%) [3.9/10,000] | — | *P* < .001 |
| **Acute Kidney Injury Treated With Dialysis** | | | | | | | | |
| Lam[140] | 2027 | 20,270 | 6.6 | 43 [34–50] | 1 (0.05%) [6.5/100,000] | 14 (0.07%) [9.4/100,000] | 0.58 (0.08–4.47) | *P* = .61 |
| **All-Cause Mortality** | | | | | | | | |
| Mjøen[70] | 1901 | 32,621 | 15.1 | 46 (11) | 224 (11.8%) | 2425 (7.4%) | 1.30 (1.11–1.52) | *P* = .001 |
| Segev[82] | 80,347 | 80,347 | 6.3 | — | –(1.5%) | –(2.9%) | — | *P* < .001 |
| Reese[141] | 3368 | 3368 | 7.8 | 59 (–) | 115 (3.4%) [4.9/1000] | 152 (4.5%) [5.6/1000] | 0.90 (0.71–1.15) | *P* = .21 |
| **Cardiovascular Mortality** | | | | | | | | |
| Mjøen[70] | 1901 | 32,621 | 15.1 | 46 (11) | 68 (3.6%) | 688 (2.1%) | 1.40 (1.03–1.91) | *P* = .03 |
| **Death or Cardiovascular Event** | | | | | | | | |
| Reese[141] | 1312 | 1312 | — | 59 (–) | — | — | 1.02 (0.87–1.20) | *P* = .70 |
| Garg[95] | 2028 | 20,280 | 6.5 | 43 [34–50] | 42 (2.1%) [2.8/1000] | 652 (3.2%) [4.1/1000] | 0.66 (0.48–0.90) | *P* = .008 |
| **Major Cardiovascular Events** | | | | | | | | |
| Garg[95] | 2028 | 20,280 | 6.5 | 43 [34–50] | 26 (1.3%) [1.7/1000] | 287 (1.4%) [2.0/1000] | 0.85 (0.57–1.27) | *P* = .43 |
| **Kidney Stones With Surgical Intervention** | | | | | | | | |
| Thomas[40] | 2019 | 20,190 | 8.4 | 43 [34–50] | 16 (0.79%) [8.3/10,000] | 179 (0.89%) [9.7/10,000] | 1.04 (0.60–1.80) | *P* = .90 |
| **Major Gastrointestinal Bleeding** | | | | | | | | |
| Thomas[142] | 2009 | 20,090 | 8.4 | 42 [34–50] | 33 (1.6%) [18.5/10,000] | 253 (1.3%) [14.9/10,000] | 1.25 (0.87–1.79) | *P* = .24 |
| **Skeletal Fractures** | | | | | | | | |
| Garg[143] | 2015 | 20,150 | 6.6 | 43 [34–50] | [16.4/10,000] | [18.7/10,000] | 0.87 (0.58–1.31) | *P* = .50 |
| **Gout** | | | | | | | | |
| Lam[42] | 1988 | 19,880 | 8.4 | 43 [35–51] | 67 (3.4%) [3.5/1000] | 390 (2.0%) [2.1/1000] | 1.6 (1.2–2.1) | *P* < .001 |
| **Gestational Hypertension or Preeclampsia** | | | | | | | | |
| Garg[130] | 85[c] | 510[c] | 11.0 | 29 [26–32] | 15 (11.5%) | 38 (4.8%) | 2.4 (1.2–5.0)[d] | *P* = .01 |

[a]Data presented as mean (standard deviation) or median [interquartile range].
[b]Living kidney donors were not matched to healthy nondonors in the comparison for end-stage kidney disease risk.
[c]In 85 donors, there were 131 pregnancies in follow-up. In 510 nondonors, there were 788 pregnancies in follow-up.
[d]Presented risk estimate is an odds ratio rather than a hazard ratio.
Modified from Lam NN, Lentine KL, Levey AS, et al. Long-term medical risks to the living kidney donor. *Nat Rev Nephrol.* 2015;11(7): 411–419.

of death among living kidney donors is cardiovascular disease, accounting for 30% to 40% of all deaths.[70,90] Although other studies have not shown a higher risk of cardiovascular mortality in donors compared with healthy matched nondonors, the Norwegian study also reported an increased risk in their donors (adjusted HR, 1.4).[70,94,95] Limitations of the Norwegian study included differences in baseline characteristics (e.g., age) and differences in accrual periods between donors and nondonors.[69,70,96,97]

## KIDNEY FUNCTION

Despite losing 50% of functioning renal mass, living kidney donors are typically left with 70% of their predonation GFR due to compensatory hyperfiltration of the remaining kidney.[36,98–100] In the first decade following donation, 40% of donors have a GFR between 60 and 80 mL/min/1.73 m$^2$, 12% of donors have a GFR between 30 and 59 mL/min/1.73 m$^2$, and 0.2% of donors have a GFR less than 30 mL/min/1.73 m$^2$.[98] Following donation, there does not appear to be an accelerated loss of function in the remaining kidney, above that expected with normal aging.[100] A prospective study of 198 living kidney donors and 194 controls from the United States reported that the linear slope of the measured GFR by iohexol clearance, between 6 and 36 months of follow-up, increased among donors (+1.47 mL/min/year) and decreased among controls (−0.36 mL/min/year).[101] Several investigators have evaluated the change in renal functional reserve (RFR) capacity in donors postnephrectomy.[102] The value of this test in predicting long-term kidney function postdonation is unclear; however, RFR capacity appears to be blunted or lost in older and obese donors.[103]

## END-STAGE KIDNEY DISEASE

Many transplantation programs and countries have reported their incidence of ESKD, typically defined as undergoing chronic dialysis or kidney transplantation.[91,104–114] A meta-analysis of 12 studies involving 108,900 living kidney donors has reported that the overall prevalence of ESKD is 0.5% in the 6 months to 5 years postdonation and 1.1% in the 10 years after that.[89] One study from Japan has reported the clinical course of eight living kidney donors who subsequently developed ESKD after a mean of 16 years.[108] For these donors, their renal function remained stable postdonation until they experienced an inciting event, such as infection, or a new comorbidity, such as hypertension or proteinuria, that led to progressive CKD.

The risk of ESKD in living kidney donors is lower than that in the general unscreened population (134 vs. 354 cases/million person-years).[114] In contrast, two studies have reported an increased risk of ESKD in living kidney donors compared with healthy matched nondonors.[70,96,115] In the previously described study from Norway, the incidence of ESKD over a median of 15 years was 0.5% ($n$ = 9) for living kidney donors and 0.07% ($n$ = 22) for healthy, matched nondonors (HR, 11.4; 95% CI, 4.4–29.6).[70] All affected donors were biologically related to their recipient. In another study of 96,217 living kidney donors from the United States, after a median follow-up of 7.6 years (maximum, 15.0 years), 99 donors (0.10%) developed ESKD after a mean of 8.6 years after donation.[115] The 15-year risk of ESKD was higher in donors who were men versus women, black versus white, and older versus younger (≥50 vs. <50 years). There was no significant difference between donors who were biologically related to their recipient versus those were unrelated to their recipient. In addition, the risk of ESKD was 86% higher among obese compared with nonobese donors (HR, 1.86; 95% CI,1.1–3.3); this risk increased by 7% for each unit increase in donor BMI above 27 kg/m$^2$ (HR 1.07; 95% CI,1.0–1.1).[116] Compared with healthy matched nondonors selected from the third NHANES study, the estimated 15-year risk of ESKD in this study was higher in living kidney donors (30.8 vs. 3.9/10,000; risk attributable to donation, 26.9/10,000).[19,115] The estimated lifetime risk of ESKD was also higher in donors compared with healthy, matched nondonors (90 vs. 14/10,000) but lower when compared with the unscreened general population (326/10,000). Despite these two studies, which reported a higher relative risk of ESKD in donors compared with healthy matched nondonors, the absolute risk of ESKD for living kidney donors is low. In a qualitative study of living kidney donors who subsequently developed ESKD, most donors did not regret their decision to donate, despite the adverse outcome.[117] Interestingly, recipients of kidneys from donors who developed ESKD also had a higher risk of graft loss (74% vs. 56%) and death (61% vs. 46%) at 20 years compared with those who received kidneys from donors who did not develop ESKD, suggesting some intrinsic risk conferred by the donor kidney.[118]

## PROTEINURIA

In the general population, a higher level of proteinuria is associated with an increased risk of CKD, ESKD, cardiovascular disease, and death, independently of the GFR.[119] In a systematic review, the pooled incidence of postdonation proteinuria was 12%.[98] The degree of proteinuria was higher in donors ($n$ = 129; 147 mg/day) compared with controls ($n$ = 59; 83 mg/day) and increased with the time from donation.[98] In a study of 3956 white living kidney donors, the incidence of proteinuria after 17 years of follow-up was 6.1% and was higher in male donors (HR, 1.6) and in donors with an increased predonation BMI (HR, 1.1).[120]

## HYPERTENSION

In addition to the increase in blood pressure that occurs with normal aging, the postdonation reduction in kidney function may contribute to a further increase in blood pressure.[121] A systematic review, which included 157 living kidney donors, has reported that after an average of 5 years, the blood pressure is 5 mm Hg higher in donors compared with nondonors (weighted mean for systolic blood pressure, 6 mm Hg; weighted mean for diastolic blood pressure, 4 mm Hg).[122] The risk of postdonation hypertension may be higher in black donors compared with white donors.[123,124] In a study of 3956 white living kidney donors, postdonation hypertension was associated with a more than twofold risk of ESKD.[120]

## CARDIOVASCULAR EVENTS

In the general population, a reduced GFR is associated with cardiovascular events.[125–127] In living kidney donors who have undergone a surgical reduction in their GFR, the risk of long-term cardiovascular events does not appear to be increased compared with healthy matched nondonors.[95] In 2028 living kidney donors from Ontario, Canada (1992–2009), the risk of death-censored cardiovascular events (including myocardial infarction, stroke, and coronary or other revascularization) was similar to 20,280 healthy matched nondonors (1.7 vs. 2.0 events/1000 person-years; HR, 0.85; median follow-up, 7 years; maximum, 18 years). However, one study from Norway did report a higher risk of cardiovascular death in donors compared with nondonors (adjusted HR, 1.4; 95% CI,1.0–1.9).[70]

## MATERNAL AND FETAL COMPLICATIONS

Compared with predonation pregnancies, postdonation pregnancies may be associated with a lower likelihood of full-term deliveries and a higher risk of fetal loss, gestational diabetes, gestational hypertension, proteinuria, and preeclampsia.[128,129] This risk may be attributed to other factors, such as maternal age at the time of pregnancy, rather than to donation. In a retrospective study of 85 female donors with 131 pregnancies from Ontario, Canada (1992–2009), the risk of gestational hypertension and preeclampsia was higher compared with 510 healthy matched nondonors with 788 pregnancies (11% vs. 5%; odds ratio, 2.4).[130] In this study, there were no significant differences in preterm births, cesarean section, postpartum hemorrhage, or low birth rate between donors and nondonors. Although most donors will have uncomplicated pregnancies and deliveries postdonation, it is recommended that pregnant donors have access to adequate perinatal care to reduce the risk of pregnancy complications.[19]

# ETHICAL, LEGAL, AND POLICY CONSIDERATIONS

In 1988, Iran became the first and only country to implement a state-regulated, government-funded program to compensate living unrelated kidney donors financially.[131] This controversial program, known as the "Iranian model," has raised concerns about the exploitation of living kidney donors who may be from vulnerable populations, such as the undereducated and impoverished. Over 100 countries support the Declaration of Istanbul, which prohibits the practice of organ trafficking and transplant tourism, although it is estimated that 5% to 10% of kidney transplants globally are the result of commercial organ transplants.[132,133] Despite this, there is growing evidence that the out of pocket costs prevent potential candidates from completing the evaluation or donating.[134] Reimbursing the costs incurred by donor candidates or reimbursing the donor's funeral costs have been well-received by the public and other stakeholders as viable options for negating financial disincentives.[135]

Local laws and regulations on living donation should be followed and communicated clearly to donor candidates. Countries and programs should be explicit regarding their legal mandate to protect vulnerable populations, respect donor candidate autonomy (to be considered as candidates or withdraw at any time from the evaluation in a way that is confidential and protected), and prohibit incentives to donation that could create undue influence on the donor candidate's decision to donate. Countries and programs should also be clear on how donor candidates may be identified (e.g., living donor "champions," use of social media to advertise the need for a donor, or independent living donor advocates), as well as the policy on postdonation follow-up.

 Complete reference list available at ExpertConsult.com.

## KEY REFERENCES


1. Murray JE. The first successful organ transplants in man. *J Am Coll Surg.* 2005;200(1):5–9. doi:10.1016/j.jamcollsurg.2004.09.033.
2. Murray JE. Ronald Lee Herrick Memorial: June 15, 1931-December 27, 2010. *Am J Transplant.* 2011;11(3):419. doi:10.1111/j.1600-6143.2011.03445.x.
3. Terasaki PI, Cecka JM, Gjertson DW, et al. High survival rates of kidney transplants from spousal and living unrelated donors. *N Engl J Med.* 1995;333(6):333–336. doi:10.1056/NEJM199508103330601.
7. Wolfe RA, Ashby VB, Milford EL, et al. Comparison of mortality in all patients on dialysis, patients on dialysis awaiting transplantation, and recipients of a first cadaveric transplant. *N Engl J Med.* 1999;341(23):1725–1730. doi:10.1056/NEJM199912023412303.
9. Tonelli M, Wiebe N, Knoll G, et al. Systematic review: kidney transplantation compared with dialysis in clinically relevant outcomes. *Am J Transplant.* 2011;11(10):2093–2109. doi:10.1111/j.1600-6143.2011.03686.x.
10. Axelrod DA, Schnitzler MA, Xiao H, et al. An economic assessment of contemporary kidney transplant practice. *Am J Transplant.* 2018;18(5):1168–1176. doi:10.1111/ajt.14702.
11. Medin C, Elinder CG, Hylander B, et al. Survival of patients who have been on a waiting list for renal transplantation. *Nephrol Dial Transplant.* 2000;15(5):701–704. http://www.ncbi.nlm.nih.gov/pubmed/10809814. Accessed May 26, 2014.
13. Habbous S, McArthur E, Sarma S, et al. Potential implications of a more timely living kidney donor evaluation. *Am J Transplant.* 2018;doi:10.1111/ajt.14732.
15. Tong A, Ralph A, Chapman JR, et al. Public attitudes and beliefs about living kidney donation: focus group study. *Transplantation.* 2014;97(10):977–985. doi:10.1097/TP.0000000000000080.
16. LaPointe Rudow D, Hays R, Baliga P, et al. Consensus conference on best practices in live kidney donation: recommendations to optimize education, access, and care. *Am J Transplant.* 2015;15(4):914–922. doi:10.1111/ajt.13173.
19. Lentine KL, Kasiske BL, Levey AS, et al. KDIGO Clinical Practice Guideline on the Evaluation and Care of Living Kidney Donors. *Transplantation.* 2017;101(8S suppl 1):S7–S105. doi:10.1097/TP.0000000000001769.
21. Andrews PA, Burnapp L, Manas D, et al. Summary of the British Transplantation Society/Renal Association U.K. guidelines for living donor kidney transplantation. *Transplantation.* 2012;93(7):666–673. doi:10.1097/TP.0b013e318247a7b7.
22. Abramowicz D, Cochat P, Claas FHJ, et al. European Renal Best Practice Guideline on kidney donor and recipient evaluation and perioperative care: FIGURE 1. *Nephrol Dial Transplant.* 2015;30(11):1790–1797. doi:10.1093/ndt/gfu216.
23. OPTN. *Policy 14: Living Donation*; 2015. http://optn.transplant.hrsa.gov/governance/policies/. Accessed August 11, 2019.
26. Habbous S, Garg AX, Lam NN. Optimizing efficiency in the evaluation of living donor candidates: best practices and implications. *Curr Transplant Reports.* 2018;5(1):55–63. doi:10.1007/s40472-018-0184-y.
27. Tong A, Chapman JR, Wong G, et al. Screening and follow-up of living kidney donors: a systematic review of clinical practice guidelines. *Transplantation.* 2011;92(9):962–972. doi:10.1097/TP.0b013e3182328276.
29. Grams ME, Sang Y, Levey AS, et al. Kidney-failure risk projection for the living kidney-donor candidate. *N Engl J Med.* 2016;374(5):411–421. doi:10.1056/NEJMoa1510491.
32. Levey AS, Inker LA. GFR evaluation in living kidney donor candidates. *J Am Soc Nephrol.* 2017;28(4):1062–1071. doi:10.1681/ASN.2016070790.
34. Gaillard F, Flamant M, Lemoine S, et al. Estimated or measured GFR in living kidney donors work-up? *Am J Transplant.* 2016;16(10):3024–3032. doi:10.1111/ajt.13908.

36. Mueller TF, Luyckx VA. The natural history of residual renal function in transplant donors. *J Am Soc Nephrol.* 2012;23(9):1462–1466. doi:10.1681/ASN.2011111080.
39. Choi SR, Sun IO, Hong YA, et al. The role of kidney biopsy to determine donation from prospective kidney donors with asymptomatic urinary abnormalities. *Transplant Proc.* 2012;44(1):11–13. doi:10.1016/j.transproceed.2011.12.008.
41. Rizkala E, Coleman S, Tran C, et al. Stone disease in living-related renal donors: long-term outcomes for transplant donors and recipients. *J Endourol.* 2013;27(12):1520–1524. doi:10.1089/end.2013.0203.
45. O'Brien B, Mastoridis S, Crane J, et al. Safety of nephrectomy in morbidly obese donors. *Exp Clin Transplant.* 2012;10(6):579–585. http://www.ncbi.nlm.nih.gov/pubmed/23216566. Accessed July 6, 2018.
48. Zhang S, Yuan J, Li W, et al. Organ transplantation from donors (cadaveric or living) with a history of malignancy: review of the literature. *Transplant Rev (Orlando).* 2014;28(4):169–175. doi:10.1016/j.trre.2014.06.002.
49. Lugo-Baruqui JA, Guerra G, Chen L, et al. Living donor renal transplantation with incidental renal cell carcinoma from donor allograft. *Transpl Int.* 2015;28(9):1126–1130. doi:10.1111/tri.12594.
51. Newell KA, Formica RN, Gill JS, et al. Integrating APOL1 gene variants into renal transplantation: considerations arising from the American Society of Transplantation Expert Conference. *Am J Transplant.* 2017;17(4):901–911. doi:10.1111/ajt.14173.
52. Dew MA, Jacobs CL, Jowsey SG, et al. Guidelines for the psychosocial evaluation of living unrelated kidney donors in the United States. *Am J Transplant.* 2007;7(5):1047–1054. doi:10.1111/j.1600-6143.2007.01751.x.
54. Tong A, Chapman JR, Wong G, et al. The motivations and experiences of living kidney donors: a thematic synthesis. *Am J Kidney Dis.* 2012;60(1):15–26. doi:10.1053/j.ajkd.2011.11.043.
56. Ferrari P, Weimar W, Johnson RJ, et al. Kidney paired donation: principles, protocols and programs. *Nephrol Dial Transplant.* 2015;30(8):1276–1285. doi:10.1093/ndt/gfu309.
58. Yuan H, Liu L, Zheng S, et al. The safety and efficacy of laparoscopic donor nephrectomy for renal transplantation: an updated Meta-analysis. *Transplant Proc.* 2013;45(1):65–76. doi:10.1016/j.transproceed.2012.07.152.
62. Liu N, Wazir R, Wang J, et al. Maximizing the donor pool: left versus right laparoscopic live donor nephrectomy–systematic review and meta-analysis. *Int Urol Nephrol.* 2014;46(8):1511–1519. doi:10.1007/s11255-014-0671-8.
64. Waterman AD, Dew MA, Davis CL, et al. Living-donor follow-up attitudes and practices in U.S. kidney and liver donor programs. *Transplant J.* 2013;95(6):883–888. doi:10.1097/TP.0b013e31828279fd.
69. Lam NN, Lentine KL, Levey AS, et al. Long-term medical risks to the living kidney donor. *Nat Rev Nephrol.* 2015;11(7):411–419. doi:10.1038/nrneph.2015.58.
70. Mjøen G, Hallan S, Hartmann A, et al. Long-term risks for kidney donors. *Kidney Int.* 2014;86(1):162–167. doi:10.1038/ki.2013.460.
77. Manyalich M, Ricart A, Martínez I, et al. EULID project: European living donation and public health. *Transplant Proc.* 2009;41(6):2021–2024. doi:10.1016/j.transproceed.2009.05.021.
78. Kasiske BL, Asrani SK, Dew MA, et al. The living donor collective: a scientific registry for living donors. *Am J Transplant.* 2017;17(12):3040–3048. doi:10.1111/ajt.14365.
80. Lentine KL, Segev DL. Understanding and communicating medical risks for living kidney donors: a matter of perspective. *J Am Soc Nephrol.* 2017;28(1):12–24. doi:10.1681/ASN.2016050571.
81. Schold JD, Goldfarb DA, Buccini LD, et al. Comorbidity burden and perioperative complications for living kidney donors in the United States. *Clin J Am Soc Nephrol.* 2013;8(10):1773–1782. doi:10.2215/CJN.12311212.
82. Segev DL, Muzaale AD, Caffo BS, et al. Perioperative mortality and long-term survival following live kidney donation. *JAMA.* 2010;303(10):959–966. doi:10.1001/jama.2010.237.
85. Lentine KL, Lam NN, Axelrod D, et al. Perioperative complications after living kidney donation: a national study. *Am J Transplant.* 2016;16(6):1848–1857. doi:10.1111/ajt.13687.
86. Mjøen G, Øyen O, Holdaas H, et al. Morbidity and mortality in 1022 consecutive living donor nephrectomies: benefits of a living donor registry. *Transplantation.* 2009;88(11):1273–1279. doi:10.1097/TP.0b013e3181bb44fd.
91. Ibrahim HN, Foley R, Tan L, et al. Long-term consequences of kidney donation. *N Engl J Med.* 2009;360(5):459–469. doi:10.1056/NEJMoa0804883.
94. Garg AX, Prasad GVR, Thiessen-Philbrook HR, et al. Cardiovascular disease and hypertension risk in living kidney donors: an analysis of health administrative data in Ontario, Canada. *Transplantation.* 2008;86(3):399–406. doi:10.1097/TP.0b013e31817ba9e3.
97. Garg AX, Boudville N. Live kidney donation was associated with increased mortality and end-stage renal disease at 15 years. *Ann Intern Med.* 2014;160(10):JC12. doi:10.7326/0003-4819-160-10-201405200-02012.
115. Muzaale AD, Massie AB, Wang MC, et al. Risk of end-stage renal disease following live kidney donation. *JAMA.* 2014;311(6):579–586. doi:10.1001/jama.2013.285141.
116. Locke JE, Reed RD, Massie A, et al. Obesity increases the risk of end-stage renal disease among living kidney donors. *Kidney Int.* 2017;91(3):699–703. doi:10.1016/j.kint.2016.10.014.
117. Halverson CME, Wang JY, Poulson M, et al. Living kidney donors who develop kidney failure: excerpts of their thoughts. *Am J Nephrol.* 2016;43(6):389–396. doi:10.1159/000446161.
130. Garg AX, Nevis IF, McArthur E, et al. Gestational hypertension and preeclampsia in living kidney donors. *N Engl J Med.* 2015;372(2):124–133. doi:10.1056/NEJMoa1408932.
134. Tushla L, Rudow DL, Milton J, et al. Living-donor kidney transplantation: reducing financial barriers to live kidney donation–recommendations from a consensus conference. *Clin J Am Soc Nephrol.* 2015;10(9):1696–1702. doi:10.2215/CJN.01000115.
137. Richardson R, Connelly M, Dipchand C, et al. Kidney paired donation protocol for participating donors 2014. *Transplantation.* 2015;99(10 suppl 1):S1–S88. doi:10.1097/TP.0000000000000918.

# PEDIATRIC NEPHROLOGY

SECTION XII

# 72 Diseases of the Kidney and Upper Urinary Tract in Children

Todd Alexander | Christoph Licht | William E. Smoyer | Norman D. Rosenblum

CHAPTER OUTLINE

## THE SPECTRUM OF KIDNEY AND URINARY TRACT DISORDERS IN CHILDREN

The spectrum of chronic pediatric kidney disorders is distinct from that observed in adults (Fig. 72.1). Congenital abnormalities of the kidneys and/or lower urinary tract are most frequent, together accounting for just less than 50% of all kidney–urinary tract disorders. Glomerular disorders constitute the next largest group, constituting approximately 25% of all disorders. Cystic disorders (autosomal dominant and recessive forms) are then most frequent followed by systemic disorders, such as vasculitis, and metabolic disorders. The prevalence of end-stage renal disease (ESRD) among children younger than 15 years in Europe is currently 34 per million age-related population (pmarp) or 5.4 per million population (pmp).[1] The annual incidence is 6.5 pmarp or 1.0 pmp. When the pediatric population is defined as those up to age 19 years, the prevalence of ESRD in children and adolescents is 80 to 90 pmp and the annual incidence is 15 pmp. This is only 10% of the incidence in young adults and fewer than 2% of that observed in the older population. Because of the preponderance of males among those with certain urinary tract abnormalities (e.g., urethral valves), renal replacement therapy (RRT) occurs almost 50% more often in males than in females. ESRD incidence is highest in adolescence (8 pmarp), lowest in middle childhood (4.6 pmarp), and intermediate in children younger than 5 years of age (6.7 pmarp). Because of the predominantly genetic origin of pediatric nephropathies, chronic kidney disease (CKD) in children is frequently associated with a variety of extrarenal abnormalities. Impaired neurodevelopment and sensory dysfunctions are among the most severe general disabilities interfering with psychosocial adjustment and integration in children with CKD.

## EVALUATION OF KIDNEY FUNCTION IN CHILDREN

During the period from birth to adulthood, body weight increases 20-fold, body length threefold to fourfold, and body surface area (BSA), the closest correlate of basal metabolic rate, eightfold. By convention, glomerular filtration rate (GFR) is normalized to the BSA of an average-sized adult—that is, 1.73 $m^2$. Although nephron formation is complete by the 34th gestational week, nephrons continue to grow in size and functional capacity after birth. In early postnatal life, nephron size and capacity increase not only in absolute terms but also relative to BSA, which results in a significant physiologic gain in normalized global renal function. The average GFR in the neonate is 20 to 30 mL/min/1.73 $m^2$ and increases rapidly in the first few months of life. From 18 months of age, the absolute increase in GFR precisely matches the growth in BSA, which results in a constant normal range of BSA-indexed GFR throughout childhood and adolescence. After 2 years of age, the conventional CKD staging system, which assigns stages of CKD based on estimated GFR (eGFR) in multiples of 15 and 30 mL/min/1.73 $m^2$, can be used.

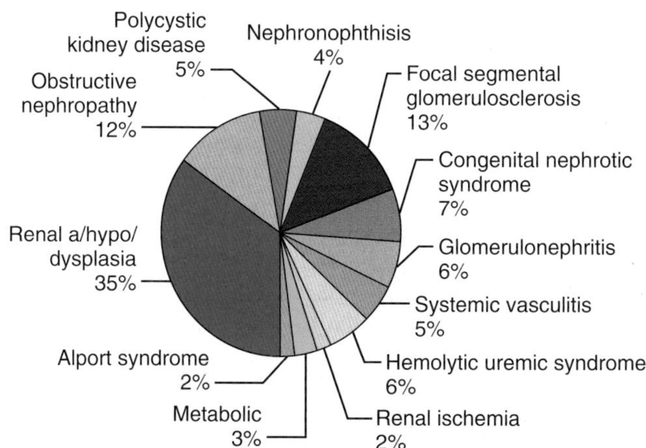


**Fig. 72.1** Spectrum of underlying renal diagnoses in 1367 children with end-stage kidney disease. (From the International Pediatric Peritoneal Dialysis Network Registry.)

The direct measurement of GFR is a challenging task in children. The most commonly used measurement in children is endogenous creatinine clearance, which requires that the child be able to provide urine samples during a defined period. Creatinine clearance accurately reflects a reasonable estimate of GFR in patients with normal or mildly impaired renal function. As GFR declines, tubular creatinine secretion increases, which results in an overestimation of true GFR. In clinical practice, prediction equations that estimate GFR from one or more serum markers are commonly used. Although many such equations exist, the most commonly used equation uses creatinine as a marker. Because creatinine generation, and consequently steady-state serum creatinine levels, depends on muscle mass, which in turn is dependent on age and gender, this equation estimates GFR from the ratio of height to serum creatinine concentration multiplied by a constant, K.[2] In the original "Schwartz" equation, K was age and gender specific. In a more recent equation, Schwartz and colleagues use a uniform K value for both genders.[3] This equation is valid in children from 1 to 16 years of age:

$$\text{eGFR} = \text{Height (cm)} \times 0.413/\text{serum creatinine (mg/dL)}$$

Most healthy children excrete small amounts of protein in their urine. Physiologic proteinuria varies with the age and size of the child. When corrected for BSA, the upper normal limit of protein excretion is 300 mg/$m^2$/day at age 1 month in full-term infants, 250 mg at 1 year, 200 mg at 10 years, and 150 mg in late adolescence. Urinary protein excretion exceeding 1.0 g/$m^2$/day is strongly indicative of inherent kidney pathophysiology. The upper limit of normal for the urine protein-to-creatinine ratio (as grams of protein/gram of creatinine) is 0.5 at age 6 months to 2 years and 0.2 in older children and adolescents.[4] A urine protein-to-creatinine ratio above 3.0 is consistent with nephrotic-range proteinuria, thought to reflect glomerular disease, and is often associated with systemic manifestations, such as salt and fluid retention and edema. Estimates of the prevalence of isolated asymptomatic proteinuria in children range between 0.6% and 6%. Orthostatic proteinuria accounts for up to 60% of all cases of asymptomatic proteinuria reported in children, with an even higher incidence in adolescents. Children with orthostatic proteinuria usually excrete less than 1 g of protein/day (urine protein-to-creatinine ratio <1.0). Although patients with orthostatic proteinuria have an excellent prognosis, the long-term prognosis for children with isolated fixed proteinuria remains unknown.

## CONGENITAL ANOMALIES OF THE KIDNEY AND URINARY TRACT

Developmental disorders of the kidney and urinary tract comprise a spectrum of malformations ranging from complete absence of kidney tissue to minor structural abnormalities. Together, these malformations are classified within the rubric Congenital Anomalies of the Kidney and Urinary Tract (CAKUT). Kidney–urinary tract structural abnormalities are an important cause of human disease; they are the most common cause of all birth defects, comprising 23% of all such defects[5] and cause 30% to 50% of all cases of ESRD in children.[6] Within the adult population, CAKUT is the cause of 2.2% of all ESRDs. Adult patients with CAKUT differ from adults with other causes of CKD in their requirement for RRT at a mean age of 30 years compared with 61 years.[7] This section is focused on the classification, epidemiology, pathogenesis, and clinical management of kidney malformations.

## CLINICAL CLASSIFICATION OF KIDNEY MALFORMATION

As a group, renal–urinary tract malformations have been grouped together under the rubric CAKUT. In support of this rubric: (1) multiple structures within one or both kidney–urinary tract units may be affected within any given affected individual, (2) mutation in a particular gene is associated with different urinary tract anomalies in different affected individuals, and (3) mutations in different genes give rise to similar renal and lower urinary tract phenotypes. A classification of kidney and urinary tract malformations within the CAKUT rubric is as follows:

- Aplasia (agenesis), defined as congenital absence of kidney tissue.
- Simple hypoplasia, defined as renal length less than 2 standard deviations (SDs) below the mean for age, a reduced number of nephrons and normal renal architecture.
- Dysplasia ± cysts, defined as malformation of tissue elements.
- Isolated dilatation of the renal pelvis ± ureters (collecting system).
- Anomalies of position including the ectopic and fused (horseshoe) kidney.

Simple renal hypoplasia is defined by the presence of a small kidney with a decrease in the number of nephrons and normal renal architecture. Viewed through the lens of embryology, normal tissue architecture indicates that patterning of renal tissue elements is normal.

Renal dysplasia is defined as an abnormality of tissue patterning (Fig. 72.2). Renal dysplasia is a polymorphic disorder. At the level of gross anatomy, the dysplastic kidney varies in size from one extreme to the other compared with the mean size for age. However, most dysplastic kidneys are small for age. Dysplastic kidneys also vary in the presence of epithelial cysts, the number of cysts, and cyst size. The multicystic dysplastic kidney (MCDK) is an extreme form of renal dysplasia in which large polymorphic cysts dominate kidney structure (Fig. 72.3). At the level of histopathology, the dysplastic kidney (Fig. 72.2) is characterized by several primary features: (1) abnormal differentiation of mesenchymal and epithelial elements, (2) decreased nephron number, (3) loss of corticomedullary differentiation, and (4) metaplastic transformation of mesenchyme to cartilage and bone. Renal tubular dysgenesis represents a particular form of renal dysplasia and is characterized by the absence or poor development of proximal tubules and is accompanied by thickening of the renal arterial vasculature from the arcuate to the afferent arteries.[8]

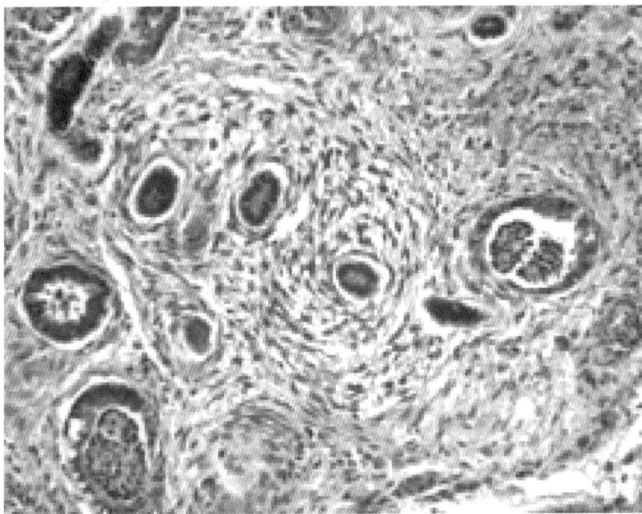

**Fig. 72.2** Histologic section of renal dysplastic tissue. Dysplastic renal tissue demonstrates a paucity of glomerular and tubular elements, disorganization of tissue elements, an abundance of stroma, and thickened and dilated renal tubules.

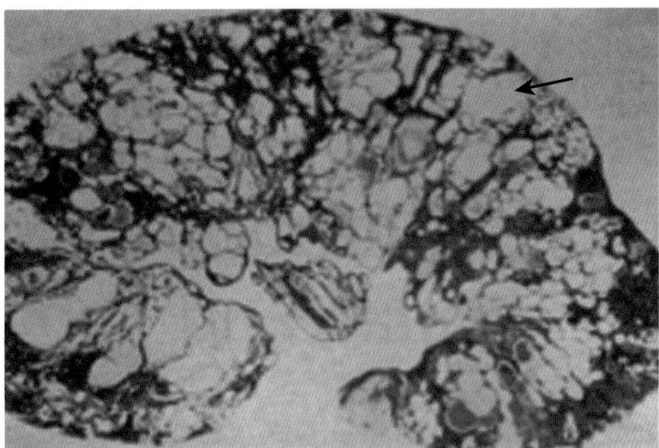

**Fig. 72.3** Histologic section of a multicystic dysplastic kidney. The kidney consists in large part of multiple polymorphic cysts *(arrow)*. Normal renal tissue elements cannot be identified.

An ectopic kidney is classified by its position and its relationship with an independent kidney unit (Fig. 72.4). Simple (nonfused) ectopy refers to a kidney that lies on the correct side of the body but lies in an abnormal position. Kidneys that cross the midline are referred to as crossed renal ectopy. Crossed renal ectopy can occur with and without fusion to

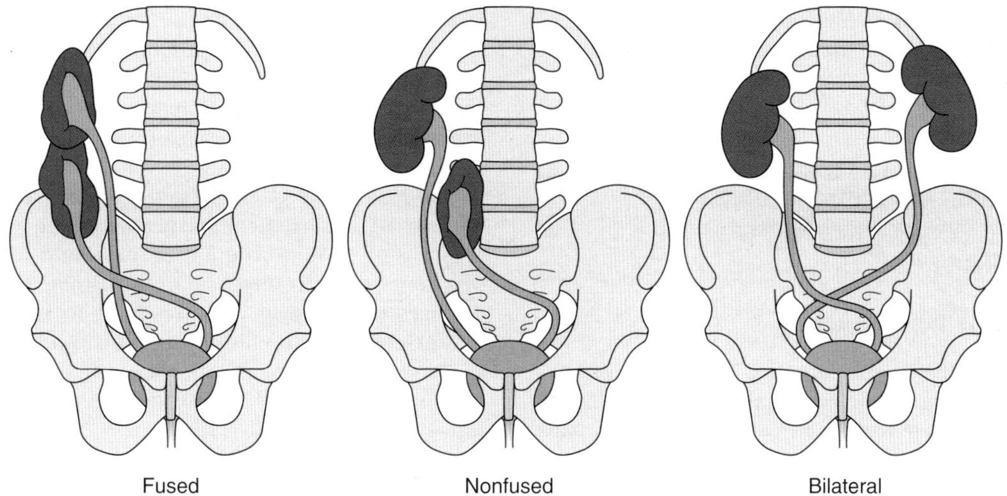


**Fig. 72.4** Crossed fused ectopia. Renal ectopia is classified as simple (nonfused), fused, and bilateral. A fused kidney migrates across the midline and fuses to the lower pole of the normally positioned contralateral kidney. A simple crossed (nonfused) kidney migrates across the midline, does not fuse with the normally positioned contralateral kidney, and is usually positioned at the rim of the pelvis. In bilateral ectopia, both kidneys are ectopic and cross the midline with their native ureters, which are inserted normally into the bladder.

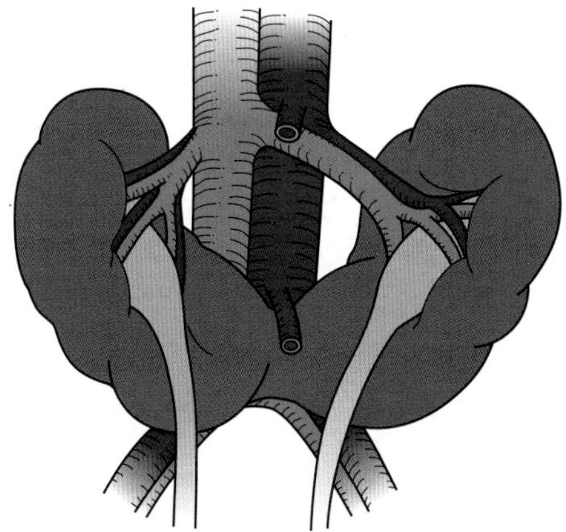

**Fig. 72.5** Horseshoe kidney. A horseshoe kidney with fusion of the lower poles. Note that the renal pelvis is positioned anteriorly and the ureter traverses the anterior aspect and the fused lower pole of each kidney.

the contralateral kidney. Ectopic kidneys that do not ascend above the pelvic brim are commonly called pelvic kidneys. Renal fusion occurs when a portion of one kidney is fused to the other. The most common fusion anomaly is the horseshoe kidney, which involves abnormal migration of both kidneys (ectopy), resulting in fusion (Fig. 72.5). This differs from crossed fused renal ectopy, which usually involves abnormal movement of only one kidney across the midline with fusion of the contralateral noncrossing kidney.

## EPIDEMIOLOGY OF CONGENITAL ANOMALIES OF THE KIDNEY AND URINARY TRACT

CAKUT is the most frequent malformation detected in utero. Using fetal ultrasound, the incidence of renal and urinary tract malformations is 0.3 to 1.6 per 1000 live-born and stillborn infants.[9] Lower urinary tract abnormalities can be identified in approximately 50% of affected patients, consistent with the common origin of the kidney and ureter from the mesonephric duct. These anomalies include vesicoureteral reflux ([VUR] 25%), ureteropelvic junction obstruction (11%), and ureterovesical junction obstruction (11%).[10] Renal malformations, other than mild antenatal pelviectasis, occur in association with nonrenal malformations in about 30% of cases.[9]

The reported incidence of particular types of renal–urinary tract malformation is no doubt dependent on the ascertainment method. Most incidence rates are not based on population-based studies during pregnancy. Rather, they are based on autopsy series or studies in selected live-born infants. Incidence rates based on methods other than population-based ascertainment may underestimate the true incidence because fetal loss may not be accounted for and CAKUT can be clinically silent in the surviving fetus.

Complete or partial duplication of the renal collecting system is the most common congenital anomaly of the urinary tract.[11] Autopsy studies report an estimated incidence of 0.8% to 5%.[12] A similar rate was reported in a study of 13,705 fetuses with antenatal ultrasounds performed in a tertiary center in Turkey.[13] However, a study that screened 132,686 Taiwanese schoolchildren (6 to 15 years of age) found a lower incidence of 1 in 5000 children.[14] Bilateral renal agenesis occurs in 1:3000 to 10,000 births. Males are affected more often than females. Unilateral renal agenesis has been reported with a prevalence of 1:1000 autopsies. The incidence of unilateral dysplasia is 1 in 3000 to 5000 births (1:3640 for the MCDK) compared with 1 in 10,000 for bilateral dysplasia.[15] The male-to-female ratio for bilateral and unilateral renal dysplasia is 1.32:1 and 1.92:1, respectively.[16] The incidence of renal ectopia is 1 in 1000 autopsies, but the clinical recognition is estimated to be only 1 in 10,000 patients.[17] Males and females are equally affected. Renal ectopia is bilateral in 10% of cases; when unilateral, there is a slight predilection for the left side. The incidence of fusion anomalies is estimated to be about 1 in 600 infants.[18] The most common fusion anomaly is the horseshoe kidney, which occurs with fusion of one pole of each kidney. The reported incidence of horseshoe kidney based upon data from birth defect registries varies from 0.4 to 1.6 to 10,000 live births.[18,19]

## PATHOGENESIS OF CONGENITAL ANOMALIES OF THE KIDNEY AND URINARY TRACT

### MECHANISMS OF INHERITANCE

The genetics of CAKUT are complex. In the majority of affected patients, congenital renal malformations occur as sporadic events. In approximately 30% of affected individuals, these malformations occur as part of a multiorgan genetic syndrome. Renal–urinary tract malformations and extrarenal malformations can go unrecognized unless a careful phenotypic examination is performed. Over 200 distinct monogenic syndromes feature some type of kidney and urinary tract malformation. Approximately 50 genes have been identified as mutant in human CAKUT, 25 with autosomal dominant inheritance and 15 with autosomal recessive inheritance (Table 72.1).[20-48] Incomplete penetrance with variable expressivity is frequent in affected families. That is, within any particular family in which affected members carry the same mutation, the renal phenotype can vary from agenesis to dysplasia to isolated abnormalities of the collecting system (e.g., hydronephrosis).[20]

The majority of CAKUT occurs without a clear Mendelian pattern of inheritance. In probands with bilateral renal agenesis or bilateral renal dysgenesis and without evidence of a genetic syndrome or a family history, 9% of first-degree relatives were shown by ultrasound to have some type of malformation in the kidney and/or lower urinary tract.[21] A study of CAKUT in asymptomatic first-degree relatives of patients with CAKUT in Turkey revealed a positive family history of CAKUT in 23% and ultrasound evidence of CAKUT also in 23% of individuals.[22] A study of 100 patients with renal hypodysplasia and renal insufficiency demonstrated a gene mutation in 16% of affected individuals.[23] Another study of 204 unrelated patients with CAKUT using target exome sequencing of 330 genes implicated in CAKUT in humans and other species demonstrated pathogenic mutations in 31/204 (17.6%) patients. The 24 pathogenic mutations were identified in seven genes associated with CAKUT: HNF1b,

**Table 72.1 Human Gene Mutations Associated With Syndromic Congenital Anomalies of the Kidney and Urinary Tract**

| Primary Disease | Gene | Kidney Phenotype | References |
|---|---|---|---|
| Alagille syndrome | *JAGGED1*<br>*NOTCH2* | Cystic dysplasia | 1170,1171 |
| Apert syndrome | *FGFR2* | Hydronephrosis | 1172 |
| Atypical DiGeorge syndrome | *CRKL* | Hypodysplasia, vesicoureteral reflux (VUR), obstructive uropathy | 1173 |
| Beckwith–Wiedemann syndrome | $p57^{KIP2}$ | Medullary dysplasia | 1174 |
| Branchio-oto-renal (BOR) syndrome | *EYA1, SIX1, SIX5* | Unilateral or bilateral agenesis/ dysplasia, hypoplasia, collecting system anomalies | 1175 |
| Campomelic dysplasia | *SOX9* | Dysplasia, hydronephrosis | 1176 |
| Duane radial ray (Okihiro) syndrome | *SALL4* | UNL agenesis, VUR, malrotation, cross-fused ectopia, pelviectasis | 1177 |
| Fraser syndrome | *FRAS1*<br>*FREM1*<br>*FREM2* | Agenesis, dysplasia | 1178,1179 |
| Isolated renal hypoplasia | *BMP4*<br>*RET* | Hypoplasia, VUR | 1180,1181 |
| Hypoparathyroidism, sensorineural deafness, and renal anomalies syndrome | *GATA3* | Dysplasia | 1182 |
| Kabuki syndrome | *KDM6A, KMT2D* | VUR, hypodysplasia, ectopia | 1183 |
| Kallmann syndrome | *KAL1, FGFR1, PROK2, PROK2R* | Agenesis | 1184 |
| Leukemia, acute B cell | *PBX1* | Hypodysplasia, VUR, ectopia, horseshoe kidney | 1185 |
| Mammary–ulnar syndrome | *TBX3* | Dysplasia | 1186 |
| Okihiro syndrome | *SALL4* | Ectopia, dysplasia | 1176 |
| Pallister–Hall syndrome | *GLI3* | Agenesis, dysplasia, hydronephrosis | 1187,1188 |
| Renal-coloboma syndrome | *PAX2* | Hypoplasia, vesicoureteral reflux | 1189 |
| Renal tubular dysgenesis | *RAS components* | Tubular dysplasia | 1190 |
| Renal cysts and diabetes syndrome | *HNF1b* | Dysplasia, hypoplasia | 1191 |
| Rubinstein–Taybi syndrome | *CREBBP* | Agenesis, hypoplasia | 1192 |
| Simpson–Golabi–Behmel syndrome | *GPC3* | Medullary dysplasia | 1193 |
| Smith–Lemli–Opitz syndrome | *7-hydroxy-cholesterol reductase* | Agenesis, dysplasia | 1194 |
| Townes–Brock syndrome | *SALL1* | Hypoplasia, dysplasia, VUR | 1195 |
| Ulnar–mammary syndrome | *TBX3* | Hypoplasia | 1186 |
| Zellweger syndrome | *PEX1* | VUR, cystic dysplasia | 1196 |

PAX2, EYA1, ANOS1, GATA3, CHD7, and KIF14. Sixteen of these 31 patients had extrarenal as well as renal abnormalities.[24] This frequency of pathogenic mutations is considerably higher than that found in a study of 453 patients in which exome sequencing of >200 candidate genes identified pathogenic mutations in 6/453 patients.[25] The difference in results likely is explained by the phenotypes studied. Although Nicolaou et al.[25] studied a wide variety of CAKUT phenotypes including unilateral malformations and lower urinary tract obstruction, Heidet et al. only included bilateral CAKUT and/or familial and/or syndromic forms of CAKUT.[24] Taken together, these results indicate that currently as many as 18% of CAKUT cases can be explained by an established monogenic cause.[20,26] The majority of mutations identified are in *TCF2* (hepatocyte nuclear factor-1β [HNF-1β]; especially in patients with kidney cysts) and PAX2. Some of the mutations are de novo, explaining the sporadic appearance of CAKUT. Careful clinical analysis of patients with *TCF2* and *PAX2* mutations revealed the presence of extrarenal symptoms in only 50%, supporting previous reports that *TCF2* and *PAX2* mutations can be responsible for isolated renal tract anomalies or at least CAKUT malformations with minimal extrarenal features.[27,28] Exome sequencing studies also identify rare heterozygous missense gene variants, some of which are predicted by bioinformatic analyses to be pathogenic.[24,25] Yet, the lack of functional validation for many of these variants underlies a lack of certainty of how such information can be applied to diagnosis and counselling of patients.

Studies suggest that polymorphic variants in genes that control renal development and copy number variants (CNVs) contribute to the pathogenesis of CAKUT. Analysis of a cohort of 168 Caucasian newborns from Montreal suggests that single-nucleotide polymorphisms (SNPs) in *PAX2* are associated with newborn kidney size at the low end of the population spectrum.[29] Analysis of the *RET* gene in the aforementioned Montreal cohort demonstrated that a reduction in newborn kidney volume by 9.7% was significantly associated with an SNP (rs1800860) that encodes an A versus G at codon 1476.[30] Analyses in vitro indicate that the amount of messenger RNA (mRNA) generated from this allele is reduced consistent with decreased *RET* expression in affected individuals. Analysis of genomic CNVs has revealed that 10% to 15% of CAKUT cases are associated with such variants. For example, a study of 522 children with renal hypodysplasia revealed genomic abnormalities in 10.5% of cases.[31] In this and other similar studies, the abnormalities detected are predominantly localized to the renal cyst and diabetes syndrome locus on chromosome 17 or the DiGeorge syndrome region on chromosome 22.

## MOLECULAR PATHOGENESIS

The morphologic and genetic events that control kidney development are detailed in Chapter 1. Briefly summarized, formation of the human kidney is initiated at 5 weeks' gestation in the human when the ureteric duct is induced to undergo lateral outgrowth from the wolffian duct and to invade the adjacent metanephric mesenchyme. The ureteric bud then undergoes repetitive branching events, so termed because each event consists of expansion of the advancing ureteric bud branch at its leading tip, division of the ampulla resulting in formation of new branches, and elongation of the newly formed branches. Beginning with the 10th–11th branch generation, the pattern of branching becomes terminally bifid. During branching morphogenesis, 65,000 collecting ducts are formed, as both cortical and medullary collecting ducts, a process that is essential to the function of the mature kidney. During the latter stages of kidney development, tubular segments formed from the first five generations of ureteric bud branching undergo remodeling to form the kidney pelvis and calyces.[32]

Genetic analyses in humans have identified mutant alleles associated with CAKUT. Studies in mice have identified more than 180 genes that are required during renal development.[20] Together, studies in humans and mice have provided complimentary information and critical insights into the likely functions of CAKUT-related genes during human renal morphogenesis. In this section, the functions of genes mutated in human CAKUT and for which a function has been elucidated are reviewed as a framework for understanding the molecular pathogenesis of CAKUT.

### URETERIC BUDDING, *ROBO2*, AND *BMP4*

The protooncogene *RET*, a tyrosine kinase receptor, and its ligand, GDNF, regulate ureteric budding and renal branching morphogenesis. RET is expressed on the surface of ureteric cells.[33] GDNF is expressed by metanephric mesenchyme cells.[34] Homozygous deletion of either *Ret* or *Gdnf* in mice causes failure of ureteric outgrowth and renal agenesis. Patients with CAKUT have mutations in the RET/GDNF signaling pathway.[35–37] A study of 122 patients with CAKUT identified heterozygous deleterious sequence variants in *GDNF* or *RET* in 6/122 patients, 5%, whereas another group screened 749 families from all over the world and identified three families with heterozygous mutations in RET.[35] Similar findings have been reported in studies of fetuses with bilateral or unilateral renal agenesis.[36,37]

The site of ureteric bud outgrowth from the wolffian duct is normally invariant and the number of outgrowths is limited to one. Outgrowth of more than one ureteric bud can result in renal malformations including a double collecting system and duplication of the ureter. The position at which the ureteric bud arises from the wolffian duct relative to the metanephric mesenchyme is critical to the nature of the interactions between the ureteric bud and the metanephric mesenchyme. Ectopic positioning of the ureteric bud is associated with renal tissue malformation (dysplasia) due to abnormal ureteric bud–metanephric mesenchyme interactions and is also thought to contribute to the integrity of the ureterovesical junction. Mackie and Stephens postulated[38] that an abnormal position of the ureteral orifice in the bladder is associated with VUR in humans. Consistent with this hypothesis, mutations in *ROBO2* are associated with VUR in humans.[39] ROBO2, a cell surface receptor, is expressed in the nephrogenic mesenchyme.[40] Mice deficient in *Robo2* exhibit ectopic ureteric bud formation, multiple ureters, and hydroureter. Interestingly, the domain of *Gdnf* expression is expanded anteriorly in these mice, suggesting that loss of inhibition of *Gdnf* expression by ROBO2-dependent signaling expands the domain of *Gdnf* expression and results in ectopic ureter budding.[41] Members of the bone morphogenetic protein (BMP) family of secreted proteins also negatively regulate GDNF signaling. *Bmp4* is expressed in stromal cells immediately adjacent to the wolffian duct and the ureteric bud. Mice heterozygous for *Bmp4* exhibit ectopic or duplicated ureteric buds, suggesting that BMP4 suppresses ureteric induction by antagonizing the local effect of GDNF-RET signaling at the normal site of induction on the wolffian duct. Indeed, exogenous BMP4 has been shown to block GDNF-induced ureteric bud outgrowth from the wolffian duct in vitro.[42] Consistent with these observations, mutations in *BMP4* have been identified in humans with CAKUT phenotypes including renal dysgenesis and VUR.[43]

## URETERIC BRANCHING, *PAX2,* AND *RET*

Branching of the ureteric bud is initiated immediately following invasion of the metanephric mesenchyme by the ureteric bud. The number of ureteric bud branches elaborated is considered to be a major determinant of final nephron number because each ureteric bud branch tip induces a discrete subset of metanephric mesenchyme cells to undergo nephrogenesis (see Chapter 1: Normal Renal Development). Regulation of ureteric branch number has been informed by complementary studies in humans and mice. These investigations have demonstrated an essential role for *PAX2,* a transcription factor of the paired-box family of homeotic genes that is expressed in the mesonephros and in the metanephros during renal development.

Mutations in *PAX2* cause renal coloboma syndrome (also named papillorenal syndrome), an autosomal dominant disorder characterized by the association of renal hypoplasia, vesicoureteric reflux, and optic nerve coloboma.[44] While the prevalence of the syndrome is unknown, approximately 100 affected families have been reported.[45] A wide range of renal malformations are observed in renal coloboma syndrome and include most frequently oligomeganephronic hypoplasia, renal dysplasia, and vesicoureteric reflux.[46] Ureteropelvic junction obstruction has also been described.[23,27,46] The ocular phenotype is extremely variable. The most common finding is an optic disc pit associated with vascular abnormalities and cilioretinal arteries, with mild visual impairment limited to blind spot enlargement.[47] In other cases, the only ocular anomaly is optic nerve dysplasia with an abnormal vessel pattern and no functional consequence.

The PAX2 gene is located on chromosome 10q24-25. It encodes a transcription factor that belongs to the paired-box family of homeotic genes. The vast majority of the mutations are located in exons 2 and 3 encoding the DNA-binding domain. In 1995, Sanyanusin and colleagues reported heterozygous mutations in two renal coloboma syndrome (RCS) families.[48] Since then, more than 30 mutations have been reported, most of them lying in the second and third exons that encode the paired domain that binds to DNA or in exons 7–9 that encode the transactivation domain.[45,49]

During renal development, *Pax2* is expressed in the wolffian duct, the ureteric bud, and the metanephric mesenchyme. Studies in the 1Neu mouse strain, which is characterized by a *Pax2* mutation, demonstrated decreased ureteric branching in association with decreased nephron number. Decreased ureteric branch number and nephron number are rescued by inhibition of apoptosis in the ureteric lineage.[50,51] Studies in normal term newborns suggest that loss of PAX2 function may also contribute to generating a lower number of nephrons within the range of nephron number (approximately 250,000–1,600,000) observed in humans.[52] Goodyer hypothesized that gene polymorphisms that generate loss of PAX2 function could contribute to mild reductions in nephron number and discovered that a *PAX2* haplotype (*PAX2*$^{AAA}$) is associated with an approximately 10% decrease in kidney volume in a cohort of newborn infants.[29]

Ureteric branching is also mediated in large part by the GDNF–RET signaling axis. During ureteric branching, RET is expressed on the surface of ureteric tip cells and controls the number and pattern of branches elaborated.[53] The observation that *Ret*$^{+/-}$ mice exhibit a 22% reduction in nephron number[54] suggested that allelic variants in *RET* associated with decreased RET function contribute to decreased nephron number in humans. Indeed, an *RET* allelic variant which generates a reduced amount of RET mRNA in vitro control with the predominant *RET* allele has been associated with an approximately 10% decrease in total kidney volume, used in this case as a quantitative trait and surrogate measure of nephron number, in a cohort of newborn infants.[30]

## CONTROL OF GDNF EXPRESSION IN THE METANEPHRIC MESENCHYME: *SALL1, EYA1,* AND *SIX1*

As discussed earlier, GDNF expression by metanephric mesenchyme cells is critical to ureteric branching. In the metanephric mesenchyme, *Sall1, Eya1,* and *Six1* positively control *Gdnf* expression. *Sall1,* a member of the Spalt family of transcriptional factors,[55] is expressed in the metanephric mesenchyme prior to and during ureteric bud invasion. Mutational inactivation of *Sall1* in mice causes renal agenesis or severe dysgenesis and a marked decrease in GDNF expression.[56] Mutations in *SALL1* are associated with Townes–Brock syndrome, an autosomal dominant malformation syndrome characterized by imperforate anus, preaxial polydactyly and/or triphalangeal thumbs, external ear defects, sensorineural hearing loss (SNHL), and, less frequently, kidney, urogenital, and heart malformations.[57,58] *SALL1* mutations have also been identified in patients that lack extrarenal features of Townes–Brock syndrome.[23]

EYA1, a DNA binding transcription factor, is expressed in metanephric mesenchyme cells in the same spatial and temporal pattern as GDNF. EYA1 functions in a molecular complex with SIX1[59] to control expression of *Gdnf.*[60] Both EYA1 and SIX1 are also expressed in developing otic and branchial tissues.[61,62] Mice with EYA1 deficiency demonstrate renal agenesis and failure of GDNF expression.[61] Mutations in *EYA1* and *SIX1* occur in humans with branchio-oto-renal (BOR) syndrome.[59,63] Classic BOR syndrome, an autosomal dominant disorder, is defined by its major features, conductive and/or SNHL, branchial defects, ear pits, and renal anomalies in 95%, 49% to 69%, 83%, and 38% to 67% patients, respectively.[64,65] Renal malformations include unilateral or bilateral renal agenesis, hypodysplasia as well as malformation of the lower urinary tract including VUR, pyeloureteral obstruction, and ureteral duplication. Different renal malformations can be observed in the same family. Many patients have only one or two of these major BOR syndrome features; these findings in the absence of renal findings are termed BO syndrome. Mutations in *EYA1* have been identified, as well, in children with CAKUT who lack any of the extrarenal features of BOR or BO syndromes.[23]

BOR syndrome is transmitted as an autosomal dominant trait with incomplete penetrance and variable expressivity. A mutation in EYA1 has been identified in approximately 40% of patients with BOR syndrome.[65] Mutations are most commonly identified in a highly conserved region called the eyes absent homologous region encoded within exons 9–16. It is estimated that 5% may have a mutation in SIX1.[66] Molecular testing can confirm the diagnosis and provide genetic recurrence risk information to families. However, variability of the phenotype even with the same mutation does not permit accurate prediction of the disease severity. Within the same family, a given mutation may be associated with renal malformation in some individuals, but not in others.

## HEDGEHOG SIGNALING, GLI3 REPRESSOR, AND CONGENITAL ANOMALIES OF THE KIDNEY AND URINARY TRACT

Studies in mice and humans have demonstrated a critical role for Hedgehog-dependent signaling during kidney development. Hedgehog ligands function within concentration gradients. Binding of Hedgehog ligand, including Sonic Hedgehog (SHH), to its cognate cell surface receptor stimulates nuclear translocation of full-length GLI transcriptional activators and inhibits proteolytic processing of full length GLI3 to a shorter transcriptional repressor.[67] Loss-of-function mutations in *SHH* have been identified in patients with holoprosencephaly and renal hypoplasia or urogenital malformations.[68] Renal malformations have also been reported in patients exhibiting deletions of chromosome 7q, encompassing the *SHH* gene locus.[69–71] Posttranslational modification of Hedgehog ligand is essential for regulated diffusion of Hedgehog proteins and signaling.[72] A Hedgehog loss-of-function phenotype, including renal agenesis and hypodysplasia, is observed in Smith–Lemli–Opitz syndrome, which is caused by heterozygous mutations in the *DHCR7* gene, encoding sterol delta-7-reductase, that is required in mammalian sterol biosynthesis to convert 7-dehydrocholesterol into cholesterol.[73] Reduced Hedgehog modification with cholesterol may be pathogenic in Smith–Lemli–Opitz syndrome.

Pallister–Hall syndrome is an autosomal dominant multiorgan disorder characterized by multiple renal abnormalities including agenesis or dysplasia, hypoplasia, and hydronephrosis.[74–76] Affected individuals carry frameshift/nonsense and splicing mutations exclusively in the second third of the *GLI3* gene. These mutations are predicted to generate a truncated protein similar in size to GLI3 repressor.[77,78] The pathogenic role of GLI3 repressor was demonstrated in mice with homozygous *Shh* deficiency in which the levels of GLI3 in kidney tissue are elevated. Remarkably, renal dysgenesis in the absence of *Shh* is completely rescued by homozygous inactivation of *Gli3*.[79] Analysis of mice with constitutive expression of GLI3 repressor demonstrated aberrant common nephric duct patterning and ureteric stalk outgrowth associated with ureteric duplication and blind ending ureter.[80] Murine deficiency of *Smo*, which encodes a cell surface protein required for Hedgehog signaling, targeted to the metanephric mesenchyme lineage causes hydronephrosis, dyskinesia of the ureter, and absent expression of cell surface markers that characterized pacemaker cells in the renal pelvis and upper ureter. Homozygous deficiency of GLI3 in these mutant mice rescues these abnormalities.[81]

## THE MEDULLA AND GLYPICAN-3

Between the 22nd and 34th week of human fetal gestation, the peripheral (cortical) and central (medullary) domains of the developing kidney are established. Glypican-3 (GPC3), a glycosyl-phosphatidylinositol–linked cell surface heparan sulfate proteoglycan, and the gene that is mutated in Simpson–Golabi–Behmel syndrome, is required for normal patterning of the medulla.[82,83] Medullary dysplasia in mice deficient in *Gpc3* is associated with increased ureteric branching and cell proliferation,[82] and subsequent destruction of medullary collecting ducts due to apoptosis.[83] The defect is thought to be caused by insensitivity to inhibitors of branching morphogenesis including BMPs and enhanced sensitivity to the stimulatory effect of other factors including FGF7. The finding of medullary dysplasia in humans and mice mutant for $p57^{KIP2}$, an inhibitor of cell proliferation, further suggests that regulation of cell proliferation and apoptosis is important in the renal medulla[84] and suggests a further link to human renal medullary dysplasia as observed in some patients with Beckwith–Wiedemann syndrome and *p57*KIP2 mutations.[85]

## *TCF2*, MODY5, AND SPORADIC FORMS OF CONGENITAL ANOMALIES OF THE KIDNEY AND URINARY TRACT

*TCF2* encodes HNF-1β, a homeotic DNA-binding transcription factor, which is required during the development of the pancreas, kidneys, liver, and intestine. During mouse kidney development, *TCF2* is expressed in the wolffian duct, ureteric bud, comma and S-shaped bodies, and proximal and distal tubules.[86] Epithelial-specific inactivation of *Tcf2* in the kidney causes renal cystic disease and downregulation of several genes, inactivation of which cause renal cystic disease.[87] In humans, heterozygous mutations in *TCF2* cause maturity-onset diabetes type 5 (MODY5).[86,88] More than 50 different *TCF2* mutations have been reported, most of which are located in the first four exons that encode the DNA-binding domain. In more than one-third of the cases, the gene is entirely deleted.[28,89] Diabetes mellitus is present in approximately 60% of all the cases reported, usually occurs before 25 years of age, and is often associated with pancreatic atrophy.[89–91] In the presence of renal cysts, the term, renal cysts and diabetes syndrome, is used.

While *TCF2* mutations were first identified in MODY5, such mutations are observed more frequently in fetuses with bilateral hyperechoic kidneys. An analysis of 62 newborns or fetuses with antenatally diagnosed bilateral hyperechogenic kidneys revealed that large genomic *TCF2* deletions were the most frequent cause (29%).[92] A complementary retrospective analysis of 377 patients with a *TCF2* mutation demonstrated that isolated hyperechogenic kidney with normal or slightly enlarged size is the most frequent phenotype observed before birth in these patients.[93] After birth, *TCF2* mutations most commonly manifest as bilateral small cortical cysts.[28] However, other manifestations of CAKUT are observed in these patients and include renal hypoplasia and dysplasia, MCDK, renal agenesis, horseshoe kidney, pelviureteric junction obstruction, and clubbing and tiny diverticula of the calyces.[90,93–96] Patients with hyperechoic kidneys as a fetus and bilateral cortical cysts after birth and found to harbor *TCF2* mutations rarely manifest extrarenal anomalies during infancy and childhood.

## TUBULAR DYSGENESIS AND MUTATIONS OF RAS SYSTEM ELEMENTS

Renal tubular dysgenesis is a severe perinatal disorder characterized by absence or paucity of differentiated proximal tubules, early severe oligohydramnios, and perinatal death. The latter is usually due to pulmonary hypoplasia and skull ossification defects.[8,97,98] This condition has also been described in clinical conditions associated with renal ischemia including the twin–twin transfusion syndrome, major cardiac malformations, severe liver diseases, and fetal or infantile renal artery stenosis[99] and in fetuses that are exposed in utero to angiotensin-converting enzyme (ACE) inhibitors or angiotensin II (Ang II) receptor antagonists.[100] All of these pathophysiologic states are postulated to lead to chronic hypoperfusion of the fetal kidneys with upregulation of the renin–angiotensin system.[101] Mutations in the genes that encode components of the renin–angiotensin system have been identified in some families.[102] Mutations in the ACE and renin genes have been identified in 65.5% and 20% of cases, respectively. Mutations in angiotensinogen (AGT) and in the angiotensinogen type I receptor occur much less frequently.[103]

## CHD1L, CHD7, AND CHARGE SYNDROME

Chromodomain helicase DNA binding protein 1-like protein, CHD1L, is a member of the SNF2 family of helicase-related ATP-hydrolyzing proteins. Like its related family member, CHD7, CHD1L contains a helicase-like region. CHD1L is expressed in early ureteric bud and comma- and S-shaped structures during human kidney development.[104] Heterozygous missense mutations in CHD1L were identified in three patients among 85 with CAKUT.[104] Mutations in CHD7 have also been identified in CHARGE syndrome with 20% of these patients affected with CAKUT phenotypes including horseshoe kidneys, renal agenesis, renal dysplasia, VUR, ureterovesical junction obstruction, posterior urethral valves, and renal cysts.[105,106]

## DSTYK AND CONGENITAL ANOMALIES OF THE KIDNEY AND URINARY TRACT

DSTYK is a dual serine–threonine and tyrosine protein kinase that is coexpressed with fibroblast growth factor receptors in the developing mouse and human kidney in both metanephric mesenchyme and ureteric bud cells. Heterozygous mutations in DSTYK have been identified in a small number of individuals (7/311) with CAKUT.[107]

### COPY NUMBER VARIANTS, CONGENITAL ANOMALIES OF THE KIDNEY AND URINARY TRACT, AND NEUROPSYCHIATRIC DISORDERS

CNVs are stretches of DNA that are larger than 1 kb in length. Rare CNVs have been implicated in neuropsychiatric and craniofacial syndromes, and in syndromes with CAKUT.[31,108] Sanna-Cherchi et al. examined the frequency of rare CNVs in individuals with CAKUT and identified such variants in 10% of affected individuals compared with 0.2% of population controls.[31] Deletions at the *HNF1* locus (chromosome 17q12) and the locus for DiGeorge syndrome (chromosome 22q11) were most frequently identified, suggesting these are "hot spots" for copy number variation. Interestingly, 90% of the CNVs associated with congenital renal malformations were previously reported to predispose to developmental delay or neuropsychiatric disease, suggesting that there are shared pathways implicated in renal and central nervous system (CNS) development. Similarly, Handrigan et al. demonstrated that CNVs at chromosome 16q24.2 are associated with autism spectrum disorder, intellectual disability, and congenital renal malformations.[108]

# THE ENVIRONMENT IN UTERO AND CONGENITAL ANOMALIES OF THE KIDNEY AND URINARY TRACT

There is an increasing body of evidence, derived from human epidemiological studies and animal models, demonstrating an important role for the intrauterine environment and fetal programming in the pathogenesis of renal hypoplasia and predisposition to later kidney disease (reviewed in[109–118]; Table 72.2) Low birth weight or intrauterine growth retardation (IUGR) is generally considered to be due to a suboptimal in utero environment. Here, the fetal kidney is particularly susceptible, leading to reduced nephron number. In humans, IUGR is most often due to uteroplacental insufficiency and maternal undernutrition. Modeling of these disorders in animals causes a significant reduction in nephron endowment.[119] Maternal dietary protein restriction results in decreased nephron number, reduced renal function, and hypertension in a variety of species including rodents and sheep.[120–123] Although the underlying mechanisms are not well defined, there is some evidence suggesting that the maternal diet programs the expression of critical genes required for embryonic kidney development, cell survival,

**Table 72.2 Factors Influencing in Utero Environment That Are Associated With Renal Hypoplasia**

| Fetal Exposure to | Renal Phenotype | References |
|---|---|---|
| Uteroplacental insufficiency | Hypoplasia | 110 |
| Vitamin A deficiency | Hypoplasia, hydronephrosis/ureter | 111 |
| Low protein diet | Hypoplasia | 112,113 |
| Hyperglycemia | Agenesis, ectopic/horseshoe, cystic/dysplasia, hypoplasia, hydronephrosis/ureter | 114 |
| Cocaine | Agenesis, hypoplasia, hydronephrosis/ureter | 115 |
| Alcohol | Agenesis, ectopia/horseshoe, cystic dysplasia, hypoplasia, hydronephrosis/ureter | 116,117 |
| Angiotensin-converting enzyme inhibitors and angiotensin II receptor blockers | Renal dysgenesis | 118 |

and renal function.[121,124,125] It is likely that such changes in gene expression are controlled by epigenetic regulation.

Studies in mutant mice have identified a requirement for vitamin A and its retinoic acid receptor signaling effectors in RET expression and ureteric branching.[126] Vitamin A deficiency during pregnancy causes renal hypoplasia and decreased glomerular number and *Ret* expression in the rodent fetus.[127] Interestingly, a single dose of retinoic acid administered at midgestation is able to normalize kidney size and nephron number in rat offspring exposed to maternal protein restriction, raising the possibility of preventative approaches in humans.[128]

Maternal diabetes and in utero exposure to drugs and alcohol are associated with renal hypoplasia in the absence of reduced birth weight. In animal models, offspring of hyperglycemic or diabetic mothers demonstrate a significant nephron deficit.[129] Exposure of human fetuses to ACE inhibitors during the first trimester is associated with an increased risk of renal dysplasia as well as cardiovascular and CNS malformations.[130] Human infants exposed to cocaine in utero have an increased risk of renal tract anomalies.[131] Similarly, infants with fetal alcohol syndrome have a higher incidence of CAKUT.[132] The pathogenic mechanisms underlying fetal alcohol exposure are beginning to be elucidated. Ethyl alcohol administration to pregnant rats at E13.5 and E14.5, stages which correspond to human E5–E7, caused a modest decrease in nephron number but no deleterious effect on fetal kidney weight or maternal weight gain. The expression of *Gdnf* and *Wnt11,* both of which are required during ureteric branching, was reduced, consistent with a decrease in nephrogenesis. Analysis of blood pressure at 6 months of age in pups exposed to ethyl alcohol in utero demonstrated a 10% increase in both males and females compared with age-matched sham-treated controls although GFR and renal vascular resistance differed between sexes.[133]

## FUNCTIONAL CONSEQUENCES OF CONGENITAL ANOMALIES OF THE KIDNEY AND URINARY TRACT

A growing body of evidence indicates that the number of functional nephrons formed by 32 to 34 weeks' gestation has important implications for short- and long-term renal function. Infants with simple renal hypoplasia or a moderate to severe degree of hypodysplasia exhibit renal insufficiency. A subtle deficiency in nephron number has been associated with adult-onset hypertension.[134] The association of decreased nephron number with hypertension is consistent with the "Barker hypothesis," which is based on epidemiologic evidence showing a correlation between birth weight and the incidence of cardiovascular diseases and proposes that adult-onset diseases such as hypertension have a fetal origin.[135,136] The human kidney does not exhibit a capacity to accelerate the rate of nephron formation in children born prematurely or to extend the period of nephrogenesis beyond the equivalent of 34 weeks' gestation.[137] Thus the integrity of nephron formation in utero is absolutely critical to postnatal life.

Growth of renal tubules and expansion of glomerular cross-sectional area in utero and after birth are critical to renal functional capacity. The general observation that tubule number, cross-sectional area, and cellular maturation are abnormal in renal dysgenesis is consistent with clinical observations that infants with moderate to severe renal hypoplasia or dysplasia demonstrate a limitation of GFR and tubular function. Here, the developmental maturation of renal structures is discussed in the context of their functions. Illustrative examples are provided for how abnormal differentiation, growth, and maturation in the malformed kidney can limit these functions. Existing knowledge has been generated, for the most part, from the study of maturing preterm and term animals. By contrast, very little data have been derived from the study of animals, such as mutant mice, with renal malformation. Thus interpretation of physiologic abnormalities in humans and experimental animals with renal malformation is largely an extrapolation from developmental studies in experimental animals with normal kidney development.

A major increase in glomerular basement surface area after birth contributes to the maturational increase in GFR during infancy, childhood, and adolescence.[138] Low GFR at birth limits excretion of free water, increasing the susceptibility of newborns to hyponatremia in association with a hypotonic fluid challenge.[139] Maximum urine concentrations achieved by preterm and term infants following fluid restriction are 600 and 800 mOsm/kg, respectively.[140] An adult level of urine concentrating capacity is attained by 6 to 12 months of age.[141] Establishment of cortical and medullary domains during the 22nd to 24th week of gestation is critical to urine concentration.[137] During embryogenesis, the renal cortex grows along a circumferential axis with a tenfold increase in its volume. The renal medulla expands 4.5-fold in thickness along a longitudinal axis, an increase that is mainly due to elongation of the outer medullary collecting ducts.[142] Longitudinal growth of the medulla contributes to lengthening of the loops of Henle such that they reach the inner renal medulla in the mature kidney. Elongation of the loops of Henle is important to the urine concentration mechanism because the magnitude of sodium and urea transport is greatest in longer loops, which generate steeper medullary tonicity gradients. The responsiveness of collecting duct cells to vasopressin is limited in newborns. This is thought to be due to high intrarenal levels of prostaglandins, which antagonize vasopressin.[143]

Maturation of sodium transport in the fetus and infant is dependent on growth and differentiation within the proximal tubule, loop of Henle, and distal tubule. Normal newborn infants are limited in their capacity to respond to sodium restriction by reducing urinary sodium excretion. Interruption of tubule generation, differentiation, and growth, hallmark features of renal dysplasia, contribute to an exaggerated limitation in the capacity to absorb sodium in affected infants and children. The proximal tubule exhibits dramatic growth and maturation during renal development. The epithelium matures from a columnar to a cuboidal epithelium, microvilli are elaborated on the apical and basal domains, and expression of the $Na^+,K^+$-ATPase and the type 3 sodium-hydrogen exchanger (NHE3) increase.[144–146] At birth, proximal tubule length is heterogeneous between the inner and outer cortex[138]; by 1 month of life proximal tubule length becomes uniform and tubule length and diameter have increased.[144] Maturation of tubule length is associated with the capacity to absorb sodium.[147]

The loop of Henle is also characterized by increased spatial expression of transporters (NKCC2, NHE3, ROMK, $Na^+,K^+$-ATPase) key to sodium transport.[148] Similarly, expression of

NCCT and epithelial sodium channel (ENaC) is low in the neonatal kidney and increases thereafter.[149]

Urinary potassium secretion is achieved predominantly by secretion of potassium in the cortical collecting duct via apical ROMK $K^+$ channels. In neonates, $K^+$ secretion is lower than in children due to the low secretory capacity of the cortical collecting duct. The postnatal increase in $K^+$ secretion is thought to be due to a developmental increase in the number of ROMK channels[150] as well as the BK potassium channel of the collecting duct.[151] Malformation of tubules in disorders such as renal dysplasia is commonly associated with limited $K^+$ secretion particularly during infancy.

## CLINICAL PRESENTATION OF CONGENITAL ANOMALIES OF THE KIDNEY AND URINARY TRACT

### CLINICAL PRESENTATION IN THE FETUS

The majority of renal malformations are diagnosed antenatally, largely because of the widespread use and sensitivity of fetal ultrasound. The fetal kidney can be visualized at 12 to 15 weeks of human gestation. A screening antenatal ultrasound is recommended between 16 and 20 weeks of gestation by which time renal anatomy can be imaged with considerable definition and anomalies can be detected with a sensitivity of approximately 80%.[152] Corticomedullary differentiation is distinct by 25 weeks of gestation and sometimes earlier. The fetal ureters are not normally detected by ultrasound. Visualization of ureters may be indicative of ureteric or bladder obstruction, or VUR. A urine-filled bladder is normally identified at 13 to 15 weeks' gestation.[153] The normal bladder wall is normally thin. If the bladder wall is thick, urethral obstruction such as posterior urethral valves in a male fetus may be present.

Development of the kidney in utero is commonly assessed using fetal renal length standardized for gestational age as a surrogate marker.[154] The volume of amniotic fluid is a surrogate measure of renal function. Fetal urine production begins at 9 weeks of gestation. By 20 weeks' gestation and thereafter, fetal urine is the primary source of amniotic fluid volume.[155] A decrease in amniotic fluid volume, termed oligohydramnios, at or beyond the 20th week of gestation is an excellent indicator of a critical defect in both kidneys, for example bilateral renal dysplasia (or a critical defect in one kidney where a solitary kidney exists), bilateral ureteral obstruction, or obstruction of the bladder outlet. Severe oligohydramnios in the second trimester can result in lung hypoplasia because an adequate amniotic fluid volume is critical for lung development.[156] In its most severe form, oligohydramnios results in Potter syndrome, which consists of a typical facies characterized by pseudoepicanthus, a recessed chin, posteriorly rotated and flattened ears, and flattened nose, as well as decreased fetal movement, clubfoot, hip dislocation and joint contractures, and pulmonary hypoplasia.

The composition of fetal urine is also used as a marker of kidney function. Urine levels of sodium and beta-2-microglobulin decrease with increasing gestational age and urine osmolality increases.[157,158] Impaired resorption occurs in fetuses with bilateral renal dysplasia or severe bilateral obstructive uropathy, resulting in abnormal high urine levels of sodium and beta-2-microglobulin and low urine osmolality.[159] In general, sodium and chloride concentration greater than 90 mEq/L (90 mmol/L) and urinary osmolality less than 210 mOsmol/kg·$H_2O$ (210 mmol/kg·$H_2O$) are indicative of fetal renal tubular impairment and poor renal prognosis.[160] In addition, urinary beta-2-microglobulin levels greater than 6 mg/L are predictive of severe renal damage with a sensitivity and specificity of 80% and 71%, respectively.[161]

### CLINICAL PRESENTATION OF SPECIFIC FORMS OF CONGENITAL ANOMALIES OF THE KIDNEY AND URINARY TRACT

#### RENAL AGENESIS

A diagnosis of unilateral renal agenesis depends on the certainty that a second kidney does not exist in the pelvis or some other ectopic location. Because absence of one kidney induces compensatory hypertrophy in the existing kidney, the presence of a large kidney on one side supports a diagnosis of unilateral renal agenesis. Unilateral renal agenesis is generally asymptomatic. A solitary kidney is most often detected either during routine antenatal ultrasonography or during the assessment of an accompanying urinary tract abnormality, the occurrence of which has been reported in 33% to 65% of cases.[162] VUR is the most commonly identified urological abnormality, occurring in approximately 37% of patients with unilateral renal agenesis and prompting investigation particularly in newborn infants. Other associated urological anomalies include obstruction of the ureteropelvic junction in 6% to 7%, and ureterovesical junction in 11% to 18% of patients.

### RENAL DYSPLASIA

The dysplastic kidney is generally smaller than normal and is characterized with ultrasound by increased echogenicity, loss of corticomedullary differentiation, and cysts of varied size and location. Large cystic elements can contribute to large kidney size. The MCDK is an extreme example of a large dysplastic kidney (Fig. 72.2). Renal dysplasia may be unilateral or bilateral and may be discovered during routine antenatal screening or postnatally when renal ultrasonography is performed in a dysmorphic infant. Bilateral dysplasia is likely to be diagnosed earlier than unilateral dysplasia especially if oligohydramnios is present. Infants with bilateral dysplasia may demonstrate impaired renal function shortly after birth. Associated urinary tract abnormalities include hydronephrosis, a duplicated collecting system, megaureter, ureteral stenosis, and VUR.[160] Clinical presentation may be related to complications such as urinary tract infection (UTI) associated with these disorders.

The MCDK is identified by ultrasound as a large cystic nonreniform mass in the renal fossa and by palpation as a flank mass. The MCDK is nonfunctional and usually unilateral. If bilateral, it is fatal. In unilateral MCDK, associated contralateral abnormalities occur in 25% of cases and can include rotational or positional anomalies, renal hypoplasia, vesicoureteric efflux, and ureteropelvic junction obstruction.[15] While hypertension rarely occurs (0.01%–0.1% of cases), blood pressure should be monitored intermittently during the first few years of life. Wilms tumor and renal cell carcinoma

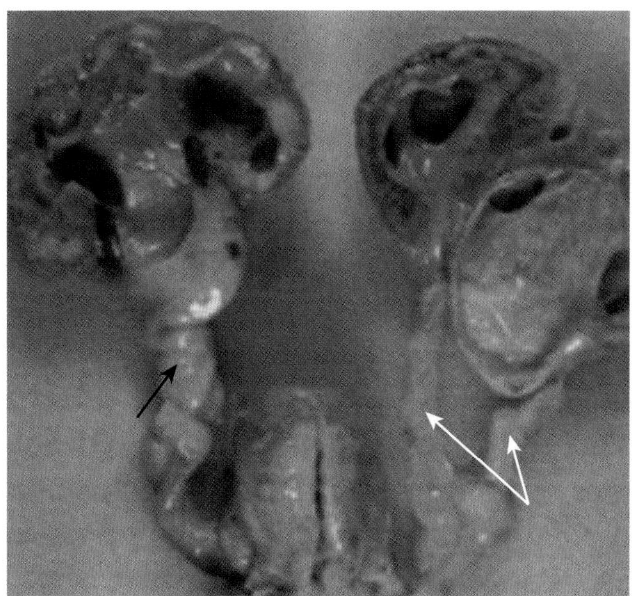

**Fig. 72.6** Duplicated collecting system. Duplicated ureters *(white arrows)* are shown on the right. A single dilated ureter *(black arrow)* is shown on the left. Each ureter is dilated due to obstruction at the level of the bladder.

have also been described but the incidence of malignant complications is not significantly different from the general population.[163] The natural history of an MCDK is gradual reduction in size such that the kidney eventually cannot be detected using noninvasive imaging. At 2 years of age, an involution in size by ultrasound occurs in up to 60% of the affected kidneys.

## DOUBLE COLLECTING SYSTEM

Complete or partial duplication of the renal collecting system is the most common congenital anomaly of the urinary tract (Fig. 72.6).[11] A double collecting system is thought to result from duplication of the ureteric bud with the superior bud associated with the upper renal pole and the inferior bud with the lower renal pole. In complete duplication, the kidney has two separate pelvicalyceal systems and two ureters. The ureter from the lower collecting system usually enters the bladder in the trigone, whereas the ureter from the upper collecting system can have a normal insertion in the trigone or be inserted ectopically in the bladder or elsewhere. In boys, insertion can occur in the posterior urethra, ejaculatory ducts, or epididymis and in girls into the vagina or uterus. Ectopic insertion of the ureter can result in obstruction or VUR. Depending upon the location of the ectopic insertion, incontinence also may be present. Partial duplication is more common than complete duplication. In these cases, the kidney has two separate pelvicalyceal systems with either a single ureter or two ureters that unite prior to insertion into the bladder.

## RENAL ECTOPY

Renal ectopy (Fig. 72.5) results from disruption of the normal embryologic migration of the kidneys. Rapid caudal growth during embryogenesis results in migration of the developing kidney from the pelvis to the retroperitoneal renal fossa. With ascension comes a 90° rotation from a horizontal to a vertical position with the renal hilum finally directed medially. Migration and rotation are complete by 8 weeks of gestation. Simple congenital ectopy refers to a low-lying kidney that failed to ascend normally. It most commonly lies over the pelvic brim or in the pelvis and is termed a pelvic kidney. Less commonly, the kidney may lie on the contralateral side of the body, a state that is termed *crossed ectopy without fusion*. Affected individuals generally have no symptoms and the condition is identified during an imaging study performed for some other indication; however, some patients develop symptoms due to complications, such as infection, renal calculi, and urinary obstruction.[154] The ectopic kidney is often characterized by decreased function. In a case study of 82 cases of unilateral renal ectopy, decreased renal function was detected by $^{99}$mTc-dimercaptosuccinic acid (DMSA) renal scan in 74 patients.[154] A high incidence of other urological abnormalities has been associated with renal ectopy. The most frequent of these is VUR, which occurs in 20% of crossed renal ectopy, 30% of simple renal ectopy, and 70% of bilateral simple renal ectopy.[154] Other associated urological abnormalities include contralateral renal dysplasia (4%), cryptorchidism (5%), and hypospadias (5%).[17]

## RENAL FUSION

Renal fusion occurs when a portion of one kidney is fused to the other (Fig. 72.5). The most common fusion anomaly is the horseshoe kidney, which involves abnormal migration of both kidneys (ectopy). The horseshoe kidney differs from crossed fused renal ectopy, which usually involves abnormal movement of only one kidney across the midline with fusion of the contralateral noncrossing kidney. In more than 90% of horseshoe kidneys, fusion occurs at the lower poles; as a result, two separate excretory renal units and ureters are maintained. The isthmus (fused portion) may lie over the midline (symmetric horseshoe kidney) or lateral to the midline (asymmetric horseshoe kidney). Depending on the degree of fusion, the isthmus can be composed of renal parenchyma or a fibrous band. Fusion is thought to occur before the kidneys ascend between the fourth to ninth week of gestation from the pelvis to their normal dorsolumbar position. If large portions of the renal parenchyma fuse, the fusion anomaly loses its horseshoe appearance and appears as a flattened disc or lump kidney. Early fusion also causes abnormal rotation of the developing kidneys. As a result, the axis of each kidney is shifted so that the renal pelvis lies anteriorly and the ureters either traverse over the isthmus of the horseshoe kidney or the anterior surface of the fused kidney. Fusion anomalies seldom ascend to the dorsolumbar position of normal kidneys and are typically found in the pelvis or at the lower lumbar vertebral level (L4 or L5). The blood supply of the fused kidney is variable and may come from the iliac arteries, aorta, and at times, the hypogastric and middle sacral arteries.

The majority of patients with renal fusion are asymptomatic. Some, however, develop urinary tract obstruction which presents with loin pain, hematuria, and may be associated with UTIs due to urinary stasis or vesicoureteric reflux. Renal calculi may occur in up to 20% of cases.[164] Other associated urological anomalies include ureteral duplication, ectopic ureter, and retrocaval ureter. Investigations can include static imaging (renal ultrasound) and functional imaging such as a $^{99}$mTc-DMSA scan and a voiding cystourethrogram (VCUG). Renal calculi are reported to occur in 20% of cases. Obstruction resulting in urinary stasis and complicating UTI have been thought to be the major contributing factors to stone formation. Patients with a horseshoe kidney appear to have an increased risk for Wilms tumor. This was illustrated in a retrospective review of 8617 patients from the National Wilms Tumor Study, between 1969 to 1998, that identified 41 patients with Wilms tumor in a horseshoe kidney.[165]

In crossed fused ectopy, the ectopic kidney and ureter cross the midline to fuse with the contralateral kidney but the ureter of the ectopic kidney maintains its normal insertion into the bladder. In most cases, the ectopic kidney is positioned inferiorly to the contralateral kidney. The contralateral kidney can either retain its normal dorsolumbar position or is positioned lower in the pelvis or lower lumbar vertebral level (L4 or L5). Most patients with crossed fused ectopy are asymptomatic and are detected coincidentally, often by antenatal ultrasonography. As is true in patients with horseshoe kidney, most patients have an excellent prognosis without need for intervention. In some cases, complications can occur, including obstructive uropathy due to extrinsic ureteric compression by aberrant blood vessels or ureteropelvic junction obstruction, renal calculi, urinary infection, and VUR.[166]

## CLINICAL MANAGEMENT OF CONGENITAL ANOMALIES OF THE KIDNEY AND URINARY TRACT

Because CAKUT play a causative role in 30% to 50% of cases of end-stage renal disease (ESRD) in children,[167] it is important to diagnose and initiate therapy to minimize renal damage, prevent or delay the onset of ESRD, and provide supportive care to avoid complications of ESRD.

### OVERALL APPROACH TO MANAGEMENT OF CONGENITAL ANOMALIES OF THE KIDNEY AND URINARY TRACT IN UTERO AND IN THE IMMEDIATE POSTNATAL PERIOD

Counseling of families during pregnancy is a key element in the management of CAKUT. Coordinated consultation among professionals in the disciplines of obstetrics, pediatric nephrology, pediatric urology, and neonatology is critical. Consistent and clear clinical information regarding diagnosis and prognosis should be provided during pregnancy and after birth. The level of certainty regarding the severity of the diagnosis and prognosis has a major impact on decision-making during pregnancy and in the immediate postnatal period. Intervention in utero has been designed to (1) reduce renal damage arising from urinary tract obstruction, and (2) rescue pulmonary development in the face of urinary tract obstruction and oligohydramnios. To date, little evidence exists that relief of urinary tract obstruction in utero prevents the development of associated renal dysplasia or renal scarring. By contrast, insertion of a bladder–amniotic cavity shunt in the fetus with obstruction below the bladder neck can rescue oligohydramnios and pulmonary hypoplasia.[166,168] Diagnostic and therapeutic management after birth should be anticipated via the coordinated actions of obstetricians, neonatologists, pediatric nephrologists, and pediatric urologists and should include an immediate assessment in the postnatal period of the need for specialized imaging, assessment of renal function, and management of nutrition and electrolytes.

After delivery, a detailed history and careful physical examination should be performed in all infants with an antenatally detected renal malformation. The examination should include the respiratory system to assess the presence of pulmonary insufficiency; the abdomen to detect the presence of a mass that could represent an enlarged kidney due to obstructive uropathy or MCDK or a palpable enlarged bladder, which could suggest posterior urethral valves; the ears, because outer ear abnormalities are associated with an increased risk of CAKUT; and the umbilicus, because a single umbilical artery is associated with an increased risk of CAKUT.

In newborns with bilateral renal malformation, a solitary malformed kidney, or a history of oligohydramnios, an abdominal ultrasound is recommended within the first 24 hours of life because an intervention such as decompression of the bladder with a transurethral catheter may be required. Newborn infants with unilateral involvement do not need immediate attention. In these infants, a renal ultrasound is generally performed after 48 hours of age and within the first week of life. Ultrasound examination before 48 hours of age may not detect collecting system dilatation because a newborn is relatively volume contracted during this period.[169] The serum creatinine estimates the extent of renal impairment and should be used when there is bilateral renal disease or an affected solitary kidney. The serum creatinine concentration at birth is similar to that in the mother (usually ≤1.0 mg/dL [88 μmol/L]). Thus serum creatinine should be measured after the first 24 hours of life. It declines to normal values [serum creatinine 0.3 to 0.5 mg/dL (27–44 μmol/L]) within approximately 1 week in term infants and 2 to 3 weeks in preterm infants.

### MANAGEMENT OF SPECIFIC TYPES OF CONGENITAL ANOMALIES OF THE KIDNEY AND URINARY TRACT

#### RENAL DYSPLASIA

Renal dysplasia is frequently associated with collecting system anomalies, particularly VUR. Thus a VCUG should be considered in all patients with renal dysplasia, particularly after detection of hydronephrosis by ultrasound and/or occurrence of a UTI. The presence of VUR or some other collecting system abnormality in the normal contralateral kidney places children with unilateral renal dysplasia at increased risk of long-term sequelae of renal scarring from recurrent UTI. A DMSA radionuclide scan can provide further information on the differential function of each kidney, which may be useful in management decisions regarding surgical interventions. The prognosis of renal dysplasia depends on whether there is unilateral versus bilateral disease. In general, the long-term outcome of unilateral renal dysplasia is excellent, particularly if there is a normal contralateral kidney. Serial ultrasonography can assess compensatory renal growth of a normal contralateral kidney and any further change in the size of the abnormal kidney.

The natural history of an MCDK is gradual reduction in size such that the kidney eventually cannot be detected using noninvasive imaging. At 2 years of age, an involution in size by ultrasound occurs in up to 60% of the affected kidneys. Renal ultrasound is generally recommended at an interval of 3 months for the first year of life and then every 6 months up to involution of the mass, or at least up to 5 years.[170] Compensatory hypertrophy of the contralateral kidney is expected and should be monitored by renal ultrasound. Hypertension is unusual; blood pressure should be monitored intermittently during the first few years of life. Medical therapy is usually effective in treating hypertension in the small number of affected patients, but nephrectomy may be curative in resistant cases. Wilms tumor and renal cell carcinoma have also been described but the incidence of malignant complications is not significantly different from the general population.[163]

### RENAL ECTOPY AND FUSION

Detection of an ectopic kidney provides a basis to determine renal function and any associated urinary tract anomalies. Reduced renal function in the ectopic kidney can be determined by radionuclide scan. An abdominal and pelvic ultrasound is indicated to determine the presence of collecting system abnormality. A VCUG should be undertaken, particularly if there is hydronephrosis and in the aftermath of a UTI to detect possible VUR or urinary tract obstruction. If VUR is detected, then prophylactic antibiotics should be considered, especially in patients who have a history of UTIs.

Further evaluation is based upon the results of a renal ultrasound, VCUG, and serum creatinine. No further evaluation is required in the patient with a normal appearing contralateral kidney and no evidence of hydronephrosis in the ectopic kidney. If the serum creatinine is elevated or if the contralateral kidney appears abnormal, a DMSA renal scan should be performed to assess differential renal function. A diuretic renogram with ($^{99}$mTc)-mercaptotriglycylglycine (MAG-3) or technetium $^{99}$mTc-diethylenetriamine pentaacetic acid (DTPA) should be performed to detect obstruction if there is severe hydronephrosis and the VCUG is normal. If the hydronephrosis is mild or moderate and the VCUG is normal, then follow-up ultrasonography should be performed 3 to 6 months later. If there is progressive hydronephrosis, then an MAG-3 or DTPA diuretic renogram should be performed to detect obstruction.

### LONG-TERM OUTCOMES OF RENAL MALFORMATION

Clinical outcomes in CAKUT vary widely from no symptoms whatsoever to CKD resulting in a need for renal replacement during a period ranging from the newborn period to the 4th and 5th decades of life. Risk factors for mortality during infancy and early childhood include coexistence of renal and nonrenal disease, prematurity, low birth weight, oligohydramnios, and severe forms of renal–urinary tract malformation (agenesis, hypodysplasia).[171] In a case series of 822 children with prenatally detected CAKUT that were followed for a median time of 43 months, Quirino et al. reported a mortality of 1.5% and morbidities including UTI, hypertension, and CKD in 29%, 2.7%, and 6% of surviving children, respectively.[172] A faster rate of decline of renal function in patients with CAKUT and CKD has been associated with a urine albumin-to-creatinine ratio greater than 200 mg/mmol compared with less than 50 mg/mmol (eGFR −6.5 mL/min/1.73 m$^2$/year vs. −1.5 mL/min/1.73 m$^2$/year), and with more than two (vs. <2) febrile UTIs (eGFR −3.5 mL/min/1.73 m$^2$/year vs. −2 mL/min/1.73 m$^2$/year). A greater decline in eGFR occurs during puberty (eGFR −4 mL/min/1.73 m$^2$/year vs. −1.9 mL/min/1.73 m$^2$/year).[173] A study examining the risk for dialysis in patients with CAKUT demonstrated a significantly higher risk for patients with a solitary kidney compared with nondisease controls.[174] These results raise the possibility that the prognosis for a solitary apparently normal kidney may not be as "normal" as previously thought. Finally, a study of CAKUT patients receiving some form of replacement therapy and registered within the European Dialysis and Transplant Association Registry showed that some of these patients only require renal replacement in the third, fourth, or fifth decade of life. The finding that the mean age at which patients with CAKUT require dialysis and/or transplantation is 31 years indicates that children with CAKUT are at risk of developing a requirement for dialysis and/or transplantation as adults.[7]

# GLOMERULAR DISEASES

## NEPHRITIC SYNDROME AND RELATED DISEASES

### DIFFERENTIAL DIAGNOSIS OF GLOMERULAR HEMATURIA

A urine sediment that consists of >5 red blood cells/high-power field together with acanthocytes, red cell casts, or mixed red and white cell casts is characteristic of glomerular hematuria and is called a nephritic urine. Hematuria, impaired kidney function, and hypertension define a nephritic syndrome.[175] The differential diagnosis of glomerular hematuria is extensive and includes, but is not limited to, structural defects of the glomerular basement membrane (GBM); (e.g., Alport syndrome [AS]); thin basement membrane nephropathy (TBMN), inflammatory/autoimmune processes affecting the GBM (e.g., Goodpasture syndrome; anti-GBM antibody disease), systemic diseases affecting the glomerular capillaries (e.g., thrombotic microangiopathy [TMA]), systemic lupus erythematosus (SLE), antineutrophil cytoplasmic antibody (ANCA) vasculitis, antiphospholipid syndrome (APS), immunoglobulin A (IgA) nephropathy (IgAN), Henoch–Schönlein purpura (HSP), membranous nephropathy (MN), immune complex membranoproliferative glomerulonephritis (IC MPGN)/C3 glomerulopathy (C3G), and postinfectious GN (PIGN), and—to a lesser extent—nephrotic syndrome (NS). Identifying the specific diagnosis underlying glomerular hematuria can be challenging and requires in addition to the obligatory microscopic urinalysis (urine sediment; see earlier discussion) a detailed review of the personal and family medical history, a thorough clinical examination with focus on extrarenal disease manifestations, and a complete laboratory workup (including blood and urine) for the parameters specific for the aforementioned differential diagnoses.

Glomerular hematuria is a common first symptom of glomerulopathy and can mark the beginning of a disease process subsequently characterized by (glomerular) proteinuria and a progressive decline in kidney function, leading to CKD, and eventually resulting in ESRD. Presently, a total of six genes are known to cause familial microscopic hematuria (FMH): CFHR5, MYH9, and FN1 (not discussed here), as well as COL4A3, COL4A4, and COL4A5.[176]

## ALPORT SYNDROME AND THIN BASEMENT MEMBRANE NEPHROPATHY

### PATHOGENESIS

AS and TBMN define a spectrum of hereditary diseases affecting collagen type IV, the major component of the GBM.[177,178] Collagen IV is made of α chains (monomers), three of which combine to form a triple helical heterotrimer, or protomer, with the following structural domains: (1) a 7S triple helical domain at the N terminus, (2) a central triple helical collagenous domain, and (3) a noncollagenous (NCl) trimer at the C terminus. The collagen IV network exists as a combination of protomers, which is stabilized via disulfide cross-links between triple helical collagenous domains of the collagen IV chains.[179]

The triple helical collagen IV protomers are composed of defined combinations of six distinct monomeric chains (α1–6). In the embryonic kidney, the GBM is composed of α1 and α2 chains in the combination of α1.α1.α2, whereas the mature kidney contains the α3, α4, and α5 chains in the combination of α3.α4.α5.[179] In contrast to the embryonic α1.α1.α2 protomer, the mature α3.α4.α5 protomer forms a higher number of disulfide bonds, thus enhancing its mechanical stability toward the hydrostatic (blood) pressure the glomerular capillary loop is constantly exposed to. Mutations in the COL4A3, COL4A4, or COL4A5 genes result in the formation of defective collagen IV protomers forming a GBM with (partial) persistence of the embryonic α1.α1.α2 chains and with decreased mechanical stability, which in turn is the cause of progressive deterioration of the GBM structure and loss of function in AS and TBMN.[177–179]

Additional factors contributing to the decreased stability and increased permeability of the GBM as well as progressive glomerulopathy in AS include compensatory overproduction of atypical laminin isoforms (laminin α1 and α5),[180,181] the production of transforming growth factor β1 by podocytes,[181,182] and matrix metalloproteinase (MMP)-mediated proteolytic removal of the embryonic collagen IV protomers (α1.α1.α2).[181,183,184] Recently, crosstalk between the podocytes and abnormal collagen IV of the GBM via the discoidin domain receptor (DDR) 1 and α2β1 integrin has been identified as critical for AS pathogenesis.[185,186] DDR1 is a tyrosine kinase transmembrane receptor with collagens I–V as its ligand.[187] DDR1 regulates extracellular matrix remodeling by controlling the adhesion and proliferation of renal mesangial cells.[188] It has been postulated that the podocyte detects altered collagen protomers via DDR1 receptors, resulting in the upregulation of various cytokines and growth factors, ultimately leading to progressive glomerulopathy via inflammation and fibrosis.[186] An additional possible pathogenic mechanism involves α2β1 integrin, present on the basolateral surface of podocytes. α2 integrin binds to a specific sequence of the collagen IV protomer.[189] α2β1 integrin can be upregulated in signaling to downstream mechanosensor proteins in the presence of abnormal collagen chains, thus resulting in overproduction of extracellular matrix by podocytes.[190,191]

### CLINICAL MANIFESTATIONS

First described in 1927 by A.C. Alport,[192,193] the triad of familial nephritis, deafness, and ocular changes was subsequently named AS.[193] The clinical manifestation of AS at disease onset in childhood is typically mild with hematuria only. Untreated, AS progresses to proteinuria, CKD, and eventually ESRD in adulthood.

AS is caused by mutations in the collagen IV α3, α4, and α5 genes (COL4A3, COL4A4, and COL4A5).[178,179] COL4A3 and COL4A4 are encoded on chromosome 2 (2q35-37); COL4A5 is encoded on the X chromosome (Xq26-48). About 65% of AS cases are inherited in an X-linked fashion via COL4A5, about 15% in an autosomal recessive fashion via mutations in COL4A3 and COL4A4, and about 20% in an autosomal dominant fashion with mutations in COL4A3 and COL4A4.[179] While male AS patients with an X-linked COL4A5 mutation are always severely affected with progression to ESRD in 50% typically during the 2nd decade of life,[194] female carriers present with a wide phenotypic spectrum ranging from microscopic hematuria to ESRD.[178] Of note, the clinical presentation is similar between males with hemizygous COL4A5 mutations and individuals with homozygous or compound heterozygous COL4A3 and COL4A4 mutations.[178] AS can vary in both severity and organ involvement (mosaicism) in females due to random inactivation of one of the two alleles of each X chromosome.[195]

Disease severity of AS is determined by the type of mutation with a strong genotype–phenotype correlation (point or missense mutations versus deletions, frame shift, or truncating mutations) and the type of inheritance. In a large cohort of X-linked AS patients, missense mutations were the most common, occurring in 51% of cases, and conferred the most favorable prognosis with a median time to ESRD of 37 years, as compared with patients with deletions, who reach ESRD by age 22 (95% confidence interval, 16–23 years).[196]

AS disease manifestation is also determined by the organ distribution pattern of the collagen IV α chains involved in the formation of the mature collagen IV protomers. Collagen IV α3.α4.α5 is not only found in the GBM, but also in the basement membrane of the renal tubules, the inner ear, and the posterior lens capsule.[197] Collagen IV α5.α5.α6 is found in the basement membrane of the eye and in visceral smooth muscle cells of the gastrointestinal (esophagus), the respiratory (trachea), and the female reproductive tract.[178,198] Thus AS is also characterized by cochlear and ocular involvement. Progressive SNHL is usually present by late childhood or early adolescence.[197,199] Ocular findings include corneal opacities, anterior lenticonus, fleck retinopathy, and temporal retinal thinning. Rarer findings include posterior dysmorphous corneal dystrophy, giant macular hole, and maculopathy—all causing loss of visual acuity.[197,200] In addition, in very rare cases AS can manifest leiomyomatosis affecting the visceral smooth muscle cells of the esophagus, the trachea, or the female genital tract.[179,201]

## THIN BASEMENT MEMBRANE NEPHROPATHY

TBMN, previously termed benign FMH, is the most common cause of persistent glomerular hematuria in adults and children, and has a prevalence of approximately 1%. TBMN is characterized by a benign clinical course with minimal or no proteinuria and normal renal function. The family history is typically positive for microscopic hematuria and ultrastructural examination of a renal biopsy specimen via electron microscopy (EM) reveals uniform thinning of the GBM to approximately half of its normal thickness.[202,203]

Approximately 40% to 50% of TBMN patients carry heterozygous mutations in COL4A3 or COL4A4. This genetic finding and the clinical observation that TBMN patients occasionally present with a more severe disease course characterized by marked proteinuria and progressive glomerulopathy have given rise to the concept of a collagen IV disease spectrum with AS at its severe end and with TBMN at its mild end. Thus TBMN patients can be considered as heterozygous carriers of autosomal-recessive AS.

## ESTABLISHING THE DIAGNOSIS OF ALPORT SYNDROME AND THIN BASEMENT MEMBRANE NEPHROPATHY

Diagnostic criteria for AS include the combination of hematuria and a positive family history of hematuria, chronic renal failure, or both, high-frequency SNHL, pathognomonic ocular anomalies (see earlier discussion), or characteristic ultrastructural changes in glomerular kidney or skin basement membranes.[204,205] A renal biopsy is diagnostic. In AS, ultrastructural examination of a renal biopsy specimen via EM reveals GBM thinning associated with early stages of disease, and thickening and multilamellation associated with late stages of the disease (Fig. 72.7).[184,206] By contrast, in TBMN, ultrastructural examination reveals uniform thinning of the GBM to approximately half of its normal thickness without thickening and multilamellation (Fig. 72.7).[202,203] Immunofluorescence (IF) staining identifies the absence of the mutant collagen IV α5 chain in the most frequent form of AS, autosomal dominant AS, affecting approximately 85% of cases. Of note, while X-mosaicism might obscure the correct diagnosis, an IF-based diagnosis can in principle also be established via skin biopsy.[207]

## TREATMENT

While originally aiming to establish the blood pressure target for optimal renal protection in children via blockade of the renin–angiotensin–aldosterone system (RAAS), the ESCAPE Study Group identified that both blood pressure control and a decrease in proteinuria in CKD were significant independent predictors of delayed progression of renal disease.[208] Groundbreaking studies in COL4A3 knockout mice[209] established the benefit of ACE inhibitor and angiotensin receptor blocker (ARB) treatment in this animal model of progressive AS. While untreated knockout mice died from ESRD after approximately 70 days (71 ± 6 days), RAAS blockade resulted in a significant delay in disease progression with an increase in life span by 100% (150 ± 21 days) using ACE inhibitors,[210] and by 40% (98 ± 16 days) in ARB-treated mice.[211]

Current guidelines for the treatment of AS suggest the initiation of ACE inhibitors and/or ARBs at the onset of overt proteinuria to prolong renal survival and delay the need for RRT. ACE inhibitors should be first line, with ARB or aldosterone inhibition used as second-line agents.[212] RAAS blockade has been studied in children with AS.[194,213] The comparison of the ARB losartan with placebo or amlodipine over 12 weeks in 30 children resulted in a significant reduction in proteinuria.[214] In a retrospective evaluation of 283 AS patients followed for 20 years in the European Alport Registry, three treatment subgroups were identified: (1) patients in whom ACE inhibitor treatment was commenced with onset of microalbuminuria, (2) with proteinuria of greater than 0.3 g/day, or (3) with CKD III–IV. ESRD with onset of dialysis treatment was delayed by 3 years in the CKD group, and by 18 years in the proteinuria group. Of note, in 15 sibling pairs, in whom treatment initiation occurred later in the older than in the younger sibling, the median age of ESRD was 27 years in the older, but 40 years in the younger sibling. Proteinuria was reduced in all patients, but treatment benefit was more sustained if treatment was commenced prior to advanced stages of CKD.[194]

Increasing evidence points toward aldosterone inhibition to have a blood pressure–independent, antiproteinuric effect

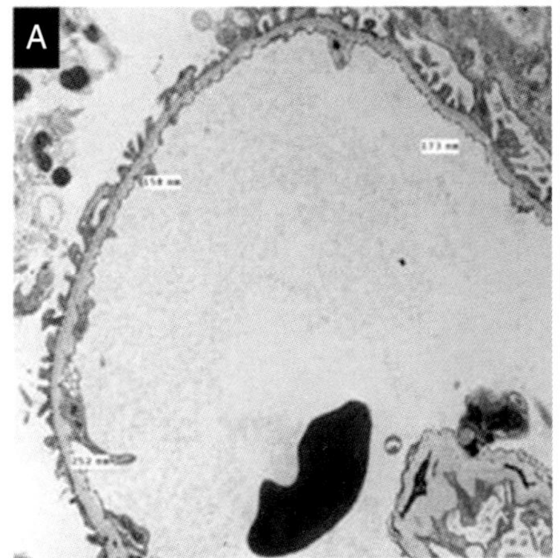


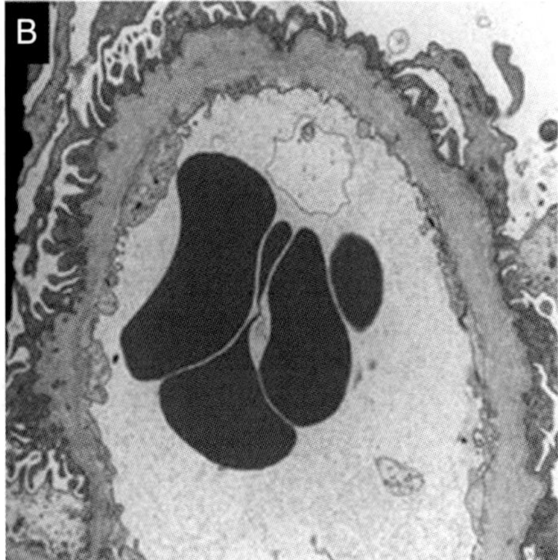


**Fig. 72.7** Electron microscopy findings in thin basement membrane disease (TBMD) and Alport syndrome (AS): (A) TBMD shows diffuse thinning of the glomerular basement membrane (GBM) lamina densa compared with that of age-matched controls (best established in the same laboratory). (B) AS shows an irregular GBM with thinning and thickening, the latter becoming more prominent over time, and with splitting/fragmentation of the lamina densa resulting in a multilaminated/basket-weave appearance often containing stubs of cellular processes with electron lucent areas and small electron dense particles. A and B: electron microscopy ×10,000.

in adults.[214–219] Aldosterone inhibition was also found to be beneficial in children: in five children with persistent proteinuria despite ACE inhibitors or ACE inhibitor/ARB combination treatment, significant improvement in proteinuria was achieved and maintained for at least 18 months via aldosterone inhibition.[220] Of note, spironolactone may offer renoprotection in pediatric CKD patients with aldosterone breakthrough.[221]

The reported experience of calcineurin inhibitors (CNIs) such as cyclosporine in AS patients involves three case series involving a total of 32 patients.[222–224] Although a significant and sustained improvement in proteinuria was found, this was associated with a significant reduction in GFR, calcineurin toxicity on renal biopsy, and hypertension. Nephrotoxicity and hypertension likely preclude the use of cyclosporine in AS, particularly in children. Whether tacrolimus could offer a more favorable profile may warrant further study.

Numerous novel treatments for AS are currently under investigation, some of which are still in the phase of preclinical development, while others are in clinical trials. These treatments include chemokine receptor 1 (CCR 1) antagonists,[225] BMP 7,[226] MMP inhibitors,[227] DDR1 and integrin $\alpha 2\beta 1$ antagonists,[186,191] and bone marrow transplant/stem cell therapy.[228–231]

## NEPHROTIC SYNDROME

NS is one of the most common types of kidney diseases occurring in children. Children with NS typically present with massive proteinuria, edema, and hypoalbuminemia, which is almost always accompanied by marked hyperlipidemia. While NS typically occurs as a primary disorder in children, it can also be associated with a variety of systemic illnesses. The clinical manifestations of NS are increasingly understood to result from structural and/or functional abnormalities in the glomerular filtration barrier. These abnormalities most often involve the podocyte, the primary target cell of injury in NS, but in some cases may result from abnormalities in the extracellular GBM. In most children, the specific cause of disease remains unknown. However, expanding genetic studies are steadily revealing greater numbers of genetic mutations that result in the aforesaid observed abnormalities.

### CLINICAL CLASSIFICATION AND DEFINITIONS

The diagnosis of NS requires the presence of edema, massive proteinuria (>40 mg/m$^2$/h, or a urine protein-to-creatinine ratio > 2.0), hypoalbuminemia (<2.5 g/dL), and hyperlipidemia.[232–236]

Clinical remission is defined by a marked reduction in proteinuria (to <4 mg/m$^2$/h, or urine albumin dipstick of 0 to trace for 3 consecutive days) in association with resolution of edema.[235,237]

Clinical relapse is defined by a recurrence of severe proteinuria (>40 mg/m$^2$/h, or urine albumin dipstick ≥ 2+ on 3 successive days), typically with a recurrence of edema.[232,233,235]

Patients who enter clinical remission in response to daily glucocorticoid treatment alone are referred to as having steroid-responsive or steroid-sensitive NS (SSNS).

A majority of children who develop NS will experience at least one relapse of their disease. While many will have only infrequent relapses (≤3 relapses per year), a significant proportion (~33%) of children who develop NS will experience multiple relapses. If a child has four or more relapses in any 12-month period, or two relapses in the first 6 months after diagnosis, he or she should be labeled as having frequent relapsing NS (FRNS).[238]

Some children respond to initial glucocorticoid treatment by entering clinical remission, but develop a relapse either while still receiving glucocorticoids, or within 2 weeks of discontinuation of treatment following a steroid taper. Such children may require continued low-dose treatment with glucocorticoids to prevent this rapid development of relapse, and thus should be labeled as having steroid-dependent NS (SDNS).[238]

Patients with either FRNS or SDNS are at slightly increased risk of developing complications of NS, as well as disease progression to CKD or ESRD (SDNS > FRNS). However, these risks are generally felt to be intermediate between those of children with SSNS and those with steroid-resistant NS (SRNS), who are at a far higher risk. In addition, children with FRNS, SDNS, and most importantly SRNS often require prolonged or more frequent glucocorticoid treatment which increases their risks for steroid-induced side effects compared with children with SSNS.

Patients with NS who fail to enter clinical remission after 4 to 8 weeks of daily glucocorticoid treatment are referred to as having SRNS.[234,235] It should be noted, however, that there are significant discrepancies in the literature regarding the definition for SRNS. While some authors define SRNS as a failure to enter clinical remission after 4 weeks of daily prednisone at a dose of 60 mg/m$^2$/day, others define it as failure to enter remission after 4 weeks of daily prednisone at a dose of 60 mg/m$^2$/day followed by 4 weeks of alternate-day prednisone at a dose of 40 mg/m$^2$/dose[239] or 4 weeks of prednisone at a dose of 60 mg/m$^2$/day followed by three intravenous pulses of methylprednisolone at a dose of 1000 mg/1.73 m$^2$/dose.[239] While several groups have to date developed evidence- and/or expert-opinion-based treatment protocols to define SRNS, these ongoing discrepancies in the definition of SRNS make direct comparisons of the efficacy of therapies for NS challenging. Indeed, development of a worldwide initial treatment protocol for new-onset NS in children could greatly enhance the nephrology community's ability to collaborate more effectively on the development and testing of novel future treatments for NS. The important implication of being diagnosed with SRNS, however, is that children who present with or develop SRNS are at significantly higher risk for the development of disease complications, as well as for progression to CKD or ESRD.[240]

### EPIDEMIOLOGY

The estimated annual incidence of NS ranges from 2 to 7 new cases per 100,000 children,[234,241–244] while the estimated prevalence is approximately 16 cases per 100,000 children, or 1 in 6000 children.[198,208] Gender differences are present in NS, but appear to be age dependent. Among younger children, boys are almost twice as likely to develop NS as girls. However, by adolescence and into adulthood the proportion of males and females developing NS becomes essentially equal.[244] Ethnic differences in NS are also well-known. While idiopathic NS is six times more common among Asian versus Caucasian children in the United Kingdom,[245] idiopathic NS is comparatively less common among African children, in whom SRNS due to structural glomerular lesions are more common.[246] By contrast, NS in the United States appears to occur relatively proportionately among children of various ethnic backgrounds.[247] Race, however, does appear to have an important correlation with the histologic lesions associated with NS. In a study performed in Kansas City, focal segmental glomerulosclerosis (FSGS) was found in 44% of African-American children, but in only 17% of Caucasian children.[243] In addition, another study reported that 47% of African-American children had FSGS, whereas only 11% of Hispanic children and 18% of Caucasian children with NS had FSGS.[247] Thus African-American children appear to be at dramatically increased risk for developing FSGS compared with other races.

Idiopathic NS is also known to occur in families. It has also been reported to occur in identical twins.[248] A very large European cohort of 1877 children reported that 3.3% of children had affected family members, typically siblings,[249] and that disease often developed in siblings at the same ages, and with similar clinical outcomes and renal biopsy findings.[250]

NS most commonly presents at 2 years of age, and almost 80% of cases of NS present in children younger than 6 years of age.[234,244] Notably, the age at presentation appears to also be predictive of the underlying histologic lesion associated with NS. The International Study of Kidney Diseases in Children (ISKDC) reported that approximately 80% of children who developed NS before 6 years of age had minimal change NS (MCNS), whereas only 50% of those with FSGS, and 2.6% of children with MPGN presented before 6 years of age.[251] In this landmark study, the median age at presentation of MCNS was 3 years versus 6 years for FSGS versus 10 years for MPGN.[251] Together, these findings suggest that the likelihood of NS being associated with MCNS decreases with increasing age at onset, whereas the likelihood for having the far less-favorable diagnoses of FSGS or MPGN increases.[251,252]

Failure to enter clinical remission of NS in response to daily glucocorticoid treatment (i.e., SRNS) has very important implications for the risk of developing progressive CKD later in life. The Southwest Pediatric Nephrology Study Group found that within 5 years of being diagnosed with SRNS, 21% of children with FSGS developed ESRD and another 23% developed CKD.[253] Thus among children diagnosed with FSGS, the risk of developing CKD or ESRD within 5 years approaches 50%.

Finally, while the overall prevalence of NS has remained relatively stable over the last 30 years, there appears to have been a dramatic increase in the incidence of FSGS and a corresponding decrease in the incidence of MCNS.[243,247] This increased incidence of FSGS must be interpreted cautiously, however, because renal biopsies are typically only performed in children with atypical presentations, older ages at presentation, or those who develop SRNS. Thus it remains possible that this apparent increase in the incidence of FSGS simply indicates that a larger percentage of children with SRNS undergo renal biopsies than in the past.

## PATHOGENESIS

The molecular pathogenesis of most forms of NS is still not clear. However, significant evolving information over the last 10 to 20 years has clarified that the primary target cell of injury during NS is the podocyte. All forms of this disease involve structural changes in podocytes, including cell swelling, as well as retraction and effacement (spreading) of the podocyte's distal foot processes, leading to the formation of a diffuse cytoplasmic sheet overlying the GBM. Additional podocyte structural changes include the formation of vacuoles, development of occluding junctions with displacement of the normal slit diaphragms that extend between podocyte foot processes, and in some areas detachment of podocytes from the underlying GBM. These podocyte structural changes, along with detachment from the GBM, have been demonstrated to result in the proteinuria that characterizes NS.[243,247,251] Table 72.3 shows the variety of podocyte structural abnormalities seen in essentially all forms of NS, as well as the variety of potential causes (some with potential overlap) that have been identified to date for the various forms of this disease.

Extensive investigations over several decades have failed to identify a single unifying cause for idiopathic NS. However, many secondary causes for disease have now been identified, which include various infections, allergies, immunizations, drugs, malignancies, and autoimmune disorders. Of note, Table 72.3 shows that there is potential overlap among some of these identified causes, which highlights that we still have only partial understanding of the molecular cause(s) of idiopathic NS. New secondary causes for idiopathic NS continue to be identified each year, particularly with regard to genetic causes. Indeed, more than 60 genes have now been identified for which mutations of various types have been found to lead to either idiopathic NS or FSGS (discussed later). Several recent publications document the growing number of gene mutations found to be associated with NS.[254–260] In general, however, the majority of mutations identified to date have been found to affect podocyte structure or function, with smaller numbers affecting the GBM or immune pathways. While the number of gene mutations associated with NS is expected to continue to grow in the future, the vast majority of patients who present with NS, particularly children, still have no identified secondary cause for their idiopathic NS. Over time it is hoped and anticipated that the list of identified secondary causes for idiopathic NS will continue to expand as we learn more about the molecular pathogenesis of this disease. For interested readers, a nice review has recently been published that provides a more comprehensive discussion of idiopathic NS.[256]

Of particular note is that almost one-third of patients who present with NS have some history of allergies, asthma, or atopy.[235,261–264] Consistent with this, allergies, immunizations, and autoimmune disorders (Table 72.3) are all known causes of NS. Together, these findings suggest a strong, but indirect, correlation between idiopathic syndrome and dysregulation of the immune system. Moreover, the fact that almost all treatments known to induce clinical remission of NS are immunosuppressants further strengthens this argument. Indeed, it has been suggested that idiopathic NS may be either an immune disorder to which the kidney

**Table 72.3 Abnormalities Underlying Nephrotic Syndrome**

| Podocyte Structural Abnormalities Seen in Nephrotic Syndrome | Potential Causes for Idiopathic Nephrotic Syndrome Identified to Date | Potential Causes for Focal Segmental Glomerulosclerosis Identified to Date |
|---|---|---|
| Cell swelling<br>Retraction (effacement) of distal foot processes<br>Formation of vacuoles<br>Development of occluding junctions between podocytes<br>Apical displacement of normal junctions (i.e., slit diaphragms) between podocytes<br>Detachment of podocytes from underlying glomerular basement membrane (GBM) | Soluble plasma factor(s)<br>Genetic predisposition (i.e., mutations)<br>Dysregulation of podocyte structure<br>Dysregulation of podocyte function<br>Dysregulation of immune system function (T cells, B cells [more recent])<br>Malignancies (i.e., Hodgkin disease, non-Hodgkin lymphoma, leukemia, etc.)<br>Drugs (i.e., nonsteroidal antiinflammatory drugs, D-penicillamine, lithium, tyrosine kinase inhibitors, captopril)<br>Infections (hepatitis B, hepatitis C, HIV, parasitic, mycoplasma, etc.)<br>Allergies (food, pollen, dust, bee stings, cat fur, etc.)<br>Immunizations<br>Autoimmune disorders (systemic lupus erythematosus, celiac disease, allogeneic stem cell transplantation, myasthenia gravis, etc.)<br>Systemic diseases (i.e., diabetes mellitus, Henoch–Schönlein purpura, sarcoidosis, etc.) | Soluble plasma factor(s)<br>(especially in recurrent focal segmental glomerulosclerosis)<br>Genetic predisposition (i.e., mutations)<br>Immunologic podocyte injury<br>(i.e., human immunodeficiency virus [HIV] nephropathy, cytomegalovirus, other viruses)<br>Toxic podocyte injury<br>(lithium, bisphosphonate, heroin, other medications?, cytokines)<br>Inflammatory podocyte injury (APOL1 variant, cytokines)<br>Hemodynamic podocyte injury (morbid obesity, low birth weight, reflux nephropathy)<br>Structural GBM abnormalities (inherited, acquired)<br>APOL1 focal segmental glomerulosclerosis |

(i.e., the podocyte) is especially susceptible, or a kidney disorder to which the systemic immune system is especially susceptible.

The pathogenesis of FSGS has been the subject of intensive study for several decades. During this time it has become clear that FSGS is not a single disease, but a pattern of glomerular injury that can represent the final outcome of a variety of mechanistically distinct pathologic processes. As shown in Table 72.3, FSGS may result from circulating plasma factors, which are most clearly seen in recurrent FSGS after renal transplantation, or due to a variety of other forms of glomerular and/or podocyte injury. These include inflammatory, immunologic, structural, or hemodynamic injury to podocytes, as well as the GBM and glomerular parietal epithelial cells. Several recent advances in our understanding of the pathophysiologic, genetic, and histologic features of FSGS have led to a more mechanistic and clinically useful proposed classification of this multifaceted disease. While the historical classification of FSGS separated this condition into primary FSGS (i.e., idiopathic) versus secondary FSGS (i.e., due to known causes),[265] integration of more robust clinical, histologic, and genetic knowledge of this disease has led to the recent proposal that FSGS be categorized into six forms: (1) primary FSGS, (2) adaptive FSGS, (3) APOL1 FSGS, (4) genetic FSGS, (5) virus-associated FSGS, and (6) medication-/toxin-associated FSGS. Among these, the most common causes are primary FSGS, adaptive FSGS, and APOL1 FSGS, which all appear to occur with similar prevalence in the United States, with lower prevalence of genetic FSGS, virus-associated FSGS, and medication-/toxin-associated FSGS.[255] In this schema, primary FSGS is thought to be due to suspected circulating plasma factor(s), whereas adaptive FSGS is thought to be due to either conditions with elevated total kidney GFR such as cyanotic congenital heart disease,[266] androgen abuse,[267] sleep apnea[268] or conditions with reduced functional nephron mass such as renal dysplasia, reflux nephropathy, repeated episodes of acute kidney injury (AKI), or premature or small-for-gestational age birth.[269]

Note that while the precise relationships among the diverse potential causes of FSGS remain uncertain, the podocyte has emerged as the final common target cell of injury for all of these causes. Moreover, any of the aforementioned forms of FSGS, and likely any chronic glomerular or interstitial disease that leads to reduced nephron mass, can potentially result in podocyte injury and glomerular changes consistent with adaptive FSGS. In this setting, progressive loss of injured or dead podocytes into the urine (i.e., podocyturia) often leads to depletion of podocytes in the glomerulus (i.e., podocytopenia), which then induces podocytes to hypertrophy to try to compensate for these losses. These (mal)adaptive changes are now thought to result in the development of podocyte sheer forces which further exacerbate podocyte injury,[270] and ultimately lead to increases in glomerular pressures and flows in the remaining intact glomeruli that, in turn, induce further glomerular injury and disease progression.[255]

## CLINICAL PRESENTATION

Most children who develop idiopathic NS present with acute or subacute onset of periorbital or generalized edema. These findings combined with the presence of 3–4+ proteinuria on a dipstick urinalysis (~300–2000 mg/dL [17.7–118 mmol/L]) typically establish a preliminary diagnosis of NS. The extent of proteinuria can be better quantified by obtaining a spot urine protein-to-creatinine ratio (typically >2.5 mg/mg), and the diagnosis can be confirmed by documenting the presence of hypoalbuminemia (typically <2.5 g/dL [<25 g/L]) and hyperlipidemia.

**Table 72.4 Primary Causes of Childhood Nephrotic Syndrome**

| |
|---|
| Minimal change nephrotic syndrome (MCNS) |
| Focal segmental glomerulosclerosis (FSGS) |
| Mesangial proliferative glomerulonephritis |
| Membranoproliferative glomerulonephritis (MPGN) |
| Membranous nephropathy (MN) |

Childhood NS is most often due to primary glomerulopathies. These include MCNS, FSGS, mesangial proliferative glomerulonephritis, MPGN, and MN (Table 72.4). However, a careful history may reveal potential secondary causes for this disease, including infections, systemic diseases, drugs, malignancies, autoimmune disorders, and allergies, as detailed in Table 72.3.

Physical examination can also often provide suggestive clues about the diagnosis. For example, while periorbital and peripheral edema, and ascites are common in most children with NS, this appears not to be similar for the presence of hypertension. In a very large international study of children with NS, the ISKDC, it was determined that hypertension was far less common in children found to have MCNS (~21%) than in children found to have either of the less favorable diagnoses of FSGS or MPGN, where the incidence was approximately 50%.[251]

The laboratory evaluation of children presenting with NS always begins with confirmation of the presence of hypoalbuminemia and hyperlipidemia, as noted earlier, and determination of the renal function. The presence of AKI is not uncommon, and is often attributed to intravascular volume depletion and renal hypoperfusion. While this may be only prerenal AKI, in more severe cases AKI may be found to be due to acute tubular necrosis, likely reflecting more severe renal hypoperfusion resulting in renal tubular injury. In the ISKDC study in 1978, 32% of children with MCNS had elevated serum creatinine, while 41% of those with FSGS and 50% of those with MPGN had elevated creatinine.[251] Of note, a recent large multicenter study of 370 children admitted to the hospital with NS performed through the Midwest Pediatric Nephrology Consortium identified a tripling of the incidence of AKI among this cohort.[271] While the cause of this dramatic increase in AKI incidence is not yet known, it is suspected that it may be related to the significant increase in the use of CNIs as alternative treatments for NS in the last decade, as these agents are well-known to have vasoconstrictive effects on the glomerular vasculature.

Microscopic hematuria is also not uncommon in children with NS. Microscopic hematuria was found in 23% of children with MCNS versus 48% of children with FSGS versus 59% of children with MPGN in the ISKDC study.[251] By contrast, the presence of macroscopic hematuria is unusual, and should prompt the suspicion of a possible renal venous thrombosis.

In addition to the aforementioned laboratory studies, serologic evaluation to screen for potential secondary causes of NS is often performed in children presenting at an older age, or who have a history or signs or symptoms of systemic illness. The finding of low serum complement levels can identify children with MPGN, SLE, or PIGN, and positive serum antinuclear antibody and antidouble-stranded DNA studies can confirm the diagnosis of SLE. Screening for viral infections can identify patients with disease due to hepatitis B (typically associated with MN), hepatitis C (typically associated with MPGN), or human immunodeficiency virus (HIV; typically associated with collapsing variant of FSGS). In addition, a complete blood count found to be abnormal could potentially identify patients with leukemia, lymphoma, or SLE.

Because immunosuppressive treatments are the mainstay of therapy for childhood NS, it is recommended to place a purified protein derivative test in all children prior to initiating treatment, to screen for possible previously undiagnosed tuberculosis. In addition, consideration should be given to obtaining varicella IgG titers to screen for immunity to this virus, which can be potentially life-threatening in immunocompromised hosts. Such knowledge can be very helpful to ensure optimal management of a nonimmune child with NS under immunosuppressive treatment with varicella zoster Ig.

Finally, while a renal ultrasound is not routinely indicated in children with NS, development of gross hematuria represents a clear indication to obtain an ultrasound with Doppler evaluation of the renal vasculature to exclude possible development of a renal venous thrombosis.

## CONSIDERATION OF RENAL BIOPSY

The role of the renal biopsy in the diagnosis and management of children with NS remains somewhat controversial. In the 1970s the ISKDC study included renal biopsies for all children with NS before treatment initiation.[278] Since that time the clinical indications have been debated, with some pediatric nephrologists reserving biopsies for older children in whom diagnoses other than MCNS are more likely to be found. Among others, renal biopsies are reserved for those children in whom there is a clinical or serologic suspicion that the child may have a glomerulonephritis. Renal biopsies are also often performed by some, but not all, nephrologists to determine baseline and follow-up levels of glomerular and interstitial scarring when a child is being transitioned to an alternative therapy with significant potential nephrotoxicity, such as the CNIs cyclosporine and tacrolimus. Despite these variations in practice patterns, however, almost all pediatric nephrologists agree that a renal biopsy should be performed in a child who presents with or subsequently develops SRNS.

## HISTOLOGICAL CLASSIFICATION

From a clinical perspective, most children who present with idiopathic NS under the age of 10 to 12 years receive empiric initial treatment with oral glucocorticoids (discussed later). Only if they present with or subsequently develop clinical steroid resistance (or steroid dependence in some cases) do such patients routinely undergo a renal biopsy. While renal biopsy findings at the level of EM almost always reveal numerous abnormalities involving the podocytes (Table 72.3), at the light microscopic level many patients have no or only minimal other histologic abnormalities. Dating back to the early days of renal biopsies when only light microscopy (LM) was available, such patients are still often referred to as having "MCNS" or "minimal change disease."

The primary glomerulopathies that comprise childhood NS include MCNS, FSGS, mesangial proliferative glomerulonephritis, MPGN, and MN (Table 72.4). The detailed histologic features of each of these diseases have been addressed elsewhere in the text, and the reader is referred to these sections for more detailed images and descriptions of these features.

The secondary glomerulopathies associated with childhood NS include systemic diseases such as SLE, HSP, diabetes mellitus, sickle cell disease, and sarcoidosis. In addition, other secondary causes of disease include infections such as HIV, hepatitis B, hepatitis C, malignancies such as leukemia and lymphoma, and drugs such as nonsteroidal antiinflammatory drugs (NSAIDs), ACE inhibitors (captopril), D-penicillamine, and gold. Finally, morbid obesity, pregnancy (preeclampsia), and allergies to food, bee stings, and even immunizations have all also been associated with the development of NS. The detailed histologic features of most of these diseases have also been presented elsewhere in the text and the reader is referred to these sections for more detailed images and descriptions of these histologic features.

## TREATMENT OF NEPHROTIC SYNDROME

The primary treatment of NS in children has remained daily oral glucocorticoids for more than 60 years. Unlike adults, in whom prolonged steroid treatment has been associated with increases in remissions of NS,[272,273] the vast majority of children respond to a 4- to 8-week course of oral glucocorticoids by entering into complete clinical remission.

Interestingly, while almost all pediatric nephrologists will initiate glucocorticoids upon diagnosis of NS, it is known that spontaneous remissions occur in approximately 5% of patients, often within the first 1 to 2 weeks.[274,275] Such findings suggest that delaying slightly the initiation of treatment in some cases could be reasonable.

Initial treatment of NS in children who present at the age of 1 year or more includes daily high-dose oral glucocorticoids (i.e., most commonly prednisone at 2 mg/kg/day with maximal dose of 60 mg/day) for 4 to 8 weeks. Most children (~75%) enter complete remission within 2 weeks, and the vast majority of children (~95%) enter remission within 4 weeks.[235,276] Continued treatment for an additional 4 weeks typically identifies only a few additional patients able to enter a complete remission, with the remainder either failing to respond or responding with only a partial resolution of their proteinuria. Such patients are then labeled as having SRNS. Children with SRNS are at a dramatically higher risk than those with SSNS for the development of progressive renal disease (see the "Outcomes" section), and almost always undergo a renal biopsy to confirm a histologic diagnosis. Regardless of the histologic diagnosis, however, treatment decisions in children are guided primarily by either the success (i.e., SSNS) or the failure (i.e., SRNS) of oral glucocorticoids to induce a complete clinical remission.

### STEROID-SENSITIVE NEPHROTIC SYNDROME

Over the last few decades, multiple protocols have been reported for the initial treatment of children presenting with NS. The initial widely accepted approach was reported by the ISKDC and suggested treatment with prednisone in divided doses for 4 weeks at 60 mg/m$^2$/day (or 2 mg/kg/day up to a maximal dose of 80 mg/day), followed by a taper to 40 mg/m$^2$/day (or 1.5 mg/kg/day up to a maximal dose of 60 mg/day) for an additional 4 weeks.[235] Since then there have been numerous subsequent reports of variations on this regimen.[277–281] Recently, a comprehensive meta-analysis has systematically compared many of these approaches.[281] Despite all of these publications over the years, however, there remains a fairly wide distribution of initial treatment practices among pediatric nephrologists in the United States,[282] as well as among pediatric nephrologists in many other countries around the world. The unfortunate result of this is that the worldwide pediatric nephrology community has yet to come to consensus on one single definition of a glucocorticoid treatment dose and duration that clearly defines when a child should be labeled as having SRNS. As noted earlier, because the vast majority of nephrologists base their treatment decisions on the distinction between SSNS and SRNS, such variations in this definition impede the ability to directly compare the effectiveness of new treatments for this disease developed primarily for children with SRNS.

Once complete remission has been achieved with one of the aforementioned protocols, many pediatric nephrologists elect to taper the prednisone to alternate days with weekly dosage reductions to discontinue the medication over about 6 weeks, although significant practice variation regarding prednisone taper also remains.[282]

### STEROID-DEPENDENT AND FREQUENT RELAPSING NEPHROTIC SYNDROME

Once diagnosed with NS, the majority of children (50%–75%) will experience one or more relapses of disease. While some relapses can be transient and remit spontaneously as noted earlier,[283] unfortunately approximately 50% of children with initial SSNS ultimately develop either frequent relapses (FRNS; see definition earlier) or steroid dependence (SDNS; see definition earlier).[277,280] Such relapses require additional courses of oral prednisone, and thus greater overall glucocorticoid exposure and risk for side effects, compared with children with fewer relapses.[278]

Several additional factors also increase the risk for relapses. Children who present with NS under the age of 5 years, as well as those who are boys, are both at greater risk for frequent relapses.[284] Perhaps the greatest risk for relapses, however, occurs during intercurrent infections. Indeed, upper respiratory infections are the single most common cause for relapses of NS in children, and approximately 70% of relapses have been reported to be preceded by an upper respiratory infection.[285] Despite this strong correlation, however, a large multicenter study of more than 200 children performed by the ISKDC failed to identify any other specific factors predictive of frequent relapses, including time to initial remission of disease, time between first remission and first relapse, MCNS histologic subtypes, clinical findings, or laboratory findings.[286] One exception to this was the identification of a strong correlation between the number of relapses in the initial 6 months of disease and the subsequent clinical course, with more early relapses predicting a continued frequent relapsing course of disease. Together, these findings suggest that earlier age at presentation, male gender, and early frequent relapses all are associated with an increased risk for more frequent future relapses.

Treatment of relapses typically involves reinitiation of oral prednisone at the standard dose of 2 mg/kg/day (maximal dose of 80 mg/day) divided twice daily until the urine protein is trace or negative for 3 consecutive days by urine dipstick. Preferably these urine samples are obtained on first-morning voids, so as to minimize the risk for confounding by possible orthostatic proteinuria, which occurs more commonly in older children. Once in remission, prednisone is typically tapered to 1.5 mg/kg on alternate mornings for 4 weeks (ISKDC protocol)[235] or gradually tapered further (~0.25 mg/kg/dose) every week until discontinuation in approximately 6 weeks. For children with FRNS, this taper can be slowed significantly to be weaned and discontinued over 5 to 6 months to try to reduce the frequency of relapses. Those children unable to remain in complete remission during this prednisone wean, or who relapse within 2 weeks of discontinuation of prednisone, should be labeled as having SDNS. Such patients can be treated generally as noted earlier, but the alternate-day prednisone tapered only to the lowest dose that has historically kept the patient in remission, and continued for 6–18 months, followed by gradual further tapering of the dose every 2 weeks until discontinuation.

For children in whom the aforementioned measures fail to adequately control the disease, or in whom significant signs and symptoms of steroid toxicity develop, there are several alternative treatments that are used. While these agents as a group can often reduce the frequency of relapses, many of them have significant toxicities of their own.

Alkylating agents, which include cyclophosphamide and chlorambucil, are historical treatments that, while still used, are used increasingly infrequently. Typical courses of oral cyclophosphamide include administration of 2 mg/kg/day for 8 to 12 weeks, while chlorambucil is typically prescribed at 0.2 mg/kg/day for 8 to 12 weeks. Both treatments have been reported to reduce the frequency of relapses in approximately 75% of children with FRNS, whereas their efficacy among children with SDNS is only 30% to 35%.[287,288] Importantly, these agents have been associated with significant toxicities, including leukopenia, hair loss, thrombocytopenia, seizures (chlorambucil only), hemorrhagic cystitis (cyclophosphamide only), severe infections, malignancies, and fatalities.[289] For these reasons, other less toxic alternatives have gained in popularity compared with these treatments in recent years.

Levamisole is another alternative treatment used to treat many children with FRNS and SDNS. Similar to most other treatments for NS, its mechanism of action in NS is not known. However, unlike all other reported treatments for NS, levamisole is known to act not as an immunosuppressant, but as an immunostimulant. Despite this, it has been widely reported to prolong remissions and reduce the overall exposure to glucocorticoids in children with both FRNS and SDNS.[290–294] Typical dosing includes administration of 2.5 mg/kg PO on alternate days, and a typical treatment duration ranges from 4 months to a year. This regimen has been reported to be generally effective and safe, although reported side effects include flulike symptoms, neutropenia, agranulocytosis, vomiting, seizures, rash, and hyperactivity. Unlike alkylating agents, the beneficial effects of levamisole (as well as most other alternative agents) do not extend beyond the period of treatment.

Mycophenolate mofetil (MMF) and its closely related compound mizoribine are additional alternative agents that have gained in popularity to treat FRNS and SDNS in recent years. Although their mechanism of action in NS remains unclear, these compounds are known to inhibit lymphocyte DNA synthesis and cellular proliferation via inhibition of inosine monophosphate dehydrogenase, a key enzyme in purine biosynthesis.[295] These agents also interfere with adhesion of activated lymphocytes to endothelial cells via inhibition of glycosylation of selected adhesion molecules.[296] From a clinical perspective, these effects are selective only for T lymphocytes and B lymphocytes, because all other cells in the body have a "salvage pathway" that enables purines to still be synthesized in the presence of these agents.[297] These drugs have been widely used to reduce the frequency of relapses in children with both FRNS and SDNS,[298–301] enabling significant reductions in overall glucocorticoid exposure and thus the incidence and severity of their side effects. A typical treatment dose is approximately 600 mg/m$^2$/dose given twice daily (maximum dose ~1000 mg BID). While most children do not have significant side effects that limit treatment, more prevalent side effects include nausea, vomiting, diarrhea, bone marrow suppression, anemia, and gastrointestinal bleeding. Notably absent for this list, however, is the induction of renal injury (see later). Given their general effectiveness, modest side-effect profiles, and lack of renal toxicity, MMF and mizoribine have become very popular alternative treatments for children with FRNS and SDNS in recent years.

CNIs include cyclosporine and tacrolimus, and have become far more widely used alternative agents in the last decade. While their exact mechanism of action in NS is not fully understood, both agents are known to inhibit T-cell activation via inhibition of calcineurin-induced interleukin-2 gene expression, an early step in T-cell activation,[302] and cyclosporine has additionally been reported to act directly on podocytes to stabilize their actin cytoskeleton.[303] Use of these agents has been widely reported to reduce the frequency of relapses,[304,305] but unlike the alkylating agents noted earlier which have beneficial effects well beyond their course of treatment, many children relapse when CNIs are tapered or discontinued. CNIs can also have several side effects. These include hypertension, mild AKI, hyperkalemia, hypertrichosis (mostly cyclosporine), gingival overgrowth (mostly cyclosporine), and most importantly an increased risk for calcineurin nephrotoxicity which manifests as irreversible interstitial fibrosis. This typically occurs in a striped pattern that is reflective of the interstitial vascularization, and its incidence and severity appear to correlate generally with the duration and dose of drug exposure. Despite this, these agents have gained much favor in recent years as perhaps the preferred alternative treatments for FRNS and SDNS.

## STEROID-RESISTANT NEPHROTIC SYNDROME

Despite optimal management, approximately 10% to 20% of children with NS will initially present with or subsequently develop SRNS. Notably, prior to labeling a child as having SRNS it is essential to exclude several potentially treatable

**Table 72.5 Current, Emerging, and Potential Future Treatment Options for Children With Steroid-Resistant Nephrotic Syndrome**

| Immunosuppressive | Immunostimulatory | Nonimmunosuppressive |
|---|---|---|
| Alkylating agents[a] (cyclophosphamide, chlorambucil) | Levamisole[a] | Angiotensin-converting enzyme inhibitors |
| Pulse intravenous methylprednisolone[a] | | Angiotensin receptor blockers (ARBs) |
| Plasmapheresis/immunoadsorption[a] | | Vitamin E (antioxidant)[a] |
| Mycophenolate mofetil (and mizoribine) | | |
| Calcineurin inhibitors (cyclosporine, tacrolimus) | | |
| Anti-CD20 monoclonal antibodies (rituximab, ofatumumab[b]) | | |
| Low-density lipoprotein apheresis[b] (LIPOSORBER) | | |
| ACTHar[b] | | |
| CTLA-4-Ig[b] (Abatacept) | | |
| ARB + endothelin type A receptor antagonist[b] (Sparsentan) | | |
| p38 mitogen-activated protein kinase inhibitor[c] (Losmapimod) | | |
| Peroxisome proliferator-activated receptor-$\gamma$ agonist[c] (Pioglitazone) | | |
| Anti-interleukin-13 monoclonal antibody[c] (Lebrikizumab) | | |

[a]Less commonly used treatment.
[b]Emerging treatment.
[c]Potential future treatment.
*ACTH,* Adrenocorticotropic hormone.

causes for treatment failure, including poor medication adherence, poor medication absorption, possible underlying infection, and possible malignancy. Once diagnosed with SRNS, a child's risk for both the development of extrarenal complications of NS and for the development of ESRD and/or CKD increases greatly. For this reason, both the alternative treatments described earlier, as well as additional alternative treatments, are often employed in an attempt to induce a complete remission of proteinuria. Although the results of the renal biopsy are helpful in guiding the clinical management of patients with SRNS, it is generally accepted that the best way to reduce an SRNS patient's risk of developing progressive CKD or ESRD is to utilize these alternative treatments, either singly or in combination, to induce a complete remission. Induction of only a partial clinical remission, however, is controversial as it provides an unproven and unclear reduction in risk for future CKD or ESRD. Despite this, most clinicians agree that achieving lower levels of proteinuria, however induced, are associated with generally better clinical outcomes and fewer disease complications.

Treatment of SRNS in children includes the use of a wider array of alternative treatments than for FRNS and SDNS. Importantly, almost all treatments used for FRNS and SDNS are notably less effective in the setting of SRNS, and it is thus not uncommon for multiple alternative treatments to be added to one another or even initiated simultaneously in an attempt to induce a complete clinical remission of NS. Unfortunately, all of the available alternative treatments are only partially effective, and many are associated with significant toxicities of their own.

Although significant advances have been made in expanding the array of alternative treatments available to treat SRNS in the last several years, most published data reporting their usage, efficacy, and toxicity remain derived from anecdotal reports and uncontrolled clinical trials, with relatively few randomized controlled trials completed that have been able to confirm the safety and efficacy of these newer treatments. This lack of high-quality clinical trial data, combined with the lack of a standardized definition for the diagnosis of SRNS, makes it difficult to directly compare the relative effectiveness of the various alternative treatments currently available, as well as to compare emerging alternative treatments with the existing ones. Despite these limitations, Table 72.5 lists the current, emerging, and several potential future treatment options for children with SRNS.

The overall management of children with SRNS can be divided into four major categories: (1) supportive therapy, (2) immunosuppressive therapy, (3) immunostimulatory therapy, and (4) nonimmunosuppressive therapy. Supportive therapy for SRNS includes the provision of general medical care, management of edema, and management of dyslipidemia (Table 72.6). General medical care includes the identification and treatment of suspected infection, which may present as pneumonia, cellulitis, peritonitis, or sepsis.[271] It also includes the identification and treatment of suspected thrombosis, which may present with gross hematuria with or without acute oliguria (renal venous thrombosis), respiratory distress (pulmonary thrombosis), asymmetric swelling of an extremity (deep venous thrombosis), or neurologic symptoms (cerebral venous thrombosis).[306–308] Additional important aspects of general care include the maintenance or restoration of the patient's intravascular volume, maintenance of adequate protein intake,[274] and alteration of immunizations while the patient remains immunosuppressed.[309–311,311a,311b]

Management of the chronic edema associated with SRNS includes use of moderate restriction of fluid intake, moderate restriction of salt intake, and the judicious use of diuretics. Severe anasarca can be reasonably effectively treated with 25% albumin at a dose 1 g/kg infused over 4 to 6 hours, followed by IV furosemide at a dose of 1 to 2 mg/kg to induce diuresis. This can be repeated every 8 to 12 hours as clinically indicated, assuming care is taken to ensure that mobilization of interstitial fluid into the intravascular space is not too rapid, which may result in pulmonary edema and possible congestive heart failure.[312] Additional approaches to control severe edema include elevation of the extremities,

**Table 72.6 Major Components of Supportive Therapy for Children With Steroid-Resistant Nephrotic Syndrome**

| General Medical Care | Management of Edema | Management of Dyslipidemia |
|---|---|---|
| Identification and treatment of suspected infection<br>• Pneumonia<br>• Cellulitis<br>• Peritonitis<br>• Sepsis<br>Identification and treatment of suspected thrombosis<br>• Gross hematuria +/-acute oliguria (renal venous thrombosis)<br>• Respiratory distress (pulmonary thrombosis)<br>• Asymmetric extremity swelling (deep venous thrombosis)<br>• Neurologic symptoms (cerebral venous thrombosis)<br>Maintenance or restoration of intravascular volume<br>Maintenance of adequate protein intake (130%–140% of recommended dietary allowances)<br>Alteration of immunizations while immunosuppressed | Avoidance of excessive fluid intake<br>Elevation of extremities<br>Moderate dietary salt restriction<br>Judicious use of diuretics for severe edema<br>Head-out water immersion | Avoidance of high fat intake<br>Regular exercise (>30 min/day of moderately intense activity)<br>Consideration of hydroxymethylglutaryl-coenzyme A reductase inhibitors (statins)<br>Consideration of low-density lipoprotein apheresis |

as well as the use of head-out water immersion, which although not commonly considered, has been reported to induce strong diuretic and natriuretic effects in patients with NS.[313]

Management of the chronic dyslipidemia that almost always accompanies SRNS includes the avoidance of high fat intake, introduction of a regular daily exercise regimen, pharmacologic therapy when the aforementioned approaches fail, and more recently the use of low-density lipoprotein (LDL) apheresis. The dyslipidemia in NS typically includes marked elevations in LDL, very-low-density lipoprotein, cholesterol, lipoprotein A, and often triglyceride levels, with variable abnormalities in high-density lipoprotein levels.[314] This chronic dyslipidemia has been clearly associated with increased risks for atherosclerosis, myocardial infarction, cardiac death, cerebral infarctions, and accelerated progression of CKD, although primarily among adults.[315–319] Conservative treatment of the dyslipidemia in SRNS is commonly ineffective, and pharmacologic treatment is thus sometimes required to control severe chronic lipid abnormalities, although none of the treatments have been approved by the Food and Drug Administration for use in children with NS to date. The most common treatment includes the use of hydroxymethylglutaryl-coenzyme A inhibitors (HMG-CoA inhibitors; i.e., statins), for which there are a few uncontrolled trials in children reporting moderate efficacy without significant toxicity.[320–322] Among adults with NS, statin usage has been generally well tolerated, with only mild elevations in liver enzymes and creatinine kinase, and rarely diarrhea, reported.[323]

Among the pharmacologic treatments for children with SRNS, the immunosuppressive alternative treatments are the most widely employed. The most widely used currently available and emerging alternative treatments for SRNS will be described briefly in the following section, highlighting their known mechanisms of action, and their popularity of usage among pediatric nephrologists. In addition, a few potential future treatments for SRNS will be briefly described.

Several alternative treatments for SRNS have already been described in detail earlier for the management of FRNS and SDNS. These treatments include cytotoxic agents, levamisole, and MMF and mizoribine. While they are sometimes still used to treat children with SRNS, their reported efficacy among children with SRNS is far lower and they are thus gradually falling out of favor among pediatric nephrologists. One notable exception is that MMF continues to be widely used in attempt to maintain remission among children with SRNS in whom complete remission has been induced with another alternative treatment.

Another alternative treatment that has gradually fallen out of favor for SRNS is the use of high-dose pulse IV methylprednisolone. Like most drugs used to treat NS, its mechanism of action in NS is not fully known. However, multiple reports have documented that in addition to their known antiinflammatory effects, glucocorticoids also act directly on podocytes to protect against and enhance recovery from NS-related cellular injury, suggesting that at least part of the beneficial effects of glucocorticoids result from direct action on the primary target cell of injury during NS.[324,325] While courses of this drug have demonstrated relatively good efficacy (38%–82% complete remission rates) among children with SRNS for many years, treatment has been associated with toxicity in 17% to 25% of children, and due to concerns about the long-term side effects of steroids, has long been controversial among pediatric nephrologists.[326–331]

Another less widely used treatment for SRNS is plasmapheresis. While it is widely used for the treatment of recurrence of NS following renal transplantation in treatment of a presumed circulating factor which induces increased glomerular permeability,[299,332–336] use of plasmapheresis in children with SRNS before renal transplantation has never become widely accepted.[337] Immunoadsorption, a related extracorporeal treatment to directly bind potential circulating factors on a column, has also been reported to have some efficacy, but has not gained as much popularity in the United States as it has in Europe.[337–339]

The CNIs cyclosporine A and tacrolimus have become among the most widely used treatments for children with SRNS over the last 10 to 15 years. Numerous reports have documented their ability to induce complete remissions in significant percentages of children with SRNS (33%–59%), as well as partial remissions in many of the remaining patients.[284,305,340–343] Their mechanism of action in NS remains uncertain, but these drugs are currently thought to exert their beneficial clinical effects via their immunosuppressive actions, as well as via direct action on podocytes to stabilize the podocyte actin cytoskeleton.[303] Despite these beneficial effects, CNIs have been associated with several potentially significant side effects that can limit their clinical usefulness. These include hypertension, mild AKI, hyperkalemia, gingival overgrowth (primarily cyclosporine), hypertrichosis (primarily cyclosporine), headaches, nausea, and vomiting. The most concerning side effect, however, is the development of irreversible interstitial fibrosis (calcineurin nephrotoxicity). This side effect appears to be generally associated with the cumulative exposure to CNIs, and thus increases with longer time of treatment and higher dosages.[284,344–348] This is especially problematic for children with SRNS, because many of whom respond well to CNIs will experience future relapses, and not infrequently become dependent on calcineurin treatment to maintain remission, thus increasing their risk for future nephrotoxicity.[349] Because SRNS is a potentially reversible disease, prolonged usage of CNIs which may induce irreversible side effects has raised important concerns about their long-term usage in children with SRNS. In this light, many pediatric nephrologists choose to perform a renal biopsy prior to initiation of a CNI to determine the baseline extent of interstitial fibrosis, as well as repeat biopsies at periodic intervals (usually about every 2 years or so) to screen for potential development or progression of interstitial fibrosis as long as a child requires continued calcineurin treatment due to his or her inability to be transitioned to another alternative treatment.

More recently, the use of anti-CD20 monoclonal antibodies (mAbs) has become increasingly popular as an alternative treatment for SRNS (and sometimes for FRNS or SDNS). Rituximab is a chimeric (i.e., combined mouse + human) mAb directed at the CD20 antigen on B lymphocytes, while its newer closely related biologic agent atumumab is a fully humanized mAb directed at this same antigenic target.[350] While originally developed to treat lymphomas, these biologics are highly effective in essentially eliminating circulating B lymphocytes, and it is thought that their mechanism of action in NS results from reductions in B lymphocyte numbers and/or function. An additional potential mechanism of action directly on podocytes has also been reported, but remains somewhat controversial.[351] Several reports have now demonstrated that anti-CD20 mAb therapy is effective in inducing remission in children with SRNS, as well as a landmark randomized controlled trial confirming rituximab's effectiveness in prolonging remission in children with FRNS.[352] Unlike most other alternative treatments for SRNS, rituximab is administered as one to four infusions over 1 to 4 weeks (usually 375 mg/m$^2$ over several hours) and has a prolonged duration of effect that lasts for approximately 5 to 9 months, when the B lymphocytes destroyed by this therapy gradually recover toward normal levels. The efficacy of this treatment has been reported in mostly small case series and uncontrolled trials, where it has been found generally to induce complete remission in approximately 25% of children with SRNS, and partial remission in another approximately 25% of children. Despite premedication, side effects of anti-CD20 mAb therapy are relatively common, occurring in 20% to 30% of cases, and include rash, flushing, and rarely acute respiratory distress. In most cases, slowing or stopping the infusion temporarily has allowed completion of most infusions, but in rare cases treatment has had to be discontinued. Because of its efficacy, long-term clinical benefits, and elimination of noncompliance due to drug infusion, anti-CD20 mAb treatment for SRNS (as well as for FRNS and SDNS) has gained wide popularity in recent years. Owing to its high price, however, its use remains restricted by private and/or public payers in some settings, and it is still unavailable in several areas of the world.

Sparsentan is an emerging alternative treatment for SRNS. It is an orally active dual-acting ARB combined with a highly selective endothelin type A receptor antagonist. A recent report of its use in a phase 2 trial in children and adults with primary FSGS is currently underway to determine how effective this treatment may be in reducing proteinuria in patients with primary FSGS.[353]

Another emerging alternative treatment for SRNS is LDL apheresis, which is not a drug but a device. This is an extracorporeal therapy that was originally developed to treat familial hypercholesterolemia, but its usage has been expanded for several years in Japan to also include the treatment of hyperlipidemia in NS. Strikingly, it has been reported to not only reduce the hyperlipidemia of NS very effectively, but also to induce complete remission in approximately 25% of adults and children diagnosed with SRNS, and to induce partial remission in another 25% of patients.[354] This efficacy is comparable with that of rituximab, and has thus raised several new questions about whether the dyslipidemia seen in NS is simply a consequence of disease, as has been historically thought, or whether it might in fact play a pathophysiologic role in the development or the progression of disease in patients with SRNS who remain clinically nephrotic.[314]

One potential future therapy for the treatment of SRNS (and possibly SSNS) is the Peroxisome proliferator-activated receptor-γ agonist pioglitazone. This drug is a member of a family of insulin-sensitizing compounds developed to treat type 2 diabetes in adults, but which has been found in recent reports in animals and humans to have potential in the treatment of glomerular disease.[355–358] Moreover, pioglitazone has recently been reported to directly protect podocytes against NS-related injury, and to both reduce proteinuria directly and enhance glucocorticoid-induced proteinuria reduction in experimental NS in rats.[324–359] Of greater clinical interest, introduction of pioglitazone to a child with multidrug-resistant NS resulted in a significant reduction in proteinuria (80%, but not complete remission) in the face of a simultaneous 64% reduction in overall immunosuppression.[360] Importantly, no toxicity related to pioglitazone treatment was reported in the first 2 years of treatment.

## OUTCOME

The long-term outcome for childhood NS is excellent overall. The vast majority of children who develop NS will have SSNS, among which approximately one-third of children will have no relapses, one-third will have infrequent relapses (i.e., <4 relapses per year), and another third will have frequent relapses (≥4 relapses per year, or FRNS). Nonetheless, the most significant predictor of a child's likelihood of outgrowing NS without the development of CKD is entry into complete clinical remission in response to glucocorticoids. By extension, with the continuing expansion of alternative treatments able to induce complete remission among children with SRNS, we now infer that induction of complete remission by any of these treatments confers similar reduction in risk for the development of CKD or ESRD. By contrast, while the risk for the development of CKD or ESRD among children with SSNS is <5%, this risk rises dramatically for children who present with or subsequently develop SRNS, where the risk of CKD and/or ESRD approaches 50% within 5 years.[240] Lastly, mortality in NS is now <5%, and is most commonly due to infection.[233,237] Importantly, this represents a dramatic drop from the 67% mortality estimated to exist 60 to 70 years ago, prior to the development of antibiotics and introduction of glucocorticoids. Despite these major advances, deaths do still occur among children with NS, most commonly among those with SRNS who remain in relapse and are often exposed to prolonged immunosuppression.

In summary, NS is among the most common forms of kidney disease in children. While significant progress had been made in recent years in developing more effective treatments for this disease, the molecular pathophysiology of the most common form of this disease, SSNS, remains unknown, as do the mechanisms of action of many of the newer treatments that have improved the clinical outcomes of children with SRNS. Additional research to better define the molecular pathophysiology of the disease is needed to enable the development of more targeted and effective and less toxic treatments for this very common kidney disease in children.

## COMPLEMENT-ASSOCIATED KIDNEY DISEASES

Complement-associated kidney diseases comprise a spectrum of conditions, which are caused by genetic mutations and/or the presence of autoantibodies disrupting regulation of the innate immune complement system.[360–363] An increasing number of diseases and conditions are linked to complement regulatory defects that result in chronic complement overactivation. Complement-associated diseases manifest in many tissues, but predominantly affect the kidneys.[364–366] Two of the most prominent examples for complement-associated kidney diseases are MPGN/C3G and atypical hemolytic uremic syndrome (aHUS).[365] In aHUS, mutations of complement regulators and inhibitory anticomplement factor H (CFH) autoantibodies are found in approximately 50% of cases resulting in complement dysregulation on endothelial surfaces.[367] By contrast, in C3G, which encompasses both C3 glomerulonephritis (C3GN) and dense deposit disease (DDD), complement dysregulation is caused by the presence of autoantibodies and/or mutations resulting in complement dysregulation in plasma (fluid phase) with subsequent deposition of C3 degradation products along and/or within the GBM.[368] The firm link of aHUS and C3G pathogenesis to complement [alternative pathway (AP)] dysregulation allows for new, specific treatment strategies directed at reestablishing complement control, and raises hopes for better patient outcomes.[266,369]

### COMPLEMENT SYSTEM

The classical pathway (CP) of complement is initiated by Igs or ICs and thus is especially involved in autoimmune diseases and the Ig/IC-mediated form of MPGN. The lectin pathway (LP) is activated by repetitive carbohydrate structures found, for example, on the surface of bacteria. By difference, the AP of complement is constitutively active via a process called "tick over" and requires tight regulation. All three activation pathways converge in the activation of the central complement component C3 to C3b. Together with complement factor B (CFB)—activated by complement factor D—and properdin (CFP), C3b forms the AP C3 convertase (C3bBb), which rapidly amplifies C3 activation. The resulting activation products are involved in inflammatory responses (C3a; anaphylatoxin) or deposit on bacterial surfaces (C3b; opsonization), rendering them a target for phagocytosis. C3b also initiates C5 activation via the formation of the C5 convertase (C3bBbC3b), thus contributing to inflammation (C5a; anaphylatoxin) and initiation of the terminal pathway (TP) of complement (C5b) with the formation of the membrane attack complex (MAC) C5b-9 (Fig. 72.8).[360–363,370]

Complement regulation is provided by soluble and membrane-anchored proteins, which limit complement activation in a timely and spatial fashion both in fluid phase and on cell surfaces. The most important complement regulator, fluid-phase CFH (FH), regulates complement via (1) limiting C3b binding to surfaces and formation of the C3 convertase, C3bBb (competition), (2) inactivating/cleaving C3b (cofactor activity), and (3) accelerating the natural decay of the C3 convertase, C3bBb (decay-acceleration activity; Fig. 72.8).

While the C-terminal region of CFH is responsible for surface recognition and binding to C3b, its N-terminal region provides cofactor and decay-accelerating function.[371] Of note, aHUS—a disease characterized by uncontrolled complement activation on endothelial cells—is associated with mutations in the C-terminal region of CFH, while in C3G—a disease associated with enhanced C3 conversion in fluid phase—mutations are found in the N-terminal region (Figs. 72.8 and 72.9).[368,372]

Besides CFH there are five proteins sharing sequence and structural homology with CFH – the CFH-related proteins (CFHR) 1–5. CFHR1 regulates complement on the level of the C5 convertase, C3bBbC3b.[373] CFHR1, CFHR2, and CFHR5 form homodimers and heterodimers via shared short consensus repeats (SCRs) 1 and 2, which compete with CFH for C3b binding, thus physiologically modulating its function.[374,375] Mutations within the CFHR locus (1q32) result in copy number variations (deletions and duplications) and the formation of fusion proteins, which more avidly than nonmutant proteins form CFHR homodimers and heterodimers. These atypical complexes compete with CFH for C3b binding in a manner exceeding physiological modulation, thus preventing CFH from executing its physiological complement regulatory functions. This "CFH deregulation" has recently been identified as disease causing in C3G patients.[374,375]

In addition, cellular surfaces are protected via complement receptor 1 (CR1) and membrane cofactor protein (MCP; CD46), both acting as cofactors to CFI, via decay-accelerating factor (DAF; CD55) and via CD59, which prevents assembly of the MAC (C5b-9; Fig. 72.8).[360–363,370]

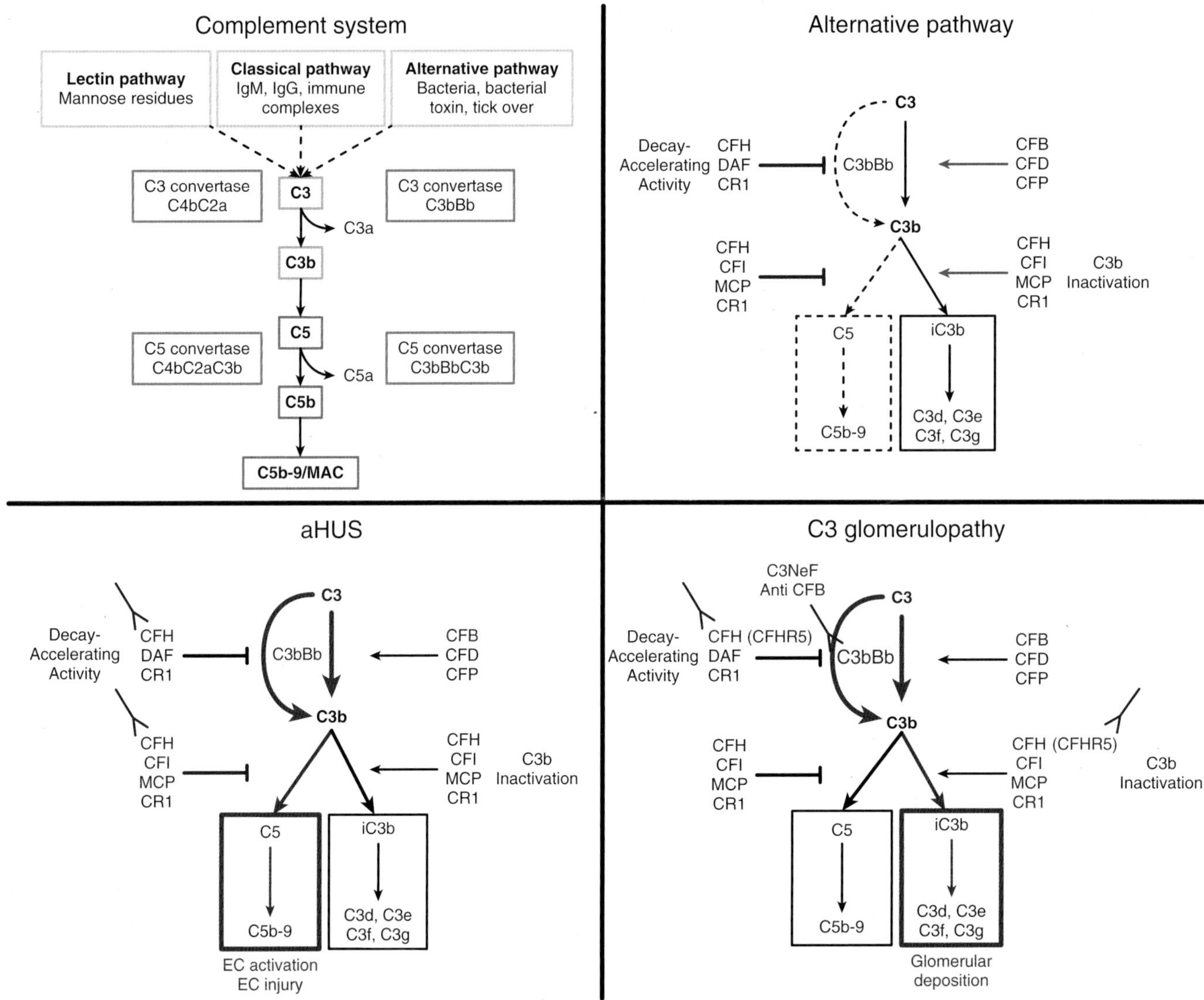


**Fig. 72.8** Complement and its link to disease. Complement activation via the lectin, classical (immune complexes), or alternative pathway (constitutively active) resulting in C3, followed by C5 activation, terminal pathway activation and formation of the MAC (Cb-9; for details, see text). Alternative pathway: a small amount of C3 is constantly activated and turned into C3b. If not inhibited, C3b leads via an amplification loop to the activation of C5 followed by the induction of the terminal pathway and the formation of the MAC, C5b-9. Physiologically, C3b is immediately inactivated via plasma or endothelial cell membrane–anchored regulators (such as CFH, CFI, MCP, CR1) and cleaved to become C3d-g. aHUS: aHUS is caused by unrestricted activation of the complement alternative pathway on vascular endothelial cells. Loss-of-function mutations in genes encoding complement regulators (such as CFH, CFI, MCP), gain-of-function mutations of complement activators (such as C3, CFB), or CFH autoantibodies result in a shift of the balance between C3 activation and inactivation toward C3 activation with subsequent induction of the terminal pathway. C3 glomerulopathy: C3 glomerulopathy is caused by an overactive C3 amplification loop, which can be caused via gain-of-function mutations in components of the C3 convertase complex, C3bBb (such as C3 and CFB), loss-of-function mutations in C3 amplification regulators (such as CFH, CFHRs, CFI, MCP), autoantibodies inhibiting complement regulators (such as CFH), or stabilizing complement activators (such as CFB, C3NeF). Accordingly, excessive amounts of C3b metabolites (C3d-g) are generated, which deposit in the glomerular filter and cause a local inflammatory response. *aHUS,* Atypical hemolytic uremic syndrome; *C3NeF,* C3 nephritic factor; *CFB,* complement factor B; *CFD,* complement factor D; *CFH,* complement factor H; *CFI,* complement factor I; *CFP,* properdin; *CR1,* complement receptor 1; *DAF,* decay-accelerating factor; *Ig,* immunoglobulin; *MAC,* membrane attack complex; *MCP,* membrane cofactor protein.

C3 inactivation results in the formation of iC3b, C3dg, and C3d, degradation products of C3b, which can be interpreted as indirect measure of complement activation, but are also of biological relevance, as they interact with the adaptive immune system and deposit within and along the GBM where they initiate the histomorphological changes typical for IC-MPGN/C3G (Fig. 72.10).[376,377]

## IMMUNE COMPLEX MEMBRANOPROLIFERATIVE GLOMERULONEPHRITIS AND C3 GLOMERULOPATHY

MPGN is characterized by the histopathological pattern of mesangial and endocapillary proliferation and thickening

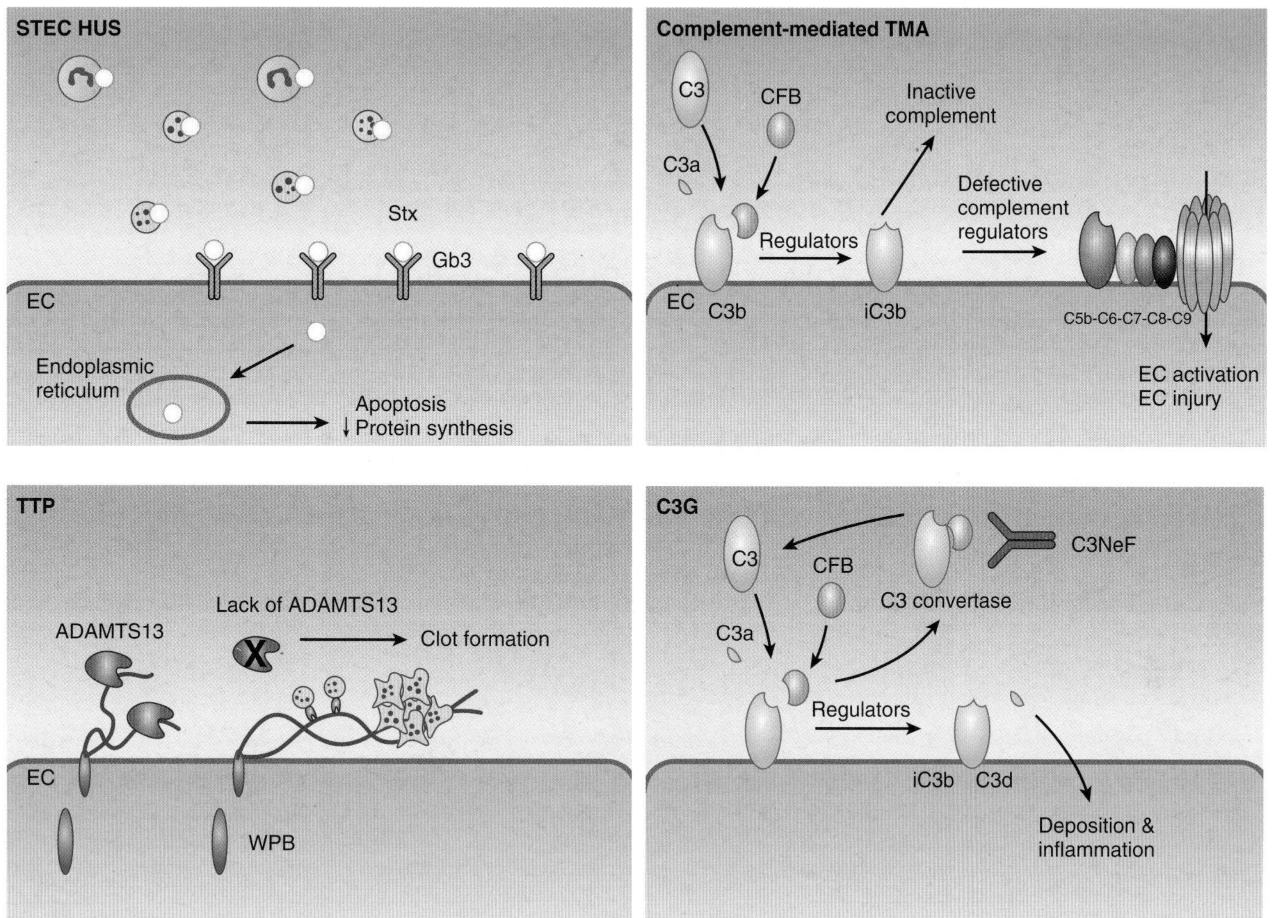


**Fig. 72.9** Mechanism of complement-mediated disease. STEC–HUS is caused by bacterial exotoxins produced, for example, by *Escherichia coli* O157:H7. Toxin binds to the endothelial expressed Gb3 receptor, is internalized, transferred to the ER, and results in apoptosis or necrosis interfering with protein translation. Complement-mediated TMA: Complement-mediated TMA is caused by unrestricted activation of the complement alternative pathway on vascular endothelial cells. In primary TMA, congenital or acquired defects in the activation or regulation of the complement alternative pathway cause unrestricted activation of the terminal pathway. In secondary TMA, complement overactivation in secondary TMA can be caused, for example, by inflammation, drug toxicity, shear stress. TTP: TTP is caused by the genetic or acquired functional defect in the serine protease ADAMTS13, which physiologically cleaves vWF multimers upon release from the vascular endothelium. With impaired ADAMTS13 function, vWF multimers persist and provide a nidus for the formation of platelet rich clots. C3G: C3G is caused by an overactive C3 amplification loop caused by mutations or autoantibodies affecting the physiological decay of the C3 convertase complex, C3bBb. Excessive amounts of activated C3 (C3b), and subsequently of C3b metabolites (C3d-g), are generated, which deposit in the glomerular filter and cause a local inflammatory response. *ER,* Endoplasmic reticulum; *STEC–HUS,* Shiga toxin *Escherichia coli*–hemolytic uremic syndrome; *TMA,* thrombotic microangiopathy; *TTP,* thrombotic thrombocytopenic purpura; *vWF,* von Willebrand factor.

of the capillary with the formation of double contours. This results from the deposition of Ig/ICs and/or complement proteins in the mesangium and/or along the capillary wall of the glomerulus.[378,379]

MPGN has recently been reclassified into (1) a primary complement-mediated C3G with predominant C3 deposition, and (2) a secondary Ig/IC-mediated glomerulonephritis with predominant IgG/IgM deposition on immunohistochemistry (IC-MPGN).[379,380] This new classification system encompasses all glomerular lesions with predominant C3 staining (≥2 orders of magnitude stronger than any other immune reactant on a scale ranging from 0 to 3),[380] and, in addition, enables the inclusion of cases with C3 deposition without a membranoproliferative pattern.[380] C3G is considered a primary complement disease, where complement deposition is a result of defective control of the AP of complement.[381,382] By contrast, IC-MPGN may be idiopathic or secondary to a spectrum of underlying diseases or conditions including infections, autoimmune diseases, malignancies, or monoclonal gammopathy (Table 72.7), and is characterized by Ig/IC deposition in the kidney with subsequent activation of the CP.[383–386] The diagnosis of C3G is based on LM and EM.[380] C3GN and DDD can present on LM as MPGN, diffuse proliferative/mesangioproliferative glomerulonephritis, and necrotizing or crescentic glomerulonephritis.[380,387] C3GN and DDD can be differentiated by EM: C3GN and DDD are characterized by discrete C3 deposits in the mesangium and along the capillary walls, DDD by C3 deposits in the mesangium and within the GBM.[380]

## PATHOGENESIS

During recent years major progress has been made in the understanding of IC-MPGN and C3G pathogenesis via the investigation of disease causing genetic and autoimmune

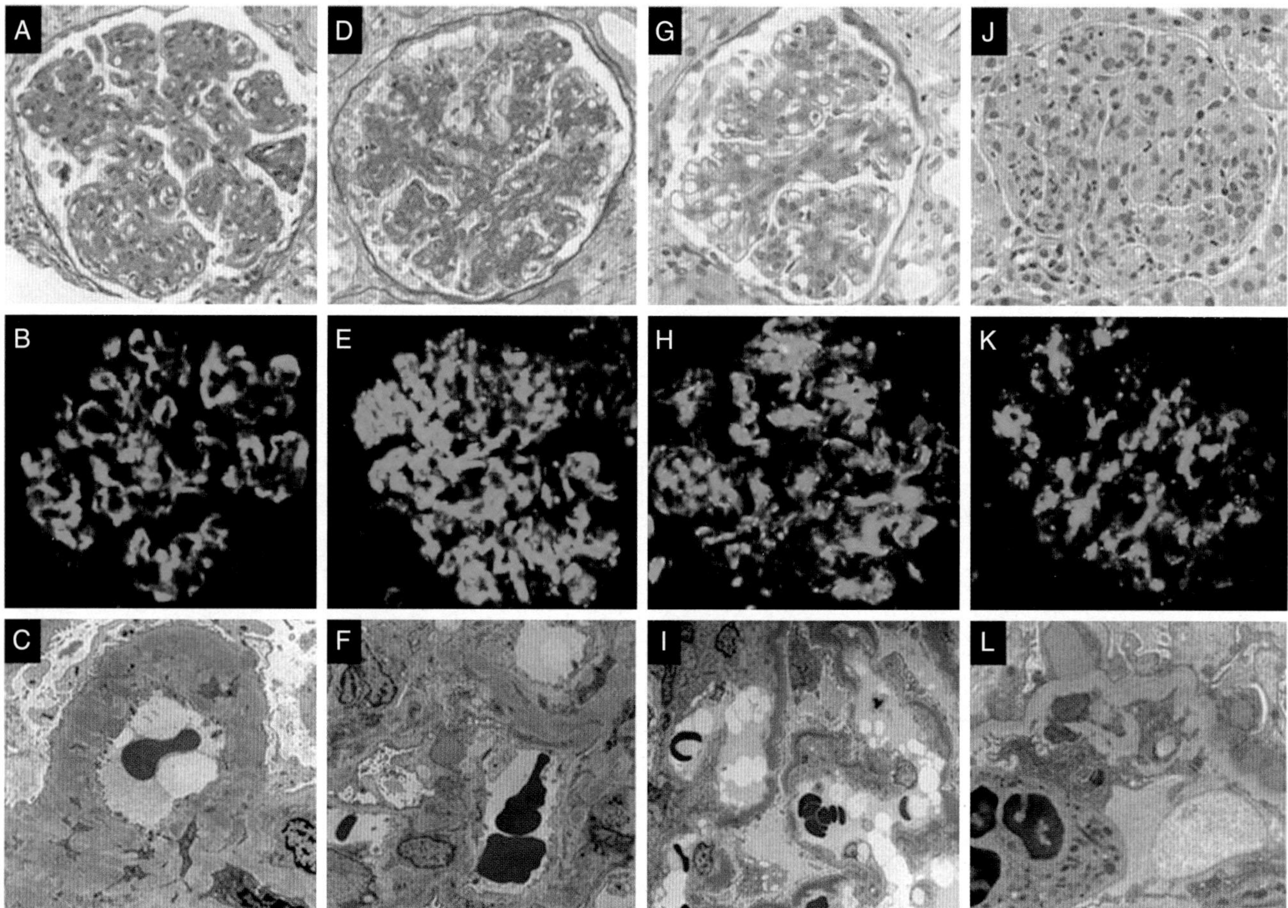


**Fig. 72.10** Histopathologic characteristics in membranoproliferative glomerulonephritis (MPGN) – immune complex-mediated (IC-MPGN) and C3 glomerulopathy (C3G). Also shown in this figure and frequently in the differential diagnosis are dense deposit disease (DDD) and postinfectious glomerulonephritis (PIGN). Panels highlight the microscopic features of (A–C) MPGN, (D–F) C3G, (G–I) DDD, and (J–L) PIGN by light microscopy *(top row)*, immunofluorescence microscopy *(middle row)*, and electron microscopy *(bottom row)*. MPGN has typical features of glomerular lobular accentuation, mesangial expansion by matrix and cells, endocapillary hypercellularity, and capillary wall double contouring (A); coarse granular peripheral capillary and variable mesangial staining for C3 (B), invariably with one or more immunoglobulins (Ig), usually IgG and/or IgM; and mesangial and subendothelial deposits with cellular interpositioning and new basement membrane formation (C). C3G often shows a membranoproliferative (D) or mesangial proliferative pattern; dominant C3 staining (with little or no staining for immunoglobulin) in the mesangium and capillary walls (E); and a combination of mesangial, subendothelial, and subepithelial deposits, and often including subepithelial hump-type deposits (F). DDD can show an MPGN pattern (G) just as commonly as a mesangial proliferative, proliferative/exudative, or crescentic pattern; dominant glomerular C3 staining, often in a pseudolinear capillary pattern with mesangial coarse granules or rings (H); and pathognomonic electron dense transformation of the basement membrane (I), often also with mesangial deposits. PIGN shows a proliferative glomerulonephritis with prominent neutrophilic infiltration (J); mesangial and often spotty granular capillary staining for C3 (K), often with IgG; and subepithelial hump-type deposits with scattered mesangial and subendothelial deposits (L). A, D, and G: Periodic acid–Schiff ×400; J: hematoxylin and eosin ×400; B, E, H, K: C3 ×400; C and L: electron microscopy ×10,000; F: electron microscopy ×6000; I: electron microscopy ×4000.

defects affecting activation and regulation of the complement system—in particular its AP—identified in patients both in vitro and in vivo, and via testing of new complement modulating drugs in animal models recapitulating such defects.[369,388,389]

Principles of C3G pathogenesis can be derived from spontaneously occurring and genetically engineered animal models.[368] A lesion consistent with MPGN II/DDD developed in pigs with complete CFH deficiency due to a spontaneously occurring truncating CFH mutation. Notably, administration of CFH (via plasma or as purified protein) delayed disease progression.[390–394] A similar phenotype developed also in genetically engineered mice ($cfh^{-/-}$) with complete CFH deficiency.[395] In both animal models, C3 accumulates along the GBM in the setting of systemic hypocomplementemia, and immune EM identified complement components (i.e., C3, C5, C5b-9) within these deposits.[390,395] An essential role for the AP in disease pathogenesis was demonstrated by the observation that the C3G phenotype in the $cfh^{-/-}$ mice could be rescued if mice were also genetically deficient in the AP activation protein, factor B.[395] Utilizing mice lacking complement factor I (CFI) ($cfh^{-/-}$; $cfi^{-/-}$), it was demonstrated that renal C3 deposition is complement factor I (FI) dependent as mice did not develop renal C3 deposition unless they were treated with FI containing serum.[396]

In humans, the phenotype associated with complete CFH deficiency was not limited to C3G but included also the TMA aHUS. Besides the differences in the complement systems of mice versus man, this observation indicates that AP defects can give rise to a spectrum of renal pathologies. aHUS-associated FH mutations typically occur within the CFH

**Table 72.7 Causes of Secondary Membranoproliferative Glomerulonephritis**

| | |
|---|---|
| Infectious diseases: bacterial/viral/ protozoal | • Hepatitis B, C, Epstein–Barr virus, human immunodeficiency virus<br>• Endocarditis/visceral abscesses<br>• Infected ventriculoatrial shunts/ empyema<br>• Malaria, schistosomiasis, mycoplasma<br>• Tuberculosis, leprosy<br>• Epstein-Barr virus infection<br>• Brucellosis |
| Systemic immune diseases | • Cryoglobulinemia<br>• Systemic lupus erythematosus<br>• Sjögren syndrome<br>• Rheumatoid arthritis<br>• Hereditary deficiencies of complement components<br>• X-linked agammaglobulinemia |
| Neoplasms/ dysproteinemias | • Plasma cell dyscrasia<br>• Fibrillary and immunotactoid glomerulonephritis<br>• Light-chain deposition disease<br>• Heavy-chain deposition disease<br>• Light- and heavy-chain deposition disease<br>• Leukemias and lymphomas (with cryoglobulinemia)<br>• Waldenstrom macroglobulinemia<br>• Carcinomas, Wilms tumor, malignant melanoma |
| Chronic liver disease | • Chronic active hepatitis (B and C)<br>• Cirrhosis<br>• Alpha-1-antitrypsin deficiency |
| Miscellaneous | • Thrombotic microangiopathy<br>• Sickle cell disease<br>• Partial lipodystrophy<br>• Transplant glomerulopathy<br>• Niemann–Pick disease (type C) |

surface recognition domains SCR18–20 (CFH C terminus). In CFH null mice with transgenic expression of a mutant FH protein functionally mimicking human aHUS-associated CFH mutations (CFHΔ16-20; *cfh*$^{-/-}$.FHΔ16-20), systemic hypocomplementemia was ameliorated as the mutant protein still had an intact complement regulatory domain (CFH N terminus). These animals spontaneously developed aHUS (not C3G), and the aHUS phenotype was dependent on C5 activation[397,398] as opposed to the C3G phenotype observed in the *cfh*$^{-/-}$; *cfi*$^{-/-}$ mice substituted with CFI containing serum (see earlier text), which was C3 dependent.[399] Mice lacking CFH expression by hepatocytes (hepatocyte *cfh*$^{-/-}$) showed significantly reduced but not absent peripheral CFH levels. At baseline, these mice did not develop C3 deposition along the GBM, but mesangial C3 accumulation consistent with C3G. However, after induction of complement activation via nephrotoxic serum they developed C5-dependent TMA.[400]

Taken together, these studies indicate that the aHUS phenotype depends on defective endothelial surface complement regulation combined with an (partially) intact complement system allowing for the presence and activation of sufficient amounts of C5 to induce the TP-mediated endothelial damage, whereas the C3G phenotype depends on

**Table 72.8 Complement Activation Markers in Serum and Tissue Biopsy**

| Measurement | Interpretation |
|---|---|
| **Markers in Serum** | |
| Increased C3 split products (C3d) | Sign for C3b inactivation |
| Decreased Bb | Sign for alternative pathway activation |
| Increased sC5b-9 | Sign for terminal pathway activation |
| **Markers in Tissue Biopsy** | |
| Increased C3(c) | Sign for complement deposition |
| Increased C3 split products (C3d) | Sign for C3b inactivation |
| Increased sC5b-9 | Sign for terminal pathway activation |

fluid phase complement (AP) dysregulation with the generation of C3-sufficient amounts of C3b split products to deposit along and within the GBM (Fig. 72.8).

In patients with IC-MPGN/C3G, a central role for complement in disease pathogenesis has long been recognized, as decreased C3 levels are a hallmark feature of the clinical presentation. Mutations or autoantibodies result in the loss of control of AP C3 convertase via one or more of the following mechanisms:

- Autoantibodies to components of the AP C3 convertase stabilizing this complex, thus prolonging its natural decay.
- Mutations in or autoantibodies to CFH resulting in the absence or loss of function of CFH.
- Mutations in C3 or CFB resulting in their gain of function with an exceedingly stable AP C3 convertase.

All these scenarios result in an enhanced rate of C3 activation with subsequent enhanced levels of MAC/C5b-9 as found in C3G patients.[372]

In further support of a complement-mediated pathogenesis, the presence of AP and TP proteins was demonstrated in the glomerulus of patients with C3G via a combination of laser microdissection and mass spectrometry.[381,382]

The association of low C3 and MPGN was first reported in 1965, leading to the hypothesis of the presence of a C3 cleavage factor in GN patients.[401] Subsequently, an antibody binding and stabilizing the AP C3 convertase (C3bBb), thus enhancing C3 activation and C3b generation, was detected and named C3 nephritic factor (C3NeF).[402] C3NeF was detected in 86% of DDD and 46% of C3GN patients, respectively, and is associated with decreased C3 levels.[372] C3NeF levels show significant intraindividual and interindividual variability and do not necessarily correlate with disease activity or treatment status.[403]

Detection of C3NeF is challenging, and current assays involve measurement of IgG binding to the C3 convertase or the detection of the ability to stabilize the AP C3 convertase.[404,405] C3NeF was also reported in SLE,[406–408] PIGN,[382] meningococcal meningitis,[409] as well as in healthy individuals.[404] The finding of C3NeF does not exclude the coexistence of complement mutations, and despite C3NeF positivity, comprehensive complement diagnostic workup (Table 72.8) is required.[410]

Recently, additional nephritic factors—autoantibodies to C4[411] and C5[412]—have been identified in rare cases of C3G patients. Other autoantibodies also detected in C3G patients include anti-CFB and anti-C3b antibodies.[413,414] Nephritic factors bind to and stabilize their respective convertase complexes, thus prolonging the natural decay and rendering them inert for CFH-mediated decay acceleration. By contrast, anti-CFH autoantibodies—frequent in aHUS—can rarely also be detected in C3G patients: while aHUS-associated anti-CFH autoantibodies recognize the C terminus of CFH,[415] C3G-associated anti-CFH autoantibodies such as the CFH mini autoantibody (i.e., antibody fragment-like λ-light chain dimer) block the interaction of CFH and C3b, thus abolishing the cofactor activity of CFH in cleaving C3b.[416,417]

To date, complement mutations have been reported in the following complement genes: CFH, CFHR5, CFI, MCP/CD46, C3, and CFB (Fig. 72.8).[372,374,418–431]. In a series of 134 patients with MPGN I, C3G, and DDD, mutations in *CFH, CFI,* and *MCP/CD46* were detected in 16.6%, 17.2%, and 19.6% patients, respectively (Fig. 72.8).[372]

More recently, genetic variants including CNVs with deletions (internal), duplications, and the formation of hybrid genes within the gene locus encoding for the CFHRs (1q32) have been associated with C3G.[432,433] CFHR5 nephropathy was defined as a specific subtype of C3G arising from an internal duplication within the *CFHR5* gene.[422] CFHR5 nephropathy presents in childhood with persistent microscopic hematuria, synpharyngitic gross hematuria, and a strong family history of ESRD. The disease has been identified and reported primarily in the Cypriot population, but also in two patients of non-Cypriotic background.[422,434–436]

Several more mutations and hybrid variants within the *CFHR* gene locus have been identified and linked to C3G (Fig. 72.8). The function of CFHR CNV and hybrid gene C3G was unclear until it was recognized that CFHR1, CFHR2, and CFHR5 via (almost) identical N-terminal SCR1 and SCR2 were naturally forming homodimers and heterodimers and as such competing with CFH for surface and C3b binding. Under physiological conditions, this competition provides a physiological balance and allows for titration of CFH function. However, in the presence of *CFHR* mutations with the resulting CNV and hybrid gene/protein formation, nonphysiological multimers with enhanced affinity for the shared binding partners form. This scenario results in the loss of CFH complement regulatory function and is termed "CFH deregulation."[401,402]

Risk haplotypes were identified in CFH, C3, and MCP/CD46, with the CFH Y402H haplotype more frequently reported in DDD and the MCP/CD46 652A4G polymorphism in C3G and MPGN I.[372,418] The presence of two or more complement haplotypes significantly increased the risk of disease manifestation.[372,418] Of note, in a recent study in 140 IC-MPGN and C3G patients, two important findings were made: (1) different from previous claims, mutations in genes encoding AP proteins were found in both subgroups regardless of their histopathological pattern (17% and 18%, respectively); (2) these mutations alone did not increase the risk of disease manifestation, unless mutations combined with specific susceptibility variants (i.e., MCP/CD46 c.-366G>A in IC-MPGN; CFH V62 and thrombomodulin [THBD]/CD141 A473V in C3G).[437]

Taken together, these findings support the central role of complement defects for IC-MPGN/C3G pathogenesis and highlight the complexity of the underlying genetic and/or autoimmune defects. They also identify the crucial role of complete genetic and biochemical analyses in the advanced management of IC-MPGN/C3G patients.

## CLINICAL MANIFESTATIONS

MPGN and C3G (C3GN and DDD) are rare diseases with an annual incidence of 1 to 2 per million (both pediatric and adult).[438,439] Once thought to be primarily pediatric diseases, a recent study noted that the mean age at diagnosis for MPGN and C3G was 20.7 ± 16.8 years, 18.9 ± 17.7 years, and 30.3 ± 19.3 years, respectively.[372] Within pediatric patients, DDD presents at a younger age with 70% of patients diagnosed prior to age 15.[440] There is a slight bias with males predominating in MPGN and C3G.[372,438]

The clinical manifestation of MPGN and C3G typically includes hematuria, proteinuria (up to nephrotic range), hypertension, and impaired kidney function with significant overlap of symptoms between disease subtypes.[441,442] NS at disease onset has been reported in 40% to 65% of patients with MPGN, 30% to 40% with DDD, and 25% to 40% with C3GN, respectively. Regardless of disease subtype, microscopic hematuria has been reported in 40% to 75%, gross hematuria in 10% to 20%, and nonnephrotic proteinuria in 30% to 40% of patients. Acute glomerulonephritis is common and is accompanied by hypertension in 30% to 60%, and impaired kidney function in 20% to 50% of patients.[372,378,438,443] Although rare, rapidly progressive glomerulonephritis (RPGN) has also been reported in patients with MPGN and C3G.

Hypocomplementemia is long considered a key feature in MPGN,[442] and differential findings in serum C3 and C4 levels were used to distinguish between MPGN I (low C3 and low C4) and other types of MPGN (low C3 and normal C4).[444] Applying the current classification, IC-MPGN as IC-mediated disease is commonly associated with depressed C3 and C4 levels, whereas C3GN and DDD as primary complement-driven diseases are associated with depressed C3 but normal C4 levels.[372,436] There were, however, important caveats noted in these studies as patients did not always follow the expected pattern of C3/C4 levels, and a significant subgroup of patients presented even with normal C3 levels.[372,438] It appears that while assessment of C3 and C4 levels is suggestive of IC-MPGN or C3G (C3GN and DDD), suppressed C3 or C4 levels are not sufficient to establish these diagnoses.[372,438] Of note, patients with CFHR5 nephropathy are also reported to have normal serum C3 levels.[445]

In addition to decreased C3 levels, C3G patients—both C3GN and DDD—were found to also present with decreased CFB levels, increased C3b breakdown products, and elevated soluble C5b-9 levels.[446]

Extrarenal manifestations of C3G are uncommon and include acquired partial lipodystrophy (aPL)[447] and ocular C3 deposits[424] similar to soft drusen seen in age-related macular degeneration (AMD). aPL is presumably caused by complement dysregulation on adipocytes and results in the breakdown of the fat tissue of the upper parts (i.e., head and trunk) of the body. aPL typically precedes the renal manifestation of MPGN and may be associated with decreased C3 levels and the presence of C3NeF.[447,448] Soft drusen consist of C3 split products and CFH,[449,450] may be associated with polymorphisms/mutations in complement genes,[391] and may

**Table 72.9 Spectrum of Thombotic Microangiopathies**

| Thrombotic Microangiopathy (TMA) | Role of Complement | Diagnostic Test |
|---|---|---|
| Thrombotic thrombocytopenic purpura | Elevated C5b-9 | Biochemistry |
| Hemolytic uremic syndrome | | |
| STEC–HUS/eHUS | Transient activation possible | Biochemistry; if persistent C activation, consider genetics |
| Atypical HUS | Continuous (mutation and abs.) | Biochemistry and genetics and antibody screen |
| Other hereditary forms of TMA<br>DGKE<br>INF2 | N/A | Biochemistry; if persistent C activation, consider genetics |
| TMA postsolid organ transplantation<br>De novo TMA<br>TMA recurrence | Transient or continuous (mutation and abs.) | Biochemistry and genetics and antibody screen |
| TMA posthematopoietic stem cell transplantation/bone marrow transplantation | Transient or continuous (mutation and abs.) | Biochemistry and genetics and antibody screen |
| TMA associated with pregnancy | Transient or continuous (mutation and abs.) | Biochemistry and genetics and antibody screen |
| TMA associated with glomerulonephritis | Continuous C activation possible (mutation and abs.) | Biochemistry and genetics and antibody screen |
| TMA associated with drugs | Transient C activation possible | Biochemistry; if persistent C activation, consider genetics |
| TMA associated with metabolic disease | C activation possible | Biochemistry; if persistent C activation, consider genetics |
| TMA associated with infections (e.g., *Streptococcus pneumoniae*, human immunodeficiency virus, influenza) | Transient C activation possible | Biochemistry; if persistent C activation, consider genetics |
| TMA associated with malignant hypertension | Transient C activation possible | Biochemistry; if persistent C activation, consider genetics |

Persistent: after initial cause has resolved; Biochemistry: Complement activation tests (see Table 72.3).
*eHUS, Escherichia coli*-induced hemolytic uremic syndrome; *STEC,* Shiga toxin *Escherichia coli*.

also be associated with the risk of developing AMD.[451] The long-term risk for visual problems is about 10%.[452]

## DIAGNOSIS

MPGN and C3G most commonly present as acute nephritis or NS. More subtle presentations are also seen, and there is considerable clinical overlap with the presentations of other forms of renal disease. Complement analysis (e.g., C3 and C4 levels, CFB levels, C3b breakdown products, soluble C5b-9) may be useful; however, normal results do not exclude the diagnosis.[372] The measurement of nephritic factors or other complement autoantibodies (e.g., anti-CFH, CFB, C3b) may also be supportive; however, these assays are neither standardized nor widely available and lack diagnostic specificity. Genetic complement testing may be valuable and is—in particular in the background of the increasing number of identified disease-causing mutations in the CFHR locus—highly recommended. Ultimately, the diagnosis is finalized by renal biopsy (Table 72.9).

The differential diagnosis of a setting of nephritic/NS with hypocomplementemia (in particular, low C3 and C4 levels) is narrow and mainly includes IC-MPGN/C3G and SLE. Extrarenal disease manifestations such as arthralgias; rashes; neurologic, hepatic, lung, or cardiac involvement combined with laboratory evidence of immune dysregulation including antibody-mediated hemolysis, leukopenia, coagulopathy, myositis, or hepatitis support a diagnosis of SLE as opposed to MPGN. Although exceedingly rare in children, cryoglobulinemia may also present with multiorgan involvement and systemic findings. IC-mediated (secondary) forms of MPGN (IC-MPGN) may present with decreased C3 and C4 levels.[453] The combination of decreased C3 and normal C4 levels points toward PIGN and shunt nephritis. The history of a recent episode of pharyngitis, possibly accompanied by elevated antistreptolysin (ASO) titer or anti-DNase titers, in combination with decreased C3 levels, defines the signature of PIGN. The differential diagnosis of C3G may be considered only if the clinical course is atypical, that is, the C3 level does not return to normal within 8 to 10 weeks of presentation.[382] In such cases—in particular, in the background of a family history of unexplained ESRD—a kidney biopsy should be considered.[382] As MPGN and C3G may present with normal complement levels, they should also be considered in any differential diagnosis for glomerular disease even if the patient's C3 and C4 levels are normal. CFHR5 nephropathy should be considered even in patients outside Cyprus for patients with persistent microscopic hematuria, and synpharyngitic gross hematuria with or without a family history of ESRD.

## TREATMENT

To date, no treatment standards exist for patients with IC-MPGN or C3G, and current treatment recommendations are mainly based on small size single-center studies and expert opinions.

ACE inhibitors or Ang II receptor antagonists (ARBs) are used in many patients with IC-MPGN/C3G due to their antiproteinuric and antihypertensive effect, and their use was associated with better renal survival.[372] Treatment of arterial hypertension and CKD/ESRD follows established standards.

Prednisone is considered the first-line agent in patients with IC-MPGN who present with (nephrotic range) proteinuria with or without renal failure. In children a beneficial effect of long-term low-dose prednisone treatment was shown for proteinuria and long-term renal outcome even though only a subgroup of patients will (partially) respond. A typical treatment regimen consists of a prednisone dose of 60 mg/m$^2$ (maximal 60 mg/day) × 4 weeks (induction) followed by 40 mg/m$^2$ on alternate-day for 6 to 12 months (maintenance). Of note, no beneficial effect was shown in patients with DDD.

MMF was administered to IC-MPGN and C3G patients alone or in combination with prednisone and was successful in achieving sustained improvement of proteinuria and renal function after 1 year.[454] In patients with primary GN, including MPGN, a partial or complete remission was achieved in 70% after 1 year.[455] In another study, in pediatric patients with MPGN I treated with MMF and prednisone for a mean of 40 months, 56% achieved complete or partial remission. However, treatment failed in all patients with decreased C3 levels.[456] In addition, no treatment benefit was found in patients with DDD. In a recent analysis, renal outcome in 22 IC-MPGN/C3G patients treated with a combination of steroids and MMF was compared with 18 patients treated with different immunosuppressive regimens including steroids alone or in combination with cyclophosphamide. While in principle immunosuppressive (as opposed to no) treatment was beneficial, renal outcome in patients commenced on the combination of steroids and MMF was significantly better than in patients commenced on any other single immunosuppressive regimen.[457]

CNIs (cyclosporine A and tacrolimus) were found to have questionable benefit in IC-MPGN/C3G patients. CNIs were used in steroid-resistant MPGN patients. One study demonstrated efficacy of the combination of low-dose steroids and CNI in patients with refractory MPGN with respect to reduction of proteinuria and decline in renal function in 94% after 2 years.[458] In five adult steroid and cyclophosphamide-resistant MPGN patients, the combination of steroids and tacrolimus resulted in complete or at least partial remission in all patients after 24 weeks or longer.[459,460] In two children with MPGN and suboptimal response to long-term prednisone, a rapid and complete remission was achieved with tacrolimus.[461] In another two patients with DDD low-dose prednisone and cyclosporine A were able to induce remission.[462,463] In another study no treatment benefit of CNI was found in DDD patients.[452]

In analogy to other autoimmune diseases, the pathogenetic role of C3NeF and other complement antibodies (see earlier discussion) has prompted the use of B-cell depleting agents such as rituximab in IC-MPGN/C3G. Several case reports of MPGN (in particular, IC-MPGN) patients describe partial or complete remission after administration of rituximab (in 50% combined with steroids).[464–468] By contrast, two DDD patients did not show any improvement in proteinuria or renal function, but were rescued by eculizumab therapy (discussed later).[469,470]

With the emerging role for the complement AP in IC-MPGN/C3G pathogenesis, complement-targeted treatment strategies are increasingly considered for such patients. Treatment strategies include plasma infusion (PI) or exchange (PLEX) as described for patients with MPGN I and DDD at first disease manifestation and recurrence in native and graft kidneys. Partial or complete remission is reported in about 80% of published cases.[466,471–483]

In one patient with IC-MPGN, despite transient improvement of renal function and proteinuria, clinical condition worsened including seizures, respiratory distress, and sustained anuria. Because of a CFHR1 deletion (without CFH antibodies), low C3 and elevated sC5b-9, indicating AP activation, and TMA-related symptoms, the patient was switched from PLEX to eculizumab. This resulted in dramatic clinical improvement including proteinuria and renal function.[473]

Three case reports, including two siblings with DDD caused by a CFH mutation (CFH SCR4), and one patient with MPGN I with an MCP/CD46 mutation were treated for more than 3 years with plasma. Fresh frozen plasma as maintenance therapy, individualized according to the patient needs (e.g., intercurrent infection), was able to prevent disease progression and stabilize kidney function.[423,427,473] However, PI might not be enough as induction therapy.[484]

Recently, the complement blocker eculizumab has become available. Eculizumab is a humanized monoclonal anti-C5 antibody, which prevents C5 activation and TP induction with the formation of the terminal complement complex (C5b-9).[485] While so far approved only for the use in paroxysmal nocturnal hemoglobinuria (PNH), aHUS, and myasthenia gravis, eculizumab has also been used in the treatment of IC-MPGN/C3G, and recently reports of its successful use for this indication were published either in context of investigator-initiated clinical trials or as (single) case reports.[470,473,486,487] IC-MPGN and C3G (C3GN and DDD) patients were treated for disease manifestation due to genetic mutations or the presence of autoantibodies such as C3NeF in native or graft kidneys at first presentation or disease recurrence. Treatment response spans from "no" to "partial" or "full" response.[486] Although a favorable treatment response seems to be associated with elevated sC5b-9 levels and shorter disease duration,[488] criteria clearly identifying individuals with the potential to respond to eculizumab treatment are still lacking.

Long-term outcome data for MPGN patients—in particular, applying the new classification—are limited. Disease progression in MPGN patients occurs regardless of the underlying MPGN subtype in 40% to 50% within 10 years of diagnosis.[441,442] Renal function (eGFR), nephrotic range proteinuria, hypertension, and age at presentation are negatively correlated with long-term renal outcome.[372,438,441,442] In addition, the presence of glomerular crescents or DDD by biopsy is an independent predictor of disease progression.[438]

Disease recurrence of MPGN and DDD in renal grafts has been well described with recurrence rates ranging from 10% to 100%. However, the impact of disease recurrence on allograft survival remains controversial. Applying the new classification, MPGN recurrence rates for renal grafts are reported as 43%, 55%, and 60% for MPGN, DDD, and C3GN, respectively. The impact on allograft survival was not reported.[372] In another study with 13 transplants all of the six DDD and four of the seven C3GN patients had disease recurrence with graft failure due to recurrence in three of the DDD, and three of the four C3GN patients with recurrence.[438] Overall, allograft survival after 5 years was 69%.

## POSTINFECTIOUS (POSTSTREPTOCOCCAL) GLOMERULONEPHRITIS

### PATHOGENESIS

The new MPGN classification (discussed earlier) also includes acute postinfectious (PIGN) or poststreptococcal glomerulonephritis as part of the MPGN disease spectrum.[380] PIGN is characterized by strong mesangial C3 with codominant IgG staining (IF), and the formation of mesangial, subendothelial, and subepithelial humps (EM).[380] Of note, some patients present with C3 deposition only without IgG deposition and/or humps.

PIGN can be diagnosed clinically without a renal biopsy.[489] It usually follows a bacterial infection—typically pharyngitis or pyoderma—with β-hemolytic group A *Streptococcus pneumoniae* with a latency of 7 to 14 days and is usually associated with an increased antistreptolysin (ASO) titer. The bacterial infection results in the formation of circulating ICs, which deposit in the kidneys and cause an inflammatory response with leukocyte recruitment and complement activation via both the CP and AP.[490,491] While numerous antigens have been considered as being responsible for streptococcal nephritogenicity,[492] currently two antigens, the nephritis-associated plasmin receptor (NAPlr) and a cationic cysteine proteinase known as streptococcal pyrogenic exotoxin B, are favored. Of note, both of these fractions are capable of activating the AP.[491]

As infections—such as streptococcal infections—are also common triggers for the manifestation of IC-MPGN/C3G, and the PIGN typical humps also occur in biopsies of patients with IC-MPGN/C3G, the differential diagnosis can be difficult and mostly relies on clinical observations.[490,491]

### CLINICAL MANIFESTATIONS

PIGN is the most common cause of acute glomerulonephritis in childhood with a median age at presentation of 6 to 8 years. Occurrence prior to age 2 is rare. The male-to-female ratio of PIGN is 2 : 1, but is not different with respect to the presence or absence of a preceding pharyngitis or pyoderma.[490] Three phases of disease manifestation can be distinguished: (1) the latent phase, that is, the phase from bacterial infection to disease manifestation (1–2 weeks); (2) the acute phase (about 2 weeks); and (3) the recovery phase, that is, the phase of resolution of edema, normalization of blood pressure, resolution of hematuria and proteinuria, and normalization of C3 levels (4–6 weeks).[490]

The clinical manifestation of PIGN is characterized by a nephritic syndrome with gross hematuria, proteinuria, edema hypertension, and low C3 levels.[490,491] PIGN usually follows a benign course and has an excellent prognosis in children, which significantly worsens in elderly patients or in individuals with preexisting renal disease.[490,491] In rare cases, PIGN can also be associated with AKI,[492] ESRD,[493,494] and death.[490]

A subgroup of patients clinically diagnosed as PIGN follows an atypical course showing ongoing C3 consumption with low C3 levels, persistent hematuria and/or proteinuria beyond the expected period of recovery, and progressive decline in renal function.[495] Motivated by the clinical similarity between IC-MPGN/C3G and atypical PIGN, and the ongoing signs of complement activation with decreased C3 levels in PIGN patients with incomplete recovery, PIGN patients were screened for complement defects, and AP mutations and autoantibodies (i.e., C3NeF) were detected in patients with "atypical" PIGN.[382,496,497]

In a recent study of 33 pediatric patients clinically diagnosed as PIGN, reassessment of the renal biopsies resulted in the reclassification of 24% of patients as IC-MPGN/C3G according to the new MPGN classification.[495] Review of the clinical course of the reclassified patients revealed that 72% of patients with typical PIGN recovered completely as compared with only 25% of IC-MPGN/C3G patients. PIGN patients had a more severe disease course at baseline but showed a more favorable long-term outcome. Of note, C3 levels of PIGN patients were significantly lower at baseline than C3 levels of IC-MPGN/C3G patients—a difference that disappeared at later follow-up with a trend toward normalization in both groups.[495] While these findings are in keeping with a disease spectrum spanning from IC-MPGN/C3G to PIGN, the study lacks information on possibly underlying complement defects. Prospective trials including full complement workup in patients with typical and atypical PIGN will be required to fully proof this new concept.

### TREATMENT

Typical PIGN takes a benign course with excellent prognosis, and thus does not require specific treatment. Supportive measures mainly include management of edema, and blood pressure control. Still controversial are a potential treatment benefit of antibiotics to treat the underlying bacterial infection, and of immunosuppressants, which are typically used in cases with RPGN and the finding of crescents on renal biopsy.[490,491]

## MEMBRANOUS NEPHROPATHY

MN, which is also sometimes referred to as membranous glomerulonephritis, is a relatively rare cause of glomerular disease among children. It may present with proteinuria, hematuria, or in more severe cases with AKI and/or NS. In contrast to the low frequency in children, MN is the most common primary cause of NS among adults, where it represents one-fourth to one-third of all adults presenting with NS.[498–502] MN can occur either as a primary disease (i.e., idiopathic MN) or as a disease secondary to a variety of causes such as infections, medications, or autoimmune diseases.

### EPIDEMIOLOGY

The incidence of MN is strikingly different between children and adults. Among adults it occurs at a frequency of about 1.2/100,000 population per year, whereas among children it occurs at only about 0.05–0.1/100,000 population per year, or approximately 10 to 20 times less commonly than in adults. Moreover, while MN represents 25% to 35% of new cases of NS among adults, it represents less than 5% of new cases of NS among children.[251,439,503–505] However, within the pediatric age group the incidence of MN is sixfold to 20-fold higher in children who present in adolescence (i.e., 13–18 years) than in children who present under the age of 12 years.[506–508]

Based on data from the US Renal Data System (USRDS), MN has a similar incidence among African-American versus Caucasian children, and occurs approximately equally among girls and boys.[509]

## PATHOGENESIS

MN can be either a primary disease, termed idiopathic MN, or secondary to a wide variety of causes. The many causes of MN in children are shown in Table 72.10. This table highlights that MN is essentially a pathologic finding that likely represents a variety of disease states.[503,510]

Idiopathic MN is characterized by IC formation associated with the GBM (Fig. 72.11). Four stages of disease have been described, which begins with subepithelial deposits on a normal GBM (stage 1), followed by the deposits extending projections into the GBM (stage 2), then incorporation of the deposits into the GBM (stage 3), and ultimately remodeling of the GBM associated with absent deposits (stage 4).[511] A more detailed discussion of the histology of MN is described elsewhere. Unfortunately, despite the variety of histologic features known to occur in MN, these features have not been able to be used to accurately predict clinical outcomes in children.[510,512,513]

Recently, the molecular cause for many cases of idiopathic MN has been identified. Investigators discovered that almost 70% of patients presenting with idiopathic MN (but not secondary MN) had antibodies directed against phospholipase A2 receptor (PLA2R), a transmembrane glycoprotein receptor on the surface of podocytes.[514] Indeed, these same antibodies could be eluted from renal biopsy samples of patients with idiopathic MN (but not secondary MN).[514] By contrast, PLA2R staining was reported in only 45% of children with MN, suggesting that the sensitivity of PLA2R staining of renal biopsies in children is lower than in adults with idiopathic MN.[515] Importantly, anti-PLA2R antibody titers have been demonstrated to be an excellent biomarker of disease activity in patients with MN, with levels being increased during relapses, absent during remissions, and rituximab-induced depletion of anti-PLA2R titers correlating with clinical responses.[516,517]

## CLINICAL MANIFESTATIONS

The clinical presentation of children with MN can range widely, from asymptomatic proteinuria to SRNS. Unfortunately, due to the very low incidence of disease in children, few data are available about the relative distribution across this clinical spectrum among children.

**Table 72.10 Causes of Membranous Nephropathy in Children**

| | Secondary | | | | |
|---|---|---|---|---|---|
| **Primary** | **Infections** | **Medications** | **Autoimmune Diseases** | **Neoplasms** | **Miscellaneous** |
| Idiopathic membranous nephropathy | Hepatitis B | Captopril | Systemic lupus erythematosus | Neuroblastoma | Sickle cell disease |
| | Hepatitis C | Nonsteroidal antiinflammatory drugs | Sjögren syndrome | Angiomatoid fibrous histiocytoma | De novo, postrenal transplantation |
| | Streptococcal infections | Penicillamine | Sarcoidosis | Ovarian tumor | Mercury exposure |
| | Syphilis | Infliximab | Autoimmune hepatitis | | |
| | Tuberculosis | Tiopronin | Primary biliary cirrhosis | | |
| | Epstein–Barr virus | Etanercept | | | |
| | Cytomegalovirus | Gold | | | |
| | Malaria | | | | |

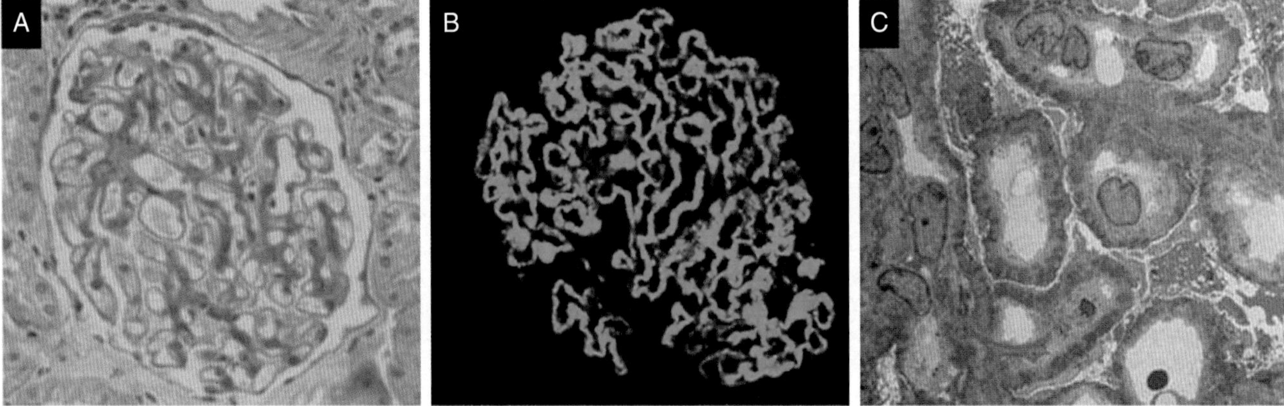


**Fig. 72.11** Histopathologic findings in membranous nephropathy (MN) on light, immunofluorescence, and electron microscopy. MN manifests as global/homogeneous glomerular capillary wall thickening, the degree of which relates to the stage of deposits, (A) from mild when early to thick when late; (B) granular capillary staining for IgG that follows the contours of the basement membrane, and almost always with C3; and (C) diffuse subepithelial deposits close to the podocyte in early stages and progressively incorporating into the basement membrane over time. A: Periodic acid–Schiff ×400; B: immunoglobulin G ×400; C: electron microscopy ×5000.

## TREATMENT

As in adults, the decision about whom and how to treat children with MN centers around determination of the relative risk versus benefit of any specific therapy. In general, because of few published pediatric studies in this area, such decisions for children with MN are usually derived from data published in adult populations. Notably, however, children typically have very different comorbid factors than adults and inherently different life expectancy potential, and these factors must be considered in making treatment decisions. As such, based primarily on adult literature, children with asymptomatic proteinuria are often treated conservatively with only close observation for potential development of more ominous risk factors of disease progression. Reported risk factors of progressive CKD include severe proteinuria (>8 g/day), baseline renal insufficiency, and the rate of decline in renal function over the initial 6 to 12 months of observation.[518] Children presenting with subnephrotic range proteinuria (urine protein-to-creatinine ratio <2.0 mg/mg), normal renal function, and minimal sclerosis on renal biopsy are often treated with ACE inhibitors and/or ARBs.[498] This approach can generally be expected to achieve only approximately 30% reduction in proteinuria, however, and thus would be insufficient for patients with more severe proteinuria.[519–521]

For children who present with NS, the risk–benefit calculation is notably altered. Given the 30% incidence of spontaneous remission reported among adults with MN, an initial 6-month period focused on antiproteinuric and antihypertensive treatment without immunosuppression has been recommended in adults without life-threatening symptoms or worsening renal function.[522] However, in children such patients may very well have already had steroid treatment started as presumed initial management of childhood NS, which complicates the decision about the use of immunosuppression early in the disease course. Although no controlled trials have examined steroid treatment of MN in children, a report from 1966 found that steroid treatment of children with MN (80% with NS) resulted in a 50% remission rate for those with NS.[523] Importantly, children diagnosed with MN on renal biopsy have almost always been selected for having steroid-resistant NS, because the standard of care for childhood SRNS is a course of oral steroids, and no biopsy is usually performed among children with steroid-sensitive NS.

While monotherapy with either steroids or alkylating agents has been reported to be generally ineffective in adults, combination treatment with these agents has been reported to have reasonably good efficacy among both adults and children.[510,524–528] In addition, combination treatment with steroids and CNIs has also been reported to have similar or better clinical efficacy in both adults and a few pediatric studies.[466,497–501,529–533] By contrast, reported studies of the use of MMF to treat MN in adults appear not to support its use, although a small case series of MMF use in children with MN reported some benefit in proteinuria reduction.[534–537] A more recently introduced treatment for MN is adrenocorticotropic hormone, which seems in adults to have relatively similar efficacy to that of steroids combined with alkylating agents, although no data are available for children.[538–540] Another more recent treatment approach has been the use of rituximab, and the results to date suggest that its efficacy may surpass earlier treatment approaches, particularly when combined with the recent use of anti-PLA2R titers to guide therapy.[516–543]

**Table 72.11 Current Treatment Options for Children With Membranous Nephropathy**

| Immunosuppressive | Nonimmunosuppressive |
|---|---|
| Oral glucocorticoids (usually in combination with other agents) | Angiotensin-converting enzyme inhibitors |
| Alkylating agents (cyclophosphamide, chlorambucil) | Angiotensin receptor blockers |
| Calcineurin inhibitors (cyclosporine, tacrolimus) | |
| Rituximab | |
| Adrenocorticotropic hormone | |
| Mycophenolate mofetil[a] (and mizoribine) | |
| Pulse intravenous methylprednisolone[a] | |

[a]Less commonly used treatment.

In summary, while there are very few data to guide the treatment of MN specifically among children, therapy combining steroids with alkylating agents or CNIs appears to be reasonably effective, and the more recent introductions of adrenocorticotropic hormone and rituximab appear to offer the potential for somewhat improved outcomes, potentially with fewer side effects. Table 72.11 shows a summary of the current treatment options for children with MN. While conservative treatment with ACE inhibitor or ARB therapy may suffice for children with modest proteinuria, immunosuppressive treatment appears necessary to induce remission in the majority of patients. The choice of the use of immunosuppression is complicated in children by the fact that most have already been treated with oral steroids prior to the renal biopsy establishing the diagnosis of MN. Unfortunately, due to the very low incidence of MN in children, there are no randomized trials to help guide optimal therapy.

## OUTCOMES

There are few data documenting long-term outcomes in children with MN. However, reports from the North American Paediatric Renal Trials and Collaborative Studies (NAPRTCS) group and the USRDS suggest that the incidence of MN among children with CKD to be 0.5%, and that MN represents approximately 0.5% of all pediatric patients with ESRD.[544,545]

# THROMBOTIC MICROANGIOPATHY

TMA defines a spectrum of diseases, which manifest clinically with microangiopathic hemolytic anemia (MAHA), nonimmune thrombocytopenia, and organ dysfunction. Central to the development of TMA is the activation and injury of the microvascular endothelium, which result in platelet and neutrophil recruitment, thrombus formation, inflammation, thromboembolic occlusion of the dependent microvasculature, and subsequent organ failure (Fig. 72.12).[366,367,546]

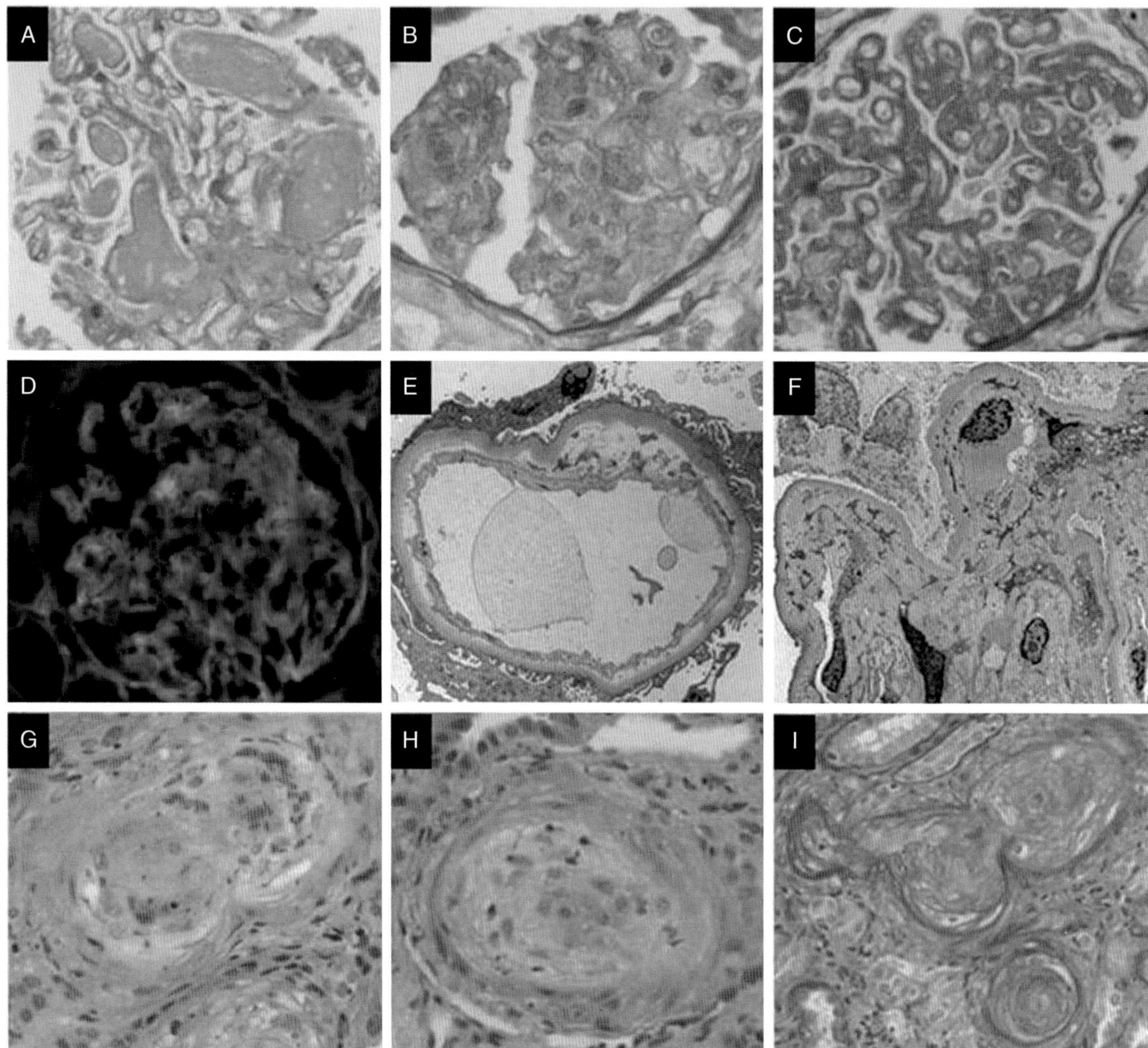


**Fig. 72.12** Histopathologic findings in thrombotic microangiopathy (TMA) within glomeruli and arterioles/small arteries in acute and chronic stages. Panels highlight the microscopic features of TMA within glomeruli by light microscopy *(top row),* immunofluorescence and electron microscopy *(middle row)* as well as light microscopic features of TMA within arterioles/small arteries *(bottom row).* Glomerular changes include (in the acute stage) (A) thrombi and/or (B) mesangiolysis and endothelial cell swelling; and (in the chronic stage) (C) capillary wall double contouring; (D) immunofluorescence microscopy shows absent staining for immunoglobulin (Ig; although some trapping can occur in the chronic stage); (E) electron microscopy shows (in the acute stage) subendothelial lucent widening, including with particulate or flocculent material, and sometimes with fibrin tactoids; and (in the chronic stage) (F) cellular interpositioning with new basement membrane formation and subendothelial expansion. Arterioles/small arteries show (in the acute stage) (G) thrombi and/or intimal fibrin and/or red cell fragments, and/or (H) intimal edema; and (in the chronic stage) (I) onion skin-type change from myointimal proliferation.

HUS defines a systemic TMA mainly targeting the kidneys but potentially also involving other organ systems such as the brain, heart, lungs, gastrointestinal tract, and skin.[366,367,546–548] HUS was initially described in 1955 by Gasser as clinical triad of hemolytic anemia, thrombocytopenia, and acute renal failure.[549] The cause of this “typical” form of HUS was unraveled in 1983 when Karmali identified Shiga toxin (ST)/Vero toxin produced by enterohemorrhagic *Escherichia coli* (EHEC) as cause of the disease (STEC or VETEC, respectively).[550–552]

Historically, HUS was defined as pathological entity strictly distinct from the clinically and pathologically almost indistinguishable thrombotic thrombocytopenic purpura (TTP).[553] TTP was first described in 1923 by Moschcowitz in a patient with acute febrile illness, anemia, petechiae, paralysis, and coma with hyaline thrombi in terminal arterioles and capillaries throughout most organs including the kidneys.[554] Subsequently, TTP was defined by the clinical pentad of fever, purpura/hemorrhage with thrombocytopenia, hemolytic anemia, neurological manifestations, and variable degrees of renal dysfunction.[555] TTP is caused by deficiency of ADAMTS13 (a disintegrin and metalloproteinase with a thrombospondin type 1 motif, member 13), a protease that cleaves von Willebrand factor (vWF) multimers upon release from endothelial cells.[555–557]

While histopathologically indistinguishable, a rare subgroup of patients presenting with familial manifestation, significantly higher rates of renal and extrarenal morbidity, and high risk of posttransplant disease recurrence was identified defining a new disease entity called aHUS.[558–560] aHUS is caused by dysregulation of the complement AP on the level of the vascular endothelium. The subsequent endothelial injury induces a sequence of inflammation and coagulation with thromboembolic events, which is shared with HUS.[561] The use of the term aHUS was later used to refer to all non-STEC-caused cases of HUS including (but not exclusively applied to) patients with recurrent disease associated with a more severe clinical course and poorer outcomes.

Today, a wide range of conditions occurring in context of an underlying disease or condition including infections, hypertension, pregnancy, transplantation, medications, and metabolic conditions are considered secondary TMA (Table 72.9).[548,562] While previously not appreciated, secondary and/or causal involvement of the complement system via underlying genetic or autoimmune susceptibility factors are now increasingly recognized to occur in patients with secondary TMA.[563,564] Thus the historical nomenclature of TMA distinguishing between HUS, aHUS, TTP, and nonrelated secondary TMAs is problematic as it emphasizes distinct differences in the individual disease pathogenesis, which today is conflicting with the increasing notion of shared pathogenetic mechanisms. These insights are critical as they have the potential to identify new therapeutic targets for these diseases which to date often poor prognosis.[369,388]

## DIAGNOSIS

The diagnosis of TMA is defined by clinical criteria including MAHA, thrombocytopenia, and renal and extrarenal disease manifestation.[563–565]

The initial assessment of a TMA patient must on one hand consider the three most likely differential diagnoses—STEC–HUS, TTP, and aHUS—and on the other hand consider the expanding spectrum of secondary TMA (Fig. 72.9; Table 72.9). Of note, while not defining, complement defects in form of mutations or anti-CFH autoantibodies can also be present in secondary TMA, or complement activation can occur transiently in the absence specific complement defects.[563–565] Although some forms of secondary TMA present undoubtedly (e.g., pregnancy-associated TMA, transplant-associated [TA] TMA, Streptococcal pneumoniae [SP] TMA) other forms will have to be actively excluded (e.g., cblC defect–associated TMA). Table 72.8 provides an overview of meaningful clinical tests relevant to the identification of diagnoses/conditions possibly underlying secondary TMA (Table 72.9).[563–565]

STEC–HUS typically follows a specific clinical sequence: diarrhea developing 2 to 12 days after ingestion of the disease causing bacteria (e.g., *E. coli* O157:H7) is initially nonbloody but becomes bloody in 90% of cases after 1 to 3 days. Microbiological identification of *E. coli* in the stool culture, detection of antilipopolysaccharide (LPS) antibodies specific for disease-causing bacteria, and ST detection in blood via polymerase chain reaction (PCR) confirm the diagnosis.[366,551,552]

TTP is typically characterized by an ADAMTS13 activity level of less than 10%. Detection of anti-ADAMTS13 autoantibodies (inhibitors) or identification of an ADAMTS13 mutation confirms the diagnosis of TTP.[553,555]

By contrast, aHUS is in the first place a diagnosis of exclusion of secondary TMA, STEC–HUS, and TTP. Global complement assays such as CH50 and AP50 allow to screen for complement and AP activation, respectively. Commercially available assays such as the Wieslab enzyme-linked immunosorbent assay (ELISA) allow for the individual assessment of the complement CP, LP, and AP.[377,566,567] The utility of in vitro/ex vivo hemolytic assays for monitoring treatment efficacy in individual patients has recently been demonstrated.[568] Similarly, the prospective eculizumab trial demonstrated full complement blockade (i.e., CH50 <20%) with the recommended treatment regimen.[569]

Additional biomarkers such as serum C3, CFB, and sC5b-9 levels have been used as surrogate markers of complement activation.[570,571] While low C3 and CFB levels indicating AP activation and complement consumption and high sC5b-9 levels indicating TP activation have been reported in aHUS patients,[572,573] C3 and sC5b-9 levels can remain normal during the acute phase of aHUS, revealing a limitation in their utility as markers to monitor disease activity and treatment efficacy.[571,574]

Diagnostic workup of patients with suspected aHUS must include genetic analysis and screening for anti-CFH autoantibodies. While in the past, genetic workup of aHUS patients consisted in Sanger sequencing of panels of target genes including the complement genes currently associated with aHUS (see earlier discussion), today genetic testing is increasingly offered via whole-exome sequencing (WES) or whole-genome sequencing (WGS), thus allowing not only for comprehensive coverage of all known complement genes but also for opening genetic testing up to include so far unknown, potentially disease-causing genes, which is of particular importance for patients without identified complement mutation. Anti-CFH autoantibodies are tested via ELISA against a positive control with international standardization efforts currently underway (Table 72.8).

As complement-mediated injury of the vascular endothelium is central to aHUS pathogenesis, biomarkers of TP activation (C5a and sC5b-9), vascular inflammation (soluble tumor necrosis factor receptor-1 [sTNFR1]), endothelial activation (soluble vascular cell adhesion molecule-1 [sVCAM1]) and damage (THBD [CD141]), coagulation (prothrombin fragment 1+2 [F1+2], D-dimer), and renal injury (clusterin, tissue inhibitor of metalloproteinases-1 [TIMP-1], liver fatty acid binding protein-1 [L-FABP-1], β2-microglobulin, cystatin-C) were assessed and found to be elevated in patients with aHUS regardless of the underlying complement defect.[575] Of note, these markers were suppressed to varying degrees in response to eculizumab therapy.[575]

Recently, an ex vivo assay determining complement activation on endothelial cells was developed to monitor disease activity and potential treatment efficacy.[571] When incubating nonactivated endothelial cells with serum of aHUS patients with active disease, endothelial C3 and C5b-9 deposition were enhanced, whereas complement deposition returned to baseline when serum of aHUS patients in remission was used. Preactivation of endothelial cells with adenosine 5′-diphosphate (ADP), however, unraveled subclinical complement activation in aHUS patients in clinical remission, as incubation of endothelial cells with their serum resulted in enhanced C3 and C5b-9 deposition. This assay became clinically useful when serum of eculizumab-treated aHUS patients was tested: serum of one patient with clinical breakthrough despite eculizumab therapy demonstrated enhanced endothelial complement deposition, which subsided upon dose increase; serum of another patient in stable remission did not result in enhanced endothelial complement deposition despite increased dosing intervals.[571]

## INFECTIOUS FORMS OF THROMBOTIC MICROANGIOPATHY

### STEC–HUS

#### PATHOGENESIS

HUS is the most common cause for childhood AKI in the Western world.[576] Infections with Shiga toxin (Stx) producing *E. coli* can cause sporadic forms of HUS or can cause regional outbreaks.[576] HUS usually affects children between the age of 2 and 10 years; however, in outbreaks adults are also affected.[577] The overall incidence of STEC–HUS is about 2/100,000, with a peak of 6.1/100,000 in children younger than 5 years of age.[578,579]

The EHEC O157:H7 serotype was worldwide the main serotype causing HUS until recently.[578] In Europe and North America, other non-O157:H7 serotypes are now found to be as frequent as O157:H7.[578] However, O157:H7 remains the predominant (>70%) serotype in Latin America, where STEC–HUS occurs up to 10 times more frequently. In 2011, a large HUS outbreak in northern Germany was linked to the consumption of raw fenugreek sprouts. The unusual *E. coli* O104:H4 strain that combined the virulence potentials of enteroaggregative *E. coli* and typical Stx-producing EHEC was the causative agent.[577,580]

The main reservoir of STEC is the intestinal tract of (healthy) cattle, raw or undercooked beef, and unpasteurized milk.[581] Cattle manure–contaminated vegetables and fruit or water are major sources of STEC infection in humans, especially in outbreaks.[578,582] Person-to-person transmission and contact with infected animals after farm or petting zoo visits have also been reported.[581,583] The production of Stx is the main virulence factor of STEC and associated with the development of HUS. HUS symptoms occur typically 6 days after the start of diarrhea.[584] Host factors are thought to contribute to the risk of developing HUS after STEC infection; however, a genetic susceptibility polymorphism has not been identified yet.[585]

EHEC is ingested and causes secretory diarrhea followed by bloody diarrhea. Injured epithelial cells allow translocation of Stx from the gut into the bloodstream. LPS developed in the gut by STEC may also enter the systemic circulation and promote an inflammatory response that contributes to renal injury. Stx and LPS are thought to bind to various blood cells in order to reach the target organs, predominantly the kidney. Stx binds to the endothelial globotriaosylceramide type 3 (Gb3) receptor, is internalized, and undergoes retrograde transport to the endoplasmic reticulum. The Stx A subunit is proteolytically processed to form a 27-kDa A1-fragment, which upon translocation to the cytosol triggers molecular damage.[582] The A1 fragment also inactivates the host ribosomes by removing a single adenosine residue from the 28*S* ribosomal RNA of the 60*S* subunit, and subsequently inhibiting protein synthesis. Furthermore, multiple stress-induced signaling pathways are activated, leading to the induction of inflammatory gene expression and apoptosis. The cumulative effect is endothelial cell activation and loss of endothelial cell function. Leukocyte adhesion is a result of upregulation of adhesion molecules on the endothelial surface. Platelet adhesion might be the result of vWF release.[586]

In vitro evidence indicates that Stx can activate complement through the AP and results in formation of soluble C5b-9 in normal human serum exposed to Stx2. Stx binds to CFH, the main complement regulator in fluid phase, which results in endothelial C3b deposition.[587] Stimulation of whole blood with Stx2 increased formation of platelet–monocyte and platelet–neutrophil complexes, and the release of blood cell–derived microparticles, with surface-bound C3 and C9.[588] Stx2 also caused the release of red blood cell–derived microvesicles coated with C5b-9, indicating that complement plays a role in the hemolytic process that occurs during STEC–HUS.[589] Patients with STEC–HUS had alternative and TP activation at disease onset, which was not observed anymore after recovery.[389]

#### CLINICAL MANIFESTATIONS

The clinical manifestation of STEC–HUS is characterized by a typical sequence of (1) ingestion of the infectious agent, (2) diarrhea, abdominal pain, fever, and vomiting, (3) bloody diarrhea, and (4) spontaneous resolution (approximately 85%) versus manifestation of HUS (approximately 15%).[551] Ninety-four percent of patients show a diarrheal prodrome, with two-thirds of them having bloody diarrhea. HUS symptoms usually appear on days 6 to 7 after EHEC ingestion. Extrarenal manifestations are possible and include CNS involvement with neurological symptoms, pancreatitis, elevated transaminases, acute respiratory distress syndrome, and cardiac involvement. The kidney is the most commonly involved organ, and dialysis is required in two-thirds of the patients, with a median treatment duration of 10 days. Mortality in the acute phase of STEC–HUS manifestation is 1% to 4% with the main reason for death being multiorgan failure. CNS involvement is reported in 30% to 40% of patients. Prognostic markers for poor clinical outcome and persistence of long-term sequelae were longer time on dialysis (median 15 days), increased leukocyte count ($>20 \times 10^9$/L), and arterial hypertension at disease onset. Interestingly, the Stx serotype has no impact on long-term outcome.[576,590] The mortality in STEC–HUS is reported as 1% to 4% in sporadic cases; however, higher mortality rates occurred in outbreaks.[581,591]

For diagnostic purposes, EHEC can be isolated from stool specimen, and the serotype can be determined by PCR or enzyme immunoassay. In addition, Ig against LPS of O157 can be detected in the serum. Infection with EHEC belonging to one of the five traditional high-risk serogroups (O157, O26, O145, O111, and O103) or Stx2-producing EHEC has been shown to be associated with a higher risk of developing HUS. Nonsorbitol-fermenting O157:H7/$H^-$ is the most common serotype (50%), but non-O157 serotypes are emerging and occur more often in patients 1 year of age.[576,590]

In patients with positive testing for EHEC, Stx, or LPS antibodies the diagnosis of STEC–HUS is confirmed and no further investigations are required. In pediatric patients with bloody diarrhea but negative EHEC, Stx, or LPS testing, STEC–HUS still remains the most likely diagnosis. In patients without bloody diarrhea and negative testing (discussed earlier) other differential diagnoses for TMA should be considered.

### TREATMENT

Supportive care is the main pillar of STEC–HUS treatment, including fluid management, treatment of arterial hypertension, RRT, and, if indicated, ventilatory support. Routine use of antibiotics is not recommended and is discouraged during the diarrheal phase often preceding the manifestation of STEC–HUS, unless secondary complications enforce such a treatment. Anticoagulants, antiplatelet drugs, plasma therapy, and steroids are of no use.[576,590,592] With more recent in vivo and in vitro data pointing toward an important role of complement in STEC–HUS pathogenesis, in 2011 three patients with STEC–HUS and severe neurological symptoms were treated with the TP inhibitor eculizumab and showed significant improvement.[593] During the 2011 STEC–HUS outbreak in Germany, eculizumab was administered in a noncontrolled trial in combination with concomitant treatments to mostly adult patients with the most severe disease course. In this instance, no clear treatment benefit was found.[594,595] Currently, there is not enough evidence to support eculizumab treatment in patients with STEC–HUS. However, individual patients with a severe disease course and signs of complement activation might benefit from complement inhibition.

Neurological sequelae are reported in 4% and proteinuria in 19% of patients after 1-year follow-up, arterial hypertension in 5% of patients after 5-years follow-up.[590] Long-term follow-up data indicate that some asymptomatic patients after 1 year will develop hypertension or proteinuria 2 to 5 years after first onset of HUS.[590] This important finding warrants yearly follow-up in all patients at least up to 5, probably up to 10 years, to monitor for proteinuria, decline in renal function, and hypertension. Patients with any sequelae need follow-up as indicated by their severity. Closer follow-up might be warranted in patients where—despite diarrhea—no EHEC or Stx was detected in stool or serum. Disease recurrence should trigger further investigations to exclude potential differential diagnoses such as aHUS and TTP (discussed later). Patients with ESRD after STEC–HUS receiving transplantation have a good long-term outcome, as no disease recurrence was reported so far.[590]

## PNEUMOCOCCAL HUS

### PATHOGENESIS

After EHEC-associated HUS, pneumococcal HUS is the most frequent form of postinfectious HUS, accounting for around 5% to 15% of all HUS cases.[366,596] TMA occurs 3 to 13 days after pneumococcal infection, with the main presenting features being pneumonia with empyema and bacteremia. Pneumococcal HUS is caused by infections with *S. pneumoniae* (SP HUS), and the most frequent serotype associated with TMA was *S. pneumoniae* 19A. *S. pneumoniae* produces neuraminidase, which cleaves N-acetyl neuraminic acid from cell surfaces and thereby exposes the so-called Thomsen–Friedenreich antigen (T-antigen) on the surface of various cell types including vascular endothelial cells and erythrocytes. Naturally occurring circulating antibodies bind the T-antigen, which results in Coombs positive hemolysis (i.e., erythrocytes), cellular injury (e.g., vascular endothelial cells), and subsequent thrombosis with the clinical picture of HUS.[366] In vitro work has also shown that neuraminidase causes desialylation, thus reducing the binding of complement regulator CFH to the endothelial surface.[597] Of note, investigation of the AP in patients with pneumococcal HUS (SP HUS) revealed mutations in complement regulators in three of five patients in one recent study.[366]

### CLINICAL MANIFESTATIONS

The overall mortality rate of SP HUS is 2% to 12%; in patients who present with meningitis, mortality rates are as high as 37%. Dialysis was needed in 50% of the patients. Extrarenal manifestations occur. ESRD occurred in 10% to 16% of patients; proteinuria and hypertension persisted in others. No disease recurrence has been reported.

### TREATMENT

Treatment of patients with pneumococcal HUS (SP HUS) includes infection-specific treatment (e.g., antibiotics, antiviral drugs) and supportive care (e.g., RRT, ventilatory support). PLEX was used in a proportion of patients and considered as beneficial. The use of complement-targeted treatment strategies such as commencing eculizumab in pneumococcal HUS (SP HUS) has not been reported, yet. However, the capacity of bacteria and viruses to enhance complement activation and induce endothelial damage, and the impaired endothelial surface binding of complement regulator CFH due to *S. pneumoniae*-induced change in the endothelial glycocalyx (discussed earlier) suggest enhanced complement activation on endothelial cell surfaces, and thus provide a rationale for the use of complement-targeted treatment strategies in patients with pneumococcal HUS (SP HUS). Immunization with the Prevnar 13 vaccine covers most of the serotypes associated with pneumococcal HUS (SP HUS), and is recommended in patients on eculizumab treatment (TP blockade), and after splenectomy.[598,599]

## NONINFECTIOUS, NONCOMPLEMENT-MEDIATED FORMS OF THROMBOTIC MICROANGIOPATHY

Over the past 20 years, extensive genetic screening has identified the underlying genetic cause in about 50% of patients with TMA. In recent years, new techniques such as WES and WGS have allowed for a broader approach to genetic screening, and several mutations in genes not associated with the complement system were discovered in patients and families with aHUS/TMA. Although their prevalence is low, genetic testing applying next-generation sequencing should be considered in patients without complement alterations, being nonresponsive to complement-targeted therapy, and in patients presenting with specific clinical characteristics. Identification of the underlying genetic defect will guide treatment decisions and inform discussions about inheritability, long-term outcome, transplantation, and posttransplant recurrence risk.

## DIACYLGLYCEROL KINASE EPSILON THROMBOTIC MICROANGIOPATHY

### PATHOGENESIS

Recently, a subgroup of aHUS patients was identified, which was characterized by the manifestation of MAHA, thrombocytopenia, and acute renal failure during the first year of life. The further disease course was typically complicated by (nephrotic range) proteinuria, and the progression to ESRD during the second or third decade of life. Of note, treatment response to complement-targeted treatments (i.e., plasma; eculizumab) was incomplete, and disease recurrences occurred despite ongoing treatment.[600] While testing of complement mutations and anti-CFH autoantibodies was negative, WES identified homozygous and compound heterozygous mutations in the gene encoding for diacylglycerol kinase epsilon (*DGKE*).[600] Subsequently, the prevalence of *DGKE* mutations among aHUS patients was determined as 2% to 3%.[601]

DGKE is an intracellular lipid kinase that phosphorylates diacylglycerol to phosphatidic acid, securing recycling of phosphatidylinositol, an important second messenger in membrane signaling.[602] So far, 44 patients with a DGKE mutation (homozygous or compound heterozygous) have been reported, 35 of whom presented with the clinical picture of TMA, 9 with an MPGN-like picture. Additional complement mutations were only observed in three patients, although biochemical evidence for mild complement activation was detected in about 25% of patients. How *DGKE* mutations render the vascular endothelium to be more procoagulant and facilitate thrombus formation in particular in the small capillaries of the kidney is still unclear.[601] However, it has been shown that endothelial cells lacking DGKE show increased platelet binding capacity, impaired angiogenic response, and increased cell death.[603]

### CLINICAL MANIFESTATIONS

As mentioned earlier, most TMA patients diagnosed with a *DGKE* mutation had a disease onset within the first year of life. Proteinuria, in most patients within nephrotic range, was a hallmark feature in the acute phase. Dialysis was needed in about 75% of patients. Disease recurrence was observed in 70% of patients. Distinctive for DGKE TMA, in 80% of patients proteinuria (up to nephrotic range in 24%) persisted beyond resolution of acute TMA. Of note, 88% of patients also showed persistent hematuria during follow-up. Progression to ESRD occurred in seven of 35 patients, with a median age of 11 years. Ten-year renal survival was reported as 89%.[601]

Nine patients with an MPGN-like picture on renal biopsy had a slightly later disease onset (median 2 years of age) with continuous nephrotic-range proteinuria in most of them. No TMA features were reported during follow-up. Three patients progressed to ESRD at a median age of 19 years.[601]

### TREATMENT

The optimal treatment for DGKE TMA is unclear. Retrospectively collected data indicate spontaneous recovery in most patients without specific therapy (plasma or eculizumab for TMA, immunosuppression for MPGN). TMA recurrence was recorded while on eculizumab. As of now, patients with DGKE mutations will likely not benefit from either complement-targeted therapy (i.e., plasma and eculizumab) or immunosuppression. Renal transplantation is a safe option, as there is no risk of posttransplant recurrence.[601]

## COBALAMIN C–ASSOCIATED THROMBOTIC MICROANGIOPATHY

### PATHOGENESIS

Cobalamin C (CblC) deficiency is the most commonly inherited error of vitamin $B_{12}$ metabolism. CblC deficiency is characterized by multisystem involvement with severe neurological, hematological, renal, and cardiopulmonary manifestations.[604,605] Mutations in the gene encoding for the methylmalonic aciduria and homocystinuria type C protein (MMACHC) are responsible for the most severe CblC disorder, which is characterized by methylmalonic academia (MMA) and hyperhomocysteinemia and can be associated with TMA.[606] Reports of CblC-associated TMA include patients with early (<4 years of age) and late-onset CblC disease, including two adults.[606–608] CblC deficiency causes hyperhomocysteinemia, which induces platelet aggregation and a procoagulant phenotype of the vascular endothelium, and is therefore thought to be the main contributor to the pathogenesis of CblC deficiency–associated TMA.[606]

### CLINICAL MANIFESTATIONS

Infantile onset of CblC disease is associated with poor outcome and has a mortality rate of 30%. CblC-associated TMA increases the mortality rate to 56%.[606] Involvement of the lungs, the need for dialysis, and very early disease onset are negative prognostic markers.[605] The classical presentation of MMA with hyperhomocysteinemia, metabolic acidosis, hyperammonemia, and encephalopathy may not always be present, especially in patients with late onset of disease.[606,609] Furthermore, despite extended newborn screening, CblC deficiency might be missed[606] and therefore a high index of suspicion needs to be maintained. In patients with late-onset CblC-associated TMA, proteinuria and/or hematuria occasionally accompanied by renal failure might be the only symptom, and diagnosis has to be made via renal biopsy. Clinical overlap with C3G has also been reported.[366]

A recent case report highlighted the diagnostic challenge of CblC-deficiency TMA[604]: A 20-year-old female patient with CKD/ESRD developed severe pulmonary arterial hypertension (PAH). Ten years before, she had first presented with acute renal failure accompanied by malignant hypertension. Renal biopsy showed TMA, and—in light of decreased ADAMTS13 activity levels and after exclusion of other etiologies—a diagnosis of TTP was established. Despite chronic plasma treatment, renal function deteriorated progressively to CKD/ESRD. When presenting with PAH, CblC deficiency was—among other differential diagnoses—considered and supported by significantly elevated homocysteine and MMA levels. Genetic analysis confirmed the diagnosis via detection of two heterozygous pathogenic MMAACHC mutations. Treatment with hydroxocobalamin, betaine, folic acid, and carnitine resulted in dramatic improvements with resolution of PAH and improvement of renal function to a level allowing for discontinuation of dialysis.[604]

As highlighted by this case, timely diagnosis and initiation of specific treatment are crucial to prevent disease manifestation or slow down disease progression. Thus urine organic acids, serum MMA levels, total plasma homocysteine levels, plasma amino acid profile, and an acylcarnitine profile should be performed in all (pediatric and adult) patients with pulmonary hypertension or TMA with unclear etiology.[366] By contrast, complement mutations were described in several patients with CblC deficiency and TMA. Therefore genetic complement testing is also warranted in CblC-deficiency patients. The detection of an additional complement defect would alter the therapeutic approach and have a significant impact on risk assessment for renal transplantation and peritransplant patient management.[366]

### TREATMENT

Treatment of patients with CblC deficiency includes systemic administration of hydroxocobalamin, folinic acid, betaine, and carnitine.[606] Complement-targeted treatment was reported to be nonbeneficial, except for patients with an additional complement abnormality.[366]

## INF2-MEDIATED THROMBOTIC MICROANGIOPATHY

Atypical HUS and posttransplant TMA were recently also reported in two families with INF2 mutations and common aHUS risk haplotypes. INF2 is a ubiquitously expressed formin protein which accelerates actin polymerization and depolymerization, thus regulating a range of cytoskeleton-dependent cellular functions including the secretory pathway.[578,610] Mutations in INF2 are the commonest cause of familial autosomal dominant NS. In a minority of these cases the mutations cause FSGS associated with the demyelinating peripheral neuropathy Charcot–Marie–Tooth (CMT). One family with TMA was also affected with CMT. Of note, patients with INF2-induced TMA do not benefit from complement-targeted therapy including plasma and eculizumab.[610]

# NONINFECTIOUS, COMPLEMENT-MEDIATED THROMBOTIC MICROANGIOPATHY

## ATYPICAL HUS

### PATHOGENESIS

The complement system (Fig. 72.8), in particular its AP, plays a critical role in the pathogenesis of aHUS. Different from IC-MPGN/C3G, where complement dysregulation mainly occurs in the fluid phase, complement dysregulation in aHUS occurs on the surface of microvascular endothelial cells and results in their activation and injury with initiation of a cascade of proinflammatory and procoagulatory events shared by all forms of HUS together with closing an amplification loop of injury to the microvasculature (Fig. 72.8).[579–581,611–613]

The constitutively active AP has the potential to cover cell surfaces with significant amounts of covalently bound C3b within seconds to minutes. Host cells, such as the vascular endothelial cells, require tight complement regulation to protect them from attack by uncontrolled complement activation and to limit complement activation to when and where needed. Complement regulation is provided by a combination of fluid-phase and membrane-bound regulators (Fig. 72.8). In principle, these regulators interfere with the progression of the complement cascade on the level of C3b activation or AP C3 convertase (C3bBb) activity. CFH is the principal fluid-phase regulator, which acts in three different ways: (1) as a cofactor for the serine protease complement factor I (CFI) in cleaving C3b to inactive C3b (iC3b), (2) by promoting disintegration (decay) and thus inactivation of the AP C3 convertase (C3bBb), and (3) by competitively preventing C3b deposition on cell surfaces.[614–617] By contrast, membrane-bound regulators include CR1 (CD35), MCP (CD46), and THBD (CD141), which serve like CFH as cofactors for CFI in C3b cleavage. DAF (CD55) facilitates the disintegration of both the AP C3 (C3bBb) and C5 (C3bBbC3b) convertases. Finally, CD59 interfering with the assembly of the MAC serves as last line of defense in the complement activation cascade.[360,618–620]

Tight regulation of complement is critical to maintain the integrity of the vascular endothelium. Loss of complement control, by contrast, results in activation and injury of the endothelial cells and induces the TMA phenotype. Complement dysregulation can be due to loss-of-function mutations and/or autoantibodies impairing the function of complement regulators, or gain-of-function mutations enhancing the level of activity of complement activators.[547,548,561] Beginning in 1998 with the seminal publication of a CFH mutation explaining for a familial case of HUS,[560] numerous reports on individual patients and registry-enrolled patient cohorts—most recently reporting on 851 patients enrolled in the global aHUS registry[621]—have identified mutations in additional complement regulators such as MCP (CD46),[622] complement factor I (CFI),[623] THBD (CD141),[624] and in complement activators such as CFB[625] and complement C3.[428,626]

Most insights in aHUS pathogenesis have been gained from the identification of complement mutations or anti-CFH autoantibodies in aHUS patients and subsequent studies unraveling their functional relevance in vitro. In-depth investigations of the aberrant functions of normal and mutant CFH[627,628] and of the nature and function of anti-CFH autoantibodies[629,630] have likely advanced our understanding of the principles of aHUS pathogenesis the most.[370] CFH is an abundant (about 200–300 μg/mL), mainly liver-made 155-kD protein composed of 20 SCRs; SCRs 1–4 (N terminus) govern the cofactor activity of CFH, and SCRs 19–20 (C terminus) govern the binding activity of CFH to C3b and to negatively charged glycosaminoglycans, phospholipids, and sialic acid residues of the plasma membrane of the vascular endothelial cells.[627–631] While IC-MPGN/C3G/CFH mutations typically impair CFH cofactor activity via mutations (e.g., affecting the CFH N terminus),[427] the vast majority of aHUS causing mutations affects the CFH C terminus, thus impairing CFH surface binding. Utilizing CFH mutant in SCR20 (truncation) purified from an aHUS patient, it was demonstrated in a seminal sequence of experiments that CFH cofactor activity was maintained in fluid phase but absent on the surface of endothelial cells, which was due to the lack of C-terminal binding of CFH to the endothelial cells.[632,633] Similarly, anti-CFH autoantibodies detected in aHUS patients exclusively recognize epitopes in the CFH C terminus, thus impairing CFH cofactor activity on surfaces via impaired binding—a scenario mimicking the presence of a C-terminal CFH mutation.[629,630,634]

Mutations in complement activators or regulators have been found in 50% to 70%, and anti-CFH autoantibodies in 10% to 20% of patients.[415,561,574,635–639] In patients with recurrent TMA postrenal transplantation complement mutations were found in up to 68% of cases[640]; in patients with a de novo TMA postrenal transplantation complement mutations were found in 29% of cases.[641]

In aHUS patients, complement mutations have also been described as combinations of two or even three defects.[621,642–646] In a US cohort, 12% of patients had mutations in more than one gene,[636] and in a Dutch (pediatric) cohort 9% of patients carried combined mutations.[645] In addition, genetic haplotypes and SNPs in complement genes have been identified in aHUS patients and may act as disease-susceptibility factors.[623] These variations can be additive,[647] and a single SNP—for example, in MCP (CD46)—is unlikely to be sufficient to cause disease.[648] Recent evidence has shown that the combination of complement gene risk haplotypes can increase disease penetrance.[637]

Complement mutations or autoantibodies have also been found in patients with secondary TMA (discussed later) in the context of hematopoietic stem cell transplantation (HSCT),[649,650] pregnancy,[651] CblC deficiency,[652] malignant hypertension,[653] exposure to certain medications,[654,655] and refractory antibody-mediated rejection (AMR).[656]

## CLINICAL MANIFESTATIONS

aHUS is an ultra-rare disease with an incidence of about 0.5 pmp. aHUS affects patients in both the pediatric and the adult age group.[643,657] Data from the global aHUS registry demonstrate a female predominance of disease manifestation from about 30 years of age onward while disease manifestation in the younger age group is dominated by males (median age at disease manifestation 10.0 years in males vs. 25.6 years in females). This biphasic pattern found in females might reflect the enhanced risk for aHUS manifestation caused by pregnancy.[621] While age at disease manifestation was independent of any identified underlying complement abnormality, analysis of individual complement defects identified specific patterns: patients with CFI mutations typically presented during adulthood, whereas patients with MCP/CD46 mutations typically presented during childhood. Within the pediatric cohort, patients with anti-CFH autoantibodies presented at a significantly older age than patients with other complement abnormalities (median age 6.4 years). Of note, between 6 and 17 years, anti-CFH autoantibodies were the most frequent cause for aHUS.[621]

As demonstrated previously,[643,657] ESRD-free survival of aHUS patients was poor, and renal outcome was impacted by the underlying complement defect: patients with CFH mutations showed poorer and patients with MCP (CD46) mutations more favorable outcomes with longer ESRD-free survival compared with individuals who tested negative for mutations in these genes. Also relatively benign were anti-CFH autoantibodies with outcomes in antibody-positive patients being only marginally inferior as compared with antibody-negative patients.[648] Renal outcome was also dependent on age at first manifestation of disease with pediatric onset of aHUS providing a significant advantage with respect to decline in kidney function.[621]

aHUS causing mutations and autoantibodies are characterized by variable/incomplete penetrance. Incomplete penetrance has been described for mutations in genes encoding for MCP (CD46)[630] and other genetic and autoimmune forms of aHUS.[643,658,659] Following a current concept, genetic and autoimmune defects present a specific but variable susceptibility risk, which combines with epigenetic and/or environmental factors to possibly cross the threshold of disease manifestation (multiple-hit hypothesis).[366] While epigenetic factors other than the aforementioned risk haplotypes are to date widely unknown, a number of "environmental" factors triggering first manifestation or disease recurrence of aHUS have been recognized: among known events preceding the onset of aHUS are respiratory and gastrointestinal tract infections[637,660] and pregnancy.[651] Posttransplant recurrence of TMA is associated with ischemia-reperfusion injury, immunosuppressive medications, and AMR.[661–663]

## TREATMENT

Treatment of aHUS includes supportive care (RRT, antihypertensive medications, fluid and electrolyte management), plasma therapy (PI, PLEX), and more specific complement-targeted therapy (anti-C5 antibody eculizumab).[563,565,664] Treatment of aHUS caused by anti-CFH autoantibodies (DEAP-HUS: deficiency of CFH-related proteins and anti-CFH autoantibody-positive HUS)[627] includes, besides eculizumab, also PLEX and immunosuppression (i.e., steroids, cyclophosphamide, MMF, rituximab, and combinations thereof).[563,565,639,665,666] Prior to the advent of eculizumab, plasma therapy was the mainstay of treatment for aHUS. However, treatment efficacy was limited (about 50%), and risk of progression to ESRD was high (about 50%).[410,561,643,657]

The advent of eculizumab marked a paradigm shift in the treatment of aHUS patients. Eculizumab is a humanized, monoclonal anti-C5 antibody, which specifically binds complement C5 and prevents its cleavage into the potent anaphylatoxin C5a, and C5b, which initiates the TP with the formation of the MAC, C5b-9.[485] While first successfully used in the treatment of PNH,[667,668] eculizumab has subsequently been commenced in pediatric and adult cases of acute and chronic aHUS, and proven highly efficient in blocking complement activation, reversing acute TMA, and preventing TMA progression and recurrence. Eculizumab was also effective in preventing disease recurrence postrenal transplantation.[669,670] Clinical trials suggest that eculizumab treatment not only results in recovery of renal function in acute TMA, but also could lead to some recovery of renal function even in chronic TMA, potentially allowing for discontinuation of dialysis.[599,671,672] Of note, success of eculizumab treatment was independent of the identification of an underlying genetic or autoimmune complement defect.[599,671,672]

The current recommended eculizumab treatment regimen consists of an induction followed by a maintenance phase. Eculizumab dosing and treatment intervals vary based on patient age and body weight, respectively. For adult aHUS patients a 4-week induction phase with weekly eculizumab doses is followed by a (timely nonlimited) maintenance phase with eculizumab doses administered every second week.[599] Of note, this treatment schedule applies regardless of an identified genetic defect. In patients with anti-CFH autoantibody-mediated aHUS, however, treatment options and recommendations are different and include (1) eculizumab monotherapy,[599,666] (2) immunosuppression via PLEX, steroids, cyclophosphamide, MMF, rituximab, or various combinations thereof,[639] and (3) a combination therapy with eculizumab and immunosuppression.[563,665] The overarching treatment principle is based on the appreciation of the autoimmune character of the disease identifying anti-CFH autoantibodies as treatment target and monitoring tool. A recent Kidney Disease Improving Global Outcomes (KDIGO) consensus conference has proposed a stepwise approach to the treatment of DEAP HUS including (1) eculizumab for the acute phase, (2) subsequent introduction of PLEX and/or immunosuppressants to remove circulating and prevent formation of new autoantibodies, and (3) discontinuation of eculizumab upon suppression of the autoantibody titer below the detection threshold.[563,665]

Eculizumab treatment is typically well tolerated with side effects being rare and mild.[599,671,672] In a small case series, liver enzyme elevation was observed resulting from eculizumab treatment—a complication, which was typically transient and on liver biopsy did not correlate with specific pathology.[673] As eculizumab-treated patients are vulnerable for infections by gram-negative encapsulated bacteria such as *Neisseria meningitides*, meningococcal vaccination is strictly required before eculizumab treatment can be safely commenced. Recently, additional chronic antibiotic prophylaxis with penicillin has been recommended to complete protection from infection with gram-negative bacteria.[599,652,674]

An international consensus has been achieved with respect to commencing complement-targeted treatment such as eculizumab in adult patients with confirmed diagnosis of aHUS in pediatric patients with suspected diagnosis of aHUS. Treatment recurrence in all confirmed cases of aHUS, and treatment of patients with a renal transplant at the time of transplantation or of aHUS recurrence as first-line treatment. However, the question of treatment duration has not yet been answered, and criteria for the safe discontinuation of eculizumab are lacking.[563,565] While successful discontinuation of eculizumab treatment has been reported in individual cases and small case series with urine testing for hematuria as reliable monitoring strategy,[675] recently the risk for aHUS recurrence after discontinuation of eculizumab varied depending on the type of the underlying genotype with MCP/CD46 versus CFH mutations spanning the risk spectrum of low versus high risk level, respectively.[547] Recent efforts aimed at defining reliable and practical biomarkers of aHUS disease activity and tests allowing for the monitoring of treatment efficacy (discussed earlier).[571,575]

## SECONDARY FORMS OF THROMBOTIC MICROANGIOPATHY WITH POSSIBLE COMPLEMENT CONTRIBUTION

### TRANSPLANT-ASSOCIATED THROMBOTIC MICROANGIOPATHY

TA-TMA can occur as de novo disease, disease recurrence, or in context of antibody-mediated recurrence.[640,641,676] Diagnostic approach and investigations are similar to the ones discussed for aHUS earlier. As complement dysregulation is central to most of these cases, complement-targeted treatment is the first choice. Weaning or treatment withdrawal needs to be carefully considered and should be guided by the evaluation of genetic findings and prior clinical presentation.

### RECURRENT ATYPICAL HUS AFTER RENAL TRANSPLANTATION

After renal transplantation, the risk of aHUS recurrence is high and graft survival is poor. A recent study in 57 aHUS patients, who received a kidney transplant, highlights that TMA recurrence occurred during the early posttransplant course with a cumulative incidence of 43% (19/44) at 1 month, and 70% (31/44) at 1 year.[640] The type of complement mutation predicted the recurrence risk, and patients with complement mutations and low C3 had the highest risk of graft loss. The risk of recurrence was high in patients carrying CFH and gain-of-function (i.e., C3 or CFB) mutations, intermediate in patients carrying CFI mutations or homozygous at-risk CFH polymorphisms, and low in patients without identified mutations.[640] Several patients with low-titer CFH antibodies were successfully transplanted without aHUS recurrence.[415] Despite evidence of endothelial toxicity of CNIs in vitro, CNI immunosuppressive treatment was not associated with a higher risk of recurrence in these patients.[677] Thus currently there is no evidence supporting the discontinuation of CNI treatment in patients with posttransplant aHUS recurrence.

Renal transplantation in patients with aHUS needs to be carefully considered, and CFH antibody screening and complement genetic testing should be performed prior to transplantation. Recently, prophylactic treatment with complement-targeted treatment has improved patient outcome and enabled transplantation in high-risk patients. Eculizumab should be considered as first-line (prophylactic) treatment in patients with high recurrence risk.[678] In case of recurrence, eculizumab is the preferred choice and should be administrated as soon as possible after a diagnosis of aHUS recurrence has been established.[679] Except for one patient who lost the graft to an arterial thrombosis on day 1 after transplantation, eculizumab treatment was successful in 13 patients treated prophylactically, and in 17 in whom treatment was initiated after recurrence.[670,679] Although patients with recurrence after transplantation showed good response, prophylactic treatment with eculizumab should be considered especially in high-risk patients.

### DE NOVO THROMBOTIC MICROANGIOPATHY AFTER RENAL TRANSPLANTATION

De novo TMA occurred in 4% to 15% of patients treated with cyclosporine, and 1% treated with tacrolimus after renal transplantation, and resulted in graft loss in one-third of the patients.[366] While not contributing to TMA recurrence, CNIs have a stand-alone role in de novo TMA after transplantation. In addition, complement mutations (i.e., CFH and CFI) were detected in 29% of patients with de novo TMA after transplantation.[641] This phenomenon remains one of the least understood of the CNI-related toxicities. CNI toxicity occurs primarily via its effects on the vascular endothelium.[645] CNIs are known to cause endothelial cell injury[680,681] related to cell mitochondrial dysfunction and reactive oxygen species formation.[682] Cyclosporine exposure also induces endothelial microparticle formation, leading to the activation of the AP.[677]

A consensus on treatment of de novo TMA after kidney transplantation does not exist. (Temporary) withdrawal of CNIs has been applied frequently.[683,684] A CNI-free, sirolimus-based immunosuppressive regimen was administered to 14 patients with aHUS or de novo TMA after transplantation. Treatment showed long-term success in 13/14 patients, but acute rejection was reported in 53% of patients.[711] Sirolimus treatment has recently also been associated with posttransplant TMA and CNI-free immunosuppressive regimens are not recommended.[366,679] Given the high rate of complement alterations in patients with de novo TMA after kidney transplantation, complement-targeted therapy is a reasonable option. Eculizumab treatment was reported in four patients with de novo TMA after combined lung–kidney or pancreas–kidney transplantation, or ABO-incompatible kidney transplantation. Administration of eculizumab led to a prompt hematologic and renal recovery.[366]

## AMR-ASSOCIATED THROMBOTIC MICROANGIOPATHY

TMA was reported in 4% to 46% of patients with AMR and was associated with increased risk for graft loss.[685] Donor-specific antibodies have the potential to activate the complement system on the endothelium via the CP, the proposed mechanism of acute AMR, and facilitate chronic inflammatory processes, the proposed mechanism in chronic AMR.[686] Anaphylatoxins promote infiltration of inflammatory cells. In addition, C5b-9 might directly injure the allograft.[686] The ability of donor-specific human leukocyte antigen antibodies to bind C1q, and initiate the CP, was recently linked to an increased risk for AMR and graft loss.[687] In one reported patient, AMR was accompanied by severe TMA on the background of a homozygous CFHR3-CFHR1 deficiency.[656]

To date, there is no definitive treatment for AMR, irrespective of the finding of TMA on biopsy. Prophylactic eculizumab treatment in 26 highly sensitized kidney transplant recipients reduced the incidence of AMR from 41% to 8%.[688] In the same study, biopsies taken 1 year after transplantation were comparable between groups, and did not prevent chronic rejection in patients with a positive cross-match and high antibody titers. Several cases of successful treatment of AMR with eculizumab were reported.[366] On the contrary, nonresponders to eculizumab were also published in the literature.[689,690]

## BONE MARROW/STEM CELL TRANSPLANT–ASSOCIATED THROMBOTIC MICROANGIOPATHY

TMA following allogeneic and autologous transplantation is estimated to occur in 0.5% to 15% and 0.1% to 0.25% of cases, respectively.[691] TMA after bone marrow transplantation (BMT)/HSCT is associated with a high mortality. Diagnosing TMA in the setting of BMT/HSCT is challenging, as thrombocytopenia, renal insufficiency, and the presence of schistocytes may also represent other complications, such as graft versus host disease (GvHD) and systemic infections.[692] It has been noted that lactate dehydrogenase, proteinuria, and hypertension are the first signs for TMA in this patient cohort, and a diagnostic risk score has been published recently.[649] Schistocytes may be absent in patients with TMA.[650]

Endothelial cell injury, induced by chemotherapy and other drugs such as cyclosporine, a general prothrombotic state, and additional risk factors such as intravenous catheters, infections, and GvHD may well contribute to TMA pathogenesis.[692] Endothelial cell regeneration is limited, as bone marrow endothelial progenitor cell populations, the source for endothelial cell repair, are depleted by conditioning treatments.[692]

Complement alterations were discovered in variants in 65% of HSCT recipients with TMA as compared with only 9% in those without TMA, including CFH antibodies and/or a heterozygous CFHR3-CFHR1 deletion and mutation in regulators. Complement alterations were associated with increased disease severity and mortality.[650] TMA after BMT or SCT might be multifactorial and requires the combination of genetic susceptibility as well as secondary endothelial cell activation.[366,650] Complement activation markers such as sC5b-9 were elevated in 70% of HSCT patients with TMA. Elevated blood sC5b-9 levels in conjunction with proteinuria are associated with the most severe TMA phenotype after HSCT, resulting in unfavorable outcomes if not treated.[649]

The optimal management of BMT/HSCT-related TMA has not been established yet. Treatment can be supportive or targeting the underlying condition. CNIs and sirolimus are discussed in the literature as important factors for endothelial injury.[650,692] Clinical decision for temporary discontinuation must balance the subsequent increased risk for GvHD and should only be considered in patients with severe kidney injury and/or severe hypertension. In patients with high risk for GvHD and well-controlled hypertension and kidney function no change in immunosuppressive regimen is needed.[650]

Historical data from two reviews involving 260 patients suggest a median response rate to plasma exchange (PE) to range from 37% to 55%, and a mortality rate of approximately 80% to 100%.[692] Prolonged time to resolution of TMA was associated with nonsurvival.[693] Other reported treatment options included rituximab, defibrotide, and intravenous Ig with variable success.[366] Recently, with the evolving role of complement, eculizumab has been used in several case reports and one single-center prospective study including 30 patients. The latter included patients with proteinuria, activated terminal complement, and multiorgan impairment. One-year survival was reported as 62% compared with 9% in patients with TMA not receiving eculizumab treatment. Patients received a median of 14 doses and were safely discontinued after resolution of the disease. Of note, these patients have a variable eculizumab clearance and need personalized drug dosing based on pharmacokinetics and treatment effect (i.e., CH50 suppression). Early treatment initiation was crucial for outcome. In the same study, patients with only hematologic signs of microangiopathy without proteinuria or elevated sC5b-9 fully recovered from TA-TMA without treatment.[649,650]

## GLOMERULOPATHY AND VASCULITIS-ASSOCIATED THROMBOTIC MICROANGIOPATHY

TMA was reported in patients with SLE, ANCA vasculitis, APS, IgAN, MN, and IC-MPGN/C3G. Only a handful of patients are reported, and in-depth genetic testing was not performed in the majority. Treatment strategies include various immunosuppressive protocols and symptomatic therapy, for example, of hypertension and impaired renal function.

## SLE-ASSOCIATED THROMBOTIC MICROANGIOPATHY

The prevalence of SLE-associated TMA is estimated as 1% to 4% with a higher prevalence in patients with renal involvement.[694,695] TMA lesions in renal biopsies of SLE patients were detected in 24%, 80% of whom were lacking the clinical diagnosis of TM.[696] Outcome (mortality rate 34%–52%) and treatment response were worse in patients with lupus nephritis and renal TM.[695,696] Infections were a major trigger of SLE-associated TMA and predicted poor outcome.[697]

Complement activation is a hallmark feature in both SLE with activation of the CP and aHUS activation of AP. In a large case–control study of 15,864 SLE patients, an association of CFHR1/CFHR3 deletions and SLE was established. Of note, different from DEAP HUS, these patients were anti-CFH autoantibody negative.[698] However, in a Swedish cohort anti-CFH autoantibodies were identified in 6.7% of patients with SLE.[697,699] Successful single case reports exist for the use of PLEX as well as eculizumab in patients with a syndrome combining TMA and SLE.

## APS-ASSOCIATED THROMBOTIC MICROANGIOPATHY

APS or life-threatening catastrophic APS is an autoimmune disease characterized by arterial and venous thrombi due to autoantibodies directed against phospholipids.[700] APS nephropathy is common (71% of cases), histopathologically often presenting as TMA.[701] APS is associated with post-transplant recurrence, presenting as TMA especially in the early posttransplant phase. Of note, antiphospholipid antibodies lead to complement activation via the CP.

In biopsies of three patients with APS nephropathy that developed TMA after renal transplantation, intense C4d and C5b-9 staining on endothelial cells of injured vessels was detected.[702] In these patients, eculizumab treatment was commenced after failing PLEX and was successful in reversing clinical and histopathological findings of TMA. Despite terminal complement inhibition, C5b-9 deposition remained persistent over several months, and chronic vascular changes could not be prevented.[702]

## IC-MPGN/C3G-ASSOCIATED THROMBOTIC MICROANGIOPATHY

Similar to aHUS, C3G is associated with AP activating (gain-of-function) and regulating (loss-of-function) mutations and—more frequently—with autoantibodies stabilizing the AP convertase C3bBb.[380] However, aHUS and C3G not only overlap pathogenetically, but also phenotypically, which became evident when patients previously diagnosed with aHUS developed C3G or vice versa, or when different individuals of one family carrying the same complement mutation developed either aHUS or C3G.[366] More recently, complement mutations and/or autoantibodies (i.e., C3NeF) were also detected in IC-MPGN patients.[437] Thus despite limited literature, there is a role for complement-targeted therapy in patients with IC-MPGN/C3G, especially with underlying complement alterations and TP activation.[487]

## ANCA-ASSOCIATED VASCULITIS-ASSOCIATED THROMBOTIC MICROANGIOPATHY

TMA was also detected in 15% of patients with ANCA-associated vasculitis (AAV), which was associated with a negative outcome.[437] In AAV, endothelial cell activation and injury are induced by activated neutrophils and subsequent complement activation, which might result in TMA.[703]

Treatment for AAV includes immunosuppressive and antiinflammatory medications coupled with antibody depleting agents such as PLEX and rituximab. Unraveling the role of complement in AAV pathogenesis has led to the investigation of complement-targeted therapies, and C5a receptor (C5aR) blockage has shown to ameliorate the disease.[432,704]

## MALIGNANT HYPERTENSION–ASSOCIATED THROMBOTIC MICROANGIOPATHY

Established nomenclature suggests a disease sequence beginning with (malignant) hypertension leading to TMA. Accumulating evidence in individual cases, however, today provides a rationale for the reversal of this concept with TMA being the initiating culprit, and being a secondary phenomenon arising secondary to microthrombus formation. In patients presenting with malignant hypertension and TMA, diagnostic and treatment algorithms should be followed as detailed for aHUS (Table 72.8). Hypertension causes endothelial cell dysfunction, platelet activation, and increased thrombin, thus generating a prothrombotic milieu.[705] While blood pressure normalization remains the main goal both in the acute and in the chronic phase, additional complement-targeted therapy was reported in some patients.[366]

## DRUG-ASSOCIATED THROMBOTIC MICROANGIOPATHY

An association of drugs and TMA was found in 13% of patients,[706] and was mainly described in patients treated with CNIs (discussed earlier), and with mammalian target of rapamycin inhibitors (e.g., sirolimus).[707] Other drugs associated with TMA include quinine, chemotherapeutic agents, vascular endothelial growth factor (VEGF) inhibitors, antiplatelet agents, and cocaine.[708–712] ADAMTS13 mutations or anti-ADAMTS13 autoantibodies are prominent in the TMA associated with the antiplatelet agent ticlopidine.[708]

Mechanisms leading to drug-induced TMA include direct injury of the endothelium, vasoconstriction, impaired vasodilatation, procoagulant activity, and antiplatelet activity.[710,711] A genetic susceptibility might exist in some patients.[366] The association of TMA and VEGF inhibitors, such as bevacizumab, suggests VEGF as a critical player for glomerular endothelial cell integrity.[713]

Treatment of drug-associated TMA includes—as far as possible—the removal of the disease-inducing agent, and complement-targeted therapy in patients with underlying complement alterations.[366]

# THROMBOTIC THROMBOCYTOPENIC PURPURA

## PATHOGENESIS

The TMA TTP must be distinguished from (a)HUS. Like (a) HUS, TTP is a potentially life-threatening thromboembolic disorder of the microvasculature, which is characterized by organ ischemia in particular of the brain, but also the heart, the gastrointestinal tract, and the kidneys, as well as thrombocytopenia (<30 × $10^9$/L) and the appearance of fragmented red blood cells on blood film.[553–555] TTP was first described in 1924 by Moschcowitz;[714] however, its pathogenesis was only unraveled in 1982 by Moake who detected a defect in the processing of vWF in cases of chronic relapsing TTP.[715] Subsequently, impaired vWF cleavage was attributed to a functional deficiency in ADAMTS13 (a disintegrin and metalloproteinase with thrombospondin motifs 13).[716,717] Of note, a decrease in ADAMTS13 activity to less than 10% is considered pathognomonic.[555–557] ADAMTS13 deficiency can result from homozygous or compound heterozygous *ADAMTS13* mutations, which constitutes the hereditary or congenital form of TTP (cTTP; Upshaw–Schulman syndrome),[717–719] or from inhibiting anti-ADAMTS13 autoantibodies, which constitutes the acquired, immune-mediated form of TTP (iTTP).[716] TTP is more common in adults and occurs with a standardized annual incidence rate of 2.88 × $10^6$ per year in adults versus 0.09 × $10^6$ per year in children.[720] Of note, while adults are more likely diagnosed with iTTP, children are more likely diagnosed with cTTP.[555,557]

vWF is synthesized by endothelial cells and megakaryocytes as monomeric pre–pro-vWF, which is modified to become pro-vWF and form the typical ultra-large vWF (ULVWF; >10,000 kDa) multimers. The molecular architecture of the vWF monomers is characterized by their multidomain structure; vWF multimers are packaged and stored in granular compartments, that is, Weibel–Palade bodies in endothelial cells, and α-granules in platelets.[721,722] Besides storage, these granules also facilitate vWF release into the circulation.[721,723] Basal vWF release occurs at a low rate in a nonstimulated fashion, whereas regulated vWF release follows a stimulus such as elevated intracellular calcium or cyclic adenosine monophosphate levels.[721] Under the shear stress of blood flow, secreted vWF unfolds and elongates to form strings of 100–500 μm, thereby exposing otherwise cryptic platelet-binding (A1 domain; glycoprotein 1b platelet and collagen-binding site)[723,724] and ADAMTS13 cleavage (A2 domain)[725] sites.

Physiologically, vWF multimers are subject to proteolytic cleavage (A2 domain) by a zinc protease[726,727] termed ADAMTS13[717,728] to prevent them from becoming excessively large.[729] Alternatively, released vWF can also bind to collagen.[730] Secreted vWF differs from that in circulation, which is present in a globular state, thus maintaining the platelet GP1b (A1 domain) and the ADAMTS13 cleavage site (A2 domain) cryptic (i.e., hidden) to prevent platelet binding and clot formation.[699,731]

vWF multimers attached to endothelial cells undergo structural changes under shear flow that enable ADAMTS13 to cleave them.[732,733] However, when ADAMTS13 activity is decreased (<10%) via an *ADAMTS13* mutation or inhibiting autoantibodies, ULVWF multimers persist in the circulation, bind, accumulate, and activate platelets, and thus initiate the formation of vWF-rich platelet thrombi, the hallmark of TTP, which occlude the microcirculation.[555,557,723,734–737]

## CLINICAL MANIFESTATIONS

The clinical manifestation of TTP is characterized by a nonimmune MAHA, thrombocytopenia, neurological symptoms (often transient; ranging from headache or mental changes to focal signs, seizures, and coma), variable degrees of renal dysfunction and fever, which together constitute the classical pentad of TTP historically found in 88% to 98% of patients.[555,557,738] Disease onset is often preceded by prodromal manifestations including fatigue, arthralgia, myalgia, and abdominal or lumbar pain. Cardiac involvement may include myocardial infarction, congestive heart failure, arrhythmias, cardiogenic shock, and sudden cardiac arrest. Digestive tract involvement may include abdominal pain, nausea, vomiting, and diarrhea. Autopsy studies revealed microvascular thrombi in almost all organs, particularly in the brain, heart, kidneys, digestive tract, spleen, pancreas, and adrenal glands. Of note, thrombi are typically rare in the lungs and liver.[555,557]

Pathognomonic are ADAMTS13 activity levels of less than 10%; the detection of inhibiting ADAMTS13 autoantibodies or genetic *ADAMTS13* mutations corroborate the diagnosis.[555,557] TTP is a chronic condition that often manifests as severe acute episodes of TMA, which are associated with a high (up to 20%) mortality and the continuing risk of relapse in survivors of a first acute disease episode.[555,557]

The clinical distinction of TTP from its major differential diagnosis (a)HUS was historically based on the involvement of the CNS and the relative sparing of the kidneys in TTP, versus the predominant renal phenotype in (a)HUS. However, although unusual in TTP, renal manifestation can also occur in up to 27% of TTP patients,[739,740] and while frequently occurring in TTP patients (up to 50%), neurological involvement has also been reported in 10% to 30% of (a)HUS patients.[741] The current standard of establishing the diagnosis of TTP involves measuring plasma ADAMTS13 activity.[742–744] ADAMTS13 activity assays using multimeric vWF substrate are difficult to perform and laborious. Today's fluorescence resonance energy transfer–based assay uses instead a minimal functional ADAMTS13 substrate composed of 73 amino acid residues (D1596–R1668) in the vWF A2 domain.[742,744] Activity levels of less than 10% are considered highly suggestive of TTP and are generally used as a diagnostic guide.[679] Additional diagnostic criteria include the degree of thrombocytopenia with platelet levels in TTP of typically less than 30 × $10^9$/L (as opposed to aHUS with >30 × $10^9$/L), and serum creatinine levels reflecting the degree of renal impairment being less elevated in TTP than in (a)HUS.[555,557]

TTP is associated with the life-long risk of disease recurrence, and recurrent episodes can be life threatening. Most relapses occur during the first or second year of the previous disease manifestation, but can occur as late as after 10 to 20 years.[740] As at first onset of disease, TTP relapses are characterized by decreased ADAMTS13 activity, an observation which points toward a potential for ongoing monitoring of ADAMTS13 activity to allow for preemptive treatment.[557]

## TREATMENT

In adult patients fulfilling the diagnostic criteria for TMA, STEC–HUS, aHUS, and TTP are—besides the numerous forms of secondary TMA—the main differential diagnoses. In the absence of clinical or diagnostic evidence for STEC–HUS and secondary TMA, TTP and aHUS remain the key differential diagnoses. In adult patients in whom the likelihood of TTP is significantly higher than in pediatric patients (in whom aHUS would be the more likely diagnosis), immediate treatment initiation is critical.[563,679,745]

Acute TTP episodes are medical emergencies and require immediate and intensive treatment.[555] The historically very poor prognosis of TTP with survival rates of <10% improved dramatically to >80% with the implementation of the consequent use of plasma treatment.[746]

Plasma treatment is appropriate for both iTTP and cTTP and can be delivered in form of PI or PLEX. While both treatment modalities were suitable to supplement or replace decreased or missing function of ADAMTS13, PLEX removes circulating inhibiting ADAMTS13 autoantibodies as well as high-molecular-weight vWF multimers. In 1991, a randomized controlled trial of PI versus PLEX for the treatment of adult TTP patients established a plasma volume-dependent response (9 days: 47% in PLEX vs. 27% in PI) and survival (6 months: 78% in PLEX vs. 49% in PI) rate.[747,748] Compared with fresh frozen (individual donors) and solvent detergent (multiple pooled donors) plasma, cryo-supernatant plasma is depleted of higher-molecular-weight proteins including high-molecular-weight vWF multimers. In iTTP, plasma treatment in form of PLEX—in the acute phase possibly even twice daily—continues until recovery of the platelet count, resolution of hemolysis, and resolution of organ dysfunction.[555,557] By contrast, in cTTP, plasma treatment in form of chronic periodical PI might be sufficient.[555,557,749]

For iTTP, additional treatment strategies include the use of immunosuppressants in the form of corticosteroids and/or biologics such as rituximab. Prior to the systematic use of PLEX, corticosteroids were reported to be successful in 55% of TTP patients with mainly hematological manifestation,[750] and the use of high-dose corticosteroids resulted in remission in 77% of patients.[751] In addition, administration of corticosteroids in combination with PLEX reduced the number of PLEX sessions required to achieve remission.[752]

The use of the monoclonal anti-CD20 antibody rituximab in iTTP patients is still controversial. As a B-cell depleting drug, the use of rituximab has been suggested for iTTP, and has been proven beneficial in several trials.[753–759] Rituximab was successful when used in combination with PLEX (daily PLEX + 4 weekly doses of rituximab) to achieve more frequent recovery of ADAMTS13 activity and more effective depletion of anti-ADAMTS13 autoantibodies, but also when used as frontline therapy in reducing number and frequency of TTP relapses.[757–760]

For TTP patients who were refractory to plasma cell depletion via rituximab, treatment strategies developed for patients with multiple myeloma were considered, and the successful use of bortezomib as rescue therapy in rituximab refractory TTP patients has been reported.[761–763]

Recently, ADAMTS13 replacement therapy in the form of recombinant ADAMTS13 has become available as a promising treatment strategy for both cTTP and iTTP. Recombinant ADAMTS13 effectively restores vWF cleaving activity in cTTP.[764] In iTTP, the required amount of recombinant ADAMTS13 was dependent on the anti-ADAMTS13 antibody titer.[765] In a recent first-in-human phase 1 clinical study of recombinant ADAMTS13 (BAX 930) in 15 cTTP patients, treatment was found to be safe, nonimmunogenic, and well tolerated. The pharmacokinetic profile of recombinant ADAMTS13 was comparable to PIs, and there was evidence for pharmacodynamic activity. A dose-related increase in ADAMTS13 antigen and activity levels was observed with a maximum effect after 1 hour. Besides, with increasing doses, a dose-dependent persistence of vWF cleavage products and reduced vWF multimeric size were observed.[745]

Other treatment approaches currently under investigation include compounds (1) modifying vWF affinity for platelets, and (2) interfering with vVF–platelet interaction.

The reducing agent *N*-acetylcysteamine has been shown to depolymerize vWF multimers and prevented clot formation in *Adamts13*$^{-/-}$ mice. In addition, *N*-acetylcysteamine reduced vWF disulfide bonds, thus inhibiting vWF–platelet interactions via GP1b.[766] *N*-acetylcysteamine was also successful in preventing clot formation in 5/8 TTP patients, and is currently tested in a clinical trial (ClinicalTrials.gov identifier NCT01808521).[555,557]

Caplacizumab is a bivalent humanized llama Ig variable region that recognizes the vWF A1 domain, thus preventing vWF–platelet binding via GP1b.[94] Caplacizumab was recently tested in a phase 2 randomized trial (TITAN) during PLEX and for 30 days afterward, and was successful in shortening the time to platelet count normalization. TTP relapse occurred quickly after caplacizumab discontinuation in patients with persistently decreased ADAMTS13 activity. A follow-up trial (HERCULES) is currently investigating the extension of caplacizumab treatment in patients with ADAMTS13 activity of 10% after 30 days of treatment.

## SYSTEMIC DISEASES WITH RENAL INVOLVEMENT

### HENOCH–SCHÖNLEIN PURPURA AND IGA NEPHROPATHY

#### INTRODUCTION

IgAN is the most common type of chronic glomerulonephritis in children,[767] while HSP is the most common type of vasculitis in children, with glomerulonephritis being its most common chronic manifestation.[768] First described by Berger and Hinglais in 1968 among patients with macroscopic hematuria during viral upper respiratory infections, IgAN is now recognized as the most common primary glomerulopathy in the world.[769,770] While early on it was considered a benign disease, subsequent studies revealed that between 20% and 50% of adults and children ultimately developed ESRD.[770–775] In contrast to IgAN which is limited to the kidneys, HSP nephritis is a multisystem disease primarily affecting the skin, joints, gastrointestinal tract, and kidneys.[776,777] Because these diseases share many pathogenic and clinical features, however, they will be discussed together.

#### EPIDEMIOLOGY

Although IgAN occurs worldwide, its incidence varies widely among different regions. In North America it accounts for only approximately 5% to 10% of all cases of primary glomerulonephritis, whereas in Europe it accounts for 20% to 30% of cases, and in the Pacific Rim it accounts for almost 50% of cases.[778] It is generally thought that both genetic and environmental factors account for much of this diversity, with differing approaches among various countries to screening urinalyses also likely playing a role in the detection of disease.[779–781] While IgAN occurs in both children and adults, it presents most commonly during the second and third decades of life.[770] Among children, IgAN appears to generally occur with a male-to-female ratio of approximately 2 : 1.[773,775,782]

In comparison to IgAN, HSP occurs almost 20 times more commonly.[767] However, because only a minority (~30%) of children with HSP develop glomerulonephritis, which is most commonly only mild, the incidence of clinically significant HSP nephritis has been estimated to be potentially lower than that of IgAN.[277,783–785] In addition, HSP appears to occur with a male-to-female ratio of approximately 1:1, although HSP nephritis has a slight male predilection with a male-to-female ratio of approximately 1.5:1.[775,786,787] While HSP affects children far more commonly than adults, with a peak incidence at approximately 4 to 5 years of age, it is rare among children younger than 2 years of age.[293,788–790] There is also a notable seasonal variation in the incidence of HSP, with its peak incidence occurring during the winter months.[310,783,787]

## PATHOPHYSIOLOGY

The molecular pathogenesis of IgAN has yet to be fully clarified, but it is understood to be an IC-mediated disease. The disease is characterized by granular electron-dense deposits in the glomerular mesangium that are comprised at least in part of IgA and C3. In addition, circulating IgA ICs have been well described, and conditions known to induce IgA ICs have been reported in patients with IgAN. The mesangial deposits have been reported to contain primarily the IgA1 subclass, and to be present in the polymeric form, rather than the monomeric form.[791,792] Although not yet proven, it is now suspected that incomplete galactosylation of O-linked glycans in the hinge region of IgA1 may lead to increased serum levels as well as a propensity for IgA1 complexes to bind to the glomerular mesangium, stimulating the production of cytokines and growth factors by both glomerular cells and circulating lymphocytes that results in the mesangial cell proliferation and deposition of extracellular matrix that characterize IgAN.[793–796] Serum levels of IgA are increased in 50% to 70% of patients with IgAN during active disease, but return to normal during recovery.[787,797,798] In addition, various IgA-derived autoantibodies and circulating ICs have been frequently reported in patients with IgAN.[799,800] More recently, microRNAs have also been suggested to have potential roles in the pathogenesis of IgAN and/or disease progression.[801–804] Lastly, the available evidence suggests that the precipitating event in IgAN, abnormal glycosylation of IgA1, appears to be an inherited trait rather than an acquired abnormality, but that different families may have differing molecular mechanisms of disease development.[805]

## CLINICAL PRESENTATION

IgAN in children initially presents with macroscopic hematuria in almost 75% of cases in the United States, although only in 26% of cases in Japan.[772,773,806,807] The hematuria usually occurs during an upper respiratory infection and resolves within 2 to 4 days. Less commonly it occurs in association with other infections associated with the mucosal system, such as sinusitis or diarrhea. Other less common presentations include microscopic hematuria with proteinuria, isolated microscopic hematuria, and isolated proteinuria. Even less commonly (~10% of cases), IgAN can present with macroscopic hematuria with reversible AKI, although it is rare for a child to present with CKD,[772,773] and even rarer to present with RPGN.[808,809] Hypertension is present in approximately 25% of children at presentation, although it is usually not severe unless AKI is also present.

Children with HSP nephritis typically present far earlier (~4–6 years) than those with IgAN (~10–30 years), although like IgAN, HSP nephritis can present at any age. The typical presentation includes a lower extremity purpuric rash, often associated with abdominal pain, and sometimes arthritis. In addition, approximately 25% of such children will also have macroscopic hematuria, although the renal manifestations of HSP nephritis at presentation may range from nonexistent to severe nephritic and/or NS.[767,810] Notably, children with HSP nephritis are approximately twice as likely to develop NS than those with IgAN.[773,810–813]

## LABORATORY EVALUATION

Because no specific serologic biomarker exists to diagnose IgAN, confirmation of the diagnosis depends on the identification of IgA deposits by renal biopsy in the glomerular mesangium. When IgAN is suspected, however, laboratory evaluation generally includes serum creatinine, serum albumin, serum C3 level, serum antinuclear antibody (to exclude possible SLE), as well as a complete urinalysis and urine protein-to-creatinine ratio determination. Diagnosis of HSP nephritis includes identifying the clinical features of HSP noted earlier in combination with evidence of renal involvement on urinalysis and urine protein-to-creatinine ratio.

Serum IgA levels are often elevated in both IgAN and HSP nephritis, but have not been found to be sufficiently sensitive and specific to serve as a clinically useful biomarker of disease.[772,814,815] Serum C3 and C4 levels are usually normal in both diseases as well, helping to distinguish IgAN from the hypocomplementemia seen in PIGN, MPGN, or SLE nephritis. Although a renal biopsy for children with HSP nephritis is usually reserved only for more severe cases, the renal biopsy findings for HSP nephritis and IgAN are virtually indistinguishable.[787,816]

## TREATMENT

Because of its variable disease progression, and its likely multifactorial pathogenesis, effective treatment of children with IgAN represents a significant challenge and remains somewhat controversial.[817] In addition, the published evidence to guide the treatment of children with IgAN differs significantly from the published evidence to guide the treatment of adults. Specifically, suggested treatments for adults with IgAN tend to be generally more passive, focusing more on nonimmunosuppressive treatment with ACE inhibitors and ARBs, whereas suggested treatments for children with IgAN tend to be more active, often including immunosuppression. In this context, Table 72.12 lists several of the current and emerging treatments reported for children with IgAN.

For children presenting with only mild IgAN or HSP nephritis, reflected by a first-morning urine protein-to-creatinine ratio of less than 0.5 mg/mg, most often no treatment is necessary. For those children who remain asymptomatic but who have more active disease, as reflected by a first-morning urine protein-to-creatinine ratio of greater than 0.5 mg/mg, initiation of ACE inhibitors and/or ARBs is generally indicated. By contrast, children who present with nephrotic-range proteinuria or NS require more aggressive treatment. This should include ACE inhibitors and/or ARBs to which oral prednisone (2 mg/kg PO daily; maximal dose = 80 mg/day) is added. If this treatment successfully induces

**Table 72.12 Current and Emerging Treatment Options for Children With IgA Nephropathy or Henoch–Schönlein Purpura Nephritis**

| Immunosuppressive | Nonimmunosuppressive |
|---|---|
| Oral glucocorticoids | Angiotensin-converting enzyme inhibitors |
| Pulse intravenous methylprednisolone | Angiotensin receptor blockers |
| Mycophenolate mofetil (and mizoribine) | Fish oil[a] (omega 3 fatty acids) |
| Alkylating agents[a] (cyclophosphamide, chlorambucil) | Tonsillectomy[a] |
| Calcineurin inhibitors[a] (cyclosporine, tacrolimus) | Chinese herbal medicine[a] (Sairei-to; TJ-114) |
| Budesonide[b] | Coagulation-modifying drugs[a] (warfarin, urokinase, antiplatelet drugs) |

[a]Less commonly used treatment.
[b]Emerging treatment.

remission of disease, the prednisone dose can be gradually tapered over 2 to 3 months and discontinued. If significant proteinuria persists, however, additional immunosuppressive treatment in indicated. Moreover, most pediatric nephrologists perform renal biopsies in children who present with NS, nephritic syndrome, or nephrotic-range proteinuria. If the biopsy reveals a significant percentage of crescents (typically >10%–20%), more aggressive immunosuppression with pulse IV methylprednisolone (typically 10–30 mg/kg over 1 hour; maximal dose = 1000 mg) is administered daily for 3 consecutive days, followed by initiation of daily oral prednisone as described earlier.

Interestingly, there is a fairly high rate of spontaneous remissions among children with mild forms of IgAN. One report of a large cohort of 555 children with only mild glomerular abnormalities on renal biopsy documented spontaneous remissions (i.e., without drug therapy) in the range of approximately 55% at 5 years and approximately 75% at 10 years from diagnosis.[818]

As noted earlier, the most widely used initial therapy for IgAN and HSP nephritis in both adults and children is treatment with ACE inhibitors and ARBs. While there are robust data demonstrating their effectiveness in reducing proteinuria and preserving renal function in adults,[819,820] there are fewer data supporting these same beneficial effects in children.[821,822] In addition, combination therapy with ACE inhibitors and ARBs has been reported to have beneficial and potentially additive effects in both adults and children.[823–826]

The second most widely used therapy for IgAN and HSP nephritis in children is treatment with oral and/or pulse IV glucocorticoids. While very widely used, the many historical variations in the reported routes of administration, as well as the doses and durations of treatment, have made it difficult in the past to accurately assess their efficacy.[785] However, there are now several randomized, controlled trials in adults and children demonstrating their effectiveness in reducing proteinuria and preserving renal function.[827–832]

In addition to ACE inhibitors/ARBs and glucocorticoids, fish oil has been utilized to treat IgAN. Notably, while randomized trials of adults have reported that fish oil for 2 years slowed the progression of renal disease, a randomized trial of children treated with omega 3 fatty acids failed to demonstrate a clear benefit in preserving renal function compared with placebo treatment.[833–836]

Additional commonly used immunosuppressive treatments for IgAN include cyclophosphamide, MMF or mizoribine, and cyclosporine. There are published reports suggesting some efficacy for each of these agents, but their use is generally less favored than the treatments described earlier, largely due to a relative lack of clear evidence to support more widespread use.[827,837–840]

There are also some nonimmunosuppressive treatments for IgAN that have reported some success. Tonsillectomy has been reported to have some marginal efficacy, although the studies were complicated by its use in combination with other simultaneous treatments, and the overall beneficial effects were uncertain.[841,842] Thus clear evidence to support its more widespread use in IgAN remains lacking. Another nonimmunosuppressive treatment is the Chinese herbal medicine Sairei-to (TJ-114). Although not widely used, a large randomized, controlled trial in children with mild IgAN by the Japanese Pediatric IgA Nephropathy Treatment Study Group reported that treatment early in disease for 2 years was more effective than no treatment.[843] In addition, coagulation-modifying treatments including warfarin, antiplatelet drugs, and urokinase have also been used to treat IgAN.[332,831,844] The data to date do not provide much support for their use as primary treatments for IgAN, although their inclusion as adjunctive treatments may have some potential.

Several new approaches to the treatment of IgAN are under investigation, at various stages of development. To date, however, only budesonide, a corticosteroid targeting the mucosal production of IgA1, has undergone a phase II trial demonstrating a reduction in proteinuria.[845]

Finally, in consideration of future clinical trials to improve the care of children with IgAN and HSP nephritis, it should be noted that given the prolonged clinical disease course for many children, the design of rigorous clinical trials to compare potential new treatments with current approaches suffers from the reality that most children will transfer their care to an adult nephrologist before a clinically meaningful endpoint for a clinical trial can be reached. Thus enhanced collaboration between pediatric and adult nephrology programs will likely be critical to demonstrate the long-term efficacy and safety of any future treatments for children with IgAN and HSP nephritis.

## OUTCOME

The long-term outcome for children with IgAN is highly variable. Historical reports show outcomes ranging from complete remission of disease to development of ESRD. While approximately one-third of children will experience a complete remission of disease, long-term studies among children have reported the development of progressive CKD in 9% at 15 years from diagnosis, and ultimately ESRD in 20% to 27% of children, whereas adult studies have reported progressive CKD among 30% to 35% of patients at 20 years from diagnosis.[298,767,770,772,806,807,846–849]

In general, poor clinical prognostic indicators have included persistent severe proteinuria and persistent hypertension, while poor histologic prognostic indicators have included higher percentages of glomeruli with crescents, adhesions or sclerosis, significant tubulointerstitial changes, subepithelial electron-dense deposits, or lysis of the GBM.[296,782,848,850–852]

For children with HSP nephritis, long-term outcomes are less clear, due to marked variability in disease severity among the reported cases. While some reports have noted ESRD developing in 22% to 25% of children, others have estimated the risk for ESRD among all children with HSP nephritis at only approximately 3%.[308,769,786,787,810,813,844,853–855]

## RENAL DISEASES WITH VASCULITIS

Vasculitis, or inflammation of the blood vessel walls, is an uncommon cause of glomerular injury in children, but can result in severe glomerulonephritis and even death. Vascular inflammation can lead to stenosis and/or aneurysm of the vessel walls, and result in various types of glomerulonephritis, depending of the size of the vessel walls and the organs most affected by disease. As such, a major effort was undertaken recently to update the nomenclature describing these various lesions.[856] Table 72.13 summarizes the current classification of vasculitides affecting children. The most common types of vasculitis seen in children are Kawasaki disease (KD) and IgA vasculitis (IgAV; i.e., HSP). IgAV and IgAN have already been discussed in detail earlier in this chapter, while the large vessel vasculitides, Takayasu arteritis, and giant cell arteritis are extremely rare in children and are thus discussed elsewhere in the text.

### MEDIUM VESSEL VASCULITIDES

The medium vessel vasculitides include two primary diseases that include KD, which is common but only rarely has renal manifestations, and polyarteritis nodosa (PAN), which is rare in both children and adults, but commonly has renal manifestations (Table 72.13).

#### KAWASAKI DISEASE

KD is a vasculitis that typically involves the mucosa and skin, and is known to also preferentially affect coronary vessels. This common vasculitis is defined by a child having at least 5 days of fever, accompanied by four of the following five criteria: (1) edema, erythema, or desquamation of the hands, feet, or perineal area, (2) bilateral nonpurulent conjunctival injection, (3) polymorphous exanthema (primarily truncal), (4) oral and pharyngeal mucosal injection, and (5) cervical lymphadenopathy (typically unilateral). KD only rarely has renal manifestations, which can include sterile pyuria, proteinuria, AKI with tubulointerstitial changes, and rarely renal artery aneurysms. NS has also been reported, although it appears to remit spontaneously without glucocorticoid therapy.[857–861]

#### POLYARTERITIS NODOSA

PAN is now defined as a necrotizing arteritis involving small or medium arteries, without evidence of antineutrophil cytoplasmic antibodies or vasculitis in venules, capillaries, or arterioles.[856] While very uncommon in both children and adults, specific criteria for diagnosing pediatric PAN have been published.[862,863] This disease is specifically distinguished from microscopic polyangiitis (MPA) pathologically by its lack of ANCAs or necrotizing glomerulonephritis, and clinically by its higher incidence of gastrointestinal symptoms and peripheral neuropathy.[864] Clinical presentation typically includes fever, skin lesions, and/or myalgia, with involvement of the kidneys, heart, and/or lungs occurring in 15% to 20% of children.[865–867] Notably, the major renal manifestations result from involvement of medium size vessels, and include renovascular hypertension and aneurysms with the potential for rupture or hemorrhage. Treatment generally includes oral and/or IV glucocorticoids combined with cyclophosphamide.[868–870]

### SMALL VESSEL VASCULITIDES

The small vessel vasculitides are now divided into two main categories (Table 72.13). The first category is AAV, and includes granulomatosis with polyangiitis (GPA; Wegener), MPA, and

**Table 72.13 Classification of Pediatric Vasculitides by Primary Vessel Involvement**

| Small Vessel Vasculitis | Medium Vessel Vasculitis | Large Vessel Vasculitis[a] |
|---|---|---|
| • Antineutrophil cytoplasmic antibody (ANCA)–associated vasculitis (AAV) (i.e., pauci-immune small vessel vasculitis)<br>• Granulomatosis with polyangiitis (Wegener, GPA; can also involve medium vessels)<br>• Microscopic polyangiitis (MPA)<br>Eosinophilic granulomatosis with polyangiitis (Churg–Strauss syndrome, EGPA)[a] | • Kawasaki disease (KD) | • Takayasu arteritis[a] |
| • Immune complex small vessel vasculitis<br>• IgA vasculitis (Henoch–Schönlein) (IgAV)<br>• Antiglomerular basement membrane (anti-GBM) disease[a]<br>• Hypocomplementemic urticarial vasculitis (anti-C1q vasculitis)[a]<br>Cryoglobulinemic vasculitis (CV)[a] | • Polyarteritis nodosa (PAN, can also involve small vessels)[a] | • Giant cell arteritis[a] |

[a]Rarely seen in children.

Modified from Jennette JC, Falk RJ, Bacon PA, et al. 2012 revised International Chapel Hill Consensus Conference nomenclature of vasculitides. *Arthritis Rheum.* 2013;65:1–11.

**Table 72.14 Clinical and Pathologic Features Distinguishing Selected Small Vessel Vasculitides**

| Feature | IgA Vasculitis (IgAV; Henoch–Schönlein Purpura Nephritis) | Granulomatosis With Polyangiitis (GPA; Wegener Granulomatosis) | Microscopic Polyangiitis | Eosinophilic Granulomatosis With Polyangiitis (EGPA; Churg–Strauss Syndrome) | Antiglomerular Basement Membrane (Anti-GBM) Disease | Systemic Lupus Erythematosus Nephritis (SLEN) |
|---|---|---|---|---|---|---|
| Vasculitis of small vessels | YES | YES | YES | YES | YES | YES |
| Immune complexes | YES | NO | NO | NO | YES (linear IgG deposits along GBM due to in situ immune complex formation) | YES |
| Necrotizing granuloma presence | NO | YES (usually extrarenal) | NO | YES (usually extrarenal) | NO | NO |
| Predominant IgA glomerular immune deposits | YES | NO | NO | NO | NO | NO |
| PR3 antibody presence | NO | Sometimes (more likely) | Sometimes (less likely) | Sometimes | NO | NO |
| MPO antibody presence | NO | Sometimes (less likely) | Sometimes (more likely) | Sometimes | Sometimes (overlap between anti-GBM and MPO-ANCA disease) | NO |
| Eosinophilia and/or asthma presence | NO | NO | NO | YES | NO | NO |

eosinophilic granulomatosis with polyangiitis (EGPA; Churg–Strauss syndrome). The second category is IC small vessel vasculitis, and includes IgAV (HSP), anti-GBM disease, hypocomplementemic urticarial vasculitis (anti-C1q vasculitis), and cryoglobulinemic vasculitis. The clinical and pathologic features that distinguish those small vessel vasculitides seen more commonly in children from each other are compared in Table 72.14. Far and away the most common of these diseases seen in children is IgAV, and this topic was discussed earlier in this chapter.

While vasculitis is an uncommon cause of glomerular injury in children, presentation with vasculitis can be associated with the development of an RPGN. This is a clinical diagnosis characterized by rapid deterioration in renal function over a few days to weeks, as measured by a consistently rising serum creatinine. In this clinical setting, consideration needs to be given to the possibility of either an AAV or an IC small vessel vasculitis (Table 72.13). The ANCA-associated vasculitides are typically "pauci-immune," meaning that there are few or no immune deposits affecting the arterioles, capillaries, or venules (i.e., small vessels). From a clinical perspective, any of the small vessel vasculitides noted in Table 72.13 may be associated with ANCAs directed against either proteinase 3 (PR3) or myeloperoxidase (MPO). However, PR3–ANCA are more commonly associated with GPA, whereas MPO–ANCA are more commonly associated with MPA. In contrast to the pauci-immune ANCA-associated vasculitides, anti-GBM disease is associated with linear IgG staining of the GBM, and is almost always associated with a positive serum anti-GBM antibody test. In very rare cases where the serum anti-GBM antibody is negative, it is suspected that disease may be due to an anti-GBM antibody not detected by the current serum anti-GBM antibody test (i.e., "atypical anti-GBM disease"). Of significant clinical interest, a recent publication from the Midwest Pediatric Nephrology Consortium of a large multicenter cohort of approximately 260 children with glomerular disease who had more than one crescent on renal biopsy has reported a significantly worse 1-year renal survival among children whose biopsies had 43% or more crescents versus those with less than 43% crescents, regardless of the specific histologic diagnosis.

## GRANULOMATOSIS WITH POLYANGIITIS (WEGENER GRANULOMATOSIS)

GPA is rare in children, with an incidence of 1 to 2 per million, compared with 1 to 2 per 100,000 adults.[848,871] It is a necrotizing granulomatous vasculitis of small- and medium-sized vessels that primarily affects the kidneys, the upper and lower respiratory tracts, and multiple other organs. Diagnosis in a child requires three of the following six features: (1) renal involvement, (2) upper airway involvement, (3) pulmonary involvement (infiltrates, nodules, or cavities), (4) laryngo-tracheobronchial stenosis, (5) granulomatous inflammation, and (6) ANCAs.[862] On renal biopsy, while granulomata are only rarely detected, approximately 90% of children have crescents, and more than half of children have crescents in more than 50% of their glomeruli.[872] Although the etiology remains unclear, recent reports have suggested that the initial injury is to endothelial cells, and that this injury is induced by inflammatory cells that have been primed with ANCAs.[873,874] However, the factor(s) precipitating the initial production of ANCAs remain unclear.[875–877]

From a clinical perspective, the vast majority of children with GPA (~90%) present initially with upper and/or lower respiratory findings, including epistaxis, sinusitis, nasal ulceration, hemoptysis, cough, subglottic stenosis (hoarseness), or dyspnea.[201,878,879] Additional common constitutional symptoms include weight loss, fever, and abdominal pain.[806] The presence of renal disease at presentation varies greatly, but can include hematuria, proteinuria, and AKI. Other organ systems that can also be affected include the eyes, CNS, skin, musculoskeletal system, and the heart. In 70% to 90% of cases, ANCAs are detected, usually with specificity for PR3 (c-ANCA).[201,862,878]

Treatment of GPA is generally separated into induction and maintenance phases. Induction phase treatment generally includes three daily initial IV methylprednisolone boluses, followed by oral glucocorticoids (1–2 mg/kg/day). In addition, IV cyclophosphamide (500–750 mg/m$^2$) is also administered every 2 to 4 weeks, although oral cyclophosphamide is sometimes used instead of IV treatments.[874] The anti-CD20 mAb rituximab has also been used as a newer alterative to cyclophosphamide for induction therapy, and has been reported to be as effective as cyclophosphamide in inducing remission in new patients, and superior to cyclophosphamide in inducing remission in relapsing patients.[880–882] Another alternative to cyclophosphamide for induction therapy is methotrexate, which has been reported to induce remission by 6 months at a similar rate in patients with mild vasculitis (serum creatinine < 150 µmol/L and without critical organ manifestations), but was associated with delayed induction of remission and more frequent relapses compared with cyclophosphamide.[861] Methotrexate should be avoided in patients with glomerulonephritis and decreased GFR. PLEX is used to treat patients with diffuse pulmonary hemorrhage, as well as those with RPGN approaching a need for dialysis, and has been reported to improve both patient survival and renal survival.[883–886] A large randomized controlled trial is ongoing to evaluate the role of plasmapheresis in patients with more moderate degrees of renal dysfunction (PEXIVAS trial, ClinicalTrials.gov identifier NCT00987389##). This trial is expected to be completed by the end of 2018. Lastly, an emerging induction treatment is the use of a C5a receptor blocker (Avacopan) as a steroid-sparing agent in addition to either cyclophosphamide or rituximab.[704] Table 72.15 summarizes the current and emerging induction phase and maintenance phase treatments used to treat GPA, which is very similar to the treatment of MPA described in the following section.

Maintenance phase treatment is initiated once a patient is declared to be in remission, and generally includes a gradual taper of prednisone, after the initial 4 weeks of therapy, over several months to a final maintenance dose of 5 to 10 mg every other morning. In addition, options for maintenance treatment also include azathioprine, methotrexate, MMF, or more recently rituximab. In a randomized controlled trial, maintenance therapy with azathioprine was found to be associated with lower rates of relapse than MMF.[887–890]

Relapses are relatively common among children with GPA, as they are among adults.[871] While the time to relapse ranges widely, from 4 months to 20 months, the median time to relapse is approximately 28 months from diagnosis.

Long-term outcomes for GPA appear to be somewhat better among children than adults. Approximately 80% to 90% of children achieve a remission of disease, although 40% of them have subsequent relapses.[891,892] Overall mortality rates are approximately 3% to 10%.[806]

**Table 72.15 Current and Emerging Treatment Options for Children With Granulomatosis With Polyangiitis and Microscopic Polyangiitis**

| Induction Phase Treatment | Maintenance Phase Treatment |
|---|---|
| Pulse intravenous (IV) methylprednisolone (daily for 3 days) | Oral glucocorticoids (taper over several months to 5–10 mg qod) |
| Oral glucocorticoids (daily at 1–2 mg/kg/day) | Azathioprine |
| IV cyclophosphamide (500–750 mg/m$^2$ every 2–4 weeks; PO dosing sometimes substituted) | Mycophenolate mofetil |
| IV rituximab | IV rituximab |
| Plasma exchange (plasmapheresis; especially indicated in pulmonary hemorrhage) | Methotrexate[a] |
| C5a receptor blocker (Avacopan) as steroid-sparing agent in addition to cyclophosphamide or rituximab[b] | |
| Methotrexate[a] | |

[a]Less commonly used treatment.
[b]Emerging treatment.

## MICROSCOPIC POLYANGIITIS

MPA is also rare in children. Like GPA, it is also a necrotizing glomerulonephritis, with arteritis involving small- and medium-sized vessels of the kidneys and lungs. Unlike GPA, however, patients with MPA do not have granulomatous lesions, and typically do not have subglottic stenosis or severe, destructive involvement of the upper respiratory tract.[862,893] Children typically present with AKI due to necrotizing crescentic glomerulonephritis, and approximately 50% of them will also present with a pulmonary–renal syndrome, making a chest X-ray mandatory in all suspected cases.[891,894–898] For diagnosis of MPA, these children also have ANCAs, which are most often anti-MPO antibodies that show a perinuclear pattern (i.e., p-ANCA positivity) by indirect IF staining.[829] While the etiology of MPA is not entirely clear, reports from several experimental studies support the concept that the anti-MPO antibodies in MPA have a pathogenic role in disease induction, and that ANCA-associated disease has a genetic component.[874,899,900]

Treatment of MPA is very similar to GPA, and indeed many of the studies developing evidence for treatment of these vasculitides have included both patients with MPA and GPA. Table 72.15 summarizes the current and emerging treatments used to treat both GPA and MPA. Like children with GPA, the long-term outcomes for children with MPA appear to be generally better than those reported in adults.

### Eosinophilic Granulomatosis With Polyangiitis (Churg–Strauss Syndrome)

EGPA, also known as Churg–Strauss syndrome, is even rarer than GPA or MPA. Like these diseases, it is a pauci-immune small vessel necrotizing vasculitis, but it is distinguished from them by the presence of extravascular granulomatous inflammation combined with asthma and hypereosinophilia.[856,901]

Clinically, children typically present with a long history of asthma, and are often found to also have histories of allergies, sinus disease, or peripheral nervous system abnormalities. In addition, vasculitic skin involvement appears to be relatively common, and similar to that seen in children with PAN.[902,903] Although relatively few data are available related to renal involvement specifically among children, renal involvement based on adult studies occurs in approximately 20% of patients, and typically manifests as acute glomerulonephritis with or without AKI.[902]

Laboratory evaluation for EGPA is generally similar to that for GPA or MPA, and children with EGPA are typically found to have ANCAs, most often p-ANCA indicating the presence of anti-MPO antibodies.[901] Histologic confirmation of disease usually includes findings of a necrotizing vasculitis of small- and/or medium-sized vessels, and granulomatous inflammation of the respiratory tract.

There are relatively few data on optimal treatment or long-term outcomes for children with EGPA, given its rarity. However, treatment is generally similar to that for the other small vessel vasculitides GPA and MPA, and is summarized in Table 72.15.

## ANTI-GLOMERULAR BASEMENT MEMBRANE (ANTI-GBM) DISEASE

Anti-GBM disease is yet another rare cause of necrotizing small vessel vasculitis. Indeed, among children presenting with RPGN, anti-GBM comprised only 12% of cases, which was far less common than either pauci-immune RPGN (42% of cases) or IC-mediated RPGN (45% of cases).[872,904] This disease results from circulating antibodies which bind the noncollagenous globular domain (NC1 domain) at the C terminus of the alpha-3 chain of type IV collagen (COL4A3) in the GBM. This is seen in IF staining of renal biopsies as intense linear IgG staining along the GBM of glomerular capillary loops, with or without the presence of C3. Notably, these autoantibodies can also cross-react with alveolar basement membranes, resulting in lung injury and pulmonary hemorrhage (Goodpasture syndrome). Such pulmonary involvement is thought to result from exposure of the alveolar basement membranes to these circulating autoantibodies as a result of prior pulmonary injury, potentially due to hydrocarbons, glue, or cigarette smoke.[905,906]

Anti-GBM disease occurs more commonly among males and can occur at any age. However, there are two known peak incidences; at 30 to 40 years and again at 70 to 80 years.[806] Children with anti-GBM often present with constitutional symptoms, and in approximately 50% of cases will also have pulmonary symptoms.[904] For those with pulmonary involvement, presenting symptoms can include cough, anemia, hemoptysis, fever, as well as pulmonary infiltrates or frank pulmonary hemorrhage. Overall, approximately 50% of children present with isolated renal disease, whereas the remaining 50% of children present with combined renal and pulmonary disease.[872,907,908] Diagnosis of anti-GBM is confirmed with a combination of intense linear IgG staining of the GBM in glomerular capillary loops noted earlier, and a positive serum anti-GBM antibody test.

Treatment of anti-GBM is generally similar to the other vasculitides described earlier, with pulse IV methylprednisolone for several days followed by daily oral prednisone during the initiation phase of treatment, in conjunction with IV cyclophosphamide (500–1000 mg/m$^2$ monthly for 3–6 months), or less commonly oral cyclophosphamide (2 mg/kg daily for several months). In addition, PLEX is also widely used in an attempt to reduce circulating anti-GBM autoantibodies and proinflammatory cytokines.[872,909] Following induction of disease remission, which occurs in as many as 90% of patients, maintenance phase treatment typically includes azathioprine, methotrexate, or MMF.

Few long-term outcome data for children with anti-GBM are available. Despite this, unlike the pauci-immune vasculitides described earlier, anti-GBM is generally not considered a relapsing disease.[806] Known poor prognostic indicators for renal survival include severe AKI and/or extensive fibrous crescents at initial clinical presentation.[872]

## SYSTEMIC LUPUS ERYTHEMATOSUS NEPHRITIS

SLE is a common systemic inflammatory autoimmune disease that can affect many organ systems. While renal involvement may not be present at the initial disease presentation, most children with SLE will develop renal involvement at some point in their disease, and SLEN often becomes among the most significant predictors of morbidity and mortality among children with SLE.[910–914] For example, data from adults have reported that approximately 10% of patients who develop SLEN will progress to ESRD.[915] In this light, this section will not address the initial diagnosis of SLE, but focus instead on the diagnosis and treatment of SLEN among children previously diagnosed with SLE.

The epidemiology of SLE is notable for its strong predilection for females, with the female-to-male ratio ranging from 1.3:1 among prepubertal children to 4.5:1 among adolescents to 8 to 15:1 among adults.[916–919] In addition, the prevalence of SLE among children has also been estimated to be as frequent as 10 per 100,000 persons.[920] Furthermore, higher risks for SLE compared with Caucasians have been reported for Asian (7×), African-American (4.5×), and Hispanic (3×) females, as well as more severe disease with poorer prognoses.[806,921]

The pathogenesis of SLEN among patients with SLE is multifactorial. While a detailed review of the genetics and pathogenesis is beyond the scope of this chapter, such a review has recently been published.[922] Briefly, recently published data suggest that the nephritis is initiated by an interferon response, possibly due to compromised clearance of apoptotic cells, that leads to differentiation of B cells into plasmablasts, which then progresses to activation of neutrophils and myeloid cells that results in both renal and systemic inflammation.[923–925] In addition, complement system activation is also common in SLEN and is thought to mediate kidney injury both directly via the terminal complement pathway and indirectly via recruitment of leukocytes to the kidney.[924]

The diagnosis of SLEN in patients with SLE may be clinically subtle, making screening urinalyses (at least yearly) of all SLE patients important. The most common clinical manifestations of SLEN include proteinuria (100%), which may range from mild to NS (50%), followed by microscopic hematuria (80%), tubular abnormalities (70%), and AKI (60%).[924] In children with SLE in whom SLEN is suspected, the renal evaluation should include a urinalysis, renal function panel, and consideration of a renal biopsy if more than mild disease appears present. The histologic classification of SLEN is described in detail elsewhere in the text.

The treatment of SLEN has been primarily guided by trials in adults due to the relatively low numbers of children with SLEN. In general, children with class I or class II SLEN generally do not need kidney-specific treatment, although close observation to ensure they do not convert to a more severe class of SLEN is important. Children who develop mild class III SLEN (<20% glomerular involvement) can usually also be managed conservatively, although more aggressive treatment is indicated when moderate or severe class III disease is present. For patients with class IV SLEN, aggressive treatment is clearly indicated, although the optimal treatment approach remains uncertain. Like some of the other small vessel vasculitides described earlier (i.e., GPA and MPA), treatment is usually divided into an induction phase and a maintenance phase. The current and emerging treatment options for each of these phases for SLEN in children are shown in Table 72.16.[926]

Induction phase treatment typically includes pulse IV methylprednisolone for 3 or more days, followed by daily oral prednisone at 1 to 2 mg/kg/day, in addition to treatment with IV cyclophosphamide (500–1000 mg/m$^2$ monthly for ~6 months), or less commonly oral cyclophosphamide (2 mg/kg daily for ~6 months). Such combined therapy has been reported to reduce the risk for subsequent disease progression, although it is not clear whether cyclophosphamide given IV is superior to oral administration.[910,927–931] A more recent alternative to cyclophosphamide for induction phase treatment has been MMF. Several reports in both children and adults have found MMF to be as or more effective than cyclophosphamide in inducing complete and partial remissions of disease, often with fewer side effects.[932–941] Dosing for MMF in children with SLEN is typically approximately 1200 mg/m$^2$/day, during both the induction phase and the maintenance phase of treatment. However, titration of dosing based on trough mycophenolic acid levels and/or area under the curve (AUC) has been associated with improved clinical efficacy.[942–944]

**Table 72.16 Current and Emerging Treatment Options for Children With Systemic Lupus Erythematosus Nephritis**

| Induction Phase Treatment | Maintenance Phase Treatment |
|---|---|
| Pulse IV methylprednisolone (daily for 3 days) | Oral glucocorticoids (taper over several months) |
| Oral glucocorticoids (daily at 1–2 mg/kg/day) | Mycophenolate mofetil |
| IV cyclophosphamide (500–1000 mg/m$^2$ monthly for ~6 months; PO dosing sometimes substituted at 2 mg/kg daily for ~6 months) | Azathioprine |
| Mycophenolate mofetil | IV cyclophosphamide[a] (500–750 mg/m$^2$ every 3 months) |
| Calcineurin inhibitors (tacrolimus [preferred], cyclosporine, voclosporin[b]) | Cyclosporine[a] |
| IV rituximab[b] | |
| Belimumab[b] (anti-BLyS mAb) (in addition to standard of care with steroids + cyclophosphamide or mycophenolate mofetil) | Hydroxychloroquine (adjunctive therapy) |
| Plasma exchange (plasmapheresis)[a] | |
| Azathioprine[a] | |

[a]Less commonly used treatment.
[b]Emerging treatment.
From Dooley MA, Houssiau F, Aranow C, et al. Effect of belimumab treatment on renal outcomes: results from the phase 3 belimumab clinical trials in patients with SLE. *Lupus*. 2013;22:63–72.

Another newer alternative to cyclophosphamide for induction phase treatment of SLEN is the use of CNIs. While tacrolimus has become preferred over cyclosporine, there have now been several uncontrolled and a few controlled studies in both children and adults that have collectively reported that tacrolimus (or cyclosporine) is as or more effective than either cyclophosphamide or MMF in inducing partial or complete remissions of disease.[945–950] For induction phase treatment, voclosporin, a new CNI with less variable plasma concentrations, is under investigation in a phase III trial (ClinicalTrials.gov identifier NCT03021499).[949]

Yet another emerging alternative to cyclophosphamide for induction phase treatment is rituximab. This anti-CD20 mAb targets B lymphocytes, which have been implicated in the pathogenesis of SLE and SLEN due to their ability to both present (auto)antigens and produce (auto)antibodies. Several uncontrolled studies in adults and children and one controlled study in adults have reported that rituximab can be relatively effective in inducing partial or complete disease remissions, although variable frequencies of serious side effects were also noted.[951–956]

A less commonly used induction phase treatment is azathioprine. Although there are relatively few data to support its use in this setting, one study reported comparable partial and compete remissions to that of cyclophosphamide, although those patients who received azathioprine experienced more relapses than those who received cyclophosphamide.[957]

Finally, PLEX has also been used infrequently as an induction phase treatment for SLEN, with the rationale that removal of circulating autoantibodies should be clinically beneficial. One randomized trial compared standard treatment with oral glucocorticoids + oral cyclophosphamide with that same treatment combined with 12 plasmapheresis treatments over 4 weeks, but found no differences in either short- or long-term outcomes compared with standard treatment.[958] To date, there is no established role for PLEX or plasmapheresis in the routine induction therapy of SLEN. PLEX may have a role in the treatment of severe SLEN associated with thrombotic microangiopathies or APS.[959–961] Whether it has a role as an adjunctive therapy for severe SLEN refractory to conventional therapy is unclear.[962,963]

Maintenance phase treatment almost always includes oral glucocorticoids, with the dosage minimized to maintain remission while reducing the risk of long-term glucocorticoid side effects. Based on the available data from primarily adult studies, MMF and azathioprine both appear to be more effective than IV cyclophosphamide in preventing relapses,

CKD, and death, with MMF being somewhat more effective than azathioprine.[964–969] Lastly, although not widely used, cyclosporine has also been used for maintenance phase treatment, where it has been reported to have similar long-term outcomes to azathioprine.[970] The optimal duration for maintenance phase treatment of SLEN remains uncertain, although suggested durations have ranged from approximately 2 years to as long as 8 years.[971]

Long-term outcomes for children with SLEN have improved significantly over the last few decades. Improved treatments have resulted in 10-year survival rates that now approach approximately 90%.[972–974] Among those patients with childhood onset of SLE, almost 50% of patients developed cumulative organ damage in one report, and those at highest risk for this were those who presented with CNS involvement and those who had more prolonged disease and received more IV cyclophosphamide.[972] Specifically among children, a recent study of long-term outcomes among 16 children with SLEN reported a cumulative 10-year renal relapse-free survival of 73%, and a cumulative probability that hospitalization would not be required of 94% at 1 year and 71% at 10 years.[975]

## TUBULAR DISORDERS

### FANCONI SYNDROMES—WITH EMPHASIS ON CYSTINOSIS

#### ETIOLOGY

Fanconi syndrome is the result of global proximal tubular dysfunction. It is characterized by the constellation of renal tubular acidosis (RTA), low-molecular-weight proteinuria, amino aciduria, glucosuria, and hypophosphatemia (secondary to renal phosphate wasting). Causes can be subdivided into primary/genetic and secondary. Table 72.17 provides a broad list of causes. Of note, Dent disease and the oculocerebral syndrome of Lowe are described in more detail in the next section discussing urolithiasis and nephrocalcinosis. The most common genetic cause of Fanconi syndrome in childhood is cystinosis, which will be focused on here. Cystinosis is a lysosomal storage disorder. It is the result of a mutation in the *CTNS* gene, encoding the protein cystinosin.[976] Defective cystinosin fails to transport cystine, a product of protein degradation, out of the lysosome into the cytoplasm.[977] Cystine therefore accumulates and precipitates in the lysosome, leading to cell toxicity and the clinical manifestations of the disease. Although cystinosis is the most common genetic cause of Fanconi syndrome, Fanconi syndrome is more likely to be seen as a consequence of drug toxicity, particularly in patients receiving chemotherapy. Finally, there are a number of rheumatological causes of acquired Fanconi syndrome that should be considered in the differential diagnosis (Table 72.17).

**Table 72.17 Causes of Fanconi Syndrome**

| Genetic | |
|---|---|
| | Cystinosis |
| | Dent disease |
| | Galactosemia |
| | Glycogen storage disease (type 1) |
| | Hereditary fructose intolerance |
| | Lowe syndrome |
| | Mitochondrial diseases |
| | Tyrosinemia |
| | Wilson disease |
| Acquired – Drugs | |
| Nucleoside reverse transcriptase inhibitors | Tenofovir, adefovir |
| Nucleoside analogs | Didanosine, lamivudine, stavudine |
| Chemotherapeutics | Ifosfamide, cisplatin, streptozocin |
| Anticonvulsants | Valproic acid |
| Antibiotics | Aminoglycosides, expired tetracyclines |
| Antivirals | Cidofovir |
| Antiparasitics | Suramin |
| Miscellaneous/toxins | Fumaric acid, paraquat |
| Acquired – Other conditions | |
| Amyloidosis | |
| Heavy metals | For example, lead, cadmium, mercury |
| Membranous nephropathy | |
| Multiple myeloma | |
| Paroxysmal nocturia | |
| Postrenal transplantation | |
| Tubulointerstitial nephritis | |
| Vitamin D deficiency | |

#### PRESENTATION

Patients with genetic causes of Fanconi syndrome typically present within the first year of life with manifestations of tubular transport dysfunction including polyuria, polydipsia, hypokalemia, metabolic acidosis, hypophosphatemia, dehydration, and subsequent failure to thrive.[978] This is also the typical presentation for the infantile form of cystinosis, the most common form of the disease. Less commonly, patients with cystinosis present later in childhood with other manifestations of the Fanconi syndrome, often rickets.[979] Because the proximal tubule is the primary site of vitamin D activation, patients with Fanconi syndrome often display vitamin D–deficient rickets.[980] This later presenting form of cystinosis has been referred to as the "late-onset" or "juvenile" form.[978,979] Although the clinical manifestations are the same, juvenile cystinosis is typically less severe, and loss of renal function proceeds less rapidly. Cystinosis is a multiorgan disease; over time patients typically develop a number of other sequalae including hypothyroidism, photophobia, chronic renal failure, myopathy including difficulty swallowing, diabetes mellitus, male hypogonadism, and pulmonary dysfunction.[978,981] Interestingly, an ocular variant of the disease typically manifests in adults[982] and is characterized by eye involvement only. Clinical manifestations include photophobia due to cystine crystal accumulation.

#### DIAGNOSIS

When the clinical features of Fanconi syndrome are identified on urine analysis and blood work (i.e., hypokalemia, hypophosphatemia, nonanion gap metabolic acidosis, low-molecular-weight proteinuria, amino aciduria, and glucosuria), patients should be screened for cystinosis by examining polymorphonuclear cell cysteine concentration.[978] Alternatively, in older patients, examination of the cornea for cystine crystals by slit lamp can be completed. Crystals are universally present after 16 years of age. Finally, molecular genetic testing demonstrating biallelic variants in the *CTNS* gene is also consistent with the diagnosis. In children presenting with Fanconi syndrome in the first year of life, the differential diagnosis should also include tyrosinemia, hereditary fructose intolerance, galactosemia, glycogen storage disease (type 1) mitochondrial disorders, Wilson disease, oculocerebral syndrome of Lowe, and Dent disease.

## TREATMENT

Therapy should be aimed at correcting metabolic abnormalities arising from tubular transport defects. This should include the administration of alkali, typically as potassium or dicitrate, volume replacement, administration of vitamin D, and phosphate replacement.[978] Children who are severely affected may require growth hormone (GH) as well. Patients with cystinosis should receive cysteamine to reduce cellular cysteine levels as soon as the diagnosis is made.[983] This can prevent/delay the onset of other symptoms and protect renal function. Cysteamine eye drops should also be administered to prevent the onset or progression of ocular disease.[984] When children progress to renal failure, renal transplantation will prevent further renal disease. However, cysteamine therapy should be continued in order to prevent nonrenal disease. Adherence to cysteamine therapy has been facilitated by the introduction of the delayed-release cysteamine bitartrate.[985,986]

# DISORDERS OF RENAL TUBULAR NACL TRANSPORT

## BARTTER SYNDROME

### Etiology

Bartter syndrome is typified by hypochloremic, hypokalemic, metabolic alkalosis, and both hyperreninemia and hyperaldosteronism secondary to volume contraction. Clinically, Bartter syndrome can be subdivided into antenatal Bartter syndrome, which presents shortly after birth; classical Bartter syndrome presenting in childhood or adolescence; and Bartter syndrome with deafness.[987] The etiology of each of these various clinical presentations is a mutation in a single gene affecting transport of sodium and chloride across the thick ascending limb (TAL) of the loop of Henle (Table 72.18). Antenatal Bartter syndrome is the result of a mutation in either the *SLC12A1* gene encoding the furosemide-sensitive sodium–potassium–chloride cotransporter, NKCC2, or *KCNJ1,* the gene encoding the renal outer medullary potassium channel, ROMK.[988–990] Classical Bartter syndrome is caused by mutations in the *CLCKNB* gene encoding the chloride voltage-gated channel CLCKb.[991] Bartter syndrome with sensorineural deafness is the result of mutations in either *BSND,* which encodes the accessory protein Barttin required for CLCKb (and CLCKa) activity or disease-causing mutations

**Table 72.18 Gene Defects and Description of Disorders of Tubular Salt Handling**

| Name | Gene Affected[a] | Clinical Description |
|---|---|---|
| **Primary Disorders of the Thick Ascending Limb** | | |
| Bartter syndrome | *SLC12A* | Polyhydramnios, premature delivery, hypokalemic metabolic alkalosis |
| | *KCNJ1* | Polyhydramnios, premature delivery, hypokalemic metabolic alkalosis, transient postnatal hyperkalemia |
| | *CLCKNB* | Childhood/adolescent presentation, hypokalemia, metabolic alkalosis |
| | *BSND*[b] | Polyhydramnios, premature delivery, hypokalemic metabolic alkalosis, and sensorineural hearing loss |
| | *CASR* | Metabolic alkalosis, hypokalemia, hypercalciuria, hypocalcemia with low parathyroid hormone |
| **Primary Disorders of the Distal Convoluted Tubule** | | |
| Gitelman syndrome | *SLC12A3* | Metabolic alkalosis, hypokalemia, hypomagnesemia |
| EAST (epilepsy ataxia sensorineural-deafness tubulopathy) syndrome | *KCNJ10* | Hypokalemic metabolic alkalosis, epilepsy, ataxia, sensorineural deafness |
| Pseudohypoaldosteronism type 2 | *WNK1, WNK4, CUL3,* and *KLH3* | Hyperkalemia, metabolic acidosis, high plasma aldosterone |
| **Primary Disorders of the Collecting Duct** | | |
| Pseudohypoaldosteronism type 1 | *SCNN1A, SCNN1B, SCNN1G* | Hyperkalemia, metabolic acidosis, high plasma aldosterone, autosomal recessive inheritance |
| | *NR3C2* | Hyperkalemia, metabolic acidosis, high plasma aldosterone, autosomal dominant inheritance |
| Liddle syndrome | *SCNN1A, SCNN1B, SCNN1G* (activating) | Hypertension, hypokalemia, suppressed renin and aldosterone |

[a]Unless stated otherwise genetic alterations are inactivating.
[b]Mutations in both *CLCKNB* and *CLCKNA* genes cause a similar phenotype.

in both CLCKa and CLCKb.[992–994] Both CLCKb and CLCKa are expressed in the inner ear and their activity is required for hearing. Activating mutations in the calcium sensing receptor (CaSR), which is expressed in the basolateral membrane of the TAL, inhibit sodium chloride reabsorption from this segment, causing a Bartter-like syndrome.[995,996] However, the phenotype of these patients also includes low plasma calcium and inappropriately low parathyroid hormone (PTH) levels. Finally, polyhydramnios and transient antenatal Bartter syndrome have been ascribed to mutations in the *MAGED2* gene.[997]

Bartter syndrome is classified as type 1 to type 6, which reflects the gene affected. Type 1 is caused by mutations in *SLC12A1*, type 2 by mutations in *KCNJ1*, type 3 by *CLCKNB* mutations, type 4 *BSND* mutations, type 5 by activating mutations in the *CASR*, and type 6 by mutations in both *CLCKNA* and *CLCKNB*. Some references refer to Bartter-like syndromes and include the previous as well as Gitelman syndrome and the EAST (epilepsy ataxia sensorineural-deafness tubulopathy) syndrome (Table 72.18).[998] As these latter two disease processes affect a different part of the nephron and can often be separated clinically by the presence of hypomagnesemia and the absence of hypercalciuria, they are discussed separately in the following sections.

### Presentation

Antenatal Bartter syndrome manifests in utero with polyhydramnios that commonly results in premature delivery. Infants typically present shortly after birth with polyuria, episodes of severe dehydration, recurrent vomiting, and failure to thrive. Significant hypercalciuria and nephrocalcinosis are often present, as 25% of filtered calcium is reabsorbed from the TAL by a process dependent on sodium chloride reabsorption. The presence of hyperkalemia in the first few weeks shortly after birth, which then changes to the classic hypokalemia typical of this syndrome, is seen in patients with mutations in *KCNJ1*.[999] This interesting phenotype has been proposed to be the result of the developmental expression pattern of potassium channels. Specifically, the BK potassium channel of the collecting duct is not expressed until approximately 6 weeks. As such, children with *KCNJ1* mutations cannot effectively excrete potassium until then and therefore become hyperkalemic until after this channel is expressed.[151]

Classical Bartter syndrome manifests itself later in infancy or throughout childhood. Presenting symptoms are varied but can include muscle weakness and cramps, fatigue, constipation, recurrent vomiting, polyuria, and/or significant volume depletion. Hypercalciuria and nephrocalcinosis are not always present. It is noteworthy that *CLCKNB* is also expressed in the basolateral membrane of the distal convoluted tubule (DCT), where it contributes to magnesium reabsorption. Thus in some cases mild hypomagnesemia has been reported.[1000]

Children with antenatal Bartter syndrome and deafness typically present in a similar fashion to antenatal Bartter syndrome, with severe polyhydramnios, premature delivery, polyuria, severe volume contraction, and failure to thrive.[993,994] Hyperkalemia is not a feature. However, auditory testing distinguishes these subtypes as sensorineural hearing is severely affected. Patients with activating mutations in the CaSR can present as previously or secondary to alterations in divalent cation handling, specifically with cramps or seizures. These patients display hypocalcemia, hypercalciuria, hypomagnesemia, and inappropriately low plasma PTH levels.[995,996]

### Diagnosis

Diagnosis is based on analysis of specific genes based on the clinical presentation. A history of significant antenatal polyhydramnios, postnatal polyuria, and typical features of hypokalemic, hypochloremic metabolic acidosis should prompt hearing testing. If this is normal, then examination of *SLC12A1* should be considered. An immediate postnatal history of hyperkalemia shifting to hypokalemia several weeks later should prompt investigation of *KCNJ1*. If abnormalities in sensorineural hearing are detected, examination of the *BSND* gene should ensue, and if normal, then *CLCKB* and/or *CLCKA*. Later presentation without a significant antenatal history should lead one to suspect isolated abnormalities in the *CLCKB* gene. Finally, if serum calcium is low in the presence of low PTH, one needs to consider abnormalities in the CaSR resulting in its inappropriate activation.

### Treatment

There is no cure for Bartter syndrome currently. Treatment should focus on replacing electrolyte losses and mitigating the effects of hyperaldosteronism and increased prostaglandin release.[998] Most patients will require potassium supplementation and younger children might need additional sodium in order to achieve adequate growth. Administration of an NSAID (2–4 mg/kg/day of indomethacin) and a potassium sparing diuretic (spironolactone or amiloride) can help to attenuate the effects of increased prostaglandin release and help to raise the serum potassium level. The addition of an ACE inhibitor should be considered to block the secondary activation of the RAAS; however, some children will have difficulty tolerating this due to blood pressure effects. Long term, approximately one-quarter of patients will develop some degree of renal impairment. However, with attention to electrolyte replacement and administration of indomethacin and amiloride, growth velocity can be recovered and maintained.[1001]

## GITELMAN SYNDROME

Gitelman syndrome is the result of a failure to reabsorb sodium and chloride from the DCT. Patients with this syndrome display hypochloremic, hypokalemic metabolic alkalosis. In contrast to Bartter syndrome–affected children, patients manifest hypocalciuria and hypomagnesemia.[1002] The only identified etiology of this disease to date is a mutation in *SLC12A3*, which encodes the sodium-chloride cotransporter (NCC), expressed in the apical membrane of the DCT (Table 72.18).[989] Presentation of Gitelman syndrome is similar to classical Bartter syndrome, although patients often present later in life, including as adults. The clinical picture varies and can range from growth retardation through milder manifestations such as muscle weakness, cramping, and electrolyte abnormalities.[997]

Molecular diagnostics should be considered in patients with typical electrolyte abnormalities, including hypomagnesemia. Treatment requires replacement of electrolytes, in particular potassium and magnesium. The long-term outcome is excellent for these patients; however, potassium and magnesium supplementation at higher doses can lead to some gastrointestinal upset.[997] Because urinary prostaglandin excretion is not elevated in this syndrome, administration of prostaglandin synthesis inhibitors is not indicated.[1003]

## EAST SYNDROME

EAST syndrome is a rare multiorgan disease that also includes renal salt losing due to a failure of sodium and chloride reabsorption from the DCT.[1004] The renal phenotype is thus very similar to Gitelman syndrome. Patients display hypokalemic metabolic alkalosis and hypomagnesemia due to renal wasting of this divalent cation. In contrast to Gitelman syndrome, patients with EAST syndrome also display epilepsy, ataxia, sensorineural deafness, and a tubulopathy. This condition is caused by mutations in the *KCNJ10* gene, which encodes the Kir4.1 potassium channel that is expressed in the basolateral membrane of the DCT (Table 72.18).[1004] This syndrome has also been referred to as the SeSAME syndrome, an acronym for seizures, sensorineural deafness, ataxia, mental retardation and electrolyte imbalance.[1005] Treatment of the renal manifestations includes replacement of electrolytes as in Gitelman syndrome.

## PSEUDOHYPOALDOSTERONISM

Pseudohypoaldosteronism (PHA) is a collection of rare heterogeneous syndromes characterized primarily by mineralocorticoid resistance, resulting in reduced potassium and proton excretion from the collecting duct.[1006] The clinical constellation of hyperkalemia, metabolic acidosis, and increased plasma aldosterone levels is universally present. In some subtypes there is also significant salt wasting. PHA has been subdivided into three subtypes, which are described in the following sections (Table 72.18).

### PHA Type I

PHA type I is characterized by presentation in infancy with life-threatening hyperkalemic metabolic acidosis and severe salt wasting tubulopathy leading to dehydration and failure to thrive.[1007] Both plasma renin and aldosterone levels are extremely high. PHA type I can be further subdivided into an autosomal recessive form that is the result of abnormalities in the genes encoding the different subunits of the ENaC, *SCNN1A*, *SCNN1B*, and *SCNN1G*.[1008] This autosomal recessive form can be distinguished from the autosomal dominant form as ENaC is also expressed in sweat glands, the lung, and the colon, and manifests as a multiorgan disease including the skin, respiratory as well as renal dysfunction.[1009] The autosomal dominant form is limited to renal resistance to mineralocorticoids and typically displays a less severe phenotype. Metabolic acidosis may be absent, but salt losing is a persistent feature. Autosomal dominant PHA type I is due to mutations in *NR3C2*, the gene encoding the mineralocorticoid receptor.[1010] Treatment of both varieties of PHA type I requires attention to sodium replacement enabling volume expansion. Potassium binders are also frequently necessary.

### PHA Type II

In contrast to PHA type 1, patients with PHA type II, which has also been called Gordon syndrome, do not display a salt-losing phenotype. Rather, patients with this disorder display hyperkalemia and hypertension.[1011] This heterogeneous disorder is the result of increased sodium chloride reabsorption from the DCT, leading to volume expansion and suppressed renin levels. It is the result of alterations in a variety of genes including *WNK1*, *WNK2*, *CUL3*, and *KLHL3*.[1012,1013] Given that this disorder consists of increased sodium chloride transport from the DCT, simply blocking this pathway with a thiazide diuretic generally ameliorates the symptoms of this disease.[1012]

## LIDDLE SYNDROME

The inappropriate increase of sodium and chloride transport from the collecting duct results in volume expansion and hypertension in the presence of suppressed renin and aldosterone levels, a syndrome referred to as Liddle syndrome. This constellation of clinical features is due to activating mutations in one of the genes encoding the ENaC, *SCNN1A*, *SCNN1B*, or *SCNN1G* (Table 72.18).[1014–1017] As in Gordon syndrome, therapy is directed at inhibiting the primary mechanism and involves treatment with the ENaC inhibitor amiloride. Although required life-long, this therapy completely prevents the manifestations of this disease.

## RENAL TUBULAR ACIDOSIS

A nonanion gap metabolic acidosis is consistent with the presence of an RTA. However, especially in young children, it is more common to demonstrate a nonanion gap metabolic acidosis as a result of diarrhea. Therefore diarrheal illnesses must first be excluded as a cause of the nonanion gap metabolic acidosis. The nephron segment affected has been used to classify different RTAs.[1018] Abnormalities in proton excretion from the distal nephron are classified as distal or type I RTA. A failure to reabsorb bicarbonate from the proximal tubule is referred to as a proximal or type II RTA. Finally, type IV, which is also called hyperkalemic RTA, is due to aldosterone resistance or absence. Type III, or mixed RTA, is a rare disease that displays both a failure to reabsorb bicarbonate from the proximal tubule and the inability to secrete protons from the distal nephron.

Examination of plasma electrolytes is useful in identifying the subtype of the RTA. Types I and II typically display normal or low serum potassium levels while patients with type IV have high serum potassium.[1019] Consideration of the etiology of the disease helps to further distinguish between proximal and distal RTAs. Patients with proximal RTA maintain an ability to secrete protons into the urine. Thus when not receiving treatment, they should display a urine pH less than 5.5. Children with proximal RTA display a bicarbonate reabsorption threshold above which they will spill bicarbonate into the urine.[1020] Thus when administered alkali they have an alkaline urine. Another approach to determine urine acidification is the urine anion gap.[1021] Protons secreted into the urine are trapped by ammonia, forming ammonium ($NH_4^+$). While ammonium is difficult to measure in the urine, a surrogate is to calculate the difference between urine cations ($Na^+ + K^+$) and urine $Cl^-$. When acidotic, the patient should be secreting protons into their urine, forming ammonium, and therefore display a negative anion gap (urine $Na^+ + K^+ - Cl^- < 0$). If this is not the case, then there is a failure to secrete protons by the distal nephron and the patient has a distal RTA. If the previous does not clarify the etiology of the disease, then more definitive testing can be employed. The traditional means of diagnosing proximal RTA is to bicarbonate load the patient in order to correct the acidosis and demonstrate a significant increase in fractional excretion of bicarbonate, that is, to greater than 15%.[1020] Distal RTA is definitively demonstrated by either an acid load with ammonium chloride (100 mg/kg), which is poorly tolerated, or by administrating furosemide and fludrocortisone and monitoring urine pH over the next 8 hours.[1022,1023] Patients with distal RTA are not able to acidify their urine below pH 5.3.

### Type I, Distal Renal Tubular Acidosis

The most common form of RTA is type I, or distal RTA. Clinically patients with this disorder display hypercalciuria, hypocitraturia, nephrolithiasis, and nephrocalcinosis.[1024] Untreated disease often results in failure to thrive, bone demineralization, and rickets.[1025] The etiology of this disorder is either primary, that is, genetic, or acquired secondarily from drug toxicity, or a rheumatological condition. Genetic causes of distal RTA include mutations in the genes encoding machinery required for the secretion of protons from alpha intercalated cells of the collecting duct, specifically the plasma membrane $H^+$ATPase, that is, *ATP6V1B1* or *ATP6V0A4*,[1026–1029] or the basolateral chloride–bicarbonate exchanger AE1 (gene name *SLC4A1*; Table 72.19).[1026,1030–1032] The gene affected results in slightly different clinical manifestations. Mutations in *SLC4A1* produce a milder phenotype, which might not manifest itself clinically until the teenage years or adulthood, and is often inherited in an autosomal dominant fashion. By contrast, patients with mutations in the subunits of the $H^+$ATPase typically have more severe disease, which often presents in infancy and is commonly associated with deafness.

### Type II, Proximal Renal Tubular Acidosis

Proximal RTA rarely occurs in isolation and is much more frequently seen as a part of the Fanconi syndrome, that is, with hypophosphatemia, glycosuria, aminoaciduria, and low-molecular-weight proteinuria. Common causes of the Fanconi syndrome in childhood have been described earlier and in Table 72.17. Patients with isolated RTA rarely have renal calculi or nephrocalcinosis, potentially due to the increased urinary citrate excretion that typically accompanies this disorder.[1024] They also tend not to display abnormalities in bone mineral density or rickets. Isolated proximal RTA is caused by mutations in the basolateral sodium-bicarbonate exchanger NBCe1 (gene name *SLC4A4*), which is essential to the reclamation of filtered bicarbonate from the proximal tubule (Table 72.19).[1033–1037] Patients with mutations in this gene also display ocular abnormalities and mental retardation.

**Table 72.19 Renal Tubular Acidosis Characteristics and Single-Gene Defects Causing Renal Tubular Acidosis**

| Gene | Inheritance | Associated Clinical Features |
|---|---|---|
| **Type I – Distal Renal Tubular Acidosis** | | |
| *ATP6V1B1* | AR | Nephrocalcinosis/ nephrolithiasis, sensorineural hearing loss |
| *ATP6V0A4* | AR | Nephrocalcinosis/ nephrolithiasis, late-onset sensorineural hearing loss |
| *SLC4A1* | AD (rarely AR) | Nephrocalcinosis, osteomalacia with AR inheritance can be associated with hemolytic anemia |
| **Type II – Proximal Renal Tubular Acidosis** | | |
| *SLC4A4* | | Cataracts, glaucoma, band keratopathy |
| **Type III – Mixed Renal Tubular Acidosis** | | |
| *CA2* | | Osteopetrosis |

Causes of type IV, hyperkalemic metabolic acidosis, are described in Table 72.1.
*AD*, Autosomal dominant; *AR*, autosomal recessive.

### Type IV, Hyperkalemic Renal Tubular Acidosis

Patients with type IV RTA display resistance to, or an absence of, aldosterone effect on the distal nephron. Patients typically display a milder degree of acidosis and hyperkalemia, which is proportionate to the degree of aldosterone deficiency. This disease can be the result of drug administration such as NSAIDs, ACE inhibitors, CNIs or potassium-sparing diuretics, obstructive uropathy, or due to a single gene defect such as occurs in PHA, which is described earlier.

### A Note on Type III, Renal Tubular Acidosis

A failure to reabsorb bicarbonate from the proximal tubule and acidify the urine is known as a mixed, or type III RTA. This rare autosomal recessive disorder is a consequence of mutations in carbonic anhydrase II (CAII, gene name *CA2*), which is required for both processes (Table 72.19).[1038,1039] Type III RTA is a complex syndrome; in addition to RTA, patients also demonstrate osteopetrosis, cerebral calcifications, and mental retardation.[1040] Further features that have been associated with the disorder include facial bone overgrowth resulting in facial dysmorphism, conductive hearing loss, and blindness.

Treatment of RTA involves supplementation with alkali to normalize plasma pH. In the hypokalemic forms of the disease this is best supplied as potassium citrate.[1041] The amount of supplementation required to treat the disease differs depending on the cause, with distal RTA requiring much less supplementation (typically 1–2 mEq/kg/day of alkali) than proximal RTA (which can require upward of 10 mEq/kg/day of alkali). In patients with distal RTA, treatment should also include minimizing the risk of stone formation and renal calcification as this can lead to renal insufficiency.[1042] To this end, thiazide diuretics and increased fluid intake should be considered.

## NEPHROGENIC DIABETES INSIPIDUS

### Etiology

A failure to respond to the action of arginine vasopressin (AVP) results in nephrogenic diabetes insipidus (NDI).[1043] AVP is released in response to increased plasma osmolarity and results in the phosphorylation and insertion of aquaporin-2 into the apical membrane of principal cells of the collecting duct, allowing water to be reabsorbed.[1044] NDI can be either congenital (i.e., genetic) or acquired. The majority (90%) of congenital diabetes insipidus is the result of mutations in the AVP receptor, V2R, encoded by the gene *AVPR2*.[1045,1046] The other roughly 10% are due to mutations in aquaporin-2, encoded by *AQP2*.[1047] *AVPR2* mutations are inherited in an X-linked recessive fashion, whereas AQP2 mutations occur in an autosomal recessive manner. Acquired NDI can be the result of renal injury (i.e., AKI, obstructive uropathy, renal dysplasia, tubulointerstitial nephritis, cystic kidney diseases, or nephronophthisis) or drug toxicity (i.e., lithium, ifosfamide, foscarnet, and amphotericin B).

#### Presentation

Congenital forms of NDI tend to be more severe and present in infancy with polyuria, hypernatremic dehydration, fever, irritability, constipation, and failure to thrive.[1048] In contrast to Bartter syndrome, polyhydramnios is not a feature. Infants who are breastfed have less severe features, likely due to their reduced solute load. Untreated patients can present later in childhood with enuresis and mental retardation.[1049] Overall the symptoms tend to improve with age.

#### Diagnosis

The diagnosis of NDI requires the demonstration that urine osmolarity cannot be concentrated in the presence of desmopressin (1-deamino-8-D-arginine vasopressin [ddAVP]). This is demonstrated by performing a ddAVP challenge, and monitoring urine concentration. ddAVP can be administered intranasally, orally, intramuscularly, or intravenously. Administration of ddAVP by the intramuscular or intranasal route requires longer monitoring than oral or IV administration (6 vs. 4 hours). A diagnosis of NDI is established by the failure of the urine osmolarity to increase above 200 mOsm in this time frame. The development of a urine osmolarity greater than 200 mOsm but less than 800 mOsm in children (and <500 mOsm in infants) is consistent with a partial NDI. It is noteworthy that activation of V2R mediates peripheral vasodilation, thus patients with mutations of *AQP2* display tachycardia and reduced blood pressure in response to IV ddAVP, in contrast to children with mutations of V2R.

#### Treatment

It is important to make the diagnosis of NDI early and treat patients aggressively to avoid complications arising from severe and frequent hypernatremia. Adequate fluid intake should be insured (at least 150 mL/kg/day), which becomes easier as children age and can respond to thirst. A thiazide diuretic (i.e., hydrochlorothiazide 2 mg/kg/day) can be employed to increase proximal sodium and consequently water reabsorption and decrease urine output. Amiloride (0.2 mg/kg/day) can also be employed to reduce urine output, via a similar mechanism. Indomethacin (1–3 mg/kg/day) has also been demonstrated to be useful in reducing urine volume, perhaps by reducing GFR. Typically, a combination of these drugs are employed initially to reduce urine output. The combination of amiloride, a potassium sparing diuretic, and hydrochlorothiazide is beneficial to maintain normal plasma potassium levels.

There are several promising new therapies for this disease. Vaptans such as tolvaptan are small-molecule agonists that bind V2R. Many mutations in V2R cause protein misfolding and intracellular retention. These membrane-permeant drugs are proposed to rescue the receptor to the cell surface, thereby ameliorating the disease.[1050] Further, as the majority of patients have functional aquaporin-2 water channels, different attempts have been made to stimulate their phosphorylation and trafficking to the cell surface by activating the pathway downstream of V2R.[1051] Most promising has been the administration of phosphodiesterase inhibitors such as sildenafil[1052] or agonists of other G-protein coupled receptors expressed in the principal cell such as the prostanoid receptor butaprost.[1053] Finally, statins have been proposed to alter the principal cell membrane cholesterol content in a way that promotes the recruitment of aquaporin-2 to the apical plasma membrane.[1054,1055]

## UROLITHIASIS AND NEPHROCALCINOSIS IN CHILDREN

### EPIDEMIOLOGY

Although a common disorder in adults, affecting up to 10% of adult males, the frequency of kidney stone formation in childhood is much lower. However, the incidence of urolithiasis in children is increasing, accounting for a greater number of emergency room visits and hospitalizations.[1056,1057] The reason for this increasing incidence is unclear, although it is speculated to be the result of increased sensitivity of radiographic techniques, the increased incidence of childhood obesity, increased consumption of processed foods contributing to increased sodium chloride consumption, or the result of a greater number of surviving premature infants who are treated with medications causing urolithiasis.[1056,1057] In contrast to adults, males are not more frequently affected; indeed, emerging evidence suggests that girls more commonly suffer from kidney stones, especially during adolescence.[1058] Ultimately, when the mechanisms preventing the precipitation of solutes in urine are overwhelmed, calculi are precipitated, causing the signs and symptoms of urolithiasis

### RISK FACTORS

#### HYPERCALCIURIA

Most kidney stones are composed of calcium oxalate, and the next most frequent type of stone is calcium phosphate. Perhaps not surprisingly then, the most common risk factor for kidney stone formation is the generation of urine containing an increased concentration of calcium.[1059,1060] Because of the difficulty in collecting a 24-hour urine in younger children, hypercalciuria is often diagnosed by a spot urine collection and then normalizing the concentration of urine calcium to urine creatinine. Importantly, urinary calcium excretion decreases with age.[1061,1062] Normal values are listed in Table 72.20.[1061,1063–1066] The majority of calcium filtered by the renal glomerulus is reabsorbed from the proximal tubule and TAL by a passive paracellular process.[1067] Therefore a common cause of hypercalciuria is excess sodium chloride ingestion. Metabolic acidosis causes hypercalciuria via liberation from bone.[1024] Multiple drugs induce hypercalciuria including loop diuretics, vitamin D (in high doses), and corticosteroids.

The most common etiology of hypercalciuria in childhood is idiopathic. However, the genetics of this “unknown” cause of hypercalciuria have begun to be unraveled with the discovery of the CaSR–claudin-14 axis (Table 72.21). This axis refers to the ability for the TAL to sense circulating plasma calcium levels via the basolaterally expressed CaSR and respond by increasing the expression of the tight junction protein claudin-14.[1068] This claudin blocks paracellular calcium reabsorption from the TAL, increasing urinary calcium excretion. Subtle variations in the *CaSR* gene as well as intronic

**Table 72.20 Normal Pediatric Values for Urinary Excretion of Solutes**

| Solute | Ratio; Solute/Creatinine | | 24-Hour Urinary Excretion |
|---|---|---|---|
| **Calcium** | **mol/mol** | **g/g** | |
| <1 year | <2.2 | <0.8 | <0.1 mmol/kg |
| 1–3 years | <1.5 | <0.53 | <4 mg/kg |
| 3–5 years | <1.1 | <0.4 | |
| 5–7 years | <0.8 | <0.3 | |
| >7 years | <0.6 | <0.2 | |
| **Citrate** | **mol/mol** | **g/g** | |
| 0–5 years | 0.12–0.25 | 0.20–0.42 | >0.8 mmol/1.73 $m^2$ |
| >5 years | 0.08–0.15 | 0.14–0.25 | >0.14 g/1.73 $m^2$ |
| **Oxalate** | **mmol/mol** | **mg/g** | |
| <1 year | 15–260 | 12–207 | <0.5 mmol/1.73 $m^2$ |
| 1–5 years | 11–120 | 9–96 | <45 mg/1.73 $m^2$ |
| 5–12 years | 60–150 | 47–119 | |
| >12 years | 2–80 | 2–64 | |
| **Uric Acid** | **mol/mol** | **g/g** | |
| <1 year | <1.5 | <2.2 | >1 year; <815 mg/1.73 $m^2$ |
| 1–3 years | <1.3 | <1.9 | |
| 3–5 years | <1.0 | <1.5 | |
| 5–10 years | <0.6 | <0.9 | |
| >10 years | <0.4 | <0.6 | |
| **Cystine** | **mmol/mol** | **mg/g** | |
| <1 month | <85 | <180 | <10 years: < 55 μmol/1.73 $m^2$ |
| 1–6 months | <53 | <112 | >10 years: < 200 μmol/1.73 $m^2$ |
| >6 months | <18 | <38 | >18 years: < 250 μmol/1.73 $m^2$ |

**Table 72.21 Genetic Conditions Displaying Hypercalciuria**

| Condition Name | Gene(s) | Clinical Features |
|---|---|---|
| Dent disease | *CLCN5* | Nephrocalcinosis, low-molecular-weight proteinuria, X-linked inheritance |
| Oculocerebral syndrome of Lowe | *OCRL* | Congenital cataracts, mental retardation, hypotonia, rickets, partial or complete Fanconi syndrome |
| Bartter syndrome | *SLC112A1, KCNJ1, CLCKNB, BSND* | Hypokalemic metabolic alkalosis, nephrocalcinosis |
| Autosomal dominant hypocalcemia and hypercalciuria | *CASR* | Hypocalcemia, suppressed parathyroid hormone, hypokalemic metabolic alkalosis |
| Familial hypomagnesemia hypercalciuria and nephrocalcinosis | *CLDN16, CLDN19* | Hypomagnesemia, hypercalciuria, nephrocalcinosis, progressive renal impairment, macular colobomata, myopia horizontal nystagmus (CCLDN19 mutations only) |
| Distal renal tubular acidosis | *ATP6V0A4, ATP6V1B1, SLC4A1* | Nephrocalcinosis, kidney stones, renal tubular acidosis |
| Williams syndrome | ??? | Cardiovascular disease, triangular facies, connective tissue abnormalities, intellectual disabilities |

variations in the *CLDN14* gene appear to inappropriately cause increased claudin-14 expression and calciuria.[1069–1072] Further, mutations in the TAL paracellular calcium pore forming claudin-16 also contribute to idiopathic hypercalciuria.[1073] Finally, there are multiple genetic syndromes, which have as a component of their phenotype hypercalciuria. They are discussed in the next section on the genetics of pediatric urolithiasis and nephrocalcinosis.

## HYPOCITRATURIA

Citrate binds calcium in the urine and prevents the precipitation of calcium salts. Thus a consequence of hypocitraturia is the formation of calcium containing urolithiasis. Although affecting approximately 10% of children with urolithiasis, the etiology of reduced urinary citrate excretion is unclear, except in specific genetic conditions such as distal RTA.[1074]

Another approach to detecting low urinary citrate excretion has been to evaluate the calcium-to-citrate ratio (rather than citrate-to-creatinine ratio). This has helped to identify children who might benefit from therapy.[1075]

### HYPERURICOSURIA

A small fraction of children with nephrolithiasis (approximately 5%) will display hyperuricosuria. Like urinary calcium excretion, urinary urate excretion is highest in infants and decreases with age. In fact, the concentration of uric acid in the urine of infants can be so high that it precipitates as crystals and can be confused with blood. Normal values for urinary uric acid excretion are presented in Table 72.20. Traditionally, uric acid stones have been seen in children with overproduction due to tumor lysis syndrome, although the frequency of this has been greatly reduced with the introduction of urate oxidases such as rasburicase. Other causes include high dietary purine intake and hemolysis.[1076] There are also a number of rare genetic disorders, which result in increased urinary uric acid secretion, which are outlined later.

### HYPEROXALURIA

After hypercalciuria, hyperoxaluria is the next most common urinary abnormality seen in children with urolithiasis.[1077] The etiology of hyperoxaluria is most frequently idiopathic, although a number of primary and secondary causes should be considered. Secondary causes are much more frequent than primary genetic disorders. Increased ingestion of oxalate or oxalate precursors such as vitamin C can lead to hyperoxaluria as can pyridoxine deficiency or ingestion of methanol. Alternatively, hyperabsorption of oxalate from the intestine, which can be due to a variety of diseases that lead to fat malabsorption including inflammatory bowel disease, post-bowel resection, pancreatic insufficiency, or biliary disease, can cause hyperoxaluria. The mechanism mediating this is via excess intestinal luminal fat binding calcium, leading to increased free oxalate in the intestinal lumen that can be more readily absorbed, and subsequently excreted in the urine. Therapies aimed at improving the underlying disorder, decreased oxalate ingestion, increasing free water intake, and added calcium administration help to treat this form of hyperoxaluria.[1040,1078]

### ALTERED URINARY FLOW AND INFECTIONS

A nonmetabolic risk factor for kidney stone formation is urinary stasis or abnormal urinary flow. Children with congenital abnormalities of the kidney and urinary tract are more likely to develop kidney stones. UTIs with urea-splitting organisms such as *Proteus* spp. can alkalinize the urine and increase ammonium production. This in turn favors the formation of struvite stones (magnesium ammonium phosphate).[1079] These stones typically fill multiple renal calyces in a staghorn configuration. Patients with neurogenic bladders who have undergone surgical procedures including ileal augmentation are at increased risk of struvite stone formation.[1076]

## PRESENTATION

Infants and younger children often do not present with typical flank pain radiating to the groin.[1058,1080] Further, a significant fraction of children may not even display hematuria. Instead young children can present with nonspecific abdominal pain, dysuria, frequency, urgency, emesis, diarrhea, or a UTI.[1081] Of note, patients with hypercalciuria are at increased risk of developing a UTI independent of urinary tract abnormalities.[1082,1083] Why hypercalciuria predisposes to UTI is not clear; perhaps crystals in the urinary tract form nidus for bacteria to adhere to. Adolescents more commonly present like adults with renal colic. However, as noted earlier, there is not a clear male preponderance.

## DIAGNOSIS

Having a high index of suspicion is key in younger children. The radiologic test of preference is a renal ultrasound as it avoids exposure to ionizing radiation. Unfortunately, despite significant advances in ultrasound technology, smaller stones and stones in the calyces, papillae, or ureter may be missed by this technique.[1084] Large radiopaque stones are visible on plain films of the abdomen; however, helical noncontrast computed tomography (CT) examination is the most sensitive test and should be considered when ultrasound is negative and there is a high index of suspicion.[1085] Helical CT has the added benefit of providing further information with regard to anatomy and obstruction.

Examining urine for the presence of crystals is also useful. Identification of colorless hexagonal crystals are diagnostic of cystinuria. Large rectangular crystals are consistent with hyperoxaluria and calcium oxalate stone formation. Further clues can be provided by urine examination for hypercalciuria, hyperoxaluria, cystinuria, and hyperuricosuria. Serum calcium, phosphorus, uric acid, and electrolytes should be measured and can help identify the underlying cause.

## TREATMENT

Renal calculi greater than 7 mm are unlikely to pass and elective surgical removal should be considered.[1080] Other indications for surgical removal include single kidney, prolonged obstruction, significant pain, or infection. Surgical options include extracorporeal shock wave lithotripsy (for stones >2 cm), percutaneous nephrolithotomy, and ureteroscopy. It may be necessary to leave a ureteral stent in some patients in order to dilate the ureter before extraction can be accomplished. For stones impacted in a ureter, medical expulsive therapy can be considered. This includes hydration and use of either an α-adrenergic blocker or a calcium channel blocker. While significant evidence of the effectiveness of these therapies exists for adults, there is only anecdotal evidence available for children.[1086,1087]

Dietary advice should otherwise be provided to decrease the risk of recurrence, which is significant in infants and children.[1088] Fluid intake should be increased to approximately 2 L/m$^2$ to both dilute precipitating solutes and help with the passage of stones in situ. In patients with hyperoxaluria, a low oxalate diet should be recommended. Hypercalciuric patients (and indeed most patients) benefit from a normal sodium diet (i.e., at the minimum <2000 mg sodium chloride per day). Restriction of calcium should be avoided,[1089] as this can be paradoxically associated with hypercalciuria due to the dissolution of calcium from bone. Instead attention should be paid to ensuring adequate calcium intake. High fructose containing beverages should be avoided.[1090] Finally, in contrast to adults, a low protein diet is not recommended due to potential adverse consequences on growth.

Medical therapy should target underlying metabolic risk factors. Patients with hyperuricosemia typically benefit from allopurinol. Patients with hypocitraturia should receive potassium citrate. It is not recommended to alkalinize the urine of all stone formers as this simply changes the forming calcium oxalate stones to calcium phosphate. Patients with hypercalciuria, besides the many dietary recommendations suggested earlier, may also benefit from administration of a thiazide (i.e., 1–2 mg/kg per day of hydrochlorothiazide). Thiazides, in blocking sodium reabsorption from the DCT, augment sodium and consequently calcium reabsorption from the proximal nephron, thereby contributing a hypocalciuric effect.[1091]

## GENETICS OF PEDIATRIC UROLITHIASIS AND NEPHROCALCINOSIS

### HYPERCALCIURIA-INDUCING CONDITIONS

#### WILLIAMS SYNDROME

Williams syndrome is characterized by a constellation of cardiovascular disease (typically peripheral pulmonary stenosis but can include supravalvular aortic stenosis or hypertension), a distinctive triangular facies, connective tissue abnormalities, intellectual disability (typically not severe), unique personality features, early puberty, and in up to 50% of cases hypercalcemia in infancy, hypercalciuria, and nephrocalcinosis.[1092] The etiology of this disorder is a 7q11.23 contiguous deletion of the Williams–Beuren syndrome critical region encompassing the elastin gene (Table 72.21). It is unclear why a deletion of this region results in hypercalcemia, hypercalciuria, and nephrocalcinosis. Hypercalcemia tends to resolve by the age of 4.[1093] The hypercalciuria responds to typical treatments including increased fluid intake, a reduced sodium diet, and thiazide diuretics, and this treatment should be considered, especially when nephrocalcinosis is present.

#### DENT DISEASE/OCULOCEREBRAL SYNDROME OF LOWE

Dent disease is typically an X-linked recessive disorder characterized by hypercalciuria, nephrocalcinosis, low-molecular-weight proteinuria, and renal insufficiency with some patients progressing to renal failure.[1094] Dent disease can also be associated with the complete Fanconi syndrome. It is most commonly caused by a mutation in *CLCN5,* which encodes a chloride-proton exchanger expressed at high levels in the kidney, with the highest levels in the proximal tubule and TAL (Table 72.21).[1095,1096] The exact molecular pathophysiology is unclear, especially with regard to the pathogenesis of hypercalciuria and nephrocalcinosis. However, defects in CLCN5 appear to cause an impairment of endocytosis, which somehow results in the clinical phenotype observed.

A smaller fraction of patients with the Dent phenotype, described earlier, do not have mutations in CLCN5, but instead display variations in the *OCRL* gene, which encodes the oculocerebral syndrome of Lowe protein 1.[1097] This protein is an inositol polyphosphate 5-phosphatase, which regulates endomembrane lysosomal sorting. More typically individuals with mutations in *OCRL* have congenital cataracts, mental retardation, muscle hypotonia, and rickets as well as evidence of partial or complete Fanconi syndrome.[1098,1099] Renal insufficiency can occur in more severely affected individuals, which are predominantly boys as this is also an X-linked disorder.

#### BARTTER SYNDROMES

Disorders of TAL sodium and chloride reabsorption are often accompanied by hypercalciuria and nephrocalcinosis. This association is the direct consequence of transcellular sodium-chloride transport being necessary for passive paracellular calcium (and magnesium) reabsorption from this nephron segment. Hypercalciuria and nephrocalcinosis tend to be more severe in neonatal Bartter syndrome patients with mutations in *SLC12A1* and *KCNJ1* than in patients with classical Bartter syndrome due to mutations in *CLCKNB.*[1100]

#### AUTOSOMAL DOMINANT HYPOCALCEMIA WITH HYPERCALCIURIA

Children with activating mutations in either the CaSR or the G protein coupled to CaSR display a phenotype characterized by hypokalemia, hypercalciuria, and hypoparathyroidism.[996,1101] Interestingly, there is at least one other gene responsible for this disease that has yet to be identified.[1102] The CaSR resides both in the parathyroid gland and in the nephron, including the basolateral membrane of the TAL. In the TAL, activation of the CaSR not only prevents paracellular calcium reabsorption by increasing claudin-14 expression in this segment, but also inhibits sodium and chloride reabsorption. Hence patients with these mutations can also demonstrate a Bartter phenotype (Table 72.21).[996] This is why these mutations have also been referred to as Bartter syndrome type 5 causing mutations. Treatment of these defects is slightly different than classical Bartter syndrome as administration of active vitamin D is required to elevate serum calcium levels as is a thiazide diuretic to reduce urinary calcium excretion. Unfortunately, this can lead to hypokalemia, which can be remedied by addition of a potassium-sparing diuretic in a combined diuretic such as aldactazide.

#### FAMILIAL HYPOMAGNESEMIA HYPERCALCIURIA AND NEPHROCALCINOSIS

The clinical constellation of hypomagnesemia (secondary to renal wasting), hypercalciuria, and nephrocalcinosis is due to a mutation in either claudin-16 or claudin-19.[1103–1105] Both these tight junction proteins are expressed in the TAL of the loop of Henle where they are essential to forming a paracellular divalent cation permeable pore. Consequently, disruption in the structure of one of these pore forming claudins prevents the reabsorption of calcium and magnesium from the TAL, leading to the clinical phenotype. Unfortunately, a majority of patients tend to progress to renal impairment with upward of 50% requiring RRT.[1106] Clinically, mutations in claudin-19 can be distinguished from claudin-16 alterations by the presence of ocular abnormalities including macular colobomata, myopia, and horizontal nystagmus.[1105] Claudin-19 is also expressed to a high level in the eye consistent with this phenotype. Interestingly, milder mutations in claudin-16 have been proposed to cause isolated hypercalciuria in the presence of only mild hypomagnesemia or without any alteration in plasma magnesium (Table 72.21).[1073]

### DISTAL RENAL TUBULAR ACIDOSIS

Type 1, or distal RTA, is due to a defect in the ability to secrete protons into the urine. This is a result of mutations in either genes encoding the plasma membrane $H^+$ATPase (i.e., *ATP6V1B1* or *ATP6V0A4*) or the basolateral chloride bicarbonate exchanger, AE1 (gene name *SLC4a1*; Table 72.21). In contrast to proximal RTA, distal RTA is often accompanied by hypercalciuria and nephrocalcinosis, perhaps due to hypocitraturia, which is not seen with proximal RTA.[1024] Nephrocalcinosis has been proposed to contribute to renal dysfunction in these patients, thus treatment of the hypercalciuria is recommended to prevent renal insufficiency. Finally, it should be considered that patients with incomplete distal RTA due to mutations in *SLC4a1* may display hypercalciuria and kidneys stones.[1107]

### HEREDITARY HYPOPHOSPHATEMIC RICKETS WITH HYPERCALCIURIA

This syndrome presents with rickets, short stature, and increased renal phosphate excretion despite hypophosphatemia and hypercalciuria. It is the result of mutations in the type 2, sodium phosphate transporter isoform C, encoded by the gene *SLC34a3*.[1108] This transporter contributes significant phosphate reabsorption from the proximal tubule, and when not functioning leads to a primary renal leak. As a consequence, serum phosphate levels are reduced, driving the suppression of PTH and increasing 1,25-dihydroxyvitamin D synthesis. This leads to increased intestinal phosphate and calcium absorption, resulting in hypercalciuria.

## NONCALCIUM WASTING DISORDERS

### CYSTINURIA

This is a rare autosomal recessive cause of kidney stone formation. The primary defect is in the reabsorption of dibasic amino acids, specifically cysteine, ornithine, arginine, and lysine.[1109] These amino acids are reabsorbed from the glomerular filtrate in the proximal tubule via the amino acid transporters encoded by the *SLC3A1* or *SLC7A9* genes. Mutations in *SLC34A1* cause type A cystinuria and *SLC7A9* type B cystinuria.[1110,1111] They are clinically indistinguishable and do not appear to correlate with disease severity or response to therapy. Moreover, compound heterozygotes with monoallelic mutations in both genes do not display altered urinary dibasic amino acid excretion.[1112]

Patients can present at any age, but typically present in the early teens. Severe cases may present in the first year of life. Diagnosis is suggested by family history and confirmed by isolation of pathognomonic hexagonal crystals on urinalysis.[1109] Incident patients with kidney stones can be screened with the cyanide-nitroprusside test. A positive result of this screening study should be confirmed with high-performance liquid chromatography for urine amino acids. Urinary cystine excretion increases with age and normal values can be found in Table 72.20. Patients with cystinuria generally display more than five times the upper limit for age. Patients with Fanconi syndrome and heterozygotes will have intermediate excretion values; however, these patients tend not to form stones with this amount of cysteine excretion.

First-line therapy should include increased fluid intake, urinary alkalization, and a lower sodium containing diet. In cases where significant cystinuria persists despite these measures a number of therapies have been proposed. Alpha-mercaptopropionylglycine forms a soluble dimer with cysteine and can be administered at a dose of 10 to 15 mg/kg/day.[1113] This therapy reduces new stone formation and may dissolve existing calculi. D-penicillamine is a chelating agent that binds to cysteine and homocysteine increasing their solubility. This compound has the potential for significant side effects including renal and monitoring is required. Other potential therapies that bind cysteine increasing its solubility include captopril and bucillamine.[1114]

### HYPERURICOSURIA (INCLUDING 2,8-DIHYDROXYADENINE UROLITHIASIS)

A number of rare single-gene defects of purine metabolism result in hyperuricosuria and uric acid lithiasis. Defects in hypoxanthine guanine phosphoribosyl-transferase (HPRT1) cause Lesch–Nyhan syndrome which is an X-linked disorder characterized by dystonia, gout (including hyperuricosuria), intellectual disability, and self-mutilation.[1115] Patients with glycogen storage disease type 1a have mutations in the enzyme glucose-6-phosphatase.[1116] They demonstrate a severe phenotype typically in the first year of life, which includes growth retardation, lactic academia, hypoglycemia, hepatomegaly, hyperlipidemia, and hyperuricemia leading to hyperuricosuria and uric acid stone formation. Another rare enzymatic deficiency is adenine phosphoribosyl-transferase deficiency, which leads to the overproduction of 2,8-dihydroxyadenine that is excreted in the urine and can precipitate causing calculi.[1117] Urolithiasis is the most common manifestation of this disorder and patients can present at any age with calculi. A urinalysis will display characteristic round, brown crystals suggestive of the disorder, which can be tested by enzymatic activity testing or demonstration of a biallelic pathogenic variant in the *APRT* gene. A low purine diet and ample food intake is the recommended treatment for the renal manifestations of these disorders. Medical therapy can include allopurinol even for patients with APRT deficiency. Alternatively, for APRT deficiency, the xanthine dehydrogenase inhibitor febuxostat can be employed.

### PRIMARY HYPEROXALURIAS

This is a group of rare autosomal recessive disorders that display increased generation and urinary excretion of oxalate (i.e., hyperoxaluria).[1064] Three different subtypes have been described and are the result of mutations in three different enzymes that participate in oxalate metabolism. Type 1 is the most severe form and type 3 the least. Type 2 can be difficult to distinguish from type 1 by clinical features alone. Instead, measurement of urinary glycolate and L-glyceric acid is beneficial. Patients with type 1 hyperoxaluria will display elevated urinary glycolate, whereas patients with type 2 will demonstrate elevated urinary L-glyceric acid. Confirmation of the diagnosis can be made by DNA analysis of the affected enzyme and demonstrating a deleterious genetic alteration.

#### Hyperoxaluria Type 1

Many patients with type 1 hyperoxaluria will develop progressive severe nephrolithiasis and nephrocalcinosis leading to renal failure. However, there is significant phenotypic variation, with some patients developing renal failure in infancy and others not developing their first renal calculi until adulthood.

The majority of patients with type 1 hyperoxaluria typically present with symptoms of their renal calculi before the age of 5 years, and in one cohort these patients accounted for 1% of children with ESRD.[1118] Mutations in alanine-glyoxalate aminotransferase are responsible for hyperoxaluria type 1.[1119] The variability of disease severity is due to mutations that permit residual enzyme activity. Importantly, residual alanine-glyoxalate aminotransferase enzyme activity in some cases can be stimulated by the cofactor pyridoxine.[1120] Patients with these mutations tend to display a more benign course. In the most severe cases infants can progress to renal failure within the first year of life; other cases might not be diagnosed until presentation of ESRD.

Systemic oxalosis occurs when plasma oxalate levels rise in patients with primary hyperoxaluria with decreasing GFR, due to reduced oxalate clearance. Systemic oxalosis results in the precipitation of calcium oxalate crystals in multiple tissues including the skeleton, heart, blood vessels, joints, retina, and skin. This is a severe disease with significant functional sequalae. Treatment is difficult and relies on aggressive dialytic therapy bridging to kidney–liver transplantation. Diagnosis is suggested by calcium oxalate nephrolithiasis, nephrocalcinosis, and significantly increased urinary oxalate excretion. Urinary glyoxalate will be elevated in the majority of patients; however, urinary glyoxalate can also be increased in patients with type 3 hyperoxaluria. Systemic oxalosis is not described in patients with a GFR greater than 60 mL/min/1.73 $m^2$, and as such there is no need to monitor plasma oxalate levels until GFR is below this level. Historically measurement of reduced alanine-glyoxalate aminotransferase activity was performed on liver biopsy to definitively demonstrate the diagnosis of primary hyperoxaluria type 1. However, this this is no longer necessary if one can demonstrate a deleterious mutation in the alanine-glyoxalate aminotransferase gene.

Therapy involves increasing fluid intake (to at least 2.5 L/$m^2$), avoidance of high oxalate-containing foods (i.e., chocolate, tea, rhubarb, and spinach), and administration of potassium citrate to both ensure adequate urinary citrate excretion and alkalinize the urine. Both of these urinary alterations tend to prevent calcium oxalate precipitation. A trial of high-dose pyridoxine (5–10 mg/kg/day) should be administered and urine oxalate followed to identify responders. Specific mutations are known to be sensitive to this therapy. Thus genetic analysis is helpful for therapeutic decision-making and prognostication. The earlier in the course of the disease therapy is instituted, the better the reported outcome and the longer renal function can be preserved.[1121] Unfortunately, even very intensive dialytic therapies (i.e., up to 40 hours of hemodialysis per week) are often ineffective at preventing the consequences of systemic oxalosis. Isolated kidney transplantation is not recommended, as it does not correct the primary metabolic problem because alanine-glyoxalate aminotransferase is expressed exclusively in the liver. However, in some patients who are responsive to pyridoxine, who present late with renal dysfunction, it might be considered.[1122] Isolated liver transplantation should be considered when GFR is greater than 40 mL/min/1.73 $m^2$.[1123] In patients with more severe renal dysfunction a combined kidney–liver transplantation is the treatment of choice.[1123] Unfortunately, administration of the oxalate degrading intestinal bacteria *Oxalobacter formigenes* has failed to demonstrate significant reduction in oxalate absorption and urinary excretion.

### Hyperoxaluria Type 2

Primary hyperoxaluria type 2 is the result of mutations in the enzyme glyoxylate reductase/hydroxypyruvate reductase (GRHPR).[1124] This form of primary hyperoxaluria is typically less severe than type 1. It traditionally presents in adolescence with repeated calcium oxalate stone formation. A minority of patients develop chronic renal impairment. Diagnosis is suggested by the demonstration of significantly elevated urinary oxalate excretion and the presence of increased urinary L-glycerate. Definitive diagnosis is made via mutation analysis of the *GRHPR* gene, or traditionally by demonstration of reduced liver GRHPR enzyme activity. Pyridoxine is not beneficial. Liver transplantation has not been demonstrated to be beneficial in patients with type 2 primary hyperoxaluria. Patients with this disease may instead benefit from isolated renal transplantation.

### Hyperoxaluria Type 3

Primary hyperoxaluria type 3 is the result of mutations of 4-hydroxy-2-oxoglutarate aldolase (*HOGA1* gene).[1125,1126] This enzyme is localized to the mitochondria in both the liver and the kidney and catalyzes 4-hydroxy-2-oxoglutarate to glyoxylate and pyruvate. Of the three subtypes, this is the most mild, clinically, and consists of recurrent calcium oxalate stone formation. Diagnosis is suspected by increased urinary oxalate excretion and can be confirmed by genetic analysis of the *HOGA1* gene. Fortunately, nephrocalcinosis and renal impairment are rarely seen.

# PEDIATRIC ASPECTS OF CHRONIC KIDNEY DISEASE

## GROWTH, NUTRITION, AND DEVELOPMENT

Childhood CKD impairs statural growth in a manner related to the age of CKD onset. Approximately 50% of children requiring RRT before their 13th birthday have a final height below the normal range.[1127] Results from the Chronic Kidney Disease in Children Study (CKiD, a US registry of children with a GFR <75 mL/min/1.73 $m^2$) demonstrated that height is below the normal range (median height standard deviation score [HtSDS] −0.55, fall in HtSDS of 0.12 to 0.16 for each decline of 10 mL/min/1.73 $m^2$) in children with predialysis CKD as well.[1128] One-third of all postnatal growth occurs during the first 2 years of life. Birth with CKD and inhibition of growth during this critical 2-year period can have major effects on the total amount of growth achieved.[1129] This particular age-related risk to final statural growth is illustrated by the 2006 North American Pediatric Transplant Cooperative Study (NAPRTCS) report, which demonstrated a mean HtSDS at under 2 years of age being −2.3 (increasing to −1.7, −1.4, and −1.0 at 2 to 6, 6–12, and >12 years, respectively).[1130] Between the second year of life and onset of puberty, growth inhibition is more subtle. Growth patterns typically remain stable along the normal percentiles as long as GFR remains greater than 25 mL/min/1.73 $m^2$ but gradually deviate from the normal range in CKD stages 4 and 5[1131] (Fig. 72.13). Even in children who appear to be growing normally successful kidney transplantation can result in accelerated or catch-up growth as metabolic homeostasis is restored, which suggests persistent suppression of growth potential in the uremic state.

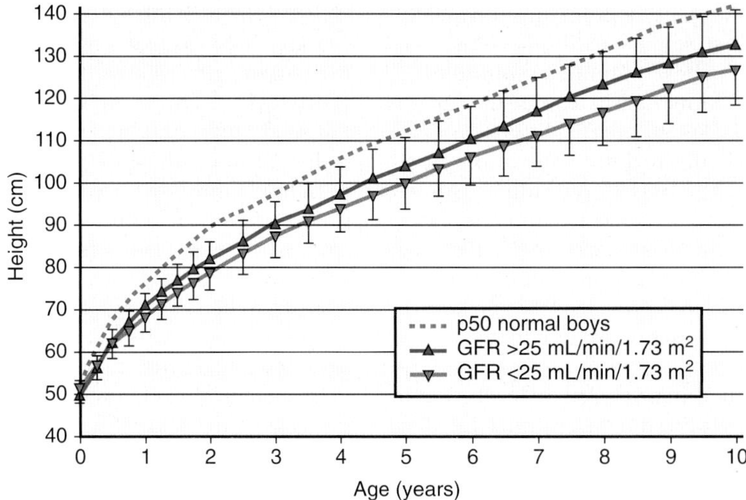


**Fig. 72.13** Glomerular filtration rate (GFR)–dependent growth pattern in children with chronic renal failure due to hypodysplastic renal disorders. Approximately 100 children per age interval were evaluated. Mean ± 1 standard deviation of height is shown for children with an average GFR more or less than 25 mL/min/1.73 m$^2$. (Modified from Schaefer F, Wingen AM, Hennicke M, et al. Growth charts for prepubertal children with chronic renal failure due to congenital renal disorders. European Study Group for Nutritional Treatment of Chronic Renal Failure in Childhood. *Pediatr Nephrol.* 1996;10:288–293.)

Renal dysfunction can also delay the onset of puberty, as well as the start of the pubertal growth spurt, in a manner dependent on the degree of renal dysfunction.[1132] Pubertal height gain is diminished by up to 50% (from 30 to 15 cm) in adolescents with advanced stages of CKD. Final adult heights below the normal range are attained by 30% to 50% of children with CKD, although a trend of improving final heights has been noted during the past decade. The duration of CKD, presence of a congenital nephropathy, and male gender are among the most important predictors of a reduced final height.[1129]

Growth failure in infants with CKD usually is caused by inadequate spontaneous intake of nutrients due to anorexia and frequent vomiting. Numerous factors contribute to anorexia in CKD. These include accumulation of circulating satiety factors, retarded psychomotor development, slow gastric emptying, fluid and electrolyte losses due to tubular dysfunction in renal dysplasia, and catabolic episodes related to intercurrent infections. Metabolic acidosis, which usually occurs when GFR is below 50% of normal, contributes to CKD associated growth failure by various mechanisms, including increased protein breakdown, suppressed secretion of GH and insulin-like growth factor-1 (IGF-1), as well as impaired GH and IGF-1 receptor expression in target tissues.[1129] Independent of metabolic acidosis, the endocrine systems show a complex dysregulation in the uremic state. Circulating GH levels are normal or increased due to impaired metabolic clearance, but the actual rate of GH secretion from the pituitary is diminished.[1133] GH-induced IGF-1 synthesis is impaired in uremia due to impaired activation of the GH-dependent JAK2/STAT5 (Janus kinase 2/signal transducer and activator of transcription-5) signaling pathway.[1134] This postreceptor signaling defect may be caused by upregulation of inhibitory suppressors of STAT signaling (SOCS [suppressor of cytokine signaling] proteins), which are induced by inflammatory cytokines in the uremic state. In addition, accumulation of IGF-1–binding proteins results in a molar excess of IGF-binding proteins relative to circulating IGFs, which results in reduced IGF bioactivity. Finally, normal or reduced GH secretion in the presence of markedly reduced IGF-1 bioactivity is consistent with an insufficient feedback activation of the somatotropic hormone axis at the hypothalamic and pituitary levels.

The gonadotropic hormone axis is subject to a similarly impaired activation in CKD.[1133] Peripubertal patients with advanced renal disease or ESRD exhibit normal or low sex steroid levels in the presence of elevated levels of circulating gonadotropins. The elevation of circulating gonadotropins is explained by impaired metabolic hormone clearance, whereas pituitary secretion rates are low, possibly due to impaired hypothalamic gonadotropin-releasing hormone (GnRH) secretion related to increased inhibitory neurotransmitter tone. In addition to deficient central nervous activation, there is accumulation of circulating factors that inhibit GnRH release from the hypothalamus and testosterone release from Leydig cells. Finally, crosstalk between gonadotropic and somatotropic hormones during puberty appears to be impaired, as evidenced by a blunted surge of GH secretion in response to rising sex steroid levels. Together, advanced stages of CKD cause a state of multiple endocrine resistance, effectively inhibiting longitudinal growth and sexual development.

## PREVENTION AND TREATMENT OF GROWTH FAILURE IN CHRONIC KIDNEY DISEASE

In infants with CKD, the most important measures for avoiding growth failure are the provision of adequate energy intake, correction of metabolic acidosis, and maintenance of fluid and electrolyte balance.[1135] Supplementary feedings via nasogastric tube or gastrostomy are frequently required to achieve these targets. Caloric intake should be targeted to provide 80% to 100% of the regular daily allowance for healthy children. Increasing caloric intake above 100% of the recommended daily allowance does not induce further catch-up growth but

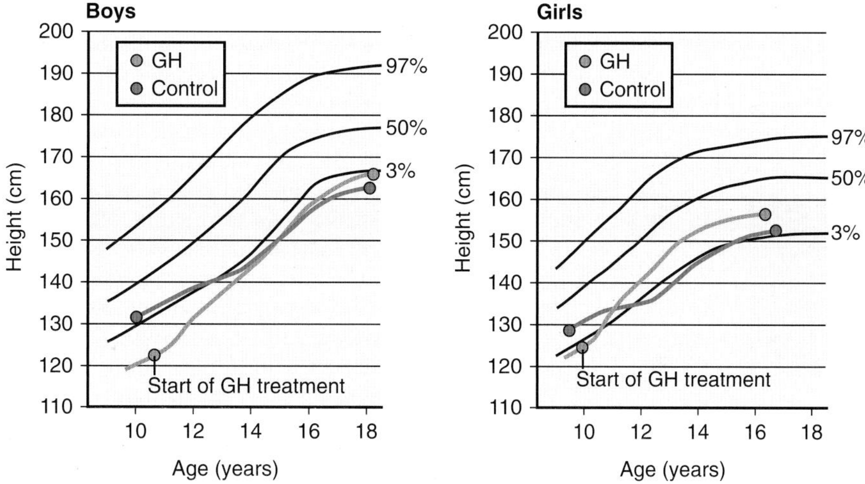


**Fig. 72.14** Favorable effects of long-term recombinant human growth hormone (GH) therapy on final adult height in children with chronic kidney disease (CKD). Synchronized mean growth curves are shown for 38 children (32 boys and 6 girls) with CKD who were treated with GH and for 50 control children with CKD who did not receive GH. Normal values are indicated by the 3rd, 50th, and 97th percentiles. The *circles* indicate the time of the first observation (the start of GH treatment in the treated children) and the end of the pubertal growth spurt. (Haffner D, Schaefer F, Nissel R, et al. Effect of growth hormone treatment on the adult height of children with chronic renal failure. German Study Group for Growth Hormone Treatment in Chronic Renal Failure. *N Engl J Med.* 2000;343:923–930.)

rather results in obesity. Protein intake should be at least 100% of the dietary reference intake but should not exceed 140% of the dietary reference intake in patients with CKD stage 2 or 3 and 120% of the reference intake in children with CKD stage 4 or 5. Excessive protein intake should be avoided in advancing CKD to limit phosphorus and acid load in patients with failing kidney function.[1136] Metabolic acidosis should be rigorously treated by oral alkaline supplementation. In addition, the supplementation of water and electrolytes is essential for children with polyuria and/or salt-losing nephropathies, as observed in tubulopathies and renal dysplasia. Early and consistent provision of supplementary nutrients, fluids, and electrolytes, with delivery ensured by enteral feeding via a nasogastric tube or percutaneous gastrostomy whenever necessary, has markedly improved the growth and development of young children with CKD.[1129,1137] In the postinfantile phase of childhood, nutrition, fluid, and electrolyte balance continue to be permissive factors for adequate longitudinal growth, but catch-up growth can rarely be provided by dietary and supplementary measures alone.

If growth failure is imminent and/or has already occurred, despite adequate provision of nutrients, salts, and fluid, then treatment with recombinant GH (rGH) may be indicated. The efficacy and safety of rGH therapy in children with CKD have been demonstrated in numerous short- and long-term trials and has been comprehensively reviewed.[846] The administration of rGH at pharmacologic dosages (0.05 mg/kg/day subcutaneously) overcomes endogenous GH resistance and markedly increases systemic and local IGF-1 production, with only a slight effect on IGF-binding proteins. This restores normal IGF-1 bioactivity and stimulates longitudinal growth. In children with predialytic CKD, height velocity typically doubles in the first treatment year, and a steady albeit less marked catch-up growth is observed during subsequent years of therapy. Long-term studies have demonstrated mean standardized height increases of −2.6 to −0.7 SD in North American children, −3.4 to −1.9 SD in German children, and −3.0 to −0.5 SD in Dutch children after 5 to 6 treatment years.[1129] The therapeutic response to rGH in CKD patients is superior to that observed in children who are undergoing dialysis or who have undergone kidney transplantation, probably due to a more marked uremic GH resistance in ESRD and the growth-suppressive effect of glucocorticoids in renal allograft recipients. In patients receiving rGH studied at around 9 to 10 years of age and followed through puberty until attainment of final height, catch-up growth was largely limited to the prepubertal period (Fig. 72.14).[1138] Final height was markedly improved in comparison with an untreated control group, with an overall benefit attributable to rGH treatment of 10 to 15 cm. Total height gain was positively correlated with the duration of rGH therapy and was negatively affected by the time spent on dialysis. These studies support a conclusion that rGH therapy should be initiated as early as possible in the predialytic CKD period, preferentially before severe growth retardation has occurred.

## CARDIOVASCULAR COMORBIDITY IN PEDIATRIC CHRONIC KIDNEY DISEASE

CKD-associated cardiovascular disease manifests relatively early in the course of CKD,[1139] leading to significant morbidity and mortality (Fig. 72.15).[1140] Among individuals younger than 19 years of age with ESRD, cardiac disease is responsible for 22 deaths/1000 patient-years, accounting for 16% of all deaths in whites and 26% in African Americans. This represents up to a 1000-fold increase in risk compared with that in the general population.

### HYPERTENSION

The prevalence of hypertension is 40% to 50% in children with CKD stages 2 to 4 and approaches 70% by the time ESRD has developed. High blood pressure is associated with target organ damage during childhood and is closely related to the rate of progression of renal failure. CKD-associated

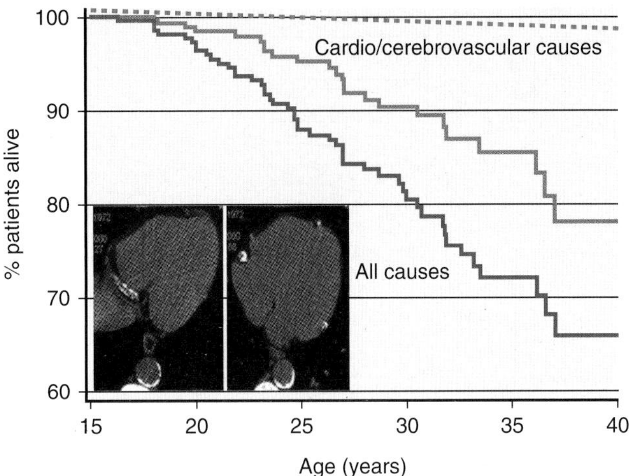


**Fig. 72.15** Long-term survival of 283 patients with childhood-onset end-stage kidney disease. *Green dotted line,* Survival rate considering all causes of death. *Red line,* Survival rate considering cardiovascular and cerebrovascular causes of death only. *Blue line,* Survival rate in the general population. *Inset,* Computed tomography sections from a 27-year-old male hemodialysis patient with extensive calcification in all three coronary arteries and aorta. (From Oh J, Wunsch R, Turzer M, et al. Advanced coronary and carotid arteriopathy in young adults with childhood-onset chronic renal failure. *Circulation.* 2002;106:100–105.)

hypertension develops by a variety of pathophysiologic mechanisms including fluid overload, increased peripheral vascular resistance, activation of the RAAS, sympathetic hyperactivation, endothelial dysfunction, and chronic hyperparathyroidism.[1141]

The American Academy of Pediatrics Fourth Report on the Diagnosis, Evaluation, and Treatment of High Blood Pressure in Children and Adolescents defines arterial hypertension in the pediatric population.[1142] According to these guidelines, childhood hypertension is defined based on the distribution of blood pressure in the general population matched for age, gender, and height. Hypertension is defined as a systolic and/or diastolic blood pressure that on at least three occasions is greater than or equal to the 95th percentile for age, sex, and height. Values from the 90th to 95th percentile at any blood pressure level at or above 120/80 mm Hg are termed prehypertension.[1142] Altered circadian blood pressure patterns, as described in adult patients with CKD, can be detected by ambulatory blood pressure monitoring in children.[1143] Analysis of the CKiD cohort showed that up to 35% of children with CKD (eGFR 30–90 mL/min/1.73 m$^2$) have so-called masked hypertension – that is, elevated blood pressure with 24-hour monitoring despite normal office readings, a condition associated with an increased prevalence of left ventricular hypertrophy (LVH).[1144,1145] Various online calculators are available to compare the blood pressure of a child of a given gender, age, and height with that in the normal population (e.g., www.pediatriconcall.com/fordoctor/pedcalc/bp.aspx).

Current management guidelines recommend regular blood pressure screening for all children with CKD.[1146] In addition to clinic measurements, ambulatory blood pressure monitoring should be performed at least once a year and within 1 to 2 months of modification of therapy in patients receiving antihypertensive medication. Children with CKD should be considered at increased risk for cardiovascular complications, and therapeutic interventions should be initiated when blood pressure exceeds the 90th percentile for age and height. The therapeutic target for blood pressure in CKD varies according to different published guidelines.[1146] The American Academy of Pediatrics Fourth Report recommends a target blood pressure of less than 90%. Both the European Society of Hypertension and KDIGO recommend a target of less than 75% for nonproteinuric CKD and less than 50% for proteinuric CKD.[1146,1147] Lifestyle changes such as increased physical activity, avoidance of salty foods, and reduction of weight in obese patients are also recommended for children with CKD but are rarely effective as sole measures.[560,1141] ACE inhibitors and ARBs should be the first choice of antihypertensive medications (see the "Progression of Chronic Renal Failure in Children" section) and, if given at appropriate dosages (e.g., ramipril 6 mg/m$^2$/day[565,1148] or candesartan 0.2–0.4 mg/kg/day[1149]), will normalize blood pressure in most patients. If the blood pressure–lowering effect is insufficient, a loop diuretic should be added (e.g., furosemide, 2–4 mg/kg/day), followed by a calcium channel antagonist (e.g., amlodipine, 0.2 mg/kg/day). The timing of drug dosing should be adapted to achieve optimal blood pressure control throughout 24 hours as verified by ambulatory blood pressure monitoring.

## ANEMIA

Anemia is a common and serious complication in both adult and pediatric patients with CKD. Severe anemia is associated with increased morbidity and mortality and development of cardiovascular disease in patients with CKD. In children, growth, neurocognitive development, school attendance, and exercise capacity are important clinical outcomes related to anemia.

Erythropoiesis-stimulating agents (ESAs) are central to the treatment of anemia. While the efficacy of ESAs is clear in childhood CKD,[1150] the desired therapeutic target of blood hemoglobin has not been defined in children via randomized trials. Studies in adults with CKD have raised important concerns regarding an increased cardiovascular morbidity and mortality in patients with hemoglobin greater than 120 g/L.[1151] A recent study[1152] provides new insights into the association of hemoglobin levels with cardiovascular morbidity in pediatric patients receiving hemodialysis. Using data from the Centers for Medicare and Medicaid Services ESRD Clinical Performance Measure project and United States Renal Data System, the authors studied 1569 children receiving hemodialysis. Examination of outcomes including mortality, hospitalization, and cardiovascular event over 1 year follow-up showed that the hazard ratio of all-cause mortality and the adjusted relative rate of all-cause hospitalization were significantly lower in the hemoglobin 12 g/dL or greater group, and cardiovascular hospitalizations were significantly higher in the hemoglobin under 10 g/dL group. Inpatient and outpatient visits for congestive heart failure, cardiomyopathy, and valvular heart disease were most common in the hemoglobin under 10 g/dL group, and the frequency of these diagnoses decreased with increasing hemoglobin level.

### INTERMEDIATE CARDIOVASCULAR ENDPOINTS IN CHILDREN WITH CHRONIC KIDNEY DISEASE

LVH and increased carotid intima-media thickness have been demonstrated in hypertensive children with advanced CKD, in whom alterations of mineral metabolism and volume

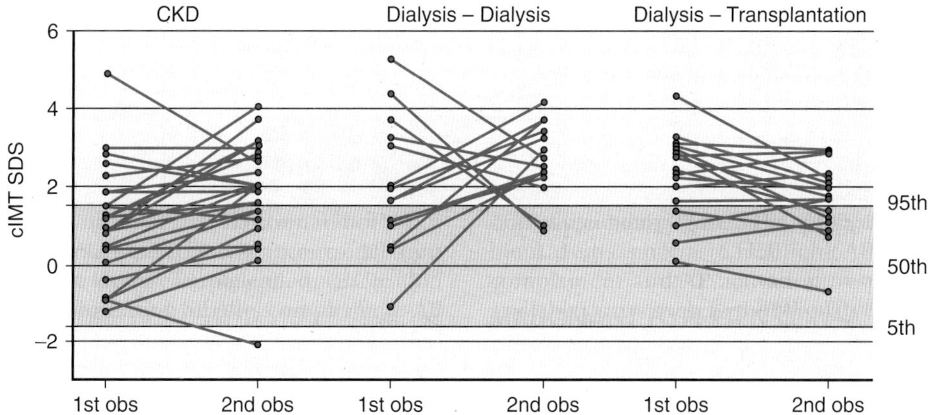


**Fig. 72.16** Change in sonographically determined carotid intima-media thickness (cIMT) in children with chronic kidney disease, children undergoing dialysis, and children who underwent kidney transplantation. Mean time interval between the first and second observations *(obs)* was 12 months. IMT is expressed as a standard deviation (SD) score normalized for age and gender. *Shaded area* denotes normal range, with SDs of −1.64, 0, and +1.64 corresponding to the 5th, 50th, and 95th percentiles. *cIMT SDS,* Change in intima media thickness standard deviation score. (From Litwin M, Wühl E, Jourdan C, et al. Evolution of large-vessel arteriopathy in pediatric patients with chronic kidney disease. *Nephrol Dial Transplant.* 2008;23:2552–2557.)

overload are important superimposed risk factors, but also in children with early essential hypertension and in children with masked hypertension. LVH is the most common identifiable cardiac alteration in CKD and the most important indicator of cardiovascular risk in adult and pediatric patients with ESRD.[1153–1156] LVH is believed to contribute to the high risk of sudden cardiac death in children with CKD due to lethal arrhythmias via underlying myocardial fibrosis and cellular hypertrophy. LVH is present in approximately 15% to 30% of children with stage 2 to 4 CKD,[1157,1158] in 50% to 75% of children undergoing dialysis,[1159,1160] and in 50% to 67% of renal allograft recipients.[1161,1162] Factors that promote LVH could include increased circulating volume, hyperactivation of the RAAS and sympathetic nervous system, hyperparathyroidism, and proinflammatory cytokines. In addition to the morphologic change of LVH, a subclinical impairment of left ventricular systolic function is found in about 25% of children with mild to moderate CKD.[1163] Systolic dysfunction is most common in patients with concentric LVH and is associated with a low GFR and anemia.

Increasing evidence in children, as in adults, has suggested that the CKD-associated bone mineral disorder and its treatment not only affects bone and mineral metabolism but also contributes to the development of calcifying uremic vasculopathy. This is a consequence of a redistribution of mineral salts from the skeleton to the large arteries and soft tissue compartments. Coronary artery calcifications are found in individual adolescent patients undergoing dialysis[1164] and in more than 90% of young adults with childhood-onset CKD.[1140] Early signs of vasculopathy, such as an increased intima-media thickness and stiffness of the carotid artery, can be detected as early as the second decade of life.[1165] Both morphologic and functional alterations are progressive over time and are most marked in adolescents undergoing dialysis, but they also may be seen in children with moderate CKD and appear to improve partially after successful renal transplantation (Fig. 72.16). Intima-media thickness and stiffness of the carotid artery correlate with the degree of hyperparathyroidism, serum calcium–phosphorus ion product, and cumulative dose of calcium-containing phosphate binders.

## PROGRESSION OF CHRONIC RENAL FAILURE IN CHILDREN

### COURSE OF RENAL FUNCTION IN CHILDREN WITH CHRONIC KIDNEY DISEASE

The course of renal function in pediatric CKD is mainly determined by the age and degree of renal failure at the time of first disease manifestation. Two-thirds of children with CAKUT progress to ESRD during the first 2 decades of life.[6] The physiologic early increase in GFR is typically extended to the first 3 to 4 years of life, which potentially reflects an adaptive hypertrophy of the reduced number of functioning nephrons.[173] In approximately 50% of children, this early incremental phase is followed by a period of stable or very slowly deteriorating renal function, which usually lasts for 5 to 8 years. Around the onset of puberty, the GFR loss tends to accelerate, typically leading to ESRD in late adolescence or early adulthood (Fig. 72.17). The reasons for this nonlinear progression of renal failure are incompletely understood and may include an insufficient capacity of the nephrons to adapt to the rapidly growing metabolic needs during the pubertal growth spurt, adverse renal effects of puberty-related increases in sex steroid production, and/or an accelerated sclerotic degeneration of a diminishing number of remnant hyperfiltering nephrons. In children with very severe renal hypoplasia, the early increase in GFR may be blunted, and early progression to ESRD may occur instead. About 20% of patients with renal hypoplasia maintain a stable GFR, even beyond puberty. Follow-up studies have shown that in patients with mild bilateral renal hypoplasia, progressive deterioration of GFR frequently ensues in the third decade of life.

### RISK FACTORS FOR PROGRESSION OF RENAL FAILURE

Among the numerous factors predicting progressive renal failure in adult populations and in animal models, hypertension and proteinuria have also been identified as consistent, modifiable risk factors in children. In the European Study

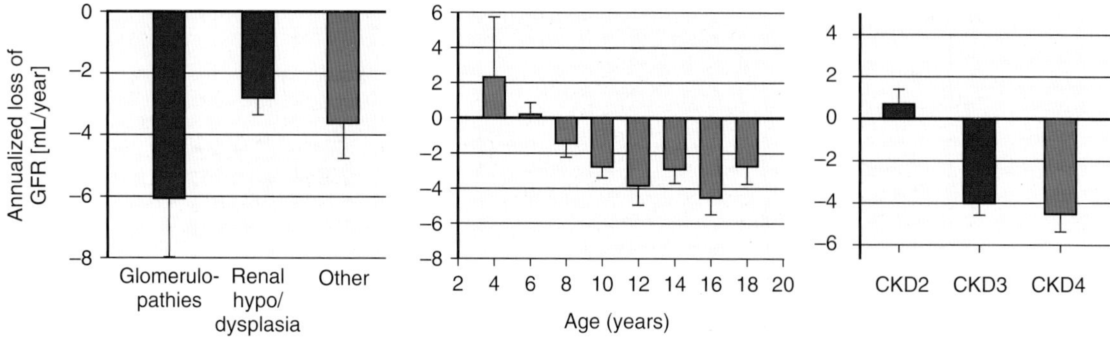


**Fig. 72.17** Mean spontaneous change in estimated glomerular filtration rate (GFR) in 385 children with chronic kidney disease (CKD) randomly assigned to treatment conditions in the ESCAPE trial (measured during the run-in period). The rate of renal failure progression in children depends on underlying renal disease, age, and CKD stage.

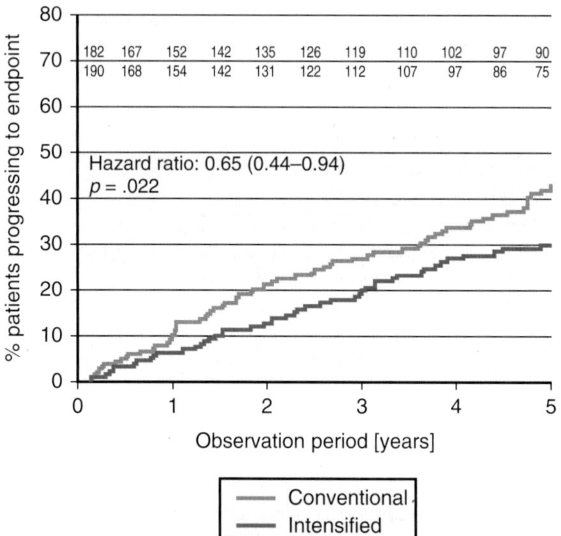


**Fig. 72.18** Effect of intensified blood pressure control on renal survival in children with chronic kidney disease. Within 5 years, 30% of patients randomly assigned to intensive control with a low-normal, 24-hour blood pressure target reached the endpoint of 50% glomerular filtration rate loss or end-stage kidney disease, compared with 42% of patients assigned to standard control with a conventional blood pressure target. (Data from Wühl E, Trivelli A, Matteucci MC, et al. Strict blood pressure control and progression of renal failure in children. *N Engl J Med.* 2009;361:1639–1650.)

for Nutritional Treatment of Chronic Renal Failure in Childhood, a systolic blood pressure greater than120 mm Hg was associated with a significantly faster decline of GFR.[1136] The randomized, prospective ESCAPE trial (Effect of Strict Blood Pressure Control and ACE Inhibition on the Progression of CRF in Pediatric Patients) demonstrated that in children with CKD due to various disorders, intensified antihypertensive treatment forcing blood pressure into the low-normal range (<50th percentile for age) was associated with improved long-term renal survival (Fig. 72.18).[208] Proteinuria is predictive of CKD progression in children, as it is in adult populations. Proteinuria predicts renal disease progression in children with renal hypodysplasia and, even in children with normal kidney function, persistent nephrotic-range proteinuria is a risk factor for progressive renal injury. In the ESCAPE trial, for children receiving fixed-dose ACE inhibitors, residual proteinuria proved to be predictive of CKD progression, despite treatment. These findings provide a strong rationale for the early and consistent application of RAAS antagonist treatment protocols.[208] Both ACE inhibitors and ARBs have been shown to be safe and effective in children with CKD. Ramipril, administered at a dosage of 6 mg/m$^2$/day, normalized blood pressure and lowered proteinuria by approximately 50% in the ESCAPE trial patients.[1148] Similar results have been obtained with the ARBs losartan,[1166,1167] valsartan,[1168] and candesartan.[1149] It should be noted, however, that the renoprotective superiority of RAAS antagonists over other antihypertensive agents has not been formally demonstrated in pediatric CKD. Data from the ItalKid registry did not show significant modification of CKD progression by ACE inhibitor treatment in children with hypodysplastic kidney disease compared with matched untreated cases.[1169] However, no information regarding the type and dosages of ACE inhibitors used and prevailing degree of proteinuria was available, and the baseline progression rate was very slow. Another important observation in the ESCAPE trial was a gradual return of proteinuria, despite ongoing ACE inhibitor treatment. This effect was dissociated from persistently excellent blood pressure control and might limit the long-term renoprotective efficacy of ACE inhibitor monotherapy in pediatric CKD.[208]

 Complete reference list available at ExpertConsult.com.

## KEY REFERENCES


7. Wuhl E, van Stralen KJ, Verrina E, et al. Timing and outcome of renal replacement therapy in patients with congenital malformations of the kidney and urinary tract. *Clin J Am Soc Nephrol.* 2013;8(1):67–74.
20. van der Ven AT, Vivante A, Hildebrandt F. Novel Insights into the Pathogenesis of Monogenic Congenital Anomalies of the Kidney and Urinary Tract. *J Am Soc Nephrol.* 2018;29(1):36–50.
26. Sanna-Cherchi S, Westland R, Ghiggeri GM, et al. Genetic basis of human congenital anomalies of the kidney and urinary tract. *J Clin Invest.* 2018;128(1):4–15.
53. Shakya R, Watanabe T, Costantini F. The role of GDNF/Ret signaling in ureteric bud cell fate and branching morphogenesis. *Dev Cell.* 2005;8(1):65–74.
80. Blake J, Hu D, Cain JE, et al. Urogenital development in Pallister-Hall syndrome is disrupted in a cell-lineage-specific manner by constitutive expression of GLI3 repressor. *Hum Mol Genet.* 2016;25(3):437–447.
106. Hwang DY, Dworschak GC, Kohl S, et al. Mutations in 12 known dominant disease-causing genes clarify many congenital anomalies of the kidney and urinary tract. *Kidney Int.* 2014;85(6):1429–1433.

254. Schell C, Huber TB. The evolving complexity of the podocyte cytoskeleton. *J Am Soc Nephrol.* 2017;28(11):3166–3174.
255. Rosenberg AZ, Kopp JB. Focal segmental glomerulosclerosis. *Clin J Am Soc Nephrol.* 2017;12(3):502–517.
256. Vivarelli M, Massella L, Ruggiero B, et al. Minimal change disease. *Clin J Am Soc Nephrol.* 2017;12(2):332–345.
314. Agrawal S, Zaritsky JJ, Fornoni A, et al. Dyslipidaemia in nephrotic syndrome: mechanisms and treatment. *Nat Rev Nephrol.* 2017; 14(1):70.
335. Shalhoub RJ. Pathogenesis of lipoid nephrosis: a disorder of T-cell function. *Lancet.* 1974;2(7880):556–560.
352. Iijima K, Sako M, Nozu K, et al. Rituximab for childhood-onset, complicated, frequently relapsing nephrotic syndrome or steroid-dependent nephrotic syndrome: a multicentre, double-blind, randomised, placebo-controlled trial. *Lancet.* 2014;384(9950): 1273–1281.
359. Agrawal S, Chanley MA, Westbrook D, et al. Pioglitazone enhances the beneficial effects of glucocorticoids in experimental nephrotic syndrome. *Sci Rep.* 2016;6:24392.
368. Riedl M, Thorner P, Licht C. C3 glomerulopathy. *Pediatr Nephrol.* 2017;32(1):43–57.
369. Ricklin D, Mastellos DC, Reis ES, et al. The renaissance of complement therapeutics. *Nat Rev Nephrol.* 2018;14(1):26–47.
378. Sethi S, Fervenza FC. Membranoproliferative glomerulonephritis–a new look at an old entity. *N Engl J Med.* 2012;366(12):1119–1131.
380. Pickering MC, D'Agati VD, Nester CM, et al. C3 glomerulopathy: consensus report. *Kidney Int.* 2013;84(6):1079–1089.
422. Gale DP, de Jorge EG, Cook HT, et al. Identification of a mutation in complement factor H-related protein 5 in patients of Cypriot origin with glomerulonephritis. *Lancet.* 2010;376(9743):794–801.
427. Licht C, Heinen S, Jozsi M, et al. Deletion of Lys224 in regulatory domain 4 of Factor H reveals a novel pathomechanism for dense deposit disease (MPGN II). *Kidney Int.* 2006;70(1):42–50.
457. Rabasco C, Cavero T, Roman E, et al. Effectiveness of mycophenolate mofetil in C3 glomerulonephritis. *Kidney Int.* 2015;88(5):1153–1160.
486. Bomback AS, Smith RJ, Barile GR, et al. Eculizumab for dense deposit disease and C3 glomerulonephritis. *Clin J Am Soc Nephrol.* 2012;7(5):748–756.
546. George JN, Nester CM. Syndromes of thrombotic microangiopathy. *N Engl J Med.* 2014;371:654–666.
547. Fakhouri F, Zuber J, Fremeaux-Bacchi V, et al. Haemolytic uraemic syndrome. *Lancet.* 2017;390(10095):681–696.
555. Kremer Hovinga JA, Coppo P, Lammle B, et al. Thrombotic thrombocytopenic purpura. *Nat Rev Dis Primers.* 2017;3:17020.
563. Goodship TH, Cook HT, Fakhouri F, et al. Atypical hemolytic uremic syndrome and C3 glomerulopathy: conclusions from a "Kidney Disease: improving Global Outcomes" (KDIGO) controversies conference. *Kidney Int.* 2017;91(3):539–551.
569. Legendre CM, Licht C, Muus P, et al. Terminal complement inhibitor eculizumab in atypical hemolytic-uremic syndrome. *N Engl J Med.* 2013;368:2169–2181.
600. Lemaire M, Fremeaux-Bacchi V, Schaefer F, et al. Recessive mutations in DGKE cause atypical hemolytic-uremic syndrome. *Nat Genet.* 2013;45(5):531–536.
621. Schaefer F, Ardissino G, Ariceta G, et al. Clinical and genetic predictors of atypical hemolytic uremic syndrome phenotype and outcome. *Kidney Int.* 2018.
805. Gharavi AG, Moldoveanu Z, Wyatt RJ, et al. Aberrant IgA1 glycosylation is inherited in familial and sporadic IgA nephropathy. *J Am Soc Nephrol.* 2008;19(5):1008–1014.
821. Coppo R, Peruzzi L, Amore A, et al. IgACE: a placebo-controlled, randomized trial of angiotensin-converting enzyme inhibitors in children and young people with IgA nephropathy and moderate proteinuria. *J Am Soc Nephrol.* 2007;18(6):1880–1888.
845. Fellstrom BC, Barratt J, Cook H, et al. Targeted-release budesonide versus placebo in patients with IgA nephropathy (NEFIGAN): a double-blind, randomised, placebo-controlled phase 2b trial. *Lancet.* 2017;389(10084):2117–2127.
876. Jennette JC, Falk RJ. Pathogenesis of antineutrophil cytoplasmic autoantibody-mediated disease. *Nat Rev Rheumatol.* 2014;10(8): 463–473.
879. Siomou E, Tramma D, Bowen C, et al. ANCA-associated glomerulonephritis/systemic vasculitis in childhood: clinical features-outcome. *Pediatr Nephrol.* 2012;27(10):1911–1920.
887. Hiemstra TF, Walsh M, Mahr A, et al. Mycophenolate mofetil vs azathioprine for remission maintenance in antineutrophil cytoplasmic antibody-associated vasculitis: a randomized controlled trial. *JAMA.* 2010;304(21):2381–2388.
923. Niaudet P, Bader-Meunier B, Salomon R. Renal involvement in children with systemic lupus erythematosus. In: Avner ED, Harmon WE, Niaudet P, et al, eds. *Pediatric Nephrology.* Vol. 1. Berlin Heidelberg: Springer-Verlag; 2016:1449–1488.
950. Tian SY, Feldman BM, Beyene J, et al. Immunosuppressive therapies for the induction treatment of proliferative lupus nephritis: a systematic review and network metaanalysis. *J Rheumatol.* 2014; 41(10):1998–2007.
976. Town M, Jean G, Cherqui S, et al. A novel gene encoding an integral membrane protein is mutated in nephropathic cystinosis. *Nat Genet.* 1998;18(4):319–324.
988. Simon DB, Karet FE, Rodriguez-Soriano J, et al. Genetic heterogeneity of Bartter's syndrome revealed by mutations in the K+ channel, ROMK. *Nat Genet.* 1996;14(2):152–156.
989. Simon DB, Karet FE, Hamdan JM, et al. Bartter's syndrome, hypokalaemic alkalosis with hypercalciuria, is caused by mutations in the Na-K-2Cl cotransporter NKCC2. *Nat Genet.* 1996;13(2):183–188.
990. Simon DB, Nelson-Williams C, Bia MJ, et al. Gitelman's variant of Bartter's syndrome, inherited hypokalaemic alkalosis, is caused by mutations in the thiazide-sensitive Na-Cl cotransporter. *Nat Genet.* 1996;12(1):24–30.
991. Simon DB, Bindra RS, Mansfield TA, et al. Mutations in the chloride channel gene, CLCNKB, cause Bartter's syndrome type III. *Nat Genet.* 1997;17(2):171–178.
1004. Bockenhauer D, Feather S, Stanescu HC, et al. Epilepsy, ataxia, sensorineural deafness, tubulopathy, and KCNJ10 mutations. *N Engl J Med.* 2009;360(19):1960–1970.
1008. Chang SS, Grunder S, Hanukoglu A, et al. Mutations in subunits of the epithelial sodium channel cause salt wasting with hyperkalaemic acidosis, pseudohypoaldosteronism type 1. *Nat Genet.* 1996;12(3):248–253.
1010. Geller DS, Rodriguez-Soriano J, Vallo Boado A, et al. Mutations in the mineralocorticoid receptor gene cause autosomal dominant pseudohypoaldosteronism type I. *Nat Genet.* 1998;19(3):279–281.

# 73 Fluid, Electrolyte, and Acid-Base Disorders in Children

Detlef Bockenhauer

CHAPTER OUTLINE



The pathophysiology of fluid and electrolyte disorders and the principles for their treatment are the same, irrespective of age. Yet, there are unique aspects to managing a child, especially in the first year of life:

- Body composition with respect to water and its distribution between extracellular and intracellular compartment changes substantially with age. In a 23-week premature baby, the relative size of the extracellular compartment is about three times larger, at 60% of body weight compared with an adult, where it is roughly 20%.[1,2]
- Similarly, the glomerular filtration rate (GFR), even when corrected for surface area, is much lower at 28 weeks' gestation, at around 10 mL/min/1.73 $m^2$ in the first week of life and increases to only around 15 mL/min/1.73 $m^2$ by 4 weeks of life.[3]
- Urinary concentrating ability is severely impaired in the neonate and reaches full potential only at around 1 year of age.[4,5]
- Childhood is especially vulnerable because of the need to facilitate growth and development. Disorders of fluid, electrolyte, and acid-base homeostasis can severely affect this, leading to rickets and stunted growth, and meticulous monitoring is required to adjust treatment to the needs of the growing body.

In this chapter, disorders of fluid, electrolyte, and acid-base homeostasis will be discussed, with particular attention to these specific aspects.

## SODIUM AND WATER DISORDERS

### NORMAL METABOLISM OF WATER AND SODIUM SPECIFIC TO PEDIATRICS

The most abundant constituent of the human body is water, but the relative amount changes with age. In newborns and infants, total body water (TBW) constitutes a greater proportion of body weight than in adults, approximately 90% at 23 weeks' gestation to 70% in term infants, and 65% at 12 months of age, compared with about 60% in an adult.[1,2]

The TBW is comprised of the intracellular fluid (ICF) and extracellular fluid (ECF), which may in turn be subdivided into intravascular and interstitial fluids. The age-dependent changes in TBW that occur during infancy and childhood are mostly attributable to variations in ECF because the ICF proportion remains essentially constant after the first year of life, at roughly 40% of the body weight. In contrast, the ECF decreases rapidly during the embryonic development stage, during the first year of life, and more slowly from 1 year of age onward.

In addition to the internal distribution of water, water and electrolyte metabolism depend on the external balance between intake and output. Children must keep a positive balance to allow body growth. A young infant gains approximately 30 g of weight/day, which includes the physiologic retention of 20 mL/day of water and 2 mEq/day of sodium. On the other hand, the ratio of surface area to weight is higher in infants than in adults, and the skin is more permeable in infants, probably due to the higher expression of water channels (aquaporins).[6,7] This means that water loss is proportionately much greater in infants than in adults, especially in children with fever.

## HYPEROSMOLALITY AND HYPERNATREMIA: PATHOGENESIS AND CLASSIFICATION

Hyperosmolality results from a deficiency of water relative to solutes in the ECF. The vast majority of situations leading to hyperosmolality are attributable to losses of body water in excess of body solutes caused by insufficient water intake, excessive water excretion, or both, although a minority of cases can occur as a result of excessive total body sodium loading.[8] A list of the causal mechanisms of hyperosmolar disorders is summarized in Table 73.1 and demonstrates the specific vulnerability of young infants for developing hypernatremia. The conjunction of several factors, such as lack of voluntary access to water, high physiologic insensible water loss because of a large body surface in relation to body weight, occurrence of acute diarrhea frequently associated with fever, vomiting, and intolerance of oral fluid intake all contribute to this potentially dangerous vulnerability.

### DEHYDRATION

It should be noted that in pediatrics the term "dehydration" is often used as the most general term, encompassing the different forms of net fluid loss, including forms in which the following are found: (1) water loss exceeds solute loss, leaving the child hypertonic; (2) water and solute loss are proportionate, leaving the child normotonic; and (3) solute loss exceeds water loss, leaving the child hypotonic. Although not as strictly rigorous as the term *net fluid volume depletion*, the term *dehydration* will be retained in this chapter to be consistent with terminology used in everyday pediatrics.

#### Hypernatremic Dehydration

Dehydration may occur as a result of inappropriately low intake (inadequate supply, anorexia, coma, fluid restriction) or excessive loss of fluids by gastrointestinal (GI; vomiting, diarrhea, fistula, or drains), renal (polyuric states), and/or cutaneous (heat, cystic fibrosis, burns, inflammatory skin disease) routes. Hypernatremic dehydration results from insufficient water intake or net loss of water in excess of solutes (see Table 73.1; i.e., the net fluid loss is hypotonic). In hypernatremic dehydration, water shifts from the ICF to the ECF, driven by an osmotic gradient. Thus, a certain degree of extracellular and intracellular volume loss coexists. In view of the fact that many of the most commonly assessed clinical manifestations are proportional to the reduction of ECF volume, the manifestations of dehydration will be less intense for the same degree of water loss in the hypernatremic dehydration state than in other forms of dehydration (see later). Therefore progressive dehydration associated with hypernatremia may be overlooked, even in babies with marked weight loss.[9]

Any form of dehydration is characterized by weight loss in the child. The magnitude of acute weight loss reflects the amount of water loss and is the best clinical indicator of the degree of dehydration. Weight losses in infants of 5%, 10%, and 15% (50, 100, and 150 /kg, respectively) classically correspond with mild, moderate, and severe degrees of dehydration. Older children and adults manifest symptoms at a somewhat lower degree of fluid loss than infants because the former have relatively smaller TBW and ECF volume, whereby weight losses of 3%, 6%, and 9% are better used as indicators of mild, moderate, and severe dehydration, respectively.[10]

In addition to weight loss, the reduction of ECF will cause a range of symptoms and physical signs, depending on the intensity and rate of the dehydration, such as decreased skin turgor, dry mucous membranes, sunken anterior fontanelle, cool and mottled skin with poor capillary refilling, oliguria, acceleration of heart rate and pulse, decrease in blood pressure and, in the most severe cases—most commonly, combined volume depletion with concomitant net sodium loss, as well—hypovolemic shock. A review of the literature to find out the precision and accuracy of symptoms, signs, and basic laboratory tests for evaluating dehydration in infants and children came to the conclusion that delayed capillary refill time, reduced skin turgor, and deep respirations, with or without an increase in rate, were the most useful clinical signs that predicted 5% hypovolemia; these parameters should be the basis of the initial assessment of dehydration in young children.[11]

In infants with hypernatremic dehydration, the reduction of the ICF volume may also cause fever and central nervous system (CNS) manifestations such as irritability, a high-pitched cry, seizures, and other neurobehavioral disturbances, reminiscent of febrile and neurologic illness. Hyperosmolality causes thirst and avidity for water. Elevations of hematocrit and plasma concentrations of total proteins, uric acid, and urea are biochemical indicators of dehydration, although they are not reliable parameters to assess its severity. Metabolic acidosis is usually present because of the frequent associated loss of bicarbonate and alkalinizing organic anions from the GI tract (non–anion gap [AG] acidosis) or anaerobic metabolism caused by poor peripheral perfusion (AG acidosis caused by lactate accumulation). A value of plasma bicarbonate below 17 mmol/L in the context of dehydration is suggestive of moderate or severe hypovolemia.[11]

**Table 73.1 Pathogenesis of Hyperosmolar Disorders**

| Disorder | Features |
|---|---|
| Insufficient water intake | • Inability to obtain water: preambulatory infants, unconscious or disabled children, lack of water<br>• Abnormalities of thirst—hypodipsia secondary to CNS disorders |
| Net loss of water in excess of solutes | • Renal losses—central and nephrogenic diabetes insipidus<br>• GI losses: vomiting, diarrhea<br>• Cutaneous losses: sweating, burns<br>• Pulmonary losses: hyperventilation |
| High sodium intake + low intake of water free of solutes | Excessive administration of NaCl or $NaHCO_3^-$—parenteral nutrition, cardiopulmonary resuscitation, seawater intake |

*CNS,* Central nervous system; *GI,* gastrointestinal.

The vast majority of cases of hypernatremic dehydration are caused by diarrheal illnesses, but two particular, albeit rare causes will be highlighted here, because they are specific to children and need to be considered in the differential diagnosis.

**The Exclusively Breast-Fed Baby.** Life-threatening hypernatremia with values up to 188 mmol/L has been reported in otherwise healthy newborn babies who were exclusively breast-fed.[12,13] These infants usually present between 10 and 21 days of age, and the spectrum of symptoms can range from minor nonspecific signs such as irritability, lethargy, and decreased urine output to jaundice, fever, anuria, and hypovolemic shock.[12] The cause is usually insufficient lactation and, even though many of these babies were regularly followed by health care professionals or even in the hospital, the extent of dehydration was typically missed until the dehydration had become severe. These babies are usually firstborns and inexperience with and sensitivities around breast-feeding, as well as early discharge from the hospital, may all be contributing factors.[13] Close attention to weight gain and feeding history during the first 2 to 3 weeks of life and support for first-time mothers may prevent or ameliorate this serious complication.

**Nephrogenic Diabetes Insipidus.** Nephrogenic diabetes insipidus (NDI) is a disease defined by renal resistance to arginine vasopressin (AVP) action, which results in an inability to concentrate urine adequately. Primary inherited NDI is discussed in detail in Chapter 44. Thus, this chapter will focus on the typical presentation and its fluid management.

***Presentation.*** The osmotic load from breast milk is very low and, for this reason, urinary concentrating ability is usually not needed in the first weeks of life. This may explain the physiologic NDI that occurs in essentially all newborns, with full urinary concentrating ability being attained only by as late as 1 year of age.[5] Thus, most babies with NDI present later during the first year of life, or even later in childhood, when changes in diet present a higher osmotic load or when intercurrent illnesses lead to increased extrarenal water losses.[14] As discussed, apparent clinical signs of hypernatremic dehydration may not be noted until dehydration is severe. When infants affected with NDI present to medical attention with nonspecific symptoms, the families are often discharged without further investigation, because the medical staff is falsely reassured by the voluminous urine output typically provided in the history. Given that NDI is a rare disease, with most emergency physicians never encountering a single patient during their entire life of practice, and whereas dehydration from GI losses with a consequently reduced urine output in an otherwise healthy infant is a common condition, this mistake is understandable. Yet, it is important to realize that a large output of dilute urine in an infant with clinical signs of dehydration should be a severe warning sign, rather than reassuring, and plasma electrolyte levels should be assessed. In older children, reports of a constant craving for water, sometimes associated with unusual drinking behavior, such as from the bathtub, toilet, or flower vase, should alert the clinician to the potential of a urinary concentrating defect.

***Fluid Management.*** Most patients with NDI maintain electrolyte homeostasis simply by drinking sufficient volumes of water to compensate for the renal losses. Problems arise when this is impaired, either because of an inability to drink sufficiently—for example, when the patient is vomiting or if oral intake is stopped, such as before a procedure requiring an anesthetic. In these cases, intravenous (IV) fluids need to be provided. Patients with NDI essentially lose pure water in the urine and thus should receive dextrose in water as IV fluid, just as they would otherwise drink water. Due to concerns over the development of hyponatremia in hospitalized children, most hospitals have discouraged or even banned hypotonic fluids for routine use.[15]

Although this makes sense for the child with a normal urinary concentrating ability, it poses a problem for the rare child with NDI. Administration of a fluid with a higher tonicity than the urine will increase the tonicity of the blood, leading to iatrogenic hypernatremia.[16] This is especially problematic if the child presents with hypernatremia. Because of concerns over rapid lowering of the plasma sodium level, with the consequent risk of brain edema and herniation, hypotonic fluids are usually avoided in hypernatremic dehydration.[17] Again, although this makes perfect sense in the child with a normal urinary concentrating ability, it can have disastrous consequences in the rare child with NDI because the administration of a fluid with a higher sodium concentration than the urine, such as 0.9% or even 0.45% saline, will worsen the hypernatremia.[18] Physicians caring for children with NDI need to be aware that the fluid needs of these children are different, and that they primarily need water, as highlighted by their own drinking habits. Concerns about the rapidity of restoring the water deficit should be accounted for by the rate of water replacement (see later), rather than by resorting to a fluid with a sodium and effective osmolality concentration that exceeds that of the child's urine. Increasing the osmotic load by provision of fluids high in sodium increases the obligate water losses needed for the kidneys to excrete this increased load.[14]

***Secondary Forms.*** The most common form of NDI in adults is lithium-induced, but this is virtually nonexistent in children.[19] Instead, secondary NDI can be seen as a complication of other kidney diseases, such as Bartter syndrome, or in cystinosis.[20] Again, awareness by the clinician is key because treatment of these disorders usually involves supplementation with large doses of salt and/or the administration of salt-containing IV fluids. The unexpected development of hypernatremia should prompt investigations into a urinary concentrating defect and consequent adjustment of treatment.[21]

### Hypernatremia From Excess Salt

The vast majority of cases of hypernatremia reflect dehydration—that is, a net water loss. However, there are rare cases of hypernatremia in children due to excess salt administration, which can occur inadvertently or with malicious intent, and recognizing these cases is important.[22] At risk are especially those children without free access to water, such as infants or tube-fed children, in whom the natural aversion to a high salt intake can be bypassed.[23] Because salt is an effective emetic and can cause osmotic diarrhea, affected children can present with GI symptoms, leading to a misdiagnosis of hypernatremic dehydration.[8] Most reported cases experienced recurrent episodes of hypernatremia, and there should be a high index of suspicion in such patients if the observed weight loss is not consistent with the expected change in weight if the hypernatremia was due to water loss.[8] Once suspected, the diagnosis is best established by calculation of the fractional excretion of sodium (FENa), and administered feeds and fluids should be ascertained.[9] Although the FENa level can also be elevated in hypernatremic dehydration, this will only be in the context of acute kidney injury.[13]

## HYPOOSMOLALITY AND HYPONATREMIA: PATHOGENESIS AND CLASSIFICATION

Hypoosmolality indicates excess water relative to solute in the ECF. Because water moves freely between the ECF and ICF, this also indicates an excess of TBW relative to total body solute. Hyponatremia (plasma sodium concentration <135 mmol/L) and hypoosmolality (plasma osmolality <280 mOsm/kg $H_2O$) are typically used synonymously. However, high or normal osmolality with a low sodium concentration may be found when effective solutes other than sodium are present in the plasma, enlarging the osmolal gap. The latter is the difference between the measured osmolality and the calculated osmolality (see earlier); normal values in children are between 0 and 10 mOsm/kg $H_2O$.[24] Pseudohyponatremia, hyponatremia with normal osmolality, can be produced by marked elevation of plasma lipid or protein levels when measured by an indirect ion-selective electrode. This method is especially popular in pediatric laboratories because it requires only a very small sample volume, which is then diluted with water. In the calculation of the original sodium concentration in the plasma from the measured diluted sample, it is assumed that 93% of the plasma sample is water. If this assumption is wrong because of a high protein or lipid content, the calculated sodium concentration will be erroneously low.[25] Although the concentration of sodium per liter of plasma water is unchanged, the concentration of sodium per liter of plasma is decreased because of the increased nonaqueous portion of the plasma occupied by lipids or protein. This does not occur when using techniques such as direct potentiometry, in which the water content of the sample does not affect the measurement of sodium concentration, but that require larger sample volumes and is thus not commonly used in pediatric laboratories.

Children are at increased risk for developing hyponatremic encephalopathy because of the relatively larger ratio of brain to intracranial volume compared with adults. The brain reaches adult size by 6 years of age, but the skull does not reach adult size until 16 years of age.[26] The average plasma sodium concentration in children with hyponatremic encephalopathy has been found to be 120 mmol/L; in adults, it is 111 mmol/L. Hypoxia is also a major risk factor for the development of hyponatremic encephalopathy because it impairs the ability of the brain to adapt to hyponatremia, and hyponatremia in turn leads to a decrease in cerebral blood flow and arterial oxygen content.[27]

Briefly, hyponatremia may result from a loss of sodium in excess of water or from a gain of water in excess of sodium. For the kidneys, volume homeostasis is the most important priority; to maintain this, normal plasma osmolality and sodium concentration can be compromised. Thus, primary sodium depletion is accompanied by some degree of secondary retention of water by the kidneys in response to the resulting intravascular hypovolemia and consequent stimulation of AVP secretion.[28] Conversely, primary water retention can lead to hypervolemia, which in turn causes sodium losses.[25] Thus, both mechanisms (sodium loss and water retention) can coexist in the same patient, leading to frequent confusion in the diagnosis (e.g., cerebral salt wasting versus the syndrome of inappropriate antidiuretic hormone [ADH] release [SIADH]). Nevertheless, identifying the primary mechanism (sodium loss vs. water gain) is critical to institute appropriate treatment, which in turn will stop the secondary compensatory attempts by the kidneys to maintain volume homeostasis.

For this reason, patients with hyponatremia are best classified according to the status of the ECF volume (Table 73.2). The presence of ECF volume contraction is consistent with a primary sodium loss, whereas euvolemia or hypervolemia suggest primary water excess. In children with primary sodium loss, the FENa can help distinguish between renal (FENa > 1%) or extrarenal losses (<1%). Yet, FENa may only be increased acutely because compensatory mechanisms such as aldosterone will reduce renal sodium losses at the expense of potassium. Consequently, the fractional excretion of chloride (FECl) may be more informative of renal salt losses because both sodium and potassium in the urine need to be accompanied by an anion. In one study, an FECl value

**Table 73.2 Clinical Classification of Hyponatremic Disorders in Children**[a]

| Contracted | Normal | Expanded |
|---|---|---|
| Renal solute loss | Administration of hypotonic solutions | Congestive heart failure |
| • Diuretics (thiazides) | SIADH | Cirrhotic liver disease |
| • Osmotic diuresis—hyperglycemia | Nephrogenic syndrome of inappropriate antidiuresis | Nephrotic syndrome |
| • Salt-wasting nephropathies | Severe hypothyroidism | Advanced oliguric renal failure |
| • Mineralocorticoid deficiency | Glucocorticoid deficiency | Excessive water intake |
| • Cerebral salt wasting | | |
| Nonrenal solute loss | | |
| • Gastrointestinal—vomiting, diarrhea, aspiration, fistula, stoma, third space | | |
| • Cutaneous—sweating, burns, cystic fibrosis | | |

[a]According to the status of extracellular fluid volume.
*SIADH,* Syndrome of inappropriate antidiuretic hormone secretion.

more than 0.5% was consistent with a renal salt-wasting disorder.[29] Obviously, normal values for fractional excretion only apply in the setting of a normal GFR.[25]

In children with primary water excess, urine osmolality can help distinguish between renal water retention (e.g., SIADH—urine osmolality >100 mOsm/kg) and water intoxication (urine osmolality <100 mOsm/kg).[25]

## TREATMENT OF HYPONATREMIA

The treatment of hyponatremia follows simple principles[30]:

- Hyponatremia due to water overload should be treated by restricting water intake and/or enhancing water excretion.
- In the rare case of hyponatremia due to sodium deficiency, sodium supplementation is appropriate.
- In a chronic case or case of unknown duration, without acute symptoms, extreme care needs to be taken to correct the hyponatremia slowly to avoid complications, such as osmotic demyelination (central pontine myelinosis).
- Regardless of the cause, in acute symptomatic hyponatremia (e.g., seizures, confusion, coma), a rapid increase in sodium concentration to a level considered acceptable (usually 125 mmol/L), and where symptoms improve, can be achieved by administering 3% saline. A simple approach of using a 2-mL/kg body weight bolus (maximal, 100 mL), which can be repeated, as needed, has been suggested.[30,31]

## SYNDROME OF INAPPROPRIATE ANTIDIURETIC HORMONE SECRETION

SIADH is characterized by hyponatremia less than 135 mEq/L, low plasma osmolality (<275 mOsm/kg $H_2O$ in typical descriptions), and urine osmolality that is not at a minimum value of less than 100 mOsm/kg $H_2O$. The diagnosis requires the absence of clinical or biochemical signs of hypovolemia, diuretic use, and other causes of impaired free water excretion by the kidneys, such as nephrotic syndrome, hypothyroidism; adrenal insufficiency; renal, cardiac, or hepatic failure. Characteristically the urinary sodium concentration is greater than 20 mmol/L, reflecting the attempts by the kidneys to maintain volume homeostasis, because the primary water retention leads to volume overload, which is corrected by sodium excretion. This increased urinary sodium concentration often leads to diagnostic uncertainty or a misdiagnosis of salt wasting, which is then treated with sodium supplementation, typically resulting in hypertension.[25,32]

It is important to emphasize that the vast majority of cases of SIADH in children is acute and transient, resolving with the passage of time or after the underlying condition improves or heals. Thus, pediatricians usually do not cope with chronic states of hyponatremia. If the SIADH resolves while the patient has hyponatremia, AVP secretion will be suppressed by the hypo-osmolality, and a water diuresis will ensue. The treatment of choice for patients with acute SIADH is water restriction, which, if adhered to, usually achieves normalization of the plasma sodium concentration within 2 or 3 days. In those with persisting hyponatremia, treatment with AVPR2 antagonists, a vaptan or urea has been reported to be successful.[32–34]

## HYPONATREMIA IN HOSPITALIZED CHILDREN

The prescription of hypotonic solutions as maintenance intravenous (IV) fluids in hospitalized children, according to the classic recommendations of Holliday and Segar,[35] has been challenged by a growing number of studies over the past 2 decades, which have drawn attention to the risk for severe neurologic complications and even death in hospitalized children who develop hyponatremia.[36] The incidence of acute hospital-acquired hyponatremia has been reported to be as high as 10% in a case-control study performed in a pediatric tertiary hospital.[37] Likewise, 11% of infants with severe bronchiolitis had serum sodium levels less than 130 mEq/L at the time of admission to the intensive care unit.[38] The retrospective incidence of postoperative hyponatremia among 24,412 pediatric patients with generally minor illnesses subjected to routine surgical procedures has been reported to be 0.34%, with a mortality rate of those so affected of 8.4%.[39]

Hospital-acquired hyponatremia is usually attributed to the administration of hypotonic fluids in the presence of simultaneous impaired free water excretion resulting from elevated AVP secretion by hemodynamic (e.g., effective circulating volume depletion) and nonhemodynamic (e.g., malignancies, CNS disorders, pulmonary diseases, medications, nausea, pain, stress) stimuli.[40] Excessive fluid administration is also considered a common contributing factor.[41] Thus, hospital-acquired hyponatremia typically reflects SIADH. To reduce the risk for hyponatremia, the British National Patient Safety Agency has recommended increasing the tonicity of IV fluids administered as maintenance therapy in children from 0.18% NaCl, as formerly used, to 0.45% NaCl, and prescribing isotonic solutions to hospitalized children with disorders entailing a high risk for elevated AVP secretion and ensuing hyponatremia.[42] Concerns that using solutions with higher salt content would result in an increased incidence of hypernatremia instead have not been confirmed.[43] Yet, considering that hyponatremia in the context of elevated ADH levels is due to an excess of water, rather than a deficiency of salt, a more physiologic measure to decrease the risk for hyponatremia would be the reduction of fluids to two-thirds of the normal recommended volume, except in dehydrated children.[44]

## NEPHROGENIC SYNDROME OF INAPPROPRIATE ANTIDIURESIS

Nephrogenic syndrome of inappropriate antidiuresis is caused by activating mutations in AVPR2, thus constituting a mirror image to NDI.[45] The spectrum of symptoms has been reported to vary within the same family, ranging from infrequent voiding to incidentally noted hyponatremia to recurrent admissions with hyponatremic seizures.[46,47] Hyponatremia can manifest as early as the neonatal period, but usually is more prominent, once urine concentrating ability develops fully during the first year of life.[48] Unsurprisingly, given the X chromosome location of *AVPR2*, males are typically more severely affected than females. Administration of oral urea as osmotic agent at a dose titrated up from 0.25 up to 2 g/kg/day, given in up to four divided doses, has been shown to be effective in these children.[49]

### Basis of Fluid Therapy for Dehydration in Children

The three steps in treating dehydration are as follows: (1) repletion of deficit, which means previous losses of fluids, and that can be estimated by the patient's weight loss; (2) maintenance therapy, which means physiologic requirements

**Table 73.3 Features of Intravenous Fluids Commonly Used in Pediatrics**

| Solution | Osmolality (mOsm/L) | Sodium (mEq/L) | Osmolality (Compared With Plasma) | Tonicity (With Reference to Cell Membrane) |
|---|---|---|---|---|
| NaCl, 0.9% | 308 | 154 | Isosmolar | Isotonic |
| NaCl, 0.45% | 154 | 77 | Hyposmolar | Hypotonic |
| Glucose, 5% | 278 | 0 | Isosmolar | Hypotonic |
| Glucose, 10% | 555 | 0 | Hyperosmolar | Hypotonic |
| NaCl, 0.9% with glucose 5% | 586 | 150 | Hyperosmolar | Isotonic |
| Lactated Ringer's solution[a] | 273 | 130 | Hyposmolar | Isotonic |
| Hartmann's solution | 278 | 131 | Isosmolar | Isotonic |
| Human albumin, 5% | 260 | 140 | Hyposmolar | Isotonic |

[a]Lactated Ringer's solution also contains 4 mEq/L of potassium as well as 1.4 mmol/L of calcium and 28 mmol/L of lactate.

of fluid and electrolytes; and (3) sustained provision of continuing extraordinary losses. Replacement of the deficit was traditionally carried out slowly, over 24 to 48 hours, particularly in the presence of hyponatremia or hypernatremia. In acute processes, usually from a GI origin, and when most of the fluid lost by the child comes from the ECF, current recommendations are more in favor of a policy of rapid repletion of the isotonic depletion to restore the ECF volume quickly on the basis of the following benefits—improved GI perfusion that allows earlier oral feeding, improved renal perfusion, and a lower morbidity and mortality rate.[44] If the child has signs of severe hypovolemia (see earlier), repletion therapy may begin with a rapid IV infusion of 10–20 mL/kg of isotonic 0.9% saline (Table 73.3), which can be repeated as needed until adequate perfusion is restored under careful monitoring of the patient. A recent large multicenter trial of fluid resuscitation in patients with septic shock, however, has cautioned against the use of fluid boluses, which was associated with a significant increase in mortality compared with children receiving only maintenance fluids without an initial bolus.[50]

Maintenance fluids used to be calculated following the Holliday-Segar method,[35] which estimates physiologic losses of water scaled to the metabolic rate. Yet, given the increased incidence of hyponatremia in children receiving IV fluids in an isotonic solution (see Table 73.3), is now considered an appropriate initial option.[15] The rate of fluid administration is determined by maintenance need, estimated fluid deficit (usually replaced over 24–48 hours), and ongoing losses. Key is ongoing close monitoring of clinical state, fluid balance, weight, and biochemistries to allow appropriate adaptation of fluid rate and composition, if needed. Under normal circumstances, the kidneys will be able to maintain volume and electrolyte homeostasis with almost any fluid administered, but problems arise when kidney function is impaired or if the kidneys receive inappropriate signals (e.g., as in SIADH).

In hypernatremic dehydration, the gravest danger is posed by a rapid decrease in plasma sodium concentration, leading to cerebral edema. A rate of decrease in the sodium concentration by 0.5 mmol/L/h or less is usually considered safe; fluid composition and/or the rate may need to be adjusted to maintain a safe normalization of sodium concentration, emphasizing again the importance of close monitoring of the patient.[17]

Rehydration therapy with oral solutions, such as the World Health Organization solution, should be attempted as an alternative to IV therapy in children with mild and moderate dehydration and good oral tolerance.[44] Even in patients with initial vomiting, the oral administration of small and frequent volumes of the solution often succeeds in correcting the dehydration.

## POTASSIUM DISORDERS

Unlike adults, infants and children need to maintain a positive balance of potassium to grow normally because cellular mass depends on potassium as the major intracellular cation. Total body potassium increases from approximately 8 mmol/cm body height at birth to greater than 14 mmol/cm body height by 18 years of age, with the rate of accumulation of body potassium per kilogram of weight being more rapid in infants than in children and adolescents.[51] In vitro and experimental studies have indicated that the capacity of the neonatal kidney to secrete potassium is less than in the adult. The immature kidneys are relatively insensitive to aldosterone, which, in the clinical setting, correlates with the higher plasma concentrations of aldosterone and potassium and the lower ratio of urinary sodium to potassium characteristic of newborns and infants.[51]

### HYPOKALEMIA

Hypokalemia is usually defined as a serum potassium concentration less than 3.5 mEq/L. Acute changes in the serum potassium concentration usually reflect modifications in the distribution of potassium between the extracellular and intracellular compartments. By contrast, alterations in the external potassium balance give rise to more chronic changes of plasma potassium concentration and lead to situations of true potassium deficit. Clinical conditions leading to sustained hypokalemia are listed in Table 73.4.

Potassium is critical for many important cell functions, so hypokalemia and potassium depletion may result in clinical manifestations in several organs and tissues (Table 73.5). In general, the same degree of hypokalemia is better tolerated when it results from a chronic potassium loss than from an acute decline, but both conditions may coexist in the same

**Table 73.4 Most Relevant Causes of Hypokalemia in Pediatric Patients**

| Acquired Causes | Inherited Causes |
|---|---|
| Acute redistribution of potassium to the intracellular compartment | Hypokalemia with normal blood pressure |
| Metabolic alkalosis | Bartter syndrome |
| Insulin administration | Gitelman syndrome |
| Hypokalemic periodic paralysis | Epilepsy, ataxia, sensorineural deafness, and tubulopathy (EAST syndrome) |
| Prolonged lack of intake | Fanconi syndrome |
| Increased renal loss | Hypokalemia with hypertension |
| Drugs—diuretics, antibiotics, aminoglycosides, penicillin, amphotericin B, capreomycin | Congenital adrenal hyperplasia |
| Metabolic acidosis, including diabetic ketoacidosis | Primary hyperaldosteronism |
| Increased gastrointestinal loss | Liddle syndrome |
| Vomiting (hypertrophic pyloric stenosis) | Apparent mineralocorticoid excess |
| Diarrhea | Hypokalemia with acidosis |
| | Renal tubular acidosis (types 1, 2, and 3) |

**Table 73.5 Primary Manifestations of Hypokalemia and Potassium Deficit in Pediatric Patients**

| Organ System | Manifestation |
|---|---|
| Neuromuscular | • Skeletal muscle weakness<br>• Muscular paralysis<br>• Paralytic ileum<br>• Muscle ischemia and rhabdomyolysis |
| Heart | • Electrocardiographic alterations<br>  • Depression of S-T segment<br>  • Low amplitude of T wave<br>  • Appearance of U wave<br>• Arrhythmias |
| Nutrition and growth | • Mild glucose intolerance<br>• Growth retardation |
| Kidney | • Hypokalemic nephropathy<br>• Polyuria-polydipsia |

patient. Arrhythmias and marked weakness or paralysis of respiratory muscles are life-threatening symptoms that require urgent therapy. Growth retardation can be seen in children with hypokalemic tubular disorders.[29,52,53] Association with growth hormone (GH) deficit has been reported in a few of these patients.[54] Yet, these patients typically have complex abnormalities, typically including alkalosis and often elevated prostaglandin levels. To what degree the hypokalemia is responsible for the impaired growth remains unresolved. In one report, response to GH was only seen after concurrent treatment with a prostaglandin synthesis inhibitor.[29] In another study, amelioration of the alkalosis was associated with improved growth.[55] Similarly, long-standing hypokalemia has been associated with so-called hypokalemic nephropathy, which includes the development of renal cysts, chronic interstitial nephritis and, in the very long term, progressive loss of renal function. However, whether it is truly the hypokalemia causing this or other factors associated with the underlying disorder, such as hypovolemia or nephrocalcinosis, remains to be clarified. In one study, no association between the degree of hypokalemia and chronic kidney disease was seen.[56] Polyuria resistant to the administration of AVP and polydipsia (secondary NDI) has also been associated with hypokalemic disorders.[20,57] Yet, patients with Gitelman syndrome typically have preserved urinary concentrating ability, whereas patients with Bartter syndrome may have hyposthenuria, despite comparable potassium levels.[29] Moreover, of all forms of Bartter syndrome, type 3 (due to mutations in CLCNKB; see later) typically have the lowest plasma potassium levels, yet the best preserved urine-concentrating ability.[29,58] This suggests, that other factors such as hypercalciuria may actually be more relevant for the impaired urinary concentration.[21]

The cause of hypokalemia is usually apparent from the clinical history and global assessment of the patient. Excessive renal wasting of potassium can be identified by measuring potassium loss in urine collected for 24 hours or by calculating urinary indices in spot samples. Thus, in a hypokalemic child, fractional excretion of potassium (K):

$$\text{Fractional excretion of potassium} = (\text{urine K}/\text{plasma K}) \times (\text{plasma creatinine} \times 100/\text{urine creatinine})$$

above 30%, or a transtubular potassium gradient (TTKG):

$$\text{TTKG} = (\text{urine K}/\text{plasma K}) \times (\text{plasma osmolality} \times 100/\text{urine osmolality}))$$

greater than 6 is consistent with renal potassium wasting. In the clinical setting, the coexistence of hypokalemia of renal origin with alkalosis indicates enhanced sodium reabsorption in the collecting duct. If accompanied by arterial hypertension, this suggests primary salt retention, either due to stimulation of the mineralocorticoid receptor (e.g., renal vascular hypertension, salt-retaining forms of congenital adrenal hyperplasia, apparent mineralocorticoid excess) or from gain-of-function mutations in the mineralocorticoid receptor (pregnancy-associated hypertension) or the epithelial sodium channel ENaC (Liddle syndrome). Conversely, if the hypokalemic alkalosis is associated with normal or low blood pressure, this suggests a salt-wasting disorder (e.g., Bartter or Gitelman syndrome or extrarenal salt losses), with secondary activation of salt reabsorption in the collecting duct. A list of inherited disorders associated with hypokalemic alkalosis is provided in Table 73.4.

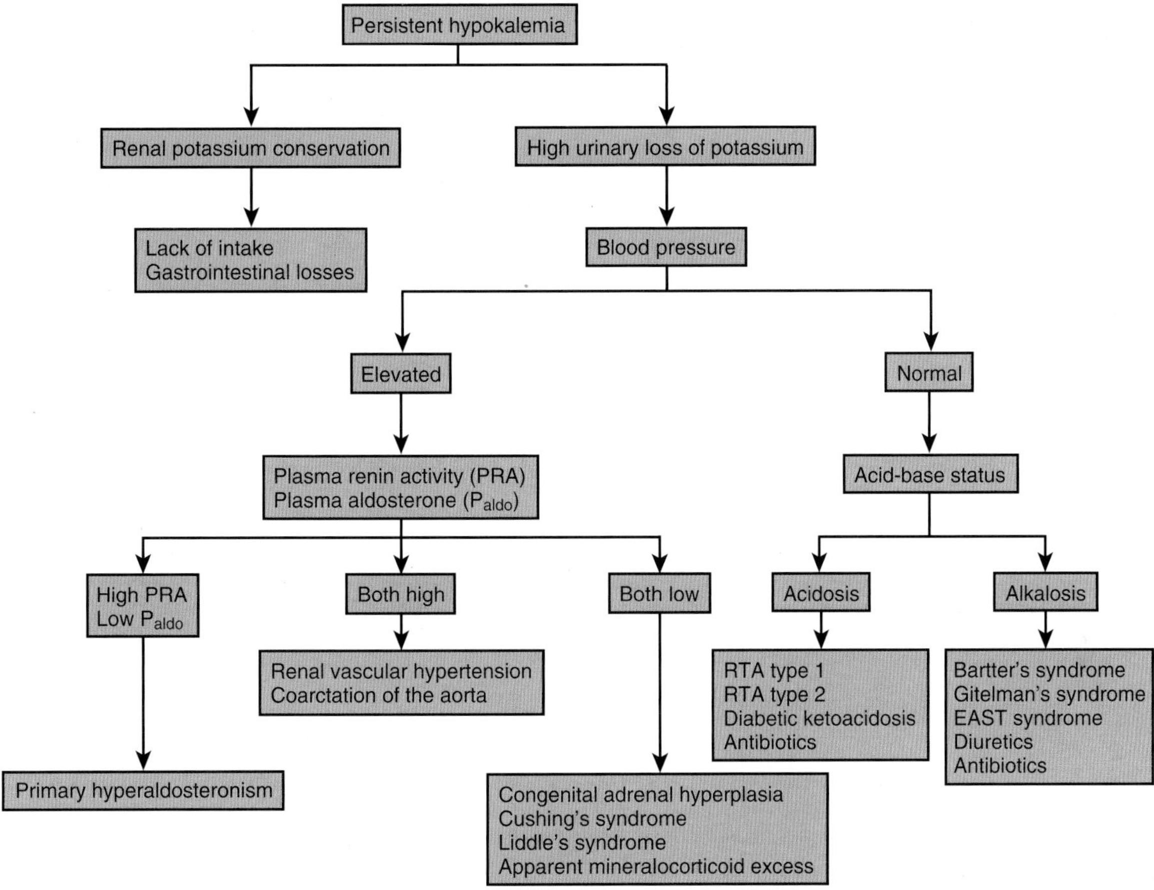


**Fig. 73.1** Diagnostic approach to persistent hypokalemia in children. Transient hypokalemias are usually secondary to transcellular shifts of potassium ion. *EAST,* Epilepsy, ataxia, sensorineural deafness, and tubulopathy; *RTA,* renal tubular acidosis.

In contrast, if hypokalemia is associated with acidosis, this suggests renal tubular acidosis (RTA; proximal or distal, inherited or acquired; Fig. 73.1).

Hypokalemia secondary to internal potassium redistribution is transient and normalizes after the underlying disorder is corrected. Potassium deficit is treated with a potassium-rich diet and, if needed, oral potassium supplements, usually potassium chloride; potassium citrate is preferred in patients with concomitant acidosis. Patients with arrhythmias, respiratory paralysis, or rhabdomyolysis or those unable to take oral medications must be treated with IV potassium chloride at a maximum rate of 0.5 mEq/hg/hr and maximum concentration of 40 mEq/L in saline solutions. A higher concentration and rate of administration can be used in life-threatening situations under intensive care control and continuous electrocardiographic monitoring.[59]

## INHERITED DISORDERS ASSOCIATED WITH HYPOKALEMIA

All disorders mentioned here are discussed in detail in the other relevant chapters; thus, mainly aspects specific to pediatric patients are considered here. We can distinguish three different forms of hypokalemia, based on the underlying pathophysiology, which leads to the following associated other homeostatic abnormalities (see Table 73.4): (1) alkalosis without hypertension; (2) alkalosis with hypertension; and (3) acidosis.

### Hypokalemic Alkalosis Without Hypertension

#### Bartter Syndrome

***Antenatal Presentation.*** The clinical manifestations of Bartter syndrome can already start during intrauterine life or immediately after birth; these include polyhydramnios, premature birth, polyuria, and loss of salt. A key aspect of Bartter syndrome is the impaired function of the juxtaglomerular apparatus (JGA), the site of tubular glomerular feedback (TGF), which acts as a "volume sensor" of the kidney.[60] Salt or, more precisely, chloride reabsorption in the macula densa, is a key signaling pathway for TGF, but is essentially short-circuited in Bartter syndrome due to the genetic knockout of salt reabsorption in the thick ascending limb of Henle's loop (TAL), which includes the macula densa.[55,61] The impaired chloride reabsorption leads to primary activation of cyclooxygenase-2 (COX-2), with the consequent formation of prostaglandin E2, hyperreninism, and afferent arteriolar dilation.[62,63] This aspect of Bartter syndrome is most prominent in types 1, 2, and 4 and is typically associated with antenatal presentation (Fig. 73.2).

It is presumed that in type 3, CLCNKA, which is also expressed in TAL, can compensate to some degree for the loss of CLCNKB function, as illustrated by the fact that combined mutations in both chloride channels are associated with a severe antenatal presentation (Bartter syndrome type 4b).[64] Yet, there is a wide spectrum of severity in all forms of Bartter syndrome and some patients with types 1, 2, or 4

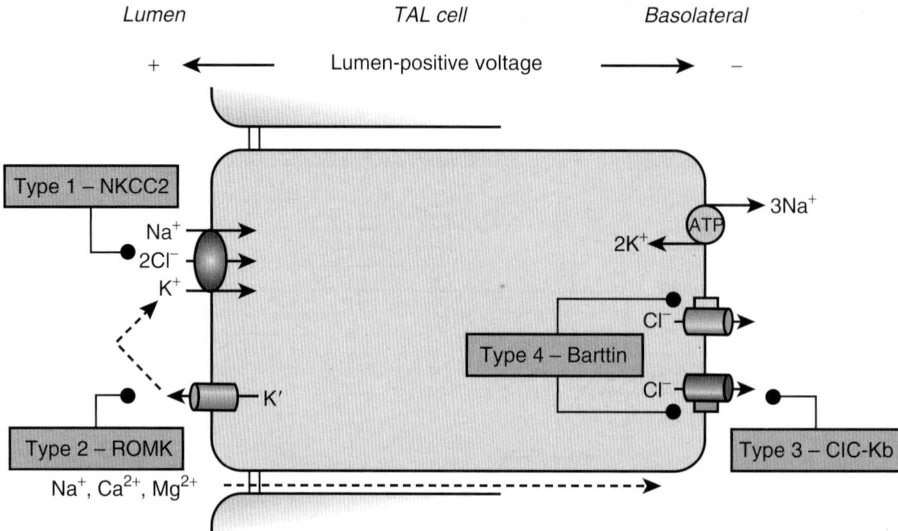


**Fig. 73.2** Schematic representation of a cell of the thick ascending limb of the loop of Henle *(TAL)* showing the transport systems disturbed in the four types of Bartter syndrome. The bumetanide-sensitive $Na^+$-$K^+$-$2Cl^-$ cotransporter *(NKCC2)* and the renal outer medullary $K^+$ channel *(ROMK)* are depicted on the luminal membrane of the cell. The $Na^+$-$K^+$-ATPase and the chloride channels ClC-Ka and ClC-Kb with their Barttin subunit are represented on the basolateral side. See text for description of types 5 and 6 Bartter syndrome. *ATP,* Adenosine triphosphate.

can have mild forms and present later in childhood or even in adulthood, whereas up to one-third of patients with type 3 can have an antenatal or neonatal presentation.[62,65] Bartter syndrome is a salt-wasting disorder, so salt supplementation is a mainstay of treatment. In the antenatal form, this may include an IV infusion of saline solutions for prolonged periods of time to avoid dehydration and even death, but this will not be sufficient to suppress the prostaglandin production due to the dysfunction of TGF. This may explain why most patients with the antenatal presentation benefit clinically from the use of cyclooxygenase inhibitors, which ameliorate the polyuria and electrolyte wasting, as already noted by Bartter.[66] Due to the potential of severe complications of indomethacin, including bowel perforation and necrotizing enterocolitis, the use of the more selective COX-2 inhibitors, such as rofecoxib and celecoxib, has been proposed.[67,68] The association of these drugs with an increased incidence of cardiovascular complications in adults taking these medications for chronic pain has, however, dampened the enthusiasm, although it is unclear to what degree this risk applies to patients with Bartter syndrome and whether it outweighs the risks of indomethacin.[62,69]

A special aspect of Bartter syndrome type 2 is an initial presentation with hyperkalemia, sometimes resulting in an erroneous initial diagnosis of pseudohypoaldosteronism type 1 (see "Hyperkalemia," later).[70] This paradoxic feature can be explained by the expression of the renal outer medullary $K^+$ channel (ROMK), also in the collecting duct, where it mediates potassium secretion. The hyperkalemia resolves typically within the first week of life, presumably due to tubular maturation with the expression of other potassium channels, which can compensate for ROMK dysfunction in the collecting duct.[51]

An interesting aspect of antenatal regulation of tubular salt transport was revealed by the identification of mutations in MAGED2 as the cause of a severe, but transient, antenatal form of Bartter syndrome, with symptoms resolving completely within the first 3 to 4 weeks of life.[71] These patients showed evidence for reduced expression of both SLC12A1 and SLC12A3, suggesting that MAGED2 is involved in the regulation of expression of these transporters in utero.[72]

Some patients, typically with Bartter syndrome types 1 or 2, can have marked hyposthenuria (secondary NDI) and present a treatment dilemma—salt supplementation helps compensate for the renal salt losses, but excess salt in NDI worsens the urinary water losses.[20] Indeed, persistent hypernatremia, leading to the cessation of salt supplementation, has been reported in such patients.[29]

***Classic Presentation.*** The patients included in Bartter's original report all presented in childhood.[73] For this reason, Bartter syndrome with a postnatal presentation is typically referred to as "classic" Bartter syndrome. It is usually associated with loss-of-function mutations in CLCNKB (type 3), but can be seen with all types, potentially due to residual function of the mutated proteins in some cases.[29,65,74,75] Despite the suggestion of a milder phenotype by the later presentation, patients with type 2 Bartter syndrome typically have the most severe electrolyte abnormalities and alkalosis. Supplementation of potassium salts rarely achieves normalization of plasma levels. Treatment with potassium-sparing diuretics can improve this, but obviously worsens the salt wasting and thus risks life-threatening hypovolemia.[55] Use of these drugs should thus be very carefully considered, especially in babies, who cannot self-regulate their salt and fluid intake, and is probably best reserved only for extreme cases with apparent complications from the electrolyte abnormalities, such as arrhythmia or paralysis.[62]

There are several other abnormalities associated with Bartter syndrome, including growth hormone deficiency, hypophosphatemia with renal phosphate wasting, and hyperparathyroidism.[54,76,77] Potentially, these are linked to the impaired electrolyte–acid-base balance and/or the elevated prostaglandin levels. Improvement of growth after treatment with celecoxib and amelioration of phosphate wasting after improvement of alkalosis has been reported in isolated cases.[29,55]

**Gitelman Syndrome.** Gitelman syndrome is arguably the most common tubulopathy, with an estimated prevalence of 1 in 40,000.[78] Although often considered primarily a disease of teenagers and adults, it is a common tubulopathy diagnosis also in children, and manifestations have been noted even in premature infants.[79,80]

Gitelman syndrome is biochemically characterized by hypokalemic metabolic alkalosis in association with hypomagnesemia and hypocalciuria, reflecting the side effects seen with thiazide treatment, consistent with the common molecular basis. Thiazides inhibit the sodium chloride cotransporter NCC, encoded by *SLC12A3*, recessive mutations which are the cause of Gitelman syndrome (Fig. 73.3).[81] Yet, the phenotype can be mimicked by mutations in *CLCNKB* (Bartter syndrome type 3) or *HNF1B*.[79,82] Moreover, there is variability in the severity of the phenotype, with some patients only showing minor electrolyte abnormalities, including normal plasma magnesium concentrations.[29,78]

Many patients are diagnosed incidentally, when blood tests are obtained for an unrelated indication. Other patients, however, present with other symptoms, including tetany, paresthesias, muscle cramps, salt craving, generalized weakness, and fatigue.[83] Interestingly, the magnitude of the electrolyte abnormalities does not necessarily correlate with the severity of symptoms as perceived by the patient. Some patients have only mild biochemical abnormalities but experience the disease as a disabling illness that disrupts their ability to have a normal life, whereas others have marked hypokalemic alkalosis and hypomagnesemia but feel well and are only occasionally troubled by symptoms, such as cramps.[84] Symptom severity, as reported by the patient, appears to be milder in children than in adults; in one pediatric study, 21% of children considered their symptoms as a moderate to big problem, compared with 45% of adults.[83,85]

There have been isolated reports of GH deficiency in Gitelman syndrome, but typically in patients without genetic confirmation of the diagnosis. It is thus unclear whether these patients had mutations in *SLC12A3* or in *CLCNKB* and thus a diagnosis of Bartter syndrome type 3, where GH deficiency has been reported recurrently.[86,87] Yet, also in molecularly confirmed series of patients, up to one-third of patients had a height less than 2 standard deviations (SD) below the norm.[85,87] Often, this is associated with pubertal delay and thus may not reflect the patient's final height.[87] As in Bartter syndrome, this may be related to the biochemical abnormalities. In one study, those patients deemed compliant with their treatment had significant improvement in growth compared with those found to be noncompliant.[85]

Gitelman syndrome is a disorder of salt reabsorption in the distal convolute. Salt transport in the TAL and thus the macula densa is intact. Therefore, in contrast to Bartter syndrome, TGF is intact, and hyperreninism should be suppressible by salt and volume expansion.[62] Patients typically have a pronounced salt craving, yet additional salt supplementation may still be beneficial.[78] Potassium chloride and magnesium supplements are often prescribed as well, depending on electrolyte abnormalities. As in Bartter syndrome, normalization of these abnormalities is frequently not achieved with oral supplementation, because increased plasma levels increase the filtered load and thus, typically, renal losses. Although severe complications of extreme electrolyte abnormalities have been reported, a stable subnormal concentration may still be safer than marked swings

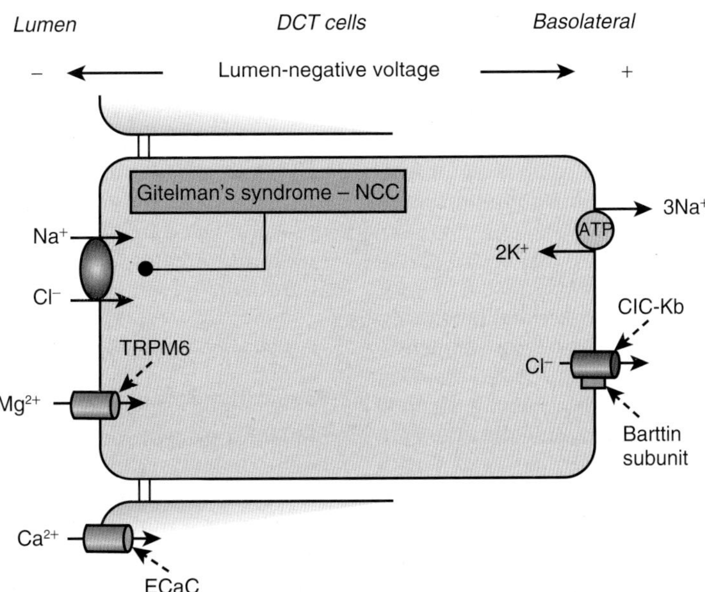


**Fig. 73.3** Schematic representation of a cell of the distal convoluted tubule *(DCT)* showing the transport systems involved in the reabsorption of NaCl. The thiazide-sensitive $Na^+$-$Cl^-$ cotransporter *(NCC)*, the magnesium-transporting channel TRPM6, and the epithelial calcium channel *(ECaC)* are depicted on the luminal membrane of the cell. The $Na^+$-$K^+$-ATPase and the chloride channel ClC-Kb with their Barttin subunit are represented on the basolateral side. NCC, ClC-Kb, and TRPM6 are expressed in the early downstream segment of the DCT, and ECaC is expressed in the late downstream portion of DCT. *TRPM6,* Transient receptor potential channel melastatin 6.

in plasma concentrations associated with large intermittent supplement doses.[78] For this reason, supplements should always be distributed in several doses throughout the day. Dissolving the salt supplements in a bottle of water, from which the patient drinks throughout the day, may help achieve more stable levels by providing frequent small doses. Moreover, a large dose can have side effects itself, such as diarrhea, vomiting (thus worsening electrolyte losses), and gastric ulcers. In an expert consensus statement, an "individual balance between improvement in blood values and side effects" was recommended, which may include target values well below the norm.[78]

**EAST Syndrome.** The EAST syndrome (*e*pilepsy, *a*taxia, *s*ensorineural deafness, and *t*ubulopathy), also known as SeSAME syndrome (*se*izures, *s*ensorineural deafness, *a*taxia, *m*ental retardation, and *e*lectrolyte imbalance) is rare, with approximately 30 patients described so far.[88–90] Mutations in the *KCNJ10* gene encoding a potassium channel expressed in the brain, inner ear, and basolateral membrane of the distal convoluted tubule in the kidney have been found in these children. Loss of function of this channel impairs salt reabsorption in the distal convolute and the renal manifestations thus mimic Gitelman syndrome, with hypokalemia, hypomagnesemia, and hypocalciuria.[88] Patients typically present in the first year of life with seizures, and blood tests at the time reveal the typical biochemical picture. Patients often receive enormous doses of potassium and magnesium supplementation out of concern that the electrolyte abnormalities are the cause of the seizures. Yet, experience so far suggests that seizures are independent of the biochemical alterations and rather reflect the important role of *KCNJ10* for potassium balance in the brain.[91] Indeed, whereas the biochemical abnormalities may worsen during school age, seizure activity spontaneously improves in most patients at this time.[92,93]

**Claudin 10.** Recessive mutations in *CLDN10*, part of the paracellular junction in the TAL, have been identified in two patients with a hypokalemic alkalotic salt-wasting phenotype, consistent with data from Cldn10 knockout mice that have shown a reduced sodium permeability in TAL.[94,95] Mutations in this gene may thus explain some patients with a Bartter-like tubulopathy yet no identified mutations in known genes.

### Hypokalemic Alkalosis With Hypertension

In contrast to the salt-wasting disorders described previously, in which hypokalemic alkalosis reflects the secondary activation of the renin-aldosterone axis, the identical biochemical picture can also be seen in disorders with primary enhanced salt reabsorption in the collecting duct. These disorders are thus salt retaining and are consequently associated with hypertension (see Table 73.4). All are associated with enhanced salt reabsorption through the epithelial sodium channel ENaC in the principal cells of the collecting duct, either directly (Liddle syndrome) or through enhanced stimulation of the mineralocorticoid receptor (MCR). Most of these disorders are inherited in a dominant fashion and often are diagnosed later in childhood or even in adulthood. The exemption is apparent mineralocorticoid excess (AME), which is caused by recessive mutations in the enzyme HSD11B, which metabolizes cortisol to cortisone and thus normally protects the MCR from activation by cortisol.[96] The enzyme is also important in the placenta, and affected patients are typically born small for gestational age.[97] Further abnormalities include hypercalciuria and hyposthenuria, and patients may initially be misdiagnosed as having Bartter syndrome or NDI.[21] Hypertension is typically severe and left untreated, patients may die from cardiovascular complications, such as stroke or heart failure.[98]

Normalization of blood pressure and electrolyte abnormalities in all these salt-retaining disorders of the collecting duct can be achieved by pharmacologic blockade of ENaC (e.g., with amiloride or triamterene) and/or the MCR (e.g., spironolactone or eplerenone). Interestingly, recovery of urine-concentrating ability with such normalization has been reported in AME.[20]

**Disorders Associated With Hypokalemia and Acidosis.** Hypokalemia with acidosis is the typical biochemical constellation seen in either proximal (type 2) or distal (type 1) RTA. It will be discussed later.

## HYPERKALEMIA

The same principles for the pathophysiology and assessment of hyperkalemia discussed in Chapter 17 apply in children, yet there are also some differences. Plasma potassium concentrations are higher in babies and young children, perhaps reflecting the increased potassium requirement for growth at this age. Consequently, the upper limit of normal is usually defined as a plasma potassium concentration of 6.5 mmol/L in newborns, which then gradually reduces to 5.5 mEq/L in older children.[99] Pseudohyperkalemia refers to those conditions in which the elevation in the measured serum potassium concentration is caused by potassium movement out of the cells during or after the blood specimen has been drawn, typically due to hemolysis caused by mechanical trauma during sample extraction. Considering the difficulties of obtaining a free-flowing blood sample, especially in premature babies, this is a complication encountered much more frequently in children than in adults. Causes of hyperkalemia are listed in Table 73.6.

The acute treatment of symptomatic hyperkalemia is discussed in Chapter 17. Typical treatment measures and doses are listed in Table 73.7. Aside from these emergency measures, treatment should focus on the underlying abnormality.

## DISORDERS ASSOCIATED WITH HYPERKALEMIA

### Pseudohypoaldosteronism

Pseudohypoaldosteronism (PHA) is a clinical syndrome caused by end-organ resistance to the effects of aldosterone, resulting in hyperkalemia, metabolic acidosis, and normal to high serum aldosterone levels. Due to the interdependence of sodium reabsorption and potassium and hydrogen ion secretion in the collecting duct, it is sometimes also referred to as type 4 RTA.[100] PHA may be primary (hereditary) or secondary (acquired).

Primary forms are subclassified into two distinct congenital syndromes, PHA type 1 (PHA1) and PHA type 2 (Gordon syndrome, or familial hyperkalemic hypertension; PHA2).

**Table 73.6 Most Relevant Causes of Hyperkalemia in Pediatric Patients**

| Disorder | Relevant Causes |
|---|---|
| Pseudohyperkalemia | Improper collection of blood<br>• Hematologic disorders—leukocytosis, thrombocytosis, spherocytosis |
| Transcellular shift of potassium | Acidosis<br>• Insulin deficiency<br>• Hyperosmolality<br>• Exercise with nonselective beta-blockers<br>• Familial hyperkalemic periodic paralysis |
| Increased potassium load | • From exogenous origin—pharmacologic supplements<br>• From endogenous origin (cellular lysis)—burns, trauma, intravascular hemolysis, rhabdomyolysis, tumor mass destruction |
| Decreased urinary excretion | Renal failure<br>Mineralocorticoid deficiency<br>• Addison disease<br>• Hypoaldosteronism<br>Mineralocorticoid resistance<br>• Types 1 and 2 pseudohypoaldosteronism<br>Hyperkalemic drugs—potassium-sparing diuretics, trimethoprim, calcineurin inhibitors, renin-angiotensin-aldosterone system blockers |

Importantly, PHA1 is a salt-wasting disorder and thus is associated with low-normal blood pressure or even hypovolemic shock. In contrast, PHA2 is a salt-retaining disorder associated with hypertension. Both disorders are discussed in detail in Chapters 17 and 44, so the focus here will be mainly on pediatric aspects of these disorders.

Secondary forms are typically associated with urinary obstruction, often in the context of a congenital urinary tract malformation and/or severe urinary tract infection.[101] Clinically, they resemble PHA1 and are typically seen in the first year of life. The electrolyte and acid-base abnormalities resolve with treatment of the obstruction or infection.

**Pseudohypoaldosteronism Type 1.** PHA1 may be renal or systemic. The renal form occurs more frequently and is caused by heterozygous inactivating mutations in the *NR3C2* gene encoding the human MCR.[102] Patients typically present in the first weeks of life, with failure to thrive and frequent episodes of vomiting and dehydration. Biochemistries reveal hyponatremia, hyperkalemia, and metabolic acidosis, although there is considerable variability in severity. Treatment consists of sodium supplementation (in the form of sodium chloride and sodium bicarbonate) in amounts sufficient to normalize the biochemistries and maintain normovolemia. Plasma electrolytes typically normalize, even without supplementation, as early as 6 months of age, although elevated concentrations of aldosterone persist.[79,103]

Systemic PHA1 follows an autosomal recessive transmission and is caused by mutations in the *SCNN1A*, *SCNN1B*, or *SCNN1G* genes encoding the α-, β-, and γ- subunits of ENaC, respectively.[104] ENaC is expressed in the epithelial cells of the renal collecting ducts, respiratory airways, colon, and salivary and sweat glands; in addition to the severe renal salt-wasting, with life-threatening hypovolemia, extreme hyperkalemia, and metabolic acidosis, patients can suffer from a cystic fibrosis-like lung involvement, as well as a miliaria rubra-like rash.[105]

Affected children typically present in the first few days of life, with failure to gain weight and inadequate feeding, and are often severely hypovolemic or even in shock, with dramatic hyperkalemia, sometimes exceeding 10 mmol/L.[105] Acute treatment focuses on volume restoration and normalization of the acidosis, with an IV infusion of saline and sodium bicarbonate. Potassium levels improve with expansion of the intravascular volume and correction of the acidosis, but in the long term, sodium exchange resins can be very helpful to provide a steady source of sodium supplementation and potassium removal. Sodium supplementation with doses up to 50 mmol/kg/day have been reported but, despite this, patients can experience acute episodes of hypovolemia, typically associated with intercurrent infections.[106] In our own clinical practice (unpublished), we typically use gastrostomies to facilitate the regular administration of supplements and feeds and sometimes use port-a-caths to ensure emergency IV access during a hypovolemic crisis. Management typically becomes easier as the child reaches school age, with episodes of hypovolemic crisis becoming rare and lung manifestations improving. Nevertheless, lifelong salt supplementation is needed.[105]

**Pseudohypoaldosteronism Type 2.** PHA2 (Gordon syndrome, or familial hyperkalemic hypertension) is characterized by hyperkalemia and hyperchloremic metabolic acidosis, with normal to high circulating levels of mineralocorticoids but suppressed levels and activity of renin. It is distinguished clinically from PHA1 by its distinct lack of sodium wasting and volume depletion. Instead, salt retention and hypertension are the hallmarks of this syndrome.[107] So far, four genes (*WNK1, WNK4, KLHL3,* and *CUL3*) have been identified as causative, all inherited in an autosomal dominant fashion. In addition, mutations in *KLHL3* can also cause a recessive form of the disorder.[108] Mutations in all four genes directly or indirectly stimulate activity of NCC (SLC12A3) the sodium-chloride cotransporter in the distal convoluted tubule (DCT).[109] In this way, PHA2 pathophysiologically and clinically constitutes the mirror image to Gitelman syndrome, caused by loss of function of NCC.

The phenotypic variability is high. Several patients are identified incidentally because of hyperkalemia noted on an unrelated blood test or because of family screening. Hypercalciuria is also frequently noted. Hypertension is present in approximately two-thirds of patients at the time of diagnosis, is often absent early in life, and is believed to develop eventually in all patients with time.[110] Less consistent features are age of apparent symptoms (neonate to adulthood), and there appears to be some genotype-phenotype correlation, with mutations in *CUL3* typically causing the most severe form, with earliest diagnosis and most severe electrolyte abnormalities.[111] In addition, patients with mutations in *CUL3* typically have

**Table 73.7 Management of Severe Hyperkalemia in Children[a]**

| Parameter | Route of Administration | Dose | Onset of Action | Comments |
|---|---|---|---|---|
| **Stabilization of Cardiac Membranes** | | | | |
| Calcium gluconate, 10% solution | IV | 0.5–1 mL/kg over 10 min | Immediate | Repeat one dose after 5 min if ECG changes persist; cardiac monitor |
| **Movement of Potassium Into Cells** | | | | |
| Glucose + Regular insulin | IV | 10% dextrose at 5 mL/kg/hr + insulin, 0.1–0.2 U/kg/hr | 15–30 min | Monitor blood glucose level at least hourly. |
| Salbutamol | Nebulized | 0.1–0.3 mg/kg | 20–30 min | Doses may be repeated as often as needed; effect lasts for up to 2 hr; tachycardia is main side effect. |
| | IV | 4 µg/kg over 10–20 min | 5–10 min | |
| Sodium bicarbonate | IV | 2–3 mEq/kg over 30 min | 15–30 min | Do not give in the same IV line as calcium; minimum effect unless the patient has acidosis. |
| **Removal of Potassium From the Body** | | | | |
| Cation exchange resins | PO | 1 mo–8 yr: 125–250 mg/kg (max, 15 g) | 1–2 hr | 3-4 times daily |
| | Rectal | Neonate to 18 yr: 125–250 mg/kg | 1–2 hr | Repeat doses every 6 hr if needed; colonic irrigation to remove resin after 6-12 hr.<br>Dilute 1 g resin with 5–10 mL methylcellulose or water.<br>Do not give within 1 wk of surgery.<br>Do not use enema with sorbitol, and keep in mind that sodium polystyrene sulfonate use, both with and without sorbitol, may be associated with fatal gastrointestinal injury. |
| Furosemide | IV | 1–2 mg/kg | 5 min | Repeat dose every 2 hr if needed; monitor fluid balance. |
| Hemodialysis or peritoneal dialysis | | | | Hemodialysis is more effective. |

[a]The measures listed here can be carried out simultaneously. The choice of therapy to be used depends on the severity of the symptoms and the particular clinical situation.
*ECG,* Electrocardiographic, *IV,* intravenous; *PO,* orally.

failure to thrive or growth impairment, and mutations are often de novo, suggesting an impaired reproductive fitness.[108] Although PHA2 is rare, diagnosis is important, not only for genetic counseling, but also to initiate appropriate treatment. A key feature of PHA2 is the complete reversal of biochemical abnormalities and hypertension by treatment with a thiazide, which, in fact, can be used as a diagnostic feature. There is also an acquired form of PHA2, associated with tacrolimus use.[112] Again, recognition of the combination of hyperkalemia and hypertension is important because patients with the acquired form also respond to thiazide treatment.

## HYDROGEN ION DISORDERS

### ACID-BASE EQUILIBRIUM IN CHILDREN

Acid-base homeostasis is maintained by the kidney by adjusting acid excretion to the acid load. The acid load is derived chiefly from the diet, specifically sulfur-containing amino acids, which are metabolized to sulfuric acid.[113] Net acid excretion (NAE) is defined as the sum of titratable acid and ammonium ($NH_4^+$) minus urine $HCO_3^-$. This emphasizes the importance of tubular reabsorption of filtered $HCO_3^-$ to enable NAE and highlights the two key factors that can lead to acidosis—net loss of $HCO_3^-$ or the net gain of acid. The AG (usually calculated as $Na^+ - (Cl^- + HCO_3^-) = AG$) can be used to distinguish between these two forms. Because $HCO_3^-$ loss has to be accompanied by a cation, typically $Na^+$, the AG is unchanged. In contrast, with net acid gain (e.g., lactic acid), the excess acid is buffered by $HCO_3^-$, leading to an increased AG because $Na^+$ and $Cl^-$ are unchanged, yet $HCO_3^-$ is decreased. Thus, net $HCO_3^-$ loss is associated with a normal AG acidosis, whereas net acid gain leads to an increased AG. A normal AG is typically 8 to 12 mmol/L, but depends mainly on the albumin concentration, the main anion missing from the calculation.[114] The AG falls approximately 2.3 mmol/L for every 10-g/L reduction in serum albumin concentration.[115] A list of causes of acidosis according to AG is given in Table 73.8.

**Table 73.8 Metabolic Acidosis in Children According to the Serum Anion Gap**

| Serum Anion Gap | Features |
|---|---|
| Normal | Loss of bicarbonate in the stool<br>• Diarrhea<br>• Digestive fistulas or surgical drainage<br>• Drugs—$CaCl_2$, $MgCl_2$, cation exchange resins<br>Loss of bicarbonate in urine<br>• Mild to moderate renal failure (greater tubulointerstitial than glomerular damage)<br>• Renal tubular acidosis<br>• Extracellular volume expansion |
| High | Advanced renal failure (uremic acidosis)<br>• Ketoacidosis<br>  ◦ Diabetes mellitus<br>  ◦ Inborn errors of metabolism<br>  ◦ Prolonged fasting<br>• Lactic acidosis<br>  ◦ Tissue hypoxia<br>  ◦ Inborn errors of metabolism<br>Toxins—salicylate, methanol, ethylene glycol |

**Table 73.9 Classification of Renal Tubular Acidosis in Children by Cause**

| Type | Features |
|---|---|
| Proximal renal tubular acidosis (RTA) (type 2) | Primary<br>• Autosomal recessive: with ocular abnormalities<br>Secondary<br>• Component of renal Fanconi syndrome<br>• Drugs and toxins (e.g., ifosfamide, carbonic anhydrase inhibitors, heavy metals) |
| Distal RTA (type 1) | Primary<br>• Autosomal dominant<br>• Autosomal recessive, with or without sensorineural deafness<br>Secondary<br>• Autoimmune diseases—Sjögren syndrome, rheumatoid arthritis, hyperglobulinemia<br>• Drugs and toxics (e.g., amphotericin B, lithium salts, amiloride, toluene) |
| Mixed proximal and distal RTA (type 3 RTA) | Deficiency of carbonic anhydrase II (associated with osteopetrosis and mental retardation) |
| Hyperkalemic RTA (type 4) | Hypoaldosteronism<br>• Pseudohypoaldosteronism<br>• Drugs and toxics (e.g., potassium salts, heparin, spironolactone, triamterene, amiloride, trimethoprim, indomethacin, ACEi, ARB, cyclosporin A, tacrolimus) |

*ACEi,* Angiotensin-converting enzyme inhibitor; *ARB,* angiotensin receptor blocker.

The NAE per kilogram of body weight is higher in infants than in adults and less in infants fed human milk than in infants fed formulas. This reflects the higher metabolism of infants associated with growth and the higher content of sulfur-containing amino acids in formula milk.[116]

Except for the few hours during and after birth, the blood pH during infancy and childhood remains relatively constant. Values are equivalent to normal adult values at 3 to 5 years of age.

Metabolic acidosis is diagnosed by a low plasma $HCO_3^-$ concentration (<22 mmol/L in children and <20 mmol/L in infants) and a low blood $P_{CO_2}$ (<40 mm Hg in children and <35 mm Hg in infants). If the pH is also low, this is termed *acidemia.*

## RENAL TUBULAR ACIDOSIS

The term *renal tubular acidosis* refers to a group of clinical entities in which normal AG hyperchloremic metabolic acidosis occurs as a result of impaired proximal tubular reabsorption of $HCO_3^-$ or distal secretion of $H^+$. Consequently, RTA can be classified as proximal (type 2) or distal (type 1; Table 73.9). In addition, there is a rare combined form (type 3) caused by recessive mutations in the gene encoding carbonic anhydrase II (see later). The so-called hyperkalemic RTA (type 4) is really a disorder of impaired salt reabsorption in the collecting duct, with consequent hyperkalemia and acidosis, and is discussed previously (see "Pseudohypoaldosteronism"). This section focuses on the primary congenital inherited forms of RTA because they are characteristic of the pediatric age; acquired forms are more prevalent in adults. As before, the focus will be primarily on aspects relevant to pediatrics; these inherited forms are discussed in more detail in Chapter 44.

### PROXIMAL TYPE 2 RENAL TUBULAR ACIDOSIS

Proximal RTA results from decreased reabsorption of $HCO_3^-$ in the proximal tubule (Fig. 73.4). Most cases in children are seen in the context of a generalized dysfunction of the proximal tubule (renal Fanconi syndrome). Thus, aside from RTA, these children typically display the whole spectrum of a proximal tubulopathy, such as renal wasting of phosphate, glucose, amino acids, and low-molecular weight proteins.[117]

RTA as the only manifestation of proximal tubular dysfunction is an exceedingly rare disorder and is caused by mutations in *SLC4A4* encoding the basolateral $Na^+$-$HCO_3^-$ cotransporter (NBC1), which also plays a major role in $HCO_3^-$ transport in the ocular lens epithelium.[118,119] Consequently, patients typically have eye abnormalities, such as band keratopathy, glaucoma, or cataract, in addition to the proximal RTA. Hence, the name "Proximal RTA with Ocular Abnormalities" (Online Mendelian Inheritance in Man [OMIM] no. 604278). Additional clinical features may include enamel defects of the permanent teeth, impaired intellectual capacity, calcification of the basal ganglia, hypothyroidism, and hyperamylasemia.[118] The mainstay of treatment of the acidosis is alkali supplementation yet, given the vast amount of physiologic $HCO_3^-$ reabsorption in the proximal tubule, the normalization of plasma $HCO_3^-$ concentration is typically impossible when

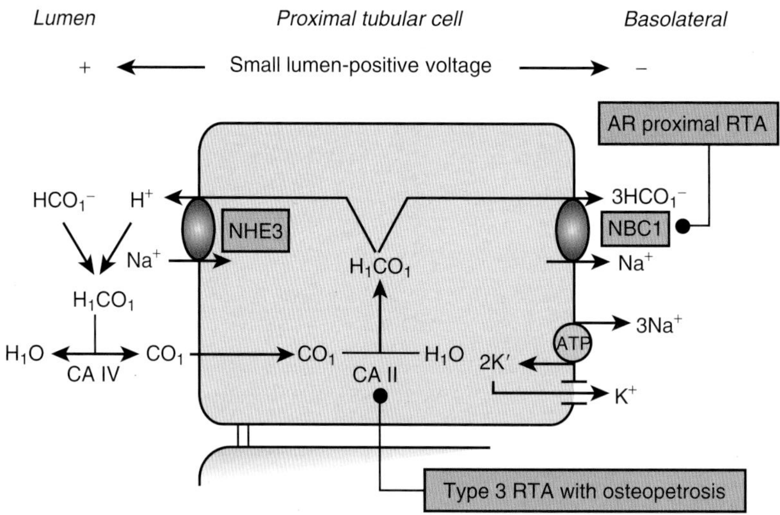


**Fig. 73.4** Schematic representation of the reabsorption of bicarbonate in a cell of the proximal tubule showing the transport systems involved in the genesis of primary proximal renal tubular acidosis *(RTA)*. The $Na^+$-$H^+$ exchanger isoform 3 *(NHE3)* is depicted on the luminal membrane of the cell. The $Na^+$-$K^+$-ATPase and $Na^+$-$HCO_3^-$ cotransporter *(NBC1)* are represented on the basolateral side. *AR,* Autosomal recessive; *ATP,* adenosine triphosphate; *ATPase,* adenosine triphosphatase; *CA II,* intracellular carbonic anhydrase; *CA IV,* luminal carbonic anhydrase.

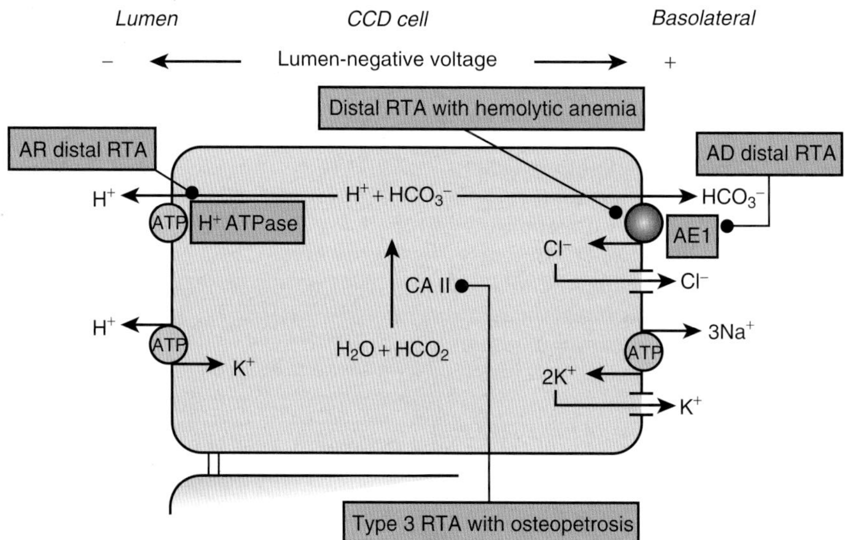


**Fig. 73.5** Schematic representation of the system of acidification and regeneration of bicarbonate in an α-intercalated cell of the cortical collecting duct *(CCD)* showing the transport systems involved in the genesis of primary distal renal tubular acidosis *(RTA)*. The $H^+$-ATPase pump and $H^+$-$K^+$-ATPase are depicted on the luminal membrane of the cell. The $Na^+$-$K^+$-ATPase and $Cl^-$-$HCO_3^-$-exchanger *(AE1)* are represented on the basolateral side. *AD,* Autosomal dominant; *AR,* autosomal recessive; *ATP,* adenosine triphosphate; *ATPase,* adenosine triphosphatase; *CA II,* intracellular carbonic anhydrase.

this is impaired. Patients with proximal RTA have a lower threshold for $HCO_3^-$ reabsorption—that is, the plasma concentration at which bicarbonate is wasted into the urine is lower than normal. Consequently, by increasing the plasma concentration with alkali supplementation, renal $HCO_3^-$ losses are augmented. Nevertheless, improvement of growth velocity with alkali supplementation has been reported.[118]

## PRIMARY DISTAL TYPE 1 RENAL TUBULAR ACIDOSIS

Primary distal type 1 RTA is the most common RTA found in children. It results from defective urinary acidification in the cortical collecting tubule secondary to mutations in genes involved in the elimination of $H^+$ and associated regeneration of $HCO_3^-$ (Fig. 73.5). Autosomal dominant distal RTA is caused by mutations in the *SLC4A1* gene, leading to loss of function by abnormal processing or trafficking of the $Cl^-$-$HCO_3^-$ exchanger (AE1) located at the basolateral surface of α-intercalated cells and in the erythrocytes.[120,121] Mutations in *SLC4A1* also cause the dominant red cell morphologic diseases of hereditary spherocytosis and ovalocytosis, although the association of these entities with distal RTA is rare.[121]

The apical proton pump $H^+$-ATPase that transfers $H^+$ into the urine (see Fig. 73.5) is composed of at least 13 different subunits.[122] Mutations in the gene *ATP6V1B1* encoding the B1 subunit of $H^+$-ATPase are responsible for a form of autosomal recessive distal RTA associated with sensorineural deafness.[123] $H^+$-ATPase containing the B1 subunit is also involved in maintaining a pH of 7.4 and low $Na^+$ and high

$K^+$ concentrations in the endolymph, explaining the concomitant deafness. Although usually congenital and severe, in some individuals hearing impairment is delayed in onset.[124] Recessive mutations in *ATP6V0A4* encoding the a4 subunit of $H^+$-ATPase are responsible for another form of autosomal recessive distal RTA.[125] It is initially associated with preserved hearing; however, long-term follow-up of patients with distal RTA caused by *ATP6V0A4* mutations has demonstrated that some of them develop hearing loss consistent with the expression of *ATP6V0A4* within the human cochlea.[126] Both *ATP6V1B1* and *ATP6V0A4* are regulated by FOXI1, a transcription factor important for the function of the inner ear, as well as the intercalated cells in the collecting duct.[127] Recessive mutations in *FOXI1* have also been associated with distal RTA (dRTA) and deafness.[128]

### Clinical Presentation

Patients with recessive forms of dRTA typically present in the first year of life, with failure to thrive and a history of polydipsia/polyuria. Nephrocalcinosis is usually present and marked.[124,129] An associated proximal tubular dysfunction, suggesting an erroneous diagnosis of renal Fanconi syndrome, is common, but disappears with treatment of the acidosis. Patients typically have a urine-concentrating defect, sometimes attributed to the hypercalciuria and/or hypokalemia, although it persists even after normalization of the biochemical abnormalities and thus may reflect the nephrocalcinosis.[21]

In contrast, patients with the dominant form are increasingly diagnosed before the development of overt symptoms by genetic screening based on the family history. With adequate treatment and compliance, complications such as nephrocalcinosis and stones can be minimized and potentially completely avoided.[129]

### Treatment

In contrast to most tubulopathies, where symptoms can only be ameliorated, treatment of dRTA is usually rewarding for patients and clinicians because oral alkali supplementation normalizes the biochemical abnormalities and induces catch-up growth. Citrate or bicarbonate supplements are typically used, ideally as a potassium salt. If given as a sodium salt, additional potassium supplementation is often needed. Large doses of up to at 9 mmol/kg/day of alkali equivalent may be needed, especially in infants at the beginning of treatment.[129] Frequent dosing, every 4 to 6 hours, is important to maintain normal values of the serum $HCO_3^-$ concentration throughout the day. In infants, distribution of the daily dose throughout all feeds is often the easiest. Development of longer acting formulations allowing twice-daily administration should facilitate treatment in the future.[130]

## HYPERKALEMIC TYPE 4 RENAL TUBULAR ACIDOSIS

Hyperkalemic (type 4) RTA is found together with aldosterone deficiency or aldosterone resistance and thus primarily reflects a disorder of sodium transport. It was discussed earlier ("Pseudohypoaldosteronism").

# MAGNESIUM DISORDERS

The regulation of serum magnesium (Mg) concentration depends primarily on the kidney. With normal magnesium intake, approximately 95% to 97% of filtered magnesium is reabsorbed along the nephron. In contrast to most other ions, the proximal tubule contributes the relatively smallest part to magnesium reabsorption, only about 5% to 15%, although it is of note that a much larger fraction of filtered magnesium is reabsorbed in the proximal tubule in newborns. About 50% to 70% is reabsorbed in the TAL, where it diffuses passively through the paracellular pathway. Finally, 5% to 10% of Mg is reabsorbed in the early DCT. This segment determines the final urinary magnesium concentration by active transcellular absorption via the TRPM6 channel.[131] The body of an adult contains approximately 24 g of magnesium, of which only a small fraction, around 60 mg, is present in the plasma, where it is available for measurement.[132]

## HYPOMAGNESEMIA

In the clinical setting, low serum magnesium concentrations indicate magnesium deficiency, although values in the normal range do not rule out the possibility of a total body deficit, compensated for by the release of magnesium from the bone.[133] In the presence of hypomagnesemia, normal kidneys retain magnesium by decreasing its excretion to as little as 0.5% of the filtered load. In clinical practice, in the context of hypomagnesemia, a fractional excretion of magnesium (FEMg) of 2% is typically considered normal, whereas more than 4% is considered pathogenic.[134] For the calculation of FEMg, the serum concentration of magnesium is usually multiplied by 0.7 to use the filtered fraction only and exclude the estimated protein-bound fraction.[131] Of note, with markedly decreased serum levels, FEMg may be falsely normal if the remaining intact pathways are able to cope with the small filtered load. Assessment while the patient is receiving magnesium supplements is better suited to determine the presence or absence of renal magnesium wasting in uncertain cases.

Known genetic causes of hypomagnesemia are listed in Table 73.10 and depicted in Fig. 73.6. Based on clinical and pathophysiologic criteria, hypomagnesemia disorders can be classified into four groups[131]:

1. Hypercalciuric hypomagnesemias, affecting magnesium reabsorption primarily in the TAL
2. Gitelman-like hypomagnesemias, affecting transport in DCT in general
3. Mitochondrial hypomagnesemias, which may affect magnesium and other transport pathways along the entire nephron and consequently can have a very variable phenotype
4. Other hypomagnesemias, which include several forms of isolated or syndromic hypomagnesemia not fitting into the previous groups

## CLINICAL MANIFESTATIONS

Hypomagnesemia is often asymptomatic, and clinical manifestations of magnesium deficiency are generally not manifested until the serum magnesium concentration decreases below 0.4 mmol/L, although the appearance of symptoms may depend on the rate of development of magnesium deficiency or on the total body deficit. Initial symptoms are often nonspecific, such as fatigue or cramps, which may not

**Table 73.10 Main Causes of Hypomagnesemia in Children**

| Type of Hypomagnesemia | Description |
|---|---|
| **Primary Inherited Disorders** | |
| 1. Hypercalciuric hypomagnesemias | Familial hypomagnesemia with hypercalciuria and nephrocalcinosis (*CLDN16,19*) |
| 2. Gitelman-like hypomagnesemias | Gitelman syndrome (*SLC12A3*)<br>Bartter syndrome (types 3 and 4, *CLCNKB, BSND*)<br>EAST syndrome (*KCNJ10*)<br>Autosomal dominant hypomagnesemia (*FXYD2*)<br>HNF1B nephropathy<br>Neonatal hyperphenylalaninemia and primapterinuria (*PCBD1*) |
| 3. Mitochondrial hypomagnesemias | Mitochondrial metabolic syndrome (*tRNA*)<br>Kearns-Sayre and Pearson syndrome (*SARS2*) |
| 4. Other hypomagnesemias | Hypomagnesemia with secondary hypocalcemia (*TRPM6*)<br>Hypomagnesemia seizures and mental impairment (*CNNM2*)<br>Autosomal dominant hypomagnesemia (*KCNA1*)<br>Hypomagnesemia with abnormalities in EGF signaling (*EGF, EGFR*)<br>Hypomagnesemia with Kenney-Caffey syndrome (*FAM111A*) |
| **Secondary Disorders** | |
| Decreased gastrointestinal absorption | Malabsorptive syndromes<br>• Vomiting and diarrhea |
| Increased urinary excretion | Drugs<br>• Diuretics<br>• Calcineurin antagonists<br>• Others—cisplatinum, aminoglycosides, amphotericin B |
| Miscellaneous | "Hungry bone," low-birth-weight newborn, infant of diabetic mother |

be presented to medical attention or not investigated. Often, patients may present with tetany. Magnesium depletion inhibits parathyroid hormone (PTH) secretion and causes resistance to PTH action, leading to hypocalcemia and consequent neuromuscular hyperexcitability and tetany or even convulsions.[135] Cardiac manifestations of hypomagnesemia can include prolongation of the QT interval and a wide range of arrhythmias.

## HYPERCALCIURIC HYPOMAGNESEMIA: FAMILIAL HYPOMAGNESEMIA WITH HYPERCALCIURIA AND NEPHROCALCINOSIS

Familial hypomagnesemia with hypercalciuria and nephrocalcinosis (FHHNC) is an autosomal recessive primary tubulopathy caused by loss-of-function mutations in *CLDN16* or *CLDN19*.[136,137] These genes encode two proteins, claudin 16 (formerly paracellin 1) and claudin 19, which are expressed in the tight junction in TAL and are critical for magnesium and calcium permeability.[138,139] Claudin 19 is also important in the eye, explaining the additional ocular involvement, such as macular colobomata, significant myopia, and horizontal nystagmus.

Most common presenting manifestations of FHHNC are recurrent urinary tract infections and polyuria and polydipsia. Hematuria, abdominal pain, urolithiasis, sterile leukocyturia, growth failure, and seizures are also frequent.[140,141]

Chronic kidney disease is often present at diagnosis, and progression is not affected by magnesium supplementation.

## GITELMAN-LIKE HYPOMAGNESEMIA

This group includes salt-wasting disorders of the DCT, such as Gitelman and EAST syndrome, as well as Bartter syndrome types 3 and 4.[131] Although not invariably present, hypomagnesemia is a typical feature in these disorders, otherwise characterized by hypokalemic hypochloremic alkalosis (see previously, "Hypokalemic Alkalosis Without Hypertension"). Dominant mutations in *FXYD2*, encoding the gamma subunit of the Na-K-ATPase in DCT, can cause a similar picture, albeit reported in only three families so far, putatively descended from a single founder.[142] *FXYD2* is regulated by the transcription factor HNF1B and, consequently, mutations in HNF1B can also cause a similar phenotype.[143] HNF1B, in turn, is regulated by *PCBD1*, which affects dimerization. *PCBD1* encodes an enzyme involved in the metabolism of aromatic amino acids, and loss-of-function mutations cause neonatal hyperphenylalaninemia and primapterinuria.[144] Reexamination of patients with such mutations has revealed the presence of maturity onset diabetes of the young (MODY) and hypomagnesemia, mimicking the HNF1B phenotype.[145]

## MITOCHONDRIAL HYPOMAGNESEMIA

An association between mitochondrial dysfunction and hypomagnesemia was first highlighted during the investigation of a large pedigree affected with metabolic syndrome and hypomagnesemia, which cosegregated with a mutation in the mitochondrial tRNA(Ile) gene.[146] Hypomagnesemia has been further recognized in other mitochondrial diseases, specifically in some patients with Kearns-Sayre and Pearson syndromes, as well as with mutations in *SARS2*.[147-149] Presumably, the impaired energy supply limits magnesium transport, explaining the renal wasting. Why hypomagnesemia is such an inconstant feature in mitochondrial cytopathies remains unclear.

## OTHER HYPOMAGNESEMIAS: FAMILIAL HYPOMAGNESEMIA WITH SECONDARY HYPOCALCEMIA

Familial hypomagnesemia with secondary hypocalcemia (HSH) is a rare autosomal recessive disorder caused by loss-of-function mutations in the *TRPM6* gene encoding the TRPM6 channel essential for the intestinal and renal reabsorption of magnesium (see Fig. 73.6).[150] Patients with HSH typically present in infancy or early childhood, with generalized convulsions associated with extremely low levels of serum magnesium, hypocalcemia, and inadequately low PTH levels. Because of the combined intestinal uptake and renal reabsorption defect, improvement of serum magnesium levels is challenging. Despite persistently low levels, however, the prognosis in HSH is favorable with oral supplementation,

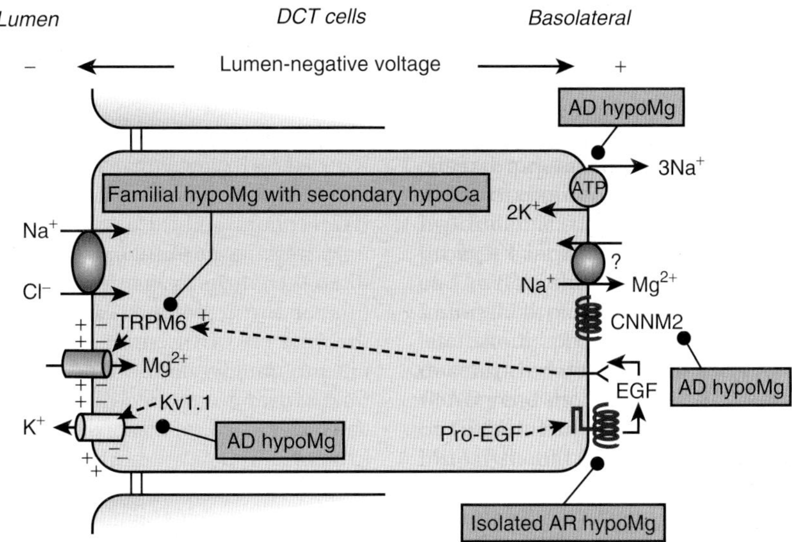


**Fig. 73.6** Schematic representation of a cell of the distal convoluted tubule *(DCT)* showing the transport systems involved in the reabsorption of magnesium and its inherited disorders. The thiazide-sensitive $Na^+$-$Cl^-$ cotransporter, the magnesium-transporting channel TRPM6, and the voltage-gated Kv1.1 potassium channel are depicted on the luminal membrane of the cell. The $Na^+$-$K^+$-ATPase, a putative $Na^+$-$Mg^{2+}$ exchanger, the cyclin M2 protein *(CNNM2)*, the receptor of epidermal growth factor *(EGF)*, and the precursor of this peptide, the membrane protein pro-EGF, are represented on the basolateral side (see text for details). *AD,* Autosomal dominant; *AR,* autosomal recessive; *ATP,* adenosine triphosphate; *ATPase,* adenosine triphosphatase; *hypoCa,* hypocalcemia; *hypoMg,* hypomagnesemia; *TRPM6,* transient receptor potential channel melastatin 6.

although persistent neurologic damage has been described in patients with delayed diagnosis and prolonged seizures.[151]

Hypomagnesemia has been described further with mutations in *CNNM2, KCNA1, EGF,* and *EGFR,* as well as *FAM111A.*[131] All these are exceedingly rare and are described in more detail in Chapters 18 and 44.

## CALCIUM AND PHOSPHATE DISORDERS

### CALCIUM AND PHOSPHATE CONCENTRATIONS IN SERUM

The normal ranges for calcium and phosphate change during the first few years of life, perhaps reflecting the high requirement for bone formation during this phase of fastest growth. The normal range for total serum calcium is 2.4 to 2.8 mmol/L (9.3–11.1 mg/dL) in a neonate and decreases slowly so that around the age of 7 years the normal range is the same as in adults at 2.2 to 2.6 mmol/L (8.8–10.4 mg/dL).[152] Similarly, the normal range for phosphate in a neonate is 1.4 to 2.3 mmol/L (4.3–7.1 mg/dL) and decreases slowly, so that around the age of 7 years, the normal range is the same as in adults, at 0.9 to 1.6 mmol/L (2.8–5.0 mg/dL).[152]

This neonatal hyperphosphatemia is linked to higher tubular reabsorption of phosphate, potentially due to a blunted tubular response to the already low circulating PTH normally encountered in neonatal life.

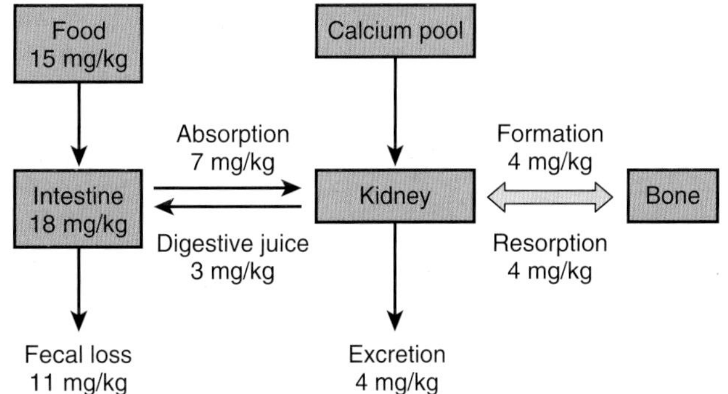


**Fig. 73.7** The calcium pool is sustained essentially by balance among dietary intake, intestinal absorption, and renal excretion of calcium. Every day, the skeletal system uses calcium at 4 mg/kg body weight per day to form new bone. This rate of calcium accretion in new bone formation is balanced by the same rate of calcium resorption from bone. Calcium in food is the most important source. Food provides calcium nutrition of 15 mg/kg body weight per day on a North American diet. Approximately 7 mg/kg is absorbed to augment the calcium pool. Digestive juice contributes 3 mg/kg to bring the total intestinal calcium content to 18 mg/kg body weight per day, out of which fecal loss is 11 mg/kg body weight per day. Finally, the renal excretion is 4 mg/kg body weight per day to maintain calcium balance.

### VITAMIN D, PARATHYROID HORMONE, CALCITONIN, AND FIBROBLAST GROWTH FACTOR 23

The control of calcium and phosphate homeostasis is complex (Figs. 73.7 and 73.8). For the purposes of this chapter, we shall focus here on four of the key regulators engaged in maintaining calcium and phosphate balance: vitamin D, parathyroid hormone, calcitonin, and fibroblast growth factor 23 (FGF-23; Fig. 73.9).

#### VITAMIN D

Vitamin D exists in two principal forms: vitamin $D_2$ (ergocalciferol) and $D_3$ (cholecalciferol). They result from the ultraviolet (UV) irradiation of ergosterol ($D_2$), which is mainly found in plants and fungi, or 7-dehydrocholesterol ($D_3$), which is

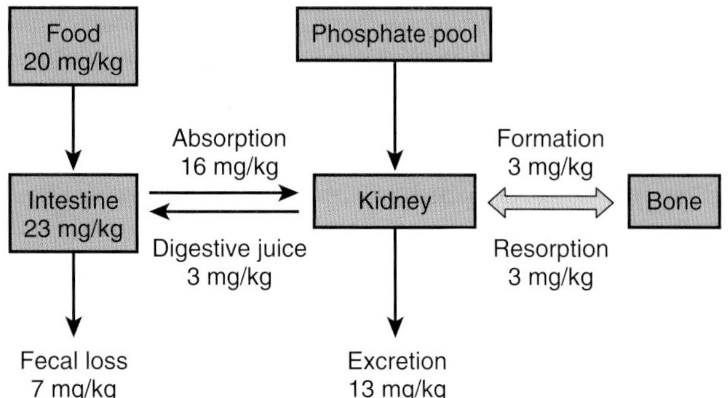


**Fig. 73.8** The phosphate pool is sustained essentially by dietary intake, intestinal absorption, and renal excretion of phosphate. Every day, the skeletal system uses phosphate at 3 mg/kg body weight per day to form new bone. This rate of phosphate used in new bone formation is balanced by the same amount of phosphate resorption from bone. Phosphate in food is the most important source. Food provides phosphate nutrition of 20 mg/kg body weight per day on a North American diet. Approximately 16 mg/kg body weight per day is absorbed to augment the phosphate pool. Digestive juice contributes 3 mg/kg body weight per day to bring the total intestinal phosphate content to 23 mg/kg body weight per day, out of which fecal loss is 7 mg/kg body weight per day. Finally, the renal excretion of phosphate is 13 mg/kg body weight per day to maintain phosphate balance.

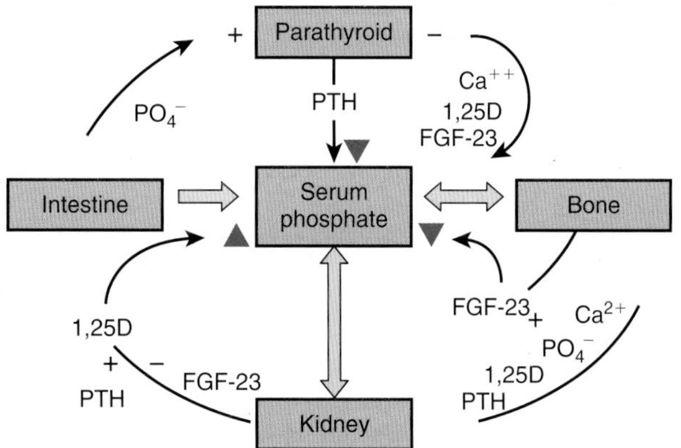


**Fig. 73.9** Serum phosphate homeostasis is conserved by three potent hormones, the parathyroid hormone *(PTH)*, fibroblast growth factor 23 (FGF-23), and 1,25-dihydroxyvitamin D (1,25D). As indicated by the *green arrowheads* in the diagram, PTH and FGF-23 lower serum phosphate concentrations and 1,25D increases serum phosphate concentrations. Secretion of these hormones is regulated by reciprocal relationships and by the interaction of calcium *($Ca^{2+}$)* and phosphate *($PO_4^-$)*. Specifically, the kidney's production of 1,25D is stimulated by low serum $PO_4^-$ and PTH and inhibited by FGF-23 levels. At the parathyroid gland, high $PO_4^-$ stimulates the production of PTH, which increases phosphaturia.

from animal sources.[153] Vitamin D is further activated in two hydroxylation reactions; the first one occurs in hepatocytes, which activate it to 25-hydroxyvitamin D (25[OH]D) by the enzymatic activity of CYP2R1 and CYP27A1. The second occurs in the proximal tubule, generating 1,25-dihydrovitamin D (1,25[OH]$_2$D).

Vitamin D in its various forms in blood is mainly bound to vitamin D–binding protein (DBP) and, to a much lower degree (~10%), to albumin. Yet, only unbound vitamin D is bioavailable and can thus bind to the vitamin D receptor.[154] Of note, common polymorphisms affect the levels of DBP, leading to ethnic differences.[155] Because the usual assays for vitamin D measure the total concentration, these can vary, despite similar levels of bioavailable vitamin D. Thus, US blacks have been shown to have lower total vitamin D levels than US whites, yet similar levels for bioavailable vitamin D.[155]

Despite its molecular weight of around 52 kDa, DBP is filtered by the glomerulus and is reabsorbed in the proximal tubular brush border via megalin (LRP2).[156] It is through this process of filtration and reabsorption that vitamin D reaches the mitochondria in the proximal tubule, where the final activation step to 1,25-dihydrovitamin D takes place via the 1α-hydroxylase (CYP27B1). The activity of this key enzyme in vitamin D activation is tightly regulated, stimulated by low concentrations of circulating 1,25(OH)$_2$D, calcium, and phosphate, as well as high concentrations of circulating PTH and inhibited by FGF-23 and Klotho.[157,158]

The key enzyme for 1,25(OH)$_2$D catabolism is CYP24A1. In a five-step progression, starting with 24-hydroxylation, CYP24A1 catabolizes 1,25(OH)$_2$D into water-soluble calcitroic acid.[159]

A high level of 1,25(OH)$_2$D inhibits 1α-hydroxylase and stimulates the production of FGF-23 and Klotho, both of which inhibit 1α-hydroxylase. Such feedback loops precisely control 1,25(OH)$_2$D production.[160]

A high extracellular ionized calcium concentration activates the calcium-sensing receptor (CaSR) in the parathyroid chief cell. CaSR belongs to the family of G protein–coupled receptors, and activation triggers a signaling cascade that suppresses PTH secretion.[161]

## CALCITONIN, FIBROBLAST GROWTH FACTOR 23, AND PARATHYROID HORMONE

Calcitonin, produced by the parafollicular cells (C cells) of the thyroid gland, inhibits calcium resorption from osteoclasts. Calcitonin operates via the same CaSR as PTH, but the action of calcitonin is opposite to that of PTH.

FGF-23 from osteocytes is a potent phosphaturic agent. In concert with calcium, phosphate, 1,25(OH)$_2$D, and parathyroid hormone, FGF-23 plays an important role in regulating phosphate homeostasis.[162]

FGF-23 decreases the serum phosphate concentration by downregulating expression of sodium phosphate transporters, both NaPi-IIa and NaPi-IIc, in the proximal tubular membrane. FGF-23 and Klotho inhibit renal 1α-hydroxylase expression. FGF-23 promotes 24-hydroxylase expression.[162] Consequently, 1,25(OH)$_2$D production is reduced, resulting in lowered phosphate absorption from the intestine and bone.

In contrast, with a low serum phosphate concentration and/or low serum PTH concentration, the kidneys increase production of 1,25(OH)$_2$D (see Fig. 73.9). Consequently, the intestinal absorption of phosphate is increased.

At the parathyroid glands, high serum phosphate concentrations stimulate PTH production, promoting phosphaturia to restore serum phosphate levels to normal concentrations. In essence, PTH and FGF-23 reduce the serum phosphate level, whereas 1,25(OH)$_2$D increases it (see Fig. 73.9). These three hormones are regulated by reciprocal interaction and calcium and phosphate levels in serum.

## HYPOCALCEMIA

The causes of hypocalcemia are listed in Table 73.11. Mild hypocalcemia is often without apparent symptoms, whereas severe hypocalcemia can present with symptoms of paresthesia, tetany, positive Chvostek and Trousseau signs, prolongation of the QT interval, QRS and ST complex changes, and eventually grand mal seizures and ventricular arrhythmias.

### TYPES AND CAUSES

#### Early Neonatal Hypocalcemia

Early neonatal hypocalcemia, presenting in the first 3 days of life, is frequently seen in premature infants of diabetic mothers and in asphyxiated neonates. The hypocalcemia is due to an inadequate parathyroid response associated with the hypomagnesemia common in diabetic pregnant mothers

**Table 73.11 Causes of Hypocalcemia**

| Type of Hypocalcemia | Causes |
|---|---|
| **Neonatal Hypocalcemia** | |
| Early neonatal hypocalcemia (first few days of life) | Maternal hyperparathyroidism<br>• Maternal diabetes mellitus<br>• Toxemia of pregnancy<br>• Sepsis<br>• SGA, IUGR, prematurity<br>• Asphyxia<br>• Transfusion (citrated blood products)<br>• Congenital rubella<br>• Hypomagnesemia<br>• Respiratory or metabolic alkalosis |
| Late neonatal hypocalcemia (4th–10th day of life) | Vitamin D deficiency—nutritional deficiency; VDR loss-of-function mutation; deficient 1α-hydroxylase activity<br>Phosphate overload—excessive intake of evaporated or whole milk<br>Nutritional calcium deficiency<br>Hypomagnesemia<br>Hypoalbuminemia (nephrotic syndrome)<br>Transfusion (citrated blood products)<br>Acute or chronic kidney insufficiency<br>Diuretics (furosemide)<br>Organic acidemia<br>Primary hypoparathyroidism—DiGeorge syndrome, familial hypoparathyroidism, pseudohypoparathyroidism, Kenny-Caffey syndrome, partial deletion of GCMB, retardation dysmorphism syndrome, Pearson syndrome, Kerns-Sayre syndrome, PTH gene defects, CaSR-activating gene mutation |
| **Hypocalcemia in Childhood** | |
| Parathyroid-related hypocalcemia | Primary hypoparathyroidism—DiGeorge syndrome, familial hypoparathyroidism, pseudohypoparathyroidism, Kenny-Caffey syndrome, Sanjad-Sakati syndrome, partial deletion of GCMB, retardation dysmorphism syndrome, Pearson syndrome, Kerns-Sayre syndrome, PTH gene defects, CaSR-activating gene mutation<br>Secondary hypoparathyroidism—radiation, surgery, infiltration (hemochromatosis, thalassemia, Wilson disease)<br>Autoimmune polyglandular syndrome type 1<br>Nutritional vitamin D deficiency<br>• Defective 1α-hydroxylase activity<br>• VDR loss-of-function mutation |
| Vitamin D–related hypocalcemia | Nutritional calcium deficiency<br>Hypomagnesemia<br>Hyperphosphatemia—kidney failure, rhabdomyolysis, tumor lysis<br>Hypoalbuminemia (nephrotic syndrome)<br>Medications—diuretics, chemotherapeutics, transfusion (citrated blood)<br>Organic acidemia (IVA, MMA, PPA) |

*CaSR,* Calcium-sensing receptor; *GCMB,* glial cell missing homolog B (a parathyroid-specific transcription factor); *IUGR,* intrauterine growth retardation; *IVA,* isovaleric acidemia; *MMA,* methylmalonic acidemia; *PPA,* propionic acidemia; *PTH,* parathyroid hormone; *SGA,* small for gestational age; *VDR,* vitamin D receptor.

and compounded by hyperphosphatemia secondary to delayed phosphaturic action of PTH.[163]

### Late Neonatal Hypocalcemia

Late neonatal hypocalcemia presents at 5 to 10 days of life and is commonly due to anticonvulsants administered to the pregnant mother.[163] Phenytoin and phenobarbital anticonvulsants amplify the hepatic clearance of vitamin D, resulting in hypovitaminosis D in the mother and neonate. The consequent impaired absorption of calcium results in the delayed hypocalcemia. Hypocalcemia can also arise from neonatal hyperphosphatemia, which is the result of three compounding factors: (1) the diminished phosphate excretion of the immature neonatal kidneys and the high circulating GH level; (2) the low circulating PTH level at this stage of life; and (3) the high phosphate load in milk.[163]

Maternal hyperparathyroidism also can be associated with late neonatal hypocalcemia in the first few weeks to as late as 1 year of life due to the suppression of fetal PTH production.[164] Similarly, familial hypocalciuric hypercalcemia (FHH) in the mother also suppresses fetal parathyroid secretion.[165]

### Infusions of Lipid or Citrate Blood Products

Infusions of lipid or citrate blood products cause hypocalcemia by complexing with ionized calcium.

### Alkalosis

Finally, alkalosis, whether respiratory or metabolic, causes hypocalcemia, by increasing the protein binding of calcium.

Most cases of mild neonatal hypocalcemia resolve after 2 to 4 weeks of life. If hypocalcemia and hyperphosphatemia persist beyond this period of time, further workup for hypocalcemia is essential to rule out vitamin D metabolic defects, isolated hypoparathyroidism, or pseudohypoparathyroidism. Finally, neonates with chronic kidney failure are expected to show hypocalcemia, hyperphosphatemia, and elevated concentrations of serum PTH, as well as urea nitrogen and creatinine.

## DIAGNOSTIC WORKUP FOR HYPOCALCEMIA

The diagnostic workup for hypocalcemia in the neonate, infant, or child follows the algorithm presented in Fig. 73.10. The initial steps are a determination of the serum albumin level, spot urine sample for the calcium-to-creatinine ratio to

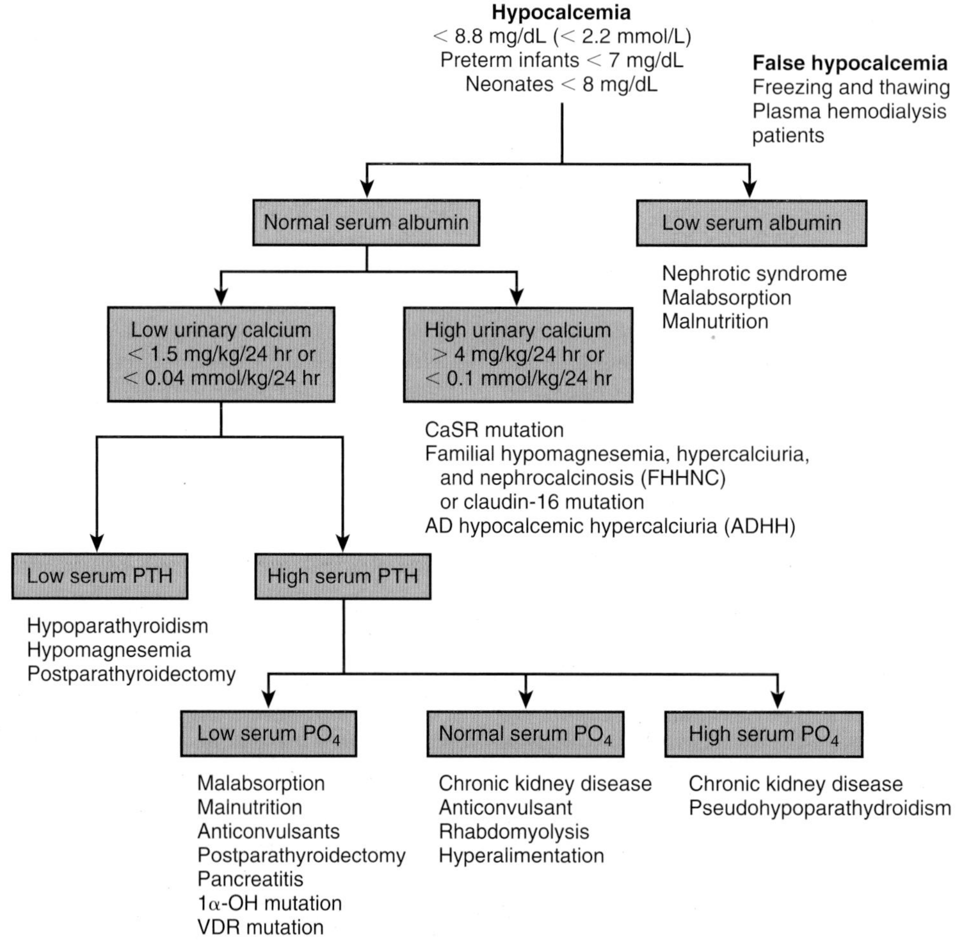


**Fig. 73.10** Algorithm for the diagnosis of hypocalcemia. After false hypocalcemia has been excluded by careful history, the first laboratory diagnostic step is to determine serum albumin concentrations. A low serum albumin concentration indicates specific disorders associated with hypocalcemia, such as nephrotic syndrome, malabsorption, and malnutrition. A normal serum albumin concentration indicates an examination of urinary calcium excretion. Low urinary calcium excretion relative to low serum parathyroid hormone *(PTH)* indicates hypoparathyroidism, hypomagnesemia, and postparathyroidectomy. A low urinary calcium excretion associated with high serum PTH relative to low, normal, and high serum $PO_4$ concentration, respectively, indicates several diagnostic conditions, as listed. *AD,* Autosomal dominant; *CaSR,* calcium-sensing receptor; *1α-OH,* 1α-hydroxylase; *$PO_4$,* phosphate; *VDR,* vitamin D receptor.

**Table 73.12 Treatment of Hypocalcemia**

| Medication | Dose | Administration |
|---|---|---|
| **Symptomatic Hypocalcemia in the Neonate** | | |
| Calcium gluconate | IV 10% solution, 1 mg/kg (9 mg elemental $Ca^{2+}$/mL); 1 mL/min over 10 min | Repeat as needed, with careful monitoring. |
| Magnesium sulfate, 50% solution | 0.1 mL/kg IV or IM | |
| **Symptomatic Hypocalcemia in the Infant** | | |
| Calcium gluconate | IV 10% solution, 1 mg/kg (9 mg elemental $Ca^{2+}$/mL), 1 mL/min over 10 min | Repeat as needed, with careful monitoring. |
| Elemental $Ca^{2+}$ continuous infusion | 1 mg elemental $Ca^{2+}$/kg/hr | |
| **Asymptomatic Hypocalcemia in the Infant** | | |
| Calcium carbonate, PO | 50 mg elemental calcium/kg/day | Divided into four doses per day |

*IM,* Intramuscularly; *IV,* intravenously; *PO,* orally.

delineate urinary calcium excretion, and then determination of values for serum PTH, magnesium, phosphate, serum creatinine, and 25-hydroxyvitamin D (25[OH]D) levels and other specific tests, as dictated by the underlying disease causing the hypocalcemia (see Table 73.11). In the presence of persistent hypocalcemia and suspected maternal hypoparathyroidism or vitamin D deficiency, the mother should be assessed.

## TREATMENT OF HYPOCALCEMIA

Treatment of acute symptomatic hypocalcemia (Table 73.12) consists of 10% calcium gluconate at a dose of 1 to 2 mL/kg body weight (9.3 mg of elemental calcium/mL) IV at a slow drip of less than 1 mL/min over 10 minutes, with electrocardiographic monitoring of the QT interval until symptoms vanish.[166] If tetany or seizures persist, calcium infusion is repeated as necessary until the resolution of severe symptoms. Alternatively, a continuous infusion of elemental calcium, 1 to 3 mg/kg body weight per hour, can be given. Extravasation of calcium-containing fluids causes tissue necrosis, and thus any calcium infusion must be monitored carefully. If the serum calcium concentration fails to rise with this therapy, primary hypomagnesemia must be considered and, if present, treated with magnesium sulfate IV at a dose of 0.1 to 0.2 mL/kg body weight (50% solution) under cardiac monitoring or given intramuscularly.

Hypocalcemic infants with hyperphosphatemia may benefit from low-phosphate formula or breast milk with an overall calcium-to-phosphate ratio of 4:1. Infants with vitamin D deficiency rickets due to maternal hypovitaminosis D respond well to oral vitamin D (1000–2000 U daily for 4 weeks) and elemental calcium (40 mg/kg body weight per day).

For early neonatal hypocalcemia, this treatment brings about normalization in 2 to 3 days, after which the calcium supplementation is reduced by half for 2 days and then discontinued. If prolonged calcium supplementation is required, hypoparathyroidism, pseudohypoparathyroidism, or defective vitamin D metabolism must be considered.

## MONITORING HYPOCALCEMIA

Monitoring of hypocalcemia during treatment includes determination of fasting total and ionized serum calcium concentration, fasting serum phosphate concentration, and spot urine examination for the calcium-to-creatinine ratio. A 24-hour urine collection at home before the clinic visit is recommended to measure calcium and creatinine excretion in continent children.

The goal is to keep 24-hour urinary calcium excretion below 4 mg (0.1 mmol)/kg body weight per day to prevent hypercalciuria and nephrocalcinosis related to the calcium supplementations and vitamin D administration. The serum PTH level is included in the monitoring if hypocalcemia is not due to PTH deficiency or resistance. Serum magnesium concentrations should be checked at least annually.

# HYPERCALCEMIA

Although the range of normal for serum calcium concentrations varies with age and among laboratories, a serum calcium concentration of 12 mg/dL (3.0 mmol/L) is usually considered mild hypercalcemia, between 12 and 14 mg/dL (3.0–3.5 mmol/L) it is considered moderate, and above 14 mg/dL (3.5 mmol/L) it is considered severe and is typically associated with symptoms.[167]

Presenting features of hypercalcemia include hypertension and GI symptoms due to its effect on increasing the contractility of cardiac and smooth muscle. Complaints of weakness, hypotonia, anorexia, nausea, colic, and constipation are common. The polyuria and dehydration are caused by hypercalcemia inhibiting the action of AVP on the collecting tubules. The vasoconstriction of hypercalcemia reduces renal blood flow and the GFR, with the fall in GFR aggravated by the dehydration. Nephrocalcinosis ensues from prolonged hypercalcemia and dehydration. Acute pancreatitis associated with hypercalcemia is related to microcalcinosis. How hypercalcemia induces somnolence, lethargy, stupor, and coma is poorly understood. Vasoconstriction reducing cerebral blood flow is considered a possible mechanism.

Table 73.13 lists the causes of hypercalcemia. This list is extensive, and many of the individual conditions are covered elsewhere in this text. Here we will focus on the following four conditions—idiopathic infantile hypercalcemia, Williams-Beuren syndrome, familial hypocalciuric hypercalcemia, and neonatal severe hyperparathyroidism.

**Table 73.13 Causes of Hypercalcemia**

| Type | Cause |
|---|---|
| Neonatal hypercalcemia | Maternal hypervitaminosis D<br>Idiopathic infantile hypercalcemia<br>Excess calcium and vitamin D intakes<br>Infantile hypothyroidism<br>• Williams-Beuren syndrome |
| PTH-dependent hypercalcemia | Primary hyperparathyroidism—adenoma, hyperplasia, carcinoma<br>Tertiary hyperparathyroidism<br>Drug-induced: lithium<br>Familial hypocalciuric hypercalcemia<br>PTH receptor gain-of-function mutation (Jansen syndrome)<br>Autoimmune hypocalciuric hypercalcemia |
| PTH-independent hypercalcemia | Immobilization<br>Vitamin D excess—ingestion or topical analogues, granulomatous disease, Williams-Beuren syndrome<br>Drug induced—thiazides, milk-alkali syndrome, estrogen, vitamin A intoxication, aminophylline<br>Kidney insufficiency—acute kidney injury, chronic kidney disease with aplastic bone disease<br>Neoplasm—multiple endocrine neoplasia types 1 and 2, lytic bone metastases, hyperparathyroidism–jaw tumor syndrome<br>PTH receptor excess (nonneoplastic)<br>Thyrotoxicosis<br>• Adrenal insufficiency |

*PTH,* Parathyroid hormone.

## IDIOPATHIC INFANTILE HYPERCALCEMIA

In Britain in the 1950s, vitamin D supplementation of infant formula and fortified milk at high doses (up to 4000 IU/day) brought about an epidemic of infantile hypercalcemia, presenting with failure to thrive, intermittent fever, vomiting, dehydration, and nephrocalcinosis. A number of fatalities occurred. Vitamin D hypersensitivity and/or defective catabolism of vitamin D was suspected, but never resolved. In response to these fatalities, a dramatic reduction in vitamin D supplementation to 400 IU/day was enforced, resulting in a significant drop in idiopathic infantile hypercalcemia in Britain.

Later evidence showed loss of function of *CYP24A1* in some of these patients, causing poor degradation of $1,25(OH)_2D$.[159] This was the first gene identified associated with autosomal recessive idiopathic infantile hypercalcemia. Subsequently and somewhat surprisingly, mutations in the gene *SLC34A1*, encoding NaPI-IIa, were identified as another cause.[168] Initial data have indicated that the primary renal phosphate wasting, with consequent hypophosphatemia, induces inappropriate 1-alpha hydroxylation of cholecalciferol, leading to hypercalcemia. Importantly, data from some patients have indicated that the hypercalcemia can be ameliorated by phosphate supplementation.[168] Thus, identification of *SLC34A1*-asscoiated infantile hypercalcemia, either by low plasma phosphate levels or by genetic testing, may have important therapeutic consequences.

## WILLIAMS-BEUREN SYNDROME

Microdeletion at chromosome 7q11.23 gives rise to the multisystem disorder known as Williams-Beuren syndrome (OMIM no. 194050; also known as Williams syndrome), which is characterized by hypercalcemia, supravalvular aortic and pulmonary stenosis, growth retardation, and variable gradations of mental retardation.[169]

Williams-Beuren syndrome (prevalence, 1/10,000) is a contiguous gene syndrome, which may reveal genetic factors underlying calcium and cardiovascular lesions, hypertension, glucose intolerance, and anxiety disorders. A critical region at 7q11.23 for this syndrome is a microdeletion of the elastin gene *(ELN)*. Interestingly, Williams-Beuren syndrome is not caused by point mutations in *ELN*. Instead, a segment of an allele of the *ELN* gene is completely lacking. The fluorescence in situ hybridization (FISH) test includes *ELN*-specific probes and has become the most widely used laboratory test to establish the diagnosis of Williams-Beuren syndrome.

Presenting features include round, elfin face and full lips, broad forehead, strabismus, flat nasal bridge, upturned nostrils, dental malocclusion, hypodontia, early graying hair, and slight premature aging. Short stature and obesity are persistent features. Hypotonia, poor balance, and reduced coordination, scoliosis, lordosis, joint laxity, and hyperreflexia, and inguinal hernia and rectal prolapse are findings described in patients with Williams-Beuren syndrome. These patients are often friendly, engaging, and endearing, with a high musical ability. Cognitive impairment varies over a wide range, with IQ scores from 40 to 100 (mean IQ, 55). Some patients suffer from hypersensitivity to sound, visuospatial weaknesses, and enormous learning difficulties, but selective language skills.

An episode of hypercalcemia is seen in 5% to 50% of cases and is usually mild but can be more severe, especially during infancy.[169] Transient hypercalciuria usually accompanies the duration of the hypercalcemic episode. Whether the hypercalcemic episode is the result of vitamin D hypersensitivity as originally proposed or of elevated $1,25(OH)_2D$ levels or defective calcitonin production has not been resolved.

## FAMILIAL HYPOCALCIURIC HYPERCALCEMIA

FHH is a rare, typically asymptomatic autosomal dominant condition, with mild to moderate elevation of total and ionized calcium concentration. Serum vitamin D concentrations are normal. Serum PTH concentrations are normal in most patients, but in 15% to 20% of patients, the PTH level is mildly elevated. Serum magnesium concentrations are normal or slightly elevated. Serum phosphate concentrations are low or normal. Bone mineral density is normal.

FHH has been regarded as a benign, albeit lifelong condition, with a small risk for pancreatitis and chondrocalcinosis. Hence, FHH is also known as *familial benign hypocalciuric hypercalcemia.*

Three variants of FHH have been identified, based on genetics, providing insights into the signaling pathways of CaSR[170]:

1. Type 1 FHH is due to loss-of-function mutations of CaSR, a guanyl nucleotide–binding protein (G protein)–coupled

receptor.[171] CaSR signals by means of a G protein subunit $\alpha 11$ ($G_{\alpha 11}$).

2. Type 2 FHH is due to loss-of-function mutations of $G_{\alpha 11}$, encoded by the *GNA11* gene, which colocalizes with the FHH type 2 loci on chromosome 19p13.3.[172]
3. Type 3 FHH is due to mutations of adaptor-related protein complex 2, $\sigma_1$-subunit (AP2S1), which modifies CaSR endocytosis.[173] Patients with this form typically have more severe hypercalcemia than in the other two forms, and some have additional features, such as intellectual impairment, consistent with the relevance of AP2S1 beyond calcium regulation.

The hypercalcemia of FHH is usually asymptomatic and does not need medical intervention. Occasionally a calcimimetic agent—for example cinacalcet—has been used successfully.

## NEONATAL SEVERE HYPERPARATHYROIDISM

Neonatal severe hyperparathyroidism is an extremely rare autosomal recessive disorder, characterized by relentlessly symptomatic hypercalcemia, elevated PTH level, severe parathyroid hyperplasia, and hyperparathyroid bone disease. It is caused by the recessive inheritance of loss-of-function mutations in the *CASR* gene. The hypercalcemia of neonatal severe hyperparathyroidism is fatal without a total parathyroidectomy. Postoperatively, the patient needs lifelong vitamin D and calcium supplementation.

## DIAGNOSTIC WORKUP FOR HYPERCALCEMIA

The diagnostic workup for hypercalcemia follows the algorithm presented in Fig. 73.11. It starts by ruling out false hypercalcemia by careful history to exclude laboratory error and phlebotomy-induced hemolysis. Further investigations include PTH and a spot urine test to determine the calcium-to-creatinine ratio. In the context of a low serum PTH concentration, examination of PTH-related protein (PTHrP), followed by serum 25(OH)$D_3$ and 1,25(OH)$_2D_3$, is indicated. It is essential to examine the family history for FHH, as shown in the algorithm; search for occult neoplasms, including multiple endocrine neoplasia syndromes; and review the history of medications (see Table 73.13) with side effects of hypercalcemia.

## TREATMENT OF HYPERCALCEMIA

Treatment of patients with symptomatic hypercalcemia (Table 73.14) consists of rehydration with normal saline to restore

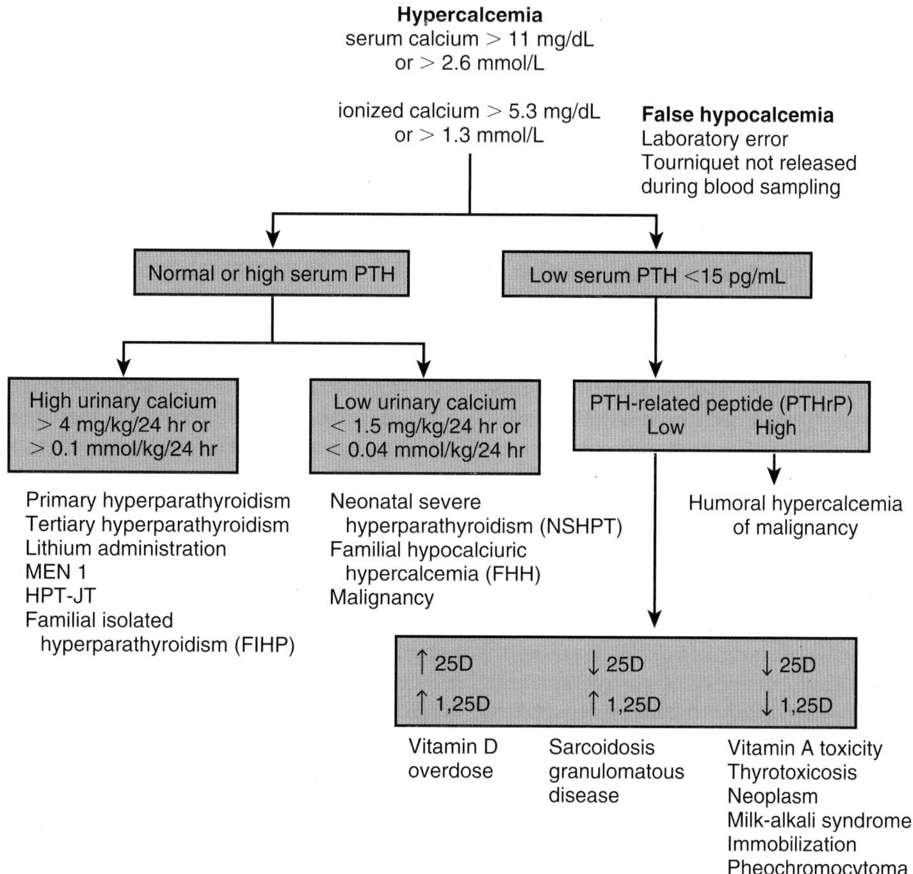


**Fig. 73.11** Algorithm for the diagnosis of hypercalcemia. After false hypercalcemia has been excluded by careful history, the first laboratory diagnostic step is to determine serum parathyroid hormone *(PTH)* concentrations. A low serum PTH level in relation to PTH-related peptide *(PTHrP)* suggests specific disorders associated with hypercalcemia and may need an examination of vitamin D metabolites—25 hydroxyvitamin D (25D) and 1,25-dihydroxyvitamin D (1,25D)—for differential diagnosis. A normal or high serum PTH concentration calls for an examination of urinary calcium excretion. High urinary calcium excretion relative to normal or high serum PTH concentration indicates several diagnostic considerations. Low urinary calcium excretion with a normal or high serum PTH concentration yields another set of diagnostic conditions, as listed in the algorithm. *HPT-JT,* Hyperparathyroidism–jaw tumor syndrome; *MEN,* multiple endocrine neoplasia.

**Table 73.14 Treatment Options for Symptomatic Hypercalcemia**

| Therapy | Dosage | Administration |
|---|---|---|
| Saline infusion | 3000 mL/m²/day IV | This is twice the daily maintenance; reduce to maintenance dose as soon as serum calcium level is <12 mg/dL. |
| Furosemide | 1 mg/kg IV | q12–24 hr |
| Severe hypercalcemia (>14 mg/dL or 3.5 mmol/L) | | |
| • Bisphosphonate (e.g., pamidronate) | 1–2 mg/kg IV over 4 hr | Once |
| • Calcitonin | 4–8 IU/kg SC | q12–24 hr |
| • Dialysis | | |

*IV*, Intravenously; *q*, every; *SC*, subcutaneously.

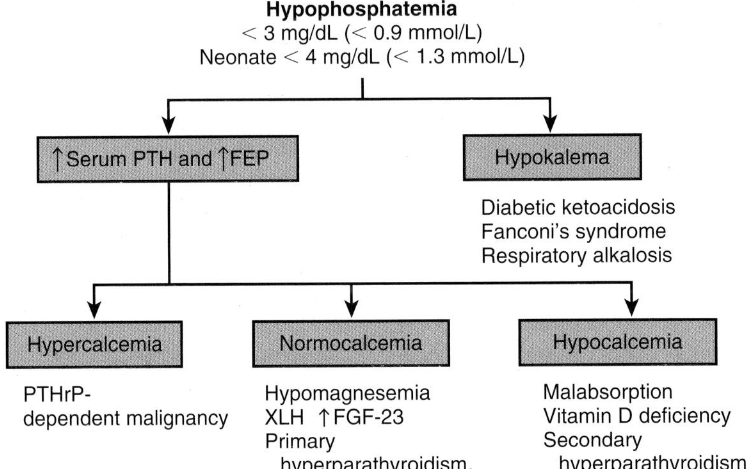


**Fig. 73.12** Algorithm for the diagnosis of hypophosphatemia. The diagnostic workup requires determination of the serum parathyroid hormone *(PTH)* level and fractional excretion of phosphate *(FEP)*, as well as serum potassium concentrations. Hypophosphatemia in the presence of increased serum PTH levels, and FEP requires a determination of the serum calcium concentrations. *FGF-23,* Serum fibroblast growth factor 23; *PTHrP,* PTH-related peptide; *XLH,* X-linked hypophosphatemia.

the normal circulating volume and improve the GFR and calcium excretion.[174] To further augment calcium excretion, furosemide can be given once the patient is euvolemic. To keep up with the furosemide-induced diuresis, additional fluid intake must be provided. Once the calcium concentration falls below 12 mg/dL (3.0 mmol/L), furosemide is no longer needed.

Severe hypercalcemia with serum values exceeding 14.0 mg/dL (3.5 mmol/L) can be treated with bisphosphonate to impair bone reabsorption. To prevent recurrent dehydration during treatment, monitoring of fluid intake and output is critical. In addition, dialysis to remove calcium has been effective. Finally, parathyroidectomy may be indicated in cases of severe hypercalcemia from primary hyperparathyroidism that fails to respond to medical therapy.

## HYPOPHOSPHATEMIA

A serum phosphate concentration of 1.5 to 3.5 mg/dL (0.48–1.12 mmol/L) is typically considered mild hypophosphatemia and asymptomatic. A serum phosphate concentration less than 1.5 mg/dL (0.48 mmol/L) in a child is severe and usually symptomatic. Clinical symptoms are related to a reduction in intracellular adenosine triphosphate level, increasing the risks for hemolysis, rhabdomyolysis, and myopathies including respiratory and cardiac failures. Paradoxically, intracellular phosphate released from cell breakdown may result in normophosphatemia or hyperphosphatemia, which may mask the true hypophosphatemia.

The causes of hypophosphatemia are listed in Table 73.15.

### DIAGNOSTIC WORKUP FOR HYPOPHOSPHATEMIA

The diagnostic workup for hypophosphatemia follows the algorithm presented in Fig. 73.12 and starts with the serum PTH concentration and urine for the determination of renal phosphate handling. The tubular maximum reabsorption of phosphate (TmP/GFR) is calculated as follows:

$$\text{TmP/GFR} = P_{\text{phosphate}} - (U_{\text{phosphate}} \times P_{\text{creatinine}} / U_{\text{creatinine}})$$

These values are all in consistent units, mmol/L or mg/dL. Age-dependent normal ranges for TmP/GFR are detailed in Table 73.16. Alternatively, the tubular reabsorption of phosphorus (TRP) can be calculated, which is the complement to the fractional excretion of phosphorus (FEP)—that is, TRP (in %) = 100 − FEP (in %). Typically, a TRP greater than 85% is considered normal, but this can be falsely normal if the serum phosphate level is so low that the impaired tubular reabsorption can cope with the decreased filtered

**Table 73.15 Causes of Hypophosphatemia**

| Cause | Features |
|---|---|
| Decreased phosphate intake | • Starvation, inadequate phosphate intake, chronic diarrhea<br>• Total parenteral nutrition with insufficient phosphate content |
| Increased loss of phosphate | Increased renal phosphate excretion<br>• Primary hyperparathyroidism<br>• Secondary hyperparathyroidism—vitamin D deficiency or resistance (including 1α-hydroxylase deficiency, VDR mutations, VDDR); imatinib<br>• Excess FGF-23 or phosphatonins, X-linked hypophosphatemia, AD hypophosphatemic rickets, tumor-induced osteomalacia, epidermal nevus, McCune-Albright syndrome<br>• Fanconi syndrome, cystinosis, Wilson disease, Dent disease, Lowe syndrome, multiple myeloma, amyloidosis, heavy metal toxicity, rewarming of hyperthermia, Na/Pi-IIa and Na/Pi-IIc mutation (HHRH)<br>• PTHrP-dependent hypercalcemia of malignancy<br>• Hypomagnesemia<br>Decreased intestinal absorption<br>• Vitamin D deficiency or resistance (VDDR types 1 and 2)<br>• Malabsorption<br>Increased intestinal loss<br>• Phosphate binding antacids used in treating peptic ulcers<br>Increased losses from other routes<br>• Skin—severe burns<br>• Vomiting |
| Phosphate shifting from extracellular compartment to cells and bones | Diabetic ketoacidosis<br>• Alcohol intoxication<br>• Acute respiratory alkalosis, salicylate intoxication, gram-negative sepsis, toxic shock syndrome, acute gout<br>• Refeeding syndromes from starvation, anorexia nervosa, hepatic failure: acute intravenous glucose, fructose, glycerol<br>• Rapid cellular proliferation—intensive erythropoietin therapy, GM-CSF therapy, leukemic blast crisis<br>• Recovery from hypothermia<br>• Heat stroke<br>• Postparathyroidectomy; "hungry bone" disease—osteoblastic metastases, antiresorptive treatment of severe Paget disease<br>• Catecholamines (e.g., albuterol, dopamine, terbutaline, epinephrine)<br>• Thyrotoxic periodic paralysis<br>• Hypocalcemic periodic paralysis |
| Miscellaneous | • Hyperaldosteronism<br>• Oncogenic hypophosphatemia<br>• Post–kidney transplantation<br>• Post–partial hepatectomy<br>• High-dose corticosteroids, estrogens<br>• Medications—ifosfamide, toluene, calcitonin, bisphosphonate, tenofovir, paraquat, cisplatin, acetazolamide and other diuretics<br>• Postobstructive diuresis |

*AD,* Autosomal dominant; *FGF-23,* fibroblast growth factor 23; *GM-CSF,* granulocyte-macrophage colony-stimulating factor; *HHRH,* hereditary hypophosphatemic rickets with hypercalciuria; *Na/Pi-II,* type II sodium-dependent phosphate cotransporter; *PTHrP,* parathyroid hormone–related peptide; *VDR,* vitamin D receptor; *VDDR,* vitamin D–dependent rickets.

load of phosphate. For this reason, Tmp/GFR is more reliable because it corrects for the filtered load.[175]

The serum calcium concentration is particularly helpful in the workup for hypophosphatemia. Because PTH is a powerful phosphaturic hormone, a low Tmp/GFR accompanied by hypercalcemia points to primary hyperparathyroidism as the cause of the hypophosphatemia. In contrast, if a low Tmp/GFR is accompanied by hypocalcemia, vitamin D deficiency and malabsorption or malnutrition must be considered.

## IMAGING STUDIES IN CHRONIC HYPOPHOSPHATEMIA

Imaging studies in chronic hypophosphatemia may include a skeletal x-ray examination to delineate osteopenia, osteomalacia, and rickets. Ultrasonography of the neck can be helpful if a parathyroid adenoma is suspected. Finally, a scan using technetium 99m–labeled sestamibi as an imaging agent may be indicated to delineate the presence of an ectopic parathyroid gland.

**Table 73.16 Age-Appropriate Reference Ranges for Tubular Maximum Reabsorption of Phosphate**

| Age | Range (mmol/L) | Range (mg/dL) |
|---|---|---|
| <1 mo | 1.48–3.43 | 4.58–10.62 |
| 1–3 mo | 1.48–3.30 | 4.58–10.22 |
| 4–6 mo | 1.15–2.60 | 3.56–8.05 |
| 7 mo–2 yr | 1.10–2.70 | 3.41–8.36 |
| 2–4 yr | 1.04–2.79 | 3.22–8.64 |
| 4 -6 yr | 1.05–2.60 | 3.25–8.05 |
| 6–8 yr | 1.26–2.35 | 3.90–7.28 |
| 8–10 yr | 1.10–2.31 | 3.41–7.15 |
| 10–12 yr | 1.15–2.58 | 3.56–7.99 |
| 12–15 yr | 1.18–2.09 | 3.65–6.47 |
| >15 yr | 0.80–1.35 | 2.48–4.18 |

Modified from Kruse, K, Kracht, U, Gopfert, G: Renal threshold phosphate concentration (TmPO4/GFR). *Arch Dis Child.* 1982;57:217-223.

**Table 73.17 Treatment of Severe Hypophosphatemia**

| Therapy | Dosage | Route of Administration |
|---|---|---|
| **Asymptomatic Severe Hypophosphatemia** | | |
| Elemental phosphate | 2.5 mg (0.1 mmol)/kg body weight | IV |
| **Symptomatic Severe Hypophosphatemia** | | |
| Elemental phosphate | 5 mg (0.2 mmol)/kg body weight | IV over 6 hr |

IV (intravenous) treatment is recommended for ventilated patients. In nonventilated asymptomatic patients, oral supplementation with 5–15 mg (0.2–0.6 mmol)/kg/day may suffice.

### TREATMENT OF HYPOPHOSPHATEMIA

The treatment of hypophosphatemia from a long-standing condition, such as starvation or diabetic ketoacidosis, is complicated by the risk for rapid progression to severe, life-threatening hypophosphatemia during refeeding, as precipitated by rehydration and glucose or insulin provision. Thus, the concurrent use of phosphate supplementation (Table 73.17) is indicated.

## HYPERPHOSPHATEMIA

As discussed earlier in this chapter, the normal range for serum phosphate changes with age, and hyperphosphatemia thus refers to a serum concentration above the age-appropriate reference range. The clinical features of hyperphosphatemia are related to hypocalcemia. In view of the reverse interrelationship between these divalent ions, a high serum phosphate concentration is chemically linked to a low serum ionized calcium concentration, and vice versa.

**Table 73.18 Causes of Hyperphosphatemia**

| Cause | Features |
|---|---|
| Impaired renal excretion of phosphate | Renal insufficiency<br>• Hypoparathyroidism, pseudohypoparathyroidism<br>• Transient parathyroid resistance of infancy<br>• Acromegaly<br>• Tumoral calcinosis<br>Hyperthyroidism<br>• Juvenile hypogonadism<br>• High ambient temperature<br>• Heparin<br>• Bisphosphonate etidronate |
| Increased phosphate intake<br>• Exogenous loads<br>• Endogenous loads | • Phosphate salts—laxatives and enemas<br>• Vitamin D intoxication<br>• Blood transfusion<br>• White phosphorus burns<br>• Liposomal amphotericin B<br>• Fosphenytoin<br>• Parenteral phosphate<br>• Crush injury<br>• Rhabdomyolysis<br>• Cytotoxic therapy of neoplasms—tumor lysis<br>• Hemolysis<br>• Malignant hyperthermia<br>• Catabolic states<br>• Lactic acidosis<br>• Fulminant hepatitis |
| Transcellular shift of phosphate | Cellular shift in diabetes ketoacidosis<br>Metabolic acidosis<br>Respiratory acidosis |
| Miscellaneous | Hyperostosis |

Thus, hyperphosphatemia becomes symptomatic from the hypocalcemia (e.g., tetany and other symptoms, discussed earlier in the section on hypocalcemia). Table 73.18 lists the causes of hyperphosphatemia.

### DIAGNOSTIC WORKUP FOR HYPERPHOSPHATEMIA

The diagnostic workup for hyperphosphatemia follows the algorithm presented in Fig. 73.13 and includes serum calcium, PTH, potassium, creatinine, and 25(OH)D concentrations. The suspected underlying disease (see Table 73.18) causing hyperphosphatemia may require other specific tests. Finally, spurious hyperphosphatemia can result from interference with the phosphate measurement by hyperlipidemia, hyperbilirubinemia, and hyperglobulinemia, requiring specific tests for each condition.[176]

### IMAGING STUDIES IN HYPERPHOSPHATEMIA

Imaging studies in hyperphosphatemia depend on the underlying disease—for example, wrist x-ray examination to delineate renal osteodystrophy and magnetic resonance imaging to rule out pituitary adenoma in acromegaly.

### TREATMENT OF HYPERPHOSPHATEMIA

The treatment of hyperphosphatemia in the context of normal kidney function includes adequate fluid intake to

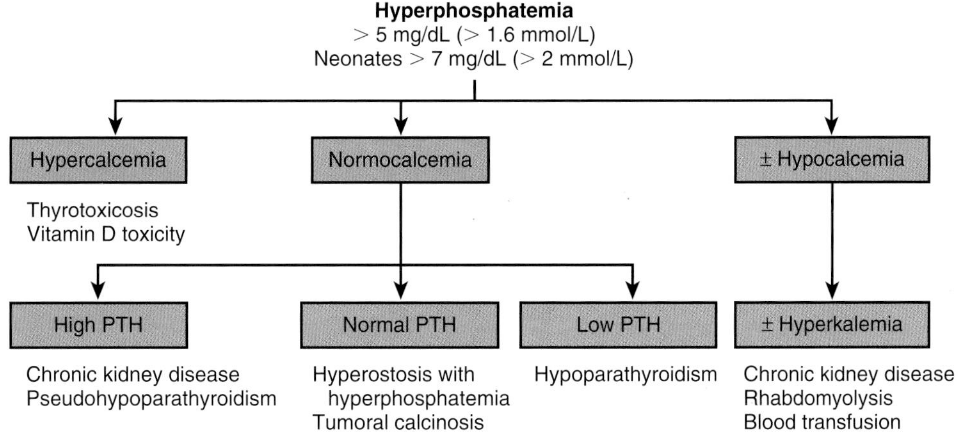


**Fig. 73.13** Algorithm for the diagnosis of hyperphosphatemia. The first step is to differentiate between conditions associated with hypercalcemia, normocalcemia, and hypocalcemia, respectively. Subsequently, serum parathyroid hormone *(PTH)* and serum potassium concentrations indicate related diagnoses.

promote diuresis and restriction of phosphate intake with the addition of phosphate binders. Finally, specific treatment for the underlying disease is discussed in other chapters in this text.

## SUMMARY AND CONCLUSION

We have highlighted the causes, clinical characteristics, and management of acid-base, water, and electrolyte disorders in pediatric patients. Although the principles of fluid, electrolyte, and acid-base homeostasis are the same as for adults, the specific requirements of the growing child lead to altered age-specific normal ranges (e.g., for calcium, phosphate) and occasionally altered tubular function, such as the impaired urine-concentrating ability during the first year of life. Moreover, the differential diagnosis of homeostatic abnormalities in children is different and much more likely to include mendelian disorders, rather than acquired diseases with secondary electrolyte abnormalities.

 Complete reference list available at ExpertConsult.com.

## KEY REFERENCES

21. Bockenhauer D, Bichet DG. Inherited secondary nephrogenic diabetes insipidus: concentrating on humans. *Am J Physiol Renal Physiol.* 2013;304:F1037–F1042.
45. Feldman BJ, Rosenthal SM, Vargas GA, et al. Nephrogenic syndrome of inappropriate antidiuresis. *N Engl J Med.* 2005;352:1884–1890.
55. Plumb LA, Van't Hoff W, Kleta R, et al. Renal apnoea: extreme disturbance of homoeostasis in a child with Bartter syndrome type IV. *Lancet.* 2016;388:631–632.
62. Kleta R, Bockenhauer D. Saltwasting tubulopathies in children: what's new, what's controversial? *J Am Soc Nephrol.* in press;2017.
73. Bartter FC, Pronove P, Gill JR Jr, et al. Hyperplasia of the juxtaglomerular complex with hyperaldosteronism and hypokalemic alkalosis. A new syndrome. *Am J Med.* 1962;33:811–828.
75. Peters M, Jeck N, Reinalter S, et al. Clinical presentation of genetically defined patients with hypokalemic salt-losing tubulopathies. *Am J Med.* 2002;112:183–190.
78. Blanchard A, Bockenhauer D, Bolignano D, et al. Gitelman syndrome: consensus and guidance from a Kidney Disease: Improving Global Outcomes (KDIGO) Controversies Conference. *Kidney Int.* 2017;91:24–33.
112. Hoorn EJ, Walsh SB, McCormick JA, et al. The calcineurin inhibitor tacrolimus activates the renal sodium chloride cotransporter to cause hypertension. *Nat Med.* 2011;17:1304–1309.
146. Wilson FH, Hariri A, Farhi A, et al. A cluster of metabolic defects caused by mutation in a mitochondrial tRNA. *Science.* 2004;306:1190–1194.

# 74

# Renal Replacement Therapy (Dialysis and Transplantation) in Pediatric End-Stage Kidney Disease

Yaacov Frishberg | Choni Rinat III | Rachel Becker Cohen

## CHAPTER OUTLINE



## KEY POINTS

- ESKD in children has broad clinical consequences, including a major impact on growth and development.
- Most common causes of ESKD in children are CAKUT, acquired glomerular disease, and genetic diseases.
- Although kidney transplantation is the preferred modality of RRT, the majority of children require at least temporary dialysis.
- Choice of dialysis modality depends on medical issues, but also on age and geographical and social considerations.
- Some complications are unique to or more severe in pediatric dialysis patients, such as catheter malfunction, vascular damage, and stenosis and infections.
- Advances in kidney transplantation over the past decades have transformed the field, enabling children with ESKD to live close to normal lives, with constantly improving outcomes.
- Posttransplantation infections may be more common in children, particularly viral infections.
- Clinical data on many medications and interventions are not available in the pediatric ESKD population and require further study.

Until the middle of the twentieth century, end-stage kidney disease (ESKD) was a lethal condition, with a life expectancy of at most weeks to months. The developments over the subsequent 2 decades in both dialysis and transplantation completely transformed the lives of patients with chronic kidney disease (CKD), dramatically reducing mortality and morbidity. As technologies and surgical techniques developed, these treatments became available for children and later infants as well.

Treating pediatric ESKD patients poses unique challenges to the medical team and the health care system, which must address not only the disease itself, but also the many manifestations that affect patients' lives and families. Reynolds et al. reported 20 years ago, that compared with the general population, adult survivors of pediatric ESKD were less socially mature, had lower educational qualifications, fewer had intimate relationships outside the family, and more were unemployed. Two decades later, changing this unfavorable state remains the major goal for providers treating children with ESKD.[1]

## EPIDEMIOLOGY OF END-STAGE KIDNEY DISEASE

There are many barriers to accurate assessment of the global epidemiology of end-stage renal disease (ESRD) in pediatric patients. Approximately 80% of pediatric renal replacement therapy (RRT) is provided to patients who live in high-income countries, who account for only 12% of the global population. Registries, such as the North American Pediatric Renal Trials and Collaborative Studies (NAPRTCS), the European Society of Paediatric Nephrology, the European Renal Association and European Dialysis and Transplant Association (ESPN/ERA-EDTA), which can provide robust information, exist only in those developed countries. The information from developing countries is derived from surveys conducted among health-care providers or from reports of patients admitted to tertiary centers. Both these methods result in underestimation of ESKD because much of the population has limited access to health services. Furthermore, in countries in which registries exist, there are differences in the age span reported as pediatric ESKD. Information from high-income countries show an incidence of ESKD of 15 per million age-related population (pmarp) in the United States, 9.5 pmarp in most West-European countries and Australia, and only 4.0 pmarp in Japan.[2–7] This is less than 10% of the incidence of ESKD in adults in the same countries. On the far end of the spectrum, Nepal, Nigeria, and some Eastern European countries report an incidence of less than 1 pmarp.[6,8] This very low incidence probably reflects underdiagnosis rather than true rarity of ESKD. The incidence, in all registries, is higher in adolescents, due to new cases of acquired kidney disease typical to this age group, as well as the accelerated progression of CKD during adolescence. Rapid physical growth and possibly also hormonal factors are responsible for the decline in kidney function observed in adolescents with CKD. Higher incidence in males, due to the higher prevalence of congenital anomalies of kidneys and urinary tract (CAKUT) in boys compared with girls, is also a finding common to all registries and reports.[9–13] The ancestry composition of each one of the registries may also affect the incidence of ESKD reported, suggesting yet undefined genetic susceptibility factors. In the United States, African-American children have a twofold increased incidence of ESKD compared with Caucasian children.[3] High-risk variants in *APOL1* gene may partially account for this observation, as they appear in about 16% of African-American children and not in other ethnic groups. CKD patients with high-risk *APOL1* variants present with later-onset focal segmental glomerulosclerosis (FSGS; 89% of CKD patients with high-risk variants, compared with 25% with low-risk genotype), with lower glomerular filtration rate (GFR) at diagnosis, rapid decline in GFR, and higher risk of uncontrolled hypertension (HTN).[14,15] Racial differences are also seen in other countries. In the United Kingdom the incidence is higher in patients who originate from Southeast Asia, and in Australia and New Zealand, the incidence was higher in indigenous populations.[16,17] In Kuwait, the incidence of CKD is high (17 pmarp), probably due to the increased frequency of autosomal recessively inherited diseases among populations with a high rate (40%–50%) of consanguineous marriages.[18] A study from Jordan showed similar findings—among children with ESKD in Jordan, 23.2% were attributed to hereditary disease, and 8% were because of autosomal recessive primary hyperoxaluria type 1 (PH1) alone (compared with the US incidence in the period of 2011–2015 of 12.5% hereditary diseases and 0.2% with PH1).[3,19] Over the years there is an increase in both incidence and prevalence of pediatric ESKD in Western countries (United States Renal Data System [USRDS], 2017).[20] This may not indicate a real biological change in disease incidence, but instead may result from the inclusion of individuals (such as infants), who in the past would not have been thought to be eligible for RRT. In addition, improved childhood RRT survival rates may increase the ESKD prevalence.

## ETIOLOGY

A major obstacle to accurately comparing the various etiologies leading to ESKD worldwide is the definition of a given entity, which may vary by reporting center (Table 74.1). This may be due to the introduction of a more accurate diagnosis based on genetic or other diagnostic study, which may be expensive and thus not widely available, or to adherence to previous dogmas that are now regarded as inaccurate. These include FSGS, which is a histological diagnosis encompassing different disease processes, or reflux nephropathy, which may be more accurately described as hypodysplastic kidneys with vesicoureteral reflux (VUR). In addition, a specific patient's diagnosis may occasionally fit more than one etiological category; for example, autosomal dominant FSGS may be recorded under FSGS or as a hereditary disorder. A strictly defined and universally accepted CKD etiologic classification is often lacking. In spite of these caveats and lack of concise etiologic definitions, CAKUT remains the leading primary diagnosis in pediatric patients with ESRD worldwide, responsible for 24% to 39.5% of patients with ESKD (Table 74.1).[3,5,7,9,20,21,24] Of note, this is proportionately lower compared with the incidence of CAKUT at earlier CKD stages, reflecting the relatively slow progression rate of this subgroup of diseases, at least during childhood and early adolescence. Hypoplastic–dysplastic kidneys with or without VUR and obstructive uropathies are the main categories of

**Table 74.1 Main Causes of End-Stage Kidney Disease in Various Registries and Reports Worldwide**

| Source | USRDS | ANZDATA | Italkid | ERA-EDTA | Iran | Japan | UK |
|---|---|---|---|---|---|---|---|
| Years of data collection | 2011–2015 | 2010–2015 | 1990–2000 | 2005–2012 | 1993–2006 | 1998 | 2015 |
| Number of patients | 7340 | 327 | 263 | 1973 | 120 | 582 | 769 |
| Age, years | <21 | <18 | <20 | <15 | <14 | <20 | <16 |
| Registry type | Incidence | Incidence | Prevalence | Incidence | Incidence | Prevalence | Prevalence |
| CAKUT (%) | 1617 (22%) | 105 (32%) | 104 (39.5%) | 680 (34.5%) | 32 (26.7%) | 208 (35.7%) | 267 (34.7%) |
| Hypodysplasia ± VUR | 905 (12.3%) | 79 (24%) | 27%[a] | | 21 (17.5%) | 198 (34.0%) | 145 (11.4%) |
| obstructive uropathy | 712 (9.7%) | 26 (7%) | 12% [a] | | 9 (7.5%) | 10 (2%) | |
| Glomerulonephritis (%) | 1603 (21.8%) | 84 (24%) | 28 (10.6%) | 320 (16.2%) | 8.3% | 177 (30.4%) | 88 (11.4%) |
| FSGS | 849 (11.6%) | 24 (7%) | 16 (6.1%) | | 5.0% | 112 (19.2%) | |
| Hereditary (%) autosomal recessive | 921 (12.5%) 470 (6.1%) | 28 (9%)–6% | 66 (25.1%) 57 (21.7%) | 410 (20.7%) | 57 (47.5%) 47.5% | 101 (17.4%) 73 (12.5%) | 139 (18.1%) |

[a]Estimated.

*ANZDATA,* Australian and New Zealand Dialysis and Transplant Registry; *CAKUT,* congenital anomalies of kidneys and urinary tract; *ERA-EDTA,* European Renal Association and European Dialysis and Transplant Association; *FSGS,* focal segmental glomerulosclerosis; *USRDS,* United States Renal Data System; *VUR,* vesicoureteral reflux.

Data adapted from ANZDATA Registry. Chapter 11: Paediatric report. In *40th Report: Australia and New Zealand Dialysis and Transplant Registry, Adelaide, Australia*. 2018. Available from http://www.anzdata.org.au/anzdata/AnzdataReport/35thReport/2012c11_paediatric_v1.9.pdf [Last accessed June 14, 2019]; ESPN ERA-EDTA. *ESPN/ERA-EDTA Registry*. Available from https://www.espn-reg.org/index.jsp?p=hom [Last accessed June 14, 2019]; Hattori M, Sako M, Kaneko T, et al. End-stage renal disease in Japanese children: a nationwide survey during 2006–2011. *Clin Exp Nephrol*. 2015;19:933–938; Ardissino G, Daccò V, Testa S, et al. Epidemiology of chronic renal failure in children: data from the ItalKid project. *Pediatrics*. 2003;111:e382-7; Hooman N, Esfahani ST, Mohkam M, et al. The outcome of Iranian children on continuous ambulatory peritoneal dialysis: the first report of Iranian national registry. *Arch Iran Med.* 2009;12:24–8; USRDS Annual Data Report. Chapter 7: ESRD among Children, Adolescents, and Young Adults. *Am J Kidney Dis*. 2018;71:S383–S416; UK Renal Registry. 18th annual report. *Nephron* 2016;132:1–366.

CAKUT, and the differences in listed diagnoses between various reports and registries are often semantic rather than biological in nature. In most countries, the second most frequent category is glomerulonephritis (8.3%–30.4%), of which the most common entity is FSGS, especially in Japan and the United States, where it is the most common cause of ESRD among adolescent African-Americans. Inherited diseases comprise the next category, although there are variations in which diseases are classified under this heading in different reports. The frequency varies from 19% (Australia and New Zealand) to 47.5% (Iran).[2,21] In countries where there is a high rate of consanguineous marriages, autosomal recessive inherited diseases comprise a much higher proportion of ESKD etiology. Specific diagnoses include cystinosis, familial steroid-resistant nephrotic syndrome (SRNS; mostly due to mutations in *NPHS1*, *NPHS2*, and *PLCE1*), autosomal recessive polycystic kidney disease, PH1, nephronophthisis, and others.

## CLINICAL CONSEQUENCES OF PEDIATRIC END-STAGE KIDNEY DISEASE

In children with ESKD, the treatment goal is not only to prolong survival and to enable a life as normal as possible, but also to promote normal long-term growth and development.

As life expectancy is much longer in a young child with ESKD, compared with a patient in his sixth or seventh decade of life, the child may go through the cycle of CKD–dialysis–transplantation more than once. This also has implications on the choice of treatment modalities (e.g., type of dialysis, vascular access) and the priority given in allocation of organs for transplantation.

Before describing the various modalities of RRT in children, the main medical issues of pediatric ESKD and their management will be discussed.

### NUTRITION AND WEIGHT

Nutrition has a critical role in childhood. It significantly affects both linear growth and neurocognitive development. Malnutrition, which is the result of poor appetite, vomiting, and decreased intestinal absorption, is common in children with ESKD. Close monitoring is crucial when the patient is younger than 1 year (every 2–4 weeks), decreasing in frequency as the patient grows. Dietary intake should be assessed periodically. In patients on a formula-based diet, this includes formula type, caloric value, protein content, volume, and duration of each meal. Height and weight are plotted on appropriate growth curves and Z-scores are calculated. Head circumference is measured regularly in children younger than 3 years. Normalized protein catabolic rate can be calculated for patients on dialysis. The individual nutritional plan is based on Kidney Disease Outcomes Quality Initiative (KDOQI) guidelines with adjustments to achieve weight gain and linear growth targets, while addressing clinical and laboratory issues. The majority of younger children fail to meet the energy and protein requirements by oral feeding alone and need supplementation by nasogastric tube or gastrostomy.

Initial recommended caloric intake is the age-related dietary reference intake (DRI) but is adjusted according to weight gain. Protein intake recommendation is 100% to 120% of the age-related DRI, with somewhat higher intake in peritoneal dialysis (PD) patients to compensate for peritoneal losses.[25] In contrast to adults, a Cochrane Review found that protein restriction has no impact on delaying progression of renal failure.[26,27] Another study raised concern about detrimental influence of protein restriction on linear growth.[28]

Dietary restrictions may include fluid, sodium, phosphorous, and potassium, and special infant formulas are adapted to the needs of patients with CKD. Human milk also has the adequate electrolyte composition for the infant with CKD, as it is relatively low in potassium and phosphorus. However, because infants' diet is fluid based, it may ultimately cause volume overload. This requires in some cases concentrating the formula to achieve a higher caloric intake in a smaller volume (80–120 Kcal/100 mL vs. the usual 67 Kcal/100 mL). It may also influence the dialytic modality selected or the frequency of the dialysis sessions. Conversely, in several renal diseases (e.g., dysplastic kidneys, nephronophthisis, and cystinosis) patients may be polyuric due to a renal concentrating defect even when they reach ESKD. This makes water handling and nutrition easier.

## LINEAR GROWTH

Growth is severely impaired in children with ESKD. Almost half of children with ESKD reach a final adult height below the third percentile if growth hormone (GH) is not prescribed.[29] A longer period with ESKD and short stature at disease onset are associated with decreased final height. Short stature affects body image and may have an impact on self-esteem. Patients, including young adults, are often treated as younger than their chronological age. In the context of chronic illness this leads to overprotection, low expectations, and delayed independence, and may subsequently affect future socioeconomic status and formation of intimate relationships.

When assessing patient height, it should be remembered that there are differences between races and in growth curves, with normal values available only for some (developed) countries. In countries with nonhomogenous population, constructing growth charts for the whole population creates inaccuracies that may lead to inappropriate clinical decisions.[30]

Many factors contribute to impaired linear growth:

- Low energy and protein intake: this is especially significant in early childhood.
- Impaired GH–IGF-1 (insulin-like growth factor 1) axis.
- Additional factors include water and electrolyte imbalance, anemia, mineral bone disease, and metabolic acidosis.[31] Correcting these abnormalities may improve the likelihood of achieving normal growth.

Beyond correction of the metabolic abnormalities and providing the best possible nutritional support, treatment includes recombinant human GH (rhGH) therapy.

The use of GH in kidney failure is based on experimental and clinical evidence demonstrating that GH insensitivity can be overcome by supraphysiologic doses of exogenous GH.[32] This treatment was proved to be effective in a study based on NAPRTCS data: of 5122 dialysis patients, 33% received rhGH treatment. Catch-up growth was achieved in 11% of the treated dialysis patients (compared with 27% of patients in earlier stages of CKD). The mean increase was 0.5 standard deviation score (0.8 standard deviation score in earlier CKD stages).[33] In addition, Cochrane database meta-analysis found increased height velocity (+3.9 cm/year after the first year), without advance in bone age.[34] In the NAPRTCS 2011 report children younger than 6 years of age had improvement in Z score of +0.63 compared with –0.1 in the untreated patients. Older children had milder improvement of +0.26 Z scores.[35]

## ELECTROLYTE IMBALANCE

Hyperkalemia is commonly found in children with ESRD, due to decreased urinary excretion. Treatment includes dietary potassium restriction and the use of sodium polystyrene sulfonate. Formula adapted for infants with CKD, low in potassium, phosphorous, and calcium, is commercially available. Further reduction in potassium content of formula-based diet can be achieved by pretreatment of the food by sodium polystyrene sulfonate.[36] This method is associated with increased sodium intake, which may lead to hypervolemia and HTN.

Patiromer, a potassium-binding polymer, has been studied in adults with CKD.[37] Pediatric data on the drug are not presently available, although studies are ongoing in children.

## METABOLIC ACIDOSIS

Chronic metabolic acidosis is treated in children because of its impact on bones' linear growth and structure. The effect of acidosis on bone health and growth is multifactorial, including increased osteoclastic and decreased osteoblastic activity; blunted action of the GH–IGF-1 axis on bones; decreased 1,25-$(OH)_2$ vitamin D production, and hence less intestinal calcium absorption; and alteration of homeostatic relationships between vitamin D, parathyroid hormone (PTH), and ionized calcium. Metabolic acidosis is treated with bicarbonate salts with target bicarbonate serum concentrations of 20 to 22 mEq/L.

## ANEMIA

Hemoglobin starts to decline in children when estimated GFR (eGFR) is lower than approximately 50 mL/min/1.73 $m^2$.[38] Diagnosis of iron deficiency may be challenging, because many patients with ESRD have low transferrin levels, due to malnutrition or chronic inflammation, causing the calculated transferrin saturation to be seemingly normal. Ferritin concentrations, by contrast, may be high as ferritin is an acute-phase reactant and increases in inflammatory states. Additional data including mean corpuscular volume, red blood cell distribution width, reticulocyte count, and a blood smear may assist in diagnosis. Other assays such as hepcidin and soluble transferrin receptor are not in routine clinical use. The physiologic hemoglobin concentrations vary with age and gender as do the recommended target levels: above the 5th percentile of the specific age. Treatment includes iron supplementation and erythropoiesis-stimulating agents (ESAs). Target iron levels are higher than in the healthy population: transferrin saturation greater than 20% and ferritin greater than 100 ng/mL (to optimize the effect of ESA). The relative ESA dose (units/kg/week) is higher in children and may even reach 1250 erythropoietin units/kg/week in infants.[39] In very young children undergoing chronic hemodialysis (HD) there is an obligatory blood loss in the dialysis tubing, which is comparable (in absolute volume units) with adults, but when calculated per kilogram body weight, it is much higher and may reach a total volume almost equivalent to three units of blood (27 mL/kg) per month.[39] Other causes for failure of ESAs include osteitis fibrosa cystica, chronic inflammation, malnutrition, hemolysis, and rarely carnitine deficiency or aluminum toxicity. Studies in adults on dialysis found that excessive correction of anemia (even within the physiologic hemoglobin level) is associated with increased mortality; therefore it is recommended not to exceed hemoglobin levels of 13 g/dL. The pathophysiology of this phenomenon is unclear and has not been validated in children.

## CHRONIC KIDNEY DISEASE–MINERAL BONE DISEASE

Although the pathophysiology of CKD–mineral and bone disorder (MBD) and the pathological subtypes in children are similar to those in adults, both the management and the consequences differ, as linear growth is an important factor in children. In addition, not all medications used in treating CKD–MBD are approved for children. Monitoring of various CKD–MBD-associated parameters includes measurement of serum calcium, phosphorous, and PTH levels every 1 to 3 months, vitamin D every 3 to 6 months, and bone radiography annually, although no single laboratory value is proven as a reliable marker of bone disease type and severity. As normal blood calcium and phosphorous concentrations and DRI are age dependent, the target levels and nutritional recommendations vary also with age. Age-adjusted hypophosphatemia should be avoided as it can result in hypophosphatemic rickets, often seen in preterm infants with insufficient phosphorous intake or in children with phosphaturia due to proximal tubulopathy. In CKD stage 5 the KDOQI 2017 guidelines recommend phosphorous restriction depending on blood levels.[40] However, there is no evidence that the restriction is effective outside the research setting. It may also be that a modest increase in PTH concentration is an appropriate adaptive response that contributes to phosphaturia in CKD and may therefore be beneficial for maintenance of normal serum phosphate levels as GFR declines. Phosphorous restriction may not only be ineffective, but also it is a goal very difficult to achieve: there is great variability in phosphate absorption in the general population, phosphate content is not stated on processed food labels, and low-phosphate food (raw, organic, unprocessed) is more expensive. Balanced phosphorous is expected to result in lower PTH and increased 1,25-dihydroxyvitamin D (calcitriol) levels, as well as better bone morphology and reduced risk for CKD-associated vasculopathy without linear growth restriction.[40–43] The choice of phosphate binders is limited in children. The first line remains calcium-based phosphate binders. Sevelamer HCL was associated with worsening of metabolic acidosis, which may impair linear growth.[44] The newer sevelamer carbonate addresses the issue of acidosis but is US Food and Drug Administration (FDA) approved for use in children only above 6 years of age (not tested at lower age).[45,46] The use of lanthanum carbonate is not recommended in children because lanthanum deposits in bones, including growth plates, and the consequences on the developing bone are yet unknown.

Vitamin D monitoring and supplementation are important in patients at all CKD stages. The use of activated vitamin D analogs, such as calcitriol, in adults is limited to CKD stage 5D, but in children their use may be considered to maintain serum calcium levels in the normal range in CKD stages 2 to 5D.[40] The ESPN CKD–MBD work group published somewhat different guidelines, in which the treatment with activated vitamin D analogs should be started if hyperparathyroidism is persistent despite therapy with vitamin D, aimed at normalizing serum calcium concentration and decreasing PTH (although the target PTH values at each CKD stage are not widely agreed upon[47,48]). There is no advantage to any analog over the other.[49] Finally, calcimimetics, which increase the sensitivity of the parathyroid calcium receptors, are not yet approved for use in children.

Deformities of the growing bone and impaired linear growth are complications that are typical in the pediatric age group, in addition to vascular calcifications (VCs) that are also well described in the adult patient population. As abnormal linear growth is due to a number of factors whose relative contribution remains to be determined, the consensus is to treat whatever is treatable. Of note, it has been shown that correcting active vitamin D metabolite deficiency alone can increase growth rate.[31] This was possibly achieved due to maintaining PTH levels at near-normal values.[50] Skeletal deformities in CKD, similar to the phenotype of vitamin D-deficient rickets, may be very debilitating but are amenable to medical therapy with marked improvement and even complete resolution (Fig. 74.1).

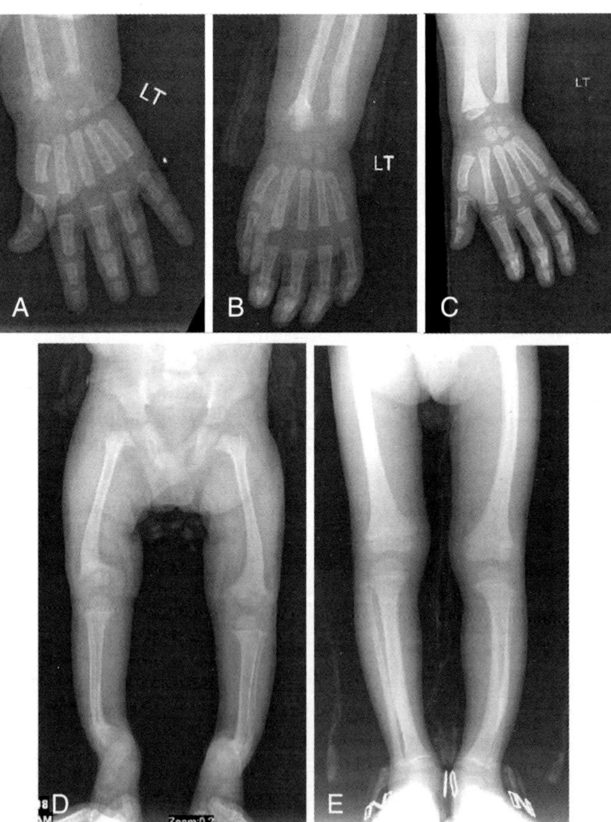


**Fig. 74.1** Severe renal osteodystrophy in a boy with end-stage renal disease with resolution obtained with medical treatment: (A) Age 1 year: severe rickets, absorption of the metaphyseal edges of the radius and ulna. Delayed bone age (6 months). (B) Age 2 years: deformation in the radius and ulna bones, widening of the metaphyseal edges, healing rickets. (C) Age 4 years: normal bone structure. Bone age is 3½ years. (D) Age 2 years: deformation with angulations of the femur, tibia, and fibula bones – healing phase. (E) Age 4 years: marked improvement, although some angulation can still be seen.

## CARDIOVASCULAR

Cardiovascular system (CVS) disease is common in children with ESRD. Because clinical entities such as ischemic heart disease and valvular heart disease are rare in children, there is an opportunity to better define the development and progression of CKD-related CVS disease. There are some distinct although interrelated clinical features.

### HYPERTENSION

HTN, defined as blood pressure (BP; systolic or diastolic) above the 95th percentile for age, gender, and height percentile or treated HTN, is found in 51% to 79% of ESRD patients.[51–54] In one of these studies 21% of the hypertensive children were not treated at all, and 74% of the treated patients had uncontrolled HTN. It was more frequent in HD patients compared with PD or transplanted children (63.8%, 54.6%, and 26.6%, respectively).[53] Other risk factors for HTN were age under 3 years, short time on RRT, acquired (as compared with congenital) kidney disease, and very low body mass index (BMI). Younger hypertensive patients are more likely to be untreated. This may be due to underestimation of the measured BP as HTN: for example, in a 2-year-old, average-height girl the 95th percentile of BP is as low as 104/59 mm Hg. Other explanations are that this group of patients tends to be hypervolemic due to a predominantly liquid diet and, in addition, correct assessment of dry weight is difficult and constantly changing with the patients' growth. Short time on RRT as a risk factor for HTN may be due to a patient not yet accustomed to fluid intake limitation or too short follow-up for adequate BP control. Patients with congenital kidney diseases (mostly dysplastic kidneys) tend to be polyuric or salt losing, and thus normotensive. The 90th percentile of BP measurements should be used as the definition of HTN as well as the treatment goal in high-risk patients, including children with CKD.[55] Using this lower cutoff, more children with CKD are defined as hypertensive and may therefore be undertreated. In conclusion, HTN, with its extremely detrimental effects (as detailed later), is frequently overlooked, undertreated, or even untreated in pediatric patients with ESRD.

### VASCULAR CALCIFICATION

Milliner et al. first noted the high prevalence of VC as part of systemic calcinosis in autopsies of pediatric patients with uremia, on dialysis, or after renal transplantation: 43 of 120 patients (36%) had systemic calcinosis; 30 of them (83%) had VC. A positive correlation was found with the use of vitamin D and peak calcium–phosphorous product (but also age and male gender), which are now well-known risk factors.[56]

In vivo, VC can be measured anatomically by duplex studies measuring carotid intima media thickness (cIMT) or by electron beam computed tomography enabling quantification of VC. Functional studies are also available and measure arterial stiffness by various modes.[57]

As opposed to adults, where two different vascular calcifying processes coexist (intimal-atherosclerotic plaque and medial), in children with CKD medial calcification is the main pathology. VC is associated with hyperphosphatemia, high calcium × phosphorous product, incremental dose of vitamin D and calcium (as phosphate binder), as well as reduced calcification inhibitors such as fetuin A, all leading to calcification and concomitant osteoblastic differentiation of vascular smooth muscle cells. There is increased vascular stiffness rather than narrowing of the arterial lumen despite the mineral deposition. These may in turn cause HTN, increased pulse pressure, and later left ventricular hypertrophy (LVH) and relative cardiac ischemia. cIMT has also been found to be thickened in children with ESRD, though not in all studies.

The primary process, endothelial dysfunction, is found in early stages of CKD in children and worsens as disease progresses. Subsequently, medial VC appears and worsens, both quantitatively and functionally, with the increase in CKD stage.[41,42,58,59,59a] In young adults with ESRD since childhood, increased arterial stiffness is found.[60]

Possible strategies to prevent VC include lowering calcium × phosphorous product, reduction of calcium-containing phosphate binder dose, lower calcitriol intake, reducing PTH levels, optimal BP control, and shortening of time on dialysis. This may be achieved by reducing dietary phosphate intake, using noncalcium-containing phosphate binders, rarely parathyroidectomy, intense antihypertensive therapy, intensified dialysis, and early transplantation.[61] The following two studies, which explored the effects of various interventions, are of special interest: Shroff et al., in an observational rather than an interventional study, showed that patients with time-integrated PTH levels of less than twice the upper normal limit had normal vessels, measured by cIMT and stiffness, compared with those with higher PTH levels.[58] Hoppe et al. demonstrated that intensified dialysis improved all variables associated with VC, in addition to improved BP control and, surprisingly, better quality of life and school attendance.[62] Anatomic and functional VC measures were not tested.

Classic atherosclerosis has an accelerated course in adults with ESRD and this disease process starts even among the healthy population in childhood. The only prevalent modifiable risk factor for atherosclerosis is HTN. The dyslipidemia observed in children with ESRD is not the typical atherosclerosis risk profile, and is characterized by high triglycerides, low high-density lipoprotein (HDL) but usually normal total and low-density lipoprotein (LDL) cholesterol in CKD patients, as opposed to low HDL and high total and LDL cholesterol.[63] Dyslipidemia of CKD also does not correlate with current CVS disease; therefore it is not clear whether lipid-lowering therapy is appropriate.[60,64] Diabetes, smoking, and obesity are all rare before transplantation in children.

### CARDIAC PATHOLOGY

#### Left Ventricular Hypertrophy

LVH is found in 30.4% to 63% of pediatric ESRD patients.[54,63,65] It is correlated (in different studies) with systolic BP, anemia, gender, and PTH levels. The pathophysiology is complicated and includes HTN, volume overload, anemia, and the uremic milieu per se. Important components of the uremic milieu are the endogenous cardiotonic steroids, digitalis-like substances whose secretion is augmented in CKD patients as an adaptation to the uremic electrolyte–water imbalance.[66] Another pathogenic factor that has been shown to induce LVH is elevated serum fibroblast growth factor-23 (FGF-23) levels.[216] LVH in itself may lead to relative ischemia and diastolic dysfunction. In adults, LVH is considered a significant risk factor for mortality, although this has not been directly proven in children.

### Diastolic Dysfunction

Diastolic dysfunction prevalence may be as high as 22.5% to 43.4% in ESRD patients.[54,59] It is associated with left ventricular mass index (left ventricular mass corrected for height to power of 2.7), calcium–phosphorus product, anemia, HTN, and PTH levels.[63,65,67] The pathophysiology may be poor compliance of the hypertrophied left ventricle, myocardial fibrosis, and myocardial ischemia.

### Arrhythmia

The common arrhythmias seen in children with CKD are ventricular and supraventricular extrasystoles, first-degree arteriovenous (AV) block, or sinus tachycardia and transiently prolonged QTc.[68–70] However, the incidence of these arrhythmias is not higher than in the general pediatric population.[69] Life-threatening arrhythmia is rare, and is usually associated with severe electrolyte abnormalities.

### Valvular Disease

Valvular disease has a reported incidence of 6% to 15%, depending on age and race.[69] The specific pathology may be not structural but secondary to overload (mitral regurgitation) or to pulmonary hypertension (PHT; tricuspid regurgitation), which are frequent findings in HD patients.[71] Aortic valve calcification, without hemodynamic significance, was found in 12% to 25% of patients in a single report.[63]

Overall, the burden of cardiovascular disease in children with ESKD may have been overestimated. According to the USRDS 2017 annual report, the 1-year cardiovascular hospitalization rate declined by approximately 30% between the periods of 2005 to 2009 and 2010 to 2014.[3] This is unlikely to be due only to improvement in treatment, but rather changes in semantic definitions (e.g., is HTN a cardiovascular problem?).

## NEURODEVELOPMENT

There are a number of reasons for neurodevelopmental compromise in children with ESRD. Some pediatric kidney diseases are a part of a syndrome or systemic disease which may have an effect on the central nervous system and on psychomotor development (e.g., syndromes such as Bardet-Biedl, Joubert, trisomy 21, Galloway Mowat, Wilms tumor, anirida, genitourinary anomalies, and intellectual disability (WAGR), and more). Chromosomal microarrays to detect genomic imbalances were performed in children enrolled in the Chronic Kidney Disease in Children study. Genomic imbalances were detected in 7.4% of children with CKD. In the vast majority of these cases, the genomic lesion was unsuspected based on clinical assessment.[72] Other pediatric kidney diseases can be associated with prematurity (Finnish-type nephrotic syndrome) or with oligohydramnios and hypoplastic lungs, and hence possible perinatal hypoxia (autosomal recessive polycystic kidney disease). Uremic toxins, HTN (or BP fluctuations during HD), and chronic anemia can cause further damage to the developing brain. Motor skills development can also be delayed because the sick infant is not free to move and play while connected to the dialysis or feeding machine. Various catheters including feeding tubes and gastrostomy may interfere with rolling over and crawling and there is less sensory stimulation during hospitalization or dialysis. Muscle tone is diminished and renal osteodystrophy may be painful and prevent the needed physical activity for normal development. Some medications frequently given to CKD patients, including aminoglycoside antibiotics (limited use, only in anuric patients) and furosemide, are potentially ototoxic. Several studies over the last 30 years showed that patients with CKD have compromised cognitive functions. This can be seen even in the early stages of CKD.[73] Specifically, studies found lower intelligence quotient (IQ) levels (~10 points), verbal or written language difficulties, impaired memory, decreased executive functions, and inefficiency in key neurocognitive domains.[74–78] Particularly affected are children who reached ESKD at a younger age (Fig. 74.2),[75,79] children with longer dialysis vintage,[76,80,81] more severe HTN or hypertensive crisis events,[80,82] as well as children with comorbidities.[83] Sensorineural hearing loss was found in 14% to 18% and ischemic lesions of variable severity on magnetic resonance imaging (MRI) were seen in 18% to 33% of the patients.[80,83] Despite this, 61% to 79% of the children with ESKD attend regular school and have academic achievement comparable with their siblings.[76,77,80] Long-term follow-up in adults treated since childhood for ESKD found impaired schooling and lower IQ (9.2–10.4 points less than controls).[84] Current ESKD treatment modality (dialysis or transplantation) was not associated with decreased IQ score. However, dialysis for more than 4 years was associated with 3.4 higher risk for decreased IQ. The authors conclude that it is not clear whether the lower IQ and achievements are the result of lower potential or lack of school attendance.

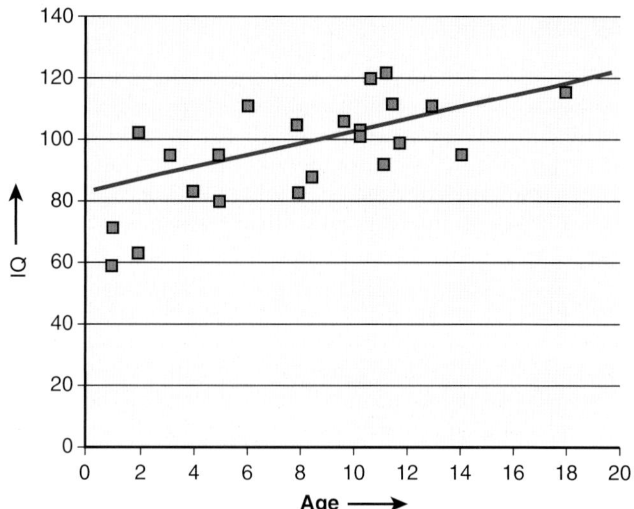


**Fig. 74.2** Distribution of intelligence quotient *(IQ)* scores by age at onset of renal failure (creatinine > 2.5 mg/dL). The earlier the onset of chronic renal failure the lower the IQ score: $R = 0.49$; $P = 0.029$. (Modified from Lawry KW, Brouhard BH, Cunningham RJ. Cognitive functioning and school performance in children with renal failure. *Pediatr Nephrol.* 1994;8:326–329.)

## QUALITY OF LIFE

Quality of life of children on RRT was assessed in only a few studies.[85] Quality of life scores are lower than the general population norms in all domains. Generally, patients perceive their quality of life as better than their parents do.[86] This may be due to the fact that patients are unaware of an alternative reality, developing a defense mechanism, or reflecting parental overprotection. The disadvantage is that parents' lower rating may decrease the patients' or their parents' motivation, and thus may adversely affect their outcomes.

## MORTALITY

Mortality rate in pediatric patients with ESRD is 30 to 74 times higher than healthy age-adjusted population,[84,87] with overall survival (in Australia) of 79% at 10 years and 66% at 20 years.[88] Factors associated with higher death rates are earlier era, younger age at initiation of RRT, and mode of treatment (dialysis mortality rate higher compared with transplantation). These factors were repeatedly confirmed in other studies.[3,4,24] Most deaths occurred within the first year of life. Similar results were presented in an all-European study and in the USRDS database: overall 5-year survival was 90% for patients beginning RRT during the years 2006 to 2010, with the worst results for patients aged 0 to 4 years (85%) and the best for the 10- to 13-year-old group (96.5%).[89] Analysis of the USRDS data by type of RRT found 5-year survival of 97% for transplanted patients, 81% for HD patients, and 83% for PD patients (all somewhat better than results achieved in the period 2001–2005). Finally, there are also racial disparities, with Hispanic children having the lowest mortality rates, followed by non-Hispanic white children, and non-Hispanic black children with the highest mortality rates.[90]

The main causes of death were documented as cardiovascular disease and infection, responsible for 45% and 21%, respectively, according to the Australian and New Zealand Dialysis and Transplant Registry (ANZDATA).[88] Similar findings in the United States showed death from cardiovascular disease of 27.1% to 39.3% and from infection of 9.7% to 22.5%.[91] A decrease over time of death rates from both these causes was demonstrated: CVS mortality decreased in patients younger than 5 years from 36.3 per 1000 person years in 1990 to 1994 to 22.6 in 2006 to 2010 (adjusted hazard ratio [HR] 0.54, confidence interval [CI] 0.47–0.63), and in older patients declined from 16.2 to 9.3 per 1000 person years (HR 0.66, CI 0.61–0.70). According to the USRDS the 1-year adjusted cardiovascular mortality rates were lower and declining over time: 7.5 per 1000 patients in 2010 to 2014, compared with 14 per 1000 patient years in 2005 to 2010 (47% reduction). This was noted in all age groups and for all treatment modalities. A similar trend was found for infection-related mortality: a decline from seven per 1000 patient years in 2005 to 2009 to four in 2010–2014. The decrease in the cardiovascular mortality is (at least in part) due to better definition of the cause of death. A different point of view was presented by Kramer et al., studying young adults who started RRT as children. The 5-year survival from the 18th birthday was 95.1% (CI 93.9–96.0), with an average life expectancy of 63 years for young adults with a functioning graft and 38 years for those remaining on dialysis.[92]

### CARDIOVASCULAR MORTALITY

Cardiovascular mortality is the most frequent reported cause of death: 14% to 41% of all pediatric deaths, depending on age and race.[52,86,88,92,93] Although CVS disease has a major impact, it is conceivable that the percentages are an overestimation and in fact, death may not be caused directly or exclusively by a disease of either the heart or blood vessels. All the studies are, by nature, retrospective and rely on physicians' report. The most frequent cause of death is "cardiac arrest" (25%–52%), a very nonspecific diagnosis, which may well be the final common pathway of various primary causes of death.[86,92] In a single study where the authors directly reviewed all patients' files, the report includes under the heading of CVS death, cerebrovascular accident (58% of cardiac deaths), congestive heart failure (15%), and other diagnoses which may be the consequence of HTN, heparinization, and volume overload.[81] In addition, most of the data available are on children who reached ESKD 2 or 3 decades ago. There is marked decrease not only in the absolute death rate but also in the percentage of deaths attributed to cardiac causes over the years: from 44.4% in 1972 to 1981 to 33.3% in 1992 to 1999. This was also shown in the period of 1990 to 2010: in patients younger than 5 years at initiation of dialysis CVS mortality decreased from 35.3% in 1990 to 1994 to 22.6% in 2005 to 2010[88] or, according to the USRDS, from 29% in 2005 to 2009 to 15% in 2010 to 2014 (same trend, lower percentages, in other age groups). A study from the Netherlands points to a shift from cardiovascular disease to infections as the main cause of death at long-term follow-up in patients with CKD—all these maybe reflecting a more accurate diagnosis.[94] However, more specific causes of death must be defined. This is not merely semantic, as accurate determination of causes of death can help focus efforts aimed at decreasing death rate.

Nevertheless, to underscore the high risk for morbidity and mortality, the American Heart Association classified pediatric CKD patients in the same high-risk group as children with homozygous familial hypercholesterolemia, type 1 diabetes mellitus, and postorthotopic heart transplantation.[55]

## MEDICATIONS

Any medication theoretically needs to be specifically approved for its use in children, after testing its pharmacokinetics, pharmacodynamics, bioavailability, efficacy, dosing, effects on growth, and development at various ages. Many routinely used drugs have not been through this process, never received such formal approval for use in children, and yet are widely used based on clinical experience accumulated and lack of alternatives. Newer medicines approved for adults are often not yet adequately tested in children, for example, some long-acting ESAs, whereas others have raised concerns over safety, such as calcimimetics. Some drugs used for treatment of patients with CKD are contraindicated in children due to possible side effects specific to children (e.g., lanthanum carbonate, which has been shown to accumulate in bone growth plates).

## RENAL REPLACEMENT THERAPY

All available RRT modalities can be used in children. Transplantation is the preferred long-term modality, but it is not always initially possible.

## ADVANTAGES OF RENAL TRANSPLANTATION OVER CHRONIC DIALYSIS IN CHILDREN

### SURVIVAL

Survival is longer following transplantation in all age groups and in both genders (from 6 months posttransplantation and on): The adjusted relative risk of death in a transplanted child compared with a child who remained on dialysis at 30 months is 0.26 (95% CI 0.11–0.46; $P < .001$; Fig. 74.3).[95] Similar results are presented in the USRDS 2017 report: in the 2010 to 2014 period the all-cause mortality rate per 1000 patient years is 24, 43, and 9 for children on HD, PD, and postrenal transplantation, respectively (a decline from the 2005–2009 period: respective rates were 51, 43, and 13 per 1000 patient years). The 5-year survival in the same report is 96% for transplanted patients, compared with 83% for PD and 81% for HD patients. In a report from the ANZDATA registry[88] HR was calculated using HD as the reference value, PD was equivalent to HD, but transplantation had reduced HR of 0.15 to 0.30 (dependent on era tested).

Several risk-associated variables are improved in transplanted children compared with children treated with dialysis: BP values above the 95th percentile were significantly more prevalent in patients on HD compared with transplant recipients (as well as those on PD) with odds ratios of 2.48 and 1.59, respectively.[53] In addition, there is slower coronary artery calcification after transplantation as compared with HD patients.[96] cIMT does not progress and sometimes regresses after kidney transplantation.[97]

### QUALITY OF LIFE

Parents of patients who underwent renal transplantation (but less so the children themselves) noted a positive impact of transplantation on almost all the domains of health-related quality of life questionnaire.[98] Another study found that patients after renal transplantation and their parents reported better health-related quality of life compared with patients on chronic HD.[99]

### NEURODEVELOPMENT

Neurodevelopment is improved following renal transplantation. This was shown as early as 1984 and later in a longitudinal study, showing improved mental processing speed and better sustained attention.[82,100] Comparative studies demonstrated better language performance and school grades in transplanted patients compared with children on dialysis.[75] Furthermore, the number of dialysis years correlated with worse neurocognitive outcome.[76,80,101]

### EXHAUSTION OF ACCESS SITES

Because life expectancy is longer than the graft survival in children, the patient may pass more than once through the cycle of dialysis–transplantation. Being exclusively on dialysis as mode of RRT will exhaust access sites (vascular and peritoneal) sooner.

### COST

Kidney transplantation is more cost effective than any other RRT modality. In a meta-analysis of articles published between 1968 and 1998, after adjusting to changing price levels, in-center HD was found to be the most expensive modality (steady over the years between $55,000 and $80,000 per life year saved [LYS]) compared with kidney transplantation ($10,000 per LYS, becoming more cost-effective over time).[102] Another study[103] calculated cost-effectiveness of RRT in Austria: the cost of the first year of treatment was €43,600 for HD, €25,900 for PD, and €51,000 for renal transplantation. In the third year of treatment, medical costs declined to €40,600 for HD, €20,500 for PD, and €12,900 for the transplanted patient. In some developing countries where most people do not have health insurance, dialysis is not a valid option

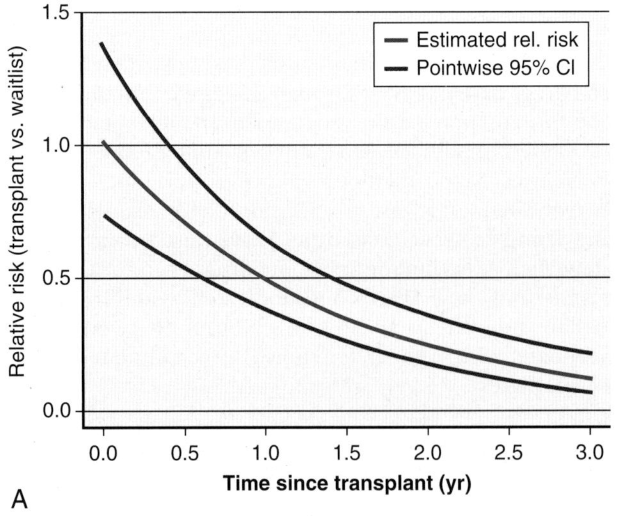


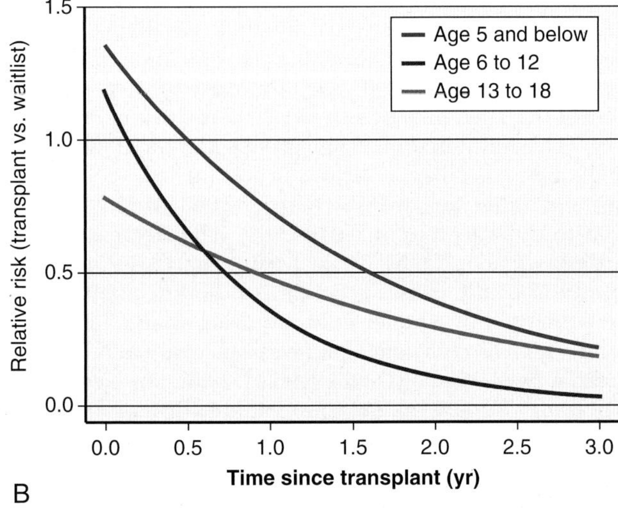


**Fig. 74.3** Estimated relative risk of mortality by time since transplantation. (A) The figure is estimated from a model including all ages. (B) Model-based estimates stratified by age. *CI,* Confidence interval. (Modified from Gillen DL, Stehman-Breen CO, Smith JM, et al. Survival advantage of pediatric recipients of a first kidney transplant among children awaiting kidney transplantation. *Am J Transplant.* 2008;8:2600–2606.)

due to its high price as well as the limited professional services. Transplantation remains the only option, although at times with catastrophic financial ramifications for the families.[104]

Usually, a minimal weight of 8.5 to 10 kg is required to achieve good surgical results, necessitating postponement of transplantation in smaller infants. Although the pediatric patient often has potential willing and suitable donors, primarily the parents, this is not always the case. Donor issues such as ABO incompatibility, positive crossmatch, medical conditions or unwillingness to donate a kidney, and sometimes patient size or medical reasons preclude or delay transplantation. For all these reasons in the great majority of children, dialysis is regarded as a necessary but temporary interim solution until transplantation is possible.

## COMPARING HEMODIALYSIS WITH PERITONEAL DIALYSIS

If preemptive transplantation is not an option, mode of dialysis (HD or PD) has to be selected. There is a notable absence of comparative studies proving superiority of one method of dialysis over another. Of special interest are infants for whom the widespread recommendation is to treat with PD preferentially and to initiate HD only if PD is not feasible. Nevertheless, in a study based on the ESPN/ERA registry in which 1063 infants were included, 13.7% were initiated on HD rather PD. The median age was 4.5 months (interquartile range [IQR] 0.7–7.9) and the median weight was 5.7 kg (IQR 3.7–7.5). The HD and PD groups had similar characteristics at initiation, and prospective mortality and time to transplantation were the same.[105] Another small study showed an advantage for daily nocturnal HD over PD.[106] The treatment burden on the patients' families is extreme, whichever dialysis mode is chosen. Parents of patients on RRT, in addition to their normal parental roles, become high level health care providers, and are required to solve problems and seek information, and provide financial resources and practical skills. Caregivers are in continuous need of emotional, psychological, and financial support.[85] These stresses cause fatigue, as well as disruption of work and social life.[107] Thus once a patient approaches ESKD, the family's abilities and socioeconomic and psychological background must be carefully evaluated by a multidisciplinary team, including nephrologist, dialysis nurse, social worker, and psychologist. PD enables more liberal fluid intake, which is especially important in infants with fluid-based nutrition. In-center HD mandates traveling at least thrice weekly to the dialysis center, which is time-consuming, costly, and not available in some places. PD enables better school attendance than HD: according to the 2011 NAPRTCS report 74% to 85% of PD patients receive full schooling in the first 3 years (the rate is steady from initiation of dialysis to 36 months later) but only 47% to 59% of HD patients attend school regularly (and the rate steadily declines the longer the patient is on HD). Sometimes, PD may be the only choice in locations where there are no available HD centers at all, as occurs often in developing countries, or if the patient lives in remote area where pediatric HD service is lacking, even in developed countries.[108,109] Rarely, in very-low-birth-weight infants PD again is the only possible option.[110] However, with PD the treatment burden is on the caregivers to be compliant and capable of performing dialysis at home, with the additional risk of parental stress and burnout. Taken together, the final decision of HD versus PD is based upon center experience, patient and family choice, socioeconomic issues, compliance, and treatment availability.

The first treatment modality used for children with ESKD in developed countries according to the registries is presented in Table 74.2. Preemptive transplantation is performed in 14% to 24.4% of patients. However, there is variability between centers; in the Norwegian RRT program, for example, 51%

**Table 74.2 First Treatment Modality for End-Stage Kidney Disease Pediatric Patients in the Main Registries Worldwide**

| | ESPN/ERA-EDTA | ANZDATA | UK Renal Registry | NAPRTCS |
|---|---|---|---|---|
| Year(s) of data collection | 2015 (incidence) | 2010–2015 (incidence) | 2015 (prevalence) | 1992–2010 (prevalence) |
| *N* | 512 | 327 | 769 | 9198[a] |
| Age limit, years | <15 | <18 | <16 | <18 |
| Preemptive transplant | 96 (18.8%) | 64 (19.6%) | 23% [b,c] | 26%[a] |
| Hemodialysis | 213 (41.6%) | 108 (33.0%) | 33%[b] | 46%[a] |
| Peritoneal dialysis | 202 (39.5%) | 155 (47.4%) | 44%[b] | 26%[a] |

[a]Approximate percentages and total number (*N*): *N* calculated from absolute preemptive transplants number plus number of first course of dialysis.

[b]Data for treatment at 3 months from initiation of renal replacement therapy (RRT).

[c]Preemptive transplantation includes both living (15%) and deceased donors (9%). Includes all living transplantations until 3 months from initiation of RRT.

*ANZDATA,* Australian and New Zealand Dialysis and Transplant Registry; *ERA-EDTA,* European Renal Association and European Dialysis and Transplant Association; *ESKD,* end-stage kidney disease; *ESPN,* European Society of Paediatric Nephrology; *NAPRTCS,* North American Pediatric Renal Trials and Collaborative Studies.

Modified from ANZDATA Registry. Chapter 11: Paediatric report. In *40th Report: Australia and New Zealand Dialysis and Transplant Registry, Adelaide, Australia*. 2018. Available from http://www.anzdata.org.au/anzdata/AnzdataReport/35thReport/2012c11_paediatric_v1.9.pdf [Last accessed June 14, 2019]; ESPN ERA-EDTA. *ESPN/ERA-EDTA Registry*. Available from https://www.espn-reg.org/index.jsp?p=hom [Last accessed June 14, 2019]; UK Renal Registry. 18th annual report. *Nephron* 2016;132:1–366; North American Pediatric Renal Trials and Collaborative Studies (NAPRTCS). *Annual Transplant Report*. Boston, MA: NAPRTCS; 2014.

of children undergo preemptive transplantations (from living donors) and the median duration of dialysis treatment before first transplantation is 3 months.[112] The cause of the disparities between the reports reflects differences in attitudes to kidney donation, traditions and religious beliefs, as well as health care system and financial issues.

The choice of selection of HD versus PD is greatly influenced by patient age: according to the NAPRTCS 2011 report, of 927 patients initiating dialysis at the age of 0 to 1 years 857 (92%) were on PD, compared with 552 of 727 (76%) in the 2- to 5-year age group, 1373 of 2125 patients (65%) in the 6- to 12-year age group, and 1648 of 3250 (51%) in the 13- to 18-year age group who were on this dialysis mode. In Australia and New Zealand similar proportions are seen: 89.8% of infants were initially treated with PD, with declining percentage to 34.5% of adolescents.[20] Similar trends were noted in the United Kingdom: at age 0 to 2 years, 80% were on PD and at age 16 to 18 years only 10.4%.

The proportion of patients under the age of 1 year at initiation of dialysis has steadily increased and doubled from 10% to around 20% of all pediatric dialysis patients from 1990 to 2010.[113] This is explained by the fact that more nephrologists were encouraged to treat younger patients as their survival improved. The same trend was found in the UK renal registry: from the 1996 to 2000 period to the 2006 to 2010 period the percentage of patients at age 0 to 2 increased from 13.7% to 17.6% (the absolute figures are from 70–104 per year) while the age group of 12 to 16 decreased by 2.3%.[4,16]

In the United States there is a steady trend of increased use of HD instead of PD, from 34% of patients treated with HD in 1991 to 54% in 2010. This trend was not found in the UK where a relatively constant percentage, around 30%, of the pediatric dialysis patient population has been on HD since 1996. Similarly, in Australia and New Zealand, 30% to 40% of all dialysis patients were on HD during the period 2006 to 2015.

## HEMODIALYSIS

Given the complexity of the treatment with HD in children, a hospital providing this service needs to have a multidisciplinary team with expertise in the various facets of this modality. This includes pediatric nephrologists, dialysis nurses, dietitians, invasive radiologists, vascular surgeons, pediatric surgeons, vascular laboratory, all the subspecialties in pediatrics, as well as social workers, educators, psychologists, and other therapists.

There are several modifications of the HD procedure distinct for children and several specific medical issues that must be addressed in addition to tailoring the dialysis prescription for every child according to size.

### VASCULAR ACCESS

The main forms of vascular access are central venous catheter (CVC), AV fistula, or rarely AV graft. AV fistula is the recommended choice because of the lower rate of complications including infection and malfunction, and longer access longevity: median survival time is 3.14 years for AV fistula (95% CI 1.22–5.06) compared with 0.6 year for a CVC (95% CI 0.2–1.00).[114] Additional advantages attributed to AV fistulas including better clearance and higher albumin and hemoglobin levels are less convincing.[115] CVCs cause more damage to blood vessels and the resulting central venous stenosis may preclude future CVC insertion or ipsilateral AV fistula creation. This is important in children, who are expected to require RRT for a longer time, often also for a second dialysis period after failure of kidney transplant, and therefore blood vessel preservation is crucial.[116] Therefore AV fistula is the preferred vascular access, with the exception of children weighing less than 20 kg, because of technical difficulties of vascular surgery. Although some exceptions exist, AV fistula is rarely created in patients weighing less than 15 kg.[117] When HD is planned for a short time, bridging for PD, or awaiting a potential living donor to complete their evaluation, CVC should be used.

In practice, reviewing the pediatric registries demonstrates a different picture. A survey in Europe found that the use of CVCs was more frequent than recommended in prevalent pediatric HD patients: 40% had AV fistula or graft versus 57% who had CVCs.[118] Only in children over 15 years of age, there were more patients with AV fistula as an access. In the ANZDATA 2009 registry all children under 9 years had CVC as their prevalent access. Although in adolescents prevalence of AV fistula was higher, there is a decreased trend over time in Australia from 78% in 2005 to only 46% in 2008 and 25% in 2014.[119] According to the NAPRTCS 2011 report, the majority of patients on HD use CVCs: 78.7% of all incident pediatric HD patients had a CVC, and a clear increase in this trend was observed, from 73% in 1992 to more than 90% in 2010. However, in many cases this is probably due to the choice of HD using CVC access by patients who are expected to require dialysis for a short time. Time on dialysis is shorter in children with CVCs: at 3 months 20.7% ± 1.0% of those with CVCs have discontinued dialysis compared with 7.2% ± 1.6% for AV fistula and 7.0% ± 2.0% for AV grafts. At 24 months the comparable figures are 71.9% ± 1.2%, 50.0% ± 3.2%, and 57.5% ± 4.3%. In addition, dialysis is terminated sooner in HD compared with PD patients: within 6 months 30.0% ± 1.0% of HD patients have discontinued treatment compared with only 18.9% ± 0.6% of PD patients.[3] Other reasons for increased use of CVC in pediatric HD include lack of venipuncture experience in small HD units, the ease of achieving an immediately functioning CVC with the advancement of invasive radiology, and the preference for painless connection to the dialysis machine. Not all centers have vascular surgeons experienced in construction and maintenance of AV fistulae in children, a factor which is crucial to fistula patency and function, and therefore CVCs may be used more often in such units.[120] AV fistula needs time to mature before it can be used, usually longer in children than adults.[121] In the majority of cases appropriate planning can overcome this issue.

CVCs should be adjusted to patient size. Catheter diameter of 8 Fr is the smallest tunneled catheter size available, and can be used even in patients as small as 3 kg of weight. This is also the smallest size that can provide long-term adequate flow to ensure sufficient solute and fluid removal, as the flow is proportional to the fourth power of the CVC diameter. The distance between the arterial and venous ends should ideally be as far as possible to reduce recirculation (and urea clearance) but close enough to ensure that both are within the right atrium, preventing sealing of the catheter ends by the venous wall. However, 8-Fr size CVC is almost the same size as the venous lumen of the small child, increasing the risk of vascular damage and stenosis. Patients weighing more than 18 to 20 kg can accommodate 10-Fr catheters. Ultrasound and fluoroscopic guidance are used to prevent catheter malposition, reducing the primary failure rate to almost zero. Although there are no published data in children, it is recommended to follow the experience in adults using the internal jugular (IJ) veins as the preferred access, as the risk of central venous stenosis is reduced in this site. Anecdotally, in newborns who need short-term HD, as in the case of inborn errors of metabolism, the umbilical vein can be used as a temporary access.

The main CVC complications are infections and malfunction. Infections are more common in younger patients, possibly due to close proximity of the exit site to the infection source: diapers and gastrostomy tubes.[122,123] Infection rate is usually 1.5 to 4.8/1000 CVC days, although an exceptionally favorable report documented a rate of 0.5/1000 CVC days.[124–128] Malfunction is the result of thrombosis, fibrin sheath formation, vascular stenosis, or mechanical damage to the CVC. If local fibrinolysis fails, the CVC must be replaced. A major complication with long-term sequelae is central venous stenosis. It occurs more often in younger patients, with small-diameter veins, with prolonged use of CVCs, with many reinsertions and possibly also depending on CVC locations. The worst outcome is for subclavian veins, followed by left IJ vein, whereas the right IJ vein has the smallest chance of becoming obstructed. Clinically, stenosis is often asymptomatic until an ipsilateral AV fistula is constructed, but sometimes superior vena cava syndrome may develop.[129]

AV fistulas, and rarely AV grafts, have a much lower complication rate, resulting in fewer hospitalizations, less revisions, and have higher access longevity.[130] In a small survey, although with significant age difference between groups, the hospitalization rate for access-related issues was 0.44% versus 3.1% per year in the AV fistula versus the CVC groups.[131] Because fistula thrombosis/malfunction is the main complication, and this is usually the result of vessel stenosis, routine surveillance of the fistula by Doppler ultrasound performed by an experienced professional should be performed. Vascular surgeons and invasive radiologists should be available to detect and treat stenosis or thrombosis.

The average AV fistula blood flow is 800–1200 mL/min. In adults, this is significant compared with the normal cardiac output (CO): normal adult CO is 5.2–8.6 L/min and the flow through an AV fistula will increase CO by 9% to 23%. A similar flow in a child, required for adequate dialysis, may increase the CO of a child with a 0.7-$m^2$ body surface area (BSA), whose normal CO is 2.1 to 3.5 L/min, by 23% to 57%. Theoretically, this may lead to high-output heart failure, especially in face of the high cardiac morbidity in dialysis patients; in practice this rarely becomes clinically significant.

PHT is another complication of adults on HD, and the presence of an AV fistula accounts, at least in part, for this process.[71] High pulmonary blood flow, a direct result of the AV fistula, may cause PHT.[132,133] Other contributing factors include endohormonal imbalances such as high endothelin-1 and low nitric oxide levels. This has not been tested in the pediatric HD population. PHT is partially reversible, after kidney transplantation, but may have significant sequelae including increased mortality.

## DIALYSIS APPARATUS

### TUBING

Tubing should be adapted to the patient's size. The extracorporeal volume, consisting of the arterial and venous segments and the dialyzer, should not exceed 10% of the patient's blood volume. For patients weighing less than 6 kg this goal cannot be achieved even with the smallest available tubing, and priming of the extracorporeal system is needed, either with whole blood or with packed red blood cells diluted with normal saline to an estimated hematocrit of 33% to 36%. Although blood units can be divided so a single unit can be used for four consecutive HD sessions, there still is a high exposure to blood products. Iron overload may occur despite the fact that at the end of each session the blood in the extracorporeal system is not routinely washed back to the patient, unless the patient requires a transfusion.

Exposing a patient to many units of blood increases the risk of viral infection and of human leukocyte antigen (HLA) sensitization. However, the incidence of sensitization in infants treated with chronic HD necessitating multiple transfusions has not been systematically studied.

In patients weighing more than 6 kg the tubing is primed with either 5% albumin solution (in smaller patients) or physiological saline solution in those weighing more than 10 kg. In those patients, the blood in the tubing is washed back to the patient at the end of each session. This procedure deserves special consideration as the blood volume filling the tubing is equivalent to 0.5 to 1 weight-adjusted blood unit. Even with the slowest possible pump speed the whole volume will be washed back within 2 to 3 minutes, which is exceptionally fast. This may cause an abrupt increase in the right atrial pressure and if the patient has a patent foramen ovale (PFO) it would increase the risk for possible microthrombi paradoxical embolism. Despite this concern, as well as the known relative cognitive deficiency in patients on dialysis and the frequent (18%–33%) finding of ischemic lesions on brain MRI studies in pediatric ESRD patients, this point has not been explored.[80,83] In adult patients there was no evidence of faster cognitive deterioration with PFO on HD compared with those without PFO, although atrial pressures during blood return at the end of dialysis may not be as high in adults.[134]

### DIALYZER

The dialyzer should also be adjusted to patient size to ensure adequate clearance with minimal extracorporeal blood volume, and therefore hollow fiber dialyzers are used. The dialyzer size is determined by the patient's BSA.

### HEMODIALYSIS MACHINE

The HD machine, to provide dialysis for children, must be compatible with the use of small tubing, be adjustable to low pump speed, and have a volumetric function. The latter is crucial as the ultrafiltrate has to be measured directly, because small inaccuracies in volumes removed that are negligible in adults can have a major hemodynamic effect on the small child.

### BLOOD FLOW

Blood flow speed is a major determinant of solute clearance, but excessively high flow can cause cardiovascular instability, which might manifest as pallor, irritability, vomiting, or altered mental status. Blood flow is determined according to body size, and is usually not higher than 10% of blood volume in milliliter/minute.

## DOSE OF DIALYSIS

According to National Kidney Foundation KDOQI 2006 guidelines, dialysis should be initiated once the eGFR falls below 15 mL/min/1.73 $m^2$, or earlier, if other metabolic derangements, volume overload, or medical signs and symptoms are refractory to conventional treatment. Practically, there are variations in eGFR at dialysis initiation among nephrologists.[135]

Once dialysis is started, the recommendation states that solute clearance should be greater than that recommended for adults (Kt/V >1.2, urea reduction ratio >65%), given that it should support higher protein intake, needed for adequate growth and development.[136] However, there is little observational information and no randomized studies regarding the correct dose of dialysis for children. Hence HD is arbitrarily delivered thrice weekly, for 3 to 4 hours each session. However, the true adequacy test is based on clinical parameters, which include in the short term, optimal balance of electrolytes, BP, and volume, and in the long term, adequate weight gain, linear growth, neurodevelopment, and quality of life. Several small studies suggest that delivering more dialysis can improve BP control, hyperphosphatemia, obviate dietary restriction, and improve appetite and general well-being, linear growth, and even school attendance.[82,137–142] Intensive dialysis may also attenuate vascular disease, which is a major concern.[61] This goal can be achieved by either nocturnal home HD, performing 5–7 sessions per week, hemodiafiltration, or a combination of both. The theoretical basis for these observations was established in a study by Daugirdas et al.[136]: In the standard calculation, the dose of dialysis is scaled to urea distribution volume (V), which is similar to total body water. If, however, dialysis is scaled to BSA, similar to calculation of GFR, because BSA is relatively higher in children, this would require increased dialysis time for smaller children. When these calculations were applied to two of the studies of intensive dialysis, the patients were indeed found to have a much higher weekly dialysis dose.[140,142] Despite this, intensive dialysis is still not widely used, and it is premature to recommend a general increase in the dose or frequency of dialysis in all pediatric patients. Randomized studies with clinical endpoints are necessary. Widespread changes in clinical practice would have substantial financial ramifications. Daily or nocturnal home HD is not available in most countries for children.

## FLUID REMOVAL

Total body water percentage changes by age: from 80% in a newborn to 65% in a 12-year-old child and to 55% to 60% in adults (female and male, respectively), and moreover the extracellular volume falls from 52% in infancy to only 18% to 20% in adults.[143] For this reason the allowance of interdialytic fluid gain is larger and also the tolerance of dialysis fluid removal is better in infants (up to 8%–10% of body weight) compared with adolescents (up to 5%). An additional challenge is that the child's weight constantly changes, so the dry weight has to be reassessed frequently, especially in the very young ages. There is no single reliable marker of correct dry weight, and thus it is estimated as the lowest weight not causing symptomatic hypovolemia.

Infants receiving fluid-based nutrition often need to have HD performed 4 to 5 days weekly in order to enable adequate caloric intake without volume overload. This also provides more clearance, as discussed earlier.

## COMPLICATIONS

Complications associated with vascular access for HD are detailed earlier, and include catheter-related infections, malfunction, and in the long term, central venous stenosis. AV fistula complications include fistula malfunction and thrombosis, or rarely high-output heart failure or PHT. In smaller children, there is obligatory exposure to multiple blood products, which may increase the risk of infection or HLA sensitization.

### HYPOTENSION

Hypotension is a common complication during dialysis. It is associated with excessive or rapid fluid removal, which often exceeds 5% of body weight, both in younger children on liquid diets and in adolescent patients who are not adherent to their fluid restriction requirements. Hypotension may appear without warning, particularly in infants, and manifest as pallor, irritability, vomiting, or altered mental status. Accurate measurement of ultrafiltration (UF) volume is crucial in small children, as small volumes constitute a relatively large percentage of their blood volume. In patients with repeated hypotensive episodes, sodium profiling, osmotic agents such as mannitol, lowering dialysate temperature, or (off-label) use of the alpha 1 receptor agonist, midodrine, can sometimes be helpful. More frequent dialysis sessions may be necessary for large interdialytic weight gain, to reach dry weight and avoid hypotension during dialysis.[144]

### DISEQUILIBRIUM SYNDROME

Disequilibrium syndrome is now a rare, yet potentially dangerous complication of HD. It is usually precipitated by overly rapid urea removal causing a discrepancy between the osmolality of the plasma and that of the brain cells, causing fluid shift into the brain.[145] Seizures are more common in children with disequilibrium syndrome than in adults. Prevention is aimed at a gradual reduction of urea, especially in new HD patients and when urea is very high. This is achieved by selection of an appropriately small dialyzer and limiting blood flow and session length for the first few treatments. Mannitol infusion, or in cases of HTN and hypervolemia, high dialysate glucose or slightly increased dialysate sodium concentration may also be helpful, by preventing the rapid decrease in plasma osmolality. Blood flow rate should be slowed if mild symptoms such as nausea, vomiting, or headache appear, and dialysis stopped if more significant neurological manifestations appear.[146]

### HYPOTHERMIA

Hypothermia may occur if the dialysate is not warmed, particularly in small children, as the dialysate flow is generally constant regardless of patient size.

### HYPOPHOSPHATEMIA

Hypophosphatemia may be caused by HD, particularly in younger children, when kidney function is normal (e.g., when HD is done as emergency treatment for inborn errors of metabolism) and when intensive dialysis is performed (for fluid removal purposes or daily dialysis for ESRD due to primary hyperoxaluria). Hypophosphatemia is attributed to excessive phosphate clearance due to high flow of dialysate relative to patient weight.[147] This can be treated either by adding phosphate (e.g., sodium phosphate in enema preparations) to the dialysate concentrate, or by slowing the dialysate flow.

### HYPOGLYCEMIA

Hypoglycemia may occur during HD as described in adults.[148] It is associated with the use of glucose-free dialysate and high dialysate flow, leading to excessive glucose clearance. Infants, especially if catabolic, may be at a higher risk for hypoglycemia and plasma glucose should be monitored during dialysis if suspected.

# PERITONEAL DIALYSIS

PD is the most common modality of dialysis treatment in children worldwide, especially at young ages.[3,8,35] The PD prescription can be individualized according to the patient's age, body size, residual renal function (RRF), nutritional intake, and growth-related metabolic needs. As stated earlier, studies comparing outcomes of children treated with HD or PD are scarce. The choice of PD is based on the assumption that PD is better adapted to the lifestyle and diet of the infant or child. Sometimes PD is the default choice due to the lack of experienced HD personnel or equipment. However, family preference and center expertise may direct even newborns to HD. In contrast to HD, PD efficacy is dependent on biologic properties of patient's peritoneal membrane rather than on a synthetic dialyzer. This means that the initial prescription must be modified according to membrane characteristics, which are determined only after initiation of PD. The peritoneum is periodically assessed and prescription modified according to findings, and it may also fail, precluding further PD. Assessing the membrane function is done by peritoneal equilibration test (PET), which is modified according to BSA of the individual as exchange volume may impact test results.

Some contraindications to performing PD are specific to the pediatric patient.[149] These include various abdominal congenital anomalies such as gastroschisis, omphalocele, diaphragmatic hernia or bladder exstrophy, and usually polycystic kidney disease where cysts may literally fill the entire abdominal cavity. In addition, medical issues including abdominal surgery, ventriculoperitoneal shunt, abdominal adhesions, and membrane failure may all preclude the use of PD. Finally, because PD depends on the availability of a compliant and competent caregiver, the lack of appropriate parental support precludes using this technique.

Infants in need of dialysis pose many challenges to the medical team and family. For this reason many nephrologists refrained from treating these patients.[150,151] However, current USRDS data show that although overall death rate among infants on PD is 20.3%, there is decline in the 2000 to 2014 era compared with the 1990 to 1999 era, with current 5-year patient survival of 74.6% for neonates and 79.3% for older infants.[152] Similar results were found in another study, showing also 92.1% 3-year graft survival for those patients.[153] As often happens when new treatment modalities or options are introduced, further options are tried and past limits are pushed: PD has been performed in very-low-birth-weight neonates (weight 825 ± 215 g) with acute kidney injury (AKI), with 20% survival.[110]

## ACCESS

A reliable access is critical for successful PD. A double-cuffed Tenckhoff catheter with downward-pointing exit site is associated with a lower infection rate. Specifically in infants or children on PD, the catheter has to be placed as far as possible from sources of infection such as diapers or gastrostomy tubes.[149]

## PERITONEAL DIALYSIS PRESCRIPTION

### TYPES OF PERITONEAL DIALYSIS

All available PD modalities can be used in children. Continuous ambulatory PD (CAPD), which is manual, is usually reserved for special circumstances. However, in many parts of the world, if dialysis is not at all available, this is the only modality used.[21] Because automated PD (APD) is easier and flexible, this is almost the exclusive modality used in developed countries. Nightly intermittent PD (NIPD), which is APD at night, with no dialysis in the daytime, can be used when there is significant RRF, because fluid removal and solute clearance are limited. The advantages are daytime convenience, lower intraperitoneal pressure (IPP), lower risk of hernia formation, less glucose absorption, and less membrane exposure to glucose. In continuous cycling PD a daytime exchange is added, thus the NIPD advantages are partially abolished, although better fluid and clearance are achieved, making it more suitable for patients with low RRF or with continuous need for efficient fluid removal (e.g., infants with fluid-based diet). Tidal PD is an option recommended when complete drainage either causes pain or is not possible. Only part of the fluid is removed in each cycle. This makes the dialysis cycle less efficient but is partially compensated for by shorter drainage time and thus more cycles.

### PERITONEAL DIALYSIS SOLUTIONS

Standard PD solutions contain buffer to control acidosis, electrolytes, an osmotic agent (usually dextrose at varying concentrations) to enable net fluid removal, and water as a carrier. However, long-term membrane exposure to lactate-acidic solution and high dextrose concentration are detrimental, leading to peritoneal fibrosis and reduced function.[154] This is more common in frequent and short cycles as used in APD. For this reason newer solutions have been developed, which have also been tested in children. In addition, there are special considerations in children at varying ages. Recommendations by the European Pediatric Dialysis Working Group include the use of the lowest glucose concentration possible, and fluids with reduced glucose degradation products (GDPs) content whenever possible.[154] In face of a paucity of studies prospectively comparing low GDP solutions or various buffers, evidence-based recommendations cannot yet be given, but it seems that correction of metabolic acidosis with pH-neutral bicarbonate-based fluids is superior to single-chamber, acidic, lactate-based solutions. Icodextrin (a high-molecular-weight glucose polymer, with high osmotic power) may be applied once daily in a long dwell, in particular in children with insufficient UF. In addition, sodium balance needs to be closely monitored as infants on PD are at risk for UF-associated sodium depletion, while anuric adolescents may have salt and water overload. Dialysate calcium should be adapted according to individual needs as the child grows to maintain positive calcium balance.[149] The use of amino acid–based PD fluids (designed to compensate for excessive protein loss during PD) in children is well tolerated but has little anabolic effect.

### EXCHANGE VOLUME

The volume of dialysate infused is adjusted to patient size, 1000 to 1200 mL/m$^2$ for patients 2 years of age or older, about two thirds of that volume for younger patients.[149] As in adults, volumes that are too small can lead to rapid solute equilibration and thus inadequate UF, and too high a volume may result in increased IPP, with increased lymphatic absorption (causing reduced UF), physical discomfort, dyspnea, hernia formation, and gastroesophageal reflux.

### DWELL TIME

The length of each exchange depends on PD modality; it is short in APD compared with CAPD. Membrane properties, as detected by PET, guide the subsequent adjustment of the initial prescription, shortening dwell time in patients with higher solute transport, to prevent loss of osmotic gradient due to solute equilibration and reduced UF.

## ADEQUACY OF DIALYSIS

No large-scale prospective studies have been performed in children that assess the correlation between solute removal and clinical outcomes. This is the result of the rarity of ESKD in children and the relatively shorter time on dialysis in children compared with adult patients. Furthermore, longer life expectancy in pediatric RRT precludes the assessment of the effect of dialysis prescription changes on survival. In areas where there are no pediatric data, adult clinical practice guidelines serve as a minimal standard. Clinical and laboratory assessment should be done at least once a month (more often if clinically necessary). Kt/V should be measured 1 month after initiating PD and subsequently at least every 6 months, and RRF is assessed by 24-hour urine collection every 3 months. Adequacy is evaluated clinically, seeking signs and symptoms of uremia: HTN, pulmonary congestion, pericarditis, hyperkalemia, hyperphosphatemia, and worsening school performance and general well-being. Additional laboratory data may indicate inadequacy of dialysis (serum solute concentrations, and hemoglobin and albumin levels), and finally, calculating Kt/V. Target Kt/V is 1.8 or greater per week, while V, or total body water, should be calculated using age- and gender-specific nomograms.[149] Prescription should be modified if needed, taking into account also preservation of RRF, patient convenience (IPP, fitting with the child's daily routine), and lowest possible dialysate dextrose concentration to achieve sufficient fluid removal.[154]

## COMPLICATIONS

### INFECTION

Peritonitis is a major complication in patients on PD, which may result in long-term membrane failure. The reported rate by NAPRTCS in 2011 is one episode per 18.8 PD months, higher in infants (1/15.3 months) compared with adolescents (1/21.2 per months), probably due to close proximity to contamination sources such as diapers or gastrostomy tubes in the young ages. Similar results were found in Australia (1/16.9 months), but with no correlation with age.[155] A report of the Italian Registry of Paediatric Chronic Dialysis found somewhat better results; 1/20.7 months in infants and 1/28.3 in older children.[156] In a survey including 47 centers in 14 countries 44% of the peritonitis events were due to gram-positive bacteria, 25% due to gram-negative bacteria, and 31% were culture negative.[157] Less than half of the patients had fever higher than 38°C, less than half had abdominal pain, and 70% had marked effluent cloudiness. Of 482 children, 420 (89%) made a full recovery, and 39 (8.1%) had to discontinue PD permanently, due to UF problems, adhesions, uncontrolled infection, and secondary fungal infection. As such, infections are the most common reason for modality change for patients on PD. In another study, including 501 peritonitis events from 44 pediatric dialysis centers in 14 countries, significant regional variability was found for both bacteria type and sensitivity.[158] This makes recommendation for global treatment guidelines more complex. Permanent discontinuation of PD varied considerably, from 0/18 episodes (Argentina) to 9/46 episodes (20%) in Eastern Europe. Of note, a recent Cochrane study assessing evidence in PD-associated peritonitis (including adults) concluded that the data available are poor. In general, review conclusions were based on a small number of studies with few events, in which risk of bias was generally high; interventions were heterogeneous, and outcome definitions were often inconsistent. There were no randomized controlled trials evaluating optimal timing of catheter removal and data for APD were absent.[159]

Other infections include exit site and tunnel infections. Preventive measures include aseptic handling of the catheter, daily cleansing, immobilization, and applying topical antibiotics and intranasal mupirocin application. Interestingly, an alternative measure of preventing exit site infection with antibacterial honey found noninferior results compared with intranasal mupirocin.[160]

### TECHNIQUE FAILURE

#### Catheter Malfunction

Catheter malfunction due to its migration or occlusion may preclude effective dialysis. Technical solutions such as the use of specific types of catheters and omentectomy at the time of catheter insertion may reduce the incidence.

#### Ultrafiltration Failure

UF failure is a main cause of technique failure and leads to volume overload. High solute transport, as detected by PET, causes rapid dissipation of the osmotic gradient needed for UF. Peritonitis events and long-term exposure to GDPs in the standard PD solutions are the main causes. Filling volume that is too high can, in addition, lead to UF failure due to lymphatic absorption, whereas low exchange volumes may falsely seem as peritoneal failure, because with low volumes there is rapid solute equilibration.

#### Fluid Leaks

Fluid leaks secondary to high IPP are more common in infants, often manifesting as hernias. Recurrent hydrothorax is due to pleura-peritoneal connections and the negative pressure produced on inhalation. Pericatheter exit site leak is usually an early event after insertion, and is usually managed by postponing start of PD or using smaller volumes initially. Leak into the abdominal wall causes subcutaneous edema.

### ENCAPSULATING PERITONEAL SCLEROSIS

Encapsulating peritoneal sclerosis (EPS) is a rare complication with high fatality rate, characterized by extensive intraperitoneal fibrosis that causes UF failure occasionally with symptoms of bowel obstruction. It was found in 14 of 712 (1.9%) pediatric PD patients registered in the Italian registry of chronic dialysis.[161] Eleven of the patients were treated with PD for longer than 5 years. Because the disease is insidious and progresses slowly, five (36%) were diagnosed when no longer on dialysis. In 71% of the patients, high dextrose solutions were used over the 6 months prior to diagnosis. Peritonitis rate was not higher than in patients without this complication. A second study found the same rate of EPS, but a higher infection rate relative to those without this complication, and no correlation with dialysate type.[162]

## ADHERENCE TO TREATMENT

Patient compliance was evaluated in 51 patients in a single-center study, using automatic PD device memory cards.[163] Variables tested were number of sessions per month, duration of each session, number of cycles per session, and volume of PD solution instilled. Only 55% were adherent in all four variables; males and African-American patients were more likely nonadherent. Nonadherent patients tended to skip whole sessions or instill reduced volumes more than shortening sessions or reducing the number of cycles. Apart from being aware of the gap between prescribed and provided PD treatment, this can shed light on the challenge of being compliant with complex treatment, the aspiration for some "treatment holidays," and the discomfort of large-volume instillation.

## WORLD DISPARITIES

Gross national income (GNI) has major impact not only on the availability but also on practices of PD. In a study of the International Pediatric Peritoneal Dialysis Network Registry close associations were found between GNI and percentage of infants on dialysis, lack of diagnosis of the primary disease, prevalence of APD, and more advanced techniques such as biocompatible solutions, enteral feeding, calcium-free phosphate binders, ESAs, and vitamin D analogs.[164] This led to higher death rate from infectious complication (although peritonitis incidence was not higher), lower hemoglobin and calcium levels, higher PTH, lower height percentile, and overall higher mortality.

## CHANGE OF DIALYSIS MODALITY

The main reasons for termination of PD are transplantation, transition to HD, death, and rarely withdrawal of treatment or recovery of renal function.

The NAPRTCS 2011 report provides information about termination of 4687 PD courses in the registry (excluding deaths): 19.4% still had a working access, 53.7% were transplanted, and 16.0% changed modality. The main reason for modality change was excessive infections (43%), 8.8% did so because of family choice, 8.2% due to access failure, and 26.7% due to other medical issues.[35] It is not clear what the percentage of UF failure was. It is interesting to note that in HD patients, reasons for modality change were mainly family choice (43.0%) and only rarely excessive infections (7.0%). As PD is much more demanding for caregivers, one would expect the opposite ratio, reflecting caregiver burnout.[35] The answer to this may be the following: half of HD patients who change modality do so within 3 months and two thirds within 6 months, over a total 36 months' observation period. PD patients, by contrast, change modality at a steady pace over the period. This implies that most modality changes from HD to PD are actually planned in advance, and only insufficient time for Tenckhoff catheter insertion and PD learning time mandated starting HD temporarily. In addition, some patients live very far from pediatric HD centers, and therefore have no option of modality change to HD.

There are several other reports from around the world demonstrating transition of pediatric PD patients to HD: In a report from Taiwan[165] eight of 29 (27.5%) changed modality—two due to refractory peritonitis, three inadequate dialysis, and three UF failure. In Turkey, of 476 children treated with CAPD, 142 converted later to APD. Ninety-five percent remained on PD at 1 year and 69% at 5 years,[166] whereas 13.7% changed to HD. In a report from Iran, outcomes improved by era but are still poor[21]: between 1998 and 2001 the annual death rate was 60%, 13% switched to HD, 11% were transplanted, and only 4% stayed on PD. In the next era (2002–2006) the death rate decreased to 23%, 15% switched to HD, 10% were transplanted, and 50% were still on PD.

# RENAL REPLACEMENT THERAPY FOR CHILDREN WITH INBORN ERRORS OF METABOLISM

Some inborn errors of metabolism manifest in early infancy and may lead to death or permanent, severe neurological damage due to accumulation of neurotoxic abnormal metabolites. Long-term outcome depends upon quick diagnosis and removal of the toxins by diet (reducing their synthesis) or medications (redirecting the toxins to alternative metabolic pathways). These modalities are frequently insufficient in the short term and necessitate more aggressive treatment to reduce metabolites to a nonhazardous range, especially in neonates. All RRT modalities have been used for metabolite clearance in various diseases, such as urea cycle defects, maple syrup urine disease, and methylmalonic acidemia. In the past, acute PD was the only technological solution for clearance of toxic metabolites, but HD, continuous venovenous HD, and continuous venovenous hemofiltration

(CVVH) are now possible even in neonates and have been found to be superior in clearance rate.[167–170] Comparison of recent outcomes with historical cohorts shows clearly better outcomes. However, due to the rarity of these diseases and their detrimental outcome, there are no comparative studies of long-term outcomes of the various treatment modalities.

## CONTINUOUS RENAL REPLACEMENT THERAPY

Over the past 2 decades, continuous RRT (CRRT) has become the preferred modality for the management of children with AKI and volume overload, who may be hemodynamically unstable.[171–173] CRRT allows provision of diffusive and convective clearance separately or in combination. Diffusion refers to the movement of molecules down a concentration gradient across a semipermeable membrane and convection describes the movement of dissolved solutes with water in response to transmembrane pressure. Both mechanisms provide similar clearance of small molecules, although larger ones would be better cleared by convection. The nomenclature of CRRT stems from the access type and the mode of clearance. Although CRRT was originally developed based on combined arterial and venous access, namely, continuous arteriovenous hemofiltration, current practice uses pump-driven venovenous access (CVVH). CVVH, in and of itself, provides convective clearance through high UF rates. In order to prevent volume depletion, most of the ultrafiltrate is replaced by electrolyte-containing fluid. Continuous venovenous hemodiafiltration combines both diffusive and convective clearance by countercurrent infusion of dialysate and net UF to maintain euvolemia. The choice of a given modality is often center dependent.

The shift in the epidemiology of AKI in developed countries impacts on the use of CRRT as it is delivered to critically ill patients with AKI. In the 1980s the leading causes of AKI were primary renal diseases, including hemolytic uremic syndrome (HUS), sepsis, and burns.[174] The Prospective Pediatric Continuous Renal Replacement Therapy (ppCRRT) registry enrolled 344 patients from 13 centers in the United States from 2001 to 2005, ranging from 1 day to 25 years. The most represented diagnoses include sepsis, stem cell transplantation, cardiac disease, liver disease, and malignancies.[172]

### INDICATIONS

In the ppCRRT, 46% received CRRT to treat fluid overload (FO) and electrolyte abnormalities, 29% for isolated volume overload, and additional 3% to obviate the need for fluid restriction and allow better intake of nutrition or the administration of blood products. An additional 6% were treated for inborn errors of metabolism, primarily hyperammonemia, or intoxications/overdose.[175] The rationale for attention to FO as a trigger for initiation of CRRT has been the understanding of the potential deleterious effect of excess fluid on pulmonary function and the need to provide critically ill children with adequate caloric intake. Several studies have recently shown an association between the degree of fluid accumulation from intensive care unit (ICU) admission to CRRT initiation and mortality.[176] Percent FO is calculated according to the following formula[177]:

$$\text{Fluid overload (\%FO)} = \frac{\text{Fluid intake (L)} - \text{Fluid output (L)}}{\text{Intensive care unit (ICU) admit weight (kg)}} \times 100$$

### COMPARISON WITH HEMODIALYSIS AND PERITONEAL DYALYSIS

Although CRRT shares similar principles with HD, both the blood and dialysate flows are significantly slower, resulting in a lower hourly clearance rate. This is compensated for by extending the clearance time: over 24 hours, CRRT provides solute clearance comparable to a 4-hour HD session. The main advantage of CRRT in the critically ill child is the ability to maintain hemodynamic stability. CRRT and PD are continuous in nature, but the former provides much greater daily clearance rates.

### TECHNICAL CONSIDERATIONS

Double-lumen catheters are usually used and the diameter size is selected based on the patient's BSA. One must reconcile the need for adequate blood pump flow rates with the desire to limit vessel trauma. Although femoral catheters are four times more often used than IJ ones, the latter result in a far better circuit survival.[178] Furthermore, femoral catheters, unless located in the inferior vena cava (IVC), are significantly affected by patient movement and may require the patient to be sedated or even paralyzed for proper use. Taken together, the preferred site for vascular access is in the right IJ vein with the distal tip of the catheter placed in the right atrium of the heart. The recommended blood flow is 3 to 10 mL/kg/h with a relatively higher flow in the very young child if an adult-size device is used. Although no prospective study has randomized pediatric patients to different effluent dose targets, the common practice is to use a dose of approximately 2000 mL/1.73 $m^2$/h to achieve good metabolic control within 24 hours of CRRT initiation.[173] One should be cautious, as a recent study has demonstrated that hypotension after the connection to CRRT occurred in 49.7% of the connections a median of 5 minutes after the beginning of therapy.[179] In previous years, lactate-based fluids were used, resulting in lactic acidosis, cardiac dysfunction, and hypotension. Bicarbonate-based dialysate and replacement fluids are currently considered standard of care.[180] Large volumes of replacement fluid, containing varying amounts of electrolytes, are administered. This requires close monitoring of the patient laboratory profile to assure stable acid–base and electrolyte balance.

Activation of the clotting cascade, impacting circuit longevity, results from the contact of blood with the artificial filter as well as from slow blood flow and small catheters used. This mandates the administration of anticoagulants: Although a single pediatric study demonstrated that heparin and citrate are equally efficacious with more bleeding episodes occurring with the former,[181] most adult studies favor regional citrate, together with systemic calcium infusion, for better longevity of the circuit and fewer bleeding episodes. Citrate is metabolized to bicarbonate in the liver and should be cautiously used in patients with liver failure. In a multicenter pediatric survey, it was shown that citrate was used in 56% of children and heparin in 37%.[175] In a recent retrospective study it was demonstrated that hemofilter survival was higher in the citrate group than in the heparin group. Bivariate analysis showed that the hemofilter coagulation risk was significantly increased when heparin was used, regardless of hemofilter size and pump flow.[182]

## DOSING OF CONTINUOUS RENAL REPLACEMENT THERAPY

There are no robust studies in children exploring optimal CRRT dosing, but the recently reached consensus in adults is that there is no benefit to delivering high-volume CRRT reaching greater than 20 to 25 mL/kg/h clearance.[183] Attention should be paid, though, to the potential discrepancy between the prescribed and the delivered doses of CRRT, particularly those that are due to technical difficulties which are prevalent among the very young patients. Higher intensity of CRRT may lead to hypophosphatemia, increased amino acid loss, and augmented drug clearance rate.

## CONTINUOUS RENAL REPLACEMENT THERAPY OUTCOMES

Patient outcomes are largely dependent on the underlying disease state and comorbid conditions. According to the ppCRRT registry, overall mortality was 42%, with higher rates in children with liver failure or liver transplant, pulmonary disease, or lung transplant and in stem cell transplant recipients, ranging from 55% to 69%.[184] FO at the initiation of CRRT is an independent risk factor for mortality: patients with greater than 20% FO were 8.5-fold more likely to expire.[177] Of note, this incremental increased risk of mortality was greater than that conferred by multiorgan failure (defined as receiving one vasoactive medication and invasive mechanical ventilation), sepsis, or malignancy, none of which were modifiable risk factors. Patients with over 20% FO demonstrated similar illness severity to those with 10% to 20%, inferring that the most severely fluid overloaded group was not sicker and there was probably no reason to administer the excessive fluid they received. A prospective multicenter study in children, addressing the effect of early initiation of CRRT on outcome measures, including mortality, is currently required.

# PEDIATRIC KIDNEY TRANSPLANTATION

Dialysis and kidney transplantation developed in parallel, and gradually became available for pediatric patients, offering long-term survival to children with ESKD. The first case series of kidney transplantation in children was described in the mid-1960s by Starzl et al.[185] Over the subsequent decades, tremendous advances in pretransplant and posttransplant patient care, operative techniques, immunosuppression, and infection prophylaxis and treatment have transformed the field, enabling children with ESKD to undergo transplantation and live a normal life with constantly improving outcomes.[186]

Although chronic dialysis provides clearance of uremic toxins, and together with medications and strict dietary limitations, enables long-term survival of patients with ESRD, renal transplantation offers significant advantages, particularly in children. A well-functioning kidney graft can provide all the functions of a normal kidney, in addition to efficient clearance of metabolic waste products and fine-tuning of water and electrolyte balance, as well as secretion of hormones involved in systemic and renal hemodynamics, erythropoietin and calcitriol. There is a significant survival advantage for children with a functioning graft, compared with children remaining on chronic dialysis, with expected life span close to the general age-matched population (Fig. 74.4).[22,187] Until the quest for tolerance in transplantation is successful, long-term immunosuppression must still be universal and close monitoring of patients is critical in order to achieve optimal outcomes, including improved growth, development, and rehabilitation.

Several national and international databases collect information on pediatric patients undergoing kidney transplantation. The NAPRTCS database has been collecting data on pediatric kidney transplantation recipients since 1987, and was later expanded to include children with CKD.[111] The Organ Procurement and Transplant Network (OPTN) has been collecting data on all organ transplantations in the United States since 1986, including pediatric renal transplantation.[188] The USRDS is the US database on ESKD, including kidney transplantation.[22] These registries provide current information about the status of pediatric renal transplantation in the United States, and extensive analysis has been performed on the data collected. Other registries providing information on pediatric renal transplantation include ESPN/ERA-EDTA in Europe, with the latest annual report providing data from 35 countries, the United Kingdom renal registry, the ANZDATA, and others.[23,187,189]

## INCIDENCE, PREVALENCE, AND ALLOCATION

In 2015, 928 children under the age of 18 years were added to the United States waiting list for a kidney, with a prevalence of 1509 children listed at the end of that year, out of a total of 97,680 patients listed (1.5%).[188] Table 74.3 shows data on age, race, gender, and ESKD etiology at time of transplant in the United States. Of the 18,597 kidney transplants performed in 2015, 718 were in children (3.8%), a significantly higher proportion than those waitlisted. Of these, 33.7% of pediatric kidney transplants were from a living donor, down from 50.1% in 2005. The most frequent living donor was a parent (78% of living donors in 2014),[111] the rest were siblings, other family members, and living unrelated donors. Whereas there was an increase in living kidney donation to pediatric patients between 1987 and 2001, with a peak of 64% of kidney transplants, there has been a gradual decrease in this trend in the years between 2001 and 2015 in the United States. Changes in allocation policy of deceased donor kidneys, which favor pediatric patients and shorten waiting times, may have resulted in a decrease in living donation. Specifically in the United States, the implementation of the "Share 35" policy in 2005 gave priority to patients under 18 years to be offered a kidney from young deceased donors. However, further analysis has shown that the decline in living donor rates, particularly parental donation, predated this policy, and may also be affected by changes in patient demographics.[190] In the United States, a new national deceased donor

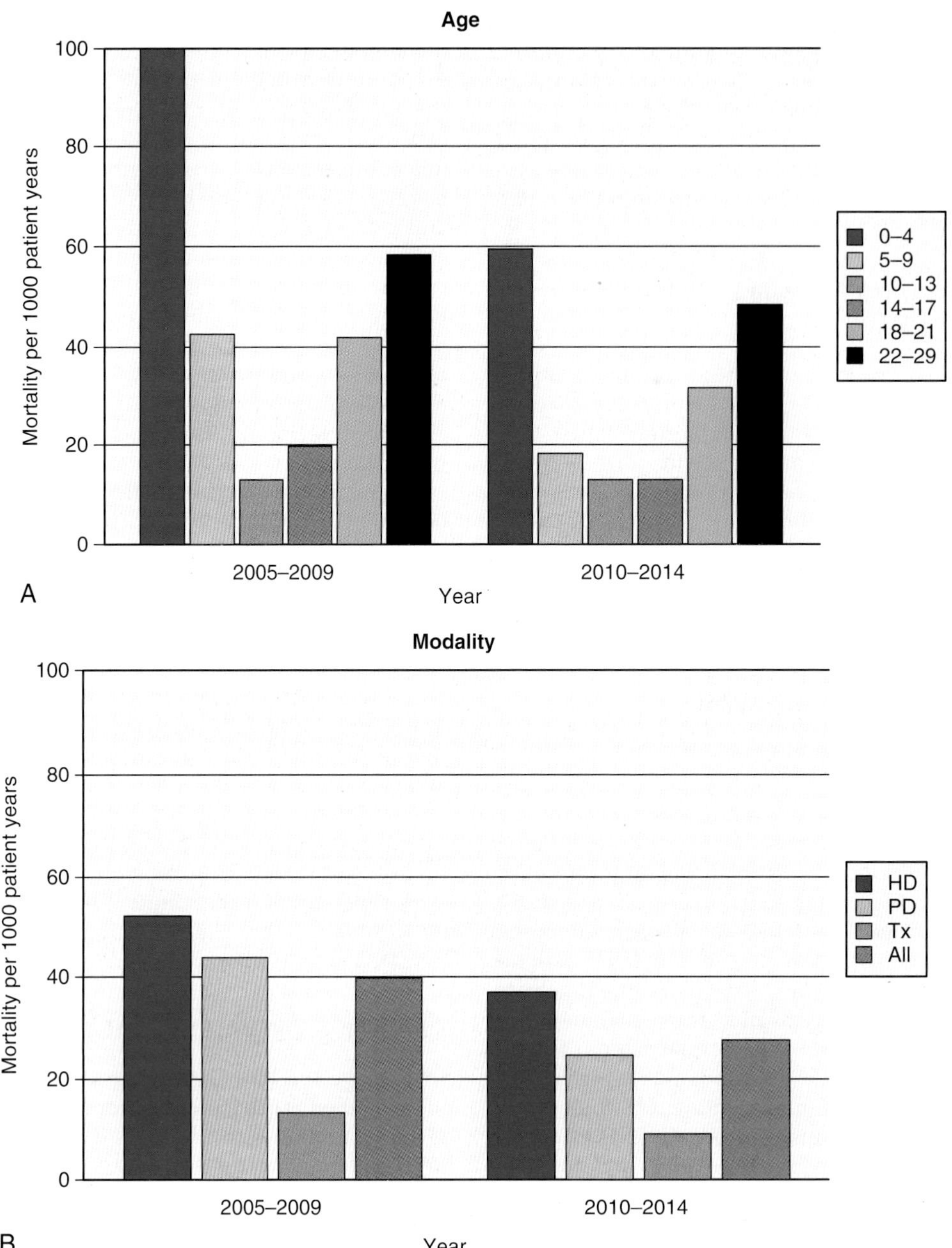


**Fig. 74.4** One-year adjusted all-cause mortality rates in incident pediatric patients with end-stage kidney disease by (A) age with comparison to young adults (aged 0–29 years), and (B) modality (aged 0–21 years only), 2005 to 2009, and 2010 to 2014. *HD,* Hemodialysis; *PD,* peritoneal dialysis; *Tx,* kidney transplantation. (From Report., U. A. 2017 USRDS Annual Data Report. Chapter 7: ESRD among children, adolscents and young adults. *Am J Kidney Dis.* 2018;71(S1):S383–S416.)

kidney allocation system was implemented in December 2014. Its major goals were to decrease disparities in transplant access and to align expected survival of the allograft with the expected survival of the recipient. This system allocates the top 20% of kidneys in the kidney donor profile index to candidates in the top 20% of expected posttransplant survival. Priority is given to pediatric candidates, as well as patients with prior living donors, zero-HLA mismatch kidneys, and calculated panel-reactive antibodies (PRAs) 98% and up.[188] The change in policy may, however, result in a reduction in transplant rate for children, but further observation of these trends is necessary before firm conclusions can be drawn.[191]

In Europe, data collected from 32 countries demonstrated that 43% of pediatric kidney transplants were from living donors. Most countries implement an allocation scheme which prioritizes pediatric patients on the waiting list, in particular with regard to younger donors.[192] The rate of pediatric kidney transplantation, waiting time, and donor source varies considerably between the different European countries. A positive correlation between the national gross domestic product per capita and the rate of pediatric kidney transplantation was noted.[193] In countries with a high pediatric priority policy the percentage of children with ESRD with a functioning graft was significantly higher.[193] Access to transplantation differed according to ethnic groups, with black and Asian children

**Table 74.3 Age, Race, Gender, and End-Stage Kidney Disease Etiology at Time of Transplant in the United States**

| | Recipient and Transplant Characteristics | N | % |
|---|---|---|---|
| Total | | 11,186 | 100 |
| Sex | Male | 6606 | 59.1 |
| | Female | 4580 | 40.9 |
| Race | White | 6605 | 59 |
| | Black | 1911 | 17.1 |
| | Hispanic | 1910 | 17.1 |
| | Other | 760 | 6.8 |
| Underlying diagnosis | Kidney aplasia/hypoplasia/ dysplasia | 1769 | 15.8 |
| | Obstructive uropathy | 1713 | 15.3 |
| | Focal segmental glomerulosclerosis | 1308 | 11.7 |
| | Reflux nephropathy | 576 | 5.1 |
| | Chronic glomerulonephritis | 344 | 3.1 |
| | Polycystic disease | 339 | 3 |
| | Medullary cystic disease | 305 | 2.7 |
| | Congenital nephrotic syndrome | 289 | 2.6 |
| | Hemolytic uremic syndrome | 288 | 2.6 |
| | Prune belly | 279 | 2.5 |
| | Familial nephritis | 247 | 2.2 |
| | Cystinosis | 225 | 2 |

As of January 1, 2014, 12,189 renal transplants had been reported for 11,186 pediatric patients. This represents 586 new transplants and 554 patients with their first registry transplant since the 2010 Annual Report. Other diagnoses, not listed, with less than 2% of total for each include idiopathic crescentic glomerulonephritis, membranoproliferative glomerulonephritis, interstitial nephritis, lupus nephritis, immunoglobulin A nephritis, granulomatosis with polyangiitis, renal infarct, oxalosis, Wilms tumor, Drash syndrome, membranous nephropathy, sickle cell nephropathy, as well as 6.2% falling into the category of unknown etiology. Kidney dysplasia, hypoplasia, reflux nephropathy, and obstructive uropathy can also be grouped together as congenital anomalies of kidneys and urinary tract.

Modified from North American Pediatric Renal Trials and Collaborative Studies (NAPRTCS). *Annual Transplant Report.* Boston, MA: NAPRTCS; 2014.

less likely to receive a kidney transplant than white patients, mostly due to decreased living donation.[194]

Preemptive kidney transplantation, meaning no dialysis performed prior to transplantation, is the modality used in 25% of pediatric ESRD patients in the United States and 27% in Europe.[111,192] Worldwide, preemptive transplantation is mostly from living donors.

Renal transplantation in infants under the age of 1 year is uncommon, reported at 0.8% of pediatric transplants in the NAPRTCS database.[111] As noted earlier, deceased donor kidneys from younger donors are often allocated preferentially to children. However, utilization of deceased donor kidneys from infants and very small children holds unique challenges, as they are more prone to vasospasm and graft thrombosis, urinary complications, and possibly glomerular hyperfiltration. Recent data have shown good results in children receiving kidneys from small pediatric donors, either a single kidney or both donor kidneys en bloc.[195–197] One study from Europe reported a significant increase in allograft size after transplantation and superior graft function in the recipients of pediatric kidneys.[196]

Although allocation systems usually try to match pediatric recipients with the best donors, a recent study showed excellent 3-year graft survival in children receiving a kidney after circulatory death of the donor.[198]

## PREPARATION OF THE RECIPIENT FOR TRANSPLANTATION

### CHOICE OF DONOR

Living donor kidney transplantation offers better graft survival than deceased donor transplantation, though other factors, such as donor age, HLA matching, and sensitization play a significant role.[199] Kidney grafts from middle-aged living donors afford improved long-term allograft survival compared with younger deceased donor kidneys.[200] However, data from the Collaborative Transplant Study showed that well-matched deceased donor kidneys compare favorably with living donor grafts with many HLA mismatches.[201] The question of whether it is advantageous to perform living or deceased donor transplantation first has been studied, as most pediatric kidney transplant patients will eventually require a second transplant. For most candidates, living donor transplantation as the first treatment option provides the best long-term benefit, except possibly for children who are highly sensitized, for whom deceased donor transplantation first, while they have priority as children on the waiting list, may be an advantage.[202]

### TIMING

When the patient approaches KDOQI stage 4 CKD, preparation of the patient for transplant, as well as evaluation of potential living donors should be pursued. However, graft survival is not indefinite, and no benefit has been demonstrated for transplantation prior to reaching ESKD.[203] Preemptive transplantation is associated with better patient and graft survival when compared with children who receive dialysis for longer than 1 year.[203] Other considerations, particularly morbidity on dialysis, neurocognitive development, and decreased linear growth also favor transplantation as the first modality of RRT. Certain situations may preclude preemptive transplantation, such as active nephrotic disease, which is also a hypercoagulable state, presenting a high risk of thrombosis during transplantation. To be a candidate for transplantation without dialysis, the patient must have some minimal residual kidney function and urine volume.

Two age groups require special consideration. Very small children may have inferior results due mainly to technical difficulties and graft thrombosis. Some specialized centers, with greater experience in this age group, have demonstrated excellent results.[199] The alternative, remaining on dialysis for a prolonged period, also carries a high morbidity and mortality, particularly in this young age group.[111] Most units refer young patients for transplantation when they reach a weight close to 10 kg, but the risks and benefits must be carefully considered in each case. The other potentially complex age group is adolescents. There is a higher rate of acute rejection episodes, shorter graft survival, and lower creatinine clearance in this group.[111] This is mostly due to nonadherence, which is more frequent in teenagers, and may manifest as missed doses of immunosuppressive medications, more extensive "drug holidays," missed clinic visits, and other high-risk behaviors.[204–206]

## CONTRAINDICATIONS

Some clinical situations may present a temporary or permanent contraindication to transplantation. Malignancy should postpone plans for transplantation until complete remission is achieved, chemotherapeutic medications are discontinued, and no relapse is evident. High-dose immunosuppressive therapy after transplantation may increase the risk of cancer recurrence due to enhanced development of micrometastases. The period between completion of therapy for cancer and listing for transplant will depend also on the type of malignancy and its characteristics.[207] Immunosuppressive medications also impair the body's ability to fight infection; therefore active infection is a temporary contraindication to transplantation and latent infections should be sought out and addressed before proceeding to transplant. Severe comorbidities or profound neurodevelopmental delay may render a child unsuitable for transplant. However, intellectual disability does not impact patient or graft survival, and should not be a barrier to transplantation in itself.[208,209] Each child should be evaluated individually to assess the impact of transplantation on life expectancy, quality of life, and rehabilitation, taking into account the wishes of the family. Recalcitrant nonadherence to medication or dialysis schedule, diet, and clinic appointments may also be a temporary contraindication to transplantation.

## RECIPIENT EVALUATION

A comprehensive evaluation of the pediatric kidney transplant candidate is crucial to achieve the best results. The goals of this workup are to provide an optimal plan for each individual patient, reduce complications, and increase long-term patient and graft survival. The main elements of the pretransplant evaluation are summarized in Table 74.4. Some of the important issues are discussed in the following sections.

### INFECTION

A history, physical signs, or laboratory findings suggesting active infection need to be addressed before subjecting the patient to major surgery and high-dose immunosuppression. The respiratory tract, teeth, skin, dialysis access exit site, and other sites of possible chronic infection should be carefully examined, as even a minor infection may be exacerbated by immunosuppressive therapy. Testing of serology for cytomegalovirus (CMV) and Epstein–Barr virus (EBV) to assess the risk of posttransplant viral disease are important in planning monitoring and antiviral prophylaxis posttransplant. Many pediatric patients are seronegative for these viruses, and should be monitored frequently while waitlisted, to avoid inadvertently transplanting during a subclinical primary infection. Vaccinations should be reviewed and completed before transplantation, as patients will be at increased risk

**Table 74.4 Evaluation of Pediatric Candidates for Renal Transplantation**

| | |
|---|---|
| Medical history | End-stage renal disease etiology, family history of renal or other disease, biopsy results, previous transplant history, dialysis access and prescription, medication list, compliance with medical regimen, urological interventions, urine output, other comorbidities, allergies, previous procedures, transfusions, growth charts |
| Physical examination | Weight, height, body mass index and percentiles, blood pressure and pulse, general well-being, complete physical examination |
| Specialist assessments | Pediatric nephrologist, transplant surgeon, urologist, anesthesiologist, transplant coordinator, nurse, social worker, dietitian, pediatric dentist. As indicated: psychologist, cardiologist, hematologist, pulmonologist |
| Laboratory tests | Blood type, complete blood count, electrolytes, blood urea nitrogen, creatinine, calcium, phosphorus, liver enzymes, protein, albumin, lipids, iron, parathyroid hormone, thyroid, fasting glucose and HbA1C, prothrombin time/ partial thromboplastin time, urinalysis, 24-hour urine collection for creatinine clearance and proteinuria |
| Serology | Epstein–Barr virus (immunoglobulin [Ig]G Epstein-Barr nuclear antigen and IgM), cytomegalovirus (IgG and IgM), hepatitis B virus (surface Ag and Ab), hepatitis C virus, human immunodeficiency virus, varicella, purified protein derivative test |
| Histocompatibility testing | Human leukocyte antigen typing – class I (A,B), class II (DR, DQ), panel-reactive antibodies, donor-specific antibodies, crossmatch with donor (T- and B-cell crossmatch, by complement-dependent cytotoxicity with antihuman globulin or flow cytometry) |
| Imaging | Chest X-ray, abdominal ultrasound including the kidneys, bladder, and postvoiding volume |
| | Cardiac echo and electrocardiogram. Doppler study of abdominal and pelvic arteries and veins |
| | Voiding cystourethrogram, urodynamic testing, or other if indicated |
| Vaccinations | Diphtheria, tetanus, pertussis (DTaP), hemophilus influenza type B (HiB), inactivated polio vaccine (IPV), hepatitis A virus (HAV), hepatitis B virus (HBV), varicella, measles, mumps, and rubella (MMR), pneumococcus conjugate and polysaccharide, influenza |
| | Selected patients: meningococcus, human papillomavirus |
| Social | Evaluation of the family, support systems, financial issues, school |

of infection after transplantation. In addition, response to vaccines may be attenuated by immunosuppressive medications, and live vaccines are not recommended posttransplant.[209a] However, even with pretransplantation vaccination, immunity may wane in some recipients when they receive immunosuppression.[210] Higher pretransplant titers of hepatitis B antibodies may protect against titer loss after transplantation.[211] The regular pediatric schedule should be given, including pneumococcus, influenza, and varicella, as well as other vaccines depending on age and exposure. Close contacts and household members of these children should complete age-appropriate vaccination schedules to increase the child's indirect protection.[212] Despite these recommendations, the vaccination coverage in pediatric kidney transplant candidates is incomplete, and efforts need to be made to improve vaccination rates before kidney transplantation.[211]

## MALIGNANCY

Although less common in children, a basic workup to rule out malignancy includes history, physical examination, chest X-ray, and abdominal ultrasound, as well as routine laboratory tests. Children with a history of cancer should be evaluated by a pediatric oncologist to assess remission and risk of recurrence and to help determine the timing of transplantation.[207]

## UROLOGICAL ISSUES

The most frequent cause of ESRD in younger children is CAKUT.[111] Structural and functional evaluation of the urinary tract is important before transplant, as the kidney allograft may be compromised by an abnormal urinary tract, with obstructed drainage, massive reflux, or a small defunctionalized bladder. Investigation should begin with an ultrasound of the kidneys and urinary tract, including imaging of the full and postvoid bladder. In patients with an abnormal urinary tract, further tests like a voiding cystourethrogram and urodynamic evaluation provide further information. When the child has prolonged anuria, it is sometimes difficult to assess bladder capacity and function. Surgical intervention to alleviate obstruction, correct massive reflux if needed, or occasionally bladder augmentation can be performed prior to or during transplantation. However, the capacity of a small defunctionalized bladder may increase after renal transplantation and enable normal voiding without compromising graft function, thus avoiding the need for bladder augmentation.[213] Nephrectomy of native kidneys is indicated in cases of persistent nephrotic syndrome of presumed immunological etiology (to enable prompt and accurate diagnosis of recurring nephrotic syndrome), chronically infected kidneys, very large kidneys in polycystic kidney disease (to enable more physical space for the graft and alleviate discomfort), and sometimes for uncontrolled HTN.[214] In cases of congenital nephrotic syndrome, particularly the Finnish type, mortality due to infection and thrombosis is high; therefore bilateral nephrectomy is usually performed when the child has reached a size compatible with transplantation, even if renal function is good or even normal.[215]

## CARDIOVASCULAR ISSUES

Congenital heart disease may coexist with CKD in some patients, which requires consultation with a pediatric cardiologist and consideration of surgical correction prior to transplantation. HTN is very common in ESKD, in many cases causing LVH, with diastolic and occasionally systolic dysfunction. Treatment with antihypertensive medications and avoiding chronic volume overload in dialysis patients are important, though optimal control of HTN is often difficult to achieve. However, FGF-23 which is elevated in CKD, induces LVH independent of BP. Therefore LVH may not be completely correctible as long as CKD persists.[216,217] Cardiomyopathy may improve significantly in children undergoing renal transplantation and LVH may improve.[218,219]

Evaluation of abdominal vasculature prior to transplantation is beneficial in planning anastomoses and anticipating significant surgical challenges. Children who have had previous abdominal or pelvic surgery, CVCs in the lower body, including neonatal umbilical arterial or venous catheterization, and patients with hypercoagulable state should have Doppler studies of the large arteries and veins prior to transplantation. Abnormal studies can be followed by formal venography.[220]

## RISK OF RECURRENCE

The disease process that caused ESKD may affect the graft. Many immune-mediated kidney diseases have a tendency to recur due to continuation of the underlying immunological process or persistence of a humoral factor (FSGS, membranoproliferative glomerulonephritis [MPGN], systemic lupus erythematosus, immunoglobulin A [IgA] nephropathy). Genetic mutations causing formation of an abnormal protein product or enzymatic deficiency are highly likely to lead to rapid disease recurrence in the transplanted kidney (atypical HUS [aHUS], primary hyperoxaluria).

Recurrence is particularly frequent in idiopathic FSGS, with a rate in children of 30% to 80%, depending on the report. Nephrotic syndrome and graft dysfunction may appear immediately after transplantation, and prompt intervention is needed. In these cases pretransplant nephrectomy of native kidneys, if the patient still has proteinuria, will assist in timely diagnosis of recurrence and enable early treatment.[214] However, FSGS is a histological diagnosis, which may be due to one of several underlying pathophysiological processes. Conversely, SRNS may have histological findings compatible with minimal change nephropathy or other nonspecific findings, and yet have clinical features indistinguishable from FSGS. The PodoNet registry, a large multinational study of childhood-onset SRNS, demonstrated posttransplant disease recurrence in only 4.5% of children with a genetic diagnosis compared with 25.8% of patients without.[221] Children who developed secondary steroid resistance were more likely to have posttransplantation recurrence than those who never responded to steroid treatment.[222] Higher risk of recurrence is seen in young children and in those who already had recurrence in a previous graft.[223,224] To help quantify the risk of recurrence, it is important to clarify, prior to transplantation, whether FSGS is genetic, due to mutations in genes encoding components of the glomerular filtration barrier.

MPGN also carries a high risk of recurrence, which affects graft survival. The risk of graft loss at 5 years is significantly higher in children with FSGS or MPGN compared with children with renal dysplasia.[225] Other glomerular diseases, such as lupus nephritis and IgA nephropathy, may recur but are not usually associated with graft loss.

aHUS can cause ESRD and has a high rate of recurrence in the graft.[226] It is often caused by various disorders of complement regulation, including mutations in complement factor H or I, membrane cofactor protein, and others. The specific cause of the disease should be investigated before considering transplantation, in order to assess the risk of recurrence and guide treatment. Living related donors should be screened for the causative mutation, if known, prior to approval for donation. Disease recurrence can be prevented or treated with eculizumab (discussed later).[227]

PH1 is a disorder of glyoxylate metabolism in which an enzymatic defect in the liver causes overproduction of oxalate and deposition of calcium oxalate in the kidneys and in other organ systems once advanced renal failure develops. Presentation in infancy is associated with nephrocalcinosis and early CKD. Renal transplantation alone usually results in massive oxalate deposition in the new kidney and early graft failure. Combined liver and kidney transplantation (or liver transplantation alone if renal function is not severely affected) is curative, correcting the underlying enzymatic defect.[228]

### SENSITIZATION

Blood type, HLA typing, PRAs should be tested in each transplant candidate. If a living donor is being considered, donor-specific antibodies (DSAs) should be identified and quantified if PRA is positive. A negative direct crossmatch by complement-dependent cytotoxicity with antihuman globulin is crucial to avoid hyperacute rejection. Crossmatch by the flow cytometry method is more sensitive, but the clinical implications of a positive test are less clear-cut. Low-level DSA may be overcome with desensitization protocols, particularly in a planned living donor transplantation.

## TRANSPLANT IMMUNOLOGY

### HLA MATCHING AND SENSITIZATION

Transplantation immunobiology is covered elsewhere in detail. The importance of HLA matching between donor and recipient was recognized in the 1960s and 1970s and became the cornerstone of deceased donor allocation policy. A clear association between number of HLA mismatches and graft survival was shown in several large studies.[229] With the introduction of more potent immunosuppression, the significance of HLA matching may have diminished, while other factors such as peak PRAs, cold ischemic time, and donor age retained their relative importance.[230] However, other recent publications have shown that HLA mismatches continue to adversely affect renal allograft outcomes in the present era, as shown by a study from ANZDATA that included children.[231] Studies that examined the effect of HLA matching specifically in children have also shown that an increase in number of HLA mismatches is associated with decreased graft survival.[201] Recently new allocation algorithms have been implemented which prioritize better HLA-matched kidneys in addition to favoring pediatric patients.[188] Both donor age and HLA matching are important in determining deceased donor graft survival and may be offset by each other.[232]

Most pediatric patients with CKD will need to undergo more than one transplant over their lifetime, and HLA matching of the first kidney graft may have an impact on subsequent transplants. More HLA mismatches at first transplant are associated with HLA sensitization, longer waiting time for a second transplant, and decreased graft survival.[233,234] However, the benefits of better HLA matching at first transplant on lifetime with graft function, although significant, are relatively small.[235]

In addition to HLA matching, PRAs are measured in renal transplant candidates, and if positive, should be characterized by solid-phase assays.[236] The presence of DSA is associated with increased risk of acute antibody-mediated rejection (AMR) as well as chronic AMR and decreased graft survival. When DSAs are further characterized, patients with complement-binding DSA after transplantation are at the highest risk of graft loss and AMR.[237] The deleterious impact of DSA has been demonstrated in children, even when the direct crossmatch between donor and recipient is negative by flow cytometry, though not in all series.[238,239] Although good HLA matching without DSA is desirable, not all patients will find an appropriate donor. Annual reports show that about 5% of children listed for deceased donor transplantation have PRA greater than 80%.[188] Desensitization protocols, including treatment with combinations of intravenous immunoglobulin (IVIG), plasma pheresis, and rituximab, have shown acceptable intermediate-term outcomes in adults undergoing living or deceased donor transplantation.[240,241] Pediatric patients are theoretically at higher risk for infectious complications after transplantation; therefore, desensitization in children may cause overimmunosuppression. There are remarkably few case series and clinical trials of desensitization in children. A recent study used IVIG and rituximab desensitization with alemtuzumab induction in highly sensitized children who underwent deceased donor kidney transplantation. Although a higher rate of acute rejection was seen in the sensitized patients, there was no significant decrease in 6-year graft survival and no increase in infectious complication.[242]

De novo DSA appears in 35% of children in the first years after transplantation, with a high prevalence of DSA to class II and specifically HLA-DQ antigens.[243] These antibodies are associated with increased risk of AMR and graft dysfunction, regardless of whether they develop in the first year after transplantation or later.[244] Serial monitoring of DSA in children after transplant may help to identify patients at risk for adverse outcomes, and guide tailoring of immunosuppression.

Although theoretically kidneys transplanted from maternal donors might be less immunogenic than paternal kidneys, due to fetal–maternal interaction, this does not seem to be the case. A recent study shows that in the current era of immunosuppression, patients receiving a kidney from their mother were slightly more likely to experience acute rejection, consistent with earlier findings from the European Collaborative Transplant Study.[245,246]

### ABO COMPATIBILITY

In the past, ABO incompatibility was considered a contraindication to transplantation, because of the high risk of hyperacute AMR. However, in the past few years there are reports of successful ABO-incompatible renal transplantation in children. ABO-incompatible transplantation in children is rare, and usually involves patients with blood type O or B and low titers of anti-A antibodies, receiving an organ from blood type A donors. No ABO-incompatible transplants took place in pediatric kidney recipients in 2015 in the United States.[188] ABO-incompatible transplantation is more common in Japan, where most transplants are from living donors. Treatment of these patients with a desensitization protocol has shown long-term outcomes equivalent to the general pediatric transplant population.[247] In Europe, data from the collaborative transplant study, which included children, reported that 1420 ABO-incompatible living donor kidney transplants were performed in 2005–2012, with similar long-term patient and graft survival. A slight increase in death due to infection was seen in the first year after ABO-incompatible transplantation.[248] Treatment protocols initially utilized pretransplant plasmapheresis, in order to remove anti-A/anti-B antibodies, together with splenectomy or rituximab. Newer regimens include immunoadsorption, using either blood group–specific columns or nonspecific columns, to remove the antibodies, together with rituximab to prevent ongoing antibody production after transplantation. Addition of other antibody induction in these patients did not result in altered graft survival.[248] The risk of AMR is associated with higher titers of anti-A/B isoagglutinins, and the intensity of desensitization may be modifiable according to pretreatment titers, thus potentially opening this option in deceased donor transplantation as well.[249] Immunoadsorption therapy for ABO-incompatible renal transplantation has been associated with surgical bleeding in some cases.[250] Late AMR in the setting of ABO incompatibility is less frequent than AMR in HLA sensitization.[236,251,252] Despite more intense immunosuppressive regimens, a study in adults did not demonstrate a higher risk of cancer in patients undergoing ABO-incompatible transplantation.[253]

## IMMUNOSUPPRESSION

The goal of immunosuppressive therapy in pediatric kidney transplantation is to prevent graft rejection while minimizing adverse effects. A wide range of immunosuppressive medications are used in pediatric renal transplantation and are a key factor in preventing rejection and enabling long-term graft function. In general, more information is available from trials in adult transplant patients, and specific data in children do not always exist. Special considerations in children include altered drug metabolism, as well as adverse effects particular to children, including effects on growth and development. The optimal immunosuppression regimen should minimize the risk of rejection, without causing over-immunosuppression or other side effects of medications.

### INDUCTION IMMUNOSUPPRESSION

The risk of acute rejection is highest in the immediate posttransplant period, which is why in addition to higher doses of maintenance immunosuppressive drugs, many transplantation protocols include a biological induction agent. These antibody preparations are aimed at depleting T cells or preventing their activation and are administered in the perioperative period.

Antilymphocyte preparations are T-cell depleting agents that can be polyclonal or monoclonal. In addition to their use for induction immunosuppression, they have a role in treatment of acute cellular rejection. The polyclonal antibody antithymocyte globulin (ATG) contains antibodies to a wide variety of lymphocyte antigens in serum of animals immunized with human lymphocytes. The most frequently used preparation today is the rabbit-derived ATG.

The first monoclonal preparation, introduced in the 1980s, was OKT3, containing antibodies to the CD3 receptor on the surface of T cells. It is no longer in use, due to some severe adverse effects. The anti-CD52 antibody preparation alemtuzumab binds to the CD52 receptor, found on both T and B cells as well as monocytes and natural killer cells, causing cell lysis.

T-cell activation induces interleukin-2 (IL-2) production causing T-cell proliferation; therefore monoclonal IL-2 receptor antibodies such as basiliximab block this pathway, preventing T-cell activation without depletion.

Antibody induction has been shown to improve outcomes in kidney transplantation in adults, compared with conventional immunosuppression alone. However, in children there are less supportive data. Patients who are highly sensitized are more likely to receive antibody-induction therapy; therefore it is difficult to compare efficacy or safety outcomes in retrospective studies. Data from earlier studies of antibody induction, which used maintenance immunosuppression agents that are rarely used today, such as azathioprine and cyclosporine, are also not necessarily pertinent today.

ATG is the most frequently used antibody induction in the United States, particularly in steroid-free protocols and in highly sensitized patients.[254,255] Alemtuzumab induction has been described in several small series of children, enabling steroid avoidance or tacrolimus monotherapy, with good results.[256–258] Alemtuzumab has also been used for highly sensitized children in combination with desensitization. Outcomes were similar to nonsensitized patients who received IL-2 receptor blockers. A significant reduction in lymphocyte counts was observed in the alemtuzumab group up to 1 year from transplantation.[242] Concerns regarding the risk for posttransplant lymphoproliferative disease (PTLD) have been raised regarding the use of lymphocyte-depleting agents, particularly alemtuzumab. In a large OPTN database study, T-cell depleting agents, alemtuzumab and ATG, were compared with nondepleting induction agents or no induction, and the incidence of PTLD without induction (0.43%) was shown not to be different from that with basiliximab (0.38%) or alemtuzumab (0.37%), but was slightly higher in patients who received ATG (0.67%).[259] The population in the study had received higher doses of ATG than employed today, higher doses of maintenance immunosuppression, and less antiviral prophylaxis, suggesting that the ATG induction may not currently be a significant risk factor for PTLD.[260]

Pediatric studies using the IL-2 receptor blocker basiliximab as induction therapy combined with triple-drug maintenance immunosuppression showed a good safety profile but minimal or no additional benefit compared with no antibody induction.[261,262] A recent large study using data from the Australia and New Zealand Dialysis and Transplant registry showed that induction with IL-2 receptor antibodies in pediatric patients was associated with at least a 40% reduction in the rate of acute rejection, though no significant decrease in graft loss was found. This was found to be consistent across donor types, initial immunosuppression, and transplant era;

propensity scoring was used to account for confounding factors.[263]

Comparing the efficacy of lymphocyte-depleting agents with IL-2 receptor blockers in a prospective trial would require a very large study population. Retrospective data from the OPTN database found that lymphocyte-depleting induction (ATG or alemtuzumab) is more effective at lowering acute rejection rates in African-American pediatric kidney transplant recipients, but no difference was found in other ethnic groups.[264]

According to the OPTN data report from 2015, most children undergoing kidney transplantation in the United States received antibody induction, approximately 60% were treated with ATG and 33% received basiliximab induction.[188] Children with elevated PRAs (HLA sensitized) were more likely to receive ATG induction.[188] In Australia and in Europe the preferred induction agent is basiliximab, used in 76% to 93% of children according to the 2016 ANZDATA, whereas 4% to 6% were treated with ATG.[189]

## MAINTENANCE IMMUNOSUPPRESSION

### CALCINEURIN INHIBITORS

#### Cyclosporine

Cyclosporine was introduced as an immunosuppressant for renal transplantation in 1982, revolutionizing the treatment of transplant recipients. Whereas in 1996, 82% of children were treated with cyclosporine 1 month after renal transplantation, consistently less than 3% received cyclosporine since 2009, as it was largely replaced by tacrolimus.[188] Recently, low-dose cyclosporine has been used in pediatric kidney transplant patients together with the proliferative signal inhibitor everolimus, with good 3-year outcomes.[265]

Cyclosporine doses in children need to be higher per body weight, as it is more rapidly metabolized than in adults. It has been suggested that cyclosporine should therefore be divided every 8 hours in young children and infants; however, this may actually result in lower dose-normalized area under the curve (AUC) throughout the day, in addition to being a drug regimen that is more difficult to follow.[265a] Drug level monitoring of cyclosporine is important to maintain therapeutic concentrations, while avoiding toxicity. Trough levels are usually kept at 150 to 300 mcg/L initially, and 75 to 125 mcg/L after the first 6 months. Monitoring AUC or 2-hour postdrug level, as an indicator of AUC, may be more effective in avoiding toxic effects. Cyclosporine is available as capsules and oral solution. Absorption of different formulations may vary, and dosing should be guided by serum drug levels.

Cyclosporine is nephrotoxic in a dose-dependent manner. It is associated with HTN, hyperlipidemia, and hyperuricemia, all of which may contribute to cardiovascular disease, as well as their deleterious effect on graft function.[267] Cosmetic side effects are a major issue in young patients, including hirsutism, gum hyperplasia, and less frequently coarse facial features, which may contribute to nonadherence, particularly in teenagers. Several drugs interact with cyclosporine, in many cases decreasing its metabolism and potentially causing toxic concentrations. Common examples in children include macrolide antibiotics or azole antifungal medications, which should be given with care, while monitoring calcineurin inhibitor levels. Ingestion of grapefruit also decreases calcineurin inhibitor metabolism and increases serum levels, mostly by inhibition of enteric CYP3A4, and should be avoided.

#### Tacrolimus

The use of tacrolimus as part of the immunosuppression regimen has continuously increased since its introduction in the 1990s. In 2015, 96.3% of pediatric kidney transplant recipients received tacrolimus initially.[188] Metabolism varies greatly between individuals, younger children may require higher doses by weight, and all patients should have regular drug level monitoring.[268] Other factors also have impact on tacrolimus dose needed to achieve trough blood concentrations. Studies have shown that frequency of various cytochrome P450 CYP3A5 allele variants may account for over 50% of variance of tacrolimus blood concentrations.[269] Moreover, the frequency of these alleles is different in African-American patients, which can explain higher doses needed to achieve therapeutic drug concentrations in this population.[270] Initial target tacrolimus levels are high (10–15 ng/mL), gradually decreasing to 3 to 6 ng/mL after the first 6 months, depending on the specific protocol.

In the first years after tacrolimus became available, several studies were published comparing tacrolimus and cyclosporine in children. An NAPRTCS study comparing tacrolimus and cyclosporine, both in combination with mycophenolate mofetil and prednisone, showed no difference in rejection or graft survival at 1 and 2 years posttransplant. However, the children in the tacrolimus group were less likely to require antihypertensive treatments, and had a higher GFR.[271] A similar multicenter study from Europe showed decreased frequency of acute rejection and a higher GFR in the tacrolimus group, with a similar safety profile for both drugs.[272] Long-term data showed better graft survival and GFR in the tacrolimus group, as well as lower cholesterol levels.[266] A comparison of protocol biopsies in children demonstrated more subclinical acute rejection in those treated with cyclosporine.[273] More recent data have shown a lower prevalence of cardiovascular risk factors in children treated with tacrolimus, compared with cyclosporine or sirolimus.[267] As tacrolimus became the standard of care for immunosuppression for pediatric kidney transplantation, large head-to-head studies were no longer performed. A study comparing children treated with tacrolimus and mycophenolate with a historical cohort treated with cyclosporine and prednisone showed superior graft survival in the tacrolimus group.[274]

Tacrolimus adverse effects are similar to cyclosporine, with a higher rate of posttransplant diabetes mellitus and neurotoxicity for tacrolimus, manifested as tremor or seizures.[275] A frequent reason for changing treatment from cyclosporine to tacrolimus in children and adolescents is the lack of cosmetic side effects of tacrolimus. A once-daily modified-release formulation of tacrolimus has been shown to improve patient compliance.[276]

### ANTIMETABOLITES

#### Azathioprine

Azathioprine was found to be effective in prevention of renal graft rejection in the early 1960s, especially when combined with corticosteroids. Subsequently, studies comparing azathioprine with mycophenolate mofetil showed a significantly lower rate of acute rejection in patients treated with mycophenolate.[277] While in the first years, most children were treated with azathioprine as part of their immunosuppression regimen, in the 2014 NAPRTCS report, only 2.5% to 3% of children received azathioprine since 2002.[111] Adverse effects of azathioprine include myelosuppression and hepatotoxicity, which might require dose reduction. Therapeutic efficacy, bone marrow toxicity, and liver toxicity of azathioprine and its active metabolite 6-mercaptopurine (6-MP) may be related to their metabolites: 6-thioguanine and 6-methylmercaptopurine. Thiopurine methyltransferase (TPMT) enzyme activity is a major factor determining azathioprine and 6-MP metabolism. Testing for TPMT genotype and enzyme activity is available and can help guide therapy. The myelosuppressive action of azathioprine is potentiated by xanthine oxidase inhibitors such as allopurinol, and if necessary, the dose of azathioprine must be reduced by 50% to 75%. Although azathioprine is still classified by the FDA as category D for use in pregnancy, suggesting positive evidence of risk to the fetus, data accumulated over the past few decades, especially from the National Transplantation Pregnancy Registry, have shown that the incidence of birth defects is similar to the general population.[278] Therefore azathioprine might present as an alternative to mycophenolate formulations for female kidney transplant recipients planning pregnancy. In addition, azathioprine is significantly less expensive than mycophenolate.

#### Mycophenolate

Mycophenolate mofetil, a reversible inhibitor of inosine monophosphate dehydrogenase that downregulates specifically T- and B-cell proliferation, was developed as an alternative antimetabolite to azathioprine, with less bone marrow toxicity. It is rapidly metabolized to mycophenolic acid in vivo. It was shown to reduce frequency of acute rejection and improve 5-year graft survival in children compared with azathioprine, in combination with cyclosporine and prednisone.[277] Some data suggest that in children with chronic allograft nephropathy (CAN), adding mycophenolate to the immunosuppressive regimen improves graft function.[279] In 2015 mycophenolate formulations were used as part of the initial maintenance immunosuppression regimen in 93.2% of pediatric kidney recipients in the United States.[188] Although initially dosing was 600 mg/m$^2$ BSA twice daily, some protocols give a lower dose (300 mg/m$^2$) to low-risk patients, with less adverse effects.[280]

The main adverse effects of mycophenolate mofetil are gastrointestinal, including abdominal discomfort, nausea, and diarrhea. Although there have been reports of mycophenolate-associated inflammatory bowel disease, a recent case series of pediatric liver or kidney transplant recipients with new-onset colitis did not show a link to mycophenolate treatment.[281] An alternative formulation, enteric-coated mycophenolic acid, has been shown to have fewer gastrointestinal adverse effects, as shown in small studies in children.[282] Mycophenolate mofetil is available as capsules, tablets, and oral suspension, as well as intravenous preparation. Enteric-coated mycophenolic acid cannot be made into a suspension, which limits its use in younger children. There is debate over whether mycophenolic acid monitoring is beneficial in prevention of acute rejection. Data suggest that mycophenolate exposure is associated with time from transplantation, graft function, and age, with younger patients requiring higher doses per BSA in order to reach therapeutic levels.[283] Lower mycophenolate exposure has been shown to be associated with de novo DSA formation.[284] Mycophenolate has been associated with neutropenia in pediatric kidney transplant recipients, often necessitating dose reduction or temporary interruption.[285] Pregnancies in patients exposed to mycophenolic acid are associated with a high rate of birth defects; therefore adolescent girls and women of childbearing potential must be cautioned to use reliable contraception if sexually active while treated with mycophenolate.[286]

### CORTICOSTEROIDS

Corticosteroids have been a cornerstone drug in prevention of rejection of transplanted organs for decades. However, chronic corticosteroid therapy is associated with many adverse effects including HTN, hyperlipidemia, cardiovascular disease, glucose intolerance, osteoporosis and aseptic bone necrosis, cataracts and glaucoma, as well as weight gain, cushingoid appearance, acne, and psychological effects. The cosmetic effects are often a cause of nonadherence in many patients, particularly adolescents. Corticosteroids also inhibit linear growth by several mechanisms of action, including interference with the action of GH and inhibition of bone formation.[287] Efforts to reduce the adverse effects of corticosteroids in children undergoing renal transplantation have included using lower doses of prednisone, alternate-day regimens, steroid-withdrawal protocols, and steroid avoidance.

According to NAPRTCS, corticosteroid use was almost universal in children undergoing renal transplantation until the year 2000. Subsequently, their use decreased to 50% to 60%, which has remained constant over the past few years, despite extensive research on steroid-sparing immunosuppression in pediatric kidney transplantation.[188] However, centers that continue to use triple immunosuppression in low-risk patients generally use lower doses than previously used, tapering corticosteroid dose within a few weeks to doses of 0.1 mg/kg or 5 mg/m$^2$ or even lower.[111]

Initial single-center studies of steroid-free pediatric kidney transplantation in low-risk patients showed promising results at the turn of the twenty-first century. Larger multicenter randomized controlled studies, in both the United States and Europe, found improved linear growth with no increase in biopsy-proven acute rejection (BPAR) in children on steroid avoidance or early steroid-withdrawal protocols.[280,288] Improvement in height standard deviation scores was significant only in prepubertal children. Other benefits of steroid avoidance, such as lower rates of HTN and posttransplant diabetes, were inconsistent. Of note, most of these studies used daclizumab induction, which is no longer available, and although small studies have shown similar results with thymoglobulin induction, prospective studies using other IL-2 receptor blockers have not been performed.[254] Late withdrawal of steroid treatment in children treated with cyclosporine–mycophenolate immunosuppression also demonstrated improved linear growth with no increase in the rate of graft rejection.[289] Two meta-analyses of steroid avoidance or withdrawal studies confirmed the findings of no increase in acute rejection episodes with improved linear growth in prepubertal children.[290,291] In addition, the pooling of data demonstrated a beneficial effect on HTN and new-onset diabetes in children in the steroid-sparing groups.[290] Corticosteroid avoidance protocols have not been well studied in high-risk pediatric transplant recipients, including non-Caucasians, retransplants, and sensitized patients.

### MAMMALIAN TARGET OF RAPAMYCIN INHIBITORS

Mammalian target of rapamycin (mTOR) inhibitors block the proliferative response of T-cells to IL-2 stimulation. This group of immunosuppressive agents also inhibit proliferation of vascular muscle and some cancer cells, and therefore can reduce transplant vasculopathy. This, together with lack of nephrotoxicity, made this group of drugs a promising treatment option for pediatric transplantation. Adverse effects of mTOR inhibitors include impaired wound healing, which can present a problem when used immediately after transplantation, hyperlipidemia, proteinuria, decreased levels of testosterone in some adolescent males, aphthous ulcers, interstitial pneumonia (including *Pneumocystis jirovecii* infections), anemia, and thrombocytopenia.[292]

#### Sirolimus

The first drug in this group was approved for use in adult solid organ transplantation in 2000. Initially it was used in an attempt to avoid calcineurin inhibitors completely, by combination with IL-2 receptor blocker induction, mycophenolate, and steroids. A higher incidence of acute rejection was seen in this protocol as well as increased adverse events.[293] Subsequently sirolimus was used in steroid-sparing protocols, together with low-dose cyclosporine in a study that was terminated due to a higher incidence of PTLD.[294] Conversion from calcineurin inhibitor to sirolimus to treat calcineurin inhibitor–induced nephrotoxicity has also been attempted with improved GFR in some children, but with an increase in adverse events.[295,296] The use of sirolimus in pediatric kidney transplantation peaked in 2002 at 25%, but subsequently decreased to less than 1% in the United States,[111] with a similar trend seen also in other registries.[189]

#### Everolimus

Everolimus has been studied in several small uncontrolled studies in children, generally instead of mycophenolate treatment and in combination with low-dose calcineurin inhibitors. A study based on data from the Cooperative European Paediatric Renal Transplant Initiative (CERTAIN) registry compared children treated with everolimus with low-dose cyclosporine and steroids with those on standard immunosuppression. There was no increase in biopsy-proven rejection and graft function was similar between the groups, although side-effect profiles differed. The everolimus group had a higher incidence of hyperlipidemia, HTN, and anemia than the control group.[297] Further analysis showed a significant decrease in CMV replication and disease in the group treated with everolimus, most likely due to the avoidance of mycophenolate.[298] Another study, with a similar treatment protocol with no control arm, also showed promising long-term results. To avoid wound healing problems, most protocols delay everolimus introduction until a few weeks after transplantation.[265]

### OTHER IMMUNOSUPPRESSIVE MEDICATIONS

In most cases, new immunosuppressive agents are studied in adults before trials in children are performed. Belatacept, a costimulation inhibitor, has shown promise in adult renal transplant patients, demonstrating improved GFR compared with cyclosporine, though with a higher incidence of acute rejection. No studies have been performed in children to date, and a specific concern might be higher frequency of PTLD in EBV-seronegative patients, particularly of the central nervous system. As more children are EBV naïve going into transplantation, the potential risk of PTLD could be even higher in this population.[299] A potential advantage is the intermittent intravenous administration, which could help overcome drug nonadherence particularly in adolescent patients.

## IMMUNOSUPPRESSION COMBINATIONS

In North America, the most common combination of immunosuppression for pediatric kidney transplantation in the past decade is tacrolimus, mycophenolate, and prednisone (42.3% at 3 years posttransplantation), followed by tacrolimus and mycophenolate without corticosteroids (22.5% at 3 years).[111] Other combinations include tacrolimus with low-dose prednisone either as dual therapy or with azathioprine. No difference was seen in the frequencies of the immunosuppression combinations between deceased versus living donor recipients.

# PERIOPERATIVE MANAGEMENT

Pediatric renal transplantation should always be managed by an experienced team which includes pediatric experts in the fields of transplant surgery, nephrology, anesthesiology, intensive care, and other specialties, to ensure an optimal outcome.

Technical causes are responsible for a higher proportion of early graft loss in young children, primarily from graft thrombosis. Although the graft kidney is usually placed extraperitoneally in the iliac fossa in adults and older children, a midline intraperitoneal approach is often used in youngest patients. Vascular anastomoses of the graft in very small children are usually to the aorta and the IVC, rather than the iliac vessels used in older children and adults, to provide sufficient renal perfusion, particularly when the graft is an adult-sized kidney. The donor renal artery may be the same size as the recipient aorta and the renal vein may be significantly larger than the recipient's IVC. A straight and direct course for each renal vessel to the aorta and vena cava will avoid kinking and decrease the risk of thrombosis. Stenosis or thrombosis of the IVC is a rare finding but may be seen in children who have had CVCs in infancy, abdominal surgery, or a hypercoagulable state, posing a problem for graft anastomosis. This should be evaluated pretransplant by Doppler study or venography, and in case of significant IVC pathology an alternative vein should be selected. There may be an advantage for transplanting a pediatric (deceased) donor kidney in such cases.[300,301]

The adult-sized kidney graft requires a major increase in CO to maintain good perfusion and avoid acute tubular necrosis or vascular thrombosis. Even with optimal maintenance of recipient intravascular volume, blood flow to the adult-sized donor kidney is significantly reduced at transplantation. Further reduction in blood flow could result in graft ischemia; therefore BP values, which may be relatively high for the young child, and high-normal central venous pressure need to be maintained during transplant surgery and postoperatively. After anastomosis is completed, release of vascular clamps will cause immediate flow of a large portion of the child's blood volume into the graft, a critical time point when intravascular volume must be controlled. Maintaining relative hypervolemia immediately posttransplant may delay weaning from mechanical ventilation for 1 to 2 days, but is nonetheless of utmost importance to preserve graft perfusion.[302] Aggressive hydration to optimize intravascular volume and graft blood flow is important in the following weeks and months, and may require fluid supplements by the nasogastric route.[300] Avoiding acute tubular necrosis in the postoperative period also enables early full dosing of calcineurin inhibitors, thus preventing early acute rejection.

## IMMEDIATE POSTOPERATIVE PERIOD

In the first few days after transplantation the child is usually treated in the ICU. Close attention is paid to vital signs and fluid management with the goal of optimizing graft perfusion. Brisk urine output, particularly in a patient previously oliguric or anuric, is a useful marker of graft function. Oligoanuria or a significant decrease in urine output, by contrast, needs to be evaluated and treated immediately. Bladder drainage must be ensured by flushing or exchanging the bladder catheter. Ultrasound can assess the kidney, the blood vessels, ureter, and bladder, and provide information on organ perfusion, the presence of a fluid collection suggesting leak or bleeding. Absent blood flow may be due to thrombosis, and necessitate prompt surgical intervention, as do significant bleeding or a urinary leak. Intravenous fluids are given to replace insensible losses and urine output, as well as additional fluids to account for third space losses and to keep central venous pressure on the high side of normal. This approach should maintain good graft perfusion, which in turn will increase urine output. However, if urine output does not increase, intravascular volume overload may result, manifesting as respiratory compromise and HTN.[302] Volume overload may respond to diuretics, but dialysis may be necessary in some patients.

Immunosuppression is started at transplantation, including intravenous corticosteroids perioperatively in most cases (except for complete steroid-avoidance protocols). Initiation of calcineurin inhibitors may be delayed for several hours or longer, if there is postoperative oliguria. Prophylactic treatment for infections is started postoperatively. Perioperative antibiotics are usually given to prevent wound infection.[303] *P. jirovecii* prophylaxis, usually with trimethoprim–sulfamethoxazole (TMP–SMX), may also decrease the incidence of urinary tract infection (UTI). Antiviral medication is given to prevent CMV disease, usually oral valganciclovir, with the duration of therapy depending upon pretransplant donor and recipient serologic status and on whether lymphocyte-depleting induction immunosuppression was given.[304] Some centers prescribe antifungal prophylaxis, especially in patients with prolonged ICU stay or antibiotic treatment. Low-molecular-weight heparin or aspirin is often given after transplantation to prevent graft thrombosis, particularly in younger patients and in patients with abnormal pretransplant coagulation workup.[305]

## EARLY COMPLICATIONS OF KIDNEY TRANSPLANTATION

### DELAYED GRAFT FUNCTION

Delayed graft function (DGF) is usually defined as the need for dialysis during the first week after renal transplantation and is sometimes referred to as acute tubular necrosis.[111] The most common cause of DGF is postischemic acute injury of the graft, which is associated with deceased donor kidney, prolonged ischemic time, and hemodynamic compromise during and immediately after transplantation. Changes in allocation policies in the United States resulted in deceased donor organs being shipped over longer distances, leading to increased cold ischemic times, with an increase in DGF rates.[306] The incidence of DGF is higher in children receiving kidneys from donors after cardiac death (DCD), although pediatric DCD kidney recipients have good renal allograft survival at 3-year follow-up.[198] DGF has been shown to adversely affect long-term graft survival and function, with children who required posttransplantation dialysis having a twofold risk of overall graft loss.[307] DGF is also associated with a higher risk of subsequent acute rejection, in both living and deceased donor pediatric kidney transplantation.[111]

Other causes of DGF include graft thrombosis, which can be diagnosed by ultrasound or radionuclide scan, and may require surgical revision. Thrombosis can be prevented by meticulous surgical technique and attention to fluid balance, as well as identifying and treating patients with thrombophilic risk factors prior to transplantation. Use of antibody induction may decrease the incidence of postischemic DGF, although the reasons for this are not clear.[308]

Urological complications such as urinary leak or obstruction may also cause DGF or acute decrease in urine output, and diagnosis is aided by ultrasound and radionuclide scan. Ureteral stents are often placed at transplantation for 4 to 6 weeks to prevent obstruction, but their use may be associated with increased risk of UTI.[309]

Hyperacute rejection or accelerated acute rejection superimposed upon postoperative acute tubular necrosis (ATN) may also present as DGF. Hyperacute rejection is usually due to preformed antidonor ABO or HLA antibodies, manifesting as irreversible rapid destruction of the graft within minutes to hours of transplantation. Because blood type and HLA matching have been routinely performed, these reactions are exceedingly rare. Pretreatment of recipients with grafts mismatched for ABO antigens or with DSA with desensitization protocols generally prevents this disastrous outcome.[310]

Recurrence of FSGS can manifest as primary nonfunction, and requires a graft biopsy for diagnosis, in order to guide treatment.[213]

### ACUTE REJECTION

Acute renal allograft rejection is a common complication of pediatric renal transplantation, though its frequency has decreased significantly from over 70% in 1987 to 1990 to 16% since 2007.[111] In NAPRTCS, a rejection episode is defined by the physician's decision to initiate specific antirejection therapy, rather than BPAR. However, in the latest cohort the frequency of biopsy in reported acute rejections has increased from 45% in 1987 to 94%. The trend away from clinical diagnosis of acute rejection to BPAR may also impact the overall frequency of reported acute rejection episodes. The probability of acute rejection 1 year after transplantation in children decreased from 52.8% in 1987 to 1991 to 9.3% between 2007 and 2013 for living donor kidneys. In patients receiving a kidney from a deceased donor the probability of acute rejection in the first year dropped from 67.4% to 13.8%.[111]

The lower incidence of acute rejection in recent years is thought to be due to newer, more potent immunosuppressive medications now used. The highest risk of acute rejection is in the first few weeks to months; however, it may occur at any time, even years after transplantation.[311] It is more frequent after deceased donor transplantation compared with living donor, suggesting susceptibility of the graft with longer ischemic time, for example, due to exposure of antigens promoting an immune reaction. Although in earlier patient cohorts risk factors for acute rejection included African-American race and no induction therapy, in the latest NAPRTCS cohort (2007–2013) these factors were no longer significant. This may be a result of differential practices in choice of immunosuppression protocol in African-American children.[264] As noted earlier, DGF due to acute tubular necrosis continues to be a significant risk factor for subsequent acute rejection.[111] Combined liver–kidney transplantation may protect the kidney from acute cellular and antibody-mediated rejection and from decline in kidney graft function.[312]

Acute rejection may often be clinically asymptomatic. Graft tenderness and fever as manifestations are unusual in the present era of immunosuppression, and acute decrease in GFR may be the only sign. GFR may decrease significantly before an increase in serum creatinine is noted, particularly when baseline creatinine is normal. A prompt workup should include urinalysis and urine culture to rule out infection and glomerular disease, BK virus (BKV) polymerase chain reaction (PCR), and ultrasound to look for obstruction, fluid collection, or vascular compromise. Biopsy should be performed whenever possible to confirm a diagnosis of acute rejection, as other causes of graft dysfunction, such as calcineurin inhibitor toxicity or viral infection including BK nephropathy, may be difficult to distinguish from acute rejection on clinical grounds alone. Graft biopsy is safely performed under ultrasound guidance, and light general anesthesia or conscious sedation is helpful in reducing anxiety and pain. The Banff criteria are utilized to grade acute rejection.[313] Acute cellular rejection is characterized by lymphocyte infiltration of tubules (tubulitis) and interstitial inflammation, with involvement of arterial walls in more severe cases. In acute antibody-mediated rejection (ABMR) there is acute tissue injury including findings of microvascular inflammation and often also acute tubular injury, arteritis, or fibrin thrombi in glomerular capillaries. In addition, there is evidence of antibody-mediated complement activation – C4d deposition in the peritubular capillaries of the allograft, although C4d-negative ABMR is recognized. The biopsy findings together with circulating DSAs complete the diagnosis of ABMR. The two types of acute rejection may coexist.[313] The question of whether to perform routine surveillance graft biopsies to help tailor immunosuppressive therapy and detect subclinical rejection is unresolved.[314] Serial monitoring of DSA may help identify high-risk patients, adjust immunosuppression, and prevent overt antibody-mediated injury.[315]

The cornerstone of therapy for acute cellular rejection is high-dose corticosteroids, most often pulse intravenous methylprednisolone. In steroid-resistant rejection, lymphocyte-depleting agents, particularly thymoglobulin, may be administered. Premedication with methylprednisolone and antihistamine usually prevents a cytokine release syndrome, which may be seen particularly with the first dose of thymoglobulin. Approximately 50% to 60% of children treated for acute rejection will have a complete response, with GFR returning to baseline, and another 30% to 40% will have a partial response. Complete reversal of acute rejection is less likely in repeated episodes.[111] When acute rejection is diagnosed, the possibility of underimmunosuppression must be addressed. This may be due to underdosing of medications, or more commonly, particularly in teenage patients, nonadherence to immunosuppressive drugs.[206] Attention must be given to maintenance immunosuppression, considering adding prednisone to a steroid-free protocol, switching cyclosporine to tacrolimus, or increasing the antimetabolite dose or the target levels of tacrolimus, in order to improve response to therapy and reduce the incidence of recurrent acute rejection.[316]

ABMR is often refractory to conventional antirejection therapy and has a high rate of graft loss. Few randomized controlled studies have been performed regarding treatment of ABMR, in adults or in children, and there is insufficient evidence to guide therapy.[317,318] The first line of treatment usually includes high-dose corticosteroids, plasma exchange, and IVIG. The goal of plasma exchange and IVIG is removal of DSA from the circulation.[319] Second-line therapies target antibody production by depleting B cells (rituximab) or plasma cells (bortezomib). Recent studies have shown stabilization of graft function in children with refractory ABMR after treatment with bortezomib.[320,321] Inhibition of complement with eculizumab to decrease the antibody-mediated injury has been described in a small number of pediatric patients.[322] Less severe cases of ABMR, for example, the presence of DSA with mild findings of ABMR on graft biopsy, but without significant deterioration of graft function, might be treated with corticosteroids and IVIG with or without rituximab. This approach avoids the need for CVC insertion and plasma exchange in lower-risk patients.[320]

Acute rejection is the most common cause of graft loss in the first year after transplantation and has a significant negative impact on long-term graft survival.[199,311,323] Close monitoring is imperative in order to avoid early acute rejection and enable its prompt detection and treatment. Serum creatinine is monitored daily in the first few days after transplantation, followed by at least twice weekly for 2 to 3 months, together with drug concentration monitoring. Later, if there are no complications, the frequency of testing is decreased to once a month after the first 6 to 12 months. DSA should be monitored regularly during the first months after transplantation, and periodically after that. This is especially important in children with pretransplantation sensitization, or at any time if there are signs of graft dysfunction. The appearance of de novo DSA, most frequently DQ antibodies, is a risk factor for subsequent ABMR, which could be prevented by timely intervention.[324] Even stable children and adolescents require regular follow-up at the pediatric transplant clinic, to help prevent nonadherence and the resulting risk of graft rejection, as well as long-term management of the many other aspects of their health.

## INFECTIONS

As more potent immunosuppressive agents were introduced into the treatment of renal transplantation, the frequency of acute rejection decreased, as did hospitalizations for rejection episodes. In the pediatric population in particular, the price for this has been a higher rate of infections and hospitalization for infection.[325] The use of antibody induction and the presence of indwelling vascular or urinary catheters and the presence of posttransplantation neutropenia increase the risk of infection.[285] Hospitalization for infection was higher in children after renal transplantation at 47% in the first 3 years, than in adults.[326] In the immediate posttransplant period, the most frequent infections are surgical, UTIs, and pneumonia. Subsequently, in the early months after transplantation viral infections are common, particularly CMV and EBV and BKV nephropathy, which cause significant morbidity and may adversely affect graft function. In pediatric kidney transplant recipients hospitalized for fever, the rate of bacterial illness is high (50%) and warrants a full workup, with consideration for empiric antibiotic treatment.[327]

### Urinary Tract Infection

UTI is a common complication in children who have undergone renal transplantation, with hospitalization of 16.8% of patients in the first 3 years.[326] The risk of UTI after pediatric kidney transplant has increased over the last 2 decades.[325] Risk factors include a pretransplant diagnosis of obstructive uropathy or VUR and bladder abnormalities.[328] Ureteral stents placed during transplantation may also increase the risk of UTI.[309] Although graft dysfunction may occur during allograft pyelonephritis, long-term graft function may not be affected.[329] TMP–SMX prophylaxis for *P. jiroveci* infection may reduce the incidence of UTI, but bacterial susceptibilities vary between medical centers and may render this strategy ineffective. Many clinics routinely culture urine from transplant patients at every visit; however, the indication for treatment of asymptomatic bacteriuria without pyuria remains unclear, as resistant organisms may emerge.[330] Recurrent UTI after kidney transplantation may be associated with VUR, which should be addressed (see the "Urological Complications" section).

### Cytomegalovirus

CMV infection in pediatric kidney transplantation has decreased significantly since the widespread use of antiviral prophylactic treatment, yet it remains an important and occasionally severe complication. Up to 20% of pediatric kidney recipients in the current era will develop CMV infection (defined as evidence of viral replication) and 3% to 10% have CMV disease (viral replication with clinical disease).[331]

The most vulnerable group is children who are seronegative for CMV pretransplant, receiving a kidney from a seropositive donor (D+/R–), who develop a primary infection. Primary infection may also be community acquired in children whose donor was seronegative for CMV.[331] Children who receive thymoglobulin induction are also at a higher risk of CMV infection.[332] According to OPTN data, over half of children undergoing kidney transplantation in 2011 to 2015 had negative CMV serology, whereas only a quarter of adults were CMV negative at transplantation.[188] Secondary infection may also occur, either as reactivation of the host strain or as infection from the donor strain, and may be less severe clinically. The risk of acute graft rejection is higher following CMV infection in kidney transplant recipients and may be associated with increased graft loss.[333] Decline in kidney graft function was more pronounced in children with CMV replication.[298]

Valganciclovir has been shown to be at least as effective as oral ganciclovir in children for CMV prevention, and has better bioavailability and easier once-daily dosing.[334] Dosing should be based on BSA and corrected for renal function.[335] There are two CMV prevention strategies: prophylaxis and preemptive antiviral treatment. In adults, the incidence of CMV infection and disease is lower in patients receiving prophylaxis; however, there is no significant difference in graft outcome or death between the strategies.[336] The proportion of CMV-naïve children who undergo transplantation is high, rendering them at higher risk for CMV disease. Most centers use prophylaxis for at least the first few weeks, to reduce viral replication within the incoming CMV-positive graft. Most prophylaxis protocols are 3 to 6 months long, depending on immunosuppression regimen and patient serostatus, but the optimal length of prophylaxis is unknown.[331] Viral monitoring is important during prophylaxis and particularly in patients being managed preemptively, or after valganciclovir discontinuation.[337] Antiviral prophylaxis should also be considered when there is intensification of immunosuppression, for example, when treating acute graft rejection. Adverse effects of valganciclovir include hematological toxicity—mainly leukopenia and neutropenia, as well as gastrointestinal discomfort or diarrhea, occasionally necessitating dose reduction or discontinuation of treatment.[338]

CMV infection is most common after cessation of prophylactic antiviral therapy. Asymptomatic CMV infection should be treated with intravenous ganciclovir; however, in stable older children and adolescents, oral valganciclovir can be used as initial therapy.[331] CMV disease is defined as viremia with clinical symptoms, most commonly fever and malaise, with tissue-invasive disease in some cases, involving the respiratory, hepatic, and gastrointestinal tracts. Allograft dysfunction as well as leukopenia and thrombocytopenia are frequently observed laboratory findings. In invasive disease, treatment is usually started with intravenous ganciclovir, followed by oral valganciclovir, when clinical improvement and reduction in viral load are seen. Although the VICTOR study demonstrated equivalent efficacy of oral valganciclovir to IV ganciclovir in adult transplant recipients, it is not clear if these findings can be extrapolated to the pediatric population. To assist in viral eradication, immunosuppression should be reduced, usually by discontinuation of antimetabolite drug – azathioprine or mycophenolate. Hyperimmune CMV globulin preparation may be given to the most severe cases, though its efficacy is questionable.[331] Treatment is continued until after viral eradication is demonstrated, followed by a prophylactic dose for several weeks. Relapse may occur after end of therapy; therefore viral monitoring should be continued for several weeks after treatment cessation, and after reintroduction of the antimetabolite, which is usually at a lower dose than before CMV infection. Failure to respond to therapy, either clinically or virologically, may be due to viral ganciclovir resistance usually due to viral UL97 mutations. Treatment options include high-dose ganciclovir or switching to foscarnet, which is nephrotoxic, though studies in children are lacking.[339]

## EPSTEIN–BARR VIRUS INFECTION

Similar to the situation with CMV serology, about half of the pediatric patients undergoing renal transplantation are seronegative for EBV, whereas only 10% of donors are EBV naïve.[188] Seronegative patients receiving grafts from EBV-positive patients are at a higher risk of infection, therefore EBV disease is more common in younger children. EBV infection may be asymptomatic, it can present as an acute viral syndrome, or may be associated with PTLD. The risk of developing PTLD is higher when primary EBV infection occurs after transplantation. Children who are EBV negative prior to transplantation have a 2.9% incidence of PTLD in the first 5 years after transplantation, compared with 0.7% in children who are seropositive.[188] Of the patients with primary EBV infection, adolescents may be more likely to develop PTLD and have a poorer prognosis.[340]

Monitoring viral load in peripheral blood by quantitative PCR, particularly in high-risk patients in the first year after transplantation, is important in order to identify infection and allow early intervention. A prospective study in Germany found that primary infection occurred in 63% of seronegative pediatric patients and reactivation or reinfection in 44% of seropositive patients in the first year, though many of the infections were asymptomatic.[341] More intensive immunosuppression is associated with a higher rate of symptomatic EBV infection. Prophylaxis with ganciclovir or valganciclovir in high-risk patients was shown to decrease the incidence of EBV, according to some but not all studies.[342–344] Clinical disease usually presents with protracted fever, lymphadenopathy, tonsillitis, and hepatosplenomegaly. Laboratory findings may include leukopenia, atypical lymphocytes, elevated liver enzymes, and IgM antibodies for EBV, and allograft dysfunction may occur. Diagnosis is confirmed by EBV viral load, which is also used to monitor the course of the disease and response to therapy.

EBV-associated PTLD appears to be due to B-cell proliferation induced by infection with EBV. There is continuum between EBV-associated diseases from mononucleosis to full-blown monomorphic lymphoma. Imaging will help in detecting lymphoid masses, which might require biopsy to rule out malignant PTLD. Other than chest X-ray and abdominal sonography, computed tomography and positron emission tomography can assist in staging of the disease and can guide biopsy.[345] The cornerstone of treatment of EBV infection and prevention of PTLD is immunosuppression reduction. Strategies include discontinuation of the antimetabolite and lowering the target levels of tacrolimus, or switching to mTOR inhibitors. Antiviral therapy for persistent EBV viremia with valganciclovir has not been proven to be effective.[344] Some children after renal transplantation may have persistent high EBV viral load without ever developing PTLD.[342]

## BK VIRUS INFECTION

BK polyomavirus infection emerged as an important clinical entity in patients undergoing renal transplantation in the late 1990s, coinciding with the introduction of more potent immunosuppression regimens. BKV infection may result in BKV-associated nephropathy (BKVAN), manifesting as tubulointerstitial nephritis with graft dysfunction and potential graft loss, as well as ureteral stenosis and hemorrhagic cystitis.[346] Although previously thought to be rare in children, recent data from NAPRTCS showed a prevalence of 4.6%, similar to that in adults.[347] Some recent studies have shown a higher incidence (10%–27%) of pediatric kidney transplant patients with BK viremia detected by screening tests, though overt nephropathy is less common.[348,349] BK transmission occurs in childhood, when the virus remains latent in the tubular epithelial cells. Immunosuppression after transplantation may cause reactivation and high-rate viral replication in the kidney graft and is therefore considered a consequence of immunosuppression. Young recipients may develop primary BK infection transmitted from the donor kidney. Risk factors for BKVAN include antibody induction, DR mismatch, or treatment for rejection.

The virus appears first in the urine, and if progression occurs, is detected in the blood by quantitative PCR for viral DNA. Histological changes are observed in patients with persistent or increasing plasma viral loads.[346] Surveillance is recommended to enable early diagnosis and intervention. Detection of viruria has questionable clinical implications, as it is not correlated with graft damage, but does identify patients at risk for subsequent viremia. Monitoring plasma quantitative PCR periodically, particularly in the early months after transplantation, after acute rejection, and at any time when there is an unexplained elevation of serum creatinine, is the accepted strategy for diagnosis in children.[350,351] Renal biopsy is performed if there is graft dysfunction. Typical findings include cytopathic changes and tubulointerstitial nephritis, which can be difficult to differentiate from other viral infections or acute cellular rejection, and may even coexist with other conditions in some cases. Immunohistochemical staining for SV40 viral antigen is highly specific for BKV nephropathy.[346] Relevant histological findings on kidney biopsy in association with high BK viral load in the blood are diagnostic.

The cornerstone of management of BKV infection is reduction of immunosuppression when significant BK viremia is detected. This is usually done by discontinuation of the antimetabolite or decrease in the target levels of the calcineurin inhibitor, with the goal of prevention of progression to overt nephropathy. The reduction of immunosuppression enables the patient's immune system to clear viremia more effectively by expanding BKV-specific cell immunity and specific immunoglobulins.[347] Treatment of established BKVAN is often less successful. Several medications with antiviral activity have been used to treat patients with BKVAN unresponsive to immunosuppression minimization, with varying degrees of success, but no randomized controlled studies have been performed.[346] These include high-dose IVIG, quinolone antibiotics, cidofovir, and leflunomide.[349,351–353]

## VARICELLA

Immunization against varicella-zoster virus is recommended before transplantation, as the use of live attenuated viral vaccine is controversial in immunocompromised patients.[212] Loss of antibody response after transplantation has been reported in 25% of children who were vaccinated before transplantation.[211] In addition, these antibodies may have lower avidity and the cellular immune response may also be decreased in solid organ transplant recipients compared with healthy controls.[354] Varicella infection in an unimmunized renal transplantation recipient may result in severe disease, with visceral involvement in some cases. Postexposure prophylaxis of unimmunized patients with varicella-zoster immunoglobulin should be administered as early as possible, and if clinical disease develops, treatment with intravenous acyclovir is initiated. Temporary discontinuation of the antimetabolite, or dose reduction, is usually recommended.[355]

## OTHER INFECTIONS

### Respiratory Viruses

Respiratory viruses, in particular influenza virus infection, may be associated with severe morbidity in the immunosuppressed host. Disease severity may be related to the degree of immunosuppression and clinical presentation may be atypical. Diagnosis of presumed respiratory viral infection can be made by nasopharyngeal swab, wash, or aspirate testing for pathogens. Neuraminidase inhibitors such as oral oseltamivir can be started empirically for suspected influenza infection before virological confirmation. Pretransplant vaccination is recommended as well as yearly seasonal inactivated influenza vaccine after transplantation. Young children (<9 years) receiving the vaccine for the first time should receive two doses, 4 weeks apart. Vaccine immunogenicity is variable, but recent data suggest that immunization reduces mortality and clinical severity as well as infection-related acute rejection.[356]

### Cutaneous Warts

Cutaneous warts, usually due to infection with human papillomavirus, are common in children after renal transplantation, as are molluscum contagiosum lesions. Although malignant potential is low, these lesions can be numerous and cause distress due to cosmetic issues. Warts may be refractory to treatment or recurrent and may respond to adjustment of the immunosuppressive regimen if possible.[357] Topical treatment is often ineffective and surgical removal may be required.

### *Pneumocystis jirovecii* Pneumonia

*P. jirovecii* pneumonia is a classic example of an opportunistic infection, which is very rare in the immunocompetent host. With the widespread use of prophylaxis, usually with TMP–SMX, the true incidence of posttransplantation infection is unknown. Intravenous pentamidine can be given if TMP–SMX is contraindicated.[358] Antipneumocystis prophylaxis is usually given for 6–12 months after kidney transplantation, after which net immunosuppression is lower. *Pneumocystis* infection may coexist with CMV or respiratory viruses, and should be considered in the immunosuppressed child with unexplained respiratory symptoms.[359]

### Infectious Diarrhea

Diarrhea is a common symptom experienced by children after kidney transplantation. In some cases it can be attributed to medication such as mycophenolate or valganciclovir, is usually mild, and resolves with a decrease in dose or change of formulation.[338] Rarely, mycophenolate may cause severe colitis, which improves with discontinuation of the drug.[360] In up to 60% of children with diarrhea, an infectious cause can be diagnosed, whether viral, bacterial, or parasitic.

Although in healthy children, diarrhea due to infection with the parasite cryptosporidium is common, it is almost always a mild self-limiting disease. In immunosuppressed patients, diarrhea may be protracted and can cause hypovolemia, perturbations in calcineurin inhibitor serum concentrations, and AKI. Treatment with nitazoxanide is often necessary as well as supportive measures.[361,362]

Organ transplant recipients can also have persistent norovirus infection. Chronic infection with viral shedding may continue for several months.[363] In many cases hospitalization for fluid therapy is necessary, and 30% still have diarrhea after 2 weeks.[364]

## RECURRENCE OF PRIMARY RENAL DISEASE

According to NAPRTCS data, 7.8% of grafts in children are lost to disease recurrence.[188] The most common recurring kidney disease is FSGS, but MPGN (type II in particular), aHUS, PH1, and others can recur in the graft. A study from the ANZDATA database demonstrated that younger patients have a higher risk of recurrence of glomerular disease after transplantation, in comparison to older adults.[365] It is important to identify patients at risk for recurrence to enable early diagnosis and therapeutic intervention (see also in "Recipient Evaluation" section above).

FSGS is responsible for approximately 10% of ESRD in children in the United States, presenting as SRNS, and carries an overall risk of 30% for recurrent nephrotic syndrome.[111] Native kidney nephrectomy before or during transplantation surgery, in children with persistent proteinuria, may enable prompt diagnosis of recurrence. Clinical presentation may include severe proteinuria immediately after transplantation or later in the course, but DGF or anuria may also be a sign of disease recurrence. Humoral factors cause damage to the glomerular barrier, which is the rationale for treatment strategies aimed at removal of such a factor. Serum soluble urokinase-type plasminogen activator receptor has been identified as a possible permeability factor responsible for recurrent FSGS, though this has not been supported in pediatric studies.[366] Preemptive and therapeutic plasmapheresis for disease recurrence, as well as treatment with anti-CD-20 antibody rituximab, have shown some efficacy in achieving remission of proteinuria.[221,367] Recurrent FSGS in the graft, particularly if unresponsive to therapy, is associated with a high rate of graft failure.

MPGN is the underlying diagnosis in 1.7% of children receiving their initial kidney transplant, may recur in 20% to 45% after transplantation, and is a cause of graft failure in many of the patients.[368] When studying MPGN type I and type II separately, the risk of 5-year graft loss was 23.5% for MPGN type I and 67.5% among patients with type II, but the number of children with MPGN type II was very small.[225] The newer classification of MPGN is based on glomerular injury mechanism rather than the location of and appearance of deposits. Under this system, most patients with MPGN had biopsies consistent with immune-complex-mediated glomerulonephritis, characterized by the presence of immune complexes and complement components, and only 12% had complement-mediated glomerulonephritis in the absence of immune complexes.[369] A recent study in adults, including some teenaged patients, showed a recurrence rate of 45% overall in MPGN patients, 55% of whom recurred in the first year after transplantation. Risk factors for recurrence included low complement level and the presence of monoclonal gammopathy, but not the subtype of the disease.[369] Treatment with plasmapheresis, rituximab (anti-CD20), and corticosteroids has been used to treat MPGN recurrence without clear evidence of benefit.[368]

aHUS may recur in up to 60% of patients undergoing kidney transplantation without specific intervention. Most will progress to graft loss unless promptly treated with plasmapheresis or complement inhibition.[370] Eculizumab, a monoclonal antibody of complement factor 5, inhibits terminal complement activation and was found to be effective in the treatment of aHUS.[227] It has become the treatment of choice both to prevent and to treat recurrence of aHUS after transplantation with excellent results, as shown in a case series from France. Three patients in whom treatment was discontinued experienced a relapse, suggesting that long-term therapy is needed.[227] Patients treated with complement inhibitors are at risk for meningococcal infection and preventive measures must be taken.[370]

In PH1 treatment of choice is combined or sequential liver–kidney transplantation. However, children who have been treated with dialysis for a long period prior to transplantation may have significant oxalate deposition, mostly in the bones. Despite the discontinuation of oxalate production, achieved by liver transplantation, mobilization of the systemic oxalate burden can cause damage to the kidney graft. Meticulous attention to hydration, use of crystallization inhibitors such as oral citrate, or even HD immediately after transplantation can help protect the new kidney.[371]

Other diseases that may recur and may cause graft dysfunction or failure include lupus nephritis, IgA nephropathy, Henoch–Schönlein nephritis, membranous nephropathy, and diabetic nephropathy.

## CHRONIC ALLOGRAFT NEPHROPATHY

The most common cause of graft loss after the first year is CAN, accounting for about 35% of failed kidney grafts, according to several pediatric databases worldwide.[111,189] The term CAN replaces previously used terms, including chronic rejection, transplant nephropathy, and chronic renal allograft dysfunction or injury. It is primarily a histopathological diagnosis, used to denote features of chronic interstitial fibrosis and tubular atrophy within the renal allograft without evidence of any specific etiology. Pathological involvement also typically includes the blood vessels with arteriolar hyalinosis and fibrointimal hyperplasia, and chronic transplant glomerulopathy.[372] The pathogenesis is not completely understood, but numerous etiological factors have been implicated, both immune and nonimmune. Clinically, CAN is suspected when there is a slow deterioration in allograft function beyond the first 3 months after transplantation, with no evidence of acute rejection, drug toxicity, infection, or other pathological process. There may also be increasing proteinuria and worsening HTN. The prevention and management of chronic renal allograft rejection remains one of the major challenges facing clinicians. Adequate long-term immunosuppression is important in prevention of immunologically mediated CAN, although chronic calcineurin inhibitor toxicity may be difficult to distinguish from CAN in some cases. Nonadherence to medical therapy in pediatric renal transplant recipients is associated with a higher rate of interstitial fibrosis and tubular atrophy.[373] Changes in immunosuppression may occasionally ameliorate CAN, for example, treatment with mycophenolate in children with CAN may improve graft function.[279] Optimal control of HTN, with possible preference for angiotensin-converting enzyme (ACE) inhibitors, and treatment of hyperlipidemia are also important. One future direction is clinical utilization of urinary biomarkers to help differentiate CAN from other graft injury phenotypes.[374]

## PATIENT SURVIVAL

Survival of children after renal transplantation has improved in 2005 to 2013 compared with 1987 to 1996, and is 96.4% for recipients of deceased donor allografts and 97.4% for recipients of living donor allografts, at 5 years. Survival is lower in infants younger than 24 months at transplantation; however, this group of patients is small, and has also shown the most significant improvement in the past 2 decades.[111] The most common cause of death is infection (28.5%), followed by cardiopulmonary causes (14.6%) and malignancy (11.5%). Overall, death was more likely in patients with failed grafts, though 48.2% of patients who died had a functioning allograft. The USRDS 2017 annual report found a 30.8% decrease in adjusted 1-year all-cause mortality rate when comparing the 2005 to 2009 and 2010 to 2014 periods. Survival after renal transplantation is higher than in children remaining on chronic dialysis. Adjusted all-cause mortality is approximately fourfold higher in children on dialysis than in children after renal transplantation.[22]

## GRAFT SURVIVAL

Graft survival has improved greatly over the past 3 decades. Five-year deceased donor graft survival in the 2005 to 2013 cohort is 83%, compared with 78.1% in the cohort of 1996 to 2004 and only 62.4% in patients transplanted in 1986 to 1995. In living donor kidney allografts, an increase in 5-year graft survival was seen up until 2004, after which the 5-year graft survival stabilized at 83% to 85%, closing the gap with deceased donor kidney transplantation.[111] Reports from several developing countries that have a pediatric kidney transplantation program (some with living donor option only) have shown 5-year graft survival of 65% to 92%.[375] Graft failure was defined by return to dialysis, retransplantation, or death. When assessing graft loss from January 2000 onward, the most common cause of graft failure was CAN or chronic rejection (40.5%), with various types of acute rejection responsible for 10.2% of graft loss. Disease recurrence was the cause of graft loss in 7.8% of pediatric patients, with FSGS accounting for almost half of these. In comparison to adults, death with functioning graft was less common (8.4%), whereas vascular thrombosis or technical difficulties were more frequent (6.6%).[111] This is due to better general health in pediatric kidney recipients on the one hand, and smaller blood vessels which make vascular anastomoses technically challenging on the other.

Prognostic factors associated with shorter graft survival include race, prior transplantations, HLA mismatching, and blood transfusions. Patients receiving their graft at age 14 to 16 years were at risk for graft failure, in particular if they were African-American or did not have private insurance.[376] It is difficult to evaluate the association of antibody induction therapy with graft outcome, due to patient selection bias. DGF (requiring dialysis) and slow-to-recover graft function are associated with a 20% reduction in 5-year graft survival in living and deceased donor kidney recipients.[111,231]

Glomerular filtration rate, estimated by serum creatinine–based formula, has improved over the last decade: 74.7% of pediatric patients who received a kidney transplant in 2015 had an eGFR greater than 60 mL/min/1.73 $m^2$ at 1 year.[111]

Irreversible graft failure may be associated with an inflammatory reaction, which may be severe enough to necessitate graft nephrectomy. This is more common in early graft loss or high-grade rejection by biopsy. The impact of graft nephrectomy on alloimmunization is difficult to determine due to multiple potential confounding factors.[377]

## LONG-TERM FOLLOW-UP OF CHILDREN WITH KIDNEY TRANSPLANT

### HYPERTENSION

BP monitoring is an integral part of regular follow-up of pediatric kidney transplant recipients. Appropriate size cuff should be used, and at least two or three measurements should be performed when the child is calm. BP measurements are compared with normal value for gender, age, and height percentile, as published in the fourth report on the diagnosis, evaluation, and treatment of high BP in children and adolescents, which provides 90th and 95th percentiles.[378] The vast majority of children reaching ESRD have HTN, defined as values above the 95th percentile, and it remains a problem for many patients after kidney transplantation. In a European study reporting data from 10 countries, about two thirds of children receiving RRT had HTN, but uncontrolled HTN was more common in children on dialysis than in transplanted patients.[53]

In the early period after transplantation HTN is common, due in part to volume overload, early graft dysfunction, higher doses of corticosteroids and calcineurin inhibitors, or kinking of the transplant renal artery. HTN may appear months or even years after transplantation and is more common in older recipients. In a study from the Netherlands, the prevalence of uncontrolled HTN, defined according to Kidney Disease Improving Global Outcomes guidelines, was 75.8% in adolescents and young adults compared with 38.3% in younger children, and was not found to be affected by transition to adult care facilities.[379] Ambulatory 24-hour BP monitoring is a useful tool in diagnosing masked or nocturnal HTN, which are phenomena frequently seen in children with kidney transplantation.[380]

Any injury of the allograft, such as acute rejection or recurrence of glomerular disease, can cause or worsen HTN. CAN, like CKD of any cause, is also strongly associated with HTN. Increased prevalence of HTN is seen with use of calcineurin inhibitors, particularly cyclosporine, but also tacrolimus.[381] The most common etiology of secondary HTN after transplantation is transplant renal artery stenosis. This entity may present as new-onset resistant HTN, occasionally with hypokalemia or worsening allograft function. A bruit may be heard over the kidney allograft and duplex ultrasonography often detects the stenosis, although computed tomography, MRI, or angiography may be needed for diagnosis. Treatment of transplant renal artery stenosis depends on the severity and response to medication; however, angioplasty with or without stenting is the definitive treatment.[381]

Although posttransplantation HTN may be partly due to native kidneys, it often improves with a well-functioning graft and only rarely warrants native nephrectomy. Obesity, which predates transplantation or develops subsequently, is also associated with HTN and metabolic syndrome.[382]

Treatment of posttransplantation HTN involves lifestyle modification including exercise, reducing salt intake, weight control, and smoking avoidance. Antihypertensive medication is prescribed as necessary, with target BP measurements under the 90th percentile for age and height, as in other high-risk pediatric groups.[380] Choice of therapeutic agent depends on the underlying cause; ACE inhibitors and angiotensin receptor blockers may be appropriate in patients with HTN, particularly associated with proteinuria, but possibly hazardous in uncorrected allograft artery stenosis. Diuretics are helpful in treatment of early volume overload–associated HTN, but are not ideal agents later, as they induce a state of relative volume depletion. Calcium channel blockers may minimize calcineurin inhibitor–related renal vasoconstriction.[380] Uncontrolled HTN may adversely affect graft function, as shown in adults in the Collaborative Transplant Study, which demonstrated that lowering systolic BP was associated with improved graft function.[383]

### CARDIOVASCULAR DISEASE

LVH is the most frequent cardiac abnormality in children after renal transplantation, with a prevalence of 10% to 50% in various studies.[384–386] LVH is correlated with HTN, and also with the presence of metabolic syndrome.[387] In most children with LVH it appears prior to transplantation, and some studies have shown improvement in left ventricular mass index after transplantation.[218]

Cardiovascular mortality is much higher in children with CKD compared with the general pediatric population. Although mortality is lower in children after kidney transplantation than in children on dialysis, it remains unacceptably high. According to the NAPRTCS database, 14.6% of mortality is due to cardiopulmonary causes, second only to infection, and ahead of malignancy.[111] Traditional risk factors such as HTN, dyslipidemia, diabetes mellitus, and obesity are more frequent due to impaired renal function as well as the adverse effects of immunosuppressive medications. Nontraditional risk factors such as abnormalities in calcium–phosphorus metabolism, anemia, hyperuricemia, and hyperhomocysteinemia are also common in children with CKD and are correlated with arterial stiffness and carotid intimal-medial thickness.[54] Some of these risk factors may persist after transplantation, particularly if graft function is impaired. While vascular lesions progress in children with CKD, kidney transplantation can bring about improvement in some measures of endothelial function. However, cIMT may remain abnormal even years after kidney function is restored.[388,389]

Interventions to reduce premature cardiovascular disease for young patients after renal transplantation must include lifestyle modification. Dietary interventions should be offered to all children, in particular to those with obesity and dyslipidemia. Encouraging physical activity is important, as is education to prevent smoking. Adherence to a healthy diet and physical activity is not straightforward, especially in adolescents. The Active Care after Transplantation (ACT) trial is investigating the effectiveness of an exercise intervention, or an exercise + diet intervention on physical functioning, weight gain, and cardiometabolic health in adults after transplantation.[390] Similar studies could be helpful in determining the role of lifestyle modification in children and adolescents.

Optimization of graft function and BP remain major factors in cardiovascular risk after kidney transplantation. One of the main goals of steroid avoidance or withdrawal protocols is mitigating risk factors for cardiovascular disease. Several studies in children have shown decrease in the frequency of posttransplant diabetes mellitus, hyperlipidemia, and HTN in children on steroid-free protocols compared with triple immunosuppression.[289,391] Children treated with tacrolimus were less hypertensive and had better lipid profiles than those on cyclosporine-based protocols.[271,392] Treatment with β-hydroxy β-methylglutaryl-coenzyme A (HMG-CoA) reductase inhibitors has been shown to be effective and safe in reducing total and LDL-cholesterol in children.[393] Although the ALERT study showed a reduction in cardiac deaths and nonfatal myocardial infarctions in adults, this has not been shown in other studies.[394] In children and adolescents, movement between study groups of CKD, dialysis, and transplantation is rapid and makes long-term study of statins challenging. Currently, there are no pediatric data on posttransplantation statin therapy with endpoints of cardiovascular events; therefore, except in special circumstances, statin treatment is not recommended.[395]

## METABOLIC SYNDROME AND DIABETES MELLITUS

Metabolic syndrome is less well defined in children and adolescents than in adults, but is based on the finding of at least three abnormalities such as obesity, elevated BP, low-HDL cholesterol, hypertriglyceridemia, and impaired glucose tolerance. It is increasingly common and its frequency correlates with age. In the United States, prevalence is estimated at 1.2% in 12-year-olds and up to 7.1% in 16- to 17-year-olds.[396] Screening and prevention of metabolic syndrome in childhood is important, as it frequently continues into adulthood and carries an increased risk for cardiovascular disease, and even in childhood, there is evidence of significant atherosclerotic changes. The frequency of metabolic syndrome in children in the United States after kidney transplantation is high, up to 37% in the first year, most of which is of new onset.[387] Dietary intervention and physical activity are the mainstay of prevention and treatment. In patients treated with corticosteroids, late steroid-withdrawal has been shown to improve metabolic parameters and decrease the frequency of metabolic syndrome from 39% to 6% 2 years later.[289]

New-onset diabetes mellitus after transplant (NODAT) is less common in children than in adult patients, with an incidence of 7.1% at 3 years. However, its frequency may be increasing. It is associated with older age (adolescents vs. younger children), higher BMI, and treatment with tacrolimus.[397] A study comparing early corticosteroid withdrawal with low-dose chronic prednisone treatment in adults did not show a significantly lower incidence of NODAT.[398] Hypomagnesemia has emerged recently as a significant risk factor for NODAT in adults and in children. Although tacrolimus is known to cause renal magnesium wasting and is also a risk factor for NODAT, it appears that hypomagnesemia is independently associated with NODAT.[399] Further studies are necessary to elucidate the effect of magnesium supplementation. Fasting blood glucose should be monitored regularly in the first months after transplantation; hemoglobin A1C is also helpful in diagnosing insidious-onset diabetes. When diabetes is diagnosed, optimizing tacrolimus levels and minimizing corticosteroid dose should be considered. Referral to a pediatric diabetes specialist clinic for patient and parent education and a combination of dietary modification and pharmacological therapy are needed. NODAT is not associated with decreased graft or patient survival in pediatric patients, and some cases may resolve spontaneously.[323]

## CANCER

Immunosuppressive therapy for prevention of rejection after solid organ transplantation carries a risk for malignancy. In children, 2.6% of renal transplants develop a malignancy, of which 85% were classified as lymphoproliferative cancers.[111] The 3-year incidence of malignancy increased from 1% in 1987 to 1991 to 2.96% in 1997 to 2001; however, in the latest cohort an improvement has been noted: 1.78% in 2007 to 2013. This trend mirrors the introduction of newer, more potent immunosuppressive agents like tacrolimus in the early 1990s, followed by the use of lower doses and immunosuppression minimization protocols in subsequent years. Another study from the United States transplant registry showed a diagnosis of malignancy in 2.18% of pediatric solid organ transplant recipients. Compared with the general pediatric population, the incidence was significantly increased for hematological malignancies, particularly non-Hodgkin lymphoma, as well as other types of cancer including of the genitourinary tract.[400] Long-term follow-up showed a sixfold increased rate of cancer compared with the general population. A larger single-center series in the United States found 13% of patients contracting some form of malignancy by 20 years after transplantation, with similar findings in a large study from the ANZDATA database – a cumulative incidence of nonskin cancer in 14% of pediatric patients at 25 years.[401,402] A higher hazard of death or graft loss was seen in patients with posttransplantation cancer, compared with those with no malignancy.

PTLD is an uncontrolled proliferation of lymphocytes in the constellation of posttransplant immunosuppression, most often associated with EBV infection. The cumulative incidence of PTLD in children in the United States is 1.7% at 5 years posttransplant, but is close to 3% in children who are EBV seronegative at transplantation.[188] The risk of PTLD is 30-fold higher than in healthy controls, and is higher in EBV-negative recipients of EBV-positive donor kidneys.[401,402] By contrast, PTLD in children infected with EBV, who were previously seronegative, is associated with better survival.[403] A high EBV viral load is correlated with the probability of developing PTLD.[404] Diagnosis is made by histological examination of involved tissue, and is classified by the World Health Organization (WHO) into four categories: early lesions, polymorphic PTLD, monomorphic PTLD, and Hodgkin lymphoma. Early lesions are usually managed by immunosuppression reduction in order to restore the host's virus-specific immunity, and by monitoring of viral loads to assess response. In CD20-positive B-cell polymorphic disease, an anti-CD20 antibody, such as rituximab, is often effective together with immunosuppression reduction. Monomorphic disease is most frequently large B-cell lymphoma and may also respond to rituximab therapy, but many patients require the addition of chemotherapy. T-cell lymphoma is often more aggressive in nature, and Hodgkin lymphoma PTLD is very rare. The source of the lymphoma is almost always the recipient rather than the donor kidney.[405] In a retrospective study of 45 consecutive PTLD patients younger than 25 years, 80% of tumors expressed EBV and 70% were CD20 positive. Both of these presented earlier after transplantation, and CD20-positive PTLD was associated with a higher 5-year survival.[406] Patients with PTLD are at risk for graft dysfunction and loss, due to acute rejection or CAN.[403]

Other types of cancer in children after renal transplantation include the urinary tract, primarily renal cell or urothelial cell carcinoma, which may arise from the native kidneys or the allograft.[407] Nonmelanoma skin cancer is common in transplant recipients, though more frequently diagnosed in young adults than in children. Regular use of high protection factor sunscreen can reduce the incidence of skin cancer, and referral for an annual dermatological examination may help in detection of malignant and premalignant lesions.[408]

## ANEMIA

Anemia is usually defined in children as hemoglobin concentration more than 2 standard deviation below mean for age, or dependency on erythropoietin therapy. Blood transfusion is necessary in up to half of pediatric kidney transplantations, predicted by pretransplant hemoglobin.[409] Anemia is common in children after renal transplantation, ranging from 25% to 50% of patients.[410–412] Incidence is highest in the early months after transplantation, after which many patients have a gradual increase in hemoglobin.[410] Decreased graft function is strongly associated with posttransplant anemia, as anemia is a marker of allograft dysfunction due to impaired erythropoietin production. However, immunosuppressive and antiviral drugs are also implicated in its pathogenesis.[413,414] Other causes of anemia include nutritional deficiencies and blood loss, particularly in the perioperative period, viral infections, chronic inflammation, severe hyperparathyroidism, and treatment with ACE inhibitors. CMV infection is associated with anemia as well as leukopenia and thrombocytopenia in some patients, and the anemia resolves with antiviral treatment. Parvovirus B19 infection has been described in pediatric kidney transplant recipients, presenting as severe anemia with reticulocytopenia and bone marrow findings compatible with pure red cell aplasia.[415] Parvovirus infection can be confirmed by bone marrow and sometimes by peripheral blood PCR testing for the virus, and treatment with IVIG is successful in viral eradication and correction of anemia.[416]

Posttransplant anemia should be treated, in order to optimize oxygen delivery to organs and improve patient well-being. It is important to avoid unnecessary blood transfusions, which may cause alloantigen sensitization. An iron-rich diet is insufficient and oral iron supplementation is usually required (often ESAs). In some patients, parenteral iron sucrose or sodium ferric gluconate may be beneficial, as it results in faster repletion of iron stores and is not dependent on patient compliance.[417] Complete blood count and iron stores parameters should be frequently monitored in pediatric kidney transplant recipients, and other causes of anemia, including $B_{12}$ and folate deficiencies, occult infection, inflammation, or blood loss, must be ruled out.

Leukopenia or neutropenia may also be seen after kidney transplantation, and are usually noted in the first few months after transplantation.[285] They are associated with immunosuppressive medications, most frequently mycophenolate, though both viral infections and antiviral prophylactic therapy may also induce neutropenia.[338] Drug withdrawal may increase the risk of rejection or viral infection, respectively, and granulocyte-colony stimulating factor therapy may accelerate recovery in severe cases.[285]

## BONE HEALTH AND GROWTH

Children are unique in that they grow, and the effect of MBD on growing bones is enhanced. Preexisting renal osteodystrophy at the time of transplantation, impaired graft function and the effects of medications, particularly corticosteroids, are the main factors associated with bone disease and growth retardation. Successful kidney transplantation corrects many of the metabolic abnormalities which characterize CKD; however, some may persist, particularly when allograft function is impaired. New mineral disturbances may appear such as hypophosphatemia, due to residual hyperparathyroidism and elevated levels of FGF-23, a phosphaturic hormone produced by osteocytes, particularly in the early posttransplant period.[418,419] Vitamin D deficiency is common among children with CKD and does not significantly improve after transplantation, whereas PTH levels decrease in most patients and are inversely correlated with 25-OH vitamin D concentrations.[420,421] Bone mineral density may be measured by dual-energy X-ray absorptiometry (DXA); however, this modality is limited in differentiating between trabecular and cortical bone in CKD–MBD and thus does not predict fracture risk well in this population.[418] Peripheral quantitative computed tomography is another modality to assess bone mineralization, which can distinguish between cortical and trabecular bone. Adjustment of DXA spine and whole-body measures for height Z-scores can provide clinically relevant data on bone health that can be monitored over time.[422] Spine bone mineral density decrease is associated with higher corticosteroid doses. Therapeutic interventions to promote bone health include steroid minimization or avoidance, promoting good nutrition, correction of metabolic abnormalities, and vitamin D deficiency. Weight-bearing physical activity can increase bone mass, especially in children and adolescents, who have not yet reached their peak bone mass, and should be encouraged in pediatric kidney transplant recipients.[423]

At the time of transplantation, most children have linear growth retardation, with a mean height deficit of −1.73 standard deviation according to NAPRTCS data.[111] After transplantation, reversal of the uremic milieu should allow normal GH/IGF-1 secretion and function; however, catch-up growth is not seen in all patients. Improved height deficit is observed in children younger than 6 years at transplantation, whereas other age groups tend to maintain a relatively normal growth rate without improvement in Z-scores. Final adult height of children undergoing kidney transplantation has improved over the past decades, with the most recent cohort (2007–2013) reaching a mean Z-score of −0.89, compared with −1.93 20 years earlier.[111] This increase of height Z-score in children undergoing kidney transplantation over the past 20 years is a result of many factors, including optimizing rhGH use prior to and after transplantation, corticosteroid minimization and avoidance, and a lower incidence of acute rejection (necessitating additional steroid therapy).

Catch-up growth is limited in patients with poor graft function. Children with ESKD often have disproportionate growth stunting, with shorter leg length, whereas after transplantation a restoration of normal body proportions is noted.[424]

Corticosteroid treatment and impaired allograft function are associated with decreased linear growth. Steroid avoidance or early steroid-withdrawal protocols have shown improved linear growth particularly in younger children.[280] Several studies have demonstrated the efficacy of rhGH treatment in pediatric kidney transplant recipients. Treatment with rhGH improves final adult height without adversely affecting graft function.[425] Prescription of rhGH after kidney transplantation varies considerably between countries, as a result of differing reimbursement policies, but also diverse clinical practices. In many countries, rhGH is significantly less often prescribed than would be expected, even when patients are eligible.[426]

## UROLOGICAL ISSUES

Ureteral stent placement at the time of transplantation has become standard of practice and may reduce early obstruction or leak.[427] The stent is usually removed within a month to 6 weeks, but earlier removal may prevent stent-related adverse events, including UTI, pain, and hematuria.[428] Late-onset ureteral obstruction is less frequent, and has been reported to be associated with BKV infection.[429] Children with ESRD due to posterior urethral valves are at a higher risk for ureteral stenosis and VUR, most likely due to abnormal bladder wall.[430,431] VUR to the allograft is not uncommon, as shown in a study in adults, which found early VUR to the graft in 40.7% of patients, despite using extravesical mucosal tunneling technique to prevent reflux. There was no increased incidence of UTI or impact on graft function.[432] In children with recurrent UTI after transplantation, voiding cystourethrography is recommended. In these patients, antibiotic prophylaxis together with behavioral treatment of voiding dysfunction, if present, may be helpful. Endoscopic correction of reflux in symptomatic children is a feasible option; however post-procedure obstruction and graft dysfunction have been reported.[433,434] Open surgical correction of VUR is an alternative approach that has been found safe.[435,436]

Boys who undergo renal transplantation due to posterior urethral valves often have ongoing bladder dysfunction. Small defunctionalized bladders can increase in capacity and compliance after transplantation, but others might develop more severe bladder dysfunction over time and require later surgical intervention.[437] Bladder dysfunction may manifest as increased postvoid volume; daytime frequency, urgency, or incontinence; and nighttime incontinence. Inadequate bladder drainage may adversely affect allograft function. Some children require intermittent catheterization, particularly if they have undergone bladder augmentation.[438]

## PUBERTY AND REPRODUCTION

Delayed onset of puberty, menstrual irregularity, and infertility are common in patients with CKD, particularly ESKD. After transplantation many of the hormonal disturbances resolve and fertility is usually restored. Most adolescents who underwent kidney transplantation in childhood have normal onset of puberty, although a minority have delayed sexual maturation.[439] No difference in growth and pubertal development was noted between patients treated with mTOR inhibitors compared with conventional calcineurin inhibitor-based immunosuppression.[440] A recent study of young men who had undergone kidney transplantation in childhood suggested that although reproductive hormone levels were normal, testicular volume and sperm counts were lower than in healthy controls, raising concerns about fertility.[439,440a]

Restoration of fertility in adolescent girls after kidney transplantation exposes them to the risk of unplanned pregnancy. Counseling regarding reproductive health is important in order to avoid unplanned pregnancy as well as sexually transmitted diseases. The form of contraception used must take into account safety and efficacy of the method and patient adherence.[441] Pregnancy after renal transplantation is high risk both to the mother and to the fetus, but with meticulous prenatal care in selected patients with stable graft function and well-controlled BP, excellent outcomes can be achieved.[278] Timing is important, as pregnancy in the first 2 years after transplantation may adversely affect graft function.[442] Changes in medications including immunosuppressive regimen may be necessary before considering pregnancy, to avoid teratogenic effects of medications, such as mycophenolate, sirolimus, ACE inhibitors, and others.[443] No increase in congenital malformations has been observed in infants fathered by kidney allograft recipients.[444]

## NONADHERENCE

Alloimmunity necessitates lifelong immunosuppression in order to preserve graft function. Nonadherence to the medical regimen remains a major barrier to long-term allograft survival. In the case of young children, parents or caregivers are responsible for medical care. Risk factors for nonadherence include health system factors such as insurance coverage for care and medications and treatment-related factors, like regimen complexity, side effects, and even taste and size of pills. Psychosocial factors such as poor social support, family distress, and lower health literacy also affect adherence.[445] In adolescent patients, additional factors include the desire to be normal, poor planning, and insufficient parental monitoring.[204] In some studies, deceased donor kidney transplantation was associated with a higher rate of nonadherence.[206]

Adherence can be measured by missed appointments, prescription-filling patterns, self-report or patient questionnaires, variance in immunosuppressive drug levels, or various electronic monitoring systems.[446] The prevalence of drug nonadherence in pediatric renal transplant recipients varies in studies between 6% and 45% depending on the group and the method used to assess adherence.[206] Adolescents are at high risk for nonadherence and have shorter graft survival; in fact, between the ages of 17 and 24 years the adjusted HR of graft loss was 1.61 compared with ages of 3 to 17 years and 1.28 compared with young adults aged older than 24 years.[205] Persistent nonadherence is associated with acute rejection, graft loss, and death as well as increased medical costs.[311,447] It is important to develop strategies to improve patient and family adherence to the medical regimen, using a multidisciplinary approach aimed at improving communication between the medical team and the family, as well as between the patient and caregivers. Attention to adverse effects and trying to minimize them, as well as simplifying the medication regimen, may help improve patient adherence. Empowering adolescents to gradually assume responsibility for their medical care, patient and family educational interventions at clinic visits, and availability of clinic staff to answer questions may all assist in improving adherence in pediatric kidney transplant recipients.

## TRANSITION

Transition of adolescents or young adults from the pediatric to adult nephrology or transplant unit is a challenging process, which may be associated with increased risk of nonadherence and graft loss.[448] Although some clinics may use chronological age alone to guide timing, other measures such as medical adherence, patient competency, and responsibility for care should be taken into account. Use of specialized transition clinics may assist in a smoother process, less medication changes, and higher patient satisfaction.[449] Practices vary between centers as to age at transition (usually 16–21 years), the utilization of specialized transition clinics, structured assessment of patient readiness, and the use of educational tools.[450] Strategies for avoiding the pitfalls of transition might include initiating the transition process early and involving the patient in an age-appropriate manner. Coordination with all members of the team and good communication, as well as transfer during a stable period are crucial for a successful process.[451]

## REHABILITATION AND QUALITY OF LIFE

Optimizing kidney transplantation in children cannot be defined only by excellent patient and graft survival rates. Measures of general health and well-being, psychosocial adjustment, school attendance, level of education, neurodevelopmental outcome, psychological morbidity, and other parameters are important in evaluating overall quality of life. Several studies have utilized various questionnaires and scales to quantify psychosocial outcomes in these patients. Although health-related quality of life is higher in pediatric kidney transplant recipients compared with those remaining on dialysis, it is still lower than in healthy controls.[452] Many issues remain pertinent, for example, distress arising from physical symptoms and body image, especially height, adverse effects of medications, nonadherence, and psychological problems such as anxiety and depression. Neurocognitive development may be impaired in children with CKD, some of whom have lower scores on IQ testing than the general population, in particular in executive function and memory domains. Although children after kidney transplantation compared favorably with their counterparts treated with dialysis, their scores were below those of matched healthy children. Mild deficits in academic skills were also found.[453] This difference persisted when children with neurological comorbidities were excluded.[454] School performance is also affected by prolonged absences for medical reasons, which impact on academic achievements as well as peer relationships.

Kidney transplantation in childhood has a long-term influence on socioeconomic rehabilitation in adulthood. Two studies report on adult outcomes of children who underwent transplantation in an earlier era (1970s and early 1980s) and reached adulthood. A study from France found a lower level of education than in the general population and a lower rate of independent living, marriage, and parenthood, although most of the patients were employed. A significant correlation was found between education level, employment, marriage, independent living, and final height.[455] A similar study from the United States found a high rate of employment, as well as education levels and overall satisfaction equivalent to the general population, despite significant physical morbidity.[456] Of note, in both these studies a large percentage of the patients were severely short, and therefore different from recent cohorts who are treated with lower doses of corticosteroids or steroid-avoidance protocols, as well as rhGH. One study compared young adults with ESKD which presented in childhood with a group with later-onset disease. Patients with later clinical presentation were more likely to have a higher educational attainment, to be employed, and to be living independently than young adults with early onset disease.[457] A recent study which looked at long-term rehabilitation in kidney-transplanted children in France found lower rates of living with a partner and of parenthood than the general population, and this was correlated with disease severity. Approximately 10% had intellectual disability and the remainder were within the normal range of intelligence. When corrected for the parental educational level, most educational levels were comparable to the general population as were professional occupational categories. Adult height was much improved in the pediatric kidney transplant recipients in comparison to the earlier cohort, and was no longer associated with most social outcomes.[458]

Although most adults with CKD who underwent kidney transplantation in childhood have good long-term outcomes, some challenges persist in integrating into work, independent living, and building a family. A multidisciplinary team approach helps provide individualized care to children and adolescents with CKD on dialysis and after kidney transplantation. The goal in these young patients is to achieve the best outcomes, not just of kidney function, but in all aspects of health maintenance and rehabilitation.

 Complete reference list available at ExpertConsult.com.

## KEY REFERENCES


2. ANZDATA Registry. *40th Report: Australia and New Zealand dialysis and transplant registry, Adelaide, Australia*; 2018, 1 1. Retrieved 7 11, 2018, from Chapter 11: Paediatric report: http://www.anzdata.org.au/anzdata/AnzdataReport/35thReport/2012c11_paediatric_v1.9.pdf.
3. United States Renal Data System. *Chapter 7: ESRD among Children, Adolescents, and Young Adults*; 2017, 12 31. Retrieved 1 28, 2018, from United States Renal Data System. 2017 USRDS annual data report: Epidemiology of kidney disease in the United States. National Institutes of Health, National Institute of Diabetes and Digestive and Kidney Diseases, Bethesda, MD.
16. Lewis MA, et al. UK Renal Registry 12th Annual Report (December 2009): chapter 14: demography of the UK paediatric renal replacement therapy population in 2008. *Nephron Clin Pract.* 2010;c279–c288.
35. North American Pediatric Renal Trials and Collaborative Studies. NAPRTCS. *NAPRTCS 2011 Annual Dialysis Report*; 2011, 1 1. Retrieved 8 1, 2018, from North American Pediatric Renal Trials and Collaborative Studies: http://www.emmes.com/study/ped/annlrept/annualrept2011.pdf.
111. *North American Pediatric Renal Trials and Collaborative Studies NAPRTCS 2014 Annual Transplant Report*; n.d.
136. Daugirdas JT, et al. Dose of dialysis based on body surface area is markedly less in younger children than in older adolescents. *Clin J Am Soc Nephrol.* 2010;821–827.
186. Van Arendonk KJ, et al. National trends over 25 years in pediatric kidney transplant outcomes. *Pediatrics.* 2014;133:594–601.
188. Hart A, et al. OPTN/SRTR 2015 annual data report: kidney. *Am J Transplant.* 2017;17 Suppl 1:21–116.
189. *ANZDATA Autstralia and New Zealand dialysis and transplantation registry, 39th Annual Report.* Chapter 11: Paediatrics; 2016.
199. Chinnakotla S, et al. Outcomes and risk factors for graft loss: lessons learned from 1,056 pediatric kidney transplants at the University of Minnesota. *J Am Coll Surg.* 2017;224(4):473–486.
445. Nevins TE, et al. Understanding medication nonadherence after kidney transplant. *J Am Soc Nephrol.* 2017;28:2290–2301.
452. Francis A, et al. Quality of life of children and adolescents with chronic kidney disease: a cross-sectional study. *Arch Dis Child.* 2019;104:134–140.

# GLOBAL CONSIDERATIONS IN KIDNEY DISEASE

SECTION XIII

# 75 Global Challenges and Initiatives in Kidney Health

Valérie A. Luyckx | Boris Bikbov | Aminu K. Bello

## CHAPTER OUTLINE



## KEY POINTS

- The global burden of chronic kidney disease (CKD) is rising. In 2015, CKD was the 10th most common cause for death globally, directly causing 1 out of every 43 deaths. CKD contributes to a similar number of deaths from cardiovascular disease.
- CKD occurs in younger individuals in lower-income regions.
- The global burden of acute kidney injury (AKI) remains unknown.
- Kidney disease is a major risk factor for cardiovascular morbidity and mortality.
- Many countries lack policies regarding kidney disease advocacy, screening, and prevention.
- Achieving universal health coverage may reduce the global burden of AKI and CKD through improved access to primary care and essential medication.
- Access to dialysis and transplantation is highly inequitable across the globe and within regions and countries, largely dictated by ability to pay.
- If dialysis and transplantation are to be provided in low-resource settings, rigorous planning must be done initially to determine affordability and ensure sustainability, and transparent criteria must be developed to achieve fairness and equitable access to RRT.

## GLOBAL CHALLENGES IN KIDNEY HEALTH

### AWARENESS OF KIDNEY DISEASE AS AN IMPORTANT PUBLIC HEALTH ISSUE

Kidney disease is an important noncommunicable disease (NCD) worldwide; however, this is not yet widely acknowledged in the global policy agenda. The World Health organization (WHO) Global Action Plan for the Prevention and Control of NCDs has focused on addressing four main disease areas—heart diseases and stroke, cancer, chronic respiratory diseases, and diabetes, with the recent addition of mental health—and has identified these diseases as the major NCD killers globally.[1] According to WHO, in 2012, 46.2% of NCD deaths (17.5 million deaths) were attributed to cardiovascular disease (CVD), 21.7% (8.2 million deaths) to cancers, 10.7% (4 million deaths) to chronic respiratory diseases, and 4% (1.5 million deaths) due to diabetes, totaling 82% of all NCD deaths. As discussed in more detail later, estimates from the Global Burden of Disease (GBD) study in 2015 have shown that around 1.2 million people were known to have died of chronic kidney disease (CKD).[2] Others have estimated that at least 2.3 million people died in 2010 because they had no access to dialysis, and 1.7 million die annually from acute kidney injury (AKI).[3,4] It is possible, therefore, that kidney disease may contribute to more deaths than diabetes, respiratory diseases, or individual forms of cancer, which are among the four main NCDs targeted by the current NCD Action Plan.[1,5] The global importance of kidney disease as a cause of mortality, as well as morbidity, has been increasing, and the Global Action Plan does acknowledge that synergies exist between NCDs, and that "conditions such as kidney disease result from lack of early detection and management of hypertension and diabetes, and therefore are closely linked to major non-communicable diseases."[1]

AKI and CKD are both of public health concern. Although their true prevalence in low-income countries (LICs) and lower middle-income countries (LMICs; collectively, LLMICs) is unknown, it is estimated that they are at least as high, if not higher, than in high-income countries (HICs).[4,6,7] Approximately 750 million adults (8%–16%) worldwide are living with CKD, of whom around 78% reside in LLMICs.[6,8] Up to 90% of those affected, however, are not aware of their condition.[8,9] The prevalence of CKD among children is unknown but may reach 1% of the pediatric population.[10] Traditional and universal risk factors for CKD include diabetes

*Text continued on page 2453*

**Table 75.1 Global Relevance of Major Risk Factors for Chronic Kidney Disease and Suggested Mitigation Strategies**

| Risk Factor | Global Prevalence | Primary Prevention | Projected Risk for CKD | Secondary Prevention of CKD | Knowledge Gaps | Relevance for HIC | Relevance for LIC | Advocacy Required | References |
|---|---|---|---|---|---|---|---|---|---|
| Diabetes type 2 | All diabetes 387 million, with largest concentrations in Western Pacific (138 million) and Southeast Asia (75 million)<br>Type 2—About 95% of overall global prevalence | Education, lifestyle, diet, exercise, weight, management | ~40% overall and >50% in most non-white populations | Glucose control, BP control, lifestyle factors (avoidance of high dietary protein), ACEI or ARB | Glucose targets, best medications, need for novel therapies for diabetic kidney disease | Obesity, DM, GDM | Increasing obesity and DM, GDM; poor facilities for diagnosis and treatment | Policy development around food content and prices of healthy food; urban planning to increase walking opportunities, tobacco; universal health care; access to diagnosis; reliable access to medication; lifestyle | 127–130 |
| Diabetes, type 1 | Type 1—about 5% of overall global prevalence | Viral exposures (?) | ~30 %<br>Not known to vary by race/ethnicity | Glucose control, BP control, lifestyle factors (avoidance of high dietary protein), ACEI or ARB | Glucose targets, novel therapies for diabetic kidney disease | Glycemic control | Glycemic control; poor facilities for diagnosis and treatment | Universal health care, access to diagnosis, reliable access to medication, lifestyle | 127 |
| Hypertension | 2010—31% of adults globally (28.5% in HICs, 31.5% LMICs); 1.39 billion people (349 million in HICs, 1.04 billion in LMICs) | Education, lifestyle, diet, exercise, weight, management, smoking, stress reduction | ~10 % | Blood pressure control, ACEI or ARB if high-level albuminuria; other medication types? | BP targets; albuminuria-based? | Obesity, dietary sodium | Obesity, dietary sodium; strokes also; high awareness, Rx, and control vs. low in LMICs | Policy development around food sodium content, tobacco, alcohol; need to increase awareness; treatment and control globally; universal health care; consider polypill strategy; awareness, access to diagnosis; reliable access to medication, lifestyle | 131 |

*Continued on following page*

**Table 75.1 Global Relevance of Major Risk Factors for Chronic Kidney Disease and Suggested Mitigation Strategies (Cont'd)**

| Risk Factor | Global Prevalence | Primary Prevention | Projected Risk for CKD | Secondary Prevention of CKD | Knowledge Gaps | Relevance for HIC | Relevance for LIC | Advocacy Required | References |
|---|---|---|---|---|---|---|---|---|---|
| Obesity (risks may vary for childhood and adult obesity) | Adult: overweight, 2013: 36.9% men, 38.0% women. Obesity 2014: 10.8% men, 14.9% women Children: in 2014, 41 million children <5 years of age were overweight or obese (48% in Asia, 25% in Africa) | Education, lifestyle, diet, exercise, weight management, stress reduction | Unknown Proteinuria or macroalbuminuria present in 4%–10% obese patients In morbidly obese risk of GFR decline ≥30% over 4 years was 48.2 per 1000 person years Adolescent obesity associated with HR of 6.9 for all ESKD and HR of 19.4 for diabetic ESKD | Diet, exercise, weight loss, bariatric surgery (HICs), ACEI, ARB for proteinuria | Risk of CKD, optimal BMI and variance by race and ethnicity and age, safe and effective weight management strategies (e.g., bariatric surgery) | Access to weight management programs | Access to weight management programs; social roots of obesity, poverty, culture; access to nutritious food | Policy development to regulate food content, food prices; urban planning to permit physical exercise; access to better diet; education, physical activity education | 132–137 |
| Medications (antibiotics, NSAIDS, PPI, counterfeit drugs, contrast media) | AKI: 24% globally related to nephrotoxins (29% HICs, 22% UMICs, 23% LLMICs) CKD: unknown | Improve awareness, prescription flagging, stop unnecessary prescriptions | 70% of children with nephrotoxin-induced AKI had CKD at 6 months CKD risk variable, by medication | Early detection, urine screening for leukocytes, stop medications early | Burden of disease; which medication may increase risk for CKD | Electronic alert systems, prescription data-sharing databases, package warnings | Reduce counterfeit drugs; regulate drug manufacture to reduce adulterants | Awareness, prescription practices, marketing | 24, 138, 139 |
| Traditional, alternative remedies | Frequent use globally, >80% in LMICs | Improve awareness Improve access to alternatives (UHC) | 35% of AKI in Africa; unknown contribution to CKD; increased risk of ESKD with consumption of some remedies | Stop medication, hydration | Burden of disease, toxic compounds | Huge market OTC and over the Internet, need regulation of the industry | Engage with communities to, for example, understand reasons for use, barriers to Western medicine | Policies to regulate manufacture and sale of alternative remedies; limit unfounded, fraudulent advertising; universal health care; awareness, collaboration with traditional healers, improve access to medical care and affordability of medication; encourage publication of case reports to build database | 21, 140, 141 |

| | | | | | | | | | |
|---|---|---|---|---|---|---|---|---|---|
| Kidney stones | Geographic variability<br>Adults: 5%–9% Europe, 12% Canada, 13%–15% United States, 1%–5% East, 20% Saudi Arabia | Increase awareness of local risks; emphasize importance of hydration, certain infections | GFR tends to be reduced in stone formers vs. controls | Hydration, diet, recurrent stone prevention, early reversal of obstruction | Regional risks | High costs | Likely unrecognized important cause of CKD and infections | Access to clean water, reduce environmental and occupational risks; increase awareness of need for follow-up for CKD, CVD in stone formers | 142–144 |
| Low birth weight, SGA, prematurity | Globally: LBW 15%, preterm 10%<br>In LMICs, 2010, 13.7 million babies preterm; 2010, 43.3 million babies LBW, SGA | Avoid obesity, healthy lifestyle | 70% increased risk | Screen for BP and proteinuria; treat early | Would reduction affect future risk? | Increased maternal age, assisted reproduction, maternal chronic illness | Preeclampsia, maternal malnutrition, poverty, war, poor antenatal care, pregnancy spacing, child marriage | Awareness, public health measures, optimize maternal and child health, avoid childhood obesity, universal health care, document birth weights, prematurity in health record; need for long-term follow-up of children at risk | 145, 146 |
| Preeclampsia, eclampsia | 2%–5% globally<br>Global prevalence, 2013—1.3 million | Optimize maternal health prepregnancy | RR, HT, 3.7;<br>RR, microalbuminuria, 4–8;<br>RR, ESKD, 4.7;<br>RR, kidney biopsy, 3.3 | Screen for BP and proteinuria treat early | How to diagnose and prevent? | Prematurity, later CVD, ESKD | Prematurity, CVD, ESKD | Maternal health, access to antenatal care, universal health care; mothers require long-term follow-up for CKD and CVD | 147–150 |
| HIV | 2013: 35 million worldwide, 24.7 million in sub-Saharan Africa | Education, condoms | Africa 6.0%–48.5%, Europe 3.5%, 18%, Hong Kong 18%, Brazil 1.1%–5.6%, India 27%, Iran 20% | PEP, HAART | Impact of HAART on all forms of renal disease, other kidney diseases in HIV-infected individuals | Competing risks of mortality | Poverty, suboptimal access to ART, ongoing infection risk<br>ApoL1 genotype with African origin | Policies around needle sharing, prostitution; universal health care; national policies for prevention education; access to ART, reduce gender and sexuality discrimination, empower women; surveillance of renal function on ART | 151 |

*Continued on following page*

**Table 75.1 Global Relevance of Major Risk Factors for Chronic Kidney Disease and Suggested Mitigation Strategies (Cont'd)**

| Risk Factor | Global Prevalence | Primary Prevention | Projected Risk for CKD | Secondary Prevention of CKD | Knowledge Gaps | Relevance for HIC | Relevance for LIC | Advocacy Required | References |
|---|---|---|---|---|---|---|---|---|---|
| Hepatitis B | Global prevalence 2013—331.0 million | Education, reduce scarification, vaccination | Hepatitis B–associated GN, 3% France, 3% China | Treatment of hepatitis B | Impact of routine vaccination on CKD burden | Reduce HCC, liver failure, transplantation | High prevalence | Policies around needle sharing, vaccination; advocacy for sexual health, drug abuse; equity in access to vaccination (vaccination reduced membranous nephropathy among Taiwanese children); equity in access to antiviral therapy | 150, 152, 153 |
| Hepatitis C | Global prevalence 2013: 147.8 million | Education | Global: 10%–16%; glomerular lesions in 54.8% of HCV-positive subjects at autopsy | Treatment of hepatitis C | Impact of treatment on disease burden | Reduce HCC, liver failure, kidney transplantation; new medication very costly | Lower prevalence, unlikely to gain access to expensive therapies | Policies around needle sharing; advocacy against drug abuse; lobby for access to therapy in HICs and LMICs | 150, 152, 154 |
| Bacterial skin diseases | Global prevalence 2013: 5–8 million | Sanitation, early treatment | Acute PSGN, 9/100,000 in LMICs<br>Higher frequency of CKD after poststreptococcal GN, worse in adults | Early detection of renal involvement; treatment and follow-up | Contribution to CKD burden in LICs unknown | Likely low | Likely high | Policies to improve child nutrition, school feeding programs; poverty, overcrowding; scabies prevention and early treatment; consider screening school children for hematuria, proteinuria | 150, 155, 156 |
| Schistosomiasis | Global prevalence, 2013: 290.6 million | Safe water Education | Obstruction, 2%–62%, chronic glomerulonephritis (hepatosplenic) in 15% | Prompt treatment; screening for obstruction | Obstruction usually not severe, renal function preserved; regional contribution to ESKD may be 3%–7% (Egypt) | Low | High regional | Public health policies, neglected tropical diseases; clean water; consider screening school children for hematuria, proteinuria; prompt access to diagnosis and treatment | 150, 157–161 |

| | | | | | | | | | |
|---|---|---|---|---|---|---|---|---|---|
| Diarrheal illnesses | Global prevalence 2013: 4.24 million | Safe water Sanitation, nutrition, vaccination | Important cause of AKI worldwide | Appropriate hydration, antibiotics when needed | Burden of CKD related to diarrhea-associated AKI, impact of vaccination on AKI, CKD | Relatively low, diarrhea-associated HUS | High, important cause of childhood AKI through volume depletion, sepsis, HUS | Public health policies, sanitation, water education, infrastructure, vaccination; advocacy to chlorinate water; handwashing, improve water safety, equitable access to vaccination, education about oral rehydration therapy | 150 |
| Malaria | Worldwide prevalence 2013: 351 million | Use of ITNs Vector control Prompt treatment with correct drugs | AKI <1%–>50% in adults with severe *Falciparum* malaria; CKD not often reported among survivors | Early screening and diagnosis and management | Contribution to CKD burden regionally unknown; possible differences among those living in endemic areas (or not?); may be associated with CKDu | Low | High regional | Public health policies: vector control, insecticide-treated nets, monitor medication resistance, combat counterfeit medication, introduce RDT; access to prevention, diagnosis, appropriate treatment | 30, 150, 162–164 |
| Tuberculosis | Worldwide prevalence 2013: 12.1 million | Healthy diet, reduce poverty, reduce HIV | Genitourinary, 27% of extrapulmonary TB (obstruction, parenchymal infection, interstitial nephritis) | Prompt diagnosis and full treatment | Low | Low, higher in immigrants, prison, indigenous, immuno-suppressed populations | High, regional; often coinfection with HIV | Public health policies about detection, supervision of therapy, GeneXpert System, management of MDR, XDR, integration with HIV services; poverty, comorbid illness, nutrition, overcrowding, occupational exposure (mining), HIV infection | 150, 165 |

Continued on following page

**Table 75.1 Global Relevance of Major Risk Factors for Chronic Kidney Disease and Suggested Mitigation Strategies (Cont'd)**

| Risk Factor | Global Prevalence | Primary Prevention | Projected Risk for CKD | Secondary Prevention of CKD | Knowledge Gaps | Relevance for HIC | Relevance for LIC | Advocacy Required | References |
|---|---|---|---|---|---|---|---|---|---|
| Leptospirosis | Global incidence: 1.03 million | Use of ITNs, vector control, prompt treatment | AKI (Weil disease) 10%–60% | Early diagnosis | Contribution to burden of CKD unknown | Little | High, regional | Public health policies, neglected tropical diseases; poverty, water quality, overcrowding | 30, 166 |
| Environmental factors | (?) Risk factor prevalence for CKDu—likely association with environment, occupation, poor fluid intake, coinfections, traditional remedies | Avoid occupation, climate, environmental hazards | Prevalence: 13%–26% in high- risk populations | Hydration; avoid nephrotoxins | Causes and pathophysiology unknown | Low | CKDu major problem in multiple LMICs | Policies around working conditions, environmental contamination | 27, 164, 167, 168 |
| AKI | 21% of hospital admissions (global data insufficient for accurate quantitation) | Early risk identification<br>Treat underlying cause early<br>Avoid nephrotoxins | Adults: 25.8/100 person-years (CKD), 8.6/100 person-years (ESKD)<br>Children: 3.1/100 person-years (proteinuria), 0.9/100 person-years (ESKD) | Early diagnosis and treatment of AKI | Actual risk of CKD after AKI in population, impact of interventions to reduce AKI on CKD prevalence | Predominantly hospital-acquired, older adults, multiple comorbidities | Predominantly community-acquired, adults younger, few comorbidities | Increase awareness of risk of AKI and need for prompt treatment; require accessible methods to diagnose AKI; awareness of risk of CKD requiring long-term follow-up after severe AKI | 4, 25, 26 |

*ACEI*, Angiotensin-converting enzyme inhibitor; *AKI*, acute kidney injury; *ARB*, angiotensin receptor blocker; *ART*, antiretroviral therapy; *BMI*, body mass index; *BP*, blood pressure; *CKD*, chronic kidney disease; *CKDu*, chronic kidney disease of uncertain cause; *CVD*, cardiovascular disease; *DM*, diabetes mellitus; *GDM*, gestational diabetes mellitus; *GFR*, glomerular filtration rate; *GN*, glomerulonephritis; *ESKD*, end-stage kidney disease; *HAART*, highly active antiretroviral therapy; *HIC*, high-income country; *HIV*, human immunodeficiency virus; *HCV*, hepatitis C Virus; *ITN*, insecticide-treated nets; *LBW*, low birth weight; *LMIC*, low middle-income country; *MDR*, multidrug resistance; *NSAID*, nonsteroidal antiinflammatory drug; *OTC*, over-the-counter; *PEP*, postexposure prophylaxis; PPI, proton pump inhibitor; *PSGN*, poststreptococcal glomerulonephritis; *Rx*, treatment; *SGA*, small for gestational age; *TB*, tuberculosis; *UHC*, universal health care; *UMIC*, upper middle-income country; *XDR*, extensive drug resistance.

Adapted from Luyckx VA, Tuttle KR, Garcia G, et al. Reducing major risk factors for chronic kidney disease. *Kidney Int Suppl* 2017;7:71–87.

and hypertension (Table 75.1).[11] Nontraditional risk factors for CKD are being increasingly recognized, including nephrotoxins (e.g., prescription medication and complementary remedies), kidney stones, fetal and maternal exposures, infections, environmental and occupational exposures, and AKI (see Table 75.1).[7,12,13] For example, the use of traditional remedies is widespread, and some are known to be nephrotoxic.[14] The contribution of such nontraditional risk factors to the burdens of AKI and CKD is unknown but may be significant, especially in LLMICs.

The public health importance of CKD lies not only in the risk of end-stage kidney disease (ESKD) requiring dialysis or transplantation, at great expense to the individual and the health system, but also because CKD is a major risk multiplier of cardiovascular risk, contributing to excess strokes and heart attacks and leading to death of many CKD patients before they ever reach ESKD.[15–17] It is frequently underappreciated that CKD alone is a stronger risk factor for coronary events than diabetes alone and, when the two conditions coexist (which occurs in one of every three patients with diabetes), the risk of cardiovascular events and overall mortality is further multiplied.[16]

AKI occurs in 7% to 21% of hospitalized patients (30%–70% of critically ill patients) worldwide, affecting around 13.3 million people/year, of whom around 85% reside in LLMICs.[4,18,19] Data for children are again relatively scarce, with estimates of 7.5% to 23.3% among hospitalized children, depending on the definition used.[20] Overall mortality has been estimated at 11% to 23% in adults and 14% in children, but varies with the population studied (up to 80% if no dialysis is available when required).[4,19,21] AKI is associated with high costs of care because many patients require intensive care management, and mortality is lower in countries with higher expenditures on health care, reflecting better access to health care and dialysis in these countries.[19] In higher-income countries, most cases of AKI are hospital-acquired, whereas in many LLMICs, community-acquired AKI is more common.[18,22,23] Sepsis, dehydration, use of nephrotoxins, and primary AKI are major universal causes of AKI.[24] In many patients with AKI, kidney function will recover, but adults and children experiencing AKI have up to an eightfold risk of developing CKD and are at increased risk of longer-term CVD and death.[12,25,26] CKD, in turn, is an important risk factor for AKI.[12]

Challenges to diagnosis of kidney disease include the necessity for access to blood and urine testing, awareness among health care workers, a degree of therapeutic nihilism in environments where access to specialist care and dialysis is limited, and the fact that kidney disease is often asymptomatic or symptoms are nonspecific until advanced stages. Proactive screening for early detection of AKI or CKD in high-risk individuals to permit interventions to delay worsening of the disease is therefore required.[8,27–29] Increased awareness of risk factors for CKD and AKI in communities and hospitalized populations is urgently needed to implement prevention strategies successfully.[12] Kidney disease also bridges communicable and NCDs. Acute infections such as malaria and leptospirosis may lead to AKI, and chronic infections such as hepatitis B and C and HIV are important causes of CKD.[12,13,30] In turn, AKI and CKD increase the risk and morbidity of infections.[31] Many people worldwide are therefore affected by kidney disease, at least some of which is preventable. Despite the best efforts at prevention, however, some people will develop either acute or end-stage kidney failure and require renal replacement therapy (RRT)—dialysis or transplantation—to remain alive.

## RENAL REPLACEMENT THERAPY AND THE CHALLENGES OF LIMITED ACCESS

Many barriers reduce access to dialysis around the globe.[3,21,32–35] Unless dialysis is covered through state coverage or insurance schemes, access to dialysis is often restricted by prohibitive out-of-pocket (OOP) expenditures, patient age or gender, geography, and lack of expertise and infrastructure (Fig. 75.1).[36,37]

The global incidence of ESKD in 2010 was 93 (95% confidence interval [CI], 90–95) per million population (pmp), but varies significantly across the globe (Fig. 75.2A).[11,17] The true incidence of ESKD in LLIMCs is unknown because existing data come only from those who have access to dialysis and where data exist. The incidence of ESKD in LLMICs is often higher than the prevalence, indicating high attrition rates, predominantly because of the inability to pay for dialysis or being too sick at presentation.[11] In 2010, the global average prevalence rate of ESKD was 284 pmp; however, individual country prevalence ranged from 0 to over 2000 pmp, reflecting large global inequities (see Fig. 75.2B).[17] Among children, the global prevalence rate is estimated to be under 100 pmp, but again is highly variable, depending on the accessibility of chronic dialysis.[10,35,38,39] It has been estimated from the literature and available registries that there are large treatment gaps between those who need and those who obtain dialysis globally, with the largest gaps in Africa (84%–91% not treated) and Asia (66%–83% not treated).[3] It has been estimated that at least 2.3 million people died prematurely in 2010 because they could not access dialysis.[3] These deaths occurred predominantly in LLMICs. Other authors have estimated that a total of 1.2 million premature deaths resulted from lack of access to RRT among people with hypertension and diabetes alone, based on prevalence and expected rates of ESKD.[40] Of major concern is the prediction that by 2030, attributable to population aging and increasing rates of diabetes and hypertension, the global need for dialysis will double, with the greatest growth occurring in LLMICs.[3]

Few data are available regarding the need for dialysis for AKI in LLMICs. In general, AKI appears more severe at diagnosis in LLMICs compared with HICs, most likely due to delays in presentation to hospital, and therefore the need for dialysis is higher, but access to dialysis is lower in LLMICs.[4,21,24] Acute peritoneal dialysis (PD) is an attractive modality for AKI because this is as effective as hemodialysis (HD), requires far less infrastructure, and can be performed with solutions and catheters adapted to local resources.[41,42] PD should be cheaper than HD, especially if solutions are manufactured locally.[43,44] However, owing to the necessity to import fluids, customs, and corruption, the costs of 5 days of PD or HD for a child in Nigeria, for example, were similar, and amounted to several times the monthly minimum wage, making OOP payment impossible for most.[45,46] In recent years, some governments (e.g., Ghana, Tanzania, Nigeria) have introduced coverage for short-term dialysis for AKI paid for by national health insurance schemes, inpatient government-funded services, or nongovernmental organizations and charities.[47–50] If renal

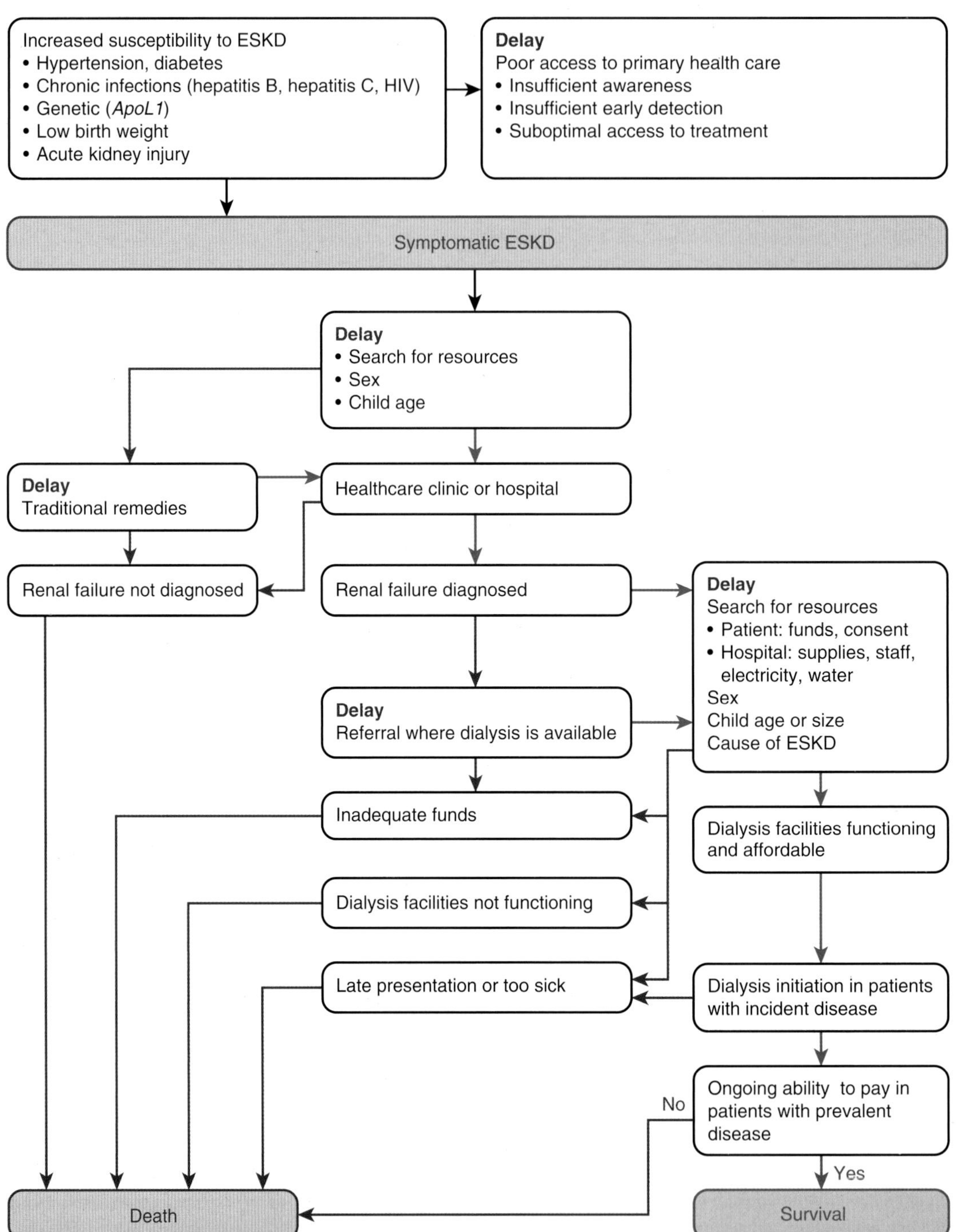


**Fig. 75.1 Barriers to care in end-stage kidney disease *(ESKD).*** This flow diagram shows barriers to access to dialysis contributing to mortality in ESKD in many sub-Saharan African countries. *Green arrows* show factors present to facilitate diagnosis of ESKD or referral for, or access to dialysis; *red arrows* show absence of these factors. Most barriers are related to access to care, access to diagnosis, out-of-pocket payments needed, and infrastructural resources. *ApoL1,* Apolipoprotein L1. (Adapted from Ashuntantang G, Osafo C, Olowu WA, et al. Outcomes in adults and children with end-stage kidney disease requiring dialysis in sub-Saharan Africa: a systematic review. *Lancet Glob Health*. 2017;5[4]:e408–e417.)

recovery does not occur within the coverage period, however, costs revert to OOP, which are unsustainable, and dialysis must then be actively discontinued.[47,48,50]

Transplantation is the most cost-effective RRT solution in the long term; however, again, if costs of the surgery and long-term medication and follow-up are not sustainably covered by governments, health insurance, or donors, accessibility and success are significantly reduced.[29,51,52] In India, for example, 72% of patients undergoing kidney transplantation reported some form of resulting financial crisis, with 10% expressing regret at having embarked on the procedure.[53] Globally, most transplantations are conducted in HICs, in part due to lack of resources and knowledge in LICs, as well as cultural practices and absence of legal frameworks governing organ donation (Fig. 75.3).[52] Worldwide, transplantation activity is directly associated with health expenditure, physicians per

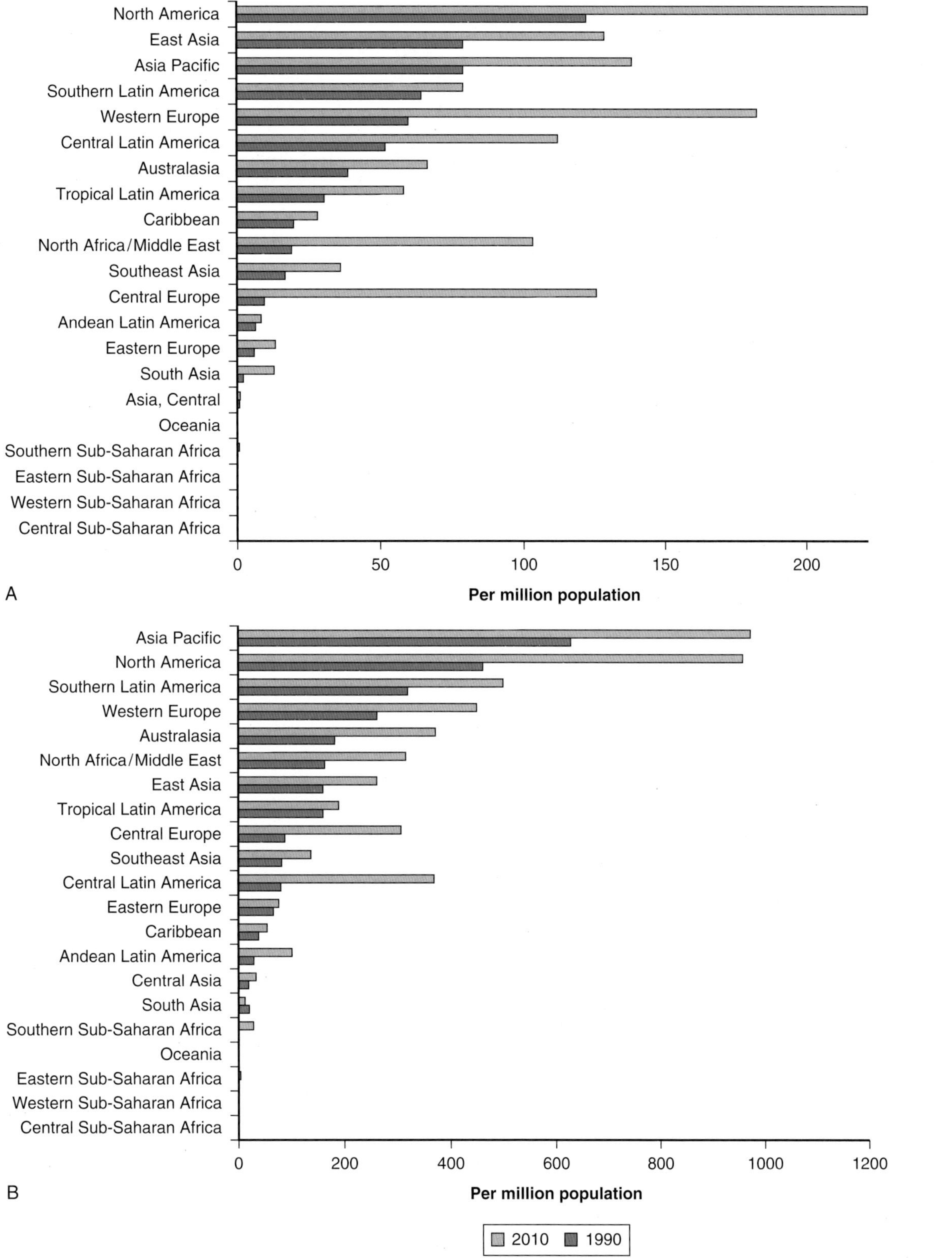


**Fig. 75.2 Age-standardized maintenance dialysis.** (A) Incidence/million population and (B) prevalence/million population for 21 world regions in 1990–2010. (From Thomas B, Wulf S, Bikbov B, et al., Maintenance dialysis throughout the world in years 1990 and 2010. *J Am Soc Nephrol.* 2015;26[11]:2621–2633.)

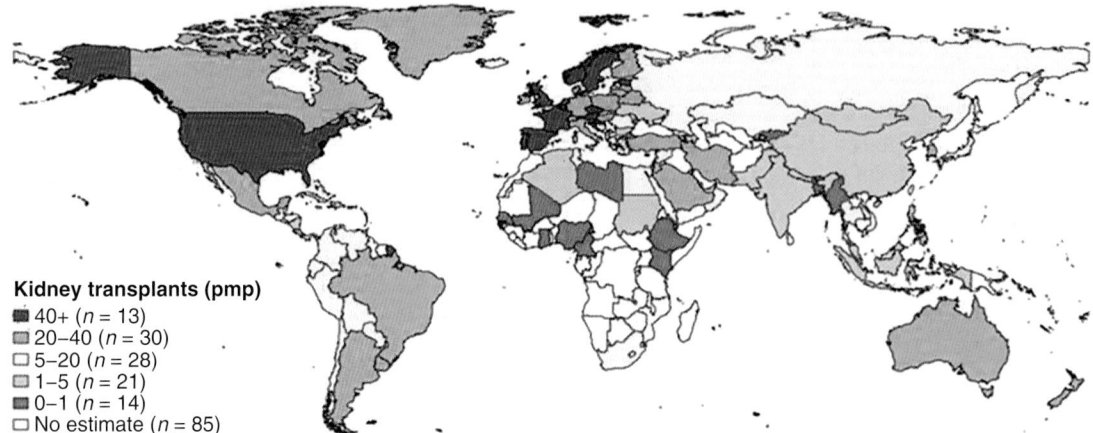


**Fig. 75.3** Global distribution of kidney transplantation rates/million population *(pmp)* in 2012. (From Muralidharan A, White S. The need for kidney transplantation in low- and middle-income countries in 2012: an epidemiological perspective. *Transplantation.* 2015;99[3]:476–481.)

capita, and life expectancy at birth and inversely associated with reliance on OOP payments and reliance on external resources for health care.[52] In some countries where the local population cannot access kidney transplantation, patients and donors travel abroad, if resources exist, for transplantation.[54,55] Organ trafficking and commercial transplantation are a global problem, not only because of the ethical dilemmas they pose, but also because they are associated with worse outcomes for the transplant recipient. Also, they put living donors at risk in low-income environments, where they are unlikely to have been well screened and cannot access routine follow-up care.[56,57]

## DILEMMAS POSED BY LACK OF SUSTAINABLE RENAL REPLACEMENT THERAPY IN LOW-RESOURCE SETTINGS

Attempting to meet dialysis costs OOP generally constitutes a catastrophic health expenditure for a patient and family. Protection from individual financial risk is one of the cornerstones of the global push for universal health coverage; however, how far a government should go to meet the needs of patients requiring dialysis, potentially at the expense of funding other programs, is a contentious issue.[58,59] The limited health budgets and current burdens of renal and nonrenal disease in LLMICs make progress toward universal access to RRT challenging.[60] Globally, on average, 0.15% of the population requires treatment for ESKD, at a cost of around 2% to 4 % of health expenditures.[9,29] These direct costs of ESKD often do not account for costs of frequent hospitalizations and management of other comorbidities; therefore, total costs are even higher.[9,29] Such disproportionate expenditures on a relatively small proportion of the population pose a challenge in terms of prioritization of health expenditure and opportunity costs. Some governments (e.g., Guinea, Cameroon, Senegal, India), alone or in partnership with private institutions or charities, have elected to subsidize the cost of chronic dialysis, requiring OOP payments of a few dollars a day.[61–63] Even these prices, which are much lower than the average unsubsidized cost of $60 to $100 for a single HD treatment, remain unsustainable for families over the long term and often do not cover the vital costs of transport, medications, or time lost from work, which can almost double the total OOP cost for a patient.[21,35,64–68] In sub-Saharan Africa and India, most patients who initiate chronic dialysis cannot sustain it and stop dialysis within days to weeks.[33,35] Even among European cohorts, mortality of children on dialysis was related to public health expenditures.[69] Sustainable and sufficient funding is therefore necessary for the successful treatment of kidney failure. It is unrealistic to imagine that in the short to medium term, all those requiring RRT will be able to access it equitably. Recognition of this fact is important to ensure that patients are still treated with dignity and have universal access to symptom relief and palliative care.

> *Clinical Relevance*
> **Catastrophic Health Expenditures**
> Out-of-pocket health expenditure amount to >10% of total household expenditures or 40% of household nonfood expenditures.[53] Such expenses risk plunging families into poverty and reduce their capacity to obtain other necessities.

> *Clinical Relevance*
> **Universal Health Coverage (UHC)**
> This is defined by WHO as "all people receiving quality health services that meet their needs without being exposed to financial hardship in paying for the services."[59] The three dimensions of UHC include expanding priority services, expanding the number of people covered, and reducing out-of-pocket payments and thereby financial hardship.

> *Clinical Relevance*
> **Opportunity Costs**
> These are health gains that could have been realized had the money been allocated to an alternative intervention.[29]

## POLICY DEVELOPMENT AND ACCESS TO RENAL REPLACEMENT THERAPY

Most states in LLMICs cannot afford to provide universal access to RRT; however, if states choose to provide some RRT, whether through sole funding or through partnership agreements, it is important that transparent and just eligibility criteria governing who will gain access to RRT are established.[58] Development of such criteria should facilitate bedside discussions and decision making and likely will involve consideration of clinical, social, and environmental realities that may affect a patient's ability to continue dialysis without incurring catastrophic health expenditures. Official criteria will also reduce moral distress among health care workers, removing the burden of individual case-by-case, life-and-death decision making.[70] Eligibility criteria may be more flexible for AKI than ESKD because the personal resources required will be less for AKI. To be effective, however, the development of such guidelines requires a transparent, consultative, and iterative development process and engagement with many different stakeholder groups. Potential policy scenarios and processes for development of dialysis guidelines are outlined elsewhere.[58,71]

Policy options would include the following: (1) provision of RRT to all; (2) provision of dialysis for AKI only; (3) provision of RRT to a restricted eligible group (i.e., rationing); and (4) no state provision of RRT and allowing market forces to determine access (Table 75.2). Major inequities are inherent in each of these scenarios:

- Where universal RRT is not covered, inequities exist between countries.
- Where AKI only is covered, inequities exist between those with AKI and those with ESKD.
- Where rationing occurs, inequities exist between those meeting and not meeting the eligibility criteria.
- Where dialysis is not covered by the state, inequities exist within countries and regions depending on ability to pay and location.

In addition, when developing RRT policies and guidelines, consideration must also be given to achievable minimum safe standards of practice realistically because patients and providers may attempt to reduce dialysis frequency and dose to curb costs at the expense of health.[35]

It is also important to recognize, however, that other inequities and health challenges in many LLMICs may be more urgent and affect many more people than kidney disease. In fact, the WHO specifically advises against the provision of dialysis in countries that have not yet met the needs of expanding priority health services (e.g., vaccinations, treatment of diarrhea, pneumonia, maternal health, hypertension, diabetes; http://www.who.int/choice/documents/making_fair_choices/en). Individual financial risk protection is, however, one of the three dimensions of universal health coverage; therefore, dialysis provision poses a dilemma—people die without it, people are impoverished because of it, and opportunity costs are extremely high. Priority setting within each country is therefore essential but requires reliable relative assessments of the disease burden, which is lacking for kidney disease in most LLMICs. Chronic dialysis for ESKD is suggested by some to be an unacceptable trade-off given that in Kenya, for example, 300 times more healthy life-years could be saved if dialysis expenditures were spent on tuberculosis control instead.[59] Once a country has made significant progress toward universal health coverage, however, the provision of acute dialysis for AKI is seen as cost-effective.[59] Whichever policies are put in place, it is crucially important to advocate for the need for prevention, early detection, and treatment of AKI and CKD as the most effective means to reduce health expenditures and the need for RRT.

## GLOBAL INITIATIVES FOR KIDNEY HEALTH

In recent years, various initiatives have been launched or supported by the global nephrology community to improve understanding of the burden of kidney disease, estimate the

**Table 75.2 Simplified Ethical Analysis of Potential Government Policies for Renal Replacement Therapy**

| Policy | Expected Health Benefits for Patients | Potential Harm and Burdens | Impact on Autonomy | Impact on Equity | Expected Efficiency |
|---|---|---|---|---|---|
| Universal coverage of dialysis for AKI and ESKD | All benefit | High opportunity costs | Good | Good | Expensive |
| Universal coverage for AKI only | AKI patients benefit | What if AKI does not recover? | Good for AKI | ESKD not considered | Less expensive |
| State coverage under limited conditions (rationing, AKI and ESKD) | Eligible patients benefit | Ineligible patients die; perception of unfairness | Need rationing | Inequity within patients with AKI and ESKD | Less expensive |
| No state coverage | Limited to rich few | Much harm, especially if problem "ignored" and no official guidelines; moral distress for health care workers needing to decide; may exacerbate brain drain | Very restricted | Very inequitable | Left to the market |

*AKI,* Acute kidney injury; *ESKD,* end-stage kidney disease.

Adapted from Luyckx VA, Miljeteig I, Ejigu AM, et al. Ethical challenges in the provision of dialysis in resource-constrained environments. *Semin Nephrol.* 2017;37(3):273–286.

resources available to tackle kidney disease, advocate for kidney health, and contribute to the development of innovative strategies to prevent or detect and treat kidney disease early. Some of these initiatives are described later.

## GLOBAL BURDEN OF DISEASE STUDY

### MORTALITY AND MORBIDITY DUE TO CHRONIC KIDNEY DISEASE

The most comprehensive assessment of the global epidemiology of CKD has been carried out within the framework of the GBD study, which has described CKD mortality and morbidity in 195 countries from 1990 to 2015 (for yearly updated data please see https://vizhub.healthdata.org/gbd-compare). The combined CKD data from the GBD study are summarized in Table 75.3. According to the latest published evidence,[72–74] global CKD stages 3 to 5 prevalence was 322.5 million (4.6% of the world's population) in 2015. This estimate is higher, or at least comparable, with the prevalence of ischemic heart disease, chronic obstructive pulmonary disease, osteoarthritis, malaria, or the number of people living with the consequences of road injury.[72]

Most cases of CKD stages 3 to 5 in 2015 were assumed to be due to diabetic nephropathy (100.8 million), followed by hypertensive nephropathy (79.0 million) and chronic glomerulonephritis (67.3 million). Notably, as many as 94.6 million people had CKD due to other causes, including unknown causes. Thus, 52.6% of CKD cases were attributed to diabetes or hypertension, whereas almost the same number of people had intrinsic kidney disease. CKD was more

**Table 75.3 Global Burden of Low GFR (Chronic Kidney Disease [CKD] Stages 3–5)**

| Parameter | CKD Stages 3–5 | Low GFR Overall[a] | CVD Due to Low GFR |
|---|---|---|---|
| **Prevalence** | | | |
| Number, 2015 | 322.5 million | | — |
| Crude rate/100,000 population, 2015 | 4375.4 | | — |
| Change in number from 1990 to 2015, % | 78.3 | | — |
| Change in crude rate from 1990 to 2015, % | 28.3 | | — |
| Change in age-standardized rate from 1990 to 2015, % | 0.4 | | — |
| **Years Lived With Disability** | | | |
| Number, 2015 | 8.2 million | 9.3 million | 1.0 million |
| Crude rate, 2015, per 100,000 population | 110.9 | 126.7 | 13.4 |
| Global rank, 2015 | 24th | 11th | — |
| Change in number from 1990 to 2015, % | 67.5% | 68.2 | 71.8 |
| Change in crude rate from 1990 to 2015, % | 20.5% | 21.0 | 23.6 |
| Change in age-standardized rate from 1990 to 2015, % | −2.3 | −3.0 | −8.8 |
| **Deaths** | | | |
| Number, 2015 | 1.2 million | 2.4 million | 1.2 million |
| Crude rate/100,000 population, 2015 | 16.7 | 32.9 | 16.2 |
| Global rank, 2015[b] | 10th | 11th | — |
| Change in number from 1990 to 2015, % | 108.3 | 69.5 | 42.0 |
| Change in crude rate from 1990 to 2015, % | 49.9 | 21.9 | 2.2 |
| Change in age-standardized rate from 1990 to 2015, % | 14.3 | −13.0 | −29.6 |
| **Years of Life Lost Due to Premature Mortality** | | | |
| Number, 2015 | 27.1 million | 45.1 million | 18.0 million |
| Crude rate/100,000 population, 2015 | 367.5 | 611.8 | 244.3 |
| Global rank, 2015[b] | 17th | 15th | — |
| Change in number from 1990 to 2015, % | 62.1 | 49.1 | 33.1 |
| Change in crude rate from 1990 to 2015, % | 16.6 | 7.3 | −4.2 |
| Change in age-standardized rate from 1990 to 2015, % | 1.2 | −14.8 | −30.2 |
| **Disability-Adjusted Life-Years[79]** | | | |
| Number, 2015 | 35.3 million | 54.4 million | 19.0 million |
| Crude rate/100,000 population, 2015 | 478.4 | 738.5 | 257.7 |
| Global rank, 2015[b] | 20th | 15th | — |
| Change in number from 1990 to 2015, % | 63.3 | 52.1 | 34.7 |
| Change in crude rate from 1990 to 2015, % | 17.5 | 9.4 | −3.1 |
| Change in age-standardized rate from 1990 to 2015, % | 0.4 | −13.0 | −29.3 |

[a]Low GFR (glomerular filtration rate) as a risk factor resulted in the burden of CKD, cardiovascular disease (CVD), and gout.
[b]Global rank for CKD stages 3–5 refers to a rank among 295 diseases and injuries; global rank for a low GFR refers to a rank among 79 risk factors expressed as a crude rate.

prevalent in females (195.4 million) than in males (127.1 million).

Almost one-third of subjects with a reduced estimated glomerular filtration rate (GFR; CKD stages 3–5) in 2015 lived in two countries: India (69.8 million, equal to 5.5% of the population) and China (47.8 million, 3,6% of the population). The United States, Brazil, and Japan each had more than 10 million people with a reduced GFR, and Russia, Germany, Pakistan, Indonesia, Bangladesh, Mexico, and Nigeria each had between 5 and 8 million. Two independent meta-analyses have also included albuminuria with a normal GFR in the definition of altered kidney function and estimated the burden of CKD to be 13.4% (with 10.6% attributed to stages 3–5) globally,[75] and 14.3% (with 9.8% attributed to stages 3–5) in geographically dispersed developing countries.[15] It must be noted that these numbers do not fully take into account differences in age structure of the studied populations, which was included in the GBD study, and may explain the lower estimates of CKD prevalence in that study. Notwithstanding these differences, even the GBD study reported significant growth in the prevalence of CKD stages 3 to 5 since 1990—by 78.3% in absolute numbers and by 28.3% in crude rate. Moreover, there is significant heterogeneity among countries and regions, and the crude CKD prevalence rate is much higher in high-income countries (Fig. 75.4). In contrast, the age-standardized prevalence rate is higher among low- and middle-income countries (Fig. 75.5). The highest age-standardized prevalence of CKD stages 3 to 5 in 2015 was found in Southern and Western sub-Saharan Africa and South Asia (7285.5, 6462.4, and 6074.6/100,000 age-standardized population, respectively). Of concern, these rates were almost 50% higher than the mean global value. One of the prominent GBD study findings is that the change in age-standardized prevalence over 25 years, accounting for the dynamics of both age structure and population number, is much higher in the developing world (Fig. 75.6), whereas many HICs showed small increases or even a decline in age-standardized CKD rates. Importantly, the age-standardized prevalence rate increased significantly for 40 countries from 1990 to 2015, including India, Brazil, Pakistan, Mexico, Thailand, South Africa, and Iran, with each having more than 2 million people with CKD.

There is a significant disproportion between the crude and age-standardized rates of CKD, which is not always considered by policy makers. The crude prevalence rate (and thus the absolute number of patients requiring treatment) is higher in HICs (Fig. 75.7), mostly due to the longer life duration and higher proportion of older individuals. The age-standardized prevalence rate, which considers not only the size but also the age structure of a country's population, however, is much higher in LMICs (with a lower sociodemographic index; see Fig. 75.7), highlighting the fact that there are more young individuals of working age affected by CKD in lower-income compared with higher-income regions. This could suggest differences in causes, progression rates, and mortality of CKD by income region or lack of access to early detection and treatment of CKD in lower-income regions. It is well recognized that important differences in access to and quality of kidney care exist among different countries[76] and, even within the same country, different populations have higher risks of late referral to nephrology services.[77] Taken together, the higher frequency among younger individuals, limited access to kidney care, and inadequate access to essential medication contribute to the CKD burden, which has important implications for national economies, especially in countries with lower socioeconomic development.[78]

It is estimated that in 2015, CKD resulted in 1.23 million deaths worldwide, being the direct cause of 1 in 43 global

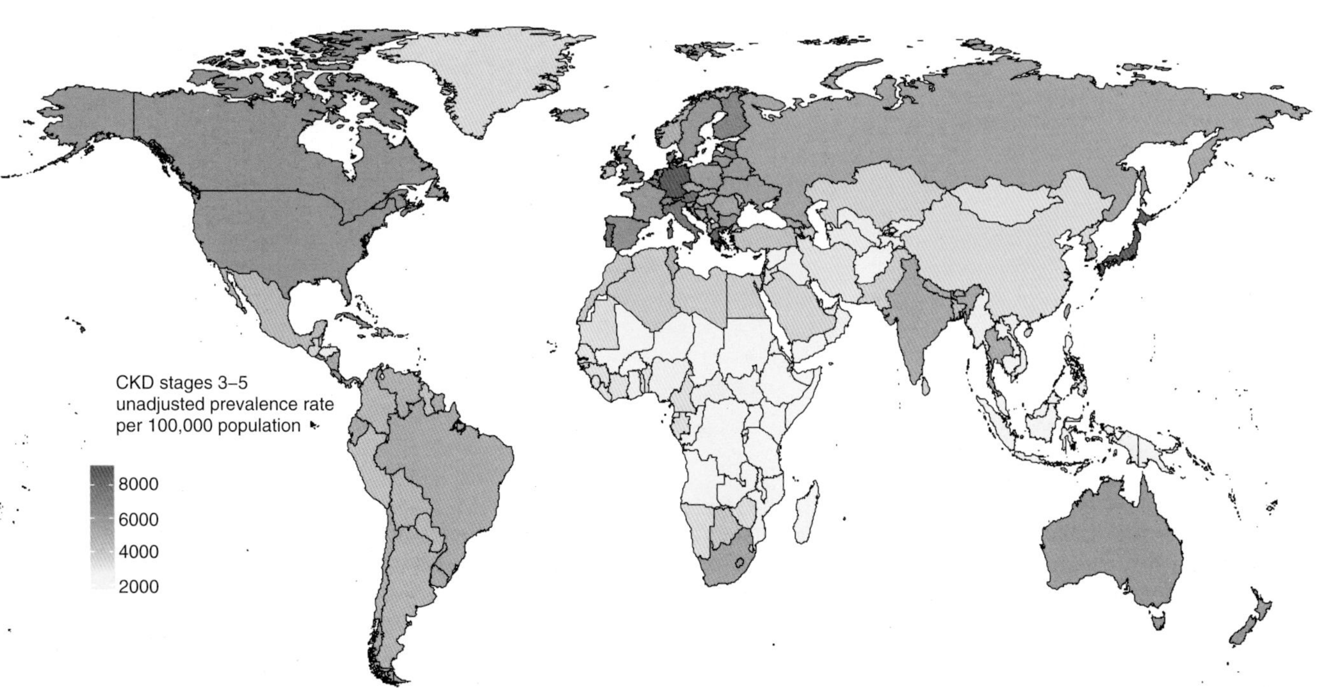


**Fig. 75.4** World map of crude prevalence rate/100,000 population for chronic kidney disease *(CKD)* stages 3–5 in 2015 (both genders combined).

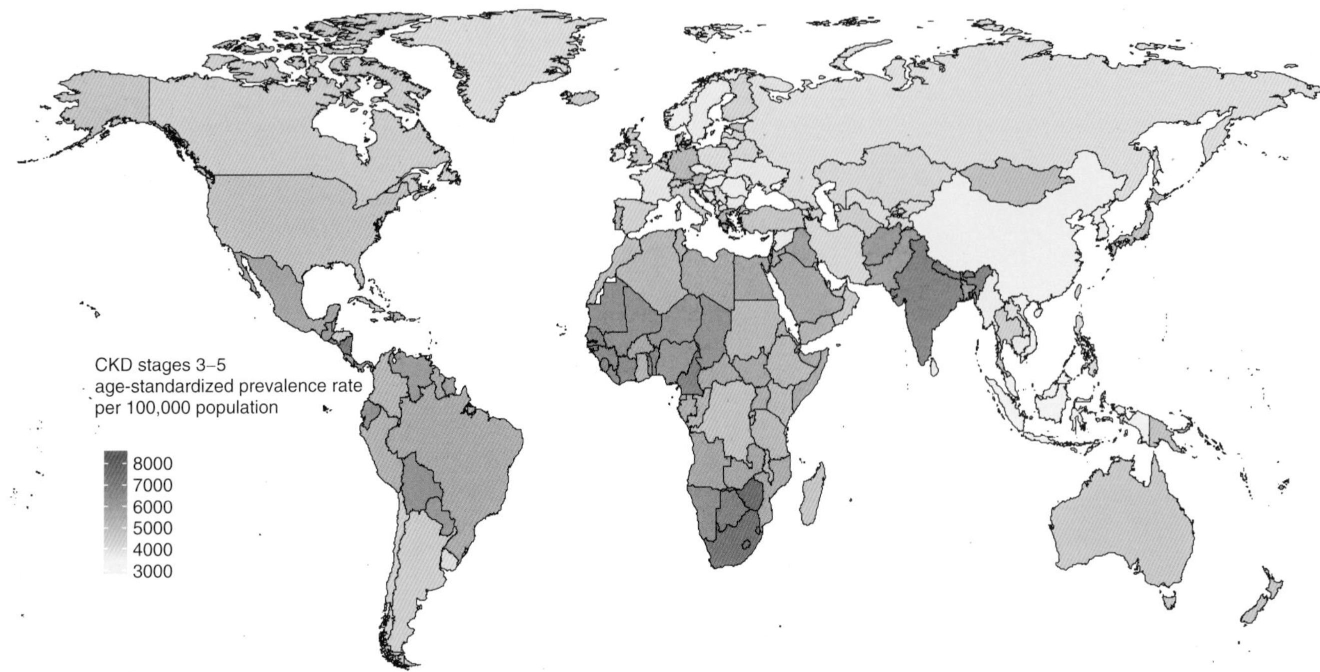


**Fig. 75.5** World map of age-standardized prevalence rate/100,000 population for chronic kidney disease *(CKD)* stages 3–5 in 2015 (both genders combined).

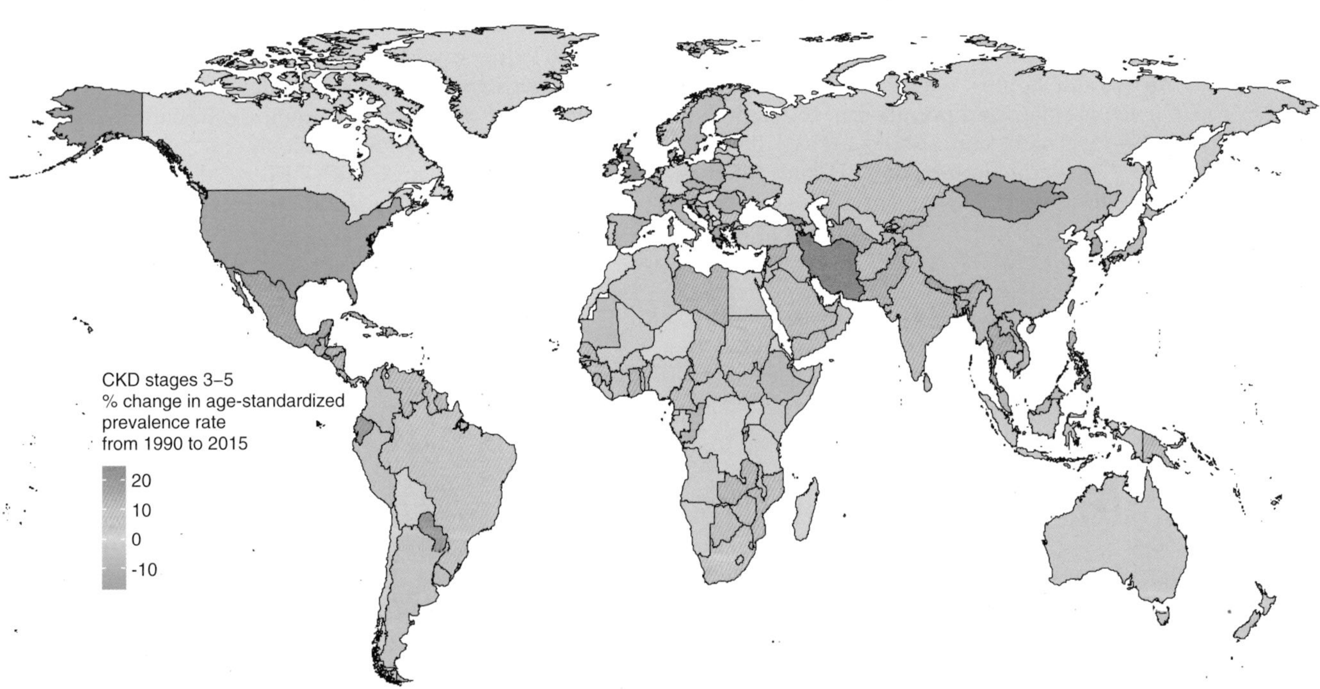


**Fig. 75.6** World map of changes from 1990 to 2015 in age-standardized prevalence rate/100,000 population for chronic kidney disease *(CKD)* stages 3–5 (both genders combined).

fatal outcomes (see Table 75.3).[2] Of note, CKD is one of the few causes of death that is still increasing (Fig. 75.8). The global mortality rate from CKD has increased by 49.8% over the past 25 years, which far exceeds the percentage change of most other NCDs, infections, and injuries. This increase made CKD the 10th leading cause of death in 2015 among over 300 causes accounted for in the GBD study, compared with its ranking of 19th in 1990. Considering the burden expressed in years of life lost (YLLs) due to premature death, the impact of CKD is somewhat lower, being the 17th leading cause of YLLs globally and accounting for 27.1 million YLLs in 2015. This observation reflects the fact that CKD affects more persons of advanced age. The aforementioned GBD study estimates of CKD mortality are based on sophisticated modeling that includes data on reported causes of death. A different approach to the estimation of CKD mortality, based

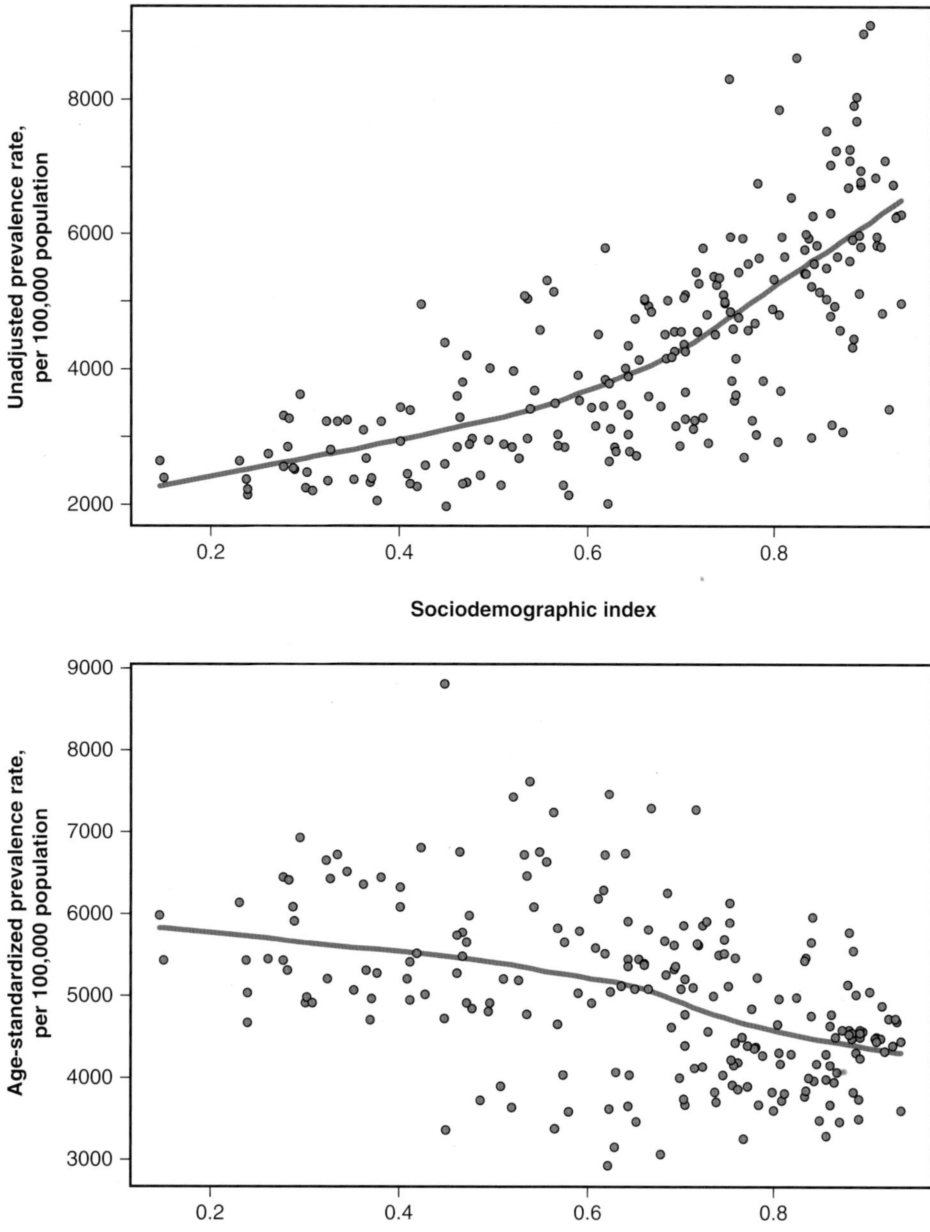


**Fig. 75.7** Country-level correlation between sociodemographic index and chronic kidney disease *(CKD)* stages 3–5 prevalence rate/100,000 population in 2015 (both genders combined). *Upper panel* shows crude prevalence rate; *lower panel* shows age-standardized prevalence rate.

on the comparison of actual provision of RRT (dialysis and transplantation) and estimated RRT need,[3] has suggested that between 2.3 and 7.1 million deaths worldwide could be attributable to death from ESKD due to lack of access to RRT. Lack of access to diagnosis of CKD in many lower-income regions hampers the accurate measurement of the true global CKD burden, which may therefore be underestimated in current studies.

Worldwide, the CKD-related number of years lived with disability (YLDs) accounted for almost 8.17 million in 2015, which corresponds to 1 of each 100 global YLDs from all diseases. This is an important number considering that the vast majority of individuals with CKD stage 3 are not included in the YLDs due to the GBD study methodology (see Table 75.3).[72] Disability-adjusted life years (DALYs),[79] as a measure of disease burden, sums YLLs and YLDs, thus accounting for both mortality and morbidity. CKD led to 35.26 million DALYs globally in 2015, reflecting a growth of 63.3% over 25 years. In contrast, the age-standardized DALY rate did not change significantly over the same period (0.4%), indicating that population growth and aging were the major drivers of global CKD DALYs.[79] However, age-standardized DALY rates did significantly increase in Oceania, Central Asia, high-income North America, and Central Latin America, highlighting a true increase in kidney disease burden, independent of demographic factors, and pointing to regions that require special attention to improve kidney health. Worldwide, the age-standardized DALY rate for CKD has increased from the 25th to the 20th position since 1990, in part because many other diseases demonstrated a decrease in this metric over the same period. All CKD burden indicators were substantially higher among those in older age groups (Fig. 75.9).

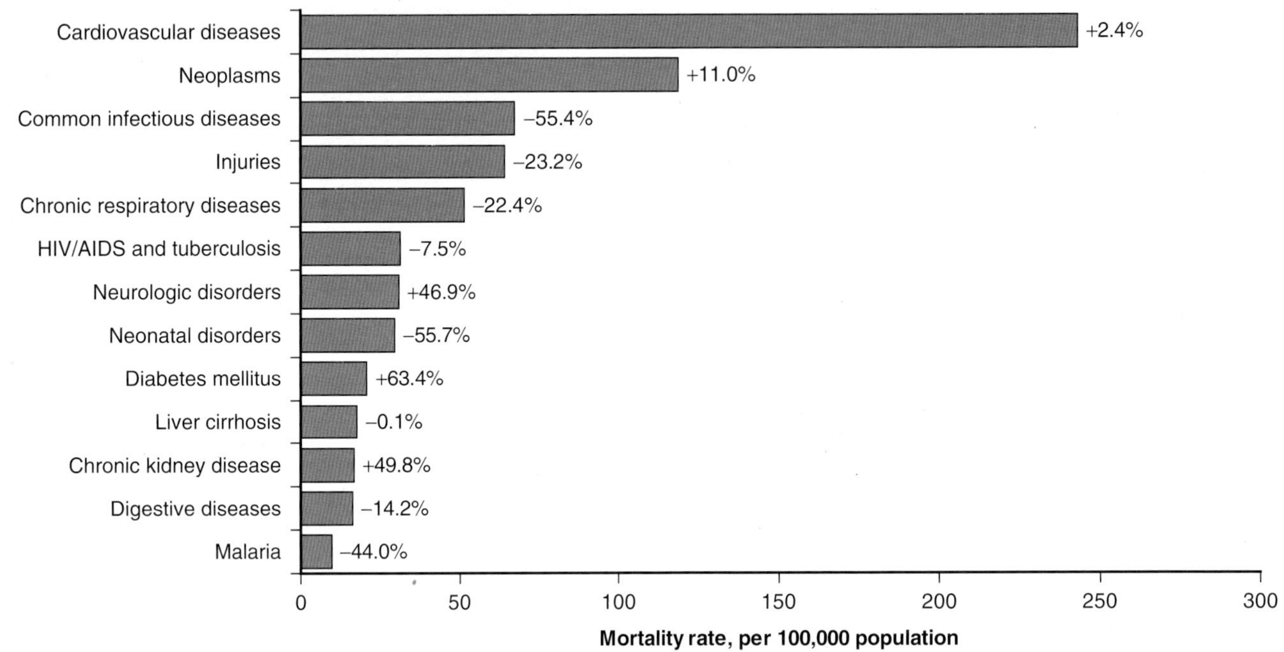


**Fig. 75.8 Mortality crude rate for major classes of diseases and injuries.** *Bars* represent mortality rate/100,000 population in 2015; numbers at the *right side of bars* represent percentage change in mortality rate between 1990 and 2015.

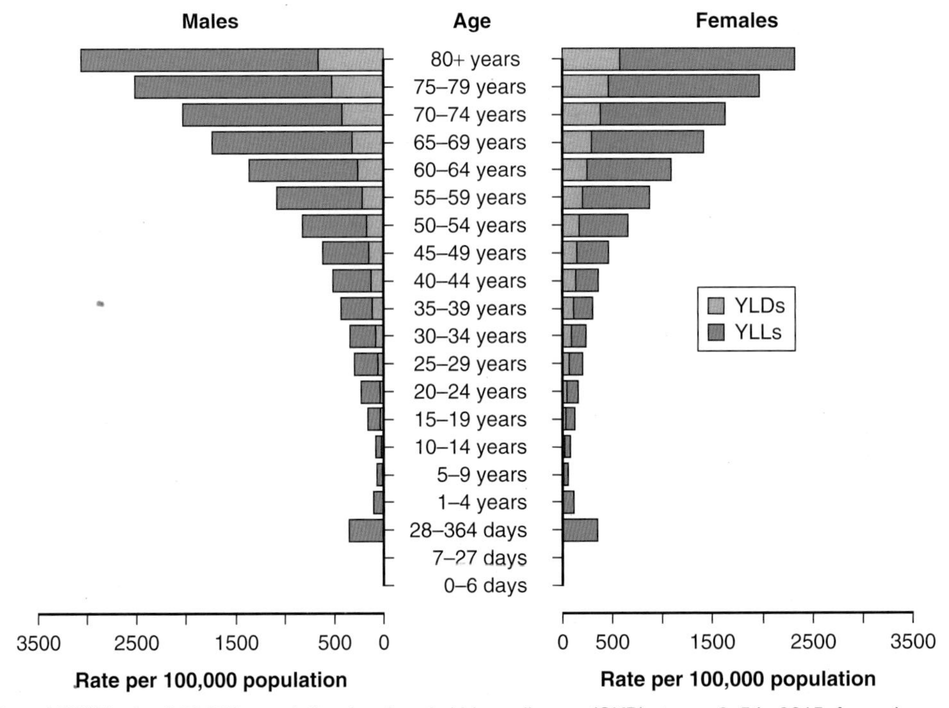


**Fig. 75.9** YLL, YLD, and DALY rates/100,000 population for chronic kidney disease (CKD) stages 3–5 in 2015, for males and females according to age group. *Orange bars* represent YLDs, *blue bars* represent YLLs; total size of the bars equal to DALYs. *DALYs,* Disability-adjusted life years; *YLDs,* years lived with disability; *YLLs,* years of life lost.

## MORTALITY AND MORBIDITY DUE TO CARDIOVASCULAR DISEASE DRIVEN BY LOW GLOMERULAR FILTRATION RATE

Importantly, kidney disease represents a direct cause of morbidity and mortality and is a risk factor for morbidity and mortality from other diseases. The GBD study has recognized this double role of kidney disease and specifically considered a low GFR as a risk factor for CVD and gout.[74] The global number of YLDs attributed to low GFR includes those accounted for by CKD itself (8.17 million), as well as for CVD (0.98 million), and a minor fraction for gout (0.18 million). Thus, in total, a low GFR accounted for 9.34 million YLDs in 2015 (see Table 75.3). Worldwide, a low GFR resulted in 27.1 million YLLs from CKD itself and 18.0 million YLLs for CVD, accounting for the total of 45.1 million YLLs in 2015. In other words, 1 of each 22 global YLDs, and 1 of each 18 YLLs from all risk factors in 2015 was attributed to a low GFR. A decreased GFR accounted for 1.19 million CVD deaths, which was almost equal to the 1.23 million deaths due to CKD itself. The number of CVD deaths attributed to a low GFR increased by 42%, whereas the number of deaths directly due to CKD stages 3 to 5 increased by 108% over 25 years. These numbers reflect less success in reducing mortality from kidney disease compared with CVD over this period. Within such growth, a low GFR became the 11th leading risk factor contributing to number of deaths in 2015 (ranked 17th in 1990). The total number of DALYs due to low GFR reached a total of 54.43 million in 2015, of which 35.26 million corresponded to CKD, 18.99 million to CVD, and 0.18 million to gout. Considering both absolute count and crude and age-standardized DALY rates/100,000 population, a low GFR ranked 15th among all 79 GBD risk factors considered, thus outranking such factors as low physical activity, drug use, unsafe sanitation, occupational injuries, and iron, vitamin A, and zinc deficiencies.[74] In total, one of each 19 DALYs in the world in 2015 was attributed to a low GFR.

The GBD study results permit expression of the burden of decreased GFR for each country and comparisons of the burden (expressed as DALY rates) of CKD and GFR-related CVD between countries (Fig. 75.10). In general, these two conditions are well correlated, but there are several countries with prominent discordance, which could be explained either by the extremely high burden of CVD (as in former socialist countries) or an exceptionally high burden of CKD morbidity and mortality (as in Mexico, El Salvador, and Thailand). On the global scale, CVD accounted for 11.3% of all age-standardized YLDs and 36.5% of all age-standardized DALYs due to a low GFR. From the cardiovascular perspective, a low GFR was responsible for 4.0% of all age-standardized YLDs and 5.7% of all age-standardized DALYs for CVD in 2015. In other words, a low GFR resulted in one of each 25 CVD age-standardized YLDs and one of each 17 CVD age-standardized DALYs. This was almost double the impact on CVD from excessive alcohol use, comparable with the impact of low physical activity, and only three times lower than the impact of high fasting plasma glucose levels or smoking as CVD risk factors.[74]

## SCOPE OF AMENABLE CHRONIC KIDNEY DISEASE MORTALITY AMENABLE TO INTERVENTION

In LLMICs, the burden of CKD is much higher as compared with high-income regions, especially if age-standardized rates are considered. The major reason for the higher burden in LLMICs is the excessive mortality due to lack of access to RRT and higher rates of fatal CVD events where health facilities are inadequate or universal health coverage is not in place. In countries where CKD-related mortality is higher, a substantial part of the population would not survive to live with disability; therefore, comparison of the ratio of YLLs to YLDs as composite indicators of mortality and morbidity would provide important information that could be used as a

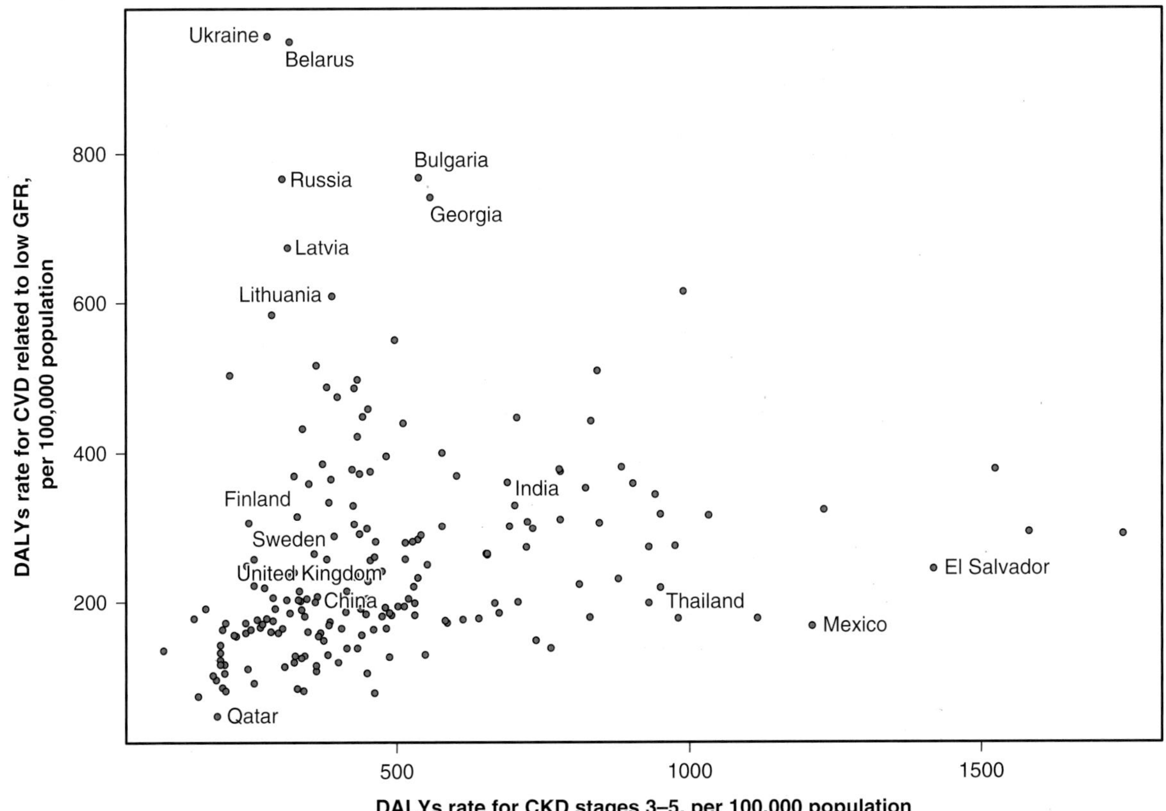


**Fig. 75.10** Country-level DALY crude rates/100,000 population for chronic kidney disease *(CKD)* stages 3–5 and cardiovascular diseases *(CVD)* attributed to low glomerular filtration rate *(GFR)* in 2015 (both genders combined). *DALY,* Disability-adjusted life-year.

surrogate marker of amenable mortality (Fig. 75.11). In HICs, the ratio of YLDs to YLLs for CKD is close to 1 (e.g., CKD in Western Europe accounted for 676.7 thousand YLDs and for 822.7 thousand YLLs in 2015). This reflects the universal provision of RRT that prevents a substantial proportion of immediate CKD deaths and the longer duration of a healthy life, which reduces both morbidity and mortality. An exception to this model, however, is the United States where, despite being the world's largest economy, the number of YLLs is almost twice as high as YLDs, indicating a greater impact of CKD mortality. This observation highlights the importance of universal health coverage because its lack leads to late referral to nephrology services and higher rates of complications and mortality.[80]

A more critical situation exists in regions with both a shortage of RRT treatment and mainly OOP health expenditures, where YLLs prominently predominate over YLDs; the ratio is close to 5 in Southern sub-Saharan Africa and to 15 in Oceania. In such emerging regions, data are sparse but, as discussed earlier, even after the start of dialysis, a vast majority of patients are forced to withdraw from this life-saving treatment (up to 85% of the incident patients) and die because of their inability to pay for RRT.[3,35] The difference between YLLs and YLDs illustrates how many lives could be saved by implementing appropriate prevention strategies, conducting early kidney disease detection programs, educating health personnel, improving access to nephroprotective treatment and RRT, and preventing CKD and CVD complications. Considering the global numbers of 27.1 million YLLs and 8.2 million YLDs due to CKD in 2015, the reduction of amenable CKD mortality in 2015 would have been expected to save almost 20 million YLLs globally.

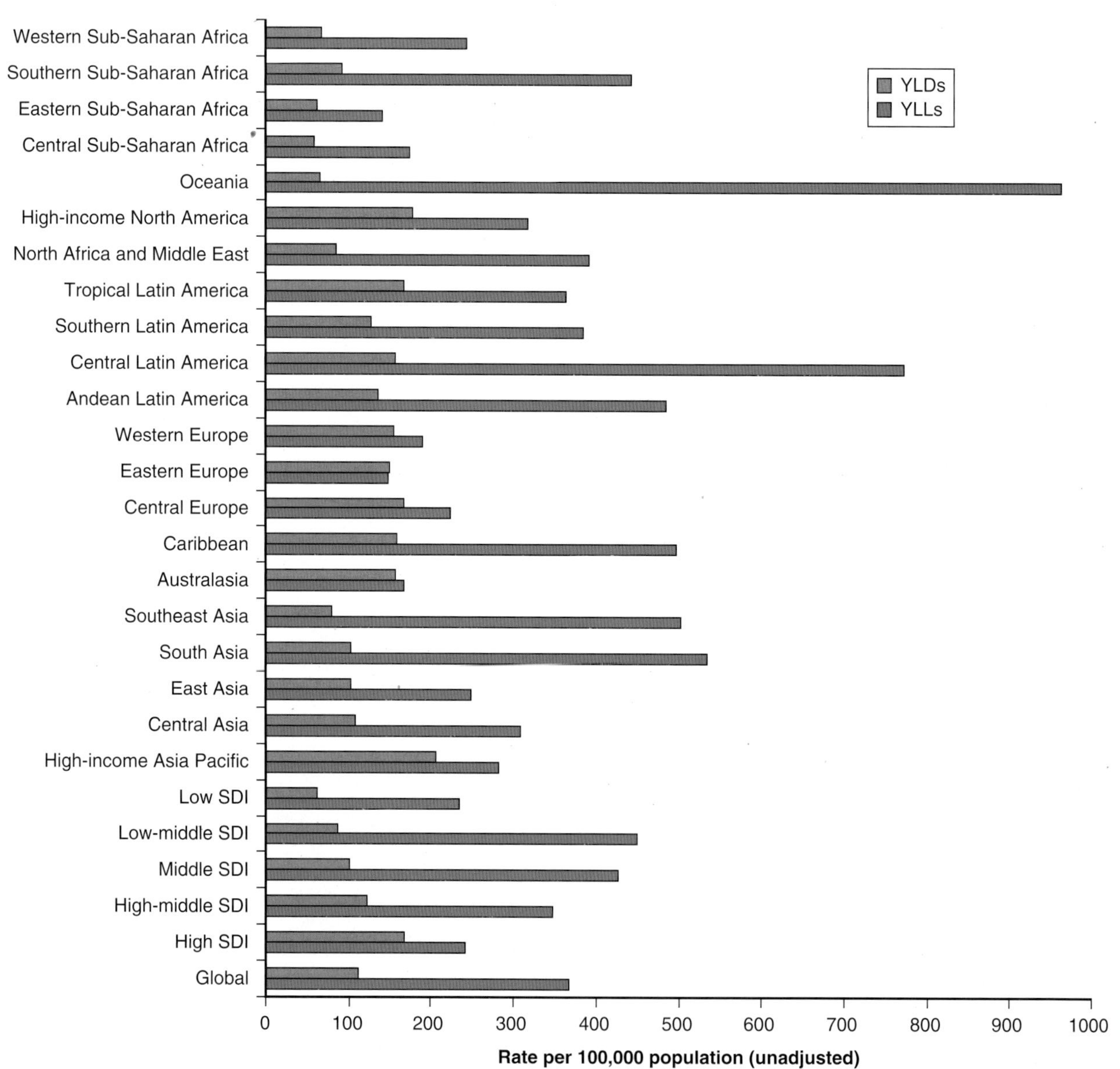


**Fig. 75.11** Global and regional burden of chronic kidney disease *(CKD)* stages 3–5 in YLLs and YLDs crude rates/100,000 population for 2015 (both genders combined). *YLDs,* Years lived with disability; *YLLs,* years of life lost.

## DRIVERS OF EPIDEMIOLOGIC TRANSITION FOR CHRONIC KIDNEY DISEASE

The changes in epidemiology of CKD over recent decades may have various causative factors. First, CKD morbidity and mortality are related to the global processes of population growth, aging, and migration. The world's population grew from 5.3 billion in 1990 to 7.3 billion in 2015. In the same period, the median global age increased from 24 to 30 years, and the proportion of urban populations increased from 43% to 53.8% (http://www.un.org/en/development/desa/population/theme/trends/index.shtml). These changes directly affect the epidemiology of CKD, with absolute counts of CKD patients increasing in proportion to population growth and aging and possibly also to improved health outcomes in the urban populations. This epidemiologic transition also drives the metabolic and nutritional risk factors for CKD development and progression. Thus, over 25 years, the CKD age-standardized DALY rates attributable to arterial hypertension have increased by 6.8%, to high fasting plasma glucose levels by 15.0%, to high body mass index by 34.2%, and to high-sodium diet by 5.6%. During the same period, however, the DALY rates attributable to these risk factors have decreased in the case of CVD.[74]

A second important driver of CKD growth, especially relevant to the increase in LMICs, is the persistent inequality among different population subgroups in exposure to risk factors, as well as access to prevention and treatment. Usually countries with lower economic development have higher rates of CKD and of NCDs in general.[81] However, even within the same country, substantial inequalities exist in access to medical care and RRT in particular.[82] Thus, in many regions, medical care for rural populations is insufficiently developed and available, and one would expect a higher mortality from CKD and ESKD, even if the prevalence of CKD risk factors might be lower in rural settings. CKD is also more prevalent among the urban poor than those of higher socioeconomic status in developed countries.[83] Other vulnerable groups include women, older persons, and children who in many societies still have reduced access to medical treatment. Women have a higher CKD prevalence but generally a lower rate of CKD progression as compared with men. In addition, there is evidence of lower access to kidney treatment for women.[84] Moreover, CKD in pregnant woman substantially increases the risk of preeclampsia, preterm delivery, small-for-gestational-age and low-birth-weight infants, all factors associated with low nephron number and increased risks of CKD and other NCDs over the life course (see Chapter 21).[85,86] Thus, persisting inequalities and lack of attention to women's health form a vicious circle that contributes to the CKD burden over generations. It could be speculated that current higher age-standardized rates of CKD burden in LLMICs may in part be affected by suboptimal fetal and early childhood nutrition and development leading to CKD in later life. Future generations may see the impact of the current humanitarian crises on fetal health and CKD epidemiology scattered worldwide over the coming decades.

A third reason underlying the CKD epidemiologic transition is the increase in CKD burden in certain countries and whole regions, independent of changes in the general population. Positive and significant dynamics of age-standardized CKD rates across regions highlight the most problematic countries where investigation is urgently needed to examine and address the factors leading to increasing age-standardized rates. An example of such an emerging CKD epidemic is "CKD of unknown cause," CKDu), which affects predominantly adult agricultural workers in subequatorial countries of Central America and South Asia. Available data have not permitted an estimate of the burden of CKDu over time, but in some regions such as Nicaragua, CKD is the primary cause of death, fueled by the epidemic of CKDu.[2] Additional evidence, not well represented in the scientific literature, has suggested that other groups of workers (e.g., metal and diamond miners, industrial paint shop workers) with high exposure to environmental or occupational hazards are also affected by nephropathies that require further investigation and efforts at prevention.[87–89] It is possible that worldwide, millions of people work or live in unsafe environments, which adds to the global CKD burden.

A fourth factor influencing CKD estimates is the precision of estimated GFR (eGFR) equations (i.e., the correspondence between measured and estimated GFR) and the availability of repetitive testing to confirm chronic persistence of abnormal kidney disease markers. Use of different GFR estimation equations may lead up to a 30% difference in CKD prevalence estimates. A meta-analysis analyzing data from 1.1 million individuals has found that the proportion of subjects with a low GFR decreased from 8.7% or 6.3% with the use of the Chronic Kidney Disease Epidemiology Collaboration (CKD-EPI) equation relative to the Modification of Diet in Renal Disease Study (MDRD) equation.[90] Because a substantial amount of data on CKD prevalence in the GBD study was obtained by using the MDRD equation, the true CKD estimates in the studied populations could be substantially lower. Of note, in the GBD study, the reference equation was MDRD until 2015, but was switched to the CKD-EPI equation as of 2016 with the application of a specific crosswalk procedure. Consequently, a decrease in CKD prevalence estimates will occur in the GBD study in comparison with the aforementioned numbers simply because of the use of a different reference eGFR equation. These observations demonstrate the importance of a good instrument to measure kidney function for both individual patient and population studies to best inform planning of the necessary health interventions.

## ACUTE KIDNEY INJURY AND THE 0BY25 INITIATIVE

The 0by25 initiative of the International Society of Nephrology (ISN), launched in 2013, aimed to raise awareness about the preventability and treatability of AKI worldwide, targeting no preventable deaths from AKI by 2025. As described earlier, AKI is associated with significant morbidity and mortality, but data have not thus far been reported by the GBD study. One aim of the 0by25 initiative was to determine the burden of AKI. Two large meta-analyses and systematic reviews were performed, which reported that AKI affected 21% of hospital admissions worldwide.[4,19,24] Most cases of AKI were Kidney Disease: Improving Global Outcomes (KDIGO) stage 1, and dialysis was required in 11% of cases.[4] Pooled mortality was 21%. The 0by25 investigators also conducted a global snapshot of AKI, inviting clinicians to enter data about patients with AKI over a 2-month period.[24] The most common causes of AKI were hypotension in HICs and dehydration in LLMICs. Dialysis requirement and mortality were higher in LMICS, likely reflecting the severity of illness (lateness) on presentation. The meta-analyses and the global snapshot are, however, inherently biased by publication availability and by elective participation in the snapshot; therefore, the true global picture of AKI remains unknown. What is clear is that the causes of AKI differ across the globe, depending on prevalence rates of diabetes and hypertension, infections, and public health interventions.[20,22,91] As with CKD, AKI in LLMICs tends to affect younger individuals and is more severe on presentation to hospital.[18,19,21,22] The 0by25 initiative has, however, served to raise awareness about AKI globally. Future iterations of the GBD study will attempt to report AKI data better, which will be an important step in achieving a more complete picture of the global burden of kidney disease.

### SAVING YOUNG LIVES INITIATIVE

There has been a global push for universal access to dialysis for AKI through the 0by25 and Saving Young Lives (SYL), given that dialysis need should be temporary because renal function can recover and therefore is less expensive per patient than lifelong treatment for ESKD.[4] The SYL initiative, launched as a combined endeavor between the International Pediatric Nephrology Association, ISN, International Society of Peritoneal Dialysis, and European Peritoneal Dialysis in 2012, has saved the lives of several hundred individuals (mostly children) over the past 5 years and has trained and mentored local physicians and nurses to perform acute PD[92] using home-made dialysis solutions and innovative use of alternative catheters (Table 75.4).[93,94] This program has remained dependent on external funding and is highly reliant on individual champions. Unexpected challenges, outlined by those implementing SYL programs, include lack of access to routine laboratory testing, staff changes, unreliability of financing sources, cultural differences, and lack of referrals to SYL centers.[94] These challenges highlight the crucial importance of program integration into existing health care system structures, which is important to avoid generation of isolated programs and contribute to strengthening of the health care system.

## THE GLOBAL KIDNEY HEALTH ATLAS

The Global Kidney Health Atlas (GKHA), as part of the "Closing the Gaps" initiative of the ISN, has provided an overview of the current state of kidney care and how it is organized and structured across the world, focusing on existing kidney care (AKI, CKD), awareness levels (based on existence of relevant policies and guidelines), care structures, and workforce for optimal care delivery.[11,95,96] A total of 125 United Nations Member States (encompassing 93% of the world's population) responded to the survey, as described in more detail elsewhere.[97–102] For comprehensiveness, the elements of the survey were evaluated within the framework of the health systems building blocks outlined by the WHO—leadership and governance, health care financing, health care workforce, medical products and technologies, information and research, and service delivery.[103] Study respondents across countries included national nephrology society leaders, policy makers, and patient organization representatives identified by the country and regional nephrology leadership through the ISN.[95] As expected, there was significant variation across countries on the key survey elements discussed later.[97–102]

### AWARENESS OF KIDNEY HEALTH AS A GOVERNMENT PRIORITY, STRATEGIES, GUIDELINES, AND ADVOCACY

CKD was recognized as a health care priority (defined as outlining principles and/or defining practices) by government in 36% of countries overall ($n$ = 42/116) and in 53% ($n$ = 9/17), 52% ($n$ = 16/31), 20% ($n$ = 6/30), and 29% ($n$ = 11/38) of low, lower middle, upper middle, and high-income countries, respectively. Overall, 42% of countries ($n$ = 49/116) reported an advocacy group at higher levels of government to raise the profile of CKD and its prevention, whereas only

**Table 75.4 Preparation of Dialysis Solution Using Commercially Available Intravenous Fluid[a]**

| Type of Fluid | $Na^+$ | $K^+$ | $Ca^{2+}$ | Mg | $Cl^-$ | $HCO_3^-$ | Lactate | pH | Osmolarity |
|---|---|---|---|---|---|---|---|---|---|
| Hartmann's solution | 131 | 5 | 2.0 | | 111 | | 29 | 7.0 | 278 |
| Ringer's lactate | 131 | 5 | 1.8 | | 112 | | 28 | 6.5 | 279 |
| Plasmalyte B | 130 | 4 | 0 | 1.5 | 110 | 27 | | 7.4 | 273 |
| Half-normal saline | 77 | | | | 77 | | | 5.0 | 154 |

[a]Preparation of dialysis solutions using the above intravenous solutions:

- 1 L Plasmalyte + 30 mL 50% dextrose (15 g) will generate a solution with the following concentrations: glucose, 1.45%; Na, 126 mmol/L; $HCO_3^-$, 2 7 mmol/L; K, 3.8 mmol/L; Mg, 1.45 mmol/L; osmolarity = 342 osm.

This is very similar to some of the bicarbonate-based solutions sold by industry:

- 1 L Ringer's lactate + 30 mL 50% dextrose (15 g) will generate a solution with the following concentrations: Na, 127 mmol/L; lactate, 27 mmol/L; Ca, 1.36 mmol/L; K, 3.8 mmol/L; glucose 1.45 %; osmolarity = 346 osm.

This is similar to lactate-based peritoneal dialysis solutions.

**NOTE:** The above solutions both contain potassium.

- 1 L half-normal saline + 40 mL 8.5% $NaHCO_3$ (40 mmol) + 40 mL 50% dextrose (20 g) + 60 mL 3% NaCl (30 mmol) will generate a solution with approximately the following concentrations: Na, ± 130 mmol/L; $HCO_3^-$, 35 mmol/L; glucose, 1.7%; osmolarity = 340 osm.

*$Na^+$*, Sodium; *$K^+$*, potassium; *$Ca^{2+}$*, calcium; *Mg*, magnesium; *$Cl^-$*, chlorine; *$HCO_3^-$*, bicarbonate.

Adapted from Cullis Abdelraheem M, Abrahams G, et al. Peritoneal dialysis for acute kidney injury. *Perit Dial Int.* 2014;34(5):494–517.

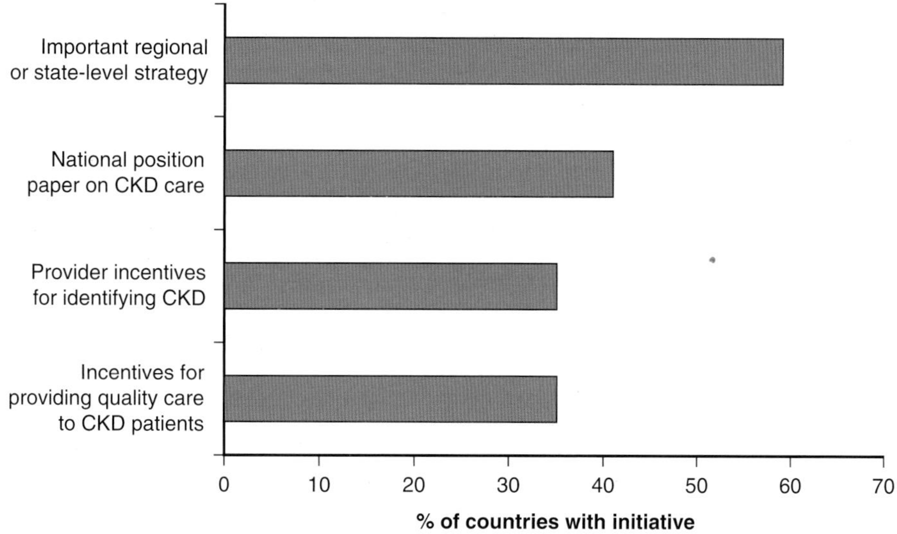


**Fig. 75.12 Reported distribution of initiatives for promoting chronic kidney disease *(CKD)* as a health care priority among countries with no national strategy for CKD.** Of the 43 countries with no CKD strategy, 34 (79%) responded to this question. Percentages do not total 100% because countries were able to select more than one option. (Data from Global Kidney Health Atlas. https://www.theisn.org/images/ISN_Biennial_Report_2011-2013/GKHAtlas_Linked_Compressed1.pdf.)

19% of countries ($n = 21/116$) reported advocacy for AKI.[95,99] A lack of government priority for kidney health could represent a lack of awareness of CKD or the prioritization of other political issues.

It is also necessary to consider that the definition of health priority differs across countries. For example, a priority in some regions could represent a focus on prevention, whereas in others it could refer to increasing access to treatment. Advocacy for AKI was less than half that for CKD. The reduced attention given to AKI has been recognized, and the 0by25 initiative is one response to this. Dissemination of this strategy aims to increase advocacy and awareness of the importance of preventing AKI. Both CKD and AKI advocacy groups were more common in LICs compared with HICs; however, details regarding the roles or actions of the advocacy groups were not reported.

Overall, 17% of countries ($n = 19/109$) reported a national strategy for improving awareness and optimal care for nondialysis CKD patients, 43% for chronic dialysis patients ($n = 45/104$), and 40% for kidney transplant patients ($n = 40/100$). Conversely, 37% of countries ($n = 43/116$) reported no national strategy for CKD care (irrespective of nondialysis CKD, chronic dialysis, or transplantation). These countries reported other initiatives that identified CKD as a health care priority, including strategies at a regional or state level, a national position paper on CKD (a document providing an overview of information and recommendations for kidney care, but not mandated by legislation), and incentives for identifying CKD and providing quality care to CKD patients (Fig. 75.12). For AKI, 49% of countries ($n = 57/116$) reported at least one strategy for improving the identification of AKI (Fig. 75.13). The most common strategies were having tools available for the detection and management of AKI (32%; $n = 37/116$) and increasing access to acute dialysis facilities (31%; $n = 36/116$); 16% of countries ($n = 19/116$) reported having a national position paper on AKI identification and care.

Overall, national strategies for enhancing awareness of kidney disease were quite low, particularly in LICs. Because of their importance in providing consistent high-quality and safe care and for standardization of metrics for evaluating quality and outcomes of care, the development of national strategies to address kidney disease should receive more attention. Professional guidelines and care frameworks are vital for enhancing the understanding of AKI and CKD care. Despite the significant work of the ISN and a related organization (KDIGO) to facilitate adoption of practice guidelines in kidney care across countries, this is not yet universal. Access to management and referral guidelines was more common for CKD (79%; $n = 92/116$) than AKI (53%; $n = 61/116$; Table 75.5). A lack of guidelines was more common among LICs compared with HICs for both AKI and CKD. AKI guidelines focused on the identification of AKI in inpatient (95%; $n = 57/60$) and outpatient (67%; n = 40/60) settings, access to dialysis treatment (93%; $n = 56/60$), timing and urgency for nephrology referral (80%; $n = 48/60$), and protocols for mitigating risk of AKI in specific situations (70%; $n = 42/60$). CKD guidelines covered complication management (86%; $n = 79/92$), identification of CKD progression (88%; $n = 81/92$), timing and urgency of nephrology referral (87%; $n = 80/92$), risk factor management (84%; $n = 77/92$), and multidisciplinary care approaches (71%; $n = 65/92$).

Of note, in 50% of countries rated, both awareness and adoption of CKD guidelines among non-nephrologist physicians was suboptimal. This may reflect an equally low level of awareness about CKD in general. Awareness of CKD among non-nephrologist specialists was reported as low or below average (based on perception of survey respondents of what they deemed to be level of awareness about CKD guidelines in their countries) by 49% of countries and as average by 35% of countries and, among primary care physicians, as low or below average by 50% of countries. With the recognition that non-nephrologist physicians have low awareness and

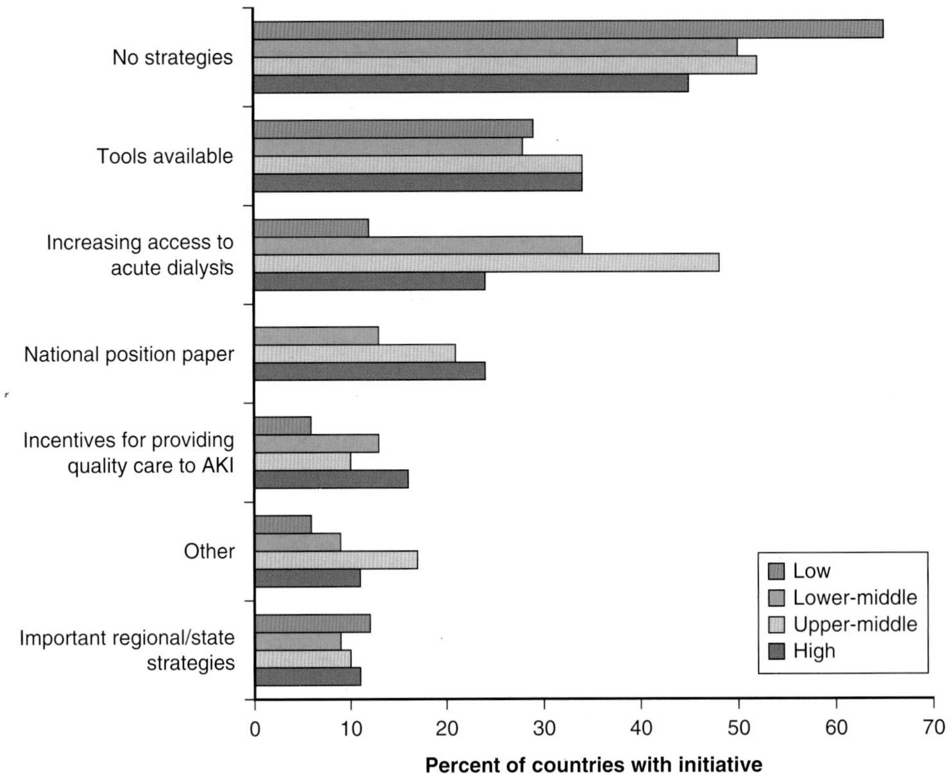


**Fig. 75.13 National policies and strategies for identifying acute kidney injury *(AKI)* by World Bank income group across 116 countries.** Percentages do not total 100% because countries were able to select more than one option. (Data from Global Kidney Health Atlas. https://www.theisn.org/images/ISN_Biennial_Report_2011-2013/GKHAtlas_Linked_Compressed1.pdf.)

**Table 75.5 Availability of and Access to Management and Referral Guidelines for Kidney Care Across 116 Countries**

| | **AKI Management and Referral Guidelines** | | | | **CKD Management and Referral Guidelines** | | | |
|---|---|---|---|---|---|---|---|---|
| **Region** | National *N* (%) | Regional *N* (%) | International *N* (%) | None *N* (%) | National *N* (%) | Regional *N* (%) | International *N* (%) | None *N* (%) |
| Overall | 8 (7) | 1 (1) | 52 (45) | 55 (47) | 31 (27) | 1 (1) | 60 (52) | 24 (21) |
| **ISN Region** | | | | | | | | |
| Africa | 2 (7) | 0 (0) | 8 (27) | 20 (67) | 4 (13) | 0 (0) | 13 (43) | 13 (43) |
| Eastern and Central Europe | 0 (0) | 0 (0) | 15 (94) | 1 (6) | 2 (13) | 0 (0) | 13 (81) | 1 (6) |
| LAC | 1 (6) | 0 (0) | 7 (44) | 8 (50) | 9 (56) | 0 (0) | 7 (44) | 0 (0) |
| Middle East | 0 (0) | 0 (0) | 5 (38) | 8 (62) | 1 (8) | 1 (8) | 8 (62) | 3 (23) |
| NIS and Russia | 2 (33) | 0 (0) | 3 (50) | 1 (17) | 1 (17) | 0 (0) | 5 (83) | 0 (0) |
| North America | 0 (0) | 0 (0) | 2 (100) | 0 (0) | 1 (50) | 0 (0) | 1 (50) | 0 (0) |
| North and East Asia | 0 (0) | 0 (0) | 2 (33) | 4 (67) | 3 (50) | 0 (0) | 3 (50) | 0 (0) |
| OSEA | 2 (15) | 1 (8) | 3 (23) | 7 (54) | 6 (46) | 0 (0) | 2 (15) | 5 (38) |
| South Asia | 0 (0) | 0 (0) | 1 (20) | 4 (80) | 0 (0) | 0 (0) | 3 (60) | 2 (40) |
| Western Europe | 1 (11) | 0 (0) | 6 (67) | 2 (22) | 4 (44) | 0 (0) | 5 (56) | 0 (0) |
| **World Bank Income Group** | | | | | | | | |
| Low Income | 0 (0) | 0 (0) | 3 (18) | 14 (82) | 1 (6) | 0 (0) | 6 (35) | 10 (59) |
| Lower middle income | 5 (16) | 0 (0) | 11 (35) | 15 (48) | 7 (23) | 0 (0) | 16 (52) | 8 (26) |
| Upper middle income | 1 (3) | 1 (3) | 14 (47) | 14 (47) | 9 (30) | 0 (0) | 16 (53) | 5 (17) |
| High Income | 2 (5) | 0 (0) | 24 (63) | 12 (32) | 14 (37) | 1 (3) | 22 (58) | 1 (3) |

*AKI*, Acute kidney injury; *CKD*, chronic kidney disease; *ISN*, International Society of Nephrology; *LAC*, Latin America and the Caribbean; *NIS*, newly independent states (of the former Soviet Union); *OSEA*, Oceania and Southeast Asia.

Adapted from GBD 2015 Mortality and Causes of Death Collaborators. Global, regional, and national life expectancy, all-cause mortality, and cause-specific mortality for 249 causes of death, 1980–2015: a systematic analysis for the Global Burden of Disease Study 2015. *Lancet.* 2016;388(10053):1459–1544; and from Global Kidney Health Atlas. https://www.theisn.org/ images/ISN_Biennial_Report_2011-2013/GKHAtlas_Linked_Compressed1.pdf.

adoption of CKD guidelines, it is important to determine if it is due to lack of distribution, accessibility, or interest. Even in cases where national or regional guidelines do not exist, international guidelines should be accessible; however, if barriers such as Internet access or language prevent the distribution or adoption of guidelines, these issues should be addressed. Similar to CKD guidelines, nearly 50% of countries rated both awareness and adoption of AKI guidelines among non-nephrologist physicians as low or below average, and this may correspond with the limited awareness of AKI in general among non-nephrologist specialists and primary care physicians. Notably, the level of awareness and level of adoption of AKI guidelines were similar, suggesting that awareness may not be as much of an issue as reasons why guidelines are not being adopted. Further efforts to increase awareness of AKI and increase adoption of guidelines are warranted.

## INFRASTRUCTURE FOR TREATMENT OF ACUTE KIDNEY INJURY AND CHRONIC KIDNEY DISEASE

The GKHA was the first initiative to assess global capacity for kidney care in terms of the key building blocks of a functional health system and to evaluate the readiness of countries and regions to enhance such care.[95,98,99,101] There were significant gaps in services, workforce, and capacity for research in some countries and regions. For example, most countries in Africa had no facilities for PD or kidney transplantation. Few countries had public funding for RRT services and medications for CKD care (including dialysis and transplant); there was a large private contribution toward payment for RRT services and medications, particularly in countries across Africa, South Asia, Oceania, and Southeast Asia.[97] More than two-thirds of countries reported the absence of capacity to participate in clinical research.[100]

### Availability of Chronic Kidney Disease Monitoring and Management Services

There has been wide variation in terms of availability of services for CKD monitoring and management at the primary, secondary, and tertiary care levels across countries based on income groups (Fig. 75.14).[95,104] LMICs, especially in Africa, had limited services for the diagnosis, management, and monitoring of CKD at the primary care level, with only 12% having serum creatinine level measurement, including eGFR, available. In LICs, 29% had access to qualitative urinalysis using urine test strips; however, no LICs had access to determining the urine albumin-to-creatinine ratio (UACR) or urine protein-to-creatinine ratio (UPCR) measurements at the primary care level (see Fig. 75.14A). Across all income groups, availability of services in the secondary/tertiary care level was considerably higher compared with the primary care level (see Fig. 75.14B).

### Availability of Renal Replacement Therapy Services

**Dialysis.** All countries reported having chronic HD services, and more than 90% of countries reported having acute HD (see Fig. 75.14C).[95,98] More than 90% of upper middle and high-income countries reported having chronic PD services, with 64% and 35% availability in LMICs and LICs, respectively. In comparison, acute PD had the lowest availability across all income groups (see Fig. 75.14B).

**Kidney Transplantation.** More than 90% of upper middle and high-income countries reported having kidney transplantation services, with more than 85% of these countries reporting the organ source as a combination of living and/or deceased donors (see Fig. 75.14D). As expected, LICs had the lowest availability of kidney transplantation services, with only 12% reporting availability and live donors as the only source.

### Workforce for Care Delivery

Considerable variation was noted in the density of nephrologists across countries. The lowest density (<5 nephrologists/million population) was very common in LICs, whereas the highest density (>15 nephrologists/million population) was mainly reported in HICs (Fig. 75.15).[95,101] Most countries reported nephrologists as primarily responsible for both CKD and AKI care. Primary care physicians (PCPs) had more responsibility for CKD care than AKI care; 64% of countries reported that PCPs were primarily responsible for CKD and 35% for AKI. Intensive care specialists were primarily responsible for AKI in 75% of countries; this is understandable because AKI is an acute condition typically treated in the hospital. However, only 45% of LICs reported that intensive care specialists were primarily responsible for AKI, compared with 90% of HICs. This discrepancy may be due to a general shortage of intensive care specialists in LIC. The appropriate number of nephrologists in a country is dependent on many factors, including need, priority, and resources and, as such, there is no global standard with respect to nephrologist density. Nevertheless, the density in LICs suggests a shortage of nephrologists, which is problematic because nephrologists are essential to provide leadership, and a lack of nephrologists may result in consequences for policy and practice. Encouragingly, the number of nephrologists and nephropathologists is rising in LICs, in part due to the existence of fellowship programs supported by international nephrology organizations.[105] Importantly, the role of a nephrologist may differ, depending on how the health care system is structured. In some regions, kidney disease patients are primarily cared for by PCPs, so the need for nephrologists may differ compared with other regions that primarily depend on a nephrologist for managing kidney disease patients.

The density statistics merely represent the number of nephrologists per million population and provide no indication of the adequacy to meet the needs of the population or quality of care, which depend on the volume of patients with kidney disease and workforce support. For the other care providers essential for kidney care, there were variations with distribution (availability and adequacy) across countries. Overall, provider shortages were highest for renal pathologists (86% of countries reported a shortage), vascular access coordinators (81%), and dietitians (78%), and shortages were more common in LICs. A minority of countries (35%) reported a shortage in laboratory technicians (Fig. 75.16).

### Capacity for Kidney Research

There were significant variations across countries regarding the infrastructure available for optimal conduct of kidney research, including availability of funding agencies and structures, capacity building and training systems, regulatory frameworks, and storage facilities.[95,100] Only 27% of countries reported a national agency for funding clinical trials, and these were more common in HICs (45%) compared with LICs (12%). Overall, 15% of countries did not participate in clinical trials on kidney disease, and LICs had lower participation across all phases (1–4) of clinical trials. Moreover, less than half of countries (46%) had formal training for physicians in clinical trial conduct, and even fewer countries (34%) had formal training for nonphysicians or research assistants and associates involved in clinical trials. Although 85% of countries had the capacity (trained workforce) to conduct observational cohort studies, fewer countries (48%) had funding to conduct the studies, particularly LICs. Nonetheless, 91% of countries had ethics approval for observational studies in CKD, 62% of which were managed by an institutional regulatory agency. Nearly half of countries (47%) had academic centers for coordinating and monitoring sites for renal clinical studies; however, this was more common in HICs (63%) compared with LICs (12%).

Similarly, the capacity for storing clinical trial medications was low across LICs. Storing medication requires equipment, electricity, facilities, and other resources. It has been

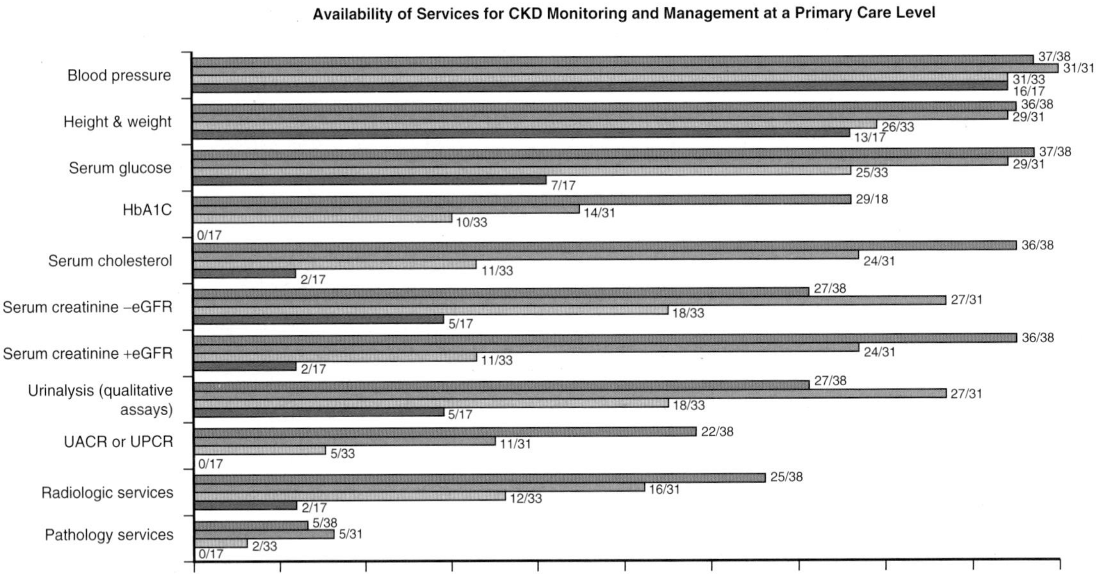


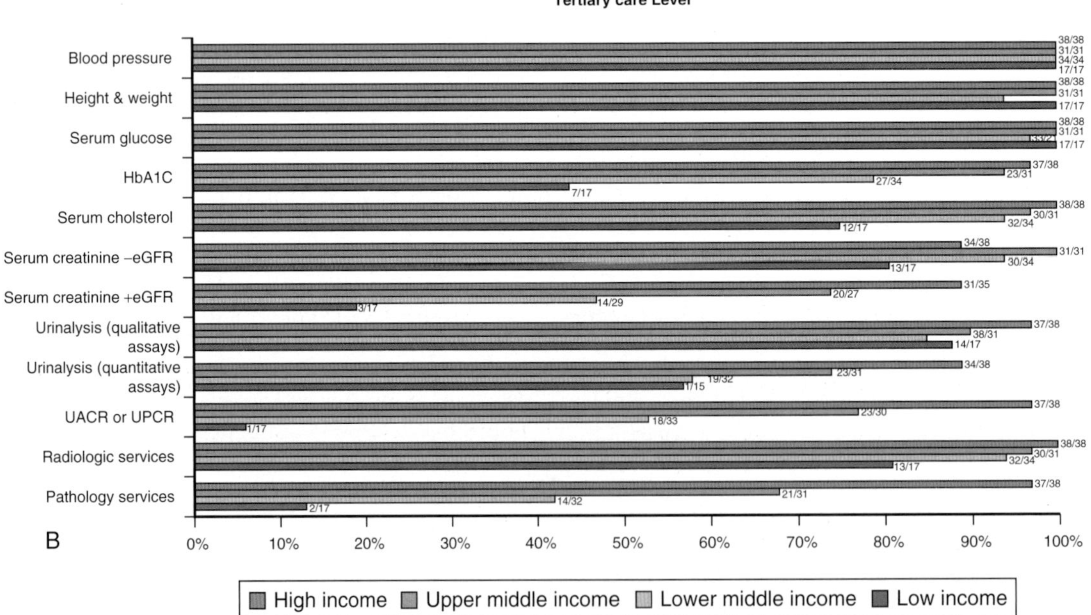


**Fig. 75.14** Availability of health care services for chronic kidney disease *(CKD)* care at primary (A) and secondary and tertiary levels (B), dialysis (C), and kidney transplantation (D), percentage of countries with available health care service. *eGFR,* estimated glomerular filtration rate; *HbA1C,* Hemoglobin A1c; *UACR,* urine albumin-to-creatinine ratio; *UPCR,* urine protein-to-creatinine ratio. (Data from Global Kidney Health Atlas. https://www.theisn.org/images/ISN_Biennial_Report_2011-2013/GKHAtlas_Linked_Compressed1.pdf.)

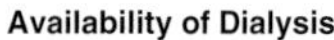

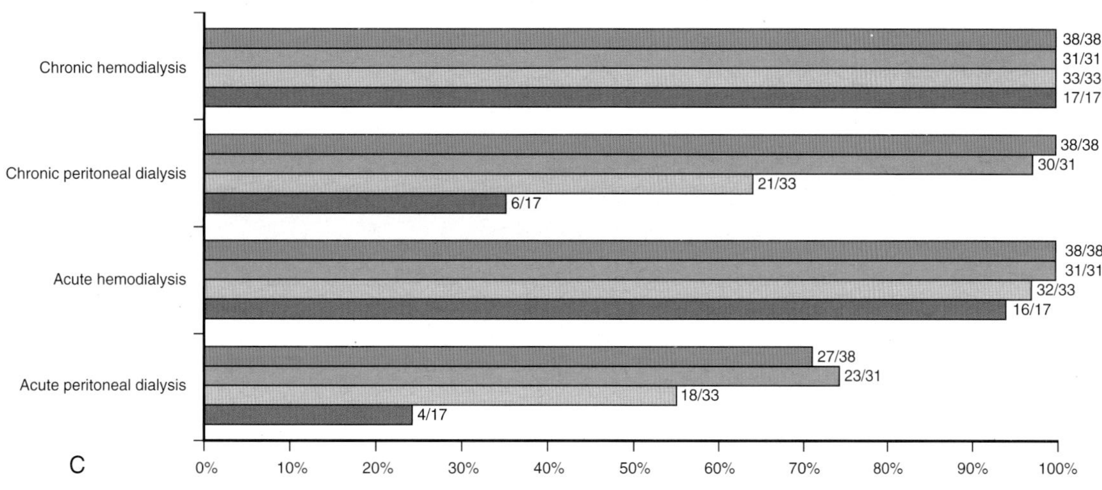


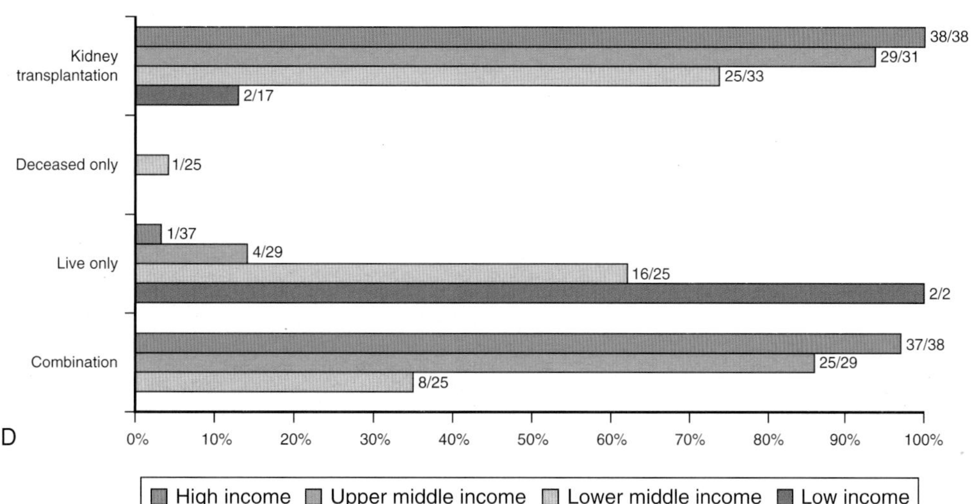


**Fig. 75.14, cont'd**

widely acknowledged that there is a shortage of randomized controlled trials guiding decision making in nephrology care. Enhancing capacity for and involvement in research globally, and especially in LICs, through improved funding of research programs and coordinating academic centers may lead to a more representative understanding of kidney disease globally.

The GKHA has demonstrated significant inter- and intraregional variability in the current capacity for kidney care across the world.[95] Important gaps in awareness, services, workforce, and capacity for research were identified in many countries and regions. The findings have implications for policy development toward the establishment of robust kidney care programs, particularly for LLMICs. Basic infrastructure for services must be strengthened at the primary care level for early detection and management of AKI and CKD across all countries.[4,32] Such information is crucial for advocacy among governmental and nongovernmental stakeholders to support countries in improving the quality of kidney care. The GKHA provides a baseline understanding of where countries and regions stand with respect to several domains of the health system, thus allowing the monitoring of progress through the implementation of various strategies targeted toward improving kidney care. The GKHA is freely available and will be updated biannually to develop country-specific score cards and facilitate identification of country-specific gaps and targets to enhance local kidney health (https://www.theisn.org/initiatives/ckd#health-atlas).

## PUBLIC HEALTH INITIATIVES AND POLICIES TO IMPROVE KIDNEY HEALTH AND ACCESS TO CARE

The public health approach to disease control must consider action at all levels of the health system and beyond:

- At the macro level, government health policy and intersectoral collaboration are key to improving population health.
- At the meso level, health administrators must translate policies into action and conduct monitoring and evaluation exercises to determine effectiveness and address problems.

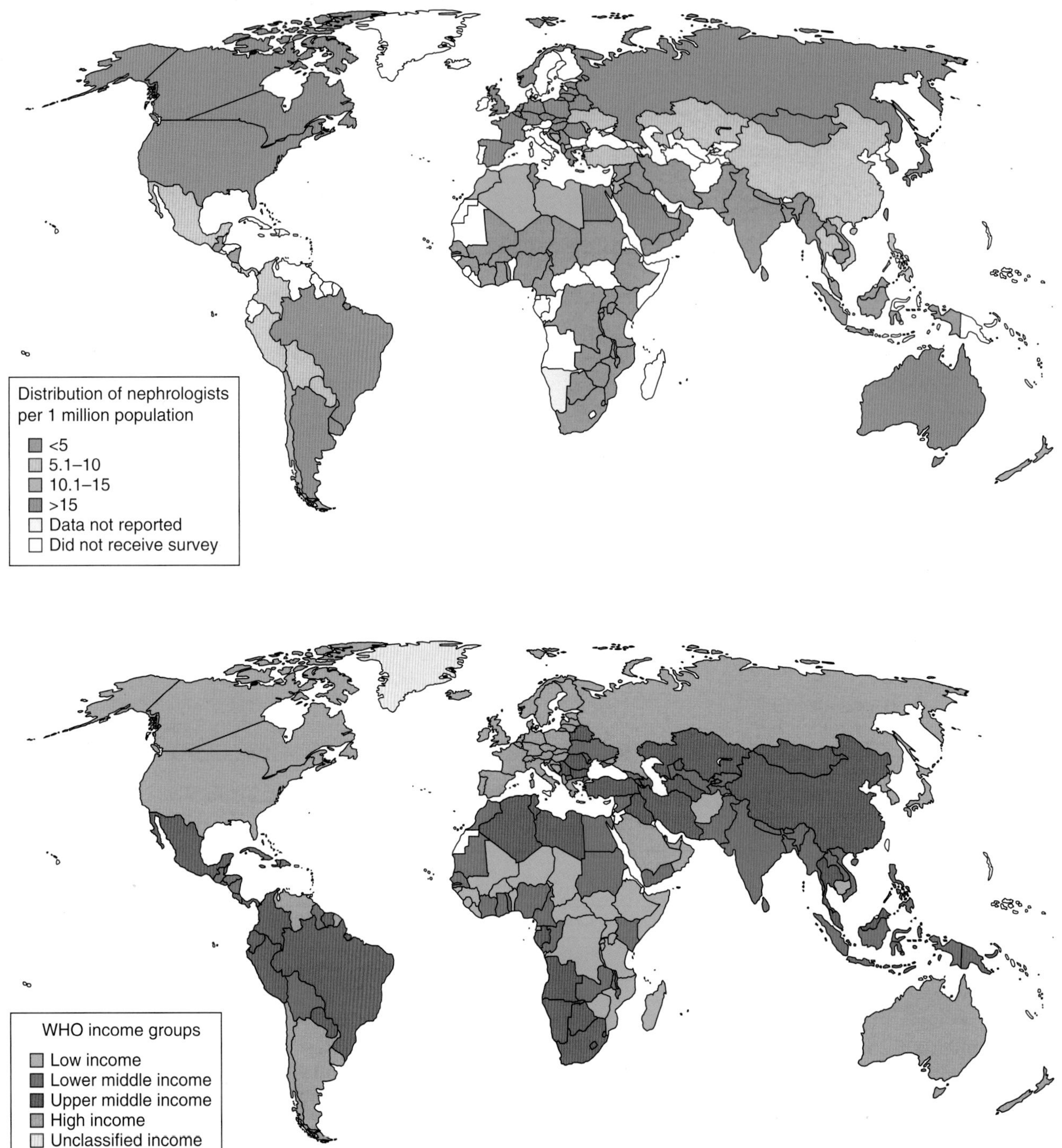


**Fig. 75.15 Distribution of the global nephrologist workforce.** The map depicts global distribution of nephrologists/1 million population by country and region. Data not available indicate that data were either not known or not provided on the questionnaire for countries that received the survey. (Adapted from Bello AK, Levin A, Tonelli M, et al. Assessment of global kidney health care status. *JAMA* 2017;317[18]:1864–1881.)

- At the micro level, individual health care workers and patients must work together to preserve health.

Kidney disease is affected by many social and structural factors and therefore is amenable to public health interventions (Table 75.6). Government policies that have proven effective in reducing the risk of NCDs include economic incentives to reduce prices of healthy food, taxation on unhealthy foods and beverages, school programs, including health and physical education, food advertising restrictions and standards, increasing safe spaces for sport and recreation, media campaigns promoting smoking cessation, health warnings on cigarette packages, restriction of tobacco advertising, increased taxes on tobacco, and prohibition of smoking in public spaces.[12,13,106,107] Implementation of public health programs such as vaccinations, health education, malaria prevention, providing access to clean water, antenatal care, ensuring safe deliveries, and optimizing child nutrition can all also reduce

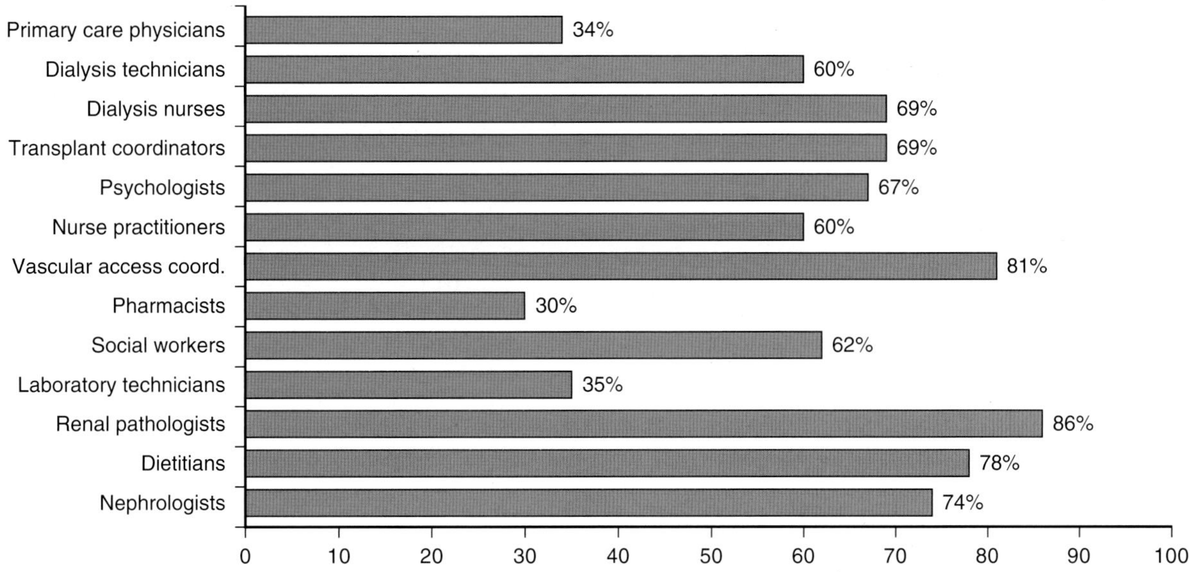


**Fig. 75.16 Overall shortage in nephrology workforce.** Shown are the percentages of countries globally reporting shortages of health care across the spectrum of kidney care (Data from Global kidney Health Atlas. https://www.theisn.org/images/ISN_Biennial_Report_2011-2013/GKHAtlas_Linked_Compressed1.pdf.)

**Table 75.6 Levels of Public Health Interventions, Specific Steps, and the Potential Impact on Kidney Health**

| Parameter | Specific Steps | Impact on Kidney Health | Comments |
|---|---|---|---|
| Socioeconomic factors | Improved livelihood, education, and sanitation; universal access to timely and affordable health care | Overall improvement in health; reduced NCD burden | Requires political will; linked to overall development and economic growth over long term; radical redesign of health systems required |
| Changing the context to make default decisions healthy | Reducing salt in packaged foods; higher taxation for tobacco, sweetened beverages, and processed foods; regulate OTC and indigenous medicine use<br>Mandate protective clothing and footwear in certain occupations (e.g., outdoor exposure); access to quality reproductive care, legalization of abortions; widespread ORS availability | Reduction in kidney disease risk factors (e.g., hypertension, diabetes, metabolic syndrome); reduction in CKDnT; slowed progression of CKD; reduction in occupation-related CKD and AKI; reduction in obstetric AKI | Requires political will; likely opposition from special interest groups and industry lobby |
| Long-lasting protective interventions | Vaccinations, improved immunization coverage for VPDs; kidney disease screening at schools and workplaces; vector control | Reduced infection-related kidney disease (AKI and CKD); reduced infections in those with kidney disease; early prevention opportunities | Can be controversial; requires multisectoral approaches |
| Clinical interventions | Treatment of risk factors and predisposing conditions; measures to improve adherence to treatment | Reduction in CKD development and progression; improvement in obstetric AKI through tracking outcomes | Needs manpower and resources; ensuring a continuum of care; effective health information systems deployment |
| Counseling and education | Increase kidney disease awareness; dietary counseling; increase physical activity | Can slow CKD progression and prevent AKI in certain situations | Least effective; requires civil society engagement and ownership |

*AKI,* Acute kidney injury; *CKD,* chronic kidney disease; *CKDnT,* chronic kidney disease of nontraditional causes; *NCD,* noncommunicable disease; *ORS,* oral rehydration solution; *OTC,* over the counter; *VPD,* vaccine-preventable disease.

From Joshi R, John O, Jha V, The potential impact of public health interventions in preventing kidney disease. *Semin Nephrol.* 2017;37(3):234–244.

the burden of AKI and CKD in the community.[12,13] The risk of kidney disease begins in fetal life and spans a lifetime, so prevention of kidney disease starts with optimization of health and education for girls, universal health coverage for antenatal care and safe deliveries, and optimizing child nutrition and growth.[85]

Targeted screening of high-risk individuals (with diabetes, hypertension, and CVD) has been shown to be cost-effective in detecting and treating CKD early and delaying progression to ESKD.[29,108] Screening and early treatment strategies require availability of the necessary resources and trained personnel at all levels of the health care system to manage kidney disease.[109] Given the broad reach required and the need for simple screening strategies, which can be integrated into existing WHO NCD strategies, task shifting may be required and desired to improve uptake and coverage, especially in countries with very large populations, such as India.[110–112] Systematic screening activities will also facilitate the generation of renal registries and provide information on local kidney disease burdens necessary for priority setting and program planning.[113] Integration of care for patients with kidney disease into communicable and NCD programs, coupled with community engagement and empowerment of patients, promises to improve quality of care with greater efficiency and at lower cost, as well as providing a more holistic approach to patient care (Fig. 75.17).[31,112,114,115]

## HEATH IN ALL POLICIES AND SUSTAINABLE DEVELOPMENT GOALS

The implementation of population-level strategies to reduce the risk of NCDs and kidney disease requires coordinated multisectoral action across government and society, as emphasized in the health in all policies strategy.[107,116,117] The health in all policies framework reflects the principles of "legitimacy, accountability, transparency and access to information, participation, sustainability and collaboration across sectors and levels of government" as important components of an equitable approach to improving population health.[117] This multisectoral approach highlights the impact of the non-health sectors, such as industry, education, housing, transportation, agriculture, and environment, in improving population health.

In recognition of this multisectoral impact on health and the negative impact of illness on communities and overall economic growth, the United Nations launched the Sustainable Development Goals (SDGs) project in 2015 with the goal of achieving healthy people living on a healthy planet.[78,118] Multiple social and structural factors affect the risk of kidney

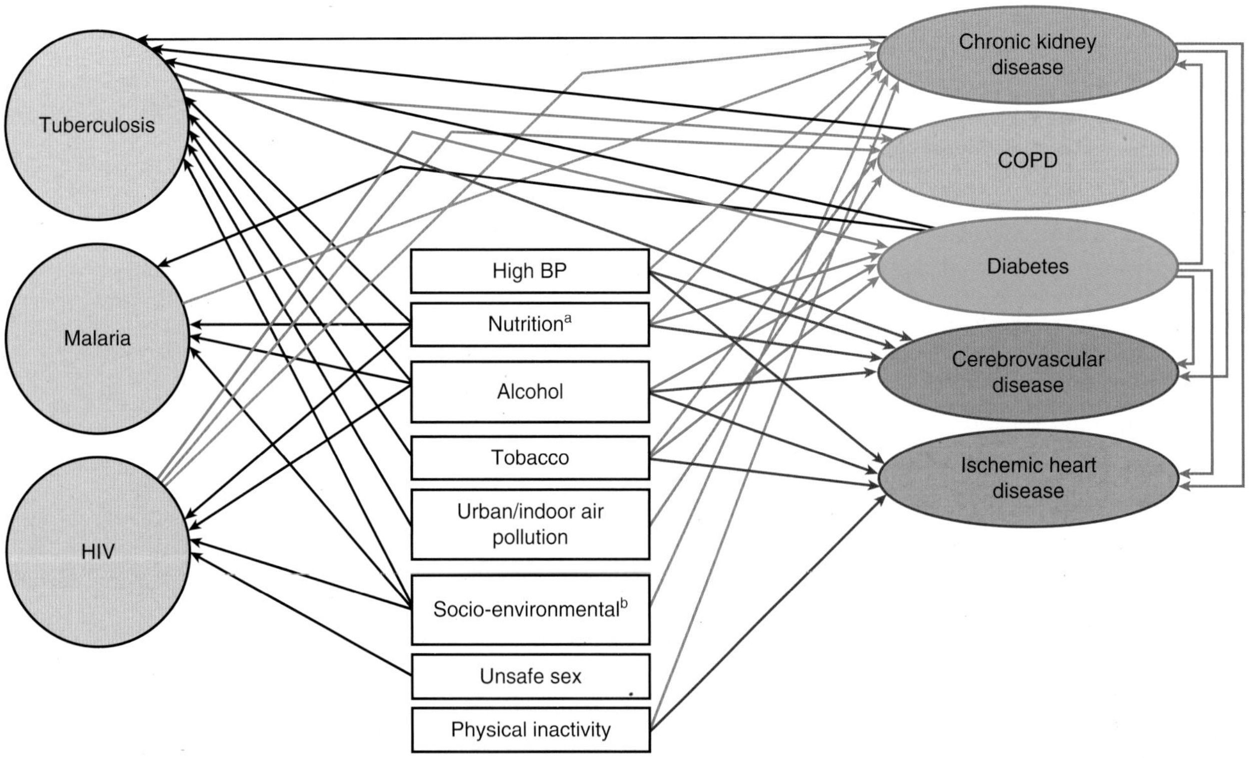


**Fig. 75.17 Interaction between tuberculosis *(TB)*, malaria, and HIV and risk factors, disease precursors, and noncommunicable diseases.** *BP,* Blood pressure; *COPD,* chronic obstructive pulmonary disease. (Adapted from Oni T, Unwin N. Why the communicable/non-communicable disease dichotomy is problematic for public health control strategies: implications of multimorbidity for health systems in an era of health transition. *Int Health.* 2015;7[6]:390–399.)

disease across the life course, including poverty, over- and undernutrition, poor education, access to public health interventions and health care, gender inequality, environmental and occupational factors, urban or rural location, violence, social disruptions and war, climate change, and the effects of globalization. Each SDG has direct or indirect relevance to kidney health, so progress toward each SGD promises to improve the global burden of kidney disease.[119] It is important to acknowledge the links with other diseases; therefore, the nephrology community has the opportunity to lead in working with public health professionals and all levels of health care workers on the ground to improve synergies and coordination between disease silos to improve overall health and thereby kidney health.

### HEALTH TECHNOLOGY ASSESSMENT: THE EXAMPLE OF THAILAND

As discussed earlier, reliance on OOP payments for RRT or rationing of dialysis access are highly inequitable and contribute to many annual deaths globally.[3,71,120] The costs of dialysis and transplantation are high for all health care systems. Even in an HIC such as the United States, which otherwise does not have universal health coverage, the need to create an exception and provide coverage for ESKD patients has long been recognized and implemented (see Chapter 82).[121] The challenge, however, is how to provide equitable access to RRT sustainably and without compromising funding for other health priorities. Systematic analyses of local circumstances in terms of disease burden, projected costs (direct, indirect, and opportunity costs), and expected benefits are required prior to developing policies around the provision of RRT. Such analyses are often not performed, leading to the provision of inadequate services that may exacerbate inequities.[58,122] The example of Thailand's approach to the provision of RRT under universal health coverage is highly instructive. Thailand is an MIC that introduced universal health coverage in 2002.[123] At that time, universal coverage for RRT was deliberately excluded because of the high anticipated costs. This meant that patients covered under two private insurers (25% of the population) had free access to RRT, but the rest did not.[124]

Over the ensuing years, policy makers conducted a comprehensive series of studies to investigate the potential demand for RRT, survey public opinion, conduct policy and cost-effectiveness analyses, and understand the impact of high OOP costs on individuals and families.[125] Specifically, it was found that many households experienced catastrophic health expenditures, with some households spending up to 70% of total income to keep one member on dialysis; often, costs were met through reduction of food consumption and dialysis frequency.[126] In the context of some favorable political circumstances, in 2008, the decision was made to include dialysis under the universal coverage scheme to reduce catastrophic expenditures and improve equity in access to dialysis across all health care schemes, despite evidence that dialysis per se is not cost-effective compared with many other interventions.[125]

Prior to implementation, much consideration was given to cost containment, including a PD-first policy (analyses had shown that PD was more cost-effective than HD); bulk negotiation for pricing of dialysis supplies and medications (e.g., 25% reduction in cost of HD, 62% reduction in cost of erythropoietin); and negotiated incentive and reimbursement strategies.[124,125] PD centers of excellence providing training and support to peripheral centers were established, and active stakeholder, community, and patient engagement programs were conducted to enhance uptake and provide support in communities to meet additional needs, such as transport costs.[124] The numbers of patients requiring RRT initially grew rapidly as services expanded but have since plateaued, and outcomes are comparable with those of other programs.[124] Thailand is a world leader in health technology assessment, as evidenced by the deliberate and systematic approach it has taken in developing dialysis policy decisions. The Thai Health Intervention and Technology Assessment Program (HITAP; globalhitap.net) provides a framework that is adaptable and is being used by other countries in their decision making around RRT.

## CONCLUSION

The global burden of kidney disease has been relatively underappreciated until rather recently. International activities are increasing to quantify this burden better, detect and address gaps in kidney care, and advocate for patients unable to access RRT.

### ACKNOWLEDGMENTS

Boris Bikbov has received funding from the European Union's Horizon 2020 research and innovation program under the Marie Sklodowska-Curie grant agreement No. 703226.

Boris Bikbov acknowledges that work related to this paper has been done on the behalf of the GBD Genitourinary Disease Expert Group supported by the International Society of Nephrology, and acknowledges the contribution of GBD Genitourinary Disease Expert Group members Professor Giuseppe Remuzzi and Dr. Norberto Perico.

Complete reference list available at ExpertConsult.com.

### KEY REFERENCES

2. GBD 2015 Mortality and Causes of Death Collaborators. Global, regional, and national life expectancy, all-cause mortality, and cause-specific mortality for 249 causes of death, 1980-2015: a systematic analysis for the Global Burden of Disease Study 2015. *Lancet.* 2016;388(10053):1459–1544.
3. Liyanage T, Ninomiya T, Jha V, et al. Worldwide access to treatment for end-stage kidney disease: a systematic review. *Lancet.* 2015;385(9981):1975–1982.
4. Mehta RL, Cerda J, Burdmann EA, et al. International Society of Nephrology's 0by25 initiative for acute kidney injury (zero preventable deaths by 2025): a human rights case for nephrology. *Lancet.* 2015;385(9987):2616–2643.
6. Mills KT, Xu Y, Zhang W, et al. A systematic analysis of worldwide population-based data on the global burden of chronic kidney disease in 2010. *Kidney Int.* 2015;88(5):950–957.
7. Stanifer JW, Muiru A, Jafar TH, et al. Chronic kidney disease in low- and middle-income countries. *Nephrol Dial Transplant.* 2016;31(6):868–874.
10. Harambat J, Ekulu PM. Inequalities in access to pediatric ESRD care: a global health challenge. *Pediatr Nephrol.* 2016;31:353–358.
12. Levin A, Tonelli M, Bonventre J, et al. Global kidney health 2017 and beyond: a roadmap for closing gaps in care, research, and policy. *Lancet.* 2017;390(10105):1888–1917.
13. Luyckx VA, Tuttle KR, Garcia Garcia G, et al. Reducing major risk factors for chronic kidney disease. *Kidney Int Suppl.* 2017;in press.

14. Stanifer JW, Kilonzo K, Wang D, et al. Traditional medicines and kidney disease in low- and middle-income countries: opportunities and challenges. *Semin Nephrol.* 2017;37(3):245–259.
15. Ene-Iordache B, Perico N, Bikbov B, et al. Chronic kidney disease and cardiovascular risk in six regions of the world (ISN-KDDC): a cross-sectional study. *Lancet Glob Health.* 2016;4(5): e307–e319.
17. Thomas B, Wulf S, Bikbov B, et al. Maintenance dialysis throughout the world in years 1990 and 2010. *J Am Soc Nephrol.* 2015;26(11): 2621–2633.
18. Lewington AJ, Cerda J, Mehta RL. Raising awareness of acute kidney injury: a global perspective of a silent killer. *Kidney Int.* 2013.
21. Olowu WA, Niang A, Osafo C, et al. Outcomes of acute kidney injury in children and adults in sub-Saharan Africa: a systematic review. *Lancet Glob Health.* 2016;4(4):e242–e250.
29. Vanholder R, Annemans L, Brown E, et al. Reducing the costs of chronic kidney disease while delivering quality health care: a call to action. *Nat Rev Nephrol.* 2017;13(7):393–409.
30. Jha V, Prasad N. CKD and infectious diseases in Asia Pacific: challenges and opportunities. *Am J Kidney Dis.* 2016.
31. Oni T, Unwin N. Why the communicable/non-communicable disease dichotomy is problematic for public health control strategies: implications of multimorbidity for health systems in an era of health transition. *Int Health.* 2015;7(6):390–399.
32. Couser WG, Remuzzi G, Mendis S, et al. The contribution of chronic kidney disease to the global burden of major noncommunicable diseases. *Kidney Int.* 2011;80(12):1258–1270.
35. Ashuntantang G, Osafo C, Olowu WA, et al. Outcomes in adults and children with end-stage kidney disease requiring dialysis in sub-Saharan Africa: a systematic review. *Lancet Glob Health.* 2017;5(4):e408–e417.
37. White SL, Chadban SJ, Jan S, et al. How can we achieve global equity in provision of renal replacement therapy? *Bull World Health Org.* 2008;86:229–237.
40. Anand S, Bitton A, Gaziano T. The gap between estimated incidence of end-stage renal disease and use of therapy. *PLoS ONE.* 2013;8(8):e72860.
42. Cullis B, Abdelraheem M, Abrahams G, et al. Peritoneal dialysis for acute kidney injury. *Perit Dial Int.* 2014;34(5):494–517.
51. Arogundade FA. Kidney transplantation in a low-resource setting: Nigeria experience. *Kidney Int Suppl.* 2013;3(2):241–245.
52. Muralidharan A, White S. The need for kidney transplantation in low- and middle-income countries in 2012: an epidemiological perspective. *Transplantation.* 2015;99(3):476–481.
58. Luyckx VA, Miljeteig I, Ejigu AM, et al. Ethical challenges in the provision of dialysis in resource-constrained environments. *Semin Nephrol.* 2017;37(3):273–286.
59. World Health Organization. Making fair choices on the path to universal health coverage. Final report of the WHO Consultative Group on Equity and Universal Health Coverage. Geneva, Switzerland: WHO; 2014. Available from: http://apps.who.int/iris/bitstream/10665/112671/1/9789241507158_eng.pdf?ua=1. Accessed June 30, 2016.
69. Chesnaye NC, Schaefer F, Bonthuis M, et al. Mortality risk disparities in children receiving chronic renal replacement therapy for the treatment of end-stage renal disease across Europe: an ESPN-ERA/EDTA registry analysis. *Lancet.* 2017;389(10084):2128–2137.
70. Defaye FB, Desalegn D, Danis M, et al. A survey of Ethiopian physicians' experiences of bedside rationing: extensive resource scarcity, tough decisions and adverse consequences. *BMC Health Serv Res.* 2015;15:467.
72. GBD 2015 Disease and Injury Incidence and Prevalence Collaborators. Global, regional, and national incidence, prevalence, and years lived with disability for 310 diseases and injuries, 1990-2015: a systematic analysis for the Global Burden of Disease Study 2015. *Lancet.* 2016;388(10053):1545–1602.
73. GBD 2015 DALYs and HALE Collaborators. Global, regional, and national disability-adjusted life-years (DALYs) for 315 diseases and injuries and healthy life expectancy (HALE), 1990-2015: a systematic analysis for the Global Burden of Disease Study 2015. *Lancet.* 2016;388(10053):1603–1658.
74. GBD 2015 Risk Factors Collaborators. Global, regional, and national comparative risk assessment of 79 behavioural, environmental and occupational, and metabolic risks or clusters of risks, 1990-2015: a systematic analysis for the Global Burden of Disease Study 2015. *Lancet.* 2016;388(10053):1659–1724.
75. Hill NR, Fatoba ST, Oke JL, et al. Global prevalence of chronic kidney disease—a systematic review and meta-analysis. *PLoS ONE.* 2016;11(7):e0158765.
79. GBD 2013 DALYs and HALE Collaborators. Global, regional, and national disability-adjusted life years (DALYs) for 306 diseases and injuries and healthy life expectancy (HALE) for 188 countries, 1990-2013: quantifying the epidemiological transition. *Lancet.* 2015;386(10009):2145–2191.
80. Smart NA, Dieberg G, Ladhani M, et al. Early referral to specialist nephrology services for preventing the progression to end-stage kidney disease. *Cochrane Database Syst Rev.* 2014;(6):CD007333.
83. Norton JM, Moxey-Mims MM, Eggers PW, et al. Social determinants of racial disparities in CKD. *J Am Soc Nephrol.* 2016;27(9):2576–2595.
84. Carrero JJ, Hecking M, Ulasi I, et al. Chronic kidney disease, gender, and access to care: a global perspective. *Semin Nephrol.* 2017;37(3):296–308.
85. Low Birth Weight and Nephron Number Working Group. The impact of kidney development on the life course: a consensus document for action. *Nephron.* 2017;136(1):3–49.
94. Smoyer WE, Finkelstein FO, McCulloch MI, et al. "Saving Young Lives" with acute kidney injury: the challenge of acute dialysis in low-resource settings. *Kidney Int.* 2016;89(2):254–256.
95. Bello AK, Levin A, Tonelli M, et al. Assessment of global kidney health care status. *JAMA.* 2017;317:1864–1881.
109. Vachharajani TJ, Bello AK, Evans R, et al. Nephrology education and continuing education in resource-limited settings. *Semin Nephrol.* 2017;37(3):224–233.
110. Joshi R, John O, Jha V. The potential impact of public health interventions in preventing kidney disease. *Semin Nephrol.* 2017; 37(3):234–244.
113. Davids MR, Caskey FJ, Young T, et al. Strengthening renal registries and ESRD research in Africa. *Semin Nephrol.* 2017;37(3):211–223.
119. Luyckx VA, Tonelli M, Stanifer JW. Reducing the global burden of kidney disease through action on the Sustainable Development Goals. *Bull World Health Org.* 2018.
123. Tantivess S, Werayingyong P, Chuengsaman P, et al. Universal coverage of renal dialysis in Thailand: promise, progress, and prospects. *BMJ.* 2013;346:f462.
130. Narayan KM, Echouffo-Tcheugui JB, Mohan V, et al. Global prevention and control of Type 2 diabetes will require paradigm shifts in policies within and among countries. *Health Aff.* 2012;31(1):84–92.
131. Mills KT, Bundy JD, Kelly TN, et al. Global disparities of hypertension prevalence and control: a systematic analysis of population-based studies from 90 countries. *Circulation.* 2016;134(6):441–450.
140. Luyckx VA. Nephrotoxicity of alternative medicine practice. *Adv Chronic Kidney Dis.* 2012;19(3):129–141.
146. Luyckx VA, Brenner BM. Birth weight, malnutrition and kidney-associated outcomes—a global concern. *Nat Rev Nephrol.* 2015;11(3):135–149.
148. Vikse BE. Pre-eclampsia and the risk of kidney disease. *Lancet.* 2013;382(9887):104–106.
157. Thomas B, Matsushita K, Abate KH, et al. Global cardiovascular and renal outcomes of reduced GFR. *J Am Soc Nephrol.* 2017;28(7):2167–2179.
167. Lunyera J, Mohottige D, Von Isenburg M, et al. CKD of uncertain etiology: a systematic review. *Clin J Am Soc Nephrol.* 2016;11(3):379–385.

# Latin America

# 76

Leonardo V. Riella | Miquel C. Riella

**CHAPTER OUTLINE**



**KEY POINTS**

- Latin America is a heterogeneous region with variable health expenditures and prevalence of kidney disease.
- Mesoamerican nephropathy is a tubulointerstitial kidney disease of unclear cause, with a high prevalence in agricultural workers along the coast of central America.
- Risk factors for Mesoamerican nephropathy may include heat stress, pesticides, heavy metals, and other environmental toxins.
- Kidney involvement in dengue fever varies from acute tubular injury and immune complex glomerulonephritis to thrombotic microangiopathy.
- Leptospirosis affects the kidneys in more than 50% of cases and is characterized primarily by acute interstitial nephritis.

## INTRODUCTION

Some 200 years after achieving political independence from European colonizers, Latin America became an area of rapid growth and great economic opportunity. Despite the unifying term, this region is very heterogeneous, consisting of 20 different countries with different languages and degrees of economic as well as social development. Even within a single country such as Brazil, different regions may have diverse levels of development and medical needs.

The total population of Latin America in 2017 was estimated at 645 million people.[1] Brazil, Mexico, Chile, Colombia, and Peru represent more than 70% of the population and account for 75% of its gross domestic product (GDP).[1] Poverty and extreme poverty are present in 29% and 11% of the population, respectively, with a predominance in rural areas.[2] Average life expectancy in Latin America is 75.7 years; it has risen from 69.7 years in 1995, about 8.6% in 20 years (Fig. 76.1),[3] although differences of more than 10 years can be seen between countries. Similar differences are observed in the infant mortality rate, ranging from 6.9 deaths/1000 live births in Chile to 50 deaths/1000 live births in Bolivia (average, 16 deaths/1000 live births).[2] Variability in other outcomes, such as maternal mortality, malnutrition, and the lack of access to safe water and sanitation, tend to be obscured by regional averages.[2] A high prevalence of certain infectious diseases, such as tuberculosis, malaria, dengue fever, and cholera, is also characteristic. Total health expenditures in Latin America rose to 7.3% of the GDP in 2014 from 6.5% in 2008,[3] although this figure is still below that of the United States (16.6%) and Europe (9%), and almost half of Latin America's population lacks health insurance (46%; Fig. 76.2).[2,4]

On the basis of its geographic location, diverse ethnic backgrounds, and socioeconomic status, Latin America is the setting for a number of unique diseases that may affect kidney function; these are reviewed in this chapter. Infections such as dengue fever, malaria, yellow fever, leptospirosis, schistosomiasis, and leprosy are prevalent, and nephrotoxicity from the venom of spiders, caterpillars, or snakes has become more frequent with changes in the environment. In addition, chronic kidney diséase (CKD) has become a major health concern with the epidemic of Western metabolic syndrome and unique obscure cases of progressive kidney disease in

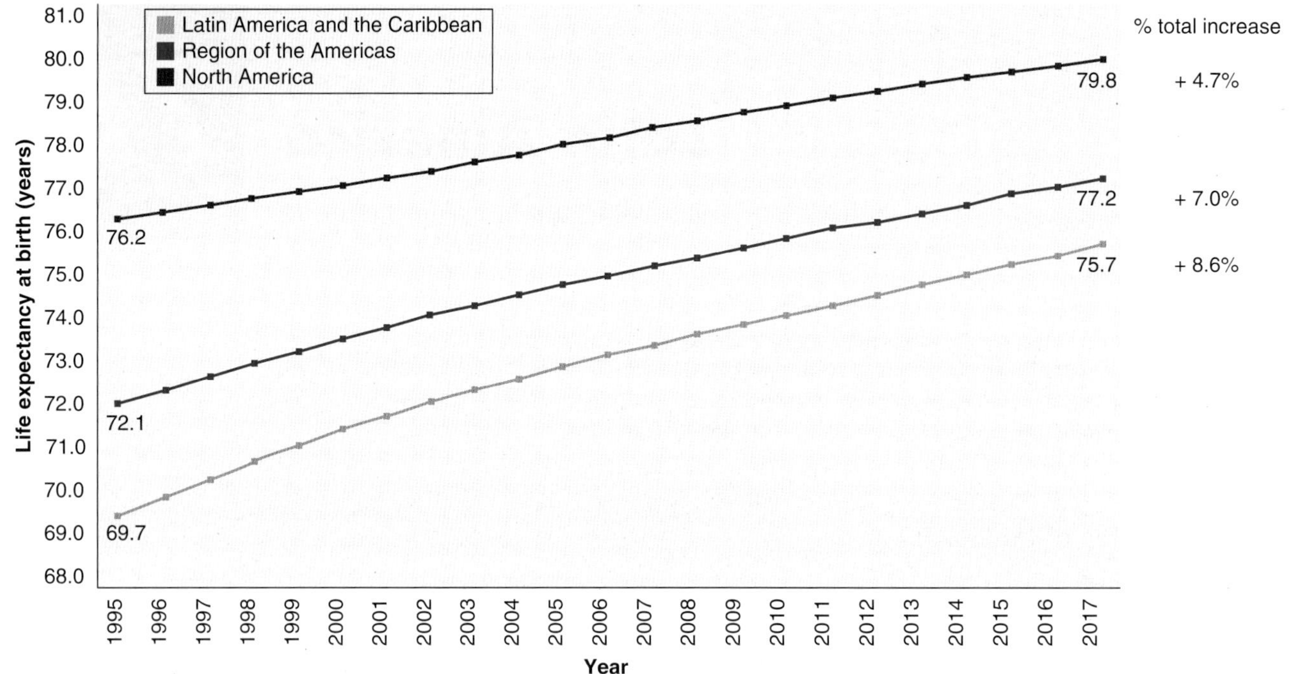


**Fig. 76.1** Life expectancy at birth in region of the Americas, North America, Latin America, and the Caribbean, 1995–2017. (Modified from Health in the Americas, 2017 Edition. Summary: Regional Outlook and Country Profiles. http://iris.paho.org/xmlui/handle/123456789/34321? show=full.)

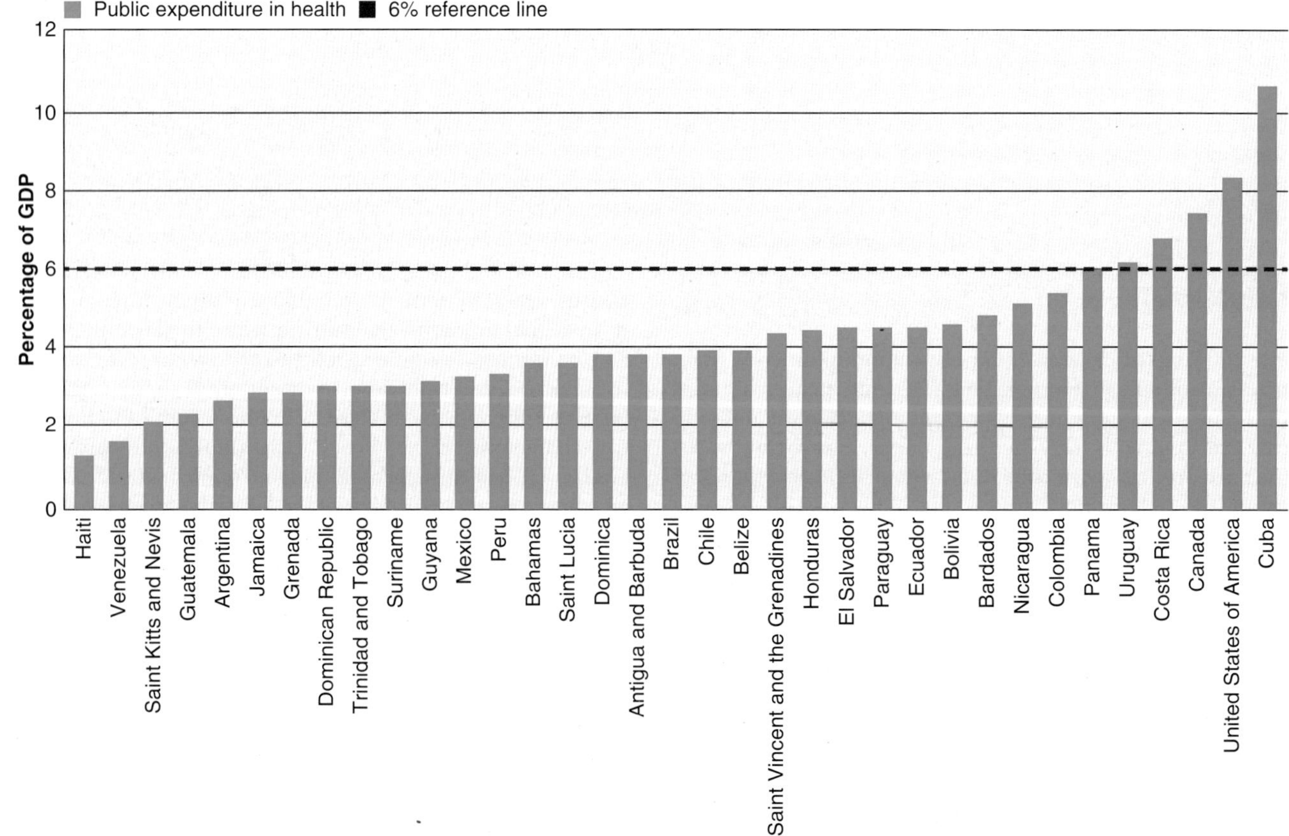


**Fig. 76.2** Public health expenditure as a percentage of gross domestic product (GDP), 2014. (Modified from Health in the Americas, 2017 Edition. Summary: Regional Outlook and Country Profiles. http://iris.paho.org/xmlui/handle/123456789/34321? show=full.)

sugar cane agricultural workers. This chapter attempts to summarize the current status of the care of patients with kidney disease in Latin America and describe some leading priorities necessary for the improvement and progress of kidney health in the region.

## TROPICAL DISEASES AND KIDNEY INJURY

### DENGUE FEVER

Dengue fever (DF) is a mosquito-borne infection that causes a severe flu-like illness and, sometimes, a potentially lethal complication called *dengue hemorrhagic fever* (DHF). The main dengue vector is the female of the *Aedes aegypti* mosquito. Male mosquitoes do not transmit the disease because they feed on plant juices. DF and DHF are primarily diseases of tropical and subtropical areas, and the four different dengue serotypes are maintained in a cycle that involves humans and the *Aedes* mosquito. The global incidence of DF has grown dramatically in recent decades.

Approximately half of the world's population lives in areas potentially at risk for DF, and 50 to 100 million cases are estimated to occur annually.[5,6] Brazil has the highest absolute number of cases and the highest incidence of the disease in Latin America.[5] The principal method for prevention of DF virus transmission is mosquito control. The high incidence of DF in Latin America has been ascribed to global warming and ecosystem modifications, facilitating the dissemination of pathogens and vectors of the disease. In addition, demographic factors, including uncontrolled migration of people and unplanned urbanization, have facilitated the increase in the occurrence of DF in urban areas and large cities.

DF is caused by one of four closely related, but antigenically distinct, virus serotypes—DEN-1, DEN-2, DEN-3, and DEN-4—of the genus *Flavivirus*. Infection with one of these serotypes provides immunity to only that serotype for life; therefore, persons living in a DF-endemic area can have more than one DF infection during their lifetimes.

Dengue virus infection may manifest clinically as an undifferentiated fever—DF, DHF, or dengue shock syndrome (DSS). DHF usually occurs in patients who have previously been infected with other serotypes of dengue virus ("secondary infection"), although it may follow primary infections, particularly in infants.[6] Classic DF is an acute febrile illness accompanied by headache, retroorbital pain, and muscle and joint pains that lasts approximately 5 days but that has no specific physical findings except a maculopapular rash in about 50% of cases. DHF is a severe form of the disease and manifests with fever, hemorrhagic phenomena, thrombocytopenia, and evidence of plasma leakage (high hematocrit, pleural effusion, ascites, and hypoalbuminemia). Malaria, leptospirosis, hantavirus infection, typhoid fever, human immunodeficiency virus (HIV) infection, enterovirus infection, influenza, and sepsis must be ruled out in the differential diagnosis. The diagnosis of acute dengue virus infection is mainly a clinical one, but serologic tests are available in specialized reference laboratories, including hemagglutination inhibition (HI) assay (considered the gold standard), immunoglobulin (Ig) G or IgM enzyme immunoassays, and reverse transcription polymerase chain reaction (RT-PCR) analysis for dengue virus RNA.

#### KIDNEY INVOLVEMENT IN DENGUE FEVER

Renal injury, comprised of acute tubular injury, glomerulonephritis, or hemolytic-uremic syndrome, has been reported in patients with DF. The clinical presentation is variable, ranging from an elevation in creatinine level, proteinuria, and active urinary sediment to thrombotic microangiopathy. The possible pathogenesis of renal involvement includes ischemic or hemoglobin-associated tubular injury, glomerular injury, secondary immune complex deposition, and thrombotic microangiopathy.[7] Lima and colleagues have described a case of DHF-induced acute kidney injury (AKI), in which renal injury occurred without hemodynamic instability, hemolysis, rhabdomyolysis, or use of nephrotoxic drugs.[5]

The prevalence of AKI in dengue infection is variable, ranging from 0.3% to as high as 15%.[7] In a series from Thailand, 51 deaths were reported among 6154 cases of DHF, with an overall incidence of AKI of 0.3%, but an incidence of 33.3% among the fatal cases. Kidney biopsies performed in patients with DHF and proteinuria, hematuria, or both revealed glomerular changes characterized by hypertrophy and hyperplasia of mesangial and endothelial cells, the presence of monocyte-like cells in some of the glomerular capillary lumens, and focal thickening of the glomerular basement membrane. Immune complexes (IgG, IgM or both, and C3) were found in glomeruli and arterioles in biopsy specimens from 10 cases that were collected 2 weeks after the onset of symptoms. Dense spherical particles were found in the 12 cases in which electron microscopy was carried out. The researchers in this series hypothesized that the particles might be nucleocapsid cores of dengue virions.[8]

Experimental studies with inoculation of the virus in mice have suggested that the dengue virus can induce glomerulopathy. In one study in which dengue virus type 2 was inoculated into mice, diffuse proliferative glomerular injury was seen 14 days after the inoculation and, in another study, enlarged glomerular volume, increased endocapillary and mesangial cellularity, and glomerular IgM deposition were observed 48 hours after virus inoculation.[9] In a case report from Brazil, the presence of proteinuria, hematuria, generalized edema, and hypertension associated with low levels of C3 and C4 suggested an immune-mediated, acute glomerular injury.[7]

There is no specific treatment for DF, so management consists of supportive care, including controlling fever (acetaminophen), preventing dehydration (oral [PO] or intravenous [IV] fluids), and managing complications such as bleeding. Aspirin and nonsteroidal antiinflammatory drugs (NSAIDs) should be avoided. There are no vaccines available, and the only mode of prevention is to protect against the mosquito bite by covering exposed skin areas and using an effective mosquito repellent, such as *N,N*-diethyl-meta-toluamide (DEET).

### YELLOW FEVER

Yellow fever (YF) is a viral hemorrhagic fever transmitted by infected mosquitoes. There are three types of transmission cycle—sylvatic, intermediate, and urban. All three cycles exist in Africa, but in South America, only sylvatic and urban yellow fever occur.[10] Sylvatic (or jungle) YF occurs in tropical rainforests, where monkeys, infected by sylvatic mosquitoes, pass the virus to other mosquitoes that feed on them; these mosquitoes, in turn, bite and thus infect humans entering the rainforest. This type of transmission produces sporadic cases, most of which affect young men working in the forest (e.g., loggers). The intermediate cycle of YF transmission, which occurs in humid or semihumid savannahs of Africa, can produce small-scale epidemics in rural villages. Semidomestic mosquitoes infect monkey and human hosts, and increased contact between human and infected mosquito leads to disease. This is the most common type of outbreak seen lately in Africa. Urban yellow fever results in large, explosive epidemics when travelers from rural areas introduce the virus into areas with a high human population density. Domestic mosquitoes, most notably *Aedes aegypti*, carry the virus from person to person. These outbreaks tend to spread outward from one source to cover a wide area.

YF transmission in the Americas continues to follow the jungle cycle. There are 14 YF-endemic countries in the region. However, only five of them (Bolivia, Brazil, Colombia, Ecuador, and Peru) reported cases of yellow fever between 2011 and 2016. As of March 2017, the Pan American Health Organization reported that Brazil, Colombia, Peru, and the plurinational state of Bolivia had suspected and confirmed yellow fever cases.[10] In Brazil, since the outbreak of December 2016, 1368 cases were reported—326 confirmed, 125 excluded, and 916 suspected cases remain under investigation—including 220 deaths (109 confirmed, 6 discarded, and 105 under investigation). The case fatality rate (CFR) is 33% among confirmed cases and 11% among suspected cases.[10]

To avoid the reurbanization of this disease *A. aegypti* vector control measures are critical, mainly in cities and in localities bordering affected areas. Such measures also facilitate the prevention of dengue outbreaks. One of the most important mechanisms for preventing YF is vaccination. The live attenuated vaccine against YF confers protective immunity in about 90% of individuals within 10 days of receiving the 0.5-mL subcutaneous dose and in nearly 100% of individuals within 3 to 4 weeks after vaccination. A booster dose is recommended every 10 years. The World Health Organization (WHO) recommends vaccination for travelers to YF-endemic areas of Africa and South America, as well as for residents of those areas. The vaccine is contraindicated in persons who have known egg allergy or are immunosuppressed (e.g., transplant recipients). YF causes epidemics that can affect 20% of the population. When epidemics occur in unvaccinated populations, case fatality rates may exceed 50%. Clinical presentation is characterized by three stages—infection, remission, and intoxication. The period of infection consists of viremia with nonspecific symptoms and signs including fever, malaise, headache, joint pain, nausea, and vomiting. This is followed by a period of remission, with resolution of symptoms for up to 2 days. The subsequent period of intoxication is characterized by hepatic dysfunction, AKI, coagulopathy (low platelets), and shock. Diagnosis is confirmed by serologic testing such as IgM enzyme immunoassays or RT-PCR analysis for the YF virus genome.

### KIDNEY INVOLVEMENT IN YELLOW FEVER

Renal complications usually occur in the severe form of the disease between the fifth and seventh days, with reduction in urine volume and albuminuria. The mechanism of kidney involvement is poorly understood, although multiple causes are possible, including ischemic tubular injury due to shock, rhabdomyolysis, glomerulonephritis, and acute interstitial nephritis.[11,12] In experimental kidney injury, during the first 24 hours, kidney dysfunction appears to be related to hypovolemia and, later, oliguria, metabolic acidosis, albuminuria, and cylindruria occur. Viral antigen has been found in glomeruli and tubules. No treatment beyond supportive care is currently available.[10]

## MALARIA

Malaria is caused by *Plasmodium* parasites, which are carried by mosquitoes and transmitted to people through their bites. In Latin America and the Caribbean, 75% of malaria infections are caused by *Plasmodium vivax* and are rarely fatal; 25% are caused by the more lethal *Plasmodium falciparum*, the dominant malaria parasite in Africa.

Between 2000 and 2015, the number of cases of malaria in Latin America declined by 62%.[13] Of the total cases, 77% were reported by Brazil, Peru, and Venezuela. During the same period, malaria-related deaths fell by 76%. At the end of 2015, malaria was still endemic in 21 countries of Latin America.[13] Venezuela saw a 50% increase in its malaria cases between 2014 and 2015. If this trend continues, it is expected that Venezuela will have the largest number of cases in the region.[3,13] Despite the achievements, there are still an estimated 108 million people at risk for malaria, of which at least 5.7 million were classified as being at high risk.[13] The progress so far is largely due to improved treatment of the most deadly form of the disease, along with more effective mosquito control.

The clinical manifestations of malaria vary according to geography and prior immunity. Following the bite of an infected female *Anopheles* mosquito, the inoculated sporozoites go to the liver within 1 hour. Individuals are asymptomatic for 2 to 3 weeks, depending on parasite species, until the erythrocytic stage of the parasite life cycle. The release of merozoites from infected red blood cells when they rupture causes fever, malaise, headache, nausea, vomiting, and myalgias. Severe cases of hyperparasitemia may be associated with shock, acute respiratory distress syndrome (ARDS), AKI, coagulopathy, and hepatic failure. Physical findings include pallor, petechiae, jaundice, hepatomegaly, and splenomegaly. Clinical suspicion should prompt a confirmatory test for the parasite, which may involve light microscopy (visualization of parasites in stained blood samples), a rapid diagnostic test (detecting antigen or antibody), or a molecular technique for detecting parasite genetic material.

### KIDNEY INVOLVEMENT IN MALARIA

AKI is one of the most dreaded complications of severe malaria. According to WHO criteria, AKI (serum creatinine level ≥ 3 mg/dL, or ≥ 265 μmol/L) occurs as a complication of *P. falciparum* malaria in less than 1% of cases, but the mortality rate in these cases may be up to 45%.[14] Malaria-induced AKI is more common in adults than children. Renal involvement varies from mild proteinuria to severe azotemia associated with metabolic acidosis. It may be oliguric or nonoliguric. AKI may occur as a component of multiorgan dysfunction or as a lone complication. AKI is seen mostly in *P. falciparum* infections, but can occasionally occur with *P. vivax* and *P. malariae*. Malarial AKI is predominantly found in nonimmune adults and older children with falciparum malaria.

Several hypotheses have been proposed to explain the pathogenesis, including mechanical obstruction of glomerular capillaries by infected erythrocytes, immune-mediated glomerular injury, and acute tubular necrosis secondary to shock and/or free hemoglobin tubular toxicity.[15] It is likely that more than one of these mechanisms may occur simultaneously to produce the clinical manifestation. The predominant lesions on biopsy are acute tubular necrosis and mild proliferative glomerulopathy. Patients with these findings tend not to progress to CKD. Excessive fluid administration, oxygen toxicity, and yet unidentified factors may contribute to pulmonary edema, ARDS, multiorgan failure, and death.[14]

The management of malaria-induced AKI includes appropriate antimalarials (parenteral artesunate or quinine), fluid and electrolyte management, and early renal replacement therapy (RRT). Currently, high-quality intensive care, early institution of RRT, and avoidance of nephrotoxic drugs are standard practice for the prevention and management of AKI. Preliminary data have suggested that albumin infusion for volume expansion may reduce mortality rates.[16]

## LEPTOSPIROSIS

Leptospirosis is a zoonosis with protean manifestations caused by the spirochete *Leptospira interrogans*. The genus *Leptospira* consists of two species, *Leptospira interrogans* and *Leptospira biflexa*, only the former of which is known to cause human disease. More than 200 serovars of *L. interrogans* have been identified.

Leptospirosis is distributed worldwide, except for the polar regions. However, most clinical cases occur in the tropics. Leptospirosis presents a greater problem in humid tropical and subtropical areas, where most developing countries are found, than in areas with temperate climates. The magnitude of the problem in tropical and subtropical regions can be largely attributed not only to climatic and environmental conditions, but also to the greater likelihood of contact with a *Leptospira*-contaminated environment caused by, for example, local agricultural practices, as well as poor housing and waste disposal, all of which give rise to many sources of infection.[17]

Human leptospirosis is endemic in Latin America and usually reaches epidemic levels after higher rainfall periods with flooding or natural disasters such as hurricanes. In Brazil, 23,574 cases were reported from 1997 through 2008, with a mortality rate of 11.2%, and with similar figures reported from 2009 to 2017.[18] The number of cases in Brazil has steadily declined: 4341 in 2015, 2870 in 2016 and, as of September 2017, 2003.[18] Similarly, the death rate has declined from 334 in 2015 to 234 in 2016 and to 231 in 2017.[19]

The natural hosts for the organism are various mammals, including rodents, dogs, pigs, cattle, and horses. Humans are only incidentally infected, typically after exposure to the environment contaminated by animal urine, contaminated water or soil, or infected animal tissue. Portals of entry include cuts and abraded skin, mucous membranes, and conjunctiva. The infection is rarely caused by the ingestion of food contaminated with urine or via aerosols. Controversy exists as to whether *Leptospira* can penetrate intact skin.[20]

Leptospirosis is a potentially serious but treatable disease. It can provoke a broad range of manifestations, from benign infection, characterized by nonspecific symptoms, to Weil disease, a severe form of the disease that causes jaundice, hemorrhagic events, and AKI. Its symptoms may mimic those of a number of other unrelated infections, such as influenza, meningitis, hepatitis, dengue, and viral hemorrhagic fever.

Leptospirosis manifests as an abrupt onset of fever, rigors, myalgias, and headache in 75% to 100% of patients after an incubation period of 2 to 26 days (average, 10 days). After the acute septicemic stage, hyperbilirubinemia occurs in 85% of cases.[21] On physical examination, conjunctival suffusion is an important sign. Most patients have muscle tenderness, splenomegaly, lymphadenopathy, pharyngitis, hepatomegaly, muscle rigidity, abnormal respiratory auscultation, and/or rash.

The most widely used method for diagnosing leptospirosis is the microscopic agglutination test (MAT), which is performed using two blood samples collected 2 weeks apart. The MAT results are considered positive when the antibody titers are fourfold higher than the normal reference value.[22] Available in some laboratories, detection of antigens by a PCR assay offers the possibility of earlier diagnosis.

### KIDNEY INVOLVEMENT IN LEPTOSPIROSIS

Renal involvement is common in leptospirosis. Clinical manifestations vary from urinary sediment changes to AKI, which is observed in 44% to 67% of patients.[21,23] Leptospirosis manifesting as AKI is a severe disease, frequently leading to multiorgan failure and death. Leptospirosis-induced AKI typically is nonoliguric and often includes hypokalemia.[22]

The renal pathologic findings in leptospirosis are characterized by acute interstitial nephritis that may be associated with acute tubular necrosis.[24] The tubular injury may reflect a direct toxic effect of leptospiral compounds on tubular epithelial cells or indirect effects of dehydration, hypovolemia, and ischemia due to ionic wasting defects and the inability to concentrate urine.[20,21] Vasculitis is also observed in the acute phase of the disease. A cellular infiltrate consisting primarily of mononuclear cells can be diffuse or focused around the glomeruli and venules.[22] Studies have suggested that inflammation is most likely a secondary feature following acute epithelial damage and is observed only in patients who survive long enough for this feature to develop.[25]

Silver and other immunohistochemical staining reveals large numbers of intact leptospires throughout the tubular basement membrane, among tubular cells, and within the tubular lumens and the interstitium, with associated interstitial nephritis.[24] In some cases, organisms are seen in limited numbers within glomeruli, but glomerular changes in general are not remarkable.

Experience with leptospirosis-associated AKI in Thailand has shown that the use of hemodialysis or hemofiltration is associated with lower mortality (0% vs. 10%), shorter recovery time (8 vs. 16 days), and faster reduction in serum levels of bilirubin, urea, and creatinine in comparison with standard peritoneal dialysis.[26] There is, however, no data from randomized clinical trials evaluating different methods of RRT in patients with leptospirosis.[20]

The vast majority of infections with *Leptospira* are self-limiting. Two small randomized, placebo-controlled trials have shown a benefit of antimicrobial therapy. In one of these trials, in which doxycycline (100 mg PO, bid) was compared with placebo, doxycycline shortened the illness by an average of 2 days and prevented shedding of the organism in the urine. In a second trial, patients with severe leptospirosis who were treated with penicillin had fewer days of fever, more rapid resolution of serum creatinine level elevations, and shorter hospital stays; penicillin therapy also prevented urinary shedding. Therefore, symptomatic patients should receive antimicrobial therapy to shorten the duration of illness and reduce shedding of organisms in the urine. For patients with mild leptospirosis a course of doxycycline, amoxicillin, or azithromycin is recommended. Severe leptospirosis is usually treated with intravenous penicillin (1,500,000 U every 6 hours). Intravenous ceftriaxone (1 g once daily) or cefotaxime (1 g every 6 hours) has efficacy equivalent to that of penicillin. Treatment must be maintained for 7 days.

Doxycycline prophylaxis appears to be protective, reducing morbidity and mortality during outbreaks.[22] Control of reservoirs is difficult, and no vaccines are available. China and Brazil, countries where leptospirosis is a major health problem, have completed the sequence of the *L. interrogans* genome. Together with new genetic tools and proteomics, novel insights have been made into the biology of *Leptospira* and the mechanisms used to adapt to host and external environments. Surface-exposed proteins and putative virulence determinants have been identified that may serve as subunit vaccine candidates.

## NEPHROTOXICITY DUE TO VENOMS

### SPIDERS

Spiders of the genus *Loxosceles* are known colloquially as recluse spiders, violin spiders, fiddleback spiders and, in South America, by the nonspecific name "brown spiders." In South America, *Loxosceles* spiders of medical importance are found in Brazil and Chile. The most common species involved in envenomations are *Loxosceles laeta, Loxosceles intermedia,* and *Loxosceles gaucho. L. laeta* is often considered the most dangerous of the recluse spiders, in part because it is the species that attains the largest body size. Recluses are found mostly inside homes, in basements, in attics, behind bookshelves and dressers, and in cupboards. As their name implies, these spiders prefer dark quiet areas that are rarely disturbed. Outdoors, they are found under objects, such as rocks and the bark of dead trees.

*Loxosceles* spider bites are the leading cause of spider envenomation and necrotic arachnidism in humans. The venom of the spiders is inoculated to paralyze and digest their prey. "Loxoscelism," the term used to describe lesions and reactions induced by bites from spiders of the genus *Loxosceles,* causes skin necrosis, rhabdomyolysis, hemolysis, coagulopathy, AKI, and systemic inflammatory response syndrome (SIRS) in humans (Fig. 76.3). Loxoscelism is currently considered a serious public health problem in southern Brazil. There are 3000 reports of *Loxosceles* bites annually, and it constitutes the third leading cause of accidents involving venomous animals in Brazil.[27]

The venom can trigger a powerful inflammatory response characterized by local and systemic production of cytokines and chemokines, as well as the activation of complement and nitric oxide production, together with inflammatory cell migration and platelet aggregation.[28] The venom also has a direct hemolytic effect on red blood cells and damages the membranes of endothelial cells in blood vessel walls.[29]

#### KIDNEY INVOLVEMENT IN LOXOSCELISM

Rhabdomyolysis and hemolysis are recognized cofactors involved in the genesis of AKI,[29] and there is also evidence of a direct nephrotoxic action. The nephrotoxic effect of

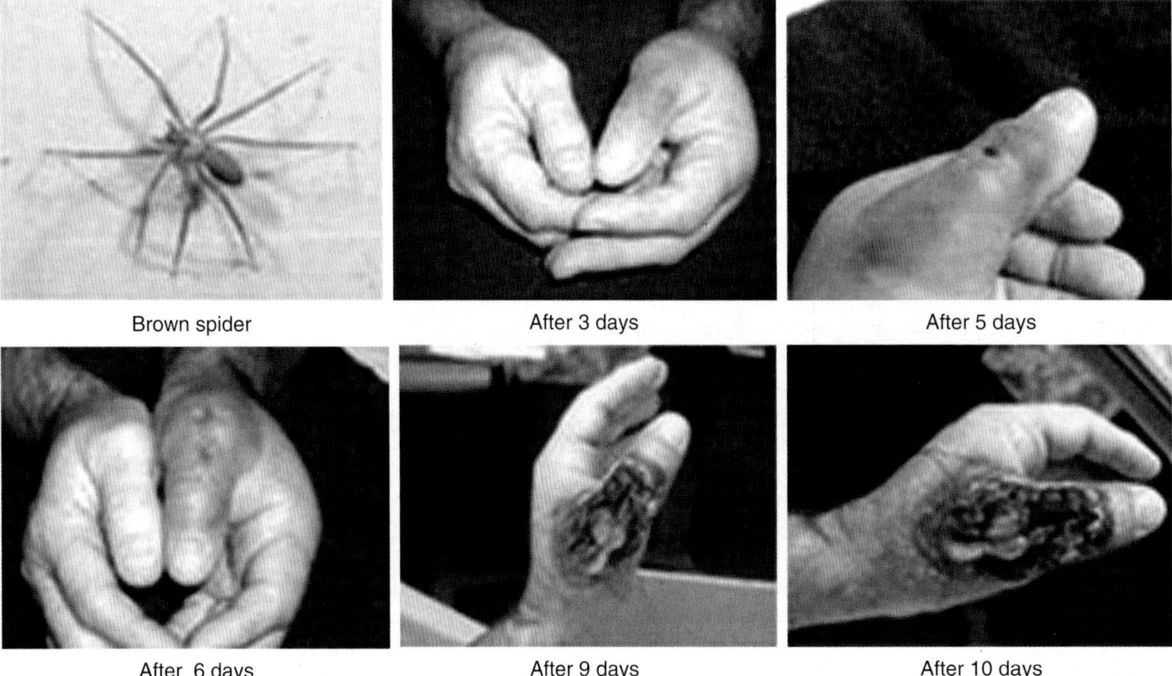


**Fig. 76.3** Evolution of skin lesions after brown spider bite.

the *Loxosceles* spider venom has been demonstrated experimentally in mice exposed to whole venom. Light microscopic analysis of kidney biopsy specimens has shown alterations, including hyalinization of proximal and distal tubules, erythrocytes in Bowman's space, glomerular collapse, tubule epithelial cell blebs and vacuoles, interstitial edema, and deposition of eosinophilic material in the tubule lumen.[30] Electron microscopic findings have indicated changes, including glomerular epithelial and endothelial cell cytotoxicity and disorders of the basement membrane. Tubule alterations include epithelial cell cytotoxicity with cytoplasmic membrane blebs, mitochondrial changes, increase in smooth endoplasmic reticulum, the presence of autophagosomes, and deposits of amorphous material in the tubules. In the same study, confocal microscopy with antibodies against venom proteins showed direct binding of toxins to renal structures, confirmed by competition assays.[30]

The treatment of a recluse spider bite involves local wound care, pain management, and tetanus prophylaxis, if indicated. Dapsone may be administered in some cases, both to prevent progression to necrosis and to reduce pain. Antivenoms for the treatment of recluse spider bites are available in Brazil, Mexico, and Peru, although not in the United States. The bites of South American *Loxosceles* species (e.g., *L. gaucho*) are more severe than those of recluse spiders found in the United States.

The results of studies involving animal models have suggested that specific types of antivenom decrease the lesion size and limit systemic illness, even when its administration is delayed. To date, the most extensive use of antivenom treatment has been in Brazil, and the Brazilian Ministry of Health has developed guidelines for its use in patients with extensive cutaneous lesions or severe systemic illness.[29] South American recluse antivenoms may help reduce the risk of dermonecrosis as well as systemic envenomation and its severe complications (e.g., hemolysis, AKI, disseminated intravascular coagulation [DIC]). The data regarding the efficacy of antivenom treatment are largely based on animal studies, and the benefit in humans has not been well established.

## *LONOMIA* CATERPILLARS

Caterpillars are the larval stage of moths and butterflies and are found worldwide.[31] *Lonomia* caterpillars (family, Saturniidae) are found in South America, and their venom affects mainly the coagulation system.[32] Accidental poisoning by caterpillars has become increasingly frequent in southern Brazil, partly owing to deforestation and the elimination of natural predators.[31] Accidental contact with caterpillars' bristles induces allergic and toxic signs and symptoms that range from a mild cutaneous reaction to severe systemic reactions, depending mainly on the number and species of the caterpillar involved. Symptoms include local irritation, urticarial dermatitis, allergy, ocular injuries, osteochondritis, hemorrhage, secondary coagulopathy, and AKI. Hemorrhagic complications, including intracerebral hemorrhage, can result in death.[22,31]

Caterpillars cluster in large numbers on tree barks and blend in very well (Fig. 76.4). Contact with large numbers of caterpillars can occur, exposing the individual to large dangerous doses of venom. Two species of *Lonomia,* the Brazilian caterpillar *Lonomia obliqua* and the Venezuelan caterpillar *Lonomia achelous,* provoke activation of the coagulation cascade through the action of several compounds that are the subject of toxicology research.[31] In *L. obliqua* bristle extract toxins have been identified, including a factor X activator named Losac and a prothrombin activator named Lopap.[33] Zannin and colleagues have reported a series of 105 patients poisoned by *L. obliqua* and found coagulation factor depletion and enhanced levels of fibrin degradation in keeping with DIC, although platelet counts were typically preserved.[34]

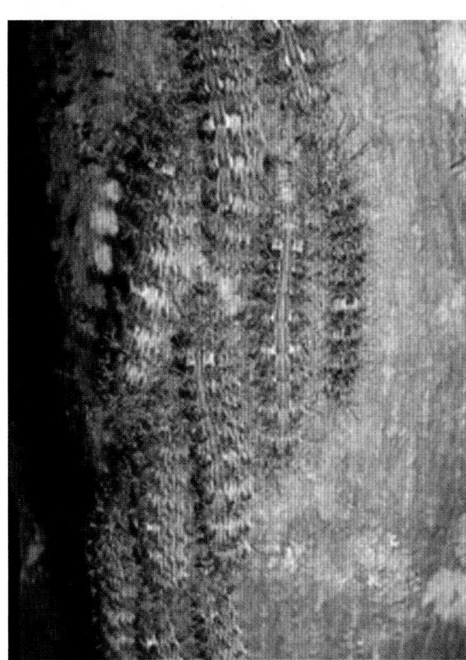

**Fig. 76.4** Cluster of caterpillars on the trunk of a tree. (Courtesy M. Vennegoor.)

Mortality in Brazil secondary to these toxins peaked at 20% before falling to less than 2% following the introduction of the anti-*Lonomia* horse serum (in Brazil) in 1995 and educational campaigns.

### RENAL INVOLVEMENT IN *LONOMIA* ACCIDENTS

Since 1989, the southern Brazilian states have reported accidental poisoning by *L. obliqua* in 2067 individuals. AKI developed in 1.9% of patients and, of these, 32% required dialysis, with 10.3% going on to have CKD.[35] Our group has reported an event with a successful outcome due to early recognition and treatment with the antivenom serum.[36] Even with anti-*Lonomia* serum, however, AKI can still occur.[37] Coagulation factors tend to be more profoundly altered in all patients with AKI, in keeping with their having more severe disease. The renal lesion appears to be secondary to massive deposition of fibrin in the glomeruli, leading to ischemia.[37,38] Some of the toxin components also cause direct toxicity to endothelium and tubular cells. The histology is poorly characterized because the coagulopathy prevents biopsies in the acute phase of the illness.

When traveling to endemic zones in Central and South America, travelers should be aware of poisonous caterpillars and avoid direct contact. Accidental poisoning should be reported immediately to the health authorities nearest the site where the poisoning took place because they are more likely to have immediate access to anti-*Lonomia* serum. Most countries do not stock this product, so timely administration and supportive measures are critical.

## SNAKES

Envenomation resulting from snakebites is a particularly important public health problem in rural areas of tropical and subtropical countries in Africa, Asia, Oceania, and Latin America. One study has estimated that at least 421,000 envenomations and 20,000 deaths occur worldwide from snakebite each year but warns that these figures may be as high as 1,841,000 envenomations and 94,000 deaths. The highest burdens of snakebites are in South Asia, Southeast Asia, and sub-Saharan Africa.[39]

There are approximately 3000 species of snakes, of which approximately 19% are venomous. Most snakebites occur in tropical regions, where they represent a serious public health burden because of the resulting morbidity and mortality. Latin America is the third most affected area after Asia and Africa. Snakebites are more common in the rainy seasons and are related to the increase in human activity in rural areas. The most affected group is 25- to 49-year-old men. Lower limbs are the most frequently injured sites.

Epidemiologic data on snakebite envenomation in Latin America are scarce. In Brazil, there are 20,000 accidents involving venomous snakes annually, an incidence of 13.5 accidents/100,000 inhabitants, and a mortality rate of about 0.45%. AKI is one of the main complications after snakebite envenomation and it is an important cause of death in affected patients. Snakebite-induced renal injury has been reported with almost all venomous snakes; however, AKI is more frequent with *Vipera russelli* in Asia, as well as *Bothrops* and *Crotalus* spp. in South America.[40]

### *CROTALUS* SNAKES

The South American rattlesnake, which belongs to the Viperidae family, Crotalinae subfamily, *Crotalus* genus, is represented in Brazil by a single species, *Crotalus durissus*, distributed into five subspecies, of which *Crotalus durissus terrificus* and *Crotalus durissus collilineatus* are the most important. *Crotalus* venom effects are multiple; the most important clinical manifestations are neurotoxicity, myotoxicity, nephrotoxicity, and coagulopathy.[41]

*Crotalus* venom induces clinical manifestations that can vary from mild local to severe systemic manifestations.[41] Neurotoxicity may manifest as eyelid ptosis, blurred and/or double vision, ophthalmoplegia, and facial paralysis. Myotoxicity is revealed by generalized myalgia and myoglobinuria due to the rhabdomyolysis. The coagulopathy caused by the thrombin-like enzyme produces blood incoagulability and afibrinogenemia in 40% to 50% of patients, although bleeding is a rare manifestation.[41]

#### Kidney Involvement in Crotalus Bites

The prevalence of AKI associated with *Crotalus* envenomation ranges from 10% to 29% and occurs within the first 24 to 48 hours after the bite. Experimental and clinical studies have suggested that the pathogenesis of *Crotalus* venom–induced AKI is likely related to rhabdomyolysis, renal vasoconstriction, and direct tubular cell toxicity.

*Crotalus* venom and probably crotoxin, the most important component of the venom, have direct and indirect actions on renal cells. Histologic injury usually found in *Crotalus* snakebite victims is acute tubular necrosis, although cases of interstitial nephritis have also been reported.[42,43] Shock, hypotension, hemolysis, sepsis, or nephrotoxic drugs can contribute to the AKI. In one report, dialysis was necessary in 24% of cases.[44] Mortality rates reported for AKI after *Crotalus* envenomation range from 8% to 17%.

### *BOTHROPS* SNAKES

In Latin America, the vast majority of snakebite envenomations are inflicted by species of the genus *Bothrops*. *Bothrops asper*, a species widely distributed in southern Mexico, Central America, and the northern areas of South America, is responsible for most cases in these regions.[45]

Snakes of the *Bothrops* genus belong to the Viperidae family and Crotalinae subfamily. There are more than 30 species distributed from southern Mexico to Argentina and Brazil. The most important species are *Bothrops asper* in Central America and *Bothrops atrox*, *Bothrops erythromelas*, *Bothrops neuwiedi*, *Bothrops moojeni*, *Bothrops jararaca*, *Bothrops jararacussu*, and *Bothrops alternatus* in Brazil.[41] These species are found in rural areas and on the outskirts of large cities and prefer humid environments, such as forests, plantation areas, and structures (e.g., barns, silos, and wood deposits), which are thought to contribute to the proliferation of snakes and rodents. These animals have nocturnal or crepuscular habits and an aggressive defensive behavior.[41]

*Bothrops* venom has proteolytic, coagulant, and hemorrhagic actions. Local manifestations at the bite site such as edema, blisters, and necrosis are caused by the venom's proteolytic action.[45] A direct nephrotoxic action of the venom has also been shown.[45] Lesions result from the activity of proteases, esterases, hyaluronidases, and phospholipases (phospholipase A2 [PLA2]), release of inflammatory mediators, action of hemorrhagins on the vascular endothelium, and procoagulant action of the venom.[41,46] The pathogenesis of these pathologic alterations has been investigated in experimental models. The observed effects result mostly from the combined action of $Zn^{4+}$-dependent metalloproteinases (snake venom metalloproteinases [SVMPs]) and myotoxic PLA2.[46] SVMPs are able to degrade extracellular matrix components, such as those present in the basement membrane of microvessels and at the dermal-epidermal junction, whereas myotoxic PLA2 disrupts the integrity of the plasma membrane of skeletal muscle fibers. In addition, a prominent inflammatory reaction of multifactorial origin develops, resulting in a pronounced edema and an inflammatory cell infiltrate.[46] The edema, in turn, contributes to hypovolemia and may promote increments in intracompartmental pressures in some muscle compartments, thus inducing further ischemia and tissue damage.

*Bothrops* venoms activate factor X and prothrombin, either alone or simultaneously.[45] They also have thrombin-like activity, converting fibrinogen into fibrin. These actions may lead to DIC. *Bothrops* venom may induce platelet function abnormalities, as well as a low platelet count.

Hemorrhagic manifestations result from the action of hemorrhagins, the metalloproteinases containing zinc described previously, in association with a low platelet count and coagulation abnormalities. Moreover, hemorrhagins are potent inhibitors of platelet aggregation.[41,46]

Early and progressive pain and edema, bruises, blisters, and bleeding are frequently observed at the venom inoculation area. In the most severe cases, there is necrosis of soft tissues with abscess formation and the development of compartment syndrome, which may result in functional or anatomic loss of the affected limb.[41] Systemic manifestations include bleeding (preexisting skin injuries, gingival bleeding, epistaxis, hematemesis, and hematuria), nausea, vomiting, excessive sweating, and hypotension. The most severe systemic complications are shock, AKI, septicemia, and a DIC-like syndrome.[41]

### Kidney Involvement in *Bothrops* Bites

AKI associated with *Bothrops* envenomation has been attributed to hemodynamic changes, myoglobinuria, hemoglobinuria, coagulation abnormalities, and direct venom nephrotoxicity.[40] Myoglobinuria is unlikely to be an important factor in the pathogenesis of renal injury because *Bothrops* venom may cause localized muscular injury but does not have a systemic myotoxic effect like *Crotalus* venom and does not induce a significant increase in the creatine kinase level.[45]

The development of hypotension or shock is a rare event after a *Bothrops* snakebite. Venom may cause hemodynamic abnormalities as a result of sequestration of fluids at the bite site, bleeding, and release of vasoactive substances. *Bothrops* venom is considered hemolytic in vitro, and there have been clinical reports of anemia and hemolysis after *Bothrops* envenomation, as well as reports of hemoglobinuria after the administration of *Bothrops* venom to rats. Hemoglobinuria might contribute to renal injury, worsening renal vasoconstriction, glomerular coagulation, and tubular nephrotoxicity.[47]

Renal dysfunction after *Bothrops* poisoning occurs early, is usually severe and oliguric, and presents the need for dialysis in 33% to 75% of cases.[47] The most frequent renal structural injury found is acute tubular necrosis, although cases of bilateral cortical necrosis, interstitial nephritis, and acute glomerulonephritis with mesangial proliferation have also been reported.[47] The mortality rate of *Bothrops* venom–induced AKI ranges from 13% to 19%.[47]

The management of snakebites involves immobilizing the injured part of the body to reduce the spread of venom and expediting transfer to an appropriate medical center. Tourniquets are not indicated because of the risk of significant ischemic damage. Expert consultation with a clinical toxicologist and/or poison control center is necessary for the timely administration of the appropriate antivenom.

## CHRONIC KIDNEY DISEASE IN LATIN AMERICA

Latin America has undergone tremendous demographic and socioeconomic development in the past few decades. Improvement in sanitation, access to clean water, and expansion of health care programs have contributed to a significant reduction in infant mortality, as well as death due to malnutrition and infectious diseases, resulting in the prolongation of life expectancy. However, urbanization and assimilation of a Western lifestyle have resulted in an increase in noncommunicable diseases, such as diabetes, obesity, and hypertension, leading to a significant rise in kidney disease prevalence.[48,49]

Currently, cardiovascular disease, diabetes, and malignancies are the leading causes of death in Latin America. Coping with this growth in noncommunicable diseases may be unsustainable and unaffordable for most countries, urging interventions to halt the trend. To achieve this goal, better characterization of the problem through data collection is critical. The Pan American Health Organization (PAHO) has developed strategies for the prevention and control of noncommunicable disease for the period 2012 to 2025, with a focus on cardiovascular diseases, cancer, diabetes and chronic respiratory diseases, their four common risk factors—tobacco use, unhealthy diet, physical inactivity, and harmful use of alcohol—and the related biologic risk factors such as hypertension and hyperglycemia.[50] Uruguay was the first country in Latin America to ban smoking in enclosed public spaces. Uruguay also has expanded access to primary health care services related to the early detection and risk factor prevention of noncommunicable diseases (NCDs). As a result, mortality linked to circulatory system diseases in the population 70 years of age and older has fallen from 75.18% in 2006 to 60.3% in 2014.[51,52] Mexico, which has one of the highest prevalence rates for diabetes, overweight, and obesity in the world, has reduced the consumption of sugar- sweetened beverages through the implementation of an excise tax of 1 peso/L on these drinks since January 2014.[53]

This section discusses the prevalence of, and risk factors and treatment strategies for, CKD in various Latin American countries, as well as the importance of the development of health programs for the earlier detection and prevention of CKD in this population.

## PREVALENCE OF CHRONIC KIDNEY DISEASE

The prevalence of CKD in Latin America is difficult to assess owing to the lack of reliable and systematically recorded data. Most information comes from voluntary registries so it may be skewed or incomplete, leading to an inaccurate picture. In addition, these records are confounded by heterogeneity in the population screened and in the methods used to determine the glomerular filtration rate (GFR) and proteinuria. A recent report from Brazil on the prevalence of CKD based on Kidney Disease: Improving Global Outcomes (KDIGO) criteria has revealed a prevalence of 11.4% in a randomly screened population.[54] In a Mexican population-based study, the prevalence rate of creatinine clearance ($C_{Cr}$) less than 15 mL/min was 1142/million population and of $C_{Cr}$ less than 60 mL/min was 80,788/million population.[55] Most of the data available have been based on advanced stages of CKD (end-stage kidney disease [ESKD]), showing that the prevalence has been growing by 7% annually during the past 10 years in Latin America. Nonetheless, the limited registry data of CKD in Latin America has revealed an average 12% prevalence of CKD compared with 11% in North America and 12% in Europe.[56,57] CKD is a major cause of death in the region, ranking as high as second in Nicaragua and Mexico (Fig. 76.5)[58]

From 1991 to 2013, the prevalence of ESKD in those undergoing RRT increased from 119 patients per million population (pmp) to 660 (hemodialysis [HD], 436 pmp; peritoneal dialysis [PD], 67 pmp; kidney transplantation, 157 pmp; Figs. 76.6 and 76.7). Only six countries have an RRT prevalence above the mean—Argentina, Brazil, Chile, Jalisco

| | Data quality rating | 1 | 2 | 3 | 4 | 5 | 6 | 7 | 8 | 9 | 10 |
|---|---|---|---|---|---|---|---|---|---|---|---|
| Argentina | ★★★★☆ | IHD (0-66) | LRI (1-93) | Stroke (0-62) | Road Inj (0-75) | Lung C (0-84) | COPD (1-1) | Self-Harm (0-79) | Congenital (1-1) | NN Preterm (1-21) | CKD (1-72) |
| Chile | ★★★★☆ | IHD (0-35) | Stroke (0-62) | Road Inj (0-69) | Self-Harm (0-78) | Stomach C (1-47) | Congenital (1-05) | Lung C (0-47) | LRI (0-77) | CKD (1-59) | Alzheimer's (0-77) |
| Uruguay | ★★★★☆ | IHD (0-58) | Stroke (0-96) | Lung C (1-5) | Self-Harm (1-17) | Road Inj (0-76) | COPD (1-47) | LRI (1-14) | Colorect C (1-73) | Alzheimer's (1-39) | Breast C (1-42) |
| Colombia | ★★★★☆ | Violence (5-37) | IHD (0-45) | Road Inj (0-62) | Stroke (0-32) | Congenital (0-75) | LRI (0-55) | NN Preterm (0-66) | COPD (0-71) | CKD (1-09) | Self-Harm (0-47) |
| Costa Rica | ★★★★★ | IHD (0-41) | Road Inj (0-67) | CKD (1-79) | Congenital (0-78) | Violence (1-34) | Stroke (0-25) | Self-Harm (0-55) | Alzheimer's (1-12) | Stomach C (1-07) | NN Preterm (0-55) |
| El Salvador | ★★★☆☆ | Violence (6-51) | IHD (0-63) | CKD (3-78) | Road Inj (0-78) | LRI (0-74) | Diabetes (1-5) | Alcohol (5-41) | Congenital (0-65) | Self-Harm (0-91) | Stroke (0-28) |
| Cuba | ★★★★★ | IHD (0-88) | Stroke (0-96) | Lung C (1-43) | LRI (1-27) | Self-Harm (0-75) | Alzheimer's (1-31) | COPD (1-01) | Colorect C (1-1) | CKD (1-73) | Prostate C (3-03) |
| Dominica | ★★★★☆ | IHD (0-57) | Diabetes (3-62) | Stroke (0-8) | CKD (3-37) | LRI (1-33) | Road Inj (0-81) | NN Enceph (3-73) | Prostate C (7-24) | Congenital (1-26) | HTN HD (3-24) |
| Dominican Republic | ★★★☆☆ | IHD (0-67) | HIV (29-32) | NN Preterm (1-7) | Stroke (0-63) | Road Inj (0-82) | Violence (2-01) | Congenital (1-1) | LRI (0-89) | NN Sepsis (6-8) | Diabetes (0-96) |
| Puerto Rico | ★★★★☆ | IHD (0-6) | Diabetes (6-21) | Violence (7-75) | Stroke (0-59) | LRI (1-95) | CKD (3-53) | Road Inj (0-98) | Alzheimer's (0-99) | COPD (1-04) | Colorect C (0-79) |
| Guatemala | ★★★★☆ | LRI (1-13) | Violence (3-49) | IHD (0-38) | NN Preterm (0-6) | Diarrhea (1-08) | Road Inj (0-54) | Diabetes (1-47) | Congenital (0-73) | CKD (1-57) | Stroke (0-31) |
| Honduras | ★★☆☆☆ | IHD (0-86) | Violence (3-17) | Stroke (0-58) | NN Preterm (0-58) | CKD (1-68) | Road Inj (0-45) | Congenital (0-52) | LRI (0-25) | Diarrhea (0-7) | NN Enceph (0-62) |
| Mexico | ★★★★☆ | IHD (0-43) | CKD (4-23) | Diabetes (2-95) | Violence (2-97) | Road Inj (0-81) | Congenital (1-28) | LRI (0-88) | Stroke (0-32) | NN Preterm (0-94) | Cirr HepC (2-91) |
| Nicaragua | ★★★☆☆ | IHD (0-41) | CKD (2-42) | LRI (0-39) | Road Inj (0-42) | Congenital (0-6) | Violence (1-03) | Diabetes (0-94) | Stroke (0-26) | NN Preterm (0-33) | Self-Harm (0-78) |
| Panama | ★★★★☆ | IHD (0-36) | Violence (3-32) | Road Inj (0-78) | Congenital (1-37) | LRI (1-18) | Stroke (0-45) | HIV (11-87) | Diabetes (1-57) | CKD (2-0) | NN Preterm (0-8) |
| Venezuela | ★★★★☆ | Violence (8-16) | IHD (0-67) | Road Inj (1-33) | Stroke (0-47) | Congenital (1-23) | NN Preterm (1-41) | CKD (2-26) | LRI (0-98) | Diabetes (1-62) | Self-Harm (0-77) |
| Bolivia | ★☆☆☆☆ | LRI (1-65) | NN Preterm (1-28) | IHD (0-54) | Congenital (1-25) | Road Inj (0-69) | Stroke (0-53) | NN Enceph (1-28) | CKD (1-66) | NN Sepsis (2-47) | Diabetes (0-95) |
| Ecuador | ★★★★☆ | Road Inj (0-98) | LRI (1-06) | IHD (0-32) | NN Preterm (1-09) | Violence (1-77) | Congenital (0-98) | CKD (1-92) | Stroke (0-35) | Diabetes (1-15) | Disaster (46-67) |
| Peru | ★★★☆☆ | LRI (1-6) | IHD (0-77) | Road Inj (0-52) | Congenital (0-85) | NN Preterm (0-64) | F Body (5-97) | Stroke (0-26) | NN Enceph (1-18) | NN Sepsis (3-16) | CKD (1-08) |
| Brazil | ★★★★☆ | IHD (0-6) | Violence (4-73) | Road Inj (1-07) | Stroke (0-7) | LRI (1-13) | Congenital (0-9) | Diabetes (1-41) | COPD (0-97) | Alzheimer's (1-14) | NN Preterm (0-68) |
| Paraguay | ★★★☆☆ | IHD (0-58) | Road Inj (1-05) | Stroke (0-68) | Violence (1-82) | Diabetes (1-71) | NN Preterm (0-97) | Congenital (1-0) | LRI (0-67) | CKD (1-72) | Self-Harm (0-57) |

**Fig. 76.5** Ranking of chronic kidney disease *(CKD)* as a cause of death in Latin America. CKD (highlighted in *green rectangle*) ranks within the top 10 causes of death in 18 of 20 countries and ranks among the top three causes of death in four countries. The Latin American rankings for CKD are the highest globally. (Modified from GBD 2016 Causes of Death Collaborators. Global, regional, and national age-sex specific mortality for 264 causes of death, 1980–2016: a systematic analysis for the Global Burden of Disease Study 2016. Lancet. 2017;390(10100):1151–1210.)

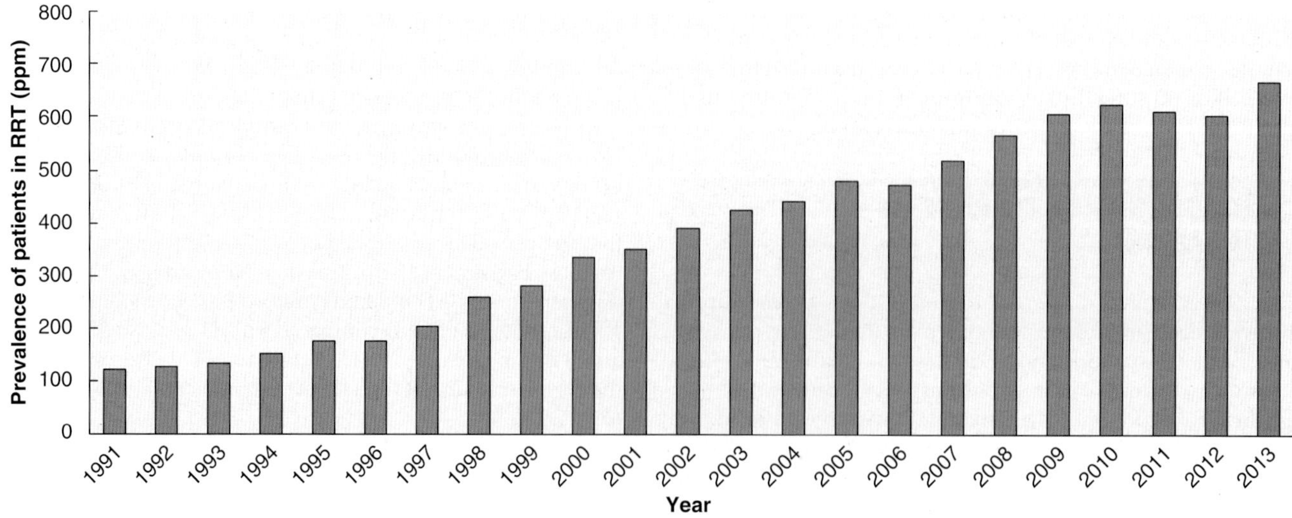


**Fig. 76.6** Prevalence of renal replacement therapy over time in Latin America 1991-2013. *RRT*, Renal replacement therapy. (From Cusumano AM, Rosa-Diez GJ, Gonzalez-Bedat MC. Latin American Dialysis and Transplant Registry: experience and contributions to end-stage renal disease epidemiology. World J Nephrol. 2016;5(5):389–397.)

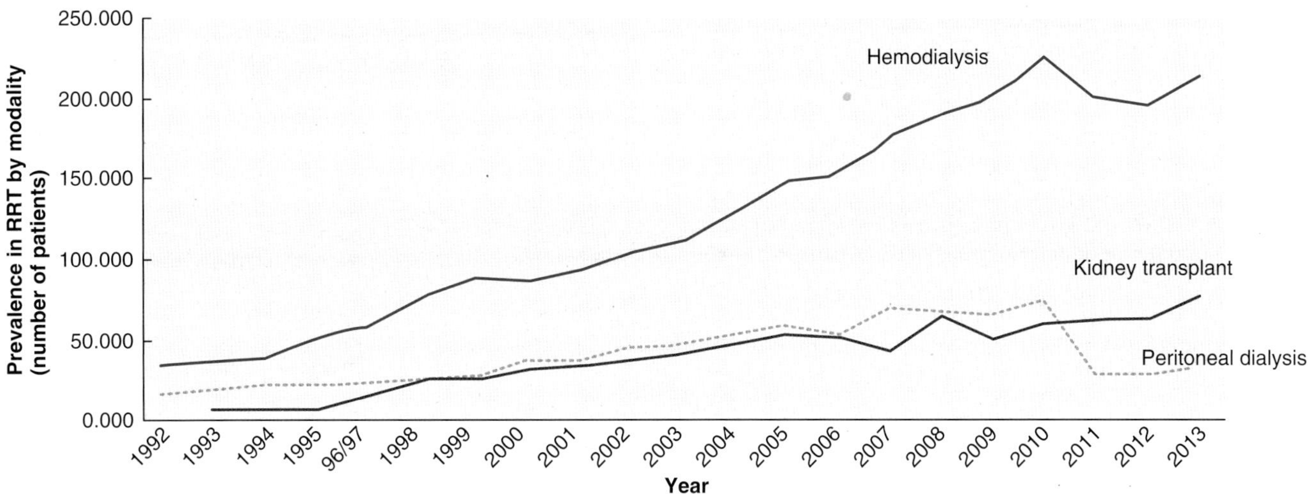


**Fig. 76.7** Prevalence of different renal replacement therapy modalities in Latin America, 1991–2013. *RRT,* Renal replacement therapy. (Modified from Cusumano AM, Rosa-Diez GJ, Gonzalez-Bedat MC. Latin American Dialysis and Transplant Registry: experience and contributions to end-stage renal disease epidemiology. World J Nephrol. 2016;5(5):389–397.)

**Table 76.1 Total Incidence Rates and Percentages of New Diabetic Renal Replacement Therapy Patients in Latin America**

| Country | Population | Incident Patients (pmp) | Incident Rate | Diabetics (%) |
|---|---|---|---|---|
| Argentina | 4,2202,935 | 6760 | 160.2 | 35.1 |
| Bolivia | 10,448,913 | 991 | 94.8 | 30.0 |
| Brazil | 202,740,000 | 36548 | 180.3 | 40.0 |
| Chile | 17,819,054 | 3230 | 182.4 | 16.7 |
| Colombia | 47,661,787 | 4274 | 89.7 | 33.5 |
| Ecuador | 161,00,000 | 2860 | 177.6 | 30.0 |
| Guatemala | 16,173,133 | 2018 | 124.8 | 30.0 |
| Jalisco (Mexico) | 7,742,303 | 3259 | 420.9 | 58.0 |
| Nicaragua | 6,146,000 | 150 | 24.4 | 41.6 |
| Paraguay | 6,783,374 | 137 | 20.2 | 45.3 |
| Peru | 30,297,279 | 910 | 30.0 | 32.2 |
| Puerto Rico | 3,615,000 | 1565 | 432.9 | 66.9 |
| Uruguay | 3,406,545 | 536 | 157.3 | 27.7 |

*pmp,* Per million population.
Modified from Cusumano AM, Rosa-Diez GJ, Gonzalez-Bedat MC. Latin American Dialysis and Transplant Registry: experience and contributions to end-stage renal disease epidemiology. World J Nephrol. 2016;5(5):389–397.

(Mexico), Puerto Rico, and Uruguay—with the reported rates ranging from 778 to 1847 pmp.[59]

## RISK FACTORS FOR CHRONIC KIDNEY DISEASE

Following the universal trend, the major risk factors for CKD in Latin America are hypertension and diabetes. Diabetic nephropathy is responsible for more than 30% of all cases of CKD in the region, although variation occurs (Mexico 40% vs. Argentina 20%) (Table 76.1).[49,60] The epidemic of diabetes is expected to continue worldwide, and an increase of more than 248% is forecast for the region from 2000 to 2030. Hypertension also is a silent cause of CKD, with a prevalence as high as 30% in the Mexican population. An evaluation of 8883 individuals in Southern Brazil, self-referred from the general population during a health fair, has shown that 16% of the population screened has a history of hypertension.[61] A family history of hypertension or diabetes was present in 42%. In addition, 30% of patients evaluated in this screening program had signs of hematuria, 6% had proteinuria, and 3% had hematuria and proteinuria.[61] In a Mexican national screening study of the general population, 9.2% of participants had proteinuria, which was strongly associated with hypertension, diabetes, obesity, and age.[62] Sedentary lifestyle, smoking, and unhealthy dietary habits, which included high-fat and high-carbohydrate consumption in Latin America, have contributed to the described comorbidities and expanding incidence of obesity.

Other important risk factors for CKD in the region include infectious complications, glomerulonephritis, and interstitial nephritis of unclear cause (discussed later in "Mesoamerican Nephropathy").

In summary, it is clear that the rising incidence of CKD is a major public health concern in Latin America, and diligent assessment of its prevalence, geographic distribution, and risk factors will be critical to establishing appropriate prevention programs for early screening and intervention. Uruguay has initiated a prevention program enrolling patients with CKD, and preliminary results have shown a significant improvement in blood pressure and glycemic control in association with a reduction in the rate of deterioration of renal function—from 3.1 mL/min per year to –0.13 mL/min per year in patients with CKD stages 2 to 3.[63] In Southern Brazil, the Pro-Renal Foundation has taken a leading role in raising awareness of CKD in the community.[61] It has also been a local pioneer in providing multidisciplinary care to patients with CKD with teams of nephrologists, nurses, social workers, dentists, podiatrists, psychologists, and dietitians.[64]

These successes demonstrate that it is possible to modify health trends in Latin America with the help of the local community. Even basic interventions, such as encouraging lifestyle changes through exercise and dietary substitutions, in combination with augmenting the awareness of blood pressure and blood glucose control, may yield significant reductions in incidence and progression of kidney disease.

**Table 76.2 Potential Causes of Mesoamerican Nephropathy**

| Cause | Examples |
|---|---|
| Toxins | Pesticides and agricultural chemicals, heavy metals, herbal toxins |
| Drugs | Nonsteroidal antiinflammatory drugs |
| Infections | Leptospirosis, pyelonephritis |
| Genetic, developmental susceptibility | Low birth weight, specific genetic predisposition of unclear origin (*APOL1*-like) |
| Heat-related volume depletion | Ischemia, repeated rhabdomyolysis, fructose-mediated injury |

## MESOAMERICAN NEPHROPATHY—CHRONIC KIDNEY DISEASE OF UNKNOWN CAUSE

The World Health Organization has demonstrated a high prevalence of CKD in regions of Nicaragua, Costa Rica, and El Salvador, with the highest mortality in El Salvador.[65]

Over the last decade, numerous reports have emerged from Central America regarding a rising prevalence of CKD, particularly among agricultural workers. CKD in this region seems to have a higher prevalence in men, favoring regions at lower altitudes, and particularly affecting workers in sugar cane plantations.[66–71]

These early reports described a clinical presentation characterized by an elevation of serum creatinine level and nonnephrotic proteinuria in young men without evidence of any known risk factors for CKD such as hypertension or diabetes, raising the possibility of a tubulointerstitial kidney disease due to an unknown environmental or occupational hazard.[72–74] Another hypothesis was an ischemic injury as a result of the heavy workload in a hot climate leading to chronic dehydration and hypovolemia. The significance of heat stress was suggested by the male preponderance and high prevalence in low-altitude farming villages close to the Pacific Ocean, where it is hotter. The combination of repeated episodes of dehydration during heavy manual work, and perhaps the concomitant use of NSAIDs, could explain the renal lesion. Nonetheless, it is clear that a second "hit" would be necessary for significant kidney injury to develop in such healthy young men. This endemic form of chronic kidney disease of unknown cause was named "Mesoamerican nephropathy" (MeN) and seemed to be endemic to Pacific coastal communities in Central America.[69]

Wijkström and colleagues presented the first study on the correlation of clinical data with biochemical and morphologic findings in patients with MeN. The investigators analyzed renal biopsy samples from eight male sugarcane workers (aged 22–57 years) from a rural area of El Salvador who had presented with impaired renal function (estimated GFR, 27–77 mL/min/1.73 m$^2$), inactive urinary sediment, and nonnephrotic proteinuria.[66,75] The morphologic picture was similar in biopsy specimens of all included patients. Chronic tubulointerstitial damage with tubular atrophy and interstitial fibrosis was found, in combination with chronic glomerular changes. The most striking and surprising finding was the presence of relatively extensive global sclerosis, involving 29% to 78% of glomeruli analyzed.[66] These biopsies confirmed the suspicion of a primary tubulointerstitial disease. Immunofluorescence and electron microscopy did not show immune complex deposits, so an immune complex disease seemed unlikely.[66]

In one study, recurrent dehydration has been shown to raise serum osmolarity and activate the polyol pathway in the kidney, leading to increased conversion of glucose to sorbitol and fructose. Fructose in turn can be metabolized by the fructokinase that is constitutively present, resulting in the generation of uric acid, oxidants, and chemokines, which can cause local tubulointerstitial injury.[76,77] The same group has also shown that repeated dehydration can cause chronic kidney injury in mice and that this injury is fructokinase-dependent, because mice with knockout of fructokinase are protected.[76] Thus, it is possible that MeN may be a kidney disease due to chronic dehydration and that recurrent dehydration is almost certainly a component of its pathogenesis, leading to tubulointerstitial injury.[78,79] However, toxins (e.g., pesticides) or heavy metals might contribute as a second factor in the development of the disease. Although originally reported in Central America, MeN could represent a larger entity, explaining CKD epidemics seen in countries such as Sri Lanka, Bangladesh, and central Australia (Table 76.2; see related discussion in Chapters 75, 77, and 79).[68]

## END-STAGE KIDNEY DISEASE IN LATIN AMERICA

The prevalence of ESKD in Latin America is extrapolated from data provided about RRT in the region. However, due to the heterogeneous availability of RRT according to the nations' health care coverage and budget, these numbers do not clearly represent the true prevalence. The best available information comes from the Latin American Dialysis and

Kidney Transplant Registry (LADKTR), a committee of the Latin American Society of Nephrology and Hypertension (SLANH), that has been collecting data since 1991 (Table 76.3). These data show a growth of more than 200% in the prevalence of ESKD in Latin America over the past 13 years (see Fig. 76.6).

Although RRT is provided to all patients with a diagnosis of ESKD in Argentina, Brazil, Chile, Cuba, Puerto Rico, Uruguay, and Venezuela, some countries may provide RRT for as few as 20% of these patients and other countries, such as Bolivia, may pay for only twice-weekly dialysis. Furthermore, Latin American middle-income countries have a disproportionally different prevalence of RRT, which seems to correlate with the type of health coverage provided. Universal RRT coverage is associated with the highest prevalence of RRT (e.g., Argentina, Brazil) compared with no universal access (e.g., Nicaragua, Guatemala, Paraguay).[81] The consequence of this heterogeneous coverage is that the prevalence rate of RRT may vary enormously among countries (see Table 76.3). Thus,the prevalence rate is more than 600 pmp in Puerto Rico, Chile, Uruguay, and Argentina; between 300 and 600 pmp in Colombia, Brazil, Mexico, Panama, and Venezuela; and significantly lower, perhaps less than 100 pmp, in the remaining countries.[81] The leading cause of ESKD in Latin America is diabetes, with the highest incidences reported in Puerto Rico (66.9%), Mexico (58.0%), Paraguay (45.3%), and Brazil (40.0%).[56]

The low prevalence of ESKD in some regions should raise the suspicion of underdiagnosis and/or lack of available resources to offer RRT. The direct correlation of the degree of development of a country with the prevalence of RRT suggests that access to ESKD care is an important component. One report has confirmed this relationship by showing that RRT prevalence and kidney transplantation rates correlate significantly with gross domestic product, health expenditure, proportion of the population older than 65 years, life expectancy at birth, and proportion of the population living in urban settings.[82] Owing to the substantial economic burden of providing dialysis in many countries that still lack essentials such as sanitation, prevention strategies to halt kidney disease progression are critical.

## TRANSPLANTATION

Renal transplantation has also developed significantly in Latin America. The data from the LADKTR indicated that the overall kidney transplantation rate increased from 3.7 pmp in 1987 to 6.9 in 1991, and then to 19.4 in 2013, although, there were remarkable disparities among the various countries in the last year—57.7 pmp in Jalisco (Mexico), 32 pmp in Uruguay, and 1.8 pmp in Nicaragua. The highest number of transplants ($n$ = 5433) was in Brazil, which had a transplantation rate of 26.8 pmp for 2013.[56] More recent data from Brazil have revealed an annual total transplant number of 5648 in 2015 (27.9 pmp), followed by Mexico, with 2707, Argentina, 1198, and Colombia, 761. In 2016, Brazil had performed 5492 kidney transplantations—4292 deceased donors, 1200 living donors (171 partners, 80 unrelated).[83] These rates are still remarkably lower than those in other developed countries, such as the United States (46 pmp) and Sweden (41 pmp). About 52% of these transplants are from deceased donors, though some countries, such as Nicaragua, Peru and El Salvador, performed solely living donor kidney transplantations.

Brazil has been one of the countries with the greatest expansion in kidney transplantation numbers, in part because of its free universal health coverage system, which includes full ambulatory and hospital medical care, along with provision of all immunosuppressive drugs for patients undergoing transplantation. A single city in Brazil (São Paulo) has developed the largest kidney transplantation program in the world.[83] In addition to increased efficiency in organ procurement, several other factors have contributed to this expansion, including the development of a dedicated hospital (Hospital do Rim) for kidney transplantations and a system for rapid workup of recipients and donors.[83] This program has approximately 5011 patients on the waiting list, and the recipient selection is based on human leukocyte antigen (HLA) matching. A significant proportion of the recipients are black and have been on dialysis for a long time. More than 700 first consultations for living donation are done every year, and most patients are followed locally after transplantation, with more than 200 appointments/day. Transplantation outcomes among living donor recipients are comparable to those reported in large registries but inferior outcomes have been observed among recipients of deceased donor organs. This is likely due to prolonged ischemia time due to poor care of critically ill potential deceased donors and logistic difficulties from a lack of financial support in organ allocation.[83,84]

The criteria for brain death have been well established and culturally accepted in all Latin American countries, and family consent is required for organ donation.[85] The regulations for living donors are also well defined, with restrictions against unrelated donors and prohibition of any kind of organ commerce. Access to transplantation is limited by the health care models of individual countries. In addition, lack of an organized organ procurement system leads to significant limitations in the number of organs available in many countries. One of the greatest challenges is to reduce the regional disparities related to access to transplantation. Furthermore, improvements and resources could be better used, with the development of a Latin American registry of outcomes of transplanted patients and living donors. Finally, clinical and experimental studies to understand the transplantation-related immune response of the ethnically diverse Latin American population better would be critical to advance the transplantation field in this region further.

## TRENDS AND THE FUTURE

The greatest challenge for the nephrology community in Latin America in the coming years will be dealing with the growing number of patients with ESKD, the lack or incompleteness of health care coverage for RRT in some countries, late referrals, shortage of trained personnel, small kidney transplantation programs, and lack of registries. In addition, the early identification and aggressive treatment of infectious diseases complicated by AKI may minimize long-term renal sequelae. In spite of the worldwide concern about the increasing number of patients with ESKD and efforts to identify risk groups, as well as the development of strategies for the

**Table 76.3 Socioeconomic Indexes, Prevalence and Incidence of Renal Replacement Therapy and Transplantation Rate in Latin America**

| Country | Population | GNI | LEB | Prevalence Rates, pmp | | | | | Incidence Rate | Kidney Tx, *n* | Tx by Deceased Donors, % | Kidney Tx, Rate | Nephrologists, *n* | Nephrologists, pmp |
|---|---|---|---|---|---|---|---|---|---|---|---|---|---|---|
| | | | | HD | PD | Total Dialysis | Lfg | Total RRT | | | | | | |
| Argentina | 42,202,935 | 13,690 | 76 | 626.6 | 36.0 | 662.7 | 197.2 | 859.9 | 160.2 | 1287 | 68.4 | 30.5 | 1150 | 27.2 |
| Bolivia | 10,448,913 | 2220 | 67 | 195.2 | 18.3 | 213.5 | 31.6 | 245.1 | 94.8 | 75 | 24.0 | 7.2 | 24 | 2.3 |
| Brazil | 202,740,000 | 11,640 | 74 | 449.6 | 45.6 | 495.2 | 212.6 | 707.8 | 180.3 | 5433 | 74.7 | 26.8 | 3300 | 16.3 |
| Chile | 17,819,054 | 14,290 | 80 | 1019.1 | 61.2 | 1080.3 | 205.1 | 1285.4 | 182.4 | 234 | 74.8 | 13.1 | 132 | 7.4 |
| Colombia | 47,661,787 | 7020 | 74 | 349.0 | 143.6 | 492.6 | 111.3 | 603.9 | 89.7 | 680 | 99.7 | 14.3 | 95 | 2.0 |
| Costa Rica | 4,773,730 | 8850 | 80 | 42.3 | 76.0 | 118.4 | 282.6 | 400.9 | ND | 105 | 48.6 | 22.0 | 24 | 5.0 |
| Cuba | 11,163,934 | 6051 | 79 | 259.1 | 10.1 | 269.3 | 78.4 | 347.6 | 103.1 | 174 | ND | 15.6 | 524 | 46.9 |
| Ecuador | 16,100,000 | 3600 | 76 | 481.8 | 48.0 | 529.8 | 20.4 | 550.2 | 177.6 | 127 | 81.1 | 7.9 | 143 | 8.9 |
| El Salvador | 6,401,240 | 5360 | 72 | 232.5 | 288.7 | 521.1 | 73.6 | 594.7 | 390.1 | 20 | 0.0 | 3.1 | 47 | 7.3 |
| Guatemala | 16,173,133 | 3130 | 72 | 157.7 | 221.3 | 379.0 | 54.0 | 433.0 | 124.8 | 90 | 13.3 | 5.6 | 54 | 3.3 |
| Honduras | 8,500,000 | 2140 | 73 | 186.9 | 14.4 | 201.3 | 8.4 | 209.6 | 176.7 | 0 | 0.0 | 0.0 | 18 | 2.1 |
| Jalisco (Mexico) | 7,742,303 | ND | ND | 599.4 | 486.7 | 1086.1 | 567.4 | 1653.5 | 420.9 | 447 | 16.1 | 57.7 | 45 | 5.8 |
| Nicaragua | 6,146,000 | 1690 | 74 | 211.5 | 24.4 | 235.9 | 21.2 | 257.1 | 24.4 | 11 | 0.0 | 1.8 | 28 | 4.6 |
| Panamá | 3,975,404 | 9030 | 77 | 495.0 | 90.3 | 585.3 | 110.7 | 696.0 | 462.1 | 48 | 73.1 | 12.1 | 25 | 6.3 |
| Paraguay | 6,783,374 | 3310 | 75 | 165.7 | 4.0 | 169.7 | 19.9 | 189.6 | 20.2 | 26 | 79.0 | 3.8 | 46 | 6.8 |
| Perú | 30,297,279 | 5680 | 72 | 272.2 | 43.1 | 315.3 | 63.2 | 378.5 | 30.0 | 184 | 75.0 | 6.1 | 301 | 9.9 |
| Puerto Rico | 3,615,000 | 18,370 | 79 | 1362.1 | 106.2 | 1468.3 | 378.4 | 1846.7 | 432.9 | 80 | 86.3 | 22.1 | 97 | 26.8 |
| Rep Dominicana | 12,000,000 | 5570 | 73 | 178.8 | 47.3 | 226.1 | 52.8 | 278.9 | 208.3 | 84 | 92.9 | 7.0 | 135 | 11.3 |
| Uruguay | 3,406,545 | 13,670 | 77 | 692.2 | 71.6 | 763.8 | 323.5 | 1087.3 | 157.3 | 105 | 91.4 | 30.8 | 173 | 50.8 |
| Venezuela | 30,389,596 | 12,460 | 74 | 505.1 | 0.0 | 505.1 | 60.8 | 565.9 | ND | 281 | 69.8 | 9.2 | 502 | 16.5 |
| Totals | 488,340,227 | 147,771 | 75 | 442.0 | 67.0 | 509.0 | 159.0 | 669.0 | 149 | 9491 | 70.4 | 19.4 | 6863 | 14.0 |

prevention of CKD, there is little activity in many Latin American countries. Dialogue between the nephrology community and government authorities in the region has to be based on data, which are lacking. Only a few countries have reliable registries of ESKD and transplantation programs. The lack of universal health care coverage in some countries and, in many cases, a restrictive renal replacement program, poses a much greater challenge because it reflects the public health agenda of a particular country and is a difficult scenario to modify. It is to be hoped that the combined efforts of scientific, nephrology and transplantation societies, kidney foundations, and patient organizations will advocate for and implement screening and prevention programs for CKD, educate the community, establish registries and more active kidney transplantation programs, and engage policy makers regarding the importance of kidney disease prevention and treatment.

 Complete reference list available at ExpertConsult.com.

## KEY REFERENCES


1. *World population review*; 2017. http://worldpopulationreview.com/continents/latin-america-population/. Accessed December 11, 2017.
5. Lima EQ, Gorayeb FS, Zanon JR, et al. Dengue haemorrhagic fever-induced acute kidney injury without hypotension, haemolysis or rhabdomyolysis. *Nephrol Dial Transplant.* 2007;22(11):3322–3326.
7. Khalil MAM, Sarwar S, Chaudry MA, et al. Acute kidney injury in dengue virus infection. *Clin Kidney J.* 2012;5:390–394.
8. Boonpucknavig V, Bhamarapravati N, Boonpucknavig S, et al. Glomerular changes in dengue hemorrhagic fever. *Arch Pathol Lab Med.* 1976;100(4):206–212.
10. Pan American Health Organization/World Health Organization. *Epidemiological Update: Yellow Fever.* 2 March, Washington, D.C.: PAHO/WHO; 2017; Accessed December 13, 2017.
11. Monath TP. Yellow fever: a medically neglected disease. Report on a seminar. *Rev Infect Dis.* 1987;9(1):165–175.
12. Lima EQ, Nogueira ML. Viral hemorrhagic fever-induced acute kidney injury. *Semin Nephrol.* 2008;28(4):409–415.
13. Pan American Health Organization. *Health in the Americas+, 2017 Edition.* Summary: Regional Outlook and Country Profiles. Washington, D.C.: PAHO; 2017.
14. Mishra SK, Das BS. Malaria and acute kidney injury. *Semin Nephrol.* 2008;28(4):395–408.
15. Barsoum RS. Malarial acute renal failure. *J Am Soc Nephrol.* 2000;11(11):2147–2154.
20. Cerqueira TB, Athanazio DA, Spichler AS, et al. Renal involvement in leptospirosis—new insights into pathophysiology and treatment. *Braz J Infect Dis.* 2008;12(3):248–252.
22. Andrade L, de Francesco Daher E, Seguro AC. Leptospiral nephropathy. *Semin Nephrol.* 2008;28(4):383–394.
23. Sitprija V, Losuwanrak K, Kanjanabuch T. Leptospiral nephropathy. *Semin Nephrol.* 2003;23(1):424–428.
24. Covic A, Goldsmith DJ, Gusbeth-Tatomir P, et al. A retrospective 5-year study in Moldova of acute renal failure due to leptospirosis: 58 cases and a review of the literature. *Nephrol Dial Transplant.* 2003;18(6):1128–1134.
25. Arean VM. The pathologic anatomy and pathogenesis of fatal human leptospirosis (Weil's disease). *Am J Pathol.* 1962;40:393–423.
27. McBride AJ, Athanazio DA, Reis MG, et al. Leptospirosis. *Curr Opin Infect Dis.* 2005;18(5):376–386.
28. de Souza AL, Malaque CM, Sztajnbok J, et al. Loxosceles venom-induced cytokine activation, hemolysis, and acute kidney injury. *Toxicon.* 2008;51(1):151–156.
33. Alvarez Flores MP, Fritzen M, Reis CV, et al. Losac, a factor X activator from Lonomia obliqua bristle extract: its role in the pathophysiological mechanisms and cell survival. *Biochem Biophys Res Commun.* 2006;343(4):1216–1223.
36. Riella M, Chula D, de Freitas S, et al. Acute renal failure and haemorrhagic syndrome secondary to toxin of caterpillars (*Lonomia obliqua*). *NDT Plus.* 2008;1:445–446.
37. Burdmann EA, Antunes I, Saldanha LB, et al. Severe acute renal failure induced by the venom of *Lonomia* caterpillars. *Clin Nephrol.* 1996;46(5):337–339.
42. Pinho FM, Yu L, Burdmann EA. Snakebite-induced kidney injury in Latin America. *Semin Nephrol.* 2008;28:354–362.
44. Pinho FM, Zanetta DM, Burdmann EA. Acute renal failure after *Crotalus durissus* snakebite: a prospective survey on 100 patients. *Kidney Int.* 2005;67(2):659–667.
47. Albuquerque PL, Jacinto CN, Silva Junior GB, et al. Acute kidney injury caused by Crotalus and Bothrops snake venom: a review of epidemiology, clinical manifestations and treatment. *Rev Inst Med Trop Sao Paulo.* 2013;55(5):295–301. Accessed June 28, 2018. online.
48. Cusumano AM, Gonzalez Bedat MC. Chronic kidney disease in Latin America: time to improve screening and detection. *Clin J Am Soc Nephrol.* 2008;3(2):594–600.
49. Jha V, Garcia-Garcia G, Iseki K, et al. Chronic kidney disease: global dimension and perspectives. *Lancet.* 2013;382(9888):260–272.
53. Colchero MA, Popkin BM, Rivera JA, et al. Beverage purchases from stores in Mexico under the excise tax on sugar sweetened beverages: observational study. *BMJ.* 2016;352:h6704.
54. Piccolli AP, Nascimento MM, Riella MC. Prevalence of chronic kidney disease in a population in southern Brazil (Pro-Renal Study). *J Bras Nefrol.* 2017;39(4):385–391.
56. Hill NR, Fatoba ST, Oke JL, et al. Global prevalence of chronic kidney disease – a systematic review and meta-analysis. *PLoS ONE.* 2016;11(7):e0158765.
57. Bello AK, Levin A, Tonelli M, et al (2017). *Global Kidney Health Atlas: A report by the International Society of Nephrology on the current state of organization and structures for kidney care across the globe.* International Society of Nephrology, Brussels,Belgium. https://www.theisn.org/images/ISN_advocacy/GKHAtlas_Linked_Compressed1.pdf. Accessed June 28, 2018.
58. GBD 2016 Causes of Death Collaborators. Global, regional, and national age-sex specific mortality for 264 causes of death, 1980-2016: a systematic analysis for the Global Burden of Disease Study 2016. *Lancet.* 2017;390(10100):1151–1210. doi:10.1016/S0140-6736(17)32152-9. PubMed PMID: 28919116. PubMed Central PMCID: PMC5605883.
59. Cusumano AM, Rosa-Diez GJ, Gonzalez-Bedat MC. Latin American Dialysis and Transplant Registry: experience and contributions to end-stage renal disease epidemiology. *World J Nephrol.* 2016;5(5):389–397.
61. Mazza Nascimento M, Riella MC. Raising awareness of chronic kidney disease in a Brazilian urban population. *Braz J Med Biol Res.* 2009;42(8):750–755.
63. Rodriguez-Iturbe B. Progress in the prevention of chronic kidney disease in Latin America. *Nat Clin Pract Nephrol.* 2008;4(5):233.
64. Riella MC. Nephrologists Sans Frontieres: a kidney foundation—advancing research and helping patients meet their needs. *Kidney Int.* 2006;69(8):1285–1287.
68. Johnson RJ, Sanchez-Lozada LG. Chronic kidney disease: mesoamerican nephropathy—new clues to the cause. *Nat Rev Nephrol.* 2013;9(10):560–561.
72. Haas M. Mesoamerican nephropathy: pathology in search of etiology. *Kidney Int.* 2018;93(3):538–540.
73. Fischer RSB, Vangala C, Truong L, et al. Early detection of acute tubulointerstitial nephritis in the genesis of Mesoamerican nephropathy. *Kidney Int.* 2018;93(3):681–690.
74. Lusco MA, Fogo AB, Wernerson AÖ, et al. AJKD atlas of renal pathology: CKD of unknown cause (CKDu); Mesoamerican nephropathy. *Am J Kidney Dis.* 2017;70(3):e17–e18.
75. Wijkström J, González-Quiroz M, Hernandez M, et al. Renal morphology, clinical findings, and progression rate in Mesoamerican nephropathy. *Am J Kidney Dis.* 2017;69(5):626–636.
76. Cirillo P, Gersch MS, Mu W, et al. Ketohexokinase-dependent metabolism of fructose induces proinflammatory mediators in proximal tubular cells. *J Am Soc Nephrol.* 2009;20(3):545–553.
77. Nakayama T, Kosugi T, Gersch M, et al. Dietary fructose causes tubulointerstitial injury in the normal rat kidney. *Am J Physiol Renal Physiol.* 2010;298(3):F712–F720.
78. Gonzalez-Quiroz M, Smpokou ET, Silverwood RJ, et al. Decline in kidney function among apparently healthy young adults at risk of Mesoamerican nephropathy. *J Am Soc Nephrol.* 2018;doi:10.1681/ASN.2018020151. pii: ASN.2018020151, Epub ahead of print.
79. González-Quiroz M, Camacho A, Faber D, et al. Rationale, description and baseline findings of a community-based prospective cohort study of kidney function amongst the young rural population of Northwest Nicaragua. *BMC Nephrol.* 2017;18:1.

81. Obrador TT, et al. The challenge of providing renal replacement therapy in developing countries: the Latin American perspective. *Am J Kidney Dis.* 2016;67(3):499–506.
82. Cusumano AM, Garcia-Garcia G, Gonzalez-Bedat Maria C, et al. Latin American Dialysis and Transplant Registry: 2008 prevalence and incidence of end-stage renal disease and correlation with socioeconomic indexes. *Kidney Int.* 2013;3:153–156.
83. Garcia VD, Abbud-Filho M, Felipe C, et al. An Overview of the Current Status of Organ Donation and Transplantation in Brazil. *Transplantation.* 2015;99(8):1535–1537.
84. Registro Brasileiro de Transplantes. *Associacao Brasileira de Transplante de Orgaos.* Ano XXII N.o 4. Dimensionamento dos Transplantes no Brasil e em cada estado. http://www.abto.org.br/abtov03/Upload/file/RBT/2016/RBT2016-10032017.pdf. Accessed December 13, 2017.
85. Medina-Pestana JO, Duro-Garcia V. Strategies for establishing organ transplant programs in developing countries: the Latin America and Caribbean experience. *Artif Organs.* 2006;30(7):498–500.

# 77

# Global Considerations in Kidney Disease: Africa

Mogamat Razeen Davids | Mohammed Benghanem Gharbi

## CHAPTER OUTLINE



## KEY POINTS

- The growing burden of renal disease in Africa is driven by the high rates of infectious diseases, noncommunicable diseases, pregnancy-related diseases, and injuries.
- In most African countries, financial and human resources are inadequate to meet this challenge.
- Most patients with end-stage renal disease cannot access renal replacement therapy and the lack of access to acute dialysis results in many potentially preventable deaths due to acute kidney injury.
- Positive initiatives that provide hope for the future include the training of nephrology healthcare professionals via the ISN and ISPD Fellowship programs, increased awareness of kidney disease resulting from World Kidney Day activities, and the Saving Young Lives and 0by25 projects, which are improving the outcomes for patients with acute kidney injury.

## INTRODUCTION

Africa is the world's second-largest and second-most-populous continent, including 55 countries and diverse ethnic groups, religions and languages. Its population in mid-2017 was estimated at 1.3 billion and it is projected to reach 2.6 billion by 2050, at which time it will account for most of the global population increase (Fig. 77.1).[1,2] Half of the world's population growth is expected to be concentrated in nine countries, and this list includes five countries from Africa: Nigeria, the Democratic Republic of the Congo, Ethiopia, the United Republic of Tanzania, and Uganda.[2]

The African population is very young, with 41% of people being under the age of 15 years old and only 3% being 65 years or older, compared with the world averages of 26% and 9%, respectively.[1] In Western Africa, the life expectancy of men is 55 years and 57 years for women, both of which are the lowest of any world region.[1] These findings are in stark contrast to many other regions of the world, where lower fertility rates and increasing life expectancy have contributed to the aging of populations. Africa's youth population is predicted to rise from 20% in 2017 to 35% of the world youth population in 2050 (Fig. 77.2).

Globally, the highest birth rates are seen in African countries, with the highest average lifetime births per woman being recorded in Niger (7.3), Chad (6.4), and Somalia (6.4).[1] Child marriages and adolescent childbearing are common in many countries of sub-Saharan Africa,[3] and pose serious consequences for the health of young girls and their offspring. Early childbearing also limits their educational and employment opportunities.

Table 77.1 summarizes the population estimates and the economic, and development indicators of African countries. Africa is by far the world's poorest region and is currently recovering from a sharp economic slowdown experienced over the last two years. There are improved outputs from the mining and agriculture sectors, which are boosting

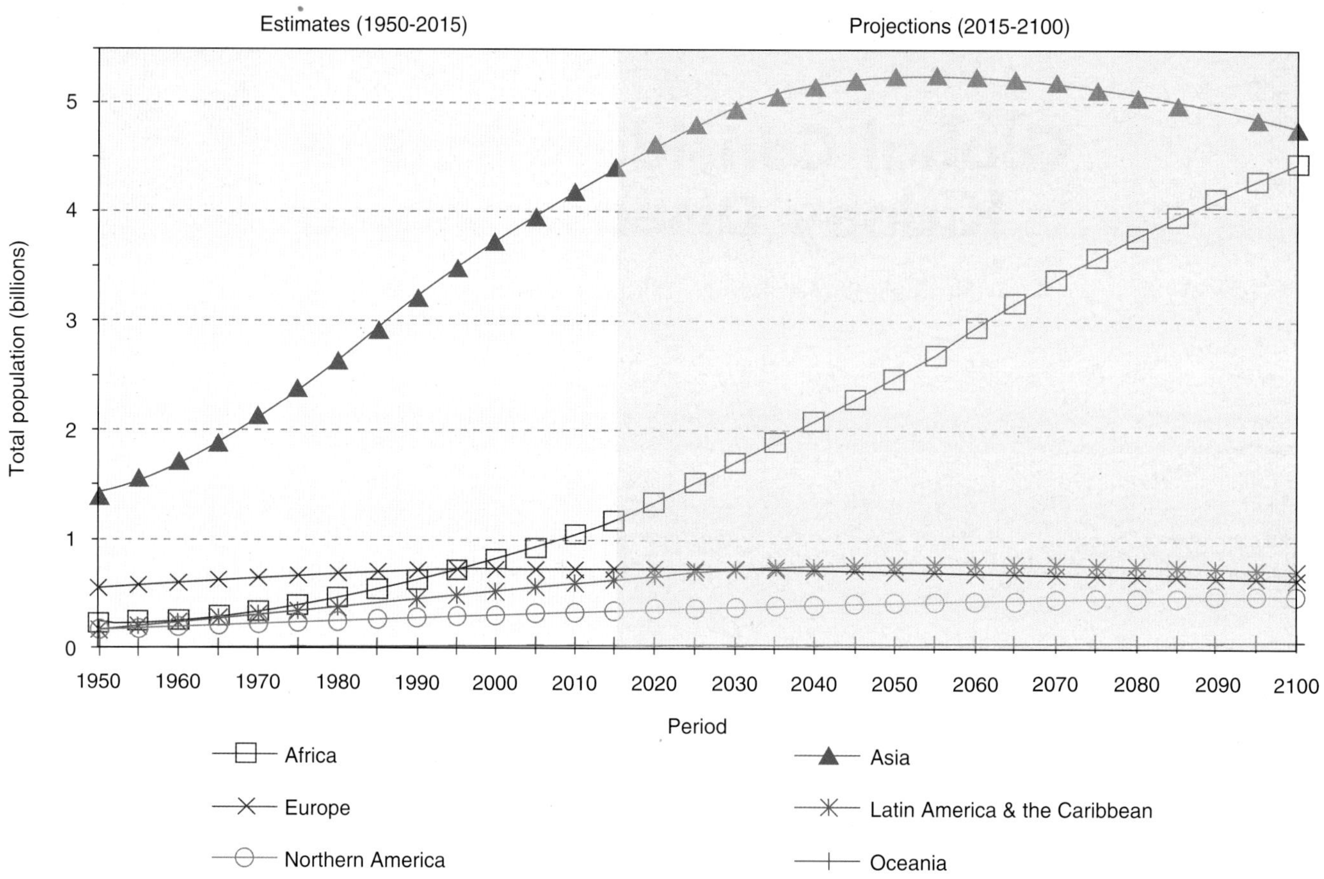

Estimates (1950-2015)
Projections (2015-2100)
Total population (billions)
0
1
2
3
4
5
1950
1960
1970
1980
1990
2000
2010
2020
2030
2040
2050
2060
2070
2080
2090
2100
Period
Africa
Asia
Europe
Latin America & the Caribbean
Northern America
Oceania

**Fig. 77.1** World population by region, with projections to 2100. (From World Population Prospects: *The 2017 revision, key findings and advance tables: United Nations, Department of Economic and Social Affairs, Population Division;* 2017.)

Population Pyramid, Africa: 2014 and 2050
Population size
2014 1,136 million
2050 2,428 million
Age
80+
75-79
70-74
65-69
60-64
55-59
50-54
45-49
40-44
35-39
30-34
25-29
20-24
15-19
10-14
5-9
0-4
2050 Males
2050 Females
2014 Males
2014 Females
Males
Females
150
100
50
0
0
50
100
150
Population (in milions)

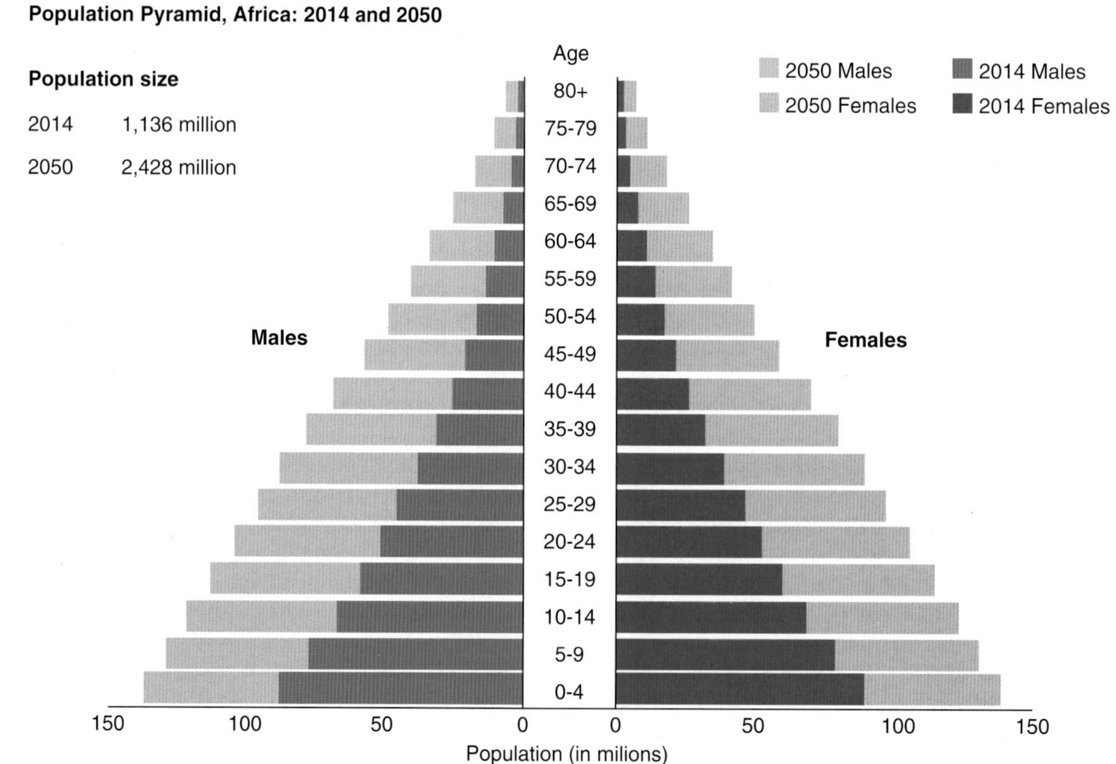

**Fig. 77.2** Population pyramid for Africa; 2014 and 2050. (From *Noncommunicable diseases among young people in Africa*. Washington, DC: Population Reference Bureau; 2015.)

**Table 77.1 Population Estimates, Economic and Development Indicators of African Countries**

| | Total Population (Thousands) | | | | | | | |
|---|---|---|---|---|---|---|---|---|
| **Subregion and Country** | **2017** | **2030** | **2050** | **GNIPC** | **Life Exp** | **MMR** | **Under 5** | **New HIV** |
| AFRICA | 1 256 268 | 1 703 538 | 2 527 557 | | | | | |
| Eastern Africa | 422 036 | 587 330 | 888 129 | | | | | |
| Burundi | 10 864 | 15 799 | 25 762 | 280 | 52.2 | 712 | 81.7 | 0.1 |
| Comoros | 814 | 1 062 | 1 463 | 760 | 55.9 | 335 | 73.5 | |
| Djibouti | 957 | 1 133 | 1 308 | [a] 1030 | 55.8 | 229 | 65.3 | 1.1 |
| Eritrea | 5 069 | 6 718 | 9 607 | [a] 520 | 55.9 | 501 | 46.5 | 0.2 |
| Ethiopia | 104 957 | 139 620 | 190 870 | 660 | 56.1 | 353 | 59.2 | |
| Kenya | 49 700 | 66 960 | 95 467 | 1 380 | 55.6 | 510 | 49.4 | 2.3 |
| Madagascar | 25 571 | 35 592 | 53 803 | 400 | 56.9 | 353 | 49.6 | 0.2 |
| Malawi | 18 622 | 26 578 | 41 705 | 320 | 51.2 | 634 | 64 | 4.5 |
| Mauritius | 1 265 | 1 287 | 1 221 | 9 760 | 66.8 | 53 | 13.5 | 0.4 |
| Mayotte | 253 | 344 | 495 | | | | | |
| Mozambique | 29 669 | 42 439 | 67 775 | 480 | 49.6 | 489 | 78.5 | 7.4 |
| Reunion | 877 | 957 | 1 014 | | | | | |
| Rwanda | 12 208 | 16 024 | 21 886 | 700 | 56.6 | 290 | 41.7 | 1.1 |
| Seychelles | 95 | 98 | 97 | 15 410 | 65.5 | | 13.6 | |
| Somalia | 14 743 | 21 535 | 35 852 | | 47.8 | 732 | 136.4 | 0.5 |
| South Sudan | 12 576 | 17 254 | 25 366 | 820 | 49.9 | 789 | 92.6 | 2.6 |
| Uganda | 42 863 | 63 842 | 105 698 | 660 | 54.0 | 343 | 54.6 | 6 |
| United Republic of Tanzania | 57 310 | 83 702 | 138 082 | 900 | 54.1 | 398 | 48.7 | 2.6 |
| Zambia | 17 094 | 24 859 | 41 001 | 1300 | 53.6 | 224 | 64 | 7.5 |
| Zimbabwe | 16 530 | 21 527 | 29 659 | 940 | 52.3 | 443 | 70.7 | 9.2 |
| Middle Africa | 163 495 | 237 771 | 384 005 | | | | | |
| Angola | 29 784 | 44 712 | 76 046 | 3 440 | 45.8 | 477 | 156.9 | 2.1 |
| Cameroon | 24 054 | 32 980 | 49 817 | 1 200 | 50.3 | 596 | 87.9 | 3.8 |
| Central African Republic | 4 659 | 6 124 | 8 851 | 370 | 45.9 | 882 | 130.1 | 2.7 |
| Chad | 14 900 | 21 460 | 33 636 | 720 | 46.1 | 856 | 138.7 | 1.5 |
| Congo | 5 261 | 7 319 | 11 510 | 1 710 | 56.6 | 442 | 45 | 1.4 |
| Democratic Republic of the Congo | 81 340 | 120 443 | 197 404 | 420 | 51.7 | 693 | 98.3 | 0.6 |
| Equatorial Guinea | 1 268 | 1 871 | 2 845 | 6 550 | 51.2 | 342 | 94.1 | 2.9 |
| Gabon | 2 025 | 2 594 | 3 516 | 7 210 | 57.2 | 291 | 50.8 | 1.4 |
| Sao Tome and Principe | 204 | 268 | 380 | 1730 | 59.1 | 156 | 47.3 | 0.1 |
| Northern Africa | 233 604 | 285 204 | 359 905 | | | | | |
| Algeria | 41 318 | 48 822 | 57 437 | 4 270 | 66.0 | 140 | 25.5 | <0.1 |
| Egypt | 97 553 | 119 746 | 153 433 | 3 460 | 62.2 | 33 | 24 | <0.1 |
| Libya | 6 375 | 7 342 | 8 124 | [a] 4730 | 63.8 | 9 | 13.4 | |
| Morocco | 35 740 | 40 874 | 45 660 | 2850 | 64.9 | 121 | 27.6 | 0.1 |
| Sudan | 40 533 | 54 842 | 80 386 | 2140 | 55.9 | 311 | 70.1 | 0.2 |
| Tunisia | 11 532 | 12 842 | 13 884 | 3 690 | 66.7 | 62 | 14 | <0.1 |
| Southern Africa | 65 143 | 74 786 | 85 800 | | | | | |
| Botswana | 2 292 | 2 800 | 3 421 | 6 610 | 56.9 | 129 | 43.6 | 14 |
| Lesotho | 2 233 | 2 608 | 3 203 | 1 210 | 46.6 | 487 | 90.2 | 20.1 |
| Namibia | 2 534 | 3 246 | 4 339 | 4 680 | 57.5 | 265 | 45.4 | 9.1 |
| South Africa | 56 717 | 64 466 | 72 755 | 5 480 | 54.5 | 138 | 40.5 | 12.7 |
| Swaziland | 1 367 | 1 666 | 2 081 | 2830 | 50.9 | 389 | 60.7 | 18.9 |
| Western Africa | 371 990 | 518 446 | 809 719 | | | | | |
| Benin | 11 176 | 15 628 | 23 930 | 820 | 52.5 | 405 | 99.5 | 0.6 |
| Burkina Faso | 19 193 | 27 382 | 43 207 | 640 | 52.6 | 371 | 88.6 | 0.5 |
| Cabo Verde | 546 | 635 | 734 | 2970 | 64.4 | 42 | 24.5 | 0.9 |
| Cote d'Ivoire | 24 295 | 33 337 | 51 375 | 1520 | 47.0 | 645 | 92.6 | 2.1 |
| Gambia | 2 101 | 3 001 | 4 562 | 440 | 53.8 | 706 | 68.9 | 1.1 |
| Ghana | 28 834 | 37 294 | 51 270 | 1 380 | 55.3 | 319 | 61.6 | 0.7 |
| Guinea | 12 717 | 17 631 | 26 852 | 490 | 51.7 | 679 | 93.7 | 1.1 |
| Guinea-Bissau | 1 861 | 2 493 | 3 603 | 620 | 51.5 | 549 | 92.5 | 2.5 |
| Liberia | 4 732 | 6 495 | 9 804 | 370 | 52.7 | 725 | 69.9 | 0.6 |
| Mali | 18 542 | 27 057 | 44 020 | 750 | 51.1 | 587 | 114.7 | 1.3 |
| Mauritania | 4 420 | 6 077 | 8 965 | 1 120 | 55.1 | 602 | 84.7 | 0.4 |
| Niger | 21 477 | 34 994 | 68 454 | 370 | 54.2 | 553 | 95.5 | <0.1 |
| Nigeria | 190 886 | 264 068 | 410 638 | 2450 | 47.7 | 814 | 108.8 | 2 |

*Continued on following page*

**Table 77.1 Population Estimates, Economic and Development Indicators of African Countries (Cont'd)**

| Subregion and Country | Total Population (Thousands) 2017 | 2030 | 2050 | GNIPC | Life Exp | MMR | Under 5 | New HIV |
|---|---|---|---|---|---|---|---|---|
| Saint Helena | 4 | 4 | 4 | | | | | |
| Senegal | 15 851 | 22 123 | 34 031 | 950 | 58.3 | 315 | 47.2 | <0.1 |
| Sierra Leone | 7 557 | 9 720 | 12 972 | 490 | 44.4 | 1360 | 120.4 | 0.7 |
| Togo | 7 798 | 10 507 | 15 298 | 540 | 52.8 | 368 | 78.4 | 1 |

[a]GNIPC data for Djibouti from 2005, Eritrea 2011, and Libya 2011.

*GNIPC*, Gross national income per capita for 2016 by the Atlas method; *Life Exp*, life expectancy at birth; *MMR*, maternal mortality rate per 100 000 live births; *Under 5*, mortality rate per 1000 children under the age of 5 years; *HIV infections*, new human immunodeficiency virus infections per 1000 adults aged 15–49 years.

Adapted from *Noncommunicable diseases among young people in Africa.* Washington, DC: Population Reference Bureau; 2015; the Global Health Observatory; and the World Bank World Development Indicators database.

**Table 77.2 Examples of Noncommunicable Diseases Which Are Linked to Poverty**

| | Condition | Risk Factors Related to Poverty |
|---|---|---|
| Cardiovascular | Hypertension | Treatment gap |
| | Pericardial disease | Tuberculosis |
| | Rheumatic valvular disease | Streptococcal diseases |
| | Cardiomyopathies | Human immunodeficiency virus (HIV), other viruses, pregnancy |
| | Congenital heart disease | Maternal rubella, micronutrient deficiency, treatment gap |
| Respiratory | Chronic pulmonary disease | Indoor air pollution, tuberculosis, schistosomiasis, treatment gap |
| Endocrine | Diabetes mellitus | Malnutrition |
| | Hyperthyroidism and hypothyroidism | Iodine deficiency |
| Neurological | Epilepsy | Meningitis, malaria |
| | Stroke | Rheumatic mitral stenosis, endocarditis, malaria, HIV |
| Renal | Chronic kidney disease | Streptococcal disease |
| Musculoskeletal | Chronic osteomyelitis | Bacterial infection, tuberculosis |
| | Musculoskeletal injury | Trauma |

Modified from Marquez PV, Farrington JL. *The challenge of non-communicable diseases and road traffic injuries in Sub-Saharan Africa: an overview.* Washington, DC: The World Bank; 2013.

economic activity but investment growth remains low and productivity growth is falling. The gross domestic product (GDP) growth in the region was expected to increase from 1.3% in 2016 to 2.4% in 2017, mainly led by the continent's largest economies: Nigeria, South Africa, and Angola.[4] However, this moderate improvement will only translate into slow gains in per capita income and will likely be insufficient to promote shared prosperity or accelerate poverty reduction. The proportion of total expenditure on health as a proportion of GDP is highly variable across the region, where universal health coverage is uncommon (Fig. 77.3). Poverty, overcrowding, and unhealthy environments persist as common social conditions that affect the occurrence of many diseases and the care available to address them (Table 77.2).

Africa labors under the quadruple burdens of communicable, noncommunicable, perinatal and maternal, and injury-related disorders. These factors are driving the current epidemic of kidney disease. Acute kidney injury (AKI) often develops in the setting of infectious diseases, complicated pregnancies, or injuries. Chronic kidney disease (CKD) may be related to human immunodeficiency virus (HIV) or other infections and is a frequent complication of noncommunicable diseases (NCDs) such as diabetes mellitus and hypertension.

Although communicable diseases have long been the leading causes of death and disease burden in Africa, the pattern of disease is changing as a result of rising incomes, population growth and aging, globalization, rapid urbanization, and Westernized lifestyles. NCDs are fast becoming the leading cause of death throughout Africa.[6] NCDs are emerging in both rural and urban areas, and most prominently in poor people living in urban settings, resulting in increasing pressure on acute and chronic healthcare services.[7] In North African countries, NCDs are already responsible for more than three-quarters of all deaths. In sub-Saharan Africa, NCDs account for more than 25 percent of deaths in 80 percent of the countries and by 2030, NCDs will be the leading cause of death even in sub-Saharan Africa. This is already the case in countries such as Mauritius and the Seychelles and in some populations, such as those over the age of 45 years.[8]

Four key risk behaviors for NCDs—tobacco and alcohol use, physical inactivity, and unhealthy diet—are on the rise among young Africans. These risk factors will need to be addressed to shift the projected trajectory of NCDs in Africa.[6]

Overweight and obesity, especially among girls, are emerging as critical public health issues even where undernutrition still remains a problem. Urbanization and globalization have

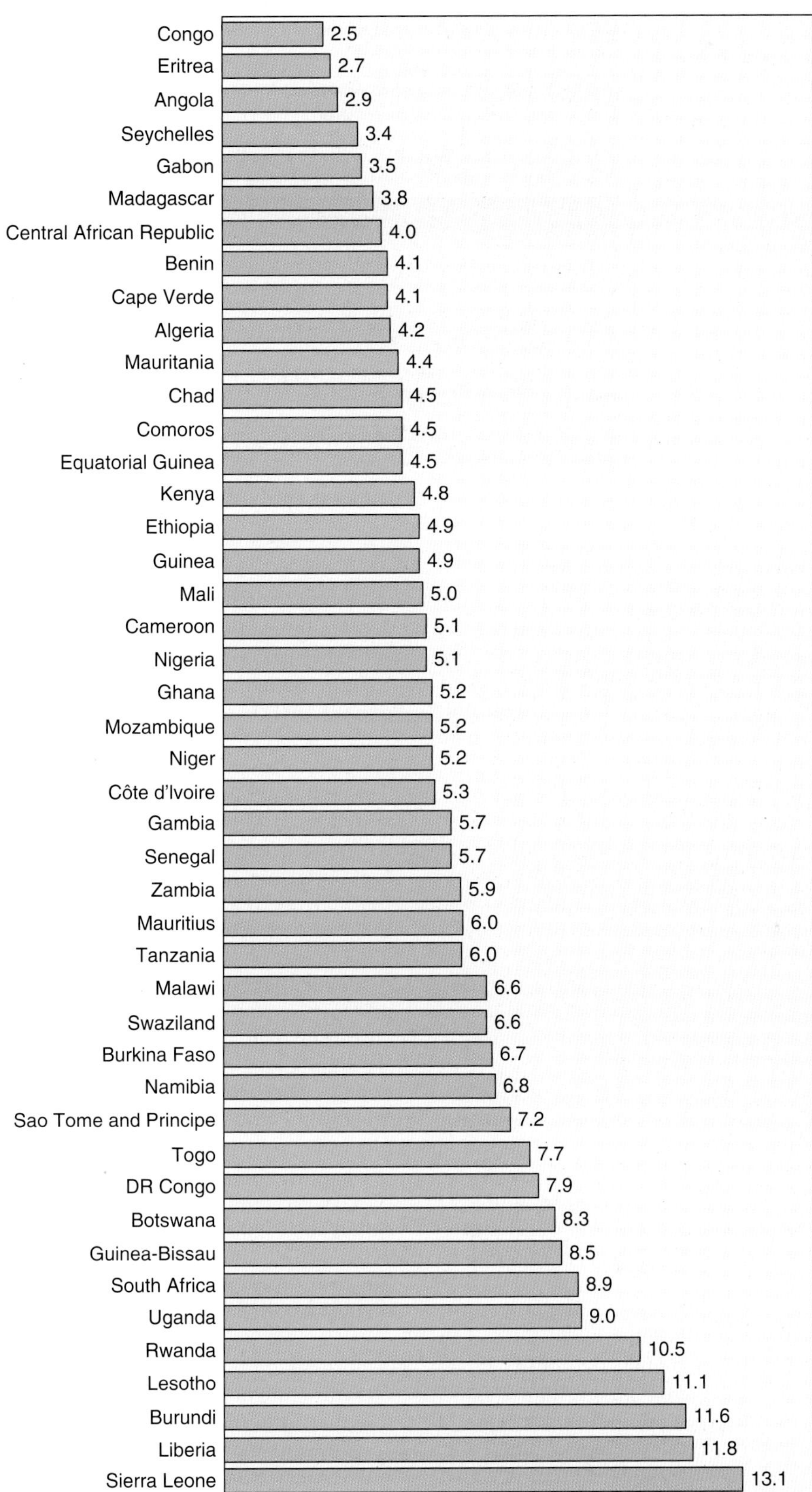


**Fig. 77.3** Total expenditure on health as percentage of gross domestic product in the African region, 2010.

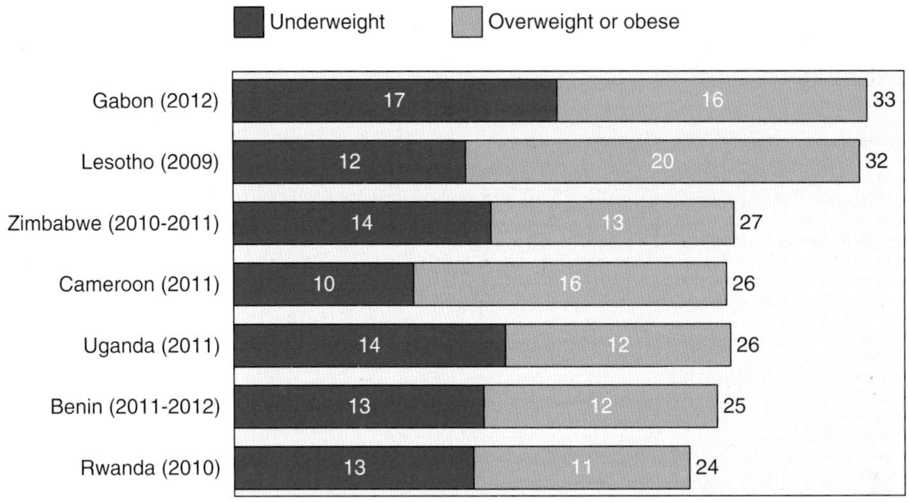


**Fig. 77.4** Overweight/obesity or underweight in young women 15–19 years old. (From *Noncommunicable diseases among young people in Africa.* Washington, DC: Population Reference Bureau; 2015.)

led to sedentary lifestyles and diets filled with calorie-dense, processed foods that are high in saturated fat, sodium, and sugar. These shifts are leading to a rise in NCDs such as type 2 diabetes, cardiovascular disease, stroke, and certain cancers.[6] Fig. 77.4 illustrates the percentage of young women with over- or undernutrition in selected African countries.

Africans are using more tobacco and are starting to smoke at younger ages, increasing their risk for NCDs (Fig. 77.5). More than 40 million people smoke in Africa. About 1 in 10 adolescents smoke cigarettes and the same proportion uses other tobacco products, such as chewing tobacco, snuff, or pipes.[6] Harmful alcohol consumption, a risk factor for NCDs and injuries, is expected to increase with further economic development.[8] Africa already has the highest prevalence of heavy episodic drinking of any region.

The burden from cancer is expected to more than double between 2008 and 2030, with annual deaths rising from 512,000 to 1.2 million over that period. The drivers for this increase include HIV and other infections, tobacco use, occupational and environmental risks, such as air pollution and exposure in mining, and the aging of the population. The proportion of elderly people is projected to double in many African countries between 2000 and 2030, accounting for a substantial proportion of the projected increase in cancer.[8]

Injuries, such as those related to violence or road traffic accidents, also contribute a substantial disease burden in Africa. Sub-Saharan Africa has the highest road traffic death rate in the world, estimated at 24.1 people per 100,000 population per year.[8,9] Conflicts are another major cause of death and disability.[5] The deadliest of these occurred in Nigeria, where the militant group, Boko Haram, is active. Sudan and South Sudan are also suffering from conflict as are a number of other African countries. Although most of the deaths and injuries affect men, there are high rates of sexual violence against women in conflict situations, as documented for the Liberian civil war and the Rwandan genocide. In conflict-affected countries, poverty levels are usually high and welfare levels low. The stability and social cohesion necessary for development are lacking and there is often breakdown of death registration and other statistical monitoring systems.

Improvements in HIV/acquired immunodeficiency syndrome (AIDS)-related mortality rates and life expectancy have been recorded in many African countries, mainly as a result of the increasing availability of antiretroviral treatments. This major public health achievement is the result of a global response involving enormous commitment and solidarity, strong partnerships, generous funding and other support, and far-sighted innovations.[10] In Southern Africa, which has the highest HIV prevalence, life expectancy at birth, which fell from 62 years in 1990 to 1995 to 53 years in 2000 to 2010, has increased to 59 years in 2010 to 2015.[2]

Major challenges still remain, however, as the coverage and quality of HIV services is insufficient in some large countries with high HIV prevalence. Although declining, the numbers of people acquiring HIV infection are still high. Young people, and especially young women, are most affected. Worldwide, an estimated 250,000 youth aged 15 to 19 years old were newly infected in 2015, with two-thirds living in sub-Saharan Africa.[1] Young women are most vulnerable because of gender-based violence and less access to educational and economic opportunities.

## HUMAN RESOURCES FOR NEPHROLOGY

According to the World Health Organization (WHO) Global Health Observatory, over 44% of WHO member states have less than one physician per 1000 population. The African region bears more than 24% of the global burden of disease but has access to only 3% of health workers.[11] The same disparity exists in the nephrology healthcare workforce. Africa has the lowest number of nephrologists per million population (PMP) in the world, and many parts of the continent have no nephrologists at all. A survey conducted by the International Society of Nephrology (ISN) Africa Regional Board in 2014 revealed that, except for North Africa and Mauritius, all African countries have less than two nephrologists PMP, and most have less than one PMP

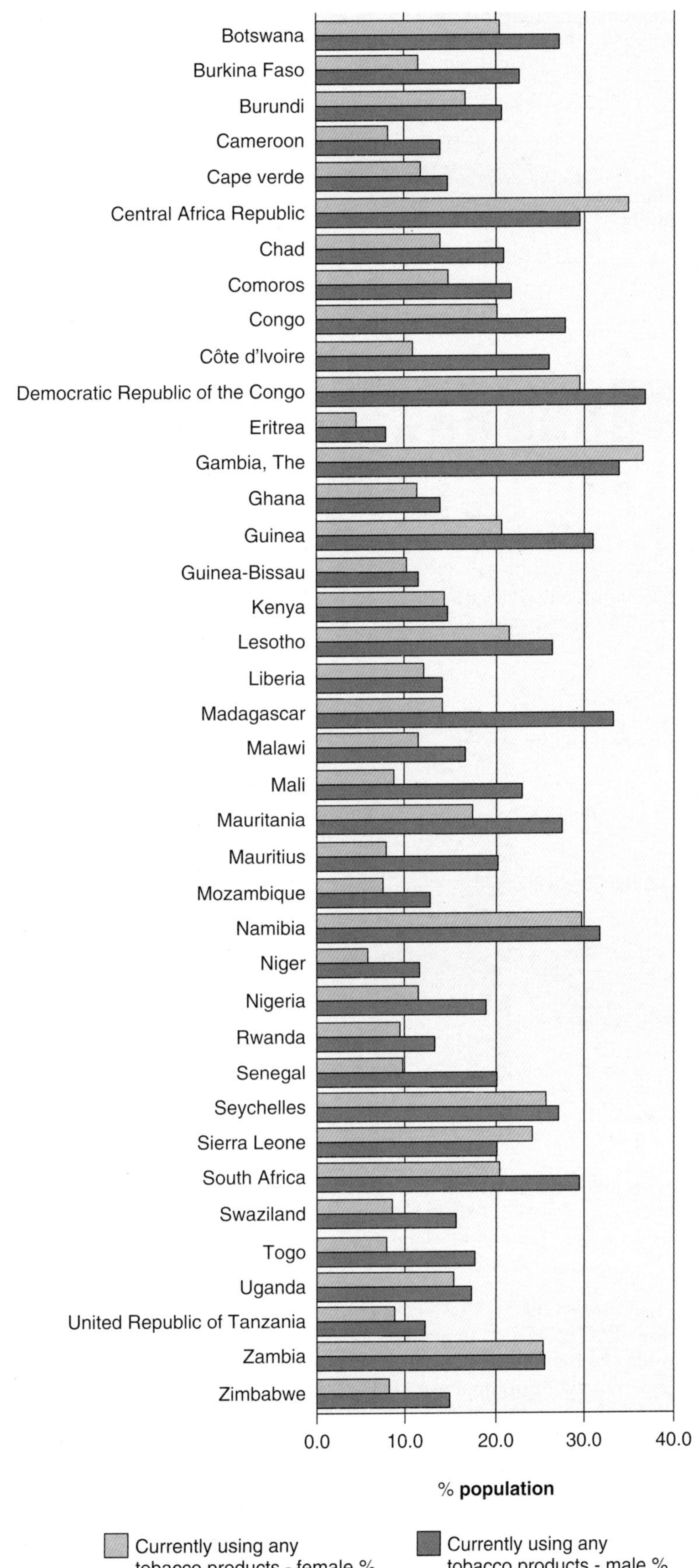


**Fig. 77.5** Use of tobacco products among African youth 13–15 years old, 2005–2010. (From Marquez PV, Farrington JL. *The challenge of non-communicable diseases and road traffic injuries in Sub-Saharan Africa: an overview.* Washington, DC: The World Bank; 2013.)

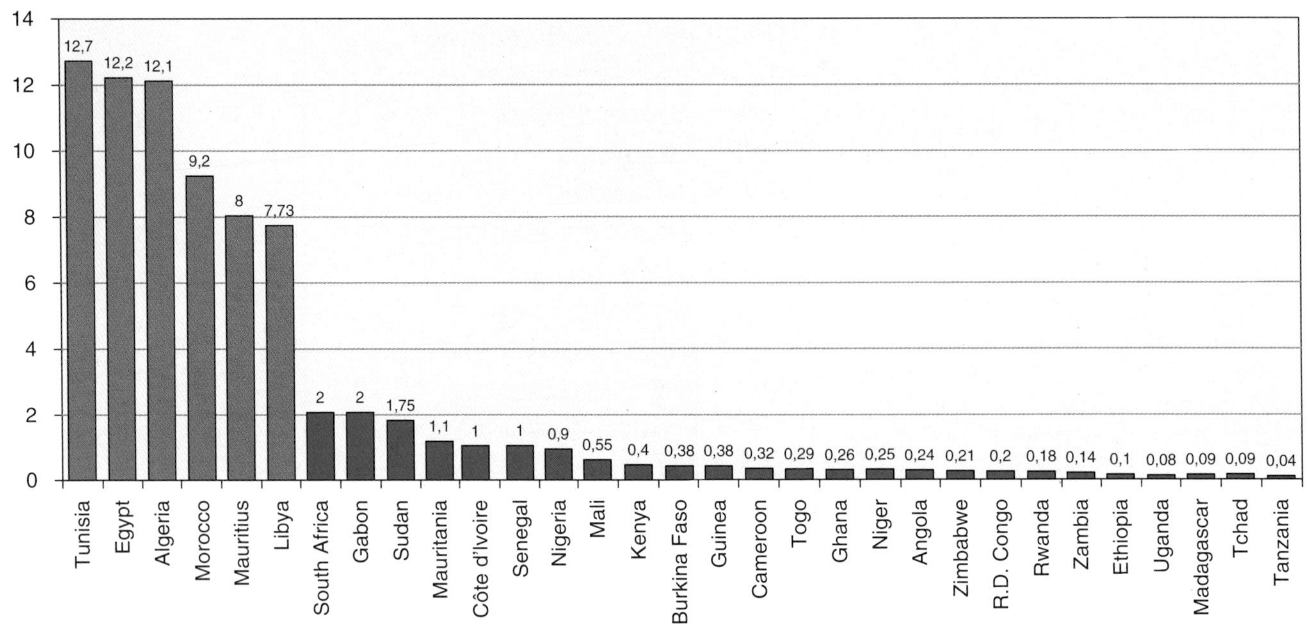


**Fig. 77.6** **Number of nephrologists per million population in African countries.** (From Benghanem Gharbi M. Chronic dialysis programs in African countries: Barriers and successes. World Congress of Nephrology; 2015; Cape Town, South Africa.)

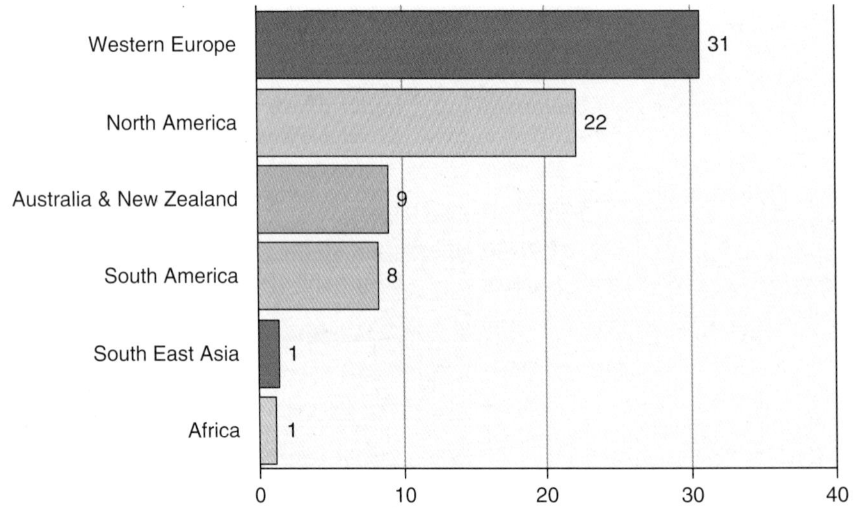


**Fig. 77.7** **Number of nephrologists per million population, by continent.** (From Sharif MU, Elsayed ME, Stack AG. The global nephrology workforce: emerging threats and potential solutions. *Clin Kidney J.* 2016;9:11–22.)

(Fig. 77.6).[12] In contrast, Western Europe and North America have more than 10 nephrologists PMP (Fig. 77.7).[13] In general, nephrologists are clustered around large, densely populated urban centers, which may actually represent optimal use of a scarce resource.[14]

Brain drain continues to pose a great threat to the limited nephrology health workforce on the African continent despite various recommendations[15] and global initiatives.[16] Some of the recommendations proposed include increasing the training of doctors in developed countries, providing assistance to developing countries to aid retention of skilled personnel, restricting the duration of training or work visas for doctors from developing countries, and strengthening specialist training within developing countries.[15]

The ISN Fellowship Program, which started in 1985, is a particularly noteworthy initiative which sponsors physicians from developing countries to undertake nephrology training in centers of the developed world. By the end of 2017, 196 fellows from Africa had been trained, with 84 of them trained in Western European centers, 74 in African centers (mainly in South Africa), and 30 in North America. In a survey conducted in 2010,[16] 90% of ISN fellows indicated that their training had high or good relevance to the needs of their home institution or country, and 85% reported having a high level or good impact on their home institution and home country. Within 10 years of completing their fellowship, 60% of responding fellows occupied a leadership position within their department or hospital, 28% within their country, and 7% at an international level. Fellows who had trained at centers within their region reported fewer difficulties with obtaining visas, more hands-on clinical training, greater relevance and impact on their home units, and less brain drain. However, there were fewer publications reported, and none of high impact.[16]

Because the most effective interventions to reduce the burden of renal disease are likely to be implemented at primary care settings, it would be logical to involve general practitioners and nurses. Providing these categories of healthcare workers with adequate training in the early diagnosis and management of renal disease, with prompt referral when appropriate, could mitigate the effect of low numbers of nephrologists and improve outcomes.[17]

## ACUTE KIDNEY INJURY

Epidemiological data for AKI is scarce in Africa. The most comprehensive study is the ISN 0by25 Global Snapshot, conducted over a 10-week period in 2014, to assess the range of AKI seen by physicians in different settings worldwide.[18] African centers contributed 13% of the cases and all the subregions of the continent were represented: North Africa (Egypt, Morocco, and Tunisia), West Africa (Ghana, Niger, Nigeria, and Senegal), Central Africa (Cameroon), East Africa (Ethiopia, Kenya, Sudan, and Tanzania), and Southern Africa (Malawi and South Africa). The mean age of the African patients was 53 years. Most of AKI cases (83.9%) were community-acquired and 19% were seen in intensive care unit (ICU) settings.[19] Dehydration was the most frequent cause of AKI (51.5%), followed by sepsis (32.1%), hypotension (31.8%), and infection (29.8%). The etiologic factors are presented in Fig. 77.8.

It is generally argued that the epidemiology of AKI differs between North Africa and sub-Saharan Africa. In 2016, Olowu et al. published an informative systematic review aiming to assess the outcomes of AKI in sub-Saharan Africa and to identify barriers to care.[20] Among the studies included in this review, 8 were prospective, 32 were retrospective, and one was cross-sectional. AKI was predominantly community-acquired, and the causes are shown in Fig. 77.9. Infection, including malaria, accounted for more than 30% of AKI cases. The other etiologies were dominated by nephrotoxins, pregnancy complications and glomerulonephritis in adults, and by glomerulonephritis, nephrotoxins, hypovolemia, and urinary tract obstruction in children. Most patients presented with severe AKI, with 70% of adults and 66% of children needing dialysis, suggesting that AKI is a more aggressive disorder in sub-Saharan Africa.[20] The likely reasons for this include late presentation to hospital and reliance on clinical criteria for the diagnosis of AKI.

From North Africa, Bourial et al.[21] conducted a 6-month, prospective, multicenter survey (September 2012 to February

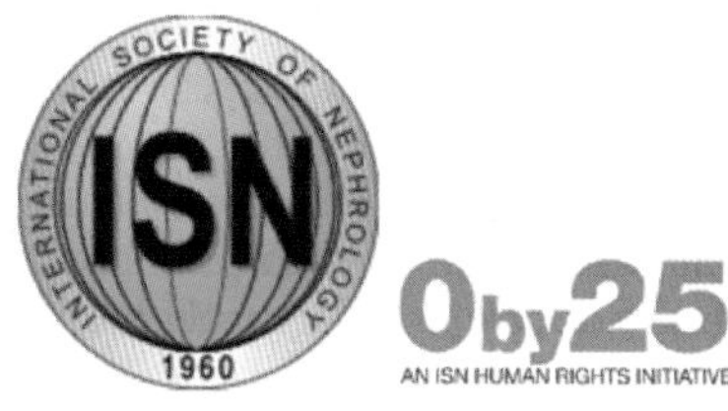


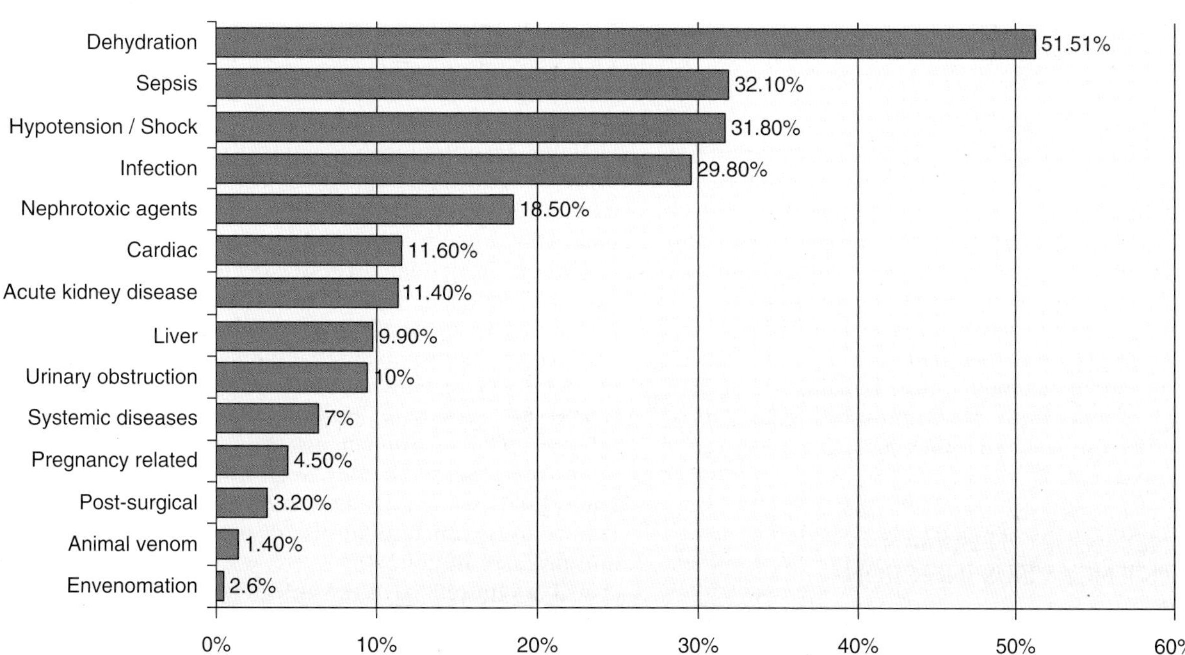


**Fig. 77.8** Etiologic factors for acute kidney injury in Africa. (From Mehta RL, Macedo E, Zhang J, ISN 0by25 Initiative Steering Committee. International Society of Nephrology 0by25 Global Snapshot. Regional report for Africa, 2015.)

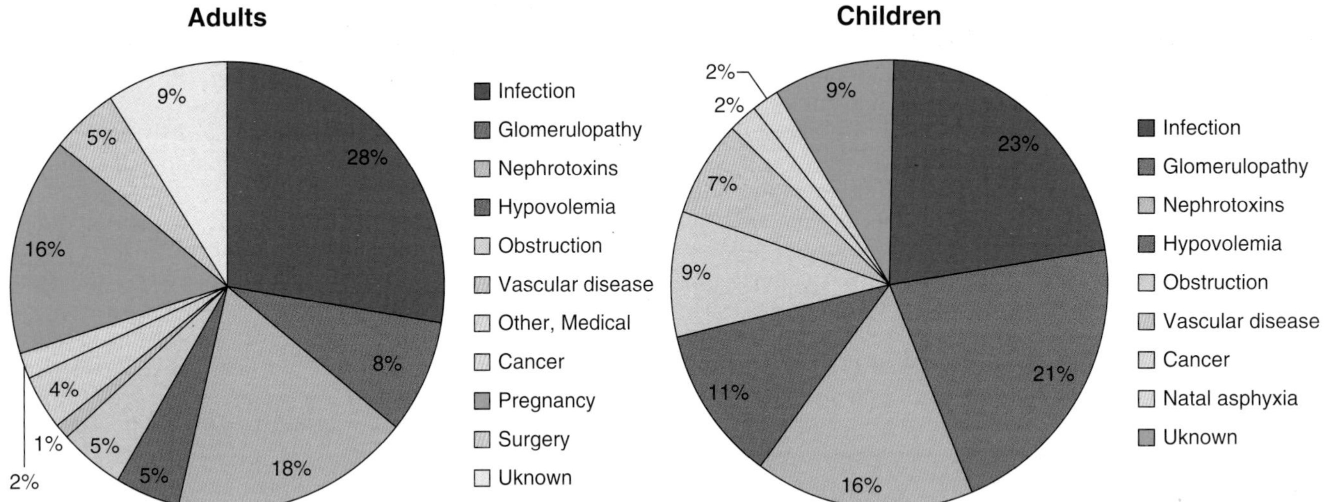


**Fig. 77.9** Prevalence of etiologic factors for acute kidney injury in adults and children in sub-Saharan Africa. (Modified from Olowu WA, Niang A, Osafo C, et al. Outcomes of acute kidney injury in children and adults in sub-Saharan Africa: a systematic review. *Lancet Glob Health.* 2016;4:e242-250.)

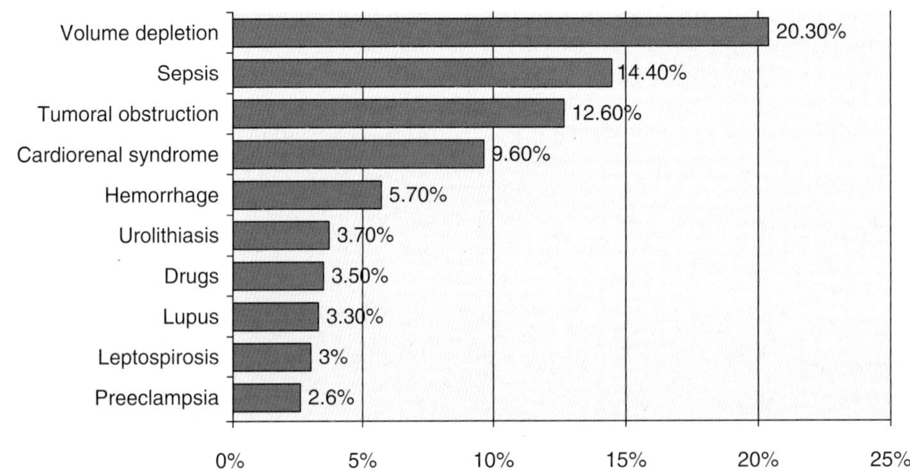


**Fig. 77.10** Prevalence of etiologic factors for acute kidney injury in Morocco. (From Bourial M. Aspects epidemiologiques de l'insuffisance renale aigue au Maroc. *Premiere enquete nationale.* Casablanca, Morocco: Université Hassan II de Casablanca; 2014.)

2013) across Morocco (the IRAM Survey) and recruited 541 cases of AKI. Most of the cases (82.4%) were community-acquired and the median age was 57 years (range 3 months–94 years). As shown in Fig. 77.10, volume depletion, sepsis, and tumor obstruction of the urinary tract were the top etiologic factors. Dialysis was required in 40.3% of patients and 21.8% of patients died. Renal function recovered in 25.1% of the cases, whereas 33.6% developed CKD.

Hypovolemia and infection therefore remain the principal causes of AKI in both North Africa and sub-Saharan Africa. Differences in the prevalence of other etiologies are apparent in some regional reports.

## ACUTE KIDNEY INJURY IN HUMAN IMMUNIDEFICIENCY VIRUS INFECTION

AKI is a common complication in HIV-infected patients compared with uninfected patients, with an odds ratio of 2.82 for those treated with ART, and 4.62 in the pre-HAART era.[22] Patients hospitalized with complications of HIV may be at increased risk of AKI due to volume depletion, hemodynamic stress, infections, malignancy, and administration of nephrotoxic medication or radiocontrast material.

Kidney injury related to ART occurs in less than 10% of patients. Tenofovir disoproxil fumarate (TDF), a first-line ART agent, is potentially nephrotoxic, as it causes mitochondrial toxicity in proximal renal tubular cells. This may result in AKI, CKD, or Fanconi syndrome. Although TDF is well tolerated by most patients, there is an increased risk of TDF-related renal injury in patients with preexisting renal impairment, older age, low body weight, advanced HIV disease, comorbidities (e.g., diabetes, hypertension and hepatitis C coinfection), concomitant use of other nephrotoxic drugs, and protease inhibitors.[23]

AKI in hospitalized HIV-infected patients is associated with a sixfold higher risk of in-hospital mortality.[23] The most important risk factors include severe levels of immunosuppression (CD4 count <200 cells/mm$^3$) and opportunistic infection. The most common causes are acute tubular necrosis and thrombotic microangiopathy. After initiation of ART, HIV-infected patients with AKI still have an increased risk of in-hospital mortality, and episodes of AKI seem to be more frequent in the first year of ART. AKI has been associated with infection, hypotension, and exposure to nephrotoxic antimicrobial agents such as aminoglycosides and amphotericin B.[23] Risk factors are low CD4 count, coinfection with hepatitis C, acute or chronic liver injury, diabetes mellitus, and underlying CKD. Glomerular disease in HIV-infected patients (HIV-associated nephropathy [HIVAN], HIV-related immune complex disease [HIV-ICD], and other pathologies)[24–26] can also manifest as AKI and may be the underlying condition upon which an additional insult has precipitated an acute decline in kidney function.

Data on AKI with HIV infection in developing countries are emerging. According to a 2005 to 2006 survey from Johannesburg, South Africa, 101 of 700 patients with kidney failure (14.8%) were HIV-positive, with a mean age of 38 years.[27] Sepsis was the cause of AKI in 60% of the HIV-positive patients. Mortality occurred in 44% of these patients and in 47% of a control group of HIV-negative patients. Hyponatremia, hyperphosphatemia and anemia were predictors of mortality in the HIV-positive patients.[27]

A review of 117 HIV-positive patients with AKI who received acute dialysis in Cape Town, South Africa, revealed that sepsis was present in over 50% at presentation. Acute tubular necrosis was diagnosed in 58%; recovery of renal function occurred in 33.3% while mortality occurred in 41%.[28] A recent study from Bloemfontein, South Africa, reported high mortality among HIV-infected ICU patients needing continuous renal replacement therapy (CRRT). These patients had a mortality rate of 60% as compared with 10% among the HIV-uninfected patients.[29]

## ACUTE KIDNEY INJURY AND MALARIA

According to the World Malaria Report, 445,000 deaths were caused by malaria in 2016 and 90% of these deaths occurred in sub-Saharan Africa.[30] Just over half of the people at risk in sub-Saharan Africa were using the primary prevention method, sleeping under an insecticide-treated mosquito net. Although this represents a significant increase, the report also documents a decline in the use of another important preventative measure, spraying the inside walls of homes with insecticides.[30]

Malaria-associated AKI is usually due to *Plasmodium falciparum* infection. The incidence of AKI approaches 60% in patients with a severe form of malaria, with risk factors including severe parasitemia, children under the age of 5 years, pregnant women, and HIV infection.[31] The mortality rate is approximately 45%, and highest in children.[32] Early antimalarial treatment with artemisinin-based therapies, good fluid and electrolyte management, and dialysis when indicated, is associated with improved patient survival and recovery of renal function in patients with malaria-induced AKI. See Chapter 79 for a detailed discussion on malaria and the kidney.

## ACUTE KIDNEY INJURY AND TOXINS

The use of traditional medicines is very common in developing countries, where its use is related to spiritual beliefs, the need for protection or cleansing, sexual potency or fertility, suspicion of conventional medicine, and poor access to medical care.[33] In sub-Saharan Africa, more than 80% of people use traditional medicines as their principal form of healthcare. Traditional medicines are used for numerous conditions, including CKD, hypertension, and diabetes, in both urban and rural settings, and by people of all socioeconomic classes (Table 77.3).[34]

These medicines are mostly used without major adverse effects; however, many have been associated with kidney injury. The use of traditional medicines may also delay patients' presentation to medical care for many conditions, including kidney disease.[34] Volume depletion is a major risk factor for the development of AKI associated with traditional medicines. In developing countries, such remedies account for up to 35% of AKI cases and the reported mortality rates range from 24% to 75%.[33] In those who survive, renal recovery is often incomplete, resulting in CKD. As the use of traditional medicines is generally underreported to physicians, it should always be considered in the differential diagnosis of any community-acquired or unexplained renal injury.[35]

Components of traditional medicines that may be associated with AKI include cancer bush (*Sutherlandia frutescens*), ysterhouttoppe (*Dodonaea angustifolia*), marking nut tree (*Semecarpus anacardium*), Bao Gong Teng (*Erycibe obtusifolia Benth*), spearmint (*Mentha spicata*), Opuntia megacantha, and Alder buckthorn bark and berry (*Rhamnus frangula*).[33] The nephrotoxicity of a remedy may also be related to contamination of the remedy, the erroneous identification or preparation of plants, incorrect use, interaction with other medications, and patient factors such as comorbid conditions, age, and sex.[33]

The mechanism of nephrotoxicity is mostly unknown. Examples where the pathophysiology has been identified include aristolochic acid (proximal tubular dysfunction due to inactivation of antioxidant enzymes),[36] atractyloside, the toxic ingredient in impila (inhibits mitochondrial oxidative phosphorylation),[37] and star fruit juice (induces apoptosis in renal tubular cells with precipitation of calcium oxalate crystals).[38] The wide range of renal pathologies reported includes glomerular injury (bladderwrack), Fanconi's syndrome (aristolochic acid), distal renal tubular acidosis (coneflower), nephrogenic diabetes insipidus (bladderwrack), papillary necrosis (willow bark), interstitial nephritis, acute tubular necrosis, kidney stones (djenkol beans), and urothelial malignancies (aristolochic acid). In renal transplant recipients, traditional medicines may also affect allograft function through immune activation (alfalfa and black cohosh) or by influencing the metabolism of immunosuppressive medications (St. John's wort, an inducer of cytochrome P450 3A4). Many electrolyte abnormalities have been associated with the use of traditional medicines, either as a result of volume overload or depletion, or as a result of renal tubular toxicity.[33]

Strategies targeting kidney diseases in LMICs require engagements with key community stakeholders, including practitioners and users of traditional medicines.[33,34] Healthcare practitioners should be proactive in obtaining a history of remedy use, in carefully documenting the clinical features, pathophysiology and renal pathology, and in reporting adverse events so that more comprehensive data can be collected.[35]

**Table 77.3 Examples of Traditional Medicines Used Across Sub-Saharan Africa That Have Known Nephrotoxic Effects**

| Nomenclature | | | |
|---|---|---|---|
| Scientific Name | Common English Name | **Common Uses or Indications** | **Nephrotoxic Effects** |
| *Aloe vera* species including ferox and secundiflora | Cape aloes<br>Aloe vera | Southern Africa: arthritis, burns/skin conditions, hypertension, purging/laxative, dyspepsia, antiinflammatory, cosmetics, eye ailments/conjunctivitis, venereal diseases, infertility, impotence<br>East Africa (Kenya, Uganda, Ethiopia, and Tanzania): malaria, purging/laxative for cleansing purposes, dyspepsia, skin ulcerations/wound healing, cosmetic, infertility, antiparasitic | Volume depletion and electrolyte imbalance<br>Acute tubular necrosis<br>Acute interstitial nephritis |
| *Euphorbia matabalensis* | Three-forked shrub (Euphorbia) | Eastern Africa (including Somalia, Kenya, Tanzania, Malawi, Mozambique, and Zimbabwe): constipation, purging, hypertension<br>Southern Africa (including Zambia, Botswana, Angola, and Namibia): Abortifacient, constipation, purging, hypertension, venereal diseases, dyspepsia, myalgias | Acute tubular necrosis: directly nephrotoxic, perhaps attributable to latex compounds |
| *Cymbopogon citrullus* | Lemongrass | South Africa: diabetes, oral thrush<br>Nigeria: fever/malaria, stimulant, antispasmodic<br>Cameroon: malaria, jaundice<br>Angola; cough, antiemetic, antiseptic, arthritis/arthralgia | Volume depletion/diarrhea<br>Chronic decrease in glomerular filtration rate: chronic interstitial nephritis |
| *Securidaca longepedunculata* | African violet tree<br>Wild wisteria | Zambia: abortifacient<br>Burkina Faso: malaria, skin disorders<br>Nigeria: abortifacient, constipation, fever, aphrodisiac<br>Botswana and Eastern Africa (including Tanzania, Malawi, Uganda, Kenya, and Zimbabwe): epilepsy, arthritis, purging, constipation, wound healing, snakebites, fever/malaria, impotence, dysmenorrhea | Acute tubular necrosis: causes cortical necrosis, volume depletion, and contains salicylates thought to contribute to renal vasoconstriction<br>Acute interstitial nephritis |
| *Crotalaria laburnifolia* | Wild sunhemp<br>Rattlepod<br>Birdflower | South Africa, Botswana, and Eastern Africa (including Mozambique and Zimbabwe): enema, purging, dysmenoritiea, abortifacient, dyspepsia, antispasmodic | Acute tubular necrosis: contains nephrotoxic alkaloids<br>Hepatorenal failure |
| *Callilepsis laureola* | Ox-eye daisy<br>Impila | Mozambique and South Africa: dyspepsia, antiparasitic, impotence/infertility, purging, evil spirits | Acute tubular necrosis and acute interstitial nephritis<br>Hepatorenal failure and chronic decrease in glomerular filtration rate<br>Hyperkalemia |

From Stanifer JW, Kilonzo K, Wang D, et al. Traditional medicines and kidney disease in low-and middle-income countries: opportunities and challenges. *Sem Nephrol*. 2017;37:245-259.

Other nephrotoxic agents encountered in some African countries, especially in East Africa and the Maghreb, include hair dye preparations that contain paraphenylenediamine.[39] Some of these dyes are added to henna, a traditional cosmetic agent applied to the upper and lower limbs, for its skin staining effect. Paraphenylenediamine can be absorbed through the skin, but more severe intoxication results from ingestion of the hair dye, mostly in suicide attempts.[40] AKI is mainly due to acute tubular necrosis caused by rhabdomyolysis. Mortality may result from other manifestations of the poisoning—for example, angioedema, which occurs early, and arrhythmias caused by direct cardiotoxicity of the chemical.[39] There is no known antidote.

Animal toxins are also a major cause of AKI in Africa. Snake venoms are a complex mix of different toxic and nontoxic proteins and peptides, nonprotein toxins, carbohydrates, lipids, amines, and other small molecules. The toxins of most importance in human envenoming include those that affect the nervous, cardiovascular, and hemostatic systems, and cause tissue necrosis.[41]

AKI developing after snake bites may be related to intravascular hemolysis, hypotension, blood hyperviscosity, myoglobinuria, and hemorrhage. Bites occur especially in plantations and commonly involve *Causus maculatus* (spotted night adder), *Naja melanoleuca* (black cobras), and *Dendroaspis* species (green mambas). In forested areas, gaboon vipers (bitis species) are common while in savanna areas *Echis* species are common and cause the greatest numbers of deaths by envenomation in Africa.[42] The range of renal pathology includes acute tubular necrosis, cortical necrosis, acute interstitial nephritis, and proliferative glomerulonephritis.

Scorpion stings are a significant public health problem in north-Saharan Africa, Sahelian Africa, and South Africa.[43] The scorpion α-toxins bind to voltage-gated sodium channels to cause neuronal excitation.[44] AKI may develop in some patients as a result of cardiac dysfunction, disseminated intravascular coagulation and hemorrhage.

## PREGNANCY-RELATED ACUTE KIDNEY INJURY

Obstetric AKI has become rare in industrialized countries, whereas it continues to be a frequent clinical problem in many African countries, mainly secondary to preeclampsia and eclampsia, septic conditions, and obstetric hemorrhage (see also Chapter 48). In Morocco, pregnancy-related AKI occurred mostly in the third trimester (66.6% of affected patients) and in the postpartum period (25%). Preeclampsia and hemorrhagic shock (25%) were reported as the major causes of AKI.[45] In a retrospective study of patients admitted to an ICU for eclampsia in Nigeria from 2001 to 2005, Okafor and Efetie[46] found a case-fatality rate of 29%, with 9.1% of deaths related to AKI. The incidence of eclampsia was inversely related to good antenatal care, standard of living, and literacy rate. In a prospective study of 178 consecutive women with eclampsia in Morocco, Mjahed et al.[47] found that the incidence of AKI was 25.8%. Dialysis was needed in one-third of the patients, and mortality rates were higher among patients with AKI than those without AKI (32.6% vs. 9.1%).

## THERAPEUTIC CHALLENGES

In most African countries, low availability of resources and inadequate health infrastructure are associated with poor recognition and treatment of AKI. As illustrated in the systematic review of Olowu et al., AKI in sub-Saharan Africa is severe, mainly because of the late presentation of patients to tertiary care centers.[20] In the studies reporting patients who needed dialysis, 66% of children and 70% of adults had indications for dialysis. However, only 64% of children (across 11 studies) and 33% of adults (four studies) received dialysis when needed. The overall mortality was 34% in children and 32% in adults but rose to 73% in children and 86% in adults when dialysis was needed but not received. Major barriers to access to care were unaffordable out-of-pocket costs, limited hospital resources, late presentation, and female sex.[20] In another review of AKI publications on Nigerian children between 1990 and 2012, dialysis access rates ranged between 15.2% and 68.2% of those with a medical indication for dialysis.[48]

This contrasts with the practice in North Africa, where dialysis for AKI is more easily accessible in hospital settings. In the Moroccan survey, dialysis was needed in 40.3% of cases and intermittent hemodialysis was the predominant prescribed modality (96%). At discharge, the mortality was 25.4%, dialysis dependence was 6.8%, residual renal failure was present in 39.2% and there was complete renal recovery in 29.3%.[21]

Two recent global initiatives have the potential to have a major impact on the outcomes of patients with AKI, especially in low-resource settings. The ISN has launched "0by25", an ambitious agenda to eliminate all preventable deaths from AKI by 2025.[49] The 0by25 project will focus on evidence and awareness, and on education and training for health workers to increase the early detection of AKI and the appropriate use of simple management, such as fluid repletion.

The second global initiative is "Saving Young Lives", which is focused on AKI in children and aims to develop sustainable acute peritoneal dialysis (PD) programs in very low-resource settings.[50,51] PD is now being increasingly utilized to manage patients with AKI and can be life-saving in situations where hemodialysis is not available. Outcomes appear to be similar when compared with treatment with extracorporeal therapies.[52,53] Support provided by organizations such as the International Society for Peritoneal Dialysis (ISPD), the International Pediatric Nephrology Association (IPNA), the ISN and the Sustainable Kidney Care Foundation (SKCF) have allowed physicians working in resource-constrained regions of Africa to develop expertise in the provision of acute PD. Practical hands-on training has already been provided to more than 50 nurses and physicians at an annual training course held at the Red Cross War Memorial Children's Hospital in Cape Town, South Africa. This course covers all aspects of acute PD, including catheter insertion, fluid prescription, and clinical problem solving.

It is important to note that a large proportion of AKI cases and their clinical consequences are potentially preventable.[54] Education regarding the avoidance of nephrotoxins, prompt treatment of infections, and fluid replacement are therefore important facets of therapy.[55] This approach is vital because many countries in Africa are still not able to provide renal replacement therapies.

# CHRONIC KIDNEY DISEASE

Chronic kidney disease (CKD) is a major public health problem, with an estimated global prevalence of 11% to 13%.[56] In Africa, the increases in NCDs, pregnancy-related disorders and injuries, and the high burden of infectious diseases may all contribute to the epidemic of CKD. People from disadvantaged communities are at particularly high risk of unrecognized and untreated CKD.[57] This includes indigenous communities, and racial and ethnic minorities.[58]

CKD is defined as the presence of abnormalities of kidney structure or function, with implications for health, for more than three months.[59] In practice, this is usually determined by finding a glomerular filtration rate (GFR) of below 60 mL/min/1.73 $m^2$ or markers of kidney damage such as proteinuria, hematuria, or abnormalities on renal imaging. The latest KDIGO guidelines[59] recommend that CKD classification be based on cause, GFR category, and degree of albuminuria. GFR should be estimated using serum creatinine and a creatinine-based prediction equation.[59]

## ISSUES IN THE DIAGNOSIS OF CHRONIC KIDNEY DISEASE

The accurate diagnosis and staging of CKD are especially important in Africa, as options for treating late complications such as ESRD are very limited. The screening of those at higher risk of developing CKD is therefore essential. The choice of methods used to assess GFR can have a major impact on determining if an individual has CKD or not, on the stage of CKD, and on the reported population prevalence.

Different assays may result in interlaboratory differences in serum creatinine and therefore estimated GFR.[60] All creatinine assays should therefore be standardized by calibration to isotope-dilution mass spectrometry (IDMS)-traceable reference material. Enzymatic methods are preferred as they have greater analytical precision than the colorimetric Jaffe reaction-based methods.

GFR prediction equations need to be validated in local populations against gold standard methods. Three African studies, two from South Africa and one from Côte d'Ivoire, have compared prediction equations with GFR measured by gold standard methods. Van Deventer et al.[61] studied 100 black South Africans and measured GFR using the plasma clearance of chromium-51-EDTA ($^{51}$Cr-EDTA). Serum creatinine was measured using an IDMS-traceable assay. Madala et al.[62] studied 91 participants of African and 57 of Indian origin, and measured GFR using technetium-99m-diethylenetriaminepentaacetic acid ($^{99m}$Tc-DTPA). Both studies reported a good performance of the 4-variable MDRD equation in black South Africans, and both concluded that the correction factor for black ethnicity should not be used. Madala et al. suggested that a new correction factor, or a new equation, is needed for South Africans of Indian origin. Sagou Yayo et al.[63] used iohexol to measure GFR in 120 blood donors in Abidjan and also found that the performance of the CKD-EPI and MDRD prediction equations was better without the "African-American" ethnicity factor.

International guidelines recommend the use of the Chronic Kidney Disease Epidemiology Collaboration (CKD-EPI) prediction equation, unless an alternative equation has been shown to improve the accuracy of GFR estimates.[59,64] This equation is considered more accurate than the previously recommended Modification of Diet in Renal Disease (MDRD) study equation, which systematically underestimates GFR at higher values.

Although current guidelines use a universal GFR threshold of 60 mL/min/1.73 m$^2$ for the diagnosis of CKD, this may not be appropriate in all cases. Pottel et al.[65] have suggested that a cut-off of 75 mL/min/1.73 m$^2$ be used for children and young adults because they may have low GFR values, below the third percentile for age and sex, but still above 60 mL/min/1.73 m$^2$. At the other end of the age spectrum, there have been calls for caution in labeling older patients as having CKD if they have mild, stable reductions in GFR (between 45 and 60 mL/min/1.73 m$^2$) without any other evidence of kidney damage or systemic disease.[66]

Many cross-sectional epidemiologic studies suffer from a common weakness in that they do not include repeat estimates of GFR or protein excretion and hence do not meet the criterion of chronicity for diagnosing CKD. People with abnormal kidney function or damage are inferred to have CKD if there is not an acute illness likely to cause acute kidney injury. When repeat measurements are done, however, this will often result in lower estimates for CKD prevalence.[67]

## CHRONIC KIDNEY DISEASE PREVALENCE IN AFRICAN COUNTRIES

The systematic review on the population prevalence of CKD in sub-Saharan Africa by Stanifer et al.[68] identified only 18 medium-quality studies and three high-quality studies for inclusion in their meta-analysis. These studies reported data from 13 African countries (Fig. 77.11). The authors reported an overall prevalence of 13.9% but highlighted the need for more studies of good quality. Country estimates ranged from 2% in Cote d'Ivoire to 30% in Zimbabwe. Nearly half of the countries represented had prevalence estimates ranging between 4% and 16%.

More recently, population prevalence studies have been published from a number of African countries. From Cape Town, South Africa, Matsha et al.[69] reported a crude prevalence of 17.3% in a geographical cohort, while Adeniyi et al.[70] reported an age-adjusted prevalence of 6.4% in a cohort of teachers. The higher estimates by Matsha et al. may at least partly be explained by the very high burden of hypertension, diabetes, obesity, and smoking in their cohort. In northern Tanzania, the CKD AFRiKA Study reported a prevalence of 7.0%, with a much higher prevalence in urban than in rural areas,[71] whereas Seck et al. reported a prevalence of 4.9% in a population-based survey in northern Senegal.[72] Kaze et al. found a CKD prevalence of 10% in an urban district of Cameroon[73] and Kalyesaluba et al. reported a prevalence of 9.8% in central Uganda.[74] In Nigeria, Wokoma et al.[75] summarized the results of 30 community-based CKD screening studies, which included more than 17,000 participants, and found an overall crude CKD prevalence of 11.7%. The prevalence was much higher in rural than in urban communities (16.4% vs. 7.0%).

The large Maremar study[67] included over 10,000 Moroccan adults and reported a population prevalence of 5.1%. This study by Benghanem Gharbi et al. is especially noteworthy in that it is one of the few studies of CKD prevalence in which particular care was taken to satisfy the criterion of chronicity in diagnosing CKD.[67,76]

Kayange et al. have published a systematic review of community-based studies describing the prevalence of renal abnormalities among children in sub-Saharan Africa.[77] Thirty-two studies from nine countries were included and these reported widely varying results. The mean prevalence of proteinuria was 32.5% (2.2%–56.0%), hematuria 31.1% (0.6%–67%), and imaging abnormalities 14.8% (0.5%–38.0%). The quality of these studies was graded as moderate to poor. Few were recent, and none included the calculation of eGFR. Most of the studies were performed in areas where schistosomiasis is endemic, and this was the main risk factor identified.

## COMMON CAUSES OF CHRONIC KIDNEY DISEASE AND END-STAGE RENAL DISEASE

In many cases where CKD or ESRD is identified in African patients, a specific diagnosis is never established. This may be because renal biopsy services are often not available or

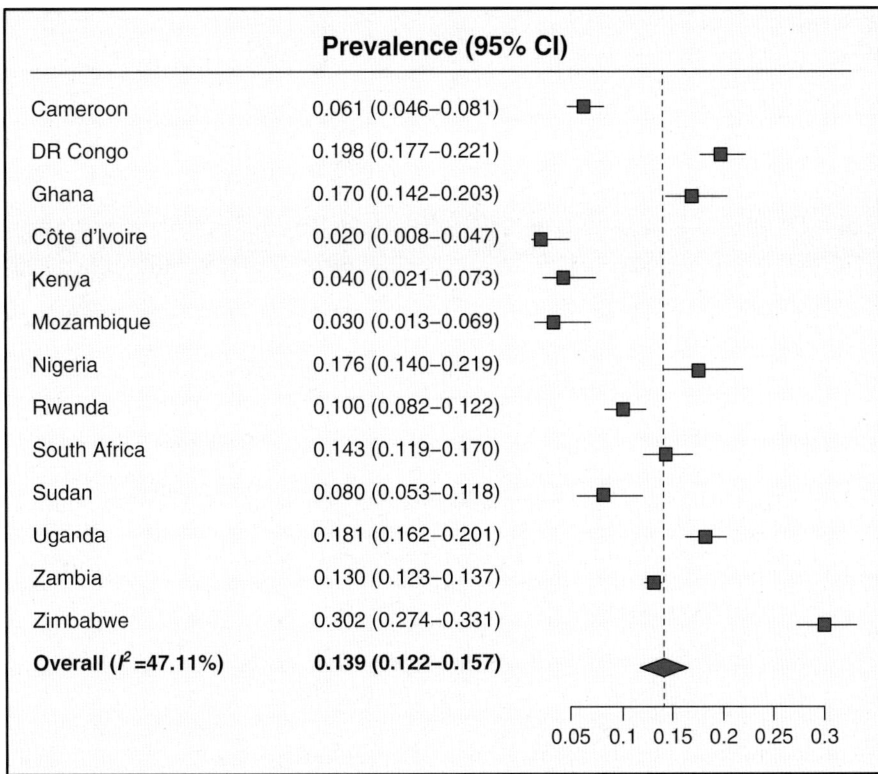


**Fig. 77.11** Forest plot of meta-analyses showing the pooled prevalence of chronic kidney disease by country. (From Stanifer JW, Jing B, Tolan S, et al. The epidemiology of chronic kidney disease in sub-Saharan Africa: a systematic review and meta-analysis. *Lancet Glob Health.* 2014;2:e174-e181.)

**Table 77.4 Etiology of End-Stage Renal Disease (% of Total) Reported in Registry Data From African Countries**

| Study | Country | Last Data | Cause Unknown | Hypertension | Diabetes | GN | Cystic Disease |
|---|---|---|---|---|---|---|---|
| Afifi, 2008[83] | Egypt | 2008 | 15.2 | 36.6 | 13.5 | 8.7 | 3.2 |
| Alashek, 2012[84] | Libya | 2010 | 7.3 | 14.6 | 26.5 | 21.2 | 6.3 |
| Albitar, 1998[85] | Reunion Island | 1996 | | 27.5 | 33.6 | 13.1 | 5.8 |
| Davids, 2017[79] | South Africa | 2015 | 34.1 | 33.7 | 14.4 | 9.5 | 2.9 |
| Elamin, 2010[80] | Sudan | 2009 | 42.6 | 26.1 | 10.4 | 5.5 | 2.6 |
| Tunisian Ministry of Health, 2011[81] | Tunisia | 2010 | 29.2 | 13.6 | 21.0 | 13.0[86] | 3.4 |
| Moroccan Society of Nephrology and Ministry of Health, 2013[82] | Morocco | 2007 | 37.9 | 10.1 | 17.8 | 8.5 | 3.4 |

*GN*, Glomerulonephritis.

because patients present late, with poor renal function, hypertension and shrunken kidneys. A presumptive diagnosis of chronic glomerulonephritis or of hypertensive renal disease is often made, without good grounds for making such a diagnosis.[78] It has been recommended that the label "CKD/ESRD etiology uncertain/unknown" be used in such cases, and whenever there is uncertainty about the renal diagnosis.

Data on the etiology of CKD/ESKD is available from renal registries for some African countries (Table 77.4). The "CKD/ESRD unknown" category was indicated as the most common renal diagnosis in reports from South Africa,[79] Sudan,[80] Tunisia,[81] and Morocco.[82]

## DIABETIC NEPHROPATHY

The International Diabetes Federation has estimated that three-quarters of people with diabetes live in low- or middle-income countries and that the number of adults with diabetes will increase from 415 million in 2015 to 642 million in 2040.[87] The Africa region is projected to experience the highest growth rates in the number of diabetic patients, with an increase of 140.7% by 2040. These increases are driven

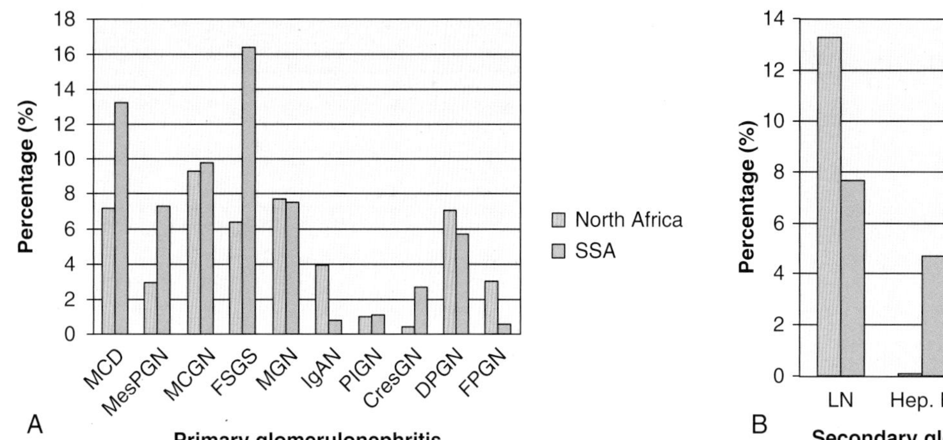


**Fig. 77.12** Differences between North Africa and sub-Saharan Africa in the prevalence of common primary (A) and secondary (B) glomerular diseases. *MCD*, Minimal change disease; *MesPGN*, mesangioproliferative GN; *MCGN*, mesangiocapillary GN; *FSGS*, focal segmental glomerulosclerosis; *MGN*, membranous GN; *IgAN*, IgA nephropathy; *PIGN*, postinfectious GN; *CresGN*, crescentic GN; *DPGN*, diffuse proliferative GN; *FPGN*, focal proliferative GN; *LN*, lupus nephritis; *Hep B*, hepatitis B virus-associated nephropathy; *HIVAN*, HIV-associated nephropathy. (From Okpechi IG, Ameh OI, Bello AK, Ronco P, Swanepoel CR, Kengne AP. Epidemiology of histologically proven glomerulonephritis in Africa: a systematic review and meta-analysis. *PLoS ONE.* 2016;11:e0152203.)

by sedentary lifestyles, unhealthy diets, obesity, population growth, and aging.

The rates of diabetes-related complications, including diabetic nephropathy, have slowed markedly over the past two decades, as a result of improved medical care for blood pressure, glycemic control, lipid management, and the use of agents that block the renin-angiotensin system. For example, in the US, the rate of patients with diabetes reaching ESRD declined by 28% between 1990 and 2010.[88] However, a large burden of disease persists because of the continued increase in the prevalence of diabetes.

Noubiap et al.[89] have published a systematic review of diabetic nephropathy in Africa that included 32 studies from 16 countries. They found that measurement of urine protein excretion was the most common method of assessing kidney damage in diabetic patients and that the reported overall prevalence of CKD in diabetics varied from 11% to 83.7%. The rate of ESRD at 5 years of follow-up was 34.7% and the mortality rate from nephropathy was 18.4% at 20 years of follow-up. Duration of diabetes, high blood pressure, advancing age, obesity, and glucose control were the common determinants of kidney disease.

## GLOMERULONEPHRITIS

Okpechi et al.[90] have conducted a systematic review of histologically-proven glomerulonephritis in Africa, which covered the period from 1980 to 2014. They noted declining renal biopsy rates and the consequent paucity of data on pathologic patterns of renal diseases from Africa. Their review included 24 studies (12,093 biopsies) from 13 countries, with 70% of the studies originating from North African countries. Nephrotic syndrome was the most common indication for renal biopsy. The frequency of common primary renal diseases reported included minimal change disease (MCD) at 16.5%, focal segmental glomerulosclerosis (FSGS) at 15.9%, mesangiocapillary GN (MCGN) at 11.8%, IgA nephropathy at 2.8%, and crescentic GN at 2.0%. Nephritis related to hepatitis B (8.4%) and systemic lupus erythematosus (7.7%) had the highest prevalence among the secondary glomerular diseases. Fig. 77.12 illustrates some of the differences between North African and sub-Saharan African countries.[90]

It is unlikely that quartan malaria due to *Plasmodium malariae* infection causes a specific glomerulopathy which presents as nephrotic syndrome in African children. Almost all of the reports of "malarial glomerulopathy" or "tropical glomerulopathy" were published before 1975; they rest mainly on circumstantial evidence and there seems to be no recent data to support the existence of this entity.[91]

## KIDNEY DISEASE ASSOCIATED WITH HUMAN IMMUNODEFICIENCY VIRUS INFECTION

A broad spectrum of renal diseases is seen in patients with HIV infection. This includes diseases directly related to the HIV infection, those related to superinfections, those related to the immune response, and those related to the treatment. HIV-associated nephropathy (HIVAN) is the classic lesion described, presenting with nephrotic-range proteinuria and decreased renal function but, because of renal salt wasting, patients often do not have hypertension or significant edema. Renal histology reveals a collapsing form of FSGS, with associated cystic tubular dilatation, interstitial inflammation, and the presence of tubuloreticular inclusion bodies. HIV RNA has been demonstrated in podocytes and tubular epithelial cells.[92]

HIVAN was first reported in 1984,[93–95] with the first reports from Africa published in the late 1980s and early 1990s.[96–98] The worldwide prevalence is highest in sub-Saharan Africa,[99] occurring especially in the absence of antiretroviral therapy and in patients with markedly reduced CD4 counts and elevated viral loads.[100]

Individuals of African descent have a genetic susceptibility to the development of HIVAN that is related to single nucleotide polymorphisms in the apolipoprotein L1 (APOL1) gene.[101] The G1 variant includes two missense mutations

(S342G, Rs73885319 and I384M, Rs60910145) that are in close linkage disequilibrium, and the G2 variant is a two-base pair deletion (N388del, Y389del, Rs71785313). These variants confer risk for HIVAN and HIV-associated FSGS, as well as other glomerular diseases and hypertensive nephrosclerosis. Kasembeli et al.[102] have demonstrated that HIV-positive, ART-naïve black South Africans with two APOL1 risk alleles are at very high risk of developing HIV-associated nephropathy. In their study, 79% of patients with HIV-associated nephropathy and only 2% of controls carried two risk alleles. Individuals carrying any combination of two risk alleles had 89-fold higher odds of developing HIV-associated nephropathy compared with HIV-positive controls. It is estimated that 50% of HIV-positive individuals who have two APOL1 risk alleles and do not receive effective ART will develop HIVAN.[103]

There is a wide variability in the prevalence of HIVAN in different African populations and this is likely related to the frequency of the APOL1 risk alleles. The highest frequency of the G1 and G2 variants is found in West Africa whereas populations in North and East Africa have a much lower frequency of the risk alleles and of HIV-related renal disease.[104] For example, in Kenya, Koech et al.[105] performed renal biopsies on ART-naïve, HIV-positive adults who had persistent proteinuria. None of the biopsies revealed HIVAN; acute interstitial nephritis was the most common histological diagnosis in this group of patients.

Renal biopsy data on African patients with HIV infection has mostly come from South African studies. In Durban, Han et al. biopsied 30 HIV-positive patients with proteinuria who were not on antiretroviral therapy and found that 83% had HIVAN. Gerntholtz et al.[24] described the findings in 99 patients from the Johannesburg area: 27% of the biopsies showed classic HIVAN, 21% had HIV-related immune complex disease (HIV-ICD), and more than half had diagnoses which were not directly related to the HIV infection. In those patients with immune complex disease, subepithelial deposits were sometimes associated with a "ball-in-cup" basement membrane reaction pattern. Also, from Johannesburg, the biopsy series of Vermeulen et al.[25] included 364 HIV-infected patients; HIVAN was present in 32.7% and HIV-ICD in 11.8% of these patients. Wearne et al.[26] reviewed the biopsies of 192 HIV-infected patients in Cape Town, reporting that HIVAN was the most common histological diagnosis (57%), with the collapsing subtype of FSGS present in 43%, and describing a "fetal variant" of FSGS in some cases. Immune complex disease was present in 8.3% and a combination of HIVAN and HIV-ICD in 21.9%.

In the absence of antiretroviral therapy, HIVAN progresses rapidly to ESRD. In many countries, the introduction of ART has led to substantial reductions in the incidence of HIVAN and HIVAN-related ESRD.[106] However, there have been conflicting reports on the benefit of ART in patients with HIV-ICD, with a study by Szczech et al.[107] finding that renal lesions other than HIVAN did not benefit from ART. Several African studies have demonstrated improvements in kidney function in patients who have initiated ART for HIV-related renal disease. These include the DART study in Uganda and Zimbabwe,[108] the study by Peters et al. in Uganda,[109] the study by Mpondo et al. in Tanzania,[110] and the South African studies by Wearne et al.[26] in Cape Town and Fabian et al.[111] in Johannesburg. The South African studies included renal biopsy data and, unlike the Szczech et al. study,[107] demonstrated benefit in both HIVAN and HIV-ICD.

**Table 77.5 Regional Access to Antiretroviral Therapy in 2015 for Africans Living With Human Immunodeficiency Virus. Figures Are Percentages With Confidence Intervals**

| | Adults (Aged 15 Years+) | Children (Aged 0–14 Years) | Pregnant Women[a] |
|---|---|---|---|
| Eastern and Southern Africa | 53% (50–57) | 63% (56–71) | 90% (82–95+) |
| Western and Central Africa | 29% (24–35) | 20% (16–25) | 48% (40–58) |
| Middle East and North Africa | 16% (12–24) | 20% (16–25) | 12% (9–18) |
| Global averages | 46% (43–50) | 49% (42–55) | 77% (69–86)[114] |

[a]Treatment to prevent mother-to-child transmission of human immunodeficiency virus.

From AIDS by the numbers. Geneva, Switzerland: Joint United Nations programme on HIV/AIDS 2016.

Globally, there has been a rapid scale-up of antiretroviral therapy. Gains have been greatest in Eastern and Southern Africa, the world's most affected region.[112] South Africa alone had nearly 3.4 million people on treatment in 2015, more than any other country in the world. The latest South African guidelines recommend initiating ART in all HIV-infected persons, irrespective of CD4 count or viral load.[113] Kenya has the next-largest program in Africa, with nearly 900,000 people on treatment. Botswana, Eritrea, Kenya, Malawi, Mozambique, Rwanda, South Africa, Swaziland, Uganda, the United Republic of Tanzania, Zambia, and Zimbabwe all increased treatment coverage by more than 25% between 2010 and 2015.[112] Table 77.5 summarizes the data from the different African regions regarding access to ART.[114] Western and Central African countries have the lowest access, with only 29% of adults, 20% of children, and 48% of pregnant women living with HIV accessing treatment. The global averages are 46%, 49%, and 77%, respectively.

## GLOMERULAR DISEASE ASSOCIATED WITH HEPATITIS B VIRUS INFECTION

Hepatitis B virus (HBV) infection is highly endemic with at least 65 million chronic HB surface antigen (HBsAg) carriers in Africa. The major transmission route is horizontal transmission between children under the age of 5 years, and sexual transmission in adolescents and young adults. Healthcare workers are also at risk for parenteral/percutaneous transmission during occupational exposures.[115]

The first case of HBV-associated membranous glomerulonephritis (MGN) was reported in 1971,[116] and the frequency of reported cases reached its peak around 1988–1994. Since then, there has been a decline in the numbers of new cases, largely linked to increasing HBV immunization.[115] Despite the high burden of HBV infection in Africa, there are relatively few reported case series of HBV-associated renal disease, and these are mainly from Southern Africa.[117–123] This is likely related to the availability of renal biopsy and pathology services, including access to electron microscopy.

In one of the larger African case series, Bates et al.[123] studied 71 South African and Namibian children with HBV-associated MGN and compared them with 12 adults who had HBV-associated MGN and 33 adults with idiopathic MGN. The children with HBV-associated MGN more frequently had prominent hematuria, raised serum transaminases, or low serum C3 and C4 levels. Their renal biopsies frequently revealed features of mesangiocapillary glomerulonephritis (MCGN) in addition to the typical subepithelial deposits of MGN. Virus-like bodies and tubuloreticular inclusion bodies were seen in more than 80% of the biopsies and HBeAg was identified in the subepithelial deposits. The remission rate in this cohort of children was 57% at four years; age of 6 years and above at presentation and prominent mesangial deposits on biopsy was associated with fewer remissions and worse renal outcome.

Bhimma et al.[122] documented a significant change in the incidence of HBV-associated MGN over the 6 years following the introduction of the HBV vaccine into the routine childhood immunization schedule in South Africa in 1995. By 2000 to 2001, the incidence of HBV-associated MGN had declined to 12% of the preimmunization rate. The latest data from the South African Renal Registry indicates that 1.3% of all patients on RRT are hepatitis B positive.[79] The prevalence is somewhat lower in public sector treatment centers (1.1% vs. 1.5%) than in private sector centers, where many patients are excluded from RRT because HBV infections are associated with adverse renal transplant outcomes and there is limited access to nucleoside/nucleotide analogues.[124]

## POSTINFECTIOUS GLOMERULONEPHRITIS

Poststreptococcal glomerulonephritis follows upper respiratory tract infections or impetigo caused by nephritogenic strains of group A beta-hemolytic streptococcus. It is currently a childhood disease of the developing world, where the burden ranges between 9.5 to 28.5 new cases per 100,000 individuals per year.[125] The condition has become rare in developed nations, where it is now seen mainly in patients over the age of 60 years, especially in association with conditions of immune system compromise such as malignancy, diabetes, alcoholism, or intravenous drug use.[125,126]

Okpechi et al.[90] reported a prevalence of postinfectious glomerulonephritis (PIGN) of 3.5% in their systematic review of biopsy-proven glomerular disease in Africa. The region with the highest reported frequency was North Africa, at 10.3%. In the study by Elzouki et al.[127] poststreptococcal glomerulonephritis was the most common renal disease seen in children admitted to a large referral hospital in Libya. Preceding streptococcal throat infections (occurring in 80%) were much more common than skin infections. In a 30-year review of histologically-proven glomerulonephritis in Tunisia, Ben Maïz et al.[128] reported that the proportion of glomerulonephritis cases with proliferative endocapillary and mesangiocapillary GN fell between the periods 1975 to 1985 and 1995 to 2005, from 15.9% and 21.6% to 6.9% and 7.7%, respectively. This change matched a drop in the incidence of acute rheumatic fever in the Tunisian population, most likely resulting from public health interventions and the widespread use of antibiotics.

The prognosis for PIGN is generally excellent, especially in children, but may be less benign in some cases where hypertension, proteinuria, and loss of renal function may persist after the initial illness or develop some years later.[129] Nasr et al.[126] reported 109 cases in patients older than 65 years, finding a male predominance, and an immunocompromised background in 61%, most commonly diabetes or malignancy. The most common site of infection was the skin, and the most common causative agent was staphylococcus (46%), followed by streptococcus (16%) and unusual gram-negative organisms. Fewer than one-quarter of the patients had full recovery of renal function.

## LUPUS NEPHRITIS

Lupus nephritis is a significant cause of mortality and morbidity in patients with systemic lupus erythematosus (SLE) and has been reported to be more aggressive in African populations. The review by Okpechi et al.[90] found lupus nephritis to have a high prevalence among the secondary glomerular diseases (7.7% of all biopsies), with the highest regional prevalence reported from North Africa (13.9%).

The management of African patients with SLE is hampered by the limited availability and high costs of renal biopsy services, immunosuppressive drugs, and laboratory facilities.[130] Ameh et al.[131] conducted a systematic review of the treatment and outcomes of lupus nephritis in Africa, including sixteen studies in their review, with one-half of these being from North Africa. All the studies reported the use of corticosteroids for induction therapy and 15/16 also used cyclophosphamide. Evidence from the Aspreva Lupus Management Study (ALMS)[132] supports the use of mycophenolate mofetil (MMF) in patients of African ancestry, but MMF is much more expensive than cyclophosphamide and there was low usage of this agent in the studies reviewed by Ameh et al. There was no consistent reporting on the use of adjuvant therapies such as chloroquine. The overall mortality ranged from 7.5% to 34.9%, with a study from Kenya reporting mortality in excess of 80% in patients with proliferative lupus nephritis.[133] The five-year renal survival was 48% to 84%, whereas five-year patient survival was 54% to 94%. Outcomes were better for the studies reported from North Africa. This systematic review has highlighted the severity of SLE and the poor outcomes for lupus nephritis in sub-Saharan Africa.[131]

A recent paper by Tannor et al.[134] examined the utility of repeat renal biopsies in South African patients with lupus nephritis. In 96 patients who had developed a disease flare, repeat biopsies infrequently revealed changes in histologic class and appeared to be of limited value especially when the first biopsy revealed proliferative disease. Even when there were changes in the histologic class, this seldom led to changes in treatment. The authors suggested that repeat biopsies be considered if the reference biopsy is nonproliferative or in the case of nonresponders or partial responders. In this study, there were poor outcomes following the repeat biopsy in patients with disease flares. There was failure to respond to induction therapy in 62.2%; end-stage renal disease developed within one year in 36.3%; and the mortality rate after one year was 23.0%.

## SCHISTOSOMIASIS

*Schistosoma haematobium* or *Schistosoma mansoni* is endemic to many countries of Africa. The disease burden of schistosomiasis in Africa may be equivalent to malaria or HIV/AIDS, and despite the fact that praziquantel is available as a simple annual treatment for less than 50 cents per person, fewer than 5% of the infected population is treated.[135] Terminal hematuria is the typical clinical presentation, usually associated with frequency and dysuria. In a large cross-sectional study in an untreated African population infected with *S. haematobium,* microhematuria was reported in 41% to 100%, and gross hematuria in 0% to 97%.[136]

Although the early renal lesions of schistosomiasis may regress with appropriate antiparasitic treatment, the chronic sequelae are irreversible.[137] Renal failure results from the deposition of ova in the genitourinary system, which causes obstruction, reflux, infection, and stone formation. Immune complexes containing worm antigens may also deposit in the glomeruli, which leads to different patterns of glomerular disease, including mesangioproliferative, exudative, and mesangiocapillary types, focal segmental sclerosing lesions, or amyloidosis.[137,138] Exudative lesions occur in the presence of salmonella coinfection. The development of mesangiocapillary GN and focal segmental sclerosis correlates with the degree of associated hepatic fibrosis; amyloidosis occurs in prolonged infection and correlates with the antigen load.

## RENAL STONES

North African countries lie within a geographical Afro-Asian stone-forming belt where renal stone disease is particularly common. In this region, all age groups are affected, with a male predominance. The high prevalence of urolithiasis may be related to high rates of consanguinity, hot climates, and dietary factors such as high intake of animal protein.[139]

There is a paucity of African data on CKD or ESRD resulting from renal stone disease. In Tunisia, 2.7% of patients on chronic dialysis have renal stones as the etiology.[81] In South Africa, only 1.5% of patients on RRT have obstruction and/or reflux as the primary renal disease.[79] Although some of these cases may have been related to renal stones, there were very few patients (24 out of 10,360) where there was specific mention of calculi, uric acid nephropathy, cystinosis, hyperoxaluria, or hypercalcaemia. From the Sudan, Abboud et al. reported that 12% of Sudanese patients with chronic renal failure had renal calculi as the etiology,[140] whereas Elsharif et al. reported obstruction as the etiology of ESRD in 11.6% of patients on chronic hemodialysis.[141] The prevalence of obstructive uropathy in ESRD patients has been reported as 5% in Libya[84] and 11% in Egypt.[142]

## SICKLE CELL DISEASE

Africa carries approximately 75% of the global disease burden of sickle cell disease, mainly due to a high prevalence of sickle cell trait in West Africa.[143] It is estimated that 25% of Nigerian adults are carriers. The presence of sickle cell trait protects against the severe complications of *Plasmodium falciparum* malaria, which is endemic in the region.

Renal involvement is common, and more severe in homozygous disease (sickle cell anemia, HbSS) than in the compound heterozygous forms; however, even sickle cell trait is associated with increased risk of CKD.[144] A Nigerian case series by Arogundade et al. reported that 37.4% of their patients with sickle cell disease had CKD as defined by persistent proteinuria, hematuria and/or reduction in GFR.[145]

Hemolysis, vasoocclusion, and ischemia-reperfusion injury are the mechanisms underlying the clinical manifestations of sickle cell disease. The pathophysiology of the renal involvement involves the coexistence of cortical hyperperfusion, medullary hypoperfusion, and an increased renal vasoconstrictive response to systemic and regional stress.[146] Red blood cells sickle in the renal medulla because of its hypoxic, acidotic and hyperosmolar conditions. Clinical manifestations are protean, ranging from hematuria and loss of concentrating ability to acute kidney injury, chronic kidney disease, and renal medullary carcinoma. The most common glomerular lesion seen is focal segmental glomerulosclerosis. Hyperfiltration and impaired concentrating ability may occur in infancy; albuminuria may develop in childhood and progress thereafter; and in older adults the risk of CKD and end-stage renal disease increases. Hematuria and acute kidney disease can occur at any age.[146]

Renal involvement contributes to the diminished life expectancy of patients with sickle cell disease, accounting for 16% to 18% of mortality. Even patients who are able to access RRT still have a mortality rate several-fold higher than patients without sickle cell disease.[146]

## HYPERTENSIVE RENAL DISEASE

In registry data from African countries, hypertension has been reported as the etiology of ESRD in 10.1% to 36.6% of patients on RRT (see Table 77.4). Egypt (36.6%) and South Africa (33.7%) have the highest percentages of patients with this primary renal diagnosis, while Morocco (10.1%) and Tunisia (13.6%) are at the lower end of the spectrum.

It is generally accepted that accelerated and malignant forms of hypertension can lead to end-stage renal failure,[147,148] although renal recovery sometimes occurs months after starting RRT, especially when patients are treated with peritoneal dialysis.[149] In a study to determine the basis of ESRD in black South Africans, Gold et al.[150] reviewed the renal histology in 65 black patients on chronic hemodialysis and reported that essential/primary malignant hypertension was the most common cause, occurring in 49%.

Nephrologists also often apply a diagnosis of "hypertensive renal disease" or "hypertensive nephrosclerosis" to nondiabetic patients, especially black patients, who present with chronic kidney disease and only mild-to-moderate hypertension.[78] It has now become clear that many of these patients have glomerular disease, which is related to the presence of renal-risk variants of the APOL1 gene and have secondarily elevated blood pressure.[151] For example, in the African American Study of Kidney Disease and Hypertension (AASK), the APOL1 association was strongest in individuals with more proteinuria and progressive nephropathy. Aggressive hypertension control and the use of angiotensin-converting enzyme inhibitors failed to halt progression, supporting the role of mechanisms other than hypertension.[152] The AASK patients predominantly had focal glomerulosclerosis with interstitial and vascular changes that did not correlate with blood pressure.[153] This new information has prompted calls for the term "hypertensive nephrosclerosis" to be abandoned.[78,154]

The South African Renal Registry has recommended that users submitting data indicate hypertensive nephropathy as the primary renal diagnosis only if there is no reason to suspect that the hypertension may be secondary to preexisting renal disease.[79] They suggest that the following criteria be met: hypertension known to precede renal dysfunction, left ventricular hypertrophy, proteinuria less than 2 g/day, and no evidence of other renal diseases.[155,156]

## GENETIC DISORDERS

To date, Africans have only participated minimally in genomics research, and then often only at the level of sample collection. The many reasons for this include a shortage of African scientists with genomic research expertise, lack of research infrastructure, limited computational expertise and resources, and inadequate support by governments.[157] Adedokun et al.[158] performed an analysis of genetics publications from sub-Saharan Africa for the period 2004 to 2013 and found that most of the publications involved populations from South Africa (31.1%), Ghana (10.6%), and Kenya (7.5%). Almost half of all the studies investigated HIV, TB or malaria, while about one-tenth related to NCDs. Less than half of the publications had a first author from an African institution. In most studies without an African first author, local authors mostly had administrative roles and were seldom involved in the conceptualization or design of the studies, data analysis, or in the writing of the manuscripts.[158]

The Human Heredity and Health in Africa (H3Africa) initiative is a large-scale collaboration between the US National Institutes of Health (NIH), the UK-based Wellcome Trust and the African Society of Human Genetics, which aims at addressing some of these issues by focusing strongly on capacity building, as well as specific scientific goals.[157] The project is training African clinical research personnel and genomic investigators, establishing genomic research laboratories in West Africa, and conducting international-level genetic and translational research. Regarding renal disease, the H3Africa Kidney Disease Research Network is currently recruiting patients in Ghana, Nigeria, Ethiopia and Kenya, and analyzing environmental and genetic factors associated with CKD. The recruitment targets are 4000 participants with CKD and 4000 controls, and 50 families with hereditary glomerular disease.[159,160]

Among the genetic disorders relevant to Africa, which are actively researched, is the association of kidney disease with African "risk" variants of the APOL1 gene (see Chapter 43)[160] and genetic factors in sickle cell disease.[161,162]

### The Role of Consanguineous Marriage

A consanguineous marriage is defined as a union between two individuals who are related as second cousins or closer. This practice is common throughout Arab countries and contributes to the increase in genetic disorders, especially autosomal recessive disorders, also seen in North Africa (see Chapter 78). For example, the high rates of renal stone disease seen in the region is at least partly due to consanguinity, which results in higher rates of predisposing conditions such as primary hyperoxaluria and cystinosis.[139] Jaouad et al.[163] studied the rates of consanguineous marriages in 176 Moroccan families with autosomal recessive diseases. Although the overall reported prevalence of consanguinity in Morocco was 15%, the rate among the families with autosomal recessive disorders was 59%.

### Cystic Kidney Disease

Worldwide, autosomal dominant polycystic kidney disease (ADPKD) is a common cause for CKD and ESRD, but the data from African populations are sparse. Bourquia[164] reported data on ADPKD in 308 Moroccan families. The mean age at diagnosis was 46 years; the most frequent symptom was pain, which led to a diagnosis. Hypertension was present in 11% of the patients, loss of renal function in 17%, and hepatic cysts in 17.8%. In Benin, Laleye et al. described 70 patients with ADPKD.[165] Their mean age was 47.2 years, a positive family history was obtained in 47%, and lumbar pain was the most common presenting symptom. Mutations in the polycystin 1 gene (PKD1) were identified, including several variants not previously described. A cohort of 53 Senegalese patients has also been described,[166] as has a case where a PKD1 mutation was identified.[167] In the Senegalese cohort, there was a high rate of ESRD at the time of diagnosis or soon thereafter, mainly due to delays in making the diagnosis and in referrals to nephrologists. In the Seychelles, ADPKD is seen almost exclusively in people of Caucasian extraction, even though they comprise only 30% of the population. This may be the consequence of a founder effect.[168]

Autosomal recessive polycystic kidney disease (ARPKD) is caused by mutations in the PKHD1 gene and has a worldwide incidence of 1:20,000, corresponding to a heterozygote frequency of 1:70. Among the Afrikaner population of South Africa, the live-birth rate and the carrier rate have been estimated at 1:11,000 and 1:53, respectively.[169] Lambie et al.[170] studied a cohort of patients from 36 Afrikaner families, finding that 27 patients, from 24 families, were homozygous for the p.M627K substitution, providing strong evidence of a founder mutation.

Nephronophthisis (NPHP) is an autosomal recessive cystic kidney disease, which is a leading genetic cause of ESRD in children. In contrast to ADPKD, the kidneys are not enlarged, cysts are present mostly at the corticomedullary junction, and there is prominent tubulointerstitial fibrosis.[171] Soliman et al.[172] studied 20 Egyptian children with NPHP, reporting a mean age at diagnosis of 88 months, and a mean age at the onset of symptoms of 44 months. Patients were categorized as 75% juvenile NPHP, 5% infantile NPHP and 20% Joubert syndrome-related disorders. Homozygous NPHP1 deletions were detected in six patients.

### Metabolic Diseases

Primary hyperoxaluria type 1 (PH1) is an autosomal recessive metabolic disease where there is an increased endogenous production of oxalate. Progressive kidney failure results from the excessive urinary oxalate excretion and renal deposition of calcium oxalate. Disease-causing mutations of the alanine glyoxylate aminotransferase (AGXT) gene have been identified in patients from Tunisia[173] and Egypt.[174]

Familial Mediterranean fever (FMF) is an autosomal recessive disease that primarily affects populations surrounding the Mediterranean and it is characterized by recurrent attacks of fever and serosal inflammation. Amyloidosis is a serious complication of the disease and may result in renal failure.

The disease is caused by mutations in the FMF gene (MEFV), which encodes pyrin, a protein involved in regulating inflammatory responses. Mutations may cause gain of function so that pyrin can initiate inflammation in the absence of a toxin or infection. MEFV mutations have been identified in Tunisian patients.[175] Amyloidosis is more common in North African patients, who are homozygous for the M694V mutation; the risk also increases in male patients and in those bearing the polymorphism a/a in the SAA1 gene.[176]

### Tubular Disorders

Familial hypomagnesemia with hypercalciuria and nephrocalcinosis caused by a novel claudin16 mutation has been reported in an Egyptian family.[177] In South Africa, new mutations of the SLC12A3 gene, which encodes the sodium-chloride cotransporter on the apical membrane of the distal convoluted tubule, have been reported in a family with Gitelman syndrome, who presented with hypokalaemia and unusual cravings for salt and vinegar.[178] Mutations of the epithelial sodium channel (ENaC) have also been identified in South African patients in association with hypertension[179,180] and preeclampsia.[181] In Tunisia, mutations of the $H^+$-ATPase pump have been identified in children with primary distal renal tubular acidosis, often associated with sensorineural deafness.[182]

### Glomerular Diseases

Mutations of the nephrin gene (NPHS1) have been discovered in North African patients with congenital nephrotic syndrome of the Finnish type.[183] A Moroccan infant with steroid-resistant nephrotic syndrome was found to have a mutation in the ARHGDIA gene, which encodes Rho-GDP dissociation inhibitor 1. This protein modulates signaling through Rho GTPases and thereby regulates cell motility.[184]

## CHRONIC KIDNEY DISEASE OF UNCERTAIN ETIOLOGY

CKD of uncertain etiology (CKDu) describes CKD not attributable to traditional risk factors, such as diabetes, hypertension, or HIV infection. CKDu is reported with increasing frequency and has reached epidemic proportions in many countries. The term CKDu is a generic one, and likely includes kidney diseases with many disparate etiologies. It serves to highlight the need for hot-spot identification through adequate surveillance and for collaborative studies to identify specific causes.

The term was first used in El Salvador to describe a disease affecting mainly agricultural communities and has subsequently been reported in many other countries, including Nicaragua, Costa Rica, and Sri Lanka.[185] Factors that have been implicated in the pathogenesis of CKDu include exposure to agricultural toxins, traditional medicines, heavy metals, and heat stress.[185] Interactions between genetic and environmental factors may also be important, as suggested by the finding that a single-nucleotide polymorphism in *SCL13A3* predisposes to CKDu in Sri Lanka.[186]

CKDu hotspots have also been reported from several African countries. For example, in Tunisia, chronic interstitial nephropathy has been linked to the contamination of food with ochratoxin,[187] while in Tanzania, urban residence was a strong risk factor for the presence of CKD.[71] In the El-Minia region of Egypt, ESRD with an unknown etiology in rural farm workers has been associated with environmental factors, such as drinking unsafe water, exposure to pesticides, and using herbal medications.[188]

## SCREENING AND PREVENTION OF CHRONIC KIDNEY DISEASE

CKD can be prevented by effective control of known etiologies and risk factors and by implementing adequate renoprotective measures. The early detection of CKD by efficient screening programs is important, especially in African countries where renal replacement therapy is not easily accessible.[189]

Various challenges need to be overcome to include CKD screening and prevention in daily clinical practice. The access to diagnostic tools is sometimes a challenge for practitioners and patients. Ensuring the accuracy of the diagnosis and confirming the chronicity of the renal abnormalities is a necessity, since the classification of a person as having CKD has major consequences.[76] In the Maremar study,[190] the investigators demonstrated that repeating eGFR after 3 months avoided a false positive diagnosis of CKD in 32% of cases. The same reasoning can be applied for albuminuria and proteinuria, the other common screening tests for CKD. Repeating dipstick testing after 1 to 2 weeks allowed positive results to be identified as false positives in 67.5% of subjects with mild proteinuria (dipstick +) and in 28.7% of those with overt proteinuria (dipstick ++ to +++).[190] Another recent African epidemiological study, which determined the prevalence of CKD in sugarcane workers in Cameroon, also included the element of chronicity in their methods, and reported a relatively low CKD rate of 3.4%.[191]

Screening mostly detects individuals with earlier stages of CKD, and therefore the CKD-EPI study equation is recommended, as it is more accurate than the MDRD equation at higher GFR values. As discussed in the Chronic Kidney Disease section previously, the ethnicity correction factor should not be used.[61–63]

Another challenge is the feasibility and the cost-effectiveness of CKD screening and prevention programs in African countries. Many epidemiological studies have shown that diseases such as diabetes, hypertension, and HIV infection are the major causes of CKD in many countries.[67,68,192] It seems reasonable to couple simple CKD screening and preventive measures with already-implemented programs for diabetes, hypertension, and HIV infection.[193] For example, the WHO STEPS method is a simple, standardized method for collecting data on NCDs and their risk factors, and could easily be adapted to include screening for CKD.[194]

Education of patients and healthcare workers regarding hypertension, diabetes, obesity, and healthy lifestyles (e.g., prudent diet, cessation of smoking, exercise) is essential for primary prevention of CKD. The programs of organizations such as the ISN and initiatives such as World Kidney Day have heightened awareness of renal disease among both medical professionals and the public in developing countries. Efforts should be made to optimize therapy for hypertension, diabetes mellitus, and renal disease, applying best practice clinical guidelines for the management of these conditions. Unfortunately, the shortage of healthcare workers and the lack of availability of pharmaceutical agents to retard progression of CKD are impediments in many African countries.[195]

## END-STAGE RENAL DISEASE AND RENAL REPLACEMENT THERAPY

Anand et al.[196] have predicted an annual ESRD incidence of 239 per million population (PMP) in people with diabetes and hypertension who live in sub-Saharan Africa. In North African countries, the annual incidence has been estimated at 150 PMP.[197,198] The wide variations in the reported prevalence of treated ESRD seen in developing countries are mainly a reflection of differing access to dialysis and transplantation rather than differences in the burden of disease,[199] and this provision of RRT is strongly associated with gross national income per capita.[200] Liyanage et al.[201] have estimated that at least 432,000 people in Africa require RRT but are not receiving it. In most countries where RRT is available, patients carry the cost, and few are able to afford dialysis beyond the first 3 months.[202]

The lack of renal registries means that there are few reliable, current statistics on RRT in Africa.[203] Estimates are often based on old registry reports and unpublished data,[204,205] but suggest that the provision of RRT services has been a low priority for the governments of most African countries. A few renal registries, mainly from North Africa, have been established in African countries but these projects have mostly not been sustainable, and reports have not been published regularly. The earliest reports were from Egypt and Tunisia in 1975, followed by South Africa in 1977, and thereafter by Libya, Algeria, and Morocco.[203]

Table 77.6 summarizes the African publications since 1996 that have most recently reported country wide data on RRT.[203] Data from North African countries also have been published in the European Renal Association–European Dialysis and Transplant Association (ERA-EDTA) Registry Annual Reports over a number of years.[203]

South Africa is the only country on the continent that has regularly reported country wide data on RRT in recent years.[79,206–208] In December 2015, the number of patients who were treated with chronic dialysis or transplantation in South Africa stood at 10,360, a prevalence of 189 PMP. The treatment modality was hemodialysis in 72.7%, peritoneal dialysis in 13.9%, and transplantation in 13.4%. The prevalence, which was 167 PMP in 2013 and 178 PMP in 2014, has been increasing due to increasing numbers of patients accessing hemodialysis in the private healthcare sector. In the public sector, which serves 84% of the South African population, the prevalence of RRT was 71.9 PMP, as compared with 799.3 PMP in the private sector. Disparities between different provinces were also identified as were disparities related to ethnicity, with Blacks being the most underserved group.[79]

The African Association of Nephrology (AFRAN) and the African Pediatric Nephrology Association (AFPNA) are now addressing this serious knowledge gap and have established the African Renal Registry, using the expanded platform of the South African Renal Registry.[209] Ghana, Zambia, Burundi, and Kenya have formally joined the African Renal Registry during this pilot phase.

Recently, data on RRT from Egypt and Morocco have been published in the International Comparisons chapter of the United States Renal Data System Annual Data Report.[210] In Egypt, the prevalence of RRT in 2015 was 624 PMP. The incidence of new patients starting RRT was 56 PMP, with diabetes the cause of the renal disease in 15%. The 2015 transplant rate was 15 PMP. In Morocco, the prevalence of RRT in 2015 was 541 PMP and the incidence 144 PMP. Diabetes was reported as the cause of the renal disease in 44% of the patients. The transplant rate was 1 PMP.

There have been few economic evaluation studies of RRT in African countries. At Muhimbili National Hospital in Tanzania, Mushi et al.[211] estimated the costs of hemodialysis for 34 patients in 2014 to be US$176 per treatment, or US$27,440 per annum. In Cameroon, Halle et al.[212] conducted a cost analysis of hemodialysis care in 154 patients at three public-sector facilities. The annual cost of hemodialysis per patient was US$13,581, with out-of-pocket payments of US$4,114, accounting for 30% of the total cost. The authors concluded that the cost of maintaining patients on hemodialysis was very high considering the national gross domestic

**Table 77.6 Most Recent Publications Reporting Countrywide Data on Renal Replacement Therapy From African Countries**

| Author and Year | Country/Region | Last Data | Key Data Reported |
|---|---|---|---|
| USRDS Report, 2017[210] | Egypt | 2015 | Incidence 56 PMP, diabetes the cause in 15%; prevalence 624 PMP. Dialysis modality: HD 100%. Transplant rate 15 PMP, all living donors. |
| Alashek et al., 2012[84] | Libya | 2010 | Dialysis-treated ESRD. Incidence 282 PMP, diabetes the cause in 28.4%; prevalence 624 PMP, diabetes the cause in 26.5%, unknown cause in 7.3%. |
| USRDS Report, 2017[210] | Morocco | 2015 | Incidence 144 PMP, diabetes the cause in 44%; prevalence 541 PMP. Transplant rate 1 PMP. |
| Albitar et al., 1998[85] | Reunion Island | 1996 | Incidence 188 PMP, prevalence 1155 PMP, cause was diabetes in 33.6%. Modality: HD 82.7%, PD 3.0%, TX 14.3%. Annual mortality 8.1%. |
| Davids et al., 2017[79] | South Africa | 2015 | Prevalence 189 PMP, cause unknown in 34.1%, hypertension in 33.7%, diabetes in 14.4%. Modality: HD 72.7%, PD 13.9%, TX 13.4%. Transplant rate 4.6 PMP. |
| Elamin et al., 2010[80] | Sudan | 2009 | Prevalence 106 PMP, no cause identified in 42.6%, diabetes in 10.4%. Modality: HD 68.9%, PD 2.9%, TX 28.2%. |
| Ministry of Health, 2010[81] | Tunisia | 2010 | Incidence 133 PMP; prevalence 806 PMP, diabetes the cause in 21.0%. Transplants performed during 2010 = 132, living donors in 77.3%. |

*ESRD,* End stage renal disease; *HD,* hemodialysis; *PD,* peritoneal dialysis; *PMP,* per million population; *TX,* transplant.

product per capita in Cameroon, and that the out-of-pocket payments were unsustainable for most patients.

The outcomes of patients requiring chronic dialysis in sub-Saharan Africa have been reviewed by Ashuntantang et al.[213] Summarizing 68 studies, they reported a treatment discontinuation rate of 59% in adults and 49% in children. This attrition usually occurred within the first two weeks of starting dialysis and was mainly the result of an inability to pay for the treatment. When studies from South Africa and Sudan were excluded, the proportions of patients who discontinued dialysis were 78% and 86% among adults and children, respectively. When patients were able to pay for long-term dialysis, outcomes were improved, with over 75% remaining on dialysis for over one year.

Several African studies have examined the quality of life (QOL) of patients on RRT. These have mainly used standardized questionnaires such as the Kidney Disease Quality of Life–Short Form (KDQOL-SF) and the KDQOL-36 questionnaire. Okaka et al.[214,215] found that patients on CAPD in Johannesburg, South Africa, had lower QOL scores than healthy controls, with better scores in patients under the age of 30 years, those with a duration on PD of less than 4 years and those with higher incomes. In Cape Town, Tannor et al.[216] used mixed methods to investigate the QOL of patients on chronic hemodialysis and peritoneal dialysis and found that PD patients experienced a heavier symptom burden and greater limitations related to their dialysis modality, especially with regards to social functioning. The fear of developing peritonitis caused many patients to sacrifice social interactions to be able do their PD exchanges at home and at the specified times. In Malawi, Masina et al.[217] found the QOL scores of their hemodialysis patients to be generally low, and particularly low in the case of physical health scores. Similar findings were reported from Kenyatta National Hospital in Nairobi, Kenya, by Kamau et al.[218] In Morocco, El Filali et al.[219] reported high rates of major depressive and anxiety disorders (34% and 25.2%, respectively) in chronic hemodialysis patients. Major depressive episodes were associated with living alone, the presence of pain, and anxiety disorders. Bouidida et al.[220] have developed a Moroccan version of the KDQOL-SF and demonstrated its validity and reliability as a measure of QOL in Moroccan hemodialysis patients. In Egypt, Abdelfatah et al.[221] studied dialysis and transplant recipients, finding that younger patients had better QOL scores and that there was no difference in overall QOL with different modalities of RRT.

## CONCLUDING REMARKS

Africa faces many health challenges as its rapidly-growing populations struggle with the multiple burdens of infections, noncommunicable diseases, pregnancy-related diseases and injuries. These factors are the driving force behind an epidemic of acute and chronic kidney disease, which often affects young, economically active individuals and has serious economic consequences for their families and communities. In most African countries, financial and human resources are inadequate to meet this challenge.

There are, however, several successful initiatives which provide hope for the future. Regarding human resources, the ISN and ISPD Fellowship programs are making a big contribution to the training of nephrology healthcare workers in Africa. Events such as World Kidney Day are creating increased awareness of kidney disease among the public and other health professionals, and the outcomes for patients with AKI are improving as a result of the Saving Young Lives and 0by25 projects. Finally, ambitious new research projects such as the H3Africa project and the African Renal Registry have the potential to improve the outcomes of people with kidney disease and provide valuable training platforms for African researchers.

 Complete reference list available at ExpertConsult.com.

## KEY REFERENCES


2. *World Population Prospects: The 2017 revision, key findings and advance tables: United Nations, Department of Economic and Social Affairs, Population Division*; 2017.
6. *Noncommunicable diseases among young people in Africa.* Washington, DC: Population Reference Bureau; 2015.
8. Marquez PV, Farrington JL. *The challenge of non-communicable diseases and road traffic injuries in Sub-Saharan Africa: an overview.* Washington, DC: The World Bank; 2013.
13. Sharif MU, Elsayed ME, Stack AG. The global nephrology workforce: emerging threats and potential solutions. *Clin Kidney J.* 2016;9:11–22.
16. Harris DC, Dupuis S, Couser WG, et al. Training nephrologists from developing countries: does it have a positive impact? *Kidney Int Suppl (2011).* 2012;2:275–278.
18. Mehta RL, Burdmann EA, Cerda J, et al. Recognition and management of acute kidney injury in the International Society of Nephrology 0by25 Global Snapshot: a multinational cross-sectional study. *Lancet.* 2016;387:2017–2025.
20. Olowu WA, Niang A, Osafo C, et al. Outcomes of acute kidney injury in children and adults in sub-Saharan Africa: a systematic review. *Lancet Glob Health.* 2016;4:e242–e250.
24. Gerntholtz TE, Goetsch SJ, Katz I. HIV-related nephropathy: a South African perspective. *Kidney Int.* 2006;69:1885–1891.
26. Wearne N, Swanepoel CR, Boulle A, et al. The spectrum of renal histologies seen in HIV with outcomes, prognostic indicators and clinical correlations. *Nephrol Dial Transplant.* 2012;27:4109–4118.
33. Luyckx VA, Naicker S. Acute kidney injury associated with the use of traditional medicines. *Nat Rev Nephrol.* 2008;4:664.
34. Stanifer JW, Kilonzo K, Wang D, et al. Traditional medicines and kidney disease in low-and middle-income countries: opportunities and challenges. *Semin Nephrol.* 2017;37:245–259.
40. Hamdouk MI, Abdelraheem MB, Taha AA, et al. Paraphenylene diamine hair dye poisoning. In: De Broe ME, Porter GA, Bennett WM, et al, eds. *Clinical Nephrotoxins.* 3rd ed. Boston: Springer; 2008:871–879.
42. Chippaux JP. Snake-bites: appraisal of the global situation. *Bull World Health Organ.* 1998;76:515–524.
45. Arrayhani M, El Youbi R, Sqalli T. Pregnancy-related acute kidney injury: experience of the nephrology unit at the University Hospital of Fez, Morocco. *ISRN Nephrol.* 2013;2013:109034.
51. Abdou N, Antwi S, Koffi LA, et al. Peritoneal dialysis to treat patients with acute kidney injury-the Saving Young Lives experience in West Africa: Proceedings of the Saving Young Lives session at the First International Conference of Dialysis in West Africa, Dakar, Senegal, December 2015. *Perit Dial Int.* 2017;37:155–158.
61. van Deventer HE, George JA, Paiker JE, et al. Estimating glomerular filtration rate in black South Africans by use of the Modification of Diet in Renal Disease and Cockcroft-Gault equations. *Clin Chem.* 2008;54:1197–1202.
62. Madala ND, Nkwanyana N, Dubula T, et al. Predictive performance of eGFR equations in South Africans of African and Indian ancestry compared with $^{99m}$Tc-DTPA imaging. *Int Urol Nephrol.* 2012;44:847–855.
63. Sagou Yayo É, Aye M, Konan J-L, et al. Inadequacy of the African-American ethnic factor to estimate glomerular filtration rate in an African general population: Results from Côte d'Ivoire. *Nephrol Ther.* 2016;12:454–459.
67. Benghanem Gharbi M, Elseviers M, Zamd M, et al. Chronic kidney disease, hypertension, diabetes, and obesity in the adult population

of Morocco: how to avoid "over"- and "under"-diagnosis of CKD. *Kidney Int.* 2016;89:1363–1371.

68. Stanifer JW, Jing B, Tolan S, et al. The epidemiology of chronic kidney disease in sub-Saharan Africa: a systematic review and meta-analysis. *Lancet Glob Health.* 2014;2:e174–e181.
77. Kayange NM, Smart LR, Tallman JE, et al. Kidney disease among children in sub-Saharan Africa: systematic review. *Pediatr Res.* 2014;77:272–281.
79. Davids MR, Marais N, Jacobs JC. South African Renal Registry annual report 2015. *Afr J Nephrol.* 2017;20:201–2013.
80. Elamin S, Obeid W, Abu-Aisha H. Renal replacement therapy in Sudan, 2009. *Arab J Nephrol Transplant.* 2010;3:31–36.
84. Alashek WA, McIntyre CW, Taal MW. Epidemiology and aetiology of dialysis-treated end-stage kidney disease in Libya. *BMC Nephrol.* 2012;13:1.
85. Albitar S, Bourgeon B, Genin R, et al. Epidemiology of end-stage renal failure in Reunion Island (results from the registry of the Indian Ocean Society of Nephrology). *Nephrol Dial Transplant.* 1998;13: 1143–1145.
86. Counil É, Cherni N, Kharrat M, et al. Trends of incident dialysis patients in Tunisia between 1992 and 2001. *Am J Kidney Dis.* 2008;51: 463–470.
89. Noubiap J, Naidoo J, Kengne AP. Diabetic nephropathy in Africa: a systematic review. *World J Diabetes.* 2015;6:759–773.
90. Okpechi IG, Ameh OI, Bello AK, et al. Epidemiology of histologically proven glomerulonephritis in Africa: a systematic review and meta-analysis. *PLoS ONE.* 2016;11:e0152203.
91. Ehrich JH, Eke FU. Malaria-induced renal damage: facts and myths. *Pediatr Nephrol.* 2007;22:626–637.
100. Rosenberg AZ, Naicker S, Winkler CA, et al. HIV-associated nephropathies: epidemiology, pathology, mechanisms and treatment. *Nat Rev Nephrol.* 2015;11:150–160.
102. Kasembeli AN, Duarte R, Ramsay M, et al. APOL1 risk variants are strongly associated with HIV-associated nephropathy in black South Africans. *J Am Soc Nephrol.* 2015.
105. Koech M, Owiti M, Owino-Ong'or W, et al. Absence of HIV-associated nephropathy among antiretroviral naïve adults with persistent albuminuria in Western Kenya. *Kidney Int Rep.* 2017;2: 159–164.
111. Fabian J, Naicker S, Goetsch S, et al. The clinical and histological response of HIV-associated kidney disease to antiretroviral therapy in South Africans. *Nephrol Dial Transplant.* 2013;28:1543–1554.
123. Bates WD *Hepatitis-B-associated glomerular disease: a clinicopathological study of hepatitis B virus associated membranous glomerulonephritis in Namibian and South African children 1974-2005 and a comparison with hepatitis B associated membranous glomerulonephritis as well as idiopathic membranous glomerulonephritis in adults.* Cape Town: Stellenbosch University; 2011.
131. Ameh O, Kengne A, Jayne D, et al. Standard of treatment and outcomes of adults with lupus nephritis in Africa: a systematic review. *Lupus.* 2016;25:1269–1277.
137. Barsoum RS. Schistosomiasis and the kidney. *Semin Nephrol.* 2003; 23:34–41.
146. Nath KA, Hebbel RP. Sickle cell disease: renal manifestations and mechanisms. *Nat Rev Nephrol.* 2015;11:161–171.
152. Freedman BI, Langefeld CD. The new era of APOL1-associated glomerulosclerosis. *Nephrol Dial Transplant.* 2012;27:1288–1291.
158. Adedokun BO, Olopade CO, Olopade OI. Building local capacity for genomics research in Africa: recommendations from analysis of publications in Sub-Saharan Africa from 2004 to 2013. *Glob Health Action.* 2016;9:31026.
160. Osafo C, Raji YR, Olanrewaju T, et al. Genomic approaches to the burden of kidney disease in Sub-Saharan Africa: the Human Heredity and Health in Africa (H3Africa) Kidney Disease Research Network. *Kidney Int.* 2016;90:2–5.
185. Lunyera J, Mohottige D, Von Isenburg M, et al. CKD of uncertain etiology: a systematic review. *Clin J Am Soc Nephrol.* 2015;11:1–7.
196. Anand S, Bitton A, Gaziano T. The gap between estimated incidence of end-stage renal disease and use of therapy. *PLoS ONE.* 2013;8:e72860.
201. Liyanage T, Ninomiya T, Jha V, et al. Worldwide access to treatment for end-stage kidney disease: a systematic review. *Lancet.* 2015;385: 1975–1982.
202. Arogundade F, Sanusi A, Hassan M, et al. The pattern, clinical characteristics and outcome of ESRD in Ile-Ife, Nigeria: Is there a change in trend? *Afr Health Sci.* 2011;11:594–601.
203. Davids MR, Caskey FJ, Young T, et al. Strengthening renal registries and ESRD research in Africa. *Semin Nephrol.* 2017;37:211–223.
209. Davids MR, Eastwood JB, Selwood NH, et al. A renal registry for Africa: first steps. *Clin Kidney J.* 2016;9:162–167.
211. Mushi L, Krohn M, Flessa S. Cost of dialysis in Tanzania: evidence from the provider's perspective. *Health Econ Rev.* 2015;5:28.
212. Halle MP, Jimkap NN, Kaze FF, et al. Cost of care for patients on maintenance haemodialysis in public facilities in Cameroon. *Afr J Nephrol.* 2017;20:230–237.
213. Ashuntantang G, Osafo C, Olowu WA, et al. Outcomes in adults and children with end-stage kidney disease requiring dialysis in sub-Saharan Africa: a systematic review. *Lancet Glob Health.* 2017;5: e408–e417.
216. Tannor EK, Archer E, Kapembwa K, et al. Quality of life in patients on chronic dialysis in South Africa: a comparative mixed methods study. *BMC Nephrol.* 2017;18:4.

# Near and Middle East 78

Suheir Assady | Rawi Ramadan | Yaacov Frishberg

## CHAPTER OUTLINE



## KEY POINTS

- Health care disparities do exist among countries of the Middle East (ME).
- Accurate and detailed epidemiologic data regarding acute and chronic kidney diseases in ME countries are still needed.
- Community-based screening programs for chronic kidney disease, risk factors, and intervention strategies are limited in most countries of the region.
- Diabetes mellitus is the major cause of end-stage kidney disease in most ME countries.
- Recessively inherited kidney diseases are prevalent in the ME, and targeted screening in populations at risk should be encouraged.
- Renal replacement therapies are available in all ME countries, and hemodialysis is mostly used.
- Hepatitis C infection is prevalent among dialysis patients in the ME. Implementation of infection control measures and introduction of new antiviral agents are of great importance to eradicate it.
- Legal kidney transplantation from both living and deceased donors should be expanded, and organ donation encouraged, in view of the positive ethical and religious authorizations.

This chapter is a discussion of the epidemiology, causes, predisposing factors, management, and prevention of kidney diseases. Future strategies for dealing with kidney diseases in the Near and Middle East are proposed. The term *Near and Middle East* is a historical, Eurocentric, and Western term that was used to describe a geographic region whose boundary is imprecise and whose internal borders are constantly changing because of political and historical evolution.[1] Therefore, the Near and Middle East, hereafter called the Middle East (ME), is defined for the purpose of this chapter as the region that encompasses the following 20 countries (in alphabetical order): Algeria, Bahrain, Egypt, Iran, Iraq, Israel, Jordan, Kuwait, Lebanon, Libya, Morocco, Oman, Palestinian Authority, Qatar, Saudi Arabia, Syria, Tunisia, Turkey, the United Arab Emirates (UAE), and Yemen (Fig. 78.1).

The ME has always been important for the following reasons: (1) its strategic location as a tricontinental hub that links Asia, Africa, and Europe; (2) its economic resources; and (3) its spiritual significance as the birthplace of the world's three major monotheistic religions—Judaism, Christianity, and Islam. Of the adherents to the three religions, Muslims constitute the largest religious population in the ME; the sizes of the Christian and Jewish populations are smaller and vary from country to country.[1] Although the ME has several cultural, linguistic, and geographic associations, considerable disparity exists among the different countries in terms of economy, resources, political systems, health care systems, health expenditure, and disease incidence and prevalence.[2]

According to data from the World Bank, the estimated population in the 20 ME countries in 2016 was 514,854,000 (Table 78.1).[3] The gross national income (GNI) per capita varies across ME countries. According to the classification system of the World Bank,[3,4] most ME countries are considered "developing countries." Egypt, Morocco, Syria, Palestinian Authority, and Yemen are considered lower middle-income countries because the GNI per capita of each is between $1006 and $3955 (USD) per annum, whereas Algeria, Iran,

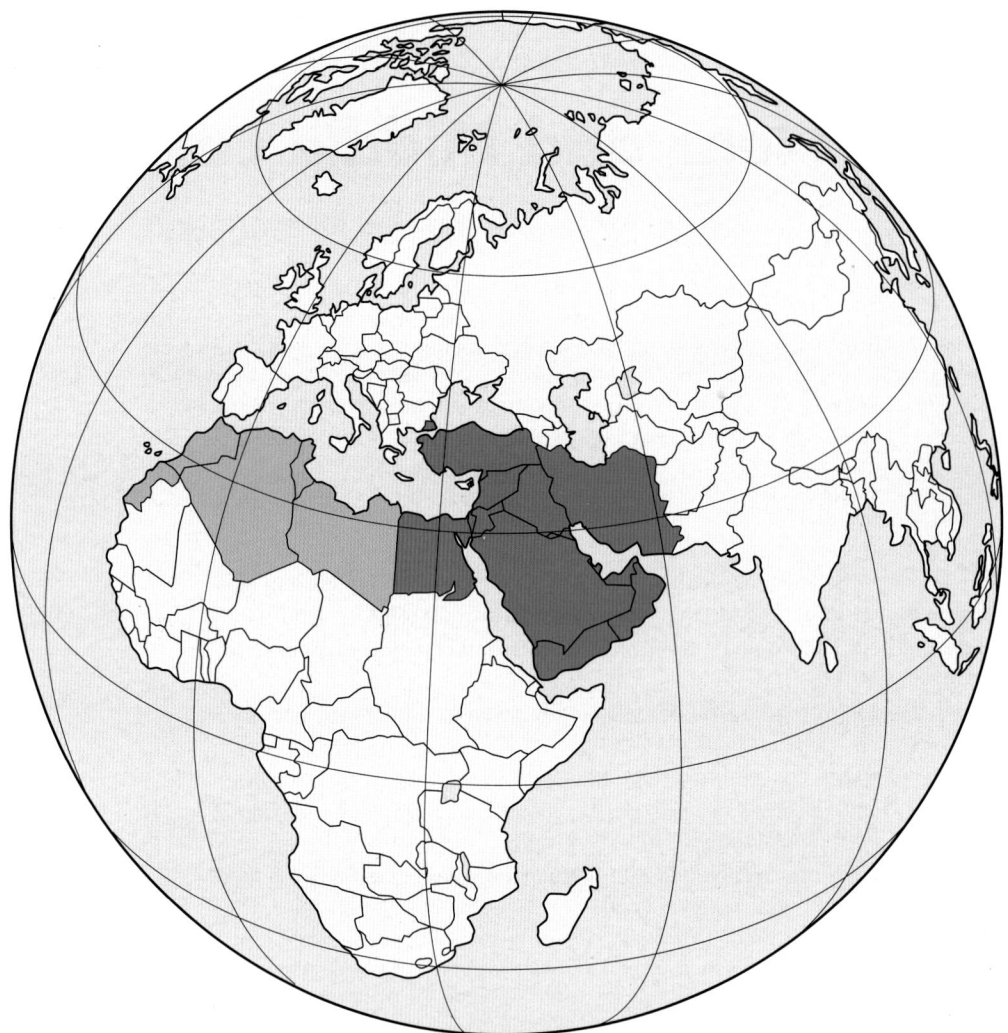

**Fig. 78.1** Map of Middle Eastern countries. Countries illustrated in *light green* are also known as "El Maghreb"; those in *dark green,* as "El Mashreq."[1] (Modified from a public domain image available at http://en.wikipedia.org/wiki/Middle_East.)

Iraq, Jordan, Lebanon, Libya, Tunisia, and Turkey are considered upper middle-income countries because the GNI per capita of each is between $3956 and $12,235 per annum. The following countries are considered high-income countries because the GNI per capita of each is more than $12,236 per annum: Bahrain, Israel, Kuwait, Oman, Qatar, Saudi Arabia, and UAE (Fig. 78.2). Inevitably, disease incidence, prevalence, course, and outcomes are affected by the different socioeconomic factors and health policies in each country (Fig. 78.2).[5–7] For example, the infant mortality rate in each ME country is concordant with the socioeconomic, political, and health status of that country;[8] and life expectancy for men is lowest in the low-income ME countries and in countries affected by man-made conflicts (see Table 78.1).[6]

The mortality rate for those younger than 5 years in Yemen, the poorest country in the ME, is at least five times higher (55/1000 live births) than that in industrialized, high-income ME countries (4–13/1000 live births; see Table 78.1).[3,8] Health disparities also exist among minority populations (ethnic groups or expatriates) who live in industrialized ME countries, as well as among individuals of ME origin who live in countries that are not in the ME.[9–19] Many developing ME countries have been affected by various types of natural disasters (e.g., earthquakes, floods, droughts) and other disasters (e.g., military conflicts). Casualties, displacement, and migration are significant consequences of such disasters and adversely affect the socioeconomic strata and health status of a country, as in the recent devastating humanitarian crises in Yemen and Syria.[2,20–23] Therefore, many ME countries and their communities need assistance to upgrade their existing health care structures to improve their ability to cope with any future disasters.[2,20,22,24,25] Consequently, the World Health Organization (WHO) and national and international nephrology societies, such as the International Society of Nephrology (ISN), have pooled their resources to enhance the resilience of nations to the effects and consequences of disasters.[9,22,23,26,28]

## ACUTE KIDNEY INJURY

As in many countries worldwide, data on the incidence and prevalence of acute kidney injury (AKI) in many ME countries are scarce and imprecise because of an inconsistent definition

**Table 78.1 Demographics, Health Indicators, and Human Development Indices in Middle Eastern and Western Industrialized Countries**

| Country | Total Population, 2016[a] | Median Age (years) | Life Expectancy at Birth (years), 2015[b] | | Rate of Mortality Before Age 5 Years (/1000 Live Births, 2016)[b] | Country Ranking in Human Development Index (of 188 Countries)[c] |
|---|---|---|---|---|---|---|
| | | | Male | Female | | |
| **Middle Eastern Countries** | | | | | | |
| Algeria | 40,606,050 | 28.1 | 74 | 78 | 25 | 83 |
| Bahrain | 1,425,170 | 32.3 | 76 | 78 | 8 | 47 |
| Egypt | 95,688,680 | 23.9 | 69 | 73 | 23 | 111 |
| Iran | 80,277,430 | 30.3 | 74 | 77 | 15 | 69 |
| Iraq | 37,202,570 | 20 | 66 | 72 | 31 | 121 |
| Israel | 8,547,100 | 29.9 | 81 | 84 | 4 | 19 |
| Jordan | 9,455,800 | 22.5 | 72 | 76 | 18 | 86 |
| Kuwait | 4,052,580 | 29.3 | 74 | 76 | 8 | 51 |
| Lebanon | 6,006,670 | 30.5 | 74 | 76 | 8 | 76 |
| Libya | 6,293,250 | 28.9 | 70 | 76 | 13 | 102 |
| Morocco | 35,276,790 | 29.3 | 73 | 75 | 27 | 123 |
| Oman | 4,424,760 | 25.6 | 75 | 79 | 11 | 52 |
| Palestinian Authority | 4,551,570 | 20 | 71 | 75 | 19 | 114 |
| Qatar | 2,569,800 | 33.2 | 77 | 80 | 9 | 33 |
| Saudi Arabia | 32,275,690 | 27.5 | 73 | 76 | 13 | 38 |
| Syria | 18,430,450 | 24.3 | 60 | 70 | 18 | 149 |
| Tunisia | 11,403,250 | 31.6 | 73 | 78 | 14 | 97 |
| Turkey | 79,512,430 | 30.9 | 73 | 79 | 13 | 71 |
| United Arab Emirates | 9,269,610 | 30.3 | 76 | 79 | 8 | 42 |
| Yemen | 27,584,210 | 19.5 | 64 | 67 | 55 | 168 |
| **Western Industrialized Countries** | | | | | | |
| Australia | 24,127,160 | 38.7 | 81 | 85 | 4 | 2 |
| Canada | 36,286,430 | 42.2 | 80 | 84 | 5 | 10 |
| France | 66,896,110 | 41.4 | 79 | 85 | 4 | 21 |
| Germany | 82,667,680 | 47.1 | 79 | 83 | 4 | 4 |
| Italy | 60,600,590 | 45.5 | 80 | 85 | 3 | 26 |
| Japan | 126,994,510 | 47.3 | 80 | 87 | 3 | 17 |
| United Kingdom | 65,637,240 | 40.5 | 79 | 83 | 4 | 16 |
| United States | 323,127,510 | 38.1 | 77 | 82 | 7 | 10 |

[a]Data from World Bank: Indicators. http://data.worldbank.org/indicator.
[b]Source data for country profiles from the World Health Organization: Countries. http://www.who.int/ countries/en.
[c]Data from the 2016 Human Development Report, published for the United Nations Development Programme: http://hdr.undp.org/sites/default/files/2016_human _development_report.pdf.

of AKI in medical reports, underreporting, seasonal dependency on the occurrence of AKI, and the frequency and location of natural and human-induced disasters.[29–32] There are large knowledge gaps about the age, number, natural history, and outcome of patients with AKI in both the community and hospitals and about the use of preventive measures in each ME country. Most published reports on AKI in ME countries are short-term studies done in tertiary-level hospitals or single-center studies and, of these studies, only a few were of the prospective type. Moreover, the definition of AKI is not consistent in these reports.[33–39] Al-Homrany has reported that the incidence of AKI among hospitalized patients is 0.6% in a 2-year prospective study in one hospital in southern Saudi Arabia.[35] Of these cases of AKI, 62% were hospital acquired and 38% were community acquired. In a 1-year retrospective cohort study from a single center in northern Israel, Shema and associates have reported that the annual incidence rate of AKI among hospitalized adult patients is 1% to 5.1%, depending on the AKI definition that was used.[36] In a case series study of the ME respiratory syndrome (MERS) coronavirus outbreak, AKI requiring renal replacement therapy (RRT) was reported in 58% of critically ill patients.[40] This percentage is high compared with that reported in equivalent critically ill patients who were treated during the severe acute respiratory syndrome (SARS) epidemic in Canada (5%).[41] The Acute Kidney Injury–Epidemiologic Prospective Investigation (AKI-EPI) study was the first multinational and cross-sectional study to investigate the epidemiology of AKI in intensive care unit (ICU) patients worldwide (33 countries) prospectively using the Kidney Disease: Improving Global Outcomes (KDIGO) definition for AKI[42] and a standardized data collection instrument.[31] AKI was found in 57.3% of

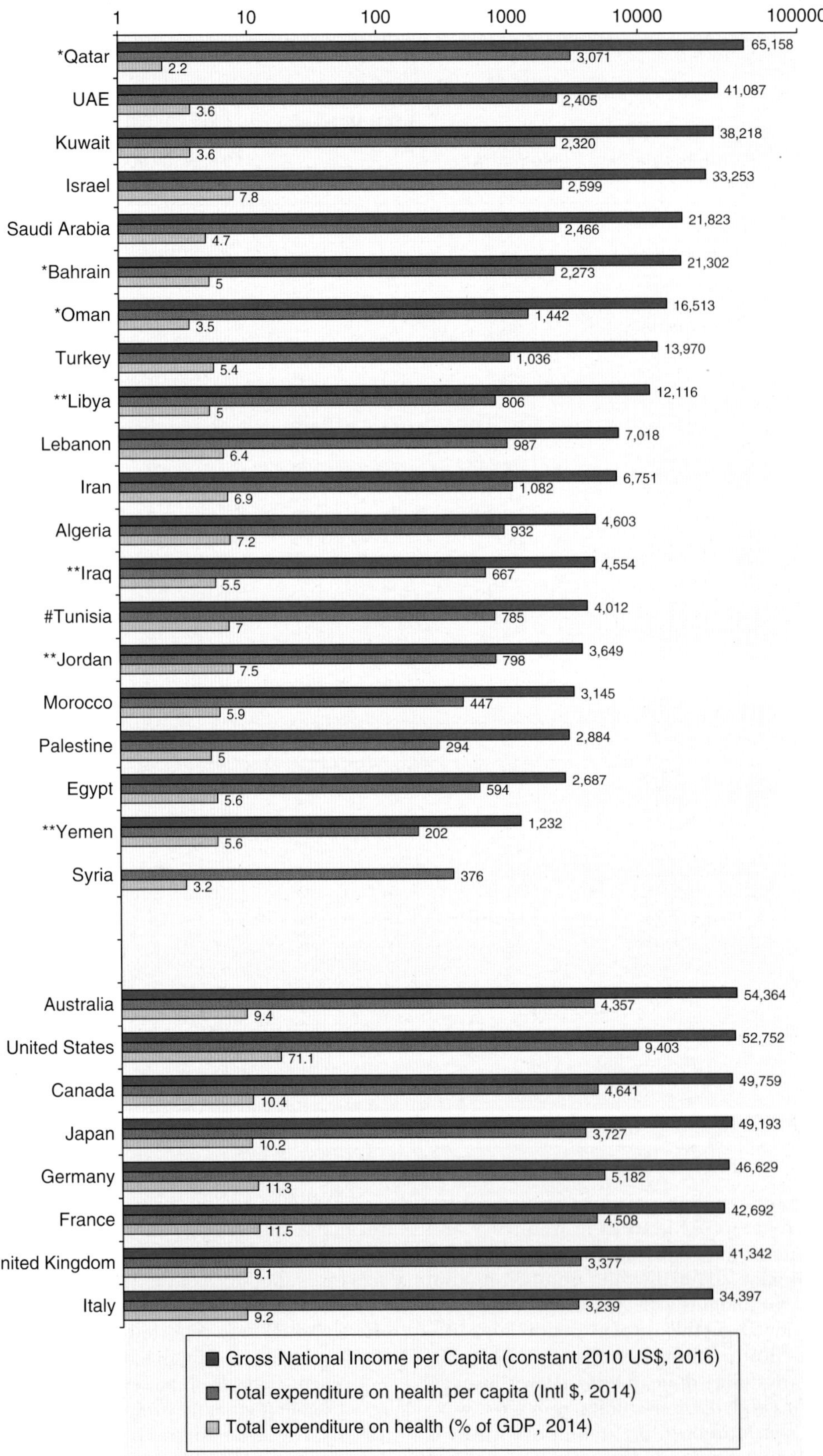


**Fig. 78.2** Indices of wealth and health care expenditures in the 20 Middle Eastern and selected Western and industrialized countries in 2014. For each country, three indices are presented—gross national income per capita, on a purchasing power parity, expressed in constant 2010 US dollars *(blue bars)*; total expenditure on health per capita, expressed in international dollars *(violet bars)*; and total expenditure on health, expressed as percentages of gross domestic product (GDP; *yellow bars).* The upper seven countries are the wealthy high-income Middle East nations. Indices from *2015; #2013; **2010. *UAE,* United Arab Emirates; *USA,* United States of America. (Data from the World Bank: Countries and economies. http://data. worldbank.org/country; and from the World Health Organization: Countries. http://www. who.int/countries/en.)

subjects. Yet, only 5 of 97 participating centers were from the ME—three ICUs from Egypt, one from Tunisia, and one from Turkey. These are low numbers from which to draw firm conclusions regarding the whole ME region.

## CAUSES

The causes of AKI have changed over time in ME countries. A nationwide prospective study, conducted by the Turkish Society of Pediatric Nephrology Acute Kidney Injury Study Group,[43] demonstrated that the cause of AKI in Turkish pediatric patients has greatly changed over the last 2 decades. Acute gastroenteritis and acute poststreptococcal glomerulonephritis have decreased significantly as causes of AKI, and prematurity, malignancy, and congenital heart disease have increased. In adults, obstructive uropathy, unspecified postsurgical complications, and crush injury were the most prevalent causes of AKI in Syria during the 1980s, according to Hadidy and colleagues.[33] In contrast, Said has reported findings similar to those from industrialized countries in 215 patients with AKI, aged between 12 and 90 years, in three Jordanian hospitals over an 18-month study period.[44] Renal parenchymal disease was the most common cause of AKI (58%), and acute tubular necrosis (ATN) and contrast-induced nephropathy were the two most prevalent causes of renal parenchymal disease. Prerenal causes (28%) and postrenal causes (14%) accounted for the remaining causes of AKI.[44] Of note, obstructive uropathy was a common cause of AKI as a result of the high prevalence of nephrolithiasis in the study patients who originally came from Yemen and Sudan. In another study from one center in Qatar, ATN was reported in 83% of all patients with AKI, who were referred mainly from ICUs.[45] Al-Homrany[35] has reported that ATN resulting from sepsis, ischemia, and rhabdomyolysis, as well as distinctive causes, such as malaria and snakebites (4.6% of all cases), were the major causes of AKI in tropical southern Saudi Arabia.

Malaria is rarely reported as a primary cause of AKI in most ME countries, with the exception of Yemen.[46] In the Hajjah and Sanaa regions of Yemen, malaria caused by *Plasmodium falciparum* was the cause of 29% of all cases of AKI. However, prerenal disorders, such as infectious diarrheal diseases, are still the predominant cause of AKI in Yemen because of the tropical climate and poor hygiene.[46] Malarial kidney injury is often a consequence of several hemodynamic, immune, and metabolic disturbances, which may also be accompanied by central nervous system sequelae and by fluid and electrolyte alterations.[47–49] Malarial kidney disease can manifest as AKI in the form of the following: (1) ATN that accompanies or occurs as a complication of severe hemolysis, hemodynamic derangements, and tissue hypoxemia; (2) interstitial nephritis; or (3) glomerular mesangial proliferative lesions with immune complex deposits.[47] In areas where malaria is not common, a high index of suspicion is required.

Reporting the cause of AKI may, however, be biased by the type of referral hospital that documents the various causes. In a retrospective 18-month study from one cancer hospital in the UAE, sepsis and drug-induced nephrotoxicity were the leading causes of AKI because 30% of the patients were immunocompromised and were receiving chemotherapy.[50] Preexisting comorbid conditions, such as diabetes, hypertension, and chronic kidney disease (CKD), were documented in approximately one-third of all patients with AKI in the UAE and Jordan[34,39,50] and in as many as 87% of all such patients in Qatar.[45]

AKI-associated mortality rates range between 12% and 77% in ME countries.[33–36,39,44,45,50–52] The ISN's 0by25 AKI initiative aims to prevent all avoidable deaths from AKI by 2025, especially in low- and middle-income countries.[53] To implement such an initiative, a clear definition of a preventable death from AKI, and a strategy to regionalize any recommendations for AKI care in terms of health care infrastructure, socioeconomic conditions, and education and training were considered.[53,54] The first global 10-week snapshot in 2014 included AKI data from 289 sites across 72 countries, mostly academic and referral centers, of which 32 centers represented ME countries—13 centers in Egypt, four in Iran, three in Saudi Arabia and three in UAE, two each in Morocco and Tunisia, and one center per country, including Israel, Kuwait, Oman, Palestinian Authority, and Syria.[52] In this study, the median age of patients from ME countries was 60 years, with a male predominance. Two-thirds of AKI cases were community acquired and, as expected, mortality increased in hospital-acquired AKI and in patients requiring the ICU or dialysis. However, many areas of the ME were underrepresented in this study, and data from Egypt and Tunisia were combined with those from Africa; those from Israel were collected with Western Europe.

Devastating earthquakes have struck some ME countries and are a constant threat because their territory encompasses the Great African Rift Valley. Clinician investigators have described and analyzed the factors that have had major implications for kidney involvement and outcomes in survivors who sustained crush syndrome in catastrophic earthquakes in Turkey and Iran.[55,56] Crush syndrome often causes profound hypovolemic shock that (1) is complicated and aggravated by gross disorders of acid-base balance and electrolytes, of which hyperkalemia is life-threatening, and (2) increases susceptibility to myoglobinuric AKI. These complications can occur within hours of the initial injury and can lead to early loss of limb or life.[28,57] According to data collected after the 1999 Marmara earthquake in Turkey and the 2003 Bam earthquake in Iran, the number of casualties, incidence of crush injury, and incidence of myoglobinuric AKI are related to several variables, including the following[55,56,58]:

1. The intensity of the earthquake and the magnitude of the aftermath.
2. The time of the day that the earthquake happened. The Turkish earthquake occurred during the night and was associated with more crush injuries than earthquakes that have occurred during the day because the victims were in the supine position. Erect subjects tend to be killed by head injuries from falling buildings.
3. The population density and type of residential area at the site of the earthquake. The population density in rural areas, where the buildings are single-storied and made from light construction materials, is less than that in urban areas, where the buildings may be multistoried and made of heavy construction materials, leading to more crush injury in urban areas.
4. The climate. Earthquake survivors suffer more volume depletion and dehydration, exacerbating AKI in hot weather compared with cold weather.

5. The time to rescue, because this reflects both the amount of time under the rubble and the magnitude of imposed pressure over a given time.
6. The extent of destruction of health care facilities at the site of the earthquake and the distance from referral hospitals.
7. The availability of medical support and the availability and efficiency of rescue teams.
8. The availability of dialysis.[28,55,56,58,59]

An important issue in these disasters is the identification of patients with AKI who need early referral to specialized nephrology facilities.

The ISN Renal Disaster Relief Task Force, in cooperation with European Renal Best Practice, has published comprehensive clinical practice guidelines for the management of crush victims in mass disasters.[58] These recommendations include medical and logistic principles and were based on lessons learned from the activities of the Renal Disaster Relief Task Force in disaster-affected areas during the past 2 decades.[28,55,56,58] Of note, vigorous fluid resuscitation, which should begin while victims are still trapped under the rubble, and the use of mannitol with proper monitoring, are now proven therapies for reducing AKI and for saving limbs by preventing the development of compartment syndrome in crush injuries, the second leading cause of death after disasters (Fig. 78.3). These therapies can also reduce the need to perform fasciotomies, which are associated with severe bleeding, sepsis, and amputations.[28,57,58,60]

In summary, it is still difficult to draw general conclusions about the epidemiology, causes, and outcomes of AKI in many ME countries because of regional variations and methodologic

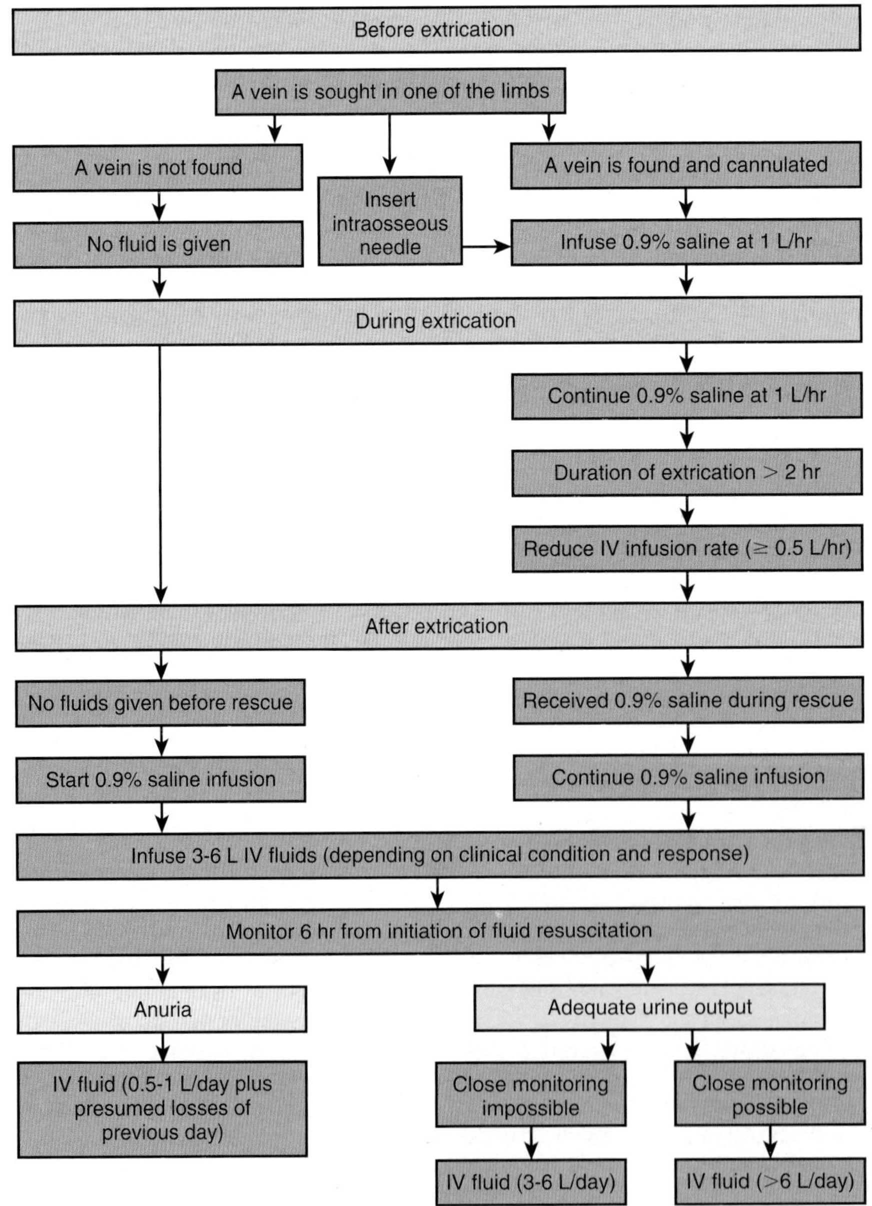


**Fig. 78.3** Algorithm for fluid resuscitation in crush victims of mass disasters before, during, and after extrication. *IV,* Intravenous. (Modified from Sever MS, Vanholder R: Management of crush victims in mass disasters: highlights from recently published recommendations. *Clin J Am Soc Nephrol.* 2013;8:328–335; Gibney RT, Sever MS, Vanholder RC: Disaster nephrology: crush injury and beyond. *Kidney Int.* 2014;85:1049–057.)

differences in the few studies that have been performed in the region. Well-conducted regional studies in which the published definition of AKI[42] is used are needed to clarify the actual occurrence of AKI. Accordingly, the results of these studies can then be used to identify the needed infrastructure and evaluate treatment strategies to prevent AKI and improve the clinical outcomes.

## CHRONIC KIDNEY DISEASE

### EPIDEMIOLOGY

The incidence and prevalence of noncommunicable diseases have been changing rapidly as a result of demographic transition, and the burden of disease has consequently shifted from infections in the pediatric population to chronic diseases of the adult population in many ME countries.[13,61–64] This demographic shift in the burden of disease is exemplified by the emerging epidemic of diabetes mellitus that is occurring globally and affects Arab and Chaldean Americans. In 2017, the International Diabetes Federation ranked Saudi Arabia, Egypt, and UAE as having the highest age-adjusted (20–79 years) comparative diabetes prevalence in the ME (17.7%, 17.3%, and 17.3%, respectively) and worldwide after countries in the Western Pacific region.[65] The International Diabetes Federation has also predicted that the prevalence of diabetes mellitus in ME countries will increase by 2045. These alarming statistics for ME countries have been attributed to a combination of increasing urbanization, aging populations, increasing obesity, and falling levels of physical activity.[7,13,63,64,66–77] Accordingly, the direct and indirect medical expenditures associated with diabetes mellitus will become a profound economic burden. As a result, ME countries with limited or scarce resources (see Fig. 78.2) will be unable to cope with the social, economic, and public health consequences of complications of diabetes mellitus, one of which is CKD.

In addition, the common practice of consanguineous marriages in ME countries has led to a high incidence of genetic disorders, some of which may lead to CKD and end-stage kidney disease (ESKD), especially in children, and has possibly altered the pattern of renal disease in these countries.[74,78–84] Genetic renal diseases and their complications in the ME are discussed further later in this chapter.

It is difficult to estimate the incidence and prevalence of CKD in most ME countries. Obtaining the epidemiologic statistics concerning CKD, ESKD, and RRT is a work in progress that is hampered by the lack of well-conducted, cross-sectional, longitudinal cohort studies and a lack of reliable registries that incorporate data on comorbid conditions. Furthermore, additional research is required to establish the best and most cost-effective approach for screening for CKD.[85,86]

Hence, the creation of a reliable and easily accessible medical registry is urgently needed in the ME countries where existing registries are lacking, unreliable, or difficult to access. The information in such registries would be essential for planning health policies and the allocation of resources. In long-term, nationwide, population-based, retrospective cohort studies, factors such as overweight, obesity, normal renal function with a history of any childhood kidney disease or persistent asymptomatic isolated hematuria detected in Israeli adolescents and young adults were found to be strongly associated with an increased cumulative incidence of treated ESKD, with crude hazard ratios of 3, 6.89, 4.19, and 18.5, respectively.[87–89] Therefore, although not yet proven, it is hoped that early detection of CKD and its risk factors will increase health awareness and permit early intervention, which in turn may modify the disease course, complexity, and costs of overall therapy.[85,90–92]

Community-based screening programs for CKD and risk factors, such as diabetes mellitus, obesity, proteinuria, and hypertension, have been launched in developing countries worldwide under the auspices of the Research and Prevention Committee of the ISN.[76,91] These programs are expected to detect CKD in populations in which the people are unaware of such chronic diseases. This initiative includes ongoing programs in Egypt and Morocco.[93] The Egypt Information, Prevention, and Treatment of Chronic Kidney Diseases (EGIPT-CKD) program was the first to report interim results. It investigated the prevalence of microalbuminuria among first-degree relatives of people with ESKD in the city of Damanhur and the surrounding towns in the Al-Buhayrah governorate, in Lower Egypt.[94] In this study, microalbuminuria was detected in 10.6% of participants. In an adjusted logistic regression analysis, smoking and a personal history of cardiovascular disease were strongly associated with microalbuminuria. The well-conducted, cross-sectional Maladie Rénale chronique au Maroc (MAREMAR) study involved 10,524 individuals from two Moroccan towns, El-Jadida (coastal and industrial) and Khemisset (inland and rural).[77] It found that the adjusted prevalence of CKD in Morocco is among the lowest in the world (5.1%), including estimated glomerular filtration rate (eGFR) under 60 mL/min/1.73 m$^2$ (1.6%), confirmed proteinuria (1.9%), and hematuria (3.4%). The low rate of CKD in this study may reflect the fact that the diagnosis was made on repeat samples and not on purely cross-sectional data, suggesting possible overestimation of CKD in studies relying on a single GFR estimate. The MAREMAR-CKD cohort was also classified according to the KDIGO eGFR stages[95]: G1,17.8%; G2, 17.2%; G3A, 40.2%; G3B, 12.3%; G4, 4.4%; and G5, 7.2%. Patients with CKD G3A-G4 will be followed for 8 years. Furthermore in Morocco, population-adjusted prevalence rates for hypertension, obesity, and diabetes mellitus were reported to be 16.7%, 23.2%, and 13.8%, respectively.[77]

According to the Chronic REnal Disease In Turkey (CREDIT) study,[75] the population-based estimated prevalence rates for CKD stages 1 to 5 among Turkish adults were 5.4%, 5.2%, 4.7%, 0.3%, and 0.2%, respectively, with an overall prevalence of 15.8%. Moreover, the frequency of concomitant cardiovascular risk factors such as diabetes, hypertension, dyslipidemia, and obesity was increased in patients with CKD, and odds ratios versus non-CKD population were 3.22, 2.86, 1.60, and 1.65, respectively. Based on analysis of one spot urine specimen per participant, 10.2% of the cohort subjects had microalbuminuria, and 2% had macroalbuminuria.[75] The causes of CKD were not detailed, but the study cohort continues to be followed longitudinally.

The actual or estimated number of patients with CKD at each eGFR stage of the KDIGO classification in other ME countries is unclear.[96] A small pilot study, which is part of the Global SEEK Project, demonstrated the feasibility of screening and early detection of CKD in a Saudi population.

Using standardized GFR prediction equations, the prevalence of CKD stages 1, 2, and 3 was relatively low—3.5%, 1.6%, and 0.6%, respectively—which may be attributed to the low mean age of the participants (37.4 ± 11.3 years).[97] In Kuwait, a 4-year prospective study from one referral center by El-Reshaid and associates[98] has reported a high incidence of CKD among Kuwaiti nationals. Specifically, they reported an average annual incidence of 366 per million population (pmp), with a higher incidence among the older population (≥60 years) of 913 pmp. Of patients with CKD who were admitted to the center, 6% presented with uremic syndrome, and 40% experienced acute deterioration of their kidney function that resulted mainly from drugs (mostly over-the-counter nonsteroidal antiinflammatory drugs [NSAIDs]), infection, and volume depletion. The authors did not report categories of eGFR or proteinuria in their patients.

In 2007, a study involving 31,999 taxi drivers in Tehran, mostly males, showed that 6.5% of drivers had an eGFR of less than 60 mL/min/1.73 $m^2$.[99] However, community-based studies revealed considerable differences in CKD prevalence between counties of Iran (10.2%–18.9%).[73,100]

In a pioneering work, Tohidi and colleagues[101] examined the incidence of CKD among a subgroup, 20 years or older, in the Tehran Lipid and Glucose Study, which is a long-term community-based prospective study. During 10-year follow-up, the cumulative incidence of CKD stages 3 to 5 among women and men was 27.8% and 14.2%, respectively. Age, hypertension, diabetes, and current smoking were found to be independent predictors of CKD stages 3 to 5 in both genders. In addition, for males, high-normal blood pressure and, for females, being single, divorced, or widowed were associated with an increased risk of incident CKD.[101] Interestingly, adherence to Mediterranean or Dietary Approaches to Stop Hypertension (DASH)–style diets had a positive impact on reducing the incidence and prevention of CKD,[102–104] which may ultimately translate into favorable survival and cardiovascular outcomes.[105]

Although the number of patients who underwent preemptive kidney transplantation might not be included, estimates of the prevalence and incidence of ESKD are more reliable in countries that have a national database in which each patient who has received RRT is registered (Tables 78.2 and 78.3). Nevertheless, patient numbers in a national registry in ME countries may be underestimated for two additional reasons: (1) the treatment of ESKD may be beyond the reach of the average citizen in low-income ME countries, such as

**Table 78.2 Epidemiology of Renal Replacement Therapy in Middle Eastern Countries**

| | Dialysis | | | | Kidney Transplantation | | |
|---|---|---|---|---|---|---|---|
| Country | First Hemodialysis[a] | No. of Hemodialysis Centers | Incidence[b] | Prevalence[b,c] | Date of Country's First Transplantation | Incidence[b] | Type |
| Algeria | 1962 | 281 | 104 | 482 | 1986 | 3.9 | C |
| Bahrain | 1971 | 5 | 62 | 410 (800) | 1995 | 6.7 | C |
| Egypt | 1958 | 1050 | NA | 609.7 | 1976 | 14.8 | L |
| Iran | 1965 | 316 | 63.8 | 332.6 | 1967 | 32 | C |
| Iraq | 1967 | 27 | NA | 83 | 1973 | 12.2 | L |
| Israel | 1948 | 79 | 191 | 783.4 | 1964 | 41.5 | C |
| Jordan | 1968 | 78 | 117.3 | 754.74 | 1972 | 29.2 | C |
| Kuwait | 1976 | 9 | 100 | 400 (960) | 1979 | 35.4 | C |
| Lebanon | 1960 | 66 | NA | 665.4 | 1972 | 19 | C |
| Libya | 1972 | 53 | 282 | 624 | 1989 | 8.6 | L |
| Morocco | 1980 | 197 | 42 | 405.8 | 1990 | 1.3 | C |
| Oman | 1983 | 21 | 60 | 365 (640) | 1988 | 16.5 | C |
| Palestinian Authority | 1997 | 13 | NA | 240.3 | 2011 | NA | L |
| Qatar | 1981 | 6 | 75 | 320 (1230) | 1986 | 22.1 | C |
| Saudi Arabia | 1971 | 187 | 136 | 513 (645) | 1979 | 24.2 | C |
| Syria | 1974 | NA | 111 | 228 | 1976 | 16.2 | L |
| Tunisia | 1963 | 146 | 142 | 812 | 1986 | 13.2 | C |
| Turkey | 1965 | 860 | 125.1 | 754.2 | 1975 | 42.8 | C |
| United Arab Emirates | 1975 | 33 | 129 | 210 (760) | 1985 | 2.3 | L |
| Yemen | 1982 | NA | 64 | 91 | 1998 | 1.4 | L |

[a]For acute kidney injury or end-stage kidney disease.
[b]Per million population.
[c]Prevalence not including expatriates—in parentheses.
*C*, Combined living and deceased kidney donors; *L*, only living kidney donors; *NA*, not available.
Adapted from Bello AK, et al: Global Kidney Health Atlas (GKHA)—country profiles; Bello AK, Levin A, Tonelli M, et al: Global kidney health atlas: A report by the International Society of Nephrology on the current state of organization and structures for kidney care across the globe. Brussels, Belgium, 2017, International Society of Nephrology; and personal communication with Dr. Bello.

**Table 78.3 Registries, Awareness, and Strategies for Kidney Care—Nephrology Workforce Capacity in Middle Eastern Countries**

| | ESKD Registries[a] | Priority and Advocacy for Kidney Care | | Presence of National Strategies For Kidney Care | | | Workforce |
|---|---|---|---|---|---|---|---|
| **Country** | **Availability of Dialysis and Kidney Transplantation** | **CKD Recognized as Health Priority by the Government** | **Presence of CKD Advocacy Group** | **Nondialysis CKD** | **Dialysis** | **Kidney Transplantation** | **Nephrology Workforce (pmp)** |
| Algeria | | | | | | | 11.3 |
| Bahrain | | | | | | | 5.9 |
| Egypt | | | | | | | 21.7 |
| Iran | | | | | | NA | 3.9 |
| Iraq | | | | | | | 1 |
| Israel | | | | | | | 9.7 |
| Jordan | | | | | | | 10.2 |
| Kuwait | | | | | | | 10.8 |
| Lebanon | | | | | | | 22.6 |
| Libya | | | | | | | 12.5 |
| Morocco | | | | | | | 10.5 |
| Oman | | | | | | | 30.4 |
| Palestinian Authority | | | | | | NA | 2.2 |
| Qatar | | | | | | NA | 11.4 |
| Saudi Arabia | | | | | | | 17.7 |
| Syria | | | | | | | 4.7 |
| Tunisia | | | | | | | 16.3 |
| Turkey | | | | | | | 6.3 |
| UAE | | | | | | | 8.7 |
| Yemen | | | | | NA | NA | 0.2 |

[a]Few countries regularly report national registry data, such as Israel,[127] Turkey,[128] Jordan,[129] and Saudi Arabia.[112,448]

*Blue and red boxes* indicate that the survey participants answered yes and no, respectively, to GKHA Questionnaire[76]; *yellow,* only dialysis registry is available.

*CKD,* Chronic kidney disease; *ESKD,* end-stage kidney disease; *pmp,* per million population; *NA,* not available; *UAE,* United Arab Emirates.

Data from Bello AK, et al: Global Kidney Health Atlas (GKHA)—country profiles; Bello AK, Levin A, Tonelli M, et al: Global kidney health atlas: A report by the International Society of Nephrology on the current state of organization and structures for kidney care across the globe. Brussels, Belgium, 2017, International Society of Nephrology; and personal communication with Dr. Bello.

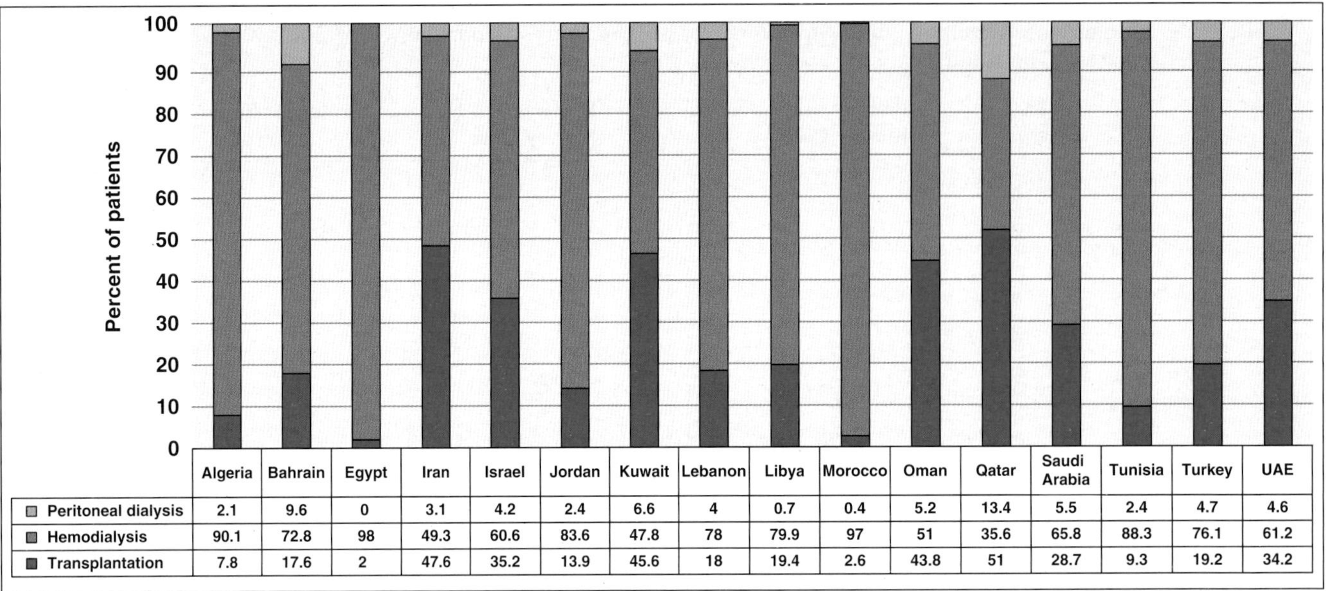


| | Algeria | Bahrain | Egypt | Iran | Israel | Jordan | Kuwait | Lebanon | Libya | Morocco | Oman | Qatar | Saudi Arabia | Tunisia | Turkey | UAE |
|---|---|---|---|---|---|---|---|---|---|---|---|---|---|---|---|---|
| Peritoneal dialysis | 2.1 | 9.6 | 0 | 3.1 | 4.2 | 2.4 | 6.6 | 4 | 0.7 | 0.4 | 5.2 | 13.4 | 5.5 | 2.4 | 4.7 | 4.6 |
| Hemodialysis | 90.1 | 72.8 | 98 | 49.3 | 60.6 | 83.6 | 47.8 | 78 | 79.9 | 97 | 51 | 35.6 | 65.8 | 88.3 | 76.1 | 61.2 |
| Transplantation | 7.8 | 17.6 | 2 | 47.6 | 35.2 | 13.9 | 45.6 | 18 | 19.4 | 2.6 | 43.8 | 51 | 28.7 | 9.3 | 19.2 | 34.2 |

**Fig. 78.4** Percentage distribution of renal replacement therapy modalities used for treating end-stage kidney disease in selected Middle Eastern countries. *UAE,* United Arab Emirates. (Adapted from US Renal Data System [USRDS]: Annual Data Report, Chapter 11: International comparisons. https://www.usrds. org/2017/ download/v2_c11_IntComp_17.pdf; and Benghanem GM: Epidemiology of ESRD in the Maghreb [lecture]. Presented at the 5th Maghrebian Congress of Nephrology, March 19–22, 2014, Djerba Island, Tunisia; data from references **107, 125, 128,** and **130.**)

Yemen; and (2) a high number of expatriates live in some ME countries that may not be included. Fig. 78.4 and Tables 78.2 and 78.3 summarize the available data on ESKD from published articles, registries, and abstracts of proceedings of international symposia in ME countries.[66,76,106–132] Of note, most investigators relied mainly on the results of limited retrospective studies and answers to questionnaires that were sent to leading nephrologists in each country and not on accurate documented statistics, registries, or results of epidemiologic studies.

Israel and Turkey have reported their ESKD data to the European Renal Association–European Dialysis and Transplantation Association registry[131] and the US Renal Data System.[132] The registry in Turkey was established in 1990.[116,133] In 2016, the prevalence of ESKD in Turkey plateaued at 933.1 pmp, and the incidence rate for new RRT patients declined to 139.9 pmp.[128,132] Diabetic nephropathy and hypertension were the two main causes of ESKD in Turkey.[128,131–134]

Data from the report of the Israeli Center for Disease Control (ICDC) have indicated that the incidence of ESKD increased by 73% during the past 25 years, from 113 to 196 pmp. The average annual increase was highest in the years 1996 to 1999, but it has stabilized since 2003. The increase in ESKD was observed mainly in the older population (≥65 years). Likewise, a 2.8-fold increase in the prevalence of ESKD was observed, from 416 pmp in 1990 to 1171 pmp in 2015. Of note, diabetes mellitus was the cause of ESKD in 11.5% of prevalent patients in 1990 and increased to 45.9% in 2015.[127,135]

The Tunisian registry was started in 1990 and has also reported an increase in the incidence and prevalence of ESKD.[136] The incidence of ESKD increased from 81.6 pmp in the period 1992 to 1993 to 158.8 pmp in 2000 to 2001; the average annual increase was 9.6%. The incidence of ESKD in older persons, women, and individuals with diabetic nephropathy has risen steeply. However, regional variations were noted among urban and rural districts.[136,137]

A comprehensive 1-year observational study, conducted by Alashek and colleagues,[66,138–141] shed light on the epidemiology of ESKD and RRT practices in Libya before the conflict. The prevalence and incidence of dialysis-treated ESKD from mid-2009 until August 2010 were 624 and 282 pmp, respectively.[66]

The Saudi Center for Organ Transplantation (SCOT) has established an open-access RRT registry that provides annual information on the epidemiology and treatment of ESKD in Saudi Arabia. In 2016, the incidence and prevalence of RRT were 178 and 741 pmp, respectively, including non-Saudis, who comprise 15% of dialysis patients.[142] Over the past 2 decades, the average annual increase in dialysis population was 6.2%.[112] In 2016, annual report of the Jordanian National Registry of End-Stage Renal Disease, established in 2007, did not include data on kidney transplantation.[129] The incidence and prevalence of dialysis were 191 and 783 pmp, respectively (excluding non-Jordanians).

In March 2011, Lebanon launched its national kidney registry, aiming to report reliable data on prevalence, incidence, patient management, practice patterns, clinical outcomes, and survival among CKD patients. In the first annual report of the registry in 2012, the incidence of ESKD and patient survival could not be accurately calculated because of incomplete data. However, the prevalence was estimated to be 855 pmp.[130] Since then, no other official report has been published. As of December 2015, 4496 dialysis patients were registered in the Lebanese registry.

In Iran, a treatment program for ESKD was introduced in 1975. The reported number of Iranians with ESKD has also increased, and this increase is mirrored in the growing number of dialysis centers and renal transplantation programs. The incidence and prevalence of ESKD were 49.9 and 238 pmp, respectively, in 2000 and increased to 63.8 and 357 pmp, respectively, in 2006.[106,143,144] By the end of 2015, 50,223 patients were undergoing RRT in Iran, with a prevalence of 635.9 pmp.[132]

In the ME countries for which detailed data are available, there is a male predominance among patients with ESKD, similar to that reported worldwide.*

The mean age of patients undergoing dialysis in each ME country varies between 42 and 68 years. Interestingly, the youngest patients with ESKD on dialysis are in the developing ME countries, and the oldest patients with ESKD on dialysis are in Israel.†

Of note, kidney diseases and risk factors or access to therapy in expatriates—who may comprise as much as 50% of the population, especially in the wealthy Gulf countries—have not been carefully investigated. This population needs to be distinguished from the resident population and may require special attention because of their different ethnic, socioeconomic, and environmental backgrounds.[19,112,144,149,150]

## CAUSES

The causes of CKD in ME countries are highly influenced by the bioecology of a particular region and the ethnic and socioeconomic background of its population. Accordingly, the various causes of CKD are ranked differently in ME countries. The populations of the five ME countries in North Africa—Morocco, Algeria, Tunisia, Libya, and Egypt—have similar ethnicity and socioeconomic backgrounds in that they are of African descent that has been intermixed with Berber, Arab, and Mediterranean population streams.[7,151] In the 1990s, interstitial nephritis and glomerulonephritis each accounted for approximately 20% of all cases of CKD in these countries.[151] The number of individuals with interstitial nephritis increased during the 2000s, possibly as a result of environmental pollution and abuse of over-the-counter drugs.[152] Most cases of glomerulonephritis are of the proliferative type, whereas immunoglobulin A (IgA) nephropathy is rare. The high prevalence of proliferative glomerulonephritis in these ME countries reflects postinfectious glomerulonephritis caused by viruses, bacteria, and parasites. In Egypt, Libya, and southern Algeria, approximately 7% of patients with CKD suffered from obstructive uropathy as a result of urinary schistosomiasis caused by *Schistosoma haematobium* or *Schistosoma mansoni.* It is noteworthy that tuberculosis, other bacterial infections, and familial Mediterranean fever (FMF) are the main causes of renal (type AA) amyloidosis in many ME countries.[151,153]

However, the frequency of causes of ESKD has changed. All ME countries except Algeria and Yemen have reported diabetes mellitus as the most frequent cause of ESKD (20%–48%) in incident patients undergoing RRT, followed by hypertension (11%–30%) and glomerulonephritis (11%–24%).[7,62,66,107,111,127,129–132,142–144,149,154,155]

### GENETIC DISORDERS

Genetic kidney diseases have received much attention in the fields of pediatric and adult nephrology because the underlying molecular defects in many of these diseases have been elucidated as a result of advances in genetics and molecular biology. The ME population is ethnically and genetically diverse.[156] The primary demographic features of Arab Muslim and Druze communities in the ME include large families, rapid population growth, and high rates of consanguinity. Among Palestinian Arabs, more than 40% of marriages are between relatives and, of these, 50% are between first cousins.[156,157] In Bedouin society, 40% of women of childbearing age are married to first cousins.[158] Nevertheless, a comprehensive recent study, conducted in a single Muslim village in Israel, has demonstrated significant sociodemographic changes during a 50-year time period.[84] A shift from the practice of marrying a first cousin to marrying a remote relative was noted. There was a significant reduction in the mean number of children born per woman and, in parallel, the mean age of first-time mothers progressively increased. The impact of these changes on the incidence of recessively inherited diseases among this population is of much interest.

In contrast, the consanguinity rate among Israeli Jews is reported to be 2.3% and, of these, first cousin marriages account for 0.8%. The highest consanguinity rate among Israeli Jews (7.1%) is found among Eastern (i.e., Asian, non-Sephardic) Jews.[159]

High consanguinity rates have also been reported in the Saudi Arabian, Kuwaiti, Lebanese, and Moroccan populations.[78,79,81,83,160–162]

> ***Clinical Relevance***
> **Inherited Kidney Disease**
> High rates of genetic kidney diseases occur in the ME because of high rates of consanguinity.

The results of an epidemiologic survey from Lebanon has revealed that 26% of patients undergoing chronic hemodialysis are the children of consanguineous parents.[79] In addition, Barbari and colleagues[79] have reported that the risk for a family history of kidney disease is particularly high among patients from consanguineous families who were undergoing hemodialysis. Populations with a high rate of consanguinity also have an increased prevalence of adulthood diseases associated with renal insufficiency, such as hypertension, metabolic syndrome, and diabetes mellitus.[80,163] A study of kidney biopsies from three pathology centers in Lebanon has shown that mesangioproliferative glomerulonephritis is significantly more frequent among Muslims and offspring of consanguineous unions, whereas focal segmental glomerulosclerosis (FSGS) is most prevalent in Christians.[82] It should be noted that mutation screening in genes known to be responsible for either of these histological diagnoses had not been performed.

A significant proportion of genetic kidney diseases are inherited in an autosomal recessive manner. It is therefore not surprising that these diseases occur most frequently in communities with high consanguinity rates.[164] The contribution of large families with many offspring, resulting in high carrier rates, to the augmented prevalence of recessively inherited disorders is also appreciated. Yet, the possibility of a higher mutation rate among consanguineous populations in the ME has thus far not been documented. Consanguinity

*References 111, 112, 128, 130, 132, 145, and 146.
†References 111–113, 127, 128, 130, 134, 144, 147, and 148.

**Table 78.4 Genetic Kidney Diseases in Southern Israel, 1994 to 2010**

| Type of Disease | Disease | OMIM No. | No. of Patients | No. of Families | No. of Bedouin Patients | No. of Jewish Patients |
|---|---|---|---|---|---|---|
| Glomerular | Alport syndrome | 301050 | 5 | 3 | 0 | 5 |
| | Benign familial hematuria | 141200 | 3 | 2 | 2 | 1 |
| Tubular | Familial hyperkalemic hypertension | 145260 | 1 | 1 | 0 | 1 |
| | Cystinuria | 220100 | 14 | 7 | 14 | 0 |
| | Distal RTA | 602722 | 4 | 3 | 2 | 2 |
| | Nephrogenic diabetes insipidus | 125800 | 18 | 11 | 17 | 1 |
| | Type 2 Bartter syndrome | 241200 | 10 | 6 | 3 | 7 |
| | Type 4 Bartter syndrome | 602522 | 20 | 13 | 20 | 0 |
| | Unclassified Bartter's syndrome | | 3 | 3 | 1 | 2 |
| | Familial hypomagnesemia | 602014 | 21 | 15 | 21 | 0 |
| | Gitelman syndrome | 263800 | 3 | 3 | 1 | 2 |
| | Hypophosphatemic rickets | 307800 | 4 | 2 | 3 | 1 |
| Cystic/NPHP | ADPKD | 173900 | 14 | 13 | 0 | 14 |
| | ARPKD | 263200 | 16 | 12 | 13 | 3 |
| | Bardet-Biedl syndrome | 209900 | 5 | 4 | 5 | 0 |
| | Juvenile nephronophthisis | 256100 | 3 | 3 | 2 | 1 |
| | Infantile nephronophthisis | 602088 | 5 | 4 | 5 | 0 |
| Metabolic | Fanconi-Bickel syndrome | 227810 | 2 | 2 | 2 | 0 |
| | Xanthinuria | 278300 | 5 | 2 | 5 | 0 |
| | Lowe syndrome | 309000 | 1 | 1 | 0 | 1 |
| | Cystinosis | 219800 | 3 | 3 | 0 | 3 |
| Other | Atypical HUS | 134370 | 8 | 4 | 8 | 0 |
| | Renal tubular dysgenesis | 267430 | 5 | 5 | 4 | 1 |
| Total | | | 173 | 122 | 128 | 45 |

*ADPKD,* Autosomal dominant polycystic kidney disease; *ARPKD,* autosomal recessive polycystic kidney disease; *HUS,* hemolytic-uremic syndrome; *NPHP,* nephronophthisis; *OMIM,* Online Mendelian Inheritance in Man catalogue (http://www.ncbi.nlm.nih.gov/omim); *RTA,* renal tubular acidosis.

Modified from Landau D, Shalev H: Childhood genetic renal diseases in southern Israel. *Harefuah.* 2010;149:180–185.

may enhance allelic and locus heterogeneity.[80,163–165] In Palestinian Arabs, 71 different autosomal recessive kidney diseases have been reported[157]; these include primary renal diseases (congenital nephrotic syndrome, nephronophthisis), metabolic and tubular defects (cystinuria, Bartter syndrome, renal tubular acidosis, primary hyperoxaluria type 1), and FMF (discussed in detail later in this chapter). The influence of genetic factors is very evident in pediatric patients with kidney diseases, particularly in Saudi Arabia and Syria, where increased numbers of congenital and hereditary kidney and urologic diseases are now being reported.[156,166] The results of an extensive study of Jewish and Bedouin populations in southern Israel have shown that genetic kidney diseases are overrepresented in the pediatric population (see Table 78.4).[81]

By combining whole-exome sequencing with a high-resolution metabolomics profiling for a highly consanguineous Arab cohort in Qatar, 21 common variant and 12 functional rare variant metabolomics quantitative trait loci (mQTLs) were discovered, of which 45% were novel altogether.[167] This project may have wide implications for precision medicine in the ME in various areas, including kidney diseases.

### Cystic Kidney Diseases

Autosomal dominant polycystic kidney disease is one of the most common genetic renal diseases in adults and occurs in 1.2% to 10% of ESKD patients in several ME communities.[127,155,168–170] Autosomal recessive polycystic disease (ARPKD; Online Mendelian Inheritance in Man [OMIM] catalogue number 263200) occurs with a proposed incidence of 1/20,000 to 1/40,000. Mortality during the first month of life is particularly high among those born with severe oligohydramnios leading to pulmonary hypoplasia. Its principal manifestations include fusiform dilation of the renal collecting ducts and distal tubules and dysgenesis of the hepatic portal triad. ARPKD is associated with mutations in the *PKHD1* gene on chromosome 6p21.1-p12, encoding fibrocystin, a membrane protein located on the primary cilium.[171] Over 700 mutations in *PKHD1* gene have been reported.[172] Several mutations were reported in Turkish and Israeli children who participated in a large international study.[173,174]

Meckel-Gruber syndrome (MKS) is a lethal, recessively inherited ciliopathy characterized by multiple congenital anomalies, including polycystic kidneys, occipital encephalocele, and polydactyly. At least 13 genes have been reported to date to underlie MKS. The incidence of this relatively rare disorder in Qatar has been reported as 1 in 500 live births for a population with over 40% consanguineous marriages.[175] The underlying genetic cause was identified in 11 of 12 Arab families residing in a distinct region in Israel, comprising mutations in seven different genes and revealing high genetic heterogeneity.[176] Likewise, other ciliopathies, including various forms of nephronophthisis (including the infantile type) with mutations in *NPHP1*, *NPHP2 (INVS)*, and *NPHP3*, encoding nephrocystin 1, inversin, and nephrocystin 3, respectively, have been reported in several ME countries[177–179] (Table 78.5). Cases of Joubert syndrome, characterized by cerebellar vermis

**Table 78.5 Rare Genetic Diseases With Renal Involvement Reported in Middle Eastern Communities**

| Country, Community | Disease | OMIM No. | Phenotype | Defect, Mutation | References |
|---|---|---|---|---|---|
| Saudi Arabs, Turks | Alström syndrome[a] | 203800 | Retinal degeneration, obesity, cardiomyopathy, sensorineural hearing loss, insulin resistance, renal impairment | *ALMS1* gene, ubiquitously expressed, encodes a protein of unknown function | 220, 247 |
| Israeli Jews of Iraqi origin | Renal hypouricemia type I | 220150 | Hypouricemia, hyperuricosuria, nephrolithiasis, exercise-induced acute kidney injury | *SLC22A12* gene, encodes uric acid transporter URAT1 | 242 |
| Israeli Arabs | Renal hypouricemia type II | 612076 | Increased renal clearance of uric acid, hypouricemia, nephrolithiasis, exercise-induced acute kidney injury | *SLC2A9* gene, encodes glucose transporter 9 (GLUT9) | 233, 237, 243 |
| Israeli Jews, Turks | Dent disease[a] | 300008 | Low-molecular-weight proteinuria, hypercalciuria, nephrocalcinosis, nephrolithiasis, rickets, renal failure, hypokalemic metabolic alkalosis, focal glomerulosclerosis | *CLCN5*, encodes the chloride/proton ClC-5 antiporter | 234, 236, 244 |
| Egyptian and Saudi Arabs, Turks, Iranians, Jordanians | Cystinosis | 219750 (adult) 219900 (juvenile) 219800 (infantile) | Failure to thrive, polydipsia, polyuria, Fanconi-like syndrome; corneal, conjunctival, and retinal deposition | *CTNS,* encodes the lysosomal cystine transporter | 232, 240, 248, 249, 251 |
| Israeli Druze | Autosomal recessive proximal tubulopathy with hypercalciuria | 138160 | Proximal tubulopathy, hypercalciuria, normal or slightly elevated urinary phosphate excretion | *SLC2A2* (*GLUT2*), encodes the glucose transporter 2[b] | 246 |
| Israeli Arabs | Autosomal recessive Fanconi syndrome and hypophosphatemic rickets | 613388 | Proximal tubulopathy, renal phosphate wasting, normocalciuria, bone mineral deficiency, decreased glomerular filtration rate | *SLC34A1*, encodes the renal sodium phosphate cotransporter IIa | 245 |
| Israeli Arabs | Familial renal glycosuria and aminoaciduria[c] | 233100 | Glycosuria, aminoaciduria | *SLC5A2*, encodes the kidney-specific $Na^+$/glucose cotransporter | 239 |
| Israeli Jews | Proximal renal tubular acidosis and glaucoma | 604278 and 603345 | Short stature, deformed teeth, bilateral glaucoma, blindness, metabolic acidosis | *SLC4A4*, encodes the sodium bicarbonate cotransporter (NBCe1) | 235 |
| Israeli Arabs and Jews | Familial autosomal recessive renal tubular acidosis | 267300 | Distal renal tubular acidosis, deafness | *ATP6V1B1*, encodes the B1-subunit of $H^+$-ATPase | 250 |
| Israeli Arabs | Familial autosomal recessive renal tubular acidosis | 259730 | Proximal and distal renal tubular acidosis, osteopetrosis, mental retardation | *CA2*, encoding carbonic anhydrase | 250 |
| Egyptian Arabs | Familial hypomagnesemia with hypercalciuria and nephrocalcinosis | 248250 | Hypocalcemia, hypomagnesemia, hypercalciuria, nephrocalcinosis, congenital cataracts | *CLDN16*, the claudin-16 gene | 241 |
| Iranians | Familial lecithin-cholesterol acyltransferase deficiency[d] | 245900 | Lower extremity edema, proteinuria, corneal opacities, hypercholesterolemia, hemolytic anemia | Lecithin-cholesterol Acyltransferase (*LCAT*) gene | 238 |

[a]X-linked.
[b]Homozygous mutations in *GLUT2* also cause Fanconi-Bickel syndrome.
[c]Autosomal recessive.
[d]Diagnosis made on the basis of family history and electron microscopic findings on kidney biopsy.
*OMIM,* Online Mendelian Inheritance in Man catalogue (http://www.ncbi.nlm.nih.gov/omim).

hypoplasia, developmental delay, seizures, retinal dystrophy, and kidney involvement, have been reported in the ME. There is genetic heterogeneity with pathogenic mutations in 33 distinct genes responsible for this disorder. Founder mutations have been identified in Iranian families and in Ashkenazi Jews.[180]

### Genetic Glomerular Diseases

A substantial number of patients in the ME with renal disease have familial glomerular diseases whose spectrum includes familial hematuria, Alport syndrome, IgA nephropathy, and familial steroid-resistant nephrotic syndrome (SRNS) with histologic findings consistent with FSGS.[81,166,181] A recessive form of SRNS has been shown to be associated with mutations in the *NPHS2* gene, which encodes the glomerular barrier protein podocin.[182] The most common phenotype is of a nephrotic syndrome that is resistant to immunosuppressive treatment in early childhood, and most patients will develop ESKD by the end of their second decade of life. In a group of children from two consanguineous families of Israeli Arab descent, mutation analysis of the *NPHS2* gene revealed homozygosity for the C412T nonsense mutation (R138X).[183] The same mutation was subsequently found in additional children who presented with SRNS from the same ethnic background, which points to the possibility of a founder effect.[183] Interestingly, cardiac anomalies, especially left ventricular hypertrophy, pulmonary stenosis, and discrete subaortic stenosis, were detected in a high proportion of the children with *NPHS2* mutations.[184] Frishberg and associates[184] have speculated that podocin may have a role in normal cardiac development because podocin messenger RNA is reported to be expressed in the human fetal heart.

At least 53 *NPHS2* mutations have also been found in Turkish children with familial and "sporadic" SRNS.[185,186] In this context, the term *sporadic* is a misnomer. As a recessively inherited disease, both parents are obligatory carriers of pathogenic mutations, and the lack of positive family history may merely represent the first case in a given nuclear family. Among Turkish patients with *NPHS2* mutations, the proportion of patients with CKD or ESKD was significantly higher (19 of 73) than that of patients without these mutations (28 of 222). Furthermore, the mean time for progression to ESKD was significantly shorter in patients with mutations compared with those without mutations.[185,186] The prevalence of *NPHS2* mutations among 49 children with SRNS and 50 children with steroid-sensitive nephrotic syndrome from Iran was 31% and 4%, respectively.[187] Of these children, 33% experienced recurrence of primary disease after kidney transplantation, none of whom had an *NPHS2* mutation.

The *NPHS1* gene encodes nephrin, an essential protein for maintaining the normal structure and function of the slit diaphragm of the visceral glomerular epithelial cell. Three mutations in the *NPHS1* gene were reported in 12 children with congenital nephrotic syndrome of the Finnish type from a large consanguineous Israeli Arab family.[165] Steroid-sensitive nephrotic syndrome is rarely reported to have a familial pattern. However, a familial pattern associated with this condition has been reported in Israeli Bedouin families with a high rate of consanguinity, and the authors of the report proposed that the increased incidence of steroid-sensitive nephrotic syndrome resulted from selective enrichment of susceptibility genes in this population.[188]

A study has evaluated causative mutations related to childhood nephrotic syndrome in 49 families from Saudi Arabia[189]; 62 patients were screened for mutations in genes associated with congenital, infantile, or childhood nephrotic syndrome, such as *NPHS1, NPHS2, LAMB2* (laminin-$\beta_2$), *PLCE1* (phospholipase C$\varepsilon_1$), *CD2AP* (CD2-associated protein), *MYO1E* (myosin 1E), *WT1* (Wilms' tumor suppressor gene 1), *PTPRO* (protein tyrosine phosphatase receptor type O), and *NEIL1* (Nei endonuclease VII-like 1).[189] A homozygous mutation in the *NPHS2* gene was found in 11 families (22%) and was the most common cause of nephrotic syndrome. Other mutations were found in *NPHS1* (12%), *PLCE1* (8%), and *MYO1E* (6%) genes. FSGS was the most common pattern of histopathologic injury, and a significant proportion of patients developed ESKD requiring RRT.[189]

The Podonet Consortium, an international registry for congenital nephrotic syndrome and childhood SRNS, has analyzed the data retrieved from 1655 patients, 9.2% of whom were from the ME (Syria, Lebanon, Iran, and the UAE). Pathogenic mutations were detected in 23.6% of the screened patients.[190] A cohort of children with SRNS from a single center in Saudi Arabia was tested for causing mutations in *NPHS1, NPHS2,* and *WT1.* All 44 children were older than 1 year, and presumably pathogenic mutations were identified in five children (11.4%), three in *NPHS2* and the remaining two in *NPHS1.*[191] None of those with an identified genetic cause showed any response to immunosuppressive treatment.

In Turkey, 25 children with SRNS underwent mutation screening in *TRPC6*, a dominantly inherited form of SRNS. Positive family history was found in nine children.[192] The results showed a variant in one patient, intronic nucleotide substitution in six patients, and previously described missense and synonymous amino acid variants in nine patients. Although the pathogenicity of all these genetic variants remains to be proven, the authors concluded that *TRPC6* mutations may play a significant role in childhood SRNS.

Galloway-Mowat syndrome (GAMOS) is an autosomal recessive disease characterized by the combination of early-onset nephrotic syndrome (SRNS) and microcephaly with brain anomalies. Recessive mutations in *OSGEP, TP53RK, TPRKB,* and X-linked mutations in *LAGE3* genes encoding the four subunits of the KEOPS complex have been recently detected in 37 individuals from 32 families with GAMOS, 6 of whom are from the ME (Iran, Turkey, Jordan, and Egypt).[193]

Coenzyme Q10 (CoQ10), also known as ubiquinone, is a lipid-soluble component of virtually all cell membranes and plays a critical role in transporting electrons along the respiratory chain of the mitochondrial inner membrane. *ADCK4* appears to have a role in CoQ10 biosynthesis; mutations in ADCK4 may cause SRNS and/or CKD of presumably unknown cause.[194] A total of 146 index patients aged 10 to 18 years from Turkey, with newly diagnosed nonnephrotic proteinuria, nephrotic syndrome, or CKD of varying severity, were screened for *ADCK4* mutations.[195] In this study, 28 individuals with a biallelic mutation were identified, and CoQ10 supplementation appeared efficacious in reducing proteinuria in a subgroup of this cohort.

The Rat sarcoma homolog gene family of small guanosine triphosphate (GTP)-ases (Rho GTPases) is associated with actin remodeling and podocyte migratory ability. Alterations in Rho GTPases signaling interfere with podocyte mobility and cause proteinuria.[196] Rho guanosine diphosphate (GDP) dissociation inhibitor 1, a regulator of Rho GTPases, is a protein that is encoded in humans by the *ARHGDIA* gene and is also expressed in podocytes. *ARHADIA* mutations, associated with SRNS progressing to ESKD during the first decade of life, have been reported in three siblings from a family of Ashkenazi Jews and in a Moroccan infant.[197]

### Genetic Metabolic Diseases and Inherited Tubular Disorders

The primary hyperoxalurias (PHs) are a group of rare autosomal recessive inborn errors of glyoxylate metabolism that result in the excessive production of oxalate.[198,199] Currently, three types of PH have been characterized genetically and phenotypically.[200] The relatively more frequent PH type 1 (OMIM number 259900) is caused by the absence, deficiency, or mistargeting to the mitochondria of the liver-specific peroxisomal enzyme alanine-glyoxylate aminotransferase (AGT), which catalyzes the conversion of glyoxylate to glycine. Accumulating glyoxylate diffuses from the peroxisome into the cytosol, where it is oxidized to oxalate, a reaction catalyzed by lactate dehydrogenase (LDH). Excessive oxalate synthesis and massive urinary excretion of the insoluble calcium oxalate crystals results in nephrocalcinosis, kidney stones, and declining kidney function. As the glomerular filtration rate (GFR) declines, the oxalate load, produced by the liver, can no longer be cleared by the kidneys, the plasma oxalate level increases, and calcium oxalate crystals are deposited in almost all tissues in a devastating process termed "systemic oxalosis." PH type 2 (OMIM number 260000) is caused by a deficiency of the mitochondrial enzyme glyoxylate reductase/hydroxypyruvate reductase (GRHPR), which catalyzes the reduction of glyoxylate to glycolate. In 2010, PH type 3 (OMIM number 613616) was described in a cohort of patients with calcium oxalate nephrolithiasis due to hyperoxaluria in whom PH1 and PH2 were excluded.[201] In affected members of nine unrelated families, Belostotsky and colleagues found biallelic loss-of-function mutations in *HOGA1*, formerly *DHDPSL*, which encodes a mitochondrial 4-hydroxy-2-oxoglutarate aldolase that catalyzes the fourth step in the hydroxyproline pathway.[201,202] A founder mutation in *HOGA1* among Ashkenazi-Jews was identified.

PH types 1 to 3 are relatively prevalent in the ME. Cases of PH1 and isolated cases of type 2 have been reported in Israeli families.[203–205] In 22 Israeli Arab families with type 1 hyperoxaluria, at least 15 different mutations in the AGT-encoding *AGXT* gene have been detected.[203,205] Marked intrafamilial phenotypic variability, with no definite genotype-phenotype correlation, was noted in these families, and the prevalent phenotype was of early onset of disease with progression to ESKD in the first decade of life.[203] The diagnosis of PH1 was confirmed in 15 of 19 children tested in a single tertiary center in Egypt.[206] Two-thirds of this cohort reached ESKD, with one-third during infancy. A large European study of 155 patients from 129 families with type 1 hyperoxaluria, including a large proportion of ME individuals, has shown that the most common mutation is *p.Gly170Arg* (allelic frequency, 21.5%). This mutation results in mistargeting of AGT into the mitochondria while the catalytic activity of the enzyme remains intact. A subgroup of these patients will respond to vitamin $B_6$ treatment, a product of pyridoxal phosphate, which is a known cofactor in all aminotransferase reactions and therefore may have a better long-term prognosis.[207]

Hyperoxaluria manifesting as kidney stone disease and/or progressive CKD has been described in the following reports from the ME. Although, systematic genetic analysis has not been performed, it is likely that PH accounts for the disease in a significant number of individuals. For example, among 260 adult patients with recurrent nephrolithiasis from a tertiary center in Israel, hyperoxaluria was detected in 24.2%.[208] Hyperoxaluria was found among 10.7% of 84 patients with CKD, treated conservatively or by hemodialysis, in Jenin district in the Palestinian Authority.[155] PH1 is the probable cause of hyperoxaluria in most of these cases. In a retrospective report from a single center in Amman, Jordan, 70 children with suspected PH were identified.[209] At the time of initial presentation, 15.7% were in ESKD and an additional 25% had impaired kidney function. Although not tested at the time of this report, PH1 may be responsible for hyperoxaluria in many of these children, particularly in those with compromised kidney function. Similarly, a high prevalence of hyperoxaluria was demonstrated among Turkish children with kidney stone disease.[210] Hyperoxaluria causing nephrolithiasis, nephrocalcinosis, and kidney failure was reported in children from other ME countries in western North Africa, Saudi Arabia, and Kuwait.[151,211,212] Primary hyperoxaluria is probably underdiagnosed because, by the time of diagnosis, advanced CKD or early graft dysfunction in kidney transplant recipients may have already developed.[199]

Cystinuria is a recessively inherited kidney stone disease, prevalent in various ethnic groups in ME countries.[151,211,213] Cystinuria is a different disorder from cystinosis, which is a recessively inherited lysosomal transport disease leading to the accumulation of cystine, presenting with renal Fanconi syndrome, and resulting in CKD, with various extrarenal manifestations (see Table 78.5). Cystinuria is caused by biallelic mutations in either one or both of two genes:

1. The *SLC3A1* gene on chromosome 2p16.3-p21 encodes rBAT, a protein required for normal trafficking of the amino acid transporter to its appropriate location in the apical membrane of affected epithelia. In its mutated form, it leads to impairment of cystine and dibasic amino acid (e.g., ornithine, lysine, arginine) transport.
2. The *SLC7A9* gene located on chromosome 19q12-13.1 encodes an amino acid transporter, $b^{0,+}$AT. When this protein is defective, its appearance at the apical membrane, assuming that rBAT is normal, does not lead to normal amino acid reabsorption.

Because parents of patients with cystinuria due to *SLC7A9* mutations have increased levels of urinary cystine excretion, they may sometimes form stones if the urine volume is low or if animal protein intake is high. Otherwise, disease manifestations caused by either mutation are similar.[214–216] Some patients may bear heterozygous digenic mutations, and they do not tend to form cystine stones unless there are mutations in two copies of a single gene. Mutations in *SCL3A1* have been detected in Turks, Muslim Arabs, Druze, and Ashkenazi and Sephardic Jews of Persian and Yemenite origin. The disease is also common among Libyan Jews, in whom the estimated prevalence is 1/2500 and the carrier rate is 1/25.

In this population, the disease is caused by a single founder mutation, V170M, in the *SLC7A9* gene.[214–220]

Fabry disease is a rare X-linked inborn error of the glycosphingolipid metabolic pathway caused by deficiency of α-galactosidase A. A mutation in the gene encoding this enzyme results in insufficient breakdown of lipids, which accumulate to harmful levels in the eyes, kidneys, autonomic nervous system, and cardiovascular system. In untreated patients, the accumulation of globotriaosylceramide (Gb3) in lysosomes may result in multiple organ damage that includes the development of ESKD between the fourth and fifth decades of life. Histologic evidence of Fabry disease has been detected in graft biopsy samples many years after successful kidney transplantation.[221,222] Although most disease features have been reported in adults, a pediatric disease phenotype that includes acroparesthesias, skin manifestations, and glomerular alterations has been described.[222,223] Fabry disease has been diagnosed in families in Israel and Turkey.[221–225] The disease may be underdiagnosed in other ME countries because of phenotypic variability of the disease, with often nonspecific signs and symptoms or insufficient awareness. However, screening of adult patients with ESKD undergoing dialysis in Turkey and in Lebanon has yielded an extremely low prevalence rate of Fabry disease.[226,227]

Bartter syndrome and Gitelman syndrome belong to a group of inherited salt-losing tubulopathies with distinct phenotypes; they are caused by inherited defects in ion transporters in the loop of Henle and distal convoluted tubule, respectively. Most cases of the variants of Bartter syndrome in the ME have been reported in Israeli Arabs, in large Bedouin communities living in southern and northern Israel, and in Kuwaiti children.[81,228,229]

Congenital anomalies of the kidney and urinary tract (CAKUT) comprise the most common cause of CKD in childhood. To understand the underlying pathogenetic mechanisms better, Vivante and associates have identified 20 Israeli pedigrees with isolated nonsyndromic renal hypodysplasia and screened for mutations in genes known to be involved in kidney development.[230] Two brothers were found to have a heterozygous *PAX2* nonsense mutation, responsible for renal coloboma syndrome, which includes kidney dysplasia, eye coloboma, and hearing impairment. Nine affected subjects from two unrelated families were found to harbor heterozygous *HNF1B* mutations, encoding the hepatocyte nuclear factor-1β. These mutations are associated with variable renal phenotypes, maturity-onset diabetes of the young (MODY5), hypomagnesemia, and hyperuricemia. In one family, two affected brothers were heterozygous for a missense mutation in *WNT4*. Functional analysis of this variant in different cell lines revealed both agonistic and antagonistic canonical WNT stimuli. In primary cultures of human fetal kidney cells, this mutation causes loss of function, resulting in diminished canonical WNT/β-catenin signaling. These findings were interpreted as suggestive of a role for heterozygous *WNT4* variants in renal hypodysplasia.[230] A three-generation Yemenite Jewish family with seven individuals who had CAKUT was investigated by whole-exome sequencing. Renal hypoplasia-dysplasia was the predominant phenotype (six individuals), together with vesicoureteral reflux (VUR; four individuals) and/or ectopia (two individuals).[231] A heterozygous truncating mutation of the nuclear receptor interacting protein 1 gene (*NRIP1*) was identified in all seven affected members. *NRIP1* encodes a nuclear receptor transcriptional cofactor that directly interacts with the retinoic acid receptors (RARs) to modulate retinoic acid transcriptional activity.

Some rare genetic kidney diseases that have been reported in ME communities are listed in Table 78.5.[232–251] Other nonrenal genetic diseases may cause glomerular and tubulointerstitial complications; an example is sickle cell anemia, a hemoglobinopathy that is prevalent in the ME countries in western North Africa and the Arabian Peninsula.[151,156,215,252,253] Inherited diseases of the kidney are discussed further in Chapters 43, 44, and 72.

#### Familial Mediterranean Fever

FMF is the most common of the hereditary periodic fever syndromes and is a prevalent recessively inherited disease in the ME. FMF is an autoinflammatory disease that is characterized by recurrent attacks of fever, serositis, arthritis, and erysipelas-like skin lesions. The disease affects several ethnic groups in the ME, including Sephardic Jews, Armenians, Turks, and Arabs.[254] The most significant complication of FMF is renal amyloidosis that progresses to nephrotic syndrome and ESKD. Renal amyloidosis is occasionally diagnosed in patients without a typical history of FMF attacks.

In the 1990s, two groups identified the *MEFV* gene by positional cloning as the underlying genetic cause of FMF.[255,256] At least 327 mutations in the *MEFV* gene have been reported, and more than 195 of these mutations have been found to be associated with FMF.[257] The *MEFV* gene encodes the protein pyrin (or marenostrin). The gene is located on the short arm of chromosome 16 (16p13.3) and includes 10 exons that encode 781 amino acids. Pyrin is expressed predominantly in polymorphonuclear cells (PMNCs), eosinophils, and monocytes, but not in lymphocytes. It is also expressed in dendritic cells and fibroblasts from the synovium, peritoneum, and skin.[258,259] Pyrin has an important role in the innate immune system, which constitutes a primary defense against external pathogens and other noxious agents.[260] Its exact role and mechanism of action appear to be in sensing changes in the Rho GTPases.[261] Rho proteins are involved in controlling GTPase activity, which in turn are important in the regulation of actin and tubulin dynamics. Actin-tubulin interactions contribute to neutrophil motility and chemotaxis. Bacterial toxin (e.g., *Clostridium difficile* toxin) may modify the effect of Rho proteins on GTPases, thereby inhibiting actin-tubulin activity and neutrophil chemotaxis. Pyrin does not directly recognize Rho modification but probably senses an event downstream of Rho modification in the actin cytoskeleton pathway and forms a caspase-1–activating inflammasome.[262,263] Therefore, pyrin-mediated innate immunity is unique in that it senses bacterial virulence rather than microbial molecules.[262]

In patients with FMF, the mutations in the *MEFV* gene lead to the production of pyrin protein, which is capable of constructing the inflammasome, even in the absence of a known external trigger such as a toxin or infectious agent. This possibility suggests that the mutations in *MEFV* gene cause gain of function of pyrin protein so that it acts without a known provocation. The outcome of this process is the secretion of interleukin (IL)-1, IL-18, and other mediators of inflammation, which enhance chemotaxis and neutrophilia and induce an attack of FMF.

The carrier frequency of mutant alleles is high, as much as one-fifth to one-third, in certain populations of the ME countries (Armenians, Jews, and Turks). The most common reported mutations are *M694V, V726A, M680I,* and *M694I* in exon 10 and *E148Q* in exon 2.[264,265] The first four mutations are believed to be pathogenic, with the M694V homozygotes having the most severe phenotype. Although the E1489Q homozygotes are asymptomatic in 50% of cases, this variant may be associated with other systemic inflammatory diseases, including Behçet disease, vasculitis, ulcerative colitis, rheumatoid arthritis, and multiple sclerosis.[266] The most frequent *MEFV* mutations in the ME populations are listed in Table 78.6.[266–294] Data from five databases encompassing whole-genome and whole-exome datasets for 2115 individuals from multiple subpopulations in the ME were available for analysis.[295] A compendium for MEFV genetic variants was also created. The carrier frequency for genetic variants in MEFV was found to be 8%, with differences in allele frequency among subpopulations. Also, three pathogenic variants were added to the four popular studied variants. The former include c.1261-11T>G, Y688X, and E148V. Mutations in the *MEFV* gene have also been reported in Spanish, Italian, Greek, Portuguese, Indian, Chinese, and Japanese populations.[296,297] Most *MEFV* mutations are single amino acid substitutions (missense), and some patients with FMF have a single *MEFV* mutation. The latter may imply a dominantly inherited trait, which may go along with a gain of function of the gene product. Alternatively, additional genes or immune factors may modulate the innate immune response in FMF.

The clinical spectrum of FMF and the elucidation of the molecular biology, structure, and regulation of pyrin and its role during inflammation have been reviewed.[263,298–301] Pyrin belongs to the large family of proteins sharing a conserved domain structure with the tripartite motif (TRIM) consisting of an N-terminal RING domain, B-box domain(s), and C-terminal coiled coil domain. In pyrin, the RING domain with the ubiquitin ligase activity is replaced by the PYD domain, which belongs to the death domain. It also carries an additional approximately 200–amino acid C-terminal B30.2/rfp/PRY/SPRY domain. Most of the disease-associated mutations are located in the C-terminal B30.2 domain. The B30.2. domain is present in primate and human pyrin, but not in rodent pyrin.[301] It includes a SPRY domain that is located in front of the C-terminal region and a SPRY extension at the N terminus. The SPRY domain is a protein interaction module, which is implicated in several biologic pathways, including those that regulate innate and adaptive immunity.[302]

During the last decade, the functions of pyrin have been the subject of intensive research. Advances in our understanding of its functionality are the result of identifying its interaction with different proteins and oligomers.[263] In particular, the PYD domain, via cognate pyrin domain association, interacts with an adapter protein termed *apoptosis-associated specklike protein with a caspase recruitment domain* (ASC)[303] and thus participates in the regulation of apoptosis, inflammation, and IL-1β processing.[304] The B30.2/rfp/PRY/SPRY domain-mediated protein interactions indicate the role of this domain as an adaptor module to assemble macromolecular complexes.[305] As a part of the pyrin inflammasome, pyrin also acts as a pattern recognition receptor, sensing pathogen modification and inactivation of Rho GTPases (see earlier).[261]

Paradoxically, pyrin also acts as a component directing the inflammasome components NLRP1, NLRP3, and pro-caspase 1 to selective autophagic degradation.[306] On its own, the dimerization of B30.2 domains by means of the CHS domain appears to be crucial for the recognition of higher order oligomers.[307] Inflammasomes contain members of the nucleotide-binding oligomerization domain, leucine-rich repeat, and PYRIN domain–containing subfamily of proteins, now known as NLRP proteins. Mutations in the gene expression of the NLRP protein, *NLRP3* (cryopyrin), are associated with monogenic autoinflammatory diseases—cryopyrin-associated periodic syndromes.[308]

**Clinical Spectrum and Renal Disease.** The wide clinical spectrum and possible genotype-phenotype correlations in FMF are influenced by genotype (extent and position of the *MEFV* mutation), ethnicity, and environmental factors. Although mutations are found throughout the entire *MEFV* gene in patients with FMF, the mutations with the most severe forms of disease are clustered in exon 10, which encodes a motif known as the B30.2/SPRY domain at the C terminus of the protein. Genetic variants found in exons 2 (e.g., E148Q) and 3 are usually associated with less severe clinical presentations of FMF or even just mild nonspecific inflammatory manifestations. Overall, M694V homozygotes have a severe phenotype and are more likely to have arthritis, renal amyloidosis, erysipelas-like skin lesions, high fever, splenomegaly, and more frequent attacks as compared with individuals with other *MEFV* mutations.[309] In addition, patients with these mutations require higher doses of colchicine to prevent attacks as compared with patients with other genotypes. Among Arab patients with FMF, the worst disease severity is associated with alleles carrying the mutations *M694V/M694V* and *M694V/M726A,* whereas the *M694I/M694I* mutation is associated with a mild form of the disease.[310] In Turkish patients with FMF, the common *M694V* mutation is associated with more severe disease but not with amyloidosis.[293,300] In contrast, the homozygous *M694V* mutation was reported to be associated with amyloidosis in Jews from North Africa, in Arabs, and in Turks and also with the protracted febrile myalgia syndrome, which is a type of myalgia that is associated with FMF in Arabs.*

FMF has traditionally been considered an autosomal recessive genetic disease, but as many as 25% of patients with clinical FMF have only one *MEFV* mutation.[292,293,299] This finding could explain the vertical transmission of the disease in some families. In patients with FMF who have a single *MEFV* mutation, an additional but less common mutation may account for the disease, but this has not yet been confirmed in carefully performed studies. A dominant segregation of a heterozygous *MEFV* mutation was reported in some families. Therefore, it was suggested that complex alleles can lead to a more severe form of disease.[311] One study has reported that heterozygous mutations at amino acid position 577 of pyrin (T577) can induce autosomal dominant autoinflammatory disease. The T577 is located in front of the C-terminal B30.2/SPRY domain and is crucial for pyrin function.[309,312] The T577 mutations were found in a family of Turkish descent with autosomal dominant FMF phenotype and also in European patients with other periodic syndromes. The impact of *MEFV* mutations has been shown in other inflammatory diseases, such as Henoch-Schönlein purpura,

*References 276, 278, 285, 287, 293, 294, and 310.

**Table 78.6 Genotype-Phenotype Correlations in Several Patient Populations With Familial Mediterranean Fever**

| Population, Community | Frequent Mutations | Phenotype | Amyloidosis (% of Patients) | Associated Syndromes and Diseases | Reference |
|---|---|---|---|---|---|
| Israeli Jews and Arabs | *M680I, M694V, M694I, V726A* | Arthritis, fever, serositis, vasculitis | 1.4% (associated with mutation in *M694V*) | NR | Brik et al[278] |
| Israeli Jews and Arabs | *M694V* (very common in Jews), *M694I* (exclusive in Arabs), *M680I, V726A, E148Q* | Arthritis, fever, serositis, vasculitis | NR | NR | Ben-Chetrit et al[276] |
| Israeli Arabs | *M694V* (associated with severe disease), *V726A* (most common) | Arthritis, fever, serositis, vasculitis | NR | NR | Shinawi et al[291] |
| Israeli Jews of North African origin and Arabs[a] | *M694I, M694V* (very common in North African Jews), *E148Q* | Synovitis, pleuritis, abdominal pain, skin rash | 95%[a] | Focal glomerulosclerosis | Ben-Chetrit and Backenroth[275] |
| Israeli Jews of North African origin, Ashkenazi Jews, Jews of Iraqi origin, Israeli Arabs, and Druze | *E148Q, M694V* (very common in North African Jews), *V726A* | FMF criteria[284] | 4.6% (most common in *M694V* homozygous) | NR | Zaks et al[294] |
| Israeli Jews (Ashkenazi and non-Ashkenazi), Arabs, and Druze | *M694V* (very common in Jews), *E148Q, M694V, V726A* (equally common in Arabs), *E148Q* (most common in Druze) | Fever, serositis | NR | NR | Sharkia et al[290] |
| Turks | *M680I, M694V, M694I, V726A, E148Q* | Abdominal pain, fever, arthralgia, chest pain, skin rash | 3% (mostly associated with *M694V*) | NR | Solak et al[292] |
| Turks | *M680I, M694V, V726A* | Abdominal pain, fever, arthralgia, pleuritis, muscle pain, skin rash | 12.9%; 0.9% as the main disease manifestation (phenotype II, associated with *M694V*) | Nonamyloid renal disease, Henoch-Schönlein purpura, polyarteritis nodosa, Behçet syndrome, rheumatic fever, uveitis, inflammatory bowel disease | Tunca et al[293] |
| Turks[b] | *M680I, M694V* (most common), *V726A, E148Q* | Abdominal pain, fever, arthralgia, chest pain, erysipelas-like lesion, vomiting, family history of renal failure | 0% | NR | Caglayan et al[279] |
| Turks | *M680I, M694V* (most common), *M694I, V726A E148Q* (common) | Abdominal pain, fever, arthritis, pleuritis, erysipelas-like erythema, peritonitis | NR | NR | Ozdemir et al[270] |
| Turks | *M680I, M694V* (most common), *V726A, E148Q* | Fever, arthritis, pleuritis, erysipelas-like erythema, peritonitis, vasculitis | 8.6% (most common in *M694V* homozygous) | NR | Kasifoglu et al[268] |
| Azeri Turks | *M680I, M694V* (most common), *M694I, V726A E148Q* | Fever, serositis, synovitis, kidney failure | NR | NR | Mohammadnejad and Farajnia[269] |
| Jordanian Arabs Palestinian Arabs | *M680I, M694V, M694I, V726A, E148Q* | Abdominal pain, fever, arthralgia, myalgia, skin rash | 1% (associated with *M694V*) | Protracted fever, myalgia syndrome; 42% homozygous for *M694V* | Langevitz et al[283]; Majeed et al[285] |

**Table 78.6 Genotype-Phenotype Correlations in Several Patient Populations With Familial Mediterranean Fever (Cont'd)**

| Population, Community | Frequent Mutations | Phenotype | Amyloidosis (% of Patients) | Associated Syndromes and Diseases | Reference |
|---|---|---|---|---|---|
| Jordanian Arabs | *M680I, M694V, V726A, E148Q* | Abdominal pain, fever, arthralgia | 9% (*M694V* in one patient, *V726A/M680I* in two patients) | Celiac disease, folliculitis | Medlej-Hashim et al[287] |
| Palestinian Arabs | *M680I, M694V, V726A, E148Q* | NR | NR | NR | Ayesh et al[273] |
| Arabs from Jordan, Egypt, Syria, Iraq, and Saudi Arabia | *M694V, V726A, E148Q* | NR | NR | NR | Al-Alami et al[272] |
| Iranian Azeris who live in Turkey | *M680I, M694V, M694I, V726A, E148Q* | Abdominal pain, fever, arthralgia, pleuritis, skin rash | 7% | NR | Esmaeili et al[282] |
| Iranians (72% Azeri) | *M680I* (most common), *M694V, V726A* | Fever, peritonitis, arthralgia, pleuritis, skin rash | 5.6% | NR | Bidari et al[277] |
| Egyptian Arabs | *M680I, M694V, V726A* | Abdominal pain, chest pain, fever, arthritis, myalgia | NR | NR | Settin et al[289] |
| Egyptian Arabs | *M680I, M694I* (most common), *M694V, V726A, E148Q* | Fever, serositis | Mostly associated with *M694V* | NR | el Gezery et al[280] |
| Egyptian Arabs | *V726A* (most common), *M694V* (common), *M680I, M694I, E148Q* | Abdominal pain, fever, arthralgia, pleuritis, skin rash, myalgia | 2.9% (associated with *M694V*) | NR | el Garf et al[267] |
| Syrian Arabs | *M680I, M694V, M694I, V726A, E148Q, A744S, R761H* | Serositis, fever, arthritis, pleuritis | 5% | NR | Mattit et al[286] |
| Lebanese Arabs | *M680I, M694V* (very frequent), *M694I, V726A, E148Q* (very frequent); minor alleles also detected | Serositis, fever, arthritis, chest pain | NR | NR | Sabbagh et al[288] |
| Algerian, Moroccan, and Tunisian Arabs | *M694V, M694I* (most common), *M680I, M680I, A744S, V726A, E148Q* | Serositis, fever, arthritis, chest pain | NR | NR | Belmahi et al[274] |
| Algerians | *M694I* (most common), *M694V, E148Q, A744S, M680I* | Abdominal pain, fever, arthritis, chest pain, erythema | 8% | NR | Ait-Idir et al[271] |
| Tunisian Arabs | *M680I* (most common), *M694V, M694I, V726A, E148Q, A744S, R761H, 1692del* | FMF criteria[284] | 3.5% | NR | Chaabouni et al[281] |

[a]Study performed in patients with end-stage kidney disease.
[b]Study performed in compound heterozygous patients.
*FMF*, Familial Mediterranean fever; *NR*, not reported.

polyarteritis nodosa, Behçet disease, rheumatic heart disease, and rheumatoid arthritis (reviewed by Guz and associates).[300] Of interest, individuals who carry a single mutated allele in the *MEFV* gene can also suffer from the syndrome of periodic fever, aphthosis, pharyngitis, and adenitis (PFAPA), ankylosing spondylitis, and Crohn disease.[313]

Secondary or reactive AA amyloidosis is the most severe complication of FMF. Before the advent of colchicine treatment, amyloidosis was reported to occur in approximately 75% of patients with FMF who were older than 40 years.[314] The disease is caused by the extracellular deposition of amyloid A fibrils. These fibrils consist of β-pleated sheet polymers of the N-terminal fragments, the products of incomplete proteolytic digestion of the acute-phase precursor serum amyloid A (SAA) protein, whose production is markedly increased in chronic inflammatory processes.[315] Amyloidosis is frequently found in Jews of North African descent, in Turks, and in Armenians. As mentioned earlier, a positive association of amyloidosis with the *M694V* mutation has been reported in patients from several ethnic groups.*

The *M694V* mutation has also been found in patients with FMF phenotype II, in which amyloidosis is detected before the onset of clinical symptoms of FMF.[293] Phenotype III is defined as the presence of two *MEFV* mutations (homozygous or compound heterozygote state) without clinical manifestation of FMF or amyloidosis. This condition, however, like phenotype II, could predispose to the development of amyloidosis in families in which one sibling is afflicted with FMF.[317] A screening study of patients with FMF from 14 countries worldwide—which included Israel, Turkey, Qatar, Jordan, and Lebanon—has revealed that amyloid nephropathy is present in 11.4% of patients with FMF.[318] In this study, however, the country of recruitment, rather than *MEFV* genotype, was found to be the leading risk factor for amyloidosis.[318] These findings underscore the relative contribution of environmental factors to the genetic background in defining the phenotypic variation and severity of the disease.[319]

Male gender, a positive family history of amyloidosis, pain flares in joints, and the SAA1 α/α genotype have been suggested as additional risk factors for amyloidosis.[311] Albuminuria is usually the first manifestation of renal involvement in patients with FMF and amyloidosis, and in untreated patients it may appear early in the course of FMF.[320] In one study, the serum cystatin C level was found to be significantly increased in patients with FMF and secondary amyloidosis. It was suggested that the cystatin C serum level may be an early marker of renal impairment, even before the onset of albuminuria.[321] Proteinuria, mostly represented by albumin, can reach the nephrotic range, with urinary protein excretion rates higher than 20 g/day. If untreated, AA amyloidosis progresses to ESKD, which ultimately necessitates RRT. Renal disease due to amyloidosis accounts for 35% and 60% of deaths in men and women, respectively, with FMF.[322] Extrarenal deposits of AA amyloid can be found in the liver, spleen, lung, thyroid, heart, adrenal glands, stomach, and testes. These deposits can be clinically significant and are associated with intestinal malabsorption and adrenal insufficiency, which are often diagnosed after the initiation of chronic hemodialysis or after kidney transplantation.[320,323,324]

The diagnosis of amyloidosis can be confirmed by tissue biopsy; the sensitivities of the rectal or bone marrow biopsy and renal biopsy are 79.5% and 88%, respectively, whereas the sensitivity of biopsy of abdominal fat is lower.[325–327] The presence of amyloid deposits is demonstrated histologically with Congo red staining of the biopsy tissue sample. Congo red–stained amyloid has an orange appearance when viewed under a light microscope and an apple green birefringence when viewed under polarized light. Another amyloid-specific stain, thioflavin T, is used less frequently than Congo red. Amyloidosis is diagnosed definitively on electron microscopy by the demonstration of characteristic amyloid fibrils. The AA protein in tissue can also be detected with antibodies against AA protein.[325]

In addition to AA amyloidosis, other kidney diseases have been diagnosed in patients with FMF. It is worth mentioning that many of the reports of systemic and inflammatory diseases in patients with FMF contain descriptions of kidney involvement.[293] In fact, the frequency of the reported nonamyloid glomerular lesions reflects the number of kidney biopsies performed in patients with abnormal findings on urinalysis or on kidney function tests. Recurrent focal and proliferative glomerulonephritis and polyarteritis nodosa were described in an early report of the disease.[328] Rapidly progressive glomerulonephritis, mesangial proliferative glomerulonephritis, IgA nephropathy, and membranous nephropathy have also been reported.[293,299,329–332]

**Treatment of Familial Mediterranean Fever.** Daily oral colchicine is the most effective therapy for patients with FMF, and its use since the 1980s has dramatically changed the course of the disease. Colchicine prevents both acute attacks of FMF and SAA amyloidosis.[333,334] The mechanism of colchicine action is not completely understood. The pathophysiology of FMF involves the recruitment and activation of neutrophils at serosal surfaces. Colchicine affects the motility of neutrophils by reducing their deformability and elasticity. These properties are crucial for their extravasation in response to inflammatory stimuli. On a cellular level, it is believed that one of its major actions is to interact with cytoskeletal structures, such as microtubules. It has been shown that colchicine accumulates in PMNCs, where it depolymerizes the microtubules and suppresses microtubule dynamics. Pyrin is also expressed in PMNCs and associates with microtubules.[335] Because colchicine also has an inhibitory effect on chemotaxis and reduces serum levels of IL-6, IL-8, and tumor necrosis factor-α (TNF-α),[336] its antiinflammatory action is thought to be related to its ability to suppress nuclear factor-kappa B (NF-κB) activation by attenuating calpain-mediated IκB kinase α degradation, which is enhanced by N-terminal cleaved pyrin.[337] Suppression of caspase-1 expression in PMNCs was also suggested to be a potential mechanism of the action of colchicine.[338]

In vitro, colchicine has been shown to have a specific effect on pyrin and pyrin-interacting protein, such as proline-serine-threonine phosphatase interacting protein 1 (PSTPIP1) and ASC. In THP-1 cells, colchicine reorganized cytoskeleton and downregulated MEFV expression. This effect, which may result in a reduction of the level of a proinflammatory mutant pyrin, may explain the suppressive mechanism of colchicine on FMF attacks.[339]

The most common adverse effects of colchicine are gastrointestinal, especially abdominal pain and diarrhea. Colchicine toxicity from overdosing is associated with hepatic, renal, muscle, and cerebral effects.[340] Approximately 5% to 10% of FMF patients are nonresponders, and 2% to 5% do not tolerate the drug, mainly due to gastrointestinal side effects. In M694V homozygotes, a significant portion of patients show a partial or minimal response to colchicine, despite being treated with appropriate doses.[341] In contrast, prolonged colchicine-free remission has been noted in some individuals, none of whom was homozygous for this mutation.[342]

One study has revealed the existence of an association between polymorphism of the adenosine triphosphate–binding cassette, subfamily B, member 1 (*ABCB1*) gene and the response to colchicine in Turkish patients with FMF. The *ABCB1* gene encodes p170—also known as multidrug resistance 1 (MDR1)—a glycoprotein that functions as a drug

*References 275, 278, 285, 287, 292, 293, and 316.

transport pump, which can cause a variety of drugs, including colchicine, to become extruded from cells. In this study, patients with FMF who had the TT genotype for the c.3435C>T variant of *ABCB1* responded better to colchicine in terms of treatment efficacy and lower dose requirements in comparison with patients who had the CT and CC genotypes.[343] These results warrant validation in further studies in patients with FMF from different ethnic populations.

Thalidomide, NSAIDs, corticosteroids, azathioprine, prazosin, and eprodisate disodium, an inhibitor of fibril formation, had occasionally been used to treat patients with FMF whose disease was refractory to colchicine.[325,344–346] Interferon-α (IFN-α) was one of the first drugs used to treat patients with FMF who were refractory to colchicine.[347] Two studies of patients with FMF who were treated with IFN-α have shown that the duration and pain intensity of most of the attacks were reduced by more than 50%.[348,349] In addition, clinical improvement has been reported in patients with FMF who were treated with the TNF-α antagonists etanercept or infliximab.[345,350,351]

Because most inflammatory manifestations of FMF are believed to be associated with the induction of IL-1β production by mutations in the C-terminal B30.2 domain of pyrin, it has been proposed that IL-1β antagonists may be an effective therapy for FMF. In fact, more studies have suggested that IL-1 inhibition seems to be a safe and effective alternative for patients with FMF who do not respond to or cannot tolerate colchicine. The IL-1β receptor antagonist anakinra has been shown to have a beneficial effect in patients with FMF and with cryopyrin-associated periodic syndromes.[344,346] Indeed, significant improvement and resolution of FMF symptoms have been reported in patients with colchicine-resistant FMF (crFMF) who were treated with anakinra.[346,352,353] Anakinra elicited a beneficial therapeutic response in individuals with FMF and chronic kidney disease, and even in a patient on maintenance hemodialysis and after kidney transplantation.[353,354] The main limitation of anakinra treatment in patients with FMF is probably the need for daily subcutaneous injections. The administration of canakinumab, a human monoclonal antibody against IL-1β, every 8 weeks has been associated with rapid remission of symptoms in FMF and cryopyrin-associated periodic syndromes.[355] In a systematic review of eight studies that included 40 patients with crFMF, rates of complete and partial response to canakinumab were 68% and 32%, respectively.[356]

Rilonacept is a dimeric fusion protein consisting of the extracellular portions of the human IL-1 receptor and the Fc region of human IgG1 that binds and neutralizes IL-1. A relatively small, randomized controlled study has shown a decrease in the attack rate, but the duration of attacks did not differ between placebo and rilonacept.[302] Similarly, a beneficial effect has been noted with the use of rilonacept in cryopyrin-associated periodic syndromes.[357]

**Familial Mediterranean Fever and End-Stage Kidney Disease.** In contrast to the poor prognosis of patients with primary (AL) amyloidosis who require RRT, most patients with FMF and secondary (AA) amyloidosis do relatively well with chronic dialysis.[358] However, the issue of which dialysis modality is ideal for the treatment of FMF-associated ESKD is still unresolved,[83] and prospective studies that compare the different modalities are still needed. Of the dialysis modalities, hemodialysis is more widely used in patients with FMF. Continuous ambulatory peritoneal dialysis (CAPD), however, has been performed successfully in selected patients. The effects of CAPD on azotemia and overall survival are similar in patients with nonamyloid diseases and patients with FMF. However, serum albumin levels are reported to be lower, and the rate of peritonitis and requirements for erythropoietin-stimulating agents (ESAs) higher, in patients with FMF who underwent CAPD than in patients with FMF who underwent hemodialysis.[359,360]

A considerable number of patients with FMF and ESKD have undergone kidney transplantation in the last few decades. The rates of survival of patients and allografts are reported to be worse or similar to those in the general population of kidney transplant recipients.[83,293,361–363] Analysis of the data from a single center in Israel has shown that graft survival is comparable between patients with FMF and controls.[364] However, FMF was associated with more than a twofold increased risk for death following transplantation. Infections and cardiovascular disease were the leading causes of death. Maintenance colchicine therapy is obligatory after kidney transplantation because it may prevent the recurrence both of FMF symptoms and of amyloidosis. However, recurrence of AA amyloidosis has been frequently reported 8 to 10 years after kidney transplantation,[365] and the rate of recurrence may be as high as 71%.[366] Adverse drug effects are seen in kidney transplant recipients with FMF who are taking cyclosporine. In addition, increased gastrointestinal complications can be observed in patients who are treated with a combination of mycophenolate mofetil and colchicine.[367]

## MANAGEMENT OF END-STAGE KIDNEY DISEASE IN THE MIDDLE EAST

Dialysis and kidney transplantation are available in all ME countries. In all industrialized and many developing ME countries, RRT is accessible to every patient with ESKD, regardless of the patient's socioeconomic status or whether the patient has health insurance (see Table 78.3 and Fig. 78.4).*

On the other hand, the number of patients offered RRT in other developing ME countries may be affected by late diagnosis and referral, the presence of comorbid conditions, the country's health system, reimbursement, and the availability of dialysis facilities.[2,151]

## DIALYSIS

### PERITONEAL DIALYSIS

Throughout the ME, hemodialysis is the preferred treatment modality for ESKD (see Fig. 78.4). Peritoneal dialysis is an underused treatment modality for ESKD, although its use has been increasing in Tunisia, Kuwait, Iran, Saudi Arabia, Qatar, and Turkey.†

Several medical and nonmedical factors play an important role in inhibiting the widespread use of peritoneal dialysis throughout the ME, including the following: (1) health care providers generally offer low or no reimbursement for

*References 19, 109, 111–113, 118, 119, 127, 128, 136, 144, 151, and 368–373.

†References 112, 121, 125, 127, 132, 374, and 375.

peritoneal dialysis; (2) the numbers of peritoneal dialysis training programs, qualified nephrologists, and skilled dialysis nurses are limited, and the salaries of attending physicians for peritoneal dialysis are low; (3) many patients have poor education and poor hygiene practices; and (4) patients and caregivers have concerns about the high rates of peritonitis.

At the end of 2006, 38,824 patients were treated with dialysis (87.4% with hemodialysis, 12.6% with peritoneal dialysis) in Turkey, and 99.7% of all patients undergoing dialysis were covered by the social security system.[370] The Turkish experience in establishing a peritoneal dialysis program has been outstanding and could be used as an example by other ME countries. The Turkish Multicenter Peritoneal Dialysis Study Group (TULIP) has established a platform for organizing peritoneal dialysis facilities and units. The group helped standardize patient records and various peritoneal dialysis treatments and maximized the number of patients with ESKD who can benefit from this treatment modality. TULIP has published clinical research that has affected peritoneal dialysis practice locally and worldwide.[370] The Turkish peritoneal dialysis program has good rates of survival of patients and technique efficacy, which are comparable with those in Western industrialized countries.[154] The peritoneal dialysis dropout rate was 21%, and the incidence of peritonitis was one episode per 35.5 patient-months in 2007. Dyslipidemia was the most common noninfectious complication[134]; cardiovascular diseases (42.3%), followed by infections (19.9%) and cerebrovascular events (13.6%), were the major causes of death among Turkish patients undergoing peritoneal dialysis.[134,154] Moreover, peritoneal dialysis has been suggested as a means of reducing the seroconversion rate for hepatitis C virus (HCV) in populations with ESKD and a high prevalence of infection[376]; such treatment thereby confers an advantage to kidney transplantation candidates.[377]

Peritoneal dialysis was started in Iran in 1978 and in Saudi Arabia and Kuwait during the 1980s with imported peritoneal dialysis solutions. The costs of this treatment are low in Turkey and Iran because peritoneal dialysis solutions began to be produced locally in Turkey in 1994 and in Iran in 1995.[125] Establishment of a peritoneal dialysis registry and a multidisciplinary approach has dramatically increased the numbers of patients undergoing peritoneal dialysis in Iran since 2001.[107,125] In 2010, the 1-, 3-, and 5-year patient survival rates in Iran were reported as 89%, 64%, and 49%, respectively, whereas death- and transplantation-censored technique survival rates were 90%, 73%, and 58%.[107] The main causes of death among Iranian patients undergoing peritoneal dialysis were cardiac events (46%), cerebral stroke (10%), and infection (8%). More recently, the rate of peritonitis has improved from one episode in 15.2 to 19.4 patient-months to one episode in 25 patient-months (in 2010).[107,125]

The use of peritoneal dialysis has been growing in Qatar since its introduction in 1997, and peritoneal dialysis is offered to approximately 23% of ESKD patients. Most of these patients are non-Qatari male expatriates, a group that favors a mode of dialysis that can be self-administered, secures the ability to work or travel, requires less dietary restrictions, and potentially decreases the hospital and medical costs.[374]

These advantages of peritoneal dialysis, which provides flexibility and ease of adjustment for lifestyle and daily schedule, has encouraged some clinically stable Muslim patients on peritoneal dialysis to fast during the holy month of Ramadan.[378] However, patients who intend to fast need to be comprehensively educated and followed up by their peritoneal dialysis units.

## HEMODIALYSIS

There are limited detailed published data on hemodialysis in the ME with regard to practice patterns and outcomes, such as the quality of dialysis, survival of patients per technique, type of vascular access, standard dialysate solutions and dialyzers, medical complications and their management, comorbid conditions, and other measures of quality assurance.*

In general, quality is ensured according to best medical practice guidelines in industrialized ME countries with more resources, easily accessible health care systems, and availability of advanced medical supplies.[111,112,128,142,386–390] In ME countries that lack resources, the quality of dialysis is dictated by nonmedical financial considerations. In these countries, dialysis may be offered only once or twice weekly because of recent conflicts, lack of skilled personnel, distance of the dialysis centers from the patient's residence, and inability of the patient to pay for more frequent treatment.[22,86,128,138,373] The number of patients who withdraw from hemodialysis therapy because of financial problems has not been documented, however. A small number of patients do seek pre-ESKD care in most ME countries.[128,381,391,392]

Practice guidelines for hemodialysis have been developed in Egypt. These included five main domains: personnel, patient care practices, infection prevention and control, facility, and documentation or records. Before distribution of the guidelines, one study had disclosed flawed compliance and variability in adoption of evidence-based hemodialysis guidelines among 16 Egyptian facilities affiliated with the Ministry of Health and Population.[379] Therefore, it is mandatory to distribute these guidelines to all hemodialysis facilities in Egypt, along with the organization of workshops to educate staff and follow-up to ensure implementation of the guidelines. In Libya, the provision of dialysis was adequate in 2010. However, several areas for improvement were identified by Alashek and associates,[138] such as lack of national dialysis practice guidelines, and few clinical practitioners were familiar with KDOQI guidelines. Because of continuous drought, many dialysis centers were obliged to dig their own wells to maintain the water supply. However, testing of water quality was not regularly practiced. In addition, wide discrepancy in methods applied to manage and monitor patients was observed among centers.[138,140]

According to the 2016 SCOT report,[112] 16,315 patients undergoing hemodialysis were treated in 243 centers in Saudi Arabia. Of these patients, approximately 17% were on active waiting lists for kidney transplantation. Bicarbonate dialysis solutions were used in all centers, and only a few centers (6.3%) still use acetate dialysis solutions.[393] The predominant type of vascular access for hemodialysis varies among the Gulf Cooperation Council (GCC) countries.[389] In Saudi Arabia, arteriovenous fistulas (71.2% of all patients) are mostly used, followed by jugular catheters (12.6%) and arteriovenous grafts (7.6%),[393] whereas in Kuwait 56% of patients undergo dialysis via catheters.[389] In Tehran, arteriovenous fistula is the type of

*References 109, 111, 112, 124, 128, 129, 138, 140, 369, and 379–390.

vascular access used most in patients receiving hemodialysis (91%); only 3% of such patients have arteriovenous grafts, and 4% have permanent catheters.[144] Arteriovenous fistula was also preferred in Turkey. In 2016, it was used in 79.1% of Turkish patients undergoing routine hemodialysis, whereas permanent tunneled catheters and temporary catheters were used in 19.4% of patients.[128]

Reuse of dialyzers is not practiced in Saudi Arabia, Libya, and Iran[138,394] and is prohibited by law in Egypt.[381] Approximately 87% of Saudi patients undergoing hemodialysis are treated with ESAs and, of these patients, approximately 23% have hemoglobin levels lower than 10 g/dL. In Turkey, ESAs are administered to 61.8% of patients undergoing hemodialysis. In comparison, 48.2% of patients undergoing hemodialysis in Tehran have anemia as a result of low-dose treatment with ESAs, and dialysis may be inadequate because the mean measured treatment adequacy for these patients was $0.97 \pm 0.25$.[144] Thus, common clinical practice for hemodialysis in Iran does not meet all the targets recommended by international guidelines.[144,382]

Limited studies have been conducted to describe the patterns, prevalence, or therapy of CKD-associated mineral bone disorders (CKD-MBDs) in patients undergoing dialysis in ME countries.[128,387] In developing ME countries, the use of aluminum-based phosphate binders, presence of high amounts of strontium in the soil, and use of dialysis acetate concentrates that are contaminated with strontium have been implicated as causes of osteomalacia in adult patients undergoing hemodialysis and of rickets in pediatric patients undergoing hemodialysis.[395,396] Hyperphosphatemia and increased serum levels of calcium-phosphorus product are serious problems in dialysis recipients in developing ME countries, and their occurrence is correlated with poor patient knowledge of an appropriate diet. In a large cross-sectional multicenter study that included 1005 patients in Egypt who were undergoing hemodialysis, two-thirds of the patients had hyperphosphatemia and one-third had an elevated serum level of calcium-phosphorus product. The patients used mainly calcium-based phosphate binders.[397] In most developing ME countries, economic considerations hinder the use of the newer non–calcium-based phosphate binders, calcium-sensing receptor agonists (calcimimetics), or vitamin D receptor agonists. Therefore, prolonged or additional dialysis sessions are frequently prescribed to control hyperphosphatemia in patients undergoing hemodialysis.[128,144,387,397]

The results of one survey have suggested that practicing Saudi nephrologists have an adequate perception of the morbidity in patients with CKD-MBDs.[398] However, the results of this survey also identified a need for creating national guidelines because the physicians' assessment of the prevalence, patterns, and results of therapeutic interventions in patients with CKD-MBDs was relatively inadequate. Approximately 25% of their patients had hyperphosphatemia (serum phosphorus levels >6 mg/dL), and 20% had hypocalcemia (serum calcium levels <8.4 mg/dL), although vitamin D was administered orally to most patients. In view of the current status of CKD-MBDs in the ME and the associated economic and logistic constraints, a committee of experienced nephrologists from the region was created. Its members examined the KDIGO guidelines and formulated recommendations that can be implemented practically for the management of CKD-MBD in the ME.[399]

## MANAGEMENT OF END-STAGE KIDNEY DISEASE WITH VIRAL HEPATITIS

Available global data have indicated that the prevalence of chronic infection with hepatitis B virus (HBV) and HCV is high in African and ME populations.[400–405] These two viral infections have considerable effects on morbidity and mortality among patients with ESKD, as well as on graft survival in kidney transplant recipients.[406–410] However, surveys are still needed to estimate the incidence and prevalence correctly of these infections in patients with CKD and ESKD in each ME country. In addition, screening will identify patients who would benefit from a number of highly efficacious, direct-acting, antiviral oral therapies.[410–412] The HCV epidemic is particularly devastating in Egypt, where its prevalence in the general population is estimated to be more than 18%. The start of the HCV epidemic in Egypt is attributed to the use of unsterilized needles and syringes during the mass anti-schistosomiasis treatment programs that were conducted during the 1960s and 1970s.[413] Several studies have reported a dismal prevalence of anti-HCV serologic findings among Egyptian patients undergoing hemodialysis and kidney transplant recipients that ranged between 46% and 100%.[404,410,413–415] Implementation of an infection control program by 60 Egyptian dialysis facilities has 3 years later resulted in improvements in infection control practices among health care workers and a subsequent decrease in the annual incidence of HCV infection among patients undergoing dialysis from 28% to 6%.[414]

Among Saudi patients undergoing hemodialysis, according to the 2016 SCOT report,[112] the prevalence of HBV positivity is 4%, whereas HCV infection continued to be problematic (12%). Nonetheless, it has decreased compared with findings in previous reports.[393] However, there is considerable variability in the prevalence of HCV infection between the various regions of Saudi Arabia (9%–16%).[112] This variability is important to consider when patients who are undergoing hemodialysis travel to other units and emphasizes the importance of screening them for seroconversion after their return.

> ***Clinical Relevance***
> **Hepatitis C in Dialysis**
> Owing to high prevalence of HCV infection in some countries in the ME, dialysis patients who travel to the ME and receive dialysis should be monitored for seroconversion after their return.

The annual rate of HCV seroconversion in Saudi patients undergoing hemodialysis is between 7% and 9%. The most common variant of the virus is HCV genotype 4, which is also prevalent in North African countries in the ME, followed by HCV genotypes 1a and 1b.[406,408,416] Implementation of strict measures of infection control and isolation of HCV-positive patients and dialysis machines has resulted in a significant drop in the annual incidence of HCV infections from 2.4% to 0.2% in one Saudi hemodialysis center.[417] A similar high prevalence of HCV was observed in neighboring GCC countries, which was associated with a higher risk of death, hospitalization, and worse quality of life scores.[111,418]

In Iran, where genotypes 3a and 1a are the common variants, impressive drops in the rates of HCV and hepatitis B surface antigen (HBsAg) positivity have been reported in patients undergoing hemodialysis. These decreases (14.4% in 1999 to 4.5% in 2006 for HCV and 3.8% in 1999 to 2.6% in 2006 for HBV) have been attributed to the introduction of several measures, such as strict isolation policies, no reuse of dialyzers, compulsory HBV vaccination in patients, and early kidney transplantation.[394] Implementation of routine virologic testing, strict isolation measures, HBV vaccination, and ESA administration with few blood product transfusion requirements have resulted in a low prevalence of both HBV (1.7%–2%) and HCV (3.7%–5.7%) infection among Israeli patients undergoing dialysis between 2005 and 2010, according to the 2012 ICDC report.[146]

Using second-generation immunoassays to detect HCV infection in 30 Turkish dialysis centers, Köhler has found that the prevalence of HCV was 49.9% in 1995.[408] Sayiner and colleagues have reported that the duration of dialysis, kidney transplantation history, and history of blood product transfusion were all related to HCV transmission and high prevalence of HCV among Turkish patients undergoing hemodialysis.[419] Turkey is also endemic for HBV infection; 10% of patients undergoing hemodialysis and 2.9% of blood donors are HBsAg-positive. Of note is that the 2008 and 2016 registry of the Turkish Society of Nephrology[128,420] has reported a progressive decline in the prevalence of HBV infection (4.5%–3.88%), HCV infection (12.7%–5.2%), and both infections (0.9%–0.3%) in Turkish patients undergoing hemodialysis. A similar trend was observed among hemodialysis patients in Lebanon, who have the lowest prevalence of HBV and HCV (1.6% and 4.7%, respectively).[421] The results of a survey conducted among Jordanian patients undergoing hemodialysis during 2003 revealed HBV positivity in 4% and HCV positivity in 21%, with annual seroconversion rates of 0.34% for HBV and 2.6% for HCV.[113] In 2007, high seropositivities for HBV (8%) and HCV (22%) were also detected in Palestinian patients undergoing hemodialysis who were residing in the Gaza Strip.[422]

Alashek and colleagues have found a remarkably high prevalence of seropositivity for HCV among Libyan patients undergoing hemodialysis (31.1%), which is 25-fold higher than the general population.[139] The overall incidence of seroconversion during this 1-year prospective study was 7.1%, with wide variation between hemodialysis units. Conversely, the prevalence of HBsAg positivity was low (2.6%), with a seroconversion incidence of 0.6%. Factors associated with seroconversions, such as duration of dialysis, history of receiving dialysis in another center in Libya, and prior kidney transplantation, possibly suggest nosocomial transmission.[139] In Jordan, 1.2% and 7.8% of prevalent dialysis patients are seropositive to HBV and HCV, respectively.[129] In comparison, the adjusted prevalence of HBV is 4.6% among patients in Germany who are undergoing hemodialysis, 4.3% in Italy, 3.7% in France, 2.1% in Spain, 2.1% in Japan, and 2.4% in the United States, and adjusted seroconversion rates range from 0.4 to 1.8/100 patient-years.[423] The adjusted prevalence of HCV also varies among these countries—22.9% in Spain, 20.5% in Italy, 10.4% in France, 3.8% in Germany, 2.6% in the United Kingdom, 14.8% in Japan, and 14% in the United States. The adjusted seroconversion rates range from 1.2 to 3.9/100 patient-years and are highest in Italy and Spain.[424]

### DIALYSIS-RELATED OUTCOMES

With regard to other dialysis-related outcomes, reports from Egypt have revealed significant center-specific effects (which were not defined) on the survival and quality of life of patients undergoing dialysis; these effects were dependent largely on funding.[381] In Syria, the 3-year survival rate among patients undergoing hemodialysis was unsatisfactory, ranging from 26% to 64% in different hemodialysis centers.[119] Regrettably, during the recent conflicts, death due to lack of dialysis or underdialysis has been common in Syria and Yemen, although the exact figures are difficult to extract from published literature.[22] In Jordan, the 1-year mortality rate among patients undergoing hemodialysis was approximately 20%,[113] although it decreased to 7% in 2016.[129] In Libya, the 1-year mortality was similar to many other countries (21.2%).[141] However, this is a poor outcome when taking into consideration the young mean age of patients undergoing hemodialysis. Although not reported, it is expected that the survival of Libyan ESKD patients was also aggravated by the conflicts in their country.[141] According to the 2018 ICDC report,[127] the unadjusted 1-, 2-, 3-, and 10-year survival rates among Israeli patients undergoing dialysis were 86.6%, 73%, 61.3%, and 15%, respectively, from 1990 to 2010. Of note, there appears to be a survival advantage for Arab patients over Jewish patients on maintenance dialysis in Israel, in contrast to the life expectancy of Arabs in the general population, which is 3 to 4 years lower than that of the Jewish population.[135] The survival of patients undergoing hemodialysis was high in Qatar, with 1-year and 5-year survival rates of 84% and 53%, respectively,[124] as well as in other GCC countries (annual mortality, 8%–14.65%).[111]

It is of interest that a health disparity exists for both legal and illegal immigrants from ME countries with CKD who live and work in Western industrialized countries and may need RRT. The ethnic and educational backgrounds of these patients are different from those of the local population. Accordingly, they face potential problems with communication, health insurance, and care.[9,27,425] Fogazzi and Castelnovo have reported their experience with these patients who were treated in an Italian dialysis unit.[426] Although the number of patients was small, they reported that those undergoing hemodialysis who came from developing countries, which included some ME countries, were younger at the initiation of dialysis (38.2 ± 7.9 years vs. 63 ± 12.6 years), were referred at a later stage of their disease, and had more infections, such as tuberculosis and viral hepatitis, than did patients from the local population who were undergoing hemodialysis. Furthermore, they also reported that a visit to their native countries was usually associated with medical complications, such as worsening of anemia.

## KIDNEY TRANSPLANTATION

In ME countries, as in all other countries, kidney transplantation is recognized as the treatment of choice for ESKD. The beneficial effects of kidney transplantation on life expectancy, quality of life, and medical expenses are greater than those associated with maintenance dialysis. However, legislative obstacles, an underdeveloped and poorly funded health care infrastructure, poor public awareness of the importance of organ donation, lack of effective kidney transplantation programs, cultural and religious barriers, and lack of trained multidisciplinary medical teams are some of the obstacles that prevent the promotion of kidney transplantation in some ME countries.[86,122,126,427–433]

Most ME countries are members of the Middle East Society for Organ Transplantation (MESOT). MESOT includes Iran, Turkey, and all the Arab countries in the ME, as well as Pakistan, Cyprus, and some countries of central Asia.[126,427] There are very few organ procurement centers in the MESOT member countries for overseeing the activities of organ donation, sharing, and transplantation at a national level. Israel is not a member of MESOT; it has its own national center for organ transplantation. The first successful living- and deceased-donor kidney transplants in the ME were performed in Israel (1964 and 1966, respectively)[117] and were reported to have been performed in Iran in 1967 and 2003, respectively.[126,434] The first successful kidney transplantation in an Arab country in the ME was performed with a kidney from a deceased donor with no heartbeat in Jordan in 1972. Most other ME countries, such as Lebanon and Turkey, started their kidney transplantation programs during the early 1970s, and Egypt and Saudi Arabia commenced their programs in 1976 and 1979, respectively. Since then, the remaining ME countries have established their own kidney transplantation programs; Libya did so in 2004. Currently, kidney transplantation programs are active in most ME countries but are relatively limited in Algeria, Yemen, the UAE, and Bahrain (see Tables 78.2 and 78.3).[86,121–123,126,435–438]

Most kidneys for transplantation are obtained from living donors. An important milestone that paved the way for organ donation for transplantation from deceased donors in Arab countries in the ME was the Amman declaration in 1986. In this declaration, Islamic theologians recognized that brain death was irreversible and could be used to declare a person legally dead, thereby making it permissible to disconnect that person from mechanical life support systems. This declaration was preceded in 1982 by a resolution of the Islamic Council in Saudi Arabia that permitted the use of organs from both living and deceased donors for transplantation.[121,439,440] Similar declarations have since been made by religious authorities in Egypt, Turkey, and Iran.[121,439] As a result of these declarations, most Arab countries in the ME, including Egypt, have now enacted laws for regulated organ donation for transplantation from both living and cadaveric donors, and transplantation programs for kidneys and other organs are beginning to expand.[108,119,441] Programs for donation after cardiac death are limited in many Arab countries because of religious, legal, ethical, and social issues.[442] Such a program has recently begun in Israel.[443]

In his code of Jewish law, the Mishneh Torah (Laws of Sanhedrin, 12: 3), the 12th century philosopher and physician Maimonides interpreted the Talmud as saying that someone who saves the life of one person is considered to have saved the entire world. This is similar to what is written in the Koran, Chapter 5, verse 32: "... if any one saved a life, it would be as if he saved the life of all mankind." Therefore, organ donation that saves a life is considered in Islam and Judaism to be a good deed. With regard to living related donors, Bulka has argued that organ donation is permissible because the danger to the donor is minimal, but it is not obligatory.[444] Likewise, Christians believe that organ donation is an act of love and nobility (e.g., as interpreted from Corinthians and from the parable of the Good Samaritan in Luke, Chapter 10, verses 25 to 37).[445]

Active deceased-donor kidney transplantation programs exist in Iran, Israel, Turkey, and 10 Arab countries (Algeria, Bahrain, Jordan, Kuwait, Lebanon, Morocco, Oman, Qatar, Saudi Arabia, and Tunisia; see Table 78.2).[86,122,446] However, deceased-donor kidney transplantation is inadequate to address the current need for allografts, and the number of patients on kidney transplantation waiting lists in these ME countries has been progressively increasing. The use of kidneys from living related donors is increasing, but the gap between demand and supply is continuously widening in all ME countries. To meet the growing demand for kidneys and the shortfall in donors, some countries have initiated kidney transplantation programs involving organs from living unrelated donors. Using emotionally related donors extends donor eligibility to include individuals who are not genetically related to recipients.

Although kidney transplantation involving organs from deceased donors has been increasing in the ME, it accounts for less than 21% of kidney transplantations in most ME countries, with large national variations.[126,447] In 2016, 3416 kidney transplantations were performed in Turkey, of which 22.8% were from deceased donors.[128] In Saudi Arabia, kidney transplantation from living unrelated donors is forbidden. SCOT reported that 798 kidney transplantations were performed in 2016, and 16% of the kidneys (125) were obtained from deceased donors[448]; the rest were obtained from living related donors. In fact, in 2006, Saudi Arabia had the highest reported rate of living-donor kidney transplantations worldwide, at 32 procedures pmp, followed by Jordan (29 procedures pmp), Iceland (26 procedures pmp), Iran (23 procedures pmp), and the United States (21 procedures pmp).[371] However, the quoted Saudi statistic should be interpreted cautiously because the rate of living related donor kidney transplantations is 10.1 pmp. According to Nöel,[449] the report by Horvat and colleagues[371] probably included "transplant tourism" activity because it incorporated data on kidney transplantation in Saudi patients from living unrelated donors that was performed in other countries.

In Egypt, approximately 7% of Egyptian patients with ESKD are offered kidney transplantation in the year of diagnosis, and no kidneys are obtained from deceased donors— 80% of the kidneys are obtained from living unrelated donors, and 20% are obtained from living related donors. In 2013, 264 kidney transplantations were performed in Israel; of the transplanted kidneys, 43.5% were obtained from deceased donors and 54.5% from living related and living unrelated donors. The ratio of deceased donors to living donors is not constant—according to the annual reports of the Israeli National Transplant Center—yet it remains higher than in most ME countries (e.g., 38.2% in 2017). This could be attributed to a high consent rate (about 60%) for organ donation after brain death.

Kidney transplantation in Syria commenced in 1976 with exclusive reliance on kidneys from living related donors. Since 2003, transplantation of kidneys from deceased donors has been allowed. As of 2010, 13.2 kidney transplantations pmp were performed, of which 22% were from deceased donors.[119,122] Unfortunately, the war in Syria destroyed the hospitals' infrastructure and decreased the kidney transplant programs from eight to four centers, along with difficulties in providing immunosuppressive therapies.[450]

In Iran, the living unrelated donor transplantation program operates under the close supervision and scrutiny of the Ministry of Health and Medical Education, Iranian Scientific Society of Organ Transplantation, Foundation for Patients with Special Diseases, and Dialysis and Transplant Patients Association (DATPA).[451] In the Iranian model, patients who need kidney transplantation are referred to the DATPA, a charity founded in 1978 by Iranian patients with ESKD, which acts as a liaison agency between patients and potential donors. The altruistic volunteers are also registered by the DATPA and undergo evaluation in the foundation's clinics. Several important features characterize the Iranian model of living unrelated donors for kidney transplantation[436]:

- No coercion is allowed.
- Written consent is obtained from the donor and the donor's parents or spouse.
- Donors are rewarded with gifts from the government.
- No commercialism is allowed.
- The medical teams receive no financial benefit.
- Recipients and donors must be Iranian citizens.
- Time on the waiting list is minimal.

Consequently, the annual number of kidney transplantations has substantially increased in Iran, from 1421 in 2000 to 2285 in 2010.[120,436] However, the 86% share of living unrelated kidney donation in 2000 (20.1 pmp) decreased to 75% in 2006 (23 pmp) and to 69% in 2010 (21.8 pmp). This change was mainly due to a substantial parallel increase in brain-dead kidney donation (2.2% in 2000, equivalent to 0.4 pmp, increasing to 26% and 7.9 pmp in 2010), after the Organ Transplantation and Brain Death Act in 2000, which legalized brain-dead organ donation.[120] Of note, 10 years after the introduction of the controlled living unrelated donor kidney transplantation program in Iran, the national waiting list for renal transplants was eliminated.[452,453]

Simforoosh and associates have reported that patient and graft survival rates of 2155 Iranian recipients of kidneys from living unrelated donors after 15 years were 76.4%, and 53.2%, respectively.[454] These results are comparable with survival data in the 2003 annual report of the US Renal Data System on living donor kidney transplantations.[455] However, the Iranian model has been criticized for ethical reasons because 85% of the vendors are very poor, a fact that may increase the risk that potential donors will withhold relevant medical information.[456] A study from the Shiraz Transplant Center has revealed that Iranian paid unrelated donors have a lower quality of life and a higher incidence of microalbuminuria compared with related donors.[457] Hence, the lack of long-term donor follow-up and the direct financial connection between donor and recipient are major weak points that should be ethically reviewed.[120,458–460]

## COMMERCIAL KIDNEY TRANSPLANTATION

The lack of deceased donors for kidney allograft transplantation, combined with other medical factors (prolonged graft survival and improved surgical techniques, including laparoscopic nephrectomy) and nonmedical factors (economic and cultural), have motivated many patients with ESKD to seek kidney transplants from living unrelated donors outside their home countries. This practice is often called commercial kidney transplantation or organ tourism[461] because the donor sells his or her kidney for a certain amount of money. These kidney transplantations are performed in many countries worldwide, such as the Philippines, Russia, India, China, Pakistan, and South Africa, as well as some ME countries, such as Turkey, Iraq, and Egypt.[428,462–464] The surgery is commonly performed in substandard conditions under the cover of secrecy. Many transplant recipients return to their homeland 1 to 2 weeks after transplantation without crucial information (e.g., a complete medical report, important information about the donor, HLA typing, and details of the medical treatment, surgery, and postoperative care). In addition, the recipients are exposed to potential risk for infection, such as HBV, HCV, or human immunodeficiency virus infection, as well as tuberculosis from inadequately evaluated donors. Thus the results of such commercial kidney transplantations are reported to be substandard.[461,463,464]

To undermine the practice of global commercial kidney transplantation, the Transplantation Society and the ISN convened an international summit meeting in Istanbul, Turkey, in April 2008. The outcome of this meeting was the "Declaration of Istanbul on Organ Trafficking and Transplant Tourism," which suggested that strategies to increase the donor pool and encourage legitimate, lifesaving transplantation programs be developed by countries to prevent organ trafficking, transplant commercialism, and transplant tourism. In addition, strategies should be aimed at stopping and prohibiting unethical activities, as well as encouraging safe and accountable practices that both meet the needs of transplant recipients and protect donors.[462,465,466] Many ME countries need to develop national self-sufficiency in organ donation to combat organ tourism and achieve global justice in transplantation.[462,465]

In 2008, two laws were approved by the Israeli parliament, the Brain-Respiratory Death Law and the Organ Transplantation Law. As a result, health insurance reimbursement for transplantation performed abroad that contravenes local Israeli laws was prohibited, and criminal penalties for brokering organ sales were introduced. Consequently, Israel has both increased organ donations from living and deceased sources and has reduced the number of transplant candidates seeking transplantation abroad (from 150 in 2006 to 44 in 2017).[446,467] In Egypt, however, in spite of the April 2010 organ transplantation law, which prohibits and penalizes organ trafficking and permits deceased donation in accord with the WHO Guiding Principles and the Declaration of Istanbul, little enforcement has been evident, and the problem of a black market in organs from living donors has increased.[428,441,462,468]

## PHARMACOLOGIC TREATMENT OF KIDNEY TRANSPLANT RECIPIENTS

In general, all approved medications that are used worldwide to treat kidney transplant recipients are also used in the ME.[120,435] In all ME countries with kidney transplantation programs, induction therapy with methylprednisolone, lymphocyte-depleting agents, or IL-2 receptor antagonists is widely used. In most of the commercial transplantation programs, induction therapy with lymphocyte-depleting agents is routinely given to reduce the frequency of acute graft rejection so that the recipient can be discharged early after the transplantation surgery. No reports have yet been published on the long-term complications of this routine treatment, such as bone marrow suppression, cytomegalovirus infections, and posttransplantation lymphoproliferative disorder.

Maintenance treatment after kidney transplantation in most ME countries consists of triple therapy with corticosteroids, azathioprine, or mycophenolate mofetil and calcineurin inhibitors. A small number of kidney transplantation centers have started prescribing rapamycin, a drug that inhibits a serine-threonine kinase called the mammalian target of rapamycin (mTOR), to prevent transplant rejection.[120,439] Treatment of acute rejection in most ME countries consists mainly of methylprednisolone (Solu-Medrol) and rabbit antithymocyte globulin (Thymoglobulin). Hyperimmune globulins and plasmapheresis are used by some centers when indicated.

## POSTTRANSPLANTATION COMPLICATIONS

There have been only a few reports in the literature on the outcomes, as well as patient and graft survival rates, after kidney transplantation in ME countries. In general, these reports claim that outcomes in Saudi Arabia, Kuwait, Egypt, and North African countries in the ME are in line with international standards, although infections remain the main reason for morbidity and mortality.[128,149,151,432,454, 464]

Distinctive infections are of special concern in some ME countries. Tuberculosis is prevalent among dialysis recipients in some countries such as Saudi Arabia, Yemen, Turkey, and the North African countries in the ME.[431,469–473] Patients in these countries are at increased risk for developing active tuberculosis after kidney transplantation, and approximately 30% have symptoms of tuberculosis in extrapulmonary organs, particularly the lymph nodes, gastrointestinal tract, and peritoneal cavity. The Mantoux test often yields negative results in kidney transplant recipients, possibly because of the suppression of cellular immunity. Tuberculosis in the graft kidney tends to manifest as granulomatous interstitial nephritis. Urinalysis results are often negative for bacilli. The diagnosis is usually made on kidney biopsy or after nephrectomy in transplant recipients, who often present with fever of unknown origin and deteriorating graft function.

Prophylactic treatment with isoniazid or rifampin for patients at high risk (Mantoux skin test reaction of >10 mm) has decreased the development of active tuberculosis. An important sequela of this treatment is the induction of cytochrome P450 enzymes by the antituberculous drugs, which results in a severe drop in the circulating therapeutic levels of calcineurin inhibitors and, consequently, severe acute rejection. Therefore, increasing the dose of calcineurin inhibitors and frequent monitoring of their circulating levels are mandatory in such cases.[431,472]

Viral hepatitis, as discussed previously, is also common in the ME, especially among patients undergoing dialysis. Eligible patients with HBV and HCV infections are offered transplantation in many ME kidney transplantation centers after appropriate presurgical workup and management.[406,472,474]

The most common types of neoplasia among kidney transplant recipients are skin malignancies, lymphoproliferative disorders, and Kaposi sarcoma. The incidence of some uncommon tumors in the general population (e.g., Kaposi sarcoma) can be 400- to 500-fold higher among kidney transplant recipients. Kaposi sarcoma is most often seen in transplant recipients of Mediterranean, Jewish, and Arabic descent. Its reported incidence is 0.5% in most Western industrialized countries and as high as 5.3% in Saudi Arabia.[472,475–478]

> ***Clinical Relevance***
> **Kaposi Sarcoma Postransplant**
>
> Kaposi sarcoma is more common in patients from the ME, potentially linked to greater rates of human herpesvirus 8 seropositivity than in Europe and North America.

The preponderance of cases of Kaposi sarcoma in certain ethnic groups appears to be linked to the geographic distribution of human herpesvirus 8 infection, inasmuch as more than 80% of transplant recipients with Kaposi sarcoma are seropositive for human herpesvirus 8 before undergoing transplantation.[478]

## SUMMARY

The ME has a strategic global location. Its fascinating geography is combined with rich national histories, cultures, and resources. In addition, the countries of the ME differ in their economics, political systems, culture, and bioecology, all of which eventually translate into disparities in their health care systems, as well as in disease epidemiologic features, causes, management, and outcomes. The burden of kidney diseases is high in all ME countries and is compounded by many risk factors in the region, although data from developing countries are possibly underestimates. Practicing nephrologists in the ME are familiar with the genetic background, social habits, and culture of their patients. However, this is not so for many individuals of ME origin who now live in non-ME countries. Nephrologists in those countries need to take these considerations into account when diagnosing or treating the kidney diseases and comorbid conditions of their patients of ME origin. Therefore, the emerging epidemic of diabetes mellitus in many ME countries is pertinent, and the prevailing genetic kidney diseases in the various population groups who live in the ME, have been reviewed in this chapter.

Moreover, the ME has experience in management of mass disasters and consequent kidney complications, which can be implemented in regions outside the ME. However, several issues still need to be addressed, and hurdles must be overcome to improve the overall management of kidney diseases in the ME. Well-conducted epidemiologic cohort studies are urgently needed, and regional and national registries must be established as sources of transparent and accurate data. The results of the studies should provide accurate estimates of the public health burden of AKI, CKD, and ESKD, their risk factors, and comorbid conditions. This information should also improve the quality of therapy provided to patients. In addition, these efforts should also focus on the special needs of refugees in countries where human-engendered and natural disasters have occurred.

The entire international nephrology community agrees that improving existing diagnostic methods and establishing preventive strategies for the detection and treatment of kidney diseases at the earliest possible stage is of utmost importance, especially in countries with limited resources or health care expenditures. Therefore, to achieve these goals, ME countries need to invest in the following: (1) training qualified nephrologists and medical personnel; (2) public education and campaigns for lifestyle modification to combat obesity and diabetes mellitus and to explain proper use of over-the-counter drugs; (3) premarital genetic counseling to decrease the burden of genetic diseases; (4) vigorous treatment of comorbid conditions, which include infectious diseases, and strategies for preventing dehydration in tropical ME countries; and (5) use of low-cost, generic medications.[52,76,86,469,479]

Because transplantation is the most cost-effective treatment for ESKD, ME countries also need to create a societal environment that motivates and encourages its population to support organ donation for transplantation in patients with ESKD. Encouraging organ donation through deceased donors, living related donors, and paired-exchange kidney transplantation programs, as well as organ sharing among the MESOT member states, will enable ME countries to reach national sufficiency for organ transplantation. The establishment of such programs will then help reduce the long waiting lists in each ME country and combat unethical commercial kidney transplantations.[76,86,96,427]

## ACKNOWLEDGMENT

The authors are deeply grateful to Dr. Dvora Rubinger who contributed to the previous versions of this chapter.

 Complete reference list available at ExpertConsult.com.

## KEY REFERENCES


1. Held CC, Cummings JT. *Middle East Patterns: Places, Peoples, and Politics*. 6th ed. Boulder, CO: Westview Press; 2014.
6. Mokdad AH, Forouzanfar MH, Daoud F, et al. Health in times of uncertainty in the eastern Mediterranean region, 1990-2013: a systematic analysis for the Global Burden of Disease Study 2013. *Lancet Glob Health*. 2016;4:e704–e713.
9. Van Biesen W, Vanholder R, Ernandez T, et al. Caring for migrants and refugees with end-stage kidney disease in Europe. *Am J Kidney Dis*. 2018;71:701–709.
27. Van Biesen W, Vanholder R, Vanderhaegen B, et al. Renal replacement therapy for refugees with end-stage kidney disease: an international survey of the nephrological community. *Kidney Int Suppl*. 2016;6:35–41.
28. Gibney RT, Sever MS, Vanholder RC. Disaster nephrology: crush injury and beyond. *Kidney Int*. 2014;85:1049–1057.
31. Hoste EA, Bagshaw SM, Bellomo R, et al. Epidemiology of acute kidney injury in critically ill patients: the multinational AKI-EPI study. *Intensive Care Med*. 2015;41:1411–1423.
47. Barsoum RS. Malarial acute renal failure. *J Am Soc Nephrol*. 2000;11: 2147–2154.
52. Mehta RL, Burdmann EA, Cerda J, et al. Recognition and management of acute kidney injury in the International Society of Nephrology 0by25 Global Snapshot: a multinational cross-sectional study. *Lancet*. 2016;387:2017–2025.
55. Hatamizadeh P, Najafi I, Vanholder R, et al. Epidemiologic aspects of the Bam earthquake in Iran: the nephrologic perspective. *Am J Kidney Dis*. 2006;47:428–438.
56. Kantarci G, Vanholder R, Tuglular S, et al. Acute renal failure due to crush syndrome during Marmara earthquake. *Am J Kidney Dis*. 2002;40:682–689.
59. Rifai AO, Murad LB, Sekkarie MA, et al. Continuous venovenous hemofiltration using a stand-alone blood pump for acute kidney injury in field hospitals in Syria. *Kidney Int*. 2015;87:254–261.
75. Süleymanlar G, Utaş C, Arinsoy T, et al. A population-based survey of Chronic REnal Disease In Turkey–the CREDIT study. *Nephrol Dial Transplant*. 2011;26:1862–1871.
77. Benghanem Gharbi M, Elseviers M, Zamd M, et al. Chronic kidney disease, hypertension, diabetes, and obesity in the adult population of Morocco: how to avoid "over"- and "under"-diagnosis of CKD. *Kidney Int*. 2016;89:1363–1371.
82. Karnib HH, Gharavi AG, Aftimos G, et al. A 5-year survey of biopsy proven kidney diseases in Lebanon: significant variation in prevalence of primary glomerular diseases by age, population structure and consanguinity. *Nephrol Dial Transplant*. 2010;25:3962–3969.
86. Bello AK, Levin A, Tonelli M, et al. Assessment of global kidney health care status. *JAMA*. 2017;317:1864–1881.
88. Vivante A, Afek A, Frenkel-Nir Y, et al. Persistent asymptomatic isolated microscopic hematuria in Israeli adolescents and young adults and risk for end-stage renal disease. *JAMA*. 2011;306:729–736.
89. Calderon-Margalit R, Golan E, Twig G, et al. History of childhood kidney disease and risk of adult end-stage renal disease. *N Engl J Med*. 2018;378:428–438.
94. Gouda Z, Mashaal G, Bello AK, et al. Egypt Information, Prevention, and Treatment of Chronic Kidney Disease (EGIPT-CKD) programme: prevalence and risk factors for microalbuminuria among the relatives of patients with CKD in Egypt. *Saudi J Kidney Dis Transpl*. 2011;22:1055–1063.
97. Alsuwaida AO, Farag YM, Al Sayyari AA, et al. Epidemiology of chronic kidney disease in the Kingdom of Saudi Arabia (SEEK-Saudi investigators) - a pilot study. *Saudi J Kidney Dis Transpl*. 2010;21: 1066–1072.
101. Tohidi M, Hasheminia M, Mohebi R, et al. Incidence of chronic kidney disease and its risk factors, results of over 10 year follow up in an Iranian cohort. *PLoS ONE*. 2012;7:e45304.
103. Yuzbashian E, Asghari G, Mirmiran P, et al. Adherence to low-sodium Dietary Approaches to Stop Hypertension-style diet may decrease the risk of incident chronic kidney disease among high-risk patients: a secondary prevention in prospective cohort study. *Nephrol Dial Transplant*. 2018;33:1159–1168.
107. Najafi I, Alatab S, Atabak S, et al. Seventeen years' experience of peritoneal dialysis in Iran: first official report of the Iranian Peritoneal Dialysis Registry. *Perit Dial Int*. 2014;34:636–642.
108. El Matri A. History of nephrology in Mediterranean Arab countries. *J Nephrol*. 2013;26:170–174.
111. AlSahow A, AlRukhaimi M, Al Wakeel J, et al. Demographics and key clinical characteristics of hemodialysis patients from the Gulf Cooperation Council countries enrolled in the dialysis outcomes and practice patterns study phase 5 (2012-2015). *Saudi J Kidney Dis Transpl*. 2016;27:S12–S23.
120. Mahdavi-Mazdeh M. The Iranian model of living renal transplantation. *Kidney Int*. 2012;82:627–634.
133. Süleymanlar G, Serdengeçti K, Altiparmak MR, et al. Trends in renal replacement therapy in Turkey, 1996-2008. *Am J Kidney Dis*. 2011;57:456–465.
134. Utaş C. The development of PD in Turkey. *Perit Dial Int*. 2008;28: 217–219.
135. Kamyar KZ, Eliezer G, Tamy S, et al. Survival Disparities within American and Israeli Dialysis Populations: Learning from Similarities and Distinctions across Race and Ethnicity. *Semin Dial*. 2010;23:586–594.
136. Counil É, Cherni N, Kharrat M, et al. Trends of incident dialysis patients in Tunisia between 1992 and 2001. *Am J Kidney Dis*. 2008;51:463–470.
141. Alashek WA, McIntyre CW, Taal MW. Determinants of survival in patients receiving dialysis in Libya. *Hemodial Int*. 2013;17:249–255.
165. Frishberg Y, Ben-Neriah Z, Suvanto M, et al. Misleading findings of homozygosity mapping resulting from three novel mutations in NPHS1 encoding nephrin in a highly inbred community. *Genet Med*. 2007;9:180–184.
167. Yousri NA, Fakhro KA, Robay A, et al. Whole-exome sequencing identifies common and rare variant metabolic QTLs in a Middle Eastern population. *Nat Commun*. 2018;9:333.
200. Ben-Shalom E, Frishberg Y. Primary hyperoxalurias: diagnosis and treatment. *Pediatr Nephrol*. 2015;30:1781–1791.
201. Belostotsky R, Seboun E, Idelson GH, et al. Mutations in DHDPSL are responsible for primary hyperoxaluria type III. *Am J Hum Genet*. 2010;87:392–399.
229. Zelikovic I, Szargel R, Hawash A, et al. A novel mutation in the chloride channel gene, CLCNKB, as a cause of Gitelman and Bartter syndromes. *Kidney Int*. 2003;63:24–32.
239. Magen D, Sprecher E, Zelikovic I, et al. A novel missense mutation in SLC5A2 encoding SGLT2 underlies autosomal-recessive renal glucosuria and aminoaciduria. *Kidney Int*. 2005;67:34–41.

245. Magen D, Berger L, Coady MJ, et al. A loss-of-function mutation in NaPi-IIa and renal Fanconi's syndrome. *N Engl J Med.* 2010;362:1102–1109.
263. Manukyan G, Aminov R. Update on pyrin functions and mechanisms of familial Mediterranean fever. *Front Microbiol.* 2016;7:456.
275. Ben-Chetrit E, Backenroth R. Amyloidosis induced, end stage renal disease in patients with familial Mediterranean fever is highly associated with point mutations in the MEFV gene. *Ann Rheum Dis.* 2001;60:146–149.
356. van der Hilst J, Moutschen M, Messiaen PE, et al. Efficacy of anti-IL-1 treatment in familial Mediterranean fever: a systematic review of the literature. *Biologics.* 2016;10:75–80.
364. Green H, Lichtenberg S, Rahamimov R, et al. Familial Mediterranean fever is associated with increased mortality after kidney transplantation–a 19 Years' single center experience. *Transplantation.* 2017;101:2621–2626.
371. Horvat LD, Shariff SZ, Garg AX. Global trends in the rates of living kidney donation. *Kidney Int.* 2009;75:1088–1098.
401. Lavanchy D. The global burden of hepatitis C. *Liver Int.* 2009;29(suppl 1):74–81.
406. Harfouche M, Chemaitelly H, Mahmud S, et al. Epidemiology of hepatitis C virus among hemodialysis patients in the Middle East and North Africa: systematic syntheses, meta-analyses, and meta-regressions. *Epidemiol Infect.* 2017;145:3243–3263.
418. Goodkin DA, Bieber B, Jadoul M, et al. Mortality, Hospitalization, and Quality of Life among Patients with Hepatitis C Infection on Hemodialysis. *Clin J Am Soc Nephrol.* 2017;12:287–297.
427. Shaheen FA. Organ donation in the Middle East countries. *Ethn Dis.* 2009;19:S1-16-17.
446. Lavee J, Ashkenazi T, Stoler A, et al. Preliminary marked increase in the national organ donation rate in Israel following implementation of a new organ transplantation law. *Am J Transplant.* 2013;13:780–785.
457. Fallahzadeh MK, Jafari L, Roozbeh J, et al. Comparison of health status and quality of life of related versus paid unrelated living kidney donors. *Am J Transplant.* 2013;13:3210–3214.
462. Danovitch GM, Chapman J, Capron AM, et al. Organ trafficking and transplant tourism: the role of global professional ethical standards-the 2008 Declaration of Istanbul. *Transplantation.* 2013;95:1306–1312.
479. Levin A, Tonelli M, Bonventre J, et al. Global kidney health 2017 and beyond: a roadmap for closing gaps in care, research, and policy. *Lancet.* 2017;390:1888–1917.

# 79 Indian Subcontinent

Vinay Sakhuja | Harbir Singh Kohli

## CHAPTER OUTLINE



## KEY POINTS

- Community-acquired AKI secondary to tropical infections, use of indigenous drugs, toxic envenomation, and obstetric factors are some of the common causes of AKI in this region.
- Peritoneal dialysis in acute settings has been used and holds promise in resource-constrained and far-off settings, where it can be used with minimal expertise and infrastructure to treat life-threatening complications of kidney failure, especially AKI.
- CKD is a major emerging noncommunicable disease in this region on account of the rapid rise in population and high prevalence of risk factors such as diabetes, hypertension, and nephrolithiasis.
- CKD of undetermined cause is common in this region and is mostly seen in young men, who are often in rural areas and work outdoors. The clinical presentation is usually late and suggests chronic tubulointerstitial involvement. It is likely that a host of environmental factors or toxins in conjunction with chronic dehydration play a role.
- Long-term renal replacement therapy is unavailable to most patients with end-stage kidney disease (ESKD) because of inaccessibility and unaffordability. However, joint public and private efforts have shown promise in establishing self-sustaining programs to provide therapy.

The Indian subcontinent occupies the southern portion of the Asian continent and includes India, Pakistan, Bangladesh, Sri Lanka, Nepal, Bhutan, and the Maldives. The subcontinent is home to well over 20% of the world's population, making it the most densely populated region in the world. These countries are all approximately at the same stage of economic development and are considered emerging and developing economies, according to the International Monetary Fund's *World Economic Outlook* report.[1,2] Most of the population of the region lives in rural areas, relies on agriculture for its livelihood, and has limited access to health care. The countries of the subcontinent fall into the category of medium human development,[3] as measured by the human development index, which takes into account not only the standard of living as determined by purchasing power parity but also the literacy rate and life expectancy.

India is the largest country in the subcontinent, with a population of more than 1 billion, and is also the largest economy in the region. It has enjoyed impressive economic growth, as a result of which India has been put into the category of "newly industrialized countries," a classification between industrialized and developing countries. The mean per capita gross national product has grown, but 0.7 billion people still continue to live on less than one U.S. dollar a day. Economic and development indicators of major countries of the region are shown in Table 79.1.[2,3] This combination of underdevelopment, plus a rapidly growing economy, is reflected in the disease spectrum. On the one hand, countries of the subcontinent are challenged with epidemics of infectious disease and on the other hand diabetes mellitus, the so-called disease of the affluent, has reached epidemic proportions. Health care in the public sector in these countries is organized in the shape of a pyramid, with primary health centers at the bottom, followed by intermediate-level hospitals and referral hospitals at the top. Specialized care for disease is usually available only at the major referral hospitals. There are only about 900 nephrologists in India. There is a thriving private sector health care industry, but treatment costs are quite high, and only the rich or patients whose expenses are covered by their employers can afford treatment in these hospitals.

The differences in living standards and availability of health care determine the variations in disease patterns, management practices, and disease outcome. The spectrum of kidney

**Table 79.1 Economic and Development Indicators on the Indian Subcontinent**

| Parameter | India | Pakistan | Bangladesh | Sri Lanka |
|---|---|---|---|---|
| Population (billions) | 1.22 | 0.193 | 0.163 | 0.021 |
| Population growth rate (%) | 1.31 | 1.55 | 1.58 | 0.91 |
| Life expectancy at birth (yr) | 67.48 | 66.7 | 70.36 | 76.15 |
| Median age (yr) | 26.7 | 22.2 | 23.9 | 31.4 |
| Percentage of total population that is elderly (>65 yr) | 5 | 4 | 5 | 8 |
| Literacy rate (%) | 64.84 (in 2011) | 55 (in 2009) | 57.7 (in 2011) | 92.5 (in 2010) |
| Infant mortality rate/1000 live births (in 2013) | 44.6 | 59.35 | 47.30 | 9.24 |
| Per capita gross domestic product purchasing power parity (U.S. $; in 2012) | 3800 | 3100 | 2000 | 6000 |
| Percentage of the population living below the national poverty line | 29.8 | 22.3 | 31.5 | 8.9 |
| Human development index | 0.554 | 0.515 | 0.515 | 0.715 |
| Country ranking by human development index (of 179 countries) | 136 | 146 | 146 | 92 |

**Table 79.2 Causes of Acute Kidney Injury in a Tertiary Referral Center on the Indian Subcontinent (%)**

| Cause | 1965–1974[a] | 1975–1980[a] | 1981–1986[a] | 2001–2006[b] |
|---|---|---|---|---|
| Medical causes | 67 | 55 | 61 | 65 |
| Diarrheal diseases | 23 | 12 | 10 | 7.3 |
| Intravascular hemolysis due to glucose-6-phosphate dehydrogenase deficiency | 12 | 12 | 6 | 1 |
| Glomerulonephritis | 11 | 9 | 9.5 | 11 |
| Copper sulfate poisoning | 12 | 12 | 6 | 1 |
| Chemical and drug exposure | 4 | 5 | 7 | 7.2 |
| Snakebites and insect stings | 3 | 3 | 2.5 | 6.5 |
| Sepsis | 0 | 3 | 4 | 17.8 |
| Miscellaneous | 7 | 11 | 17 | 13.2 |
| Obstetric causes | 22 | 21 | 9 | 5 |
| Surgical causes | 11 | 24 | 30 | 30 |

[a]Adapted from Chugh KS, Sakhuja V, Malhotra HS, et al. Changing trends in acute renal failure in third world countries–Chandigarh study. *Q J Med*. 1989;73:1117–1123.
[b]Authors' unpublished data.

diseases in this region is characterized by a mix of conditions that are globally encountered and those specific to the subcontinent. The latter can be secondary to a genetic predisposition in specific ethnic groups or related to exposure to environmental factors, such as climatic conditions, infectious agents, envenomation, and chemical toxins. Genetic factors that predispose to kidney disease in the tropics include glucose-6-phosphate dehydrogenase (G6PD) deficiency, which gives rise to intravascular hemolysis and pigment-induced acute kidney injury (AKI). Indigenous health care systems are still popular in rural areas, and patients are frequently treated with herbs and potions that could add to the burden of kidney disease.

## ACUTE KIDNEY INJURY

Reliable statistics on the patterns and prevalence of AKI in this region are not available, but it is the most commonly encountered renal emergency.[4-6] For example, about 0.1% to 0.25% of all admissions to the authors' hospital admissions are for AKI. In a study of 536 patients admitted in a pediatric intensive care unit (ICU) in a large tertiary care hospital in North India, AKI was seen in 42.9% of subjects.[7] However, it was lower, at 25.1%, in South India under similar clinical settings.[8] Most of the causes of AKI described elsewhere in the world are encountered in the Indian subcontinent as well. Several causes, however, either are unique or are seen with increased frequency in this part of the world. Compared with industrialized countries, in which AKI is mainly a disease of the elderly and is seen primarily in hospitalized patients, community-acquired AKI in otherwise healthy individuals is common in countries in this region, a characteristic they share with other developing countries.[9] Patients with AKI are younger in this region than their counterparts in the West. The median age of patients with AKI in the West increased from 41.2 years in the 1950s to 60.5 years in the 1980s[10]; the average age of patients with AKI in India is 37.1 years.[9] Hospital-acquired AKI is more common in the older population than in the young.[11]

Over the years, there has been a change in the spectrum of AKI (Table 79.2).[12] In urban areas, the causes of AKI are similar to those in the industrialized world, but in rural areas, AKI is mainly the result of diarrheal illnesses, chemicals, snake bite, and insect stings.[13] Renal failure after the suicidal ingestion of copper sulfate has shown a significant decline,[14,15] possibly because of the easy availability of other poisons, such as organophosphate insecticides.[16] At a large tertiary care center in Pakistan, paraphenyline diamine poisoning was the most common cause for poisoning associated with AKI.[17] Data from a large tertiary care referral institute in India has shown that sepsis as a cause of AKI has increased almost seven times, from just 1.57% from 1983 through 1995 to 11.43% from 1996 to 2008.[18]

Treatment facilities are grossly inadequate. Patients are referred late, only after renal failure becomes severe and complications set in. They often require immediate dialysis and, therefore, the mortality rate is high. Intermittent peritoneal dialysis (PD) is still used in several areas[19-21] because hemodialysis (HD) facilities are limited to bigger cities. The outcome of AKI is worse in the elderly than in the younger population.[22] Conditions causing AKI that are specific to the Indian subcontinent are discussed in the following sections.

## PREGNANCY-ASSOCIATED ACUTE KIDNEY INJURY

Improvements in obstetric care have led to the virtual disappearance of pregnancy-related AKI in the industrialized world. Data from a large tertiary care hospital in the eastern part of India have shown that the proportion of obstetric AKI cases has remained more or less similar at 11.8% and 12.8% of total cases of AKI over two 13-year time periods (1996–2008 vs. 1983–1995, respectively).[23] However, some investigators have described a decline in the rate of obstetric AKI in India from 22% to 5% of all cases of AKI over the past 4 decades (Table 79.2).[19] The frequency distribution of AKI is bimodal in terms of the duration of gestation.

The first peak, seen between 8 and 16 weeks of gestation, is associated chiefly with induced septic abortions. The abortion practices include the use of sticks, the insertion of abortifacient chemicals, pastes, and soap solutions, and dilation and curettage performed under unhygienic conditions and by untrained personnel.[24] Postabortal sepsis has remained the most common cause for obstetric AKI over the past 3 decades.[23] The incidence of AKI has decreased since the legalization and regulation of abortions and the wider availability of medical facilities,[24,25] although heterogenous, limited data from other countries have also suggested that postabortal or puerperal sepsis is the leading cause of obstetric AKI.[26]

The second peak in obstetric AKI occurs after 34 weeks of gestation and is related to preeclampsia, eclampsia, abruptio placentae, postpartum hemorrhage, and puerperal sepsis. The incidence of preeclampsia in the Indian population has been reported to be 28.7% in a population-based study.[27] Data from Pakistan, Bangladesh, and Nepal have also suggested sepsis related to abortion or puerperium, hemorrhage, hypotension, and preeclampsia as main associations of pregnancy-related AKI.[26] Acute cortical necrosis has been observed in about 25% of patients with obstetric AKI in parts of India.[23,24,27] The provision of institutional care and early referral for patients with complicated pregnancies to specialized centers is important to ensure better prevention and management of AKI in such settings. Community-based education and awareness are required, so that patients seek proper medical attention as soon as possible. AKI in pregnancy is managed along the usual lines, with additional cause-specific interventions, if any.[26] Those women who do not recover kidney function usually undergo contrast-enhanced computed tomography (CT) of the kidneys to look for acute cortical necrosis. If this is absent, a renal biopsy is done in such individuals. Pregnancy and kidney disease are further discussed in Chapter 48.

## ACUTE KIDNEY INJURY ASSOCIATED WITH SURGICAL CAUSES

The proportion of AKI from surgical causes has increased from 11% to 30% (see Table 79.2). Obstructive nephropathy constitutes a major cause of surgical AKI.[28] The high incidence of nephrolithiasis contributes and is related to inherited metabolic disorders, dietary factors, and fluid losses. A high prevalence of nephrolithiasis in some areas, aggravated by dehydration caused by a combination of exposure to high ambient temperatures and a high prevalence of diarrheal diseases, is an example. Faith in the efficacy of indigenous medicines to dissolve stones causes delay in surgical intervention and hastens the development of renal failure.

## ACUTE KIDNEY INJURY DUE TO INFECTIONS

### DIARRHEAL DISEASES

AKI secondary to diarrhea is encountered not only in children but also in adults. In adults, diarrheal diseases cause 30% of all AKI,[9] whereas 35% to 50% of all children undergoing dialysis for AKI have preceding diarrhea and dehydration.[28-30] This problem is common in rural areas and urban slums inhabited by poverty-stricken individuals, where sanitation is poor and potable water is not available. The incidence increases during summer and the rainy season. Associated vomiting is an early feature of rotavirus infection. Loose watery stools indicate infection with enterotoxigenic *Escherichia coli* or *Vibrio cholerae*. Fever, cramps, tenesmus, and blood and mucus in stools suggest *Shigella, Salmonella,* or enteroinvasive *E. coli* infection. The diagnosis of cholera can be confirmed by microscopic demonstration of the highly motile *V. cholerae* organisms in a hanging drop preparation; culture is necessary to confirm the presence of other organisms.

Early and adequate fluid replacement is the cornerstone of therapy. Widespread use of the oral rehydration solution recommended by the World Health Organization (WHO) has led to a significant decline in the mortality rate from this condition. Intravenous rehydration with lactated Ringer solution may be required in patients with severe dehydration, persistent vomiting, or paralytic ileus. Hypokalemia may worsen as the metabolic acidosis is corrected, and large amounts of potassium may be required to prevent life-threatening cardiac arrhythmias. Because peritoneal dialysis fluid is potassium-free, potassium should be replaced through an intravenous (IV) or intraperitoneal route in patients with severe AKI treated with this modality. Volume depletion secondary to acute gastroenteritis is presumed to be the most common cause of kidney injury; occasionally, acute cortical necrosis can also occur.[31]

### HEMOLYTIC-UREMIC SYNDROME

Hemolytic-uremic syndrome was responsible for 25% to 55% of all cases of pediatric AKI in some parts of the subcontinent, but the proportion has decreased.[8,32-34] In one report, diarrhea-related, hemolytic-uremic syndrome accounted for only 3.8% of pediatric AKI cases at a pediatric ICU in South India.[8] This condition is seen mainly in preschool-aged children and is less common in adults. The main feature is oliguric renal failure, preceded by a diarrheal prodrome in about 70% of cases. Neurologic involvement is seen in 30% to 50% of cases. Examination shows pallor and mild icterus. Renal failure is severe and requires prolonged dialysis. Diagnosis is confirmed by the demonstration of fragmented erythrocytes on blood smear, as well as thrombocytopenia. Supportive evidence includes unconjugated hyperbilirubinemia and increased plasma lactate dehydrogenase levels. The causative organism in the Indian subcontinent is usually *Shigella* and not *E. coli*.[35,36] The histologic hallmark of this condition is thrombotic microangiopathy in the renal vasculature. Histologic examination shows frequent involvement of arterioles and small arteries, with severe intimal proliferation and luminal stenosis. Patchy or diffuse renal cortical necrosis develops in up to 40% of patients.[32] The treatment is mainly supportive. Plasma infusions or plasma exchange are used infrequently; the outcome is poor, with a mortality rate of 60%.[37] Of those who recover, a significant proportion are left with residual renal dysfunction and eventually progress to ESKD. The management of thrombotic microangiopathies is discussed in detail in Chapter 34.

## MALARIA

Malaria is caused by the protozoan *Plasmodium* and is transmitted by the *Anopheles* mosquito. Of the four *Plasmodium* species, AKI is seen most frequently with *Plasmodium falciparum* infection. A few reports have described an association of AKI with *Plasmodium vivax* infection.[38,39] Multiple organ dysfunctions have been also associated with *P. vivax* malaria.[40]

These forms of malaria predominate in warmer regions closer to the equator in the subcontinent (parts of India, Pakistan, Bangladesh, and Sri Lanka) and are associated with intense, year-round transmission. In addition to being a burden to the native communities, malaria is a danger to nonimmune travelers to endemic areas.[41] The Southeast Asian region has the highest burden of malaria after Africa. India, Indonesia, Pakistan, and Myanmar are the leading countries that are affected.[41] A more than 50% reduction in incidence is expected over the next few years as compared with the incidence in 2000.[42] In 2016, Sri Lanka was declared malaria-free by WHO.[43] Preventive measures are directed at reducing exposure and preventing transmission of disease by better vector control and sanitation. Travelers from nonendemic areas should be aware of the risks and encouraged to seek treatment or chemoprophylaxis whenever indicated.

The contribution of malaria to overall hospital admissions for AKI varies from 2% to 39%.[44] The incidence of malarial AKI among those living in endemic areas is 2% to 5%, but 25% to 30% of nonimmune visitors with malaria experience renal failure.[45] Among those with severe parasitemia, as many as 60% have AKI.[46] In Pakistan, malaria-induced AKI also contributes significantly to the total AKI burden.[47]

### Clinical Features

Malaria causes classic paroxysms of spiking fever, along with malaise, myalgia, headache, and chills, and the disease can be confused with a viral illness. Nausea, vomiting, and hypotension are common in nonimmune individuals. Severe infection may involve several vital organs, including the central nervous system, manifesting as deep coma and seizures, noncardiogenic pulmonary edema, shock, and disseminated intravascular coagulation (DIC). AKI usually is seen by the end of the first week and is nonoliguric in 50% to 75% of cases.[45] In more than 75% of cases, AKI is associated with cholestatic jaundice. It is usually associated with a hypercatabolic state, with a rapid increase in creatinine levels. In a study from India, of a total of 101 patients with malarial AKI over a 1-year period, about 37% required dialytic support, and hospital mortality was around 10%.[48] Other manifestations include nonnephrotic proteinuria, microscopic hematuria, hemoglobinuria, and electrolyte abnormalities.

Diagnosis can be established by the demonstration of asexual forms of the parasite in peripheral blood smears stained with Giemsa stain. Staining with the fluorescent dye acridine orange allows more rapid diagnosis. Also, simple but specific antibody-based card tests that detect *P. falciparum*–specific histidine-rich protein 2 or lactate dehydrogenase antigens in fingerstick blood samples have been introduced. Most patients present with fever and nonspecific symptoms and are often treated empirically, depending on which are the most common local causes for acute febrile illness. These simple card-based tests allow rapid bedside diagnosis and early institution of therapy. They allow differentiation of *P. falciparum* from non–*P. falciparum* malarias, but results can remain positive for several weeks after acute infection. A scoring system based on the number of organ systems involved has been suggested for judging the severity and predicting outcomes in *P. falciparum* malaria.[49]

### Histologic Features

Acute tubular necrosis is the most common lesion found on histologic analysis. Pigment casts may be seen in tubular lumina in patients with intravascular hemolysis. Varying degrees of interstitial edema and mononuclear cell infiltrate are common accompaniments.[49]

### Pathogenesis

Disease severity is related to the intensity of infection.[50] The most important pathogenetic factor is the hemodynamic change caused by altered erythrocyte rheology. The infected cell becomes more spherical and less deformable as a result of the formation of membrane protuberances or knobs on the cell surface. These knobs extrude a strain-specific adhesive variant protein of high molecular weight that mediates attachment to receptors on venular and capillary endothelium, causing a phenomenon called "cytoadherence." The major adhesive protein family is known as "*P. falciparum* erythrocyte membrane protein." The cell surface receptors for these knobs include complement receptor 1, glycosaminoglycans, intercellular adhesion molecule-1, chondroitin sulfate B, CD36, platelet endothelial cell adhesion molecule 1/CD31, thrombomodulin, E- and P-selectins, and vascular cell adhesion molecule-1. Some of these receptors are expressed constitutively, whereas others are induced by inflammatory mediators released in severe disease. Infected erythrocytes also adhere to uninfected red cells, platelets, monocytes, and lymphocytes. These aggregated and sequestered red blood cells interfere with microcirculatory flow in the kidneys and other organs.[51] This phenomenon is unique to *P. falciparum* infection and has not been observed in infection with other species.

#### Treatment

Mortality from malarial AKI varies between 15% and 50%.[46] Severe *P. falciparum* malaria requires intensive nursing and close multidisciplinary care.[46] Prompt assessment of volume status, blood glucose level, and acid–base status is essential. All patients with *P. falciparum* infection should be presumed to have chloroquine-resistant infection. The cinchona alkaloids (quinine or quinidine) are the mainstay of treatment because of their activity against chloroquine-resistant strains. Quinine often causes hyperinsulinemia and hypoglycemia, and many centers recommend the administration of a continuous infusion of 5% to 10% dextrose to all patients.[52] Compounds derived from artemisinin (isolated from the Chinese herb *Artemisia annua*) such as artesunate, artemether, and arteether are particularly valuable in areas with quinine resistance and in patients with recurrent quinine-induced hypoglycemia.

All patients should also receive gametocidal therapy (tetracycline or pyrimethamine–sulfadoxine). Mefloquine, halofantrine, atovaquone, artemisinin, and pyrimethamine–sulfadoxine (Fansidar) derivatives are possible alternatives for resistant *P. falciparum* malaria. Patients with evidence of hemolysis should receive adequate hydration and parenteral sodium bicarbonate to alkalinize the urine to a pH of more than 7.0. AKI is usually associated with a hypercatabolic state, and frequent dialysis may be needed.[53] Hyperkalemia should be watched for and adequately treated. The peritoneal microcirculation is impaired as a result of clogging with infected erythrocytes and vasoconstriction, reducing the efficacy of PD. Despite these limitations, PD has been shown to improve survival by 16%, with early institution of manual, immediate PD in AKI due to *P. falciparum* malaria.[54] Exchange transfusion has also been tried in patients with severe parasitemia.

## LEPTOSPIROSIS

Leptospirosis, the most widespread zoonosis in the world,[55] is particularly prevalent in parts of southern and western India.[56,57] The animal hosts include rats, mice, gerbils, hedgehogs, foxes, dogs, cattle, sheep, pigs, and rabbits. Even asymptomatic animals carry a high number of organisms ($>10^{10}$/g) in their kidneys and shed *Leptospira* in urine for years.[58] Human infection occurs incidentally, either directly through contact with the urine or tissue of an infected animal or indirectly through contaminated water, soil, or vegetation. The usual portals of entry are abraded skin and exposed mucosae. Leptospirosis is an occupational hazard for coal miners and sewage, abattoir, and farm workers, as well as workers in the aquaculture industry. The genus *Leptospira* includes the pathogenic *Leptospira interrogans* strains and the saprophytic *Leptospira biflexa*. The disease occurs throughout the year, with an increase in incidence during or soon after the rainy season, especially after floods. Adult men are affected most frequently.

#### Clinical Features

The manifestations of leptospirosis vary from subclinical infection or a self-limited anicteric febrile illness to severe and potentially fatal disease.[55,56] Symptoms appear 1 to 2 weeks after exposure and are typically biphasic in character. The leptospiremic phase is characterized by high fever, with chills, headache, and severe muscle aches and tenderness. Renal failure develops in the second, immune phase, when patients also have progressive jaundice, epistaxis, hemoptysis, gastrointestinal bleeding, hemorrhagic pneumonia, and bleeding into the adrenal glands. The triad of acute renal failure, cholestatic jaundice, and bleeding constitutes Weil syndrome caused by Leptosirosis. AKI occurs in 20% to 85% of cases.[57,59,60] In about 50% of cases of AKI, renal failure is associated with polyuria and hypokalemia, along with increased fractional excretion of potassium. Renal failure is mild and nonoliguric in patients without icterus. Hypotension is noted in more than 60% of cases and is often unresponsive to volume expansion and inotropic support. Hypotensive patients are also more likely to have adult respiratory distress syndrome.[61]

Diagnosis is based on culture or serologic testing. Organisms can be isolated in blood cultures during the first phase and later from urine. However, growth takes up to 4 weeks in Fletcher or Stuart semisolid medium. The macroscopic agglutination test can be used as a screening test but is not specific. The benchmark is the microscopic agglutination test, but this is a complex procedure that requires maintenance of live *Leptospira* cultures. An immunoglobulin M (IgM)–specific dot enzyme-linked immunosorbent assay has been found to be specific in diagnosing leptospirosis in endemic areas. Urinalysis during the leptospiremic phase reveals mild proteinuria, as well as hyaline and granular casts.

#### Histologic Features

The kidneys typically are swollen and may be bile-stained. The main lesions seen on light microscopy are interstitial edema and infiltration with mononuclear cells and eosinophils. Mild and transient mesangioproliferative glomerulonephritis with C3 and IgM deposition may sometimes be observed.[62]

#### Pathogenesis

Renal involvement results from direct invasion of the renal tissue by the organism, which leads to liberation of enzymes, metabolites, and endotoxins, as well as complement activation. Ultrastructural studies after inoculation of *Leptospira pomona* into mice have shown the organism infiltrating the glomerular capillary lumen at day 2, the interstitium at days 4 to 8, the proximal tubular cells by day 10, and the tubular lumen by day 14.[63] Several leptospiral outer membrane proteins have been localized to the proximal tubules and interstitium of infected animals. The addition of *Leptospira* endotoxin to human macrophages induces tumor necrosis factor-α (TNF-α). The glycoprotein component of endotoxin could inhibit renal $Na^+$-$K^+$–adenosine triphosphatase ($Na^+$-$K^+$-ATPase), in turn affecting the apical Na-K-2Cl cotransporter and leading to potassium wasting.[64] An upregulation of nuclear factor kappa B binding to DNA was noted on the addition of outer membrane extracts from pathogenic serovars to cultured medullary thick ascending limb cells; this was accompanied by an increase in inducible nitric oxide synthase, monocyte chemoattractant protein-1, and TNF-α. Alterations in intravascular volume, hemoglobinuria, and myoglobinuria also contribute.[62] The tubules become insensitive to the action of antidiuretic hormone.

#### Treatment

Leptospirosis is a self-limiting disease, and patients with mild cases recover spontaneously. The emphasis is on symptomatic measures, together with correction of hypotension and fluid and electrolyte imbalances. Administration of crystalline penicillin or doxycycline shortens the duration of fever and hospital stay and may hasten amelioration of leptospiruria. In a meta-analysis of controlled trials, the role of various antibiotics for the treatment of leptospirosis was found to be uncertain; this finding could be attributed to a lack of adequate clinical trials.[65] The role of penicillin in the treatment of leptospirosis can be debated.[65] Patients with renal failure need close monitoring and dialysis when necessary. Poor prognostic indicators include increasing age and the presence of jaundice, pulmonary complications, hyperbilirubinemia, diarrhea, hyperkalemia, pulmonary rales, and hypotension on admission.[66] Internal hemorrhage and myocarditis are common causes of death.

## ZYGOMYCOSIS

Zygomycosis is a rare opportunistic infection caused by fungi of the order Mucorales and genera *Rhizopus, Absidia,* and *Rhizomucor.* Organ involvement occurs through vascular invasion, which leads to thrombosis of large and small arteries and infarction and necrosis of the affected organ. The major presentations have rhinocerebral, pulmonary, gastrointestinal, and disseminated forms. Renal mucormycosis involving the major renal vessels has been reported primarily in northern India in the past decade and may occur as isolated renal involvement or as part of disseminated disease.[67] The administration of IV fluids contaminated with fungus may be responsible in some patients. Bilateral renal arterial involvement leads to oliguric AKI. The condition usually develops in otherwise immunocompetent individuals; presentation is with fever, lumbar pain, pyuria, and oliguria. CT reveals enlarged nonenhancing kidneys with perirenal collections and/or intrarenal abscesses (Fig. 79.1).[68] The diagnosis can be confirmed by demonstration of hyphae in the material obtained by aspiration or percutaneous biopsy. The only definitive treatment is extensive débridement of affected tissue, which may include bilateral nephrectomy, and systemic antifungal therapy with amphotericin B. Bilateral renal mucormycosis carries an extremely poor prognosis.[67]

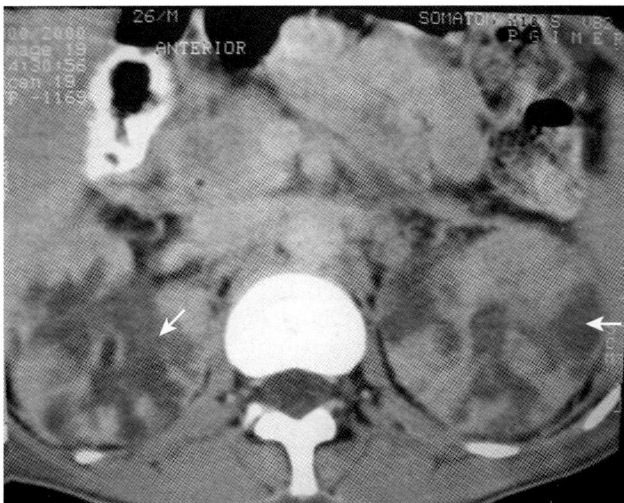


**Fig. 79.1 Renal mucormycosis.** This contrast-enhanced computed tomography scan shows bulky kidneys, with large nonenhancing areas *(arrows)* involving the cortex and medulla and with no contrast in the pelvicalyceal system.

## DENGUE FEVER

Dengue fever is the most prevalent mosquito-borne viral disease. There are four closely related but serologically distinct dengue viruses—DENV-1, DENV-2, DENV-3, and DENV-4, of the genus *Flavivirus.* The infection is primarily transmitted by *Aedes* mosquitoes, particularly *Aedes aegypti.* Dengue fever is a self-limiting illness, with symptoms including fever, headache, and muscle and joint pain. However, a life-threatening dengue hemorrhagic fever (DHF) develops in a small minority of patients, with low platelet count, bleeding, and capillary plasma leakage.[69] In severe cases, patients may have dengue shock syndrome. The cardinal features of DHF are increased vascular permeability (plasma leakage syndrome), marked thrombocytopenia, hemorrhagic tendency (as demonstrated by a positive tourniquet test result), and spontaneous bleeding.

In a study from South India, AKI was seen in 10.8% of patients with dengue fever. Of these, 12 (5.4%) had mild AKI, 7 (3.1%) had moderate AKI, and 5 (2.2%) had severe AKI according to Acute Kidney Injury Network (AKIN) criteria.[70] Proposed mechanisms for AKI are capillary leak, shock resulting in hypoperfusion, and acute tubular necrosis. Also, hemolysis or rhabdomyolysis contribute to AKI. Of 198 patients with dengue admitted to an ICU, 15 (7.6%) required dialytic support.[71] The presence of dengue hemorrhagic and dengue shock syndrome, neurologic involvement, and prolonged activated partial thromboplastin time have been found to be independent predictors of AKI. Mortality is about 6% to 9% in patients with dengue fever and AKI. AKI during hospitalization for dengue fever is a predictor of death.[72] Vector control, improvements in sanitation, and preventing exposure are the main strategies for prevention of this disease.

# ACUTE KIDNEY INJURY DUE TO SNAKE BITE AND INSECT STINGS

## SNAKE BITE

Snake bite is an occupational hazard and occurs when people are working barefoot in the fields.[73,74] On the Indian subcontinent, AKI develops after bites by snakes of the viper family, such as Russell's viper, the saw-scaled viper *(Echis carinatus),* and pit vipers. The incidence of AKI varies from 13% to 32% in India after Russell's viper or *E. carinatus* bites[75-77] and is 27% in Sri Lanka after bites of unidentified vipers.[78]

### Clinical Features

The severity of the symptoms and signs is related to the type of venom, as well as to the dose injected during the bite. Severely envenomed patients experience DIC, which frequently results in spontaneous bleeding and coagulopathy. The latter features often dominate the clinical course until coagulation returns to normal.[79] Many viper-envenomed patients have hypotensive shock as a consequence of hypovolemia from significant blood loss. Blood can ooze continuously from the fang marks, and severe hemorrhage may manifest as hematemesis, melena, hemoptysis, or bleeding into the muscles, fascial compartments, serous cavities, and subarachnoid space.[80] Pain and swelling of the bitten part are generally the earliest symptoms, appearing within a few minutes. The swelling may spread to involve the whole limb and is due to exudation of plasma or extravasation of blood into the subcutaneous tissues. Blistering or local necrosis is observed in one-third to one-half of patients.

In patients with AKI, oliguria often develops rapidly, within the first 24 hours, but it may be delayed until 2 to 3 days after the bite. Some patients become anuric, whereas occasional patients remain nonoliguric. Urine may show gross or microscopic hematuria. Some patients complain of pain in the renal angle preceding oliguria, which may be a useful clue to impending renal failure. Jaundice and hemoglobinuria resulting from intravascular hemolysis are not infrequent after Russell's viper or *E. carinatus* bites and have been reported in India and Sri Lanka.[77]

Laboratory investigations reveal varying degrees of anemia, resulting from a combination of intravascular hemolysis and blood loss. Hemolysis results in unconjugated hyperbilirubinemia, reticulocytosis, elevated plasma free hemoglobin level, and hemoglobinuria. In some patients, the peripheral blood smear may show fragmented erythrocytes, suggesting microangiopathic hemolysis. The blood fails to coagulate normally, and features of DIC are often present.[80] Thrombocytopenia may occur, however, even in the absence of a consumptive coagulopathy.

The mortality rate for patients with snake bite–associated AKI varies with the nature of the renal lesion. According to one report, although only 16% of those with acute tubular necrosis died, as many as 80% of those with cortical necrosis had a fatal outcome.[77]

### Histologic Features

Renal histologic examination shows acute tubular or cortical necrosis. Glomerular changes have been described in rare cases, but their significance is not known.

**Acute Tubular Necrosis.** Acute tubular necrosis is the predominant lesion seen in 70% to 80% of patients with snake bite–associated AKI. On light microscopy, the tubules appear dilated and lined by flattened epithelium. Severe cases exhibit cell necrosis and desquamation of necrotic cells from the basement membrane. Hyaline, granular, or pigment casts are seen in tubular lumina. Varying degrees of interstitial edema, hemorrhage, and inflammatory cell infiltration are present. Later biopsy specimens reveal regenerating tubular epithelium. Intrarenal blood vessels are usually unaffected.

On ultrastructural examination, proximal tubules show dense intracytoplasmic bodies that represent degenerating organelles or protein resorption droplets.[81] Small areas of basement membrane are denuded. Distal tubular cells have a dilated endoplasmic reticulum and many degenerating organelles. Apoptosis, a prominent feature in the distal tubules, indicates a high cell turnover. In the interstitium, fibroblasts appear active, with increased numbers of organelles and cytoplasmic processes. Mast cells and eosinophils show both granulated and partially degranulated forms.

**Acute Cortical Necrosis.** Bilateral diffuse or patchy cortical necrosis has been observed in 20% of patients with snake bite–induced AKI.[77] The presence of fibrin thrombi in the arterioles is a prominent feature in these patients. A narrow subcapsular rim of cortex often escapes necrosis. The area underlying this rim, however, shows necrosis of glomerular as well as tubular elements. The necrotic zone is often bordered by an area of hyperemia and leukocytic infiltration.

### Pathogenesis

The exact pathogenesis of AKI following snake bite is not well established because of the lack of a reproducible animal model. However, a number of factors may contribute, including bleeding, hypotension, circulatory collapse, intravascular hemolysis, DIC, microangiopathic hemolytic anemia, and the direct nephrotoxicity of the venom. Bleeding either into tissues or externally and loss of plasma into the bitten extremity can produce hypotension and circulatory collapse. These effects are caused by venom metalloproteinases that degrade basement membrane proteins surrounding the vessel wall, leading to loss of integrity. Hemorrhagic toxins have been isolated from the venom of many snakes of the Viperidae and Crotalidae families.[79] In addition, vasodilation and increased capillary permeability can aggravate the circulatory disturbances of shock.

Hemolysis results from the action of phospholipase $A_2$, which is present in almost all snake venoms. Phospholipase $A_2$ causes hemolysis directly by hydrolysis of red blood cell membrane phospholipids or indirectly via the production of the strongly hemolytic lysolecithin from plasma lecithin.[82] The human hemostatic system is regulated through a number of critical interactions involving blood proteins, platelets, endothelial cells, and subendothelial structures. Snake venoms, particularly those from the viper and pit viper families, contain many proteins that interact with members of the coagulation cascade and the fibrinolytic pathway.[82]

### Treatment

The therapeutic approach to renal failure after snake bite is the same as that for AKI from any other cause. Early administration of antivenom is vital; delay results in a steep increase in the dose requirements. Indications include prolonged coagulation time or failure of blood coagulation, spontaneous systemic bleeding, intravascular hemolysis, and local swelling involving more than two segments of the bitten limb. Knowledge of the offending snake species allows administration of monovalent antivenom, if available. Immunodiagnostic techniques are helpful in the identification of the venom antigen. The enzyme-linked immunosorbent assay has been used extensively in rural Thailand for this purpose.[83] The currently available test, however, is not quick enough for clinical application. Because only polyvalent antivenom is available in most parts of Asia, precise identification of the snake is not essential for management.

Indian studies recommend initial administration of 20 to 100 mL of antivenom, followed by repeated doses of 25 to 50 mL every 4 to 6 hours until the effects of systemic envenomation disappear.[80,84] A simple way to monitor antivenom treatment efficacy is by monitoring whole blood clotting time three or four times daily. Coagulation is generally restored within 6 hours of an adequate dose. Coagulation testing must be performed for at least 3 more days, because delayed absorption of the venom can lead to recurrence of the coagulopathy. Immunoassays permit serial estimation of venom levels and are useful in guiding antivenom therapy.

Other therapeutic measures include replacement of lost blood with fresh blood or plasma, maintenance of electrolyte balance, administration of tetanus immunoglobulin, and treatment of pyogenic infection with antibiotics. The prognosis is good in patients who receive adequate doses of antivenom. One study has shown the outcome for venom-induced AKI to be better after HD than after PD.[85] The overall mortality rate is about 30%.[77]

### BEE, WASP, AND HORNET STINGS

Honeybees, yellow jackets, hornets, and paper wasps are stinging insects belonging to the order Hymenoptera. An isolated sting causes just a local allergic reaction, but attack by a swarm of insects introduces a large dose of the venom, sufficient to cause systemic symptoms.[86-88] These include vomiting, diarrhea, hypotension, loss of consciousness, and AKI. Patients with AKI have been reported to have received from 22 to more than 1000 stings.[89] AKI is secondary to hemolysis and/or rhabdomyolysis.[89] Hemolysis results from the action of a basic protein fraction, as well as melittin and phospholipase A present in the venom. Rhabdomyolysis has been attributed to polypeptides, histamine, serotonin, and acetylcholine. A direct nephrotoxic role for these venoms has also been suggested. Renal biopsy specimens reveal acute tubular necrosis.

## ACUTE KIDNEY INJURY DUE TO CHEMICAL TOXINS

### COPPER SULFATE POISONING

Copper sulfate is a strong corrosive that produces symptoms within minutes of ingestion, usually with suicidal intent. Metallic taste, excessive salivation, burning retrosternal and epigastric pain, nausea, and repeated vomiting are the initial features. The vomitus is blue-green and turns deep blue on the addition of ammonium hydroxide, which allows it to be differentiated from bile. Diarrhea, hematemesis, and melena follow. Jaundice, hypotension, convulsions, and coma may develop in severe cases. Acute pancreatitis, myoglobinuria, and methemoglobinemia have also been reported. AKI is seen in 20% to 25% of cases and is invariably oliguric.[90] Hemoglobinuria may be seen in about 40% of cases. Diuresis ensues after 7 to 10 days and is usually followed by complete renal recovery.[14]

Copper can produce considerable oxidative stress and interferes with the activity of several key enzymes, such as $Na^+$-$K^+$-ATPase, G6PD, glutathione reductase, and catalase.[90] Direct nephrotoxicity, severe hemolysis, and hypovolemia secondary to fluid loss are the main factors responsible for kidney injury. In experimental animals, copper sulfate causes toxic damage to the proximal tubules.[90] Histologic examination usually shows acute tubular necrosis, with predominant involvement of the proximal tubules. Hemoglobin casts may be seen in patients with intravascular hemolysis.[90,91] Acute cortical necrosis has been seen rarely.

Management entails gastric lavage using 1% potassium ferrocyanide, which leads to the formation of insoluble cupric ferrocyanide. Egg whites or milk can be administered as an antidote. Emesis should not be induced. Any volume deficit should be corrected quickly. Hyperkalemia may be severe and sustained because of the ongoing hemolysis and requires early and frequent dialysis.

### ETHYLENE GLYCOL POISONING

Diethylene and polyethylene glycols have been used as cheap substitutes for propylene glycol as vehicles in pediatric syrup preparations. Epidemics of diethylene glycol–induced AKI have been reported in India and Bangladesh.[92-94] In one large study, 236 deaths were recorded among 339 children with unexplained AKI in a children's hospital in Dhaka, Bangladesh.[92] A total of 51 children had ingested a brand of acetaminophen (paracetamol) known to contain diethylene glycol, whereas 85% of the remaining patients had ingested an unknown elixir for fever.[92] The likelihood of hepatomegaly, edema, hypertension, severe acidosis, higher serum creatinine level, and in-hospital mortality was higher in patients with suspected poisoning.[92] In another report, 14 patients died of AKI after the administration of glycerol to decrease intracranial or intraocular pressure.[93] Analysis of this preparation showed it to be 70% ethylene glycol. Autopsy revealed acute cortical necrosis as the most frequent lesion.

### ETHYLENE DIBROMIDE POISONING

Ethylene dibromide (EDB), a pesticide fumigant, is absorbed from the skin, gastrointestinal tract, and intestinal mucosa. Both accidental and suicidal poisonings with EDB have been reported. AKI and hepatocellular injury are the chief manifestations.[95,96] The mortality remains very high, despite all supportive measures.[97] EDB is postulated to lead to the generation of free oxygen radicals through the cytochrome P450 pathway, causing lipid peroxidation and membrane damage. Dimercaprol has been suggested as an antidote on the basis of the structural similarities of the two compounds.

### CHROMIC ACID POISONING

Chromic acid ($H_2CrO_7$) and its salts (chromates and dichromates) are used in the electroplating, leather tanning, and anticorrosive metal treatment industries. Renal lesions have been reported after the acute ingestion of large quantities of these substances.[98,99] Ingestion is most often with suicidal intent and is followed by severe abdominal pain, vomiting, gastrointestinal bleeding, and circulatory collapse. Dichromate is directly nephrotoxic and causes extensive proximal tubular necrosis.[100] Hypotension and hemolysis also contribute to tubular damage. Management entails gastric lavage with alkaline solutions such as sodium bicarbonate to prevent absorption and IV fluids to combat hypotension. Forced diuresis enhances renal excretion of the compound. Reducing agents such as vitamin C have been shown to prevent chromic acid–induced acute tubular necrosis in experimental animals.[101]

### HAIR DYE–RELATED ACUTE KIDNEY INJURY

Hair dye and its constituent, paraphenylenediamine (PPD), have been reported as an accidental and intentional cause of poisoning on the Indian subcontinent.[102,103] Acute poisoning with PPD due to accidental or intentional consumption causes edema of the face and neck, resulting in severe respiratory distress that requires tracheostomy. The preceding manifestations are followed by rhabdomyolysis and AKI. In one study, AKI was seen in 32% of patients consuming hair dye.[102,103] The mean nephrotoxic dose was 79 mL.[102] Mechanisms of AKI are direct nephrotoxicity, myoglobinuria, hemoglobinuria, hypovolemia, and hypotension.[102,103] The renal lesions are usually found to be acute tubular necrosis or acute interstitial nephritis in patients undergoing biopsy. Renal replacement therapy (RRT) is required in 82% of patients in whom AKI develops.[102] The overall mortality rate is about 26%, and death is attributed mainly to acute respiratory distress, cardiac arrhythmias, and shock.[103]

## ACUTE KIDNEY INJURY DUE TO INTRAVASCULAR HEMOLYSIS AND GLUCOSE-6-PHOSPHATE DEHYDROGENASE DEFICIENCY

G6PD is a key enzyme that protects erythrocytes from oxidative stresses. Deficiency caused by mutations in the *G6PD* gene causes intravascular hemolysis.[104] The gene is located on the X chromosome, and hence males carrying the affected gene have more severe hemolysis. The severity also depends on the nature of the genetic defect. The G6PD variant (Mediterranean) in parts of India and Pakistan leads to hemolysis only in response to oxidative stress.[105] Individuals deficient in the enzyme cannot maintain an adequate level of reduced glutathione, leading to the precipitation of oxidized hemoglobin in red blood cells, which are then sequestered and lysed. Hemolytic crisis develops within hours of exposure to the stress, usually in the form of drugs, toxins, or infections. Specific causes include pharmacologic agents such as primaquine, sulfonamides, acetylsalicylic acid, nitrofurantoin, nalidixic acid, furazolidone, niridazole, doxorubicin, and phenazopyridine, toxic compounds such as naphthalene balls, infections such as viral hepatitis, rickettsiosis, typhoid fever, and urinary tract infections, and severe metabolic acidosis of any cause. Passage of dark urine followed by oliguria is the most common presentation.[106]

Haemolysis resulting from G6PD deficiency may contribute to 5% to 10% of AKI, precipitated by multiple medications and/or infections.[6] Estimation of the G6PD level in the erythrocytes by the fluorescent spot test confirms the deficiency. Normally, the enzyme activity decreases as the cells age, and older cells with the lowest enzyme activity are destroyed first in a crisis. This process can result in a false-negative test result during a hemolytic episode when the surviving red blood cell population consists of younger erythrocytes, especially in an individual with mild deficiency. The test should, therefore, be repeated after the patient has recovered from the acute episode to confirm the diagnosis. In practice, patients are routinely screened for G6PD deficiency before prescribing a drug that is known to cause hemolysis in such patients, at least in larger centers. Prevalence has been reported to be 8.5% and 7.7% in Indian and selected tribal populations, respectively.[107,108]

## ACUTE CORTICAL NECROSIS

Acute renal cortical necrosis is the most catastrophic of all types of AKI. Of more than 2900 patients with AKI treated with dialysis over 28 years in a study in northern India, 3.8% were found to have acute cortical necrosis.[109] It can develop after a variety of conditions, with the most common being obstetric complications and snake bite. Obstetric complications were responsible in 56% of all cases of acute cortical necrosis, whereas snake bite accounted for 14%. In children, the most common cause is hemolytic-uremic syndrome. The most striking feature of this condition is prolonged oliguria or anuria. This phase may extend for weeks to months, and patients with diffuse cortical necrosis may never enter a diuretic phase.[110,111]

Renal recovery depends on the amount of viable cortical tissue and can be slow and incomplete as the surviving nephrons hypertrophy to compensate for the lost nephron mass. In the study in northern India, only 17% of patients could discontinue dialysis by the end of 3 months.[109] Kidney function deteriorates with time in patients who have achieved partial functional recovery. The longest recorded dialysis-free survival has been 12 years.[109]

The gold standard for establishing the diagnosis is renal biopsy, although CT has emerged as a reliable noninvasive imaging modality for the early diagnosis of acute cortical necrosis.[112,113] The characteristic findings include a lack of enhancement of the renal cortex, except for the subcapsular rim after injection of a contrast agent, medullary enhancement, and absence of pelvicalyceal excretion.[109] Cortical tram-track or eggshell calcification develops later and may be detected on a plain radiograph, ultrasonogram, or CT scan. Histologic examination shows a variable degree of necrosis of all elements of the renal parenchyma, especially the cortical region.[109] Some cortical tissue in the subcapsular and juxtamedullary regions may be spared, and its hypertrophy is responsible for the partial recovery of renal function. Other findings include fibrin thrombi in the glomerular capillaries, fibrinoid necrosis of vessel walls, calcification of the necrotic areas, and cortical hemorrhages. The lesions may be classified into patchy and diffuse types, depending on whether the entire parenchyma or only a part of the renal tissue examined shows features of acute cortical necrosis.[109] Needle biopsy can at best give only an approximate idea of the extent of the lesions and can underestimate or overestimate the extent of lesions because of sampling error.

The pathogenesis of acute cortical necrosis remains unclear. The main hypotheses are vasospasm of small vessels and toxic capillary endothelial damage.[109] Prolonged vasospasm of both cortical and medullary vessels induces cortical necrosis in experimental animals. The reasons for increased propensity for renal cortical necrosis during pregnancy are not clear. Renal vasculature in pregnancy may be more prone to vasoconstriction secondary to the effect of sex hormones. Similarities between acute cortical necrosis and the generalized Shwartzman reaction induced in experimental animals by the injection of endotoxin have also been noted.[114] Unlike in nonpregnant animals, in which two small doses of endotoxin administered 24 hours apart cause this phenomenon, only one injection is sufficient in pregnant rabbits.[115]

The presence of fibrin thrombi in the vasculature of patients with acute cortical necrosis has led to consideration of intravascular coagulation as the initial event. A role for endothelium-derived vasoactive substances in the genesis of acute cortical necrosis has also been proposed.[110] The increased endothelin-1 levels in women with preeclampsia could contribute to renal ischemia, and a potential role for polymorphisms in the endothelin-1 gene has been suggested.[116] However, more studies are needed to establish the exact role of endothelin in the pathogenesis of acute cortical necrosis.

## ACUTE PERITONEAL DIALYSIS FOR ACUTE KIDNEY INJURY

As with all AKI, supportive care and removal or reversal of the cause are the mainstay of treatment; however, some patients will recover kidney function in time to avoid dialysis. Where resources are scare, acute dialysis may not be available, and these patients will die.

PD becomes important in such resource-constrained settings because it requires minimal infrastructure and expertise. Whether peritoneal dialysis is similar or inferior to hemodialysis has been the subject of a Cochrane review protocol, but appears to be noninferior.[117,118]

However, when required, and if available, PD is likely to be lifesaving. There have been several success stories of acute PD being lifesaving in desperate and emergency circumstances.[119] Rigid temporary catheters, which are inserted over a stylet at the bedside, and PD fluid are easily available and inexpensive. Performance of acute PD is a skill that is easily taught and acquired. In fact, many general physicians, especially in the armed forces, who might be posted to far-off places or places where hemodialysis is not available around the clock, routinely carry out acute PD whenever required. Because facilities may be inadequate and overloaded, and delay is inevitable, the timing of dialysis is also an issue. A single-center, open-label, randomized controlled trial has investigated the early initiation of dialysis versus traditional indication-based initiation of dialysis in 208 subjects with community-acquired AKI in India. The investigators did not find any differences in mortality or dialysis dependence at 3 months between the two groups.[120]

# CHRONIC KIDNEY DISEASE

## INCIDENCE AND PREVALENCE OF CHRONIC KIDNEY DISEASE

An accurate estimate of the number of patients on the Indian subcontinent who have CKD or need RRT is not available owing to the lack of nationwide registry data.[121] A countrywide cohort study of early-stage CKD patients has been started in India. Over the next 5 years, approximately 5000 patients would be enrolled and followed up for the next 5 years. The study aims to describe the epidemiology of CKD progression and the development of complications such as cardiovascular disease in CKD in developing countries. In India, Mani has reported a prevalence of CKD of 1.1% among a rural population of 25,000 who were subjects of a universal screening program in which the serum creatinine concentration was measured only in those with hypertension or proteinuria.[122] Agarwal and colleagues screened 4700 adults in an urban community and found a point prevalence of 7852/million individuals with a serum creatinine level higher than 1.8 mg/dL.[123]

Another cross-sectional study that screened 5588 adults from different parts of India reported a CKD prevalence of 17.2%, with about 6% having CKD stage 3 or worse.[124] The prevalence of early stages of CKD (stages 1–3) was reported to be about 13.1% to 15% using the Chronic Kidney Disease Epidemiology Collaboration (CKD-EPI) or Modification of Diet in Renal Disease study (MDRD) equation in a cohort of 3398 otherwise healthy adults.[125] Studies from Pakistan,[126] Nepal,[127] and Bangladesh[128] have reported a CKD prevalences of 25.3%, 10.7%, and 13.1% to 16%, respectively, in the general population. These figures must be interpreted with caution because of the wide variations in the definition of CKD, study methodology, and sampled population. Despite a high prevalence of CKD, there is a low awareness of the disease; only 7.9% and 2.3% of subjects were aware of the disease in the studies from India[124] and Pakistan,[126] respectively. Lack of both health care resources and education is possibly responsible for the low awareness of disease.

Commonly used formulas for the estimation of the glomerular filtration rate (GFR), such as the MDRD equation, have been validated only in small population-based studies in the Indian subcontinent.[129,130] Differences in body habitus and dietary habits make it likely that these formulas may require further validation and possibly correction factors for the accurate assessment of GFR in this population.[130] Two of the later studies showed the mean measured GFR in healthy Indian adults (kidney donors) to be only 81 mL/min, substantially lower than values reported in the West.[131,132] This finding raises the question of whether the thresholds used to define CKD should be modified. The crude and age-adjusted incidences of ESKD in India have been estimated to be 151 and 232/million population, respectively.[133] This means that 250,000 to 300,000 new patients need RRT every year. Data on the prevalence of ESKD are not available.

## DEMOGRAPHICS OF CHRONIC KIDNEY DISEASE AND END-STAGE KIDNEY DISEASE

In the past, glomerulonephritis was reported to be the most common cause of ESKD in the Indian subcontinent.[134] The high prevalence of glomerular diseases was linked to the prevalence of bacterial and viral infections. The causative spectrum, however, has been changing in the past decade (Table 79.3).

Diabetic nephropathy, previously restricted to high-income urban residents and older individuals, has now emerged as the most important cause of CKD in this region (see discussion

**Table 79.3 Causes of Chronic Kidney Disease and End-Stage Kidney Disease in India and Pakistan (%)**

| Cause | India (*N* = 57,273)[a] | Pakistan (*N* = 6127)[b] |
|---|---|---|
| Diabetic nephropathy | 31.3 | 40.35 |
| Hypertension | 12.9 | 28.89 |
| Chronic glomerulonephritis | 13.8 | 11.57 |
| Chronic interstitial nephritis, calculus disease, obstructive nephropathy | 10.4 | 7.6 |
| Other, unknown | 31.8 | 11.48 |

[a]Adapted from Rajapurkar MM, John GT, Kirpalani AL, et al. What do we know about chronic kidney disease in India: first report of the Indian CKD registry. *BMC Nephrol.* 2012;13:10.
[b]Data from The Kidney Foundation. Dialysis Registry of Pakistan 2007–2008. Karachi, Pakistan: The Kidney Foundation; 2008.

on diabetic nephropathy in Chapter 39). According to the Indian CKD Registry, which has information on more than 57,000 patients, diabetes was listed as the primary diagnosis in 31% of cases of the CKD.[135] The frequency increased to 40% in incident ESKD cases.[133] In older adults (>60 years), diabetic nephropathy accounted for about 58% of all cases of CKD[136]; however, this is not a nationwide registry. According to the Dialysis Registry of Pakistan, more than 40% of cases of ESKD are due to diabetic nephropathy.[137] In Sri Lanka and Bangladesh also, diabetic nephropathy is an important cause of CKD.[138,139] This change has paralleled the increase in the prevalence of type 2 diabetes in the general population, especially in the areas undergoing rapid urbanization.[140] The projected increase in the prevalence of diabetes in the region suggests that these numbers will rise further over the next 15 years.[141]

The role of the intrauterine environment in the development of chronic disease in adults, particularly systemic arterial hypertension and CKD, has come to the fore and could explain the link between poverty and malnutrition in the mother and the subsequent development of CKD in the offspring. Low birth weight and early malnutrition, followed by overnutrition in adult life, have been shown to be associated with the development of metabolic syndrome, diabetes, and diabetic nephropathy in an Indian cohort.[142] Whether nephrogenesis is influenced by intrauterine malnutrition and/or any adverse intrauterine environment is a matter of ongoing investigation (see discussion of nephron endowment and developmental programming of blood pressure and renal function in Chapter 21). The finding of a high prevalence of proteinuria and high blood pressure in southern Asian children could be part of this jigsaw puzzle.[143,144] Also not investigated has been the role of dietary habits and indigenous medicines. Whether any of these factors has an adverse effect on kidney function remains unknown. Infections such as chronic hepatitis B or C, HIV, and tropical infectious diseases are prevalent in this part of the world, and renal involvement is not uncommon in these infections. Although there are no credible data that support these infections as a significant cause of CKD, this possibility cannot be rule out because it is likely that this is missed in practice and hence not recorded.[145]

The mean age of patients with CKD, including those requiring RRT, is generally lower in this region than in other parts of the world. The mean age of Indian patients with CKD is 50.1 ± 14.6 years; 70.3% are males and 29.7% females, according to the Indian CKD Registry.[135] This lower mean age is likely related to unique environmental exposures at a younger age and the poor availability of health care, which delays diagnosis and leads to a loss of opportunities to institute timely preventive measures, culminating in faster progression to ESKD. Dialyzer reuse offers cost savings and is common.[146] Social and infrastructural limitations lead to poor compliance, even when dialysis is offered free of cost.[147] Certain causes of CKD have been shown to predominate in specific geographic locations, as discussed later.

## CHRONIC KIDNEY DISEASE DUE TO GLOMERULONEPHRITIS

In the absence of a biopsy registry, the exact spectrum of glomerulonephritis cannot be known. However, a large study of more than 5400 kidney biopsy specimens at a south Indian tertiary care center that treats not only patients from India but also those from neighboring countries has provided an insight into the range of glomerulonephritis in the region.[148] Primary glomerulonephritis was diagnosed in 71% of all the biopsy specimens. Mesangioproliferative glomerulonephritis without IgA was the most common lesion (20.2%), followed by idiopathic focal segmental glomerulosclerosis (FSGS) (17%), minimal change disease (11.6%), membranous nephropathy (9.8%), IgA nephropathy (8.6%), and membranoproliferative glomerulonephritis (3.7%). Postinfectious glomerulonephritis accounted for 12.3% of all lesions.

To ascertain changing trends, biopsy data collected between 1971 and 1985 were compared with later data in the same study. The later data showed significant increases in FSGS (17% vs. 8.6%) and membranous glomerulonephritis (9.8% vs. 6.4%) during the period 1986 to 2002, whereas minimal change disease (11.6% vs. 16.5%) and membranoproliferative glomerulonephritis (3.7% vs. 7.2%) decreased significantly during the same period. Thus, in comparison with other registries, the prevalence of IgA nephropathy is much lower than that in East Asians, whereas FSGS is more common. Similar trends have been reported in another study from the northern region of the subcontinent.[149] The analysis of data for adults presenting with nephrotic syndrome due to primary glomerular disease has revealed that FSGS is the most common lesion in both India and Pakistan. The frequency of occurrence of other primary glomerular diseases in these patients is presented in Table 79.4.[149-151] The morphologic categories of FSGS in the Indian population have been described and are different from those in the West.[152] There is a lower prevalence of the perihilar and collapsing variants and a higher prevalence of tip and cellular variants. Secondary amyloidosis is an important cause of glomerular disease on the subcontinent and is much more common than primary amyloidosis. Tuberculosis is the main cause of secondary amyloidosis in India, accounting for two-thirds of cases, whereas rheumatoid arthritis is responsible in only 6% of cases.[153,154]

## CHRONIC KIDNEY DISEASE DUE TO VASCULAR DISORDERS

The most common causes of renovascular hypertension worldwide are fibromuscular dysplasia in the young and atherosclerosis in older adults. On the Indian subcontinent, however, Takayasu arteritis or nonspecific aortoarteritis is the main cause of renovascular hypertension in young adults, as well as in children, accounting for 59% to 80% of all cases in these groups.[155,156] In older adults, as elsewhere, atherosclerosis is the most common cause.

Takayasu arteritis is an inflammatory vascular disease of unknown cause predominantly affecting young females in their second and third decades. There is a potential association described with tuberculosis.[157] Takayasu arteritis involves the large elastic arteries and results in occlusive or ectatic changes, mainly in the aorta and its major branches. The average age of Indian patients is between 25 and 30 years.[158]

Aortoarteritis has been classified into the following types, according to the site of involvement[159,160]:

- Type I affects the branches of the aortic arch.
- Type IIa affects the ascending aorta, aortic arch, and its branches.

**Table 79.4 Spectrum of Primary Glomerular Lesions Causing Nephrotic Syndrome on the Indian Subcontinent[a]**

| Disorder | India (*N* = 324)[b] | Pakistan (*N* = 316)[c] | Nepal (*N* = 137)[d] |
|---|---|---|---|
| Focal segmental glomerulosclerosis | 99 (30.6) | 126 (39.9) | 11 (8.0) |
| Membranous nephropathy | 79 (24.4) | 84 (26.6) | 58 (42.3) |
| Membranoproliferative glomerulonephritis | 58 (17.9) | 14 (4.4) | 30 (21.9) |
| Minimal change disease | 48 (14.8) | 50 (15.8) | 14 (10.2) |
| Postinfectious glomerulonephritis | 9 (2.8) | 9 (2.8) | 4 (2.9) |
| Immunoglobulin A nephropathy | 6 (1.8) | 8 (2.5) | 3 (2.2) |
| Other | 25 (7.7) | 25 (8.0) | 17 (12.4) |

[a]Numbers in parentheses indicate percentages.
[b]Data from Rathi M, Bhagat RL, Mukhopadhyay P, et al. Changing histologic spectrum of adult nephritic syndrome over five decades in Northern India: a single center experience. *Ind J Nephrol.* 2014;24:13–18.
[c]Data from Kazi JI, Mubarak M, Ahmed E, et al. Spectrum of glomerulonephritides in adults with nephrotic syndrome in Pakistan. *Clin Exp Nephrol.* 2009;13:38–43.
[d]Data from Garyal, Kafle RK. Histopathological spectrum of glomerular disease in Nepal: a seven-year retrospective study. *Nepal Med Coll J.* 2008;10:126–128.

- Type IIb affects the ascending aorta, aortic arch, and its branches and the descending thoracic aorta.
- Type III affects the thoracic aorta, abdominal aorta, and/or renal arteries.
- Type IV affects the abdominal aorta and/or renal arteries.
- Type V is a combination of types IIb and IV.

Involvement of a coronary or pulmonary artery is indicated by appending the suffix *C*(+) or *P*(+) to any of the types.[161] Involvement of the abdominal aorta and/or renal arteries is more common in India and other Southeast Asian countries and South America than in Japan, where the aortic arch and its branches are more commonly involved. In Indian and Bangladeshi patients, type III disease is the most common, accounting for 53% to 76% of all cases.[162]

In a large study of 650 cases in India, clinical manifestations of aortoarteritis included unequal pulses (96%), hypertension (72%), oliguria due to renal failure (30%), intermittent claudication (25%), neurologic symptoms (e.g., amaurosis fugax, syncope, transient ischemic attacks; 22.5%), eye changes (8.1%), and skin manifestations (e.g., erythema nodosum, Raynaud phenomenon, leg ulcers; 3.8%).[162] It is important to record blood pressure in all four limbs because arteries supplying the upper limbs are often involved in the disease process.

The renal artery is narrowed at its ostium and in the proximal third. Bilateral renal artery stenosis is seen in about 50% of all patients (Fig. 79.2). Histologic findings in affected vessels vary according to the stage of the disease. In the early stages, granulomatous inflammation and infiltration with polymorphs, mononuclear cells, and multinucleated giant cells are seen in all the layers but are more marked in the adventitia than in the media or intima.[163] These features may also be seen around the vasa vasorum, which show endothelial proliferation and obliteration of the vessel lumen. In more advanced disease, the inflammatory process is less evident, but adventitial fibrosis and intimal smooth muscle proliferation and fibrosis result in marked luminal narrowing.

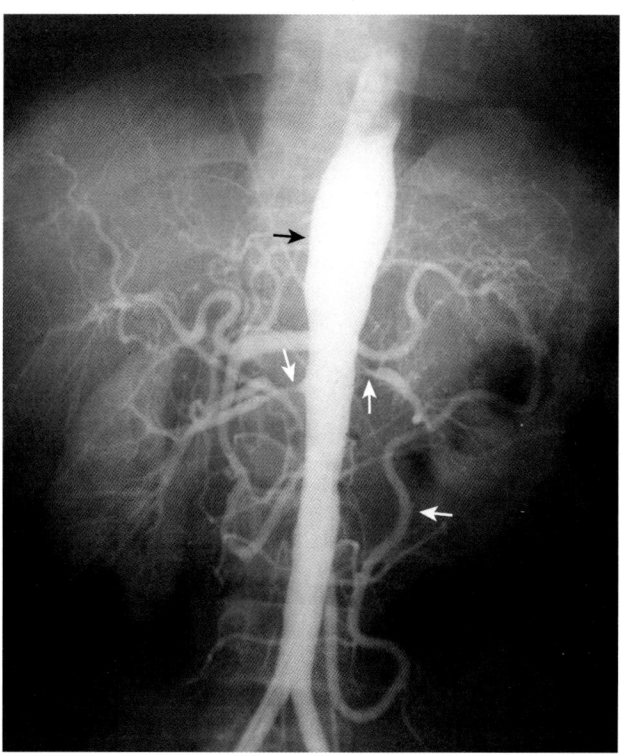

**Fig. 79.2** Takayasu arteritis. Shown is bilateral renal artery narrowing *(vertical arrows)* with poststenotic dilation on the left side, dilation and irregularity of the abdominal aorta *(black arrow)*, and a large collateral vessel *(horizontal arrow)* arising from the inferior mesenteric artery.

Nonspecific ischemic glomerular lesions resulting from arterial narrowing and hypertension are frequently observed in patients with renal artery involvement. Rarely, glomerular lesions, such as mesangioproliferative, focal proliferative, membranoproliferative, and crescentic forms of glomerulonephritis, have been reported. Renal amyloidosis in association with Takayasu arteritis has also been reported in rare cases.[164]

Prednisolone, at a dosage of 1 mg/kg body weight per day, tapered to 15 mg/day by 3 months,[165] often dramatically improves the constitutional symptoms, halts disease progression in patients with inflammatory stage disease, and lowers the erythrocyte sedimentation rate (ESR) toward normal. However, even the ESR is not a reliable marker of disease activity. If progression of disease is seen in patients undergoing steroid therapy, cytotoxic drugs such as cyclophosphamide or azathioprine may be used.[166] Alternatively, low-dose methotrexate may enhance the efficacy of steroid therapy and facilitate steroid sparing.[166] The results of balloon angioplasty with stent placement in narrowed arteries are highly encouraging.[166] In patients in whom stents cannot be implanted, surgical reconstruction may be carried out after the disease becomes inactive.

## CHRONIC KIDNEY DISEASE DUE TO RENAL CALCULI

Obstructive nephropathy due to urolithiasis is common in Pakistan and contiguous parts of northern India. This constitutes what has been referred to as a "renal stone belt,"[167] where nephrolithiasis is responsible for 5% of all cases of ESKD.[167]

The available literature on urinary calculi shows a different stone pattern across the world, highlighting different geographic and causative factors. Studies in northern India have shown that the vast majority of calculi (>90%) are calcium oxalate stones, predominantly calcium oxalate monohydrate (80%).[168] Apatite, struvite, and uric acid stones account for less than 2% each. This incidence of calcium oxalate monohydrate stones is significantly higher than that in Western countries, where such stones constitute up to 55% of the total.[169] Typically, staghorn calculi are composed of calcium magnesium ammonium phosphate. However, in Indian studies, even staghorn calculi are found to be made up predominantly of calcium oxalate. Reasons for the high incidence of calcium oxalate calculi in this region could include the oxalate-rich vegetarian diet, along with its high carbohydrate content and the high mineral and fluoride content of drinking water. Fluoride is thought to promote stone formation by increasing oxaluria and insoluble calcium fluoride in urine.[170]

## CHRONIC KIDNEY DISEASE DUE TO INDIGENOUS THERAPIES

### HERBAL MEDICINE TOXICITY

On the subcontinent, a combination of ignorance, poverty, nonavailability of health care facilities, high cost of modern medicines, and the widespread belief in indigenous systems drives people to turn to indigenous drugs. It is commonly believed that these remedies are gentler and have no side effects. Herbal remedies are often classified as dietary supplements for regulatory and marketing purposes and hence are exempt from rigorous safety testing. However, adulteration of herbal medicines is common in many countries. A state government report has cited finding undeclared pharmaceuticals or heavy metals in 32% of Asian patent medicines sold in California.[171] The high heavy metal content of indigenous herbal drugs could be due to heavily polluted soil or irrigation water. Dwivedi and Dey have found high lead and cadmium levels in the leaves of medicinal plants from India.[172]

The medical community has increasingly recognized the potential role of these remedies in causing harm to various organ systems, including the kidneys. Indigenous therapies may cause AKI as well as CKD. In AKI, the cause-and-effect relationship is easier to establish because there is a temporal relation between the intake of the agents and the injury. However, physicians often do not seek the history of intake of natural medicines. Moreover, a chemical analysis of such drugs is seldom carried out. Prakash and colleagues have described the case of a 60-year-old man who had unexplained kidney failure.[173] Investigation revealed that he had been taking an herbal medicine from India containing a large amount of lead. After discontinuation of the herbal medicine and several sessions of lead chelation therapy, his creatinine level declined. Lead poisoning should be considered as a consequence of traditional remedy-induced kidney injury.[174] As of now, supporting alternative drugs without any scientific evidence is not recommended. However, trying to find reasons for their use in community and discovering their beneficial effects, if any, could be an area for research.

### TOXICITY OF NATURAL MEDICINES FROM ANIMAL SOURCES

The raw gallbladder or bile of freshwater and grass carp is used in parts of eastern India to reduce fever, treat cough, decrease hypertension, improve visual acuity, treat rheumatism, and promote general health.[175] A syndrome of acute hepatic and renal failure has been reported in exposed patients.[175] Symptoms appear minutes to hours after ingestion and include abdominal pain, nausea, vomiting, and watery diarrhea. Hepatocellular jaundice is observed in more than 60% of patients. AKI sets in within 48 hours and is oliguric in most patients, and more than 75% also show microscopic hematuria. The duration of AKI ranges from 2 to 3 weeks. The variation in symptomatology is likely to be related to differences in the varieties of fish or amount of bile ingested, as well as in individual susceptibility. Renal histologic examination reveals tubular necrosis and interstitial edema.

The mechanism whereby AKI develops is not well understood and may include bradycardia and hypotension owing to the cardiotoxic effect of the bile salts.[175] Bile salts also inhibit intestinal $Na^+$-$K^+$-ATPase, which increases mucosal permeability and leads to diarrhea.[175] Bile produces diuresis, excessive salt loss, and cardiac depression in rats.[176] Hypotension and hemolysis may also contribute to renal failure. Recovery has been universal among patients who have sought medical attention in a timely manner, and death has occurred only in those who reported late and had multiorgan failure.

## CHRONIC KIDNEY DISEASE OF UNCERTAIN CAUSE

A large proportion of Indian patients with ESKD come for treatment with a relatively short history of kidney problems and advanced renal failure with no previous health records.[167] This makes the task of determining the primary disease difficult. Thus there is a large proportion of patients with ESKD of unknown cause (CKDu), which accounts for over one-third of all patients at our center. Reports of CKD of CKDu have also emerged from the north central provinces of Sri Lanka. A detailed epidemiologic investigation has suggested that potential exposure to cadmium through local food chains might be associated with CKDu. The mean concentration of cadmium in urine was found to be significantly higher in those with CKDu as compared with controls in the endemic and nonendemic areas (1.039 μg/g vs. 0.646 μg/g, $P < .001$; 1.039 μg/g vs. 0.345 μg/g, $P < .05$, respectively).[177] Also, dietary selenium deficiency and genetic factors have also been proposed as possible risk factors for development of CKDu.[177,178] In a recent systematic review, positive family history, male gender, farming occupation, middle age, snake bite, and possible heavy metal exposure were found to be associated with CKDu.[179] Most of the affected individuals were male paddy farmers of low socioeconomic status who had progressive nonproteinuric CKD.[180,181] Biopsy specimens showed tubulointerstitial nephritis, with minimal inflammation and extensive fibrosis. The disease bears a strong resemblance to Balkan nephropathy and Chinese herbal nephropathy. CKDu is discussed further in Chapter 76.

## END-STAGE KIDNEY DISEASE

### FINANCIAL AND REIMBURSEMENT ISSUES

Unlike in Western nations, the concept of health insurance (both government-funded and private) is still in a primitive stage on the Indian subcontinent. The costs of RRT, therefore, have to be borne by most patients out of their own funds.[182] Some government and private organizations cover the cost of treatment of employees and their dependents as part of employment benefits. The overall cost of RRT is less in dollar terms than in the industrialized countries because of the lower staff salaries and the low cost of drugs. Nevertheless, it is still several times higher than the per capita gross national product and remains out of reach for most of the population.

One Indian study has reported that about two-thirds of patients who needed RRT obtained financial assistance from employers or accepted charity, one-third sold property or family valuables, and one-quarter took out loans to cover the cost.[122] Many patients raised funds in more than one way. Only 4% were able to cover the cost using their family resources.

According to the Indian CKD Registry, about 57% of patients with ESKD are not receiving any replacement therapy.[135] Among those who started dialysis in one unit in India, 28% were able to sustain treatment beyond 3 months.[183] Among older adults, one study has reported that of those who started HD, only 18% were still receiving dialytic support at the end of 1 year.[136] Similar high dropout rates (18%) were observed at the Sindh Institute of Urology and Transplantation, which provides free dialysis in Pakistan,[147] illustrating that the provision of free dialysis is not enough to overcome the access barriers in the region. The cost of dialysis is also influenced by late presentation, with resulting poor clinical status that necessitates hospitalization. Poor hygiene, hot and humid climate, and overcrowding predispose to a variety of life-threatening infections. It has been reported that 12% to 18% of all patients undergoing dialysis eventually have tuberculosis.[184]

### HEMODIALYSIS

There are about 5500 dialysis centers in India, with over 90% in the private sector.[185] Pakistan had 140 dialysis centers in 2004, which increased to 175 in 2009.[185] They are spread over 53 cities—about 30% are government-funded, and 45% are under private management. The rest are run by community support or charitable agencies. In both countries, a large number of dialysis units are small minimal care facilities, owned and looked after by non-nephrologists or even technicians.[185]

Decisions on the frequency and duration of HD sessions are based on patient symptomatology, financial considerations, and the availability of dialysis slots. Most patients undergo one or two 4-hour sessions every week. Dialyzer reuse is practically universal, and reprocessing is often performed manually. The absence of regulation by the government or professional societies has prevented standardization of dialysis procedures, including the establishment of minimum standards for dialysis machines, water quality, type of dialyzers, and reuse policies.[182]

Viral hepatitis is among the most common viral infections encountered in patients undergoing dialysis. Hepatitis B vaccination, despite low seroconversion rates, has reduced the prevalence from 32% to 4.7% among patients in India.[186] Hepatitis C virus (HCV) has emerged as the predominant cause of viral hepatitis in patients undergoing maintenance HD. The annual incidence of HCV infection as detected by anti-HCV antibodies among patients at an Indian HD center was reported to be as high as 18%, compared with about 2% in patients receiving continuous ambulatory PD.[187] The prevalence of HCV was found to be 27.7% when HCV RNA was tested in patients receiving HD at a tertiary care hospital.[188] The high incidence of HCV in HD units could be related to the high prevalence of HCV seropositivity in patients undergoing HD, total transfused blood volume, lack of enforcement of universal precautions, high comorbid illness burden, and greater frequency of intervention. It has been shown that the isolation of HCV-infected patients during HD significantly decreases the HCV seroconversion rate, from 36.2% to 2.7%.[189]

Malnutrition affects most patients receiving dialysis in this region; the reported frequency is 44% to 77%.[190] The imposition of protein restriction in patients who are already consuming a calorie-deficient diet, delay in initiation of dialysis, and delivery of inadequate dialysis contribute to this problem. In fact, in one study, protein malnutrition was found to increase in as many as 86% of Indian patients after the initiation of dialysis.[191]

### PERITONEAL DIALYSIS

Facilities for HD are available only in the larger cities. Because PD can be done at home, it could be regarded as the preferred form of dialysis for most patients who live in rural areas and small towns. Despite this advantage, PD continues to be grossly underused. The major reason is its higher cost in comparison with HD on the subcontinent. Other reasons include delayed presentation to dialysis units, which gives insufficient time for patient education and preparation, and the fact that many nephrologists are not adequately trained to provide PD. Concerns are often raised on the grounds that poorly educated patients are likely to be nonadherent to therapy and would be at greater risk of peritonitis owing to the hot humid climate and poor hygienic conditions.

Although PD has been available for almost 25 years in India, at our center this modality is used in fewer than 20%

of patients. In 2008, the number of patients treated with long-term PD in India and Pakistan was only about 6500 and 100, respectively.[192] Patients are assigned to PD not as a matter of choice but mainly because they have contraindications for other modalities of RRT. In one large hospital, only 8% of PD recipients were started on PD directly; 92% were shifted after receiving HD for a mean duration of about 6 months. Of those, two-thirds were switched because they tolerated HD poorly, 30% because of comorbid conditions and vascular access problems, and 3% because of lifestyle issues.[193] Patients who initially underwent PD were more likely to have diabetes mellitus and coronary artery disease.[193] Their average age was 63 years, compared with 34 years for the HD population.

The patient's economic status also determines the PD prescription. The most common practice is to start patients on three 2-L exchanges daily.[194] It is not uncommon for patients to reduce the number of exchanges as their financial resources dwindle and eventually die of complications of underdialysis. Cycler-assisted PD and the use of newer solutions remain the exclusive privilege of the rich.

In addition to factors directly related to PD, cardiovascular disease is an important killer. Patients often do not undergo cardiovascular evaluation, having already exhausted their resources on PD. This scenario is similar to that seen in the early years of PD practice in Mexico, where aggressive marketing led non-nephrologists to start PD without attention to quality.[195]

Peritonitis remains the major problem associated with PD on the Indian subcontinent. The initial rate of peritonitis was one episode every 5 to 6 patient-months,[196] but this has declined significantly as training has improved and patients have been switched to the double-bag system. Some programs reported a higher incidence of infections in the summer months.[196] Peritonitis rates are now around 0.39 to 0.41 episodes/patient-year.[197-201] Two unique features of PD-related infections in Indian patients are a high rate of culture-negative cases and a predominance of gram-negative peritonitis, mainly in northern India. Culture-positive peritonitis was found in only 63% to 72% of episodes.[197,198]

Gram-negative bacteria constitute 60% to 66% of all organisms found on culture of patients undergoing PD.[202-205] *E. coli* is usually found. Other organisms are *Klebsiella pneumoniae, Acinetobacter calcoaceticus, Pseudomonas aeruginosa,* and *Enterobacter* spp. Overall, organisms of fecal origin are more common than those of skin origin. This finding could be related to the unique habit of ablution after defecation in the region, which facilitates the transfer of fecal organisms to the hand. Patients with gram-negative peritonitis require more frequent hospitalization and have higher rates of catheter loss, switch to HD, and death.[198]

In southern India, Pakistan, and Nepal, gram-positive infections are predominant, in contrast to the pattern of infections seen in North India.[202,205] Fungal peritonitis is noted in about 10% to 14% of all peritonitis episodes.[203] More than 90% of these are *Candida* infections. Most episodes are preceded by bacterial peritonitis. Prompt catheter removal improves outcomes. Despite the high frequency of mycobacterial infections in the community, tuberculous peritonitis has not emerged as a significant problem in the Indian PD population.

Malnutrition is a major problem in these patients. Prasad and associates have shown that nutritional status at the time of PD initiation was predictive of peritonitis rates. Malnourished patients experienced significantly more peritonitis episodes than patients with normal nutritional status (1.0 vs. 0.2 annually).[206]

## KIDNEY TRANSPLANTATION

Constraints in operating an effective maintenance dialysis program leave renal transplantation as the only viable option for patients with ESKD. However, transplantation activity falls woefully short of demand; lack of finances, lack of an organized cadaver-donor transplant program, and social issues are the major stumbling blocks. Despite these limitations, community participation coupled with strong public and private sector efforts can establish a free and self-sustaining RRT program, as has been demonstrated in Karachi, Pakistan; 1- and 5-year graft survival rates of 92% and 85%, respectively, have been reported, which are highly encouraging.[207]

Cadaver donors are seldom used because of absence or ineffectiveness of an organ procurement network, lack of facilities for taking care of potential donors, and poor public education. The process depends on the initiative of individual transplant physicians, surgeons, and cooperating ICUs. Even though more than 70,000 road fatalities were recorded annually in India in 2014,[208] lack of prompt transport and unavailability of life support services preclude organ donation, even in situations in which the families could be approached for consent.[209] Of around 4000 renal transplantations performed annually in India, only 2% use organs from cadaveric donors. For transplantations involving living related donors in India, the proportion of spousal donors (mainly wives) has increased over the past decade; they constitute about 40% of all donors.[210]

Affordability is another major barrier. Even though patients do not have to bear hospitalization costs in state-subsidized hospitals, the cost of immunosuppressive therapy is not reimbursed. In a prospective analysis of 50 kidney transplant recipients in India, direct expenses for kidney transplantation—physician fees, cost of drugs and disposables, dialysis, and costs of laboratory investigations and hospitalization—were estimated to range from $2151 to $23,792 and indirect expenses—travel, food, stay, and loss of income—from $226 to $15,283 (all in U.S. dollars).[211] Overall, about 54%, 8%, and 10% of families suffered from severe, moderate, and some financial crisis, respectively.[211] Antibody induction therapy and prophylaxis for cytomegalovirus infection are therefore rarely used. Pretransplantation HCV infections also often go untreated. Patients are nonadherent with regimens of expensive drugs such as calcineurin inhibitors, leading to high rates of graft loss. The cost of treating steroid-resistant rejections is prohibitive. Cost reduction strategies that are frequently used include limiting induction therapy to high-risk patients, using cytochrome P450 inhibitors (e.g., ketoconazole, non–dihydropyridine calcium channel blocker), using azathioprine instead of mycophenolate mofetil, continuing prednisolone long term, and using bioequivalent generic drugs.

The worldwide shortage of organs for transplantation has given rise to the practice of the purchase of kidneys from poor donors by affluent persons in India in the 1980s and early 1990s.[212] The buyers came from both within and outside the country—hence, the term "transplant tourism." The exploitation of donors and substandard medical care provided to recipients were widely condemned and prompted the enactment of a law by the Indian Parliament in 1994 officially banning this practice. Since then, it has been carried out only clandestinely in India; it is more common in some parts of Pakistan, although exact numbers are not known.[213,214] The Human Organ and Tissue Transplantation Ordinance, which was passed in September 2007 in Pakistan, explicitly and unambiguously makes the buying and selling of human organs a crime and prohibits transplantation of organs from Pakistanis into foreigners.[215] Of late, more transplants from unrelated living donors are being done in Sri Lanka, as reported in the lay press.

Infections complicate the course in 50% to 75% of kidney transplant recipients in the region, with mortality ranging from 20% to 60%.[190] Rubin has categorized these infections as those occurring within the first month after transplantation, those occurring within 2 to 6 months, and those occurring thereafter.[216] The reported 6-month milestone of a decrease in the susceptibility to infections after a step-down of immunosuppression is not seen in these patients. This reflects an altered susceptibility pattern caused by coexisting infections in immunosuppressed patients in the region, together with a higher prevalence of endemic infections.[217]

Tuberculosis affects 10% to 13% of renal transplant recipients in India[218-220] and results from the reactivation of a quiescent focus. It manifests in the first year after transplantation in more than 50% of patients. Although pleuropulmonary involvement is the most common, disseminated disease occurs in about 30% of patients. Unusual sites of involvement include the skin, tonsils, vocal cords, and prostate.

Renal transplant recipients with tuberculosis present numerous diagnostic difficulties. The Mantoux test is generally unhelpful, classic radiologic findings are seen only in a minority, examination of a sputum smear for acid-fast bacilli has a low yield, and culture takes 4 to 6 weeks. Bronchoalveolar lavage, bone marrow biopsy, and liver biopsy must be used to make a diagnosis of tuberculosis.

There are also problems with the treatment of tuberculosis in transplant recipients, specifically in selecting antituberculous drugs and determining the duration of therapy. Rifampicin is a well-known hepatic P450 microsomal enzyme inducer that increases the clearance of both prednisolone and calcineurin inhibitors. The dosage of calcineurin inhibitors needs to be increased threefold to fourfold to maintain therapeutic blood levels. This change raises the cost of therapy and is unacceptable to the vast majority of patients. An alternative regimen that has been successfully used consists of a combination of isoniazid, ethambutol, pyrazinamide, and ofloxacin or ciprofloxacin.[221] The optimal duration of therapy is a matter of debate. For combinations using rifampicin and isoniazid, 9 months of treatment have been recommended.[221] However, the duration is increased to 18 months for patients who are not receiving rifampicin.[218] Such patients generally receive two drugs, usually a fluoroquinolone and isoniazid for 18 months. The initiation of isoniazid chemoprophylaxis during dialysis prevents the development of tuberculosis after transplantation. However, isoniazid can cause hepatic dysfunction, for which it often must be discontinued.[222] Drug-resistant mycobacterial strains are also of concern, and the incidence of primary isoniazid resistance has been increasing steadily.[223] The role of isoniazid prophylaxis thus remains controversial.[224]

Other common infections in transplant recipients are hepatitis B and hepatitis C, both of which are highly prevalent in patients undergoing dialysis. Hepatitis B is encountered in about 5%, whereas hepatitis C is seen in 15% to 20%. The cost of interferon therapy and indirect expenses (including dialysis) during therapy for HCV infection have been so prohibitive that the majority (≈75%) of HCV-positive patients undergo kidney transplantation without receiving anti-HCV treatment.[225] With the availability of new directly acting antiviral drugs, however, the paradigm is rapidly changing. Most patients now receive treatment and enter sustained remission. Although patient and graft survivals at 5 years were reported to be similar in HCV-positive and HCV-negative patients, serious bacterial infections were significantly more common in HCV-positive patients.[226,227] The rate of cytomegalovirus infection was found to increase from 4% in the years before calcineurin inhibitors were widely used to 17% in the calcineurin inhibitor era in one autopsy series.[184] Primary infection is seldom seen because the vast majority of both donors and recipients are seropositive.[184] Opportunistic fungal infections occur in 4% to 7% of recipients, but these carry a high mortality rate, more than 65%.[228,229] Malaria and leishmaniasis are also encountered.[230]

## SUMMARY

The spectrum of both acute and chronic kidney disease on the Indian subcontinent differs significantly from that encountered in the industrialized world and other developing countries. Community-acquired AKI in otherwise healthy individuals continues to be common in the region. Although glomerulonephritis has been the most common cause of ESKD, it is being replaced by diabetic nephropathy. The lack of an adequate number of nephrologists and the high cost of treatment pose the biggest challenges to the management of patients with kidney disease in this region of the world.

 Complete reference list available at ExpertConsult.com.

## KEY REFERENCES

9. Jayakumar M, Prabahar MR, Fernando EM, et al. Epidemiologic trend changes in acute renal failure—a tertiary center experience from south India. *Ren Fail.* 2006;28:405–410.
11. Kohli HS, Madhu C, Muthu Kumar T, et al. Treatment related acute renal failure in the elderly: a hospital based prospective study. *Nephrol Dial Transplant.* 2000;15:212–217.
13. Cerda J, Bagga A, Kher V, et al. The contrasting characteristics of acute kidney injury in developed and developing countries. *Nat Clin Pract Nephrol.* 2008;4(3):138–153.
16. Murali R, Bhalla A, Singh D, et al. Acute pesticide poisoning: 15 years experience of a large north-west Indian hospital. *Clin Toxicol (Phila).* 2009;47:35–38.
22. Kohli HS, Bhat A, Aravindan AN, et al. Predictors of mortality in elderly patients with acute renal failure in a developing country. *Int Urol Nephrol.* 2007;39(1):339–344.
25. Prakash J, Kumar H, Sinha DK, et al. Acute renal failure in pregnancy in a developing country: twenty years of experience. *Ren Fail.* 2006;28:309–313.
34. Jamal A, Ramzan A. Renal and post-renal causes of acute renal failure in children. *J Coll Physicians Surg Pak.* 2004;14:411–415.
40. Mehndiratta S, Rajeshwari K, Dubey AP. Multiple-organ dysfunction in a case of *Plasmodium vivax* malaria. *J Vector Borne Dis.* 2013;50(1):71–73.

48. Shukla VS, Singh RG, Rathore SS, et al. Outcome of malaria-associated acute kidney injury: a prospective study from a single center. *Ren Fail.* 2013;35(6):801–805.
49. Mishra SK, Mohanty S, Satpathy SK, et al. Cerebral malaria in adults—a description of 526 cases admitted to Ispat General Hospital in Rourkela, India. *Ann Trop Med Parasitol.* 2007;101:187–193.
57. Ittyachen AM, Krishnapillai TV, Nair MC, et al. Retrospective study of severe cases of leptospirosis admitted in the intensive care unit. *J Postgrad Med.* 2007;53:232–235.
67. Gupta KL, Joshi K, Sud K, et al. Renal zygomycosis: an under-diagnosed cause of acute renal failure. *Nephrol Dial Transplant.* 1999;14:2720–2725.
70. Mehra N, Patel A, Abraham G, et al. Acute kidney injury in dengue fever using Acute Kidney Injury Network criteria: incidence and risk factors. *Trop Doct.* 2012;42(3):160–162.
76. Sharma N, Chauhan S, Faruqi S, et al. Snake envenomation in a north Indian hospital. *Emerg Med J.* 2005;22:118–120.
79. Kohli HS, Sakhuja V. Snake bite and acute renal failure. *Saudi J Nephrology.* 2003;14(2):165–176.
86. Vikrant S, Patial RK. Acute renal failure following multiple honeybee stings. *Indian J Med Sci.* 2006;60:202–204.
97. Singh N, Jatav OP, Gupta RK, et al. Outcome of sixty four cases of ethylene dibromide ingestion treated in tertiary care hospital. *J Assoc Physicians India.* 2007;55:842–845.
102. Sandeep Reddy Y, Abbdul Nabi S, Apparao C, et al. Hair dye related acute kidney injury—a clinical and experimental study. *Ren Fail.* 2012;34(7):880–884.
105. Khan M. Glucose 6 phosphate dehydrogenase deficiency in adults. *J Coll Physicians Surg Pak.* 2004;14:400–403.
109. Chugh KS, Jha V, Sakhuja V, et al. Acute renal cortical necrosis—a study of 113 patients. *Ren Fail.* 1994;16:37–47.
113. Jha V, Sakhuja V. Postpartum renal cortical necrosis. *Nephrol Dial Transplant.* 2005;20:1010.
124. Singh AK, Farag YM, Mittal BV, et al. Epidemiology and risk factors of chronic kidney disease in India—results from the SEEK (Screening and Early Evaluation of Kidney Disease) study. *BMC Nephrol.* 2013;14:114.
125. Varma PP, Raman DK, Ramakrishnan TS, et al. Prevalence of early stages of chronic kidney disease in apparently healthy central government employees in India. *Nephrol Dial Transplant.* 2010;25(9):3011–3017.
126. Saeed ZI, Hussain SA. Chronic kidney disease in Pakistan: an under-recognized public health problem. *Kidney Int.* 2012;81(11):1151.
127. Sharma SK, Dhakal S, Thapa L, et al. Community-based screening for chronic kidney disease, hypertension and diabetes in Dhahran. *JNMA J Nepal Med Assoc.* 2013;52(189):205–212.
128. Huda MN, Alam KS, Harun-Ur R. Prevalence of chronic kidney disease and its association with risk factors in disadvantageous population. *Int J Nephrol.* 2012;267–329.
130. Jessani S, Levey AS, Bux R, et al. Estimation of GFR in South Asians: a study from the general population in Pakistan. *Am J Kidney Dis.* 2014;63:49–58.
131. Barai S, Bandopadhayaya GP, Patel CD, et al. Do healthy potential kidney donors in India have an average glomerular filtration rate of 81.4 ml/min? *Nephrol Physiol.* 2005;101:21–26.
133. Modi GK, Jha V. The incidence of end-stage renal disease in India: a population-based study. *Kidney Int.* 2006;70:2131–2133.
135. Rajapurkar MM, John GT, Kirpalani AL, et al. What do we know about chronic kidney disease in India: first report of the Indian CKD registry. *BMC Nephrol.* 2012;13:10.
136. Kohli HS, Bhat A, Aravindan AN, et al. Spectrum of renal failure in elderly patients. *Int Urol Nephrol.* 2006;38(3–4):759–765.
137. *Dialysis Registry of Pakistan 2007-2008.* Karachi: The Kidney Foundation; 2008.
148. Narasimhan B, Chacko B, John GT, et al. Characterization of kidney lesions in Indian adults: towards a renal biopsy registry. *J Nephrol.* 2006;19:205–210.
149. Rathi M, Bhagat RL, Mukhopadhyay P, et al. Changing histologic spectrum of adult nephritic syndrome over five decades in Northern India: a single center experience. *Ind J Nephrol.* 2014;24:13–18.
152. Nada R, Kharbanda JK, Bhatti A, et al. Primary focal segmental glomerulosclerosis in adults: is the Indian cohort different? *Nephrol Dial Transplant.* 2009;24(12):3701–3707.
162. Panja M, Mondal PC. Current status of aortoarteritis in India. *J Assoc Physicians India.* 2004;52:48–52.
173. Prakash S, Hernande GT, Dujaili I, et al. Lead poisoning from an Ayurvedic herbal medicine in a patient with chronic kidney disease. *Nat Rev Nephrol.* 2009;41:297–300.
181. Wanigasuriya KP, Peiris-John RJ, Wickremasinghe R, et al. Chronic renal failure in north central province of Sri Lanka: an environmentally induced disease. *Trans R Soc Trop Med Hyg.* 2007;101:1013–1017.
182. Jha V. Current status of end-stage renal disease care in India and Pakistan. *Kidney Int Suppl.* 2013;3:157–160.
187. Johnson DW, Hannah D, Qiang Y, et al. Frequencies of hepatitis B and C infections among haemodialysis and peritoneal dialysis patients in Asia-Pacific countries: analysis of registry data. *Nephrol Dial Transplant.* 2009;24:1598–1603.
188. Jasuja S, Gupta AK, Choudhry R, et al. Prevalence and association of hepatitis C viremia in hemodialysis patient at a tertiary care hospital. *Indian J Nephrol.* 2009;19:62–67.
189. Agarwal SK, Dash SC, Gupta S, et al. Hepatitis C virus infection in haemodialysis: the "no-isolation" policy should not be generalized. *Nephron Clin Pract.* 2009;111:133–140.
193. Mahajan S, Tiwari SC, Kalra V, et al. Factors affecting the use of peritoneal dialysis among the ESRD population in India: a single-center study. *Perit Dial Int.* 2004;24:538–541.
198. Prasad KN, Singh K, Rizwan A, et al. Microbiology and outcomes of peritonitis in northern India. *Perit Dial Int.* 2014;34:188–194.
202. Abraham G, Pratap B, Sankarasubbaiyan S, et al. Chronic peritoneal dialysis in South Asia-challenges and future. *Perit Dial Int.* 2008;28:13–19.
210. Mittal T, Ramachandran R, Kumar V, et al. Outcomes of spousal versus related donor kidney transplants: a comparative study. *Indian J Nephrol.* 2014;24:58–63.
211. Ramachandran R, Jha V. Kidney transplantation is associated with catastrophic out of pocket expenditure in India. *PLoS ONE.* 2013;8(7):e67812.
215. Akhtar F. Organ transplantation law in Pakistan to curb kidney trade: chance for global reflection. *NDT Plus.* 2008;1(2):128–129.
217. John GT. Infections after renal transplantation in India. *Indian J Nephrol.* 2003;13:14–19.
225. Duseja A, Choudhary NS, Gupta S, et al. Treatment of chronic hepatitis C in end stage renal disease: experience at a tertiary care centre. *Trop Gastroenterol.* 2012;33(3):189–192.

# The Far East

# 80

Tak Mao Daniel Chan

CHAPTER OUTLINE



KEY POINTS

- Along with rapid economic development, diabetic nephropathy is fast becoming the leading cause of chronic kidney disease and end-stage kidney disease in many Asian countries. Data from major kidney biopsy registries show that immunoglobulin A nephropathy (IgAN) is the leading diagnosis among primary glomerular diseases and lupus nephritis is the leading diagnosis among secondary glomerulonephritides.
- Treatment of active severe lupus nephritis with corticosteroids and mycophenolate is effective and associated with fewer adverse effects compared with prior treatment regimens combining corticosteroids with cyclophosphamide; and recent data showed that maintenance therapy with low-dose corticosteroids and mycophenolate was associated with a relatively low flare rate.
- Results from recent major clinical trials in IgAN highlight the potential risks of high-dose corticosteroid treatment and the critical importance of judicious balance between potential benefit versus risk in treatment decisions.
- Experience with aristolochic acid nephropathy and endemic (Balkan) nephropathy highlights the importance of awareness of potential pathogenic contributions by environmental toxins in patients presenting with acute kidney injury or chronic kidney disease of known or unknown etiology.
- In contrast to Caucasian populations in which granulomatosis with polyangiitis and antiproteinase 3 antibodies are more common, antineutrophil cytoplasmic antibody–associated vasculitis in East and Northeast Asia is characterized by a high percentage of patients presenting with microscopic polyangiitis and antimyeloperoxidase antibodies and more chronic lesions in the kidney biopsy.
- In the current era with effective nucleoside/tide therapy for hepatitis B, the short- and medium-term survival of hepatitis B surface antigen (HBsAg)-positive kidney transplant recipient is comparable with those without hepatitis B virus infection.

## INTRODUCTION

The term "Far East" refers to East Asia (including Northeast Asia), part of North Asia, and Southeast Asia (Fig. 80.1).[1,2] In addition to its vast geographical extent and big population, Asia is characterized by marked variations in socioeconomic development, ethnicity, and culture, both between countries and within big countries. Such heterogeneity is associated with marked differences in epidemiology of kidney diseases including both causes of acute kidney injury (AKI) and chronic kidney disease (CKD), and access to health care, the latter with direct implications on clinical outcomes especially patient and kidney survival rates. The disease pattern in developed areas such as Japan, Korea, Singapore, and Hong Kong largely resembles that of the West, with diabetic nephropathy being the major cause of end-stage kidney disease (ESKD) and immunoglobulin A (IgA) nephropathy being

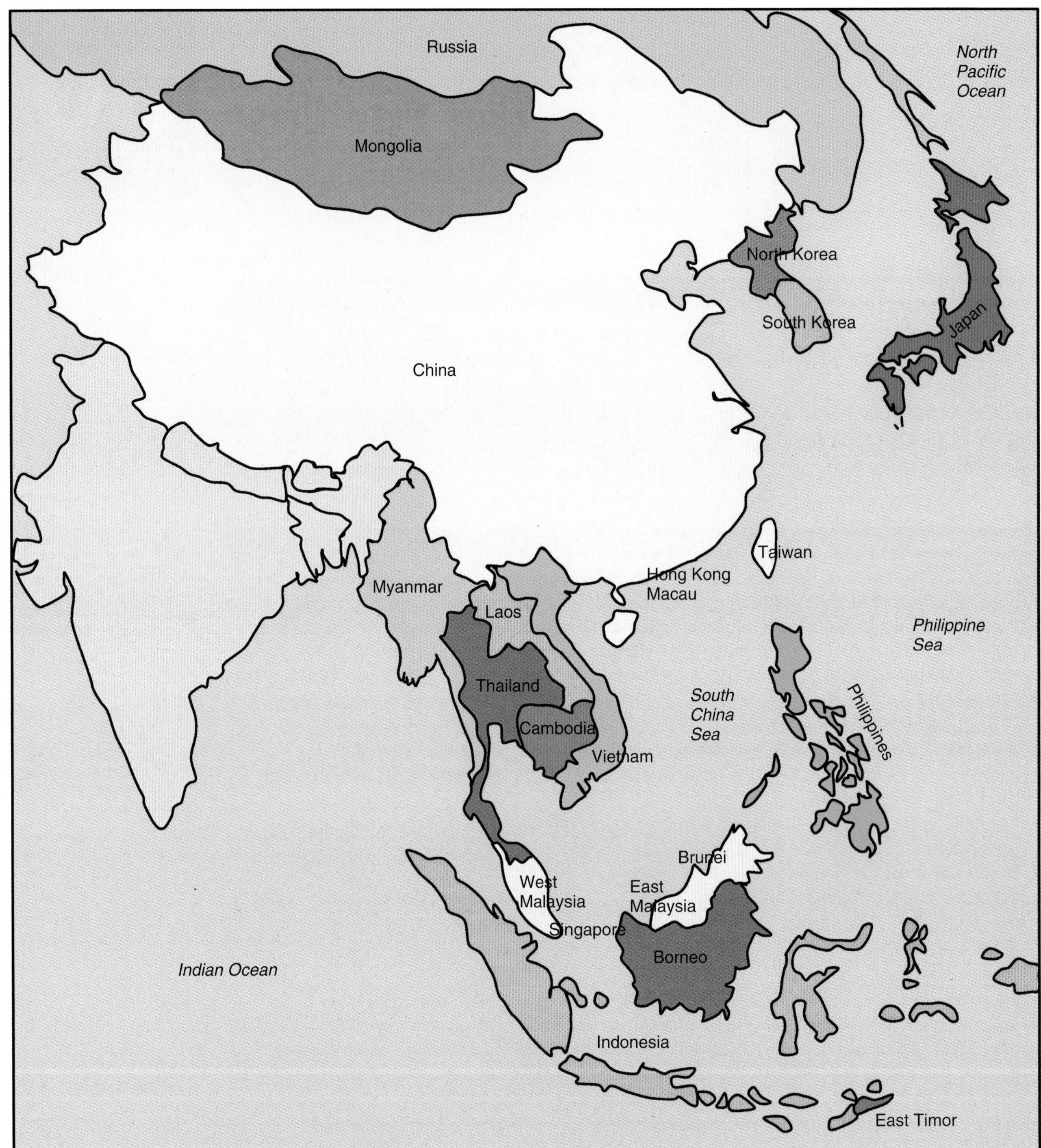


**Fig. 80.1** Countries and territories that constitute the Far East. (Modified from Wikipedia, https://en.wikipedia.org/wiki/Geography_of_Asia.)

the leading primary renal parenchymal disease. With rapid economic development, the major cities in China are moving toward the same pattern with diabetic nephropathy quickly becoming the leading cause of ESKD. Some conditions are more common in Asia, for example, IgA nephropathy (IgAN), lupus nephritis, chronic hepatitis B, and aristolochic acid (AA) nephropathy. Conditions that are typically found in the tropics or subtropics such as malaria or dengue fever could present as imported cases in other Asian countries, while AKI associated with infections such as leptospirosis, scrub typhus, or hemorrhagic fever with renal syndrome (HFRS) due to hantavirus is still present in some countries. The massive volume of international travel and commuting by humans and traffic of commodities between nations, and the climate change associated with global warming have all contributed to the spread of certain diseases such as dengue fever to previously less afflicted areas.

While kidney diseases, especially AKI and CKD, constitute a major public health problem with increasing cost to communities globally, the data on disease varieties and burden, and also on the kidney health-care structure and delivery systems for treatment and prevention, remain fragmented. The International Society of Nephrology (ISN) has undertaken the Global Kidney Health Atlas project, which was a multinational cross-section survey to gather information on the current capacity for kidney care over all world regions, and the findings showed marked diversity in nephrologist density and institutional kidney care provision within Asia and also considerable knowledge gaps in some Asian countries.[3] For example, data on patients receiving maintenance dialysis are available only in countries or areas with national health insurance or renal registries such as Japan, Korea, Taiwan, Singapore, and Hong Kong, and few countries have data on AKI or nondialysis CKD. Renal replacement therapies are costly, and hemodialysis (HD) facilities may not be immediately available to patients with AKI in rural areas. The outcome of patients with AKI would thus be adversely affected due to financial disadvantage or inconvenient social setting. It is against this background that the ISN has launched the 0by25 initiative to prevent death related to AKI through the promulgation of knowledge and advocacy to facilitate early diagnosis and the building of sustainable capacities for timely clinical management.[4] The benefits of this project extend beyond the areas of direct impact such as some South Asian countries to other parts of Asia, such as the less developed regions in China, through enhancing awareness and promoting proactivity and preparedness.

Health expenditure and health-care funding models, which have a direct impact on the access to health care, vary widely between Asian countries. Economic development varies markedly within the Far East region, ranging from high-income economies such as Japan, South Korea (Republic of Korea), Singapore, Hong Kong, and Taiwan, to low- or lower-middle income economies such as North Korea (Democratic People's Republic of Korea), the Philippines, Indonesia, Vietnam, Cambodia, Lao People's Democratic Republic, Myanmar, and Mongolia.[5] Among Asian countries Japan has the highest health expenditure, amounting to 10.2% of gross domestic product (GDP) in 2014, compared with 17.1% in the United States of America.[6] Health-care systems in places such as Japan, South Korea, Singapore, and Taiwan are based on national insurance and are well developed, while the health insurance coverage is being expanded in other areas such as China and Hong Kong.

## TRADITIONAL MEDICINE

Many countries in Asia have a long history of traditional systems of medicine, and the use of traditional herbal medicine is still very common among Chinese in different countries and in other Asian counties such as Korea, Thailand, and Japan. Traditional medicines have served a significant role in providing health-care access to patients in less developed regions and in relatively low-income economies. For example, it has been reported that traditional Chinese medicine accounted for >20% of health-care services and treated approximately 200 million people annually in China.[7] Traditional medicine is covered to variable extents by national health insurance schemes in China, Taiwan, South Korea, and Japan, and there are formal education systems for traditional medicine in China and Korea.[8] Regulatory systems are in place in some areas, such as the State Traditional Chinese Medicine Administration in China, the Ministry of Health and Welfare in Korea, the Ministry of Health and Welfare in Taiwan, and the Department of Health in Hong Kong, which include compliance requirements with regard to good manufacturing practice.[9] However, due to the complexities in plant taxonomy and the components that are related to medicinal effects or toxicities, adverse effects related to intentional or inadvertent exposure to herbal medicines are not uncommon. Nephrotoxicity of *Tripterygium wilfordii*, a traditional Chinese medicine used in the treatment of lupus, rheumatoid diseases, and psoriasis, is well recognized,[10] and the etiology, modes of exposure, and pathogenic mechanisms in AA nephropathy serve as illustrative examples.[11] A study in Taiwan reported a 20% increase in the risk of developing CKD in subjects who took herbal medicine regularly.[12] While the heritage of traditional medicine has its values and undeniable contributions, such as the case of artemisinin (from the plant qing hao) in the treatment of malaria, care and caution must be exercised especially in view of the commercial interest and its increasing use globally.

This chapter discusses the renal diseases that are more common, or of special interest, in the Far East, focusing on recent data and developments.

# ACUTE KIDNEY INJURY AND CHRONIC KIDNEY DISEASE

## ACUTE KIDNEY INJURY

AKI can be induced by a diverse range of endogenous or environmental factors. AKI affects >13 million people per year, although few countries maintain a record or have a registry for AKI patients.[4] AKI is an important cause of hospital admission in Asian countries, and the leading causes of AKI vary according to the socioeconomic development status and the living standard of the general population in different countries.[4,13] In areas with less developed building infrastructure and where the majority of the population is engaged in agriculture, community-acquired AKI is common and the causes include infections and animal or plant toxins (Table 80.1).[14] Some of the causes are related to culture or folklore, for example, accidental exposure to toxin in the grass carp fish bladder used by merchants to replace the more costly snake gallbladder or ingestion of raw or dried cyprinid fish gallbladder as a health tonic or for the treatment of rheumatism,[15] followed by the development of AKI which is sometimes accompanied by hepatotoxicity and myopathy due to the 5-alpha-cyprinol sulfate nephrotoxin/hepatotoxin.[16] Another example of great public health importance is the exposure to AA present in herbs used in traditional medicine, which leads to not only CKD but also to AKI and multifocal urological malignancies.[17,18] In more developed high-income countries such as Japan, Korea, or Singapore, causes such as toxin- or infection-associated AKI are much less common, while AKI is often a complicating factor in hospitalized critically ill patients with cardiovascular compromise, surgical conditions, and severe infections. In large countries with rapid economic development, such as China, the epidemiology of AKI varies according to geographical and topographical location.[19] Knowledge of locally prevalent causes of AKI is thus crucial to timely therapeutic intervention.

**Table 80.1 Secondary Renal Diseases Presenting as AKI in East, Southeast, and Northeast Asia**

| Causes | Examples |
|---|---|
| Autoimmunity | • Lupus nephritis<br>• ANCA vasculitis<br>• Antiglomerular basement membrane disease<br>• Miscellaneous glomerulonephritis |
| Infections | • Leptospirosis<br>• Dengue fever<br>• Hantaviruses (hemorrhagic fever with renal syndrome)<br>• Scrub typhus<br>• Malaria<br>• Severe fever with thrombocytopenia syndrome virus |
| Toxins | • From plant (e.g., aristolochic acid, djenkolic acid)<br>• From animal or insect (e.g., snake venom, grass carp fish gallbladder)<br>• Chemical (e.g., ketamine abuse presenting with CKD or AKI due to obstructive uropathy) |

*AKI,* Acute kidney injury; *ANCA,* antineutrophil cytoplasmic antibody; *CKD,* chronic kidney disease.

## CHRONIC KIDNEY DISEASE

CKD affects 10%–15% of the adult population worldwide.[20–22] A meta-analysis reported in 2016 showed that the prevalence rate of Stage 1–5 CKD was approximately 13% in China, Japan, Korea, and Taiwan, whereas that for Stage 3–5 CKD was approximately 10%–12%.[21] An earlier study in China reported a CKD prevalence rate of 10.8%, implying that approximately 120 million adults in China had reduced kidney function and/or albuminuria.[23] It was estimated that, in the year 2010 and for the whole of Asia, 218 patients per million population (pmp) were receiving dialysis and 232 patients pmp were receiving renal replacement therapy (RRT). In comparison, 1839 patients pmp were on renal replacement therapies in the United States in the same period.[24]

A report from South Korea in 2016, based on the results of the Korean National Health and Nutritional Examination Survey in 2011–2013 that involved 23,280 subjects showed that the prevalence rate of CKD as defined by urine albumin-to-creatinine ratio ≥30 mg/g or estimated glomerular filtration rate (eGFR) < 60 mL/min/1.73 m$^2$ with the Chronic Kidney Disease-Epidemiology Collaboration equation was 8.2% in adults at or above the age of 20 years, with respective proportions in Stages 1, 2, 3a, 3b, and 4–5 being 3.0%, 2.7%, 1.9%, 0.4%, and 0.2%.[25] Factors associated with increased risk of CKD included older age, diabetes, hypertension, cardiovascular disease, body mass indexes ≥25 kg/m$^2$ or below 18.5 kg/m$^2$, and residence in a rural area. The KoreaN Cohort Study for Outcomes in Patients With Chronic Kidney Disease (KNOW-CKD) investigated the factors that impact the progression of CKD, based on data from 2238 subjects enrolled in 2011–2015.[26,27] The age of the cohort was 53.7 ± 12.2 years and 61.2% were men. eGFR was 50.5 ± 30.3 mL/min/1.73 m$^2$, and lower eGFR values were associated with older age, comorbidities, higher systolic blood pressure, greater pulse pressure, lower income level, and lower education attainment. Glomerulonephritis, diabetic nephropathy, hypertensive nephropathy, and polycystic kidney disease accounted for 36.2%, 23.2%, 18.3%, and 16.3% of cases, respectively. The overall prevalence of previous cardiovascular disease was 14.4%, and the rate was highest in those with diabetes. The diabetic cohort also showed more adverse cardiovascular risk profiles including higher systolic blood pressure, higher levels of cardiac troponin T, higher left ventricular mass index, higher coronary calcium score, and higher brachial-ankle pulse wave velocity than the others.[27]

The relationship between kidney function and survival was investigated in the population-based China National Survey of Chronic Kidney Disease study, which recruited adult subjects in 13 provinces starting from 2007.[23] Data from 47,204 subjects over a median follow-up duration of 6.1 years showed that all-cause and cardiovascular mortality increased with increasing severity of CKD and also albuminuria.[28] Baseline albumin-to-creatinine ratio ≥300 mg/g was associated with a hazard ratio (HR) of 2.07 for all-cause mortality and 2.32 for cardiovascular mortality compared with subjects with a ratio <30 mg/g. Interestingly, reduced eGFR was not identified as a death risk predictor in multivariate analysis, although there was interaction between eGFR and age.[28]

Health-care economics has a direct impact on access to clinical care and the availability and/or choice of therapies. This is particularly relevant to CKD care and renal replacement therapies, which are costly especially in Asia where the rate of organ transplantation is low and many patients remain on dialysis for years.[3,29] Not surprisingly, large treatment gaps with regard to RRT have been noted in low-income countries in Asia.[24] Data from the International Society of Nephrology Global Kidney Health Care Status survey showed a variety of financing models ranging from total government funding to a mixture of public and private facilities for dialysis service in North and East Asia, with marked variations in the availability of services for CKD monitoring and management at the primary care level.[3,30] In addition, very few countries have a registry for nondialysis CKD (or AKI) patients.[3,31] In this context, a cost-effectiveness study from Japan published in 2015 showed that, based on 29 maintenance HD patients (eight had diabetes mellitus) with mean age of 59.9 years, the estimated total medical cost for HD treatment was approximately 45,200 USD annually, and the incremental cost utility ratio was 6.88 ± 4.47 × 10$^4$ USD per quality-adjusted life-year, being higher for patients with diabetes mellitus (8.17 ± 6.28 × 10$^4$ USD) per quality-adjusted life-year.[32] The challenge to health-care financing for CKD is compounded when economic development often brings about increasing life expectancy and a growing prevalence of CKD.[24] Heterogeneities in health-care spending, the developmental status of nephrology care and personnel, and sociocultural background result in marked variations in practice across Asian countries. For example, the health expenditure as a percentage of GDP in 2014 was 10.2% in Japan, highest among Asian countries, and was 7.373% in Korea, 5.548% in China, 4.710% in the Philippines, and 4.122% in Thailand, compared with 9.4% in Australia, 9.1% in the United Kingdom, 11.3% in Germany, and 17.1% in the United States.[6] National health-care insurance in places such as Japan, Taiwan, Korea, and Singapore provides coverage for dialysis therapy of residents. In places such as Hong Kong, Thailand, and Vietnam, economic or facility considerations have led to peritoneal dialysis (PD) being promoted or preferred to HD for the treatment of patients with ESKD as public health-care policies.[33–38] Similarly, government-sponsored reimbursement schemes have led to an increase in PD utilization in some provinces in China, so that the number of PD patients in China increased from 37,942 in 2012 to 62,589 in 2015.[39,40] Twice weekly or incremental HD has also been used in patients of small body size or with residual renal function to limit health-care expenditure.[41,42]

In Japan, maintenance HD for patients with ESKD started in 1963.[43] A report from the Japanese Society for Dialysis Therapy Renal Data Registry in 2015, which covered 304,856 prevalent dialysis patients in 2011 (97% on HD), showed a progressive increase in the number of dialysis patients over the years, primarily due to increased number of patients above the age of 65 years, so that the mean age of prevalent dialysis patients was 66.6 years in 2011, compared with 46.2 years in 1981.[44,45] Diabetes mellitus was the leading cause of ESKD, accounting for approximately 40% of incident patients and 45% of prevalent cases. By contrast, glomerular diseases accounted for 75% of incident patients in 1983, decreasing to around 35% in 2011. Cardiovascular disease was the leading cause for mortality, accounting for around 40%. In addition, approximately 30% of dialysis patients were above the age of 75 years, and 8% of patients had been on dialysis for >20 years.[44]

While kidney transplantation offers the best potential for rehabilitation and is associated with lower long-term treatment costs, the current transplantation rate only meets approximately 10% of the demand globally.[46] Asia is the most populated region in the world but it also has the lowest rate of organ transplantation.[46] Socioeconomic, cultural, political, legislative, and developmental issues contribute to the overall low organ donation rate, development of organ transplantation facilities, and access to such treatment.[47] Attempts to overcome some of the challenges have resulted in the development of kidney transplantation across ABO blood group barrier,[48] exchange donor kidney transplantation,[49] improvements in the management of hepatitis B after kidney transplantation so that hepatitis B virus (HBV)-infected renal failure patients can be included for kidney transplantation,[50,51] and the use of hepatitis B surface antigen (HBsAg)-positive kidney donors.[52]

## SPECIFIC KIDNEY DISEASES

### IGA NEPHROPATHY

IgAN is the most common primary glomerulonephritis worldwide, and the condition is common in Asia (Fig. 80.2).[53] Data from renal biopsy registries in China showed that IgAN accounted for >45% of primary glomerular diseases.[54,55] The pathogenesis of IgAN is related to the overproduction of aberrantly glycosylated IgA1, which shows a relative deficiency of galactose at some hinge-region *O*-linked glycans, coupled with glycan-specific IgA and IgG autoantibodies that recognize the undergalactosylated IgA1 molecule.[53] Nephritogenic IgA1 molecules are produced by B cells following mucosal infections such as tonsillitis, and IgA and IgG that recognize the autoantigen IgA1 in IgAN are typically also reactive against antigens from microorganisms involved in recurrent upper respiratory and gastrointestinal mucosal infections. Glomerular deposition of immune complexes thus formed leads to activation of mesangial cells and overproduction of cytokines,

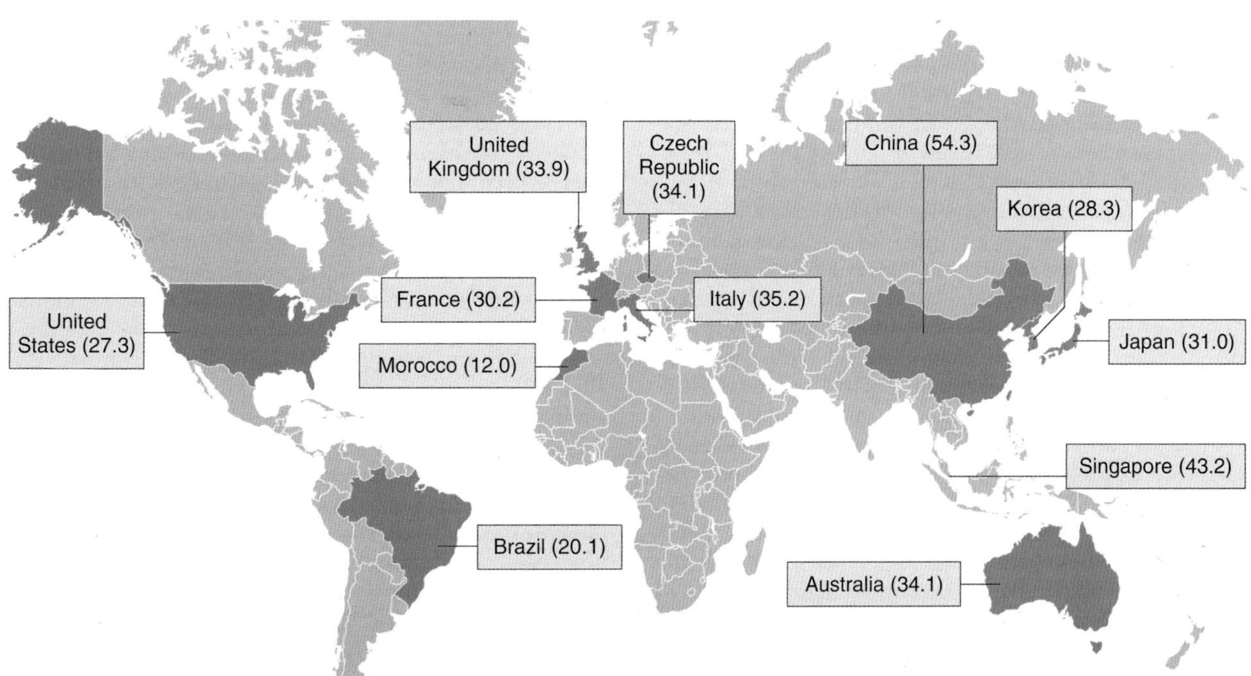


**Fig. 80.2** Prevalence rates of immunoglobulin A nephropathy in different parts of the world. (Reprinted by permission from Macmillan Publishers Ltd. From Lai KN, Tang SCW, Schena FP, et al. IgA nephropathy. *Nat Rev Dis Primers* 2016;2:16001.)

chemokines, and other proinflammatory and profibrotic mediators locally, resulting in injury to normal parenchyma and replacement with fibrous tissue.

Results from linkage and genome-wide association study (GWAS) analyses have shown susceptibility loci of IgAN.[56,57] Studies of familial IgAN in Chinese using whole-exome sequencing identified six deleterious variants in four genes, namely, defensin alpha 4 (*DEFA4*), MYC target 1 (*MYCT1*), caspase recruitment domain family member 8 (*CARD8*), and zinc-finger protein 543 (*ZNF543*).[58] Disease susceptibility has also been associated with genes involved in antigen processing and presentation such as the major histocompatibility complex locus or the mucosal defense system (the *DEFA* gene cluster), and also the alternative complement pathway.[56,59]

Clinical presentation of IgAN is variable, ranging from asymptomatic microscopic hematuria with or without proteinuria or renal impairment to rapidly progressive renal impairment associated with abundant proliferative features and crescent formation in the glomeruli. Overall, about 30%–40% of patients reach ESKD in 20–30 years after initial presentation, but the prognosis and the rate of progression varies considerably between patients.[53] There is no specific blood or urine biomarker for the diagnosis of IgAN. The diagnosis is based on renal biopsy features and the detection of IgA in the mesangial area. Pathogenic polymeric IgA1 immune complexes, with IgG or IgM in some patients, deposit or form in situ in the glomerular mesangium and are associated with mesangial cell proliferation; increased synthesis of extracellular matrix; and variable infiltration of macrophages, monocytes, and T cells. The Oxford classification for IgAN was established in 2009 and updated in 2016 with the objective of identifying specific pathologic features that more accurately predict risk of progression of renal disease.[60–62] According to the classification, renal biopsies of IgAN are scored according to mesangial hypercellularity (M0 or M1), segmental glomerulosclerosis (S0 or S1), endocapillary hypercellularity (E0 or E1), tubular atrophy/interstitial fibrosis (T0, T1, T2), and crescents (C0, C1, or C2) (MEST C Score), items that were shown to have independent value in predicting renal outcome. Analysis of pooled data from 3096 patients, including 700 patients from Japan and 1017 from China, showed that crescents predicted a higher risk of the combined renal endpoint, which was at least 50% eGFR decline or ESKD, in patients not treated with immunosuppression. Having crescents in at least one-sixth or one-fourth of glomeruli was associated with an HR of 1.63 or 2.29, respectively, for the combined renal endpoint, and having crescents in at least one-fourth of glomeruli was independently associated with a combined event irrespective of immunosuppression.[63] The T score in the Oxford classification and the Japanese Histologic Classification score have been shown to be associated with renal outcome in a series that included 86 Japanese patients with IgAN.[64]

Based on the Oxford classification, the European Validation study of the Oxford classification of IgAN (VALIGA) study examined 1147 patients from 13 European countries encompassing different clinical and pathologic manifestations of IgAN.[65] Over a median follow-up of 4.7 years, 86% received renin–angiotensin–aldosterone system (RAAS) blockade and 42% immunosuppressive treatment. The results showed that M, S, and T lesions independently predicted the loss of eGFR and a lower renal survival. The addition of M, S, and T lesions to clinical variables significantly enhanced the ability to predict progression only in patients not treated with immunosuppression.[65] In addition, applying the Oxford classification in 261 European patients below the age of 23 years with mean follow-up of 4.9 (range 2.5–8.1) years, investigators of the VALIGA cohort found that the rate of renal function decline was −0.2 mL/min/1.73 m$^2$ per year (interquartile range −2.7 to 0.5 mL/min/1.73 m$^2$ per year), and that the MEST M, S, and T scores predicted survival to the combined endpoint of ESKD and 50% loss of eGFR in the overall cohort but not in the subgroup of 174 children below the age of 18 years.[66] Applying the Oxford classification, investigators in Singapore showed that mesangial hypercellularity and tubular atrophy/interstitial fibrosis scores (M1 and T1/T2 lesion) of the Oxford classification independently predicted ESKD over long-term follow-up.[67]

Treatment decisions take into account clinical and histological parameters. Patients with normal blood pressure, insignificant proteinuria, normal renal function, and renal histology demonstrating the absence of poor prognostic features may need only periodic monitoring of blood pressure, proteinuria, and renal function. Optimal treatment of hypertension and the use of RAAS inhibition or blockade, with the objective of minimizing proteinuria and the rate of renal function deterioration, form the mainstay of management strategy in other patients. The Kidney Disease Improving Global Outcomes (KDIGO) 2012 guidelines suggest optional use of fish oil in patients with persistent proteinuria of >1 g/day despite standard of care therapy, but its impact on long-term renal outcome remains uncertain.[68] A recent study in Japan showed that mizoribine treatment conferred no benefit on proteinuria.[69] The role of mycophenolate therapy remains controversial, and this is not recommended in the 2012 KDIGO guidelines, and the factors contributing to the conflicting conclusions from different studies include inadequate sample size, race and ethnicity, and histological variations.[70–75]

Results from the Supportive Versus Immunosuppressive Therapy for the Treatment of Progressive IgA Nephropathy (STOP-IgAN) trial, which included 162 patients in Germany, showed that the addition of immunosuppressive therapy in the form of corticosteroids with or without cyclophosphamide or azathioprine in patients who showed persistent proteinuria of at least 0.75 g/day while on standard of care reduced proteinuria but did not reduce the rate of eGFR decline (24% in the supportive-care group and 22% in the immunosuppression group had a decrease in eGFR of at least 15 mL/min) >3 years of follow-up, and immunosuppression was associated with more infections (resulting in one death), impaired glucose tolerance, and weight gain.[76] The Therapeutic Evaluation of Steroids in IgA Nephropathy Global (TESTING) trial investigated the efficacy and safety of corticosteroids in 262 patients (251 patients in China) with IgAN and persistent proteinuria of >1 g/day despite standard therapy.[77] Corticosteroid treatment was in the form of oral methylprednisolone 0.6–0.8 mg/kg daily for 2 months then tapered by 8 mg/day each month, with a total treatment duration of 6–8 months. The trial was stopped early due to significantly higher incidence of serious adverse events in the methylprednisolone group (14.7% vs. 3.2%), primarily due to infections. In patients treated with methylprednisolone, 8.1% developed serious infections with two fatalities, whereas there was no serious infection in the placebo group. At trial termination with median follow-up of 2.1 years, the primary efficacy outcome, which was a composite of ESKD, death due to kidney failure, or a 40% decrease in eGFR, favored methylprednisolone over placebo (5.9% vs. 15.9%; HR: 0.37).[77] In a trial that included 176 Chinese patients with IgAN and cellular/fibrocellular crescents in ≥10% of glomeruli or endocapillary hypercellularity or glomerular necrosis, treatment with high-dose prednisone alone was comparable with mycophenolate combined with reduced-dose prednisone with regard to proteinuria reduction, and approximately 50% of patients in each group achieved complete renal remission with the latter group showing a lower incidence of treatment-related adverse effects.[78] Overall, the data from the trials that involved big samples of Chinese patients suggest potential renal benefit of immunosuppression, especially in patients whose renal histology shows active proliferative features, and that treatment decisions need to take into consideration the balance between risk and potential benefit according to the characteristics of individual patients. The data to date are insufficient to conclude that race or ethnicity has an impact on the response of IgAN to immunosuppressive treatments, due to the marked heterogeneity in histological manifestations and clinical disease severity, and the variable timing of diagnosis in the natural course of disease between different studies.

Microbial pathogens can multiply in the tonsillar crypts, and tonsillar lymphocytes of patients with IgAN showed increased production of dimeric IgA1 with altered glycosylation compared with controls.[79,80] In addition, tonsillar germinal center B cells are implicated in pathogenesis.[81] The role of tonsillectomy in the management of IgAN remains controversial. Tonsillectomy has been associated with more favorable renal outcome,[82,83] and is considered a standard of care treatment for IgAN in Japan.[84,85] A randomized controlled trial in Japan showed lower proteinuria in patients treated with tonsillectomy plus corticosteroids.[86] A recently reported long-term retrospective study in 227 Japanese patients showed possible benefit of tonsillectomy in patients presenting with lower levels of proteinuria and serum creatinine, but some of the patients also received corticosteroid treatment.[87] By contrast, analysis of data from the VALIGA cohort of 1147 European patients with IgAN showed no association between tonsillectomy and renal function decline over a follow-up of 4.7 years.[88]

## LUPUS NEPHRITIS

Lupus nephritis is common in Asia. Previous studies showed that not only is systemic lupus erythematosus (SLE) more common in Asian populations compared with Caucasians, but also renal involvement is more common among these patients.[89,90] Data from renal biopsy registries showed that lupus nephritis is the leading cause of secondary glomerular diseases, accounting for >50% in countries such as China, Korea, and Japan.[54,55,91–93]

A recent meta-analysis of GWAS data showed substantial commonality in shared risk variants between European and Chinese patients with SLE, with overall higher risk variant frequencies in the Chinese, suggesting a greater SLE genetic risk burden in East Asia.[94] Compared with other race or ethnicity, Asian patients may also develop more severe nephritis, resulting in lupus nephritis being an important cause of ESKD in Asia.[95] Genetic association studies have identified >50 polymorphisms associated with lupus nephritis susceptibility or pathogenesis, encompassing functional abnormalities such as altered programmed cell death, defective immune clearance of programmed cell death debris, altered innate or adaptive immunity, and kidney-specific effector mechanisms.[96] An example is the reported association between variants of CCR6, a surface marker for Th17 effector cells, and susceptibility to lupus nephritis in a study that involved >1100 Chinese patients with lupus nephritis compared with 900 healthy controls and 1063 nonrenal lupus patients.[97]

Clinical manifestation and the diagnosis of lupus nephritis in Asian patients are no different from other parts of the world.[98] However, within Asia there is marked variation in the timing of presentation due to variations in health-care delivery systems and primary care setup between countries. This has important implications on treatment and patient outcomes, because earlier presentation is in general associated with less severe disease that requires less immunosuppressive exposure for treatment. Earlier presentation is usually associated with less chronic irreversible damage. Reduced exposure to immunosuppressive medications, especially corticosteroids, leads to a more favorable efficacy versus risk balance and a lower risk of infective and other complications, whereas a lower level of damage in the kidneys implies a more favorable long-term renal survival. Except in some developing South Asian countries and disadvantaged populations in less developed areas in China and other Asian countries, the standard diagnostic facilities including blood and urine tests and lupus serology are available, though there may be economic barriers to kidney biopsy and regular serological tests. High baseline serum creatinine and significant chronic damage shown in the kidney biopsy portend an unfavorable long-term renal prognosis, whereas histologic features such as vascular or endothelial abnormalities and crescents signify aggressive disease.[99–103] Studies from China have implicated antineutrophil cytoplasm antibodies in the pathogenesis of crescentic lupus nephritis,[99,104,105] while a study in Korea reported that anti-Sm antibody was detected in 48.8% of patients with biopsy-proven lupus nephritis, and was associated with worse renal prognosis.[106] Furthermore, data from Korea showed that patients presenting after the age of 50 years showed higher renal chronicity features and had inferior outcomes during follow-up compared with those with disease onset at a younger age.[107] Renal histology of lupus nephritis is presently assessed according to the 2003 ISN/Renal Pathology Society classification,[108] although evaluation of individual lesions according to the specified diagnostic criteria may not be always easy.[109]

While instituting prompt and effective treatment in Asian patients with severe lupus nephritis is intuitively important in view of the high disease prevalence in the region, this presents a challenge in some Asian regions due to insufficient knowledge of disease and management by patients, great variations in socioeconomic status of patients, variations in health-care financing and access to diagnosis and treatment, susceptibility to treatment-related adverse effects, access to and standard of general medical care and management of severe life-threatening complications, compliance, and follow-up issues.[110–112]

Immunosuppressive treatment for lupus nephritis has evolved considerably since the 1980s, resulting in improved clinical outcomes and significantly reduced treatment-associated adverse effects, and a shift from corticosteroids combined with cyclophosphamide to corticosteroids combined with mycophenolate therapy.[113] Initial results demonstrating treatment efficacy and tolerability of combined prednisolone and mycophenolate therapy in Chinese lupus nephritis patients were subsequently confirmed by data from a Food and Drug Administration (FDA)-supported trial in the United States, data from a trial in Malaysia, and the industry-led international multicenter Aspreva Lupus Management Study, in which 123 of the 370 randomized patients were Asians.[114–119] The reduced incidence of adverse events with mycophenolate treatment compared with cyclophosphamide was associated with improved quality of life.[120] Results from these trials showed racial variation in response to treatment, with inferior efficacy rates observed in patients of African descent and in Latin America while high response rates were observed in Chinese patients.[114,115,121] The high short-term response rates in Chinese patients translated into relatively favorable long-term patient and renal survival, and are associated with a relatively low rate of nephritic flares.[122–124]

Mycophenolic acid pharmacokinetics vary markedly between patients, and therapeutic drug monitoring is increasingly used in the management of organ transplant recipients treated with various preparations of mycophenolate.[125–127] Studies in Thai patients with lupus nephritis showed that with the commonly adopted daily mycophenolate mofetil dose of 1.5–2 g the mycophenolic acid exposure of most patients was in the desired therapeutic range.[128–130] However, while selected single time point drug levels correlated with area-under-curve data overall, drug exposure with the same single time point level can vary considerably between patients. In view of the generally high efficacy and tolerability in Asian lupus nephritis patients treated with mycophenolate, and the cost and availability of drug level monitoring, therapeutic drug level monitoring should preferably be reserved for patients who show unsatisfactory treatment response, including multiple relapses, or who develop marrow suppression, and in pediatric patients.[131] The accumulating data on tacrolimus in the treatment of lupus nephritis have largely come from Asia. Owing to its distinct effect on podocytes in addition to potent immunosuppressive actions, calcineurin inhibitors have demonstrated efficacy in the treatment of lupus nephritis, especially when there were membranous features.[132–139]

Investigators in China have reported the results with a 'multitarget therapy' with triple immunosuppression comprising corticosteroids, tacrolimus (4 mg/day), and reduced-dose (1.0 g/day) mycophenolate mofetil, showing that the multitarget regimen was associated with a higher short-term complete remission rate (65%) compared with corticosteroids and intravenous (IV) cyclophosphamide (15%) in patients with combined class IV and class V lupus nephritis,[140] a higher complete remission rate (45.9%) compared with IV cyclophosphamide (25.6%) at 24 weeks in patients with class III/IV/V lupus nephritis,[141] and a similar renal flare rate (5.47%) compared with azathioprine (7.62%) as maintenance therapy for 18 months with the latter showing more adverse events.[142]

Investigators in Japan have performed a pilot study in 15 patients with lupus nephritis to investigate another 'multitarget' immunosuppressive treatment regimen that included prednisolone, IV cyclophosphamide for 3 months, and tacrolimus at a standard dose of 3 mg daily, and reported a complete remission rate of 80% at 6 months, with three patients showing a transient increase of serum creatinine level initially, one cytomegalovirus antigenemia, and one death related to thrombotic microangiopathy.[143] Overall, the results with tacrolimus in the treatment of lupus nephritis are promising, especially with regard to reduction of proteinuria. In view of potential nephrotoxicity which could be subclinical initially, and also its effects on blood pressure, lipids, and glucose metabolism, long-term safety data are required and further studies are warranted to delineate which are the patients most likely to benefit from this treatment.

In Japan, mizoribine is the first drug approved (in 1990) for the indication of lupus nephritis treatment. The mechanism of action is similar to mycophenolic acid, and the drug has been largely used during the maintenance therapy for steroid sparing, with generally acceptable tolerability. A recently reported postmarketing surveillance study on long-term mizoribine treatment in 559 patients with lupus nephritis showed that overall there was a continued decline in disease activity and 26.5% of patients were in complete remission at 24 months, yet progressive deterioration of kidney function was observed after 12 months of follow-up. Serious adverse drug reactions occurred in 3.6% of patients. In addition, nearly all patients were on concomitant corticosteroid treatment, whereas 51.2% of patients were also receiving tacrolimus.[144]

The data on Asian patients with lupus nephritis show that the clinical outcomes with regard to response to treatment of active disease, long-term patient and renal survival, morbidities related to disease or treatment, disease flare rate, and quality of life of patients have improved over the past few decades due to advances in immunosuppressive management and improvements in general medical care. There are still questions and challenges with regard to optimal treatment regimens and durations for novel and existing therapies including calcineurin inhibitors, socioeconomic barriers to appropriate and timely diagnosis and treatment, and the prevention and management of infections.[110,111]

## DIABETIC NEPHROPATHY

Diabetic nephropathy, mostly due to type 2 diabetes in Asia, has become a major cause of ESKD in many Asian cities, in parallel with economic development. In Japan, diabetic nephropathy has overtaken glomerulonephritis as the leading underlying cause of ESKD in dialysis patients since 1997, and the proportion continues to increase (Fig. 80.3).[44] In China, among hospitalized patients, diabetic nephropathy has been the leading cause of CKD surpassing glomerulonephritis (Fig. 80.4).[145] The association between diabetes mellitus and CKD has similarly been demonstrated in Korea and Singapore.[146,147] In a cross-sectional survey that included 1861 patients with type 2 diabetes in Singapore, 53% were found to have concomitant CKD, and variables significantly associated with CKD included retinopathy or neuropathy, age, blood pressure of ≥140/80 mm Hg, history of cardiovascular disease, and duration of diabetes.[147]

Around 30%–40% of type 2 diabetic patients develop diabetic nephropathy, the pathogenesis of which involves genetic and environmental factors.[148,149] The genes related to the initiation and progression of diabetic nephropathy remain to be investigated. Previous studies have adopted the candidate gene approach, based on pathophysiologic considerations, or GWASs. Data to date show that the RAAS plays an important role in the progression of diabetic nephropathy, and RAAS blockers are now standard therapy to reduce proteinuria and the rate of renal function deterioration.[150] Among candidate genes, genetic polymorphism of angiotensin-converting enzyme (ACE) gene has been studied intensively. The ACE gene 287-bp Alu repetitive sequences in intron 16 show genetic variations that create insertion (II) or deletion (DD) homozygous or insertion/deletion (ID) heterozygous genotypes, and that the D allele is associated with high ACE enzymatic activity not only in sera but also in renal tissues, and data from single-center studies and meta-analyses showed that the D allele and DD genotype were associated with higher susceptibility to ESKD.[151–153] In addition, an association with acetyl coenzyme A carboxylase β (ACACB) gene, which may be related to proinflammatory responses in renal tubular epithelial cells, has been reported in Japanese and Chinese patients.[154,155] Considering the role of inflammation in pathogenesis, data from Chinese patients in Henan Province showed that the AA genotype and A allele of interleukin-10 (IL-10) –1082G/A was associated with increased susceptibility to diabetic nephropathy with adjusted odds ratios of 2.52 and 1.51 compared with wild-type genotype and the G allele, respectively.[156]

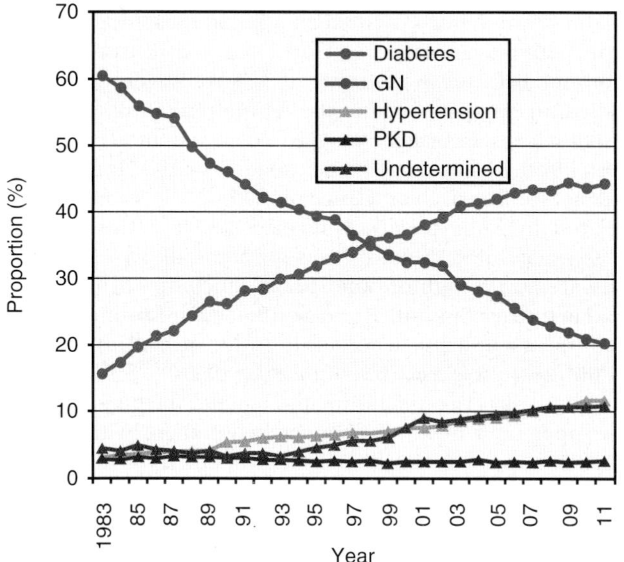


**Fig. 80.3** Proportion of primary diagnoses of end-stage renal disease in prevalent patients on dialysis in Japan. *GN,* Glomerulonephritis; *PKD,* polycystic kidney disease. (Reprinted with permission from Elsevier. From Hanafusa N, Nakai S, Iseki K, et al. Japanese Society for Dialysis Therapy Renal Data Registry – a window through which we can view the details of Japanese dialysis population. *Kidney Int Suppl.* 2015;5:15–22.)

Data from 568 Chinese patients with type 2 diabetes in Taiwan showed that IL-6 gene polymorphisms rs1800796 and rs1524107 predicted progression of nephropathy.[157] An association between diabetic nephropathy and intercellular adhesion molecule-1 (ICAM1) K469E(A/G) polymorphism (rs5498) has been reported in Malaysian patients.[158] In another study in Singapore that included 1950 Asians with type 2 diabetes, a higher plasma level of vascular cell adhesion molecule-1 (VCAM1), but not ICAM1, was associated with worse renal function and proteinuria.[159] With regard to the role of lipids in disease progression, higher levels of lipoprotein(a) has been associated with the development of CKD in Korean patients with type 2 diabetes,[160] and recent data from Chinese patients with type 2 diabetes suggested an association between diabetic nephropathy and apolipoprotein E isoforms, with the ApoE ε2 allele being more prevalent and the ApoE ε4 allele less prevalent in diabetic patients with nephropathy compared with those without renal abnormality.[161] Dietary salt intake and serum uric acid level have been reported as independent risk factors, with odds ratios of 1.15 and 2.00,

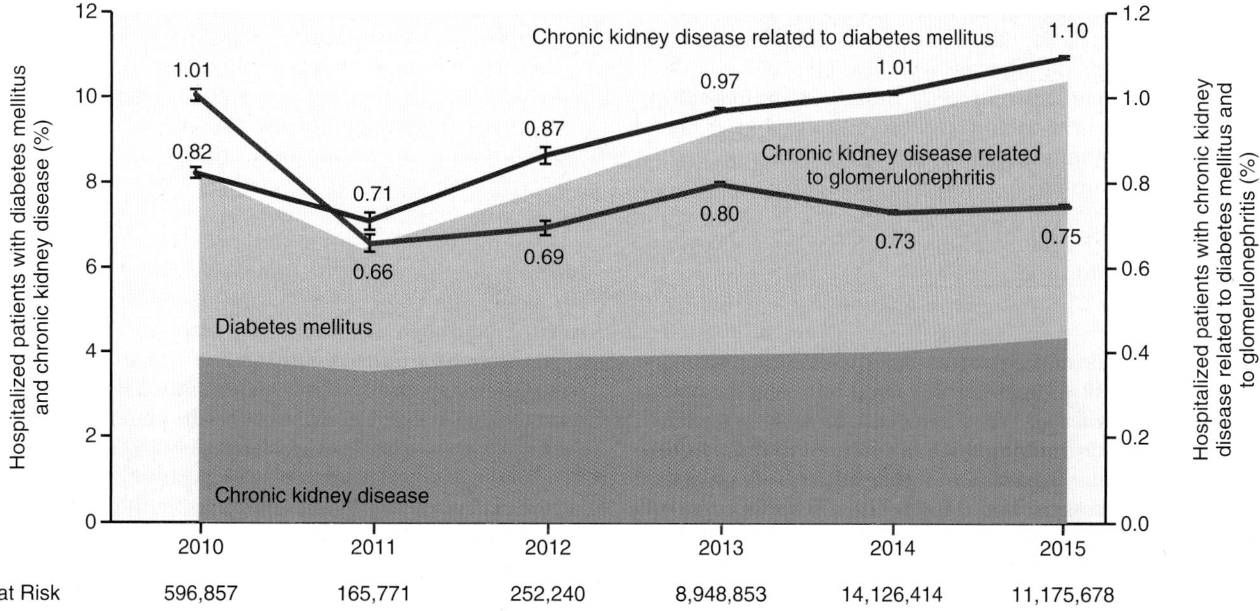


**Fig. 80.4** Trends in chronic kidney disease related to diabetes and to glomerulonephritis among hospitalized patients in China. (Reprinted from Zhang L, Long J, Jiang W, et al. Trends in chronic kidney disease in China. *N Engl J Med.* 2016;375:905–906. Copyright (2016) Massachusetts Medical Society, with permission from the Massachusetts Medical Society.)

respectively, associated with renal impairment in Japanese patients with type 2 diabetes.[162] Examples of other genetic polymorphisms implicated in susceptibility or progression of diabetic nephropathy include that of ELMO1 in Chinese,[163] 5,10-methenyltetrahydrofolate synthetase in Taiwan,[164] and 2184AG polymorphism in the gene for the receptor for advanced glycation end product in China.[165] In the field of epigenetics, data from Taiwan showed higher levels of miR-21, miR-29a, and miR-192 in diabetic patients with heavier proteinuria, and an association between miR-21, miR-29a, miR-29b, and miR-29c with progressive renal failure.[166]

As in other parts of the world, Asian patients with diabetic nephropathy also show markedly increased cardiovascular risk and thus control of vascular risk factors is important in patient management.[167] Data from the West showed that combined use of ACE inhibitor (lisinopril) and angiotensin receptor blocker (losartan) compared with single-agent treatment may reduce proteinuria but did not reduce cardiovascular mortality and was potentially risky with regard to hyperkalemia and AKI.[168] Adding the direct renin inhibitor (aliskiren) to diabetic nephropathy patients already on angiotensin receptor blocker losartan reduced proteinuria and might better preserve the renal function.[169,170] Subsequently, the Aliskiren Trial in Type 2 Diabetes Using Cardio-Renal Disease Endpoints (ALTITUDE) trial was stopped prematurely when interim analysis showed that adding aliskiren 300 mg daily to an ACE inhibitor or an angiotensin receptor blocker, though resulted in reduction of blood pressure and proteinuria, was associated with significantly higher occurrence rates of hyperkalemia of ≥6 mmol/L (11.2% vs. 7.2% in the placebo group) and hypotension (12.1% vs. 8.3% in controls; $P < .001$ for both).[171] Caution is thus advised when considering dual blockade in the RAAS pathway. The balance between potential benefit versus risk is affected by the characteristics of individual patients.

In a study that included 563 patients with diabetic nephropathy from Japan and Hong Kong, with 73.5% already receiving treatment with an ACE inhibitor, treatment with the angiotensin receptor blocker olmesartan was shown to reduce proteinuria independent of ACE inhibitor and also reduce adverse cardiovascular outcomes (HR: 0.65, $P = .042$), but had no effect on adverse renal outcomes compared with placebo.[172] Another post hoc analysis of this trial investigated the impact of systolic blood pressure on renal and cardiovascular outcomes.[173] A total of 566 Asian patients were followed for a mean of 3.2 years, and the results showed that in patients with proteinuria ≥1 g/gCr, a mean follow-up systolic blood pressure of >130 mm Hg was associated with an HR of 2.33 (1.62–3.36) for renal composite outcome comprising doubling of serum creatinine, ESKD, or death, compared with patients whose mean follow-up systolic blood pressure was ≤130 mm Hg. In patients without a history of cardiovascular disease, a follow-up mean systolic blood pressure of >140 mm Hg was associated with an HR of 2.04 (1.23–3.40) for cardiovascular outcomes compared with those whose systolic blood pressure was <140 mm Hg. The median slopes of eGFR were −3.27, −4.53, and −7.13 dL/mg/year in patients with systolic blood pressure ≤130, 131–140, and >140 mm Hg, respectively ($P = .008$ between ≤130 and 131–140, $P < .001$ between ≤130 and >140 mm Hg). The investigators thus concluded that in Asian type 2 diabetic patients with CKD and heavy proteinuria, blood pressure control should be individualized and a systolic blood pressure not >130 mm Hg was associated with renoprotection.[173]

## ARISTOLOCHIC ACID NEPHROPATHY

The story of AA nephropathy began in the early 1990s when a group of young females in Belgium was noted to develop tubulointerstitial nephritis with rapidly progressive deterioration of kidney function following the intake of slimming medications containing herbal ingredients.[11,174] Subsequently the causative nephrotoxic agent was identified as AA,[175] present in the Chinese herb Guang Fang Ji, and poisoning occurred when this was mistaken as Han Fang Ji, a diuretic herb in traditional Chinese medicine.[176] It was also noted that AA exposure predisposed to the development of urothelial malignancies, so that AA was classified as a human carcinogen class I by the World Health Organization (WHO) International Agency for Research on Cancer in 2002.[18,177,178] Kidney disease related to AA exposure is termed AAN. In the following years, cases of AAN have been reported all over the world, and areas with high prevalence rates include China, Taiwan, and countries in Eastern and Southeastern Europe near the Danube tributaries, where the entity of Balkan endemic nephropathy was recognized since the 1950s.[179,180] After noting the similarities in renal histopathology and the high incidence of upper tract urothelial cancer between AAN and Balkan endemic nephropathy, the etiological link to environmental exposure to AA has been confirmed,[181,182] and the evidence includes the detection of AA-DNA adducts and the hallmark A:T to T:A base transversion in renal cortical and urothelial malignant tissues.[183]

> ***Clinical Relevance***
> **Aristolochic Acid Nephropathy**
> Pathogenesis in aristolochic acid nephropathy involves (i) injury to renal tubular cells with altered oxidative pathways and mitochondrial damage, followed by apoptosis, resulting in interstitial fibrosis and tubular atrophy; (ii) aristolactams activated by peroxidase at the urothelium, forming adducts with DNA, resulting in A:T to T:A base transversion in the TP53 tumor suppression gene, thereby affecting cell-cycle checkpoints, DNA repair, and apoptosis, leading to carcinogenesis.

AA is present in plants of the *Aristolochia* genus containing nitrophenanthrene carboxylic acids, of which 8-methoxy-6-nitro-phenanthro-(3,4-d)-1,3-dioxolo-5-carboxylic acid (aristolochic acid I, AAI) and 6-nitro-phenanthro-(3,4-d)-1,3-dioxolo-5-carboxylic acid (AAII) are the predominant components.[184] In Asia, exposure to AA is mostly related to intake of herbal remedies, whereas in patients with Balkan endemic nephropathy the data to date suggest that AA might have been ingested via bread made with flour contaminated by *Aristolochia clematitis*.[185–187] AA has been identified in different Chinese medicinal herbs (Table 80.2).[186] Pathogenesis involves injury to renal tubular cells with altered oxidative pathways and mitochondrial damage, followed by apoptosis and impaired regenerative potential, resulting in interstitial fibrosis and tubular atrophy.[188–190] Human urothelium is rich in peroxidases; the aristolactams activated by peroxidase then

**Table 80.2 Chinese Medicinal Herbs That Contain Aristolochic Acids**

| Name of Chinese Herb | Botanical Name |
|---|---|
| Guang Fang Ji (Fangchi) | *Aristolochia fangchi* |
| Xixin | Radix et Rhizoma Asari |
| Guan Mu Tong | *Aristolochia manshuriensis* |
| Qing Mu Xiang | *Aristolochia cucurbitifolia* |
| Ma Dou Ling | *Aristolochia debilis* |
| Tian Xian Teng | *Aristolochia contorta* |

Modified from Yang HY, Chen PC, Wang JD. Chinese herbs containing aristolochic acid associated with renal failure and urothelial carcinoma: a review from epidemiologic observations to causal inference. *Biomed Res Int.* 2014;2014:569325.

form adducts with DNA, which have been associated with A:T to T:A base transversion in the TP53 tumor suppression gene.[184,187,191,192] TP53 is involved in cell-cycle checkpoints, DNA repair, and apoptosis,[193] thereby explaining the carcinogenic effect of AA. Characteristic AA-DNA adducts in the renal tissue such as 7-(deoxyadenosin-N6-yl) aristolactam I (dA-AAI) can serve as biomarkers of prior AA exposure.[18,184,187,194] This deoxyadenosine adduct causes characteristic A–T transversion mutations and such mutations were found in the TP53 tumor suppressor gene in tumors from AAN and patients with Balkan endemic nephropathy.[181,195] More recently, using whole-genome and exome sequencing analysis, A:T transversion mutations were also observed in other gene loci.[196–198]

AAN is characterized by extensive cortical interstitial fibrosis with relative sparing of glomeruli and urinary tract urothelial carcinomas. Most cases presented with renal failure, moderate hypertension, and severe anemia, and approximately 70% showed rapid progression to ESKD.[188,199] Some patients presented with Fanconi syndrome.[200,201] Proteinuria was relatively mild due to its tubular origin.[202] Kidney biopsies showed extensive interstitial fibrosis and tubular atrophy, often starting from the peripheral cortex.[11,174] Only in the late stage did the glomeruli show collapse of the capillaries and wrinkling of the glomerular basement membrane. Interstitial infiltrating cells were mostly not prominent, though inflammatory infiltration was observed in some renal biopsies, suggesting that immune-mediated injury could not be totally excluded.[180] While there is no pathognomonic diagnostic feature, the pattern of injury in the absence of other diseases would suggest the diagnosis of AAN. In a series of 300 Chinese patients with AAN, 13 patients presented with AKI, 7 patients presented with tubular dysfunction with relatively normal serum creatinine, and 280 patients presented with CKD.[203] It is noteworthy that AKI was associated with a high level of AA exposure and they progressed to kidney failure over 1 to 7 years. By contrast, patients presenting with predominantly tubular dysfunction and relatively normal serum creatinine showed slow CKD progression rates. These observations suggested a dose-dependent relationship between AA exposure and the severity of renal injury.[204] In this regard, cumulative exposure to 61–100 g of Mu Tong or Fangchi (herbs that contain AA) had been associated with increased risk of ESKD with odds ratios of 1.47 and 1.60, respectively, and the odds ratios increased to 5.82 and 1.94, respectively, when the exposure was >200 g.[205]

The causative link between AA exposure and urothelial malignancies emerged from clinical and animal studies.[17,18,191,206–210] Some patients first developed upper urinary tract urothelial carcinoma followed by subsequent bladder cancer, and it must be remembered that malignancies may develop at variable periods after the diagnosis of AAN, when patients are already on long-term dialysis or after kidney transplantation.[18,211] The risk for malignancies is related to the cumulative dose of AA exposure, and cumulative exposure to >200 g of Guang Fang Ji was associated with increased risk of urothelial carcinoma.[18] Prophylactic removal of native kidneys and ureters is recommended for some patients, especially those planned for kidney transplantation or with high-level prior exposure.[18] The incidence of upper tract urothelial cancer appears particularly high in Eastern European patients diagnosed with Balkan endemic nephropathy and in patients with AAN in Taiwan, the latter especially in females.[212,213]

Ultra-high-performance liquid chromatography–multistage fragmentation mass spectrometry can be used to detect AAI and AAII in herbal products,[214] and a hollow fiber liquid-phase microextraction technique in conjunction with high-performance liquid chromatography has been used for the extraction and quantitation of AAI in human urine.[215] AA-DNA adducts in the renal cortex or urothelial tissues can serve as biomarkers of prior AA exposure,[18,184,194] using $^{32}P$ labeling or liquid chromatography–mass spectrometry, or ultraperformance liquid chromatography–triple quadruple mass spectrometry of exfoliated urothelial cells.[216–219]

Continued exposure to AA should be stopped. Patients with tubular dysfunction or CKD should be managed accordingly. Standard algorithms for diagnosis and management have been devised for subjects at increased risk of Balkan endemic nephropathy based on geographical location or family history.[179] Whether similar approaches could be applicable to Asian subjects with AAN remains to be investigated. In view of the inflammatory cell infiltration in the renal interstitium,[220] the effect of corticosteroid therapy has been investigated. There are data in Caucasian AAN patients to suggest that corticosteroid therapy may reduce the rate of progression to ESKD.[221,222] In a trial that included 43 Chinese patients with AAN, 25 patients were treated with prednisolone at 0.5 mg/kg body weight daily for 1–3 months, which was then reduced by 0.05 mg/kg every month and maintained at 10 mg daily, and the results suggested slower rate of CKD progression in the steroid-treated group.[223] Subjects who have taken AA-containing herbal remedies, or those with occupational or environmental AA exposure, should have regular follow-up for the monitoring of kidney function and manifestations suggestive of uroepithelial malignancies. Patients with histopathologic features of endemic nephropathy and those in CKD stage 3 or above, including those on dialysis or after kidney transplantation, are considered at increased risk for developing upper tract urothelial cancer and are recommended to have urine cytology and imaging every 6 months according to the European consensus on endemic nephropathy.[179] This also applies to patients with previous bladder cancer. In view of the high incidence of urothelial carcinoma in patients with ESKD due to endemic nephropathy, prophylactic bilateral nephroureterectomy has been recommended with determination of the level of AA-DNA adducts in the resected renal cortical tissue, especially in kidney transplant recipients before or after transplantation.[179,224]

## ANCA-ASSOCIATED VASCULITIDES

Antineutrophil cytoplasmic antibody (ANCA)–associated vasculitis (AAV) comprises granulomatosis with polyangiitis (GPA), eosinophilic GPA, microscopic polyangiitis (MPA), and the renal-limited variant of MPA.[225] ANCAs are serologic hallmarks of these small-vessel vasculitides. Proteinase 3 (PR3) and myeloperoxidase (MPO) are two major target antigens of ANCA in AAV. The histopathologic hallmark of ANCA-associated glomerulonephritis (ANCA-GN) is pauci-immune necrotizing glomerulonephritis, often with abundant crescents. While the typical finding is little or no glomerular staining for immunoglobulins by immunofluorescence microscopy, immune complexes could be detected in renal biopsies of some patients.[226]

Pathogenesis involves the interaction between genetic predisposition, environmental triggers such as infection, and effector mechanisms in the innate and adaptive immune system. Acute vascular inflammation is induced when resting neutrophils that have ANCA autoantigens sequestered in cytoplasmic granules are exposed to priming factors such as cytokines and proinflammatory mediators induced by infection or complement activation, triggering the appearance of ANCA antigens on the surface of neutrophils and their release into the surrounding microenvironment. ANCA then bind to these ANCA antigens on the primed neutrophils, resulting in neutrophil activation and the release of neutrophil extracellular traps.[227] This and other mediators released by activated neutrophils activate the alternative complement pathway, which generates C5a, that acts as a chemoattractant for neutrophils and also primes the neutrophils for activation by ANCA. Activated neutrophils also adhere to and penetrate vessel walls and release oxygen radicals and destructive enzymes that induce local damage in the form of necrotizing inflammation of small vessels.[228]

AAV is a common autoimmune disease in Caucasians, with an annual incidence rate of 10–20 pmp and peak age of disease onset of 65–74 years.[229] In Asia, AAV is an important glomerular disease in elderly patients presenting with AKI.[230] In contrast to Caucasian populations, where GPA and anti-PR3 are more common, data from China and Japan showed a preponderance of MPA and anti-MPO disease, often associated with more chronic lesions in the kidney biopsy.[231–236] MPA or GPA mostly occurs in older adults, although it has been reported at all ages. A series that included 234 Chinese patients with AAV showed that >40% of patients were above the age of 65 years at diagnosis and 94.9% of the elderly patients had anti-MPO antibodies.[237] Data from Japan also showed that the annual incidence of MPA was approximately 10 times higher in subjects above the age of 65 years than in younger adults.[235] In addition, compared with younger patients, older patients had more pulmonary involvement and a higher risk of infections. The typical presentation of ANCA-GN in Asia is rapidly progressive glomerulonephritis, often in an elderly patient. A retrospective study in China showed that 27 (12.1%) of 223 patients with ANCA-GN showed concomitant membranous nephropathy, and these patients were characterized by a higher level of proteinuria and more severe renal injury and tubulointerstitial disease compared with those without membranous features in the kidney biopsy, and a relatively low seropositive rate for anti-PLA2R antibodies compared with patients with primary membranous nephropathy (12.5% vs. 65.0%).[238]

The 2015 European League Against Rheumatism and European Renal Association–European Dialysis and Transplant Association (EULAR/ERA-EDTA) recommendations for the management of AAV suggest that glucocorticoids combined with either cyclophosphamide or rituximab be used for remission-induction treatment of severe organ-threatening disease, with the additional consideration of plasma exchange in patients presenting with serum creatinine ≥500 μmol/L due to rapidly progressive glomerulonephritis or those with alveolar hemorrhage, and that low-dose glucocorticoids combined with azathioprine, rituximab, methotrexate, or mycophenolate mofetil be used for remission maintenance.[239] Corticosteroids combined with cyclophosphamide is still the most commonly used treatment for remission induction.[240–242] In view of the predilection for elderly subjects and a high incidence of infective complications, treatment decisions with regard to the dose of immunosuppression entail a delicate balance between efficacy and potential treatment-related adverse effects. Data from a study in China that included 398 patients with AAV showed that 135 (33.9%) died during follow-up, with 83 deaths occurring within the first 12 months after diagnosis and infection being the leading cause of death (39 cases). Besides, older age, pulmonary involvement, and poor renal function at presentation predicted mortality.[243] In patients presenting with rapidly progressive glomerulonephritis that required dialysis, infection (47.4%) and active vasculitis (26.3%) were the leading causes of death.[244] The high incidence and poor outcome of infections in this patient population have also been reported from Japan, and the excessive mortality was attributed to cyclophosphamide, so that many patients are treated with corticosteroids alone and a starting dose of prednisolone <0.8 mg/kg per day has been recommended especially for elderly patients.[245,246] In this context, data from a retrospective study in 82 Japanese patients with ANCA-positive MPA, 29 of whom were treated with corticosteroids plus cyclophosphamide while 53 were treated with corticosteroids alone, showed similar remission rates of >90% in both groups but a lower 5-year survival rate in those given cyclophosphamide (50% vs. 73% in the noncyclophosphamide group, $P = .041$).[247] Another study reported that disease severity at presentation was associated with both the risk of relapse and infective complications during follow-up.[248]

The clinical outcomes including the survival of patients with AAV have improved substantially over the past decade. In a study of 398 patients >30% died after mean follow-up of approximately 2 years.[243] Data from Japan showed improved renal and patient prognosis in patients presenting with ANCA-positive MPA with rapidly progressive glomerulonephritis in recent years, which was attributed to earlier diagnosis and improved treatment.[246,249]

## HEPATITIS B/C-ASSOCIATED RENAL DISEASES

Infection with HBV or hepatitis C virus (HCV) may be associated with a variety of glomerular diseases due to immune complex deposition or immune complex–mediated vasculitis,[250–253] with or without cryoglobulinemia,[254] the latter being more common in the case of HCV infection.

HBV, a hepadnavirus with the virion consisting of a 42-nm spherical, double-shelled particle composed of small spheres and rods and with an average width of 22 nm, is partially double-stranded DNA. In endemic areas the transmission of HBV is mostly vertical from infected mother to child, followed by horizontal transmission within families or horizontal infection of adults who do not have protective immunity. In areas of intermediate prevalence transmission is mostly horizontal, affecting older children, adolescents, and adults. In areas of low prevalence, HBV is primarily a disease of adolescents and young adults, through sexual or parenteral acquisition.[255] In the Far East prior to the advent of vaccination programs, vertical maternal–infant transmission of HBV during the perinatal period had been the predominant route of infection accounting for persistent endemicity.[256] The age of presentation for HBV-associated kidney diseases thus varies according to the time of infection. Mass HBV vaccination programs markedly reduced the HBsAg carriage rate and the consequent HBV-associated liver complications including hepatocellular carcinoma.[257] For example, the nationwide HBV vaccination program of Taiwan that was introduced in 1984 reduced the HBsAg carrier rate in children from 9.8% to <1% in 2 decades.[258] The frequency of HBV-associated membranous nephropathy among children infected with HBV also decreased from 11.6% in the period 1974–1984 to 2.1% in 1994–2004, and to 0% in 2004–2009.[259] A similar impact of immunization program on HBV-associated membranous nephropathy, reducing the incidence by approximately 90%, had previously been observed in South Africa.[260]

Extrahepatic manifestations such as glomerulonephritis, vasculitis, or reactive arthritis can occur with either acute or, more commonly, chronic HBV infection. Pathogenesis is related to the formation of immune complexes followed by complement activation. Renal diseases secondary to HBV can take the form of membranous glomerulonephritis, membranoproliferative glomerulonephritis, polyarteritis nodosa, or mesangial proliferative glomerulonephritis. The low molecular weight of HBeAg ($3 \times 10^5$ Da) has been speculated to account for its ability to traverse the glomerular basement membrane and form subepithelial immune deposits. In a report from China that included 5935 kidney biopsies performed in 2010–2015, of which 1038 (17.5%) were diagnosed as secondary glomerular diseases, HBV-associated glomerulonephritis accounted for 9.2% of the secondary cases.[261] The most common pattern of renal involvement in renal biopsy is membranous nephropathy, followed by membranoproliferative glomerulonephritis, polyarteritis nodosa, IgAN, and focal segmental glomerulosclerosis, although the latter two categories might represent coincidental findings.[251] HBV-associated membranous nephropathy is more common in children and in many cases resolves spontaneously when seroconversion from HBeAg seropositivity to anti-HBe seropositive status occurs, but spontaneous resolution of HBV-related glomerulonephritis is uncommon in adults, and some patients show progressive renal deterioration over time.[262] Confirmation of HBV etiology is by the demonstration of HBV antigens in the kidney biopsy, although this may not be positive in all cases and positive staining needs to be interpreted in the context of appropriate histopathologic features.[263]

Much of the data on the treatment of HBV-associated glomerular diseases are derived from patients with membranous nephropathy. Treatment with interferon or nucleoside analogs has been reported to lead to a reduction of proteinuria in patients with HBV-related membranous nephropathy. Interferon treatment given for 4–12 months was associated with sustained remission of proteinuria in 20%–100% of patients, usually occurring within 6 months of clearance of HBeAg.[262]

The M-type phospholipase A2 receptor (PLA2R) on the surface of podocytes has been identified as the major autoantigen in primary membranous nephropathy, and autoantibodies directed against PLA2R are mostly of IgG4 subclass.[264,265] Up to 80% of patients with primary membranous nephropathy, including patients in Asia, have circulating anti-PLA2R antibodies.[266–271] Data from a recent study in China that included 179 patients with primary membranous nephropathy, 40 patients with membranous lupus nephritis, and 26 patients with HBV-associated membranous nephropathy showed glomerular PLA2R expression, in a fine granular pattern along the glomerular capillary wall, in 92.2% of patients with primary membranous nephropathy and 7.7% of patients with HBV-associated membranous nephropathy.[272] In addition, 93.3% of the primary membranous nephropathy cases showed prominent glomerular IgG4 deposition, while IgG3 was the predominant subclass in patients with HBV-associated membranous nephropathy, with IgG4 present in 11.5%.[272]

While more often associated with HCV than HBV,[254,273–275] cryoglobulinemic renal disease has been reported in China, which has an HBV prevalence rate of 7.18% in the general population.[276] A series of 12 patients diagnosed with HBV-associated cryoglobulinemia in 2008–2015 showed that renal involvement, characterized by nephrotic range proteinuria with microscopic hematuria, affected 75% of patients while 58.3% presented with skin rash.[277] All patients showed reduced complement level and tested positive for rheumatoid factor. Kidney biopsies showed membranoproliferative glomerulonephritis, but HBV antigens were not demonstrable in all patients. All the patients were treated with glucocorticoids alone or in combination with other immunosuppressive agents, and 50% died or reached end-stage renal failure.[277]

The body of data to date suggests that antiviral therapy improves HBV-associated membranous nephropathy. However, this conclusion is based on a relatively small number of subjects and not from randomized controlled trials.[278–280] A recent meta-analysis included 325 Asian patients with HBV-associated glomerulonephritis.[281] A total of 219 (215 Chinese and 4 Thai) patients had received treatment and were compared with 106 controls (96 Chinese and 10 Thai). The results showed an overall efficacy of nucleoside/tide in reducing proteinuria, resulting in a 3.6-fold increased rate of proteinuria remission.[281] Another meta-analysis that included 127 patients also yielded results supportive of treatment efficacy, applicable to both interferon and nucleoside/tide analogs.[282] The generalizability of these results to other patient populations is unclear.

Based on available data, and considering the safety of entecavir, which is a recommended standard of care treatment for HBV, antiviral therapy is recommended in patients with HBV-associated renal disease and evidence of active viral replication as indicated by the level of HBV DNA.[283,284]

According to prevailing HBV treatment recommendations, nucleoside/tide analog treatment is continued for at least 12 months after seroconversion of HBeAg (to anti-HBe), whereas patients who are HBeAg negative at the start of treatment often require lifelong therapy.[285] In patients with HBV-associated renal disease, immunosuppression should be reserved to those with rapidly progressive glomerulonephritis or severe polyarteritis nodosa, with plasmapheresis considered in cryoglobulinemic cases.

Recent epidemiological reports showed a prevalence rate of approximately 3%–4% for HCV infection in the general population across Asia, varying from 0.08% in Hong Kong, 0.37% in Singapore, 0.47% in the Philippines, 0.49% in Japan, 0.6%–1.3% in Korea, 1.6%–3.2% in China, 2.2% in Thailand, to 1.8%–4.4% in Taiwan.[286–289] The predominant genotypes also vary, with 1b accounting for around 70% in China and around 40% in Korea, whereas genotype 3 accounts for up to 80% of cases in India and Pakistan, and genotype 6 restricted to a few places such as Hong Kong and Thailand.[287] Prevalence is higher with increasing age, among injecting drug users (48%–90%), and those with coinfection by human immunodeficiency virus (32%–85%). Annual incidence of HCV in China was estimated as 6.01/100,000.[288]

Extrahepatic manifestations occur in 38%–76% of patients with chronic HCV infection, mostly as immune-mediated diseases such as mixed cryoglobulinemia, Sjögren syndrome, autoimmune thyroiditis, and B-cell lymphoproliferative disorders.[290] Renal involvement, mostly as membranoproliferative glomerulonephritis, occurs in approximately 20% of patients with mixed cryoglobulinemia.[291] For extrahepatic manifestations of HCV, including glomerulonephritis and cryoglobulinemic vasculitic syndromes, treatment with direct-acting antiviral agents has demonstrated efficacy and is recommended.[291,292] Antiviral efficacy and improvement of renal abnormalities have been demonstrated in Asian patients with HCV-associated cryoglobulinemic membranoproliferative glomerulonephritis.[293,294] However, a recent case report from the United States described a patient with recurrent mixed cryoglobulinemia syndrome despite sustained virologic response after treatment with direct-acting antiviral agent.[295] In addition, the high cost of direct-acting antiviral agents presents a substantial financial barrier to treatment access in many Asian countries, as is the case with rituximab for the treatment of HCV-associated cryoglobulinemic vasculitis.

## KIDNEY INJURY RELATED TO INFECTIONS

### LEPTOSPIROSIS

Leptospirosis is the most widespread zoonosis and is endemic worldwide, being most prevalent in tropical, humid, and rural environments, particularly in warm and humid regions.[296] The disease is caused by the spirochete *Leptospira*, which enters the human body through direct cutaneous or mucosal transmission or by aerosolization.[297] Rodents and small mammals are reservoirs for *Leptospira*, and infected animals shed the spirochete in their urine into water or soil, which then infect humans through occupational (as occurs in farmers, sewage workers, and miners), household environmental, or recreational exposure. Increased risk of exposure to *Leptospira* after flooding has been observed.[298] Each *Leptospira* serovar is frequently associated with a particular maintenance host. Results of genotype investigation using multiple-locus variable-number tandem repeat analysis, including 11 loci in 110 *Leptospira interrogans* serogroups from Japan, the Philippines, Taiwan, and Vietnam, and 4 loci in 52 *Leptospira borgpetersenii* isolates from Japan, the Philippines, and Taiwan, showed variable genetic diversity in different serogroup strains and a wider host range for *L. borgpetersenii* compared with *L. interrogans*.[299]

Approximately 90% of *Leptospira* infections are subclinical or associated with mild self-limited disease. A study in India that included serum samples from 244 miners detected antibodies to leptospires in 38.5% of subjects, compared with 13% in nonminer controls, and serogroup analysis showed concordance with carrier animals in the region.[300] Leptospirosis is an important topic in travel medicine because the disease can present as an imported case in Western countries in travelers returning from Asia.[301] However, it can also occur in subjects with no recent travel history and in urban settings,[302] especially in areas with a large population of rodents. For example, it has been reported that 65% of live-trapped rats in Baltimore (USA) had antibodies to *L. interrogans*.[303] Leptospirosis occurring in an endemic setting or presenting as epidemic outbreaks, especially in developing areas and crowded urban areas, occurs in different parts of the world including Thailand, the Philippines, and China.[304–307] It has been recognized as a reemerging infectious disease in Japan,[308] and a high prevalence rate of up to 50% of pathogenic *Leptospira* has been detected in wild and domesticated animals including rats and dogs in an endemic area in Jiangxi Province of China.[309]

Symptoms develop after an incubation period of 5 to 14 days. Mild disease has nonspecific symptoms that are indistinguishable from other febrile illnesses. Severe and potentially fatal disease characterized by fever; headache; myalgia; AKI due to acute interstitial nephritis, jaundice, and hemorrhagic complications; and multiorgan failure occurs in up to 10% of patients, and is associated with a mortality rate of 5% to 15%.[297] Typical clinical manifestations of leptospirosis fall into four categories: 1. mild influenza-like illness; 2. Weil syndrome characterized by jaundice, renal failure, hemorrhage, and myocarditis with arrhythmias; 3. meningitis/meningoencephalitis; and 4. pulmonary hemorrhage with respiratory failure.[310] Infection with icterohemorrhagiae serogroups has been reported to be associated with an increased risk of severe disease or death.[296,311] Cardinal features of severe leptospirosis include nonoliguric AKI, marked hyperbilirubinemia of >30 mg/dL (512 μmol/L) with less severe elevation of aminotransferase levels, thrombocytopenia, and lung involvement.[296] AKI as a result of acute tubulointerstitial nephritis is an early manifestation.[312] Oliguria, cardiac arrhythmia, and pulmonary involvement portend a poor prognosis.[313] Urinary sodium and potassium loss due to proximal renal tubular dysfunction resulting in electrolyte abnormalities is common.[314] Proximal tubular dysfunction such as bicarbonaturia, glycosuria, decreased proximal sodium reabsorption, phosphaturia, magnesuria, and uricosuria can occur.[315] Rhabdomyolysis can also contribute to the AKI.[316] The manifestation of severe disease can be variable. In some patients after the initial septicemic phase there is a period of transient symptomatic improvement before an immune phase in which critical disease manifestations can occur, whereas in other patients there is progressive symptomatic deterioration to fulminant disease.[296] The triad of fever, jaundice, and AKI in an acutely ill patient should alert the clinician of possible leptospirosis.

*Leptospira* reach the kidneys via hematogenous spread and finally localize in the proximal tubular lumen.[317] Guinea pigs infected with *Leptospira* showed renal tubular cell injury, interstitial nephritis, and associated microvascular injury, particularly at the corticomedullary junction.[318] Ultrastructural studies in mice showed the entry of *Leptospira* from the capillary lumen to the renal interstitial tissue inducing interstitial edema and cellular infiltration after 4–8 days.[319] Leptospiral antigens are found in the proximal tubule cells and infiltrating macrophages, and also in the form of large extracellular clumps in the interstitium.[320] Expression of leptospiral glycolipoprotein in renal tubules and vascular lumen has been implicated in the pathogenesis of acute tubulointerstitial nephritis and chronic tubulointerstitial lesions in chronically infected rats.[318,321] *Leptospira* outer membrane proteins (OMPs) may elicit tubular injury and inflammation through Toll-like receptor (TLR)-dependent pathways involving activation of nuclear transcription factor kappa B and mitogen-activated protein kinases, with downstream induction of chemokines and cytokines relevant to tubular inflammation.[312] LipL32, a 32-kDa lipoprotein, is a prominent leptospiral protein that is highly conserved among pathogenic *Leptospira* species.[322] LipL32 has been shown to induce inflammatory cytokines and stimulate extracellular matrix production in cultured renal tubular epithelial cells through transforming growth factor-β1 (TGF-β1)/Smad-dependent pathway,[323,324] and these proinflammatory steps involved Toll-like receptor 2 (TLR2) but not TLR4 in cultured renal tubular cells.[325–327] LipL32 also recognized and adhered to components of extracellular matrix including laminin, collagen I, and collagen V.[328,329] *Leptospira santarosai* serovar Shermani OMP increased the secretion of active TGF-β1 by proximal renal tubular epithelial cells and increased nuclear translocation of Smad3, accompanied by increased type I and type IV collagen messenger RNA and protein expression.[324] In chronic infection *Leptospira* may colonize and persist in the proximal renal tubule, and this has been associated with chronic tubulointerstitial nephritis and fibrosis.[330] Results from a recent epidemiological study showed an association between previous *Leptospira* exposure and impaired kidney function, suggesting that previous or chronic leptospiral infection is a risk factor for CKD.[331]

The diagnosis of leptospirosis depends mainly on serologic methods such as microscopic agglutination test to detect antibody to *Leptospira*, polymerase chain reaction (PCR) to detect *Leptospira* DNA, or culture of the microorganism.[297] The diagnosis of leptospirosis can be challenging to confirm, as the organism requires specialized culture media and grows over a period of weeks.[296,297] Serologic testing is often negative early in the course of the disease,[332] and suboptimal sensitivity and specificity rates have been reported with an IgM enzyme-linked immunosorbent assay (ELISA) for the diagnosis of acute leptospirosis.[333] PCR-based nucleic acid amplification testing of blood, urine, or cerebrospinal fluid is much more sensitive than culturing and can be performed early in the course of the disease, but such testing is not widely available.[302] Given these limitations, most diagnoses are still confirmed by serologic testing. A single indirect hemagglutination titer of at least 1:200 but <1:800 is suggestive of *Leptospira* infection, and infection is confirmed by either a single titer of ≥1:800 or by a fourfold or higher increase in titer in the convalescent serum specimen.[334]

Guidelines and expert opinion support prompt treatment with antibiotics in suspected and confirmed cases.[310,313] A review of seven randomized trials showed insufficient evidence for or against antibiotic therapy, but the duration of disease appeared shorter in patients treated with antibiotics though the difference did not reach statistical significance.[335] Clinical studies have demonstrated the effectiveness of early antibiotic treatment for leptospirosis.[336] It has been shown that serum creatinine level improved after 2.7 ± 2.2 days of IV penicillin therapy.[337] Treatment with effective antibiotics should be initiated as soon as leptospirosis is suspected based on clinical features before microbiological confirmation. Delayed initiation of antibiotics by ≥2 days was associated with more severe disease.[311] While a trial comparing ceftriaxone (1 g daily) with penicillin (1.5 million units every 6 hours) for 7 days showed no significant difference in the time to resolution of fever, in general IV penicillin is used to treat severe disease and oral doxycycline is used to treat mild disease.[338] Adults with severe disease should receive either penicillin (1.5 million units IV every 6 hours), doxycycline (100 mg IV twice daily), ceftriaxone (1–2 g IV once daily), or cefotaxime (1 g IV every 6 hours) for a duration of at least 7 days. Pregnant women with severe leptospirosis may be treated with IV penicillin, ceftriaxone, cefotaxime, or azithromycin, but not doxycycline. Patients with mild disease can be treated with doxycycline (adults: 100 mg orally twice daily) or azithromycin (adults: 500 mg orally once daily for 3 days), and pregnant women should be treated with either azithromycin or amoxicillin. Jarisch–Herxheimer reactions may occur following effective treatment. In addition, it is advisable to follow the kidney function of these patients in view of the recent data suggesting an association between prior leptospirosis and CKD.[331]

***Clinical Relevance***

**Leptospirosis**

Localization of leptospiral antigens and glycolipoprotein in the proximal tubular cells, infiltrating macrophages, and vascular lumen, or in the form of extracellular clumps in the interstitium, are implicated in the pathogenesis of acute tubulointerstitial nephritis and chronic tubulointerstitial lesions. *Leptospira* outer membrane proteins such as LipL32 may elicit tubular injury and inflammation through pathways dependent on Toll-like receptors and involving the activation of nuclear transcription factor kappa B and mitogen-activated protein kinases, with downstream induction of chemokines and cytokines such as the transforming growth factor-β1 (TGF-β1)/Smad-dependent pathway that are relevant to inflammation and fibrosis. Chronic *Leptospira* colonization in the proximal renal tubule is associated with chronic tubulointerstitial nephritis and fibrosis. These findings, together with data from a recent epidemiologic study in Taiwan, suggest potential contribution of previous or persistent *Leptospira* exposure to chronic kidney disease.

## DENGUE VIRAL INFECTION

Dengue is a common arthropod-borne viral (arbovirus) disease in tropical and subtropical regions.[339–341] While the annual incidence is estimated as 50 to 200 million by the WHO,[342] this could be an underestimate because the symptoms and signs are nonspecific, with fever being one of the most common clinical manifestations.[343] It is endemic in >100 countries, and an estimated 2.5 billion of the world's population are at risk of dengue infection.[344,345] The incidence of dengue fever has increased 30-fold in the past 50 years, and factors such as global warming, increased air travel and globalization, urbanization, and ineffective mosquito control have resulted in the spread of Dengue virus and the introduction of multiple viral serotypes into permissive areas, resulting in most tropical regions becoming hyperendemic with multiple viral serotypes cocirculating (Fig. 80.5).[346–352] The disease is common in South and Southeast Asia in countries such as Malaysia, Thailand, Indonesia, Vietnam, and Singapore,[339,353–355] and is spreading to other parts of Asia such as Japan, Korea, China, Taiwan, and Hong Kong.[343,347–351,356]

Dengue is transmitted by *Aedes* mosquitoes, principally *Aedes aegypti,* and is caused by four viral serotypes of the genus *Flavivirus* (DENV-1 to DENV-4).[344] Infection with one serotype confers lifelong immunity to that type but only short-term immunity to the others, and subsequent infection with a different serotype is associated with increased risk of severe complications. The female mosquito becomes infected when she takes a blood meal from an infected subject during the acute febrile and viremic phase of illness. During the extrinsic incubation period, the virus first infects midgut cells and then disseminates to replicate in numerous mosquito tissues, ultimately infecting the salivary glands after 8–10 days. Once the salivary glands are infected, the mosquito is infective and can transmit the virus to another person. The mosquito remains infective for life. There is no specific antimicrobial therapy. DENV vaccines are currently under development, including some in phase III safety and efficacy testing. Prevention is primarily by reducing the habitat and the number of mosquitoes, and limiting exposure to bites.

The time from infection to onset of illness, termed the intrinsic incubation period in humans, ranges from 3 to 14 days, with an average of 4 to 7 days. The symptoms that may appear include fever (often the first manifestation and can be the only manifestation in children), headache, myalgia, joint pain, and a measles-like skin rash which lasts up to 7 days. Slight abdominal pain and diarrhea can occur. Leukocyte

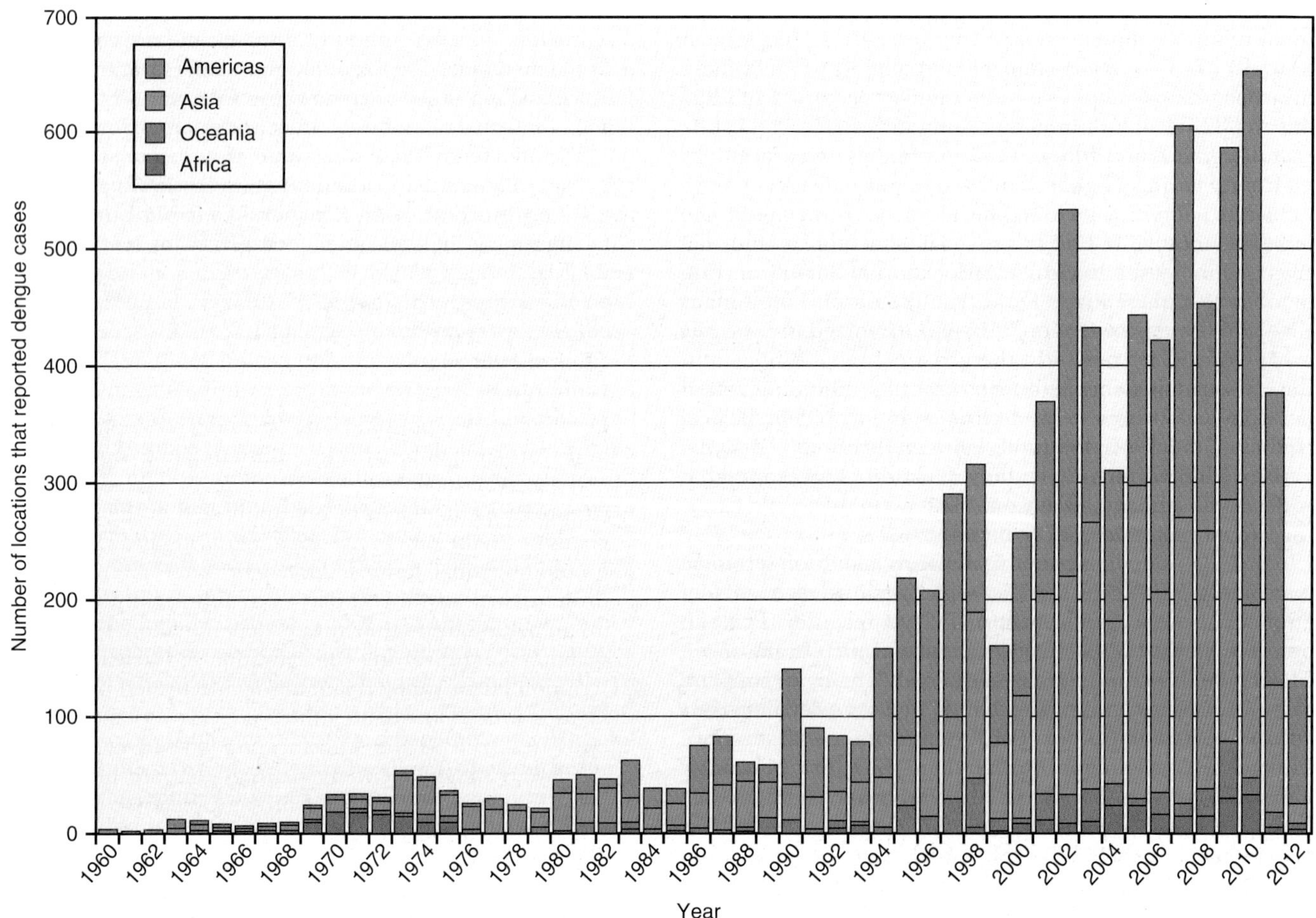


**Fig. 80.5** **Changing epidemiology of dengue over time.** (Reprinted by permission from Macmillan Publishers Ltd. Guzman MG, Gubler DJ, Izquierdo A, et al. Dengue infection. *Nat Rev Dis Primers* 2016;2:16055; adapted from Messina JP, Brady OJ, Pigott DM, et al. A global compendium of human dengue virus occurrence. *Sci Data* 2014;1:140004.).

counts are usually decreased. Patients can become better or deteriorate after 2–5 days. A small proportion of patients develop life-threatening dengue hemorrhagic fever (DHF), with features of thrombocytopenia, petechiae or ecchymosis, disseminated intravascular coagulation, and plasma leak resulting in hemoconcentration, hypoproteinemia, pleural effusion, and ascites. More severe cases are termed dengue shock syndrome (DSS), in which systemic vascular leak and severe hypotension occur.[343] There can be concomitant hepatitis, neurologic disorders, and myocarditis. Mortality rate in untreated cases could reach 20%, while supportive treatment including IV hydration can reduce the mortality rate to <1%.[344] In 2009, the WHO revised the classification as dengue with or without warning signs, and severe dengue, with the objective of facilitating the identification of patients at risk of severe disease.[346] It has been suggested that severe manifestations such as DHF and DSS occur as a result of antibody-dependent enhancement when a dengue-immune subject acquires infection by a different DENV serotype.[357] The facilitation of DENV lineage dispersal by air traffic of humans and/or mosquitoes thus has potential clinical and public health implications, and recent investigations showed that large transportation hubs such as Thailand could act as central points of DENV lineage movement in Asia.[352]

Proteinuria is common in severe dengue, and a detection rate of 74% has been reported.[358] The underlying pathogenesis of renal abnormalities in dengue is probably multifactorial. AKI is an infrequent complication of dengue infection, occurring in up to 13% of patients depending on the severity of infection, but is associated with increased morbidity and mortality, and a mortality rate of 64% has been reported.[359–362] In severe dengue infection hemodynamic disturbance, acute hemolysis, and rhabdomyolysis may contribute to direct kidney injury.[363–366] Immunologic mechanisms might also play a role, as suggested by renal abnormalities in the absence of shock, the demonstration of immune complex–mediated mesangial proliferation in human and animal models, and association with reduced levels of complement components.[367,368]

Anti-DENV IgM antibody detection with ELISA is most commonly used for diagnosis of acute disease, while patients in convalescence are identified through IgM and IgG seroconversion.[346] For patients suspected of dengue, a presumptive diagnosis can be made by the detection of IgM antibodies in samples collected at day 6 of acute symptoms. DENV viremia is detectable 24–48 hours before fever onset and continues for 5–6 days. During this period, infective virus, its specific RNA, and the NS1 protein can be detected in patient blood, serum, and plasma, and also in tissues from fatal cases. If the acute-phase sample obtained within the first 3 days after onset of symptoms is negative for IgM antibodies, testing for dengue viral RNA or NS1 antigen can be performed. DENV RNA detection provides a rapid, sensitive, and specific method for virological diagnostic confirmation. NS1 protein detection provides a window of opportunity for early etiological diagnosis. The sensitivity and specificity of DENV NS1 detection depend on the infecting serotype, the timing of sample collection, and the parity of DENV infection. Antibody cross-reaction is observed between DENV and Zika virus because both are Flaviviridae. Specific detection of DENV, chikungunya, and Zika viral RNA can be done by real-time PCR in acute samples. Under appropriate circumstances, IgM serology on serum samples collected from individuals with clinically suspected DENV infection or Zika virus infection should be performed by IgM Capture ELISA for both DENV and Zika virus. If positive to both viruses, a secondary *Flavivirus* infection should be considered.

Supportive care and careful monitoring are essential, as there is no specific treatment for dengue. Treatment with corticosteroid or chloroquine was shown to be not beneficial.[369,370] Fluid intake during the 24 hours before being seen by a clinician has been significantly associated with decreased risk for hospitalization.[371] Analgesic and antipyretic drugs such as paracetamol can be prescribed at the usual dosage for children and adults. Neither aspirin nor nonsteroidal antiinflammatory drugs should be taken. Vector control to avoid mosquito bites should be used to prevent disease transmission.

Fluid therapy is key to dengue management and is applied based on disease severity, and fluid lost due to capillary leakage must be replaced with IV crystalloid solutions (volume-expanding fluid replacements such as lactated Ringer's solution) or physiological (normal) saline solution. The subsidence of fever could portend clinical deterioration, and thus patients need to be carefully monitored.

## MALARIA

Malaria is a protozoan disease caused by four main *Plasmodium* species (*Plasmodium falciparum, Plasmodium vivax, Plasmodium malariae,* and *Plasmodium ovale*) and the zoonotic parasite *Plasmodium knowlesi* found in many Southeast Asian countries.[372,373] Over 200 million cases of malaria occurred in 2015 and the number of deaths exceeded 420,000.[372] The majority of infections occur in Africa (90%), followed by South/Southeast Asia (6%), and the eastern Mediterranean region (2%). Morbidity and mortality due to malaria have decreased globally secondary to malaria control programs over the last few decades, while a high level of transmission continues in some regions. In addition, the emergence of artemisinin-resistant *P. falciparum* malaria in Southeast Asia and the lack of a highly protective vaccine present challenges to continued progress.[374]

Malaria is transmitted by *Anopheles* mosquito. Infection in an individual without prior exposure almost invariably produces a febrile illness. The accompanying symptoms are nonspecific and often include rigors, headache, nausea, and muscle pains. If treated with appropriate drugs at this stage the symptoms remit over a few days, though often with considerable exhaustion. In the case of *P. falciparum*, complete treatment will eradicate the infection, and any return of symptoms reflects incomplete treatment, resistance to the drugs used, or new infection. In the case of *P. vivax* and *P. ovale*, subsequent infections may recur at intervals as a result of reactivation of the dormant liver-resident hypnozoite stage, unless this is cleared by a prolonged treatment with an 8-aminoquinoline drug.[375–377] Clinical and laboratory criteria are used to establish the diagnosis of severe malaria, which requires aggressive treatment especially for travelers who have no prior immunity.[376,378] The clinical features of malaria can simulate other febrile illnesses. Therefore the WHO recommends that diagnosis be established with a parasite-specific laboratory test in patients suspected to have malaria based on clinical grounds.[376] Laboratory testing options vary based on the geographic, clinical, and socioeconomic setting.

The most commonly used methods for laboratory diagnosis include microscopic examination of stained blood films and detection of parasite antigen or nucleic acid,[379] of which microscopic examination of thick and thin blood films remains the gold standard. Rapid antigen detection methods and molecular amplification tests are used increasingly as adjunctive tests. Tests for antiplasmodial antibodies are commercially available but are not recommended for diagnosis of acute disease.

About 120 types of *Plasmodium* species have been reported, although only five are accepted as human malaria parasites. Notably, *P. falciparum* and *P. vivax* cause most of the human infections worldwide. The most virulent species *P. falciparum* is also the most prevalent parasite in Africa, whereas *P. vivax* is the most widely distributed parasite outside of Africa, for example, in India.[380,381] *P. malariae* and *P. ovale* spp are much less prevalent. *P. malariae* is more or less sympatric with *P. falciparum* in distribution, mainly found in sub-Saharan Africa and southwest Pacific.[382] *P. ovale* spp were thought to have a limited distribution, mostly found in Africa and some Pacific Islands.[383] However, the prevalence of these two species is probably underestimated, due to low parasitemia, morphological resemblance with *P. vivax,* and occurrence as mixed infections.[384] *P. malariae, P. ovale,* and *P. vivax* may cause febrile attacks years after exposure.[385] Delayed clinical disease due to *P. ovale* or *P. vivax* is due to the existence of hypnozoites, a minority of parasites that remain in the liver instead of inducing a blood stage like the majority. These dormant microorganisms can remain viable for many years, thereby causing late onset of disease. For *P. malariae* a low level of parasitemia may persist for years, sometimes below the level of detection on a thick film, and disease can emerge more than a decade after primary infection.[382] Chronic *P. malariae* infection can result in immune complex formation, leading to membranoproliferative or mesangioproliferative glomerulonephritis and proteinuria (quartan malarial nephropathy).[386,387] Molecular testing and genotyping have yielded more accurate data on distribution.[388] In the Greater Mekong Subregion of Southeast Asia, including the countries of Cambodia, China, Laos, Myanmar, Thailand, and Vietnam, where there is a plan for regional malaria elimination by 2030, all five *Plasmodium* parasites infecting humans coexist and *P. vivax* and *P. falciparum* are the predominant parasite species.[389] A recent study of 2701 blood samples collected from the China–Myanmar border region using nested PCR to detect the protozoan genome identified 561 malaria cases, including 161 *P. falciparum,* 327 *P. vivax,* 66 *P. falciparum–P. vivax* mixed infections, 4 *P. malariae,* and 3 *P. ovale* spp. *P. vivax* and *P. falciparum* accounted for >60% and approximately 30% of all malaria cases, respectively.[390] In addition to South Asian countries, *P. malariae* infections have been described in China,[391] Thailand,[392,393] and Vietnam,[394] and may exhibit high genetic diversity.[395] *P. ovale* spp have been found in South Asian and neighboring countries including Cambodia, Laos, Myanmar, Thailand, and Vietnam.[392] Most *P. ovale* spp reported in China have been imported, mainly from Africa.[396] Indigenous malaria cases decreased significantly after the National Malaria Elimination Action Plan was initiated in China in 2010.[397] A recent report from Jiangsu province in China showed that of the 1268 cases of malaria reported in the province in 2011–2014, 83.4% were imported *P. falciparum* cases, while 13.0% were due to *P. ovale,* and 2.8% were due to *P. malariae,* many of which were imported from countries in Africa and South Asia.[398]

In Korea, *P. falciparum* infection was once present among IV drug abusers, while indigenous falciparum malaria has not been reported since 1945.[399] *P. malariae* was also present before 1945, but has not occurred since. Vivax malaria had been prevalent in Korea for many centuries, but its incidence decreased rapidly from the 1970s. The Republic of Korea (South Korea) was once declared as malaria free in the late 1970s, but vivax malaria reemerged in 1993. Initially localized to the area bordering North Korea it has subsequently spread from west to east.[400–402]

In the nonendemic setting of Singapore, a retrospective analysis of 214 patients with smear-positive malaria treated at a tertiary hospital in 2000–2010 showed that *P. vivax* accounted for 59.3% of cases, whereas *P. falciparum, P. malariae,* and mixed infections accounted for 38.8%, 0.3%, and 1.4% of cases, respectively.[403] Most patients presented with fever and thrombocytopenia was common. The 43 severe cases were characterized by older patient age and higher level of parasitemia. All the patients survived.

*P. knowlesi* has emerged as the most common cause of malaria infection in Malaysia.[404,405] Owing to its 24-hour erythrocytic stage, *P. knowlesi* replicates quickly.[406,407] It can cause severe and fatal disease and thus it is important to diagnose and treat early.[408–411] Knowlesi malaria shows a fatality rate that is comparable with, if not higher than, that of falciparum malaria.[409,410] The severity of knowlesi malaria, including the complication of AKI, is significantly associated with high parasitemia level.[410,412,413] Diagnosis with blood film microscopy may be associated with misidentification because the *P. knowlesi* ring stages resemble *P. falciparum* and later trophozoites resemble *P. malariae.* Newer methodologies such as loop-mediated isothermal amplification are being investigated.[414]

Previous reports from India showed that the clinical presentation of severe falciparum malaria has more complications, including multiorgan failure often including AKI, which was associated with a higher mortality rate.[415–417] Disease severity is usually lower with vivax malaria compared with falciparum malaria. However, there are marked variations and there have been increasing reports of severe vivax malaria, including respiratory distress,[418] AKI,[419] and cerebral malaria,[420] and also reports of disease occurring in temperate regions.[421] In a series that included 341 Korean patients diagnosed in 2005–2009, including six recurrent cases, the common manifestations included fever (98.8%), thrombocytopenia (99.7%), chills (62.5%), transaminasemia (54.8%), leukopenia (43.4%), headache (33.7%), anemia (28.5%), and myalgia (24.9%). Less common but severe complications included hypotension (4.1%), altered mentation (0.9%), AKI (0.9%), spleen infarction (0.6%), and spleen rupture (0.3%).[421] Another series that included 210 Korean patients diagnosed with vivax malaria in 2006–2012 showed that 11 (5.2%) required intensive care unit admission and among these patients five required mechanical ventilation and one was treated with extracorporeal membrane oxygenation.[399] Overall, the disease was categorized as severe in 21.0%, with pulmonary complications being most common (21.9%), followed by cerebral (2.4%), shock (1.9%), and bleeding complications (1.4%), and AKI occurred in 1.0% of patients. None of the patients died.

Pathogenesis leading to organ injury in severe malaria involves a complex interplay between direct damage due to parasite sequestration in microcirculation and host response with the release of various cytokines.[422–425] Parasitized red cells adhere to vascular endothelial cell surface markers such as ICAM1.[426] In this regard, cerebral malaria and multiorgan dysfunction (including AKI) have been associated with distinct profiles of cytokines and chemokines involving IL-17, IL-10, and human interferon-inducible protein 10 (IP-10).[427] The incidence of AKI can be up to 60%.[428] AKI complicating *P. falciparum* seems to have increased over the past decade.[429–431] In addition, AKI has been associated with vivax malaria.[419,432] AKI complicating *P. falciparum* malaria is associated with acute tubular necrosis with renal tubular cells showing variable degrees of cloudy swelling, degeneration, and necrosis. A recent report from Thailand showed predilection of injury at the distal tubule and a correlation between the degree of tubular injury and serum creatinine level. Changes in the renal tubules included cell vacuolation and degeneration, necrosis of individual tubular cells or tubular segments, scattered or diffused detachment of the renal tubular cells from the basement membrane, deposition of hemosiderin pigments, and minimal chronic inflammatory cell infiltration.[433]

## SCRUB TYPHUS

Scrub typhus is a mite-borne infectious disease caused by the intracellular gram-negative bacteria *Orientia tsutsugamushi* (former name *Rickettsia tsutsugamushi*). Rodents are the main reservoir, and their mites act as both the reservoir and the vector. Human infection occurs when the larvae of the trombiculid mite infected with *O. tsutsugamushi* bite to suck human tissue fluid.[434,435] An estimated 1 million cases occur each year,[436] and the disease is common in Southeast Asia, Japan, China, and South Korea.[437,438] Disease manifestations vary from mild or asymptomatic infection to severe potentially fatal illness, with clinical features of high fever, skin rash, headache, myalgia, lymphadenopathy, gastrointestinal symptoms, and cough. Most patients have a relatively benign course. A typical eschar occurs at the site of the bite, but is not always present. According to organ involvement, patients could present with pneumonitis, meningitis, encephalitis, myocarditis, acute pulmonary edema, pericarditis, hepatitis, or multiorgan failure.[439] Severe disease is characterized by acute respiratory distress syndrome, AKI, bleeding, coagulation disorders, meningoencephalitis, and shock.[440–444] Respiratory distress and encephalitis are the major causes of death.[445] Renal involvement is common. Urinary abnormalities, such as hematuria, proteinuria, pyuria, and granular casts, occur in up to 80% of patients, and AKI occurs in 8%–60%.[441–444,446–450] Pathogenic mechanisms include direct renal tubular cell injury with or without tubulointerstitial inflammatory cell infiltration.[451,452] A higher serum level of neutrophil gelatinase–associated lipocalin has been shown to be associated with the development of AKI in scrub typhus.[453] Intravascular hemolysis in patients with glucose-6-phosphate dehydrogenase deficiency, rhabdomyolysis, hypoperfusion, and vasculitis are other contributing factors to kidney injury.[446,454] Histopathology shows acute tubular necrosis, interstitial nephritis, and mesangial proliferation.[451,455–457] A retrospective study of 510 Korean patients with scrub typhus diagnosed in 2001–2013 showed that 35.9% developed AKI, and that risk factors for AKI included older age and concomitant comorbidities such as diabetes mellitus and preexisting CKDs.[458] Furthermore, the complication of AKI was associated with higher rates of intensive care unit admission and death. All except one patient with AKI recovered. Serologic diagnosis of acute scrub typhus infection is based on a fourfold or higher increase in titer in paired samples drawn at least 14 days apart.[459] Serum or eschar PCR to detect bacterial genome may also be used for diagnosis.[460,461] Prompt treatment with doxycycline results in rapid improvement, including that of renal function.[442,455] Elderly patients are at risk of more complications and poor clinical outcome, which could be related also to delayed presentation.[462]

## SEVERE FEVER WITH THROMBOCYTOPENIA SYNDROME

Severe fever with thrombocytopenia syndrome (SFTS) was initially recognized in the Henan and Hubei provinces of China around 2007,[463] and was subsequently reported in other provinces in China such as Zhejiang and Liaoning,[464,465] South Korea,[466] and Japan.[467] The syndrome is caused by the SFTS virus (SFTSV; genus *Phlebovirus*, family Bunyaviridae), and ticks (e.g., *Rhipicephalus microplus*) in domestic animals are the vector.[463,468–470] Investigations showed that SFTSV was common throughout different parts of Korea and China, especially in the warmer areas where ticks were more prevalent, and the disease mostly occurred in the months between April and October with farmers at higher risk due to occupational exposure.[470–473] Patients infected with SFTSV presented with fever, thrombocytopenia, leukocytopenia, hemorrhagic features, and in severe cases multiorgan failure. Mortality rate was reported as 8.7%–47.2%.[472,474] AKI occurred in about 20% of cases and was associated with a higher mortality rate of 12%–30%.[463] Studies from China reported hemorrhagic features in >70% of patients, including gastrointestinal bleeding in 10% of patients, liver dysfunction in the majority, AKI requiring dialysis in 23%, and a 27% mortality rate.[475,476] In a study that included 129 cases from Zhejiang province, China, the death rate was 12.4% and extremes of body mass index and delayed diagnosis were associated with increased risk of death.[477] Clinical features of SFTS are nonspecific and overlap with those of human granulocytic anaplasmosis (caused by *Anaplasma phagocytophilum*), HFRS due to leptospirosis, or Hanta virus infection,[471] while lymphadenopathy has been reported as more common in SFTSV and AKI more common in Hanta virus infection (>80%).[478] CD3- and CD4-positive T lymphocytes were lower than normal in patients, while natural killer cell counts were increased.[479] Impaired β-interferon production and induction of a proinflammatory cytokine storm contributed to disease pathogenesis.[464,480] Recent investigations showed that nonstructural proteins of SFTSV could suppress exogenous type I interferon–induced Janus kinase/signal transducer and activator of transcription (Jak/STAT) signaling to facilitate the virus evading host immune surveillance.[481] Diagnosis can be made by serological testing with ELISA or detection of viral genome using reverse transcription-PCR or reverse transcription–cross-priming amplification.[482–485] Supportive therapy and treatment of various complications are currently the mainstay of management.[465]

## HANTAVIRUSES AND HEMORRHAGIC FEVER WITH RENAL SYNDROME

Hantaviruses are single-stranded, enveloped, negative-sense RNA viruses that belong to the Bunyaviridae family.[486] Hantavirus is named after the Hantaan River in South Korea around which an outbreak occurred. The virus was isolated in the late 1970s.[487] The zoonosis is endemic in East Asia, including China, Korea, and part of Russia.[488–490] These viruses normally infect rodents, the field mouse *Apodemus agrarius* being the major animal reservoir, and do not cause disease in these hosts. Humans may become infected with hantaviruses through aerosolized excreta inhalation and contact infection by rodent urine, saliva, or feces, and human-to-human transmission has been reported with the Andes virus in South America.[491] Some strains of hantaviruses cause potentially fatal diseases in humans, such as hantavirus HFRS and hantavirus pulmonary syndrome – also known as hantavirus cardiopulmonary syndrome.[487]

HFRS (also termed Korean hemorrhagic fever, epidemic hemorrhagic fever, or nephropathia epidemica) is a group of clinically similar illnesses caused by species of hantaviruses. HFRS can thus be caused by the Hantaan virus (HTNV), Amur virus (AMV), Seoul virus (SEOV), Dobrava virus (DOBV), or Puumala virus (PUUV), with variable disease severity (often more severe with HTNV and DOBV).[492] HTNV and SEOV are found in China, with the main natural hosts being *A. agrarius* and *Rattus norvegicus,* respectively.[493] SEOV is globally widespread and may cause moderate HFRS, whereas PUUV is endemic in northern Europe and may cause a generally mild form of HFRS, also called nephropathia epidemica. About 100,000 cases of HFRS are documented annually,[494] most of which are in China, Korea, and Russia, though the disease has also been reported in Europe, Africa, and the Americas.[495] PUUV is found in Scandinavia, Western Europe, and western part of Russia. DOBV is found primarily in the Balkans, and SEOV is found worldwide. Saaremaa virus is found in central Europe and Scandinavia.

Hantavirus mainly infects human vascular endothelial cells and causes extensive damage to capillaries and small vessels. Viral entry in target cells is mediated via integrins and CD55, and pathogenic virus strains appear to utilize beta 3 integrins while beta 1 integrin is utilized by nonpathogenic strains.[496] Immune-mediated mechanisms including cytokines and complement activation are involved in the pathogenesis of organ injury.[497–499] Clinical manifestations include AKI, increased vascular permeability, and coagulation abnormalities. Typical kidney biopsy findings include acute tubulointerstitial nephritis, hemorrhage into medullary tissues, interstitial edema, renal tubular cell necrosis, and in some cases podocyte injury with foot process effacement associated with mislocalization of junctional proteins thereby resulting in glomerular proteinuria.[500,501] While there is no gross cytopathic effect, changes of subcellular structures are accompanied by cellular dysfunction, and typical disruption of cell–cell contact, as occurs in glomerular endothelial cells.[496] Data from in vitro studies also showed that hantavirus-infected vascular endothelial cells were sensitized to the action of vascular endothelial growth factor in increasing permeability.[502] AKI was associated with increased mortality, especially in elderly patients who also had more severe hypotension.[503] In HFRS, the clinical picture is characterized by AKI, often with massive proteinuria due to tubular and glomerular involvement.[486] Infection with hantavirus is associated with significant morbidity and mortality worldwide. Approximately a quarter of infected patients have a severe course. A mortality rate of 5%–10% has been reported from Korea, whereas in Europe the mortality rate appeared lower at 0.5%.[486]

Symptoms usually develop 1–2 weeks after exposure to infectious material, but can be delayed for weeks. Initial symptoms begin suddenly and include severe headache, back, and abdominal pain, fever, chills, nausea, facial flushing, conjunctival injection, and skin rash. Severe manifestations include hypotension, vascular leakage, and AKI.

HFRS follows a typical clinical course (Table 80.3).[486,504] In the initial "febrile phase," which lasts for 3–7 days, symptoms often include facial redness, fever and sweating, headache, malaise, abdominal and back pain, nonspecific respiratory symptoms, and gastrointestinal symptoms such as nausea and diarrhea. This is followed by the "hypotensive and hemorrhagic phase," lasting for about 2 days, which is associated with increased vascular permeability. Tachycardia occurs and

**Table 80.3 Typical Clinical Phases of Hemorrhagic Fever With Renal Syndrome Due to Hantavirus Infection**

| Phase of Illness | Time of Occurrence | Principal Features | Signs and Symptoms | Complications |
|---|---|---|---|---|
| 1. Febrile | 1–7 days | Fever | • Headache<br>• Vomiting<br>• Abdominal pain<br>• Back pain<br>• Visual disturbance | • Acute encephalomyelitis<br>• Bleeding<br>• Shock<br>• Multiorgan failure<br>• Pituitary hemorrhage |
| 2. Hypotensive | 1–3 days | Hypotension | • Capillary leak<br>• Pulmonary symptoms | • Renal<br>• Pulmonary edema |
| 3. Oliguric | 2–6 days | ↓ urine output | • Severe oliguria can occur<br>• Fluid retention | • Acute respiratory distress syndrome |
| 4. Polyuric | 2 weeks | ↑ urine output | • Decrease of body weight | • Disseminated intravascular coagulation |
| 5. Convalescent | 3–6 months | | • Weakness<br>• Fatigue | |

Modified from Jiang H, Du H, Wang LM, et al. Hemorrhagic fever with renal syndrome: Pathogenesis and clinical picture. *Front Cell Infect Microbiol.* 2016;6:1.

patients can develop hypoxemia. Leukocytosis occurs with thrombocytopenia, elevated C-reactive protein, and lactate dehydrogenase levels. The next stage is the "kidney phase," which lasts 3–7 days, characterized by AKI with frequent oliguria, hematuria, proteinuria, and hypoalbuminemia. The severity of AKI has been associated with the severity of thrombocytopenia and also the presence of glomerular proteinuria.[486,503,505] This initial oliguria is followed by subsequent polyuria and convalescence.

Diagnosis is by serological testing of IgM against hantavirus by various means such as reverse transcription-PCR.[506,507] Supportive therapy is still the mainstay of care for patients with hantavirus infection.[508] Careful attention to fluid management and hemodynamics is necessary, with RRT by intermittent HD or continuous RRT in unstable subjects. The role of ribavirin remains controversial, with recent results showing a lack of efficacy and safety.[509–511]

## DIALYSIS IN ASIA

Dialysis, while life-saving for patients with ESKD, is a high-cost treatment, and the access to dialysis in developing countries or those with less developed national health-care insurance systems is fraught with economic and ethical issues. It has been reported that >2.6 million people received RRT worldwide in 2010, while an estimated 2.3 million people might have died prematurely due to limited access to RRT, with the largest treatment gaps in low-income countries in Asia and Africa, which affected populations amounting to 1.9 million and 0.4 million, respectively.[24] Over the period of 2000–2013 the incidence of ESKD increased 13 times in Thailand, two to three times in the Philippines, Malaysia, and South Korea, and the reported figures were affected by the variable improvements in the access to RRT between different countries.[512] While close to 1 million people are on maintenance dialysis in Asia, the prevalence varies considerably within the region, owing to differences in the status of development of health-care systems in different regions. Access to dialysis therapy is not restricted by personal financial means in Japan, Taiwan, South Korea, Singapore, and Hong Kong, and there is ongoing expansion of health-care insurance coverage for dialysis in other places such as Thailand, Malaysia, and many parts in China; and dialysis registries have been established in Japan, South Korea, Taiwan, Malaysia, Hong Kong, Shanghai, Thailand, and Singapore.[31] The incidence and prevalence rates of treated ESKD are highest in Japan, Taiwan, South Korea, and Singapore, at approximately 300–450 pmp and 1800–3000 pmp, respectively, and are much lower in areas with lower income such as the Philippines and Indonesia.[512] With the size of the ESKD population predicted to increase to 5.4 million by 2030, the financial implications of the RRT program are daunting.[24]

### PERITONEAL DIALYSIS

Insufficient HD facilities, draconian selection criteria for RRT, cost containment, and clinical outcomes that were at least comparable with HD in the short-term were factors that led to the establishment of a PD-First policy for publicly funded dialysis service in Hong Kong in the mid-1980s, and to this date Hong Kong continues to report the highest PD utilization rate in the world (73% of all dialysis patients).[513–516] A similar PD-First policy has been implemented since 2008 in Thailand, which presently has approximately 60% of dialysis patients in the public health-care system on PD and 40% on HD, and the policy has been shown to facilitate cost containment (health-care cost reduced by approximately 1500 USD per patient per year) and increase dialysis utilization by the general public (prevalence rate of ESKD increased from 420 pmp in 2007 to 1073 pmp in 2013).[517] A recent study from Indonesia based on economic modeling reported an equal number of 5.93 life-years saved by either a PD-First or an HD-First policy, while a PD-First policy would be associated with a slightly higher quality-adjusted life-years of 4.40 (compared with 4.34 for HD-First), a lower total lifetime treatment cost of 700 million IDR (51,800 USD) per patient (compared with 54,400 USD for HD-First), and a substantial health-care budget saving in the long term.[518] From a clinical and patient-focused perspective, PD would be more suitable than HD in patients with unstable cardiovascular status or vascular access problems, or those who live far from dialysis facilities. Care should be exercised to ensure adequate dialysis dose and ultrafiltration in patients of large body size, especially those with minimal residual kidney function.[519] The incidence rate of PD-associated peritonitis has decreased significantly consequent to improvements in connectology, with peritonitis rates of <0.3 episode per patient-year reported by some centers, below the 0.5 episode per patient-year as recommended by the International Society for Peritoneal Dialysis.[520,521] Despite the advent of PD solutions with improved biocompatibility,[522,523] progressive peritoneal membrane fibrosis and deterioration of dialytic functions of the peritoneum remain unresolved problems limiting the long-term application of PD and also having an adverse impact on patient outcomes.[524–526] In addition, although the number of affected patients accounts for a relatively small percentage of all PD patients, with reported incidence rates of 0.7%–3.3%, encapsulating peritoneal sclerosis is a severe and often devastating complication with no effective therapy, which can present during dialysis or after kidney transplantation, and lead to much patient suffering often over long durations and eventually a high mortality rate of >50%.[527] Duration of PD is a significant risk factor, because encapsulating peritoneal sclerosis predominantly affects patients on PD for >5 years, and the incidence rate increases with further time on PD.[528] The implementation of health-care policies that place a large proportion of patients on long-term PD must therefore incorporate long-term perspectives, and measures, to minimize the occurrence of complications consequent to peritoneal fibrosis after prolonged PD, which incur not only patient suffering but also high treatment costs.

### HEMODIALYSIS

The HD service in Japan is characterized by a high proportion of in-center HD (>85%), which is related to the progressive establishment of accessible HD centers over the past decades, and clinical outcomes that are deemed very favorable by international standards including both early and long-term survival rates.[512] The low rate of kidney transplantation in Japan has contributed to the progressive expansion of the dialysis population, especially the elderly age group and those with diabetes mellitus.[529] Unadjusted 5-year survival rate was

60% in Japan compared with 39% in USA in 2004–2008.[530] Studies from the Dialysis Outcomes and Practice Patterns Study (DOPPS) were launched in the USA in 1996 and extended to Japan in 1998–2002, and to China in 2010. Results from DOPPS and Japan Dialysis Outcomes and Practice Patterns Study (J-DOPPS) showed that, compared with Western countries, HD patients in Japan showed a high utilization rate (>90%) of arteriovenous fistula, less intensive anemia management with lower target hemoglobin and lower doses of erythropoietin-stimulating agent as well as IV iron, lower parathyroid hormone levels, and lower levels of C-reactive protein; and treatment time was >4 hours in approximately 80% of Japanese patients, compared with 40% in the United States.[512,531] Similar to earlier findings in the Hemodialysis Study and DOPPS, results from the MONDO database, which included data of HD patients from different networks globally including the Asian-Pacific region, showed that failure to convert from central venous catheter access to noncatheter vascular access within 6 months of commencing HD was associated with a higher mortality rate.[532–534] Twice-weekly HD is not uncommon in Asian countries especially those with insufficient access to HD or where patients are required to pay for the treatment. In this regard, use of twice-weekly HD is <3% in Japan, Europe, and North America, but is approximately 20% in China.[535] Data from serial phases of J-DOPPS also showed a U-shaped relationship between blood pressure and all-cause mortality, with lowest mortality in patients with baseline systolic blood pressure of 140–159 mm Hg and diastolic blood pressure of 65–74 mm Hg,[536] an association between vascular access failure and high intradialytic ultrafiltration (HR: 1.41 when ultrafiltration was 5.1%–13.7% of body weight),[537] an inverse relationship between employment and mortality or hospitalization,[538] and improved prediction of cardiovascular events using a new model which incorporated six variables (age, diabetes mellitus, history of cardiovascular events, dialysis time per session, serum phosphorus level, and serum albumin level) compared with the Framingham Risk Score.[539] Recent data on 1350 patients from the China Dialysis Outcomes and Practice Patterns Study (C-DOPPS) showed that 21% had hemoglobin <9 g/dL, and attributed the relatively high percentage to less frequent HD and financial barrier.[540]

## KIDNEY TRANSPLANTATION—SPECIAL ISSUES IN ASIA

### KIDNEY TRANSPLANTATION ACROSS ABO BLOOD GROUP BARRIER

Presently there are >0.3 million Japanese patients on long-term dialysis.[44] Due to the rarity of deceased-donor organ transplantation, kidney transplantation across ABO blood group barrier has developed in Japan. The first case of ABO-incompatible (ABO-I) kidney transplantation from a live donor in Japan was reported in 1991.[541] Subsequently >3500 ABO-I kidney transplantations have been performed, with outcomes now comparable with ABO-compatible (ABO-C) procedures.[542–544] The success is attributed to continued improvements in preoperative desensitization therapy, which prevents posttransplant serious acute antibody-mediated rejection.[544,545] ABO-I kidney transplantation programs are now well established in many transplant centers in Japan, and account for approximately 30% of live-donor kidney transplant operations in Japan.[544] The numbers of centers and patients undergoing ABO-I kidney transplantation have also increased rapidly in Korea, and ABO-I kidney transplantation accounted for 10% and >20% of all live-donor kidney transplantations in 2010 and 2014, respectively.[546–548] ABO-I kidney transplantation is also performed in selected patients in Thailand, Malaysia, China, and Hong Kong.

Antiblood group antibody-mediated acute rejection ceases to appear after accommodation is induced a few weeks after kidney transplantation.[549] Therefore the most important elements in the pretransplant desensitization protocol are removal of preformed antibodies and inhibition of antibody production by B cells. Previously, this could only be achieved with splenectomy.[550,551] Rituximab has been used in ABO-I kidney transplantation in Japan since 2002, and is now an integral element in standard desensitization protocols.[552,553] The incorporation of tacrolimus and mycophenolate into the immunosuppressive regimen has also contributed to improved clinical outcomes.[554] The 5-year graft survival rates of ABO-I kidney transplantation in Japan improved from 68% in 1989–1994 to 90% in 2001–2006, and further improved after the introduction of rituximab.[543,545] The 5-year graft survival rates of ABO-C, ABO-I with splenectomy, and ABO-I with rituximab were reported as 88.4%, 90.3%, and 100%, respectively.[555] An analysis of single-center data from 1032 live-donor kidney transplantations performed in 1989–2013, of whom 247 were ABO-I, showed that ABO-I and ABO-C cases had comparable 9-year graft survival rates (86.9% and 92.0%, respectively), and that the graft survival was better in 2005–2013 compared with 1998–2004 (HR: 0.30).[48]

A desensitization protocol comprising mycophenolate mofetil and low-dose corticosteroids started 28 days pretransplant, preoperative plasmapheresis, and two doses of rituximab at 375 mg/m$^2$ on day −14 and day −1, and postoperative immunosuppression with basiliximab, corticosteroids, and tacrolimus or cyclosporine was investigated in a prospective 1-year study that included 18 patients who underwent ABO-I kidney transplantation, and the results showed high tolerability of the treatment protocol and high efficacy with no anti-A/B antibody-mediated rejection.[556] One patient developed anti-HLA antibody-mediated rejection, which was successfully managed with standard antirejection therapy. Patient and graft survival were both 100% after 1 year.

In a retrospective series of 327 Japanese patients who underwent live-donor kidney transplantation, comparison of protocol graft biopsies performed at 3 and 12 months after transplantation between 226 ABO-C and 101 ABO-I patients showed comparable allograft histology overall, with subclinical acute rejection detected in 6.9% and 9.9% of patients in the ABO-C and ABO-I groups at 3 months ($P$ = .4) and in 12.4% and 10.1% at 12 months, respectively ($P$ = .5), and no between-group difference with regard to the rate of infections (including BK nephropathy) and patient or graft survival.[557]

Worldwide, the Collaborative Transplant Study reported outcomes from 1420 ABO-I kidney transplantations performed at 101 transplant centers from 2005 to 2012.[558] The 3-year graft survival rate of ABO-I transplants did not differ from matched ABO-C cases (89.9% vs. 90.1%). Patient survival in ABO-I cases was lower initially due to infection-related deaths, but 3-year patient survival rates were similar between the two groups (95.6% in ABO-I vs. 96.3% in ABO-C). Data from 125 Korean patients who underwent ABO-I kidney transplantation in 2007 to 2010 showed 2-year graft and patient survival rates of 97.5% and 99.2%, respectively.[546]

## HEPATITIS B IN KIDNEY TRANSPLANT RECIPIENTS

One-third of the world's population shows serological evidence of HBV infection, and >350 million people are chronic HBV carriers, with a worldwide seroprevalence rate of 3.61% for HBsAg.[559–561] Endemicity of HBV infection varies between Asian countries, with HBsAg seroprevalence rates ranging from <1% to >10% (Table 80.4).[561]

Hepatitis B vaccination and matching of HBV status between donor and recipient are measures to prevent HBV infection in kidney transplant recipients. Hepatitis B vaccination at birth was introduced in some Asian countries since the late 1980s but is still not universally practiced, especially in less developed areas. EASL clinical practice guidelines recommend vaccination in HBV seronegative patients with end-stage renal disease.[562] The efficacy of hepatitis B vaccination is significantly lower in patients with moderate to severe renal impairment and in immunosuppressed patients,[563,564] and thus patients with CKD should receive vaccination early. Maintaining an anti-HBs titer of ≥100 IU/L with booster is in general recommended, although hepatitis B reactivation could still occur, albeit uncommonly, in anti-HBc-positive subjects upon heavy immunosuppression.[565,566] Donor–recipient matching with regard to HBV serological status aims to prevent transmission of HBV from the kidney donor to the recipient. An organ from an HBsAg-positive donor must not be transplanted into a recipient who is seronegative for both HBsAg and anti-HBs except when the transplant is deemed urgent and antiviral treatment is available. The risk of HBV transmission from HBsAg-negative anti-HBc-positive donors to HBsAg-negative recipients appeared low, especially when the recipient is anti-HBs-positive,[567] and transplanting a kidney from an HBsAg-positive donor into an anti-HBs-positive recipient with immunoglobulin cover appeared safe,[52] although in both cases surveillance of de novo HBV infection with HBsAg and HBV DNA monitoring is advisable.

Immunosuppression enhances viral replication, leading to reactivation of hepatitis B and progressive liver disease.[568,569] Without treatment, reactivation of HBV infection occurs in patients who receive immunosuppressive agents for the treatment of diseases or the prevention of rejection after transplantation. Before the availability of antiviral prophylaxis, the rates of HBV reactivation in HBsAg-positive kidney transplant recipients were reported as 50%–94%, and HBV infection was associated with significantly increased morbidity and mortality, related to liver complications and nonliver complications, especially infections.[50,568,570–573] Clinical manifestations of HBV-related liver complications after kidney transplantation can present as acute hepatitis, fibrosing cholestatic hepatitis, chronic hepatitis with fulminant reactivation, chronic hepatitis, cirrhosis and its complications, or hepatocellular carcinoma.[50,51,573–578] The 10- and 20-year patient survival rates in HBsAg-positive kidney transplant recipients without antiviral therapy were 85% and 71%, respectively (vs. 98% and 95% at 10 and 20 years in HBsAg-negative patients).[51] Prior to the availability of antiviral treatment, HBsAg-positive kidney transplant recipients showed a 9.7-fold increased risk of death and 68-fold increase in liver-related mortality rate compared with HBsAg-negative controls, while the survival of these patients is similar to subjects without HBV infection in the present era of effective antiviral nucleoside/tide analog therapies.[50]

Interferon as a therapy for hepatitis B precipitates allograft dysfunction and rejection and is thus contraindicated in kidney allograft recipients except for life-saving indications.[579] The advent of effective antiviral nucleoside/tide analog therapies has markedly improved posttransplant outcomes of patients infected with HBV. Antiviral treatment can be given prophylactically at the time of kidney transplantation or preemptively when increasing level of circulating HBV DNA indicate impending reactivation, although the former is more convenient especially in the context of a busy clinical setting. Salvage therapy, given after the onset of clinically evident liver exacerbation, is associated with inferior outcome.[580] A study that included 26 HBsAg-positive Chinese patients who received lamivudine therapy preemptively based on increasing HBV DNA levels showed effective suppression of viral replication and normalization of liver biochemistry,

**Table 80.4 HBsAg Seroprevalence and the Number of People Living With Chronic HBV in the General Population in Some Asian Countries**

| Country | Prevalence Estimates (%, 95% CI) | Population Size Per Country | HBsAg-Positive Population |
|---|---|---|---|
| China | 5.49 (5.47–5.50) | 1,359,821,465 | 74,601,204 |
| Japan | 1.02 (1.01–1.02) | 127,352,833 | 1,294,431 |
| Malaysia | 0.74 (0.70–0.77) | 28,275,835 | 208,540 |
| Mongolia | 9.07 (8.41–9.78) | 2,712,738 | 246,070 |
| The Philippines | 4.63 (4.53–4.73) | 93,444,322 | 4,326,212 |
| Singapore | 4.09 (3.87–4.33) | 5,078,969 | 207,943 |
| South Korea | 4.36 (4.36–4.37) | 48,453,931 | 2,111,914 |
| Thailand | 6.42 (6.37–6.47) | 66,402,316 | 4,260,008 |
| Vietnam | 10.79 (10.29–11.31) | 89,047,397 | 9,607,438 |

*CI,* Confidence interval; *HBsAg,* hepatitis B surface antigen; *HBV,* hepatitis B virus.

Modified from Schweitzer A, Horn J, Mikolajczyk RT, et al. Estimations of worldwide prevalence of chronic hepatitis B virus infection: a systematic review of data published between 1965 and 2013. *Lancet* 2015;386:1546–1555.

and improved survival rate to that approaching HBsAg-negative patients.[50] The high incidence of drug resistance associated with lamivudine was tackled with newer antiviral agents including adefovir, entecavir, and tenofovir.[581,582] Adefovir is nephrotoxic and its role has been superseded by newer agents. At present, entecavir and tenofovir are the recommended first-line antiviral therapies.[285] Entecavir is preferred in the kidney transplant setting especially in patients with suboptimal graft function as tenofovir has been associated with renal tubular toxicity.[583] A 20-year patient survival rate of 69% has been reported for HBsAg-positive kidney transplant recipients transplanted in the recent era of antiviral treatment, which was superior to 40% in patients transplanted before the advent of antiviral drugs.[582] Overall, the short- and medium-term survival rates of HBsAg-positive kidney transplant patients are now comparable with subjects not infected with HBV.[50,584,585] Nevertheless, while antiviral therapy prevents severe exacerbation due to heavy immunosuppression, liver-related deaths can still occur during long-term follow-up due to progressive liver disease. Data from a retrospective study of 74 Korean patients who had received antiviral treatment showed comparable renal allograft survival between HBsAg-positive and HBsAg-negative patients, while seropositivity for HBsAg was associated with 2.19-fold increased risk of death, with one-third of the deaths related to HBV, during a mean follow-up of 75.7 months.[586] In another multicenter study that included 160 Korean kidney transplant recipients with HBV infection, transplanted after 1999, HBV infection was associated with 2.37-fold increased risk of death, and mortality correlated with the severity of inflammation in the prekidney transplant liver biopsy.[587] Surveillance measures including monitoring of liver function and the development of malignancy by alpha-fetoprotein measurement and liver ultrasound are thus important elements in the clinical care of kidney transplant recipients infected with HBV in Asia.

B-cell depletion with rituximab is often included in desensitizing immunosuppressive protocols for patients with antiblood group or anti-HLA antibodies prior to kidney transplantation.[588] However, rituximab is associated with a high rate of hepatitis B reactivation, not only in HBsAg-positive subjects but also in subjects with apparent clinical resolution of prior infection as denoted conventionally by seronegativity for HBsAg and seropositivity for anti-HBc.[589–592] The rate of hepatitis B reactivation in HBsAg-negative/anti-HBc-positive patients who received rituximab-containing chemotherapy was reported as 11.3%–41.5%.[593–595] Patients with autoimmune diseases treated with rituximab are similarly at risk.[596,597] In this regard, a study in 49 HBsAg-negative anti-HBc-positive kidney transplant recipients in Korea showed hepatitis B reactivation in five patients (10.2%), in whom two were regarded clinically severe, resulting in one mortality.[598]

Prior to the advent of effective and safe antiviral treatment, patients with cirrhosis were largely declined for kidney transplantation in view of the unacceptably high rate of liver-related mortality.[599] In the present era patients with compensated cirrhosis and no evidence of portal hypertension can be considered for kidney transplantation. Data from a retrospective study in Korea of 12 kidney transplant recipients with prior HBV-associated liver cirrhosis showed liver deterioration after kidney transplantation in one patient and stable liver status in the other 11 patients.[600] Patient survival rate at 5 years was similar in patients with or without prior cirrhosis, at 100% and 94%, respectively. Patients with decompensated cirrhosis and those with compensated cirrhosis and portal hypertension are not eligible for kidney transplantation, but may be considered for combined liver and kidney transplantation.[599]

## CONCLUDING STATEMENTS

Clinical nephrology has advanced significantly over the past half a century in the Far East. Variations in geotopography and genetic background, and rapid changes in the urban environment and socioeconomic development, have contributed to the marked diversity of disease spectra and multiplicity of challenges to the prevention and treatment of kidney diseases in the region. By contrast, the relatively low facility costs in many parts of Asia and the abundance of patients and biomedical samples present invaluable research opportunities to address knowledge gaps that are critical in the strive to continue to improve clinical outcomes.

Complete reference list available at ExpertConsult.com.

## KEY REFERENCES

3. *ISN Global Kidney Health Atlas*; 2017. Available at: www.theisn.org/global-atlas.
13. Susantitaphong P, Cruz DN, Cerda J, et al. World incidence of AKI: a meta-analysis. *Clin J Am Soc Nephrol*. 2013;8:1482–1493.
19. Yang L, Xing G, Wang L, et al. Acute kidney injury in China: a cross-sectional survey. *Lancet*. 2015;386:1465–1471.
23. Zhang L, Wang F, Wang L, et al. Prevalence of chronic kidney disease in China: a cross-sectional survey. *Lancet*. 2012;379:815–822.
24. Liyanage T, Ninomiya T, Jha V, et al. Worldwide access to treatment for end-stage kidney disease: a systematic review. *Lancet*. 2015;385:1975–1982.
44. Hanafusa N, Nakai S, Iseki K, et al. Japanese society for dialysis therapy renal data registry–a window through which we can view the details of Japanese dialysis population. *Kidney Int Suppl*. 2015;5:15–22.
50. Chan TM, Fang GX, Tang CS, et al. Preemptive lamivudine therapy based on HBV DNA level in HBsAg-positive kidney allograft recipients. *Hepatology*. 2002;36:1246–1252.
52. Jiang H, Wu J, Zhang X, et al. Kidney transplantation from hepatitis B surface antigen positive donors into hepatitis B surface antibody positive recipients: a prospective nonrandomized controlled study from a single center. *Am J Transplant*. 2009;9:1853–1858.
53. Lai KN, Tang SC, Schena FP, et al. IgA nephropathy. *Nat Rev Dis Primers*. 2016;2:16001.
76. Rauen T, Eitner F, Fitzner C, et al. Intensive supportive care plus immunosuppression in IgA nephropathy. *N Engl J Med*. 2015;373:2225–2236.
77. Lv J, Zhang H, Wong MG, et al. Effect of oral methylprednisolone on clinical outcomes in patients with IgA nephropathy: the TESTING randomized clinical trial. *JAMA*. 2017;318:432–442.
113. Chan TM. Treatment of severe lupus nephritis: the new horizon. *Nat Rev Nephrol*. 2015;11:46–61.
114. Chan TM, Li FK, Tang CS, et al. Efficacy of mycophenolate mofetil in patients with diffuse proliferative lupus nephritis. Hong Kong-Guangzhou Nephrology Study Group. *N Engl J Med*. 2000;343:1156–1162.
118. Appel GB, Contreras G, Dooley MA, et al. Mycophenolate mofetil versus cyclophosphamide for induction treatment of lupus nephritis. *J Am Soc Nephrol*. 2009;20:1103–1112.
119. Dooley MA, Jayne D, Ginzler EM, et al. Mycophenolate versus azathioprine as maintenance therapy for lupus nephritis. *N Engl J Med*. 2011;365:1886–1895.
141. Liu Z, Zhang H, Liu Z, et al. Multitarget therapy for induction treatment of lupus nephritis: a randomized trial. *Ann Intern Med*. 2015;162:18–26.
142. Zhang H, Liu Z, Zhou M, et al. Multitarget therapy for maintenance treatment of lupus nephritis. *J Am Soc Nephrol*. 2017; In Press.

145. Zhang L, Long J, Jiang W, et al. Trends in chronic kidney disease in China. *N Engl J Med.* 2016;375:905–906.
150. Molitch ME, Adler AI, Flyvbjerg A, et al. Diabetic kidney disease: a clinical update from Kidney Disease: Improving Global Outcomes. *Kidney Int.* 2015;87:20–30.
173. Imai E, Ito S, Haneda M, et al. Effects of blood pressure on renal and cardiovascular outcomes in Asian patients with type 2 diabetes and overt nephropathy: a post hoc analysis (ORIENT-blood pressure). *Nephrol Dial Transplant.* 2016;31:447–454.
180. Jadot I, Decleves AE, Nortier J, et al. An integrated view of aristolochic acid nephropathy: update of the literature. *Int J Mol Sci.* 2017;18:297.
186. Yang HY, Chen PC, Wang JD. Chinese herbs containing aristolochic acid associated with renal failure and urothelial carcinoma: a review from epidemiologic observations to causal inference. *Biomed Res Int.* 2014;2014:569325.
228. Xiao H, Hu P, Falk RJ, et al. Overview of the pathogenesis of ANCA-associated vasculitis. *Kidney Dis (Basel).* 2016;1:205–215.
235. Fujimoto S, Watts RA, Kobayashi S, et al. Comparison of the epidemiology of anti-neutrophil cytoplasmic antibody-associated vasculitis between Japan and the U.K. *Rheumatology (Oxford).* 2011;50: 1916–1920.
239. Yates M, Watts RA, Bajema IM, et al. EULAR/ERA-EDTA recommendations for the management of ANCA-associated vasculitis. *Ann Rheum Dis.* 2016;75:1583–1594.
250. Shah AS, Amarapurkar DN. Spectrum of hepatitis B and renal involvement. *Liver Int.* 2017; In Press.
252. Ferri C, Giuggioli D, Colaci M. Renal manifestations of hepatitis C virus. *Clin Liver Dis.* 2017;21:487–497.
261. Wang P, Tang L, Yao J, et al. The spectrum of biopsy-proven secondary glomerular diseases: a cross-sectional study in China. *Clin Nephrol.* 2017; In Press.
270. Akiyama S, Akiyama M, Imai E, et al. Prevalence of anti-phospholipase A2 receptor antibodies in Japanese patients with membranous nephropathy. *Clin Exp Nephrol.* 2015;19:653–660.
283. Chan TM, Lok ASF. Renal disease associated with hepatitis B virus infection. *UpToDate.* 2017. Available at: https://www.uptodate.com/home.
285. Lok AS, McMahon BJ, Brown RS Jr, et al. Antiviral therapy for chronic hepatitis B viral infection in adults: a systematic review and meta-analysis. *Hepatology.* 2016;63:284–306.
302. Mixter S, Sedighi Manesh R, Keller SC, et al. Spiraling out of control. *N Engl J Med.* 2017;376:2183–2188.
316. Abdulkader RC, Silva MV. The kidney in leptospirosis. *Pediatr Nephrol.* 2008;23:2111–2120.
332. Haake DA, Levett PN. Leptospirosis in humans. *Curr Top Microbiol Immunol.* 2015;387:65–97.
343. Simmons CP, Farrar JJ, Nguyen vV, et al. Dengue. *N Engl J Med.* 2012;366:1423–1432.
346. Guzman MG, Gubler DJ, Izquierdo A, et al. Dengue infection. *Nat Rev Dis Primers.* 2016;2:16055.
374. Daily JP. Malaria 2017: update on the clinical literature and management. *Curr Infect Dis Rep.* 2017;19:28.
376. World Health Organization. *Guidelines for the treatment of malaria - 3rd edition.* Available at: www.who.int.
377. Cowman AF, Healer J, Marapana D, et al. Malaria: biology and disease. *Cell.* 2016;167:610–624.
446. Attur RP, Kuppasamy S, Bairy M, et al. Acute kidney injury in scrub typhus. *Clin Exp Nephrol.* 2013;17:725–729.
458. Hwang K, Jang HN, Lee TW, et al. Incidence, risk factors and clinical outcomes of acute kidney injury associated with scrub typhus: a retrospective study of 510 consecutive patients in South Korea (2001-2013). *BMJ Open.* 2017;7:e013882.
477. Sun J, Gong Z, Ling F, et al. Factors associated with Severe Fever with Thrombocytopenia Syndrome infection and fatal outcome. *Sci Rep.* 2016;6:33175.
486. Krautkramer E, Zeier M, Plyusnin A. Hantavirus infection: an emerging infectious disease causing acute renal failure. *Kidney Int.* 2013;83:23–27.
504. Jiang H, Du H, Wang LM, et al. Hemorrhagic fever with renal syndrome: pathogenesis and clinical picture. *Front Cell Infect Microbiol.* 2016;6:1.
512. Robinson BM, Akizawa T, Jager KJ, et al. Factors affecting outcomes in patients reaching end-stage kidney disease worldwide: differences in access to renal replacement therapy, modality use, and haemodialysis practices. *Lancet.* 2016;388:294–306.
514. Chan MK. Peritoneal dialysis - a review with consideration of the role of CAPD in renal replacement therapy in developing countries. *Singapore Med J.* 1984;25:212–215.
516. Li PK, Chow KM, Van de Luijtgaarden MW, et al. Changes in the worldwide epidemiology of peritoneal dialysis. *Nat Rev Nephrol.* 2017;13:90–103.
548. Koo TY, Yang J. Current progress in ABO-incompatible kidney transplantation. *Kidney Res Clin Pract.* 2015;34:170–179.
553. Aikawa A, Saito K, Takahashi K. Trends in ABO-incompatible kidney transplantation. *Exp Clin Transplant.* 2015;13(suppl 1):18–22.
580. Han DJ, Kim TH, Park SK, et al. Results on preemptive or prophylactic treatment of lamivudine in HBsAg (+) renal allograft recipients: comparison with salvage treatment after hepatic dysfunction with HBV recurrence. *Transplantation.* 2001;71:387–394.

# 81 Oceania Region

Yeoungjee Cho | Suetonia C. Palmer | David W. Johnson

CHAPTER OUTLINE



KEY POINTS

- The burden of chronic kidney disease is increasing across the Oceania region, largely driven by growth in noncommunicable chronic illnesses such as diabetes mellitus.
- Access to health care, ranging from primary preventative management to renal replacement therapy, is limited in many nations of the Oceania region outside of Australia and New Zealand, especially for those who are unable to afford care.
- In response to growth in chronic kidney disease prevalence, countries such as Fiji are currently in the process of expanding their capacity to care for these patients with financial support from their government.

## INTRODUCTION

Oceania is a collective name for the land masses scattered throughout most of the Pacific Ocean. It is the term originally conceived by the French explorer Dumon d'Urville (1790–1842) in 1812 as "Océanie," which is a French word derived from the Latin word *oceanus,* meaning ocean. In its broadest sense, the term *Oceania* embraces the entire insular region between Asia and the Americas. The most commonly used definition of the term, however, excludes Ryukyu, Kuril, Aleutian islands, Japan archipelago, Indonesia, Taiwan, and the Philippines, because the people and cultures of those islands are more closely related historically to Asia. Oceania then, in its most commonly defined terms, includes >10,000 islands, with a total area of 8.526 million km$^2$ and estimated population of >40 million people. Oceania can be divided into four geopolitical subregions: Australasia, Melanesia, Micronesia, and Polynesia (Fig. 81.1), formed by 14 countries and 25 sovereign states and dependent territories, including Australia (population, 23 million), Papua New Guinea (8 million), New Zealand (4.5 million), and other island nations with populations ranging from <100 to >450,000 (Table 81.1).

Indigenous Australians are the original inhabitants of the Australian continent and nearby islands. Although disagreeing on details, scientists generally support a theory that calls for a Southeast Asian origin of the island people in other regions of Oceania. Over the years, many cultures have been influenced by migration, invasion, and colonization with resultant diversity in cultures, economy, language, and religions. Increased influence of the Western world in the region of Oceania has led to an increased urbanization and witnessed a growing burden of adverse health outcomes including obesity, hypertension, diabetes, and chronic kidney disease (CKD).

Kidney disease is one of the major socially transmitted diseases that contributes to higher health-care utilization, poor quality of life, and serious adverse outcomes including cardiovascular disease (CVD), need for renal replacement therapy (RRT), and death.[1,2] Although the exact incidence and prevalence across the Oceania region are incompletely known, reported deaths and years lost due to disability resulting from CKD range up to 4.28% and 2.24%, respectively (Table 81.1). Quantification of the burden of kidney disease is least well understood in the lowest income countries, and given the need for higher health-care utilization, there is an associated cost of kidney disease, which needs to be understood in the context of local government health-care expenditure.

The per capita income [gross domestic product (GDP) nominal per capita], not accounting for the cost of living, ranges widely in Oceania from those countries among the highest incomes in the world (Australia, US$44,820; New Zealand US$38,399) to under US$10,000 in many smaller island countries, states, and territories. The proportion of government expenditure spent on health also ranges from 4% (Papua New Guinea, Vanuatu) to 29% [French Polynesia

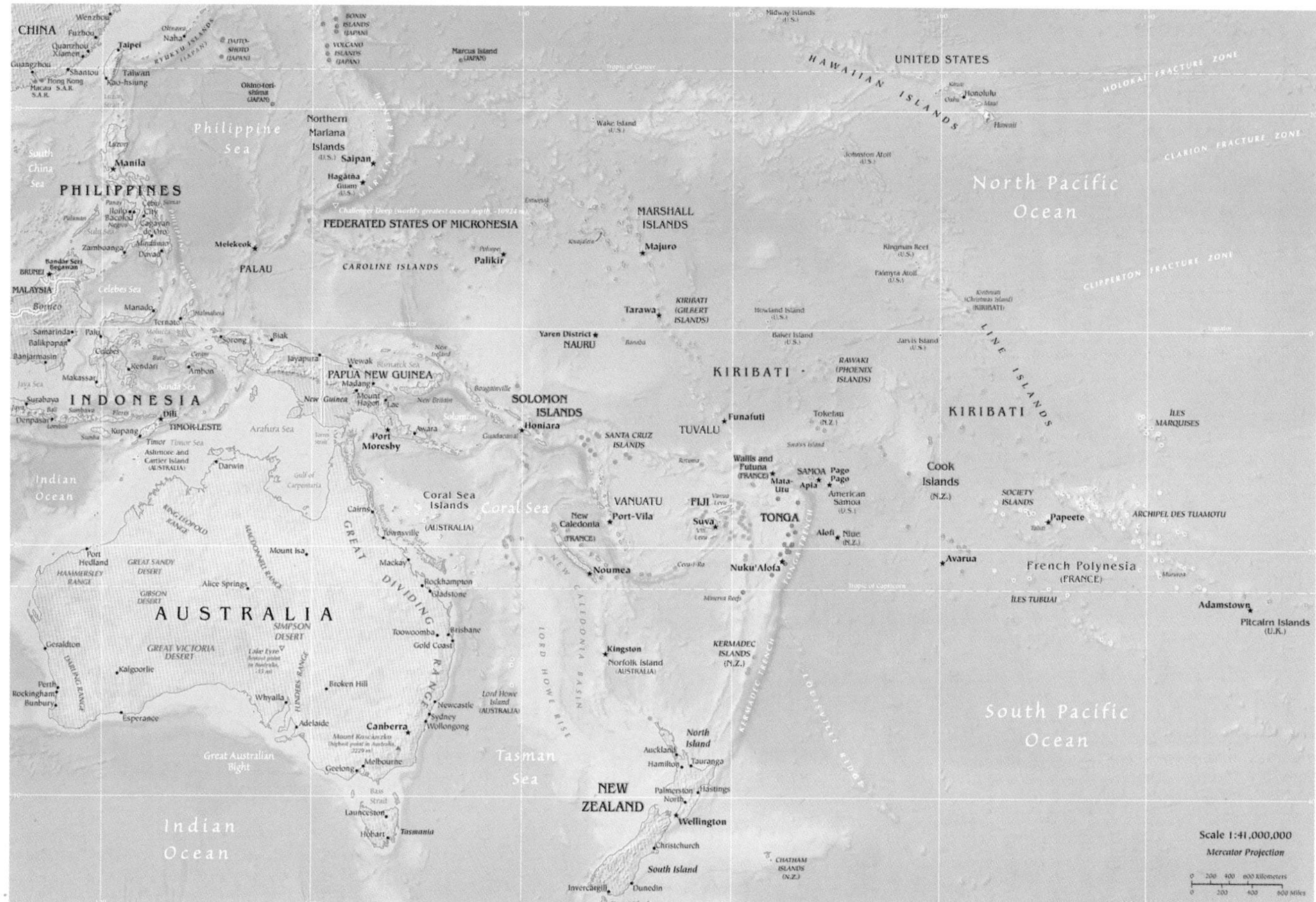


**Fig. 81.1** Map of Oceania region. (From Geographic Guide. Available from: http://www.geographicguide.com/oceania-map.htm. Last accessed January 24, 2019.)

(France Protectorate)]. Unsurprisingly, there is considerable variation in health outcomes and risk factors for long-term conditions (Table 81.1). This chapter discusses the burden of kidney disease, both acute and chronic, in Australia, New Zealand, and the island nations of Oceania. However, due to the relative paucity of information and data available from the island nations of Oceania, the main focus of this chapter will be on Australia and New Zealand.

## AUSTRALIA

### BURDEN OF DISEASE

In Australia, >1.7 million adults over the age of 18 years have indicators of CKD, such as reduced estimated glomerular filtration rate (eGFR) or proteinuria.[3] This equates to 1 in 10 Australian adults, with even higher incidence amongst indigenous Australians (1 in 5)[4] who make up approximately 3% of the total Australian population (estimated to be 669,900 people as of June 2011).[5] In contrast to the nonindigenous population where the CKD burden appears to be predominantly situated in major cities, the highest CKD burden in the indigenous population is found in the remote and very remote areas (remote 34% vs. nonremote 13%).[4,6] A small proportion of these patients will progress to end-stage kidney disease (ESKD), requiring RRT. With the growth in CKD burden, the number of patients with ESKD has doubled in Australia over the past decade and is currently >20,000 patients.[7] This growth is not surprising, and is an inevitable consequence of background increase in both behavioral (e.g., inactive/insufficiently active: 56%; smoking on daily basis: 16%) and biomedical [e.g., overweight or obese: 63%; high blood pressure: 32% (including 22% with uncontrolled high blood pressure)] risk factors for CKD in the Australian general population.[6] For instance, the prevalence of diabetes mellitus has tripled between 1989–90 and 2014–15 (1.5% vs. 4.7%), affecting >1.2 million Australian adults.[8] It is the fastest growing chronic disease and diabetic nephropathy has become the most common cause of ESKD in Australia (37%) as a result.[9] Patients with CKD stages 1–5 exhibit risk factors for both CKD and CVD more frequently than people without CKD, including diabetes mellitus (14.2% vs. 6.6%), high blood pressure (39.1% vs. 27.8%), smoking (17.6% vs. 15.7%), and obesity (25.7% vs. 20.0%).[10] Inherently, the burden of CKD relates not only to the health-care requirements of patients who progress to ESKD, but also to broader public health through its close association with CVD, which affects 22% of Australian adults.[11] CKD was estimated to cause 2.6% of the total burden of disease and injury in Australia in 2003,

**Table 81.1 Population and Gross Domestic Product (GDP) per Capita of Oceania Countries[176–178]**

| Country | Population (in thousands)[a] | GDP per Capita (US$ per person/ year) | General Government Expenditure on Health as % of Total Government of Expenditure | Life Expectancy at Birth (Years) | Under-Five Mortality Rate (Probability of dying by age 5 per 1000 live births) | Raised Blood Pressure (%)[b] | Obesity (%)[b] | Deaths Attributable to CKD (%) | Years Lost Due to Disability Attributable to CKD (%) | Disability Adjusted Life-Years Attributable to CKD |
|---|---|---|---|---|---|---|---|---|---|---|
| American Samoa (USA) | 57 | 9164 | 14 | 73 | 9.4 | n/a | n/a | n/a | n/a | n/a |
| Australia | 23,470 | 44,820 | 17 | 73 | 4.0 | 21.4 | 26.8 | 2.38 (1.99–3.45) | 2.05 (1.63–2.57) | 1.85 (1.6–2.21) |
| Cook Islands (NZ) | 15 | 19,659 | 14 | 72 | 10.3 | 32.4 | 63.7 | n/a | n/a | n/a |
| Federated States of Micronesia | 103 | 2223 | 20 | 70 | 39.0 | n/a | n/a | n/a | n/a | n/a |
| Fiji | 859 | 6557 | 9 | 68 | 17.9 | 28.9 | 30.6 | 2.97 (2.64–3.92) | 1.07 (0.84–1.38) | 2.42 (2.09–3.16) |
| French Polynesia (France) | 270 | 16,803 | 29 | 75 | 2.2 | n/a | n/a | n/a | n/a | n/a |
| Guam (USA) | 175 | 22,991 | 9 | 79 | 0.7 | n/a | n/a | n/a | n/a | n/a |
| Kiribati | 109 | 1701 | 10 | 75 | 47.3 | 23.6 | 46.0 | 2.97 (1.55–6.43) | 0.92 (0.71–1.19) | 2.24 (1.24–4.53) |
| Marshall Islands | 54 | 2851 | 17 | 72 | 6.0 | 22.8 | 45.4 | 4.28 (1.74–12.16) | 1.01 (0.79–1.31) | 3.12 (1.4–8.12) |
| Nauru | 11 | 5462 | 10 | 61 | 37.0 | 31.1 | 71.1 | n/a | n/a | n/a |
| New Caledonia (France) | 260 | 36,637 | 10 | 77 | 5.0 | n/a | n/a | n/a | N/a | n/a |
| New Zealand | 4242 | 38,399 | 10 | n/a | 6.6 | 21.6 | 28.3 | 2.43 (1.98–3.19) | 2.24 (1.74–2.84) | 2.14 (1.86–2.52) |
| Niue (NZ) | 1 | 21,043 | 18 | 74 | 16.1 | n/a | n/a | n/a | n/a | n/a |
| Northern Mariana Islands (USA) | 56 | 11,719 | 25 | n/a | 8.2 | n/a | n/a | n/a | n/a | n/a |
| Palau | 18 | 8423 | 11 | 64 | 12.2 | 26.6 | 48.9 | n/a | n/a | n/a |
| Pitcairn Islands (UK) | 0.05 | n/a | n/a | n/a | n/a | n/a | n/a | n/a | n/a | n/a |
| Papua New Guinea | 7275 | 2133 | 4 | 62 | 75 | 16.7 | 16.2 | 1.55 (1.05–2.18) | 0.92 (0.7–1.21) | 1.2 (0.82–1.68) |
| Samoa | 188 | 408 | 7 | 74 | 19.4 | 30.6 | 54.1 | 3.66 (1.22–9.81) | 1.18 (0.95–1.47) | 2.63 (1.18–6.09) |
| Solomon Islands | 611 | 1954 | 9 | 67 | 15.5 | 21.2 | 30.0 | 2.09 (1.59–2.98) | 1 (0.78–1.28) | 1.71 (1.28–2.35) |
| Tokelau (NZ) | 1 | 1007 | 10 | n/a | 0.0 | n/a | n/a | n/a | n/a | n/a |
| Tonga | 103 | 7738 | 5 | 71 | 23.0 | 30.0 | 57.6 | 1.69 (0.94–4.03) | 1.11 (0.92–1.4) | 1.27 (0.85–2.57) |
| Tuvalu | 11 | 3348 | 17 | 70 | 10.3 | n/a | n/a | n/a | n/a | n/a |
| Vanuatu | 265 | 295,349 | 4 | 71 | 30.7 | 33.8 | 27.5 | 1.39 (0.93–2.12) | 1 (0.76–1.29) | 1.17 (0.81–1.77) |
| Wallis and Futuna (France) | 12 | 3800 | 24 | 76 | n/a | n/a | n/a | n/a | n/a | n/a |

[a]Data from World Health Organization, Health Information and Intelligence Platform (HIIP). Available from: http://hiip/wpro/who.int/portal/Countryprofiles.aspx. [Accessed December 2016].
[b]Data from World Health Organization, Noncommunicable diseases and mental health. Available from: http://www.who.int/nmh/countries/en/. [Accessed December 2016].
*CKD,* Chronic kidney disease; *n/a,* not available.

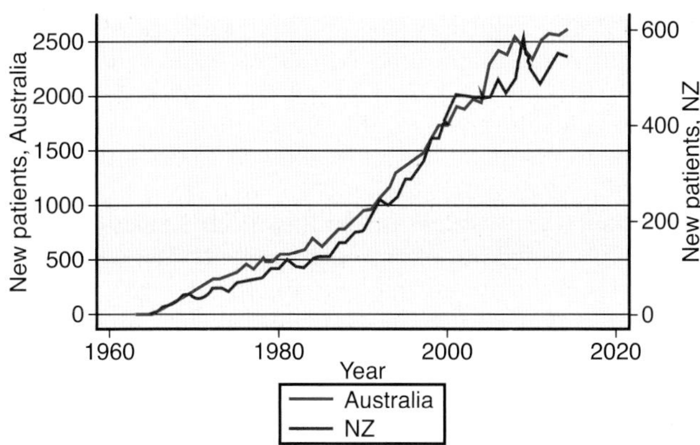


**Fig. 81.2** Number of patients starting renal replacement therapy in Australia and New Zealand (NZ). (From ANZDATA Registry. Chapter 1: Incidence of end-stage kidney disease. In: *38th Report*. Adelaide, Australia; 2015. Available from: http://www.anzdata.org.au. Last accessed December 10, 2018.)

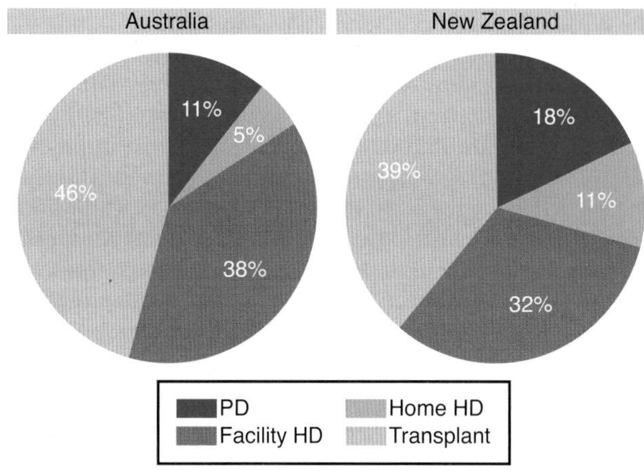


**Fig. 81.3** Overall distribution of renal replacement therapy (RRT) modality in Australia and New Zealand at the end of 2015. *HD,* Hemodialysis; *PD,* peritoneal dialysis. (From ANZDATA Registry. Chapter 2: Prevalence of end-stage kidney disease. In: *39th Report*. Adelaide, Australia; 2016. Available from: http://www.anzdata.org.au. Last accessed December 10, 2018.)

with nearly 95% of this burden attributed to years of life lost due to premature death.[10] Patients with CKD incur 85% higher health-care costs and 50% higher government subsidies than individuals without CKD. In 2012, the total costs attributable solely to predialysis CKD were estimated at $4.1 billion, made up of $2.5 billion in direct health-care costs, $700 million in direct non–health-care costs, and $900 million in government subsidies.[12,13] The cost of treating patients with ESKD with dialysis and transplantation are estimated to cost >$1 billion/year.[13]

## DIALYSIS

According to the Australia and New Zealand Dialysis and Transplant (ANZDATA) Registry, there were 2654 new RRT patients in Australia in 2015 (Fig. 81.2), with an overall incidence rate of 112 per million population (pmp). Although this rate has remained stable for several years, the number of prevalent patients has continued to climb with 23,012 (968 pmp) patients receiving RRT at the end of 2015.[9] This figure contrasts with the large variation in ESKD prevalence across the world, which is highest in Taiwan (3170 pmp), followed by Japan (2620 pmp), and then the United States (2080 pmp). In the 28 countries that form the European Union, it averages to 1090 pmp with the global average of 450 pmp.[14] A large discrepancy in prevalence of ESKD across regions may relate to variation in population characteristics, but also suggests limited access to treatment in many countries.

The mean ages of female and male patients commencing RRT were 55.7 years and 60.9 years, respectively. The most common cause of ESKD amongst incident RRT patients in Australia is diabetes mellitus (37%), followed by glomerulonephritis (18%), hypertension (13%), polycystic kidney disease (6%), reflux nephropathy (2%), and others.[9] In 2015, over half (54%) of ESKD patients received dialysis (Fig. 81.3), which comprised facility hemodialysis (38%), peritoneal dialysis (PD; 11%), and home hemodialysis (5%).[15]

The first dialysis in Australia took place at the Royal Brisbane Hospital on February 10, 1954, under the supervision of Dr. Dique, who developed a dialysis machine consisting of cellophane tubing wound around wooden slats.[16] The number of patients receiving hemodialysis has grown over the years. In 2015, there were a total of 9947 patients who received hemodialysis as their RRT, with 2195 patients who were new to hemodialysis.[17] In Australia, hemodialysis can be accessed in two main settings: facility (88%) or at home (12%).[15] Facility hemodialysis can be accessed either in hospital (also known as in-center) or in a satellite unit, which is often a regional hospital or community-based dialysis unit distant from the tertiary hospital unit. Increases in the growth of satellite units and PD have contributed to a gradual reduction in the proportion of patients undertaking home hemodialysis in Australia (50% of dialysis patients on home hemodialysis in the mid-1970s, to about 10% from the early 2000s).[18] Although it appears to be relatively small compared with the proportion of patients undergoing facility hemodialysis, the prevalence of home hemodialysis in Australia is second in the world after New Zealand (15.6%).[19] There are regional differences in the uptake of home hemodialysis programs in Australia, whereby the numbers are greatest in the state of New South Wales (including Australian Capital Territory, $n = 2700$), followed by Queensland ($n = 284$), Victoria ($n = 214$), and Western Australia ($n = 81$). The numbers of prevalent home hemodialysis in other states were <40 patients.[17] The reasons behind such large disparities remain unclear.[18]

There are also opportunities to help facilitate travel on dialysis across Australia, including prearrangement with the dialysis unit near the travel destination, or participating in programs such as "Big Red Kidney Bus" holiday dialysis program, which provides a mobile dialysis service. The bus travels to popular holiday destinations where it is located for up to 6 weeks at a time, and is staffed by experienced dialysis nurses and renal technicians. This is an initiative of the Kidney Health Australia currently available in two states of Australia (Victoria and New South Wales).[20]

Hemodialysis patients in Australia most frequently undergo treatment ≤3 sessions/week (86%), 5 hours/session (26%).[17]

This equates to a mean treatment duration of 271.57 minutes/session, which is the longest amongst countries (compared with US 217.42 minutes/session) contributing data to the Dialysis Outcomes and Practice Patterns Study (DOPPS).[21] Analysis of the DOPPS data has shown lower mortality risk for patients undergoing longer dialysis treatment duration – hazard ratio for every 30 minutes: all-cause mortality: 0.94 [95% confidence interval (CI): 0.92–0.97], cardiovascular mortality: 0.95 (95% CI: 0.91–0.98), sudden death: 0.93 (95% CI: 0.88–0.98).[22] Over the years, the uptake of hemodiafiltration has increased markedly, now taking up almost 21% of hemodialysis treatment[17] (Fig. 81.4). Using these treatment measures and dialysis prescription, 90.9% of patients achieve a urea reduction ratio ≥65% as a measure of dialysis adequacy. This achievement has been relatively stable over the years.[17]

Most prevalent hemodialysis patients (about 85%) in Australia dialyze via either arteriovenous fistula or graft.[17,23] Disappointingly, however, the majority of incident ESKD patients start hemodialysis with a catheter, which is associated with poorer patient outcomes including increased infection, hospitalization, and mortality rates compared with arteriovenous fistula or graft.[24] The risk was greater in patients who were female, young (age <25 years), and first seen by nephrologists <3 months prior to starting hemodialysis (late referrals).[17] Several clinical networks at a state level (e.g., Victoria and South Australia) have set permanent vascular access at dialysis initiation as one of the measured key performance indicators to increase its rates.[25,26]

Patient survival on hemodialysis has remained relatively unchanged over the last few years, with unadjusted survival rates of 91% (95% CI: 90–92), 71% (95% CI: 70–73), and 54% (95% CI: 52–56) at 1, 3, and 5 years, respectively.[17]

The ongoing costs of caring for a patient with ESKD on dialysis are significant, and are greatest for in-center hemodialysis ($76,881/person per year), followed by satellite hemodialysis ($63,505), PD ($51,640), and home hemodialysis ($47,775).[27] With the growth in the prevalent ESKD population, facility hemodialysis capacity has been saturated, and attention has been drawn to enhancing the capacity of home dialysis, particularly PD, which makes up 68% of all home dialysis patients in Australia. The number of prevalent PD patients has grown over time from 93 pmp in 2011 to 106 pmp in 2015.[28] This rate is lower than Hong Kong (488.5 pmp) but greater than many other developed countries (e.g., Germany 38.8 pmp, UK 74.8 pmp, US 87.1 pmp).[29] PD is an attractive dialysis modality due to its technical simplicity, cost-effectiveness, and ability to allow patients to dialyze at home. The ability to independently dialyze at home in a country such as Australia is highly desirable given its large geographic distribution in which patients may live quite distantly from their renal unit. The majority of patients starting PD are incident patients (74%), with smaller proportions transitioning from hemodialysis (24%) or failed kidney transplant (2%).[28] Automated PD (APD) is the most commonly utilized form of PD (70%), and is higher than average APD utilization amongst developed countries (42.4%, 95% CI: 34.4–50.5).[29] Other notable PD practices include a growing usage of icodextrin (46% in 2015 compared with 37% in 2010) and neutral pH, low glucose degradation product PD solutions (18% in 2015 compared with 4% in 2010).[28,30]

Although patient survival on PD is comparable with hemodialysis [1 year 96% (95% CI: 95%–96%), 3 years 79% (95% CI: 75%-81%), 5 years 63% (95% CI: 60%–65%)], further uptake of PD has been hampered by relatively poor technique survival [3 years 49% (95% CI: 45%–53%)].[28] Technique survival has improved slowly over the years, but remains relatively low, and is driven by infection (22%; e.g., peritonitis) and inadequate dialysis (13%; e.g., inadequate fluid ultrafiltration, solute clearance). In recognition of the high burden from peritonitis, the Australian Peritonitis Registry was set up in October 2003 as part of the ANZDATA Registry. This initiative, in conjunction with augmentation of the existing evidence by conducting investigator-initiated clinical trials, ongoing analysis of the data from the ANZDATA registry, improvement in existing guidelines, development of key performance indicators to meet evidence-based practice, and reinforcement of PD training, has witnessed a significant improvement in PD peritonitis rates[31] (Fig. 81.5). However, there remains a large (sevenfold) variation in peritonitis rates amongst PD units and up to twofold variation between states (Fig. 81.6). Although some of these differences relate to patient-level risk factors (e.g., living distantly from PD unit,[32] indigenous[33]), the majority of the risk has been shown to be associated with modifiable center-level characteristics

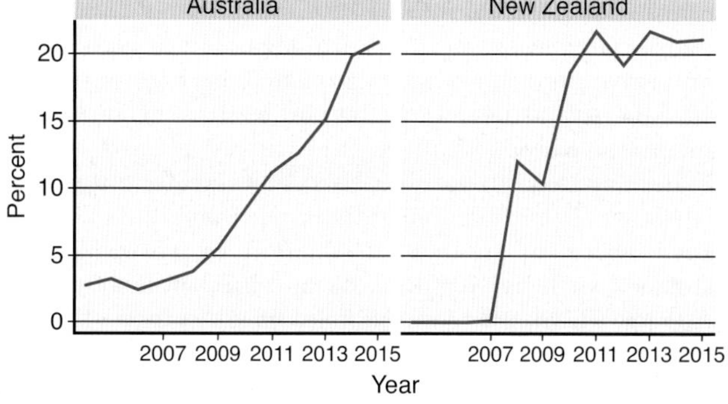


**Fig. 81.4** Proportion of maintenance hemodialysis patients receiving hemodiafiltration in Australia and New Zealand 2006–2015. (From ANZDATA Registry. Chapter 1: Incidence of end-stage kidney disease. In: *39th Report*. Adelaide, Australia; 2016. Available from: http://www.anzdata.org.au. Last accessed December 10, 2018.)

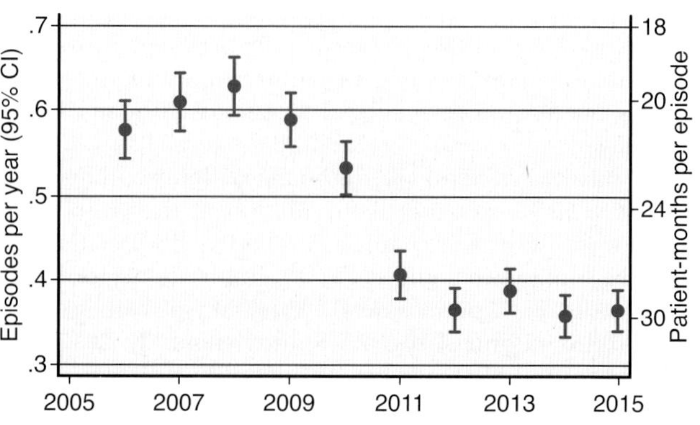


**Fig. 81.5** Peritoneal dialysis (PD) peritonitis rates in Australia. *CI*, Confidence interval 2006–2015. (From ANZDATA Registry. Chapter 5: Peritoneal dialysis. In: *39th Report*. Adelaide, Australia; 2016. Available from: http://www.anzdata.org.au. Last accessed December 10, 2018.)

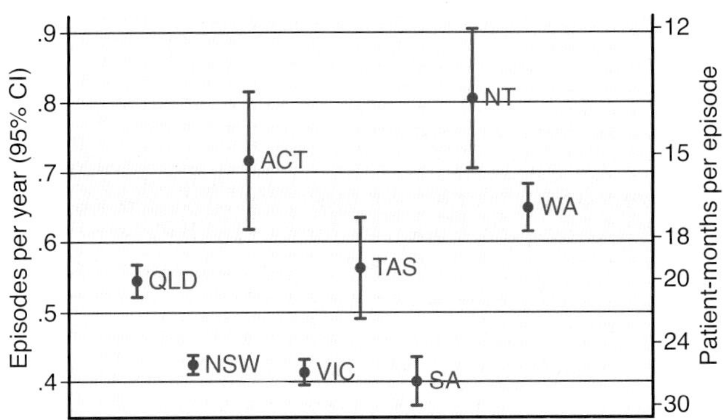


**Fig. 81.6** Peritoneal dialysis (PD) peritonitis rates across states and territories in Australia 2006–2015. *ACT,* Australian Capital Territory; *CI,* confidence interval; *NSW,* New South Wales; *NT,* Northern Territory; *QLD,* Queensland; *SA,* South Australia; *TAS,* Tasmania; *VIC,* Victoria; *WA,* Western Australia. (From ANZDATA Registry. Chapter 5: Peritoneal dialysis. In: *39th Report.* Adelaide, Australia; 2016. Available from: http://www.anzdata.org.au. Last accessed December 10, 2018.)

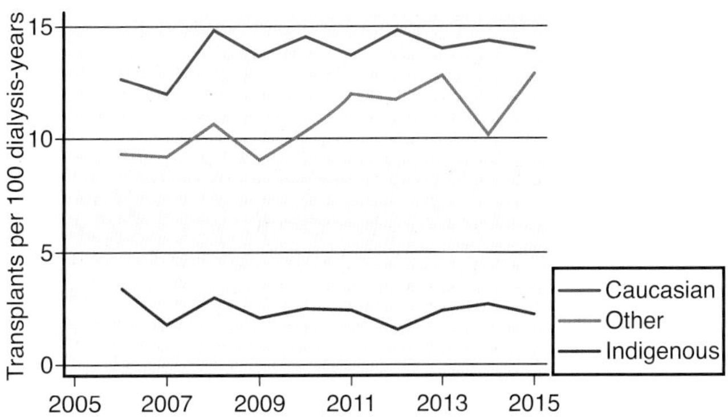


**Fig. 81.7** Transplant rate of dialyzed patients in Australia aged 15–64 years by race from 2006 to 2015. (From ANZDATA Registry. Chapter 8: Transplantation. In: *39th Report.* Adelaide, Australia; 2015. Available from: http://www.anzdata.org.au. Last accessed December 10, 2018.)

(e.g., center size, proportion of PD, peritoneal equilibration test use at PD start).[34]

## KIDNEY TRANSPLANTATION

In 2015, 949 transplants were performed in Australia, which is the highest number ever performed [40 pmp, which is still only about 30% of the rate of incident ESKD patients (112 pmp)[9]].[35] The transplant rate in Australia is higher than the global average (11.08 pmp) and the highest amongst Western Pacific countries (average 5.82 pmp).[36] Approximately 26% of cases were living-donor transplants ($n$ = 242).[35]

The first renal transplant in Australia took place on February 21, 1965, in Adelaide, South Australia. The number of renal transplants has consistently increased since then (2004: 650 patients; 2015: 949 patients), largely from an increase in the rate of deceased-donor renal transplantation in the context of a national reform program "Donate Life" led by the Australian Organ and Tissue Donation and Transplant Authority (AOTDTA) to increase organ donation rate (www.donatelife.gov.au). With the growing burden of CKD and patients with ESKD requiring RRT, there has been a focus on increasing transplant rates as it confers benefits at both patient (e.g., improved survival)[35] and government levels [e.g., cost-effective treatment, estimated cost in the first year $65,375 (deceased-donor renal transplant) to $70,553 (live-donor renal transplant), with ongoing cost from the years thereafter of $10,749/year)].[10] An increase in transplant rate has disproportionately increased in Caucasian patients, while the rate has remained relatively static for indigenous dialysis patients (Fig. 81.7).[35] Similar within-country disparities in transplant rates involving ethnic minorities have been reported previously in Canada[37] and the United States.[38]

Another initiative of the AOTDTA to increase the number of living-donor kidney transplants is the Australian paired kidney exchange program. A paired kidney exchange occurs when a live donor wants to donate to a spouse, friend, or relative but is unable to due to blood or tissue incompatibilities. The program aims to increase living-donor kidney transplants by finding compatible donors among other registered pairs, enabling transplants to occur. The Australian kidney exchange started enrolling donor–recipient pairs in August 2010 and, up until December 2015, 154 people had received a transplant through the program.[39]

An increased rate of kidney transplantation has translated into a growth in the prevalence of patients with functioning grafts to 10,551 patients (444 pmp) in 2015 compared with 6981 patients (341 pmp) in 2005.[35] Similar to dialysis data, there is a variation in prevalence of transplant patients across states ranging from 385 pmp (Western Australia) to 571 pmp (South Australia/Northern Territory). The proportion of patients receiving living-donor grafts was greatest in the younger age group (5–14-year-old group: 66% living donor; 34% deceased donor). For the first time for recipients of kidney transplants in Australia the 1-year graft survival rate was excellent, especially for living-donor kidney transplantation recipients (98% vs. 94% in deceased-donor recipient).[35] The 5-year survival rates for primary transplants performed during 2000 to 2004 were around 87.7% for living-donor transplants and 80.9% for deceased-donor transplants.[27] By 2010–2014, these rates had slightly improved to 89% and 83%, respectively.[35] Although the long-term outcomes (i.e., >10-year graft survival) have also improved gradually, the trend has been less evident compared with short-term outcomes.[35,40] These results similarly mirror data from the United States[41] and the United Kingdom.[42]

According to the ANZDATA Registry, the most common cause of graft loss during the years 2011–2015 was death with a functioning graft ($n$ = 1049, 46%), followed by chronic allograft nephropathy ($n$ = 832, 37%). The most common cause of death was cancer ($n$ = 309, 29%), followed by CVD ($n$ = 268, accounting for 26% of deaths).[35] In contrast to a decreasing trend in cardiovascular deaths over the last 20 years from 1.8 deaths/100 patient-years in the mid-1980s to 0.9 deaths/100 patient-years in the mid-2000s, deaths from cancer have progressively increased, which is now the most common cause of death in renal transplant recipients.[43] This result is not surprising as recipients of solid organ transplants have been reported to experience cancer rates similar to nontransplant people 20–30 years older.[44] Reasons for the increased risk of cancer posttransplant have been attributed to several factors, including exposure to new and previously acquired viral infections and ongoing exposure to immunosuppression.[44] Although the patient survival rates are superior after transplant compared with remaining on dialysis, the risk of death remains significantly greater than in the general population by up to tenfold.[40]

## NONDIALYSIS SUPPORTIVE CARE FOR ESKD

As aforementioned, the number of ESKD patients is growing in Australia. It is, however, important to note that the growth in the past decade has been the greatest amongst those who are elderly with multiple comorbidities.[45,46] This change has led to an increase in the age of prevalent ESKD patients receiving RRT in Australia, with patients over the age of 65 years making up 39% of the total RRT population.[15] However, the exact number and characteristics of patients who choose not to dialyze when they reach ESKD is unknown, as the ANZDATA registry does not capture information on patients not receiving RRT. The Patient Information about Options for Treatment (PIVOT) study observed that 14% of incident stage V CKD patients chose a nondialysis pathway[47]; however, this is likely to be an underestimate of true disease burden, as it did not account for patients who were never referred to nephrology services in the first instance. Although incompletely understood, it has been suggested that for every patient who dies while receiving RRT, there is another patient who has died without accessing RRT.[10,48]

## ACUTE KIDNEY INJURY

Acute kidney injury (AKI) is a condition where an abrupt loss of kidney function occurs to a point where the body accumulates waste products and becomes unable to maintain electrolyte, acid–base, and water balance. Although it has a broad range of causes, it is most commonly diagnosed in general hospitalized patients in developed countries such as Australia (e.g., critically ill patients admitted to intensive care units in the context of sepsis, or following exposure to radiographic contrast agents). Another cause of AKI relatively unique to Australia includes snakebite caused by hemotoxic or myotoxic snakes, such as brown snakes, which account for over half of all hospitalized snakebites in Australia.[49–51] There have been reports of thrombotic microangiopathy-like presentations following brown snakebites with resultant severe AKI requiring temporary treatment with hemodialysis and plasma exchange.[49]

Although CKD is a risk factor for AKI,[52] AKI is also recognized to be an independent risk factor for CKD.[53] In Australia, hospitalizations due to AKI have more than doubled between 2000–2001 and 2012–2013 (from 8050 to 18,010), representing an increase of 6%/year.[54] Even though the deaths due to AKI have remained relatively similar over the past decade (an average of 4670 deaths/year between 2000 and 2012), the average length of stay in AKI hospitalizations was about twice as long as the average length of stay for hospitalizations overall (11.4 days vs. 5.6 days).[54] People living in remote areas, in socioeconomically disadvantaged areas, and with Aboriginal and Torres Strait Islander status were associated with higher rates of hospitalizations and mortality.[54]

## INDIGENOUS AUSTRALIANS

Disparity in the risk of renal disease and poorer outcomes are uniformly seen across all phases of disease and treatment in indigenous Australians.[55] For instance, even though indigenous Australians make up only 3% of the total Australian population, almost 11% of new cases of treated ESKD in 2015 were indigenous Australians. The growth in the number of ESKD patients from 2011 to 2015 was almost threefold when compared with nonindigenous Australians (25.7% vs. 8.7%).[55] The hospitalization rate for regular dialysis treatment in indigenous Australians was 11 times as high as for other Australians,[55] which reflects a higher proportion of patients receiving facility hemodialysis (12.7% vs. 51.0%).[56] By contrast, the proportion of prevalent indigenous Australian patients with functioning transplants was only about 2% of all Australian patients (241 patients vs. 10,310 patients).[35] Within indigenous Australians, the risk of CKD-related hospitalizations not involving dialysis was significantly higher in those living in remote and very remote areas (hospitalization rate ratio for indigenous vs. nonindigenous Australians: major city: 2.9; inner regional: 3.8; outer regional: 6.9; remote/very remote: 12.8).[56] Previous studies have shown that remoteness of residence is associated with pervasive socioeconomic disadvantage, including poverty, poor nutrition and food insecurity, poor housing, unemployment, and impaired access to services of all kinds.[57] Furthermore, indigenous Australians were almost four times as likely to die with CKD as a cause of death than nonindigenous Australians.[55]

AKI is also significantly more common in indigenous Australians, with hospitalization rates almost three times higher than those of nonindigenous Australians (males 158 vs. 71 per 100,000 population, respectively; females 229 vs. 70 per 100,000 population).[54] Similarly, AKI death rates are 1.8 times higher in indigenous Australians (35 vs. 19 per 100,000 population) and are considerably higher in indigenous females than indigenous males (2.1-fold vs. 1.6-fold higher than nonindigenous males and females, respectively).[54] As with CKD, there is a complex interaction between indigenous status, remoteness, and socioeconomic status that impacts upon AKI occurrence and outcome in Australia.

## ETHNIC INEQUITIES

The burden of kidney disease (AKI, CKD, and ESKD) in indigenous Australians is disproportionately greater compared with that in nonindigenous Australians[55] and affects these patients at an earlier age. For instance, of all the patients who commenced RRT for treatment of ESKD in Australia between the years 2010 and 2014, 59% of indigenous patients were aged less than 55 years, compared with 31% of nonindigenous patients.[58] Although the most common cause of ESKD in Australia is diabetic nephropathy for both groups, the proportion of indigenous patients with diabetic nephropathy is more than double that of nonindigenous patients (70% vs. 33%).[59] Differences in the causes of CKD and AKI across these two groups are more challenging to describe in detail as data are not as readily available due to a lack of established CKD and AKI registries (the ANZDATA only includes ESKD patients[54,58] who received dialysis or kidney transplantation). The reasons for ethnic inequality in the burden of kidney disease amongst indigenous Australians have been attributed to higher levels of socioeconomic disadvantage,[60,61] residence in "remote" and "very remote" areas of Australia,[54] and a high burden of chronic diseases, such as diabetes mellitus which is an important cause of kidney disease.[58] There are also many other contributory factors, including poorer nutrition, higher tobacco use and alcohol consumption, and lower levels of education attainment, employment, social support, and housing.[58] Moreover, there is a greater proportion of indigenous patients who reside in remote and very remote areas of Australia where access to and use of health services are more challenging.[58] In recognition of a significant deficit in health outcomes of indigenous patients in Australia, on December 20, 2007, the Council of Australian Governments agreed to work with indigenous communities to achieve the target of "closing the gap" on indigenous disadvantage. The Closing the Gap campaign aims to address not only gaps in the areas of health, but also in education and employment. One of the three main health goals includes targeting main components of the life expectancy gap and chronic diseases, such as CKD and diabetes mellitus. Some of the listed targets to improve outcomes in this area include attainment of blood pressure targets in patients with type 2 diabetes mellitus, and stabilization of all-cause incidence of ESKD within 5–10 years.[62] In order to help support access to appropriate medications, indigenous patients with chronic diseases or at risk of developing chronic diseases, such as CKD, are eligible to access the Closing the Gap Pharmaceutical Benefits Scheme co-payment measure to help access most prescription medications at a lower price or free of charge, depending on eligibility criteria (http://www.humanservices.gov.au/). Following implementation of the scheme, improvements in health-care access and a declining trend in indigenous mortality rate from chronic diseases have been observed.[63]

## DOMAINS OF KIDNEY DISEASE CARE IN AUSTRALIA

### HEALTH FINANCE

Australia's health-care system is complex with a multifaceted network of public and private providers. Medical providers deliver a plethora of services across many levels, from public health and preventive services in the community, to primary health care, emergency health services, hospital-based treatment, and palliative care. For most Australians, their first contact with the health system is a visit to a general practitioner (GP) who may identify risk factors or features of renal impairment through clinical assessment. The GP may then refer them to a specialist based in private practice or a public hospital based on clinical findings.

Public sector health services are funded by the state, territory, and Australian governments, but managed by state and territory governments. By contrast, private hospitals are owned and operated by the private sector. Patients who are cared for in public hospitals (e.g., for AKI and CKD) are able to access all investigations and treatments for free if they are eligible for Medicare. Medicare is a scheme administered by the federal government that provides a range of medical services; lower cost prescriptions and free care as a public patient in a public hospital. All eligible Australian residents and certain categories of visitors to Australia can enroll in Medicare and access these services. The Department of Health is responsible for developing Medicare policy, and the fund is partly contributed to by Australian taxpayers, who pay a Medicare levy of 2% of their taxable income (with exceptions for low-income earners), with the balance being provided by government from general revenue. An additional levy of 1% is imposed on high-income earners without private health insurance policies. If patients are treated as a private patient in public or private hospitals, Medicare will cover 75% of the Medicare schedule fee for services and procedures, such as dialysis. However, Medicare will not cover hospital accommodation, or fees such as theater costs. If patients are insured privately through a private health insurance provider, part or all of these costs may be subsidized through the insurance policy in place, including RRT.

### ESSENTIAL MEDICATIONS AND TECHNOLOGY ACCESS

As well as Medicare, Australia has a separate Pharmaceutical Benefits Scheme (PBS; www.pbs.gov.au), also funded by the federal government, which subsidizes a range of prescription medications. These two schemes jointly facilitate delivery of universal health-care system in Australia. Eligible indigenous patients who are living with, or at risk of, chronic disease, such as CKD, are able to additionally benefit from the Closing the Gap PBS Co-payment measure which improves access to medicines by further lowering or forgoing patient co-payment for PBS-subsidized medicines. Nonetheless, being a large country with the vast majority of large cities located along the coast where major health facilities reside, there is a significant proportion of the population living in regional areas with limited access to medical services, such as general practitioners (GPs), nephrologists, and renal replacement therapies (RRT), including dialysis and transplantation. According to the ANZDATA Registry, 5.9% of incident PD patients ($n$ = 749) were living in remote and very remote regions, as defined by Accessibility and Remoteness Index of Australia (E. See, personal communication). In recognition of the great need for medical workforce in rural and regional Australia, the Australian government has introduced several initiatives to date, including the Australian General Practice Training Program with rural training pathway, Bonded Medical Places Scheme (i.e., a percentage of all first-year Commonwealth Supported Places in Australian medical schools are allocated to the scheme where successful applicants commit to working in a district of workforce shortage during their return of service period) and 5-Year Overseas Trained Doctor Scheme (which allows a reduction in the 10-year moratorium for overseas-trained doctors by encouraging them to work in remote or difficult-to-recruit locations).[64] These schemes, however, do not address limited access to specialist care or access to RRT closer to home. Patients living remotely,[33] and further from their dialysis providers,[32] have been shown to experience worse outcomes than others with easier access to specialist care. Moreover, if patients require facility hemodialysis treatment, they need to relocate closer to their dialysis unit if the distance is not feasible to travel thrice weekly, which results in significant social dislocation and disruption (see the *Dialysis Unit Guide* by Kidney Health Australia, www.kidney.org.au/your-kidneys/support/dialysis/dialysis-unit-guide).

### DETECTION AND MONITORING OF KIDNEY DISEASE

One of the main predictors of poor patient outcomes in those with ESKD has included late referral, defined as less than 3 months between referral and RRT commencement.[9] Although there are cases where prevention or early recognition may not be possible, the majority of CKD cases should have been able to be recognized in primary care and reviewed by a nephrologist prior to imminently requiring RRT. In appreciation of the importance of early recognition of CKD, several initiatives have been developed and evolved over the years in Australia. These have focused on empowering health-care providers to recognize risk factors for CKD to trigger screening, optimally manage risk factors to retard progression of disease, and know when a specialist referral is indicated.

An Australasian Creatinine Consensus Working Group developed recommendations to commence automatic reporting of an eGFR from each serum creatinine measurement performed in pathology laboratories.[65] This was to increase the likelihood of early detection of CKD and indeed witnessed a significant growth in the number of patients diagnosed with CKD since its implementation.[66] There have also been studies to help guide how and who to screen for CKD, such as a pilot program Kidney Evaluation for You.[67] The aim of this study was to establish community-based screening protocols by targeting people identified to be at an increased risk of CKD (i.e., those with diabetes mellitus, hypertension, a first-degree relative with kidney disease, or age >50 years), and to assess efficacy in promoting changes in risk-factor management and to understand the CKD awareness amongst participants. Of 402 high-risk individuals recruited, 20.4% of participants exhibited features of CKD with a large proportion having risk factors for CKD including hypertension (69%), diabetes (30%), and dyslipidemia (40%). Outcomes from such projects have led to recommendations such as the "Kidney Health Check" through Kidney Health Australia, whereby patients with diabetes, hypertension, or other established CKD risk factors are recommended to undergo three tests every year (i.e., blood test to check eGFR, urine test to evaluate for proteinuria or hematuria, and blood pressure measurement).[68]

There has also been a huge focus on augmenting resources and support for GPs who are often the first health-care providers to manage patients with CKD in the community. For example, the Primary Care Education Advisory Committee for Kidney Health Australia formed by nephrologists, GPs, primary health nurses, educators, and government representatives provides free accredited education to GPs to increase their awareness and implementation of best practice detection and management of CKD (www.kcat.org.au). These education sessions are delivered through various platforms, including interactive face-to-face workshops, active learning modules, online learning, and conference sessions.[69] Other strategies to improve quality of care delivery in primary care settings include development of customized software programs to integrate with primary care electronic health-care records to allow real-time promotion of detection and management of CKD according to best practice recommendations (eMAP:CKD),[70] provision of decision support tools for health-care providers (Health Tracker, George Institute),[71] and development of quality improvement programs through the Australian Primary Care Collaborative (http://apcc.org.au).

Although clear guidelines exist on indications for referral to a nephrologist in Australia (e.g., eGFR <30 mL/min/1.73 $m^2$),[72] some remote living patients are unable to be reviewed easily by nephrologists. In areas where telehealth facilities are available, nephrologists from the nearest renal units have managed selected patients with CKD via telehealth with local nursing support and coordination.[73] These practices have received additional funding support from the Commonwealth Department of Health by reimbursements for telehealth services under the Medical Benefit Scheme. Supporting patients and health-care providers through telehealth has been extended to cover patients receiving RRT in Australia, including those undergoing home dialysis. For example, several renal units have developed phone apps to provide ongoing support, communication, and monitoring for home hemodialysis patients.[74] Renal transplant units may also elect to provide regular telehealth transplant clinic support to regional centers to help improve management of patients and provide support to their clinicians.

## HEALTH WORKFORCE

In 2005, the Australian and New Zealand Society of Nephrology (ANZSN) reported 171 full-time–equivalent adult nephrologists (136 full time and 82 part-time) in clinical practice.[75] This equated to 8.6 pmp (or 1 nephrologist for every 116,000 residents) or 1 nephrologist for every 79.5 patients with ESKD.[75] Subsequently, the Australian Nephrology Workforce Survey completed in 2007 identified several factors that could influence the size of the nephrology workforce in future years, including a desire of young nephrologists to retire early, a large proportion of nephrologists who are greater than 55 years of age, and workload and clinical demands that were perceived to exceed personal capacity.[76] Based on these findings, several recommendations were made, including the need to improve recruitment strategies, and to have greater emphasis on regular workforce and workload predictions. Since the release of the report, there has been more than a twofold increase in the number of nephrology training positions in Australia (106 positions in 2014 compared with 56 in 2008). In fact, the projection has overshot the number of nephrologists required to an extent that by year 2018, there will be 94 excess nephrologists (Dialysis Nephrology & Transplant Workshop, Launceston, Tasmania, March 2015).

## HEALTH INFORMATION SYSTEMS AND STATISTICS

Information on patients with ESKD receiving RRT is well described through the ANZDATA registry, which collects a wide range of statistics relating to the outcomes of treatment of those with ESKD from all renal units in Australia and New Zealand (www.anzdata.org.au). Its main results are published annually in the form of a report, with interim analyses and publications that occur throughout the year as conference papers or research projects designed to answer specific questions. The data relating to CKD are also collected through the Australian Institute of Health and Welfare (AIHW) through the National Centre for Monitoring Vascular Diseases (www.aihw.gov.au), and Australian Health Survey from the Australian Bureau of Statistics (http://www.abs.gov.au/australianhealthsurvey). The AIHW has also started providing information on AKI burden in Australia, and their official first report was published in 2015.[54] In order to further enhance understanding in disease and outcomes, several newer registries have been developed over the past decade, including statewide collaborative multidisciplinary research and practice programs in various states across Australia, such as CKD.QLD (Chronic Kidney Disease in Queensland, www.ckdqld.org), the Registry of Kidney Diseases (Victoria; http://rokd.org.au), and for specific disease groups, such as for glomerulonephritis (QLD. GN Registry). One of the main criticisms of these existing health information systems has been an unduly long lag period between an event and its being reported. As the health system increases uptake of technology, including adoption of digital hospitals, the data are increasingly likely to be captured and reported in real-time to more efficiently assist planning.

### STRATEGIES AND POLICY FRAMEWORKS

Data collected from health information systems help formulate guidelines and direct strategies and policies to improve patient care. In Australia, one of the most well-recognized national guidelines is the Kidney Health Australia – Caring for Australasians with Renal Impairment (KHA-CARI; www.cari.org.au), which lists a broad range of recommendations on caring for predialysis, dialysis, and transplant patients. To ensure the appropriate usage of KHA-CARI guidelines in clinical practice, the group has also launched several implementation projects, in areas such as iron therapy, hemodialysis vascular access, and prevention of infection in PD patients. Kidney Health Australia has been an active advocate to initiate other national policies including the national renal action plan to reduce Australia's kidney disease burden,[77] and is one of the four members of the National Vascular Disease Prevention Alliance committed to reduce the burden of CVD in Australia. The Australian Government also recognizes the growing burden of CKD and has listed it as one of the chronic conditions in the National Strategic Framework for Chronic Conditions, which aims to reduce the impact of chronic conditions in Australia.[78] At a national level, various working groups have published seminal position statement papers to direct clinical practice, such as the Australasian Creatinine and eGFR Consensus,[65] Australasian Proteinuria Consensus,[79] and Home Dialysis Favored Position.[80] Within each state of Australia, there also exist separate statewide renal networks to inform more relevant practice at a local level.

### CAPACITY FOR RESEARCH AND DEVELOPMENT

Australia is a major contributor to research and development amongst countries in Oceania. In order to further strengthen its capacity, a collaborative research program, the Better Evidence and Translation – Chronic Kidney Disease (www.beatckd.org), funded by a National Health and Medical Research Council Program Grant was initiated, which aims to improve the lives of CKD patients by generating high-quality research evidence to inform health-care decisions. The program supports four existing national research and translation platforms, including the ANZDATA Registry, KHA-CARI guidelines, Cochrane Kidney and Transplant Group, and the Australasian Kidney Trials Network (AKTN). Cochrane Kidney and Transplant was initially established in 1997 and the editorial base moved to Sydney, Australia, in 2000. It forms one of 53 Cochrane Review Groups that constitute the Cochrane Collaboration, which is an independent organization dedicated to providing up-to-date, accurate information about the effects of health care. The AKTN is also a not-for-profit collaborative research group that designs, conducts, and supports investigator-initiated clinical trials with the aim of improving life for people living with CKD (www.aktn.org.au).[81] Since its inception in 2004 and endorsement by ANZSN and KHA, the AKTN has successfully completed eight trials with ongoing growth in productivity. More recently, there has been a growing focus on priorities from all involved in caring for patients with CKD, including patients, caregivers, clinicians, researchers, policy makers, and other stakeholders. This has led to the Standardised Outcomes in Nephrology (SONG) initiative, which aims to establish a set of core outcomes and outcome measures across the spectrum of kidney disease for trials and other forms of research (www.songinitiative.org). Currently, core outcomes for hemodialysis (SONG-HD),[82–84] transplantation (SONG-Tx), PD (SONG-PD), children and adolescents (SONG-Kids),[85] and polycystic kidney disease (SONG-PKD) are being developed.

## NEW ZEALAND

Aotearoa/New Zealand is situated 2000 km southeast of Australia. Comprising two large islands and several smaller islands, New Zealand was first settled following migration across the Pacific Ocean in the late 13th century by Māori, the indigenous population. Māori settled throughout Aotearoa, living within iwi (tribes), hapū (subtribes), and whānau (extended families). Abel Tasman was the first European explorer known to have reached New Zealand in 1642. Progressive settlement by European settlers occurred in the 18th century for whaling and sealing. Progressive colonization in the 19th century by the British Crown resulted in the signing of the Treaty of Waitangi in 1840 between the Crown and iwi. Following World War II, extensive migration to New Zealand by people in the Pacific occurred. Currently, of the 4.6 million people living in New Zealand, 3.3 million (71%) identify as New Zealand European, 692,000 (15%) as Māori, 344,000 (7%) as Pacific people, and 541,000 (12%) as Asian.[86]

### ACCESS TO HEALTH CARE

The New Zealand health-care system is predominantly publicly funded by taxes. Twenty District Health Boards (DHBs) are responsible for funding health-care services to their catchment population within a geographical region, providing acute care services, and promoting the health of the population. All public hospital and specialist outpatient services within the public system are free, while attendance in primary care incurs some payment, based on income. Prescriptions provided by hospitals for inpatients and outpatient care in a hospital setting are fully subsidized by the government. RRT (dialysis or kidney transplantation) is provided nearly entirely within the public health-care system. Renal specialists provide dialysis and transplantation care through hospital-based remuneration and are not incentivized to provide specific dialysis treatment modalities. Citizens or permanent residents of New Zealand and dependencies (Niue, the Cook Islands, and Tokelau) receive treatment for ESKD within the tax-funded public health system in New Zealand.

### BURDEN OF CHRONIC KIDNEY DISEASE

In Aotearoa/New Zealand, the proportion of the population who have CKD is unknown, as census or systematic observational data have not been reported. Based on 2011–2012 Australian data showing albuminuria present in 7.7% of people aged 18 years or older and 3.6% with an eGFR < 60 mL/min/1.73 $m^2$,[87] it can be estimated that 361,300 New Zealand adults may have indicators of CKD. The frequency of albuminuria is approximately twofold to fivefold lower for New Zealand European than for Māori and Pacific adults with[88] and without[89] diabetes.

Approximately 500 New Zealand patients (including 20 children and adolescents) commence dialysis for treatment of ESKD each year and 150 receive a kidney transplant, while 472 patients are actively on the waiting list for kidney transplantation.[90] The incidence of RRT in New Zealand increased threefold from 30 pmp in 1986 to 120 pmp in 2001; the incidence has largely plateaued in the last 15 years, with currently 4500 patients receiving treatment. There is considerable regional variation in the incidence of treated ESKD across the country with higher rates in Northern regions, excluding higher-income areas of Auckland.

Diabetes is the most frequent cause of treated ESKD in Aotearoa/New Zealand, with 54% of patients treated with dialysis and 22% of kidney transplant recipients having a diagnosis of diabetes. This proportion is increasing by about 1% each year in the dialysis population and 0.5% each year in the kidney transplant setting. Risk factors for CKD frequently coexist including socioeconomic deprivation, obesity, dyslipidemia, and hypertension.

The burden of disease in New Zealand has become decoupled from disease frequency, reflecting the predominant impact of multiple long-term conditions (multimorbidity) on health burden rather than the presence of individual conditions such as diabetes. About one-third of health lost by New Zealanders is caused by known risk factors for long-term conditions including CKD; high blood pressure accounts for 8.3% of disability-adjusted life years, while low physical activity accounts for 3% of health loss, dietary risks for 9.4%, high body mass index (BMI) for 9.2%, and glucose intolerance for 5.7%. CKD accounts for approximately 2.1% of health loss in New Zealand, ranking 16 in the top 20 leading major specific conditions contributing to health loss for both men and women. CKD is a key outcome from the burden of high BMI, mediated in part through type 2 diabetes.[91]

The annual health expenditure in Aotearoa/New Zealand has risen on average 5.1% compared with annual population growth of 1.3% between 1990 and 2010. The total health expenditure was NZ$19.9 billion in 2009/2010, and in 2016 accounted for 9.2% of real GDP, similar to many peer nations in the Organization for Economic Co-operation and Development (OECD).[92,93] The estimated health costs attributable to CKD in New Zealand have not been specifically reported. Previous studies have estimated the direct costs of diabetes in New Zealand to account for NZ$0.6 billion with an additional indirect cost estimate of NZ$0.6 billion, accounting for 6% of the annual health expenditure.[94] The provision of dialysis is estimated to cost 1% of New Zealand's health expenditure.[95]

## INEQUITY BASED ON ETHNICITY

The incidence of treated ESKD in New Zealand is not equitable, with an incidence of 62 pmp for New Zealand European patients, compared with incidences of 216 pmp for Māori and 272 pmp for Pacific patients, giving a 3.5-fold difference in the incidence of treated ESKD. There is considerable regional variation in the incidence of treated ESKD across the country with higher rates in Northern regions, excluding higher-income areas of Auckland. Notably, the age of onset for diabetes diagnosis is 10 years younger among non-European ethnicities in New Zealand, in parallel with the premature onset of treated ESKD at younger age groups for Māori and Pacific patients.

The incidence of dialysis in New Zealand varies over fourfold by ethnicity, with an incidence of 62 pmp for New Zealand European patients, 76 pmp for those identifying as Asian, 216 pmp for Māori, and 272 for Pacific patients. The most common cause of treated ESKD for incident patients in New Zealand is diabetes (39%), followed by glomerulonephritis (17%), hypertension (11%), polycystic kidney disease (5%), and reflux nephropathy (2%).

There is marked inequity in kidney transplantation rates in New Zealand based on ethnicity. Despite an age-standardized risk of ESKD for Māori and Pacific patients, approximately 2 to 10 times that for New Zealand European patients, the rate of kidney transplantation is markedly lower. In 2015, 28 Māori patients received a kidney transplant (38 pmp) while 21 Pacific patients received a kidney transplant (54 pmp), compared with dialysis incidences of 216 pmp and 272 pmp for those populations, respectively. In addition, recent increases in preemptive kidney transplantation appear to be favoring New Zealand European patients. This phenomenon of increased disparity in transplantation rates during periods of improved access through better service delivery has been similarly observed in Australia, Canada, and the United States (Fig. 81.8). In addition, there is considerable variation between

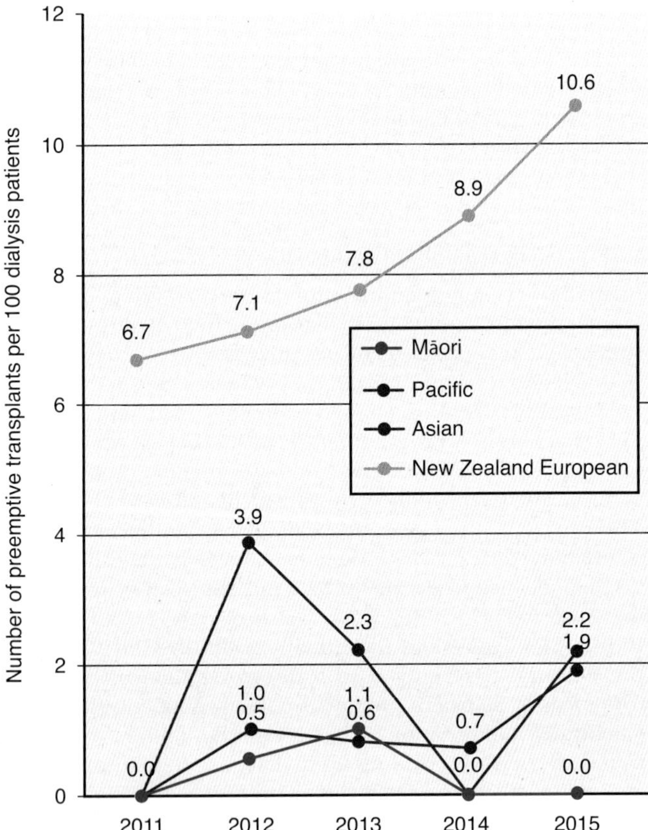


**Fig. 81.8** Preemptive kidney transplantation rates in New Zealand by ethnicity, 2011–2015. (From Ministry of Health National Renal Advisory Board. *New Zealand Nephrology Activity Report 2015*. Wellington, New Zealand: Ministry of Health; 2015. Available from: http://www.health.govt.nz/about-ministry/leadership-ministry/expert-groups/national-renal-advisory-board/papers-and-reports. Last accessed December 10, 2018.)

New Zealand renal centers in the rate of transplantation, varying between 9 pmp and 46 pmp in 2015.

## DIALYSIS

The population with treated ESKD in Australia and New Zealand has been documented and described within the ANZDATA registry since 1978 (www.anzdata.org.au). Based on the ANZDATA registry, 508 adults and 19 children and young adults started RRT in New Zealand in 2015, with 503 starting dialysis, comprising an incidence rate of 115 pmp (Fig. 81.9).[9,96] The incidence of treated ESKD in New Zealand is similar to that of neighboring Australia (111 pmp in 2015) and has remained relatively unchanged over the last 15 years. The incidence of dialysis varies markedly by DHB catchment area with the highest rate for counties Manukau (including South Auckland; 611 pmp) and Waikato (496 pmp) and the lowest for Southern (45 pmp) and Canterbury (78 pmp) regions, with differences between regions related in part to ethnicity and socioeconomic opportunity.

Overall, 2674 people were treated with dialysis in New Zealand in 2015, accounting for a prevalence of 582 pmp. Together with kidney transplantation (369 pmp), the overall prevalence of RRT for Aotearoa/New Zealand in 2015 was 950 pmp, which is nearly identical to neighboring Australia (947 pmp), and comparable with the average of the nation states of the European Union (1090 pmp).

Older age groups have the highest incidence of RRT [311 pmp for the 65- to 74-year-old age group and 260 pmp for the 75- to 84-year-old age group (compared with 77 pmp for the 25- to 44-year-old age group)]. Children and young adults (0 to 25 years old) experienced an incidence of 13 pmp. The proportion of adults older than 85 years of age starting dialysis has fallen over time; zero patients over 85 years commenced dialysis in 2015.

The first RRT occurred in New Zealand in Wellington Hospital in 1954, performed by Dr. Neil Turnball and Dr. Dave Reid, in which PD was carried out.[97] The first hemodialysis was also performed in Wellington in 1958 by Dr. Verney Cable using a Kolff dialysis machine. The first home dialysis was done in 1968 in Auckland and the first home dialysis training program was established in Christchurch under the leadership of Dr. Peter Little.[98]

Overall, most prevalent patients with treated ESKD in New Zealand are treated with dialysis (61.2%; Fig. 81.9). New Zealand has the highest global rate of home-based dialysis therapy, although this is falling due to falling rates of PD (Fig. 81.10). In 2015, 18.0% of patients treated with dialysis in New Zealand did home hemodialysis, 29.6% did PD, and 52.5% received hospital hemodialysis.

In New Zealand, hemodialysis is accessed in three principal settings: facility (hospital or satellite), community house, or home.[99] Community house hemodialysis involves patients performing their hemodialysis independently without direct nursing or medical supervision in an unstaffed nonmedical community homelike setting, and is used in two DHB regions (Counties Manukau and Hawke's Bay), serving approximately 650,000 people. In a 10-year analysis between 2000 and 2010, 113 patients commenced dialysis in a community house setting.

New Zealand has the highest rate of home hemodialysis in the world (18.0%), which is similar to the rate in Australia (15.6%). The rate of home hemodialysis in New Zealand appears to have been stable over the last decade, despite a progressively more dependent dialysis population with increasing medical comorbidity. The principal secular change in dialysis modalities in New Zealand has been reducing utilization of PD (falling from 38.3% to 29.6% over 10 years) in favor of center-based hemodialysis (increasing from 45.4% to 52.5%; see Fig. 81.10). There is marked regional variation in home hemodialysis uptake, ranging from 12% of all dialysis patients treated at Capital and Coast District Health Board to 58% at the Southern District Health Board. Regional variation is likely related to policy (two DHBs, Canterbury and Southern, maintain a universal home dialysis program), remoteness, comorbidity, and socioeconomic factors. Home-based hemodialysis among children is rare.

As with modality practices, the hemodialysis prescription varies across regions related to the uptake and utilization of home-based therapy. The majority of New Zealand hemodialysis

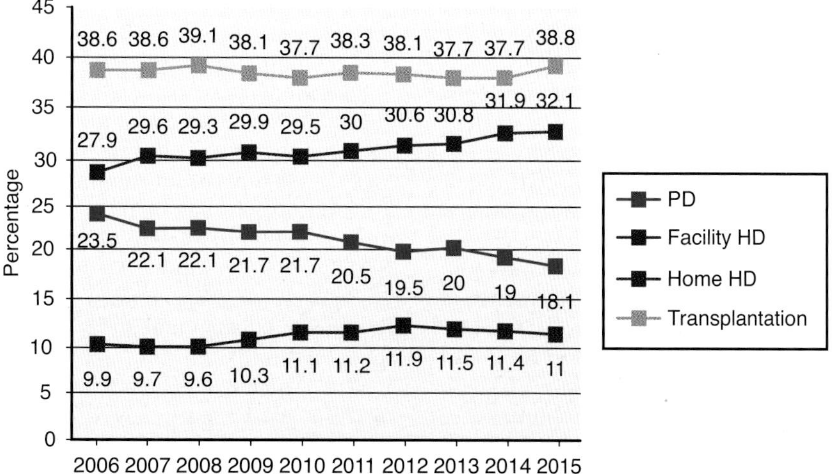


**Fig. 81.9** Prevalence of renal replacement therapy modality in New Zealand 2006–2015. (From Ministry of Health National Renal Advisory Board. *New Zealand Nephrology Activity Report 2015*. Wellington, New Zealand: Ministry of Health; 2015. Available from: http://www.health.govt.nz/about-ministry/leadership-ministry/expert-groups/national-renal-advisory-board/papers-and-reports. Last accessed December 10, 2018.)

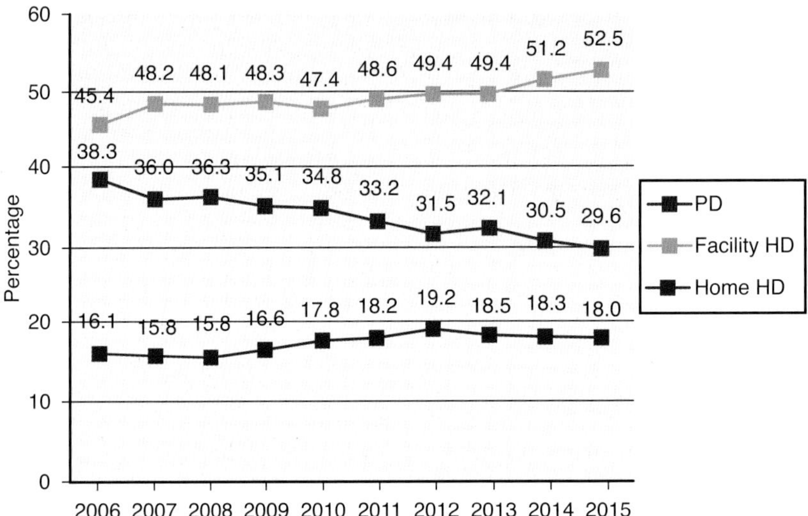


**Fig. 81.10** Prevalence of dialysis modality in New Zealand 2006–2015. *HD,* Hemodialysis; *PD,* peritoneal dialysis. (From Ministry of Health National Renal Advisory Board. *New Zealand Nephrology Activity Report 2015*. Wellington, New Zealand: Ministry of Health; 2015. Available from: http://www.health.govt.nz/about-ministry/leadership-ministry/expert-groups/national-renal-advisory-board/papers-and-reports. Last accessed December 10, 2018.)

patients do hemodialysis 3 days a week (ranging from 51.6% of unit patients to >95%). At most centers, >90% of patients undergo three dialysis sessions each week. In centers with high uptake of home dialysis, 40%–50% of patients do dialysis either on alternate days or more frequently, while the national average is 18% for more frequent hemodialysis. The vast majority of New Zealand patients (>90%) undergo ≥4.5 hours of hemodialysis at each session. The most frequent blood flow rate used in New Zealand for patients with an arteriovenous fistula is 300–349 mL/min (59%), with smaller fractions prescribed 250–299 mL/min (16.7%) or 350–399 mL/min (16.6%). Hemodiafiltration practices have changed markedly since 2007, with a sharp increase from nearly zero to 20% in 2010, and with a subsequent plateau between 2010 and 2014. As the urea reduction ratio or Kt/V is not measured routinely at some centers, particularly those with a high prevalence of home dialysis, this measure of dialysis adequacy is not reliably ascertained for New Zealand hemodialysis patients.

About one-third of New Zealand patients commence hemodialysis with permanent arteriovenous vascular access (either fistula or graft), even when assessed by a nephrologist >3 months before starting RRT. About 80% of prevalent hemodialysis patients have permanent vascular access, although the prevalence decreases with age; approximately 40% of patients in the >75-year-old age group have a tunneled or nontunneled central venous catheter for dialysis access. The National Renal Advisory Board in New Zealand—the national leadership body advising on and monitoring renal care—has set the quality care standard for permanent vascular access at dialysis start (late referrals excluded) at 80% and prevalent permanent vascular access at 70%; however, these targets continue not to be achieved across the country.[100]

Median patient survival on hemodialysis in New Zealand varies with modality, age, and ethnicity.[101] The median survival for those aged 25 to 44 years is 8 years, 45 to 64 years is 5.5 years, 65 to 74 years is 3.7 years, 75 to 84 years is 2.8 years, and 85+ years is 2.2 years. There is a 52% lower risk of mortality with home dialysis during the first 3 years of dialysis and beyond, although this difference may not be present for Pacific patients.[102]

PD was utilized by 791 (30%) patients treated with dialysis in New Zealand in 2015. Unlike Australia (105 pmp), the prevalence of PD is decreasing, although at 172 pmp it remains higher than peer nations such as Germany (39 pmp), the United Kingdom (75 pmp), and the United States (87 pmp), likely driven by treatment policies in some regions (home dialysis) and geographical remoteness. Most patients (>50%) commencing PD are aged between 55 and 84 years, in parallel with the age groups with the highest incidence of treated ESKD (Fig. 81.11). In contrast to Australia, in which APD is utilized by 65% of those treated with PD, the use of APD in New Zealand is approximately 50%, at the upper end of the range of utilization reported among higher income countries (42.4%, 95% CI: 34.4 to 50.5).[29] Most (72%) of the 291 patients starting PD in New Zealand in 2015 were incident dialysis patients, while 27% transferred from hemodialysis, and 1% commenced PD after a failed transplant.

The median survival for PD in New Zealand is 3.92 years (95% CI: 2.11 to 6.34), although it varies substantially by age, comorbidity, and time.[102] PD is associated with a 20% lower mortality risk in the first 3 years of treatment in New Zealand, which may be offset by a 33% increased mortality during treatment >3 years. The survival benefit observed with PD may be lower among Māori and Pacific patients. Current 1-, 3-, and 5-year survival for PD is 92%, 63%, and 37% in those with diabetes, and 95%, 78%, and 63% in those without diabetes.[28]

While uptake of PD among incident patients has increased over the last 10 years in New Zealand (from 32% to 40% of all incident dialysis patients), the overall prevalence of the modality has been falling, hampered principally by technique survival and a consequent shift to hospital-based hemodialysis care.[103] Current estimates of technique survival for PD in New Zealand are 95%, 86%, 46%, and 16% at 6 months, 1,

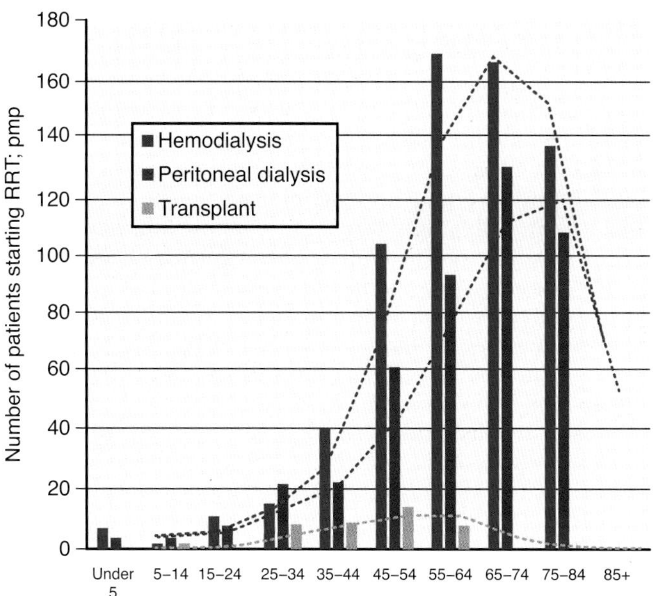


**Fig. 81.11** Incidence of RRT by age group and modality in New Zealand, 2015. *pmp,* per million population; *RRT,* renal replacement therapy. (From Ministry of Health National Renal Advisory Board. *New Zealand Nephrology Activity Report 2015*. Wellington, New Zealand: Ministry of Health; 2015. Available from: http://www.health.govt.nz/about-ministry/leadership-ministry/expert-groups/national-renal-advisory-board/papers-and-reports. Last accessed December 10, 2018.)

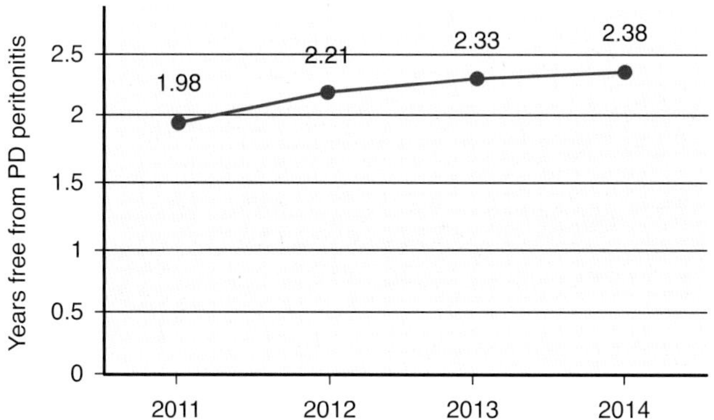


**Fig. 81.12** National average years free from peritoneal dialysis (PD) infection in New Zealand between 2011 and 2014. *PD,* Peritoneal dialysis. (From Ministry of Health National Renal Advisory Board. *New Zealand Nephrology Activity Report 2015*. Wellington, New Zealand: Ministry of Health; 2015. Available from: http://www.health.govt.nz/about-ministry/leadership-ministry/expert-groups/national-renal-advisory-board/papers-and-reports. Last accessed December 10, 2018.)

3, and 5 years. Infection has been the most frequent cause of technique failure (44%), followed by failure of dialysis function (23%), technical issues (19%), and change in modality due to patient preference (7%). Unlike in Australia, in which the rate of PD-related peritonitis has fallen since 2009 as a result of several quality improvement initiatives,[20] the rate of PD peritonitis in New Zealand has improved at a smaller rate over time (Fig. 81.12) and remains somewhat higher than for Australia.

The costs of dialysis are not publicly available. Estimations of dialysis and transplant treatment costs are available from the Auckland Regional Renal Report in 2002–2004. In that report, annual costs (including routine dialysis treatments, hospitalizations, physician assessment not related to dialysis, and transportation) were estimated at US$44,053 for hospital hemodialysis, US$32,995 for satellite hemodialysis, US$25,078 for continuous APD, and US$23,003 for home hemodialysis.[95] Costs of APD are not available.

## TRANSPLANTATION

Three centers perform kidney transplantation in New Zealand: Auckland, Wellington, and Christchurch. Simultaneous kidney and pancreas transplants are performed in Auckland, as are combined solid organ transplants. The first organ to be transplanted in New Zealand was a kidney at Auckland Hospital on May 28, 1965, about 3 months after Australia's first kidney transplant. Lung transplantation started in 1993 and liver and pancreas transplantation in 1998. Organ Donation New Zealand arose from an expanded and renamed national Transplant Donor Coordination Office in 2005 and is the national deceased-organ donation agency. In 2012, the New Zealand Government provided NZ$4 million for initiatives to increase living and deceased donation rates by funding Organ Donation New Zealand, the Counties Manukau District Health Board "Live Kidney Donation Aotearoa" project, and the Auckland District Health Board to formalize the Kidney Exchange Program. An additional NZ$4 million was allocated in 2014 for the establishment of the National Renal Transplant Service to increase and improve transplantation processes, increase donor liaison coordinator capacity, and provide further funding for the New Zealand Kidney Exchange program (NZKX).

In 2015, there were 147 kidney transplants in New Zealand, which is the highest number ever performed in 1 year in the country (Fig. 81.13), and represents a rate of 32 pmp. The number of transplant operations each year has sharply increased in the last 2 years and is likely to be related to the quality improvement initiatives arising from government funding over the previous decade.[104]

The transplantation rate (32 pmp) remains substantially lower than the overall incidence of ESKD (115 pmp), and somewhat lower than the transplantation rate for Australia (40 pmp). The number of kidney transplants each year in New Zealand (147 in 2015) represents 31% of the 472 patients who are active on the kidney transplantation waiting list. Unlike Australia, in which most transplants were from deceased donors (70%), 50% of kidney donors in New Zealand in 2015 were deceased. In 2015, there were 19 preemptive kidney transplants, representing 4.6% of all patients starting RRT. The preemptive transplantation rate has changed little over the last decade but does vary by ethnicity (see Fig. 81.8).

As in Australia, recent developments in New Zealand transplantation services have included the NZKX and ABO-incompatible kidney transplantation. In 2015, there were two kidney exchange chains providing four kidney transplants and nine ABO blood group–incompatible kidney transplants were performed.

During the last 5 years and consequent to increasing transplantation rates, the prevalence of patients living with a functioning kidney transplant has increased in New Zealand from 1483 patients (338 pmp) to 1694 patients (369 pmp). There continues to be marked variation between DHBs in the overall prevalence of kidney transplantation, ranging from 238 pmp to 508 pmp. This variation reflects local transplantation practices, patient comorbidity, and the underlying rates of ESKD. Transplantation most commonly occurred in the 55–64-year-old age group, consistent with a higher incidence of ESKD at this age. As a proportion of all patients with treated ESKD, the age group with the highest prevalence of transplantation was the 5–14-year age group. Over 90% of children and adolescents live with a functioning transplant, with most receiving a kidney transplant from a living donor.

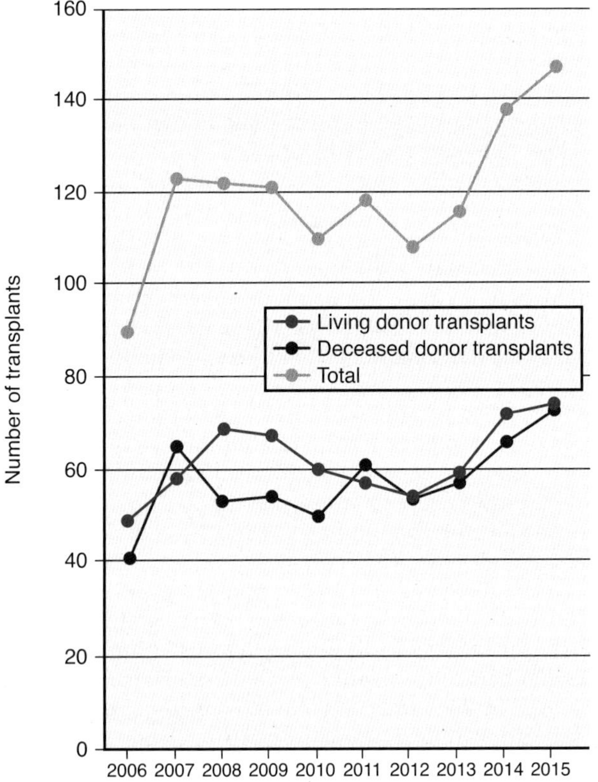


**Fig. 81.13** Living and Deceased donor kidney transplantation in New Zealand during 2006 and 2015. (From Ministry of Health National Renal Advisory Board. *New Zealand Nephrology Activity Report 2015*. Wellington, New Zealand: Ministry of Health; 2015. Available from: http://www.health.govt.nz/about-ministry/leadership-ministry/expert-groups/national-renal-advisory-board/papers-and-reports. Last accessed December 10, 2018.)

Graft survival rates in New Zealand for first grafts are presented in Table 81.2. The 1-year patient and graft survivals have remained stable across recent transplantation eras (2008–2015) for both recipients of a deceased-donor transplants and living-donor transplants. The patient and graft survivals remain approximately 90% and 80%–85%, respectively, for living- and deceased-donor transplant recipients in New Zealand, although data are susceptible to variation due to the relatively small numbers of transplants performed.

As is observed in Australia, the most frequent cause of graft loss is death with a functioning transplant (185 patients during 2011–2015; 51.3%), followed by chronic allograft nephropathy (113 patients; 31.3%). The most common causes of death for transplant recipients are cancer (59 patients accounting for 32% of all deaths) and CVD (also accounting for 32% of all deaths). Increased risks of cancer are observed at numerous body sites after kidney transplantation, principally representing cancers of known or suspected viral etiology, suggesting a role for impaired immunological surveillance.[105]

## NONDIALYSIS SUPPORTIVE CARE FOR ESKD

Increasing recognition of nondialysis care for ESKD has led to the emergence of nondialysis supportive care services within hospital-based nephrology care in New Zealand, as has been similarly observed in many higher-income countries. Nondialysis supportive care can offer patients information and support when considering whether or not to commence dialysis or withdrawing from dialysis care, and for management of symptoms related to ESKD. Supportive care services in New Zealand are not coordinated at a national level and represent local care initiatives related to existing capacity and expertise.[100] Supportive care practices frequently include multidisciplinary teams including palliative care and community nursing services. For many patients in primary care, palliative management of ESKD is coordinated within general practice without the involvement of secondary nephrology services.

## ACUTE KIDNEY INJURY

Few systematic data exist for the incidence and outcomes related to AKI in Aotearoa/New Zealand in adults. AKI occurred in 5.2% of patients at the time of or during the first 24 hours of intensive care unit admission, with a rising

**Table 81.2** Patient and Graft Survival for First Grafts in Aotearoa/New Zealand by Donor Type for Transplants Occurring in 2010–2011

| Outcome | 1 Month | 6 Months | 1 Year | 5 Years |
|---|---|---|---|---|
| **Patient Survival** | | | | |
| Deceased donor ($n$ = 103) | 99 (93–100) | 99 (93–100) | 98 (92–100) | 88 (79–93) |
| Living donor ($n$ = 111) | 100 | 99 (94–100) | 97 (92–99) | 90 (82–94) |
| **Graft Survival** | | | | |
| Deceased donor ($n$ = 103) | 96 (90–99) | 95 (89–98) | 94 (87–97) | 82 (73–89) |
| Living donor ($n$ = 111) | 97 (92–99) | 96 (91–99) | 95 (88–98) | 81 (72–87) |

Data are shown with 95% confidence interval.

incidence noted during the years of 1996 to 2005. Incidence increases with age and comorbidity, and is more frequent for patients with liver disease (12.1%) or hematological malignancy (10.5%) admitted to intensive care. Crude hospital mortality for patients admitted to intensive care with AKI (42.7%) is substantially higher than for those patients without AKI (13.4%), although in the decade through to 2006, mortality decreased among patients with AKI.[106] AKI is associated with a hospital stay of 19.8 days on average for those patients surviving to discharge, and patients with AKI are more likely to be transferred to further acute care or rehabilitation.

For children, the annual incidence of AKI between 2001 and 2006 was 4.0 per 100,000 children under 15 years of age, most commonly associated with cardiac surgery (58%), hemolytic uremic syndrome (17%), and sepsis (13%).[107] Survival of AKI to hospital discharge for children was 89%, with evidence of ongoing kidney impairment in 40%. Māori and Pacific children are treated for AKI more often than New Zealand European children.

## KIDNEY DISEASE CARE IN NEW ZEALAND

### HEALTH FINANCE

Before World War II, the health care in New Zealand was predominantly privately funded, with around 57% of total health funding from the private sector in 1925.[92] Public contributions to health funding increased, such that in 1945, 74% of health expenditure was from public sources, with a peak in the 1980s of 88%. Direct funding from the government, through the Ministry of Health, is the largest source of funding of the health and disability sector.

In 2000, the New Zealand Public Health and Disability Act allowed the implementation of DHBs. There are currently 20 DHBs in New Zealand that are responsible for planning, and providing or purchasing health and disability services within their geographical region, including acute hospital services.

CKD and AKI are managed collaboratively across the health sector in primary, secondary, and tertiary care. At present, hospital-based dialysis services are provided by 11 DHBs to their own regions and other DHBs. CKD is most commonly identified within primary care settings, and referral is made to nephrology services for virtual or in-person consultation.

New Zealand's total health expenditure in 2016 was NZ$15.6 billion, representing approximately 9.5% of GDP in 2013.[108] Growth in health spending slowed following the global financial crisis and greater use of pharmaceutical spending on generic medications (accounting for 34% of pharmaceuticals in 2013). New Zealand ranked 12th in OECD nations for spending on health as a share of GDP in 2013.

Total expenditure on ESKD care is about 1% of total health expenditure. ESKD treatment is nearly entirely funded through the tax-funded health system. All inpatient and outpatient secondary-level health-care services including hospital-based care are free to patients, as are pharmaceuticals prescribed within secondary services. Primary care services are subsidized, although patients may be required to pay for services above any subsidy they receive. Similarly, prescriptions in the primary care setting accrue direct costs to the patient.

DHBs are provided a budget weighted according to the services they provide and the demographic and socioeconomic characteristics of their population. Budgetary constraints occur, such that DHBs are incentivized to manage funds within their allocation including dialysis and transplantation care. Private insurance can enable patients to recoup costs for pharmaceuticals and consultation within primary care, but cannot be applied to dialysis or transplantation care. A recent law change resulted in the Compensation for Live Organ Donors Act 2016, which provides financial assistance for lost income and childcare assistance for 12 weeks after living donation of kidney or liver tissue.

### ESSENTIAL MEDICATIONS AND TECHNOLOGY ACCESS

Pharmaceutical Management Agency (Pharmac) is the government agency that determines which pharmaceuticals are publicly funded in New Zealand. Pharmac manages the Combined Pharmaceutical Budget which is set each year by the Minister of Health, and includes funding for community medicines, some hospital medicines, and some devices. The funding decisions of Pharmac are listed in the Pharmaceutical Schedule that defines subsidies for specific medicines and devices. A copayment for pharmaceutical items is set by the government and is free for children under the age of 13 years and about NZ$5 per item for the first 20 items prescribed to a family each year.

Many New Zealand patients live considerable distances from dialysis and transplant units, and for children, there is a single hospital in Auckland that provides in-patient and outpatient pediatric nephrology care in New Zealand. A National Travel Assistance program provides funding for transport and accommodation for patients required to travel and live in regions distant from their home for specialist care. Qualitative research has documented the considerable social disruption arising from dialysis treatment in New Zealand because of living remotely from dialysis and transplantation care.[109]

### DETECTION AND MONITORING OF KIDNEY DISEASE

Late assessment by a specialist nephrologist (within 3 months of requiring RRT) is associated with poorer clinical outcomes and reduces the likelihood of preemptive transplantation.[110] Timely assessment for RRT requires detection of progressive kidney disease particularly within primary care practice, and collaborative management between primary and secondary care. In New Zealand, approximately 13% of patients experience late assessment, although this proportion is decreasing.[90] Younger adults and children are at particularly higher risk of late referral to specialist care; 26% of children and adults younger than 25 years old were referred within 3 months of RRT in 2015. Early detection of kidney disease and appropriate referral of patients who are likely to progress to ESKD may improve clinical outcomes, although empirical data suggest that large-scale implementation of global referral guidelines (Kidney Disease Improving Global Outcomes guidelines) may not be feasible under usual clinical practice models.[111]

There have been some nationwide programs in New Zealand to guide primary and secondary care practitioners in assessment and referral of patients with CKD. In 2015, a national consensus statement on managing CKD in primary care was released by the Ministry of Health[112] intended to articulate best practice in identification and management of CKD in primary care. This statement included systematic screening in primary care linked to existing diabetes and CVD screening programs, management of cardiovascular risk, and enablers of monitoring and recall systems for CKD care.

Strategies to support primary care of CKD include HealthPathways, which are agreements between primary and specialist services on how patients with specific health conditions will be managed within the local health service context. HealthPathways are principally designed to support primary care clinicians to manage patients in the community and guide referral practices for specialist assessment (www.healthpathwayscommunity.org). Decision aids for patients and clinicians making choices about treatment for ESKD have been developed by Kidney Health New Zealand an established patient advocacy group.[113]

A randomized clinical trial of community-based visits by nurse-led health-care assistants for medication adherence and algorithm-guided blood pressure care in Māori and Pacific patients led to greater use of medications, lower blood pressure, and reductions in proteinuria, suggesting an effective model of primary care for CKD.[114] Challenges to wider adoption of newer primary care practices to prevent ESKD include limited resourcing for nursing, availability of secondary care services to upskill primary care clinicians, and adequate protocols to integrate medical management across primary and secondary care. A recent systematic review of studies examining the effectiveness of chronic disease management programs of indigenous people in Australia, New Zealand, and Canada demonstrated that effective and acceptable programs were those that were integrated in existing health services, were nurse led, provided intensive follow-up, had governance structures supporting local leadership, included robust clinical systems for communication, and involved indigenous health workers as central to practice.[115] Use of telehealth within secondary nephrology services in New Zealand is not systematic. Telehealth-based services for long-term conditions in Australia and New Zealand lack high-level evidence of effectiveness.[116]

## HEALTH WORKFORCE

At present, there are 423 medical graduates each year in New Zealand. Increased funding for medical education has led to a forecast expansion in numbers, which are expected to plateau in 2022 at 553 each year.[117] Reductions in international medical graduates suggest that additional training opportunities for New Zealand graduates within the health workforce will increase.

Recent workforce estimates in New Zealand indicate there are 230 full-time equivalent nurses providing care in hospital dialysis units and 21.5 full-time-equivalent nurses in home hemodialysis roles (R. Walker, personal communication). It was estimated in 2009 that there was one nurse for every 6.3 patients compared with 1 nurse for every 4.2 patients in Australia.[118] Nurses supporting CKD services specifically within secondary services are rare, with 2.5 full-time equivalents in hospital care in New Zealand. There are currently 6.1 full-time equivalent transplant coordinators and 3.9 full-time pharmacist equivalents.

In 2015, there were 45.4 full-time nephrologists (11.3 pmp), equivalent to 1 nephrologist for every 96 patients with ESKD (similar to 1 specialized nephrologist per 102 patients with ESKD reported in March 2004) and compares with 1 specialized nephrologist for every 80 patients with ESKD in Australia.[95] Historically, there have been insufficient New Zealand-trained nephrologists for workforce requirements, such that nephrologists have received prioritization within immigration processes. The nursing workforce in New Zealand is anticipated to be insufficient for an aging population, attributed to an older nursing workforce, reduced arrival of overseas-trained nurses, and increasing complexity of health services with multimorbidity.[119] The existing participation of Māori and Pacific practitioners in the New Zealand health workforce is low. In 2009, Māori and Pacific clinicians represented 3.1% and 1.5% of medical practitioners and 6.3% and 1.8% of the nursing workforce, respectively.[120] Specific programs have been established to increase Māori and Pacific participation in the medical workforce, which is considered to be a factor in reducing inequitable outcomes for Māori and Pacific communities.[121]

## HEALTH INFORMATION SYSTEMS AND STATISTICS

Health-related information for patients with treated ESKD has been systematically collated in the ANZDATA Registry since 1978. Data about the incidence and prevalence of dialysis and transplantation treatment, together with information about treatment practices and clinical outcomes, are reported annually and as individual reports to DHBs. While comprehensive, ANZDATA does not include health information about untreated ESKD or earlier stages of CKD.

New Zealand has a National Health Index that assigns a unique number to each person in New Zealand who receives health care. This includes information on name, address, date and place of birth, gender, resident and citizen status, ethnicity, and (if appropriate) date of death.[122] The National Health Index number can be linked to other national and international health information repositories. An important aspect of health information used to drive health-care improvement is the accurate recording of ethnicity data. Specific protocols for the collection, recording, and output of ethnicity data are described for the Health and Disability Sector, with a specific focus to improve health outcomes and reduce health inequity.[123] Key requirements include ethnicity as self-identification, ethnicity is context specific and can change, that more than one ethnicity can be recorded, and that a standardized approach increases the accuracy of ethnicity data for decision-making.

At present, the number of people in New Zealand with CKD is unknown, as these data are not systematically recorded. Similarly, there is no existing framework for measurement of AKI or untreated ESKD in New Zealand. It is likely, due to increasing availability of large data sets, routine capture of diagnostic codes, and the National Health Index, that additional census data for kidney diseases will become available in the future.

## STRATEGIES AND POLICY FRAMEWORKS

The New Zealand Ministry of Health has a Long-Term Conditions Program that provides support to the Ministry, health sector, and nongovernmental organizations to provide leadership, evaluate progress, and support clinical quality initiatives.[124] CKD is included in this framework as a condition that leads to an ongoing, long-term, and recurring impact on well-being. A National Health Strategy, released in 2016, has outlined higher-level direction and actions to improve the New Zealand health system between 2016 and 2026.[125]

Specifically, for CKD, the Ministry of Health provides leadership through the National Renal Advisory Board comprising clinical and managerial leaders in DHBs and professional and consumer groups.[100] The board holds responsibility for national strategy, projecting treatment demand, and defining service specifications for conditions involving the renal and urinary tract, and reporting the health activities and outcomes in nephrology services to the Ministry of Health. As discussed earlier in this chapter, the National Renal Transplant Service was established in 2014, and is implementing quality improvement metrics for transplantation. Quality improvement metrics include 1. the proportion of donor–recipient pairs who undergo transplantation surgery should receive surgery within 4 months of being accepted by the transplant service and are ready to proceed; and 2. the proportion of kidney transplants from living donors occurring as preemptive or early kidney transplants. In addition, the New Zealand Kidney Allocation Scheme was developed in 2016 as an algorithm for allocation of deceased-donor kidneys and nondirected live-donor kidneys to maximize equity, accountability, and transparency.[126]

In addition to national bodies and practice frameworks, clinical practice guidelines for care of dialysis, transplant, and earlier stages of CKD are provided through the KHA-CARI.

### CAPACITY FOR RESEARCH AND DEVELOPMENT

Health research in New Zealand is predominantly conducted within tertiary education institutions and DHBs. New Zealand spent 1.2% of GDP on research and development in 2014, which is substantially lower than the average among OECD countries of 2.4%. The New Zealand Government spending on research was 0.27% of GDP in the same period, and represents considerably lower investment than in other small advanced economies, such as Israel (>4%), Denmark and Finland (>3%), and Singapore (>2%).[127] A New Zealand Health Research Strategy developed by the Ministry of Health and the Ministry of Business, Employment and Innovation, together with the primary governmental health research funder, the Health Research Council, has recently been released, and is designed to increase implementation of health research findings and retain clinicians with an interest in health research.[128]

There is limited coordination in research for kidney disease in New Zealand with a range of researchers and small research aggregates drawing funding from private and public sources. The AKTN is a nonprofit collaborative research group that supports the collaborative development of trials in kidney disease in both Australia and New Zealand and which supports funding applications for trial conduct. The New Zealand Institute for Pacific Research is aimed to promote and support excellence in Pacific Research, although to date there are no specific collaborative research projects with Pacific and New Zealand researchers specifically for kidney disease.[129]

## SAMOA

Samoa is made up of six islands, and is a member of the Commonwealth of Nations. From the end of World War I until 1962 when Samoa attained independence, it was under the control of New Zealand. Similar to other island nations in the Pacific, diabetes is highly prevalent in Samoa, and CKD is listed within the top 10 causes of deaths in the country (ranked fourth in 2015).[130] Samoa's health system is made up of public and private health sectors and the first hemodialysis unit (12 dialysis machines) opened in 2002 with assistance from the Singapore National Kidney Foundation.[131] There are currently two centers located in two main islands (Upolu and Savaii), providing treatment for 88 patients who are on a waiting list to access the service. The government of Samoa has acknowledged the strain imposed by the growing burden of CKD, and is currently working on public awareness campaigns and evaluating methods to promote healthier lifestyle measures to lower risk factors for CKD, such as hypertension and diabetes.[132]

### NEW ZEALAND DEPENDENCIES (COOK ISLANDS, NIUE, TOKELAU)

Cook Islands, Niue, and Tokelau are all self-covering island countries in the South Pacific Ocean in free association with New Zealand. Cook Islands is the most populous of the group, which comprises 15 islands. Tourism is the country's main industry as it lacks major natural resources (makes up approximately 67.5% of GDP).[133] Although Cook Islands is thought to perform better than other Pacific island nations in relation to health indicators, there has been a 40%–50% increase in the prevalence of diabetes followed by increasing number of CKD patients (expected to more than double in the next 10 years).[134] Noncommunicable diseases such as CKD are reported to be the leading causes of mortality in the Cook Islands (responsible for 75% of deaths).[135] According to a report generated in 2012, there were 26 physicians working in Cook Islands, but whether this includes a nephrologist is uncertain.[136] Patients with ESKD, as New Zealand citizens, receive dialysis treatment within the New Zealand tax-funded public health system presently, as there is no capacity for RRT within the Cook Islands. The majority of patients receive hospital-based hemodialysis in New Zealand, driven by patient preference.[131]

Niue is located 2400 km northeast of New Zealand and west of Cook Islands, with the population made up predominantly of Polynesians (around 1612 as of November 2016). Over 90% of Niuean people live in New Zealand, and Niue was the first country in the world to offer free wireless Internet to all its inhabitants.[137] Similarly, about 1400 people are thought to reside in Tokelau, which is another island country located north of the Samoan Islands. It is known as the first 100% solar-powered nation in the world.[138] Given their small population with limited data available on health, there is no known information pertaining to the burden of AKI or CKD in either of these two nations.

## PAPUA NEW GUINEA

Papua New Guinea is classified as a low- to middle-income country with close to 90% of the population living in rural areas. Primary health-care facilities are the main point of access to the health system, but access to these services faces many geographic, cultural, financial, and systemic challenges.[139] Many villages can only be reached via air or foot, where over 90% of existing roads are unpaved.[140] Over the past 20 years, there has been a deterioration in the availability of primary health-care services,[141] with up to 40% of aid posts closing, thereby restricting access to health care. Moreover, in spite of a predominant public funding base supplemented in some areas with church-run facilities supported by grants from the National Department of Health, many facilities charge a user fee, which creates further barriers to health care for those who cannot afford the service.[142]

The exact prevalence of CKD in Papua New Guinea is unknown, however CKD was ranked as the eighth most common cause of death in 2015.[143] Increase in the burden of CKD is likely to be driven by growth in prevalence of diabetes mellitus, which is thought to affect 12.9% of the adult population in Papua New Guinea.[144] This is concerning, as access to RRT is inadequate. Although PD is available, a limited number of hemodialysis machines are available (reported to be two in 2014),[145] with no capacity for renal transplantation.

## PACIFIC ISLANDS

### FRENCH PROTECTORATES (FRENCH POLYNESIA, NEW CALEDONIA, WALLIS AND FUTUNA)

French Polynesia, New Caledonia, Wallis and Futuna form French protectorates within Oceania. French Polynesia is made up of 118 islands scattered over 2000 km of ocean, divided into five groups of islands, with 67 islands that are inhabited.[146] Tahiti is the most populated island of the group and serves as the capital of the collectivity. Although the Government of France directs justice, university education, security, and defense, the local government controls health.[146] French Polynesia has a moderately developed economy with modest GDP per capita amongst countries within Oceania (Table 81.1). Health facilities are considered to be of reasonable standard, however access to medical services, including dialysis, is restricted in less-populated islands. There is only one hemodialysis unit, located in Tahiti.[147] The medical practitioners operate in private practice, with consultation costs up to 3500 Comptoirs Français du Pacifique Franc to see a GP with a higher cost for a specialist review.[148] Diabetic nephropathy is a major cause of CKD in this region,[149] with relatively high background prevalence of diabetes mellitus (7.3%).[150] Another important cause of ESKD in French Polynesia is Alport syndrome, which affects 18% of the patients receiving dialysis[151] (compared with 1%–2% of ESKD patients in Europe, and 2.3% of renal transplant patients in the United States[152]). It is the most prevalent monogenic inherited disorder found within French Polynesia.[151]

New Caledonia is another special collectivity of France, located within the Melanesia subregion, formed by several islands, including the main island of Grand Terre. It has one of the largest economies in the South Pacific, with GDP per capita similar to New Zealand (Table 81.1). According to a retrospective renal biopsy study, which included 202 renal biopsies from 181 patients in New Caledonia, the most prevalent primary glomerular disease was focal segmental glomerulosclerosis and the most prevalent systemic glomerulopathy was amyloidosis. Other common pathological findings included postinfectious glomerulonephritis, minimal change disease, and diabetic nephropathy.[153] In 2009, the most common conditions requiring long-term treatment included diabetes (9509 cases, 17.6%) and 1198 cases of renal failure (2.2%) requiring treatment. Given the growing burden of diabetes in the community, CKD from diabetic nephropathy is likely to have also increased over time. The local government has endorsed the "Health for All" principle, with provision of public and private health-care services (with 2.9 hospital beds available for every 1000 people). Economic growth of New Caledonia and improvement in quality of health-care coverage have led to unfettered access to health services by the whole population.[154] Access to both hemodialysis and PD is available.[147]

The Territory of the Wallis and Futuna Islands is made up of three main islands with a smaller number of tiny islets. The vast majority of the population is of Polynesian ethnicity, with a small minority of French descent. A large proportion of Wallisians and Futunians live as expatriates in New Caledonia due to limited resources on their homelands, which has led to a decreasing trend in population over time (14,166 in 1996 vs. 12,197 in 2013).[155] The Health Agency for the Territory of the Wallis and Futuna Islands is a French national public administrative agency with the aim to ensure health protection in the Territory. There is a high prevalence of risk factors for chronic noncommunicable diseases, including cigarette smoking (49.1%), obesity (59.5%), hypertension (34.1%), diabetes mellitus (17.1%), and dyslipidemia (16.1%) according to a study, which comprised 560 people from the Territory (representing 6.71% of the adult population living in Wallis and Futuna).[156] In the studied population, moderate CKD, defined as an eGFR of 30–59 mL/min/1.73 $m^2$, was present in 5.8% of the participants.[156] At present, there is no dialysis unit in the Territory.

### US PROTECTORATES (AMERICAN SAMOA, GUAM)

American Samoa is an unincorporated territory of the United States consisting of five main islands. It has a small developing economy with two main sources of income, the United States Government and tuna canning, which make up 93% of the economy together.[157] The most significant health problems relate to the increase in chronic diseases associated with lifestyle, due to poor nutrition and physical inactivity, such as hypertension, CVD, and type 2 diabetes mellitus.[158] According to the American Samoa noncommunicable STEPwise approach to Surveillance (STEPS) survey, conducted between June and August 2004, 74.6% of American Samoans were obese (defined as BMI $\geq$ 30 kg/$m^2$) and 93.5% were classified as overweight (BMI 25–29.9 kg/$m^2$) or obese, whilst hypertension and diabetes were present in 34.2% and 47.3% of the adult population, respectively.[159] Although the exact burden of CKD is uncertain, it is likely to be significant and growing in the context of increasing burden of risk factors for CKD. There is one hemodialysis unit at the Lyndon B. Johnson Tropical Medical Center in Pago Pago, which has 16 dialysis chairs,[159] where 160 patients with ESKD receive hemodialysis treatment each week.[160] The number of patients receiving hemodialysis in American Samoa has increased by 33% from 2006 to 2010.[159]

Guam is another unincorporated and organized territory of the United States. However, unlike American Samoa, Guamanians are American citizens by birth. Guam has a land area of 544 km$^2$ (75% the size of Singapore), and is the largest island in Micronesia. The largest ethnic group is the native Chamorros (37.3%), followed by Filipinio (26.3%), White (7.1%), and Chuukese (7%) ethnicities. Guam's economy depends primarily on tourism.[161] Similar to other Pacific Island nations, the most common cause of ESKD is diabetic nephropathy, particularly amongst Pacific Islanders.[162] US board–certified medical practitioners serve the people of Guam in all specialties and health care is available through public and private sectors.[161] There were four dialysis units and six nephrologists in 2014,[163] and there is no transplant program in place.

## NORFOLK ISLAND (AUSTRALIAN PROTECTORATE)

Norfolk Island is located between Australia, New Zealand, and New Caledonia, which forms part of the Commonwealth of Australia. Given close ties with Australia and New Zealand, with a small economy, there has been a growth in emigration that has led to a decreasing trend of population (1796 people in 2011 compared with 2601 in 2001).[164] Norfolk Island Hospital is the only medical center on the island with three medical practitioners.[165] Medicare and PBS cover medical treatments, analogous to mainland Australia. However, the hospital is not equipped to treat any serious emergencies. In situations where health conditions deteriorate in residents of Norfolk Island, many are forced to leave their homes and relocate to New Zealand or Australia to receive medical care, including RRT.[164]

## PITCAIRN ISLAND (BRITISH COLONY)

The Pitcairn Islands is the last British Overseas Territory of the Pacific. Of the four islands (Pitcairn, Henderson, Ducie, and Oeno), only Pitcairn is inhabited by approximately 50 permanent people including one government-employed medical practitioner, and is the least populous national jurisdiction in the world.[166] The island can only be accessed by yachts or ships and receives a scheduled supply boat at 3-monthly intervals.[167] Its remote location with a lack of access to services including hospital and reliable power has been blamed as a major barrier to growth. Like other island nations of the Pacific, diabetes mellitus is reported to be highly prevalent,[168] but the burden of CKD is unknown.

## FIJI

Fiji is an island country in Melanesia formed by >330 islands, of which 110 are permanently inhabited. Over 80% of the population resides on the two main islands: Viti Levu and Vanua Levu. Fiji has one of the most developed economies in the Pacific due to an abundance of natural resources and an active tourism sector. CKD has been identified as the fourth most common cause of death in 2015 (increase by 34.0% since 2005).[169] A recent STEPS survey has reported 30% of Fiji's adult population as diabetic and the incidence of stage 5 CKD is estimated to be the highest in the world, at around 680 pmp.[170] Fiji suffers from an underdeveloped health system, and there is only one formally trained nephrologist in Fiji (1.1 pmp). This has led to difficulties to screen and treat early-stage CKD and the urgent need to address noncommunicable diseases including CKD has been recognized by the government. Although chronic hemodialysis is available in three units (Suva, Labasa, and Nadi), it is only accessible to those who are able to afford the service, and long-term treatment is rare due to financial constraints. In 2016, there were 107 dialysis patients in Fiji. PD and kidney transplant programs are currently unavailable in Fiji. Living-donor kidney transplants are performed in India.[170] There are plans to expand capacity to support patients with ESKD in Fiji, especially those who could not previously afford RRT, with recent government announcement of allocating $1 million for the establishment of the National Kidney Research and Treatment Centre and an additional $300,000 for dialysis treatment.[171] In addition to three chronic hemodialysis units, two of the three public hospitals are able to perform dialysis for treatment of AKI (A. Krishnan, personal communication). One of the important causes of AKI in Fiji has included leptospirosis, which is identified as one of the four priority climate-sensitive diseases of major public health concern.[172] Outbreaks of leptospirosis have frequently occurred in the setting of floods, which resulted in 576 reported cases and 40 deaths (7% case fatality) in 2012.[173] Some of the identified risk factors have included male gender, indigenous Fijian status, young adults (15 to 45 years of age), living in rural areas, and abattoir workers, with peak seasons following rainy months and cyclones.[174,175]

## CONCLUSION

Oceania is a region which comprises >10,000 islands with an estimated population of >40 million people with a large variation in the level of economic status. The burden of CKD is increasing across the region, driven by inexorable growth in noncommunicable chronic illnesses, such as diabetes mellitus. Access to health care and data on health outcomes or burden of disease are highly variable and mostly very limited in many nations of the Oceania region outside of Australia and New Zealand. Even within affluent countries, such as Australia and New Zealand, there exist inequities in health outcomes affecting indigenous patients. In response to growth in the prevalence of CKD and its associated adverse health outcomes, various governments are currently expanding their capacities to improve care for these patients. Implementing infrastructure to capture the true disease burden and health outcomes will be an important component of strategies to achieve better health outcomes.

## ACKNOWLEDGMENTS

The authors gratefully acknowledge the substantial contributions of the entire Australia and New Zealand nephrology community in providing information for and maintaining the ANZDATA database. We also thank the ANZDATA executive for granting permission to use figures from the ANZDATA Registry annual report.

 Complete reference list available at ExpertConsult.com.

## KEY REFERENCES

1. Couser WG, Remuzzi G, Mendis S, et al. The contribution of chronic kidney disease to the global burden of major noncommunicable diseases. *Kidney Int.* 2011;80(12):1258–1270.

6. AIHW. *Cardiovascular Disease, Diabetes and Chronic Kidney Disease-Australian Factors: Aboriginal and Torres Strait Islander People.* Canberra: Australian Institute of Health and Welfare; 2015.
7. AIHW. *Projections of the Prevalence of Treated End-Stage Kidney Disease in Australia 2012-2020.* Canberra: Australian Institute of Health and Welfare; 2014.
9. Australia and New Zealand Dialysis and Transplant Registry. The 39th Annual Report, *Chapter 1: Incidence of End stage kidney disease.* Adelaide, Australia 2016, available at www.anzdata.org.au.
10. AIHW. *An Overview of the Chronic Kidney Disease in Australia.* Canberra: AIHW: Australian Insititute of Health and Welfare; 2009.
12. Wyld ML, Lee CM, Zhuo X, et al. Cost to government and society of chronic kidney disease stage 1-5: a national cohort study. *Intern Med J.* 2015;45(7):741–747.
13. Kidney Health Australia. *Station of the Nation: 2016 Kidney Health Week.* Chronic Kidney Disease Hot Spots *KHA*; 2016.
15. Australia and New Zealand Dialysis and Transplant Registry. The 39th Annual Report, *Chapter 2: Prevalence of end stage kidney disease.* Adelaide, Australia 2016, available at www.anzdata.org.au.
27. AIHW. *Dialysis and Kidney Transplantation in Australia: 1991-2010.* Canberra: AIHW; 2012.
28. Australia and New Zealand Dialysis and Transplant Registry. The 39th Annual Report, *Chapter 5: Peritoneal Dialysis.* Adelaide, Australia 2016, available at www.anzdata.org.au.
29. Jain AK, Blake P, Cordy P, et al. Global trends in rates of peritoneal dialysis. *J Am Soc Nephrol.* 2012;23(3):533–544.
31. Cho Y, Johnson DW. Peritoneal dialysis-related peritonitis: towards improving evidence, practices, and outcomes. *Am J Kidney Dis.* 2014;64(2):278–289.
34. Nadeau-Fredette AC, Johnson DW, Hawley CM, et al. Center-Specific factors associated with peritonitis Risk-A Multi-Center Registry Analysis. *Perit Dial Int.* 2016;36(5):509–518.
36. WHO. *Global Observatory on Donation and Transplantation*; 2015. Available at: http://www.transplant-observatory.org/summary/. Accessed January 02, 2017.
40. Chapman JR. What are the key challenges we face in kidney transplantation today? *Transplant Res.* 2013;2(suppl 1):S1.
44. Chapman JR, Webster AC, Wong G. Cancer in the transplant recipient. *Cold Spring Harb Perspect Med.* 2013;3(7).
54. AIHW. *Acute Kidney Injury in Australia: A First National Snapshot.* Canberra: Australian Institute of Health and Welfare; 2015.
55. AIHW. *Chronic Kidney Disease in Aboriginal and Torres Strait Islander People.* Canberra: Australian Institute of Health and Welfare; 2011.
56. Hoy WE, Mott SA, McDonald SP. An expanded nationwide view of chronic kidney disease in Aboriginal Australians. *Nephrology (Carlton).* 2016;21(11):916–922.
57. Hoy WE. Kidney disease in Aboriginal Australians: a perspective from the Northern Territory. *Clin Kidney J.* 2014;7(6):524–530.
68. Kidney Health Australia. *Kidney Health Check*; 2017. http://kidney.org.au/health-professionals/detect/kidney-health-check. Accessed January 23, 2017.
70. Pefanis A, Botlero R, Langham RG, et al. eMAP:CKD: electronic diagnosis and management assistance to primary care in chronic kidney disease. *Nephrol Dial Transplant.* 2016.
71. Institute TG *Health Tracker - Decision support for primary care professionals*; 2017. http://www.georgeinstitute.org.au/projects/healthtracker-decision-support-for-primary-care-professionals. Accessed January 23, 2017.
72. KHA. *Chronic Kidney Disease (CKD) Management in General Practice.* In: Australia KKH, ed. Vol 3rd Edition 2015 KHA; 2015.
74. Chow J, Donaldson P, Fortnum D, et al. Beyond dialysis - telehealth initiatives. *Renal Society Australasia J.* 2016;12(1):18–25.
77. Kidney Health Australia. *Tackling kidney disease: a national action plan to reduce Australia's kidney disease burden*; 2016. http://kidney.org.au/cms_uploads/docs/checklist-for-change–kidney-health-australia.pdf. Accessed January 23, 2017.
90. New Zealand Society of Nephrology. *New Zealand Nephrology Annual Data Report 2015.* New Zealand; 2015.
91. Ministry of Health. *Health loss in New Zealand 1990-2013: A report from the New Zealand Burden of Diseases, Injuries, and Risk Factors Study.* Wellington, New Zealand; 2016.
94. Ministry of Health. *Report on New Zealand Cost-of-Illness Studies on Long-Term Conditions.* Wellington, New Zealand; 2009.
95. Ashton T, Marshall MR. The organization and financing of dialysis and kidney transplantation services in New Zealand. *Int J Health Care Finance Econ.* 2007;7(4):233–252.
96. Australia and New Zealand Dialysis and Transplant Registry. The 39th Annual Report, *Chapter 13: End stage kidney disease in Aotearoa/New Zealand.* Adelaide: ANZDATA Registry; 2016. Available at www.anzdata.org.au.
98. McGregor D, Buttimore A, Robson R, et al. Thirty years of universal home dialysis in Christchurch. *N Z Med J.* 2000;113(1103):27–29.
100. Ministry of Health. *National Renal Advisory Board*; 2017. http://www.health.govt.nz/about-ministry/leadership-ministry/expert-groups/national-renal-advisory-board. Accessed July, 2017.
103. Mudge DW, Boudville N, Brown F, et al. Peritoneal dialysis practice in Australia and New Zealand: a call to sustain the action. *Nephrology (Carlton).* 2016;21(7):535–546.
112. Ministry of Health. *Managing Chronic Kidney Disease in Primary Care: National Consensus Statement.* Wellington, New Zealand; 2015.
113. Fortnum D, Smolonogov T, Walker R, et al. 'My kidneys, my choice, decision aid': supporting shared decision making. *J Ren Care.* 2015;41(2):81–87.
114. Hotu C, Bagg W, Collins J, et al. A community-based model of care improves blood pressure control and delays progression of proteinuria, left ventricular hypertrophy and diastolic dysfunction in Maori and Pacific patients with type 2 diabetes and chronic kidney disease: a randomized controlled trial. *Nephrol Dial Transplant.* 2010;25(10):3260–3266.
115. Reilly R, Evans K, Gomersall J, et al. Effectiveness, cost effectiveness, acceptability and implementation barriers/enablers of chronic kidney disease management programs for Indigenous people in Australia, New Zealand and Canada: a systematic review of mixed evidence. *BMC Health Serv Res.* 2016;16:119.
121. Russell L, Smiler K, Stace H. *Improving Maori health and reducing inequalities between Maori and non-Maori: Has the Primary Health Care Strategy worked for Maori? A report for the Health Research Council of New Zealand.* New Zealand; 2013.
124. Ministry of Health. *Long-term conditions*; 2017. http://www.health.govt.nz/our-work/diseases-and-conditions/long-term-conditions, Accessed July 2017.
125. Ministry of Health. *New Zealand Health Strategy: Future direction*; 2016. http://www.health.govt.nz/publication/new-zealand-health-strategy-2016, Accessed July 2017.
141. Janovsky K, Travis P. *Non-State Providers of Health Care in Papua New Guinea: Governance, Stewardship and International Support.* Geneva: World Health Organization; 2007.
150. Nanditha A, Ma RC, Ramachandran A, et al. Diabetes in Asia and the Pacific: implications for the global epidemic. *Diabetes Care.* 2016;39(3):472–485.
153. Painter D, Clouston D, Ahn E, et al. The pattern of glomerular disease in New Caledonia: preliminary findings. *Pathology.* 1996;28(1):32–35.
159. Ichiho HM, Roby FT, Ponausuia ES, et al. An assessment of non-communicable diseases, diabetes, and related risk factors in the territory of American Samoa: a systems perspective. *Hawaii J Med Public Health.* 2013;72(5 suppl 1):10–18.
162. Safabakhsh S, Charfauros A, Chargualaf J, et al *Diabetic end stage renal disease in the Indigenous population of Guam.* Pacific Regional Medical Conference 2011; 2011; Guam.
176. Collaborators GBDRF, Forouzanfar MH, Alexander L, et al. Global, regional, and national comparative risk assessment of 79 behavioural, environmental and occupational, and metabolic risks or clusters of risks in 188 countries, 1990-2013: a systematic analysis for the global burden of disease study 2013. *Lancet.* 2015;386(10010):2287–2323.
177. DALYs GBD, Collaborators H, Murray CJ, et al. Global, regional, and national disability-adjusted life years (DALYs) for 306 diseases and injuries and healthy life expectancy (HALE) for 188 countries, 1990-2013: quantifying the epidemiological transition. *Lancet.* 2015; 386(10009):2145–2191.
178. Mortality GBD, Causes of Death C. Global, regional, and national age-sex specific all-cause and cause-specific mortality for 240 causes of death, 1990-2013: a systematic analysis for the global burden of disease study 2013. *Lancet.* 2015;385(9963):117–171.

# CHALLENGES IN NEPHROLOGY

# SECTION XIV

# 82 Ethical Dilemmas Facing Nephrology: Past, Present, and Future

Alvin H. Moss | Catherine R. Butler

## CHAPTER OUTLINE



## KEY POINTS

- The ethical issues facing nephrology played a fundamental role in the early development of the field of bioethics. Because the life-sustaining therapies of dialysis and kidney transplantation predated many parallel therapies in other fields, the ethical issues that inevitably accompany these highly specialized medical treatments were first addressed by nephrologists.
- The criteria for dialysis patient selection used by the Seattle Artificial Kidney Center Admissions and Policy Committee in the 1960s were widely criticized. It was deemed unacceptable to make life and death decisions based on a narrow definition of social worth.
- The US Medicare End-Stage Renal Disease (ESRD) program quickly grew beyond initial projected number of covered patients in part because the dialysis community began treating older patients with more comorbidities. These included patients with other life-threatening illnesses such as end-stage cardiovascular disease, debilitating pulmonary disease, dementia, or untreatable cancer.
- Advance care planning with the completion of advance directives is especially important for dialysis patients. About half of the dialysis population is elderly. The elderly population have the shortest life expectancy on dialysis and are the most likely to withdraw from dialysis. Prior discussion of advance directives has been shown to help dialysis patients and their families approach death in a reconciled fashion.
- The concept of a "time-limited trial" of dialysis is a way to avoid a sense of inflexible commitment to a treatment strategy when the benefit of the treatment to the particular patient is uncertain. Dialysis may be initiated with a planned reevaluation of whether goals are being met with continuation or withdrawal based on this assessment.
- Prior to implementation of the 2014 United Network for Organ Sharing Kidney Allocation System, troubling disparities had been noted in the kidney transplant program. Studies had found that blacks were less likely than whites to be deemed appropriate candidates for transplantation, to be referred for transplant evaluation, to complete a transplant evaluation, to be added to a transplant waiting list, and to receive a kidney transplant.
- Cherry picking, patient solicitation, and other forms of acting in favor of physician or medical group interest rather than patient welfare compromise a physician's fiduciary responsibility and the very foundation of medicine and the doctor–patient relationship.
- Because ESRD Seamless Care Organizations are financed based on a shared risk model, large dialysis organizations have a strong incentive to cherry pick healthy patients because a large percentage of their income is at stake. Older and sicker dialysis patients require more dialysis center staff time and resources and are more frequently hospitalized. Both detract from a large dialysis organization's income in a shared risk model. There is a need for nephrologists and large dialysis organizations to exercise professional ethics and maintain their fiduciary obligation to all patients including those who are the sickest.

# PAST: THE EVOLUTION OF DIALYSIS AND TRANSPLANT ETHICS IN THE UNITED STATES

## NEPHROLOGY'S CONTRIBUTION TO THE BIRTH OF BIOETHICS

Any review of the ethical issues facing nephrology should start by acknowledging the fundamental role that nephrology played in the early development of the field of bioethics. Because the life-sustaining therapies of dialysis and kidney transplantation predated many parallel therapies in other fields, the ethical issues that inevitably accompany these highly specialized medical treatments were first addressed by nephrologists. This chapter focuses on ethical developments with regard to dialysis and transplantation in the United States, because many innovations and associated ethical challenges occurred first in the United States. These experiences were instructive to other countries. A global perspective on the ethical challenges in treating patients with advanced kidney disease in low-resource countries and those with differing health-care systems is addressed later in this chapter.

Although dialysis had been used to save lives from acute kidney injury for years, chronic dialysis was only possible in 1960 with the invention of the arteriovenous shunt. Amid the excitement of this substantial medical advance, nephrologists were quickly confronted by the unprecedented ethical problem of determining which patients should be granted access to chronic hemodialysis (HD) given the limited availability of expensive machines. It was apparent that this decision required more than medical facts, and that value judgments would have a large influence. The Seattle Artificial Kidney Center invited a group of citizens to make allocation decisions, a role that was previously well within the guarded realm of physician autonomy. Historian David Rothman heralded this engagement of the lay population as the event that signaled the entrance of bioethics into medicine.[1] Bioethics scholar Albert Jonsen similarly believed that the field of bioethics emerged in response to the nationwide controversy that ensued.[2]

In his 1964 presidential address to the American Society of Artificial Internal Organs, Dr. Belding Scribner, one of the early fathers of nephrology, identified four major ethical problems that he and his colleagues were facing: 1. patient selection for dialysis; 2. termination of dialysis, which he called "dialysis suicide," but is now referred to as "stopping" or "withdrawing" dialysis; 3. "death with dignity," which involved the treatment of patients with end-stage renal disease (ESRD) who were having dialysis withheld or withdrawn; and 4. donor selection for transplantation.[3] Dr. Scribner anticipated many of the ethical challenges that would face nephrology and in parallel, many other fields of medicine. Other challenges were yet to be conceived.

Ethical issues arising in treating patients with advanced chronic kidney disease (CKD) can be unpacked using a principlist structure. Principlism is a widely accepted framework for identifying and analyzing ethical problems by applying four ethical principles: respect for autonomy, beneficence, nonmaleficence, and justice.[4] Fig. 82.1 presents a time line for the relative salience of these principles throughout the history of the ESRD program.[4] The fourth principle, justice, is particularly relevant to the first ethical challenge that Dr. Scribner identified in his address, patient selection for dialysis, and questions of distributive justice continue to arise in other settings through the evolution of nephrology health care.

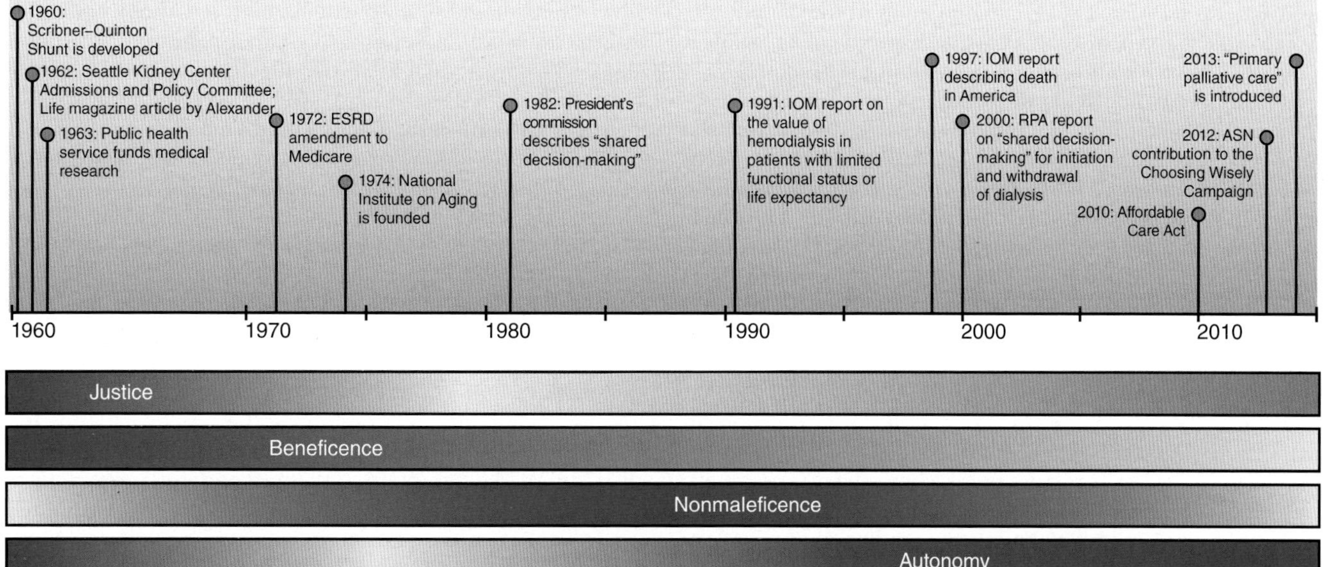


**Fig. 82.1** Time line of important events and publications related to the development of dialysis. Although there is significant overlap, the relative salience of each of the four principles varies over this course. *ASN,* American Society of Nephrology; *ESRD,* end-stage renal disease; *IOM,* Institute of Medicine; *RPA,* Renal Physicians Association. Used with permission of the American Society of Nephrology. Prior publication in the *Clinical Journal of the American Society of Nephrology*: Butler CR, Mehotra R, Tonelli MR, Lam DY. The evolving ethics of dialysis in the United States: A principlist bioethics approach. *Clin J Am Soc Nephrol.* 2016;11:704–709.

## RATIONING OF HEMODIALYSIS AND PATIENT SELECTION CRITERIA AT THE BEGINNING OF CHRONIC DIALYSIS IN THE UNITED STATES

The invention of the Quinton–Scribner arteriovenous shunt expanded the patient population who could potentially benefit from HD. When the first US chronic dialysis center, the Seattle Artificial Kidney Center, opened in 1962, the number of patients seeking dialysis treatment far outweighed the center's ability to provide it. Physicians used medical criteria to narrow the group to otherwise healthy patients aged 18 to 45 years, but there remained more candidates than could be accommodated and no established criteria to decide who amongst them would receive the life-sustaining treatment. The ethical principle of justice requires distribution of benefits and burdens in a way that is most fair and/or useful, and that each patient receives that to which she is entitled. In 1962 the ethical problem confronting the Seattle Artificial Kidney Center was one of distributive justice, because they did not have enough dialysis machines or trained personnel to provide dialysis to all patients with ESRD.

Health-care rationing is when a treatment that may benefit a patient is withheld because of resource limitation. The Seattle Artificial Kidney Center was challenged with how to ration dialysis. In response, the Seattle group appointed the Admissions and Policy Committee. The group was composed of a dozen citizens intended to represent a broad swath of the local community and who were tasked with selecting between medically suitable dialysis candidates in the state of Washington. The committee considered choosing patients by lottery, but rejected this idea, believing that more ethical decisions could be made by active selection based on a patient's ability to be rehabilitated and eventually return on society's investment in their health. Factors taken into consideration included age and sex, marital status and number of dependents, income, net worth, emotional stability, educational background, occupation, and future potential contribution. As the selection process evolved, a pattern emerged in which committee decisions weighed heavily on a narrow definition of a favorable personal character and valuable contribution to society.[5]

Journalist Shana Alexander called national attention to the committee in her *Life Magazine* article, "They Decide Who Lives, Who Dies: Medical Miracle Puts Moral Burden on Small Committee."[5] Once public, the Seattle dialysis patient selection process was subjected to harsh criticism. The committee was castigated for using upper middle-class values and social-worth criteria to make decisions.[6] Critics wrote, "The prejudices and mindless clichés that pollute the committee's deliberations ... [rule out] creative non-conformists, who rub the bourgeoisie the wrong way but who historically have contributed so much to the making of America. The Pacific Northwest [where Seattle is located in the US] is no place for a Henry David Thoreau with bad kidneys."[7] The increasingly complex ethical structure on which medicine is practiced was exposed to the public, making several points clear. First, the public has a moral stake in how medical decisions are made. Further, in situations requiring rationing, it is unacceptable to make life and death decisions based on a narrow definition of social worth, though a clear set of guidelines was yet to be developed. Policy decisions over the following years emphasized the country's preference to avoid rationing altogether if possible, even at great financial cost.

### US HEALTH-CARE COVERAGE FOR DIALYSIS AND AN EXPANDING DIALYSIS PATIENT DEMOGRAPHIC

The prevailing distaste for health-care rationing practices was reflected by Senator Russell Long of Louisiana following contentious policy debates in the United States, who remarked, "We are the greatest nation in the world, the wealthiest per capita. Are we so hard pressed that we cannot pay for...a life extended for 10–15 years?"[8] In 1972, passage of the ESRD Amendment to Medicare, Section 2991 of Public Law 92-603, virtually eliminated the need to ration dialysis. The US Congress passed this legislation because of the clear life and death urgency of chronic dialysis for patients with ESRD and the expectation that the number of patients who would need this treatment would be limited. This legislation classified ESRD patients who were otherwise eligible for Social Security as disabled and authorized a Medicare entitlement covering dialysis and transplantation.[9] Neither Congress nor physicians thought it necessary or proper for the government to further direct which patients were appropriate candidates for dialysis. Although in the early days of dialysis, medical criteria for acceptance to the dialysis program had limited patients to those who were young and relatively healthy, many believed that it was morally unjustified to deny dialysis treatment to any patient with ESRD.[6] A decade later, the first report of the US Renal Data System documented the progressively greater acceptance rate of patients for dialysis treatment,[10] explained in part by the inclusion of patients who had poor prognoses, especially the elderly and those with diabetic nephropathy.[11] By 2000, 48% of new patients starting dialysis were 65 years of age or older and 45% had ESRD from diabetes. Observers raised concerns about the appropriateness of treating patients with a limited life expectancy and quality of life.[9,12] Others questioned the utility of providing dialysis to patients with life-threatening illnesses such as end-stage cardiovascular disease, debilitating pulmonary disease, or untreatable cancer. Benefit was also unclear in patients with severe neurologic disease which rendered them unable to engage with others, such as those in a persistent vegetative state, with severe dementia, or with debilitating cerebrovascular disease.[13]

In 1991, the Institute of Medicine Committee for the Study of the Medicare ESRD Program emphasized that the existence of the public entitlement for treatment of ESRD does not obligate physicians to treat all patients who have kidney failure with dialysis or transplantation.[9] For some, the burden of dialysis substantially outweighed the benefit. The provision of dialysis to these patients would violate the medical maxim, "Be of benefit and do no harm." In other words, the decision to institute a life-sustaining therapy required a balance of beneficence and nonmaleficence. Systematic differences amongst providers and regional variation in gauging the resultant balance of these factors risked causing health-care disparity.[14,15] The committee recommended that guidelines be developed for identifying such patients but with continued respect for physicians' discretion in individual assessment. Such guidelines were intended to help nephrologists make dialysis decisions more uniformly, with greater ease, and in a way that promoted patient benefit. The first edition of the clinical practice guidelines on *Shared Decision-Making in the Appropriate Initiation of and Withdrawal from Dialysis* was published in 2000.[16]

### WITHDRAWAL FROM DIALYSIS

In the 1960s, patients felt fortunate to be among the few chosen by dialysis selection committees to receive a rationed therapy. No one anticipated that a patient might choose to forgo this sought-after treatment knowing that they would shortly die. Practitioners grappled with whether this so-called dialysis suicide was a form of psychopathology or whether, given the unprecedented nature of the life-sustaining therapy, requests to "stop the machine" should be interpreted differently. Physicians and ethicists drew on Catholic moral theology that makes a distinction between ordinary and extraordinary measures, the latter not being morally obligatory. They concluded that patients may refuse or stop aggressive interventions such as dialysis, because they represent extraordinary attempts to sustain life.[17]

In its 1983 report, *Deciding to Forego Life-Sustaining Treatment*, the President's Commission for the Study of Ethical Problems in Medicine and Biomedical and Behavioral Research considered ethical and legal issues raised by life-sustaining treatments such as dialysis. The commission understood that "biomedical developments ... have made death more a matter of deliberate decision. ... Matters once the province of fate have now become a matter of human choice."[18] The President's Commission reached two major conclusions that provide justification for withholding and withdrawing dialysis: "the voluntary choice of a competent and informed patient should determine whether or not life-sustaining therapy will be undertaken; and health-care professionals serve patients best by maintaining a presumption in favor of sustaining life, while recognizing that competent patients are entitled to choose to forgo any treatments, including those that sustain life."[18]

Similarly, in its 1993 annual report, the End-Stage Renal Disease Data Advisory Committee to the US Renal Data System articulated ethical justifications and general and specific principles to be used in making decisions about withholding or withdrawing dialysis. This report reflected the deliberations of an ad hoc committee composed of nephrologists, ethicists, and health policy experts. The report described two ethical justifications for forgoing dialysis: 1. the right of patients to refuse dialysis based on the ethical principle of respect for autonomy and the legal right of self-determination; and 2. a judgment that dialysis does not offer a reasonable expectation of medical benefit based on the ethical principles of beneficence and nonmaleficence.[19]

An early study attempting to describe how these principles were adopted in practice noted that dialysis withdrawal accounted for 22% of deaths in one large dialysis program,[20] ranking behind cardiovascular disease and infection as the most common cause of death in this population. Subsequent research found that older patients (those aged 65 years or older) and patients with diabetes were the most likely to stop dialysis. According to a survey of dialysis units performed in 1990, at least one and on average three patients withdrew from dialysis in the preceding year.[14]

The recommendations of these regulatory bodies emphasize the importance of optimizing benefit and reducing harm while introducing the emerging concept of respect for autonomous choice. However, the process of arriving at a balance between these values incorporating input from the nephrologist, patient, and family remained opaque. Simple answers were not forthcoming as individual patients evaluate benefits and burdens differently and enter discussion with varying cognitive abilities and social backgrounds.

## PRESENT

### ADVANCE DIRECTIVES AND DIALYSIS PATIENTS

By the 1990s, studies showed that 90% of nephrologists would stop dialysis at the request of a patient with decision-making capacity.[14,15] Nephrologists also expressed a willingness to stop dialysis of "irreversibly incompetent" patients who had previously documented their wish to stop in such a condition. However, they disagreed about how to treat these patients in the absence of clear advance directives.[15] Following a precedent set in the earliest days of dialysis, there was a strong default toward continued treatment for patients who could not or had not expressed their wishes. Therefore, a patient's right to forgo dialysis was difficult to exercise in these circumstances.

The Patient Self-Determination Act, which required institutions participating in Medicare and Medicade to educate patients about the importance of completing advance directives, became effective in December 1991.[21] Although the ESRD program was almost entirely funded by Medicare, dialysis units were inadvertently left out of the law. This was a problematic omission given that advance care planning is especially important for dialysis patients for several reasons[22]: 1. about half of the dialysis population is elderly, and the elderly have the shortest life expectancy on dialysis and are the most likely to withdraw or be withdrawn from dialysis; 2. prior discussion of advance directives has been shown to help dialysis patients and their families approach death in a reconciled fashion[23]; 3. patients who discuss and complete written advance directives are significantly more likely to have their wish to die at home respected; 4. unless a specific directive to withhold cardiopulmonary resuscitation is obtained—which can be done in the framework of advance care planning—it will be automatically provided, even though it rarely leads to extended survival in dialysis patients.[24]

It had already been established that many dialysis patients have a personal threshold at which point they would choose to stop aggressive care. Discussions and documentation to specify these situations in advance protect autonomy and personal preferences when patients are unable to advocate for themselves. For these reasons, nephrologists have been encouraged to discuss the circumstances under which patients would want to discontinue dialysis and forgo cardiopulmonary resuscitation and to urge patients to complete written advance directives.[25] When patients lack decision-making capacity and have not completed advance directives, ethically complex issues often arise in discussion about whether to start or stop dialysis. In these situations, many nephrologists indicate that they would consult an ethics committee for assistance.[14] See Chapter 62 for more discussion on the practical aspects of decision-making in this context.

## FINANCING DIALYSIS CENTERS AND CONFLICTS OF INTEREST

Conflict of interest occurs when there is a clash between a physician or medical group's interests and the welfare of a patient. These conflicts represent a serious challenge to a physician–patient relationship, which is based on open disclosure of patient information under the assumption of a physician's fiduciary responsibility to prioritize the patient's goals over their own. Fee-for-service medicine will always involve some conflict of interest, but nephrology has encountered particularly problematic situations when physicians share ownership in for-profit dialysis centers in which they treat patients. In these cases, nephrologists are financially rewarded for reducing costs. While not inherently problematic, cost reduction can compromise patient welfare if it entails decreasing dialysis time, purchasing less effective equipment, or hiring fewer nurses, social workers, and dietitians.

For-profit dialysis companies flourished under the early ESRD program and, by 1990, they accommodated two-thirds of ESRD patients.[26] Physicians were paid per-patient and centers paid per-treatment. Although this incentive structure does not necessitate unethical practice, trends in care suggested that compensation may have driven some aspects of care. The United States quickly developed the highest dialysis patient acceptance rate in the world.[11] Short dialysis times, which are associated with increased mortality, were found disproportionately in for-profit dialysis units. Patients treated in these units had a 20% higher mortality rate and a 26% lower rate of referral for renal transplantation.[27]

In order to hold dialysis units accountable for the quality of care they provided, the Medicare ESRD program, through the 18 ESRD networks, established quality indicators to measure the performance of dialysis units both individually and regionally. Metrics included adequacy of dialysis, anemia management, vascular access placement, and standardized mortality ratios. Despite the intention to improve care, some raised concerns that a focus on metrics could lead practitioners to "cherry pick" healthier patients who would improve their units' aggregate numbers while restricting access to sicker or more socially complex patients.[28] Cherry picking, patient solicitation, and other forms of acting in favor of physician or medical group interest rather than patient welfare compromise a physician's fiduciary responsibility and the very foundation of medicine and the doctor–patient relationship.

## CKD CARE AND DIALYSIS OF THE OLDER AND/OR MULTIMORBID PATIENT

Old age and medical comorbidity are no longer seen as contraindications to dialysis. Far from it, as the population ages and diabetes and other chronic conditions become more prevalent, the number of very elderly patients (those aged 75 years or older) has become the fastest growing patient population on dialysis.[29] Deciding whether to start elderly patients with CKD on dialysis involves an understanding and consideration of factors common to this group including reduced life span, complex comorbidities, heterogeneous personal values, and varied quality of life.[30]

Between 1996 and 2003, rates of dialysis initiation among octogenarians and nonagenarians nearly doubled.[31] At the same time, median survival for patients aged 85 to 89 beginning dialysis was only 8.4 months compared with 24.9 months for patients aged 65 to 70.[31] Clinical characteristics such as older age, nonambulatory status, poor nutritional status, and presence of comorbid conditions were associated with shorter life span.[31] Amongst US veterans with CKD stage 3 to 5, those older than 75 were far more likely to die than to develop ESRD.[32] In a study comparing dialysis with conservative treatment in a population of patients greater than 75 years old with advanced CKD, there was a 2.9-fold greater survival on dialysis.[30] However, in a multivariate subgroup analysis of these older patients, dialysis offered no survival benefit for patients with ischemic heart disease or those with the highest comorbidity scores. This finding has since been replicated.[33,34] Moreover, researchers have found that comorbid conditions do not influence the decision to initiate dialysis treatment despite the fact that comorbidity strongly influences CKD patients' prognosis.[35]

Trends toward higher medical resource use among the older population despite uncertain benefits have led some to be concerned about the "biomedicalization of aging" in which technology is used for its own sake rather than as merely a means to support individual life goals.[36] Medical anthropologist Sharon Kaufman identified indiscriminant use of dialysis in the elderly as a prime example. She describes the "routinization" of starting dialysis for older patients, and the impact of societal expectations in which there is no age limit to the use of standard medical treatments. She writes that nephrologists report they feel obligated to dialyze very old patients even if they have personal moral concerns about whether the patient is likely to benefit.[37]

Given the unique aspects of caring for an older and multimorbid population, the Renal Physicians Association and American Society of Nephrology clinical practice guideline emphasized the importance of discussing prognosis and advance care planning with elderly patients and their families to make individualized decisions.[16,31] These data argue against an "age-neutral" approach to the management of CKD and emphasized the need for prognostic tools that enable clinicians to identify the subgroup of older patients who are most likely to benefit from dialysis.[32] An integrated prognostic tool to estimate 6-month mortality in dialysis patients was developed and validated with a C-statistic of 0.80. It considers age, serum albumin, dementia, peripheral vascular disease, and the nephrologist's response to the surprise question ("Would I be surprised if this patient died in the next six months?")[38] The accuracy of this tool in the stage 5 CKD population remains to be studied. One observer raised the possibility that the standard content of informed consent for dialysis warrants an age-sensitive approach that is attuned to the different balance of advantages and harms of dialysis for older patients with multiple comorbidities.[39] The American Geriatrics Society has developed a structure for approaching the medical evidence base recognizing that it is often difficult to extrapolate results from trial data to an elderly population.[40] See Chapter 84 for more discussion of decision-making and clinical management of elderly patients with CKD.

*Clinical Relevance*

Clinical characteristics of advanced chronic kidney disease patients such as older age, nonambulatory status, poor nutritional status, and presence of comorbid conditions are associated with shorter life span. In a multivariate subgroup analysis of older patients, dialysis offered no survival benefit for patients with ischemic heart disease or those with the highest comorbidity scores.

## ETHICAL ISSUES IN ESRD END-OF-LIFE CARE

The Robert Wood Johnson Foundation ESRD Peer Work Group stated in 2002 that "most patients with ESRD, especially those who are not candidates for renal transplantation, have a significantly shortened life expectancy."[41] In the wake of public dissatisfaction with end-of-life care practices across the breadth of chronic disease, nephrology physician groups, including the Renal Physicians Association and American Society of Nephrology, recognized that they have a particular ethical responsibility to improve patients' experience of the end of life. Given the shortened life expectancy and high symptom burden of this population, they noted it was especially important that nephrologists and dialysis staff learn primary palliative care techniques and also have the ability to refer to palliative specialists. Nephrology fellowships generally have yet to respond to this need with specialized training in primary palliative care and end-of-life care, but trainees report a sense of moral obligation to provide such care.[42]

Palliative care strategies can promote the autonomy of CKD patients. Although notoriously difficult for clinicians, prognostication is critically important for patients planning their remaining time. The "surprise" question identifies dialysis patients at high risk for early mortality. The odds of a patient dying within a year were shown to be 3.5 times higher if the nephrologist or nephrology nurse practitioner answered "No" than for those patients about whom the provider answered "Yes."[43] Nephrologists have been encouraged to implement the surprise question monthly on dialysis rounds to screen for patients who might benefit from palliative care intervention.

When dialysis is deemed not beneficial, it is critical to have alternative care options available. Physicians struggle with the decision against dialysis when there seems to be "nothing else to offer." Patients similarly feel that they are not adequately counseled on alternatives to dialysis and express a sense of "powerlessness" when faced with ESRD.[44] "Comprehensive conservative care" as defined by a Kidney Disease Improving Global Outcomes (KDIGO) consensus group includes interventions to delay progression, control symptoms, and promote social support, but excludes treatment with dialysis.[45] In order for this approach to be viable, further research and evidence are needed, as well as established pathways to mirror the multidisciplinary coordinated care that is already built into the dialysis network (see Chapter 62: Supportive Care in Advanced Chronic Kidney Disease).

Even with effective communication and preparation, it is often difficult for patients to fully anticipate the impact of dialysis on their life. The concept of a "time-limited trial" is a way to avoid a sense of inflexible commitment to a treatment strategy when the benefit of the treatment to the particular patient is uncertain.[46] Dialysis may be initiated with a planned reevaluation of whether goals are being met with continuation or withdrawal based on this assessment.

## SHARED DECISION-MAKING AND CLINICAL PRACTICE GUIDELINE ON APPROPRIATE USE OF DIALYSIS

In an effort to reduce the variation in dialysis practices between physicians and across regions of the United States, clinical practice guidelines have been established over the last decades. By the early 1990s, demographics of the ESRD population had changed greatly from earlier years. Nephrologists reported being asked to provide dialysis to patients for whom it seemed of marginal benefit including patients who were elderly and with multiple comorbidities. The US Renal Data System confirmed highest incident treatment rates for 75- to 79-year-old patients.[47] By contrast, research found that some patients regret their decision to start dialysis, but felt they had no other choice.[48,49] In 1991, the Institute of Medicine recommended development of an evidence-based, clinical practice guideline "for evaluating patients for whom the burdens of renal replacement therapy may substantially outweigh the benefits."[13]

A paradigm of "shared decision-making" was developed to address these questions, and has become the ethical standard for health-care practice. Through this process, physicians and patients agree on a specific course of action based on a common understanding of treatment goals and the risks and benefits of each option. However, there are acknowledged limits to this process in cases where the patient's preferences and medical team's sense of beneficial course cannot be reconciled. In these cases, a patient has the right to refuse dialysis even if the renal care team disagrees with the decision. Similarly, the renal care team has the right to refuse to offer dialysis when the expected benefits do not justify the risks.

In 2000 the Renal Physicians Association and the American Society of Nephrology published the clinical practice guideline *Shared Decision-Making in the Appropriate Initiation of and Withdrawal from Dialysis.*[16] These guidelines were intended to help those involved in care of CKD and ESRD patients including nephrologists, intensivists, primary-care physicians, nephrology nurses, advanced practice nurses, and nephrology social workers. The guidelines are also potentially useful to patients and their families, renal dietitians, dialysis technicians, renal administrators, clergy, and policy makers.

In the following years, an extensive evidence base was developed regarding dialysis decision-making, including 1. the poor prognosis of some elderly stage 4 and 5 CKD patients, many of whom are likely to die prior to initiation of dialysis or for whom dialysis may not provide a survival advantage over medical management without dialysis; 2. the prevalence of cognitive impairment in dialysis patients and the need to periodically assess them for decision-making capacity; 3. the underrecognition and undertreatment of pain and other symptoms in dialysis patients; 4. the underutilization of hospice in dialysis patients; and 5. the distinctly different treatment goals of ESRD patients based on their overall condition and personal preferences. In 2010 the Renal Physicians Association developed a second edition of the guideline to provide

**Box 82.1 Systematic Evaluation of a Patient or Family Request to Stop Dialysis**[50]

1. Determine the reasons or conditions underlying the patient/surrogate desires regarding withdrawal of dialysis. Such assessment should include specific medical, physical, spiritual, and psychological issues, as well as interventions that could be appropriate. Some of the potentially treatable factors that might be included in the assessment are as follows:
   a. Underlying medical disorders, including the prognosis for short- or long-term survival on dialysis
   b. Difficulties with dialysis treatments
   c. The patient's assessment of his or her quality of life and ability to function
   d. The patient's short- and long-terms goals
   e. The burden that costs of continued treatment/medications/diet/transportation may have on the patient/family/others
   f. The patient's psychological condition, including depression and conditions or symptoms that may be caused by uremia
   g. Undue influence or pressure from outside sources, including the patient's family
   h. Conflict between the patient and others
   i. Dissatisfaction with the dialysis modality, the time, or the setting of treatment
2. If the patient wishes to withdraw from dialysis, did he or she consent to referral to a counseling professional (e.g., social worker, spiritual advisor, psychologist, or psychiatrist)?
3. If the patient wishes to withdraw from dialysis, are there interventions that could alter the patient's circumstances that might result in his or her considering it reasonable to continue dialysis?
   a. Describe possible interventions.
   b. Does the patient desire the proposed intervention(s)?
4. In cases in which the surrogate has made the decision to either continue or withdraw dialysis, has it been determined that the judgment of the surrogate is consistent with the stated desires of the patient?
5. Questions to consider when a patient asks to stop dialysis:
   a. Is the patient's decision-making capacity diminished by depression, encephalopathy, or other disorder?
   b. Why does the patient want to stop dialysis?
   c. Are the patient's perceptions about the technical or quality-of-life aspects of dialysis accurate?
   d. Does the patient really mean what he or she says or is the decision to stop dialysis made to get attention, help, or control?
   e. Can any changes be made that might improve life on dialysis for the patient?
   f. Would the patient be willing to continue dialysis while the factors responsible for the patient's request are addressed?
   g. Has the patient discussed his or her desire to stop dialysis with significant others such as family, friends, or spiritual advisors? What do they think about the patient's request?

From Shared Decision-Making in the Appropriate Initiation of and Withdrawal From Dialysis. 2nd ed. Rockville, MD: Renal Physicians Association; 2010.

clinicians, patients, and families with 1. the most current evidence about the benefits and burdens of dialysis for patients with diverse conditions; 2. recommendations for quality in decision-making about treatment of patients with acute kidney injury, CKD, and ESRD; and 3. practical strategies to help clinicians implement the guideline recommendations.[50] Box 82.1 presents a practical approach from the guideline on how to systematically evaluate a patient's request to stop dialysis.

This second edition also made explicit recommendations to integrate palliative care into the treatment of CKD and ESRD patients and to develop quality metrics for dialysis patients whose goals of care focus on comfort that are distinct from those whose goals are to aggressively prolong life and function. It noted that good communication improves patients' adjustment to illness, increases adherence to treatment, and results in higher patient and family satisfaction. The second edition called on nephrologists and other members of the interdisciplinary team to communicate prognostic information, allowing patients to reach more informed decisions about dialysis and transplantation options. It urged nephrology fellowship programs to incorporate training in effective, empathetic communication skills so that patients' decisions can be based on an accurate understanding of their overall condition and the pros and cons of treatment options.[50] The roles of supportive or palliative care and incorporation of these options into treatment planning are discussed further in Chapter 62.

The objectives for both editions of this guideline are listed in Box 82.2. The second edition provides 10 recommendations with regard to decision-making about withholding or withdrawing dialysis and the care of patients who forgo dialysis

**Box 82.2 Objectives of the Clinical Practice Guideline Shared Decision-Making in the Appropriate Initiation of and Withdrawal From Dialysis**[50]

- Synthesize available research evidence regarding patients with acute kidney injury and end-stage renal disease (ESRD) as a basis for making recommendations about withholding and withdrawing dialysis.
- Enhance understanding of the principles and processes useful for and involved in making decisions to withhold or withdraw dialysis.
- Promote ethically as well as medically sound decision-making in individual cases.
- Recommend tools that can be used to promote shared decision-making in the care of patients with acute kidney injury or ESRD.
- Offer a publicly understandable and acceptable ethical framework for shared decision-making among health-care providers, patients, and their families.

From Shared Decision-Making in the Appropriate Initiation of and Withdrawal From Dialysis. 2nd ed. Rockville, MD: Renal Physicians Association; 2010.

(Box 82.3). These guidelines have been widely quoted in the nephrology and palliative care literature, and studies have documented their effectiveness.[51–53] More than half of US nephrologists in 2005 reported awareness and use of these guidelines and surveys, and a comparison of nephrologist

## Box 82.3 Renal Physicians Association Clinical Practice Guideline Recommendations for Shared Dialysis Decision-Making[50]

### Establishing a Shared Decision-Making Relationship

***Recommendation No. 1***

**Develop a physician–patient relationship for shared decision-making.**

Shared decision-making is the recognized preferred model for medical decision-making because it addresses the ethical need to fully inform patients about the risks and benefits of treatments, as well as the need to ensure that patients' values and preferences play a prominent role. Because of the number and complexity of decisions involved in treating kidney failure, a shared decision-making relationship is particularly important for patients with acute kidney injury (AKI), stage 4 and 5 chronic kidney disease (CKD), and stage 5 CKD requiring dialysis end-stage renal disease (ESRD). Participants in shared decision-making should involve at a minimum the patient and the physician. In addition, patients should identify and include a person who could serve as their decision-maker in the event they lose decision-making capacity. If a patient lacks decision-making capacity, decisions should involve the person legally authorized to make health-care decisions on behalf of the incapacitated patient. This person is often (though not always) a family member and will be called "the legal agent" in the remainder of this document (see Glossary for a full description). With the patient's consent, shared decision-making may include family members or friends and other members of the health-care team.

### Informing Patients

***Recommendation No. 2***

**Fully inform AKI, stage 4 and 5 CKD, and ESRD patients about their diagnosis, prognosis, and all treatment options.**

In the setting of critical illness many patients with CKD will require urgent dialysis and the vast majority of patients with AKI will have multiple medical problems, in addition to kidney failure. The concept of shared decision-making necessitates a multidisciplinary approach including nephrologists, intensivists, and others as appropriate and decisions about acute renal replacement therapy should be made in the context of other life-sustaining treatments. For example, a decision to withhold dialysis in a patient agreeing to and receiving multiple other forms of life-sustaining therapy could represent discordant treatment in the same way that offering dialysis to a patient who has decided to forgo other forms of life-sustaining therapy might be inappropriate. Intensive care physicians need to be included in shared decision-making for kidney patients in the intensive care unit (ICU).

For ESRD patients, the shared decision-making options include:

1. available dialysis modalities and kidney transplantation if applicable
2. not starting dialysis and continuing medical management
3. a time-limited trial of dialysis
4. stopping dialysis and receiving end-of-life care.

Choices among options should be made by patients or, if patients lack decision-making capacity, their designated legal agents. Their decisions should be informed and voluntary. The renal care team, in conjunction with the primary care physician, should insure that the patient or legal agent understands the benefits and burdens of dialysis and the consequences of not starting or stopping dialysis. Research studies have identified a population of CKD patients for whom the prognosis is particularly poor. This population has been found to include patients with two or more of the following characteristics: (1) elderly (defined by research studies identifying poor outcomes in patients who are aged 75 years and older); (2) patients with high comorbidity scores (e.g., modified Charlson Comorbidity Index score of ≥8); (3) marked functional impairment (e.g., Karnofsky Performance Status Scale score of < 40); and (4) severe chronic malnutrition (e.g., serum albumin level < 2.5 g/dL using the bromocresol green method). Patients in this population should be informed that dialysis may not confer a survival advantage or improve functional status over medical management without dialysis and that dialysis entails significant burdens that may detract from their quality of life.

***Recommendation No. 3***

**Give all patients with AKI, stage 5 CKD, or ESRD an estimate of prognosis specific to their overall condition.**

To facilitate informed decisions about starting dialysis for AKI, stage 5 CKD, or ESRD, all patients should have their prognosis estimated and discussed, with the realization that the ability to predict survival in the individual patient is limited. Depending on the setting, a primary care physician, intensivist, or nephrologist who is familiar with estimating and communicating prognosis should conduct these discussions (see Recommendation No. 10 for communication strategies). For patients with ESRD, the "surprise" question "Would I be surprised if this patient died in the next year?" can be used together with known risk factors for poor prognosis: age, comorbidities, severe malnutrition, and poor functional status. For patients with stage 5 CKD predialysis, the estimate of prognosis should be discussed with the patient or legal agent, patient's family, and among the medical team members to develop a consensus on the goals of care and whether dialysis or active medical management without dialysis should be used to best achieve these goals. These discussions should occur as early as possible in the course of the patient's kidney disease and continue as the kidney disease progresses. For ESRD patients on dialysis who experience major complications that may substantially reduce survival or quality of life, it is appropriate to reassess treatment goals, including consideration of withdrawal from dialysis.

### Facilitating Advance Care Planning

***Recommendation No. 4***

**Institute advance care planning.**

The purpose of advance care planning is to help the patient understand his/her condition, identify his/her goals for care, and prepare for the decisions that may have to be made as the condition progresses over time. For chronic dialysis patients, the interdisciplinary renal care team should encourage patient–family discussion and advance care planning and include advance care planning in the overall plan of care for each individual patient (see Section 10: Glossary for definition of renal care team). The renal care team should designate a person to be primarily responsible for ensuring that advance care planning is offered to each patient. Patients with decision-making capacity should be "strongly" encouraged while they have capacity to talk to their legal agents to ensure that the legal agent knows the patient's wishes and agrees to make decisions according to these wishes.

The renal care team should attempt to obtain written advance directives from all dialysis patients. Where legally accepted, Physician Orders for Life-Sustaining Treatment or similar state-specific forms, also should be completed as part of the advance care planning process. At a minimum, each dialysis patient should be asked to designate a legal agent in a state-specific advance directive. Advance directives should be honored by dialysis centers,

*Continued on following page*

**Box 82.3 Renal Physicians Association Clinical Practice Guideline Recommendations for Shared Dialysis Decision-Making** (Continued)

nephrologists, and other nephrology clinicians except possibly in situations in which the advance directive requests treatment contrary to the standard of care (see Recommendation No. 8 on conflict resolution).

**Making a Decision to Not Initiate or to Discontinue Dialysis**

***Recommendation No. 5***[a]

**If appropriate, forgo (withhold initiating or withdraw ongoing) dialysis for patients with AKI, CKD, or ESRD in certain, well-defined situations.**

These situations include the following:

- Patients with decision-making capacity, who being fully informed and making voluntary choices, refuse dialysis or request that dialysis be discontinued.
- Patients who no longer possess decision-making capacity who have previously indicated refusal of dialysis in an oral or written advance directive.
- Patients who no longer possess decision-making capacity and whose properly appointed legal agents/surrogates refuse dialysis or request that it be discontinued.
- Patients with irreversible, profound neurological impairment such that they lack signs of thought, sensation, purposeful behavior, and awareness of self and environment.

***Recommendation No. 6***

**Consider forgoing dialysis for AKI, CKD, or ESRD patients who have a very poor prognosis or for whom dialysis cannot be provided safely.**

Included in these categories of patients are the following:

- Those whose medical condition precludes the technical process of dialysis because the patient is unable to cooperate (e.g., advanced dementia patient who pulls out dialysis needles) or because the patient's condition is too unstable (e.g., profound hypotension).
- Those who have a terminal illness from nonrenal causes (acknowledging that some in this condition may perceive benefit from and choose to undergo dialysis).
- Those with stage 5 CKD older than age 75 years who meet two or more of the following statistically significant very poor prognosis criteria (see Recommendation Nos 2 and 3): 1. clinicians' response of "No, I would not be surprised" to the surprise question; 2. high comorbidity score; 3. significantly impaired functional status (e.g., Karnofsky Performance Status score < 40); and 4. severe chronic malnutrition (i.e., serum albumin < 2.5 g/dL using the bromocresol green method).

**Resolving Conflicts About What Dialysis Decisions to Make**

***Recommendation No. 7***

**Consider a time-limited trial of dialysis for patients requiring dialysis, but who have an uncertain prognosis, or for whom a consensus cannot be reached about providing dialysis.**

If a time-limited trial of dialysis is conducted, the nephrologist, the patient, the patient's legal agent, and the patient's family (with the patient's permission to participate in decision-making) should agree in advance on the length of the trial and parameters to be assessed during and at the completion of the time-limited trial to determine whether dialysis has benefited the patient and whether dialysis should be continued.

***Recommendation No. 8***

**Establish a systematic due process approach for conflict resolution if there is disagreement about what decision should be made with regard to dialysis.**

Conflicts may occur between the patient/legal agent and the renal care team about whether dialysis will benefit the patient. Conflicts also may occur within the renal care team or between the renal care team and other health-care providers. In sitting down and talking with the patient/legal agent, the nephrologist should try to understand their views, provide data to support his/her recommendation, and correct misunderstandings. In the process of shared decision-making, the following potential sources of conflict have been recognized: 1. miscommunication or misunderstanding about prognosis; 2. intrapersonal or interpersonal issues; or 3. special values. If dialysis is indicated emergently, it should be provided while pursuing conflict resolution, provided the patient or legal agent requests it.

**Providing Effective Palliative Care**

***Recommendation No. 9***

**To improve patient-centered outcomes, offer palliative care services and interventions to all AKI, CKD, and ESRD patients who suffer from burdens of their disease.**

Palliative care services are appropriate for people who choose to undergo or remain on dialysis and for those who choose not to start or to discontinue dialysis. With the patient's consent, a multiprofessional team with expertise in renal palliative care, including nephrology professionals, family, or community-based professionals, and specialist hospice or palliative care providers, should be involved in managing the physical, psychological, social, and spiritual aspects of treatment for these patients, including end-of-life care. Physical and psychological symptoms should be routinely and regularly assessed and actively managed. The professionals providing treatment should be trained in assessing and managing symptoms and in advanced communication skills. Patients should be offered the option of dying where they prefer, including at home with hospice care, provided there is sufficient and appropriate support to enable this option. Support also should be offered to patients' families, including bereavement support where appropriate. Dialysis patients for whom the goals of care are primarily comfort should have quality measures distinct from patients for whom the goals are aggressive therapy with optimization of functional capacity.

***Recommendation No. 10***

**Use a systematic approach to communicate about diagnosis, prognosis, treatment options, and goals of care.**

Good communication improves patients' adjustment to illness, increases adherence to treatment, and results in higher patient and family satisfaction with care. Patients appreciate sensitive delivery of information about their prognosis and the ability to balance reality while maintaining hope. In communicating with patients, the critical task for clinicians is to integrate complicated biomedical facts and conditions with emotional, social, and spiritual realities that are equally complex but not well described in the language of medicine. This information must be communicated in a way that patients, legal agents, and families can understand and use to reach informed decisions about dialysis and transplantation options. Patients' decisions should be based on an accurate understanding of their condition and the pros and cons of treatment options. To facilitate effective communication,

**Box 82.3 Renal Physicians Association Clinical Practice Guideline Recommendations for Shared Dialysis Decision-Making** (Continued)

reliance upon a multidisciplinary approach including nephrologists, intensivists, and others as appropriate is warranted. Decisions about acute renal replacement therapy in AKI should be made in the context of other life-sustaining treatments. Intensive care physicians should be included in shared decision-making for kidney patients in the ICU to facilitate discussions on global disease or injury prognosis. Fellowship programs should incorporate training to help nephrologists develop effective, empathetic communication skills, which are essential in caring for this patient population.

[a]Medical management incorporating palliative care is an integral part of the decision to forgo dialysis in AKI, CKD, or ESRD, and attention to patient comfort and quality of life while dying should be addressed directly or managed by palliative care consultation and referral to a hospice program (see Recommendation No. 9 on palliative care services).

From *Shared Decision-Making in the Appropriate Initiation of and Withdrawal From Dialysis*. 2nd ed. Rockville, MD: Renal Physicians Association; 2010.

knowledge and attitudes between 1991 and 2005 showed increasing alignment with their recommendations. More homogeneity has been noted in practices on withholding care in patients with permanent cognitive deficits. More US dialysis centers had written policies on cardiopulmonary resuscitation and dialysis withdrawal. Nephrologists were more likely to honor a dialysis patient's do-not-resuscitate order (66% in 1990 and 83% in 2005) and to consider consulting an ESRD network ethics committee (39% in 1990 and 52% in 2005).[53] Although these results are promising, recent research continues to show that shared decision-making remains poorly integrated into the practice of predialysis counseling of advanced CKD patients about their treatment options.[54]

Because of the early recognition of heterogeneity in practice causing potential health-care disparity and issues of justice, clinical practice guidelines have focused on practice and process of withdrawing and withholding dialysis. A recent meta-analysis draws attention to the breadth of ethical issues in nephrology with many related to heterogeneous practice including referral from primary care to nephrology, referral to transplantation, delivery of prognosis, and availability of alternative treatment options.[55] The authors recognize the success of guidelines in dialysis care and suggest that development of a broader scope of clinical practice guidelines may address these growing concerns. Shared-decision making is challenging because it requires robust and recurring discussion of core patient values and treatment options, but if done well, it may significantly improve patient-centered care for dialysis patients.[54]

***Clinical Relevance***

A paradigm of shared decision-making has become the ethical standard for health-care practice. Through this process, physicians and patients agree on a specific course of action based on a common understanding of treatment goals and the risks and benefits of each option. Shared decision-making prior to the initiation of dialysis has been recommended by the American Society of Nephrology and the Renal Physicians Association.

## ACCESS TO RENAL TRANSPLANTATION IN THE UNITED STATES

Dr. Scribner was prescient in 1964 when he identified donor selection for transplantation as one of the major ethical problems facing nephrologists. There is little disagreement that the quality of life for ESRD patients is often better after transplantation, and most patients prefer this strategy to continuing dialysis.[56] Research also shows that transplantation is associated with lower costs to the health-care system. In recent times, organ shortage has replaced immunologic barriers as the major hurdle to transplantation.[57] Because the growth in the number of transplantations has not kept pace with the growth in the incidence of ESRD, the rate of transplantations per 100 dialysis patient-years has actually fallen annually since the 1990s.[29] In its 2016 Annual Report, the US Renal Data System indicated that 88,231 people were on the kidney transplant waiting list. In many parts of the country the average waiting time was >5 years.[29]

Ethical issues arise in both attempts to increase the donor pool and appropriate allocation of available donor kidneys. As was discovered during the early days of dialysis, criteria for appropriate distribution of a limited resource are difficult and can be fraught with the biases of those making allocation decisions. Transplantation carries with it additional ethical issues related to respecting the unique gift of an organ whether from a living or deceased donor.

The majority of transplanted kidneys come from deceased donors. In an attempt to expand this donor pool, new policies allow use of a greater breadth of types of deceased donor kidneys including grafts from older donors and donors after cardiac death. The Institute of Medicine committee recently considered a variety of additional approaches to expand the pool (Box 82.4).[58] However, even given a larger number of donors, the medical community is unlikely to close the gap between supply and demand.[59] This absolute limitation on resources necessitates rationing, and the proper strategy to distribute organs most fairly while also using them to their greatest benefit remains an ongoing debate. At its core, the United Network for Organ Sharing allocation system is a waiting line in which candidates are prioritized by how long they have been listed. This egalitarian strategy intends to give equal weight to all-comers. In an attempt to also satisfy the other value of distributive justice – utility – other criteria match kidneys with patients who may benefit most from them. For example, priority is given to a particularly good immunological match. Although there are benefits and drawbacks to all criteria, they are openly published and available for debate and change. In 2014, the New Kidney Allocation System incorporated a strategy of "longevity matching" in attempts to fit young, healthy recipients with more robust kidneys while matching older recipients with grafts that would

**Box 82.4 Institute of Medicine Recommendations With Regard to Increasing Postmortem Organ Donations**

**Recommended Against the Following Approaches**

- Provision of financial incentives
- Assignment of priority to persons who registered for postmortem organ donation if they ever need an organ transplant
- Requirement for mandated choice forcing people to commit with regard to their willingness to be a postmortem organ donor
- Presumption of consent to postmortem organ donation with an opt-out provision

**Recommended in Favor of the Following Approaches**

- Enhanced public education about organ donation
- Influencing of the sociocultural atmosphere to support an expectation of donation
- Simplification of ways for people to register to be organ donors
- Expansion of the efforts of state donor registries
- Improvement in organ procurement organizations' systems so that best practices result in a higher percentage of families' giving consent for organ donation

Data from Childress JF, Liverman CT, eds. *Organ Donation: Opportunities for Action.* Washington, DC: National Academies Press; 2006.

likely still be sufficient for their lifetime, thereby optimizing overall kidney years without sacrificing aggregate recipient life-years.[60]

Although they were not intended or explicit, troubling disparities have resulted from the transplant allocation system. Studies have found that blacks are less likely than whites to be deemed appropriate candidates for transplantation, to be referred for transplant evaluation, to complete a transplant evaluation, to be added to a transplant waiting list, and to receive a kidney transplant.[61] Socioeconomically disadvantaged patients may be delayed in applying for the waiting list, so spend many more years on dialysis. In an effort to reduce these inequalities, the system continues to adjust its allocation criteria. The New Kidney Allocation system amended the definition of wait time to start at the time of listing or retroactively starting at the time of dialysis initiation.[60] Initial data show that under the new Kidney Allocation system African Americans and Hispanics are receiving a more equitable proportion of transplants.[60,62]

Transplant of a kidney from a living donor leads to better patient and graft survival than transplant from a deceased donor. However, living-organ donation presents a unique ethical dilemma in that a surgeon must risk the safety of a healthy person to improve the life of a patient. There are three categories of organ donation by living persons: 1. directed donation to a loved one or a friend, 2. nondirected donation to a general pool of patients on a waiting list, and 3. directed donation to a stranger. Each strategy raises ethical concerns. In directed donation, there is the concern that a family member or friend may feel pressured or coerced into donation. Although sometimes admirably altruistic, there is often concern that nondirected donation may be triggered by ethically fraught motivations such as seeking to compensate for depression, hoping for media attention, or the anticipation of being a part of the recipient's life. There will always be concern about compensation – financial or otherwise – for donation to strangers, especially as there is no national organization to regulate it.[63] Although the United Network for Organ Sharing bars directed donation based on race, sex, religion, or national origin, there are many examples of infringements on these directives.[63,64]

In an attempt to address some of these concerns, a statement from the Live Organ Donor Consensus Group includes requirements for the circumstances of live donation. The donor must be competent, willing to donate, free from coercion, and medically and psychosocially suitable. He or she must also be fully informed of the risks and benefits of being a donor, as well as the risks, benefits, and alternative treatment options for the recipient. Further, the benefits to both the donor and the recipient must outweigh the risks associated with the donation and transplantation.[65] In 2006, an Institute of Medicine committee cited the need for scientific evidence about long-term risks to donors to help inform this consent process.[66]

The economic pressure inherent in a limited resource of high value caused patients to seek new markets abroad. This created a "transplant tourism" culture in which wealthy patients purchase organs from vulnerable populations of lower-resourced countries. The Declaration of Istanbul on Organ Trafficking and Transplant Tourism strictly prohibited the sale of organs as well as travel to a country for the purpose of obtaining an organ citing violation of the principles of justice and respect for human dignity.[67] With the notable exception of Iran, organ sale is now illegal across the world. Despite this prohibition, black markets flourish. Poor, indebted donors are subjected to dangerous and unregulated surgeries with frequent infectious complications and long-term poor health. They often receive less compensation than advertised, which is rarely sufficient to create lasting changes in their economic situation. Studies on recipient outcomes are more equivocal, but some have shown more severe infection and more frequent hospitalization.[68] In 1988, Iran adopted a regulated living-unrelated donor program with a resulting rapid increase in transplants and elimination of the waiting list by 1999.[69] The system addressed some ethical issues by replacing a black market with regulated practice and by the provision of health care for donors. Charitable contributions limit the disparity between rich and poor recipients. However, donations continue to be from a vulnerable lower socioeconomic group and the financial incentive is still rarely translated into lifelong benefit.

Renal transplantation remains a field rife with active ethical challenge. With unsettled questions of how to best ration limited but life-saving organ resources, and the uncertain territory of a physician's moral stance toward subjecting a healthy donor to a surgical procedure, it is likely to continue to drive ethical debate.

## THE "DIFFICULT" DIALYSIS PATIENT AND CONFLICT MANAGEMENT

In recent years, dialysis units have been treating an increasing number of disruptive patients. These patients may be verbally or physically abusive, nonadherent to medical advice, or have substance abuse problems. Their behaviors may interfere

**Box 82.5 Strategies for Dealing With the Disruptive or Difficult Dialysis Patient**[73]

**Strategies for Working With the Patient**

1. Learn the patient's story and seek to understand his or her perspective.
2. Identify the patient's goal for treatment.
3. Share control and responsibility for treatment with the patient.
   - Educate the patient so that he or she can make informed decisions.
   - Involve the patient in the treatment as much as possible.
   - Negotiate a behavioral contract.
4. Appoint a patient advocate.

**Strategies for Preparing the Staff**

1. Teach the staff not to criticize patients and call them names.
2. Have the staff use "reflective listening" to show that the patient has been heard.
3. Deal directly with problem behavior; involve the patient, build on the patient's strength, and be clear about who is to do what and when.
4. Take a nonjudgmental approach.
5. Focus on the issue that started the disagreement.
6. Detail the consequences of aberrant behavior in terms that are comprehensible.
7. Prepare a behavior contract that specifies what is to be done by the patient and renal team.
8. Prepare in advance to manage anger.
9. Be patient and persistent.
10. Do not tolerate verbal abuse.
11. Outline for the staff step by step means of coping with agitated and disruptive patients.
12. Establish and publicize a grievance procedure.
13. After effective resolution of a conflict, follow up with the patient to monitor the patient's progress and demonstrate to the patient the commitment to resolve a conflict.
14. Contact law enforcement officials when physical abuse is threatened or occurs.
15. As a last resort consider transfer of the patient to another facility or discharge.
16. Consult with legal counsel before proceeding with plans for discharge and do not discharge the patient without advance notice and disclosure of future treatment options.
17. Contact the end-stage renal disease network if satisfactory resolution has not occurred with the use of these strategies.

From Johnson CC, Moss AH, Clarke SA, Armistead NC. Working with noncompliant and abusive dialysis patients: Practical strategies based on ethics and the law. *Adv Ren Replace Ther.* 1996;3:77–86.

with their own treatment, affect the welfare of other patients and staff, or disrupt the smooth running of the center.[70,71] The medical community acknowledged the strong ethical and legal obligations toward the patient who requires life-sustaining dialysis treatment. At the same time, the ethical principles of respect for patient autonomy, beneficence, nonmaleficence, and justice command an equal moral weight with respect to other patients and staff on the unit. Dialysis center caregivers report that they feel undertrained and that they lack guidelines to address these situations, causing moral distress and fatigue.[70] As early as 1990, the "difficult" dialysis patient was identified as one of the top three ethical challenges facing nephrologists.[72] In 1998 when the Renal Physicians Association and the American Society of Nephrology were developing their Shared Decision-Making clinical practice guideline, the Centers for Medicare and Medicaid Services (CMS) advocated for an entire chapter devoted to such patients (Box 82.5).[50]

The first step in approaching a clash between obligations toward a difficult or disruptive dialysis patient and other values of a dialysis center is to try to change the situation to reduce ethical conflict. The ESRD community collaborated in the Decreasing Dialysis Patient–Provider Conflict project to develop resources promoting understanding, education, and ability to cope with patient–provider conflict in an effort to improve staff–patient relationships and create safer dialysis facilities. The goal was to increase awareness and improve skills to ameliorate conflict including creating a common language to describe and classify conflicts.[71]

At times, despite efforts to reduce conflict, the ethical pull to respect a patient's preferences and health continues to compete with the duty to protect welfare and rights of other patients and staff. Nephrologists and other dialysis personnel must use their judgment to balance their moral obligations as they affect multiple stakeholders. A spectrum of disruptive or difficult dialysis patients ranges from the patient whose behavior harms only himself to one whose behavior endangers other patients and staff in the dialysis unit.[73] Ethical obligation will vary depending on where a patient's behavior falls on this spectrum. Mere nonadherence should not usually lead to denial of treatment or discharge from the dialysis unit. Even in cases involving verbally or physically abusive patients, discharge from a dialysis unit should be undertaken only as a last resort after the other strategies presented in Box 82.5 have been exhausted.[74] This approach allows health-care professionals to identify the limited situations in which involuntary patient discharge from a dialysis unit is ethically justified.[74]

*Clinical Relevance*

Dialysis units have been treating an increasing number of disruptive and difficult-to-treat patients. Even in cases involving verbally or physically abusive patients, discharge from a dialysis unit should be undertaken only as a last resort.

# FUTURE

## FINANCIAL STRESSES AND COST-CONTAINMENT STRATEGIES IN NEPHROLOGY

At the time of its implementation in the 1970s, the ESRD program was expected to incur modest costs compared with the value of a life-saving treatment. However, early cost expectations were quickly outpaced by an expanding dialysis population, and optimism for the treatment effects was tempered by increasingly apparent limitations on the quality of life that could be restored to ESRD patients on dialysis. Since the establishment of the Medicare ESRD program, high costs throughout the entirety of Medicare became a more pressing concern. In the context of rising health-care costs in the late 1980s in the United States, critics wondered if more good could be done by investing resources in other chronic disease programs.[75] They raised concern that the ESRD program was not sufficiently fair and was not the best use of limited financial resources. In other words, it satisfied neither of the first principles of distributive justice: equality and utility. First, it was unclear why governmental support should privilege one group of patients with chronic illness—those with ESRD—while there was no comparable program for failure of the heart, lungs, or liver.[75,76] It was difficult to justify the use of 7.2% of the total 2013 Medicare budget for <1% of the Medicare population while millions of Americans go without basic health-care insurance.[29] From a cost-effectiveness perspective, mounting data showing that dialysis was not the rehabilitating therapy that it had been hoped was discouraging. For many, life on dialysis was synonymous with physical incapacitation, dependency, chronic depression, and disrupted family functioning.[77] Further, the 3-year adjusted survival rate for an HD patient in 2011 had increased slowly to only 59%.[29]

Short of dismantling the program, the Centers for Medicare and Medicaid proposed significant payment cuts to dialysis facilities in 2013 and a variety of strategies for cost containment have been subsequently suggested.[78] The Affordable Care Act established ESRD Seamless Care Organizations (ESCOs) giving dialysis providers and centers an incentive to promote value and cost containment by their sharing in the financial benefits of savings and burdens of spending.[79] (The ethical challenges of ESCOs are discussed in more detail later.) Others have pointed to the extreme waste in the medical system as a focus for future cost reduction.

Given high potential savings, the prospect of rationing has also emerged in discussions of cost containment. Age-based rationing has been suggested because elderly patients are a growing portion of the dialysis population, their care is more expensive, and they have a shortened survival.[80] However, rationing by age is prohibited by the Age Discrimination Act and regardless is not thought justifiable by most ethicists.[81] Covert age rationing of dialysis by the British National Health Service raised the ire of the British public, with resultant regulations to improve dialysis services provided to the elderly to be more consistent with neighboring European countries.[82] While overt rationing seems unlikely to gain public or political traction, an increased cost awareness necessitates creative thinking on how to integrate financial considerations into health care without sacrificing quality. In the United States, Medicare's National Quality Strategy advocates a balance of multiple values by endorsing three aims: 1. better care for the individual, 2. better health for populations, and 3. reduced health-care costs.[83] An example of such a strategy includes starting dialysis later in the disease course, which has been shown to have similar patient outcomes and to be more cost-effective. Others have advocated greater adoption and support for peritoneal dialysis (PD) given that it has been shown to have comparable rates of survival and complications, and is less expensive compared with HD.[84]

## ESCOS AND CHERRY PICKING OF DIALYSIS PATIENTS

In a new effort to improve quality and control the cost of the Medicare ESRD Program, the CMS have implemented the Comprehensive ESRD Care Model.[85] CMS is partnering with large dialysis organizations to test the effectiveness of a new payment and service delivery model in providing beneficiaries with person-centered, high-quality care. This ESCO model is built on the Accountable Care Organization (ACO) experience from the Pioneer ACO Model, Next Generation ACO Model, and the Medicare Shared Savings Program. However, while the attempt to improve quality of care and respect for cost is laudable, potential conflicts of interest arise. Under the existing system of value-based purchasing, in which dialysis centers are held accountable for their achievements on quality metrics, there has been a temptation to enrich one's pool with relatively healthy dialysis patients. Because ESCOs are financed based on a shared risk model, large dialysis organizations have an even stronger incentive to cherry pick healthy patients as a large percentage of their income is at stake. Older and sicker dialysis patients require more dialysis center staff time and resources and are more frequently hospitalized. Both detract from a dialysis organization's income in a shared risk model. Under the current program, patients already established with a dialysis unit cannot be excluded when it becomes an ESCO, but nephrologists and unit administrators may be tempted to encourage older, sicker, and therefore more expensive patients to withdraw from dialysis. Commentators have called for "ethically transparent" approaches for deciding who does and does not start dialysis and for meaningful shared decision-making based on evidence-based guidelines to resist the temptation to cherry pick.[86]

## PROFESSIONAL ETHICS IN DIALYSIS

A significant portion of many nephrologists' income comes from practice in dialysis centers and often a share in ownership. Ownership offers the opportunity for a nephrologist to direct the mission of a center toward patient goals, but also brings conflict of interest and potential breach of professional ethics. Decades ago, nephrologist and then *New England Journal of Medicine* editor Arnold Relman anticipated this predicament. He warned that the private enterprise system—the so-called new medical–industrial complex—had a particularly striking effect on the practice of dialysis, and he urged physicians to separate themselves totally from any financial participation so as to maintain professional integrity.[87]

As dialysis centers expand and the market becomes saturated, there is intense pressure to recruit patients. A nephrologist who encounters a patient during a hospital admission might encourage the patient to transfer to a different dialysis center in which he has a financial interest. She may suggest that her own dialysis center is better when there are no objective quality measures to support the assertion. This practice of patient solicitation disrespects the physician–patient relationship, informed consent, continuity of care, and is an example of clear conflict of interest. It has been roundly criticized as falling short of professional ethical conduct.[88,89]

Dr. Relman's strict entreaty to completely separate practice from financial interests may not be entirely achievable because both nephrologists and dialysis centers do need to maintain healthy financing to continue to provide care. However, medicine as a professional practice is held to a different ethical standard than behavior in other marketplaces. As compared with businessmen engaging in a free-market enterprise, professionals have a fiduciary duty to prioritize the well-being of the customer-patient. With this in mind, nephrology societies have established recommendations around professional ethics in dialysis practice. Nephrologists have a duty to give patients evidence-based information about the quality of dialysis centers and treatment options as well as fully disclose their personal interests which might interfere with professional judgment.[88]

## A GLOBAL PERSPECTIVE ON NEPHROLOGY HEALTH CARE

Patterns and norms directing dialysis use in the United States are all the more stark in contrast to other developed countries. For example, in comparing practices between a population in the United States and Australia, rates of treatment in patients aged under 45 years were similar, but rates of treatment for patients greater than 85 years of age were 41% in the United States compared with 6.8% in Australia.[35] Japan, Taiwan, and Singapore also manifest a pattern of higher rates of dialysis in the elderly ESRD population, whereas other comparably high-income countries have lower prevalence.[90] These differences emphasize the context and value-dependent nature of what is considered ethical policy and practice.

As life expectancy increases through social and medical advances worldwide, chronic diseases including diabetes and hypertension become more prevalent. The rate of ESRD has similarly risen sharply. One systematic review estimates that in 2010, 2.6 million people received dialysis worldwide, but that nearly the same number died without access to the treatment.[90] They further anticipate a doubling of the global prevalence of ESRD by 2030, with growth largely in regions with limited access. KDIGO guidelines on supportive care draw attention to low-income populations as a distinct group with "choice restriction," emphasizing the importance of developing policy aligned with the realities of differing resources in high- and low-income countries.[45] One strategy of cost containment while maintaining quality is the "PD first initiative" exemplified by Hong Kong. Patients are informed and free to choose either PD or HD, but only PD will be reimbursed if there is no contraindication to this therapy. This practice makes Hong Kong one of the only countries to have a greater proportion of PD than HD patients.[91] Given the similar quality of life and efficacy of PD there are many reasons the modality is better suited to resource-limited settings. It is simpler, requires fewer trained staff, does not require electricity or large volumes of filtered water, and is importantly potentially cost saving in comparison with HD.[91] As individual nations develop a more connected global community, disparities between resource-rich and resource-poor countries are more apparent, and the question of the ethical responsibilities of a resource-rich country to a resource-poor country becomes more poignant.

## ETHICAL CHALLENGES POSED BY GENETIC ADVANCES IN CKD

Better understanding of the genetic factors that predispose to particular diseases has revolutionized detection and counseling for high-penetrance genetic disorders such as autosomal dominant polycystic kidney disease. However, with this information come complex questions about how to convey risk information to presymptomatic carriers, the duty to warn genetically related family members, and how this information should inform reproductive choices. In 1997, the World Health Organization (WHO) proposed international guidelines on many ethical issues in medical genetics. These include protocols for informed consent for testing, disclosure and confidentiality, and presymptomatic testing.[92] They highlight the unique aspect of genetic testing which involves people beyond the patient. For example, family members may not have personally sought out medical information, but their lives might be changed by it nonetheless. Unfortunately, recent U.S. history gives examples of mishandling of genetic information that led to social stigma and mistrust of the healthcare community. In the 1970s, sickle cell screening was implemented before a clear understanding of any clinical significance of carrier status, and it caused stigmatization of many patients of African descent, seeding distrust of medical providers within this community. The WHO emphasizes the imperative to never use genetic data to stigmatize or discriminate.[92]

Genome-wide sequencing technology has the potential to identify new genetic risk factors for kidney disease. As an example, certain APOL1 alleles have been associated with a 1.8 hazard ratio of progressive kidney disease among the African American population.[93] While the prospect of genetic tests moving from laboratory bench to clinical practice is exciting, it also raises ethical concerns. For example, should genetic testing be performed if the prognostic significance and/or therapeutic options have yet to be clarified? Potential genetic risk factors that are more prevalent in particular populations such as APOL1 in those of African descent risk causing health-care disparity. For example, APOL1 has been proposed as a screening tool for transplant donor candidates to protect those who are at higher risk for future kidney disease. However, because the risk allele is found exclusively in those of African descent, a selected exclusion of many black donor candidates could cause disparity in black donors' ability to offer organs to friends and family. Further, as the medical utility of the concept of race comes into question, it will be ethically challenging to design population-level uses for genes that are shown to cosegregate by distant genetic heritage. Anticipating that new advances will bring novel ethical dilemmas, the WHO-proposed guidelines emphasize the importance of interval modification over the years.[92] Collectively, these concerns remind us that medicine is not practiced by healthcare providers in ethical isolation, and it continues to be important to incorporate diverse community perspectives in defining research priorities, policy development, and clinical practice.

## CONCLUSION

The ethical issues facing nephrologists in the 1960s ushered in the field of bioethics. Despite being decades old, the ESRD program in the United States is still confronted with new ethical challenges including uncertainty about what is a fair proportion of federal funding for the Medicare ESRD program to receive, how to counter unintended incentives to cherry pick dialysis patients amid new funding structures, what are appropriate responses to difficult patients, and how to care for an increasingly elderly and multimorbid population at the end of life. With the growth in the CKD and ESRD population, the changes in its demographics, and the economic challenges to the Medicare ESRD program posed by a large federal government budget deficit, sustainable and equitable financing strategies are needed. In transplantation, the intricate considerations related to putting a living kidney donor's health at risk for the benefit of a kidney transplant recipient continue to be ethically complex. As the demand for transplantation donors continues to rise and as waiting times on the deceased donor transplant list lengthen, new strategies to increase the number of donors while being careful to regulate equitable distribution stretch our ethical foundation. Given new challenges posed by scientific discoveries, there is every expectation that nephrologists will continue to be at the forefront among those facing ethical challenges in medicine.

 Complete reference list available at ExpertConsult.com.

## KEY REFERENCES


1. Rothman D. *Strangers at the Bedside: A History of How Law and Bioethics Transformed Medical Decision Making.* New York: Aldine Transaction; 1991.
2. Jonsen A. *The New Medicine and the Old Ethics.* Cambridge, MA: Harvard University Press; 1990.
3. Scribner BH. Ethical problems of using artificial organs to sustain human life. *Trans Am Soc Artif Intern Organs.* 1964;10:209–212.
4. Butler CR, Mehrotra R, Tonelli MR, et al. The evolving ethics of dialysis in the United States: a principlist bioethics approach. *Clin J Am Soc Nephrol.* 2016;11(4):704–709.
5. Alexander S. They decide who lives, who dies: medical miracle puts a moral burden on a small committee. *Life.* 1962;53:102–104, 106, 108, 110, 115, 117-108, 123-124.
6. Fox R, Swazey J. *The Courage to Fail: A Social View of Organ Transplants and Dialysis.* Chicago: The University of Chicago Press; 1974.
7. Sanders D, Dukerminier J. Medical advance and legal lag: hemodialysis and kidney transplantation. *UCLA Law Rev.* 1968;15: 357–413.
8. Rettig RA. The policy debate on patient care financing for victims of end-stage renal disease. *Law Contemp Probl.* 1976;40(4): 196–230.
9. Levinsky NG, Rettig RA. The Medicare end-stage renal disease program. A report from the Institute of Medicine. *N Engl J Med.* 1991;324(16):1143–1148.
10. *United States Renal Data System: USRDS 1989 Annual Data Report.* Bethesda, MD: National Institutes of Health, National Institute of Diabetes and Digestive and Kidney Diseases; 1989.
11. Hull A, Parker T III. Introduction and summary. Proceedings from the morbidity, mortality and prescription of dialysis symposium, Dallas, Tx, September 15 to 17, 1989. *Am J Kidney Dis.* 1990;15(5): 375–383.
12. Fox RC. Exclusion from dialysis: a sociologic and legal perspective. *Kidney Int.* 1981;19(5):739–751.
13. Rettig R, Levinsky N. *Kidney Failure and the Federal Government.* Washington, DC: The National Academy of Sciences; 1991.
14. Moss AH, Stocking CB, Sachs GA, et al. Variation in the attitudes of dialysis unit medical directors toward decisions to withhold and withdraw dialysis. *J Am Soc Nephrol.* 1993;4(2):229–234.
15. Singer PA. Nephrologists' experience with and attitudes towards decisions to forego dialysis. The End-Stage renal Disease Network of New England. *J Am Soc Nephrol.* 1992;2(7):1235–1240.
17. Jonsen AR. *The Birth of Bioethics.* New York: Oxford University Press; 1998.
18. *Deciding to Forego Life-Sustaining Treatment.* Washington, DC: Presidents Commission for the Study of Ethical Problems in Medicine and Biomedical and Behavioral Research; 1983:1–3.
19. *ESRD Data Advisory Committee 1993 Annual Report.* Washington, DC: US Department of Health and Human Services; 1993.
20. Neu S, Kjellstrand CM. Stopping long-term dialysis. An empirical study of withdrawal of life-supporting treatment. *N Engl J Med.* 1986;314(1):14–20.
22. Moss AH. Dialysis decisions and the elderly. *Clin Geriatr Med.* 1994;10(3):463–473.
23. Swartz RD, Perry E. Advance directives are associated with "good deaths" in chronic dialysis patients. *J Am Soc Nephrol.* 1993;3(9): 1623–1630.
24. Lehrich RW, Pun PH, Tanenbaum ND, et al. Automated external defibrillators and survival from cardiac arrest in the outpatient hemodialysis clinic. *J Am Soc Nephrol.* 2007;18(1):312–320.
25. Moss AH, Holley JL, Upton MB. Outcomes of cardiopulmonary resuscitation in dialysis patients. *J Am Soc Nephrol.* 1992;3(6):1238–1243.
27. Levinsky NG. Quality and equity in dialysis and renal transplantation. *N Engl J Med.* 1999;341(22):1691–1693.
28. Parker JC. Cherry picking in ESRD: an ethical challenge in the era of pay for performance. *Semin Dial.* 2011;24(1):5–8.
30. Murtagh FE, Marsh JE, Donohoe P, et al. Dialysis or not? A comparative survival study of patients over 75 years with chronic kidney disease stage 5. *Nephrol Dial Transplant.* 2007;22(7):1955–1962.
31. Kurella M, Covinsky KE, Collins AJ, et al. Octogenarians and nonagenarians starting dialysis in the United States. *Ann Intern Med.* 2007;146(3):177–183.
32. O'Hare AM, Choi AI, Bertenthal D, et al. Age affects outcomes in chronic kidney disease. *J Am Soc Nephrol.* 2007;18(10):2758–2765.
35. Wong SP, Hebert PL, Laundry RJ, et al. Decisions about renal replacement therapy in patients with advanced kidney disease in the US Department of Veterans Affairs, 2000-2011. *Clin J Am Soc Nephrol.* 2016;11(10):1825–1833.
36. Estes CL, Binney EA. The biomedicalization of aging: dangers and dilemmas. *Gerontologist.* 1989;29(5):587–596.
38. Cohen LM, Ruthazer R, Moss AH, et al. Predicting six-month mortality for patients who are on maintenance hemodialysis. *J Am Soc Nephrol.* 2010;5(1):72–79.
40. Guiding principles for the care of older adults with multimorbidity: an approach for clinicians: American Geriatrics Society Expert Panel on the Care of Older Adults with Multimorbidity. *J Am Geriatr Soc.* 2012;60(10):E1–E25.
41. *Promoting Excellence in End-of-Life Care program, End-Stage Renal Disease Workgroup: Recommendations to the field. Robert Wood Johnson Foundation.*
43. Moss AH, Ganjoo J, Sharma S, et al. Utility of the "surprise" question to identify dialysis patients with high mortality. *Clin J Am Soc Nephrol.* 2008;3(5):1379–1384.
51. Davison SN, Jhangri GS, Holley JL, et al. Nephrologists' reported preparedness for end-of-life decision-making. *Clin J Am Soc Nephrol.* 2006;1(6):1256–1262.
52. Holley JL, Carmody SS, Moss AH, et al. The need for end-of-life care training in nephrology: national survey results of nephrology fellows. *Am J Kidney Dis.* 2003;42(4):813–820.
53. Holley JL, Davison SN, Moss AH. Nephrologists' changing practices in reported end-of-life decision-making. *Clin J Am Soc Nephrol.* 2007;2(1):107–111.
54. O'Hare AM, Armistead N, Schrag WL, et al. Patient-centered care: an opportunity to accomplish the Three Aims of the National Quality Strategy in the Medicare ESRD program. *Clin J Am Soc Nephrol.* 2014;9(12):2189–2194.
55. Kahrass H, Strech D, Mertz M. The full spectrum of clinical ethical issues in kidney failure. Findings of a systematic qualitative review. *PLoS ONE.* 2016;11(3):e0149357.
57. Matas AJ, Sutherland DE. The importance of innovative efforts to increase organ donation. *JAMA.* 2005;294(13):1691–1693.
60. OPTN/UNOS. *The New Kidney Allocation System (KAS): The First Year.* https://www.transplantpro.org/wp-content/uploads/sites/3/KAS_12month_analysis.pdf. Accessed May 7, 2017.
75. Moskop JC. The moral limits to federal funding for kidney disease. *Hastings Cent Rep.* 1987;17(2):11–15.
76. Rettig R. *Biomedical Politics: Origins of the Medicare Kidney Disease Entitlement: The Social Security Amendments of 1972.* Washington, DC: National Academies Press; 1991.
80. Andersen MJ, Friedman AN. The coming fiscal crisis: nephrology in the line of fire. *Clin J Am Soc Nephrol.* 2013;8(7):1252–1257.
83. CMS Quality Strategy. *Centers for Medicare & Medicaid Services*; 2016.
87. Relman AS. The new medical-industrial complex. *N Engl J Med.* 1980;303(17):963–970.
88. Ozar DT, Kristensen C, Fadem SZ, et al. Nephrologists' professional ethics in dialysis practices. *Clin J Am Soc Nephrol.* 2013;8(5):840–844.

# 83

# Health Disparities in Nephrology

Yoshio N. Hall

## CHAPTER OUTLINE



## KEY POINTS

- In the United States, significantly lower incidence of end-stage kidney disease (ESKD) and smaller health insurance–related gaps in care access were recently observed in states with broader as compared with narrower health insurance coverage for the poor.
- Targeted efforts by the US Indian Health Service to improve screening and management of diabetes mellitus and hypertension have led to a 54% decline in the incidence of diabetes-related ESKD among American Indians over the past 2 decades: the age-adjusted incidence rate of diabetes-related ESKD is now the same as that for non-Hispanic white Americans.
- Emerging evidence suggests that the dialysis center may play an influential role in promoting and facilitating access to kidney transplant, particularly among racial–ethnic minority patients.
- Gap programs aimed at increasing kidney donation in the United States particularly among black Americans have yielded a 30% increase in the donation rate of deceased-donor kidneys (from 18.1 per 1000 deaths in 2000 to 23.6 per 1000 deaths in 2014) from this racial group.
- In the early months following implementation of a new Kidney Allocation System, incidence rates of deceased-donor kidney transplantation improved by 13% for Hispanic and 19% for black patients in the United States.
- The black–white disparity in renal allograft loss after both deceased- and living-donor kidney transplantation has steadily declined over the past 2 decades due to differential improvements in 5-year graft survival among black as compared with white Americans.

Disparities in the incidence, progression, and treatment of kidney diseases according to socioeconomic status, race–ethnicity, and geographic location have been documented for many years. These relative differences arise and persist via multiple intermediaries, including biologic susceptibility, differential access to high-quality health care, and contextual impediments to healthy living. This chapter provides a framework for evaluating systematic differences in health, describes what is known about root causes of disparities in nephrology and nephrology care, and highlights broad strategies for addressing key determinants of these inequities.

## DISPARITY

The term "health disparity" often refers to suboptimal health processes or outcomes experienced by demographically defined groups that occur in the context of social or economic inequality. The United States National Library of Medicine defines a "health status disparity" as variation in rates of disease occurrence and disabilities between (among) socioeconomic and/or geographically defined population groups.[1] By contrast, a "health-care disparity" refers to a difference in access to or availability of health-care facilities and services.[1] Health status and health-care disparities relate to systematic inequalities in health among social groups that are deemed to be preventable by reasonable means.

This chapter covers five broad areas of health status and health-care disparities in nephrology observed in socially disadvantaged groups: 1. disparities in the incidence and prevalence of risk factors for chronic kidney diseases (CKDs); 2. disparities in the treatment of these risk factors and in progression of CKD; 3. disparities in the incidence of end-stage kidney disease (ESKD); 4. disparities in the treatment of ESKD; and 5. initiatives to reduce these disparities.

Global estimates of ESKD incidence vary widely and are strongly influenced by the availability of funding for the treatment of kidney diseases and associated risk factors.[2] Worldwide approximately 2.6 million people received treatment for ESKD in 2010; however, estimates suggest that roughly 2.3 to 6.1 million people may have died from ESKD because renal replacement therapy was declined or not accessed.[3] In fact, prior to passage of US Public Law 92-603 in 1972, access to maintenance dialysis in the United States was commonly based on the candidate's financial health and social worth criteria such as occupation.[4] Such biases remain operative in many countries, where people of low socioeconomic status and members of socially disadvantaged minority groups experience disproportionately high incidence of ESKD.[5–8] For example, in the United States, approximately 25% of black Americans reside in poverty as compared with less than 10% of non-Hispanic white Americans.[9] Black Americans also experience disproportionately high rates of ESKD,[2,7] and yet for over 2 decades they have been consistently less likely than their white counterparts to receive a living- or deceased-donor kidney transplant.[2,10,11] Although much less is known about people with kidney diseases who do not require or pursue dialysis, reports suggest that compared with US adults with earlier stages of CKD, those with more advanced CKD are younger and more likely to be nonwhite, poor, and uninsured.[2,12] Similar disparities in the incidence, treatment, and risk factors of ESKD have been observed among indigenous people from North America, Australia, and New Zealand.[13–21] The magnitude and persistence of these disparities have prompted some governments to prioritize elimination of the disparities while also attempting to reduce the overall burden and costs attributed to kidney diseases.[22,23]

## HEALTH JUSTICE

In 1966, Dr. Martin Luther King, Jr. proclaimed, "Of all the forms of inequality, injustice in health care is the most shocking and inhumane." The pursuit of equal health outcomes or equal access to health care plays a prominent role in contemporary debates on health care.[24,25] Examples of equal access and equal outcomes with respect to health care reflect the Aristotelian principles of horizontal and vertical equity.[26] However, such debates in health care often include conflicting views of justice. For example, a medical model of justice focuses attention at a point in time when someone who is already ill seeks access to scarce and/or an expensive service such as dialysis or kidney transplantation. (Many credit the birth of bioethics in the United States to the introduction of the arteriovenous shunt by Belding Scribner in 1960 which allowed for long-term hemodialysis to treat patients with ESKD.) By contrast, a social model of justice highlights how social determinants such as access to education, employment, preventative care, safe neighborhoods, and nutritional foods affect the health of a population.[25,27] In other words, the social model focuses on how a person's need for health care arose in the first place. Although inequities in distributive justice (e.g., in kidney transplantation) persist in many areas of medicine, health status and health-care disparities in nephrology have focused growing attention on the link between social conditions and risk factors that place people at risk for progressive diseases of the kidney such as low birth weight, obesity, type 2 diabetes mellitus, and hypertension.[24,28]

## SOCIAL ORIGINS OF DISPARITIES IN NEPHROLOGY

Link and Phelan originally referred to social conditions, including social class, race, income, and education level, as "fundamental causes of disease because these conditions govern access to resources that influence health and disease."[29] Prior studies have reported that the incidence of progressive CKD and ESKD is highest among persons living in the most impoverished neighborhoods.[6,30,31] Additional US-based studies have reported lack of health insurance coverage and residence in a high-poverty area as exposures linked with worse kidney-related biochemical abnormalities at dialysis initiation and marked delays in receipt of a kidney transplant.[32–34] Although these disparities arise from a variety of mechanisms, including biologic susceptibility and economic vulnerability, environmental exposures such as contextual impediments to healthy living likely play a central role. Discussion of the hypothesized influences of social conditions on disparities in nephrology through various life stages uses the framework shown in Fig. 83.1.

### PRENATAL ENVIRONMENT AND DISPARITIES IN RISK FACTORS FOR KIDNEY DISEASES

In 1990, Barker noted, "The womb may be more important than the home" in terms of the origins of adult disease.[35] Worldwide, every year approximately 15 million newborns (10 per 100 live births) are born prematurely and 22 million (16 per 100) weigh <2500 g (i.e., low birth weight).[36,37] While intrauterine growth retardation and low birth weight are invariably linked with measures of maternal poverty,[38–40] much debate surrounds the influence of early fetal programming on subsequent risk of chronic diseases including those of the kidney (see Chapter 21 for a detailed discussion). The "critical periods" model is one of three models that has been proposed to explain how socioeconomic position over the life course may influence subsequent health.[41] The "fetal programming" hypothesis is based on the critical periods model and states that intrauterine growth retardation results in permanent alterations in fetal physiology that become deleterious later in adult life.[35] Brenner hypothesized that

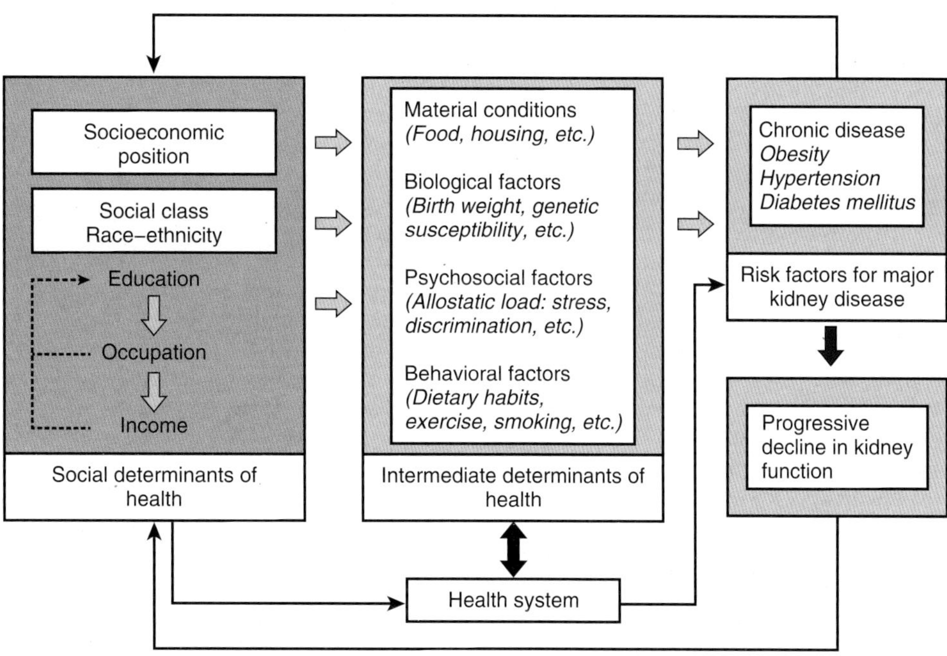


**Fig. 83.1** Social determinants of health disparities framework.

retardation of renal development as occurs in individuals of low birth weight both increases postnatal risks for systemic and glomerular hypertension and predisposes an individual to further nephron loss and the development of progressive kidney injury.[42–44] This hypothesis draws support from reports of 1. a direct relationship between birth weight and nephron number,[45] 2. an inverse relation between birth weight and hypertension later in life,[35,46–48] and 3. an inverse relation between nephron number and blood pressure.[49]

In addition to hypertension, low birth weight has been variably linked with risk factors such as diabetes and obesity and has been directly associated with later-life onset of microalbuminuria, reduced estimated glomerular filtration rate (eGFR), and ESKD.[50–53] One study conducted on a cohort of term singletons born around the time of the 1944–1945 Dutch famine found that midgestational exposure to famine was associated with microalbuminuria and that late gestational exposure was associated with glucose intolerance.[51] Notably, a rapid increase in nephron number occurs in midgestation, which is a critical period for determining nephron endowment at birth.[51] Moreover, rapid growth and weight gain during infancy and childhood that occur after intrauterine growth restriction (and/or low birth weight) are associated with increased risks of insulin resistance, obesity, diabetes, and hypertension.[42,53,54]

Because low birth weight is strongly linked to indices of parental poverty and occurs more commonly among socially or economically disadvantaged groups, researchers have posited that low birth weight may partly account for socioeconomic and racial–ethnic disparities in congenital, hypertensive, and hyperfiltrative kidney diseases.[55,56] For example, Australian Aboriginals experience higher rates of poverty and an approximate tenfold higher risk of ESKD than nonindigenous Australians.[8] One study conducted in a remote Australian Aboriginal community (where low-birth-weight infants compose approximately 25% of live births) observed that low as compared with high birth weight was significantly associated with lower kidney volumes, higher blood pressure, and later in life, higher levels of urinary albumin excretion.[49] In a recent study of 447 Japanese children, low as compared with normal birth weight was associated with a nearly fivefold higher risk of having moderate or severe elevations in serum creatinine levels during childhood (mostly due to congenital anomalies of the kidney and urinary tract).[57] In the Bogalusa Heart Study, a biracial prospective cohort study of cardiovascular risk factors in children and adolescents in the Southern United States, the prevalence of low birth weight was higher among black than white infants.[58] Subsequent reports have linked lower birth weight in this cohort with higher blood pressure levels later in life. These reports have also noted that the magnitude of the association between lower birth weight and higher blood pressure appears to increase with advancing age.[46,47,58]

Globally, many high- and medium-income countries now face rising incidence of maternal overnutrition.[59–61] In some countries, maternal obesity has replaced tobacco smoking as the most important preventable risk factor for adverse pregnancy outcomes including preterm births.[59,61] In addition to preterm delivery, excessive weight gain during pregnancy is associated with increased risk for development of obesity, diabetes, and hypertension in the offspring.[59] Less is known, however, about the pathways through which excessive weight gain during pregnancy and maternal obesity affect later-life CKD risk factors. The degree to which maternal obesity and excessive weight gain during pregnancy contribute to socioeconomic and racial–ethnic disparities in kidney disease incidence is likewise unknown. The trend toward increasing survival of low-birth-weight infants further underlines the importance of intrauterine fetal environment and timing of insults in future risk for development of precursors to progressive kidney disease.[55]

## POSTNATAL ENVIRONMENT AND DISPARITIES IN RISK FACTORS FOR KIDNEY DISEASES

Over the past 2 decades, the nephrology community has paid increasing attention to how a person's living environment may influence his or her downstream risk of chronic diseases. This heightened attention is evidenced by the growing body of literature examining the complex influences of individual- and area-level measures on important processes and outcomes related to the care of people with CKDs.[31,62–64] People residing in impoverished neighborhoods experience more crime, less access to high-quality educational and employment opportunities, and poorer health outcomes in comparison with persons from less distressed areas.[63,65] Several contemporary studies have described higher incidence of ESKD as well as higher prevalence of albuminuria and reduced eGFR in areas of high residential poverty than in areas of low residential poverty.[31,62,64] However, much debate surrounds how and how much adverse social conditions in childhood and early adult life influence a person's subsequent risk of developing chronic diseases of the kidney.[28] Many writers posit that social conditions act through a host of intermediaries such as education, housing, and diet, thereby molding health-related behaviors, which in turn influence risk for kidney diseases.[28,29,63] Prior studies suggest that education may influence disparities in health behaviors through its effects on lifestyle, social support, and social norms, whereas income may drive disparities in health outcomes through access to resources and services, including health care.[66,67] The social distribution of important risk factors for progressive diseases of the kidney, including the higher prevalence of smoking, low birth weight, type 2 diabetes mellitus, hypertension, and obesity within poor as compared with less impoverished areas, lends evidence to these claims.[24,28] This unequal distribution of intermediary exposures linked to progressive kidney injury is further compounded by the vulnerability of certain groups (i.e., persons of low socioeconomic position) to health-compromising illnesses such as ESKD. Poor health then exerts potent feedback on an individual's socioeconomic position through lost income or medical costs associated with a major illness (Fig. 83.1).[68]

The concept of "allostatic load," the accumulation of physiologic insults due to repeated insults or chronic stressors experienced in daily life, has gained increasing interest as a model for explaining socioeconomic (and racial–ethnic) disparities in the processes and outcomes of chronic diseases.[69,70] Specific measures of allostatic load include levels of hormones secreted in response to stress and biomarkers that reflect the effects of these hormones on the body.[69,71] This concept, which is based on the cumulative exposures theory, posits that stress may accumulate from early life and manifest as an accumulation of physiologic dysregulation.[69,72] Chronic stressors such as food insecurity, discrimination, living in substandard housing, inadequate access to health care, and exposure to violence are more pronounced among persons of lower socioeconomic status than among those of intermediate or higher socioeconomic status.[70,71] Such psychosocial stressors may lead to hypertension and autonomic dysregulation (e.g., diminished heart rate variability), which in turn are linked to increased risk of incident ESKD.[70,71,73] Accordingly, higher levels of exposure and adaptation to life stressors experienced more commonly by the poor or members of some racial–ethnic minority groups may put them at higher risk for kidney disease through the aforementioned pathways than their less impoverished or white counterparts.[74–76]

Similarly, contemporary debates in many industrialized countries have increasingly focused on the role of nutrition and childhood obesity in later-life risks for development of chronic disease.[77,78] Estimates suggest that more than a third of children in North America and Europe, and approximately a quarter in the western Pacific and southeast Asia, are overweight or obese.[79,80] In the United States, the prevalence of childhood obesity is markedly higher among black and Hispanic children than among non-Hispanic white children.[77] Public health policy and nutrition experts attribute the marked growth in childhood obesity to the widespread availability of energy-dense, inexpensive foods and the low energy requirements of modern daily life.[79]

Several studies have also linked residence in impoverished areas with higher levels of processed food consumption (rich in sodium and phosphorus), lower levels of physical activity, and increased risk for chronic diseases such as cardiovascular disease, diabetes, and hypertension in comparison with residence in more affluent areas.[63,81–84] In addition to offering fewer options for affordable, nutritious foods, poorer neighborhoods tend to have fewer (or less attractive) areas to promote physical activity such as parks and community centers.[83,84] The undue influence of crime, poor housing quality, and suboptimal educational and medical infrastructure may also render poor communities less supportive of healthy lifestyles than less distressed neighborhoods.[65] One study linked racial–ethnic disparities in childhood obesity with differential exposure to risk factors during early life, such as gestational diabetes, rapid infant weight gain, excessive television viewing, and high intake of sugar-sweetened beverages or fast food.[78] The strong relation between childhood obesity and later-life antecedents of hypertensive and hyperfiltrative kidney diseases (obesity, hypertension, metabolic syndrome, type 2 diabetes mellitus) suggests that interventions targeting the early life period may contribute substantially to reducing socioeconomic and racial–ethnic disparities in kidney and other chronic diseases.[85]

Perhaps the strongest evidence that neighborhood socioeconomic distress may influence downstream risk factors and lead to health status disparities in certain types of kidney disease emanates from the Moving to Opportunity Study.[86,87] During the period 1994–1998, the US Department of Housing and Urban Development conducted this "randomized social experiment" in five cities (Baltimore, Boston, Chicago, Los Angeles, and New York City) to examine the extent to which relocating from a more to a less distressed neighborhood might influence downstream health outcomes. Collectively, 4498 women (90% were either black or Hispanic) with children from high-poverty neighborhoods were randomly assigned to one of three groups: 1788 were assigned to receive housing vouchers that were redeemable only if they relocated to a low-poverty area, 1312 received unrestricted vouchers, and 1398 were assigned to a control group that offered neither of these opportunities. In terms of risk factors for kidney diseases, the study found that participants who received a voucher to relocate to a low-poverty neighborhood experienced absolute risk reductions of 5% and 4% for extreme obesity and diabetes mellitus, respectively, 10 to 15 years

communities strongly influences the frequency and quality of care received.[14,15,17] Several United States–based studies have now demonstrated that socioeconomic and racial–ethnic disparities in care may be partly explained by differences in where and by whom patients are treated, leading to systematic differences in the care environment, provider quality, and access to care.[127–129] For example, Bach and associates[127] found that black and white Medicare beneficiaries were treated for the most part by different physicians. Strikingly, 80% of all outpatient primary-care visits by black patients in this study were accounted for by only 22% of physicians. Moreover, the primary-care physicians who cared primarily for black patients were less likely to be board certified, more likely to be in training, and more likely to report encountering system barriers to providing high-quality care to their patients (e.g., securing referrals to specialists). Varkey and colleagues[128] further found that clinics serving higher proportions of patients from racial–ethnic minority groups were more chaotic than and had different organizational characteristics from those of other clinics. Recent qualitative studies of nephrology and primary-care providers have identified system-level factors such as referral process delays, insufficient time to build patient partnerships, and poorly integrated nephrology and primary care as major barriers to optimal preparation for renal replacement therapy in diverse health-care settings.[130,131] Such systematic barriers may also account for the historically lower utilization of home dialysis and preemptive kidney transplantation among black and Hispanic patients than among white patients in the US.[132,133] In short, several key factors linked to the provision of high-quality medical care, such as coordination of care, subspecialist access, and provider experience differ markedly according to the health system. Such health system–level determinants may delay or restrict the access of poor and underserved patients to receiving adequate management of common kidney diseases and their antecedent risk factors.

## DISPARITIES IN THE TREATMENT OF CHRONIC KIDNEY DISEASES

Blood pressure control is a central target to reduce morbidity and mortality in CKD.[114] Hypertension as a contributing cause of ESKD is blamed for more than a quarter of incident cases in the United States.[2] Hypertension is also the most common modifiable risk factor for disease progression among uninsured American adults with CKD, affecting approximately 57% of this population as compared with obesity (40%), diabetes (22%), and overt albuminuria (13%).[12] However, several United States–based studies have described marked disparities in blood pressure control in CKD according to measures of socioeconomic status and health system access. For example, data from the US National Health and Nutrition Examination Surveys indicated that hypertensive adults with reduced eGFR (15–59 mL/min/1.73 m$^2$) and/or albuminuria (≥30 mg/g) who lacked health insurance were far less likely to be receiving treatment for their hypertension than insured counterparts.[12] Moreover, among hypertensive adults with reduced eGFR and/or albuminuria, those who lacked health insurance coverage were 55% less likely to be receiving treatment with an angiotensin inhibitor than insured adults (Table 83.1).[12] Similarly, Olomu and associates[116] reported

**Table 83.1 Odds Ratio (OR) of Hypertension Treatment and Renin–Angiotensin Antagonist Use Among Uninsured as Compared With Insured US Adults With Chronic Kidney Diseases and Hypertension**

| Outcome | Unadjusted OR (95% CI) | Adjusted OR (95% CI) |
|---|---|---|
| Hypertension treatment[a] | 0.44 (0.31–0.62) | 0.59 (0.40–0.85) |
| Renin–angiotensin–aldosterone inhibitor use | 0.34 (0.20–0.59) | 0.45 (0.26–0.77) |

[a]Treated: We considered participants with hypertension to be "treated" if they reported that they were currently taking medications to lower blood pressure.

*CI*, Confidence interval.

that only 38% of hypertensive patients achieved target blood pressure control in a federally qualified health clinic in Michigan; the US average is 54%.[134] Even fewer (31%) hypertensive patients with diabetes achieved target blood pressure control in the same clinic.[116]

In addition to experiencing reduced access to high-quality care, low-income and racial–ethnic minority groups may harbor risk factors that heighten their susceptibility to further morbidity and mortality. While observing a high (10%–35%) prevalence of moderately or severely reduced eGFR (<60 mL/min/1.73 m$^2$) among ambulatory users of a large safety net health system, we found that the prevalence of "socially determined" risk factors that might influence medical outcomes—such as chronic viral diseases, substance abuse, homelessness, and mental illness—was far higher than observed in other health-care settings.[97,135] In one safety net setting, >7% of persons with moderate-to-advanced CKD progressed to ESKD and 16% died during median follow-up of 6.6 years.[97] Notably, nearly 30% of patients were never assessed for proteinuria, and fewer than 20% were ever seen by nephrology specialists during follow-up.[97] The elusive nature of this population, their frequent loss to follow-up, reduced access to specialty care, and limited provider accountability further complicate patient–provider interactions, highlighting a critical need for more effective strategies to optimize surveillance and management of common risk factors for kidney diseases in traditionally underserved populations in order to mitigate health status and health-care disparities.

## DISPARITIES IN THE TREATMENT OF END-STAGE KIDNEY DISEASE

Conservative estimates suggest that ESKD affects at least 4.9 million people worldwide at considerable cost to society.[3] In some high-income countries with universal access to ESKD treatment, there are persistent racial–ethnic and socioeconomic disparities in access to certain types of renal replacement therapies.[2,3] In most medium- and low-income nations, access to ESKD treatment remains limited and is governed predominantly by socioeconomic position and occupation.[3,5]

## DIALYSIS: PROCESS AND OUTCOME

In terms of access to maintenance dialysis, socioeconomic disparities are evident at several levels, from the country's health region and system to the individual patient. Regular access to maintenance dialysis remains, for the most part, limited to patients receiving care in high-income and upper-middle-income nations.[2,3,5] In most low-income and lower-middle-income countries, the majority of patients who initiate dialysis either die or stop treatment within the first 3 months because of cost restraints.[5,23] While the numbers who do not receive treatment for ESKD is unknown, estimates suggest that at least 2.2 million people might have died prematurely in 2010 because renal replacement therapy could not be accessed, with the largest treatment gaps occurring in low-income countries in Asia and Africa.[3] Within high-income nations, an increasing number of studies have focused on differences in dialysis process measures as indicators of the quality of dialysis care received.[133,136–139] A large fraction of these studies emanate from the United States, likely reflecting incorporation of specific measures for anemia management and dialysis adequacy into facility performance assessment and care reimbursement.[138,140]

As noted previously, there are prominent and persistent racial–ethnic disparities in process measures at dialysis initiation that largely reflect the presence and quality of care leading up to ESKD.[33,139,141] However, data from the US Centers for Medicare and Medicaid Services (CMS) suggest that these disparities attenuate and may even reverse for some racial–ethnic groups over time.[142,143] In two studies from the CMS's ESRD Clinical Performance Measures Project, Frankenfield and associates reported that Hispanic and Asian patients undergoing hemodialysis experienced process measures (e.g., arteriovenous fistula use and serum albumin, hemoglobin, and dialysis adequacy targets) that were equivalent, and in some cases superior, to those of non-Hispanic whites 1 year after dialysis initiation; and that black patients receiving hemodialysis continued to experience the worst process measures of all racial–ethnic groups surveyed.[136,142] While the first study did not elucidate specific mechanisms by which racial–ethnic differences in process measures abated, it seems plausible that the establishment of a regular site of care with access to wraparound services (i.e., social work, dietician, primary nephrology care) may have offset the lack of, or variation in, medical care received prior to ESKD onset. Whether achievement of specified targets for these measures actually reflects dialysis-related quality of care remains a source of substantial debate.[133,138] Recent voices have called for additional metrics such as kidney transplant referral rates to provide further insight into the overall quality of dialysis care delivered.[144] Regardless, in the setting of universal access to dialysis services, more research is needed to determine how quality improvement methods can be effectively targeted to reduce health disparities without misprioritizing low-value care and creating unwarranted and wasteful incentives that might also exclude vulnerable patients.[133,145]

## KIDNEY TRANSPLANTATION: PROCESS

In terms of survival and quality of life, kidney transplantation is the optimal treatment for most patients who progress to ESKD. However, significant disparities in receiving a transplant according to socioeconomic status, race–ethnicity, and geography persist worldwide.[2,11,13,146–148] In the United States, transplantation rates are significantly lower among the poor and among most racial–ethnic minority groups than among less disadvantaged groups and whites, respectively.[2] Racial–ethnic disparities are also present in Canada despite uniform health insurance coverage, where kidney transplantation rates in Aboriginal, African, Indo Asian, and East Asian Canadians range from one-half to two-thirds those of white Canadians.[146] In Australia, transplantation rates in Aboriginal Australians are 77% lower than those in nonindigenous Australians, and in New Zealand, Maori/Pacific Islanders are similarly disadvantaged.[8] Although key mediators of, and their relative contributions to, racial–ethnic disparities in transplant access vary by population and health system, many are directly linked to social conditions described previously.

For example, in the United States, American Indian and black patients encounter delays in accessing the kidney transplant waiting list that are partly attributable to lower socioeconomic status and a higher prevalence of diabetes mellitus in comparison with white patients.[19,34,149,150] Similarly, contextual poverty and health insurance coverage account for the largest fraction of the disparity in live-donor kidney transplantations among American Indians, Alaska Natives, and black and Hispanic Americans in comparison with white Americans.[148] By contrast, geographic differences (primarily attributed to organ availability) account for substantial fractions of the disparity in receiving a deceased-donor kidney from the waiting list among US Hispanics, Pacific Islanders, and American Indians/Alaska Natives.[34]

Additional studies have identified differences in attitudes and knowledge about kidney transplantation among black and Hispanic Americans in comparison with white Americans.[151] Providers may also be less likely to recommend kidney transplantation to minority patients owing to impaired communication and misconceptions regarding its benefits relative to prolonged dialysis.[151,152] Emerging evidence further suggests that the dialysis center may play an influential role in promoting and facilitating access to kidney transplant, particularly among racial–ethnic minority patients.[153,154] The influence of cultural and/or linguistic isolation on delays in accessing the transplant waiting list or in receiving a kidney transplant remains understudied.[34]

Specific mechanisms by which social disadvantage influences access to transplantation include low educational attainment, suboptimal health insurance coverage, and contextual impediments to healthy living. Poor or uninsured patients appear to encounter more difficulty than less disadvantaged patients in navigating the complex steps required to successfully receive a kidney transplant, and this vulnerability appears to have changed little over time.[149,155,156] This may be a direct effect of low educational attainment, inadequate insurance coverage, suboptimal patient–provider communication, and lack of support and information about transplant from dialysis centers, all of which have been linked with delays in accessing the transplant waiting list, in completing the transplant evaluation, and in successful receipt of a transplant.[100,146,149,150,152,157,158] Nephrology providers also appear reticent to refer poor patients for transplant because of concerns about inadequate coverage for prescription and procedural costs.[152,159] In a national survey of US transplant programs, >70% responded that they frequently or occasionally exclude patients from the kidney transplant waiting list owing to concerns that the patients will not be able to afford the immunosuppressive medications.[160]

Although socioeconomic status and contextual poverty are linked with disparities in transplantation rates in the United States,[30,78,149] the magnitude of such disparities is markedly higher in middle-income nations such as in Mexico, where transplantation rates are more than tenfold higher among insured patients than among uninsured patients.[161] As concerning is the unethical practice of organ trafficking and exploitation of disadvantaged populations for profit that occurs in many low- and middle-income nations.[161] This pervasive commercialization of live donor transplantation is supported by reports of affluent foreigners undergoing large fractions of the kidney transplantations performed in some low- and middle-income countries.[162] Although some writers justify paying persons to donate a kidney as mutually benefitting recipient and donor, one study conducted in India showed that such transactions do not lead to long-term economic benefit and may be associated with a decline in health for the donor.[163]

Historically, racial–ethnic differences in the distribution of ABO blood type and antibodies to human leukocyte antigens (HLAs) have been linked with disparities in receiving a deceased-donor kidney transplant among patients who have successfully accessed the waiting list.[34,164,165] In particular, black candidates have encountered marked delays in receiving a deceased-donor kidney owing partly to their higher frequencies of ABO types that are associated with longer waits.[10,22,165–167] Such factors may account for marked delays in kidney transplantation among black as compared with nonblack children, which persisted even when accounting for socioeconomic measures.[91] However, the influence of biologic perpetrators of racial–ethnic disparities in transplantation access, such as the distribution of blood type and HLA, has progressively declined as a result of major changes in the deceased donor allocation policy. Recognizing the contribution of HLA matching to racial disparities in receiving a deceased-donor kidney, US policy makers eliminated the HLA-B locus as a priority for the allocation of deceased kidney donors on May 7, 2003.[168] This change led to an increase in the proportion of deceased-donor organs directed to minority candidates on the waiting list. Specifically, in the 6 years after the policy change, deceased-donor transplantation in racial–ethnic minority recipients rose 40%, compared with an 8% rise for non-Hispanic whites and a 23% increase overall.[169] Moreover, this improved access to transplantation for minority groups has not been accompanied by declines in short-term graft survival during the initial period after the policy change.[169]

In 2013, the US Organ Procurement and Transplantation Network approved additional amendments to the kidney allocation policy that included changes to promote greater equity in accessing deceased-donor kidneys.[166] In particular, there were two amendments, one that allows for blood type B recipients to receive kidney offers from donors with certain subtypes of blood type A and another that calculates waiting time from the start of dialysis (or qualifying eGFR ≤ 20 mL/min). In the first 9 months under the new allocation system, incidence rates of deceased-donor kidney transplantation improved by 13% and 19% for Hispanic and black patients (as compared with rates under the old allocation system), respectively, but these improvements in transplant access for racial–ethnic minorities were tempered by higher rates of delayed graft function.[166,170,171]

Over the past decade, kidney exchange has gained substantial momentum in the US and has prompted forward thinking on how the global nephrology community might leverage this approach to mitigate racial–ethnic and socioeconomic inequities in kidney transplantation. Additional strategies to promote greater racial–ethnic and social equity in rates of assigning patients to the waiting list and in living-donor kidney transplantation remain areas of heightened investigation.[154]

## KIDNEY TRANSPLANTATION: OUTCOMES

Socioeconomic and racial–ethnic disparities in kidney transplantation extend to outcomes after receipt of a functional allograft. Similar to transplant access, specific causes of these disparities in allograft survival may differ by population and health system, but the root causes commonly reflect differential social conditions and access to high-quality health care. For example, adherence to posttransplantation immunosuppressive therapy remains a critical determinant of long-term allograft survival. Regrettably, the inability to afford immunosuppressive medications appears to be a primary mechanism that restricts disadvantaged patients from not only receiving a kidney transplant but also in maintaining one.[170,172] In the United States, for example, federal prescription drug coverage for immunosuppressive medications extends to only 36 months after kidney transplantation, with few exceptions.[173] For this reason, disadvantaged patients are particularly vulnerable to the long-term financial burden of maintaining a functional allograft.[174] In one study, >40% of transplant recipients reported financial difficulty after transplantation, with health-related out-of-pocket expenses averaging approximately $475 per month.[172] In a recent single-center study of 1171 kidney transplant recipients, lower socioeconomic status was associated with an 11% higher risk of acute rejection and 77% higher risk of graft loss among black Americans.[175] Socioeconomic disparities in maintaining a transplant are magnified in medium-income countries such as Mexico and Pakistan, where excellent long-term results for allograft survival are offset by the prohibitive cost of immunosuppressive and antiviral medications. In these countries, transplant access and allograft maintenance for the average citizen often require a state-sponsored model.[5,47,161]

In terms of the disparity in allograft loss between black and white Americans, the gap has steadily declined over the past 2 decades. Recent data from the US organ transplant registry point to differential improvements in 5-year graft survival after deceased-donor kidney transplantation among black (from 49% to 69%) as compared with white (from 63% to 75%) Americans. Similar gains (63% to 79% among blacks vs. 79% to 86% among whites) have led to a narrowing of the black–white gap in allograft survival following living-donor kidney transplantation.[176] Temporal changes in deceased donor allocation, immunosuppressive agents, and desensitization strategies have been credited as major contributors to these observations.

Racial differences in biologic factors such as age at transplantation, HLA mismatching, and APOL1 genotype status may account to some degree for the remaining disparity in allograft survival between some racial–ethnic groups, such as between black and white Americans.[10,177,178] The transplant community is now seeking ways to integrate the APOL1 genotype into clinical practice in order to enhance evaluation of donor organs and better align this assessment with recipient need.[179] Although prevailing beliefs attribute reduced graft survival among black recipients to heightened immune responsiveness and poorer immunologic matching, remarkably few reports have actually linked better HLA matching with improved graft survival in this racial group.[10,164,180] In addition, Asian recipients enjoy the longest graft survival of all racial–ethnic groups despite the presence of suboptimal HLA matching comparable with that observed in black recipients.[10,181] Alternatively, pharmacokinetic studies report greater clearance and/or lower bioavailability of certain immunosuppressive agents among black than among white transplant recipients.[182–184] However, the influence of these biologic factors on racial disparities in allograft survival is likely mediated at least in part through differences in immunosuppressive medication regimens and nonadherence.[173,185–187] In the United States, nonadherence strongly correlates in turn with social factors such as household income, presence and type of health insurance coverage, and history of drug abuse.[10,173,188,189]

Lastly, studies have raised concerns regarding inequities in the quality of transplanted organs based on recipient socioeconomic status and race–ethnicity.[190] Emerging data on provision of comparatively "lower quality organs" to black, low-income, or less educated recipients than to white, more affluent, or college-educated counterparts have cast additional light on the complex nuances that underlie this social gap in allograft access and survival.[190,191]

## MOVING TOWARD MORE EQUITABLE CARE

Currently, global cost estimates of treating kidney diseases remain elusive. In the United States alone, treatment of CKD costs the federal government >$50 billion annually, including $33 billion for ESKD.[2] Hence, there is an urgent need to identify cost-effective strategies to address risk factors for major kidney diseases, particularly among populations that bear a disproportionate burden of disease.[2] Strategies to reduce disparities in chronic diseases include three general approaches: (1) targeted programs, (2) gap programs, and (3) gradient programs.[68,192] "Targeted programs" comprise strategies aimed at improving the health of groups that are particularly disadvantaged in terms of disease burden or treatment access. Such targeted programs are advantageous in that they focus on a well-defined, often small segment of the population. This aspect provides for ease in monitoring and assessing results. However, the targeted approach is similarly weakened by its narrow focus and its lack of commitment to reduce the disparity between the most and least disadvantaged groups. In some instances, health gains in the targeted groups may still lag behind those observed in less disadvantaged groups, leading to widening of the disparities.[68] An example is programs that attempt to promote live-donor kidney transplantation among patients of low socioeconomic status. Although such programs may increase live-donor kidney transplantation rates among the poor, the disparity between patients of lower and those of intermediate or higher socioeconomic status may actually increase owing to the differential effects of other programs (e.g., paired donation) or resource-mediated advances (e.g., Internet use and social networking).

Strategies that aim to target the health gap address the issue of disparities, but these programs are more challenging than those that seek to improve the health status of targeted groups. In order to succeed, "gap programs" must achieve absolute improvements in health status among, for example, persons in the lowest socioeconomic position at a rate of improvement that exceeds that observed in the comparison group. Like targeted programs, gap programs often focus solely on the most disadvantaged groups and largely ignore gradients in health and the health status of those in the intermediary groups.[68] For example, over the past 14 years, collective efforts to increase kidney donation in the United States among black Americans have yielded a 30% increase in the donation rate of deceased-donor kidneys (from 18.1 per 1000 deaths in 2000 to 23.6 per 1000 deaths in 2014) from this racial group. By comparison, the donation rate from white donors remains higher (29.8 per 1000 deaths in 2014), but this rate has been relatively stagnant over the same period (note: donation rates from deceased donors of American Indian and Asian descent have increased substantially during the same period, but the small number of traumatic deaths occurring in these racial–ethnic groups provides less stable estimates).[2]

Addressing socioeconomic gradients in health relies on comprehensive strategies that involve the entire population. In contrast to targeted and gap programs, "gradient strategies" address the effect of socioeconomic inequality on health across the socioeconomic hierarchy. In other words, a gradients model addresses not only intermediaries of health disparities among the disadvantaged but also systematic inequities in life course exposures (educational and occupational opportunities, nutrition, living standards, and health-care access) that strongly influence an individual's position in the socioeconomic hierarchy.[68] Needless to say, gradient strategies must often contend with conflicting political agendas, major logistical challenges, and prohibitive costs.[193] Moreover, such strategies commonly yield results only in a prolonged time frame. These three strategies (targeted, gap, and gradient) for reducing disparities are intended to complement one another and can often provide sequential layers for addressing socioeconomic (and racial–ethnic) inequities.[68]

On the basis of the framework shown in Fig. 83.1, researchers have identified four major intervention areas for addressing socioeconomic and racial–ethnic disparities in kidney disease.[68] First, reducing inequalities in the distribution of structural determinants such as education, occupation, and income may alter social stratification and mitigate its effects on health outcomes. Second, addressing specific intermediary determinants that mediate the effects of socioeconomic position on health (e.g., consumption of high-calorie foods and beverages, lack of physical exercise, unhealthy living conditions, and cigarette smoking) may reduce specific health-damaging exposures that disproportionately affect disadvantaged groups; in other words, changing the distribution of risk factors related to socioeconomic position may attenuate long-term health consequences for underprivileged groups.[28] Third, reversing the effect of health status on socioeconomic position may lessen the vulnerability of disadvantaged groups to the health-damaging conditions they face[24]; examples include programs to keep persons with chronic diseases such as diabetes and CKD within the workforce.[174] Lastly, targeting the delivery of health care to socially disadvantaged groups may reduce the unequal consequences of illness and prevent further disease progression and economic loss; such strategies might offer additional care or health coverage to members of disadvantaged groups who have conditions (obesity, diabetes, hypertension, homelessness) that are linked to the excess burden of progressive CKD in these groups.[68]

## INITIATIVES TO REDUCE DISPARITIES

Successful initiatives to reduce socioeconomic and racial–ethnic disparities in CKD risk factors might reference the US government–sponsored Vaccines for Children Program, the Standards of Care for Diabetes and Kidney Disease Programs administered by the US Indian Health Services, and the US National Health Service Corps' scholarship and loan repayment programs. A generation ago, fatal outbreaks of measles in predominantly poor, minority communities in several US cities underscored marked disparities in vaccination coverage that placed disadvantaged children at increased risk for disease. In direct response to these disparities, the US government initiated the Vaccines for Children Program, which now purchases and provides vaccines for children who are particularly vulnerable to lapses in vaccination coverage (i.e., those who were uninsured, on Medicaid, or of American Indian or Alaska Native ancestry, or who had health insurance that did not cover universally recommended vaccines). From 2000 to 2010, racial–ethnic disparities in vaccination series completion rates in the United States decreased from 6% to 4% (for minority groups vs. non-Hispanic white children), and poverty-related inequalities from 8% to 3%.[194]

Several decades ago, in response to rising concerns over the burden of ESKD due to diabetes in many American Indian communities, the Indian Health Service established the Standards of Care for Diabetes Program (followed later by the Kidney Disease Program) in order to improve the screening of and the management of patients with diabetes and CKD.[18] Based on the Chronic Care Model, these two programs implemented routine reporting of eGFR, annual monitoring of protein excretion, utilization of renin–angiotensin system antagonists, and aggressive control of glucose and blood pressure in association with enhanced patient and provider education (Fig. 83.2).[18,195] By 2001, age-adjusted ESKD incidence among American Indians with diabetes had decreased by 31% from that in 1990. By 2006, 82% of American Indians with hypertension and diabetes were receiving a renin–angiotensin–aldosterone system inhibitor. Remarkably, among American Indians, age-adjusted incidence rates of diabetes-related ESKD have decreased by 54%, from 573 per million population in 1996 to 265 per million population in 2013, and are now the same as those for non-Hispanic whites (Fig. 83.3).[2,18,196] A similar gap initiative by the Australian government, the Medical Outreach–Indigenous Chronic Disease Program, aims to close the disparity in life expectancy between indigenous and nonindigenous Australians by improving access of indigenous people to best-practice chronic disease management.[23] Notably, the five areas of highest priority include diabetes mellitus and CKDs.

In terms of addressing disparities in kidney transplantation, recent efforts have targeted dialysis facilities with substantial racial disparities in transplant referral while others have aimed to streamline the cumbersome medical work-up. The Reducing Disparities in Access to kidNey Transplantation (RaDIANT) Community Study, an ESKD network–led, randomized, pragmatic trial of 134 dialysis facilities, tested the effectiveness of a 1-year multicomponent intervention (a combination of outreach, education, and quality improvement) targeting dialysis facility patients, staff, and leadership on rates of kidney

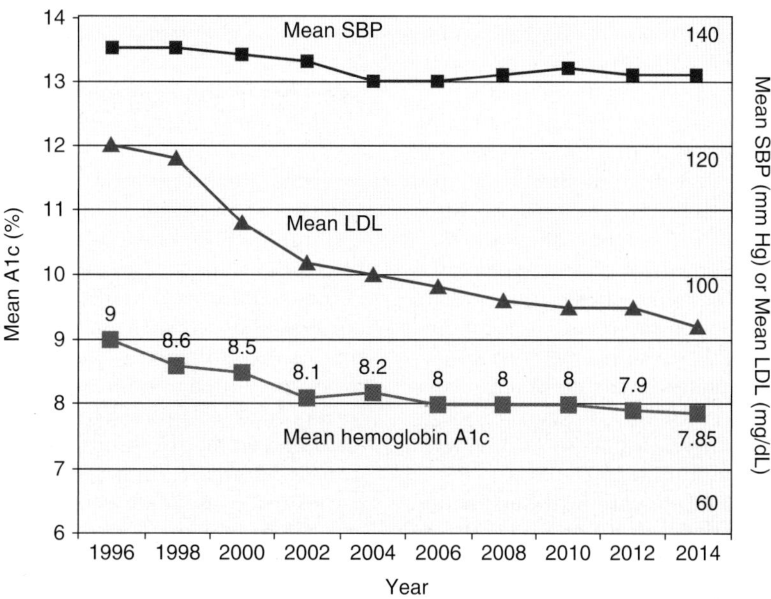


**Fig. 83.2** Risk factor control among American Indians with diabetes mellitus within the Indian Health Service. *LDL,* Low-density lipoprotein; *SBP,* systolic blood pressure. (Data from Indian Health Service website at http://info.ihs.gov/Diabetes.asp.)

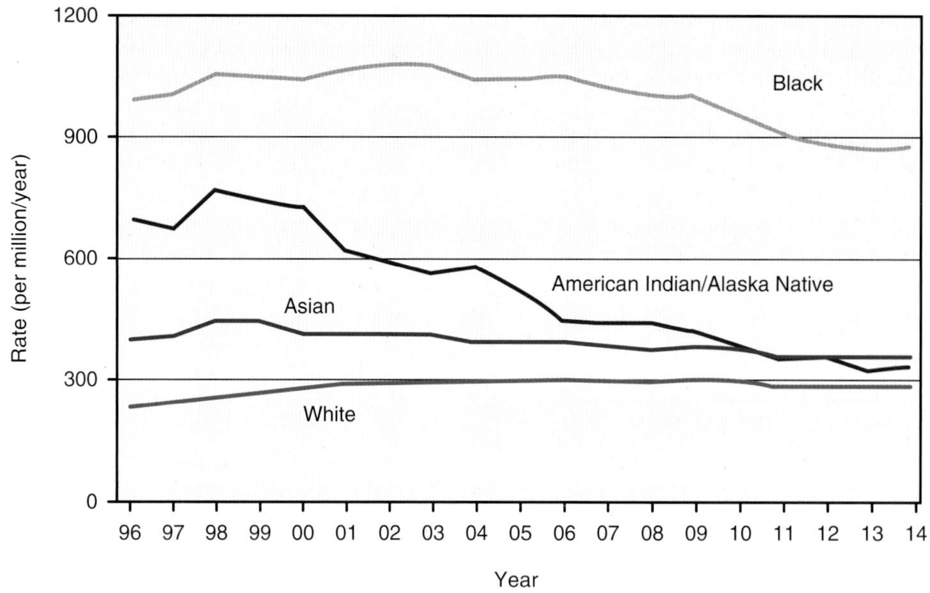


**Fig. 83.3** Trends in age- and sex-adjusted incidence rate (per million/year) of end-stage kidney disease by race in the United States. (Data from US Renal Data System. *USRDS 2016 Annual Data Report: Atlas of Chronic Kidney Disease and End-Stage Renal Disease in the United States*. Bethesda, MD: National Institutes of Health, National Institute of Diabetes and Digestive and Kidney Diseases; 2016.)

transplant referral.[154] After adjustment for time and clustering, the percentage of patients referred for transplant evaluation 1 year after intervention start was 7.3% (95% confidence interval, 5.5% to 9.2%) higher in intervention as compared with control facilities. Notably, the adjusted increase in transplant referrals in the intervention as compared with the control facilities was more pronounced for black (6.4%) as compared with white (3.7%) patients.[154] A second study, The Kidney Transplant Fast Track – Talking About Live Kidney Donation study, aims to address a major factor contributing to racial disparities in kidney transplantation, lower rates of live-donor kidney transplantation. This study will test the effectiveness of a 1-day, streamlined evaluation process combined with a randomized controlled trial of the Talking About Live Kidney Donation intervention, a validated, culturally sensitive program to support consideration of live-donor kidney transplantation among patients and their families.[197–199]

In 1970, the US government established the National Health Service Corps to help underserved communities across the nation receive critically needed primary medical, oral, and mental and behavioral health care. Through the National Health Service Corps, clinicians receive scholarships and loan repayment in return for committing to practice in underserved areas for a defined period. More than 40,000 primary-care clinicians have participated in this program since its inception. Later reports suggest that 82% of clinicians continue to practice in underserved communities 1 year after their service completion and that 55% remain for 10 years. Notably, long-term retention rates are higher for those who serve in rural as opposed to urban communities.[200]

Many US policy makers and health-care providers lauded passage of the Affordable Care Act as a fundamental step toward achieving equitable access to health care for all Americans. However, uncertainty surrounding its legislative future continues to shroud robust gains in health-care coverage since enactment.[120] Furthermore, as Schrag[201] noted in 1983, the ability to pay for health services does not necessarily guarantee their availability. In order to address socioeconomic and racial–ethnic disparities in treatment of kidney disease and its antecedent risk factors, US policy makers will need to work with health systems to tackle the unequal distribution of resources including experienced health-care providers situated in areas of low and high poverty. In terms of kidney transplant, efforts to reduce economic vulnerability by providing medication prescription benefits to disadvantaged groups at risk for nonadherence to posttransplantation regimens may partially address socioeconomic and racial–ethnic inequities in transplant access as well as in long-term allograft survival.[173] To date, lobbying efforts have failed to convince the US Congress to extend support for immunosuppressive medications beyond 3 years after transplantation.

## SUMMARY AND CHALLENGES

Socioeconomic and racial–ethnic disparities in the incidence and treatment of kidney diseases and their risk factors occur worldwide. They occur within and between countries, and the reader is referred to the Global Considerations in Kidney Disease section of this edition (Chapters 75 through 81) for consideration of particular constituencies. Growing recognition of these disparities has fueled additional research and programs aimed at addressing gaps between persons of low socioeconomic status and their less impoverished counterparts, and between racial–ethnic minority groups and white majority groups. However, despite in-depth knowledge of the root causes and consequences of these disparities, including their social determinants, progress remains slow and the structural elements that allow these disparities persist. Marked differences in education, living conditions, and employment opportunities combined with inequitable access to high-quality health care and genetic susceptibility act in tandem to promote and maintain disparate milieus for chronic diseases. In the setting of such widespread inequities, we should anticipate that disparities in health outcomes such as kidney diseases will continue to plague the nephrology community for the foreseeable future. The persistence of, and costs attributed to, potentially preventable disparities in nephrology mark our field as one that remains in crisis.

Fortunately, several countries including the United States have now prioritized initiatives aimed to reduce socioeconomic gaps in health insurance coverage, maternal prenatal care, vaccinations, smoking, nutrition, and childhood obesity in order to improve the overall quality of health care to, and mitigate the effects of social conditions that disproportionately afflict, socially disadvantaged populations. Within nephrology, targeted efforts over the past 2 decades have yielded substantial declines in diabetes-related ESKD incidence among American Indians and improved access to deceased-donor kidneys among black and Hispanic Americans. However, for the long term, reducing disparities rooted in social inequity will likely improve health and health-care quality more than would technical advances in overall medical care.[194] The social distribution of prematurity, low birth weight, diabetes mellitus, hypertension, and obesity and their indelible link to progressive declines in kidney function provides further evidence in favor of this approach to address disparities in nephrology.[28] Unfortunately, many high- and medium-income countries continue to witness stagnant or reduced social mobility, increased social unrest, and widening inequities in living conditions. Needless to say, even in the presence of astute public policies aimed to address marked differences in social conditions, reducing long-standing disparities in nephrology will remain a major challenge for the foreseeable future.

 Complete reference list available at ExpertConsult.com.

## KEY REFERENCES


2. *U.S. Renal Data System, USRDS 2016 Annual Data Report: Atlas of Chronic Kidney Disease and End-Stage Renal Disease in the United States,* National Institutes of Health, National Institute of Diabetes and Digestive and Kidney Diseases, Bethesda, MD, 2016. Available at https://www.usrds.org/2016/view/Default.aspx. Accessed April 24, 2017.
5. Garcia-Garcia G, Renoirte-Lopez K, Marquez-Magana I. Disparities in renal care in Jalisco, Mexico. *Semin Nephrol.* 2010;30(1):3–7.
6. Grace BS, Clayton P, Cass A, et al. Socio-economic status and incidence of renal replacement therapy: a registry study of Australian patients. *Nephrol Dial Transplant.* 2012;27(11):4173–4180.
12. Hall YN, Rodriguez RA, Boyko EJ, et al. Characteristics of uninsured Americans with chronic kidney disease. *J Gen Intern Med.* 2009;24(8):917–922.
15. Wang Z, Hoy WE. Diabetes and lifetime risk of ESRD in high-risk remote-dwelling Australian Aboriginal people: a 20-year cohort study. *Am J Kidney Dis.* 2013.
17. Hoy WE, Kondalsamy-Chennakesavan S, Scheppingen J, et al. A chronic disease outreach program for Aboriginal communities. *Kidney Int Suppl.* 2005;98:S76–S82.
18. Narva AS, Sequist TD. Reducing health disparities in American Indians with chronic kidney disease. *Semin Nephrol.* 2010;30(1):19–25.
26. Beever A. Aristotle on equity, law, and justice. *Legal Theory.* 2004; 10(01):33–50.
27. Macintyre SA, Ellaway A. *Neighborhoods and Health.* New York: Oxford University Press; 2003.
28. Braveman PA, Cubbin C, Egerter S, et al. Socioeconomic disparities in health in the United States: what the patterns tell us. *Am J Public Health.* 2010;100(suppl 1):S186–S196.
29. Link BG, Phelan J. Social conditions as fundamental causes of disease. *J Health Soc Behav.* 1995;Spec No:80-94.
31. Volkova N, McClellan W, Klein M, et al. Neighborhood poverty and racial differences in ESRD incidence. *J Am Soc Nephrol.* 2008; 19(2):356–364.
32. Kausz AT, Obrador GT, Arora P, et al. Late initiation of dialysis among women and ethnic minorities in the United States. *J Am Soc Nephrol.* 2000;11(12):2351–2357.
34. Hall YN, Choi AI, Xu P, et al. Racial ethnic differences in rates and determinants of deceased donor kidney transplantation. *J Am Soc Nephrol.* 2011;22(4):743–751.
35. Barker DJ. The fetal and infant origins of adult disease. *BMJ.* 1990;301(6761):1111.
49. Hoy WE, Hughson MD, Bertram JF, et al. Nephron number, hypertension, renal disease, and renal failure. *J Am Soc Nephrol.* 2005;16(9):2557–2564.
50. Luyckx VA, Bertram JF, Brenner BM, et al. Effect of fetal and child health on kidney development and long-term risk of hypertension and kidney disease. *Lancet.* 2013;382(9888):273–283.
52. White SL, Perkovic V, Cass A, et al. Is low birth weight an antecedent of CKD in later life? A systematic review of observational studies. *Am J Kidney Dis.* 2009;54(2):248–261.
63. Diez Roux AV, Merkin SS, Arnett D, et al. Neighborhood of residence and incidence of coronary heart disease. *N Engl J Med.* 2001;345(2):99–106.
65. Sampson RJ, Raudenbush SW, Earls F. Neighborhoods and violent crime: a multilevel study of collective efficacy. *Science.* 1997; 277(5328):918–924.
70. Lynch JW, Kaplan GA, Shema SJ. Cumulative impact of sustained economic hardship on physical, cognitive, psychological, and social functioning. *N Engl J Med.* 1997;337(26):1889–1895.
73. Brotman DJ, Bash LD, Qayyum R, et al. Heart rate variability predicts ESRD and CKD-related hospitalization. *J Am Soc Nephrol.* 2010;21(9):1560–1570.
86. Ludwig J, Sanbonmatsu L, Gennetian L, et al. Neighborhoods, obesity, and diabetes–a randomized social experiment. *N Engl J Med.* 2011;365(16):1509–1519.
87. Ludwig J, Duncan GJ, Gennetian LA, et al. Neighborhood effects on the long-term well-being of low-income adults. *Science.* 2012; 337(6101):1505–1510.
90. Wilson WJ. *The Truly Disadvantaged: The Inner City, the Underclass, and Public Policy.* Chicago: University of Chicago Press; 1987.
93. Shoham DA, Vupputuri S, Diez Roux AV, et al. Kidney disease in life-course socioeconomic context: the Atherosclerosis Risk in Communities (ARIC) Study. *Am J Kidney Dis.* 2007;49(2):217–226.
94. Vart P, Gansevoort RT, Crews DC, et al. Mediators of the association between low socioeconomic status and chronic kidney disease in the United States. *Am J Epidemiol.* 2015;181(6):385–396.
97. Hall YN, Choi AI, Chertow GM, et al. Chronic kidney disease in the urban poor. *Clin J Am Soc Nephrol.* 2010;5(5):828–835.
98. Genovese G, Friedman DJ, Ross MD, et al. Association of trypanolytic ApoL1 variants with kidney disease in African Americans. *Science.* 2010;329(5993):841–845.
103. Karter AJ, Ferrara A, Liu JY, et al. Ethnic disparities in diabetic complications in an insured population. *JAMA.* 2002;287(19): 2519–2527.
110. Donabedian A. The quality of medical care. *Science.* 1978; 200(4344):856–864.
117. Kurella-Tamura M, Goldstein BA, Hall YN, et al. State medicaid coverage, ESRD incidence, and access to care. *J Am Soc Nephrol.* 2014;25(6):1321–1329.
120. Glied S, Jackson A. The future of the Affordable Care Act and insurance coverage. *Am J Public Health.* 2017;107(4):538–540.
121. Williams DR, Collins C. Racial residential segregation: a fundamental cause of racial disparities in health. *Public Health Rep.* 2001; 116(5):404–416.
127. Bach PB, Pham HH, Schrag D, et al. Primary care physicians who treat blacks and whites. *N Engl J Med.* 2004;351(6):575–584.
128. Varkey AB, Manwell LB, Williams ES, et al. Separate and unequal: clinics where minority and nonminority patients receive primary care. *Arch Intern Med.* 2009;169(3):243–250.
130. Greer RC, Ameling JM, Cavanaugh KL, et al. Specialist and primary care physicians' views on barriers to adequate preparation of patients for renal replacement therapy: a qualitative study. *BMC Nephrol.* 2015;16:37.
132. Mehrotra R, Soohoo M, Rivara MB, et al. Racial and ethnic disparities in use of and outcomes with home dialysis in the United States. *J Am Soc Nephrol.* 2016;27(7):2123–2134.

133. Hall YN, Xu P, Chertow GM, et al. Characteristics and performance of minority-serving dialysis facilities. *Health Serv Res.* 2014;49(3):971–991.
141. Hall YN, Sugihara JG, Go AS, et al. Differential mortality and transplantation rates among Asians and Pacific Islanders with ESRD. *J Am Soc Nephrol.* 2005;16(12):3711–3720.
149. Alexander GC, Sehgal AR. Barriers to cadaveric renal transplantation among blacks, women, and the poor. *JAMA.* 1998;280(13):1148–1152.
154. Patzer RE, Paul S, Plantinga L, et al. A randomized trial to reduce disparities in referral for transplant evaluation. *J Am Soc Nephrol.* 2017;28(3):935–942.
156. Patzer RE, Plantinga LC, Paul S, et al. Variation in dialysis facility referral for kidney transplantation among patients with end-stage renal disease in Georgia. *JAMA.* 2015;314(6):582–594.
169. Ashby VB, Port FK, Wolfe RA, et al. Transplanting kidneys without points for HLA-B matching: consequences of the policy change. *Am J Transplant.* 2011;11(8):1712–1718.
171. Massie AB, Luo X, Lonze BE, et al. Early changes in kidney distribution under the new allocation system. *J Am Soc Nephrol.* 2016;27(8):2495–2501.
176. Purnell TS, Luo X, Kucirka LM, et al. Reduced racial disparity in kidney transplant outcomes in the United States from 1990 to 2012. *J Am Soc Nephrol.* 2016;27(8):2511–2518.
193. Bloche MG. Health care disparities–science, politics, and race. *N Engl J Med.* 2004;350(15):1568–1570.
194. Woolf SH, Johnson RE, Phillips RL Jr, et al. Giving everyone the health of the educated: an examination of whether social change would save more lives than medical advances. *Am J Public Health.* 2007;97(4):679–683.
196. Bullock A, Burrows NR, Narva AS, et al. Vital signs: decrease in incidence of diabetes-related end-stage renal disease among American Indians/Alaska natives - United States, 1996-2013. *MMWR Morb Mortal Wkly Rep.* 2017;66(1):26–32.

# 84

# Care of the Older Adult With Chronic Kidney Disease

Gabrielle Lafreniere | Sarbjit Vanita Jassal

## CHAPTER OUTLINE



## KEY POINTS

- Common equations used to estimate the glomerular filtration rate (GFR) have wider margins of error when applied to older adults. These may misclassify individuals as having chronic kidney disease (CKD), resulting in debate about whether it is appropriate to label individuals, in their eighth and ninth decade, as having a chronic disease based on current criteria.
- Older individuals with CKD appear to have an unexpectedly high burden of geriatric syndromes (GSs) such as frailty, cognitive impairment, functional limitation, depression, incontinence, sensory deficits, malnutrition, and falls.
- Patients with CKD often use polypharmacy. Polypharmacy in older adults is further complicated by the altered pharmacokinetics and pharmacodynamics in the setting of advancing age and presence of CKD.
- A complete evaluation (known as a comprehensive geriatric assessment; CGA) is recommended for all older individuals. This should include a detailed medical history (including treatment targets); assessment of the home environment and social support structure, functional history, and assessment of personal values and lifestyle preferences.
- Although it is often assumed that treatment with dialysis will extend life and alleviate the signs and symptoms of advanced kidney disease, there is growing evidence that these benefits may not always accrue in older adults.
- Several studies have suggested that dialysis initiation may exacerbate or accelerate functional and cognitive decline, resulting in a 1.6-fold higher risk of serious fall injuries and a higher risk of requiring professional nursing care.
- It is important to distinguish among younger and older individuals, robust or frail, and those with renal-limited CKD and those with complex clustering of multiple chronic diseases while engaging in shared decision-making processes.
- Most studies have shown that dialysis is associated only with a modest survival advantage over comprehensive conservative renal care.

## INTRODUCTION

Although chronic kidney disease (CKD) is a significant public health issue for patients of all ages, there is a limited body of literature addressing the management of CKD in older adults. Most health care practitioners would agree, however, that caring for older adults with CKD presents unique challenges because of the substantial differences between older and younger patients with this condition. In this chapter, we will provide an overview of a broad number of issues related to providing care for the older adult with CKD. We have included discussions about the emerging debate rejecting current definitions used to define CKD, detailed information about common geriatric syndromes (e.g., falls, functional decline, cognitive impairment) and their relationship with renal disease and treatment, and introduced the role of palliative dialysis and comprehensive conservative renal care (CCRC).

## CHRONIC KIDNEY DISEASE AND AGE-RELATED CHANGES IN ESTIMATED GLOMERULAR FILTRATION RATE

Kidney Disease Improving Global Outcomes (KDIGO) clinical guidelines define CKD based on measured serum creatinine level and estimated glomerular filtration rate (eGFR). Traditionally, the presence of an eGFR of less than 60 mL/min/1.73 $m^2$ for longer than 3 months is considered consistent with CKD. Using this definition, CKD prevalence in those aged 65 years and older is approximately 10-fold higher than that seen in those younger than 50 years (40% vs. 4%, respectively).[1] Estimates of prevalence, however, vary widely from study to study and appear to be highly dependent on the method used to evaluate renal function and on the population under study. One uniform observation, however, is that older age is associated with lower renal function than that seen in younger patients. Using creatinine-based estimates, more than 75% of the older population identified as having kidney disease fall into the CKD stage 3a category (eGFR = 45–59 mL/min/1.73 $m^2$).[1,2]

The high prevalence of CKD in older adults is attributed to multiple factors, including improved longevity despite chronic diseases such as diabetes, hypertension, and cardiovascular disease, newer population screening strategies and kidney damage resulting from newer drugs or medical interventions used for revascularization, and cancer management or organ failure.[3] The rate of renal decline varies among individuals. In general, however, older individuals have a lower rate of renal function decline than younger people, particularly at lower levels of eGFR. In an observational study of 4562 patients older than 65 years of age, Arora et al. have found that 62% of patients with CKD stage 3b and 69% of patients with CKD stage 4 progressed at an annual rate of <1 mL/min/1.73 $m^2$.[4] Similar findings have been reported elsewhere[5,6] and likely reflect the fact that relatively few older patients with an eGFR < 45 mL/min have albuminuria.[7,8]

### EVALUATION OF RENAL FUNCTION IN OLDER ADULTS

In most cases, kidney function in routine clinical practice is estimated based on serum creatinine or cystatin C concentration, rather than determined using exogenous filtration markers such as inulin, iothalamate, or other radiocontrast clearance measures. This is discussed in detail in Chapter 23. Formal evaluation of renal function, using inulin or iothalamate, is impractical and costly in the clinical setting. Similarly, 24-hour urine collections can be cumbersome for older individuals to collect and are more likely to be unreliable due to inappropriate collection, incontinence, or accidental spills. Current KDIGO guidelines[9] recommend reporting the eGFR using the 2009 Chronic Kidney Disease Epidemiology Collaboration (CKD-EPI) creatinine-based equation with the use of additional tests such as cystatin C or a clearance measurement for confirmatory testing only in specific circumstances. European guidelines, specific to the older population,[10] allow more flexibility and do not recommend one equation over the other. Neither guideline, at present, distinguishes among different age groups, or among robust, vulnerable, and frail individuals. In older adults, however, the margins of error associated with eGFR estimates may be wider than in younger populations, and commonly used formulae may overestimate or underestimate the true GFR in older adults. Although beyond the scope of this chapter to give a detailed discussion of the attributes of the various methods for GFR estimation, several clinical factors can affect serum creatinine and cystatin C levels, independent of the GFR. These non-GFR determinants are more common among older rather than younger individuals. They include, among other factors, a low dietary intake of protein and reduced muscle mass (both factors specific to creatinine levels), subclinical inflammation, and a change in body habitus with increased adiposity. Even in the absence of overt disease, older individuals are more likely to be frail or have chronic inflammation arising from normal age-related conditions (sometimes referred to as "inflammaging"). This causes a systematic bias, resulting in wider margins of error when commonly used formulae are applied to older adults. Use of the CKD-EPI equation[11] has superseded the Modification of Diet in Renal Disease (MDRD) Study equation[12] in many parts of the world because it is less likely to misclassify individuals as having CKD[13]—although it is unclear if the improved accuracy is clinically meaningful in older adults. Other formulae, including those using cystatin C[14–16] and those specific to the older population, have been recently proposed but further validation, in external data sets, is awaited (Table 84.1).

Albuminuria is known to be an important clinical finding that is associated with increased mortality, vascular events, and progression to end-stage renal disease (ESRD) across all ages and levels of eGFR.[17–19] In the Berlin Initiative Study (BIS), the albuminuria rate among 2069 adults 70 years of age and older was 26%. Unlike younger individuals, only a small percentage had macroalbuminuria (3.6% had an albumin-to-creatinine ratio [ACR] ≥ 300 mg/g).[20] Similar results were found in the National Health and Nutrition Examination Survey (NHANES) III population, where 21% presented with albuminuria at 70 years of age and older and 32.7% at 80 years and older.[21] The prevalence of albuminuria in older individuals seems substantially lower than that of abnormal eGFR; more than 50% of the 75+ years group are diagnosed with CKD based on an eGFR < 60 mL/min/1.73 $m^2$ in the absence of albuminuria (Fig. 84.1).[22] This further adds doubt to current definitions of CKD in older patients that

**Table 84.1 Estimated Glomerular Filtration Rate (eGFR) Equations**

| Research Group | Endogenous Filtration Marker (units) | Equation | Development Population | Limitations |
|---|---|---|---|---|
| Cockcroft-Gault[301] | Creatinine (mg/dL) | CrCl = [(140 – age) × weight) / (72 × $S_{Cr}$)] × 0.85 (if female) | *N* = 505 (236 for training sample)<br>whites, 4% women<br>hospitalized pts<br>Age range: 18–92 yr (only 17 pts > 80 yr) | Values not adjusted for BSA<br>Developed to predict CrCl instead of GFR<br>Underestimates GFR in older adults, especially at higher GFRs |
| MDRD[302] | Creatinine (μmol/L) | eGFR = 175 × $(S_{Cr})^{-1.154}$ × $(age)^{-0.203}$ × (0.742 if female) × (1.212 if black) | *N* = 1628 whites and blacks; 40% women<br>Nondiabetic pts with CKD<br>Mean age: 51 ± 13 yr (age range, 18–70 yr) | Tends to underestimate renal function in those with a normal eGFR<br>Not validated in pts >70 yr, at extremes of body weight, and in some ethnic groups (e.g., Asian ethnic groups) |
| CKD-EPI[11,303] | CKD-EPIcr—creatinine (mg/dL) | eGFR = 141 × $\min(S_{cr/\kappa,1})^{\alpha}$ × $\max(S_{Cr/\kappa,1})^{-1.209}$ × $0.993^{age}$ [×1.018 if female] [×1.159 if black] where κ is 0.7 for females and 0.9 for males | *N* = 8254 nonblacks and blacks, 44% women<br>Mean age: 47 ± 15 yr (only 216 pts > 70 yr and 41 > 80 yr) | Developed in a population with few pts > 70 yr and almost none > 80 yr<br>Less accurate in men with BMI ≥ 35 kg/m$^2$ |
| | CKD-EPIcys—cystatin C (mg/L) | eGFR = 133 × $\min(S_{cys/0.8,1})^{-0.499}$ × $\max(S_{cys/0.8,1})^{-1.328}$ × $0.996^{age}$ [×0.932 if female] where min indicates the minimum of $S_{Cr/\kappa}$ or 1 and max indicates the maximum of $S_{Cr/\kappa}$ or 1 | *N* = 5352 nonblacks and blacks; 42% women<br>Mean age: 47 ± 15 yr (719 pts > 65 yr) | |
| LMR[304] | Creatinine (μmol/L) | eGFR = $e^{X-0.0158 \times age + 0.438 \times \ln(age)}$<br>Female: pCr < 150 μmol/L:<br>X = 2.50 + 0.0121 × (150 – pCr)<br>Female: pCr ≥ 150 μmol/L:<br>X = 2.50 –0.926 × ln(pCr/150)<br>Male: pCr < 180 μmol/L:<br>X = 2.56 + 0.00968 × (180 – pCr)<br>Male: pCr ≥ 180 μmol/L:<br>X = 2.56 –0.926 × ln(pCr/180) | *N* = 3495 Swedish whites; 47% women<br>Mean age: 63 yr (age range, 21–86 yr; 756 pts 70–79 yr and 342 pts ≥ 80 yr) | Difficult to apply<br>Overestimation in pts with BMI < 20 kg/m$^2$, especially males<br>Not validated in other racial and ethnic groups (e.g., black, Asian)<br>Lack of external validation |
| FAS[305,306] | Creatinine (mg/dL) | $eGFR = \frac{107.3.}{(SCr/Q_{crea})} \times 0.988^{(age-40)}$<br>Equation for age > 40 yr, where $Q_{crea}$ = 0.7 mg/dL for females and 0.9 mg/dL for males | *N* = 6870 nonblacks; 47% women<br>Mean age: 74 yr (1764 pts ≥ 70 yr). | May perform better in healthy and general population than in the CKD population<br>Needs further external validation (e.g., blacks, Asians)<br>Clinical utility needs to be confirmed in further studies |
| | Cystatin C (mg/L) | $eGFR = \frac{107.3.}{(S_{cysC}/Q_{cysC})} \times 0.988^{(age-40)}$<br>where $Q_{cysC}$ = 0.82 mg/L when age 40–70 yr and 0.95 mg/L when age ≥ 70 yr | *N* = 6132 nonblacks; 7% women<br>Mean age: 58 ± 18 yr (1469 pts ≥ 70 yr) | |
| BIS[307] | BIS1—creatinine (mg/dL)<br>BIS2—cystatin C (mg/L) | BIS1: 3736 × $creatinine^{-0.87}$ × $age^{-0.95}$ × 0.82 (if female)<br>BIS2: 767 × cystatin $C^{-0.61}$ × $creatinine^{-0.40}$ × $age^{-0.57}$ × 0.87 (if female) | *N* = 570 (for equation development; whole cohort, *N* = 2073)<br>White German participants; 43% women<br>Community-dwelling older adults ≥ 70 yr<br>Mean age: 78 yr (208 pts ≥ 80 yr) | Needs further external validation (e.g., blacks, Asians) |

*BIS,* Berlin Initiative Study equation; *BMI,* body mass index; *BSA,* body surface area; *CKD-EPI,* Chronic Kidney Disease-Epidemiology Collaboration equation; *FAS,* Full Age Spectrum equation; *LMR,* revised Lund-Malmö equation; *MDRD,* Modification of Diet in Renal Disease Study equation; *pts,* patients.

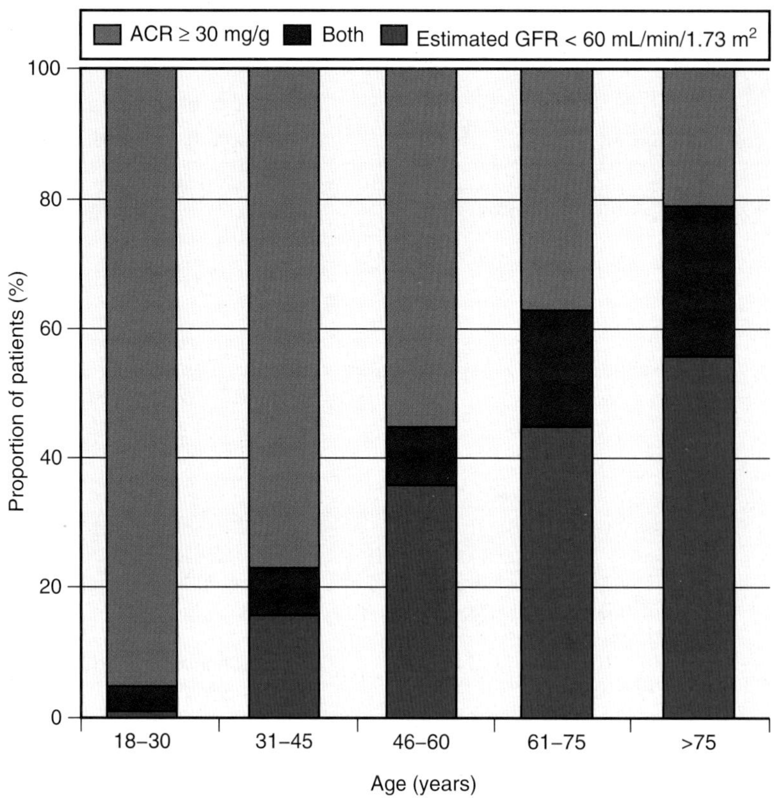


**Fig. 84.1** Proportions of patients with chronic kidney disease identified by the albumin-to-creatinine ratio (ACR), estimated glomerular filtration rate (GFR), or both in the US population. (Adapted from James, MT, Hemmelgarn BR, Tonelli M. Early recognition and prevention of chronic kidney disease. *Lancet.* 2010;375(9722):1296–1309.)

only include a low eGFR without consideration of albuminuria or proteinuria.

In addition to the relationship between albuminuria and vascular health, there is a strong association between the presence of CKD and vascular events.[17,23–25] In the Cardiovascular Health Study, a community-based cohort of US adults aged 65 years and older, individuals with CKD had more than twice the prevalence of coronary artery disease compared with those without CKD.[26,27] In three large cohorts, the Kidney Early Evaluation Program (KEEP; $N$ = 27,017), NHANES, 1999 to 2006 ($N$ = 5,538), and the Medicare 5% sample ($N$ = 1,236,946), the prevalence of diabetes in those with CKD ranged from 21.4% to 46.2% and that of hypertension was 90% or higher.[25] High rates of concomitant high cholesterol, coronary artery disease, congestive heart failure, cardiovascular disease, and cancer were also seen in the KEEP and NHANES cohorts (Fig. 84.2). This relationship remained consistent across age groups.

The lower rate of renal decline observed in older individuals, especially those older than 75 years, means that older adults are more likely to die than to develop ESKD, even when eGFR is severely reduced. In a large Veterans Administration (VA) cohort, the risk of death exceeded that of dialysis in adults older than 85 years, regardless of eGFR (Fig. 84.3).[5] In a community-dwelling population of 1268 older individuals (mean age, 75 years) with an eGFR < 60 mL/min/1.73 m$^2$ followed for 9.7 years, death was 13 times more likely than progression to ESKD, and 25 times more likely for those between 76 and 85 years of age. Even among those who had more advanced CKD (eGFR < 45 mL/min/1.73 m$^2$), the risk of death remained more than sixfold higher than the risk of ESKD.[28] Clinical prediction models to assess risk of death among older patients with CKD are rare and not widely used.[29–31] Instead, prediction models that predict the likelihood that an individual will progress to ESKD are increasingly being used in clinical practice. Using two large Canadian cohorts of patients with CKD stages 3 to 5 defined using eGFR, Tangri et al. developed, and subsequently validated in diverse global cohorts ($N$ = 721,357), two risk equations, termed the eight- and four-variable kidney function risk equation (KFRE).[32,33] The more popular four-variable KFRE uses age, gender, eGFR, and urinary ACR and performs sufficiently well for use in older patients with an eGFR < 45 mL/min/1.73 m$^2$.[10] One criticism of the four-variable KFRE is that it does not address the risk, particularly in older populations, that an acute illness may be associated with an acute precipitous drop in renal function. In fact, between 25% and 50% of those starting dialysis do so after an episode of acute kidney injury (AKI)[34,35] and it has been suggested that future modeling equations include the patient's competing risk of death prior to dialysis requirements, rate of renal function decline, and information about the AKI risk.[36]

## NORMAL AGING VERSUS DISEASE: IS THERE A NEED FOR CHANGE IN HOW WE DEFINE CHRONIC KIDNEY DISEASE?

Inaccuracies around eGFR estimation, and the observation that older patients have less albuminuria and slower deterioration rates, have been fueling debate about whether it is appropriate

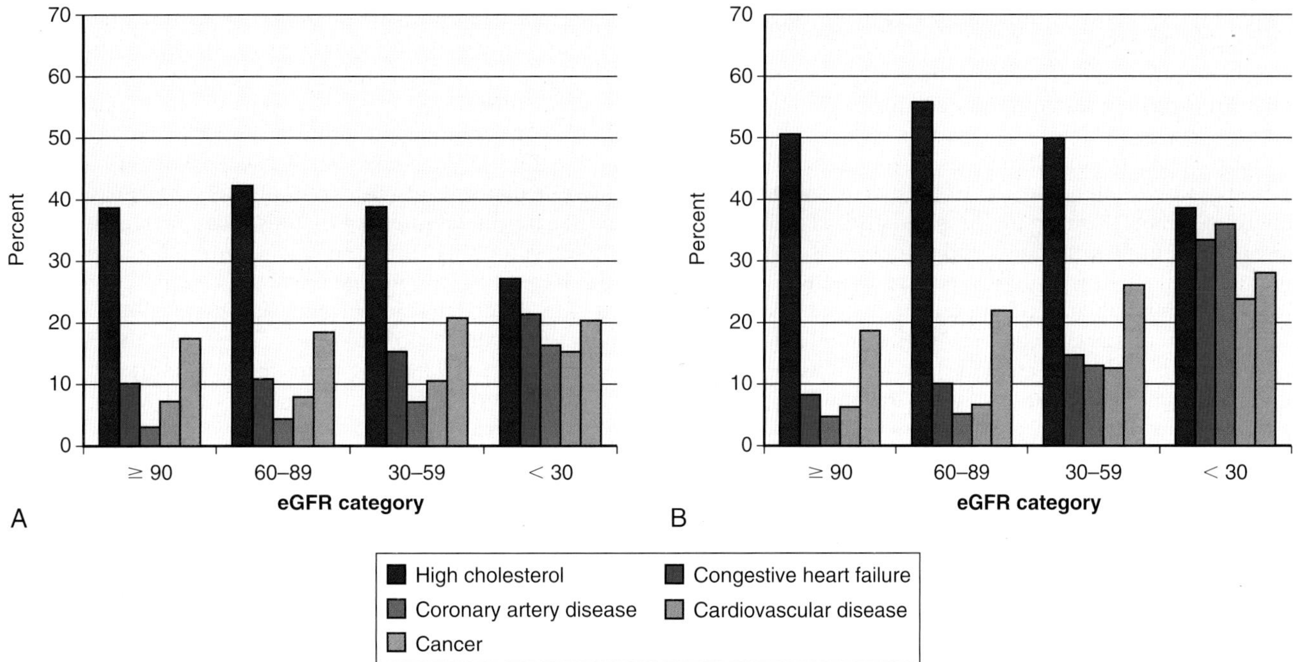


**Fig. 84.2** Comorbid conditions by level of estimated glomerular filtration rate (eGFR) in the Kidney Early Evaluation Program (A) and National Health and Nutrition Examination Survey (B). (From Stevens LA, Li S, Wang C, et al: Prevalence of CKD and comorbid illness in elderly patients in the United States: results from the Kidney Early Evaluation Program (KEEP). *Am J Kidney Dis.* 2010;55(Suppl 2):S23–S33.)

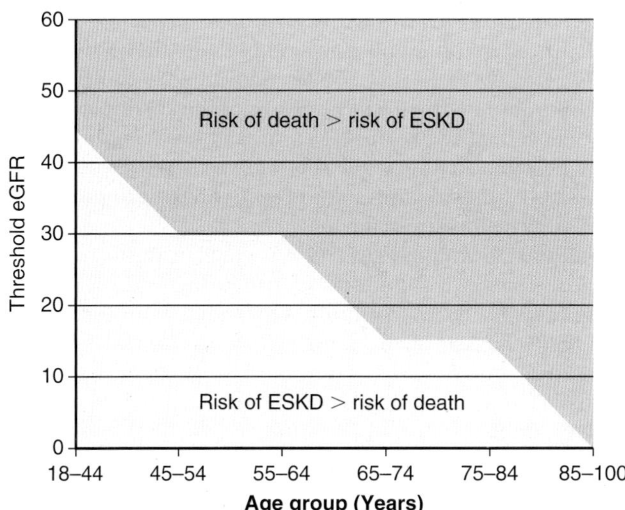


**Fig. 84.3** Baseline estimated glomerular filtration rate (eGFR) threshold below which the risk for end-stage kidney disease (ESKD) exceeded the risk for death for each age group. (From O'Hare AM, Choi AI, Bertenthal D, et al. Age affects outcomes in chronic kidney disease. *J Am Soc Nephrol.* 2007;18:2758–2765.)

to label individuals, in their 8th and 9th decades, as having a chronic disease based on current criteria. More recently, several authors have suggested that the prevalence of CKD is greatly overestimated in older individuals.[37,38] They note that a decline in renal function is a normal component of aging and suggest that the nomenclature used to define CKD be modified, and based on age.[39–41] Contemporary definitions of CKD do not differentiate between older and younger adults and likely result in a number of older individuals being mislabeled and potentially overtreated for CKD.[42–45]

Several studies have suggested that the GFR declines steadily with healthy aging, often at a slow rate and in the absence of albuminuria. Although these changes are often attributed to fibrotic changes in the kidney, there is insufficient evidence to suggest that pathologic findings parallel changes in renal function. In an evaluation of 1203 healthy potential kidney donors, Rule and colleagues[46] have correlated the degree of renal fibrosis on histology with the GFR measured using iothalamate clearance across a number of age groups. This reduction in renal function appeared to begin in the 3rd decade, but was most discernible by the 6th or 7th decade.[47] Fibrosis was more common with advancing age, and the measured GFR fell with age (estimated at 4.6 mL/min/1.73 $m^2$ per decade in men and 7.1 mL/min/1.73 $m^2$ per decade in women), but there was substantial heterogeneity in GFR values among patients with similar degrees of fibrosis and of the same age, and the resulting correlation between the GFR and degree of fibrosis was weak.[48] (See Chapter 22 for further discussion on the physiology and pathophysiology of the aging kidney.)

## COMORBIDITIES AND GERIATRIC SYNDROMES AMONG OLDER INDIVIDUALS WITH CHRONIC KIDNEY DISEASE

"Geriatric syndromes" (GSs) is the term used to describe a group of common health conditions in older people that do not fit into discrete disease categories. These conditions include frailty, functional limitation, falls, depression, polypharmacy, malnutrition, and cognitive impairment. Collectively, the GSs arise from a complex interplay between age-related physiologic changes, chronic disease, and functional stressors in older adults. Each interacts with the other, and often the syndromes co-occur.

Emerging data in older individuals with CKD have suggested an unexpectedly high burden of GSs. It is important for nephrology teams to recognize these geriatric issues for several reasons. The appropriateness and effectiveness of medical interventions, such as dialysis care, are dependent on the overall patient well-being, GSs, and general health. Moreover, from the patient's perspective, the presence of one or more GSs almost invariably affects their lifestyle, as well as that of their family and social circle. Timely recognition of these syndromes can help with treatment decision making, and trigger discussions around goals of care and advance care planning.

The formal evaluation of a patient, using a geriatric lens to recognize GSs and incorporate findings into clinical care, is referred to as a comprehensive geriatric assessment (CGA). Ideally, the CGA assessment is conducted over several visits, in the home and in the clinic, by a variety of health care professionals in addition to the physician, including nursing, physiotherapy, occupational therapy, and social work. Evaluation includes a detailed medical history, including treatment targets, assessment of the home environment and social support structure, functional history, and an assessment of personal values and lifestyle preferences. This information is then coupled with the medical issues and assessment of strength, balance, sensory function, cognition, depression, nutrition, and communication skills and used to identify potential areas of concern. Multidisciplinary teams use the results of the assessment to develop a coordinated plan that maximizes health while minimizing the impact of the geriatric impairments, or the treatments being initiated, on the individual and his or her caregivers. This multidimensional and multidisciplinary approach to GSs has been shown to be effective in the general population[49–51] and across multiple renal clinical settings.[52–55] Awareness of GSs can improve outcomes and well-being,[52,55] and routine CGA has been recommended by the American Society of Nephrology, Geriatric Advisory Group, for all older CKD patients.[56]

## FRAILTY

In the clinical realm, frailty is a complex syndrome (or state) associated with increased vulnerability. It often results from a combination of problems occurring across different domains of daily functioning, including physical, sensory, psychological, and social domains. Frailty has multiple causes and contributors and is characterized by diminished strength and endurance and by reduced physiologic function that leave the individual vulnerable to developing increased dependency and/or death.[57,58] Operational definitions for determining frailty vary, and a multitude of validated measurement scales have been used.[59] This contributes to much of the variability in estimated prevalence. The sole use of the physical domain as a surrogate measure for the global assessment of frailty, such as the Fried et al. classification,[60] in which definitions are based on five physical components—unintentional weight loss, decreased strength, decreased exercise tolerance, reduced gait speed, and fatigue, may be an inadequate metric for frailty, particularly in CKD. Social determinants of frailty, such as those associated with environmental and mental well-being, are also of importance and may be recognized through more holistic assessments.[61,62] The Clinical Frailty Scale is an example of a simple and clinically applicable validated tool that can be used to assess global frailty status. The scale uses several grades of frailty (Fig. 84.4) based largely on the clinical judgment of the physician, making it an easily applied screening instrument to identify those who would most benefit from a formal CGA.

Frailty is of clinical importance because it is associated with an increased risk of both morbidity (e.g., falls, hospitalization, dependence, need for long-term care) and mortality.[63–65] Risks of mortality are twice as high in those with frailty, compared with nonfrail individuals, across the complete spectrum of CKD. For example, in CKD patients enrolled in the MDRD study, frailty determined from self-reported questionnaires was associated with a 1.7-fold increase in mortality over time (hazard ratio (HR) 1.7; 95% confidence interval [CI], 1.3–2.3)[66] and, in frail patients starting dialysis in a special US Renal Data System (USRDS) study, mortality was 1.8-fold higher over a 3-year period (HR, 1.8; 95% CI, 1.4–2.2).[65]

The prevalence of frailty appears to increase as renal function declines[66,67] and is estimated to be two- to fourfold higher in the renal population, compared with those with normal renal function.[67–69] Recent prevalence estimates have suggested that between 40% and 60% of those on dialysis have frailty characteristics.[63,70,71] Although more prevalent in those with increased age, there is also an unexpectedly high burden of frailty in younger individuals on dialysis.[72,73] This high prevalence may be partly explained by concomitant CKD-related conditions such as protein-energy wasting (PEW), anemia, inflammation, acidosis, and hormonal disturbances.[74] There is also an increasing awareness of how renal care and treatments may inadvertently promote the sick role and create barriers to routine participation in exercise programs and other positive health behaviors.[63]

Frailty is a dynamic process in which transitions across states of frailty are common but, on average, transition to a worse state is more common than to a better state.[75–77] Although characterized by a decline in physical function, including physical activity and exercise capacity, it is often also associated with reduced social participation and self-care abilities, depression, and cognitive impairment and should trigger open discussions reviewing the current goals of care, prognosis, and more frequent evaluation of symptoms. To date, there are no simple one-step interventions that reverse frailty, but multidisciplinary care, nutritional supplementation, exercise, and rehabilitation may attenuate the morbidity associated with frailty, particularly when applied early.[24,74]

## FUNCTIONAL IMPAIRMENT

Functional status describes an individual's ability to perform tasks associated with personal care and maintaining a household. In contrast to leisure activities (e.g., gardening, sports), functional tasks are often regarded as fundamental for daily life, and loss of independence is associated with reduced quality of life (QOL) for patients and their caregivers. Although patients with frailty characteristics have a high burden of functional dependence, both frailty and functional loss may occur independently of each other.

## Clinical Frailty Scale

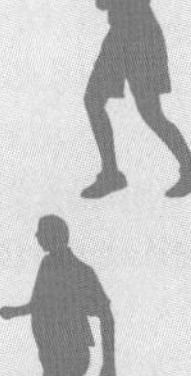

**1. Very Fit** – People who are robust, active, energetic and motivated. These people commonly exercise regularly. They are among the fittest for their age.

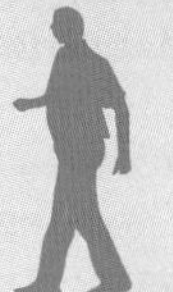

**2. Well** – People who have no active disease symptoms but are less fit than category 1. Often, they exercise or are very active occasionally, e.g., seasonally.

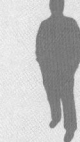

**3. Managing Well** – People whose medical problems are well controlled, but are not regularly active beyond routine walking.

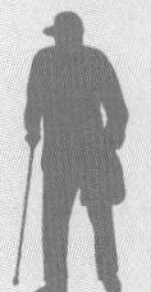

**4. Vulnerable** – While not dependent on others for daily help, often symptoms limit activities. A common complaint is being "slowed up", and/or being tired during the day.

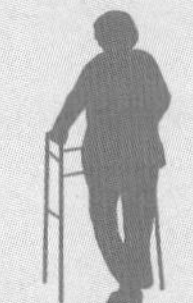

**5. Mildly Frail** – These people often have more evident slowing, and need help in high order IADLs (finances, transportation, heavy housework, medications). Typically, mild frailty progressively impairs shopping and walking outside alone, meal preparation and housework.

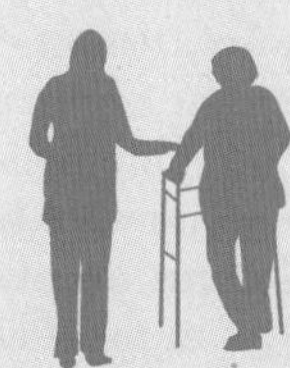

**6. Moderately Frail** – People need help with all outside activities and with keeping house. Inside, they often have problems with stairs and need help with bathing and might need minimal assistance (cuing, standby) with dressing.

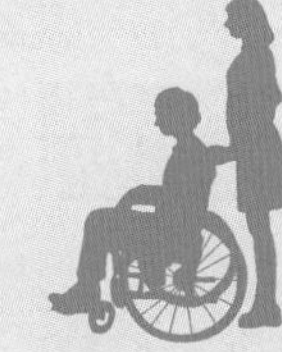

**7. Severely Frail** – Completely dependent for personal care, from whatever cause (physical or cognitive). Even so, they seem stable and not at high risk of dying (within ~ 6 months).

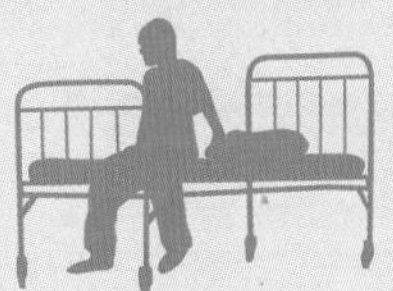

**8. Very Severely Frail** – Completely dependent, approaching the end of life. Typically, they could not recover even from a minor illness.

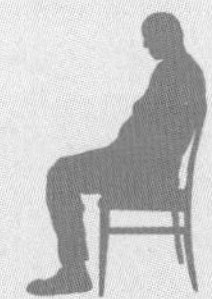

**9. Terminally Ill** – Approaching the end of life. This category applies to people with a life expectancy <6 months, who are not otherwise evidently frail.

**Scoring frailty in people with dementia**

The degree of frailty corresponds to the degree of dementia. Common **symptoms in mild dementia** include forgetting the details of a recent event, though still remembering the event itself, repeating the same question/story and social withdrawal.

In **moderate dementia**, recent memory is very impaired, even though they seemingly can remember their past life events well. They can do personal care with prompting.

In **severe dementia**, they cannot do personal care without help

**Fig. 84.4** Clinical frailty scale. *IADLs,* Instrumental activities of daily living. (From Rockwood K, Song X, MacKnight C, et al. A global clinical measure of fitness and frailty in elderly people. *CMAJ.* 2005;173(5):489–495.)

Recent estimates have shown that individuals with CKD stage 3b have a threefold increased risk of developing dependence in daily activities such as bathing, dressing, and personal care compared with individuals without renal impairment.[78] Although causation cannot be proven, several studies have suggested that dialysis initiation may exacerbate or accelerate functional decline (Fig. 84.5).[79–81] Most at risk are those with multiple comorbidities, those of older age, and those with a functional loss at the time of dialysis initiation. In a representative, cross-sectional sample of patients on maintenance hemodialysis (HD), followed by the Dialysis Outcomes and Practice Patterns Study (DOPPS), 77% of noninstitutionalized patients 70 years or older reported dependency[82] in contrast to 15% of older adults (≥65 years) in the Cardiovascular Health Study.[83]

In the general geriatric literature, functional dependence is recognized as a contributor to subsequent disability, recurrent hospitalization, and increased mortality.[84–89] Several studies have shown an association between poor mobility status (i.e.,requiring assistance with or total dependency for transfers and ambulation) and mortality risk among incident dialysis patients (Table 84.2).[90–96] Functional dependency (increased need for nursing care, less participation in social societal roles) is associated with a twofold increase in mortality (HR, 2.4; 95% CI, 1.9–2.9) for those with the highest degree of functional loss.[82]

Many factors contribute to the high rate of functional dependencies among older patients with advanced CKD. High rates of depression, cognitive impairment, poor physical functioning, multimorbidity, and the need for repeated hospitalizations may all contribute to the patient's reduced overall health and self-care ability. Early identification of functional impairment in CKD patients may provide an opportunity to ensure adequate management of modifiable contributing factors, provide support and referral to geriatric rehabilitation services, and trigger discussions, with the family

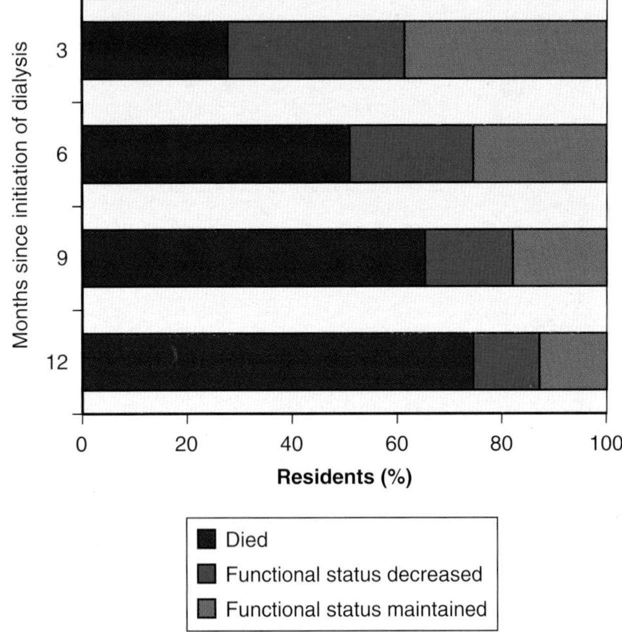


**Fig. 84.5** Survival and functional status after the initiation of dialysis among nursing home residents. (From Kurella Tamura M, Covinsky KE, Chertow GM, et al: Functional status of elderly adults before and after initiation of dialysis. *N Engl J Med.* 2009;361:1539–1547.)

and patient, around the prognosis and identification of the trajectory of functional decline in older patients starting dialysis with limitations.

## FALLS

As noted previously, several GSs tend to occur concomitantly. Accidental falls are more common in individuals with other GSs, such as concomitant frailty and functional decline, although this relationship is not absolute.[97] Falls are common among older adults and are a leading cause of injury-related hospitalizations, often with prolonged hospital stays, functional decline, long-term care admission, and mortality.[98–102] Up to one-third of community-dwelling individuals older than 65 years fall annually, often recurrently.[103] Injurious falls, such as those causing fractures, head injuries, or cuts, occur in one out of five falls,[104,105] although usually one fall will trigger a cycle of fear of falling (>25% of cases) and a reduction in activity levels, furthering the risk of subsequent falls and the ability to care for oneself.[106]

Falls are almost twofold more common in the dialysis population, both in those maintained on HD and those on peritoneal dialysis (PD).[107,108] Although there are multiple common risk factors for falls (Table 84.3), one of the less appreciated complications of HD that may contribute to falls is the effect of forced immobility. The long time during which patients are sitting relatively still in the dialysis chair may lead to changes in balance, lack of sensory stimulation, and, over time, muscle atrophy. More concerning, however, is the 1.6-fold higher risk of serious fall injuries (i.e., resulting in fractures, head injury, or joint dislocation) that occurs in the year after dialysis initiation, compared with the year prior to dialysis care.[109] Clinical data also support the suggestion that dialysis itself may be causative. In a small single-center study of community-dwelling seniors, falls were more common on dialysis days than on nondialysis days (1.45 vs. 1.35 falls/person, respectively) and, if occurring on dialysis days, threefold more common after dialysis than before dialysis.[102] The association between falls and earlier stages of kidney disease has been less well studied, but some authors have suggested that a reduction in eGFR may be a marker of higher fall risk and that elevated ACR may be an independent predisposing factor associated with serious fall injuries, such as fractures.[98]

Routine clinical questioning about previous falls and conducting simple tests for gait and balance may be a key strategy to identify at-risk individuals who warrant a more detailed evaluation and referral for a CGA. Multidisciplinary risk assessment, followed by tailored multifactorial interventions, such as exercise, treatment of pain, assistive devices, medication review, and home hazard modifications, may be effective in reducing fall risk.

## DEPRESSION

Depressive symptoms and clinical depression are common in patients across the complete spectrum of CKD. The prevalence of depression varies, depending on the assessment tools used and the population studied, but, using self-report or screening questionnaires, it is estimated that close to 40% of those undergoing maintenance dialysis have some depressive symptomatology, even if they do not fulfill all criteria for a major depressive episode. Prevalence estimates of major depressive episodes, using formal psychiatrist interview assessments, are lower, ranging from 21% in earlier stages of CKD to 23% in those undergoing maintenance dialysis.[110] These estimates may, however, be influenced by the observation, from a number of studies, that patients on dialysis are often unwilling to undergo formal psychiatric evaluation or treatment. Age-specific data are not available, but depression is often more common in socially isolated individuals and those with functional or cognitive impairment placing frail older individuals at increased risk. In addition often co-occurring with other GSs, depression can be associated with a high burden of pain, fatigue, poor sleep, pruritus, and nausea.[111]

The recognition of depression in the older individual is important for several reasons. In addition to the well-recognized impact on QOL,[112–115] individuals who are maintained on dialysis and are older than 75 years are among those at highest risk of suicide.[116] Furthermore, depression is associated with increased hospitalization and mortality in both CKD and ESKD.[117–122]

The approach to treating depression in older patients is the same as for younger patients. The mainstay treatments are depression-specific psychotherapies, such as cognitive-behavioral therapy (CBT) or interpersonal therapy, and pharmacologic treatment with an antidepressant.

Several studies have shown CBT to be successful in patients with ESKD[123–125] and, where possible, it should be considered the first-line treatment for patients with mild to moderate depression.[126] However, little is known about the influence of physical diseases, frailty, and cognitive impairment on the efficacy or feasibility of psychotherapy. Despite the high prevalence and clinical implications of depression, many patients remain untreated. Several studies have shown low

**Table 84.2 Association of Functional Impairment at Time of Dialysis Initiation With Adverse Health Outcomes**

| Study, Date of Study | Patients | Study Setting | Functional Assessment | Outcome | Association |
|---|---|---|---|---|---|
| Arai et al.,[91] 2014 | *N* = 202<br>Mean age, 80 yr | Single-center study, incident to dialysis<br>Age ≥ 75 yr | Mobility (ability or lack of ability to walk without assistance) | 6-mo mortality | Higher mortality if unable to walk without assistance; 6-mo mortality risk: aHR, 4.9; 95% CI, 1.4–17.1 |
| Couchoud et al.,[92] 2009 | *N* = 2500<br>Mean age, 81 yr | French REIN Registry data, incident to dialysis<br>Age ≥ 75 yr | Mobility (walk without help, assistance with or total dependency for transfers) | 6-mo mortality | Higher mortality if fully dependent for transfers; 6-mo mortality risk: aOR, 1.7; 95% CI, 1.4–2.0 |
| Couchoud et al.,[93] 2015 | *N* = 12,500<br>Age (median), 81 yr | French REIN Registry data, incident to dialysis<br>Age ≥ 75 yr | Mobility (walk without help, assistance with or total dependency for transfers) | 3-mo mortality | Higher mortality if requiring assistance for transfers; 3-mo mortality risk: aOR, 2.5; 95% CI, 2.1–2.9<br>Higher mortality if totally dependent for transfers; 3-mo mortality risk: aOR, 6.5; 95% CI, 5.4–7.9 |
| Dusseux et al.,[90] 2015 | *N* = 8955<br>Age (median), 78 yr | French REIN Registry data, incident to dialysis<br>Age ≥ 70 yr | Mobility (walk without help, assistance with or total dependency for transfers) | 3-yr mortality | Higher mortality if requiring assistance for transfers; 3-yr mortality risk: aOR, 1.7; 95% CI, 1.5–1.9<br>Higher mortality if total dependency for transfers; 3-yr mortality risk: aOR, 3.0; 95% CI, 2.3–3.8 |
| Glaudet et al.,[94] 2013 | *N* = 557<br>Mean age, 71 yr | French REIN Registry data, incident to dialysis | Mobility (walk without help, assistance with or total dependency for transfers) | 4-yr mortality | Higher mortality if requiring assistance for transfers; 4-yr mortality risk: aHR, 1.4; 95% CI, 1.2–1.7<br>Higher mortality if total dependency for transfers; 4-yr mortality risk: aHR, 1.4; 95% CI, 1.0–2.0 |
| Kurella et al.,[96] 2007 | *N* = 83,996<br>Mean age, 84 yr | USRDS Registry data, incident to dialysis<br>Age ≥ 80 yr | Mobility (inability to walk or transfer) | Mortality | Higher mortality if unable to walk or transfer<br>Overall mortality risk: aRR, 1.5; 95% CI, 1.5– .6 |
| Thamer et al.,[95] 2015 | *N* = 52,796<br>Mean age, 77 yr | USRDS Registry data, incident to dialysis<br>Age ≥ 67 yr | Assistance with daily living (requiring assistance with daily living, inability to ambulate, or has an amputation) | 3-mo mortality | Higher mortality if requiring assistance with daily living or for walking; 3-mo mortality risk: aOR, 1.4; 95% CI, 1.3–1.5 |

*aHR,* Adjusted hazard ratio; *aRR,* adjusted relative risk; *aOR,* adjusted odds ratio.

treatment acceptance and, on average, only one-third of patients who may benefit actually receive antidepressant medication.[127–131]

Pharmacologic therapies have been used in patients with CKD or ESKD; however, there is little information on safety, efficacy, and optimal dosing.[132,133] Most antidepressant medications are highly protein-bound and are not removed by dialysis. Although they commonly undergo hepatic metabolism, the active metabolites are excreted via the kidney, and consequently dosing should be adjusted to the eGFR level (Table 84.4). Based on current data, selective serotonin reuptake inhibitors (SSRIs), such as sertraline, escitalopram, and paroxetine, should be considered first-line for pharmacologic treatment for depression in patients with kidney disease.[134,135] Tricyclic antidepressants (TCAs) and monoamine oxidase inhibitors (MAOIs) should be avoided in older patients with (or without) kidney disease because of cardiac and central nervous system side effects, including prolonged QTc, arrhythmia, anticholinergic effects, and orthostatic hypotension. Paroxetine may be useful when treating a depressed patient with concomitant intractable pruritus because of its antipruritic actions; drugs such as duloxetine may be prescribed, off-label for those with concomitant pain. Treatment doses of duloxetine need to be adjusted and, based on data from a small pharmacokinetic study in HD patients,[136] ideally given at 48-hour intervals. It is important to note that in many regions of the world, this is an off-label prescription, with current US product labeling recommending that the drug not be administered if creatinine clearance (CrCl) is < 30 mL/min. Mirtazapine, a noradrenergic and specific

**Table 84.3 Common Risk Factors for Falls in Older Patients With Chronic Kidney Disease**

| Risks | Details | References |
|---|---|---|
| Previous falls | One or more falls during the previous 12 mo | 99, 102, 308 |
| Fear of falling | Fearful anticipation of a fall; detectable on screening using the Falls Efficacy Scale (high scores) | 106 |
| Frailty | Predisposes to falls for multiple reasons (see text) | 108, 309 |
| Balance and gait problems | Increased postural sway, failed walking test; can be exacerbated by arthritic changes or neuropathy | 310 |
| Pain | Pain may lead to guarding and abnormal posture due particularly to lower limb and foot pain | |
| Depression and antidepressants | Fall risk worsened by insomnia and sleep fragmentation, impaired attention and psychomotor slowing, and/or exacerbated by the use of sedatives and antidepressants | 308, 310 |
| Number of prescribed oral drugs | Increased fall risk, particularly with benzodiazepines, antidepressants, beta-blockers, other antihypertensive agents, opiate derivatives | 310-312 |
| Cognitive impairment | Falls precipitated by decreased awareness of environmental risks; altered judgment and reduced executive functioning result in less effective compensation for age- or disease-associated changes in gait and balance | 313 |
| Sensory deficits | Poor vision and/or hearing affect environmental awareness, balance, and compensation strategies | |
| Diabetes | Impaired vision due to retinopathy, peripheral neuropathy and hypoglycemic episodes increase the risk of falls | 310, 314 |
| Anemia | May result in low energy, poor exercise tolerance, and postural hypotension | |
| Protein energy wasting and sarcopenia | Loss of muscle mass and strength result in less effective strategies to compensate and prevent falling; reduced exercise capacity | 308, 315 |
| HD therapy | Increased risk of transient or rapid fluid and electrolyte shifts, hypotension, arrhythmias; stiffness and muscle weakness exacerbated by forced mobility | 316 |
| PD therapy | Environmental risks—connected to a cycler machine overnight, tubing around the bed area may pose trip risk; mechanical factors—changes in the center of gravity due to large volumes of intraabdominal fluid | 107 |

*HD*, Hemodialysis; *PD*, peritoneal dialysis.

serotonergic antidepressant medication, has hypnotic, appetite stimulant, and antipruritic effects and can be used at reduced doses in older renal patients with concomitant anorexia, sleep disturbance, and/or pruritus.

## POLYPHARMACY

Polypharmacy is often defined as a medication count of five or more medications.[137,138] Because patients with CKD take on average 8 medications, and those on dialysis take between 10 and 12, polypharmacy is possibly one of the largest issues in renal medicine. In older populations, polypharmacy is associated with increased mortality, adverse drug events and drug interactions, falls and other GSs, low medication adherence, and greater health care costs.[139] Safe medication prescribing in older adults with CKD is complicated not only by the number of medications and presence of comorbidities, but also by the altered pharmacokinetics and pharmacodynamics in the setting of advancing age and presence of CKD. The combination of age-related changes and CKD places older patients at increased risk of drug accumulation and higher potential for adverse drug effects.[140,141] Evidence to guide prescribing is severely limited because a large proportion of clinical trials excluded those older than 65 years, and therefore treatment decisions were often based on evidence extrapolated from other patient groups.[142–144] As a general guide, clinicians are advised to consider multiple factors listed in Table 84.5. Drugs that have a narrow therapeutic index and/or high toxicity levels should only be used when other alternatives are not available, and individuals should be monitored carefully.[145]

Several tools can identify medications in which the risks of use in older adults often outweigh the benefits or identify medications that have been omitted but are likely to benefit the individual. The most widely used tools include the Beers Criteria,[146] Screening Tool to Alert doctors to the Right Treatment (START),[147] and Screening Tool of Older Person's potentially inappropriate Prescriptions (STOPP).[148] START focuses on ensuring that medications that are indicated, and likely to provide benefit, are not omitted in error, whereas the Beers Criteria and STOPP focus more on minimizing the exposure to medications for which the risks outweigh potential benefits. The 2015 Beers Criteria are divided into five sections—medications to avoid in most older adults, medications to avoid in older adults with specific diseases or syndromes, medications to be used with caution in older adults, potentially clinically important drug-drug interactions, and medications to avoid or adjust dose in older adults based on kidney function. The combined STOPP-START criteria, recently updated,[149] have been shown to improve medication appropriateness significantly and reduce adverse outcomes from potentially inappropriate medications.[150] Incorporating the Beers criteria and STOPP-START criteria into a daily drug prescription review process can maximize the efficiency and safety of pharmacotherapy and minimize the number of errors in the administration of drugs to older patients with CKD.

**Table 84.4 Safety, Dosing, and Efficacy of Common Antidepressant Medications Used in Chronic Kidney Disease (CKD) and End-Stage Kidney Disease**

| Drug Class, Generic | Dose Adjustment in CKD[132] | Comment | Efficacy Studies | Class Adverse Effects[132,133,317] |
|---|---|---|---|---|
| **Selective Serotonin Reuptake Inhibitor (SSRI)** | | | | |
| Sertraline | CKD stages 1–4: no dosage adjustment required; 50–200 mg/day<br>CKD stages 5–5D: start at 25 mg/day, consider decreasing max dose | Less than 1% excreted unchanged in urine<br>Pharmacokinetics in CKD are unchanged in single-dose studies, but no published data on multiple dosing<br>Likely not dialyzed | Three prospective efficacy studies[129,318,319]: sertraline significantly improved BDI scores | Common: insomnia, restlessness, nausea, headache, GI upset, sexual dysfunction, activation (mainly with fluoxetine and sertraline)<br>Rare: SIADH, increased bleeding risk, extrapyramidal symptoms, serotonin syndrome (in combination with other serotonergic drugs), and QT prolongation (seen with dose > 40 mg of citalopram) |
| Paroxetine | IR: 10–40 mg/day<br>CR: 12.5–50 mg/day | <2% excreted in urine<br>Increased plasma concentration found when GFR < 30 mL/min<br>If GFR < 30 mL/min, start at 10–20 mg/day, increase slowly<br>Likely not dialyzed | One study among HD patients ($N$ = 34)[320]: paroxetine significantly improved depressive symptoms and nutritional markers | |
| Citalopram | No dosage adjustment required: 10–40 mg/day | <15% excreted in urine<br>Manufacturer does not recommend use if GFR < 20 mL/min<br>Dose adjustment normally not required in renal impairment, but use with caution when GFR < 10 mL/min<br>Only 1% of drug removed by HD | One randomized study (citalopram versus psychological training) in HD population ($N$ = 44)[321]: both citalopram and psychological training significantly reduced HADS scores at the end of 3 mo | |
| Escitalopram | No dosage adjustment required: 10–20 mg/day | <10% excreted in urine<br>Manufacturer does not recommend use if GFR < 20 mL/min<br>Likely not dialyzed | One randomized study[322] (escitalopram vs. placebo) in 58 ESKD patients—escitalopram significantly improved HADS scores compared with placebo | |
| Fluoxetine | No dosage adjustment required: 20–60 mg/day | 5%–10% excreted in urine<br>Long half-life.<br>If GFR < 20 mL/min, consider using on alternate days or low dose<br>Likely not dialyzed | Two small prospective efficacy studies—fluoxetine improved depressive symptoms by more than 25% in six HD patients[323] and, compared with placebo, improved depression at 4 wk but not 8 wk in 14 HD patients[324] | |
| **Serotonin-Norepinephrine Reuptake Inhibitor (SNRI)** | | | | |
| Venlafaxine | Normal dosage: 75–225 mg/day<br>eGFR 10–70: consider reducing dose by 25%–50%. Dialysis: reduce total daily dose by 50% | 5% excreted in urine, clearance decrease and half-life prolonged in renal impairment<br>Manufacturer advises to avoid use if GFR < 10 mL/min<br>Accumulation of toxic metabolite can occur, rhabdomyolysis and renal failure have been reported, but rare | No efficacy data | Similar to SSRIs plus increased blood pressure<br>Liver toxicity seen with duloxetine |
| Duloxetine | No adjustment required if eGFR > 30: 40–120 mg/day; use not recommended with eGFR < 30 | Off-label use in patients with advanced CKD and on maintenance dialysis | No efficacy data | |

Continued on following page

**Table 84.4 Safety, Dosing, and Efficacy of Common Antidepressant Medications Used in Chronic Kidney Disease (CKD) and End-Stage Kidney Disease (Cont'd)**

| Drug Class, Generic | Dose Adjustment in CKD[132] | Comment | Efficacy Studies | Class Adverse Effects[132,133,317] |
|---|---|---|---|---|
| **Noradrenergic and Specific Serotonergic Antidepressant** | | | | |
| Mirtazapine | No dosage adjustment recommended for eGFR 10–50: 15–45 mg/day<br>GFR < 10: consider dose reduction | 75% excreted unchanged in urine<br>Clearance reduced by 50% in those with GFR <10 mL/min<br>Has been used to treat pruritus caused by renal failure | No efficacy data | Appetite stimulation, weight gain, sedation |
| **Norepinephrine-Dopamine Reuptake Inhibitor** | | | | |
| Bupropion | Consider reduced dose and/or frequency: 150–450 mg/day | | No efficacy data | Increased risk of seizures, insomnia, anxiety, decreased appetite |
| **Tricyclic Antidepressant (TCA)** | | | | |
| Nortriptyline | No dosage adjustment required: 35–150 mg/day<br>Not recommended for older adults, especially those with CKD | <5% excreted in urine<br>All metabolites are highly lipophilic. | No efficacy data | Anticholinergic effects, orthostatic hypotension, sedation, cardiotoxicity |
| Amitriptyline | No dosage adjustment required: 10–200 mg/day<br>Not recommended for older adults, especially those with CKD | <2% excreted in urine | No efficacy data | |

*BDI,* Beck Depression Inventory; *CR,* controlled release; *HADS,* Hospital Anxiety and Depression Scale; *IR,* immediate release; *SIADH,* syndrome of inappropriate antidiuretic hormone.

## MALNUTRITION AND PROTEIN-ENERGY WASTING

Depending on the definitions used, anywhere between 25% and 75% of older patients maintained on dialysis have evidence of uremic malnutrition, muscle wasting, and body fat loss.[151] In the renal literature, the term "protein-energy wasting" (PEW) is used in preference to malnutrition because CKD-related factors contribute to the development of wasting, independent of the nutrient intake.[152] A full review of PEW is beyond the scope of this chapter; however, it is important to recognize PEW in the older patient because it is associated with weakness, falls, and increased mortality and remains largely unrecognized and undertreated.[153,154]

Appetite loss is relatively common in older patients with ESKD, with an estimated one-third to one-half of patients experiencing a progressive, spontaneous decrease in food intake as CKD progresses.[155,156] This change in appetite often drives the initial changes in nutrient intake[152]; however, the spiral of decline in overall nutrition is compounded by multiple factors common among older individuals (Fig. 84.6). In renal medicine, the introduction of dietary restrictions affects variety, flavor, and palatability of food and further increases the undernutrition. In many cases, the loss of the social pleasures of eating leads to a low QOL, in addition to PEW.

Special attention should be given to nutritional status in older individuals, and personalized support from a renal dietitian is imperative when PEW is noted—both the subjective global assessment (SGA) and malnutrition inflammation score (MIS) are reliable screening tools. Interventions to improve PEW are often limited to supplementation, with little evidence to support changes in dialytic interventions. Symptoms of constipation and/or dry mouth should be aggressively treated and, where possible, the use of drugs known to reduce appetite should be avoided. Although not evidence-based, mirtazapine and/or other pharmacologic stimulants, together with relaxation of all dietary restrictions, have been tried.

## COGNITIVE IMPAIRMENT

Cognitive impairment affects patients negatively by contributing to functional dependence and behavioral symptoms, which in turn have important effects on patient well-being and QOL. Impaired cognition potentially affects multiple areas of patient care, including patient adherence with treatment plans and medication, and may lead to premature institutionalization and death.[157–159] Pathophysiology, prevalence, and treatments of neurologic conditions in kidney disease are discussed elsewhere in this text (see Chapter 57). Screening is important for all individuals, and relatively quick

**Table 84.5 Key Elements in Considering Risks and Benefits When Prescribing for Older Adults With Kidney Disease**

| Risk Considerations | Benefit Considerations |
|---|---|
| **Medication-Associated Risks** | |
| • Is the medication cleared in whole or in part by the kidney? Does the medication have a narrow therapeutic window?<br>• Is the medication thought to be of high risk in the general older population or in individuals with comorbidities similar to those of the patient in question?<br>• Does the medication have potential central nervous system effects?<br>• Are data available to guide dosing in patients with kidney disease (e.g., pharmacokinetic studies, drug level monitoring)?<br>**Patient-Associated Risks**<br>• Is the patient already taking multiple medications?<br>• Does the patient have cognitive dysfunction, poor vision, frailty? Risk of additional medications may be higher in this group.<br>• Does the patient have a history of adherence problems, and what would be the consequences of patient-related erratic dosing? | • What is the population in which this medication has been studied? Does it include older adults or those with kidney disease? Is there observational or clinical trial evidence that benefits extend to those with kidney disease?<br>• If patients with kidney disease have not been studied, does the medication have a track record of safety in postapproval studies?<br>• Would benefits of the medication be due to improvement in symptoms or in decrease in risk from asymptomatic disease? What are the patient's preferences in adding new medications?<br>• Does the medication address a problem for which the patient is at significant risk (e.g., cardiovascular disease in patients with kidney disease)? Is the patient likely to accrue significant absolute risk reduction from the new medication? |

From Rifkin DE, Winkelmayer WC: Medication issues in older individuals with CKD. *Adv Chronic Kidney Dis.* 2010;17:320–328.

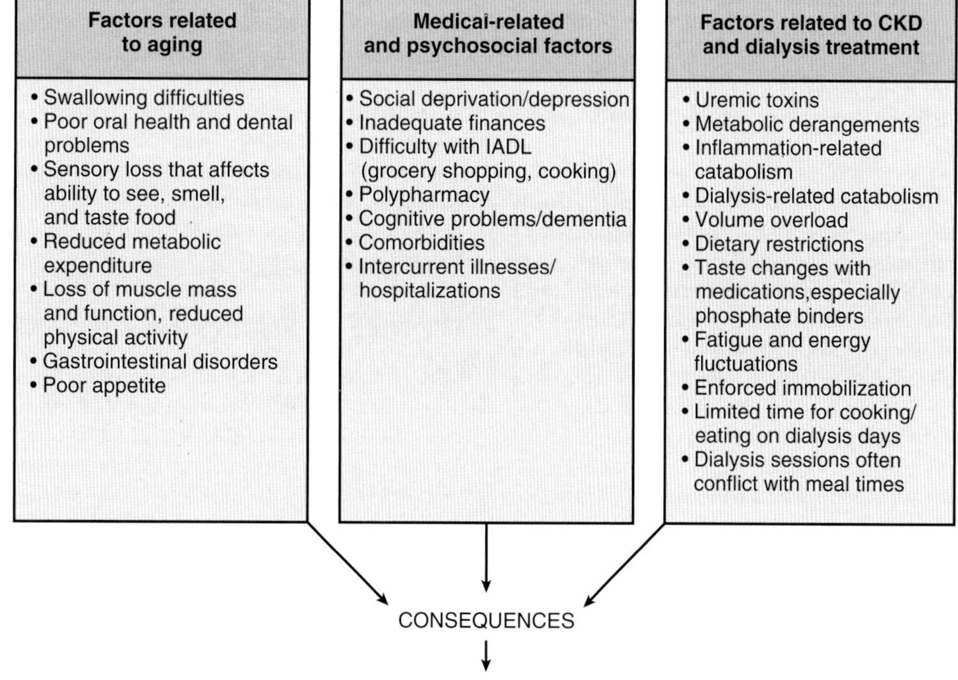


**Fig. 84.6** Common factors related to aging and dialysis leading to malnutrition and protein-energy wasting (PEW). *CKD,* Chronic kidney disease; *IADL,* instrumental activities of daily living; *QOL,* quality of life.

tests such as the Mini-Cog (three-word recall and clock drawing) or the Mini-Mental State Exam (MMSE) may be useful in a busy practice. Because cognitive impairment deteriorates over time, particularly after dialysis initiation,[160] it is important to recognize and discuss any features of cognitive impairment that are present and introduce the patient and family to the high likelihood of further progression to dementia. Implementation of adequate social support and planning for future patient care is a critical part of these discussions.

## CONTROVERSIES AND COMPLEXITY IN THE MANAGEMENT OF OLDER PATIENTS WITH CHRONIC KIDNEY DISEASE

Over the last decade, multiple clinical practice guidelines have emerged, creating an evidence-based structure that is currently used to guide clinical CKD care. Clinical practice guidelines help standardize care and ensure a consistent approach, across all patients, that includes the interventions most likely to reduce mortality and cardiovascular events and to slow disease progression. Guidelines incorporate data from large population studies and consequently their strength—the ability to create a simplified model to guide consistent high-quality care—is also, in some respects, their greatest weakness. Individual patients bring their own complexities, values, and goals and, particularly when applied to frail older individuals approaching the end of life, guidelines may lead to care that is poorly aligned with the individual's needs. Clinicians are encouraged to solicit individual patient goals and values, distinguish between younger and older individuals, robust or frail, and between those with renal-limited CKD and those with complex clustering of multiple chronic diseases.

Within the renal sphere, guidelines have given rise to several discussions around whether adaptation is required when treating an older frail patient. These controversial issues are introduced in the subsequent sections.

### HYPERTENSION IN THE FRAIL OLDER PATIENT WITH CHRONIC KIDNEY DISEASE: TARGETING BLOOD PRESSURE

Decades of research have unequivocally shown that antihypertensive treatment reduces the risk of cardiovascular (CV) outcomes in several populations, including older and very old patients. Currently, however, there is uncertainty about how strict blood pressure (BP) control should be in older individuals with advanced kidney disease.[161,162] Although a discussion of all hypertensive trials is beyond the scope of this chapter and is well covered elsewhere (see Chapter 49), data pertinent specifically to older individuals with CKD are included later.

Newer guidelines, such as those in Canada and Australia, have incorporated data from the Systolic Blood Pressure Intervention Trial (SPRINT)[163] published in 2015 promoting systolic BP targets < 120 mm Hg.[164–166] SPRINT is a prospective randomized controlled trial, funded by the National Institutes of Health, that has randomized 9361 patients with high CV risk to standard treatment targeting systolic BP < 140 mm Hg or to intensive BP-lowering targeting systolic BP < 120 mm Hg. SPRINT included adults aged 50 years or older who were at modest risk of vascular disease but who were free of diabetes mellitus and did not have a recent stroke, CV event, or heart failure. SPRINT showed that in this select population, lowering systolic BP to a goal of <120 mm Hg resulted in significantly lower rates of fatal and nonfatal CV events and death from any cause. The benefits of stricter BP goals were also confirmed in a prespecified subgroup analysis of 2636 subjects aged 75 years or older.[167] Of interest, although the overall rate of serious adverse events was not different between groups (38.3% in intensive vs. 37.1% in the control group; $P = .25$), more patients in the intensive arm developed AKI, syncope, electrolyte abnormalities, and hypotension (but had no injurious falls).

However, there is concern that the data from SPRINT may not be applicable to the older, frail patient population with advanced CKD.[161,162,168] Although a proportion of those aged 75 years or older recruited in SPRINT had elevated creatinine levels (16% had an eGFR < 45 mL/min/1.73 m$^2$), few had other features of progressive kidney disease (see earlier discussion on controversies around defining older adults as having a disease based on eGFR thresholds alone).[167] Patients with proteinuria > 1 g/day and those with polycystic kidney disease were actively excluded. Unlike many CKD patients, BP was easily controlled with a minimal number of medications. Furthermore, patients with dementia, unintentional weight loss > 10%, or residence in a nursing home were excluded, as were individuals with medical conditions limiting life expectancy to less than 3 years (including cancer).

The benefits of treating hypertension have been confirmed in a recent meta-analysis incorporating data from almost 45,000 patients across all ages.[169] The evidence for which BP targets to use is less clear. Weiss et al.[161] have shown robust evidence that BP targets of less than 150/90 mm Hg led to a reduction in mortality, cardiac events, and stroke but only low to moderate evidence that a BP lower than 140/85 mm Hg was beneficial in adults aged 60 years or older. In addition, they found lower BP targets to be associated with an increase in syncope and medication burden but not higher rates of falls or cognitive decline. Although the rate of adverse effects seemed similar across all BP targets, the impact of an adverse event is likely higher in older patients, particularly those residing in a nursing home,[170] and consequently caution is advised. At least, at present, as data continue to emerge, the reader is best advised to integrate the results of a CGA into decision making and adapt treatments to align with individual patient complexity.

### THE ROLE OF STATINS IN OCTOGENARIANS

CKD is associated with an increased risk of major CV events and mortality and is sometimes considered a coronary risk equivalent to diabetes and hypertension.[171] Although dyslipidemia is an important modifiable risk factor for CV disease in the general population, particularly in those older than 50 years, its role and relevance in the older CKD population are less clear. Current KDIGO guidelines recommend the initiation of statin therapy, either alone or in combination with ezetimibe, for all nondialysis patients aged 50 years or older with an eGFR < 60 mL/min/1.73 m$^2$, irrespective of age or baseline lipid profile.[172] Much of the evidence is based on high quality data from the Study of Heart and Renal Protection (SHARP) discussed later.[173] Unlike contemporary guidelines for the general population, published by the American College of Cardiology and American Heart Association,[174] that apply only to those aged 20 to 79 years, there is, however, no upper age limit included in the KDIGO guidelines. As a result, it may be appropriate to take a more cautious approach, particularly in those with multimorbidity, using guiding principles published by the American Geriatric Society.[175]

The SHARP trial, published in 2011, randomized patients with CKD to 20 mg simvastatin plus 10 mg ezetimibe or placebo.[173] Patients were followed prospectively for a median of 5 years, and results showed a lower incidence of cardiac death, stroke, nonfatal myocardial infarction, and cardiac revascularization (11.3% vs. 13.4%, respectively). A number of participants were aged 70 years and older (28% of SHARP participants), and the effectiveness of the interventions, simvastatin and ezetimibe, was similar. There was little evidence from the data presented that suggested any increased risk of adverse events in these older participants. The dilemma, however, arises from what, and who, was not included in the study. A number of patients were excluded because their physician did not think that participation was appropriate. Many of these may have been older individuals with social or other characteristics not captured in the study data. In an eloquent piece, Butler et al. have argued that application of current KDIGO guidelines advocating for the use of statins in those of any age with CKD may not be appropriate.[176] They suggested that the older patients recruited into the study were likely not representative of many of those attending our clinics; they referred specifically to patients with a history of myocardial infarction, cognitive impairment, or functional limitations who would have been excluded, but also allude to those with social or psychological frailty. Also, they remind us of the need to elicit treatment preferences and goals, especially because both pill burden and cost are often more important to older individuals than to younger patients, and the impacts of any adverse drug effects are higher.

Whereas the benefits of lipid lowering have been shown for patients with nondialysis CKD, the benefits do not appear to extend to dialysis patients. Several large randomized trials and high-quality meta-analyses have suggested that statin therapy has little or no effect on cardiovascular outcomes among adults undergoing maintenance dialysis.[173,177–183] Furthermore, emerging evidence has suggested that statins may accelerate vascular calcification in the dialysis population.[184] As a result, the indication for use in older patients, particularly those with frailty or multimorbidity in whom the life expectancy is a few years, is weak. At present, the 2014 KDIGO Lipid Guidelines[172] and 2016 Canadian Cardiovascular Society Guidelines[185] recommend statins not be started in adults receiving dialysis, but that they be continued in patients already receiving them at the time of dialysis initiation. Although not supported by evidence or by guidelines, discontinuation of statins may have a role in older individuals maintained on dialysis who present with increasing frailty, multimorbidity, polypharmacy, or malnutrition and those entering the end of life.

## ANTICOAGULATION IN ATRIAL FIBRILLATION

The prevalence of atrial fibrillation (AF) in patients with impaired kidney function is considerably higher than that seen in the general population.[186,187] Adults aged 65 to 74 years, undergoing maintenance dialysis, have a prevalence of AF of 13%. This increases to 23% among those 85 years or older.[188] A large proportion of these patients are treated with oral anticoagulants, specifically warfarin, with the intention to reduce the risk of stroke and systemic embolism.

There is mounting evidence that the benefit-risk ratio of warfarin may not be extrapolated to patients with ESKD. At the center of the controversy is the question if, when used in patients with AF undergoing dialysis, warfarin is less effective at stroke risk reduction and is associated with increased bleeding risk.[189,190] Recent observational studies have shown high rates of early discontinuation (47% stop after 8 months)[191] and physician uncertainty.[192,193] At present, there are conflicting guidelines across the world. Both the 2012 KDIGO[9] and 2016 Canadian Cardiovascular Society Guidelines[194] recommend against anticoagulation in patients with a creatinine clearance < 15 mL/min with AF (including patients on dialysis); the 2014 American College of Cardiology/American Heart Association Practice Guidelines[195] suggest anticoagulation with warfarin to an international normalized ratio (INR) target of 2.0 to 3.0 in patients with nonvalvular AF, with a CHA2DS2-VASc score of 2 or higher. The 2012 American College of Chest Physicians[196] and 2016 European Society of Cardiology[197] have made no specific recommendation for patients with ESKD. For older patients, particularly those with one or more GSs, the risks appear to equal or outweigh benefits[198,199] and, at least until results of ongoing trials are available,[200,201] caution is advised when prescribing warfarin for stroke prevention, especially in frail older patients, those with a history of major bleeding and those with known vascular calcification.

Currently, there is optimism that non–vitamin K antagonist oral anticoagulants (NOACs) will offer an alternative anticoagulant for the dialysis population.[189] Dabigatran, rivaroxaban, apixaban, and edoxaban have been studied in large phase III trials in the setting of nonvalvular AF in the general population and were found to have an overall favorable risk-benefit profile versus warfarin.[202] However, only a limited number of small controlled trials of NOACs have included patients with severe CKD (CrCl < 25–30 mL/min), and little is still known about the influence of HD on their pharmacokinetics. Nevertheless, the use of these drugs has become more prevalent, with an estimated 12% of dialysis patients on anticoagulation being treated with NOACs.[203,204]

## ANTIRESORPTIVE TREATMENT: BONE HEALTH

Bone health remains a challenging aspect of renal care, amplified in the older population by the attendant high risk of fragility fractures, adynamic bone disease, and polypharmacy. In this section, we review the data (or lack thereof) supporting the use of antiresorptive therapies in older patients who have recently had a fracture.

Fragility fractures, fractures that occur as a result of a low-energy trauma such as a fall from standing height or lower, are common in older people and are associated with excess mortality, prolonged rehabilitation, long-term pain, and high medical costs. This is particularly the case with hip fractures, which have a substantial impact on an older individual's health, QOL, and abilities, with only 50% of patients regaining their prefracture level of mobility and independence.[205] In 2000, an estimated 1.6 million hip fractures occurred worldwide.[206] This number is expected to increase to 6.3 million by 2050.[207] The risk of fracture increases with CKD progression, resulting in risks 1.5 to 4 times higher in older individuals versus those with normal renal function (Fig. 84.7).[208,209,300] Hip fractures occurring in dialysis patients are particularly concerning because the 1-year mortality after hip fracture in the dialysis population is close to 65% versus 20% in the general US population.[210]

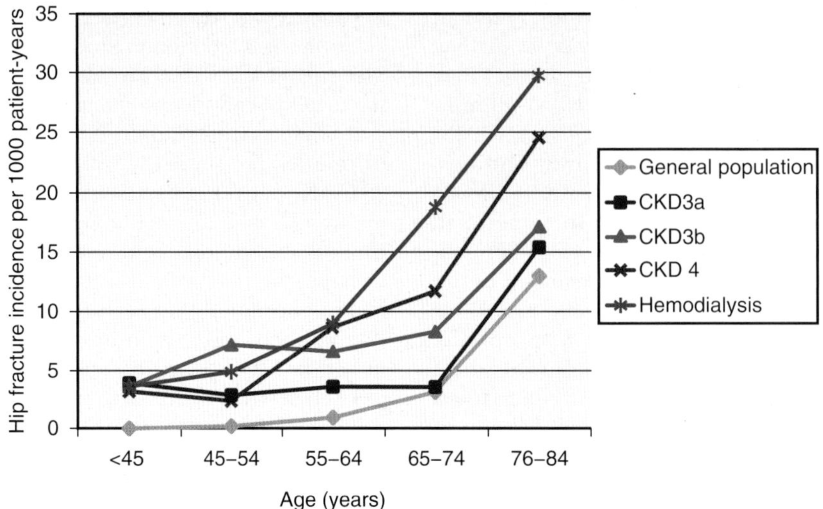


**Fig. 84.7** Hip fracture incidence increases with progressive chronic kidney disease (CKD). (From Moe SM, Nickolas TL. Fractures in patients with CKD: time for action. *Clin J Am Soc Nephrol.* 2016;11(11):1929–1931.)

Despite these alarming numbers, there are sparse data to guide clinicians providing postfracture care to older patients with CKD. Older patients with CKD stages 4 to 5D have been uniformly excluded from clinical trials evaluating pharmacotherapies. The uniqueness and complexity of CKD in the pathogenesis of fractures, mixed with age-related and postmenopausal causes of bone loss, render this population very challenging in terms of diagnosis and management of osteoporosis. Active management of hyperparathyroidism and phosphate-lowering therapies may have an effect on fracture risk, but may also negatively affect other predisposing risks such as falls, malnutrition, and aging itself.

There have been few studies regarding the use of bisphosphonates or denosumab in patients with CKD stages 4 to 5D. Clinical experience is limited, and the theoretic risks of administering antiresorptives must be carefully weighed against unknown benefits, particularly because bone pathology can be difficult to determine accurately. Consequently, the widespread use of osteoporosis therapies in patients with advanced CKD and/or with evidence of CKD–mineral and bone disorder (MBD) is discouraged, especially in frail older individuals who, despite an increased risk of recurrent fractures, are likely to suffer equally from adverse effects and potential harm.[211] Antiresorptives and other osteoporosis therapies can be used in patients with modest reductions in eGFR (≥30 mL/min/1.73 $m^2$) and a parathyroid hormone (PTH) level within the normal range.[212] However, for individuals with severe CKD (stages 4–5D) and those maintained on dialysis, there are limited therapeutic interventions that are known to reduce fracture recurrence. Standard therapies for osteoporosis may be ineffective or possibly harmful in this population. For example, antiresorptives may worsen low bone turnover, osteomalacia, and mixed uremic osteodystrophy and exacerbate hyperparathyroidism; denosumab may induce significant hypocalcemia.[213] In the 2017 KDIGO guideline update, treatment recommendations are discretionary and recommended only after "taking into account the magnitude and reversibility of the biochemical abnormalities and the progression of CKD, with consideration of a bone biopsy."[212]

Nephrologists should continue to pay careful attention to emerging information in this relatively new field while prospective studies, specifically designed for CKD patients, are performed.

## VASCULAR ACCESS CREATION

Vascular access creation in older patients undergoing hemodialysis has remained a topic of ongoing discussion over several years.[214–217] In the older patient, it is more important to prioritize the choice of dialysis access based on the treatment goals. Although high-quality studies have shown that dialysis through an arteriovenous fistula (AVF) is associated with a lower infection risk and remains optimal for patient survival,[218–220] there is little doubt that in the field of geriatric nephrology, there are several situations in which a fistula may not be the most appropriate approach.

Earlier studies comparing AVFs with arteriovenous grafts (AVGs) or central venous catheters (CVCs) have likely overestimated the survival benefits for those dialyzed via an AVF. By comparing outcomes of patients who underwent an unsuccessful fistula attempt with those who did not have fistula creation attempted, it appears that the observed survival gains are attributable to residual confounding factors, arising from the inherent bias that individuals undergoing surgery are likely healthier than those for whom surgery is not attempted.[221,222] Furthermore, although the relative gains may be similar regardless of age, the absolute gains, in terms of survival days, are likely to be small because overall survival on dialysis is lower in older individuals. DeSilva and colleagues[223] analyzed data from 115,425 incident US patients on hemodialysis aged 67 years and older. They assessed mortality outcomes based on the first vascular access placed but found no difference in mortality for patients with an AVG as the first access compared with those who started with an AVF. Similar results were reported by Drew et al.[224] using decision analytic techniques to combine current knowledge of the risks and benefits of different access strategies. Although their study has faced minor criticism for the assumption that most patients initiate dialysis with a CVC, the methodology used was robust, valid, and widely generalizable across the world. Results have shown that the mean estimated survival benefit for those aged 80 years is modest when patients are dialyzed using a fistula strategy. For example, life expectancy gains were maximal in men and in nondiabetic patients, with the estimated prolongation of life for an 80-year-old nondiabetic male estimated at 8 months when a fistula strategy was preferred over a CVC strategy and 6 months when compared with AVG. Survival for an 80-year-old diabetic female was best with an AVG and, when comparing AVF with CVC, survival differed by only 3 weeks.[224]

Access-related morbidity is also known to be high. Patients with an AVF or an AVG are more likely to be bothered by pain, bleeding, bruising, and swelling than those with a CVC.[225] Cannulation-related complications are more common, in part due to fragile skin and in part related to the higher use of antiplatelet or anticoagulant medications.[226] Access creation is also associated with reduced grip strength and impaired arm and hand function.[227] In patients with marginal functional status, creation of AVFs or AVGs may affect personal independence and limit dressing, bathing, and other activities of daily living. Furthermore, in studies of octogenarians who underwent fistula creation during the predialysis period, one third to one half died before they needed renal replacement therapy (RRT).[223,228] Other studies have shown fistula failure rates to be high in older patients, with some suggesting up to 60% of older adults will have a fistula that fails to mature.[229–231] Of those that do function, several will require interventions, particularly early in the clinical course, causing a high clinical and economic burden when overall survival and gains are limited.[217]

The ideal clinical scenario is when results of the individual's CGA help inform the choice of vascular access.[232] AVGs in predialysis patients placed closer to the time of HD initiation have been shown to be an effective CVC-sparing strategy[233] and to be less costly than placing an AVF.[217] Although we await the results of ongoing randomized controlled trials comparing access approaches in an older patient population,[234] we recommend a patient-first approach that identifies "the right access for the right patient" based on patient preferences, priorities, life expectancy, and QOL.

## CARE FOR OLDER ADULTS WITH END-STAGE RENAL DISEASE

### DIALYSIS

The demographics of the dialysis population have been changing over time. Compared with the early 2000s, patients are older and more medically complex[235] with more than 50% being older than 65 years and 25% older than 75 years.[236] Until recently, the adjusted ESKD prevalence has also been rising, with steeper increases among older age groups compared with those younger than 65 years. These trends, however, have started to change, and data from USRDS have suggested more conservative dialysis practice patterns, with pronounced declines in the number of older people starting dialysis resulting in 2016 incidence rates being the lowest among those aged 65 years and older since the late 1990s.[236]

Although it is often assumed that treatment with dialysis will extend life and alleviate the signs and symptoms of advanced kidney disease, there is growing evidence that these benefits may not always accrue in older adults. The median life expectancy after the initiation of chronic dialysis in the United States is comparable to (or worse than) many cancers, and is estimated to be less than 2 years for patients aged 75 years or older. However, considerable heterogeneity exists and, although almost 25% of those aged 70 years or older survive less than 6 months, a similar proportion survive for more than 4 years.[79,96] For all ages, the relative median life expectancy after starting dialysis is close to 25% that of age-matched individuals from the general population,[236] and therefore older adults are most likely to have the smallest absolute gain measured in months or years. Among factors that predict early mortality are the presence of frailty, impaired functional status, low body weight or serum albumin concentration, and need for nursing care at the time of dialysis initiation.[90,95,237–241] There are several prognostic tools,[92,93,237,242] but these are limited to use in individuals who initiate dialysis and do not help prognosticate survival in those who are already established on dialysis or who opt for a comprehensive conservative renal care approach. A recent review has highlighted the limits and deficiencies of the most commonly used prognostic tools.[243]

### DIALYSIS MODALITY SELECTION

Among patients 65 years of age and older initiating dialysis in the United States, most of them (92%) will start in-center HD as their initial modality choice, followed by PD (7%) and preemptive transplantation (1%),[236] as shown in Fig. 84.8. Until recently, one of the main arguments favoring HD was based on the overall mortality rates seen in the older patient population treated with PD. In a recent meta-analysis

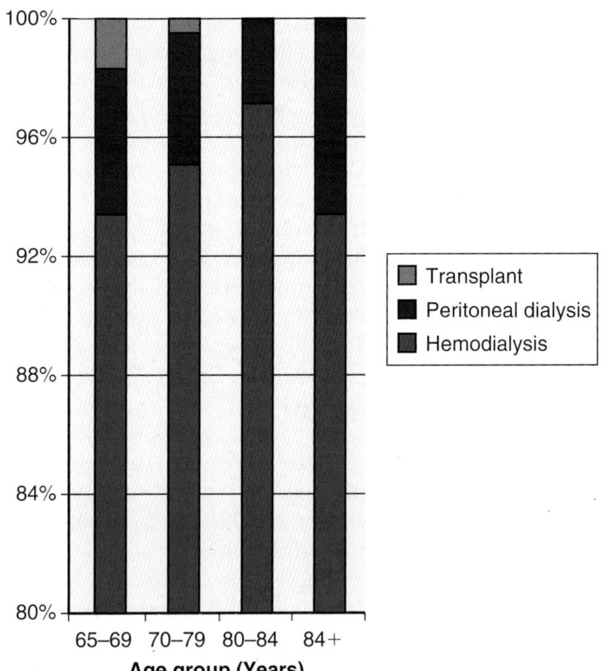


**Fig. 84.8** Initial kidney replacement therapy modality in the United States in 2008, according to age group. (From Tamura MK, Tan JC, O'Hare AM: Optimizing renal replacement therapy in older adults: a framework for making individualized decisions. *Kidney Int.* 2012;82:261–269.)

involving 631,421 older patients, the mortality was higher in those undergoing PD compared with HD (HR, 1.10; 95% CI, 1.01–1.20).[244] However, particularly within the field of geriatric nephrology, it is important to recognize that the flexibility and gentle nature of PD offers much to an older individual, and many individuals forfeit a longer time alive but feeling unwell for a shorter time feeling well. Patients may be attracted to several other aspects of PD, such as increased dietary freedom, decreased hospital visits, control over one's own care, and a feeling of personal autonomy.[245] In those with a guarded prognosis but high symptom level, PD may be an ideal alternative to comprehensive conservative renal care because it can be adapted to patients' needs as they transition along their disease course until they reach end of life.[246] For example, in a patient with progressively worsening limb ischemia, who is experiencing a deterioration in his or her health combined with increasing pain and frustration, dialysis exchange frequency can be reduced, and the solution volume and concentration adapted, to improve comfort, prevent shortness of breath, and enhance the feeling of control and freedom. Frail older patients who are unable to perform their own PD exchanges can be successfully supported by assisted PD.[247] With assisted PD, home care workers, family members or staff in long-term care facilities are trained to perform the exchanges and supervise the dialysis. Different models have been used across different countries, and currently neither functional dependence nor cognitive impairment are considered absolute barriers to PD.[248–250]

In-center HD may be preferred over home-based PD treatment by some individuals because their day can be structured around scheduled and fixed times, facilitating coordination for family members or staff providing support. Others benefit from socialization with staff and other patients at the dialysis facility and from having frequent contact with the dialysis staff to provide both medical and psychosocial support.[245,251] HD in frail older patients is, however, more likely to precipitate episodic postural hypotension and possibly accelerate cognitive decline from myocardial and cerebral stunning. Additional challenges include the creation and maintenance of vascular access, problems associated with postdialysis recovery time, such as fatigue, and the risk of falls after dialysis.[252]

As a result, there is no one dialysis modality of choice for the frail older patient. Clinicians are advised to use information from the CGA to build a framework of total care, focusing on the needs of the individual patient and the goals of care in the context of her or his life experience.

## KIDNEY TRANSPLANTATION

Patients aged 65 years or older currently comprise almost 25% of all kidney transplant wait-listed patients; 19% of all recipients are older adults.[253] Over the past 2 decades, there has been a fivefold increase in the number of patients aged 65 years and older undergoing kidney transplantation in the United States.[253] Although advanced age is no longer a barrier to kidney transplantation, age remains an important surrogate factor when assessing suitability for transplantation. Chronologic age is less important than the patient's level of frailty, burden of coexisting conditions, and overall prognosis.[254,255] Often, transplantation assessments include more rigorous assessment of cardiac and cancer risk.[256]

Transplantation offers survival benefits across all ages, although due to the attendant risks of the surgery itself and side effects associated with immunosuppressive drugs, patients have an increased mortality risk in the initial few months. Survival equivalence, as compared with maintenance dialysis, is seen approximately 8 months after the surgery is performed in younger patients[257] but not seen in those aged 70 years and older until more than 10 months have elapsed from the date of transplantation.[258] As a result, there is little survival advantage in the initial 18 months posttransplantation.[258] Several strategies have been used to maximize kidney transplantation success, including the use of expanded criteria donor (ECD) kidneys and pairing organs harvested from older donors with older recipients.[259] These systems offer advantages and disadvantages, but overall the most beneficial and commonly used strategy in North America is to offer ECD kidneys to the older patient.[260]

The most common cause of graft loss in older kidney transplant recipients remains death with a functioning graft.[261,262] Death-censored graft failure risk remains lowest, across all age groups, in patients aged 65 years or older likely because of a shorter life span and lower risk of acute rejection. Older patients are at higher risk of medication-related adverse events and higher rates of opportunistic infections and neoplasia.[263,264]

## COMPREHENSIVE CONSERVATIVE RENAL CARE

Although the change in dialysis utilization is captured across several regions of the world through dialysis registries, little is known about how often patients with advanced stages of CKD choose not to undergo dialysis or are not offered dialysis. Single-center studies from Europe and Australia have suggested that a substantial number of older patients with advanced kidney disease are treated conservatively and do not receive dialysis.[265–270] Other studies, using administrative data, also found that a notable number of older patients do not undergo dialysis. These studies identified patients with advanced CKD who were likely at risk of dialysis by selecting those who had two or more creatinine levels determined at least 3 months apart that met criteria for a low eGFR. In one study, from Canada, the clinical course of all individuals with creatinine values consistent with CKD were tracked over a 2-year period (Fig. 84.9).[271] In the second study, from the VA, detailed data were extracted from electronic charts data and used to identify whether patients either underwent dialysis or were being prepared for dialysis.[272] In both studies, older adults were found to be less likely to undergo dialysis than their younger counterparts, implying that there may be a relatively large "reservoir" of older adults with high creatinine levels (and, by implication, very low levels of eGFR) who, for a number of reasons, do not get started on dialysis (Fig. 84.10). Similar patterns have been reported for the incidence of hospitalized patients with AKI treated with dialysis.[273] Although provocative, these data cannot distinguish between those who did not meet clinical criteria or a need for dialysis from those who did not get offered or who chose not to undergo dialysis.

Although registry data serve as a valuable source of information about outcomes in older adults with ESKD who are treated with dialysis, less is known about outcomes among those who are not treated with dialysis. What little is known

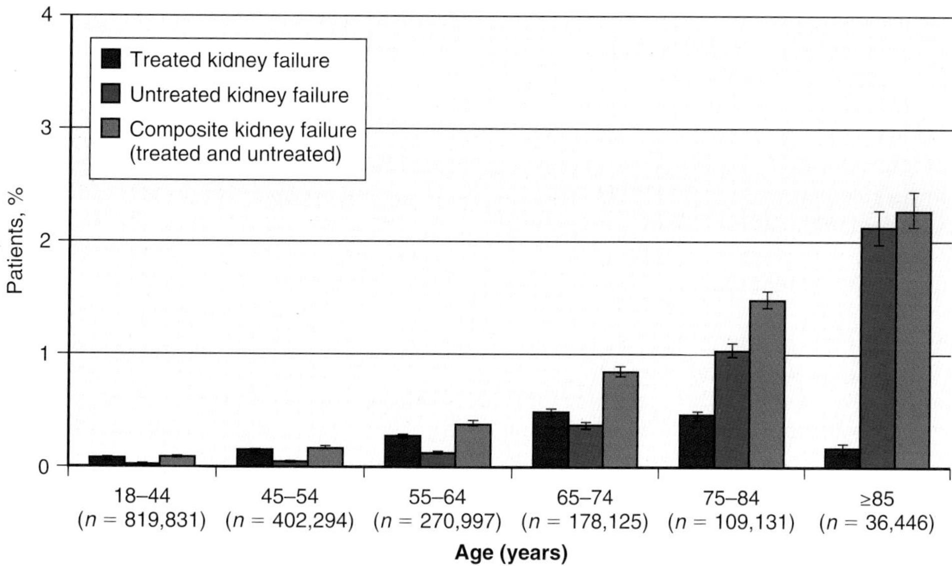


**Fig. 84.9** Treated and untreated kidney failure as a function of age in Alberta, Canada. (From Hemmelgarn BR, James MT, Manns BJ, et al: Rates of treated and untreated kidney failure in older vs. younger adults. *JAMA.* 2012;307:2507–2515.)

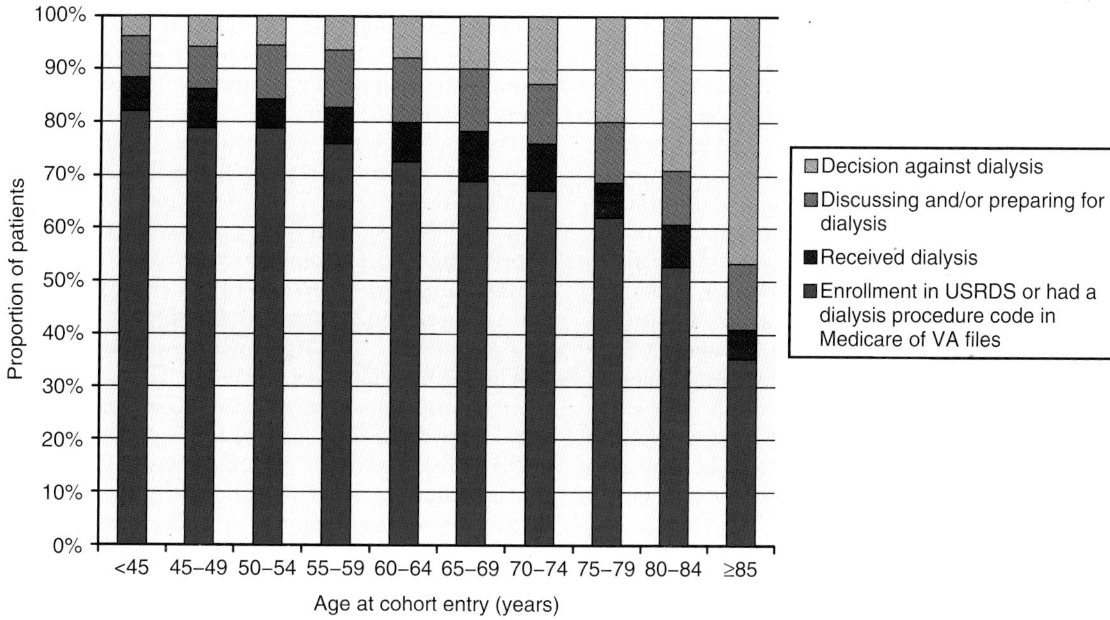


**Fig. 84.10** Age differences in treatment decisions and practices for advanced kidney disease. These are based on the basis of a chart review of a random sample of patients who were not enrolled in the US Renal Data System (USRDS) and did not have a dialysis procedure code in Medicare or Department of Veteran Affairs (VA) administrative files during follow-up. (From Wong SP, Hebert PL, Laundry RJ, et al. Decisions about renal replacement therapy in patients with advanced kidney disease in the US Department of Veterans Affairs, 2000-2011. *Clin J Am Soc Nephrol.* 2016;11(10):1825–1833.)

about this group comes from a number of small, single-center studies that have examined outcomes among patients with advanced kidney disease who were managed with comprehensive conservative renal care (CCRC).

Most studies have shown that dialysis is associated with a modest survival advantage over CCRC; however, the magnitude of this effect varies across studies, and the potential advantage seems to be lost for a subgroup of older patients with a high burden of comorbidity.[274–276] The comparisons, however, between patients managed with CCRC and those initiating dialysis are challenging because there is no clear starting point for analysis. It is often difficult to know when dialysis would have been started in those who chose a CCRC pathway, and it is possible that studies suffer from a lead time bias. Robust patients and those with rapid declines in renal function are more likely to undergo dialysis; those who are frail or have slowly progressing renal declines are more likely to undergo CCRC. Thus, the use of time points determined from the eGFR, to set a time when dialysis may have been otherwise started, is likely to lead to further systematic biases.

Evolving literature has recognized that a number of older patients may benefit equally from dialysis as from CCRC. Particularly in older adults with a high burden of geriatric syndromes, small gains in longevity that are potentially achieved with dialysis care need to be balanced against high risk of increased symptom burden, worsening dependency, and often a negative effect on QOL.[252,277,278] The overall gains are modest, particularly in those who have recently undergone one or more life-prolonging procedures, such as intubation, feeding tube placement, and cardiopulmonary resuscitation.[279]

Patients who opt for a CCRC pathway tend to fare well for several months. Their symptom burden and QOL remain stable until the last 1 or 2 months of life, at which time palliative care interventions are often beneficial.[276] Functional status is often maintained until the last months of life and, overall, patients are more likely to die in their home environment or in hospice compared with those starting RRT.[274] Further information on the trajectories seen in those initiating dialysis have been emerging, although insufficient information is currently available to make clear distinctions between patient groups.

## IMPORTANCE OF SHARED DECISION MAKING IN END-STAGE RENAL DISEASE

Shared decision making is a critical component of renal care, particularly for older patients and their families. See Chapters 62 and 82, but remember that discussions should be open, collaborative, and structured. Ideally a multidisciplinary renal team, patient, and family should be present and information shared about the potential benefits and harms of the various treatment options. Discussions should be specific to the individual and his or her lifestyle and values. Prognosis should be integrated with the results of the CGA, allowing clinicians to share information about the possible positive and negative effects on daily living and symptom burden. It is important that patients and key individuals in their social network have realistic expectations of life with the different treatment options. Helping patients and families to be part of a problem-solving approach to individualized management will maximize treatment benefits.

## DIALYSIS TREATMENTS UNIQUE TO OLDER PATIENTS

### DIALYSIS AND GERIATRIC REHABILITATION PROGRAMS

Geriatric rehabilitation programs are designed to optimize the functioning of older adults and often premorbidly frail individuals who have experienced loss of independence due to acute illness or injury, often superimposed on chronic functional and medical problems.[280] Geriatric rehabilitation provides evaluative, diagnostic, and therapeutic interventions to restore functional ability or enhance residual functional capacity in older people with disabling impairments.[281] Physical deterioration occurs in predialysis CKD prior to the commencement of RRT.[282,283] Once patients start RRT, they appear to decrease their levels of physical activity further,[284] leading to increased skeletal muscle wasting and poorer overall physical function.[285,286] This vulnerable state is exacerbated by multiple or recurrent periods of illness or hospitalization, which, even if short-lived, may lead to persistent disability.[287] Over a span of 6 months, vulnerable individuals experience increased dependency in a number of aspects of daily living, which may eventually result in a nursing home placement.[79,80,288] Timely referral for geriatric rehabilitation may reverse recent onset dependence and disability and increase the likelihood that patients return home or to a community residential setting following rehabilitation.[289]

Specialized dialysis rehabilitation programs integrate active rehabilitation with dialysis care. An interdisciplinary team consisting of multiple professionals, including physicians, nurses, pharmacists, physiotherapists, occupational therapists, speech-language pathologists, social workers, psychologists, dietitians, and recreation therapists, work together, often with overlapping roles, to provide interventions such as therapeutic exercises, fall prevention plans, education on ways to conserve energy during activity, and recommendations of assistive devices.[290] Geriatric dialysis rehabilitation often occurs at a turning point in a patient's disease trajectory and can allow a patient to recover personal function after a complicated course in hospital or a recent multisystem illness. It is also an opportune moment to initiate or pursue discussions around goals of care and advance care planning. Providing dialysis in short daily sessions, if feasible, may improve the success of the program. Short daily dialysis (6 times/week for 2 hours) is well tolerated, limits scheduling conflicts and interference between medical and rehabilitation treatments, and may lead to improved nutrition and better participation in therapy sessions. Patients report less fatigue and fewer symptoms associated with rapid fluid shifts.[291]

Limited effectiveness data exist, with the largest information coming from a single-center report of 164 patients. In this series, more than 70% of patients met functional goals and showed clinically meaningful improvements in personal independence.[289,292] Other models of geriatric rehabilitation, including outpatient rehabilitation, community rehabilitation, and fall prevention programs, have not been well studied in the older renal population but have been shown to benefit other clinical geriatric populations and thus warrant further investigation in the CKD population. A practical first step is for nephrology teams to consider if rehabilitation would be beneficial using information gathered through the CGA—for example, at dialysis initiation, after hospitalization or accidental fall(s), or if there is a change in social status (e.g., changing residence or the death of a caregiver or key family member). Nephrologists may collaborate with the rehabilitation team to reevaluate health targets at this time.

### PALLIATIVE DIALYSIS

There has been an emerging dialogue around the role of a palliative approach to care for those on maintenance dialysis.[270,293–296] The palliative approach to dialysis care can be defined as a:

> *transition from a conventional disease-oriented focus on dialysis as rehabilitative treatment to an approach prioritizing comfort and alignment with patient preferences and goals of care to improve QOL and reduce symptom burden for maintenance dialysis patients in their final year of life.*[294]

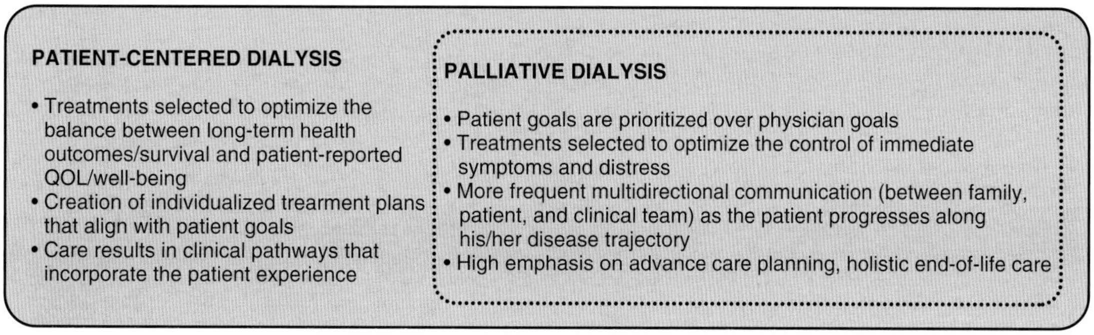

**PATIENT-CENTERED DIALYSIS**

- Treatments selected to optimize the balance between long-term health outcomes/survival and patient-reported QOL/well-being
- Creation of individualized trearment plans that align with patient goals
- Care results in clinical pathways that incorporate the patient experience

**PALLIATIVE DIALYSIS**

- Patient goals are prioritized over physician goals
- Treatments selected to optimize the control of immediate symptoms and distress
- More frequent multidirectional communication (between family, patient, and clinical team) as the patient progresses along his/her disease trajectory
- High emphasis on advance care planning, holistic end-of-life care

**Fig. 84.11** Conceptualizing palliative dialysis. In patient-centered dialysis, treatments are chosen to align with patient goals. In palliative dialysis, a subset within patient-centered care, treatments are chosen so that if needed, patient goals are prioritized over physician goals. *QOL*, Quality of life.

One approach is to classify patients into one of three treatment groups, each with a different expected outcome:

1. Dialysis as a bridging treatment or long-term maintenance treatment, when the patient is expected to return to usual life activities
2. Dialysis as a final destination, when dialysis treatment is used to alleviate symptoms but it is expected that the CKD and/or non-CKD disease will continue to deteriorate
3. Active medical management without dialysis.[297]

Those with high levels of comorbidity, ongoing concomitant nonrenal disease, or an unclear prognosis likely best fit within the second final destination group, and are those who are most likely to benefit from a palliative approach to dialysis care. After shared decision making, dialysis treatments can be customized to alleviate the individual's symptoms and minimize treatment-related distress.[298]

Palliative dialysis is often, incorrectly, thought of as being equivalent to less dialysis or a precursor to dialysis discontinuation. Although it is often necessary to adapt dialysis timings and prescriptions, and dialysis discontinuation may be a component, these interventions are rarely sufficient to ameliorate symptoms and suffering.[293] Ongoing symptom assessment and therapeutic interventions (discussed briefly later) are required. When taking a palliative approach to renal care, advance care planning becomes of paramount importance. As the patient continues along the disease trajectory, he or she, together with the immediate family, will increasingly need support as they learn to accept death as a natural consequence. As death approaches, the focus becomes more consistent with interventions that improve the dying process and end-of-life care. At this point, patients' goals of care tend to shift to focus almost exclusively on QOL and minimizing suffering rather than survival, with a strong emphasis on emotional, social, and family support.[299] Palliative dialysis is a form of patient-centered dialysis in that it continues to align care with patient preferences. In palliative dialysis, the focus of care is on the prevention and relief of suffering. Treatments are adapted to the issues that matter most to the patient and are adjusted so that the individual patient can achieve goals for the remaining life. This approach, also termed "patient-centered care," requires setting a balance between issues important to the clinician (e.g., survival, laboratory targets) with those affecting the individual (restrictions affecting quality of life, symptom control, and physical function; Fig. 84.11).[293] The clinician may therefore need to forgo traditional treatment targets and disease-oriented guidelines in favor of the patient's symptom management and individualized goals of care. This can mean that less emphasis is placed on maximizing long-term health outcomes, such as optimal control of BP, phosphate levels, and other laboratory results, unless they result in immediate symptom improvement.

Common symptoms associated with advanced CKD include fatigue, nausea and vomiting, sleep disorders, restless legs syndrome, depressive symptoms, and pruritus.[293] Many occur in complex clusters and treatments are primarily to ease symptoms sufficiently to maximize comfort because it is not always possible to alleviate them completely.[277,278] Less dialysis rarely provides benefits and may result in increased symptoms and postdialysis fatigue, especially if greater ultrafiltration is required to manage troublesome shortness of breath. However, it can be an option for those in whom fluid management is not a big problem and who favor spending more time at home, with reduced transportation to and from the dialysis facility over symptoms related to underdialysis. Engaging patients and families in discussions often leads to identification of the issues and symptoms that lead to a request to reduce dialysis. Some patients will feel stressed when rushing to prepare for an early morning dialysis session or when they have to change their routine to eat their midday meal earlier and their evening meal later when attending afternoon dialysis. Dosing and timing of dialysis can then be adjusted accordingly to improve dialysis tolerance. A number of symptoms can also be mitigated by more frequent, but shorter, dialysis sessions, such as sleep disorders, respiratory distress, and postdialysis fatigue. This option may be acceptable for some patients who are not distressed by the dialysis procedure itself.

## CONCLUSION

Care of the older patient with CKD has increasingly become a subspecialty in nephrology due to the challenge of balancing efficient, high-quality medical care with a personalized and humane approach to the older individual. Multiple areas of increased information and knowledge have been emerging in the field of geriatric nephrology, heralding a new era of personalized quality care. At the core is appreciation of the need for a better and deeper understanding of the individual to whom we are providing care before offering treatment suggestions or evaluations.

 Complete reference list available at ExpertConsult.com.

## KEY REFERENCES


10. Farrington K, Covic A, Aucella F, et al. Clinical Practice Guideline on management of older patients with chronic kidney disease stage 3b or higher (eGFR <45 mL/min/1.73 m2). *Nephrol Dial Transplant.* 2016;31(suppl 2):ii1–ii66.
20. Ebert N, Jakob O, Gaedeke J, et al. Prevalence of reduced kidney function and albuminuria in older adults: the Berlin Initiative Study. *Nephrol Dial Transplant.* 2017;32(6):997–1005.
36. Rosansky SJ, Schell J, Shega J, et al. Treatment decisions for older adults with advanced chronic kidney disease. *BMC Nephrol.* 2017;18(1):200.
37. Glassock RJ, Warnock DG, Delanaye P. The global burden of chronic kidney disease: estimates, variability and pitfalls. *Nat Rev Nephrol.* 2017;13(2):104–114.
40. Glassock R, Delanaye P, El Nahas M. An age-calibrated classification of chronic kidney disease. *JAMA.* 2015;314(6):559–560.
43. Rule AD, Cornell LD, Poggio ED. Senile nephrosclerosis–does it explain the decline in glomerular filtration rate with aging? *Nephron Physiol.* 2011;119(suppl 1):6–p11.
50. Stuck AE, Siu AL, Wieland GD, et al. Comprehensive geriatric assessment: a meta-analysis of controlled trials. *Lancet.* 1993; 342(8878):1032–1036.
52. Hall RK, Haines C, Gorbatkin SM, et al. Incorporating geriatric assessment into a nephrology clinic: preliminary data from two models of care. *J Am Geriatr Soc.* 2016;64(10):2154–2158.
61. Bowling CB, Booth JN 3rd, Safford MM, et al. Nondisease-specific problems and all-cause mortality in the REasons for Geographic and Racial Differences in Stroke study. *J Am Geriatr Soc.* 2013;61(5):739–746.
62. Bowling CB, Muntner P, Sawyer P, et al. Community mobility among older adults with reduced kidney function: a study of life-space. *Am J Kidney Dis.* 2014;63(3):429–436.
70. Johansen KL, Delgado C, Bao Y, et al. Frailty and dialysis initiation. *Semin Dial.* 2013;26(6):690–696.
79. Kurella Tamura M, Covinsky KE, Chertow GM, et al. Functional status of elderly adults before and after initiation of dialysis. *N Engl J Med.* 2009;361(16):1539–1547.
80. Jassal SV, Chiu E, Hladunewich M. Loss of independence in patients starting dialysis at 80 years of age or older. *N Engl J Med.* 2009;361(16):1612–1613.
84. Covinsky KE, Palmer RM, Fortinsky RH, et al. Loss of independence in activities of daily living in older adults hospitalized with medical illnesses: increased vulnerability with age. *J Am Geriatr Soc.* 2003;51(4):451–458.
92. Couchoud C, Labeeuw M, Moranne O, et al. A clinical score to predict 6-month prognosis in elderly patients starting dialysis for end-stage renal disease. *Nephrol Dial Transplant.* 2009;24(5):1553–1561.
93. Couchoud CG, Beuscart JB, Aldigier JC, et al. Development of a risk stratification algorithm to improve patient-centered care and decision making for incident elderly patients with end-stage renal disease. *Kidney Int.* 2015;88(5):1178–1186.
96. Kurella M, Covinsky KE, Collins AJ, et al. Octogenarians and nonagenarians starting dialysis in the United States. *Ann Intern Med.* 2007;146(3):177–183.
102. Cook WL, Tomlinson G, Donaldson M, et al. Falls and fall-related injuries in older dialysis patients. *Clin J Am Soc Nephrol.* 2006;1(6):1197–1204.
109. Plantinga LC, Patzer RE, Franch HA, et al. Serious fall injuries before and after initiation of hemodialysis among older ESKD patients in the United States: a retrospective cohort study. *Am J Kidney Dis.* 2017;70(1):76–83.
110. Palmer S, Vecchio M, Craig JC, et al. Prevalence of depression in chronic kidney disease: systematic review and meta-analysis of observational studies. *Kidney Int.* 2013;84(1):179–191.
111. Shirazian S, Grant CD, Aina O, et al. Depression in chronic kidney disease and end-stage renal disease: similarities and differences in diagnosis, epidemiology, and management. *Kidney International Reports.* 2017;2(1):94–107.
121. Farrokhi F, Abedi N, Beyene J, et al. Association between depression and mortality in patients receiving long-term dialysis: a systematic review and meta-analysis. *Am J Kidney Dis.* 2014;63(4):623–635.
132. Nagler EV, Webster AC, Vanholder R, et al. Antidepressants for depression in stage 3-5 chronic kidney disease: a systematic review of pharmacokinetics, efficacy and safety with recommendations by European Renal Best Practice (ERBP). *Nephrol Dial Transplant.* 2012;27(10):3736–3745.
144. Rifkin DE, Winkelmayer WC. Medication issues in older individuals with CKD. *Adv Chronic Kidney Dis.* 2010;17(4):320–328.
146. By the American Geriatrics Society Beers Criteria Update Expert P. American Geriatrics Society 2015 updated beers criteria for potentially inappropriate medication use in older adults. *J Am Geriatr Soc.* 2015;63(11):2227–2246.
149. O'Mahony D, O'Sullivan D, Byrne S, et al. STOPP/START criteria for potentially inappropriate prescribing in older people: version 2. *Age Ageing.* 2015;44(2):213–218.
153. Obi Y, Qader H, Kovesdy CP, et al. Latest consensus and update on protein-energy wasting in chronic kidney disease. *Curr Opin Clin Nutr Metab Care.* 2015;18(3):254–262.
161. Weiss J, Freeman M, Low A, et al. Benefits and harms of intensive blood pressure treatment in adults aged 60 years or older: a systematic review and meta-analysis. *Ann Intern Med.* 2017;166(6):419–429.
169. Xie X, Atkins E, Lv J, et al. Effects of intensive blood pressure lowering on cardiovascular and renal outcomes: updated systematic review and meta-analysis. *Lancet.* 2016;387(10017):435–443.
175. Guiding principles for the care of older adults with multimorbidity: an approach for c. Guiding principles for the care of older adults with multimorbidity: an approach for clinicians: American Geriatrics Society Expert Panel on the Care of Older Adults with Multimorbidity. *J Am Geriatr Soc.* 2012;60(10):E1–E25.
184. De Vriese AS. Should statins be banned from dialysis? *J Am Soc Nephrol.* 2017;28(6):1675–1676.
189. De Vriese AS, Caluwe R, Raggi P. The atrial fibrillation conundrum in dialysis patients. *Am Heart J.* 2016;174:111–119.
217. Al-Balas A, Lee T, Young CJ, et al. The clinical and economic effect of vascular access selection in patients initiating hemodialysis with a catheter. *J Am Soc Nephrol.* 2017.
221. Brown RS, Patibandla BK, Goldfarb-Rumyantzev AS. The survival benefit of "fistula first, catheter last" in hemodialysis is primarily due to patient factors. *J Am Soc Nephrol.* 2017;28(2):645–652.
223. DeSilva RN, Patibandla BK, Vin Y, et al. Fistula first is not always the best strategy for the elderly. *J Am Soc Nephrol.* 2013;24(8): 1297–1304.
224. Drew DA, Lok CE, Cohen JT, et al. Vascular access choice in incident hemodialysis patients: a decision analysis. *J Am Soc Nephrol.* 2015;26(1):183–191.
232. O'Hare AM, Allon M, Kaufman JS. Whether and when to refer patients for predialysis AV fistula creation: complex decision making in the face of uncertainty. *Semin Dial.* 2010;23(5):452–455.
237. Cohen LM, Ruthazer R, Moss AH, et al. Predicting six-month mortality for patients who are on maintenance hemodialysis. *Clin J Am Soc Nephrol.* 2010;5(1):72–79.
245. Brown EA, Finkelstein FO, Iyasere OU, et al. Peritoneal or hemodialysis for the frail elderly patient, the choice of 2 evils? *Kidney Int.* 2017;91(2):294–303.
258. Rao PS, Merion RM, Ashby VB, et al. Renal transplantation in elderly patients older than 70 years of age: results from the Scientific Registry of Transplant Recipients. *Transplantation.* 2007;83(8): 1069–1074.
270. Brown MA, Collett GK, Josland EA, et al. CKD in elderly patients managed without dialysis: survival, symptoms, and quality of life. *Clin J Am Soc Nephrol.* 2015;10(2):260–268.
276. Murtagh FE, Burns A, Moranne O, et al. Supportive care: comprehensive conservative care in end-stage kidney disease. *Clin J Am Soc Nephrol.* 2016;11(10):1909–1914.
279. Wong SP, Kreuter W, O'Hare AM. Treatment intensity at the end of life in older adults receiving long-term dialysis. *Arch Intern Med.* 2012;172(8):661–663, discussion 663–664.
290. Farragher J, Jassal SV. Rehabilitation of the geriatric dialysis patient. *Semin Dial.* 2012;25(6):649–656.
293. Davison SN, Jassal SV. Supportive care: integration of patient-centered kidney care to manage symptoms and geriatric syndromes. *Clin J Am Soc Nephrol.* 2016;11(10):1882–1891.

295. O'Hare AM, Song MK, Kurella Tamura M, et al. Research priorities for palliative care for older adults with advanced chronic kidney disease. *J Palliat Med.* 2017;20(5):453–460.
296. Romano TG, Palomba H. Palliative dialysis: a change of perspective. *J Clin Med Res.* 2014;6(4):234–238.
297. Vandecasteele SJ, Kurella Tamura M. A patient-centered vision of care for ESKD: dialysis as a bridging treatment or as a final destination? *J Am Soc Nephrol.* 2014;25(8):1647–1651.
305. Pottel H, Delanaye P, Schaeffner E, et al. Estimating glomerular filtration rate for the full age spectrum from serum creatinine and cystatin C. *Nephrol Dial Transplant.* 2017;32(3):497–507.
306. Pottel H, Hoste L, Dubourg L, et al. An estimated glomerular filtration rate equation for the full age spectrum. *Nephrol Dial Transplant.* 2016;31(5):798–806.

# 85 Stem Cells, Kidney Regeneration, and Gene and Cell Therapy in Nephrology

Benjamin S. Freedman

CHAPTER OUTLINE



KEY POINTS

- Nephron loss is a major cause of chronic and end-stage kidney disease, which current therapies are insufficient to prevent.
- Recent advances in cell culture and reprogramming make it possible to derive new nephron progenitor cells from patients, which can be expanded and differentiated into kidney organoids.
- Stem cell therapies can be delivered by intravenous administration, cortical injection, or beneath the kidney capsule, but these methods require further optimization to demonstrate safety and efficacy.
- Larger functional units including metanephric implants, xenografts, and bioartificial kidneys are being tested for their capacity to substitute whole kidneys.
- Gene transfer techniques have improved in safety and efficacy, and are beginning to reach the clinic for nonkidney disorders, usually in combination with cell therapies.
- CRISPR and related technologies enable precision editing of genetic elements and control of gene expression, but remain relatively inefficient and unpredictable in therapeutic settings.
- Combinatorial use of stem cell therapy and gene therapy will provide an expanded menu of treatment options for the nephrologist of the future.

A critical mass of nephrons is required to perform the kidney's daily tasks. Reductions in nephron number are associated with increased risk of hypertension and kidney disease.[1,2] The postnatal mammalian kidney lacks any clinically significant capacity to grow new nephrons to replace those that have been permanently lost.[3–8] The loss of nephron subunits may therefore be considered a principal cause of chronic kidney disease (CKD) and end-stage renal disease (ESRD).

Kidney transplantation, first successfully introduced over 60 years ago, remains the gold standard for treatment of ESRD. However, demand for transplantable kidneys far exceeds supply. In the United States, ~80% of patients that meet eligibility criteria for a kidney transplant do not receive one every year.[9] Among those fortunate enough to receive a kidney, a transplant is not a cure. Allograft recipients—even those receiving a so-called "perfect match"—must receive sustained immunosuppression for the lifetime of the transplant, which can have serious side effects. Acute rejection occurs within a year of transplant in ~10% of recipients, whereas the long-term graft longevity is ~12 years.[9–11]

Dialysis can be used as an alternative to kidney transplantation, and it does not require immunosuppression but it is associated with higher rates of mortality.[9] Dialysis machines clean the blood by equilibrating it with a balanced salt solution through a membrane, which does not substitute completely the complex filtration, reabsorption, secretion, and metabolic functions of kidney nephrons. Furthermore, dialysis is expensive, time-consuming and requires repeated access to the bloodstream, which can affect quality of life. In addition to kidney transplantation and dialysis, a limited number of pharmaceutical drugs are approved for use in individuals with kidney disease, including angiotensin-converting enzyme inhibitors, which reduce blood pressure and slow further deterioration of renal function, and corticosteroids, which reduce inflammation. However, these drugs are relatively few and primarily treat advanced stages of disease progression rather than root causes.[12]

The limitations of current therapies have inspired research and development of alternative approaches with the potential to prevent or treat kidney disease. Several emerging technologies have substantial promise to combat nephron loss, including stem cell therapy, gene therapy, and kidney regeneration. This chapter summarizes the state of the art in applying these strategies, both in the preclinical laboratory, and, where available, in the clinic.

## KIDNEY STEM CELLS

A stem cell is an ancestor cell capable of producing a larger and more complex multicellular lineage. The process whereby stem cells change into more mature cell types is called differentiation. Alternatively, stem cells may duplicate themselves to produce two identical daughter cells, a process known as self-renewal. The balance between self-renewal and differentiation determines the fraction of stem cells versus mature cells in a tissue or organ. The ability of stem cells to generate many differentiated descendants makes them an attractive potential source of replacement tissue for the kidneys and other organs.

"Stem cell" is a general term that is not restricted to any specific biological entity or lineage.[13] A wide variety of unrelated cell types, with distinct origins and abilities, may be labeled stem cells. Various types of developmental stem cells arise transiently in the body at specific stages of embryonic development, proliferating and differentiating in a coordinated process to produce the bodily organs. In contrast, adult stem cells persist throughout postnatal life and contribute to the continuous renewal of rapidly growing organs such as blood, skin, hair, and intestine. Here, we summarize what is known about both developmental and adult stem cells for the kidney.

### PLURIPOTENT STEM CELLS (ES AND IPS)

Pluripotent stem cells (PSC) can differentiate into all other cell types of the body, i.e., they have the potential for many different cell fates. PSC that arise during the natural development of an embryo are called embryonic stem (ES) cells. Vertebrate ES cells are a transient population that appears shortly after fertilization, and disappears after gastrulation, when the three embryonic germ layers have been established. ES cells can be cultured and expanded outside of the body in specialized growth media that sustain their self-renewal.[14–16] ES cells from different species have distinct cell culture requirements, morphological characteristics, and gene expression patterns. Mouse ES cells resemble the inner cell mass of the blastocyst-stage embryo, which is a tightly compacted ball of cells.[14,15] Human ES cells resemble the early embryonic epiblast, a disc-like, columnar epithelium that derives from the inner cell mass and is therefore further along in development.[16]

The nucleus of an adult cell can be reprogrammed (converted) to an ES cell-like state by forcibly altering its gene expression patterns. This can be accomplished by implanting the nucleus within an enucleated egg cell, a procedure known as somatic cell nuclear transfer (SCNT). The reconstructed cell resembles a fertilized egg (zygote) and can undergo embryonic development to produce an entire organism, which possesses genomic DNA identical to the donor's, and closely resembles the donor phenotypically. This process is called reproductive cloning.[17,18]

The first mammal to be successfully cloned from an adult cell was Dolly the sheep in 1996.[17] Reproductive cloning has since been successfully performed in a variety of species, including dogs and monkeys,[19,20] endangered animals,[21] and even from mice that have been deceased for decades.[22] However, cloning is highly inefficient, and successfully cloned animals frequently suffer from a variety of congenital maladies, which likely result from incomplete reprogramming of the somatic nucleus. These safety issues must be resolved before reproductive cloning can be ethically attempted in human beings.

In many species, including humans, ES cells can be derived in vitro from an SCNT blastocyst.[23,24] This process is called therapeutic cloning, because the resultant ES cells are expected to be highly immunocompatible with the donor, and could be used for cell therapy applications in that individual. However, therapeutic cloning remains an inefficient process and depends on the availability of human eggs, which are precious and can only be obtained from a female donor of reproductive age.[23,24] This has greatly limited the practicality of using SCNT for therapeutic purposes.

Induced pluripotent stem (iPS) cells are somatic cells that have been directly reprogrammed to an ES cell-like pluripotent state, without requiring eggs or SCNT. To generate iPS cells, a primary culture of mature, differentiated cells from any organ is forced to express a set of master regulatory genes that are normally expressed in ES cells.[25,26] When these cells are cultured under conditions that promote ES cell self-renewal, a small minority is "induced" (reprogrammed) into PSC.[25,26] Once reprogrammed, iPS cells are stable in the undifferentiated state and do not require forced expression of ES cell genes to sustain pluripotency.[25-29] iPS cells and ES cells are highly similar cell types, to the point that genome-wide gene expression analysis cannot easily distinguish between them.[30]

iPS cells can be utilized to produce a variety of differentiated cells, using protocols that work similarly for ES cells.[31–35] Compared with ES cells derived from SCNT, iPS cells are a much more convenient source of autologous PSC, because they can be generated using conventional cell culture techniques, and do not depend on the availability of human eggs. iPS cells have been generated from hundreds of patients.[36,37] With respect to immunocompatibility, the mitochondria of iPS cells are genetically identical to those of the original donor cell, unlike SCNT-derived ES cells, whose mitochondria derive from the host egg.[23,24]

Because iPS cells are derived directly from the original patient, they are predicted to be immunocompatible and would not require immunosuppression upon transplantation. Studies in mice support this prediction.[31,32] In a recent study in humans, a patient with wet (neovascular) macular degeneration was administered a graft of retinal pigmented epithelial cells derived from her own iPS cells.[38,39] After 25 months, the graft did not show any signs of rejection despite the complete absence of immunosuppressive medication.[38] Notably, a second patient from whom iPS cells were derived was not transplanted, due to concerns about potentially oncogenic somatic DNA mutations that arose in the iPS cells during the reprogramming process.[38] This highlights the importance of characterizing each new cell line to make sure that it is safe for transplant.

Collectively, ES cells and iPS cells are the two main types of PSC currently in use in the research laboratory and the clinic. PSC in culture represent a later stage of development than the zygote and cannot form a blastocyst on their own. In mice, however, PSC can be combined with extraembryonic stem cells to produce a blastocyst, which can develop into a whole, fertile mouse.[40,41] This demonstrates that PSC are truly pluripotent and can give rise to the entire body, including the kidneys. When cultured PSC are implanted into immunodeficient animals, they grow and differentiate into large tumors called teratomas, which contain tissues representing the three germ layers of the embryo.[16,25] A remarkable feature of PSC is that they can be cultured extensively in the undifferentiated state, for hundreds of passages, and still appear and function similar to earlier passages.[16,26]

Even after extensive passaging, PSC can be readily differentiated in vitro into a variety of somatic cell types, including cardiomyocytes, intestinal cells, cartilage, pancreatic cells, endothelial cells, and other lineages. Detailed regimens of specific growth factors are required to enrich PSC differentiation for specific cell types, which in some cases can form functional grafts in laboratory animals.[33–35] A number of PSC lines have now been generated from individuals with kidney disorders, including polycystic kidney disease (PKD), Alport syndrome, Wilms tumor, focal segmental glomerulosclerosis (FSGS), and systemic lupus erythematosus.[42–52] An immediate use of these cell lines has been to elucidate molecular and cellular mechanisms of human kidney disease, which was initially explored in nonrenal cell types.[42,52] Recently, it has also become possible to successfully differentiate PSC into the kidney lineage, as described later.

## NEPHRON PROGENITOR CELLS AND ORGANOIDS

During embryonic development, ES cells differentiate into the three germ layers of the embryo, namely the endoderm, ectoderm, and mesoderm. The kidneys arise through an iterative series of reciprocal interactions between two stem cell populations, the ureteric bud (UB) and the metanephric mesenchyme (MM).[53,54] The UB differentiates into collecting ducts, while the MM differentiates into the tubules, podocytes, vasculature, and interstitial (stromal) cells.

Nephron progenitor cells (NPC) are a specialized subset of MM cells that differentiate into the podocytes, proximal tubules, and distal tubules of the nephron (Fig. 85.1A). In mammals, NPC are a transient population, like PSC. NPC express specific genes, such as SIX2, which balance self-renewal and differentiation during embryonic kidney development.[6,8] The final wave of differentiation is completed approximately at the time of birth, after which nephrogenesis ceases for the rest of the organism's life.[3–8]

In some fish species, a reservoir of NPC resides within a specialized niche even during adult life and becomes activated after kidney injury.[55] This differs from adult mammals, which lack NPC and the capacity to generate new nephrons. Under certain circumstances, however, NPC can persist in the postnatal mammalian kidney. An example of this is Wilms tumor, a pediatric renal cancer that contains structures that resemble developing kidneys, expresses NPC genes, and grows via a process that mimics nephrogenesis.[56–58] In transgenic mice, overexpression of the RNA-binding protein LIN28 in NPC results in the formation of Wilms tumors, which cause the kidneys to grow to massive proportions.[59] Using techniques such as these, it may be possible to sustain NPC postnatally, to augment kidney tissue. However, it is not clear yet whether the developmental program of nephrogenesis can be reactivated in adult cells, or how to control nephrogenesis in adult kidneys to produce healthy, functional kidney tissue, rather than tumors.

NPC have specialized requirements for survival and growth. For many years, long-term cultures of NPC could not be established in the laboratory. Recently, however, specific culture conditions have been identified that enable the stable propagation of mouse and human NPC in vitro, in some cases for over fifty passages, or approximately six months (Fig. 85.1B).[60–62]

Although there was no way to derive kidney cells from ES or iPS cells for many years, recent work by a number of groups has established methodologies to induce NPC differentiation from PSC.[50,63–65] Treatment of PSC with specific combinations of growth factors or chemical activators is sufficient to upregulate transcription factors associated with primitive streak mesendoderm, intermediate mesoderm, and NPC.[66,67] For human PSC, this involves activation of the canonical WNT signaling pathway. Optimization of these protocols has resulted in the successful differentiation of PSC into NPC.[50,63–65] Thus by reprogramming somatic cells to an iPS cell intermediate, it is now possible to differentiate and expand new NPC from any individual.

Kidney organoids are multicellular units in vitro containing structures that resemble nephrons, including tubular and podocyte components.[61,62] Kidney organoids are the products of NPC differentiation in vitro. Conversely, the ability to differentiate into kidney organoids is a litmus test for the presence of bona fide NPC. Kidney organoids in culture contain translucent, tubular structures that can be discerned by phase-contrast microscopy (see Fig. 85.1B).[50,60–65] At least three major nephron segments are present in kidney organoids: proximal tubules, distal tubules, and podocytes.[50,61–65] These segments form a continuum within the kidney organoid tubules and appear in a proximal-to-distal order that matches the nephron. Their appearance is a common denominator between different protocols and a defining characteristic of kidney organoids (Fig. 85.1C).[50,61–65]

Kidney organoids can be generated from primary and PSC-derived NPC, and they are similar with regards to marker expression and culture requirements.[50,60–65] Depending on the protocol used, organoids can range from smaller adherent structures enriched for nephron cell types (~200 µm diameter),[50] to unpurified aggregates containing both kidney and nonkidney cells (~3 mm diameter).[63–65] When injured with cisplatin or gentamicin, two well-characterized nephrotoxins, kidney organoids exhibit dose-dependent toxicity and express kidney injury molecule 1, a specific biomarker of acute kidney injury.[50,62,64,65] Tubular segments in kidney organoids furthermore absorb specific cargoes typical of kidney tubules.[50,65]

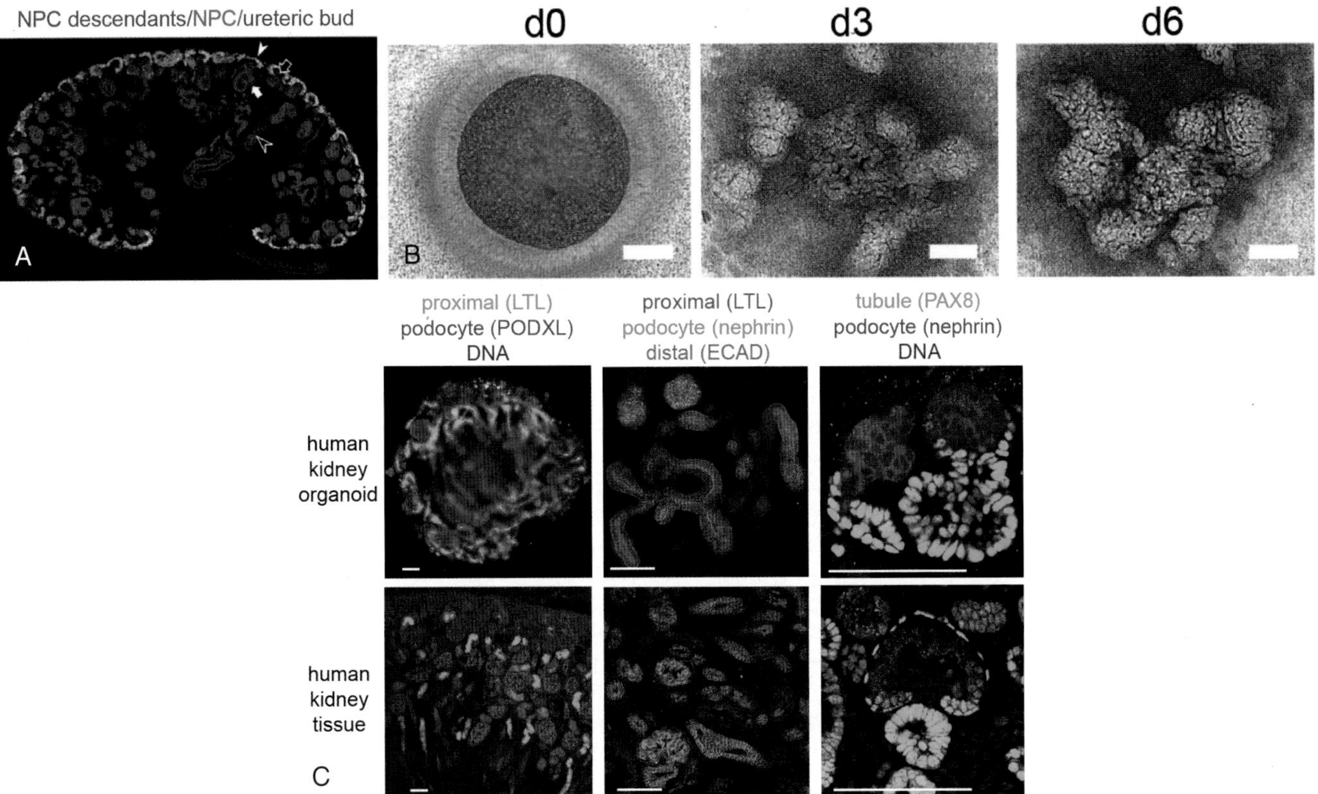


**Fig. 85.1 Differentiation of mouse and human nephron progenitor cells (NPC)** (A) Embryonic mouse kidney showing lineage tracing of NPC in differentiating nephrons. (From Kobayashi A, Valerius MT, Mugford JW, et al. Six2 defines and regulates a multipotent self-renewing nephron progenitor population throughout mammalian kidney development. *Cell Stem Cell* 2008;3:169–181.) (B) Nephron differentiation from human NPC cultures for 43 passages (~6 months). Scale bar, 200 μm. (From Li Z, Araoka T, Wu J, et al. 3D culture supports long-term expansion of mouse and human nephrogenic progenitors, *Cell Stem Cell.* 2016;19:516–529.) (C) Nephron segment profiles in human kidney organoids derived from PSC compared with developing kidneys. Scale bars, 100 μm. *LTL,* Lotus tetragonolobus lectin; *ECAD,* E-cadherin; *PODXL,* podocalyxin; *PAX8,* paired box 8. (From Freedman BS, Brooks CR, Lam AQ, et al. Modelling kidney disease with CRISPR-mutant kidney organoids derived from human pluripotent epiblast spheroids. *Nat Commun* 2015;6:8715; Cruz NM, Song X, Czerniecki SM, et al. Organoid cystogenesis reveals a critical role of microenvironment in human polycystic kidney disease. *Nat Mater.* 2017;16:1112–1119; and Kim YK, Refaeli I, Brooks CR, et al. Gene-edited human kidney organoids reveal mechanisms of disease in podocyte development. *Stem Cells* 2017;35(12):2366–2378.)

Importantly, these biomarker and transporter characteristics differ from those of undifferentiated PSC epithelia (epiblast), indicating that they are lineage-specific.[50] Most impressively, kidney organoids can recapitulate three-dimensional phenotypes of genetic kidney disease, including polycystic kidney disease and podocyte disorders.[50,68,69] The organoids therefore mimic essential properties of kidney tissue in vivo.

Kidney organoids in their current form also have limitations. Although several groups have shown that kidney organoids contain podocytes, proximal tubules, and distal tubules, all of which derive from NPC,[50,61–65] there are differences in opinion over whether these cultures also contain UB and a collecting duct network, which would represent a major advance over MM derivatives alone.[65,70] Complicating this question, PSC from different individuals exhibit substantially different abilities to form kidney organoids, depending on the protocol used for differentiation.[68] This variability, which is not unusual for PSC derivatives, poses a significant technical challenge for using these techniques for patient-specific kidney regeneration and disease modeling. There are also concerns regarding the maturity of the epithelial cells within kidney organoids. There is no source of nephron perfusion, and the tubules do not form expansive lumens or brush borders.[50,64] Podocytes do not form bona fide foot processes with secondary and tertiary interdigitations and appear to be arrested at the capillary loop stage of glomerular development.[50,69,71] Development of the mammalian kidney proceeds via a series of successive phases: the pronephros, mesonephros, and metanephros. The pronephros is the most primitive form of kidney, while the metanephros is the most developed. The metanephros forms the definitive adult kidney. It is not yet clear whether organoids derived from PSC represent pronephric, mesonephric, or metanephric kidneys.

In addition to kidney epithelial lineages, other cell types also arise within kidney organoid cultures. For primary NPC, the identity of these nonepithelial cell types is not yet clear.[60–62] For PSC-derived organoid cultures, several nonepithelial cell types have been identified, including endothelial cells, fibroblast-like stromal cells, and neurons.[50,65] Contamination with nonkidney cell types is to be expected given that these protocols begin with PSC, which can naturally differentiate into any cell type. The presence of these nontubular cell types could be advantageous; for instance it has been observed that endothelial cells within these cultures interact with kidney tubular cell types and podocytes.[50,65] However, the presence of nonkidney cells also has disadvantages, in that it decreases the purity and yield of the resultant kidney structures, which cannot be easily separated from the contaminants.

One promising strategy that remains to be fully developed is to directly reprogram patient cells into NPC or UB, rather than into PSC. Direct reprogramming approaches have succeeded to a varied degree for other cell types, such as cardiomyocytes and neurons.[72,73] As culture conditions for culturing NPC are now established, and many of the major transcription factors are known, the field is primed for such an advance. Efforts in this direction have succeeded in inducing changes to cells that partially resemble NPC or kidney tubules, although sustained expression of the transgenes was required to maintain the phenotype, and no kidney organoids were generated, indicating that reprogramming was insufficient to induce bona fide NPC.[74,75] Achieving the goal of directly reprogramming somatic cells into NPC could be an important step in establishing a more reproducible and practical strategy for kidney cell therapy. A limitation of this approach, however, is that NPC or UB have a more limited potential than PSC and cannot generate entire kidneys on their own.

## ADULT STEM CELLS

Adult stem cells are specialized resident cells that continuously repopulate a specific organ throughout life. They typically reside within a specialized structure, or niche, within the tissue. Examples of adult stem cells are intestinal stem cells, epidermal stem cells, and muscle satellite cells. Adult stem cells are typically found in tissues or organs that have a high turnover rate at homeostasis. They first arise during fetal development, and persist into old age, for the lifetime of the organism.

Although mammalian kidneys are incapable of wholly regenerating new nephrons, they do possess the ability to replace cells within existing nephrons. When subjected to acute tubular damage, such as after ischemia-reperfusion injury, new tubular epithelial cells arise within the kidney to heal the wounded epithelium.[76,77] Evidence from mice carrying specific lineage reporters indicates that the new epithelial cells derive from older epithelial cells, which appear to dedifferentiate and repopulate the basement membrane in a segment-specific manner.[76–79]

Subsets of epithelial cells can exhibit an increased propensity to proliferate and repopulate injured tubules.[77,80] Nevertheless, in contrast to classic adult stem cells in tissues such as skin, blood, and intestine, no specialized stem cell niche can be readily discerned in the mature, quiescent epithelium of the kidney nephron. Furthermore, this epithelium does not undergo rapid and constant self-renewal under conditions of homeostasis. For these reasons, kidney tubular epithelial cells do not completely represent a classic adult stem cell. Rather, they may more closely resemble the beta cells of the pancreas, which grow and maintain their number via a process of self-duplication of other terminally differentiated beta cells.[81]

Unlike tubular epithelial cells, podocytes in the adult kidney permanently exit the cell cycle and are incapable of repopulating their own epithelium after injury.[82] Rather, the primary response of podocytes to injury is hypertrophy, an increase in the size of individual cells.[83] However, recent work suggests that podocytes increase in number by up to 20% during human adolescence, suggesting a progenitor source.[84] Furthermore, patients with kidney disease shed podocytes into their urine at a faster rate than would be expected based on clinical progression, which suggests that the body may harbor an innate capacity to replace lost podocytes.[85,86] Lineage tracing experiments in animals suggest that the new podocyte-like cells do not derive from other podocytes.[87–89]

One possible reservoir of replacement cells resides within the population of parietal epithelial cells (PEC) that lines Bowman's capsule. A subpopulation of cells in this compartment coexpress podocyte and PEC markers, and has been referred to as "glomerular epithelial transitional cells" or "parietal podocytes" for their proposed ability to transdifferentiate into podocytes during adolescence or after injury.[86,88–93] However, there is also evidence that podocytes can transition into the parietal compartment in injury states, therefore the role of the transitional podocytes in glomerular repair has not yet been settled.[94] A second possible reservoir of replacement cells for podocytes are cells of renin lineage (CoRL), which are vascular smooth muscle cells in the juxtaglomerular compartments which produce renin.[95] Like parietal podocytes, CoRL can migrate into the glomerulus and adopt features of podocytes, including the expression of podocyte-specific markers and the elaboration of foot processes.[96,97]

Nonrenal adult stem cells have also been investigated for their potential to contribute to kidney repair after injury. Hematopoietic stem cells (HSC) naturally reside in the bone marrow and have the ability to repopulate the entire blood lineage. HSC can also be found in other sites, such as amniotic fluid and umbilical cord blood. Initially, it was surmised that circulating HSC might also be capable of differentiating into kidney cells. However, a series of studies has now established that HSC do not differentiate into tubular epithelial cells after injury.[98,99]

Mesenchymal stem cells (MSC), also called multipotent stromal cells, are populations of interstitial cells with expansive proliferative potential. A hallmark of MSC is that they can be induced to differentiate in vitro into fat, cartilage, and bone. MSC were first identified in the bone marrow but are now recognized to reside within a variety of different organs. The kidney contains a reservoir of MSC in the peritubular interstitium and vasculature, which enact fibrotic scarring after injury.[100,101] Human MSC can be similarly purified from the renal artery.[102] Ablation of MSC from mouse kidneys induces acute tubular necrosis and capillary rarefaction but can also be protective from vascular calcification in chronic disease.[103,104]

## KIDNEY REGENERATION

Transplantation experiments in several organs, including the heart, liver, and pancreas, suggest that somatic cells and tissues derived from stem cells can engraft and function in animal models.[33–35] Whether such approaches might also be efficacious to treat kidney disease is currently being investigated in experimental models, which are optimizing the delivery of kidney stem cells and testing their potential for clinical kidney regeneration.

## STEM CELL THERAPY

Cell therapy involves the direct administration of cells into the body for healing purposes. The units of therapy in this approach are single cells. For regenerative medicine, the ultimate objective of cell therapy is to establish a long-term graft with the capacity to perform organ functions. A practical example is bone marrow transplantation, in which HSC are the units of therapy, engraft in the bone marrow, and repopulate the entire blood lineage.[105]

Intravenous administration describes the direct injection of dissociated cells into the bloodstream using a syringe. It is the simplest delivery route for cell therapies and is used for HSC therapy in the clinic. Kidney cells, however, are different from blood cells and do not typically circulate throughout the body. The kidney is furthermore a densely-packed organ with no obvious route for stem cells to traverse from the bloodstream into the nephrons. Whether kidney stem cells have the ability to engraft and regenerate the kidney after intravenous administration therefore needs to be tested in preclinical animal models. In these experiments, the kidneys are typically subjected to acute injury. This damages the glomerular filtration barrier, which can enhance penetration of cells into the kidney and subsequent engraftment.

In one example, human iPS cell-derived cells expressing a variety of NPC and adult kidney cell markers were injected into the mouse tail vein 24 hours after administration of the nephrotoxic drug cisplatin.[106] Extensive engraftment was reported in proximal tubules, which coincided with a 55% reduction in urea levels in treated mice, compared with control animals administered with saline or undifferentiated iPS cells.[106] These experiments suggest a possible benefit of iPS-derived kidney cells on kidney injury. However, the isolated cells were not shown to demonstrate the ability to form kidney organoids with segmented nephrons. It is therefore unclear whether the implanted cells contained bona fide NPC or whether new nephrons were actually formed.

Intravenous administration has also been applied to adult kidney cell populations. Human glomerular epithelial transitional cells (see earlier), administered intravenously into a mouse model of chemically-induced podocytopathy, were found in glomeruli, and were associated with a decrease in proteinuria.[107] These cells also contributed to tubules after acute injury.[80] As these cells cannot form new nephrons, this approach seeks to repair and replace, rather than to completely regenerate.

MSC can be readily obtained, for instance from a patient's adipose tissue. Intravenous administration of MSC in experimental models can have a beneficial effect on ischemia-reperfusion injury.[99,102,108] This benefit can be obtained even in the absence of MSC engraftment, likely via a paracrine effect. However, MSC administered to injured kidneys do not contribute tangibly to new nephron formation and can differentiate ectopically into undesirable fat cells or fibroblasts within glomeruli.[108,109] Collectively, these findings suggest that intravenous administration of cell therapeutics may provide some benefit in cases where the glomerular filtration barrier has been compromised but may also have unwanted side effects.

In the technique of parenchymal injection, cell therapies are directly delivered into the kidney cortex using a syringe. In one study, $5 \times 10^5$ primary NPC were purified from human fetal kidneys, and injected directly into kidney parenchyma of immunodeficient mice subjected to 5/6 nephrectomy.[110] Follow-up revealed engraftment of the NPC, which was associated with a modest improvement in serum creatinine.[110] In another instance, newborn mouse kidneys were implanted with dissociated cultures of kidney organoids derived from human ES cells.[50] Three weeks later, human proximal tubular structures were observed alongside mouse proximal tubules within the cortex.[50] In a similar model, mouse primary NPC injected into newborn mouse kidneys formed chimeric tubules and glomeruli with the host mouse, which could be distinguished based upon expression of a fluorescent tracer (Fig. 85.2A).[62]

Parenchymal injection has the advantage of placing the cells in direct physical contact with other nephrons. However, the kidney parenchyma is tightly packed with blood vessels and nephrons. This limits the ability to introduce large numbers of stem cells and target them to specific locations. In addition, injection of cells is likely to damage existing kidney tissues. Illustrating this, human iPS cells were differentiated into cells expressing the NPC markers OSR1 and SIX2, treated with growth factors, and injected into the kidney parenchyma immediately after induction of ischemia-reperfusion injury.[111] Although some engraftment was observed, the authors noted difficulty administering a large number of cells directly into the parenchyma, and were concerned about causing damage to the kidneys using this method.[111]

Subcapsular implantation describes insertion of cells in between the kidney cortex and the renal capsule, a thin, fibrous membrane surrounding the kidneys.[111] This space can accommodate a large number of cells. Subcapsular implantation of stem cells into the mouse kidney has been performed by several groups.[63,66,111] Using this method, the foreign growth can be distinguished from existing kidney structures, from which it is largely separated geographically, and analyzed side-by-side.

Using protocols that produce kidney organoids, mouse or human NPC were implanted beneath the capsule of immunodeficient mice.[63,71] These growths contained a variety of stromal and epithelial structures. Some of these resembled primitive nephrons, including both tubules and glomerulus-like rosettes, both of which appeared more diffuse and eosinophilic than the neighboring kidney tissue (Fig. 85.2B).[63,71] These growths also contained endothelial structures, derived from the mouse host.[63,71] Notably, most of the growth area appeared stromal. Similarly, subcapsular implantation of kidney-like cells derived from human ES cells resulted in large growths that expressed AQP1 at similar levels to neighboring kidney cortical cells.[66] However, these growths did not morphologically resemble the neighboring parenchyma histologically and appeared instead to contain diffusely staining stroma instead of tubular structures.[66]

In a functional test, NPC-like cells derived from human iPS cells subjected to subcapsular implantation appeared to significantly ameliorate the effects of kidney ischemia-reperfusion injury prior to the transplant, as determined by serum creatinine and urea levels as well as by histological injury scores, compared with mice receiving grafts of undifferentiated iPS cells or mock injections.[111] Because the capsule is a distinct location from the rest of the kidney, with no

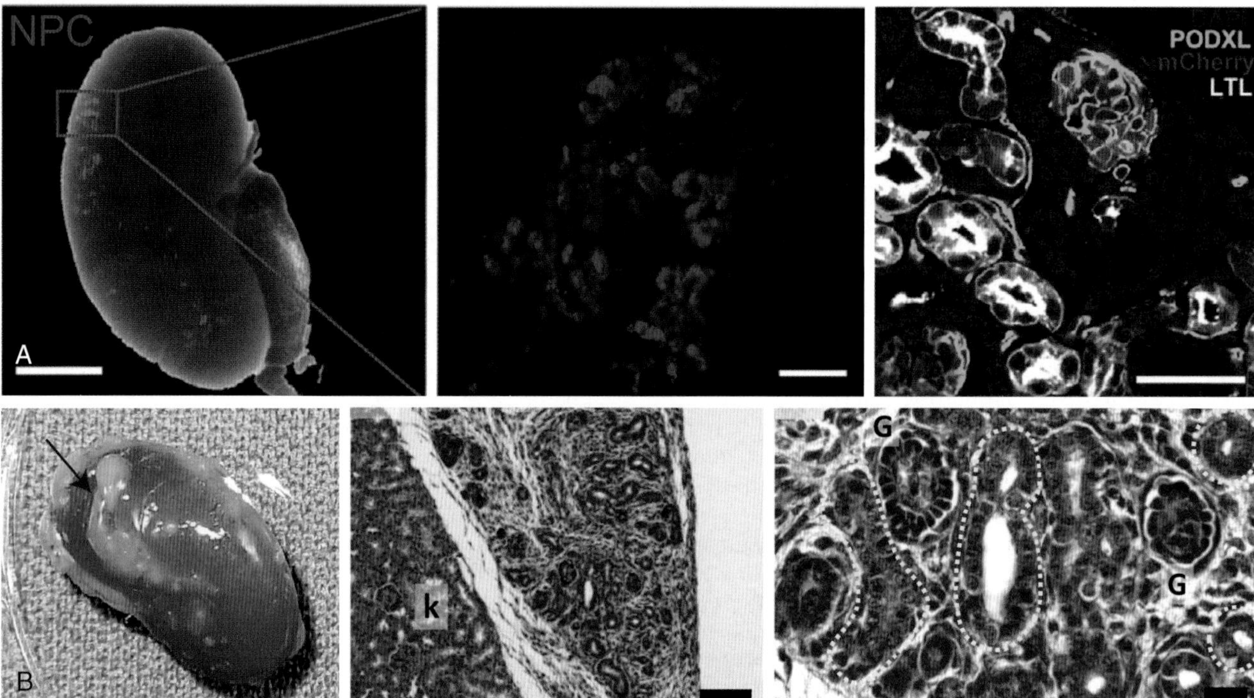


**Fig. 85.2 Delivery of kidney cell therapies** (A) Eight-day-old mouse kidney 1 week after cortical injection of mCherry-labeled nephron progenitor cells (NPC; *red*). Chimeric nephrons are observed by immunofluorescence. Scale bars are 1 mm, 100 μm, and 50 μm *(from left)*. (From Li Z, Araoka T, Wu J, et al. 3D culture supports long-term expansion of mouse and human nephrogenic progenitors, *Cell Stem Cell.* 2016;19:516–529). (B) Growths of human NPC derived from pluripotent stem cells (PSC) and implanted beneath the mouse kidney capsule. *Arrow* indicates NPC-derived mass. Nascent tubules are outlined in histology images. *k,* Host kidney; *G,* glomerulus-like structures. Scale bars, 100 μm (low magnification) and 20 μm (higher magnification). (From Lam AQ, Freedman BS, Morizane R, et al. Rapid and efficient differentiation of human pluripotent stem cells into intermediate mesoderm that forms tubules expressing kidney proximal tubular markers. *J Am Soc Nephrol.* 2014;25:1211–1225, and Taguchi A, Kaku Y, Ohmori T, et al. Redefining the in vivo origin of metanephric nephron progenitors enables generation of complex kidney structures from pluripotent stem cells. *Cell Stem Cell* 2014;14:53–67.)

obvious way to connect with the kidney, this functional improvement is hypothesized to be a paracrine effect.[111] The NPC-like cells expressed a variety of paracrine factors such as VEGF and HGF that might promote functional recovery.[111] A limitation of this study is that the iPS-derived cells were not shown to form kidney organoids, therefore it is unclear whether they were true NPC.

Because kidney disease has systemic causes and effects, implantation of nonrenal cells may also be therapeutically beneficial. For instance, subcapsular implantation of erythropoietin-expressing liver cells derived from iPS cells improves renal anemia in a mouse model.[112] Similarly, implantation of human beta cells derived from PSC, optimized to secrete insulin in response to glucose, rapidly reduced hyperglycemia in a small cohort of diabetic mice.[113] Whether the kidney capsule will provide a suitable microenvironment for engraftment of nonrenal cells in human beings is not yet clear.

To summarize, based on the studies mentioned earlier, implantation of NPC can result in the differentiation of new nephron-like structures in mammalian kidneys in vivo. However, tissues derived from kidney cell therapies in their present form appear disorganized and immature, and it is unclear whether they can integrate into the extant collecting duct or vascular networks. Only in a limited number of these cell therapy studies has any beneficial effect been shown in animal models of kidney disease.[106,107,110,111] Safety must also be considered, as immature kidney cells or contaminating nonkidney cells could be harmful or tumorigenic. This is illustrated by recent cases in which administration of autologous adipose stem cells caused deterioration instead of improvement in the kidneys or the eyes.[109,114] Further preclinical studies in animal models is therefore required to establish therapeutic proof of principle, compared with the gold standard of kidney transplant.

***Clinical Relevance***

Over 700 clinics across the United States offer stem cell therapies that are unproven and have not been FDA approved. Treatments typically involve intravenous or intramuscular administration of nonrenal adult stem cells. These therapies are being advertised for an assortment of maladies, including kidney disease. Patients should be reminded that these unproven stem cell treatments are associated with significant risks, including damage to glomeruli, unexpected immune responses, and tumorigenesis, and may compromise insurance claims. In many cases, the physicians involved in these practices may be under investigation by the local or state medical board.

## BIOARTIFICIAL KIDNEYS

Biomedical engineering or bioengineering is the construction of artificial tissues and organs. This may include, for instance, the combination of natural and synthetic materials to create a patterned scaffold onto which cells are layered in specific arrangements. Bioengineering is typically performed outside of the body, in a lab dish or on a silicon chip. Strategies are currently being developed to generate artificial devices with kidney-like functionalities.

One approach is to utilize existing organs as scaffolds for cells. Whole kidneys are perfused with a detergent agent, which decellularizes the organ, leaving only the extracellular matrix intact in its original shape (Fig. 85.3A). Cells are then reintroduced into the kidney to recellularize it, either through the vasculature (anterograde) or from the ureter (retrograde). Decellularized rodent kidneys can be partially recellularized from primary kidney cells or PSC.[115,116] However, there is no clear way to target specific cell types to designated segments within the nephron, and it is unclear whether recellularization confers upon the scaffold the ability to function like a kidney, or filter urine.[117,118]

A "kidney on a chip" device consists of a synthetic scaffold seeded with kidney cells and subjected to continuous perfusion from a reservoir, which is attached to the device via tubing.[119–121] The scaffold itself may be molded from a synthetic material, naturally occurring extracellular matrix, or a combination of these. These devices tend to be small, about the size of a credit card, and are limited to specific segments of the nephron, such as the proximal tubule (Fig. 85.3B). Toxicity and transport assays indicate that these "three-dimensional" cell culture devices recapitulate nephron functions more accurately than monolayer cultures.[119–121] Currently, the primary application of these systems is to model injury responses in human kidney cells.

To bioengineer larger structures appropriate for transplantation, an emerging technology is 3D bioprinting. This approach utilizes robotic automation to seed cells in patterned layers of biomaterials, resulting in the manufacture of macroscopic, complex tissue constructs.[122–124] To maintain structural integrity, the cells are embedded in biodegradable (sacrificial) hydrogels of sufficient stiffness to withstand transplantation. The mold for bioprinted constructs can be based on a digitalized image, and microchannels can be included to enhance diffusion and cell survival.[122] This technique has primarily been applied to structural and connective tissues, which are relatively simple, and nevertheless remain less mature or organized than the corresponding tissues in vivo. Moreover, bioprinted tissue constructs have not been demonstrated to exhibit long-term functionality. Due to the intricate nephron infrastructure of the kidney, 3D bioprinting of this organ has not yet been attempted and represents an important frontier for this line of research.

Artificial kidneys are medical devices capable of performing renal replacement therapy. Conventional artificial kidneys (dialysis machines) are limited to intense periods of therapy, interspersed with periods of nonuse. In contrast, a wearable artificial kidney (WAK) is a miniaturized, mobile machine that continuously dialyzes the blood, based on dialysate-regenerating sorbent technology (Fig. 85.3C).[125,126] A recent WAK trial suggested that the device could achieve effective uremic solute clearance over a 24-hour period, and no serious adverse events were observed. Patients reported greater satisfaction with the WAK, compared with conventional dialysis, but technical difficulties and performance variabilities were also observed.[126]

A bioartificial kidney, also known as a renal assist device (RAD), consists of a hollow tubular scaffold lined with kidney tubular epithelial cells (similar to a kidney-on-a-chip device) that is designed to simulate the reabsorption and secretion functions of the nephron tubule. The epithelial cells perform vectorial transport of nutrients or toxins between the luminal (inner) and peritubular (outer) filtrates, which are confined to separate compartments. The luminal filtrate can then be discarded or recycled, while the peritubular filtrate is returned to the patient, enriched with nutrients and cleansed of uremic solutes.

A prototype RAD, consisting of approximately one billion porcine kidney cells grown to confluence along the inside of the hollow fibers of a conventional hemodialysis filter cartridge, was effective in curtailing acute uremia in a canine model.[127] The device also provided kidney metabolic functions, which are not provided by conventional dialysis. Subsequently, a similar device lined with human cells was investigated in clinical trials, which suggested both safety and efficacy.[128,129] However, a follow-up phase II study was not completed, and further work is necessary to reproduce these findings.

An ambitious proposal is to make bioartificial kidneys implantable in the body (Fig. 85.3D).[130,131] It is envisioned that such a device could use specialized hemofiltration membranes that have been optimized to mimic glomerular slit diaphragms.[132,133] The filtrate from these membranes would pass along to a bioreactor that would be sustained inside the body. Major technical and conceptual challenges for this approach include: 1. Keeping the cells inside the device alive, protected from the patient's immune system, and in an intact tubular conformation that supports function; 2. Achieving suitable pump power and sufficient water supply, as extracorporeal dialysis can use up to 200 L of water over four hours, whereas water in the implanted bioartificial kidney would be restricted to that which can be supplied by drinking; 3. Designing a nephron-like device of sufficient complexity and organization to properly balance secretion, reabsorption, and concentration functions, resulting in hemofiltrates of appropriate composition and volume. Overcoming these challenges could produce a radically different form of renal replacement from conventional therapies.

***Clinical Relevance***

Efforts to generate WAK devices began in the 1970s, but have recently accelerated, due in part to advances in miniaturization. The new generation of wearable or implantable artificial kidneys is envisioned as the renal equivalent of the cardiac pacemaker or pancreatic insulin pump. The continuous operation of the device is predicted to have a stabilizing effect on blood volume and composition, while its mobility affords patients with a greater sense of agency, compared with conventional hemodialysis. However, these devices remain in the prototype form, and require further optimization and testing before they are fit for regular use in patients.

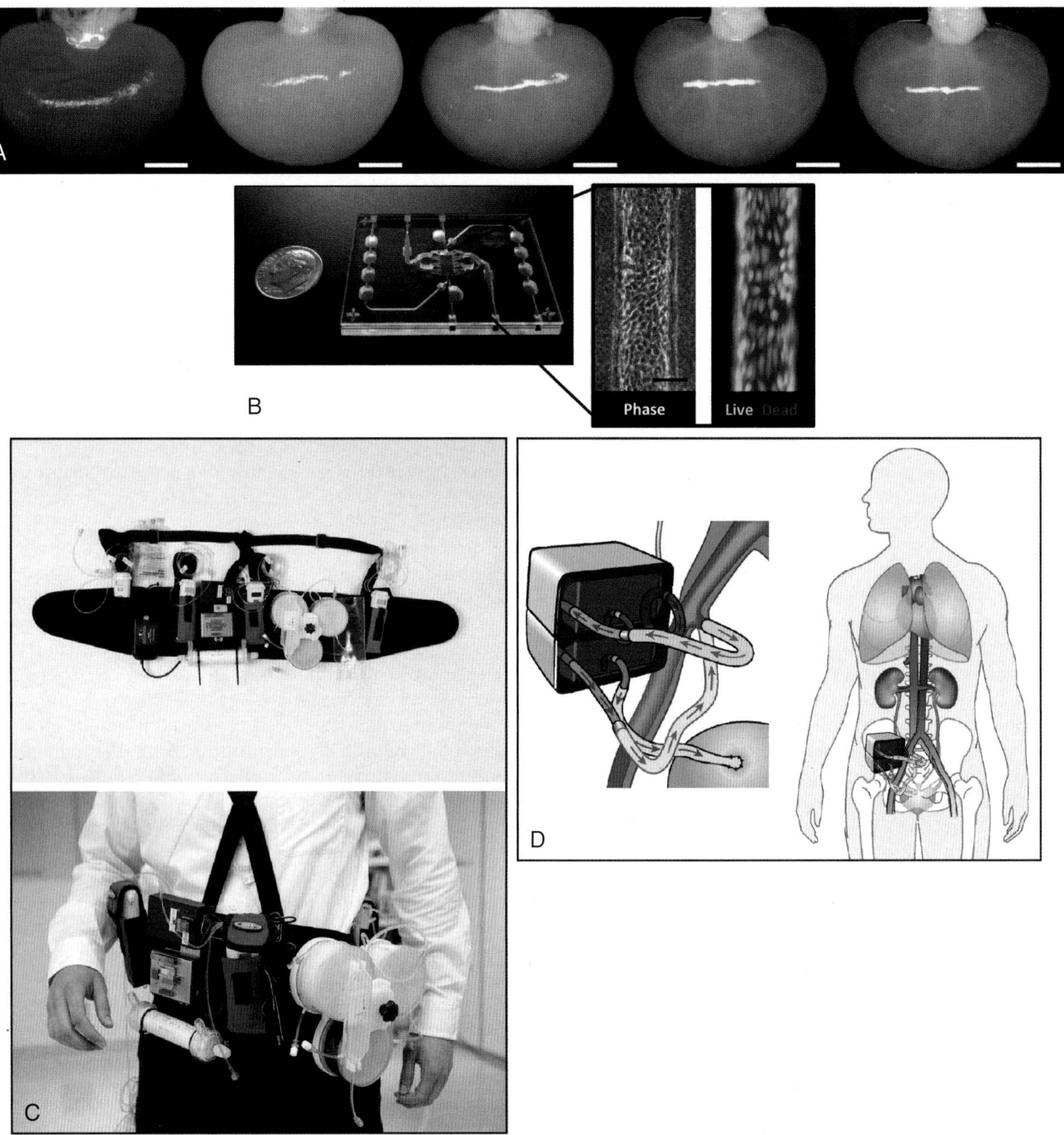


**Fig. 85.3 Kidney bioengineering** (A) Rat kidney subjected to progressive decellularization. Scale bars, 5 mm. (From Caralt M, Uzarski JS, Iacob S, et al. Optimization and critical evaluation of decellularization strategies to develop renal extracellular matrix scaffolds as biological templates for organ engineering and transplantation. *Am J Transplant.* 2015;15:64–75.) (B) Kidney-on-a-chip device, with dime for scale. Inset shows central tubule lined with kidney tubular epithelial cells. Scale bar, 50 μm. (From Weber EJ, Chapron A, Chapron BD, et al. Development of a microphysiological model of human kidney proximal tubule function. *Kidney Int.* 2016;90:627–637.) (C) Prototype wearable artificial kidney tested in patients. (From Gura V, Rivara MB, Bieber S, et al. A wearable artificial kidney for patients with end-stage renal disease. *JCI Insight.* 2016;1(8):e86397.) (D) Theoretical schematic of implantable bioartificial kidney, using iliac vessels for blood supply, and with ultrafiltrate draining to the bladder. (From Fissell WH, Roy S, Davenport A. Achieving more frequent and longer dialysis for the majority: wearable dialysis and implantable artificial kidney devices. *Kidney Int.* 2013;84:256–264.)

## METANEPHRIC IMPLANTS

A limitation of cell therapy and bioengineering approaches is that they involve relatively simple cell populations and configurations, which do not recapitulate the intricate architecture of the kidney. The goal of metanephros implantation is to grow whole kidney organs in situ inside living hosts. The metanephros first appears during the fifth week of human development and contains NPC, UB, vascular cells, and stromal cells organized within a growing, branching cortex (Fig. 85.4A).[7,134] When multiple metanephroi (also called kidney analgens, rudiments, or primordia) are implanted into adult hosts, they can grow and differentiate into kidney-like masses.[135–139]

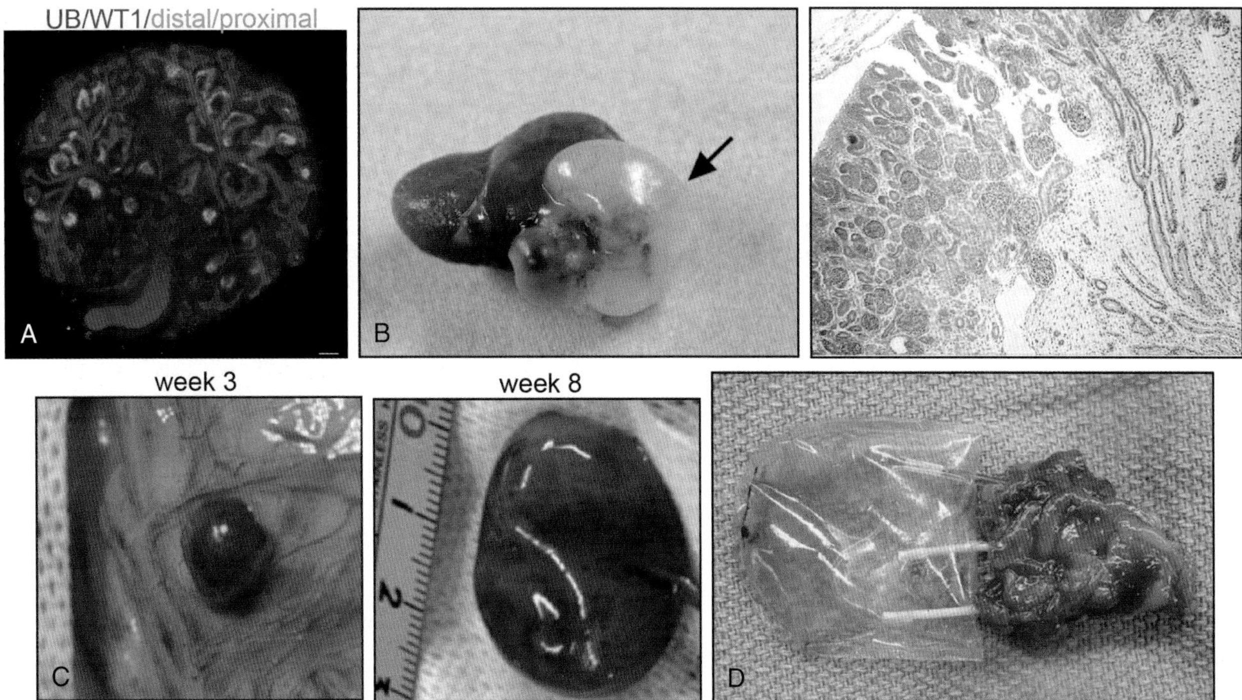


**Fig. 85.4 Ectopic growth of metanephroi.** (A) Mouse metanephros cultured in vitro, delineating nephron lineages naturally present in these structures. *UB,* Ureteric bud; *WT1,* Wilms tumor 1. Scale bar, 100 μm. (From Barak H, Boyle SC: Organ culture and immunostaining of mouse embryonic kidneys. *Cold Spring Harb Protoc.* 2011;2011:pdb prot5558.) (B) Human growth *(arrow)* arising from metanephric tissues implanted beneath the kidney capsule of an immunodeficient mouse, 8 weeks after transplant. Histology of the growth is shown at right. (From Dekel B, Burakova T, Arditti FD, et al. Y: Human and porcine early kidney precursors as a new source for transplantation. *Nat Med.* 2003;9:53–60.) (C) Pig metanephroi implanted in the omentum of a syngeneic host, 3 weeks *(left)* and 8 weeks *(right)* posttransplant. Hydronephrosis is observed at later time points. (From Yokote S, Matsunari H, Iwai S, et al. Urine excretion strategy for stem cell-generated embryonic kidneys. *Proc Natl Acad Sci U S A.* 2015;112:12980–12985.) (D) Bioengineered renal construct seeded with the metanephric cells of a cloned cow, retrieved from the SCNT donor 12 weeks after histocompatible transplant. (From Lanza RP, Chung HY, Yoo JJ, et al. Generation of histocompatible tissues using nuclear transplantation. *Nat Biotechnol.* 2002;20:689–696.)

Metanephric implants can grow in a variety of bodily locations, including beneath the kidney capsule, the anterior chamber of the eye, and the omentum. Implantation of allogeneic rat metanephroi beneath the kidney capsule or into the anterior chamber of the eye resulted in the rapid vascularization of the grafts within 10 days.[135] The grafts, which contained metanephric mesenchyme and ureteric buds when implanted, differentiated extensively into nephron structures, which accumulated intravenously-injected IgG. However, the rapidly-growing allografts also provoked a strong immune response and were rejected after 2 weeks.[135] Matching of rat recipient and host strain allowed implanted metanephroi to survive for up to four weeks. The resultant metanephric implant grew to several times its original size, although the graft never approached the size of an actual adult kidney.[136]

Metanephroi grown in the omentum allow for efficient anastomosis of the metanephric ureter to the ureter of a nephrectomized kidney of the host animal (ureteroureterostomy).[136,137] When the contralateral kidney was subsequently removed, urine production and prolongation of life was observed in the recipient rats, although the effects were relatively modest and insufficient to replace kidney function.[136,137] Although this model involved matching of rat strains, an immune response was still observed, and tolerance was limited to metanephroi whereas adult kidneys transplanted in a similar way were rapidly rejected.[136]

Immunodeficient mice have been used as graft recipients to study the formation of metanephric implants from other species, including pigs and humans.[138] Graft success was dependent on gestational age, with younger grafts (embryonic week 7) growing much more successfully compared with older metanephric tissues or adult kidneys.[138] Under these conditions, and over approximately 8 weeks of growth, both human and porcine metanephroi grew to large sizes in the mouse kidney capsule, forming grafts that rivaled the size of the attached mouse kidneys and that included regions of well-formed cortex (Fig. 85.4B).[138]

Even if the metanephric implant grows to an appropriate size, it is important to provide it with conditions where it might be able to function properly. This is necessary both to confer the desired functional benefit to the host, and also to ensure that the graft develops without disease. Comparison of porcine metanephric implants with and without the associated cloaca (bladder primordial) revealed that inclusion of a bladder component was important for establishing a drain for the implant (Fig. 85.4C).[139] In the absence of cloaca, the implants grew but showed signs of hydronephrosis, whereas inclusion of the cloaca reduced tubular dilation and fibrosis, and increased both the quantity and concentration of uremic solutes within the urine produced by the grafts.[139] Anastomosis of the graft ureter to the host ureter also resulted in improved graft health in both rats and pigs, and prolonged survival of anephric rats.[139]

Implantation of metanephroi can also be combined with bioengineering and stem cell approaches to produce immunocompatible tissue constructs. To investigate such a strategy, the metanephros of a 56-day-old bovine calf embryo produced by reproductive cloning was harvested, seeded onto a scaffold of polycarbonate and collagen, and reimplanted back into the original donor cow. The resultant renal constructs secreted yellow, "urine-like" fluid containing urea nitrogen and creatinine, which accumulated in an attached reservoir over the next twelve weeks (Fig. 85.4D).[140] Thus there is significant potential for combining iPS cells, metanephroi, and bioartificial kidney technologies.

For such approaches to become a realistic option, a reliable source of metanephroi is needed. Human metanephroi appear early in development and cannot be obtained for transplantation. Older kidneys may be less suitable for transplantation, compared with metanephroi.[136,138] Therefore, the possibility of using metanephroi from other species, which can be farmed, is being investigated.

## XENOTRANSPLANTS AND CHIMERAS

Xenotransplantation refers to implantation of grafts from a different species than the recipient. The ability to harvest organs from other species, if successful, would present a possible solution to the current shortfall of donor organs. In early clinical trials of xenotransplantation in the 1960s, chimpanzees were used as donors but the recipients did not survive beyond 2 months. Subsequently, pigs have emerged as the leading potential donor species for such a procedure because they are domesticated, inexpensive, readily available, and their kidneys resemble human kidneys in size, architecture, and physiology.[141,142]

Historically, xenotransplantation approaches have been stymied by safety issues. First, the body's immune system will rapidly reject cells from other species, due to an abundance of nonself antigens. Xenograft rejection is therefore more rapid and severe than allograft rejection. Pig cells are particularly vulnerable, because they express specific carbohydrate antigens such as galactosyl-α1,3,-galactose (Gal) that provoke hyperacute (within minutes) and acute (within days) rejection responses in humans and other primates, which can cause graft failure shortly after transplant (Fig. 85.5A).[143,144]

Progress has been made toward mitigating these acute rejection responses. Miniature pigs lacking Gal have been generated, by genetic engineering in a cultured cell line followed by reproductive cloning to produce the animals.[145] Kidneys from these minipigs provoke a reduced hyperacute rejection response, but are nevertheless rejected in the weeks following transplant.[143,146] Combination of Gal-deficient kidneys with nonconventional immunosuppression regiments that block the costimulatory complement cascade further increases the maximum survival of porcine renal xenotransplants to greater than seven months.[147,148] These experiments have been performed in nonhuman primates, but have not yet been attempted in humans.

An alternative approach that has been proposed is to grow human organs in animals. A technique called interspecies blastocyst complementation (IBC) has recently been developed, as a step towards this goal.[149,150] In IBC, PSC from a donor species are implanted into blastocyst-stage embryos of a recipient species deficient in their ability to grow a specific organ. As a result, the donor cells "complement" the deficiency and form an organ that is largely donor-derived in an otherwise foreign host. Because the resultant animal comprises a mixture of host and donor tissues, it is called a chimera. IBC is still in its infancy and has not yet been successfully used with human PSC. In proof of principle experiments, however, researchers have grown a variety of rat organs in mice, including pancreas, heart, and eyes, which grow to the size of the recipient's organ (Fig. 85.5B).[149,150]

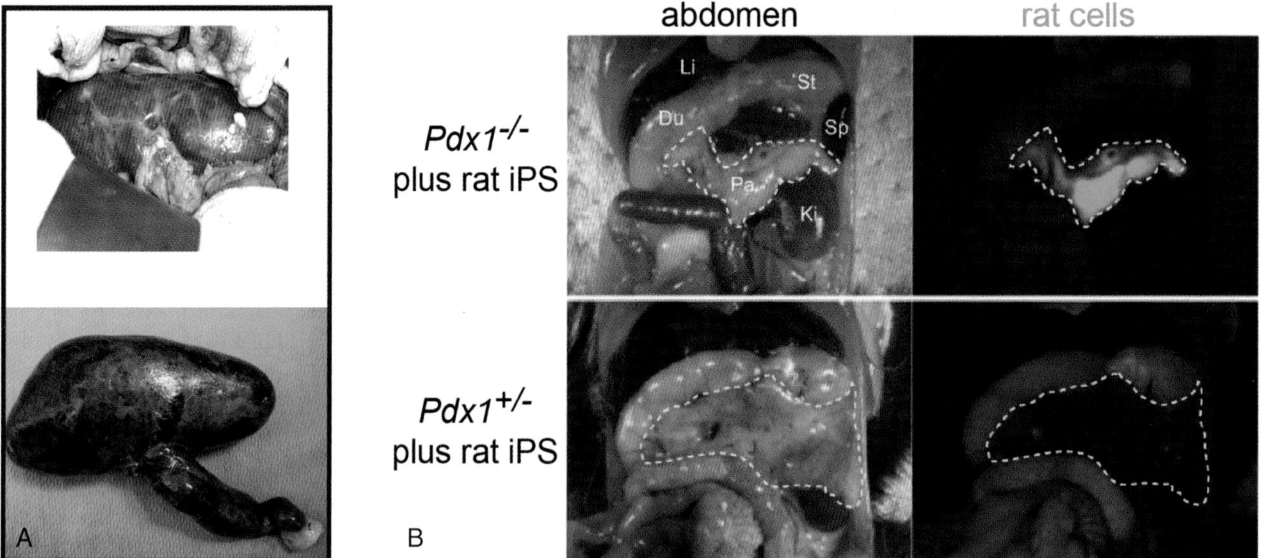


**Fig. 85.5 Xenotransplantation challenges and solutions.** (A) Pig kidney immediately after transplant into a baboon recipient *(top)*, and 10 minutes later after hyperacute rejection *(bottom)*. (From Cooper DK, Ezzelarab MB, Hara H, et al. The pathobiology of pig-to-primate xenotransplantation: a historical review. *Xenotransplantation* 2016;23:83–105.) (B) Rat pancreas grown in a mouse. Abdominal organs are indicated in shorthand notation. The homozygous mutant is permissive for engraftment of rat cells *(green)* to form a pancreas. (From Kobayashi T, Yamaguchi T, Hamanaka S, et al. Generation of rat pancreas in mouse by interspecific blastocyst injection of pluripotent stem cells. *Cell* 2010;142:787–799.)

Several significant technical hurdles need to be overcome, however, before IBC can be utilized successfully to farm human organs.[151] Although IBC organs are highly enriched for donor cells, the organs are still chimeric, containing a mixture of host and donor cells. One reason for this is that organs arise from many different cell populations; for instance, kidneys arise from UB, MM, nerves, vasculature, and interstitial stem cells. Genetic techniques typically establish a niche in only one of these populations, but it would be necessary to target all of them in order to create a "pure" human organ inside an animal that would not provoke an extreme immune rejection response. Another problem is that cells from one species may be poorly compatible with cells from another species during development, resulting in defects during organogenesis.

In addition to these technical concerns, human cells could potentially contribute to brains or gonads in chimeras, raising issues of human rights and dignity. Although chimerism is very low (<1%) in organs that are not targeted for complementation,[149,150] it is nevertheless important to perform these experiments in the most ethically responsible way possible. For this reason, research involving the creation of human-animal chimeric embryos is subject to a funding moratorium by the United States National Institutes of Health. Thus both ethical and technical challenges must be overcome before IBC can be tested in humans.

## GENE THERAPY

Genetics contribute significantly to an individual's risk of kidney disease. Approximately 15% of kidney disease is caused directly by single-gene mutations.[152] Polycystic kidney disease (PKD), which is commonly caused by autosomal dominant mutations in either the *PKD1* or *PKD2* genes, accounts for the primary diagnosis of renal failure in ~10% of all patients.[153–155] In addition to Mendelian disorders such as PKD, a substantial portion of kidney disease genetics is complex, involving sequence variants that contribute in a combinatorial fashion to a patient's risk, such as *APOL1*.[156,157] Gene tools are furthermore emerging as powerful modulators of the immune system, with relevance to systemic kidney disorders and transplantation. A deeper understanding of disease genetics is therefore of increasing relevance for nephrology.

### PREIMPLANTATION GENETIC DIAGNOSIS

Risk of hereditary kidney disease may be predictable based on family history. For instance, autosomal dominant PKD (ADPKD) is inherited as a single mutant allele from one affected parent, and therefore has a 50% chance of affecting any child of that parent. Alternatively, disease risk may be detected by prenatal screening for genetic mutations that predispose toward a variety of congenital diseases affecting the kidneys, such as Alport syndrome, autosomal recessive PKD (ARPKD), maple syrup urine disease, Fabry disease, and ciliopathy disorders.

If risk for a genetic disease is detected, prospective parents may elect to undergo preimplantation genetic diagnosis (PGD). PGD is an in vitro fertilization (IVF) technique used by parents to avoid passing on a known disease gene to their offspring. In PGD, a genetic diagnosis is made on each of several IVF embryos, based on a biopsy sample consisting of a single blastomere cell.[158] Embryos that do not carry the genetic mutation are selected for uterine implantation, while embryos with the mutation are not implanted. In this way it is possible to interrupt the transmission of disease genes from generation to generation.

Although PGD can be used to prevent any kidney disease in which genetic inheritance can be predicted, it is most commonly used for diseases that have a severe effect early in life, such as ARPKD.[159] The putative mutation that causes the disease must be known ahead of the PGD analysis, which is performed on a small sample of DNA. Sequencing of the mutation locus may be costly or require specialized techniques.[160] As PGD is a prophylactic approach, when it is successful it completely prevents the disease. However, as genotyping does not always correctly identify the mutation, the success of PGD may only become clear after the time when symptoms typically begin to present.

> ***Clinical Relevance***
> Many patients who are considering starting a family may not know about PGD. It is therefore appropriate to present PGD as an option to patients that are at risk for genetic forms of kidney disease, for instance, if both of the parents are carriers of a recessive risk allele. Some patients who might otherwise choose not to have children under these circumstances might elect to have children through PGD. Others may not feel comfortable with PGD, either for religious or practical reasons, and may opt to forego it even in cases where it would be strongly recommended. Ultimately, the choice to undergo PGD is a personal one that should be made by prospective parents in an informed way, in careful consultation with their physicians.

### GENE TRANSFER

In postnatal patients with genetic disease, PGD is no longer an option. Most genetic diseases result from insufficient expression levels of a functional gene. For such disorders, a straightforward strategy is to introduce a healthy copy of the gene into cells. This approach has been the cornerstone of gene therapy efforts for the past 30 years. During this time, major advances have been made with regard to the safety and efficacy of these products. Today, gene therapies are in clinical trials for a wide variety of ailments, and the United States Food and Drug Administration has approved a few of these for clinical use.

Delivery is a major challenge for all gene therapies. As small pieces of DNA are not efficiently absorbed in most tissues, successful gene therapies typically require a vector to deliver genes into cells, a process known as gene transfer. The two vectors most commonly used for gene transfer are retroviruses (including lentiviruses), which integrate into the genome and can accommodate up to 8 kb of DNA, and AAV, which are more limited in packaging size and mostly propagate as nonintegrating episomes, which have a shorter half-life than retroviral vectors. The safety and efficacy profiles of AAV and retroviral vectors are constantly improving, with advantages and disadvantages to each, depending on the context. For the kidneys, intravenous administration of lentiviral or AAV vectors is technically challenging and inefficient, at least in rodents, whereas parenchymal and retrograde (ureteral) injections may be effective if carefully performed.[161–163] AAV can be used successfully to elicit transient gene expression and is the generally preferred vector for renal gene therapy.

In certain cases, gene therapy vectors can be administered directly into the body. For instance, an AAV-based therapy for hemophilia B, encoding the factor IX gene, was administered intravenously into ten human patients, resulting in its sustained expression and the cessation of prophylactic infusions of recombinant factor IX in most of the trial subjects.[164] To date, however, most gene therapies rely upon a combination of gene and cell therapy, in which cells from the patient are first treated ex vivo and subsequently delivered back into the body. Although more laborious than direct administration, this approach overcomes certain technical hurdles in gene delivery, and presents greater opportunities for quality control checks to mitigate safety risks. Gene transfer is typically performed in adult stem cells, which can be harvested from the body and are capable of extensive self-renewal. In a recent example, large epidermal grafts were constructed from a keratinocyte clone transduced with a healthy copy of a laminin isoform, resulting in substantial remission of severe blistering disease in one patient (Fig. 85.6A).[165]

For certain renal conditions, gene therapy in an extrarenal stem cell may constitute a viable strategy to treat or prevent disease. For instance, in a mouse model of cystinosis, lentivirus gene transfer of the missing CTNS gene into HSC decreased the formation of cystine crystals in the kidneys, and moderately improved kidney function.[166] More generally, in the setting of kidney transplantation, transfer of immunomodulatory genes into HSC may improve immune tolerance of the graft. In a pig model, kidney allograft recipients first received bone marrow transplants from autologous HSC modified to express donor-specific major histocompatibility complex class II molecules, resulting in increased tolerance or acceptance of the graft in the absence of sustained immunosuppression.[167] Dendritic cells have likewise been shown to be modifiable to express immunoregulatory cytokines or receptors, which can enhance the survival of renal grafts.[168]

In contrast to skin and blood, the kidneys do not contain adult stem cells that can be modified ex vivo and subsequently used to regenerate the entire organ. Kidneys are, however, isolated ex vivo in preparation for transplant, which presents an opportunity to perform gene therapy on the entire organ. Thus gene therapy is being explored as a means of protecting donor kidneys from ischemia-reperfusion injury and immune rejection. In rat models, animal kidneys can be efficiently transduced ex vivo with AAV encoding immunomodulatory receptors, which can result in less severe outcomes after transplantation.[169–171] These studies are building towards improved graft survival rates.[9,10]

For Mendelian disorders that are intrinsic to the kidney and do not necessarily involve transplantation, such as ADPKD or Alport syndrome, gene therapy strategies remain to be tested. In addition to restoring the deficient gene, it is important to also express it at the appropriate levels, as overexpression can have deleterious effects. For instance, overexpressing *Pkd1* and *Pkd2* genes in transgenic animals can paradoxically cause PKD.[172,173] Even when employed responsibly, gene transfer carries inherent risks of side effects. For instance, retroviral gene transfer in HSC initially appeared be both safe and efficacious in treating X-linked severe combined immunodeficiency, but leukemias subsequently developed in some patients due to clonal proliferation of T-cells, in which the gene had integrated into an undesired location in the genome.[174] Cases such as these have sparked interest in more controllable, and therefore safer, gene therapy methods.

## GENE EDITING

Gene editing differs from gene transfer in that it involves the deliberate alteration of a specific genetic sequence within a genome. Since the 1980s, a variety of different gene editing techniques have been developed, including site-directed homologous recombination, zinc-finger nucleases, transcription activator-like effector nucleases, piggyBac transposons, and adeno-associated viruses.[175–179] The latest and most widely

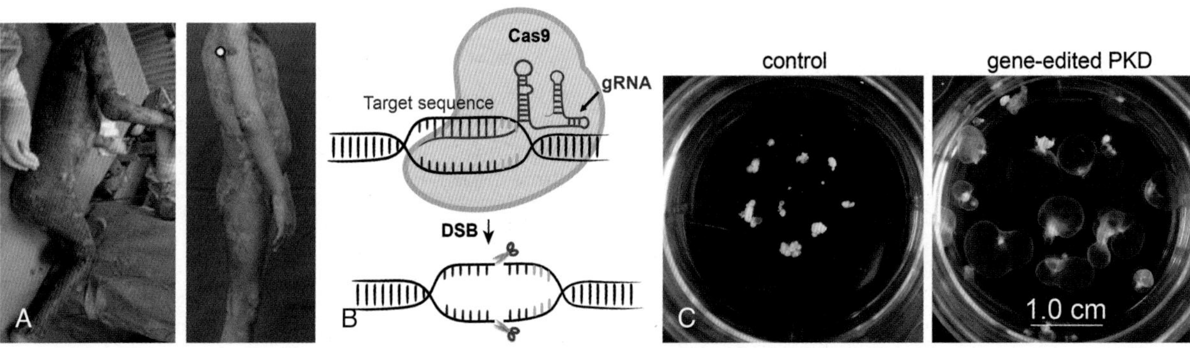


**Fig. 85.6 Gene therapy and gene editing.** (A) Patient with junctional epidermolysis bullosa before *(left)* and after *(right)* receiving a skin graft treated with gene therapy. White circle indicates a rare patch of non-regenerated skin. (From Hirsch T, Rothoeft T, Teig N, et al. Regeneration of the entire human epidermis using transgenic stem cells. *Nature* 2017;551:327–332.) (B) Schematic of CRISPR-Cas complex initiating DSB at a targeted site. (From Cruz NM, Freedman BS. CRISPR Gene Editing in the Kidney. *Am. J. Kidney Dis.* 2018;71(6):874–883.) (C) Kidney organoids with gene-edited PKD mutations, compared with control organoids of identical genetic background. (From Cruz NM, Song X, Czerniecki SM, et al. Organoid cystogenesis reveals a critical role of microenvironment in human polycystic kidney disease. *Nat Mater.* 2017;16:1112–1119.)

adopted of these techniques is the clustered regularly interspaced short palindromic repeats (CRISPR) system. Gene editing with this system requires the transient expression of two components: a CRISPR-associated system (Cas) endonuclease and a guide RNA (gRNA).[180,181] The gRNA combines an invariant "scaffold" sequence that binds to Cas and a variable "spacer", approximately 20 base pairs in length, which determines sequence specificity. There are four possible nucleotides for each of the positions in the spacer, providing up to $4^{20}$ possible sequence combinations. This exceeds the number of nucleotides in any known genome and provides sufficient sequence specificity to target unique DNA sequences complementary to the spacer.

To initiate gene editing, Cas associates with the gRNA at matching sites and introduces double-stranded breaks (DSB) in genomic DNA. Such lesions are predominantly repaired by the cell via nonhomologous end joining (NHEJ), in which the DNA ends are severed and subsequently ligated together (Fig. 85.6B). Such events frequently introduce small insertion or deletion mutations (indels). Less commonly, DSB can be corrected based on a DNA template of similar sequence, a mechanism known as homology-directed repair (HDR). This DNA template may reside elsewhere in the genome, or can be supplied artificially, providing an opportunity to introduce specific edits into DNA.[182–184]

Although CRISPR can induce DSB in a site-specific way, its effects remain relatively inefficient and unpredictable. In human PSC, for instance, the efficiency of NHEJ using CRISPR ranges from 4%–25%, and the efficiency of HDR is approximately 1% or less.[183,185] Inherent to the use of CRISPR and other gene editing methods is the risk of inadvertent edits to nuclear DNA sequences elsewhere in the genome that are similar to the target. A variety of measures can be taken to reduce the likelihood of such "off-target" effects, including the use of computational algorithms that maximize sequence specificity,[182,183] minimizing the genome's exposure to Cas, and more complex strategies that merely "nick" DNA,[186] although none of these completely eliminates the risk. Whole-genome sequencing can also be performed to verify that only the desired modifications have been made,[187,188] although this may not be economically feasible.

Despite these limitations, CRISPR and related techniques are being used to develop a new wave of gene therapies, starting with animal models. In rodent models, CRISPR has been used to inactivate pathogenic viral (HIV) or genetic (Huntington disease) sequences, by disrupting them with NHEJ.[189,190] CRISPR-induced HDR has similarly been applied to correct genetic deficiencies in muscular dystrophy[191–193] and retinal degeneration.[194–197] These studies suggest promise for application of CRISPR directly in vivo.

In many organs, including the kidneys, clinical trials have been initiated to study the potential of CRISPR-mediated gene therapy, particularly immunotherapies, which show great promise for treating certain cancers. In most of these trials, CRISPR is being used to construct T-lymphocytes that express chimeric antigen receptors (CAR-T cells), which can recognize and attack specific types of tumor cells. As such treatments can have strong side effects, they are currently restricted to patients with cancer, including metastatic renal carcinoma. Improved safety profiles might render such approaches suitable for other types of kidney diseases with an immunomodulatory component, such as lupus nephritis.[198]

CRISPR can also be applied to human embryos at the single-cell stage. Because the zygote gives rise to every other cell type in the body, a successful edit at this stage will be transmitted to the entire organism. However, due to the unpredictability of CRISPR, zygotic gene editing may be more likely to produce off-target mutations and mosaic embryos containing both modified and unmodified cells.[199–201] The efficiency of gene correction may be increased if the DSB can be repaired from a second, healthy allele, although additional studies are required to reproduce this.[184] In any case, use of CRISPR in human zygotes raises ethical concerns, and the benefits of such a therapy must outweigh the risks. PGD is almost always likely to be safer and more practical than CRISPR in human embryos, although there may be rare cases where PGD is not an option, for instance in an autosomal recessive disease where both parents are affected.

## DESIGNER THERAPEUTICS

The ability to edit the genome, in combination with stem cell technology, is providing new tools for evaluation and treatment of human kidney disease. For instance, it has traditionally been challenging to study disease phenotypes in human cells, because these cultures are highly heterogeneous and do not recapitulate the complexity of the kidney. Kidney organoids provide more physiologically relevant structures for disease modeling, but PSC from patients are limited to naturally occurring mutations and exhibit substantial variability in their ability to differentiate into the kidney lineage, for reasons that are unrelated to disease.[68] Gene editing presents a possible solution to these problems by providing a way of introducing custom mutations on an otherwise identical (isogenic) genetic background. To establish a human cellular model of PKD, CRISPR was used to introduce loss-of-function mutations into *PKD1* or *PKD2* in human ES cells. Kidney organoids derived from these cells formed cysts from kidney tubules, which were not observed in isogenic controls.[50] Removal of adherent cues greatly increased the rate of cystogenesis in these organoids, resulting in their expansion into macroscopic cysts that could be observed by eye (Fig. 85.6C).[68] These experiments indicate that the essential hallmark of PKD can be reconstituted in a human cellular system in vitro, which can be used to unveil mechanisms of disease and test candidate therapeutics.

Due to the size and complexity of the human genome, inheritance mapping and genome sequencing is insufficient to conclusively identify many rare mutations as disease-causative.[202] Gene editing provides a functional strategy to rapidly validate such genes. For instance, CRISPR-mediated knockout of *GANAB*, a candidate gene for rare cases of genetically unresolved ADPKD, caused specific trafficking defects in human renal cortical tubular epithelial cells, a molecular phenotype associated with ADPKD.[203] Similarly, CRISPR knockout of *PODXL*, a candidate gene for focal segmental glomerulosclerosis,[204] caused defects in junctional migration, microvillus formation, and cell-cell spacing between podocytes in kidney organoids, similar to those observed in knockout mice.[50,69,205] Biallelic, loss-of-function mutations in *PODXL* were subsequently described in a rare patient with congenital nephrotic syndrome, consistent with the predictions of the organoid and mouse models.[206]

The use of CRISPR is not limited to the targeted editing of individual candidate genes. Genome-wide libraries of CRISPR gRNA can be applied to collections of cells in vitro, which can then be selected and analyzed for disease-relevant phenotypes.[207] Performing these screening techniques can reveal novel candidate genes for kidney disease, which can subsequently be validated in genetically unresolved family cohorts, reversing the traditional process of disease gene discovery.[208] An example of this is *PODXL*, for which the organoid phenotype preceded the case study.[69,206] Using a screening approach, modifier genes could also be identified, whose activation or inhibition can rescue kidney disease phenotypes. Noncutting variants of CRISPR-Cas have also been developed that can silence or activate genes by binding to DNA without modifying it.[209,210] In a recent example relevant to the kidney, CRISPR was used to activate expression of *Klotho* or *IL10* in the liver, which conferred renoprotection from subsequent acute kidney injury.[211]

CRISPR can also be used to more rapidly and economically manufacture regenerative therapeutics. For instance, a single zygotic injection of CRISPR can be used to generate transgenic mice and miniature pigs with mutations in multiple distinct genes.[182,212,213] This approach has been used to knock out three surface antigens that provoke acute rejection of pig cells, as well as three class I major histocompatibility complex genes, to generate pigs more immunocompatible with humans.[214,215] CRISPR has furthermore been applied in pigs to disrupt over 60 DNA sequences required for porcine endogenous retrovirus activity, resulting in virus-deficient pigs with reduced hazard of viral transmission across species lines.[216,217] Gene editing can also be combined with IBC, described earlier, to more rapidly construct chimeric embryos with organs from other species.[150]

For the kidney, a frontier is to use gene editing to produce designer human stem cells that would be immunocompatible. For instance, disease mutations could be corrected in iPS cells and rescue of phenotypes confirmed in kidney organoids in vitro, prior to implantation of NPC into a patient.[42] As generation of iPS cells and derived NPC for each individual patient may not be practical or economical,[218] an alternative strategy is to use gene editing to engineer "universal donor" cells lacking major histocompatibility genes and expressing specific immunoregulatory molecules, resulting in improved immunotolerance in humanized mice.[219,220] Although the safety and efficacy of these cells has not yet been demonstrated, such cells might provide "off-the-shelf" solutions for regenerative medicine applications with reduced need for immunosuppression. This could represent a significant improvement in the safety and availability of cell therapies for patients with kidney disease.

## CONCLUSION

The survey of new technologies described earlier suggests both promise and caution with regard to renal medicine. Gene therapy and regenerative medicine remain exciting prospects, which are closer to clinical translation than ever before. In many ways, these new technologies are combinatorial and complementary—for instance, nuclear transfer techniques from the stem cell field have been critical in generating gene-edited animals for enhanced xenotransplantation. As these fields mature, efforts towards clinical translation are providing a more realistic and nuanced understanding of these technologies, revealing technical challenges and side effects that must be overcome, as illustrated by gene therapy trials. Radical changes to the practice of nephrology, where the gold standards of kidney transplantation and dialysis are well established, are therefore unlikely in the short term. To first do no harm, it is important to carefully characterize these new approaches in the research setting, before implementing them in the clinic.

With cautious and gradual adaptation of these technologies, however, it is likely that the nephrology clinic of the future will appear dramatically different from the clinic of today. The kidney has been a testing ground for many of the exciting discoveries in both the stem cell and gene editing fields and is viewed as a challenging and important frontier. New inventions, such as human kidney organoids, which did not exist only years ago, have already changed the research landscape in significant ways. Advances are being made in parallel on multiple fronts, including dialysis, transplant, and gene therapy. These accomplishments are the integrated product of decades of research by multiple groups, building toward a common vision of what care could be, rather than what it is. In practical terms, the nephrologist of the future will need to select carefully from an expanded menu of treatment options. This will require the development of new expertise with regard to stem cells, genetics, immunology, and the molecular pathophysiology. These efforts will be rewarded with increased prevention of kidney disease at early stages, and improved treatment outcomes at later stages, to prolong and enhance the lives of millions of patients.

## ACKNOWLEDGMENTS

The Freedman laboratory is supported by NIH Awards K01DK102826, R01DK117914, UG3TR002158, an Allen Institute Translational Science Grant, a Regular Award from the United States–Israel Binational Science Foundation, an Institute for Stem Cell and Regenerative Medicine Innovation Pilot Award, a gift from the Northwest Kidney Centers to the Kidney Research Institute, and start-up funds from the University of Washington. Dr. Freedman is an inventor on patent applications related to human kidney organoid differentiation.

 Complete reference list available at ExpertConsult.com.

## KEY REFERENCES

6. Kobayashi A, Valerius MT, Mugford JW, et al. Six2 defines and regulates a multipotent self-renewing nephron progenitor population throughout mammalian kidney development. *Cell Stem Cell*. 2008;3:169–181.
7. Barak H, Huh SH, Chen S, et al. FGF9 and FGF20 maintain the stemness of nephron progenitors in mice and man. *Dev Cell*. 2012;22:1191–1207.
16. Thomson JA, Itskovitz-Eldor J, Shapiro SS, et al. Embryonic stem cell lines derived from human blastocysts. *Science*. 1998;282:1145–1147.
17. Wilmut I, Schnieke AE, McWhir J, et al. Viable offspring derived from fetal and adult mammalian cells. *Nature*. 1997;385: 810–813.
22. Wakayama S, Ohta H, Hikichi T, et al. Production of healthy cloned mice from bodies frozen at -20 degrees C for 16 years. *Proc Natl Acad Sci USA*. 2008;105:17318–17322.

23. Tachibana M, Amato P, Sparman M, et al. Human embryonic stem cells derived by somatic cell nuclear transfer. *Cell.* 2013;153: 1228–1238.
26. Takahashi K, Tanabe K, Ohnuki M, et al. Induction of pluripotent stem cells from adult human fibroblasts by defined factors. *Cell.* 2007;131:861–872.
32. Araki R, Uda M, Hoki Y, et al. Negligible immunogenicity of terminally differentiated cells derived from induced pluripotent or embryonic stem cells. *Nature.* 2013;494:100–104.
33. Chong JJ, Yang X, Don CW, et al. Human embryonic-stem-cell-derived cardiomyocytes regenerate non-human primate hearts. *Nature.* 2014;510:273–277.
38. Mandai M, Watanabe A, Kurimoto Y, et al. Autologous induced stem-cell-derived retinal cells for macular degeneration. *N Engl J Med.* 2017;376:1038–1046.
40. Boland MJ, Hazen JL, Nazor KL, et al. Adult mice generated from induced pluripotent stem cells. *Nature.* 2009;461:91–94.
42. Freedman BS, Lam AQ, Sundsbak JL, et al. Reduced ciliary polycystin-2 in induced pluripotent stem cells from polycystic kidney disease patients with *PKD1* mutations. *J Am Soc Nephrol.* 2013; 24:1571–1586.
50. Freedman BS, Brooks CR, Lam AQ, et al. Modelling kidney disease with CRISPR-mutant kidney organoids derived from human pluripotent epiblast spheroids. *Nat Commun.* 2015;6:8715.
54. Rosines E, Sampogna RV, Johkura K, et al. Staged in vitro reconstitution and implantation of engineered rat kidney tissue. *Proc Natl Acad Sci USA.* 2007;104:20938–20943.
55. Diep CQ, Ma D, Deo RC, et al. Identification of adult nephron progenitors capable of kidney regeneration in zebrafish. *Nature.* 2011;470:95–100.
59. Urbach A, Yermalovich A, Zhang J, et al. Lin28 sustains early renal progenitors and induces Wilms tumor. *Genes Dev.* 2014;28:971–982.
62. Li Z, Araoka T, Wu J, et al. 3D culture supports long-term expansion of mouse and human nephrogenic progenitors. *Cell Stem Cell.* 2016;19:516–529.
63. Taguchi A, Kaku Y, Ohmori T, et al. Redefining the in vivo origin of metanephric nephron progenitors enables generation of complex kidney structures from pluripotent stem cells. *Cell Stem Cell.* 2014;14:53–67.
64. Morizane R, Lam AQ, Freedman BS, et al. Nephron organoids derived from human pluripotent stem cells model kidney development and injury. *Nat Biotechnol.* 2015;33:1193–1200.
65. Takasato M, Er PX, Chiu HS, et al. Kidney organoids from human iPS cells contain multiple lineages and model human nephrogenesis. *Nature.* 2016.
66. Lam AQ, Freedman BS, Morizane R, et al. Rapid and efficient differentiation of human pluripotent stem cells into intermediate mesoderm that forms tubules expressing kidney proximal tubular markers. *J Am Soc Nephrol.* 2014;25:1211–1225.
68. Cruz NM, Song X, Czerniecki SM, et al. Organoid cystogenesis reveals a critical role of microenvironment in human polycystic kidney disease. *Nat Mater.* 2017;16:1112–1119.
69. Kim YK, Refaeli I, Brooks CR, et al. Gene-edited human kidney organoids reveal mechanisms of disease in podocyte development. *Stem Cells.* 2017.
70. Taguchi A, Nishinakamura R. Higher-order kidney organogenesis from pluripotent stem cells. *Cell Stem Cell.* 2017;21:730–746 e736.
74. Hendry CE, Vanslambrouck JM, Ineson J, et al. Direct transcriptional reprogramming of adult cells to embryonic nephron progenitors. *J Am Soc Nephrol.* 2013;24:1424–1434.
76. Humphreys BD, Valerius MT, Kobayashi A, et al. Intrinsic epithelial cells repair the kidney after injury. *Cell Stem Cell.* 2008;2:284–291.
77. Rinkevich Y, Montoro DT, Contreras-Trujillo H, et al. In vivo clonal analysis reveals lineage-restricted progenitor characteristics in mammalian kidney development, maintenance, and regeneration. *Cell Rep.* 2014;7:1270–1283.
86. Appel D, Kershaw DB, Smeets B, et al. Recruitment of podocytes from glomerular parietal epithelial cells. *J Am Soc Nephrol.* 2009;20: 333–343.
87. Kaverina NV, Eng DG, Schneider RR, et al. Partial podocyte replenishment in experimental FSGS derives from nonpodocyte sources. *Am J Physiol Renal Physiol.* 2016;310:F1397–F1413.
89. Lasagni L, Angelotti ML, Ronconi E, et al. Podocyte regeneration driven by renal progenitors determines glomerular disease remission and can be pharmacologically enhanced. *Stem Cell Reports.* 2015;5:248–263.
99. Duffield JS, Park KM, Hsiao LL, et al. Restoration of tubular epithelial cells during repair of the postischemic kidney occurs independently of bone marrow-derived stem cells. *J Clin Invest.* 2005;115:1743–1755.
100. Kramann R, Schneider RK, DiRocco DP, et al. Perivascular Gli1+ progenitors are key contributors to injury-induced organ fibrosis. *Cell Stem Cell.* 2015;16:51–66.
106. Imberti B, Tomasoni S, Ciampi O, et al. Renal progenitors derived from human iPSCs engraft and restore function in a mouse model of acute kidney injury. *Sci Rep.* 2015;5:8826.
107. Ronconi E, Sagrinati C, Angelotti ML, et al. Regeneration of glomerular podocytes by human renal progenitors. *J Am Soc Nephrol.* 2009;20:322–332.
110. Harari-Steinberg O, Metsuyanim S, Omer D, et al. Identification of human nephron progenitors capable of generation of kidney structures and functional repair of chronic renal disease. *EMBO Mol Med.* 2013;5:1556–1568.
111. Toyohara T, Mae S, Sueta S, et al. Cell therapy using human induced pluripotent stem cell-derived renal progenitors ameliorates acute kidney injury in mice. *Stem Cells Transl Med.* 2015;4:980–992.
117. Caralt M, Uzarski JS, Iacob S, et al. Optimization and critical evaluation of decellularization strategies to develop renal extracellular matrix scaffolds as biological templates for organ engineering and transplantation. *Am J Transplant.* 2015;15:64–75.
119. Weber EJ, Chapron A, Chapron BD, et al. Development of a microphysiological model of human kidney proximal tubule function. *Kidney Int.* 2016;90:627–637.
126. Gura V, Rivara MB, Bieber S, et al. A wearable artificial kidney for patients with end-stage renal disease. *JCI Insight.* 2016;1.
130. Humes HD, Buffington D, Westover AJ, et al. The bioartificial kidney: current status and future promise. *Pediatr Nephrol.* 2014;29: 343–351.
138. Dekel B, Burakova T, Arditti FD, et al. Human and porcine early kidney precursors as a new source for transplantation. *Nat Med.* 2003;9:53–60.
139. Yokote S, Matsunari H, Iwai S, et al. Urine excretion strategy for stem cell-generated embryonic kidneys. *Proc Natl Acad Sci USA.* 2015;112:12980–12985.
143. Chen G, Qian H, Starzl T, et al. Acute rejection is associated with antibodies to non-Gal antigens in baboons using Gal-knockout pig kidneys. *Nat Med.* 2005;11:1295–1298.
147. Higginbotham L, Mathews D, Breeden CA, et al. Pre-transplant antibody screening and anti-CD154 costimulation blockade promote long-term xenograft survival in a pig-to-primate kidney transplant model. *Xenotransplantation.* 2015;22:221–230.
149. Kobayashi T, Yamaguchi T, Hamanaka S, et al. Generation of rat pancreas in mouse by interspecific blastocyst injection of pluripotent stem cells. *Cell.* 2010;142:787–799.
165. Hirsch T, Rothoeft T, Teig N, et al. Regeneration of the entire human epidermis using transgenic stem cells. *Nature.* 2017;551: 327–332.
169. Tomasoni S, Trionfini P, Azzollini N, et al. AAV9-mediated engineering of autotransplanted kidney of non-human primates. *Gene Ther.* 2017;24:308–313.
181. Jinek M, Chylinski K, Fonfara I, et al. A programmable dual-RNA-guided DNA endonuclease in adaptive bacterial immunity. *Science.* 2012;337:816–821.
216. Niu D, Wei HJ, Lin L, et al. Inactivation of porcine endogenous retrovirus in pigs using CRISPR-Cas9. *Science.* 2017;357:1303–1307.
220. Gornalusse GG, Hirata RK, Funk SE, et al. HLA-E-expressing pluripotent stem cells escape allogeneic responses and lysis by NK cells. *Nat Biotechnol.* 2017;35:765–772.

# Index



Note: Page numbers followed by “f” refer to illustrations; page numbers followed by “t” refer to tables; page numbers followed by “b” refer to boxes.

## B

## C

## D

## F

## G

## J



## K

## L

## M

## N

## Q



## R

## S

## V